T0315393

THE MERCK VETERINARY MANUAL

ELEVENTH EDITION

Dedicated to all veterinarians and their colleagues in animal health worldwide.

THE MERCK VETERINARY MANUAL

ELEVENTH EDITION

Editor-in-Chief: Susan E. Aiello, DVM, ELS
Executive Editor: Michael A. Moses

Published by

MERCK & CO., INC.
KENILWORTH, NJ, USA

2016

Editorial and Production Staff

Editor-in-Chief: Susan E. Aiello, DVM, ELS
Executive Editor: Michael A. Moses

Publisher: Melissa Adams
Partnership Manager: Michael Wisniewski
Subsidiary Rights Coordinator: Sheryl Olinsky-Borg
Sales and Service Specialist: Leta S. Bracy

Associate Director, Merck Digital Publications: Michael DeFerrari
Business and Operations Manager: Jennifer A. Doyle

Library of Congress Control Number: 2016905370
ISBN-13: 978-0911910612
ISSN Number: 0076-6542

Printed in China

Designer: Jerilyn Bockorick, Cenveo® Publisher Services

Composition by Cenveo® Publisher Services
Fort Washington, Pennsylvania

Printed and bound at RR Donnelley Asia

THE MERCK VETERINARY MANUAL

Previous Editions

First Edition	1955
Second Edition	1961
Third Edition	1967
Fourth Edition	1973
Fifth Edition	1979
Sixth Edition	1986
Seventh Edition	1991
Eighth Edition	1998
Ninth Edition	2005
Tenth Edition	2010

Foreign Language Editions

Chinese
China Agriculture Press, Beijing

Croatian/Slovakian
Komora Vetarinarnich Lekarov, Brno

French
Editions d'Apres, Paris

Italian
Cristiano Giraldi Editore, Bologne

Japanese
Gakusosha, Tokyo

Portuguese
Editora Roca, São Paulo

Spanish
Editorial Oceano, Barcelona

OTHER
MERCK BOOKS

The Merck Index
First Edition, 1889

The Merck Manual of Diagnosis and Therapy
First Edition, 1899

The Merck Manual of Medical Information
Home Edition
First Edition, 1977

The Merck Manual of Health and Aging
First Edition, 2004

The Merck/Merial Manual for Pet Health
First Edition, 2007

The Merck Manual of Patient Symptoms
First Edition, 2008

The Merck Manual Go-To Home Guide for Symptoms
First Edition, 2013

Merck books are published as a service to the scientific community and the public.

FOREWORD

Merck & Co., Inc., has a long history of providing medical information to both human and animal health care professionals. For more than 60 years, the *Merck Veterinary Manual* (MVM) has provided veterinarians and other animal health professionals with concise and authoritative information on diseases and management of food-producing, companion, laboratory, and exotic animals. The 11th edition carries on this proud tradition.

This new edition has been completely updated and revised to continue to address the many diverse aspects of veterinary medicine. The first half of the book covers all body systems, including discussions of disease etiology, diagnosis, treatment, control, and prevention. The second half addresses special topics, including behavior, clinical pathology, management and nutrition, pharmacology, toxicology, and poultry medicine. Although the contents of the book have expanded with each edition, the MVM remains true to its original objective: a concise, easy-to-use, comprehensive reference that covers the diversity of species and animal diseases worldwide. Coverage is straightforward and practical, with explicit recommendations given for treatment whenever possible. The succinct discussions also serve to give readers a strong foundation for seeking out and understanding more detailed information available elsewhere.

The MVM covers all the basics, but it is also often relied on for areas not commonly encountered in the daily routine of most animal health professionals. This is no more evident than in the growing responsibility of veterinarians to society, in which general practitioners and specialists alike must vigilantly embrace their role in the international movement of animals, maintaining a safe food supply, and minimizing the spread of infectious animal disease and zoonotic agents. In this vein, a new section is dedicated to public health, covering public health functions and agencies, epidemiologic principles, disease outbreak investigations, food safety, and an extensive table of zoonoses.

Other significant new information has been added on heart disease, diagnostic imaging, emergency medicine, wound management, and pharmacology, including drug resistance. The emerging area of aquaculture is reflected in new chapters on aquaculture, aquatic systems, and aquarium fish. Veterinary responsibilities under the new Veterinary Feed Directive rule are also summarized. Additional timely new topics have been added throughout, covering subjects as diverse as backyard poultry, equine arboviral encephalomyelitis, neonatal management, smoke inhalation, rhodococcosis, scorpion bites, spider flies, xylitol toxicity, toxicologic hazards in the workplace, and the human-animal bond and service animals. And as medical knowledge of exotic and laboratory animals continues to increase, so does the MVM's coverage of pet birds, rabbits, reptiles, rodents, fish, and other nontraditional species.

The contents of the MVM are available online and as an app for handheld devices, providing enhanced capability to quickly access needed information. Digital versions are updated more frequently and include thousands of additional images and other multimedia offerings.

As always, we are deeply grateful to the authors and reviewers who have contributed to the current and past editions of the MVM. The 11th edition of the MVM is an extensive collaboration of the MVM Editorial Board and nearly 400 veterinary experts from academia, government, research organizations, and specialty practices, representing more than 20 countries worldwide. It is only through their dedication to animal health and their efforts and willingness to share their time and expertise that the MVM is possible.

Acknowledgment and thanks are also due to the following individuals for their assistance in the 11th edition of the MVM: Jennifer A. Doyle for business operations and technical troubleshooting, Lisa P. Glinski for index entry coding and other critical tasks, Jean L. Perry for general project administrative support, and Michelle A. Steigerwald for image processing. Appreciation is also expressed to Robert S. Porter, MD, for his management support.

Lastly, there is nothing more rewarding than hearing directly from our readers. Please continue to share your many thoughts, experiences, and stories about the MVM so that the book and its legacy can continue to improve, evolve, and endure.

Susan E. Aiello, DVM, ELS, Editor-in-Chief

Michael A. Moses, Executive Editor

GUIDE FOR READERS

- The Contents shows the title of each section of the *Merck Veterinary Manual* (MVM) and the corresponding thumb tab abbreviation.
- Each section has its own Table of Contents that lists chapter and subchapter titles in that section.
- Many cross-reference page numbers are found throughout the text to enable the reader to quickly find discussions of related material elsewhere in the book.
- A number of abbreviations and symbols used routinely throughout the text are listed beginning on p xiii. Other abbreviations used in the text are defined at their first use.
- Generic (nonproprietary) names of drugs are used in most instances.
- Running heads on left-hand pages correspond to the chapter title of the text appearing at the top of that page. Running heads on right-hand pages correspond to the chapter title of the text appearing at the bottom of that page. In other words, running heads are used as in a standard dictionary.
- The Index is the best way to locate specific discussions of a disease, condition, or syndrome for which the name is known.
- The first half of the MVM is arranged into anatomic systems, and specific conditions are located in the system that is primarily affected. Conditions that may affect more than one system are covered in the section Generalized Conditions (GEN). The second half of the MVM covers special topics or disciplines.
- The authors, reviewers, editors, and publisher have made extensive efforts to ensure that treatments, drugs, dosage regimens, and withdrawal times are accurate and conform to the standards accepted at the time of publication. **However, constant changes in information resulting from continuing research and clinical experience, reasonable differences in opinions among authorities, unique aspects of individual clinical situations, and the possibility of human error in preparing such an extensive text require that the reader exercise individual judgment when making a clinical decision and, if necessary, consult and compare information from other sources**. In particular, the reader is advised to check the product information currently provided by the manufacturer of each drug before prescribing or administering it, especially if the drug is unfamiliar or is used infrequently. Many of the drug dosages given are considered extra-label usages, which require a valid veterinarian-client-patient relationship. Veterinarians should also be familiar and comply with the regulations set forth by the Veterinary Feed Directive.

CONTENTS

CONTENTS

ABBREVIATIONS AND SYMBOLS

ad lib	as much as desired
ADP	adenosine diphosphate
ALT	alanine aminotransferase
AST	aspartate aminotransferase
ATP	adenosine triphosphate
bid	twice a day
bpm	beats per minute
BUN	blood urea nitrogen
C	Celsius (Centigrade)
cal	calorie(s)
CBC(s)	complete blood count(s)
CDC	Centers for Disease Control and Prevention
CFU	colony-forming unit
cm	centimeter(s)
CNS	central nervous system
CK	creatine kinase (CPK, creatine phosphokinase)
CSF	cerebrospinal fluid
CT	computed tomography
cu	cubic
DIC	disseminated intravascular coagulation
dL	deciliter(s)
DNA	deoxyribonucleic acid
ECG	electrocardiogram
eg	for example
ELISA	enzyme-linked immunosorbent assay
EPA	Environmental Protection Agency
EPG	eggs per gram (of feces)
et seq	and the following one(s)
EU	European Union
F	Fahrenheit
FDA	Food and Drug Administration
fL	femtoliter(s)
ft	foot, feet
g	gram(s)
gal.	gallon(s)
GI	gastrointestinal
GnRH	gonadotropin-releasing hormone
H&E	hematoxylin and eosin
Hgb	hemoglobin
hr	hour(s)
ie	that is
Ig	immunoglobulin (with class following: A, D, E, G, or M)
IL	interleukin
IM	intramuscular(ly)
in.	inch(es)
IP	intraperitoneal(ly)
IU	international unit(s)
IV	intravenous(ly)
kcal	kilocalorie(s)
kg	kilogram(s)
L	liter(s)
LDH	lactate dehydrogenase
lb	pound(s)
m	meter(s)
M	molar
Mcal	megacalorie(s)
mcg	microgram
ME	metabolizable energy
mEq	milliequivalent(s)
mg	milligram(s)
min	minute(s)
mL	milliliter(s)
mm	millimeter(s)
mo	month(s)
mol	mole(s)
mOsm	milliosmole(s)
nm	nanometer(s)
MRI	magnetic resonance imaging
NRC	National Research Council
NSAID(s)	nonsteroidal anti-inflammatory drug(s)
OIE	Office International des Épizooties
oz	ounce(s)
p/pp	page/pages
PCR	polymerase chain reaction
PCV	packed cell volume
pH	negative logarithm of hydrogen ion activity
PO	per os, orally
ppb	part(s) per billion
ppm	part(s) per million
qid	four times a day
qs ad	quantity sufficient to make
RBC(s)	red blood cell(s)
RNA	ribonucleic acid
SC	subcutaneous(ly)
sec	second(s)
SI units	International System of Units
SPF	specific pathogen free
sq	square
tbsp	tablespoon(s)

TDN	total digestible nutrients
tid	three times a day
tsp	teaspoon(s)
U	unit(s)
UK	United Kingdom
USDA	United States Department of Agriculture
USA	United States of America
USSR	Union of Soviet Socialist Republics (former)
WBC(s)	white blood cell(s)
wk	week(s)
wt	weight
yr	year(s)

α	alpha
β	beta
δ	delta
ϵ	epsilon
γ	gamma
λ	lambda
μ	micro, mu
κ	kappa
σ	sigma

EDITORIAL BOARD

EDITORIAL BOARD

CONTRIBUTORS

Tahseen Abdul-Aziz, BVMS, MS, PhD, DACPV
Veterinary Pathologist, Rollins Animal Disease Diagnostic Laboratory, North Carolina Department of Agriculture and Consumer Services, Raleigh, NC

Avian Encephalomyelitis; Botulism; Listeriosis

Stephen B. Adams, DVM, MS, DACVS
Professor of Surgery, Department of Veterinary Clinical Sciences, School of Veterinary Medicine, Purdue University, West Lafayette, IN

Arthroscopy; Lameness in Horses: Introduction; Musculoskeletal System: Introduction; The Lameness Examination

Andrew J. Allen, DVM, PhD, DACVIM
Assistant Professor, Department of Veterinary Clinical Sciences, Washington State University, Pullman, WA

Disorders of Calcium Metabolism: Parturient Paresis in Cows; Metabolic Disorders: Introduction; Transport Tetany in Ruminants

Dana G. Allen, DVM, MSc, DACVIM
Professor Emeritus, Ontario Veterinary College, University of Guelph, Ontario, Canada

Congenital and Inherited Anomalies; Systemic Pharmacotherapeutics of the Cardiovascular System: Drugs Acting on the Blood

Kelly E. Allen, MS, PhD
Lecturer, Department of Veterinary Pathobiology, Center for Veterinary Health Sciences, Oklahoma State University, Stillwater, OK

Blood Parasites: Old World Hepatozoonosis and American Canine Hepatozoonosis

Sandra Allweiler, DVM, DACVA
Assistant Professor, Department of Clinical Sciences, College of Veterinary Medicine and Biomedical Sciences, Colorado State University, Fort Collins, CO

Pain Assessment and Management

Glen W. Almond, DVM, PhD
Professor, Swine Health and Production Management, North Carolina State University, Raleigh, NC

Postpartum Dysgalactia Syndrome and Mastitis in Sows

Gary C. Althouse, BS, MS, DVM, PhD, DACT
Professor of Reproduction and Swine Health; Marion Dilley and David George Jones Endowed Chair in Animal Reproduction, Department of Clinical Studies, New Bolton Center, University of Pennsylvania, Kennett Square, PA

Management of Reproduction: Pigs

Claire B. Andreasen, DVM, PhD, DACVP
Associate Dean for Academic and Student Affairs and Professor, College of Veterinary Medicine, Iowa State University, Ames, IA

Staphylococcosis

Frank M. Andrews, DVM, MS, DACVIM (Large Animal)
Louisiana Veterinary Medical Association Equine Committee Professor and Director, Equine Health Studies Program, Department of Veterinary Clinical Sciences, School of Veterinary Medicine, Louisiana State University, Baton Rouge, LA

Gastrointestinal Ulcers in Large Animals: Gastrointestinal Ulcers in Horses

John A. Angelos, DVM, PhD, DACVIM
Associate Professor, Department of Medicine and Epidemiology; Livestock Medicine and Surgery, School of Veterinary Medicine, University of California, Davis, CA

Infectious Keratoconjunctivitis

David A. Ashford, DVM, MPH, DSc
Attaché, US Department of Agriculture, Office of Agricultural Affairs, Port au Prince, Haiti

Foot-and-Mouth Disease

Clarke Atkins, DVM, DACVIM
Jane Lewis Seaks Distinguished Professor, Professor Emeritus, College of Veterinary Medicine, North Carolina State University, Raleigh, NC

Heartworm Disease

Rick Atwell, BVSc, PhD, FACVSc
Honorary Professor, School of Veterinary Science, University of Queensland, Brisbane, Queensland, Australia

Tick Paralysis

David G. Baker, DVM, MS, PhD, DACLAM
Director and Professor, Division of Laboratory Animal Medicine, School of Veterinary Medicine, Louisiana State University, Baton Rouge, LA

Eyeworm Disease

Lora R. Ballweber, MS, DVM
Professor, Clinical Parasitology, College of Veterinary Medicine and Biomedical Sciences, Colorado State University, Fort Collins, CO

Fluke Infections in Ruminants; Gastrointestinal Parasites of Pigs; Lungworm Infection

Alejandro Banda, DVM, MSc, PhD, DACPV, DACVM
Associate Clinical Professor of Avian Virology, Poultry Research and Diagnostic Laboratory, College of Veterinary Medicine, Mississippi State University, Mississippi State, MS

Duck Viral Enteritis

Gad Baneth, DVM, PhD, DECVCP
Professor, Koret School of Veterinary Medicine, Hebrew University, Rehovot, Israel

Leishmaniosis

Lisa G. Barber, DVM
Assistant Professor, Department of Clinical Sciences, Cummings School of Veterinary Medicine, Tufts University, North Grafton, MA

Antineoplastic Agents

George M. Barrington, DVM, PhD, DACVIM
Professor, Food Animal Medicine and Surgery, College of Veterinary Medicine, Washington State University, Pullman, WA

Congenital Erythropoietic Porphyria; Photosensitization

Robert B. Beckstead, PhD
Associate Professor, Department of Poultry Science, University of Georgia, Athens, GA

Hexamitiasis; Histomoniasis

Daniela Bedenice, DVM, DACVIM, DACVECC
Assistant Professor, Department of Clinical Sciences, Cummings School of Veterinary Medicine, Tufts University, North Grafton, MA

Hypoxic Ischemic Encephalopathy; Management of the Neonate: Large Animals; Sepsis in Foals

Sylvia J. Bedford-Guaus, DVM, PhD, DACT
Animal Reproduction Consultant, Barcelona, Spain

Breeding Soundness Examination of the Male

James K. Belknap, DVM, PhD, DACVS
Professor of Equine Surgery, Department of Veterinary Clinical Sciences, College of Veterinary Medicine, The Ohio State University, Columbus, OH

Lameness in Horses: Disorders of the Foot

William G. Bickert, PhD
Deceased
Professor Emeritus, Biosystems and Agricultural Engineering, Michigan State University, East Lansing, MI

Ventilation

Rob Bildfell, DVM, MSc, DACVP
Professor, Department of Biomedical Sciences, College of Veterinary Medicine, Oregon State University, Corvallis, OR

Collection and Submission of Laboratory Samples; Pyrrolizidine Alkaloidosis

Patrick Joseph Blackall, BSc, PhD
Principal Research Fellow, Queensland Alliance for Agriculture and Food Innovation, The University of Queensland, Brisbane, Queensland, Australia

Infectious Coryza

Barry R. Blakley, DVM, PhD
Professor, Department of Veterinary Biomedical Sciences, Western College of Veterinary Medicine, University of Saskatchewan, Saskatoon, Canada

Copper Poisoning; Fluoride Poisoning; Lead Poisoning; Mercury Poisoning; Metaldehyde Poisoning; Molybdenum Poisoning; Quercus Poisoning; Sorghum Poisoning

Shauna L. Blois, DVM, DVSc, DACVIM
Assistant Professor, Clinical Studies, Ontario Veterinary College, University of Guelph, Ontario, Canada

Diseases of the Stomach and Intestines in Small Animals: Gastrointestinal Neoplasia, Gastrointestinal Ulcers, Helicobacter Infections

Dawn Merton Boothe, DVM, PhD
Professor, Department of Anatomy, Physiology, and Pharmacology, College of Veterinary Medicine, Auburn University, Auburn, AL

Antibacterial Agents; Antifungal Agents; Antiviral Agents; Chemotherapeutics Introduction; Pharmacology Introduction

Manuel Borca, DVM, PhD
Research Microbiologist, Foreign Animal Disease Research, USDA, Orient Point, NY

Classical Swine Fever

Jane C. Boswell, MA, VetMB, CertVA, CertES (Orth), DECVS, MRCVS
The Liphook Equine Hospital, Liphook, Hampshire, UK

Lameness in Horses: Disorders of the Stifle, Disorders of the Tarsus and Metatarsus

Joan S. Bowen, DVM
Bowen Mobile Veterinary Practice, Wellington, CO

Health-Management Interaction: Goats; Lameness in Goats

Perle E. Boyer, DVM
Lecturer, North Carolina State University, Raleigh, NC

Postpartum Dysgalactia Syndrome and Mastitis in Sows

R. Keith Bramwell, BS, MS, PhD
Extension Poultry Specialist, Cooperative Extension Service, and Associate Professor, Department of Poultry Science, University of Arkansas, Fayetteville, AR

Artificial Insemination (Poultry)

Matthew T. Brokken, DVM, DACVS
Clinical Assistant Professor, Department of Veterinary Clinical Sciences, College of Veterinary Medicine, The Ohio State University, Columbus, OH

Lameness in Horses: Disorders of the Carpus and Metacarpus, Disorders of the Fetlock and Pastern

Scott A. Brown, VMD, PhD, DACVIM
Josiah Meigs Distinguished Professor and Head, Department of Small Animal Medicine and Surgery, College of Veterinary Medicine, University of Georgia, Athens, GA

Infectious Diseases of the Urinary System in Small Animals; Noninfectious Diseases of the Urinary System in Small Animals

Cecil F. Brownie, DVM, PhD, DABVT, DABFE, DABFM, FACFEI
Professor Emeritus, College of Veterinary Medicine, North Carolina State University, Raleigh, NC

Poisonous Mushrooms; Poisonous Plants

Glenn F. Browning, BVSc, DVCS, PhD
Professor in Veterinary Microbiology, Asia-Pacific Centre for Animal Health, Faculty of Veterinary Science, The University of Melbourne, Werribee, Victoria, Australia

Infectious Bronchitis

David Bruyette, DVM, DACVIM
Medical Director, VCA West Los Angeles Animal Hospital, Los Angeles, CA

The Adrenal Glands; The Pancreas

Marie S. Bulgin, DVM, MBA, DACVM
Emerita, Caine Veterinary Teaching Center, University of Idaho, Caldwell, ID

Health-Management Interaction: Sheep; Lameness in Sheep; Scrapie

Kristine E. Burgess, DVM, DACVIM (Oncology)
Assistant Professor, Department of Clinical Sciences, Cummings School of Veterinary Medicine, Tufts University, North Grafton, MA

Antineoplastic Agents

Amanda Burling, DVM
Maddie's Shelter Medicine Program, College of Veterinary Medicine, University of Florida, Gainesville, FL

Feline Leukemia Virus and Related Diseases

Raymond Cahill-Morasco, MS, DVM
SeaPort Veterinary Hospital, Gloucester, MA

Zinc Toxicosis

Robert J. Callan, DVM, MS, PhD, DACVIM
Professor, Department of Clinical Sciences, College of Veterinary Medicine and Biomedical Sciences, Colorado State University, Fort Collins, CO

Bluetongue; Congenital and Inherited Anomalies: Border Disease; Malignant Catarrhal Fever; Sporadic Bovine Encephalomyelitis

John Campbell, DVM, DVSc
Professor, Large Animal Clinical Sciences, Western College of Veterinary Medicine, University of Saskatchewan, Saskatoon, Saskatchewan, Canada

Respiratory Diseases of Cattle

Wayne W. Carmichael, PhD
Professor of Aquatic Biology/Toxicology, Wright State University, Dayton, OH

Algal Poisoning

James W. Carpenter, MS, DVM, DACZM
Professor, Zoological Medicine, Department of Clinical Sciences, College of Veterinary Medicine, Kansas State University, Manhattan, KS

Hedgehogs

Phillip D. Carter, BVSc, MVS
Queensland Department of Agriculture, Fisheries and Forestry, Tick Fever Centre, Wacol, Queensland, Australia

Blood Parasites: Babesiosis

Samuel C. Cartner, DVM, PhD, DACLAM
Assistant Vice President for Animal Research Services and Director, Animal Resources Program, University of Alabama, Birmingham, AL

Euthanasia

Christopher K. Cebra, VMD, MA, MS, DACVIM
Professor, Large Animal Medicine, College of Veterinary Medicine, Oregon State University, Corvallis, OR

Hepatic Lipidosis: Pregnancy Toxemia in Cows

Sharon A. Center, BS, DVM, DACVIM
Professor, Department of Clinical Sciences, College of Veterinary Medicine, Cornell University, Ithaca, NY

Hepatic Disease in Small Animals

Jens Peter Christensen, DVM, PhD
Associate Professor, Department of Veterinary Disease Biology, Faculty of Life Sciences, University of Copenhagen, Denmark

Fowl Cholera; Riemerella anatipestifer Infection

Edwin Claerebout, DVM, PhD, DEVPC
Professor, Department of Virology, Parasitology and Immunology, Faculty of Veterinary Medicine, Ghent University, Merelbeke, Belgium

Anthelmintics

Peter Clegg, MA, Vet MB, DECVS, PhD, MRCVS
Professor of Equine Surgery, Veterinary Teaching Hospital, School of Veterinary Sciences, University of Liverpool, Neston, UK

Lameness in Horses: Disorders of the Back and Pelvis, Disorders of the Hip

Johann (Hans) F. Coetzee, BVSc, CertCHP, PhD, DACVCP
Department of Veterinary Diagnostic and Production Animal Medicine, College of Veterinary Medicine, Iowa State University, Ames, IA

Systemic Pharmacotherapeutics of the Ruminant Digestive System

Stephen R. Collett, BSc, BVSc, MMedVet
Clinical Associate Professor, Department of Population Health, College of Veterinary Medicine, University of Georgia, Athens, GA

Biosecurity; Sudden Death Syndrome of Broiler Chickens

Michael T. Collins, DVM, PhD, DACVM
Professor of Microbiology, Department of Pathobiological Sciences, School of Veterinary Medicine, University of Wisconsin, Madison, WI

Paratuberculosis

Peter D. Constable, BVSc (Hons), MS, PhD, DACVIM
Dean, College of Veterinary Medicine, University of Illinois, Urbana, IL

Abdominal Fat Necrosis; Acute Intestinal Obstructions in Large Animals; Bovine Secondary Recumbency; Coccidiosis; Cryptosporidiosis; Diseases of the Abomasum; Disorders of Potassium

Metabolism; Diseases of the Ruminant Forestomach: Bloat in Ruminants, Grain Overload, Simple Indigestion, Traumatic Reticuloperitonitis, Vagal Indigestion Syndrome; Infectious Diseases of the Urinary System in Large Animals: Bovine Cystitis and Pyelonephritis

Rhian B. Cope, BVSC, PhD, DABT, ERT, FACTRA
Toxicology Section, Office of Scientific Evaluation, Therapeutic Goods Administration of Australia, Symonston, Australian Capital Territory, Australia

Cyanide Poisoning; Smoke Inhalation; Toxicologic Hazards in the Workplace

Robert W. Coppock, DVM, MS, PhD, DABVT, DABT
President and CEO, Robert W. Coppock, DVM, Toxicologist and Associate Ltd., Vegreville, Alberta, Canada

Persistent Halogenated Aromatic Poisoning

Susan M. Cotter, DVM, DACVIM (Small Animal, Oncology)
Distinguished Professor of Clinical Sciences Emerita, Cummings School of Veterinary Medicine, Tufts University, North Grafton, MA

Blood Groups and Blood Transfusions; Hematopoietic System Introduction; Hemostatic Disorders

Laurent L. Couetil, DVM, PhD, DACVIM (Large Animal)
Professor, Department of Veterinary Clinical Sciences, College of Veterinary Medicine, Purdue University, West Lafayette, IN

Pulmonary Emphysema

Kate E. Creevy, DVM, MS, DACVIM
Associate Professor of Internal Medicine, Department of Small Animal Medicine and Surgery, College of Veterinary Medicine, University of Georgia, Athens, GA

Canine Distemper; Canine Herpesviral Infection; Infectious Canine Hepatitis

Rocio Crespo, DVM, MSc, DVSc, DACPV
Associate Professor and Director, Avian Health and Food Safety Laboratory, Washington Animal Disease Diagnostic Laboratory, Washington State University, Pullman, WA

Miscellaneous Conditions of Poultry: Urate Deposition (Gout)

Gary L. Cromwell, PhD
Professor, Department of Animal and Food Sciences, University of Kentucky, Lexington, KY

Iron Toxicity in Newborn Pigs; Nutrition: Pigs

Suzanne M. Cunningham, DVM, DACVIM (Cardiology)
Assistant Professor of Cardiology, Department of Clinical Sciences, Cummings School of Veterinary Medicine, Tufts University, North Grafton, MA

Cardiovascular System Introduction; Thrombosis, Embolism, and Aneurysm

Andrew Dart, BVSc, PhD, DACVS, DECVS
Director of the Research and Clinical Training Unit, Faculty of Veterinary Science, The University of Sydney, New South Wales, Australia

Congenital and Inherited Anomalies

Autumn P. Davidson, DVM, MS, DACVIM
Clinical Professor, School of Veterinary Medicine, University of California, Davis, CA

Management of Reproduction: Small Animals; Management of the Neonate: Small Animals; Reproductive Diseases of the Male Small Animal

Peter R. Davies, BVSc, PhD
Professor, Swine Health and Production, Department of Veterinary Population Medicine, College of Veterinary Medicine, University of Minnesota, St. Paul, MN

Exudative Epidermitis; Parakeratosis; Pityriasis Rosea in Pigs; Swine Vesicular Disease; Vesicular Exanthema of Swine

Sherrill Davison, VMD, MS, MBA, DACPV
Associate Professor, Laboratory of Avian Medicine and Pathology, School of Veterinary Medicine, University of Pennsylvania, Kennett Square, PA

Salmonelloses (Poultry)

Scott A. Dee, DVM, MS, PhD
Director of Research, Pipestone Applied Research, Pipestone Veterinary Services, Pipestone, MN

Infectious Diseases of the Urinary System in Large Animals: Porcine Cystitis-Pyelonephritis Complex; Porcine Reproductive and Respiratory Syndrome; Pseudorabies; Respiratory Diseases of Pigs

Alice Defarges, DVM, MSc, DACVIM
Assistant Professor in Internal Medicine, Department of Clinical Studies, Ontario Veterinary College, University of Guelph, Ontario, Canada

Diseases of the Stomach and Intestines in Small Animals: Colitis in Small Animals, Constipation and Obstipation in Small Animals, Inflammatory Bowel Disease in Small Animals

Sagi Denenberg, DVM, DACVB, DECAWBM (Behaviour), MACVSc (Behaviour)
North Toronto Veterinary Behaviour Specialty Clinic, Thornhill, Ontario, Canada

Normal Social Behavior and Behavioral Problems of Domestic Animals

R. Page Dinsmore, DVM
Associate Professor, Department of Clinical Sciences, College of Veterinary Medicine and Biomedical Sciences, Colorado State University, Fort Collins, CO

Health-Management Interaction: Dairy Cattle

Stephen J. Divers, BVetMed, DZooMed, DACZM, DECZM (Herpetology), FRCVS
Professor of Zoological Medicine, Department of Small Animal Medicine and Surgery, College of Veterinary Medicine, University of Georgia, Athens, GA

Reptiles

Thomas J. Divers, DVM, DACVIM, DACVECC
Professor of Medicine, Department of Clinical Sciences, College of Veterinary Medicine, Cornell University, Ithaca, NY

Leptospirosis: Horses, Ruminants, Swine; Noninfectious Diseases of the Urinary System in Large Animals

Thomas M. Donnelly, BVSc, DVP, DACLAM, DABVP (ECM)
The Kenneth S. Warren Institute, Ossining, NY; Adjunct Associate Professor, Cummings School of Veterinary Medicine, Tufts University, North Grafton, MA

Rodents

Patricia M. Dowling, DVM, MSc, DACVIM, DACVCP
Professor, Veterinary Clinical Pharmacology, Western College of Veterinary Medicine, University of Saskatchewan, Saskatoon, Canada

Systemic Pharmacotherapeutics of the Monogastric Digestive System; Systemic Pharmacotherapeutics of the Muscular System; Systemic Pharmacotherapeutics of the Respiratory System; Systemic Pharmacotherapeutics of the Urinary System

Michael W. Dryden, DVM, PhD, DACVM
University Distinguished Professor of Veterinary Parasitology, Diagnostic Medicine/Pathobiology, College of Veterinary Medicine, Kansas State University, Manhattan, KS

Ectoparasiticides: Ectoparasiticides Used in Small Animals; Fleas and Flea Allergy Dermatitis; Mange: Mange in Dogs and Cats

J. P. Dubey, MVSc, PhD
Microbiologist, Animal Parasitic Diseases Laboratory, Beltsville Agricultural Research Center, USDA, Beltsville, MD

Toxoplasmosis

Rebecca S. Duerr, DVM, MPVM, PhD
Staff Veterinarian, International Bird Rescue Research Center, Cordelia, CA

Management of the Neonate: Care of Orphaned Native Birds and Mammals

John Dunn, DVM, PhD
Veterinary Medical Officer, Avian Disease and Oncology Laboratory, USDA-ARS, East Lansing, MI

Neoplasms (Poultry)

Jack Easley, DVM, MS, DABVP (Equine)
Equine Veterinary Practice, LLC, Shelbyville, KY

Dentistry: Dentistry in Large Animals

Scott H. Edwards, BSc, BVMS, PhD, MANZCVSc
Senior Lecturer, Veterinary Pharmacology, Charles Sturt University, Wagga Wagga, New South Wales, Australia

Anti-inflammatory Agents

Steve M. Ensley, DVM, PhD
Veterinary Toxicologist, Veterinary Diagnostic and Production Animal Medicine, College of Veterinary Medicine, Iowa State University, Ames, IA

Toxicology Introduction

Ronald J. Erskine, DVM, PhD
Professor, Large Animal Clinical Sciences, College of Veterinary Medicine, Michigan State University, East Lansing, MI

Mastitis in Large Animals

Paul Ettestad, DVM, MS
State Public Health Veterinarian, Epidemiology and Response Division, New Mexico Department of Health, Santa Fe, NM

Plague

Timothy M. Fan, DVM, PhD, DACVIM
Associate Professor, Department of Veterinary Clinical Medicine, College of Veterinary Medicine, University of Illinois, Urbana, IL

Canine Lymphoma

Susan E. Fielder, DVM, MS, DACVP (Clinical Pathology)
Clinical Assistant Professor, Department of Pathobiology, Center for Veterinary Health Sciences, Oklahoma State University, Stillwater, OK

Reference Guides

Scott D. Fitzgerald, DVM, PhD, DACVP, DACPV
Professor, Department of Pathobiology and Diagnostic Investigation, College of Veterinary Medicine, Michigan State University, East Lansing, MI

Congenital and Inherited Anomalies of the Urinary System; West Nile Virus Infection in Poultry

Sherrill A. Fleming, DVM, DACVIM, DABVP
Associate Professor, Food and Animal Medicine, College of Veterinary Medicine, Mississippi State University, Mississippi State, MS

Pasteurellosis of Sheep and Goats

Janet E. Foley, DVM, PhD
Professor, Department of Medicine and Epidemiology; Co-Director, Center for Vector-Borne Disease, School of Veterinary Medicine, University of California, Davis, CA

Tularemia

Jonathan H. Foreman, DVM, MS, DACVIM (Large Animal)
Associate Dean, Professor, College of Veterinary Medicine, University of Illinois, Urbana, IL

Hepatic Disease in Large Animals

Mark T. Fox, BVetMed, PhD, DEVPC, FHEA, MRCVS
Professor of Veterinary Parasitology, Department of Pathology and Pathogen Biology, The Royal Veterinary College, University of London, UK

Gastrointestinal Parasites of Ruminants

Ruth Francis-Floyd, DVM, MS, DACZM
Professor, Department of Large Animal Clinical Sciences, College of Veterinary Medicine, University of Florida, Gainesville, FL

Aquaculture; Aquarium Fishes; Aquatic Systems

Robert M. Friendship, DVM, MSc, DABVP
Professor, Department of Population Medicine, Ontario Veterinary College, University of Guelph, Ontario, Canada

Gastrointestinal Ulcers in Large Animals: Gastric Ulcers in Pigs; Health-Management Interaction: Pigs

Laurie J. Gage, DVM, DACZM
Big Cat and Marine Mammal Specialist, USDA APHIS Animal Care, Center for Animal Welfare, Napa, CA

Management of the Neonate: Care of Orphaned Native Birds and Mammals

Maricarmen García, PhD
Associate Professor, Poultry Diagnostic and Research Center, Department of Population and Health, University of Georgia, Athens, GA

Infectious Laryngotracheitis

Tam Garland, DVM, PhD, DABVT
Veterinary Medical Diagnostic Laboratory, Texas A&M University, College Station, TX

Arsenic Poisoning; Gossypol Poisoning

Jack M. Gaskin, DVM, PhD, DACVM
Associate Professor Emeritus, Department of Infectious Disease and Pathology, College of Veterinary Medicine, University of Florida, Gainesville, FL

Encephalomyocarditis Virus Infection

Kirk N. Gelatt, VMD, DACVO
Emeritus Distinguished Professor, Department of Small Animal Clinical Sciences, College of Veterinary Medicine, University of Florida, Gainesville, FL

Neoplasia of the Eye and Associated Structures; Ophthalmic Emergencies; Ophthalmology

Richard W. Gerhold, DVM, MS, PhD
Department of Biomedical and Diagnostic Sciences, College of Veterinary Medicine, University of Tennessee, Knoxville, TN

Coccidiosis (Poultry); Cryptosporidiosis (Poultry); Trichomonosis

E. Paul J. Gibbs, BVSc, PhD, FRCVS
Professor Emeritus, College of Veterinary Medicine, University of Florida, Gainesville, FL

Pox Diseases

Thomas W. G. Gibson, BSc, BEd, DVM, DVSc, DACVS
Assistant Professor of Small Animal Surgery, Department of Clinical Studies, Ontario Veterinary College, University of Guelph, Ontario, Canada

Diseases of the Stomach and Intestines in Small Animals: Gastric Dilation and Volvulus in Small Animals, Gastrointestinal Obstruction in Small Animals

Robert O. Gilbert, BVSc, MMedVet, DACT, MRCVS
Professor, Reproductive Medicine, Department of Clinical Sciences, College of Veterinary Medicine, Cornell University, Ithaca, NY

Metritis in Large Animals; Retained Fetal Membranes in Large Animals; Systemic Pharmacotherapeutics of the Reproductive System; Uterine Prolapse and Eversion; Vaginal and Cervical Prolapse; Vulvitis and Vaginitis in Large Animals

Sabine Gilch, PhD
Assistant Professor, Veterinary Medicine, University of Calgary, Alberta, Canada

Chronic Wasting Disease

Eric Gonder, DVM, MS, PhD, DACPV
Veterinarian, Butterball LLC, Goldsboro, NC; Adjunct Professor, Department of Population Health and Pathobiology, College of Veterinary Medicine, North Carolina State University, Raleigh, NC

Miscellaneous Conditions of Poultry: Pendulous Crop

Sonya G. Gordon, DVM, DVSc, DACVIM (Cardiology)
Associate Professor, Department of Small Animal Clinical Sciences, Texas A&M University, College Station, TX

Systemic Pharmacotherapeutics of the Cardiovascular System

Louis Norman Gotthelf, DVM
Animal Hospital of Montgomery; Montgomery Pet Skin and Ear Clinic, Montgomery, AL

Tumors of the Ear Canal

Marcelo Gottschalk, DVM, PhD
Professor, College of Veterinary Medicine, University of Montreal, St-Hyacinthe, Quebec, Canada

Streptococcal Infections in Pigs

Gregory F. Grauer, DVM, MS, DACVIM
Professor and Jarvis Chair of Small Animal Internal Medicine, Department of Clinical Sciences, College of Veterinary Medicine, Kansas State University, Manhattan, KS

Ethylene Glycol Toxicity

Deborah S. Greco, DVM, PhD, DACVIM
Senior Research Scientist, Nestle Purina PetCare, New York, NY

The Pituitary Gland

Paul R. Greenough, FRCVS
Professor Emeritus of Veterinary Surgery, Western College of Veterinary Medicine, University of Saskatchewan, Saskatoon, Canada

Lameness in Cattle

Tara L. Grinnage-Pulley, DVM, PhD
Adjunct Lecturer and Postdoctoral Research Fellow, Department of Epidemiology, College of Public Health, University of Iowa, Iowa City, IA

Blood Parasites: Trypanosomiasis

Walter Gruenberg, DMV, MS, PhD, DECAR, DECBHM
Assistant Professor, Department of Farm Animal Health, Utrecht University, Utrecht, The Netherlands

Colisepticemia; Disorders of Phosphorus Metabolism; Dystrophies Associated with Calcium, Phosphorus, and Vitamin D; Hepatic Lipidosis: Fatty Liver Disease of Cattle; Intestinal Diseases in Ruminants; Salmonellosis

P. K. Gupta, PhD, Post Doc (USA), PGDCA, MSc VM & AH BVSc, FNA VSc, FASc, AW, FST, FAEB, FACVT (USA), Gold Medalist
Editor-in-Chief, *Toxicology International*, Bareilly-India

Herbicide Poisoning; Pentachlorophenol Poisoning

Ramesh C. Gupta, DVM, MVSc, PhD, DABT, FACT, FACN, FATS
Professor and Head, Toxicology Department, Breathitt Veterinary Center, Murray State University, Hopkinsville, KY

Insecticide and Acaricide (Organic) Toxicity

James S. Guy, DVM, PhD
Professor, Department of Population Health and Pathobiology, College of Veterinary Medicine, North Carolina State University, Raleigh, NC

Coronaviral Enteritis of Turkeys; Viral Encephalitides

Sharon M. Gwaltney-Brant, DVM, PhD, DABVT, DABT
Toxicology Consultant, Veterinary Information Network and Adjunct Faculty, College of Veterinary Medicine, University of Illinois, Urbana, IL

Food Hazards; Household Hazards; Snakebite; Toad Poisoning

Carlton L. Gyles, DVM, PhD
Professor Emeritus, Department of Pathobiology, Ontario Veterinary College, University of Guelph, Ontario, Canada

Edema Disease

Caroline N. Hahn, DVM, MSc, PhD, DECEIM, DECVN, MRCVS
Senior Lecturer in Veterinary Clinical Neuroscience, Royal (Dick) School of Veterinary Studies, University of Edinburgh, Midlothian, UK

Dysautonomia

Edward J. Hall, MA, VetMB, PhD, DECVIM-CA
Professor of Small Animal Internal Medicine, Department of Clinical Veterinary Science, University of Bristol, Bristol, UK

Diseases of the Stomach and Intestines in Small Animals: Malabsorption Syndromes in Small Animals

Jean A. Hall, DVM, PhD, DACVIM
Professor, Department of Biomedical Sciences, College of Veterinary Medicine, Oregon State University, Corvallis, OR

Disorders of Calcium Metabolism: Puerperal Hypocalcemia in Small Animals

Jeffery O. Hall, DVM, PhD, DABVT
Professor and Head of Diagnostic Toxicology, Utah State University, Logan, UT

Selenium Toxicosis

R. Reid Hanson, DVM, DACVS, DACVECC
Professor of Equine Surgery, Department of Clinical Sciences, College of Veterinary Medicine, Auburn University, Auburn, AL

Congenital and Inherited Anomalies of the Musculoskeletal System; Equine Emergency Medicine: Thermal Injuries

Joseph Harari, MS, DVM, DACVS
Veterinary Surgeon, Veterinary Surgical Specialists, Spokane, WA

Arthropathies and Related Disorders in Small Animals; Lameness in Small Animals; Myopathies in Small Animals; Osteopathies in Small Animals

Billy M. Hargis, DVM, PhD
Professor and Director, JKS Poultry Health Research Laboratory, University of Arkansas; Tyson Sustainable Poultry Health Chair, Department of Poultry Science, University of Arkansas, Fayetteville, AR

Miscellaneous Conditions of Poultry: Ascites Syndrome; Necrotic Enteritis; Spontaneous Cardiomyopathy of Turkeys

D. L. Hank Harris, DVM, PhD
Professor, Department of Animal Science, Iowa State University, Ames, IA

Intestinal Diseases in Pigs

Lynette A. Hart, PhD
Professor, Population Health and Reproduction, School of Veterinary Medicine, University of California, Davis, CA

The Human-Animal Bond

Joe Hauptman, DVM, MS, DACVS
Professor of Surgery, College of Veterinary Medicine, Michigan State University, East Lansing, MI

Diaphragmatic Hernia

Jan F. Hawkins, DVM, DACVS
Associate Professor, Veterinary Clinical Sciences, School of Veterinary Medicine, Purdue University, West Lafayette, IN

Diseases of the Esophagus in Large Animals; Diseases of the Mouth in Large Animals; Pharyngeal Paralysis; Pharyngitis

Marcus J. Head, BVetMed, MRCVS
Senior Associate, Rossdales Equine Hospital and Diagnostic Centre, Newmarket, UK

Lameness in Horses: Disorders of the Shoulder and Elbow

J. Jill Heatley, DVM, MS, DACZM, DABVP (Avian)
Associate Professor, Zoological Medicine, College of Veterinary Medicine, Texas A&M University, College Station, TX

Vaccination of Exotic Mammals

Charles M. Hendrix, DVM, PhD
Professor, Department of Pathobiology, College of Veterinary Medicine, Auburn University, Auburn, AL

CNS Diseases Caused by Helminths and Arthropods; Diagnostic Procedures for the Private Practice Laboratory: Parasitology; Flies; Venomous Arthropods

Thomas H. Herdt, DVM, MS, DACVN, DACVIM
Professor, Department of Large Animal Clinical Sciences and Diagnostic Center for Population and Animal Health, College of Veterinary Medicine, Michigan State University, East Lansing, MI

Ketosis in Cattle; Nutrition: Dairy Cattle

Laurie Hess, DVM, DABVP
Veterinary Center for Birds & Exotics, Bedford Hills, NY

Sugar Gliders

Michael Hess, DMV
Clinic for Poultry and Fish Medicine, Department for Farm Animals and Veterinary Public Health, University of Veterinary Medicine, Vienna, Austria

Avian Spirochetosis; Miscellaneous Conditions of Poultry: Fluke Infections

Hugh Hildebrandt, DVM
Medford Veterinary Clinic, Medford, WI

Mink

W. Mark Hilton, DVM, DABVP
Clinical Associate Professor, Veterinary Clinical Sciences, School of Veterinary Medicine, Purdue University, West Lafayette, IN

Health-Management Interaction: Beef Cattle; Nutrition: Beef Cattle

Katrin Hinrichs, DVM, PhD, DACT
Professor and Patsy Link Chair in Mare Reproduction, Department of Veterinary Physiology and Pharmacology, College of Veterinary Medicine and Biomedical Sciences, Texas A&M University, College Station, TX

Cloning of Domestic Animals

Frederic J. Hoerr, DVM, PhD, DACVP, DACPV
Pathologist, Veterinary Diagnostic Pathology, LLC, Fort Valley, VA

Aspergillosis; Miscellaneous Conditions of Poultry: Breast Blisters, Breast Buttons, Cannibalism; Mycotoxicoses (Poultry)

Timothy N. Holt, DVM
Associate Professor, Clinical Sciences, Livestock Medicine and Surgery, College of Veterinary Medicine and Biomedical Sciences, Colorado State University, Fort Collins, CO

Bovine High-Mountain Disease

Sharman M. Hoppes, DVM, ABVP (Avian)
Clinical Associate Professor, Zoological Medicine, Department of Veterinary Small Animal Clinical Sciences, Texas A&M University, College Station, TX

Pet Birds

Michael J. Huerkamp, DVM, DACLAM
Director, Division of Animal Resources; Professor, Pathology and Laboratory Medicine, Emory University, Atlanta, GA

Laboratory Animals

Martin E. Hugh-Jones, VetMB, MPH, PhD, MRCVS
Professor Emeritus, School of Veterinary Medicine, Louisiana State University, Baton Rouge, LA

Anthrax

Staci Hutsell, DVM
Resident, Maddie's Shelter Medicine Program, College of Veterinary Medicine, University of Florida, Gainesville, FL

Feline Infectious Peritonitis

Basil O. Ikede, BVetMed, DVM, PhD, FCVSN
Retired Professor and Chair, Department of Pathology and Microbiology, Atlantic Veterinary College, University of Prince Edward Island, Charlottetown, Prince Edward Island, Canada

Bovine Petechial Fever

Peter G. G. Jackson, MA, BVM&S, DVM&S, FRCVS
St. Edmund's College, University of Cambridge, Cambridge, UK

Prolonged Gestation in Cattle and Sheep

Daral J. Jackwood, PhD
Professor, Department of Veterinary Preventive Medicine, Ohio Agricultural Research and Development Center, The Ohio State University, Wooster, OH

Infectious Bursal Disease

Mark W. Jackwood, PhD
Professor, Department of Population Health, College of Veterinary Medicine, University of Georgia, Athens, GA

Bordetellosis

Eugene D. Janzen, DVM, MVS
Professor, Production Animal Health, Faculty of Veterinary Medicine, University of Calgary, Alberta, Canada

Histophilosis; Lightning Stroke and Electrocution; Trichomoniasis

LaRue W. Johnson, DVM, PhD
Professor Emeritus, College of Veterinary Medicine and Biomedical Sciences, Colorado State University, Fort Collins, CO

Llamas and Alpacas

Richard C. Jones, BSc, PhD, DSc, FRCPath
Emeritus Professor, School of Veterinary Science, University of Liverpool, Leahurst, Neston, Wirral, UK

Malabsorption Syndrome; Viral Arthritis

Maureen H. Kemp, BVMS, MVM, PhD, DCHP, MRCVS
Wern Veterinary Surgeons, Wales, UK

Laryngeal Disorders

Robert J. Kemppainen, DVM, PhD
Professor, Department of Anatomy, Physiology & Pharmacology, College of Veterinary Medicine, Auburn University, Auburn, AL

Endocrine System Introduction; Neuroendocrine Tissue Tumors

Safdar A. Khan, DVM, MS, PhD, DABVT
Director of Toxicology Research, ASPCA Animal Poison Control Center, Urbana, Illinois

Rodenticide Poisoning; Strychnine Poisoning; Toxicities from Human Drugs

Peter D. Kirkland, BVSc, PhD
Senior Principal Research Scientist, Officer-in-Charge, Virology Laboratory, Elizabeth Macarthur Agricultural Institute, Menangle, New South Wales, Australia

Congenital and Inherited Anomalies: Akabane Virus Infection

Mark D. Kittleson, DVM, PhD, DACVIM (Cardiology)
Professor Emeritus, School of Veterinary Medicine, University of California, Davis, CA

Heart Disease and Heart Failure

Kirk C. Klasing, BS, MS, PhD
Professor of Animal Biology, Department of Animal Science, University of California, Davis, CA

Nutrition and Management: Nutritional Requirements of Poultry

Thomas R. Klei, PhD
Boyd Professor and Associate Dean for Research and Advanced Studies, School of Veterinary Medicine and Louisiana Agricultural Experiment Station, Louisiana State University, Baton Rouge, LA

Gastrointestinal Parasites of Horses; Helminths of the Skin

Nick J. Knowles, MPhil
Head of Molecular Epidemiology Section, Vesicular Disease Reference Laboratory, The Pirbright Institute, Woking, Surrey, UK

Teschovirus Encephalomyelitis

Alexandre Kreiss, BVSc, PhD
Research Fellow, Menzies Research Institute Tasmania, University of Tasmania, Australia

Tasmanian Devils

Janice E. Kritchevsky, VMD, MS, DACVIM
Professor, Large Animal Medicine, Department of Veterinary Clinical Sciences, School of Veterinary Medicine, Purdue University, West Lafayette, IN

Equine Metabolic Syndrome; The Pituitary Gland: Hirsutism Associated with Adenomas of the Pars Intermedia; The Thyroid Gland: Non-neoplastic Enlargement of the Thyroid Gland

Thomas G. Ksiazek, DVM, PhD
Professor, Department of Pathology, University of Texas Medical Branch, Galveston, TX

Crimean-Congo Hemorrhagic Fever; Nipah Virus Infection

Ned F. Kuehn, DVM, MS, DACVIM
Section Chief, Internal Medicine, Michigan Veterinary Specialists, Southfield, MI

Respiratory Diseases of Small Animals; Respiratory System Introduction

Mahesh C. Kumar, BVSc, MS, PhD, DACPV
Consultant, Poultry Health & Food Safety, St. Cloud, MN

Dissecting Aneurysm in Turkeys

Nina Yu-Hsin Kung, PhD, MSc, BVSc, BVM
Principal Veterinary Epidemiologist, Animal Biosecurity and Welfare Program, Department of Agriculture, Fisheries and Forestry, Biosecurity Queensland, Queensland, Australia

Hendra Virus Infection

Michelle A. Kutzler, DVM, PhD, DACT
Banfield Professor of Companion Animal Industries, Department of Animal and Rangeland Sciences, Oregon State University, Corvallis, OR

Canine Transmissible Venereal Tumor; Mammary Tumors; Prostatic Diseases

Natalie A. Kwit, DVM, MPH

Foot-and-Mouth Disease

Gary M. Landsberg, BSc, DVM, MRCVS, DACVB, DECAWBM
Veterinary Behaviourist, North Toronto Veterinary Behaviour Specialty Clinic, Thornhill, Ontario, Canada

Behavioral Medicine Introduction; Normal Social Behavior and Behavioral Problems of Domestic Animals

Thomas J. Lane, BS, DVM
Professor Emeritus, University of Florida, Gainesville, FL

Health-Management Interaction: Horses

Jimmy C. Lattimer, DVM, MS, DACVR, DACVRO
Associate Professor (Radiology and Radiation Oncology), Veterinary Medicine and Surgery, College of Veterinary Medicine, University of Missouri, Columbia, MO

Diagnostic Imaging; Radiation Therapy

D. Bruce Lawhorn, DVM, MS
Relief Veterinarian; Veterinary Information Network Swine Consultant, College Station, TX

Potbellied Pigs

Andrea S. Lear, DVM
Clinical Instructor, Department of Large Animal Clinical Sciences, College of Veterinary Medicine, The University of Tennessee, Knoxville, TN

Bluetongue; Congenital and Inherited Anomalies: Border Disease; Malignant Catarrhal Fever; Sporadic Bovine Encephalomyelitis

Margie D. Lee, DVM, PhD
Professor of Population Health, Poultry Diagnostic and Research Center, College of Veterinary Medicine, University of Georgia, Athens, GA

Avian Campylobacter Infection

Steven Leeson, PhD
Professor Emeritus, University of Guelph, Ontario, Canada

Fatty Liver Hemorrhagic Syndrome; Nutrition and Management: Nutritional Deficiencies in Poultry

Michael L. Levin, PhD
Medical Entomology Laboratory Director, Rickettsial Zoonoses Branch, Centers for Disease Control and Prevention, Atlanta, GA

Ticks

Julie K. Levy, DVM, PhD, DACVIM
Department of Small Animal Clinical Sciences, College of Veterinary Medicine, and Director, Maddie's Shelter Medicine Program, University of Florida, Gainesville, FL

Feline Infectious Peritonitis; Feline Leukemia Virus and Related Diseases

Michel Lévy, DVM, DACVIM
Professor, Department of Veterinary Clinical and Diagnostic Sciences, University of Calgary, Alberta, Canada

Polioencephalomalacia

Alicja E. Lew-Tabor, BSc (Hons), PhD
Principal Research Fellow, Queensland Alliance for Agriculture & Food Innovation, The University of Queensland, Brisbane, Queensland, Australia

Blood Parasites: Anaplasmosis; Enteric Campylobacteriosis

David H. Ley, DVM, PhD
Professor, Department of Population Health and Pathobiology, College of Veterinary Medicine, North Carolina State University, Raleigh, NC

Mycoplasmosis

HuiChu Lin, DVM, MS, DACVAA
Professor, Large Animal Anesthesia, Department of Clinical Sciences, College of Veterinary Medicine, Auburn University, Auburn, AL

Malignant Hyperthermia

Dana Lindemann, DVM
Resident, Illinois Zoological and Aquatic Animal Residency Program, Wildlife Epidemiology Laboratory, College of Veterinary Medicine, University of Illinois at Urbana-Champaign, IL

Hedgehogs

Andrew Linklater, DVM, DACVECC
Clinical Instructor, Lakeshore Veterinary Specialists, Glendale, WI

Emergency Medicine Introduction; Evaluation and Initial Treatment of the Emergency Patient; Fluid Therapy; Monitoring the Critically Ill Animal; Specific Diagnostics and Therapy

Jeanne Lofstedt, BVSc, MS, DACVIM (Large Animal)
Professor of Large Animal Internal Medicine, Department of Health Management, Atlantic Veterinary College, University of Prince Edward Island, Charlottetown, Prince Edward Island, Canada

Caprine Arthritis and Encephalitis

Maureen T. Long, DVM, PhD, DACVIM
Associate Professor, Department of Infectious Diseases and Pathology, College of Veterinary Medicine, University of Florida, Gainesville, FL

Equine Arboviral Encephalomyelitis; Meningitis, Encephalitis, and Encephalomyelitis

Michael R. Loomis, DVM, MA, DACZM
Chief Veterinarian, North Carolina Zoological Park, Asheboro, NC

Zoo Animals

Ingrid Lorenz, DMV, DMVH, DECBHM
Lecturer in Bovine Medicine, School of Agriculture, Food Science and Veterinary Medicine, University College Dublin, Ireland

Diseases of the Ruminant Forestomach: Ruminal Drinking, Ruminal Parakeratosis, Subacute Ruminal Acidosis

Jodie Low Choy, BVSc, BVMS, IVAS Cert
Menzies School of Health Research; University Avenue Veterinary Hospital, Durack, Northern Territory, Australia

Melioidosis

Katharine F. Lunn, BVMS, MS, PhD, MRCVS, DACVIM
Associate Professor, Department of Clinical Sciences, College of Veterinary Medicine, North Carolina State University, Raleigh, NC

Fever of Unknown Origin; Leptospirosis

Robert J. MacKay, BVSc, PhD
Professor, Large Animal Medicine, Department of Large Animal Clinical Sciences, College of Veterinary Medicine, University of Florida, Gainesville, FL

Equine Protozoal Myeloencephalitis

Charles Mackenzie, BVSc, PhD, ACVM, AO
Professor, Department of Pathobiology and Diagnostic Investigation, Michigan State University, East Lansing, MI

Besnoitiosis

Kenneth S. Macklin, MSc, PhD
Associate Professor, Department of Poultry Science, Auburn University, Auburn, AL

Helminthiasis

John E. Madigan, DVM, MS
Distinguished Professor, Department of Medicine and Epidemiology, School of Veterinary Medicine, University of California, Davis, CA

Equine Granulocytic Ehrlichiosis

Richard A. Mansmann, VMD, PhD (Hon), DACVIM (Large Animal)
Equine Podiatry & Rehabilitation Practice; Clinical Professor Emeritus, College of Veterinary Medicine, North Carolina State University, Raleigh, NC

Prepurchase Examination of Horses

Steven L. Marks, BVSc, MS, MRCVS, DACVIM
Clinical Professor of Emergency and Internal Medicine; Associate Dean and Director of Veterinary Medical Services, College of Veterinary Medicine, North Carolina State University, Raleigh, NC

Anemia; Health-Management Interaction: Small Animals

Bret D. Marsh, DVM
Indiana State Veterinarian, Indiana State Board of Animal Health, Indianapolis, IN

Prepurchase Examination of Ruminants and Swine

Joerg Mayer, DMV, MSc, DABVP (ECM), DECZM (Small Mammal)
Associate Professor of Zoological and Exotic Animal Medicine, Department of Small Animal Medicine & Surgery, College of Veterinary Medicine, University of Georgia, Athens, GA

Rabbits

Milton M. McAllister, DVM, PhD, DACVP
Associate Professor, School of Animal and Veterinary Sciences, University of Adelaide, Roseworthy, South Australia, Australia

Neosporosis

C. Wayne McIlwraith, BVSc, PhD, DSc, FRCVS, DACVS, DACVSMR
Department of Clinical Sciences, College of Veterinary Medicine and Biomedical Sciences, Colorado State University, Fort Collins, CO

Arthropathies in Large Animals; Lameness in Horses: Tendinitis

Thomas St. C. McKenna, DVM, PhD
Assistant Director for New England, Surveillance, Preparedness and Response Services, District 1, USDA, APHIS, Veterinary Services, Sutton, MA

African Horse Sickness

Jennifer H. McQuiston, DVM, MS
Epidemiology Team Leader, Rickettsial Zoonoses Branch, Centers for Disease Control and Prevention, Atlanta, GA

Rickettsial Diseases

Mushtaq A. Memon, BVSc, PhD, DACT
Theriogenologist, Department of Veterinary Clinical Sciences, College of Veterinary Medicine, Washington State University, Pullman, WA

Reproductive Diseases of the Female Small Animal

Paula I. Menzies, DVM, MPVM, DECS-RHM
Professor, Ruminant Health Management Group, Department of Population Medicine, Ontario Veterinary College, University of Guelph, Ontario, Canada

Disorders of Calcium Metabolism: Parturient Paresis in Sheep and Goats; Hepatic Lipidosis: Pregnancy Toxemia in Ewes and Does; Management of Reproduction: Sheep; Posthitis and Vulvitis in Sheep and Goats

Sandra R. Merchant, DVM, DACVD
Professor of Dermatology, Department of Veterinary Clinical Sciences, School of Veterinary Medicine, Louisiana State University, Baton Rouge, LA

Dermatophytosis

Joanne B. Messick, VMD, PhD, DACVP
Associate Professor of Veterinary Clinical Pathology, Department of Comparative Pathobiology, College of Veterinary Medicine, Purdue University, West Lafayette, IN

Blood Parasites: Hemotropic Mycoplasmas

Samia A. Metwally, DVM, PhD
Senior Animal Health Officer (Virologist), AGAH, AGA Division, Food and Agriculture Organization of the United Nations, Rome, Italy

Nairobi Sheep Disease

Patti J. Miller, DVM, PhD
Veterinary Medical Officer, Exotic and Emerging Avian Viral Diseases Research, USDA Agricultural Research Service, Athens, GA

Newcastle Disease and Other Paramyxovirus Infections: Newcastle Disease

Kelly D. Mitchell, BSc, DVM, DVSc, DACVIM
Toronto Veterinary Emergency Clinic, Scarborough, Ontario, Canada

Diseases of the Stomach and Intestines in Small Animals: Canine Parvovirus, Feline Enteric Coronavirus, Gastritis in Small Animals, Hemorrhagic Gastroenteritis in Small Animals

Harry W. Momont, DVM, PhD, DACT
Clinical Associate Professor, Department of Medical Sciences, School of Veterinary Medicine, University of Wisconsin, Madison, WI

Reproductive System Introduction

Donald R. Monke, DVM, MBA
Vice President, Production Operations, Select Sires, Inc., Plain City, Ohio

Seminal Vesiculitis in Bulls

James N. Moore, DVM, PhD
Distinguished Research Professor, Department of Large Animal Medicine, College of Veterinary Medicine, University of Georgia, Athens, GA

Colic in Horses

Gastón A. Moré, MV, DVM
Facultad de Ciencias Veterinarias, Laboratorio de Inmunoparasitología, Universidad Nacional de La Plata, Buenos Aires, Argentina

Sarcocystosis

Karen A. Moriello, DVM, DACVD
Professor of Dermatology, Department of Medical Sciences, School of Veterinary Medicine, University of Wisconsin, Madison, WI

Acanthosis Nigricans; Atopic Dermatitis; Congenital and Inherited Anomalies of the Integumentary System; Cuterebra Infestation in Small Animals; Dermatophilosis; Hygroma; Integumentary System Introduction; Interdigital Furunculosis; Otitis Externa; Otitis Media and Interna; Pyoderma

Teresa Y. Morishita, DVM, MPVM, MS, PhD, DACPV
Professor of Poultry Medicine & Food Safety, College of Veterinary Medicine, Western University of Health Sciences, Pomona, CA

Enterococcosis; Streptococcosis

James K. Morrisey, DVM, DABVP (Avian)
Service Chief, Companion Exotic Animal Medicine Service, Department of Clinical Sciences, College of Veterinary Medicine, Cornell University, Ithaca, NY

Ferrets

W. Ivan Morrison, PhD, BVMS
Professor, The Roslin Institute, Royal (Dick) School of Veterinary Studies, University of Edinburgh, Scotland, UK

Blood Parasites: Theileriasis

Derek A. Mosier, DVM, PhD, DACVP
Professor, Department of Diagnostic Medicine/Pathology, College of Veterinary Medicine, Kansas State University, Manhattan, KS

Hemorrhagic Septicemia

Amelia S. Munsterman, DVM, MS, DACVS, DACVECC
Clinical Instructor, Equine Emergency and Critical Care, College of Veterinary Medicine, Auburn University, Auburn, AL

Equine Emergency Medicine; Fatigue and Exercise

Jeffrey Musser, DVM, PhD
Clinical Associate Professor, Department of Veterinary Pathobiology, College of Veterinary Medicine, Texas A&M University, College Station, TX

Vaccination of Exotic Mammals

Sofie Muylle, DVM, PhD
Faculty of Veterinary Medicine, Department of Morphology, Ghent University, Salisburylaan, Merelbeke, Belgium

Dental Development

Dusty W. Nagy, DVM, MS, PhD, DACVIM
Associate Teaching Professor, Department of Veterinary Medicine & Surgery, College of Veterinary Medicine, University of Missouri, Columbia, MO

Bovine Leukosis

T. Mark Neer, DVM, DACVIM
Professor and Hospital Director, Center for Veterinary Health Sciences, Oklahoma State University, Stillwater, OK

Demyelinating Disorders; Motion Sickness

Robin A. J. Nicholas, MSc, PhD, FRCPath
Animal Health and Veterinary Laboratories Agency, Addlestone, Surrey, UK

Contagious Agalactia

Paul Nicoletti, DVM, MS, DACVPM
Deceased
Professor Emeritus, College of Veterinary Medicine, University of Florida, Gainesville, FL

Brucellosis in Dogs; Brucellosis in Large Animals

Michelle Nic Raghnaill, PhD
Research Fellow, National Academy of Science, Canberra, Australia
Pharmacology Introduction: Dosage Forms and Delivery Systems, Drug Action and Pharmacodynamics, Nanotechnology

Joeke Nijboer, PhD
Nutritionist, Rotterdam Zoo, Rotterdam, The Netherlands
Nutrition: Exotic and Zoo Animals

Donald L. Noah, DVM, MPH, DACVPM
Associate Professor, Public Health, College of Veterinary Medicine, Midwestern University, Glendale, AZ
Public Health Primer

Lisa K. Nolan, DVM, PhD
Dr. Stephen G. Juelsgaard Dean, College of Veterinary Medicine, Iowa State University, Ames, IA
Colibacillosis

Kenneth Opengart, MS, DVM, PhD, DACPV
Vice President, Live Operations, Keystone Foods, Huntsville, AL
Gangrenous Dermatitis

Tanja Opriessnig, DMV, PhD
The Roslin Institute, University of Edinburgh, Scotland, UK; Professor, Department of Veterinary Diagnostic and Production Animal Medicine, Iowa State University, Ames, IA
Erysipelothrix rhusiopathiae Infection

Stephanie R. Ostrowski, DVM, MPVM, DACVPM
Associate Professor, Department of Pathobiology, College of Veterinary Medicine, Auburn University, Auburn, AL
Public Health Primer

Gary D. Osweiler, DVM, MS, PhD
Professor Emeritus, Veterinary Diagnostic and Production Animal Medicine, College of Veterinary Medicine, Iowa State University, Ames, IA
Coal-Tar Products Poisoning; Mycotoxicoses; Petroleum Product Poisoning

Raul E. Otalora, DVM
Production Manager/Veterinarian, Quail International, Inc., Greensboro, GA
Ulcerative Enteritis

Chris Oura, BVetMed, MSc, PhD, MRCVS
Senior Lecturer in Veterinary Virology, School of Veterinary Medicine, University of the West Indies, Champ Fleurs, Trinidad
African Swine Fever

Rebecca A. Packer, MS, DVM, DACVIM (Neurology)
Assistant Professor, Neurology/Neurosurgery, Department of Veterinary Clinical Sciences, and Department of Basic Medical Sciences, School of Veterinary Medicine, Purdue University, West Lafayette, IN
Congenital and Inherited Anomalies of the Nervous System

Terri Parrott, DVM
Veterinarian, St. Charles Veterinary Hospital, Davenport, FL
Nonhuman Primates

Sharon Patton, MS, PhD
Professor, Department of Comparative Medicine, College of Veterinary Medicine, University of Tennessee, Knoxville, TN
Amebiasis; Giardiasis

Susan L. Payne, PhD
Associate Professor, Veterinary Pathobiology, Texas A&M University, College Station, TX
Vaccines and Immunotherapy

Lisa K. Pearson, DVM, MS, PhD, DACT
Clinical Instructor, Comparative Theriogenology, Department of Veterinary Clinical Sciences, College of Veterinary Medicine, Washington State University, Pullman, WA
Congenital and Inherited Anomalies of the Digestive System

Angela Pelzel-McCluskey, DVM
National Epidemiologist for Equine Diseases, USDA, APHIS Veterinary Services, Fort Collins, CO
Vesicular Stomatitis

Maurice B. Pensaert, DVM, MS, PhD
Emeritus Professor of Animal Virology, Faculty of Veterinary Medicine, Ghent University, Merelbeke, Belgium
Porcine Hemagglutinating Encephalomyelitis

Andrew S. Peregrine, BVMS, PhD, DVM, DEVPC, DACVM
Associate Professor, Department of Pathobiology, Ontario Veterinary College, University of Guelph, Ontario, Canada
Gastrointestinal Parasites of Small Animals

Donald Peter, DVM, MS, DACT
Veterinarian/Owner, Frontier Genetics, Hermiston, OR

Bovine Genital Campylobacteriosis; Equine Coital Exanthema

Christine Petersen, DVM, PhD
Associate Professor, Department of Epidemiology, University of Iowa, Iowa City, IA

Blood Parasites: Trypanosomiasis

Mark E. Peterson, DVM, DACVIM
Director of Endocrinology and Nuclear Medicine, Animal Endocrine Clinic, New York, NY

The Parathyroid Glands and Disorders of Calcium Metabolism; The Thyroid Gland: Hyperthyroidism, Hypothyroidism

Barbara D. Petty, DVM
North Florida Aquatic Veterinary Services, Fort White, FL

Aquarium Fishes

James R. Philips, PhD
Associate Professor of Science, Math/ Science Division, Babson College, Babson Park, MA

Air Sac Mite; Ectoparasites of Poultry

Carlos R. F. Pinto, MedVet, PhD, DACT
Associate Professor, Theriogenology Section, Department of Veterinary Clinical Sciences, School of Veterinary Medicine, Louisiana State University, Baton Rouge, LA

Embryo Transfer in Farm Animals

Paul J. Plummer, DVM, PhD, DACVIM (Large Animal), DECSRHM
Department of Veterinary Diagnostic and Production Animal Medicine, College of Veterinary Medicine, Iowa State University, Ames, IA

Coxiellosis

Robert E. Porter, DVM, PhD, DACVP, DACPV
Clinical Professor, Veterinary Population Medicine, College of Veterinary Medicine, University of Minnesota, St. Paul, MN

Perirenal Hemorrhage Syndrome of Turkeys; Poisonings (Poultry)

Karen W. Post, DVM, MS, DACVM
Director of Laboratories, Veterinary Bacteriologist, North Carolina Veterinary Diagnostic Laboratory System; Consumer Services, Rollins Animal Disease, Diagnostic Laboratory, Raleigh, NC

Diagnostic Procedures for the Private Practice Laboratory: Clinical Microbiology

David G. Pugh, DVM, MS, MAg, DACT, DACVN, DACVM
Department of Pathobiology, College of Veterinary Medicine, Auburn University, Auburn, AL

Nutrition: Goats; Nutrition: Sheep

Sarah L. Ralston, VMD, PhD, DACVN
Professor, Department of Animal Sciences, School of Environmental and Biological Sciences, Rutgers University, New Brunswick, NJ

Nutrition: Horses

John F. Randolph, DVM, DACVIM
Professor, Department of Clinical Sciences, College of Veterinary Medicine, Cornell University, Ithaca, NY

Erythrocytosis and Polycythemia

Silke Rautenschlein, DVM, PhD
Professor, Clinic for Poultry, University of Veterinary Medicine, Hannover, Germany

Avian Metapneumovirus

Willie M. Reed, DVM, PhD, DACVP, DACPV
Dean, College of Veterinary Medicine, Purdue University, West Lafayette, IN

Quail Bronchitis; Turkey Viral Hepatitis

Philip T. Reeves, BVSc (Hons), PhD, FANZCVS
Chief Regulatory Scientist, Veterinary Medicines and Nanotechnology, Australian Pesticides and Veterinary Medicines Authority, Canberra, Australia

Pharmacology Introduction: Chemical Residues in Food and Fiber, Dosage Forms and Delivery Systems, Drug Action and Pharmacodynamics, Nanotechnology

Mason V. Reichard, PhD
Associate Professor, Department of Veterinary Pathobiology, Center for Veterinary Health Sciences, Oklahoma State University, Stillwater, OK

Cattle Grubs; Mange in Large Animals

Hugh W. Reid, MBE, BVM&S, DTVM, PhD, MRCVS
Moredun Research Institute, Pentlands, Science Park, Penicuik, UK

Louping Ill

Douglas J. Reinemann, PhD
Professor and Chair, Department of Biological Systems Engineering, College of Agricultural and Life Sciences, University of Wisconsin, Madison, WI

Stray Voltage in Animal Housing

Christopher D. Reinhardt, BS, MS, PhD
Assistant Professor and Extension Feedlot Specialist, Animal Sciences and Industry, Kansas State University, Manhattan, KS

Growth Promotants and Production Enhancers

Petra Reinhold, DVM, PhD
Friedrich-Loeffler-Institute, Federal Research Institute for Animal Health, Jena, Germany

Chlamydiosis

Alexander M. Reiter, DT, DMV, DAVDC, DEVDC
Chief, Dentistry and Oral Surgery Service, Ryan Veterinary Hospital, School of Veterinary Medicine, University of Pennsylvania, Philadelphia, PA

Dentistry: Dentistry in Small Animals; Diseases of the Mouth in Small Animals

Márcio Garcio Ribeiro, DVM, PhD
Professor, Infectious Diseases of Domestic Animals, Department of Veterinary Hygiene and Public Health, School of Veterinary Medicine and Animal Sciences, São Paulo State University – UNESP, Botucatu, São Paulo, Brazil

Nocardiosis; Rhodococcosis

Franklin Riet-Correa, PhD
Professor, Veterinary Hospital, Federal University of Campina Grande, Patos, Paraíba, Brazil

Cattle Grubs: Lechiguana

Yasuko Rikihisa, PhD
Professor, Veterinary Biosciences, The Ohio State University, Columbus, OH

Rickettsial Diseases: Salmon Poisoning Disease and Elokomin Fluke Fever

Guillermo R. Risatti, MV, MS, PhD
Associate Professor, Department of Pathobiology and Veterinary Science, University of Connecticut, Storrs, CT

Classical Swine Fever

Narda G. Robinson, DO, DVM, MS
College of Veterinary Medicine and Biological Sciences, Colorado State University, Fort Collins, CO

Complementary and Alternative Veterinary Medicine

Kursten V. Roderick, DVM
Cardiology Resident, Cummings School of Veterinary Medicine, Tufts University, North Grafton, MA

Cardiovascular System Introduction; Thrombosis, Embolism, and Aneurysm

Camille Roesch, PhD
Nanosafety Pharmacist Consultant, Australian Pesticides and Veterinary Medicines Authority, Symonston, Australia

Pharmacology Introduction: Dosage Forms and Delivery Systems, Drug Action and Pharmacodynamics, Nanotechnology

Peter Rolls, BVSc, MVS
Veterinary Officer, Tick Fever Centre, Department of Agriculture, Fisheries and Forestry, Biosecurity Queensland, Wacol, Queensland, Australia

Blood Parasites: Babesiosis

Juan E. Romano, DVM, MS, PhD, DACT
Associate Professor, Department of Large Animal Clinical Sciences, College of Veterinary Medicine, Texas A&M University, College Station, TX

Hormonal Control of Estrus

A. Gregorio Rosales, DVM, MS, PhD, DACPV
Vice President of Veterinary Services, Aviagen Inc., Huntsville, AL

Disorders of the Reproductive System (Poultry)

Stanley I. Rubin, DVM, MS, DACVIM
Clinical Professor, Department of Veterinary Clinical Medicine, College of Veterinary Medicine, University of Illinois, Urbana, IL

Digestive System Introduction; Diseases of the Rectum and Anus

Pamela L. Ruegg, DVM, MPVM
Professor, Department of Dairy Science, College of Agricultural and Life Sciences, University of Wisconsin, Madison, WI

Udder Diseases

Charles E. Rupprecht, VMD, MS, PhD
Director, LYSSA LLC, Lawrenceville, GA

Rabies

Bonnie R. Rush, DVM, MS, DACVIM
Professor, Equine Internal Medicine, College of Veterinary Medicine, Kansas State University, Manhattan, KS

Respiratory Diseases of Horses

Y. M. Saif, DVM, PhD
Professor Emeritus, Food Animal Health Research Program, The Ohio State University, Wooster, OH

Rotaviral Infections in Chickens, Turkeys, and Pheasants

Jeremiah T. Saliki, DVM, PhD, DACVM
Professor and Director, Athens Veterinary Diagnostic Laboratory, University of Georgia, Athens, GA

Peste des Petits Ruminants; Rinderpest

Jean E. Sander, DVM, MAM, DACPV
Dean, Center for Veterinary Health Sciences, Oklahoma State University, Stillwater, OK

Candidiasis; Disposal of Carcasses and Disinfection of Premises; Omphalitis

Sherry Lynn Sanderson, BS, DVM, PhD, DACVIM, DACVN
Associate Professor, Physiology and Pharmacology, College of Veterinary Medicine, University of Georgia, Athens, GA

Nutrition: Small Animals; Urinary System Introduction

Yuko Sato, DVM, MS, DACPV
Assistant Professor, Veterinary Diagnostic & Production Animal Medicine, Poultry Extension and Diagnostics, Iowa State University, Ames, IA

Backyard Poultry

Ashley B. Saunders, DVM, DACVIM (Cardiology)
Associate Professor of Cardiology, Department of Small Animal Clinical Sciences, College of Veterinary Medicine and Biomedical Sciences, Texas A&M University, College Station, TX

Systemic Pharmacotherapeutics of the Cardiovascular System

Charles M. Scanlan, DVM, PhD
Professor, Department of Veterinary Pathobiology, College of Veterinary Medicine and Biomedical Sciences, Texas A&M University, College Station, TX

Meat Inspection

Karel A. Schat, DVM, PhD
Professor, Department of Microbiology and Immunology, College of Veterinary Medicine, Cornell University, Ithaca, NY

Chicken Anemia Virus Infection

Mary M. Schell, DVM, DABVT, DABT
Senior Toxicologist, ASPCA Animal Poison Control Center, Urbana, Illinois

Rodenticide Poisoning

David G. Schmitz, DVM, MS, DACVIM (Large Animal)
Visiting Associate Professor, Department of Veterinary Large Animal Clinical Sciences, College of Veterinary Medicine, Texas A&M University, College Station, TX

Cantharidin Poisoning

Thomas Schubert, DVM, DACVIM, DABVP
Clinical Professor and Chief of Neurology Service, Small Animal Clinical Sciences, College of Veterinary Medicine, University of Florida, Gainesville, FL

Facial Paralysis; Limb Paralysis; Nervous System Introduction

James Schumacher, DVM, MS
Professor, Large Animal Clinical Sciences, College of Veterinary Medicine, University of Tennessee, Knoxville, TN

Lameness in Horses: Regional Anesthesia

John Schumacher, DVM, MS
Professor, Department of Clinical Sciences, College of Veterinary Medicine, Auburn University, Auburn, AL

Lameness in Horses: Regional Anesthesia

Philip R. Scott, BVM&S, MPhil, DVM&S, DSHP, DECBHM, FHEA, FRCVS
Veterinary Clinical Sciences, University of Edinburgh, Midlothian, UK

Aspiration Pneumonia; Contagious Ecthyma; Listeriosis; Mycotic Pneumonia; Respiratory Diseases of Sheep and Goats; Ulcerative Dermatosis of Sheep

Joaquim Segalés, DVM, PhD, DECVP, DECPHM
Facultat de Veterinària, Departament de Sanitat i d'Anatomia Animals and Centre de Recerca en Sanitat Animals, Universitat Autònoma de Barcelona, Bellaterra, Barcelona, Spain

Glässer's Disease; Porcine Circovirus Diseases

Patricia L. Sertich, MS, VMD, DACT
Associate Professor-Clinician Educator, Department of Clinical Studies, New Bolton Center, School of Veterinary Medicine, University of Pennsylvania, Kennett Square, PA

Management of Reproduction: Horses

Torsten Seuberlich, DMV
Professor, NeuroCentre, Division of Neurological Sciences, OIE Reference Laboratories for BSE and Scrapie; Vetsuisse Faculty, Department of Clinical Research and Veterinary Public Health, University of Berne, Berne, Switzerland

Bovine Spongiform Encephalopathy

A. S. Shakespeare, BSc (Eng) (Natal), BVSc (Hons) (Pret), MMedVet (Med) (Pret)
Onderstepoort Veterinary Faculty, University of Pretoria, South Africa

Heartwater

Linda Shell, DVM, DACVIM (Neurology)
Professor, Small Animal Internal Medicine, Ross University School of Veterinary Medicine, Basseterre, Saint Kitts and Nevis

Systemic Pharmacotherapeutics of the Nervous System

Clifford F. Shipley, DVM, DACT
Clinical Associate Professor, Agricultural Animal Care and Use Program and College of Veterinary Medicine, University of Illinois, Urbana, IL

Management of Reproduction: Goats

Michael Shipstone, BVSc, FACVSc, DACVD
Queensland Veterinary Specialists, Brisbane, Queensland, Australia

Systemic Pharmacotherapeutics of the Integumentary System

H. L. Shivaprasad, BVSc, MS, PhD, DACPV
Professor, California Animal Health and Food Safety Laboratory System, University of California, Tulare, CA

Hemorrhagic Enteritis/Marble Spleen Disease

Wayne Simpson, MSc (Microbiology), BHort Sc, DHort
Scientist, Endophyte Mycology, Forage Improvement Section, AgResearch Limited, Palmerston North, New Zealand

Ryegrass Toxicity

Annette N. Smith, DVM, MS, DACVIM
Professor, Department of Clinical Sciences, College of Veterinary Medicine, Auburn University, Auburn, AL

Neoplasia of the Nervous System; Paraneoplastic Disorders of the Nervous System

Geof W. Smith, DVM, PhD
Associate Professor of Ruminant Medicine, Department of Population Health and Pathobiology, College of Veterinary Medicine, North Carolina State University, Raleigh, NC

Actinobacillosis; Actinomycosis

Joan A. Smyth, PhD
Director, Connecticut Veterinary Medical Diagnostic Laboratory, Department of Pathobiology and Veterinary Science, University of Connecticut, Storrs, CT

Egg Drop Syndrome '76

Victoria Smyth, PhD
Senior Scientific Officer for Avian Virology, Veterinary Sciences Division, Agri-Food and Biosciences Institute, Belfast, UK

Avian Nephritis Viral Infections

Arthur M. Spickett, BSc (Hons) Zoology
Parasites, Vectors and Vector-borne Diseases Programme, ARC-Onderstepoort Veterinary Institute, South Africa

Sweating Sickness

Anna Rovid Spickler, DVM, PhD
Veterinary Specialist, Center for Food Security and Public Health, College of Veterinary Medicine, Iowa State University, Ames, IA

Zoonoses

Sharon J. Spier, DVM, PhD, DACVIM
Professor, Department of Medicine and Epidemiology, School of Veterinary Medicine, University of California, Davis, CA

Disorders of Calcium Metabolism: Hypocalcemic Tetany in Horses; Lymphadenitis and Lymphangitis: Corynebacterium pseudotuberculosis Infection of Horses and Cattle

Richard A. Squires, BVSc (Hons), PhD, DVR, DACVIM, DECVIM-CA, GCertEd, MRCVS
Head of Veterinary Clinical Sciences, School of Veterinary and Biomedical Sciences, James Cook University, Townsville, Australia

Feline Panleukopenia

Henry R. Stämpfli, DVM, DMV, DACVIM
Professor, Large Animal Medicine, Department of Clinical Studies, Ontario Veterinary College, University of Guelph, Ontario, Canada

Clostridial Diseases

Jonathan Statham, MA, VetMB, DCHP, MRCVS
Veterinarian, Bishopton Veterinary Group, North Yorkshire, UK

Cystic Ovary Disease; Management of Reproduction: Cattle

Bryan L. Stegelmeier, DVM, PhD, DACVP
Veterinary Pathologist, Poisonous Plant Research Laboratory, USDA-ARS, Logan, UT

Bracken Fern Poisoning; Sweet Clover Poisoning

Jörg M. Steiner, DMV, PhD, DACVIM, DECVIM-CA, AGAF
Associate Professor and Director, Gastrointestinal Laboratory, Department of Small Animal Clinical Sciences, College of Veterinary Medicine and Biomedical Sciences, Texas A&M University, College Station, TX

The Exocrine Pancreas

Allison J. Stewart, BVSC (Hons), MS, DACVIM (Large Animal), DACVECC
Professor of Equine Internal Medicine, Department of Clinical Sciences, College of Veterinary Medicine, Auburn University, Auburn, AL

Disorders of Magnesium Metabolism; Intestinal Diseases in Horses and Foals

Jamie Lynn Stewart, DVM
Department of Veterinary Clinical Medicine, College of Veterinary Medicine, University of Illinois, Urbana, IL

Management of Reproduction: Goats

Bruce Stewart-Brown, DVM, DACPV
Senior Vice President of Food Safety, Quality, and Live Operations, Perdue Farms, Salisbury, MD

Nutrition and Management Poultry: Feeding and Management Practices

Roger W. Stitch, MS, PhD
Professor of Parasitology, Department of Veterinary Pathobiology, College of Veterinary Medicine, University of Missouri, Columbia, MO

Ectoparasiticides: Ectoparasiticides Used in Large Animals

Michael K. Stoskopf, DVM, PhD, DACZM
Professor of Wildlife and Aquatic Health, Director of the Environmental Medicine Consortium, College of Veterinary Medicine, North Carolina State University, Raleigh, NC

Marine Mammals

George M. Strain, PhD
Professor of Neuroscience, Comparative Biomedical Sciences, School of Veterinary Medicine, Louisiana State University, Baton Rouge, LA

Deafness

Reinhard K. Straubinger, DMVH, PhD
Professor and Head for Bacteriology and Mycology, Institute for Infectious Diseases and Zoonoses, Faculty of Veterinary Medicine, Ludwig-Maximilians University, Munich, Germany

Lyme Borreliosis

Bert E. Stromberg, PhD
Professor, Veterinary and Biomedical Sciences, College of Veterinary Medicine, University of Minnesota, St. Paul, MN

Infectious Diseases of the Urinary System in Large Animals: Swine Kidney Worm Infection; Trichinellosis

David E. Swayne, DVM, PhD, DACVP, DACPV
Laboratory Director, USDA-ARS, Southeast Poultry Research Laboratory, Athens, GA

Avian Influenza; Newcastle Disease and Other Paramyxovirus Infections: Other Avian Paramyxovirus Infections

Thomas W. Swerczek, DVM, PhD
Professor, Department of Veterinary Science, University of Kentucky, Lexington, KY

Tyzzer Disease

Jane E. Sykes, BVSc (Hons), PhD, DACVIM
Professor of Small Animal Medicine, Department of Medicine and Epidemiology, School of Veterinary Medicine, University of California, Davis, CA

Chlamydial Conjunctivitis

Joseph Taboada, DVM, DACVIM
Professor and Associate Dean, Office of Student and Academic Affairs, School of Veterinary Medicine, Louisiana State University, Baton Rouge, LA

Fungal Infections

Jaime L. Tarigo, DVM, PhD, DACVP
Assistant Professor, Veterinary Clinical Pathology, University of Georgia, Athens, GA

Blood Parasites: Cytauxzoonosis

Marcel Taverne, PhD
Emeritus Professor of Fœtal and Perinatal Biology, Department of Farm Animal Health, Faculty of Veterinary Medicine, Utrecht University, Utrecht, The Netherlands

Pseudopregnancy in Goats

Charles O. Thoen, DVM, PhD
Deceased
Professor, Veterinary Microbiology and Preventive Medicine, College of Veterinary Medicine, Iowa State University, Ames, IA

Tuberculosis and other Mycobacterial Infections; Tuberculosis in Poultry

Jennifer E. Thomas, DVM
Post-Doc Fellow, Department of Veterinary Pathobiology, Center for Veterinary Health Sciences, Oklahoma State University, Stillwater, OK

Lice; Mange in Large Animals

William B. Thomas, DVM, MS, DACVIM (Neurology)
Professor, Neurology and Neurosurgery, Department of Small Animal Clinical Sciences, University of Tennessee, Knoxville, TN

Diseases of the Peripheral Nerves and Neuromuscular Junction; Diseases of the Spinal Column and Cord

Sara M. Thomasy, DVM, PhD, DACVO
Vision Researcher, Department of Surgical and Radiological Sciences, School of Veterinary Medicine, University of California, Davis, CA

Equine Recurrent Uveitis

Larry J. Thompson, DVM, PhD, DABVT
Senior Research Scientist, Nestlé Purina PetCare, St. Louis, MO

Nitrate and Nitrite Poisoning; Nonprotein Nitrogen Poisoning; Salt Toxicity

Peter N. Thompson, BVSc, MMV, PhD
Professor of Veterinary Epidemiology, Faculty of Veterinary Science, University of Pretoria, South Africa

Rift Valley Fever; Wesselsbron Disease

Ahmed Tibary, DMV, PhD, DACT
Professor, Comparative Theriogenology, Department of Veterinary Clinical Sciences, College of Veterinary Medicine, Washington State University, Pullman, WA

Abortion in Large Animals; Congenital and Inherited Anomalies of the Reproductive System

John F. Timoney, MVB, PhD, Dsc, MRCVS
Keeneland Chair of Infectious Diseases, Gluck Equine Research Center, Department of Veterinary Science, University of Kentucky, Lexington, KY

Glanders

Peter J. Timoney, MVB (Hons), MS, PhD, FRCVS
Professor; Frederick Van Lennep Chair in Equine Veterinary Science, Gluck Equine Research Center, University of Kentucky, Lexington, KY

Equine Infectious Anemia; Equine Viral Arteritis

Ian Tizard, BVMS, PhD, DACVM
University Distinguished Professor of Immunology; Director, Richard M. Schubot Exotic Bird Health Center, Department of Veterinary Pathobiology, College of Veterinary Medicine and Biomedical Sciences, Texas A&M University, College Station, TX

Amyloidoses; Immunologic Diseases; The Biology of the Immune System; Vaccines and Immunotherapy

Sheila M. F. Torres, DVM, MS, PhD, DACVD
Associate Professor, Dermatology, College of Veterinary Medicine, University of Minnesota, St. Paul, MN

Diseases of the Pinna

Jerry L. Torrison, DVM, PhD, DACVPM
Swine Veterinarian, Zinpro Corporation; Adjunct Professor, College of Veterinary Medicine, University of Minnesota, St. Paul, MN

Lameness in Pigs

Sandra P. Tou, DVM, DACVIM
Assistant Clinical Professor of Cardiology, Department of Clinical Sciences, College of Veterinary Medicine, North Carolina State University, Raleigh, NC

Congenital and Inherited Anomalies of the Cardiovascular System

Josie L. Traub-Dargatz, DVM, MS, DACVIM
Professor of Equine Medicine, Department of Clinical Sciences, College of Veterinary Medicine and Biomedical Sciences, Colorado State University, Fort Collins, CO

Vesicular Stomatitis

Robert Tremblay, DVM, DVSc, DACVIM
Bovine/Equine Specialist, Boehringer Ingelheim (Canada) Ltd, Burlington, Ontario, Canada

Management and Nutrition Introduction

Deoki N. Tripathy, DVM, MS, PhD, DACVM, DACPV
Professor Emeritus, Department of Veterinary Pathobiology, College of Veterinary Medicine, University of Illinois, Urbana, IL

Fowlpox

Thomas N. Tully, Jr., BS, DVM, MS, DABVP (Avian), DECZM (Avian)
Professor, Zoological Medicine, School of Veterinary Medicine, Louisiana State University, Baton Rouge, LA

Ratites

Tracy A. Turner, DVM, MS
Anoka Equine Veterinary Services, Elk River, MN

Lameness in Horses: Imaging Techniques

Stephanie J. Valberg, DVM, PhD, DACVIM, ACVSMR
Professor, Department of Veterinary Population Medicine, University of Minnesota Equine Center, St. Paul, MN

Myopathies in Horses; Myopathies in Ruminants and Pigs

Arnaud J. Van Wettere, DVM, MS, PhD, DACVP
Assistant Professor of Veterinary Pathology, Utah Veterinary Diagnostic Laboratory, Utah State University, Logan, UT

Avian Chlamydiosis; Bloodborne Organisms; Disorders of the Skeletal System (Poultry); Myopathies (Poultry)

Jozef Vercruysse, DVM
Professor, Faculty of Veterinary Medicine, Ghent University, Merelbeke, Belgium

Anthelmintics; Blood Parasites: Shistosomiasis

Alice E. Villalobos, DVM, DPNAP
Director, Animal Oncology Consultation Service; Director, Pawspice, Hermosa Beach, CA

Tumors of the Skin and Soft Tissues

Pedro Villegas, DVM, MS, PhD, DACVM, DACPV
Professor Emeritus, Department of Population Health, College of Veterinary Medicine, Poultry Diagnostic & Research Center, University of Georgia, Athens, GA

Inclusion Body Hepatitis/Hydropericardium Syndrome

Patricia S. Wakenell, DVM, PhD, DACVP
Head, Avian Diagnostics, Animal Disease Diagnostic Laboratory; Associate Professor, Department of Comparative Pathobiology, School of Veterinary Medicine, Purdue University, West Lafayette, IN

Backyard Poultry; Erysipelas

Peter J. Walker, BSc, PhD, DSc
CSIRO Biosecurity, Australian Animal Health Laboratory, Victoria, Australia

Bovine Ephemeral Fever

Patricia Walters, VMD, DACVIM, DACVECC
New England Animal Medical Center, West Bridgewater, MA

Diseases of the Esophagus in Small Animals

Kevin Washburn, DVM
Professor, Large Animal Clinical Sciences, College of Veterinary Medicine, Texas A&M University, College Station, TX

Lymphadenitis and Lymphangitis: Caseous Lymphadenitis

Nick Whelan, BVSc, MVSc, MACVSc, DACVCP, DACVO
Animal Eye Clinic of Waterloo Region, Cambridge, Ontario, Canada

Systemic Pharmacotherapeutics of the Eye

Brent R. Whitaker, MS, DVM
Vice President of Biological Programs, National Aquarium, Baltimore, MD

Amphibians

Trevor J. Whitbread, BSc, BVSc, MRCVS, DECVP
Pathologist, Abbey Veterinary Services, Devon, UK

Diagnostic Procedures for the Private Practice Laboratory: Clinical Biochemistry, Clinical Hematology, Cytology, Serology, Urinalysis

Stephen D. White, DVM, DACVD
Professor and Chief of Service, Dermatology, Department of Medicine and Epidemiology, School of Veterinary Medicine, University of California, Davis, CA

Eosinophilic Granuloma Complex; Food Allergy; Miscellaneous Systemic Dermatoses; Nasal Dermatoses of Dogs; Saddle Sores; Seborrhea; Urticaria

Chris Whitton, BVSc, FANZCVS, PhD
Associate Professor, Equine Centre, University of Melbourne, Victoria, Australia

Lameness in Horses: Developmental Orthopedic Disease

Mark L. Wickstrom, DVM, MS, PhD
Associate Professor, Department of Veterinary Biomedical Sciences, Western College of Veterinary Medicine, University of Saskatchewan, Saskatoon, Canada

Antiseptics and Disinfectants

Kevin P. Winkler, DVM, DACVS
Surgeon, Georgia Veterinary Specialists, Atlanta, GA

Wound Management

Thomas Wittek, Univ.-Prof. Dr.med. vet., DECBHM
University Clinic for Ruminants, University of Veterinary Medicine, Vienna, Austria

Malassimilation Syndromes in Large Animals; Peritonitis

Zerai Woldehiwet, DVM, PhD, DAgric, MRCVS
Professor, Institute of Infection and Global Health and School of Veterinary Science, University of Liverpool, Wirral, UK

Tick Pyemia; Tickborne Fever

R. Darren Wood, DVM, DVSc, DACVP
Associate Professor, Department of Pathobiology, Ontario Veterinary College, University of Guelph, Ontario, Canada

Leukocyte Disorders

Peter R. Woolcock, BSc, MSc, PhD
Professor, Clinical Diagnostic Virology, California Animal Health and Food Safety Laboratory System, School of Veterinary Medicine, University of California, Davis, CA

Duck Viral Hepatitis

Mariko Yamamoto, PhD
Department of Population Health and Reproduction, School of Veterinary Medicine, University of California, Davis, CA

The Human-Animal Bond

Roy P. E. Yanong, VMD
Associate Professor and Extension Veterinarian, Tropical Aquaculture Laboratory, Fisheries and Aquatic Sciences Program, School of Forest Resources and Conservation, Institute of Food and Agricultural Sciences, University of Florida, Gainesville, FL

Aquaculture

Laszlo Zsak, DVM, PhD
Research Leader, USDA-Agricultural Research Center, South Atlantic Area, Southeast Poultry Research Laboratory, Athens, GA

Goose Parvovirus Infection

CIRCULATORY SYSTEM

CIR

THE BLOOD AND LYMPHATICS

THE HEART AND VESSELS

HEMATOPOIETIC SYSTEM INTRODUCTION

Blood supplies cells with water, electrolytes, nutrients, and hormones and removes waste products. The cellular elements supply oxygen (RBCs), protect against foreign organisms and antigens (WBCs), and initiate coagulation (platelets). Because of the diversity of the hematopoietic system, its diseases are best discussed from a functional perspective. Function may be classified as either normal responses to abnormal situations (eg, leukocytosis and left shift in response to inflammation) or primary abnormalities of the hematopoietic system (eg, pancytopenia from marrow failure). Furthermore, abnormalities may be quantitative (ie, too many or too few cells) or qualitative (ie, abnormalities in function).

RED BLOOD CELLS

The function of RBCs is to carry oxygen to the tissues at pressures sufficient to permit its rapid diffusion. This is accomplished through the following mechanisms: a carrier molecule, hemoglobin (Hgb); a vehicle (RBC) capable of bringing the intact Hgb to the cellular level; and a metabolism geared to protect both the RBC and the Hgb from damage. Interference with synthesis or release of Hgb, production or survival of RBCs, or metabolism causes disease.

Hgb is a complex molecule, formed of four heme units attached to four globins (two α and two β globins). Iron is added in the last step by the ferrochelatase enzyme. Interference with the normal production of heme or globin leads to anemia. Causes include copper or iron deficiency and lead poisoning. Hemoglobinopathies such as thalassemias and sickle cell anemia, important genetic diseases of people, have not been seen in other animals. In these diseases, the production of globins (α or β or both) does not balance heme production, and the Hgb is not functional. The only known hemoglobinopathy of animals is porphyria. Although described in several species, it is most important as a cause of photosensitivity in cattle (*see* p 976).

Red cell mass, and thus oxygen-carrying capacity, remains constant over time in healthy animals. Mature RBCs have a finite life span; their production and destruction must be carefully balanced, or disease ensues.

Erythropoiesis is regulated by erythropoietin, which increases in the presence of hypoxia and regulates RBC production. In most species, the kidney is both the sensor organ and the major site of erythropoietin production, so chronic renal failure is associated with anemia. Erythropoietin acts on the marrow in concert with other humoral mediators to increase the number of stem cells entering RBC production, to shorten maturation time, and to cause early release of reticulocytes. Other factors that affect erythropoiesis are the supply of nutrients (eg, iron, folate, or vitamin B_{12}) and cell-cell interactions between erythroid precursors, lymphoid cells, and other components of the hematopoietic microenvironment. Factors that may suppress erythropoiesis include chronic debilitating diseases and endocrine disorders (such as hypothyroidism or hyperestrogenism).

Two mechanisms exist for removal of senescent RBCs; both conserve the principal constituents of the cell for reuse. Removal of aged RBCs normally occurs by phagocytosis by the fixed macrophages of the spleen. As the RBC ages it may change antigenically, acquiring senescent antigens and losing its flexibility due to impaired ATP production. Both of these changes increase the risk that the cell will become trapped in the spleen and removed by macrophages. After phagocytosis and subsequent disruption of the cell membrane, Hgb is converted to heme and globin. Iron is released from the heme moiety and either stored in the macrophage as ferritin or hemosiderin or released into the circulation for transport back to the marrow. The remaining heme is converted to bilirubin, which is released by the macrophages into the systemic circulation, where it complexes with albumin for transport to the hepatocytes; there, it is conjugated and excreted into the bile. In extravascular hemolytic anemias, RBCs have a shortened life span, and the same mechanisms occur at an increased rate.

Approximately 1% of normal aging RBCs are hemolyzed in the circulation, and free Hgb is released. This is quickly converted to Hgb dimers that bind to haptoglobin and are transported to the liver, where they are metabolized in the same manner as products from RBCs removed by phagocytosis. In intravascular hemolytic anemia, more RBCs are destroyed in the circulation (hemoglobinemia) than can be bound to haptoglobin. The excess Hgb and, therefore, iron are excreted in the urine (hemoglobinuria).

The principal metabolic pathway of RBC is glycolysis, and the main energy source in most species is glucose. Glucose enters the RBC by an insulin-independent mechanism, and most is metabolized to produce ATP and reduced nicotinamide adenine dinucleotide (NADH). The energy of ATP is used to maintain RBC membrane pumps so as to preserve shape and flexibility. The reducing potential of the NADH is utilized via the methemoglobin reductase pathway to maintain the iron in Hgb in its reduced form (Fe^{2+}).

The glucose not used in glycolysis is metabolized via a second pathway, the hexose monophosphate (HMP) shunt. No energy is produced via the HMP shunt; its principal effect is to maintain reducing potential in the form of reduced nicotinamide adenine dinucleotide phosphate (NADPH). In conjunction with the glutathione reductase/peroxidase system, NADPH maintains the sulfhydryl groups of globin in their reduced state.

Some disorders are the direct result of abnormal RBC metabolism and interference with glycolysis. Inherited deficiency of pyruvate kinase, a key glycolytic enzyme, causes ATP deficiency, which leads to reduced RBC life span and hemolytic anemia. Excessive oxidant stress may overload the protective HMP shunt or methemoglobin reductase pathways, causing Heinz body hemolysis or methemoglobin formation, respectively. Hemolytic anemia caused by a drug, such as acetaminophen in cats, is an example of this mechanism. (*See also* ANEMIA, p 7.)

A decreased RBC mass (anemia) may be caused by blood loss, hemolysis, or decreased production. In acute blood loss anemia, RBCs are lost, but mortality is usually related to loss of circulating volume rather than to loss of RBC. Iron is the limiting factor in chronic blood loss. Hemolysis may be caused by toxins, infectious agents, congenital abnormalities, or antibodies directed against RBC membrane antigens. Decreased RBC production may result from primary marrow diseases (eg, aplastic anemia, hematopoietic malignancy, or myelofibrosis) or from other causes such as renal failure, drugs, toxins, or antibodies directed against RBC precursors. Malignancy of RBCs or their precursors may be acute (eg, erythroleukemia) or chronic (eg, polycythemia vera). Animals with erythroleukemia are anemic despite having a marrow filled with rubriblasts, whereas those with polycythemia vera have erythrocytosis.

WHITE BLOOD CELLS

Phagocytes: The principal function of phagocytes is to defend against invading microorganisms by ingesting and destroying them, thus contributing to cellular inflammatory responses. There are two types of phagocytes: mononuclear phagocytes and granulocytes. Mononuclear phagocytes arise primarily from the marrow and are released into the blood as monocytes. They may circulate for hours to a few days before entering the tissues and differentiating to become macrophages. Granulocytes have a segmented nucleus and are classified according to their staining characteristics as neutrophils, eosinophils, or basophils. Neutrophils circulate for only a few hours before travelling to the tissues.

Five distinct stages in the process of phagocytosis have been identified: 1) attraction of phagocytes (chemotaxis) to microorganisms, antigen-antibody complexes, and other mediators of inflammation; 2) attachment to the organism; 3) ingestion; 4) fusion of cell lysosomes with ingested microorganisms and bacterial killing; and 5) digestion. In addition, many phagocytes have other specialized functions. Monocytes form a link to the specific immune system by processing antigen for presentation to lymphocytes and by producing substances such as interleukin-1, which initiates fever and lymphocyte activation and stimulates early hematopoietic progenitors.

Eosinophils, while having a role as phagocytes, also have more specific functions that include providing a defense against metazoan parasites and modulating the inflammatory process. They respond chemotactically to histamine, immune complexes, and eosinophil chemotactic factor of anaphylaxis, a substance released by degranulating mast cells. Basophils are not true phagocytes but contain large amounts of histamine and other mediators of inflammation. Eosinophilia and basophilia may be seen in response to systemic allergic reactions and invasion of tissues by parasites.

As with the RBCs, the production and circulating numbers of phagocytes are tightly regulated and controlled by various humoral factors, including colony-stimulating factors and interleukins. Unlike the RBCs, which remain circulating in the blood, the phagocytes use this compartment as a pathway to the tissues. Consequently, the number of phagocytes in the blood reflects circumstances in the tissues (eg, inflammation) as well as the proliferative function of the bone marrow. The sensitivity with which phagocytes reflect these conditions varies from species to species. Abnormal response, such as neutropenia from marrow failure, infections, drugs, or toxins, is likely to result in secondary bacterial infections. Some cases of "idiopathic" neutropenia in dogs may have an immune-mediated cause. Finally, phagocyte precursors may undergo malignant transformation, which results in acute or chronic myelogenous leukemia.

Lymphocytes: Lymphocytes are responsible for both humoral and cellular immunity. Cells of the two branches of the immune system cannot be differentiated morphologically, but they differ in their dynamics of production and circulation. Lymphocyte production in mammals originates in the bone marrow. Some of the lymphocytes destined to be involved in cellular immunity migrate to the thymus and differentiate further under the influence of thymic hormones. These become T cells and are responsible for a variety of helper or cytotoxic immunologic functions. Most circulating lymphocytes are T cells, but T cells are also present in the spleen and lymph nodes. The B cells migrate directly to organs without undergoing modification in the thymus and are responsible for humoral immunity (antibody production).

Thus, lymphoid organs have populations of both B and T lymphocytes. In the lymph nodes, follicular centers are primarily B cells, and parafollicular zones are primarily T cells. In the spleen, most of the lymphocytes of the red pulp are B cells, whereas those of the periarteriolar lymphoid sheaths are T cells. Close association of T cells and B cells within lymphoid organs is essential to immune function.

Lymphocyte function in the cellular immune system features both afferent (receptor) and efferent (effector) components. Long-lived T cells of the peripheral blood are the receptors. In response to antigens to which they have been previously sensitized, they leave the circulation and undergo blast transformation to form activated T cells, which in turn cause other T cells to undergo blast transformation, both locally and systemically. Stimulated T cells produce lymphokines with a wide range of activities, such as attraction and activation of neutrophils, macrophages, and lymphocytes.

The humoral immune system is composed of B cells that produce antibodies of several classes. When sensitized B cells encounter antigen, they divide and differentiate into plasma cells that produce antibody. Therefore, each initially stimulated B cell produces a clone of plasma cells, all producing the same specific antibody.

Antibody molecules (immunoglobulins) fall into several classes, each with its own functional characteristics. For example, IgA is the principal antibody of respiratory and intestinal secretions, IgM is the first antibody produced in response to a newly recognized antigen, IgG is the principal antibody of the circulating blood, and IgE is the principal antibody involved in allergic reactions.

Antibodies perform their function by combining with the specific antigens that stimulated their production. Antigen-antibody complexes may be chemotactic for phagocytes, or they may activate complement, a process that produces both cell lysis and substances chemotactic for neutrophils and macrophages. In this manner, the humoral immune system is related to, and interacts with, the nonspecific immune system.

The humoral immune system also is related to both the nonspecific immune system and the cellular immune system in other ways. Both "helper" (CD4) and "cytotoxic" (CD8) T-cell classes have been described. Helper T cells recognize processed antigen and activate the humoral immune response. Cytotoxic T cells, after sensitization by antigen, are effector cells, which are especially important in antiviral immunity. Natural killer cells, which are a class of lymphocyte distinct from T cells and B cells, destroy foreign cells (eg, neoplastic cells) even without prior sensitization. Antigen processing by macrophages precedes recognition of an antigen by lymphocytes. These complex processes are involved in routine surveillance against neoplastic cells and recognition of "self."

Lymphocyte response in disease may be appropriate (activation of the immune system) or inappropriate (immune-mediated disease and lymphoproliferative malignancies). (*See also* THE BIOLOGY OF THE IMMUNE SYSTEM, p 811.) Immune-mediated disease results from failure of the immune system to recognize host tissues as self. For example, in immune-mediated hemolytic anemia, antibodies are produced against the host's own RBCs. Another inappropriate response of the immune system is allergy. In allergic individuals, IgE antibodies to allergens are bound to the surface of basophils and mast cells. When exposure to the allergen occurs, antigen-antibody complexes are formed, and degranulation of the mast cells and basophils releases vasoactive amines. Reaction to this may be mild (as in urticaria or atopy) or life-threatening (as in anaphylaxis).

Lymphocytosis occurs in some species, especially the cat, as a response to epinephrine secretion. Atypical lymphocytes may be seen in the blood in response to antigenic stimulation (eg, vaccination). Persistent lymphocytosis in cattle infected with bovine leukemia virus is a benign polyclonal increase in lymphocyte numbers. Lymphoproliferative malignancies include lymphomas and acute lymphoblastic and chronic lymphocytic leukemias. Lymphopenia may occur most commonly as a response to glucocorticoid secretion.

PLATELETS

Platelets form the initial hemostatic plug whenever hemorrhage occurs. They also are the source of phospholipid, which is needed for the interaction of coagulation factors to form a fibrin clot. Platelets are produced in the bone marrow from megakaryocytes, under the influence of thrombopoietin. Platelet production begins with invagination of the megakaryocyte cell membrane and the formation of cytoplasmic channels and islands. The cytoplasmic islands produce platelets by fragmentation from the megakaryocyte.

Mature circulating platelets are packed with dense granules containing ATP, adenosine diphosphate (ADP), and calcium, as well as serotonin, lysosomes, glycogen, mitochondria, and an intracellular canalicular system. The mitochondria and glycogen are involved in energy production, and the canalicular system serves both as a transport system for granule components and as a source of phospholipid, which is found in high concentration in the membrane lining of the canals.

When vessel walls are damaged, collagen and tissue factor are exposed, and circulating platelets adhere via von Willebrand factor and undergo a change in shape with the accompanying release of ADP. Local platelet aggregation is stimulated by ADP, with the ultimate formation of the primary platelet plug. The local accumulation of fibrin and platelets is known as a hemostatic plug. The fibrin clot that then forms is consolidated by the action of platelet contractile proteins.

Platelet disorders are either quantitative (thrombocytopenia or thrombocytosis) or qualitative (thrombocytopathy). Thrombocytopenia is one of the most common bleeding disorders of animals. In general, platelet counts must fall to $<30,000/\mu L$ before the risk of hemorrhage increases. Consumption, destruction, or sequestration of platelets causes thrombocytopenia associated with increased production by the bone marrow. Consumptive thrombocytopenia occurs with massive hemorrhage or with disseminated intravascular coagulation, secondary to a variety of diseases. Destruction occurs in immune-mediated thrombocytopenia, in which platelets become coated with antiplatelet antibodies and are removed from the circulation by the fixed phagocyte system. Excessive sequestration of platelets by an enlarged spleen (hypersplenism) may occur in conditions such as myeloproliferative diseases.

Decreased production of platelets in the marrow may be caused by drugs, toxins, or by primary marrow disorders such as aplasia, fibrosis, or hematopoietic malignancy. In primary marrow disorders, more than one hematopoietic cell line is often decreased, resulting in pancytopenia.

Thrombocytosis is rare and often idiopathic. It may be associated with primary marrow disease such as in megakaryocytic leukemia. It is often associated with chronic blood loss and iron deficiency because of increased platelet production in the marrow reacting to continued consumption and loss.

Thrombocytopathies comprise a poorly defined group of diseases in which platelet numbers are normal but their function is impaired. Von Willebrand disease is characterized primarily by a defect in platelet adhesion to the endothelium. The platelets themselves are normal. Other hereditary disorders of platelet function have been described but are relatively rare. Probably the most common platelet function defect is the irreversible inhibition of thromboxane (which is necessary for platelet aggregation) caused by aspirin administration.

ANEMIA

Anemia is defined as an absolute decrease in the red cell mass as measured by RBC count, hemoglobin concentration, and/or PCV. It can develop from loss, destruction, or lack of production of RBCs. Anemia is classified as regenerative or nonregenerative.

With regenerative anemia, the bone marrow responds appropriately to the decreased red cell mass by increasing RBC production and releasing reticulocytes. With nonregenerative anemia, the bone marrow responds inadequately to the increased need for RBCs. Anemia caused by hemorrhage or hemolysis is typically regenerative. Anemia caused by decreased erythropoietin or an abnormality in the bone marrow is nonregenerative.

Clinical Findings: Clinical signs in anemic animals depend on the degree of anemia, the duration (acute or chronic), and the underlying cause. Acute anemia can result in shock and even death if more than a third of the blood volume is lost rapidly and not replaced. In acute blood loss, the animal usually presents with tachycardia, pale mucous membranes, bounding or weak peripheral pulses, and hypotension. The cause of the blood loss may be overt, eg, trauma. If no evidence of external bleeding is found, a source of internal or occult blood loss must be sought, eg, a ruptured splenic tumor, other neoplasia, coagulopathy, GI ulceration, or parasites. If hemolysis is present, the animal may be icteric. Animals with chronic anemia have had time to accommodate, and their clinical presentation is usually more indolent with vague signs of lethargy, weakness, and anorexia. These animals may have similar physical examination findings such as pale mucous membranes and weak peripheral pulses. The lack of expected clinical signs may alert the clinician to the time frame involved. Splenomegaly, abdominal distention, and/or heart murmur may be present, depending on the underlying cause of anemia.

Diagnosis: A complete history is an important part of the evaluation of an anemic animal. Questions might include duration of clinical signs, history of exposure to toxins (eg, rodenticides, heavy metals, toxic plants), drug treatments, vaccinations, travel history, and any prior illnesses.

A CBC, including a platelet and a reticulocyte count, will provide information on the severity of anemia and degree of bone marrow response, and also allow for evaluation of other cell lines. A blood smear should be evaluated for abnormalities in RBC morphology or size and for RBC parasites. The RBC indices (measures of size and hemoglobin concentration) are calculated by automated cell counters calibrated for the species in question. RBC size is expressed by the mean corpuscular volume (MCV) in femtoliters and can reflect the degree of regeneration. Macrocytosis (an increase in the MCV) usually correlates with a regenerative anemia. Macrocytosis can be a heritable condition in Poodles without anemia and may be seen in anemic cats infected with feline leukemia virus. Microcytosis (a decrease in the MCV) is the hallmark of iron-deficiency anemia. The hemoglobin concentration of each RBC, measured in g/dL, is defined as the mean corpuscular hemoglobin concentration (MCHC). Terms used for description of abnormalities with MCHC include normochromia and hypochromia. Abnormalities in RBC morphology, such as basophilic stippling, can indicate lead intoxication. Heinz body formation indicates oxidative injury to the RBCs, secondary to toxin exposure (*see* TABLE 1). Cats are more susceptible to Heinz body formation than other species, and cats without anemia can have a small number of Heinz bodies. The presence of schistocytes or spherocytes may also help identify the pathophysiology associated with the cause of anemia.

The reticulocyte count is usually reported as a percent of the RBC mass. This value should be corrected for the degree of anemia to evaluate the degree of regeneration. An absolute reticulocyte count (measured by RBCs/μL × reticulocyte percentage) of >50,000/μL in cats or >60,000/μL in dogs is considered regenerative. To correct the percent reticulocytes, the formula (*see* below) can be applied. A corrected reticulocyte percent >1% indicates regeneration in dogs and cats. After acute blood loss or hemolytic crisis, reticulocytosis usually takes 3–4 days to become evident.

A serum chemistry panel and urinalysis evaluate organ function. If GI blood loss is suspected, an examination of the feces for occult blood and parasites can be useful. Radiographs can help identify occult disease, such as a penny (zinc toxicity) in the stomach of a puppy with hemolytic anemia. Bruising or bleeding may be signs of a coagulopathy and indicate the need for a coagulation profile. Presence of petechiae or ecchymotic hemorrhage suggest significant thrombocytopenia or thrombocytopathy. If hemolytic disease is suspected, blood can be evaluated for autoagglutination, or a direct Coombs' test might be indicated. A test for autoagglutination can be done by placing a

$$\text{corrected reticulocyte \%} = (\text{observed reticulocyte \%}) \times \frac{\text{PCV of the patient}}{\text{normal PCV for that species}}$$

TABLE 1 TOXIC CAUSES OF ANEMIA

Pathogenic Mechanism	Drugs	Plants, Foods	Toxins, Chemicals	Heavy Metals
Oxidation	Acetaminophen, benzocaine, dapsone, nitrofurans, primaquine, propofol, quinacrine	Fava beans, oak, onions, propylene glycol, red maple	Crude oil, naphthalene	Copper, zinc
Blood loss	Aspirin, naproxen	Bracken fern, sweet clover	Dicoumarol	
Immune-mediated hemolysis	Cephalosporins, levamisole, penicillin, propylthiouracil, sulfonamides		Pirimicarb	
Hemolysis	Fenbendazole, heparin		Indole	Lead, selenium
Decreased marrow production	Amphotericin, azidothymidine, cephalosporins, chloramphenicol, estrogen, fenbendazole, griseofulvin, meclofenamic acid, phenobarbital, phenothiazine, phenylbutazone, propylthiouracil, quinidine, recombinant human erythropoietin, sulfonamides, thiacetarsamide	Bracken fern	Benzene, trichloro ethylene	Lead

drop of saline on a slide with a fresh drop of the animal's blood; the slide should be gently rotated to mix the drops together, then evaluated grossly and microscopically for macro- and microagglutination. If autoagglutination is present, there is no need to perform a Coombs' test. Serology or PCR for infectious agents such as feline leukemia virus, *Ehrlichia*, equine infectious anemia virus, and *Babesia* may also help define the cause of anemia (*see* TABLE 2).

Bone marrow evaluation by aspiration and/or biopsy (*see* p 14) is indicated in any animal with an unexplained, nonregenerative anemia. If the CBC reveals a decrease in more than one cell line, possibly indicating hypoplastic marrow, a biopsy would be indicated along with an aspirate. Biopsies and aspirates are complementary: biopsies are better to evaluate the architecture and degree of cellularity of the marrow, and aspirates allow for better evaluation of cellular morphology. Aspirates also allow for an evaluation of orderly maturation of the red and white blood cell lines, the ratio of myeloid to erythroid precursors (M:E ratio), and the number of platelet precursors. Iron stores can also be evaluated by Prussian blue staining. An M:E ratio of <1 indicates that red cell production is greater than white cell production; with an M:E ratio >1, the opposite is likely. The M:E ratio is always interpreted in light of a recent CBC, because changes in the ratio could also be due to suppression of one cell line compared with the other.

REGENERATIVE ANEMIAS

BLOOD LOSS ANEMIA

Acute blood loss can lead to shock and even death if >30%–40% of blood is lost and the hypovolemia that develops is not treated aggressively with IV fluids or compatible blood (*see* p 17), or both. Causes of acute loss can be known (eg, trauma, surgery) or occult. Coagulopathies, bleeding tumors, gastric ulceration, and external or internal parasites should be excluded as causes. GI parasites, such as *Haemonchus* in ruminants and hookworms in dogs, can lead to severe blood loss, especially in young animals. Low-grade, chronic blood loss eventually results in iron-deficiency anemia, although some degree of reticulocytosis may persist even after iron stores become depleted. The hallmark of an iron-deficiency anemia is microcytic, hypochromic anemia. This chronic blood loss can be due to some type of parasitism in young animals (eg, fleas, lice, intestinal parasitism), but in older animals, bleeding from GI ulcers or tumors is more common.

TABLE 2 INFECTIOUS CAUSES OF ANEMIA

Infectious Agent	Species Affected	Hemolytic	Marrow Affected
	BACTERIA		
Clostridium perfringens A	Cattle, sheep	Yes	No
Clostridium haemolyticum	Cattle, sheep	Yes	No
Leptospira interrogans	Cattle, pigs, sheep	Yes	No
Mycoplasma spp	Cats	±	Rarely
Haemobartonella spp	Cattle, cats	±	No
	VIRUSES		
Equine infectious anemia virus	Horses	±	Rarely
Feline leukemia virus	Cats	±	Yes
Feline immuno-deficiency virus	Cats	No	Yes
	RICKETTSIA		
Mycoplasma spp	Cattle, goats, llamas, pigs, sheep[a]	Yes (piglets only)	No
Anaplasma spp	Cattle, goats, sheep	Yes	No
Ehrlichia spp	Dogs	Yes	Yes
	PROTOZOA		
Babesia spp	Cattle, cats, dogs, horses, sheep	Yes	No
Theileria spp[b]	Cattle, goats, sheep	±	No
Cytauxzoon spp	Cats	No	Yes
Trypanosoma spp	Cattle, horses, pigs	Yes	No
Sarcocystis cruzi	Cattle	Yes	No

[a] In adults, only clinically relevant in splenectomized or critically ill animals.

[b] Pathogenic species of *Theileria* are found in Africa, the Mediterranean, the Middle East, Asia, and Europe. Species found in North America are nonpathogenic.

HEMOLYTIC ANEMIA

Hemolytic anemias are typically regenerative and result from lysis of RBCs in either the intra- or extravascular space. Intravascular hemolysis results in hemoglobinemia and hemoglobinuria, whereas extravascular hemolysis does not. Both types of hemolysis can result in icterus. In dogs, the most common cause of hemolytic anemia is immune mediated (60%–75%), although toxins, RBC trauma, infections, and RBC membrane defects can also cause hemolysis.

Immune-mediated Hemolytic Anemia: Immune-mediated hemolytic anemia (IMHA, *see* p 826) can be primary or secondary to neoplasia, infectious agents, drugs, or vaccinations. In IMHA, the immune system no longer recognizes RBCs as self and develops antibodies to circulating RBCs, leading to RBC destruction by macrophages and complement. In some cases, antibodies are directed against RBC precursors in the marrow, resulting in nonregenerative anemia. Animals with IMHA are usually icteric, sometimes febrile, and may have splenomegaly. Hematologic hallmarks of IMHA are regenerative anemia, hyperbilirubinemia, spherocytosis, autoagglutination, or a positive Coombs' test.

Another methodology to evaluate dogs for anti-RBC antibodies is flow cytometry. Flow cytometry allows for detection and quantitation of red cell surface–bound IgG and IgM. Flow cytometry was found to be 88%–100% specific for diagnosing dogs with anti-RBC antibodies. One report suggests using flow cytometry to assess response to treatment for dogs, because there is a decrease in surface anti-RBC antibodies before reticulocytosis or increase in RBC count. Flow cytometry may not be readily available to all veterinary hospitals.

Animals with IMHA can show mild, indolent signs or be in an acute crisis. It is important to tailor treatment to the animal's signs, including treating any underlying infections. Transfusion with packed RBCs is usually required. The goal of therapy is to stop the destruction of RBCs by treating with immunosuppressive drugs; supportive care is also a priority. Prednisone or prednisolone at a dosage of 1–2 mg/kg, bid, is considered first-line therapy, with azathioprine at 2 mg/kg/day (azathioprine is contraindicated in cats and may be replaced by chlorambucil) or cyclosporine at 5–10 mg/kg/day considered as a possible second agent. In one study, low-dose aspirin at 0.5 mg/kg/day improved survival times in dogs treated with azathioprine and prednisone. The veterinary literature is ambiguous on choice of second agent or when to introduce a second agent. Other immunosuppressive agents that have been used include mycophenolate and leflunomide.

In the acute hemolytic crisis, drugs such as cyclosporine (10 mg/kg/day, initially) or human intravenous immunoglobin (IVIG, 0.5–1.5 g/kg as a single dose) may also have benefit because of rapid onset of action.

Pulmonary thromboembolism is a risk in dogs with IMHA. These dogs are often hypercoagulable, which can be documented with thromboelastography. Dogs documented to be in a hypercoagulable state should be anticoagulated with heparin, which may be used in combination with antiplatelet therapy (aspirin 0.5 mg/kg/day with or without clopidogrel 1–2 mg/kg/day) if the platelet count is >40,000/μL. The dosing range for heparin is wide and variable, and dosage also depends on whether fractionated or unfractionated heparin is used. Heparin therapy can be monitored using activated partial thromboplastin time (APTT) or antifactor Xa concentrations (low-molecular-weight heparin).

Mortality rates for IMHA range from 20%–75%, depending on the severity of clinical signs. Negative prognostic indicators may include a rapid drop in PCV, high bilirubin concentration, moderate to marked leukocytosis (28,000 to >40,000 cells/μL), increased BUN, petechiae, intravascular hemolysis, autoagglutination, disseminated intravascular coagulation, and thromboembolic complications. Moderate to marked leukocytosis has been reported to be associated with tissue necrosis, most likely secondary to tissue hypoxia or thromboembolic disease. Referral to tertiary care facilities may improve survival.

Alloimmune Hemolysis: Neonatal isoerythrolysis (NI) is an immune-mediated hemolytic disease seen in newborn horses, mules, cattle, pigs, cats, and rarely dogs. NI is caused by ingestion of maternal colostrum containing antibodies to one of the neonate's blood group antigens. The maternal antibodies develop to specific foreign blood group antigens during previous pregnancies, unmatched transfusions, and from *Babesia* and *Anaplasma* vaccinations in cattle. Cats are unique in that blood type B cats have naturally occurring anti-A antibodies without prior exposure, and their kittens that are type A develop hemolysis after nursing. In horses, the antigens usually involved are A, C, and Q; NI is most commonly seen in Thoroughbreds and mules. Neonates with NI are normal at birth but develop severe hemolytic anemia within 2–3 days and become weak and icteric. Diagnosis is confirmed by screening maternal serum, plasma, or colostrum against the paternal or neonatal RBCs. Treatment consists of stopping any colostrum while giving supportive care with transfusions. If necessary, neonates can be transfused with triple-washed maternal RBCs. NI can be avoided by withholding maternal colostrum and giving colostrum from a maternal source free of the antibodies. The newborn's RBCs can be mixed with maternal serum to look for agglutination before the newborn is allowed to receive maternal colostrum.

Microangiopathic Hemolysis: Microangiopathic hemolysis is caused by RBC damage secondary to turbulent flow through abnormal vessels. In dogs, it can be seen secondary to severe heartworm infection, vascular tumors (hemangiosarcoma), splenic torsions, and disseminated intravascular coagulation; in other species, causes include hemolytic uremic syndrome in calves, equine infectious anemia, African swine fever, and chronic classical swine fever. Schistocytes are common in blood smears from these animals. Treatment involves correction of the underlying disease process.

Metabolic Causes of Hemolysis: Hypophosphatemia (*see* p 1000) causes postparturient hemoglobinuria and hemolysis in cattle, sheep, and goats. It can occur 2–6 wk after parturition. Hypophosphatemia with secondary hemolysis is seen in dogs and cats secondary to diabetes mellitus, hepatic lipidosis, and refeeding syndrome. Treatment with either oral or IV phosphorus is indicated, depending on the degree of hypophosphatemia. Cattle that drink too much water (water intoxication) are at risk of developing hemolysis secondary to hypotonic plasma. This is seen in calves 2–10 mo old and causes respiratory distress and hemoglobinuria. Clinical signs can progress to convulsions and coma. Hemolytic anemia, hyponatremia and hypochloremia, decreased serum osmolality, and low urine specific gravity in a calf would support the diagnosis of water intoxication. Treatment consists of hypertonic fluids (2.5% saline) and diuretics (eg, mannitol).

Toxins: Toxins and drugs can cause anemia by many mechanisms. Those implicated most frequently in animals and their pathogenic mechanisms are listed (*see* TABLE 1).

Infections: Many infectious agents—bacterial, viral, rickettsial, and protozoal—can cause anemia by direct damage to RBCs, leading to hemolysis, or by direct effects on precursors in the bone marrow (*see* TABLE 2).

Heritable Diseases: Several heritable RBC disorders cause anemia. Pyruvate kinase deficiencies are seen in Basenjis, Beagles, West Highland White Terriers, Cairn Terriers, and other breeds, as well as Abyssinian and Somali cats. Phosphofructokinase deficiency occurs in English Springer Spaniels. Deficiencies in these enzymes lead to shortened RBC life span and regenerative anemia. In dogs with phosphofructokinase deficiency, the hemolytic crises are set off by alkalosis secondary to excessive excitement or exercise. If such situations are minimized, these dogs may have a normal life expectancy. There is no treatment for pyruvate kinase deficiency, and affected dogs will have a shortened life span due to myelofibrosis and osteosclerosis of the bone marrow. Affected cats will have chronic intermittent hemolytic anemia, which is sometimes helped by splenectomy and steroids. Unlike dogs, cats have not been reported to develop osteosclerosis. A hereditary hemoglobinopathy, porphyria (*see* p 986), leads to build-up of porphyrins in the body and has been described in cattle, cats, and pigs. It is most prevalent in Holstein cattle and can lead to a hemolytic crisis. Affected calves fail to thrive and are photosensitive. Diagnosis is made by finding increased levels of porphyrins in bone marrow, urine, or plasma. Teeth of affected animals fluoresce under ultraviolet light.

NONREGENERATIVE ANEMIAS

NUTRITIONAL DEFICIENCIES

Nutritional deficiency anemias develop when micronutrients needed for RBC formation are not present in adequate amounts. Anemia develops gradually and may initially be regenerative but ultimately becomes nonregenerative. Starvation causes anemia by a combination of vitamin and mineral deficiencies as well as a negative energy and protein balance. Deficiencies most likely to cause anemia are iron, copper, cobalamin (B_{12}), B_6, riboflavin, niacin, vitamin E, and vitamin C (important only in primates and guinea pigs).

Iron deficiency is the most common deficiency seen in dogs and piglets but occurs less commonly in horses, cats, and ruminants. Iron deficiency is rarely nutritional in origin—it most commonly occurs secondary to blood loss (*see* p 9). Young animals have minimal iron stores, and milk contains very little iron. This can be especially important for piglets that grow rapidly and are often raised indoors with no access to iron. Oral iron supplementation is indicated as treatment for iron deficiency; any source of blood loss must be eliminated.

Copper deficiency can develop in ruminants fed forage grown in copper-deficient soil. Copper is necessary for the metabolism of iron. Copper deficiency may occur secondary to high dietary molybdenum or sulfate in cattle and can develop in pigs fed whey diets. Low blood copper concentrations or low copper concentrations in liver biopsies (more definitive) are diagnostic. Treatment is oral or injectable copper supplementation.

B vitamin deficiencies are rare. Certain drugs (anticonvulsants, drugs that interfere with folate metabolism) have been associated with development of folate or cobalamin deficiency, leading to a normocytic, normochromic, nonregenerative anemia. Cobalamin malabsorption has been reported in Giant Schnauzers (their enterocytes are unable to absorb cobalamin). These dogs respond to parenteral supplementation with cobalamin. Ruminants also develop a secondary cobalamin deficiency when grazing on cobalt-deficient pasture. Treatment with oral cobalt or parenteral cobalamin is indicated.

ANEMIA OF CHRONIC DISEASE

Anemia of chronic disease can be characterized as mild to moderate, nonregenerative, normochromic, and normocytic. It is the most common form of anemia seen in animals. The anemia can be secondary to chronic inflammation or infection, neoplasia, liver disease, hyper- or hypoadrenocorticism, or hypothyroidism. The anemia is mediated by cytokines produced by inflammatory cells, which lead to decreases in iron availability, RBC survival, and the marrow's ability to regenerate. Treatment should be directed at the underlying disease and often results in resolution of the anemia. The anemia may be reduced by treatment with recombinant human erythropoietin, but the risk of antibody formation to endogenous erythropoietin may outweigh benefit. Darbepoetin appears to have less impact to induce reactive antibodies.

RENAL DISEASE

Chronic renal disease is a common cause of nonregenerative anemia in animals. Erythropoietin is normally produced by the peritubular endothelial cells in the renal cortex. Animals with renal disease produce less erythropoietin, leading to anemia. Recombinant human erythropoietin (44–132 U/kg, three times/wk, with most animals starting at 88 U/kg) has been used for treatment. PCV is monitored weekly until the desired improvement is reached (this will vary with the initial degree of anemia), after which the dosage is decreased. Animals receiving recombinant human erythropoietin require supplemental iron to support RBC production. (*See also* HEMATINICS, p 2540.) Darbepoeitin also has been found to be valuable in management of anemia associated with chronic kidney disease.

PRIMARY BONE MARROW DISEASES

Primary bone marrow disease or failure from any cause can lead to nonregenerative anemia and pancytopenia. With diffuse marrow involvement, granulocytes are affected first, followed by platelets and finally RBCs.

Aplastic anemia has been reported in dogs, cats, ruminants, horses, and pigs with pancytopenia and a hypoplastic marrow, replaced by fat. Most cases are idiopathic, but reported causes include infection (feline leukemia virus, *Ehrlichia*, parvovirus), drug therapy (methimazole, chemotherapeutic agents, antibiotics [trimethoprim-sulfa, chloramphemicol], fenbendazole), toxin ingestion (estrogen), and total body irradiation (*see* TABLES 1 and 2). There may also be an immune-mediated component to this disease. Diagnosis is confirmed by bone marrow aspiration and core biopsy. Treatment consists of eliminating the underlying cause and providing supportive measures such as broad-spectrum antibiotics and transfusions. Immunosuppressive agents such as prednisone, cyclosporine, mycophenolate, or azathioprine may be considered. Recombinant human erythropoietin and granulocyte colony-stimulating factor (5 mcg/kg/day, PO) can be used until the marrow recovers. If the disease is idiopathic or if marrow recovery is unlikely (eg, phenylbutazone toxicity in dogs), bone marrow transplantation is beneficial if a suitable donor is available (investigational and limited availability).

In **pure red cell aplasia** (PRCA), only the erythroid line is affected. It is characterized by a nonregenerative anemia with severe depletion of red cell precursors in the bone marrow. It has been reported in dogs and cats and may be primary or secondary. Primary cases are most commonly immune mediated and may respond to immunosuppressive therapy. Supportive care, including transfusion, may be indicated when anemia is severe. Feline leukemia–positive cats can have PRCA. Recombinant human erythropoietin has been reported to cause PRCA in dogs and horses. Discontinuation of therapy may eventually lead to RBC recovery in some animals.

Primary leukemias are uncommon to rare in domestic species but have been reported in dogs, cats, cattle, goats, sheep, pigs, and horses. Retroviruses are a cause in some cattle, cats, primates, and chickens. Leukemias can develop in myeloid or lymphoid cell lines and are further classified as acute or chronic. Most affected animals have nonregenerative anemia, neutropenia, and thrombocytopenia, with circulating blasts usually present. Acute leukemias, characterized by infiltration of the marrow with blasts, generally respond poorly to chemotherapy. In animals that do respond, remission times are usually short. In acute lymphoblastic leukemia in dogs, the response rate to chemotherapy is ~30%, with a median survival of 4 mo. Acute myeloblastic leukemias are less common and even less responsive to treatment than acute lymphoblastic leukemia. In acute leukemias, the cell lineage is often difficult to identify morphologically, so cytochemical stains or immunologic evaluation of cell surface markers may be necessary for definitive diagnosis. Chronic leukemias, characterized by an overproduction of one hematopoietic cell line, are less likely to cause anemia and more responsive to treatment.

Myelodysplasia (myelodysplastic syndrome, MDS) is considered a preleukemic syndrome characterized by ineffective hematopoiesis, resulting in a nonregenerative anemia or other cytopenias. MDS has been described in dogs, cats, and people. The disease can be primary or secondary and is commonly seen in cats with feline leukemia. Primary syndromes probably arise from mutations in stem cells. Secondary syndromes are caused by other neoplasia or drug therapy. Some cats and dogs respond to treatment with recombinant human erythropoietin and prednisone. Supportive care with transfusions may be helpful. Survival is variable because MDS can progress to leukemia; many animals are euthanized or die of sepsis, bleeding, or anemia.

Myelofibrosis causes bone marrow failure secondary to replacement of normal marrow elements with fibrous tissue. It has been seen in dogs, cats, people, and goats. It can be a primary disorder or secondary to malignancies, immune-mediated hemolytic anemia, whole body irradiation, and congenital anemias (eg, pyruvate kinase deficiency). Diagnosis can be made by bone marrow biopsy. Treatment varies with the underlying cause but usually consists of immunosuppressive therapy.

Bone Marrow Aspiration and Biopsy: Bone marrow aspiration and biopsy are techniques used to evaluate the bone marrow in domestic animal species. The basic technique involves introducing a hollow needle into the bone marrow to obtain a sample for evaluation. Bone marrow aspiration provides a sample for cytologic evaluation, and bone marrow biopsy provides a sample for histopathologic evaluation.

Specific clinical indications to evaluate bone marrow include but are not limited to investigation of nonregenerative anemia, thrombocytopenia, leukopenia, bicytopenia, pancytopenia, abnormal circulating cells of any type, monoclonal gammopathy, suspected osteomyelitis, suspected bone neoplasia, infectious disease affecting the bone, and clinical staging of neoplastic processes such as lymphoma and mast cell disease.

The conventional anatomic sites used for bone marrow aspiration include the iliac crest, the trochanteric fossa of the femur, the tibial crest, and the greater tubercle of the humerus. Some clinicians have also used the rib (costochondral junction) or sternabrae. The humerus is the most common site for bone marrow biopsy.

For bone marrow aspiration, cats and dogs generally require sedation, although some cats may require general anesthesia. General anesthesia is required for bone marrow biopsy. The animal is positioned in lateral recumbency when using the trochanteric fossa or the greater tubercle, and in sternal recumbency when using the iliac crest. The area to be accessed is shaved and aseptically prepared. The site, including the periosteum, is infiltrated with local anesthetic. A #11 scalpel blade is then used to make a stab incision through the skin.

The equipment used for these procedures may differ slightly. Most bone marrow aspiration needles (eg, Rosenthal, Illinois) are very similar and have a removable stylet. With the stylet in place, the needle is advanced with a back and forth screw-like motion until the needle is well seated in the bone. The stylet is then removed, and a syringe (6–12 mL) attached for aspiration. If the animal feels any discomfort, this is when it will occur. Only a small sample is required, ie, enough to fill the syringe hub, which should be put onto slides for cytologic evaluation. The needle can then be removed.

Bone marrow biopsy generally requires a Jamshidi needle, which is rigid and hollow with a stylet. The Jamshidi needle has a cutting edge at its end, designed to obtain a core marrow sample (although it can also be used to obtain a bone marrow aspirate). The needle is driven into the bone with a back and forth, screw-like motion. Once the needle is well seated, the cap is unscrewed and the stylet removed. An aspirate can be obtained similar to the technique described above. To obtain a core sample for histopathology, the needle is advanced further (about ¼ in.) into the marrow and twisted in one direction. The needle is then moved in a wide, circular motion to try to dislodge a core sample. The needle is removed by twisting in the opposite direction in which it was advanced. A blunt stylet is then passed retrograde to remove the core sample. The core can be gently rolled onto a slide for cytology and then placed into formalin for histopathology.

BLOOD GROUPS AND BLOOD TRANSFUSIONS

Blood groups are determined by genetically controlled, polymorphic, antigenic components of the RBC membrane. The allelic products of a particular genetic locus are classified as a blood group system. Some of these systems are highly complex, with many alleles defined at a locus; others consist of a single defined antigen. Blood group systems, in general, are independent of each other, and their inheritance conforms to Mendelian dominance. For polymorphic blood group systems, an animal usually inherits one allele from each parent and thus expresses no more than two blood group antigens of a system. An exception is in cattle, in which multiple alleles, or "phenogroups," are inherited. Normally, an individual does not have antibodies against any of the antigens present on its own or against other blood group antigens of that species' systems unless they have been induced by transfusion, pregnancy, or immunization. In some species (people, sheep, cattle, pigs, horses, cats, and dogs), so-called "naturally occurring" isoantibodies, not induced by transfusion or pregnancy, may be present in variable but detectable titers. For example, Group B cats have naturally occurring anti-A antibody. Also, circulating antibodies to animal blood group antigens may be induced by transfusion. With random blood transfusions in dogs, there is a 30%–40% chance of sensitization of the recipient, primarily to blood group antigen DEA 1, but risk is also present for development of antibody to any other antigen lacked by the recipient. In horses, transplacental immunization of the mare by an incompatible fetal antigen inherited from the sire may occur. Immunization also may result when some homologous blood products are used as vaccines (eg, anaplasmosis in cattle). In dogs, prior pregnancy does not result in sensitization of the bitch to foreign blood group antigens.

The number of major recognized blood group systems (*see* TABLE 3) varies among domestic species, with cattle being the most complex and cats the simplest. Animal

TABLE 3 MAJOR BLOOD GROUPS OF CLINICAL INTEREST

Species	Blood Group
Canine	DEA 1.1 and 7
Feline	A, B, *mic*
Equine	A, C, Q
Bovine	B, J
Ovine	B, R

blood groups are typed to aid in the matching of donors and recipients and, especially in horses, to identify breeding pairs potentially at risk of causing hemolytic disease in their offspring. Because expression of blood group antigens is genetically controlled and the modes of inheritance are understood, these systems also have been used to substantiate pedigrees in cattle and horses; however, in most cases, DNA testing has replaced blood typing for paternity testing.

BLOOD TYPING

Antisera used to identify blood groups (typing reagents) usually are produced as isoimmune sera. Their in vitro serologic characteristics vary with the species. Many reagents are hemagglutinins; others are hemolytic and require complement to complete the serologic reaction, such as in cattle (because RBCs do not readily agglutinate) and horses (because RBC rouleaux are a problem). Other typing reagents, neither hemagglutinating nor hemolytic, combine with RBC antigens in an "incomplete" reaction because they lack additional combining sites to agglutinate other RBCs; addition of species-specific antiglobulin is required for agglutination.

The diversity of blood groups in animals and the lack of commercially available blood-typing reagents to all antigens make complete typing difficult but should not preclude the clinical use of transfusions. In horses and dogs, the blood group antigens most commonly implicated in transfusion incompatibilities are known; by selecting donor animals that lack these groups, or that match the recipient, the risk of sensitization of the recipient to the most important antigens can be minimized. For dogs and cats, commercially available, point-of-care testing for major antigens is available in either gel or card testing kits. Reagents are available for only some antigens, generally those that are most likely to sensitize a recipient, or those for which naturally occurring antibodies, primarily in cats, might be present. For example, dogs have more than 12 blood group systems but generally are typed for only one (DEA 1.1). An additional blood group antigen (dal) was discovered when a dal-negative, previously transfused Dalmatian reacted to many potential donors, and only a few Dalmatians were found to be compatible. It is a common antigen in most dogs but is lacking in some Dalmatians. Because multiple blood group antigens are present, it is likely that an animal receiving a transfusion might be exposed to some antigens that are not present on its RBCs.

CROSSMATCHING

Previously sensitized recipients or those with naturally occurring antibodies can be detected by crossmatching, which is done to preclude administration of incompatible blood. In the USA, >99% of cats are of blood group A, so the risk of incompatible transfusion is low. However, certain breeds, including Abyssinian, Birman, British Shorthair, Devon Rex, Himalayan, Persian, Scottish Fold, and Somali, have a higher frequency of blood group B. Any incompatible transfusion in cats results in rapid destruction of transfused cells, so typing and crossmatching should be done before any transfusion. The *mic* antigen is present in some cats, and naturally occurring antibodies are present in cats that lack the *mic* antigen. For that reason, crossmatching should be performed for cats before the first transfusion, even if they will receive A or B matched blood.

The direct crossmatch procedure, with appropriate controls, is effective for all species. The **major crossmatch** detects antibodies already present in recipient plasma that could cause a hemolytic reaction when donor RBCs are transfused; it will not detect the potential for sensitization to develop. Anticoagulant (calcium disodium edetate or citrate) is added to blood samples from donor and recipient; the donor RBCs are washed 3 times with 0.9% saline, and a 4% RBC suspension in saline is made from the washed cells. The major crossmatch consists of combining equal volumes (0.1 mL) of the donor RBC suspension and recipient plasma. The control tube contains recipient RBCs and recipient plasma. The samples are incubated, centrifuged, and evaluated for hemolysis or agglutination. Hemolysis is evaluated by comparing the color of the supernatant in the test sample with that of the control sample. Each sample is then gently shaken until all cells in the "button" at the bottom of the tube have returned to suspension. Again, the degree of cell clumping of the test sample is compared with that of the control sample. The test is negative, or compatible, when the plasma is clear and the RBCs are readily suspended. A positive, or incompatible, test can have hemolysis or hemagglutination or both. All tests judged macroscopically to be negative for hemagglutination should be confirmed microscopically at low power. Some newer crossmatching systems that use a gel technique are becoming available. This is particularly important in horses, because their RBCs tend to form rouleaux.

The **minor crossmatch** is the reverse of the major crossmatch, ie, recipient cells are combined with donor plasma. The minor crossmatch is important only in species such as cats with clinically significant naturally occurring isoantibodies or if the donor has been previously transfused or, in horses, those with previous pregnancies.

BLOOD TRANSFUSIONS

Frequently, the need for blood transfusions is acute, as in acute hemolysis or hemorrhage; transfusions are also appropriate in treatment of acute or chronic anemias. Animals with hemostatic disorders often require repeated transfusions of whole blood, red cells, plasma, or platelets. Blood transfusions must be given with care, because they have the potential to further compromise the recipient.

Whole blood frequently is not the ideal product to be administered. If the need is to replace the oxygen-carrying capability of the blood, then packed RBCs are more appropriate; if replacement of circulatory volume is needed, crystalloid or colloid solutions may be used, with packed RBCs added as needed. Platelet numbers rise rapidly after hemorrhage, so replacement is rarely needed. Plasma proteins equilibrate from the interstitial space, so plasma is not needed except in massive hemorrhage (>1 blood volume in 24 hr). Animals that require coagulation factors benefit most from administration of fresh-frozen plasma or cryoprecipitate if the need is specifically for factor VIII, von Willebrand factor, or fibrinogen. Platelet-rich plasma or platelet concentrates may be of value in thrombocytopenia, although immune-mediated thrombocytopenia usually does not respond to administration of platelets because they are removed rapidly by the spleen.

The decision to transfuse RBCs is determined by clinical signs, not by any pre-selected PCV. Animals with acute anemia show signs of weakness, tachycardia, and tachypnea at a higher PCV than animals with chronic anemia. The amount of RBCs required to relieve clinical signs will generally increase the PCV above 20%. Domestic animals have blood volumes of 7%–9% of their body weight; cats have a slightly lower volume of ~6.5%. By determining the recipient's blood volume and knowing the animal's PCV, the required replacement RBC volume can be calculated. For example, a 25-kg dog has a total blood volume of ~2,000 mL; with a PCV of 15%, the RBC volume is 300 mL; if the PCV is to be increased to 20%, that equals an RBC volume of 400 mL. Therefore, 100 mL of RBCs or 200 mL of whole blood (with PCV of 50%) would be required to increase the recipient's PCV to the desired level. These calculations assume no ongoing losses of RBCs through hemorrhage or hemolysis. Obviously, the post-transfusion PCV is the most important measure of adequacy of red cell dose. No more than 20% of a donor animal's blood should be collected at one time.

Collection, storage, and transfusion of blood must be done aseptically. The anticoagulant of choice is citrate phosphate dextrose adenine (CPDA-1). Commercial blood bags containing the appropriate amount of anticoagulant for a "unit" (500 mL) are available. Heparin should not be used as an anticoagulant, because it has a longer half-life in the recipient and causes platelet activation; also, heparinized blood cannot be stored.

Blood collected in CPDA-1 with added RBC preservation or nutrient solutions may be safely stored at 4°C for 4 wk. If the blood will not be used immediately, the plasma can be removed and stored frozen for later use as a source of coagulation factors or albumin for acute reversible hypoalbuminemia. Plasma must be frozen at –20° to –30°C within 6 hr of collection to assure that levels of factor VIII are adequate and will remain so for 1 yr. Chronic hypoproteinemia is not helped by plasma, because the total body deficit of albumin is so large that it could not be improved by the small amount contained in plasma. Colloid solutions such as hetastarch are more effective for treatment of hypoalbuminemia. Human albumin has been used in dogs; however, the risk of sensitization and allergic reactions is significant.

Risks of Transfusion: The most serious risk of transfusion is acute hemolysis. Fortunately, this is rare in domestic animals. Dogs rarely have clinically significant preformed antibodies, so only those that have received repeated transfusions are at risk. The most common hemolytic reaction in dogs that have received multiple transfusions is delayed hemolysis, seen clinically as shortened survival of transfused RBCs and a positive Coombs' test. Even crossmatch-compatible RBCs given to horses or cattle survive only 2–4 days. Nonimmune causes of hemolysis include improper collection or separation of blood, freezing or overwarming of RBCs, and infusing under pressure through a small needle.

Other complications include sepsis from contaminated blood, hypocalcemia from too much citrate, and hypervolemia (especially in animals with preexisting heart disease or in very small animals). Urticaria, fever, or vomiting are seen occasionally. Transfusions can also spread disease from donor to recipient, such as RBC parasites (eg, *Mycoplasma* in cats or *Babesia* in dogs) and viruses (eg, retroviruses in cats, horses, or cattle). Other diseases, such as those caused by rickettsia or other bacteria, can also be spread if the donor is bacteremic. Donors should be tested periodically for infectious diseases that are prevalent locally. Flea and tick prevention is also important to prevent vector-borne infections in donors.

BLOOD SUBSTITUTES

(Hemoglobin-based oxygen carrier solutions)

Because of problems associated with finding compatible donors and disease transmission by transfusion, the search for a red cell substitute has been ongoing for >50 yr. An ideal substitute would carry and deliver oxygen like red cells, be easy to produce in large quantities, be nonantigenic, and persist in the circulation at least long enough for resuscitation.

One hemoglobin-based oxygen carrier of bovine origin is currently licensed for use in dogs. The hemoglobin is collected aseptically, filtered to remove all red cell stromal elements, and polymerized to allow the product to persist in the circulation for a half-life of ~36 hr. This product has been shown to carry and deliver oxygen efficiently, can be used immediately without need for typing or crossmatching, and has a 3-yr shelf life at room temperature. Because the structure of the hemoglobin molecule is similar between species, bovine hemoglobin is minimally antigenic. Although currently licensed for use only in dogs, it has been used in cats, horses, llamas, birds, and people. Its colloidal effects are especially useful in resuscitation after trauma with acute blood loss. Because the cost of hemoglobin solution is often higher, and duration of effect is shorter than that of blood, the main value of hemoglobin is in emergency situations when blood is not immediately available. Volume overload is a potential risk if hemoglobin is given too rapidly. Another concern with hemoglobin solutions is that nitric oxide is scavenged and removed by the product. This paradoxically might cause vasoconstriction and decrease oxygen delivery to ischemic tissues.

BLOOD PARASITES

ANAPLASMOSIS

Anaplasmosis, formerly known as gall sickness, traditionally refers to a disease of ruminants caused by obligate intraerythrocytic bacteria of the order Rickettsiales, family Anaplasmataceae, genus *Anaplasma*. Cattle, sheep, goats, buffalo, and some wild ruminants can be infected with the erythrocytic *Anaplasma*. Anaplasmosis occurs in tropical and subtropical regions worldwide (~40°N to 32°S), including South and Central America, the USA, southern Europe, Africa, Asia, and Australia.

The *Anaplasma* genus also includes *A phagocytophilum* (compiled from species previously known as *Ehrlichia phagocytophila*, *E equi*, and human granulocytic ehrlichiosis agent, *see* p 803), *A bovis* (formerly *E bovis*), and *A platys* (formerly *E platys*), all of which invade blood cells other than erythrocytes of their respective mammalian hosts. Bovine anaplasmosis is of economic significance in the cattle industry.

Etiology and Pathogenesis: Clinical bovine anaplasmosis is usually caused by *A marginale*. An *A marginale* with an appendage has been called *A caudatum*, but it is not considered to be a separate species. Cattle are also infected with *A centrale*, which generally results in mild disease. *A ovis* may cause mild to severe disease in sheep, deer, and goats. *A phagocytophilum* has recently been reported to infect cattle; however, natural infection is rare and it does not cause clinical disease.

Transmission and Epidemiology: Up to 17 different tick vector species (including *Dermacentor*, *Rhipicephalus*, *Ixodes*, *Hyalomma*, and *Argas*) have been reported to transmit *Anaplasma* spp. Not all of these are likely significant vectors in the field, and it has been shown that strains of *A marginale* also coevolve with particular tick strains. *Rhipicephalus* (*Boophilus*) spp are major vectors in Australia and Africa, and *Dermacentor* spp have been incriminated as the main vectors in the USA. After feeding on an infected animal, intrastadial or trans-stadial transmission may occur. Transovarial transmission may also occur, although this is rare, even in the single-host *Rhipicephalus* spp. A replicative cycle occurs in the infected tick. Mechanical transmission via biting dipterans occurs in some regions. Transplacental transmission has been reported and is usually associated with acute infection of the dam in the second or third trimester of gestation. Anaplasmosis may also be spread through the use of contaminated needles or dehorning or other surgical instruments.

There is a strong correlation between age of cattle and severity of disease. Calves are much more resistant to disease (although not infection) than older cattle. This resistance is not due to colostral antibody from immune dams. In endemic areas where cattle first become infected with *A marginale* early in life, losses due to anaplasmosis are minimal. After recovery from the acute phase of infection, cattle remain chronically infected carriers but are generally immune to further clinical disease. However, these chronically infected cattle may relapse to anaplasmosis when immunosuppressed (eg, by corticosteroids), when infected with other pathogens, or after splenectomy. Carriers serve as a reservoir for further transmission. Serious losses occur when mature cattle with no previous exposure are moved into endemic areas or under endemically unstable situations when transmission rates are insufficient to ensure that all cattle are infected before reaching the more susceptible adult age.

Clinical Findings: In animals <1 yr old anaplasmosis is usually subclinical, in yearlings and 2-yr-olds it is moderately severe, and in older cattle it is severe and often fatal. Anaplasmosis is characterized by progressive anemia due to extravascular destruction of infected and uninfected erythrocytes. The prepatent period of *A marginale* is directly related to the infective dose and typically ranges from 15–36 days (although it may be as long as 100 days). After the prepatent period, peracute (most severe but rare), acute, or chronic anaplasmosis may follow. Rickettsemia approximately doubles every 24 hr during the exponential growth phase. Generally, 10%–30% of erythrocytes are infected at peak rickettsemia, although this figure may be as high as 65%. RBC count, PCV, and hemoglobin values are all severely reduced. Macrocytic anemia with circulating reticulocytes may be present late in the disease.

Animals with peracute infections succumb within a few hours of the onset of clinical signs. Acutely infected animals lose condition rapidly. Milk production falls. Inappetence, loss of coordination, breathlessness when exerted, and a rapid bounding pulse are usually evident in the late stages. The urine may be brown but, in contrast to babesiosis, hemoglobinuria does not occur. A transient febrile response, with the body temperature rarely exceeding 106°F (41°C) occurs at about the time of peak rickettsemia. Mucous membranes appear pale and then yellow. Pregnant cows may abort. Surviving cattle convalesce over several weeks, during which hematologic parameters gradually return to normal.

Bos indicus breeds of cattle appear to possess a greater resistance to *A marginale* infection than *B taurus* breeds, but variation of resistance of individuals within breeds of both species occurs. Differences in virulence between *Anaplasma* strains and the level and duration of the rickettsemia also play a role in severity of clinical manifestations.

Lesions: Lesions are typical of those found in animals with anemia due to erythrophagocytosis. The carcasses of cattle that die from anaplasmosis are generally markedly anemic and jaundiced. Blood is thin and watery. The spleen is characteristically enlarged and soft, with prominent follicles. The liver may be mottled and yellow-orange. The gallbladder is often distended and contains thick brown or green bile. Hepatic and mediastinal lymph nodes appear brown. There are serous effusions in body cavities, pulmonary edema, petechial hemorrhages in the epi- and endocardium, and often evidence of severe GI stasis. Widespread phagocytosis of erythrocytes is evident on microscopic examination of the reticuloendothelial organs. A significant proportion of erythrocytes are usually found to be parasitized after death due to acute infection.

Diagnosis: *A marginale*, together with the hemoprotozoa *Babesia bovis* and *B bigemina*, are the causative agents of tick fever in cattle. These three species have similar geographic distributions, except that anaplasmosis occurs in the absence of babesiosis in the USA. Microscopic examination of Giemsa-stained thin and thick blood films is critical to distinguish anaplasmosis from babesiosis (*see* p 21) and other conditions that result in anemia and jaundice, such as leptospirosis (*see* p 646) and theileriosis (*see* p 33). Blood in anticoagulant should also be obtained for hematologic testing. In Giemsa-stained thin blood films, *Anaplasma* spp appear as dense, homogeneously staining blue-purple inclusions 0.3–1 μm in diameter. *A marginale* inclusions are usually located toward the margin of the infected erythrocyte, whereas *A centrale* inclusion bodies are located more centrally. *A caudatum* cannot be distinguished from *A marginale* using Giemsa-stained blood films. Special staining techniques are used to identify this species based on observation of characteristic appendages associated with the bacteria. *A caudatum* has been reported only in North America and could possibly be a morphologic form of *A marginale* and not a separate species. Inclusion bodies contain 1–8 initial bodies 0.3–0.4 μm in diameter, which are the individual rickettsiae. The percentage of infected erythrocytes varies with the stage and severity of disease; maximum rickettsemias in excess of 50% can occur with *A marginale*. Microscopically, the infection becomes visible 2–6 wk after transmission. During the course of infection, the rickettsemia can double each day for up to 10 days and then decreases. Severe anemia can persist for weeks after parasites cannot be detected in blood smears.

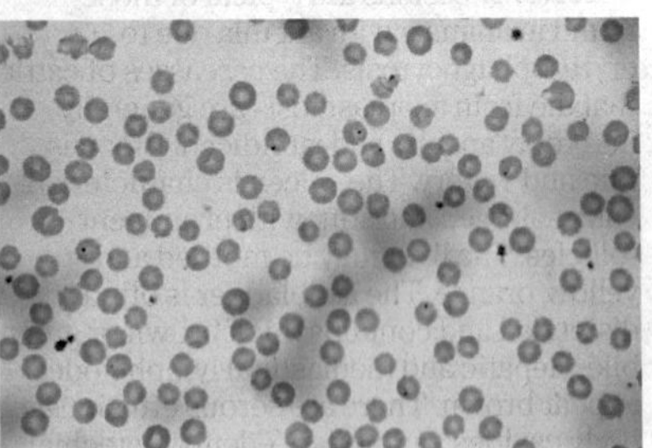

Anaplasma marginale in bovine blood, Wright-Giemsa, 100× oil immersion. Intracellular organisms appear as basophilic, spherical inclusions generally located near the margin of erythrocytes. Echinocytes are frequently present. *Courtesy of Ms. Sue Anderson, Tick Fever Centre, Wacol, Queensland, Australia.*

Chronically infected carriers may be identified with a fair degree of accuracy by serologic testing using the msp5 ELISA, complement fixation, or card agglutination tests. Nucleic acid–based detection methods are most useful, because species and strain differentiation tests may not detect carrier levels.

At necropsy, thin blood films of liver, kidney, spleen, lungs, and peripheral blood should be prepared for microscopic examination.

Treatment, Control, and Prevention: Tetracycline antibiotics and imidocarb are currently used for treatment. Cattle may be sterilized by treatment with these drugs and remain immune to severe anaplasmosis subsequently for at least 8 mo.

Prompt administration of tetracycline drugs (tetracycline, chlortetracycline, oxytetracycline, rolitetracycline, doxycycline, minocycline) in the early stages of acute disease (eg, PCV >15%) usually ensures survival. A commonly used treatment consists of a single IM injection of long-acting oxytetracycline at a dosage of 20 mg/kg. Blood transfusion to partially restore the PCV greatly improves the survival rate of more severely affected cattle. The carrier state may be eliminated by administration of a long-acting oxytetracycline preparation (20 mg/kg, IM, at least two injections with a 1-wk interval). Withholding periods for tetracyclines apply in most countries. Injection into the neck muscle rather than the rump is preferred.

Imidocarb is also highly efficacious against *A marginale* as a single injection (as the dihydrochloride salt at 1.5 mg/kg, SC, or as imidocarb dipropionate at 3 mg/kg). Elimination of the carrier state requires the use of higher repeated doses of imidocarb (eg, 5 mg/kg, IM or SC, two injections of the dihydrochloride salt 2 wk apart). Imidocarb is a suspected carcinogen with long withholding periods and is not approved for use in the USA or Europe.

In South Africa, Australia, Israel, and South America, infection with live *A centrale* (originating from South Africa) is used as a vaccine to provide cattle with partial protection against the disease caused by *A marginale*. *A centrale* (single dose) vaccine produces severe reactions in a small proportion of cattle. In the USA, where live vaccines cannot be used, vaccines comprising nonliving *A marginale* purified from infected bovine erythrocytes and adjuvant have been used in the past but may not currently be available. Immunity generated by using multidose killed vaccine protects cattle from severe disease on subsequent infection, but cattle can still be susceptible to challenge with heterologous strains of *A marginale*. Instances of isoerythrolysis in suckling calves have occurred due to prior vaccination of dams with preparations that contained bovine erythrocytic material. Long-lasting immunity against *A marginale* is conferred by preimmunization with live rickettsia, combined with the use of chemotherapy to control severe reactions. The use of attenuated strains of *A marginale* as a live vaccine has been reported, with instances of severe reactions also occurring. *A marginale* grown in tick cell cultures are being investigated as an alternative live vaccine source. Subunit vaccines to control bovine anaplasmosis are also under investigation. In some areas, sustained stringent control or elimination of the arthropod vectors may be a viable control strategy; however, in other areas immunization is recommended.

BABESIOSIS

Babesiosis is caused by intraerythrocytic protozoan parasites of the genus *Babesia*. Transmitted by ticks, babesiosis affects a wide range of domestic and wild animals and occasionally people. Although the major economic impact of babesiosis is on the cattle industry, infections in other domestic animals, including horses, sheep, goats, pigs, and dogs, assume varying degrees of importance throughout the world.

Two important species in cattle—*B bigemina* and *B bovis*—are widespread in tropical and subtropical areas and are the focus of this discussion. However, because there are many common features of the diseases caused by different *Babesia*, much of this information can be applied to other species.

Transmission and Epidemiology: The main vectors of *B bigemina* and *B bovis* are 1-host *Rhipicephalus (Boophilus)* spp ticks, in which transmission occurs transovarially. Although the parasites can be readily transmitted experimentally by blood inoculation, mechanical transmission by insects or during surgical procedures has no practical significance. Intrauterine infection has also been reported but is rare.

In *Rhipicephalus* spp ticks, the blood stages of the parasite are ingested during engorgement and undergo sexual and asexual multiplication in the replete female, infecting eggs and subsequent parasitic stages. Transmission to the host occurs when larvae (in the case of *B bovis*) or nymphs and adults (in the case of *B bigemina*) feed. The percentage of larvae infected can vary from 0–50% or higher, depending mainly on the level of parasitemia of the host at the time the female ticks engorge. Under field conditions, the rate of tick transmission is generally higher for *B bigemina* than for *B bovis*.

In endemic areas, three features are important in determining the risk of clinical disease: 1) calves have a degree of immunity (related both to colostral-derived antibodies and to age-specific factors) that persists for ~6 mo, 2) animals that recover from *Babesia* infections are generally immune for their commercial life (4 yr), and 3) the susceptibility of cattle breeds to ticks and *Babesia* infections varies; eg, *Bos indicus* cattle tend to be more resistant to ticks and the effects of *B bovis* and *B bigemina* infection than *Bos taurus*–derived breeds. At high levels of tick transmission, virtually all calves become infected with *Babesia* by 6 mo of age, show few if any clinical signs, and subsequently become immune. This situation can be upset by either a natural (eg, climatic) or artificial (eg, acaricide treatment or changing breed composition of herd) reduction in tick numbers to levels such that tick transmission of *Babesia* to calves is insufficient to ensure all are infected during this critical early period. Other circumstances that can lead to clinical outbreaks include the introduction of susceptible cattle to endemic areas and the incursion of *Babesia*-infected ticks into previously tick-free areas. Strain variation in immunity has been demonstrated but is probably not of practical significance in the field.

Clinical Findings and Pathogenesis: *B bovis* is a much more virulent organism than *B bigemina*. With most strains of *B bigemina*, the pathogenic effects relate more directly to erythrocyte destruction. With virulent strains of *B bovis*, a hypotensive shock syndrome, combined with generalized nonspecific inflammation, coagulation disturbances, and erythrocytic stasis in capillaries, contribute to the pathogenesis.

The acute disease generally runs a course of ~1 wk. The first sign is fever (frequently ≥106°F [41°C]), which persists throughout, and is accompanied later by inappetence, increased respiratory rate, muscle tremors, anemia, jaundice, and weight loss; hemoglobinemia and hemoglobinuria occur in the final stages. CNS involvement due to adhesion of parasitized erythrocytes in brain capillaries can occur with *B bovis* infections. Either constipation or diarrhea may be present. Late-term pregnant cows may abort, and temporary infertility due to transient fever may be seen in bulls.

Animals that recover from the acute disease remain infected for a number of years with *B bovis* and for a few months in the case of *B bigemina*. No clinical signs are apparent during this carrier state.

Lesions: Lesions (particularly with *B bovis*) include an enlarged and friable spleen; a swollen liver with an enlarged gallbladder containing thick granular bile; congested, dark-colored kidneys; and generalized anemia and jaundice. Most clinical cases of *B bigemina* have hemoglobinuria, but this is not invariably the case with *B bovis*. Other organs, including the brain and heart, may show congestion or petechiae.

Diagnosis: Clinically, babesiosis can be confused with other conditions that cause fever, anemia, hemolysis, jaundice, or red urine. Therefore, confirmation of diagnosis by microscopic examination of Giemsa-stained blood or organ smears is essential. From the live animal, thick and thin blood smears should be prepared, preferably from capillaries in the ear or tail tip.

Smears of heart muscle, kidney, liver, lung, brain, and from a blood vessel in an extremity (eg, lower leg) should be taken at necropsy.

Microscopically, the species of *Babesia* involved can be determined morphologically, but expertise is required, especially in *B bovis* infections in which few organisms are present. *B bovis* is small, with the parasites in paired form at an obtuse angle to each other and measuring ~1–1.5 × 0.5–1 µm. *B bigemina* is larger (3–3.5 × 1–1.5 µm), with paired parasites at an acute angle to each other. Single forms of both parasites are also commonly seen.

A number of serologic tests have been described for detection of antibodies to *Babesia* in carrier animals. The most commonly used are the indirect fluorescent antibody test and ELISA. A commercially produced ELISA for *B bigemina* is available. PCR and real-time PCR assays capable of detecting extremely low parasitemias, as occur in carrier animals, and differentiating isolates have also been described. A procedure that may occasionally be justified to confirm infection in suspected carrier animals is the subinoculation of blood (~500 mL) into a fully susceptible animal, preferably a splenectomized calf, and subsequent monitoring of the recipient for infection.

Treatment and Control: A variety of drugs have been used to treat babesiosis in the past, but only diminazene aceturate and imidocarb dipropionate are still in common use. These drugs are not available in all endemic countries, or their use may be restricted. Manufacturers' recommendations for use should be followed. For treating cattle, diminazene is given IM at 3.5 mg/kg. For treatment, imidocarb is given SC at 1.2 mg/kg. At a dosage of 3 mg/kg, imidocarb provides protection from babesiosis for ~4 wk and will also eliminate *B bovis* and *B bigemina* from carrier animals.

Supportive treatment is advisable, particularly in valuable animals, and may include the use of anti-inflammatory drugs, corticosteroids, and fluid therapy. Blood transfusions may be life-saving in very anemic animals.

Vaccination using live, attenuated strains of the parasites has been used successfully in a number of countries, including Argentina, Australia, Brazil, Israel, South Africa, and Uruguay. The vaccine is provided in either a chilled or frozen form. One vaccination produces adequate immunity for the commercial life of the animal; however, vaccine breakdowns have been reported. Several recombinant antigens have been shown experimentally to induce some immunity, but commercial vaccines are not yet available.

Although controlling or complete eradication of the tick vector can break the transmission cycle, this approach is rarely feasible in the longterm and can lead to large, susceptible populations in endemic areas with consequent risk of outbreaks of disease in naive animals.

Zoonotic Risk: A number of cases of human babesiosis have been reported. The rodent parasite *B microti* and the cattle parasite *B divergens* are the most commonly implicated species in North America and Europe, respectively. However, *B duncani*, *B venatorum*, *B conradae*, and some less well-defined species have also been incriminated. The reservoir hosts and vectors of some of these species are not necessarily known with any certainty. Human *Babesia* infections are acquired via bites from infected ticks or through contaminated blood from an infected transfusion donor. Cases reported in splenectomized or otherwise immunocompromised individuals are often fatal.

Other Important *Babesia* of Domestic Animals

More than 100 species of *Babesia* have been isolated from domestic animals and wildlife. The following are indicative of those affecting domestic animals, but the list is far from complete.

Cattle: *B divergens* and *B major* are two temperate-zone species with features comparable to those of *B bovis* and *B bigemina*, respectively. *B divergens* is a small, pathogenic *Babesia* of considerable importance in the British Isles and northwest Europe, whereas *B major* is a large *Babesia* of lower pathogenicity. *B divergens* is transmitted by *Ixodes ricinus*, and *B major* by *Haemaphysalis punctata*.

Horses: Equine babesiosis is caused by *Theileria* (formerly *Babesia*) *equi* or *B caballi*. *T equi* is a small parasite and is more pathogenic than *B caballi*. *T equi* was reclassified as a *Theileria* (*see* p 33) in 1998. Equine babesiosis is found in Africa, Europe, Asia, South and Central America, and the southern USA. It is transmitted by ticks of the genera *Rhipicephalus*, *Dermacentor*, and *Hyalomma*. Intrauterine infection, particularly with *T equi*, is also relatively common.

Sheep and Goats: Although small ruminants can be infected by several species of *Babesia*, the two most important species are *B ovis* and *B motasi*, transmitted by *Rhipicephalus bursa* and *Haemaphysalis* spp, respectively. Infection is of importance in the Middle East, southern Europe, and some African and Asian countries.

Pigs: *B trautmanni* has been recorded as causing severe disease in pigs. This parasite has been reported from Europe and Africa. Another species, *B perroncitoi*, is of similar pathogenicity but apparently has a limited distribution in the areas mentioned above. The vectors of these *Babesia* have not been clarified, although *Rhipicephalus* spp have been shown to transmit *B trautmanni*.

Dogs and Cats: *Babesia* species have been reported in dogs from most regions. These include *B canis*, *B vogeli*, and *B rossi*. *B canis* is transmitted by *Dermacentor reticularis* in Europe, *B vogeli* by *Rhipicephalus sanguineus* in tropical and subtropical countries, and *B rossi* by *Haemaphysalis leachi* in South Africa. Consequences of *Babesia* infection vary from a mild, transient illness to acute disease that rapidly results in death.

B gibsoni is the other important *Babesia* of dogs and is a much smaller parasite. It has a more limited distribution and characteristically causes a chronic disease with progressive, severe anemia that is not readily treated with normal babesiacides.

Illness of varying severity due to *B felis* in domestic cats has mostly been reported in southern Africa. Sporadic cases associated with other *Babesia* species have been reported elsewhere. An unusual feature of *B felis* is its lack of response to the normal babesiacides. However, primaquine phosphate (0.5 mg/kg, IM, twice with a 24-hr interval) is reported to be effective.

CYTAUXZOONOSIS

Cytauxzoonosis is an emerging, life-threatening infectious disease of domestic cats (*Felis catus*) caused by the tick-transmitted protozoan parasite *Cytauxzoon felis*. *Cytauxzoon* spp are apicomplexan parasites within the family Theileriidae along with their closest relatives of *Theileria* spp. *C felis* is transmitted to domestic cats by the lone star tick (*Amblyomma americanum*). The natural host for *C felis* is the bobcat (*Lynx rufus*); reservoir hosts of the parasite include bobcats and domestic cats that survive infection.

Since the discovery of feline cytauxzoonosis in Missouri in the mid-1970s, the distribution of *C felis* has been expanding. *C felis* has been reported in domestic cats in Missouri, Arkansas, Florida, Georgia, Louisiana, Mississippi, Oklahoma, Texas, Kentucky, Kansas, Tennessee, North Carolina, South Carolina, Nebraska, Iowa, and Virginia. Anecdotal reports of *C felis* infection in domestic cats in additional states include Alabama, southern Illinois, and Ohio.

Aberrant and Natural Hosts: The domestic cat has been considered an aberrant or dead-end host of *C felis* given the acute and fatal course of disease; however, there are reports of domestic cats surviving natural infection with and without treatment. As a natural host, the bobcat typically experiences subclinical infection, followed by a chronic parasitemia. Rare cases of fatal cytauxzoonosis in bobcats have been reported. Cytauxzoonosis has been reported in several other wild felids in the USA and other countries, with both fatal and nonfatal outcomes. Infection has been reported in cougars, panthers, and tigers in the USA, in addition to two suspected but unconfirmed cases in cheetahs. *C felis* infections of wild felids reported in other countries include lions, jaguars, pumas, ocelots, and little spotted cats. In the early 1980s, interspecies transmission of *C felis* was investigated to identify additional potential natural and aberrant hosts among 91 wildlife, laboratory, and domestic farm animals. Bobcats and domestic cats were the only animals confirmed to be susceptible to *C felis*.

Transmission and Risk Factors: *C felis* is transmitted by the lone star tick, *A americanum*. Cytauxzoonosis is typically diagnosed during April through September, which correlates with climate-dependent seasonal tick activity. Cats living near heavily wooded, low-density residential areas particularly close to natural or unmanaged habitats where both ticks and bobcats may be in close proximity are at highest risk of infection. Experimental infections have been induced with parenteral injection of tissue homogenates (SC, IP, and IV) from acutely infected cats. However, infection was not induced when these tissues were administered intragastrically or when noninfected cats were housed together with infected cats in the absence of arthropod vectors, suggesting that oral and "cat-to-cat" transmission does not occur. One recent study failed to document perinatal transmission of *C felis* from 2 chronically infected dams to 14 healthy kittens, suggesting that vertical transmission may not occur commonly, if at all.

Life Cycle and Pathogenesis: After transmission from the tick into the cat, *C felis* undergoes two major stages: schizogony and merogony. First, sporozoites infect WBCs (mononuclear phagocytes) and undergo schizogony (asexual reproduction) to form schizonts. Schizont-infected WBCs have been detected ~12 days after experimental infection and increase in size from 15 µm to up to 250 µm in diameter. They are most commonly detected in lymph node, spleen, liver, lung, and bone marrow but have been documented in many organs and are occasionally seen on blood smears.

Schizont-infected WBCs are the principal cause of disease and death; they are found predominantly lining and often occluding blood vessels. These "parasitic thrombi" result in ischemia and tissue necrosis. Schizont-infected WBCs then rupture and release piroplasms (merozoites), which infect RBCs. The piroplasms in RBCs are fairly innocuous, with parasitemias ranging from 1%–4% on average; however, higher parasitemias (ie, >10%) have been documented. During acute infection, detection of merozoite-infected RBCs is variable and has been correlated with an increase in body temperature and a decrease in leukocytes. Without treatment, survivors typically remain chronically parasitemic, and at least one cat has been shown experimentally to be solidly immune to subsequent infections. Chronic parasitemia has been established via inoculation with merozoite-infected RBCs. These chronically parasitemic cats did not develop overt clinical disease but were not immune to subsequent challenge with infection of sporozoites/schizonts, suggesting that the schizogenous tissue phase is required to establish immunity in domestic cats.

Clinical Findings and Lesions: Onset of clinical signs for cats infected with *C felis* usually occurs 5–14 days (~10 on average) after infection by tick transmission. Nonspecific signs such as depression, lethargy, and anorexia are the most common presenting problems. Pyrexia and dehydration are the most common findings on physical examination; body temperature, which increases gradually, can be as high as 106°F (41°C). Other findings include icterus, lymphadenomegaly, and hepatosplenomegaly. In extremis, cats are often hypothermic, dyspneic, and vocalize as if in pain. Without treatment, death typically occurs within 2–3 days after peak in temperature. At necropsy, splenomegaly, hepatomegaly, enlarged lymph nodes, and renal edema are usually seen. The lungs show extensive edema and congestion with petechial hemorrhage on serosal surfaces and throughout the interstitium. There is progressive venous distention, especially of the mesenteric and renal veins and the posterior vena cava. Hydropericardium is often seen with petechial hemorrhage of the epicardium.

When first described, mortality of *C felis* infection was reported to be nearly 100%. A study of *C felis* in northwestern Arkansas and northeastern Oklahoma indicated survival of natural infection in 18 cats with and without treatment; these cats seemed "less sick" initially, did not have temperatures >106°F (41°C), and never became hypothermic. Similar sporadic reports in other areas exist. Some hypotheses for survival in these cats have included the following: 1) an atypical route of infection, 2) innate immunity in certain cats, 3) increased detection of carriers, 4) decreased virulence with strain attenuation or occurrence of a new strain, 5) dose of infectious inoculum, and 6) timing and type of treatment.

Diagnosis: The most common abnormalities on the CBC in animals with cytauxzoonosis include leukopenia with toxic neutrophils and thrombocytopenia with a normocytic, normochromic anemia seen at later stages. The most common biochemical abnormalities are hyperbilirubinemia and hypoalbuminemia but may vary depending on organ systems affected by parasitic thrombosis and ischemia with tissue necrosis. Other, less consistently detected abnormalities include increased liver enzyme concentrations and azotemia.

Rapid diagnosis requires microscopic observation of piroplasms or schizonts. Observation of piroplasms on blood smears is variable; they are seen in association with increasing body temperature and typically become apparent approximately 1–3 days before death. There are anecdotal reports of a higher level of sensitivity when blood is collected from smaller vessels (eg, ear vein prick) to prepare blood smears. On a well-prepared, well-stained (Wright-Giemsa, Giemsa, Romanowsky most commonly) blood smear, when detectable, merozoites may be seen ranging from 1%–4% on average, with extremely high percentages (ie, >10%) reported in some cases. They are pleomorphic and may be round, oval, anaplasmoid, bipolar (binucleated), or rod-shaped; however, the round and oval piroplasm forms are most commonly seen. The round forms are 1–2.2 μm in diameter, whereas oval forms are 0.8-1 μm × 1.5–2 μm. They are pale centrally and contain a small, magenta, round to crescent-shaped nucleus on one side. Once the parasitemia is ~0.5%, Maltese cross and paired piriforms may be seen. Smears must be examined carefully to exclude *Mycoplasma haemofelis*, Howell-Jolly bodies, stain precipitate, and water artifact.

The schizont tissue stage precedes the formation of the RBC phase. Occasionally, schizonts may be seen in peripheral blood smears, particularly at the feathered edge, and may be mistaken for large platelet clumps at low power. In the absence of detection of RBC piroplasms or schizonts on blood smear, a rapid diagnosis should be pursued by performing fine-needle aspiration of a peripheral lymph node, spleen, or liver to identify schizonts cytologically. These phagocytes are 15–250 μm in diameter and contain an ovoid nucleus with a distinctive, prominent, large, dark nucleolus. The cytoplasm is often greatly distended, with numerous small deeply basophilic particles representing developing merozoites.

In the absence of these observations, a diagnostic PCR test with greater sensitivity and specificity than microscopy can be done. This test is recommended in suspect cases in which the parasite is not observed, as well as to confirm identification of piroplasms or schizonts.

Treatment and Control: Historically, attempts to treat cytauxzoonosis with a variety of antiparasitic drugs (parvaquone, buparvaquone, trimethoprim/sulfadiazine, sodium thiacetarsamide) have been met with little success. In one study, five of six cats and one additional cat were successfully treated with diminazene aceturate (not approved in the USA) and imidocarb dipropionate (2 mg/kg, IM, two injections 3–7 days apart), respectively.

The most consistent successful treatment in a large case series resulted in survival of 64% of cats given a combination of atovaquone (15 mg/kg, PO, tid for 10 days) and azithromycin (10 mg/kg/day, PO, for 10 days) and supportive care. Atovaquone is a ubiquinone analogue that binds cytochrome b. In one study of *C felis*–infected cats treated with atovaquone and azithromycin, a *C felis* cytochrome b subtype (cytb1) was identified that was associated with increased survival in the cats infected with this subtype compared with other subtypes. Future development of a rapid means to identify the cytb1 *C felis* subtype in infected cats may help better predict the likelihood of survival with treatment.

Supportive care, including IV fluid therapy and heparin (100–200 U/kg, SC, tid) should be instituted in all cases. Nutritional support via an esophageal or nasoesophageal feeding tube is recommended, which also facilitates administration of oral medications (eg, atovaquone and azithromycin). Oxygen therapy and blood transfusions should be administered when necessary. Anti-inflammatory drugs may be warranted in cases with unrelenting fever; however, the use of NSAIDs is contraindicated in cats with azotemia or dehydration.

Once a diagnosis is achieved and treatments have begun, minimal stress and handling are recommended. Recovery, including resolution of fever, is often slow and may take as long as 5–7 days. Cats that survive have a complete clinical recovery, including resolution of hematologic and biochemical abnormalities within 2–3 wk. Some survivors remain persistently infected with piroplasms and may represent a reservoir of infection. In one study, dose-intense diaminazene diaceturate (4 mg/kg/day, IM, for 5 consecutive days) failed to reduce the severity of parasitemia in cats chronically infected with *C felis* and resulted in adverse drug reactions.

Prevention: Routine application of a tick preventive is recommended to prevent cytauxzoonosis; however, disease has occurred in cats despite this treatment. In one study, a tick-repellent collar for cats containing imidacloprid 10%/flumethrin 4.5% prevented *A americanum* ticks from attaching, feeding, and transmitting *C felis* in 10 cats infested with infected ticks after application of the collar. In the same study, ticks attached and fed on 10 of 10 control cats not treated with a collar, and 9 of the 10 control cats were infected with *C felis*. Exclusion of cats from areas likely to be infested with the tick vector (ie, indoor only) is still considered the best method of prevention.

HEMOTROPIC MYCOPLASMAS

(Hemoplasmas)

Eperythrocytic parasites previously known as *Haemobartonella* and *Eperythrozoon* and formerly classified as rickettsial organisms are now understood to be more closely related to the order Mycoplasmatales. This affiliation is based on their lack of a cell wall, use of the codon UGA to encode tryptophan, and 16S rRNA gene sequences. Although the reassignment of *Eperythrozoon* and *Haemobartonella* to the genus *Mycoplasma* is still under debate, referral to this genus has been embraced, and they are commonly referred to as hemotropic mycoplasmas or hemoplasmas. Several of these previously described red cell parasites, now also having supporting genetic data, have been renamed *Mycoplasma*, whereas newly described hemoplasmas are given the designation "*Candidatus*." The hemoplasmas infect a wide variety of vertebrates throughout the world, including several reports of human infection. They share similar characteristics and morphologic features such as rod, coccoid, and ring-shaped structures found individually or in chains on the red cell and gram-negative staining because of the lack of a cell wall; none of the hemoplasmas have been cultured outside their hosts. It is well established that the hemoplasmas attach to the surface of the red cell but may under certain conditions penetrate this host cell.

Several hemoplasmas are of veterinary importance (*see* TABLE 4). These organisms vary in their ability to cause clinically significant hemolytic anemia, but infected animals may remain carriers despite antibiotic therapy. Parasitemia may reemerge if the animal is stressed or immunocompromised. Once an initial infection is controlled, either naturally or after antibiotic treatment, protective immunity develops against repeat

TABLE 4 HEMOPLASMAS OF VETERINARY IMPORTANCE

Species	Hemoplasma
Dogs	*Mycoplasma haemocanis* (formerly *Haemobartonella canis*) "*Candidatus Mycoplasma haematoparvum*"
Cats	*Mycoplasma haemofelis* (formerly *Haemobartonella felis*) "*Candidatus Mycoplasma haemominutum*" "*Candidatus Mycoplasma turicensis*"
Pigs	*Mycoplasma suis* (formerly *Eperythrozoon suis*) *Mycoplasma parvum* (formerly *Eperythrozoon parvum*)
Cattle	*Mycoplasma wenyonii* (formerly *Eperythrozoon wenyonii*)
Sheep and goats	*Mycoplasma ovis* (formerly *Eperythrozoon ovis*)
Llamas and alpacas	"*Candidatus Mycoplasma haemolamae*"

M haemofelis infection; how long this immunity will last and whether this applies to other hemoplasma infections is unknown.

Transmission: Hemoplasmas may be transmitted by transfer of infected blood (blood transfusion or use of contaminated needles, surgical instruments, herd or flock management equipment) or via arthropod vectors such as lice, flies, ticks, and mosquitoes. Vertical transmission from mother to offspring has been reported in cats, swine, and camelids. Direct transmission associated with fighting is suspected in cats and supported by studies reporting presence of hemoplasma DNA in saliva, on gingiva, and on claw beds of infected cats.

Clinical Findings: Hemoplasmas are capable of causing a hemolytic anemia, but the severity varies greatly. In general, asymptomatic infections tend to occur in healthy adult animals, and more severe acute anemias are associated with splenectomy, immunocompromise, concurrent diseases (such as feline leukemia virus or feline immunodeficiency virus in cats), or coinfection with multiple hemoplasma species. The main exception is *M haemofelis*, which causes acute hemolytic anemia in healthy cats. The anemia may be severe and occasionally fatal. Typical clinical signs include lethargy, anorexia, and fever, with splenomegaly and icterus occurring less often.

M haemocanis causes acute hemolysis in dogs that are splenectomized, but infections are usually asymptomatic in healthy dogs. *M suis* causes hemolytic anemia accompanied by icterus in neonatal pigs, feeder pigs, and pregnant sows. Chronic infection is associated with poor growth rates, decreased conception rates, reproductive failure, and decreased milk production. *M wenyonii* infection in cattle is usually asymptomatic, but a syndrome of mammary gland and hindlimb edema, decreased milk production, fever, and lymphadenopathy has been described in young, nonanemic, primiparous heifers. Infection in young bulls has been reported to cause scrotal and hindlimb edema. *M ovis* infection in sheep and goats is often asymptomatic, but hemolytic anemia can occur in young animals, especially those with heavy intestinal worm burdens. Chronic infection may result in poor weight gain, exercise intolerance, decreased wool production, and mild anemia. Hemoplasma infection in camelids can cause a severe hemolytic anemia in young crias. The prevalence of chronic infection in sheep, pigs, and kennel-raised dogs is high, and outbreaks of acute disease have been reported in animals during research studies. Whether the infection is chronic or acute, it may affect experimental results and lead to misinterpretation of data.

The hemolysis caused by hemoplasma infections is typically extravascular and results in a regenerative anemia. Erythrocyte agglutination may be present, and Coombs' test results are often positive in cats infected with *M haemofelis*. Splenectomized dogs with acute hemolysis due to *M haemocanis* may have agglutination, spherocytosis, and a positive Coombs' test. Hypoglycemia secondary to glucose consumption by the bacteria has been reported in heavily parasitized pigs, sheep, llamas, and calves; however, rapid bacterial glycolysis in vitro may also cause artifactually decreased blood glucose concentrations.

Diagnosis: Historically, diagnosis has been made based on detection of organisms on routine Wright-stained blood smears, on which they appear as small (0.5–3 μm), basophilic, round, rod, or ring-shaped structures present on erythrocytes individually or in chains, or sometimes seen free in the background. However, parasitemia in chronic infections can be cyclic, and organisms can disappear from circulation in as little as 2 hr. In addition, hemoplasmas dissociate from erythrocytes and die after a variable amount of time in EDTA, hampering detection of organisms in aged samples. Recent development of sensitive PCR assays capable of discriminating between various hemoplasmas has greatly enhanced diagnosis of these parasites and has led to identification of several new *Mycoplasma* species.

Treatment and Control: For acute infections, tetracyclines (doxycycline, oxytetracycline) have been the mainstay of treatment; enrofloxacin and marbofloxacin have also been effective against *M haemofelis*. Glucocorticoids may be useful to decrease erythrophagocytosis in cases of severe hemolysis; some animals may require blood transfusion. Treated animals remain carriers and may experience periodic clinical relapses. Blood donors should be screened using PCR-based DNA assays to prevent transmission to transfusion recipients. Iatrogenic transmission can be avoided by using properly sterilized needles and equipment. Control of arthropod vectors is recommended, as is minimizing stress in herd and flock situations.

Zoonotic Risk: Hemoplasma infections are usually species specific, except for *M ovis*, which infects both sheep and goats, and "*Candidatus M haemolamae*," which infects both llamas and alpacas. There are reports of human eperythrozoonosis from Inner Mongolia, China, but supporting evidence is not compelling. However, there have been rare reports of hemoplasma infections in immunocompromised people in which molecular methods were used for confirmation. One report documented an HIV-positive human patient coinfected with *Bartonella henselae* and a hemoplasma genetically similar to *M haemofelis*. This individual owned five cats and had multiple scratch and bite wounds. All five cats were PCR positive for *Bartonella* spp and two were positive for *M haemofelis*, suggesting the possibility of zoonotic transmission. The coinfection of a veterinarian in Texas with *B henselae* and *M ovis* also has been reported.

Feline Infectious Anemia

(Hemoplasmosis)

In cats, hemotropic mycoplasmosis can produce a disease called feline infectious anemia (FIA), previously known as hemobartonellosis. Most cases are in outdoor, male cats. *M haemofelis* (previously the Ohio strain, or large form, of *Haemobartonella felis*) is the most pathogenic organism causing FIA, and it can cause hemolytic anemia in immunocompetent cats. "*Candidatus M haemominutum*" (previously the California strain, or small form, of *H felis*) is the most common hemoplasma in cat populations worldwide, but it has not been clearly associated with disease in immunocompetent cats. "*Candidatus M turicensis*" has never been seen on blood smears, and its pathogenicity is not well understood. Both *Candidatus* species may be capable of inducing anemia in cats with underlying immunosuppressive disease, such as feline leukemia virus infection.

In the case of *M haemofelis* infection, an incubation period of 2–30 days is followed by anemia, with some cats developing cyclical changes in PCV that coincide with the appearance of large numbers of organisms on blood smears. In untreated cats, this acute phase lasts for 3–4 wk, after which some cats may remain chronically infected despite normal or near normal PCV values. It has been suggested that recrudescence of anemia may occur when these chronically infected cats are subject to debilitating disease, stress, or immunosuppressive therapies.

Any anemic cat, especially an anemia showing evidence of regeneration (polychromasia and/or reticulocytosis), may be suspected of having FIA. The severity of clinical signs correlates with the rapidity of onset of anemia. Clinical findings include weakness, pallor of the mucous membranes, tachypnea, tachycardia, and occasionally collapse. Acutely ill cats may be febrile, and moribund cats may be hypothermic. Other physical examination abnormalities may include cardiac murmurs, splenomegaly, and icterus. In chronic or slowly developing cases, there may be normal or subnormal body temperature, weakness, depression, and weight loss or emaciation.

Expected laboratory abnormalities include a moderate to marked regenerative anemia, increased numbers of nucleated RBCs, polychromasia, anisocytosis, Howell-Jolly bodies, and an increased reticulocyte count. Coombs' tests can become positive 7–14 days after organisms appear in the blood and remain positive throughout the acute phase, reverting to negative in chronically infected carrier cats.

Laboratory confirmation has traditionally been based on identification of organisms in the peripheral blood using light microscopy, although *M haemofelis* is visible <50% of the time in acutely infected cats. Some laboratories offer PCR assays that are considerably more sensitive and specific than blood-smear evaluation. Detection of *M haemofelis* via PCR is more significant than detection of other hemoplasma species ("*Candidatus M turicensis*" and "*Candidatus M haemominutum*"), which are not as strongly associated with anemia.

Without treatment, one third of acutely ill cats may die. Treatment involves both supportive therapies, such as oxygen and blood transfusions, and specific therapy with doxycycline (10 mg/kg/day, PO, for a minimum of 2 wk). Because of the potential for esophagitis and esophageal strictures, administration of doxycycline hyclate preparations should be followed by administration of a bolus of several milliliters of water. Enrofloxacin (5 mg/kg/day, PO) is a suitable alternative to doxycycline. Treatment of PCR-positive, healthy cats is currently not recommended, because no regimen has yet been identified that completely eliminates the organism. The use of immunosuppressive dosages of glucocorticoids to suppress immune-mediated RBC injury is controversial but may be used in cats that do not respond to antimicrobial therapy alone, or when primary immune-mediated hemolytic anemia is a possible cause.

OLD WORLD HEPATOZOONOSIS AND AMERICAN CANINE HEPATOZOONOSIS

Etiology, Epidemiology, and Transmission: Old World hepatozoonosis is a tickborne disease of wild and domestic carnivores caused by the protozoal agent *Hepatozoon canis*. It is unclear whether infections in wild and domestic Felidae are caused by *H canis* or by another species of *Hepatozoon*. This organism is transmitted by the brown dog tick, *Rhipicephalus sanguineus*. In the late 1990s, unique features of the clinical presentation in North American dogs suggested that a different strain or species of *Hepatozoon* might be responsible for the disease in North America than in other parts of the world; in 1997, this suspicion was confirmed based on parasite morphology, tissue tropism, and pathogenesis. The disease in North America is caused by *H americanum*, which is transmitted by the Gulf Coast tick, *Amblyomma maculatum*, rather than by the brown dog tick. Accordingly, the disease in North America is now recognized as a separate entity, American canine hepatozoonosis (ACH). Genetic and antigenic differences now documented between the North American and Old World organisms further support their classification as distinct species.

The mode of transmission of hepatozoonosis is not typical in the classical sense of a tickborne disease; like other species in the genus, *H canis* and *H americanum* infections occur when an infected tick, the definitive host, is ingested by the dog (or other vertebrate intermediate host). Sporozoites released from the mature oocysts in the tick's hemocoel enter the vertebrate host via the gut. Dogs can also acquire ACH by eating paratenic (transport) hosts that contain cystozoites, a resting stage of *H americanum* encysted in their tissues. Experimentally, cystozoite-engendered infection results in the same disease manifestations seen in dogs that ingest sporulated oocysts. It is unknown at present whether a similar path of infection may occur in *H canis* infections, although monozoic cyst stages have been reported in the spleen of both experimentally and naturally infected dogs. It is possible that canids may serve as both transport and definitive hosts of *H canis*.

In much of the world (India, Africa, southeast Asia, the Middle East, southern Europe, and islands in the Pacific and Indian Oceans), dogs with hepatozoonosis usually have subclinical infections or only mild clinical signs. In these areas, immunosuppression caused by concurrent disease or other factors appears to play an important role in the manifestation of significant clinical signs. In the USA, immunosuppression or concurrent disease does not appear necessary to induce the more severe clinical signs typically seen with ACH.

ACH is an emerging disease that has primarily spread north and east from the Gulf Coast of Texas, where it was originally detected in 1978. The distribution of this parasite parallels the distribution of the Gulf Coast tick. Most cases in the USA have been diagnosed in Texas (primarily along the Gulf Coast), Oklahoma, and Louisiana; numerous cases have been reported from Alabama, and cases have been seen as far east as Tennessee, Georgia, and Florida. Sporadic cases have been reported from such disparate geographic locations as California, Washington, and Vermont; it is assumed these dogs were relocated from enzootic areas, because the Gulf Coast tick has not become established in such distant locations. *H americanum* may be present in Central and South America, as is *A maculatum*, but to date, no autochthonous transmission of *H americanum* has been reported from these regions. *A ovale* has been identified as a vector for *H canis* in South America. It was previously thought that *H canis* did not infect canids in North America, despite the presence of *R sanguineus*, but molecular evidence has recently emerged that suggests otherwise. Still, ACH remains the more severe and more common form of hepatozoonosis in the New World.

In general, immunocompetent dogs appear to tolerate infection with *H canis* very well. Although life-threatening infections have been reported, clinical signs associated with *H canis* infection are most often subclinical to mild. However, *H americanum* causes severe clinical signs in most dogs, with death often occurring within 1–2 yr without supportive therapies.

Clinical Findings: The tissue phases of the hepatozoonosis organism, especially those of *H americanum*, induce pyogranulomatous inflammation, which results in clinical signs. These signs, which may be intermittent, include fever, depression, weight loss, poor body condition, muscle atrophy, soreness, stiffness, and weakness; mucopurulent ocular discharge is common, and bloody diarrhea occurs occasionally. Surprisingly, many dogs maintain a normal appetite if food is placed directly in front of them, but they often will not move to eat, apparently owing to intense pain. Severe hyperesthesia or pain over the paraspinal region is a common finding on physical examination; cervical, joint, or generalized pain is also seen. Hyperesthesia, presumably due to severe inflammation within muscle and sometimes along bone, manifests as stiffness and reluctance to move, as well as cervical and/or truncal rigidity. Fever, which may fluctuate with the waxing and waning of clinical signs, ranges from 102.7°–106°F (39.3°–41°C) and is unresponsive to antibiotics. Longterm sequelae include glomerulonephritis and amyloidosis. *H canis* tissue stages reside within bone marrow, lymph nodes, and spleen. Unlike in dogs with ACH, dogs infected with *H canis* typically do not appear painful at presentation; in dogs with overt disease, nonspecific symptoms including fever, lethargy, and depression may be seen.

Diagnosis: In dogs with ACH, the most consistent laboratory abnormality is a neutrophilic leukocytosis, with counts ranging from 20,000–200,000 cells/μL. This is typically a pronounced, mature neutrophilia, although a left shift may be present. A mild to moderate normocytic, normochromic, nonregenerative anemia is also common. The platelet count is typically normal to high. Mildly increased alkaline phosphatase, hypoalbuminemia, and increased CK may also be seen. Although profound hypoglycemia has been reported, this finding is thought to be an in vitro sampling artifact that results from increased metabolism of glucose by the overly abundant leukocytes. On radiographs, periosteal reactions may be seen involving any bone, including the skull and vertebrae. These periosteal reactions resemble those of hypertrophic osteoarthropathy, except that lesions tend to be proximal rather than distal with ACH, often markedly obvious in long bones. The physiologic basis of the bone lesions has not been determined. Definitive diagnosis of ACH is made by finding rare gamonts in peripheral blood leukocytes (using Romanowsky-type stains) or identifying pathognomonic "onion skin" cysts or pyogranulomas in stained sections of biopsied muscle sample. Muscle biopsy, although invasive, is considered the gold-standard method for diagnosing ACH, because parasite and parasite-induced lesions are often extensively distributed throughout muscle tissue (especially in areas with observable atrophy). However, in some dogs, multiple or sequential biopsies may be necessary to detect the organism.

Unlike in *H americanum* infections, parasitemia in dogs with clinical *H canis* infection is often quite high, and a diagnosis can readily be achieved by microscopic examination of stained blood films to visualize parasite-containing leukocytes. The most common abnormality on bloodwork in dogs infected with *H canis* is anemia. Serum chemistry abnormalities may be similar to those seen in dogs with ACH. Hepatitis, pneumonia, and glomerulonephritis associated with *H canis* meronts have been reported postmortem in some animals with extremely high parasitemia. Although experimental serologic assays have been developed to detect both *H americanum* and *H canis* infections, none is available commercially. PCR methods developed to detect circulating *Hepatozoon* are available through several different institutions (including Auburn University and North Carolina State University), although they may lack sensitivity in *H americanum* infections because of typically low levels of parasitemia. These molecular tests have led to the realization that classical hepatozoonosis caused by *H canis* is more common in North America than previously known. Moreover, recognized variation in an 18S rDNA sequence from infected dogs has raised new questions about canine hepatozoonosis. It may be that still more species (or strains) that vary in pathogenicity and/or life cycle patterns will be found to cause disease in dogs.

Treatment: Hepatozoonosis is generally considered a lifelong infection in dogs. No known therapeutic regimen completely clears the body of the organism. In the past, treatment of ACH has been frustrating, because most dogs showed only temporary improvement with frequent relapses within 3–6 mo and death within 2 yr of diagnosis. Remission of clinical signs can usually be achieved through a 14-day course of combination therapy, referred to as TCP, which consists of trimethoprim-sulfadiazine

(15 mg/kg, PO, bid), clindamycin (10 mg/kg, PO, tid), and pyrimethamine (0.25 mg/kg/day, PO). Unfortunately, remission with this therapy has often been short-lived, and dogs frequently relapse within 2–6 mo. However, an adjunctive treatment using decoquinate has been useful. Decoquinate does not resolve active clinical disease but may prevent clinical relapses; it is given after resolution of clinical signs as an adjunct to TCP therapy. The recommended dosage of decoquinate is 10–20 mg/kg, PO, bid continuously for 2 yr. The advent of TCP combination therapy followed by daily decoquinate therapy has resulted in marked improvement in the prognosis for dogs with ACH. NSAIDs may be the best treatment for control of fever and pain, especially during the first few days of TCP therapy. Glucocorticoid administration should be avoided because, although steroids may provide temporary relief, longterm use can exacerbate the disease.

H canis infections are treated with imidocarb dipropionate, twice monthly, at 5–6 mg/kg, SC, until the parasite is no longer evident in blood smears for 2–3 consecutive months. Prognosis often depends on the degree of parasitemia; dogs with low parasitemia typically respond well to treatment, whereas those with high parasitemia may not, especially if afflicted by concurrent illness.

Preventing access to ticks and discouraging predation are the most effective forms of control for hepatozoonosis. Predation presents a dual risk for acquiring ACH: prey captured/ingested by dogs could have infected ticks on their coats that would provide a source of sporozoites; additionally, the prey could contain cystozoites (at least in the case of *H americanum*) that are also infectious. Additionally, dogs diagnosed with hepatozoonosis should not be bred because transplacental transmission of *H canis* has been documented, and although vertical transmission of *H americanum* has not been reported, the possibility should not be disregarded.

There is no known zoonotic risk with hepatozoonosis.

SCHISTOSOMIASIS

Schistosomiasis is a common parasitic infection in cattle and rarely in other domestic animals in Africa and Asia. Although schistosomes may act as important pathogens under rare conditions favoring intensive transmission, most infections in endemic areas are subclinical. However, high prevalence rates of subclinical infections cause significant losses due to longterm effects on growth and productivity and increased susceptibility to other parasitic or bacterial diseases.

Schistosomes are members of the genus *Schistosoma*, family Schistosomatidae. Adult worms are obligate parasites of the vascular system of vertebrates. Schistosomes are dioecious. The mature female is more slender than the male and normally is carried in a ventral groove, the gynaecophoric canal, that is formed by ventrally flexed lateral outgrowths of the male body.

Of the 19 species reported to naturally infect animals, 8—all parasites of ruminants—have received particular attention, mainly because of their recognized veterinary significance: *S mattheei*, *S bovis*, *S curassoni*, *S spindale*, *S indicum*, *S nasale*, *S incognitum*, and *S japonicum*. *S mattheei* is found in southeastern Africa, from the Cape Province in South Africa northward to Tanzania and Zambia. *S bovis* is found in the Mediterranean region and Middle East, and is common in northern, western, and eastern Africa (except Egypt) extending southward to Central Angola, southern Congo, and possibly northern Zambia. *S curassoni* has been found in ruminants in Senegal, Mauritania, Mali, Niger, and Nigeria. *S spindale* has been recorded from India, Sri Lanka, Indonesia, Malaysia, Thailand, and Vietnam. The distribution of *S indicum* appears confined to the Indian subcontinent. *S nasale* is found in India, Sri Lanka, Bangladesh, and Myanmar. *S incognitum* has been reported from India, Thailand, and Indonesia. *S japonicum* is endemic in several countries of the Far East. Some of these species are known to interact in areas where they coexist, and instances of interspecific hybridization have been reported, eg, the cattle parasites *S bovis* and *S curassoni*. Novel molecular tools have also provided evidence for the natural hybridization between *S haematobium*, a parasite of people, and *S mattheei*, *S bovis*, and *S curassoni*. The hybridization between human and ruminant schistosomes is of particular interest, because for this to occur, host switching must have taken place of *S mattheei*, *S bovis*, or *S curassoni* into people or of *S haematobium* into domestic livestock.

To differentiate the different *Schistosoma* spp, egg morphology (size, shape) can be used. The species can also be differentiated through such taxonomic features as morphologic (adult worms), life-cycle, or behavioral characteristics; chromosomes; host specificity; or enzyme and DNA studies.

Life Cycle, Transmission, and Epidemiology: Schistosomes live in the mesenteric and hepatic veins of the host (except for *S nasale*, which lives in the nasal veins), where they feed on blood and produce eggs with a characteristic terminal or lateral spine. Eggs passed in the feces must be deposited in water if they are to hatch and release miracidia, which invade suitable water snails and develop through primary and secondary sporocysts to become cercariae. When fully mature, the cercariae leave the snail and swim freely in the water, where they remain viable for several hours. Ruminants are usually infected with cercariae by penetration of the skin, although infection may be acquired orally while animals are drinking. During penetration, cercariae develop into schistosomula, which are transported via the lymph and blood to their predilection sites. The prepatent period varies according to the species but is generally 45–70 days.

The occurrence of cattle schistosomes within their range is discontinuous, depending on the presence of intermediate snail hosts, their level of infection, and the frequency of water contacts. In areas where conditions are favorable, prevalence rates of infections in cattle may be 40%–70% and commonly higher.

The increased host range of the hybrid parasites and changes in host distribution seen in Africa may have a direct impact on transmission of these schistosomes. Laboratory hybrids have been observed to acquire enhanced characteristics such as infectivity, fecundity, and growth rates.

There is strong evidence that acquired immunity to schistosome infection in cattle exists. This immunity mainly acts through suppression of worm fecundity. Examination of naturally infected animals has shown that partial protection against reinfection also occurs, and acquired resistance to schistosomes is of major importance in the regulation of infection intensity in the field.

Clinical Findings and Lesions: In the great majority of cases, **visceral schistosomiasis** in endemic areas is subclinical and characterized by a high prevalence of low to moderate worm burdens in the cattle population. Although few or no overt clinical signs may be recognized in the short term, high prevalence rates of chronic schistosome infections cause significant losses on a herd basis. These losses are due to less easily recognizable effects on growth and productivity, as well as increased susceptibility to other parasitic and bacterial diseases.

Occasional outbreaks of clinical intestinal schistosomiasis due to *S mattheei*, *S bovis*, or *S spindale* have been reported. They are usually restricted to young livestock and adult animals undergoing relatively heavy primary infections under conditions of intensive transmission. The disease is characterized by diarrhea, weight loss, anemia, hypoalbuminemia, hyperglobulinemia, and severe eosinophilia that develop after the onset of egg excretion. Severely affected animals deteriorate rapidly and usually die within a few months of infection, while those less heavily infected develop chronic disease with growth retardation.

In the intestinal and hepatic forms, adult flukes are found in the portal, mesenteric, and intestinal submucosal and subserosal veins. However, the main pathologic effects are associated with the eggs. In the intestinal form, passage of eggs through the gut wall causes the lesions, while in the hepatic form, granulomas form around eggs trapped in the tissues. Other hepatic changes include medial hypertrophy and hyperplasia of the portal veins, development of lymphoid nodules and follicles throughout the organ, and periportal fibrosis in more chronic cases. Extensive granuloma formation also is seen in the intestine. In severe cases, numerous areas of petechiation and diffuse hemorrhage are seen in the mucosa, and large quantities of discolored blood may be found in the intestinal lumen. Frequently, the parasitized blood vessels are dilated and tortuous. Vascular lesions also may be found in the lungs, pancreas, and bladder of heavily infected animals.

The hybridization events reported between animal and human schistosomes may result in phenotypic characteristics that influence pathology (and drug sensitivity).

Nasal schistosomiasis is associated with cauliflower-like growths on the nasal mucosa, causing partial obstruction of the nasal cavity and snoring sounds when breathing. Hemorrhagic and/or mucopurulent nasal discharge is a common feature. Adult flukes are found in the blood vessels of the nasal mucosa, but again, the main pathogenic effects are associated with the eggs, which cause abscesses in the mucosa. The abscesses rupture and release eggs and pus into the nasal cavity, which eventually leads to extensive fibrosis. In addition, large granulomatous growths are common on the nasal mucosa and occlude the nasal passages and cause dyspnea.

Diagnosis: Because signs and history alone are insufficient to distinguish visceral schistosomiasis from other debilitating diseases, diagnosis should be confirmed by the presence and identification of eggs in the feces of the infected animal. At necropsy, macroscopic examination of the mesenteric veins for the presence of adult worms or microscopic examination of scrapings of the intestinal mucosa or of crushed liver tissue (both for eggs) may prove easier.

Eggs of *S bovis*, *S curassoni*, and *S mattheei* are spindle-shaped. Because of the interspecific hybridization between *S bovis* and *S curassoni* and the natural hybridization between *S haematobium* and *S mattheei*, *S bovis*, and *S curassoni*, eggs of intermediate morphology may be seen. The eggs of *S spindale* are more elongated and flattened on one side, and those of *S nasale* are boomerang-shaped. The oval eggs of *S japonicum* are relatively small, with a rudimentary spine.

Very low fecal egg excretion is commonly seen in chronic infections; therefore, it may be preferred to use quantitative miracidial hatching techniques which, in addition to being more sensitive, also provide information on the viability of the eggs excreted in the feces.

Treatment and Control: Praziquantel (25 mg/kg) is highly effective, although two treatments 3–5 wk apart may be required. However, for practical and economic reasons, schistosomiasis in domestic stock is rarely treated. Only in China, where infected livestock constitute important reservoirs of human infection, have mass treatments with praziquantel been practiced widely.

The most effective way to control cattle schistosomiasis in endemic areas is to prevent contact between the animals and the parasite by fencing of dangerous waters and supplying clean water. Unfortunately, this is not always possible in parts of the world where nomadic conditions of management prevail. Other methods of control include destruction of the snail intermediate host population at transmission sites, either by chemical or biologic methods, or their removal by mechanical barriers or snail traps. Ecologic measures against the snails that aim to render their habitat unsuitable for survival, such as drainage, removal of water weeds, and increased water flow, have also proved valuable. These measures not only help reduce the transmission of schistosomiasis but also help control other parasitic trematodes such as *Fasciola gigantica* and paramphistomes, which also have water snails as intermediate hosts and frequently are found in the same localities as schistosomes.

THEILERIASES

Theileriases are a group of tickborne diseases caused by *Theileria* spp. A large number of *Theileria* spp are found in domestic and wild animals in tick-infested areas of the Old World. The most important species affecting cattle are *T parva* and *T annulata*, which cause widespread death in tropical and subtropical areas of the Old World. *T lestoquardi*, *T luwenshuni*, and *T uilenbergi* are important causes of mortality in sheep.

Both *Theileria* and *Babesia* are members of the suborder Piroplasmorina. Although *Babesia* are primarily parasites of RBCs, *Theileria* use, successively, WBCs and RBCs for completion of their life cycle in mammalian hosts. The infective sporozoite stage of the parasite is transmitted in the saliva of infected ticks as they feed. Sporozoites invade leukocytes and, within a few days, develop to schizonts. In the most pathogenic species of *Theileria* (eg, *T parva* and *T annulata*), parasite multiplication occurs predominantly within the host WBCs, whereas less pathogenic species multiply mainly in RBCs. Development of the schizont stage of pathogenic *Theileria* causes the host WBC to divide; at each cell division, the parasite also divides. Thus, the parasitized cell population expands and, through migration, becomes disseminated throughout the lymphoid system. Later in the infection, some of the schizonts undergo merogony, releasing merozoites that infect RBCs, giving rise to piroplasms. Uptake of piroplasm-infected RBCs by vector ticks feeding on infected animals is the prelude to a complex cycle of development, culminating in transmission of infection by ticks feeding in their next instar (trans-stadial transmission). There is no transovarial transmission as occurs in *Babesia*. Occurrence of disease is limited to the geographic distribution of the appropriate tick vectors. In some endemic areas, indigenous cattle have a degree of innate resistance. Mortality in such stock is relatively low, but introduced cattle are particularly vulnerable. Unlike in babesiosis, in theileriasis there is no evidence of increased resistance in calves <6 mo old.

East Coast Fever

East Coast fever, an acute disease of cattle, is usually characterized by high fever, swelling of the lymph nodes, dyspnea, and high mortality. Caused by *Theileria parva*, and transmitted by the tick vector *Rhipicephalus appendiculatus*, it is a serious problem in east and southern Africa.

Etiology and Transmission: The African buffalo (*Syncerus caffer*) is an important wildlife reservoir of *T parva*, but infection is asymptomatic in buffalo. *T parva* transmitted by ticks from either cattle or buffalo cause severe disease in cattle, but buffalo-derived parasites differentiate poorly to merozoites in cattle and generally are not transmitted by ticks. Hence, buffalo *T parva* are maintained as a separate population. Buffalo *T parva* were previously considered a separate subspecies (*T parva lawrencei*), but DNA typing indicate that the cattle and buffalo parasites are a single species. *T parva* is usually highly pathogenic, causing high levels of mortality, although some less pathogenic isolates have been identified.

Pathogenesis, Clinical Findings, and Diagnosis: *T parva* sporozoites are injected into cattle by infected vector ticks. An occult phase of 5–10 days follows before infected lymphocytes can be detected in Giemsa-stained smears of cells aspirated from the local draining lymph node. Subsequently, the number of parasitized cells increases rapidly throughout the lymphoid system, and from about day 14 onward, cells undergoing merogony are observed. This is associated with widespread lymphocytolysis, marked lymphoid depletion, and leukopenia. Piroplasms in RBCs infected by the resultant merozoites assume various forms, but typically they are small and rod-shaped or oval.

Clinical signs vary according to the level of challenge, and they range from inapparent or mild to severe and fatal. Typically, fever occurs 7–10 days after parasites are introduced by feeding ticks, continues throughout the course of infection, and may be >106°F (41°C). Lymph node swelling becomes pronounced and generalized. Lymphoblasts in Giemsa-stained smears of needle aspirates from lymph nodes contain multinuclear schizonts. Anorexia develops, and the animal rapidly loses condition; lacrimation and nasal discharge may occur. Terminally, dyspnea is common. Just before death, a sharp decrease in body temperature is usual, and pulmonary exudate pours from the nostrils. Death usually occurs 18–24 days after infection. The most striking postmortem lesions are lymph node enlargement and massive pulmonary edema and hyperemia. Hemorrhages are common on the serosal and mucosal surfaces of many organs, sometimes together with obvious areas of necrosis in the lymph nodes and thymus. Anemia is not a major diagnostic sign (as it is in babesiosis) because there is minimal division of the parasites in RBCs, and thus no massive destruction of them.

Animals that recover are immune to subsequent challenge with the same strains but may be susceptible to some heterologous strains. Most recovered or immunized animals remain carriers of the infection.

Treatment and Control: Treatment with parvaquone and its derivative buparvaquone is highly effective when administered in the early stages of clinical disease but is less effective in the advanced stages, in which there is extensive destruction of lymphoid and hematopoietic tissues. Immunization of cattle against *T parva* using an infection-and-treatment procedure is practical and continues to gain acceptance in some regions. The components for this procedure are a cryopreserved sporozoite stabilate of the appropriate strain(s) of *Theileria* derived from infected ticks and a single dose of long-acting oxytetracycline given simultaneously; although oxytetracycline has little therapeutic effect when administered after development of disease, it inhibits development of the parasite when given at the outset of infection. Cattle should be immunized 3–4 wk before being allowed on infected pasture. Parasitized bovine cells containing the schizont stage of *T parva* and *T annulata* can be cultivated in vitro as continuously growing cell lines. In the case of *T annulata*, cattle can be infected with a few thousand cultured cells. Attenuated strains produced by serial passage of such cultures form the basis of live vaccines used in several countries, including Israel, Iran, India, and the former USSR.

Incidence of East Coast fever can be reduced by rigid tick control, but this is not feasible in many areas because of cost and the high frequency of acaricidal treatment required.

Tropical Theileriosis

Theileria annulata, the causal agent of tropical theileriosis, is widely distributed in north Africa, the Mediterranean coastal area, the Middle East, India, the former USSR, and Asia. It is transmitted by several species of ticks of the genus *Hyalomma*. *T annulata* can cause mortality of up to 90%, but strains vary in their pathogenicity. The kinetics of infection and the main clinical findings are similar to those produced by *T parva*, but unlike in East Coast fever, anemia is often a feature of the disease. Characteristic signs include fever and swollen superficial lymph nodes. If the disease progresses, cattle rapidly lose condition. The schizonts and piroplasms are morphologically similar to those of *T parva*. Animals that recover from infection are immune to subsequent challenge. Treatment and control are as described for East Coast fever (*see* p 34).

Other Theileriases of Cattle

The *Theileria orientalis* group, consisting of the closely related parasites *T orientalis*, *T buffeli*, and *T sergenti*, has a worldwide distribution. These parasites are transmitted by ticks of the genus *Haemaphysalis*. The piroplasms are larger than those of *T parva* and *T annulata*, and they multiply principally by intraerythrocytic division. Mortality, particularly in indigenous cattle, is rare, but infection can sometimes result in progressive chronic anemia.

T mutans and *T velifera* are found in Africa, where they are transmitted by ticks of the genus *Amblyomma*. Multiplication occurs mainly by intraerythrocytic division. The piroplasms are morphologically indistinguishable from those of *T orientalis* and *T taurotragi* (an African parasite of eland and cattle), but the parasites can be differentiated by serologic tests such as indirect fluorescent antibody and by DNA typing. Some strains of *T mutans* are pathogenic as well. In addition, concurrent infection may add to the pathogenicity of *T parva*.

Ovine and Caprine Theileriases

Theileria lestoquardi (formerly *T hirci*) causes a disease in sheep and goats similar to that produced in cattle by *T annulata*, with which it is closely related. *T lestoquardi* is transmitted by ticks of the genus *Hyalomma*. The limited available epidemiologic data indicate that *T lestoquardi* has a more restricted geographic distribution than that of *T annulata*, being particularly prevalent in the Middle East and northeast Africa. Mortality can approach 100%. Schizonts can readily be demonstrated in Giemsa-stained smears of needle biopsies from swollen superficial lymph nodes.

Recently, two species of *Theileria*, *T luwenshuni* and *T uilenbergi*, have been identified as the causal agents of a severe disease in sheep in China. These species are morphologically indistinguishable and cause similar disease but can be distinguished by DNA typing methods. They are transmitted by ticks of the genus *Haemaphysalis*. Schizonts are detected in a range of tissues, but later and in smaller numbers than in other pathogenic *Theileria* spp. Piroplasms are consistently detected in RBCs. Morbidity and mortality rates of up to 65% (*T luwenshuni*) and 75% (*T uilenbergi*) have been seen in susceptible animals introduced into endemic areas. Affected animals show sustained fever and anemia.

Several other nonpathogenic *Theileria* spp (eg, *T ovis*) are also widely distributed. Piroplasms of these species are polymorphic.

Equine Theileriasis

Babesia equi was reclassified as *T equi* in 1998, based on DNA analysis and other biologic data (*see* p 21).

TRYPANOSOMIASIS

Tsetse-transmitted Trypanosomiasis

This group of diseases caused by protozoa of the genus *Trypanosoma* affects all domesticated animals. The major veterinary species are *T congolense*, *T vivax*, *T brucei brucei*, and *T simiae*. *T brucei rhodesiense* and *T brucei gambiense* are zoonotic, with people as the predominant host. For the animals mainly affected by these tsetse-transmitted trypanosomes and the geographic areas where tsetse-transmitted trypanosomiasis occurs, *see* TABLE 5.

Cattle, sheep, and goats are infected, in order of importance, by *T congolense*, *T vivax*, and *T brucei brucei*. In pigs, *T simiae* is the most important. In dogs and cats, *T brucei* is probably the most important. It is difficult to assign an order of importance for horses and camels. *T vivax* is found outside tsetse-infested areas of sub-Saharan Africa, carried mechanically by biting flies.

The trypanosomes that cause tsetse-transmitted trypanosomiasis (sleeping sickness) in people, *T brucei rhodesiense* and *T brucei gambiense*, closely resemble *T brucei brucei*, and suitable precautions should be taken when working with such

TABLE 5 TSETSE-TRANSMITTED TRYPANOSOMES

Trypanosoma spp	Animals Mainly Affected	Major Geographic Distribution
T congolense	Cattle, sheep, goats, dogs, pigs, camels, horses, most wild animals	South and eastern Africa
T vivax	Cattle, sheep, goats, camels, horses, various wild animals	Africa, Central and South America, West Indies[a]
T brucei brucei	All domestic and various wild animals; most severe in dogs, horses, cats	South and eastern Africa
T brucei rhodesiense	Cattle, wild hooved stock, people	South and eastern Africa
T brucei gambiense	Cattle, sheep, goats, people	West and central Africa, including Uganda
T simiae	Domestic and wild pigs, horses, camels	South and eastern Africa

[a] In non-tsetse areas, transmission is by biting flies.

isolates. Domestic animals act as reservoirs of human infections.

Transmission and Epidemiology: Most tsetse transmission is cyclic and begins when blood from a trypanosome-infected animal is ingested by the fly. The trypanosome alters its surface coat, multiplies in the fly, then alters its surface coat again, and becomes infective. *T brucei* spp migrate within the tsetse from the gut and eventually to the salivary glands; the cycle for *T congolense* stops at the hypopharynx, and the salivary glands are not invaded; the entire cycle for *T vivax* occurs in the proboscis. Therefore, the location within the tsetse can be useful in identifying the parasite species. The animal-infective form in the tsetse salivary gland is referred to as the metacyclic form. The life cycle in the tsetse may be as short as 1 wk with *T vivax* or extend to a few weeks for *T brucei* spp.

Tsetse flies (genus *Glossina*) are restricted to Africa from about latitude 15°N to 29°S. The three main species inhabit relatively distinct environments: *G morsitans* usually is found in savanna country, *G palpalis* prefers areas around rivers and lakes, and *G fusca* lives in high forest areas. All three species transmit trypanosomes, and all feed on various mammals.

Mechanical transmission can occur through tsetse or other biting flies. In the case of *T vivax*, *Tabanus* spp and other biting flies seem to be the primary mechanical vectors outside tsetse-endemic areas, as in Central and South America. Mechanical transmission requires only that blood containing infectious trypanosomes be transferred by bite from one animal to another.

Pathogenesis: Infected tsetse inoculate metacyclic trypanosomes into the skin of animals, where the trypanosomes reside for a few days and cause localized inflammation (chancres). They enter the lymph and lymph nodes, then the bloodstream, where they divide rapidly by binary fission. In *T congolense* infection, the organisms attach to endothelial cells and localize in capillaries and small blood vessels. *T brucei* species and *T vivax* invade tissues and cause tissue damage in several organs.

The immune response is vigorous, and immune complexes cause inflammation, which contributes to fever and other signs and lesions of the disease. Antibodies against the surface-coat glycoproteins kill the trypanosomes. However, trypanosomes have a large family of genes that code for variable surface-coat glycoproteins that are switched in response to the antibody response, evading immunity. This antigenic variation results in persistence of the organism. Antigenic variation has prevented development of a protective vaccine and permits reinfections when animals are exposed to a new antigenic type.

Clinical Findings and Lesions: Severity of disease varies with species and age of the animal infected and the species of trypanosome involved. The incubation period is usually 1–4 wk. The primary clinical signs are intermittent fever, anemia, and weight loss. Cattle usually have a chronic course with high mortality, especially if there is poor nutrition or other stress factors. Ruminants may gradually recover if the number of infected tsetse flies is low; however, stress results in relapse.

Necropsy findings vary and are nonspecific. In acute, fatal cases, extensive petechiation of the serosal membranes, especially in the peritoneal cavity, may occur. Also, the lymph nodes and spleen are usually swollen. In chronic cases, swollen lymph nodes, serous atrophy of fat, and anemia are seen.

Diagnosis: A presumptive diagnosis is based on finding an anemic animal in poor condition in an endemic area. Confirmation depends on demonstrating trypanosomes in stained blood smears or wet mounts. The most sensitive rapid method is to examine a wet mount of the buffy coat area of a PCV tube after centrifugation, looking for motile parasites. Other infections that cause anemia and weight loss, such as babesiosis, anaplasmosis, theileriosis, and haemonchosis, should be excluded by examining a stained blood smear.

Various serologic tests measure antibody to trypanosomes, but their use is more suitable for herd and area screening than for individual diagnosis. Rapid agglutination tests to detect circulating trypanosome species-specific antigens in peripheral blood are available for both individual and herd diagnosis, although their reliability remains varied. Molecular techniques for trypanosome detection and differentiation have been developed, but they are not generally available for routine field use.

Treatment and Control: Several drugs can be used for treatment (*see* TABLE 6). Most have a narrow therapeutic index, which makes administration of the correct dose essential. Drug resistance occurs and should be considered in refractory cases.

Control can be exercised at several levels, including eradication of tsetse flies and use of prophylactic drugs. Tsetse flies can be partially controlled by frequent spraying and dipping of animals, aerial and ground spraying of insecticides on fly-breeding areas, use of insecticide-impregnated screens and targets, bush clearing, and other habitat removal methods. The Sterile Insect Technique (SIT) has been used with success in Zanzibar and may be used in other area-wide control operations after suppression of tsetse populations by insecticides.

TABLE 6 DRUGS COMMONLY USED FOR TRYPANOSOMIASIS IN DOMESTIC ANIMALS

Drug	Animal	*Trypanosoma*	Main Action
Diminazene aceturate	Cattle	*vivax, congolense, brucei*	Curative
Homidium bromide	Cattle	*vivax, congolense, brucei*	Curative, some prophylactic activity
Homidium bromide	Equids	*vivax*	Curative, some prophylactic activity
Homidium chloride	Equids	*vivax*	Curative, some prophylactic activity
Isometamidium chloride	Cattle	*vivax, congolense*	Curative and prophylactic
Quinapyramine sulfate	Horses, camels, pigs, dogs	*vivax, congolense, brucei, evansi, equiperdum, simiae*	Curative
Quinapyramine dimethylsulfate	Horses, camels, pigs, dogs	*vivax, congolense, brucei, evansi, equiperdum, simiae*	Prophylactic
Suramin	Horses, camels, dogs	*brucei, evansi*	Curative, some prophylactic activity
Melarsomine dichlorhydrate	Camels	*evansi*	Curative

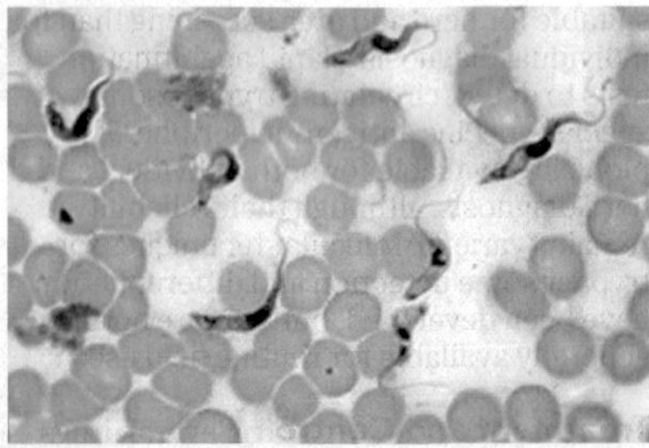

Trypanosoma vivax, blood smear of a cow.
Courtesy of Dr. Corrie Brown.

There is renewed international interest in large-scale tsetse eradication through the Pan African Tsetse and Trypanosomiasis Eradication Campaign (PATTEC) supported by the African Union. Animals can be given drugs prophylactically in areas with a high population of trypanosome-infected tsetse. Drug resistance must be carefully monitored by frequent blood examinations for trypanosomes in treated animals.

Several breeds of cattle and water buffalo have been identified that have innate resistance to trypanosomiasis and could play a valuable role in reducing the impact of the disease in these areas. However, resistance may be lost because of poor nutrition or heavy tsetse challenge.

Control is ideally achieved by combining methods to reduce the tsetse challenge and by enhancing host resistance with prophylactic drugs.

Surra

(*Trypanosoma evansi* infection)

Surra is usually transmitted by other biting flies that are found within and outside tsetse fly areas. It occurs in North Africa, the Middle East, Asia, the Far East, and Central and South America. The distribution of *T evansi* in Africa extends into the tsetse areas, where differentiation from *T brucei* is difficult. It is essentially a disease of camels and horses, but all domestic animals are susceptible. The disease can be fatal, particularly in camels, horses, and dogs. *T evansi* in other animals appears to be nonpathogenic, and these animals serve as reservoirs of infection.

Transmission is primarily by biting flies, probably resulting from interrupted feedings. A few wild animals are susceptible to infection and may serve as reservoirs.

Pathogenesis, clinical findings, lesions, diagnosis, and treatment are similar to those of the tsetse-transmitted trypanosomes (*see* p 35).

Dourine

Dourine is a chronic venereal disease of horses that is transmitted during coitus and caused by *T equiperdum*. The disease is recognized on the Mediterranean coast of Africa and in the Middle East, southern Africa, and South America; distribution is probably wider.

Signs may develop over weeks or months. Early signs include mucopurulent discharge from the urethra in stallions and from the vagina in mares, followed by gross edema of the genitalia. Later, characteristic plaques 2–10 cm in diameter appear on the skin, and the horse becomes progressively emaciated. Mortality in untreated cases is 50%–70%.

Demonstration of trypanosomes from urethral or vaginal discharges, skin plaques, or peripheral blood is difficult unless the material is centrifuged. Infected horses can be detected with the complement fixation test but only in areas where *T evansi* or *T brucei* are not found because they have common antigens. An ELISA test may become available for diagnosis.

In endemic areas, horses may be treated (*see* TABLE 6). When eradication is required, strict control of breeding and elimination of stray horses has been successful. Alternatively, infected horses may be identified using the complement fixation test; euthanasia is mandatory.

Chagas' Disease

(*Trypanosoma cruzi* infection)

Chagas' disease, or American trypanosomiasis, is a zoonotic, vectorborne disease transmitted by triatomine bugs and caused by *T cruzi*. All mammals are considered susceptible to infection, with infection demonstrated in >100 mammalian species. Avian species are not susceptible. The disease is best recognized in dogs and people, with dogs serving as a major domestic reservoir. Domestic pigs and cats can also be infected, but their role as reservoirs for human infection is limited. Wildlife reservoirs include opossums, armadillos, raccoons, woodrats, and nonhuman primates.

Transmission and Epidemiology:

Chagas' disease is endemic in 21 countries of South America, Central America, and Mexico, and is increasingly reported in the southern USA. Chagas' was once confined to the Americas, but human and animal migration has resulted in distribution to Europe, where it is an emerging disease of Spain, Switzerland, France, Italy, Germany, and England. Seropositivity in dogs in endemic regions can vary from 5%–92%. In some areas such as Venezuela, the seropositivity of dogs is similar to that of people, whereas in other areas, such as Campeche, Mexico, seropositivity can be higher in dogs than people.

The nocturnal and hematophagous triatomine insects of the *Triatoma*, *Rhodnius*, and *Panstrongylus* genera serve as vectors for *T cruzi*. Common names include the "kissing bug," "assassin bug," "cone-nosed bug," "vinchuca," "chinche," and "barbeiro." There are >130 species of triatomines in the Americas, and most are considered competent vectors. Insects take an infected blood meal ingesting extracellular *T cruzi* trypomastigotes. These differentiate in the midgut to epimastigotes and divide. Epimastigotes travel to the hindgut, where they differentiate back into metacyclic trypomastigotes. Infective metacyclic trypomastigotes are shed in insect feces. In insectivorous animals, including dogs, consumption of infected bugs or materials contaminated with infected triatomine feces is a major mode of transmission. The opossum (*Didelphis* species) is a unique host for *T cruzi*, because the parasite can complete its entire life cycle without the need for a vector. *T cruzi* maturation occurs in the anal odoriferous glands, and infective trypomastigotes can be shed in feces or urine and ingested. Additional methods of transmission include transplacentally or via blood transfusions and organ transplant.

Pathogenesis: Once metacyclic trypomastigotes enter the bloodstream, they actively invade many cell types, exiting the parasitophorous vacuole and becoming nonflagellated amastigotes. Intracellular amastigotes divide every 15–18 hr for 5–6 days. *T cruzi* transforms back into trypomastigotes and lyses the cell. Released trypomastigotes invade new cells. *T cruzi* has a tropism for cardiac and smooth muscle but can be found in numerous other tissues.

Clinical Findings and Lesions: Chagas' disease is divided into acute and chronic phases, with the chronic phase further subdivided into latent and symptomatic chronic disease. Incubation ranges from 5–42 days before acute disease. Acute infections may be asymptomatic or consist of nonspecific febrile illness with a chancre at the site of parasitic entry. Dogs may also present with regional or generalized lymphadenopathy, anorexia, lethargy, vomiting, diarrhea, and hepatomegaly or splenomegaly. Rarely, acute clinical myocarditis is seen. Parasitemia peaks 2–3 wk after infection and dissipates after the first month as the organism moves to predominantly tissue-borne disease.

The latent phase can last for months to years. Chronic disease symptoms can include generalized weakness or sudden death. Symptomatic dogs commonly present with right-side congestive heart failure. This can progress to myocarditis, with arrhythmias and bilateral cardiac dilation. Histologic examination of cardiac muscle may contain unruptured pseudocysts without inflammation or contain ruptured pseudocysts with lymphocytic, monocytic, and/or neutrophilic inflammation. Death secondary to heart failure is common.

Diagnosis: Diagnosis of Chagas' disease can be made by visualization of the organism, detection of DNA, or antibody detection. Parasitemia during the acute phase allows for detection on a microscopy of a routine peripheral blood smear. Although samples can be tested for *T cruzi* DNA by PCR or cultured, these diagnostic tests are uncommon in the field. On Giemsa stain, *T cruzi* is an extracellular, C-shaped protozoan with a single flagellum.

Antibody testing is of primary importance during the chronic phase. Whole blood, plasma, or serum can be submitted. Testing methodologies include immunochromographic "dipstick," immunofluorescent antibody, or ELISA. Notably, cross-reaction with antibodies to *Leishmania* species, another tryponsomatid, can occur. Because of cross-reactivity of serologic tests, testing with at least two different methodologies or antigens is recommended. Additionally, cardiac tissue in the chronic phase can be analyzed by PCR for *T cruzi* DNA or by immunohistochemical analysis for amastigotes.

Treatment and Control: Benznidazole is the drug of choice for treatment, but nifurtimox can also be used. In dogs, benznidazole is administered at 5–10 mg/kg/day, PO, for 2 mo. In the USA, both of these drugs lack FDA approval, and their use requires permission from the CDC as investigational protocols. Symptomatic treatment for heart failure and arrhythmias is also recommended.

No vaccine is available; thus, control focuses on preventing disease transmission.

Vector control methods include pesticide application to eliminate triatomine vectors and decreasing vector attraction to dwellings at night by turning off outdoor lighting. Breeding of positive bitches is discouraged. Screening of blood donors is recommended. To avoid iatrogenic transmission, disinfection with 10% bleach or 70% ethanol is suggested for contaminated surfaces. Dead infected insects can remain a source of infective *T cruzi* for up to 6 days at 10°C or up to 2 mo at 26°–30°C.

Nonpathogenic Trypanosomes

Trypanosoma theileri or markedly similar trypanosomes have been detected in peripheral blood from cattle on every continent. Infection with similar trypanosomes also has been detected in domestic and wild buffalo and various other wild ungulates. In the few areas studied, transmission is by contamination after a cycle of development in species of tabanid flies. Although most parasitemias are subpatent, the trypanosomes may be seen in a blood smear being examined for pathogenic protozoa or in a hemocytometer chamber. Pathogenicity has never been proved experimentally.

T melophagium of sheep also has a worldwide distribution and is transmitted by the sheep ked. *T theodori*, reported in goats, may be a synonym for the same trypanosome.

CANINE LYMPHOMA

Canine lymphoma is a disease term comprising a heterogeneous group of malignancies with varying biologic aggressiveness derived from the uncontrolled and pathologic clonal expansion of lymphoid cells of either B- or T-cell immunophenotype. Although neoplastic transformation of lymphocytes is not restricted to specific anatomic compartments, canine lymphoma most commonly involves organized primary and secondary lymphoid tissues, including the bone marrow, thymus, lymph nodes, and spleen. In addition to these lymphoid-rich organs, extranodal sites affected by lymphoma include the skin, intestinal tract, liver, eye, CNS, and bone. Lymphoma is reported to be the most common hematopoietic neoplasm in dogs, with an incidence reported to approach 0.1% in susceptible dogs. Despite the prevalence of malignant lymphoma, the underlying causes for its development remain poorly characterized; however, advanced genetic studies have revealed that canine lymphoma can be molecularly distinguished and categorized into discrete groups that correlate with biologic aggressiveness. Hypothesized causes include retroviral infection with Epstein-Barr virus–like viruses, environmental contamination with phenoxyacetic acid herbicides, magnetic field exposure, chromosomal abnormalities, and immune dysfunction. With the completion of the dog genome, it is anticipated that genome-wide association studies will identify specific genetic and chromosomal signatures involved in the pathogenesis of lymphoma.

Clinical Findings: Canine lymphoma is a heterogeneous cancer, with variable clinical signs, responses to therapy, and survival times. The heterogeneity associated with canine lymphoma is influenced in part by several tumor and host factors, including anatomic involvement, extent of disease, morphologic subtype, host constitution, and immunocompetence. In dogs, the most common clinical variants of lymphoma are high-grade T- or B-cell variants, and four conventionally recognized anatomic forms of lymphoma have been described: multicentric, alimentary, mediastinal, and extranodal (renal, CNS, cutaneous, ocular, bone, etc). Multicentric lymphoma is by far the most common anatomic form, accounting for ~80%–85% of all diagnosed cases. The most common and overt clinical manifestation of multicentric lymphoma is the rapid and nonpainful development of generalized lymphadenopathy. In addition to peripheral lymphadenopathy, most affected dogs will have malignant lymphocytes that are detectable by sensitive diagnostic tests, including flow cytometry or PCR for antigen receptor rearrangement

(PARR) that involve internal organs, including the spleen, liver, bone marrow, and other extranodal sites. In dogs with significant tumor burden, systemic constitutional signs, including profound lethargy, weakness, fever, anorexia, and dehydration, may become evident.

Alimentary lymphoma accounts for <10% of all canine lymphomas. Dogs with focal intestinal lesions may exhibit clinical signs consistent with partial or complete luminal obstruction (eg, vomiting, constipation, abdominal pain). With diffuse involvement of the intestinal tract, dogs with alimentary lymphoma may show significant and debilitating GI signs, including anorexia, vomiting, diarrhea, hypoproteinemia, and weight loss secondary to malabsorption and maldigestion.

Exclusive involvement of the cranial mediastinum with lymphoma comprises only a small fraction of diagnosed cases; however, sternal lymph node enlargement is frequently observed in dogs with multicentric disease. Mediastinal lymphoma is typically characterized by enlargement of the cranial mediastinal lymph nodes, thymus, or both. Mediastinal lymphoma arising from the thymus is predominantly comprised of high-grade malignant T lymphocytes, and with advanced disease, clinical signs may include respiratory distress associated with pleural fluid accumulation, direct compression of adjacent lung lobes, or caval syndrome. In addition to respiratory signs, some dogs with mediastinal lymphoma may have primary polyuria with secondary polydipsia resulting from humoral hypercalcemia of malignancy, a paraneoplastic syndrome seen in 10%–40% of dogs with lymphoma. Confirmation of humoral hypercalcemia of malignancy can be documented through the measurment of ionized calcium, parathyroid hormone, and parathyroid hormone–related peptide within circulating blood.

The clinical signs associated with various high-grade extranodal lymphomas (which may involve the skin, lungs, kidneys, eyes, CNS, etc) are often variable and dictated by the organs infiltrated. The most common extranodal form of lymphoma involves the skin, referred to as cutaneous lymphoma. Cutaneous lymphoma (epitheliotropic and nonepitheliotropic) may appear as solitary, raised, ulcerative nodules or generalized, diffuse, scaly lesions. Involvement of peripheral lymph nodes and mucocutaneous junctions is frequent. Clinical signs associated with lymphoma involving other extranodal sites may include respiratory distress (lungs), renal failure (kidneys), blindness (eyes), seizures (CNS), and skeletal pain or pathologic fracture (bone).

Although high-grade lymphoma of either B- or T-cell origin is most commonly diagnosed in dogs, low-grade or indolent lymphoma is a recently described molecular variant of canine lymphoma and comprises up to 30% of all lymphoma diagnoses. Like high-grade lymphoma, indolent lymphoma consists of several histopathologic subtypes, including marginal zone, follicular, mantle cell, and T-zone lymphoma. Collectively, indolent lymphomas are slowly progressive, and dogs often remain asymptomatic for a prolonged time regardless of therapy.

Lesions: Commonly, peripheral and various internal lymph nodes are 3–10 times normal size (multicentric form) and nonpainful on digital palpation. Affected nodes are freely movable, firm, and gray-tan; they bulge on cut surface and have no cortical-medullary demarcation. Frequently, there is hepatosplenomegaly with either diffuse enlargement or multiple, pale nodules of variable size disseminated in the parenchyma. In the alimentary form, any part of the GI tract or mesenteric lymph nodes may be affected. Involvement of the bone marrow, CNS, kidney, heart, tonsils, pancreas, and eyes can be seen but is less common.

Diagnosis:

The definitive diagnosis of lymphoma is often uncomplicated and can be obtained by either cytologic or histopathologic evaluation of the affected organ system. Fine-needle aspiration of enlarged peripheral lymph nodes or affected visceral organs usually provides specimens of adequate cellular content and detail to make a definitive diagnosis. Cytologically, lymph node or tissue aspirates may identify a monomorphic population of lymphoid cells, either of large (lymphoblastic), intermediate, or small size. Despite the ease of diagnosis, conventional cytology is limited for differentiating or categorizing the heterogeneous spectrum of lymphomas with regard to morphologic subtype (diffuse versus follicular, cleaved versus noncleaved) and histologic grade (high versus low). Specialized cytology utilizing lineage-specific antibodies can differentiate between B- and T-cell lymphomas and can provide some information regarding prognosis based on immunophenotype. However, because of the inherent limitations associated with cytology, histopathologic tissue evaluation remains the gold standard for the diagnosis of lymphoma, providing additional morphologic information required for definitive classification, as well as guiding therapeutic decisions.

In rare situations when cytology or histopathology fails to confirm the diagnosis of lymphoma, more advanced molecular techniques are available for definitive diagnosis, including flow cytometry for specific cell surface markers called cluster of differentiation (CD) antigens and PCR for PARR. The use of PCR allows for the amplification of DNA sequences that confirms or denies the presence of lymphocytes of either clonal, oligoclonal, or polyclonal origin. Because most neoplastic outgrowths result from the clonal expansion of one malignantly transformed cell, PCR techniques can differentiate lymphocyte expansion as a consequence of cancer (lymphoma) versus inflammation (reactive or hyperplastic lymphocytosis). Although PCR techniques are highly sensitive, the methodology should be reserved for cases in which conventional cytology and histopathology prove nondiagnostic, or when results are discordant with clinical signs and disease progression.

Treatment: Treatment of high-grade, multicentric canine lymphoma with aggressive, multi-agent chemotherapy protocols is often rewarding, with >90% of all dogs achieving complete reduction of tumor burden, termed complete remission. The most common chemotherapeutic agents used in combination protocols are vincristine, doxorubicin, cyclophosphamide, L-asparaginase, and prednisone. Individual treatment protocols vary with respect to dosage, frequency, and duration of treatment; advantages and disadvantages of each treatment protocol can be found in medical oncology textbooks. With combination chemotherapy, the expected survival time for dogs with B-cell lymphoma is ~12 mo, whereas for dogs with T-cell lymphoma, expected survival times are often in the range of 6 mo. Although immunophenotype (B- versus T-cell) provides a general guideline for treatment prognosis, multiple factors (tumor and host) contribute to the overall response duration and survival time of dogs diagnosed with lymphoma. Dogs that do not respond to traditional combination chemotherapy or that relapse may achieve disease remission, added survival times, or both with the use of various rescue protocols (eg, lomustine, MOPP, ADIC, DMAC).

Although systemic chemotherapy remains the cornerstone to treat high-grade lymphoma, the idea that both induction and maintenance phases of chemotherapy are necessary to achieve durable remission times has changed. Shorter and more dose-intense chemotherapy protocols (eg, Madison Wisconsin protocol) without maintenance provide disease-free intervals and survival times equivalent to protocols that include chronic maintenance therapy. Additionally, the use of half-body radiation in replacement of maintenance chemotherapy has been demonstrated to be safe and clinically efficacious, providing another option to achieve durable remission times without the need for chronic chemotherapy. For select cases, autologous canine bone marrow transplant after systemic chemotherapy and whole-body radiation can afford some dogs extended, progression-free intervals and survival times.

Despite the favorable outcomes expected in treating high-grade multicentric lymphoma, the successful management of other anatomic forms of lymphoma is often more difficult and less rewarding. Alimentary lymphoma, if focal, can be treated effectively with surgical resection and combination chemotherapy. However, with diffuse involvement of the intestinal tract, low constitutional reserve, severe malabsorption of nutrients, and loss of proteins often result in poor clinical responses and short survival times (ie, <3 mo). The use of combination chemotherapy with or without palliative radiation therapy can afford dogs with mediastinal lymphoma considerable improvement in survival times and quality-of-life scores. Lymphoma involving other extranodal sites (such as the skin) can be managed with either single-agent oral lomustine or combination systemic chemotherapies (eg, CHOP); however, the development of refractory and progressive disease is common and ultimately life limiting.

Clinical prognosis for dogs diagnosed with low-grade, indolent lymphoma tends to be good. The institution of low-intensity oral chemotherapy protocols (chlorambucil and prednisone) often provides prolonged survival times (>2 yr), and in specific dogs with localized and low-grade disease (eg, splenic involvement), splenectomy can be an effective and durable treatment option without the necessity of adjuvant chemotherapy administration. (*See also* TREATMENT OF CANINE LYMPHOMA, p 40.)

ERYTHROCYTOSIS AND POLYCYTHEMIA

Erythrocytosis is a relative or absolute increase in the number of circulating RBCs, resulting in a PCV increased above reference ranges. Polycythemia is frequently used synonymously with erythrocytosis; however, polycythemia may imply leukocytosis and thrombocytosis, as well as erythrocytosis.

Relative Erythrocytosis: Relative erythrocytosis is an increase in RBC numbers without an increase in total RBC mass. Usually, this is caused by loss of plasma volume with resultant hemoconcentration, as seen in severe dehydration attributable to vomiting and diarrhea. Alternatively, a mild, transient form of relative erythrocytosis unassociated with clinical signs may develop in dogs when fear or excitement causes splenic contraction with release of RBCs into the circulation.

Absolute Erythrocytosis: Absolute erythrocytosis, defined as increased RBC numbers because of increased RBC mass, develops from primary or secondary causes. **Primary erythrocytosis (polycythemia vera)** is a myeloproliferative disease of unknown cause that has been reported in dogs, cats, cattle, and horses. RBC production is dramatically increased, while serum erythropoietin (EPO) activity typically is low or low-normal. **Secondary erythrocytosis**, in contrast, generally develops from excessive production of EPO. If EPO is secreted because of systemic hypoxia, then the resultant erythrocytosis is an appropriate compensatory response. This may be seen with severe pulmonary disease or heart anomalies resulting in right-to-left shunting with blood bypassing the lungs (eg, reversed patent ductus arteriosus, tetralogy of Fallot). If EPO production increases without systemic hypoxia, then the response is inappropriate. EPO-secreting tumors of the kidneys or other organs, or non-neoplastic renal disorders resulting in local hypoxia with EPO production, may cause inappropriate erythrocytosis. Another type of secondary erythrocytosis, called **endocrinopathy-associated erythrocytosis**, results from hormones other than EPO (eg, cortisol, androgen, thyroxine, growth hormone) that stimulate erythropoiesis. The mild erythrocytosis in dogs with adrenocortical hyperactivity or in cats with hyperthyroidism or acromegaly is insufficient to cause clinical signs.

Clinical Findings: Clinical signs of absolute erythrocytosis include red mucous membranes, bleeding tendencies, polyuria, polydipsia, and neurologic disturbances (ataxia, weakness, seizures, blindness, behavioral change). On retinal examination, dilated, tortuous vessels may be visualized. These collective clinical features are attributed to hyperviscosity from the increased RBC mass.

Diagnosis: The dehydration and hemoconcentration of relative erythrocytosis may be identified by clinical findings (dry mucous membranes, loss of skin turgor), laboratory variables (hyperproteinemia, prerenal azotemia), and response to rehydration. Excitable dogs with mild erythrocytosis attributed to splenic contraction usually have normal PCV on subsequent blood samples collected less stressfully. Sighthounds (eg, Greyhounds) normally have mild erythrocytosis compared with standard canine reference ranges.

With absolute erythrocytosis, serum EPO determinations have been recommended to differentiate primary from secondary causes. Unfortunately, considerable overlap exists in EPO activity among normal animals, animals with primary erythrocytosis, and animals with secondary erythrocytosis. Furthermore, current availability of validated EPO assays for companion animals is limited. Routine examination of bone marrow is not useful to distinguish primary from secondary erythrocytosis because both conditions show erythroid hyperplasia. As a result, primary erythrocytosis usually is diagnosed by eliminating secondary causes.

To investigate types of secondary erythrocytosis, assessment of tissue oxygenation may be helpful. Arterial blood pO_2 <80 mmHg and pulse oximetry oxygen saturation <90%–95% are consistent with the hypoxemia and tissue hypoxia of appropriate secondary erythrocytosis. Examination of heart and lungs by auscultation, radiographs, electrocardiography, and echocardiography may reveal the underlying problem. Selective angiography or contrast echoaortography may be needed to confirm right-to-left cardiac shunting. If systemic hypoxia is not present, then locating the potential source of inappropriate EPO production is facilitated by physical and neurologic examinations, abdominal ultrasonography, IV urography, and CT or MRI.

Treatment: For relative erythrocytosis due to dehydration, therapy consists of rehydration with IV fluids and treating the underlying cause.

For polycythemia vera, treatment initially consists of phlebotomy (5–20 mL/kg to reduce the PCV to ~50%–60%) with simultaneous fluid replacement. Periodic phlebotomy with or without administration of hydroxyurea (30 mg/kg/day, PO, for 7–10 days, then 15 mg/kg/day, PO, titrated) has been advocated in affected dogs and cats. RBC, WBC, and platelet counts should be monitored during hydroxyurea treatment.

For inappropriate secondary erythrocytosis, EPO-secreting tumors should be managed with surgery, chemotherapy, or radiation therapy. Phlebotomy to normalize the PCV helps reduce hyperviscosity.

For appropriate secondary erythrocytosis, the underlying problem should be addressed. If corrective treatment of that disease process is not feasible, clinical signs associated with hyperviscosity may be alleviated by judicious phlebotomy (5–10 mL/kg) and hydroxyurea therapy. However, because this type of erythrocytosis is a compensatory response to hypoxia, the PCV should be maintained at values above normal reference ranges.

HEMOSTATIC DISORDERS

Effective hemostasis depends on an adequate number of functional platelets, an adequate concentration and activity of plasma coagulation and fibrinolytic proteins, and a normally responsive blood vasculature. The diagnosis, treatment, and monitoring of hypo- and hypercoagulable animals is difficult with regard to both progression of disease and monitoring blood component and/or anticoagulation therapy. Citrated plasma samples are often used in veterinary medicine to determine fibrinogen concentration, activated partial thromboplastin time (APTT), prothrombin time (PT), and D-dimer or fibrinogen degradation product (FDP) concentration. The introduction of the cell-based, tissue factor (TF)/Factor VII–dependent model of hemostasis has increased understanding of the complex biochemistry of physiologic hemostasis, leading to reevaluation of the traditional understanding of physiologic hemostasis divided into the intrinsic and extrinsic pathways of coagulation. Although citrated plasma contains many of the factors involved in coagulation, whole blood contains both the soluble factors and intravascular cells active in physiologic and pathologic hemostasis, incorporating TF and phospholipid-bearing cells, such as platelets and leukocytes.

Physiologic Understanding of Hemostasis

A cell-based model of hemostasis has been introduced that explains physiologic hemostasis through a complex process in which the interaction of vascular tone, blood flow, endothelial cells, platelets, leukocytes, coagulation factors, and fibrinolytic factors and their cofactors and inhibitors result in balanced hemostasis and formation of a clot at the injured site. This dynamic model involves cellular regulation of coagulation in three phases: initiation, amplification, and propagation.

TF-bearing cells initiate hemostasis. TF is a transmembrane glycoprotein receptor found in extravascular tissues, including organ capsules and the adventitia of blood vessel walls. It is constitutively expressed on fibroblasts and, on cellular activation, on vascular smooth muscle cells, monocytes, and neutrophils. The TF-bearing cells and platelet surfaces act as the main cellular surfaces for assembly of the procoagulant complexes. Any vessel injury leads to TF exposure. Factor VII binding to TF results in activation to Factor VIIa. Factor VIIa bound to TF on the cell surface activates Factor IX to Factor IXa and Factor X to Factor Xa. Initially, the formed Factor Xa is limited to the TF-bearing cell, because Factor Xa that diffuses away from the cell is rapidly inhibited by TF pathway inhibitor (TFPI) or antithrombin.

Together with formed Factor Va, Factor Xa is assembled into the prothrombinase complex on the surface of the TF-bearing cell. An initial small amount of thrombin close to the cell independent of the presence of platelets is generated and is responsible for activation of platelets, release of Factor V from the platelets, activation of Factor V, activation of Factor VIII and release of Factor VIII from von Willebrand factor, and activation of Factor XI. Platelets also are activated by other mechanisms, including vessel wall collagen and von Willebrand factor, leading to adhesion and aggregation at the injured site.

As an essential part of the platelet activation process, the procoagulant phospholipid phosphatidylserine becomes available. The initially generated Factor IXa binds to the activated platelet surfaces, promoting formation of the "tenase" complex; this results in major Factor Xa formation and amplification of the coagulation process. The formed Factor IXa diffuses to the platelets, because it is not inhibited by TFPI and is inhibited slowly by antithrombin. The formed Factor Xa complexes with Factor Va on the activated platelet surface, forming the "prothrombinase" complex that leads to cleavage of prothrombin and to the major subsequent burst of thrombin responsible for cleaving fibrinogen and forming the hemostatic plug. Additional Factor IXa is supplied by Factor XIa on the platelet surface. Factor XIa activates the antifibrinolytic pathway.

The second wave of thrombin activates plasmin, thereby initiating fibrinolysis. This keeps the clot controlled at the site of injury. To control fibrinolysis, the antifibrinolytic pathway is activated by thrombin activation of thrombin-activatable fibrinolysis inhibitor (TAFI). TAFI slows the fibrinolytic process by inhibiting plasmin activity; this prevents premature clot lysis and allows clot propagation. The balance of fibrin formation and fibrinolysis regulates the size and quality of the fibrin plug and localizes it to the site of injury. The quality of the clot has a significant impact on how effectively it provides hemostasis.

Clinical Approach to Hemostasis

Although the traditional division between primary and secondary hemostasis is not biologically accurate, it is still a useful diagnostic approach to hemostasis in animals with acquired or hereditary hemostatic disorders. Primary hemostasis is accomplished by interaction of platelets with exposed subendothelial surfaces. Simultaneously, plasma coagulation proteins are activated in a sequential cascade that depends on the phospholipid provided by the activated platelets and calcium ions from plasma to form a stable clot (secondary hemostasis). Circumstances that activate platelets and the coagulation proteins also activate plasma fibrinolytic proteins, which ensure localization of the clot and its timely dissolution.

Hemostatic capabilities are traditionally assessed by tests of primary hemostasis (platelet count and buccal mucosal bleeding time) and secondary hemostasis through plasma-based assays designed to further localize defects, such as the APTT (intrinsic and common pathway) and PT (extrinsic and common pathway). The fibrinolytic system is traditionally evaluated with measurements of degradation products such as FDP and D-dimer, and endogenous anticoagulant ability has been evaluated through antithrombin, protein C, and protein S. Additional specialized individual coagulation factor tests can further localize congenital defects. Thus, plasma-based coagulation screening tests can help identify the defective or deficient coagulation protein. Although this traditional approach makes it possible to effectively and systematically localize the cause of bleeding, it may be difficult from a clinical perspective to evaluate general hemostatic capability and to predict or monitor the effect of anticoagulant or procoagulant treatment. This may partially be because plasma-based tests of the secondary and fibrinolytic systems target specific elements of the hemostatic system, thus potentially ignoring other factors that may contribute significantly to overall hemostatic capability in acquired disorders. Another plausible reason is the low sensitivity of APTT and PT; usually, activity of a coagulation protein must be <30% and sometimes <10% of normal before an abnormality is detected.

Tests for increased risk or tendency toward thrombosis are generally available only through some academic and research laboratories. Measurement of antithrombin activity is being offered by increasing numbers of laboratories. Tests for measurement of activities of plasminogen, protein C, α_2-antiplasmin, tissue plasminogen activator, and plasminogen activator inhibitor have been established in some domestic animals.

Assessment of Hemostatic Function in Whole Blood

Because whole blood contains all the intravascular factors and cells involved in physiologic and pathologic hemostasis, incorporating TF and phospholipid-bearing cells, whole blood assays may provide a more accurate reflection of in vivo hemostasis than traditional plasma-based hemostasis assays. However, few whole blood assays to assess both primary and secondary hemostasis have been used in veterinary studies to date.

PFA-100: The platelet function analyzer, PFA-100, is a method for quantitative, simple, and rapid in vitro assessment of primary platelet-related hemostasis at high shear stress. The test requires a small volume (0.8 mL) of citrated whole blood, which is drawn under vacuum through a 200-μm diameter stainless steel capillary and a 150-μm diameter aperture in a nitrocellulose membrane coated with collagen and epinephrine (CEPI) or collagen and ADP (CADP). In response to the high shear rates and the agonists, a platelet aggregate forms that blocks blood flow through the aperture; the time taken to occlude the aperture is reported as the closure time. Prolonged closure times with only the CEPI cartridge are seen with mild inherited platelet function disorders (eg, storage pool disorders) and with aspirin ingestion, while prolonged closure times with both CEPI and CADP cartridges are seen with more severe inherited platelet dysfunctions and with von Willebrand disease. The PFA-100 also has the ability to monitor response to treatment with both desmopressin acetate and glycoprotein IIb/IIIa antagonists. The quality of blood bank platelet concentrates for transfusion can be evaluated, as well as response to platelet transfusion. The PFA-100 is a good screening method to detect platelet function defects. It also has been evaluated in many other studies for its use in assessing drug effects or for evaluation of overall primary hemostasis in various clinical disorders or during surgical procedures.

Thromboelastography (TEG): TEG allows for rapid assessment of hemostatic function in whole blood. It evaluates all of the steps in hemostasis, including initiation, amplification, and propagation, as well as fibrinolysis, including the interaction of platelets and leukocytes with the proteins of the coagulation cascade. Thus, TEG combines evaluation of the traditional plasma components of coagulation with the cellular components. TEG is performed on unstabilized fresh whole blood within 4–6 min of taking the blood sample. This is generally not practical in a routine clinical setting, and using citrated stabilized whole blood (with recalcification immediately before analysis) has been proposed to increase the time span from sampling to analysis. A TF-activated TEG assay on citrated whole blood has been validated in dogs and shown to have a low analytical variation and good correlation to clinical signs of bleeding compared with many traditional plasma-based coagulation assays.

TEG is the first modality available to clinicians that can evaluate hypercoagulability. It is especially useful in dogs with disseminated intravascular coagulation, neoplasia, sepsis, and parvoviral infection, and to evaluate platelet dysfunction in dogs with hypothermia. TEG analysis is a valuable aid in the diagnostic evaluation of animals with abnormal hemostasis and a supplement to traditional coagulation tests such as PT, APTT, D-dimer, and fibrinogen assays.

COAGULATION DISORDERS

Bleeding diatheses may be caused by congenital or acquired defects in the vasculature, platelets, or the coagulation proteins. Congenital or acquired defects or deficiencies of platelets usually manifest as superficial petechial and ecchymotic hemorrhages (especially of mucous membranes), epistaxis, melena, or prolonged bleeding at injection and incision sites, whereas congenital or acquired deficiencies in coagulation proteins usually manifest clinically as delayed deep tissue hemorrhage, hematoma formation, and bleeding into joints and body cavities.

Pathologic thrombosis may occur because of primary or inherited disorders of anticoagulant protein factors or because of secondary or acquired disorders. Collectively, these conditions are called hypercoagulable states. Systemic syndromes, such as disseminated intravascular coagulation, that enhance platelet responsiveness to agonists and alter the balance between anticoagulant and procoagulant protein factors or that increase the reactivity of endothelium are more common in animals than inherited disorders.

PLATELET DISORDERS

Disorders of platelets can be divided into acquired or congenital thrombocytopenias and acquired or congenital functional disorders (thrombocytopathias), with acquired thrombocytopenia being the most common.

Congenital Thrombocytopenia

Hereditary Macrothrombocytopenia in Cavalier King Charles Spaniels: This benign, inherited giant platelet disorder affects ~50% of dogs in the breed. It is characterized by thrombocytopenia with macrothrombocytes in 30% of cases and variable platelet aggregation in response to adenosine diphosphate, depending on the platelet count. No correlation has been found between macrothrombocytopenia and age, gender, neuter status, coat color, weight, or heart murmur status. The disorder is detected by a routine CBC. Affected dogs have normal coagulation protein activity.

Cyclic Hematopoiesis in Gray Collie Dogs: This autosomal recessive disorder is characterized by 12-day cycles of cytopenia. All marrow stem cells are affected, but neutrophils are most affected because of their short half-life (usually <24 hr). Mild to severe thrombocytopenia can be seen, and excessive bleeding is a potential complication. The disorder is fatal; affected dogs usually die from fulminating infections before 6 mo of age. Even dogs that receive intensive antibiotic therapy usually die by 3 yr of age with amyloidosis (*see* p 592) secondary to chronic antigenic stimulation from recurrent infections. Treatment with recombinant granulocyte colony-stimulating factor has been temporarily successful in alleviating the neutropenic cycles until antibodies are produced against the noncanine proteins.

Fetal and Neonatal Alloimmune Thrombocytopenia: This disorder occurs when maternal antibodies are produced against a paternal antigen on fetal platelets. It has been reported in a 1-day-old Quarter horse foal. Immunoglobulins bound to the foal's platelets were identified in the mare's plasma, serum, and milk by indirect assays. The immunoglobulins were further shown to recognize platelets from the foal's full brother, born 1 year earlier. This diagnosis should be considered for foals with severe thrombocytopenia when other causes can be excluded.

A group of lambs artificially reared and fed bovine colostrum had prolonged bleeding from puncture wounds from ear tag placement, subcutaneous bruising, weakness, and pale mucous membranes. All affected lambs died within 48 hr of birth. Thrombocytopenia was seen in whole blood, and platelets were markedly decreased on blood smears. The presence of antibodies directed against platelets was suspected because the cows from which colostrum was obtained had been used in a previous experiment in which they had been immunized against sheep blood.

Acquired Thrombocytopenia

Acquired thrombocytopenias are reported frequently in dogs and cats, less often in horses, and rarely in other species. Numerous causes have been identified, most involving immunologic or direct destruction of platelets.

Primary Immune-mediated Thrombocytopenia: This condition (also called idiopathic thrombocytopenia or idiopathic thrombocytopenic purpura is characterized by immune-mediated destruction of either circulating platelets or, less commonly, marrow megakaryocytes. It has been seen in dogs, horses, and rarely cats. Clinical signs include petechiae of the gingivae or skin and ecchymosis, melena, or epistaxis. Platelet concentration is usually <50,000/μL and often <10,000/μL at the time of diagnosis. Evaluation of megakaryocytes (by bone marrow aspiration) helps determine whether circulating platelets or marrow megakaryocytes are targeted by antibody. A test for platelet factor 3 released from damaged platelets has been unreliable or not readily available commercially. A megakaryocyte immunofluorescence assay that detects antibodies on megakaryocytes has been done, but an adequate bone marrow aspiration sample must be obtained. A direct test for the presence of antiplatelet antibodies—an ELISA that detects platelet-bound antibodies—has been reported to have good sensitivity (94%) but is not highly specific for primary immune-mediated thrombocytopenia. A negative test result likely excludes primary immune-mediated thrombocytopenia as the cause of thrombocytopenia; however, a positive test result could indicate either primary immune-mediated thrombocytopenia or secondary immune-mediated thrombocytopenia (eg, thrombocytopenia associated with autoimmune hemolytic anemia, lymphoproliferative diseases, systemic lupus erythematosus).

Affected animals should be kept at rest, and treatment is based on administration of corticosteroids, starting at a high dose and then tapering (as in the treatment of IMMUNE-MEDIATED HEMOLYTIC ANEMIA, p 10). Transfusion with fresh whole blood should be performed in animals with a PCV <15%; however, whole blood transfusion to replenish platelets is often futile with regard to normalization of primary hemostasis, because the platelets are removed from circulation within a couple of hours. Splenectomy should be reserved as a treatment for animals that have recurrent episodes of thrombocytopenia. Vincristine has been used to enhance the release of platelets from marrow megakaryocytes. It also coats platelets and has a cytotoxic effect on macrophages that ingest coated platelets. A single dose of vincristine at the time corticosteroids are started shortens the time to recovery of the platelet count.

Rickettsial Diseases: *Anaplasma platys*, *A phagocytophilum*, or *Ehrlichia canis* infections cause mild to severe thrombocytopenia in dogs. *A platys* infection (*see* p 803) usually is characterized by mild, often cyclic thrombocytopenia in the acute stages of disease. Chronic infections often have constant mild to moderate thrombocytopenia. Morula (single to multiple, round to oval basophilic inclusions) can sometimes be identified in platelets of infected dogs. The thrombocytopenia is seldom severe enough to result in clinical bleeding tendencies. Ticks are the likely vectors. *E canis* infections are characterized by variable alterations in total WBC count, PCV, and platelet count. In acute infections, there is usually thrombocytopenia and possibly anemia or leukopenia. In chronic infections, there may or may not be thrombocytopenia or anemia; however, there is often leukocytosis and sometimes hyperglobulinemia (monoclonal or polyclonal). Infected dogs may have epistaxis, melena, gingival bleeding, retinal hemorrhage, hematoma formation, and prolonged bleeding after venipuncture or surgery.

A phagocytophilum infection has been documented in a wide variety of domestic and wild animals. It is characterized by fever, lethargy, and a reluctance to move. Changes in blood parameters include thrombocytopenia and lymphopenia accompanied by increased serum alkaline phosphatase and hypoalbuminemia.

Neoplasia: Hemangiosarcoma, lymphoma, and adenocarcinoma may be associated with consumptive thrombocytopenia due to disseminated intravascular coagulation. Immunologic and inflammatory mechanisms cause increased platelet consumption and decreased platelet survival. However, bleeding tendencies without thrombocytopenia occasionally exist. Altered platelet function due to an acquired membrane defect has been associated with hyperglobulinemia. Vasculitis also may contribute to the hemostatic disorder.

Vaccine-induced Thrombocytopenia: Dogs vaccinated repeatedly with modified-live adenovirus and paramyxovirus vaccines may develop thrombocytopenia 3–10 days after repeat vaccination. The thrombocytopenia is usually transient and may be sufficiently mild that a bleeding tendency will not be evident unless superimposed on another platelet or coagulation disorder. Studies have failed to confirm an association between recent vaccination and development of idiopathic thrombocytopenic purpura; however, it might still occur rarely.

Drug-induced Thrombocytopenia: Thrombocytopenia associated with administration of certain drugs has been reported in dogs, cats, and horses. One mechanism is marrow suppression of megakaryocytes or generalized marrow stem cell suppression (after administration of estrogen, chloramphenicol, phenylbutazone, diphenylhydantoin, and sulfonamides). Another mechanism is increased platelet destruction and consumption (after administration of sulfisoxazole, aspirin, diphenylhydantoin, acetaminophen, ristocetin, levamisole, methicillin, and penicillin). Drug reactions are idiosyncratic and therefore unpredictable. Platelets usually return to normal shortly after the drug is discontinued. Drug-induced bone marrow suppression may be prolonged. The chemotherapy drug lomustine has sometimes caused prolonged thrombocytopenia that persists after the drug is stopped.

Other: Quantitative platelet disorders have been reported in liver disease with or without coagulation protein deficiencies. In two studies of cats with thrombocytopenia, 29%–50% had infectious diseases, including feline leukemia, feline infectious peritonitis, panleukopenia, or toxoplasmosis. The mechanism of thrombocytopenia has not been identified in many cases. Feline leukemia virus replicates and accumulates in megakaryocytes and platelets; aplasia or hypoplasia of marrow stem cells, immune destruction of infected platelets, or extravascular sequestration of platelets within lymphoid tissues may contribute to thrombocytopenia in this disease.

Congenital Platelet Function Disorders

Congenital disorders of platelet function affect platelet adhesion, aggregation, or secretion. They can be either intrinsic or extrinsic to platelets. Testing of intrinsic platelet function requires careful handling of samples and specialized equipment that is not routinely available in diagnostic laboratories; therefore, the incidence of intrinsic functional defects in platelets is not known accurately. However, if a bleeding disorder (especially mucosal bleeding or superficial petechiation) exists in an animal that has not received any medication and that has normal coagulation screening test results, platelet concentration, and von Willebrand factor concentration, then an intrinsic platelet defect should be suspected.

There is no specific treatment for any of the intrinsic platelet function disorders. In instances of severe hemorrhaging, fresh, platelet-rich plasma can be administered. Whole blood may be administered if the affected animal is anemic.

Von Willebrand Disease: This disorder, caused by a defective or deficient von Willebrand factor (vWF, also called Factor VIII-related antigen), is the most common inherited bleeding disorder in dogs (reported in nearly all breeds and in mixed breeds). It has also been reported in cats, rabbits, cattle, horses, and pigs. It is relatively frequent (10%–70% prevalence) in several breeds of dogs: Doberman Pinschers, German Shepherds, Golden Retrievers, Miniature Schnauzers, Pembroke Welsh Corgis, Shetland Sheepdogs, Basset Hounds, Scottish Terriers, Standard Poodles, and Standard Manchester Terriers. Canine von Willebrand disease is classified into three subtypes based on clinical severity, plasma vWF concentration, and vWF multimer composition. Type 1 is the most common form and is characterized by mild to moderate clinical signs, low vWF concentration, and a normal multimer distribution. Type 2 is characterized by moderate to severe clinical signs, low vWF concentration, and a loss of high-molecular-weight multimers. Type 3, seen most often in Shetland Sheepdogs and Scottish Terriers, is a severe disorder characterized by total absence of vWF. Two modes of inheritance are known. In the less common autosomal recessive pattern of inheritance, homozygosity is usually fatal, and heterozygosity results in asymptomatic carriers. In the more common inheritance pattern of autosomal dominant with incomplete penetrance, homozygotes and heterozygotes can have variable bleeding tendencies. Affected animals may have gingival bleeding, epistaxis, and hematuria. Some puppies may bleed excessively only after injection, venipuncture, or surgery, such as tail docking, ear cropping, and dewclaw removal.

vWF circulates as a complex with coagulation Factor VIII (also called Factor VIII-coagulant) and mediates platelet adhesion to subendothelial surfaces—the first step in clot formation. Defective or deficient vWF mimics disorders caused by thrombocytopenia or intrinsic platelet defects. Von Willebrand disease should be suspected in animals with clinical signs of a bleeding disorder that have normal results on coagulation screening tests (APTT and PT) and adequate platelet concentrations, long buccal mucosa bleeding time, and prolonged platelet function analysis closure times. Quantitative tests of vWF are diagnostic. Diagnosis is confirmed by identifying low vWF concentration in plasma or via DNA screening. Occasionally, affected animals may have decreased Factor VIII-coagulant and therefore have prolonged APTT and activated clotting time (ACT). Drugs known to interfere with normal platelet function should be avoided in animals with suspected disease. Transfusion of cryoprecipitate, fresh plasma, or fresh whole blood effectively alleviates a bleeding episode. Type 1 von Willebrand disease may respond to treatment with desmopressin acetate, which causes Weibel-Palade release (high-molecular-weight multimers) from the endothelium through an unknown method of action. Desmopressin may also be used in these dogs before surgery to minimize bleeding complications.

Concomitant hemostatic abnormalities may exacerbate von Willebrand disease. Hypothyroidism (*see* p 553) previously had been thought to be associated with von Willebrand disease; both conditions are prevalent in many of the same breeds of dogs, eg, Doberman Pinschers and Golden Retrievers. In one study, administration of thyroid supplementation to hypothyroid dogs without deficiency of vWF did not increase vWF activity; in fact, in most of the tested dogs, vWF activity actually decreased. Therefore, administration of levothyroxine as a treatment of von

Willebrand disease cannot be recommended and may even exacerbate the disease.

Chédiak-Higashi Syndrome: This autosomal recessive disorder is characterized by abnormal granule formation in leukocytes, melanocytes, and platelets (*see* p 59). The defect appears to be in microtubule formation; therefore, granules, which are abnormally large but reduced in number, are evident in numerous types of cells. Diluted coat color results from the defect in the melanocytes. Leukocytes may have decreased functional ability to phagocytize and kill organisms (an inconsistent finding in animals), and platelets have decreased aggregation and release reactions. Platelets are almost devoid of dense granules and have markedly decreased storage quantities of adenosine diphosphate and serotonin. Prolonged bleeding in affected blue smoke Persian cats occurs after venipuncture or surgery. The syndrome has been diagnosed in mink, cattle, and beige mice with similar bleeding tendencies.

Canine Thrombopathia: This disorder has been described in Basset Hounds. Affected dogs have epistaxis, petechiation, and gingival bleeding. Results of studies suggest that inheritance is autosomal with variable penetrance. Platelets have abnormal fibrinogen receptor exposure and impaired dense granule release. Basset Hounds with mucosal bleeding and petechiation and normal concentrations of platelets and vWF should be suspected of having thrombopathia. Specific diagnosis of this disorder requires specialized platelet function testing. Results of the clot retraction test are usually normal.

Bovine Thrombopathia: This autosomally inherited platelet function defect is seen in Simmental cattle. Bleeding can be mild to severe in affected cattle and is exacerbated by trauma or surgery. Platelets have impaired aggregation responses. Bovine viral diarrhea virus (*see* p 1436) may cause thrombocytopenia in cattle.

Glanzmann Thrombasthenia: This autosomally transmitted disorder, previously thrombasthenic thrombopathia, has been diagnosed in Otterhounds and Great Pyrenees dogs, and in Thoroughbred-cross, Quarter horse, and Oldenburg filly horses. Affected animals have prolonged bleeding times and form hematomas at sites of venipuncture or injury. Numerous (30%–80% of all platelets), bizarre, giant platelets are seen on blood smears. Due to a decreased synthesis of either glycoprotein IIb or IIIa, the membrane receptor glycoprotein IIb-IIIa is reduced or lacking on the surface of platelets. All affected animals to date have had a defect in IIb synthesis.

Blood from affected animals does not have normal clot retraction, and the platelets do not aggregate normally after stimulation with adenosine diphosphate, collagen, or thrombin.

Acquired Platelet Function Disorders

Dogs with immune-mediated thrombocytopenia also may have an acquired platelet functional defect. Dogs can have excessive bleeding tendencies without severely decreased platelet concentrations. In dogs with immune-mediated thrombocytopenia, abnormal platelet function in addition to decreased platelet concentration may contribute to their bleeding tendency.

Several diseases have been associated with acquired platelet function disorders. Hyperglobulinemia associated with multiple myeloma induces a platelet membrane defect resulting in impaired hemostatic function. In uremia associated with any form of renal disease, platelet adhesion and aggregation are decreased.

Numerous drugs can impair platelet function. Drugs reported to block platelet receptor binding or to change platelet membrane charge or permeability include furosemide, penicillin, carbenicillin, lidocaine, phentolamine, and chlorpromazine. Drugs that inhibit transduction of messages received at the platelet surface include caffeine, theophylline, dipyridamole, and papavarine. Drugs that inhibit execution of platelet responses (aggregation, secretion, or thromboxane production) include aspirin, indomethacin, acetaminophen, phenylbutazone, ticlopidine, pentobarbital, and sulfinpyrazone. Clinical bleeding problems may not be caused by drug-induced impairment of platelet function unless another disorder associated with a hemostatic defect is also present.

VASCULAR DISORDERS

Congenital Vascular Disorders

Cutaneous asthenia (Ehlers-Danlos syndrome, rubber puppy disease) is caused by a defect in the maturation of type I collagen. This causes weak structural support of blood vessels and can result in hematoma formation and easy bruising. The disorder has been reported in dogs, cats, mink, horses, cattle, sheep, and people but is rare in domestic animals. The most striking clinical abnormality is loose, hyperextensible skin that tears easily. No treatment is available.

Acquired Vascular Disorders

Several diseases cause severe, often generalized vasculitis and are characterized by bleeding disorders.

Rocky Mountain spotted fever (*see* p 806) is caused by *Rickettsia rickettsii*, which is transmitted by the ticks *Dermacentor variabilis* and *D andersoni*. The rickettsial organisms invade endothelial cells and cause cellular death with resultant perivascular edema and hemorrhage. Variable degrees of coagulation cascade activation can occur along with thrombocytopenia. Infected dogs may have epistaxis, petechial and ecchymotic hemorrhages, hematuria, melena, or retinal hemorrhages. In severely affected dogs, disseminated intravascular coagulation may occur.

Canine herpesvirus generally affects puppies 7–21 days old. Generalized necrotizing vasculitis is accompanied by perivascular hemorrhage. The disease is usually rapidly fatal, and most puppies die within 24 hr after showing signs.

COAGULATION PROTEIN DISORDERS

Congenital Coagulation Protein Disorders

In a severe deficiency or functional defect of coagulation proteins, clinical signs appear at an early age. Marked reductions in activity of coagulation proteins essential to hemostasis are usually fatal. Animals may be stillborn if there is <1% of normal activity or die shortly after birth owing to massive hemorrhage. Insufficient production of coagulation proteins or limited access to vitamin K by the immature neonatal liver may exacerbate a coagulation defect. If activity of any particular coagulation protein is 5%–10% of normal, the neonate may survive, but signs usually appear before 6 mo of age. It is during this time, when numerous routine procedures (eg, vaccination, declawing, tail docking, dewclaw removal, ear cropping, and castration or ovariohysterectomy) are usually done, that a bleeding tendency may become apparent.

Most of the congenital coagulation protein disorders reported in domestic animals are deficiencies or abnormalities of a single factor.

Congenital afibrinogenemia (Factor I deficiency) has been reported in a family of Saanen dairy goats but not in dogs or cats. **Hypofibrinogenemia**, accompanied by severe bleeding, has been reported in Saint Bernards and Vizslas and in one mixed-breed dog; the ACT, APTT, PT, and thrombin time (TT) were prolonged. **Dysfibrinogenemia** has been reported in an inbred family of Russian Wolfhounds (Borzois). The ACT, APTT, PT, and TT were prolonged, but fibrinogen was present by quantitative testing. Affected dogs had mild bleeding episodes with epistaxis and lameness, but trauma or surgery resulted in life-threatening bleeding. IV administration of fresh-frozen plasma or cryoprecipitate is the best treatment to stop the bleeding.

Factor II (prothrombin) disorders are rare. Boxer dogs have been reported to have abnormally functioning prothrombin but normal concentrations; the defect was inherited as an autosomal recessive trait. A disorder of Factor II has been reported in English Cocker Spaniels; clinical signs in affected puppies (epistaxis and gingival bleeding) decrease with age, and adults bruise easily or have dermatitis. In affected puppies, TT is normal, while ACT, APTT, and PT are prolonged. Treatment is by transfusion of fresh-frozen plasma or fresh whole blood if RBCs are needed.

Factor VII deficiency has been reported in Beagles, English Bulldogs, Alaskan Malamutes, Alaskan Klee Kai, Miniature Schnauzers, Boxers, and mixed-breed dogs. It is inherited in an autosomal pattern with incomplete dominance. Usually, it is not associated with spontaneous clinical bleeding, but affected dogs may have bruising or prolonged bleeding after surgery. Prolonged postpartum hemorrhaging has been reported. Factor VII deficiency is most often diagnosed coincidentally when coagulation screening tests are performed; the PT is prolonged, while APTT and other test results are normal.

Factor VIII deficiency (hemophilia A) is the most common inherited bleeding disorder in dogs and cats; it has also been reported in several breeds of horses, including Arabians, Standardbreds, Quarter horses, and Thoroughbreds. There is an X-linked pattern of inheritance, so usually females are asymptomatic carriers and males are affected. Rarely, in highly inbred families, a carrier female mated with an affected male can produce affected female offspring.

In affected puppies, prolonged bleeding is seen from the umbilical vessels after birth; from the gingiva during tooth eruption; and after surgery such as tail docking, dewclaw removal, or ear cropping. Hemarthrosis accompanied by intermittent lameness, spontaneous hematoma formation, and hemorrhagic body cavity effusions also are common clinical findings in dogs with <5% of normal Factor VIII activity. Animals with 5%–10% of normal activity often do not bleed spontaneously but exhibit prolonged bleeding after trauma or surgery. Affected cats and sometimes small dogs may show prolonged bleeding after surgery or trauma but rarely bleed spontaneously, probably because of their agility and light weight. Affected animals usually have very low concentrations of Factor VIII (<10%) and prolonged ACT and APTT. Von Willebrand factor (Factor VIII–related antigen) concentrations are normal or greater than normal. Carrier animals have intermediate concentrations of Factor VIII (40%–60%), and results of coagulation screening tests are usually normal. Care should be taken in diagnosis if animals are <6 mo old because of possible low production of coagulation factors by an immature liver. Usually, results of coagulation screening tests are normal in carrier animals.

Treatment of bleeding diatheses requires repeated transfusions of cryoprecipitate or fresh-frozen plasma (10 mL/kg) 2–3 times/day until bleeding has been controlled. Fresh-frozen plasma or cryoprecipitate is preferable to whole blood because of the possible sensitization of the animal to RBC antigens with repeated transfusions.

Factor IX deficiency (hemophilia B) is diagnosed less often than Factor VIII deficiency. It has been reported in several breeds of purebred dogs, a mixed-breed dog, Himalayan cats, a family of Siamese-cross cats, and a family of British Short-haired cats. The defect is X-linked with carrier females and affected males, although affected females can be seen in closely inbred families. Clinical presentation is similar to that of animals with Factor VIII deficiency. Animals with extremely low Factor IX activity (<1%) usually die at birth or shortly thereafter. Animals with 5%–10% of normal Factor IX activity may spontaneously form hematomas, hemarthroses, hemorrhagic body cavity effusions, or organ hemorrhage. Gingival bleeding during tooth eruption or prolonged bleeding after tail docking or dewclaw removal can occur. Some animals are asymptomatic until trauma or surgery. The ACT and APTT are prolonged. Carrier animals with 40%–60% of normal Factor IX activity are usually asymptomatic, and results of coagulation screening tests are normal. Treatment requires transfusion with fresh-frozen plasma (10 mL/kg), bid, until bleeding resolves. Often, internal hemorrhage into the abdomen, thorax, CNS, or between muscle fascial planes occurs and may be undetected until a crisis.

Factor X deficiency has been reported in a single family of American Cocker Spaniels and a mixed-breed dog. In the former, the inheritance pattern was autosomal dominant with variable penetrance. Homozygotes usually die early in life or are stillborn because of massive internal hemorrhage. Heterozygotes have mild to severe bleeding problems. The ACT, APTT, and PT are usually prolonged when animals have <30% normal activity of Factor X. Transfusions with fresh or fresh-frozen plasma are required to control hemorrhage.

Factor XI deficiency has been recognized in Kerry Blue Terriers, a female English Springer Spaniel, a Great Pyrenees dog, Weimaraners, and Holstein cattle. Mild deficiencies usually go undetected. In severe deficiencies with Factor XI at 30%–40% or less of normal activity, mild prolonged bleeding may occur after trauma or surgery. Bleeding tendencies usually are not immediate but delayed for 3–4 days. The ACT and APTT are usually prolonged. Transfusion with fresh-frozen plasma (10 mL/kg) is sufficient to stop the bleeding for up to 3 days. Inheritance is autosomal, but it has not been determined whether the gene is dominant or recessive. A single case involving an adult cat with epistaxis and diagnosed with systemic lupus erythematosus was attributed to the presence of a circulating inhibitor against Factor XI.

Factor XII (Hageman) deficiency has been reported in German Shorthaired Pointers, Standard Poodles, a family of Miniature Poodles, and in cats. Affected animals do not have clinical bleeding problems. The deficiency is usually diagnosed coincidentally when coagulation screening tests are performed and the APTT is prolonged. People with Factor XII deficiency do not have bleeding problems but are predisposed to thrombosis or infections, which is attributed to the normal role of Factor XII in fibrinolysis and complement activation. Tendencies for thrombosis or infection have not been reported in animals. Factor XII deficiency has been found to coexist with von Willebrand disease in a dog and with Factor IX deficiency in a cat, but bleeding tendencies were not exacerbated. Factor XII is not present in the plasma of birds, marine mammals, and reptiles, with no untoward effects.

Deficiency of Factors II, VII, IX, and X has been described in Devon Rex cats that experienced bleeding, most commonly after surgery. The bleeding can be controlled by vitamin K administration, and some of these cats appear to overcome the bleeding tendency as adults.

Prekallikrein deficiency has been reported in Poodles, a family of miniature horses, and a family of Belgian horses. Clinical bleeding problems are not usually apparent. One horse bled excessively after castration. The diagnosis is usually made coincidentally when coagulation screening tests are performed. The ACT and APTT are usually prolonged.

Poor clot strength in Greyhounds has been found to cause delayed postoperative bleeding. An abnormal maximum amplitude is observed on TEG in these dogs. Epsilon aminocaproic acid is effective to prevent or stop bleeding in affected dogs.

Acquired Coagulation Protein Disorders

Liver Disease: Most coagulation proteins are produced primarily in the liver. Therefore, liver disease characterized by necrosis, inflammation, neoplasia, or cirrhosis often is associated with decreased production of coagulation proteins, anticoagulants, and fibrinolytic proteins. Because the various coagulation proteins have a relatively short half-life (4 hr to 2 days), mild to marked deficiencies can result in secondary to severe hepatopathies. The APTT and/or PT are prolonged in 50%–85% of dogs with severe liver disease, meaning that the factor activity is <30% of normal. Nevertheless, <2% actually develop hemorrhage and, when bleeding does occur, it is usually associated with concurrent disease. Coagulation tests are often performed before liver biopsy.

Severe hepatic diseases can also lead to disseminated intravascular coagulation. Fibrinogen, an acute phase reactant, and von Willebrand factor, which is produced extrahepatically, can be increased in liver disease.

Vitamin K Deficiency: Vitamin K is solubilized in mixed micelles before passive diffusion across the brush border. Fat malabsorption associated with inadequate amounts of bile salts (eg, biliary obstruction), lymphangiectasia, or severe villous atrophy may result in vitamin deficiency and coagulopathy owing to the lack of production of the functional vitamin K–dependent Factors II, VII, IX, and X.

Ingestion of Anticoagulant Rodenticides: Ingestion of certain rodenticides by dogs and cats causes a coagulopathy owing to the lack of production of functional vitamin K–dependent factors (*see* p 3165). Inactive precursor coagulation Factors II, VII, IX, and X are still produced by the liver, but γ-carboxylation of the inactive precursors does not occur, because the rodenticide inhibits the epoxide-reductase enzyme required for recycling of active vitamin K. There are two general classes of anticoagulant rodenticides: the coumarin compounds (warfarin, coumafuryl, brodifacoum, and bromadiolone) and the indanedione compounds (diphacinone, pindone, valone, and chlorophacinone). The anticoagulant rodenticides are further divided into first- and second-generation based on their toxicity and half-life. In general, the half-life of the coumarins (up to 55 hr) is much shorter than that of the indanedione compounds (15–20 days). Various concurrently administered drugs and coexisting disease may exacerbate the toxicity of the ingested anticoagulant.

Affected animals may have hematoma formation (especially over pressure points) and bruising of superficial and deep tissues. Often, the animals do not bleed within the first 24 hr after ingestion of the toxin. The APTT, PT, and ACT are usually prolonged. Factor VII has the shortest half-life of the vitamin K–dependent coagulation proteins; therefore, the PT is often abnormal before other tests and can be used to monitor response to treatment. With acute ingestion, emetics, absorbents, and cathartics are used to minimize absorption. Vitamin K therapy is often initiated even in asymptomatic animals. Vitamin K_1, 2.5–5 mg/kg, SC, divided between several injection sites, is recommended for initial treatment of coumarin toxicity, followed by 1.25–2.5 mg/kg, PO, bid for 4–6 days if the ingestion is thought to be minimal. PT should be measured 48 hr after termination of treatment, and if prolonged, treatment should be continued for another 14 days. If the initial PT is normal, another PT should be performed in 48 hr. If that test is normal, treatment can be discontinued. Dosages of vitamin K_1 as high as 5 mg/kg, PO, for 3–6 wk may be required for treatment of indanedione toxicity; however, these high dosages should be administered cautiously, because Heinz body anemia has been reported in dogs given 4 mg/kg for 5 days. IV administration of vitamin K_1 is not recommended, because anaphylactic reactions can result. Administration of vitamin K_3 is not useful.

Disseminated Intravascular Coagulation (DIC): DIC is not a primary disease but occurs secondary to numerous underlying diseases, such as bacterial, viral, rickettsial, protozoal, or parasitic diseases; heat stroke; burns; neoplasia; or severe trauma. The underlying disease causes an uncontrolled systemic inflammatory response characterized by massive activation and consumption of coagulation proteins, endogenous inhibitors, fibrinolytic proteins, and platelets.

In the initial stage of DIC, the animal is hypercoagulable because of circulating inflammatory mediators that cause activation of hemostasis through increased exposure of TF and inhibitor consumption. With time, consumption of coagulation factors, if not compensated by increased production, may lead to a hypocoagulable state with overt clinical symptoms. Because of the progressive nature of DIC, the clinical findings vary considerably and range from no overt signs of disease, accompanied by no or perhaps only subtle changes in traditional hemostasis parameters (APTT, PT, D-dimer, fibrinogen, and platelet count), to clinical signs of organ failure, associated with microvascular thrombosis in vital organs, finally culminating in overt bleeding symptoms. The latter presentation is traditionally thought of as the characteristic DIC patient, in which there are also pronounced alterations in hemostasis parameters and a drop in the platelet count.

Thromboelastography can differentiate the stage of DIC in dogs. Dogs diagnosed in the hypercoagulable stage have a much better chance of survival than dogs diagnosed in the hypocoagulable stage. This is likely because of early and aggressive intervention through supportive and/or antithrombotic therapy while the underlying disease is treated. Aggressive treatment likely minimizes thromboembolic complications and delays or even prevents progression to overt signs.

In veterinary medicine, the laboratory diagnosis of DIC is not standardized and the hemostatic function tests used are not consistent, but DIC is often diagnosed based on three or more abnormal hemostatic parameters such as APTT, PT, fibrinogen, D-dimer, platelet count, and RBC morphology, along with predisposing disease, which is a sensitive but unspecific approach. Postmortem fibrinolysis makes necropsy an insensitive diagnostic criterion.

Therapy is often empirically directed at correcting the imbalance in the hemostatic system while treating the underlying disease aggressively. Administration of balanced electrolyte solutions and plasma expanders to maintain effective circulating volume is imperative. The response to treatment with fresh-frozen plasma and heparin is unpredictable, and their use is controversial.

PATHOLOGIC THROMBOSIS

Primary or Inherited Anticoagulant Disorders

Congenital deficiency of any anticoagulant protein has not been recognized in domestic animals. If such a condition exists in animals, it is probably incompatible with life.

Secondary or Acquired Procoagulant Disorders

The presence of hypercoagulability is difficult to assess antemortem in dogs, and the importance of hypercoagulability and thromboembolic disease has not been well defined in veterinary medicine. Thromboelastography (TEG, *see* p 46) enables global assessment of hemostatic function in whole blood; advantages of TEG include the evaluation of the viscoelastic properties of the developing blood clot (including clot formation, kinetics, strength, stability, and resolution) and immediate detection of hyper- and hypocoagulable states.

Certain diseases in animals have been associated with increased risk of thrombosis. Cats with cardiomyopathy, more commonly the dilated form but also the hypertrophic and restrictive forms, can develop large thromboemboli in the aorta or brachial artery. Thrombosis has been seen in dogs with protein-losing nephropathies, hyperadrenocorticism, neoplasia, chronic hypothyroidism accompanied by atherosclerosis, and instances of autoimmune hemolytic anemia. Thrombi and thromboemboli have been seen in horses with systemic inflammatory diseases (such as colic, laminitis, or equine ehrlichial colitis) and in instances of prolonged jugular catheter placement and infusion of drugs that irritate the vasculature.

Neoplasia is a risk factor for hypercoagulability and likely associated complications, such as thromboembolic disease. Many of the cells and proteins involved in maintaining hemostasis are also involved in the processes of cancer growth, invasion, metastasis, and angiogenesis. Deep venous thrombosis is a significant clinical complication in human cancer patients, but whether this is true in dogs with cancer is unknown.

In protein-losing nephropathies (eg, glomerulopathies, nephrotic syndrome, renal amyloidosis), a deficiency of antithrombin has been well documented. Antithrombin has a molecular weight of 57,000 kilodaltons (kD), which is similar in size to albumin (60,000 kD); therefore, glomerular lesions sufficient to result in albumin loss also result in loss of antithrombin. Other abnormalities identified in renal disease include increased responsiveness of platelets to agonists, increased procoagulant activities, and decreased antiplasmin activity. Currently, the cause of thrombosis is thought to be multifactorial.

Hypercholesterolemia has been associated with increased risk of thromboembolism. It is hypothesized that endothelial and platelet membrane phospholipid concentrations are altered, which leads to damaged vasculature and increased platelet responsiveness to agonists, respectively. Increased production of thromboxane via the cyclooxygenase pathway in platelets has been seen. Diseases characterized by hypercholesterolemia include hyperadrenocorticism, diabetes mellitus, nephrotic syndrome, hypothyroidism, and pancreatitis. All have been associated with increased risk of thrombus formation, often pulmonary thrombosis.

Cats with cardiomyopathy have increased risk of thromboembolism. Endomyocardial lesions and turbulent blood flow through the heart chambers and valves secondary to altered myocardial functioning are thought to initiate thrombus formation. Specific deficiencies of anticoagulant or fibrinolytic proteins have not been seen. Interestingly, antithrombin is markedly increased but does not provide protective benefits. Cats with cardiac disease secondary to hyperthyroidism are often treated with drugs (eg, propranolol, atenolol, or diltiazem) that abate clinical signs of cardiac dysfunction. These drugs appear to protect against increased risk of thrombosis by altering platelet responsiveness to agonists.

Horses with colic associated with endotoxemia have decreased plasminogen activity and protein C antigen concentration. These horses have increased mortality and risk of thrombus formation. Laminitis is thought to be the end result of several diverse systemic disorders. Microthrombi in the vasculature of the hoof lamina have been identified in the early stages of laminitis. One theory is that endotoxin has direct effects on the vasculature and activates contact factors in the coagulation cascade. Ischemia of the lamina secondary to edema, vascular compression, and possible blood shunting at the level of the coronet also damage endothelium. When circulation is reestablished, reperfusion injury results, and the exposed subendothelial collagen promotes thrombosis.

The most appropriate treatment of an animal with thrombi or thromboemboli is diagnosis and management of the underlying disease process, along with good supportive care. Maintenance of adequate tissue perfusion is critical. Dissolution of clots and prevention of clot recurrence by administration of anticoagulants (eg, heparin and coumarin) has had mixed success. Heparin facilitates the action of antithrombin, but to be effective, adequate antithrombin must be present. In dogs with protein-losing nephropathies or in horses with endotoxemia, plasma transfusion may be necessary before heparin therapy is effective. Coumarin has been most useful for control or prevention, rather than for treatment. Fibrinolytic compounds have been administered to animals to enhance dissolution of clots. Tissue plasminogen activator (TPA) has more fibrin specificity than does streptokinase or urokinase and, therefore, provides more localized fibrinolytic effects (although not totally). The main deterrent to use of TPA is its high cost. One study of cats with aortic thrombosis treated with TPA found a risk of reperfusion injury after the clot dissolved. Streptokinase is more available and less expensive, but the therapeutic dose is difficult to determine. Many animals have naturally occurring antibodies to streptokinase as a result of previous streptococcal infections. Administration of streptokinase must be sufficient to neutralize all antibodies but not produce a systemic fibrinolytic state with resultant bleeding diathesis.

LEUKOCYTE DISORDERS

Leukocytes, or WBCs, in the blood of healthy mammals include segmented neutrophils, band neutrophils, lymphocytes, monocytes, eosinophils, and basophils. Abnormal leukocytes include neutrophils less mature than bands (eg, metamyelocytes, myelocytes, progranulocytes), blast cells of any hematopoietic lineage, mast cells, and other neoplastic cells. WBCs vary in their site of production, their duration of circulation, and the stimuli that affect their release into and migration out of the vascular system. Differences in leukocyte physiology account for species differences in normal blood cell concentrations and their responses in disease.

The leukogram, a component of the CBC, is an organized tabulation of the total nucleated cell concentration, along with the concentrations of specific WBC types present in the sample, also known as the differential. Knowledge of species-specific WBC physiology and the influence of disease processes form the basis for interpreting abnormalities of the leukogram into diagnostic information. Most leukogram interpretations define a process rather than a specific diagnosis. Processes generally fall into four groups: 1) transient physiologic responses that alter vascular hemodynamics; 2) inflammatory, infectious, and immunologic responses; 3) bone marrow responses to injury; and 4) hematopoietic cell neoplasia. (*See also* WHITE BLOOD CELLS, p 1612.)

PHYSIOLOGY OF LEUKOCYTES

Blood Vascular System

The blood vascular system is conceptually divided into two compartments: the central pool and the marginal pool. The marginal pool consists of the microcirculation at the capillary–tissue interface. The central pool consists of larger vessels. Blood samples taken by venipuncture are inherently most representative of the central pool. Flow rate, fluid movement to the extravascular space, and selective WBC adhesion to endothelium are factors that may contribute to marked differences in cell concentration in the two pools. Furthermore, these pools are in hemodynamic equilibrium with each other and the extravascular space. Therefore, WBC concentration may change appreciably because of movement of cells and/or fluid from one pool to the other as a result of a change in equilibrium. In most species, WBCs are roughly equally distributed between the two pools. Cats have a greater distribution of leukocytes within the marginal pool. WBCs in the circulating pool can be increased by certain mechanisms: epinephrine can redistribute WBCs from the marginal pool to the circulating pool, and corticosteroids can inhibit neutrophil endothelial adherence and tissue migration.

Granulocytes

Granulocytes include neutrophils, eosinophils, and basophils, all of which are produced in the bone marrow from a common stem cell. Granulopoiesis is the term used to describe production of these cells. The proliferative (or mitotic) stages of development consist of myeloblasts, promyelocytes, and myelocytes. Promyelocytes have azurophilic primary granules (lysosomes) that become inapparent in later stages. The storage (or maturation) pool consists of metamyelocytes, band neutrophils, and segmented neutrophils that are functionally mature. Specific granules, which define final cell types, are first produced at the myelocyte stage. Cell types are recognized by characteristic granule staining affinity, eg, basophilic granules for basophils, eosinophilic granules for eosinophils, and neutral or nonstaining granules for neutrophils. The population of segmented and band neutrophils in the bone marrow can be substantial in some species and is referred to as the marrow granulocyte reserve.

Neutrophils: In blood, neutrophils typically are mature (segmented), with occasional more immature band forms. Neutrophils from bone marrow enter the blood, where they remain for an average of 8 hr. They tend to adhere to the microcirculatory endothelium and then unidirectionally enter tissues, where they may participate in host defense. Given the short lifespan of neutrophils in blood, maintenance of blood neutrophil concentration depends on a relatively high, steady delivery from bone marrow. This balance may change dramatically when there is either increased tissue demand associated with the development of an inflammatory process or a stem-cell injury that reduces the marrow production rate. During initiation of an inflammatory lesion, local mononuclear cell release of specific stimulating factors rapidly stimulates bone marrow to release neutrophil reserve and accelerate granulopoiesis. When the tissue demand is intense, marrow production and release may accelerate dramatically, resulting in a left shift and toxic changes (*see* p 57).

Eosinophils: Eosinophils function in parasite killing and also contain enzymes that modulate products of mast cells released in response to antigen-IgE receptor mast cell degranulation in allergic disease. For example, histamine released by mast cells is modulated by histaminase in eosinophils. Eosinophilia is primarily induced by allergic inflammatory responses and tissue invading parasitic infestations. Less commonly, neoplasia may be associated with paraneoplastic induction of eosinophilia. Localized eosinophilic tissue lesions do not necessarily produce a peripheral eosinophilia, eg, the eosinophilic granuloma dermatopathies and oral lesions of cats. Eosinopenia is a component of corticosteroid-induced (stress) leukograms.

Basophils: Basophils are rare in all common domestic animals. Basophil granules contain histamine, heparin, and sulfated mucopolysaccharides; understanding of their function is limited. As a result, there is no clear interpretation for basophilia. Basophilia is uncommon but may accompany eosinophilia, and it is the latter that is interpreted. Although blood basophils and tissue mast cells have similar enzymatic contents, basophils do not become mast cells. They appear to arise from separate marrow stem cells.

Monocytes

Monocytes are formed in the bone marrow from monoblasts and then develop to promonocytes and finally mature monocytes. Monocytes enter the peripheral blood for ~24–36 hr and exit into tissues to mature into tissue macrophages. Monocytes and macrophages perform phagocytosis of organisms and cellular debris at sites of inflammation or tissue injury. They may form multinucleated giant cells, particularly in response to foreign bodies or complex organisms that elicit granuloma formation, such as *Mycobacterium* spp. Monocytes and macrophages are a major source of colony-stimulating factors and cytokines that regulate inflammatory responses, and they function as antigen-processing cells.

Lymphocytes

Lymphocytes originate from a bone marrow stem cell and mature in lymph nodes, spleen, and other subepithelial lymphoid tissues. Mature lymphocytes consist of two major subpopulations, B cells and T cells. **B cells** (for bone marrow or bursa equivalent) are potential precursors of plasma cells that produce antibodies for humoral immunity. **T cells** (for thymus) engage in cellular immunity (eg, histocompatibility and delayed-type hypersensitivity). Lymphocytes in tissue may return to the vascular system and recirculate. Some lymphocytes are very long-lived compared with other WBC types.

LEUKOGRAM ABNORMALITIES

Abnormalities of the leukogram include quantitative or numerical concentration abnormalities and WBC morphologic abnormalities.

Numerical Abnormalities: WBC concentration values are interpreted by comparison with species-specific reference values. Interpretations should be made only by considering the absolute numbers. For reference values for total WBC and differential WBC concentrations in absolute numbers for common domestic species, *see* TABLE 6, p 3176. The total WBC concentration is more variable and often higher in neonates than in adults. Age-related reference values should be used to evaluate leukograms in young animals, especially species in which lymphocytes are more numerous (and neutrophils less numerous) in adults, such as ruminants. Generally, differential WBC patterns of adults are reached at about the age of sexual maturity.

Abnormality in the total WBC concentration is useful only to alert the clinician to look for and interpret abnormalities in the cell distributions in the differential. When the total WBC is abnormal, one or more distributional abnormalities in the differential are likely. When the total WBC is normal, there still may be one or more distributional abnormalities in the differential. As a result, evaluation of the differential absolute values is the most important component of the leukogram.

Leukocytosis is an increase in the total WBC concentration, whereas leukopenia is a decrease in the total WBC concentration. Changes in the concentrations of specific leukocyte types are more important for clinical interpretation purposes.

Neutrophilia or neutrophilic leukocytosis is an increase in neutrophil concentration. Lymphocytosis is an increase in lymphocyte concentration. Monocytosis is an increase in monocyte concentration. Eosinophilia refers to an increase in eosinophil concentration, and basophilia to an increase in basophil concentration. Metarubricytosis is an increase in nucleated RBCs (nRBCs) in blood. Mastocytosis is an increase in mast cells in blood.

Decreases in concentration of a cell type are indicated by the suffix "penia." This is applied only to cell types in which a decrease is possible. It does not apply to cell types for which the concentration may be 0, such as monocytes, basophils, nRBCs, and any other abnormal cell type. Hence, neutropenia is a decrease in neutrophil concentration, lymphopenia is a decrease in lymphocyte concentration, and eosinopenia is a decrease in eosinophil concentration. Cytopenia is a nonspecific term indicating a decrease in cell concentration(s), but the cell type is not specified. Pancytopenia indicates all cell types are decreased, often to a severe degree.

Terms used to describe or qualify abnormalities most often associated with inflammatory responses include various left shifts and leukemoid response. A left shift is an increase in concentration of immature, nonsegmented neutrophils, typically bands, but may also include metamyelocytes or even more immature forms. A regenerative left shift describes leukocytosis characterized by the combination of neutrophilia and a left shift. In this situation, the segmented neutrophils will be greater in concentration than bands and less mature forms. A **degenerative left shift** describes a neutrophil pattern characterized by normal to decreased total neutrophil concentration, but with a left shift in which the concentration of bands and less mature forms is greater than segmented neutrophils. This is an indication of maximal release from bone marrow in response to inflammation and signifies the presence of an acute, severe lesion. A **leukemoid response** describes a marked neutrophilia of a magnitude sufficient to indicate chronicity of an inflammatory response and corresponding substantial increase in granulopoiesis in the bone marrow. The magnitude is also such that myeloproliferative disease becomes a diagnostic consideration. Guidelines for neutrophilic leukocytosis considered to indicate a leukemoid response are >70,000/μL (70×10^9/L) for dogs, >50,000/μL (50×10^9/L) for cats, >30,000/μL (30×10^9/L) for horses, and >20,000/μL (20×10^9/L) for ruminants.

Morphologic Abnormalities: Abnormalities of morphology may be associated with either acquired or inherited disease.

Toxic changes are identified only in neutrophils. The term originates from historical observation that certain cell features were associated with general, usually overwhelming, toxic states, such as systemic bacterial infections and severe, acute inflammatory lesions. The term is misleading in that it implies neutrophil injury. The cells are not injured and have normal function. Toxic change is best defined as a set of morphologic changes observed on the blood smear that occur as a result of accelerated marrow production of neutrophils. The accelerated production is in response to relatively severe inflammatory states that maximally stimulate the bone marrow. Morphologic changes include (in order of frequency) diffuse cytoplasmic basophilia, Döhle bodies, and fine cytoplasmic vacuolation. More rare changes include increased prominence of cytoplasmic azurophilic granules, cellular gigantism, and binucleation. Toxic change is almost always associated with the concurrent presence of a left shift. It is graded as mild, moderate, or severe by subjective evaluation of the more common changes noted on examination of a blood smear. Döhle bodies, blue-gray cytoplasmic inclusions, are aggregates of endoplasmic reticulum. They are unique in that they may be found in clinically healthy cats and therefore are not interpreted as toxic change in this species unless accompanied by other features.

Reactive lymphocytes have increased, distinctly basophilic cytoplasm and may have irregular or clefted nuclei. They may vary considerably in diameter. They have condensed chromatin and therefore are not blasts. They are interpreted as immunologically stimulated B cells.

Granular lymphocytes have condensed chromatin and increased pale blue-gray cytoplasm that contains several small pink or azurophilic granules. The nucleus may be round to clefted. These are large granular lymphocytes and may be either natural killer (NK) lymphocytes or T lymphocytes.

Blast cells are usually an indication of hematopoietic cell neoplasia if they are reproducible or present in large numbers.

Their lineage may be tentatively identified by morphologic criteria, but flow cytometric analysis is required to definitively identify lineage.

Many of the following morphologic changes are uncommon.

Chédiak-Higashi syndrome (*see* p 50) described in Persian cats, people, mink, foxes, Hereford and Brangus cattle, mice, and killer whales is an autosomal recessive defect involving lysosomal granules. There is hyperfusion of granules resulting in large, eosinophilic cytoplasmic inclusions. Susceptibility to bacterial infections is increased, as is the tendency to bleed because of both neutrophil and platelet function abnormalities. Partial oculocutaneous albinism due to abnormal melanin granule formation may occur.

The **mucopolysaccharidoses** are a group of lysosomal storage disorders in which there is a defect in degradation of glycosaminoglycans. Both neutrophils and lymphocytes may contain accumulated mucopolysaccharide product in the form of purple or metachromatic intracytoplasmic granules. Lymphocytes may also be vacuolated. These disorders are associated with a variety of systemic clinical abnormalities and are seen in dogs and cats.

Another group of lysosomal storage disorders recognized in dogs and cats may result in **cytoplasmic vacuoles** predominantly in lymphocytes and occasionally in neutrophils. These disorders include gangliosidoses, α-mannosidosis, Niemann-Pick disease variants, acid-lipase deficiency, and fucosidosis. Most of these disorders result in severe, progressive neurologic disorders resulting from accumulated product in neuronal tissue.

Locoweed toxicity is regarded as an acquired form of lysosomal storage defect in large animals. It is due to toxic principle from the plant that inhibits one or more enzymes of oligosaccharide metabolism. This may result in vacuolation in lymphocytes.

Pelger-Huët anomaly is a nuclear hyposegmentation defect of granulocytes in people, cats, rabbits, horses, and dogs that are heterozygous for the anomaly. Neutrophils have normal function but a near absence of segmented nuclear morphology. Most or all of the neutrophils appear as bands and metamyelocytes and may appear as a marked left shift in an otherwise normal leukogram. Eosinophils and basophils, if present, also exhibit nuclear hyposegmentation. Affected heterozygote animals are clinically normal; the homozygous inheritance of the trait is lethal.

Hypersegmentation is an increased degree of nuclear segmentation resulting in multiple lobes connected by nuclear filaments. It is a nonspecific indication of increased time in circulation and is normal aging of the cell. This may be seen with stress leukograms or corticosteroid administration.

Leukocyte agglutination may occur with either neutrophils or lymphocytes. This is seen on low magnification as aggregates of 5–15 tightly clumped leukocytes. Avid agglutination may result in a markedly false low total WBC concentration on some cell counting instruments. This is likely due to the presence of a naturally occurring cold agglutinin that is operative only in vitro at laboratory temperature. There is no known clinical significance.

Infectious disease inclusions are occasionally recognized. Canine distemper inclusions may be seen in neutrophils, monocytes, and lymphocytes, as well as in newly produced erythrocytes. The ehrlichioses of various animal species and canine hepatozoonosis may have cytoplasmic inclusions of respective organisms of these tickborne diseases.

Specific Interpretative Leukogram Responses

The abnormal leukogram is typically interpreted into one of several responses, each of which may consist of one or more abnormalities in the differential. Some may also be associated with concurrent changes in erythrocytes and platelets. Important species differences in leukogram responses are described below.

Corticosteroid-induced or Stress Response: In this very common leukocyte response, endogenous steroid release from stress or treatment with exogenous corticosteroids results in a leukogram with multiple changes. Lymphopenia is the most consistent change, and mature neutrophilia is usually present. Monocytosis and eosinopenia are expected changes in dogs but are more variable in other species. Neutrophilia is due to decreased adherence to the vascular endothelium, which inhibits margination and increases circulating time. As a result, neutrophils may also become hypersegmented. There may also be increased marrow release of neutrophils. Lymphocytes become redistributed to lymphoid tissues instead of remaining in circulation. This response may be misinterpreted as inflammation, but a left shift is not usually present.

Excitement or Epinephrine Response: Leukocytosis may occur as a result of exercise or excitement; this response is mediated by increased epinephrine concentration and may be thought of as a transient physiologic response. Epinephrine flushes cells from the marginal to the central pool. The effect may double the total WBC concentration within minutes. In addition, splenic contraction releases WBCs and RBCs into the peripheral circulation. The leukocytosis is usually due to a mature neutrophilia without a left shift. Lymphocytosis may be present, especially in young horses or cats. The effect in cats is often recognized as a prominent lymphocytosis—as much as two times the upper reference value. The excitement response is relatively uncommon in dogs.

Inflammatory Response: The concentration of neutrophils in blood in response to inflammatory disease is highly variable and dynamic. It is best viewed as a balance between tissue demand and bone marrow production at all phases of the response. There are important species differences in this balance that are related to bone marrow storage reserve and proliferative capacity.

At the beginning of an inflammatory process, the bone marrow responds by delivery of its reserve of late-stage maturing neutrophils, including band cells. If consumption exceeds marrow delivery during this acute stage, neutropenia with a prominent left shift will develop. In dogs and cats, this is an indication of severity of the inflammatory lesion.

Subsequently, it takes 2–4 days for the marrow to accelerate neutrophil production by increased stem-cell entry and expansion of proliferative stages that feed the maturation stages and amplify neutrophil delivery to blood. In dogs, the acute stage of the inflammatory response is usually characterized by mild to moderate neutrophilia, with the left shift being somewhat proportional to severity of demand.

After a few days, accelerated bone marrow production adds to the picture. Neutrophilia may increase along with left shift and toxic changes. As the process becomes chronic, the balance between increased marrow output and consumption may favor the development of even higher magnitudes of neutrophilia. The most chronic form, present for weeks or even months, is described as a "closed cavity" inflammatory process. The lesion becomes somewhat walled off and therefore consumes fewer neutrophils, yet it still stimulates maximal marrow production. Examples of closed cavity processes are pyometra in dogs and traumatic reticuloperitonitis (hardware disease) in cattle. In these conditions, the magnitude of the total WBC concentration, consisting of neutrophilia, may be as high as 100,000/μL (100×10^9/L) of blood in dogs.

Extreme neutrophilia, exceeding upper limits usually seen in inflammation, may be associated with leukemia, *Hepatozoon canis* infections, and rarely other neoplasms that produce colony-stimulating factors.

In contrast, cattle and most other ruminants have a relatively low reserve of bone marrow neutrophils and a lower capacity for accelerating granulopoiesis. This is reflected in the relatively low neutrophil concentration in normal ruminant blood. As a result, acute inflammation in cows is characterized by neutropenia that can be profound. Therefore, neutropenia in cattle does not reveal the degree of inflammatory severity. After several days, the bone marrow response may establish a return of blood neutrophils in modest concentration, characterized by a marked left shift and toxic changes. Chronic, closed cavity inflammatory lesions are associated with magnitudes of neutrophilia that rarely exceed 25,000/μL of blood. Cats and horses are intermediate in these responses, with cats being more like dogs and horses being more like cattle. Pigs have an inflammatory leukogram similar to that of dogs.

Bovine leukocyte adhesion deficiency is a lethal, autosomal recessive disorder of Holstein cattle. It is associated with marked neutrophilia; the neutrophils have a deficiency of the glycoproteins (integrins) that are essential for normal leukocyte adherence and emigration from the vasculature. Recurrent bacterial infections, persistent neutrophilia (often >100,000/μL [100×10^9/L]), lymphocytosis, and death (usually between 2 wk and 8 mo of age) are characteristic. Calves often are stunted and have recurrent pneumonia, ulcerative stomatitis, enteritis, and periodontitis. On examination of tissues, there are few neutrophils, except within vessel lumens, because they persist in the circulation and have impaired entry into the tissues. Testing is available to detect carriers. A similar defect has also been reported in some Irish Setter dogs.

Neutropenia may develop because of excessive tissue demand for neutrophils or reduced granulopoiesis. It may be seen with overwhelming bacterial infections, especially gram-negative septicemia or endotoxemia, in all species. Immune-mediated destruction of neutrophils is diagnosed by exclusion of other consumptive processes. Stem-cell injury may occur from many causes such as certain viral infections (*see* TABLE 7), chemical injury, and idiosyncratic drug reactions, eg, sulfonamides, penicillins, cephalosporins, and chloramphenicol in cats. These reactions typically affect all bone marrow cell lines but are recognized initially as neutropenia because of the relatively short lifespan of this cell type.

Neutropenia is seen in the now rare **cyclic hematopoiesis syndrome of gray Collie dogs**, also known as canine cyclic neutropenia. It is an inherited, autosomal recessive disease characterized by a profound periodic neutropenia, associated overwhelming recurrent bacterial infections, bleeding, and coat color dilution. The defect is due to a mutation in a protein that may regulate neutrophil elastase activity. Neutrophil maturation is arrested at regular intervals of 11–14 days; the peripheral blood neutropenia lasts 3–4 days and is followed by neutrophilia. All other hematopoietic cells, including lymphocytes, also have cyclic production that is minimally evident because of the relatively long circulation time of other cell types. Affected puppies often die at birth or during the first week and rarely live >1 yr. Surviving dogs may be stunted and weak and develop serious recurrent bacterial infections during periods of neutropenia.

Monocytosis may be seen in the inflammatory pattern at any stage of its progression. Monocytosis is more likely, and tends to be of greater magnitude, when the process becomes chronic.

Combined Corticosteroid-induced and Inflammatory Response: Inflammatory disease processes commonly induce a concurrent endogenous corticosteroid response, recognized by the presence of lymphopenia in conjunction with an inflammatory neutrophil response (left shift). The neutrophil response to inflammation overrides and may be additive to the corticosteroid influence on neutrophils.

Lymphocytosis: Mild lymphocytosis and reactive lymphocytes may occur after vaccination. Modest lymphocytosis, in the range of 7,000–20,000/μL (7–20 × 10^9/L), should prompt consideration of a possible physiologic excitement response, particularly in cats. If that is excluded, then a lymphoproliferative disorder should be considered. If examination of lymphocyte morphology reveals prolymphocytes and/or blast cells, then lymphocytic leukemia is the working interpretation. If the cells are all small with normal appearing chromatin, then chronic lymphocytic leukemia is a consideration requiring further evaluation. Chronic ehrlichiosis may result in lymphocytosis of this magnitude in dogs. At higher concentrations, the lymphocytosis may be regarded as conclusive evidence of leukemia.

Persistent lymphocytosis in cattle is defined by lymphocyte concentrations consistently >7,500/μL (7.5 × 10^9/L). It is due to a B-cell proliferation that occurs in a subset of animals infected with bovine leukemia virus (BLV). Affected cattle are usually asymptomatic. The finding of persistent lymphocytosis is regarded as a positive indication of BLV infection in the individual. A smaller subset of BLV-infected cattle, either with or without lymphocytosis, may progress to develop lymphoma or lymphocytic leukemia.

Lymphopenia: Lymphopenia is a common leukogram abnormality most commonly associated with endogenous (stress) or exogenous corticosteroid administration. The most likely cause is steroid-induced apoptosis of lymphocytes. Lymphopenia also rarely occurs due to

TABLE 7 VIRAL INFECTIONS THAT MAY CAUSE TRANSIENT NEUTROPENIA

Species	Infection
Dogs	Parvovirus, canine distemper (acute phase)
Cats	Panleukopenia (parvovirus), feline leukemia virus
Horses	Equine influenza, equine viral arteritis (acute phase), equine herpesvirus
Cattle	Bovine viral diarrhea virus
Pigs	Classical swine fever virus, African swine fever virus

other causes, such as extravasation of lymph (eg, lymphangiectasia, chylous effusion), some viral infections with tropism for rapidly dividing cells (eg, parvoviral infections), and hereditary immunodeficiency disease (eg, combined immunodeficiency disease of Arabian foals).

Stem-cell Injury and Pancytopenia: A number of factors may cause reversible or irreversible stem-cell injury. These injuries may affect erythrocyte, platelet, lymphocyte, and/or granulocyte production. Because of short circulating lifespan, neutropenia is often the first abnormality seen. When chronic or irreversible, these injuries result in decreases in all three major blood cell lines, with the hemogram demonstrating leukopenia, nonregenerative anemia, and thrombocytopenia. General causes include 1) overdoses of radiation and antineoplastic drugs, 2) drug or plant toxicities (eg, estrogen toxicity in dogs, bracken fern toxicity in cattle, phenylbutazone toxicity in species other than horses), 3) hematopoietic cell neoplasia involving bone marrow (myelophthisis), and 4) viral infections that injure rapidly dividing cells and may cause transient neutropenia (*see* TABLE 7).

Eosinophilia and Basophilia: Eosinophilia, or the combination of eosinophilia and basophilia, prompts the consideration of the following processes: allergic-based inflammation, parasitic infestation, subepithelial (skin, respiratory, GI) inflammation that is likely allergic in nature, and less commonly, paraneoplastic induction. Eosinophilia is seen in most dogs with heartworm disease and may be seen in dogs and cats with flea infestation.

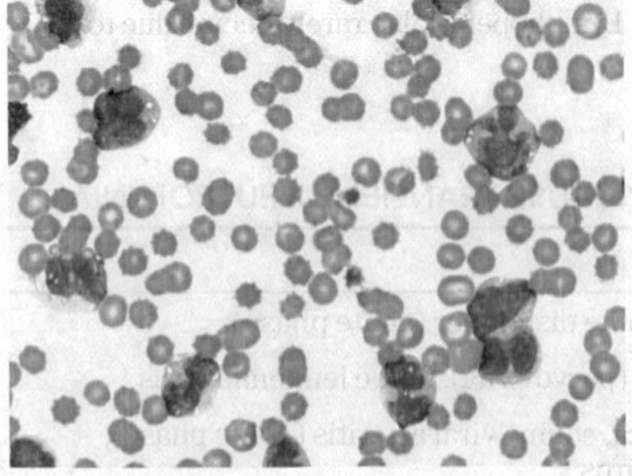

Leukemia, canine blood smear; note several atypical large cells of hematopoietic origin with convoluted nuclei. *Courtesy of Dr. Darren Wood.*

Hypereosinophilic syndrome has been reported in cats, dogs, and ferrets. This poorly understood syndrome is characterized by consistent marked eosinophilia and eosinophil tissue infiltration with associated organ dysfunction. Decreased concentration of these cell types in blood has no pathologic relevance.

Prominent Metarubricytosis: Although typically absent, metarubricytes occasionally become a major component of the total nucleated cell count. The magnitude may be 10%–50% of the nucleated cell population or more, with absolute numbers reaching 5,000–10,000/µL ($5–10 \times 10^9$/L). This may occur rarely in early phases of an intense regenerative response to anemia. It may also be associated with endothelial injury (eg, heat stroke) resulting in abnormal release rate of nRBCs from marrow. Most nRBCs will be counted as lymphocytes on cell counters with differential capability. This may result in a preliminary result of lymphocytosis being corrected later only by examination of the blood smear.

Hematopoietic Cell Neoplasia and Leukemia: Most cases of hematopoietic cell neoplasia of either lymphocytic or bone marrow origin will have some abnormal cells in blood. Sometimes, neoplastic cells are present in low numbers and are detected only by scanning the blood smear under low magnification. Finding abnormal hematopoietic precursor cells in blood in small numbers prompts investigation of bone marrow and/or other hematopoietic tissues (such as the spleen) for possible neoplastic disease.

The opposite extreme is marked leukocytosis with a predominance of the abnormal (neoplastic) cell population. In this situation, the blood sample is diagnostic for leukemia. If poorly differentiated, the cells are classified as blasts, with possible cell lineage determined based on morphologic appearance. If well differentiated, the cell lineage is usually more clear, because the cells are mature.

Lymphocytic leukemias are more common in domestic animals than are myeloproliferative disorders (ie, leukemias of granulocytes, erythrocytes, or platelets). Myelodysplasia is a term used to describe peripheral blood cytopenias, a hyperplastic response in bone marrow, and dysplastic features in developing cells. This can occur with a toxic insult to the bone marrow but may also indicate a preleukemic phase, and serial hemograms should be monitored.

A distinction is often made between an "acute" or "chronic" leukemia. The terms are more in reference to the clinical course of the disease rather than the duration of the tumor. An acute leukemia of leukocytes often causes systemic signs of illness and a poor short-term prognosis. These animals have variable numbers of poorly differentiated blast cells in circulation, as well as cytopenias in other cell lines. In contrast, a chronic leukemia of leukocytes often causes few to no clinical signs, may be discovered incidentally, and can have a long clinical course. These animals usually have large numbers of well-differentiated cells in circulation and lack cytopenias.

Considerable progress is being made in the use of monoclonal antibody labeling and flow cytometric analysis to better establish cell lineage, particularly when the morphology is equivocal. This is particularly useful for poorly differentiated leukemias, in which morphology alone is unreliable. The distinction between well-differentiated or chronic myelogenous leukemia and extreme neutrophilic leukocytosis can be difficult.

LYMPHADENITIS AND LYMPHANGITIS

CASEOUS LYMPHADENITIS OF SHEEP AND GOATS

Caseous lymphadenitis (CL) is a chronic, contagious disease caused by the bacterium *Corynebacterium pseudotuberculosis*. Although prevalence of CL varies by region and country, it is found worldwide and is of major concern for small ruminant producers in North America. The disease is characterized by abscess formation in or near major peripheral lymph nodes (external form) or within internal organs and lymph nodes (internal form). Although both the external and internal forms of CL occur in sheep and goats, the external form is more common in goats, and the internal form is more common in sheep. Economic losses from CL include death, condemnation and trim of infected carcasses, hide and wool loss, loss of sales for breeding animals, and premature culling of affected animals from the herd or flock. Once established on a farm or region (endemic), it is primarily maintained by contamination of the environment with active draining lesions, animals with the internal form of the disease that contaminate the environment through nasal discharge or coughing, the ability of the bacteria to survive harsh environmental conditions, and lack of strict biosecurity necessary to reduce the number and prevent introduction of new cases. Although CL is typically considered a disease of sheep and goats, it also occurs more sporadically in horses, cattle, camelids, swine, wild ruminants, fowl, and people. Because of its zoonotic potential, care should be taken when handling infected animals or purulent exudate from active, draining lesions.

Etiology and Pathogenesis: *C pseudotuberculosis* is a gram-positive, facultative, intracellular coccobacillus. Two biotypes have been identified based on the ability of the bacteria to reduce nitrate: a nitrate-negative group that infects sheep and goats, and a nitrate-positive group that infects horses. Isolates from cattle are a heterogeneous group. All strains produce an exotoxin called phospholipase D that enhances dissemination of the bacteria by damaging endothelial cells and increasing vascular permeability. The bacterium has a second virulence factor which is an external lipid coat that provides protection from hydrolytic enzymes in host phagocytes. Replication of bacteria occurs in the phagocytes, which then rupture and release bacteria. The ongoing process of bacterial replication, followed by attraction and subsequent death of inflammatory cells, forms the characteristic abscesses associated with CL.

To establish infection, *C pseudotuberculosis* must penetrate skin or mucous membranes. The most common site of entry is the skin after an injury that may result from shearing, tagging, tail docking, castration, or other environmental hazards resulting in skin trauma. Contact with purulent material draining from open, active lesions most commonly serves as the source of bacteria through these breaches in the skin. Although less common, entry across mucous membranes from inhalation or ingestion of the bacteria also serves as a means of infection.

Once the bacteria have entered the body, they move to the lymph nodes via the regional draining lymphatic system.

Internally, the bacteria establish infection not only in the lymph nodes but also in the viscera. The incubation period varies from 1 to 3 mo, culminating in development of encapsulated abscesses. *C pseudotuberculosis* is hardy in the environment and can survive on fomites such as bedding and wood for 2 mo and in soil for 8 mo. The presence of organic material, shade, and moisture favor and enhance survival.

Clinical Findings: The hallmark clinical finding in cases of external CL is the development of abscesses in the region of peripheral lymph nodes. Common sites of development include the submandibular, parotid, prescapular, and prefemoral nodes. Less commonly, abscessation of supramammary or inguinal lymph nodes occurs, in addition to an occasional ectopic location along the lymphatic chain. If left untreated, these lesions eventually mature into open draining abscesses. The purulent material from these lesions has no odor and varies in consistency from soft and pasty (more common in goats) to thick and caseous (more common in sheep). Once natural draining occurs, the skin lesion heals with scarring. Recurrence is common, which can be months later. CL should be highly suspected in a sheep or goat with abscessation in these regions. Although other bacteria may also cause abscessation in these locations (and in other animals), because of the ramifications of the presence of this disease within a herd or flock, these cases should be handled as CL until proved otherwise.

The internal form of CL most commonly presents as chronic weight loss and failure to thrive. The presence of other clinical signs depends on the organs of involvement, which may include any of the major organ systems. Lung abscessation is a common site of visceral involvement in internal CL; therefore, signs of chronic ill thrift with cough, purulent nasal discharge, fever, and tachypnea with increased lung sounds may be noted. The internal form is more common in sheep and has been termed the "thin ewe syndrome."

The incidence of abscesses and development of clinical disease with either the external or internal form increases with age.

Lesions: In sheep, abscesses often have the classically described laminated "onion-ring" appearance in cross section, with concentric fibrous layers separated by inspissated caseous exudate. In goats, the abscesses are less organized, and the exudate is usually soft and pasty.

Diagnosis: The presence of an external abscess on a small ruminant is highly suggestive of CL, especially in locations of peripheral lymph nodes. However, definitive diagnosis is only by bacteriologic culture of purulent material from an intact abscess. Although other pyogenic organisms such as *Trueperella pyogenes* (formerly *Arcanobacterium pyogenes*), *Staphylococcus aureus*, *Pasteurella multocida*, and anaerobes such as *Fusobacterium necrophorum* can cause abscessation, affected animals should be kept isolated pending culture results. Animals with visceral abscesses pose a greater diagnostic challenge. Radiography and ultrasonography can be useful to detect internal lesions. Culture of a transtracheal aspirate obtained from an animal with pneumonia can help determine whether CL is the cause. Excluding other causes of chronic weight loss and ill thrift in the face of proper nutrition and good appetite such as Johne's disease, parasitism, and poor dentition further raise suspicion.

In the absence of accessible abscesses for bacterial culture, definitive diagnosis of active cases of CL is challenging. Although many diagnostic tools are available, results of these tests must be interpreted with caution and with consideration of herd or flock history, the presence or absence of active infection within the herd or flock, and vaccination status. A synergistic hemolysin inhibition (SHI) test that detects antibodies to the phospholipase D exotoxin is available at many diagnostic laboratories. Positive titers indicate past resolved infections, recent exposure, recent vaccination, or active lesions or their development. Titers of 1:256 or higher have been correlated in past studies with the presence of active, developing abscesses; however, in a recent

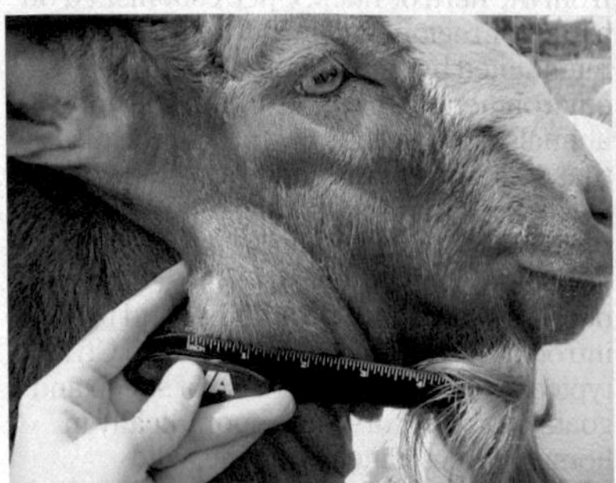

Caseous lymphadenitis lesions, external form, submandibular lymph node in a goat. *Courtesy of Dr. Kevin Washburn.*

study, a high titer was poorly correlated with presence or development of abscesses over an 18-mo period. When the status of an animal with a positive titer is in doubt, the titer should be repeated in 2–4 wk. If the titer is rising and clinical signs of abscesses are noted, then CL can be assumed to be the cause. False-negative results can occur if testing is done in the first 2 wk after exposure before the animal has seroconverted. Also, animals with chronic, walled-off abscesses can have a false-negative result. Colostral titers usually disappear by 3–6 mo of age, so serologic testing of lambs or kids <6 mo old should be interpreted with caution.

Treatment and Control: Once a diagnosis of CL has been established, owner education stressing the persistent, recurrent nature of the disease is necessary. The most practical approach for commercial animals infected with CL is to cull them from the herd or flock. However, animals with draining abscesses should not be sent through sale barns until draining has ceased and the wound has healed. Treatment of individual animals should be undertaken with the understanding that CL is not considered a "curable" disease. Animals with genetic or emotional value are treated mainly for aesthetic reasons and to limit their infectivity to the rest of the herd or flock. Treatment options have included lancing and draining, surgical excision, formalin injection of lesions, systemic antibiotics, and intralesional antibiotics.

If external abscesses are lanced and drained, the cavity should be lavaged with dilute iodine solution and the animal isolated in an area that can be disinfected until the lesion stops draining and heals. Drained purulent material should be carefully collected and disposed of. Dilute bleach and chlorhexidine solutions are effective disinfectants of hard surfaces and fomites, but the presence of organic material on these surfaces inactivates them and drastically reduces or prohibits effectiveness. Intact accessible abscesses can be surgically removed; however, this option is more expensive, and undetected abscesses are often present and continue to develop. Recurrence rates with either lancing or surgical removal are high.

The practice of injecting abscesses with formalin should be strongly discouraged, because the FDA has zero tolerance for extra-label use of a potent carcinogen in food-producing animals. The efficacy of systemic antimicrobial therapy and, more recently, intralesional antimicrobial therapy has been investigated. However, use of any antimicrobial for treatment of CL is extra-label; therefore, strict adherence to published guidelines on withdrawal times and an established veterinarian-client-patient relationship are mandatory. Longterm administration of procaine penicillin G and rifampin has been efficacious in some cases. Penicillin alone, although efficacious in vitro, is unlikely to effectively penetrate the capsule of developed abscesses, as are many, if not most, of the water-soluble or moderately lipid-soluble antimicrobials. However, recent studies have shown that administration of one dose of tulathromycin at 2.5 mg/kg, either SC directly into the abscess cavity, or two doses at 2.5 mg/kg, administered at the same time, one SC and one intralesionally, can resolve the lesions without lancing the abscess. Further, effective concentrations of tulathromycin can be achieved within walled-off abscesses caused by *C pseudotuberculosis* after a single dose at 2.5 mg/kg, SC. The highly lipid-soluble property of tulathromycin may be particularly helpful in cases of internal CL, when abscesses are not accessible for other forms of treatment. Despite the efficacy of intralesional and parenteral administration of tulathromycin in many cases, recurrence remains a problem. Therefore, use of these drugs cannot be considered curative but rather an acceptable alternative to manage cases of CL when culling from the herd or flock is not an acceptable option for the owner.

Because of the nature of the causative organism, common means of exposure, chronicity of the disease, and difficulty in completely eliminating the organism from individual animals, control of CL revolves around strict biosecurity measures. The overriding goals of any control program are to eliminate the disease from the herd or flock and to reduce the number of new cases either from the spread of disease or introduction to the farm.

Ideally, animals identified as infected should immediately be culled. If immediate removal is not possible, infected animals should be isolated from the rest of the herd or flock. Diligence in this practice will eventually result in decreased prevalence as animals that develop active cases are identified and removed, and given there are no new animals incubating the disease introduced to the premises.

When elimination through culling is not a viable option for the owner, control of CL is challenging at best. Dividing the herds or flocks into "clean" and "infected" groups and eliminating older and less genetically valuable animals over time is one control strategy.

Lambs and kids from infected dams can be raised on pasteurized colostrum and milk away from infected animals. However, the internal form of CL and animals incubating the disease can maintain infection within the "asymptomatic clean" group and limit the success of this approach.

Commercial CL vaccines are currently licensed for use in sheep and goats. These vaccines should only be used in the species they are labeled for, because adverse reactions have been reported in goats given vaccine labeled for sheep. Rigidly adhering to vaccination schedules according to the manufacturer's labeling can help reduce the prevalence and incidence of CL within herds or flocks. However, it is important to emphasize that efficacy of these vaccines is not 100%, and vaccination will not clear infected animals. Vaccination of young replacement stock should be considered, and older infected animals should be gradually culled as economics allow. Once the disease is at a low prevalence rate, vaccination should be stopped and all seropositive unvaccinated animals culled. In "clean" herds or flocks that have no history of CL, vaccination is not recommended.

The risks of disease transmission among animals should be recognized when shearing or dipping, and management practices should be adjusted accordingly. Animals with noted lesions should be shorn last, and clipper blades disinfected between animals. Shearers should recognize the hazards associated with contact with purulent material and the possibility of acting as mechanical vectors, either on clothing or via equipment, for spread of the bacteria to new animals. Further, dipping tank solutions should be kept as fresh as possible, because *C pseudotuberculosis* can survive within them and serve as a source of infection of freshly shorn sheep that have skin abrasions.

Owners should remove hazardous items (barbed wire, exposed nails, rough feeders) from the environment to decrease injury and potential CL transmission from the presence of bacteria on these fomites.

One of the most common ways CL can be introduced into a previously "clean" herd or flock, or reintroduced to one in which CL has been reduced or eliminated, is through the addition of replacement stock. Often, animals from other farms that are asymptomatic on arrival are incubating the disease and then manifest infection weeks to months later. Purchasing animals from sources with unknown histories is hazardous to maintaining a "clean" herd or flock. Newly arrived animals should be examined thoroughly for signs of CL such as abscesses or scars near peripheral lymph nodes. They should remain isolated from the rest of the herd or flock until their serologic status is determined, and only animals that are seronegative with no evidence of present or past CL lesions should be allowed to enter the herd or flock.

CORYNEBACTERIUM PSEUDOTUBERCULOSIS INFECTION OF HORSES AND CATTLE

(Pigeon fever, Dry land distemper)

In horses, *Corynebacterium pseudotuberculosis* causes ulcerative lymphangitis (an infection of the lower limbs) and chronic abscesses in the pectoral region and ventral abdomen. It is one of the most common and economically important infectious diseases of horses in California and Texas and is increasing in prevalence in other western and Midwestern states of the USA. In cattle, the bacteria most commonly cause cutaneous excoriated granulomas. Large, ulcerative skin lesions resembling infected granulation tissue and lymphangitis may occur in 2%–5% of cows. Location on the animal is variable but is often associated with skin trauma. Healing often occurs without treatment or with limited topical treatment in 2–4 wk. Abortion and mastitis may also occur. Rarely, visceral involvement has been reported.

Pathogenesis and Clinical Findings: The onset of ulcerative lymphangitis in horses is variable and usually manifests as painful inflammation, nodules, and ulcers, especially in the region of the lower limb, or lameness and edematous swelling can extend up the entire limb. The exudate is odorless, thick, tan, and blood tinged. Usually, only one leg is involved. If the animal is not treated aggressively with antimicrobials, lesions and swelling usually progress and become chronic with relapses.

In the southwestern USA, *C pseudotuberculosis* infection in horses is seasonal, with a peak incidence in summer and fall. Infection results in abscessation of the pectoral region or ventral abdominal region with secondary dissemination to internal organs. Clinical signs include diffuse or localized swellings, ventral pitting edema, ventral midline dermatitis, lameness, draining abscesses or tracts, fever, weight loss, and depression. Leukocytosis and neutrophilia may be present. A marked or prolonged fever, anorexia, or weight loss indicates untoward sequelae such as deep or recurring abscesses, internal abscessation, or systemic infection with abortion. Abscesses can be large, up to 20 cm in diameter before rupturing, and take weeks to months to resolve. Weight loss, colic, splinted abdomen, or lethargy may be signs of internal abscesses. Dermatitis lesions are painful and mildly pruritic with alopecia, exudation, crusting, and ulceration.

The bacteria enter via skin wounds by arthropod vectors such as stable flies, horn flies, and house flies, or by contact with contaminated fomites or soil.

Diagnosis: Isolation of *C pseudotuberculosis* from lesions is necessary for confirmation. In all forms of lymphangitis in horses, samples for culture include aspirates of abscesses, swabs of purulent exudate beneath crusts associated with folliculitis, and punch biopsies. Differential diagnoses include pyoderma, abscesses, lymphangitis from other bacteria (eg, *Staphylococcus aureus*, *Rhodococcus equi*, *Streptococcus* spp, or *Dermatophilus* spp), dermatophytosis, sporotrichosis, equine cryptococcosis, North American blastomycosis, and onchocerciasis.

Abdominal ultrasonography is useful for detection of internal infection of the liver, spleen, or kidneys. Ultrasonography is also useful for detection and drainage of deep abscesses causing lameness, particularly in the triceps musculature. Transtracheal aspirates are required to confirm pneumonia caused by *C pseudotuberculosis*. Serologic testing with the synergistic hemolysis inhibition test, which detects IgG to the phospholipase D exotoxin, is a useful adjunct for diagnosis of internal infection in the absence of external infection.

Treatment: Lymphangitis and internal infection should be treated with longterm antimicrobials (1 mo duration or as directed by follow-up ultrasonography). The organism is susceptible to most commonly administered antimicrobials; however, antimicrobial treatment of uncomplicated external abscesses may prolong the disease by delaying abscess maturation. External abscess swellings are treated with hot packs, poultices, or hydrotherapy until they rupture or are drained surgically. Abscesses are lanced and flushed with dilute antiseptic solutions. Deep abscesses in the triceps or quadriceps region require ultrasonography to guide placement of an indwelling drain. Phenylbutazone relieves pain and swelling. General supportive and nursing care is indicated.

If treatment is successful, the swelling gradually recedes over days or weeks. Internal infection has a 30%–40% mortality rate, even with appropriate treatment. Severe or untreated lymphangitis cases often become chronic, and fibrosis and induration of the leg occur. Isolation of infected horses, fly control, and good sanitation are recommended for prevention.

CARDIOVASCULAR SYSTEM INTRODUCTION

The cardiovascular system comprises the heart, the veins, and the arteries. The atrioventricular (mitral and tricuspid) and semilunar (aortic and pulmonic) valves keep blood flowing in one direction through the heart, and valves in large veins keep blood flowing back toward the heart. The rate and force of contraction of the heart and the degree of constriction or dilatation of blood vessels are determined by the autonomic nervous system and hormones produced either by the heart and blood vessels (ie, paracrine or autocrine) or at a distance from the heart and blood vessels (ie, endocrine).

Slightly >10% of all domestic animals examined by a veterinarian have some form of cardiovascular disease. Similar to many chronic diseases of other organ systems, cardiovascular diseases generally do not resolve but progress and become more limiting over time, which may ultimately lead to death. Evaluation of the heart is performed via assessment of heart sounds and murmurs, arterial pulses, degree of jugular vein distention, strength and location of the apex beat, electrocardiography, radiography, cardiac biomarkers, echocardiography, and other advanced imaging techniques.

Heart Rate and the Electrocardiogram

The heart beats because of a wave of depolarization that originates in the sinoatrial (SA) node at the juncture of the cranial vena cava and the right atrium. At rest, the SA node discharges ~30 times/min in horses, >120 times/min in cats (typically 180–220 times/min in a hospital setting), and 60–120 times/min in dogs, depending on their size. In general, the larger the species, the slower the rate of SA node discharge and the slower the heart rate. Birds can have a resting heart rate of ~115–130 beats/min, with active heart rates up to 670 beats/min, depending on size and species. Hummingbirds can have an active heart rate of >1,200 beats/min.

The rate of SA nodal discharge increases when norepinephrine is released from the sympathetic nerves and binds to the β_1-adrenoreceptors on the SA node. This cardioacceleration may be blocked by β-adrenergic blocking agents (eg, propranolol, atenolol, metoprolol, esmolol, carvedilol). The rate of SA nodal discharge decreases when acetylcholine released by the parasympathetic (vagus) nerves binds to the cholinergic receptors on the SA node. This vagally mediated cardiodeceleration may be blocked by a parasympatholytic (vagolytic) compound (eg, atropine, glycopyrrolate). When the SA node discharges and the wave of depolarization traverses the atria, the P wave of the ECG is produced. Subsequently, the atria contract, ejecting a small volume of remaining blood into the respective ventricles (atrial kick).

In quiet, healthy dogs, the variation of the heart rate with respiration is termed **respiratory sinus arrhythmia** (RSA); it results from decreased vagal activity during inspiration and increased vagal activity during expiration. Therefore, vagolytic compounds, as well as excitement, pain, fever, and congestive heart failure (CHF), usually abolish or diminish RSA. Heart rate variability synchronized with respirations is a good indicator of cardiac health. It is rare to find an animal that has active CHF with RSA; however, comorbid conditions that increase vagal activity (such as primary respiratory or neurologic disease) may cause RSA to persist.

Heart rate is also inversely related to systemic arterial blood pressure. When blood pressure increases, heart rate decreases; when blood pressure decreases, heart rate increases. This relation is known as the **Marey reflex** and occurs by the following mechanism. When high-pressure arterial baroreceptors in the aortic and carotid sinuses detect increases in blood pressure, they send increased afferent volleys to the medulla oblongata, which increases vagal efferents to the SA node and causes the heart rate to decrease. In heart failure, the baroreceptors (laden with Na^+/K^+-ATPase) become fatigued, which reduces the afferent signals to the medulla oblongata. This results in less vagal efferent signaling. Thus, dogs in CHF have a decrease in heart rate variability and frequently present with an underlying sinus tachycardia.

Once the wave of depolarization reaches the atrioventricular (AV) node, the speed of conduction is slowed through the nodal tissue, giving the atria time to contract and eject more blood into the ventricles, allowing for atrioventricular synchrony. The depolarization then travels rapidly to the subendocardium of the ventricles and to the ventricular septum. From these points, it travels slowly through the ventricular myocardium, producing the QRS complex of the ECG with subsequent ventricular contraction. The delay between the electrical activity visualized on ECG and mechanical function accounts for transmission of impulses, which allows contraction of myocytes to occur in synchrony. Under rare conditions, there may be depolarization without contraction; this is called **electromechanical dissociation.**

The interval on an ECG between the onset of the P wave and the onset of the QRS complex is termed the PQ or PR interval. It is a measure of the time it takes for the electrical wave of depolarization to begin at the SA node and reach the ventricles (lastly traversing the AV node). Factors that speed or slow the rate of discharge of the SA node (chronotropy) also speed or slow conduction through the AV node (dromotropy). Thus, as the heart rate increases, the PR interval shortens; when heart rate slows, the PR interval lengthens.

The T wave of the ECG represents repolarization of the ventricles. It is affected by electrolyte imbalance (eg, hypo- or hyperkalemia, hypo- or hypercalcemia), myocardial injury, or ventricular enlargement. Repolarization of the atria (Ta wave) is rarely seen, because it occurs during the much larger QRS complex. Occasionally, it can be seen with AV nodal disease (AV block) or in horses with slow heart rates, appearing as a "hammock" after the P wave.

Force of Ventricular Contraction

The force with which the ventricles contract is determined by many factors, including the end-diastolic volume (preload), which is the volume of blood within the ventricles just before they begin to contract, and myocardial contractility (inotropy), which is the rate of cycling of the microscopic contractile units of the myocardium.

The preload is determined by the difference in end-diastolic pressure between the ventricle and the pleural space, divided by the stiffness of the ventricular myocardium. The end-diastolic pressure of the ventricle is determined by the ratio of blood volume and the compliance of the myocardium. Preload is regulated predominantly by low-pressure volume receptors in the heart and large veins. When these receptors are stimulated by an increase in blood volume or by distention of the structures the receptors occupy, the body responds by making more urine and by dilating the veins—an attempt to decrease blood volume and lower the pressures in the veins responsible for venous distention. An increase in end-diastolic volume (preload) stretches the ventricular wall, resulting in a more forceful contraction as per the Frank-Starling mechanism, or Starling's law of the heart. Stretching of receptors in the atria and ventricles causes them to release natriuretic proteins: brain natriuretic peptide (BNP) primarily from the ventricles and atrial natriuretic peptide (ANP) from the atria. These peptides are natriuretic, relax smooth muscle, and in general oppose vasopressin and angiotensin II. A correlation between BNP and NT-proBNP levels and degree of stretch of the heart has been identified in dogs.

Myocardial contractility is determined by the availability of ATP and calcium, which allows myosin-actin cross-bridging to occur. The rate of liberation of energy from ATP is determined, in part, by the amount of norepinephrine binding to β_1-adrenergic receptors in the myocardium. One of the most important factors in heart failure is the down-regulation (decreased number) of myocardial β_1-receptors.

Oxygen and the Myocardium

Oxygen is essential for the production of energy that permits all body functions. The amount of oxygen available for production of this energy is termed the **tissue oxygen content**. The myocardial oxygen content is a balance between how much oxygen is delivered to the heart minus how much oxygen is consumed by the heart.

The amount of oxygen delivered to the heart depends on how well the lungs function, how much Hgb is present to carry the oxygen, and how much blood carrying the Hgb flows through the heart muscle via the coronary arteries. If pulmonary function is normal and there is sufficient Hgb, coronary blood flow will determine how much oxygen is delivered to the myocardium. Coronary blood flow is determined by the difference in mean pressure between the aorta (normally 100 mmHg) and the right atrium (normally 5 mmHg), into which coronary blood empties. Because coronary flow is greatest during diastole, slower heart rates (which preferentially increase diastolic interval) are associated with improved myocardial oxygen delivery.

The amount of oxygen consumed by the heart is termed **myocardial oxygen consumption**. It is determined, principally, by wall tension and heart rate. Wall tension is expressed by the law of LaPlace, in which tension increases with increases in pressure or diameter of the ventricle, and tension decreases with increases in wall thickness of the ventricle. Tension increases with conditions that increase afterload (pressure), such as pulmonic stenosis, subaortic stenosis, systemic or pulmonary hypertension, or preload (volume), including mitral valve insufficiency, left-to-right shunting defects, and dilated cardiomyopathy. In the absence of a stenotic lesion, afterload is determined by the relative stiffness of the arteries and by the degree of constriction of the arterioles. The tone of vascular smooth muscle depends on many factors, some of which constrict the muscle (eg, adrenergic agonists, angiotensin II, vasopressin, endothelin) and some of which relax the muscle (eg, norepinephrine, atriopeptin, bradykinin, adenosine, nitric oxide). Afterload is often increased in heart failure, and therapy is often directed at decreasing it.

Increases in heart rate result in increasing myocardial oxygen consumption while decreasing time for diastole when coronary blood flow is greatest. The combination can set the stage for an imbalance in myocardial oxygen demand and supply, leading to myocardial ischemia. Cardiac failure is characterized by an increase in sympathetic tone and relative increases in heart rate; the ultimate impact is an inefficient myocardium that can result in deleterious remodeling.

Oxygen is responsible for the production of the vast majority of ATP, which fuels both contraction and relaxation of the myocardium. Calcium must rapidly be released by intracellular stores (sarcoplasmic reticulum) via calcium-induced calcium release to allow for excitation-contraction coupling, while equally rapid removal of calcium back into the sarcoplasmic reticulum is necessary for relaxation. Both processes of calcium cycling are energy dependent.

In heart failure and cardiomyopathy, inappropriate handling of calcium may result in arrhythmogenesis and may also be the most important factor that leads to both reduced force of contraction and reduced rate of relaxation (ie, reduced systolic as well as diastolic function).

Hindrance to Blood Flow

Blood flow from the heart, termed **cardiac output**, is via both the left and right ventricles. Cardiac output is determined by the heart rate and ventricular stroke volume. Blood flows through the systemic arterial (left ventricular) or pulmonary arterial (right ventricular) trees and is critical to satisfactory function of the heart and consequent perfusion of organs with adequate quantities of blood and the oxygen it contains. Most (>90%) of the hindrance to blood flow is from the degree of constriction of the arterioles, termed **vascular resistance**; however, some interference is from the stiffness of the portion of the great arteries closest to the ventricles, termed **impedance**. The ventricles eject a stroke volume into the proximal portion of the great arteries, which expand to accommodate the stroke volume; when the ventricles are relaxed, the distended great arteries recoil and keep blood moving through the arterioles into the capillaries. The aortic and pulmonic valves close and prevent the stroke volume from returning to the ventricle that ejected it. Systemic vascular resistance is the opposing blood flow that must be overcome to push blood through the peripheral circulation and is calculated by:

(mean arterial pressure – mean venous pressure)/cardiac output

Pulmonary vascular resistance is similarly calculated and is increased in cases of pulmonary vascular obstruction or pulmonary hypertension.

One of the most important features of heart failure that leads to morbidity is increased resistance of arterial, arteriolar, and venous smooth muscle because of increased angiotensin II, vasopressin, and endothelin. If the left ventricle is unable to eject a normal stroke volume or cardiac output, it is reasonable that ventricular function might be improved by decreasing vascular resistance. Decreasing afterload (arterial vasodilation) is one therapeutic goal in heart failure therapy.

ABNORMALITIES OF THE CARDIOVASCULAR SYSTEM

The following mechanisms can result in abnormalities of the cardiovascular system: 1) the cardiac valves fail to close or open properly (valvular disease); 2) the heart muscle pumps inefficiently or relaxes inadequately (myocardial disease); 3) the heart beats too slowly, too rapidly, or irregularly (arrhythmia); 4) the systemic vessels offer too great an interference to blood flow (vascular disease); 5) there may be abnormal communications between chambers of the left side and right side of the heart (cardiac shunts) or between the systemic and pulmonary circulations (extracardiac shunts); 6) there is too little or too much blood compared with the ability of the blood vessels to store that blood; and 7) there is parasitism of the cardiovascular system (eg, heartworm disease). Cardiac diseases can be either congenital defects or acquired. The diseases of greatest importance, because of their prevalence, are mitral regurgitation in dogs, hypertrophic cardiomyopathy in cats, dilated cardiomyopathy (DCM) in dogs, arrhythmogenic right ventricular cardiomyopathy in Boxers, and heartworm disease.

Valvular Disease: Inadequate closure (coaptation) of valves leads to regurgitation (back flow of blood), which occurs most commonly as mitral regurgitation, or mitral and tricuspid regurgitation (concurrent tricuspid regurgitation occurs in ~30% of cases with mitral regurgitation). Regurgitation through the mitral and/or tricuspid valves due to myxomatous degeneration of the valve leaflets constitutes >75% of all heart disease in dogs. As blood regurgitates through either set of AV valves, a typical holosystolic murmur is heard between the first and second heart sounds. A mid-systolic click, secondary to mitral valve prolapse, may precede development of a murmur in the early stages of disease. When blood regurgitates through the mitral or tricuspid valves, an excessive amount of blood moves back and forth between the ventricle and atrium. Thus, with mitral regurgitation, it is common to see dilation of the left atrium and left ventricle. The degree of left atrial enlargement, documented by either radiography or echocardiography, may predict disease severity. Mitral or tricuspid regurgitation is most common in older small-breed dogs and older horses that have valve leaflets thickened by myxomatous degeneration (infiltration with glycosaminoglycans). Mitral regurgitation occurs more often in Cavalier King Charles Spaniels, and at a younger age, than in any other breed; however, there is not a significant difference in the time frame of progression to onset of CHF.

Aortic regurgitation occurs most often in older horses due to calcification or noninflammatory degeneration of the aortic valve. It may also develop secondary to aortic endocarditis (infection of the valve leaflets), most often in large-breed dogs. The left ventricle and atrium can become dilated due to the aortic regurgitation, but this is proportional to the degree of regurgitation. The murmur produced by blood regurgitating from the aorta into the left ventricle is always a diastolic murmur, heard immediately after the second heart sound. In horses, the murmur of aortic regurgitation can be described as "blowing" due to the regurgitant blood flow, or as "buzzing" due to the aortic leaflets vibrating as the blood flows past. The buzzing murmur is almost always associated with a relatively small amount of regurgitant flow.

Inadequate opening of valves is termed stenosis. Pulmonic stenosis is most prevalent, valvular aortic stenosis is uncommon, and mitral or tricuspid stenosis is rare. However, subaortic stenosis, produced by a fibrous or fibromuscular band of tissue just beneath the aortic valves, is prevalent, especially in certain breeds (eg, Newfoundlands, Golden Retrievers, Boxers, Rottweilers, and German Shepherds). If a valve opens inadequately, a greater pressure must be generated to maintain the normal volume of blood flowing through it. The ventricle responsible for pumping blood through the stenotic valve concentrically hypertrophies (thickens) proportionally to the degree of tightness of the stenosis. The systolic ejection quality murmurs produced by pulmonic or subaortic stenosis are heard between the first and second heart sound; typically, they are shorter in duration than the holosystolic murmur of mitral regurgitation and are heard best over the left heart base and thoracic inlet (subaortic stenosis). In general, the louder the murmur, the greater the stenosis, although the severity of stenosis is not always predicted by the intensity of the murmur. The velocity of blood flowing through a stenosis correlates with the severity of the stenosis, which can be estimated by spectral Doppler echocardiography. Medications (β-blockers) or interventional procedures (balloon valvuloplasty) may be recommended in cases of severe subaortic or pulmonic stenosis, respectively.

Myocardial Disease: Impaired force of contraction is termed reduced systolic function (pump failure), which occurs most commonly with DCM—primary DCM in large-breed dogs, DCM-phenotype with Boxer cardiomyopathy, and in cats that are typically either taurine deficient or in the end-stages of other types of cardiomyopathy and in longstanding mitral regurgitation. When this occurs, the cardiac muscle is said to be in a reduced inotropic state, or to have reduced contractile function. In large-breed dogs, this is usually termed idiopathic DCM, because the origin is unknown.

Impaired ventricular relaxation is termed reduced diastolic function, which occurs most commonly when the cardiac muscle suffers oxygen debt and the consequent lack of energy to fuel relaxation. Diastolic dysfunction is seen in most cardiac diseases as they progress to heart failure. The ventricular myocardium also relaxes poorly in hypertrophic cardiomyopathy (ie, when the muscle is too thick), or with pericardial disease when either the thickened pericardium or fluid contained within the pericardial sac interferes with relaxation. Hypertrophic cardiomyopathy is most common in cats. Probably >85% of cats with heart disease have hypertrophic cardiomyopathy. A smaller number of cats will have so-called restrictive cardiomyopathy, in which the heart fills poorly because the walls are stiffer than normal, unclassified cardiomyopathy, or valvular disease. Pericardial disease is most common in older, large-breed dogs with tumors bleeding into the pericardial sac (eg, hemangiosarcoma or chemodectoma).

Arrhythmias: Any cardiac rhythm falling outside the normal sinus rhythm is termed an arrhythmia. An arrhythmia that is too fast, too slow, or too irregular can result in reduced cardiac output, thereby causing clinical signs that could include exercise intolerance, syncope, or exacerbation of CHF. The most common arrhythmias are atrial fibrillation (seen commonly in horses and giant-breed dogs, or in any size dog with advanced cardiac disease and severe left atrial enlargement), ventricular premature depolarizations (seen most commonly in

Boxers and Doberman Pinschers), sick sinus syndrome (seen mainly in aged Miniature Schnauzers), persistent atrial standstill (seen in Labrador Retrievers and English Springer Spaniels), and third-degree AV block.

In atrial fibrillation, depolarization of the atria is not coordinated, stimulation of the AV node is frequent but random, and the heart rate is rapid and irregular. Ventricular premature contractions (also called ventricular premature beats or depolarizations) arise from irritated regions of the ventricles. Such irritations commonly result from chronic stretch of the fibers, as well as from oxygen debt or drug effects. A single premature beat does not typically cause clinical signs and can be relatively benign, but premature beats may evolve into short paroxysms (bursts) or long runs (ventricular tachycardia) that lead to hemodynamic impairment and syncope, or even to a complete loss of coordination of ventricular activity (ventricular fibrillation) and sudden death. Ventricular tachycardia commonly occurs in Doberman Pinschers with DCM and in Boxers with arrhythmogenic right ventricular cardiomyopathy (previously termed Boxer cardiomyopathy) and warrants immediate treatment with antiarrhythmics. With either sick sinus syndrome (ie, transient arrest of discharge of the SA node alternating with periods of tachycardia) or complete heart block (in which no atrial depolarization enters the ventricles), the ventricular rate is exceptionally slow and may lead to hemodynamic impairment (low cardiac output failure, hypoperfusion, hypoxemia), exercise intolerance, syncope, or sudden death. A pacemaker is indicated in all dogs with persistent high-grade AV block or persistent atrial standstill and in dogs that are symptomatic for sick sinus syndrome.

Vascular Disease: Interference to blood flow through systemic arterioles (systemic hypertension) is most common in aging animals with impaired renal function (dogs and cats), hyperadrenocorticism (dogs), or hyperthyroidism (cats). The exact underlying cause is usually unknown, but suspected causes include sodium retention and plasma volume expansion, hyperaldosteronism, increased sympathetic tone, and possibly increased angiotensin II. Regardless of the cause, a loss in arteriolar compliance may persist even with adequate treatment of the associated clinical condition. Arterial vasodilators, such as angiotensin-converting enzyme (ACE) inhibitors and amlodipine, are a mainstay of antihypertensive therapy.

Cardiac Shunts: Abnormal communications between the left and right side of the circulation are termed cardiovascular shunts. These take the form of (in decreasing prevalence) patent ductus arteriosus (between the aorta and pulmonary trunk), ventricular septal defect (between the left and right ventricles), or atrial septal defect (between the left and right atria). When blood crosses these defects from the left side to the right side, which is most common, these defects are termed left-to-right shunts. They result in overcirculation of the lungs and dilatation of the cardiac chambers required to pump or to carry the shunted blood. Chronic dilatation ultimately leads to myocardial failure. *See also* CONGENITAL AND INHERITED ANOMALIES OF THE CARDIOVASCULAR SYSTEM, p 76.

Tetralogy of Fallot (*see* p 83) is a complex congenital anomaly that consists of a hypoplastic right ventricular outflow tract and/or pulmonary trunk, an aorta that overrides the interventricular septum (therefore arising from both ventricles), ventricular septal defect, and right ventricular hypertrophy. Poorly oxygenated blood enters the systemic circulation (right-to-left shunt) and produces a bluish tinge (cyanosis) to the mucous membranes and increased numbers of RBCs (polycythemia). Tetralogy of Fallot is the most common form of a right-to-left shunt, although any large atrial or ventricular septal defect can result in right-to-left shunting (Eisenmenger physiology) secondary to pulmonary hypertension from chronic pulmonary overcirculation. Right-to-left shunting patent ductus arteriosus is also seen infrequently and typically results from persistent pulmonary hypertension from birth. Any cardiac or extracardiac shunt can also originate as a left-to-right shunt and reverse in direction if the pressure within the pulmonary circulation or right heart becomes greater than the pressure in the aorta or left heart.

Heartworm Disease: Heartworm disease (*see* p 127) is seen predominantly in dogs but also in cats and is transmitted via mosquitoes. In heartworm disease, adult heartworms in the pulmonary vessels and the pulmonary arterial changes they induce impede flow through the lungs. Severe, persistent pulmonary hypertension may result in right ventricular hypertrophy, increased right-side filling pressure, and eventual development of right-side CHF (cor pulmonale). The disease progresses at a varying rate in dogs but usually lasts <2 yr in cats. Both species may develop syncope or cor pulmonale from pulmonary hypertension or may develop pulmonary thromboembolism from in situ thrombus formation or adult worm death. Antigenic stimulation from the heartworms may also cause changes in the lungs, resulting in eosinophilic pneumonitis. The death of adult worms secondary to adulticide therapy always results in some degree of pulmonary thromboembolism. Strict cage rest is necessary in the month after adulticide therapy, and pretreatment with doxycycline and ivermectin to kill *Wolbachia* organisms before adulticide treatment may also mitigate the pulmonary pathology resulting from worm death.

Common Endpoints of Heart Disease

Signs associated with any of the above diseases are due either to inadequate organ perfusion (eg, exercise intolerance, weakness, syncope, azotemia) or to blood damming up in organs in which the venous effluent is emptied inadequately (eg, pulmonary edema, ascites, pitting edema, other effusions). An animal showing signs due to relative inadequacy of the cardiovascular system to deliver enough blood to sustain normal function is said to be in low output, or forward heart failure. An animal showing signs caused by blood damming up in poorly drained organs is said to be in CHF. When inadequate amounts of oxygen are present in systemic arterial blood and there is too much unoxygenated Hgb, the mucous membranes appear cyanotic and polycythemia may develop.

Animals with heart failure may deteriorate gradually, due most often to pulmonary edema, or they may die suddenly, due to arrhythmias, chordal rupture, or left atrial tear.

Heart Failure, Congestive Heart Failure, and the Failing Heart

Systolic myocardial failure is described as reduced myocardial contractile function, characterized by a reduced force of contraction from any given preload. More objectively, a failing heart can be described as one with a reduced rate of liberation of energy from the breakdown of ATP, or with a reduced velocity of fiber shortening when the heart contracts during the imaginary situation of contracting against no load. It is difficult to directly measure myocardial contractility and to identify myocardial failure. Almost any animal with heart disease leading to chamber enlargement or increased wall thickness has a degree of myocardial failure on the cellular level, but such animals may remain compensated without clinical signs of heart failure for a prolonged time.

Low output heart failure and CHF (*see* p 87) are clinical syndromes in which an animal manifests signs referable to a complex interaction between a failing heart and the blood vessels. In low output heart failure, cardiac output is insufficient to perfuse organs with enough oxygenated blood for the organs to function properly either at rest or during periods of exertion. In CHF, blood dams up in or around organs—usually the lungs but occasionally in the systemic organs—and causes the congested organs to function abnormally, become edematous, or both. The functional classification of heart failure is expressed when, during graded exercise, the animal shows signs (eg, dyspnea, cough, collapse) due to the heart disease. There are several classifications of heart failure, the most recent and perhaps most practical of which is based on the course of heart disease expressed in four basic stages (A, B1, B2, C, D) described in the ACVIM Consensus Statement on canine chronic valvular heart disease.

DIAGNOSIS OF CARDIOVASCULAR DISEASE

Diagnosis of cardiovascular disease is based on history and signalment, physical examination (eg, inspection, auscultation, palpation), cardiac biomarkers (NT-proBNP, BNP, ANP, troponin I), radiography, electrocardiography, and echocardiography. Clear images must be obtained for radiography, electrocardiography, and echocardiography, or accurate, valid interpretation will not be possible. Most cardiovascular diseases (eg, mitral regurgitation, dilated cardiomyopathy) can be highly suspected based on the results of physical examination and radiography. Electrocardiography is specific for diagnosis of rhythm disturbances (eg, atrial fibrillation, sick sinus syndrome). Echocardiography is excellent to confirm tentative diagnoses, assess severity of valvular regurgitations and stenotic lesions, evaluate chamber enlargement and quantify systolic and diastolic myocardial function, characterize the form of cardiomyopathy in cats, detect cardiac tumors or pericardial disease, diagnose pulmonary hypertension or heartworm caval syndrome, and identify congenital cardiac defects. Thoracic radiographs are the best diagnostic tool to evaluate the lungs for evidence of active CHF. Heartworm disease is diagnosed best by detecting antigens of mature, female heartworms circulating in the blood (dogs). In cats, diagnosis of heartworm disease may entail heartworm antigen and antibody testing, supplemented by thoracic radiographs and echocardiography.

Many heart diseases have specific breed prevalences. Any older Cavalier King Charles Spaniel with a cough, labored breathing, and exercise intolerance should be suspected to have left-side CHF due to mitral regurgitation; however, chronic obstructive pulmonary disease with fibrosis may produce nearly identical signs and thoracic radiographs; echocardiography and NT-proBNP testing may be needed to differentiate. Any middle-aged, depressed, coughing, exercise-intolerant Doberman Pinscher with a rapid, irregular heart rate likely has dilated cardiomyopathy. Any middle-aged to older Miniature Schnauzer with fainting likely has sick sinus syndrome. Any Boxer who faints intermittently should be suspected to have arrhythmogenic right ventricular cardiomyopathy; however, Boxers can also develop neurocardiogenic syncope or sick sinus syndrome, and Holter monitoring may be needed to diagnose the underlying cause of syncope and to formulate the best treatment plan. A middle-aged cat with labored breathing and reluctance to lie down probably has myocardial disease (most commonly hypertrophic cardiomyopathy), whereas an older cat with weight loss and behavioral changes is likely to have hyperthyroidism, which can result in systemic hypertension and exacerbate cardiac disease.

Heart disease should be considered if any of the following are identified on physical examination: 1) the heart rate is rapid, slow, or irregular (and not due to respiratory sinus arrhythmia); 2) respiratory sinus arrhythmia is absent even when the animal is at rest (this also occurs due to pain, fever, or excitement); 3) more than two heart sounds are heard (eg, producing a "gallop" rhythm) in any animal but a horse (most common in cats with cardiomyopathy); 4) a loud murmur is heard; 5) heart sounds are muffled in the absence of obesity (may indicate pericardial or pleural effusion); 6) arterial pulsations are rapid, feeble, or irregular with more heart beats than arterial pulsations (pulse deficits); 7) the animal faints or has reduced exercise tolerance in the absence of skeletal muscle disease or obesity; 8) the mucous membranes are acutely cyanotic in the absence of primary pulmonary disease.

Echocardiography is more effective than radiography, which is more effective than electrocardiography, to detect enlargement of chambers of the heart and great vessels. In general, the degree of chamber enlargement parallels disease severity. The degree of pulmonary infiltrates detected radiographically, or the degree of impairment of left ventricular wall motion or thinning of the left ventricular walls, may predict the severity of heart failure. Unfortunately, the correlation between hemodynamic or echocardiographic measurements and either signs or likelihood of death is not always good. There appears to be a better correlation between increase in heart and respiratory rates and exercise incapacity to severity of heart disease. NT-proBNP testing may also help in the prognostication of heart disease and heart failure.

Diagnosis of specific cardiovascular diseases are discussed in their respective chapters.

PRINCIPLES OF THERAPY

See also SYSTEMIC PHARMACOTHERAPEUTICS OF THE CARDIOVASCULAR SYSTEM, p 2525.

Although therapy is disease-specific, there are some general goals of therapy for heart disease: 1) Chronic stretch on myocardial fibers should be minimized, because chronic stretch injures and irritates fibers, causes them to consume excess quantities of oxygen, and leads to their death and replacement by fibrous connective tissue (remodeling). 2) Edema fluid should be removed because it makes the lungs wet, heavy, and stiff and causes ventilation-perfusion inequalities, impairs oxygen diffusion, and fatigues muscles of ventilation. 3) Cardiac output should be improved, and the amount of regurgitation (most often mitral regurgitation) decreased. Improved cardiac output enhances blood flow to important organs, and reducing mitral regurgitation decreases stretch and reduces pressures in the left atrium and pulmonary veins, thus reducing pulmonary capillary pressure and edema formation. 4) Heart rate and rhythm should be regulated. A heart beating too slowly fails to eject enough blood, whereas a heart beating too rapidly does not have time to fill adequately and consumes too much oxygen at a time when there is too little coronary blood flow. A heart beating too irregularly may deteriorate into ventricular fibrillation and sudden death. 5) Oxygenation of the blood should be improved. Inadequate oxygenation leads to inadequate energy to fuel both contraction and relaxation of the myocardium. Inadequate oxygenation of the myocardium may also lead to myocardial fibrosis and arrhythmia. 6) The likelihood of thromboembolism should be minimized. Cats with hypertrophic cardiomyopathy may shed emboli from the enlarged left atrium, which may block major arterial branches and lead to ischemia and death. 7) Mature heartworms and microfilariae should be killed. Mature heartworms may initiate severe changes in the pulmonary arteries that ultimately impede blood flow through the lungs.

The ultimate goals of therapy for cardiovascular disease are achieved when treatment resolves the presenting clinical signs, the respiratory and heart rates are not increased at rest, and quality of life is good for both pet and owner.

Common Therapeutic Agents

Furosemide is a loop diuretic that decreases resorption of sodium, chloride, and potassium in the thick ascending limb of the loop of Henle. It is also a venodilator when used IV. It is the most important and effective means to remove edema fluid from animals with heart failure and frequently is lifesaving in the short term. Diuresis with furosemide may be augmented by using thiazide diuretics (eg, hydrochlorothiazide). Thiazides suppress resorption of sodium and water at the distal renal tubules. When using a loop diuretic and a diuretic that works at the distal tubules, the ability of the kidneys to conserve water is reduced dramatically, so dehydration and hypokalemia may develop. This may be signaled by worsening azotemia, and renal values must be monitored closely in animals on multiple diuretics. Torsemide is a loop diuretic that is 10 times more potent than furosemide; it is reserved for refractory CHF or in cases of suspected diuretic resistance to furosemide.

Spironolactone is a potassium-sparing diuretic that blocks the effects of aldosterone. Like thiazides, it exerts its effect principally at the distal convoluted tubule. Although spironolactone effectively maintains potassium levels, data suggest that it does not induce a significant diuretic effect. However, spironolactone minimizes remodeling of both blood vessels and the heart, and like angiotensin-converting enzyme (ACE) inhibitors and β-blockers, has been shown to decrease symptoms and to prolong the lives of people and perhaps dogs with heart failure. Aldactazide, a combination diuretic consisting of spironolactone and hydrochlorothiazide, may be used in cases of refractory CHF. Renal values should be monitored closely because of the risk of worsening azotemia and renal failure with aldactazide therapy. Amiloride and triamterene are also potassium-sparing diuretics; however, these drugs are not typically used in veterinary medicine.

Digitalis glycosides exert their effects by inhibiting membrane Na^+/K^+-ATPase. This increases intracellular sodium, which activates the sodium-calcium pump that increases intracellular calcium. Digoxin increases the force of myocardial contraction (to a minor degree), slows the heart rate, and improves baroreceptor function. Digoxin has a narrow therapeutic index; thus, serum levels should be monitored, and animals should be watched for signs of toxicosis (vomiting, diarrhea, inappetance, arrhythmogenesis).

Enalapril, benazepril, lisinopril, and ramipril are ACE inhibitors commonly used in heart failure management in dogs. They are all equally effective at blocking the conversion of angiotensin I to angiotensin II. They minimize remodeling of both blood vessels and myocardium. They are part of the mainstay treatment regimen for advanced cardiac disease and heart failure.

Amrinone and milrinone, analogues of theophylline that deactivate other forms of phosphodiesterase, are potent IV inodilators. That is, they are both positive inotropes and vasodilators. However, they have been associated with worse outcomes in people with CHF and are not commonly used. Pimobendan, a calcium-sensitizing agent and phosphodiesterase inhibitor, is another inodilator shown to improve the quality of life and improve survival in dogs with CHF. Pimobendan is not approved for use in cats but may be beneficial in cats with heart failure (that do not have evidence of outflow tract obstruction). Sildenafil is a potent phosphodiesterase inhibitor used to treat moderate to severe pulmonary hypertension in dogs. Sildenafil has been shown to improve exercise intolerance and quality of life in people and dogs with pulmonary hypertension via pulmonary arterial vasodilation. There may also be additional beneficial effects on vascular remodeling and cardiac function.

Both procainamide and quinidine, class IA antiarrhythmics used formerly to manage ventricular arrhythmias, have been superseded by the class III antiarrhythmics sotalol and amiodarone, and the class IB antiarrhythmic mexiletine for treatment of malignant ventricular arrhythmias. Sotalol is used to treat both supraventricular and ventricular tachyarrhythmias, and it is particularly effective in treatment of Boxers with arrhythmogenic right ventricular dysplasia, either alone or in combination with mexiletine. Amiodarone is useful to manage all forms of arrhythmias, including ventricular arrhythmias, and rate control or conversion of atrial fibrillation. Increased liver enzymes and hepatotoxicity are potential adverse effects of amiodarone; thus, liver enzymes and serum amiodarone levels should be monitored periodically throughout therapy. Lidocaine, a class IB antiarrhythmic, is used only IV for emergency ventricular arrhythmias such as sustained ventricular tachycardia or R-on-T morphology.

Atenolol, propranolol, and metoprolol are oral β-blockers, and esmolol is an IV β-blocker, that slow the heart rate, suppress arrhythmias, and up-regulate adrenergic receptors. Carvedilol is a β- and α-adrenergic blocker that scavenges oxygen-free radicals. Like ACE inhibitors and spironolactone, carvedilol has been shown to both prolong life and decrease symptoms in people with heart failure; however, β-blockers are not generally advised for use in animals with active CHF. β-blockers are often used to treat dogs with subaortic stenosis, and for dynamic outflow obstruction in cats with hypertrophic cardiomyopathy.

Diltiazem is a calcium-channel blocker used to slow ventricular rate in animals with atrial fibrillation or supraventricular tachycardia. It is also used occasionally in cats with hypertrophic cardiomyopathy and outflow tract obstruction.

Atropine and glycopyrrolate block the effects of the vagus nerve on the SA node. Because the vagus nerve slows discharge of the SA node and heart rate, these compounds speed heart rate and may be useful when the heart beats too slowly. Nitroglycerin is a venodilator usually applied in a paste form to the skin inside the earflap or the mucous membranes; venodilation causes blood to pool in the dilated peripheral veins and splanchnic organs, decreasing left ventricular preload and pulmonary edema. Sodium nitroprusside is another nitrate that is a veno- and arterial dilator. Nitroprusside can be administered IV to treat acute fulminant CHF. These two medications should never be given simultaneously. Aspirin, clopidogrel, dalteparin, enoxaparin, and coumadin are antithrombotics that may prevent thromboembolism in cats with cardiomyopathy. Rivaroxaban is an oral factor Xa inhibitor that may prove useful for thromboprophylaxis in cats and dogs, although further studies are needed to evaluate its dosing and safety. Taurine and L-carnitine are amino acids used to prevent dilated cardiomyopathy in cats and in a limited number of dogs, respectively. Melarsomine is used to kill mature heartworms; ivermectin, milbemycin, and selamectin are used to kill microfilariae. Doxycycline should be administered to target *Wolbachia*, an intracellular bacteria that has a symbiotic relationship with heartworms.

Pimobendan and ACE inhibitors have been proved to be safe and effective to treat dogs with heart failure. Furosemide and digoxin are approved but without data proving either safety or efficacy. Use of other agents to manage heart failure or rhythm disturbances is based on anecdotal evidence or unblinded, uncontrolled reports and clinical experience.

CONGENITAL AND INHERITED ANOMALIES OF THE CARDIOVASCULAR SYSTEM

Congenital anomalies of the cardiovascular system are defects that are present at birth and can occur as a result of genetic, environmental, infectious, toxicologic, pharmaceutical, nutritional, or other factors or a combination of factors. For several defects, an inherited basis is suspected based on breed predilections and breeding studies. Congenital heart defects are significant not only for the effects they produce but also for their potential to be transmitted to offspring through breeding and thus affect an entire breeding population. In addition to congenital heart defects, many other cardiovascular disorders have been shown, or are suspected, to have a genetic basis. Diseases such as hypertrophic cardiomyopathy, dilated cardiomyopathy, and degenerative valvular disease of small breeds of dogs may have a significant heritable component.

In dogs, the prevalence of congenital heart disease is estimated at <1%. In multiple large studies of congenital heart disease in dogs, the three most common defects are aortic stenosis, pulmonic stenosis, and patent ductus arteriosus (PDA). Less common defects include ventricular septal defect, atrial septal defect, mitral valve dysplasia, tricuspid valve dysplasia, tetralogy of Fallot, cor triatriatum, and persistent right aortic arch. However, because of regional differences, the most common congenital cardiac defects in dogs in the USA vary from those reported in the UK and may likely differ from those in Europe and other regions.

In cats, the prevalence of congenital heart disease has been estimated to be 0.2%–1% and includes atrioventricular (AV) septal defects (including ventricular septal defect, atrial septal defect, and endocardial cushion defects), AV valve dysplasia, endocardial fibroelastosis, PDA, aortic stenosis, and tetralogy of Fallot.

The most common defects in other species are as follows: cattle—ventricular septal defect, ectopic heart, and ventricular hypoplasia; sheep—ventricular septal defect; pigs—tricuspid valve dysplasia, atrial septal defect, and subaortic stenosis; horses—ventricular septal defect, PDA, tetralogy of Fallot, and tricuspid atresia. Arabian horses have a relatively higher incidence of congenital defects than other breeds; a variety of defects have been reported for this breed.

Detection, Diagnosis, and Clinical Significance: The early detection of a congenital heart defect is critical for several reasons. Certain defects are surgically correctable, and treatment should be performed before the onset of congestive heart failure (CHF) or irreversible cardiac damage; recently purchased animals may be returned to avoid economic loss; pets with congenital heart defects are likely to die prematurely, causing emotional distress; and animals purchased for performance have limited potential and will likely be unsatisfactory. Early detection also prevents incorporation of genetic defects into breeding lines.

The evaluation of most animals with a congenital cardiac defect usually consists of a physical examination, electrocardiography, radiography, and echocardiography. This allows for a definitive diagnosis and an assessment of the severity of the defect. The use of Doppler echocardiography has supplanted the use of invasive cardiac catheterization studies in the evaluation of most cardiac defects. Once the diagnosis has been made and severity determined, treatment options can be developed and a prognosis given.

The clinical significance of congenital heart disease depends on the particular defect and its severity. Mildly affected animals may exhibit no ill effects and live a normal life span. Defects causing significant circulatory derangement will likely cause neonatal death. Such defects, many incompatible with life, also cause fetal death and reduced litter size. Medical or surgical management is most likely to benefit animals with congenital cardiac defects of moderate or greater severity. Left-to-right shunting PDA is one notable exception in which surgical correction is indicated in nearly all affected animals.

Pathophysiology: Congenital heart defects produce signs of cardiac failure through a variety of pathophysiologic mechanisms. Defects such as pulmonic stenosis and subaortic stenosis cause ventricular outflow obstruction and may result in right- and left-side failure, respectively. Outflow obstruction also leads to concentric hypertrophy of the respective ventricle, increasing the risk of ischemia-induced arrhythmias and sudden death. PDA and septal defects are examples of abnormal communications between the systemic and pulmonary circulatory systems and typically result in left-to-right shunting of blood. The recirculation of blood through the pulmonary circulation and into the left-side chambers often precipitates signs of left-side CHF (eg, pulmonary edema, cough, fatigue). Larger defects typically result in a greater degree of volume overcirculation to the left-side chambers. PDA is a possible exception, with very large defects sometimes contributing to pulmonary hypertension and right-to-left shunting (*see* p 83), also called a reversed PDA. Animals with right-to-left shunting defects (tetralogy of Fallot, reversed PDA) may develop right heart failure but more often have clinical signs associated with polycythemia (*see* p 43), which develops subsequent to renal perfusion with deoxygenated blood. This results in an increase in erythropoietin production by the kidneys and consequent polycythemia.

Innocent Murmurs: It is imperative to appreciate that the presence of a heart murmur in a young animal is not pathognomonic for a congenital heart defect. Many young animals will have a low-grade systolic murmur (often grade II/VI or less) that is the result of mild turbulence and is not associated with a congenital heart defect. These murmurs usually disappear by 6 mo of age in dogs and cats. Innocent murmurs are heard in the absence of any other demonstrable evidence of cardiovascular disease. High-grade systolic murmurs (grade IV/VI or greater) and diastolic murmurs are indicative of cardiac disease and should prompt further investigation.

OUTFLOW TRACT OBSTRUCTIONS

This group of congenital cardiac defects includes aortic stenosis, pulmonic stenosis, and coarctation of the aorta. All involve obstruction to either right or left ventricular outflow.

AORTIC STENOSIS

Aortic stenosis impedes normal left ventricular emptying and is caused by a narrowing at one of three locations: 1) below the aortic valve (subvalvular or subaortic), 2) at the aortic valve (valvular), or 3) above the aortic valve (supravalvular). The most common form of aortic stenosis in dogs is subaortic stenosis, caused by fibrous nodules or a ridge or ring of fibrous tissue within the left ventricular outflow tract just below the aortic valve. Subaortic stenosis is generally seen in large-breed dogs. Predisposed breeds include Boxers, Golden Retrievers, Rottweilers, German Shepherds, and Newfoundlands.

Pathophysiology: Aortic stenosis induces left ventricular concentric hypertrophy, the degree of which depends on the severity of the stenosis. In severe cases, left ventricular output may be decreased, especially during exercise. The major ramification of left ventricular hypertrophy is the risk of myocardial ischemia secondary to inadequate perfusion. Myocardial ischemia is a major factor in the development of life-threatening ventricular arrhythmias.

Clinical Findings and Treatment: Clinical signs do not consistently parallel the severity of stenosis. Inadequate output can result in lethargy, exercise intolerance, and syncope. Animals with no history of illness may die suddenly, with the defect first detected at necropsy. Affected animals have an ejection-type systolic murmur heard best at the aortic valve area. The intensity of the murmur correlates fairly well with the degree of stenosis and may increase as animals mature, reflecting progressive stenosis. Puppies without detectable murmurs should not be considered free of disease until they reach maturity (~1 yr of age). In moderate to severe cases, femoral pulse strength is diminished. Electrocardiography may show left ventricular enlargement (tall R waves in lead II) and ventricular premature complexes that may increase in frequency with exercise. Holter monitoring is indicated in syncopal animals or in animals with severe disease to define the presence of any arrhythmias, assess arrhythmia severity, and help determine the risk of sudden death. A recheck Holter monitor may be considered after initiation of antiarrhythmic therapy to assess efficacy. Radiographically, there is variable left ventricular enlargement and poststenotic dilatation of the aorta. Doppler echocardiography can generally provide a definitive diagnosis of aortic stenosis and exclude other cardiac abnormalities. A visible subaortic ridge or ring may be visible, and the velocity of systolic blood flow through the defect determines the severity of the stenosis. Dogs with more significant stenosis may show left ventricular concentric hypertrophy and hyperechoic areas within the myocardium consistent with myocardial ischemia and fibrosis.

Treatment options include medical management, balloon valvuloplasty, and open surgical correction. Medical management generally consists of the use of a β-blocker (eg, atenolol) for its potential to decrease myocardial oxygen demand, prolong diastole, and reduce left ventricular wall stress. Antiarrhythmic therapy is indicated in dogs with significant ventricular ectopy. Balloon valvuloplasty, although potentially effective short term, is unlikely to offer consistent longterm benefits. Open surgical resection is costly, limited to facilities offering cardiopulmonary bypass, and associated with higher morbidity/mortality. Mildly affected animals commonly require no treatment, and the prognosis can be fair to good in animals very mildly affected. Affected animals should not be bred.

PULMONIC STENOSIS

Pulmonic stenosis is common in dogs and infrequent in cats. It results in obstruction to right ventricular outflow due, in most cases, to dysplasia of the pulmonic valve cusps. Although the valvular form is most common, stenosis can also occur in the subvalvular region (infundibulum) or in the supravalvular area. Breed predilections for valvular pulmonic stenosis include English Bulldogs, Boxers, Beagles, Boykin Spaniels, and terriers. Supravalvular pulmonic stenosis is uncommon and may be most often seen in Giant Schnauzers.

Pathophysiology: The right ventricle must generate increased pressure during systole to overcome the stenosis, which in moderate to severe cases can lead to dramatic right ventricular concentric hypertrophy and dilatation. As the right ventricle hypertrophies, ventricular compliance diminishes, leading to increased right atrial pressure and venous congestion. The turbulent jet of blood flow across the stenosis deforms the wall of the main pulmonary artery, resulting in a poststenotic dilatation. In severe cases, right-side congestive failure may be noted. Concurrent tricuspid valve dysplasia is sometimes noted in animals with pulmonic stenosis. Anomalous coronary artery development has been documented in some affected animals with pulmonic stenosis such as English Bulldogs and Boxers. Most commonly, the left main coronary artery originates from the right coronary artery and encircles the right ventricular outflow tract.

Clinical Findings and Treatment: Affected animals may have a history of exercise intolerance and failure to thrive. Right-side CHF may be present and is characterized by ascites or peripheral edema. A prominent ejection-type systolic murmur is present and heard best at the pulmonic valve area (left base). A corresponding precordial thrill may be present. Jugular distention and pulsations may also be present. Electrocardiography will demonstrate evidence of right ventricular enlargement (deep S waves in lead II) in many cases. Radiographic abnormalities include right ventricular enlargement, dilatation of the main pulmonary artery, and diminished pulmonary perfusion. Echocardiography is indicated to obtain a definitive diagnosis and may demonstrate right ventricular hypertrophy and dilatation, thickened and relatively immobile pulmonic valve cusps, and turbulent blood flow across the stenosis. In a few cases, supravalvular or discrete subvalvular stenosis can be noted. Pulmonic insufficiency can sometimes be seen in dogs with pulmonic stenosis. The velocity of blood flow across the stenosis is used to assess the severity of disease and determine the need for intervention. Animals with moderate or severe pulmonic stenosis can benefit from balloon valvuloplasty or surgical intervention (valvulotomy, patch grafting, partial valvulectomy, or conduits). Balloon valvuloplasty is a minimally invasive and highly effective treatment option. Some animals are medically managed with a β-blocker (eg, atenolol) alone or in conjunction with balloon valvuloplasty. Congestive heart failure should be medically managed if present. Similarly, the presence of supraventricular or ventricular arrhythmias warrants therapy with the appropriate antiarrhythmic drug(s).

COARCTATION OF THE AORTA

This rare condition of dogs and cats involves narrowing of the aorta distal to the subclavian artery, typically in the area of the ductus arteriosus. Similar to other stenotic lesions, this leads to increased pressure proximal to the narrowing, resulting in concentric hypertrophy of the left ventricle. Other uncommon congenital abnormalities of the aorta include tubular hypoplasia of the ascending aorta and aortic interruption. Surgical correction has been reported.

LEFT-TO-RIGHT SHUNTS

PATENT DUCTUS ARTERIOSUS

In fetal life, blood entering the right heart largely bypasses the nonfunctional lungs through either the foramen ovale or the ductus arteriosus. The ductus arteriosus effectively shunts blood from the pulmonary artery into the descending aorta (right-to-left shunt). At birth, several factors mediate closure of the ductus to separate the systemic and pulmonary circulatory systems. Inflation of the lungs and remodeling of the fetal pulmonary vasculature allows the pulmonary circulation to change from a high-pressure, high-resistance system to a low-pressure, low-resistance system. Closure of the ductus occurs shortly after birth, leading to formation of the ligamentum arteriosum.

Pathophysiology: Persistence or patency of the ductus with an otherwise normal systemic and pulmonary circulatory system results in significant shunting of blood from the descending aorta to the pulmonary artery (left to right). Because systolic and diastolic aortic pressures normally exceed pulmonary artery pressures, shunting is continuous throughout the cardiac cycle. The result is a continuous murmur and volume overload of the pulmonary arteries and veins, left atrium, and left ventricle. Left atrial and left ventricular dilatation may result in cardiac arrhythmias. Diastolic flow (also called diastolic run-off) through the ductus leads to a decrease in diastolic and mean systemic blood pressures. The widened difference between systolic and diastolic pressures creates an increased pulse pressure and bounding femoral pulses. Chronic volume overload and dilatation of the left-side cardiac chambers usually result in development of left-side CHF in most untreated cases within the first 1–2 years of life. Animals with a small ductus and minimal shunting may reach adulthood, although most affected dogs have evidence of volume overload even at a young age. In some animals with a large PDA, increased pulmonary blood flow may induce pulmonary vasoconstriction and development of pulmonary hypertension. In cases of severe pulmonary hypertension in which pulmonary pressures exceed systemic pressures, blood flow through the ductus can reverse and result in right-to-left shunting. This "reverse PDA" causes disappearance of the classic machinery murmur and results in caudal hypoxemia. Delivery of oxygenated blood to the head and neck results in pink mucous membranes cranially, while delivery of hypoxemic blood caudally results in cyanotic mucous membranes caudally (vulva and prepuce). Differential cyanosis is a characteristic examination finding in animals with reverse PDA. In addition, perfusion of the kidneys with deoxygenated blood causes excessive release of erythropoietin and subsequent polycythemia.

Clinical Findings and Treatment: In animals with a left-to-right PDA, a prominent, continuous, machinery-like murmur is present. The murmur is usually loudest at the left base of the heart and is often associated with a precordial thrill. In some cases, the ductus remains open for several days after birth, so a continuous murmur may be detected during examination of the neonate. Femoral pulses are typically bounding. Most young animals do not demonstrate clinical signs. Those with a large shunt and older animals often have signs of left-side CHF. Electrocardiography frequently demonstrates tall R waves in lead II, indicative of left ventricular enlargement. A spectrum of cardiac arrhythmias may also be seen, including both atrial and ventricular premature complexes. Radiographic abnormalities depend on the size of the ductus and may demonstrate left atrial and left ventricular enlargement, prominent pulmonary vessels, aortic and pulmonic aneurysmal dilatations (ductal bump), and variable degrees of pulmonary edema. Echocardiography is valuable in excluding concurrent congenital cardiac defects, as well as documenting presence of the PDA. Continuous turbulence in the main pulmonary artery is characteristic of a left-to-right shunting PDA. Left ventricular and left atrial dilatation are typically noted, and mild mitral regurgitation may be present secondary to annular dilation.

Because of the high risk of CHF early in life for animals with a PDA, closure is generally recommended. There are two major treatment options for PDA closure: interventional transcatheter occlusion and surgical ligation. Catheter-based occlusion is minimally invasive and typically involves placement of an occlusion device through a peripheral vessel (most commonly the femoral artery). The Amplatz canine ductal occluder is used most often and is highly successful with minimal complications. The use of other occlusion devices such as Gianturco coils and vascular plugs has also been described. The major limitations to a transcatheter approach are ductal size and patient size. Surgical ligation of the ductus is also usually curative and considered most often for small dogs and cats. If present, CHF should be medically managed before anesthesia and surgery are performed.

In animals with a reverse PDA, there is usually a history of lethargy, exercise intolerance, and collapse that relates to severe pulmonary hypertension and venous admixture. Careful examination may reveal differential cyanosis. The second heart sound may be split, and there may be a soft diastolic murmur of pulmonic insufficiency. A continuous murmur is not present, and femoral pulses are not bounding. The finding of polycythemia in a young animal with the above clinical signs should prompt further diagnostic evaluation of the heart. Electrocardiography demonstrates severe right ventricular enlargement and occasional arrhythmias. In reverse PDA, right ventricular enlargement and aneurysmal dilatation of the descending aorta can be noted on radiographs. Echocardiography is indicated in these cases and will demonstrate abnormalities associated with pulmonary hypertension (right ventricular dilatation and hypertrophy, septal flattening pulmonary artery dilatation). Contrast echocardiography using agitated saline can be used to confirm the diagnosis. After the injection of agitated saline into a peripheral vein, microbubbles will be seen within the right heart, pulmonary artery, and abdominal aorta, suggesting a right-to-left shunt between the pulmonary artery and the aorta. Occlusion or ligation of the ductus is contraindicated with reverse PDA, because this results in an increase in pulmonary hypertension (by causing an increase in flow through the pulmonary arteries), right heart failure, and death. Therapy in these cases involves medical management of pulmonary hypertension and control of polycythemia through periodic phlebotomy. Longterm prognosis is poor.

VENTRICULAR SEPTAL DEFECTS

Ventricular septal defects are most commonly located in the perimembranous portion of the septum, high in the ventricular septum immediately beneath the right and noncoronary aortic valve cusps on the left and just below the cranioseptal tricuspid valve commissure on the right. They vary in size and hemodynamic significance. Doubly committed juxtaarterial septal defects (located beneath the aortic valve on the left and beneath the pulmonic valve on the right) and muscular septal defects (located at any site along the muscular septum) may also be seen. Ventricular septal defects may be seen with other congenital cardiac anomalies. This defect is heritable in miniature swine.

Pathophysiology: Shunting of blood from the left ventricle into the right ventricle or right ventricular outflow tract occurs in most animals because of the pressure gradient between the two ventricles. The magnitude of the shunt depends on the size of the defect, the ratio of pulmonary to systemic vascular resistance, and the relative compliance of the two ventricles. Blood shunted into the right ventricle is recirculated through the pulmonary vessels and left cardiac chambers, which causes dilatation of these structures. The right ventricle may dilate as well, especially in animals with large ventricular septal defects (which are rare). Small defects limit the volume of shunted blood and minimize hemodynamic effects, whereas large defects usually result in severe circulatory derangements and clinical signs. Most ventricular septal defects are restrictive, in which the degree of shunting is small, allowing the left and right ventricles to maintain normal pressures and a normal pressure gradient. Significant shunting through the pulmonary arteries can induce vasoconstriction and pulmonary hypertension. As resistance rises, the shunt may reverse and result in right-to-left shunting of blood, cyanosis, and polycythemia. The reversal of shunt flow (right-to-left) through a septal defect as a consequence of pulmonary hypertension is referred to as Eisenmenger syndrome.

Clinical Findings and Treatment: Clinical findings depend on the severity of the defect and the shunt direction. A small, restrictive defect usually causes minimal or no signs. Larger defects may result in left-side CHF. Cattle are prone to developing signs of right-side failure. The development of Eisenmenger syndrome is indicated by cyanosis, fatigue, and exercise intolerance. Most animals with a restrictive ventricular septal defect have a loud holosystolic murmur heard best over the right thorax that may be accompanied by a palpable thrill. This murmur is often absent or faint when a very large defect is present or when shunting is right to left. On occasion, aortic valvular insufficiency develops secondarily, because the defect may disrupt aortic valve apposition. In these cases, a concurrent diastolic murmur may be present, and the combination systolic/diastolic murmur ("to-and-fro" murmur) may be mistaken as that of a PDA. Thoracic radiographs can demonstrate generalized cardiomegaly with overcirculation of the pulmonary vessels. The defect can usually be visualized by echocardiography, although small defects may be missed. Doppler echocardiography can often confirm the presence of a shunt.

Therapy depends on use of the animal, severity of clinical signs, and direction of the shunt. Animals with small ventricular septal defects do not typically require therapy and have a good longterm prognosis if significant aortic insufficiency is not present. Animals with a moderate to severe ventricular septal defect and secondary volume overload to the left heart more commonly develop clinical signs, and treatment should be considered. Surgical closure of the defect requires cardiopulmonary bypass and is often limited by expense and availability. Percutaneous transcatheter closure can be considered for muscular septal defects and involves placement of an occluder or coil. Pulmonary artery banding to increase right ventricular outflow tract resistance, and thus decrease left-to-right shunting, can be considered. Medically, the use of drugs to reduce systemic vascular resistance (eg, vasodilators) may help to decrease the degree of left-to-right shunting. With right-to-left shunting, surgical closure of the defect is generally contraindicated. Phlebotomy to relieve the effects of polycythemia or use of hydroxyurea may be considered to relieve clinical signs; however, the prognosis is poor to guarded. Animals diagnosed with a ventricular septal defect should not be bred; the defect has been demonstrated to be heritable in at least one breed (English Springer Spaniels).

ATRIAL SEPTAL DEFECTS

A communication between the atria may be the result of a patent foramen ovale or a true atrial septal defect. During fetal life, the foramen ovale, a flapped oval opening of the interatrial septum, allows shunting of blood from the right atrium to the left atrium to bypass the nonfunctional lungs. This flapped oval opening develops between two septa that make up the interatrial septum: the septum primum and septum secundum. At birth, the drop in right atrial pressure and rise in left atrial pressure cause the foramen ovale to close and shunting to cease. Increased right atrial pressure may prevent closure of the foramen ovale and lead to persistent shunting through a patent foramen ovale. This does not represent a true atrial septal defect, because the septa have formed normally. A true atrial septal defect is an opening or hole within the interatrial septum, which allows blood to shunt from the atrium with the greater pressure. Septum secundum defects occur high in the interatrial septum, near the foramen ovale, and are the most common type. Septum primum defects are located in the most apical portion of the interatrial septum, near the AV junction, and are often a component of AV septal (AV canal) defects. Sinus venosus defects are most often located at the junction of the right atrium and cranial vena cava.

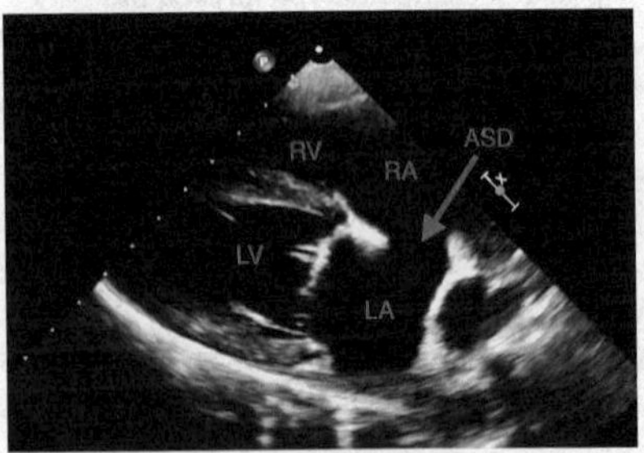

Echocardiographic image of a secundum-type atrial septal defect (ASD) in a dog. RA = right atrium, LA = left atrium, RV = right ventricle, LV = left ventricle. *Courtesy of Dr. Sandra Tou.*

Pathophysiology: In most cases, blood shunts from the left atrium to the right atrium, causing a volume overload of the right-sided chambers. The magnitude of shunting depends on the size of the defect, the ratio of pulmonary to systemic vascular resistance, and the relative compliance of the two ventricles. Excessive blood flow through the right-side chambers results in their dilation and hypertrophy. Pulmonary vasoconstriction and development of pulmonary hypertension may occur as a consequence of excessive pulmonary blood flow and may precipitate right-side CHF. In conditions associated with high right atrial pressure (eg, pulmonic stenosis), shunting may occur from right-to-left across a patent foramen ovale or atrial septal defect, potentially resulting in cyanosis and polycythemia.

Clinical Findings and Treatment: Signs of right heart failure (eg, ascites, jugular venous distention) may be present. A soft ejection-type systolic murmur is usually present over the pulmonic valve area, reflecting increased blood flow through the pulmonic valve. Blood flow through the defect itself does not produce a murmur due to the low velocity of shunt flow. Prolonged ejection time of the right ventricle may result in a split second heart sound. Electrocardiography may reveal evidence of right ventricular or right atrial enlargement (right axis shift, deep S waves, tall P waves). Right bundle-branch block and arrhythmias can also be noted. Radiographically, there are variable degrees of right ventricular enlargement and prominence to the pulmonary vessels indicating pulmonary overcirculation. Echocardiography is indicated and demonstrates varying degrees of right atrial and right ventricular dilatation, as well as identification of the defect as a loss of echogenicity at the interatrial septum. The normal loss of echogenicity of the fossa ovale (artifactual drop out) should not be interpreted as an atrial septal defect. Doppler evaluation confirms shunting through the defect and increased ejection velocities across the pulmonic valve. Surgical correction may be attempted but is associated with high expense and mortality. Animals with small or medium-sized septum secundum defects can tolerate the defects well, and many of these defects are noted as an incidental finding in older animals. Larger defects, such as noted with septum primum defects or endocardial cushion defects, are more likely to cause right-side CHF. The prognosis is guarded to poor in these cases, although many dogs show no clinical signs for years. For dogs with large defects and significant volume overload, surgical or interventional correction is possible. Surgical closure of the defect requires cardiopulmonary bypass and is often limited by expense and availability. Transcatheter closure using a septal occluder has been reported for secundum and muscular defects.

RIGHT-TO-LEFT SHUNTS

TETRALOGY OF FALLOT

Tetralogy of Fallot is the most common defect that produces cyanosis. It results from a combination of four components: pulmonic stenosis, large ventricular septal defect, right ventricular hypertrophy, and dextropositioning (overriding) of the aorta. A single conotruncal malformation (cranially displaced formation of the upper portion of the interventricular septum) is believed to result in narrowing of the right ventricular outflow tract (pulmonic stenosis), overriding of the aorta, and the ventricular septal defect. The right ventricular concentric hypertrophy is simply a consequence of the pulmonic stenosis. The pulmonic stenosis may be valvular, infundibular, or both. Breeds predisposed to tetralogy of Fallot include Keeshonds, English Bulldogs, and Wirehaired Fox Terriers. The trait is inherited in Keeshonds and presumably in other breeds. This defect has been recognized in other breeds of dogs and in cats.

Pathophysiology: The hemodynamic consequences of tetralogy of Fallot depend primarily on the severity of the pulmonic stenosis, the size of the ventricular septal defect (which is typically large and nonrestrictive), and the ratio of pulmonary to systemic vascular resistance. The direction and magnitude of the shunt through the septal defect depends in large part on the relative resistances to flow between the pulmonic circulation (obstructed by the pulmonic stenosis) and the systemic circulation. Consequences include reduced pulmonary blood flow (resulting in fatigue, shortness of breath) and generalized cyanosis (resulting in polycythemia and weakness) caused by the mixing of deoxygenated blood from the right ventricle with oxygenated blood from the left ventricle. Because of venous admixture, the kidneys release erythropoietin, resulting in polycythemia (*see* p 43). The increased blood viscosity associated with polycythemia can lead to sludging of blood and poor capillary perfusion. Consequences of polycythemia include ocular changes, bleeding diathesis, and neurologic abnormalities (ataxia, seizures).

Clinical Findings and Treatment: Typical historical features include stunted growth, exercise intolerance, cyanosis, collapse, and seizures. A precordial thrill may be felt in the area of the pulmonic valve, and in most cases, a murmur of pulmonic stenosis is present. The intensity of the murmur is attenuated when severe polycythemia is present, and in some affected animals, a cardiac murmur is not present. Electrocardiographically, a pattern of right ventricular enlargement is usually seen (deep S waves in lead II, right axis shift), and arrhythmias are infrequent. Radiographs demonstrate variable right heart enlargement and undersized pulmonary vessels. Echocardiography confirms the diagnosis. Overriding (rightward displacement) of the aortic root, right ventricular hypertrophy, and a ventricular septal defect are evident. The left-side chambers may be small as a result of decreased pulmonary venous return. Routine contrast echocardiography demonstrates right-to-left shunting at the level of the ventricular septal defect. Flow through the defect can also be detected by Doppler echocardiography.

β-adrenergic blockade has been used to reduce the dynamic component of right ventricular outflow obstruction and to attenuate β-adrenergic–mediated decreases in systemic vascular resistance. Increases in systemic vascular resistance lower the magnitude of shunting. Polycythemia should be controlled by periodic phlebotomy to resolve clinical signs of polycythemia. The prognosis is guarded, but animals with mild to moderate shunting may reach adulthood.

Treatment options include surgical and medical management. Corrective surgery has been reported in dogs but is rarely performed. Palliative surgical techniques to relieve clinical signs associated with tetralogy of

Fallot are also rarely performed and include techniques to produce systemic to pulmonary anastomoses such as a modified Blalock-Taussig shunt. These procedures increase blood flow to the lungs to reduce signs of pulmonary hypoperfusion and systemic hypoxia. In some cases, reducing pulmonic stenosis is palliative. Surgical valvuloplasty or balloon valvuloplasty of the pulmonic stenosis are also options.

OTHER CYANOTIC HEART DISEASES

PDA, ventricular septal defect, and atrial septal defect with Eisenmenger syndrome are described previously. Other cyanotic heart diseases, including truncus arteriosus, ventricular septal defect with pulmonary atresia, double-outlet right ventricle, and D-transposition of the great arteries, are rare in dogs and cats.

CONDITIONS OF THE ATRIOVENTRICULAR VALVES

MITRAL VALVE DYSPLASIA

Congenital malformation of the mitral valve complex (mitral valve dysplasia) is a common congenital cardiac defect in cats. Canine breeds predisposed are Bull Terriers, German Shepherds, and Great Danes. Mitral valve dysplasia results in mitral insufficiency and systolic regurgitation of blood into the left atrium. Any component of the mitral valve complex (valve leaflets, chordae tendineae, papillary muscles) may be malformed, and often more than one component is defective.

Pathophysiology: Malformation of the mitral valve complex results in significant valvular insufficiency. Chronic mitral regurgitation leads to volume overload of the left heart, which results in dilatation of the left ventricle and atrium. Severe mitral regurgitation can subsequently result in pulmonary venous congestion and left-side CHF. Dilatation of the left-side chambers predisposes affected animals to arrhythmias. When mitral regurgitation is severe, cardiac output decreases and signs of poor cardiac output may occur (weakness, syncope). In some cases, malformation of the mitral valve complex causes a degree of valvular stenosis as well as insufficiency (*see* p 85).

Clinical Findings and Treatment: Clinical signs correlate with the severity of the defect. Affected animals may display signs of left-side CHF. A holosystolic murmur of mitral regurgitation is prominent at the left cardiac apex. A diastolic heart sound (gallop rhythm) is present in some cases. Affected animals may have a precordial thrill over the left cardiac apex. Electrocardiography may demonstrate atrial arrhythmias (atrial premature complexes, atrial fibrillation), especially in severely affected animals with left atrial dilatation. There may also be evidence of both left atrial (widened P waves) and left ventricular enlargement. Thoracic radiographs may demonstrate severe left atrial enlargement. Left ventricular enlargement and pulmonary venous congestion can also be noted. Echocardiography demonstrates malformation of the mitral valve complex (fused chordae tendineae and thickened, immobile valve leaflets, abnormal appearance to the papillary muscles) and left atrial and ventricular dilatation. Doppler echocardiography demonstrates severe mitral regurgitation. Evidence of mitral stenosis can be identified on the echocardiogram (*see* p 85).

Prognosis for animals with clinical signs and severe disease is poor. Mildly affected animals may remain free of clinical signs for several years. Animals with CHF should be treated medically. For therapy of progressive left-side CHF, *see* MANAGEMENT OF HEART FAILURE, p 103.

TRICUSPID VALVE DYSPLASIA

Congenital malformation of the tricuspid valve complex is seen in dogs and cats. Breeds predisposed are Labrador Retrievers and German Shepherds. Tricuspid dysplasia results in tricuspid insufficiency and systolic regurgitation of blood into the right atrium. Rarely, tricuspid valve stenosis can be noted. Chordae tendineae are commonly shortened or absent, and tricuspid valve leaflets may be thickened or adhered to the ventricular or interventricular septal wall. Other concurrent congenital anomalies such as mitral valve dysplasia, septal defects, subaortic stenosis, or pulmonic stenosis may be present. In Ebstein anomaly, a variant of tricuspid dysplasia, the tricuspid valve is displaced toward the cardiac apex.

Pathophysiology: Malformation of the tricuspid valve results in significant valvular insufficiency. Chronic tricuspid regurgitation leads to volume overload of the right heart, dilating the right ventricle and atrium. Pulmonary blood flow may be decreased, resulting in fatigue and tachypnea. As the pressure in the right atrium increases, venous return is impaired, causing signs of right heart failure (ascites, jugular venous distention, and possibly pleural effusion).

Clinical Findings and Treatment: Clinical signs correlate with the severity of the defect. Affected animals may display signs of right-side CHF. A holosystolic murmur of tricuspid regurgitation is prominent at the right cardiac apex. Atrial arrhythmias, especially paroxysmal atrial tachycardia, are common. Electrocardiography and radiography typically demonstrate right ventricular and right atrial enlargement. The caudal vena cava may be significantly enlarged. Echocardiography demonstrates malformation of the tricuspid valve and varying degrees of right atrial and ventricular dilatation. Doppler echocardiography demonstrates tricuspid regurgitation.

Prognosis for animals with clinical signs is highly dependent on the severity of disease and the degree of tricuspid regurgitation. For dogs with right heart failure, CHF therapy and periodic abdominocentesis may be needed to control peritoneal effusion.

MITRAL VALVE STENOSIS

Mitral valve stenosis is a narrowing of the mitral valve orifice caused by abnormalities of the mitral valve, resulting in obstruction to left ventricular inflow. This congenital abnormality is rare in dogs and cats and can occur together with other congenital defects such as subaortic stenosis, mitral valve dysplasia, and pulmonic stenosis.

Pathophysiology: The disease results in increased resistance to left atrial outflow, creating a pressure gradient between the left atrium and left ventricle. This leads to left atrial enlargement and increases in pulmonary venous and capillary wedge pressures. Pulmonary edema can develop as a consequence, and syncope occurs in some cases.

Clinical Findings and Treatment: Mitral stenosis can result in a diastolic heart murmur that is typically low-grade (I-II/VI). If concurrent mitral valve dysplasia is present, a systolic murmur with maximum intensity at the left cardiac apex may be heard. Radiographs demonstrate varying degrees of left atrial enlargement and pulmonary edema in animals with left-side CHF. Electrocardiography may demonstrate widened P waves (indicating left atrial enlargement) and supraventricular arrhythmias. Echocardiography provides a definitive diagnosis. Doming of the mitral valve leaflets toward the left ventricle during diastole, left atrial enlargement, and thickening of the mitral valve leaflets can be noted. Doppler echocardiography demonstrates turbulent diastolic flow across the mitral valve, beginning at the mitral valve and extending into the left ventricle. A pressure gradient is documented between the left atrium and left ventricle in early diastole.

Medical management of animals with mitral valve stenosis involves use of diuretics and dietary sodium restriction. Excessive diuresis should be avoided, because this can reduce cardiac output severely. Surgical or interventional therapy options include closed commisurotomy (disruption of the stenosis without the use of bypass), open commisurotomy, mitral valve replacement, and balloon valvuloplasty.

VASCULAR RING ANOMALIES

Pairs of embryonic aortic arches exist during early fetal development and subsequently give rise to the carotid arteries (third arches), the aortic arch (left fourth arch), and the pulmonary arteries and ductus arteriosus (sixth arches). The other aortic arches regress, although the first aortic arches also become part of the maxillary arteries. Congenital defects may arise if development or dissolution of the aortic arches is disrupted. Multiple vascular ring anomalies have been reported in dogs, including persistent right aortic arch, double aortic arch, left aortic arch with right ligamentum arteriosum, and retroesophageal subclavian arteries.

PERSISTENT RIGHT AORTIC ARCH

Persistent right aortic arch is the most common vascular ring anomaly in dogs (German Shepherds and Irish Setters in particular) and has also been reported in cattle, horses, and cats. The right aortic arch fails to regress normally, resulting in entrapment of the esophagus and trachea at the level of the heart base. The structures are encircled by the persistent arch on the right, by the ligamentum arteriosum on the left and dorsally, and by the base of the heart ventrally. The esophagus is typically compressed, leading to the most common clinical sign of regurgitation (often noted at weaning). Aspiration pneumonia is common in affected animals. Surgery is recommended to transect the ligamentum arteriosum to free the esophagus from entrapment. Radiographically, leftward deviation of the trachea on dorsoventral or ventrodorsal view is highly sensitive and specific for the diagnosis of persistent right aortic arch. CT can confirm the diagnosis before surgery and assist surgical planning.

MISCELLANEOUS CONGENITAL CARDIAC ABNORMALITIES

Peritoneopericardial diaphragmatic hernia is the most common congenital pericardial disease in dogs and cats. It results from abnormal development of the dorsolateral septum transversum or from failure of the lateral pleuroperitoneal folds and the ventromedial pars sternalis to unite. The result is herniation of abdominal viscera into the pericardial sac. The liver is the most commonly herniated organ, followed by the small intestine, spleen, and stomach. Clinical signs are highly variable, with many animals remaining asymptomatic and the defect being discovered on postmortem examination. Thoracic radiographs can demonstrate lack of a visible diaphragmatic border and small-intestinal loops or liver crossing the diaphragm into the pericardial sac. The suspicion of peritoneopericardial diaphragmatic hernia is heightened when abdominal organs are seen adjacent to the heart on echocardiogram. A contrast radiographic examination using oral barium may also identify small-intestinal loops or stomach in the pericardial sac. CT can usually confirm the diagnosis before surgery. In animals with respiratory signs or signs relatable to organ entrapment, the hernia should be surgically reduced.

Cor triatriatum sinister and dexter result from a fibrous membrane dividing the left or right atrium, respectively. Cor triatriatum sinister is a rare defect of cats. It occurs when the common pulmonary vein fails to regress normally; as a result, a fibrous membrane persists within the left atrium, dividing the left atrium into two subchambers. There are commonly one or more perforations in the separating membrane, allowing communication between the two portions of the atrium. The proximal, high-pressure subchamber receives pulmonary venous return, while the distal, low-pressure subchamber is adjacent to the mitral valve and contains the left auricular appendage. Affected cats can present in left heart failure, with pulmonary edema, pleural effusion, or both. Surgical resection and balloon dilation of the membrane using a surgical approach have been reported.

Cor triatriatum dexter is a rare defect of dogs. It is caused by persistence of the right valve of the sinus venosus. The remaining fibrous membrane partitions the right atrium into two subchambers; the cranial vena cava and tricuspid valve are associated with the low-pressure subchamber (true right atrium), whereas the caudal vena cava and coronary sinus are typically associated with the high-pressure subchamber. The membrane may contain one or more perforations, or be imperforate. The degree of blood flow between the subchambers determines the severity of disease. Dogs with more severe septation often present with right heart failure (typically ascites). Surgical resection and transcatheter balloon dilation of the membrane are treatment options. CHF should be medically managed before surgery.

Double chamber right ventricle is an uncommon defect in which an anomalous muscle bundle divides the right ventricle into two chambers. The muscle bundle leads to obstruction of the right ventricular outflow tract, creating a high-pressure proximal subchamber (receiving inflow through the tricuspid valve) and a low-pressure distal subchamber distal to the obstruction. Increased pressure in the proximal subchamber leads to left atrial dilatation and subsequent right heart failure. A systolic ejection murmur is often evident on auscultation. Definitive therapy requires open-heart surgery to resect the muscle bundles, which requires cardiopulmonary bypass. Balloon valvuloplasty has not proved to be a successful treatment option.

Anomalous pulmonary venous connection is a congenital abnormality in which varying numbers of pulmonary veins (from one to all) attach to the right atrium or a systemic vein.

Endocardial cushion defects (AV canal defects, persistent AV ostium, AV septal defects) involve abnormalities of endocardial cushion development and can produce septum primum defects, AV valve abnormalities, and ventricular septal defects.

Dextrocardia, positioning of the heart in the right hemithorax, can be seen as a congenital cardiac defect and by itself is typically benign. It can also be seen in combination with **situs inversus** (an abnormal orientation of the organs of the body). The combination of these defects is typically noted in animals with other concurrent abnormalities such as sinusitis, bronchitis, and bronchiectasis.

HEART DISEASE AND HEART FAILURE

Heart disease is defined as any functional, structural, or electrical abnormality of the heart. It encompasses a wide range of abnormalities, including congenital abnormalities (*see* p 76) as well as anatomic and physiologic disorders of varying causes. Heart disease can be classified by various characteristics, including whether the disease was present at birth or not (eg, congenital or acquired), cause (eg, infectious, degenerative, genetic or heritable), duration (eg, chronic or acute), clinical status (eg, left heart failure, right heart failure, or biventricular failure), by anatomic malformation (eg, ventricular septal defect), or by electrical disturbance (eg, atrial fibrillation, ventricular premature complexes).

Heart failure is usually the end result of severe, overwhelming systolic and/or diastolic cardiac dysfunction that most commonly results in the formation of edema or effusion (eg, pulmonary edema, pleural effusion, ascites) severe enough to cause clinical signs (eg, tachypnea, dyspnea, abdominal distension). It may also produce signs referable to poor perfusion (low cardiac output). This most commonly happens in late-stage chronic heart failure; rarely, it may be due to acute heart failure (eg, ruptured chorda tendineae). The most common abnormalities in systole that lead to heart failure are decreased contractility (eg, dilated cardiomyopathy), severe valvular regurgitation (eg, mitral regurgitation), and left-to-right shunting cardiac defects (eg, ventricular septal defect, patent ductus arteriosus). Myocardial fibrosis is the most common abnormality that causes severe diastolic dysfunction, as seen in cats with hypertrophic cardiomyopathy. Heart disease can be present without ever leading to heart failure. Heart failure, however, can occur only if severe heart disease is present.

DIAGNOSIS OF HEART DISEASE

The diagnosis of heart disease typically involves evaluating the signalment, history, and physical examination findings, as well as results of diagnostic tests such as radiography, electrocardiography, and echocardiography. Rarely, more specialized tests such as cardiac catheterization, CT, MRI, or nuclear studies are necessary.

History and Signalment

For animals with suspected heart disease, the signalment (age, breed, sex) helps formulate a differential diagnosis list. The signalment influences the relative importance of possible heart diseases (eg, endocarditis is rare in cats and small dogs but more common in cows and large dogs) as well as many specific abnormalities (eg, breed predispositions for certain congenital defects, dilated cardiomyopathy (DCM), myxomatous valve degeneration, etc).

Animals presenting with heart disease may have no clinical signs or have a history of tachypnea, dyspnea, abdominal distention (ascites), subcutaneous edema, weakness, syncope (fainting), cyanosis, exercise intolerance, or weight loss. A few historical findings are more species specific, including peripheral or ventral (subcutaneous) edema in horses and cattle. Cats rarely cough with heart failure and more commonly present with a history of tachypnea/dyspnea (which may be subtle and go unnoticed by the owner) and anorexia. In dogs, coughing can occur due to pulmonary edema, but many more dogs that cough do so because of lung disease (eg, chronic bronchitis), so extreme care must be taken when evaluating dogs (especially older, small-breed dogs) with a cough and a heart murmur because most are not in heart failure.

Physical Examination

A complete physical examination should be performed on any animal being evaluated for heart disease or that presents with signs that could be attributable to heart disease. The cardiac physical examination should start with auscultation of the heart. Auscultation should be done in as quiet of an environment as possible. In all cats, small dogs, and small mammals, a pediatric stethoscope should be used and only the diaphragm of the stethoscope needs to be used, because heart sounds, including gallop sounds, in animals this size are not low enough in frequency to require the bell. In large dogs and large animals, the bell should also be used. In general, the left apex beat should first be located by palpation, then the head of the stethoscope placed over it (mitral area). The stethoscope head then should be inched forward and upward to the left base (pulmonic and aortic area).

In any young animal, care should also be taken to place the stethoscope head farther forward (left axillary region) to listen for a continuous murmur (patent ductus arteriosus). Then the right apical region should be ausculted. In a young animal suspected of having congenital heart disease, the right base and along the neck should also be ausculted.

In addition to auscultation of the thorax, palpation of the ventral thorax should be performed to assess for the presence of a thrill (vibration created by turbulent blood flow that can be palpated with the fingertips) and alterations in intensity or location of the apex beat. Concurrent auscultation and palpation of the pulse should also be performed to identify pulse deficits (premature beats, atrial fibrillation) and to assess the strength and character of the systemic arterial pulse. Pulmonary auscultation should be performed (*see* below). Mucous membrane color and refill time should be assessed but are often normal even in animals with severe heart failure. Cyanosis may be present if the animal is severely hypoxemic. Limbs should be examined for the presence of edema, and the abdomen should be assessed for presence of ascites (palpation and ballottement). The jugular veins should be examined with the animal in a standing or sitting position for presence of abnormal distention and pulsation. A normal jugular vein will be distended and may pulsate when an animal is laterally recumbent.

Heart Sounds: Heart sounds are generated by the rapid acceleration and deceleration of blood and secondary vibrations in the cardiohemic system and are associated with valve closure. Four heart sounds can potentially be ausculted. The first heart sound (S_1) is associated with closure of the atrioventricular (mitral and tricuspid) valves, and the second heart sound (S_2) with closure of the semilunar (aortic and pulmonic) valves. The third heart sound (S_3) occurs in early diastole and is a result of the ventricles vibrating at the frequency heard at the time of rapid cessation of ventricular filling, and the fourth heart sound (S_4) is in late diastole and associated with atrial systole (atrial contraction). All four sounds can be heard in a healthy horse. In healthy cattle, typically only S_1 and S_2 are audible, although S_3 or S_4 can sometimes be heard. IV fluid administration in cattle can be used to accentuate S_3 and/or S_4. In dogs, cats, and ferrets, S_1 and S_2 are the only heart sounds normally audible. Less is known about heart sounds in goats, sheep, and pigs; however, only S_1 and S_2 are believed to be audible in these species.

Three-Heart-Sound Rhythms (Gallop Heart Sounds and Systolic Clicks): A gallop heart sound (rhythm) is the presence of S_1 and S_2 accompanied by an interceding sound or sounds in diastole (between S_2 and S_1) that is either an accentuated third heart sound (S_3) or fourth heart sound (S_4), or both. These are classified as protodiastolic (S_3), presystolic (S_4), or summation gallop heart sounds (fusion of S_3 and S_4). The most common gallop heart sound noted in dogs is a result of an accentuated S_3 and typically occurs secondary to a normal quantity of blood "dumping" into a stiff left ventricle (eg, DCM), or a massive amount of blood "dumping" into a normal left ventricle in early diastole (eg, mitral regurgitation and patent ductus arteriosis). An S_4 gallop heart sound is caused by atrial contraction pushing blood into a stiff left ventricle. In cats with cardiomyopathy, especially hypertrophic cardiomyopathy, the left ventricle is stiff, so both third and fourth heart sounds can be heard. However, because the heart rate commonly exceeds 160–180 bpm in cats in an examination room, it is usually impossible via auscultation to determine whether the gallop sound is due to an S_3 or S_4 gallop; often, it is a summation of the two.

Gallop rhythms are not the only three-heart-sound rhythms that can be ausculted. Systolic clicks also occur in dogs and cats and are much more common than gallop rhythms in dogs. A systolic click is a short, sharp sound that occurs during mid to late systole. In dogs, they occur mostly in middle-aged to older small-breed dogs and are thought to be evidence of early myxomatous AV valve degeneration causing mitral valve prolapse (as they are in people). A systolic murmur may or may not also be present. Although systolic clicks are reasonably easy to distinguish from a gallop sound in a dog (they are usually relatively loud and high pitched whereas a gallop sound is soft and low-pitched), they often sound identical to a gallop sound in a cat. Thoracic radiographs can be used to help make the distinction between the two. In cats, gallop sounds are heard only in those with severe heart disease. Systolic clicks are usually heard in cats with an otherwise normal heart. So if the heart is not enlarged, the sound is more likely a systolic click. Systolic clicks usually are single but may be multiple and can vary in intensity (even completely disappearing) depending on cardiac loading conditions. Rarely, a three-heart-sound rhythm can be caused by a bigeminal rhythm.

Splitting of S_1 or S_2: Splitting of S_1 is caused by discordant closure of the mitral and tricuspid valves, which can occur when there is asynchronous contraction of the ventricles as in left or right bundle-branch block, cardiac pacing, and ectopic premature ventricular beats. Splitting of S_1 can also occur in healthy, large-breed dogs and in large animals. Delayed closure of the pulmonic valve (in relation to the aortic valve) results in splitting of S_2. Splitting of S_2 can be a normal finding in horses during respiration. Abnormal splitting of S_2 has been associated with pulmonary hypertension, as in pulmonary emphysema of horses and severe heartworm disease in dogs. Other possible causes include a large atrial septal defect, right bundle-branch block, or premature ventricular ectopic beats of left ventricular origin. Delayed closure of the aortic valve (paradoxical splitting of S_2) might be heard with left bundle-branch block or premature ventricular ectopic beats of right ventricular origin. A split second heart sound is a subtle finding that usually must be heard several times before it can be appreciated.

Heart Murmurs: Heart murmurs are audible vibrations (sound) emanating from the heart or major blood vessels. The vast majority are due to turbulent blood flow brought on by high velocity blood flow that produces a mixed-frequency murmur. Much less commonly, they are due to vibrations of cardiac structures such as part of a valve leaflet or chordal structure that produces a single frequency (musical) murmur. Murmurs are typically defined relative to timing (systole, diastole, continuous), intensity (grade I-VI), and location (eg, left apex, left base) but can also be characterized by frequency (pitch), quality (eg, musical), and configuration (eg, crescendo-decrescendo).

A systolic murmur is classically described as either ejection (crescendo-decrescendo) or regurgitant (holosystolic, plateau). However, making this distinction is often difficult, even for an experienced examiner, especially when the heart rate is fast. Ejection-quality systolic murmurs typically demonstrate the greatest intensity during mid-systole and appear diamond-shaped on phonocardiography. They are most commonly produced by stenotic lesions at the semilunar valves (eg, pulmonic stenosis or subaortic stenosis). A classic regurgitant systolic murmur demonstrates a constant intensity throughout systole and is commonly caused by mitral or tricuspid regurgitation (eg, myxomatous degeneration of the mitral valve) or a ventricular septal defect. However, these murmurs may also change intensity during systole. Diastolic murmurs are typically decrescendo (decreasing in intensity through diastole) and usually the result of aortic insufficiency (such as that caused by aortic valve infective endocarditis in dogs or degenerative disease in horses). In horses, the murmur of aortic insufficiency is most commonly musical, although "musical" in this context is a technical term (single frequency). They may sound like a dive-bomber or grunting. A continuous murmur is most commonly the result of patent ductus arteriosus and occurs throughout systole and diastole. A continuous murmur varies in intensity over time, typically being most intense at the end of ventricular ejection (second heart sound) and then decreasing in intensity through diastole. A to-and-fro murmur describes a murmur that occurs both in systole and in diastole (eg, in an animal with subaortic stenosis and aortic insufficiency).

In horses, early systolic and diastolic murmurs can be noted in the absence of heart disease or anemia. The point of maximal intensity is typically located over the left heart base. A short, high-pitched, squeaking, early diastolic cardiac murmur is sometimes heard in healthy, young horses. Often, a systolic heart murmur is heard in a cat without cardiac disease. Some of these systolic murmurs are due to an increase in right outflow tract flow velocity (dynamic right ventricular outflow tract obstruction). Innocent cardiac murmurs are also sometimes noted in immature cats and dogs (<3 mo old) and may be the result of a relative increase in stroke volume (stroke volume/aortic cross-sectional area).

Heart murmur intensity is classified as follows: Grade I—the lowest intensity murmur that can be heard, typically detected only while auscultation is performed in a quiet room; Grade II—a faint murmur, easily audible, and restricted to a localized area; Grade III—a murmur immediately audible when auscultation begins; Grade IV—a loud murmur immediately heard at the beginning of auscultation but not accompanied by a thrill; Grade V—a very loud murmur with a palpable thrill; and Grade VI—an extremely loud murmur with a thrill and that can be heard when the stethoscope is just removed from the chest wall.

Arrhythmias: Arrhythmias are abnormalities of the rate, regularity, or site of cardiac impulse formation and are noted during auscultation. Other terms such as dysrhythmia and ectopic rhythm are also used to describe arrhythmias. The presence of a cardiac arrhythmia does not necessarily indicate the presence of heart disease; some arrhythmias are normal, such as sinus arrhythmia in a dog and second-degree AV block in a horse; many cardiac arrhythmias are clinically insignificant and require no specific therapy. Some arrhythmias, however, may cause severe clinical signs, such as syncope, or lead to sudden death. Numerous systemic disorders may be associated with abnormal cardiac rhythms. (For discussion of specific arrhythmias, *see* p 94.) Common auscultatory findings in animals with an arrhythmia are a rate that is too slow (bradycardia), a rate that is too fast (tachycardia), premature beats (a beat is heard too early), an irregular rhythm, and pauses in the rhythm. Whenever an abnormal rhythm is heard, an ECG should be performed.

Pulses: The arterial pulse is the rhythmic expansion of an artery that can be digitally palpated (or visualized) during physical examination. Physiologically, the pulse pressure is the systolic pressure minus the diastolic pressure. The arterial pulse can be felt best in several different locations. For example, in dogs and cats, the arterial pulse is typically palpated at the femoral artery. In horses, the facial artery is usually used. To feel the maximum pulse, an examiner must first occlude the artery with his or her fingers and then gradually decrease the digital pressure until the maximum pulse is felt. A weak pulse (a reduction in pulse pressure) is usually caused by a decrease in systolic pressure and can be noted with decreased stroke volume in animals in heart failure, hypovolemic shock, or cardiac tamponade, as well as with subaortic stenosis. However, a weak pulse can also be felt in a healthy animal if the artery is not palpated appropriately or in an obese or heavily muscled animal. A bounding pulse (an increase in pulse pressure) is usually caused primarily by a reduced diastolic pressure and can be noted with aortic insufficiency and patent ductus arteriosus. However, the pulse in a thin, athletic dog may also feel stronger than expected. The pulse felt with mitral regurgitation is often normal but at times may be termed "brisk." A pulse deficit is an absent pulse despite auscultation of a heart beat and is thus detected during simultaneous auscultation and pulse palpation. This often occurs as the result of a premature beat that occurs so early that the ventricles are unable to fill sufficiently, resulting in a reduced stroke volume that produces either a weak pulse or no pulse. Atrial fibrillation also produces pulse deficits as well as alternating pulse strength.

Dogs with severe subaortic stenosis may have a pulse pressure that slowly increases during ventricular systole and reaches a peak pressure late in systole called pulsus parvus et tardus. Pulsus paradoxus is a decrease in pulse pressure during inspiration and an increase in pulse pressure during expiration. This is a normal occurrence in animals, but it is too subtle to observe on physical examination. Animals with cardiac tamponade (severe pericardial effusion), however, demonstrate an exaggeration of this finding, so it becomes detectable. Pulsus alternans is an alternating strong and weak pulse while the animal is in sinus rhythm; it can be noted (albeit rarely) in animals with severe (usually terminal) myocardial failure or tachyarrhythmias. Pulsus bigeminus is an alternating strong and weak pulse caused by an arrhythmia such as ventricular bigeminy. The weaker pulse (during the ventricular premature contraction) typically follows a shorter time interval than the stronger pulse.

Jugular venous pulsation can be noted in normal animals but typically does not extend beyond the thoracic inlet.

Respiratory Sounds: Pulmonary edema may develop as a result of congestive heart failure (CHF). Animals with pulmonary edema will be hyperpneic (increased rate and depth of respiration) and may be dyspneic. The increased depth of respiration may increase bronchovesicular sounds. Fine, and less commonly, coarse crackles might be ausculted in animals with pulmonary edema, but fine crackles are usually heard only at the end of a deep inspiration. Coarse crackles in dogs are most commonly heard with chronic bronchitis. Pulmonary edema is often silent (no auscultatory abnormality). Respiratory sounds may be absent in animals with pleural effusion, especially ventrally.

Ascites: Abdominal distention may occur as a result of gas, soft tissue, or fluid accumulation. Animals with right heart failure (eg, due to severe heartworm disease, severe tricuspid valve dysplasia, cardiac tamponade) can develop ascites. Because there are many causes of ascites, it is important to evaluate the jugular veins in every case in which ascites is present. If right heart failure is the cause of the ascites, the jugular veins may be distended (but often are not in dogs and cats) by the increase in right atrial pressure. If the jugular veins are not distended in a dog or cat with ascites, a hepatojugular reflux test should be performed. To do this, one person examines the jugular veins with the animal standing or sitting, while another places firm and steady pressure on the abdomen. In a dog or cat in right heart failure, the jugular veins should distend well up the neck with this maneuver. If ascites is present without jugular venous distension and with a negative hepatojugular reflux test, then extracardiac causes of the ascites should be considered.

Synchronous Diaphragmatic Flutter: The diaphragm may contract synchronously with the heart to produce loud thumping noises on auscultation and usually visible contraction in the flank area. The syndrome results from stimulation of the phrenic nerve by atrial depolarization and occurs primarily when there is a marked electrolyte or acid-base imbalance, particularly with hypocalcemia. It is most common in horses and dogs. It is seen most commonly in dogs in association with hypocalcemia and electrolyte disturbances induced by GI disease. Similarly, in horses it is seen with hypocalcemia and in endurance horses that are dehydrated and electrolyte depleted.

Radiography

Thoracic radiographs frequently provide valuable information in the assessment of animals with or suspected of having heart disease. However, thoracic radiography is rarely performed in horses or cows to evaluate heart disease because of the animal's large size and body conformation, which reduces the quality of the images. In dogs, in which numerous different body types must be dealt with, chest conformation must always be assessed before attempting to evaluate cardiac size. On the lateral view, dogs can be normal, shallow-chested, or deep-chested. On the dorsoventral (DV) or ventrodorsal (VD) views, they can be normal, narrow-chested, or barrel-chested. Many small breeds of dogs are shallow-chested. This makes the cardiac silhouette appear to be enlarged on the lateral view and often necessitates relying on the DV view to obtain an accurate assessment of size and shape. In deep-chested breeds, even severe cardiomegaly can look normal on the lateral view and, because the heart sits more upright in the chest, can also mask its presence on the DV view (eg, in Doberman Pinschers with DCM). Obesity also interferes with accurate reading of cardiac size by the presence of intrapericardial fat or by pushing the diaphragm forward, reducing the size of the thoracic space and pushing the heart into the cranial and narrower aspect of the thoracic cavity. Because of the marked variation in chest conformation, the changes seen between inspiration and expiration, and the changes seen between systole and diastole, only relatively dramatic changes in overall cardiac size can be identified in most dogs. Consequently, conditions such as mild generalized cardiomegaly cannot be identified on thoracic radiographs. The one chamber where mild, moderate, and severe enlargement can be relatively accurately identified is the left atrium. Finding enlargement of specific cardiac chambers and great vessels makes the presence of heart disease more likely and may also provide clues as to the specific disease present.

Cardiogenic pulmonary edema is a common finding in animals with CHF and may be associated with pulmonary venous congestion. However, the identification of pulmonary edema is often difficult and may not be possible in some dogs and even some cats. Cardiogenic pulmonary edema in dogs is typically found in the caudodorsal aspects of the lungs. In many cases, this region has an interstitial density that is enhanced by age and by expiration, giving a false impression that pulmonary edema is present or masking the presence of pulmonary edema. Digital radiography units, especially if not set up perfectly (to match analog units), have made the diagnosis even harder in many cases. In animals with chronic left heart failure, the left atrium is usually severely and always at least moderately enlarged. In acute heart failure (eg, chorda tendineae rupture), the left atrium may not be enlarged. Pleural effusion can usually be readily identified radiographically. In most species, this is seen with right or biventricular heart failure. However, in cats it is seen most commonly with left heart failure. Resolution of these abnormalities on subsequent thoracic radiographs can be used as one indication of efficacy of therapy. The presence of pulmonary edema or pleural effusion does not definitively confirm a cardiogenic origin or exclude another origin.

Overall cardiac size can be assessed using the vertebral heart scale or score. This is most commonly done using the lateral projection. The maximal diameter of the cardiac silhouette from cranial to caudal is measured, as well as the distance from the carina to the apex of the cardiac silhouette (dorsal to ventral). These lengths are added together and measured in terms of thoracic vertebral bodies, so they are normalized for the size of the animal. The vertebral bodies are measured from the fourth thoracic vertebra caudally. The normal range is 8.5–10.5 vertebral bodies in dogs and 6.9–8.1 in cats. In many cases, it is more important to try to accurately assess the size of the left atrium than the overall size of the cardiac silhouette.

Electrocardiography

Electrocardiography is the recording of cardiac electrical activity from the body surface (surface ECG). It should primarily be used to identify cardiac arrhythmias. It can also identify conduction disturbances that do not alter rhythm and has been used to identify chamber enlargement in dogs and cats. However, its inaccuracy in identifying chamber enlargement and the advent of diagnostic ultrasound have diminished this role. As opposed to small animals in which the Purkinje fibers penetrate only ~ ⅓ of the way into the myocardium, Purkinje fibers in horses and cattle penetrate throughout the myocardium, resulting in "burst" depolarization of the ventricles and reduced waveform production and complexes on the surface ECG. Consequently, there is no relationship between complex height on a surface ECG and chamber enlargement. The most common ECG lead used in large animals is a base-apex that produces large deflections and is used for rhythm analysis. ECGs should be used only to characterize an arrhythmia in an animal with an auscultatory arrhythmia and to monitor rhythm during anesthesia; they should never be used as screening tools, as they are in human medicine (primarily for changes secondary to coronary artery disease).

Waveform Abnormalities: Chamber enlargement can be indicated by waveform abnormalities in dogs and cats, but these abnormalities are commonly absent when there is chamber enlargement and are sometimes present when the heart is normal. In lead II in dogs and cats, wide or notched P waves suggest left atrial enlargement, whereas tall P waves suggest right atrial enlargement. Tall R waves in leads that have the positive electrode on the left and/or caudal aspect of the body (leads I, II, aVF, CV6LL, and CV6LU) are evidence of left ventricular enlargement. Deep S waves in the same leads in which the positive electrode is on the left side of the heart or the presence of a right-axis deviation suggest right ventricular enlargement. Wide QRS complexes can be seen in animals with either right or left ventricular enlargement; however, they can also be due to conduction disturbances (*see* p 93). The ECG is very insensitive at identifying mild to moderate changes in chamber size and unacceptably insensitive for detecting severe enlargement. Although false-positive findings are less frequent than false-negative findings, they do occur. Consequently, the accuracy is unacceptable, especially when compared with echocardiography and even with thoracic radiography.

Sinus Rhythm and Sinus Node Abnormalities: The sinus node initiates depolarization of the rest of the heart in a healthy animal, sets the normal rate and rhythm, and is called the normal pacemaker of the heart. It functions as the pacemaker because it is automatic (depolarizes on its own) and does so at a rate faster than the other automatic sites in the heart (AV node and Purkinje fibers). Normal sinus rhythm is regular and originates at the sinus node, indicated on the ECG by a P wave that precedes each normal QRS complex. The rate at which the sinus node fires varies tremendously from species to species and situation to situation. For example, a healthy horse can have a heart rate of 30 bpm at rest and 250 bpm during maximal exercise. Similarly, a healthy dog can have a heart rate in the teens when asleep and ≥250 bpm during maximal exercise. A healthy cat can have a heart rate of 240 bpm at rest in an examination room.

Sinus bradycardia is a regular sinus rhythm that is slower than expected for that species and for the situation the animal is in. Sinus bradycardia may be noted in animals overdosed with anesthesia or agents that can result in increased vagal tone (primary or secondary) or reduced sympathetic tone (eg, xylazine, β-adrenergic blocker), hypothermic animals, hypothyroid animals, animals with sick sinus syndrome, or in animals with increased vagal tone secondary to systemic disease (such as respiratory, neurologic, ocular, GI, or urinary tract disease). Treatment for sinus bradycardia is typically not needed unless clinical signs associated with the bradycardia, such as exercise intolerance, weakness, or collapse, are noted. In dogs and cats, atropine (0.04 mg/kg, IV, IM, or SC) may be considered for treatment of bradycardia. The initiating cause should also be corrected.

Sinus tachycardia is the finding of a regular sinus rhythm at a rate faster than normal but generally appropriate for the situation the animal is in (eg, stress, exercise, heart failure). If the rate is inappropriately high (eg, 200 bpm in an otherwise healthy dog at rest at home), another form of tachycardia (eg, atrial or ventricular) should be considered. Causes include stress (resulting in high sympathetic drive), exercise, hyperthyroidism, fever, pain, hypovolemia, cardiac tamponade, heart failure, or administration of agents that can increase the rate of sinus node discharge (eg, catecholamines). Treatment involves resolving the underlying cause.

Sinus arrhythmia occurs as a result of irregular discharge of the sinus node most commonly associated with the respiratory cycle. The site of impulse formation remains the sinus node; however, the frequency of the discharge varies. Sinus arrhythmia is a normal finding in dogs and horses; it is abnormal in cats in the hospital setting, although it appears to be more common in cats in their home environment. Respiratory sinus arrhythmia is characterized by an increase in heart rate with inspiration and a decrease with expiration. In dogs, sinus arrhythmia can also be seen that is not in sync with respiration. The variation in heart rate is associated with variation in the intensity of vagal tone. It is abolished by reduced vagal tone resulting from excitement, exercise, or administration of vagolytic drugs such as atropine. It may be associated with a wandering pacemaker, which is characterized on the ECG by taller P waves during faster rates and smaller P waves during slower rates.

Sinoatrial (SA) block occurs when the impulse from the SA node fails to be conducted through the surrounding tissue to the atria and ventricles. Thus, no P waves or QRS complexes are noted on the ECG, and the P-P interval surrounding the break in sinus rhythm is an exact multiple of the normal P-P interval. This is often difficult to diagnose in dogs because sinus arrhythmia is common, resulting in a variable normal P-P interval.

Sinus arrest (sinoatrial arrest, sinus pause) is the absence of P waves on the ECG for a short period (typically accepted as a pause exceeding twice the normal P-P interval). Sinus arrest is caused by excessive vagal tone, inherent sinus node disease, or both. This is usually due to some form of sick sinus syndrome (*see* below).

Atrial standstill is characterized as the complete absence of P waves on the ECG and occurs as a result of the atria being unable to be depolarized from the SA node discharge. This occurs either because the atrial myocardium is functionally unable to be depolarized (usually due to hyperkalemia), or because it has been destroyed by a cardiomyopathy or myocarditis (persistent atrial standstill). In hyperkalemia, the sinus node continues to depolarize, and the electrical tracts from the sinus node to the AV node (internodal tracts) continue to function, so the sinus node controls the rate (albeit at a slower rate). With persistent atrial standstill, the sinus node is destroyed, so the animal usually has an AV nodal (junctional) escape rhythm with a heart rate in the 40–65 bpm range (dog).

Sick sinus syndrome is a constellation of abnormalities, including ECG changes (sinus arrest, junctional or ventricular escape complexes, and possibly supraventricular tachycardia) and possible weakness or syncope from the bradycardia (usual) or tachycardia (rare). With this clinical syndrome, the principal problem either lies within the SA node or perinodal tissue, or is due to increased vagal tone, or both. In some instances, other portions of the specialized conduction tissue of the myocardium, including the AV node, can also be affected. Therefore, evidence for AV block may also be seen (*see* below). This condition is commonly noted in geriatric dogs, including Miniature Schnauzers and American Cocker Spaniels. Medical therapy consisting of parasympatholytics (eg, propantheline bromide, 0.25–0.5 mg/kg, PO, bid-tid) or sympathomimetics (eg, extended-release theophylline, 10 mg/kg, PO, bid; terbutaline, 0.14 mg/kg, PO, bid-tid in dogs) to increase heart rate can be tried, but these are often ineffective or are effective for only a relatively short time or with unacceptable adverse effects. These drugs may also worsen supraventricular tachyarrhythmias that can occur with sick sinus syndrome. The most effective treatment for the bradycardia is pacemaker implantation.

AV Conduction Disturbances: Atrioventricular (AV) block refers to alteration of impulse conduction through the AV node from the atria to the ventricles. In first-degree AV block (prolonged conduction), the conduction time is increased and is recognized on an ECG as an increased PR interval. This is clinically silent. In second-degree AV block (intermittent conduction), occasional impulses fail to be conducted through the AV node, bundle of His, or both bundle branches and is characterized by occasional P waves not followed by QRS complexes. During the block, there is no S_1 or S_2 and no arterial pulse. In horses, the sound associated with atrial contraction (S_4) is commonly heard, and the occurrence of S_4 not followed by other heart sounds is diagnostic for second-degree heart block. S_4 may also be audible in dogs with second-degree AV block, but this is much less common. When the PR intervals preceding the dropped beat progressively lengthen, the condition is known as Mobitz type I second-degree AV block or Wenckebach phenomenon. This is usually due to high vagal tone and is the most common type of second-degree AV block seen in horses and puppies. No treatment is indicated. If the PR intervals do not change, the condition is known as a Mobitz type II second-degree AV block. Again, no treatment is indicated, but closer surveillance may be warranted to see whether the block progresses to a more severe form. A third type of second-degree AV block, high-grade second-degree AV block, refers to the situation when the block occurs with every other beat (2:1 [ie, two P waves for every QRS complex]) or more (3:1, 4:1, etc). High-grade second-degree AV block is distinguished from third-degree AV block by identifying an association between the QRS complexes and the P wave preceding each one (same PR interval for each). Dogs with high-grade second-degree AV block can have signs the same as dogs with third-degree AV block (eg, syncope) and are also at increased risk of sudden death.

In third-degree AV or complete heart block, none of the impulses is conducted from the atria to the ventricles. The atrial rhythm (P waves) occurs more rapidly and independently from the ventricular rhythm (QRS complexes; a form of AV dissociation), which originates from subsidiary pacemakers (AV node or Purkinje fibers in the ventricles; nodal and ventricular escape beats, respectively). The heart and pulse rates are usually regular but slow and generally unresponsive to factors or agents that usually increase heart rate (eg, exercise, excitement, atropine). The difference in timing between atrial and ventricular contractions results in variation in ventricular filling and consequent variation in intensity of S_1 (bruit de canon) and possibly arterial pulse pressure. Periodically, the atria contract when the ventricle is in systole, which results in a pulsation in the jugular vein (cannon A wave).

The significance of the AV block varies by species. Both first- and second-degree AV block may be present without outward evidence of cardiac disease. First-degree AV block may result from excessive vagal tone and usually is not significant in dogs or horses unless other evidence of heart disease or pathologic cause of increased vagal tone (eg, CNS or pulmonary disease) or AV nodal disease is present. In all species, second-degree AV block may be indicative of heart disease. However, in horses, Mobitz type I is common and is a normal physiologic response resulting from increased vagal tone. Mobitz type II second-, high-grade second-, and third-degree (complete) AV blocks are always abnormal in all species.

Second- and third-degree AV blocks may be caused by fibrosis, neoplasia, or injury to the AV node, or by hypoxia, increased vagal tone, or electrolyte abnormalities. The ideal treatment would be to correct the underlying cause, although this is not usually possible. High-grade second-degree AV block and third-degree AV block can cause exercise intolerance or, more commonly, weakness, collapse, and syncope. Oral therapy with extended-release theophylline (10 mg/kg, PO, bid), terbutaline (0.14 mg/kg, PO, bid-tid in dogs), or propantheline bromide (0.25–0.5 mg/kg, PO, bid-tid) may occasionally be useful in animals with second-degree AV block, but more aggressive therapy (pacemaker implantation) is usually indicated in symptomatic (eg, syncopal) animals. Third-degree heart block is usually associated with irreversible lesions; the only effective treatment in dogs is pacemaker implantation. Dogs with third-degree AV block are at risk of sudden death and so should have a pacemaker implanted regardless of clinical signs. In cats, third-degree AV block often produces no clinical signs and so requires no therapy. However, problems can arise if it is not identified before anesthesia, and some cats will faint and thus require pacemaker implantation. Third-degree AV block is rare in horses and other species. Pacemakers have been implanted successfully in species other than dogs and cats but has rarely been done.

Common Tachyarrhythmias: Tachyarrhythmias can be divided into supraventricular and ventricular based on their site of origin. Supraventricular premature complexes are premature complexes (as seen on an ECG) that originate from ectopic (nonautomatic) sites above the ventricles (eg, atrial myocardium and AV node). They may also be called atrial or nodal premature complexes/depolarizations/contractions/beats. Possible sites for ectopic depolarizations include the SA node (rare), atrial myocardium (very common), and AV node (AV junction). Electrocardiographically, supraventricular premature complexes are identified by a QRS complex that usually appears relatively normal but occurs earlier than the next expected normal QRS complex. Variable P wave morphologies may be noted before or after the supraventricular premature complex or may be hidden in the preceding sinus complex or within the premature complex. Supraventricular premature complexes are most commonly a result of atrial enlargement or disease, stress, or other causes of increased sympathetic tone. Supraventricular tachycardia (SVT) is a series of supraventricular premature complexes occurring consecutively. It may be short (nonsustained) or occur for prolonged periods (called sustained when >30 sec). SVT most commonly ranges in rate from 200–350 bpm in dogs. At rates closer to 200 bpm, it may be indistinguishable from sinus tachycardia on a surface ECG. Vagal maneuvers (ocular pressure, carotid sinus massage), precordial blow (chest thump), and IV drug administration (eg, diltiazem) often "break" an SVT into sinus rhythm and either do not change or more gradually slow a sinus tachycardia. Diltiazem (0.5–4 mg/kg, PO, tid) is the most common drug used to treat SVT long-term, but it can also be used IV to break the SVT into sinus rhythm (0.25 mg/kg, IV bolus administered over 2 min, followed 15 min later by up to 0.35 mg/kg, IV bolus administered over 2 min, if needed). Digoxin and β-blockers are also used. An accessory pathway (bypass tract) is a congenital abnormality that forms an electrical connection between an atrium and a ventricle outside the normal connection (AV node/bundle of His). These pathways have been recognized in dogs and cats and may result in supraventricular tachycardia (eg, orthodromic reciprocating tachycardia). Treatment may include radiofrequency catheter (heat) ablation of the bypass tract or, more commonly, oral medications such as procainamide, sotalol, or diltiazem.

Atrial flutter is a rare arrhythmia that often progresses to atrial fibrillation. It is most commonly caused by a reentrant loop within the atria and is classically characterized on the ECG by a "saw-toothed" baseline with relatively normal QRS complexes that can appear in a regular or irregular rhythm. The atrial rate of discharge is very rapid (>400 bpm). Only intermittent atrial impulses are conducted through the AV node because of its normal long refractory period, so the ventricular rate is slower than the atrial rate.

In dogs and cats, atrial fibrillation is an even more rapid (>600–700 atrial depolarizations/min) atrial rhythm that results in a slower (in the 80–300 bpm range in dogs) and always irregular ventricular rhythm. As in atrial flutter, the AV node is bombarded by frequent atrial depolarizations. The AV node acts as a filter, allowing only some of the depolarizations to reach the ventricles but always in an irregular fashion. In dogs and cats, atrial fibrillation is characterized on the ECG by a supraventricular (normal-appearing QRS complexes) and an irregular ventricular rhythm that is most commonly fast. Once those characteristics are identified, the next thing to look for is the absence of P waves and an undulating baseline that can appear almost flat (fine) or very rough (coarse). The irregular rhythm results in variation in the diastolic filling period of the ventricles, resulting in variability in stroke volume and thus variability in pulse character, including pulse deficits. This also causes variation in the intensity of the heart sounds, especially the second heart sound, creating a heart that sounds like "tennis shoes in a dryer" on auscultation in dogs. In dogs, atrial fibrillation is most commonly associated with underlying cardiac disease. The notable exception occurs in some giant dog breeds, such as Irish Wolfhounds, Scottish Deerhounds, Great Danes, and others, in which the rhythm can develop with an otherwise normal heart (so-called lone or primary atrial fibrillation). Lone atrial fibrillation is the most common form seen in horses (*see* below). All cats in atrial fibrillation have severe underlying heart disease.

The goal of treatment of atrial fibrillation in most dogs and all cats is control of the ventricular rate, ie, the frequency with which QRS complexes are generated from the fibrillatory depolarization waves. Rate control is usually accomplished with digoxin alone, diltiazem alone, or a combination of the two. Diltiazem alone is generally more effective then digoxin alone, and the combination is generally more effective than either alone. A β-blocker, such as atenolol, may also be used but never in combination with diltiazem. These drugs prolong the refractory period of the AV node and slow AV nodal conduction, resulting in fewer atrial depolarizations crossing the AV node to the ventricles. Amiodarone has also been used to control the ventricular response rate, but its adverse effects (hepatic and thyroid toxicities) limit its use to second-line therapy in animals refractory to the digoxin and diltiazem/atenolol protocol. In rare instances, electrical cardioversion (defibrillation of the heart that is synced to the ECG to prevent causing ventricular fibrillation) is used to convert atrial fibrillation to sinus rhythm. This is generally more rational in a dog with lone atrial fibrillation but has also been done in dogs with severe cardiac disease. In those instances, sinus rhythm commonly reverts back to atrial fibrillation within weeks to months, necessitating reconversion or rate control. Cardioversion is frequently combined with amiodarone administration in an attempt to prolong the time until reversion to atrial fibrillation.

In ruminants, atrial fibrillation is usually paroxysmal and associated with GI tract disorders (eg, vagal indigestion), but it also may be persistent and occur as a sequela of cor pulmonale or with other cardiac diseases.

In horses, atrial fibrillation can usually be diagnosed by identifying an undulating baseline. It most often occurs in the absence of underlying cardiac disease (primary or lone atrial fibrillation) and is associated with the normally high vagal tone found in horses that most likely have some predisposition for the arrhythmia. However, it may also occur secondary to cardiac disease such as mitral insufficiency, aortic insufficiency, myocarditis, pericarditis, or untreated congenital cardiac defects. The resting heart rate is usually within the normal range when there is no underlying cardiac disease, whereas it is typically increased with underlying disease; this may help identify the cause of the arrhythmia on physical examination. Most horses with primary atrial fibrillation exhibit no clinical signs at rest or with moderate exercise or work; however, more strenuous exercise or work may result in evidence of reduced cardiac output. This can be seen in racehorses who are evaluated for a sudden reduction in race performance. In this setting, the clinical signs could also be due to paroxysmal atrial fibrillation, which can be identified only during the exercise period. In horses with primary atrial fibrillation, conversion to sinus rhythm with quinidine at a dosage of 22 mg/kg, PO, every 2 hr until conversion, is still the treatment of choice. The success rate for conversion is greatest in horses with atrial fibrillation of shorter duration. The chance for success is considered excellent if the duration is <4 mo and relatively good if >4 mo, although conversion may take longer and quinidine toxicity is more likely to develop. Horses with atrial fibrillation can also be successfully converted to sinus rhythm electrically (cardioversion). This requires the careful placement of electrode catheters in a pulmonary artery and the right atrium (via the jugular vein) of an awake horse followed by anesthesia and then delivery of electrical shocks of increasing intensity through the catheters. This method is very successful but is time-consuming and expensive. Most horses can return to successful racing performance after conversion. However, some will revert to atrial fibrillation over time. Conversion to sinus rhythm is not indicated in horses with severe underlying cardiac disease, because the likelihood of conversion, or maintenance of sinus rhythm if converted, is very low.

Ventricular premature complexes arise from a site within the ventricular myocardium or specialized conduction system. On the ECG, the QRS complex usually appears wide and is followed by a large T wave that is opposite in polarity to the QRS complex. This produces a large, bizarre complex when compared with normally sinus-driven QRS complexes, occurs earlier than the next expected sinus-driven QRS complex (ie, premature), and does not have an associated preceding P wave, although unassociated P waves going at a slower rate (AV dissociation) may be seen. Most commonly, these complexes occur from noncardiac causes such as anesthesia, age, electrolyte abnormalities, acute toxicities, neoplasia (eg, splenic hemangiosarcoma in dogs), gastric distention (eg, gastric dilation and volvulus syndrome in dogs), or trauma. They may also be associated with ventricular myocardial diseases such as DCM, arrhythmogenic right ventricular cardiomyopathy (Boxer cardiomyopathy), and myocarditis.

Ventricular tachycardia is the occurrence of three or more sequential ventricular premature complexes. These can again be nonsustained or sustained (>30 sec). They can also be divided into slower, benign ventricular tachycardias and faster, malignant ones. A slower, benign ventricular tachycardia is called an accelerated idioventricular rhythm (AIVR) and is commonly seen in dogs in the intensive care unit secondary to systemic (often intra-abdominal) disease or trauma. It is characterized on the ECG by the presence of a ventricular tachycardia that is relatively slow (usually <200 bpm). Sinus rhythm may be interspersed with the AIVR, with one rhythm taking control of the rhythm whenever it is slightly faster than the other.

Fusion beats (hybrid sinus beat and premature ventricular contraction [PVC]) can also be seen. This arrhythmia does not result in sudden death and usually dissipates on its own within 48–72 hr. As such, it only needs to be treated (eg, lidocaine) if it is causing hemodynamic instability.

Malignant ventricular tachycardia is most commonly found in dogs with severe underlying cardiac disease, usually either a cardiomyopathy (eg, DCM or arrhythmogenic right ventricular cardiomyopathy) or severe semilunar valve stenosis (eg, subaortic stenosis, pulmonic stenosis). Malignant ventricular tachycardia predisposes the animal to sudden death due to the tachycardia degenerating into ventricular fibrillation. Frequently, this arrhythmia is not identified, so the first clinical sign seen is sudden death. Some dogs (especially Boxers and Doberman Pinschers) will experience syncope as the result of a very fast (often >400 bpm) ventricular tachycardia that spontaneously reverts back to sinus rhythm within seconds (must last >6 sec and usually lasts no more than 1 min) of its onset. Sotalol or a combination of atenolol and mexiletine effectively controls the arrhythmia in Boxers and usually stops the syncope and presumably prevents sudden death. β-blockers are frequently administered to dogs with severe subaortic stenosis and to some with severe pulmonic stenosis in an attempt to prevent sudden death. Proof of efficacy is lacking. Sotalol may be a more logical choice. Ventricular tachycardia must be distinguished from ventricular escape rhythm, as seen with third-degree AV block, and from idioventricular rhythm, a terminal ventricular escape rhythm. A ventricular escape rhythm is a slow rhythm (20–40 bpm) that occurs because higher pacemakers (SA and AV nodes) have failed. Suppression of a ventricular escape rhythm by drug therapy (eg, lidocaine) results in cessation of all cardiac electrical activity (ie, death).

Ventricular fibrillation is a result of microreentrant circuits within the ventricular myocardium, resulting in the absence of effective ventricular contractions; thus, it is a terminal rhythm. The only effective treatment is electrical defibrillation.

Antiarrhythmics: A detailed discussion of antiarrhythmic therapy is covered elsewhere (*see* p 2535). Most antiarrhythmic drugs are administered to suppress ectopic premature depolarizations (eg, atrial and ventricular premature complexes, atrial and ventricular tachycardia) or to slow the ventricular rate in animals with atrial flutter or fibrillation. Many of these drugs are being supplanted by automatic implantable defibrillators in human medicine, so the manufacture of these drugs is waning. Some of the antiarrhythmics have negative inotropic effects, with the potential to worsen active CHF. This is most likely to occur with the use of β-blockers in the treatment of supraventricular tachyarrhythmias and with sotalol.

Atrial fibrillation is one of the most commonly treated tachyarrhythmias; it is imperative to decrease the ventricular rate to ≤160 bpm if the rate is faster than that in the clinic. In experimental situations, pacing the heart of a dog at a rate ≥180 bpm results in myocardial failure severe enough to cause CHF within weeks. Consequently, leaving the rate this high will cause further cardiac disease and decompensation. There are no firm data to suggest that keeping the heart rate even lower than 160 bpm is beneficial in dogs. Diltiazem (0.5–2 mg/kg, PO, tid) or a combination of diltiazem and digoxin are generally the preferred methods of controlling the ventricular rate in dogs with atrial fibrillation. A low dose of a β-blocker, such as atenolol (0.25 mg/kg, PO, bid), may also be used instead of diltiazem, but its use is uncommon. (*See also* ANTIARRHYTHMICS, p 2535.)

Ventricular tachycardia can degenerate into ventricular fibrillation and cause sudden death. Fast ventricular tachycardia (>250 bpm) and ventricular tachycardia in animals with severe underlying cardiac disease, such as subaortic stenosis, DCM, and arrhythmogenic right ventricular cardiomyopathy ([ARVC] Boxers), are most vulnerable to dying suddenly from ventricular tachycardia. In Boxers with ARVC, sotalol (0.5–3 mg/kg, PO, bid; most commonly 80 mg/dog, PO, bid) or a combination of mexiletine (5–8 mg/kg, PO, tid) and atenolol (0.5–1 mg/kg, PO, bid) can effectively reduce or, more commonly, stop the syncope (usually due to a ventricular tachycardia firing at a rate of >400 bpm) seen in these dogs. It also obviously decreases the incidence of sudden death and so commonly results in years of survival. A minority of Boxers with ARVC develop true DCM and are also prone to sudden death. Doberman Pinschers with DCM also commonly die suddenly due to ventricular tachycardia. In these instances, the negative inotropic effects of sotalol can either push a dog into heart failure or make existing heart failure worse. Consequently, if sotalol is to be used in either of these patient populations, the dose must be started low and titrated upward carefully, with pimobendan administered concurrently. Mexiletine can also be used alone but, at least in theory, is not as effective at preventing sudden death. Amiodarone (12–15 mg/kg/day, PO, for 2 wk [loading dose] followed by 5–7 mg/kg/day, PO) is probably more efficacious at preventing sudden death than mexiletine but has many more adverse effects. Doberman Pinschers appear to be particularly susceptible to the hepatotoxic effects of the drug.

Animals with chronic bradyarrhythmias as seen with AV block (high-grade second or third degree) or sick sinus syndrome most commonly present with weakness, episodic weakness/collapse, and syncope. Pacemaker implantation is the treatment of choice. If pacemaker implantation is not a viable option, anticholinergics, phosphodiesterase (PDE) inhibitors, or sympathomimetics may be administered. Propantheline is a mild anticholinergic dosed at 0.25–0.5 mg/kg, PO, bid-tid. The parenteral formulation of atropine may be administered PO but must be diluted 10:1 with corn syrup at a dosage of 0.04 mg/kg, PO, tid-qid. Adverse effects include mydriasis, dry mucous membranes, tachycardia, and GI stasis. Theophylline is a nonselective PDE inhibitor with modest positive chronotropic effects. Extended-release tablets or capsules can be given at 10 mg/kg, PO, bid. If no adverse effects are seen and the desired clinical effect is not achieved, the dosage in dogs can be increased to 15 mg/kg, PO, bid, while monitoring for adverse effects, and in cats to 20 mg/kg, PO, every 24–48 hr. Adverse effects may include restlessness, excitability, tachycardia, or GI upset. Terbutaline is a β-agonist that has more potent positive chronotropic effects but with similar adverse effects to those seen with theophylline. It is dosed to effect at 1.25–5 mg/dog (not per kg), PO, tid, and 0.625 mg/cat, PO, bid. Attempts to overcome clinically significant bradyarrhythmias with oral therapy are often unrewarding, although overall clinical signs may improve in some animals.

Echocardiography

Echocardiography, the use of diagnostic medical ultrasound to evaluate the heart and proximal great vessels, complements other diagnostic procedures by quantifying chamber dimensions, wall thicknesses, and the dynamic events of the cardiac cycle; it also allows visualization of the anatomy and motion of valves and visualization of congenital abnormalities ranging from a defect in the interventricular septum to a stenotic pulmonary valve. Blood flow velocity is also commonly measured, and turbulent blood flow is identified using Doppler echocardiography. Pressure gradients, blood flow volumes, and several indices of cardiac function can be calculated. Echocardiography can also identify changes in myocardial tissue texture indicative of ischemia and fibrosis and delineate masses, valvular vegetations, pericardial effusion, and many other features previously verifiable only with cardiac catheterization or at necropsy.

There are four main types of echocardiography: three-dimensional, two-dimensional, M-mode (one-dimensional), and Doppler. Two-dimensional echocardiography provides a wedge-shaped, two-dimensional image of the heart in real-time. Several standard long-axis and short-axis views obtained from standard imaging windows on the thorax have been developed for dogs, cats, horses, and cows. M-mode echocardiography is produced by a one-dimensional beam of ultrasound that penetrates the heart, providing an “ice-pick view” over time. The tissue interfaces that are encountered by the beam are then plotted on a screen. This mode of evaluation has been typically used to measure chamber dimensions, wall thickness, valve motion, and great vessel dimensions but, as frame rate of two-dimensional echocardiography has improved, this mode has lost some of its usefulness. Three-dimensional echocardiography is the newest modality and is still in its infancy. Doppler echocardiography uses the principle of changing frequency of the ultrasonic beam after it contacts a moving structure (eg, RBCs, cardiac wall) to measure velocity. Doppler echocardiography is further divided into spectral (pulsed and continuous wave), color flow, and tissue Doppler echocardiography. Color flow Doppler echocardiography is a form of pulsed Doppler echocardiography prone to aliasing when high velocity flow is encountered, allowing high velocity (and therefore turbulent) flow in the heart and great vessels to be detected. Continuous wave Doppler is used to quantitate high velocity flow and thus used to calculate pressure gradients, most commonly across the regions of valves, using the modified Bernoulli equation ($4 \times \text{velocity}^2$). Tissue Doppler imaging is used to measure the lower velocity motion of cardiac structures, most commonly ventricular walls, in an attempt to quantitate regional myocardial function. Variations include measuring strain and strain rate.

Cardiac Catheterization

Cardiac catheterization involves the placement of catheters into cardiac chambers and surrounding great vessels to measure pressure, inject contrast agents, and place devices. The latter is commonly termed interventional cardiology. Indications include diagnostic evaluation (eg, when other diagnostic tests are insufficient to identify specific cardiac abnormalities or are unable to identify the severity of a lesion), presurgical evaluation (eg, to help diagnose constrictive pericarditis before surgery), therapeutic intervention, and clinical research. Diagnostic and presurgical cardiac catheterization, however, have largely been replaced by echocardiography. Currently, most cardiac catheterizations are interventional procedures to address cardiac defects (eg, closure of a patent ductus arteriosus).

HEART FAILURE

Heart failure is a clinical syndrome that occurs secondary to severe, overwhelming cardiac disease. It occurs because the heart is no longer able to maintain normal venous/capillary pressures, cardiac output, and/or systemic blood pressure. It is most commonly caused by a chronic disease that results in a severe decrease in myocardial contractility, severe regurgitation or shunting, or severe diastolic dysfunction. However, it is common to have all three abnormalities present simultaneously (but with one predominating). By far, the most common clinical manifestations seen with heart failure are directly due to edema and effusion (congestive or backward heart failure). Much less commonly, animals present because of signs referable to a decrease in cardiac output (forward heart failure). Very rarely, they present in cardiogenic shock (low blood pressure due to decreased cardiac output). This occurs because the cardiovascular system operates under a system of priorities. Its three primary functions are to maintain a normal blood pressure and normal cardiac output, both at a normal venous/capillary pressure. When the system is overwhelmed, it allows venous/capillary pressure to increase first (and so allows edema or effusion to form) and then allows cardiac output to fall. Only after cardiac output has fallen remarkably does cardiogenic shock occur. In acute heart failure, before any compensation has occurred, cardiogenic shock may predominate, but even in this situation, acute chordal rupture is the most common cause of acute heart failure in animals and results in an increased left atrial pressure and thus pulmonary edema.

Initial changes in cardiac chamber dimension (volume) or wall thickness that occur are best understood in relation to preload (the tension imposed by venous return on the ventricular walls at end-diastole) and afterload (the tension imposed on the ventricular walls at end-systole). Alterations in preload or afterload may be caused by structural cardiac abnormalities, systemic compensatory mechanisms, or both. Volume overload states, such as those that occur with chronic valvular disease/valvular insufficiencies, patent ductus arteriosus, atrial or ventricular septal defects, peripheral left-to-right shunts, anemia, or hyperthyroidism, cause an increase in preload that leads to ventricular growth and chamber enlargement (euphemistically called dilation) via eccentric myocyte hypertrophy. Pressure overload states, such as those that occur with pulmonary or systemic hypertension, and pulmonic or aortic stenosis, cause an increase in afterload (systolic intraventricular pressure) that leads to ventricular wall thickening via concentric hypertrophy. Neither volume nor pressure overload is synonymous with heart failure; either state may result in heart failure, depending on the severity of the overload and the degree of compensation.

Systolic Dysfunction

Systolic function is a broad classification of cardiac function that encompasses all of the entities in systole that are capable of altering blood flow into the aorta. It includes (but is not limited to) heart rate, myocardial contractility, preload, afterload, hypertrophy (volume and pressure overload), leaks, and shunts. Diseases that alter systolic cardiac function can become severe enough to overwhelm the ability of the cardiovascular system to compensate for the systolic dysfunction (primarily renal sodium and water retention, leading to hypervolemia, leading to increased venous return to the heart, leading to increased stretch on the myocardium, leading to myocardial growth and a larger left ventricular chamber [eccentric or volume overload hypertrophy]) and thus cause heart failure. The most common disease that alters systolic function is mitral regurgitation. Here, in systole, a portion of the blood flow that should be ejected into the aorta is ejected backward through the mitral valve from the left ventricle into the left atrium. When the regurgitation is mild (<50% of the blood flow goes backward) to moderate (50%–75% goes backward), the left ventricle is able to compensate for the leak by growing larger (volume overload hypertrophy) and increasing the total stroke volume it ejects. When regurgitation is severe (>75% backward flow), the compensatory mechanisms may become overwhelmed, resulting in an increase in left atrial pressure and so pulmonary edema. The classic example of systolic dysfunction is dilated cardiomyopathy (DCM), in which an inherent myocardial disease results in a decrease in myocardial contractility (myocardial failure). The decrease in myocardial contractility results in an increase in the end-systolic diameter/volume of the left ventricular chamber (muscle is weaker and cannot contract down as far in systole) and a decrease in myocardial contraction (the amount of wall motion [shortening fraction or fractional shortening] seen on an echocardiogram). Again, the left ventricle grows larger to compensate for this disease, but when the myocardial failure is severe, compensation can no longer maintain a normal diastolic pressure in the left ventricle (kidneys continue to retain sodium and water) and this increased pressure backs up into the left atrium, pulmonary veins, and pulmonary capillaries, creating pulmonary edema.

Diastolic Dysfunction

Diastole can be roughly divided into early myocardial relaxation and late filling that is altered primarily by compliance (1/stiffness). Most ventricular diastolic dysfunction severe enough to cause heart failure is due to myocardial fibrosis, thus due to a decrease in ventricular compliance (an increase in stiffness). When a ventricle is less compliant or stiffer than normal, for any given volume of blood that fills the chamber in diastole, the pressure is higher. This increase in diastolic pressure (when the AV valves are open) is transmitted back up into the atrium, veins, and capillary beds behind the affected ventricle, resulting in transudation of fluid and signs referable to edema or effusion. The classic example of a disease that primarily causes heart failure due to diastolic dysfunction is hypertrophic cardiomyopathy. Diastolic function is compromised to some degree by the thickening of the myocardium itself but more so by the myocardial fibrosis that builds up over time when severe disease is present. Restrictive cardiomyopathy is another classic example of diastolic dysfunction, but it is much less common. Diastolic dysfunction also occurs in pericardial diseases that cause cardiac compression (pericardial effusion, constrictive pericarditis). With pericardial disease, right heart failure (eg, ascites) predominates because systemic (eg, hepatic) capillaries leak more easily (leak profusely at a pressure of 10 mmHg) than pulmonary capillaries (which can generally withstand a pressure up to 20 mmHg without leaking).

CHF may also occur if a tumor or other anatomic obstruction impedes venous return to one or both atria. Pericardial disease or effusion leading to decreased ventricular filling may also be thought of as an extracardiac cause of CHF. Iatrogenic volume overload (ie, aggressive IV fluid therapy) can lead to edema formation in the absence of primary heart disease.

Compensatory Mechanisms

Systemic blood pressure and blood flow (and thus oxygen delivery to peripheral tissues and organs) is under strict neuroendocrine control. Compensatory mechanisms act rapidly to correct any decreases in blood flow and/or pressure. Acute compensatory mechanisms, such as increased sympathetic tone, are generally short-lived and useful only for situations that demand an acute change in cardiac function (eg, hypovolemia). Chronic mechanisms of cardiac compensation generally take over within days of the onset of a cardiac disease and are viable for years. They are responsible for the heart's ability to compensate for chronic disease. These remarkable mechanisms allow for an animal to compensate for mild, then moderate, and then even severe disease, often for years. Only at the very end of a chronic disease do they contribute to the formation of heart failure and require medical intervention.

When a decline in stroke volume occurs secondary to cardiac dysfunction, cardiac output decreases. The acute response is an increase in sympathetic tone leading to peripheral vasoconstriction, increased heart rate, and increased cardiac contractility that serve to restore cardiac output and maintain systemic blood pressure. This effect fades within days as events such as β-receptor down-regulation occur. Chronically, the renin-angiotensin-aldosterone system (RAAS) is activated. Activation is initiated by events such as decreased renal perfusion, leading to decreased sodium delivery to the macula densa (which interacts with the juxtaglomerular apparatus). The juxtaglomerular cells release renin, which converts angiotensinogen (synthesized in the liver) to angiotensin I. Angiotensin-converting enzyme (ACE) converts angiotensin I to angiotensin II, chiefly in the lungs. A separate tissue RAAS exists in the brain, vascular, and myocardial tissues, which can generate angiotensin II independently of the renal, or systemic, RAAS.

Angiotensin II has widespread effects, including stimulation of aldosterone synthesis and release from the adrenal glands, increased thirst via stimulation of antidiuretic hormone (ADH) release, increased norepinephrine and endothelin release, and stimulation of cardiac hypertrophy. Aldosterone forces the renal distal tubules to retain sodium and water. This, plus the effect of ADH, causes an increase in circulating blood volume. The increased blood volume leads to an increase in venous return to the affected ventricle. This chronic increase in preload stimulates the myocytes to add in new sarcomeres (contractile elements), leading to the growth of longer myocytes. This creates a larger ventricle (larger chamber with normal wall thickness [volume overload or eccentric hypertrophy]).

In response to these compensatory mechanisms, counter-regulatory systems are in place such as the release of atrial natriuretic peptide (ANP) from the atria, and B-type natriuretic peptide (BNP) from the atria and ventricles. ANP and BNP are released in response to stretch of the atrial and ventricular chambers. Both hormones serve to increase natriuresis (with subsequent diuresis) and decrease systemic vascular resistance, thus countering the effects of the RAAS. The effects of ANP and BNP are greatly outweighed by those of the RAAS and other systems in animals with chronic disease. Again, this is beneficial up until the end, when the RAAS continues to force sodium and water retention despite the presence of edema and effusion.

In situations when the heart must deal with higher than normal systolic intraventricular pressures (eg, subaortic stenosis, pulmonic stenosis, systemic arterial hypertension), the affected ventricle must contract against a greater force. Much like skeletal muscle when it is forced to lift a heavier weight, cardiac muscle undergoes concentric or pressure overload hypertrophy. In this situation, sarcomeres again replicate within cardiac myocytes but in parallel (side by side), to grow a wider myocyte and a thicker ventricular wall.

Cardiac Biomarkers

A biomarker is a measurable characteristic that reflects the severity or presence of some disease state. Blood pressure, cholesterol, gamma-glutamyl transferase, and BUN are all biomarkers. Studies in dogs and cats have shown that increased blood concentrations of BNP (most commonly N-terminal pro-B-type natriuretic peptide [NT-proBNP]), ANP, and endothelin-1 are indicators of cardiac disease that increase proportionately with progressive cardiac disease and CHF. Cardiac troponin I (cTnI), which is released after cardiomyocyte death, has also been evaluated as a biomarker for cardiac disease but found to be less sensitive than those mentioned above. ANP, BNP, and cTnI have also been evaluated as screening tools for occult DCM (before onset of CHF) in dogs. Increased levels of BNP were found to be highly sensitive for the detection of occult DCM, whereas ANP and cTnI were relatively less sensitive. NT-proBNP is cleaved from BNP in equal amounts in response to increased cardiac filling pressures (myocardial stretch) and ischemia, and its greater stability and longer half-life make it more suitable for use as a diagnostic biomarker. Several studies have demonstrated the usefulness of NT-proBNP in differentiating between cardiac and primary respiratory causes of dyspnea in dogs and cats. A rapid assay is available for this use in cats. Biomarkers such as NT-proBNP and troponin I should never be evaluated in isolation, because they are not 100% accurate. Instead, they should be used in concert with other diagnostic modalities.

Clinical Manifestations

The hemodynamic changes that occur in heart failure are relatively limited, as are the clinical syndromes resulting from these changes. Much depends on the location(s) of cardiac chamber failure, as well as on species differences.

Left Heart Failure: The pulmonary veins drain into the left atrium. Left atrial pressure increases as left heart diseases worsen (eg, from regurgitant blood flow and increased circulating blood volume). An increase in left atrial pressure is transmitted to the pulmonary veins and to the pulmonary capillaries. Pulmonary capillary hydrostatic pressure continues to increase, promoting the transudation of fluid out of the capillaries and first into the lung interstitium and then into the alveoli as the pressure increase becomes more severe. Simply put, pulmonary edema develops and becomes worse as heart failure progresses. In animals, this first causes tachypnea and then dyspnea. Most owners do not notice the tachypnea and so do not seek veterinary attention until dyspnea is present. This often makes it look like the onset of the heart failure was acute, when, in fact, it was chronic.

Some dogs and a few cats and horses will cough with cardiogenic pulmonary edema. Cough is a much more common manifestation of primary lung disease in all species. Coughing is always present in dogs with chronic bronchitis. One manifestation of chronic bronchitis is airway collapse (tracheomalacia and bronchomalacia) on radiographs. Bronchomalacia appears to be evidence of chronic bronchitis in dogs. When the left atrium is enlarged, a collapsed left mainstem bronchus can often be seen above the left atrium, because the large left atrium highlights this finding. It does not appear that the large left atrium actually compresses this bronchus.

Animals with heart failure may also be exercise intolerant due to lower than normal cardiac output during exercise and/or hypoxemia, which is caused by pulmonary edema or pleural effusion. This is a rare presenting complaint in cats, because they usually do not exercise. The same is true for many dogs. In dogs, most true exercise intolerance (fatigue with marked tachypnea or dyspnea) is due to respiratory failure rather than heart failure. However, most "exercise intolerance" ends up being due to something else and is not true exercise intolerance. Instead, it is frequently an unwillingness to exercise because of other conditions, such as orthopedic disease or obesity. A dog that is truly exercise intolerant looks and sounds "out of breath." A severe decrease in cardiac output results in cold extremities (paws, ears) and can lead to total body hypothermia, especially in cats. Although syncope (transient loss of consciousness due to a transient decrease in cerebral metabolic substrate, most commonly oxygen) is not a sign of or directly due to heart failure, it may also be noted in dogs in heart failure, especially in small-breed dogs with chronic valvular disease. In many instances, the cause is unknown. However, syncope often improves once pulmonary edema is treated. In some, it is associated with coughing and is most likely a vagally mediated event (transient asystole). The syncope is frightening to the owner, but sudden death is rare unless associated with DCM or subaortic stenosis.

The diagnosis of congestive left heart failure (cardiogenic pulmonary edema) in dogs is classically made radiographically. However, the inability to take a radiograph during a deep inspiration is a diagnostic obstacle. Consequently, the caudodorsal lung fields on a lateral radiograph, where cardiogenic pulmonary edema is usually identified, often have an interstitial density that is either mistaken for pulmonary edema or hides pulmonary edema. This is exacerbated in older dogs. Most dogs with severe pulmonary edema can be identified radiographically, but those with mild to moderate edema are often problematic. In these dogs, it is often beneficial to send the dog home (if it is stable) to have the owner count the dog's sleeping respiratory rate (SRR). The owner must be taught how to count respiratory (breathing) rate and then count the rate preferably while the dog is sound asleep and in a cool environment. A normal dog has an SRR <30 breaths/min, so a rate greater than that is abnormally high (ie, the dog has tachypnea). All dogs with pulmonary edema have an increased SRR (are tachypneic). However, dogs with respiratory disease/failure can also have an increased SRR. Therefore, once an increased SRR is documented, the dog should be started on furosemide at a dosage of at least 2 mg/kg, PO, bid. If the SRR decreases, then the diagnosis of left heart

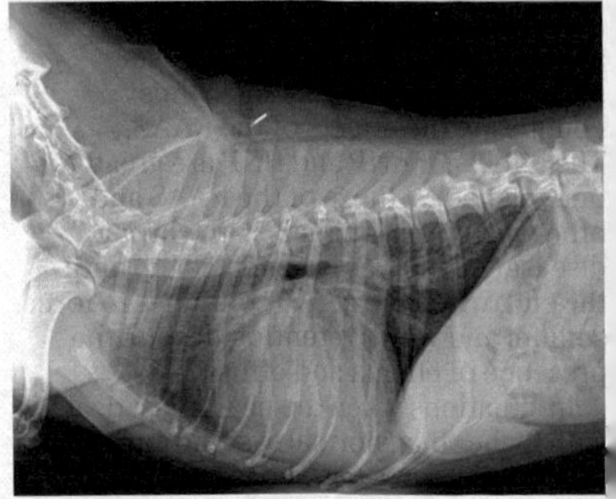

Lateral radiograph of a dog with cardiogenic pulmonary edema due to severe mitral regurgitation. Note the large body of the left atrium almost touching the spine. *Courtesy of Dr. Mark D. Kittleson.*

failure is confirmed. The same can be done in cats for both pulmonary edema and pleural effusion. All healthy cats have an SRR <40 breaths/min, with most <30 breaths/min. Once the diagnosis is established, the owner should continue to count the SRR daily and titrate the furosemide dosage to keep the SRR within the normal range. In dogs thought to be in an impending stage of heart failure (large left atrium but no pulmonary edema), the owner can also be instructed to count the SRR daily to weekly in an attempt to identify heart failure at an early stage. Owners should also always be instructed to keep a log and bring it with them at each recheck.

In cats, left heart failure also commonly manifests as pleural effusion. The visceral pleural veins (veins on the surface of the lung) drain into the left heart rather than the right heart. This also occurs in people and dogs. The exact reason for this phenomenon is not fully understood. The pleural effusion may be a modified transudate, pseudochylous, or chylous in cats with left heart failure. A small volume of pericardial effusion can also be seen in cats with heart failure and is generally of no hemodynamic consequence (pericardiocentesis is not required). Cats also often stop eating and may stop drinking when in heart failure.

Right Heart Failure: The right atrium receives systemic and cardiac venous and lymphatic drainage via the cranial and caudal vena cavae and the coronary sinus. Right atrial pressure increases as right heart disease worsens due to diseases such as tricuspid valve insufficiency and pulmonary hypertension. Clinical manifestations of right heart failure include jugular venous distention, hepatomegaly, pleural effusion, pericardial effusion, ascites, and peripheral edema. Dogs and cats are more likely to develop ascites (although right heart failure is uncommon in cats). Horses and cows more commonly develop subcutaneous edema ventrally. In dogs and cats, jugular venous distention may not be evident without intervention. A hepatojugular reflux test is often useful (*see* p 91).

Management

Management of heart failure is primarily directed at controlling clinical signs related to the presence of organ edema and cavity effusion (eg, pulmonary edema, pleural or pericardial effusion, and ascites). In some animals, decreased cardiac output, and even cardiogenic shock, need to be addressed. These are accomplished through reducing preload and/or afterload (diuretics and vasodilators), improving cardiac performance (positive inotropes, positive lusitropes, antiarrhythmics), and using neurohormonal modulators (ACE inhibitors, and potentially β-blockers, aldosterone antagonists, and angiotensin II receptor blockers).

Diuretics: The **loop diuretics** are the single most effective agents used to decrease circulating blood volume and reduce signs referable to edema and effusion in animals in heart failure. They act via inhibition of the $Na^+/K^+/2\ Cl^-$ cotransporter in the thick ascending loop of Henle. This leads to increased renal sodium and chloride excretion, with subsequent free water loss. Furosemide is the most widely used loop diuretic. When administered IV, it also directly reduces pulmonary capillary wedge pressure (before onset of diuresis) via local prostaglandin synthesis, which has a vasodilatory effect. The onset of action after IV administration is 5 min, with effects peaking at 30 min and lasting ~2 hr. The onset of action after oral administration is 60 min, with peak effects seen at 1–2 hr and lasting ~6 hr.

Emergency therapy of pulmonary edema often requires high doses of IV or IM furosemide (4–8 mg/kg for dogs; 2–4 mg/kg for cats), repeated at 60- to 120-min intervals until clinical signs, usually referable to pulmonary edema (ie, tachypnea, dyspnea), are controlled. Because of the concern for dehydration, azotemia, and significant electrolyte disturbances with overzealous furosemide administration, tapering to a lower dosage as soon as the respiratory rate decreases is mandatory. Once the pulmonary edema is controlled, the dosage that keeps the sleeping respiratory rate (SRR) normal is recommended. Mild to moderate prerenal azotemia and electrolyte and acid-base disturbances (hyponatremia, hypokalemia, and a hypochloremic metabolic alkalosis) are common and are generally well tolerated, so can be safely ignored (albeit monitored carefully) as long as the animal is eating and drinking. Oral doses used to manage chronic CHF may vary significantly between animals; in theory the lowest possible dosage should be used, but care must be exercised, again via monitoring SRR, not to lower the dosage too far. In dogs, CHF is often initially controlled at dosages of 1–2 mg/kg, bid; cats are more sensitive to the development of adverse effects and generally require lower dosages

(0.5–2 mg/kg every 12–24 hr). The maximal dosage in dogs is generally 4 mg/kg, PO, tid. In cats, it may be closer to 2 mg/kg, PO, tid, but dosages as high as 4 mg/kg, tid, may be required. Use of furosemide or other diuretics as sole therapy in long-term management of CHF increases RAAS activation; thus, combination with an ACE inhibitor is generally recommended.

Furosemide resistance, typically defined by persistent signs of heart failure despite dosages of 4 mg/kg, PO, tid, often develops in advanced cases of CHF. There are many causes of diuretic resistance, including remarkably severe cardiac disease, decreased delivery of the drug to the nephron (low cardiac output), activation of the RAAS (which counteracts the effects of diuresis), and hypertrophy of the distal convoluted tubular cells with consequent increases in ion transport in this region of the nephron. GI edema secondary to right CHF may decrease absorption of orally administered diuretics and contribute to diuretic resistance. Animals with resistance to chronic high doses of oral furosemide may thus have an improved diuretic response from parenteral (eg, SC) administration of the drug or from addition of other diuretic agents ("diuretic stacking"). In other cases, switching to torsemide (*see* below) may be the best option.

Adverse effects seen with furosemide administration are generally related to dehydration from volume depletion, reduced cardiac output and glomerular filtration rate (GFR), and electrolyte and acid-base abnormalities. Less common adverse effects include vomiting, pancreatitis, and idiosyncratic deafness with rapid IV administration. Animals with preexisting renal disease are more likely to develop adverse effects, and furosemide therapy should be reduced or temporarily withdrawn accordingly. Renal values should be monitored frequently when starting diuretic therapy (on initiation and at least 1 wk later) and should be reassessed at least every 3–6 mo during chronic administration. Some animals may remain mild to moderately azotemic (usually with a greater increase in BUN than in creatinine), which is generally tolerated provided they are eating and drinking adequately.

Torsemide is a newer loop diuretic that has better and more consistent bioavailability (better and more consistent GI absorption), has a longer duration of action (can be administered less frequently), and is more potent (requires a lower dose) than furosemide in dogs. Although there is less experience with this agent, it can be useful in management of refractory heart failure in which furosemide resistance has been documented or when furosemide is not tolerated. The starting dosage is approximately one-tenth that of the current furosemide dose (take total daily current dose of furosemide, multiply times 0.1, and divide that dose bid). Most commonly that translates into a dosage of 0.1–0.3 mg/kg, bid. However, dosages as high as 1 mg/kg, bid, have been used in a few dogs with ascites but only using careful upward titration.

Thiazide diuretics (eg, hydrochlorothiazide, chlorothiazide) decrease sodium resorption via inhibition of the Na^+/Cl^- cotransporter in the distal convoluted tubule. This results in increased sodium and water delivery to the collecting ducts and subsequent increased hydrogen and potassium excretion. Although the thiazides are relatively weak diuretics, they do exert a synergistic effect when administered with loop diuretics and can cause profound electrolyte abnormalities (particularly hypokalemia) and dehydration when used in combination if not used judiciously. Hydrochlorothiazide is more commonly used, with a recommended dosage of 1–4 mg/kg, PO, 1–2 times/day. It is also used as a combination product with the potassium-sparing diuretic spironolactone (*see* below), which may be dosed at 1–4 mg/kg, PO, 1–2 times/day. Many animals do not tolerate dosages at the higher end of this range, and the lowest effective dosage should be used. Chlorothiazide is dosed at 20–40 mg/kg, PO, 1–2 times/day. Thiazide diuretics are generally reserved for those cases in which resistance to furosemide has developed.

Potassium-sparing diuretics are the weakest of the diuretic class, exhibiting little to sometimes undetectable diuretic effect at standard dosages, especially when used alone in healthy dogs. Although they may produce more diuresis in a dog in heart failure, they should never be relied on to produce diuresis in an animal in heart failure. They should also never be used to replace a loop diuretic; they are used only as adjunctive (add-on) agents. Drugs in this class include the aldosterone inhibitors spironolactone and eplerenone and those that block sodium resorption at the distal tubules, triamterene and amiloride. Spironolactone is currently the only one used clinically in veterinary medicine. A large-scale clinical trial in people with heart failure in the 1990s demonstrated significant improvement in morbidity and mortality in patients with myocardial infarction administered spironolactone versus placebo, in addition to standard heart failure therapy. It was subsequently shown that the beneficial effect was all due to spironolactone's antifibrotic effects in the myocardium, not its diuretic properties. Only one discredited study from Europe has suggested benefit in dogs in heart failure. In theory, spironolactone may be of benefit in dogs with DCM, because myocardial fibrosis is a component of this disease. It is unlikely that myocardial fibrosis and diastolic dysfunction are important components of the pathophysiology of primary mitral regurgitation. In one study, spironolactone had no benefit in cats with hypertrophic cardiomyopathy before the onset of heart failure, another disease with myocardial fibrosis. Eplerenone has demonstrated a myocardial protective effect in dogs with experimentally induced myocardial infarction and heart failure.

Spironolactone is used by many veterinary cardiologists for its theoretical benefits. It may be beneficial in some dogs with refractory ascites or in those in which clinically significant hypokalemia has developed. It is dosed at 1–3 mg/kg, PO, 1–2 times/day.

Positive Inotropes: **Pimobendan** is a novel inodilator (inotropic drug and vasodilator) approved by the FDA in 2007 for use in dogs with CHF related to atrioventricular valve insufficiency or DCM. It is classified as a calcium sensitizer and a phosphodiesterase (PDE) III inhibitor. The parent compound (pimobendan) is responsible for the calcium sensitization, while an active metabolite (desmethylpimobendan) is a PDE III inhibitor (~100 times more potent than pimobendan). Pimobendan sensitizes cardiomyocyte contractile proteins (mostly troponin C) to calcium, and desmethylpimobendan increases cyclic AMP and calcium cycling within the cell. Myocardial oxygen consumption is increased, as for any positive inotropic agent, in healthy dogs. Vasodilation occurs via vascular PDE III inhibition, leading to endothelial smooth muscle relaxation and calcium efflux. Vasodilation includes coronary artery vasodilation, which leads to increased coronary blood flow and increased myocardial oxygen delivery. Additional beneficial effects may include improved myocardial relaxation, anti-inflammatory and anticytokine effects, and neurohumoral modulation.

Pimobendan is not approved for use in dogs before the onset of heart failure. With regard to mitral regurgitation due to myxomatous mitral valve degeneration, a study in Beagles with mild, naturally occurring mitral regurgitation demonstrated increased valvular lesions in dogs treated with pimobendan compared with dogs treated with benazepril. Preclinical studies by the manufacturer suggest the same thing might occur in healthy dogs. A clinical study is nearing completion that looks at pimobendan vs placebo in small dogs with mitral regurgitation before onset of heart failure to determine whether it prolongs the time to onset of heart failure. A study in Doberman Pinschers with DCM but no heart failure suggested that low-dose pimobendan administration may prolong the time until the onset of heart failure or sudden death. Neither of these disparate endpoints was statistically significant on its own, but the combined endpoint was.

The combination of increased inotropy with mild afterload reduction results in improved cardiac output and reduced cardiac filling (diastolic) pressures in dogs in heart failure due to either mitral regurgitation or DCM. Clinical improvements seen with pimobendan may include improved quality of life, improved clinical scores, and a longer survival time. It is not unusual for a dog to improve clinically more than expected, and it is theorized that the drug may also have nonspecific phosphodiesterase-inhibiting properties (possibly similar to those of caffeine). Consequently, the clinical improvement seen may not always be because of improvement in heart failure. No studies to date have investigated the effects of combining pimobendan with an ACE inhibitor, but most veterinary cardiologists feel that this combination may confer additional clinical benefits. The inotropic effect of pimobendan is significantly greater than that seen with digoxin, and pimobendan has supplanted digoxin for inotropic support in CHF in dogs.

Pimobendan effectively decreases calculated pulmonary artery systolic pressure (tricuspid regurgitant jet velocity) in dogs with pulmonary hypertension secondary to mitral regurgitation. Whether this decrease is due to the expected decrease in left atrial pressure, pulmonary arterial vasodilation, or both, is unknown. There are no studies that have shown that pimobendan is beneficial in dogs with pulmonary hypertension due to causes other than left heart failure.

There is ongoing debate regarding the use of pimobendan in cats. Pimobendan is not approved for use in cats, and the package insert states that it is contraindicated in cats with hypertrophic cardiomyopathy, although several studies have suggested that the drug is safe in cats, even those with hypertrophic cardiomyopathy, when administered at the same dosage as in dogs. However, a pharmacokinetic study showed that the serum concentration of pimobendan in cats given a canine dose results in a serum pimobendan concentration 10 times that seen in dogs. Cardiac pathology is found in dogs administered 3–5 times the recommended dose. It is unlikely any species that experienced a similar calcium sensitization effect as dogs could survive a dose 10 times the recommended dose, which suggests that cats are somehow very different. This requires more investigation before rational recommendations can be made with regard to using pimobendan in cats. However, anecdotally and in one retrospective study, pimobendan has been used in cats with CHF from any cause and has been beneficial clinically. Consequently, if a cat is no longer responding to conventional heart failure drug therapy, pimobendan (1.25 mg/kg/cat, bid) may be tried.

Pimobendan is dosed at 0.2–0.3 mg/kg, PO, bid, in dogs. With progression of heart failure, many veterinary cardiologists increase the dosing frequency in dogs to tid or double the dose. Adverse effects are rare and generally seen at high dosages but may include GI upset (anorexia, diarrhea). There is no clinical evidence supporting a significant increase in arrhythmias in animals treated with pimobendan; although some studies demonstrated such a trend, others refuted this. There clearly was no increase in the incidence of sudden death in the aforementioned study of Doberman Pinschers with subclinical DCM.

The **sympathomimetic amines** (eg, dobutamine, dopamine) improve contractility and cardiac output via β-adrenergic agonist effects and can be valuable in the acute management of cardiogenic shock or CHF secondary to myocardial failure. Stimulation of the membrane-bound β receptor activates adenyl cyclase, leading to the production of cAMP and subsequent phosphorylation of membrane-bound calcium channels on both the sarcolemma (myocyte membrane) and sarcoplasmic reticulum. These cellular actions increase myocardial contractility and relaxation, as well as oxygen consumption. Effects on ion channels in cardiac pacemaker cells and conduction fibers lead to decreased depolarization threshold, increased heart rate, and increased conduction velocity, all of which predispose to cardiac arrhythmias. In the peripheral vasculature, mixed β_1 and β_2 stimulation has a negligible effect on vascular resistance, although α-adrenergic stimulation (as occurs with dopamine at higher doses) can lead to vasoconstriction.

Dobutamine is administered IV as a continuous-rate infusion at 2.5–20 mcg/kg/min diluted in 5% dextrose. Dosages >15 mcg/kg/min are rarely required and can be associated with increased tachyarrhythmias. Starting at a lower dosage with uptitration every 15–30 min as required is recommended. Concurrent ECG monitoring is strongly recommended, and if arrhythmias worsen, the dosage of dobutamine should be reduced or dobutamine should be discontinued. Because dobutamine increases conduction through the AV node, additional caution is advised in atrial fibrillation. Dobutamine may preferentially increase myocardial flow, as compared with dopamine, which tends to increase renal and mesenteric flow. Dobutamine also tends to cause less tachycardia than dopamine. Dopamine is administered as a continuous-rate infusion at 2–8 mcg/kg/min; higher dosages (>10 mcg/kg/min) are associated with vasoconstriction and tachycardia. Gradual uptitration is recommended, as with dobutamine. Both dopamine and dobutamine may cause GI upset. These agents are less commonly used in cats, although the same general treatment strategy may be followed, but starting at more conservative infusion doses (~1 mcg/kg/min) for both dobutamine and dopamine.

The **bipyridine compounds** (milrinone, amrinone, or inamrinone) are PDE III inhibitors. Inhibition of PDE III reduces the degradation of cAMP, with subsequent effects similar to those seen with sympathomimetic amines. These agents are generally reserved for animals with severe refractory myocardial failure, because their use is associated with a higher level of mortality than that seen with the sympathomimetic amines. Because of lack of dependence on β-receptor stimulation, PDE III inhibitors are unaffected by β-receptor downregulation or uncoupling that may occur with progressive cardiac disease and may be useful in clinical situations when benefits of sympathomimetic therapy are less than expected. Additionally, vascular PDE III inhibition and lack of α-adrenergic stimulation results in vasodilation. Adverse effects noted with PDE III inhibitors include tachycardia, tachyarrhythmias, thrombocytopenia, GI upset, and hypotension at higher dosages. Amrinone is dosed at 1–3 mg/kg, IV, or as a constant-rate infusion at 10–80 mcg/kg/min. Milrinone is dosed at 30–300 mcg/kg (loading dose), followed by 1–10 mcg/kg/min constant-rate infusion (start low and titrate).

Cardiac Glycosides: The **digitalis glycosides** (eg, digoxin) are relatively weak positive inotropes (inhibit sodium-potassium ATPase pumps on cell surface membrane) that increase vagal tone to the heart (primarily to supraventricular regions), have a narrow therapeutic range, and are associated with significantly more adverse effects than pimobendan when administered in doses that produce toxicity. Digitoxin is no longer commercially available. Although used infrequently for its inotropic effects since the introduction of pimobendan, digoxin still plays an important role in cardiac disease, particularly in atrial fibrillation or supraventricular tachycardia with concurrent CHF, because it is the only available pharmacologic agent that slows AV nodal conduction without concurrent negative inotropic effects. (For a complete discussion, *see* p 2529.)

Rapid (IV) digitalization commonly results in toxicity and is not recommended. Digoxin may be administered at a conservative starting dosage of 0.003–0.005 mg/kg, PO, bid. Adequate serum concentration is not achieved until the second day of administration, and a serum digoxin concentration should be checked 4–7 days after initiation of therapy, 6–8 hr after the last dose is given. The therapeutic serum concentration is in the range of 0.5–2 ng/mL. There is no added benefit to a higher serum concentration within that range, so trying to keep it in the lower end of the range is recommended. Dosage adjustments should be based on the animal's serum digoxin concentration and clinical response. If digoxin is used in cats, it may be started at one-fourth of a 0.125-mg tablet every third day for cats <5 kg and every other day for cats >5 kg. Some larger cats may ultimately tolerate doses as high as one-fourth of a 0.125-mg tablet daily. An alcohol-based elixir form is available, although cats generally dislike the taste.

Adverse effects are increasingly likely at higher serum concentrations and generally occur in order of GI (anorexia, vomiting), cardiac (bradycardia, AV block, premature ventricular contractions), and CNS derangements. Because of its ability to slow electrical conduction as well as increase intracellular calcium, digoxin can cause almost any cardiac arrhythmia, and it is contraindicated in cases of AV block, significant bradycardia, and rapid ventricular tachycardia. If adverse effects are noted, the drug should be temporarily discontinued (usually for at least 1–2 days) and the dosage subsequently reduced by at least 50%.

Angiotensin-Converting Enzyme (ACE) Inhibitors: ACE inhibitors competitively inhibit ACE, which converts angiotensin I to angiotensin II. This blunts the increase in systemic vascular resistance, hypertrophy, and aldosterone release caused by angiotensin II. ACE inhibitors are mild balanced vasodilators. They may reduce systemic vascular resistance up to 25%, improving cardiac output and reducing regurgitant fraction in mitral regurgitation, although these effects are rarely clinically apparent. Additional benefits include a reduction in left ventricular filling pressure and thus pulmonary edema. It is thought that the beneficial effects of ACE inhibitors are primarily due to neurohormonal modulation, in addition to hemodynamic benefits. Studies in dogs with CHF have demonstrated improved clinical scores when an ACE inhibitor was added to standard therapy (diuretics with or without digitalis glycoside), although those benefits have generally been mild and apparent only for short times. Improvements have generally been more apparent in dogs with DCM than in those with myxomatous mitral valve degeneration. A trend toward prolonged survival has been seen in some studies.

In general, veterinary cardiologists agree that an ACE inhibitor is indicated in dogs with CHF. The benefit of ACE inhibitor therapy before the onset of CHF is more controversial, although two prospective studies and one retrospective study have shown no benefit in dogs with mitral regurgitation due to myxomatous mitral valve degeneration. One retrospective study has suggested mild benefit in Doberman Pinschers with DCM. Studies of ACE inhibition in cats are limited, and none has shown a true statistical benefit of ACE inhibition beyond what is gained from standard diuretic therapy in cats with CHF. These studies had low patient numbers, however, and most cardiologists do prescribe an ACE inhibitor in addition to appropriate background therapy for cats with CHF. No benefit has been shown in delaying the progression of occult hypertrophic cardiomyopathy.

The primary serious adverse effect of ACE inhibition is related to excessive efferent glomerular arteriolar vasodilation due to an acute decrease in plasma angiotensin II concentration, resulting in a functional azotemia due to a reduced glomerular filtration rate (GFR). This is relatively rare but can happen in any animal given an ACE inhibitor. There are no known predictors in cats or dogs. Anorexia, vomiting, and lethargy (uremia) may occur, so owners should be warned to watch for these clinical signs. Renal function tests (BUN, creatinine) should be measured before starting an ACE inhibitor and again 3–7 days later. Many clinicians wait until a dog is hemodynamically stable before starting an ACE inhibitor. Although cough is a common adverse effect of ACE inhibitor therapy in people, this is not seen in dogs and cats.

Enalapril is the only approved ACE inhibitor in the USA for dogs with CHF. It is generally dosed at 0.5 mg/kg, PO, bid. ACE inhibitors are "all-or-nothing" drugs, so giving a lower or less frequent dose probably produces no effect. Long-term dosing in cats is recommended at 0.5 mg/kg/day (most commonly 2.5 mg/cat), PO. ACE inhibitors are not emergency drugs. Clinical benefits, if any, are not commonly seen before 2–3 wk. Renal values should be monitored periodically (at least every 6 mo) while on long-term ACE inhibitor therapy.

Other ACE inhibitors used for treatment of heart failure include benazepril (0.25–0.5 mg/kg/day, PO), captopril (0.5–2 mg/kg, PO, tid), and lisinopril (0.5 mg/kg, PO, 1–2 times/day). Unlike enalapril and other ACE inhibitors that are renally excreted, benazepril undergoes significant hepatobiliary elimination (as much as 50% in dogs and 85% in cats). This does not appear to reduce the incidence of functional azotemia. Whether benazepril is safer in animals with renal insufficiency is unknown.

Vasodilators: Vasodilators exert a positive effect in CHF through dilating systemic arterioles (reduce resistance to blood flow) or systemic venodilation. The **nitrates** (sodium nitroprusside, nitroglycerin ointment, isosorbide dinitrate) act via the common end pathway of increased nitric oxide production, with subsequent activation of cyclic guanosine monophosphate (cGMP) and endothelial smooth muscle relaxation. Sodium nitroprusside (administered IV) is a potent mixed vasodilator, acting on both the arterial and venous systems. The combination of sodium nitroprusside with dobutamine may be especially useful in cases with cardiogenic shock and severe pulmonary edema. Although sodium nitroprusside dramatically and acutely reduces preload and afterload, its use is limited by the need for close monitoring and administration as a constant-rate infusion. The major adverse effect is systemic hypotension (with or without weakness, tachycardia, or vomiting); thus, concurrent blood pressure monitoring is recommended. However, its duration of effect is very short (1–2 min) so if problems arise, they dissipate rapidly once the infusion is stopped. Sodium nitroprusside is diluted in 5% dextrose and can be started at 1–3 mcg/kg/min, with careful uptitration every 5–10 min to desired effect, or started at 5 mcg/kg/min and the animal and/or blood pressure more carefully monitored. A dosage of 5–10 mcg/kg/min is usually sufficient to control clinical signs, and rarely is >10 mcg/kg/min required. Prolonged administration (>16 hr) increases the risk of cyanide toxicity (see the package insert).

If nitroprusside therapy is unavailable or undesired, nitroglycerin ointment and isosorbide dinitrate (venodilation only) might be tried, but neither is usually clinically beneficial. However, they are extremely unlikely to produce harm. Nitroglycerin is absorbed transcutaneously by the person administering the drug, so gloves must be worn during administration. It is applied at ~¼ in. per 5 kg (dogs and cats) every 6–8 hr on a hairless region such as the inner pinna or inguinal region. The latter may be preferable in animals with poor peripheral perfusion, in which the pinnae and extremities may be cool to the touch. The drug should be wiped or cleaned off after 8–12 hr or before the next dose is given. Isosorbide dinitrate is almost never used. In the one study designed to look for benefits in dogs in heart failure, none was identified when isosorbide was administered at 0.2–1 mg/kg, PO, tid. Another study showed acute benefit in dogs with mitral regurgitation when isosorbide was administered at 5 mg/kg (effect lasted 4 hr) and 10 mg/kg (effect lasted 11 hr). The largest pill size is 40 mg. Tolerance to nitrates has been demonstrated in many experimental canine models.

Hydralazine is a potent systemic arteriolar vasodilator typically reserved for dogs with mitral regurgitation due to myxomatous mitral valve degeneration that are refractory to conventional therapy, or in acute CHF when nitroprusside is unavailable. Its presumed mechanism of action is via production of vasodilatory prostaglandins. Hydralazine may reduce systemic vascular resistance up to 50%. This reduction in resistance results in the left ventricle pumping more blood flow forward through the systemic vasculature and less blood flow backward through the mitral valve into the left atrium. This decreases left atrial and pulmonary capillary pressures, reducing development of pulmonary edema. Approximately 30% of dogs vomit when receiving hydralazine; the drug generally needs to be discontinued when this happens. The recommended starting dosage in a dog in chronic heart failure is 0.5 mg/kg, PO, bid, if the animal is already on an ACE inhibitor, and 1 mg/kg, PO, bid, if not, with gradual (every 1–3 days) uptitration to effect, as high as 3 mg/kg, PO, bid. The drug is effective within 30 min, peaks in 1–3 hr, and maintains that peak for 11–13 hr. In a dog in acute, severe heart failure, a dosage of 2 mg/kg, PO, can be administered. Hydralazine is an "all-or-nothing" drug, so the primary danger is in giving too low of a dose and producing no beneficial effect. Approximately 90% of dogs respond to a dosage of 2 mg/kg. A small percentage of those dogs become weak for ~12 hr and then recover. In a dog with chronic heart failure due to mitral regurgitation, a good target would be a decrease in systolic blood pressure of 10–15 mmHg, but given the inaccuracy of blood pressure measurement in dogs this type of documentation may not be feasible. Other evidence that the dose being given is adequate is the presence of bright red mucous membranes and a decrease in murmur intensity. In cats, hydralazine can be given at a starting dose of 2.5 mg/cat, PO, bid.

Amlodipine is a calcium channel blocker with only peripheral vascular effects (no cardiac effects) and moderate to marked vasodilatory effects on systemic arterioles. Its actions are very similar to those of hydralazine (decreased mitral regurgitation and pulmonary edema) but without the adverse effects of vomiting and tachycardia. Amlodipine has a relatively slow onset of action, so its effects take 1–2 days to be noticeable. It is typically reserved for animals refractory to conventional heart failure drug therapy or for those with moderate to severe systemic hypertension. Adverse effects are generally related to hypotension and are uncommon when uptitration is done gradually. In dogs, therapy is initiated at 0.3 mg/kg/day, PO, and uptitrated every 2–3 days to a maximal dosage of 1 mg/kg/day (if needed). In cats, therapy is generally started at 0.625 mg/day (¼ of a 2.5-mg tablet) and gradually uptitrated to effect, up to as much as 1.25 mg, bid, in some cases. Because amlodipine reduces the amount of regurgitation, it may also effectively slow the progression of mitral regurgitation to heart failure in dogs. Gingival hyperplasia can occur in dogs administered amlodipine, which often necessitates discontinuation of the drug.

Phosphodiesterase type 5 (PDE 5) inhibitors (eg, sildenafil, tadalafil) are used to relax the smooth muscle in pulmonary arterioles. Their mechanism of action is somewhat similar to that seen with nitrates, with a common increase in the second messenger cGMP. PDE 5 inhibitors are used in the treatment of moderate to severe pulmonary arterial hypertension. Studies in dogs have demonstrated modest clinical improvement (reduction or cessation of syncope, improved right heart failure) with usually minimal improvement in pulmonary artery pressures, at least at lower dosages (eg, 1 mg/kg, PO, bid-tid). Anecdotally, PDE 5 inhibitors seem to provide the most notable clinical benefit to animals with syncope secondary to pulmonary hypertension. Anecdotal success has also been reported in dogs with right-to-left shunting cardiac defects in which the shunt is due to the increase in pulmonary vascular resistance. Adverse effects are uncommon but may include GI upset and hypotensive-related effects (especially when combined with nitrates, which is contraindicated). A major drawback regarding clinical use of PDE 5 inhibitors is expense, particularly in larger animals. Fake (85% in one study) sildenafil is commonly sold online. Sildenafil is administered at 1–3 mg/kg, PO, bid-tid in dogs, and at 1 mg/kg, PO, tid in cats. Tadalafil is administered at 1 mg/kg, PO, once to twice daily in dogs.

β-Adrenergic Blockers: In people with myocardial failure (eg, DCM), β-blocker administration, with a very low starting dose titrated upward over months, results (seemingly paradoxically) in an improvement in myocardial function. To date, all attempts to replicate this phenomenon in client-owned dogs have failed. Dogs with experimentally induced heart failure have shown measurable improvements in cardiac performance after administration of metoprolol, but these were models of ischemic cardiomyopathy, which is a rare cause of DCM in dogs. Large dogs (>20 kg) with experimentally induced mitral regurgitation also have had lesser decreases in contractility over time when administered atenolol when compared with placebo.

β-Blockers are commonly administered to cats with hypertrophic cardiomyopathy, primarily to reduce systolic anterior motion of the mitral valve. However, evidence that this results in clinical improvement, biochemical improvement, or prolonged survival is lacking. Atenolol (6.25–12.5 mg/cat, PO, bid) is the β-blocker most commonly used in cats. There are limited and preliminary data associating the use of atenolol in cats with hypertrophic cardiomyopathy and CHF with a shorter survival, and consideration might be given to dosage reduction or withdrawal if CHF develops.

Nutritional Considerations: Important metabolic changes may occur in animals with heart failure. Upregulation of the RAAS leads to increased plasma volume, largely mediated by increased sodium retention. Increased production of inflammatory cytokines such as tumor necrosis factor and interleukin 1 may promote increased metabolic demand and contribute to anorexia, thus worsening "cardiac cachexia." Studies in people and a study in dogs have shown that patients with CHF who lost weight during the course of these studies had a poorer prognosis. In some patients, nutrient deficiencies (taurine, carnitine) have been shown to cause DCM. Decreased levels of circulating fatty acids have been documented in people and dogs with heart failure. The overall nutritional goals in the management of animals with heart failure should therefore include supplying adequate calories, modulating the production of proinflammatory cytokines, managing sodium balance, and supplementing nutrients that may be deficient.

The idea that **sodium restriction** reduces circulating plasma volume and preload is well established. However, sodium restriction is known to activate the RAAS, and there is continued debate as to the role of sodium restriction in animals, especially those with asymptomatic cardiac disease or mild to moderate CHF. In contrast, moderate to severe sodium restriction may be indicated in animals with severe CHF, especially in those refractory to drug therapy. It is also important to counsel owners to avoid foods and treats with high sodium content, because an acutely high sodium load (as can be seen in animals fed human snacks or table foods) may precipitate CHF in animals with compensated heart disease. For animals in mild to moderate heart failure (ISACHC Class II), moderate sodium restriction (50–80 mg/100 kcal) may be tried if the dog or cat will readily eat such a diet. In animals with severe refractory CHF, more aggressive sodium restriction (<50 mg/100 kcal) may be tried. This becomes even more of a therapeutic challenge with some animals in which cardiac cachexia is present, because lower sodium foods are often less palatable. In general, maintaining adequate caloric intake is more important than sodium restriction.

Supplementation with **n-3 fatty acids** has shown multiple benefits in people with CHF, and a study in dogs suggests antiarrhythmic benefits as well. These fatty acids may reduce circulating inflammatory cytokine levels and seem to improve appetite in some dogs with cardiac cachexia. Daily doses of eicosapentaenoic acid at 40 mg/kg and docosahexaenoic acid at 25 mg/kg can be tried.

Taurine supplementation is indicated in animals with documented taurine deficiency and DCM. The incidence of DCM has declined dramatically in cats since taurine deficiency was identified as a primary cause in the late 1980s. Taurine deficiency is still documented in some cats with DCM fed noncommercial diets (especially chicken, dog food, and vegetarian diets) and rarely a commercial cat food diet. Supplementation at 250 mg, PO, bid, can be started in cats while awaiting results of plasma and whole blood taurine concentrations. Dogs are able to synthesize more endogenous taurine than cats and do not have an obligatory loss in bile, so deficiency is less common in this species. However, American Cocker Spaniels with DCM uniformly have a low plasma taurine concentration and respond to taurine or taurine and carnitine supplementation. Newfoundlands are relatively predisposed to taurine deficiency, especially when fed lamb and rice or high-fiber, low-protein/taurine diets. Rarely, other breeds (mostly breeds not usually thought of as being predisposed to developing DCM) with DCM will be taurine deficient/responsive. Whole blood and plasma taurine concentrations should be obtained in any dog suspected of having a taurine-deficient cardiomyopathy, and supplementation can be started at 500–1,000 mg, PO, bid-tid, while awaiting results. Clinical improvement occurs within weeks of starting taurine supplementation in cats or dogs with DCM due to taurine deficiency. Echocardiographic improvement takes longer (2–3 mo).

L-Carnitine plays an important role in fatty acid metabolism and energy production. Carnitine deficiency has been documented in one family of Boxers and myocardial carnitine deficiency is common in dogs with DCM, but it is most likely that this deficiency is a result of cardiomyopathy, not the cause, in these dogs. Carnitine has been supplemented in other breeds with DCM but with little success. Diagnosis of carnitine deficiency is difficult and requires an endomyocardial biopsy. Supplementation is also expensive, and given our limited knowledge of the role carnitine plays in canine cardiomyopathy, supplementation is not routinely recommended. Nevertheless, supplementation can be offered at 50–100 mg/kg, PO, bid-tid, to dogs with DCM.

Coenzyme Q_{10} is involved with mitochondrial energy production and possesses general antioxidant properties. Anecdotal benefits of supplementation in people and dogs with DCM have been reported, but well-controlled studies are lacking, and reports are conflicting. Consequently, there is no known benefit. The dosage in dogs is 30–90 mg, PO, bid.

Oxygen Therapy: The presence of pulmonary edema in animals with CHF increases the alveolar-arterial diffusion distance for oxygen to pulmonary capillaries and disturbs ventilation/perfusion matching. Supplemental oxygen administration increases the alveolar-arterial diffusion gradient and thus increases arterial oxygen content. Oxygen may be administered via oxygen cage, flow-by method (least preferred), nasal cannula, or oxygen collar (constructed by covering the ventral 50%–75% of an Elizabethan collar with plastic wrap and taping oxygen tubing along the ventral aspect of the collar). The oxygen cage is least stressful for the animal but is expensive, because high flows of oxygen are required to achieve therapeutic concentrations (>40% inspired oxygen). The oxygen collar has the potential to achieve a very high concentration of inspired oxygen (as much as 80%) but may require light sedation to increase patient tolerance.

Thoracocentesis: Pleural effusion decreases the available area for alveolar ventilation and arterial oxygenation. Pleural effusion should always be excluded as the cause of dyspnea in animals in heart failure, especially cats. This is best accomplished using ultrasound. If ultrasound is unavailable, radiographs can be taken, but extreme care must be taken to avoid stressing the animal (especially cats), because stress in a dyspneic animal often results in death. If radiographs cannot be taken, a diagnostic thoracocentesis should be done. This can often be done in cats in the examination room using a butterfly catheter with the cat in sternal recumbency. If fluid is present, as much as possible should be removed. Thoracocentesis is the most effective treatment in animals with respiratory distress due to a significant volume of effusion. However, caution again should be taken in particularly stressed animals, which may require pretreatment with oxygen and light sedation. Diuretic therapy is ineffective at acutely resolving a large volume of pleural effusion.

Abdominocentesis: Ascites may produce abdominal discomfort and worsen dyspnea by reducing available lung capacity in animals in right heart failure. Abdominocentesis should be performed at the time of initial diagnosis of right heart failure if the ascites is severe. In animals with recurrent ascites refractory to diuretic therapy, abdominocentesis may be performed every 1–4 wk to improve patient comfort and quality of life. Every attempt should be made to remove all or as much fluid as possible on each visit to prolong the time between repeat abdominocenteses. This does not result in hypoalbuminemia. Fluid can be removed manually using either a fenestrated catheter and large syringe or a suction device.

Ancillary Therapy: **Bronchodilators** (theophylline, terbutaline) are generally reserved for animals with chronic airway disease, which is common in older small-breed dogs. Caution should be taken in animals with CHF, especially with tachyarrhythmias, because of the sympathomimetic effects of these agents. In dogs with cardiovascular disease and syncope, theophylline has been used with some success for its positive chronotropic effects. Dosages of theophylline and terbutaline are as previously described under treatment of bradyarrhythmias (*see* above).

Cough suppressants generally should not be used if a cough is truly due to cardiogenic pulmonary edema. Instead, they are reserved for dogs with chronic bronchitis and airway collapse (malacia) and, even then, generally reserved for dogs not responsive to a corticosteroid and/or doxycycline with or without theophylline. It is common for dogs with CHF to have concomitant chronic bronchitis. Common antitussive agents used for dogs with cardiac disease include butorphanol at 0.05–0.3 mg/kg, PO, tid-qid, or hydrocodone at 0.22 mg/kg, PO, bid-tid.

Anxiolytic therapy may be used for some animals with severe respiratory distress secondary to CHF. Morphine has traditionally been recommended to alleviate anxiety in dogs with acute CHF because of its concurrent sedative and venodilating (and thus preload reducing) properties, but it also can produce respiratory depression, which can be catastrophic. The dosage of morphine in dogs is 0.1–0.25 mg/kg, SC. It may also cause nausea or vomiting. Morphine is generally avoided in cats, because it may induce agitation and dysphoria. Butorphanol is a partial opiate agonist/antagonist with minimal cardiovascular effects. A sedative dosage of 0.2–0.5 mg/kg administered IM or IV can be used in cats and dogs. Butorphanol may also be combined with a benzodiazepine (midazolam or diazepam), with the latter also dosed at 0.2–0.5 mg/kg, IM or IV. Phenothiazine tranquilizers (eg, acepromazine) may be used to alleviate severe anxiety and have the potential added benefit of producing mild systemic arteriolar dilation; however, they should be used cautiously in animals with severe hemodynamic compromise or systemic hypotension. A low dosage of 0.01–0.1 mg/kg, IM or IV, can be used.

SPECIFIC CARDIAC DISEASES

Myxomatous AV Valve Degeneration

(Degenerative AV valvular disease, Endocardiosis)

Myxomatous degeneration is a process of the fibrous layer of an AV valve breaking down to cause mitral valve prolapse (hooding) and the spongiform layer proliferating to cause nodular thickening of the cardiac valve leaflets, most severely at their tips. Myxomatous degeneration commonly affects the mitral and tricuspid valves in dogs. Chordae tendineae are also affected by the degenerative process, making them prone to rupture. The exact cause is unknown, but in Cavalier King Charles Spaniels and Dachshunds it is an inherited trait. Myxomatous degenerative valve disease is the most common cardiac disease in dogs and accounts for ~75% of cardiovascular disease in this species; ~60% of affected dogs have only the mitral valve affected, 30% have lesions in both the tricuspid and mitral valves, and 10% have only tricuspid valve disease. In dogs, the disease is age- and breed-related, with older, small-breed dogs demonstrating a much higher incidence. Horses and cats are also affected by this disease (most commonly affecting the mitral valve leaflets); however, it is uncommon in these species. In horses, a degenerative valve disease can also affect the aortic valve cusps and consists of valvular nodules or fibrous bands at the free borders of the valve. This condition is most common in older horses. It causes aortic regurgitation, which is heard as a diastolic murmur on the left side. The murmur is often "musical," meaning it has one frequency caused by the valve structures vibrating at the frequency heard. The murmur may be high-pitched and sound truly musical, or it may be low-pitched and sound like a grunt or a dive bomber. The murmur is often loud, but the aortic regurgitation is usually mild. Clinical signs (eg, heart failure) are usually not seen, because severe aortic regurgitation is uncommon.

Insufficiency of an AV valve results in turbulent, systolic (ie, during ventricular contraction) flow through the affected valve from a ventricle into an atrium. This regurgitation results in an increase in volume within the atrium and thus to an increase in atrial chamber size. When regurgitation is severe, atrial pressure may also increase. If the mitral valve is affected, the increased left atrial pressure results in increased pulmonary capillary pressures and, if the increase is high enough (ie, >20 mmHg), in cardiogenic pulmonary edema (ie, left heart failure). If the tricuspid valve is affected, severe regurgitation can result in an increased systemic venous pressure and signs of right heart failure (most commonly ascites in dogs). The constant, high-velocity, regurgitant jet of blood through the affected mitral valve physically damages the endocardium of the left atrium, resulting grossly in jet lesions. In cases with severe regurgitation, the chronic increase in left atrial size and pressure can also result in left atrial rupture and acute cardiac tamponade, often resulting in death.

Pathophysiologically, the body compensates for valvular regurgitation primarily by renal sodium and water retention, causing an increase in blood volume and in venous return to the heart. This results in an enlargement in ventricular chamber size and a left ventricle capable of ejecting a larger total stroke volume with each beat. That way, even though some percentage of blood flow is going backward into the left atrium, a normal or near normal amount can be ejected forward into the aorta. Multiple mechanisms exist for sodium and water retention, but the renin-angiotensin-aldosterone system (RAAS, *see* p 100) is one of the most active and best studied. Renin release by the juxtaglomerular apparatus in the kidneys cleaves angiotensinogen into angiotensin I, and angiotensin-converting enzyme then cleaves angiotensin I into angiotensin II. One of the main effects of angiotensin II is to stimulate aldosterone release by the adrenal glands. Aldosterone stimulates the cells in the distal renal tubules to bring sodium back into the vascular space, and water follows the sodium. The increase in blood volume and venous return to the heart places chronic stretch on cardiac myocytes, resulting in sarcomere replication within the myocytes and growth of longer myocytes. This allows the affected ventricle to develop a larger chamber (ie, eccentric or volume overload hypertrophy). This is the primary compensatory mechanism for valvular regurgitation. It is highly efficient and allows the heart to compensate not only for a valvular leak for years but also for an extreme amount of regurgitation. For example, a small dog can completely compensate for regurgitation in which as much as 75% of the blood flow from the left ventricle goes into the left atrium, while only 25% goes forward into the aorta.

Activation of the RAAS and other compensatory mechanisms are commonly seen as dysfunctional and increases of various neurohormones as detrimental, because overt increases are often seen in dogs that are in heart failure when compensatory mechanisms are overwhelmed. However, these mechanisms are detrimental for only a few months at the end stage of the disease.

Only ~30% of dogs with mitral regurgitation ever develop left heart failure. In dogs, there are no clinical signs in the early and middle stages of the disease, although a systolic murmur (grade I–VI) is heard with maximal intensity at the left apex. The heart murmur intensity often does not correlate with disease severity, although most soft murmurs are heard in dogs with mild mitral regurgitation. Some dogs may also develop a systolic click before developing a heart murmur. A systolic click is heard as a three-heart-sound rhythm and may be mistaken for a gallop sound (rhythm). A three-heart-sound rhythm in a middle-aged to older small-breed dog is almost always a systolic click rather than a gallop sound. A gallop sound may be heard in a dog with severe mitral regurgitation but is usually difficult to auscult because of the loud heart murmur also present. When the mitral regurgitation becomes severe and overwhelming, left heart failure (pulmonary edema) becomes evident, producing increases in respiratory rate (tachypnea) and effort (dyspnea), and cough. Syncope may also occur. Although syncope is not a sign of heart failure, it may be present when heart failure is evident and may improve when heart failure is controlled. Sudden death is rare but may occur secondary to left atrial rupture or rupture of a primary mitral valve chord. Physical examination findings in animals that have developed left heart failure are primarily referable to the increased respiratory rate and effort. Some dogs may have respiratory crackles and wheezes; however, these are much more common and more obvious in dogs with chronic bronchitis, and many dogs with pulmonary edema have no demonstrable abnormal pulmonary sounds. If tricuspid valve degeneration is significant, signs of right heart failure may be noted (eg, ascites, jugular distention/pulses).

A CBC, serum chemistry profile, and urinalysis are usually within normal limits. Left atrial enlargement is the characteristic finding on thoracic radiographs of an animal with myxomatous degeneration of the mitral valve, and the size of the left atrium correlates directly with the severity of the regurgitation in small dogs. Other changes include enlargement of the left ventricle and pulmonary veins. As left heart failure develops, increased interstitial density to the pulmonary parenchyma occurs, and as severity increases, an alveolar pattern with air bronchograms (ie, severe pulmonary edema) appears. In dogs, these changes are classically seen in the caudodorsal lung fields and may be more prominent on the right side. In older dogs, it is common to have an increased interstitial density in the lungs and to have radiographs taken at or near end-expiration. This commonly creates the illusion of pulmonary edema and therefore the misdiagnosis of left heart failure. This can be avoided by remembering that for a dog to be in chronic left heart failure, the regurgitation must be severe and overwhelming so the left atrium is usually severely enlarged. The exception to this rule is in dogs with acute heart failure due to a ruptured chord and a left atrium that is not severely enlarged. If the respiratory rate in the examination room is normal (<30 breaths/min), the dog cannot be in left heart failure. If there is doubt regarding the diagnosis of pulmonary edema in a dog that is not in critical condition, it is usually best to send the dog home and have the owner count the dog's respiratory rate when it is sound asleep in a cool environment. If pulmonary edema is present, the sleeping respiratory rate (SRR) will always be increased. If the rate is increased, the dog should be administered furosemide at a dosage of at least 2 mg/kg, PO, bid. If the SRR then decreases, the diagnosis of left heart failure can be made. In cats, the radiographic pattern is more diverse and often is not caudodorsal. A heavy interstitial to alveolar pattern in the accessory lung lobe on a lateral view is one of the more common findings. Cats in left heart failure also commonly have pleural effusion.

Echocardiography demonstrates thickened and irregular valve leaflets of normal to increased echogenicity. Chordae tendineae may be ruptured, causing the AV leaflets to flail (ie, leaflet tips to protrude) into the atrium during ventricular contraction. Mitral valve prolapse (hooding), in which the body of a leaflet (not the tip) protrudes into the left atrium in systole, may also be present. The size of the left atrium increases in direct correlation with the severity of the mitral regurgitation in small dogs. Left ventricular chamber enlargement (ie, eccentric or volume overload hypertrophy) also occurs in correlation to disease severity. In small dogs, left ventricular myocardial contractility or function is often normal as evidenced by a normal end-systolic diameter or volume. The increase in end-diastolic diameter coupled with the normal end-systolic diameter results in the left ventricular fractional shortening (ie, the amount of contraction [not contractility]) being increased. Myocardial contractility is decreased in some small dogs and many large dogs at the onset of heart failure and may become decreased in small dogs when being treated for heart failure.

Electrocardiographically, animals with mild to moderate degenerative valve disease have a normal sinus arrhythmia or normal sinus rhythm. When CHF develops, the increase in sympathetic tone often results in loss of sinus arrhythmia and usually in an increase in heart rate (ie, sinus tachycardia). Left atrial enlargement promotes the development of atrial arrhythmias such as atrial premature complexes and atrial fibrillation. Ventricular tachyarrhythmias are uncommon. There may be evidence of left atrial enlargement (P mitrale or widened P waves) and left ventricular enlargement (tall and widened R waves) on an ECG, but these changes are unreliable indicators of chamber enlargement.

Measurement of the plasma or serum concentration of NT-proBNP may be useful in dogs with mitral regurgitation. It is usually not increased in dogs with mild mitral regurgitation, may be increased in some dogs with moderate to severe mitral regurgitation, and is increased in most dogs with left heart failure secondary to mitral regurgitation. It would be most useful in dogs presented with severe tachypnea/dyspnea if a rapid assay (bedside test) were available. It might be useful for differentiating dogs with chronic lung disease from dogs in chronic left heart failure, but this can often be accomplished with less expense and greater accuracy by having the owner count the dog's SRR and doing a furosemide response test if the rate is increased. NT-proBNP often decreases after successful treatment of left heart failure but frequently does not decrease to a value within the normal range. Predicting which dogs with mitral regurgitation will go into heart failure is difficult. As populations, dogs with a larger left ventricular diastolic dimension, larger left atrial size, and a higher NT-proBNP are at greater risk of developing heart failure, but translating that to an individual dog is often fraught with error. The same is true for predicting cardiac death (ie, from heart failure or sudden death) from severe mitral regurgitation. Higher dosages of furosemide are required in dogs with more severe heart failure, so higher furosemide dosages predict decreased survival.

Studies in dogs with degenerative mitral valve disease that are not yet in heart failure have failed to convincingly demonstrate a reduction in time to onset of CHF with use of ACE inhibitors. Thus, treatment in small-breed dogs should be reserved for dogs with clinical signs of heart failure, ie, those demonstrating cardiogenic pulmonary edema on thoracic radiographs and resting/sleeping tachypnea in the absence of other severe pulmonary disease. Treatment of CHF includes administration of a diuretic (almost always furosemide) and an ACE inhibitor as adjunctive therapy. Cardiogenic pulmonary edema should not be treated with an ACE inhibitor alone. Pimobendan (0.25–0.3 mg/kg, bid) is also indicated in dogs in heart failure. Spironolactone might have chronic, long-term benefits in dogs with heart failure due to myxomatous mitral valve degeneration, but there is no convincing evidence of this in dogs with mitral regurgitation, and it should not be relied on to produce clinically relevant diuresis. Dogs refractory to administration of a maximal dosage of furosemide (4 mg/kg, tid) can be treated with several additional drugs or a change in strategy. The pimobendan dosage can be increased to tid, or the bid dosage can be doubled. Amlodipine and hydralazine decrease the amount of regurgitation and improve perfusion and can be very effective. A thiazide diuretic combined with furosemide is another effective means of treating dogs with refractory heart failure, but care must be taken to not produce clinically relevant dehydration and hypokalemia. Torsemide may be used to replace furosemide. Torsemide is more bioavailable (better absorbed) and has a longer and more consistent half-life. The starting dose is determined by multiplying the total daily dose of furosemide by 0.1 and dividing that dose bid. Care must be taken to have the owner closely monitor the SRR when this is done. If the SRR increases, the dose of torsemide must be increased promptly.

Surgical treatment of mitral regurgitation is routine in human medicine and most commonly consists of mitral valve repair. Successful mitral valve repair has also been accomplished in dogs, but the only currently truly successful program is in Japan. Replacement of the mitral valve with a prosthetic valve is almost uniformly unsuccessful.

Abnormal arrhythmias such as atrial fibrillation or other severe and sustained supraventricular arrhythmias, if present, should either be resolved or the rate controlled with digitalis glycosides and diltiazem or a β-blocker (eg, atenolol) to prevent tachycardia-induced myocardial failure. Optimal therapy should be planned for each stage of disease. In acute and severe CHF, oxygen and aggressive parenteral furosemide administration are warranted. Nitroprusside can also be beneficial.

Some affected dogs can live for >1 yr with appropriate therapy. However, survival time is highly variable, and no firm estimates should be provided. If a dog has been treated for left heart failure for >2 yr, the diagnosis should be reassessed.

Valvular Blood Cysts or Hematomas

These benign valvular lesions are present in as many as 75% of calves <3 wk of age. They are most commonly located on the AV valves.

Cardiomyopathies

Cardiomyopathy is defined as any disease involving primarily and predominantly the heart muscle. Most of the cardiomyopathies of animals are idiopathic diseases that are not the result of any systemic or other primary cardiac disease. In several instances, a mutational cause has been identified. In others, a genetic cause has been identified. In animals (primarily dogs and cats), they are classified as dilated cardiomyopathy, hypertrophic cardiomyopathy, arrhythmogenic right ventricular cardiomyopathy, and restrictive or unclassified cardiomyopathy. If a disease process has been identified as the cause of myocardial dysfunction, these are more correctly identified as secondary myocardial diseases or with a descriptive term preceding the term cardiomyopathy (eg, taurine-responsive dilated cardiomyopathy).

Dilated Cardiomyopathy (DCM): This disease is characterized by the progressive loss of myocyte number and/or function and a decrease in cardiac contractility. Several forms of secondary DCM exist (eg, taurine deficiency in cats, doxorubicin- or parvovirus-induced in dogs). In some Doberman Pinschers (primarily those in the USA), the disease is caused by a mutation in the gene that encodes for pyruvate dehydrogenase kinase 4 (PDK4), an enzyme in mitochondria required for ATP production. A small percentage of Boxers with arrhythmogenic right ventricular cardiomyopathy (*see* below) develop DCM. These dogs have a mutation in the gene that encodes for striatin, a desmosomal protein. DCM has a protracted subclinical phase in dogs, with clinical signs evident for a relatively short time. During the subclinical phase, compensatory mechanisms, primarily volume overload or eccentric hypertrophy, maintain normal hemodynamics. As cardiac contractile function is progressively lost, cardiac output, and so renal blood flow, decreases and then is normalized again as renal sodium and water retention increase blood volume and venous return and the affected ventricle is stimulated to grow larger. The increased activation of the sympathetic nervous system and the RAAS, after years of initial benefit, cause deleterious effects during the late phases of the disease (*see* p 100). Excessive stimulation of the myocardium by the sympathetic nervous system may stimulate ventricular arrhythmias and myocyte death, while excessive activation of the RAAS causes vasoconstriction and continued retention of sodium and water in the presence of edema/effusion.

DCM is most prevalent in dogs and is especially prevalent in certain breeds. It most commonly affects large-breed dogs and far less commonly small-breed dogs (with a few exceptions such as American Cocker Spaniels, Springer Spaniels, and English Cocker Spaniels). Doberman Pinschers, Boxers, Great Danes, German Shepherds, Irish Wolfhounds, Scottish Deerhounds, Newfoundlands, Saint Bernards, and Labrador Retrievers, among other large-breed dogs, are particularly at risk. In Portuguese Water Dogs, a juvenile form of the disease is seen. The disease is typically seen in middle-aged to older dogs; males are either affected more frequently or more severely than females. The incidence in cats has decreased dramatically since the discovery in 1987 that taurine deficiency was responsible for most cases (taurine-responsive DCM). Since then, taurine has been added to all commercial cat foods. Most cases today are not taurine responsive and reflect primary (or idiopathic) disease, although the disease is seen occasionally in cats fed noncommercial diets (eg, vegetarian, baby food, home-cooked food).

Doberman Pinschers typically develop concurrent and progressive ventricular arrhythmias along with progressive systolic dysfunction. Syncope and sudden death occur in as many as 20% of Doberman Pinschers, and signs of left heart failure eventually develop. Most Doberman Pinschers demonstrate evidence of myocardial failure at the time syncopal episodes are noted. In other breeds, such as Great Danes and Newfoundlands, sudden death and collapse are far less likely. Signs of left heart failure, including tachypnea and dyspnea due to pulmonary edema, weakness, and exercise intolerance often predominate, but signs of right heart failure (ascites) may also be present. Pleural effusion may be present, most commonly in dogs with both left and right heart failure. Ascites was noted in 35% of Newfoundlands with DCM in one study. Cats with DCM typically present with severe respiratory signs due to pulmonary edema and/or pleural effusion, and clinical signs are often rapidly progressive and refractory to therapy.

A soft systolic heart murmur, best heard at the left cardiac apex, is often present. A gallop sound may also be present but is subtle and usually identified in dogs only by an experienced examiner. It is often more obvious in cats. The femoral pulse may be weak, and an arrhythmia with associated pulse deficits may be noted. The arrhythmia is most commonly ventricular ectopy (eg, premature ventricular contractions, ventricular tachycardia) in Doberman Pinschers and Boxers, and atrial fibrillation in giant-breed dogs. Ascites, tachypnea, dyspnea, or cough may also be noted, depending on the type of heart failure that develops.

Blood work may demonstrate prerenal azotemia (increased BUN, creatinine). Thoracic radiographs typically demonstrate moderate to marked cardiomegaly. However, this finding may be masked by chest conformation (eg, a deep chest in a Doberman Pinscher). If left heart failure is present, pulmonary edema is more commonly evident in a large dog than it is in a small dog with mitral regurgitation, and the left atrium is moderately to markedly enlarged. Echocardiography is the best test to definitively diagnose DCM. In dogs with severe DCM that are in heart failure, there is a dramatic decrease in left ventricular fractional shortening caused by an increase in left ventricular end-systolic diameter. Cardiac chambers, especially the left atrium and left ventricle, are dilated. Mitral insufficiency typically develops as progressive left ventricular chamber dilation results in separation of the valve leaflets. Abnormal ECG findings may include ventricular premature complexes and ventricular tachycardia (especially in Doberman Pinschers and Boxers), and atrial fibrillation (especially giant breeds). There may be electrocardiographic evidence of left atrial enlargement (P mitrale or widened P waves) and left ventricular enlargement (tall and wide R waves). The occurrence of ventricular premature complexes on a routine ECG in a presumed healthy Doberman Pinscher is highly suggestive of DCM.

The objectives of therapy are to lessen edema/effusion formation (eg, with diuretics), improve contractility (eg, with pimobendan), and reduce adverse effects of angiotensin II and other neurohormonal changes (eg, with an ACE inhibitor). Taurine-responsive myocardial failure occurs in some breeds, particularly American Cocker Spaniels, and anecdotally in a few Golden Retrievers, Dalmatians, Welsh Corgis, Tibetan Terriers, and other breeds. In many of these breeds, taurine deficiency can be diagnosed by low plasma or whole blood concentrations. Response to taurine supplementation (which may take 2–4 mo) can be dramatic and may obviate the need for other cardiac medications. Carnitine-responsive cardiomyopathy, although reported, is almost a nonentity. Coenzyme Q_{10} supplementation is an unproven and, many say, irrational approach to the disease. Administration of fish oil might reduce the severity of cardiac cachexia in animals with DCM.

CHF, which may be severe, should be treated as discussed elsewhere (*see* p 99). As severe pulmonary edema resolves, furosemide can be administered orally, with oxygen continued until clinical signs are controlled. Pimobendan and an ACE inhibitor (eg, enalapril, benazepril) should be started. Pimobendan may be indicated in Doberman Pinschers with DCM before the onset of heart failure. Antiarrhythmic therapy is frequently indicated, especially for Doberman Pinschers with severe ventricular arrhythmias. Holter monitoring is the ideal method to evaluate both the severity of an arrhythmia and therapeutic efficacy. Mexiletine (5–10 mg/kg, tid) may be useful in animals with ventricular arrhythmias and concurrent heart failure, because negative inotropy is less than with sotalol (1–3 mg/kg, bid); however, sotalol can be used if therapy is initiated with a low dose carefully titrated upward and if pimobendan is used concurrently. Amiodarone may be a more effective drug than mexiletine to prevent sudden death in Doberman Pinschers, but its use is associated with a relatively high incidence of hepatotoxicity in this breed.

The prognosis is grave for cats with DCM (not taurine responsive), with a median survival time of 2 wk. Cats that are taurine responsive also have an initial high risk of death. However, cats that survive long enough for taurine to become effective (2–3 wk) have an excellent prognosis, because the disease is completely reversible. Dogs that are taurine responsive also have a fair to good prognosis once signs of CHF abate. The short-term prognosis for other dogs with DCM depends primarily on the severity of the heart failure on presentation. Longterm prognosis is poor, with survival time measured in months. The prognosis is poor in most Doberman Pinschers: in the past, ~25% died within 2 wk of presenting with heart failure, and 65% died within 8 wk. Pimobendan apparently prolongs survival, sometimes dramatically (months). The prognosis in other breeds is better but remains guarded; 75% die within 6 mo of diagnosis. As expected, dogs with severe heart failure, particularly left heart failure, have a worse prognosis than those with milder signs or signs of right heart failure at presentation.

Arrhythmogenic Right Ventricular Cardiomyopathy: Arrhythmogenic right ventricular cardiomyopathy (ARVC) is seen almost exclusively in Boxers and is also known as Boxer cardiomyopathy. It is rarely seen in cats. ARVC is characterized by a fatty or fibrofatty infiltrate of the right ventricular myocardium. In Boxers, the most common manifestation of the disease is syncope caused by a very fast (>400 bpm) nonsustained ventricular tachycardia. It takes 6–8 sec of no blood flow to the brain to result in unconsciousness, so the tachycardia must last for that long for syncope to occur and then must stop spontaneously for sudden death not to occur. The diagnosis is based on the number of premature ventricular complexes (PVCs) on a Holter monitor (>100–300 PVCs in 24 hr is generally considered diagnostic of ARVC in this breed). The QRS complexes of the PVCs are most commonly upright in the leads where the QRS complex is usually upright, meaning they originate from the right ventricle. The heart looks normal on thoracic radiographs and an echocardiogram in most Boxers with ARVC, although some will develop a true DCM and go into heart failure. Boxers presented for syncope without DCM are treated with sotalol (1–3 mg/kg, PO, bid) or a combination of mexiletine (5–10 mg/kg, PO, tid) and atenolol (12.5–25 mg/dog, PO, bid). Dogs refractory to sotalol may have mexiletine added. In Boxers with ARVC that do not have DCM, the prognosis is often good, and many live for several years on antiarrhythmic therapy. The longterm prognosis for dogs with DCM that are in heart failure is poor. Most live only several months.

In cats, the disease usually manifests as right ventricular and atrial enlargement and right heart failure, usually along with some supraventricular and ventricular tachyarrhythmias. Dyspnea and tachypnea due to pleural effusion, ascites, and nonspecific clinical signs such as anorexia and lethargy are reported in affected cats. Treatment is similar to that of DCM. Longterm prognosis is generally poor.

Hypertrophic Cardiomyopathy: Hypertrophic cardiomyopathy (HCM) is characterized by primary concentric left ventricular hypertrophy (ie, thick walls) resulting from an inherent myocardial disorder rather than pressure overload (such as caused by aortic stenosis), hormonal stimulation (such as hyperthyroidism or acromegaly), infiltration of the myocardium (eg, lymphoma), or other noncardiac disease. It is primarily seen in domestic cats and rarely in small dogs. It has also been reported in cattle. Papillary muscle enlargement is a consistent feature of the disease in cats. In people, HCM is caused by mutations in a number of sarcomeric genes. Mutations in one sarcomeric gene, the cardiac myosin binding C gene, have been identified in Maine Coon and Ragdoll cats. These mutations are thought to result in the production of dysfunctional sarcomeres within myocytes. The myocardium then produces new sarcomeres to help the dysfunctional ones, resulting in hypertrophy that may be mild to severe. Severe hypertrophy is often accompanied by cellular necrosis and resultant replacement fibrosis (myocardial scarring).

Increased fibrosis coupled with severe wall thickening results in a stiffer than normal left ventricle in diastole, which increases diastolic pressure for any given diastolic volume. The increased pressure is transmitted backward into the left atrium in diastole, resulting in left atrial enlargement and, if severe enough, in left heart failure. Left heart failure manifests as pulmonary edema and pleural effusion in cats. Myocardial contractility is normal, but left ventricular end-systolic diameter is usually less than normal and may become zero (end-systolic cavity obliteration) due to the increased wall thickness resulting in a decrease in systolic wall stress (ie, afterload). Severe left atrial enlargement can develop, which causes blood flow to stagnate. This can lead to the formation of a left atrial thrombus and the potential for systemic thromboembolism.

A cranial displacement of the anterior mitral valve leaflet during ventricular systole, a phenomenon termed systolic anterior motion of the mitral valve, is a common finding in cats with HCM and is due to marked enlargement of the papillary muscles that drag the mitral valve leaflet into the left ventricular outflow tract in systole. This phenomenon produces two turbulent jets—one of dynamic subaortic stenosis and the other of mitral regurgitation. Systolic anterior motion is the most common cause of a heart murmur in a cat with HCM. Gross pathology includes increased cardiac weight (>20 g), increased left ventricular wall thickness, papillary muscle hypertrophy, and often left atrial enlargement. The myocardium often contracts after death (ie, undergoes rigor), so the postmortem diagnosis of HCM often cannot be made based on left ventricular wall thickness alone.

HCM is the most common primary heart disease diagnosed in cats, but it is rare in dogs. It is familial in many breeds of cats, including Persians, Sphynx, Norwegian Forest Cats, Bengals, Turkish Vans, and American and British Shorthairs. As in Maine Coons and Ragdolls, the mode of inheritance is thought to be autosomal dominant. The disease is seen in cats from 3 mo to 17 yr of age, although most cats are middle aged at presentation. It is not present at birth but develops over time. Penetrance is often <100%. Male and female cats are equally predisposed, but males tend to develop more severe disease at an earlier age. In Maine Coon and Ragdoll cats, cats that are homozygous for the mutation often develop HCM earlier (often before 1 yr of age) and often develop a more severe form of the disease.

Many affected cats have no clinical signs, especially those with mild to moderate disease. Cats that develop severe disease may also have no clinical signs but will usually go on to develop left heart failure, systemic thromboembolism, or sudden death. Cats in heart failure have signs of tachypnea and dyspnea secondary to pulmonary edema or pleural effusion. Owners frequently do not note tachypnea and so do not present the cat for examination until dyspnea, often marked, is present. Cats with systemic thromboembolism most commonly have an acute onset of hindlimb paresis/paralysis coupled with acute pain, pulselessness, and poikilothermia. Cough is uncommon in cats with heart failure.

Physical examination frequently demonstrates abnormal heart sounds, including a soft to prominent systolic cardiac murmur and/or a gallop sound. The murmur is often dynamic, increasing in intensity with excitement and decreasing as the cat relaxes. A murmur is not present in at least one-third of cats with HCM. Increased respiratory sounds may suggest pulmonary edema, and decreased respiratory sounds may indicate pleural effusion, but auscultation of the lungs is often normal. The femoral pulse may be normal or weak, or absent if distal aortic thromboembolism has developed. Radiographically, there may be pronounced left atrial enlargement, especially in a cat in left heart failure, and variable left ventricular enlargement. The cardiac silhouette can appear relatively normal even in the presence of moderate to severe left ventricular hypertrophy if the left atrium is not enlarged. Echocardiography allows confirmation of the diagnosis and assessment of additional therapy needed (eg, anticoagulants may be more beneficial in cats with severe left atrial enlargement). Left ventricular wall thickening (≥6 mm; generalized or regional), along with papillary muscle hypertrophy are noted. Systolic anterior motion of the mitral valve may be present. ECG abnormalities may include supraventricular premature complexes, ventricular premature complexes, and ventricular tachycardia. With severe atrial enlargement, atrial fibrillation may rarely develop. An electrical axis deviation may be present. However, many cats with HCM have a normal ECG. The plasma concentration of NT-proBNP is often increased in cats with severe disease and particularly in those in heart failure (*see* p 101).

Treatment is directed at controlling signs of CHF, improving diastolic function, and reducing the incidence of systemic thromboembolism. Furosemide (2–4 mg/kg, IV or IM, as needed) administration and oxygen are needed when acute CHF is present. For chronic heart failure, furosemide and an ACE inhibitor, eg, enalapril (0.5 mg/kg/day, PO), are indicated. For cats not in heart failure, no drug strategy has been shown to alter the natural history of the disease. Diltiazem (7.5 mg, PO, tid), a calcium channel blocker, may improve diastolic function, but its effects are generally negligible and its use has diminished. Use of β-blockers such as atenolol (6.25–12.5 mg, PO, 1–2 times/day) may also be considered, but proof of benefit is lacking. People with HCM have shown improvement in exercise-induced angina and dyspnea, and exercise intolerance when given β-blockers. Cats rarely exert themselves, so those indications do not apply. However, a β-blocker does reduce systolic anterior motion of the mitral valve and should be considered when this abnormality is severe (pressure gradient across the dynamic subaortic stenosis is >80 mmHg). ACE inhibitors have no apparent beneficial effect before the onset of heart failure.

Prevention of left atrial thrombus formation and systemic thromboembolism is often a goal. Clopidogrel (18.75 mg/day/cat) is the only drug shown to decrease the incidence of systemic thromboembolism in cats. Warfarin (0.2–0.5 mg/day, PO) is probably ineffective and produces bleeding in some cats. Aspirin (80 mg, PO, every third day) is also believed to be ineffective. Clopidogrel plus aspirin is a common therapeutic strategy in people. A low-molecular-weight heparin such as enoxaparin (1 mg/kg, bid) might be efficacious but is expensive and must be administered parenterally.

The prognosis for cats with HCM is highly variable. Many mildly affected cats have a good longterm prognosis. Cats in CHF have a poor prognosis, with a median survival time of 3 mo. However, as many as 20% of cats with CHF might survive for a more prolonged period.

Restrictive/Unclassified Cardiomyopathy: A less common form of cardiomyopathy in cats is characterized by a relatively normal-appearing left ventricle with left atrial enlargement. Although it is logical to believe that these cats have diastolic dysfunction, many do not. Those that do have diastolic dysfunction have some form of restrictive cardiomyopathy. However, because that diagnosis cannot be made using standard two-dimensional echocardiography, it is better to term this type of disease unclassified cardiomyopathy unless diastolic dysfunction can be documented, usually by using tissue Doppler imaging echocardiography. Restrictive cardiomyopathy is characterized by a stiff, noncompliant left ventricle, usually due to increased collagen (ie, scar) formation in the left ventricle. The increased stiffness increases diastolic pressure for any given diastolic volume. As in hypertrophic cardiomyopathy, this results in an increase in left atrial size and left heart failure. In some cats that have obvious endomyocardial thickening or partial cavity obliteration, the diagnosis of restrictive cardiomyopathy can be readily made using two-dimensional echocardiography. A left atrial thrombus may be evident. Systolic function is usually preserved. Color flow Doppler echocardiography may demonstrate mitral regurgitation.

Clinical signs of and treatment for heart failure are similar to those for HCM (*see* p 117); however, prognosis seems to be worse, especially in cats with CHF. The cause of restrictive/unclassified cardiomyopathy is unknown.

Myocarditis

Myocarditis is a focal or diffuse inflammation of the myocardium with myocyte degeneration and/or necrosis. Myocarditis is rare in companion animals, although there are numerous causes, including several viruses and bacteria. Canine parvovirus (*see* p 373), encephalomyocarditis virus (*see* p 718), and equine infectious anemia virus (*see* p 699) can cause myocarditis. Myocardial degeneration is seen in lambs, calves, and foals with white muscle disease and in pigs with mulberry heart disease or hepatosis dietetica. *Streptococcus* spp are the most common cause of bacterial myocarditis in horses. *Salmonella*, *Clostridium*, equine influenza, *Borrelia burgdorferi*, and strongylosis are other recognized causes. Mineral deficiencies (eg, iron, selenium, copper) can also result in myocardial degeneration (not myocarditis). Deficiencies of vitamin E or selenium may cause myocardial necrosis. Cardiac toxins include ionophore antibiotics such as monensin and salinomycin, cantharidin (blister beetle toxicosis, *see* p 3157), *Cryptostegia grandiflora* (rubber vine), and *Eupatorium rugosum* (white snakeroot). These diseases cause typical signs of CHF. In horses, signs of right heart failure are common and include ventral edema, ascites, venous congestion, and jugular pulsations. A heart murmur of mitral or tricuspid regurgitation is usually audible as well as an irregular rhythm. Atrial fibrillation is common, and ventricular or atrial premature complexes may also be seen. Echocardiography reveals chamber dilation and poor contraction with essentially normal valves. Neutrophilic leukocytosis and hyperfibrinogenemia are common. Cardiac isoenzymes (CK, troponin, and lactate dehydrogenase) are often increased.

Treatment should be aimed at improving cardiac contractility, relieving congestion, and reducing vasoconstriction. Pimobendan and digoxin are used most commonly to improve contractility. Furosemide is indicated to control signs of pulmonary edema. Corticosteroids are often used when cardiac isoenzymes are increased and a viral infection is deemed unlikely.

Chagas' Myocarditis: *Trypanosoma cruzi*, a flagellate protozoa, causes Chagas' disease (*see* p 38). Acutely, ECG abnormalities such as first-, second-, or third-degree AV block; right bundle-branch block; sinus tachycardia; and depressed R wave amplitude are noted. There are usually no echocardiographic abnormalities during the acute phase; however, sudden death is a concern. An asymptomatic latent phase then develops for 27–120 days in dogs, followed by a chronic stage demonstrating systolic dysfunction indistinguishable from DCM. Treatment for the chronic phase is as for DCM but is typically ineffective at controlling signs of progressive myocardial failure. The disease is most commonly identified in southern states (eg, Texas) but may be spreading.

Tickborne Myocarditis: Lyme disease (*see* p 659) is caused by the spirochete *Borrelia burgdorferi*; infection might result in myocardial disease. In people, it causes a usually reversible third-degree AV block. Animals developing myocardial disease secondary to Lyme infection may, at least in theory, have ECG abnormalities such as ventricular arrhythmias or conduction disturbances such as first-, second-, or transient third-degree AV block. However, a recent study failed to identify evidence of any tickborne organism in a group of dogs presented for third-degree AV block. Two dogs with severe ventricular tachyarrhythmias with a high antibody titer to *Anaplasma phagocytophilum* required prednisone and azathioprine to control the arrhythmias. There are no reports of DCM due to these organisms in dogs or cats.

Other Causes of Myocardial Failure

In addition to the diseases listed below, histophilosis in cattle (*see* p 754) can result in myocardial infarcts and abscesses.

Persistent Atrial Standstill: A form of cardiomyopathy resulting in destruction of the atrial myocardium (that may also affect the ventricular myocardium) has been reported in dogs. Affected breeds include English Springer Spaniels, Old English Sheepdogs, Shih Tzus, German Shorthaired Pointers, and mixed-breed dogs. The disease has also been reported in some cats with concurrent cardiomyopathy. Initially, atrial myocardial destruction leading to atrial standstill and an AV nodal escape rhythm is noted. Mitral regurgitation that may be severe is often seen at this stage. Eventually, myocardial failure may ensue. Clinical signs are similar to those in animals with DCM, with right or left heart failure being noted. Pacemaker implantation may improve heart rate and cardiac output. Other treatment aims to relieve signs of CHF. This treatment typically is ultimately unrewarding, similar to treatment results in other animals with myocardial failure.

Doxorubicin-induced Myocardial Failure: Doxorubicin is a common chemotherapeutic agent that causes well-recognized cardiotoxicity. Cardiotoxicity tends to be dose dependent, but rare patients show toxicity at far lower dosages than others. Abnormalities include isolated ventricular premature complexes (which develop in 80% of dogs administered 80 mg/m^2/day for 2 days or 25 mg/m^2/wk for 4–11 wk) and periods of ventricular tachycardia. Myocardial failure may also develop and has been documented in 100% of dogs experimentally administered 25 mg/m^2/wk for 20 wk. (Sudden death and heart failure were noted in 65% of dogs after administration of ~17 wk of therapy.) The cardiotoxic effects are irreversible. Severe cardiotoxicity is rare with current chemotherapeutic protocols but depends on how aggressive the chemotherapeutic protocol is.

Endocardial Fibroelastosis: Endocardial fibroelastosis,a disease of unknown cause, is characterized by diffuse thickening of the left atrial, left ventricular, and/or mitral valve endocardium. It is a rare cause of myocardial failure in young dogs and cats. Affected animals are usually <6 mo old and present with clinical signs of left heart failure. Breeds reported include Labrador Retrievers, Great Danes, English Bulldogs, Springer Spaniels, Boxers, Pit Bulls, and Siamese and Burmese cats (in which the disease is believed to be inherited). Echocardiography demonstrates dilation of the left ventricular and atrial chambers, decreased left ventricular fractional shortening due to an increased left ventricular end-systolic diameter, and possibly diffuse endocardial thickening. Clinical signs, treatment, and prognosis are similar to those of DCM.

Duchenne Cardiomyopathy: Duchenne cardiomyopathy is an inherited, X-linked neuromuscular disorder reported in dogs, particularly Golden Retrievers. A similar disease called X-linked muscular dystrophy has been reported in Irish Terriers, Samoyeds, and Rottweilers. These diseases may result in myocardial as well as neuromuscular disease. ECG abnormalities include deep and narrow Q waves, a shortened PR interval, sinus arrest, and ventricular tachyarrhythmias. Echocardiography may demonstrate focal hyperechoic lesions affecting primarily the left ventricular and papillary muscle myocardium. This usually develops by 6–7 mo of age, with the lesions decreasing in size throughout the next 2 yr. The lesions result from calcification and fibrosis. In animals that survive, myocardial failure may develop.

Infective Endocarditis

Infection of the endocardium typically involves one of the cardiac valves, although mural endocarditis may occur. Endothelial damage is a predisposing factor for infective endocarditis to develop, although in dogs it is most common for endocarditis to form on a normal valve. When the endothelium is partially eroded and underlying collagen exposed, platelets adhere and produce a microthrombus. Immune deficiency may also be a predisposing factor. Bloodborne bacteria may become enmeshed in this thrombic lattice, resulting in a localized infection that causes a progressive destruction of the valve and results in valvular insufficiency. Vegetative lesions are the most common finding on cardiac valves and can create valvular stenosis (eg, aortic stenosis) but more commonly produce valvular insufficiency. In dogs, horses, and cats, the aortic and mitral valves are most commonly affected. The tricuspid valve is rarely affected, and pulmonic valve infective endocarditis is exceedingly rare. In contrast, the tricuspid valve is the most commonly affected valve in cattle. Infective endocarditis is rare in cats, and there are no breed predilections. In dogs, middle-aged, large-breed dogs are predisposed; <10% of dogs diagnosed with infective endocarditis weigh <15 kg. Most affected dogs are >4 yr old, and males are more commonly affected than females. Dogs with subaortic stenosis are at greater risk of developing infective endocarditis.

Infected thrombi released from the infected aortic or mitral valves enter the systemic circulation and can embolize other organs and limbs; therefore, infective endocarditis can produce a wide spectrum of clinical signs, including primary cardiovascular effects or signs related to the nervous system, GI tract, urogenital system, or joints. A chronic, intermittent or continuous fever is usually present. Shifting leg lameness may be reported, and weight loss and lethargy are frequently present. Acute to subacute mitral or aortic valve regurgitation can result in left heart failure (ie, pulmonary edema) and clinical signs of tachypnea, dyspnea, and cough. If the tricuspid valve is affected, ascites and jugular pulsations may be present. Mastitis and decreased milk production can be noted in affected cattle. Hematuria and pyuria may also be noted. A cardiac murmur is present in most cases; the exact type depends on the valve involved. When the aortic valve is affected, a low-intensity diastolic heart murmur is present, with maximal intensity over the left cardiac base. A soft systolic heart murmur caused by increased stroke volume may also be noted. In this instance, the arterial pulse is bounding (ie, increased pulse pressure) due to diastolic run-off and increased stroke volume. Mitral valve endocarditis results in a heart murmur similar to that caused by degenerative valve disease—a low- to high-intensity systolic heart murmur heard best over the left cardiac apex.

Bacteria most often isolated from affected dogs and cats include *Streptococcus*, *Staphylococcus*, *Klebsiella* spp, and *Escherichia coli*, although a host of other bacterial species may be involved. *Bartonella* is also a recognized cause of aortic valve infective endocarditis in dogs. In people, 60%–80% of patients with infective endocarditis have a predisposing cardiac lesion that facilitates bacterial attachment. In dogs, however, infection appears to develop commonly in those with no evidence of valve abnormalities. *Streptococcus* and *Actinobacillus* spp are the most common isolates in horses, and

Trueperella pyogenes is most commonly cultured from cattle.

A CBC often shows a neutrophilic leukocytosis. Active infection may be associated with the presence of band neutrophils, and chronic infection with a monocytosis (90% of cases in one series). Anemia of chronic disease is frequently present. Serum analysis abnormalities reflect organ involvement secondary to infective emboli and may include increases in liver enzymes, BUN, and creatinine. In animals that develop immune complex glomerulonephritis, significant urinary protein loss and hypoalbuminemia may develop. Blood cultures with antibiotic sensitivity should be obtained in affected animals. It is preferable to draw two or three blood samples, each 1–2 hr apart, in a 24-hr period. Strict aseptic technique is required. However, blood culture results are frequently negative (and are positive in other types of septicemia) and cannot be used alone to make the diagnosis of endocarditis.

Radiography may demonstrate cardiac chamber enlargement, depending on the location and degree of insufficiency of the involved valve. If the aortic or mitral valve is severely affected, there will be left atrial and left ventricular chamber dilation. Evidence of left heart failure may be seen as an increase in interstitial density or, in severe CHF, an alveolar pattern in the pulmonary parenchyma. If the tricuspid or pulmonic valve is affected, right-side chamber enlargement is expected. Echocardiography is the diagnostic test of choice, because blood cultures are positive in only 50%–90% of dogs. The affected valve is usually easily detected—the involved area is hyperechoic (bright), thickened, and often vegetative (ie, looks like a cauliflower). The vegetative lesion may oscillate. Erosive lesions may predominate in some animals. Doppler echocardiography will confirm insufficiency of the valve, and chamber enlargement on the side of the affected valve is expected when significant insufficiency is present. Electrocardiography may demonstrate atrial and ventricular premature complexes. Infrequently, other arrhythmias such as atrial fibrillation or conduction disturbances are found.

Therapy is directed at controlling clinical signs of CHF, resolving any significant arrhythmias, sterilizing the lesion, and eliminating the spread of infection. The heart failure may be severe and intractable if the aortic valve is significantly involved; the prognosis is grave in these cases. The prognosis is much more favorable when infection is mild and limited to one of the AV valves. Controlling heart failure requires the use of diuretics such as furosemide, an ACE inhibitor, and when myocardial failure is present, pimobendan. Initially in dogs, parenteral antibiotics are indicated for 1–2 wk (which may be cost prohibitive), followed by oral antibiotics for at least 6–8 wk. Initial broad-spectrum bactericidal antibiotics (a combination of ampicillin plus gentamicin or enrofloxacin, or cephalothin plus gentamicin) should be used and changed, if needed, based on antibiotic sensitivity studies. Renal function should be monitored when gentamicin is used, because it is nephrotoxic. The prognosis is poor in most dogs. Those that respond to therapy often require longterm medications for heart failure (eg, diuretics, vasodilators, pimobendan) and frequent reevaluations. In large animals, rifampin (5 mg/kg, PO, bid), together with another broad-spectrum antibiotic, has been demonstrated to improve short-term outlook. Aspirin (100 mg/kg/day in ruminants and 17 mg/kg every other day in horses) or heparin (30 U/kg, SC, bid in ruminants and horses) may prevent further thrombus and vegetative growth in large animals.

Antibiotic prophylaxis is indicated in dogs with subaortic stenosis when any type of procedure that can result in significant bacteremia is performed. Routine antibiotic prophylaxis for dental procedures is not warranted with other types of cardiac disease and especially not in dogs with myxomatous mitral valve degeneration, because there is no evidence these dogs are at increased risk of infective endocarditis.

Pericardial Disease

Pericardial disease most commonly causes an accumulation of fluid within the pericardial sac (ie, pericardial effusion). This accumulation can be acute or chronic, but chronic is much more common in veterinary medicine. When the fluid accumulation is severe enough to markedly increase the intrapericardial pressure, cardiac tamponade occurs. Acute cardiac tamponade (eg, due to left atrial rupture or thoracic trauma) primarily results in decreased cardiac filling and an abrupt decrease in cardiac output. Chronic cardiac tamponade primarily increases the diastolic intraventricular pressures. This causes signs of CHF. Right-side diastolic—and so systemic venous and capillary pressure—only have to increase from a normal of 5 mmHg to 10–15 mmHg to produce signs of right heart failure, whereas left-side pressures must increase from a normal of <10 mmHg to >20 mmHg to produce left heart failure. Thus, signs of right heart failure predominate.

Pericardial effusion is a relatively common form of acquired cardiovascular diseases in dogs, is uncommon in cattle, and is rare in horses and cats. In dogs, cases involving middle-aged, predominantly male, large breeds are most frequent. Idiopathic pericarditis and cardiac neoplasia are the most common causes of pericardial effusion in dogs. Hemangiosarcoma and heart base tumors (chemodectoma, ectopic thyroid carcinoma) are the most frequently seen cardiac neoplasms. Mesothelioma is a less common form of pericardial neoplasia. Using echocardiography, hemangiosarcoma is most frequently identified on the right auricle, in the right AV groove, and in the right atrial chamber in dogs. Heart base tumors usually are identified between the aorta and main pulmonary artery. In cats, the most common cardiac neoplasia is lymphoma, but the most common cause of mild pericardial effusion is heart failure. Most cases of pericardial effusion in cats are not severe enough to cause cardiac tamponade. Less common causes of pericardial effusion in dogs are infections (eg, coccidioidomycosis), trauma, left atrial rupture, and CHF. Cattle most often develop pericardial effusion secondary to traumatic reticulopericarditis (*see* p 230) or cardiac neoplasia (lymphoma). Lymphoma in cattle can also result in valvular insufficiencies. In horses, septic pericarditis and idiopathic pericarditis are most commonly reported.

The severity of clinical signs depends on the rate of pericardial fluid accumulation. In dogs, ascites is by far the most common clinical manifestation. Collapse and vomiting may be seen. The femoral pulse may be weak or decrease on inspiration and increase on expiration (pulses paradoxus). In horses, there is often a history of respiratory tract infection, fever, anorexia, and depression. Physical examination findings, in addition to abdominal distention, include generalized weakness, jugular venous distention, muffled heart sounds, and occasionally a pericardial friction rub. With slow development of pericardial fluid, the pericardial sac is able to stretch or enlarge, and clinical signs of right heart failure may not develop until severe pericardial effusion is present.

CBC, serum chemistry profile, and urinalysis results are usually normal. Mild anemia, neutrophilic leukocytosis, hyperfibrinogenemia, and hyperproteinemia may be seen in horses with septic pericarditis and effusion. In horses with suspected septic pericarditis, culture and sensitivity of the fluid should be performed. In septic pericarditis, there will be a large number of neutrophils, with some being degenerate. Protein content of the fluid will be high, and bacteria may be seen. Cytologic features of idiopathic pericardial effusion in horses are variable, with neutrophils, eosinophils, and macrophages present in variable numbers. Cytologic evaluation of the pericardial fluid usually does not provide a definitive cause for the pericardial effusion in dogs unless an infection is present, which is uncommon. Rarely a tumor (most commonly a hemangiosarcoma) will acutely bleed, producing an effusion with a PCV similar to that of blood.

Radiographs often show an increase in the size of the cardiac silhouette, which often takes on a rounded (globoid) appearance. However, this classic appearance is not always present. If the cause is a cardiac tumor, especially a heart base tumor, the cardiac silhouette may have a bulge at the top of the heart cranial to the carina or at the region of the cranial waist if no or only slight effusion is present. The caudal vena cava may be dilated if cardiac tamponade is present. Pleural effusion may also be present, more commonly if mesothelioma is the cause of the pericardial effusion. The ECG in most cases shows normal sinus rhythm to sinus tachycardia.

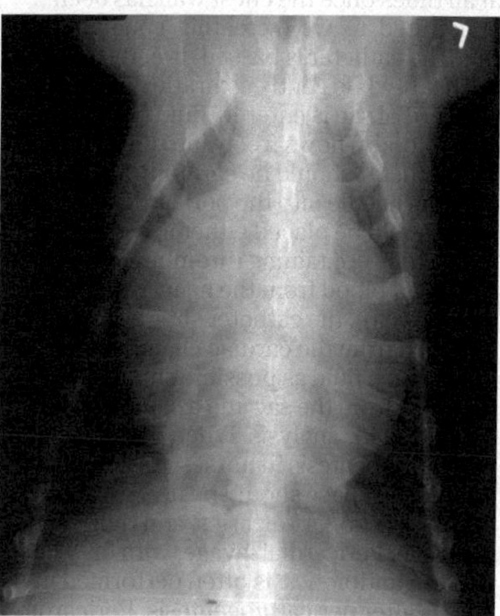

Severe pericardial effusion in a dog, dorsoventral projection. *Courtesy of Dr. Mark D. Kittleson.*

Occasional atrial premature and ventricular complexes may occur. The height of the R wave is often decreased (<1 mV in dogs), and there may be a pattern of alternating variation in R wave amplitude, referred to as electrical alternans, when there is a large amount of effusion present. This results from the swinging motion of the heart within the fluid-filled pericardial sac. Echocardiography is the most sensitive and specific test for detection of pericardial effusion. A tumor can be visualized in most cases of neoplastic effusion. When cardiac tamponade is present, the walls of the right atrium and right ventricle may collapse in systole or diastole.

Animals with cardiac tamponade require mechanical drainage of the pericardial space (pericardiocentesis) using a catheter. Medical therapy is typically ineffective at reducing pericardial effusion. Diuretics are contraindicated in acute cardiac tamponade because they decrease blood volume and cause a further decrease in cardiac output. Pericardiocentesis in dogs and cats is done by placement of a catheter through the chest wall on the right side, just above the costochondral junction at the fourth to fifth intercostal space. Echocardiography can be used to guide catheter placement at the point where the pericardial sac is closest to the thoracic wall and most distended with fluid, but it is not necessary. Fenestrating the catheter helps prevent blockage. A syringe or extension set with stopcock and syringe (preferred) is attached to the catheter. The system must be closed to air at all times once the chest wall has been penetrated, to avoid creating a pneumothorax. The catheter is passed directly toward the heart while gently aspirating. When the pericardial sac is entered, fluid (usually quite bloody) flows freely into the syringe. The catheter should be carefully advanced over the needle into the pericardial sac. The fluid should be placed either in a glass tube or in a tube containing thrombin to cause clotting if blood from the heart is aspirated; if it does clot, the catheter should be removed from the cardiac chamber it is in. As much fluid as possible should be removed from the sac and a sample submitted for analysis. When performing pericardiocentesis in horses, the left fifth intercostal space should be used to avoid the atria, coronary arteries, and right ventricle. Pericardial lavage, with or without antibiotics, is often performed in horses after pericardiocentesis. Pericardiocentesis is relatively easy to perform in dogs, and serious complications are rare. However, confirming the presence of pericardial effusion by echocardiography is advisable before performing pericardiocentesis.

Parenteral fluids may be given immediately before and after pericardiocentesis. Corticosteroids have not been shown to be beneficial in idiopathic pericarditis (benign pericardial effusion) in dogs, although they have been used with success in horses. Most tumors that cause neoplastic effusion do not respond well to chemotherapy. A heart base tumor can be surgically debulked, but only by a highly skilled surgeon. Rarely, a hemangiosarcoma can be surgically removed if it is confined to the right auricle and no metastatic disease is present. Chemotherapy (eg, adriamycin) might be beneficial in some dogs with hemangiosarcoma, although survival times are generally measured in months.

When idiopathic pericarditis is suspected (ie, no mass visible by echocardiography), the owner should be instructed to carefully monitor the animal for any signs of recurrence. Should this occur, a repeat pericardiocentesis is indicated. A subtotal pericardectomy is generally recommended after the third pericardiocentesis. Heart base tumors only rarely metastasize in dogs, although they can grow to be quite large and may compromise function of surrounding structures. If recurrent pericardial effusion secondary to a heart base tumor is diagnosed, subtotal pericardectomy should be considered. A dog can survive as long as 2 yr after successful subtotal pericardectomy. The prognosis for right atrial hemangiosarcoma is poor to grave. Many dogs have metastasis or micrometastasis (most commonly to the lungs and not visible on radiographs) at the time of diagnosis.

Constrictive and constrictive/effusive pericarditis is rare and primarily seen in dogs. It is thought to be an end result of chronic idiopathic pericarditis. A dog with constrictive pericarditis usually presents with ascites, no murmur, normal heart sounds, normal cardiac silhouette on thoracic radiographs, a positive hepatojugular reflux test, and distended hepatic veins on ultrasound. Diagnosis can be difficult and may require cardiac catheterization. Treatment is surgical. With constrictive/effusive pericarditis, there is still a fluid layer between the pericardial sac and the surface of the heart, so surgical removal of the pericardium is relatively easy. With constrictive pericarditis, the pericardium and epicardium are fused into one fibrous layer that must be painstakingly removed surgically.

Systemic and Pulmonary Hypertension

Systemic hypertension is an increase in systemic arterial blood pressure. There are two major types of systemic hypertension. Essential hypertension, which is idiopathic (primary) hypertension, is rare (essentially nonexistent) in dogs and cats but common in people. Secondary hypertension results from a specific underlying disease. In dogs, the most common cause of hypertension is renal disease/failure; in cats, the most common causes are renal disease/failure and hyperthyroidism. Hyperadrenocorticism, diabetes mellitus, and pheochromocytoma are other causes of systemic hypertension in dogs.

The diagnosis of systemic hypertension is made by measurement of systemic blood pressure. The most accurate assessment method is direct measurement via arterial puncture, which is impractical in most instances. The next most accurate method (although still often inaccurate) is indirect measurement using a Doppler probe to assess blood flow in an artery (typically the superficial palmar arterial branch of the radial artery) distal to pressure cuff placement (typically on the forelimb). Cuff width should be 30% of the circumference of the forelimb in cats and 40% of the forelimb circumference in dogs. Shaving the hair just proximal to the palmar metacarpal pad for application of the Doppler probe allows for more accurate results. The hindlimb can also be used, in which case the superficial plantar arterial branch of the caudal tibial artery is assessed. The disadvantage of Doppler blood pressure measurement is that only systolic blood pressure is reliably measured. Other methods to measure systemic blood pressure, such as the oscillometric method, are even less accurate than the Doppler method, especially in small dogs and cats. Although indirect blood pressure measurement is less accurate than direct assessment, it can detect acute trends in blood pressure during anesthesia. In conscious animals, normal values vary with patient stress; values higher than expected for a healthy animal often are caused by the stress of examination. With certain exceptions, systolic pressures >180 mmHg are likely to be truly increased in an animal that appears calm, and values >200 mmHg should be strongly considered evidence of systemic hypertension. Because of the inaccuracy of noninvasive blood pressure measurement and the influence that stress has on blood pressure, blood pressure measurements should be done only in dogs and cats that have a disease that causes hypertension or that have a clinical problem referable to systemic hypertension (eg, detached retina). Blood pressure measurement is not a screening tool in veterinary medicine as it is in human medicine, except in patient populations that have a disease that causes systemic hypertension (eg, dogs with renal failure should be screened for systemic hypertension). Even in an animal with a disease that causes hypertension that has an increased blood pressure measurement, documenting end-organ damage (eg, presence of hypertensive retinopathy) is recommended before instituting therapy.

Dogs and cats with severe systemic hypertension often have no clinical signs. Acute blindness is the most common clinical sign. Retinal lesions (eg, retinal hemorrhage, retinal detachment, arterial tortuosity, focal or diffuse retinal edema) were found in 80% of hypertensive cats in one study. Blood tests may demonstrate abnormalities consistent with the cause of hypertension (eg, increased T_4 levels in hyperthyroid cats, increased BUN and creatinine in animals with renal failure). Treatment should be initiated in animals with consistently measurable hypertension that are documented to have an underlying cause such as renal disease/failure and evidence of end-organ damage. Systemic hypertension in cats and dogs appears to be due to constriction of systemic arterioles, because only potent systemic arteriolar dilators are reasonably effective to decrease systemic blood pressure to a clinically significant degree. The treatment for cats is amlodipine (0.625–1.25 mg/day, PO). Other drugs, such as enalapril, diltiazem, β-blockers (eg, atenolol), and diuretics (eg, furosemide) are generally ineffective. In dogs, amlodipine (0.2–1 mg/kg/day) and hydralazine (1–3 mg/kg, bid) are the only consistently effective drugs. Some clinicians have had success with prazosin (1–4 mg [total dose], PO, 1–2 times/day) in dogs. Phenoxybenzamine (0.25–2 mg/kg, PO, bid) is expensive but can also be effective in dogs. It is most often used in dogs with a pheochromocytoma but can also be effective in dogs with systemic hypertension due to other causes.

Pulmonary hypertension is increased blood pressure in the pulmonary arterial circulation. Possible causes include increased pulmonary blood flow (eg, ventricular septal defect, patent ductus arteriosus), increased pulmonary vascular resistance due to decreased overall cross-sectional area of the pulmonary vascular bed (such as caused by pulmonary arterial wall hypertrophy, pulmonary thromboembolism, and pulmonary vasoconstriction), or both. Primary pulmonary hypertension is rare in any species other than people. In cattle, the most common cause is hypoxia-induced pulmonary vasoconstriction caused by high altitude (*see* p 137). Chronic ingestion of locoweed (*Oxytropis* and *Astragalus* spp) or chronic pulmonary disease caused by bronchopneumonia or lungworm infestation can also result in pulmonary hypertension severe enough to result in right heart failure. In horses, pulmonary hypertension may occur secondary to left heart failure. In dogs, pulmonary hypertension most commonly occurs secondary to heartworm disease, pulmonary thromboembolism, severe hypoxemia due to primary pulmonary disease, and left heart failure.

Clinical signs are typically those of right heart failure (ascites, exercise intolerance) and episodic collapse or syncope, usually after exercise or excitement. Physical examination findings may include evidence of ascites in dogs and ventral edema in cattle and horses along with jugular vein distention and pulsation. Definitive diagnosis requires direct measurement of pulmonary arterial pressure (rarely performed), or estimation of pulmonary pressures by Doppler echocardiography (via measuring the velocity of a tricuspid or pulmonary regurgitant jet). Echocardiography may demonstrate flattening of the interventricular septum in systole, right ventricular chamber dilatation and/or free wall thickening, and right atrial enlargement. Treatment is typically unrewarding, and the prognosis is often poor, depending on the cause. In heartworm disease, successful clearance of adult worms from the pulmonary arterial vasculature often results in a reduction in pulmonary artery pressure and resolution of right heart failure. Dogs with a right-to-left shunting PDA can live for several years despite severe pulmonary hypertension if their polycythemia is adequately controlled. Sildenafil (1–3 mg/kg, bid-tid), a phosphodiesterase V inhibitor, is probably the most effective drug to lower pulmonary artery pressure and improve clinical signs in dogs with pulmonary hypertension, but it is expensive. It is primarily warranted in dogs with clinical signs due to pulmonary hypertension, most commonly syncope and right heart failure. In these patient populations, sildenafil often will reduce or stop syncope and allow easier control of ascites. Exercise tolerance may be improved. There is limited experience with tadalafil (1 mg/kg, PO, 1–2 times/day) but, in theory, it should have the same effects. Pimobendan reduces pulmonary artery pressure in dogs with pulmonary hypertension secondary to left heart failure. The best chance for a successful longterm outcome is when the underlying disease can be identified and treated, but this is rare.

Arterial Thromboembolism

Overt intravascular thrombus formation is rare with heart failure in most species other than domestic cats and people. Cats frequently form a thrombus in a severely enlarged left atrium, most commonly in the left auricle. This thrombus then commonly breaks loose and flows into the systemic circulation. Although this occurs most commonly in a cat with a large left atrium due to cardiomyopathy, it can also occur without left atrial enlargement, sometimes even happening in an otherwise healthy cat. In a cat with severe left atrial enlargement, it is assumed that the primary reason the thrombus develops is because of blood flow stasis. Red cells aggregate when blood flow decreases below a critical velocity. When the left atrium enlarges, blood flow velocity decreases (assuming no mitral regurgitation). The area of lowest velocity is the left auricle. In some cats, red cell aggregation can be visualized as so-called spontaneous contrast or "smoke" within the left atrium. In a few cats, both a thrombus and spontaneous contrast can be noted. However, in most cats, the thrombus has already become an embolus by the time an echocardiogram is done.

The site the thromboembolus lodges once it has broken loose from its site of attachment in the left atrium depends on the size of the thrombus and blood flow patterns. A very small thrombus can gain entrance to a coronary artery and cause myocardial infarction. A mid-sized thrombus can exit into a branch coming off the aorta, such as the brachiocephalic trunk (and then most commonly to the right subclavian) or an intestinal branch. Most of these thrombi, however, are large and so cannot exit off any branch of the aorta and end up at the terminal aorta. Here, they occlude aortic flow and release vasoactive amines that shut down collateral circulation. Consequently, they cause acute cessation of blood flow to the hindlimbs. This results in pulselessness (no femoral pulse), pallor (pale or purple foot pads), poikilothermia (decreased rectal temperature and cold hindlimbs), and initially extreme pain. The gastrocnemius muscles are often very firm. The cat can often move the legs above the stifles, and the tail is commonly unaffected. In some cats, only one hindlimb is affected.

Diagnosis is most commonly based on clinical signs, physical examination findings, and Doppler blood flow readings of the hindlimbs. Ultrasound can also be used to identify the thromboembolus. Misdiagnosis of neurologic abnormalities as an arterial thromboembolus in cats is common. In some cats, the clot will lyse on its own over time (1–72 hours). However, some of these cats have residual problems (eg, dry gangrene). Numerous treatments, including surgery, thrombolytic agents, and rheolytic thrombectomy, have been tried but are largely unsuccessful when compared with waiting for the thromboembolus to lyse on its own. Euthanasia is common. Clopidogrel (18.75 mg/day/cat) has been shown to be effective at preventing recurrence of these events in cats and so is assumed to be effective at preventing first occurrence also; however, it is, by no means, 100% effective. Aspirin is believed to be ineffective.

HEARTWORM DISEASE

(Dirofilarosis, Dirofilariasis)

Heartworm (HW) disease is caused by the filarial organism, *Dirofilaria immitis*. At least 70 species of mosquitoes can serve as intermediate hosts; *Aedes*, *Anopheles*, and *Culex* are the most common genera acting as vectors. Patent infections are possible in numerous wild and companion animal species. Wild animal reservoirs include wolves, coyotes, foxes, California gray seals, sea lions, and raccoons. In companion animals, HW infection is diagnosed primarily in dogs and less commonly in cats and ferrets. HW disease has been reported in most countries with temperate, semitropical, or tropical climates, including the USA, Canada, Australia, Latin America, and southern Europe. In companion animals, infection risk is greatest in dogs and cats housed outdoors. Although any dog or cat, indoor or outdoor, is capable of being infected, most infections are diagnosed in medium- to large-sized, 3- to 8-yr-old dogs living outside.

Infected mosquitoes are capable of transmitting HW infections to people, but there are no reports of such infections becoming patent. Maturation of the infective larvae may progress to the point where they reach the lungs, become encapsulated, and die. The dead larvae precipitate granulomatous reactions called "coin lesions," which are visible with thoracic radiographs and significant because they mimic lung cancer.

HW infection rates in other companion animals such as ferrets and cats tend to parallel those in dogs in the same geographic region. No age predilection has been reported in ferrets or cats, but male cats have been reported to be more susceptible than females. Indoor and outdoor ferrets and cats can be infected. Other infections in cats, such as those caused by the feline leukemia virus or feline immunodeficiency virus, are not predisposing factors.

Life Cycle: Mosquito vector species acquire microfilariae (a neonatal larval stage) while feeding on an infected host. Once ingested by the mosquito, microfilariae develop into the first larval stage (L_1). They then actively molt into the second larval stage (L_2) and again to the infective third stage (L_3) within the mosquito in ~1–4 wk, depending on environmental temperatures. This development phase requires the shortest time (10–14 days) when the average ambient temperature is >81°F (27°C) and the relative humidity is 80%. When mature, the infective larvae migrate to the labium of the mosquito. As the mosquito feeds, the infective larvae erupt through the tip of the labium with a small amount of hemolymph onto the host's skin. The larvae migrate into the bite wound, beginning the intramammalian phase of the life cycle. A typical *Aedes* mosquito is capable of surviving the complete development of only small numbers of HW larvae, usually <10 larvae per mosquito.

In canids and other susceptible hosts, infective larvae (L_3) molt into a fourth stage (L_4) in 3–12 days. After remaining in the subcutaneous tissue, abdomen, and thorax for ~2 mo, L_4 undergo their final molt at day

50–70 into young adults, arriving in the heart and pulmonary arteries ~70–120 days after initial infection. Only 2.5–4 cm in length on arrival, worms rapidly grow in the pulmonary vasculature to adult worms (males ~15 cm long, females ~25 cm). When juvenile heartworms first reach the lungs, blood flow forces them into the more distal small pulmonary arteries of the caudal lung lobes; as the parasites grow, they occupy larger and larger pulmonary arteries, moving into the right ventricle and atrium when the worm burden is high. Gravid females produce microfilariae as early as 6 mo after infection but more typically at 7–9 mo after infection.

Microfilariae are detectable in most infected canids (~80%) not receiving macrolide prophylaxis and occasionally in those dogs placed on macrolide preventives when a HW infection was already present. The number of circulating microfilariae does not correlate well to the adult female HW burden. Adult worms typically live 3–5 yr, whereas microfilariae may survive for up to 2 yr in the dog, while awaiting arrival of a mosquito intermediate host.

Most dogs are highly susceptible to HW infection, and most (an average of 56%) experimentally administered infective larvae (L_3) develop into adults. Ferrets and cats are susceptible hosts, but the rate of infective larvae developing into adults is low (an average of 6% in cats and 40% in ferrets). In cats, the adult burden is often only one to three worms. It appears that early death of juvenile worms on arrival at the pulmonary vasculature is largely responsible for the heartworm-associated respiratory disease (HARD) syndrome in cats. HARD does not require maturation of heartworms but is due to the body's response to the dying/dead heartworms. When maturation does occur, adult worm survival in cats is typically not longer than 2–3 yr. In all animals capable of being infected, aberrant larval migration may occur, resulting in parasitic lesions in the CNS, systemic arterial system, and in visceral and subcutaneous sites.

Pathogenesis: The severity of cardiopulmonary pathology in dogs is determined by worm numbers, host immune response, duration of infection, and host activity level. Live adult heartworms cause direct mechanical trauma, and other suspected factors (eg, antigens and excretions) are thought to directly irritate or to stimulate the hosts' immune system to damage vessel intima, leading to proliferative endarteritis and perivascular cuffing with inflammatory cells, including infiltration of high numbers of eosinophils. Live worms seem to have an immunosuppressive effect; however, the presence of dead worms leads to more severe vascular reactions and subsequent lung pathology, even in areas of the lung not directly contacting the dead heartworms. Longterm infections, due to all of the factors noted (ie, direct irritation, worm death, and immune response) result in chronic lesions and subsequent scarring. Active dogs tend to more often develop pulmonary hypertension than inactive dogs for any given worm burden. Frequent exertion increases pulmonary arterial pathology and pulmonary artery resistance (with resultant pulmonary hypertension) and thereby may precipitate overt clinical signs, including congestive heart failure (CHF). High worm burdens are most often the result of infections acquired from numerous mosquito exposures. High exposures in young, naive dogs in temperate climates can result in severe infections, possibly precipitating vena cava syndrome the year after. In general, because of the worm size and smaller dimensions of the pulmonary vasculature, small dogs do not tolerate infections and treatment as well as large dogs.

The role of the endosymbiotic bacteria *Wolbachia pipiens*, which live intracellularly within the filarid parasite, is still being determined. However, these bacteria have been implicated as playing a role in the pathogenesis of filarial diseases, possibly through endotoxin production. Furthermore, studies have demonstrated that a primary surface protein of *Wolbachia* (WSP) induces a specific IgG response in hosts infected by *D immitis*. For veterinarians, the most important aspect of *Wolbachia* is its symbiotic relation with *D immitis*. This bacterium is necessary for normal maturation, reproduction, and infectivity of the heartworm. If *Wolbachia* are eradicated, the heartworm gradually dies, after first becoming sterile. This can be accomplished with doxycycline therapy.

HW-associated inflammatory mediators that induce immune responses in the lungs and kidneys (eg, immune complex glomerulonephritis) cause vasoconstriction and possibly bronchoconstriction. Leakage of plasma and inflammatory mediators from small vessels and capillaries causes parenchymal lung inflammation and mild, noncardiogenic edema formation. Pulmonary artery disease compromises vascular compliance, and this, with reduced ability to adequately vasodilate, results in increased flow velocity, especially with exertion, and resultant shear stresses further damage the endothelium. The process of endothelial damage, vascular dysfunction, increased flow velocity, and local ischemia is a vicious cycle. Inflammation with ischemia can result in irreversible interstitial fibrosis.

Pulmonary arterial pathology in cats and ferrets is similar to that in dogs, although the small arteries develop more severe muscular hypertrophy. Despite this, pulmonary hypertension with CHF is less common in cats than in dogs or ferrets. Arterial thrombi, thromboemboli, and living or dead worms become lodged within pulmonary arteries or arterioles, resulting in complete or partial obstruction. In cats, parenchymal changes associated with dead heartworms differ from those observed in dogs and ferrets. Rather than type I alveolar cell damage, as found in dogs, cats develop type II alveolar cell hyperplasia, which can act as a significant barrier to oxygenation. Most significantly, because of restricted pulmonary vascular capacity and subsequent pathology, ferrets and cats are more likely than dogs to die as a result of HW infection.

Clinical Findings: In dogs, infection is ideally identified by serologic testing before onset of clinical signs; however, at the earliest, HW antigenemia and microfilaremia do not appear until ~5 and 6.5 mo after infection, respectively. When dogs do not receive preventive medication and are not appropriately tested, infection and disease progress undetected. Clinical signs of HW infection, such as coughing, exercise intolerance, unthriftiness, dyspnea, cyanosis, hemoptysis, syncope, epistaxis, and ascites (right-side CHF) may develop. The frequency and severity of clinical signs correlate to lung pathology and level of animal activity. Signs are often not observed in sedentary dogs, even though the worm burden may be relatively high. Infected dogs experiencing a dramatic increase in activity, such as during hunting seasons, may develop overt clinical signs. Likewise, worm death and thromboemboli precipitate clinical signs.

A dog may be classified as low- or high-risk for developing clinical signs, based on assessment of potential worm burden, the health and age of the dog, and its lifestyle. There is also a more complex classification system in which dogs are classified from I to IV, based on severity of signs. Class I dogs are minimally affected clinically. Class II dogs exhibit cough. Class III dogs are severely affected and variably present with cough, hemoptysis, weight loss, lethargy, exercise intolerance, dyspnea, heart failure (ascites), and radiographic findings suggestive of HW disease (large main pulmonary artery and lobar pulmonary arteries, truncated and tortuous pulmonary arteries, pulmonary infiltrate, and hilar lymphadenopathy). Class IV includes dogs with caval syndrome. Dogs 5–7 yr old are at higher risk of having a heavy worm burden, presumably because of increased time of exposure and for disease development. Other concurrent health factors (eg, concurrent cardiopulmonary or other organ system disease) affect risk assessment. The degree to which exercise can be restricted during the recovery period is another important consideration.

Infected cats may be asymptomatic or exhibit intermittent coughing, dyspnea, heart failure, vomiting, lethargy, anorexia, or weight loss. When evident, signs usually develop during two phases of the HW life cycle: 1) the arrival of juvenile worms in the pulmonary vasculature ~3–4 mo after infection, and 2) death of adult heartworms. The early signs are associated with an acute vascular and parenchymal inflammatory response to the newly arriving young worms and the subsequent death of many or all of these juveniles. This initial phase is often misdiagnosed as asthma or allergic bronchitis. However, this is now considered to be part of HARD. Antigen tests in such cats are negative (measured antigens are associated with mature female worms) during the early eosinophilic pneumonitis syndrome, although antibody tests typically are positive. Although not yet well characterized, it is believed that clinical signs often resolve and may not reappear for months. HARD has been postulated to contribute to longterm lung damage. Cats harboring mature worms may exhibit intermittent vomiting, lethargy, coughing, or episodic dyspnea. Death of even one adult heartworm can lead to acute respiratory distress and shock, which may be fatal and appears to be the consequence of pulmonary thrombosis and/or anaphylactic-like shock.

Ferrets, more so than cats, mimic canine HW infection in terms of clinical signs. The large parasite:host body weight ratio dictates that ferrets (and cats) develop clinical signs with relatively small worm burdens. Ferrets with HW disease may demonstrate one or more of the following: weight loss, fatigue, rapid and/or labored breathing, heart murmur, distended and pulsatile jugular veins, cough, grey and cold mucous membranes, ascites, pleural effusion, fainting, and sudden death. *See* TABLE 8.

TABLE 8 DIAGNOSTIC TESTS, CLINICAL SIGNS, AND TREATMENT FOR HEARTWORMS IN DOGS, CATS, AND FERRETS

	Diagnosis (Test Utility)			
Host	Microfilaria	Ag or Ab Test	Thoracic Radiographs	Echocardiography
Dog	****	***** (Ag)	*** MPA, PA, RHE, PTE, PIE	**
Cat	*	** (Ag) **** (Ab)	** PA, PIE	****
Ferret	*	*** (Ag)	* RH	***

[a]Imidacloprid-moxidectin is the only approved microfilaricide.
* = rarely useful; ** = somewhat useful; *** = moderately useful; **** = often useful; ***** = excellent test; Ag = antigen; Ab = antibody; MPA = main pulmonary artery enlargement; PA = pulmonary artery enlargement; PTE = pulmonary thrombus/thromboembolus; PIE = pulmonary infiltrate with eosinophils; RH = right heart enlargement; NA = not applicable

Adapted from McCall, JW. *Clin Tech Small Anim Pract.* 1998;13(2):112.

Diagnosis: The antigen detection test is the preferred diagnostic method for routine screening of asymptomatic dogs or when seeking verification of a suspected HW infection. Antigen testing is the most sensitive and specific diagnostic method available to veterinary practitioners. Even in areas where the prevalence of HW infection is high, ~20% of infected dogs are not microfilaremic, which diminishes the utility of screening by testing for microfilariae. This figure is even higher for dogs infected with adult heartworms and that are consistently administered monthly macrolide prophylaxis, because this kills microfilariae and induces embryo stasis in mature female dirofilariae.

Timing of antigen testing is critical. A pre-detection period must be considered, because these tests detect only adult, female worms. This takes into account the time from exposure to seroconversion to a positive antigen test. A reasonable interval is 7 mo after last possible exposure. There is no value in testing a dog for antigen or microfilariae before ~7 mo of age. To ensure that a previously acquired infection does not exist in these young dogs, they should be tested 6–7 mo after beginning HW prophylaxis. For dogs >7 mo old, testing should be performed when preventive therapy is started and 7–12 mo later. Subsequently, annual antigen detection tests are recommended.

The terminology for HW antigen tests has changed, with the word negative being replaced by "below detectable limits" to underscore the possibility of HW-infected pets being antigen negative and that a negative test may become positive as worms mature.

The level of antigenemia is directly related to the number of mature female worms present. Most dogs harboring more than two adult female worms will test positive with most available tests. For low-burden suspects, commercial laboratory–based microwell titer tests are the most sensitive. There is, however, no test that can determine worm burden. Testing for microfilariae may be useful as an adjunctive test in suspect cases that have negative antigen test results.

In dogs, echocardiography is relatively unimportant as a diagnostic tool. Visualization of worms in the right heart and vena cava is associated with high-burden infection with or without caval syndrome. Severe, chronic pulmonary hypertension causes right ventricular hypertrophy, septal flattening, underloading of the left heart, and high-velocity tricuspid and pulmonic regurgitation. The ECG of infected dogs is usually normal. However, right ventricular hypertrophy patterns are seen when there is severe, chronic pulmonary hypertension, often associated with overt or impending

TABLE 8 DIAGNOSTIC TESTS, CLINICAL SIGNS, AND TREATMENT FOR HEARTWORMS IN DOGS, CATS, AND FERRETS *(continued)*

		Treatment	
Clinical Signs	**Prevention**	**Adults**	**Microfilariae**
Respiratory, weight loss, exercise intolerance	Ivermectin, milbemycin, selamectin, moxidectin	Melarsomine, doxycycline, symptomatic treatment	Moxidectin[a], ivermectin + doxycycline, milbemycin
Respiratory, vomiting, sudden death	Ivermectin, milbemycin, selamectin, moxidectin	Symptomatic treatment, worm extraction	NA
Heart failure, respiratory, sudden death	Topical imidacloprid-moxidectin	Symptomatic treatment, moxidectin?	NA

right-side CHF (ascites). Cardiac rhythm disturbances are usually absent or mild, but atrial fibrillation is an occasional complication in dogs.

The diagnosis of HW disease in cats is based on historical and physical findings, index of suspicion, thoracic radiographs, echocardiography, and serologic test results. Cats may develop a positive antigen test 7–8 mo after L_3 inoculation. However, antigen tests alone are considered too unreliable (insensitive, missing 25%–50% of mature infections) as the initial screening test for cats. This occurs with unisex (all male) infections, infections with insufficient numbers of mature females to be detectable, and in cats with HARD. Cats with HARD may remain antigen negative if no adults develop, in all-male infections, or when only one adult female matures. These cats can also be only temporarily negative if tested before detectable antigenemia develops. The antigen test is strongly recommended in cats in which HW infection is suspected.

Antibodies to heartworms, produced by 90% of infected cats, often appear by 2–3 mo after L_3 infection and are generally present by 5 mo. However, antibodies can persist for several months after worm death. Also, antibodies induced by larvae can persist in aborted infections and after macrolide prophylaxis has been instituted, killing the early larval stages. Thus, a positive antibody test indicates infection by HW larval stages, and possibly HARD, but not necessarily of a mature infection. In conjunction with other provocative findings, antibody seropositivity is useful in making a clinical diagnosis of HW disease in cats, and it certainly identifies cats at risk. False-positive results from cross-reactivity with other parasites have not been seen. A negative antibody test indicates ≥90% probability of the absence of mature infection. Microfilariae are rarely detected by modified Knott's tests (<10%) in cats. Annual screening of cats is not necessary but may yield information for concerned cat owners. For this purpose, the antibody test is preferred in that it detects cats with heartworms and those at risk. The antigen test is not appropriate for screening in cats because of its low sensitivity.

In cats, worms can often be imaged using echocardiography. This is because of the relative sizes of the heartworm(s) and the right heart and pulmonary arterial system of cats. Heartworms, particularly the females, are long enough to occupy the pulmonary arteries as well as the right heart, where they can be easily imaged. Parallel hyperechoic lines, produced by the HW cuticle, may be seen in the right heart and pulmonary arteries. Echocardiography is more important in cats than in dogs because of the increased difficulty of diagnosis in cats (low antigen test sensitivity and low antibody test specificity for mature infection) and the relatively high sensitivity of the test in experienced hands.

In addition to special diagnostic tests in cats and dogs, a CBC, chemistry profile, urinalysis, and particularly thoracic radiographs are indicated. Laboratory data are often normal. Eosinophilia and basophilia alone or together may occur in dirofilariasis. Eosinophilia is most often seen at the time that stage 5 (young adult) larvae arrive in the pulmonary arteries. Subsequently, eosinophil counts vary but are usually high in dogs with immune-mediated occult infections, especially if eosinophilic pneumonitis develops (<10% of total infections).

Hyperglobulinemia due to antigenic stimulation may be present in dogs and cats. Hypoalbuminemia in dogs can be associated with proteinuria in severe immune-complex glomerulonephritis or with severe emaciation/cardiac cachexia. Serum ALT and alkaline phosphatase are occasionally increased but do not correlate well with abnormal liver function, efficacy of adulticide treatment, or risk of drug toxicity. Urinalysis may reveal proteinuria that can be quantitated by a urine protein:creatinine ratio. Occasionally, severe glomerulonephritis can lead to hypoalbuminemia and nephrotic syndrome. Dogs with hypoalbuminemia, secondary to glomerular disease, also lose antithrombin III and are at risk of thromboembolic disease. Hemoglobinuria is associated with caval syndrome and occurs when RBCs are lysed in the circulation.

In dogs, thoracic radiography provides the most information on disease severity and is a necessary screening tool to assess the clinical status of dogs with dirofilariasis, particularly when symptomatic. High-risk infections are characterized by a large main pulmonary artery segment and dilated, tortuous caudal lobar pulmonary arteries. Right ventricular enlargement may also be seen and, along with enlarged pulmonary arteries, is indicative of pulmonary hypertension. With pulmonary thromboembolism and pulmonary infiltrate with eosinophils (pneumonitis), ill-defined parenchymal infiltrates surround the caudal lobar arteries, typically most severe in the right caudal lobe.

In cats, cardiac changes and pulmonary hypertension are less common. In ~50% of infected cats, caudal lobar arteries are larger than the corresponding vein and >1.6 times the diameter of the ninth rib at the ninth intercostal space. Patchy parenchymal infiltrates may also be present in cats with respiratory signs. The main pulmonary artery segment usually is not visible because of its relatively midline location.

In ferrets, the diagnosis is less readily made with thoracic radiographs, because only the right ventricle tends to be enlarged. However, the commercial antigen tests have detected HW antigen experimentally, as early as 5 mo after infection, and have been shown to be effective in clinical situations. False-negative results may occur, especially in species that harbor lower worm burdens (cats and ferrets). Furthermore, although microfilaria testing is only rarely helpful, adult worms can often be seen with echocardiography and nonselective angiography.

Treatment in Dogs: The extent of the preadulticide evaluation varies, depending on the clinical status of the dog, the likelihood of coexisting diseases that may affect the outcome of treatment, the owner's ability to restrict the dog's exercise, and cost considerations. Clinical laboratory data should be collected selectively to complement information obtained from a thorough history, physical examination, antigen test, and thoracic radiography.

Two important variables known to directly influence the probability of thromboembolic complications after adulticide treatment and the outcome of treatment are the extent of concurrent pulmonary vascular disease and the current worm burden. Assessment of cardiopulmonary status is indispensable for evaluating a dog's prognosis. Pulmonary thromboembolic complications after adulticide treatment are most likely to occur in heavily infected dogs already exhibiting clinical and radiographic signs of severe pulmonary vascular disease, especially when severe pulmonary hypertension and CHF are present.

Before adulticide therapy, HW-infected dogs are assessed and rated for risk of postadulticide thromboembolism. Dogs can be categorized as follows: 1) low risk of thromboembolic complications, light worm burden, and no evidence of parenchymal and/or pulmonary vascular lesions; or 2) high risk of thromboembolic complications. Dogs in the low-risk category would ideally fulfill the following conditions: no clinical signs, normal thoracic radiographs, a low level of circulating antigen or a negative antigen test with circulating microfilariae, no worms visualized by echocardiography, no concurrent disease, and with owners capable of completely restricting exercise. The low-risk group would also include dogs having previously undergone adulticidal therapy but that remain antigen positive. Dogs with near-normal thoracic radiographs may develop severe thromboembolic disease, occurring most often when exercise is not restricted. Dogs at high risk of thromboembolic complications include those with signs related to HW infection (eg, coughing, dyspnea, ascites), abnormal thoracic radiographs, high level of circulating antigen, worms visualized by echocardiography, concurrent disease, and little or no possibility that the owners will restrict exercise.

The only approved heartworm adulticide is melarsomine dihydrochloride, which is variably effective against mature (adult) and immature heartworms of both sexes, with male worms being more susceptible. Melarsomine is given at 2.5 mg/kg, deep IM in the belly of the epaxial (lumbar) musculature in the area of the third to fifth lumbar vertebrae, using a 22-gauge needle (1 in. long for dogs <10 kg or 1.5 in. for dogs >10 kg). Pressure at the injection site is applied and maintained for 5 min to prevent drug migration. Approximately one-third of dogs will exhibit local pain, swelling, soreness with movement, or sterile abscessation at the injection site. Local fibrosis is not uncommon (and is the reason for targeting the belly of the epaxial musculature). In standard use, the procedure is repeated on the opposite side 24 hr later for dogs at low risk of treatment complications. However, to reduce the danger of thromboembolism, a two-phase (also termed "split-dose" or "three-dose" method) treatment is highly recommended for at-risk dogs and, indeed, for all patients, unless cost considerations prohibit this approach. Using this protocol, a single injection of melarsomine is given, followed by two injections 24 hr apart, after an interval of at least 30 days. The American Heartworm Society recommends this three-dose alternative regimen, regardless of the stage of disease or risk category. Exercise restriction is essential once treatment is started to minimize the risk of pulmonary thromboembolism due to dead and dying adult worms.

An approach to adulticidal therapy in which preventive is started at time of diagnosis is doxycycline (10 mg/kg, bid for 30 days) and monthly HW preventive, at the standard preventive dosage. After 2 mo, adulticidal injections (melarsomine at 2.5 mg/kg, IM) are initiated, as the dog's condition allows. Daily corticosteroids, using a tapering dosage, may also be administered during this period to reduce pulmonary inflammatory lesions from dying worms and from melarsomine. Although exercise is minimized from the day of diagnosis, cage rest must be enforced from the day of each initial injection for 4–6 wk. If the dog's condition allows, melarsomine injections are repeated in 1 mo (2 injections 24 hr apart), with the same regimen of prescribed exercise restriction. If, after the first injection, the dog has suffered significant pulmonary damage from the resultant worm death, the second and third injections can be withheld indefinitely.

Dogs with high worm burdens are at risk of severe respiratory complications. Because only ~50% of heartworms are destroyed after the first injection, the cumulative impact of worm emboli on severely diseased pulmonary arteries and lungs is reduced. Furthermore, if serious thromboembolism develops, the second two-dose part of the regimen can be delayed, allowing the lungs to heal from the first insult. Lastly, this approach destroys a higher percentage of adult heartworms than the standard two-dose protocol. For the utility and advisability of various therapeutic protocols, *see* TABLE 9.

Doxycycline has become an important part of treatment of HW infection in dogs. Through its negative action on *Wolbachia*, it provides benefits to the canid host and works to the detriment of *D immitis*. Doxycycline is indicated in preadulticide therapy (at 10 mg/kg, bid, for 30 days) in HW-infected dogs. It is given in conjunction with ivermectin at the preventive dosage (6–12 mcg/kg/mo). This combination reduces the severity of lung injury after adulticidal therapy, probably through reducing the amount of *Wolbachia* antigen and the proteins released from the HW uterus as the bacteria die and the uterus degenerates. Doxycycline at this dosage hastens worm death when the "slow-kill" approach is used, thereby presumably reducing the negative impact of worms on the host. Doxycycline with ivermectin also clears the host of microfilariae. Therefore, in dogs undergoing slow-kill treatment, this combination decreases risk of macrolide resistance, which is a concern in the slow-kill method using ivermectin alone. Doxycycline is advocated in treating dogs with HW infection regardless of severity classification or protocol.

The American Heartworm Society recommends administration of prophylactic doses of macrolides for 2 mo before administration of melarsomine, with the first dose given concurrently with the first dose of doxycycline (day 1) and a second dose given after the end of the doxycycline treatment (day 30). A third dose is then given concurrently with the first dose of melarsomine (day 60). Macrolide administration is continued monthly thereafter at the preventive dosage. The rationale for this approach is to eliminate susceptible migrating *D immitis* larvae and to allow nonsusceptible 2–4 mo old larvae to age to a point at which they are more susceptible to melarsomine. This approach of a 2-mo

TABLE 9 GUIDE TO CHOOSING HEARTWORM THERAPEUTIC PROTOCOL

	Protocol	Advantages	Disadvantages	Utility[a]
1	Split dose (3 injections), melarsomine and doxycycline; thoracic radiographs, CBC, UA, chemistry panel, coagulation profile	↑ efficacy, ↓ risk of PTE, safety of phased worm kill, no resistance concern	Cost $$$$; exercise restriction for 2 mo	Appropriate for all; best approach for severe HW disease
2	Standard dose (2 injections), melarsomine and doxycycline; thoracic radiographs, CBC, UA, chemistry panel, coagulation profile	↓ cost, ↓ risk of PTE (vs standard dose), exercise restriction only 1 mo, no resistance concern	Cost $$$; ↑ risk of PTE (vs split dose); ↓ kill efficacy (vs split dose)	Appropriate when financial constraints and mild to moderate HW disease
3	Standard dose (2 injections), melarsomine	↓ cost; exercise restriction only 1 mo, no resistance concern, easier for shelters	Cost $$; ↑ risk of PTE (vs standard dose); ↓ kill efficacy (vs split dose); cage rest imperative	Appropriate when financial constraints and mild HW disease
4	Slow kill with ivermectin, doxycycline	↓ cost, no injections, no hospitalization, shorter treatment duration than slow kill	Cost $; ↑ risk of resistance, not approved by AHS, ~12-mo course, lung disease progression, time of HW death unknown	Appropriate only when severe financial or other constraints
5	Slow kill with ivermectin	Inexpensive; no injections	↑ risk of resistance, 30-mo course, lung disease progression, time of HW death unknown	Should be avoided

[a]None of these is appropriate for initial management of caval syndrome but may be used to complete therapy after worm removal.

UA = urinalysis; PTE = pulmonary thromboembolism; AHS = American Heartworm Society; $ = relative cost

pretreatment with macrolides has become less compelling with the recent knowledge that doxycycline kills developing larvae (L_3>L_4>young adults) when administered at 10 mg/kg, bid, for 30 days, thereby closing the gap during which developing larvae are not susceptible to melarsomine treatment.

High-risk dogs should be stabilized before melarsomine administration. Stabilizing treatment includes cage confinement, oxygen, corticosteroids, and possibly heparin (75–100 U/kg, SC, tid) for 1 wk before the alternative (split-dosage) melarsomine treatment protocol.

Dogs with right-side CHF should be treated with furosemide (1–2 mg/kg, bid), an angiotensin-converting enzyme (ACE) inhibitor such as enalapril (0.5 mg/kg/day, increased to 0.5 mg/kg, bid, after 1 wk pending renal function test results), moderate dietary sodium restriction, and abdominal paracentesis, as needed.

The inodilator, pimobendan, is also indicated at 0.25 mg/kg, bid, to support myocardial function and reduce cardiac work. Sildenafil can be used initially at 1 mg/kg, tid, as a pulmonary vasodilator. Caution is warranted with this and other vasodilators to avoid the adverse effect of systemic hypotension.

After melarsomine injection(s), exercise must be severely restricted for 4–6 wk to minimize pulmonary thromboembolic complications. Adverse effects of melarsomine are otherwise limited to local inflammation, cough, brief low-grade fever, and salivation. Hepatic and renal toxicity are seldom, if ever, seen.

Laboratory findings associated with adulticidal therapy may include an inflammatory leukogram, thrombocytopenia, and prolonged activated clotting time or prothrombin time. A postinjection increase in serum CK may be noted. Local or disseminated intravascular coagulopathy may occur when platelet counts are <100,000/μL. Treatment for severe thromboembolism should include oxygen, cage confinement, a corticosteroid at an anti-inflammatory dosage (eg, prednisone at 1 mg/kg/day, PO), and low-dose heparin (75–100 U/kg, SC, tid) for several days to 1 wk. Severe lung injury is likely present if, after 24 hr of oxygen therapy, no improvement is noted and partial pressures of oxygen remain <70 mmHg.

The standard melarsomine protocol (two-dose, 24-hr treatment regimen) kills most adult worms, clearing 50%–85% of dogs. Antigen testing should be performed 8–12 mo after the third dose of the split-dose (alternative) protocol. If a positive test result is obtained at this time, consideration can be given to abbreviated retreatment (two injections, 24 hr apart). A "slow-kill" approach with ivermectin (0.6 mcg/kg, every 2 wk for 6 mo) can be substituted for repeated melarsomine injection but should definitely be preceded by 30 days of doxycycline therapy (10 mg/kg, bid) because this minimizes the reaction to dead and dying worms, enhances the kill rate to ~1 yr (vs 2.5 yr with ivermectin alone) versus the standard slow-kill approach, and is thought to decrease the risk of resistance (*see* above). The standard "slow-kill" approach with ivermectin alone is against the current recommendations of the American Heartworm Society. Longterm use of macrolides, rather than melarsomine, to kill adult worms allows pulmonary pathology to progress during the lengthy period in which worms are dying and being processed.

Caval syndrome results from worms migrating retrograde to the right atrium and great veins and is usually the result of a precipitous fall in cardiac output, as might occur with pulmonary thrombosis. Severe pulmonary hypertension is then complicated by worm-induced tricuspid valve leakage, hemolysis, and damage to liver and kidneys. In caval syndrome, removal of worms from the right atrium and orifice of the tricuspid valve is typically necessary to save the life of the dog. This may be accomplished by using light sedation, local anesthesia, and either a rigid or flexible alligator forceps, or an intravascular retrieval snare, introduced preferentially via the right external jugular vein. With fluoroscopic guidance, if available, the instrument should continue to be passed until worms can no longer be retrieved. Immediately after a successful operation, the clinical signs should lessen or disappear. Fluid therapy may be necessary in critically ill, hypovolemic dogs to restore hemodynamic and renal function. After full recovery from surgery, adulticidal therapy is undertaken to eliminate remaining worms. Particular care should be taken if many worms are still visible echocardiographically.

Microfilaricide Treatment: At specific preventive dosages, the macrolide preventive drugs are effective microfilaricides, although not approved by the FDA for this purpose. Adverse reactions may occur in dogs with high microfilarial counts (>40,000/μL), depending on the type of macrolide given. However, the microfilarial count is usually lower, and mild adverse reactions occur in ~10% of dogs. Most adverse reactions are limited to brief salivation and defecation, occurring within hours and lasting up to several hours. Dogs, especially small dogs (<10 kg), with high microfilariae counts (>40,000/μL) may develop tachycardia, tachypnea, pale mucous membranes, lethargy, retching, diarrhea, and even shock. Treatment includes an IV balanced electrolyte solution and a soluble corticosteroid. Recovery is usually rapid when treatment is administered quickly. Microfilarial counts are not routinely performed, and thus severe reactions are seldom expected. Treatment specifically targeting circulating microfilariae has historically been undertaken 3–4 wk after adulticide administration. More commonly, microfilariae are eventually eliminated, even from dogs not treated with adulticide, after several months of treatment with prophylactic doses of the macrocyclic lactones. The current practice is to start a macrocyclic lactone for prevention and microfilarial eradication at the time of diagnosis. Although all macrocyclic lactones have microfilaricidal activity and are the safest and most effective drugs available, this characteristic varies within this drug group. Only the combination topical product containing imidacloprid and moxidectin is FDA approved as a microfilaricide. Livestock preparations of these drugs should not be used to achieve higher doses for the purpose of obtaining more rapid results. Performance of a microfilaria test is recommended at the time of diagnosis and 1–3 mo after microfilaricidal therapy has begun.

Treatment in Cats: There is currently no satisfactory treatment approach for heartworm infection in cats. Infection often is lethal. Thus, all cats in regions endemic for canine HW disease should receive drug prophylaxis. The lifespan of adult heartworms in cats has traditionally been thought to be 2 yr, so spontaneous recovery is possible. Cats may remain asymptomatic, experience episodic vomiting and/or episodic dyspnea (resembling asthma), may die suddenly from pulmonary thromboembolism or an anaphylactoid reaction, or rarely, develop CHF.

Because there is no safe or approved adulticide for cats, many are managed conservatively with restricted activity and corticosteroid therapy, such as prednisolone (1–2 mg/kg, PO, every 24–48 hr). Steroids reduce the severity of vomiting and respiratory signs. The hope is that episodes of pulmonary complications will not prove fatal as the worms die. Barring consecutive, additional infection, 25%–50% of cats may survive with this approach. Serial antigen and antibody testing (at intervals of 6–12 mo) can be used to monitor status. Although there are no supportive data, administration of doxycycline (10 mg/kg, bid for 30 days) and ivermectin (24 mcg/kg/mo) to an infected cat could be theorized to cause worm degradation and contracture, thereby lessening the potential for catastrophic consequences when the worms die. Of course, the macrocyclic lactone would also protect the cat from a new infection, if more exposure is encountered.

Surgical retrieval of worms from the right atrium, right ventricle, and vena cavae via jugular venotomy can be attempted in cats with high worm burdens detected by echocardiography. An endoscopic basket, snare, or horsehair brush can also be advanced via the right jugular vein under fluoroscopy. Cats in CHF have been cured by worm removal.

Treatment in Ferrets: Treatment in ferrets is, likewise, difficult, because there is no approved agent for this purpose. Adulticidal therapies (thiacetarsemide and melarsomine) have resulted in ~50% mortality in ferrets. Moxidectin (injectable and topical formulations) has been widely thought to be adulticidal for heartworms in ferrets and is given at the same dosage and frequency as in dogs. Moxidectin and imidacloprid (combination) is approved by the FDA for use in ferrets to prevent HW infection and to prevent and treat flea infestations.

Prevention: Heartworm infection is generally completely preventable with macrolide prophylaxis. Year-round prevention is advised. Preventive therapy in dogs is recommended beginning at 6–8 wk of age. No testing is necessary at this age, because the presence of mature female heartworms is required to produce a positive heartworm test (antigen or microfilaria). When prophylaxis is started after 7 mo of age, an antigen test and a test for presence of microfilariae is recommended, followed by another antigen test 6–7 mo later. This series of tests will help to avoid unnecessary delay in detecting subclinical infections, as well as potential confusion concerning effectiveness of the preventive program, because it cannot be determined until the second test whether infection existed before beginning chemoprophylaxis.

Formulations of the macrolide preventives ivermectin, milbemycin oxime, moxidectin, and selamectin are safe and effective, as prescribed, for all breeds of dogs. Currently marketed products have additional chemicals and parasite spectra, including GI and ectoparasites: ivermectin (hookworms), ivermectin/pyrantel pamoate (hookworms and roundworms), ivermectin/pyrantel pamoate/praziquantel (hookworms, roundworms, and tapeworms), milbemycin/lufenuron (hookworms, roundworms, whipworms, and sterilizes fleas), milbemycin/lufenuron/praziquantel (hookworms, roundworms, whipworms, tapeworms, and sterilizes fleas), selamectin (fleas, ticks, ear mites, sarcoptic mites), moxidectin injectable (hookworms), moxidectin/imidacloprid (roundworms, hookworms, whipworms, adult fleas, microfilariae), milbemycin/spinosad (hookworms, roundworms, whipworms, fleas).

At the approved dosage, milbemycin kills microfilariae quickly, and in the face of high microfilarial concentrations a shock reaction may occur. Thus, milbemycin should not be administered without close monitoring and/or prophylactic pretreatment (steroids and/or antihistamine) as a preventive in dogs with high numbers of microfilariae.

HW prevention is also recommended for all cats in endemic regions, regardless of housing status, because of the potential for severe consequences with infection. Performing microfilaria testing in cats before starting preventive therapy is not required, because cats have small microfilarial numbers and the presence of microfilaria is typically transient. Ivermectin for cats is safe and effective at 24 mcg/kg, PO, once monthly. At this dosage, the formulation is also effective against *Ancylostoma tubaeforme* and *A braziliense*. Preventive treatment should be started in kittens at 6 wk of age and continued lifelong. There is currently no milbemycin product marketed for use in cats in the USA.

Formulations of selamectin and a combination of imidacloprid/moxidectin are labeled for both dogs and cats. Selamectin is administered topically at a monthly dosage of ~6 mg/kg and also kills adult fleas and prevents flea eggs from hatching for 1 mo. It also is indicated for treatment and control of *Otodectes cynotis* in dogs and cats, sarcoptic mange, *Dermacentor variabilis* infestations in dogs, *Ancylostoma tubaeforme*, and *Toxocara cati* in cats. A topical combined formulation of imidacloprid and moxidectin administered at dosages of 10 mg/kg for imidacloprid and 1 mg/kg for moxidectin is also effective against HW infection and flea infestations. Although all currently marketed preventives are likely effective in ferrets, only imidacloprid with moxidectin is approved by the FDA. Importantly, the preventive dosage for ferrets is the same as that for dogs (not cats).

Sporadic resistance of heartworms to the macrocyclic preventive class has been recognized since 2013. All the current molecules used to prevent heartworm disease have been implicated. However, some formulations appear to be more effective against resistant isolates than others. There have been isolates from six dogs with varying degrees of resistance. There is little evidence of spread out of the Mississippi Delta region, where resistance was first recognized. It is important to realize that the current preventives are effective in the vast majority of cases and should not be abandoned. Emphasis should be placed on owner compliance and year-round preventive therapy, as well as on alternative methods of HW prevention, including topical and oral mosquito repellants, indoor/screened housing, especially at night, and mosquito abatement programs. The role of slow-kill macrolide adulticidal therapy has been questioned in the development of resistance and should be avoided. If such therapy is unavoidable, it should absolutely be accompanied by 30 days of doxycycline treatment at the outset, with assurance that microfilariae are eradicated.

BOVINE HIGH-MOUNTAIN DISEASE

("Brisket" disease, Big brisket, Dropsy, High-altitude disease, Pulmonary hypertension, Congestive right heart failure)

Bovine high-mountain disease (BHMD) is characterized by a noncontagious swelling of edematous fluid in the ventral parasternal muscles (brisket region), the ventral aspect of the body including the abdomen, and the submandibular region in cattle raised in high-altitude regions (>5,000 ft [1,524 m]) in the western USA most commonly and substantially affecting Colorado, Wyoming, New Mexico, and Utah. It also affects cattle in mountainous ranges of the world, most commonly at elevations >6,500 ft (1,981 m) in western Canada and South America. BHMD affects cattle of all ages and breeds, but not necessarily equally.

BHMD is a result of pulmonary arterial hypertension induced by pulmonary hypoxia occurring at high altitude. Hypoxia-induced pulmonary arterial vasoconstriction and arterial hyperplasia reduce the diameter of the pulmonary arterioles, resulting in pulmonary hypertension and subsequent right ventricular (RV) hypertrophy. Without intervention to reduce the hypoxia-induced pulmonary hypertension, the disease will eventually progress to RV congestive/dilatory cardiac failure. Rarely, similar lesions have been described in severely stressed and parasitized sheep and deer. Etiologically similar hypoxia-related heart failure has also been described in chickens in the Andes Mountains and in people living at extreme elevations. The incidence in cattle on high mountain pastures averages 3%–5% with variations from 0.5%–10% but has been as much as 65% in a genetically susceptible calf crop. A 25% calf loss is not uncommon in the high elevations of Colorado and Wyoming.

Although most commonly associated with altitude, other genetic, physiologic, environmental, and toxic factors play important roles in disease development and progression. Any pulmonary disease, acute or chronic, that hinders pulmonary function can result in a hypoxic condition similar to altitude-induced BHMD.

Etiology: Although many factors may contribute to the incidence of BMHD, the pathogenesis is directly related to the hypoxic condition that results from high altitude. Pulmonary vascular shunting is a normal physiologic response to hypoxic conditions and is seen in all animals. Strong responses are seen in cattle, horses, and pigs, whereas people, dogs, guinea pigs, and llamas are less responsive. These findings and the high incidence of disease in cattle indicate they are uniquely susceptible. The vasoconstriction mechanism of shunting is a way to divert unoxygenated blood to oxygen-rich regions of the lungs (dorsal aspect) and away from poorly oxygenated regions (ventral aspect). Exaggerated shunting in response to hypoxia, the anatomic pattern of the bovine lobulated lung, and the small lung-size/body-weight ratio all contribute to a severe loss of functional pulmonary capacity.

Pulmonary vascular shunting is initially mediated through pulmonary arteriole constriction in the acute stages of hypoxia. Vascular hypertrophy and thickening of the medial layers of the pulmonary arterioles (medial hypertrophy) and adventitial tissues occurs with chronic hypoxic exposure (>3 wk). Vascular remodeling leading to loss of peripheral pulmonary arteries also contributes to increased pulmonary resistance. This combination of events causes significant pulmonary hypertension, which leads to a progression of cardiac pathology: RV hypertrophy, followed by RV dilation, and finally right congestive heart failure (CHF).

This pathogenesis of exaggerated vasoconstrictive shunting, arterial medial and adventitial hypertrophy, and vascular obliteration resulting in pulmonary hypertension appears to be characteristic of some cattle and is highly heritable. Some cattle appear to be more naturally resistant to this process, both on an individual and breed basis. There is marked individual and interspecies variability in hypoxia-induced increases in pulmonary vascular resistance. The role of genetics in BHMD is supported by high familial incidence with marked variation in susceptibility between individual animals, breeds, and other species of animals. There is strong evidence that the susceptibility of cattle to hypoxia-induced pulmonary hypertension is inherited. In addition to underlying genetic predisposition, altered chemoreceptor activity or myocardial metabolism may also play a role. Acute viral or bacterial respiratory disease can exacerbate pulmonary hypoxia of high altitude, resulting in a rapid onset of RV failure.

Various range plants, both browse and non-browse types, have been associated with increased incidence of BHMD, but only locoweed has been experimentally shown to induce the disease. When consumed by cattle at high elevation, locoweed (certain *Oxytropis* and *Astragalus* spp that contain the alkaloid swainsonine) markedly increase the prevalence and severity of CHF, which develops relatively quickly (within 1–2 wk) with an incidence as high as 100%. Swainsonine, the toxin in locoweed, is excreted in milk, thereby predisposing nursing calves to developing CHF. Locoweed-poisoned cows often abort, and many develop severe hydrops amnii in addition to showing signs of BHMD. Locoweed poisoning directly contributes to increased pulmonary vascular resistance and hypertension; immunohistochemistry and electron microscopy studies have shown that poisoning causes severe swelling and cytoplasmic vacuolation of pulmonary intravascular macrophages and endothelial cells. The myocardium also is compromised by locoweed, seen as extensive vacuolation of the myocardial interstitial cells. Finally, swainsonine has systemic endocrine and paracrine effects due to altered glycoprotein metabolism, which may also contribute to the pathogenesis of BHMD.

Clinical Findings: The clinical changes of RV CHF of high-mountain disease usually develop slowly over several weeks, commonly within the first 3–4 wk after cattle are moved from lower to higher elevations. This 3–4 wk period may be an average time, but clinical signs and death from pulmonary hypertension and right CHF have been seen within 24 hr after altitude exposure and have also been seen in animals that have lived in higher elevations for years. In those areas in North America where cattle spend summer and fall grazing at high altitudes and return to lower elevations later in the fall, the disease is usually manifest in late summer and early fall and seems to be associated with weather and environmental conditions as seen in high elevations with cold nights and hot days. Pulmonary hypertension and right CHF seem to follow respiratory disease seen with these same climatic influences. In areas where cattle live year round at high altitudes, the disease incidence is greatest in late fall, winter, or early spring. Periods of severe cold or other environmental stress (eg, pregnancy, change in nutrition) appear to precipitate the onset of signs. Affected animals initially appear depressed and reluctant to move. As the syndrome progresses, subacute edema develops in the brisket region and extends cranially to the intermandibular space and caudally to the ventral abdominal wall. Pleural effusion and ascites are usually abundant. Marked distention and pulsation of the jugular veins are usually prominent. Appetite may be decreased. Profuse diarrhea may develop as a result of intestinal venous hypertension. Respiration is labored, and animals may appear cyanotic. As the disease progresses, affected cattle become more reluctant to move and may become recumbent. With forced exertion, severely affected animals may collapse and die. In the terminal stages, the animal is often anorexic, recumbent, and unable to rise. To the rancher and cattlemen, an animal experiencing "brisket disease" is most often characterized by severe brisket and abdominal edema and swelling, jugular enlargement and pulsation, bulging eyes, exophthalmos (secondary to venous congestion), ventral abdominal distention (ascites), bloating, recumbency or inability to travel with the herd, and profuse diarrhea.

Lesions: Generalized edema is especially severe in the ventral subcutaneous tissues, skeletal musculature, perirenal tissues, mesentery, and wall of the GI tract. Ascites, hydrothorax, and hydropericardium are consistent findings. Fluid characteristics include low cellularity and low to normal protein, consistent with a transudate secondary to cardiac failure. The liver lesions, due to chronic passive congestion, vary from an early "nutmeg" appearance to severe lobular and vascular fibrosis. The lungs may have varying degrees of atelectasis, interstitial emphysema, edema, and pneumonia. The heart has marked RV hypertrophy and dilatation; the cardiac apex is displaced to the left, making the enlarged heart appear round. The right atrium is often 2–3 times larger than the left and is flaccid. Pulmonary arterial thrombosis is a frequent finding. Microscopically, there is hypertrophy of the media of small arteries and arterioles in the lungs. Acute rupture of the pulmonary artery (aneurysm) secondary to the severe pulmonary hypertension is often seen as a reason for acute death without clinical signs of RV CHF.

Diagnosis: There is no definitive diagnostic test for BHMD. A diagnosis may be based on clinical findings related to CHF in cattle kept at high altitudes. Body temperature and CBC are generally normal unless there is other underlying inflammatory pathology. Recent studies in elevations ≥9,000 ft (2,743 m) found body temperatures in calves experiencing pulmonary hypertension to be increased (>104°F [40°C]). This is hypothesized to be secondary to an increased metabolic demand and tachypneic response to the hypoxic condition. Thoracic auscultation may reveal a decreased intensity of breath sounds in the ventral thorax and muffled heart sounds if pleural effusion is present. The heart and respiratory rates are generally increased, and a systolic cardiac murmur may be auscultated if RV enlargement has resulted in right atrioventricular or pulmonic valve insufficiency. In end-stage CHF, a gallop rhythm is often detected. Although jugular distention is a characteristic clinical sign, an abnormal jugular pulse may or may not be seen. The common clinical pathologic changes are increases in hepatic enzymes, particularly AST and L-iditol dehydrogenase. Clinically affected animals may be azotemic because of decreased renal perfusion secondary to heart failure and dehydration/hypovolemia.

BHMD should be differentiated from other causes of CHF, including pericarditis, traumatic reticulopericarditis, cardiac lymphosarcoma, valvular endocarditis, viral or bacterial myocarditis, cardiomyopathy (nutritional, hereditary, or idiopathic), pulmonary arterial obstruction from embolic pneumonia, or chronic hypoxia and cor pulmonale due to other primary pulmonary disease. Brisket edema may not always be present in animals with peracute RV CHF; this can result in BHMD in calves being mistaken for acute viral or bacterial pneumonia.

Treatment and Control: Affected animals should be moved to a lower altitude with minimal restraint, stress, and excitement. General supportive therapy, including diuretics, thoracocentesis, antibiotics, and appetite stimulators such as vitamin B complex, may be beneficial. Thoracocentesis is the single treatment that most dramatically improves an affected animal's chance of survival. At high elevations, use of oxygen or a hyperbaric chamber may be considered for valuable animals. Because the disease may recur, affected animals should not be returned to high altitudes.

Affected cattle should not be retained for breeding because of heritability. Treatment of concurrent diseases, including respiratory/cardiac disease, GI disease, parasitism, and plant toxicosis, should be addressed. Because locoweed poisoning has been directly linked to the development of CHF in cattle, the exposure of susceptible animals to locoweed should be minimized by ensuring that animals have a good selection of forages. Animals should be moved to pastures free of locoweed as soon as poisoning is recognized to prevent severe and irreversible damage.

Treatment of BHMD can be expensive and unrewarding, so prevention is preferred. Genetic selection through the use of pulmonary arterial pressure (PAP) measurements to select cattle resistant to the effects of hypoxia is a more effective way to control BHMD. Identifying animals highly susceptible to the effects of altitude hypoxia (those with high PAP measurements) and eliminating them from the breeding pool are practical methods to reduce the prevalence of BHMD in a herd. The PAP measurement procedure involves passing flexible polyethylene catheter tubing (1.19 mm internal diameter × 1.7 mm external diameter) through a large-bore needle (12 or 13 gauge, 3.5 in.) inserted into the jugular vein. The catheter is advanced through the jugular vein to the right atrium, into the right ventricle, and then into the pulmonary artery.

At altitudes of 5,000–7,000 ft (1,524–2,133 m), a normal mean PAP measurement should be 34–41 mmHg. In cattle displaying signs of pulmonary artery hypertension, the PAP can range from 48–213 mmHg. The PAP and the RV pressure may be normal to subnormal in cattle with end-stage right CHF because of the failing myocardium. Cattle with ventricular septal or atrial septal defects often have mean systolic and diastolic measurements in the hundreds. Any animal with a PAP measurement >48 mmHg is considered at risk of developing BHMD and may be a potential genetic carrier and should not be maintained or used in breeding programs at high altitude. These animals should also be auscultated for cardiac murmurs and evaluated for possible congenital cardiac defects. In general, cattle >1 yr old that have a PAP <41 mmHg at an elevation >5,000 feet (1,524 m) are likely to maintain an acceptable PAP at high altitude and serve as good breeding stock for herds at high elevation. PAP measurements between 41 and 49 mmHg are difficult to interpret consistently; these animals should be used with caution at high elevation.

Multiple factors contribute to the variation of PAP in cattle, including breed, gender, age, body condition, concurrent illness, environmental conditions, elevation, and genetics. Based on tests of >300,000 head of cattle, it appears that no one breed is resistant to the effects of high-altitude hypoxia, although some breeds, and pedigrees within breeds, appear to be more naturally resistant. It is not unusual to see a difference in PAP measurements between heifers and bulls because of husbandry practices. Bulls are often pushed nutritionally for faster growth and muscling, which may affect pulmonary function and give rise to pulmonary hypertension. Pregnant cattle have been noted to have a higher PAP measurement than nonpregnant cattle. The age of the animal at the time of PAP testing should always be considered, because there is greater variation and less predictability in cattle ≤1 yr old. Testing animals at ≥16 mo of age appears to be the most consistent and accurate at predicting susceptibility to pulmonary hypertension induced by high altitude. Any concurrent illness, especially respiratory disease, or any cause of temporary or permanent pulmonary hypoxia can influence the PAP measurement.

Some cattle appear to be prone to developing right CHF, whereas others live at high altitude with a documented increased PAP and never have a clinical problem. Even though these animals may not develop clinical BHMD, they can pass the genetic predisposition to their offspring. This variable expression of clinical disease and the variable penetrance of the gene makes PAP testing challenging at all elevations and becomes an even greater concern at elevations <5,000 ft (1,524 m) where the hypoxic conditions needed to stimulate a pulmonary response are not sufficient. PAP measurements taken at low elevations (<5,000 ft [1,524 m]) should not be used as a positive selection tool but only to identify animals highly susceptible to hypoxic conditions and hypertensive even at elevations <5,000 ft (1,524 m). Cattle moved from low elevations to high elevations should remain at the altitude for ≥3 wk before PAP testing.

Future advancements in the research of pulmonary hypertension in cattle are concentrating on identifying DNA markers for recognition of genetic carriers of pulmonary hyperresponders to hypoxic conditions. Other areas of interest and research are being directed at and addressing the alarming increase in incidence of RV CHF at lower elevations as seen in heavy feedlot cattle at elevations ≤4,000 ft (1,219 m). These fat cattle at this elevation seem to have the same postmortem lesions as those seen at higher elevations.

THROMBOSIS, EMBOLISM, AND ANEURYSM

A **thrombus** is an aggregation of platelets and fibrin that may form when certain conditions exist. Historically, these have included some combination of Virchow's triad such as blood stasis (reduced flow), endothelial injury, and/or an existing hypercoagulable state. A thrombus can develop in a cardiac chamber and be attached (mural) or less likely free floating (ball), or can originate *in situ* within a blood vessel where it can cause a partial or complete obstruction. The thrombus can be classified based on its location and the clinical signs it produces (eg, jugular venous thrombosis in large animals associated with prolonged venous catheterization, pulmonary arterial thromboembolism associated with heartworm disease in dogs).

All or part of a thrombus may break off and be carried through the bloodstream as an **embolus** that lodges distally at a point where the size of the embolus exceeds the vascular diameter. Poor injection or catheterization techniques along with inferior catheter material can result in vascular thrombosis. However, clinically significant vascular thrombosis is more commonly seen in animals with underlying diseases that result in a hypercoagulable state, such as systemic inflammation, endotoxemia, neoplasia, or antithrombin deficiency. If left untreated or uncontrolled, systemic thrombosis can result in hemorrhagic diathesis or disseminated intravascular coagulation (DIC), a life-threatening disorder of hemostasis with deposition of microthrombi and consumption of coagulation factors that results in concurrent hemorrhage.

Thrombus formation can occur in both large and small arteries and veins. Horses and cattle are more likely to develop venous thrombi, whereas in dogs and cats, arterial thrombi appear to be more clinically important. Arterial thrombosis or embolization results in ischemia of the tissues supplied by the infarcted vessel (eg, cats with cardiac disease and subsequent arterial thromboembolism). Emboli from infective conditions such as endocarditis are classified as septic (bacteria contained in the embolus). Septic emboli can result in bacterial dissemination and infection of distal capillary beds. Neoplastic emboli can also occur and may contribute to metastasis. Systemic arterial thromboembolism is more important in cats, whereas dogs and large animals appear to develop *in situ* arterial thrombosis more commonly. Thrombosis of limb arteries causing lameness and gangrene has been reported in adult horses and foals. This occurs secondary to hypercoagulation and systemic inflammation (eg, septicemia in foals).

An **aneurysm** is a vascular dilation caused by weakening of the tunica media of blood vessels. The weakness might be primary or caused by degenerative or inflammatory changes progressing from an intimal lesion. False aneurysms (pseudoaneurysms) are caused by damage to all three layers of the arterial wall and result in extravascular accumulation of blood. Disruption of the endothelium associated with a true aneurysm can cause formation of a thrombus with subsequent embolization; thus, aneurysms, thrombi, and emboli may be recognized simultaneously. Aneurysms are rare in domestic animal species, although they have been reported in dogs, cats, horses, primates, and turkeys.

Clinical Findings and Diagnosis: Acute onset of dyspnea is often associated with pulmonary thromboembolism, although some animals may develop hemoptysis; the latter is most associated with pulmonary arterial disease such as that resulting from heartworm infection (*see* p 127). Septic cardiac thrombi are associated with endocarditis; nonseptic cardiac thrombi are associated with myocardial disease (most commonly in cats), or rarely with cardiac or pulmonary neoplasia. Infarction within the genitourinary system can present with hematuria, abdominal pain, and splinting. Splanchnic infarction usually results in abdominal pain, with vomiting seen in small animals.

Aneurysms cause no clinical signs unless hemorrhage occurs or an associated thrombus develops. Except for dissecting aneurysm in turkeys (*see* p 2787), aortic or sinus of Valsalva rupture in horses with sudden death, hemorrhage associated with guttural pouch mycosis in horses (*see* p 1463), or pulmonary arterial aneurysm in cattle, spontaneous aneurysmal hemorrhage is rare, and clinical signs usually relate to thrombosis. An aneurysm of the abdominal aorta and its branches in large animals may be palpated rectally as a fixed firm swelling with a rough, irregular surface that pulsates with the heart beat. Fremitus may be present. In excess thrombus formation, the pulse may be delayed distally and have a slow rate of rise in pressure, or it may be absent. Other helpful diagnostic modalities include ultrasonography and angiography.

Cattle: Thrombosis of the caudal vena cava occurs in association with hepatic abscessation and vascular erosion of the abscess. Embolic pneumonia with secondary pulmonary abscessation, thromboembolism, and pulmonary arterial aneurysms are common sequelae. Affected animals may present with coughing, tachypnea, dyspnea, and abnormal lung sounds. Aneurysms in pulmonary arteries that contain septic emboli may rupture and cause intrapulmonary hemorrhage, or pulmonary abscesses may erode into bronchi and result in hemorrhage into the airways. The sequelae to these disorders may include epistaxis, hemoptysis, and death. Clinical pathologic data usually support a diagnosis of vena caval syndrome but are not specific. Increased fibrinogen, anemia, and in cases with an active abscess process, increased liver enzymes may be seen. Pulmonary arterial embolism and embolic pneumonia are also frequent complications of tricuspid or pulmonic valvular endocarditis in cattle, but aneurysms rarely develop. Intermittent fever and anorexia due to bacteremia at times of embolic showering are often present, and the animal typically has a history of a chronic active infection (eg, foot abscess, reticular abscess) as well as chronic weight loss with poor body condition score. Most cases of right heart endocarditis in cattle are bacterial and are commonly associated with a cardiac murmur, with a point of maximal intensity over the tricuspid valve. Echocardiography and blood cultures help identify right heart vegetative lesions and the causative bacterial agent, respectively. Thrombosis of the cranial vena cava in cattle produces bilateral jugular engorgement; edema of the head, submandibular area, and brisket; and pronounced oral mucosal hyperemia. However, similar clinical signs are seen with right-side congestive heart failure, which could be a sequela of tricuspid valve endocarditis. Significant lingual, pharyngeal, or laryngeal edema may develop and result in dysphagia and dyspnea.

Horses: Cranial vena cava thrombosis may result from extension of a jugular thrombus. Jugular vein thrombosis in horses is often associated with phlebitis following catheterization or extravasation of injected material and will cause swelling, heat, and pain of the affected area. Bilateral jugular vein thrombosis can cause edema and swelling of the head and neck, mimicking cranial caval thrombosis. Ultrasonographic examination of the affected vein can determine the extent of the thrombus and degree of occlusion. Doppler ultrasound is a more sophisticated method to determine blood flow and vessel patency. If a catheter-associated thrombophlebitis is suspected, blood culture and catheter-tip culture can be performed. Horses with colitis and other GI disorders are at increased risk of developing jugular thrombosis; ruminants are much less prone to jugular thrombosis than horses. Caudal vena cava–like syndrome has been described in a Quarter horse with respiratory signs. Hepatic abscesses, caudal vena cava thrombosis, pulmonary thromboembolism, and embolic pneumonia were identified at necropsy.

Migrating *Strongylus vulgaris* larvae (*see* p 316) can cause arteritis with development of thrombi and verminous aneurysms in the aorta, cranial mesenteric, or iliac artery. In some horses, emboli develop and partially or completely occlude terminal branches of the mesenteric arteries. Affected intestinal segments show changes ranging from ischemia to hemorrhagic infarction. Clinical signs are those of colic, constipation, or diarrhea. The colic usually is recurrent, and attacks may be severe and prolonged. Newer anthelmintics and improved therapeutic regimens have resulted in verminous arteritis becoming an uncommon disorder.

Thrombosis with or without aneurysm of the terminal aorta and proximal iliac arteries produces a characteristic syndrome in horses. Although associated with parasitism, other causes are possible. Affected horses appear normal at rest; however, graded exercise results in an increasing severity of weakness of the hindlimbs with unilateral or bilateral lameness, muscle tremor, and sweating. Severely affected animals may show signs of exercise intolerance, weakness, and atypical lameness that resolves after a short rest. Subnormal temperature of the affected limbs may be detectable, along with decreased or absent arterial pulsations and delayed and diminished capillary filling. Rectal palpation may show variation in pulse amplitude of the internal or external iliac arteries (or both) and asymmetric vasculature. In severe cases, the hindquarter muscles atrophy, and lameness may become evident with only mild exercise. Complete embolic or thrombotic occlusion of the distal aorta may produce acute bilateral hindlimb paralysis and recumbency in horses. Affected animals are anxious, appear painful, and rapidly go into shock. The hindlimbs are cold, and rectal palpation reveals an absence of pulsation in either iliac artery. Transrectal ultrasound can help determine bloodflow in the aorta and iliac arteries.

Aneurysm of the aortic root has been reported in horses, commonly noted at the right aortic sinus with or without concurrent endocarditis. Similar to those in people, aneurysms of the sinuses of Valsalva in horses can be congenital or acquired. Rupture of an aortic aneurysm typically leads to sudden death, a scenario most commonly seen in breeding stallions during live cover.

Dogs and Cats: In dogs, and less commonly in cats, heartworm disease may lead to pulmonary arterial thromboembolism that commonly results in dyspnea and tachypnea. Affected animals are often reportedly healthy until sudden onset of coughing, hemoptysis, respiratory distress, or sudden death. Clinical signs most commonly develop in the weeks after treatment with adulticide; however, pulmonary thromboembolism may also develop from spontaneous worm death, or pulmonary thrombosis can form *in situ* secondary to pulmonary endothelial damage. Chest radiographs in affected animals may be normal or show underperfusion of the affected lung lobe, interstitial to alveolar infiltrates, or pleural effusion. Arterial blood-gas analysis typically demonstrates hypoxemia with a normal or low level of CO_2 in the blood. Ventilation/perfusion scanning with radionuclide-labeled macroaggregated albumin and gases or pulmonary CT angiography can confirm the diagnosis. Other diseases associated with pulmonary thromboembolism in dogs and cats include protein-losing nephropathy or enteropathy, hyperadrenocorticism, immune-mediated hemolytic anemia, and neoplasia.

In cats, cardiogenic embolism (arterial thromboembolism) is a devastating complication of cardiac disease. Although hypertrophic cardiomyopathy is the most common type of cardiac disease in cats (*see* p 117), any condition that results in left atrial enlargement, including other cardiomyopathies, hyperthyroidism, or congenital heart disease, can predispose to arterial thromboembolism. Intracavitary thrombi typically form in the dilated left atrium where stagnant flow exists or, less commonly, within abnormal areas in the left ventricle. Although the condition is poorly understood, these cats most likely possess some degree of concurrent hypercoagulability, because all cats with cardiomyopathy do not develop cardiogenic embolism. Portions of these intracavitary thrombi can break off and form emboli that infarct arterial branches, most commonly the aortic trifurcation (saddle emboli). Clinical signs include pain and paresis or lower motor neuron paralysis of the hindlimbs. The arterial pulse (either femoral or pedal) is reduced to absent in the affected limbs, which are cooler than normal and have firm, swollen gastrocnemius muscle bellies. These clinical signs can be unilateral, bilateral, or bilateral but asymmetric. Emboli may also infarct other arterial beds, including the right forelimb, renal, splanchnic, cerebral, or myocardial circulation. Decompensation of the underlying myocardial disease is not uncommon and may result in congestive heart failure (pulmonary edema or pleural effusion). Ischemia and necrosis of infarcted pelvic limb musculature results in increases in serum CK and AST, and subsequent reperfusion of affected muscles can result in life-threatening hyperkalemia and acidosis. Echocardiography is the imaging modality of choice to assess cardiac structure, function, and presence of an intracardiac thrombus, whereas chest radiographs are used to diagnose left-side congestive heart failure. Nuclear perfusion studies, using the unbound radioisotope ^{99m}Tc can give sensitive information regarding the degree of perfusion of the hindlimbs and areas that may require amputation in select cases, although this is rarely done.

Systemic hypertension in cats and patent ductus arteriosis, aortic coarctation, degenerative processes, and infections in dogs have been associated with aortic aneurysms.

Cranial vena caval thrombosis and subsequent chylothorax and acute respiratory distress has been reported in dogs and cats with transvenous pacemakers and other indwelling jugular devices/catheters. Successful treatment of caval thrombosis in affected animals has been described using a combination of anticoagulants, thrombolytics, and balloon venoplasty.

Treatment: Treatment of endocarditis includes longterm antibiotics (several weeks to months) and in some cases intermittent administration of antipyretic, anti-inflammatory, or antithrombotic drugs. Antibiotic choice should be based on culture and sensitivity results obtained from blood cultures. The prognosis for recovery is poor to guarded at best, and persistent debilitating cardiac disease is common even if the active infection can be controlled.

Treatment of venous thrombosis in horses and cattle is usually limited to supportive care, including hydrotherapy of accessible veins, anti-inflammatory agents, and systemic antimicrobials to control secondary sepsis. Surgical removal of thrombosed jugular veins has been performed successfully in horses, but unless both veins are severely affected, inflammation will resolve with medical treatment, and formation of collaterals will usually result in sufficient venous circulation. Thrombosis of the cranial or caudal vena cava results in more severe clinical signs and requires more aggressive therapy, which could include thrombolytic drugs and/or intravascular/surgical removal followed by aggressive anticoagulation. Response to anticoagulation therapy alone is generally inadequate.

Measures to minimize trauma to, and bacterial contamination of, veins remain the best means to prevent venous thrombosis. Extreme care should be taken when placing catheters or giving IV injections. The effectiveness of antiplatelet therapy (aspirin 0.5–5 mg/kg/day or clopidogrel 1–3 mg/kg/day), anticoagulant therapy (unfractionated heparin, 40–80 IU/kg, SC, bid-tid, or low-molecular-weight heparin [enoxaparin at 1 mg/kg, SC, bid, or dalteparin at 150–200 IU, SC, bid]) to facilitate intrinsic thrombus resolution is unknown but should at least prevent further thrombus formation.

In horses, aneurysms due to *Strongylus vulgaris* rarely rupture; the chief concern is thromboembolism of intestinal vasculature with subsequent colic. Generally, the arterial wall is sufficiently involved that thrombus removal is impractical. Antibacterial treatment and anthelmintics to kill the migrating larvae are of considerable value. The most rational approach to cranial mesenteric and aortic-iliac thrombosis in horses is prevention and control of strongylosis (*see* p 316).

Acute management of aortic emboli in cats can be approached in several ways. More than 50% of cats that survive a cardioembolic event will regain some function of the hindlimbs over 4–6 wk with conservative medical therapy. More aggressive therapy aimed at dissolution of the thrombus through thrombolytic drugs or rheolytic intervention may result in improved short-term functional outcome, but survival is no better than that from conservative therapy and, in some cases, may actually be worse. Conservative therapy usually consists of initial pain management (hydromorphone, 0.1 mg/kg, SC, IM, or IV every 4–6 hr; or buprenorphine HCl, 0.01–0.03 mg/kg, SC, IM, or IV, every 6–8 hr) and anticoagulant therapy (heparin, 250–300 U/kg with first dose IV if animal is in shock, followed by administration SC, tid-qid; or dalteparin 150–170 IU/kg, SC, bid-tid). The activated partial thromboplastin time can be used to monitor heparin therapy, with a goal of 1.5–1.7 × the pretreatment value. The use of antiplatelet therapy (clopidogrel, 75 mg, PO, once on admission, then 18.75 mg/day, PO) should be considered to further reduce the thrombotic potential; in addition, it may have a beneficial effect on collateral circulation. Thrombolytic therapy, although not routinely recommended, could include streptokinase (90,000 IU/cat, IV over 20 min, followed by 45,000 IU as a continuous infusion for 2–24 hr), recombinant tissue-type plasminogen activator (tPA, 0.25–1 mg/kg/hr, IV, up to a total dose of 1–10 mg/kg), or urokinase (4,400 IU/kg, IV over 10 min, then 4,400 IU/kg/hr for 12 hr). These drugs promote thrombolysis by converting plasminogen to plasmin, which subsequently breaks down fibrin strands. Streptokinase is considered a nonspecific activator of plasminogen, because it activates circulating fibrin as well as fibrin contained within thrombi/emboli, which can lead to a systemic proteolytic state and bleeding. Although urokinase and tPA are more fibrin-specific than streptokinase, bleeding can also be seen with these agents. Moreover, all of these agents are prohibitively expensive and difficult to obtain. The use of antiplatelet agents such as clopidogrel has been shown to hasten thrombus dissolution and reduce acute arterial rethrombosis in experimental studies and human clinical trials, respectively. However, an in vitro feline study did not identify a significant difference in thrombolysis rates. It is not known whether these results can be applied to the natural clinical disease. Thrombolytic therapy appears to have the best response in cats with acute onset of clinical signs and incomplete or unilateral infarction. However, these cats may respond similarly well to conservative therapy, without the risk of reperfusion injury or expense of these agents. Although a severe complete infarction is more likely to develop reperfusion injury with thrombolytic therapy, these cats are also less likely to recover with conservative therapy alone. The reported survival rates for initial aortic infarction events are similar whether conservative (35%–39%) or thrombolytic (33%) therapy is used. Cats with single limb infarction do much better (68%–93%) than cats with bilateral hindlimb infarction (15%–36%) regardless of therapy used. Aspirin (25 mg/kg, PO, every 48–72 hr; or 5 mg/cat, PO, every 48–72 hr) has historically been the most widely used preventive therapy for cardioembolic disease in cats. Although aspirin appears relatively safe in cats (up to 20% GI adverse effects) and is inexpensive unless compounding is done, the antiplatelet efficacy of aspirin in cats has been called into question, and currently there is no evidence that aspirin prevents first-time or recurrent cardioembolism. Clopidogrel may be a more effective antiplatelet drug in this species.

Clopidogrel (18.75 mg/cat/day, PO) inhibits both primary and secondary platelet aggregation. These effects are more potent than those induced by aspirin. Clopidogrel also impairs the platelet-release reaction, decreasing the release of pro-aggregating and vasoconstrictive agents. Adverse effects are rare but can include vomiting in up to 10% of cats; this appears to be ameliorated by giving the drug with food. A combination protocol of aspirin and clopidogrel has been used previously. Although this protocol has not been studied objectively, it seems to be well tolerated despite a theoretical increased risk of bleeding. A multicenter, randomized, prospective study revealed that clopidogrel was associated with a significantly prolonged survival time compared with aspirin in cats that presented with cardiogenic arterial thromboembolism. The time to recurrence of arterial thromboembolism or death in the clopidogrel group was >365 days versus 192 days in the aspirin group.

Warfarin (0.25–0.5 mg/day/cat, PO) has also been used for prevention of primary or secondary cardioemboli. Dosing is adjusted to prolong the prothrombin time to 1.5–1.7 × the pretreatment value. Because warfarin decreases the anticoagulant proteins C and S before reduction in factors II, VII, IX, and X, joint treatment with heparin is recommended for the first 5–7 days of warfarin therapy. Problems with warfarin therapy include large inter- and intra-individual variability, difficult dosing because of tablet size, and bleeding, including fatal hemorrhage. Because of these limitations and lack of objective clinical data demonstrating efficacy, warfarin is not a first-line antithrombotic for cardioembolic prevention in cats.

The low-molecular-weight heparins (LMWHs) are smaller in size than unfractionated heparin but maintain the ability to inhibit factor Xa, with a greatly reduced inhibition of IIa. The reduced anti-IIa activity translates into a negligible effect on the activated partial thromboplastin time, but measurement of anti-Xa activity can be used to monitor dosing efficacy. Enoxaparin (1–1.5 mg/kg, SC, once or twice daily) and dalteparin (150–170 IU/kg, SC, bid-tid) have both been used in cats. These drugs have been well tolerated with only rare bleeding reported, but objective clinical studies evaluating their efficacy have not been performed. These agents have been frequently combined with clopidogrel in an attempt to provide a more complete antithrombotic effect. This protocol appears to be well tolerated, although some minor bleeding has been seen. Reported recurrence rates for cats receiving some form of antithrombotic prevention are 17%–75%, with a 1-yr recurrence rate of 25%–50%. Long-term median survival times after an initial cardioembolic event have ranged from 51–376 days. Although these numbers may seem daunting, many of these cats can do well. If owners are willing to treat, they should be encouraged to give cats 24–72 hr of supportive care before deciding on euthanasia, unless severe infarction, severe CHF, or reperfusion injury are present.

Arterial thrombosis in dogs is most commonly associated with protein-losing nephropathy and neoplasia, though idiopathic thrombosis is also seen. There is very little clinical experience with arterial thromboembolism in dogs, but thrombolytic therapy using streptokinase, urokinase, and tPA have been reported in isolated cases with variable success. There are no clinical trials evaluating the efficacy of antithrombotic therapy for prevention of arterial thromboembolism in dogs, but dosing protocols for aspirin (0.5–5 mg/kg, PO, once or twice daily), clopidogrel (1–3 mg/kg/day, PO), warfarin (0.1–0.22 mg/kg/day, PO), dalteparin (150 IU/kg, SC,bid-tid), enoxaparin (1–1.5 mg/kg, SC, once or twice daily), and rivaroxaban (0.5–1 mg/kg/day, PO) have been reported.

Treatment recommendations for pulmonary embolism in dogs are similar to those for cardioembolic disease in cats. Aspirin (0.5 mg/kg/day, PO) has improved survival in dogs with immune-mediated hemolytic anemia when added to standard immunosuppressive therapy.

DIGESTIVE SYSTEM

SMALL ANIMALS

DIGESTIVE SYSTEM INTRODUCTION

The digestive tract includes the oral cavity and associated organs (lips, teeth, tongue, and salivary glands), the esophagus, the forestomachs (reticulum, rumen, omasum) of ruminants and the true stomach in all species, the small intestine, the liver, the exocrine pancreas, the large intestine, and the rectum and anus. Gut-associated lymphoid tissue (tonsils, Peyer's patches, diffuse lymphoid tissue) is distributed along the GI tract. The peritoneum covers the abdominal viscera and is involved in many GI diseases. Fundamental efforts to manage GI disorders should always be directed toward localizing disease to a particular segment and determining a cause. A rational therapeutic plan can then be formulated.

Function

The primary functions of the GI tract include prehension of feed and water; mastication, ensalivation, and swallowing of feed; digestion of feed and absorption of nutrients; maintenance of fluid and electrolyte balance; and evacuation of waste products. There are four primary functions—digestion, absorption, motility, and evacuation—and, correspondingly, four primary modes of dysfunction.

Normal GI tract motility involves peristalsis, muscle activity that moves ingesta from the esophagus to the rectum; segmentation movements, which churn and mix the ingesta; and segmental resistance and sphincter tone, which retard aboral progression of gut contents. In ruminants, these movements are of major importance in normal forestomach function.

Pathophysiology

Abnormal motor function usually manifests as decreased motility. Segmental resistance is usually reduced, and transit rate increases. Motility depends on stimulation via the sympathetic and parasympathetic nervous systems (and thus on the activity of the central and peripheral parts of these systems) and on the GI musculature and its intrinsic nerve plexuses. Debility, accompanied by weakness of the musculature, acute peritonitis, and hypokalemia, produces atony of the gut wall (paralytic ileus). The intestines distend with fluid and gas, and fecal output is reduced. In addition, chronic stasis of the small intestine may predispose to abnormal proliferation of microflora. Such bacterial overgrowth may cause malabsorption by injuring mucosal cells, by competing for nutrients, and by deconjugating bile salts and hydroxylating fatty acids.

Vomiting is a neural reflex act that results in ejection of food and fluid from the stomach through the oral cavity. It is always associated with antecedent events such as premonition, nausea, salivation, or shivering and is accompanied by repeated contractions of the abdominal muscles.

Regurgitation is characterized by passive, retrograde reflux of previously swallowed material from the esophagus, stomach, or rumen. In diseases of the esophagus, swallowed material may not reach the stomach.

One of the major consequences of subnormal motility is distention with fluid and gas. Much of the accumulated fluid is saliva and gastric and intestinal juices secreted during normal digestion. Distention causes pain and reflex spasm of adjoining gut segments. It also stimulates further secretion of fluid into the lumen of the gut, which exacerbates the condition. When the distention exceeds a critical point, the ability of the musculature of the wall to respond diminishes, the initial pain disappears, and paralytic ileus develops in which all GI muscle tone is lost.

Dehydration, acid-base and electrolyte imbalance, and circulatory failure are major consequences of GI distention. Accumulation of gut fluids stimulates additional secretion of fluids and electrolytes in the anterior segments of the intestine, which can worsen the abnormalities and lead to shock.

Abdominal pain associated with GI disease usually is caused by stretching of the intestinal wall. Contraction of the gut causes pain by direct and reflex distention of neighboring segments. Spasm, an exaggerated segmenting contraction of one section of intestine, results in distention of the immediately anterior segment when a peristaltic wave arrives. Other factors that may cause abdominal pain include edema and failure of local blood supply, eg, in local embolism or twisting of the mesentery.

Specific diseases cause diarrhea by varied and characteristic mechanisms, the recognition of which is useful in understanding, diagnosing, and managing GI diseases. The major mechanisms of diarrhea are increased permeability, hypersecretion, and osmosis. Disorders of motility are often secondary. In healthy animals, water and electrolytes continuously transfer across the intestinal mucosa. Secretions (from blood to gut) and absorptions (from gut to blood) occur simultaneously. In clinically healthy animals, absorption exceeds secretion, ie, there is net absorption. Inflammation in the intestines can be accompanied by an increase in "pore size" in the mucosa, permitting increased flow through the membrane ("leak") down the pressure gradient from blood to the intestinal lumen. If the amount exuded exceeds the absorptive capacity of the intestines, diarrhea results. The size of the material that leaks through the mucosa varies, depending on the magnitude of the increase in pore size. Large increases in pore size permit exudation of plasma protein, resulting in protein-losing enteropathies (eg, lymphangiectasia in dogs, paratuberculosis in cattle, nematode infections). Greater increases in pore size result in the loss of RBCs, producing hemorrhagic diarrhea (eg, hemorrhagic gastroenteritis, parvovirus infection, severe hookworm infection).

Hypersecretion is a net intestinal loss of fluid and electrolytes that is independent of changes in permeability, absorptive capacity, or exogenously generated osmotic gradients. Enterotoxic colibacillosis is an example of diarrheal disease due to intestinal hypersecretion; enterotoxigenic *Escherichia coli* produce enterotoxin that stimulates the crypt epithelium to secrete fluid beyond the absorptive capacity of the intestines. The villi, along with their digestive and absorptive capabilities, remain intact. The fluid secreted is isotonic, alkaline, and free of exudates. The intact villi are beneficial because a fluid (administered PO) that contains glucose, amino acids, and sodium is absorbed, even with hypersecretion.

Osmotic diarrhea is seen when inadequate absorption results in a collection of solutes in the gut lumen, which cause water to be retained by their osmotic activity. It develops in any condition that results in nutrient malabsorption or maldigestion or when an animal ingests a large amount of osmotically active substances that are not absorbed, eg, an overeating puppy.

Malabsorption (*see* p 353 and *see* p 373) is failure of digestion and absorption due to some defect in the villous digestive and absorptive cells, which are mature cells that cover the villi. Several epitheliotropic viruses directly infect and destroy the villous absorptive epithelial cells or their precursors, eg, coronavirus, transmissible gastroenteritis virus of piglets, and rotavirus of calves. Feline panleukopenia virus and canine parvovirus destroy the crypt epithelium, which results in failure of renewal of villous absorptive cells and collapse of the villi; regeneration is a longer process after parvoviral infection than after viral infections of villous tip epithelium (eg, coronavirus, rotavirus). Intestinal malabsorption also may be caused by any defect that impairs absorptive capacity, such as diffuse inflammatory disorders (eg, lymphocytic-plasmacytic enteritis, eosinophilic enteritis) or neoplasia (eg, lymphosarcoma).

Other examples of malabsorption include defects of pancreatic secretion that result in maldigestion. Rarely, because of failure to digest lactose (which, in large amounts, has a hyperosmotic effect), neonatal farm animals or pups may have diarrhea while they are being fed milk. Reduced secretion of digestive enzymes at the surface of villous tip cells is characteristic of epitheliotropic viral infections recognized in farm animals.

The ability of the GI tract to digest food depends on its motor and secretory functions and, in herbivores, on the activity of the microflora of the forestomachs of ruminants, or of the cecum and colon of horses and pigs. The flora of ruminants can digest cellulose; ferment carbohydrates to volatile fatty acids; and convert nitrogenous substances to ammonia, amino acids, and protein. In certain circumstances, the activity of the flora can be suppressed to the point that digestion becomes abnormal or ceases. Incorrect diet, prolonged starvation or inappetence, and hyperacidity (as occurs in engorgement on grain) all impair microbial digestion. The bacteria, yeasts, and protozoa also may be adversely affected by the oral administration of drugs that are antimicrobial or that drastically alter the pH of rumen contents.

Clinical Findings of GI Disease

Signs of GI disease include excessive salivation, diarrhea, constipation or scant feces, vomiting, regurgitation, GI tract hemorrhage, abdominal pain and distention, tenesmus, shock and dehydration, and suboptimal performance. The location and nature of the lesions that cause malfunction often can be determined by recognition and analysis of the clinical findings. In addition, abnormalities of prehension, mastication, and swallowing usually are associated with diseases of the oral mucosa, teeth, mandible or other bony structures of the head, pharynx, or esophagus. Vomiting is most common in single-stomached animals and usually is due to gastroenteritis or nonalimentary disease (eg, uremia, pyometra, endocrine disease). The vomitus in a dog or cat with a bleeding lesion (gastric ulcer or neoplasm) may contain frank blood or have the appearance of coffee grounds. Horses and rabbits do not vomit. Regurgitation may signify disease of the oropharynx or esophagus and is not accompanied by the premonitory signs seen with vomiting.

Large-volume, fluid diarrhea usually is associated with hypersecretion (eg, in enterotoxigenic colibacillosis in newborn calves) or with malabsorptive (osmotic) effects. Blood and fibrinous casts in the feces indicate a hemorrhagic, fibrinonecrotic enteritis of the small or large intestine, eg, bovine viral diarrhea, coccidiosis, salmonellosis, or swine dysentery. Black, tarry feces (melena) indicate hemorrhage in the stomach or upper part of the small intestine. Tenesmus of GI origin usually is associated with inflammatory disease of the rectum and anus.

Small amounts of soft feces may indicate a partial obstruction of the intestines. Abdominal distention can result from accumulation of gas, fluid, or ingesta, usually due to hypomotility (functional obstruction, adynamic paralytic ileus) or to a physical obstruction (eg, foreign body or intussusception). Distention may, of course, result from something as direct as overeating. A "ping" heard during auscultation and percussion of the abdomen indicates a gas-filled viscus. A sudden onset of severe abdominal distention in an adult ruminant usually is due to ruminal tympany. Ballottement and succussion may reveal fluid-splashing sounds when the rumen or bowel is filled with fluid. Varying degrees of dehydration and acid-base and electrolyte imbalance, which may lead to shock, are seen when large quantities of fluid are lost (eg, in diarrhea or sequestered in intestinal obstruction) or in gastric or abomasal volvulus.

Abdominal pain is due to stretching or inflammation of the serosal surfaces of abdominal viscera or the peritoneum; it may be acute or subacute, and its manifestation varies among species. In horses, acute abdominal pain is common (*see* p 248). Subacute pain is more common in cattle and is characterized by reluctance to move and by grunting with each respiration or deep palpation of the abdomen. Abdominal pain in dogs and cats may be acute or subacute and is characterized by whining, meowing, and abnormal postures (eg, outstretched forelimbs, the sternum on the floor, and the hindlimbs raised). Abdominal pain may be difficult to localize to a particular viscus or organ within the abdomen.

Examination of the GI Tract

A complete, accurate history and routine clinical examination can often determine the diagnosis. In outbreaks of GI tract disease in farm animals, the history and epidemiologic findings are of prime importance. In small animals, travel history or other details such as recent adoption from a shelter or recent kenneling or exposure to other animals in dog parks might give clinical suspicion to certain infectious diseases. If the history and epidemiologic and clinical findings are consistent with GI disease, the lesion should be localized within the system, and the type of lesion and its cause determined.

The abnormality may sometimes be localized to the large or small intestine by history, physical examination, and fecal characteristics (*see* TABLE 1). The distinction is important because it narrows the differential diagnoses and determines the direction of further investigation. However, the clinician should appreciate that in some instances the disorder can involve the entire bowel, with one set of localizing signs overshadowing the other.

The clinical and laboratory techniques and their applications include the following: 1) visual inspection of the oral cavity and of the contour of the abdomen for distention or contraction; 2) palpation through the abdominal wall or per rectum to evaluate shape, size, and position of abdominal viscera; 3) abdominal percussion to detect "pings," which suggest gas-filled viscera; 4) auscultation to determine the intensity, frequency, and duration of GI movements, as well as fluid-splashing sounds associated with fluid-filled stomachs and intestines and fluid-rushing sounds associated with diarrheal disease; 5) succussion to reveal fluid-splashing sounds; 6) ballottement to evaluate density and size of abdominal organs by their movement away from and back to the abdominal wall; and 7) gross examination of feces to assess bulk, consistency, color, and presence of mucus, blood, or undigested food particles.

Microscopic studies include examination for parasites. Cytology of a rectal or colonic mucosal smear stained with new methylene blue or Wright stain for fecal leukocytes is useful to detect inflammatory bowel disease or the presence of intracellular fungal organisms in the case of infection with *Histoplasma capsulatum*. The following may be useful (or necessary): 1) bacterial culture and virus isolation; 2) endoscopy to visualize the mucosal surface of the esophagus, stomach, duodenum, colon, and rectum; 3) abdominocentesis to collect fluid from distended viscera or from the peritoneal cavity for examination; 4) radiography (contrast) to diagnose obstructive disease; 5) abdominal ultra-

TABLE 1 DIFFERENTIATION OF SMALL-INTESTINAL FROM LARGE-INTESTINAL DIARRHEA

Clinical Sign	Small Intestine	Large Intestine
Frequency of defecation	Normal or slightly increased	Very frequent
Fecal volume	Normal to increased	Decreased
Urgency	Absent	Usually present
Tenesmus	Absent	Usually present
Mucus in feces	Usually absent	Frequent
Blood in feces	Dark black (melena)	Red (fresh)
Weight loss	May be present	Rare

sonography to evaluate the wall thickness of the stomach and intestines and to detect abdominal masses, intussusceptions, and mesenteric lymphadenopathy in small animals, and to investigate abdominal disorders in horses and cows; 6) biopsy (endoscopic, laparoscopic, ultrasound-guided, surgical) to obtain samples for microscopic examination (samples of intestines and liver are useful to diagnose chronic enteritis and liver disease); and 7) tests for digestion and absorption to estimate and differentiate malabsorption and maldigestion. Common absorption tests include the measurement of the serum concentrations of cobalamin (vitamin B_{12}) and folate. In addition, in small animals, an increased serum folate concentration in conjunction with a decreased cobalamin is consistent with antibiotic-responsive diarrhea. Exocrine pancreatic function can be evaluated by the determination of serum trypsin-like immunoreactivity and by measurement of serum canine and feline pancreas-specific lipase, which are sensitive and specific markers for the diagnosis of pancreatitis; laparotomy and biopsy may be indicated in cases in which the diagnosis is not clear or in which surgical correction may be required.

INFECTIOUS DISEASES

The GI tract is subject to infection by many pathogens, which are a major cause of economic loss due to illness, suboptimal performance, and death (*see* TABLE 2). These infections spread by direct contact or the fecal-oral route. Many of the pathogens are part of the normal intestinal flora, and disease develops only after a stressful event, eg, salmonellosis in horses after transportation, extended anesthesia, or surgery. The intestinal flora becomes established within a few hours after birth, which emphasizes the importance of the early ingestion of colostrum to provide protection against septicemia and intestinal infection.

TABLE 2 COMMON PATHOGENS OF THE GASTROINTESTINAL TRACT

Pathogen	Cattle, Sheep, and Goats	Pigs
Viruses	Bovine viral diarrhea, rotavirus, coronavirus, rinderpest, malignant catarrhal fever, bluetongue, foot-and-mouth disease	Transmissible gastroenteritis, porcine circovirus type II, porcine epidemic diarrhea virus, rotavirus, foot-and-mouth disease, vesicular stomatitis, vesicular exanthema
Rickettsiae		
Bacteria	Enterotoxigenic *Escherichia coli*, *Salmonella* spp, *Mycobacterium paratuberculosis*, *Fusobacterium necrophorum*, *Clostridium perfringens* (types B, C, and D), *Actinobacillus lignieresii*, *Yersinia enterocolitica*, *Campylobacter jejuni*	Enterotoxigenic *E coli*, *Salmonella* spp, *Brachyspira hyodysenteriae*, *Clostridium perfringens* types B and C, *Lawsonia intracellularis*, *Clostridium difficile*
Protozoa	*Eimeria* spp, *Cryptosporidium* spp	*Eimeria* spp, *Isospora suis*
Fungi	*Candida* spp (cattle)	*Candida* spp
Algae	*Prototheca* spp	*Prototheca* spp
Parasites (helminths)	*See* GASTROINTESTINAL PARASITES OF RUMINANTS, p 303.	*See* GASTROINTESTINAL PARASITES OF PIGS, p 320.

Definitive etiologic diagnosis of infectious disease of the GI tract depends on demonstrating the pathogen in the tract or in the feces of the affected animal. In herd epidemics, such as an outbreak of acute undifferentiated diarrhea in newborn calves or piglets, the best opportunity to establish a diagnosis is in the earliest stage of the disease by selecting untreated animals and submitting them for necropsy and detailed microbiologic examination of the intestinal flora. When selective necropsy is not an option, a series of carefully collected daily fecal samples should be submitted to a diagnostic laboratory with a request for special culture techniques, depending on the infectious disease suspected. Molecular technologies, including ELISA and PCR, have been developed to demonstrate the presence of viral, bacterial, or protozoal proteins or nucleic acids within the feces, which can provide a definitive diagnosis (eg, canine parvovirus, salmonellosis, cryptosporidiosis).

Overview of Gastrointestinal Parasitism

The GI tract may be inhabited by many species of parasites. Their cycles may be direct, in which eggs and larvae are passed in the feces and stadial development occurs to the infective stage, which is then ingested by the final host. Alternatively, the immature stages may be ingested by an intermediate host (usually an invertebrate) in which further development occurs, and infection is acquired when the intermediate host or free-living stage shed by that host is ingested by the final host. Sometimes, there is no development in the intermediate host, in which case it is known as a transport or paratenic host, depending on whether the larvae are encapsulated or in the tissues. Clinical parasitism depends on the number and pathogenicity of the parasites, which

TABLE 2 COMMON PATHOGENS OF THE GASTROINTESTINAL TRACT *(continued)*

Horses	Dogs and Cats
Rotavirus, vesicular stomatitis, coronavirus	Canine parvovirus, canine coronavirus, feline panleukopenia virus, feline enteric coronavirus, canine and feline rotaviruses, canine and feline astroviruses
Neorickettsia risticii (Potomac horse fever [equine monocytic ehrlichiosis])	*Neorickettsia helminthoeca* (salmon poisoning in dogs)
Enterotoxigenic *E coli*, *Salmonella* spp, *Rhodococcus equi*, *Actinobacillus equuli*, *Clostridium perfringens* types B and C, *Clostridium difficile*, *Lawsonia intracellularis*	*Salmonella* spp, *Yersinia enterocolitica*, *Campylobacter jejuni*, *Clostridium* spp, *Clostridium piliforme*, *Mycobacterium* spp, *Shigella* spp, adherent invasive *E coli*, *Brachyspira* spp
Eimeria spp, *Cryptosporidium* spp	*Isospora* spp, *Sarcocystis* spp, *Besnoitia* spp, *Hammondia* sp, *Toxoplasma* sp, *Giardia* sp, *Tritrichomonas* spp, *Entamoeba histolytica*, *Balantidium coli*, *Cryptosporidium* spp, *Neospora* sp
Aspergillus fumigatus	*Histoplasma capsulatum*, *Aspergillus* spp, *Candida albicans*, phycomycetes
Prototheca spp	*Prototheca* spp
See GASTROINTESTINAL PARASITES OF HORSES, p 315.	*See* GASTROINTESTINAL PARASITES OF SMALL ANIMALS, p 412.

depend on the biotic potential of the parasites or, when appropriate, their intermediate host and the climate and management practices. In the host, resistance, age, nutrition, and concomitant disease also influence the course of parasitic infection. The economic importance of subclinical parasitism in farm animals is also determined by the above factors, and it is well established that lightly parasitized animals that show no clinical evidence of disease perform less efficiently in the feedlot, dairy, or finishing house.

Feed conversion in light to moderate parasitism is adversely affected and is primarily due to reduced appetite and poor use of absorbed protein and energy. Carcass quality and size also are reduced, which further reduce financial returns. Endoparasites of companion animals can cause severe disease or unthriftiness and are aesthetically undesirable. Furthermore, some of these parasites also infect people.

Because parasitism is easily confused with other debilitating conditions, diagnosis depends heavily on the seasonal character of parasitic infection; previous farm history; and examination of feces for evidence of oocysts, worm eggs, or larvae. Increased serum pepsinogen levels can support the diagnosis of some abomasal infections, as can increased serum liver enzymes for liver fluke infection. ELISA are being used, and other serologic (including monoclonal antibody) techniques are under development; serodiagnosis will likely be used more frequently as the specificity of the tests improves. These tests should be particularly useful in companion animals harboring parasites incriminated in zoonoses.

Advances in epidemiology (particularly regarding factors affecting seasonal development of the free-living stages and their survival), coupled with the discovery of highly efficient broad-spectrum anthelmintics, have made successful treatment and control of GI parasites both possible and practical. Response to therapy is usually rapid, and single treatments usually suffice unless reinfection occurs or the lesions are particularly severe. Preventive control in large animals is generally achieved by integrating grassland management with the use of anthelmintics. Improved methods of administering anthelmintics (eg, the pour-on method or sustained or pulsed-release devices) have also helped. Strategies to prevent parasitism and related production losses are part of any modern herd-health, flock, or stud program. Similar preventive programs are equally important in controlling parasitism in pet animals. Control by vaccination is limited to lungworms; vaccine for cattle is available in several European countries, and vaccine for sheep is available in parts of eastern Europe and in the Middle East.

To estimate parasite load, *see* p 1620.

Treatment of Infectious Diseases

Antimicrobial agents are used for the treatment of bacterial diseases, and anthelmintics for parasitic diseases. There is no specific therapy for treatment of viral diseases. Antimicrobials are commonly given PO daily for several days until recovery is apparent, but there is little objective evidence of efficacy. There is evidence that overdosage or prolonged oral treatment may be detrimental (eg, bacterial overgrowth, villous atrophy). Parenteral administration of antimicrobials is indicated when septicemia is apparent or may occur. The choice of antimicrobial agent depends on the suspected disease, previous results, and cost. In herd epidemics, antimicrobials may be added to the feed or water supplies at therapeutic levels for several days, followed by preventive levels for an extended period, depending on the infection pressure in the population. The feed and water supplies of in-contact animals also may be medicated in an attempt to prevent new cases from developing. (*See also* SYSTEMIC PHARMACOTHERAPEUTICS OF THE DIGESTIVE SYSTEM, p 2544.)

Control of Infectious Diseases

Effective control of the common infectious diseases of the GI tract depends on practicing good sanitation and hygiene, developing and maintaining nonspecific resistance in the animal, and in certain cases, providing specific immunity by vaccinating the pregnant dam or susceptible animal.

Effective sanitation and hygiene is achieved primarily by providing adequate space for animals and by regular cleaning of pens and efficient removal of manure from the immediate environment. Development and maintenance of nonspecific resistance depends on the genetic selection of animals that have a reasonable degree of inherent resistance and on the provision of adequate nutrition and housing, which minimizes stress and allows the animals to grow and behave normally. The development of infected but clinically healthy animals, which can shed pathogens for weeks or months, is a major problem with some infectious diseases of the GI tract, eg, salmonellosis. Ideally, these carrier animals should be identified by microbiologic means and isolated from the rest of the herd until free of the infection or culled.

Certain diseases (eg, enterotoxigenic colibacillosis in calves and piglets) can be controlled by vaccination of the pregnant dam several weeks before parturition. This method depends on achieving a protective level of antibodies in the colostrum. There are exceptions but, in most cases, systemic immunity provides little protection against the infectious enteritides; effective immunity against GI disease depends on stimulation of local intestinal immunity after the neonatal period. During the neonatal period, protection can be provided through the local action of maternally derived antibodies. For example, secretory IgA progressively increases in sow's milk from the time of farrowing until weaning, which provides the piglet with daily protection during the nursing period.

NONINFECTIOUS DISEASES

The major causes of noninfectious disease of the GI tract include dietary overload or indigestible feeds, chemical or physical agents, obstruction of the stomach and intestines caused by the ingestion of foreign bodies or by any physical displacement or injury to the GI tract that interferes with the flow of ingesta, enzyme deficiencies, abnormalities of the mucosa that interfere with normal function (eg, gastric ulcers, inflammatory bowel disease, villous atrophy, neoplasms), and congenital defects. GI manifestations such as vomiting and diarrhea may develop secondary to systemic or metabolic diseases such as uremia, liver disease, and hypoadrenocorticism. The causes are uncertain in several diseases, including abomasal ulcers in cattle, gastric ulcers in pigs and foals, gastric torsion in dogs, and acute intestinal obstruction and displacement of the abomasum in cattle. In noninfectious diseases of the GI tract, usually only a single animal is affected at one time; exceptions are diseases associated with excessive feed intake or poisons, in which herd outbreaks are common.

PRINCIPLES OF THERAPY

See also SYSTEMIC PHARMACOTHERAPEUTICS OF THE DIGESTIVE SYSTEM, p 2544, and THE RUMINANT DIGESTIVE SYSTEM, p 2561.
Although eliminating the cause of the disease is the primary objective, the major part of treatment is supportive and symptomatic, aimed at relieving pain, correcting abnormalities, and allowing healing to occur.

Elimination of the primary cause may involve antimicrobials, coccidiostats, antifungal agents, anthelmintics, antidotes for poisons, or surgical correction of displacements.

Correction of excessive or depressed motility appears rational, but often the nature and degree of abnormal motility are uncertain; in addition, available drugs may not give consistent results. There is little clinical evidence to recommend the routine use of anticholinergic or opioid drugs to slow intestinal transit. Slowing intestinal transit may be counterproductive to the defense mechanism of diarrhea, which acts to evacuate harmful organisms and their toxins. In general, anticholinergic drugs probably are justified only for short-term symptomatic relief of pain and tenesmus associated with inflammatory diseases of the colon and rectum. In some disorders of gastric or colonic motility, prokinetic drugs (eg, metoclopramide, erythromycin) may be useful.

Replacement of fluid and electrolytes is necessary when dehydration and electrolyte and acid-base imbalance occur as in diarrhea, persistent vomiting, intestinal obstruction, or torsion of the stomach(s), in which large amounts of fluid and electrolytes are sequestered.

Relief of distention medically by stomach tube (as in bloat in ruminants) or surgically (as in acute intestinal obstruction, or in torsion of the abomasum in ruminants or of the stomach in monogastric animals) may be required. The GI tract may become distended with gas, fluid, or ingesta at any level due to physical or functional obstruction.

Relief of abdominal pain by administration of analgesics should be done when the pain is reflexly affecting other body systems (eg, cardiovascular collapse) or when it is causing the animal to injure itself because of rolling, kicking, or throwing itself. Animals treated with analgesics must be monitored regularly to ensure that the relief of pain does not provide a false sense of security; the lesion may be progressively worsening while the animal is under the influence of the analgesic.

Reconstitution of ruminal flora should be done in situations in which the ruminal flora may be seriously depleted (eg, in prolonged anorexia or acute indigestion). Transfaunation (ruminal fluid transfer; *see* p 2562) involves oral administration of ruminal contents from a healthy animal that contains rumen bacteria and protozoa and volatile fatty acids.

CONGENITAL AND INHERITED ANOMALIES OF THE DIGESTIVE SYSTEM

MOUTH

Congenital Oronasal Fistulas (Cleft Palate and Cleft Lip): Congenital oronasal fistulas are the result of failure of fusion of the palatine shelves during gestation (which occurs at 25–28 days of gestation in dogs). Clefts can be either of the primary palate (involving the lip and incisive bone) causing cleft lip (harelip), or of the secondary palate (involving the hard and soft palate) causing cleft palate. The conditions can occur singly or together. In dogs, CT studies have shown association of cleft palate with other craniofacial abnormalities, including hypoplastic tympanic bullae, hypoplastic nasal turbinates, and maxillary malocclusions, mostly of the incisors. Neurologic examination should be performed in affected animals, because concurrent hydrocephalus has also been described. Animals are typically diagnosed at, or shortly after, birth by oral examination, by observation of dysphagia or milk from the nares after nursing, and/or by respiratory compromise and aspiration pneumonia. Many affected neonates are euthanized or die early in life.

Cleft palate and cleft lip have been described in most domesticated animal species, including dogs, cats, ruminants, horses, and camelids. In dogs, brachycephalic breeds are overrepresented, with up to 30% risk factor. Other breeds with higher incidence include Beagles, Cocker Spaniels, Dachshunds, German Shepherds, Labrador Retrievers, Schnauzers, Old Spanish Pointers, and Shetland Sheepdogs. The most commonly affected cat breed is the Siamese. Etiologies include genetic, teratogenic, and nutritional causes. Modes of inheritance are monogenic autosomal recessive or incomplete dominant in several breeds. In Brittany Spaniels, Pyrenean Shepherds, Beagles, Old Spanish Pointers, and Boxers, it is believed to be an autosomal recessive trait, whereas in Bulldogs (French and English) and Shih Tzus, an autosomal dominant with incomplete penetrance mode of inheritance is suspected. Autosomal recessive inheritance patterns are seen in Angus cattle with arthrogryposis multiplex, in Charolais cattle with cleft palate and arthrogryposis, and in Texel sheep with cleft lip. Teratogens and nutritional causes during pregnancy include high levels of vitamin A in the diet, administration of griseofulvin, folic acid deficiency, and ingestion of toxic plants. In cattle, ingestion of lupine during days 40–100 of gestation results in arthrygryposis and cleft palate, due to the effects of anagyrine found in *Lupinus sericeus* and *L caudatus*. Ingestion of poison hemlock (*Conium maculatum*), which contains the toxic principle coniine, results in similar signs in both cattle and goats, whereas ingestion of *Veratrum californicum* in sheep, goats, and cattle all result in cleft lip and/or palate in the fetus.

For puppies and kittens in which euthanasia is not elected, medical management is required until surgical options are explored. Animals are fed via orogastric intubation until dry food can be tolerated. Water can be offered by overhead dispenser. A custom-molded palate guard has been described in experimental settings to allow adult dogs to eat and drink normally. Aspiration pneumonia should be quickly identified and treated. Surgical correction is recommended after at least 12 wk of age, although some studies have shown higher success when performed at >20 wk, or as adults. Surgical correction has a high failure rate because of continued growth of puppies or kittens postoperatively, the size of the patient, and irritation of the surgery site by the tongue and feed material. Surgical techniques depend on the location and size of the cleft defect. For secondary palate defects, sliding mucoperiosteal flaps or overlapping flaps are most commonly used.

Extensive involvement of the soft palate carries a poor prognosis, even with surgical intervention. Surgical repair should be attempted only after ethical questions have been addressed, and the affected animal should be surgically sterilized or removed from breeding stock to prevent reproducing the anomaly in future offspring.

Occlusal Anomalies: Occlusal abnormalities due to abnormal lengths of the maxilla and mandible are common in animals. **Brachygnathia**, also called overbite, overshot, overjet, short lower jaw, or parrot mouth in horses, is manifest when the mandible is shorter than the maxilla. It can be found, with varying severity and incidence, in all species of animals and is diagnosed by oral examination. In Red Angus cattle, it is inherited in a recessive manner through a deletion mutation on chromosome 4, which results in stillborn calves with osteopetrosis (*see* p 1044), brachygnathism, and impacted molars. In Simmental cattle, brachygnathism can be seen in calves as an autosomal recessive trait, or in combination with trisomy 17, a lethal condition. A lethal, autosomal recessive disorder of Merino sheep results in brachygnathism, cardiomegaly, and renal hypoplasia. Brachygnathism is common in horses, due to either a lengthened maxilla or shortened mandible. Modes of inheritance are unknown. It may occur in utero due to treatment of the mare with griseofulvin. Most horses do not experience dysphagia; however, cheek teeth malocclusions are common, and regular dental care is required. Correction can be attempted in foals via surgical placement of tension band wires around the maxillary incisors to inhibit maxillary growth.

In small animals, mild forms may be of no clinical significance; however, more severe forms may result in trauma to the hard palate or the restriction of normal mandibular growth secondary to erupting adult mandibular canine teeth. Treatment varies from none to various orthodontic or endodontic procedures, depending on severity. The mandibular canine teeth are often removed or a crown reduction procedure performed, with concurrent pulpotomy or root canal. Intervention early in life is recommended and improves both short- and longterm outcomes.

Prognathia, also called undershot, underjet, or monkey or sow mouth in horses, is identified when the mandible is longer than the maxilla. It is diagnosed by oral examination. In brachycephalic dogs and Persian cats, it is considered a normal breed characteristic. In horses, it is more commonly seen in miniature and Arabian breeds. The degree of severity is variable and may not require treatment. In severe cases in foals, surgical placement of tension band wires can allow for continued maxillary growth. The most severe consequences are the result of malocclusions. Affected foals may have difficulty nursing, and older animals may experience difficulty grazing. Cheek teeth malocclusions should be addressed with regular dental care.

Chondrodysplasia, a simple dominant trait of Dexter cattle, is a lethal defect that can result in "bulldog calves," with severe skeletal malformation and craniofacial dysplasia that has the appearance of prognathism.

Tongue Anomalies: **Ankyloglossia**, also called "tongue-tie," is a disorder of Anatolian Shepherd dogs characterized by a short, thickened lingual frenulum that inhibits normal movements of the tongue. By unknown mechanism, the normal fetal apoptosis of the cranial ⅔ of the frenulum does not occur. Clinically, the tongue appears notched or with a "W" shape. Animals may experience dysphagia; difficulty suckling, drinking, or licking; trouble vocalizing; and impedence of panting and therefore thermoregulation. Frenuloplasty is corrective. Breeding of affected animals is not recommended.

Microglossia is a congenital defect characterized by missing or underdeveloped lateral and rostral thin portions of the tongue that result in prehensile and motility disturbances. It is often referred to as "bird tongue" in dogs and may be a component of the fading puppy syndrome, because affected puppies have difficulty nursing and swallowing and can aspirate or quickly become dehydrated. In cattle, excessive salivation has been seen. Even with supportive dietary measures, the prognosis is poor.

Macroglossia, or large tongue, has been described in association with nasopharyngeal dysgenesis in Dachshunds. It has also been seen in double-muscled cattle breeds, such as the Belgian Blue, and can inhibit nursing of calves.

Epitheliogenesis imperfecta is a disorder of the skin in which the epithelium is absent, revealing the dermis. Commonly affected areas include the limbs, back, and oral mucosa and tongue. It is inherited by a simple recessive manner and is well described in cattle and horses, particularly Saddlebreds. Euthanasia is typically elected.

Tight-lip Syndrome of Chinese Shar-Pei: A small or absent lower anterior lip vestibule is a congenital defect of some Shar-Pei dogs. The lower lip covers the mandibular incisors and canines, disrupting normal occlusion, inhibiting mandibular growth, and leading to the dog biting on the lip (which presents welfare issues). In extreme cases, the mandibular incisors become lingually directed. Surgical correction by chelioplasty has been described using several different mucosal flap techniques. Any animals that have undergone surgical correction should not be presented for conformation showing and should not be bred.

TEETH

Abnormal Number: Deviation from the dental formula has been seen in several species. Complete lack of development of teeth, or **anodontia**, is rare. **Hypodontia** or **oligodontia** has been described as inherited by a recessive manner in Kerry Blue Terriers and associated with X-linked hypohidrotic ectodermal dysplasia in other breeds. Most cases appear to affect the premolars. **Hyperdontia**, also called polyodontia or supernumerary teeth, is seen most often in the permanent teeth and can affect the incisors, premolars, or molars. Presumably, these teeth arise from overproliferation of the dental lamina during development. Supernumerary teeth tend to cause crowding and malocclusions, which can cause dysphagia, dental disease, and discomfort. In horses, supernumerary incisors are typically not extracted and are managed with regular reduction. For supernumerary cheek teeth, diastema and sinusitis due to oromaxillary sinus fistula formation are possible sequelae. Teeth are either extracted or reduced often to prevent complications.

Irregularities of Shedding: Retention of the deciduous teeth in horses is common. The incisors tend to retain rostrally to the permanent incisors; however, radiographs will help to discern their identity. Incisors retained in other orientations can result in malocclusion and/or displacement of permanent incisors. Retained cheek teeth are called "caps," which are typically shed as the permanent tooth erupts underneath them. Loose caps can cause discomfort to the horse, manifest as headshaking, inappetence, quidding, and training issues. Caps can be extracted if they are loose, if the contralateral cap has already been shed, or if there is space between the cap and the permanent tooth below.

Retained deciduous teeth are common in dogs and secondary to the failure of the periodontal ligament to detach from the deciduous tooth, with the permanent canine teeth erupting rostrally. One study showed highest incidence in dogs <2 yr old, with small breeds overrepresented, particularly Toy Poodles. Retention may cause permanent tooth displacement, which can result in malocclusion or food entrapment and subsequent periodontal disease. Therefore, retained deciduous teeth should be removed as soon as possible, taking care not to damage the underlying permanent tooth bud.

Retained deciduous incisors in a horse.
Courtesy of Dr. Gordon Baker.

Abnormalities in Position, Shape, and Direction: Displacement or rotation of teeth has been described in many species. In horses, the cheek teeth are affected more commonly than the incisors, with the permanent teeth most often affected rather than the deciduous teeth. Most displacements are due to crowding during eruption. Sequelae include malocclusion, uneven wear and development of sharp points, and diastema with associated feed packing. Treatment includes regular floating of unopposed surfaces, or extraction if severe. Diastema can be addressed by mechanical widening. In dogs, rotation has been described commonly in brachycephalic and large breeds, with the first mandibular premolar or upper third premolar often affected. Abnormally located or directed teeth can result in malocclusions or affect the positioning of adjacent teeth. Extraction can be performed in severely affected animals; many cases are considered incidental findings.

Enamel Lesions: Enamel hypoplasia, hypomineralization, or dysplasia is seen in both large and small animals. Common causes are pyrexia, trauma, malnutrition, toxicosis (eg, fluorosis in cattle), congenital disorders (eg, epitheliogenesis imperfecta in Saddlebred foals), and infections (eg, distemper virus in dogs or bovine viral diarrhea virus in calves) that affect ameloblast and odontoblast activity. Lesions vary, depending on the severity and duration of the insult, from pitted enamel to the absence of enamel with incomplete tooth development. Affected teeth are prone to plaque and tartar accumulation and subsequent bacterial penetration and formation of caries. In small animals, resin restoration has been used to cover defects, although diligent dental hygiene and home care is critical to reduce the incidence of complications. Enamel may also develop discoloration. In small animals, administration of tetracyclines to pregnant females or to puppies <6 mo old may result in a permanent brownish yellow discoloration of the teeth. In ruminants, the enamel of some teeth may demonstrate flecks of varying color. The condition is thought to have a genetic etiology but generally is of no clinical significance; however, some believe affected teeth may be prone to more rapid wearing.

CYSTS AND SINUSES OF THE HEAD AND NECK

Congenital cysts, sinuses, or fistulae of the branchial arch apparatus or thyroglossal duct have been reported in horses, dogs, cats, and ruminants, yet are very rare. These structures arise from persistent embryologic pharyngeal pouches, arches, or clefts, or the thyroglossal duct. Animals typically present with nonpainful, fluid-filled masses in the cervical region. Clinical signs are typically due to the space-occupying mass and include dyspnea, respiratory stridor, intermittent esophageal obstruction, and coughing. Animals may present later in life; it is not known why a cyst may suddenly enlarge but may be associated with respiratory infection. Diagnostic imaging includes radiography, ultrasonography, video endoscopy, and contrast CT to determine whether there is communication with the pharynx. **Branchial cysts** (also called lateral cervical cysts) in horses are typically seen on the right side, although a bilateral case has been reported. Surgical excision is curative, although complications include right laryngeal hemiplegia, seroma formation, and pneumonia. Alternatively, some horses have been treated with marsupialization and iodine sclerotherapy with good results. In dogs and cats, few complications have been noted. Embryologic origin of branchial cysts has been mostly of the third pharyngeal pouch, although anatomic location has also suggested origin of the fourth and sixth pouches in some cases.

Thyroglossal duct cysts appear similar in appearance to branchial cysts; differentiation is often made histologically by demonstration of thyroid follicles containing colloid or immunohistochemistry for presence of thyroglobulin. These cysts arise from the thyroglossal duct, which in the embryo is present from the base of the tongue to the eventual location of the thyroid and which is normally absent by birth. The cyst is solitary and usually located on ventral midline, although a case of a mediastinal thyroglossal duct cyst with ectopic thyroid tissue was reported in a cat and a case of subepiglottic thyroglossal duct cyst was reported in a dog. It is hypothesized that subepiglottic cysts in horses are also of thyroglossal duct origin and may be associated with epiglottic entrapment. In Damascus goats, thyroglossal duct cysts are heritable by an unknown genetic mechanism. Aspiration of the cyst for measurement of thyroxine has not been reliably diagnostic. Surgical resection is curative.

In horses, congenital cystic lesions of the esophagus are typically of two types: **intramural inclusion cysts** and **esophageal duplication cysts**. Both have been described in yearling horses that presented for recurrent choke, dysphagia, and aspiration pneumonia. Both occur in the cervical esophagus and result in compression of the esophageal lumen and its function. Diagnosis is aided by imaging, including video endoscopy, contrast radiography, and ultrasonography. Described treatments include surgical resection and marsupialization with sclerotherapy. Complications after excision have included left laryngeal hemiplegia and esophageal fistula formation. Histologically, esophageal duplication cysts include a layer of muscle, whereas inclusion cysts contain only keratinized squamous epithelium.

Heterotopic polyodontia, or teeth outside the dental arcade, includes both dentigerous cysts, which have been described in most domestic animal species, and the **ear teeth**, or temporal teratoma, of horses. **Dentigerous cysts** contain all or part of at least one tooth (including the crown). The cysts are lined by epithelium and often cause facial swelling or draining tracts, if fistulated. In horses, dentigerous cysts are often seen in association with the wolf teeth or canine teeth of mares; in dogs, commonly of the brachycephalic breeds, with the mandibular first premolars; and in sheep, with the mandibular incisors. They may be bilateral.

Surgical removal of the cyst(s) is required, with definitive diagnosis based on subsequent histopathologic examination. Curettage of extremely large cysts with compromise of the mandible may require bone grafts.

ESOPHAGUS

Clinically significant esophageal disorders generally manifest themselves as swallowing dysfunction and regurgitation, especially when puppies or kittens are weaned and begin to eat solid food. These disorders, found predominantly in small animals, can be classified as congenital megaesophagus, vascular ring entrapment anomalies, and achalasia. **Congenital megaesophagus** is thought to result from developmental anomalies in esophageal neuromuscular innervation that controls dilation and peristalsis. In dogs, incidence is increased in Chinese Shar-Pei, Fox Terriers, German Shepherds, Great Danes, Irish Setters, Labrador Retrievers, Miniature Schnauzers, and Newfoundlands. In Fox Terriers, it is an autosomal recessive trait, whereas in Miniature Schnauzers, it is autosomal dominant. It is also seen in Siamese cats and Friesian horses. Megaesophagus may also be a component of a more diffuse congenital neuropathy, such as congenital myasthenia gravis. A laryngeal paralysis-polyneuropathy complex that often includes megaesophagus has been reported in Dalmatians and Pyrenees Mountain Dogs. Secondary megaesophagus may develop in association with hypoadrenocorticism, neoplasia, or GI or neuromuscular disorders. **Vascular ring anomalies** occur due to errors in development of the third, fourth, or sixth aortic arch and result in entrapment of the thoracic esophagus and trachea, which lead to the clinical signs. They have been described in dogs, cats, horses, cattle, and camelids. The most common anomaly is persistent right aortic arch, but aberrant right and left subclavian arteries, right ligamentum arteriosum, and double aortic arch have also been reported. In dogs, Boston Terriers, German Shepherds, and Irish Setters have higher breed incidences. In cats, a report associated persistent right aortic arch with axial skeletal abnormalities. Advanced imaging, including 3-D CT, is useful for diagnosis of specific anomalies and surgical planning. **Cricopharyngeal achalasia** is a failure of the upper esophageal sphincter (specifically, the cricopharyngeal muscle) to relax during swallowing, thereby preventing the normal passage of a food bolus from the caudal pharynx to the cranial esophagus. Cocker and Springer Spaniels appear to be at increased risk. Treatment of congenital achalasia is cricopharyngeal myectomy. Acquired achalasia is treated by addressing the inciting cause and implementing dietary management. **Lower esophageal sphincter achalasia** is considered to be a component of a more generalized esophageal motor disturbance (ie, megaesophagus) and no longer a distinct entity.

Diagnosis of an esophageal disorder is generally based on characteristic clinical signs (eg, regurgitation, ptyalism, dysphagia, aspiration pneumonia) and contrast imaging. Radiography may identify a distended, gas-filled esophagus, or fluoroscopy may identify alterations in esophageal peristalsis and swallowing. Diagnosis of the specific underlying etiology may require further testing, such as endoscopy, endocrine function testing, and elimination of myasthenia gravis. Treatment is directed at the primary etiology. Some mildly affected animals may improve over time; however, in general the prognosis is poor. Aspiration pneumonia is a frequent and often lethal complication. Frequent, elevated feedings of small quantities of a highly digestible, soft diet may be helpful. For horses, feeding a mash at chest height or full-time pasture grazing have been suggested. Owner compliance is essential for successful management. Surgical correction of vascular ring anomalies had an overall survival rate of 72% in dogs in one study, whereas all horses and camelids died or were euthanized in others. In dogs, only 30% were free of clinical signs after surgery. Persistent clinical signs included regurgitation and aspiration pneumonia. Dietary modification is often required for life.

Esophageal diverticula may involve the cervical esophagus just cranial to the thoracic inlet or be epiphrenic (just cranial to the diaphragm). Small diverticula may not cause any clinical signs. In more severe cases, clinical signs may include impaction, esophagitis, and rarely rupture and pyothorax. Treatment (if necessary) is by surgical resection. Esophageal diverticulae just cranial to the thoracic inlet may be seen in English Bulldogs due to thoracic shortening and external compression of the esophagus by other thoracic structures.

HERNIAS

A true hernia is defined as having a hernia ring, sac, and contents. Hernias of the abdominal wall are common in all domestic species and include umbilical hernias and inguinal or scrotal hernias. Hernias may be direct (through a rent in the body wall) or indirect (through an already existing ring, such as the inguinal ring or umbilical ring). Congenital hernias tend to be indirect, although direct, traumatic hernias may arise during dystocia or obstetrical manipulations. **Umbilical hernias** vary in size and may contain only fat or omentum, or in more severe cases, intestinal loops. In dogs, Weimaraners, Pekingese, Basenjis, and Airedale Terriers are overrepresented. In many cases, umbilical hernia is seen in dogs with concurrent cryptorchidism. Hereditary etiology is suspected but not proved. In cattle, the Holstein Friesian breed is overrepresented. Diagnosis in all animals is by observation of the hernia sac, palpation, ultrasonography, and possibly radiographs. Surgical closure of the body wall defect is indicated in most cases to reduce risk of future intestinal incarceration.

Inguinal or **scrotal hernias** are common in pigs, horses (particularly draft breeds and warmbloods), and many breeds of dogs and are suspected to be hereditary. Inguinal hernias can occur in bitches and may involve the uterus. Clinical signs vary from nonpainful inguinal or scrotal swelling to acute colic in horses or vomiting in dogs, particularly if the small intestine is strangulated. In horses, palpation per rectum can diagnose intestinal loops in the vaginal ring, which can be gently removed to provide relief before transport to a surgical facility. Any devitalized bowel is resected via midline celiotomy. In stallions, testis-sparing laparoscopic closure of the inguinal rings has been performed in both standing and recumbent horses with good outcome and subsequent fertility. In foals and calves, medical management through reduction of the hernia and placement of a figure-eight bandage has been successful in some cases. Hernias that do not spontaneously resolve early in life should be surgically corrected to prevent later complications.

Hernias between the abdominal and thoracic cavities that involve the diaphragm are of several types and can be congenital or acquired (traumatic) in origin. Congenital **pleuroperitoneal hernias** have been described in small animals, horses, and calves. In horses, a specific type of hernia, a retrosternal or Morgani hernia, has been described in which a hernial sac protrudes into the thorax in the left dorsal tendinous portion of the diaphragm. The sac is characterized by a pleural covering and a peritoneal lining. In described cases, the presenting complaint was colic, and the diagnosis was made during exploratory celiotomy. Defects can be surgically repaired using mesh products to reduce risk of recurrence. The hernial sac is usually left in situ. In cases of direct herniation, clinical signs include dyspnea, exercise intolerance, lethargy, and weight loss. In cattle, herniation of the reticulum into the thorax has been described, with a right-side diaphragmatic defect. Clinical signs include anorexia, scant manure, tympani, and decreased or no rumination. Diagnosis is by radiography or ultrasonography. **Peritoneopericardial hernias** are defined as an embryologic defect in the failure of fusion of the septum transversum during diaphragmatic development, allowing communication between the abdominal cavity and pericardial sac. Weimaraners and domestic long-haired cats were overrepresented in one study. Clinical signs reflect the contents of the hernia, which may include omentum, liver, gallbladder, or small intestinal loops, and include cardiac tamponade, dyspnea, tachypnea, exercise intolerance, coughing, vomiting, and GI obstruction. In many cases, the diagnosis was an incidental finding during imaging or celiotomy for other reasons. Other congenital defects were found in many cases, including umbilical hernia, cryptorchidism, cleft palate, portosystemic shunt, and sternal or vertebral abnormalities. Animals with clinical signs were treated with surgical herniorrhaphy, whereas animals with no clinical signs tended to be closely monitored. **Hiatal hernias** occur through the esophageal hiatus and are classified into four types. Type I, the sliding hernia, is the most common in small animals and is characterized by intermittent displacement of the lower esophageal sphincter and gastric fundus into the thoracic cavity. Type II is less common and involves only the displacement of the gastric fundus. Brachycephalic breeds are overrepresented, with a hereditary nature suspected in Shar-Pei. Clinical signs include dysphagia, regurgitation, vomiting, ptyalism, and esophagitis due to decreased function of the lower esophageal sphincter. Diagnosis is by radiography or fluoroscopy; however, the intermittent nature can make diagnosis challenging. Medical treatment of esophagitis is required. Surgical correction is by combination of hiatal plication, esophagopexy, and left-side gastropexy.

STOMACH

Besides hiatal hernia, the most common abnormality involving the stomach with a suspected heritable etiology is **pyloric stenosis**, which affects brachycephalic dog breeds (Boxers, Boston Terriers, English Bulldogs) and Siamese cats. Pyloric stenosis or pyloric muscular hypertrophy results from muscular thickening of the pyloric sphincter, which obstructs pyloric outflow. Clinical signs reflect delayed gastric emptying and usually manifest as vomiting of food several hours after a meal but may also include poor weight gain, aspiration pneumonia, depression, and dehydration. Diagnosis is aided by contrast imaging and endoscopy, which is often combined with biopsy to exclude neoplasia. Surgical treatment is recommended to relieve the obstruction. Medical treatment of esophagitis, acid-base abnormalities, and dehydration should be instituted before surgery.

Abomasal emptying defect of sheep is a dysautonomia characterized by functional obstruction of the pyloric sphincter, possibly due to neurotoxicity of the celicomesenteric ganglia. It is well described in Suffolk sheep with few cases reported in Hampshire, Dorset, and Texel breeds. The etiology is unknown; it may be hereditary or that certain genotypes predispose to the condition. Pedigree analysis of affected flocks does not show a simple inheritance pattern. Clinical signs include weight loss, anorexia, depression, dyspnea, decreased rumen motility, and progressive distention of the right ventral abdomen. Even with abomasotomy, the prognosis is poor to grave.

SMALL AND LARGE INTESTINE

Maldigestion or malabsorption disorders usually manifest as chronic, persistent GI signs, including vomiting, weight loss, small- and/or large-intestinal diarrhea, or a combination of the above. There are many potential etiologies, both heritable and acquired, and most are associated with inflammatory bowel disease (IBD). Congenital conditions may have specific breed predilections.

Soft-coated Wheaten Terriers have a high incidence of **protein-losing enteropathy (PLE)**, which may be seen alone or in association with **protein-losing nephropathy (PLN)**. Although the mode of inheritance is not clear, the etiopathogenesis of PLN is likely different than that of PLE, due to podocytopathy. Dogs with PLE have both food hypersensitivities and IBD, although the pathogenesis is not clear. The demonstration of increased fecal α_1-protease inhibitor concentrations can help confirm abnormal protein loss through the intestinal tract, although this is more useful as a screening test in animals <3 yr old. A definitive diagnosis is based on intestinal and renal histopathology. Despite hypoallergenic diet trials and immunosuppressive therapy directed at IBD and/or glomerulonephritis, prognosis is poor.

Gluten-sensitive enteropathy has been shown to be inherited by an autosomal recessive manner in Irish Setters. However, the pathogenesis in dogs appears to be different than that of celiac disease in people. One case has also been described in a horse. The wheat sensitivity is both confirmed and treated through use of gluten-free diets.

Basenjis have been diagnosed as carriers of a severe form of lymphocytic-plasmacytic enteritis called **Basenji enteropathy**, although the mode of inheritance is not known. The stomach may also be affected. Clinical signs include diarrhea and weight loss, with hyperglobulinemia. Diagnosis is based on histopathologic examination of GI biopsies, usually obtained through endoscopy. Treatment trials with immunosuppressive drugs and hypoallergenic diets are usually unsuccessful unless aggressively initiated early in the disease.

Lymphangiectasia is a malformation of the intestinal lymphatic system that results in a protein-losing enteropathy that may be congenital or acquired, with a 50% incidence in Norwegian Lundehunds in the USA. Other affected breeds include Yorkshire Terriers, Maltese, Rottweilers, and Shar-Pei. Lymph vessels become dilated, secreting lymph into the intestines, which results in hypoproteinemia, lymphopenia, and lipogranulomatous inflammation of surrounding tissues. It is diagnosed through exclusion of other protein-losing diseases and confirmed by histopathology of the small-intestinal wall. Most affected animals respond to a combination of dietary manipulation and anti-inflammatory doses of glucocorticoids. Diets should contain minimal fat, be energy dense, and easily digestible. Although remission of clinical signs may be achieved, the longterm outcome is usually poor.

Exocrine pancreatic insufficiency (EPI) has a higher incidence in German Shepherds and Rough Collies, although it has been diagnosed in many breeds. Disease is due to pancreatic acinar atrophy, which is due to immune-mediated destruction and infiltration of lymphocytes. In German Shepherds and Pembroke Welsh Corgis, genome-wide association studies have identified several major histocompatibility complex haplotypes associated with EPI in affected animals, suggesting a complex mode of inheritance. The lack of pancreatic enzymes results in an osmotic diarrhea, in which steatorrhea is a prominent feature.

Affected animals either fail to gain weight or, if EPI is acquired later in life, show a dramatic weight loss. Diagnosis is through measurement of serum trypsin-like immunoreactivity; validated tests are available for both dogs and cats. Treatment involves exogenous replacement of pancreatic enzymes and use of highly digestible diets.

Granulomatous colitis, previously called histiocytic ulcerative colitis, has been diagnosed in Boxers and French Bulldogs, with sporadic cases in a few other breeds. The disease is characterized by granulomatous inflammation of the colonic mucosa in association with infection with adherent and invasive *Escherichia coli*. An autosomal recessive defect in the immune system that predisposes to *E coli* infection is suspected. Clinical signs arise in animals <4 yr old and include diarrhea, hematochezia, tenesmus, and weight loss. Diagnosis is by histologic examination of colonic mucosal biopsies. Successful remission has been achieved in animals treated with enrofloxacin; however, treatment has been unsuccessful in cases in which the *E coli* was resistant to fluoroquinolones.

Ileocolonic agangliosis, or overo lethal white syndrome, occurs in white foals with blue eyes produced by Overo-Overo matings. The condition is fatal. It is due to mutation in the endothelin B receptor and is inherited in an autosomal recessive manner. Although the foals appear normal at birth, they rapidly develop signs of colic and meconium impaction due to hypoinnervation of the intestinal tract, which causes lack of motility. Diagnosis can be confirmed at necropsy by the lack of ganglia in the colon. Adult Overo horses can be screened for genetic status before breeding to reduce incidence. Congenital atresias of either the small- or large-intestinal tracts have been described in most domesticated animal species. **Atresia coli** has been reported in several foals of differing breeds. **Atresia ilei** in Swedish Highland cattle, and **atresia jejunae** in Jersey cattle are likely due to autosomal recessive inheritance. These conditions are invariably fatal. Aggressive manipulation of the bovine conceptus by transrectal palpation early in gestation (<45 days) has been implicated as a cause, although a reduction in incidence through selective breeding indicates a potential genetic predisposition as well.

Atresia ani results when the dorsal membrane separating the rectum and anus fails to rupture. Clinical signs are apparent at birth and include tenesmus, abdominal pain and distention, retention of feces, and absence of an anal opening. It is rare in dogs but has been reported in several breeds, including Toy Poodles and Boston Terriers, with an increased incidence in females. Concurrent rectovaginal fistula may occur. Euthanasia is recommended in large animals. In small animals, postoperative fecal incontinence may be a complication of surgical intervention.

Segmental aplasia of the rectum (rectal atresia) is seen when the rectum terminates in a blind pouch before reaching the anus. Surgical correction is difficult because the location of the terminal section varies, and iatrogenic damage to nerves in the area may occur.

Enteric duplications are very rare, with only a few cases described in several species, and may include the colon or rectum. Duplications may communicate with the lumen of the patent tract or be separate (duplication cyst). Affected animals may be diagnosed by identification of an abdominal mass, or they may show GI signs. Diagnosis is by ultrasonography or contrast CT. Correction is via surgical removal of the duplication, although some cases have multiple concurrent abdominal developmental anomalies that preclude complete surgical correction.

Rectourethral fistula has been reported primarily in English Bulldogs and is diagnosed clinically as simultaneous urination from both the urogenital and anal orifices along with a history of chronic urinary tract infections. Diagnosis is via cystourethroscopy with concurrent colorectal infusion of contrast material, or by contrast CT. Surgical correction is curative.

Rectovaginal fistula is a fistulous tract that connects the vagina and rectum and usually is seen in conjunction with imperforate anus. Passage of feces through the vulva is suggestive. Diagnosis may be confirmed by barium enema, which outlines the extension of the defect into the vagina, or video endoscopy. Identification of the fistula, surgical correction, and reestablishment of the normal anatomic structures are imperative. Prognosis is usually guarded. Complications are common and include fecal and urinary incontinence.

Urinary and fecal incontinence is often seen in Manx cats as a sequela of heritable spina bifida.

LIVER

Portosystemic shunts (PSSs) are the most common congenital liver anomaly (*see* p 446). PSSs typically involve single extra-hepatic or intrahepatic vessels, with extrahepatic shunts more common in toy breeds (Yorkshire Terriers, Cairn Terriers, Havanese, Maltese, Pugs, and Miniature Schnauzers), and intrahepatic shunts more common in large breeds (Irish Wolfhounds, Labrador and Golden Retrievers, Australian Cattle Dogs, and Old English Sheepdogs). They have also been reported in Himalayan and Persian cats. Commonly, extrahepatic shunts occur between the portal vein or its branches, and the caudal vena cava or azygous vein, whereas intrahepatic shunts may be due to failure of closure of the ductus venosus or connections between the portal vein branches and hepatic veins. Clinical signs generally manifest as neurologic disturbances (hepatic encephalopathy) and are usually seen in young animals. Cats may show ptyalism. In the later stages, GI signs (including vomiting, anorexia, and diarrhea) as well as ascites may develop secondary to portal hypertension. Other concurrent clinical findings may include renomegaly and urate urolithiasis. Laboratory tests may show increased liver enzymes and erythrocytic microcytosis. Abdominal ultrasonography is reported to be 100% sensitive for intrahepatic PSSs (although some what less for extrahepatic PSSs), but sensitivity depends on the skill of the ultrasonographer. Definitive diagnosis via positive-contrast portography can identify shunt location and whether the shunt is single or multiple. This procedure also allows assessment of feasibility for surgical correction. Multiple shunts have a poor prognosis, because they are often secondary to an underlying, progressive hepatic parenchymal disease (eg, cirrhosis).

Hepatoportal microvascular dysplasia is an intrahepatic circulatory disorder that results in the shunting of portal blood to the systemic circulation yet no discernible large vessel shunt is identified. The disorder has been classified as a variation of primary hypoplasia of the portal vein, which results in noncirrhotic portal hypertension. The syndrome is well defined in Cairn Terriers and Yorkshire Terriers, although it has also been reported in Maltese, Dachshunds, Toy and Miniature Poodles, Bichon Frise, Pekingese, Shih Tzus, Norfolk and Norwich Terriers, Tibetan Spaniels, Havanese, and Lhasa Apsos. Animals may be asymptomatic or show clinical signs similar to those of PSSs. Dogs that progress to clinical disease are treated medically as described for PSSs. Because there is no macroscopic shunting vessel, surgery is not a therapeutic option.

Copper-associated hepatopathy results either from a metabolic derangement of hepatic copper storage or secondary to hepatobiliary disease (mostly cholestatic disease). In Bedlington Terriers it has been identified as an autosomal recessive disorder, whereas in other breeds that have been identified as susceptible (Dalmatians, Skye Terriers, West Highland White Terriers, and Doberman Pinschers) no genetic basis has been identified. Primary copper toxicosis is very rare in cats. Affected animals may be asymptomatic or show acute signs of hepatobiliary disease, including vomiting, anorexia, depression, hemolytic anemia, and icterus. Older, chronically affected animals may show progressive end-stage liver disease. Treatment is based on dietary reduction of copper and either treatment with zinc salts to prevent GI absorption of copper in asymptomatic animals, or copper chelators to reduce copper in animals with clinical signs. Because copper chelators are not without adverse effects, treatment should be closely monitored.

Congenital hepatic cysts or **congenital hepatic fibrosis** is seen in both Persian and Persian-cross cats as an autosomal dominant trait and in the Swiss Freiberger horse (also called the Franches-Montagnes horse) as an autosomal recessive trait that can be traced back to one stallion. Both are features of a larger, polycystic organ syndrome that affects the kidneys, liver, and/or pancreas. Clinical signs in cats may not be apparent or manifest as chronic renal insufficiency. In horses, affected foals present in the first year of life with weight loss, jaundice, hepatic encephalopathy, abdominal distention, fever, and colic signs. A report of dogs with congenital hepatic fibrosis described ascites, vomiting, seizures, and portal hypertension but did not draw inferences on heritability.

Primary or idiopathic **hyperlipidemias** of dogs and cats have been reported. Miniature Schnauzers have a high prevalence of **hypertriglyceridemia**, up to 33% of animals in one study, with or without concurrent hypercholesterolemia and chylomicronemia. There was an effect of age, with higher prevalence in older animals, and a genetic basis is suspected. **Hypercholesterolemia** has been reported in Briards, Rough Collies, Shetland Sheepdogs, Doberman Pinschers, and Rottweilers. Also in dogs, a syndrome of idiopathic **hyperchylomicronemia** has been reported, with hypertriglyceridemia and normal serum cholesterol. Clinical signs may be absent or may include vomiting, diarrhea, pancreatitis, lipemia retinalis, seizures, peripheral neuropathies, and abdominal pain. Hyperlipidemias also occur secondary to other diseases, including hypothyroidism, diabetes mellitus, and hyperadrenocorticism, and treatment is aimed at the inciting disease as well as dietary modifications.

In cats, familial hyperlipidemia due to hyperchylomicronemia has been identified as due to an autosomal recessive defect in lipoprotein lipase. Secondary to this disorder, cutaneous and systemic xanthomatosis have been described, with deposition of lipid-laden macrophages in the dermis, usually around the head and ears. Peripheral neuropathy may develop secondary to nerve compression by the xanthomas, particularly on the limbs and paws.

DENTAL DEVELOPMENT

All domestic animals have a diphyodont dentition, ie, a deciduous and a permanent set of teeth. The morphology as well as the dental formula (*see* TABLE 3) of mammalian teeth, however, are variable and closely related to the animal's alimentation.

Identification of teeth was formerly based on an anatomic system in which incisors were designated as I, canines as C, premolars as P, and molars as M. Veterinary dentists now most often use the modified Triadan system, which assigns a 3-digit number to a specific tooth. The animal's head is divided into four quadrants, with the upper right quadrant labeled "1" and the remaining quadrants numbered in a counterclockwise direction. Numbers 1–4 are used to identify the quadrant for permanent teeth, and 5–8 are used for the temporary dentition. The second and third digits identify the specific tooth number; eg, in horses, the left lower second premolar is tooth "306" and the last molar on the right mandible is "411."

ESTIMATION OF AGE BY EXAMINATION OF THE TEETH

In horses, which have a hypsodont dentition, age can be estimated by the eruption times and general appearance of the (lower incisor) teeth. In other species with brachydont incisors, such as cattle and dogs, age determination is less accurate and is mostly based on dental eruption times.

Horses: The most appropriate teeth to estimate age in horses are the (lower) incisors. It must be emphasized, however, that dental appearances are subject to individual and breed variations and to differences in environmental conditions. The deciduous incisors are smaller than the permanent ones, and the surfaces of their crowns are whiter and have several small longitudinal ridges and grooves. Eruption times are listed in TABLE 4. Permanent incisors are larger and more rectangular in shape. Their crown surfaces are largely covered with cement and have a yellowish appearance. The upper incisors have two distinct longitudinal grooves on their labial surface, while the lower incisors have only one.

Equine incisor teeth develop certain wear-related macroscopic features traditionally used to estimate age. The dental star consists of yellowish brown secondary dentin that fills up the pulp cavity and appears at the occlusal surface as the tooth wears. Its shape and position, as well as the appearance of the "white spot" in its center, are related to age. The shape, size, and time of disappearance of both the infundibula or "cups" (funnel-like infoldings in the occlusal surface) and the "marks" (enamel infundibular bottoms) are additional but more variable indicators of age. Progressive dental wear causes an alteration of the occlusal shape of the incisors. The occlusal surfaces of recently erupted incisors are elliptical, but with age they subsequently become trapezoid, round, and then triangular, with the apex toward the lingual side. The curvature of the dental

TABLE 3 DENTAL FORMULAS

	Deciduous	Permanent
Horse	$2\left(\mathrm{Di}\frac{3}{3}\mathrm{Dc}\frac{0}{0}\mathrm{Dp}\frac{3}{3}\right) = 24$	$2(\mathrm{I}\frac{3}{3}\ \mathrm{C}\frac{1}{1}\ \mathrm{P}\frac{3}{3}\ \mathrm{M}\frac{3}{3}) = 36(-44)$[a,b]
Cow[c] Sheep Goat	$2\left(\mathrm{Di}\frac{0}{3}\mathrm{Dc}\frac{0}{1}\mathrm{Dp}\frac{3}{3}\right) = 20$	$2(\mathrm{I}\frac{0}{3}\ \mathrm{C}\frac{0}{1}\ \mathrm{P}\frac{3}{3}\ \mathrm{M}\frac{3}{3}) = 32$
Pig	$2\left(\mathrm{Di}\frac{3}{3}\mathrm{Dc}\frac{1}{1}\mathrm{Dp}\frac{3}{3}\right) = 28$	$2(\mathrm{I}\frac{3}{3}\ \mathrm{C}\frac{1}{1}\ \mathrm{P}\frac{4}{4}\ \mathrm{M}\frac{3}{3}) = 44$
Dog	$2\left(\mathrm{Di}\frac{3}{3}\mathrm{Dc}\frac{1}{1}\mathrm{Dp}\frac{3}{3}\right) = 28$	$2(\mathrm{I}\frac{3}{3}\ \mathrm{C}\frac{1}{1}\ \mathrm{P}\frac{4}{4}\ \mathrm{M}\frac{2}{3}) = 42$
Cat	$2\left(\mathrm{Di}\frac{3}{3}\mathrm{Dc}\frac{1}{1}\mathrm{Dp}\frac{3}{2}\right) = 26$	$2(\mathrm{I}\frac{3}{3}\ \mathrm{C}\frac{1}{1}\ \mathrm{P}\frac{3}{2}\ \mathrm{M}\frac{1}{1}) = 30$

[a] The canine teeth are usually regressed or absent in mares.

[b] Small premolars 1 (wolf teeth) are often present, especially in the upper jaw.

[c] The canine tooth of domestic ruminants has commonly been counted as a fourth incisor.

arch formed by the lower incisive tables is also age related. In young horses this arch is semicircular, whereas in older horses it forms a straight line. Additionally, the arch formed by the incisors of the opposing jaws (as they meet) changes as the teeth advance from their alveoli and undergo attrition. In young horses, the upper and lower incisors are positioned in a straight line. With increasing age, the angle between upper and lower incisors becomes more acute. The Galvayne's groove and the "7-year hook," which have traditionally been used as age indicators, are variable, inconsistent, and thus of little value for age determination in horses. The more useful signs are arranged chronologically in the following list:

Birth to 5 yr: *See* TABLE 4.

5 yr: The corners are erupting. Dental star in the central incisors.

6 yr: Dental star in the middle incisors. Cups gone from the central incisors.

7 yr: Dental star in the corners.

8 yr: The central incisors are trapezoidal and have a white spot in the dental star.

9 yr: The middle incisors are trapezoidal and have a white spot in the dental star.

10 yr: Cups gone from the middle incisors. Marks on the central incisors are oval-triangular.

11 yr: White spot in the dental star on the corners. Both the central and middle incisors have a lingual apex. The corners are triangular with a labial apex.

12 yr: Cups gone from all lower incisors.

14 yr: Marks on the central and middle incisors are small and round.

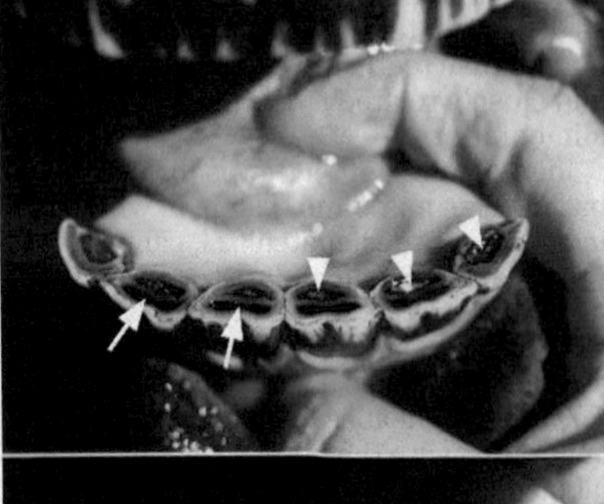

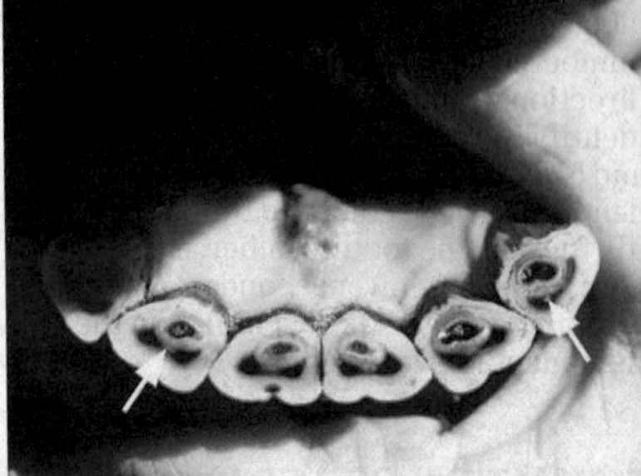

Top: occlusal view on lower incisors of a 6-yr-old mare. Dental stars are visible on I1 and I2 (arrows); cups are present as large elliptical infoldings (arrowheads). Occlusal surfaces of the incisors are oval, and curvature of the dental arch is semicircular. Bottom: occlusal view on the lower incisors of a 12-yr-old mare. In the center of the dental stars, a white spot is clearly visible (arrows). Cups have become smaller and more shallow. Occlusal surfaces are more triangular. *Courtesy of Dr. Sofie Muylle.*

TABLE 4 ERUPTION OF THE TEETH[a]

	Horse	Cow	Sheep and Goat	Pig	Dog	Cat
Di 1	0–1 wk	Before birth	0–1 wk	3–4 wk	4–5 wk	2–3 wk
Di 2	4–6 wk	Before birth	1–2 wk	2–3 mo	4–5 wk	3–4 wk
Di 3	6–9 mo	0–1 wk	2–3 wk	Before birth	3–4 wk	3–4 wk
I 1	2½ yr	2 yr	1–1½ yr	12–15 mo	4 mo	4–7 mo
I 2	3½ yr	2½ yr	1½–2 yr	16–20 mo	4½ mo	4–7 mo
I 3	4½ yr	3½ yr	2–2½ yr[b]	8–10 mo	5 mo	4–7 mo
Dc	Does not erupt	0–2 wk	3–4 wk	Before birth	3–4 wk	3–4 wk
C	4–5 yr	3½–4 yr	2½–4 yr[c]	6–10 mo	5–6 mo	4–7 mo
Dp 2	0–2 wk	0–3 wk	0–4 wk	4–6 wk	4–6 wk	5–6 wk (upper only)
Dp 3	0–2 wk	0–3 wk	0–4 wk	1½ mo	4–6 wk	5–6 wk
Dp 4	0–2 wk	0–3 wk	0–4 wk	1–5 wk	4–6 wk	5–6 wk
P 1	5–6 mo (wolf tooth)	—	—	5 mo	4–5 mo	—
P 2	2½ yr	2–2½ yr	1½–2 yr	12–15 mo	5–6 mo	4–7 mo (upper only)
P 3	3 yr	2–2½ yr	1½–2 yr	12–15 mo	5–6 mo	4–7 mo
P 4	4 yr	2½–3 yr	1½–2 yr	12–15 mo	5–6 mo	4–7 mo
M 1	9–12 mo	5–6 mo	3–6 mo[d]	4–6 mo	4–5 mo	4–7 mo
M 2	2 yr	1–1½ yr	9–12 mo	8–12 mo	5–6 mo	—
M 3	4 yr	2–2½ yr	1½–2 yr	18–20 mo	6–7 mo	—

[a] Average data, subject to considerable variation

[b] 2 yr in goats

[c] 2½–3 yr in goats

[d] 3–4 mo in sheep

18 yr: Marks disappear from the central incisors.

20 yr: Marks are gone from the middle incisors and the corners.

Cattle: Eruption times of incisors are the most reliable feature for age determination in cattle (*see* TABLE 4). Although breed-related, eruption dates are more reliable for estimation of age than signs of wear, because macroscopic age-related dental features are scarce (dental stars) or absent (cups and marks) and because rate of wear is largely influenced by nutrition.

Birth to 5 yr: *See* TABLE 4.

5 yr: All incisors in wear. Occlusal surface of the central incisors beginning to level.

6–7 yr: Central incisors are leveled and neck is visible.

8 yr: Middle incisors are leveled and neck is visible.

9–10 yr: Corners are leveled and neck is visible.

As cattle continue to age, the teeth wear shorter and more neck becomes visible; they loosen in the sockets and eventually drop out.

Dogs: The following data were found reliable in ~90% of large dogs. There is more variation in small dogs (especially toy breeds) and in dogs with undershot or overshot jaws. Even, or level, bites usually result in excessive wear.

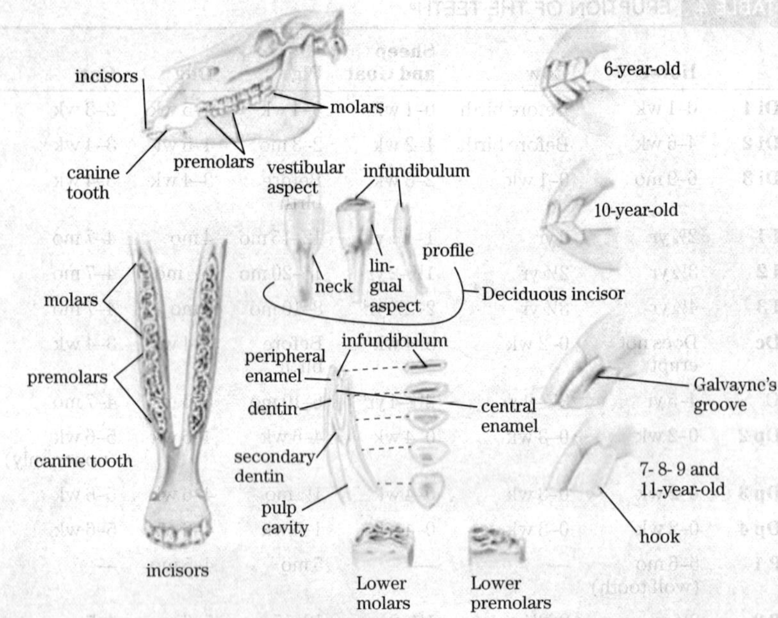

Dentition of the horse. *Illustration by Dr. Gheorghe Constantinescu.*

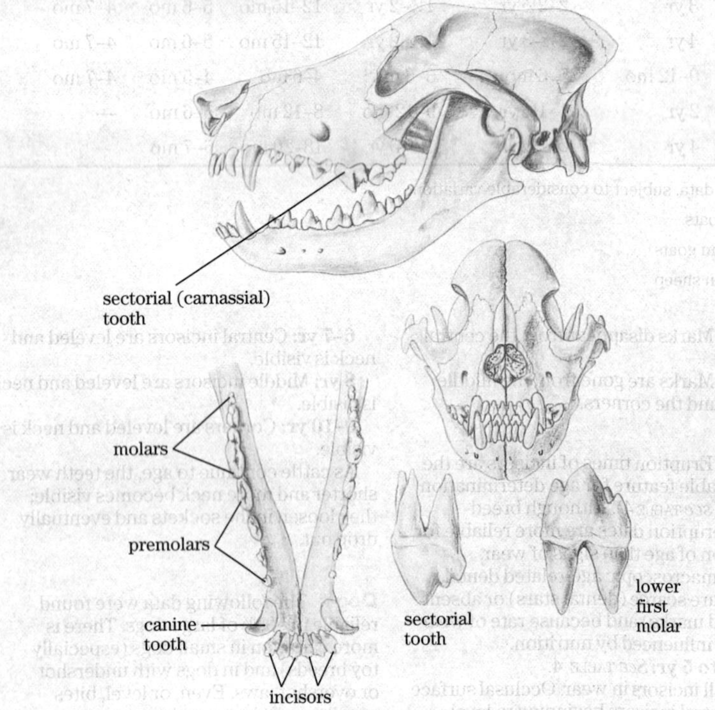

Dentition of the dog. *Illustration by Dr. Gheorghe Constantinescu.*

1½ yr: Cusps worn off lower central incisors.

1½–2½ yr: Cusps worn off lower middle incisors.

3½ yr: Cusps worn off upper central incisors.

4½ yr: Cusps worn off upper middle incisors.

5 yr: Cusps of lower corners slightly worn. Occlusal surface of lower central and middle incisors is rectangular. Slight wear of canines.

6 yr: Cusps worn off lower corners. Canines worn blunt. Lower canine shows impression of upper corner.

7 yr: Occlusal surface of lower central incisor becomes elliptical with the long axis sagittal.

8 yr: Occlusal surface of lower central incisor is inclined forward.

10 yr: Lower middle and upper central incisors have elliptical occlusal surfaces.

DENTISTRY

LARGE ANIMALS

Most large animals are herbivores, and efficient dental function is the key to food intake and to the maintenance of normal body condition. The variations in anatomic structure, dental formula, and eruption schedule for deciduous and permanent teeth is fundamental veterinary knowledge and should be reviewed before performing dentistry on any species (*see* TABLE 3).

The deciduous and permanent dental formula of cows, sheep, and goats are similar. All ruminants lack upper incisor teeth, with the mandibular brachydont (short-crowned) incisors meeting with a maxillary cornified dental pad. In many herbivore species, the forces of almost continuous grazing or rumination leads to dental attrition. Dental crown wear has been matched by the development of hypsodont (long-crowned) teeth with the continuous eruption of the reserve crown. The dental arcades in the horse consist of at least nine teeth (three incisors separated by a diastema [the interdental space], three premolars, and three molars) in each quadrant of the mouth. These hypsodont teeth have regular serrations that expose sharp enamel edges for shredding and crushing cellulose material. At the same time, the brittle nature of the enamel of the tooth is protected by the surrounding dentin and peripheral cementum. In the normal course of masticating forage, the rate of tooth eruption is matched by the rate of occlusal crown wear. Adult male horses have large permanent canine teeth situated in the interdental space. These are absent or very small in mares (sexual dimorphism).

Of the common domestic large animals, horses generally require the most dental care. In the swine industry, removal or amputation of deciduous canine teeth in piglets and tusk amputation in breeding boars may be part of routine management. In New World camelids (llamas, etc), blunting the fighting teeth (ie, the upper single incisor and canine and the lower canine teeth) is done to reduce the danger and consequences of fighting. (*See also* LLAMAS AND ALPACAS, p 1844, for additional information on dental care.) Exotic species may also have various dental conditions, eg, impacted tusks in young elephants or maxillary dental periostitis and actinomycosis in wallabies and kangaroos.

Signs of Dental Disease

Dental disease (eg, broken teeth, periodontal disease, irregular dental arcade wear) is a common underlying cause of unthriftiness, loss of condition, or poor breeding or nursing performance. The classic signs of dental disease in horses include difficulty or slowness in feeding and a reluctance to drink cold water. During the chewing process, the horse may stop for a few moments and then start again. Sometimes, the head is held to one side as if the horse were in pain. Occasionally, the horse may quid, ie, it may pick up its food, form it into a bolus but drop the bolus from the mouth after it has been partially chewed. Occasionally, the semi-chewed mass of feed may become packed between the teeth and the cheek or become lodged in the esophagus, leading to choke. To avoid using a painful tooth or a sore mouth, the horse may bolt its food and subsequently suffer indigestion, choke, or colic. There may be a lack of desire to eat hard grain accompanied by uncrushed grain in the feces. Other signs of dental disease in horses include excessive salivation and blood-tinged mucus in the mouth, accompanied by the fetid breath of dental decay. Extensive dental decay and accompanying periostitis and root abscessation may lead to empyema of the paranasal sinuses and intermittent unilateral nasal discharge. There may be facial or mandibular swelling and development of mandibular fistulas from apical infections of the lower cheek teeth.

Horses may be reluctant to take the bit, shake their head when being ridden, or resist training techniques because of irregularly worn cheek teeth and sharp edges on the maxillary cheek teeth and accompanying buccal mucosa laceration. The presence of small upper first premolar "wolf" teeth in horses may or may not be associated with resistance to the bit.

Dental Examination

In most cases, history, age, and clinical signs are correlated. A thorough physical examination should always be performed, followed by a detailed and thorough oral and dental examination. In most large animals, including horses, this may involve the use of sedation; certain animals may require general anesthesia. A thorough oral examination is facilitated by rinsing the mouth with warm water and illuminating the oral cavity with a bright headlamp while using an oral speculum. Most mouth speculums designed for horses or ponies can be modified by replacing the upper incisor plate with a flat padded gum plate for use in ruminants. A dental mirror or endoscopic camera greatly increases the quality of oral examination. The oral dental examination is often aided by radiography or other advanced imaging such as CT, scintigraphy, or MRI.

Routine Dental Prophylaxis and Extractions

Routine dental prophylaxis consisting of a complete oral dental examination and odontoplasty of sharp enamel points is important in the health care of horses. Enamel edges should be removed twice yearly during the establishment of the permanent dentition and thereafter as frequently as needed, depending on the management of the horse. Horses that graze on free range or grass usually require a yearly dental prophylaxis; horses that are stall confined and essentially fed hay and grain may require twice yearly oral examinations and dental prophylaxis.

The objective of dental prophylaxis is to remove sharp enamel edges of cheek teeth that might be causing soft-tissue irritation and any occlusal surface elongations. This odontoplasty procedure is often referred to as "floating" the teeth. By maintaining the normal occlusal surface, development of irregularities of wear on the dental arcades is inhibited. Dental prophylaxis can usually be done with simple restraint and/or the use of sedatives and analgesics. Power equipment is now being used more frequently than handheld rasps to grind, balance, and realign the occlusal surfaces of the incisors and cheek teeth. Motorized dental instruments should be used carefully to avoid thermal and pressure trauma to dentin and pulp. This means using low-speed grinders (6,000–12,000 rpm) with short contact times, light pressure, and intermittent water irrigation, while removing no more than 3–5 mm of occlusal surface every 3–6 mo.

Sharp edges on wolf teeth have been incriminated as a cause of bit resistance in horses. These small teeth, located just rostral to the upper cheek tooth row, are often extracted in performance horses. This procedure can be done in the standing, sedated horse with the aid of local infiltration anesthesia. The gingival attachment to the tooth is elevated, and a dental luxator or elevator is used to loosen the tooth. A small extraction forceps can grasp the crown and pull the tooth from its socket. Minimal aftercare or diet and work restriction are required for socket healing.

Most dental procedures can be performed on the standing, sedated horse with or without regional anesthesia, but some major dental procedures (eg, repulsions and fracture repairs) usually require general anesthesia. Radiographic evaluation and protection of the airway from debris are necessary in most cases. Some decayed teeth can be extracted per os using molar separators, extraction forceps, and elevators. However, in some cases, surgical exposure and tooth repulsion or sectioning and elevation is preferred. Tooth preservation by root end resection and endodontic therapy has demonstrated that extraction is not required in all cases of dental decay in horses.

CONGENITAL AND DEVELOPMENTAL ANOMALIES

In horses, the most commonly diagnosed oral congenital deformity is parrot mouth (class 2 malocclusion), in which the maxilla is relatively longer than the mandible. In early embryonic development, the first branchial arch extends as a solid hyaline cartilaginous rod surrounded by a fibrocellular capsule from the temporal region to the midline of the fused mandibular processes. If the first branchial arch fails to close properly in the equine fetus, tooth germ can displace and result in the formation of a dentigerous cyst in the temporal region and a draining tract from the rostral pinna of the ear. In equids and cattle, many anomalies of dental development may result from exposure to teratogenic toxins. However, underlying genetic factors should always be considered.

Dental irregularities accompany systemic fluorosis in both cattle and sheep. In the milder forms of fluorosis, only the dentition may be involved. In extreme fluorosis (eg, 40 ppm in the diet for several years), other skeletal abnormalities may be seen (phalanx fracture). (*See also* FLUORIDE POISONING, p 3075.)

Supernumerary teeth (polyodontia) are seen occasionally. In both horses and cattle, double rows of incisor teeth or extra cheek teeth may be seen. Missing teeth (oligodontia) in a dental arcade is less common and can be developmental or secondary to trauma or previous tooth removal. Treatment is determined on a case-by-case basis and may require extraction or frequent crown reduction of the unopposed teeth.

See also CONGENITAL AND INHERITED ANOMALIES OF THE TEETH, p 164.

ABNORMAL TOOTH ERUPTION

Shedding deciduous teeth can be a source of oral irritation in horses that are 2–5 yr old. Deciduous tooth caps can become loosened, displaced, or fractured, leading to problems with mastication and biting. Abnormal eruption of permanent teeth is commonly a sequela of mandibular or maxillary trauma, eg, incisor avulsion fractures in cattle and horses in which the developing dental bud of the permanent tooth is damaged by the fracture itself or by the repair process. In horses, delayed eruption or impaction of cheek teeth is a common cause of periapical infection. This particularly affects the second and third cheek tooth (premolar 3 [Triadan 07s] and premolar 4 [Triadan 08s]) in both the upper and lower arcades and is a sequela of dental overcrowding. Medial displacement of the third cheek tooth is another form of abnormal eruption due to overcrowding.

IRREGULAR WEAR OF THE DENTITION

Except for pigs, most large animals have an intermandibular space that is narrower than the intermaxillary space; ie, they are anisognathic. In horses, this, together with limited natural movement of the mandible, results in the development of enamel points on the buccal edges of the upper arcades and on the lingual edges of the lower arcades. In cattle and sheep, because the temporomandibular joint affords greater lateral movement of the mandible, such irregularities do not develop as frequently. Extreme forms of disease, however, are seen in all species and may be influenced by other skeletal deformities of the face or accompanying infections (eg, *Actinomyces* sp). Gross shear mouth may result, with exaggerated obliquity of the molar tables. It may be seen in older horses, and treatment is usually unsatisfactory. Dental care should be supplemented by special diets.

Enamel points are best treated by regular dental equilibration in horses (ie, floating). This should be done twice annually while the permanent dentition is developing; at the same time, retained caps should be removed if they cause oral ulceration or discomfort.

Wave mouth, step mouth, and rostral and caudal hooks are dental overgrowths caused by uneven wear of the teeth and are the result of local pain, dental or jaw malalignment, or missing or damaged teeth. In time, this can lead to abnormal spaces forming between the teeth (diastema), which have been shown to cause feed entrapment and secondary gum and socket disease (ie, periodontitis). Such conditions are best prevented by regular, routine dental prophylaxis. Once dental wear abnormalities are severe, results of dental procedures are usually incomplete. Although occlusal surfaces may be realigned, dental care needs to be supplemented by special dietary regimens.

PERIODONTAL DISEASE

In all animals, a degree of inflammatory change occurs during the eruption of both the deciduous and permanent teeth. However, if malocclusion occurs, severe periodontal disease is inevitable. In horses, this is a common sequela of diastema formation, oral trauma, dental fractures, and impactions, and it is usually accompanied by irregular wear.

In sheep, periodontal disease of the mandibular rostral teeth (incisors) is often referred to as broken mouth. Sometimes, the viability of grazing sheep is affected dramatically. The productive life of many farm-fed sheep is often 2 yr longer than that of range-fed animals. Little can be done to alter the progress of this disease, although dental prophylaxis and restoration of occlusal regularity of the incisor teeth has been recommended. This can be done by use of a dental grinder or a fine-bladed tooth float.

DENTAL CARIES

Infection may be introduced into the pulp chamber of the teeth by various routes, eg, hematogenous (anachoretic pulpitis), periodontal, or from direct crown insult. In horses, hypoplasia of the cementum in the enamel lakes (infundibulae) of the upper cheek teeth may predispose to infundibular caries and subsequent pulpitis and apical osteitis. Depending on the site of the infected tooth, there may be accompanying signs of maxillary sinusitis, local cellulitis, periostitis, alveolar periodontitis, and fistula formation. The pathologic features of dental decay are nonspecific. Consequently, the cause of the apical infection in a draining mandibular dental fistula in a horse or llama may be obscure. Many animals are not examined until the infection is advanced, and tooth fractures may well be secondary rather than primary. It has been suggested that, in some species (eg, the horse), the initiating feature of the establishment of apical osteitis and pulpitis is abnormal eruption and dental impaction. The cause of apical osteitis in cattle and New World camelids may be similarly influenced.

When dental decay is advanced, extraction of the affected tooth is recommended. In horses, this usually has been achieved by surgical exposure of the decayed tooth and then repulsion into the mouth. Recent experience has shown that oral extraction is possible, with careful technique, sedation, and nerve blocks, thus avoiding serious complications associated with repulsion and the use of general anesthesia. After exodontia, the socket should be cleaned carefully to remove all fragments of diseased bone and tooth. Dental acrylics, dental waxes, and wound packs should be used to ensure that the socket can heal properly by protecting it from food material. After dental extractions, the adjacent teeth gradually move to close the gap in the dental arcade. However, this process is never complete, and the occluding arcade will form a step elongation opposite the missing teeth and hooks at the ends of the opposing arcades (both rostral and caudal). Such irregularities in horses can be corrected by grinding and realigning the arcades every 6–12 mo.

Because of such complications, surgical techniques that preserve the teeth should be considered, at least for horses. The age of the animal and the specifics of local disease should be considered before contemplating root-end resection and endodontic therapy in large animals.

SMALL ANIMALS

PERIODONTAL DISEASE

Periodontal disease is infection and inflammation of the periodontium (the tissues that surround and support the teeth) due to plaque bacteria and the host's response to the bacterial insult. Gingivitis is common in dogs and cats and refers to inflammation of the gingiva in response to plaque antigen. Periodontitis is a more severe disease that involves inflammation of the periodontal ligament and alveolar bone, eventually causing loss of attachment (periodontal pocketing, gingival recession, bone resorption). Periodontitis is much more common in certain dog and cat breeds, but it can affect any individual.

Etiology and Pathogenesis: The oral cavity supports a rich bacterial microflora, much of which thrives in plaque on tooth surfaces. Bacterial plaque on the crown surface of a tooth constantly presents antigen to the marginal gingiva, stimulating an inflammatory response and resulting in gingivitis. The bacteria in plaque are predominantly nonmotile, gram-positive aerobes, including *Staphylococcus* spp and *Streptococcus* spp, but many others are also present. Although this microbiota does stimulate an immune response, the bacteria in an otherwise healthy mouth exist in relative commensal harmony with the host. They may even be beneficial by helping to limit the numbers of periodontopathogenic bacteria. If the plaque becomes very thick because of poor oral hygiene and oxygen within the plaque is depleted, the bacterial population can become more pathogenic, with a higher percentage of nonmotile, gram-negative anaerobic rods. The bacteria found in the presence of teeth with periodontal disease include *Bacteroides fragilis*, *Peptostreptococcus*, *Porphyromonas gulae*, *Porphyromonas salivosa*, *Porphyromonas denticanis*, *Prevotella intermedia*, *Treponema* spp, *Bacteroides splanchnicus*, and many others. Interestingly, some of the common human periodontopathogens such as *Haemophilus* (formerly *Actinobacillus*) *actinomycetemcomitans* are notably absent in animals. Subgingival plaque (plaque on the tooth surface below the gingival margin) is also commonly inhabited by these more periodontopathogenic species of bacteria. Periodontitis is caused by the host's response to subgingival plaque. Inflammatory mediators produced by the host directly result in bone and tissue damage around the root. The bacteria themselves and their metabolic products also contribute to the bone damage. Development of periodontitis is also affected by other intrinsic (eg, genetics, tooth crowding, thin alveolar bone, age) and extrinsic (eg, diet, stress, concurrent disease, oral hygiene) factors.

Clinical Findings and Lesions: Periodontal disease is classified in stages. In teeth with healthy periodontal tissues, no gingivitis or periodontitis is evident.

Stage 1: There is gingivitis only, without attachment loss; the height and architecture of the alveolar margin are normal.

Stage 2: There is early periodontitis with <25% of attachment loss or, at most, there is a stage 1 furcation involvement in multirooted teeth (*see* below). There are early radiographic signs of periodontitis. The loss of periodontal attachment is <25% as measured by probing of the clinical attachment level or by radiographic determination of the distance of the alveolar margin from the cementoenamel junction relative to the length of the root.

Stage 3: There is moderate periodontitis, with 25%–50% of attachment loss as measured by probing of the clinical attachment level or by radiographic determination of the distance of the alveolar margin from the cementoenamel junction relative to the length of the root, or there is a stage 2 furcation involvement in multirooted teeth (*see* below).

Stage 4: There is advanced periodontitis, with >50% of attachment loss as measured by probing of the clinical attachment level or by radiographic determination of the distance of the alveolar margin from the cementoenamel junction relative to the length of the root, or there is a stage 3 furcation involvement in multirooted teeth (*see* below).

A stage 1 furcation involvement exists when a periodontal probe extends less than halfway under the crown in any direction of a multirooted tooth with attachment loss. A stage 2 furcation involvement exists when a periodontal probe extends greater than halfway under the crown of a multirooted tooth with attachment loss but not through and through. A stage 3 furcation involvement exists when a periodontal probe extends under the crown of a multirooted tooth, through and through from one side of the furcation out the other.

A stage 0 mobility up to 0.2 mm is physiologic. A stage 1 mobility is present when tooth mobility is increased in any direction other than axial over a distance of >0.2 mm and up to 0.5 mm. A stage 2 mobility is present when tooth mobility is increased in any direction other than axial over a distance of >0.5 mm and up to 1 mm. A stage 3 mobility is present when tooth mobility is increased in any direction other than axial over a distance >1 mm or any axial movement.

Treatment: Removal of the bacterial plaque on the tooth surfaces is of utmost importance. This can reverse gingivitis, returning the gingiva to a healthy, uninflamed state. This is achieved through professional dental cleaning (scaling and polishing) with power and hand instruments under general anesthesia. Dental cleaning on an awake animal improves the cosmetic appearance of the tooth crowns but does not improve periodontal health. The owner might falsely believe the condition has been treated, while periodontal disease continues to thrive. If the gingivitis does not resolve, further examination should be performed to identify additional complicating conditions such as persistent subgingival plaque and calculus or the presence of predisposing factor(s). Some less common causes of gingivitis, including systemic disease (eg, uremic stomatitis), autoimmune disease, juvenile gingivitis, etc, may require more than only plaque removal.

Periodontitis requires more aggressive periodontal treatment. Root scaling (removing plaque and calculus on exposed root surfaces) and planing (smoothing the root surfaces by removing textural irregularities and diseased cementum) are performed, followed by gingival curettage that removes the infected and inflamed inside layer of a periodontal pocket. Shallow periodontal pockets are treated in a closed fashion, but pockets >6 mm deep require open surgery (creation of a periodontal flap) to expose the root surface and alveolar bone for adequate treatment (root scaling/planing and alveoloplasty). The connective tissue side of the flap needs to be debrided before wound closure to avoid contact of infected and inflamed granulation tissue with the planed root surfaces. Local placement of a gel containing antibiotics (eg, doxycycline) into cleaned periodontal pockets may be helpful. Extraction is often the best treatment for teeth with increased mobility that have a guarded to poor prognosis. Periodontitis is not as readily reversible as gingivitis. Lost bone may be augmented by use of bone grafts or bone graft substitutes. Barrier membranes should be placed between the bone defect and gingival tissues to achieve guided tissue regeneration. Maxillary canine teeth with pockets on their palatal side that have already progressed to form an oronasal fistula require extraction and oronasal fistula repair. Deep infrabony defects in multirooted teeth with bone loss that undermines a furcation can infect the pulp through a furcation canal, resulting in secondary endodontic disease. Similarly, if periodontitis has progressed apically and reached the apex of the root of a tooth, secondary endodontic disease will develop. Saving such teeth also requires endodontic therapy (*see* below), and the prognosis is determined by the extent of periodontal disease.

Teeth that have become mobile because of loss of attachment should be extracted. They can sometimes be saved through major periodontal surgery procedures, but disease will recur without drastic changes in home oral hygiene. Extraction allows the tissues to heal. A pet dog or cat can function perfectly fine without teeth.

Prevention: Prevention of gingivitis is the same as its treatment: plaque removal and control. Plaque is a typical biofilm, composed of many microorganisms that differ from their planktonic forms. In a biofilm, microorganisms are more resistant to antibiotics, disinfectants, and antibacterial agents. However, biofilms are easily and effectively removed mechanically with a toothbrush. Even large accumulations of supragingival plaque are easily removed by toothbrushing. The teeth should be brushed daily to remove plaque and prevent calculus (tartar) accumulation. Some dogs and cats may not allow regular toothbrushing, so the plaque should be removed by wiping with a gauze pad at least every second or third day. Only the outside (labial and buccal) surfaces of the teeth may be approachable for brushing in most dogs and cats. Plaque that remains on the tooth surface for >3 days mineralizes to form calculus that cannot be removed by brushing. Although calculus gives the appearance of unhealthy teeth, its contribution to periodontal disease is minor.

Texture of the diet, toys, and treats can affect the self-cleansing mechanisms of the teeth. Firm, fibrous items that allow tooth penetration can wipe plaque from the tooth surfaces during chewing. In addition to texture, some diets are formulated to include ingredients that help decrease oral bacteria or slow plaque mineralization.

Products that slow or prevent the attachment of pellicle or the adhesion of pioneering plaque bacteria may provide some benefit. The Veterinary Oral Health Council website (www.vohc.org) provides further information about products that meet certain requirements for plaque and/or calculus control.

Prevention of periodontitis is more complicated. Regular oral hygiene to remove supragingival plaque provides some protection to help prevent development of subgingival plaque and to minimize the number of periodontopathogens in the mouth. More importantly, predisposing factors should be identified and removed. Severe crowding can be relieved through selective extractions, predisposing anatomy can be modified, diabetes or renal failure can be treated and controlled, and inappropriate behaviors or parafunctional habits that damage the tissues can be addressed.

ENDODONTIC DISEASE

Etiology and Pathogenesis: Endodontic disease occurs when the dental pulp (odontoblasts, fibroblasts, undifferentiated mesenchymal cells, blood vessels, and nerves in the center of the tooth) becomes infected and/or inflamed. The pulp is protected from bacteria by the impervious enamel covering the dentin of the crown. Damage to the enamel, either through trauma or from a developmental abnormality that allows bacteria to reach the pulp, will result in pulpitis and possibly pulp necrosis. Blunt trauma can also injure the pulp beyond its ability to heal. A tooth with direct exposure of the pulp at a fracture site requires endodontic treatment or extraction. Teeth are fractured from external trauma (eg, catching rocks, automobile impacts, aggressive play) or from biting on inappropriate objects (eg, real bones regardless of the state of processing, hooves, antlers, hard nylon toys, rocks, fences, or cages). An inflamed or dead pulp releases inflammatory mediators into the periradicular tissues (through furcation canals into the periodontal ligament at the furcation of a multirooted tooth, through lateral canals into the periodontal ligament at the mid-root level, and through apical foramina into the periapical tissues). The tissues surrounding the apex of a tooth develop a periapical granuloma, cyst, or abscess.

Clinical Findings and Lesions: A discolored tooth (pinkish, purple, or gray) is evidence of previous trauma and hemorrhage from the pulp into the dentinal tubules. An inflamed pulp can heal after a minor injury. However, more severe trauma will cause irreversible pulpitis, eventually leading to pulp necrosis. Because dental pulp has no collateral circulation, injuries heal less readily, and extravasated blood remains in the dentin, where it deteriorates rather than being removed. The most obvious indication of endodontic disease is a fractured tooth with exposure of the pulp chamber. The exposed pulp bleeds for only a short time. After the initial injury, it may appear as a red dot at the site of the exposure if the pulp remains vital, or as a black hole if it becomes necrotic. Either way, treatment is required. Drainage is most commonly through the fracture site. However, a periapical abscess can occur if the site becomes occluded. The skin ventral to the medial canthus of the eye is a common site for swelling and purulent drainage from a fistula due to an endodontically diseased maxillary fourth premolar. This can also cause an intraoral red draining fistula near the mucocutaneous junction adjacent to the tooth. An abscessed maxillary canine tooth in dogs can cause swelling along the side of the nose; in cats, the swelling is often immediately rostral to the eye. Veterinary patients often do not give an indication of discomfort, even for conditions that cause severe orofacial pain in people.

On a radiograph of a tooth with a periapical granuloma or cyst, the typical lesion presents as a periapical lucency, ie, an irregular circular lesion with decreased radiopacity around a root tip. A tooth with an acute periapical abscess (painful accumulation of pus around the apex of a nonvital tooth) may not show distinct radiographic signs. Throughout life, the pulp produces dentin on the inside surface of the pulp cavity, resulting in a constantly decreasing cross-sectional width of the pulp chamber in the crown and root canal in the root of the tooth. A necrotic pulp discontinues its normal dentin production, and thus it falls behind that of a normally maturing tooth adjacent to it or on the contralateral side. Conversely, an inflamed pulp produces dentin at an accelerated rate. If there is generalized pulpitis, the effect can be an apparent accelerated aging of the entire tooth with an abnormally narrow root canal space and pulp chamber. Generally, when evaluating a tooth with endodontic and/or periapical disease, the focus should be on structural defects at its crown and root apex, the width of its pulp cavity, and the appearance of the periapical tissues.

Treatment: Teeth with irreversible pulpitis or pulp necrosis require either endodontic treatment (root canal therapy) or extraction. Except in very young animals, one of these options is indicated for every tooth in which a fracture has exposed the pulp chamber. Canine teeth in dogs and cats and carnassial teeth (maxillary fourth premolars and mandibular first molars) in dogs are considered strategic teeth. Root canal therapy of these teeth is much more comfortable for the animal than extraction; it also allows continued function. Military, police, and assistance dogs may require fabrication and placement of a full or partial prosthodontic crown.

TOOTH RESORPTION

(Resorptive lesion, Cervical lesion, Neck lesion, Feline odontoclastic resorption lesion)

Resorption of tooth structure occurs through the action of odontoclasts—cells virtually identical to osteoclasts. It can occur on the external or internal tooth surface (external or internal resorption). Odontoclast activity can be stimulated by inflammation, pressure from adjacent structures, orthodontic tooth movement, as a result of normal processes such as exfoliation of deciduous teeth, or in the absence of these processes (idiopathic). This idiopathic tooth resorption occurs sporadically in many species (including people), but it is most frequently seen in domestic cats.

Etiology and Pathogenesis: Tooth resorption in cats begins with a loss of the normal periodontal ligament architecture and focal damage to the cementum that covers the root surface. Microscopic areas of root resorption often repair uneventfully in cats. Tooth resorption from any cause occurs through the action of odontoclasts that remove tooth structure, creating a resorptive lacuna. In many but not all lesions, concomitant osteoblast and cementoblastic activity replaces the lost tooth with bone or cementum. If repair does not occur, the resorption progresses into dentin and extends coronally into the crown of the tooth where it undermines the enamel to cause clinically apparent defects on the tooth surface (at the "neck" of the tooth). Inflammation from periodontitis is known to cause external resorption and is most likely responsible for tooth resorption in areas of periodontal disease. However, the etiology of idiopathic tooth resorption affecting multiple (possibly all) teeth in cats has not yet been proved. Excessive intake of dietary vitamin D has been hypothesized as one possible cause among many others.

Clinical Findings and Lesions: The clinical appearance of tooth resorption greatly varies. In cats, the mandibular third premolar (the first cheek tooth) is often the first tooth affected. In dogs, premolar and molar teeth are most commonly involved. Small lesions on the enamel of the tooth crown usually begin somewhere on the root surface but can progress coronally and then appear at the gingival margin as inflamed granulation tissue filling a defect. The margin of the defect has a sharp ledge of enamel. At this stage, the visible part of the lesion is small, with most of the defect affecting the roots. Tooth resorption is characterized by severity (stage) and radiographic appearance (type).

Stage 1 lesions affect the cementum or cementum and enamel but have not yet progressed into the dentin.

Stage 2 lesions affect the dentin but have not yet progressed into the pulp cavity.

Stage 3 lesions affect the pulp cavity, but most of the tooth retains its integrity.

Stage 4 lesions have significant crown or root damage, with most of the tooth having lost its integrity.

Stage 5 lesions have remnants of dental hard tissue visible only as irregular radiopacities, and gingival covering is complete.

Lesions are categorized radiographically as type 1 when a focal or multifocal radiolucency is present in the tooth with otherwise normal radiopacity and normal periodontal ligament space (inflammatory resorption), type 2 when there is narrowing or disappearance of the periodontal ligament space (dentoalveolar ankylosis) in at least some areas and decreased radiopacity of part of the tooth (replacement resorption, moth-eaten "ghost" roots), or type 3 when features of both type 1 and type 2 are present in the same tooth.

Tooth resorption lesions exposed to the oral cavity may cause discomfort. Lesions limited to root surfaces only are unlikely to cause discomfort or other clinical signs unless they are associated with resorption of bone adjacent to the tooth resorption (eg, resorption caused by painful inflammation from periodontal or endodontic disease).

Diagnosis: Marginal gingivitis of individual teeth in the absence of periodontitis may indicate an early subgingival lesion. Lesions under the gingival margin can be identified by sharp dental exploration. Larger lesions are identified by their typical appearance on the tooth surface. Internal resorption may sometimes appear as pinkish discoloration of the crown but usually is only identifiable radiographically as round to oval-shaped areas of decreased radiopacity.

Treatment and Prevention: Most teeth affected with resorptive lesions should be extracted. Surgical crown amputation with intentional retention of already resorbing dental tissues can be performed on teeth that are radiographically confirmed to be type 2 lesions in the absence of periodontitis, endodontic disease, and stomatitis (*see* p 361). Oral hygiene prevents inflammatory lesions caused by marginal periodontitis, and root canal therapy or extraction of endodontically involved teeth prevents resorption caused by apical periodontitis. Idiopathic lesions cannot be prevented, because their etiology is unknown.

DEVELOPMENTAL ABNORMALITIES

Proper growth and development of the oral cavity depends on a series of events that must occur normally and in the proper sequence. Genetic abnormalities or trauma that affects either the developing tissues or the timing of their development can cause abnormalities. Defects that decrease comfort, health, or function require treatment; those that result in only an esthetic problem do not. Common developmental problems include persistent deciduous teeth, unerupted teeth, malformed teeth, malocclusion, and malformed jaws.

Persistent Deciduous Teeth

Deciduous teeth of kittens and puppies are designed to function in a small mouth (fewer in number and smaller in size) and for a temporary period. Dental trauma during this time of energetic oral exploration is often compensated for by the exfoliation of the damaged teeth as the permanent teeth erupt. The permanent teeth are larger and more numerous, erupting as the jaws lengthen to accommodate them.

Exfoliation of deciduous teeth is a complex process, part of which involves pressure exerted by the crown of the subjacent permanent tooth against the root of the deciduous tooth. If the permanent tooth does not erupt in the correct position, the deciduous tooth may remain firmly in position. This may be due to hypodontia with no succedaneous permanent tooth, a genetically malpositioned permanent tooth bud, or traumatic displacement of the tooth bud. Persistence of a deciduous tooth in areas of wide tooth spacing may not cause a problem. However, if the deciduous tooth causes crowding with the permanent tooth (often the case with canine teeth in dogs), then the area is predisposed to periodontitis. Additionally, the displaced permanent tooth can itself result in traumatic occlusion that requires treatment. Timing of deciduous tooth exfoliation and permanent tooth replacement are genetically determined. In rare cases, trauma during tooth development can cause displacement of a tooth bud that affects exfoliation.

Most commonly, two canine teeth (one deciduous and one permanent) are present at the same time. The permanent maxillary canine tooth erupts mesial ("rostral") to the deciduous one, giving the appearance of a wider and more blunt canine tooth rostral to a narrower one with a sharper cusp. The permanent mandibular canine tooth erupts lingual ("medial") to the deciduous one, giving the appearance of a wider and more blunt canine tooth toward the tongue next to a narrower one with a sharper cusp positioned toward the lip. In the premolar area, it is common to *see* a deciduous tooth in an area with no simultaneous permanent tooth. A smaller than normal premolar should be radiographed for evaluation of its anatomy and root structure to determine whether it is a deciduous tooth.

A deciduous tooth should be extracted when it remains firmly attached (no mobility) after its successor permanent tooth has erupted. Persistent deciduous teeth that do not have a permanent tooth replacement may be left in place if the roots are strong. However, radiographs should be taken to verify there are no embedded or impacted permanent teeth at the site and that the roots are not being resorbed.

Because most persistent deciduous teeth are genetic, pets with this problem should not be bred unless the condition is known to have been caused by trauma.

Unerupted Teeth

Tooth eruption is genetically programmed. Some breeds, particularly small breeds (eg, Maltese), are predisposed to delayed or incomplete eruption. Some brachycephalic breeds are predisposed to malpositioned first premolar teeth that remain unerupted because of their abnormal position. Trauma can also move a tooth bud into a position in which it is unable to erupt because of impact against another structure.

In some breeds (particularly the terrier breeds), missing premolars are considered a variation of normal. But in most animals, an edentulous area where there should be a tooth is an indication for radiography. An unerupted tooth is easily identified. Embedded refers to an unerupted tooth covered in bone, the eruption of which is compromised by lack of eruptive force. Impacted refers to an unerupted or partially erupted tooth, the eruption of which is prevented by contact with a physical barrier.

Teeth that are incompletely erupted with a persistent gingival covering can be treated with operculectomy (a form of gingivectomy) to sculpt the tissue to a normal architecture. Individual teeth that are completely unerupted after maturity may remain quiet and require only monitoring. However, they can also form dentigerous cysts that can destroy large areas of the jaws. Mandibular first premolars are significantly predisposed to cyst formation, particularly in brachycephalic breeds. For that reason, any missing mandibular first premolar should always be radiographed; any that are discovered should be removed or closely monitored with periodic radiographs. Other unerupted teeth should be removed if they cause a problem. Surgical removal of deeply unerupted mandibular canine teeth can be challenging.

Animals with unerupted teeth should not be bred unless it is known the condition was caused by trauma.

Malformed Teeth

Any interruption during tooth formation can result in a deformed tooth. The insult can be traumatic, metabolic, infectious, or rarely genetic. Insults to epitheliogenesis (eg, parvovirus, distemper virus, high fever) that occur during amelogenesis causes enamel hypoplasia or hypomineralization. Insults to dentin formation can cause deformed or missing roots.

Enamel abnormalities can be regional, with circumferential lines of missing enamel (rough surface with staining), or generalized with complete loss of enamel. Radicular dysgenesis can present with relatively normal appearing crowns that are mobile. The lack of roots is readily identified on radiographs. An interesting individual tooth abnormality that appears to be genetic is convergent roots of the mandibular first molar. This anomaly less commonly affects other teeth. The crown may appear normal, or it may have a small developmental groove on the buccal surface extending from the gingival margin. On a radiograph, the roots converge apically instead of having their normal divergent position. The crown sometimes appears too large in relation to the size of the roots. The convergence causes the floor of the pulp chamber to arch dorsally into the main pulp chamber, giving it the radiographic appearance of a "dens-in-dente" or dens invaginatus. These teeth commonly have a communication from the periodontal ligament to the pulp chamber in the furcation area, resulting in an extremely high rate of endodontic disease. Many other individual tooth anomalies are seen occasionally, such as supernumerary teeth, twinning and fusion of teeth, supernumerary roots, and "peg" teeth (short cylindrical teeth).

Enamel hypoplasia or hypomineralization is treated with early dentin sealant to prevent bacterial ingress to the pulp. Composite resin veneers can also protect the softer dentin from abrasion and provide a smooth surface on which plaque is less able to form, but they will eventually wear or chip. Root dysgenesis carries a poor longterm prognosis. The teeth can be maintained for years with strict oral care and avoidance of any dental trauma or overuse. Individual anomalous teeth should be evaluated for associated pathology; many cause no problem and do not require treatment.

Malformed teeth are the result of trauma, infections, or genetics. Routine caution and care during tooth development prevents most of them.

Malocclusion and Malformed Jaws

Malocclusion is nearly always genetic; however, trauma during development can interfere with normal growth. Maxillary length is easier to manipulate than mandibular length through selective breeding. As a result, a preference for longer faces and noses inadvertently selects for mandibular distocclusion (ie, overbite, or lower jaw appears shorter than upper jaw), whereas selecting for a "blockier" head or shorter nose results in mandibular mesioclusion (ie, underbite, or lower jaw appears longer than upper jaw). The upper and lower jaws develop at different rates, making the timing of tooth eruption critical. If the jaws have an abnormal relationship to each other at the time the permanent teeth gain enough height to occlude, then the dentition is locked into the abnormal position. If this occurs unilaterally, it can allow continued jaw lengthening on one side while arresting it on the other side, resulting in a mismatch of the central incisor midlines (ie, asymmetric skeletal malocclusion such as "wry" bite).

The most common maxillary-mandibular discrepancy is a horizontal symmetric skeletal malocclusion, resulting in mandibular mesioclusion (class 3 malocclusion) or mandibular distoclusion (class 2 malocclusion). The latter problem often causes traumatic occlusion when the mandibular canine teeth impact against the most rostral hard palate. Linguoversion of the mandibular canines often accompanies this problem, because they can be directed palatally as they erupt along the palatal surface of the maxillary canines. Individual tooth malposition (dental malocclusion or class 1 malocclusion) can also be genetic, such as mesioversion of the canine teeth (ie, "lance projection") in Dachshunds and Shetland Sheepdogs.

During the deciduous dentition period, interceptive orthodontics can be performed by selectively extracting deciduous teeth. If there is dental interlock, then extracting locked teeth can allow the jaws to grow to their genetic potential. Deciduous rostral crossbite can be treated by extraction of the deciduous maxillary incisors. This not only relieves the interlock but also encourages the permanent incisors to erupt in a more labial angle (they normally erupt on the palatal side of the deciduous incisors) to help correct the malocclusion. Likewise, deciduous mandibular distoclusion can be treated by extraction of the deciduous mandibular canine teeth. Again, this not only relieves the dental interlock but also encourages the permanent mandibular canine teeth to erupt in a more labial angle (they normally erupt on the lingual side of the deciduous canines) to help correct the malocclusion. Whenever deciduous teeth are extracted, touching the tooth bud of the developing permanent teeth must be avoided so as not to damage the enamel organs or developing enamel. This damage can cause brown spots on the crowns of permanent teeth due to focal enamel defects. Instruments should not be inserted on the palatal side of deciduous maxillary incisors or on the lingual side of deciduous mandibular canines. Even with proper technique, enamel damage can occur, because the enamel epithelium can be tugged as the deciduous tooth is extracted from the alveolus.

Mandibular mesioclusion in the permanent dentition is considered normal for many brachycephalic breeds and does not require treatment unless it results in traumatic occlusion. If the mandibular canines impact against the palatal aspect of the third or second maxillary incisors, then extraction of the maxillary incisors in contact will create a wide diastema into which the canine tooth can fit, resolving the problem. The rostral crossbite (ie, maxillary incisors positioned lingual to the mandibular incisors) rarely causes discomfort or health problems. In contrast, mandibular distoclusion often requires orthodontic or surgical intervention. Canine teeth can be moved into a nontraumatic (not always normal) position that is comfortable and functional. Alternatively, the tooth can be shortened and the pulp treated with vital pulp therapy. This approach requires sterile technique to avoid introduction of infection into the pulp and followup radiographs throughout life to monitor the need for definitive endodontic treatment.

Only animals with a normal, healthy occlusion should be bred.

DENTOFACIAL TRAUMA

Teeth and jaws play a prominent role in the interaction of animals with their environment. This predisposes them to traumatic injury, most commonly fights with other animals, automobile impacts, getting caught on fences, or falling onto hard surfaces. Mandibles can also suffer spontaneous pathologic fractures due to severe periodontitis around the mandibular first molars or to neoplasia.

A fractured tooth with a red or black spot in the center of an irregular crown surface indicates pulp exposure. A missing tooth after trauma might be avulsed or may be fractured with retained root fragments, which can be determined radiographically. Fractured mandibles cause acute malocclusion and inability to eat. The midline of the mandible is usually displaced toward the side of the fracture. The mouth may be held open, particularly in bilateral mandibular fractures.

Fractured teeth are treated as described above (*see* p 181). Avulsed teeth can be replaced if treated promptly (within hours). The owner should immediately place the tooth in a tooth transport medium or milk, without touching the root. The alveolus and root surface should be gently flushed with lactated Ringer's solution to remove dirt, and then the tooth placed into the alveolus and stabilized for 1 mo with interdental wiring. Rigid stabilization with acrylic or composite is less ideal for the periodontal ligament repair because it encourages ankylosis, but it may be a good idea to protect against abuse of the recently replaced tooth. Root canal therapy is done when the fixator is removed.

Soft-tissue trauma is repaired using primary closure with absorbable sutures. Oral soft tissues are vascular and heal quickly. Oral flushes with dilute chlorhexidine solution every 2 days helps decrease oral bacteria during healing.

Maxillary fractures can be stabilized with wire and sutures. Mandibular fractures can be more challenging; when possible, they can be repaired with interdental wiring and an intraoral splint made of bis-acryl composite resin. Other options include tape muzzling, cerclage wiring, interarch splinting, intraosseus wiring, external skeletal fixation, or miniplates. Preserving normal occlusion is important. With rigid stabilization, the pet can usually readily eat soft food until the appliance is removed in 6–8 wk.

Caudal mandibular body fractures in the area of or caudal to diseased molars requiring extraction are much more problematic because of the lack of teeth on both sides of the fracture and the thinner bone caudal to the body of the mandible. Plates can be used, but the prognosis is guarded. Interarch splinting (ie, between the upper dental arch to the lower dental arch) can be successful, but there is a risk of aspiration while the splint is in place if the animal vomits. A feeding tube is used until the splint is removed.

DENTAL CARIES

Dental caries, or bacterial infections of the teeth, are common in people, uncommon in dogs, and essentially nonexistent in cats. This may be related to the fact that human saliva is more acidic, human teeth contain many pits and fissures, and the human diet is rich in highly refined carbohydrates. The saliva of dogs and cats is more alkaline than that of people, their teeth contain fewer pits and fissures, and their diet is less rich in carbohydrates. Furthermore, cariogenic bacteria are less common in the mouths of dogs and cats than in those of people. The initial lesion of caries is acidic demineralization of the enamel. This is accomplished by cariogenic bacteria that ferment sugar, thus releasing acids onto the tooth surface.

In dogs, caries usually occurs on the occlusal surfaces of molar teeth. It has the appearance of a brown to black cavitated lesion with a soft surface into which a sharp explorer tip can penetrate and "stick."

The carious tooth structure must be removed using a dental bur until healthy dentin is reached. A radiograph should be taken to determine whether the infection has spread to the pulp, in which case the tooth also requires root canal therapy. The missing tooth structure is then restored using either composite or amalgam.

Dogs that have had dental caries are predisposed to additional lesions; topical treatment with a stannous fluoride product every 2 wk may help prevent future caries in these animals. Because dogs do not expectorate, they swallow any medications used. Therefore, only small amounts should be placed on the occlusal surfaces of the teeth. Fluoride can cause gastritis, and it can be nephrotoxic if significant amounts are ingested.

PHARYNGEAL PARALYSIS

Pharyngeal paralysis may be the result of a central or peripheral nervous system disorder or may develop secondary to severe local disease that may cause collapse, obstruction, or malfunction of the pharynx. Of the CNS disorders, rabies (*see* p 1302) is the most important of the viral causes of encephalomyelitis, although perhaps not the most frequent. CNS intoxication, lead poisoning, cranial trauma, intracranial abscessation, and neoplasia may also result in pharyngeal paralysis in many species.

Peripheral causes of pharyngeal paralysis include pharyngeal trauma and abnormalities of the pharyngeal adnexa, particularly involving the guttural pouch of horses. Disorders of the guttural pouch resulting in pharyngeal paralysis include guttural pouch mycosis, guttural pouch empyema, guttural pouch neoplasia, and osteoarthropathy of the temporohyoid joint. Equine protozoal myeloencephalitis (*see* p 1309) can also cause pharyngeal paralysis in some horses. The degree of pharyngeal paralysis ranges from complete to incomplete, depending on whether the abnormality is unilateral or bilateral or central versus peripheral. Unilateral lesions may result in partial pharyngeal malfunction. For example, horses with guttural pouch disease may be able to swallow but may still develop clinical signs of dysphagia (eg, nasal discharge of food or water, coughing).

Clinical Findings and Lesions: Clinical signs of pharyngeal paralysis include dysphagia with oral or nasal discharge of food, water, or saliva. Other clinical signs include coughing, dyspnea, ptyalism, or bruxism. Affected animals are at risk of inhalation pneumonia, dehydration, and cardiovascular and respiratory shock. Affected animals frequently have one or more signs, including pyrexia, coughing, retching, and signs compatible with esophageal obstruction. Severely affected animals may die or should be considered for euthanasia. Animals with dyspnea may require an emergency tracheostomy before any clinical diagnostic techniques can be performed.

Diagnosis: The history and clinical signs are usually indicative of pharyngeal paralysis. A baseline CBC and biochemistry profile should be performed. Affected animals typically may be hemoconcentrated, have electrolyte and acid-base disturbances, and may exhibit prerenal azotemia. Serology, skull radiographs, thoracic radiographs to evaluate for aspiration pneumonia, endoscopy, ultrasonography, CT, and MRI (if available) are all valuable aids to determine whether the underlying cause is central or peripheral. The use of CT and MRI has particular value in evaluating CNS causes of pharyngeal paralysis in small animals. Animals suspected of having rabies should be handled appropriately (*see* p 1302).

Treatment: Treatment protocols for pharyngeal paralysis vary depending on the underlying cause. Treatment generally includes the administration of antimicrobial and anti-inflammatory medications. Because of the inability to swallow normally, IV administration is preferred. Animals with hemoconcentration should be administered IV fluids. If the animal is unable to eat without aspiration, extraoral or parenteral nutrition should be strongly considered. Extraoral alimentation with pharyngostomy, esophagostomy, or nasogastric tubes or temporary rumenostomy in ruminants can be an economical and effective way to provide nutritional support. Other treatments include local therapy for pharyngeal abscesses.

The prognosis for pharyngeal paralysis varies with the instigating cause. The prognosis for pharyngeal abscessation can be favorable, whereas the prognosis for guttural pouch disease can be guarded. If affected animals do not improve after 4–6 wk of symptomatic therapy, the prognosis is poor and euthanasia should be considered.

DISEASES OF THE RECTUM AND ANUS

ANAL SAC DISEASE

Anal sac disease is the most common disease entity of the anal region in dogs. Small breeds are predisposed; large or giant breeds are rarely affected. In cats, the most common form of anal sac disease is impaction.

Etiology and Pathogenesis: Anal sacs may become impacted, infected, abscessed, or neoplastic. Failure of the sacs to express during defecation, poor muscle tone in obese dogs, and generalized seborrhea (which produces glandular hypersecretion) lead to retention of sac contents. Such retention may predispose to bacterial overgrowth, infection, and inflammation.

Clinical Findings and Lesions: Signs are related to pain and discomfort associated with sitting. Scooting, licking, biting at the anal area, and painful defecation with tenesmus may be noted. Induration, abscesses, and fistulous tracts are common. In impaction, hard masses are palpable in the area of the sacs; the sacs are packed with a thick, pasty, brown secretion, which can be expressed as a thin ribbon only with a large amount of pressure. When the sacs are infected or abscessed, severe pain and often discoloration of the area are present. Fistulous tracts lead from abscessed sacs and rupture through the skin; these must be differentiated from perianal fistulas. Anal sac neoplasms are usually nonpainful and are associated with perineal edema, erythema, induration, or fistula formation. Apocrine gland adenocarcinomas of the anal sac are typically seen in older female dogs. These dogs may be presented for signs secondary to hypercalcemia, such as polyuria and polydipsia, or for problems related to the perineal mass.

Diagnosis of impaction, infection, or abscessation is confirmed by digital rectal examination, at which time the sacs can be expressed. Microscopic examination of the contents from infected sacs reveals large numbers of polymorphonuclear leukocytes and bacteria. A tumor should be suspected (anal sac apocrine adenocarcinoma) in anal sacs that are firm, enlarged, and nonexpressible even with irrigation. Ultrasonographic examination may be useful to determine whether a firm, nonexpressible anal sac is due to infection/abscessation or neoplastic disease. In the case of a suspected tumor, the diagnosis should be confirmed by biopsy. Regional and systemic metastasis should be evaluated, and serum calcium measured.

Treatment: Impacted anal sacs should be gently, manually expressed. A softening or ceruminolytic agent or saline can be infused into the sac if the contents are too dry to express effectively. Infected sacs should be cleaned with antiseptic, followed by local and systemic antibiotic therapy. Hot compresses, applied every 8–12 hr for 15–20 min each, are beneficial for abscesses. Repeated weekly flushings combined with infusion of a steroid-antibiotic ointment may be needed. Adding supplemental fiber to the diet may increase fecal bulk, facilitating anal sac compression and emptying. If medical treatment is ineffective, or if neoplasia is present, surgical excision of the sac is indicated. The closed technique for excision is preferred and has the lowest complication rate. However, fecal incontinence, a common complication of anal sac surgery, may result from damage to the caudal rectal branch of the pudendal nerve and may be complete if damage is bilateral. Chronic fistula formation may be seen when sac removal is incomplete or when the sac ruptures. Scar formation in the external anal sphincter may result from surgical trauma and result in tenesmus. (*See also* APOCRINE GLAND TUMORS OF ANAL SAC ORIGIN, p 950.)

PERIANAL FISTULA

Perianal fistula is characterized by chronic, purulent, malodorous, ulcerating, sinus tracts in the perianal tissues. It is most common in German Shepherds and is also seen in Setters and Retrievers. Dogs >7 yr old are at higher risk.

Etiology and Pathogenesis: The cause is unknown, although many theories have been proposed. Contamination of the hair follicles and glands of the anal area by fecal material and anal sac secretions may result in necrosis, ulceration, and chronic inflammation of the perianal skin and tissues. Affected animals may be predisposed to generalized skin problems. Hypothyroidism, an immunologic defect, or an immune-mediated component may contribute to susceptibility. The likelihood of contamination is greater in dogs with a broad-based tail; deep anal folds may cause feces to be retained within rectal glands and play a major role. The draining tracts are lined with chronic inflammatory tissue and often extend to the lumen of the rectum and anus. Infection may spread to deeper structures involving the external anal sphincter and, therefore, should be treated promptly.

Clinical Findings: In dogs, signs include attitude change, tenesmus, dyschezia, anorexia, lethargy, diarrhea, and attempts to bite and lick the anal area. Signs in cats are similar to those in dogs but may include matting of fur and sitting in the litter box.

Treatment: Historically, management of perianal fistulae was frustrating for both veterinarians and pet owners. Surgical therapy traditionally included anal sacculectomy, in addition to destroying the diseased tissues. Surgical techniques included excision, debridement, fulguration, and cryosurgery. Amputation of the tail at its base was once advocated alone or adjunctively with other therapy. Surgery is now only recommended for fistulae resistant to medical therapy. Sequelae of surgery include fecal incontinence, rectal stricture, and recurrence.

Cyclosporine has been an effective treatment at a dosage of 5–10 mg/kg, bid for 10–20 wk and then for an additional 4 wk after all fistulae appear to be healed. Concurrent administration of ketoconazole (8 mg/kg/day) allows the dosage (and cost) of cyclosporine therapy to be reduced (1–3.5 mg/kg/day). Prompt treatment is recommended early in the course of the disease to reduce the likelihood of recurrence. However, some dogs are intolerant of ketoconazole. Cyclosporine at a dosage of 5 mg/kg/day can effectively decrease the severity of lesions. In one study, the combination of cyclosporine therapy for 12 wk followed by surgical excision of any remaining draining tracts, along with cryptectomy and anal sacculectomy, successfully resolved disease with minimal recurrence. Topical tacrolimus (0.1% ointment applied once to twice daily) in combination with a tapering course of prednisone (2 mg/kg/day for 2 wk, 1 mg/kg/day for 4 wk, and then 1 mg/kg every 2 days for 10 wk) with metronidazole (10 mg/kg, bid for 2 wk) and a novel-protein diet has also been found to be effective in some dogs. Other aspects of medical management include the use of fecal softeners to reduce dyschezia. Perianal cleansing and antibiotics may reduce inflammation.

PERIANAL TUMORS

See HEPATOID GLAND TUMORS, p 951, and APOCRINE GLAND TUMORS OF ANAL SAC ORIGIN, p 950.

PERINEAL HERNIA

Perineal hernia is a lateral protrusion of a peritoneally lined hernial sac between the levator ani and either the external anal sphincter muscle or the coccygeus muscle. Incidence in intact 6- to 8-yr-old male dogs is disproportionately high, and Welsh Corgis, Boston Terriers, Boxers, Collies, Kelpies and Kelpie crosses, Dachshunds and Dachshund crosses, Old English Sheepdogs, and Pekingese are at higher risk.

Etiology and Pathogenesis: Many factors are involved, including breed predisposition, hormonal imbalance, prostatic disease, chronic constipation, and weakness of the pelvic diaphragm due to chronic straining. The higher incidence among sexually intact males is evidence that hormonal influences probably play a primary role. Prostatic hypertrophy attributed to sex-hormone imbalance has been strongly implicated. Both estrogens and androgens have been cited as causative agents.

Clinical Findings and Diagnosis: Common signs include constipation and obstipation, tenesmus, and dyschezia. Stranguria and urinary obstruction may develop secondary to retroflexion of the bladder and prostate. Visceral strangulation may be seen. A perineal swelling ventrolateral to the anus is evident. Herniation may be bilateral, but two-thirds are unilateral and >80% of these are on the right side.

The mass is soft and fluctuant and may be reduced digitally. A firm, painful swelling may be compatible with retropulsion of the bladder and prostate. Determination of contents is often made by rectal examination and perineal centesis (to determine whether urine is present). More than 90% of perineal hernias contain a rectal deviation, which is a sacculation of the rectum into the hernial sac, where the layers of the rectal wall remain intact.

Treatment: Perineal hernia is rarely an emergency, except when the bladder has strangulated and the animal is unable to urinate. If catheterization cannot be done, the urine should be removed by cystocentesis and an attempt made to reduce the hernia. An indwelling urinary catheter may be necessary to ensure urethral patency and prevent recurrence of obstruction.

Surgical correction is always indicated, and concurrent castration to reduce recurrence is recommended. The prognosis is guarded because of the high incidence of recurrence (10%–46%) and postoperative complications such as infection, rectocutaneous fistula, anal sac fistula, ischiatic and pudendal nerve entrapment, and rectal prolapse.

RECTAL AND ANORECTAL STRICTURES

Strictures are a narrowing of the lumen due to cicatricial tissue. Injury may result from foreign bodies or trauma (eg, bite wounds, accidents) or as a complication of inflammatory disease (eg, perianal fistula disease, histoplasmosis, inflammatory bowel disease, anal sacculitis).

Neoplasia, enlarged prostate, and scar tissue after perianal fistula or anal sac abscess may all predispose to extraluminal constriction. In small animals, anorectal stricture is more common than rectal strictures, but neither is frequent. Strictures are more common in German Shepherds, Beagles, and Poodles.

Rectal stricture in cattle may result from trauma, neoplasia, or fat necrosis impinging on or within the lumen, or from defects associated with rectal and vaginal strictures. Rectal strictures in pigs are seen secondary to enterocolitis, after repair of rectal prolapse, and as a sequela of ulcerative proctitis induced by salmonellae. Treatment in small animals includes general anesthesia followed by balloon dilation of the stricture, combined with intralesional injections of long-acting corticosteroids (triamcinolone). Treatment in large animals may include resection of the strictured area or rectal pull-through.

RECTAL NEOPLASMS

Malignant rectal neoplasms are usually adenocarcinomas in dogs and lymphosarcomas in cats. Adenocarcinomas are slow growing and infiltrative. Local or systemic metastasis may develop before tenesmus, dyschezia, hematochezia, or diarrhea is seen. Surgery is the treatment of choice for adenocarcinomas, but it may be unrewarding because metastasis has usually occurred before the diagnosis. Cats and dogs with rectal lymphosarcoma are treated medically with antineoplastic drugs.

RECTAL POLYPS

Rectal adenomatous polyps are an infrequent, usually benign disease, primarily of small animals. The larger the polyp, the greater the potential for malignancy. Signs include tenesmus, hematochezia, and diarrhea. The polyp is usually palpable per rectum and bleeds easily with surface ulceration. Periodically, the polyp may prolapse through the anal orifice. Surgical excision is usually followed by rapid clinical recovery and lengthy survival time. New polyps may develop after surgery. A biopsy should always be submitted for histopathologic diagnosis.

RECTAL PROLAPSE

In rectal prolapse, one or more layers of the rectum protrude through the anus due to persistent tenesmus associated with intestinal, anorectal, or urogenital disease. Prolapse may be classified as incomplete, in which only the rectal mucosa is everted, or complete, in which all rectal layers are protruded.

Etiology: Rectal prolapse is common in young animals in association with severe diarrhea and tenesmus. Causal factors include severe enteritis, endoparasitism, disorders of the rectum (eg, foreign bodies, lacerations, diverticula, or sacculation), neoplasia of the rectum or distal colon, urolithiasis, urethral obstruction, cystitis, dystocia, colitis, and prostatic disease. Perineal hernia, or other interruption of normal innervation of the external anal sphincter, may also produce prolapse.

Animals of any age, breed, or sex may be affected. Rectal prolapse is probably the most common GI problem in pigs due to diarrhea or weakness of the rectal support tissue within the pelvis. In cattle, it may be associated with coccidiosis, rabies, or vaginal or uterine prolapse; occasionally, excessive "riding" and associated traumatic injury may be causative in young bulls. It is common in sheep with short tail docking and especially in feedlot lambs, in which high-concentrate rations may be causative. The use of estrogens as growth promotants, or accidental exposure to estrogenic fungal toxins, may also predispose large animals to rectal prolapse.

Clinical Findings, Lesions, and Diagnosis: An elongated, cylindrical mass protruding through the anal orifice is usually diagnostic. However, it must be differentiated from prolapsed ileocolic intussusception by passing a probe, blunt instrument, or finger between the prolapsed mass and the inner rectal wall. In rectal prolapse, the instrument cannot be inserted because of the presence of a fornix.

Ulceration, inflammation, and congestion of the rectal mucosa is common. Early, there is a short, nonulcerated, inflamed segment; later, the mucosal surface darkens and may become congested and necrotic.

Treatment: In all animals, identifying and eliminating the cause of prolapse is of primary importance.

In **small animals**, treatment includes prompt replacement of viable prolapsed tissue to its proper anatomic location, or amputation if the segment is necrotic. Small or incomplete prolapses can be manually reduced under anesthesia by using a finger or bougie. Warm saline lavage and lubrication with a water-soluble gel should be applied to the prolapsed tissue before reduction. Alternatively, hypertonic sugar solution (50% dextrose or 70% mannitol) applied topically may be used to relieve edematous mucosa. The placement of a loose, anal purse-string suture for 5–7 days is indicated. Straining may be prevented by applying a topical anesthetic (1% dibucaine ointment) or by administering a narcotic epidural injection before or after reduction or correction. Postoperatively, a moistened diet and a fecal softener (eg, dioctyl sodium sulfosuccinate) are recommended. Diarrhea after surgery may require treatment.

When questionable viability of tissue prohibits manual reduction, rectal resection and anastomosis are required. When rectal tissue is viable but not amenable to manual reduction, celiotomy followed by colopexy is indicated to prevent recurrence. As in medical management, epidural anesthesia may be used to reduce straining.

In **large animals**, caudal epidural anesthesia is suggested to reduce straining, facilitate repositioning of the prolapse, and permit surgical manipulations. Reduction and retention with a purse-string suture is recommended. The suture should be loose enough to leave a one-finger opening into the rectum in pigs and sheep, and slightly larger in cattle and horses. Rectal prolapse in mares, if neglected, can lead to prolapse of the small colon. The blood supply to the small colon is easily disrupted. Replacement of a rectal prolapse with prolapse of the small colon followed by purse-string suture of the anus has a poor prognosis. More aggressive treatment of the prolapse is dictated by the condition of the rectum. In general, the prolapse may be salvaged by conservative measures, unless obvious deep necrosis or trauma to the tissue exists, or the everted tissue is firm, indurated, and cannot be reduced. Under these circumstances, submucosal resection or amputation should be considered. Amputation of the rectum should be reserved for severe cases. Complete amputation has a higher incidence of rectal stricture formation, especially in swine. A prolapse ring, syringe case, or plastic tubing may be used as an alternative to surgical amputation in pigs and sheep. Postoperatively, the animal should receive antibiotics. Fecal softeners may be used in horses. Usually, it is not economically feasible to repair rectal prolapses in lambs ready for market.

RECTAL TEARS

A separation, rent, or tear in the rectal or anal mucosa is seen as a result of a laceration inflicted within the lumen. Foreign bodies (eg, sharp bones, needles, and other rough material) have been implicated. Bite wounds and, in large animals, trauma from rectal palpation are common causes. The tear may involve only the superficial layers of the rectum (partial tear) or penetrate all layers (complete tear).

Clinical Findings and Diagnosis: Constipation and reluctance to defecate are usually attributed to pain. Diagnosis is based on tenesmus and hemorrhage, perineal discoloration, and inspection of the rectum and anus; fresh blood found on a glove or on feces after rectal examination is good evidence of a rectal tear. Edema may be present when the injury has persisted. The integrity of the external anal sphincter should be evaluated carefully.

Treatment: In all species, treatment should be initiated immediately. The anorectal area should be cleaned thoroughly and systemic broad-spectrum antibiotics administered. IV fluids and flunixin meglumine may be given to prevent or treat septic and endotoxic shock. In small animals, lacerations should be debrided and may be sutured through the anal orifice, via laparotomy, or through a combination of both depending on the location and degree of the tear. Antibiotics and fecal softeners should be administered postoperatively.

In cattle and horses, accidental perforation during rectal examination necessitates immediate treatment to reduce the risk of peritonitis and death. Exploration throughout the abdomen should be slow, deliberate, and smooth. The temptation to use the fingertips excessively or to push the arm through a region of resistance must be avoided. Rectal tears in horses have been classified according to the tissue layers penetrated. Grade I tears involve the mucosa or submucosa. Grade II tears involve rupture of the muscular layers only. Grade III tears involve mucosa, submucosa, and muscular layers, including tears that extend into the mesorectum. Grade IV tears involve perforation of all layers of the rectum and extension into the peritoneal cavity.

Grade I tears may be treated conservatively with broad-spectrum antibiotics and IV fluids. Flunixin meglumine may be given to prevent or treat endotoxic shock. Mineral oil is given via stomach tube to soften feces, and the diet should consist of pasture grasses or alfalfa. Grade II and III tears require immediate and more extensive surgery. A consultation with a specialist is suggested immediately after diagnosis. Grade IV tears carry a grave prognosis; they should be repaired only if small and if treatment is instituted before the peritoneal cavity is grossly contaminated.

ENTERIC CAMPYLOBACTERIOSIS

Campylobacter spp are spiral, microaerobic, gram-negative bacteria that cause gastroenteritis in people and animals. Several *Campylobacter* spp are zoonotic. Many domestic animals develop acute gastroenteritis after ingestion of *Campylobacter* spp, including dogs, cats, calves, sheep, pigs, ferrets, mink, monkeys, and several species of laboratory animals. (*See also* BOVINE GENITAL CAMPYLOBACTERIOSIS, p 1347, AVIAN CAMPYLOBACTER INFECTION, p 2806, and ZOONOTIC DISEASES, p 2419.) Infection with *C jejuni* is one of the most common causes of gastroenteritis in people worldwide and is the most extensively studied *Campylobacter* species.

Etiology: *Campylobacter* spp are spiral or curved rods that exhibit a characteristic corkscrew darting motility, mediated by a single polar flagellum. These are slow growing, with a generation time of ~90 min, fastidious, and require enriched medium and microaerobic conditions with increased CO_2 (3%–15% O_2, 3%–10% CO_2, 85% N_2) for growth.

The family Campylobacteraceae consists of three genera, including *Campylobacter* and *Arcobacter* associated with animal and human diseases. Certain species are present commensally in animals as suspected reservoirs for human infections. The thermophilic *Campylobacter* spp, *C jejuni*, or *C coli* have the highest prevalence and disease impact. *Campylobacter* species causing diseases in livestock include *C jejuni* subsp *jejuni* (enteritis and abortion), *C coli*, *C mucosalis* (porcine enteritis), *C upsaliensis*, *C helveticus* (companion pet enteritis), *C hyointestinalis* subsp *hyointestinalis* (porcine and bovine enteritis), *C sputorum* (abortions in sheep), and *C fetus* subsp *fetus* (isolated from intestinal tracts of sheep and cattle, sporadic abortions). Certain species such as *C jejuni*, *C hyointestinalis*, and *C fetus* possess closely related subspecies with different disease foci. Initially, *Arcobacter* spp were considered to be aerotolerant campylobacters and are implicated in reproductive disorders, mastitis, gastric ulcers, and/or diarrhea in livestock, including *A cryaerophilus* (previously *C cryaerophila*), *A skirrowii*, *A thereius*, and *A butzleri*.

Transmission and Epidemiology: Transmission is food- or waterborne or via fecal-oral spread. Animals serve as reservoir hosts for *Campylobacter* spp infections in both animals and people throughout the world. The predominant ecologic niche for *Campylobacter* spp is the GI tract of a wide variety of domesticated and wild vertebrates, and zoonotic transmission from animals to people in meat of animal origin, especially chicken, is a food safety issue. *Campylobacter* spp are also commonly isolated from free-living birds, including migratory birds and waterfowl, crows, gulls, and domestic pigeons, which can contaminate environments of grazing animals. Wild rodents and insects such as flies have also been reported to harbor and transmit *C jejuni*. Fecal contamination of the environment provides a ubiquitous source of these organisms under appropriate conditions for their survival. *Campylobacter* spp can persist for long periods in feces, milk, water, and urine, especially at temperatures close to 4°C. In adverse conditions, *C jejuni jejuni* converts to a viable nonculturable form that can be reactivated when ingested.

Human foods documented as contaminated with *Campylobacter* include chicken, turkey, beef, pork, fish, and milk. Domesticated poultry are the most significant reservoir of *C jejuni jejuni* for people, causing 50%–70% of cases; chicken meat is the number one source. Dogs and cats are commonly infected similar to their owners when they ingest undercooked poultry.

Pathogenesis: Bacterial motility, mucus colonization, toxin production, attachment, internalization, and translocation are among the processes associated with *C jejuni jejuni* virulence. Infection begins with ingestion of *C jejuni jejuni* in contaminated foods or water. Gastric acid provides a barrier, and the bacteria must reach the small and large intestines to multiply; *C jejuni* invades both epithelial cells and cells within the lamina propria.

Clinical Findings: Abdominal pain, fever, diarrhea, blood in feces, and inflammatory cells in feces demonstrate the inflammatory nature of the infection. Natural infections with *C jejuni jejuni* resulting in enteritis have been reported in juvenile macaques, weaning-age ferrets, dogs, cats, and swine. Chickens, rodents, ferrets, primates, rabbits, and pigs have been inoculated experimentally by various routes with *C jejuni* and subsequently developed enteritis. Clinical reports describe primary infections with systemic spread, infection with mucosal disease, infection without disease but with short-term bacterial persistence, and infection with resistance and no bacterial persistence. These reports support the idea that *C jejuni jejuni* produces a spectrum of disease scenarios, depending on the immune status of the host, bacterial virulence, gene expression, and other factors.

C jejuni jejuni, *C coli*, *C jejuni*, *C upsaliensis*, and *C helveticus* are the *Campylobacter* spp that have been associated with intestinal disease in **companion animals**. *C jejuni jejuni* causes diarrhea in dogs and cats, which are considered a significant source of the bacterium for the human population. Diarrhea is usually acute but can be recurrent. Diarrhea lasting 515 days is the most common clinical sign in dogs <6 mo old. It may be watery to bloody with mucus and is sometimes bile-stained. Occasionally, the diarrhea becomes chronic and may be accompanied by fever and increased WBC count. Cats <6 mo old commonly have diarrhea, which may be bloody. Some infected cats show no signs. Additionally, *C jejuni jejuni* has been isolated in the profuse and odorless hemorrhagic vaginal discharge from late-pregnancy abortions in dogs.

In **cattle and sheep**, *Campylobacter* spp can cause enteritis and abortion, including *C jejuni jejuni*, *C fetus* subsp *fetus*, *C hyointestinalis* subsp *hyointestinalis*, and *C sputorum* (abortions in sheep). However, in studies that compared *C jejuni* prevalence in healthy cattle and in cattle considered "sick" because of diarrhea, the frequency of *Campylobacter* spp was not significantly different. Beef and dairy cattle can have significant levels of *Campylobacter*, with prevalences of 2.5%–60%. In a number of studies, cattle checked at slaughter harbored *Campylobacter* in gallbladders, large and small intestines, and liver. Fecal shed in cattle leads to contamination of milk and beef.

Campylobacters can contribute to colitis in weaning aged **pigs**. Swine commonly carry *C coli* and *C jejuni jejuni* as intestinal commensals, and studies in the USA, Netherlands, Great Britain, and Germany show that more than half of commercially raised pigs excrete the organisms. *C coli* strains comprise most isolates from pigs, causing first watery, then inflammatory diarrheal disease. Pigs have anorexia, fever, and diarrhea for 1–5 days followed by remission of clinical signs but continue to shed *C jejuni jejuni* in the feces. *C hyointestinalis hyointestinalis* and *C mucosalis* are also implicated as causes of enteritis in pigs. Concurrent infections with viruses, other bacteria (eg, *Escherichia coli*), and parasites increase the disease and pathology caused by *Campylobacter* spp in swine. *C hyointestinalis* subsp *lawsonii* has been isolated from pig stomachs; however, this subspecies has not been implicated in disease.

Birds, including intensively farmed poultry, appear to have a higher infection rate and carriage of *Campylobacter* spp, especially *C jejuni jejuni*, than other animals. In broilers, the organism may colonize the palatine lymphoid tissues and the crop, leading to extremely rapid transmission through communal water troughs and standard fecal-oral spread. However, the organism has been isolated from the small intestines of clinically ill birds, especially psittacines (parrots) and passeriforms (finches and canaries), with hepatitis, lethargy, loss of appetite, weight loss, and yellow diarrhea. Mortality may be high. *Campylobacter* spp have also been isolated from free-living birds, including migratory birds and waterfowl, crows, gulls, and domestic pigeons; however, disease due to *C jejuni jejuni*, for example in naturally infected birds, is rare.

Campylobacter GI disease has been reported in **exotic pets** (eg, ferrets, mink, primates, hamsters, guinea pigs, mice, and rats). Although clinical signs vary in these species, they generally include mucoid, watery, bile-streaked diarrhea (sometimes with blood), anorexia, vomiting, and fever. Prolonged infections are possible but uncommon; most infections are self-limiting with mild signs.

The following species have been isolated from birds, shellfish, reptiles, marine mammals, and livestock not known to be associated with disease symptoms: *C avium*, *C hyointestinalis lawsonii*, *C fetus* subsp *testudinum*, *C canadensis*, *C peloridis*, *C insulaenigrae*, *C subantarcticus*, *C volucris*, and *C ureolyticus* (previously *Bacteroides ureolyticus*). Several of these are implicated in human diseases.

Arcobacter spp infecting animals include *A cryaerophilus* (livestock abortion), *A butzleri* (livestock diarrhea, bovine and porcine abortions), *A skirrowii* (sheep diarrhea, livestock abortions), and *A thereius* (porcine abortion). Disease status is unknown, although these species have been isolated from food animals: *A cibarious* (chicken meat, piggery effluent), *A trophiarum* (fattening pigs), and *A suis* (pork meat). Approximately 11 additional *Arcobacter* spp found in shellfish, sewage, seawater, sediments, and salt marsh plants are not known to cause diseases in animals or people.

Lesions: *C jejuni* can stably colonize the small and large intestines, although most animals show cecal and colonic lesions with typhlocolitis. In swine and mice, gross lesions observed in *C jejuni* enteritis include enlarged and fluid-filled ceca and proximal colons with thickened walls. Lymph nodes (ileocecocolic and mesenteric) draining infected sites become significantly enlarged. Infection with particular strains of *C jejuni* produces bloody exudates with mucus. Histopathologic features include a marked inflammation of the lamina propria, dominated by neutrophilic polymorphonuclear cells and mononuclear cells that sometimes extend into submucosa. Immune cells such as plasma cells, macrophages, and mononuclear cells have been found in smaller numbers in the lamina propria. Damage to, sloughing of, and ulceration of the epithelial surface and edema have also been seen in most infected species. In pigs and mice, damage to the epithelial surface is associated with the presence of *C jejuni* at the basolateral surface of the epithelium, in paracellular junctions of the epithelium, and in erosive and ulcerative lesions of the epithelium; there is often a mucopurulent neutrophilic exudate with sloughed and lysed epithelial cells and erosive or ulcerative lesions where *C jejuni* is associated with the basolateral aspect of sloughing villous tip cells in the colon. Crypt abscesses and damage to the crypt epithelium are also common findings.

Diagnosis: *Campylobacter* spp can be found in both healthy and diarrheic animals; thus, clinical signs and postmortem findings depend on the species and the host animal and its age. Diagnosis of enteric campylobacteriosis relies on isolation of the causative agent using selective media under microaerophilic conditions. Fresh fecal samples should be collected and transported to the laboratory preferably on the same day and within at least 2 days for processing. If transport to the laboratory is delayed, transport media and storage at 4°C produce the best results. Campylobacters are very sensitive to environmental conditions, including dehydration, atmospheric oxygen, sunlight, and increased temperature. Organisms are thin (0.2–0.8 μm × 0.3–5 μm), gram-negative, motile, curved rods. The cells are S-shaped or curved but are occasionally long (8 μm) spiral rods. They exhibit a typical spiraling motility. In unfavorable growth conditions, spiral rods undergo a degenerate conversion to coccoid forms. Campylobacters can be quickly outgrown by contaminating microbes during prolonged transport to the laboratory, and isolation of pure colonies for downstream testing can be difficult. Filtration using 0.45 μm filters can help because campylobacters will pass through.

Enrichment is required for most clinical sampling unless material can be transported to the laboratory immediately.

When samples are collected in swabs, the use of commercially available transport tubes containing medium, such as Amies, is recommended. The medium can be plain agar or charcoal-based. Several transport media have been described for transport of fecal specimens, including Cary-Blair, modified Cary-Blair, modified Stuart medium, Campy thioglycolate medium, alkaline peptone water, and semisolid motility test medium. Other media are recommended for the isolation of campylobacters associated with reproductive losses.

Campylobacter spp do not ferment carbohydrates, and other biochemical characteristics are thus used to identify different species. Thermophilic/thermotolerant *Campylobacter* spp, including *C jejuni jejuni*, *C coli*, *C upsaliensis*, *C lari*, *C mucosalis*, *C sputorum*, *C hyointestinalis*, and *C helveticus* grow best at 42°C, although they are capable of growth at 37°C. *C fetus* do not grow or grow poorly at 42°C. Alternatively, this species grows well at 25°C, whereas the thermophilic campylobacters do not (except *C mucosalis*, which can grow at 42° and 25°C, weak growth for *C hyointestinalis* at 25°C). *C jejuni* is differentiated on its ability to hydrolyze hippurate, and *C upsaliensis* has negative or weak catalase production and is differentiated from other campylobacters because of its sensitivity to nalidixic acid. *C helveticus* is also catalase negative but can be difficult to differentiate biochemically from *C upsaliensis* relying on distinctive colony morphologies.

Differentiation of subspecies can be necessary for identification of significant pathogens. *C jejuni* subsp *jejuni* is the main cause of enteritis, whereas *C jejuni* subsp *doylei* has been isolated only from enteritis cases of children and not animals. They can be differentiated by the ability of *C jejuni doylei* to reduce nitrate. Similarly, *C hyointestinalis* subsp *hyointestinalis* can cause bovine and porcine enteritis; however, *C hyointestinalis* subsp *lawsonii* has been isolated from the porcine stomach, but it is not known to cause disease. The subspecies can be differentiated by testing the intolerance of *C hyointestinalis lawsonii* to 1.5% bile and/or 0.1% potassium permanganate.

Arcobacter spp (previously known as aerotolerant campylobacters) can also be associated with human and animal diarrhea and with animal abortions. Arcobacters are usually not thermophilic but can be confused with the nonthermophilic *Campylobacter* spp if aerotolerance is confirmed using standardized suspensions of organisms. Although most cases of human enteritis are attributed to *C jejuni jejuni*, *C coli*, *C lari*, and *C upsaliensis*, it has been suggested that the importance of other species also associated with GI illness may be significantly underdiagnosed as a consequence of inappropriate isolation and identification methods.

Immunodiagnosis (ELISA) is unsuitable to diagnose intestinal *Campylobacter* infections.

PCR-based methods effectively identify infection, especially if cultivation is difficult or if the sample has been somewhat mishandled. However, a positive test is not sufficient evidence to determine causation and must be considered in conjunction with clinical signs.

Treatment and Control: Clindamycin, gentamicin, tetracyclines, erythromycin, cephalosporins (eg, cephalothin), and fluoroquinolones (eg, nalidixic acid) are effective against *C jejuni*, *C helveticus*, and *C upsaliensis*. *C fetus*, *C hyointestinalis*, *C mucosalis*, and *C sputorum* are usually resistant to the fluoroquinolones yet sensitive to cephalosporins. *C coli* are sensitive to fluoroquinolones but resistant to cephalosporins. Susceptibilities to penicillins and trimethoprim are variable across *Campylobacter* spp. Resistance to the fluoroquinolones, tetracycline, kanamycin, and some other antibiotics has been documented among the *Campylobacter* spp, mediated by both chromosomal and plasmid mechanisms. Culture-dependent diagnosis can provide isolates for antibiotic sensitivity testing. However, some animals remain colonized and become persistent shedders despite antibiotic therapy. If the goal of treatment is to decrease the risk of zoonotic transmission to a susceptible household member, antibiotic treatment alone may be inadequate. Control involves treatment, removal to a clean environment, and prospective fecal testing to ascertain shedding status; even so, low infective doses and the ubiquitous distribution of the organism pose significant challenges.

SALMONELLOSIS

Salmonella, a rod-shaped gram-negative bacterium belonging to the family Enterobacteriaceae, is the causative agent of salmonellosis. Salmonellosis in warm-blooded vertebrates is in most cases associated with serovars of *Salmonella enterica*. The most common type of infection is the carrier state, in which infected animals carry the pathogen for a variable period of time without showing any clinical signs. Clinical disease is characterized by two major syndromes: a systemic septicemia (also termed as typhoid) and an enteritis. Other less common clinical presentations include abortion, arthritis, respiratory disease, necrosis of extremities, and meningitis.

Only a few serotypes produce clinical salmonellosis in healthy animals and typically have a narrow range of host species, a phenomenon termed serovar-host specificity. *Salmonella enterica* serovar Typhi (*S* Typhi) and *S* Paratyphi produce typhoid in people, *S* Gallinarum produces a similar disease in poultry, *S* Abortusovis in sheep, *S* Choleraesuis in pigs, *S* Dublin in cattle, etc.

The remaining serovars (serotypes) rarely produce clinical systemic disease in healthy, adult, nonpregnant animals. However, they colonize in the gut of many species of animals, enter the human food chain, and produce gastroenteritis in people (food poisoning). *S* Typhimurium and *S* Enteritidis are the most frequent causes of enteritis in people (nontyphoidal salmonellosis) but are also able to produce typical typhoid infections in mice; hence, the basis of pathogenicity is unclear. Strains from this latter group may also produce more severe disease, with systemic involvement resembling typhoid in very young animals if they have received insufficient protective antibody from their dam or when they are particularly susceptible, eg, as a result of old age, disease, or pregnancy. The host species from which a serotype is characteristically isolated is not necessarily the only species that can act as a host; thus, epidemiologic factors are important in determining prevalence.

Young calves, piglets, lambs, and foals may develop both the enteritis and septicemic form (*see* DIARRHEA IN NEONATAL RUMINANTS, p 275, DIARRHEAL DISEASE IN FOALS, p 289, and INTESTINAL SALMONELLOSIS, p 296). Adult cattle, sheep, and horses commonly develop acute enteritis, and chronic enteritis may develop in growing pigs and occasionally in cattle (*see also* the chapters on intestinal diseases in each of the major domestic species, p 266, et seq). Pregnant animals may abort. The clinically normal carrier animal is a serious problem in all host species. Salmonellosis is seen infrequently in dogs and cats and is characterized by acute diarrhea with or without septicemia.

Etiology and Pathogenesis: Salmonellosis has been recognized in all parts of the world but is most prevalent in regions with intensive animal husbandry. Although this facultative intracellular pathogen is primarily an intestinal bacterium, it is commonly found in an environment subject to fecal contamination. Feces of infected animals can contaminate feed and water, milk, fresh and processed meats from abattoirs, plant and animal products used as fertilizers or feedstuffs, pasture and rangeland, and many inert materials. The organisms may survive for months in wet, warm areas such as in feeder pig barns and poultry houses or in water dugouts, but they survive <1 wk in composted cattle manure. Rodents and wild birds are also sources of infection for domestic animals. Pelleting of feeds reduces the level of contamination by salmonellae largely as a result of the heat treatment involved.

Although many other *Salmonella* spp may cause enteric disease, the more common ones (to some extent varying according to geographic location) in each species are as follows: **cattle**—*S* Typhimurium, *S* Dublin, and *S* Newport; **sheep and goats**—*S* Typhimurium, *S* Dublin, *S* Abortusovis, *S* Anatum, and *S* Montevideo; **pigs**—*S* Typhimurium and *S* Choleraesuis; **horses**—*S* Typhimurium, *S* Anatum, *S* Newport, *S* Enteritidis, and *Salmonella* serovar IIIa 18:z_4:z_{23}; and **poultry**—*S* Enteritidis, *S* Typhimurium, *S* Gallinarum, and *S* Pullorum.

Although their resulting clinical patterns are not distinct, different species of salmonellae do tend to differ in their epidemiology. Plasmid profile and drug-resistance patterns are sometimes useful markers for epidemiologic studies. The prevalence of infection varies among host species and countries and is much higher than the incidence of clinical disease, which in food animals is commonly precipitated by stressful situations such as sudden deprivation of feed, transportation, drought, crowding, parturition, surgery, and administration of certain drugs, including oral antibiotics. Greater susceptibility in the very young may be the result of high gastric pH, absence of a stable intestinal flora, and limited immunity.

The usual route of infection in enteritis is fecal-oral, although infection through the upper respiratory tract and the conjunctiva have also been reported. After ingestion, the organism colonizes the digestive tract and invades and multiplies in enterocytes and tonsillar lymphoid tissue. Penetration of bacteria into the lamina propria contributes to gut damage and diarrhea. The complex process involves attachment through fimbrial appendages and the injection by the attached *Salmonella* organisms into epithelial cells of proteins, which induce changes in the actin cytoskeleton that induce membrane ruffling at the cell surface. This entraps the *Salmonella* bacteria and results in fluid secretion and their ingestion by the cell. The cellular infection results in activation of a host alarm process through signalling molecules as a result of the detection of bacterial surface proteins, which in turn induces a strong inflammatory response that generally is able to restrict the bacteria to the intestine. Some serotypes also become localized in the reproductive tract. Serotypes that are able to cause typhoid can modulate the initial host response and suppress the inflammatory response. Cell destruction follows, and the bacteria are ingested by phagocytic cells such as macrophages and neutrophils. Although neutrophils are generally able to kill *Salmonella*, the bacteria can survive and multiply within macrophages, which represent the main host cell type during infection.

As infection progresses, a true septicemia may follow, with subsequent localization in brain and meninges, pregnant uterus, joints and distal aspects of the limbs, and tips of the ears and tails, which can result, respectively, in meningoencephalitis, abortion, osteitis, and dry gangrene of the feet, tail, or ears. The organism also frequently localizes in the gallbladder and mesenteric lymph nodes, and survivors intermittently shed the organism in the feces.

Calves rarely become carriers but virtually all adults do for variable periods—up to 10 wk in sheep and cattle and up to 14 mo in horses. Adult cattle infected with *S* Dublin may excrete the organism for years. Infection may also persist in lymph nodes or tonsils, with no salmonellae in the feces. Latent carriers may begin shedding the organism or even develop clinical disease under stress. A passive carrier acquires infection from the environment but is not invaded, so that if removed from the environment, it ceases to be a carrier.

Epidemiology: In **cattle**, *S* Typhimurium is commonly associated with outbreaks of enteritis in calves <2 mo old, whereas *S* Dublin has been associated with the same condition in older calves and adult cattle. In calves and lambs, *S* Dublin is usually endemic on a particular farm, whereas *S* Typhimurium is frequently associated with introduction of calves from infected farms and may cause sporadic explosive outbreaks. Subclinical infection with occasional herd outbreaks may be seen in adult cattle. Stressors that precipitate clinical disease include deprivation of feed and water, minimal levels of nutrition, long transport times, calving and antibiotic prophylaxis, and mixing and crowding in feedlots.

Outbreaks of septicemic salmonellosis in **pigs** are rare and usually can be traced to a purchased, infected pig. Purchase of feeder pigs from *Salmonella*-free herds and use of the "all-in/all-out" policy in finishing units minimize exposure. Increasing use of extensive outdoor rearing increases the risk of exposure to environmental sources of infection. Passerines, gulls, and pigeons can present a direct source of infection or a source of contamination of feed and water.

Most cases in adult **horses** develop after the stress of surgery or transport related to sales yards and deprivation of feed and water followed by overfeeding at their destination. Mares may be inapparent shedders and shed the bacteria at parturition, infecting newborn foals. Septicemic salmonellosis may occur in **foals**, which may be endemic, or there may be outbreaks. (*See* INTESTINAL DISEASES IN HORSES AND FOALS, p 281.)

Many **dogs and cats** are asymptomatic carriers of salmonellae. Clinical disease is uncommon, but when it is seen, it is often associated with hospitalization, another infection or debilitating condition in adults, or exposure to large numbers of the bacteria in puppies and kittens, in which enteritis may be common.

Clinical Findings: Infection with localization of the pathogen in tonsils or the GI tract that is not associated with clinical disease is a common form of salmonellosis termed as the carrier state. Carrier animals are chronically infected and may shed salmonellae intermittently into the environment. Carrier animals can develop clinical disease whenever the immune function is compromised or concurrent infection with another pathogen occurs.

Enteritis with septicemia is the usual syndrome in newborn calves, lambs, foals, fowl, and piglets, and outbreaks may occur in pigs up to 6 mo old. When systemic disease occurs with enteritis as a result of insufficient immunity, illness may be acute, with depression, fever (105°–107°F [40.5°–41.5°C]), and death in 24–48 hr. Nervous signs and pneumonia may be seen in calves and pigs. Mortality may reach 100%, depending on the host genetic background and strain virulence.

Acute enteritis without extensive systemic involvement is more common in adults as well as in young animals ≥1 wk old. Initially, there is fever (105°–107°F [40.5°–41.5°C]), followed by severe watery diarrhea, sometimes dysentery, and often tenesmus. In a herd outbreak, several hours may lapse before the onset of diarrhea, at which time the fever may disappear. The feces, which vary considerably in consistency, may have a putrid odor and contain mucus, fibrinous casts, shreds of mucous membrane, and in some cases, blood. Rectal examination causes severe discomfort and tenesmus. Milk production often declines precipitously in dairy cows. Abdominal pain is common and may be severe (colic) in horses. Mortality is variable but may reach 100% depending on strain virulence. A marked leukopenia and neutropenia are characteristic of the acute disease in horses. In dogs and cats, clinical disease takes the form of acute diarrhea with septicemia and is seen occasionally in puppies and kittens or in adults stressed by concurrent disease. Pneumonia may be evident. When the enteritis becomes more chronic, abortion may occur in pregnant dogs, cats, cattle, horses, and sheep, and live progeny may have enteritis as well. Conjunctivitis is sometimes seen in affected cats.

Fur-bearing and zoo carnivores may be affected. Contaminated feed is often the source of infection. Several rodent species (eg, guinea pigs, hamsters, rats, and mice) and rabbits are susceptible. Rodents commonly act as a source of infection on farms where the disease is endemic. Pet turtles were once a common source of infection in people that has been virtually eliminated by the curtailment of commercial trafficking.

Diagnosis: Diagnosis of salmonellosis depends on clinical signs and isolation of the pathogen from feces, blood, or tissues of affected animals. The presence of organisms may also be sought in feed, water supplies, and feces from wild rodents and birds that may inhabit rearing premises to determine the source of the organism. Bacteria are usually identified by a range of biochemical tests. Identification to serotype may be done, followed by further subdivision on the basis of susceptibility to selected bacteriophages (phage typing).

Serologic tests are available and are increasingly used as a diagnostic tool in salmonellae surveillance and control programs. These tests are normally developed to identify a limited spectrum of salmonellae serovars and serogroups. Serologic tests are difficult to interpret in individual animals, because a seropositive animal may no longer be infected. Furthermore, specificity issues mean that in countries with low infection prevalence, many positive results are false-positive.

The clinical syndromes usually are characteristic but must be differentiated from several similar diseases in each species as follows: **cattle**—diarrhea due to enterotoxigenic *Escherichia coli*, dysentery due to verotoxigenic *E coli*, coccidiosis, cryptosporidiosis, the alimentary tract form of infectious bovine rhinotracheitis, bovine viral diarrhea, hemorrhagic enteritis due to *Clostridium perfringens* types B and C, arsenic poisoning, secondary copper deficiency (molybdenosis), winter dysentery, paratuberculosis, ostertagiosis, and dietetic diarrhea; **sheep**—enteric colibacillosis, septicemia due to *Haemophilus* sp or pasteurellae, and coccidiosis; **pigs**—enteric colibacillosis and *Clostridium difficile* of newborn pigs and weanlings, swine dysentery (*Brachyspira hyodysenteriae*), campylobacteriosis, and the septicemias of growing pigs (which include erysipelas, *Lawsonia intracellularis*, classical swine fever, and pasteurellosis); **horses**—septicemia (due to *E coli*, *Actinobacillus equuli*, or streptococci);

poultry—coliform enteritis and *Yersinia pseudotuberculosis*.

Lesions: Lesions are most severe in the lower ileum, cecum, and spiral colon and vary from shortening of villi with loss of the epithelium to complete loss of intestinal architecture. There is infiltration of the lamina propria with neutrophils and later with macrophages, and thrombi may be seen in capillaries in this region. Hemorrhage and fibrin strands are usually seen, and there may be a fibrinonecrotic crust on the surface of the intestinal mucosa. Culture techniques that involve suppression of fecal *E coli* are usually necessary, and several daily fecal cultures may be necessary to isolate the organism. A nonselective enrichment stage may be required for samples in which bacteria may be present in low numbers, as in foodstuffs. This may be followed by enrichment in selective broth and plating for colonies on a variety of selective agars that suppress other enteric bacteria likely to be present in the gut. Blood cultures in septicemic animals may be rewarding but are costly.

Treatment: Early treatment is essential for septicemic salmonellosis, but there is controversy regarding the use of antimicrobial agents for intestinal salmonellosis. Oral antibiotics may be ineffective and may deleteriously alter the intestinal microflora, thereby interfering with competitive antagonism and prolonging shedding of the organism. There is also concern that antibiotic-resistant strains of salmonellae selected by oral antibiotics may subsequently infect people. By suppressing antibiotic-sensitive components of the normal flora, antibiotics may also promote transfer of antibiotic resistance from resistant strains of *E coli* to *Salmonella*. Use of chemotherapeutic antibiotics for growth stimulation has been banned in many countries for this reason.

Broad-spectrum antibiotics administered systemically are indicated for treatment of septicemia. Initial antimicrobial therapy should be based on knowledge of the drug resistance pattern of the organisms previously found in the area. Nosocomial infections may involve highly drug-resistant organisms. Trimethoprim-sulfonamide combinations may be effective. Alternatives are ampicillin, fluoroquinolones, or third-generation cephalosporins. Resistance to ampicillin, trimethoprim, sulfonamide, tetracyclines, and aminoglycosides is generally plasmid mediated and transfers readily between different bacteria. Resistance to quinolones is mutational, but random mutations may be selected by antibiotic use and may be transferred by bacteriophages. Treatment should be continued daily for up to 6 days.

If oral medication is chosen, it should be given in drinking water and not mixed into solid feed, because affected animals are thirsty due to dehydration and their appetite is generally poor. Fluid therapy to correct acid-base imbalance and dehydration may be necessary. Calves, adult cattle, and horses need large quantities of fluids. Antibiotics such as ampicillin or cephalosporins lead to lysis of the bacteria with release of endotoxin, and NSAIDs or flunixin meglumine may be used to reduce the effects of endotoxemia.

The intestinal form is difficult to treat effectively in all species. Although clinical cure may be achieved, bacteriologic cure is difficult, either because the organisms become established in the biliary system and are intermittently shed into the intestinal lumen, or because the animals are reinfected from the environment at a time when their normal gut flora, which is inhibitory to colonization by pathogens, is depleted by antibiotic therapy. A concern with antimicrobial therapy is that it may increase the risk of creating carrier animals; in people and other animal species, antimicrobial therapy prolongs the period after clinical recovery during which the pathogen can be retrieved from the GI tract.

Control and Prevention: Carrier animals and contaminated feedstuffs and environment are major problems. Drain swabs or milk filters may be cultured to monitor the salmonellae status of a herd. The principles of control include prevention of introduction and limitation of spread within a herd. In many countries and in the EU, government-backed programs have been introduced to control and reduce levels of infection in food animals, especially poultry and pigs.

Prevention of Introduction: Every effort must be made to prevent introduction of a carrier; ideally, animals should be purchased directly only from farms known to be free of the disease and should be isolated for ≥1 wk while their health status is monitored. Ensuring that feed supplies are free of salmonellae depends on the integrity of the source. Some countries also test for contamination of and regulate importation and home production of feedstuffs and feed components.

Limitation of Spread Within a Herd: In an outbreak of salmonellosis, the following procedures should be implemented: 1) Carrier animals should be identified and either culled or isolated and treated vigorously. Treated animals must be rechecked several times before there can be confidence they are not carriers. 2) The prophylactic use of antibiotics in feed or water supplies may be considered (the hazards are mentioned earlier). 3) Movement of animals around the farm should be restricted to limit infection to the smallest group. Random mixing of animals should be avoided. 4) Feed and water supplies must be protected from fecal contamination. 5) Contaminated buildings must be vigorously cleaned and disinfected. 6) Contaminated material must be disposed of carefully. 7) All persons should be aware of the hazards of working with infected animals and the importance of personal hygiene. A strict farm management program should be introduced. 8) Use of a vaccine should be considered, particularly in an outbreak involving pregnant cattle, pigs, or laying poultry. Commercial killed bacterins or autogenous bacterins may be used. Live attenuated vaccines show considerable promise, but few are available commercially (*see* below). 9) Stresses should be minimized.

***Salmonella* Vaccines:** Salmonellae are facultative intracellular bacteria, and a live vaccine is therefore expected to be necessary for optimal immune protection against disease; however, there is some evidence that inactivated bacterins can induce a lower level of protection. In several studies, live attenuated *Salmonella* vaccines in pigs, cattle, and chickens stimulated a strong cell-mediated immune response and protected animals against both systemic disease and intestinal colonization. A live attenuated *S* Choleraesuis vaccine licensed for use in swine appears to effectively reduce colonization of tissues and protect pigs from disease after challenge with virulent organisms and under field conditions. This vaccine also protected calves against experimental challenge with *S* Dublin and serogroup C1 salmonellae after intranasal or SC administration. A live *S* Gallinarum vaccine has been shown to be effective not only against *S* Gallinarum (fowl typhoid) but also in significantly reducing the infection of laying hens challenged with *S* Enteritidis.

Zoonotic Risk: Infections with *Salmonella* in food-producing animals present a serious public health concern, because food products of animal origin are considered to be a significant source of human infection. Most common sources of infection are eggs and related products, and meat from poultry and other food animal species (*see* p 2865). Milk and dairy products have also been associated with outbreaks of salmonellosis in people. In addition, contamination of fruit and vegetables by infected water may also be a source of infection. In Europe, *S* Enteritidis and *S* Typhimurium, and in the USA, *S* Typhimurium are the most prevalent serovars associated with human disease.

TYZZER DISEASE

Tyzzer disease is an enterohepatic syndrome of a wide range of animals (*see* p 1948) and is seen worldwide. Tyzzer disease was first described in mice in 1917. Several years later, it was reported in laboratory rabbits and then in other small laboratory mammals, including guinea pigs, hamsters, gerbils, and rats. It is a highly fatal disease of young foals. The disease is rare in other domestic animals, including dogs, cats, and calves. It has been reported in a variety of wildlife, including muskrats, cottontail rabbit, coyote, gray fox, lesser panda, snow leopard, raccoon, marsupials, and white-tailed deer.

The disease primarily affects young, well-nourished animals, especially those fed high-protein diets, during periods of stress. Some species appear resistant unless stressed or immunosuppressed, whereas others appear to be susceptible without immunosuppression. Dietary factors, including excessive nitrogenous diets fed to laboratory animals and to nursing mares, seemingly may cause immunosuppression and may predispose susceptible animals to the disease. Other immunosuppressive agents and drugs and some antibacterials, especially sulfonamides, may also predispose animals to the disease.

Under laboratory conditions, stress is created by immunosuppressive drugs or other factors that can be easily identified. With many experiments, stress may be involved as part of the protocol, and when the disease develops, it is devastating.

Etiology and Pathogenesis: The disease is caused by *Clostridium piliforme*, a motile, spore-forming, rod-shaped, flagellated, obligate, intracellular bacterium. It does not grow in cell-free media but can be cultured in the yolk sac of chick embryos or tissue culture cells. The vegetative phase is very labile; spores may survive in soiled bedding at room temperature for >1 yr and are resistant to heating up to 60°C for 30 min, or exposure to 70% ethanol, 3% cresol, 4% chlorhexidine, and 0.037% formaldehyde; however, they are sensitive to 0.4% peracetic acid, 0.015% sodium hypochlorite, 1% iodophor, and 5% phenol.

C piliforme appears to be common in the environment, but because it is difficult to culture, very little knowledge has been accumulated on the epidemiology, pathogenesis, and immunity. Infection most likely results from oral exposure to spores from the environment. The feces of infected and carrier animals are the primary source of spores that contaminate the environment.

C piliforme infections are often subclinical or asymptomatic but may be severe in many animal species. There may be differences in susceptibility within animal species. B lymphocytes, T lymphocytes, and natural killer cells may play a role in mediating strain susceptibility. Seroanalysis using monoclonal antibody-based competitive inhibition ELISA suggests that Tyzzer disease may be relatively common in horses, which are susceptible to at least two distinct strains.

Some isolates of *C piliforme* produce toxins, whereas others do not. The role of these toxins in the pathogenesis of infection is unknown, but the toxic isolates are generally more virulent than nontoxic isolates. The toxigenic strains appear more likely to induce hepatic lesions in mice, whereas the nontoxigenic strains do not.

The primary site of infection is the lower intestinal tract with subsequent dissemination via the blood or lymphatics to the liver and heart. The bacterium has an affinity for the epithelial and smooth muscle cells of the intestines, hepatocytes, and cardiac myocytes. Stress factors such as capture, overcrowding, shipping, and poor sanitation appear to be predisposing. Sulfonamide administration predisposes rabbits to the disease. Mortality is highest at weaning age in rabbits. The disease in foals occurs most often between 1 and 6 wk of age, with most cases occurring between 1 and 2 wk of age. In some species, the disease has been identified concurrently with other diseases, eg, feline infectious peritonitis in cats, distemper and mycotic pneumonia in dogs, and cryptosporidial and coronaviral enteritis in calves.

The disease in foals is more common during the spring when nursing mares are exposed to lush, high-protein pastures. The increase in the availability of nutrients from pasture forages and supplemental diets may encourage the overgrowth of *C piliforme* in the gut of nursing mares; this seemingly predisposes neonatal foals to the disease when they are exposed to massive numbers of the bacterium after consuming the feces of their dams soon after birth as a mechanism to establish their normal intestinal flora. The immature gut is likely more permeable to pathogens like *C piliforme*.

The disease in young foals primarily affects the liver, where it induces a massive multifocal necrosis and hepatitis, and foals die of acute liver failure. In contrast, in other animals, which generally are older when infected, the bacterium affects the intestinal tract and to a lesser extent the liver and heart.

Older foals up to 6 wk of age become more resistant to the disease as the gut becomes more mature and immune factors may be involved. The disease is not recognized in older foals and adults, but they carry the bacterium in their gut.

Immune factors appear to be involved with the disease in horses, because many adults have antibodies for *C piliforme* yet do not develop Tyzzer disease. Only young foals up to 6 wk old develop lesions. The disease is more common in foals when young nursing mares are introduced to a farm where the disease is endemic and is less common in suckling foals on older mares; this suggests that older mares are immune to the disease and may be secreting *C piliforme* antibodies in the colostrum that protects young foals.

Clinical Findings: The disease often affects apparently healthy, fast-growing foals without previously observed clinical signs. The incubation period in experimentally infected foals is 4–7 days after oral exposure to bacterial spores. Most foals are found in a coma or dead. Clinical signs, if seen, are of short duration, from a few hours to up to 2 days. Signs are variable but may include depression, anorexia, pyrexia, jaundice, diarrhea, and recumbency. Terminally, there are convulsions and coma. Clinical signs vary between animal species. Laboratory animals may be found dead at the start of an outbreak. As the disease progresses, animals may show depression, ruffled coat, and varying degrees of watery diarrhea.

Clinicopathologic tests are of little value in laboratory animals, because they die so rapidly. In foals, the serum enzymes sorbitol dehydrogenase, AST, alkaline phosphatase, lactate dehydrogenase, and γ-glutamyltransferase are increased. There is also hyperbilirubinemia, leukopenia, hemoconcentration, and terminally profound hypoglycemia.

Lesions: Characteristic lesions are seen in the liver, myocardium, and intestinal tract. In the liver, white, gray, or yellowish foci of necrosis, 2 mm in diameter, are few to disseminated. The hepatic necrosis is most marked and disseminated in foals in which the multiple necrotic foci with slightly depressed hemorrhagic centers appear to infect almost every hepatic lobule. In addition, there is marked hepatomegaly, and the hepatic lymph nodes are edematous and hyperplastic. In rabbits, severe lesions develop in the intestines and heart. The terminal ileum, cecum, and proximal colon are diffusely reddened. Diffuse ("paintbrush") hemorrhage is frequently seen on the serosa of the cecum. Patchy areas of mucosal necrosis are present in the cecum and colon, together with marked edema of the wall of the cecum. Mesenteric lymph nodes may be enlarged and edematous. White streaks in the myocardium may be present, especially near the apex. Intestinal and heart lesions are generally milder or absent in other animal species.

Microscopically, there are numerous widespread multifocal areas of necrosis and hepatitis. In foals, the hepatic lesions are more pronounced than in other animals. Often the necrotic foci are so numerous that two or more coalesce. The hepatocytes in the center of the necrotic foci are destroyed and replaced by a mixture of mononuclear cells, neutrophils, and red blood cells. The causative bacteria are found in a crisscross pattern in viable hepatocytes at the periphery of the necrotic foci. In the cecum and colon of rabbits, patchy areas of necrosis extend as deep as the muscularis externa with associated mucosal and submucosal infiltrates of neutrophils. Organisms may be found within the epithelium, muscularis mucosa, and muscularis externa of the affected intestine. When cardiac lesions are present, they consist of foci of fiber fragmentation, vacuolation, loss of cross-striations, and minimal inflammatory cell infiltration.

Diagnosis: Serology of the blood and PCR assay of the feces of suspect infected animals may be used clinically to test for *C piliforme*. However, clinical signs in addition to the commonly available diagnostic methods must be interpreted together for a presumptive clinical diagnosis.

In postmortem specimens, a diagnosis is based on demonstration of organisms in tissue sections with special stains. *C piliforme* stains poorly with H&E and Gram stains. With Giemsa stain, the bacillus stains well in the liver and intestinal epithelium and in smears of infected organs but poorly in smooth muscles and cardiac muscle cells. The Warthin-Starry or Levaditi silver stains are preferable to other stains, because the bacillus stains well in the cytoplasm of all infected cells. In addition to special histochemical stains, the PCR assay can be used to detect *C piliforme* gene sequences in liver tissues from infected animals.

Treatment and Control: Little is known about the effectiveness of antibiotics for treatment. Some antibiotics are known to aggravate the disease. *C piliforme* is sensitive to tetracycline and partially sensitive to streptomycin, erythromycin, penicillin, and chlortetracycline. It is resistant to sulfonamides and chloramphenicol.

In neonatal foals, the disease seems to be nearly 100% fatal, although it is likely that older foals less severely affected may survive. Once the disease is present on a farm, it may be seen sporadically year after year. Animals suspected of being infected have been treated IV initially with 50% dextrose, followed by 10% dextrose, other fluid therapy, and antibiotics. Most foals respond dramatically to the dextrose therapy but relapse into a coma and die in a few hours. A few presumptive cases of Tyzzer disease in foals have been treated successfully by intensive administration of IV dextrose, sodium bicarbonate, potassium chloride, penicillin, and sulfamethoxazole-trimethoprim.

Because the disease in foals is sporadic and not highly contagious, specific preventive measures are usually not indicated. In areas where endospores are present in the environment, many foals may be exposed; however, only a few that are immunosuppressed become acutely affected. On premises where the disease is prevalent, overfeeding of mares, especially with high-protein diets seemingly predispose neonatal foals. Reducing the nitrogenous dietary compounds, including protein and nitrate in the diet that may induce immunosuppression in neonatal foals, may lessen the incidence of the disease. In general, factors that cause stress and immunosuppression should also be reduced. When the disease is seen in a colony of laboratory animals, treatment is not recommended because it prolongs the disease and possibly produces carrier animals. It is best to destroy all animals in the colony, decontaminate the environment, and restock with disease-free animals.

AMEBIASIS

(Amebiosis)

Amebiasis is an acute or chronic colitis, characterized by persistent diarrhea or dysentery, that is prevalent in tropical and subtropical areas worldwide. Its prevalence has declined in the USA over the past several decades, but the disease is still important in many tropical areas, particularly in times of disasters. It is common in people and nonhuman primates, sometimes seen in dogs and cats, and rare in other mammals. Several species of amebae are found in mammals, but the only known pathogen is *Entamoeba histolytica*. People are the natural host for this species and the usual source of infection for domestic animals. Mammals become infected by ingesting food or water contaminated with feces containing infective cysts. *E dispar* is a noninvasive, nonpathogenic ameba that is molecularly distinct but morphologically indistinguishable from the pathogenic species *E histolytica*. *E invadens* of reptiles is also morphologically identical to *E histolytica*, but it is not transmissible to mammals.

Clinical Findings: *E histolytica* is a pathogen with variable virulence. It lives in the lumen of the large intestine and cecum and may produce no obvious clinical signs, or it may invade the intestinal mucosa and produce mild to severe, ulcerative, hemorrhagic colitis. In acute disease, fulminating dysentery may develop, which may be fatal, progress to chronicity, or resolve spontaneously. Chronic cases may show weight loss, anorexia, tenesmus, and chronic diarrhea or dysentery, which may be continual or intermittent. In addition to the colon and cecum, amebae may invade perianal skin, genitalia, liver, brain, lungs, kidneys, and other organs. Signs may resemble those of other colonic diseases (eg, trichuriasis, balantidiasis). Invasive amebiasis is exacerbated by immunosuppression.

Diagnosis: Definitive diagnosis depends on finding *E histolytica* trophozoites or cysts in feces. Trophozoites are best seen in direct saline smears or in stained sections of affected colonic tissue. These parasites are difficult to find, because many animals with extraintestinal amebiasis have no concurrent intestinal infection. Colonoscopy with scraping or biopsy of ulcerations is more effective than fecal examination in diagnosing amebic colitis. In intestinal infections, repeated examinations may be necessary, because parasites may be passed periodically in the feces.

Trophozoites range in size from 10 to 60 μm but usually are >20 μm in diameter, have a single vesicular nucleus (usually with a central karyosome), are motile, and may contain ingested RBCs. Feces should be examined promptly, because the trophozoites die quickly once outside the body. Fecal leukocytes may be mistaken for amebae, so fixed and stained fecal smears (iodine, trichrome, iron hematoxylin, or periodic acid-Schiff reaction) may be necessary for identification.

Cysts range from 10 to 20 µm in diameter; the usual size is 12–15 µm. Mature cysts have four nuclei, whereas immature cysts may have one or two. In primates, the cysts may be recovered and identified on zinc sulfate flotations or in fixed and stained preparations (iodine, trichrome, or iron hematoxylin); however, *E histolytica* cysts are seldom, if ever, excreted by dogs or cats. An ELISA-based antigen test, available for diagnosis in people, may also aid diagnosis in other mammals. Immunostaining may also be useful.

Treatment: Scant information on treatment in animals is available. Metronidazole (10–25 mg/kg, PO, bid for 1 wk) or furazolidone (2–4 mg/kg, PO, tid for 1 wk) has been suggested. Dogs may continue to shed trophozoites after therapy. Treatment recommendations for people are available from the CDC Web site. For asymptomatic infections in people, the CDC lists iodoquinol, paromomycin, or diloxanide furoate (not commercially available in the USA) as drugs of choice, and for symptomatic intestinal disease or extraintestinal infections in people (eg, hepatic abscess), the drugs of choice are metronidazole or tinidazole, immediately followed by treatment with iodoquinol, paromomycin, or diloxanide furoate.

COCCIDIOSIS

Coccidiosis is usually an acute invasion and destruction of intestinal mucosa by protozoa of the genera *Eimeria* or *Isospora*. Clinical signs include diarrhea, fever, inappetence, weight loss, emaciation, and in extreme cases, death. However, many infections are subclinical. Coccidiosis is an economically important disease of cattle, sheep, goats, pigs, poultry (*see* p 2791), and also rabbits, in which the liver as well as the intestine can be affected (*see* p 1952). In dogs, cats, and horses, coccidiosis is less often diagnosed but can result in clinical illness. Other genera, of both hosts and protozoa, can be involved (*see* CRYPTOSPORIDIOSIS, p 209, SARCOCYSTOSIS, p 1058, and TOXOPLASMOSIS, p 685).

Etiology and Epidemiology: *Eimeria* and *Isospora* typically require only one host in which to complete their life cycles. Some species of *Isospora* have facultative intermediate (paratenic or transfer) hosts, and a new genus name, *Cystoisospora*, has been proposed for these species of *Isospora*. Coccidia are host-specific, and there is no cross-immunity between species of coccidia.

Coccidiosis is seen universally, most commonly in young animals housed or confined in small areas contaminated with oocysts. Coccidia are opportunistic pathogens; if pathogenic, their virulence may be influenced by various stressors. Therefore, clinical coccidiosis is most prevalent under conditions of poor nutrition, poor sanitation, or overcrowding, or after the stresses of weaning, shipping, sudden changes of feed, or severe weather.

In general, for most species of farm animals, the infection rate is high and rate of clinical disease is low (5%–10%), although up to 80% of animals in a high-risk group may show clinical signs. Most animals acquire *Eimeria* or *Isospora* infections of varying severity when between 1 mo and 1 yr old. Older animals usually are resistant to clinical disease but may have sporadic inapparent infections. Clinically healthy, mature animals can be sources of infection to young, susceptible animals.

Pathogenesis: Infection results from ingestion of infective oocysts. Oocysts enter the environment in the feces of an infected host, but oocysts of *Eimeria* and *Isospora* are unsporulated and therefore not infective when passed in the feces. Under favorable conditions of oxygen, humidity, and temperature, oocysts sporulate and become infective in several days. During sporulation, the amorphous protoplasm develops into small bodies (sporozoites) within secondary cysts (sporocysts) in the oocyst. In *Eimeria* spp, the sporulated oocyst has four sporocysts, each containing two sporozoites; in *Isospora* spp, the sporulated oocyst has two sporocysts, each containing four sporozoites.

When the sporulated oocyst is ingested by a susceptible animal, the sporozoites escape from the oocyst, invade the intestinal mucosa or epithelial cells in other locations, and develop intracellularly into multinucleate schizonts (also called meronts). Each nucleus develops into an infective body called a merozoite; merozoites enter new cells and repeat the process. After a variable number of asexual generations, merozoites develop into either macrogametocytes (females) or microgametocytes (males). These produce a single macrogamete or a number of microgametes in a host cell. After being fertilized by a microgamete, the macrogamete develops into an oocyst. The oocysts have resistant walls and are discharged unsporulated in the feces. Oocysts do not survive well at temperatures below ~30°C or above 40°C; within this temperature range, oocysts may survive ≥1 yr.

Of the numerous species of *Eimeria* or *Isospora* that can infect a particular host, not all are pathogenic. Concurrent infections with two or more species, some of which may not normally be considered pathogenic, also influence clinical disease. Within pathogenic species, strains may vary in virulence.

Clinical Findings: Clinical signs of coccidiosis are due to destruction of the intestinal epithelium and, frequently, the underlying connective tissue of the mucosa. This may be accompanied by hemorrhage into the lumen of the intestine, catarrhal inflammation, and diarrhea. Signs may include discharge of blood or tissue, tenesmus, and dehydration. Serum protein and electrolyte concentrations (typically hyponatremia) may be appreciably altered, but changes in Hgb or PCV are seen only in severely affected animals.

Diagnosis: Oocysts can be identified in feces by salt or sugar flotation methods. Finding appreciable numbers of oocysts of pathogenic species in the feces is diagnostic (>100,000 oocysts/g of feces in severe outbreaks), but because diarrhea may precede the heavy output of oocysts by 1–2 days and may continue after the oocyst discharge has returned to low levels, it is not always possible to find oocysts in a single fecal sample; multiple fecal examinations of one animal or single fecal examinations of animals housed in the same environment may be required. The number of oocysts present in feces is influenced by the genetically determined reproductive potential of the species, the number of infective oocysts ingested, stage of the infection, age and immune status of the animal, prior exposure, consistency of the fecal sample (free water content), and method of examination. Therefore, the results of fecal examinations must be related to clinical signs and intestinal lesions (gross and microscopic). Furthermore, the species must be determined to be pathogenic in that host. The finding of numerous oocysts of a nonpathogenic species concurrent with diarrhea does not constitute a diagnosis of clinical coccidiosis.

Treatment: The life cycles of *Eimeria* and *Isospora* are self-limiting and end spontaneously within a few weeks unless reinfection occurs. Prompt medication may slow or inhibit development of stages resulting from reinfection and, thus, can shorten the length of illness, reduce discharge of oocysts, alleviate hemorrhage and diarrhea, and lessen the likelihood of secondary infections and death. Sick animals should be isolated and treated individually whenever possible to ensure delivery of therapeutic drug levels and to prevent exposure of other animals. However, the efficacy of treatment for clinical coccidiosis has not been demonstrated for any drug, although it is widely accepted that treatment is effective against reinfection and should therefore facilitate recovery.

Most coccidiostats have a depressant effect on the early, first-stage schizonts and are therefore more appropriately used for control instead of treatment. Soluble sulfonamides are commonly administered orally to calves with clinical coccidiosis and are perceived to be more effective than intestinal sulfonamide formulations (boluses). Amprolium is also administered orally to calves, sheep, and goats with clinical coccidiosis. Preventive treatment of healthy exposed animals as a safeguard against additional morbidity is an important consideration when treating individual animals with clinical signs. The FDA is changing the marketing status of drugs, such as the sulfonamides that are used in human medicine, from over-the-counter to (veterinary) prescription for water medication or Veterinary Feed Directive (VFD) for feed medication. Drugs, such as the ionophores, that are not used in human medicine will continue to have an over-the-counter marketing status.

Prevention: Prevention is based on limiting the intake of sporulated oocysts by young animals so that an infection is established to induce immunity but not clinical signs. Good feeding practices and good management, including sanitation, contribute to this goal. Neonates should receive colostrum. Young, susceptible animals should be kept in clean, dry quarters. Feeding and watering devices should be clean and must be protected from fecal contamination; this usually means feed is placed in troughs above the ground and positioned so that it is difficult for fecal contamination of feed to occur. Stresses (eg, weaning, sudden changes in feed, and shipping) should be minimized.

Preventive administration of coccidiostats is recommended when animals under various management regimens can be predictably expected to develop coccidiosis. In virtually all cases, *Eimeria* spp are implicated. Decoquinate and ionophorous antibiotics are widely used for this purpose in young ruminants. Continuous low-level feeding of decoquinate, lasalocid, monensin, or amprolium during the first month of feedlot confinement has been reported to have preventive value. Ionophorous antibiotics and amprolium have been reported to be effective in goat kids, as have sulfonamides and amprolium in pigs.

COCCIDIOSIS OF CATTLE

Twelve *Eimeria* spp have been identified in the feces of cattle worldwide, but only three (*E zuernii*, *E bovis*, and *E auburnensis*) are most often associated with clinical disease. The other *Eimeria* spp have been shown experimentally to be mildly or moderately pathogenic but are not considered important pathogens.

Coccidiosis is commonly a disease of young cattle (1–2 mo to 1 yr) and usually is sporadic during the wet seasons of the year. "Summer coccidiosis" and "winter coccidiosis" in range cattle probably result from severe weather stress and crowding around a limited water source, which concentrates the hosts and parasites within a restricted area. Although particularly severe epidemics have been reported in feedlot cattle during extremely cold weather, cattle confined to feedlots are susceptible to coccidiosis throughout the year. Outbreaks usually occur within the first month of confinement. Cows may contribute to environmental contamination of *E bovis* oocysts through a periparturient increase in fecal oocyst counts. Time to onset of diarrhea after infection is 16–23 days for *E bovis* and *E zuernii* and 3–4 days for *E alabamensis*; clinical disease due to coccidiosis does not typically occur in the first 3 wk of life. Coccidiosis is therefore not considered part of the neonatal diarrhea complex in calves.

The most typical syndrome of coccidiosis is chronic or subclinical disease in groups of growing animals. Calves may appear unthrifty and have fecal-stained perineal areas. In light infections, cattle appear healthy and oocysts are present in normally formed feces, but feed efficiency is reduced. The most characteristic sign of clinical coccidiosis is watery feces, with little or no blood, and animals show only slight discomfort for a few days. Severe infections are rare. Severely affected cattle develop thin, bloody diarrhea that may continue for >1 wk, or thin feces with streaks or clots of blood, shreds of epithelium, and mucus. They may develop a fever; become anorectic, depressed, and dehydrated; and lose weight. Tenesmus is common because the most severe enteritis is confined to the large intestine, although pathogenic coccidia of cattle can damage the mucosa of the lower small intestine, cecum, and colon. During the acute period, some calves die; others die later from secondary complications (eg, pneumonia). Calves that survive severe illness can lose significant weight that is not quickly regained or can remain permanently stunted. Calves with concurrent enteric infections (eg, *Giardia*) may be more severely affected than calves with coccidia infections alone. In addition, management factors, such as weather, housing, feeding practices, and how animals are grouped, are important in determining the expression of clinical coccidiosis in cattle.

Nervous signs (eg, muscular tremors, hyperesthesia, clonic-tonic convulsions with ventroflexion of the head and neck, nystagmus) and a high mortality rate (80%–90%) are seen in some calves with acute clinical coccidiosis. Outbreaks of this "nervous form" are seen most commonly during, or after, severely cold weather in midwinter in Canada and the northern USA; there are no reports of the "nervous form" outside this geographic location. Affected calves may die <24 hr after the onset of dysentery and nervous signs, or they may live for several days, commonly in a laterally recumbent position with a mild degree of opisthotonos. Nervous signs have not been reported in experimental clinical coccidiosis in calves, which suggests that the nervous signs may be unrelated to the dysentery or, indeed, even to coccidiosis.

Diagnosis of coccidiosis is by finding oocysts on fecal flotation or direct smear or by the McMaster technique. Quantitative oocyst counts on individual rectal samples from at least five calves in a pen are helpful to confirm coccidiosis as a cause of clinical disease. Differential diagnoses include salmonellosis, bovine viral diarrhea, malnutrition, toxins, or other intestinal parasites.

Coccidiosis is a self-limiting disease, and spontaneous recovery without specific treatment is common when the multiplication stage of the coccidia has passed.

Drugs that can be used for therapy of clinically affected animals include sulfaquinoxaline (6 mg/lb/day for 3–5 days) and amprolium (10 mg/kg/day for 5 days). Sulfaquinoxaline is particularly useful for weaned calves that develop bloody diarrhea after arrival at a feedlot. For prevention, amprolium (5 mg/kg/day for 21 days), decoquinate (22.7 mg/45 kg/day for 28 days) and lasalocid (1 mg/kg/day to a maximum of 360 mg/head/day), or monensin (100–360 mg/head/day) can be used. The major benefits of coccidiostats are through improved feed efficiency and rate of gain.

In an outbreak, clinically affected animals should be isolated and given supportive oral and parenteral fluid therapy as necessary. The population density of the affected pens should be reduced. All feed and water supplies should be high enough off the ground to avoid fecal contamination. Mass medication of the feed and water supplies may be indicated in an attempt to prevent new cases and to minimize the effects of an epidemic. Cattle with coccidiosis and nervous signs should be brought indoors, kept well-bedded and warm, and given fluid therapy orally and parenterally. However, the case fatality rate of calves with coccidiosis and nervous signs is high despite intensive supportive therapy. Parenteral sulfonamide therapy may be indicated to control development of secondary bacterial enteritis or pneumonia, which may be seen in calves with coccidiosis during very cold weather. Corticosteroids are contraindicated, because they increase shedding of oocysts and have induced clinical disease in subclinically infected calves.

Coccidiosis has been difficult to control reliably. Overcrowding of animals should be avoided while they develop an immunity to the coccidial species in the environment. Calving grounds should be well drained and kept as dry as possible. All measures that minimize fecal contamination of hair coats and fleece should be practiced regularly. Feed and water troughs should be high enough to avoid heavy fecal contamination. Control of coccidiosis in feeder calves brought into a crowded feedlot depends on management of population density, presence of appropriate feed bunks, or use of chemotherapeutics, to control the numbers of oocysts ingested by the animals while effective immunity develops.

Coccidiostats are used to control naturally occurring coccidiosis. The ideal coccidiostat suppresses the full development of the life cycle of the coccidia, allows immunity to develop, and does not interfere with production performance. Sulfonamides in the feed at 25–35 mg/kg for ≥15 days are effective to control coccidiosis in calves. Monensin is an effective coccidiostat and growth promotant in calves. Postweaning coccidiosis in beef calves has been controlled using monensin administered via intraluminal continuous-release devices. Lasalocid is related to monensin and is also an effective coccidiostat for ruminants. Mixing lasalocid in the milk replacer of calves beginning at 2–4 days of age is an effective way to control coccidiosis. Lasalocid is also effective as a coccidiostat when fed free-choice in salt at a level of 0.75% of the total salt mixture. A level of 1 mg/kg is the most effective and rapid and is recommended when outbreaks of coccidiosis are imminent. Decoquinate in the feed at 0.5–1 mg/kg suppressed oocyst production in experimentally induced coccidiosis of calves. Decoquinate is most effective in preventing coccidial infections when fed continually in dry feed at 0.5 mg/kg. Monensin, lasalocid, and decoquinate at the manufacturer's recommended levels are equally effective. Toltrazuril administered at 15 mg/kg as a single oral dose, 14 days after animals are moved into group housing, effectively prevents diarrhea due to coccidiosis. Diclazuril (5 mg/kg) is being investigated as an oral anticoccidial in calves.

Control of infection should include changes in management factors that contribute to development of clinical disease. Inadequate housing and ventilation should be corrected, feeding practices adopted that avoid fecal contamination of feed, calves grouped by size, and an "all-in/all-out" method of calf movement from pen to pen adopted.

COCCIDIOSIS OF SHEEP

Infection with *Eimeria* is one of the most economically important diseases of sheep. Historically, some *Eimeria* spp were thought to be infectious and transmissible between sheep and goats, but the parasites are now considered host-specific. The names of some species of goat coccidia are still erroneously applied to species of similar appearance found in sheep.

E crandallis and *E ovinoidalis (ninakohlyakimovae)* are pathogens of lambs (usually 1–6 mo old); *E ovina* appears to be somewhat less pathogenic. Older sheep serve as sources of infection for the young. All other *Eimeria* of sheep are essentially nonpathogenic, even when large numbers of oocysts are present in feces.

Signs include diarrhea (sometimes containing blood or mucus), dehydration, fever, inappetence, weight loss, anemia, wool breaking, and death. The ileum, cecum, and upper colon are usually most affected and may be thickened, edematous, and inflamed; sometimes, there is mucosal hemorrhage. Thick, white, opaque patches containing large numbers of *E ovina* oocysts may develop in the small intestine. Because oocysts are prevalent in feces of sheep of all ages, coccidiosis cannot be diagnosed based solely on finding oocysts. Peak oocyst counts of >100,000/g of feces have been reported in 8- to 12-wk-old lambs that appeared healthy. However, diarrhea with oocyst counts of a pathogenic species of >20,000/g is characteristic of coccidiosis in sheep. Immune complex glomerulonephritis has also been attributed to coccidiosis. Fly strike and secondary bacterial enteric infections may accompany coccidiosis in lambs.

Lambs 1–6 mo old in lambing pens, intensive grazing areas, and feedlots are at greatest risk as a result of shipping, ration change, crowding stress, severe weather, and contamination of the environment with oocysts from ewes or other lambs. Because occurrence of coccidiosis under these management systems often becomes so predictable, coccidiostats should be administered prophylactically for 28 consecutive days beginning a few days after lambs are introduced into the environment. A concentrated ration containing monensin at 15 g/tonne can be fed to ewes from 4 wk before lambing until weaning, and to lambs from 4–20 wk of age. The toxic level of monensin for lambs is 4 mg/kg. Lasalocid (15–70 mg/head/day, depending on body wt) may be effective. A combination of monensin and lasalocid at 22 and 100 mg/kg of diet, respectively, is an effective prophylactic against naturally occurring coccidiosis in early weaned lambs under feedlot conditions.

Treatment of affected sheep once coccidiosis has been diagnosed is not effective, but severity can be reduced if treatment is begun early. A single treatment of toltrazuril (20 mg/kg) can significantly reduce the oocyst output in naturally infected lambs for ~3 wk after administration. Diclazuril (1 mg/kg) is an effective oral anticoccidial in lambs and is administered once at ~6–8 wk of age (most common) or twice (at 3–4 wk of age and again 3 wk later). Sulfaquinoxaline in drinking water at 0.015% concentration for 3–5 days may be used to treat affected lambs. In groups of lambs at pasture, frequent rotation of pastures for parasite control also helps control coccidial infection. However, when lambs are exposed to infection early in life as a result of infection from the ewe and a contaminated lambing ground, a solid immunity usually develops and problems are seen only when the stocking density is extremely high.

COCCIDIOSIS OF GOATS

Numerous species of *Eimeria* are found in goats in North America and elsewhere. The *Eimeria* spp are host specific and are not transmitted from sheep to goats.

E arloingi, *E christenseni*, and *E ovinoidalis* are highly pathogenic in kids. Clinical signs include diarrhea with or without mucus or blood, dehydration, emaciation, weakness, anorexia, and death. Some goats are actually constipated and die acutely without diarrhea. Usually, stages and lesions are confined to the small intestine, which may appear congested, hemorrhagic, or ulcerated, and have scattered pale, yellow to white macroscopic plaques in the mucosa. Histologically, villous epithelium is sloughed, and inflammatory cells are seen in the lamina propria and submucosa. In addition, there have been several reports of hepatobiliary coccidiosis with liver failure in dairy goats. Diagnosis of intestinal coccidiosis is based on finding oocysts of the pathogenic species in diarrheal feces, usually at tens of thousands to millions per gram of feces. It is not unusual to find oocyst counts as high as 70,000/g of feces in kids without overt disease, but weight gain may be affected.

Angora and dairy goats, raised under different management practices, may have similar patterns of exposure of kids. Just after parturition, nursery pens and surrounding areas may be heavily contaminated with oocysts from does. Resistance to infection is decreased just after shipping, changing rations, introducing new animals, or mixing young with older animals. Coccidiostats can be administered to a herd immediately after diagnosis or as a preventive in predictable situations such as those mentioned above.

Diagnosis and treatment are similar to those for cattle and sheep. Sulfadimidine at 55 g/tonne is also effective for control of coccidiosis in goats. In nonlactating goats, adding monensin to the feed at 18 g/tonne is preventive.

COCCIDIOSIS OF PIGS

Eight species of *Eimeria* and one of *Isospora* infect pigs in North America. Piglets 5–15 days old are characteristically infected with only *I suis*, which produces enteritis and diarrhea. These agents must be differentiated from viruses, bacteria, and helminths that also cause scours in neonatal pigs.

I suis is prevalent in neonatal pigs. Infection is characterized by a watery or greasy diarrhea, usually yellowish to white and foul smelling. Piglets may appear weak, dehydrated, and undersized; weight gains are depressed, and sometimes piglets die. A contributing factor to mortality is that piglets become covered with diarrheic feces and stay damp. Oocysts are usually shed in the feces and can be identified by their size, shape, and sporulation characteristics; however, in peracute infections, diagnosis must be based on finding stages of the parasite in impression smears or histologic sections of the small intestine, because pigs can die before oocysts are formed. In severely affected piglets, histologic lesions confined to the jejunum and ileum are characterized by villous atrophy, blunting of villi, focal ulceration, and fibrinonecrotic enteritis with parasite stages in epithelial cells.

Preventive control by feeding anticoccidials to sows from 2 wk before farrowing through lactation or to neonatal pigs from birth to weaning has been reported; however, effectiveness of the latter has not been confirmed. Although the sow is a logical source of infection for piglets, this has not been well documented. Thorough removal of feces and disinfection of farrowing facilities between litters greatly decreases infection. Piglets that recover from infection are highly resistant to reinfection.

Although less commonly associated with clinical coccidiosis, *E debliecki*, *E neodebliecki*, *E scabra*, and *E spinosa* have been found in pigs ~1–3 mo old with diarrhea. Illness may last 7–10 days, with pigs remaining unthrifty.

Treatment of coccidiosis may include sulfamethazine in drinking water. The control of coccidiosis in newborn piglets infected with *I suis* has been unreliable. The use of coccidiostats in the feed of the sow for several days or a few weeks before and after farrowing has been recommended and used in the field, but the results are variable. Amprolium and monensin are ineffective for prevention of experimental coccidiosis in piglets. A control program designed to decrease the number of oocysts has been recommended and consists of proper cleaning, disinfection, and steam cleaning of the farrowing housing. Amprolium (25% feed grade) at the rate of 10 kg/tonne of sows' feed started 1 wk before farrowing and continued until the piglets are 3 wk of age has been recommended, but the results are unsatisfactory. A single dose of toltrazuril (20 mg/kg, PO) decreased oocyst excretion, the incidence of diarrhea, and weight gain impairment in piglets with experimentally induced coccidiosis. Diclazuril (5 mg/kg) is being investigated as an oral anticoccidial in piglets.

COCCIDIOSIS OF CATS AND DOGS

Many species of coccidia infect the intestinal tract of cats and dogs. All species appear to be host-specific. Cats have species of *Isospora*, *Besnoitia*, *Toxoplasma*, *Hammondia*, and *Sarcocystis*. Dogs have species of *Isospora*, *Hammondia*, and *Sarcocystis*. Neither dogs nor cats have *Eimeria*.

Hammondia has an obligatory two-host life cycle with cats or dogs as final hosts and rodents or ruminants as intermediate hosts, respectively. *Hammondia* oocysts are indistinguishable from those of *Toxoplasma* and *Besnoitia* but are nonpathogenic in either host. (*See also* BESNOITIOSIS, p 597, SARCOCYSTOSIS, p 1058, and TOXOPLASMOSIS, p 685.)

The most common coccidia of cats and dogs are *Isospora*. Some *Isospora* spp of cats and dogs can facultatively infect other mammals and produce in various organs an encysted form that is infective for the cat or dog. Two species infect cats: *I felis* and *I rivolta*; both can be identified easily by oocyst size and shape. Almost every cat eventually becomes infected with *I felis*. Four species infect dogs: *I canis*, *I ohioensis*, *I burrowsi*, and *I neorivolta*. In dogs, only *I canis* can be identified by the oocyst structure; the other three *Isospora* overlap in dimensions and can be differentiated only by endogenous developmental characteristics.

Clinical coccidiosis, although not common, has been reported in kittens and puppies. In kittens, it is seen primarily during weaning stress. The most common clinical signs in severe cases are diarrhea (sometimes bloody), weight loss, and dehydration. Usually, coccidiosis is associated with other infectious agents, immunosuppression, or stress.

Treatment may be unnecessary in cats, because they usually spontaneously eliminate the infection. In clinically affected cats, trimethoprim-sulfonamide (30–60 mg/kg/day for 6 days) can be used.

In kennel conditions when the need for prophylaxis might be predicted, amprolium is said to be effective, although it is not approved for use in dogs. In severe cases, in addition to supportive fluid therapy, sulfonamides such as sulfadimethoxine (50 mg/kg the first day and 25 mg/kg/day for 2–3 wk thereafter) can be used. Sanitation is important, especially in catteries and kennels, or where large numbers of animals are housed. Feces should be removed frequently. Fecal contamination of feed and water should be prevented. Runs, cages, and utensils should be disinfected daily. Raw meat should not be fed. Insect control should be established.

CRYPTOSPORIDIOSIS

Cryptosporidiosis is recognized worldwide, primarily in neonatal calves but also in lambs, kids, foals, and piglets. Cryptosporidia cause varying degrees of naturally occurring diarrhea in neonatal farm animals. The parasites commonly act in concert with other enteropathogens to produce intestinal injury and diarrhea.

Etiology and Epidemiology: There are currently 19 species and 40 genotypes of *Cryptosporidium*. *C hominis* (formerly *C parvum* type I) is a specific human pathogen. *C parvum* (formerly *C parvum* type II) is zoonotic and infective to many animals, including people and calves. Four cryptosporidial species have been isolated from cattle (*C parvum*, *C andersoni*, *C bovis*, and *C ryanae*). *C andersoni* infects the abomasum of older cattle; *C bovis* and *C ryanae* are cattle adapted (cattle are the major host). *C parvum* is a common cause of calf diarrhea, and cryptosporidial oocysts have been detected in the feces of 70% of 1- to 3-wk-old dairy calves. Infection can be detected as early as 5 days of age, with the greatest proportion of calves excreting organisms between days 9 and 14. Many reports associate infection in calves with diarrhea occurring at 5–15 days of age.

C parvum is also a common enteric infection in young lambs and goats. Diarrhea can result from a monoinfection but more commonly is associated with mixed infections. Infection can be associated with severe outbreaks of diarrhea, with high case fatality rates in lambs 4–10 days old and in goat kids 5–21 days old. Cryptosporidial infection in pigs is seen over a wider age range than in ruminants and has been seen in pigs from 1 wk old through market age. Most infections are asymptomatic, and the organism does not appear to be an important enteric pathogen in pigs, although it may contribute to postweaning malabsorptive diarrhea. Cryptosporidial infection in foals appears less prevalent and is seen at a later age than in ruminants, with excretion rates peaking at 5–8 wk old. Infection is not usually detected in yearlings or adults. Most studies indicate that cryptosporidiosis is not a common disease in foals; infections in immunocompetent foals are usually subclinical. Persistent clinical infections are seen in Arabian foals with inherited combined immunodeficiency. Cryptosporidiosis is also recorded in young deer and can be a cause of diarrhea in artificially reared orphans.

Transmission: The source of cryptosporidial infection is oocysts that are fully sporulated and infective when excreted in the feces. Large numbers are excreted during the patent period, resulting in heavy environmental contamination. Transmission may occur directly from calf to calf, indirectly via fomite or human transmission, from contamination in the environment, or by fecal contamination of the feed or water supply. A periparturient rise in the excretion of oocysts may occur in ewes. *C parvum* is not host-specific, and infection from other species (eg, rodents, farm cats) via contamination of feed is also possible.

Oocysts are resistant to most disinfectants and can survive for several months in cool and moist conditions. Oocyst infectivity can be destroyed by ammonia, formalin, freeze-drying, and exposure to temperatures <32°F (0°C) or >149°F (65°C). Ammonium hydroxide, hydrogen peroxide, chlorine dioxide, 10% formol saline, and 5% ammonia are effective in destroying oocyst infectivity. Infectivity in calf feces is reduced after 1–4 days of drying.

Concurrent infections with other enteric pathogens, especially rotavirus and coronavirus, are common, and epidemiologic studies suggest that diarrhea is more severe in mixed infections. Immunocompromised animals are more susceptible to clinical disease than immunocompetent animals, but the relationship between disease and failure of passive transfer of colostral immunoglobulins is not clear. Age-related resistance, unrelated to prior exposure, is seen in lambs but not calves. Infection results in production of parasite-specific antibody, but both cell-mediated and humoral antibody are important in protection, as well as local antibody in the gut of the neonate.

Case fatality rates in cryptosporidiosis are generally low unless complicated by other factors (eg, concurrent infections, energy deficits from inadequate intake of colostrum and milk, chilling from adverse weather conditions).

Pathogenesis: The life cycle of *Cryptosporidium* consists of six major developmental events. After ingestion of the oocyst, there is excystation (release of infective sporozoites), merogony (asexual multiplication), gametogony (gamete formation), fertilization, oocyst wall formation, and sporogony (sporozoite formation). Oocysts of *Cryptosporidium* spp can sporulate within host cells and are infective when passed in the feces. Infection persists until the host's immune response eliminates the parasite. In natural and experimentally produced cases in calves, cryptosporidia are most numerous in the lower part of the small intestine and less common in the cecum and colon. Prepatent periods are 2–7 days in calves and 2–5 days in lambs. Oocysts are usually passed in the feces of calves for 3–12 days.

Clinical Findings: Calves with cryptosporidiosis usually have a mild to moderate diarrhea that persists for several days regardless of treatment. The age at onset is later, and the duration of diarrhea tends to be a few days longer than are seen in the diarrheas caused by rotavirus, coronavirus, or enterotoxigenic *Escherichia coli*. Feces are yellow or pale, watery, and contain mucus. The persistent diarrhea may result in marked weight loss and emaciation. In most cases, the diarrhea is self-limiting after several days. Varying degrees of apathy, anorexia, and dehydration are present. Only rarely do severe dehydration, weakness, and collapse occur, in contrast to findings in other causes of acute diarrhea in neonatal calves. Case fatality rates can be high in herds with cryptosporidiosis when the calf feeder withholds milk and feeds only electrolyte solutions during the episode of diarrhea. The persistent nature of the diarrhea leads to a marked energy deficit in these circumstances, and the calves die of inanition at 3–4 wk old.

Lesions: Calves with persistent diarrhea have villous atrophy in the small intestine. Histologically, large numbers of the parasite are embedded in the microvilli of the absorptive enterocytes. In low-grade infections, only a few parasites are present, with no apparent histologic changes in the intestine. The villi are shorter than normal, with crypt hyperplasia and a mixed inflammatory cell infiltrate.

Diagnosis: Diagnosis is based on detection of oocysts by examination of fecal smears with Ziehl-Neelsen stains, fecal flotation techniques, ELISA, fluorescent-labeled antibodies, a rapid immunochromatographic test, and PCR. Sheather's flotation sedimentation staining is the most sensitive (83%) and specific (99%) of these techniques, with a relatively low cost per test. This technique requires centrifuging a fecal sample in Sheather's solution, aspirating the top layer and diluting the fluid in phosphate buffer saline, centrifuging, and placing the sediment on the slide and performing a modified Ziehl-Neelsen technique to look for cryptosporidial oocysts. It has been suggested that if the diarrhea is caused by cryptosporidia, there should be 10^5–10^7 oocysts/mL of feces. The oocysts are small (5–6 mm in diameter) and relatively non-refractile. They are difficult to detect by normal light microscopy but are readily detected by phase-contrast microscopy.

Treatment: There are no currently licensed therapeutics available in the USA for *C parvum* infection in food animals. Anecdotal reports of success with extra-label use of various compounds have not been replicated in controlled trials. Experimental treatments have for the most part been toxic or ineffective. Halofuginone is reported to markedly reduce oocyst output in experimentally infected lambs and naturally and experimentally infected calves; therapy was also reported to prevent diarrhea. Paromomycin sulfate (100 mg/kg/day, PO, for 11 days from the second day of age) proved successful in preventing natural disease in a controlled clinical field trial in goat kids.

Affected calves should be supported with fluids and electrolytes, both orally and parenterally, as necessary until recovery occurs. Cows' whole milk should be given in small quantities several times daily (to the full level of requirement) to optimize digestion and to minimize weight loss. Several days of intensive care and feeding may be required before recovery is apparent. Parenteral nutrition may be considered for valuable calves.

Control: The disease is difficult to control. Reducing the number of oocysts ingested may reduce the severity of infection and allow immunity to develop. Calves should be born in a clean environment, and adequate amounts of colostrum should be fed at an early age. Calves should be kept separate without calf-to-calf contact for at least the first 2 wk of life, with strict hygiene at feeding. Diarrheic calves should be isolated from healthy calves during the course of the diarrhea and for several days after recovery. Great care must be taken to avoid mechanical transmission of infection. Calf-rearing houses should be vacated and cleaned out on a regular basis; an "all-in/all-out" management system, with thorough cleaning and several weeks of drying between batches of calves, should be used. Rats, mice, and flies should be controlled when possible, and rodents and pets should not have access to calf grain and milk feed storage areas.

Hyperimmune bovine colostrum can reduce the severity of diarrhea and the period of oocyst excretion in experimentally infected calves. Protection is not related to circulating levels of specific antibody but requires a high titer of *C parvum* antibody in the gut lumen for prolonged periods. Many research groups have attempted to develop effective vaccines against cryptosporidia. Unfortunately, to date, vaccinations have not been effective.

Zoonotic Risk: Infections in domestic animals may be a reservoir for infection of susceptible people. *C hominis* and *C parvum* are considered to be relatively common nonviral causes of self-limiting diarrhea in immunocompetent people, particularly children. In immunocompromised people, clinical disease may be severe. The infection is transmitted predominantly from person to person, but direct infection from animals and waterborne infection from contamination of surface water and drinking water by domestic or wild animal feces can also be important. Animal handlers on a calf farm can be at high risk of diarrhea due to cryptosporidiosis transmitted from infected calves. Immunocompromised people should be restricted from access to young animals and possibly from access to farms.

GIARDIASIS

(Giardosis, Lambliasis, Lambliosis)

Giardiasis is a chronic, intestinal protozoal infection seen worldwide in most domestic and wild mammals, many birds, and people. Infection is common in dogs, cats, ruminants, and pigs. *Giardia* spp have been reported in 0.44%–39% of fecal samples from pet and shelter dogs and cats, 1%–53% in small ruminants, 9%–73% in cattle, 1%–38% in pigs, and 0.5%–20% in horses, with higher rates of infection in younger animals. Farm prevalences in production animals vary between 0% and 100%, with the highest prevalence in younger animals. The cumulative incidence on a farm where *Giardia* has been diagnosed is 100% in cattle and goats and nearly 100% in sheep.

Three major morphologic groups have been described: *G muris* from mice, *G agilis* from amphibians, and a third group from various warm-blooded animals. There are at least four species in this third group, including *G ardeae* and *G psittaci* from birds, *G microti* from muskrats and voles, and *G duodenalis* (also known as *G intestinalis* and *G lamblia*), a species complex with a wide mammalian host range infecting people and domestic animals. Molecular characterization has shown that *G duodenalis* is in fact a species complex, comprising seven assemblages (A to G), some of which have distinct host preferences (eg, assemblage C/D in dogs, assemblage F in cats) or a limited host range (eg, assemblage E in hoofed livestock), whereas others infect a wide range of animals, including people (assemblage A and B). There is increasing evidence that some assemblages (A and B) that infect domestic animals can also infect people, although transmission patterns are not totally understood. Dogs have mainly assemblages C and D, cats have assemblages A1 and F, and people are infected with assemblages A2 and B; however, some studies have identified human assemblages of *Giardia* in canine fecal samples.

Cycle and Transmission: Flagellate protozoa (trophozoites) of the genus *Giardia* inhabit the mucosal surfaces of the small intestine, where they attach to the brush border, absorb nutrients, and multiply by binary fission. They usually live in the proximal portion of the small intestine. Trophozoites encyst in the small or large intestine, and the newly formed cysts pass in the feces. There are no intracellular stages. The prepatent period is generally 3–10 days. Cyst shedding may be continual over several days and weeks but is often intermittent, especially in the chronic phase of infection. The cyst is the infective stage and can survive for several weeks in the environment, whereas trophozoites cannot.

Transmission occurs by the fecal-oral route, either by direct contact with an infected host or through a contaminated environment. Characteristics that facilitate infection include the high excretion of cysts by infected animals and the low dose needed for infection. *Giardia* cysts are infectious immediately after excretion and are very resistant, resulting in a gradual increase in environmental infection pressure. High humidity facilitates survival of cysts in the environment, and overcrowding favors transmission.

Pathogenesis: *Giardia* infections cause an increase in epithelial permeability, increased numbers of intraepithelial lymphocytes, and activation of T lymphocytes. Trophozoite toxins and T-cell activation initiate a diffuse shortening of brush border microvilli and decreased activity of the small-intestinal brush border enzymes, especially lipase, some proteases, and dissacharidases. The diffuse microvillus shortening leads to a decrease in overall absorptive area in the small intestine and an impaired intake of water, electrolytes, and nutrients. The combined effect of this decreased resorption and the brush border enzyme deficiencies results in malabsorptive diarrhea and lower weight gain. The reduced activity of lipase and the increased production of mucin by goblet cells may explain the steatorrhea and mucous diarrhea that has been described in *Giardia*-infected hosts.

Clinical Findings and Lesions: *Giardia* infections in dogs and cats may be inapparent or may produce weight loss and chronic diarrhea or steatorrhea, which can be continual or intermittent, particularly in puppies and kittens. Feces usually are soft, poorly formed, pale, malodorous, contain mucus, and appear fatty. Watery diarrhea is unusual in uncomplicated cases, and blood is usually not present in feces. Occasionally, vomiting occurs. Giardiasis must be differentiated from other causes of nutrient malassimilation (eg, exocrine pancreatic insufficiency [*see* p 409] and intestinal malabsorption [*see* p 400]). Clinical laboratory findings usually are normal.

In calves, and to a lesser extent in other production animals, giardiasis can result in diarrhea that does not respond to antibiotic or coccidiostatic treatment. The excretion of pasty to fluid feces with a mucoid appearance may indicate giardiasis, especially when the diarrhea occurs in young animals (1–6 mo old). Experimental infection of goat kids, lambs, and calves resulted in a decreased feed efficiency and subsequently a decreased weight gain.

Gross intestinal lesions are seldom evident, although microscopic lesions, consisting of villous atrophy and cuboidal enterocytes, may be present.

Diagnosis: The motile, piriform trophozoites (12–18 × 7–10 μm) are occasionally seen in saline smears of loose or watery feces. They should not be confused with yeast or with trichomonads, which have a single rather than double nucleus, an undulating membrane, and no concave ventral surface. The oval cysts (9–15 × 7–10 μm) can be detected in feces concentrated by the centrifugation-flotation technique using zinc sulfate (specific gravity 1.18). Sodium chloride, sucrose, or sodium nitrate flotation media may be too hypertonic and distort the cysts. Staining cysts with iodine aids identification. Because *Giardia* cysts are excreted intermittently, several fecal examinations should be performed if giardiasis is suspected (eg, three samples collected throughout 3–5 days). *Giardia* may be underdiagnosed, because the cysts are intermittently shed.

For the detection of parasite antigen, immunofluorescence assays and ELISA are commercially available. An in-house ELISA available for use in dogs and cats is a useful tool for clinical diagnosis, particularly when coupled with a centrifugal flotation examination of feces. It is best to test symptomatic animals with a combination of a direct saline smear of feces, fecal flotation with centrifugation, and a sensitive, specific ELISA optimized for use in the animal being tested (eg, ELISA for dogs and cats).

Treatment: No drugs are approved for treatment of giardiasis in dogs and cats in the USA. Fenbendazole (50 mg/kg/day for 5–10 days) effectively removes *Giardia* cysts from the feces of dogs; no adverse effects are reported, and it is safe for pregnant and lactating animals. This dosage is approved to treat *Giardia* infections in dogs in Europe. Fenbendazole is not approved in cats but may reduce clinical signs and cyst shedding at 50 mg/kg/day for 5 days. Albendazole is effective at 25 mg/kg, bid for 4 days in dogs and for 5 days in cats but should not be used in these species, because it has led to bone marrow suppression and is not approved for use in these species. A combination of praziquantel (5.4–7 mg/kg), pyrantel (26.8–35.2 mg/kg), and febantel (26.8–35.2 mg/kg) also effectively decreases cyst excretion in infected dogs when administered for 3 days. A synergistic effect between pyrantel and febantel was demonstrated in an animal model, suggesting that the combination product may be preferred over febantel alone.

Metronidazole (extra-label at 25 mg/kg, bid for 5 days) is ~65% effective in eliminating *Giardia* spp from infected dogs but may be associated with acute development of anorexia and vomiting, which may occasionally progress to pronounced generalized ataxia and vertical positional nystagmus. Metronidazole may be administered to cats at 10–25 mg/kg, bid for 5 days. Metronidazole benzoate is perhaps better tolerated by cats. Safety concerns limit the use of metronidazole in dogs and cats. A possible treatment strategy for dogs would be to treat first with fenbendazole for 5–10 days or to administer both fenbendazole and metronidazole together for 5 days, being sure to bathe the dogs to remove cysts. If clinical disease still persists and cyst shedding continues, the combination therapy should be extended for another 10 days.

Currently, no drug is licensed for the treatment of giardiasis in ruminants. Fenbendazole and albendazole (5–20 mg/kg/day for 3 days) significantly reduce the peak and duration of cyst excretion and result in a clinical benefit in treated calves. Paromomycin (50–75 mg/kg, PO, for 5 days) was found to be highly efficacious in calves.

Oral fenbendazole may be an option for treatment in some birds.

Control: *Giardia* cysts are immediately infective when passed in the feces and survive in the environment. Cysts are a source of infection and reinfection for animals, particularly those in crowded conditions (eg, kennels, catteries, or intensive rearing systems for production animals). Feces should be removed as soon as possible (at least daily) and disposed of with municipal waste. Infected dogs and cats should be bathed to remove cysts from the hair coat. Prompt and frequent removal of feces limits environmental contamination, as does subsequent disinfection. Cysts are inactivated by most quaternary ammonium compounds, steam, and boiling water.

To increase the efficacy of disinfectants, solutions should be left for 5–20 min before being rinsed off contaminated surfaces. Disinfection of grass yards or runs is impossible, and these areas should be considered contaminated for at least a month after infected dogs last had access. Cysts are susceptible to desiccation, and areas should be allowed to dry thoroughly after cleaning.

DISEASES OF THE MOUTH IN LARGE ANIMALS

LIP LACERATIONS

Wounds of the lips and cheeks occur frequently in horses. The most common cause is external trauma or secondary to the use of inappropriate bits or restraint devices. Lip lacerations may be accompanied by mandibular or incisive bone fractures with or without dental fractures and tooth avulsions. These occur when a horse grasps objects with its mouth and then pulls back when startled. Lip lacerations without bone or teeth involvement can be sutured, usually with a good result. Healing is rapid because of the good blood supply to the head. Lacerations left to heal by second intention can result in orocutaneous fistula, which may require resection and primary wound closure. Rarely, skin grafts or mucosal flaps are required to manage orocutaneous fistula.

GLOSSOPLEGIA

Glossoplegia, or paralysis of the tongue, is uncommon. Causes in horses include incorrect placement of obstetric snares in neonates during forced extraction, strangles, upper respiratory tract infections, meningitis, botulism, encephalomyelitis, leukoencephalomalacia, equine protozoal encephalomyelitis, and cerebral abscessation. Any condition that damages the hypoglossal nerve (cranial nerve XII), which is the major motor nerve to the muscles of the tongue, can result in glossoplegia. Neonates with glossoplegia must be monitored carefully to ensure they are able to eat. If necessary in affected foals, a nasogastric tube should be placed for administration of colostrum or IV plasma administered to prevent failure of passive transfer. Foals unable to maintain hydration may require IV fluid therapy and anti-inflammatory medication (eg, phenylbutazone, flunixin meglumine, or dexamethasone). Prophylaxis against gastric ulceration is also indicated. If the condition persists for >10 days after birth, the prognosis for regaining normal function is guarded. Inflammatory diseases and trauma may also result in transient glossoplegia. Occasionally, horses undergoing prolonged dental procedures involving excessive traction on the tongue can develop temporary glossoplegia. The prognosis of glossoplegia depends on the horse's response to treatment for the primary condition.

In cattle, glossoplegia may accompany severe actinobacillosis (*see* p 589). There may be complete paralysis of the tongue accompanied by necrosis of the tip. Such conditions are occasionally seen in outbreaks in feedlot cattle and may follow a bout of viral stomatitis.

NEOPLASIA

Neoplasia of the mouth and lips other than viral papillomas are uncommon and include melanomas, sarcoids, and squamous cell carcinoma. In gray horses, melanomas may develop and infiltrate the commissures of the mouth and cause hard, thickened, tumorous plaques that may not be detected until well advanced. Verrucose, fibroblastic, and sessile or flat forms of equine sarcoid can involve the mouth and lips.

Carbon dioxide laser removal of oral and lip melanomas should be considered. Complete removal of oral and lip melanomas is not necessary for a successful outcome. In addition, some horses may respond to oral cimetidine therapy. Surgical resection of sarcoids can be performed successfully with the carbon dioxide laser. Along with laser resection, intratumoral administration of cisplatin can be considered to lessen the chances for recurrence. Cryosurgery is another acceptable method of treatment. Squamous cell carcinoma can be difficult to treat because of its invasive nature. Surgical debulking with the carbon dioxide laser followed by intratumoral injection of cisplatin can be effective in select cases. Regardless of treatment, the prognosis for complete resolution of oral squamous cell carcinoma is guarded to poor. (*See also* TUMORS OF THE SKIN AND SOFT TISSUES, p 942.)

SLAFRAMINE TOXICOSIS

Causes of slaframine toxicosis include the ingestion of forages, particularly clovers, infected with the fungus *Rhizoctonia leguminicola*, which produces the toxic alkaloid slaframine. Profuse ptyalism is often the only clinical sign. Affected animals have no evidence of oral ulceration or other oral lesions. Ptyalism resolves once the animal is removed from the affected forage. The differential diagnoses for large animals (particularly ruminants) include bluetongue, vesicular stomatitis, vesicular exanthema, and foot-and-mouth disease.

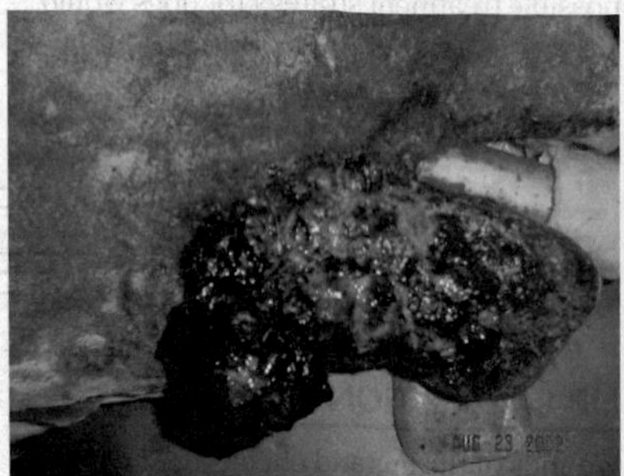

An extensive sarcoid involving the lower lip of a horse. *Courtesy of Dr. Jan Hawkins.*

STOMATITIS

Stomatitis is a clinical sign of many diseases in large animals. Oral trauma or contact with chemical irritants (eg, horses that lick at their legs after having been blistered with caustic agents) may result in transient stomatitis. Traumatic injury from the ingestion of the awns of barley, foxtail, porcupine grass, and spear grass, as well as feeding on plants infested with hairy caterpillars, also will result in stomatitis in horses and cattle.

Clinical signs commonly associated with acute active stomatitis include ptyalism, dysphagia, or resistance to oral examination. Oral examination is facilitated by sedation, after which the mouth can be examined carefully with the aid of a mouth speculum and a light source. Ulcers should be visually and digitally evaluated to determine whether embedded foreign material (eg, grass awns) is present. If the etiology is ingestion of foreign material, changing the quality and quantity of the hay or removing the animal from a pasture with grass awns may effect recovery.

Differential diagnoses include actinobacillosis, foot-and-mouth disease, malignant catarrhal fever, and bovine viral diarrhea. Epidemic diseases such as bluetongue in ruminants, swine vesicular disease, and vesicular stomatitis in horses must be differentiated from other forms of acute noninfectious or contagious stomatitis.

PAPULAR STOMATITIS

Viral papillomas are found around the lips and mouths of young animals, particularly in cattle from 1 mo to 2 yr old. In some herds, the rate of occurrence may be 100%. The lesions are characteristically white to pink, raised, and appear proliferative. Most papillomas resolve spontaneously. However, in some cases, the lesions may coalesce to form cosmetically unacceptable masses, and owners may request therapy.

Surgical removal of larger masses can be cosmetically acceptable and lessen recovery time. Small masses can also be manually debrided or crushed to stimulate the immune system. Other therapies, including cryosurgery and the use of autologous vaccines, may also be effective. Most papillomas eventually disappear if given time.

DISEASES OF THE ESOPHAGUS IN LARGE ANIMALS

ESOPHAGEAL OBSTRUCTION

(Choke)

Esophageal obstruction (choke) occurs when the esophagus is obstructed by food or foreign objects. It is the most common esophageal disease in large animals. Horses most commonly obstruct on grain, beet pulp, or hay. Esophageal obstruction can also occur after recovery from standing chemical restraint or general anesthesia. Cattle tend to obstruct on a single solid object, eg, apples, beets, potatoes, turnips, corn stalks, or ears of corn.

Clinical Findings: In **horses**, clinical signs associated with esophageal obstruction include nasal discharge of feed material or saliva, dysphagia, coughing, or ptyalism. The horse may appear anxious and/or appear to "retch" by stretching and arching the neck. Affected horses may continue to eat or drink, worsening the clinical signs.

In **cattle**, clinical signs include free-gas bloat, ptyalism, or nasal discharge of food and water. Ruminants may be bloated and in distress or recumbent, or there may be protrusion of the tongue, extension of the head, bruxism, and ptyalism. Acute and complete esophageal obstruction is an emergency because it prohibits eructation of ruminal gases, and free-gas bloat develops. Severe free-gas bloat may result in asphyxia, because the expanding rumen puts pressure on the diaphragm and reduces venous return of blood to the heart.

Diagnosis: The clinical signs of esophageal obstruction are usually diagnostic. Physical examination findings compatible with esophageal obstruction include nasal discharge of feed material and water, bruxism, ptyalism, and palpable enlargement of the esophagus; in some instances, foreign objects lodged in the cervical esophagus may be located via palpation. Subcutaneous emphysema, cervical cellulitis, and fever may be associated with esophageal rupture. The inability to pass a stomach (ruminants) or nasogastric tube (horses) can also confirm the diagnosis.

An endoscopic examination helps localize the site of esophageal obstruction, type of obstructing material, and extent of esophageal ulceration. Because of the risk of aspiration pneumonia, the respiratory tract should be evaluated carefully, including auscultation of the heart and lungs and thoracic radiography. In complicated or chronic cases, a CBC and serum biochemistry profile should be performed. CBC abnormalities include leukocytosis, left shift, toxic neutrophils, and hyperfibrinogenemia. Biochemical abnormalities include hyponatremia, hypochloremia, and hypokalemia secondary to excessive loss of saliva.

Treatment: In **horses**, many cases of esophageal obstruction may resolve spontaneously if feed and water are withheld. Spontaneous resolution can be aided by IV administration of sedatives (such as xylazine and detomidine). Oxytocin (0.11–0.22 mg/kg, IV) has proved useful to relax esophageal smooth muscle. To ensure that the esophageal obstruction has resolved completely, all horses with suspected obstruction should have a nasogastric tube passed into the stomach or an endoscopic examination.

Waiting >4–6 hr before passing a nasogastric tube is not recommended because of the risk of esophageal mucosal ulceration and aspiration pneumonia. Horses that do not respond to conservative management (withdrawal of feed and water, IV sedation or oxytocin) should be initially treated with esophageal lavage as follows: After IV sedation, a nasogastric tube is inserted to the level of the obstruction. Water is delivered to the obstruction site with a stomach pump, and the tube is slowly inserted and withdrawn to lavage the esophagus. The head must be lower than the torso to minimize aspiration of water into the lungs. Lavage via nasogastric tube is successful in at least 90% of cases.

For horses unresponsive to standing esophageal lavage, general anesthesia should be considered, with the horse positioned in lateral recumbency and orotracheally intubated. Again, the head must be positioned lower than the torso to prevent water passing into the lungs. A cuffed endotracheal tube (18–22 mm) is inserted into the esophagus as far as possible or to the level of the esophageal obstruction, and the cuff inflated. A nasogastric tube is inserted through the endotracheal tube, and the esophagus is lavaged as previously described. Again, resolution of obstruction should be confirmed with endoscopy or passage of the nasogastric tube into the stomach. An esophagotomy to resolve esophageal obstruction is rarely required.

All chronic cases of esophageal obstruction should be evaluated endoscopically after successful resolution. These horses frequently have esophageal ulceration that can be circumferential. Severe mucosal ulceration can result in esophageal stricture and repeat obstruction. Endoscopy is also useful to exclude esophageal diverticula, which can predispose to esophageal obstruction. Esophageal diverticula can also be diagnosed with contrast esophagograms.

Horses without mucosal ulceration should be fed water-soaked, complete pelleted feed for at least 7–14 days to minimize the likelihood of repeat esophageal obstruction. Horses with mucosal ulceration should be fed this diet for 60 days, after which follow-up endoscopy should be performed to evaluate whether mucosal ulceration has resolved and esophageal stricture has occurred. Horses with chronic mucosal ulceration with stricture may require surgical management.

Aspiration pneumonia should be managed with IV or oral antimicrobials and anti-inflammatory drugs. Commonly used antimicrobials include potassium or procaine penicillin G (22,000 U/kg, IV [potassium] or IM [procaine], bid-qid), trimethoprim sulfamethoxazole (30 mg/kg, PO, bid), and gentamicin sulfate (6.6 mg/kg/day, IV or IM). Metronidazole (15 mg/kg, PO, qid) is useful for management of anaerobic infections. The most common anti-inflammatory drugs used are phenylbutazone (2.2–4.4 mg/kg, PO or IV, bid) and flunixin meglumine (1.1 mg/kg, IV, bid).

In **cattle**, esophageal obstruction accompanied by ruminal tympany is an emergency, and if clinical signs of distress indicate, the bloat (*see* p 227) must be relieved by trocarization through the left sublumbar fossa. Once tympany has been relieved, solid objects (eg, potatoes) may often be massaged free or spontaneously dislodge as their outer surfaces are softened by saliva. Caution should be used if any attempt is made to push an offending object down the esophagus using a probang; esophageal rupture and fatal septic mediastinitis may result.

Esophageal obstruction in ruminants can be managed with standing esophageal lavage via orogastric tube or while under general anesthesia (*see* p 215). Large foreign bodies can often be pushed into the rumen without further problems. Rare cases of esophageal obstruction with foreign bodies may be treated with esophagotomy.

Complications of Esophageal Obstruction

In horses and cattle, aspiration pneumonia (*see* p 1417) and septic pleuropneumonia may be complications of esophageal obstruction, especially in chronic cases. Chronic esophageal obstruction (>24 hr) may be associated with pressure necrosis of the esophageal mucosa due to prolonged contact with the foreign body. Circumferential mucosal damage may contribute to esophageal stricture.

An often fatal complication of chronic esophageal obstruction is esophageal rupture. Cervical esophageal rupture can lead to localized cervical cellulitis or septic mediastinitis or pleuropneumonia. Intrathoracic esophageal rupture is typically fatal. Cervical esophageal rupture can be managed by local drainage, wound lavage, and insertion of a nasogastric tube into the rupture site. A traction diverticulum is allowed to form, and the nasogastric tube is removed. Esophageal rupture managed with extraoral alimentation rarely results in esophageal stricture. In cases of septic mediastinitis or pleuropneumonia, euthanasia should be considered because of the difficulty in successfully resolving the bacterial infection.

Esophageal Obstruction Secondary to Extraesophageal Disease

Cervical and prethoracic trauma may result in periesophageal or esophageal fibrosis involving the muscular layer. This can result in esophageal stricture and intermittent or recurrent esophageal obstruction. In some cases, there is no external evidence of cervical or prethoracic trauma. In cases of suspected extraesophageal trauma, endoscopic examination of the esophagus and a contrast esophagogram can be useful diagnostic tools. Once the site of esophageal stricture is identified, some cases of muscular stricture can be resolved with esophageal myotomy or removal of fibrous connective tissue surrounding the esophagus.

ESOPHAGEAL STRICTURES

Idiopathic esophageal strictures can occur in foals. Initial diagnosis based on clinical signs may be delayed because of other more frequent causes of dysphagia, including idiopathic dorsal displacement of the soft palate or nasal reflux of milk, cleft palate, or pharyngeal cysts. All cases of nasal discharge of milk in foals should be evaluated with endoscopy. Esophageal stricture in older horses or ruminants typically results from mucosal ulceration secondary to esophageal obstruction. Appropriate treatment depends on whether the stricture is mucosal or mural (involving the muscular wall). Mucosal strictures can be treated conservatively with dietary management (*see* p 215), bougienage with a cuffed endotracheal tube, or surgery. Mural strictures are best managed with esophageal myotomy. Surgical treatment of mucosal strictures may involve esophagotomy through the strictured area with insertion of a nasogastric tube, resulting in a traction diverticulum, mucosal resection and anastomosis, or full-thickness esophageal resection and anastomosis.

ESOPHAGEAL NEOPLASIA

The most common neoplasia of the esophagus in horses is squamous cell carcinoma, which carries a guarded prognosis. Focal neoplastic masses can be managed with esophageal resection and anastomosis. Unfortunately, most cases of squamous cell carcinoma are not amenable to surgery, and euthanasia should be considered.

In ruminants, bovine viral papillomas (ie, warts) occasionally develop in the cranial esophagus and pharynx and, in the presence of other agents, may result in development of esophageal carcinoma. In some areas of the world (eg, Scotland and South America), such disease may follow ingestion of natural bracken fern toxins. There is also a causal relationship between such bracken fern tumors and bladder cancers in cattle. (*See also* BRACKEN FERN POISONING, p 3089.)

GASTROINTESTINAL ULCERS IN LARGE ANIMALS

Gastric ulcers are important in adult horses, foals, and pigs. Abomasal ulcers (*see* p 241) in mature cattle and calves appear to be increasing in importance.

GASTRIC ULCERS IN HORSES

(Equine gastric ulcer syndrome)

Gastric ulcers (equine gastric ulcer syndrome [EGUS]) are common in horses and foals. This syndrome is most closely associated with horses involved in performance disciplines; changes in housing or social interaction; and illness. Prevalence in unmedicated racehorses in active training is at least 90%, whereas that in non-racing performance disciplines exceeds 60%. Neonatal foals are at significant risk for development of perforating peptic ulcers until they are several weeks old, because their gastric mucosa is not developed to full thickness at birth. Although spontaneous healing of peptic ulcer lesions has been noted, if the horse is maintained in the circumstances inciting EGUS, the lesions are unlikely to heal without medical intervention.

EGUS describes a spectrum of inflammatory and disruptive mucosal pathophysiology affecting tissues of the distal esophagus, stomach, and entrance into the duodenum. Endoscopic surveys indicate that ~80% of these lesions are found in the nonglandular squamous mucosa of the stomach, especially on the lesser curvature just proximal to the margo plicatus. However, significant portions of the squamous mucosa along the greater curvature and up into the fundus may also be involved, along with lesions in the antrum or pylorus. Duodenal ulceration in adult horses and foals is considered part of EGUS and, hence, a peptic (acid-induced) disorder. Duodenal ulceration, perforation, and stricture can occur, and it is not known whether these problems develop solely as a result of enteritis (duodenitis) or whether peptic factors have a role. However, once a stricture occurs, gastric and esophageal ulcers are often present and severe, secondary to delayed gastric emptying.

Etiology: Ulcers in the nonglandular squamous mucosa are associated with repeated direct insult from ultra-low pH fluid normally found in the glandular region of the stomach. Pressure increases inside the abdomen (associated with exercise), collapsing the stomach and forcing the acid gastric contents upward. The more fluid (and highly acidic) contents of the lower stomach come in contact with the nonglandular squamous mucosa, causing inflammation and, potentially, erosions to varying degrees.

The causes of ulcers in the glandular mucosa of the stomach are less well defined. Use of nonselective NSAIDs are known to reduce blood flow to the GI tract, causing decreased production of the mucobicarbonate matrix by the gastric glandular mucosa and resulting in ulceration. This is not a consistent finding, however. Additionally, attempts have been made to isolate and/or correlate evidence of *Helicobacter* spp organisms from the stomach of horses with and without gastritis and ulcers. Results of these studies have been equivocal or negative, and the role of this organism in glandular equine gastric ulcers has not been determined.

Clinical Findings: Most foals with gastric ulcers do not exhibit clinical signs. Clinical signs become apparent when the ulceration is widespread or severe. The classic clinical signs for gastric ulcers in foals include diarrhea, bruxism, poor nursing, dorsal recumbency, and ptyalism. These signs are vague and not specific for gastric ulcers. In fact, ptyalism is a sign of esophagitis, which in most foals is secondary to gastric outflow obstruction and gastroesophageal reflux. Other causes, including esophageal obstruction and *Candida* infection, should be considered. Importantly, when a foal exhibits clinical signs, the ulcers are severe and should be diagnosed and treated immediately. Sudden gastric perforation without prior signs occurs sporadically in foals.

Adult horses with ulcers display nonspecific signs, including abdominal discomfort (colic), poor appetite, mild weight loss, poor body condition, and attitude changes. Horses with severe abdominal pain or colic may have gastric ulcers, but they are unlikely to be the primary cause of the abdominal pain. No strong correlation between the extent of ulceration and the severity of clinical signs has been seen.

Complications related to gastric ulcers are most frequent and severe in foals and include perforation, delayed gastric emptying, gastroesophageal reflux and esophagitis, and megaesophagus secondary to chronic gastroesophageal reflux. Ulcers in the proximal duodenum or at the pylorus can cause fibrosis and stricture. Duodenal and pyloric stricture can lead to delayed gastric emptying in foals and adult horses. In rare cases, severe gastric ulceration causes fibrosis and contracture of the stomach.

Diagnosis: Neither clinical signs nor clinicopathologic laboratory tests are specific for gastric ulcers, and an abnormality in a laboratory test does not preclude the possibility that another disorder may be present. Gastric ulcers can develop secondary to stress due to problems in many organ systems or as a result of hospitalization or stall confinement. Endoscopy and visualization of the ulcers in an empty stomach is the only definitive method of diagnosis. Endoscopes with light sources that can be varied in wavelength may be used to more easily visualize inflammatory stages of this disease before breaching of the epithelium by outright ulceration. A presumptive diagnosis can be reasonably made from significant reduction in clinical signs after several days of treatment with a medication known to be effective in raising gastric pH and allowing healing of gastric mucosa.

Treatment: Suppression of gastric acidity and maintenance of a pH between 4 and 5 are the primary treatment objectives. Studies have examined the use of surface-coating agents, antacids, histamine type-2 receptor antagonists (ranitidine and cimetidine), and the proton pump inhibitor omeprazole in a carrier designed to aid passage through the acid stomach into the small intestine for absorption. Sucralfate binds to the gastric glandular mucosa and may promote healing there, although studies using sucralfate have not shown it to be efficacious in the treatment of gastric ulcers in horses or foals. Thus, its use in horses is questionable. Antacids have yet to be proved effective in either healing or preventing gastric ulcers. They must be administered in relatively high volumes every 2 hr to neutralize stomach acid. Ranitidine (6.6 mg/kg, PO, tid) has been shown to be effective in healing gastric ulcers when horses were removed from training. Studies have not shown cimetidine to be effective. Omeprazole is the only medication approved by the FDA for treatment (4 mg/kg/day, PO) or prevention (1 mg/kg/day, PO) of gastric ulcers in horses, and it has been shown to allow gastric ulcers to heal in horses that continue their normal training.

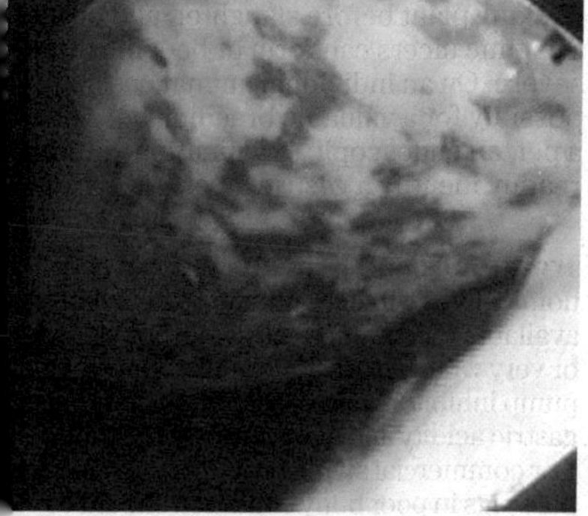

Gastric ulcers on endoscopy in a foal. *Courtesy of Dr. Thomas Lane.*

GASTRIC ULCERS IN PIGS

Ulcers affect the pars esophagea in pigs and cause sporadic cases of acute gastric hemorrhage, resulting in death or slow growth due to chronic ulceration.

Etiology: Ulcers result when the unprotected stratified squamous epithelium of the pars esophagea is subjected to insult from the mixture of acid, bile, and digestive enzymes present in the distal region of the stomach. The mucosa that surrounds the esophageal opening is not protected by mucus and therefore relies on maintenance of a pH gradient between the proximal and distal regions of the pig stomach. Many risk factors are associated with the development of ulcers, most of which are associated with an increase in fluidity of the stomach contents. The most important of these factors relate to feed, particularly the use of finely ground feed (<700 microns average particle size). Consumption of finely ground pelleted feed results in rapid stomach transit time and fluid stomach content. Other important factors tend to be associated with disruption in feed intake, eg, an outbreak of respiratory disease, hot weather, or management errors that lead to empty feeders. Disruption in feed intake results again in fluid stomach contents and lack of a physical barrier between the acidic distal contents and the sensitive pars esophageal region. It is possible that factors that cause increased acid production may influence the prevalence and severity of ulcers, but in general there is little evidence that hyperacidity is a primary cause. Similarly, *Helicobacter*-like organisms can often be identified under the mucus on the surface of the glandular mucosa of the distal stomach, but evidence that these bacteria are a cause of ulcer development in the pars esophagea is lacking, and epidemiologic studies showing an association are inconsistent. The presence of the bacteria in the glandular region and the lesion in the pars esophagea is difficult to explain from a biological standpoint.

Clinical Findings: Sudden death usually involving only a small number of pigs in a grower-finisher barn is a common presentation, but higher numbers can occur sporadically and are usually associated with a triggering event such as feed disruption. Death is caused by acute hemorrhage from the ulcer into the stomach, so the carcass appears notably pale but generally in good body condition. If bleeding is less severe, the clinical signs are those associated with anemia, such as paleness; if bleeding is prolonged, the pig will become weak, lose body condition, and grow slower than its pen-mates. Scant amounts of black tarry feces indicating digested blood may be noted. Vomiting may be seen but diarrhea is generally not present, which helps to differentiate gastric ulceration from other conditions. Other causes of blood loss or anemia need to be excluded. The most common age group to show clinical signs are pigs 2–6 mo old, as well as sows. Most pigs reared in modern confinement systems develop lesions in the pars esophagea. Lesions can both develop and heal quickly. This makes it difficult to determine whether erosions of the pars esophageal mucosa cause slow growth rate if blood loss is minimal and anemia is not present. Scarring can occur and, if severe, can result in narrowing of the esophageal-gastric opening. Clinical signs of esophageal stenosis include regurgitation of a meal shortly after consumption and loss of body condition.

Lesions: Gastric ulcers in pigs involve the mucosa near the esophageal opening in a rectangular area of white, glistening, nonglandular, squamous epithelium. In a pig that has died suddenly from a gastric ulcer, it is common to find a crater ≥2.5–5 cm in diameter encompassing the entrance of the esophagus. The crater appears as a cream or gray, punched-out area and may contain blood clots or debris. In acute hemorrhage, the stomach and upper small intestine contain dark blood. Earlier lesions are characterized by hyperkeratosis and parakeratosis of the squamous epithelium in the area of the esophageal opening into the stomach. It is assumed that the thickening of the epithelial surface is a defense against insult. Cracks and erosions can occur, particularly near the pars esophageal border. A deep erosion may result in acute and severe blood loss even while most of the surface of the pars esophagea remains intact. The healed ulcer appears as a stellate scar. Erosion and healing may occur over and over. Severe scarring can create stenosis of the esophageal opening.

Diagnosis: Appearance in a pen of one or two listless, anorectic pigs that show weight loss, anemia, dark feces, and sometimes dyspnea is suggestive of gastric ulceration, as is the sudden death of an apparently healthy pig. Differential diagnoses include hemorrhagic bowel syndrome, porcine proliferative enteropathy (*Lawsonia intracellularis* infection), porcine circovirus-associated disease, and swine dysentery. Gross lesions at necropsy are usually sufficient to confirm a diagnosis of gastric ulceration. Abattoir examination has been used to evaluate the prevalence of stomach lesions but must be interpreted with caution. Pigs are generally held without feed before shipping and may be held overnight at the packing plant before slaughter, and during this time ulcers can form or become more severe. On an individual animal basis, possibly for a valuable breeding boar or a pet, an endoscopic examination could readily identify a gastric ulcer.

Treatment and Prevention: No economically feasible treatments are currently available for commercial swine. For pet pigs or very valuable breeding animals, proton-pump inhibitors have been shown to reduce gastric acidity and allow mucosal healing. For commercial swine production, weak, pale pigs in poor body condition should be euthanized, and milder cases might respond to palliative care. Placing the affected pig in a hospital pen and initially coaxing it to eat using a highly palatable feed, and possibly administering analgesics, can be attempted. Early marketing of affected pigs should be considered.

Preventing, or reducing the incidence of gastric ulcers should focus on maintaining good feed intake, including management steps such as ensuring feeders do not run out of feed, sufficient feeder space is available, and mixing of pigs is minimized. During hot weather, it is important to make the pigs as comfortable as possible using cooling methods such as water spraying or high ventilation rates. Vaccination and other steps to minimize respiratory and systemic diseases are important to prevent gastric ulcer deaths. Attention to feed milling practices has a major impact on reducing ulcers. Feed produced using a roller mill is regarded to be less ulcerogenic than feed made with a hammer mill. Fine particle size is associated with more likelihood of ulcers but is also associated with improved feed efficiency, so economic considerations must be understood before a drastic change in particle size is recommended. In general, a coarse feed that will protect pigs from stomach lesions may not be an acceptable solution because of the added feed cost, but in an outbreak situation a short-term feed change may be necessary.

DISEASES OF THE RUMINANT FORESTOMACH

SIMPLE INDIGESTION

(Mild dietary indigestion)

Simple indigestion is a minor disturbance in ruminant GI function that occurs most commonly in cattle and rarely in sheep and goats. Simple indigestion is a diagnosis of exclusion and is typically related to an abrupt change in the quality or quantity of the diet.

Etiology: Almost any dietary factor that can alter the intraruminal environment can cause simple indigestion. The disease is common in hand-fed dairy and beef cattle because of variability in the quality and quantity of their feed. Dairy cattle may suddenly eat excessive quantities of highly palatable feeds such as corn or grass silage; beef cattle may eat excessive quantities of relatively indigestible, poor-quality roughage during winter. During drought, cattle and sheep may be forced to eat large quantities of poor-quality straw, bedding, or grain. Simple indigestion can result from suddenly changing the feed, using spoiled or frozen feeds, introducing urea to a ration, turning cattle onto a lush cereal grain pasture, or introducing feedlot cattle to a high-level grain ration.

Simple indigestion is usually associated with a sudden change in the pH of the ruminal contents, such as a decrease in ruminal pH due to rapid fermentation of ingested carbohydrates or an increase in ruminal pH due to forestomach hypomotility and putrefaction of ingested feed. It can also result from accumulation of excessive quantities of relatively indigestible feed that may physically impair rumen function. Multiple animals are usually simultaneously affected because simple indigestion has a nutritional basis, although the severity of the clinical signs can vary among animals.

Clinical Findings: Clinical signs depend on the type of animal affected and cause of the disorder. Overfeeding of silage causes anorexia and a moderate drop in milk production in dairy cattle. The rumen is usually full, firm, and doughy; primary contractions are decreased in rate or absent, but secondary contractions may be present although usually decreased in strength. Temperature, pulse, and respiration are normal. The feces are normal to firm in consistency but reduced in amount. Recovery usually is spontaneous within 24–48 hr.

Simple indigestion due to excessive feeding of grain results in anorexia and ruminal hypomotility to atony (stasis). The rumen is not necessarily full and may contain excessive fluid. The feces are usually soft to watery and foul smelling. The mechanism for diarrhea formation is uncertain but is most likely due to increased luminal osmolality as a result of the rapid degradation of ingested carbohydrates. The affected animal is bright and alert and usually begins to eat within 24 hr. A more severe digestive upset due to excessive feeding of grain is described as grain overload (*see* below).

Diagnosis: A diagnosis of simple indigestion is based on a history of an abrupt change in the nature or amount of the diet, multiple animals being affected, and most importantly the exclusion of other causes of forestomach dysfunction. The diagnosis is confirmed by collection and examination of ruminal fluid, which may have an abnormal pH (<6 or >7), decrease in the numbers and size of protozoa, or prolonged methylene blue reduction time (a measure of bacterial metabolic activity).

The systemic reaction and painful responses to deep palpation of the xiphoid in traumatic reticuloperitonitis are not seen. The history and the absence of ketonuria help eliminate clinical ketosis from consideration. The possibility of left displaced abomasum usually can be eliminated by simultaneous percussion and auscultation.

Vagal indigestion, abomasal volvulus, and cecocolic volvulus become more readily detectable as they progress. Grain overload is differentiated from simple indigestion by its greater severity and the pronounced fall in the pH of the rumen contents to <5.5.

Treatment: Treatment is aimed at correcting the suspected dietary factors. Spontaneous recovery is usual when animals are fed a typical ruminant diet. Administration of ~20 L of warm water or saline via a stomach tube, followed by vigorous kneading of the rumen, may help restore rumen function in adult cattle. Magnesium hydroxide PO may be useful when excessive amounts of grain have been ingested, but magnesium hydroxide should only be administered to cattle documented to have low ruminal pH (<6); otherwise, excessive forestomach and systemic alkalinization can result. Purported rumenatorics (eg, nux vomica, ginger, tartar emetic, parasympathomimetics) are not recommended as ancillary treatments. If too much urea (*see* p 3043) or protein has been ingested, vinegar (acetic acid) may be administered PO to return rumen pH to the normal range. If the number or activity of ruminal microbes is reduced, administration of 4–8 L of ruminal fluid from a healthy cow will help. (*See also* RUMINAL FLUID TRANSFER, p 2562.) Oral or intravenous electrolyte solutions may be needed to correct electrolyte and acid-base abnormalities, particularly in dehydrated cattle.

GRAIN OVERLOAD

(Lactic acidosis, Carbohydrate engorgement, Rumenitis)

Grain overload is an acute disease of ruminants that is characterized by rumen hypomotility to atony, dehydration, acidemia, diarrhea, depression, incoordination, collapse, and in severe cases, death.

Etiology and Pathogenesis: The disease is most common in cattle that accidentally gain access to large quantities of readily digestible carbohydrates, particularly grain. Grain overload also is common in feedlot cattle when they are introduced to heavy grain diets too quickly. Wheat, barley, and corn are the most readily digestible grains; oats are less digestible. Less common causes include engorgement with apples, grapes, bread, batter's dough, sugar beets, potatoes, mangels, or sour wet brewer's grain that was incompletely fermented in the brewery. The amount of feed required to produce acute illness depends on the kind of grain, previous experience of the animal with that grain, the nutritional status and condition of the animal, and the nature of the ruminal microflora. Adult cattle accustomed to heavy grain diets may consume 30–45 lb (15–20 kg) of grain and develop only moderate illness, whereas others may become acutely ill and die after eating 20 lb (10 kg) of grain.

Ingestion of toxic amounts of highly fermentable carbohydrates is followed within 2–6 hr by a change in the microbial population in the rumen. The number of gram-positive bacteria (such as *Streptococcus bovis*) increases markedly, which results in the production of large quantities of lactic acid. The rumen pH falls to ≤5, which destroys protozoa, cellulolytic organisms, and lactate-utilizing organisms, and impairs rumen motility. The low pH allows the lactobacilli to utilize the carbohydrate and to produce excessive quantities of lactic acid. The superimposition of lactic acid and its salts, L-lactate and D-lactate, on the existing solutes in the rumen liquid causes osmotic pressure to rise substantially, which results in the movement of excessive quantities of fluid into the rumen, causing fluid ruminal contents and dehydration.

The low ruminal pH causes a chemical rumenitis, and the absorption of lactate, particularly D-lactate, results in lactic acidosis and acidemia. In addition to metabolic (strong ion) acidosis and dehydration, the pathophysiologic consequences are hemoconcentration, cardiovascular collapse, renal failure, muscular weakness, shock, and death. Animals that survive may develop mycotic rumenitis in several days and hepatic abscesses several weeks or months later. They may have evidence of ruminal epithelial damage at slaughter. The relationship between grain overload and chronic laminitis in cattle is unclear.

Clinical Findings: Carbohydrate engorgement results in conditions ranging from simple indigestion (*see* p 221) to a rapidly fatal acidemia and strong ion (metabolic) acidosis. The interval between overeating and onset of signs is shorter with ground feed than with whole grain, and severity increases with the amount eaten. A few hours after engorgement, the only detectable abnormality may be an enlarged rumen and possibly some abdominal pain (manifest by belly kicking or treading of the hindlimbs). In the mild form, the rumen movements are reduced but not entirely absent, the cattle are anorectic but bright and alert, and diarrhea is common. The animals usually begin eating again 3–4 days later without any specific treatment.

Within 24–48 hr of the onset of severe overload, some animals will be recumbent, some will be staggering, and others will be standing quietly; all will be completely off feed. Immediately after consuming large quantities of dry grain, cattle may gorge themselves on water, but once ill they usually do not drink at all.

Body temperature is usually below normal, 98°–101°F (36.5°–38.5°C); however, in animals exposed to the sun in hot weather, it may be increased to 106°F (41°C). Respirations tend to be shallow and rapid, up to 60–90/min. The heart rate usually is increased in accordance with severity of the acidemia; the prognosis is poor for cattle with heart rates >120 bpm. Diarrhea is common and usually profuse and malodorous. The feces are soft to liquid, yellow or tan, and have an obvious sweet-sour odor. The feces frequently contain undigested kernels of the feed that has induced the overload. In mild cases, dehydration equals 4%–6% body wt, but losses may reach 10%–12% in severe cases.

In severe grain overload, the primary contractions of the rumen are completely absent, although the gurgling sounds of gas rising through the large quantity of fluid are usually audible on auscultation. Ballottement and auscultation of the left flank may elicit fluid-splashing sounds in the rumen. The contents of the rumen, as palpated through the left paralumbar fossa, may feel firm and doughy in cattle that were previously on a roughage diet and have consumed a large amount of grain. In cattle that have become ill on smaller amounts of grain, the rumen will feel not necessarily full, but rather resilient because of the excessive fluid. Severely affected animals stagger and may bump into objects; their palpebral reflex is sluggish or absent, and the pupillary light reflex is usually present but slower than normal. The extent of depression of the palpebral reflex is associated with the plasma D-lactate concentration and provides a useful clinical method to categorize severity of lactic acidosis and monitor response to treatment. Affected animals commonly lie quietly, often with the head turned into the flank, and their response to any stimulus is much decreased so that they resemble cases of parturient paresis.

Acute laminitis may be present and is most common in those animals not severely affected; chronic laminitis may develop weeks or months later. Anuria is a common finding in acute cases, and diuresis after fluid therapy is a good prognostic sign.

Death may occur in 24–72 hr, and rapid development of acute signs, particularly recumbency, indicates a need for aggressive treatment. A decrease in heart rate, increase in temperature, return of ruminal movement, and passage of large amounts of soft feces are more favorable signs. However, some animals appear to improve temporarily but become severely ill again 3–4 days later, probably because of severe bacterial and fungal rumenitis; death from acute, diffuse peritonitis usually follows in 2–3 days. In pregnant cattle that survive the severe form of the disease, abortion may occur 10–14 days later.

Diagnosis: The diagnosis is usually obvious if the history is available and multiple animals are affected. The diagnosis can be confirmed by the clinical findings, a low ruminal pH (<5.5 in cattle unaccustomed to a high grain diet), and examination of the microflora of the rumen for presence of live protozoa. When only one animal is involved and there is no history of engorgement, the diagnosis is less obvious, but the clinical signs—a static rumen with gurgling fluid sounds, diarrhea, ataxia, and a normal temperature—are characteristic. Rumen fluid analysis in these animals is required to confirm the diagnosis of grain overload.

Although parturient paresis (*see* p 988) may resemble rumen overload, diarrhea and dehydration are not typical, the intensity of heart sounds is reduced, and the response to calcium injection is usually dramatic. Peracute coliform mastitis and acute diffuse peritonitis may also resemble overload, but usually a careful examination will reveal the cause of the toxemia.

To avoid an increase in pH on exposure to air, the pH of rumen fluid obtained by ororuminal stomach tube or ruminal paracentesis should be checked promptly. Normally, the pH in cattle on roughage is 6–7; in those on a high grain diet, 5.5–6. Values <5.5 are strongly suggestive of grain overload, and a rumen pH <5 indicates severe acidemia and metabolic acidosis. Wide-range (2–11) pH indicator paper is suitable for field use. Ruminal fluid should also be examined microscopically if access to a laboratory is available; fluid from affected cattle will have decreased numbers of protozoa (particularly large and medium-sized protozoa). In grain overload, a Gram stain of ruminal fluid will reveal a change from predominantly gram-negative bacteria (normal) to predominantly gram-positive bacteria, with a concomitant loss in bacterial diversity.

Increased blood D-lactate and L-lactate and inorganic phosphate concentrations, mild hypocalcemia, and reduced urinary pH are also seen, but it is seldom necessary to check such values to make a firm diagnosis. The diagnostic problem is to properly assess which animals require vigorous therapy (or slaughter), which require supportive therapy, which have only a mild indigestion that will correct itself if water and grain intake are restricted and hay and exercise are provided, and which need nothing beyond their routine care and ration. In an outbreak of overload involving several animals, it is necessary to identify those animals that need the most intensive therapy and those that will recover with minimal medical therapy.

If the cattle are found while still eating, it is possible that some of the group will fall into each category, and close monitoring is necessary to minimize losses. Cattle found while engorging or shortly thereafter should be allowed no more concentrate but plenty of good hay for up to 24 hr and should be forced to walk periodically. Cattle that appear normal at the end of the first day are probably in good health, although if even one is ill, all should be monitored closely for 48 hr. Most of those that have eaten enough concentrate to be affected seriously show signs within 6–8 hr.

Treatment: For all cattle suspected of having eaten large quantities of concentrate, it is believed that restricting water intake for the first 18–24 hr is helpful, although this has not been proved. If overload is serious, slaughter for salvage should be considered; in feeders nearing the end of their feeding period, it may well be the most economic choice. Mortality is high in severely affected animals unless aggressive therapeutic measures are started early. In such animals, removal of rumen contents and replacement with ingesta taken from healthy animals is necessary. In animals still standing, rumenotomy is preferred to rumen lavage, because animals may aspirate during the lavage procedure and only rumenotomy ensures that all ingested grain has been removed. Rumen lavage may be accomplished with a large stomach tube if sufficient water is available. A large-bore tube (2.5 cm inside diameter, 3 m long) should be used, and enough water added to distend the left paralumbar fossa; gravity flow is then allowed to empty out what it will. Repeating this 15–20 times achieves the same results (and requires about as much time) as using rumenotomy to empty and wash out the rumen with a siphon.

Emptying the rumen should be followed by rumen inoculation (*see* p 2561) and, if not accomplished before signs of severe illness are evident, by rigorous fluid therapy to correct the metabolic acidosis and dehydration and to restore renal function. Initially, over a period of ~30 min, 5% sodium bicarbonate solution should be given IV (5 L/450 kg). During the next 6–12 hr, a balanced electrolyte solution, or a 1.3% solution of sodium bicarbonate in saline, may be given IV, up to as much as 60 L/450 kg body wt. Urination should resume during this period. Usually, it is unnecessary and even undesirable to also administer antacids PO (or intraruminally), particularly if IV sodium bicarbonate has been administered. Procaine penicillin G (22,000 U/kg/day) should be administered IM to all affected animals for at least 5 days to minimize development of bacterial rumenitis and liver abscesses. Thiamine should also be administered IM to facilitate metabolism of L-lactate via pyruvate and oxidative phosphorylation; animals with grain overload also have low concentrations of thiamine in rumen fluid because of increased production of thiaminase by ruminal bacteria. There is no effective preventive treatment for mycotic rumenitis.

Emptying the rumen is unnecessary in less severe cases. In these cattle, magnesium hydroxide (500 g/450 kg body wt) should be added to warm water, pumped into the rumen, and mixed therein via kneading the flank. This may be all that is necessary if the rumen pH is >5 and the animal is still standing and reasonably alert several hours after the engorgement. A heart rate of 70–85 bpm, weak ruminal contractions, normal body temperature, and especially willingness to eat are additional reassurances that this therapy will suffice. If any question remains, additional fluids should be given. During the convalescent period, which may last 2–4 days, good-quality hay and no grain should be given, and the grain then reintroduced gradually. If good appetite returns within 3 days, the prognosis is good. However, if treatment was not started early enough to prevent acidification of the ruminal contents, and mycotic infection of the rumen wall ensues, relapse is likely within 3–5 days and the prognosis is grave.

Prevention: Accidental access to concentrates for which cattle have developed an appetite, in quantities to which they are unaccustomed, should be avoided. Feedlot cattle should be introduced gradually to concentrate rations over a period of 2–3 wk, beginning with a mixture of ≤50% concentrate in the milled feed containing roughage.

SUBACUTE RUMINAL ACIDOSIS

(Chronic ruminal acidosis, Subclinical ruminal acidosis)

Ruminant animals are adapted to digest and metabolize predominantly forage diets; however, growth rates and milk production are increased substantially when ruminants consume high-grain diets. One consequence of feeding excessive amounts of rapidly fermentable carbohydrates in conjunction with inadequate fiber to ruminants is subacute ruminal acidosis, which is characterized by periods of low ruminal pH that resolve without treatment and is rarely diagnosed. Dairy cows, feedlot cattle, and feedlot sheep are at risk of developing this condition.

Etiology and Pathophysiology: Ruminal pH fluctuates considerably during a 24-hr period (typically between 0.5–1 pH units) and is determined by the dynamic balance between the intake of fermentable carbohydrates, buffering capacity of the rumen, and rate of acid absorption from the rumen. In general, subacute ruminal acidosis is caused by ingestion of diets high in rapidly fermentable carbohydrates and/or deficient in physically active fiber. Subacute ruminal acidosis is most commonly defined as repeatedly occurring prolonged periods of depression of the ruminal pH to values between 5.6 and 5.2. The low ruminal pH is caused by excessive accumulation of volatile fatty acids (VFAs) without persistent lactic acid accumulation and is restored to normal by the animal's own physiologic responses.

The ability of the rumen to rapidly absorb organic acids contributes greatly to the stability of ruminal pH. It is rarely difficult for peripheral tissues to utilize VFAs already absorbed from the rumen; however, absorption of these VFAs from the rumen can be an important bottleneck.

Ruminal VFAs are absorbed passively across the rumen wall. This passive absorption is enhanced by finger-like papillae, which project away from the rumen wall and provide massive surface area for absorption. Ruminal papillae increase in length when cattle are fed higher-grain diets; this presumably increases ruminal surface area and absorptive capacity, which protects the animal from acid accumulation in the rumen. Dairy cows are especially at risk in the transition period, because the ruminal mucosa needs several weeks to adjust to high-grain diets, and in peak lactation, when high levels of easily fermentable carbohydrates are fed to avoid excessive negative energy balance.

One mechanism by which affected animals resolve ruminal acidosis and return ruminal pH to normal is by selecting long forage particles, either by choosing to preferentially consume long dry hay or by sorting a mixed ration in favor of longer forage particles. Another mechanism is by reducing overall feed intake. Depressed dry-matter intake becomes especially evident if ruminal pH falls below ~5.5. Intake depression may be mediated by pH receptors and/or osmolality receptors in the rumen. Inflammation of the ruminal epithelium (rumenitis) could cause pain and also contribute to intake depression during subacute ruminal acidosis.

Absorption of VFA inherently increases as ruminal pH drops. These acids are absorbed only in the protonated state. Because they have a pK_a of ~4.8, the proportion of these acids that is protonated increases dramatically as ruminal pH decreases below 5.5. Lactate levels in the ruminal fluid of cattle with subacute ruminal acidosis, if measured, are usually not increased; however, the pathogenesis of excessive lactate production in the rumen is well described. Ruminal carbohydrate fermentation shifts to lactate production at lower ruminal pH (mostly due to *Streptococcus bovis* proliferating and shifting to lactate instead of VFA production); this can offset gains from VFA absorption. Ruminal lactate production is undesirable, because lactate has a much lower pK_a than VFAs (3.9 vs. 4.8). For example, lactate is 5.2 times less protonated than VFAs at pH 5. As a result, lactate stays in the rumen longer and contributes to the downward spiral in ruminal pH.

Additional adaptive responses are invoked if lactate production begins. Lactate-utilizing bacteria, such as *Megasphaera elsdenii* and *Selenomonas ruminantium*, begin to proliferate. These beneficial bacteria convert lactate to other VFAs, which are then easily protonated and absorbed. However, the turnover time of lactate utilizers is much slower than that of lactate synthesizers. Thus, this mechanism may not be invoked quickly enough to fully stabilize ruminal pH. Periods of very high ruminal pH, as during feed deprivation, may inhibit populations of lactate utilizers (which are sensitive to higher ruminal pH) and leave them more susceptible to severe ruminal acidosis.

Besides disrupting microbial balance, feed deprivation causes cattle to overeat when feed is reintroduced. This creates a double effect in lowering ruminal pH. Cycles of feed deprivation followed by overconsumption greatly increase the risk of subacute ruminal acidosis.

Low ruminal pH during subacute ruminal acidosis also reduces the number of species of bacteria in the rumen, although the metabolic activity of the bacteria that remain is very high. Protozoal populations are particularly limited at lower ruminal pH; the absence of ciliated protozoa in ruminal fluid is often observed during bouts of subacute ruminal acidosis. When fewer species of bacteria and protozoa are present, the ruminal microflora are less stable and less able to maintain normal ruminal pH during periods of sudden dietary change. Thus, periods of subacute ruminal acidosis leave animals more susceptible to future episodes of ruminal acidosis.

The pathophysiologic consequences of ruminal acidosis have mainly been described in feedlot cattle and in cattle surviving acute ruminal acidosis. Low ruminal pH may lead to rumenitis, erosion, and ulceration of the ruminal epithelium. Once the ruminal epithelium is inflamed, bacteria may colonize the papillae and leak into the portal circulation. These bacteria may cause liver abscesses, which may eventually lead to peritonitis around the site of the abscess.

Caudal vena cava syndrome is caused by the release of septic emboli from liver abscesses; this septic material then travels via the caudal vena cava to the lungs. These bacteria proliferate in lung tissue and may ultimately invade pulmonary vessels, causing them to rupture. This is observed clinically as hemoptysis and even peracute deaths due to massive pulmonary hemorrhage.

Subacute ruminal acidosis has traditionally been associated with claw horn lesions, assumed to be caused by subacute laminitis. However, this pathophysiologic mechanism has not been experimentally characterized or reproduced. In recent years, alternative explanations for the development of claw horn lesions have been suggested.

Clinical Findings: The main clinical signs attributed to subacute ruminal acidosis are reduced or cyclic feed intake, decreased milk production, reduced fat, poor body condition score despite adequate feed intake, and unexplained diarrhea. High rates of culling or unexplained deaths may be noted in the herd. Sporadic cases of caudal vena cava syndrome may also be seen. The clinical signs are delayed and insidious. Actual episodes of low ruminal pH are not identified; in fact, by the time an animal is observed to be off-feed, its ruminal pH has probably been restored to normal. Diarrhea may follow periods of low ruminal pH; however, this finding is inconsistent and may be related to other dietary factors as well.

Diagnosis: Subacute ruminal acidosis is diagnosed on a group rather than individual basis. Measurement of pH in the ruminal fluid of a representative portion of apparently healthy animals in a group has been used to help make the diagnosis of subacute ruminal acidosis in dairy herds. Animal selection should be from highest-risk groups: cows between ~15–30 days in milk in component-fed herds and cows between ~50–150 days in milk in herds fed total mixed rations. Ruminal fluid is collected by rumenocentesis, and its pH is determined on a pH meter. Twelve or more animals are typically sampled at ~2–4 hr after a grain feeding (in component-fed herds) or 6–10 hr after the first daily feeding of a total mixed ration. If >25% of the animals tested have a ruminal pH <5.5, then the group is considered to be at high risk of subacute ruminal acidosis. This type of diagnostic tool should be used in conjunction with other factors such as ration evaluation, evaluation of management practices, and identification of health problems on a herd basis.

Milk fat depression is a poor and insensitive indicator of subacute ruminal acidosis in dairy herds.

Treatment and Prevention: Because subacute ruminal acidosis is not detected at the time of depressed ruminal pH, there is no specific treatment for it. Secondary conditions may be treated as needed.

The key to prevention of subacute ruminal acidosis is allowing for ruminal adaption to high-grain diets, as well as limiting intake of readily fermentable carbohydrates. This requires both good diet formulation (proper balance of fiber and nonfiber carbohydrates) and excellent feed bunk management. Animals consuming well-formulated diets remain at high risk of this condition if they tend to eat large meals because of excessive competition for bunk space or after periods of feed deprivation.

Field recommendations to feed component-fed concentrates to dairy cattle during the first 3 wk of lactation are usually excessive. Feeding excessive quantities of concentrate and insufficient forage results in a fiber-deficient ration likely to cause subacute ruminal acidosis. The same situation may be seen during the last few days before parturition if the ration is fed in separate components; as dry-matter intake drops before calving, dry cows preferentially consume concentrates instead of forage and develop acidosis.

Subacute ruminal acidosis may also be caused by errors in delivery of the rations or by formulation of rations that contain excessive amounts of rapidly fermentable carbohydrates or a deficiency of fiber. Recommendations for the fiber content of dairy rations are available in the National Research Council report, *Nutrient Requirements of Dairy Cattle* (*see* p 2250). Dry-matter content errors in total mixed rations are commonly related to a lack of adjustment for changes in moisture content of forages.

Including long-fiber particles in the diet reduces the risk of subacute ruminal acidosis by encouraging saliva production during chewing and by increasing rumination after feeding. The provision of adequate long-fiber particles reduces the risk of ruminal acidosis but cannot eliminate it. If a total mixed ration is fed, it is important that the long-fiber particles not be easily sorted away from the rest of the diet; this could delay their consumption until later in the day or cause them to be refused completely. Sorting can be prevented by providing long-fiber particles less than ~5 cm in length, by having adequate (~50%–55%) moisture in the mixed ration, and by including ingredients such as liquid molasses that help ration ingredients stick together.

Ruminant diets should also be formulated to provide adequate buffering. This can be accomplished by feedstuff selection and/or by addition of dietary buffers such as sodium bicarbonate or potassium carbonate. The dietary cation-anion difference (DCAD) is used to quantify the buffering capacity of a diet; diets for animals at high risk of ruminal acidosis should be formulated to provide a DCAD of >250 mEq/kg of diet dry matter, using the formula (Na + K) – (Cl + S) to calculate DCAD.

Supplementing the diet with direct-fed microbials that enhance lactate utilization in the rumen may reduce the risk of subacute ruminal acidosis. Yeasts, propionobacteria, lactobacilli, and enterococci have been used for this purpose. Ionophore (eg, monensin sodium) supplementation may also reduce the risk by selectively inhibiting ruminal lactate producers and by reducing meal size.

BLOAT

(Ruminal tympany)

Bloat is an overdistention of the rumenoreticulum with the gases of fermentation, either in the form of a persistent foam mixed with the ruminal contents, called primary or frothy bloat, or in the form of free gas separated from the ingesta, called secondary or free-gas bloat. It is predominantly a disorder of cattle but may also be seen in sheep. The susceptibility of individual cattle to bloat varies and is genetically determined.

Death rates as high as 20% are recorded in cattle grazing bloat-prone pasture, and in pastoral areas, the annual mortality rate from bloat in dairy cows may approach 1%. There is also economic loss from depressed milk production in nonfatal cases and from suboptimal use of bloat-prone pastures. Bloat can be a significant cause of mortality in feedlot cattle.

Etiology and Pathogenesis: In **primary ruminal tympany**, or **frothy bloat**, the cause is entrapment of the normal gases of fermentation in a stable foam. Coalescence of the small gas bubbles is inhibited, and intraruminal pressure increases because eructation cannot occur. Several factors, both animal and plant, influence the formation of a stable foam. Soluble leaf proteins, saponins, and hemicelluloses are believed to be the primary foaming agents and to form a monomolecular layer around gas rumen bubbles that has its greatest stability at about pH 6. Salivary mucin is antifoaming, but saliva production is reduced with succulent forages. Bloat-producing pastures are more rapidly digested and may release a greater amount of small chloroplast particles that trap gas bubbles and prevent their coalescence. The immediate effect of feeding is probably to supply nutrients for a burst of microbial fermentation. However, the major factor that determines whether bloat will occur is the nature of the ruminal contents. Protein content and rates of digestion and ruminal passage reflect the forage's potential for causing bloat. Over a 24-hr period, the bloat-causing forage and unknown animal factors combine to maintain an increased concentration of small feed particles and enhance the susceptibility to bloat.

Bloat is most common in animals grazing legume or legume-dominant pastures, particularly alfalfa, ladino, and red and white clovers, but also is seen with grazing of young green cereal crops, rape, kale, turnips, and legume vegetable crops. Legume forages such as alfalfa and clover have a higher percentage of protein and are digested more quickly. Other legumes, such as sainfoin, crown vetch, milk vetch, fenugreek, and birdsfoot trefoil, are high in protein but do not cause bloat, probably because they contain condensed tannins, which precipitate protein and are digested more slowly than alfalfa or clover. Leguminous bloat is most common when cattle are placed on lush pastures, particularly those dominated by rapidly growing leguminous plants in the vegetative and early bud stages, but can also be seen when high-quality hay is fed.

Frothy bloat also is seen in feedlot cattle, and less commonly in dairy cattle, on high-grain diets. The cause of the foam in feedlot bloat is uncertain but is thought to be either the production of insoluble slime by certain species of rumen bacteria in cattle fed high-carbohydrate diets or the entrapment of the gases of fermentation by the fine particle size of ground feed. Fine particulate matter, such as in finely ground grain, can markedly affect foam stability, as can a low roughage intake. Feedlot bloat is most common in cattle that have been on a grain diet for 1–2 mo. This timing may be due to the increase in the level of grain feeding or to the time it takes for the slime-producing rumen bacteria to proliferate to large enough numbers.

In **secondary ruminal tympany**, or **free-gas bloat**, physical obstruction of eructation is caused by esophageal obstruction due to a foreign body (eg, potatoes, apples, turnips, kiwifruit), stenosis, or pressure from enlargement outside the esophagus (as from lymphadenopathy or sporadic juvenile thymic lymphoma). Interference with esophageal groove function in vagal indigestion and diaphragmatic hernia may cause chronic ruminal tympany. This also occurs in tetanus. Tumors and other lesions, such as those caused by infection with *Actinomyces bovis*, of the esophageal groove or the reticular wall are less common causes of obstructive bloat. There also may be interference with the nerve pathways involved in the eructation reflex. Lesions of the wall of the reticulum (which contains tension receptors and receptors that discriminate between gas, foam, and liquid) may interrupt the normal reflex essential for escape of gas from the rumen.

Ruminal tympany also can be secondary to the acute onset of ruminal atony that occurs in anaphylaxis and in grain overload; this causes a decrease in rumen pH and possibly an esophagitis and rumenitis that can interfere with eructation. Ruminal tympany also develops with hypocalcemia. Chronic ruminal tympany is relatively frequent in calves up to 6 mo old without apparent cause; this form usually resolves spontaneously.

Unusual postures, particularly lateral recumbency, are commonly associated with secondary tympany. Ruminants may die of bloat if they become accidentally cast in dorsal recumbency or other restrictive positions in handling facilities, crowded transportation vehicles, or irrigation ditches.

Clinical Findings: Bloat is a common cause of sudden death. Cattle not observed closely, such as pastured and feedlot cattle and dry dairy cattle, usually are found dead. In lactating dairy cattle, which are observed regularly, bloat commonly begins within 1 hr after being turned onto a bloat-producing pasture. Bloat may develop on the first day after being placed on the pasture but more commonly develops on the second or third day.

In primary pasture bloat, the rumen becomes obviously distended suddenly, and the left flank may be so distended that the contour of the paralumbar fossa protrudes above the vertebral column; the entire abdomen is enlarged. As the bloat progresses, the skin over the left flank becomes progressively more taut and, in severe cases, cannot be "tented." Dyspnea and grunting are marked and are accompanied by mouth breathing, protrusion of the tongue, extension of the head, and frequent urination. Rumen motility does not decrease until bloat is severe. If the tympany continues to worsen, the animal will collapse and die. Death may occur within 1 hr after grazing began but is more common ~3–4 hr after onset of clinical signs. In a group of affected cattle, there are usually several with clinical bloat and some with mild to moderate abdominal distention.

In secondary bloat, the excess gas is usually free on top of the solid and fluid ruminal contents, although frothy bloat may be seen in vagal indigestion when there is increased ruminal activity. Secondary bloat is seen sporadically. There is tympanic resonance over the dorsal abdomen left of the midline. Free gas produces a higher pitched ping on percussion than frothy bloat. The distention of the rumen can be detected on rectal examination. In free-gas bloat, the passage of a stomach tube or trocarization releases large quantities of gas and alleviates distention.

Lesions: Necropsy findings are characteristic. Congestion and hemorrhage of the lymph nodes of the head and neck, epicardium, and upper respiratory tract are marked. The lungs are compressed, and intrabronchial hemorrhage may be present. The cervical esophagus is congested and hemorrhagic, but the thoracic portion of the esophagus is pale and blanched—the demarcation known as the "bloat line" of the esophagus. The rumen is distended, but the contents usually are much less frothy than before death. The liver is pale because of expulsion of blood from the organ.

Diagnosis: Usually, the clinical diagnosis of frothy bloat is obvious. The causes of secondary bloat must be ascertained by clinical examination to determine the cause of the failure of eructation.

Treatment: In life-threatening cases, an emergency rumenotomy may be necessary; it is accompanied by an explosive release of ruminal contents and, thus, marked relief for the cow. Recovery is usually uneventful, with only occasional minor complications.

A trocar and cannula may be used for emergency relief, although the standard-sized instrument is not large enough to allow the viscous, stable foam in peracute cases to escape quickly enough. A larger bore instrument (2.5 cm in diameter) is necessary, but an incision through the skin must be made before it can be inserted through the muscle layers and into the rumen. If the cannula fails to reduce the bloat and the animal's life is threatened, an emergency rumenotomy should be performed. If the cannula provides some relief, an antifoaming agent can be administered through the cannula, which can remain in place until the animal has returned to normal, usually within several hours.

When the animal's life is not immediately threatened, passing a stomach tube of the largest bore possible is recommended. A few attempts should be made to clear the tube by blowing and moving it back and forth in an attempt to find large pockets of rumen gas that can be released. In frothy bloat, it may be impossible to reduce the pressure with the tube, and an antifoaming agent should be administered while the tube is in place. If the bloat is not relieved quickly by the antifoaming agent, the animal must be observed carefully for the next hour to determine whether the treatment has been successful or whether an alternative therapy is necessary.

A variety of antifoaming agents are effective, including vegetable oils (eg, peanut, corn, soybean) and mineral oils (paraffins), at doses of 250–500 mL. Dioctyl sodium sulfosuccinate, a surfactant, is commonly incorporated into one of the above oils and sold as a proprietary antibloat remedy, which is effective if administered early. Poloxalene (25–50 g, PO) is effective in treating legume bloat but not feedlot bloat. Placement of a rumen fistula provides short-term relief for cases of free-gas bloat associated with external obstruction of the esophagus.

Control and Prevention: Prevention of **pasture bloat** can be difficult. Management practices used to reduce the risk of bloat include feeding hay, particularly orchard grass, before turning cattle on pasture, maintaining grass dominance in the sward, or using strip grazing to restrict intake, with movement of animals to a new strip in the afternoon, not the early morning. Hay must constitute at least one-third of the diet to effectively reduce risk of bloat. Feeding hay or strip grazing may be reliable when the pasture is only moderately dangerous, but these methods are less reliable when the pasture is in the pre-bloom stage and the bloat potential is high. Mature pastures are less likely to cause bloat than immature or rapidly growing pastures.

The only satisfactory method available to prevent pasture bloating is continual administration of an antifoaming agent during the risk period. This is widely practiced in grassland countries such as Australia and New Zealand. The most reliable method is drenching twice daily (eg, at milking times) with an antifoaming agent. Spraying the agent onto the pasture is equally effective, provided the animals have access only to treated pasture. This method is ideal for strip grazing but not when grazing is uncontrolled. The antifoaming agent can be added to the feed or water or incorporated into feed blocks, but success with this method depends on adequate individual intake. The agent can be "painted" on the flanks of the animals, from which it is licked during the day, but animals that do not lick will be unprotected.

Available antifoaming agents include oils and fats and synthetic nonionic surfactants. Oils and fats are given at 60–120 mL/head/day; doses up to 240 mL are indicated during dangerous periods. Poloxalene, a synthetic polymer, is a highly effective nonionic surfactant that can be given at 10–20 g/head/day and up to 40 g/head/day in high-risk situations. It is safe and economical to use and is administered daily through the susceptible period by adding to water, feed grain mixtures, or molasses. Pluronic agents facilitate the solubilization of water-insoluble factors that contribute to formation of a stable foam. A pluronic detergent (Alfasure®) and a water-soluble mixture of alcohol ethoxylate and pluronic detergents (Blocare 4511) also are effective but are not approved by the FDA. Ionophores effectively prevent bloat, and a sustained-release capsule administered into the rumen and releasing 300 mg of monensin daily for a 100-day period protects against pasture bloat and improves milk production on bloat-prone pastures.

The ultimate aim in control is development of a pasture that permits high production, while keeping incidence of bloat low. The use of pastures of clover and grasses in equal amounts comes closest to achieving this goal. Bloat potential varies between cultivars of alfalfa, and low-risk LIRD (low initial rate of digestion) cultivars are available commercially. The addition of legumes with high condensed tannins to the pasture seeding mix (10% sainfoin) can reduce the risk of bloat where there is strip grazing, as can the feeding of sainfoin pellets.

To prevent **feedlot bloat**, rations should contain ≥10–15% cut or chopped roughage mixed into the complete feed. Preferably, the roughage should be a cereal, grain straw, grass hay, or equivalent. Grains should be rolled or cracked, not finely ground. Pelleted rations made from finely ground grain should be avoided. The addition of tallow (3%–5% of the total ration) may be successful occasionally, but it was not effective in controlled trials. The nonionic surfactants, such as poloxalene, have been ineffective in preventing feedlot bloat, but the ionophore lasalocid is effective in control.

TRAUMATIC RETICULOPERITONITIS

(Hardware disease, Traumatic gastritis)

Traumatic reticuloperitonitis develops as a consequence of perforation of the reticulum. It is important as a differential diagnosis of other diseases marked by stasis of the GI tract, because it causes similar signs. Traumatic reticuloperitonitis is most common in mature dairy cattle, occasionally seen in beef cattle, and rarely reported in other ruminants.

Cattle commonly ingest foreign objects, because they do not discriminate against metal materials in feed and do not completely masticate feed before swallowing. The disease is common when green chop, silage, and hay are made from fields that contain old rusting fences or baling wire, or when pastures are on areas or sites where buildings have recently been constructed, burned, or torn down. The grain ration may also be a source because of accidental addition of metal.

Etiology: Swallowed metallic objects, such as nails or pieces of wire, fall directly into the reticulum or pass into the rumen and are subsequently carried over the ruminoreticular fold into the cranioventral part of the reticulum by ruminal contractions. The reticulo-omasal orifice is elevated above the floor, which tends to retain heavy objects in the reticulum, and the honeycomb-like reticular mucosa traps sharp objects. Contractions of the reticulum promote penetration of the wall by the foreign object. Compression of the ruminoreticulum by the uterus in late pregnancy and straining during parturition increase the likelihood of an initial penetration of the reticulum and may also disrupt adhesions caused by an earlier penetration.

Perforation of the wall of the reticulum allows leakage of ingesta and bacteria, which contaminates the peritoneal cavity. The resulting peritonitis is generally localized and frequently results in adhesions. Less commonly, a more severe diffuse peritonitis develops. The object can penetrate the diaphragm and enter the thoracic cavity (causing pleuritis and sometimes pulmonary abscessation) and the pericardial sac (causing pericarditis, sometimes followed by myocarditis). Occasionally, the liver or spleen may be pierced and become infected, resulting in abscessation, or septicemia can develop.

Clinical Findings: The initial penetration of the reticulum is characterized by the sudden onset of ruminoreticular atony and a sharp fall in milk production. Fecal output is decreased. The rectal temperature is often mildly increased. The heart rate is normal or slightly increased, and respiration is usually shallow and rapid. Initially, the cow exhibits an arched back; an anxious expression; a reluctance to move; and an uneasy, careful gait. Forced sudden movements as well as defecating, urinating, lying down, getting up, and stepping over barriers may be accompanied by groaning. A grunt may be elicited by applying pressure to the xiphoid or by firmly pinching the withers, which causes extension of the thorax and lower abdomen. The grunt can be detected by placing a stethoscope over the trachea and applying pressure or pinching the withers at the end of an inspiration. Tremor of the triceps and abduction of the elbow may be seen.

In chronic cases, feed intake and fecal output are reduced, and milk production remains low. Signs of cranial abdominal pain become less apparent, and the rectal temperature usually returns to normal as the acute inflammation subsides and peritoneal contamination is walled off. Some cattle develop vagal indigestion syndrome (*see* p 233) because of the adhesions that form after foreign body perforation, particularly those on the ventromedial reticulum.

Cows with pleuritis or pericarditis due to foreign body perforation usually are depressed, tachycardic (>90 bpm), and pyrexic (104°F [40°C]). Pleuritis is manifest

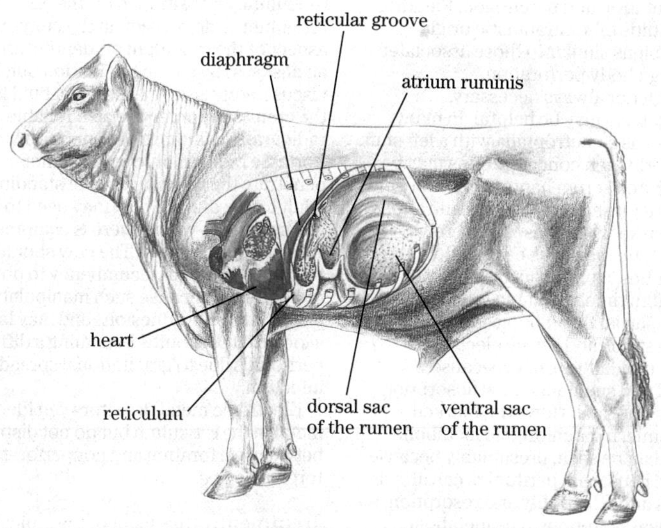

The relationship between the reticulum, diaphragm, and heart and pericardium in large ruminants. *Illustration by Dr. Gheorghe Constantinescu.*

by fast, shallow respiration; muffled lung sounds; and possibly pleuritic friction rubs. Thoracentesis may yield several liters of septic fluid. Traumatic pericarditis is most commonly characterized by muffled heart sounds; however, early in the disease process pericardial friction rubs or gas and fluid splashing sounds (washing machine murmur) can be heard on auscultation. Jugular vein distention and congestive heart failure with marked submandibular and brisket edema is a frequent sequela of traumatic reticulopericarditis. Prognosis is grave with these complications. Penetration through the pericardium into the myocardium usually results in extensive hemorrhage into the pericardial sac or ventricular arrhythmias and sudden death.

Diagnosis: This can be based on history (when available) and clinical findings if the cow is examined when signs initially appear. Without an accurate history and when the condition has been present for several days or longer, diagnosis is more difficult. Other causes of peritonitis, particularly perforated abomasal ulcers, can be difficult to distinguish from traumatic reticuloperitonitis. Differential diagnoses should include conditions that can produce variable or nonspecific GI signs, eg, indigestion, lymphosarcoma, or intestinal obstruction. Abomasal displacement or volvulus should be excluded by simultaneous auscultation and percussion. Pleuritis or pericarditis of nontraumatic origin produces signs similar to those associated with foreign body perforation.

Although not always necessary, laboratory tests may be helpful. In many cases, there is a neutrophilia with a left shift. Plasma fibrinogen concentrations may be increased, and serum haptoglobin, amyloid A, and total plasma protein concentrations may be markedly increased. Severely affected cattle may have coagulation abnormalities, as evidenced by prolonged prothrombin time, thrombin time, and activated partial thromboplastin time. The acid-base status and serum electrolyte levels are typically normal, because abomasal and small-intestinal absorption can remain normal. However, marked hypokalemic, hypochloremic metabolic alkalosis can be seen, presumably because adynamic ileus from peritonitis can affect abomasal and GI motility and resorption of abomasal secretions. The metabolic alkalosis can be created or exacerbated by treatment with alkalinizing agents such as magnesium hydroxide used as a laxative. Peritoneal fluid analysis can help determine whether peritonitis is present, particularly the concentration of D-dimer and the neutrophil percentage in the peritoneal fluid. However, the peritonitis frequently becomes walled off, and in these cases peritoneal fluid may be within the reference range unless obtained from within the lesion. The presence of a magnet in the reticulum can be determined by movement of a magnetic compass in the region of the cranioventral abdomen; the presence of a magnet in the reticulum makes traumatic reticuloperitonitis very unlikely unless the penetrating object is not magnetic.

Ultrasonography of the ventral abdomen using a 3-MHz transducer is the most accurate way to diagnose localized peritonitis near the reticulum and characterize the reticular contraction frequency. It rarely identifies the presence of a penetrating object. Ultrasonography of the heart and thorax is very useful in the diagnosis of pleuritis and pericarditis as a sequelae of traumatic reticuloperitonitis and has replaced radiography in the diagnosis of reticuloperitonitis.

Lateral radiographs of the cranioventral abdomen can detect metallic material in the reticulum but should be taken only after oral administration of a magnet. To determine whether the reticulum is currently perforated, the foreign body must be visible beyond the border of the reticulum, unattached to the magnet in the reticulum, or positioned off the floor of the reticulum. A depression in the cranioventral aspect of the reticulum or identification of an abscess (by gas accumulation outside a viscus), soft-tissue masses, or a fluid line in the cranial abdomen are also reliable radiographic findings of penetration. Portable radiographic units cannot penetrate the reticular area of standing adult cattle, and the cow may need to be transported to where there is equipment with sufficient power. The cow should not be placed in dorsal recumbency to obtain radiographs, because such manipulation places stress on adhesions and may lead to a localized peritonitis becoming a diffuse peritonitis due to gravitational spread of infection.

Electronic metal detectors can identify metal in the reticulum but do not distinguish between perforating and nonperforating foreign bodies.

Treatment: Treatment of the typical case seen early in its course may be surgical or medical. Either approach improves the chances of recovery from ~60% in untreated cases to 80%–90%. Surgery involves rumenotomy with manual removal of the object(s) from the reticulum; if an abscess is adhered to the reticulum, it should be aspirated (to confirm it is an abscess) and then drained into the reticulum. Antimicrobials should be administered perioperatively. Medical treatment involves administration of antimicrobials to control the peritonitis and a magnet to prevent recurrence. Because of the mixed bacterial flora in the lesion, a broad-spectrum antimicrobial agent such as oxytetracycline (16 mg/kg/day, IV) should be used. Penicillin (22,000 IU/kg, IM, once to twice daily) is widely used and effective in many cases despite its limited spectrum. Affected cows should be confined for 1–2 wk; placing them on an inclined plane (elevated in front) is believed by some to limit further penetration of the foreign object, but supporting studies are lacking. Supportive therapy, such as oral or occasionally IV fluids and SC calcium borogluconate or calcium gluconate, should be administered as needed. Rumen inoculation (4–8 L of ruminal fluid from a healthy donor) is beneficial in some cases with prolonged ruminal stasis and loss of normal flora.

More advanced cases, those with obvious secondary complications, or those that do not respond to initial medical or surgical therapy should be evaluated from an economic perspective; if the cow is of limited value, slaughter should be considered if the carcass is likely to pass inspection.

Prevention: Preventive measures include avoiding the use of baling wire, passing feed over magnets to remove metallic objects, keeping cattle away from sites of new construction, and completely removing old buildings and fences. Additionally, bar magnets may be administered PO, preferably after fasting for 18–24 hr. Usually, the magnet remains in the reticulum and holds any ferromagnetic objects on its surface. There is good evidence that giving magnets to all herd replacement heifers and bulls at ~1 yr of age minimizes the incidence of traumatic reticuloperitonitis.

VAGAL INDIGESTION SYNDROME

(Chronic indigestion)

Vagal indigestion syndrome is characterized by the gradual development of abdominal distention secondary to rumenoreticular distention. The distention was originally thought to be the result of lesions affecting the ventral vagus nerve. Vagal indigestion syndrome is seen most commonly in cattle but has been reported in sheep.

Etiology and Pathogenesis: Diseases that result in injury, inflammation, or pressure on the vagus nerve can result in clinical signs of vagal indigestion syndrome. However, vagal nerve damage is not present in most cases of vagus indigestion, and the most common cause is traumatic reticuloperitonitis (*see* p 230). Conditions resulting in mechanical obstruction of the cardia or reticulo-omasal orifice (eg, papillomas or ingested placenta) can also result in vagal indigestion if ruminoreticular distention is present and the condition is subacute to chronic.

Historically, there were four types of vagal indigestion described based on the purported site of the functional obstruction. Type I was failure of eructation or free-gas bloat, type II was a failure of omasal transport, type III was secondary abomasal impaction, and type IV was indigestion of late gestation. Types I and IV are rare, and this categorization system has minimal clinical relevance.

Type I vagal indigestion, or failure of eructation, results in free-gas bloat and has been attributed to inflammatory lesions in the vicinity of the vagus nerve, such as localized peritonitis, adhesions (usually after an episode of traumatic reticuloperitonitis), or chronic pneumonia with anterior mediastinitis. Other potential causes for type I vagal indigestion include pharyngeal trauma, which affects a more proximal part of the vagus nerve, and esophageal compression by abscesses or neoplasia, such as lymphosarcoma. Vagal indigestion can develop in cattle after abomasal volvulus without abomasal impaction. These cases would presumably fall into the category of type I vagal indigestion with damage to the vagal nerve near the reticulum and omasum.

Type II vagal indigestion, more correctly termed failure of omasal transport, develops as a result of any condition that prevents ingesta from passing through the omasal canal into the abomasum. Adhesions and abscesses (reticular or single liver abscesses) are the most common cause of failure of omasal transport and are usually located on the right or medial wall of the reticulum near the route of the vagus nerve. Reticular abscesses and adhesions are almost invariably the result of traumatic reticuloperitonitis. Mechanical obstruction of the omasal canal by ingested material (eg, plastic bags, rope, placenta) or masses (eg, lymphosarcoma, squamous cell carcinoma, granulomas, or papillomas) can also cause chronic ruminoreticular distention due to failure of omasal transport.

Type III vagal indigestion is a secondary abomasal impaction. Primary abomasal impaction develops due to feeding of dry, course roughage, such as straw, in a chopped or ground form with restricted access to water and usually during extremely cold temperatures (*see* p 244). Secondary abomasal impaction is seen most commonly after an episode of traumatic reticuloperitonitis or occasionally as a sequela of abomasal volvulus. Mechanical fixation of the reticulum to the ventral abdominal floor in cows with reticuloperitonitis interferes with the normal sieving action of the reticulum, with passage of large fiber particles (>2 mm long) into the abomasum. The abomasum has difficulty in emptying the larger particles of food because of the increased viscosity, and they accumulate in the abomasum, resulting in abomasal impaction.

Type IV vagal indigestion, or partial forestomach obstruction, is poorly defined. It typically develops in cattle during gestation and is more appropriately termed indigestion of late gestation. The condition is thought to be related to the enlarging uterus shifting the abomasum to a more cranial position, which inhibits normal abomasal emptying.

Clinical Findings: The clinical signs vary to some extent with the location of the obstruction. In all cases, there is a gradual development (over days to weeks) of abdominal distention secondary to ruminoreticular distention. Distention of the dorsal and ventral sacs of the rumen results in an "L-shaped" rumen on rectal examination. Left dorsal and left and right ventral distention of the abdomen causes a "papple" (pear plus apple) shape as viewed from behind.

Cattle with vagal indigestion syndrome have a diminished appetite, which typically improves temporarily if distention is relieved. Milk production gradually decreases, fecal output is reduced, and the rumen develops a "splashy" fluid consistency. The feces are characteristically very scant and sticky and may contain longer than normal particles. The strength of rumen contractions is decreased; however, rumen motility is often increased (3–4 contractions/min). It is commonly possible to see movements of the left abdominal wall that mirror the movements of the hyperactive rumen. However, rumen contraction sounds are not audible because the contents have become frothy due to the prolonged contractions and failure of the rumen to empty.

Temperature and respiratory rate are usually normal; however, these can be increased depending on the cause. Bradycardia is present in 25%–40% of cases and is due to decreased feed intake rather than a direct stimulation of the vagus nerve. Tachycardia develops as the disease progresses and cattle become dehydrated. Over time, the animal develops a rough hair coat, loses condition, and becomes weak (in some cases to the point of recumbency), with marked clinical signs of dehydration.

On rectal palpation, the rumen is distended with gas or froth that occupies the entire left abdomen, pushing the left kidney to the right of the midline. The ventral sac of the rumen is enlarged and palpable to the right of the midline (the characteristic "L-shaped" rumen). It is important to recognize that diagnosis of vagal indigestion syndrome requires the presence of a markedly increased ruminoreticular volume. Palpation of the lower half of the right side of the abdomen below the costochondral junction may detect an impacted abomasum that feels doughy. Hematologic findings vary. The PCV can be increased because of dehydration or decreased because of bone marrow depression (anemia of chronic disease). The WBC may be normal, increased, or decreased. If an inflammatory condition such as peritonitis is present, the neutrophil to lymphocyte ratio is typically reversed, and a neutrophilia may be present. Lymphocytosis can be seen with vagal indigestion due to lymphosarcoma. Leukopenia may be present with diffuse peritonitis. Increased serum globulin and total protein can be seen with abscesses.

Metabolic status is normal, or metabolic alkalosis may be present. The serum chloride concentration varies with the site of the obstruction. It is usually normal if the lesion is proximal to the abomasum. A low serum chloride concentration is consistent with reflux of chloride from the abomasum into the rumen (internal vomiting) and obstruction at the level of the abomasum (type III). Metabolic alkalosis is typically present if serum chloride is decreased. Rumen chloride concentration is increased in type III vagal indigestion and provides a useful method to differentiate type II from type III vagal indigestion. The serum potassium concentration is usually low due to decreased potassium intake in the feed. Serum calcium concentration is often moderately decreased because of ongoing milk production, but it is rarely low enough to cause recumbency. Serum urea and creatinine concentrations increase with dehydration due to prerenal azotemia.

Diagnosis: Diagnosis is based on the presence of subacute to chronic ruminoreticular and abdominal distention. Because vagal indigestion is by definition a subacute to chronic disease, this diagnosis should not be made in cattle that have not been sick for at least several days, which excludes acute rumen tympany and acute frothy bloat. Other causes of abdominal distention, such as ascites and uterine enlargement, are included in the differential diagnosis and can almost invariably be excluded by rectal palpation because of the absence of ruminoreticular distention. Occasional cases of longstanding obstruction of the cecum or small intestine can cause severe ruminoreticular and abdominal distention; however, palpable cecal or small-intestinal distention is also palpable rectally. In addition, the rumen is distended but not L-shaped, and a characteristic ping is present in the case of cecocolic volvulus.

Diagnosing the specific cause of vagal indigestion is more difficult but is important because of differences in treatment and prognosis. Physical examination, rectal examination, CBC, blood acid-base determination, and serum biochemical values are often useful. Peritoneal fluid analysis can support the diagnosis of peritonitis if total protein or nucleated cells are increased. Lateral radiographs of the reticulum should be taken to identify an opaque linear foreign body (eg, wire) or reticular abscess. Ultrasonography of the cranioventral abdomen can indicate the presence of focal peritonitis and the reticular contraction rate. Definitive diagnosis often requires exploratory surgery (left paralumbar fossa laparotomy and rumenotomy).

Treatment and Prognosis: If the value of the animal justifies treatment, surgery is almost always needed to identify and potentially correct the underlying cause. Medical management alone is usually ineffective. A left paralumbar fossa laparotomy and rumenotomy provides the opportunity for definitive treatment in some cases. Emptying the rumen at the time of surgery may help restore normal rumen motility. Stimulation of low-threshold tension receptors in the reticulum occurs under normal circumstances and causes reflex reticuloruminal contractions. However, severe distention causes stimulation of high-threshold receptors that have the opposite effect and inhibit contractions.

Supportive or symptomatic therapy should be provided in all cases, which typically involves correcting dehydration as well as calcium and electrolyte deficits, commonly with oral fluids and electrolytes. Severely dehydrated animals and those with longstanding disease require IV fluids. Fresh water and normal feed should be available. Transfaunation at surgery or via oroesophageal intubation may help reestablish normal rumen flora in cattle with chronic anorexia. Antimicrobials (procaine penicillin or oxytetracycline) should be given if the underlying cause is infectious or if a rumen fistula is created.

Treatment of type I vagal indigestion (failure of eructation) also typically involves creating a rumen fistula to allow free gas to escape. If surgery is not economically feasible and the underlying cause of vagal indigestion has been identified and treated, a rumen trocar can be placed temporarily. Such trocars are commercially available and must be secure and self-retaining to prevent potentially fatal leakage of rumen contents into the peritoneal cavity. The trocar should not be removed for at least 2 wk to allow firm adhesions to form between the rumen and body wall.

The prognosis for animals with type I vagal indigestion is usually favorable. After creation of a rumen fistula, the signs of vagal indigestion resolve in nearly all cases. However, animals with chronic respiratory disease or pharyngeal trauma may not recover from the underlying condition. Leakage of ingesta from fistulas can cause off-flavored milk. Peritonitis can develop from leakage around the fistula or after rumenotomy; however, this should not happen with good surgical technique.

Type II vagal indigestion (failure of omasal transport) rarely responds to supportive or symptomatic therapy without surgical intervention. Left paralumbar fossa laparotomy and rumenotomy can be used to identify adhesions in the vicinity of the reticulum, reticular or hepatic abscesses, or obstruction of the omasal canal. Removal of foreign bodies, wires, and some masses at surgery and lancing of perireticular abscesses into the reticulum affords a fair to good prognosis. A diagnosis of lymphosarcoma at surgery warrants a grave prognosis. Reticular abscesses identified at surgery should be cautiously drained into the reticulum, and antibiotics given for 10–14 days. Reportedly, 83% of cattle with reticular abscesses respond favorably to treatment. Identification of adhesions in the vicinity of the reticulum warrants a fair to good prognosis with surgery, antibiotic therapy, and appropriate supportive treatment. Hepatic abscesses must be drained by a second surgery. Large-bore cannulas placed through the body wall, through the adhesions, and into the abscess will drain the purulent material. However, recurrence is more of a problem with hepatic abscesses than with reticular abscesses.

Animals with type III vagal indigestion (secondary abomasal impaction) diagnosed without surgery usually do not receive further treatment because of the poor prognosis, particularly if there is a history of traumatic reticuloperitonitis or abomasal volvulus. If the diagnosis is made at surgery or if the abomasal impaction is thought to be dietary, dioctyl sodium sulfosuccinate can be infused directly into the abomasum via the reticulo-omasal orifice after emptying the rumen. A nasogastric tube can be passed into the abomasum via the reticulo-omasal orifice at surgery and left in place for continued treatment (3–4 L of mineral oil daily for 3–5 days). If possible, impacted material should be removed manually through the reticulo-omasal orifice. Other lesions, such as abscesses in the medial wall of the reticulum, should be identified and drained. Abomasotomy and removal of abomasal contents, using a right paracostal approach with the cow in left lateral recumbency, can be performed as a last resort. However, recurrence of the impaction is common. Pyloric obstruction in cattle is rare and is most often due to a foreign body obstructing the lumen. Pyloromyotomy is almost never effective in resolving abomasal impactions.

Type III vagal indigestion has a poor prognosis regardless of the cause or the treatment. However, cattle with mild to moderate primary abomasal impactions will respond to therapy, although severely affected animals will not (*see* p 244). Cattle with secondary impactions due to traumatic reticuloperitonitis or as a sequela of abomasal volvulus seldom recover. Animals with foreign bodies (eg, trichobezoars) obstructing the pylorus have a good prognosis if the obstruction is removed.

Therapeutic induction of parturition has been recommended for treatment of cattle with type IV vagal indigestion (indigestion of late gestation), and some cows have improved with this treatment; however, because type IV vagal indigestion is a poorly defined condition, the prognosis is always guarded. A more specific prognosis is based on response to therapy and identification of a specific lesion at exploratory celiotomy and rumenotomy.

Prevention: The most common cause of vagal indigestion syndrome is traumatic reticuloperitonitis, which causes adhesions and abscesses that interfere with both reticular motility and the appropriate stratification of feed particles for passage through the abomasum. Therefore, prevention of traumatic reticuloperitonitis is important. Good management practices may prevent some cases of vagal indigestion associated with chronic pneumonia. Early diagnosis of abomasal volvulus, with same-day surgical correction, may prevent some cases.

RUMINAL DRINKING

"Ruminal drinking" is caused by failure of the reticular groove reflex, and it results in ruminal acidosis in calves on a liquid diet. The disorder presents as primary chronic disease (ruminal drinking syndrome) in veal calves, and in its acute form as a complication secondary to different neonatal diseases, most commonly neonatal diarrhea. It has also been described in artificially fed lambs.

The reticular groove is a muscular structure extending from the cardia to the reticulo-omasal orifice. Its correct closure is a precondition for the direct passage of ingested milk or milk replacer into the abomasum. When the reticular groove partially or completely fails to close, milk spills into the reticulorumen and is fermented to short-chain fatty acids and/or lactic acid. The subsequent drop in the pH of the ruminal contents to values that occasionally fall below 4 leads to variable degrees of inflammation of the mucosa of the forestomachs and the abomasum. In chronic cases, hyperkeratosis or parakeratosis of the ruminal mucosa can lead to impairment of ruminal motility with chronic or recurrent tympany. Additionally, atrophy of the intestinal villi and a decrease in brush border enzyme activity with maldigestion and malabsorption have been seen.

Systemic consequences of acute ruminal drinking are mainly due to absorption of organic acids from the digestive tract. In particular, the L- and D-isomers of lactic acid may lead to metabolic acidosis with the accumulation of D-lactate because of an absence of a specific enzyme for its metabolism in mammals. This accumulation of D-lactate has recently been found to be responsible for clinical signs such as depression, ataxia, and general weakness.

Primary dysfunction of the reticular groove occurs as a result of stressful situations (prolonged transport, grouping, change in feeding techniques), especially in bucket-fed veal calves. Clinical signs usually appear some weeks after the arrival of the calves at the fattening units and are characterized by inappetence, depression, poor growth, hair loss, recurrent tympany, ventral abdominal distention, and passing of clay-like feces. Fluid-splashing sounds can be heard on succussion of the left flank. Recovery of fermented ruminal contents via stomach tube is diagnostic. In these advanced, chronic cases the prognosis is poor. If the disease is detected early enough, feeding small volumes of milk from a nipple-bottle or bucket may be successful. Additionally, the closure of the reticular groove can be triggered by allowing the calf to suck a finger before the milk feed is offered.

Acute ruminal acidosis secondary to other disorders is most commonly seen in calves with neonatal diarrhea but occurs also in other painful or weakening diseases. In these cases, the clinical picture is usually dominated by the underlying disease. In cases of severe rumenitis, calves may exhibit teeth grinding, arching of the back, and slight abdominal distention. Force-feeding of inappetent or primarily anorectic calves can also cause ruminal acidosis or worsen the situation by providing substrate for further fermentation.

The prognosis for secondary ruminal drinking depends mainly on the success of treatment of the underlying disease. Calves with metabolic acidosis and dehydration due to neonatal diarrhea usually recover spontaneously from ruminal drinking after adequate treatment, and the condition will in general remain unrecognized. In calves that were force-fed or that do not respond to treatment as expected, ruminal drinking should be considered, and an examination of the ruminal fluid performed. Removal of the contents and lavage with warm water via stomach tube may be beneficial, especially after prolonged force-feeding. Prophylaxis of ruminal drinking consists of early treatment of diseased calves, adequate feeding techniques, and minimizing stress in purchased calves.

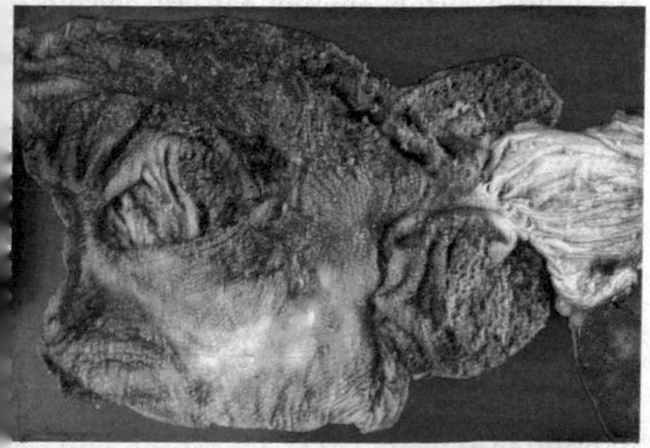

Severe rumenitis in a 10-day-old calf after a prolonged course of ruminal drinking. *Courtesy of Dr. Ingrid Lorenz.*

RUMINAL PARAKERATOSIS

Ruminal parakeratosis is a disease of cattle and sheep characterized by hardening and enlargement of the papillae of the rumen. It is most common in animals fed a high-concentrate ration during the finishing period. It also is seen in cattle fed rations of heat-treated alfalfa pellets, as well as in calves with prolonged ruminal acidosis due to ruminal drinking. It does not appear to be related to the feeding of antibiotics or protein concentrates. Incidence in a group may be as high as 40%. The lesions are thought to be caused by the lowered pH and the increased concentration of volatile fatty acids (VFAs) in the ruminal fluid, and do not usually develop in cattle fed unprocessed whole grain (on which animals gain weight as readily). This may be related to the higher pH and higher concentration of acetic acid than those of the longer chain VFAs in the ruminal contents.

Many of the papillae are enlarged and hardened, and several may adhere together to form bundles. The papillae of the anterior ventral sac are commonly affected. In cattle, the roof of the dorsal sac may show multiple foci (each 2–3 cm^2) of parakeratosis. In sheep, abnormal papillae may be visible and palpable through the wall of the intact rumen. Affected papillae contain excessive layers of keratinized epithelial cells, particles of food, and bacteria. The rumens of affected cattle are difficult to clean in the preparation of tripe. The abnormal epithelium, by interfering with absorption, may reduce efficiency of feed utilization and rate of gain, although there is little evidence to support this theory.

Ruminal parakeratosis may be prevented by finishing animals on rations that contain unground ingredients in the proportion of 1 part roughage to 3 parts concentrate. The necessity and economics of prevention are not well defined.

DISEASES OF THE ABOMASUM

Abomasal disorders include left displaced abomasum (LDA), right displaced abomasum (RDA), abomasal volvulus (AV), abomasal ulceration, and impaction. Displacement or volvulus is seen most commonly in dairy cows but can also be seen in dairy bulls and calves. Except for AV, abomasal displacement is rare in beef cattle and essentially undiagnosed in small ruminants. Abomasal ulcers are seen in dairy and beef cattle and in calves and lambs; they are rarely diagnosed in small ruminants. Impactions can be primary, which is most frequent in beef cattle, or secondary, which develop most often in dairy cows as a form of vagal indigestion. Impactions may have a hereditary basis in some black-faced sheep.

LEFT OR RIGHT DISPLACED ABOMASUM AND ABOMASAL VOLVULUS

Because the abomasum is suspended loosely by the greater omentum and lesser omentum, it can be moved from its normal position on the right ventral part of the abdomen to the left or right side (LDA, RDA), or it can rotate on its mesenteric axis while displaced to the right and lateral to the liver (AV). The abomasum can shift from its normal position to left displacement or to right displacement over a relatively short period. AV can develop rapidly or slowly from an uncorrected RDA.

Etiology: Although LDA, RDA, and AV (previously incorrectly referred to as right torsion of the abomasum) are often considered separately, there is evidence of a common underlying etiology; they may be different manifestations of the same or a similar disease process.

The etiology is multifactorial, although abomasal hypomotility and dysfunction of the intrinsic nervous system are thought to play an important role in development of displacement or volvulus. Important contributing factors include abomasal hypomotility associated with hypocalcemia and possibly hypokalemia, as well as concurrent diseases (mastitis, metritis) associated with endotoxemia and decreased rumen fill, periparturient changes in the position of intra-abdominal organs, and genetic predisposition, particularly in deep-bodied cows. Genetic predisposition is correlated with milk yield, indicating that current selection practices for milk production are increasing the incidence of abomasal displacement. Hypomotility is also related to ingestion of high-concentrate, low-roughage diets, which reduce abomasal motility through a poorly defined mechanism that may involve hyperinsulinemia or increased concentrations of volatile fatty acids. One of the mechanisms of excessive gas accumulation in cattle with abomasal displacement is reticulum-mediated inflow of ruminal gas into the abomasum that is hypomotile. In addition, high-concentrate diets result in increased gas production in the abomasum (mostly carbon dioxide, methane, and nitrogen). Finally, subclinical and clinical ketosis increase the risk of abomasal displacement through an unknown mechanism that may be associated with decreased rumen fill.

Approximately 80% of displacements are seen within 1 mo of parturition; however, they can be seen at any time. LDA is much more common than RDA (30 LDA to 1 RDA); cases of AV are also more common than RDA (10 LDA to 1 AV). AV is preceded by RDA.

Pathogenesis: In LDA, as a result of abomasal hypomotility and gas production, the partially gas-distended abomasum becomes displaced upward along the left abdominal wall lateral to the rumen. The fundus and greater curvature of the abomasum are primarily displaced, which in turn causes displacement of the pylorus and duodenum. The omasum, reticulum, and liver are also rotated to varying degrees. The abomasal obstruction is partial, and although the segment contains some gas and fluid, a certain amount can still escape, and the distention rarely becomes severe. Because there is minimal interference with blood supply unless the gas distention is marked, the effects of displacement are entirely due to interference with digestion and passage of ingesta, which lead to decreased appetite and dehydration.

A mild metabolic alkalosis with hypochloremia and hypokalemia are common. The hypochloremic metabolic alkalosis is due to abomasal hypomotility, continued secretion of hydrochloric acid into the abomasum, and the partial abomasal outflow obstruction, with sequestration of chloride in the abomasum and reflux into the rumen. Hypokalemia is due to decreased intake of feeds high in potassium, sequestration of potassium in the abomasum, and dehydration. Secondary ketosis is common and may be complicated by development of hepatic lipidosis (fatty liver disease; *see* p 1018).

In RDA, hypomotility, gas production, and displacement of the partially gas-filled abomasum occur as in LDA. Mild hypokalemic, hypochloremic, metabolic alkalosis develops as well. After this dilatation phase, rotation of the abomasum on its mesenteric axis leads to volvulus and local circulatory impairment and ischemia (hemorrhagic strangulating obstruction). The volvulus is usually in a counterclockwise direction when viewed from the rear and the right side of the animal. The omasum is displaced medially and can be involved in the volvulus with occlusion of its blood supply (called an omasal-abomasal volvulus) and displacement of the liver and reticulum. In rare cases, the reticulum can be involved (called a reticular-omasal-abomasal volvulus).

A large quantity of chloride-rich fluid (up to 50 L) accumulates in the abomasum, and hypochloremic, hypokalemic metabolic alkalosis develops. The blood supply to the abomasum, and often the omasum and proximal duodenum, is compromised, eventually resulting in ischemic necrosis of the abomasum and proximal duodenum as well as dehydration and circulatory failure. As circulatory failure progresses, a metabolic acidosis due to hyper-L-lactatemia and azotemia can become superimposed on the preexisting metabolic alkalosis.

Clinical Findings: The typical history of abomasal displacement includes anorexia (most commonly a lack of appetite for grain with a decreased or normal appetite for roughage) and decreased milk production (usually significant but not as dramatic as with traumatic reticuloperitonitis or other causes of peritonitis). In AV, anorexia is complete, milk production is more markedly and progressively reduced, and clinical deterioration is rapid. In abomasal displacement, temperature, heart rate, and respiratory rate are usually normal. The caudal part of the rib cage on the side of the displacement may appear "sprung." Hydration appears subjectively normal with displacements except in some chronic cases. Rumen motility may be normal but often is reduced in frequency and strength of contraction. Feces are usually reduced in quantity and more fluid than normal.

The most important diagnostic physical finding is a ping on simultaneous auscultation and percussion of the abdomen, which should be performed in the area marked by a line from the tuber coxae to the point of the elbow, and from the elbow toward the stifle. The ping (detected during simultaneous percussion and auscultation) characteristic of an LDA is most commonly located in an area between ribs 9 and 13 in the middle to upper third of the left abdomen; however, the ping can be more ventral or more caudal, or both. Pings associated with a rumen gas cap are usually more dorsal, less resonant, and extend more caudally through the left paralumbar fossa. Rectal examination can confirm a gas-filled rumen or an extremely empty rumen that correlates with the rumen ping in these cases. Pings associated with pneumoperitoneum typically are less resonant, present on both sides of the abdomen, and are inconsistent in location on repeated evaluation. Frequently, secondary ketosis develops, and ketones are present in the urine or milk. Ketosis that develops in association with abomasal displacement responds only transiently to treatment and recurs (versus in primary ketosis, which develops early in lactation in high-producing cows and responds to therapy permanently if instituted early). (*See also* KETOSIS IN CATTLE, p 1024.)

The ping associated with RDA also is most commonly located in the area between ribs 10 and 13 on the right abdomen. Differentiation between various causes of a right-side ping can be difficult in some cases, although a ping cranial to rib 10 usually indicates the presence of AV because the liver is displaced medially by the distended viscus. A small, right-side ping underlying ribs 12 or 13 and extending as far forward as rib 10 is common in cows with functional ileus from a number of causes. This ping is most often associated with gas in the ascending colon and resolves with correction of the underlying condition. Cecal dilatation and rotation are characterized by a right-side ping. The ping extends through the dorsal paralumbar fossa in cecal dilatation and usually is located more caudally (well into the paralumbar fossa) in cecal rotation than the ping of RDA. Palpation per rectum is helpful in differentiating an RDA from cecal dilatation or rotation. Other right-side pings are produced by pneumoperitoneum or gas in the rectum, descending colon, duodenum, or uterus.

Spontaneous fluid splashing or gas tinkling sounds may be heard on auscultation of the area of the ping or on simultaneous ballottement and auscultation of the

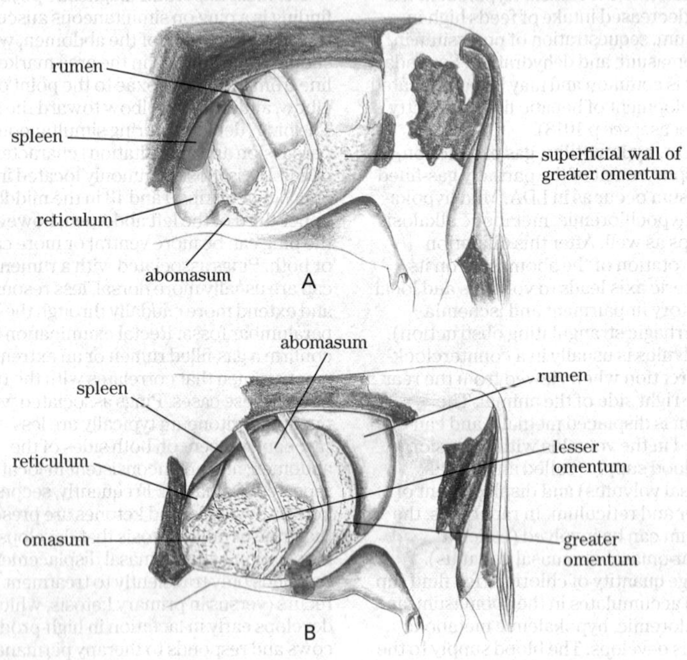

A) Normal topography of left abdominal viscera, cow. B) Left displacement of abomasum. *Illustration by Dr. Gheorghe Constantinescu.* Adapted, with permission, from DeLahunta and Habel, *Applied Veterinary Anatomy*, W.B. Saunders, 1986.

abdomen (succussion). The characteristic rectal examination findings with LDA include a medially displaced rumen and left kidney. The abomasum is rarely palpable in LDA and only occasionally in RDA.

The clinical signs associated with abomasal volvulus are more severe than with simple displacements because of the vascular compromise. However, an early abomasal volvulus can be difficult to distinguish from an RDA except by the presence of a right-side ping cranial to rib 10 (indicating medial displacement of the liver by the abomasal volvulus) and the anatomic position identified at surgery. In contrast to cases of displacement, an animal with AV has tachycardia proportional to the severity of the condition. The area of the ping is usually larger (extending as far forward as rib 8), and the amount of succussible fluid is greater. The animal is more depressed, and signs of weakness, toxemia, and dehydration develop as the disease progresses. The caudal extent of the abomasum is usually palpable per rectum. Without therapy, the animal often becomes recumbent within 48–72 hr after developing volvulus. Death occurs from shock and dehydration and is sudden if the ischemic abomasum ruptures.

Diagnosis: For displacement or volvulus, diagnosis is based on the presence of the characteristic ping on simultaneous auscultation and percussion and exclusion of other causes of left- or right-side pings. Ultrasonography may be helpful in confirming a diagnosis of LDA, RDA, or AV, but it cannot reliably differentiate RDA from AV. Recent parturition, partial anorexia, and decreased milk production suggest displacement. A ketosis that is only temporarily responsive to treatment is consistent with abomasal displacement, which may be intermittent. The typical signs on physical examination (in addition to the ping), rectal examination, and laboratory evaluation also support the diagnosis. Melena or signs of peritonitis (eg, fever, tachycardia, localized abdominal pain, pneumoperitoneum) with an LDA may indicate a bleeding or perforated abomasal ulcer, respectively. In cattle with AV, blood L-lactate concentrations ≤2 mmol/L indicate a positive outcome with surgical correction, whereas cattle with blood L-lactate concentrations ≥6 mmol/L have a high probability of a negative outcome.

Treatment: Open (surgical) and closed (percutaneous) techniques can be used to correct abomasal displacements. Rolling a cow through a 180° arc after casting her on her right side corrects most LDAs; however, recurrence is very likely. LDA can be corrected surgically using right flank pyloric omentopexy, right paramedian abomasopexy, left paralumbar abomasopexy, combined left flank and right paramedian laparoscopy (two-step procedure), or left flank laparoscopy (one-step procedure). Blind suture techniques (toggle-pin fixation or the "big needle" [blind-stitch] method), performed in the right paramedian area, are percutaneous methods for correction of LDA; however, the exact location of the suture is not known. Potentially fatal complications can develop after blind suture techniques, and the reported success rate is less than that of surgical correction by right flank pyloric omentopexy. With toggle-pin fixation, the pH can be checked to confirm that the pin is in the abomasum, which reduces the likelihood of attaching rumen, small intestine, or omentum to the body wall rather than the abomasum. RDA and AV are corrected surgically (using right paralumbar fossa omentopexy) when economically feasible. The right paramedian abomasopexy should be used only to correct RDA and AV in cattle unable to stand.

Ancillary treatment of animals with abomasal displacement include treating any concurrent disease (eg, metritis, mastitis, ketosis). Calcium borogluconate or calcium gluconate SC or calcium gels PO help restore normal abomasal motility in many cases. Administration of erythromycin (10 mg/kg, IM) at the time of surgery increases abomasal emptying rate and milk production in the immediate postoperative period. Because surgical correction of abomasal displacement or volvulus is frequently done on the farm, the prokinetic effect of erythromycin suggests that it might be preferred if antimicrobials are administered to control intraoperative infection. However, administration of an antimicrobial for a nonantimicrobial effect should not be promoted.

In simple displacement, fluid and electrolyte abnormalities correct spontaneously with access to water and a salt block. Providing electrolyte water (60 g sodium chloride and 30 g potassium chloride in 19 L of water) via stomach tube is helpful in cases of longer duration. Animals with significant dehydration and metabolic derangement require IV therapy, typically administered as hypertonic saline (7.2% NaCl, 5 mL/kg, IV over 5 min).

Occasionally, animals with abomasal displacement or volvulus have atrial fibrillation, thought to be of metabolic origin and primarily due to concurrent hypokalemia and metabolic alkalosis. Correction of the displacement or volvulus almost always results in correction of the atrial fibrillation within 5 days.

Aggressive treatment of ketosis plays an important role in successful treatment of abomasal displacement, because most of the cattle that die after surgical correction of LDA and RDA do so from the metabolic consequences of prolonged anorexia.

The prognosis after correction of simple LDA or RDA is good, with survival rates of 95%. AV has a variable and less favorable prognosis (average survival rate of 70%); a high heart rate, moderate to severe dehydration, a longer period of illness, a large quantity of fluid in the abomasum, increased blood or plasma L-lactate concentration, and the presence of omasal-abomasal or reticulo-omasal-abomasal volvulus are associated with a poorer prognosis.

Prevention: The incidence of abomasal displacements can be decreased by ensuring a rapid increase in rumen volume after calving, feeding a total mixed ration rather than feeding grain twice daily ("slug feeding"), avoiding rapid dietary changes, maintaining adequate roughage in the diet, avoiding postparturient hypocalcemia, and minimizing and promptly treating concurrent disease and ketosis.

ABOMASAL ULCERS

Abomasal ulcers affect mature cattle and calves and have several different manifestations.

Etiology and Pathogenesis: Except for lymphosarcoma of the abomasum and the erosions of the abomasal mucosa that develop in viral diseases such as bovine viral diarrhea and bovine malignant catarrhal fever, the causes of abomasal ulceration are not well understood. Many different causes have been suggested. Although abomasal ulcers can be seen any time during lactation, they are common in high-producing, mature dairy cows within the first 6 wk after parturition. The most likely cause is prolonged inappetence, which results in sustained periods of low abomasal pH; hence, the adage "no acid, no ulcer."

Abomasal ulcers may also arise in association with lymphosarcoma, abomasal disorders (displacement or volvulus), or increased luminal pressure causing ischemia of abomasal mucosa; they may also appear to be unrelated to other disease.

Abomasal ulcers are very common in milk-fed calves after they have consumed milk or milk replacer for 4–12 wk. Most of these ulcers are subclinical and nonhemorrhagic. Occasionally, milk-fed calves <2 wk old are affected by acute, hemorrhagic abomasal ulcers that may perforate and cause rapid death. Well-nourished suckling beef calves, 2–4 mo old, may be affected by acute abomasal ulcers. Abomasal trichobezoars are common in these calves but do not appear to increase risk of ulcer formation.

Clinical Findings: The syndrome varies, depending on whether ulceration is complicated by hemorrhage or perforation and by the severity of such hemorrhage or peritonitis.

A system of classification is based on the depth of penetration or the degree of hemorrhage or peritonitis caused by the ulcer: Type I is an erosion or ulcer without hemorrhage, Type II is hemorrhagic, Type III is perforated with acute localized peritonitis, Type IV is perforated with acute diffuse peritonitis, and Type V is perforated with peritonitis within the omental bursa. There may be only a single ulcer or many acute and chronic ulcers.

Cattle with bleeding abomasal ulcers may be asymptomatic except for intermittent occult blood in the feces, or they can die acutely from massive hemorrhage. Common clinical signs include mild abdominal pain, bruxism, sudden onset of anorexia, tachycardia (90–100 bpm), and fecal occult blood or melena that may be intermittent. Signs of blood loss are seen with major hemorrhage and may include tachycardia (100–140 bpm), pale mucous membranes, weak pulse, cool extremities, shallow breaths, tachypnea, and melena. More severe signs include acute rumen stasis, generalized abdominal pain with a reluctance to move and an audible grunt or groan with each breath, weakness, and dehydration. Melena may not be present in peracute cases, because it takes at least 8 hr for abomasal blood to be detected in the feces. As the condition progresses, body temperature drops, and the animal becomes recumbent and dies within 6–8 hr.

In general, bleeding ulcers do not perforate, and perforating ulcers do not bleed into the GI tract sufficiently to produce melena. However, hemorrhage and perforation are seen together occasionally, usually in cases that are chronic or associated with abomasal displacement.

Calves with abomasal ulceration and hairballs may have a distended gas- and fluid-filled abomasum that is palpable behind the right costal arch. Deep palpation may reveal abdominal pain associated with local peritonitis due to a perforated ulcer. In calves, perforating ulcers are more common than bleeding ulcers.

Lesions: Ulceration is most common in the fundic region in adult cattle and in the pyloric antrum in milk-fed calves. The single or multiple ulcers measure from a few millimeters to 5 cm in diameter. The affected artery is usually visible after ingesta and necrotic tissue are removed from a bleeding ulcerated area. Most cases of perforation are walled off by the omentum, which forms a cavity 12–15 cm in diameter that contains degenerated blood and necrotic debris. Material from this cavity may infiltrate widely through the omental fat. Adhesions may form between the ulcer and surrounding organs or the abdominal wall.

Diagnosis: In cases with only slight bleeding and mild clinical signs, diagnosis of abomasal ulcer is difficult and may require repeated fecal evaluations for occult blood. Other conditions that can cause partial anorexia and decreased milk production should be excluded by physical examination and laboratory tests, including abdominocentesis. In cases with melena, the diagnosis can be based on physical examination alone. The PCV can help to determine the degree of hemorrhage, although it takes at least 4 hr after an acute hemorrhage before the PCV decreases. An occult blood test of the feces can confirm melena. Other conditions that result in blood in the feces should be eliminated. Blood from portions of the GI tract distal to the abomasum reacts on fecal occult blood tests; it is usually bright red if from the large intestine or raspberry-colored if from the small intestine. Animals with abomasal lymphosarcoma can have a bleeding syndrome similar to that associated with abomasal ulcers but do not respond to therapy. Occasionally, oral, pharyngeal, and laryngeal lesions bleed, and the swallowed blood appears in the feces. Similarly, pulmonary abscesses that form as a sequela of rumenitis by embolization to the lungs and liver can erode blood vessels and result in hemoptysis; if the blood is swallowed, this can also result in melena. Fecal occult blood may also be due to AV or rarely to bloodsucking helminths.

Diagnosis of perforating abomasal ulcers is based on physical examination and excluding other causes of peritonitis. Abomasal ulceration with perforation and local peritonitis may be indistinguishable from chronic traumatic reticuloperitonitis (*see* p 230). A magnet in the reticulum (confirmed by use of a compass) or an accurate history of having given the cow a magnet before the onset of signs decreases the likelihood of traumatic reticuloperitonitis. Reticular radiographs may confirm or exclude the presence of radiopaque foreign bodies in the reticulum. In some cases, there is a neutrophilia, possibly with a left shift. Evaluation of peritoneal fluid will confirm peritonitis if total protein or D-dimer concentration and nucleated cell count are increased. Intracellular bacteria or degenerate neutrophils are rarely seen because, in most cases, the infection is rapidly walled off. The diagnosis of diffuse peritonitis due to perforation is based on physical examination and excluding other causes. Rupture of a distended viscus, such as can occur with AV or cecal rotation, produces similar signs. Regardless of the cause of diffuse peritonitis, the prognosis is grave because of overwhelming infection and cardiovascular deterioration. There is neutrophilia with a marked left shift and hemoconcentration. Abdominal fluid is usually readily obtainable in large quantities, and the protein level is increased; the nucleated cell count may be increased, or it may be normal due to dilution or utilization.

Treatment: Most cases of abomasal ulcers are undiagnosed and therefore untreated. Occasionally, a presumptive diagnosis is made and medical treatment instituted. The most important treatment is to get the animal to eat, because food is an excellent buffer and continual flow of forestomach contents (pH 6.0–7.0) into the abomasum helps increase abomasal pH. Broad-spectrum antimicrobial therapy (given for ≥5 days or until the rectal temperature is normal for 48 hr) is indicated for perforating ulcers. Antacids effectively increase abomasal pH in milk-fed calves when administered at 4- to 6-hr intervals in a manner that induces esophageal groove closure; however, their efficacy is extremely questionable in adult ruminants because of dilution by the large rumen volume. H_2-receptor antagonists effectively increase abomasal pH in milk-fed calves; however, the oral dosages required for cimetidine (100 mg/kg, tid) and ranitidine (50 mg/kg, tid) are high, making treatment expensive. Proton pump inhibitors, such as omeprazole (2 mg/kg, IV) effectively increase luminal pH, but again treatment is expensive. The efficacy of oral omeprazole (4 mg/kg) in adult ruminants is unknown, but it has some efficacy in milk-fed calves. Because NSAIDs can contribute to ulceration, their use is contraindicated. The prognosis for localized peritonitis associated with perforating abomasal ulcers is good with medical therapy and dietary alteration. Recovery generally takes 1–2 wk, and animals fully recovered for 1–2 wk generally do not experience recurrence. Surgery is indicated for perforating abomasal ulcers only when the abomasum is displaced; however, significant abdominal contamination can occur in the process of breaking down adhesions and resecting or oversewing the ulcer.

Animals with diffuse peritonitis after perforation of an abomasal ulcer rarely respond to therapy, and the prognosis is grave. Treatment consists of rapid and continued IV fluid therapy (based on the current metabolic status) and IV broad-spectrum antibiotics. The few animals that recover from diffuse peritonitis usually have massive abdominal adhesions.

For bleeding ulcers, blood transfusions and fluid therapy may be necessary in addition to dietary management, stall confinement, and oral antacids. If hemorrhage is acute, the PCV may not reflect the severity because equilibration between intravascular and extravascular fluid after blood loss takes at least 4 hr. Generally, a blood transfusion is required whenever weakness and lethargy are present; a decision regarding transfusion should be based on clinical signs rather than PCV. Cross-matching is not usually necessary; a single transfusion of 4–6 L of blood is required. Some cattle require more than one transfusion over the course of several days. Complete recovery usually takes 1–2 wk. The prognosis is good if weakness and lethargy have not developed before treatment is started.

Prevention: Animals should be encouraged to keep eating to avoid prolonged periods of inappetence and low abomasal pH.

DIETARY ABOMASAL IMPACTION

Impaction of the abomasum develops in pregnant beef cows during cold winter months when cattle have decreased water intake and are fed poor-quality roughage. Impaction also has been seen in feedlot cattle fed a variety of mixed rations containing chopped or ground roughage (straw, hay) and cereal grains and in late-pregnancy dairy cows on similar feeds. Impaction of the pyloric antrum is an underdiagnosed condition in dairy cows in early lactation.

Etiology and Pathogenesis: The cause of dietary abomasal impaction is unknown but considered to be consumption of excess roughage low in both digestible protein and energy. Impaction with sand can occur if cattle are fed hay or silage on sandy soils, or root crops that are sandy or dirty. Outbreaks may affect up to 15% of all pregnant cattle on individual farms when the ambient temperature drops to –14°F (–26°C) or lower for several days. The cause in postparturient dairy cows is probably related to abomasal hypomotility.

The pathogenesis is unknown but is related to diet. Once the abomasum becomes impacted, subacute obstruction of the upper GI tract develops. Ions of hydrogen and chloride are continually secreted into the abomasum in spite of the impaction, and atony and alkalosis with hypochloremia result. Varying degrees of dehydration develop, because fluids are not moving beyond the abomasum into the duodenum for absorption. Sequestration of potassium ions in the abomasum results in hypokalemia. Dehydration, alkalosis, electrolyte imbalance, and progressive starvation are seen. Impaction of the abomasum may be severe enough to cause irreversible abomasal atony.

Clinical Findings and Lesions: Complete anorexia, scant feces, moderate distention of the abdomen, weight loss, and weakness are usually the initial signs of dietary abomasal impaction. Body temperature is usually normal but may be subnormal during cold weather. A mucoid nasal discharge tends to collect at the external nares and on the muzzle; the muzzle is usually dry and cracked, caused by both the failure of the animal to lick its nostrils and the effects of dehydration. The heart rate may be increased, and mild dehydration is common.

Most often, the rumen is static and distended with dry contents, but it may contain excess fluid if the cow has been fed finely ground feed. The pH of the ruminal fluid is usually normal (6.5–7). Protozoal activity in the rumen ranges from normal to a marked reduction in numbers and activity (assessed microscopically under low power). The impacted abomasum is usually in the right lower quadrant on the floor of the abdomen. Deep palpation and strong percussion of the right flank may indicate the presence of a large, firm mass (impacted abomasum) and elicit a grunt (as is common in acute traumatic reticuloperitonitis), probably because of distention of the abomasum and stretching of its serosa.

Severely affected cattle die 3–6 days after the onset of signs. The abomasum ruptures in some cases, and death from acute, diffuse peritonitis and shock occurs precipitously in a few hours. In sand impaction, there is considerable weight loss, chronic diarrhea with sand in the feces, weakness, recumbency, and death in a few weeks.

Metabolic alkalosis, hypochloremia, hypokalemia, and hemoconcentration are common, as are total and differential WBC counts within the normal range. At necropsy, the abomasum is commonly enlarged (up to 8 times normal size) and impacted with dry rumen-like contents. The omasum may be similarly enlarged and impacted. The rumen is grossly enlarged and filled with dry contents or fluid. The GI tract beyond the pylorus is characteristically empty and has a dry appearance. Varying degrees of dehydration and emaciation are also present. If the abomasum has ruptured, lesions of acute diffuse peritonitis are present. In dairy cattle in early lactation, typically only the pyloric antrum is impacted.

Diagnosis: Clinical diagnosis of dietary abomasal impaction is based on the nutritional history, clinical evidence of impaction, and laboratory results. The disease must be differentiated from secondary abomasal impaction as a form of vagal indigestion.

Impaction of the abomasum as a complication of traumatic reticuloperitonitis usually is seen in late pregnancy, and commonly only in one animal. A mild fever may or may not be present, and there may be a grunt on deep palpation of the xiphoid. The rumen is enlarged and may be hypermotile (early) or atonic (late). In many cases, it is impossible to distinguish between the two causes of impacted abomasum, and a right flank laparotomy may be necessary to explore the abdomen for peritoneal lesions.

Treatment: The challenge is to recognize the cases of dietary abomasal impaction that will respond to treatment and those that will not, ie, to determine those animals that should be slaughtered immediately for salvage. Cows that are weak, have a severely impacted abomasum, and have a marked tachycardia (100–120 bpm) are poor treatment risks. Medical treatment usually requires a confirmed diagnosis via right-side laparotomy. In cows that are treated, the metabolic alkalosis, hypochloremia, hypokalemia, and dehydration should be corrected. Lubricants can be used in an attempt to move the impacted material; it is necessary to empty the abomasum surgically only in cattle with severe impaction. Balanced electrolyte solutions are infused IV continuously for up to 72 hr at a daily rate of 80–120 mL/kg. Some cows respond well to this therapy and begin ruminating and passing feces in 48 hr.

Mineral oil should be administered at 4 L/day for 3 days. Additionally, dioctyl sodium sulfosuccinate (DSS) can be injected once into the abomasum during standing right flank laparotomy at 60–100 mL of a 25% solution for a 1,000-lb (450-kg) animal. This dose rate should not be administered PO because DSS kills rumen protozoa. A beneficial response cannot be expected in <24 hr; in cattle that respond, improvement is usually seen by the end of day 3 after treatment begins. Erythromycin (10 mg/kg, IM, once to twice daily) can be administered as a prokinetic in cattle that do not improve after surgery, provided that mineral oil has been administered and physical obstructions were not identified at surgery.

Surgery may be considered, but results are often unsuccessful, probably because of abomasal atony, which appears to worsen after surgery. An alternative may be a rumenotomy to empty the rumen and infuse mineral oil directly into the abomasum through the reticulo-omasal orifice in an attempt to soften and promote evacuation of the abomasal contents. Cattle with secondary impactions that develop as a sequela of traumatic reticuloperitonitis or AV usually show signs of vagal indigestion, and abomasal impaction may be diagnosed at the time of exploratory surgery.

The induction of parturition using dexamethasone (20 mg, IM) may be indicated in affected cattle within 2 wk of term and in which the response to treatment for a few days has been unsuccessful. Parturition may assist recovery because of a reduction in intra-abdominal volume. For sand impaction, affected cattle should be moved off the sandy soil and fed good hay and a grass mixture containing molasses and minerals. Severely affected cattle should be treated with mineral oil (4 L/day for 3 days).

Prevention and Control: Prevention of dietary abomasal impaction is possible by providing the necessary nutrient requirements for wintering pregnant beef cattle. When low-quality roughage is used, it should be analyzed for crude protein and digestible energy. Based on the analysis, grain is usually added to the ration to meet energy and protein requirements.

The nutrient requirements of beef cattle (*see* p 2248) are guidelines for use under average conditions; higher nutrient levels than those indicated may be necessary, particularly during periods of severe cold stress. Adequate fresh drinking water should be supplied at all times; the practice of forcing wintering cows to obtain their water requirements by eating snow while on low-quality roughage is hazardous.

ACUTE INTESTINAL OBSTRUCTIONS IN LARGE ANIMALS

Intestinal obstructions are seen in all large animal species but are most common in horses. Cattle are the most commonly affected ruminants; diagnosis in sheep and goats is rare, except for intestinal volvulus in lambs. Other than inguinal hernias, intestinal obstructions are infrequently recognized in pigs.

Obstructions interrupt the flow of ingesta and can be mechanical or functional in nature. Mechanical intestinal obstructions are characterized as being luminal or extraluminal. Extraluminal obstructions include hemorrhagic strangulating obstructions in animals with volvulus of the GI tract, or simple extraluminal compression in animals with an expanding abdominal mass such as lymphosarcoma or fat necrosis. Functional obstructions have no gross abnormality but are characterized by a generalized hypomotility or ileus. In general, functional obstructions occur more often than mechanical obstructions, and they are commonly identified in horses after abdominal surgery.

Etiology and Pathogenesis: The inciting cause of a functional intestinal obstruction often is not determined. Functional obstructions are associated with altered intestinal motility, often due to dietary or management factors, phytobezoars, parasite infection, enteritis, peritonitis, or electrolyte abnormalities. Mechanical obstructions (physical blockage of ingesta) occur due to abnormalities in the bowel lumen, in the wall, or outside the tract. Mechanical obstructions include congenital obstructions (atresia jejuni, coli, recti, and ani in calves; atresia ani in lambs and pigs) that result in the lack of passage of feces since birth.

In horses, transient functional obstructions are common, as are feed impactions, which usually involve the pelvic flexure of the left colon. Parasite infection or migration, dental abnormalities, and dietary or management factors are often implicated in the development of functional obstruction. Impactions and other luminal obstructions can result from coarse feeds, reduced water intake, enteroliths, or ingested foreign material. Sites of impaction other than the pelvic flexure are the small colon, transverse colon, right dorsal colon, cecum, and ileum. Other causes of intestinal obstruction in horses are volvulus (twist on the mesenteric axis), torsion (twist along the long axis of the bowel), displacement of the ascending (large) colon, and volvulus of part or all of the small intestine. Altered motility and possibly strenuous exercise and rolling may be initiating causes. Broodmares may be predisposed to volvulus, torsion, or displacement of the ascending colon during gestation and shortly after parturition. Obstruction occurs either due to incarceration of the intestine (usually small) by herniation through the inguinal canal, diaphragm, mesenteric defects, umbilicus, or epiploic foramen; or because of fibrous bands (adhesions, mesodiverticular bands, or stalks of pedunculated lipomas). Standardbred stallions and colts develop inguinal and scrotal hernias more commonly than other breeds. Diaphragmatic hernias and mesenteric defects may be congenital or traumatically induced. Adhesions in horses are most often the sequela of parasite migration or abdominal surgery; however, most adhesions are clinically silent. Pedunculated lipomas are common in older horses. Ileocecal, cecocecal, cecocolic, and small-intestinal intussusceptions also are seen. Lymphosarcoma and other abdominal neoplasms as well as abdominal abscesses can cause intestinal obstruction.

In cattle, specific causes of intestinal obstruction include volvulus of the duodenal sigmoid flexure; intussusception of the jejunum and ileum; volvulus of the jejunoileal flange of the small intestine; volvulus at the root of the mesentery; luminal occlusion of the jejunum due to a blood clot secondary to hemorrhagic jejunitis; obstruction of the small intestine or spiral colon due to phytobezoars; cecocolic volvulus; and atresia coli, recti, and ani. Intussusceptions are thought to be the result of irregular peristaltic movements related to enteritis, intestinal parasitism, dietary disorders, and mural masses. Altered intestinal motility due to ingestion of a rapidly fermentable substrate may cause intestinal volvulus. Obstructions of the small intestine can develop due to a variety of fibrous bands (eg, adhesions, parovarian bands, falciform ligament, spermatic cord retraction into the abdomen after surgical castration), mural thickening (eg, intestinal adenocarcinoma), extramural masses (eg, lymphosarcoma, fat necrosis, abdominal abscesses), herniation (omental, inguinal, or umbilical), or hemorrhagic jejunitis (which results in luminal blood clots and obstruction). Adhesions and abdominal abscesses can form subsequent to peritonitis, intraperitoneal injections, or previous abdominal surgery. Decreased motility caused by accumulation of volatile fatty acids, possibly related to high-concentrate rations or an abrupt increase in the concentrate:forage ratio, have been suggested as causes of cecocolic volvulus in cattle. They also are associated with advanced pregnancy and ileus from concurrent disease. Atresia coli develops most commonly in Holstein-Friesian calves secondary to in utero ischemia of the developing spiral colon.

Clinical Findings and Diagnosis: Intestinal obstruction in horses generally manifests as abdominal pain, which is termed colic (*see* p 248). In cattle, signs of abdominal pain include treading of the hindlimbs, stretching, restlessness, and kicking at the abdomen; rolling and bellowing are rarely seen. The signs of intestinal obstruction in cattle are generally more subtle than in horses and are usually referable to small-intestinal distention, tension on the intestinal mesentery (by the weight of distended bowel), or vascular impairment. Signs of pain are relatively consistent but often transient with intussusceptions and are seen in some cases of cecocolic volvulus. Cattle with volvulus of the small intestine at the root of the mesentery are severely affected.

Usually, cattle with intestinal obstruction are anorectic and pass few or no feces, and milk production in lactating cows drops suddenly. The feces that are passed may be covered with mucus, or mixed or coated with blood. Thick, raspberry-colored blood mixed with scant feces is characteristic of small-intestinal bleeding, particularly that associated with intussusception or hemorrhagic jejunitis. Blood from the colon or rectum is generally brighter red. Melena is typical of abomasal bleeding. Calves with atresia coli are healthy at birth but have progressive abdominal distention and decreased appetite during the first few days of life. (*See also* CONGENITAL AND INHERITED ANOMALIES OF THE DIGESTIVE SYSTEM, p 162.)

Abdominal distention, usually with a ping on simultaneous auscultation and percussion, in the upper right caudal abdominal quadrant occurs with cecocolic volvulus. Cecal dilatation does not produce abdominal distention, but a ping is generally present in the caudal dorsal paralumbar fossa. In cecocolic volvulus, one or more large, distended loops of large intestine are identified on palpation per rectum. Rumen hypomotility is usually present, and metabolic and cardiovascular derangement tend to be mild except in cecocolic volvulus of long duration.

Abdominal distention in the lower right abdominal quadrant is sometimes seen with small-intestinal distention. Distended loops of bowel may be palpable on rectal examination, and fluid may be heard on simultaneous ballottement and auscultation of the right side of the abdomen. Small areas of tympanic resonance may be heard on simultaneous auscultation and percussion. Intussusceptions and fibrous bands that cause small-intestinal obstruction can be palpated per rectum in ~25% of cases. Ultrasonographic examination of the abdomen via the right paralumbar fossa or per rectum may help identify the presence of small-intestinal distention, ileus, and an increased peritoneal fluid volume. Occasionally, ultrasonography can identify an intussusception.

Profound changes in cardiovascular parameters, such as tachycardia, abnormal color of the mucous membranes, prolonged capillary refill time, and dehydration, are most commonly associated with hemorrhagic strangulating obstructions such as volvulus of the jejunal-ileal flange of the small intestine. Volvulus of the jejunal-ileal flange and volvulus at the root of the mesentery are characterized by acute onset and rapid cardiovascular deterioration. This is in contrast with cecocolic volvulus or intussusception, which can continue for several days in cattle.

Metabolic derangements range from hypokalemic, hypochloremic metabolic alkalosis in longstanding small-intestinal and duodenal obstructions to severe metabolic acidosis with hemorrhagic strangulating obstructions. Usually, there are no metabolic derangements in mild functional obstructions and early (simple) mechanical obstructions, particularly if a relatively distal part of the intestinal tract is involved. Hypocalcemia can develop, presumably due to decreased calcium absorption from the duodenum.

Peritoneal fluid changes reflect the degree of peritonitis and may aid in the diagnosis in both cattle and horses, although results are more variable in cattle. Hemorrhagic strangulating obstructions are characterized by an increase in the total protein concentration and nucleated cell counts of peritoneal fluid due to extravasation through the bowel wall. Neutrophils become degenerative, and intracellular gram-positive and gram-negative bacteria are seen in peritoneal fluid as the integrity of the bowel wall is lost. Plant material in the peritoneal cavity is indicative of bowel rupture or inadvertent enterocentesis. Peritoneal fluid analysis is normal with most simple mechanical and functional obstructions. When neoplasms are present and causing an extraluminal obstruction, neoplastic cells are sometimes identified in peritoneal fluid.

Treatment: Treatment of intestinal obstruction in horses is covered elsewhere (*see* p 253). Treatment of functional intestinal obstruction in cattle is generally symptomatic and supportive after identifying and eliminating the inciting cause (eg, hypocalcemia, hypokalemia, excessive grain intake) and allowing time for normal intestinal motility to return. If present, dehydration and electrolyte imbalances should be corrected by appropriate fluid therapy (PO or IV). Lactating cows often benefit from calcium chloride gels administered orally or calcium borogluconate or calcium gluconate administered SC, and oral potassium chloride (120–240 g twice at 12-hr intervals). Secondary ketosis should be treated if present. Erythromycin (10 mg/kg, IM, bid) is the most effective pharmacologic method to increase abomasal emptying rate in cattle (and presumably increasing intestinal motility), but studies documenting efficacy in functional intestinal obstruction are lacking. Prokinetics should not be administered to cattle with a mechanical obstruction because of the increased risk of intestinal rupture proximal to the obstruction. The prognosis with most functional obstructions is good with appropriate supportive therapy, particularly if the inciting cause is identified and eliminated.

Mechanical obstructions almost always require surgery. Antimicrobial therapy should be started preoperatively; supportive therapy, such as fluids, electrolytes, and calcium, should be administered as needed.

Horses that require exploratory laparotomy to correct an intestinal obstruction have an overall longterm survival rate of 50%. The survival rate is lower for horses with hemorrhagic strangulating obstructions and small-intestinal lesions than for horses with simple obstructions, but early surgical intervention can improve the prognosis.

In cattle, 70%–80% of those with cecocolic volvulus survive, although 10% of cases recur. For cows with small-intestinal obstruction amenable to resection and anastomosis, 30%–40% survive and lead a productive life. For cows with volvulus of the jejunal-ileal flange of the small intestine or at the root of the mesentery, ~50% survive if surgical correction is performed within a few hours of onset. Less than 30% of calves with atresia coli survive to adulthood. Surgical correction of atresia coli is not recommended in Holstein-Friesian calves because the condition is probably inherited in this breed, although vascular damage secondary to amniotic vesicle palpation in the first 6 wk of embryonic development can also lead to intestinal ischemia and atresia in calves.

Prevention: Prevention of all, or even most, cases of intestinal obstruction is not possible. However, abrupt changes in feeding and management; inadequate water intake; parasite infection; dental abnormalities; and access to coarse feeds, highly fermentable feedstuffs, and foreign material should be avoided or corrected.

COLIC IN HORSES

In its strictest definition, the term “colic” means abdominal pain. Throughout the years, it has become a broad term for a variety of conditions that cause a horse to exhibit clinical signs of abdominal pain. Consequently, it is used to refer to conditions of widely varying etiologies and severity. To understand these etiologies, make a diagnosis, and initiate appropriate treatments, veterinarians must first appreciate the clinically relevant aspects of equine GI anatomy, the physiologic processes involved in movement of ingesta and fluid along the GI tract, and the extreme sensitivity of the horse to the deleterious effects of the structural components of the bacteria that reside within the lumen of the intestine.

GI Anatomy

The horse is a monogastric animal, with a relatively small stomach (capacity 8–10 L) that is located on the left side of the abdomen beneath the rib cage. The junction of the distal esophagus and the cardia is a functional 1-way valve, permitting gas and fluid to move into the stomach but not out. Consequently, conditions that impede the normal aboral movement of gas and fluid through the small intestine may result in severe dilation and rupture of the stomach. Because of its position, the stomach is difficult to visualize with radiography or ultrasonography in large adult horses. The smaller size of the foal, however, permits assessment of gastric emptying by contrast radiography.

The small intestine comprises the duodenum, jejunum, and ileum, with the latter joining the cecum at a distinct ileocecal junction. The duodenum is positioned primarily dorsally on the horse's right side, where it is suspended from the dorsal body wall by a short mesentery of 3–5 cm.

Consequently, the duodenum is not involved in small-intestinal displacements involving the mesentery (volvulus). At the base of the cecum in the right paralumbar fossa region, the duodenum turns toward the midline. It is at this point that the duodenum, if distended with gas or fluid (eg, in horses with proximal enteritis), can be felt on rectal examination.

As the small intestine reaches the dorsal midline, it turns anteriorly, its mesentery lengthens, and it becomes known as the jejunum. The characteristic long mesentery allows loops of the jejunum to rest on the contents of the ventral portion of the abdomen. The jejunum is ~65 ft (19.5 m) long; its length, coupled with its long mesentery, allow it to be involved in small-intestinal volvulus and incarcerations. At the end of the jejunum, the wall of the intestine becomes more muscular, the lumen is narrowed, and an additional mesenteric attachment becomes apparent. The last 18 in. (45 cm) of the small intestine, the ileum, joins the cecum at its dorsal medial aspect. This junction is identified by the attachment of the ileocecal fold from the ileum to the dorsal band of the cecum. This ileocecal fold is used as a landmark to locate the ileum during abdominal surgery.

From the ileum, the ingesta enters the cecum, a large, blind-ended fermentation vat situated primarily on the horse's right side, extending from the region of the paralumbar fossa to the xiphoid cartilage on ventral midline. The cecum is 4–5 ft (1.2–1.5 m) long and can hold 27–30 L of feed and fluid. Under the influence of the cecal musculature, the ingesta in the cecum is massaged, mixed with microorganisms capable of digesting cellulose, and eventually passed through the cecocolic opening into the right ventral colon. The attachment of the cecum to the dorsal body wall is wide, thus minimizing the likelihood the cecum can become displaced or twisted on its own.

The right ventral colon is divided into sacculations that help mix and retain plant fibers until they are digested. It is positioned on the ventral aspect of the abdomen, extending from the flank region to the rib cage. The ventral colon then turns toward the left, becoming the sternal flexure and then the left ventral colon. The left ventral colon, which also is large and sacculated, passes caudally to the left flank area. Near the pelvic region, the diameter of the colon decreases markedly, and the colon folds back on itself. This region, called the pelvic flexure, is the initial portion of the unsacculated left dorsal colon. Presumably because of the abrupt decrease in diameter, the junction between the left ventral colon and pelvic flexure is the most common location for impactions.

The diameter of the dorsal colon is largest either at its diaphragmatic flexure or in the right dorsal colon. There are no sacculations in either the left or right portion of the dorsal colon. The right dorsal colon is closely attached to the right ventral colon by a short intercolic fold and to the body wall by a tough, common mesenteric attachment with the base of the cecum. In contrast, neither the left ventral nor left dorsal colons are attached directly to the body wall, allowing these portions of the colon to become displaced or twisted.

Ingesta moves from the large right dorsal colon into the short transverse colon, which has a diameter of ~10 cm and is fixed firmly to the most dorsal aspect of the abdominal cavity by a strong, short, fibrous mesentery. The transverse colon is located cranial to the cranial mesenteric artery. Finally, the ingesta enters the sacculated descending colon, which is 10–12 ft (3–3.6 m) long.

Blood Supply to the GI Tract

The celiac and cranial mesenteric arteries (branches of the abdominal aorta) supply blood to the GI tract. The celiac artery supplies arterial blood to the stomach, pancreas, liver, spleen, and the first portion of the duodenum. The cranial mesenteric artery supplies arterial blood to the remaining portion of the duodenum; to all of the jejunum, ileum, cecum, large colon, and transverse colon; and to the first portion of the descending colon. Because the large colon is attached to the body wall only in the region near the cranial mesenteric artery, the blood supplying all portions of the colon must traverse the entire length of the colon. The pelvic flexure receives its blood supply from two branches of the cranial mesenteric artery; one branch supplies the right and left dorsal colons before reaching the pelvic flexure, and the other branch supplies the right and left ventral colons before reaching the pelvic flexure. Thus, volvulus of the large colon near the junction of the colon and cecum may impede the flow of blood to the entire left colon.

The major branches of the cranial mesenteric artery can be damaged by the migrating forms of *Strongylus vulgaris* (*see* p 316).

Natural Openings in the Abdomen

There are several natural openings or spaces within the abdominal cavity that can be important in conditions causing colic.

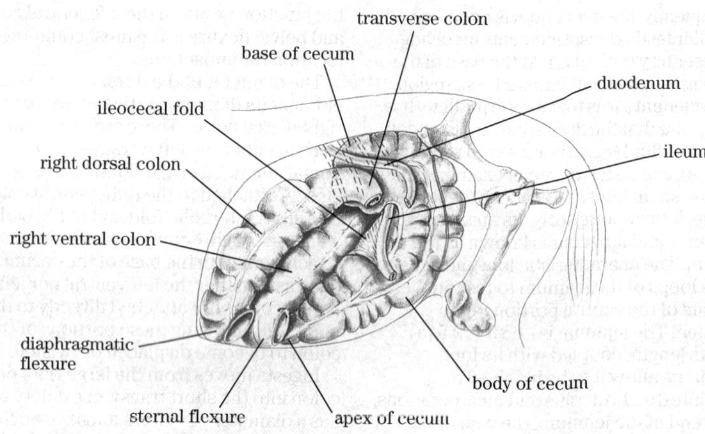

Left medial view of cecum and right colon, horse. *Illustration by Dr. Gheorghe Constantinescu.*

The inguinal canal provides an opening through which intestine might pass and become trapped. Although inguinal hernias are common in young foals, they rarely cause clinical problems; the situation is considerably different in stallions. Similarly, if the ventral abdominal wall fails to form properly around the umbilicus, an opening remains and the potential exists for intestinal problems to develop secondary to an umbilical hernia. The epiploic foramen, a natural opening between the portal vein, the caudal vena cava, and the caudate lobe of the liver, can be the site of intestinal incarcerations. Finally, there is a natural space between the dorsal aspect of the spleen and the left kidney. This space is bounded by the renosplenic ligament, a strong band of tissue that connects the dorsomedial aspect of the spleen with the fibrous capsule of the left kidney. This ligament provides a "shelf" over which large colon can be displaced.

Colonic Motility Patterns

Normograde peristalsis in the left ventral colon moves ingesta toward the left dorsal colon, and the muscles in the wall of the left dorsal colon contract to move the ingesta toward the diaphragmatic flexure. There is evidence, however, that the muscles in the left ventral colon contract in a retrograde fashion, from the pelvic flexure region toward the sternal flexure. Furthermore, these contractions appear to originate from a pacemaker region in the pelvic flexure. It has been hypothesized that this pacemaker senses either the size or the consistency of the feed particles in the ingesta and then initiates the appropriate motility pattern. If the ingesta has been digested sufficiently, it is moved in a normograde direction; if additional digestion is necessary, the ingesta is moved in a retrograde direction to retain it in the ventral colon. This theory has been proposed to help account for the common clinical occurrence of obstruction at or near the pelvic flexure.

Clinical Findings

Numerous clinical signs are associated with colic. The most common include pawing repeatedly with a front foot, looking back at the flank region, curling the upper lip and arching the neck, repeatedly raising a rear leg or kicking at the abdomen, lying down, rolling from side to side, sweating, stretching out as if to urinate, straining to defecate, distention of the abdomen, loss of appetite, depression, and decreased number of bowel movements. It is uncommon for a horse with colic to exhibit all of these signs. Although they are reliable indicators of abdominal pain, the particular signs do not indicate which portion of the GI tract is involved or whether surgery will be needed.

Diagnosis

A diagnosis can be made and appropriate treatment begun only after thoroughly examining the horse, considering the history of any previous problems or treatments, determining which part of the intestinal tract is involved, and identifying the cause of the particular episode of colic.

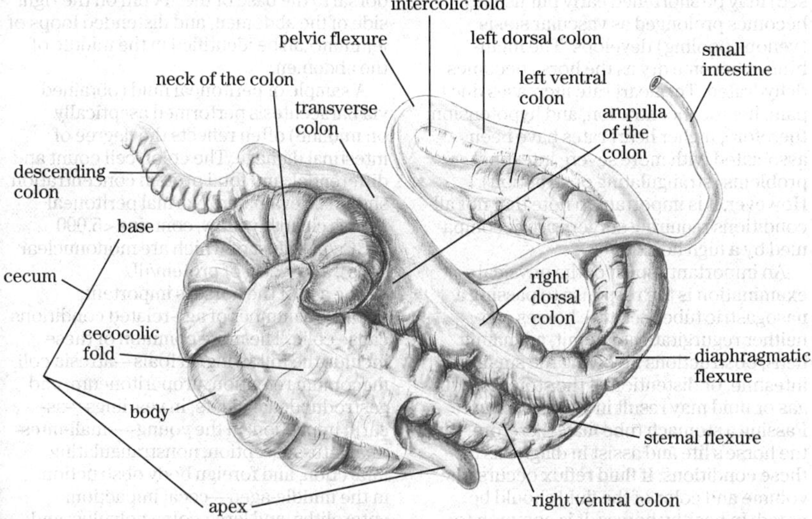

The large intestine of the horse. *Illustration by Dr. Gheorghe Constantinescu.*

In most instances, colic develops for one of four reasons: 1) The wall of the intestine is stretched excessively by either gas, fluid, or ingesta. This stimulates the stretch-sensitive nerve endings located within the intestinal wall, and pain impulses are transmitted to the brain. 2) Pain develops due to excessive tension on the mesentery, as might occur with an intestinal displacement. 3) Ischemia develops, most often as a result of incarceration or severe twisting of the intestine. 4) Inflammation develops and may involve either the entire intestinal wall (enteritis) or the covering of the intestine (peritonitis). Under such circumstances, proinflammatory mediators in the wall of the intestine decrease the threshold for painful stimuli.

The list of possible conditions that cause colic is long, and it is reasonable first to determine the most likely type of disease and begin appropriate treatments and then to make a more specific diagnosis, if possible. The general types of disease that cause colic include excessive gas in the intestinal lumen (flatulent colic), simple obstruction of the intestinal lumen, obstruction of both the intestinal lumen and the blood supply to the intestine (strangulating obstruction), interruption of the blood supply to the intestine alone (nonstrangulating infarction), inflammation of the intestine (enteritis), inflammation of the lining of the abdominal cavity (peritonitis), erosion of the intestinal lining (ulceration), and "unexplained colic." In general, horses with strangulating obstructions and complete obstructions require emergency abdominal surgery, whereas horses with the other types of disease can be treated medically.

The history of the present colic episode and previous episodes, if any, must be considered to determine whether the horse has had repeated or similar problems or whether this episode is an isolated event. The duration of the present episode, the rate of deterioration of the horse's cardiovascular status, the severity of pain, whether feces have been passed, and the response to any treatments are important pieces of information. It is also critical to determine the horse's deworming history (schedule, treatment dates, drugs used), when the teeth were floated last, if any changes in feed or water supply or amount have occurred, whether or not the horse is a "cribber," and whether the horse was at rest or exercising when the colic episode started.

The physical examination should include assessment of the cardiopulmonary and GI systems. The oral mucous membranes should be evaluated for color, moistness, and capillary refill time. The mucous membranes may become cyanotic or pale in horses with acute cardiovascular compromise and eventually hyperemic or muddy as peripheral vasodilation develops later in shock. The capillary refill time (normal ~1.5

sec) may be shortened early but usually becomes prolonged as vascular stasis (venous pooling) develops. The membranes become dry as the horse becomes dehydrated. The heart rate increases due to pain, hemoconcentration, and hypotension; therefore, higher heart rates have been associated with more severe intestinal problems (strangulating obstruction). However, it is important to note that not all conditions requiring surgery are accompanied by a high heart rate.

An important aspect of the physical examination is the response to passing a nasogastric tube. Because horses can neither regurgitate nor vomit, adynamic ileus, obstructions involving the small intestine, or distention of the stomach with gas or fluid may result in gastric rupture. Passing a stomach tube may, therefore, save the horse's life and assist in diagnosis of these conditions. If fluid reflux occurs, the volume and color of the fluid should be noted. In healthy horses, it is common to retrieve <1 L of fluid from the stomach.

The abdomen and thorax should be auscultated and the abdomen percussed. The abdomen should be auscultated over several areas (cecum on the right, small intestine high on the left, colon lower on both the right and left). Intestinal sounds associated with episodes of pain may indicate an intraluminal obstruction (eg, impaction, enterolith). Gas sounds may indicate ileus or distention of a viscus. Fluid sounds may indicate impending diarrhea associated with colitis. A complete lack of sounds is usually associated with adynamic ileus or ischemia. Percussion helps identify a grossly distended segment of intestine (cecum on right, colon on left) that may need to be trocarized. The respiratory rate may be increased due to fever, pain, acidosis, or an underlying respiratory problem. Diaphragmatic hernia is also a possible cause of colic.

The most definitive part of the examination is the rectal examination. The veterinarian should develop a consistent method of palpating for the following: aorta, cranial mesenteric artery, cecal base and ventral cecal band, bladder, peritoneal surface, inguinal rings in stallions and geldings or the ovaries and uterus in mares, pelvic flexure, spleen, and left kidney. The intestine should be palpated for size, consistency of contents (gas, fluid, or impacted ingesta), distention, edematous walls, and pain on palpation. In healthy horses, the small intestine cannot be palpated; with small-intestinal obstruction, strangulating obstruction, or enteritis, the distended duodenum can be palpated dorsal to the base of the cecum on the right side of the abdomen, and distended loops of jejunum can be identified in the middle of the abdomen.

A sample of peritoneal fluid (obtained via paracentesis performed aseptically on midline) often reflects the degree of intestinal damage. The color, cell count and differential, and total protein concentration should be evaluated. Normal peritoneal fluid is clear to yellow, contains <5,000 WBCs/μL (most of which are mononuclear cells), and <2.5 g of protein/dL.

The age of the horse is important, because a number of age-related conditions cause colic. The more common of these include the following: in foals—atresia coli, meconium retention, uroperitoneum, and gastroduodenal ulcers; in yearlings—ascarid impaction; in the young—small-intestinal intussusception, nonstrangulating infarction, and foreign body obstruction; in the middle-aged—cecal impaction, enteroliths, and large-colon volvulus; and in the aged—pedunculated lipoma and mesocolic rupture.

Ultrasonographic evaluation of the abdomen may help differentiate between diseases that can be treated medically and those that require surgery. The technique also can be applied transrectally to clarify findings noted on rectal palpation. In foals, echoes from the large colon and small intestine are commonly identified from the ventral abdominal wall, whereas only large-colon echoes are usually seen in adult horses. The large colon can be identified by its sacculated appearance. The duodenum can be identified in the tenth intercostal space and traced around the caudal aspect of the right kidney. The jejunum is rarely identified during transabdominal ultrasonographic examination of normal adult horses, whereas the thick-walled ileum can be identified by transrectal examination.

The most common abnormalities identified by ultrasonography include inguinal hernia, renosplenic entrapment of the large colon, sand colic, intussusception, enterocolitis, right dorsal colitis, and peritonitis. Stallions with inguinal hernia have incarcerated intestine on the affected side; it is possible to identify the intestine and to obtain information concerning the thickness of its wall as well as the presence or lack of peristalsis. In horses with renosplenic entrapment of the large colon, the tail of the spleen or the left kidney cannot be imaged, or the gas-filled large colon is present in the caudodorsal aspect of the abdomen in the region of the renosplenic space. Horses with sand colic have granular hyperechoic echoes originating from the affected portion of the colon. The characteristic finding in horses with intussusception is the "bull's eye" appearance of the affected portion of the small intestine. Very often the intestine proximal to the intussusception is distended, and the strangulated portion is thickened. Horses with enterocolitis frequently have evidence of hyperperistalsis, thickened areas of the bowel wall, and fluid distention of the intestine. In contrast, horses with right dorsal colitis commonly have marked thickening of the wall of the right dorsal colon. In horses with peritonitis, the peritoneal fluid may be anechoic, or there may be evidence of flocculent material and fibrin between serosal surfaces of the viscera.

Treatment

Horses with colic may need either medical or surgical treatments. Almost all require some form of medical treatment, but only those with certain mechanical obstructions of the intestine need surgery. The type of medical treatment is determined by the cause of colic and the severity of the disease. In some instances, the horse may be treated medically first and the response evaluated; this is particularly appropriate if the horse is mildly painful and the cardiovascular system is functioning normally. Ultrasonography can be used to evaluate the effectiveness of nonsurgical treatment. If necessary, surgery can be used for diagnosis as well as treatment.

If evidence of intestinal obstruction with dry ingesta is found on rectal examination, a primary aim of treatment is to rehydrate and evacuate the intestinal contents. If the horse is severely painful and has clinical signs indicating loss of fluid from the bloodstream (high heart rate, prolonged capillary refill time, and discoloration of the mucous membranes), the initial aims of treatment are to relieve pain, restore tissue perfusion, and correct any abnormalities in the composition of the blood and body fluids (*see* TABLE 5). If damage to the intestinal wall (as a result of either severe inflammation or a displacement or strangulating obstruction) is suspected, steps should be taken to prevent or counteract the ill effects of bacterial endotoxins that cross the damaged intestinal wall and enter the bloodstream. Finally, if there is evidence the colic episode is caused by parasites, one aim of treatment is to eliminate the parasites.

Pain Relief: In most cases of colic, pain is mild, and analgesia is all that is needed. In these instances, the cause of colic is presumed to be spasm of intestinal muscle or excessive gas in a portion of the intestine. If, however, the pain is due to an intestinal twist or displacement, some of the stronger analgesics may mask the clinical signs that would be useful in making a diagnosis. For these reasons, a thorough physical examination should be completed before any medications are given. However, because horses with severe colic or pain may hurt themselves and become dangerous to people nearby, analgesics often must be given first. Additionally, many horses with less severe problems may need pain relief until the other treatments have time to be effective. An analgesic that has the fewest adverse effects and causes the least alteration in the horse's attitude should be selected.

Medications used commonly for abdominal pain are NSAIDs that reduce the production of prostaglandins. When these drugs are used as recommended, their toxic effects on the kidneys and GI tract occur infrequently. Clinical experience suggests that flunixin meglumine may mask the early signs of conditions that require surgery and, therefore, must be used carefully in horses with colic.

The most commonly used sedative for colic is xylazine, an α_2-agonist. Within a few minutes after administration, the horse stands quietly and is less responsive to pain. Unfortunately, the effects of xylazine are short-lived, and it inhibits intestinal muscular activity; it also decreases cardiac output and thus reduces blood flow to the tissues. Detomidine, a more potent α_2-agonist that is much longer acting, is used successfully in similar circumstances.

Of the narcotic analgesics, butorphanol is used most often in horses with colic. Butorphanol has few adverse effects on the GI tract or heart. However, when given in large doses, narcotics can cause excitement, and the horse may become unstable. Butorphanol is frequently combined with an α_2-agonist to produce a more prolonged period of analgesia.

Although pain relief usually is provided by analgesics, there are other important ways to reduce the degree of pain. For example, passing a nasogastric tube (also an important part of the diagnostic evaluation) may remove any fluid that has accumulated in the stomach because of an obstruction of the small intestine. The removal of this fluid not only relieves pain from gastric distention but also prevents rupture of the stomach.

Horses with displacement of the colon over the renosplenic ligament (ie, left dorsal displacement of the colon) may benefit from administration of phenylephrine. This drug is given to contract the spleen and often is followed by light exercise on a lunge line in an effort to dislodge the entrapped colon. It is important to note that this treatment may cause fatal hemorrhage due to hypertension in horses >15 yr old.

Fluid Therapy: Many horses with colic benefit from fluid therapy to prevent dehydration and maintain blood supply to the kidneys and other vital organs. The fluids may be given either through the nasogastric tube or IV, depending on the particular intestinal problem (*see* TABLE 5). Horses with strangulating obstruction or enteritis must be given fluids IV, because absorption of fluids from the diseased intestine is impaired and fluid may be secreted into the lumen of the intestine. The latter mechanism causes a buildup of fluid in the intestine, which must be removed from the stomach through a nasogastric tube. This abnormal movement of body fluids into the intestine contributes to the development of circulatory shock, which is often the ultimate cause of death.

In healthy horses, most of the fluid in the intestinal tract is reabsorbed in the cecum and colons. In fact, ~95% of the fluid that normally enters the lumen of the large intestine is returned to the bloodstream. Therefore, horses with intestinal obstructions near the pelvic flexure usually require relatively small amounts of IV fluids, whereas horses with small-intestinal obstructions need extremely large amounts.

The volume and type of fluid to be given are determined by the severity and cause of the problem. Laboratory tests to determine the degree of hemoconcentration and whether concentrations of electrolytes are abnormal are critical for accurate treatment of horses with severe colic. The balance of body fluids can be reestablished by administering IV fluids formulated to replenish the deficient electrolyte(s). In most instances, however, fluid therapy must be started before laboratory results are available, particularly when the horse is showing clinical signs of circulatory shock.

When IV fluids are needed but the clinical signs are mild to moderate, the horse is usually given 8–10 L of a sterile replacement fluid that contains electrolytes in concentrations similar to those that normally exist in the blood. This volume is administered throughout 1–2 hr, and the horse is reevaluated to determine whether additional fluids are needed. Horses in circulatory shock require much larger volumes of IV fluids, given as rapidly as possible; as much as 20 L in 1 hr may be needed to reestablish tissue perfusion. In severe cases, hypertonic saline (7% NaCl) may be given to rapidly increase plasma volume. Depending on the cause of colic, IV fluids may be needed for several days until intestinal function has returned, electrolyte concentrations are balanced, and the horse can maintain its fluid needs by drinking. Under such circumstances, the daily IV fluid requirements may range from 30 to 100 L.

Fluids are sometimes given through the nasogastric tube as part of the treatment of impactions of the colon. Many clinicians believe the same result can be accomplished by giving large volumes of fluids IV. If the horse will not drink voluntarily and there is no obstruction in the small intestine, hydration may be maintained

TABLE 5 GENERAL CONCEPTS REGARDING FLUID NEEDS IN DEHYDRATED HORSES

Determining Factor	Formula Used	Amount for a 500-kg Horse
Fluid deficit	% dehydration × body weight (kg)	4%–10% × 500 = 20–50 L
Maintenance	50 mL/kg/24 hr	50 × 500 = 25 L/24 hr
Fluid losses	Estimate reflux or diarrhea volume	
Rate of administration	50% in 1–2 hr; 50% throughout rest of day	20–35 L in first 1–2 hr; remainder distributed throughout next 23 hr

Adapted, with permission, from Zimmel DN, Management of pain and dehydration in horses with colic. In *Current Therapy in Equine Medicine*, 5, 2003, Robinson, NE, (ed), Elsevier.

by administering fluids through the tube. Fluids or medications should not be given through the nasogastric tube if fluid reflux is being removed from the stomach, because this indicates either the stomach or the small intestine is not emptying properly.

Protection Against Components of Enteric Bacteria: In healthy horses, the mucosal lining of the GI tract restricts enteric bacteria and their structural components (eg, endotoxins, lipoproteins, nucleic acids, flagellin) to the intestinal lumen. These bacterial components exist in high concentrations in the intestinal lumen, because they are released when the bacteria die or, in some cases, when bacteria multiply rapidly. However, when this mucosal barrier is disrupted, as occurs with intestinal ischemia or inflammation, the bacterial components can move into the peritoneal cavity and then be absorbed into the systemic circulation. Based on recent research studies, equine leukocytes are most sensitive to endotoxins but also respond strongly to other components, most notably flagellin. Most studies performed to date have focused on endotoxins, because they are assumed to be the primary triggers for the systemic inflammatory responses that occur in many horses with GI disease. These responses can include fever, depression, hypotension, reduced tissue perfusion, and coagulation abnormalities. In fact, many equine practitioners refer to these physiologic responses as "endotoxemia." Thus, minimizing the inflammatory responses to endotoxemia is a vital part of colic therapy.

Prostaglandins are involved in causing many of endotoxin's early ill effects. Flunixin meglumine reduces the cellular production of prostaglandins and can help prevent some of their effects. Because flunixin can help prevent some of the early effects of endotoxemia at dosages less than the recommended dosage (1.1 mg/kg), smaller dosages (0.25 mg/kg) can be administered without masking clinical signs associated with conditions that require surgery.

There is considerable controversy regarding the efficacy of plasma or serum that contains antibodies designed to neutralize endotoxin. These antibodies are directed against the components of endotoxins that are consistent among different gram-negative bacteria. The results of clinical studies using such antibodies have been conflicting, with evidence of protection being seen in some studies and no positive effects identified in others. This apparent lack of efficacy of anti-endotoxin antibodies also may indicate that some of the systemic inflammatory responses encountered are triggered by other bacterial components. Because endotoxin itself stimulates the generation of a wide array of inflammatory substances that ultimately produce the pathophysiologic effects, neutralizing antibodies should be used as early as possible in the course of the disease.

As an alternative approach, polymyxin B has been used to prevent endotoxin from interacting with the horse's inflammatory cells. Polymyxin B has well-documented nephrotoxicity; however, concentrations of polymyxin B that bind endotoxin are far less than those that cause toxic effects. Polymyxin B has been evaluated in several experimental studies of endotoxemia and is being used in clinical cases at 1,000–5,000 U/kg, bid-tid. This form of therapy should be started as early as possible in the clinical course of the disease. In addition, fluid replacement therapy should be maintained in hypovolemic horses, and serum creatinine concentration should be closely monitored. This latter concern is especially relevant for azotemic neonatal foals, because they appear to be more susceptible to the nephrotoxic adverse effects of polymyxin B.

Intestinal Lubricants and Laxatives: A common cause of colic in horses is simple obstruction of the large colon by dehydrated ingesta, sometimes mixed with sand. These impactions generally develop near the pelvic flexure or in the right dorsal colon but may involve any portion of the large colon, descending colon, or cecum. In most instances, lubricants or fecal-softening agents given through a nasogastric tube soften the impacted ingesta, allowing it to be passed. This form of therapy can be aided by the simultaneous administration of IV fluids. Keeping the horse muzzled is advised to prevent further impaction of feed material while the obstruction is softening.

Mineral oil is the most commonly used medication in the treatment of a large-colon impaction. It coats the inside of the intestine and aids the normal movement of ingesta along the GI tract. It is administered through a nasogastric tube, as much as 4 L, once or twice daily, until the impaction is resolved. Although mineral oil is safe, it is not highly effective in treating severe impactions or sand impactions, because it may simply pass by the obstruction without softening it.

Dioctyl sodium sulfosuccinate (DSS) is a soap-like compound that acts by drawing water into the dry ingesta. It is more effective than mineral oil in softening impactions; however, it may interfere with the normal fluid absorptive functions of the colon and can be toxic. Thus, DSS can be given safely only in small quantities two times 48 hr apart.

A safe and useful compound to treat impactions, especially those containing sand, is psyllium hydrophilic mucilloid. When mixed with water, it forms a gelatinous mass that carries ingesta along the GI tract. Although usually given through a nasogastric tube to horses with impactions, psyllium also may be used as a preventive by mixing the dry powder into the feed. Horses that live in a sandy environment or that persistently develop impactions may be given psyllium powder, 400 g/500 kg/day, in their feed for 7 days. This treatment is repeated 2–3 times each year in an effort to prevent development of sand impactions.

Strong laxatives that stimulate intestinal contractions are not commonly used to treat impactions and, in fact, may worsen the problem. Occasionally, horses with extremely hard impactions are treated with magnesium sulfate, which draws body fluids into the GI tract. Adverse effects include dehydration and an increased risk of diarrhea.

Fluid therapy, whether the fluids are administered through a nasogastric tube or IV, is an important and effective part of treating horses with colonic or cecal impactions. If an impaction does not start to break down within 3–5 days, surgery may be necessary to evacuate the intestine and help restore normal motility.

Larvicidal Deworming: The normal migratory routes of the larvae of large bloodworms, particularly *Strongylus vulgaris*, have been implicated in many cases of colic. In response to the migratory and maturation processes of the larvae in the cranial mesenteric artery, the wall of the artery becomes thickened and forms loose plaques of inflammatory tissue. It has been hypothesized that these plaques activate coagulation, resulting in thromboembolism. The blood supply to the intestine may be reduced, resulting in altered intestinal motility, a change in the absorption of nutrients from the intestine, or death of the intestine. Thus, thromboembolism has been presumed to be a cause of recurrent episodes of colic and weight loss.

Modern deworming medications, such as ivermectin and moxidectin, have activity against migrating *S vulgaris* larvae. Fenbendazole kills migrating strongyles if given at twice the recommended dosage daily for 5 days or at 10 times the recommended dosage daily for 3 days. As a result of common use of these anthelmintics, chronic intermittent colic once thought to be caused by thromboembolism or parasite larval migration has largely been eliminated from equine practice.

There is considerable evidence that damage caused by cyathostomins causes colic, diarrhea, and loss of condition, particularly in young horses. These signs are seen on a seasonal basis and are synchronous with the emergence of large numbers of encysted larvae into the lumen of the large colon. In temperate areas of the Northern hemisphere, the larvae encyst during the winter months and emerge in the late winter and spring, causing ulceration, edema, and inflammation of the mucosa of the large colon. This may result in diarrhea, protein loss, weight loss, and mild intermittent colic and fever. Horses with cyathostomosis require treatment with larvacidal dosages of anthelmintics such as ivermectin, moxidectin, and fenbendazole. Some horses require analgesics, supportive care, and proper nutritional support.

See also p 316 for a detailed discussion of treatment for large and small strongyles.

Surgery: Surgery usually is necessary if there is a mechanical obstruction to the normal flow of ingesta that cannot be corrected medically or if the obstruction also interferes with the intestinal blood supply. The latter conditions result in death of the horse unless surgery is performed quickly. Occasionally, surgery is indicated as an exploratory diagnostic procedure for horses with chronic colic that have not responded to routine medical therapy.

Under most circumstances, horses exhibiting signs of severe abdominal pain nonresponsive to analgesic therapy require emergency abdominal surgery. Generally, the lumen of the intestine is completely obstructed, such as occurs with a strangulating obstruction, enterolithiasis, or severe displacement. Similarly, horses with an abnormally distended intestine on rectal examination and peritoneal fluid with an increased total protein concentration and number of erythrocytes probably have a strangulating lesion that requires surgical correction. However, these classic findings that characterize horses requiring emergency surgery do not always exist. Some horses with mild or moderate pain may also require surgery, and a judgment must be based on a thorough physical examination and other methods of evaluation, including abdominal ultrasonography. Some of the more commonly used indications for surgery in horses with colic include uncontrollable pain; >4 L of fluid reflux from the stomach; no borborygmi on auscultation; peritoneal fluid with increased protein, erythrocytes, and toxic neutrophils; and a tightly distended intestine, displaced colon, or enterolith or foreign body identified on rectal examination.

Performing surgery (if indicated) early is critical to success and improves the prognosis for survival. Therefore, it is more important to decide whether the horse should be referred to a clinic where surgery could be performed if needed than to determine whether emergency surgery is definitively required. It is generally prudent to refer the following types of cases: 1) a horse that responds initially to an analgesic but requires additional analgesic therapy a few hours later, 2) a horse that continues to exhibit signs of pain despite administration of analgesics, 3) a horse that remains painful but has normal peritoneal fluid, 4) a horse with distended loops of small intestine on rectal examination, or 5) a horse with large quantities of fluid removed from the stomach but no distended small intestine palpable on rectal examination.

When surgery is required, in most instances, the horse is anesthetized and positioned in dorsal recumbency, and the surgical incision is made on the ventral midline. Once the peritoneal cavity is entered, portions of the intestine should be examined to determine the definitive cause of the colic. Correction may involve repositioning a displaced portion of intestine, removing an obstruction, or resecting devitalized intestine. When devitalized segments of intestine must be removed or an enterotomy performed, postoperative care may include antibiotics, IV fluids, polymyxin B, antibodies directed against endotoxin, and NSAIDs to combat endotoxemia. When a displaced segment of intestine is simply returned to its normal location, the postoperative care is much less intense. Each horse must be handled individually, and its treatment needs are based on the response to surgery and development of complications.

Prognosis

A large retrospective study in the USA documented an overall survival rate of 60% for horses with colic and a survival rate of 50% for those horses undergoing abdominal surgery, including those euthanized during surgery for inoperative conditions. Survival rates for horses with strangulating obstruction and inflammatory diseases were only 24% and 42%, respectively. In contrast, horses with an undefined cause for the colic episode had a survival rate of 94%. When the segment of the GI tract was considered, the survival rates for conditions affecting the small intestine and stomach were poorer than for those affecting the large colon. In addition, conditions that interfered with both the passage of ingesta and the intestinal blood supply dramatically decreased the chances of survival. The results of more recent studies are far more promising, with survival rates for horses undergoing emergency abdominal surgery often >80%. Furthermore, there have been reports documenting survival rates of 70% for horses requiring resection of strangulated small intestine or correction of large-colon volvulus. In earlier retrospective studies, these conditions were associated with survival rates ≤30%. Although data on longterm survival (ie, the horse returning to its intended use) are more difficult to obtain, recent findings indicate that most horses that die or are euthanized because of serious problems do so within 3 mo after surgery.

Values obtained from several variables are often combined to predict survival in horses with colic. Prognostic indicators include pain assessment, intestinal distention, mucous membrane color, and cardiovascular system function. Survival rates are highest for horses with mild abdominal pain and are lowest for horses with severe pain. Horses with palpable intestinal distention have lower survival rates than horses lacking evidence of intestinal distention, and survival rates are even lower if no intestinal sounds are audible on auscultation of the abdomen. Red mucous membranes are frequently associated with endotoxemia, which decreases the survival rate. Cardiovascular system function reflects the degree of shock and, therefore, correlates with the prognosis for survival. For instance, horses with low systolic blood pressure or a high heart rate have a decreased chance of survival.

Of the laboratory analyses used to predict survival, blood lactate concentration and the anion gap are used most often. Measurement of blood lactate has been used as an indicator of tissue perfusion, with increasing concentrations of lactic acid corresponding with poor tissue perfusion. In recent studies, changes in blood lactate concentration over time have been particularly useful to determine the prognosis for survival, with increasing concentrations being associated with a poor prognosis. Furthermore, changes in peritoneal fluid lactate concentrations over time have been used to help identify horses that require emergency abdominal surgery. Similarly, the anion gap (the calculated difference between the measured cations and the measured anions) reflects the generation of organic anions, most notably lactic acid, due to reduced tissue perfusion. The concentration of protein in the peritoneal fluid also has been used to predict survival, with higher concentrations associated with a poorer prognosis.

DISEASES ASSOCIATED WITH COLIC BY ANATOMIC LOCATION

Stomach

Gastric Dilatation and Gastric Rupture: The most common cause of gastric dilatation in horses is excessive gas or intestinal obstruction. Gastric dilatation may be associated with overeating fermentable feedstuffs such as grains, lush grass, and beet pulp. Presumably, the large increase in production of volatile fatty acids inhibits gastric emptying. If untreated, gastric dilatation associated with overeating can rapidly lead to gastric rupture. If intestinal obstruction is the cause, the obstruction most often involves the small intestine. The fluid from the obstructed small intestine accumulates in the lumen of the stomach, causing dilatation of the stomach and retrieval of gastric reflux on passage of the nasogastric tube. Gastric dilatation also may develop in some horses with certain colonic displacements, most notably right dorsal displacement of the colon around the cecum (*see* p 265). It is presumed that the displaced colon obstructs duodenal outflow. Gastric dilatation with fluid and gastric reflux also are characteristic findings in horses with proximal enteritis-jejunitis.

Rupture of the stomach is a fatal complication of gastric dilatation. The stomach generally tears along its greater curvature. Approximately two-thirds of all gastric ruptures occur secondary to mechanical obstruction, ileus, and trauma; the remaining cases are due to overload or to idiopathic causes.

Clinical signs associated with gastric dilatation include severe abdominal pain, tachycardia, and retching. The mucous membranes may be pale. Classically, these acute signs are replaced by relief, depression, and toxemia after the stomach has ruptured. The prognosis for survival may be excellent in most cases of gastric dilatation, but gastric rupture is fatal.

Gastric Impaction: Impaction of the stomach is an uncommon cause of colic. Although it may be associated with ingestion of certain feedstuffs (eg, beet pulp, pelleted feeds, persimmon seeds, straw, barley), contributing factors (eg, diseased teeth, inadequate intake of water, and rapid eating) should also be considered. Because the incidence of this condition is low, it is difficult to determine which factors may be most important. The most striking clinical sign associated with gastric impaction is severe abdominal pain. Because of the lack of other characteristic findings, the diagnosis most often is made at surgery, and the decision for surgery is based on unrelenting pain. Use of a 3-m endoscope has made it possible to identify this problem without surgery.

Treatment usually involves repeated intragastric administration of saline carbonated drinks ("soft drinks") if the condition has been identified without surgery. If the gastric impaction has been identified at surgery, saline or water can be infused into the mass through a needle passed through the wall of the stomach. After the fluid has been injected into the mass, the stomach then is massaged and the obstruction is broken down. If a nasogastric tube is in place at the time of surgery, water may be pumped into the stomach and the mass massaged. Gavage is continued after surgery with the hopes of removing some of the impacted material, and this can be followed by feeding slurries and pasture grazing once the impaction begins to resolve. The prognosis is favorable if the diagnosis has been made without surgery or if decision to perform exploratory surgery is made early and the impaction can be broken down manually at surgery.

Small Intestine

Clinical signs of colic may arise due to obstruction, inflammation, or strangulating obstruction of the small intestine. The prognosis for conditions affecting the small intestine is often guarded. Hence, rapid diagnosis and appropriate treatment are critical.

Ileal Impaction: The most common condition producing simple obstruction of the lumen of the small intestine is ileal impaction. It is most common in the southeastern USA, Germany, and the Netherlands. The results of clinical studies in the UK indicate that infection with the intestinal tapeworm *Anoplocephala perfoliata* and ileal impaction are strongly associated. In a similar study performed in the USA, two risk factors for ileal impaction were identified: 1) the feeding of Coastal Bermuda hay, and 2) the lack of administration of pyrantel pamoate, an anthelmintic with some efficacy against *A perfoliata*, within the 3 mo preceding development of the impaction. Further, it has been suggested that the impaction develops secondary to spastic contractions of the ileal musculature against ingesta.

Clinical signs include the onset of mild to severe abdominal pain followed by reduced intestinal sounds, gastric reflux, and tachycardia. Although early rectal examination may permit identification of the impaction in the ileum low in the right caudal abdominal quadrant, subsequent distention of the jejunum may make this identification difficult or impossible. The most common differential diagnosis is proximal enteritis-jejunitis, and distinguishing the two conditions can often be difficult. Because the horse's condition initially may remain stable and the degree of abdominal pain may be mild, many horses with this condition are not referred for intensive care or surgery for >18 hr. The protein concentration of the peritoneal fluid may increase if the impaction has persisted for this long.

Horses with ileal impaction respond to treatment with fluids and mineral oil if the impaction has been identified early (ie, before gastric reflux has developed). If surgery is indicated, the impacted mass may be mixed with saline or carboxymethylcellulose and massaged into the cecum, or an enterotomy may be performed in the distal jejunum and the ingesta removed through the incision. Ileus may develop after surgery. Depending on the degree of damage to the serosal surface of the small intestine at the time of surgery, complications may develop several weeks after surgery due to intra-abdominal adhesions (*see* below).

Adhesions: Intra-abdominal adhesions generally affect the small intestine and usually cause obstruction of the intestinal lumen, although they may cause strangulating obstruction. These adhesions develop in response to peritoneal injury and, most often, are the result of previous small-intestinal surgery, chronic small-intestinal distention, peritonitis, or larval parasite migration. The tissue response to ischemia, traumatic tissue handling, foreign material, hemorrhage, or dehydration results in the formation of fibrinous (and subsequently fibrous) adhesions. Clinical signs are seen if the adhesion causes kinking, compression, or stricture of the intestine.

Adhesions should be considered if the horse has had prior abdominal surgery and a more recent history of recurrent abdominal pain. Clinical signs associated with intra-abdominal adhesions range from mild, recurrent colic to severe unrelenting pain. Most commonly, intra-abdominal adhesions cause clinical signs within 60 days of the initial surgery if they are going to be a significant problem for the horse.

Surgical treatment involves transection of the adhesion, resection of the affected intestine, and anastomosis to achieve normal flow of ingesta. Therapeutic agents purported to reduce the subsequent formation of additional adhesions then are used. These include the systemic administration of antimicrobials, NSAIDs, and instillation of sterile carboxymethylcellulose into the abdomen at the time of closure. The owner should be informed that adhesions are likely to recur and that the longterm prognosis for horses with extensive adhesions is poor.

Ascarid Impaction: Young horses, particularly those on farms with inadequate parasite control programs, may develop ascarid impactions of the small intestine. These impactions are seen after administration of an anthelmintic with high efficacy against *Parascaris equorum*. The anthelmintics most commonly associated with this condition are ivermectin, piperazine, and organophosphates. These drugs paralyze the ascarids, resulting in accumulation of masses of the worms in the small-intestinal lumen. It has been suggested that disruption of the surface of the ascarid releases antigenic fluids that inhibit intestinal muscular activity, thereby increasing the likelihood of intestinal obstruction.

Clinical signs range from mild to severe abdominal pain, evidence of toxemia, and gastric reflux that may contain ascarids. Ascarid impaction should be suspected if the affected horse is a weanling or yearling, in poor condition, and has a recent history of deworming. Medical treatment with fluids and intestinal lubricants may be successful in some cases. Other horses may require surgical intervention and removal of the ascarids through multiple enterotomies. The prognosis is guarded if surgery has to be performed. The owner should be advised that other young horses on the premises should be treated with anthelmintics that have lower efficacy against ascarids, such as fenbendazole. These initial treatments can then be followed with more efficacious compounds.

Proximal Enteritis–Jejunitis: This poorly understood disease affects the proximal portion of the small intestine and has various names, including proximal enteritis–jejunitis, anterior enteritis, and duodenitis–jejunitis. The condition has been recognized in the southeastern and northeastern USA, England, and on the European continent. The cause is unknown. The affected intestine contains lesions varying from hyperemia to necrosis and infiltration of the submucosa with inflammatory cells. Often, there is edema and hemorrhage in the various layers of the intestinal wall.

Varying degrees of abdominal pain, ranging from mild to severe, are characteristic. When the prevalence of the condition peaked in the 1980s, it was characterized by voluminous amounts of gastric reflux, progression from pain to depression, and moderate to severe distention of the small intestine on rectal examination. In addition, the distended duodenum often was palpated as it coursed around the base of the cecum. The peritoneal fluid often contained an increased concentration of protein (>3 g/dL) with a normal number of WBCs, but this finding did not consistently distinguish the condition from other causes of small-intestinal disease. Based on anecdotal reports, the prevalence and clinical severity of the condition have decreased, at least in regions of the USA where the condition characteristically had a more severe course and was accompanied by a high incidence of laminitis.

Treatment may be either medical or surgical. Medical treatment includes continued gastric decompression until the gastric reflux abates, IV fluids, and analgesics, as required. Many clinicians administer penicillin and low doses of flunixin meglumine; some also administer neostigmine, lidocaine, or metoclopramide to stimulate small-intestinal motility. Some surgeons, particularly in the UK, believe exploratory laparotomy and intestinal decompression result in a more rapid recovery. The survival rate associated with proximal enteritis–jejunitis is reported to be 44%. The horse's feet should receive particular attention because acute laminitis has been reported as a common complication, with a prevalence of ~25%.

Intussusception: Most intussusceptions that develop in horses are jejuno-jejunal, ileal-ileal, or ileocecal. The length of intestine that has become invaginated (the intussusceptum) into the more distal segment of intestine (the intussuscipiens) may range from a few centimeters to as much as a meter. Although the precise cause of most intussusceptions remains speculative, alterations in peristalsis due to enteritis, surgical trauma, parasite damage, anthelmintics, and *Anoplocephala perfoliata* infection have been suggested. Horses <3 yr old are affected most commonly.

Abdominal pain may be either acute due to complete obstruction of the intestinal lumen or chronic due to partial occlusion of the lumen. If the occlusion of the intestinal lumen is complete, the horse is acutely painful and has gastric reflux, and distended loops of small intestine are palpable per rectum. It may be possible to palpate the turgid intussusception, especially if the ileum is involved. Because the strangulated intussusceptum is contained within the intussuscipiens, the WBC count in the peritoneal fluid may not reflect the degree of intestinal damage.

Treatment requires surgery to reduce the intussusception, if possible, followed by resection and anastomosis. Because of the edema and hemorrhage in the wall of the affected intestine, it may be difficult to assess the viability of the bowel. Additionally, the damage to the intussusceptum may result in the development of adhesions. If the jejunum is involved, a jejuno-jejunal anastomosis must be performed. If the intussusception involves only the ileum, the affected intestine must be resected and a jejuno-cecal anastomosis performed. If the ileum has invaginated into the cecum, the terminal portion of the ileum should be transected close to the cecum and a jejuno-cecal anastomosis performed. The prognosis for survival is good if surgery is performed before the intussusception has become irreducible. The prognosis is fair to poor in the latter case because of the development of peritonitis, ileus, adhesions, and abscess formation.

Volvulus: A small-intestinal volvulus is seen when the intestine rotates on its mesenteric axis >180°. As the degree of the rotation increases, the vascular supply to the intestine is lost. Presumably because of its attachment to the cecum, the distal aspect of the volvulus is the ileum in most cases.

Horses with small-intestinal volvulus have acute pain and an increased heart rate, a prolonged capillary refill time, and gastric reflux. Because of the loss of fluid into the intestine and stomach, these horses rapidly become dehydrated and have increased PCV and plasma protein concentrations. The horse's status may deteriorate rapidly because of hypovolemia and endotoxemia. Rectal examination generally reveals turgid distended loops of small intestine, and the peritoneal fluid contains increased numbers of WBCs and protein.

Treatment involves surgical correction of the volvulus via a ventral midline celiotomy. If the intestine is nonviable, it must be resected and an anastomosis performed. The prognosis for survival depends on the duration of illness and amount of intestine that must be resected. Prognosis is good with early detection and surgery. Horses with a longer period of illness preoperatively, or those that develop postoperative ileus and peritonitis, are at increased risk of adhesion formation. It has been suggested that euthanasia is warranted if >50% of the length of the small intestine must be removed. However, results of an experimental study in ponies indicated that removal of 70% of the small intestine did not result in malabsorption provided the ponies were fed several (8) small pelleted meals each day.

Pedunculated Lipomas: Colic due to pedunculated lipomas is seen in horses >10 yr old. Pedunculated lipomas are suspended from the mesentery by a stalk or pedicle, which wraps around a segment of intestine, occluding the lumen of the intestine and interfering with its blood supply. The lipoma frequently forms a knot with the pedicle.

Clinical signs range from depression to severe abdominal pain, gastric reflux, and rapid deterioration in metabolic status. Distended loops of small intestine are palpable on rectal examination and can be identified with abdominal ultrasonography; the lipoma can be felt per rectum in rare cases. The peritoneal fluid contains an increased number of WBCs and RBCs and an increased protein content.

Treatment requires transection of the pedicle and, if necessary, resection of the devitalized intestine. The prognosis depends on the time between onset of clinical signs and surgery. If surgery is performed early, the prognosis is good; however, if surgery is not performed until signs of cardiovascular deterioration are present, the prognosis for survival is fair to poor.

Internal Incarceration: The most common sites for internal incarcerations are mesenteric rents and the epiploic foramen. **Mesenteric rents** are defects in the small-intestinal mesentery. Problems develop when a segment of small intestine passes through the mesenteric defect, and the intestine becomes incarcerated. Because the intestine distends with fluid and blood, volvulus of the affected segment frequently occurs. Mesenteric rents causing intestinal incarceration occur in horses of all ages.

The **epiploic foramen** is a natural opening bounded by the caudate lobe of the liver, the portal vein, and the caudal vena cava. The distal jejunum and ileum are the most common portions of the intestine that become incarcerated through the epiploic foramen. Although generally the intestine passes through the epiploic foramen from left to right, tearing the omentum in the process, it also may pass in the opposite direction to enter the omental bursa. It has been reported that horses >7 yr old are affected most frequently by epiploic foramen entrapment. However, the condition also often develops in horses <7 yr old.

Clinical signs may be vague and similar to those of horses with proximal enteritis or pedunculated lipomas. The diagnosis may have to be made at surgery. Furthermore, in some cases, because of the position of the affected intestine within the omental bursa, the peritoneal fluid available for analysis may be normal.

Treatment of horses with either mesenteric rents or epiploic foramen entrapments is surgical. The affected segment of intestine must be exteriorized, its viability evaluated, and, if necessary, a

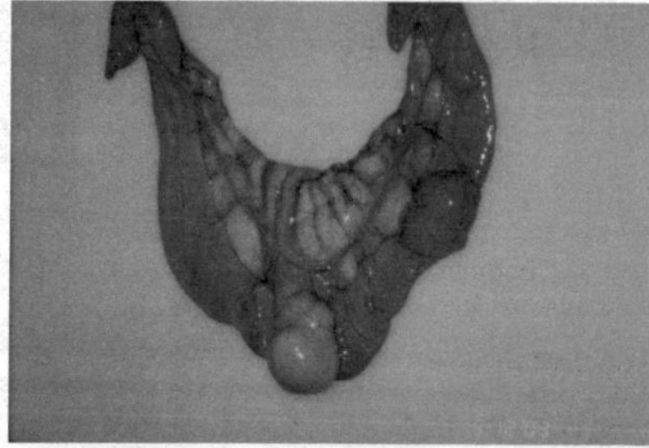

Pedunculated lipoma in a horse. *Courtesy of Dr. Sameeh M. Abutarbush.*

resection and anastomosis performed. The prognosis for survival depends on the time between onset and surgery. If surgery is performed early in the course of the disease, the prognosis is good. However, because the clinical signs may be vague, the decision to perform surgery may be delayed, worsening the prognosis.

Inguinal Hernia: Inguinal hernias generally develop in stallions after breeding a mare, trauma, or a hard workout. Hernias appear to be most common in Tennessee Walking Horses, American Saddlebreds, and Standardbreds. In most cases, the hernia results in acute colic. The intestine descends through the vaginal ring in most cases and lies next to the testis and epididymis. Physical examination reveals a swollen testis that is firm and cool to the touch. If the hernia has occurred within hours, the intestine may be palpated in the inguinal canal. In this situation, an attempt may be made to reduce the hernia by pulling down on the testis to tighten the boundaries of the inguinal canal and then forcing the intestine up toward the vaginal ring. Once the incarcerated intestine, which frequently includes the ileum, has become edematous, it is not possible to reduce the hernia manually. Rectal examination will reveal distended loops of small intestine, with one of the loops tracing to the vaginal ring on the affected side. There will be gastric reflux, and the horse's condition will deteriorate rapidly. Peritoneal fluid generally reflects the degree of ischemia.

Surgery involves a ventral midline celiotomy and inguinal approach to reduce the hernia. Often, the testicle on the affected side must be removed, and the affected intestine resected. The prognosis for survival seems to be breed-dependent, with Standardbred horses having a good prognosis and Tennessee Walking Horses having a fair to poor prognosis. Presumably, this reflects the fact that many Tennessee Walking Horse stallions with inguinal hernias show little evidence of pain, which delays the decision for surgery.

Cecum and Large Intestine

Impaction: The most common sites of impaction are the pelvic flexure region of the left colon, the junction of the right dorsal colon with the transverse colon, and the base and body of the cecum. The pelvic flexure and transverse colon regions are anatomically predisposed to obstruction because of the dramatic changes in size. The underlying reason for impaction of the cecum is unknown, although it has been speculated that cecal muscular activity is abnormal in affected horses. Other predisposing factors include feed that is too coarse, diseased or poorly managed teeth, and insufficient water intake. In one clinical study, Morgan, Arabian, and Appaloosa breeds were overrepresented among horses with cecal impaction, and it has been proposed that the condition may develop secondary to infection with the tapeworm *Anoplocephala perfoliata*. Impactions also may develop secondary to other intestinal diseases and may be associated with prolonged hospitalization. Consequently, the fecal output of horses being treated for

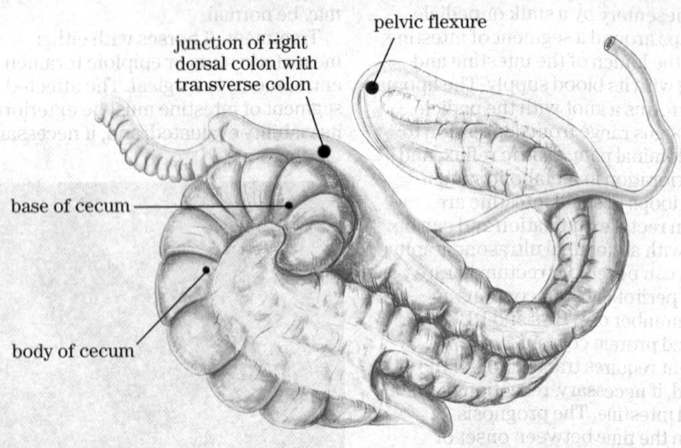

Most common sites of impaction, cecum and large intestine, in a horse (larger dots indicate more frequent impaction at that site). *Illustration by Dr. Gheorghe Constantinescu.*

other abnormalities should be assessed on a routine basis. This is especially important in horses receiving NSAIDs on a daily basis.

Horses with simple impactions of the cecum or large colon exhibit mild intermittent signs of colic, and there is minimal evidence of systemic deterioration unless the impaction has a prolonged course. Generally, the heart rate is only slightly increased. Intestinal sounds are usually heard on auscultation of the abdomen and may be associated with the onset of pain as the affected portion of the intestine contracts against the obstruction. Diagnosis is made on rectal examination. Although the most common site of obstruction is considered to be the pelvic flexure region of the large colon, the impacted ingesta actually fills much or all of the left ventral colon. The impacted mass may be felt extending cranially in the abdomen, and the affected segment of bowel is identified by palpating the longitudinal bands on the surface of the ventral colon. Impaction of the cecum is relatively easy to identify, because the mass is situated in the right paralumbar region. The cecum can be definitively identified by palpating the taut ventral cecal band and the fat and blood vessels overlying the medial cecal band. Peritoneal fluid analysis may be normal, or the total protein concentration may be increased as the course becomes more prolonged.

Cecal impactions tend to cause colic in horses >8 yr old. Alternatively, impactions may be seen in horses hospitalized for other reasons and are often associated with abrupt rupture of the cecum in these cases. Consequently, there is some controversy regarding the best method of treatment. Because medical therapy in some clinical studies has been unsuccessful in 50% of the cases, surgical removal of the impacting mass followed by an ileocolostomy has been strongly recommended. Other veterinarians report good results with aggressive medical therapy, particularly if abdominal pain associated with the cecal impaction was the primary reason the horse required veterinary attention.

Medical treatment of horses with cecal or large-colon impaction involves the administration of analgesics as necessary, large volumes of balanced IV fluids, and intragastric administration of either mineral oil or dioctyl sodium sulfosuccinate and water. Feed should be restricted until the impaction is relieved. Many veterinarians consider aggressive fluid therapy to be the mainstay of treatment. Balanced electrolyte solutions are administered to induce movement of fluid from the plasma into the lumen of the intestine. This form of treatment may require administration of >50 L of fluid/day to a 450-kg horse until the impaction is resolved. Interest has increased in using enteral fluid therapy to treat horses with impactions, primarily because enteral fluid therapy is significantly less expensive than IV fluid therapy. The clinical results with enteral fluid therapy have been rewarding, and the results of experimental work in healthy horses have shown that enteral fluid therapy is more effective than IV fluid therapy in promoting hydration of colonic contents.

If the large-colon impaction does not resolve with medical management, surgery can be performed. Generally, the impaction is approached via a ventral midline celiotomy, with the affected portion of the colon gently exteriorized and positioned on a sterile colon tray. An enterotomy then is made in the pelvic flexure and the contents of the colon removed.

Surgery for treatment of cecal impactions requires general anesthesia, a ventral midline celiotomy, isolation of the cecum from the celiotomy site, and removal of the contents of the cecum via an enterotomy. Because impactions have recurred after simple evacuation, some surgeons prefer to bypass the cecum with an ileocolostomy.

The prognosis associated with impactions involving the large colon is excellent, with a survival rate of >95%. The survival rate associated with cecal impactions is ~80% for those horses that can be treated medically and 60%–70% for those horses requiring surgical intervention.

In some geographic areas, the offending material may be sand, especially if the amount of pasture grass is insufficient and the horses are fed on the ground. The sand accumulates in the right dorsal colon and transverse colon. Intermittent signs of abdominal pain may occur because of the weight of the sand in the intestine. More severe signs of pain occur when the impaction occludes the lumen of the transverse colon. Under such circumstances, the colon proximal to the obstruction distends with gas, resulting in extreme pain. It may not be possible to distinguish this condition from an intestinal displacement or volvulus. Sand also may be identified in the feces by mixing fecal material with water in a plastic rectal examination sleeve.

Treatment of sand impaction may be either medical or surgical. Medical treatment generally involves intragastric administration of psyllium (400 g/500 kg body wt, daily for 7 days) to purge the sand from the lumen. The psyllium flakes are added to 7.5 L of warm water and rapidly pumped into the stomach. These treatments are accompanied by analgesics as needed and IV fluids to promote movement of fluid into the intestinal lumen.

Surgery via a ventral midline celiotomy is necessary if the sand completely obstructs the lumen of the transverse colon. The left colon is exteriorized on a sterile colon tray, and the sand is removed via an enterotomy. The prognosis is usually good. Problems sometimes develop during surgery if the colon was damaged due to the extensive weight of the sand or while the sand is being removed from the intestine (*see* p 287).

Enterolithiasis: Enteroliths are concretions composed of magnesium ammonium phosphate crystals around a nidus (eg, wire, stone, nail). Enteroliths may be seen singly or in groups and are commonly found in horses in certain parts of the USA, including California, the southwest, Indiana, and Florida. Enterolithiasis commonly affects Arabian horses, but the fact that these horses are extremely popular in the aforementioned areas confounds the question regarding breed association. Most horses with enteroliths are ~10 yr old; enterolithiasis rarely is seen in horses <4 yr old. Although not all factors that contribute to the formation of enteroliths have been identified, results of clinical studies indicate that large-colon contents from horses with enteroliths have higher mineral (magnesium, calcium, and phosphorus) concentrations and pH than contents from horses with colic not due to enteroliths. A common factor associated with enterolithiasis is the consumption of alfalfa hay, which results in a higher pH and increased concentrations of calcium, magnesium, and sulfur in the large colon.

Many horses with enterolithiasis have a history of recurring colic, presumably indicating that the enterolith(s) had caused partial or temporary obstruction of the colonic lumen. If the enterolith becomes lodged at the origin of the transverse colon, the colon proximal to the obstruction distends with gas and the pain is severe. Distention of the abdomen may be marked. Heart and respiratory rates are increased, and the mucous membranes may be pale or pink. Generally, colonic and cecal distention is evident on rectal examination, but the mass rarely is palpable because the transverse colon is cranial to the cranial mesenteric artery. Analysis of the peritoneal fluid is usually within normal limits unless ischemia of the colonic wall has developed over the enterolith. In areas where the problem is endemic, radiography may be used to identify the enteroliths.

Treatment involves surgery via a ventral midline celiotomy to decompress the colon and cecum and then to remove the stone(s). The left portion of the large colon is exteriorized and positioned on a sterile colon tray, the ingesta removed via an enterotomy, and then the enterolith(s) removed. If the stone has a flat side or a polyhedral shape, this is indicative of the presence of one or more additional enteroliths. Consequently, the rest of the large and small colons must be thoroughly checked for other stones. The prognosis is excellent, with practices in endemic areas reporting survival rates of 95%.

Left Dorsal Displacement: Left dorsal displacement of the colon is seen when either the pelvic flexure or the entire left colon becomes displaced over the renosplenic ligament. Because the renosplenic ligament is not attached to the most dorsal aspect of the spleen, a natural cleft exists between the spleen and left kidney. Although all ages and sexes of horses are affected equally, results of a clinical study indicate that the displacement is common in young horses.

Because left dorsal displacement results in simple obstruction of the colon at the point where it hangs across the ligament, the condition usually is associated with moderate abdominal pain or a prolonged course of intermittent painful episodes. The mucous membranes remain normal, and the heart rate is increased only slightly. The diagnosis usually is made on rectal examination (palpating the pelvic flexure over the ligament, palpating the bands of the left ventral colon running dorsocranially to the left kidney, and detecting that the spleen is displaced toward the middle of the abdomen). The condition also may be identified using ultrasonography. A paracentesis may yield blood if the spleen is displaced toward the midline.

Four forms of treatment have been used: 1) withholding feed to determine whether evacuation of the intestinal contents will allow the colon to return to its normal position, 2) rolling the horse to dislodge the colon from the ligament, 3) administering phenylephrine and/or jogging the horse to cause splenic contraction and correction of the displacement, or 4) performing surgery to return the colon to its correct position. The rolling procedure involves short-term anesthesia (generally xylazine or detomidine and ketamine), elevation of the horse's hindlimbs, and rolling the horse 360°. Surgery is performed via a ventral midline celiotomy. The advantage of surgery is that the viability of the colon can be assessed. Phenylephrine should not be administered to horses >15 yr old because of the increased risk of fatal hemorrhage in aged horses given this drug. If left dorsal displacement of the colon recurs, the renosplenic space may be sutured closed laparoscopically. Overall, the prognosis is good, with most studies reporting survival rates >80%.

Right Dorsal Displacement: The left colons move laterally around the base of the cecum to lie between the cecum and the right body wall. With the most common form of this displacement, the pelvic flexure ends up positioned near the diaphragm. In many instances, the displacement may be complicated by twisting of the colon near the base of the cecum. Although there may be some interference with venous drainage from the affected colon, usually the arterial supply remains intact.

Most horses with right dorsal displacements exhibit moderate degrees of pain, and there is slow development of systemic deterioration. In some cases, however, the pain may be severe. Rectal examination may reveal the taenia of the colon running transversely across the pelvic inlet. It may not be possible to palpate the ventral cecal band on rectal examination. Some horses with this condition have gastric reflux, presumably due to occlusion of the lumen of the duodenum.

Some horses with this condition appear to be stable and may show intermittent signs consistent with mild abdominal pain. Treatment may be conservative, involving attention to fluid needs and administration of mild analgesics. For painful horses, however, surgery must be performed to locate the pelvic flexure, to exteriorize and decompress the left portion of the colon, if possible, and then to relocate the colon to its normal position by rotating it around the cecal base. The twisting of the colon must be identified and corrected. The prognosis for survival is good, provided that the colonic wall is not damaged during surgery.

Right Dorsal Colitis: Right dorsal colitis has been recognized with increasing regularity in recent years, particularly in, but not limited to, horses receiving excessive amounts of NSAIDs. Because the condition has been identified in horses receiving recommended doses of these drugs, it appears that some horses are particularly sensitive to their toxic effects. The drug most commonly associated with right dorsal colitis is phenylbutazone, but this may reflect the common and often chronic use of this drug. The most common lesions reported in horses with right dorsal colitis are ulceration and thickening and/or fibrosis of the wall of the right dorsal colon.

Horses commonly present with abdominal pain, anorexia, and lethargy. In many cases, the signs are consistent with severe abdominal pain, fever, endotoxemia, and diarrhea. Horses with the more chronic form of the disease present with intermittent abdominal pain, weight loss, lethargy, and anorexia. In most cases, hypoproteinemia is a common finding on hematology and may account for ventral edema in some horses with the chronic form of the disease. The diagnosis is usually based on the history, clinical signs, and hematologic findings. In some cases, ultrasonographic evaluation of the colon via the twelfth to fifteenth intercostal spaces may provide evidence of marked thickening of the colonic wall.

Treatment of affected horses includes discontinuation of NSAIDs, rest, and a change in diet to a complete pelleted feed that contains ≥30% dietary fiber. Some clinicians recommend the feeding of many small meals daily, many recommend the inclusion of psyllium to promote mucosal healing, and some administer sucralfate or metronidazole. Horses with uncontrollable pain may require surgery to resect or bypass the affected portion of the right dorsal colon. The prognosis for horses with right dorsal colitis is guarded.

Volvulus of the Large Colon: Although the term "torsion" has been used for years to indicate that the colon has twisted on itself, the involvement of the mesentery between the ventral and dorsal colons indicates that the condition is a volvulus. When viewed from the most common site of the volvulus (the junction between the right ventral colon and the cecum), the volvulus most often occurs in a clockwise direction; the cecum may or may not be involved. If the volvulus is <270°, there may be obstruction of the bowel lumen without ischemia. If the volvulus is >360°, there is strangulating obstruction of the entire left colon.

The onset of colic is sudden, and the degree of pain may be mild to moderate if the volvulus results only in obstruction of the intestinal lumen. When the twist is more extensive, the pain is severe and the horse may not respond to analgesics. The colon is extremely enlarged, and the mesentery between the dorsal and ventral colons is edematous on rectal examination. The heart rate is rapid, the horse's condition deteriorates rapidly, and there is poor peripheral perfusion. Distention of the abdomen usually is marked. Generally, results of peritoneal fluid analysis and the degree of colonic involvement are poorly correlated.

Although the cause of colonic volvulus remains unknown, it is presumed to be associated with a disproportionate amount of gas in the colon. On broodmare farms, the condition frequently is associated with recent (within 90 days) or impending parturition, a grass diet, or highly fermentable feeds. The presence of a foal at the mare's side (recent history of parturition) is an additional risk factor.

Treatment of colonic volvulus requires surgery to correct the volvulus and remove affected bowel, if necessary. Although the technique for removal of 90% of the colon has been perfected in healthy horses, extreme difficulty can be encountered if the colon is edematous. Because the recurrence rate has been estimated to be as high as 20% in some clinical studies, colopexy procedures have been devised to reduce the recurrence of the condition in broodmares. Although the results of a study involving several university hospitals reported a 27% survival rate, survival rates >85% are common for practices situated near broodmare farms.

Impaction and Foreign Body Obstruction of the Descending Colon: Abnormalities involving the descending (small) colon are infrequent, accounting for <5% of conditions characterized by colic in one study. The more common causes include meconium retention, impaction, and foreign body obstruction. Meconium retention is seen in newborn male foals within the first 24 hr of life. Affected foals swish their tails from side to side, strain to defecate, and roll. The diagnosis is made by careful digital examination. Treatment involves gentle administration of a warm, soapy water enema. The prognosis is excellent.

Impaction of the descending colon is seen in ponies, miniature horses, and adult horses with limited access to drinking water or with other causes of intestinal stasis. Most recently, the condition has been associated with salmonellosis, although a cause and effect relationship has not been proved. Pain may be severe if the obstruction is complete. In such cases, tympany of the colon occurs secondarily, and ileus results. The diagnosis is made in adult horses by palpating the obstructing mass in the ventral portion of the abdomen on rectal examination. Foreign body obstruction of the descending colon must be considered if the horse is <3 yr old; the offending material may be rubber fencing, nylon fibers from halters or lead shanks, hay net, or feed sacks. Horses with impactions may be treated medically with analgesics, IV fluids, and gentle enemas. Often, however, surgery is required to evacuate the colon due to severity of pain and gas distention. The prognosis associated with impaction of the descending colon is fair, unless it is complicated by severe colitis after the obstruction has been removed. The prognosis associated with foreign body obstruction is good.

INTESTINAL DISEASES IN RUMINANTS

INTESTINAL DISEASES IN CATTLE

Determination of the cause of intestinal disease in cattle is based on clinical, epidemiologic, and laboratory findings. Nonspecific therapy includes oral and parenteral fluid therapy to restore the fluid, electrolyte, and acid-base homeostasis. Specific therapy and prevention are detailed under the individual disease headings. Intestinal diseases of neonates are discussed separately, although some of the causes also affect older animals.

Bovine Viral Diarrhea and Mucosal Disease Complex

Bovine viral diarrhea (BVD) is most common in young cattle (6–24 mo old). The clinical presentation can range from inapparent or subclinical infection to acute and severe enteric disease to the highly fatal mucosal disease complex characterized by profuse enteritis in association with typical mucosal lesions. BVD must be distinguished from other viral diseases that produce diarrhea and mucosal lesions. These include malignant catarrhal fever (*see* p 758), which usually is a sporadic disease in more mature cattle, bluetongue (*see* p 738), and rinderpest (*see* p 771), which is currently considered to be eradicated worldwide.

Bovine viral diarrhea virus (BVDV), the causal agent of BVD and mucosal disease complex, is classified in the genus *Pestivirus* in the family Flaviviridae. Although cattle are the primary host for BVDV, several reports suggest most even-toed ungulates are also susceptible. Classically, isolates of BVDV are separated into noncytopathic and cytopathic biotypes based on their ability or lack of ability to cause overt cytopathic change and cell death in cell cultures. Noncytopathic BVDV is the predominant viral biotype in nature, whereas cytopathic BVDV is relatively rare and of little epidemiologic relevance. The cytopathic biotype arises in cattle that are persistently infected with noncytopathic biotype of the same or a genetically similar BVDV strain. The switch in biotype is the result of mutations that often involve recombination of noncytopathic viral RNA with itself, with heterologous viral RNA, or with host cell RNA.

Based on comparisons of nucleotide sequence in the viral RNA, there are at least two viral genotypes (distinct genetic groups) of BVDV that can be further divided into subgenotypes or genogroups. The viral genotypes are termed BVDV type 1 and BVDV type 2, and both cytopathic and noncytopathic BVDV are represented in each viral genotype. In recent years, a new group of atypical pestiviruses, apparently forming a separate species, of which cattle are the most likely host species, have been recognized. Virus of this third *Pestivirus* genotype are designated as 'HoBi"-like pestiviruses. The subgenotypes are clusters of viruses within a viral genotype that are highly similar in nucleotide sequence of the viral RNA. (Subgenotypes are designated by lower case letters; thus, subgenotypes of BVDV genotype 1 are represented as 1a, 1b, 1c, etc). Currently, at least 12 subgenotypes for BVDV-1 (BVDV-1a to BVDV-1l) and two subgenotypes for BVDV-2 (BVDV-2a and BVDV-2b) are recognized.

BVDV type 1 and type 2 appear to be distributed worldwide; however, the prevalence of each type of virus varies considerably among regions. The distribution of viral subgenotypes is more restricted, with many viral subgenotypes being found only in certain regions of the world and, in some cases, only certain regions of a country. All BVDV, regardless of genotype or subgenotype, are antigenically related. However, serologic assays that use serum obtained from convalescent cattle can distinguish BVDV type 1 from type 2. The extent of antigenic variation among BVDV of different genotypes and subgenotypes remains unknown, but there is concern that the antigenic differences among BVDV may be sufficient to affect protection conferred by vaccination.

Etiology and Epidemiology: Serologic surveys conducted throughout the world suggest that BVDV is endemic in the cattle population of most cattle-producing countries. In some countries, BVD is considered the single most important viral infection of cattle. The prevalence of antiviral antibody in cattle varies greatly among countries and geographic regions because of differing cattle housing practices, population densities, vaccination practices, and implementation of different control or eradication programs. Prevalence of antiviral antibody may be >90% if vaccination is practiced commonly in a geographic region. Although cattle of all ages are susceptible, most cases of overt clinical disease are seen in cattle between 6 mo and 2 yr old.

Cattle persistently infected with noncytopathic BVDV serve as a natural reservoir for virus. Persistent infection develops when noncytopathic BVDV is transmitted transplacentally during the first 4 mo of fetal development. The calf is born infected with virus, remains infected for life, and usually is immunotolerant to the resident noncytopathic virus. Transplacental infection that occurs later in gestation can result in abortion, congenital malformations, or birth of healthy calves that have antibody against BVDV. The prevalence of persistent infection varies among countries and between regions within a country. The estimated mean animal prevalence of persistent infection with BVDV is

~1%–2% but may approach 4% on dairy farms with endemic BVDV infection. On a given farm, persistently infected cattle are often found in cohorts of animals that are approximately the same age. Persistently infected cattle can shed large amounts of BVDV in their secretions and excretions and readily transmit virus to susceptible herdmates. Clinical disease and reproductive failure often are seen after healthy cattle come in contact with a persistently infected animal. Although persistently infected cattle are important in transmission of BVDV, the virus also may be spread by biting insects, fomites, semen, biologic products, and other animals, including swine, sheep, goats, camelids, and possibly wild ruminants.

Clinical Findings and Lesions: Disease induced by BVDV varies in severity, duration, and organ systems involved. Infection of immunocompetent susceptible animals with either noncytopathic or cytopathic BVDV is termed acute or transient BVD. Inapparent or subclinical infection without any clinical signs that is followed by seroconversion is the most common form of infection in the field. Acute clinical disease may range from mild disease of high morbidity and low mortality to severe enteric disease with considerable mortality. Biphasic fever (~104°F [40°C]), depression, decreased milk production, transient inappetence, rapid respiration, excessive nasal secretion, excessive lacrimation, and diarrhea are typical signs of acute clinical BVD. Clinical signs of disease usually are seen 6–12 days after infection and last 1–3 days. Transient leukopenia may be seen with onset of signs of disease. Recovery is rapid and coincides with production of viral neutralizing antibody. Gross lesions seldom are seen in cases of mild disease. Lymphoid tissue is a primary target for replication of BVDV, which may lead to immunosuppression and enhanced severity of intercurrent infections.

Some isolates of BVDV (BVD type 2) have been associated with severe clinical disease that manifests as high fever (~107°F [41°–42°C]), oral ulcerations, eruptive lesions of the coronary band and interdigital cleft, diarrhea, dehydration, leukopenia, and thrombocytopenia. In thrombocytopenic cattle, petechial hemorrhages may be seen in the conjunctiva, sclera, nictitating membrane of the eyes, and on mucosal surfaces of the mouth and vulva. Prolonged bleeding from injection sites also occurs. Swollen lymph nodes, erosions and ulcerations of the GI tract, petechial and ecchymotic hemorrhages on the serosal surfaces of the viscera, and extensive lymphoid depletion are associated with severe forms of acute BVD. The duration of overt disease may be 3–7 days. High morbidity with a mortality of ≥25% is common. Severity of acute BVD is related to the virulence of the viral strain infecting the animal and does not depend on viral biotype.

In pregnant cattle, BVDV may cross the placental barrier and infect the fetus. The consequences of fetal infection usually are seen several weeks to months after infection of the dam and depend on the stage of fetal development and on the strain of BVDV. Infection of the dam near the time of fertilization may result in reduced conception rates. Infection during the first 4 mo of fetal development may lead to embryonic resorption, abortion, growth retardation, or persistent infection. Congenital malformations of the eye and CNS result from fetal infections that occur between months 4–6 of development. Fetal mummification, premature birth, stillbirth, and birth of weak calves also are seen after fetal infection.

Persistent infection is an important sequela of fetal infection with noncytopathic BVDV. Persistently infected calves may appear healthy and normal in size, or they may show stunted growth and be prone to respiratory or enteric ailments. They often have a short life span, and death before 2 yr of age is common. Persistently infected cows always give birth to persistently infected calves, but most calves sired by a persistently infected bull will not be infected with virus in utero. Lesions attributable to BVDV often are not seen in persistently infected cattle at necropsy. Antibody against BVD seldom is detected in persistently infected cattle in the absence of vaccination or superinfection with an antigenically heterologous BVDV. Persistently infected cattle exposed to BVDV that is antigenically different from their resident noncytopathic virus can produce antiviral antibody. Therefore, screening for persistent infection using serologic tests to identify animals that lack antiviral antibody may not detect some persistently infected cattle.

Mucosal disease is an uncommon but highly fatal form of BVD occurring in persistently infected cattle and can have an acute or chronic presentation. Mucosal disease is induced when persistently infected cattle become superinfected with cytopathic BVDV. The origin of the cytopathic BVDV is usually internal, resulting from a mutation of the resident persistent, noncytopathic BVDV. In those cases, the cytopathic virus is antigenically similar to the resident noncytopathic virus. External origins for cytopathic BVDV include other cattle and modified-live virus vaccines. Cattle that develop mucosal disease due to exposure to a cytopathic virus of external origin often produce antiviral antibody. Prevalence of persistent infection usually is low, and many persistently infected cattle do not develop mucosal disease, regardless of exposure. Acute mucosal disease is characterized by fever, leukopenia, dysenteric diarrhea, inappetence, dehydration, erosive lesions of the nares and mouth, and death within a few days of onset. At necropsy, erosions and ulcerations may be found throughout the GI tract. The mucosa over Peyer's patches may be hemorrhagic and necrotic. Extensive necrosis of lymphoid tissues, especially gut-associated lymphoid tissue, is seen on microscopic examination.

Clinical signs of chronic mucosal disease may last several weeks to months and are less severe than those of acute mucosal disease. Intermittent diarrhea and gradual wasting are common. Coronitis and eruptive lesions on the skin of the interdigital cleft cause lameness in some cattle. Lesions found at necropsy are less pronounced than, but similar to, those seen in acute mucosal disease. Often, the only gross lesions seen are focal ulcerations in the mucosa of the cecum, proximal colon, or rectum, and the mucosa over Peyer's patches of the small intestine may appear sunken.

Diagnosis: BVD is diagnosed tentatively from disease history, clinical signs, and gross and microscopic lesions. Diagnostic laboratory support is required when clinical signs and gross lesions are minimal. Laboratory support also is required in some outbreaks of mucosal disease or clinically severe acute BVD, because either disease may appear similar to rinderpest (*see* p 771) or malignant catarrhal fever (*see* p 758).

Laboratory tests for BVDV include isolation of virus or viral antigen in clinical specimens and tissues, and assays that detect anti-BVDV antibody in serum or milk. Because antibody against BVDV can be highly prevalent in regions with high infection prevalence and/or common use of BVD vaccines, a single serologic test is seldom sufficient for diagnosis of recent infection. A >4-fold increase in antibody titer in paired serum samples obtained ≥2 wk apart is necessary to verify recent infection. Isolation of BVDV from blood, nasal swab specimens, or tissues confirms active infection. Identification of persistent infection requires detection of virus in clinical specimens obtained at least 3 wk apart. Colostral antibody can impair the sensitivity of virus isolation in blood during the first weeks of life. At necropsy, tissues of choice for viral isolation include spleen, lymph node, and ulcerated segments of the GI tract.

Alternatives to viral isolation include antigen-capture ELISA to detect virus in blood, serum, or tissue biopsies; immunohistochemistry to detect viral protein in frozen or fixed tissues; PCR to detect viral RNA in clinical specimens; and PCR or in situ hybridization to detect viral RNA in fresh or fixed tissues. Differentiation of viral genotypes and subgenotypes may be accomplished by PCR assays alone, or by PCR assays followed by analysis of nucleotide sequence, restriction fragment analysis, or palindromic nucleotide substitution analysis. Monoclonal antibody binding assays and viral neutralization assays also differentiate viral genotypes.

Treatment and Control: Treatment of BVD remains limited primarily to supportive therapy. Control is based on sound management practices that include use of biosecurity measures, elimination of persistently infected cattle, and vaccination. Replacement cattle should be tested for persistent infection before entry into the herd. Quarantine or physical separation of replacement cattle from the resident herd for 2–4 wk should be considered, and vaccination of replacement cattle for BVD should be done before commingling with the resident herd. Embryo donors and recipients also should be tested for persistent infection. If vaccination of embryo donors or recipients is warranted, it should be done at least one estrous cycle before embryo transfer is performed. Because BVDV is shed into semen, breeding bulls should be tested for persistent infection before use. Artificial insemination should be done only with semen obtained from bulls free of persistent infection.

Screening cattle herds for persistent infection can be done by PCR assays using skin biopsies, blood, or milk; by classical virus isolation methods using serum or buffy coat cells; by antigen-capture ELISA using serum, buffy coat, milk, or skin biopsies; or by antigen detection using immunochemical methods on tissue or skin biopsies. Several strategies, based on herd size, type of herd being screened, financial limitations of the herd owner, and testing ability of the diagnostic laboratory being used, are available to screen herds for persistent infection. When identified, persistently infected cattle should be removed from the herd as soon as possible, and direct or indirect contact with pregnant cattle should be prevented.

Inactivated and modified-live virus vaccines are available. They contain a variety of strains of BVDV representing both viral biotypes and viral genotypes 1 and 2. Antigenic diversity among BVDV may affect the efficacy of a given vaccine if the vaccine virus or viruses differ significantly from the challenge virus. Proper and safe immunization of cattle with either inactivated or modified-live virus vaccines requires adherence to the manufacturer's instructions. Because BVDV is fetotropic and immunosuppressive, use of modified-live virus vaccines is not recommended in cattle that are pregnant or showing signs of disease. Inactivated viral vaccines may be used in pregnant cattle. Protection conferred by inactivated vaccines may be of short duration, and frequent vaccination may be necessary to prevent disease or reproductive failure. Colostral antibody confers partial to complete protection against disease in most calves for 3–6 mo after birth. Vaccination of neonatal cattle that have acquired colostral antibody may not stimulate a protective immune response, and revaccination at 5–9 mo of age may be necessary. A booster dose of vaccine is often administered before first breeding, and additional booster doses of vaccine may be administered in subsequent years before breeding.

Jejunal Hemorrhage Syndrome

(Hemorrhagic bowel syndrome of cattle)

Jejunal hemorrhage syndrome is a sporadic disease of uncertain etiology that is observed with increasing frequency in cattle. It is manifest by sudden onset of abdominal pain, progressing to sternal recumbency, shock, and death.

Etiology and Pathogenesis: The etiology of jejunal hemorrhage syndrome is uncertain but is believed to be multifactorial. *Clostridium perfringens* type A, a normal inhabitant of the bovine digestive tract, has been incriminated as an important causative agent, because this organism is isolated from the intestines of naturally occurring cases at a higher frequency and in higher numbers than from cattle with other intestinal diseases. Another proposed potential causative agent is *Aspergillus fumigatus*, a common fungus in feed and forages. The primary lesion is similar to that caused by *C perfringens* in young, rapidly growing animals and consists of an acute, localized, necrotizing, hemorrhagic enteritis of the small intestine that leads to development of an intraluminal blood clot. The clot causes a physical obstruction, with proximal accumulation of intestinal fluid and gas and development of hypochloremia, hypokalemia, dehydration, and varying degrees of anemia. The hemorrhagic enteritis is progressive. Ischemia and necrosis extends through the intestinal wall, and within 24–48 hr, there is a fibrinous peritonitis, continued electrolyte imbalance, profound toxemia, and death.

Epidemiology: Jejunal hemorrhage syndrome occurs sporadically, primarily in mature lactating dairy cows in North America and Europe, but it has also been recorded in beef cattle. Most cases occur in mature dairy cattle in the first 3 mo of lactation, with highest incidence rates during the cold months of the year. Possible risk factors for disease are those associated with management practices aimed at achieving high milk production, such as high fermentable carbohydrate content of the diet and feeding a total mixed ration. The animal-level disease incidence rate is estimated to be 1%–2%, but outbreaks in a herd can be associated with morbidity rates of ≥10%. Mortality in general is high, with 80%–100% of affected animals dying within 48 hr.

Clinical Findings: Cattle affected by jejunal hemorrhage syndrome have a history of sudden anorexia and depression, a pronounced reduction in milk production, abdominal distention and pain with kicking at the abdomen, and weakness progressing to recumbency. Clinical findings include depression, dehydration, increased heart and respiratory rates, and pale mucous membranes. The abdomen may be moderately distended on the right side, the rumen is atonic, and fluid sounds may be elicited by succussion over the right abdomen. Dark red blood clots may be found in the feces and rectum. Distended and firm loops of intestine may be palpable on deep rectal examination. On laparotomy, a segment of the small intestine is dark red and distended, with a serosal surface covered by tags of fibrin. The small intestine proximal to the affected segment and the abomasum are distended with gas and fluid. Ultrasonography may aid in diagnosis.

Most affected cattle die within 2–4 days despite intensive fluid and electrolyte therapy. Sudden death without prior clinical findings may occur. The hemogram is variable; serum biochemistry reflects obstruction of the upper small intestine and sequestration of abomasal secretions with resultant hypokalemia and hypochloremia.

Lesions: Necrohemorrhagic jejunitis with intraluminal hemorrhage is severe. The affected segment of intestine is dark red and dilated, with tags of fibrin on the serosal surface. The lumen contains a firm blood clot adherent to the mucosa, and the affected segment of intestine is necrotic.

Diagnosis: Diagnosis of jejunal hemorrhage syndrome can be made either during an exploratory laparotomy or at necropsy and is based on the presence of a characteristic focal necrohemorrhagic enteritis of the distal small intestine. Differential diagnoses include other causes of physical or functional obstruction of the small intestine such as intussusception (*see* p 245), cecal dilatation and volvulus, and diffuse peritonitis (*see* p 670), from right-sided torsion of the abomasum (*see* p 238) and torsion at the root of the mesentery, and from diseases with melena such as abomasal ulcer (*see* p 241).

Treatment and Control: Fluid and electrolyte therapy and laparotomy with massage of affected bowel loops to break down obstructing blood clots and, in advanced stages, resection of the affected segment of the intestine are treatment options for jejunal hemorrhage syndrome. Even with such treatment, the fatality rate is very high, and the prognosis is grave. No preventive strategies have been identified. A short-term protective effect of a *C perfringens* type C and D vaccine against hemorrhagic bowel syndrome in some herds has been reported anecdotally, but there is currently no corroborating scientific evidence.

Winter Dysentery

Winter dysentery is an acute, highly contagious GI disorder that affects housed adult dairy cattle, primarily during winter. Clinical features include explosive diarrhea (sometimes accompanied by dysentery), a profound drop in milk production, variable anorexia and depression, and mild respiratory signs such as coughing. The disease has a high morbidity but low mortality, and spontaneous recovery within a few days is typical.

Etiology: Although the precise etiology of winter dysentery has not been conclusively confirmed, an increasing body of evidence implicates a bovine coronavirus (BCoV), closely related to the virus that causes diarrhea in neonatal calves. Evidence for BCoV as the cause of winter dysentery includes the following: 1) clinical signs and pathologic findings are consistent with disease induced by BCoV, 2) seroconversion to BCoV has been demonstrated in affected cattle, 3) the virus is frequently isolated from diarrheic feces of cattle that exhibit clinical signs of winter dysentery, and 4) the disease has been reproduced by briefly exposing BCoV seronegative, lactating cows to a calf experimentally infected with feces from cows with winter dysentery. Notwithstanding, it has not been possible to consistently reproduce winter dysentery through oral inoculation of adult cattle with BCoV. Concurrent risk factors, such as changes in diet, cold temperatures, closed confinement with high animal density, poor ventilation, and presence of other microorganisms, may be required before BCoV causes clinical disease in adult cattle.

Transmission, Epidemiology, and Pathogenesis: BCoV is transmitted via the fecal-oral route through ingestion of feed or water contaminated with feces from clinical cases or clinically healthy carrier animals. Viral particles present in respiratory secretions of affected animals may further enhance transmission. Transmission of disease is promoted by close confinement. Winter dysentery is highly contagious and easily introduced to barns by visitors, carrier animals, and fomites. Winter dysentery is common in northern climates where animals are housed indoors for extended periods during the winter months. It is seen frequently in the northern USA, Canada, the UK, Europe, Australia, New Zealand, Israel, and Japan. Coronaviruses survive best at low temperatures and at low ultraviolet light intensities, which can lead to a buildup of virus in the environment during the colder months. Adult lactating cows that have recently calved are most severely affected, but the disease can affect younger or older animals and males. Mortality rates associated with winter dysentery are generally low (1%–2%), but morbidity in affected herds is high, with 20%–50% of the animals in a herd exhibiting clinical signs within a few days, and close to 100% of animals in the herd exhibiting signs within a week. Some degree of immunity to winter dysentery appears to develop, because recurrences, if seen in the same herd, are noted at 1- to 5-yr intervals.

Inflammatory mediators that cause hypersecretion in the small intestine and colon are thought to contribute to the voluminous diarrhea seen in cattle with winter dysentery. In addition, destruction of epithelial cells in the colonic crypts results in transudation of extracellular fluid and blood, explaining the hemorrhagic nature of the diarrhea in some cases.

Clinical Findings: Winter dysentery is characterized clinically by an acute onset of fluid diarrhea and a profound decrease in milk production (25%–95% production loss). Feces are liquid and homogenous with little odor, dark green to black, and may contain blood (typically in first-lactation heifers) or mucus. A sweet, musty, unpleasant odor is reported in barns with large numbers of affected cattle. Nasolacrimal discharge or cough may accompany or precede the diarrhea. Other signs include mild colic, dehydration, depression, a brief period of anorexia, and some decrease in body condition. Occasionally, animals exhibit more severe signs such as passage of feces with variable amounts of blood, severe dehydration, and weakness. Fatalities are rare. Diarrhea in individual animals has a short course, and feces return to normal in 2–3 days in most animals. Disease in the herd typically subsides in 1–2 wk, but milk production may take weeks to months to return to normal.

Lesions: The small intestine may be dilated and flaccid. Lesions are primarily seen in the large intestine and consist of cecal and colonic mucosal hyperemia, linear streaks or pinpoint-sized hemorrhages mostly along the colonic mucosal ridges, and blood in the lumen of the large intestine. Histologic findings may include widespread degeneration and necrosis of colonic glandular epithelium.

Diagnosis: A diagnosis of winter dysentery can be confirmed by demonstrating coronaviral particles in fecal samples via ELISA or electron microscopy. Seroconversion to coronavirus in acute and convalescent serum samples, taken 8 wk apart, also helps confirm the diagnosis.

Differential diagnoses for acute diarrhea in adult cattle include bovine viral diarrhea (BVD), enteric salmonellosis, and coccidiosis. These diseases can be excluded by absence of mucosal lesions (BVD), negative fecal cultures (*Salmonella* spp), and negative fecal flotation (coccidiosis), as well as by the characteristic clinical presentation of winter dysentery (rapid onset of diarrheal disease of short duration in a herd with high morbidity but low mortality).

Treatment and Control: Most cattle affected by winter dysentery recover spontaneously. Fresh water, palatable feed, and free-choice salt should be available at all times. The use of astringents, protectants, and adsorbents is controversial. IV fluid therapy or blood transfusions may be required in severely affected cattle.

There is no vaccine for winter dysentery. Isolation of newly introduced cattle for 2 wk and isolation of any adult cow with diarrhea is advised to decrease the likelihood of disease introduction into a herd. In an outbreak, access to the premises should be restricted, and all persons in contact with affected cattle should ensure that their footwear and clothing are clean before leaving an affected farm.

Other Intestinal Diseases of Cattle

Infection with *Salmonella* spp (*see* p 195) can produce diarrhea in animals of all ages, especially those that are stressed, closely stocked, or exposed to a heavily contaminated feed or water supply. In older animals, the disease is manifest by dysentery and toxemia, and mortality can be significant.

Rotavirus and coronavirus occasionally cause outbreaks of diarrhea in suckling calves up to 2–3 mo old. The feces are voluminous and may contain mucus. Toxemia is not evident and mortality is negligible, but growth is decreased. (*See also* DIARRHEA IN NEONATAL RUMINANTS, p 275.)

Necrotic enteritis of unknown etiology is seen in beef cattle 5–12 wk old, commonly affecting several calves within the herd. There is sudden onset of fever, depression, and profuse diarrhea. The feces are initially dark green, contain blood, and frequently stain the perineum. Circular erosions may be present in the oral mucosa. A proportion of calves recover after a clinical course of 3–5 days. The clinical course is longer in fatal cases; animals have scant mucohemorrhagic feces that are passed with tenesmus and develop a severe nonregenerative leukopenia. A secondary fibrinous broncho pneumonia may develop. Mortality is high despite intensive antibiotic treatment. At necropsy, there is ulcerative necrosis of the terminal small intestine and the large intestine.

Coccidiosis (*see* p 205) usually is seen in calves >2 mo old but <1 yr old, especially in situations of heavy stocking density and overgrazing. It is characterized by dysentery and tenesmus and may be accompanied by nervous signs. Intestinal helminthiasis, particularly ostertagiosis (*see* p 308), is seen in cattle of the same age group. Type I ostertagiosis is seen in cattle on pasture, but Type II ostertagiosis may be seen in housed animals.

Explosive outbreaks of diarrhea in mature cattle are associated most commonly with winter dysentery (*see* p 271) but also with salmonellosis when there is heavy contamination of feed or water.

Chronic diarrhea and wasting often in combination with good appetite, occurring as a sporadic disease in adult cattle is typical for paratuberculosis (*see* p 762). Chronic diarrhea and wasting also occurring in younger animals may be caused by chronic salmonellosis and chronic BVD infection. Other possible causes of chronic diarrhea include congestive heart failure, uremia, and chronic peritonitis. Persistent diarrhea with unthriftiness, and occasionally wasting in yearling and mature cattle, can be associated with a secondary copper deficiency due to excess molybdenum in the pastures. Diarrhea may also accompany selenium-responsive ill-thrift syndromes in growing cattle.

Individual cases or outbreaks of diarrhea may be associated with dietary indiscretions. Diarrhea may follow cases of simple indigestion and is common in grain overload (*see* p 222). It also follows ingestion of toxic amounts of chemicals (eg, arsenic, copper, zinc, and molybdenum) or certain poisonous plants and mycotoxicoses; dipyridyl and organophosphate poisoning can also cause diarrhea.

Cattle may also harbor organisms such as *Escherichia coli* O157:H7, *Yersinia enterocolitica*, and *Campylobacter jejuni* in the intestine; although these are rarely associated with clinical disease in cows, fecal contamination of milk may lead to outbreaks of gastroenteritis in people who consume unpasteurized milk or cheese products. Retail meat products can also be infected if there has been fecal contamination of the carcass at slaughter.

Intestinal adenocarcinoma, commonly seen in association with bovine enzootic hematuria, is believed to result from the interaction of a carcinogen (ptaquiloside) in bracken fern (*Pteridium* spp, *see* p 3089) and papilloma virus.

Intestinal obstructions are seen sporadically (*see* p 245). Cecal dilatation and volvulus are seen predominantly in adult cattle in the postparturient period. Intussusception occurring at the distal jejunum or proximal ileum is the most common cause of complete obstruction in both adult cattle and calves. Ileocecocolic, cecocolic, and colonic intussusceptions are seen less frequently in calves and not at all in adult cattle because of the greater strength of the ileocecal ligament and the presence of mesenteric fat, which stabilize this region of the bowel in older cattle. Intestinal volvulus and volvulus around the mesenteric root are seen sporadically at all ages. Rarely, intestinal obstruction is caused by incarceration and entrapment of the small intestine by persistent urachal or umbilical remnants, by obstruction of the small intestine or descending colon by phytobezoars and enteroliths, or by compression from fat necrosis or lipoma. Intestinal obstruction can also be caused by congenital disease (*see* p 168), most commonly by atresia coli (which is seen both sporadically and in clusters on a farm and may be caused by rectal palpation of the amniotic vesicle at 35 and 41 days of pregnancy) but also by atresia ani (which may be accompanied by urogenital defects and defects of the tail).

INTESTINAL DISEASES IN SHEEP AND GOATS

The causes and circumstances of diarrhea in neonatal lambs and kids are similar to those in newborn calves. Intensive lambing practices and shed-lambing increase the potential for disease and buildup of infectious agents and can be associated with serious outbreaks of diarrhea. The serotypes of enteropathogenic *Escherichia coli* that cause secretory diarrhea in calves also do so in lambs, and the approach to diagnosis, treatment, and control is similar. Similarly, rotavirus, coronavirus, and cryptosporidia (*see* p 209) also cause outbreaks of diarrhea in lambs. (*See also* DIARRHEA IN NEONATAL RUMINANTS, p 275.) Lamb dysentery caused by *Clostridium perfringens* type B (*see* p 609) is a distinct intestinal disease of lambs in the first week of life. It is seen principally in hill breeds of sheep in the UK and is characterized by sudden death or diarrhea, dysentery, and toxemia. In the USA, *C perfringens* type C causes a similar syndrome. Watery mouth or rattle belly (*see* below), a disease of uncertain etiology associated with failure of transfer of passive immunity, is seen predominantly in the UK. Coccidiosis (*see* p 206) and GI helminthiasis (*see* p 312), except for haemonchosis, are important causes of diarrhea in older nursing and weaned sheep. Terminal ileitis and villous atrophy, both of unknown etiology, are often present in the intestine of lambs culled because of poor growth.

GI helminthiasis is the most common cause of diarrhea in pastured sheep. Coccidiosis develops in association with overstocking or intensive indoor housing and poor sanitation. Salmonellosis (*see* p 195) can cause diarrhea in all ages; the circumstances in young lambs are similar to those in calves. It also can cause outbreaks of diarrhea late in pregnancy and is frequently accompanied by abortion. Salmonellosis is more common when sheep or goats are congregated intensively or stressed, particularly by shipping. *Yersinia pseudotuberculosis* and *Y enterocolitica* have both been associated with enterocolitis and diarrhea in young sheep at pasture that are debilitated from factors such as starvation and cold weather. Diarrhea may be present in bluetongue in sheep (*see* p 738) and is accompanied by typical mucosal lesions. In goats, diarrhea is often prominent in enterotoxemia associated with *C perfringens* type D (*see* p 610). This is not a feature of the clinical disease in sheep but may be present in flockmates of affected sheep. In feedlot sheep, diarrhea most commonly is associated with grain overload, salmonellosis, or coccidiosis.

Other intestinal diseases of adult sheep may manifest with diarrhea. Infection with *C perfringens* type C (struck, *see* p 609) manifests with abdominal pain, tenesmus, and rapid death. Intestinal obstruction due to intestinal accidents occurs sporadically but is usually not seen clinically. Sheep with paratuberculosis (*see* p 762) usually show progressive emaciation without diarrhea. Progressive emaciation also is the primary sign in adult sheep with intestinal adenocarcinoma, which can be prevalent in certain areas, associated with ingestion of bracken fern (*see* p 3089).

Watery Mouth Disease in Lambs

(Slavery mouth, Slavers, Rattle belly)

Watery mouth disease is a condition of intensively reared lambs occurring during the first days of life. Morbidity in a flock can be as high as 30%, and the mortality rate may exceed 80%.

Etiology and Pathogenesis: Watery mouth disease has been associated with ingestion of gram-negative bacteria, particularly *E coli*, that survive in the neonatal GI tract and translocate from the gut to the bloodstream. The strains involved are K99 antigen negative and regarded normally as nonenteropathogenic and nonenterotoxigenic. The resultant bacteremia may be tolerated by the lamb, but >10^4 colony-forming units/mL are associated with release of free endotoxin, and endotoxic shock develops rapidly.

Lambs 12–72 hr old with inadequate or delayed access to colostrum are at greatest risk. Other risk factors that have a negative effect on colostrum intake include being born in larger litters, being born to a dam with poor body condition, and stressors such as early castration.

Clinical Findings: Lambs affected with watery mouth disease are hypothermic, dull, stop feeding, and, classically, have long strings of saliva drooling from the mouth. Less obvious cases may have a wet muzzle; others may show no external signs of excess salivation, but the mouth may be cold to the touch and contain frothy saliva. Lacrimation may also be seen. The abomasum may become distended with gas and liquid, giving the deceptive appearance of a well-fed lamb, but if these lambs are lifted and shaken gently, a noise associated with the alternative name of "rattle belly" may be heard. Although scours occasionally occur, this is not a characteristic feature of the condition.

Lesions: Necropsy may reveal a bloated and inflamed GI tract, retained meconium, pale kidneys and muscle, dehydration, and enlarged and reactive mesenteric lymph nodes.

Diagnosis: Biochemical and hematologic changes and necropsy findings in lambs affected with watery mouth disease are consistent with endotoxemia and the clinical diagnosis of endotoxic shock. Terminally, lambs develop endotoxemia, leukopenia, severe hypoglycemia, lactic acidemia, and metabolic acidosis. Differential diagnoses include joint ill or navel ill, hypothermia, primary starvation, and infectious enteritis.

Treatment: There is no specific treatment for watery mouth disease. Parenteral antimicrobial and anti-inflammatory therapy combined with oral rehydration are essential; 50–200 mL of an electrolyte and 5%–10% glucose solution containing a water-soluble antibiotic (neomycin and/or streptomycin) given tid by stomach tube will help maintain hydration and provide energy. Systemic antimicrobial therapy with a gram-negative spectrum and anti-inflammatory therapy with NSAIDs or corticosteroids to counteract the effects of endotoxemia should also be administered. Purgatives or enemas may help overcome gut stasis and expel the infecting bacteria. Treatment should be continued until signs resolve and the lamb is sucking again. Boosting body temperature by external warming may also be required. However, such care is time-consuming and expensive and carries no guarantee of success.

Prevention: Ewes should be well nourished to ensure a plentiful supply of colostrum. Yards, pens, ewes, and equipment should be kept as clean as possible throughout lambing to help control the buildup of *E coli* and keep the incidence of disease low. Supplementary feeding of lambs using stored colostrum (ewe, cow, or goat) or commercial colostrum substitute should provide a minimum of 50 mL/kg within 6 hr of birth. Lambs should not be castrated in the first 24 hr because this depresses colostrum intake.

In controlled experiments, a single dose of oral antibiotic given within 2 hr of birth to colostrum-deprived lambs delivered into a contaminated indoor environment was as effective as ewe colostrum in preventing neonatal disease and death in all lambs up to 3 days old, despite the absence of maternal antibodies. Thus, antibiotic treatment can provide simple, quick, and inexpensive protection against watery mouth disease and is an attractive option for the busy sheep farmer. However, it is important that such treatment be targeted to lambs in the high-risk categories specified above, because indiscriminate dosing may encourage antibiotic resistance.

DIARRHEA IN NEONATAL RUMINANTS

(Scours)

Diarrhea is common in newborn calves, lambs, and kids. The clinical presentation can range from mild diarrhea without systemic disease to profuse, acute diarrhea associated with rapid dehydration, severe disturbance of acid-base and electrolyte balance, and death, sometimes in as few as 12 hr. This discussion emphasizes the disease in calves, but the principles of pathophysiology and treatment apply to lambs and kids as well.

Etiology: Several enteropathogens are associated with diarrhea in neonates. Their relative prevalence varies geographically, but the most prevalent infections in most areas are *Escherichia coli*, rotavirus, coronavirus, and *Cryptosporidium parvum*. Cases of neonatal diarrhea are commonly associated with more than one of these agents, and the cause of most outbreaks is multifactorial. Determining the particular agents associated with an outbreak of diarrhea can be important, because specific therapy and prophylaxis are available for some. Also, some agents have zoonotic risk. Diarrhea is also present in septicemic colibacillosis.

Bacteria: *E coli* is the most important bacterial cause of diarrhea in calves during the first week of life; at least two distinct types of diarrheal disease are produced by different strains of this organism. One type is associated with enterotoxigenic *E coli*, which has two virulence factors associated with production of diarrhea. Fimbrial antigens enable them to attach to and colonize the villi of the small intestine of neonatal calves in the first days of life. Strains in calves most commonly possess K99 (F5) or F41 fimbrial antigens, or both. These antigens are the focus of immunologic protection. Enterotoxigenic *E coli* also elaborate a thermostable, nonantigenic enterotoxin (Sta) that influences intestinal ion and fluid secretion to produce a noninflammatory secretory diarrhea. Diarrhea in calves and lambs also has been associated with enteropathogenic *E coli* that adhere to the intestine to produce so-called attaching and effacing lesions, with dissolution of the brush border and loss of microvillous structure at the site of attachment, a decrease in enzyme activity, and changes in ion transport in the intestine. These enteropathogens are also called "attaching and effacing *E coli*." Some produce verotoxin, which may be associated with a more severe hemorrhagic diarrhea. The infection most frequently is in the cecum and colon, but the distal small intestine can also be affected. The damage in severe infections can result in edema and mucosal erosions and ulceration, leading to hemorrhage into the intestinal lumen.

Salmonella spp, especially *S* Typhimurium and *S* Dublin, but occasionally other serovars, cause diarrhea in calves 2–12 wk

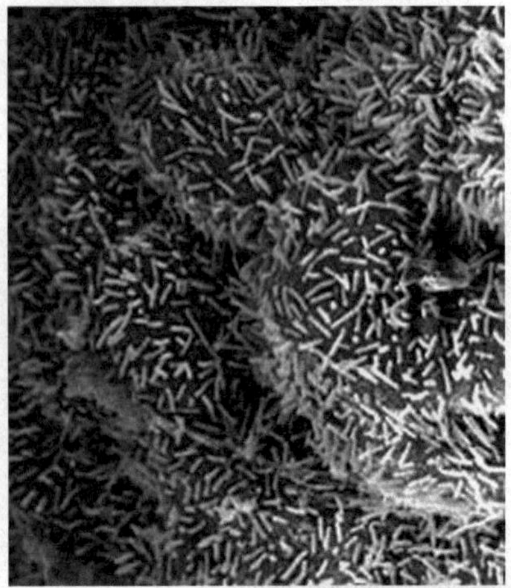

Enterotoxigenic *Escherichia coli* adhering to the intestine of a 2-day-old calf. *Courtesy of Dr. J. J. Hadad and Dr. Carlton Gyles.*

old. Salmonellae produce enterotoxins but are also invasive and produce inflammatory change within the intestine. In calves, infection commonly progresses to a bacteremia. (*See also* SALMONELLOSIS, p 195.)

Clostridium perfringens types A, B, C, and E produce a variety of necrotizing toxins and cause a rapidly fatal hemorrhagic enteritis in calves. The disease in calves is rare and usually sporadic. Infection with type B or C is a common cause of enteritis and dysentery in lambs (*see* p 609).

Campylobacter jejuni and *Yersinia enterocolitica* may be present in the feces of calves and lambs with diarrhea but also may be found in the feces of healthy animals.

Viruses: Rotavirus is the most common viral cause of diarrhea in calves and lambs. Groups A and B rotavirus are involved, but group A is most prevalent and clinically important and contains several serotypes of differing virulence. Rotavirus replicates in the mature absorptive and enzyme-producing enterocytes on the villi of the small intestine, leading to rupture and sloughing of the enterocytes with release of virus to infect adjacent cells. Rotavirus does not infect the immature cells of the crypts. With virulent strains of rotavirus, the loss of enterocytes exceeds the ability of the intestinal crypts to replace them; hence, villous height is reduced, with a consequent decrease in intestinal absorptive surface area and intestinal digestive enzyme activity.

Coronavirus is also commonly associated with diarrhea in calves. It replicates in the epithelium of the upper respiratory tract and in the enterocytes of the intestine, where it produces similar lesions to rotavirus but also infects the epithelial cells of the large intestine to produce atrophy of the colonic ridges.

Other viruses, including Breda virus (torovirus), a calici-like virus, astrovirus, and parvovirus, have been demonstrated in the feces of calves with diarrhea and can produce diarrhea in calves experimentally. However, these agents have also been found in the feces of healthy calves. The importance of these agents in the syndrome of diarrhea in neonates has yet to be determined. The viruses of bovine virus diarrhea and infectious bovine rhinotracheitis are reported to cause calf diarrhea, but this is not a common manifestation of these infections.

Protozoa: *Cryptosporidium parvum* (*see* p 209) is a common cause of diarrhea in calves and lambs. The parasite does not invade but adheres to the apical surface of enterocytes in the distal small intestine and the colon. This results in loss of microvilli, decreased mucosal enzyme activity with villous blunting and fusion (leading to a reduced villous surface absorptive area), and inflammatory changes in the submucosa. Mammalian cryptosporidia lack host specificity.

Giardia duodenalis is a common asymptomatic infection in the intestine of young calves and lambs. It has been found in the feces of poorly growing calves that have a chronic mucoid diarrhea, but there is little evidence for a causative association of this organism with diarrhea in calves or lambs.

Other Causes: Calves fed large amounts of milk or inappropriately formulated milk replacers produce a large volume of feces with a greater than normal fluid content but do not have a fluid diarrhea with weight loss. Similarly, calves sucking high-producing beef cows grazing lush pasture may have loose feces. Milk replacers with poor quality, heat-denatured proteins or with excessive amounts of soybean or fish protein or carbohydrates of nonmilk origin have a higher risk of producing diarrhea.

There is some evidence that oral administration of chloramphenicol, neomycin, or tetracycline to young calves for 3–5 days can result in villous change with resultant malabsorption and mild diarrhea. Prolonged and high-dose antibiotic treatment of calves can lead to diarrhea associated with bacterial superinfection of the intestine. Colisepticemia (*see* p 749) and ruminal drinking (*see* p 236) can also be accompanied by diarrhea.

Epidemiology and Transmission: Enteropathogens associated with diarrhea are commonly found in the feces of healthy calves; whether intestinal infection leads to diarrhea depends on a number of determinants, including differences in virulence of different strains of a pathogen and the presence of more than one pathogen. The resistance of the calf is of major importance and is largely determined by successful passive transfer of colostral immunoglobulins. Colostrum-deprived calves are highly susceptible to infection with enteropathogens and develop severe and often fatal disease.

The progression of infection, the severity of lesions produced, and the severity of the diarrhea can be modulated by immunoglobulins received via colostrum. Immunoglobulins act directly on pathogens in the intestinal lumen during the period of colostrum ingestion as well as after, because significant amounts of circulating immunoglobulins are re-secreted into the intestine, especially when the concentration of circulating immunoglobulin is high. The lack of specific antibodies in dams that have not been exposed to specific pathogens, and the use of specific vaccines, further modulate this influence. Stress caused by a poor environment, inadequate protection from the weather, or an insufficient or inappropriate diet also increases the risk of disease.

With all of the enteropathogens, healthy adult cattle may be carriers and periodically excrete the organism in feces. Excretion may increase around parturition and be more frequent in primiparous cows. This can lead to contaminated calving areas and infection of the udder and perineum of the dam. Other sources of infection include the feces of healthy calves and the feces of diarrheic calves, which contain large numbers of organisms early in the course of infection. A few scouring calves can result in severe contamination of the calf-rearing area. Transmission is by fecal-oral contact, fecal aerosol, and, in the case of coronavirus, by respiratory aerosol.

Pathogenesis: Diarrhea in neonatal ruminants is usually associated with disease of the small intestine and can be caused by hypersecretion or malabsorption. Hypersecretory diarrhea develops when an abnormal amount of fluid is secreted into the gut, exceeding the resorptive capacity of the mucosa. In malabsorptive diarrhea, the capacity of the mucosa to absorb fluid and nutrients is impaired to the extent that it cannot keep up with the normal influx of ingested and secreted fluids. This is usually the result of villous atrophy, in which the loss of mature enterocytes at the tips of the villi results both in a decrease in villous height (with a consequent decrease in the surface area for absorption) and in loss of the brush border digestive enzymes. The extent and distribution of villous atrophy varies with different pathogens and can explain variation in the severity of clinical disease. Malabsorptive diarrhea may be aggravated by the colonic fermentation of nutrients that normally would have been absorbed in the small intestine. Fermentation products, especially lactic acid, appear to draw water into the colon osmotically, which contributes to the severity of diarrhea.

Inflammation contributes to the pathophysiology of diarrhea in most intestinal infections, and mediators of inflammation can affect ion flux within the intestine. Inflammation also leads to vascular and lymphatic damage and to structural damage of the crypt-villus unit. Most infectious forms of diarrhea have hypersecretory, inflammatory, and malabsorptive components, although one usually predominates. These lead to a net loss of water, sodium, potassium, and bicarbonate; if severe, the calf develops hypovolemia, hyponatremia, acidemia, and prerenal azotemia.

Enterotoxigenic *E coli* produce the enterotoxin Sta, which stimulates marked hypersecretion by activating guanylate cyclase and by inducing a net secretion of sodium and chlorine. The membrane-bound sodium-glucose cotransport system remains functional but cannot compensate for the increased secretory activity. Salmonellae also elaborate enterotoxins. Inflammation, leading to necrosis of the enterocyte, submucosal inflammatory infiltration, and villous atrophy, is also a major component of the pathophysiology of diarrhea produced by salmonellae, as well as of diarrhea produced by enteropathogenic *E coli* and by toxigenic *C perfringens*. Infections with verotoxin-producing enteropathogenic *E coli* result in accumulation of fluid within the large intestine and extensive damage to the large intestinal mucosa, with edema, hemorrhage, and erosion and ulceration of the mucosa, which results in blood and mucus in the lumen.

Viruses usually produce a malabsorptive diarrhea by destroying the absorptive cells of the mucosa, thus shortening the intestinal villi. The mechanism by which cryptosporidia produce diarrhea is not completely understood, but it appears to have both malabsorptive and inflammatory components.

Inappropriately formulated milk replacers produce diarrhea by two mechanisms, both associated with malabsorption. Vegetable (especially soybean) products are commonly used as protein sources in the manufacture of milk replacers. Depending on the degree of refinement, these products may contain carbohydrates that are indigestible in young calves. Such carbohydrates are not absorbed in the small intestine and may contribute to diarrhea via colonic fermentation. In addition, most calves <3 wk old appear to have an allergic reaction to soy proteins that results in villous atrophy, leading to diarrhea that is probably malabsorptive.

Clinical Findings: The major signs are diarrhea, dehydration, profound weakness, and death within one to several days of onset.

Diarrhea due to enterotoxigenic (K99-bearing) *E coli* is seen in calves <3–5 days old, rarely later. However, the age of susceptibility may be extended in the presence of other pathogens. Onset is sudden. Profuse amounts of liquid feces are passed, and the calves rapidly become depressed and recumbent. Calves may lose >12% of body weight in fluid, and hypovolemic shock and death may occur in 12–24 hr. Body temperature may be increased but is commonly normal or subnormal. If fluid and electrolyte therapy is administered early, response is usually good. Disease produced by attaching and effacing *E coli* is seen predominantly in calves from 4 days to 2 mo old and may manifest with diarrhea or primarily as dysentery with blood and mucus in the feces. The clinical course is short.

Diarrhea due to *Salmonella* spp usually is not seen in calves <14 days old. It is characterized by feces that are foul smelling and contain blood, fibrin, and copious amounts of mucus. Septicemia, with high fever and depression progressing to prostration and coma, is the salient manifestation of salmonellosis in calves and, although diarrhea is present, death is usually from septicemic rather than from hypovolemic shock. Calves with salmonellosis usually lose weight rapidly and often die despite vigorous therapy.

Hemorrhagic enterotoxemia due to *C perfringens* type B or C is characterized by acute onset of depression, weakness, bloody diarrhea, abdominal pain, and death within a few hours. It usually develops in vigorous calves just a few days old that have large appetites and a ready source of milk. Calves affected with *C perfringens* usually die before treatment can be instituted.

Diarrhea due to rotavirus, coronavirus, and other viruses usually is seen in calves 5–15 days old but can affect calves up to several months of age. Affected calves are only moderately depressed and often continue to suck or drink milk. The feces are voluminous, soft to liquid, and often contain large amounts of mucus. Diarrhea commonly persists for 3 to several days, with some cases of coronaviral diarrhea becoming chronic. Cases of viral diarrhea that are uncomplicated by other pathogens commonly respond within a few days to fluid and electrolyte therapy and adequate nutritional support.

Cryptosporidiosis (*see* p 209) is seen in calves 5–35 days old but most commonly in the second week of life. It is characterized by persistent diarrhea that does not respond to therapy. Diarrhea due solely to *Cryptosporidium* spp is often mild and self-limiting, although the severity may be related to the general strength of the calf and to the intensity of challenge with the organism. Combination infections with cryptosporidia, rotavirus, and coronavirus are common and result in persistent diarrhea often characterized by emaciation and death. Death from hypoglycemia also occurs as a sequela of cryptosporidiosis in calves 3–4 wk of age that have recovered from diarrhea but are still emaciated. Death often occurs during a bout of cold weather and is more likely to occur on farms where there is a policy of reducing the amount of milk fed to calves during periods of diarrhea.

Dietary diarrheas are seen in calves <3 wk old and are characterized by voluminous feces of pasty to gelatinous consistency. Initially, the calves are bright and alert and have good appetites. Eventually, however, they become weak and emaciated if the diet is not corrected. Infectious forms of diarrhea are often complicated by poor-quality diets or insufficient nutritional intake.

Diagnosis: It is difficult to make a definite etiologic diagnosis for diarrhea based solely on clinical findings. However, the history, age of the animal(s) affected, and clinical signs may permit a presumptive diagnosis.

Fecal samples can be submitted for isolation and characterization of the common enteropathogens. Samples should be taken from several untreated calves in the early stages of diarrhea. Special techniques are necessary for the demonstration of viruses, cryptosporidia, and K99-bearing *E coli*. The interpretation of fecal microbiology can be difficult because of mixed infections and because enteropathogens are commonly present in the feces of healthy calves.

The best diagnostic information is usually obtained by submitting untreated, acutely affected animals for necropsy. This allows examination of intestinal mucosa for evidence of diagnostic lesions and for the presence of enteropathogens such as cryptosporidia. It may be the only way that disease such as that associated with attaching and effacing strains of *E coli* can be diagnosed. The diagnostic value of a necropsy diminishes quickly with time after death; important lesions can disappear within minutes due to autolysis.

Complete laboratory examination can be expensive, and it has also been argued that there is little value in expending large amounts of money on diagnosis unless there are specific control procedures that can be implemented based on the information gained. In all cases, information on total milk or milk replacer consumption should be obtained. When milk replacer is being fed, the composition of the diet should be evaluated. Nonspecific immunity should be assessed by determining immunoglobulin and vitamin A concentrations in serum.

Treatment: Many of the factors involved in disease resistance are nonspecific; thus, important preventive measures can be taken and therapy can be started before an etiologic diagnosis has been established. Treatment includes fluid therapy for water and electrolyte replacement and correction of acid-base disturbances, alteration of the diet, and antimicrobial and anti-inflammatory therapy.

Fluid and electrolyte therapy is most important and should be started as soon as possible regardless of whether clinical evidence of dehydration has developed (clinical signs of dehydration are not apparent until the calf has lost at least 6% of its body weight in fluid). Calves still able to stand and willing and able to suck can often be treated with oral electrolyte solutions alone. Fluids for oral rehydration should promote the cotransport of sodium with glucose and amino acids and should contain sodium, glucose, glycine or alanine, potassium, and either bicarbonate or citrate or acetate as alkalinizing agents. Several commercial preparations are available. These can be administered by nipple bottle or, if necessary, by stomach tube. The solutions should be used liberally until the animal is rehydrated.

Whether milk should be fed during the rehydration period remains controversial. Feeding milk may increase fecal volume, but it provides energy to the calf and may promote gut healing. Calves have large energy requirements and little reserve. Electrolyte solutions do not meet calf energy requirements, and milk should not be withheld for >24 hr, if at all.

Calves that are recumbent, weak, and show evidence of water loss of ≥8% of their body weight require IV fluid therapy. These calves are usually acidotic, and the fluid and base deficits can be corrected initially by rapidly administering a hypertonic solution of sodium bicarbonate (either 500 mL of a 4.2% solution, or 250 mL of an 8.4% solution), followed by a physiologically balanced electrolyte solution administered at up to 40 mL/kg/hr until the volume deficit is corrected. Because diarrheic calves are frequently hypoglycemic, adding 25–50 g of dextrose to the electrolyte solution is often beneficial in the initial treatment phase. Oral electrolyte solutions should be used concurrently with and after IV fluid therapy to compensate for ongoing fluid and electrolyte losses.

Although mild diarrhea without systemic disease is not an indication for antimicrobial therapy, use of parenteral antibiotics should be considered whenever calves are systemically ill or recumbent. Field studies revealed that at least 30% of diarrheic calves with systemic disease are bacteremic—a clear indication for parenteral antimicrobial therapy. Because the large majority of cases of bacteremia and septicemia in neonatal calves are associated with *E coli*, the chosen antibiotic should be effective against gram-negative bacteria.

In several studies, severely affected diarrheic calves treated with NSAIDs in conjunction with fluid therapy showed fewer signs of pain, made a faster recovery, and had better weight gains in the reconvalescent period. These effects reported for several NSAIDs have been attributed to their analgesic, anti-inflammatory, antipyretic, and antisecretory properties.

The use of drugs to reduce intestinal motility such as hyoscine-N-butylbromide or atropine is sometimes advocated, because they decrease fecal output. Although reducing fecal production may be interpreted as a positive treatment outcome, it can also be seen as sequestration of gut fluid containing bacteria, toxins, and undigested nutrients in the intestinal tract. The literature does not provide any strong supportive evidence for or against the use of antimotility drugs.

Intestinal gels and adsorbents, such as kaolin and pectin, are in general use, but their only established effect is to increase fecal consistency; they do not reduce the loss of water and ions.

Prevention and Control: Because of the complex nature of diarrhea in neonates, it is unrealistic to expect total prevention—economical control is the major objective. The incidence of clinical disease and the case fatality rate depend on the balance between the levels of exposure to infectious agents and the resistance in the calf. Differences in herd size; availability of facilities, land, and labor; and general management objectives make it impossible to recommend specific management procedures applicable to all situations. However, three broad principles apply in all herds: 1) the degree of exposure of neonates should be reduced by isolating diseased animals or by moving calving and calf rearing to a separate area, and by practicing good general hygiene; 2) nonspecific resistance should be maximized by providing good nutrition to the dam and neonate and assuring that newborn calves consume ≥5% of their body wt of high-quality colostrum, preferably within 2 hr and certainly within 6 hr of birth, followed by equivalent amounts at 12-hr intervals for the next 48 hr; and 3) the specific resistance of the newborn should be increased by vaccinating the dam or the newborn. A significant portion of both naturally sucking dairy calves and calves handfed colostrum do not acquire adequate amounts of immunoglobulin because of delayed sucking or feeding, ingestion of an inadequate volume of colostrum, or ingestion of colostrum of inferior immunoglobulin concentration. When time constraints on labor preclude an ensured intake of colostrum by nipple-bottle feeding, administration of 4 L of colostrum by esophageal feeder within the first 2 hr of life can be the best colostrum feeding policy. (*See also* MANAGEMENT OF REPRODUCTION: CATTLE, p 2171.)

Immunization of calves against colibacillosis by vaccination of pregnant dams can control enterotoxigenic colibacillosis. The pregnant dam is vaccinated 6 and 2 wk before parturition to stimulate antibodies to strains of enterotoxigenic *E coli*; these antibodies are then passed on to the newborn through the colostrum (provided the calf ingests it). A single booster is given in subsequent years. Monoclonal K99 *E coli* antibody is commercially available for oral administration to calves immediately after birth. It is an effective substitute for the K99-specific antibody in the colostrum of vaccinated cows, although calves that receive this product should also receive colostrum for its nonspecific protection.

Vaccination of pregnant cows with rotavirus and coronavirus vaccines increase the amount of specific antibody in colostrum and milk, but the concentration of antibodies in milk may be insufficient to provide local antibody in the intestinal lumen during the period of peak prevalence of infection, which, in calves, is 5–15 days of age. Controlled trials of commercial vaccines have shown variable results. The addition of small amounts of immune colostrum to milk fed during the period of susceptibility can provide some protection against disease.

Zoonotic Risk: Several of the agents that produce diarrhea in calves can also produce diarrheal disease in people. *Cryptosporidium parvum* and *S* Typhimurium can produce serious disease, particularly in immunocompromised individuals. These organisms are commonly present as subclinical infections in the gut of calves and lambs; immunocompromised people should avoid contact with young ruminants and possibly all farm animals.

Cattle, including calves, are one of the reservoirs for the verotoxic *E coli* serotype O157:H7 associated with human hemorrhagic colitis and the hemolytic uremic syndrome. Infection in people is usually acquired by consumption of contaminated food, but the infective dose is low and the possibility of infection by direct contact exists. Other verotoxic *E coli* associated with human disease can also be isolated from the feces of healthy cattle. Human disease from infection with enteric livestock pathogens has occurred after seemingly trivial contact associated with visits to livestock fairs, petting zoos, and farm educational tours. Hand cleansing and disinfection should be a component of these visits.

INTESTINAL DISEASES IN HORSES AND FOALS

Intestinal disease in horses and foals is suggested by diarrhea, weight loss, hypoproteinemia, and abdominal pain. (*See also* COLIC IN HORSES, p 248.)

DIARRHEAL DISEASE IN HORSES

A definitive cause of diarrhea can be determined in <50% of cases. Yet, treatment of most horses and foals with diarrhea is similar and thus allows supportive therapeutic management despite the lack of a definitive diagnosis.

Diarrhea in adult horses can be acute or chronic. Infectious agents that have been cited as potential causes of acute diarrhea in adult horses include numerous *Salmonella* serovars, *Neorickettsia risticii*, *Clostridium difficile*, *C perfringens*, *Aeromonas* spp, coronavirus, and cyathostomiasis. Other differential diagnoses for acute diarrhea in horses include ingestion of a toxicant(s), antimicrobial-induced colitis, NSAID toxicity, and sand enterocolopathy. An acute, fatal diarrheal disease of unknown etiology is known as colitis-X. Diarrhea that persists >1 mo is considered chronic and is often a diagnostic challenge. Chronic diarrhea can be caused by inflammatory or neoplastic conditions involving the intestine or by disruption of the normal physiologic process in the bowel. Differential diagnoses include sand enterocolopathy and infiltrative lesions, such as those associated with inflammatory bowel disease or intestinal lymphosarcoma. The body's response to certain components of feed may play a role in chronic diarrhea of horses due to bowel inflammation but has not frequently been established as a cause.

Noninflammatory conditions of the colon can also result in diarrhea. These include altered fermentation in the large colon, which is potentially the result of altered intestinal flora or milieu secondary to antimicrobial treatment, alteration in diet, or unknown etiologies. Nonintestinal causes of chronic diarrhea include congestive heart failure and chronic liver disease. The diagnostic approach to these cases is aimed at differentiation of infiltrative diseases of the intestine from physiologic causes of diarrhea.

Because of the large volume of the colon and cecum of horses, massive fluid losses can occur in a short time. Thus, diarrhea in adult horses can be an explosive event with morbidity and mortality exceeding that associated with diarrheal diseases in other animals and people.

SALMONELLOSIS

Salmonellosis (*see* p 195) is one of the most commonly diagnosed infectious causes of diarrhea in adult horses. Clinical manifestations range from no abnormal clinical signs (subclinical carrier) to acute, severe diarrhea and even death. The disease is seen sporadically but may become an epidemic, depending on the virulence of the organism, level of exposure, and host factors. Infection can occur via contamination of the environment, feed, or water or by contact with animals actively shedding the bacteria. Stress appears to play an important role in the pathogenesis—a history of surgery, transportation, or change in feed; concurrent disease, particularly GI disorders (colic); or treatment with broad-spectrum antimicrobial drugs often precedes the diarrhea.

Salmonella enterica of the serogroup B includes *S enterica* serovar Typhimurium and *S enterica* Agona, two of the most frequently isolated serovars from horses with clinical disease. Knowing the serovar and antibiogram can help track or monitor the type of serovar of salmonellae affecting any given group or population of horses (eg, tracking nosocomial spread within a veterinary hospital). The emergence of multidrug-resistant *S enterica* isolates is concerning both in dealing with nosocomial infections and zoonosis.

Clinical Findings: Three forms of salmonellosis have been recognized in adult horses. One is the subclinical carrier, which may or may not be actively shedding the organism but has the potential to transmit the bacteria to susceptible animals either by direct contact or by contamination of the environment, water, or feed sources. Multiple fecal cultures may be necessary to identify carriers, because the organism is shed in the feces intermittently and in small numbers. If stressed, the carrier may develop clinical disease. The national prevalence of fecal shedding of *S enterica* by normal horses in the USA is estimated to be <2%; however, the proportion of hospitalized horses shedding is much higher (~8%). The most common serovars identified among the general population of horses were *S enterica* Muenchen and *S enterica* Newport (both serogroup C2).

The second form of the disease is characterized by a mild clinical course, with signs of depression, fever, anorexia, and soft but not watery feces. Affected horses may have an absolute neutropenia. Clinical disease may last 4–5 days and usually is self-limiting, and *S enterica* can be isolated from the feces. Recovered horses may continue to excrete the organism in their feces for days to months; therefore, isolation of the shedding horse and thorough cleaning and subsequent disinfection of the contaminated area are recommended.

The third form of salmonellosis is characterized by an acute onset of severe depression, anorexia, profound neutropenia, and frequently abdominal pain. Diarrhea develops 6–24 hr after the onset of fever; feces are fluid and foul smelling. Affected horses dehydrate rapidly, and metabolic acidosis and electrolyte losses occur as the horse deteriorates. Clinical signs of sepsis and hypovolemic shock can progress rapidly. There may be signs of abdominal discomfort, straining, or severe colic secondary to ileus, gas distension, and colonic inflammation and possible infarction. Protein-losing enterocolopathy can occur with plasma protein concentrations becoming dangerously low (albumin <2 g/dL) after a few days of diarrhea. These horses can become bacteremic because of bacterial translocation of enteric organisms, and coagulation abnormalities resulting in disseminated intravascular coagulation can occur. If untreated, this form of salmonellosis is often fatal.

Salmonella bacteremia can occur in neonatal foals, especially from farms with endemic salmonellosis (*see* p 289).

Diagnosis: Diagnosis is based on clinical signs, severe neutropenia, and isolation of salmonellae from feces, blood, or tissues. Submission of 10–30 g of feces for culture has been more successful in identifying salmonellae than has culturing fecal swabs. It is important to collect and submit feces based on the recommendations of the laboratory performing the culture. Working with a diagnostic laboratory that uses enrichment techniques along with agars specifically selected to optimize recovery of *S enterica* is advisable. Because salmonellae cannot be consistently cultured from feces, multiple daily samples (generally 3–5) should be collected from each horse. Culturing of rectal mucosal biopsies increases the probability of isolating the organism; however, the technique is not without risk to the horse. Fecal samples that must be mailed should be placed in transport media suitable for enteric pathogens at the time of collection and shipped on ice. A PCR test is available and, depending on the primers used, appears to be more sensitive than routine bacterial culture for detection of salmonellae.

Treatment: Treatment of the severe form of salmonellosis is based on IV fluid and electrolyte replacement and efforts to control the host's responses initiated by the systemic inflammatory response. A polyionic isotonic fluid is used for volume replacement. Because of active secretion of fluid and electrolytes into the lumen of the intestine, IV fluid volumes of 40–80 L/day may be necessary. Electrolyte and acid-base deficiencies are common and are corrected by use of oral and/or IV fluids supplemented with electrolytes. It is difficult to predict the electrolyte status of affected horses. Deficits should be determined by serum biochemical analysis; supplementation with sodium chloride, potassium chloride, calcium gluconate, magnesium sulfate, and occasionally sodium bicarbonate may be indicated.

Antimicrobial treatment in adult horses with salmonellosis is controversial and does not appear to alter the course of the colitis or decrease shedding of salmonellae; however, it may reduce the likelihood of bacteremia. Selection of an antimicrobial is not easy and should ideally be based on the sensitivity of the organism isolated. Resistance patterns vary among *Salmonella* isolates and can change over the course of an outbreak. There is potential nephrotoxicosis from aminoglycoside antibiotics in volume-depleted horses; therefore, the hydration status of the horse should be considered when selecting an antimicrobial The ideal antibiotic should also be lipid soluble.

The use of GI protectants (eg, biosponge, bismuth subsalicylate, activated charcoal) may be beneficial. These substances may bind bacterial toxins. NSAIDs, such as flunixin meglumine, help counteract the effect of endotoxin, control pain, and possibly help prevent laminitis. The dosage of NSAID used has been quite variable. Serious adverse effects, such as gastric and colonic ulceration and renal nephrotoxicosis, can result from NSAID treatment, so the minimum effective dosage should be used. Equine plasma may be administered to correct hypoproteinemia and to supply coagulation factors and, depending on the source of the plasma, specific antibodies to endotoxin and *Salmonella*. Colloidal plasma substitutes such as hetastarch may be necessary to maintain oncotic pressure in horses with substantial protein loss into the GI tract. These colloidal plasma substitutes may be less expensive and better tolerated than equine plasma in some horses. Often, equine plasma and colloidal plasma substitutes are both used in horses with hypoproteinemia due to colitis.

Low-dose polymyxin B (6,000 units/kg, bid) has also been advocated to bind circulating endotoxin. In controlled trials, polymyxin B ameliorated some of the known effects of endotoxemia in horses. Antimicrobial doses of polymyxin B are substantially higher than the dose used to bind endotoxin and may be nephrotoxic. Low-dose polymyxin B therapy is unlikely to be nephrotoxic in adequately hydrated horses receiving IV fluids.

Prevention: Prevention of salmonellosis is difficult, because the organism is present in the environment as well as in the feces of some healthy animals. In a hospital environment where horses are stressed, may be off feed, and are often receiving antimicrobial treatment, aggressive identification and strict isolation of salmonellae-infected horses is indicated. Biosecurity practices to minimize cross-contamination between hospitalized horses are also advisable. Serotyping, antimicrobial susceptibility profiles and genotyping by pulse field electrophoresis, plasmid profile analysis, and phage typing can be used to determine whether isolates are genetically related and help determine whether infection is nosocomial.

Owners should be made aware of the zoonotic risk of *S enterica* infection. People working with infected animals should practice strict hygiene.

POTOMAC HORSE FEVER

(Equine monocytic ehrlichiosis, Ditch fever, Shasta River crud, Equine ehrlichial colitis)

Potomac horse fever (PHF) is an acute enterocolitis syndrome producing mild colic, fever, and diarrhea in horses of all ages, as well as abortion in pregnant mares. The causative agent is *Neorickettsia ristícii*. The infection of enterocytes of the small and large intestine results in acute colitis, which is one of the principal clinical signs of PHF. The disease is seen in spring, summer, and early fall and is associated with pastures bordering creeks or rivers. The epidemiology of PHF has been shown to involve a trematode vector. Sporadic disease caused by *N risticii* has been reported in dogs and cats; cattle appear to be resistant to infection. PHF has been reported in many areas of the USA and Canada using an indirect fluorescent antibody test as evidence of exposure; however, recent studies indicate a high rate of false-positive titers with this test, and the true geographic range of distribution is not known. Isolation or detection of the causative agent from clinical cases of PHF using conventional cell culture or PCR assay has been reported only from California, Illinois, Indiana, Kentucky, Maryland, Michigan, New York, New Jersey, Ohio, Oregon, Pennsylvania, Texas, and Virginia.

Etiology and Pathogenesis: *N risticii* is a gram-negative obligate intracellular bacterium with a trophism for monocytes. Initial morphologic studies of this organism isolated from cell culture, as well as the serologic responses of *N risticii*, caused this bacterium to be assigned to the genus *Ehrlichia*. However, DNA analyses have shown *N risticii* is most closely related to *N helminthoeca*, the agent of salmon poisoning in dogs, and *Ehrlichia sennetsu*, a disease of people in Japan. The organism is not visible in monocytes in blood films from clinical cases, in contrast to *Anaplasma phagocytophilum*, which is readily identifiable in granulocytes of infected horses.

N risticii has been identified in freshwater snails and isolated from trematodes released from the snails. *N risticii* DNA was detected in 13 species of immature and adult caddisflies (Trichoptera), mayflies (Ephemeroptera), damselflies (Odonata, Zygoptera), dragonflies (Odonata, Anisoptera), and stoneflies (Plecoptera). Transmission studies using *N risticii*–infected caddisflies have reproduced the clinical disease. One route of exposure is believed to be inadvertent ingestion of hatched aquatic insects that carry *N risticii* in the metacercarial stage of a trematode. The incubation period is ~10–18 days. The causative organism is present in the feces of experimentally infected horses, but the biologic significance of this is unknown. Clinically ill horses are not contagious and can be housed with susceptible horses. Additional studies are needed to determine the exact role of the vector and helminth hosts in the complex maintenance cycle of *N ristícii*.

Clinical Findings and Lesions: The clinical features of PHF are typified initially by mild depression and anorexia, followed by a fever of 102°–107°F (38.9°–41.7°C). At this stage, intestinal sounds may be decreased. Within 24–48 hr, a moderate to severe diarrhea, with feces ranging in consistency from that usually seen in cows to watery, develops in ~60% of affected horses. The onset of diarrhea is often accompanied by mild abdominal discomfort. Some horses develop severe signs of sepsis and dehydration. Clinical signs can be indistinguishable from those of *Salmonella* and other infectious causes of enterocolitis. Laminitis can supervene as a severe complication of PHF in 20%–30% of affected horses. Hematologic findings vary in the early stage of PHF from leukopenia (characterized by neutropenia and lymphopenia) and thrombocytopenia to a normal hemogram, despite evidence of systemic illness. A common finding in cases of PHF is a marked leukocytosis, which is normally seen within a few days of onset. PHF may present with all or any combination of these clinical signs.

Several months after clinical disease in pregnant mares, abortion due to fetal infection with *N risticii* may occur. Experimentally, pregnant mares infected at 100–160 days of gestation abort at 190–250 days of gestation. The abortion is accompanied by placentitis and retained placenta. Fetal lesions include colitis, periportal hepatitis, and lymphoid hyperplasia of mesenteric lymph nodes and spleen. Necropsy findings in nonpregnant horses with enterocolitis are nonspecific and reveal diffuse inflammation, mainly in the large intestines.

Diagnosis: A provisional diagnosis of PHF often is based on the presence of typical clinical signs and on the seasonal and geographic occurrence of the disease. A definitive diagnosis should be based on isolation or identification of *N risticii* from the blood or feces of infected horses by cell culture or PCR. Serologic testing is of limited value as a diagnostic tool, although many infected horses have high antibody titers at the time of infection. Because of the high prevalence of false-positive titers, interpretation of the indirect fluorescent antibody test in individual horses is difficult. Rising paired titers can be helpful. Isolation of the agent in cell culture, although possible, is time-consuming and not routinely available in many diagnostic laboratories. A real-time PCR assay that allows detection of *N risticii* DNA within 2 hr is a much more feasible test for routine diagnostic examination. To enhance the chances of detection of *N risticii*, the assay should be performed both on blood and fecal samples, because the presence of the organism in blood and feces may not necessarily coincide.

Treatment: Horses with PHF can be treated successfully with oxytetracycline (6.6 mg/kg, IV, bid), if given early in the clinical course of the disease. A response to treatment is usually seen within 12 hr. This is associated with a drop in rectal temperature, followed by an improvement in demeanor, appetite, and borborygmal sounds. If therapy is begun early, clinical signs frequently resolve by the third day of treatment. Generally, antimicrobial therapy is for no more than 5 days. In animals that exhibit signs of enterocolitis, fluids and NSAIDs should be administered. Laminitis is more common than in other causes of enterocolitis, and if it develops, is usually severe and often refractory to treatment. The overall case fatality rate is 5%–30%.

Prevention: Several inactivated, whole-cell vaccines based on the same strain of *N risticii* are commercially available. Although vaccination has been reported to protect 78% of experimentally infected ponies, it has been marginally protective in the field. Vaccine failure has been attributed to antigenic and genomic heterogeneity among the >14 different strains of *N risticii* isolated from naturally occurring cases. Furthermore, vaccine failure may also be due to lack of antibody protection at the site of exposure, because the natural route of transmission has been determined to be oral ingestion of the agent. Minimizing insect ingestion in stabled horses by turning off barn lights at night, which normally attract the insects, has been suggested.

No zoonotic risk is known.

CLOSTRIDIA-ASSOCIATED ENTEROCOLITIS

Clostridium difficile and *C perfringens* are common causes of enterocolitis in horses and foals. Antimicrobial administration has been associated with *C difficile* diarrhea. Some reports attribute 50% of cases of foal diarrhea to *C perfringens*. *C difficile* produces toxin A and/or toxin B, which cause fluid secretion and lead to intestinal inflammation. It is common for the GI tract of newborn foals to be rapidly colonized by *C difficile*, which can be cultured from feces using sensitive anaerobic techniques. Nontoxin-producing strains are considered commensals. *C difficile* can be isolated from various segments of the small and large intestine and rectum of a large proportion of healthy horses, and from fecal samples of as many as 8% of healthy horses. Approximately one-third of healthy broodmares and >90% of foals in the general population shed *C perfringens* in their feces; therefore, it is important to determine the presence of a toxin-producing strain.

Strains of *C perfringens* are classified by the toxins they produce. However, toxins and toxin-producing strains of *C perfringens* and *C difficile* can be detected in healthy as well as in diarrheic horses and foals. The most common type of *C perfringens* identified is type A, which can be detected in the feces of as many as 8% of healthy horses. Type C is rarely identified in the feces or environment of healthy broodmares and their foals but is associated with the highest mortality. Antimicrobial use, food deprivation, and other stressors have been suggested to predispose horses to the overgrowth of either or both *C perfringens* and *C difficile*, leading to GI disease. In one report, mares whose foals were being treated with erythromycin developed fatal enterocolitis associated with *C difficile*. Clostridial spores can persist in the environment and can be resistant to many disinfectants; therefore, nosocomial infection can occur in contaminated environments.

Clinical Findings: Clinical signs include sudden death, diarrhea with or without blood, colic, fever, reduced feed intake, and lethargy. Disease can range from subclinical to severe enterocolitis to peracute death before the development of diarrhea. With advanced diagnostic techniques, clostridial infections account for a large proportion of the previously undiagnosed cases known as "colitis-X." Because of the loss of mucosal integrity, bacterial translocation across the GI tract can occur, resulting in bacteremia due to clostridial or other enteric bacterial species. Clinical signs of sepsis or systemic inflammatory response are often present and consistent with other causes of enterocolitis. Clostridiosis cannot be clinically distinguished from salmonellosis. Foals affected at <3 days of age with *C perfringens*–associated enterocolitis often have bloody diarrhea and colic. Fluid and gas-filled intestine is often identified on ultrasound or radiography. In severe cases, necrotizing enterocolitis occurs with thickening and even intramural gas evident within the wall of the intestine. Several foals on a particular farm may be affected, but the disease is typically sporadic.

The role of *C perfringens* type A in enterocolitis in neonatal foals is less clear; it has been reported that >90% of foals at 3 days of age shed this organism in their feces and that *C perfringens* type A is likely one of the first bacteria to colonize the intestinal tract of newborn foals, irrespective of hygiene protocols.

C difficile has been associated with enterocolitis in newborn foals as well as in adult horses. It has been identified as a nosocomial infection in people, and this may also be seen in horses.

The mortality rate associated with *C difficile* and *C perfringens* enterocolitis, especially type C, can be high, even with intensive medical treatment.

Diagnosis: Diagnosis is based on identification of toxigenic clostridia from fresh fecal samples, reflux, intestinal contents, or tissue. Blood culture is indicated in foals and adults with severe enterocolitis. Fecal samples for culture and detection of toxins or toxin-producing genes should be delivered directly to the laboratory, or shipped overnight, chilled (not frozen) on ice. Samples for culture must be maintained in an anaerobic environment. Isolation of clostridial organisms requires anaerobic conditions and, depending on the organism, special growth media. *C difficile* is inherently difficult to culture, hence its name. Communicating to the laboratory that clostridial enterocolitis is a differential diagnosis is critical, because many veterinary laboratories do not routinely culture fecal samples anaerobically unless specifically requested to do so.

Because nonpathogenic serovars are common, a positive culture for *C difficile* or *C perfringens* must be confirmed by identification of toxins or their genes. A PCR test, available at selected laboratories, allows differentiation of *C perfringens* types A, B, C, D, and E based on combinations of α, β, ε, or ι toxins, as well as on identification of the gene coding for the β2 toxin. Commercially available tests for clostridial toxins include an ELISA for *C difficile* toxin A and *C perfringens* enterotoxin, and a latex agglutination test for *C perfringens* enterotoxin. Toxin tests can be performed in-house, are rapid, and for *C difficile* are both sensitive and specific. Diagnosis of clostridial enterocolitis is often made at necropsy and is based primarily on identification of intestinal necrosis associated with large gram-positive rods in intestinal smears. Tissue and fecal specimens must be taken immediately after death to avoid degradation of toxins or an overgrowth of clostridial organisms.

Treatment: Treatment with metronidazole (15–20 mg/kg, PO, tid-qid) appears to be beneficial in treating enteric clostridial infections. Pharmacokinetic studies have not been performed in foals, but oral and even IV metronidazole appears generally safe. In some geographic regions, metronidazole-resistant *C difficile* strains have emerged that appear sensitive to vancomycin; however, metronidazole should be used whenever possible.

Supportive care is similar to that for other causes of equine enterocolitis, often requiring large volumes of IV polyionic fluids, with supplemental electrolytes (potassium, magnesium, and calcium), plasma or synthetic colloids for low oncotic pressure, anti-inflammatories such as flunixin meglumine, and broad-spectrum antibiotics if the horse is leukopenic and at risk of bacterial translocation across the compromised GI tract. Polymyxin B may aid in binding systemic endotoxin. Total or partial parenteral nutrition to provide nutritional support can be useful in foals if milk is withheld or decreased to allow gut rest. Foals with colic or profuse diarrhea often benefit from milk withdrawal. Continuous infusion of IV fluids and parenteral nutritional support is optimal but labor intensive and requires separation of the foal and mare. However, the course of diarrhea appears to be dramatically shortened, thus justifying the more intensive approach in some severe cases.

The yeast *Saccharomyces boulardii* has been shown to be protective in clostridial diarrhea in other species, and there is some evidence of beneficial effects in the treatment of horses with colitis. It produces a protease that specifically degrades *C difficile* toxins A and B. Orally administered DTO smectite powder also blinds clostridial toxins and may be useful in horses with diarrhea.

Specific antitoxin for *C perfringens* type C and D has also been used in foals; however, it is not approved for this use. The benefit of type C and D antitoxin in disease associated with type A or β2 toxin is unknown, but based on production methods, the α and β2 toxins are unlikely to be present in high levels in this toxoid.

Prevention: No proven effective biologic products are available to immunize horses or foals against clostridial enterocolitis. When the disease is a problem in multiple foals on a farm, preventive measures have been implemented, but the efficacy and safety of these interventions have yet to be critically evaluated. These measures include vaccinating pregnant mares twice at 2- to 4-wk intervals at least 1 mo before foaling with *C perfringens* type C and D toxoid (bacterin products and those with oil adjuvants should be avoided); using *C perfringens* type C and D antitoxin prophylactically, PO, in newborn foals; and administering antimicrobials (eg, metronidazole) prophylactically to foals for the first 3–5 days of life. The *C perfringens* type C and D toxoid and antitoxin are not approved for use in horses; however, these products have been used by some owners because of the high mortality rate in foals with clostridial enterocolitis on problem farms. Adverse reactions to the *C perfringens* type C and D toxoid have been reported in broodmares.

The most important strategy for prevention is good farm hygiene. Clostridial spores are extremely resilient in the environment and resistant to many disinfectants. Keeping the foaling area and mare as clean as possible during the perinatal period and ensuring rapid ingestion (by stomach tube if necessary) of colostrum within 1 hr of birth have reduced incidence of disease on some contaminated farms. The mare's hindlegs, tail, and udder can also be washed in soapy water immediately after foaling to decrease ingestion of fecal material by newborn foals. Affected animals should be isolated to limit cross-infection and contamination of pastures and stalls.

COLITIS-X

Colitis-X is not actually a disease but a historic term used to describe undiagnosed causes of peracute, fatal enterocolitis in horses characterized by sudden onset of profuse, watery diarrhea and development of hypovolemic shock. Many affected horses have a history of stress. Differential diagnoses include peracute salmonellosis, clostridial enterocolitis, *Aeromonas* spp colitis, and coronavirus. *Salmonella* spp and *Clostridia difficile* can be difficult to culture from fluid fecal material, and a diagnosis of salmonellosis or clostridial enterocolitis can easily be missed. Culture of GI tissue samples and mesenteric lymph nodes is recommended in addition to intestinal contents from necropsy cases. Negative cultures and toxin tests for clostridia do not necessarily exclude these conditions; therefore, thorough disinfection of the premises, hospital facilities, and trailers is recommended in all cases.

Clinically, there may be a short febrile period, but body temperature soon returns to normal or subnormal. Tachypnea, tachycardia, and marked depression are present. An explosive diarrhea develops, followed by extreme dehydration. Sometimes death occurs before diarrhea becomes evident, with severe enterocolitis observed at necropsy. Hypovolemic and endotoxic shock are manifest by poor capillary refill time, purplish mucous membranes, and cold extremities. Death may occur within 3 hr of onset of clinical signs. In less acute cases, death occurs within 24–48 hr. At necropsy, edema and hemorrhage in the wall of the large colon and cecum are pronounced, and the intestinal contents are fluid and often blood-stained.

Typically, the PCV is >65% even shortly after the onset of clinical signs. The leukogram ranges from normal to neutropenia with a degenerative left shift. Metabolic acidosis and electrolyte disorders are also present.

Disease onset is often closely associated with stress, eg, surgery or transport. Signs are similar to those of other diarrheal diseases, including peracute salmonellosis, toxemia caused by *Clostridium* spp, Potomac horse fever, experimental endotoxic shock, and anaphylaxis. A similar condition may be seen after administration of lincomycin to horses. Colitis-X is the term reserved for those cases in which no definitive diagnosis can be made and the horse dies.

Treatment for colitis-X usually is not effective (by definition) but would be similar to that for salmonellosis (*see* p 281). Large volumes of IV fluids are needed to counter the severe dehydration, and electrolyte replacement is often necessary. Plasma or synthetic colloids are required to maintain plasma oncotic pressure if hypoproteinemia occurs secondary to protein-losing enteropathy. Flunixin meglumine may decrease inflammation, and polymyxin B can help bind endotoxin. Broad-spectrum antibiotics are indicated to treat bacteremia that often occurs secondary to bacterial translocation across the damaged GI tract.

CORONAVIRUS

Coronavirus has been identified in the feces of normal foals and those with intestinal disease. However, there have been recent outbreaks of diarrhea and colic in adult horses attributed to coronavirus. Clinical signs include anorexia, lethargy, and fever. Colic and changes in fecal consistency are seen in some cases. Occasionally, rapid progression leads to death (or euthanasia), but most cases resolve with supportive care.

Diagnosis is by detection of the organism in feces by real-time PCR, electron microscopy, and virus isolation. Leukopenia due to neutropenia and lymphopenia are the most common hematologic abnormalities.

PARASITISM

Both large and small strongyles have been incriminated as a cause of chronic diarrhea in horses and foals. The condition associated with small strongyles in horses is termed cyathomostomiasis and has been reported to result in recurrent colic, diarrhea, and weight loss. (*See* GASTROINTESTINAL PARASITES OF HORSES, p 315.)

Giardiasis (*see* p 211) has been reported in a limited number of cases as a cause of intermittent diarrhea in horses. However, *Giardia* can also be found in the feces of a small number of healthy horses and is rarely recognized as a cause of diarrhea in horses. Cryptosporidia (*see* p 209) have been identified in the feces of both healthy and diarrheic foals. There is evidence that *Cryptosporidium* spp can cause diarrhea and even death in immunocompetent foals; cryptosporidia have been described as a cause of outbreaks of foal diarrhea on some farms.

SAND ENTEROCOLOPATHY

Consumption of large amounts of sand, which then accumulates in the large intestine, can produce diarrhea, weight loss, or colic. Sand is ingested when horses or foals are kept on sandy pasture or are fed hay or grain in a sandy area (paddock, stall, or pasture). Some horses or foals preferentially eat dirt and sand if it is in their environment. A diagnosis is based on history of a sandy environment, the presence of sand in the feces, "sand sounds" on auscultation of the ventral abdomen, and (if available) abdominal radiographs that reveal the presence of sand in the large colon. Treatment involves use of a hemicellulose product (psyllium seed hull) administered via nasogastric tube or added to the grain daily. Diarrhea generally resolves within 2–3 days of initiation of treatment. Generally, 3–4 wk of treatment is necessary to remove most of the sand and may need to be repeated if the horse or foal is not removed from the source of sand. Preventive psyllium treatment (daily for 1 wk each month) has been used where sand enterocolitis is common. Several psyllium products are on the market; many horses prefer the pelleted over the powdered form. (*See also* p 262.)

RECURRENT DIARRHEA

Some horses develop semiformed feces when first introduced to lush pastures, alfalfa hay, or a temporarily stressful situation (eg, trailer ride, racing, showing, visit to a veterinary hospital). This change in fecal consistency is not of medical significance as long as the horse is healthy in all other regards, but owners may be concerned. It is important that horses with diarrhea have a physical examination and appropriate laboratory tests to exclude infectious causes and to determine whether treatment is required. Usually, the fecal consistency returns to normal when the horse adapts to its new diet or the stressful situation resolves.

INFILTRATIVE COLONIC DISEASE

Any process that causes a thickening of the wall of the large colon may interfere with absorption of fluid and result in chronic diarrhea, weight loss, and sometimes hypoproteinemia. Thickening may be due to neoplasia, inflammatory cells (such as lymphocytes, plasma cells, macrophages, or eosinophils), or scar formation from previous acute colitis.

Rectal palpation may help detect bowel thickening and mesenteric lymphadenopathy. Abdominal fluid cytology may reveal neoplastic cells. Ultrasonography can be used to determine the degree of thickening of the bowel wall (if the affected area of bowel can be imaged) and may reveal masses in the liver or spleen or on the peritoneal surfaces; a percutaneous biopsy could provide a histopathologic diagnosis of neoplasia or inflammatory cell infiltrate. A biopsy of the rectal mucosa and duodenal mucosa (via 3-m endoscope) may be beneficial in diagnosis of inflammatory bowel disease and should also be cultured for *Salmonella*. Full-thickness jejunal, cecal, and colonic biopsies are more reliable for diagnosis of inflammatory bowel disease (*see* p 291) and can be obtained surgically either by standing flank laparotomy or recumbent ventral midline celiotomy. Surgical exploratory laparotomy can provide valuable information but is expensive and involves substantial risks of poor postoperative healing because of hypoproteinemia.

Treatment of abdominal neoplasia or inflammatory bowel disease is often unrewarding, but sometimes remission of clinical signs can be obtained with dexamethasone, especially with inflammatory bowel disease. Improvement of clinical signs and laboratory parameters with high-dose dexamethasone (0.1 mg/kg/day) treatment has been reported in three horses with clinical signs of GI tract lymphoma of T-cell origin. In two horses, the high-dose dexamethasone was followed by a lower dose (0.01–0.95 mg/kg/day) once clinical improvement occurred. Favorable responses persisted for >9 mo. The third horse had to be maintained on the higher dose of dexamethasone throughout treatment, because signs recurred whenever the dose was lowered. Clinical signs recurred despite high doses of dexamethasone, and after 2 mo of treatment the horse was euthanized. The mechanism of action of the steroid is speculated to be control of inflammation associated with the condition, as opposed to glucocorticoid-induced apoptosis.

MISCELLANEOUS CAUSES OF DIARRHEA

Other causes of diarrhea or semiformed to watery feces in horses include grain overload, thromboembolic disease of the colon, peritonitis, antibiotic treatment, renal failure, numerous toxicoses (eg, blister beetles [cantharidin], salt poisoning, slaframine, amitraz, propylene glycol, phosphorus, selenium, nicotine, reserpine, arsenic, mercury, monensin, organophosphates, oleander, Japanese yew, castor bean, avocado, thorn apple, potatoes, heath, algae, acorn or oak, *Hypericum*, corn cockle, mycotoxicoses, horse tail [scouring rush]), hyperlipidosis, and resolving impaction of the large intestine after treatment with oral cathartics such as magnesium sulfate.

DIARRHEAL DISEASE IN FOALS

FOAL HEAT DIARRHEA

From 4–14 days after birth, foals often develop a mild, self-limiting diarrhea. During this time, the dam is usually undergoing her first estrous cycle, hence the name "foal heat diarrhea." However, diarrhea can also occur at this time in orphan foals; therefore, hormonal activity in the mare is unlikely to be involved in the pathogenesis. Although the cause is unknown, it may be associated with alterations in the foal's intestinal microbial flora or alteration in diet as the foal begins to eat small amounts of hay and grain. Coprophagy may also have a role.

The foal remains active and alert and has a normal appetite. Vital signs remain normal. Feces are semiformed to watery and not malodorous. Monitoring is important to ensure the foal's condition does not deteriorate. Specific treatment is usually not necessary, but application of a protectant to the skin around the perineum helps prevent scalding of the buttocks.

BACTERIAL DIARRHEA IN FOALS

Bacterial enterocolitis in neonatal foals can be a component of neonatal septicemia, and diarrhea can be seen with bacteremia of any cause. Organisms commonly involved in neonatal bacteremia and subsequent diarrhea in neonatal foals include *Salmonella* spp, *Escherichia coli*, and *Actinobacillus* spp. Although *E coli* is the most important mediator of systemic sepsis in newborn foals, it is not as common as a primary cause of diarrhea in foals as it is in calves and piglets.

Intensive antimicrobial treatment, correction of fluid loss and electrolyte abnormalities, and nursing care are needed. Foals should be evaluated to determine whether adequate passive transfer of colostral antibodies has occurred; if not, a plasma transfusion is indicated. (*See also* SEPSIS IN FOALS, p 1728.) Markedly hypoproteinemic foals will benefit from plasma transfusion and/or administration of a plasma substitute such as hetastarch to improve oncotic pressure. IV fluid treatment without correction of the severe hypoproteinemia may induce pulmonary or peripheral edema.

An acute, fulminant, hemorrhagic diarrhea syndrome with high mortality in young foals <10 days old and commonly <3 days old has been associated with *Clostridium perfringens* type C infection (*see* p 285). Enterocolitis has also been associated with *C perfringens* type A with or without β2 toxin gene. The significance of this association is less clear than with type C, because type A has been identified in the feces in >90% of healthy neonatal foals in a farm-based study. It is possible that the number of bacteria and the phase of growth predispose to disease from type A. Infections may be sporadic or seen as outbreaks in multiple foals on a farm. Severe lethargy and rapid deterioration of cardiovascular status is followed by death in 24–48 hr in many cases. Intraluminal hemorrhage and extensive mucosal necrosis of the small intestine and, in some cases, the colon are found on necropsy.

Other bacteria that have been associated with diarrhea in foals are *Bacteroides fragilis*, *C difficile* (*see* p 285), *Aeromonas hydrophila*, and *Rhodococcus equi*. Although *R equi* primarily causes respiratory disease (*see* p 1451), both acute and chronic enteritis can cause diarrhea in foals 1–4 mo old. The diagnosis is more straightforward if pneumonia is also present. When cultured from tracheal wash fluid, *R equi* is considered a pathogen; however, a positive fecal culture is not as helpful because *R equi* can be found in the feces of healthy foals. Clarithromycin combined with rifampin is the treatment of choice for *R equi* infection in foals. Other macrolides such as azithromycin or erythromycin can be used, but erythromycin can predispose to diarrhea and hyperthermia.

Equine Proliferative Enteropathy

(*Lawsonia intracellularis* infection)

Enteric infection with *Lawsonia intracellularis* causes proliferative enteropathy, resulting in outbreaks of diarrhea, rapid weight loss, colic, lethargy, subcutaneous edema, and protein-losing enteropathy in weanling foals. *Lawsonia* has a worldwide distribution and can affect many other species, including pigs, rodents, and ratites; it can survive in the environment for 2 wk, and a fecal-oral route of infection is speculated. *L intracellularis* enters the enterocytes, avoiding lysosomal destruction. Infected cells continue to divide, resulting in hyperplastic crypts of immature epithelial cells that have a poorly developed brush border, leading to decreased enzymatic activity and absorptive function. Decreased disaccharide activity results in maldigestion with subsequent overload of carbohydrates to the large colon and osmotic diarrhea. Hypoproteinemia results from a combination of malabsorption of amino acids and increased small-intestinal permeability and leads to low plasma oncotic pressure and subsequent ventral edema. Maldigestion and absorption of nutrients and protein-losing enteropathy result in weight loss and failure to thrive.

Affected foals range from 3–12 mo old, but those 4–6 mo old are most commonly infected. Stress may be a predisposing factor. Because of their debilitated state, infected foals are predisposed to secondary GI, skin, and respiratory infections. Morbidity and mortality rates are low if animals are treated appropriately, although sudden death has been reported. Marked hypoproteinemia (<4 mg/dL) with hypoalbuminemia (<1.5 g/dL) are the most common laboratory findings. The WBC count and fibrinogen concentrations tend to be normal to moderately increased. Anemia, hyponatremia, hypochloremia, and hypocalcemia may be seen. CK concentration is often mildly increased.

Diagnosis can be confirmed at necropsy with characteristic intracellular bacteria observed in silver-stained tissues. *L intracellularis* can be confirmed using PCR analysis and immunohistochemistry on tissues collected at necropsy. Because *Lawsonia* is an intracellular organism, it does not grow on standard microbiologic culture media, and permissive cell lines are required for isolation. PCR can be used to detect *L intracellularis* DNA in feces, but false-negative results can occur. Serology to detect antibodies to *L intracellularis* is more sensitive than fecal PCR, but discrimination between infected foals and exposed foals can be difficult. Indirect fluorescent antibody test and immunoperoxidase monolayer antibody tests are currently the best serologic tests available. An ELISA is also available. Both fecal PCR and serologic testing are recommended. If either test is positive in the presence of hypoproteinemia, then treatment is warranted. Foals can remain seropositive for 6 mo after clinical signs resolve. Frequently, transabdominal ultrasonography reveals a markedly thickened small-intestine wall.

Differential diagnoses for proliferative enteropathy include salmonellosis, clostridiosis, *Neorickettsia risticii*, *R equi*, parasitic infections, and any cause of infiltrative/inflammatory bowel disease. Response to treatment is considered confirmation of the diagnosis. Lack of response to therapy after 7–10 days should prompt reassessment of the diagnosis.

Lawsonia is an intracellular pathogen, so antimicrobials must be lipophilic or amphoteric to concentrate within the host cytoplasm. Treatment with oxytetracycline (6.6 mg/kg, IV, bid for 3–7 days) followed by doxycycline (10 mg/kg, bid for 14 days) has been successful. Mild cases respond to oral doxycycline alone. Alternatives include erythromycin (alone or in combination with rifampin) for 3–4 wk or chloramphenicol. Plasma transfusions are required only in the most severely affected foals. Glucocorticoids are not recommended. Response to therapy is indicated by improvement in attitude, appetite, and weight gain. Resolution of hypoproteinemia may take 4–5 wk and small-intestinal thickening 4–8 wk. With treatment, ~90% of foals usually survive.

VIRAL DIARRHEA IN FOALS

Viruses appear to cause diarrhea in foals but rarely affect adult horses. Rotavirus is the main cause of viral diarrhea in foals; however, other viruses (eg, coronavirus) have been implicated. Diarrhea induced by rotavirus is characterized by depression, anorexia, and profuse, watery, malodorous feces. It is usually seen in foals <2 mo old; younger foals typically have more severe clinical signs. The diarrhea usually lasts 4–7 days, although it can persist for weeks.

Rotavirus destroys the enterocytes on the tip of the villi in the small intestine, which results in malabsorption. Lactase becomes deficient, so lactose passing into the large intestine induces an osmotic diarrhea. Diagnosis is made by identification of virus in the feces by electron microscopy or commercial immunoassay kits designed for detection of human rotavirus. Requesting that the laboratory test specifically for rotavirus, collecting feces early in the course of disease, and sampling several foals improve the chances of virus detection.

Treatment is generally supportive. Certain farm management practices and disinfection techniques have effectively limited the spread of rotavirus during outbreaks. Sick foals are highly contagious and should be isolated in the stall in the barn in which the foal originally became ill or moved to a designated isolation facility. Personnel should wear disposable gloves and cleanable boots and wash their hands with soap before and after handling diarrheic foals. Foot dips containing phenolic disinfectants outside the stalls of sick foals should also be used. Specific stall-cleaning equipment should be designated only for cleaning the stalls of diarrheic foals. Once the stall has been vacated, it should be cleaned of particulate material, washed with detergent, and then disinfected with phenolic compounds that meet EPA standards. Bleach, chlorhexidine, and quaternary compounds do not appear to be effective disinfectants for rotavirus. Fecal material of sick foals removed from stalls should not be spread on pastures used for horses and foals, and care should be taken to avoid fecal contamination of alleyways. All stall-cleaning equipment should be disinfected. Stalls with dirt floors are difficult to adequately clean and disinfect. Removal of the top layers of dirt may be required.

Arriving horses and foals, including those returning from veterinary hospitals, should be isolated for ≥7 days before being introduced to the resident population. A vaccine for pregnant mares to induce colostral antibodies directed at reducing the risk of rotavirus infection in their foals is available.

MISCELLANEOUS CAUSES OF DIARRHEA IN FOALS

Nutritional diarrhea can result from overfeeding (eg, when a foal is reunited with the mare after a period of separation) and improper nutrition (eg, orphan foals being fed calf milk replacer or sucrose). Lactose intolerance in foals is rare and can be determined by lactose tolerance challenge tests or clinical response to supplemental lactase. Diarrhea can also develop when foals consume indigestible substances such as roughage, sand, dirt, and rocks. Diarrhea in foals has been reported to be associated with infection by *Strongyloides westeri*, *Parascaris equorum*, and *Cryptosporidium* spp. (*See also* GASTROINTESTINAL PARASITES OF HORSES, p 315.)

WEIGHT LOSS AND HYPOPROTEINEMIA

The causes for weight loss in horses are numerous and can involve many body systems. This discussion is confined to diseases of the GI tract. Protein loss may or may not be associated with weight loss. The disorders commonly associated with either of these signs are neoplasia, inflammatory bowel disease, and toxicosis from treatment with NSAIDs.

GASTROINTESTINAL NEOPLASIA

Squamous cell carcinoma of the stomach and the alimentary form of lymphosarcoma are the most common forms of neoplasia involving the GI tract in horses. Chronic weight loss may be the primary clinical sign. Chronic diarrhea and hypoalbuminemia may develop when lymphosarcoma has infiltrated the wall of the intestine.

Because the incidence of GI neoplasia is low, other causes of weight loss should be investigated first. Diagnosis is usually made by exclusion of other causes of weight loss and by histopathologic examination of the tissue collected by duodenal or rectal mucosal biopsy during exploratory laparotomy or at necropsy. Squamous cell carcinoma of the stomach can be diagnosed by gastroscopy. An endoscope 2–3 m long is necessary to examine the gastric mucosa of adult horses. In horses with lymphosarcoma, enlarged mesenteric lymph nodes or thickened bowel may be detected by rectal palpation or by ultrasonographic examination. Occasionally, neoplastic cells are identified by cytologic examination of abdominal fluid. Ultrasonography may reveal masses in the liver or spleen, as well as facilitate percutaneous biopsy of the masses. An exploratory laparotomy with biopsy of intestinal or other masses can provide a definitive diagnosis.

Treatment of GI neoplasia in horses is generally not attempted, and the prognosis is grave. There have been a few reports of surgical removal of the affected segment of bowel. Chemotherapy may be an option for some horses, and corticosteroid therapy may prolong survival time in some cases.

INFLAMMATORY BOWEL DISEASE

This collection of diseases includes granulomatous enteritis (GE), lymphocytic-plasmacytic enterocolitis (LPE), multisystemic eosinophilic epitheliotropic disease (MEED), and idiopathic focal eosinophilic enterocolitis (IFEE). Disease is characterized by infiltration of the small and large intestine with inflammatory cells, including lymphocytes, plasma cells, macrophages, and eosinophils. The inflammatory condition may be limited to only a short segment of the bowel or be more diffuse. Malabsorption and a protein-losing enterocolopathy result. Diarrhea may or may not be a clinical feature. Inflammatory bowel disease should be considered in the differential diagnosis of horses with weight loss, recurrent colic, or hypoproteinemia, as well as in some horses with generalized skin disease.

Diagnosis is based on clinical signs, low serum protein concentration, possible thickened bowel (identified by ultrasonography or on rectal palpation), malabsorption, and intestinal or rectal biopsy. Malabsorption of carbohydrates occurs secondary to severe villous atrophy throughout the small intestine. Failure to absorb oral glucose or D-xylose verifies malabsorption from the small intestine.

Histologic diagnosis is subjective and should be performed by a pathologist experienced in reading equine intestinal biopsies. Rectal mucosal biopsy is useful in the diagnosis of ~50% of cases of GE and MEED but is rarely helpful in the diagnosis of LPE and IFEE. High numbers of eosinophils and lymphocytes can be identified in the intestinal wall of normal horses, but overinterpretation should be avoided. The presence of eosinophilic granulomas, vasculitis, and fibrinoid necrosis of intramural vessels is diagnostic of MEED. Horses with MEED may have severe dermatitis, eosinophilic infiltrations in the liver or pancreas, and sometimes marked eosinophilia. Horses with IFEE have eosinophilic infiltration restricted to the intestine and have a better prognosis for survival. Full-thickness intestinal biopsies can be obtained by using a laparoscopic procedure via a flank incision or by ventral midline celiotomy. Because most of the horses have severe hypoproteinemia at the time of diagnosis, incisional healing can be problematic.

The pathophysiology of the various syndromes is not well understood. An altered immune response to a common intestinal factor (eg, feed, parasites, bacteria) has been suggested. Histopathologic similarities exist between GE in horses, Johne's disease in cattle, and Crohn's disease in people. Standardbreds seemed to be predisposed to GE and MEED, which suggests possible genetic predisposition.

Various medical treatments have been tried with limited success. Corticosteroids, dietary alterations, metronidazole, and the antimetabolite azathioprine have been used. Hypereosinophilic syndrome in people often responds to hydroxyurea or vincristine, and sometimes interferon-α and cyclosporine are used. Supportive nutritional care should involve frequent feeding of good-quality, high-energy feeds. The prognosis is grave. If only a limited and accessible section of the bowel is affected, surgical removal may be successful. This is more common in IFEE, in which horses commonly present with colic rather than weight loss. Focal thickening, sometimes restricted to circumferential mural bands, is detected via exploratory laparotomy or necropsy; a diagnosis can be made by subsequent histopathology. Horses with IFEE respond to surgical resection of the diseased segment of intestine. Medical treatment with corticosteroids and feeding small frequent meals has also led to resolution of clinical signs after small-intestinal decompression without resection.

NSAID TOXICOSIS

The toxicity of NSAIDs is related to COX selectively, dosage, and duration (*see* p 2110). It is hypothesized that nonselective COX inhibitors have greater risk of toxicity than COX-selective drugs. COX inhibitors also cause delayed GI healing. The GI tract and kidneys are most commonly affected by NSAID toxicity. NSAID-induced injury can occur anywhere in the GI tract, but the large colon (especially the right dorsal colon) and gastric mucosa appear to be the most sensitive. The ulcerogenicity of phenylbutazone is greater than that of flunixin meglumine, which has greater ulcerogenicity than ketoprofen. The COX-2 selective inhibitor firocoxib appears to be safer. Ulcerative lesions in the large colon lead to a protein-losing enteropathy, often with clinical signs of ventral edema, anorexia, lethargy, weight loss, diarrhea, and colic. Scarring of the right dorsal colon can occur leading to large-colon impactions, sometimes requiring large-colon resection.

Phenylbutazone administered at high doses or for prolonged periods causes a protein-losing enterocolopathy in horses. However, some horses are inherently sensitive to NSAIDs, and right dorsal colitis can occur at lower than recommended dosages. Toxicosis can develop from oral or parenteral administration of NSAIDs. Hypoproteinemia (hypoalbuminemia and hypoglobulinemia) is seen due to loss of protein into the intestinal lumen, which can occur without visible ulceration. Renal papillary necrosis may also be seen. Administration of flunixin meglumine at high doses or for prolonged periods can result in a similar toxicosis.

Clinical signs of NSAID toxicity include difficulty in mastication due to oral and lingual ulceration, hypersalivation, and signs of pain when swallowing due to esophageal ulceration. Gastric ulceration can result in recumbency after eating, signs of colic, and anorexia. Horses with colonic ulceration can have soft feces, diarrhea, and ventral edema. Intestinal ulceration can be severe enough to allow endotoxin and bacterial translocation and signs of systemic inflammation and septicemia. Dehydration, fever, and tachycardia can occur in severe cases. Clinical signs can occur days to weeks after NSAID therapy. More chronic cases present with recurring colic, weight loss, and soft feces.

A tentative diagnosis can be made based on history of NSAID administration, clinical signs, and presence of hypoproteinemia. Severe cases may have hyponatremia, hypochloremia, hypocalcemia, and acidemia in addition to hypovolemia. Ultrasonography may detect thickening of the colon. Gastric ulceration can be confirmed by gastroscopy but requires an endoscope 2–3 m long.

Treatment includes discontinuing use of phenylbutazone or any other NSAID. In acute toxicosis, administration of 1 gal. of mineral oil repeated after 2 hr may be beneficial to decrease drug absorption. To help prevent gastric ulceration, reducing production of gastric acid with an H_2-receptor blocker (eg, ranitidine) or a proton pump inhibitor (eg, omeprazole) may be beneficial; sucralfate may be indicated as well. Administration of misoprostol (a synthetic prostaglandin analogue) may be beneficial but can cause additional signs of diarrhea and colic. IV fluid therapy is indicated in cases of hypovolemia, especially with concurrent azotemia. Plasma transfusion or synthetic colloids can be used to increase plasma oncotic pressure.

Longterm dietary management consisting of a low-fiber complete pelleted ration fed several times throughout the day, and elimination of roughage is recommended. Corn oil can be given to provide supplemental calories and may help heal damaged intestinal mucosa. Psyllium mucilloid can also promote colonic healing by increasing the concentration of short-chain fatty acids. Surgery may be required if scarring of the bowel has resulted in partial obstruction of the intestine.

Prevention of NSAID toxicity involves limiting the dose and duration of NSAID treatment, using a COX-2 selective NSAID, or relying on alternative analgesic therapy. Monitoring for fecal consistency and serum albumin concentrations are easy methods to detect the development of right dorsal colitis in horses receiving NSAIDs.

SMALL-INTESTINAL FIBROSIS

Extensive fibrosis of the submucosa of the small intestine has been associated with weight loss and recurrent colic in adult horses on pasture in northern Colorado. All affected horses died or were euthanized because of their deteriorating condition. The cause is unknown.

INTESTINAL DISEASES IN PIGS

Pigs of all ages are susceptible to intestinal diseases, and diarrhea is the sign common to nearly all such disorders. Transmission of infectious agents that cause enteropathies is by the fecal-oral route. At least 16 different etiologic agents, including bacteria, viruses, and parasites, can cause primary intestinal disease. Porcine circovirus type 2 (PCV 2) virus may be isolated from the intestines of pigs with diarrhea. PCV 2 is the cause of several multisystemic diseases in pigs, including postweaning multisystemic wasting syndrome (*see* p 723). Diarrhea in a herd may be due to a single agent, but concurrent infections are common. Because some diseases are age-dependent, differential diagnosis is best considered by age group (*see* TABLE 6).

CLOSTRIDIUM DIFFICILE ENTERITIS

C difficile is an important emerging pathogen that causes diarrhea primarily in neonatal swine. The agent was first recognized as a cause of antibiotic-associated diarrhea in people. It most commonly causes disease in piglets 1–7 days old and in other domestic and laboratory animals.

Etiology and Pathogenesis: *C difficile* is an anaerobic, gram-positive, sporeforming rod that is more oxygen-sensitive than *C perfringens*. The organism can be demonstrated in the intestine by direct Gram stain of smears. Survival of *C difficile* in the environment and shedding by carrier sows is believed to be important in transmission.

TABLE 6 AGE DISTRIBUTION OF DIARRHEAL DISEASES IN PIGS

	Age Group		
	Nursing	Weaning	Growing-finishing or Breeding
BACTERIAL DISEASES			
Clostridium difficile enteritis	+ + +	+	+
C perfringens type A enteritis	+ +	+	–
C perfringens type C enteritis	+ +	–	–
Enteric colibacillosis	+ + +	+ + +	–
Intestinal spirochetosis	–	+ +	+ + +
Porcine proliferative enteritis	–	+ +	+ + +
Salmonella enteritis	+	+ +	+ + +
Swine dysentery	+	+ +	+ + +
PARASITISM			
Cryptosporidium sp	+	+	–
Isospora suis	+ + +	+	–
Strongyloides ransomi	+	+	+
Trichuris suis	–	–	+ +
VIRAL DISEASES			
Porcine circovirus diarrhea	+	+ +	+
Porcine epidemic diarrhea	+++	+ ++	++
Rotaviral enteritis	+ + +	+ + +	+
Transmissible gastroenteritis	+ + +	+ + +	+ +

– Rare or does not occur; + Uncommon; + + Common; + + + Very common

C difficile produces "large clostridial toxins" A and B, which are thought to be involved in lesion production. Toxin A is an enterotoxin that causes fluid secretion into the gut lumen, and toxin B is a cytotoxin.

Clinical Findings: Affected piglets may have dyspnea, abdominal distention, and scrotal edema. Diarrhea may not be present in all pigs affected.

Lesions: Ascites, hydrothorax, and edema of the ascending colon have been reported. Urates are commonly present in the kidneys. Pasty to watery colonic contents may be seen. Microscopically, the colon is primarily affected with multifocal exudation of mucus and fibrin plus submucosal edema.

Diagnosis: Gross lesions are not pathognomonic, and diagnosis must be confirmed by culture or demonstration of either toxin A or B and histopathology. *C difficile* can be cultured on selective media containing cefoxitin, cycloserine, taurocholate, and fructose under anaerobic conditions. The genes of toxins A and B are identified readily by PCR. The toxins can also be detected directly in suspensions of intestinal contents by commercially available enzyme immunoassays.

Treatment and Control: Based on minimum inhibitory concentration determinations, it has been suggested that erythromycin, tetracycline, and tylosin may be useful for treatment of suckling piglets, and tiamulin and virginiamycin may help to reduce levels of the organism in adult swine. No controlled studies on the effect of antibiotics on clinical disease have been reported.

CLOSTRIDIUM PERFRINGENS TYPE A ENTERITIS

Infection of the small intestine by type A strains of *C perfringens* is a milder condition and rarer than disease caused by *C perfringens* type C (*see* below). Suckling and sometimes weaned pigs are affected and exhibit yellow-colored feces with mucous and flecks of blood. Growth rates are suppressed but with low to no mortality. The lesions at necropsy are milder and blood-free as compared with those of *C perfringens* type C enteritis. Diagnosis, treatment, and control are as for *C perfringens* type C enteritis.

CLOSTRIDIUM PERFRINGENS TYPE C ENTERITIS

Infection of the small intestine by type C strains of *C perfringens* causes a highly fatal, necrohemorrhagic enteritis. It most commonly affects piglets 1–5 days old but may be seen in pigs up to 3 wk old (and in other species, *see* p 609).

Etiology and Pathogenesis: The organism penetrates between the absorptive cells of the upper jejunum and elaborates β toxin, a potent, heat-labile, trypsin-sensitive exotoxin that causes necrosis of all structural components of the villi. Necrotizing inflammation usually extends to the mucosal crypts. The infection may continue caudally and involve the ileum, but it rarely affects the colon. Necrosis of the mucosa is accompanied by blood loss into the intestinal wall and lumen.

Clinical Findings: Sudden onset of hemorrhagic diarrhea followed by collapse and death is characteristic in piglets 1–3 days old. In less acute cases, brownish liquid feces develop at 3–5 days. Infrequently, pigs develop a persistent, pasty, gray diarrhea and become progressively emaciated. In peracute cases, the perineal region is blood stained.

Lesions: The small intestines are dark red, hemorrhagic, and filled with hemorrhagic liquid. Less acute cases at 3–5 days may have gas bubbles in the wall of the jejunum and necrosis of the mucosa of the jejunum and ileum. More chronic cases have a thickened small intestine lined by a pale yellow or gray necrotic membrane tightly adhered to the submucosa.

Diagnosis: Necropsy is usually sufficient to establish the diagnosis in the peracute hemorrhagic form and in the acute form with jejunal emphysema. A rapid presumptive diagnosis can be made by demonstrating large rod-shaped bacteria in gram-stained mucosal impression smears. Histologic demonstration of villous necrosis with mucosal colonization by numerous large gram-positive rods is adequate for confirmation. Subacute and chronic forms of the disease in piglets 6–14 days old are easily confused at necropsy with *Isospora suis* enteritis, but diagnosis is usually possible by histologic examination of the jejunum and ileum or by observation of clostridia in mucosal smears (Gram or Giemsa stain). Isolates of *C perfringens* may be genotyped for the presence of genes that code for β toxin.

Treatment and Control: Treatment of pigs with clinical signs is of little benefit because lesions usually are irreversible at the onset of diarrhea. In an acute outbreak, prophylactic administration of type C antitoxin or antibiotic (or both) parenterally or PO is protective if given to piglets within 2 hr of birth. The disease tends to recur on infected premises. Vaccination of gestating sows at 6 and 3 wk before parturition with type C bacterin-toxoid confers some passive lactogenic immunity to subsequent litters, if piglets consume colostrum soon after birth. Once immunized with two doses of bacterin-toxoid, sows should receive one dose ~3 wk before each subsequent farrowing.

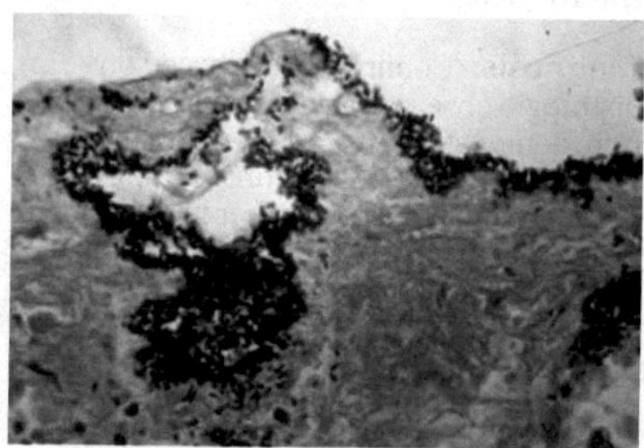

Clostridium perfringens enteritis in a piglet. Note the large numbers of gram-positive rods adhering to the necrotic jejunal epithelium. *Courtesy of Dr. John Prescott.*

EDEMA DISEASE

(*Escherichia coli* enterotoxemia)

Edema disease is an acute, highly fatal, neurologic disorder usually seen 5 days to 2 wk after weaning and possibly accompanied by diarrhea (*see* p 716).

ENTERIC COLIBACILLOSIS

Enteric colibacillosis is a common disease of nursing and weanling pigs caused by colonization of the small intestine by enterotoxigenic strains of *Escherichia coli*.

Etiology and Pathogenesis: Certain strains of *E coli* possess fimbria or pili that allow them to adhere to or colonize the absorptive epithelial cells of the jejunum and ileum. The common antigenic types of pili associated with pathogenicity are K88, K99, 987P, and F41. Pathogenic strains produce enterotoxins that cause fluid and electrolytes to be secreted into the intestinal lumen, which results in diarrhea, dehydration, and acidosis. Infection in neonates is commonly caused by K88 and 987P strains, whereas postweaning colibacillosis is nearly always due to the K88 strain.

Clinical Findings: Profuse watery diarrhea with rapid dehydration, acidosis, and death is common. Rarely, pigs may collapse and die before diarrhea begins.

Lesions: Dehydration and distention of the small intestine with yellowish, slightly mucoid fluid is characteristic. The colon contains similar fluid. The fundic portion of the gastric mucosa is often reddened. Pigs dying suddenly may have patchy cutaneous erythema. Histologically, the villi are usually of normal length and have many small bacterial rods adhered to the absorptive enterocytes.

Diagnosis: Confirmation is based on histologic observation of villous colonization; demonstration of K88, K99, 987P, or F41 pilus antigens in intestinal scrapings by immunofluorescence or other immunologic procedures; and isolation of the organism from the small intestine. Because *E coli* is a common secondary agent, the possibility of involvement of other agents such as viruses or coccidia should be considered.

Treatment and Control: Therapy includes prompt treatment with antibacterials and restoration of fluid and electrolyte balance. Bacterial antibiotic sensitivity testing is helpful to identify effective medication. Prevention includes reducing predisposing factors, such as dampness and chilling; improving sanitation, such as by replacing solid or slatted concrete flooring with wire-mesh flooring; and vaccinating gestating sows with pilus-specific vaccines. Pigs lacking receptors for K88 have been shown to be resistant to disease caused by enterotoxin-positive K88-positive *E coli*.

HEMORRHAGIC BOWEL SYNDROME

(Mesenteric torsion of the small intestine)

Hemorrhagic bowel syndrome affects rapidly growing swine 4–6 mo old. Pigs die suddenly without evidence of diarrhea, but the small intestine is thin-walled on necropsy and filled with either clotted or unclotted blood. The large intestine usually contains tarry fecal material but no lesions suggestive of swine dysentery, salmonellosis, proliferative enteritis, or intestinal spirochetosis. The condition can be prevented by the administration of either bacitracin or chlortetracycline in the feed. When performing a necropsy, the mesenteric root should be palpated before opening the abdomen. A peracute form of proliferative enteritis may have similar clinical and gross lesions; however, histology and culture of the intestine will discern the presence or absence of epithelial proliferation and *Lawsonia intracellularis*.

The cause in most cases is believed due to intestinal volvulus. Predisposing factors may include vigorous exercise, handling, fighting, piling, or irregular feeding. Long-loined pigs may be more likely to develop mesenteric torsion than shorter pigs. Rotation of the entire intestine, including the posterior part of the duodenum and the anterior part of the rectum, around the root of the mesentery obstructs venous outflow of blood, which causes blood to pool and stagnate in the intestine and soon results in infarction. Rotation may be only partial and difficult to demonstrate at necropsy, which makes diagnosis more challenging.

INTESTINAL SALMONELLOSIS

Enteropathogenic salmonellae cause inflammation and necrosis of the small and large intestines, resulting in diarrhea that may be accompanied by generalized sepsis. All ages are susceptible, but the disease is most common in weaned and growing-finishing pigs.

Etiology and Pathogenesis: *Salmonella* Choleraesuis kunzendorf (*S* Choleraesuis) is one of the most common *Salmonella* species affecting pigs. It sometimes produces necrotizing enterocolitis but far more common is a septicemic disease characterized by hepatitis, pneumonia, and cerebral vasculitis. *S* Typhisuis infection of the intestine results in necrotizing, nonsuppurative inflammation of the mucosa and submucosa of the ileum, cecum, and colon; frequently, the mucosa is ulcerative. Usually, there is extension to regional lymph nodes and, occasionally, generalized septicemia. Sources of infection for *S* Choleraesuis and *S* Typhisuis are primarily asymptomatic carrier pigs but also may include rodents and contaminated feed and premises. (*See also* SALMONELLOSIS, p 195.)

Numerous other serotypes of salmonellae are seen in pigs, some of which have been associated with human foodborne illness. Common serotypes seen in pigs are *S* Typhimurium, *S* Derby, *S* Heidelberg, *S* Worthington, and *S* Infantis. These serotypes may cause mild to moderate diarrhea in swine and may be resistant to multiple drugs.

Clinical Findings: Nursing pigs may develop diarrhea but usually succumb to generalized septicemia. Weanling or growing-finishing pigs are febrile and have liquid feces that may be yellow and contain shreds of necrotic debris.

Lesions: Pigs infected with *S* Choleraesuis have an inflamed, slightly thickened ileum and colon, usually with necrotic debris on the mucosal surface. Mesenteric lymph nodes are enlarged, edematous, and sometimes red. Mucosal ulceration may or may not be evident. A small amount of hemorrhage may be seen in acute cases. Occasionally, rectal strictures (*see* p 300) may develop. Other enteropathogenic salmonellae, except for *S* Typhisuis, produce lesions similar to but less severe than those of *S* Choleraesuis. Lesions of *S* Typhisuis enteritis are distinctive, typically yellow, round (button) ulcers in the colon, cecum, and less commonly the ileum.

Diagnosis: Culture of feces or intestinal mucosa in a selective medium may yield the organism. However, salmonellae often are isolated (and more reliably) from enlarged mesenteric lymph nodes by direct streaking on a selective medium such as brilliant green agar or by inoculation of enrichment media. Histologic examination of affected intestine and liver to differentiate salmonellosis from proliferative enteritis and swine dysentery is a valuable adjunct procedure.

Treatment and Control: Live avirulent vaccines administered either intranasally or via the water are very effective for prevention of disease caused by *S* Choleraesuis. Avirulent vaccines may also effectively reduce levels of salmonellae in the tissues of swine at slaughter. Parenteral administration of antibacterials to acutely ill pigs and medication of the affected group via water or feed may decrease the severity of the outbreak. Neomycin and lincomycin-spectinomycin are the most often used water medications. Carbadox in the feed is often used as a preventive. Susceptibility testing of the isolated organism is useful to select an appropriate antibacterial. Thorough cleaning and disinfection of contaminated facilities and elimination of the source of the organism decrease the likelihood of repeated epidemics.

INTESTINAL SPIROCHETOSIS

Intestinal spirochetosis is a disease of the large intestine seen in the absence of *Brachyspira hyodysenteriae* (*see* SWINE DYSENTERY, p 301). This disease syndrome is being recognized more frequently worldwide.

Etiology and Pathogenesis: The primary cause of intestinal spirochetosis is *Brachyspira pilosicoli*. Other weakly β-hemolytic *Brachyspira* associated with the condition are *B intermedia* and *B murdochi*. *B innocens* appears not to cause disease at all. *B pilosicoli* is emerging as a significant pathogen of people, especially in indigenous populations, homosexuals, and immunosuppressed patients. The organism is transmitted orally and survives extremely well in the environment. *B pilosicoli* has been isolated from a wide variety of animals, including waterbirds, rodents, and dogs. It has been shown to cause diarrheal disease in pigs, chickens, and people by experimental inoculation and in natural occurrence. The pathogenesis is not well studied, but apparently the end-on attachment of the spirochete to the mucosal surface interferes with the absorptive capacity of the colon, resulting in diarrhea.

Clinical Findings: Pigs initially have sticky feces on the perineum. The feces will appear as wet cement, and a mild diarrhea may result. Affected pigs may be inappetent and grow slowly.

Lesions: The lesions in the large intestine are milder than those caused by *B hyodysenteriae* in swine dysentery. The volume of the large intestine may be increased and distended with thickening of the mucosa. In some pigs, a mucohemorrhagic colitis develops in association with enlarged mesenteric lymph nodes. Microscopically, spirochetes may be seen attached end-on to the mucosal surface and give the appearance of a false brush border. The mucosal surface has focal erosions with mild catarrhal exudate. Colonic crypts are often dilated, containing numerous spirochetes.

Diagnosis: Important differential diagnoses include salmonellosis, proliferative enteritis, swine dysentery, and whipworm infection. *B pilosicoli* and other weakly β-hemolytic *Brachyspira* can be isolated on selective agar under anaerobic conditions. Biochemical tests and preferably PCR should be performed on *Brachyspira* isolates to confirm species identification.

Treatment and Control: Treatment and prevention of intestinal spirochetosis is similar to that of swine dysentery. Drugs such as tiamulin, lincomycin, and carbadox are effective. It is unknown whether the agent can be eradicated without total depopulation, as in swine dysentery, but because of the reservoir hosts and environmental survival it is doubtful.

PARASITISM

See also p 320 and *see* p 208.

Ascaris suum is the most common intestinal nematode of pigs. Adults in the intestine reduce feed efficiency, and heavy infections cause emaciation. Larval migration incites inflammation in the liver and lungs.

Cryptosporidium sp is a coccidium that attaches to the mucosal epithelium of the intestine of pigs ≥10 days old. It causes villous atrophy in the lower small intestine. Malabsorption and diarrhea may result.

Eimeria spp are common in pigs, but overt disease is seldom seen. Heavy infections may cause significant enterocolitis in young growing pigs.

Hyostrongylus rubidus is the common stomach worm found in pasture-raised pigs. It usually causes little harm.

Isospora suis is a common and important cause of coccidiosis in piglets 6 days to 3 wk old. Infection causes necrosis and villous atrophy of the ileum and jejunum. Secondary bacterial infection of the injured intestinal mucosa is common. Mortality often is 20%–25%, and many pigs are stunted. Diagnosis can be based on identification of immature coccidial forms in the intestinal mucosa by direct mucosal smear (Giemsa stain) or by histologic examination of the affected intestine. Successful prevention most commonly depends on thorough cleaning of farrowing facilities to minimize the number of oocysts. After cleaning, thorough disinfection with 50% bleach has been useful. Coccidiostats are sometimes fed to sows 2 wk before farrowing or administered PO to pigs from birth to 3 wk of age.

Adult nodular worms of *Oesophagostomum* spp in the large intestine cause little harm, but heavy infection by larvae encysted in the intestinal wall may lead to emaciation.

Strongyloides ransomi (intestinal threadworm) larvae can be transmitted via colostrum or acquired from contaminated skin of the dam. Heavily infected piglets develop severe diarrhea when 10–14 days old, with high mortality. Diagnosis is based on direct microscopical observation of mucosal scrapings.

Trichuris suis (whipworms) penetrate the mucosa of the cecum and colon and cause multifocal inflammation. Heavy infections cause diarrhea and emaciation. The feces are hemorrhagic; therefore, heavy whipworm infections may be confused clinically with swine dysentery or proliferative enteritis. Diagnosis is based on direct observation of whipworms in the large intestine or on fecal flotation.

PORCINE EPIDEMIC DIARRHEA

This coronaviral diarrhea affects pigs of all ages and clinically resembles transmissible gastroenteritis (TGE, *see* p 302) in several respects.

Etiology and Epidemiology: The porcine epidemic diarrhea (PED) virus is not related to any other member of the Coronaviridae. Pigs are the only known host. Antibodies to the virus have not been found in wild pigs or in other animal species. Infections have been seen in most European countries and in China. In April 2013, disease due to PEDV was diagnosed in the USA for the first time. Large epidemics occurred in Europe in 1969; no antibodies have been found in sera collected before 1969. Since then, the virus has become widespread and endemic in several European countries, and acute outbreaks have become rare. On large breeding farms, the virus persists in consecutive litters of pigs after weaning and after they lose their immunity from antibody in the milk. On these farms, the virus may be associated with weaning diarrhea. In Belgium, the virus is most frequently associated with diarrhea in feeder pigs, which develops shortly after they are gathered from different breeding farms and assembled in large fattening units. The virus was demonstrated in fecal material in 80% of these groups. Outbreaks in the USA caused 60%–100% mortality in suckling pigs and mild to severe diarrhea in all pigs of all ages; they were initially believed to be outbreaks of TGE. Spread of the virus mainly occurs directly through infected pigs and indirectly through virus-contaminated fomites and via transport trucks.

Pathogenesis: The pathogenesis and immune mechanisms are similar to those reported for TGE. Oral infection results in viral replication in the epithelial cells of the small intestinal villi. Cells on colonic villi also become infected. No other tissue tropisms have been shown. Virus is excreted in the feces.

Clinical Findings: Diarrhea is the only direct virus-induced clinical sign seen. An acute outbreak on a susceptible breeding farm resembles a TGE outbreak and is characterized by watery diarrhea in pigs of all ages. However, as compared with TGE, the incubation period is longer (3–4 days), not all the litters of suckling pigs may become sick, and mortality in neonatal pigs is lower (average 50%). Also, the disease within the farm spreads more slowly. In all outbreaks, signs are most consistently seen in feeders, finishers, and adults, which appear to be most susceptible because outbreaks often start in these age groups. Older pigs are more lethargic and depressed with PED than with TGE. Sick pigs appear to have colic.

Acute outbreaks in susceptible finishing pigs are characterized by watery diarrhea, but a markedly increased number of acute deaths may be seen, particularly in pigs infected toward the end of the finishing period and in stress-sensitive breeds. Death may even occur during the incubation period.

Lesions: Macroscopic lesions are confined to the small intestine, with villous shortening as the main characteristic. These lesions closely resemble those seen with TGE. No lesions have been described in the colon. A consistent finding is acute necrosis of back muscle.

Diagnosis: Clinical differentiation from TGE is difficult. TGE in its typical epidemic form causes a rapidly spreading diarrhea in animals of all ages, with high mortality in neonates. With PED, the diarrhea spreads at a slower rate, and although diarrhea is seen in most of the litters, some litters may remain healthy even in the absence of immunity. Morbidity is 100% in older pigs, and they are severely sick. Acute deaths in adults and finishing pigs due to muscle necrosis and that occurs during an outbreak of diarrhea are typical of PED and are not seen with any other infectious diarrhea.

Laboratory diagnosis in neonates is made by PCR and/or direct immunofluorescence on cryostat sections of small intestine or colon. ELISA to detect viral antigens in feces or intestinal contents is more useful for older pigs. Antibodies can be detected in paired serum samples through ELISA-blocking.

Control: No specific treatment is available. Measures taken during an outbreak are of a general nature. Pigs with diarrhea should have free access to water, and finishing pigs should have feed withheld for 1–2 days.

PED virus can be eliminated from herds without total depopulation by maximizing immunity with planned infection of the sow herd; an "all-in/all-out" management of farrowing, nursery, and grower rooms; and good sanitation.

Because PED virus is easily spread during an epidemic by people, animals, and fomites, special care should be taken to prevent spread to unexposed groups of pigs and to neighboring herds. The use of vacines for prevention has not been well documented.

PORCINE PROLIFERATIVE ENTERITIS

(Porcine intestinal adenomatosis, Proliferative hemorrhagic enteropathy, Ileitis)

Porcine proliferative enteritis is a common diarrheal disease of growing-finishing and young breeding pigs characterized by hyperplasia and inflammation of the ileum and colon. It often is mild and self-limiting but sometimes causes persistent diarrhea, severe necrotic enteritis, or hemorrhagic enteritis with high mortality.

Etiology and Pathogenesis: The etiology is *Lawsonia intracellularis*, an intracellular, gram-negative, small rod-shaped bacterium. The organism has been cultivated only in cell cultures, and attempts to propagate it in cell-free medium have failed. Koch's postulates have been fulfilled by inoculation of pure cultures of *L intracellularis* into conventionally reared pigs; typical lesions of the disease were produced, and *L intracellularis* was reisolated from the lesions. Inoculation of *L intracellularis* into gnotobiotic pigs does not cause the disease; therefore, other factors in the conventionally reared pig may contribute to development of lesions.

Clinical Findings: The more common, nonhemorrhagic form of the disease often affects 40- to 80-lb (18- to 36-kg) pigs and is characterized by sudden onset of diarrhea. The feces are watery to pasty, brownish, or faintly blood stained. After ~2 days, pigs may pass yellow fibrinonecrotic casts that have formed in the ileum. Most affected pigs recover spontaneously, but a significant number develop chronic necrotic enteritis with progressive emaciation. The hemorrhagic form is characterized by cutaneous pallor, weakness, and passage of hemorrhagic or black, tarry feces. Pregnant gilts may abort.

Lesions: Lesions may be seen anywhere in the lower half of the small intestine, cecum, or colon but are most frequent and obvious in the ileum. The wall of the intestine is thickened, and the mesentery may be edematous. The mesenteric lymph nodes are enlarged. The intestinal mucosa appears thickened and rugose, may be covered with a brownish or yellow fibrinonecrotic membrane, and sometimes has petechial hemorrhages. Yellow necrotic casts may be found in the ileum or passing through the colon. Diffuse, complete mucosal necrosis in chronic cases causes the intestine to be rigid, resembling a garden hose. Proliferative mucosal lesions often are in the colon but are detected only by careful inspection at necropsy. In the profusely hemorrhagic form, there are red or black, tarry feces in the colon and clotted blood in the ileum.

Diagnosis: Confirmation is based on histologic observation of characteristic proliferation and inflammation of mucosal crypts. *L intracellularis* (comma-shaped, resembling *Campylobacter*) can usually be demonstrated by silver stains. A PCR test has been developed and is useful for confirmation of the presence of *L intracellularis* in lesions. Bacterial culture of intestine and lymph nodes to exclude *Salmonella* infection, together with histologic examination and culture of cecum and colon to exclude swine dysentery, are essential additional procedures. The colon also should be examined for whipworms. *L intracellularis* is present in most swine herds, so demonstration of the organism in feces by PCR or the presence of antibody in clinically normal pigs is of little diagnostic value.

Treatment and Control: Various antibacterials administered parenterally to acutely affected pigs and by feed or water to the remainder of the group help reduce severity of the enteritis and prevent development of chronic, irreversible, necrotic enteritis. Porcine proliferative enteritis is one of the first diseases to be seen in new herds established by surgical derivation. A live avirulent vaccine administered via the water is highly effective. It should be administered to gilts and boars during acclimatization before introduction into a herd.

RECTAL STRICTURES

In growing pigs, rectal strictures are sequelae of severely traumatized rectal prolapses (*see* p 189) or of infections that interfere with rectal blood supply. The former cause sporadic cases; the latter may be epidemic. One cause is *Salmonella* Typhimurium infection (*see* p 296), which produces an ulcerative proctitis that heals in such a manner that normal function is not restored. The stricture is reportedly the result of fibrosis of the rectal tissue due to persistent ischemia caused by infection in an area of limited blood supply.

Clinical Findings: Several bloated pigs in varying stages of emaciation are generally seen in a group of growing pigs. Other clinical signs, including prior outbreaks of severe debilitating diarrhea, are common but not always reported. An index finger rarely can be passed into the rectum without considerable resistance.

Lesions: At necropsy the colon is grossly distended, and the intestine is filled with gas and green feces. The predominant lesion is a narrowed rectal canal, due to annular fibrotic ulcers or rectal strictures found 2–5 cm cranial to the anus.

Diagnosis: An epidemic of rectal strictures without prior rectal prolapses is indicative of *S* Typhimurium infection. Culture of feces and regional lymph nodes usually yields *S* Typhimurium. However, it is not possible to determine whether the lesion or the infection occurred first.

Treatment and Control: Early diagnosis and treatment of diarrhea is imperative for control. Good housing, management, and sanitation, with "all-in/all-out" movement of pigs is the best method to prevent further outbreaks. Surgery is not thought to be economically feasible.

ROTAVIRAL ENTERITIS

Rotaviral enteritis is a common disease of the small intestine of pigs. All ages are susceptible, but significant diarrheal disease usually is seen in nursing or post-weaning pigs.

Etiology and Pathogenesis: The causal rotavirus infects and destroys villous enterocytes throughout the small intestine, but lesions are most severe in the middle third of the intestine. Loss of villous epithelium results in partial villous atrophy, malabsorption, and osmotic diarrhea. Four antigenic groups (A, B, C, E) of rotavirus are found in pigs. They are easily spread by direct contact. Healthy carrier sows may be fecal shedders during the periparturient period, thereby exposing their litters to infection.

Clinical Findings: If neonatal pigs do not receive protective levels of maternal antibody, they are likely to develop profuse watery diarrhea in 12–48 hr. More commonly, the infection is endemic in a herd, and sows have varying levels of antibody in the colostrum and milk, which provide varying degrees of passive protection to nursing pigs. Diarrhea often begins in pigs 5 days to 3 wk old or immediately after weaning. The feces of nursing pigs often are yellow or gray and pasty in the early stages and progress to gray and pasty after ~2 days. Diarrhea persists for 2–5 days. Diarrheic pigs become gaunt and rough-haired, but mortality usually is low. Weaned pigs have watery feces that contain poorly digested feed. Weaners become inappetent and noncompetitive, which results in emaciation, stunting, and probably predisposition to pneumonia and other diseases.

Lesions: The small intestine appears thin walled, and the cecum and colon contain liquid feces.

Diagnosis: Laboratory procedures are required. Confirmation is based on histologic demonstration of villous atrophy in the jejunum, electron microscopic demonstration of virions in the intestinal contents, PCR, and immunodiagnostic procedures to demonstrate viral antigen in the intestinal mucosa or feces. Differential diagnoses include endemic transmissible gastroenteritis, porcine epidemic diarrhea, *Isospora suis* enteritis, and enteric colibacillosis.

Treatment and Control: There is no specific treatment. Minimizing heat loss and providing adequate water to maintain hydration are helpful. Concurrent infection by enterotoxigenic *Escherichia coli* is common; therefore, antibiotic therapy may reduce mortality. Providing diarrheic weaned pigs with a warm, dry, draft-free environment and frequent limited feedings help prevent starvation, secondary diseases, and permanent stunting. Vaccine for group A rotavirus appears beneficial when given to sows before farrowing. Vaccines for groups B, C, and E have not been developed because of difficulty in virus propagation. A serotyping scheme based on virus neutralization indicates a lack of cross-protection between isolates within groups.

SWINE DYSENTERY

(Bloody scours)

Swine dysentery is a mucohemorrhagic diarrheal disease of pigs that affects the large intestine.

Etiology and Pathogenesis: The essential causal agent is *Brachyspira hyodysenteriae*, an anaerobic spirochete that produces a hemolysin, although other organisms may contribute to the severity of lesions. *B hyodysenteriae* produces strong β hemolysis on blood agar under anaerobic incubation conditions. Other strongly β-hemolytic *Brachyspira* have been described that produce lesions of swine dysentery when inoculated into pigs, namely *B suanatina*, some strains of *B intermedia*, *Brachyspira* sp SASK 30446, and *B hampsonii*. The *Brachyspira* proliferate in the large intestine and cause degeneration and inflammation of the superficial mucosa, hypersecretion of mucus by mucosal epithelium, and multifocal bleeding points on the mucosal surface. The organism does not penetrate beyond the intestinal mucosa. Decreased ability of the mucosa to reabsorb endogenous secretions from the unaffected small intestine results in diarrhea.

Clinical Findings: The first signs are partial anorexia, passage of soft feces, and possibly fever. The course is variable. Some pigs die peracutely. More commonly, a mucoid diarrhea with flecks of blood and mucus develops and progresses to a watery mucohemorrhagic diarrhea. After several days, the feces are brown and contain flecks of fibrin and debris. Diarrheic pigs are dehydrated, profoundly weak, gaunt, and emaciated.

Lesions: The diffuse lesions are confined to the cecum, spiral colon, and rectum. The affected mucosa is covered with a layer of transparent or gray mucus, often with suspended flecks of blood in early stages, with a mixture of blood, fibrin, and necrotic debris in more advanced cases, and a yellow, necrotic debris late in the course.

Diagnosis: Clinical signs and necropsy findings are usually sufficient for a presumptive diagnosis. Confirmation is based on demonstration of typical histologic lesions in the large intestine and isolation of strongly β-hemolytic *Brachyspira* by anaerobic culture. Concurrent diseases are not uncommon. Differential diagnoses include intestinal spirochetosis, proliferative enteritis, salmonellosis, and heavy whipworm infections.

Treatment and Control: Therapeutic use of antibacterials is effective if started early. Water medication is preferred at first. Because drug-resistant strains are prevalent, it is essential to choose a drug to which the organism is sensitive. Bacitracin, carbadox, lincomycin, tylosin, tiamulin, and virginiamycin are commonly used. The disease may be eradicated from infected premises without total depopulation by a persistent and carefully planned program that includes treatment of carrier pigs with bactericidal drugs and thorough cleaning and disinfection of vacated facilities. Mice are an important reservoir of infection for *B hyodysenteriae*, and any eradication attempt must include elimination/reduction of the mouse population on the farm. In addition, *B hyodysenteriae* will survive >60 days in pig waste at refrigerator temperatures.

TRANSMISSIBLE GASTROENTERITIS

Transmissible gastroenteritis (TGE) is a common viral disease of the small intestine that causes vomiting and profuse diarrhea in pigs of all ages.

Etiology and Pathogenesis: The causal coronavirus infects and destroys villous epithelial cells of the jejunum and ileum, which results in severe villous atrophy, malabsorption, osmotic diarrhea, and dehydration. The incubation period is ~18 hr. The infection spreads rapidly by aerosol or contact exposure. Severe epidemics are more common during winter because of survival of the virus in colder temperatures.

Clinical Findings: In nonimmune herds, vomiting often is the initial sign, followed by profuse watery diarrhea, dehydration, and excessive thirst. Feces of nursing pigs often contain curds of undigested milk. Mortality is nearly 100% in piglets <1 wk old, whereas pigs >1 mo old seldom die. Gestating sows occasionally abort, and lactating sows often exhibit vomiting, diarrhea, and agalactia. Diarrhea in surviving nursing piglets continues for ~5 days, but older pigs may be diarrheic for a shorter period.

In large herds with endemic TGE, clinical signs are variable, depending on the level of immunity and magnitude of exposure. Immunity from antibody in the sow's milk usually is sufficient to protect piglets until they are 4–5 days old. As the antibody level in milk decreases, infection and mild disease may occur. Depending on the level of immunity and exposure, diarrhea may be mild in some litters but severe in others. If passive protection is sufficient to protect pigs throughout the nursing period, diarrhea often develops during the first few days after weaning.

Lesions: Piglets dying of TGE are severely dehydrated, and the skin is soiled with liquid feces. The stomach usually contains milk curd but may be empty. The small intestine is thin walled, and the entire intestine contains greenish or yellow watery fluid and clumps of undigested milk. Older pigs have few remarkable lesions, except that the colon contains liquid rather than formed feces. Villous atrophy can be seen by examining the mucosa of the small intestine with a hand lens.

Diagnosis: Clinical signs in the epidemic form of TGE usually justify a presumptive diagnosis. In the mild endemic form, laboratory procedures are required. Histologic and immunofluorescent examinations of the small intestine to demonstrate typical lesions and the presence of TGE viral antigen provide confirmatory evidence. In some outbreaks, hemagglutinating encephalomyelitis (*see* p 728) may cause similar signs.

Treatment and Control: There is no specific treatment. Increasing farrowing room temperature to minimize loss of body heat and providing electrolyte solutions to combat dehydration are helpful. Administration of swine immunoglobulins has been reported to be beneficial. Weaning older nursing pigs that are consuming creep feed may reduce mortality.

Protective immunity depends on presence of antibody in the small intestine. Passive protection of piglets is provided by continual nursing of immune sows. Active, protective immunity develops after infection of the intestinal mucosa with virulent TGE virus. Active infection of the intestine with virulent virus provides protective immunity for 6–18 mo due to a secretory IgA response. Vaccination of naturally immune sows boosts immunity sufficiently to protect neonates and is particularly useful in endemically infected herds. Vaccination of swine in herds free of TGE may not be economically beneficial because vaccines do not induce complete immunity.

Planned infection of pregnant sows at least 2–4 wk before farrowing in herds known to be infected with virulent virus usually provides adequate immunity. This may be accomplished by mixing ground, TGE virus–infected intestine and feces in the gestation ration. Because of the obvious hazards associated with this procedure, it should be undertaken only if a later epidemic in the farrowing house seems inevitable. The infectious material should be used only in the same herd from which it was collected, and the tissues should be as free as possible from other pathogens of pigs. TGE virus can be eliminated from herds without total depopulation by maximizing immunity with planned infection of the sow herd; an "all-in/all-out" management of farrowing, nursery, and grower rooms; and good sanitation.

Because TGE virus is easily spread during an epidemic by people, animals, and fomites, special care should be taken to prevent spread to unexposed groups of pigs and to neighboring herds.

OTHER INTESTINAL VIRUSES OF PIGS

Other viruses have been isolated from the intestines of pigs but appear not to be associated with economically significant disease. These include adenovirus and enterovirus.

GASTROINTESTINAL PARASITES OF RUMINANTS

Clinical Findings and Diagnosis: The clinical signs associated with GI parasitisms are shared by many diseases and conditions; however, a presumptive diagnosis based on signs, grazing history, and season is often justified. Infection usually can be confirmed by demonstrating nematode eggs or tapeworm segments on fecal examination. However, in clinical evaluation of fecal examinations, two points should be remembered: 1) a fecal worm egg count (number of worm eggs per gram (EPG) of feces is not always an accurate indication of the number of adult worms present, and 2) specific identification of certain nematode eggs (eg, "strongyles") is impractical except in specialized laboratories. EPG counts can be negative or deceptively low in the presence of large numbers of immature worms; even when many adult parasites are present, the count can be low if egg production has been suppressed by host immune reaction or recent anthelmintic treatment. Variations in the egg-producing capability of different worms (significantly lower for *Trichostrongylus*, *Ostertagia*, and *Nematodirus* than for *Haemonchus*) may also distort the true picture. The ova of *Nematodirus*, *Bunostomum*, *Strongyloides*, and *Trichuris* are distinctive, but reliable differentiation of the more common species of ruminant strongyle ova is difficult. Fecal culture of strongyle eggs can produce distinctive third-stage larvae if differentiation is important premortem.

The advent of safe and effective broad-spectrum anthelmintics has largely reduced the need to differentiate the genera and species of these parasites. In areas where *Ostertagia* spp predominate, the analysis of sera for increased plasma pepsinogen levels is a useful diagnostic aid. Generally, increased levels of pepsinogen activity (tyrosine levels >3 IU) are associated with clinical abomasal parasitism. Problems of interpretation may arise in immune animals under challenge, in which there are no clinical signs but the pepsinogen levels may be increased because of a hypersensitivity-type reaction in the abomasal mucosa. Where *Haemonchus* spp predominate, the traditional estimation of PCV as an indicator of anemia has been largely replaced by use of the FAMACHA test (*see* below). In some countries, serologic diagnosis (ELISA) of important species, such as *Ostertagia* in cattle, is also used and based on antibody titers in bulk tank milk samples in dairy herds. Such information is used as an indicator of pasture challenge at a herd level, as an indirect indicator of productivity, and is linked with the effectiveness of parasite control strategies.

In many management situations, high levels of infection can be expected, particularly after favorable temperature and rainfall conditions. "Diagnostic drenching" may be recommended when eggs are few or absent, yet history and signs suggest infections, although care should be taken not to treat animals indiscriminately to minimize the risk of anthelmintic resistance developing.

Routine postmortem examinations can provide valuable parasitologic data about the status of the rest of the herd or flock. On necropsy, *Haemonchus*, *Bunostomum*, *Oesophagostomum*, *Trichuris*, and *Chabertia* adults (or advanced immature worms) can be seen easily. *Ostertagia*, *Trichostrongylus*, *Cooperia*, and *Nematodirus* are difficult to see except by their movement in fluid digesta, and clinically important infections are easily overlooked. In such cases, the total contents and all washings should be combined to a known volume, and a worm count established to evaluate the severity of the infection. The number of worms found in aliquots of the gut contents and scrapings of the mucosa will enable the total worm count to be calculated. However, the smaller nematodes may be difficult to see against a background of digesta, so they can be stained (5 min) with a strong iodine solution. Once the digesta and any tissue have been decolorized with 5% sodium thiosulfate, the iodine-stained worms can be seen easily. The significance of the numbers of worms present varies according to worm and host species. For example, only 100 *Haemonchus* are of clinical significance in lambs, whereas 5,000–10,000 *Ostertagia* are typically required before clinical signs are seen. If the animals have been diarrheic for a few days, worms may have been expelled and so the location, type, and severity of gross lesions may also be of considerable diagnostic value.

Mixed parasite infections should be considered when evaluating clinical, laboratory, and necropsy findings, because grazing animals rarely have mono-specific infections in the field.

The diagnosis of ostertagiosis in cattle during the period of larval inhibition (aka arrested development, hypobiosis, diapause) presents technical problems, particularly for the feedlot industry in the USA. Fecal egg counts and plasma pepsinogen analysis do not provide useful information because inhibition occurs within a few days of larval ingestion, before either the egg-laying adult stage has been reached or plasma pepsinogen levels increase. Predisposing factors for inhibition of larvae include age and geographic source of cattle, time of year or season of arrival, previous grazing history and management, weather conditions prevailing during the last grazing period, and prevalence of *Ostertagia ostertagi* in the source region.

Information on such factors is not usually available for feedlot cattle. If cattle have arrived after spring grazing in the south of the USA or fall grazing in the north, they could have heavy burdens of inhibited larvae. Lighter calves from areas where prevalence of parasites is high may also have such a problem. It is becoming more widely accepted that a significant cause of clinical disease or feed efficiency problems in feedlot cattle is parasitism, possibly ostertagiosis. When cattle are brought in from a suspect area and at a suspect time of year, it may be advisable to treat the new arrivals promptly with an anthelmintic effective against inhibited larvae.

Treatment: Effective worm control cannot always be achieved by drugs alone; however, anthelmintics play an important role. (*See also* ANTHELMINTICS, p 2637.) They may be used to reduce pasture contamination, particularly at times when seeding of the pasture with parasite eggs is a prerequisite for development of an infective challenge necessary to cause clinical parasitism. Coordination with other methods of control, such as alternate or mixed grazing with different host species, integrated rotational grazing of different age groups within a single host species (including creep grazing), inclusion of tannin-rich forages in pasture, and alternation of grazing and cropping, are other management techniques that can help to provide safe pasture and give economic advantage when combined with anthelmintic treatment.

The "ideal" anthelmintic should be safe, highly effective against adult and immature stages (including inhibited larvae) of the important worms, available in convenient formulations, economical, and compatible with other commonly used compounds.

Broad-spectrum anthelmintics currently available belong to five different chemical groups: 1) benzimidazoles (white drenches), 2) imidazothiazoles (yellow drenches), 3) macrocyclic lactones (clear drenches), 4) amino-acetonitrile derivatives, and 5) spiroindoles. The benzimidazoles include thiabendazole, the forerunner of modern broad-spectrum anthelmintics, which set a new standard in efficacy and is still widely used today.

Thiabendazole's ineffectiveness against inhibited *Ostertagia* larvae in cattle and one or two specific worm species led to the development of other benzimidazoles (such as fenbendazole, oxfendazole, and albendazole) and the probenzimidazoles (thiophanate, febantel, and netobimin). These compounds are effective against most of the major GI parasites of ruminants and have varying levels of activity against inhibited larvae. The imidazothiazoles include levamisole, morantel, and pyrantel, which also are highly effective, safe, broad-spectrum anthelmintics but have little activity against inhibited larvae in cattle. The macrocyclic lactones, which include the avermectins and milbemycins, often administered as pour-on products or by injection, are highly effective against adult and larval stages, including inhibited larvae of all the common GI nematodes of ruminants and some of the important ectoparasites. The latter group may persist in some ruminant species for several weeks after a single subcutaneous or topical administration and confer protection against reinfection during this period. Moxidectin is also persistent after oral administration. Unlike many other anthelmintics, eprinomectin may also be used in lactating cows without the need for a milk withdrawal period. The amino-acetonitrile derivatives (monepantel) and the spiroindoles (derquantel) are given as oral drenches in sheep, the latter in combination with abamectin in New Zealand. Both of these drugs have been used in the control of multiresistant GI nematode populations, although they require careful administration if their useful life is to be preserved.

Some narrow-spectrum anthelmintics, such as the salicylanilides, closantel, and rafoxanide, bind strongly to plasma proteins and have excellent activity against *Haemonchus contortus* in sheep and remain in the host for a long time, conferring prolonged prophylactic activity after administration.

Routes of administration other than drenching or injection (eg, incorporating into feed, drinking water, and mineral or energy blocks) are used to reduce labor costs and may be useful under drylot conditions or when grazing animals are being given supplemental feed. Another advantage of these "in-feed" routes is that continual low-level administration of a drug can be achieved and pasture contamination reduced during periods that are optimal for free-living development of the parasites. Disadvantages include erratic consumption of anthelmintic, tissue residues (requiring observance of recommended withdrawal periods), and possible encouragement of drug resistance by continual exposure. Another labor-saving route of administration is the "pour-on" topical treatment, used for some of the organophosphates (eg, trichlorfon), levamisole, and avermectins. A number of bolus preparations (eg, morantel, levamisole, ivermectin, or benzimidazoles) release drug in a sustained fashion or in pulses at intervals approximately equal to the prepatent period of the most important GI parasites. The boluses used in cattle have been designed to give entire grazing season protection in temperate areas if administered at turn-out to set-stocked herds. Boluses are also available that provide treatment and subsequent prophylaxis of animals already exposed to contaminated pasture and harboring parasites. Boluses in sheep may be used to reduce the periparturient rise in fecal egg output and thus the pasture contamination responsible for disease in their offspring later in the grazing season. Despite their efficacy, some boluses used in either cattle or sheep have been withdrawn from the market because they are not commercially viable.

Niclosamide, morantel, praziquantel, and the newer benzimidazoles (albendazole, fenbendazole, and oxfendazole) are effective against tapeworms (*Moniezia* spp) in cattle and sheep. Successful treatment of the fringed tapeworm, *Thysanosoma actinioides*, has been reported using either fenbendazole or praziquantel.

When treating clinically affected animals, the following should be considered: 1) provide adequate nutrition; (2) treat all animals in the group, as a preventive measure and to reduce further pasture contamination; and 3) either house or move stock to "clean" pastures to minimize reinfection. The definition of safe pastures varies in different climates and depends on local knowledge of the seasonal mortality of infective larvae. Some authorities have suggested treating only the most severely affected animals in a flock or herd, ie, targeted selective treatment (TST). Where *Haemonchus* is a problem in sheep or goats, animals most likely to benefit from such treatment can be identified using the FAMACHA score card. This links the color of the ocular mucous membranes, measured using a color chart, with the degree of anemia associated with the blood-sucking parasite. Animals with the palest mucous membranes are those likely to have the heaviest worm burdens and be chosen for treatment. The severity of diarrhea and/or the quantitative fecal egg count for parasitic gastroenteritis in sheep or cattle can also be used to determine the need for individual treatment. The rationale behind TST is that a very large proportion of worm egg output (and thus pasture contamination) is produced by a relatively small proportion of the host animal population. Treatment of only these animals significantly reduces pasture contamination and reduces the overall selection pressure, exerted by the use of an anthelmintic, for resistant parasite genes. Untreated animals will continue to pass low numbers of worm eggs onto the pasture and so maintain a "susceptible" parasite gene pool "in refugia" (ie, unexposed to anthelmintic treatment). In contrast, the established practice of blanket treatment and movement of stock onto a clean pasture may encourage emergence of anthelmintic resistance. Any worms carrying resistance genes surviving the treatment will then seed the previously clean pasture with a largely resistant parasite population.

Finally, the development of multiple drug resistance in populations of *Haemonchus contortus*, *Trichostrongylus* spp, and *Ostertagia* spp in sheep and goats to benzimidazoles, levamisole, and avermectins/milbemycins has been demonstrated. Although such resistance is currently a problem only in certain areas, it should be considered when other factors have been excluded, such as improper dosage, rapid reinfection, poor nutrition, or some disease state other than parasitism. Drug resistance in parasites of cattle has been demonstrated, although much less frequently than in small ruminants; overuse and otherwise indiscriminate treatment should be avoided.

If anthelmintic resistance is suspected on a farm, a fecal egg count reduction test may be conducted onsite that will indicate the likelihood of resistance. Fifteen to twenty animals should be randomly selected and assigned to either control or treatment groups, one for each anthelmintic group selected. Fecal samples are collected before treatment from all groups and then again either 7 days (after levamisole treatment) or 14 days (after benzimidazole or macrocyclic lactone treatment) later. Pre- and post-treatment fecal worm egg counts are then compared and anthelmintic resistance suspected if the reduction in output after dosing is <95%.

The high cost of developing new anthelmintic drugs has encouraged researchers to look for alternative approaches to GI parasite control, such as development of a "hidden antigen" vaccine against *Haemonchus*; the use of tannin-rich forages (such as clover and lucerne or alfalfa), which have some anthelmintic action; and nematophagous fungi.

General Control Measures

"Control" generally implies the suppression of parasite burdens in the host below that level at which economic losses occur. To do this effectively requires a comprehensive knowledge of the epidemiologic and ecologic factors that govern pasture larval populations and the role of host immunity in combating infection.

The goals of control are as follows: 1) prevent heavy exposure in susceptible hosts (recovery from heavy infection is always slow), 2) reduce overall levels of pasture contamination, 3) minimize the effects of parasite burdens, and 4) encourage the development of immunity in the animals (less important in fattening animals than in those to be kept for breeding purposes).

The strategic use of anthelmintics is designed to reduce the build up of worm burdens and, as a result, pasture contamination. The timing of anthelmintic treatment is based on knowledge of the seasonal changes in infection and the regional epidemiology of the various helminthoses. Prompt recognition of circumstances likely to favor development of parasitic disease, eg, weather, grazing behavior, and loss of weight and condition, is essential.

For example, in the UK, where the pattern of disease caused by *Nematodirus battus* infection in sheep is clearly defined, strategic treatments with two or three doses of an anthelmintic at 2- to 3-wk intervals, beginning just before the disease characteristically appears, are recommended. The timing of these treatments is designed to coincide with peak numbers of *Nematodirus* larvae on pasture in the spring; timing of the latter can be predicted accurately using a simple formula that incorporates soil temperatures 1 ft below the surface during March. Similarly, in the northern USA, Canada, and western Europe, pasture levels of *Ostertagia* and other parasites increase substantially after mid-July, ie, the general pattern of infectivity is minimal in spring but increases rapidly to peak levels in late summer and early fall. Current practices in these areas indicate the effectiveness of two or more carefully timed anthelmintic treatments given during the first grazing season after turnout in the spring. Calculating the interval between treatments requires knowledge of the parasite's prepatent period (3 wk in the case of *Ostertagia* in cattle) and the duration of residual (or prolonged) activity of the anthelmintic being used, ie, the period of protection provided after a single treatment; the treatment interval is calculated as the sum of the two. For example, treatment with a macrocyclic lactone with a 5-wk period of residual activity at turnout and again 8 wk later should result in highly effective control of worm egg output and minimal numbers of larvae appearing on pasture during the fall. No further treatment is likely to be required, because any larvae surviving on pasture from the previous year would have died by the time the prophylactic effect of the second treatment had worn off.

In other countries, with either a cool or warm temperate climate, similar controls may be used if the seasonal pattern of the disease is known, but in most regions a tactical use of anthelmintics is used, eg, during warm, moist conditions.

Cattle—Special Considerations

Worm problems are seen most frequently in young beef cattle from time of weaning and several months thereafter, and in segregated groups of dairy calves during the first season at grass. Immunity to GI nematodes is acquired slowly; two grazing seasons may be required before a significant level is attained. In endemic areas, cows may continue to harbor low burdens, which may contribute to suboptimal production on some farms. GI parasitism in young stock may be controlled by use of broad-spectrum anthelmintics in conjunction with pasture management to limit reinfection; the latter includes a move to "clean" pastures (eg, grass conservation areas or silage or hay aftermath, although anthelmintic resistance concerns should be noted [above]), alternate grazing with other host species, or integrated rotational grazing in which susceptible calves are followed by immune adults. Alternate grazing with other host species may be ineffective in areas where parasite species (eg, *Nematodirus*) infect both hosts; simple pasture rotation is not effective, because the bovine fecal mass can protect larvae from adverse environmental conditions for several months, infecting rotating calves at a later date.

In beef herds, anthelmintic treatment at weaning is of value, particularly if the young cattle are to be retained, eg, as replacement heifer stock or as steers to be fed. Cattle finished on grass should receive treatment at weaning and at intervals throughout the next 12 mo and, if possible, should be moved to safe pastures to maximize liveweight gain.

When cattle cannot be moved readily to other pastures, strategic treatments (described earlier) may be given to limit contamination of pastures and rapid reinfection. Alternatively, intraruminal boluses may be used in countries where approved. In warm temperate regions of the world, such as Australia and New Zealand, the southern USA, and the large cattle-raising regions of southern Brazil, Uruguay, and Argentina, young cattle may be given two or more treatments from late summer and into fall for prevention of large increases in pasture contamination and infection during winter and spring. Two or three strategic treatments, administered with a short interval, from the time of weaning in such regions could be just as effective as spring treatments in cool temperate regions. However, survival of infective larvae on pasture from the time of fall weaning in warm temperate regions is most often persistent, and longer intervals between treatments (eg, at weaning, during winter, and in late spring) may be more applicable. In many areas, anthelmintics are simply given at regular intervals after weaning. Intervals between treatments must necessarily vary according to local parasite epidemiology and the duration of prolonged activity exhibited by the anthelmintic. When Type II ostertagiosis is a problem, treatment with an anthelmintic effective against inhibited larvae is recommended before the expected time of outbreak.

Sheep—Special Considerations

A special strategic treatment is required in most regions to counter the postparturient relaxation of immunity (resulting in the periparturient rise in worm egg output) seen in breeding ewes. The precise timing of such treatment varies between regions and for different species of parasites and will, in temperate regions, depend on whether ewes and lambs are turned out onto clean or contaminated pasture. On clean grazing, only the ewes (with an existing parasite burden) act as a source of worm eggs and, therefore, require treatment to prevent pasture contamination and subsequent infection of their lambs. Ewes treated during the month before lambing should not only exhibit a drop in worm egg output but may also show improved productivity. On contaminated pasture, both ewes and lambs pass worm eggs in their feces (ewes from their existing worm burden and lambs from larvae overwintering on pasture). The aim of treating ewes should be to prevent fecal worm egg output; this can be achieved by treating with an albendazole or ivermectin anthelmintic bolus (available in some countries), injectable long-acting moxidectin, or medicated feed blocks. In temperate areas, lambs should be dosed at weaning before a move to clean grazing.

A treatment 2 wk before breeding, as part of a "flushing" program, is another strategic application of anthelmintics. Supportive management after treatment includes movement of sheep from contaminated pastures to cattle pastures, grass conservation areas, root crops, or pasture not grazed by sheep for several months. The latter period varies according to the seasonal pattern of larval mortality in different countries and may be as long as 1 yr in some temperate countries.

Sheep are more consistently susceptible to the adverse effects of worms than other livestock, and clinical disease is more common. Immunity to the parasites is acquired slowly and is generally incomplete. Frequent treatments may be required, particularly during the first year of life, although a good understanding of local parasite epidemiology will ensure that such treatments are appropriately timed.

GASTROINTESTINAL PARASITES OF CATTLE

Haemonchus, Ostertagia, and *Trichostrongylus* spp

The common stomach worms of cattle are *Haemonchus placei* (barber's pole worm, large stomach worm, wire worm), *Ostertagia ostertagi* (medium or brown stomach worm), and *Trichostrongylus axei* (small stomach worm, *see* p 319). In some tropical countries, *Mecistocirrus digitatus*, a large worm up to 40 mm long, is present. *H placei* is primarily a parasite in tropical regions, whereas *O ostertagi* and, to a lesser extent, *T axei* are found in more temperate climates. Adult male *Haemonchus* are up to 18 mm long, females up to 30 mm. *Ostertagia* adults are 6–9 mm long, and *Trichostrongylus*, ~5 mm.

The preparasitic life cycles of the three groups are generally similar. Larvae hatch shortly after the eggs are passed in the feces and reach the infective stage in ~2 wk under optimal temperatures (~75°F [24°C]). Development to the infective stage is delayed during cold weather. In areas with narrow diurnal temperature variations, those months with a mean maximum temperature of 65°F (18°C) and with rainfall >2 in. (5 cm) are favorable for development of the free-living stages of *H placei*, but where wide fluctuations occur, a mean minimum temperature of 50°F (10°C) may effectively limit development. The preparasitic forms of *O ostertagi* and *T axei* develop and survive better in cooler conditions, and their upper limits for survival are lower than those for *H placei*. If the temperature is unfavorable or drought conditions exist, infective larvae may remain dormant in the feces for weeks until conditions become favorable again, eg, after heavy rainfall, when large numbers of infective larvae emerge onto the surrounding grass.

The prepatent period of *O ostertagi* is normally ~3 wk. Ingested larvae enter the lumen of the abomasal glands and molt by the fourth day; they remain there during the prepatent period, growing and undergoing a final molt before emerging as young adult

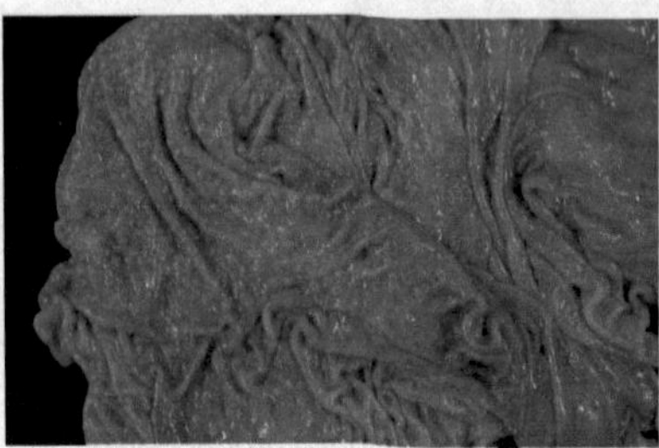

Abomasal lesions due to *Ostertagia*. Courtesy of Dr. Sameeh M. Abutarbush.

worms from the gastric glands onto the abomasal mucosa. During this time, the specialized cells (pepsinogen-producing zymogen cells, acid-producing parietal cells) lining parasitized glands are lost and replaced by hyperplastic, undifferentiated cuboidal cells, resulting in nodules that may be discrete or confluent. Around the time of worm emergence, the changes seen in parasitized glands also appear in neighboring nonparasitized glands, rapidly extending the effects of the parasite burden. As a result, in heavy infections, abomasal pH may rise from 2 to >6; from a clinical viewpoint, when pH rises above 4.5, digestion in the abomasum ceases. A protein-losing gastropathy results and, together with anorexia and impaired protein digestion, leads to hypoproteinemia and weight loss. Diarrhea is persistent. In **Type I ostertagiosis**, which results from recent infection, most worms present are adults, and the response to anthelmintic treatment is good. Type I disease is seen primarily in calves 7–15 mo old. It is most common from time of weaning and ensuing months in warm temperate regions and in young cattle during summer and early fall in cool temperate regions.

In **Type II ostertagiosis**, large numbers of larvae, which had become dormant or inhibited in development at the early fourth larval stage, emerge from the glands weeks or months later. This is seen primarily in cattle 12–20 mo old. In warm temperate regions, inhibition-prone larvae are acquired in spring, and disease may result when large numbers of larvae resume development to the adult stage in late summer or fall. In cold temperate regions, inhibition-prone larvae are acquired during late autumn and mature during late winter or early spring.

Larval inhibition in *O ostertagi* and other nematodes is thought to be analogous to diapause in insects. It has been interpreted as a survival mechanism in which the preparasitic stages on pasture avoid the adverse conditions of winter in cool regions and of hot and dry (or hot and alternately wet and dry) conditions of many warm regions. The factors that cause and later "switch off" inhibition are not completely known, but prolonged experimental cold conditioning of infective larvae was found to be important in a cool temperate region. In warm regions of both northern and southern hemispheres, conditioning of preparasitic stages to inhibition develops principally during spring before the hot and dry conditions of summer. The resumed development or maturation of the parasites is likely to be genetically predetermined and may be influenced by parturition, nutrition, concurrent infection, and host immune response.

H placei may also become inhibited over winter; they then resume development in the spring and infect the pastures with eggs at a time suitable for their development. Both the larval and adult stages are pathogenic because of their blood-sucking ability. *T axei* causes gastritis with superficial erosion of the mucosa, hyperemia, and diarrhea. Protein loss from the damaged mucosa and anorexia cause hypoproteinemia and weight loss. Inhibition does not occur to the same degree.

Clinical Findings: Young animals are more often affected, but adults not previously exposed to infection frequently show signs and succumb. *Ostertagia* and *Trichostrongylus* infections are characterized by profuse, watery diarrhea that usually is persistent. In haemonchosis and *Mecistocirrus* infection, there may be little or no diarrhea but possibly intermittent periods of constipation. Anemia of variable degree is a characteristic sign of both these infections.

Concurrent with the diarrhea of *O ostertagi* and *T axei* infections, and with the anemia of heavy *Haemonchus* infection, there is often hypoproteinemia and edema (rare in *O ostertagi* infections), particularly under the lower jaw (bottle jaw) and sometimes along the ventral abdomen. Heavy infections can result in death before clinical signs appear. Other variable signs include progressive weight loss, weakness, rough coat, and anorexia.

Lesions: Worms can readily be seen and identified in the abomasum, and small petechiae may be visible where the worms have been feeding. The most characteristic lesions of *Ostertagia* infection are small, umbilicated nodules 1–2 mm in diameter. These may be discrete, but in heavy infections they tend to coalesce and give rise to a "cobblestone" or "morocco leather" appearance. Nodules are most marked in the fundic region but may cover the entire abomasal mucosa and may be accompanied by a rise in gastric pH to 6–7. As a result, pepsinogen will no longer be converted to pepsin and may leak across the damaged epithelium, leading to high plasma levels. There is also evidence that adult *Ostertagia* can cause direct hypersecretion of pepsinogen. The increased abomasal pH may also stimulate production of gastrin and thus hypergastrinemia, which is closely associated with the inappetence that may accompany infection. This parasite-associated drop in intake has been shown to be largely responsible for impaired weight gain. Edema is often marked and, in severe cases, may extend over the abomasum and into the small intestine and omentum.

In *T axei* infections, the mucosa of the abomasum may show congestion and superficial erosions, which are sometimes covered with a fibrinonecrotic exudate.

Diagnosis, Treatment, and Control: *See* p 303 et seq.

Cooperia spp

Several species of *Cooperia* are found in the small intestine of cattle; *C punctata*, *C oncophora*, and *C pectinata* are the most common. The red, coiled adults are 5–8 mm long, and the male has a large bursa. They may be difficult to observe grossly. Their life cycle is essentially the same as that of other trichostrongylids. These worms apparently do not suck blood. Most of them are found in the first 10–20 ft (3–6 m) of the small intestine. The prepatent period is 12–15 days.

The eggs usually can be differentiated from those of the common GI nematodes by their practically parallel sides, but a larval culture of the feces is necessary to definitively diagnose *Cooperia* infection in the living animal. In heavy infections with *C punctata* and *C pectinata*, there is profuse diarrhea, anorexia, and emaciation, but no anemia; the upper small intestine shows marked congestion of the mucosa with small hemorrhages. The mucosa may show a fine lace-like superficial necrosis. *C oncophora* produces a milder disease but can be responsible for weight loss and poor productivity. It is usually necessary to make scrapings of the mucosa to demonstrate *Cooperia* spp, which must be differentiated from *Trichostrongylus* spp, *Strongyloides papillosus*, and immature *Nematodirus* spp.

For diagnosis, treatment, and control, *see* p 303 et seq.

Bunostomum sp

The adult male *Bunostomum phlebotomum* is ~15 mm long and the female ~25 mm. Hookworms have well-developed buccal capsules into which the mucosa is drawn; cutting plates at the anterior edge of the buccal capsule are used to abrade the mucosa during feeding. The prepatent period is ~2 mo. Infection is by ingestion or skin penetration; the latter is more common in animals kept in poor conditions.

Larval penetration of the lower limbs may cause uneasiness and stamping, particularly in stabled cattle. Adult worms cause anemia and rapid weight loss. Diarrhea and constipation may alternate. Hypoproteinemic edema may be present, but bottle jaw is rarely as severe as in haemonchosis. During the patent period, a diagnosis may be made by demonstrating the characteristic eggs in the feces.

On necropsy, the mucosa may appear congested and swollen, with numerous small hemorrhagic points where the worms were attached. The worms are readily seen in the first few feet of the small intestine, and the contents are often blood-stained. As few as 2,000 worms may cause death in calves. Local lesions, edema, and scab formation may result from penetration of larvae into the skin of resistant calves.

For diagnosis, treatment, and control, *see* p 303 et seq.

Strongyloides sp

The intestinal threadworm *Strongyloides papillosus* has an unusual life cycle. Only the female worms are found in the intestine. They are 3.5–6 mm long and are embedded in the mucosa of the upper small intestine. Small, embryonated eggs are passed in the feces, hatch rapidly, and develop directly into infective larvae or free-living adults. The offspring of these free-living adults may develop into another generation of infective larvae or free-living adults. The host is infected by penetration of the skin or by ingestion; infective larvae can be transmitted in colostrum as in other species of the genus. The prepatent period is ~10 days.

Infections are most common in young calves, particularly dairy stock. Although signs are rare, they may include intermittent diarrhea, loss of appetite and weight, and sometimes blood and mucus in the feces. Large numbers of worms in the intestine produce catarrhal enteritis with petechiae and ecchymoses, especially in the duodenum and jejunum.

For diagnosis, treatment, and control, *see* p 303 et seq.

Nematodirus spp

Nematodirus helvetianus is generally recognized as the most common bovine species, although other species, eg, *N spathiger* and *N battus*, can also infect cattle. The adult males of *N helvetianus* are ~12 mm long and the females 18–25 mm. The eggs develop slowly; the infective third stage is reached within the egg in 2–4 wk and may remain within the egg for several months. Eggs may accumulate on pasture and hatch in large numbers after rain to produce heavy infections over a short period. The eggs are highly resistant, and those passed by calves in one season may remain viable and infect calves the next season. After ingestion of infective larvae, the adult stage is reached in ~3 wk. Worms are most numerous 10–20 ft (3–6 m) from the pylorus.

Signs, which include diarrhea and anorexia, usually develop during the third week of infection before the worms are sexually mature; clinical infections may be seen in dairy calves from 6 wk onward. Diagnosis is difficult during the prepatent period, but during the patent period it is easily made on the basis of the characteristic eggs. Relatively small numbers of eggs are produced. Fecal sampling of both healthy and sick calves in an affected group will increase the chance of making a diagnosis. Immunity to reinfection develops rapidly. Necropsy may show only a thickened, edematous mucosa.

For diagnosis, treatment, and control, *see* p 303 et seq.

Toxocara sp

The ascarid *Toxocara vitulorum* is a stout, whitish worm (males 20–25 cm, females 25–30 cm) found in the small intestine of calves <6 mo old; older calves are resistant. Larvae hatching from ingested eggs pass to the tissues and, in pregnant cows, are mobilized late in pregnancy and passed via the milk to calves. Eggs appear in the feces of calves from 3 wk of age and are easily recognized by their thick, pitted shells and dark brown center. In some parts of the world, the infection is considered serious, particularly in buffalo calves.

For diagnosis, treatment, and control, *see* p 303 et seq.

Oesophagostomum sp

Adults of *Oesophagostomum radiatum* (nodular worm) are 12–15 mm long, and the head is bent dorsally. Because the eggs are very similar to those of *Haemonchus placei*, they are often grouped together on routine fecal examination. The life cycle is direct. The larvae penetrate primarily into the wall of the lower 10–20 ft (3–6 m) of the small intestine but also into the cecum and colon, where they remain for 5–10 days and then return to the lumen as fourth-stage larvae. The prepatent period in susceptible animals is ~6 wk. However, in subsequent reinfections, larvae become arrested for some time, and many never return to the lumen (host encystment).

Young animals suffer from the effects of adult worms, whereas in older animals, the effect of nodules enclosing larval worms is more important. Infection causes anorexia; severe, constant, dark, persistent, fetid diarrhea; weight loss; and death. In older, resistant animals, the nodules surrounding the larvae become caseated and calcified, thus decreasing the motility of the intestine. Stenosis or intussusception occasionally occurs. Nodules can be palpated per rectum, and the worms and nodules can be seen readily at necropsy.

For diagnosis, treatment, and control, *see* p 303 et seq.

Chabertia sp

Adults of the large-mouth bowel worm, *Chabertia ovina*, are ~12 mm long and bent ventrally at the anterior end. There is a typical direct life cycle. The larvae penetrate the mucosa of the small intestine shortly after ingestion and later emerge and pass to the colon. The prepatent period is ~7 wk. Larvae and adults may cause small hemorrhages with edema in the colon and passage of feces coated with mucus. Clinical chabertiosis is seldom, if ever, seen in cattle.

For diagnosis, treatment, and control, *see* p 303 et seq.

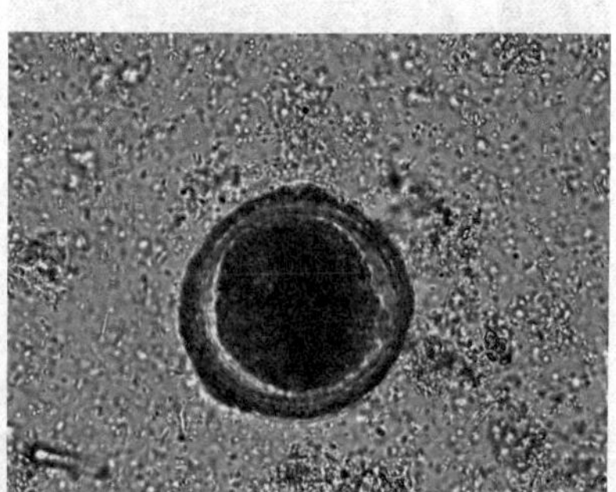

Toxocara canis egg. Courtesy of Dr. Mark Fox.

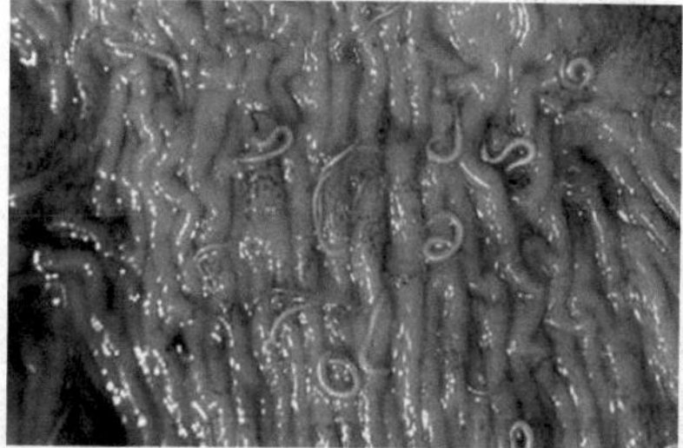

Trichuris ovis attached to intestinal wall of a sheep. Courtesy of Dr. Raffaele Roncalli.

Trichuris spp

Trichuris spp infections are common in young calves and yearlings, but the numbers of worms are seldom large. The eggs are resistant, and infections are likely to persist on problem premises. Clinical signs are unlikely, but in occasional heavy infections, dark feces, anemia, and anorexia may be seen.

For diagnosis, treatment, and control, *see* p 303 et seq.

Tapeworms

The anoplocephalid tapeworms *Moniezia expansa* and *M benedeni* are found in young cattle. The worms of this group are characterized by the absence of a rostellum and hooks, and the segments are wider than they are long. The eggs are triangular or rectangular and are ingested by the intermediate host, free-living oribatid mites, which live in the soil and grass. After 6–16 wk, infective cysticercoids are present in the mites. Infection occurs after ingestion of infected mites; the prepatent period is ~5 wk. *Moniezia* are commonly considered nonpathogenic in calves, but intestinal stasis has been reported.

For diagnosis, treatment, and control, *see* p 303 et seq.

GASTROINTESTINAL PARASITES OF SHEEP AND GOATS

Many species of nematodes and cestodes cause parasitic gastritis and enteritis in sheep and goats. The most important of these are *Haemonchus contortus*, *Teladorsagia (Ostertagia) circumcincta*, *Trichostrongylus axei*, intestinal species of *Trichostrongylus*, *Nematodirus* spp, *Bunostomum trigonocephalum*, and *Oesophagostomum columbianum*. *Cooperia curticei*, *Strongyloides papillosus*, *Trichuris ovis*, and *Chabertia ovina* also may be pathogenic in sheep; these and related species are discussed under GI parasites of cattle (*see* p 308).

Haemonchus, *Ostertagia*, and *Trichostrongylus* spp

The principal stomach worms of sheep and goats are *Haemonchus contortus*, *Teladorsagia (Ostertagia) circumcincta*, *Ostertagia trifurcata*, *Trichostrongylus axei* (*see* GASTROINTESTINAL PARASITES OF CATTLE, p 308), and in some tropical regions, *Mecistocirrus digitatus*. Cross-transmission of *Haemonchus* between sheep and cattle can occur but not as readily as transmission between homologous species. Sheep are more susceptible to the cattle species than cattle are to the sheep species. For descriptions and life cycles, *see* p 308.

Haemonchus is most common in tropical or subtropical areas or in those areas with summer rainfall, whereas *Ostertagia* and *T axei* are more common in cooler winter rainfall areas. The latter species predominate in temperate zones.

Haemonchosis in sheep may be classified as hyperacute, acute, or chronic. In the hyperacute disease, death may occur within 1 wk of heavy infection without significant signs. The acute disease is characterized by severe anemia accompanied by generalized edema; anemia is also characteristic of the chronic infection, often of low worm burdens, and is accompanied by progressive weight loss. Diarrhea is not a sign of pure *Haemonchus* infection; the lesions are those associated with anemia. In cases in which diarrhea is present, there may be mixed infection with other worm genera. The abomasum is edematous and, in the chronic phase, gastric pH increases, which causes abomasal dysfunction. Mature sheep may develop heavy, even fatal, infections, particularly during lactation.

The lesions, pathogenesis, and signs of *Ostertagia* and *T axei* infections are similar to those found in cattle. Even subclinical infection depresses appetite, impairs gastric digestion, and reduces use of metabolizable energy and protein. *Ostertagia* is the principal genus involved in the peripartu-

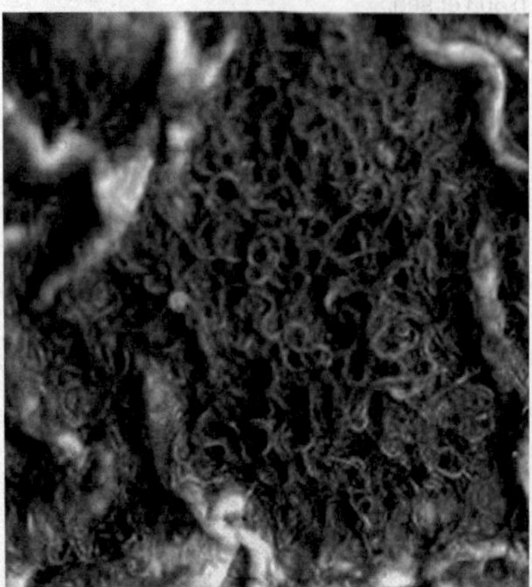

Haemonchus contortus, heavy infestation, abomasum of a sheep. Courtesy of Dr. Raffaele Roncalli.

ent rise in fecal egg counts in sheep, and heavy infections may cause diarrhea and depress milk production in ewes. This output of eggs serves as the main source of contamination for the lambs. The same type of inhibited development seen in cattle has been seen with both *Ostertagia* and *Haemonchus* in sheep.

For diagnosis, treatment, and control, *see* p 303 et seq.

Intestinal Trichostrongylosis

The life cycle of intestinal *Trichostrongylus* (*T colubriformis*, *T vitrinus*, *T rugatus*) is direct. The developing larvae burrow superficially in the crypts of the mucosa and develop to egg-laying adults in 18–21 days.

Anorexia, persistent diarrhea, and weight loss are the main signs. Villous atrophy (or stunting of villi) results in impaired digestion and malabsorption; protein loss occurs across the damaged mucosa. There are no diagnostic lesions; a total worm count should be done to evaluate the condition.

For diagnosis, treatment, and control, *see* p 303 et seq.

Bunostomum and *Gaigeria* spp

Adult *Bunostomum trigonocephalum* (hookworm) are found in the jejunum. The life cycle and clinical findings are essentially the same as for the cattle hookworm (*see* p 310), with as few as 100 worms causing clinical signs. *Gaigeria pachyscelis* is found in Africa and Asia and resembles *Bunostomum* in size and form (2–3 cm). Larvae of *G pachyscelis* infect the host only by skin penetration. *G pachyscelis* is a voracious bloodsucker and probably the most pathogenic hookworm.

For diagnosis, treatment, and control, *see* p 303 et seq.

Nematodirus spp

The species of *Nematodirus* found in the small intestine of sheep are similar in morphology and life cycle to *N helvetianus* (*see* p 310). Clinical infections are of considerable importance in the UK, New Zealand, and Australia, where lamb mortality may reach 20% in affected flocks if animals are untreated. The parasites are also endemic in some parts of the Rocky Mountain states of the USA, where they occasionally cause clinical disease in lambs.

In areas where clinical infections are common, the disease has a characteristic seasonal pattern. Many of the eggs passed by affected lambs lie dormant through the remainder of the grazing season and the winter, with large numbers of larvae appearing during the early grazing period of the following year. Thus, the lambs of one season contaminate the pastures for the next season's lambs; fortunately, the life cycle can be broken if the same area is not used for lambing each year. Most clinical infections are seen in lambs 6–12 wk old.

N battus is seen in the UK and other parts of Europe and also in North America. Eggs hatch after a period of chill and then a rise in ambient temperature to a day/night mean of 10°C (50°F). This occurs in late spring in temperate areas. The hatching requirements mean that there is generally one generation of *N battus* per year, although in the UK, occasional outbreaks in the autumn have been reported. The parasite can be highly pathogenic, because large numbers of larvae hatch over a short period at a time when young lambs are beginning to take in significant quantities of grass. Disease may be associated with developing larval stages and may be seen within 2 wk of challenge, ie during the prepatent period (15 days). Other *Nematodirus* spp often are found in low-rainfall regions (eg, the Karroo in South Africa and inland Australia) where other parasites are rarely seen.

Nematodirosis is characterized by sudden onset, "loss of bloom," unthriftiness, profuse diarrhea, and marked dehydration, with death as early as 2–3 days after an outbreak begins. Nematodirosis is commonly confined to lambs or weaner sheep, but in low-rainfall country where outbreaks are sporadic, older sheep may have heavy infections. The lesions usually consist of dehydration and a mild catarrhal enteritis, but acute inflammation of the entire small intestine may develop. Counts of ≥10,000 worms, together with characteristic signs and history, are indicative of clinical infections. Affected lambs may pass large numbers of eggs, which can be identified easily; however, because the onset of disease may precede the maturation of the female worms, this is not a constant finding.

For diagnosis, treatment, and control, *see* p 303 et seq.

Oesophagostomum sp

The nodular worm of sheep, *Oesophagostomum columbianum*, has a similar morphology and life cycle to those of the nodular worm of cattle (*see* p 311).

Diarrhea usually develops during the second week of infection. The feces may contain excess mucus as well as streaks of blood. As the diarrhea progresses, sheep become emaciated and weak. These signs often subside near the end of the prepatent period, but the continuing presence of numerous adult worms may result in a chronic infection in which signs may not develop for several months. The sheep become weak, lose weight despite a good appetite, and show intermittent diarrhea and constipation.

As immunity develops, nodules form around the larvae; they may become caseated and calcified. Nodule formation usually is more pronounced in sheep than in cattle. Affected sheep walk with a stilted gait and often have a humped back. Stenosis and intussusception may develop in severe cases. Diagnosis is difficult during the prepatent period, at which time it must be based largely on clinical signs.

For diagnosis, treatment, and control, *see* p 303 et seq.

Chabertia sp

Adult worms cause severe damage to the mucosa of the colon, with resulting congestion, ulceration, and small hemorrhages. Infected sheep are unthrifty; the feces are soft, contain much mucus, and may be streaked with blood. Immunity develops quickly, and outbreaks are seen only under conditions of severe stress.

For diagnosis, treatment, and control, *see* p 303 et seq.

Strongyloides sp

Heavy infections with adult worms cause a disease resembling trichostrongylosis. Infection is usually by skin penetration but can also occur via the milk. Damage to the skin between the claws, produced by skin-penetrating larvae, resembles the early stages of footrot and may aid penetration of the causal agents of footrot. Most infections are transitory and inconsequential.

For diagnosis, treatment, and control, *see* p 303 et seq.

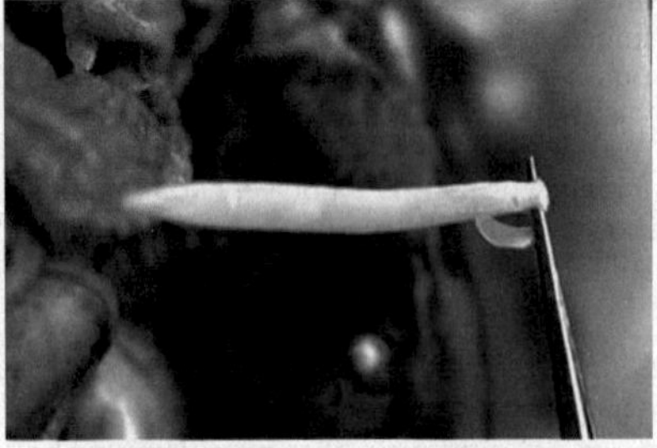

Thysanosoma actinioides, adult, in a sheep.
Courtesy of Dr. Raffaele Roncalli.

Trichuris spp

Heavy infections with whipworms are not common but may be seen in very young lambs or during drought conditions when sheep are fed grain on the ground. The eggs are very resistant. Congestion and edema of the cecal mucosa, accompanied by diarrhea and unthriftiness, are seen.

For diagnosis, treatment, and control, *see* p 303 et seq.

Tapeworms

The pathogenicity of *Moniezia expansa* in sheep has long been debated. Many earlier observations, which associated this infection with diarrhea, emaciation, and weight loss, did not accurately differentiate between tapeworm infections and infection with certain small nematodes (eg, *Trichostrongylus colubriformis*). Tapeworms are relatively nonpathogenic, but heavy infections can result in mild unthriftiness and GI disturbances. Diagnosis may be made by finding individual segments (which are much wider than long) in the feces or lengths of adult tapeworm protruding from the anus or by demonstrating the characteristic eggs on fecal examination. The life cycle involves an oribatid mite that lives in the pasture mat. The prepatent period is 6–7 wk. Infections are seasonal, in accordance with mite activity, and unusual in animals older than ~4–5 mo of age.

Thysanosoma actinioides, the "fringed tapeworm," inhabits the small intestine, the bile ducts, and the pancreatic ducts. It is commonly found in sheep from the southern and western parts of the USA and also South America. Although it has not been associated with clinical disease, it is of economic importance because livers are condemned when tapeworms are found in the bile duct.

For diagnosis, treatment, and control, *see* p 303 et seq.

GASTROINTESTINAL PARASITES OF HORSES

GASTEROPHILUS SPP

Horse bots, which are found in the stomach, are the larvae of bot flies, *Gasterophilus* spp. Three major species are distributed worldwide, and a number of minor species are found in parts of Europe, Africa, and Asia. The adult flies are not parasitic and cannot feed; they survive long enough to mate and lay eggs and die as soon as the nutrients remaining from the larval stage are used, usually in ~2 wk. The three important species can be differentiated in any stage of their development. The eggs of *G intestinalis* (the common bot) are glued to the hairs of almost any part of the body but especially the forelimbs and shoulders. The larvae hatch in ~1 wk when stimulated, usually by the animals' licking. The eggs of *G haemorrhoidalis* (the nose or lip bot) are attached to the hairs of the lips. The larvae emerge in 2–3 days without stimulation and crawl into the mouth. *G nasalis* (the throat bot) deposits eggs on the hairs of the submaxillary region. They hatch in ~1 wk without stimulation.

The larvae of all three species apparently stay embedded in the tongue or the mucosa of the mouth for ~1 mo, after which they pass to the stomach, where they attach themselves to the cardiac or pyloric portions and, in the case of *G nasalis*, to the mucosa of the first part of the small intestine. After development for ~8–10 mo, they pass out in the feces and pupate in the soil for 3–5 wk, after which the adult emerges. The main pathogenic effect is caused by larvae, which attach by oral hooks to the lining of the stomach. This induces erosions and ulcerations at the site of attachment and a hyperplastic reaction around it. However, oral stages may cause sinus tracts in which mucopurulent discharges form, especially along the lingual border of the upper, more posterior cheek teeth.

Clinical Findings and Diagnosis: Bots cause a mild gastritis, but large numbers may be present with no clinical signs. The first instars migrating in the mouth can cause stomatitis and may produce pain on eating. The adult flies may annoy horses when they lay their eggs. Specific diagnosis of *Gasterophilus* infection is difficult and can be made by demonstrating larvae as they pass in the feces. In the USA, the presence of gastric infections during the winter months is often assumed. History of the individual horses, knowledge of the local seasonal cycle of the fly, and observation of the yellow to cream-white bot eggs (1–2 mm) on the horse's hairs all help identify the presence of the parasite in a given herd.

Treatment: In temperate areas, it is assumed that most animals are infected by the end of summer. Ivermectin is effective against oral and gastric stages of bots and, when used as part of a routine parasite control program, provides effective bot control throughout the season. In subtropical or tropical areas, some transmission may occur throughout the year. Moxidectin is effective against gastric stages. Current recommendations for control include at least one treatment annually, at the end of the bot fly season. In some locations where the bot fly season is long, additional treatments may be necessary. Although there is no satisfactory method to protect exposed horses from attack by the adult flies, bot control programs, when applied on a regional basis to all horses, markedly reduce fly numbers and larval infections.

HABRONEMA SPP

The stomach worms *Habronema muscae*, *H microstoma*, and *Draschia megastoma* are widely distributed. The adults are 6–25 mm long. *Draschia* are found in tumor-like swellings in the stomach wall along the margo plicatus. The other species are free on the mucosa. The eggs or larvae are ingested by larvae of house or stable flies, which serve as intermediate hosts. Horses are infected by ingesting flies that contain infective larvae or by free larvae that emerge from flies as they feed around the lips. (*See also* CUTANEOUS HABRONEMIASIS, p 904.)

A catarrhal gastritis may result from heavy infections with adult worms. *Draschia* produces the most severe lesions—tumor-like enlargements up to 10 cm in diameter. These are filled with necrotic material and a large number of worms and are covered by intact epithelium, except for a small opening through which the eggs pass. Rarely, these nodules rupture and cause fatal peritonitis. Larvae of

Habronema spp and *Draschia* have been found in the lungs of foals associated with *Rhodococcus equi* abscesses (*see* p 1451). Clinical signs usually are absent except when, rarely, granulomas associated with *Draschia* infection lead to mechanical obstruction or rupture.

Antemortem diagnosis is difficult, because the eggs are not easily detected using standard fecal flotation methods. Molecular methods have recently been developed for this purpose but would not be useful for routine use. Worms and eggs may be found by gastric lavage. Most anthelmintics have not been tested against *Habronema* spp or *Draschia* sp, although ivermectin is effective against their cutaneous larvae and against adults of *H muscae*. Moxidectin is also effective against adult *H muscae*.

OXYURIS SP

Adult pinworms, *Oxyuris equi*, are more common in horses <18 mo old and are found primarily in the terminal portion of the large intestine. The females are 7.5–15 cm long; males are smaller and fewer in number. The gravid females pass toward the rectum to lay their eggs, "cementing" them to the perineum around the anus. Masses of eggs and cement around the anus appear as a white to yellow, crusty mass. The eggs, which are flattened on one side, become embryonated in a few hours and are infective in 4–5 days.

Adult pinworms are of little significance in the intestine but cause perineal irritation after egg laying. Rubbing of the tail and anal regions, with resulting broken hairs and bare patches around the tail and buttocks, is characteristic and suggests the presence of pinworms. Fecal examination may or may not reveal a pinworm infection. Samples collected around the perineal region may contain dried female worms or eggs. Application of cellophane tape to the skin of the perineum or scraping the area with a tongue depressor may recover ova for microscopic examination, but false-negative tests are common.

Most of the broad-spectrum drugs recommended for treatment of strongyles (*see* below) are effective against pinworms.

PARASCARIS SP

Adult *Parascaris equorum* are stout, whitish worms, up to 30 cm long, with three prominent lips. The life cycle is similar to that of *Ascaris suum* (the roundworm of pigs, *see* p 320), with a prepatent period of 10–12 wk. Large numbers of infective eggs can remain viable for years in contaminated soil. Adult animals usually harbor very few if any worms. The principal sources of infection for young foals are pastures, paddocks, or stalls contaminated with eggs from foals of the previous year.

In heavy infections, the migrating larvae may produce respiratory signs ("summer colds"). In heavy intestinal infections, foals show unthriftiness, loss of energy, and occasionally colic. Intestinal obstruction and perforation have been reported. Intestinal stages compete for absorption of essential amino acids. Diagnosis is based on demonstration of eggs in the feces. If disease due to prepatent infection is suspected, diagnosis may be confirmed by administration of an anthelmintic, after which large numbers of immature worms may be seen in the feces.

On farms where the infection is common, most foals become infected soon after birth. As a result, most of the worms are maturing when the foals are ~4–5 mo old. Treatment should be started when foals are ~8 wk old and repeated at 6- to 8-wk intervals until they are yearlings. All broad-spectrum equine anthelmintics are effective against the adult and immature worms in the small intestine and, therefore, ascarids are readily controlled by routine anthelmintic administration. However, there have been reports of resistance of *P equorum* to ivermectin and moxidectin in North America and Europe. Efficacy on any given farm should be monitored using a fecal egg count reduction test. In cases in which verminous pneumonia due to *Parascaris* migration has developed, therapeutic benefit may be achieved by treatment with ivermectin or fenbendazole (the latter at 10 mg/kg/day for 5 consecutive days) concurrent with appropriate antimicrobial therapy. *Parascaris* infection can be effectively prevented by daily administration of pyrantel tartrate once foals are eating grain regularly.

LARGE STRONGYLES

The large strongyles of horses are also known as blood worms, palisade worms, sclerostomes, or red worms. The three major species are *Strongylus vulgaris* (up to 25 mm), *S edentatus* (up to 40 mm), and *S equinus* (up to 50 mm). (*See also Triodontophorus* spp, below.) Under favorable conditions, the larvae develop to the infective stage within 1–2 wk after the eggs are passed. Infection is by ingestion of infective larvae, which exsheath in the intestine and migrate extensively before developing to maturity in the large intestine. The prepatent period is 6–11 mo. The larvae of *S vulgaris* migrate extensively in the cranial mesenteric artery and its branches, where they may cause parasitic thrombosis and arteritis. Larvae of the other two species may be found in various parts of the body, including the liver, perirenal tissues, retroperitoneal tissues, and pancreas. These species do not produce lesions in the mesenteric arteries. Mixed infections of large and small strongyles are the rule.

Clinical Findings: Adult large strongyles have large buccal capsules and are active blood feeders; they ingest mucosal plugs as they move about in the intestine. The associated blood loss may lead to anemia. Weakness, emaciation, and diarrhea are also common. *S vulgaris* is important because of the damage it does to the cranial mesenteric artery and its branches. As a result of the interference with the flow of blood to the intestine and thromboembolism, any of several conditions may follow, including colic; gangrenous enteritis; or intestinal stasis, torsion or intussusception, and possibly rupture. Cerebrospinal nematodiasis (*see* p 1312) can cause a variety of lesions and signs depending on the part of the CNS affected.

Diagnosis and Treatment: Diagnosis of mixed strongyle infection is based on demonstration of eggs in the feces. Specific diagnosis can be made by identifying the infective larvae after fecal culture. Serologic diagnosis based on a rise in β-globulins has been recommended but is not specific for *S vulgaris*. Parasitic arterial lesions have been demonstrated using arteriography in ponies and small horses. Efforts have been made to utilize molecular methods and antibody measurements for prepatent diagnosis of *S vulgaris* infections, but these techniques are not yet available for standard use.

Colic due to arterial lesions has been successfully controlled by anthelmintic treatments. Ivermectin and moxidectin at standard dosages are effective against the larval stages (L_4 and L_5) of *S vulgaris*; fenbendazole and oxfendazole, at dosages higher than that for adult parasites, are also effective against larval infections. Daily administration of pyrantel tartrate effectively prevents establishment of arterial stages of *S vulgaris*. A number of anthelmintics, including the benzimidazoles, pyrantel, and ivermectin, are active against adult large strongyles. Large strongyle infections have been eliminated from closed herds with ivermectin treatment.

Parasite control programs are designed to minimize the level of pasture contamination and thereby reduce the risks associated with migrating larvae. Routine anthelmintic treatments do this by preventing fecal excretion of strongyle eggs. (*See also* SMALL STRONGYLES, below.)

SMALL STRONGYLES

More than 40 species of small strongyles in several genera have been found in the cecum and colon of domestic equids, each with its own site of preference. They have been referred to as trichonemes, cyathostomes, and currently cyathostomins. They belong to the subfamily Cyathostominae of the family Strongylidae, and ~10 species are particularly prevalent. Most are appreciably smaller than the "large strongyles," but *Triodontophorus* spp (sometimes classified as nonmigratory large strongyles) are almost as long as *Strongylus vulgaris*.

Unlike the large strongyles, small strongyles do not migrate extraintestinally, because early development is confined to the wall of the intestine. Third-stage larvae may progress to the fourth stage without interruption, or they may undergo hypobiosis and resume development only after prolonged periods of dormancy or hypobiosis. When L_4 emerge from the gut wall, they feed superficially on the mucosa and may rupture capillaries but are less pathogenic than the large strongyles. They molt to the adult stage. An exception is *T tenuicollis*, which is found in clusters and can produce severe ulcers in the wall of the colon. Generally, however, the resulting erosions of the mucosa are slight and hard to visualize. Consequently, it is common to recover thousands of adult worms from apparently healthy horses that have received limited anthelmintic treatment. In heavier infections, however, disruption may be extensive enough to disturb digestive and absorptive function, resulting in loss of condition and even a catarrhal enteritis of the large intestine.

Larval Cyathostominosis: An acute syndrome of sudden weight loss, often with severe diarrhea, is seen in temperate areas in late winter and spring, particularly in young ponies and horses (<5 yr old). This is associated with mass emergence of previously hypobiotic larvae from the intestinal wall as L_4. Although of relatively low incidence, larval cyathostominosis is nevertheless of concern because response to treatment is variable, and prognosis must be guarded even with intensive therapy. It is reported more frequently in the UK and Europe than in the USA.

Horses with larval cyathostominosis generally have a neutrophilia and hypoalbuminemia. Hyperglobulinemia, particularly involving the β-globulin fraction described as characteristic in some reports, has been a less consistent finding. Eosinophilia is not a consistent finding. Often, strongyle eggs are not seen on fecal examination. However, gross observation of L_4 or L_5 larvae, which are often bright red, in the feces is helpful in making a diagnosis. Biopsy of large intestine via laparotomy also may assist in diagnosis; rectal biopsy is less reliable. Gross pathologic findings include typhlitis or colitis with mucosal hyperemia, hemorrhage, congestion, ulceration, or necrosis; in protracted cases, there may be only mucosal thickening. At necropsy, cyathostomin larvae can be seen as small, gray dots (1–2 mm) in the mucosa, giving it a gritty sensation on palpation. Transillumination of the mucosa from the serosal surface may help in visualizing the larvae.

Treatment: Adult cyathostomins are easily removed from the gut lumen by a wide range of anthelmintics, provided that the worm population is susceptible to the chosen drug. Benzimidazole-resistant strains of small strongyles are common in some regions, and pyrantel resistance has been demonstrated in some locations. Resistance to the macrocyclic lactones has yet to be demonstrated, but concerns exist. Drug efficacy and the presence of anthelmintic resistance may be determined by comparing the worm egg count at the time of treatment and 10–14 days later. An effective drug should reduce the egg count to zero or to very low levels. If resistance is present, a different anthelmintic class must be used, because side resistance occurs within chemical groups.

Small-strongyle larvae in the intestinal mucosa are much more difficult to effectively remove with anthelmintics. Ivermectin has been used with mixed results; lack of efficacy has been reported at and above label dosages. Treatment with large dosages of fenbendazole (10 mg/kg for 5 consecutive days) or with moxidectin has been reported as effective and can be used during the winter to reduce the risk of larval cyathostominosis. Horses already suffering from this disease may not respond to treatment if submucosal inflammation is too severe. Consequently, treatment must be augmented by corticosteroids and other appropriate supportive therapy.

Prevention: Routine or interval treatments are traditional and are intended to minimize the level of pasture contamination, thereby reducing the risks associated with accumulation of mucosal larvae and adult worms. Alternatively, infection may be prevented by daily administration of pyrantel tartrate. The interval between routine treatments depends on the duration a particular drug keeps the feces free of eggs and varies from 4–13 wk. The frequency of treatment is also influenced by the value of the horses and the perceived level of risk, which varies with access to pasture, stocking density, and management practices. In most cases, these procedures are ineffective in the face of widespread drug resistance to most compounds except ivermectin and moxidectin. Control measures should be designed to minimize the risk of resistance developing in the worm population. This includes preserving the refugia population of the worms, ie, worms not exposed or affected by the anthelmintic, and thus reducing the drug selection pressure. These populations are the arrested L_3 found in the mucosa and L_3 larvae on the pasture. Fewer treatments may be effective if given strategically according to local epidemiologic and climatic considerations. Most adult horses >3–4 yr old have developed some immunity to reinfection; thus, only a small portion of the herd harbors the adult worm populations and is responsible for contamination of the pasture with eggs. Selective treatment of only these infected horses will also reduce the exposure of the worm population to anthelmintics and selection for resistance. Removal of feces from paddocks and pastures aids in control and may also reduce the number of anthelmintic treatments required.

Generally in parasite control programs, all horses on a farm should be treated at some time, and those commingled on the same pasture or paddock should be treated at the same time. Boarded horses or horses returning after having been off the premises for an extended time should be quarantined and dewormed before being admitted to the herd. In administering the anthelmintic, all horses should receive the proper dose, as determined by body weight or an accurate estimation. Rotating different classes of anthelmintics in a fast rotation scheme (eg, every few months) or a slow rotation scheme (annually) is widely practiced to prevent development of resistant parasite strains, but there is little evidence to support the utility of this procedure. Whatever program is used, fecal samples should be examined periodically to monitor the effectiveness of the program and the presence of drug resistance. Treatment can be restricted to those horses in a group that routinely have positive egg counts >100–200 eggs per gram of feces.

STRONGYLOIDES SP

Strongyloides westeri is found in the small intestine in foals. Adult horses rarely harbor patent infections, but mares often have larval stages within their tissues that are activated by parturition to move into the mammary tissue and, subsequently, are transmitted to foals in the milk. However, the relationship of *S westeri* infection with diarrhea in foals from 10 days of age has not been clearly established. The life cycle of the worm in horses is not known to differ significantly from that of *Strongyloides* in pigs (*see* p 323). Diagnosis can be made based on observation of eggs somewhat more oval and about one-third the length of strongyle eggs that contain larvae. Ivermectin and oxibendazole effectively remove *S westeri*. Transmission of larvae to foals via mare's milk may be prevented by routine treatment of mares with ivermectin within 24 hr after foaling.

TAPEWORMS

Three species of tapeworms are found in horses: *Anoplocephala magna*, *A perfoliata*, and *Paranoplocephala mamillana*. They are 8–25 cm long (the first usually being the longest, and the last the shortest). *A magna* and *P mamillana* usually are in the small intestine; *A perfoliata* is found mostly at the ileocecal junction, in the cecum, and in the ileum. The life cycle is similar to that of *Moniezia* spp in ruminants (*see* p 312) and involves free-living oribatid mites as intermediate hosts. Diagnosis is by demonstration of the characteristic eggs in the feces, but because the discharge of proglottids is sporadic, a single fecal examination may not be diagnostic. In light infections, no signs of disease are present; in heavy infections, GI disturbances may be seen. Unthriftiness and anemia have been reported. Ulceration of the mucosa is quite common in the area of attachment of *A perfoliata* and has been suggested as one cause of intussusception. Intestinal perforation, peritonitis, and subsequent colic have been associated with *Anoplocephala* infections. Colic from disturbances of the ileocecal area is more likely in horses with tapeworm infections than in those not infected. Colic associated with tapeworm infections often recurs. The site of attachment of tapeworms frequently becomes secondarily infected or abscessed. *Anoplocephala* spp can be effectively treated with pyrantel salts; normal dosages (6.6 mg/kg) of pyrantel pamoate are 87% effective, while double the normal dosage is >93% effective. Daily administration of pyrantel tartrate (2.65 mg/kg) removes *Anoplocephala* spp. Praziquantel (0.75–1 mg/kg) is 89%–100% effective in the removal of *A perfoliata*. Praziquantel (at 1 mg/kg) appears to effectively remove *P mamillana*; pyrantel salts do not. Mixtures of the macrocyclic lactones ivermectin or moxidectin with praziquantel are available and are highly effective against *A perfoliata*.

On facilities where tapeworms are prevalent, clinical signs of tapeworm infections can be prevented by pyrantel salts administered daily during the grazing season, or by administration of effective oral anthelmintics within an interval deworming program. Treatment of horses according to the latter program immediately before turn out and at the end of the grazing season is likely to be most beneficial.

TRICHOSTRONGYLUS SP

The small stomach worm (hairworm) of horses, *Trichostrongylus axei*, is also found in ruminants (*see* p 308) and, consequently, is generally a clinical problem only in horses commingled or rotated on pasture with ruminants. Adult *T axei* are slender and measure up to 8 mm long. Details of the life cycle in Equidae have not been carefully studied, but it is known that the larvae penetrate the mucosa. These worms produce a chronic catarrhal gastritis, which may result in weight loss. The lesions comprise nodular areas of thickened mucosa surrounded by a zone of congestion and covered with a variable amount of mucus. The lesions may be rather small and irregularly circumscribed, or they may coalesce and involve most or all of the glandular portion of the stomach, and erosions and ulcerations may be seen.

Definitive diagnosis based on fecal examination is difficult, because the eggs are similar to strongyle eggs. The feces can be cultured and, in ~7 days, the infective larvae identified. Some of the benzimidazoles and ivermectin are effective against *T axei*.

GASTROINTESTINAL PARASITES OF PIGS

See also COCCIDIOSIS OF PIGS, p 208.

In pigs, GI helminths are almost always present; their main effects are loss of appetite, reduction in daily gain, poor feed utilization, and potentiation of other pathogens. Only rarely do they cause death. Adequate nutrition helps reduce the adverse effects of parasitism on feed efficiency and average daily gain.

Management and control of GI helminths depends entirely on the production system in place, with individual programs developed for the circumstances of the specific farm, including the knowledge of which parasites are present. Maintaining pigs on concrete or entirely on slatted floors, as on intensive farms, can successfully control those parasites that have intermediate hosts or that require pasture conditions for transmission. Steam cleaning is highly effective in killing eggs and larvae. The management approach for outdoor situations and nonconcrete floors is aimed at avoiding a buildup of eggs and larvae within the area. Good sanitation is critical because fecal-oral transmission, through the contamination of food, soil, or bedding, is the primary route by which pigs become infected. Direct sunlight or dry conditions shorten the survival of some eggs and larvae because moisture and warmth are needed for their development and survival, which probably accounts for decreased transmission during hot and cold months. Thermophilic composting of feces and/or bedding before use as fertilizer inactivates *Ascaris suum* and *Trichuris suis* eggs. Both can survive for a few hours at 50°C but only a few minutes at 55°C. Most disinfectants in use on farms, unfortunately, are not effective against parasite eggs, especially those of *A suum* and *T suis*. Moving "clean" animals to safe pastures will help reduce parasite buildup, but it must be remembered that eggs of *A suum* and *T suis* are capable of surviving 6–9 and 5–11 yr, respectively, in the environment, and reinfection will occur even with 2–3 yr of pasture rest. If it is not possible to rotate pastures, pigs may occupy uncleanable ground for many years. In these situations, parasites can build up quickly, and control may be impossible without the regular use of anthelmintics. Anthelmintic treatments can be incorporated into any broader program as needed but should not be the sole basis of a control program.

Various anthelmintics are available, although not all are available in every country. Benzimidazoles, including fenbendazole and flubendazole, are available for in-feed administration. Flubendazole is available for in-water and top dressing use, whereas fenbendazole has an oral formulation. Two avermectin compounds, ivermectin and doramectin, are available as injectables, whereas only ivermectin can be used in-feed. Both pyrantel tartrate and levamisole are available as in-feed formulations, but only levamisole can be used in water. Dichlorvos, an organophosphate compound, was the first broad-spectrum dewormer available for pigs and is still in use as an in-feed formulation. Piperazine salts are an older generation of anthelmintic. Despite its narrow spectrum of activity, it is still widely used, available as an in-feed or in-water formulation.

Although anthelmintic-resistant populations of *Oesophagostomum* sp were identified as early as 1987, resistance does not appear to be a widespread problem. In addition, there is no justification for routinely rotating classes of dewormers; rather, choice of product should be made on the expected efficacy against the parasites present (including ectoparasites).

ASCARIS SUUM

Adults of the large roundworm, *Ascaris suum*, are found in the small intestine and transitorily in the large intestine during expulsion of the worms. Males are up to 25 cm and females up to 40 cm long, whitish, and quite thick. Large numbers of eggs are produced (as many as 200,000 to 1 million/day/female) although shed intermittently; they can develop to the infective stage (eggs containing L_3 larva) in 3–4 wk under optimal conditions. In temperate regions, the eggs stay dormant in winter (<15°C) and resume development when temperature rises in the spring. The eggs are highly resistant to chemical agents, but conditions with low humidity, heat, or direct sunlight reduce their survival significantly. Under optimal conditions, eggs may survive for 5–11 yr. When the eggs are ingested, the larvae hatch in the intestine, penetrate the wall, and enter the portal circulation. After a short period in the liver, they are carried by the circulation to the lungs, where they pass through the capillaries into the alveolar spaces. Approximately 9–10 days after ingestion, the larvae pass up the bronchial tree, are swallowed, and return to the small intestine by ~10–15 days after infection, where they mature into adult worms. The first eggs are passed ~6–7 wk after infection. Lifespan is ~6–9 mo. Earthworms and dung beetles can serve as paratenic hosts.

Distribution and Host Range: *A suum* is found in pigs worldwide. Occasionally, nematodes may establish in sheep; however, ingestion of infective eggs while grazing generally results in pneumonia and liver lesions in sheep. Infections can also be seen in cattle and manifest as an acute, atypical interstitial pneumonia. Whether the human nematode *Ascaris lumbricoides* and *A suum* of pigs are the same is still debated. Current evidence indicates there is a single interbreeding population of *Ascaris*, and the populations occurring in pigs or people have only slight phenotypical and genotypical adaptive changes. Regardless, it is clear the pig ascarid is zoonotic, having been found in people from various areas of the world, particularly those in close contact with pigs. Visceral larva migrans due to migrating larvae has been described.

Clinical Findings: Adult worms may significantly reduce the growth rate of young pigs; in rare cases, they may cause mechanical obstruction of the intestine. Migration of larvae through the liver causes hemorrhage, fibrosis, and accumulation of lymphocytes seen as white spots (called "milk spots") under the capsule and leading to condemnation of the liver at slaughter. These lesions become visible 7–10 days after infection and will regress within 1–4 wk; therefore, their presence indicates recent infection/reinfection. In resistant pigs, only a few larvae will reach the liver and the number of white spots will be low, despite continual reinfection. Therefore, the number of white spots and the liver condemnation rate are both poor measures of herd infection level. In heavy infections, the larvae can cause pulmonary edema and consolidation, as well as exacerbate swine influenza and endemic pneumonia. Heavily exposed susceptible pigs show abdominal breathing, commonly referred to as "thumps." In addition to the respiratory signs, marked unthriftiness and weight loss may be seen. Infection generally induces development of acquired resistance to reinfection, and prevalence is highest in young growing pigs. If the treatment rate is very low and the level of herd immunity is also low, prevalence may be highest in breeding animals.

Diagnosis: During the patent period, diagnosis can be made by demonstrating the typical eggs (golden brown, thick pitted outer wall, 50–70 × 40–60 μm) by fecal analysis or by observation of large worms in feces. Pigs are coprophagic; thus, low egg counts (<200 eggs/g) may indicate coprophagy rather than actual infection. A presumptive diagnosis can be made at necropsy based on demonstration of the typical milk spots; however, other migrating parasites (eg, larvae of *Toxocara canis*, *Stephanurus dentatus*) may cause similar lesions. Worms may be demonstrated in the lungs (small immatures) and the small intestine (large immatures, adults) at necropsy.

Treatment: Supportive therapy, including treatment for secondary bacterial invaders, may be necessary during the respiratory phase of infection. Many drugs have been used to remove adult ascarids. Piperazine preparations have low toxicity and are moderately priced. The benzimidazoles and probenzimidazoles, dichlorvos, ivermectin, levamisole, and pyrantel are effective and have a broader spectrum of activity than piperazine. Hygromycin is active against ascarids when administered as a low-level additive to the feed. Less information is available concerning the control of migratory stages; pyrantel and fenbendazole show activity.

MACRACANTHORHYNCHUS SP

Adult *Macracanthorhynchus hirudinaceus* (thorny-headed worms) are usually seen in the small intestine. They are 10 cm (males) to 65 cm (females) long, 3–9 mm thick, and slightly pink with a transversely wrinkled outer covering; superficially, they resemble ascarids. However,unlike ascarids, the anterior end bears a spiny, retractable proboscis or rostellum used for firm attachment to the intestinal wall. There is a granulomatous inflammation at the site of attachment resulting in nodule formation, which will regress ~1 mo after the parasite is no longer present. The eggs (dark brown, embryonated, with three embryonic envelopes, 90–110 × 50–65 μm) passed in the feces are ingested by the grubs of various beetles that serve as intermediate hosts. Pigs become infected by ingesting either grubs or adult beetles, and the infection is thus restricted to pigs with pasture access. The prepatent period is 2–3 mo, and longevity is ~1 yr. The female can lay ~260,000 eggs/day for several months.

Signs are generally absent; when present, they are nonspecific. Antemortem diagnosis is difficult, because the ova do not float reliably in many conventional salt solutions and thus should be looked for in the sediment if using solutions of low specific gravity. At necropsy, nodules usually can be seen through the serosa. Because the proboscis is longer than the jejunal wall is thick, perforations may occur; however, the inflammatory response generally seals off any perforation. Clinical signs are not generally present; however, when perforations do occur a fatal peritonitis can result.

Levamisole and ivermectin are effective for treatment. Control depends on avoiding use of contaminated hog lots or pastures or by regular removal of feces when pigs are kept in sties or small runs.

OESOPHAGOSTOMUM SPP

Oesophagostomum spp are prevalent worldwide; *O dentatum* is the most common species, whereas *O quadrispinulatum* appears to be slightly more pathogenic. The adults are found in the lumen of the large intestine; they are 8–15 mm long, slender, and white or gray. The life cycle is direct. Eggs are passed in the feces; infective L_3 are found on pasture within 1 wk and can survive for ~1 yr under optimal conditions. Infection results from ingestion of L_3, which penetrate the mucosa of the large intestine within a few hours after ingestion and return to the lumen in 6–20 days. The prepatent period is ~3-6 wk. A periparturient rise in worm egg output has been observed in sows from 2 wk before parturition to weaning; however, this phenomenon is far less constant in pigs than sheep and its epidemiologic importance is questionable. Most infections are asymptomatic, but heavily infected pigs may show anorexia, emaciation, and GI disturbances.

The serosa shows small nodules, their size reflecting species and previous exposure. In severe cases, the intestinal wall may be thickened and necrotic. Heavy infections may reduce the lactation capacity of sows and the body weight of growing pigs. Infection induces only moderate immunity; hence, prevalence of nodular worms tends to be higher in the older age groups (sows, boars). In patent infections, typical strongyle eggs (66–80 × 38–47 μm) are found in feces, often in large numbers. These can be differentiated from those of *Hyostrongylus* by larval culture. At necropsy, the worms and lesions are readily visible. The benzimidazoles, levamisole, piperazines, dichlorvos, pyrantel tartrate, and ivermectin are effective, but anthelmintic resistance has been observed for benzimidazoles, levamisole, and pyrantel. A diet composed of highly degradable carbohydrates may support worm control by creating unfavorable conditions, which decrease worm establishment and fecundity.

STOMACH WORMS

Five genera of nematodes are found within the stomach of pigs. The trichostrongylid *Hyostrongylus* is relatively common, whereas the other four spirurids (*Ascarops*, *Gnathostoma*, *Physocephalus*, *Simondsia*) are less common or geographically limited. Although some (eg, *Ascarops strongylina*, *Physocephalus sexalatus*) are more obvious grossly, only *Hyostrongylus rubidus* is considered to be pathologically significant. *H rubidus* (the red stomach worm) is ~6 mm long, quite slender, and has a direct life cycle, features similar to those of *Ostertagia ostertagi* of cattle. The prepatent period is ~3 wk unless larval inhibition occurs; this may be induced by seasonal changes or repeated infections, explaining why hypobiotic larvae are usually found in older animals. As with *Haemonchus contortus* of sheep, relaxation of immunity associated with parturition allows inhibited larvae to resume development, leading to a periparturient rise in fecal egg counts. *A strongylina* and *P sexalatus*, the thick stomach worms, are 10–20 mm long, are much stouter than *H rubidus*, and have coprophagous beetles as intermediate hosts. The prepatent periods for the spirurids are in the range of 4–6 wk. Because of the free-living larval requirements (*H rubidus*) or the need for an intermediate host (all others), infections are confined to animals with pasture access or those kept in straw yards.

Clinical Findings: The pathogenesis of hyostrongylosis is similar to that of ostertagiosis of cattle, including the replacement of parietal cells by rapidly dividing undifferentiated cells, giving rise to nodules on the mucosal surface. Gastric pH increases as does mucus production, resulting in a catarrhal gastritis. Occasionally, gastric ulcerations of the glandular stomach occur but whether this is a direct result of the nematode infection is unclear. Light infections are usually asymptomatic. However, when present in large numbers or when the host's condition is reduced by poor nutrition or other factors, these worms may cause variable appetite, anemia, diarrhea, or weight loss, and may contribute to a thin sow syndrome. *H rubidus* characteristically is found under a heavy catarrhal or mucous exudate. Resumed development of inhibited larvae may cause severe gastritis and, in addition, contaminate the environment of the young pigs. Egg excretion per female *Hyostrongylus* worm is generally much lower than that of other nematode genera.

Diagnosis: Clinical signs other than unthriftiness are not obvious. Fecal examinations may show the distinctive ova of *Physocephalus* and *Ascarops*—small (35–40 × 17–20 mm), thick-shelled eggs containing active larvae. *Hyostrongylus* ova resemble those of other strongyle worms (eg, *Oesophagostomum*), and fecal cultures are required to obtain infective larvae for differential diagnosis.

At necropsy, adult worms, especially *Physocephalus* and *Ascarops*, are readily seen. Mucosal scrapings for microscopic examination are essential for detection of immature *Hyostrongylus*.

Treatment and Control: The same principles used for control of parasitic gastroenteritis of ruminants apply to the control of hyostrongylosis and should not depend solely on anthelmintic use. As an example, in temperate climates, an annual rotation of pastures with other livestock or crops would reduce pasture contamination. Care must be taken with rotating livestock if the pigs also harbor ascarid infections. Integration of anthelmintics depends on their availability and the season, as well as on other farming activities. The newer benzimidazoles, probenzimidazoles, and ivermectin are highly effective against adult and immature stages (including hypobiotic larvae) of *Hyostrongylus*. Implementing measures to control the intermediate hosts of the spirurid nematodes is usually not required or unproductive. Treatment for most has not been reported, although ivermectin has activity against adult *Ascarops*.

STRONGYLOIDES SP

Strongyloides ransomi (pig threadworm) is a ubiquitous and common nematode parasite of pigs; it is particularly pathogenic in suckling pigs, especially in tropical and subtropical climates. It is of less importance in adults. Threadworms are unique among helminths, having both parasitic generations (females in the small intestine) and free-living generations (males and females in the surrounding environment). Transmission occurs either by skin penetration, emphasizing the importance of good hygiene, or via infective larvae in the colostrum of lactating sows. Lactogenic transmission is highly efficient in infecting newborn piglets. Even without reinfection of the sow, dormant larvae in the udder may be transmitted to several consecutive litters of piglets. The adult female worms burrow into the wall of the small intestine, being found in tunnels in the epithelium at the base of the villi. The prepatent period is 4–9 days, depending on the mode of infection. In light and moderate infections, the pigs usually show no signs. In heavy infections, diarrhea, anemia, and emaciation may be seen, and death may result. Infection induces strong immunity; hence, older pigs are usually not clinically affected.

Diagnosis is determined by demonstration of the characteristic small, thin-shelled, embryonated eggs (20–35 × 40–55 μm) in the feces. It is important that feces are collected from the rectum, because fecal droppings often are contaminated by free-living nematodes, which may have eggs indistinguishable from the *Strongyloides* eggs. Furthermore, feces must be cooled immediately to prevent hatching. At necropsy, adults may be found in scrapings from the intestinal mucosa, and immature worms may be recovered from minced tissues using the Baermann techniques.

The benzimidazoles and levamisole are effective against intestinal infections. If administered in the feed for several days before and after parturition, they reduce lactogenic transmission to suckling piglets. Ivermectin is effective against adults and, if given to the sow 1–2 wk before farrowing, suppresses larval excretion in the milk. A high level of hygiene is necessary to diminish larval development as well as multiplication of free-living generations in the pens.

TRICHURIS SP

Trichuris suis is found worldwide in pigs. The adult worms are 5–6 cm long and whip-shaped; the anterior slender portion embeds within the epithelial cells of the large intestine, especially the cecum, with the thickened posterior third lying free in the lumen. Infection is by ingestion of eggs containing an infective first-stage larva. The larva hatches and penetrates the distal ileum, cecal, and colonic mucosa. The nematodes complete all four molts, after which the posterior end begins to protrude into the lumen. The prepatent period is 6–8 wk; longevity is 4–5 mo. Light infections, with no clinical signs, are generally the case. Heavy infections may cause inflammatory lesions in the cecum and adjacent large intestine and may be accompanied by diarrhea and unthriftiness. Clinical infection is most often seen in young animals; resistance is both acquired and age-related. The double-operculated brown eggs (50–68 × 21–31 mm) are diagnostic. Eggs are heavy; thus, good technique with media of proper specific gravity is essential. Trichurids have a short period of egg-laying (2–5 wk) before the worms are expelled by immune-mediated reactions, and thus little significance can be given to percentage of egg excreters and numbers of eggs per gram of feces. Clinical trichurosis is usually associated with the larval stages before eggs are passed in the feces; in these cases, examining mucosal scrapings taken at necropsy for smaller stages of the parasite is recommended. Mature parasites are easily found after ingesta is washed away and can be identified by their size and whip-like form. Dichlorvos, levamisole, some benzimidazoles, ivermectin, and doramectin are effective against the adult worms. Biologically, the eggs are comparable to *Ascaris* eggs—they are highly resistant to chemicals and may remain infective for 3–4 yr; control relies on thorough cleaning of the affected area and moving the animals to clean plots. *Trichuris* eggs develop rather slowly (10–12 wk under optimal conditions), and because they do not develop at temperatures <16°C, there is only one generation per year in temperate regions.

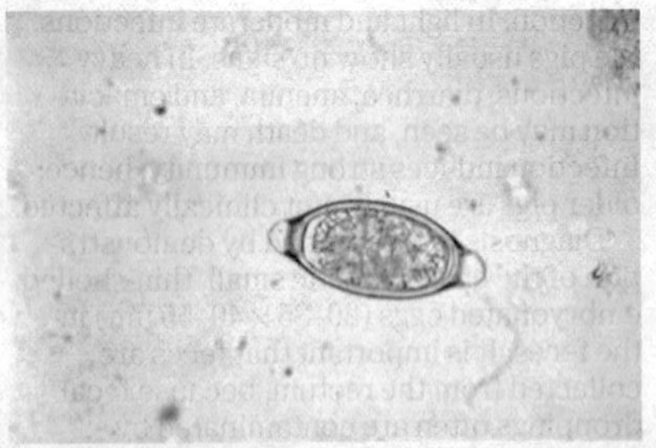

Trichuris suis egg. Courtesy of Dr. Bruce Lawhorn.

T suis larvae may hatch in the large intestine of people, in which the larvae seem to be able to establish transiently. It is this feature that has led to intense research interest in the treatment of inflammatory bowel disease, including ulcerative colitis and Crohn's disease, of people through administration of infective *T suis* eggs.

FLUKE INFECTIONS IN RUMINANTS

Fasciola hepatica, the most important trematode of domestic ruminants, is the most common cause of liver fluke disease in temperate areas of the world. In the USA, it is endemic along the Gulf Coast, the West Coast, the Rocky Mountain region, and other areas. It is present in eastern Canada, British Columbia, and South America and is of particular economic importance in the British Isles, western and eastern Europe, Australia, and New Zealand. *Fasciola gigantica* is economically important in Africa and Asia and is also found in Hawaii. *Fascioloides magna* has been reported in at least 21 states (USA) and in Europe. In North America, *Dicrocoelium dendriticum* is confined mainly to New York, New Jersey, Massachusetts, and the Atlantic provinces of Canada. It is also widespread in some areas in Europe and Asia. *Eurytrema* spp, the pancreatic flukes, parasitize sheep, pigs, and cattle in Brazil and parts of Asia. Several species of paramphistomes or rumen flukes are found throughout much of the world.

FASCIOLA HEPATICA

(Common liver fluke)

Etiology: *Fasciola hepatica* (30 × 2–12 mm and leaf-shaped) is distributed worldwide and has a broad host range, including people. Economically important infections

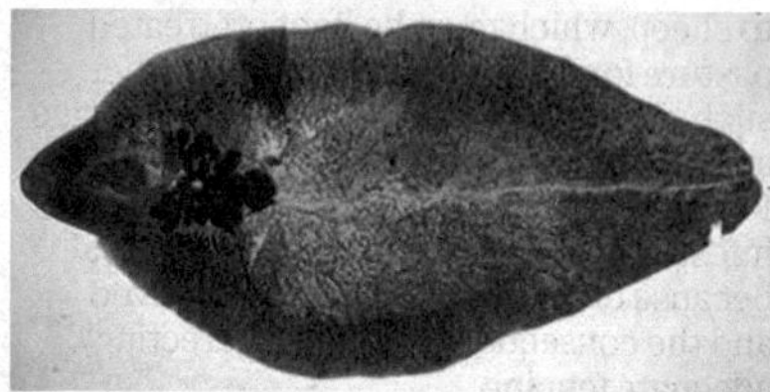

Adult *Fasciola hepatica* (Corazza stain). *Courtesy of Dr. Raffaele Roncalli.*

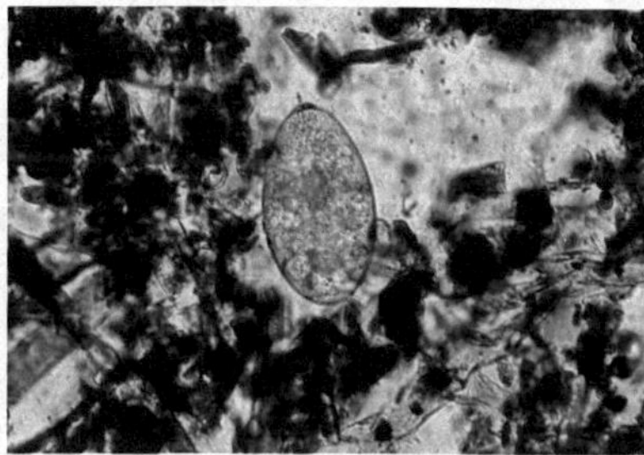

Fasciola hepatica egg found on sedimentation. Adding a drop of methylene blue to the sediment provides contrasting background, making the eggs easier to see. *Courtesy of Dr. Lora Ballweber.*

are seen in cattle, sheep, alpacas, and llamas in three forms: chronic, which is rarely fatal in cattle but often fatal in sheep, alpacas, and llamas; subacute or acute, which is primarily in sheep, alpacas, and llamas, and often fatal; and in conjunction with "black disease" (INFECTIOUS NECROTIC HEPATITIS, *see* p 603), which is most common in sheep and usually fatal.

Eggs are passed in the feces, and miracidia develop within as little as 9–10 days (at 22°–26°C [71.6°–78.8°F]; little development occurs below 10°C [50°F]). Hatching only occurs in water, and miracidia are short-lived (~3 hr). Miracidia infect lymnaeid snails, in which asexual development and multiplication occur through the stages of sporocysts, rediae, daughter rediae, and cercariae. After 6–7 wk (or longer if temperatures are low), cercariae emerge from snails, encyst on aquatic vegetation, and become metacercariae. Snails may extend the developmental period by hibernating during the winter. Metacercariae may remain viable for many months unless they become desiccated.

After ingestion by the host, usually with herbage, young flukes excyst in the duodenum, penetrate the intestinal wall, and enter the peritoneal cavity, where they migrate to the liver. The time required for this transit can vary and results in delayed development rates, which affects the efficacy of some treatments because many are effective against flukes only later in their development. The young flukes penetrate the liver capsule and tunnel through the parenchyma for 6–8 wk, growing and destroying tissue. They then enter small bile ducts and migrate to the larger ducts and, occasionally, the gallbladder, where they mature and begin to produce eggs. The prepatent period is usually 2–3 mo, depending on the fluke burden. The minimal period for the completion of one entire life cycle is ~17 wk. Adult flukes may live in the bile ducts of sheep for years; most are shed from cattle within 5–6 mo.

Clinical Findings: Fasciolosis ranges in severity from a devastating disease in sheep, alpacas, and llamas to an asymptomatic infection in cattle. The course usually is determined by the number of metacercariae ingested. Acute disease occurs 2–6 wk after the ingestion of large numbers of metacercariae (usually >2,000) over a short period. In sheep, acute fasciolosis occurs seasonally and is manifest by a distended, painful abdomen; anemia; and sudden death occurring 2–6 wk after infection. The acute syndrome can be complicated by concurrent infections with *Clostridium novyi*, resulting in "black disease" (clostridial necrotic hepatitis), although this is now less common due to vaccination against clostridial diseases. In subacute disease, large numbers (500–1,500) of metacercariae are ingested over longer periods of time; survival is longer (7–10 wk), even in cases with significant hepatic damage, but deaths occur due to hemorrhage and anemia. Chronic fasciolosis can be seen in all seasons but manifests primarily in late fall and winter. It occurs as a result of ingesting moderate numbers (200–500) of metacercariae over longer periods of time; signs include anemia, unthriftiness, submandibular edema, and reduced milk production, but even heavily infected cattle may show no clinical signs although their immunity to other pathogens (eg, *Salmonella* spp) may be reduced and reactions to the single intradermal test for tuberculosis modified. Heavy chronic infection is fatal in sheep, alpacas, and llamas.

Sheep do not appear to develop resistance to infection, and chronic liver damage is cumulative over several years. In cattle, a partial acquired resistance develops beginning 5–6 mo after infection.

Lesions: Severity depends on the number of metacercariae ingested, the phase of development in the liver, and the species of host involved. During the first phase, immature, wandering flukes destroy liver tissue and cause hemorrhage. The second phase occurs when the flukes enter the bile ducts, where they ingest blood and damage the mucosa with their cuticular spines. In acute fasciolosis, damage is extensive; the liver is enlarged and friable with fibrinous deposits on the capsule. Migratory tracts can be seen, and the surface has an uneven appearance. In chronic cases, cirrhosis develops. The damaged bile ducts become enlarged, or even cystic, and have thickened, fibrosed walls. In cattle but not sheep, the duct walls become greatly thickened and often calcified. Aberrant migrations occur more commonly in cattle, and encapsulated flukes may be found in the lungs. Mixed infections with *Fascioloides magna* can be seen in cattle.

Tissue destruction by wandering flukes may create a microenvironment favorable for activation of clostridial spores.

Diagnosis: The oval, operculated, golden brown eggs (130–150 × 65–90 μm) must be distinguished from those of paramphistomes (rumen flukes), which are larger and clear. Eggs of *F hepatica* cannot be demonstrated in feces during acute fasciolosis. In subacute or chronic disease in cattle, the number varies from day to day, and repeated fecal sedimentation may be required. Diagnosis can be aided by an ELISA (commercially available in Europe) that enables detection ~2–3 wk after infection and well before the patent period. Plasma concentrations of γ-glutamyltransferase, which are increased with bile duct damage, are also helpful during the late maturation period when flukes are in the bile ducts. At necropsy, the nature of the liver damage is diagnostic. Adult flukes are readily seen in the bile ducts, and immature stages may be squeezed or teased from the cut surface.

Control: Control measures for *F hepatica* ideally should involve removal of flukes in affected animals, reduction of the intermediate host snail population, and prevention of livestock access to snail-infested pasture. In practice, only the first of these is used in most cases. Although molluscicides can be used to reduce lymnaeid snail populations, those that are available all have disadvantages that restrict their use. Copper sulfate, if applied before the snail population multiplies each year, is effective but toxic to sheep, which must be kept off treated pasture for 6 wk after application. Other such chemicals are generally too expensive and have ecologically undesirable effects. Prevention of livestock access to snail-infested pasture is frequently impractical because of the size of the areas involved and the consequent expense of erecting adequate fencing.

Several drugs are available to treat infected ruminants, including triclabendazole, clorsulon (cattle and sheep only), albendazole, netobimin, closantel, rafoxanide, and oxyclozanide. Not all are approved in all countries (eg, only clorsulon and albendazole are approved in the USA; none are approved for alpacas and llamas), and most have long withdrawal periods before slaughter if used in meat-producing animals and before milk from treated livestock can be used for human consumption. Anthelmintic resistance by *F hepatica* to various compounds, including albendazole, clorsulon, and triclabendazole, has been demonstrated, further complicating control programs based only on anthelmintic usage. The timing of treatment is also important so that the pharmacokinetics of the drug used will result in the optimal removal of flukes—each flukicide has varying efficacy against different ages of fluke. Timing of treatments is determined by local epidemiologic factors and additional treatments by unusually suitable conditions for parasite multiplication. For example, in the Gulf Coast states of the USA, cattle should be treated before the fall rainy season and again in the late spring. In northwestern USA and in northern Europe, cattle should be treated at the end of the pasture season and, if not housed, again in late January or February. In European countries with large susceptible sheep populations, computerized prediction systems based on rainfall, evapotranspiration, number of wet days per month, and/or prevalence are used to predict the timing and severity of disease. In areas where heavy infections are expected, sheep may require treatment in September or October, January or February, and again in April or May to reduce both the chances of acute or chronic infections and the output of fluke eggs for development of future disease.

FASCIOLA GIGANTICA

(Giant liver fluke)

Fasciola gigantica is similar in shape to *Fasciola hepatica* but is longer (75 mm), with less clearly defined shoulders, and is

12 mm wide. It is found in warmer climates (Asia, Africa) in cattle and buffalo, in which it is responsible for chronic fasciolosis, and in sheep, in which the disease is frequently acute and fatal. The life cycle is similar to that of *F hepatica*, except most parasitic phases are longer, the prepatent period is 10–16 wk, and the species of snail intermediate hosts are different. The pathology of infection, diagnostic procedures, and control measures are similar to those for *F hepatica* (*see* p 324).

FASCIOLOIDES MAGNA

(Large American liver fluke, Giant liver fluke)

Fascioloides magna is up to 100 mm long, 2–4.5 mm thick, 11–26 mm wide, and oval; it is distinguished from *Fasciola* spp by its large size and lack of an anterior projecting cone. It is found in domestic and wild ruminants; deer are the reservoir host. The life cycle resembles that of *Fasciola* spp.

Although flukes will mature in cattle, the intense encapsulation response forms a closed cyst, so eggs rarely pass out of the animal. Pathogenicity is low, and losses are confined primarily to liver condemnations. In sheep and goats, encapsulations do not occur, and the parasites migrate in the liver and other organs, causing tremendous damage. A few parasites can cause death due to extensive migrations. Infection with *F magna* appears to be rare in alpacas and llamas, in which the response mirrors that seen in cattle. In deer, there is little tissue reaction, and the parasites are enclosed in thin, fibrous cysts that communicate with bile ducts. Histologically, infected livers of all species show black, tortuous tracts formed by migrations of young flukes.

While the eggs of *F magna* resemble those of *Fasciola hepatica*, this is of limited use; eggs usually are not passed by cattle and sheep and probably not by alpacas and llamas. Recovery of the parasites at necropsy as well as differentiation of *F hepatica* is necessary for definitive diagnosis. When domestic ruminants and deer share the same grazing, the presence of disease due to *F magna* should be kept in mind. Mixed infections with *F hepatica* are seen in cattle.

Oxyclozanide has been reported to be effective against *F magna* in white-tailed deer, and triclabendazole has been used in captive and free-ranging red deer. Rafoxanide has been used successfully against natural infections in cattle. Albendazole (7.5 mg/kg), clorsulon (15 mg/kg), and closantel (15 mg/kg) have shown efficacy against this fluke in sheep. Currently, no products are approved for use against this fluke in the USA. Deer are required for completion of the life cycle; if they can be excluded from the areas grazed by cattle and sheep, control may be effected. Control of the intermediate host (lymnaeid snails) may be possible once it has been identified in a region and the nature of its habitat examined. However, environmental concerns are the same as those for *F hepatica*.

DICROCOELIUM DENDRITICUM

(Lancet fluke, Lesser liver fluke)

Dicrocoelium dendriticum is slender (6–10 mm long × 1.5–2.5 mm wide). It is found in many countries and infects a wide range of definitive hosts, including domestic ruminants. Another species, *D hospes*, is common in West Africa.

The first intermediate host is a terrestrial snail (*Cionella lubrica*, in the USA), from which cercariae emerge and are aggregated in a mass of sticky mucus (slimeball). The slimeballs of cercariae are ingested by the second intermediate host, which is an ant (*Formica fusca*, in the USA), with metacercariae forming in the abdominal cavity. One or two metacercariae in the subesophageal ganglion of the ant cause abnormal behavior in which the ants climb up and remain on the tips of the herbage where they attach themselves, which increases the probability of ingestion by the definitive host. Once ingested, the metacercariae excyst in the small intestine, migrate up the main bile duct, and then on to smaller ducts. They begin laying eggs ~10–12 wk after infection. The total life cycle takes ~6 mo.

In cattle, sheep, and goats there appears to be no immunity, and heavy infections may accumulate (up to 50,000 flukes in a mature sheep) with minimal pathologic or clinical changes. Cirrhosis can develop, and the bile ducts may be thickened and distended. Economic loss is due primarily to condemnation of livers. Clinical signs are not obvious but may be seen in massive infections. Infections in alpacas and llamas are associated with an acute decline in condition, recumbency, hypothermia, and anemia. Liver enzyme values tend to be within normal limits. Severe pathologic changes occur within the liver and bile ducts, including cirrhosis, abscesses, and granulomas.

The eggs contain a miracidium and are very small (40 × 25 μm), lopsided, and yellowish brown. Fecal flotation with a solution of high specific gravity (1.30–1.45) is recommended to detect *D dendriticum*.

The complex life cycle makes control of intermediate hosts almost impossible, because widespread chemical use has damaging ecologic effects on other similar organisms. However, keeping ducks, turkeys, or chickens to eat the snails can effectively reduce the intermediate host populations in small areas. Because infected ants are usually found within 30–50 cm of the base of the nest, covering nests with tree branches to keep animals away from the base can also be useful. Effective anthelmintic treatments are available, but most must be administered at dosages higher than those recommended for *F hepatica*. Effective anthelmintic treatments in both cattle and sheep are albendazole at 15–20 mg/kg in a single dose or two doses of 7.5 mg/kg on successive days, or netobimin at 20 mg/kg. Praziquantel (50 mg/kg) has been shown to decrease egg shedding by ~90% in llamas.

EURYTREMA SPP

(Pancreatic fluke)

Pancreatic flukes have a thick body and are 8–16 mm long × 6 mm wide. They are parasites of the pancreatic ducts and occasionally of the bile ducts of sheep, pigs, and cattle in Brazil and Asia. Three species, *Eurytrema pancreaticum*, *E coelomaticum*, and *E ovis* are recognized. The first intermediate hosts are terrestrial snails (*Bradybaena* spp), and the cercariae are released onto herbage and ingested by grasshoppers (*Conocephalus* spp) or tree crickets (*Oecanthus* spp), which are the second intermediate host. After the animal ingests a metacercarial-infected grasshopper, the immature flukes excyst in the duodenum and migrate to the pancreatic duct, where they mature. The prepatent period of *E coelomaticum* in cattle is 3–4 mo.

There are no obvious clinical signs, but a general weight loss may occur in heavy infections. *Dicrocoelium*-like eggs can be demonstrated in feces. Light infections cause proliferative inflammation of the pancreatic duct, which may become enlarged and occluded. In heavy infections, fibrotic, necrotic, and degenerative lesions develop. These result in increased plasma concentrations of γ-glutamyl transpeptidase and AST. Losses are reported due to condemned pancreas, but the pathogenesis suggests an additional loss of production.

The control of intermediate hosts may not be practical. Treatment with praziquantel (20 mg/kg, for 2 days) or albendazole (7.5 mg/kg for sheep, 10 mg/kg for cattle) have reportedly been effective.

PARAMPHISTOMES

(Amphistomes, Rumen flukes, Conical flukes)

There are numerous species of paramphistomes (*Paramphistomum*, *Calicophoron*, *Cotylophoron*) in ruminants worldwide. The adult parasites are pear-shaped, pink or red, up to 15 mm long, and attach to the lining of the rumen. Immature forms are found in the duodenum and are 1–3 mm long.

Eggs are passed in the feces, and miracidiae hatch in the water and infect planorbid or bulinid snails. Development in the snail is similar to that in the life cycle of *Fasciola hepatica*, with the snail shedding cercariae that encyst on the herbage. In the ruminant host, the young flukes excyst and remain in the small intestine for 3–6 wk before migrating forward through the reticulum to the rumen. Eggs are produced 7–14 wk after infection.

Adult flukes do not cause overt disease, and large numbers may be encountered. The immature flukes attach to the duodenal and, at times, the ileal mucosa by means of a large posterior sucker and cause severe enteritis, possibly necrosis, and hemorrhage. Affected animals exhibit anorexia, polydipsia, unthriftiness, and severe diarrhea. Extensive mortality may occur, especially in young cattle and sheep. Older animals can develop resistance to reinfection but may continue to harbor numerous adult flukes.

The large, clear, operculated eggs are readily recognized, but in acute paramphistomosis there may be no eggs in the feces. Examination of the fluid feces may reveal immature flukes, many of which are passed in these cases. Diagnosis is commonly made at necropsy.

Control measures to reduce the host snail population are as for control of fasciolosis (*see* p 326). Treatments with reported success (efficacies >90%) are oxyclozanide (two doses 3 days apart) and the combination of bithional and levamisole.

HEPATIC DISEASE IN LARGE ANIMALS

Hepatic disease is common in large animals. Increases in serum hepatic enzymes and total bile acid concentration may indicate hepatic dysfunction, insult, disease, or failure. Although liver disease is especially common in horses and foals, progression to liver failure is not.

Diseases that frequently result in hepatic failure in horses include Theiler disease, Tyzzer disease (foals), pyrrolizidine alkaloid toxicosis, hepatic lipidosis, suppurative cholangitis or cholangiohepatitis, cholelithiasis, and chronic active hepatitis. Obstructive disorders (biliary stones, right dorsal colon displacement, neoplasia, duodenal ulceration and stricture, hepatic torsion, portal vein thrombosis), aflatoxicosis, leukoencephalomalacia, pancreatic disease, kleingrass or alsike clover poisoning, portal caval shunts, hepatic abscess, and perinatal herpesvirus 1 infections sporadically result in hepatic failure. Less frequently, hepatic failure is associated with endotoxemia, steroid administration, inhalant anesthesia, systemic granulomatous disease, drug-induced amyloidosis, hyperammonemia in Morgan foals, parasite damage, iron toxicity, or after neonatal isoerythrolysis.

In ruminants, hepatobiliary disease is associated with hepatic lipidosis, hepatic abscesses, endotoxemia, pyrrolizidine alkaloid and other plant toxicoses, certain clostridial diseases, liver flukes, mycotoxicosis, and mineral toxicosis (copper, iron, zinc) or deficiency (cobalt). Vitamin E or selenium deficiency (hepatosis dietetica), aflatoxicosis, ascarid migration, bacterial hepatitis, and ingestion of toxic substances (eg, coal tar, cyanamide, blue-green algae, plants, gossypol) are associated with hepatic injury in swine.

Although the exact incidence of hepatic disease in camelids (llamas, alpacas) is unknown, it appears to be common in North America. Hepatic lipidosis (secondary more often than primary) is reportedly the most common liver disease in llamas and alpacas, occurring in both crias and adults. Bacterial (*Salmonella* spp, *Escherichia coli*, *Listeria* spp, *Clostridium* spp) cholangiohepatitis, adenoviral hepatitis and pneumonia, fungal hepatitis (coccidioidomycosis), toxic hepatopathy (copper), halothane-induced hepatic necrosis, hepatic neoplasia (lymphosarcoma, hemangiosarcoma, adenoma), and liver fluke infestation have also been reported in camelids.

The liver can respond to insult in only a limited number of ways. Fat droplets in the liver may be an early and often reversible change. Biliary hyperplasia is also reversible if the insult is removed early. Necrosis of hepatocytes indicates more recent damage. The dead cells are removed by an inflammatory process and replaced with either new hepatocytes or fibrosis. Unless the dysfunction is acute and hepatocellular regeneration is evident, prognosis for animals with liver failure is usually unfavorable. Early hepatic fibrosis may be reversible with prompt recognition and intervention. Chronic disease with extensive loss of hepatic parenchyma and fibrosis, especially with portal bridging, warrants a poor prognosis.

Clinical Findings: Clinical signs of hepatic disease may not be evident until >60%–80% of the liver parenchyma is nonfunctional or when hepatic dysfunction is secondary to disease in another organ system. Clinical signs may vary with the course of the disease (acute or chronic), primary site of injury (hepatocellular, biliary), and specific cause. Onset of signs of hepatic encephalopathy and liver failure is often acute regardless of whether the hepatic disease process is acute or chronic. Clinical signs and severity of hepatic pathology reflect the degree of compromise of one or more of the liver's vital functions, including blood glucose regulation; fat metabolism; production of clotting factors, albumin, fibrinogen, nonessential amino acids, and plasma proteins; bile formation and excretion; bilirubin and cholesterol metabolism; conversion of ammonia to urea; polypeptide and steroid hormone metabolism; synthesis of 25-hydroxycholecalciferol; and metabolism and/or detoxification of many drugs and toxins.

Icterus, weight loss, or abnormal behavior are common in horses with liver disease and hepatic failure. CNS signs are often the initial and predominant sign in horses with acute hepatic failure, whereas weight loss is a prominent sign in most but not all horses with chronic liver disease and failure. Photosensitization and, less commonly, bilateral pharyngeal paralysis, causing inspiratory stridor, diarrhea, or constipation, may be present. Affected cattle usually show inappetence, decreased milk production, and weight loss. Tenesmus and ascites are seen in cattle but are not common in affected horses. Weight loss may be the only sign associated with liver abscesses. Icterus, which is most pronounced when the biliary system is diseased, is also common in horses with acute liver failure. It is more variably present in horses with chronic liver failure or in ruminants. Fasting hyperbilirubinemia is a more common cause of icterus in horses and is not associated with hepatic disease. Occasionally, persistent hyperbilirubinemia (primarily indirect or unconjugated bilirubin) may be seen in healthy horses (especially Thoroughbreds) without evidence of hemolysis or hepatic disease. In ruminants, icterus is more commonly due to hemolysis and primarily involves increases in indirect bilirubin. Hyperbilirubinemia caused by obstructive biliary conditions is rare in goats and sheep.

Hepatic encephalopathy is associated with behavioral changes in horses, ruminants, and swine. The severity of hepatic encephalopathy often reflects the degree of hepatic failure but does not differentiate between acute or chronic liver failure. Signs of hepatic encephalopathy range from nonspecific depression and lethargy to head pressing, circling, aimless walking, dysphagia, ataxia, dysmetria, persistent yawning, pica, increased friendliness, aggressiveness, stupor, seizures, or coma. Pharyngeal or laryngeal collapse with loud, stertorous inspiratory noises and dyspnea occurs in some cases of hepatic failure, especially in ponies. The pathogenesis of hepatic encephalopathy is unknown, but proposed theories include ammonia as a neurotoxin, alterations in monoamine neurotransmission (serotonin, tryptophan) or catecholamine neurotransmitters, imbalance between aromatic and short branch chain amino acids resulting in increased inhibitory neurotransmitters (γ-aminobutyric acid, L-glutamate), neuroinhibition due to increased cerebral levels of endogenous benzodiazepine-like substances, increased permeability of the blood-brain barrier, and impaired CNS energy metabolism. Although the signs can be dramatic, hepatic encephalopathy is potentially reversible if the underlying hepatic disease can be resolved.

Photosensitization, which may be seen secondary to acute or chronic liver failure, must be differentiated from primary photosensitization (*see* p 976). Hepatogenous photosensitization develops when compromised hepatic function results in phylloerythrin, a photodynamic metabolite of chlorophyll, entering the skin. Phylloerythrin in the skin reacts with ultraviolet light and releases energy, causing inflammation and skin damage. Signs of photosensitization are varied but include uneasiness, pain, pruritus, mild to severe dermatitis with erythema, extensive subcutaneous edema, skin ulceration, sloughing of skin and ophthalmia with lacrimation, photophobia, and corneal cloudiness. Dermatitis and edema are particularly evident on nonpigmented, light-colored or hairless areas of the body and areas exposed to sun. Mucocutaneous junctions and patches of white hair are the most common sites of photosensitization in cattle. Occasionally, the underside of the tongue may be affected. Blindness, pyoderma, loss of condition, and occasionally death are possible sequelae. Pruritus may result from photosensitization or from deposition of bile salts in the skin secondary to alterations in hepatic excretion.

Diarrhea or constipation may be seen in animals with hepatic disease. Diarrhea is more commonly seen in cattle than in horses with chronic liver disease or in animals with chronic fascioliasis and hepatotoxic plant poisonings. Ponies and horses with hyperlipemia and hepatic failure may develop diarrhea, laminitis, and ventral edema. Some animals with liver disease have alternating diarrhea and constipation. Horses with liver failure and hepatic encephalopathy frequently develop colonic impaction due to decreased water intake. Constipation is characteristic of *Lantana* poisoning in goats and other ruminants.

Recurrent colic, intermittent fever, icterus, weight loss, and hepatic encephalopathy may be seen in horses with choleliths that obstruct the common bile duct. Infectious or inflammatory hepatic disease or failure of the liver to prevent endotoxin from gaining access to the systemic circulation may also result in intermittent fever and colic. Abdominal pain, due to pressure on the liver capsule from parenchymal swelling, often is seen in animals with acute diffuse hepatitis or trauma to the capsule itself. Affected animals stand with an arched back, are reluctant to move, or show signs of colic. In ruminants, pain may be localized to the liver by palpation over the anterior ventrolateral aspect of the abdomen or the last few ribs on the right side. Tenesmus followed by rectal prolapse is seen in some ruminants with liver disease. It may be associated with diarrhea, hepatic encephalopathy, or edema of the bowel from portal hypertension.

Hypoalbuminemia is not as frequently associated with liver disease in horses as previously thought. Due to the long half-life (~19–20 days in horses, ~16 days in cows) and liver reserve for albumin production, hypoalbuminemia is usually a very late event in the disease process. Serum total protein concentrations may be normal or increased because of an increase in β-globulins in horses with liver disease. Hypoalbuminemia and hypoproteinemia most commonly develop in chronic liver disease, and they are common findings in llamas with liver disease. Generalized ascites or dependent edema may result. Ascites is related to portal hypertension caused by venous blockage and increased hydrostatic pressure and to protein leakage into the peritoneal cavity. The abdominal fluid present with liver disease usually is a modified transudate. Hypoalbuminemia can aggravate the ascites, but if it is seen alone, it more likely will cause intermandibular, brisket, or ventral edema. Ascites is difficult to appreciate in horses and adult cattle unless it is extensive. Ascites is a common finding in calves with liver cirrhosis.

Anemia may be seen in animals with liver dysfunction due to parasitic diseases, chronic copper toxicity (in ruminants), some plant poisonings, or chronic inflammatory disease. Anemia in acute fasciolosis results from severe hemorrhage into the peritoneal cavity as the larvae penetrate the liver capsule. Trauma and feeding activity of adult flukes within the bile ducts cause anemia and hypoproteinemia in animals with chronic fasciolosis. Chronic inflammatory disease (eg, hepatic abscesses, neoplasia) may cause anemia without accompanying hypoproteinemia.

Clinical signs of severe or terminal hepatic failure include coagulopathies and hemorrhage due to decreased production of clotting factors by the liver and possibly increased utilization in septic or inflammatory processes. A prolonged prothrombin time is usually seen first because factor VII has the shortest plasma half-life. Horses may develop a terminal hemolytic crisis caused by increased RBC fragility. This has not been reported in ruminants.

Fecal color rarely changes in adult herbivores with liver disease. In young ruminants and monogastric animals, cholestasis may result in lighter color feces being passed because of loss of stercobilin, a metabolite of bilirubin.

Liver disease should always be considered when nonspecific clinical signs, such as depression, weight loss, intermittent fever, and recurrent colic, are present without an apparent cause. Differentiation between acute and chronic hepatitis or failure based on the duration of clinical signs before presentation may be misleading, because the disease process is often advanced before clinical signs are evident. Early vague signs of depression and decreased appetite may be overlooked. Liver biopsy to determine the type of pathology, degree of hepatic fibrosis present, and the regenerative capabilities of the liver parenchyma is necessary to develop a treatment plan and give an accurate prognosis.

Diagnostic Testing: Laboratory tests often detect liver disease or dysfunction before hepatic failure occurs. Routine biochemical tests such as serum enzyme concentrations are sensitive indicators of liver disease, but they do not assess hepatic function. Dynamic biochemical tests that assess hepatic clearance provide quantitative information regarding hepatic function. Tests of hepatic function are useful diagnostic and prognostic tools and provide a guide for the modification of drug-dosing regimens.

Serum Enzyme Concentrations: Serum concentrations of liver-specific enzymes are generally higher in acute liver disease than in chronic liver disease. They may be within normal limits in the later stages of subacute or chronic hepatic disease. The magnitude of increases in hepatic enzymes (especially γ-glutamyl transpeptidase) should not be used to determine prognosis. Hepatic enzymes are used to determine the presence of disease but not necessarily the degree of hepatic dysfunction. Careful interpretation of laboratory values in conjunction with clinical findings is essential.

Sequential measurements of serum γ-glutamyl transpeptidase or transferase (GGT), sorbitol dehydrogenase (SDH; also called iditol dehydrogenase [IDH]), AST, bilirubin, and bile acids are commonly used to assess hepatic dysfunction and disease in large animals. Serum GGT, bilirubin and total bile acid concentrations, and sulfobromophthalein (BSP®) clearance are not sensitive indicators of liver disease in young calves. Although GGT is primarily associated with microsomal membranes in the biliary epithelium, it is also present in the canalicular surfaces of the hepatocytes, pancreas, kidneys, and udder. Because of urinary and milk excretion of GGT and the rarity of pancreatitis in large animals, increased serum GGT concentrations most commonly indicate bile duct or liver disease. Some consider GGT to be the single test of highest sensitivity for liver disease in adult large animals. Increase of GGT is most pronounced with obstructive biliary disease. In acute hepatic disease in horses, GGT may continue to increase for 7–14 days despite clinical improvement and return toward normal of other laboratory tests. Reportedly, serum GGT concentrations become increased within a few days of liver damage and remain increased until the terminal phase. Chronic hepatic fibrosis is the only liver disease in which an abnormal increase in GGT might not be seen. Neonatal foals have higher GGT concentrations due to GGT present in colostrum and milk. Younger adult horses, especially those in active training, may show a nonspecific increase in GGT that is not associated with liver disease or other increases in liver enzymes or serum bile acid concentration. GGT is of little value in diagnosing liver disease in neonatal calves or lambs, because it is present in colostrum and milk. GGT activity may also be increased with colonic displacement or administration of drugs (eg, corticosteroids, rifampin, benzimidazoles, anthelmintics). Some liver-derived enzymes are higher in young calves (GGT, alkaline phosphatase [AP], glutamate dehydrogenase, lactate dehydrogenase) and foals (AP, GGT, SDH, AST), because they are transiently increased or come from sources other than the liver. Serum levels of hepatic enzymes also vary in goats with age, breed, and sex. Reference ranges must be appropriate for the species and age group being evaluated.

SDH, arginase, ornithine carbamoyltransferase (OCT), AST, isoenzyme 5 lactate dehydrogenase (LDH-5), glutamate dehydrogenase (GLDH), and AP are also used to assess hepatic dysfunction and disease. Arginase, SDH, and OCT are liver-specific enzymes in horses, most ruminants, and swine. SDH is most predictive for active hepatocellular disease, with marked increases in enzyme activity after hepatocellular damage. Mild increases in SDH can also occur with obstructive GI lesions, endotoxemia, anoxia from shock, acute anemia, hyperthermia, and anesthesia. Because of their short half-lives, SDH and LDH-5 are useful in assessing resolution or progression of liver insult. Both enzymes usually return to near-normal values 4 days after liver insult, and neither is usually increased in chronic liver disease. Rarely, in severe cases of hepatic failure, SDH may return to normal in spite of a fatal outcome. Arginase and GLDH are considered specific for acute liver disease, because both have high tissue concentrations in the liver and short half-lives in the blood. AST is highly sensitive for liver disease but lacks specificity, because high concentrations come from both liver and skeletal muscle. Other AST sources include cardiac muscle, erythrocytes, intestinal cells, and the kidneys. When CK is simultaneously measured to exclude muscle disease and the serum is not hemolyzed, increases in AST and LDH-5 are caused by hepatocellular disease. AST may remain increased 10–14 days or longer after an acute, transient insult to the liver. AST values are often normal in chronic hepatic disease. SDH and AST may be markedly increased with intrahepatic cholestasis and mildly increased with extrahepatic cholestasis. Increases in AP and GGT are associated with irritation or destruction of biliary epithelium and biliary obstruction. AP comes from the placenta, bone, macrophages, intestinal epithelium, and liver. AP is increased in very young calves and foals, probably because of the placental or bone source. In young calves, AP concentrations up to 1,000 IU/L at birth and 500 IU/L at several weeks of age are considered normal. AP concentrations of 152–2,835 IU/L are reported in foals (<12 hr old), and AP activity may remain high compared with adult levels for 1–2 mo. In calves (<6 wk old), none of the common tests (bilirubin, GGT, GLDH, AP, LDH, AST, or alanine transaminase) for liver damage or function are clinically useful for detection of hepatic disease when used alone. AST and GLDH are the most sensitive of the enzymes for hepatic injury, but AST also increases with muscle damage. AST concentrations in foals may be high compared with values of adults for many months. This increase is also likely related to muscle development. Transient and mild increases in SDH activity may be noted in some foals <2 mo old.

Serum Total Bile Acid Concentration: Serum concentration of bile acids is highly specific for liver dysfunction but does not define the type of insult or disease present. Serum bile acid concentrations increase with hepatocellular damage, cholestasis, or shunts from the portal system to the vena cava. Increases are highest with biliary obstruction and portosystemic shunts. Serum bile acid concentrations rise early in liver disease and often remain high through the later stages.

Total bile acid concentration remains increased in **horses** with chronic liver disease. In horses, there is no diurnal variation, no postprandial rise, and no significant hour-to-hour variation in bile acid concentrations. Serum total bile acid concentration in most healthy horses is <10 μmol/L. Concentrations of serum or plasma bile acids >20 μmol/L have a high sensitivity and positive predictive value for determining liver disease in horses but not in ruminants. Although bile acid concentrations >30 μmol/L can be an early predictor of liver failure, caution must be used in interpretation of mild increases, because bile acid concentrations up to 20 μmol/L may be seen in horses with anorexia. Prolonged, but not short-term (<14 hr), fasting may cause increased serum bile acid concentrations in horses.

Interpretation of total bile acid concentrations is difficult in **foals** <1 wk old. Compared with those in healthy adult horses, serum bile acid concentrations in healthy foals are considerably greater during the first 6 wk of life. When measuring serum bile acid concentrations in sick foals, it is particularly important to have healthy, age-matched controls or age-dependent clinical pathology values for reference.

In **dairy cattle**, serum bile acid measurement is of little value in recognizing fatty liver or liver disease or failure because of significant hour-to-hour variations. In recently freshened cows, serum total bile acid concentrations are significantly higher than in cows in mid-lactation or in 6-mo-old heifers.

Total bile acid concentration may be the best single test for hepatic disease in young **calves**. In calves, concentrations >35 μmol/L may indicate liver disease, bile obstruction, or a portosystemic shunt.

Reported reference intervals for serum concentration of bile acids are 1.1–22.9 μmol/L for **llamas** >1 yr old and 1.8–49.8 μmol/L for llamas <1 yr old. Bile acid concentrations in individual llamas may vary with feeding or sampling time of day, remaining within the reference interval.

Serum Bile Pigments: Evaluation of serum bilirubin (direct and indirect) concentration is useful to determine hepatic dysfunction in horses and ruminants. Increases in bilirubin result from hemolysis, hepatocellular disease, cholestasis, or physiologic causes. Anorexia in horses causes a physiologic increase in total serum bilirubin to usually <6–8 mg/dL and rarely as high as 10.5–12 mg/dL, accumulating at a rate of ~1 mg/dL for each day of anorexia. The indirect bilirubin increases 2- to 3-fold, while the direct bilirubin remains within the reference range. In foals, indirect more than direct bilirubin may be increased with prematurity, neonatal isoerythrolysis, septicemia, or a portocaval shunt. Enteritis, umbilical infection, intestinal obstruction, and certain drugs (corticosteroids, heparin, halothane) may also cause hyperbilirubinemia. Mild, transient physiologic hyperbilirubinemia and icterus may be seen in newborn foals and calves. Although the mechanism(s) is not fully known, proposed causes include prebirth "loading of hepatocytes," naturally high RBC destruction at or around birth, inefficiency in bilirubin excretion, or lower hepatocellular ligandin concentrations in neonatal foals than in adult horses. In healthy calves <72 hr old, total bilirubin may be as high as 1.5 mg/dL and up to 0.8 mg/dL in 1-wk-old calves. Direct bilirubin is usually <0.3 mg/dL in young calves. In healthy foals (<2 days old), total bilirubin concentrations may range from 0.9–4.5 mg/dL, with most being unconjugated bilirubin (0.8–3.8 mg/dL). Prematurity or illness (without liver disease) may increase unconjugated bilirubin fraction in young foals. Bilirubin concentrations in healthy foals should be within adult reference ranges by the time they are 2 wk old. Normal values for total bilirubin in goats are 0–0.1 mg/dL.

Horses with hepatic disease and failure most often have significant increases in both indirect and direct bilirubin. With liver damage in horses or ruminants, most of the retained bilirubin is indirect (unconjugated), and the direct-to-total ratio usually is <0.3 (more than two-thirds is indirect). Acute liver failure caused by hepatic necrosis results in increases in both indirect and direct bilirubin fractions. In horses with acute liver failure, the increase in bilirubin is primarily because of an increase in the indirect fraction. Hepatocellular disease should be considered when the indirect bilirubin fraction is >25% of the total bilirubin value. Direct-reacting bilirubin rarely exceeds 25%–35% of the total bilirubin in horses. Increases of this magnitude suggest predominant biliary disease or obstruction. With bile blockage or intrahepatic cholestasis, the direct-to-total ratio may be >0.3 in horses or 0.5 in cows. Increases in direct bilirubin may be seen in septic foals with intestinal ileus and minimal evidence of hepatocellular dysfunction.

In chronic liver disease, bilirubin concentrations are often within normal limits. Adult cattle and calves may have severe liver disease without any increase in serum bilirubin. In cattle, goats, and sheep, circulating bilirubin concentrations increase only modestly with severe, generalized hepatic disease. The most dramatic increases in serum or plasma bilirubin concentrations are due to hemolytic crises rather than to liver dysfunction. In the absence of hemolysis, total serum bilirubin concentrations >2 mg/dL indicate impaired hepatic function in ruminants.

Urobilinogen: Urobilinogen may be detected by dipstick analysis in healthy horses. Increased concentrations of urobilinogen in urine without hemolysis are suggestive of a hepatic dysfunction, portosystemic shunting, or increased production by intestinal bacteria. Urobilinogen in the urine indicates the presence of a patent bile duct. Absence of urobilinogen may indicate complete biliary blockage, liver disease, or failure to excrete bilirubin into the intestine, reduce it by intestinal bacteria, or absorb it from the ileum. The correlation between urobilinogen and hepatocellular disease in animals is poor. Urobilinogen is unstable in urine; thus, analysis must be done within 1–2 hr, or the amount will be decreased or undetectable.

Serum and Plasma Proteins: Serum albumin and protein concentrations are variable in horses and cattle with hepatic disease. Hypoproteinemia is not common in horses with acute liver disease. Serum albumin is most likely to be reduced in chronic liver disease due to decreased functional hepatic parenchyma. In one study of 84 horses, 13% were hypoalbuminemic. Albumin concentrations were below minimum reference values in 18% of horses with chronic liver disease and 6% with acute liver disease. Globulin concentrations were increased in 64% of the horses. Hyperproteinemia due to hyperglobulinemia (polyclonal gammopathy or increase in β-globulins) may develop in horses with severe acute or chronic liver disease. Total plasma protein concentration is often normal, but the albumin to globulin ratio may be decreased.

Plasma fibrinogen concentration may not be a sensitive test in horses with hepatic insufficiency. Low fibrinogen concentrations may result from parenchymal insufficiency or disseminated intravascular coagulopathy. A high fibrinogen concentration is associated with an inflammatory response in horses with cholangiohepatitis.

Prothrombin Time: Abnormalities in prothrombin time (PT) are often the first detected because factor VII, a liver-synthesized vitamin K–dependent factor, has the shortest half-life. Serum PT may be rapidly prolonged with hepatic failure and is one of the first function tests to return to normal with recovery from acute hepatic disease. A normal PT determination, however, does not exclude coagulopathy due to vitamin K deficiency. Prolonged activated partial thromboplastin time (APTT) or other indications of coagulopathy may be noted in animals with severe hepatic disease. Because a number of factors may influence PT or APTT values in horses, the ratio of clotting time of the horse with suspected hepatic disease to that of a healthy horse's value should be >1.3 for the test to be interpreted as abnormal.

Urea, Glucose, Ammonia, and Other Alterations: Serum concentration of urea may be decreased in both acute and chronic liver failure. Hypoglycemia is common in foals with hepatic failure. Blood glucose concentrations in adult horses with hepatic dysfunction are frequently normal or increased. Hypoglycemia, while less common in adult horses and ruminants with hepatic dysfunction, is more likely in chronic liver disease. Plasma triglyceride concentrations are markedly increased in ponies, miniature horses, donkeys, and adult horses with hepatic lipidosis. The magnitude of increase in serum triglycerides may correlate with prognosis in horses. Alterations in triglycerides, very-low-density lipoproteins, and esterified cholesterol levels are more common in ruminants than in horses with hepatic insufficiency. Neonatal foals have higher blood cholesterol and triglyceride concentrations than adult horses.

Plasma ammonia concentrations may be increased with hepatic insufficiency but do not correlate well with severity of hepatic encephalopathy except during portocaval shunts. Increased concentrations of blood ammonia and signs of hepatic encephalopathy without hepatic failure are reported in Morgan weanlings with hyperornithinemia, hyperammonemia, and normocitrullinuria syndrome and in adult horses with primary or idiopathic hyperammonemia. Ingestion of urea or ammonium salts is more likely to cause increases of blood ammonia and encephalopathy in cattle than in horses.

PCV and serum iron concentrations are often high in horses with severe liver disease. An increased PCV may persist in the face of fluid therapy and normal hydration status until the underlying liver disease is resolved. Secondary erythrocytosis (with or without increased erythropoietin concentration) has been noted in some horses with hepatic neoplasia. Increased serum iron concentration is commonly seen in horses with either hepatic and/or hemolytic disease.

Dye Excretion and Clearance Tests: Sulfobromophthalein (BSP®) or indocyanine green dyes can be used to assess hepatobiliary transport. The BSP half-life is prolonged when >50% of hepatic function is lost. The normal clearance half-life of BSP is <3.7 min in horses, 2.13 ± 0.19 min in goats, and ≤4 min in sheep. BSP clearance is longer in calves (5–15 min) than in adult cattle (≤5 min). Although dye excretion tests are usually prolonged with hepatic dysfunction, they may still be within the normal range. Hyperbilirubinemia, decreased hepatic blood flow, and significant cholestasis may falsely prolong BSP clearance, and hypoalbuminemia may falsely shorten it. BSP clearance in goats is most often prolonged with generalized hepatic lipidosis secondary to pregnancy toxemia. Determination of BSP clearance time, rather than half-life, reportedly is more useful in detection of liver disease. BSP clearance time in healthy fed and 3-day fasted horses is 10 mL/min/kg and 6 mL/min/kg, respectively. These tests, however, are of limited use in clinical practice because of the lack of commercially available pharmaceutical-grade BSP. Expense, procedural limitations, and equipment requirements for quantitation of indocyanine green clearance have limited its use as a diagnostic test.

Scintigraphy: Biliary patency and hepatocyte function, structure, and blood flow may be evaluated by hepatobiliary scintigraphy. Radionucleotide liver scans and biliary scans can detect alterations in blood flow or hepatic masses and biliary obstruction (atresia, cholangitis, cholelithiasis), respectively. Scintigraphy has been used in pigs, foals, and lambs to differentiate biliary obstruction from other causes of hyperbilirubinemia.

Ultrasonography: Ultrasonography can be used to evaluate liver size, appearance (shape, texture), and location in horses and ruminants for diagnosis of hepatomegaly, hepatolithiasis, biliary dilatation, cholelithiasis, or focal lesions. Tumors, cysts, abscesses, and granulomas may be seen. Diffuse diseases are harder to detect than focal processes, because the former cause less distortion of normal hepatic architecture. Diagnosis of diffuse liver disease should be substantiated by biopsy and histopathology. Ultrasound can be used to guide collection of liver biopsy specimens and to perform cholecystocentesis and aspiration of abscesses, masses, or bile samples (fluke eggs, bile acids, culture). It is also an accurate, noninvasive way to monitor the progression or resolution of disease. In horses, the liver should be imaged from both the right and left sides of the animal.

Liver Biopsy: Percutaneous liver biopsy is the definitive way to diagnose hepatic disease. Histologic evaluation of the liver provides valuable information regarding cause and severity of the disease process. Most cases of liver disease are diffuse, so the sample will be representative of the disease. Samples can be obtained blindly, but ultrasonographic guidance decreases the risk of complications (peritonitis due to bile leakage or intestinal puncture, hemorrhage, or pneumothorax). Liver biopsies can also be obtained during laparoscopy, which offers the additional advantage of being able to visualize the surface of the liver and other abdominal organs for evidence of disease.

Samples should be placed in media for bacterial culture and sensitivity and in formalin for histologic evaluation. Coagulation profiles (prothrombin time, partial thromboplastin time, fibrinogen, fibrin degradation products, and optional platelet count) may be performed before liver biopsy to reduce the risk of hemorrhage. Liver biopsy may not be advised in an animal with clinical or clinicopathologic evidence of a coagulopathy or a hepatic abscess, because hemorrhage or contamination of the peritoneal cavity may result.

Radiography: Contrast abdominal radiography in foals may help diagnose gastroduodenal obstructions and secondary cholangiohepatitis. Portosystemic shunts in foals or young calves can be identified with mesenteric portovenography by injecting radiopaque contrast solution into a jejunal mesenteric vein, followed by fluoroscopy or sequential survey radiographs to monitor the hepatic blood flow.

Treatment and Management: Initial treatment of animals with signs of hepatic disease or insufficiency is often supportive and started before the underlying cause and extent of hepatic damage is known. History, clinical signs, and laboratory data may give some clue as to the nature of the hepatic disease process, but liver biopsy is usually required to make a definitive diagnosis and to determine the degree of hepatic injury.

Specific therapies for hepatic disease depend on cause, presence of liver failure, chronicity, degree of hepatic fibrosis or biliary obstruction, and species affected. Increases in hepatic enzymes without hepatic disease may not require specific therapy for the liver but rather for the primary disease.

Therapy is most successful when intervention is early, hepatic fibrosis is minimal, and evidence of regeneration in the liver exists. Horses with severe or bridging fibrosis respond poorly because of inadequate potential for liver regeneration. The goals for treatment of large animals with hepatic disease or insufficiency are to control hepatic encephalopathy, to treat the underlying disease process, to provide supportive care to allow time for liver regeneration, and most importantly, to prevent injury to the animal and those working with the animal. Animals with hepatic encephalopathy often show aggressive and unpredictable behavior that can result in injury to self or handlers.

Hepatic Encephalopathy and Hepatic Failure: Horses with hepatic encephalopathy may be aggressive or demonstrate repetitive behaviors that make restraint difficult. To ensure safety of the animal and handlers, sedation is required. Because most sedatives and tranquilizers are metabolized by the liver, their elimination half-life may be prolonged in animals with hepatic failure; therefore, dosages should be minimized initially until it is determined how the animal responds to lower dosages. Xylazine or detomidine given in small doses to effect can be used to control horses exhibiting abnormal behavior. Diazepam should be avoided in animals with hepatic encephalopathy, because it may enhance the effect of γ-aminobutyric acid on inhibitory neurons and worsen neurologic signs. Acepromazine should also be avoided, because it may lower the seizure threshold.

Dehydration, acid-base and electrolyte imbalances, and hypoglycemia should be corrected with appropriate IV fluids. Initially, a balanced polyionic solution is administered for rehydration. Potassium supplementation is added (10–40 mEq/L, depending on infusion rate) if the animal is hypokalemic or hypophagic. If IV infusion is not possible in ruminants, rehydration may be attempted by oral administration of fluids if rumen motility is normal. Rarely, some horses with hepatic disease have polycythemia, making evaluation of hydration status by PCV difficult. Severe acidosis may be present. Because rapid correction of the acidosis may exacerbate neurologic signs, acidosis should be corrected gradually by IV administration of fluids with a high concentration of electrolytes. If this fails or if blood pH is <7.1 (bicarbonate <14 mEq/L), bicarbonate may be administered cautiously. Supplemental vitamins are optional. Adequate fresh water should be available if the animal can swallow normally.

Factors that may contribute to the hepatic encephalopathy should be eliminated. Glucose as a 5%–10% solution is given to correct hypoglycemia if present. In addition, glucose supplementation helps decrease blood ammonia concentrations and reduces catabolic gluconeogenesis, protein catabolism, and need for hepatic gluconeogenesis. Unless the animal is hyperglycemic, a continuous IV infusion of glucose (5% at 2 mL/kg/hr or 10% at 1 mL/kg/hr) should be given, even to animals that are not hypoglycemic. The infusion rate should be adjusted so that euglycemia is maintained. Induction of moderate to severe hyperglycemia, rapid changes in glucose level, and glucosuria should be avoided. IV glucose should be used in combination with balanced electrolyte fluids and not as the sole fluid source.

Therapies directed toward decreasing either ammonia production in or absorption from the bowel include administration of mineral oil, neomycin, lactulose, and metronidazole. Administration of mineral oil decreases absorption and facilitates removal of ammonia. Passing a nasogastric tube in an animal with hepatic encephalopathy must be done cautiously, because nasal bleeding caused by decreased clotting factors may be difficult to control. Oral administration of neomycin (10–30 mg/kg, bid-qid for 1–2 days) has been used to decrease ammonia-producing bacteria in the intestine. Lactulose (0.2 mL/kg, bid; 0.3 mL/kg, PO, qid; or 90–120 mL/450 kg, tid-qid) is metabolized to organic acids by bacteria in the ileum and colon. Reduction in colonic pH reportedly fosters an increased bacterial assimilation of ammonia, decreased ammonia production, ammonia trapping in the bowel, intestinal microflora changes, and osmotic catharsis. Reportedly, oral administration of vinegar (acetic acid) has the same effect on colonic pH and ammonia concentration in the gut. Metronidazole (10–15 mg/kg, PO, bid-qid) decreases ammonia-producing organisms in horses but should not be used in food animals. If the animal can swallow, oral drugs can be mixed with corn syrup or molasses and given via dose syringe to avoid trauma and the risk of inducing hemorrhage during passage of a nasogastric tube. Neomycin, lactulose, and metronidazole may all potentially induce mild to severe diarrhea (salmonellosis) because of disruption of GI flora. Use of the drugs in combination is more likely to induce diarrhea than any one of the drugs given alone. Because metronidazole is metabolized by the liver, caution must be used when administering the drug to horses with hepatic failure. Neurologic signs due to metronidazole toxicosis may mimic hepatoencephalopathy.

Until the nature of the underlying hepatic disease is known, treatment with broad-spectrum antimicrobials is warranted if infectious hepatitis is suspected. A trimethoprim-sulfa combination is a good empiric choice because of its activity against gram-negative bacteria and its high concentration in bile. Penicillin in combination with an aminoglycoside has a broad spectrum of action and may be of benefit if a *Streptococcus* sp or an anaerobic or gram-negative coliform is suspected. Enrofloxacin has also been recommended. First- and second-generation cephalosporins have been used in foals and in other species. Ceftiofur sodium also has an enterohepatic cycle, with ~15% of active drug recycled through the liver and excreted out the biliary tree. Ceftiofur has a broader spectrum than most early generation cephalosporins and has proved useful to treat acute or recurrent ascending bacterial cholangiohepatitis. Metronidazole may be administered when anaerobic infection is suspected in horses. Specific antimicrobial therapy based on culture and sensitivity of a liver biopsy is ideal.

Pain may be controlled with appropriate doses of an NSAID (eg, flunixin meglumine, 1.1 mg/kg, IV, bid, or phenylbutazone 4.4 mg/kg, IV or PO, bid). Vitamin K_1 (up to 1 mg/kg, SC; 40–50 mg/450 kg, SC) and plasma transfusions (1–2 L/100 kg) may be given when coagulopathies develop or hypoalbuminemia is present. In some horses with acute hepatic disease and failure, antioxidant (dimethyl sulfoxide, acetylcysteine, vitamin E, S-adenosylmethionine [SAMe]), and anti-inflammatory (flunixin meglumine, phenylbutazone) therapy may be useful. Mannitol has been recommended for treatment of suspected brain edema in fulminant hepatoencephalopathy. Horses with hepatic disease should be protected from sunlight.

Dietary Management: Dietary management is essential for management of animals with hepatic encephalopathy or acute or chronic hepatopathy. Affected animals should be fed carefully, because dysphagia may be a problem. Relatively small amounts should be fed frequently, although this recommendation may prove impractical in the longterm for many clients. The diet should meet energy needs with readily digestible carbohydrates, provide adequate but not excessive protein, have a high ratio of branched-chain amino acids to aromatic amino acids, and be moderate to high in starch to decrease need for hepatic glucose synthesis. Fat and salt should not be added to the diet. Feeds used successfully in horses include grass or oat hay, corn, and sorghum. Small amounts of molasses may be added to improve palatability and add energy. Linseed meal and soybean meal have an excellent branched-chain to aromatic amino acid ratio and may be used as a protein supplement in small quantities. Beet pulp may be substituted for oat or grass hay. Beet pulp may be soaked first to allow full expansion before being fed. Choke may be a problem in some animals eating beet pulp.

The feeding of alfalfa hay, alfalfa-containing feeds, or other legume hays to horses with hepatic disease is controversial. Although alfalfa hay has a better branched-chain to aromatic amino acid ratio than grass hay, it may have too high a protein content. Feeding grass hay is preferred for animals with hyperammonemia or signs of hepatic encephalopathy. A mixed grass/alfalfa hay can be fed to horses without central neurologic signs if weight loss is a problem and the added protein is tolerated. Grazing grass pastures is allowable as long as signs of hepatic encephalopathy are controlled and exposure to sunlight is avoided.

Other feeds high in branched-chain amino acids include sorghum, bran, or milo. Parenteral or enteral supplement with branched-chain amino acids helps restore the normal ratio of branched-chain to aromatic amino acids. Supplementation with vitamins A, D, E, and K might be indicated, because these fat-soluble vitamins are not stored effectively or readily available from a diseased liver. Vitamin K_1 may be indicated in animals with a coagulopathy. Large amounts of fat should not be fed to meet energy requirements; excessive fat may lead to a fatty liver.

Transfaunation (*see* p 2562) with rumen fluid from a healthy cow may help reestablish normal ruminal flora and enhance the appetite of affected cattle. Animals that will not eat voluntarily must be force fed. A gruel may be given by nasogastric tube in horses and swine or by orogastric tube or rumen fistula in ruminants. In ruminants, forced feeding of alfalfa meal (15% protein) and dried brewer's grain or beet pulp with potassium chloride and normal rumen fluid has been recommended. Alfalfa hay and alfalfa-containing feeds may be better tolerated by cattle than by horses with hepatic disease. IV polyionic fluids with 5% dextrose, potassium chloride, and B vitamins may also be needed in animals not consuming adequate amounts.

ACUTE HEPATITIS

Acute hepatitis can have an infectious, toxic, or undefined cause. Clinical signs may appear suddenly, with horses appearing lethargic, anorectic, and icteric. Photosensitization, diarrhea, and clotting abnormalities also may be seen. Neurologic signs resulting from hepatic encephalopathy and/or hypoglycemia can be most severe in animals with acute fulminant liver disease. Signs of endotoxemia may be present, depending on the underlying cause and the ability of the Kupffer cells to remove endotoxin from the systemic circulation. Increases in serum sorbitol dehydrogenase (SDH) and AST activities indicate acute hepatocellular injury. Serum γ-glutamyl transpeptidase or transferase (GGT) is increased with cholestasis secondary to hepatocyte swelling. Cholestasis results in hyperbilirubinemia, with the direct (conjugated) fraction ranging from 15%–35% of total in horses. Increased serum total bile acid concentration, decreased glucose and BUN concentrations, and prolonged coagulation times become evident as hepatic function progressively worsens. Anorexia can lead to hypokalemia. The CBC is variable, because it may reflect an inflammatory response with a neutrophilia or endotoxemia with a neutropenia, increased band neutrophils, and toxic changes.

Idiopathic Acute Hepatic Disease

(Theiler disease, Serum hepatitis, Postvaccinal hepatitis)

Idiopathic acute hepatic disease (IAHD) is the most common cause of acute hepatitis in horses. It is primarily a disease of adult horses.

Etiology and Epidemiology: Frequently, horses with IAHD show clinical signs of hepatic failure 4–10 wk after receiving an equine origin biologic, such as tetanus antitoxin (TAT). In some cases, the affected horse may not have received TAT but may have been in contact with another horse that received TAT. Reportedly, IAHD may develop as a potential complication of administration of any equine plasma or serum product that includes commercial equine plasma. However, other affected horses have no prior history of exposure to such a product. Subclinical IAHD can also develop after administration of TAT. Most commonly, only one horse on the premises is affected, although outbreaks may occur or other horses on the farm may have evidence of liver disease (increased enzyme levels) without clinical signs. Occurrence of the disease in groups of adult horses during the late summer or early fall (August to November) suggests an infectious (viral) or vector-spread etiology, although supporting evidence is lacking. The seasonal occurrence could reflect the fact that many foaling mares receive TAT in the spring of the year along with their newborn foals. Lactating mares that receive TAT at foaling seem to be more susceptible. A Type III (immune complex–mediated) hypersensitivity reaction also has been proposed. Recent evidence suggests a viral cause, with a "Theiler disease–associated virus" of the Flaviviridae documented in association with a naturally occurring outbreak of Theilier disease. The offending virus was identified from diseased horses and was characterized as very similar to human hepatitis viruses B and C. The newly identified virus was then administered experimentally to previously naive research horses, which developed signs of Theiler disease, proving that it could be passed from one horse to another via serum administration and resulting in similar disease.

Clinical Findings: Onset of clinical signs is acute. Acute mortality may be 50%–60%, with overall mortality as high as 88% in affected horses. Horses with IAHD typically present with anorexia, hepatic encephalopathy, and icterus. The CNS signs are variable, ranging from lethargy to aggression or maniacal behavior, central blindness, and ataxia. Photosensitivity and discolored urine due to high bilirubin concentrations may be seen. Fever is present in ~50% of cases. Weight loss (uncommon), ventral edema, jugular pulses, ileus, and acute respiratory distress have been seen in some horses with IAHD. These findings suggest there may be a subclinical phase before development of overt hepatic failure. Intravascular hemolysis with hemoglobinuria may be seen in some terminal cases. Most cases are sporadic, but outbreaks with several horses involved have been reported. Recognition of IAHD in one horse indicates horses on the same premises should be carefully monitored for clinical or serum biochemical signs of hepatic disease.

Serum concentrations of GGT, AST, and SDH are increased. GGT is frequently further increased during the first few days of illness, despite clinical improvement and eventual recovery in an affected horse. Horses with AST values >4,000 IU/L have a poor prognosis. AST concentrations decrease within 3–5 days in horses that improve, and SDH concentrations decrease even more rapidly. Total serum bilirubin concentration is generally higher in horses with IAHD than in horses with anorexia. Hyperbilirubinemia is common, with the unconjugated form being >70% of the total. Serum total bile acid concentrations are increased. Moderate to severe acidosis, hypokalemia, polycythemia, increased plasma aromatic amino acids, and hyperammonemia may also be present.

Lesions: At necropsy, icterus and varying degrees of ascites are present. The liver is usually small to normal in size but may be enlarged (peracute cases), with a mottled and bile-stained surface. Histologically, there is marked centrilobular-to-midzonal hepatocellular necrosis and mild to moderate mononuclear infiltrate. Mild to moderate bile duct proliferation may be seen in some animals with more chronic disease.

Diagnosis: Diagnosis is based on history, abrupt onset of clinical signs, and laboratory alterations suggestive of hepatic insufficiency. In some cases, the liver is shrunken and difficult to visualize with ultrasonographic examination. A definitive diagnosis can be made only by liver biopsy. Differential diagnoses include acute pyrrolizidine toxicosis, hepatotoxins, acute infectious hepatitis, acute mycotoxicosis, cerebral disease, and hemolytic disease.

Treatment and Prognosis: There is no specific therapy for IAHD. Supportive therapy (IV crystalloid fluids with glucose and potassium added) and treatment of the hepatic encephalopathy may be successful. Stressful situations, such as moving the animal or weaning the mare's foal, may exacerbate the clinical signs of hepatic encephalopathy and should be avoided. Sedation should be used only to control behavior that could lead to injury of the animal or handlers and to allow therapeutic procedures.

Recovery depends on the degree of hepatocellular necrosis. Affected horses that remain stable for 3–5 days and that continue to eat often recover. Decreases in SDH concentration and prothrombin time along with improvement in appetite are the best positive predictive indicators of recovery. Horses with rapid progression of clinical signs, uncontrollable encephalopathy, hemorrhage, or hemolysis have a poor prognosis. For affected horses that do recover, the longterm prognosis is good. In some horses, progressive weight loss and death may occur during the months after the initial clinical signs.

Prevention: Use of TAT is not without risk. Routine administration of TAT to parturient mares is strongly discouraged. Use of TAT should be restricted to situations necessitating tetanus prophylaxis and in which a history of active tetanus toxoid immunization is absent or unknown.

Acute Hepatic Necrosis in Cattle

Epidemiology and Pathogenesis: Acute hepatic disease and failure in cattle most commonly results from a toxic insult. Hepatocellular necrosis with clinical and laboratory evidence of hepatic failure may develop in cattle after mastitis or metritis with clinical signs of endotoxemia. Endotoxin induces hepatocellular necrosis through both direct and indirect effects on the liver. Endotoxin can cause Kupffer cells to release lysosomal enzymes, prostaglandins, and collagenase that damage hepatocytes, or it may interact directly with the hepatocytes, causing lysosomal damage, decreased mitochondrial function, and necrosis. Endotoxin-related hepatocellular necrosis may be due in part to decreased hepatic blood flow and liver hypoxia.

Clinical Findings and Lesions: Clinical signs include weight loss, anorexia, and cessation of milk production. Photosensitization and mild icterus are variable. Serum SDH, GGT, and AST concentrations are mildly to severely increased. Fatty liver or ketosis is not characteristic. The liver may be normal in size or mildly enlarged. Histologically, there is marked hydropic change with varying degrees of hepatic necrosis.

Diagnosis: Diagnosis is based on a history of hepatic-related signs developing concurrently or after a primary disease and endotoxemia. Increases in hepatic and biliary enzymes and absence of ketosis support the diagnosis. Definitive diagnosis is based on liver biopsy and by excluding other infectious, toxic, and inflammatory causes of hepatic dysfunction. Differential diagnoses include other causes of subacute or chronic liver disease (eg, hepatotoxins, hepatic lipidosis) and conditions causing weight loss and hypophagia.

Treatment: Nutritional and fluid support is often successful in affected cows with acute hepatic necrosis after transient insults. Forced feeding of alfalfa meal (15% protein) and dried brewers' grain or beet pulp with potassium chloride and normal rumen fluid is recommended. IV polyionic fluids with 5% dextrose, potassium chloride, and B vitamins may also be needed. Control of endotoxemia and treatment of the primary disease condition are essential.

INFECTIOUS HEPATITIS AND HEPATIC ABSCESSES

Tyzzer Disease

Tyzzer disease, due to *Clostridium piliforme* (previously *Bacillus piliformis*), causes an acute necrotizing hepatitis, myocarditis, and colitis in foals 8–42 days old. (*See also* p 199.) It has been reported in two calves: a 1-wk-old Jersey bull calf with enteritis and multifocal necrotizing hepatitis and a second calf with concurrent cryptosporidiosis and coronaviral enteritis. In the latter animal, *C piliforme* was identified in hepatocytes and epithelium and smooth muscle cells of the ileum and cecum. Clinical signs included hypophagia, generalized weakness, dullness, and decreased fecal passage.

Cholangiohepatitis

Cholangiohepatitis is a severe inflammation of the bile passages and adjacent liver, which sporadically causes hepatic failure in horses and ruminants. It occasionally occurs secondary to cholelithiasis, duodenitis, intestinal obstruction, neoplasia, parasitism, and certain toxins in horses. The fungal toxin sporidesmin from *Pithomyces chartarum* may cause cholangiohepatitis in sheep and cattle.

Etiology: Bacteremia due to an organism (eg, *Salmonella* spp) eliminated in the bile, an ascending infection of the biliary tract after intestinal disturbance, or ileus is thought to be related to the development of cholangiohepatitis. In foals, duodenal ulceration and duodenitis may result in bile stasis, hepatic duct obstruction, and cholangiohepatitis. Parasite migration through the liver may predispose to cholangiohepatitis in some animals. Gram-negative organisms, including *Salmonella* spp, *Escherichia coli*, *Pseudomonas* spp, and *Actinobacillus equuli* are frequently isolated from the liver. *Clostridium* spp, *Pasteurella* spp, and *Streptococcus* spp are less frequently recovered.

Clinical Findings: Depending on the severity of infection and virulence of the organism, clinical signs may be acute with severe toxemia, subacute, or chronic. Most typically, cholangiohepatitis is a subacute or chronic disease process, with affected animals showing signs of weight loss, anorexia, intermittent or persistent fever, or colic. Icterus, photosensitivity, and signs of hyperammonemic hepatic encephalopathy are variable. Sorbitol dehydrogenase (SDH), AST, γ-glutamyl transpeptidase or transferase (GGT), conjugated bilirubin, and total bile acid concentrations are usually increased. Peripheral WBC counts are variable, depending on the degree of inflammation and endotoxemia present. Acute, suppurative cholangiohepatitis may occasionally result in severe septicemia and death.

Lesions: In acute cases, the liver is swollen, soft, and pale. Suppurative foci may be visible beneath the capsule or on cut surface. Lesions in other systems may reflect septicemia and jaundice. Microscopically in acute cases, neutrophils are present in the portal triads and degenerate parenchyma. Purulent exudate is evident in the ducts. In subacute or chronic cholangiohepatitis, the inflammation is more proliferative and bile duct proliferation more pronounced. Areas of atrophy, regenerative hyperplasia, and periportal fibrosis may be evident.

Diagnosis: Liver biopsy should be performed to confirm the diagnosis and to obtain a liver sample for aerobic and anaerobic culture and sensitivity. Differential diagnoses include other causes of acute to chronic hepatic disease, weight loss, colic, or sepsis. If neurologic signs are present, cerebral diseases must be considered. Because cholangiohepatitis is frequently associated with cholelithiasis in horses, the presence of one or more calculi must be excluded; ultrasonography of the liver may prove valuable in this case.

Treatment: Treatment based on culture and sensitivity results from liver tissue often gives favorable results. Therapy consists of longterm (≥4–6 wk) antimicrobial administration, supportive therapy with IV fluids, and management of hepatoencephalopathy, if present. Initially, broad-spectrum antimicrobials effective against gram-negative, gram-positive, and anaerobic organisms should be administered. A combination of penicillin with either a trimethoprim-sulfa or an aminoglycoside or enrofloxacin may be used. Ampicillin or a cephalosporin can be used instead of penicillin. Ceftiofur sodium has an enterohepatic cycle and broader spectrum and may prove valuable in treatment. Metronidazole can be used in horses to treat anaerobic bacteria. Antimicrobial therapy can be altered pending results of culture of tissue obtained by liver biopsy. Prognosis is good if fibrosis is not severe, but it is poor if severe periportal or bridging fibrosis is present.

Equine Rhinopneumonitis

Equine rhinopneumonitis due to equine herpesvirus 1 is a sporadic cause of interstitial pneumonia, hepatic disease, and often death in newborn foals. *See* p 1452 for clinical findings, diagnosis, and treatment.

Infectious Necrotic Hepatitis

(Black disease)

Infectious necrotic hepatitis, caused by *Clostridium novyi* type B, affects primarily sheep but also cattle, horses, and pigs. *See* p 603 for clinical findings, lesions, and control.

Bacillary Hemoglobinuria

(Red water disease, Icterohemoglobinuria)

Clostridium novyi type D (*C haemolyticum*) is the anaerobic organism that causes bacillary hemoglobinuria in cattle, other ruminants, and rarely horses. *See* p 601 for clinical findings, diagnosis, and control.

Hepatic Abscesses

Hepatic abscesses are generally polymicrobial infections; anaerobes are common. The primary etiologic agent of liver abscesses in cattle is *Fusobacterium necrophorum*. In goats, most abscesses are due to *Corynebacterium pseudotuberculosis*, *Trueperella pyogenes*, and *Escherichia coli*. Organisms less frequently isolated include *Proteus* sp, *Mannheimia haemolytica*, *Staphylococcus epidermidis*, *S aureus*, *Rhodococcus equi*, *Erysipelothrix rhusiopathiae*, and the yeast *Candida krusei*. In horses, hepatic abscesses often contain *Streptococcus* spp (*S equi equi*, *S equi zooepidemicus*), *C pseudotuberculosis*, or enterobacteria after ascending cholangiohepatitis or intestinal disease, and anaerobes. In pigs, hepatic abscesses develop after migration of ascarids into the bile ducts.

The liver is particularly susceptible to abscess formation, because it receives blood from the hepatic artery, the portal system, and the umbilical vein in the fetus and the newborn. Hepatic abscesses are most prevalent in ruminants and uncommon in horses. Abscesses are associated with rumenitis (rumenitis-liver abscess complex), bacteremia, septic portal vein thrombosis, and parasite migration or extension from intestinal disease. They can also occur as sequelae of abdominal surgery. In neonates and young animals, abscesses may develop secondary to ascarid migration, bacterial septicemia, or ascending infection of the umbilical vein. In horses and cattle, signs may be similar to those seen with other abdominal abscesses and include intermittent colic, intermittent fever, and weight loss. Often, liver abscesses are subclinical in cattle. Hepatic ultrasound may prove diagnostic. Prognosis is generally poor because of lack of response to antimicrobial therapy or incomplete resolution. (*See also* LIVER ABSCESSES IN CATTLE, p 352.)

HEPATOTOXINS

Hepatotoxins manifest their toxicity by one or more mechanisms: periacinal (centrilobular) necrosis, midzonal necrosis, periportal necrosis, cholestasis, biliary hyperplasia, fatty or hydropic change near necrotic zones, or venous occlusion. Fatal hepatic insufficiency may result if the initial injury is acute and severe. More commonly, the hepatic damage from toxins is subacute or chronic. In chronic processes, the longterm result may be cirrhosis. Many hepatotoxins, especially those in plants, exert toxic effects on multiple organs, particularly the kidneys, lungs, and GI tract.

Definitive diagnosis may be difficult. Careful history, inspection of the environment, laboratory evaluations, liver biopsy, or necropsy may be needed to determine the offending agent. With acute plant toxicities, evidence of hepatotoxic plants may be seen in the stomach contents or rumen.

Specific antidotes for hepatotoxins are limited. Removal of the animals from the source is essential to decrease additional exposure. Administration of an absorbent (eg, activated charcoal, mineral oil) or laxatives (eg, mineral oil, magnesium sulfate) or rumenotomy may decrease absorption of toxic elements in acute poisonings. These may not be helpful in chronic intoxications (ie, pyrrolizidine alkaloid toxicity), in which the toxic agent has been ingested over weeks to months before signs of toxicosis are evident. Supportive care includes correction of electrolyte, metabolic, and glucose disorders via fluid therapy and dietary management. Hepatic encephalopathy must be controlled. Sunlight should be avoided if photosensitization is present. Antimicrobials may be considered to prevent secondary pyoderma. Prognosis is guarded and depends on the particular hepatotoxin.

Chemical and Drug-related Causes of Toxic Hepatopathy

For COAL-TAR POISONING, *see* p 3045.

Iron Toxicosis: Newborn foals (<3 days old) are especially sensitive to iron overload because of their high serum iron concentrations, increased ability to absorb iron, and oversaturation of transferrin at birth. In adult horses, injectable iron increases body iron concentration more substantially than most oral supplements; liver biopsy will document increased iron stores, but these are rarely if ever associated with clinical signs of liver disease. Iron toxicosis has been reported in calves and young bulls injected with a ferric ammonium citrate alone or in combination with ferrous gluconate.

Foals given iron at birth, especially before receiving colostrum, may develop acute toxicity with clinical signs of hepatic encephalopathy in 2–5 days and a fatal outcome. Serum bilirubin and blood ammonia concentrations are high, and prothrombin time is prolonged. Alterations in serum hepatic enzymes are variable. In adult horses, acute toxicosis, although less common, may cause enteric irritation and cardiovascular collapse with sudden death. Signs of more chronic hepatic failure, including weight loss, icterus, and depression, may be seen with repeated oral administration of iron. Possible sources of excess iron include inappropriate supplementation, forages high in iron, injectable iron, and leaching of iron into water or feed. Calves with iron toxicosis have trembling, vocalizing, bruxism, colic, and convulsions.

Hepatic lesions are variable. Most livers are friable and are swollen or shrunken. The liver is pale tan or mottled red-brown in color. Hemorrhages may be present in the stomach, intestines, and bladder.

Diagnosis is based on history of iron supplementation, clinical signs, and necropsy lesions. Serum and liver iron concentrations may be normal or increased. Normal iron concentrations in horses are 66–204 mcg/dL in serum and 100–300 ppm in liver tissue. Because serum iron concentration correlates poorly with total iron stores, serum ferritin levels are better used as an estimate of total iron.

Treatment is generally supportive with fluids and nutritional supplementation. Chelation therapy with deferoxamine is unlikely to be successful in either acute iron toxicosis or chronic hemochromatosis. Repeated phlebotomy has been attempted for hemochromatosis. The prognosis is poor.

Copper Toxicosis: Acute copper toxicosis with severe hepatic necrosis and death may be seen in cattle 1–4 days after injection of copper salt. Copper toxicosis is seen in sheep and young calves after excess dietary intake of copper and in young goat kids fed calf milk replacer containing copper. The primary conditions associated with copper toxicosis are hemolytic anemia and liver damage. In camelids, ingestion of inappropriate dietary copper concentrations resulted in acute death with few premortem signs and no evidence of hemolytic crisis. (*See also* COPPER POISONING, p 3073.)

Miscellaneous Chemicals and Drugs Associated with Hepatotoxicity: Exposure to carbon tetrachloride, chlorinated hydrocarbons, hexachlorethane, carbon disulfide, arsenic, monensin, pentachlorophenols, phenol, paraquat, halothane (goats, llamas), isoflurane, phenobarbital, tannic acid, copper disodium edetate, and high doses of ivermectin may cause centrilobular necrosis and hepatic failure. Phosphorus causes primarily periportal changes. Active hepatitis to cirrhosis may be seen after use of isoniazid, nitrofuran, halothane, aspirin, or dantrolene in large animals. Erythromycin, rifampin, anabolic steroids, phenothiazine tranquilizers, some diuretics, quinidine sulfate, and diazepam have been associated with cholestasis and icterus.

Mycotoxicoses

Aflatoxins and fumonisins can cause hepatic injury and failure in ruminants, swine, and horses. Fusarium toxicosis is the most common mycotoxicosis causing liver failure in horses, whereas aflatoxins only sporadically cause hepatic failure in this species. (*See* MYCOTOXICOSES, p 3005.)

Blue-green Algae Intoxication

Acute hepatotoxicosis may be seen after ingestion of hepatotoxic cyanobacteria. (*See* ALGAL POISONING, p 2956.)

Hepatotoxic Plants

Pyrrolizidine Alkaloid Toxicity: Pyrrolizidine alkaloid toxicity most commonly is a chronic, progressive hepatopathy, but acute intoxication can occur. (*See* PYRROLIZIDINE ALKALOIDOSIS, p 3150.)

Kleingrass Toxicosis: Kleingrass (*Panicum coloratum*) can produce toxicosis in horses and ruminants. Kleingrass toxicosis is a problem in the southwestern USA from late spring to early fall. Young growing plants are most hazardous because of their high sapogenin content, believed to be the toxic principle. A similar syndrome is seen in horses in the eastern USA grazing pasture or fed hay containing high concentrations of fall *Panicum*.

Clinical signs include icterus, photosensitivity, intermittent colic and fever, weight loss, and hepatic encephalopathy. Photosensitivity may develop around the coronary band and cause lameness. Lesions include hepatic and portal fibrosis and biliary hyperplasia. Bilirubin, γ-glutamyl transpeptidase or transferase (GGT), and blood ammonia concentrations are increased. Sheep with photosensitivity caused by kleingrass ingestion commonly have a crystalline material in the bile ducts, canaliculi, and macrophages.

Presumptive diagnosis of plant-induced hepatopathy is based on history of exposure to plants and multiple affected animals on a farm or in an area. Affected animals should be removed from the kleingrass source, fed good-quality hay, and protected from sunlight. Local treatment of the photodermatitis with antimicrobial or softening creams may be needed in severe cases.

Alsike Clover Toxicosis: Alsike clover (*Trifolium hybridum*) causes two syndromes in horses in the USA and Canada: photosensitivity (trifobiasis) and Alsike clover poisoning ("big liver disease"). Alsike clover grows well on heavy clay soil, and an increased incidence of toxicosis is reported during wet seasons. The disease is seen mostly when the blossom of the plant is eaten and the predominant forage being fed is the Alsike clover. The toxic principle is an unidentified phototoxin. Photosensitivity has been reported in horses, sheep, cattle, and pigs.

Alsike photosensitivity is also known as "dew poisoning" because it is seen mostly when pastures of clover are wet and horses' skins are moist. It is characterized by reddened skin after exposure to sun, followed by dry necrosis of the skin or edema and serous discharge. The muzzle, tongue, and feet are frequently affected. If the stomatitis is severe, anorexia and weight loss develop.

Alsike clover poisoning may be fatal, with progressive loss of condition and signs of hepatic failure and neurologic disturbances. Colic, diarrhea, and other signs of GI disturbances have been noted. Affected horses may be markedly depressed or excited. Prolonged exposure is usually required before signs of hepatic insufficiency are evident. Serum chemistry alterations include increased GGT and AST activities and hyperbilirubinemia, with direct bilirubin frequently being ≥25% of the total.

Presumptive diagnosis of plant-induced hepatopathy is based on history of exposure to plants and multiple animals on a farm or in an affected area. Horses in which photosensitivity is the primary finding may recover quickly after being removed to Alsike-free pasture. Those with severe stomatitis or dermatitis require supportive care and local treatment of the stomatitis until they heal.

Mycotoxic Lupinosis: Mycotoxic lupinosis is a worldwide disease of sheep and cattle that consume lupines containing a hepatic mycotoxin produced by the fungus *Phomopsis leptostromiformis*. *See* p 3018 for clinical findings, diagnosis, and control.

***Xanthium* (Cocklebur) Toxicosis:** Cockleburs, including *Xanthium strumarium*, may be found throughout the world. Poisoning is most frequent after ingestion of the palatable two-leaf seedling stage or ground seeds. The burs are highly toxic but rarely eaten. The mature plant is less toxic and generally unpalatable. The toxic principle is carboxyatractyloside, which directly affects the liver.

Within hours of toxin ingestion, swine, cattle, and horses develop signs of depression, nausea, weakness, ataxia, and subnormal temperature. Spasms of the cervical muscles, vomiting, dyspnea, and convulsions may occur. Death may occur within hours of the onset of signs. Animals that survive initial acute poisoning frequently develop chronic liver disease.

Affected animals require intensive supportive care. Mineral oil or activated charcoal may be given orally to delay absorption of the toxic principle. Physostigmine (5–30 mg, IM) has also been recommended.

Miscellaneous Plant Hepatotoxicosis: Hepatotoxins are found in numerous plants, including *Nolina texana*, *Agave lechuguilla*, *Phyllanthus abnormis*, and *Lantana camara*. (*See* RANGE PLANTS OF TEMPERATE NORTH AMERICA, p 3103.)

CHOLELITHIASIS, CHOLEDOCHOLITHIASIS, AND HEPATOLITHIASIS

Etiology and Epidemiology: Cholelithiasis in horses may cause biliary obstruction and concurrent liver disease or may be an incidental finding at necropsy. It most commonly affects middle-aged (6–15 yr old) horses with no sex or breed predilection. Solitary or multiple calculi may be present in the common bile duct (choledocholithiasis), intrahepatic bile ducts (hepatolithiasis), or bile duct or gallbladder in ruminants (cholelithiasis). In large animals, choledocholithiasis is the most common cause of biliary obstruction, with horses more frequently affected. The cause of cholelith formation in horses is not known. Ascending biliary tract inflammation (cholangiohepatitis), intestinal bacterial infection resulting in bile stasis, and a change in bile composition or cholesterol concentration have been proposed. Choleliths formed around a foreign body or parasites may occlude the common bile duct. Cholelithiasis and hepatolithiasis reportedly are not well recognized as a clinical problem in sheep and goats. Incidence in camelids is unknown.

Clinical Findings: Clinical signs commonly seen in horses with choleliths or cholangiohepatitis include weight loss, abdominal pain, icterus, depression, and intermittent fever. Signs of hepatic failure, including encephalopathy, photosensitivity, and coagulopathy, occur less frequently. Clinical signs are often intermittent. Complete obstruction of the common bile duct often is accompanied by persistent abdominal pain. Laboratory abnormalities include hyperbilirubinemia with increased direct (conjugated) bilirubin, a marked increase in serum γ-glutamyl transpeptidase or transferase (GGT) activity, and increased serum total bile acid concentration. Sorbitol dehydrogenase (SDH) and AST activities are increased but to a lesser degree. BUN, glucose, and potassium concentrations may be decreased. Metabolic tests indicate reduced hepatic function. Activated partial thromboplastin time and one-stage prothrombin time may be prolonged. Leukocytosis, anemia of chronic disease, hyperproteinemia, hyperglobulinemia, and hyperfibrinogenemia are often present due to inflammation. Histologic changes include periportal and intralobular fibrosis, moderate bile duct dilatation and proliferation, and cholestasis. Culture of the liver may reveal a bacterial infection.

Lesions: At necropsy, the liver may be enlarged or shrunken. The liver is red to green-brown and firmer than normal. Hepatic ducts and the common bile duct are dilated and may contain one or more calculi.

Diagnosis: Cholelithiasis should be considered in horses with a history of fever, icterus, and recurrent abdominal pain. Other signs of hepatic failure (encephalopathy, photodermatitis, weight loss) are less consistently seen with cholelithiasis. A marked increase in serum GGT with hyperbilirubinemia (direct bilirubin >25%) is supportive. Increases in SDH, AST, and alkaline phosphatase are often also present, but when absent despite an increased serum GGT make the presumptive diagnosis of biliary stasis more justified. Neutrophilic leukocytosis with inconsistent increase in globulin and fibrinogen concentrations are noted on leukograms. Ultrasonographic examination may reveal hepatomegaly with increased echogenicity of the liver, thickened distended bile ducts, and hyperechoic regions suggestive of choleliths. Choleliths in horses are most often visualized in the most cranioventral portion of the right lobe of the liver, especially in the sixth to eighth intercostal spaces. Choleliths may be hyperechoic, casting an acoustic shadow, or sonolucent. Stones may be seen as discrete calculi or less discrete sludge deposits within the biliary tract. The thickened distended bile ducts may appear as dilated channels adjacent to portal veins. Because of the large lung field of horses, choleliths may be missed on ultrasound examination.

Treatment: Although biliary obstruction in horses is often fatal, choledocholithotripsy and choledocholithotomy have been performed successfully. Prognosis in cases requiring choledocholithotomy depends on the severity of concurrent cholangiohepatitis and on the size of the horse. The procedure is difficult because of limited exposure and poor visibility of the common hepatic duct. Complications include bile contamination, bile peritonitis, dehiscence, bile duct stricture, cholelith reformation, and enterocolitis (eg, stress-induced, salmonellosis). The prognosis is better if the obstruction is corrected by choledocholithotripsy.

When small calculi or less discrete sludge deposits are present, resolution by medical therapy may be successful. In addition, dissolution of bilirubinate stones, which are common in horses, may be facilitated by concurrent administration of IV dimethyl sulfoxide (<20% solution at 0.5–1 mg/kg). Dimethyl sulfoxide should be used cautiously or avoided in horses with coagulopathies or signs of hemolysis. Anti-inflammatory agents are administered to reduce inflammation and provide analgesia. Because cholangitis is often present, longterm broad-spectrum antimicrobial therapy is indicated. Antimicrobial choice is best guided by culture and sensitivity of the bacteria from a liver biopsy, bile duct aspirate, or from the cholelith. Supportive care is provided to manage any degree of accompanying hepatic insufficiency.

CHRONIC ACTIVE HEPATITIS

Chronic active hepatitis describes any progressive inflammatory process within the liver. It is a histopathologic diagnosis in which there is evidence of sustained, aggressive, chronic liver disease. The histologic diagnosis is often cholangiohepatitis, because the inflammatory response is mainly in the periportal areas.

Etiology: The exact etiology of chronic active hepatitis is not known. Infectious, immune-mediated, or toxic processes are thought to be involved. The early stages are associated with inflammation of the bile ducts and portal areas of the liver. Extension of bacterial infection through the bile duct or portal venous drainage may be responsible for the lesions in animals with suppurative cholangiohepatitis. When lymphocytes and plasma cells predominate in the cellular infiltrate, an immune-mediated process is more likely. Many causes of acute hepatic failure can progress to chronic active hepatitis.

Clinical Findings: The predominant clinical signs of chronic active hepatitis are weight loss, anorexia, depression, and lethargy. Icterus, behavioral changes, diarrhea, photosensitization, and hemorrhage are variably present. Fever may be persistent or intermittent, depending on the degree of cholangiohepatitis and fibrosis present. Dermatitis of the coronary band with regional sloughing of skin may develop. Recent or concurrent abdominal disease is often reported. Duration of clinical signs is variable, extending over days to months. Neurologic signs may seem to appear abruptly, even though there is histologic evidence of chronic disease. Alkaline phosphatase and γ-glutamyl transpeptidase or transferase (GGT) are moderately increased, as are sorbitol dehydrogenase (SDH) and glutamate dehydrogenase, which indicates ongoing hepatocyte damage. In chronic cases with marked hepatic fibrosis, enzyme activity may be normal, and BUN and albumin concentrations may be decreased. Serum total protein is either increased or normal. Globulins are usually increased. Serum total bile acid concentration is increased, and BSP® clearance prolonged. Cholestasis may cause hyperbilirubinemia, with >25% of total bilirubin being direct. With diminishing hepatic function, serum glucose and coagulation factors decrease, and one-stage prothrombin time and activated partial thromboplastin time become prolonged. Blood ammonia concentrations may be increased. There may be a neutrophilia or neutropenia with a left shift if endotoxemia develops. Anorexia can lead to hypokalemia. Ultrasonography generally reveals increased echogenicity in the liver, indicative of hepatic fibrosis. The liver may be smaller than normal, so much so it may be difficult to identify on ultrasonography.

Lesions: Grossly, the liver is firm, pale brown to green in color, and often small. Irregular markings may be seen on the cut surface. Histologic lesions are predominantly in the periportal areas. Inflammatory cell infiltration may consist primarily of mononuclear cells, neutrophils with bacteria (often coliforms), or lymphocytes and plasma cells. The character of the infiltrate may indicate the nature of the primary disease process. Biliary hyperplasia may be marked if there is cholangiohepatitis. Variable degrees of necrosis and fibrosis are present.

Diagnosis: Histologic examination of a liver biopsy is needed for a definitive diagnosis. The tissue should also be cultured, although in most cases significant isolates are not identified.

Treatment: Supportive care should be provided, including fluid therapy with potassium chloride, glucose, and vitamin supplementation; dietary management (a diet low in protein and high in branched-chain amino acids and carbohydrates); and prevention of exposure to the sun if photodermatitis is present.

Corticosteroid therapy has been used successfully in horses with a lymphocytic-plasmacytic infiltrate on liver biopsy. Reportedly, steroids act to enhance appetite, stabilize cell membranes, and reduce inflammation and connective tissue formation. Different therapeutic regimens using prednisolone and dexamethasone have been recommended. One recommended regimen involves initial administration of dexamethasone at 0.04–0.08 mg/kg for 4–7 days, followed by a gradual reduction in dosage over 2–3 wk depending on response to therapy. Prednisolone (0.5–1 mg/kg/day, PO) may be required for an additional 2–4 wk. The risk of inducing laminitis or abortion in pregnant animals with corticosteroids must be discussed with the owner before initiating therapy. Alternatively, an antifibrotic agent, colchicine (0.03 mg/kg/day, PO), has been recommended, but its efficacy in hepatic failure and safety in pregnant animals is unproved. Possible adverse reactions to colchicine in horses include laminitis, diarrhea, and rarely bone marrow suppression affecting all cell lines. Malaise, vomiting, diarrhea, abdominal pain, myopathy, alopecia, and bone marrow suppression have been reported in people and other species. Other drugs recommended for arresting or slowing fibrosis include pentoxifylline (7.5 mg/kg, PO, bid) and SAMe (5 g/day, PO). In cases complicated with septic cholangiohepatitis, broad-spectrum antimicrobials are indicated. Ideally, antimicrobial therapy should be based on bacterial culture and sensitivity from the biopsy specimen.

Prognosis: Prognosis is variable and is best based on liver biopsy and response to therapy. Prognosis is fair to good in animals with less severe lesions, especially those with a lymphocytic-plasmacytic cellular infiltrate that responds well to corticosteroid therapy; however, it is poor in horses with hepatic failure, widespread fibrosis (or severe bridging fibrosis), and disruption of normal hepatic parenchyma.

HYPERLIPEMIA AND HEPATIC LIPIDOSIS

Epidemiology and Pathogenesis: Poor feed quality or decrease in feed intake, particularly during a period of high-energy requirement (eg, pregnancy, systemic disease), may result in hyperlipemia syndrome. Hyperlipemia is seen most commonly in ponies, miniature horses, and donkeys and less frequently in standard-size adult horses. Pathogenesis of hyperlipemia is complex, with a negative energy balance triggering excessive mobilization of fatty acids from adipose tissue, leading to increased hepatic triglyceride synthesis and secretion of very-low-density lipoproteins, concomitant hypertriglyceridemia, and fatty infiltration of the liver. The biochemical etiology of hyperlipemia is overproduction of triglyceride rather than failure of triglyceride catabolism.

Onset of disease is associated with stress, decreased feed intake, fat mobilization and deposition in the liver, and overproduction of triglycerides, which may be precipitated by insulin resistance. In ponies, hyperlipemia is usually a primary disease process associated with obesity, pregnancy, lactation, stress, or transportation. Hyperlipemia may develop secondary to any systemic disease that results in anorexia and a negative energy balance. Secondary hyperlipemia is more common than primary hyperlipemia in miniature breeds. Hyperlipemia secondary to a systemic disease can be seen in horses of any age and in any condition. Female, stressed, and obese donkeys are at highest risk of developing hyperlipemia regardless of pregnancy status. Hyperlipemia is most commonly seen in winter and spring.

Alpacas and llamas may develop hyperlipemia and ketonuria in late stages of gestation or secondary to disease states. Adult camelids and even young crias are susceptible to hepatic lipidosis during disease states.

Fatty liver disease is a complex metabolic disease seen primarily in dairy cattle. *See* p 1018.

In goats, hepatic lipidosis has been associated with cobalt deficiency. Histologic lesions are consistent with those characteristic of white liver disease in sheep.

Clinical Findings: Signs of hyperlipemia are nonspecific and variable and may not relate to loss of liver function. They include lethargy, weakness, inappetence, decreased water intake, and diarrhea. Often, there is a history of prolonged anorexia, rapid weight loss, and previous obesity. Emaciation, ventral edema, colic, and trembling may be seen. Serum biochemical values and coagulation testing in miniature horses and ponies with hyperlipemia indicate that impaired hepatic function is common. Affected animals have grossly opalescent blood and lipemic plasma. The blood concentrations of all lipids are increased, especially triglycerides, nonesterified fatty acids, and very-low-density lipoproteins. Donkeys have higher plasma triglyceride concentrations than do other equids. Hypoglycemia is a common finding in ponies but not in miniature horses with hyperlipemia. Total bile acid concentration and BSP® clearance are often normal, but BSP clearance may be prolonged in some animals. Activated partial thromboplastin time and one-stage prothrombin time may be prolonged. AST and sorbitol dehydrogenase (SDH) may be normal or increased. Increased creatinine, isosthenuria, and metabolic acidosis may develop secondary to renal disease. BUN and creatinine concentrations are variable. Anorexia can lead to hypokalemia. Animals may become neutropenic with increased band neutrophils. Concurrent pancreatitis has been reported.

Prolonged increase in serum triglyceride concentrations is associated with lipid accumulation in the liver, kidneys, myocardium, and skeletal muscles, impairing function of these organs. The liver and kidneys become friable, and death may result from acute hepatic rupture.

Alpacas and llamas may develop hyperlipemia and ketonuria in late stages of gestation, during lactation, or secondary to disease states. Nonspecific clinical signs include lethargy, anorexia, and recumbency. Hypertriglyceridemia, hypercholesterolemia, increased SDH activity, metabolic acidosis, azotemia, and ketonuria may be seen. Secondary renal failure may develop. Camelids appear to be similar to both horses (hyperlipidemia) and cattle (ketosis) in their response to severe energy imbalance in late gestation. Hepatic lipidosis is the most common liver disease found in llamas and alpacas. Camelids of various ages and energy requirements are susceptible, and the pathogenesis is multifactorial. Common clinical findings include anorexia; weight loss; high concentrations of bile acids, nonesterified fatty acids, and β-hydroxybutyrate; high activities of γ-glutamyl transpeptidase or transferase (GGT) and AST; and hypoproteinemia.

Lesions: The liver and kidneys are often pale, swollen, and friable with a greasy texture. Microscopically, there is variable fat deposition within the hepatocytes and epithelium of the bile ducts. The hepatic sinusoids may appear compressed and anemic with severe fatty infiltration. Gross and microscopic lesions of the primary disease process in ponies and horses may predominate.

Diagnosis: Clinical diagnosis of hyperlipemia is often based on the signalment, history, clinical signs, and gross observation of a white to yellow discoloration of the plasma in equids. Plasma or serum triglyceride >500 mg/dL confirm the diagnosis. Cholesterol may be increased, indicating an increase in lipoprotein. Nonesterified fatty acids, very-low-density lipoproteins, and β-hydroxybutyrate (camelids) may also be increased. Laboratory evidence of hepatic dysfunction is supportive.

Treatment: Correction of the underlying disease, IV fluids, and nutritional support are the most essential factors in treatment of hyperlipemia. Nutritional support reverses the negative energy balance, increases serum glucose concentrations, promotes endogenous insulin release, and inhibits mobilization of peripheral adipose tissue. A polyionic electrolyte solution containing supplemental dextrose (50 g/hr/450 kg) and potassium (potassium chloride at 20–40 mEq/L) should be given IV to hypoglycemic, hypokalemic horses. Glucose administration may cause refractory hyperglycemia in animals with insulin resistance. Glucose concentrations, renal function, urine output, and serum electrolyte concentrations should be monitored closely. IV fluids and glucose must be administered cautiously in camelids with hepatic lipidosis, because many are already hypoproteinemic, and glucose regulation in camelids is often challenging. Intermittent bolus administration of polyionic IV fluids rather than continuous infusion may more effectively maintain hydration without exacerbating existing hypoproteinemia.

Voluntary enteral nutrition is preferred if the affected animal will consume adequate quantities of nutritionally valuable feeds; however, most will not. Frequent feedings of a high-carbohydrate, low-fat diet are preferred. In animals with inadequate oral intake, supplemental tube feeding is necessary. Commercially available high-calorie enteral formulations provide adequate short-term nutritional support. Recipes for home-prepared, liquid tube-feeding diets for horses are also available. Small frequent feedings are required to meet caloric needs without overloading the GI tract. Animals should be observed after each feeding for signs of abdominal discomfort. Body weight, total fluid intake, and fecal consistency should be monitored daily. In animals that survive, hyperlipemia usually resolves in 5–10 days, but enteral feeding should be continued until voluntary feed intake is adequate. Enteral nutritional supplementation and treatment of the primary disease often reverses hyperlipemia in miniature horses and donkeys but less frequently in ponies.

For totally anorectic horses, partial parenteral nutrition may be used. The lipid portion of the solution is omitted. Blood glucose concentration should be monitored at least twice daily to ensure that euglycemia is maintained and that substantial hyperglycemia (≥180 mg/dL) is avoided.

In camelids, partial parenteral nutrition with enteral supplementation can be used to maintain adequate energy intake and minimize further fat mobilization. Because of the distinct metabolism of camelids, parenteral nutrition products must contain higher amounts of amino acids (relative to nonprotein calories) than traditional formulations used in other species. Glucose concentrations must be carefully monitored, because camelids do not assimilate exogenous glucose well.

Exogenous insulin administration is recommended for treatment of iatrogenic hyperglycemia and hyperlipemia, especially when these conditions are resistant to more conventional therapies. Insulin decreases mobilization of peripheral adipose tissue by stimulating lipoprotein lipase activity and by inhibiting adipocyte hormone–sensitive lipase activity. The appropriate dosage of insulin to be used in horses has not been well established. When insulin is used, response to therapy, including blood glucose concentrations, must be closely monitored and the insulin dosage adjusted accordingly. Insulin administration may fail to lower serum triglyceride or glucose concentrations in hyperlipemic animals when an *insulin*-resistant state is present. Insulin treatment in camelids has reportedly been effective in treatment of hepatic lipidosis.

Heparin is used in treatment of hyperlipemia because it promotes peripheral utilization of triglycerides and enhances lipogenesis via stimulation of lipoprotein lipase activity. Heparin may be given IV or SC, with recommended dosages of 40–100 IU/kg, bid. Use of heparin is questionable in affected animals with increased hepatic production of triglycerides and without impaired peripheral removal of triglycerides. Heparin administration may potentiate bleeding complications and is contraindicated in animals with coagulopathies from liver dysfunction.

Nutritional supplementation to prevent hyperlipemia is indicated in miniature horses and donkeys, ponies, horses, and camelids with systemic disease associated with hypophagia and high metabolic demands.

Prognosis: Clinical biochemical variables are not useful prognostic indicators of survival in ponies with hyperlipemia. In most instances, survival depends on the ability to successfully treat the primary disease. Prognosis is often poor in ponies, standard-size horses, and camelids.

HEPATIC NEOPLASIA

Primary hepatic tumors are uncommon in horses and ruminants. They include hepatocellular carcinoma, cholangiocarcinoma, and rarely lymphoma, hepatoblastoma (foals, young horses, alpaca crias), and mixed hamartoma. Cholangiocarcinoma is the most common and is primarily found in middle-aged or older horses. Hepatic carcinomas arise from hepatocytes, bile ducts, or metastasis. Hepatocellular carcinomas generally are found in yearlings to young adult horses and have also been reported in llamas and goats. Adenomas or adenocarcinomas of the liver have been reported in cattle. Hepatic fibrosarcoma and bile duct carcinoma with metastasis to the lungs have been reported in goats. Erythrocytosis, large areas of extramedullary hematopoiesis, and metastasis to the thoracic cavity have been reported in horses with hepatoblastoma.

Lymphosarcoma is the most common neoplasia of the hematopoietic system in horses. As many as 37% of horses with lymphosarcoma have neoplastic involvement of the spleen, and 41% have neoplastic involvement of the liver. Metastasis of lymphosarcoma of the liver has been reported in cattle, llamas, alpacas, and goats.

The predominant clinical findings with hepatic carcinoma are lethargy and weight loss. A progressively enlarging abdomen, erythrocytosis, persistent hypoglycemia, icterus, and hepatic failure may also be seen. Cholangiocarcinoma causes pronounced weight loss before the onset of hepatic failure. Liver hepatocellular and biliary enzymes may be increased with hepatic carcinoma or cholangiocarcinoma. Serum γ-glutamyl transpeptidase or transferase (GGT) activity in affected horses is usually very high. Hepatocellular carcinomas are characteristically uniform in appearance on ultrasonographic examination.

Clinical manifestations of lymphosarcoma in horses are variable. Early in the disease, nonspecific signs such as weight loss, anorexia, and lethargy are seen. Lymphoma occasionally may diffusely infiltrate the liver and produce signs of hepatic failure, jaundice, and severe depression. Laboratory findings include hypoglycemia, mild to moderate increases in liver enzymes, hyperbilirubinemia, and abnormally low levels of IgM. Ultrasonographic examination helps to detect splenic and hepatic neoplasia. In ruminants, signs produced by tumor growth in other organs (lymph nodes, abomasum, heart, uterus, spinal cord) are often most predominant.

The presence and character of the hepatic neoplasia can be confirmed by liver biopsy and microscopic examination of the tissue. Atypical lymphocytes or lymphoblasts may be seen in peritoneal fluids and peripheral blood of some affected animals. Increased serum α-fetoprotein concentration may support hepatoblastoma; however, this is not conclusive because concentrations may also be increased with hepatocellular carcinoma.

MISCELLANEOUS HEPATIC DISORDERS

Cholangitis

Diseases of the gallbladder are rare in ruminants. Obstruction may be associated with liver fluke infestation, foreign bodies, abscesses, neoplasia, suppurative cholecystitis, or abdominal fat necrosis. Rupture of the gallbladder has been reported in a cow. Cholangitis (inflammation of the biliary system) has been reported in horses with chronic active liver disease. Mild behavior changes, weight loss, variable colic, icterus, and alterations in hepatic enzyme activity may be seen in affected horses. Treatment consists of longterm antimicrobial and supportive therapy as indicated.

Hepatic Failure in Foals

Hepatic failure in neonatal foals may follow septicemia (especially *Actinobacillus equuli*), endotoxemia, perinatal asphyxia, *Leptospira* Pomona infection, equine herpesvirus 1, hepatic duct obstruction secondary to gastroduodenal obstruction, biliary atresia, and iron toxicity. Gastric ulcers and duodenitis in foals can cause strictures of the duodenum and subsequent cholangiohepatitis due to bile stasis. Neonatal isoerythrolysis and hemolysis may cause hypoxic and cholestatic hepatic disease. Administration of total parenteral nutrition may cause cholestasis and concurrent hepatic disease.

Biliary Atresia

Biliary atresia (extrahepatic) has been reported in foals and in a neonatal lamb. Affected foals presented for anorexia, depression, lethargy, poor growth, colic, polydipsia, polyuria, pyrexia, and icterus at 1 mo of age. Markedly increased serum γ-glutamyl transpeptidase or transferase (GGT) and bilirubin with mildly increased sorbitol dehydrogenase (SDH) supported a diagnosis of biliary obstruction. Diagnosis of biliary atresia was confirmed at necropsy.

Hemochromatosis

Hemochromatosis is an iron storage disease in which hemosiderin is deposited in the parenchymal cells, causing damage and dysfunction of the liver and other tissues. The disease is either primary (idiopathic) or secondary. It is reported in people, Mynah birds, Salers cattle, and horses.

Etiology: In Salers cattle, the condition appears to be a homozygous recessive condition with inappropriate intestinal absorption of iron, excessive hepatic storage, and eventual loss of hepatic function. In horses, there is no evidence of a familial tendency or of excessive iron being consumed in the diet. Rather, it appears there is cirrhosis of the liver with secondary iron overload. In horses and cattle, increased iron is deposited in the liver.

Clinical Findings and Lesions: In horses, primary clinical signs are weight loss, lethargy, and intermittent anorexia. In cattle, signs include decreased weight gain, poor body condition, dull hair coat, and diarrhea. In both species, serum liver enzyme concentrations, including GGT, alkaline phosphatase, AST, and SDH, are increased. Serum total bile acid concentrations are increased in horses, and serum iron, total iron binding capacity (TIBC), and percent saturation of the TIBC are usually normal. In some cases, serum iron and ferritin may be increased, but TIBC is not saturated. In cattle, total serum iron, TIBC, and saturation of transferrin are increased. Iron content of the liver tissue is greatly increased in horses (normal 100–300 ppm) and cattle (normal 84–100 ppm). Hepatomegaly and hemosiderin accumulation in the liver, lymph nodes, pancreas, spleen, thyroid, kidney, brain, and glandular tissue are typically present.

Diagnosis: Diagnosis is based on history, clinical signs, and laboratory findings. Finding abundant hemosiderin in the hepatocytes on histopathologic examination of a liver biopsy supports the diagnosis. High liver iron concentrations in animals with no history of excess iron intake help confirm the diagnosis. Differential diagnoses include iron toxicosis from exogenous sources and diseases causing chronic weight loss and hepatic dysfunction or disease.

Treatment: Phlebotomies to remove blood and reduce the iron stores have been used in treatment of people with hemochromatosis. Similar treatment in horses and cattle has been unsuccessful. Deferoxamine is also used in people to induce a negative ion balance and reduce the rate at which iron accumulates. The effect in cattle and horses has not been evaluated.

Right Hepatic Lobe Atrophy in Horses

The right lobe of the liver is the largest lobe in young horses but frequently atrophies in older animals and becomes fibrous. Right hepatic lobe atrophy was previously considered an incidental postmortem finding, but some consider it to be a pathologic condition.

Right hepatic lobe atrophy has been proposed to result from chronic compression of this portion of the liver by the right dorsal colon and base of the cecum. Feeding horses high-concentrate, low-fiber diets may contribute to atony of the right dorsal colon with resultant distention; this compresses the right hepatic lobe against the visceral surface of the diaphragm. Although there is no morphologic evidence of direct vascular impairment to the right hepatic lobe, vascular compromise may result secondary to compression. With chronicity, the portal circulation to the right lobe is impaired, resulting in hepatic anoxia, deprivation of nutrients, and gradual atrophy of the right lobe of the liver. No evidence of biliary tract disease has been noted. Colic may be seen. Some horses may have signs not related to the GI tract.

Hepatic Lobe Torsion

Hepatic lobe torsion can cause colic in horses. Liver enzymes and fibrinogen are increased, but abdominal fluid analysis is variable. Bacteria, including *Clostridium* spp, may be found in the necrotic portion of liver. Exploratory celiotomy may be required for diagnosis.

Hepatic Amyloidosis

Amyloidosis refers to disease characterized by the extracellular deposition of amyloid, a proteinaceous fibril substance, in the tissue. Deposition of amyloid within an organ distorts normal tissue architecture and possibly function. In horses, the liver and spleen are the most common organs affected by systemic amyloidosis. Reactive or secondary systemic amyloidosis with deposition of amyloid A (AA) fibrils in the liver has been associated with severe parasitism and chronic infection or inflammation in horses. (*See also* AMYLOIDOSES, p 592.)

Congenital Hepatic Fibrosis

In a retrospective study of the records from the University of Berne, Institute of Animal Pathology, 30 Swiss Freiberger foals with pathologic lesions compatible with congenital hepatic fibrosis were identified. Affected foals were 1–12 mo old (average 3.7 mo). Most showed signs and had clinicopathologic changes reflecting severe liver damage. Pedigree analysis traced the disease back to one stallion. Results suggest that congenital hepatic fibrosis in Swiss Freiberger horses is a recessively inherited autosomal genetic defect. A similar condition has been reported in a calf.

Primary Hyperammonemia of Adult Horses

In this syndrome of hyperammonemia, blindness and severe neurologic signs are seen in adult horses. The etiology is unknown, but a primary intestinal problem with overgrowth of urease-producing bacteria within the intestine is suspected.

The syndrome is nearly always associated with enteric disease, diarrhea, or colic. Diarrhea and, in some cases, protein-losing enteropathy may persist for several days. In most cases, diarrhea or colic precedes the neurologic signs by 24–48 hr. Laboratory abnormalities include increased blood ammonia concentrations (200–400 mcmol/L), severe metabolic acidosis, low plasma bicarbonate (≤12 mEq/L) concentration, and profound hyperglycemia (250–400 mg/dL). Serum concentrations of liver enzymes, total bile acids, and bilirubin are normal.

In most horses, neurologic signs resolve within 2–3 days with supportive treatment (IV fluids, potassium chloride, glucose, sodium bicarbonate) and administration of drugs to reduce ammonia absorption (lactulose, neomycin).

Portosystemic Shunts

Portosystemic shunts are seen in foals and calves. Hyperammonemia and neurologic signs result from liver dysfunction with little laboratory or microscopic evidence of liver disease.

Clinical Findings and Lesions: Clinical signs are first seen when affected foals are ~2 mo old and start to ingest larger amounts of grain and forage. Neurologic signs include staggering, wandering, blindness, circling, and seizures. Poor growth and intermittent neurologic signs (ataxia, weakness, depression, bruxism, tenesmus) have been reported in affected 2- to 3-mo-old calves. Serum concentrations of hepatic enzymes are often normal. Blood ammonia and total bile acid concentration are increased, and BSP® clearance is prolonged.

The liver is often small, with a smooth surface, and normal in color and texture. Microscopically, the hepatocytes are small. Portal veins in the triads may be small or absent. Hepatic arteries are often prominent and multiple.

Diagnosis: A portosystemic shunt should be suspected in foals or calves exhibiting repeated episodes of cerebral signs without obvious reasons. Signs may be most pronounced and associated with feedings. Catheterizing the mesenteric vein and performing a portogram or nuclear scintigraphy can confirm and locate the shunt. In some cases, the shunt may be seen on ultrasonographic examination of the liver.

Treatment: Surgical repair may be attempted in animals in which the site of the shunt can be identified, but the prognosis is guarded. Clinical signs in some foals may be controlled by restricting protein intake and by careful dietary management. Neomycin or lactulose are given orally to decrease ammonia production within the bowel. Supportive care with polyionic fluids, potassium, and dextrose may be needed to help decrease neurologic signs.

Hyperammonemia of Morgan Foals

A syndrome of depression, ill thrift, and hyperammonemia with a variable degree of hepatic involvement is seen in Morgan foals. Affected foals have been related, but the cause of the syndrome is undetermined. Clinical signs are usually first seen around weaning time. Encephalopathy may temporarily improve with aggressive supportive therapy but recurs after withdrawal of treatment. Liver enzymes and blood ammonia concentrations are increased. Bilirubin concentration is often normal. Pathologic hepatic lesions include portal and bridging fibrosis, bile duct hyperplasia, karyomegaly, and cytomegaly. The disease is fatal.

HYPERBILIRUBINEMIA SYNDROMES

Gilbert Syndrome

Gilbert syndrome is a congenital hyperbilirubinemia seen in people (inherited as an autosomal dominant trait) and in Southdown sheep. It is an unconjugated hyperbilirubinemia in the presence of normal erythrocyte life span. A defect in carrier proteins or conjugating enzyme is suspected. Affected Southdown sheep have increased conjugated and unconjugated plasma bilirubin concentrations. Hepatic bilirubin clearance is defective, and affected sheep cannot excrete BSP® into the bile. Icterus is variable. Histopathologic lesions are absent except for pigment in the hepatocytes.

Dubin-Johnson Syndrome

Dubin-Johnson syndrome is seen sporadically in people and Corriedale sheep. It is a failure of conjugated bilirubin to enter the bile canaliculi. Excretion of bilirubin and other conjugated organic anions may be impaired. Affected sheep may be icteric or hyperbilirubinemic. Serum conjugated and unconjugated bilirubin concentrations are increased, and BSP® clearance and bile acid excretion may be delayed in affected Corriedale sheep. Histologically, the hepatocytes contain a black, melanin-like pigment.

LIVER ABSCESSES IN CATTLE

Liver abscesses are seen in all ages and breeds of cattle wherever cattle are raised. They are most common in feedlot and dairy cattle fed rations that predispose to rumenitis. Cattle with liver abscesses have reduced production efficiency. Affected livers are condemned at slaughter, and adhesions to surrounding organs or the diaphragm may necessitate carcass trimming. Liver abscesses can also lead to disease syndromes associated with posterior vena caval thrombosis.

Etiology and Pathogenesis: *Fusobacterium necrophorum*, a gram-negative, obligate anaerobic bacterium, and a component of normal rumen microflora, is the primary etiologic agent. Infection in the liver usually originates from a necrobacillary rumenitis. Two biovars have been implicated. Biovar A (*F necrophorum necrophorum*), the more virulent, is the predominant biovar in the rumen microflora and is isolated, usually in pure culture, from most cases of liver abscessation. Biovar B (*F necrophorum funduliforme*) is commonly isolated from microabscesses in the rumen wall but is less commonly isolated from liver abscesses, in which it is always found in mixed culture with biovar A or other bacterial species. *Trueperella pyogenes*, streptococci, staphylococci, and *Bacteroides* spp are most frequently recovered from mixed cultures.

Rumenitis is usually the result of rapid intraruminal fermentation of dietary carbohydrate with subsequent production of lactic acid and increased acidity of the ruminal fluid ("grain overload"). Rations with high levels of carbohydrate are the principal cause in both dairy and feedlot cattle, but the texture of the feed and method of feeding can be modifying factors. The incidence of rumenitis in feedlot cattle is significantly higher when the cattle are transferred directly from a roughage ration to a finishing ration, and when there is poor feed bunk management. *F necrophorum*, alone or with other bacteria, colonizes through the area of superficial necrosis produced by the acid rumen contents. Leukotoxin may facilitate resistance to phagocytosis. Bacterial emboli from the lesions invade the hepatic portal venous system and are transported to the liver, where they can establish infectious foci of necrobacillosis that eventually develop into abscesses.

Other sources of infection in liver abscesses include foreign body penetration from the reticulum, direct extension of infection from omphalophlebitis in neonatal calves, and bacteremic diseases.

Clinical Findings, Lesions, and Diagnosis: Cattle with liver abscesses seldom exhibit clinical signs. Detailed clinical examination may show periodic fever, inappetence, and evidence of pain when pressure is applied to the xiphisternum and posterior rib cage on the right side. Grunting and other signs of pain may occur with movement or when the animal lies down. An episodic drop in milk production occurs in dairy cattle. Clinical signs of omphalophlebitis are commonly present when there is liver abscessation resulting from extension of omphalophlebitis. Acute-phase proteins are increased early in the course of the disease, and serum sialic acid concentrations have been used for antemortem diagnosis. When there are several abscesses or a large abscess, leukocytosis with neutrophilia and increased fibrinogen levels develop, and serum globulin concentrations may increase. Ultrasonography is an aid to diagnosis, but abscesses in the left side of the liver may not be visualized. Feedlot cattle with abscessed livers have reduced feed efficiency, and those with severely abscessed livers gain 5%–15% less per day than cattle without abscesses. Most liver abscesses are occult lesions that regress to a sterile scar. Untoward sequelae include peritonitis after abscess rupture into the peritoneal cavity, and sudden death from an anaphylactic or toxic reaction when there is rupture of an abscess into hepatic blood vessels. Rupture into hepatic veins can also lead to thrombophlebitis of the posterior vena cava with thromboembolic disease, endocarditis, pulmonary thromboembolism, multiple pulmonary abscesses, and chronic suppurative pneumonia. Aneurysms of the pulmonary artery consequent to pulmonary thromboembolism may rupture into airways to result in hemoptysis, epistaxis, and death. Caudal vena caval thrombosis may also lead to portal hypertension with a resulting syndrome of hepatomegaly, ascites, and diarrhea.

The ruminal lesions are characterized by a marked inflammatory reaction and necrosis. Occasionally, abscesses are found in the deeper layers of the rumen wall. Hepatic necrobacillosis lesions of <6 days duration are pale yellow and spherical with irregular outlines; they are characterized by coagulation necrosis of the hepatocytes with a surrounding intense zone of hyperemia and inflammation. Older abscesses have a core that is progressively encapsulated by fibrous connective tissue. Abscesses are usually 4–6 cm in diameter. Affected livers usually have 3–10 abscesses but may have up to 100.

Liver condemnation rates as high as 40% were recorded in a large survey of cattle slaughtered in the USA. Culture is seldom done to confirm the diagnosis. Occasionally, liver abscesses due to *F necrophorum* must be distinguished from those resulting from traumatic reticuloperitonitis (*see* p 230).

Treatment and Control: Tylosin phosphate fed at 10 g/ton of feed significantly reduces the number of liver abscesses and increases feed efficiency and weight gain but has little, if any, effect on prevalence of ruminal lesions. Virginiamycin fed at 16 g/ton of feed or chlortetracycline fed continually at 70 mg/head/day during the finishing period is also used. With dairy cattle, percutaneous drainage and longterm therapy with procaine penicillin G (22,000 IU/kg) can be attempted, but the prognosis is poor. A vaccine consisting of the leukotoxoid of *F necrophorum* combined with a bacterin of *T pyogenes*, given when cattle enter the feedlot, reduces abscess incidence and severity.

The primary control is by managing ruminal acidosis through the method of feeding, diet composition, diligent feed bunk management, and use of buffers in the diet. Fewer ruminal lesions develop when the ratio of concentrate to roughage is decreased and when the transition period from a roughage to a finishing ration is lengthened. Increased roughage in the ration and multiple daily feedings increase the time of mastication and saliva flow; this increases buffer to the rumen and provides a continuous and uniform fermentation that reduces intraruminal acidity, which in turn lowers the number of ruminal lesions and, indirectly, the number of liver abscesses.

MALASSIMILATION SYNDROMES IN LARGE ANIMALS

Malassimilation is a decreased ability of the GI tract to incorporate nutrients into the body, either due to maldigestion or malabsorption. Maldigestion is the failure of adequate degradation of dietary constituents within the GI tract, which is required to facilitate absorption due to defects in pancreatic exocrine function, bile acid content, or brush border enzymes. Malabsorption is the failure of passage of nutrients from the intestinal lumen into the bloodstream. Some disease processes involve both maldigestion and malabsorption, such as is seen in young animals with lactase deficiency. Maldigestion alone is an infrequent cause of malassimilation in large animals. In horses, diseases causing malabsorption are much more common than diseases causing maldigestion. In cattle, small ruminants, and camelids, the forestomach bacteria and protozoa contribute to nutrient degradation, which makes maldigestion a very rare condition.

Etiology and Pathogenesis: Maldigestion syndromes are uncommon and poorly understood in large animals. They may be due to alterations in gastric function or activity of rumen microflora, abnormal bacterial proliferation in the small intestine, or a decrease or lack of small-intestinal brush border enzyme activity (eg, lactase deficiency). Less likely causes include drug-induced alteration in secretion or excretion of bile salts, or deficiency or inactivation of pancreatic lipase. Changes in bile salt concentration may not impair digestion in adult herbivores but may exacerbate diarrhea in milk-fed neonates. Surgical resection or bypass of the distal small intestine may facilitate bacterial overgrowth with associated bile salt abnormalities.

Lactose is a disaccharide composed of glucose and galactose. The enzyme lactase, which catalyzes the degradation of lactose into its components, is localized in the small-intestinal brush border of foals and calves. The degradation is necessary to facilitate absorption. Primary lactase deficiency is inherited as an autosomal recessive trait in people, but its occurrence and mode of inheritance in large animals is poorly documented. Acquired or secondary lactase deficiency seems to be more common in large animals. It is seen in foals, calves, and crias as a result of intestinal mucosal changes induced by viral, protozoal, and bacterial enteritis. Sloughing of the small-intestinal epithelial cells, loss of villous tips, and loss of some or all of the crypt cells result in some degree of lactase deficiency because of loss of lactase-secreting epithelial cells. Morphologic changes may include partial villous atrophy, crypt hyperplasia, and infiltration of the lamina propria. Osmotic diarrhea in lactase-deficient foals and calves occurs due to increased undigested/unabsorbed nutrients entering the caudal intestinal parts, subsequently increasing bacterial fermentation, concentration of osmotically active particles, and retention of water and electrolytes in the intestine.

A number of diseases may induce a malabsorption syndrome by altering the normal absorptive mechanisms of the small intestine. Malabsorption is commonly seen in animals with GI disease. It may arise from structural or functional disorders of the small intestine or have a multifactorial etiopathogenesis. Malabsorption is often seen concurrently with enteric protein loss. Either may cause loss of nutrients in the feces and subsequent weight loss. Malabsorption is not synonymous with diarrhea in any species, although diarrhea may be a common clinical feature. Function of the large intestine may be secondarily altered because of changes in the small intestine. Transient diarrhea may occur as abnormal quantities of carbohydrates, protein, fatty acids, and bile acids enter the large intestine in the ileal effluent. These substances can directly or indirectly enhance intestinal secretion or decrease absorption rates. Malabsorption of nutrients may result from insufficient absorptive surface area, an intrinsic defect in the mucosal or submucosal morphology of the intestinal wall, or obstruction of blood and lymphatic vessels. Rotavirus infection in younger animals may cause destruction of intestinal villous epithelial cells, which results in maldigestion due to decreased activity of brush border disaccharidase enzymes and in malabsorption due to decreased absorptive surface area. Coronavirus and cryptosporidia may have similar effects. A decreased absorptive surface area can also result from small-intestinal resection (short-bowel syndrome) or from villous atrophy due to granulomatous enteritis. Local infiltrative or inflammatory disease, edema, or lymphatic obstruction (granulomatous enteritis, lymphosarcoma) secondary to local or systemic causes may interfere with the ability of the intestinal wall to absorb nutrients. Inefficient absorption also may develop due to increased mucosal permeability caused by cellular damage. Metabolic abnormalities may alter the epithelial cells and decrease the available energy for active transport and maintenance of the carrier proteins or brush border enzymes. Congenital deficiencies of enzymes normally present on the microvilli are not well recognized in large, domestic animals. However, neonates and ruminants have low levels of maltase, and ruminants especially lack sucrase. In most mammalian species, lactase activity declines with age.

In **horses**, malabsorption is commonly caused by the following: 1) inflammatory or infiltrative disorders—diffuse lymphosarcoma of the small intestine (alimentary lymphoma); enteritis due to eosinophilic, lymphocytic-plasmacytic, or basophilic infiltrate; multisystemic eosinophilic epitheliotropic enterocolitis; granulomatous enteritis (inflammatory bowel disease); *Lawsonia intracellularis* (weanling foals, yearlings); intestinal ischemia and damage due to migration of *Strongylus vulgaris* larvae, small strongyles, or *Strongyloides westeri* (foals) infection; cryptosporidia; postinfarction inflammation; amyloid-associated gastroenteropathy; multiple abscessation in the bowel; tuberculosis; histoplasmosis; intestinal *Rhodococcus equi* infection; invasive enterocolitis (*Salmonella* spp); 2) biochemical or genetic abnormalities—congenital or acquired lactase deficiency (lactose intolerance), dietary-induced enteropathy, monosaccharide transport defect, pancreatic exocrine insufficiencies; 3) diseases causing inadequate absorptive area—villous damage or atrophy due to viral infection (rotavirus, coronavirus) or bacterial enteritides in foals, cryptosporidiosis, intestinal resection; 4) cardiovascular disorders—congestive heart failure, intestinal ischemia; 5) lymphatic obstruction—lymphosarcoma, mesenteric lymphadenopathy, intestinal lymphangiectasia, abscessation, thoracic duct obstruction; and 6) miscellaneous—drug-induced, heavy metal toxicosis, zinc deficiency.

In **cattle**, malabsorption syndromes are less frequently documented but likely are seen most often in calves with diarrhea. Diseases that cause malabsorption syndromes in ruminants include diarrhea caused by viruses, bacteria, or protozoa in calves and young stock. These inflammatory changes often result in maldigestion and malabsorption. Another major group of cattle suffering from malabsorption syndrome is older cattle with *Mycobacterium avium* subsp *paratuberculosis* infection (Johne's disease). Rare underlying reasons for malabsorption in ruminants are local or generalized ischemia, protein malnutrition, congestive heart failure, lymphatic obstruction, parasitism (eg, trichostrongylosis of sheep and cattle), or tuberculosis. Oral antibiotics may cause an imbalance in GI tract flora and interfere with digestion and intestinal absorption of nutrients. Treatment with high doses of ampicillin, neomycin, or tetracycline significantly decreases and delays glucose absorption during oral glucose tolerance tests in calves.

New World camelids can be affected by most conditions that cause malabsorption syndrome in ruminants. Virus-caused diarrhea (coronavirus) is particularly a problem in young crias. Intestinal protozoa infection (eg, *Eimeria macusaniensis*) may result in weight loss and hypoproteinemia due to malabsorption during either the prepatent or patent phase of infection. Severe debilitation caused by coccidiosis is typically seen in young animals; however, chronic malabsorption caused by chronic enteritis can also be found in adult llamas and alpacas, which typically shed high numbers of the pathogen.

In **swine**, malabsorption is poorly documented; however, proliferative enteropathy (*L intracellularis*) can result in malabsorption. In piglets, an amylase deficiency may result in starch malabsorption during the immediate postweaning period. Diarrhea of other origin (eg, *Escherichia coli*) may cause malabsorption syndrome in piglets.

Clinical Findings: Clinical signs of malassimilation syndrome are variable, depending on the underlying disease condition and the presence or absence of concurrent protein-losing enteropathy. Malassimilation syndromes frequently result in a negative energy balance, and subsequently in weight loss, muscle wasting, and possibly low serum protein concentrations. Therefore, chronic weight loss or reduced growth rate is a typical clinical sign.

Appetite of affected animals may be normal, increased, or decreased and is, therefore, not very helpful as a diagnostic parameter. Polyphagia may be seen due to insufficient nutrient absorption to stimulate the satiety centers. In small-intestinal malabsorption, decreased feed intake or anorexia is present more commonly, because the primary disease process causes loss of appetite.

Feces are frequently normal in consistency and volume. Diarrhea may be present but is not a consistent feature. In adult animals, small-intestinal disease must be rather extensive before diarrhea develops, because the colon can compensate and absorb the increased fluid load. This is especially the case in llamas and alpacas. In adult horses and ruminants, diarrhea indicates involvement of the large intestine. In young animals in which colonic function is not yet fully developed, diarrhea is seen with small-intestinal and large-intestinal disease.

Clinical signs of malassimilation may also include exercise intolerance, lethargic attitude, and variable thirst. Vital signs are usually normal until late in the disease. Pyrexia may be seen with inflammatory and neoplastic conditions. Abdominal pain may result from bowel inflammation, mesenteric or mural abscesses or adhesions, or partial obstruction. Ascites, dependent edema, and weakness may develop later in the disease process, especially if enteric protein loss is present. Skin and ocular lesions, vasculitis, arthritis, hepatitis, and renal disease may indicate immunologic reactions, particularly with inflammatory bowel disease. Skin lesions seen with malabsorption-related dermatosis include a thin hair coat, patchy alopecia, and focal areas of scaling and crusting that are often symmetrically distributed.

Foals and calves with lactose intolerance commonly show diarrhea, poor growth rate, and an unthrifty appearance. Some may experience flatulence, mild abdominal discomfort, or bloating after intake of milk. In young animals with acquired lactase deficiency, clinical signs (eg, diarrhea, dehydration, weight loss) and clinicopathologic alterations (eg, acidosis, hypoglycemia. and electrolyte abnormalities) are indistinguishable from those of the primary enteropathy. The condition of the animal may improve quickly, and diarrhea may resolve when milk is withdrawn.

Lesions: The carcass is thin to emaciated, depending on the duration and severity of the malassimilation disease. Specific lesions depend on the primary underlying disease process. Overt signs of malabsorption do not always correlate with gross and histopathologic changes, emphasizing the importance of functional disorders.

Diagnosis: Small-intestinal malabsorption cannot be determined by clinical examination or by routine laboratory data. However, clinical examination may lead to a presumptive diagnosis after more common causes of weight loss have been excluded. Determination of the primary underlying pathologic process is necessary to establish an appropriate treatment regimen and prognosis.

A complete history should focus on duration of condition, precipitating factors, nutritional history, deworming and routine health care program, previous or concurrent diseases, as well as the number, age, and proximity of other affected animals. A thorough physical examination is performed to correlate physical findings with clinical signs and history. In adult horses and cattle, rectal palpation is performed to determine the presence of intra-abdominal masses, enlarged lymph nodes, adhesions, abnormal positioning or thickening of bowel segments, or abnormalities in the cranial mesenteric artery. The kidneys, bladder, and related structures should also be evaluated.

A CBC and serum biochemical parameters (eg, total protein, albumin, fibrinogen, glucose, cholesterol, bilirubin, ketones, fatty acids, CK, AST, glutamate lactate dehydrogenase) help determine general health status of the animal; presence of inflammation or an infectious process; involvement of body systems; and metabolic, electrolyte, and serum protein status. Urinalysis, abdominocentesis, and fecal examination for parasite ova, larvae, protozoa, and occult blood should also be performed to exclude more common causes of weight loss. Additionally, urinalysis should be performed to assess whether glucose or protein is being excreted via urine, which could be a further cause for chronic weight loss.

Evaluation of plasma protein electrophoresis, fecal pH, bacteriologic culture, and immunologic studies may be indicated. Intracolonic fermentation of malabsorbed carbohydrates will often reduce the fecal pH in foals and calves. Protein-losing enteropathy can be diagnosed presumptively by excluding other causes of protein loss, such as renal disease or loss into a third space (peritoneum, pleural space), and by excluding the possibility of decreased albumin production due to another condition such as liver disease. Standard and contrast radiography of the bowel may be feasible in foals and small ponies, calves, and New World camelids. Abdominal ultrasonography is a useful diagnostic tool to determine bowel-wall thickness and intestinal motility, as well as the presence of excess fluid in the abdominal cavity, masses, adhesions, abnormal positioning of bowel in the abdominal cavity, and vascular lesions in the cranial mesenteric artery.

When malassimilation is suspected, a carbohydrate absorption test may be performed to assess small-intestinal function. In horses, a gastroscopy to diagnose lesions in the stomach (eg, granulomas, tumor, ulcers) and duodenum or retention of ingesta should be accomplished before absorption tests are performed. For absorption tests, the intestinal disorder must be diffuse and/or must affect the delivery to and transit through the small intestine to be diagnostic. An abnormal or flattened absorption curve is suggestive of small-intestinal dysfunction. However, a flattened absorption curve can also be caused by other conditions. Although absorption tests may indicate the presence of malassimilation, an etiologic diagnosis requires a biopsy of intestinal mucosa and possibly lymph node. In some cases, rectal biopsy may reveal focal or diffuse inflammatory infiltration. Bacteriologic culture of the feces, biopsy samples, and fecal examination for leukocytes and epithelial cells may confirm the presence of salmonellae or other invasive organisms. In some cases, laparoscopy or exploratory celiotomy is required to obtain the intestinal or lymph node biopsies. Surgery may not be advisable in a debilitated animal, because wound healing is poor and dehiscence is a potential problem. If undertaken, intestinal and lymph node biopsies should be obtained for culture, histopathology, enzymology, and immunology. Because of the risk and cost of obtaining appropriate tissue samples, malassimilation syndrome is often presumptively diagnosed with the aid of absorption tests.

Clinically applicable absorption tests include D-glucose and D-xylose. These tests may help assess small-intestinal function in preruminant calves, foals, crias, and mature horses. Indications for an oral D-xylose absorption test in foals, calves, and possibly crias include persistent diarrhea not attributable to infectious agents, poor growth despite normal intake, and other signs of maldigestion (repeated episodes of gas colic, bloating, ileus). In monogastric animals, the test solution is administered into the stomach. In ruminants and New World camelids, the forestomachs must be bypassed (esophageal groove, abomasocentesis), because otherwise the sugars are metabolized by the forestomach flora; however, oral carbohydrate tolerance studies are not frequently used in ruminants. The D-glucose absorption test has the advantages of being easy and inexpensive, and methods to determine blood glucose concentrations are available in most clinical laboratories. The main disadvantage is that results are not only a function of intestinal absorption, but also are strongly influenced by the intensive cellular uptake and metabolism of glucose after it has been absorbed. The D-xylose absorption test more directly measures intestinal absorptive capacity and is not influenced by endogenous factors and intestinal enzymatic activity, respectively. Disadvantages are that D-xylose is more expensive, and availability of commercial laboratories that perform plasma xylose determinations is limited. However, D-xylose concentrations can be measured using classic photometric techniques, which do not require special equipment and can be performed in a clinical laboratory.

Glucose or galactose may inhibit the absorption of D-xylose; therefore, fasting is necessary before the test is performed in horses and preruminant calves. The protocols of both tests require prolonged fasting, which may be deleterious to sick young foals and calves. The results of both tests are also affected by gastric emptying rate (D-xylose has also been used to estimate abomasal emptying rate in cattle), small-intestinal transit time, diet, and length of fasting period before testing. The shape of the absorption curve is influenced by renal clearance, hypoxia, anemia, systemic and intestinal bacterial infections, and IgG concentrations in foals. The age of the animals also affects absorption and digestion of glucose, lactose, and D-xylose. Therefore, the control animals must be within a few days of age of the affected animal if reference ranges are not available for its age group.

A delayed peak in the absorption curve of both the D-glucose and D-xylose test may result from delayed gastric emptying resulting from hypertonicity of the glucose or xylose solution, excitement, pain, retained gastric contents, changes in GI transit time and motility, or partial obstruction. Further sedation of the animal decreases GI motility and secondarily the absorption. A flat absorption curve may be also seen in animals with normal absorptive capacity due to a transient decrease in intestinal blood flow or to bacteria in the lumen of the small intestine metabolizing the test sugar. The test substance rapidly equilibrates with many body fluids (eg, ascites), which lowers the blood concentration of xylose and may result in a flat curve.

D-Xylose Absorption Test: D-xylose is a pentose also known as wood sugar; only trace amounts are found in feedstuffs of plant origin. The D-xylose absorption test measures absorptive capacity of the small-intestinal mucosa because functional enterocytes actively transport D-xylose across the mucosa and into the bloodstream. Subnormal absorption supports a diagnosis of malabsorption. Age and diet also affect D-xylose absorption in healthy horses. Foals <3 mo old have a higher peak concentration of D-xylose after administration than adults. Adult horses maintained on a high-roughage, low-energy diet have a higher peak concentration of D-xylose after administration than those fed a high-energy diet. Food deprivation can alter D-xylose absorption in horses without overt GI tract disease, which must be considered when interpreting results in horses that are anorectic regardless of cause.

D-Xylose (0.5–1 g/kg in a 10% solution) is administered via nasogastric tube to a horse that has been fasted overnight (18–24 hr). Heparinized venous blood samples are collected before D-xylose administration (time 0) and at 30-min intervals afterward for 4 hr (±6 hr sample). Expected peak values (20–25 mg/dL) should occur between 60 and 120 min after dosing. The normal curve should have a bell shape or inverted V shape with a definable peak plasma xylose concentration 1–2 hr after administration. Peak absolute plasma values should be ≥15 mg/dL above baseline values in healthy horses. In adult cattle the D-xylose (0.5 g/kg in a 50% solution) must be administered by abomasocentesis to bypass the rumen. Similar to that in horses, the curve is almost bell shaped in high-yielding dairy cattle; peak values of 1.1–1.3 mmol/L (16–20 mg/dL) occur ~90 min after the solution is administered.

D-Glucose Absorption Test: Glucose absorption curves are steeper in pasture-fed horses than in those fed a higher energy ration. Lower peak values are seen in horses on a high-concentrate ration. The length of the pretest fast influences the absorption curve. Prolonged fasting may delay or decrease peak glucose concentration, thus giving a false-positive result. In two studies, >90% of adult horses with evidence of "total" glucose malabsorption had severe infiltrative lesions of the small intestine. The majority of horses (18/25) classified with "partial" glucose malabsorption also had obvious pathologic abnormalities of the small intestine.

Performance of the D-glucose absorption test is similar to that of the D-xylose absorption test except samples are collected into sodium fluoride tubes. In healthy horses, blood glucose concentrations should peak 90–120 min after administration. This peak should be >85% above the resting glucose level. Reportedly complete malabsorption is defined as a peak <15% above resting concentrations; partial malabsorption is defined as a peak 15%–85% above resting levels. One of the major disadvantages to the oral glucose absorption test is that when using the conventional protocol sampling is over a 6-hr period. One reported modified protocol requires only two test samples at 0 and 120 min after administration. This modification reportedly did not affect the reliability of the test result.

Oral Lactose Tolerance Test: Diagnosis of acquired lactase deficiency is usually presumptive based on history, clinical signs, and confirmation of presence of associated pathogens. Definitive diagnosis can be achieved with an oral lactose tolerance test. Lactose is hydrolyzed within the brush border of the small-intestinal enterocytes by lactase to constituent D-glucose and galactose before these monosaccharides can be absorbed. Oral lactose tolerance testing is directed specifically at assessing whether lactase activity is present. Adult horses (>3 yr old) are lactose intolerant, and the test is unsuitable for adult ruminants and adult New World camelids. The oral lactose tolerance test is of value in evaluating young foals and preruminant calves with diarrhea or poor growth. Lactose intolerance has been documented in foals, calves, and kids.

An oral lactose tolerance test does not distinguish maldigestion from malabsorption and requires fasting for several hours. Feeding enzymatically treated milk (lactose-free milk) to animals suspected of being lactose intolerant may be tried before subjecting animals to the lengthy fast (12–18 hr) required before this test is performed. Before performing an oral lactose intolerance test, grain and hay should be withheld for 18 hr. The calf or foal should be prevented from nursing (muzzled) for ≥4 hr before administering D-lactose at 1 g/kg as a 20% solution via nasogastric tube; the muzzle should be kept in place for the duration of the test. Blood samples are collected into tubes containing fluoride oxalate for determination of blood glucose concentrations at 30 min, and immediately before and at 30-min intervals for 3–4 hr after dosing. Blood glucose concentration should be double that of the resting values within 60–90 min of lactose administration. Peak glucose concentrations should be ≥35 mg/dL higher than the baseline in healthy foals. Abnormal results suggestive of lactose intolerance include a delayed, prolonged, or lack of increase in blood glucose concentration from baseline.

Lack of an appropriate increase in blood glucose concentration after lactose administration may be due to maldigestion or malabsorption. Therefore, if the lactose tolerance test is abnormal, a D-glucose or D-xylose absorption test should be performed to determine whether malabsorption or maldigestion alone is the problem. Casein hypersensitivity is distinguished from lactose intolerance by assessing the animal's response to enzymatically treated and untreated milk. Definitive confirmation of lactase deficiency is through direct measurement of mucosal lactase activity in the intestinal tissue. However, this is rarely undertaken in the clinical setting, because a surgical biopsy of the mucosa is required.

A hydrogen breath test has also been described for detection of carbohydrate malabsorption in horses. In a clinical study, diseased horses showed higher fasting breath hydrogen levels than did healthy horses. However, because of the expensive laboratory procedures, the test is not widely used.

Treatment: The etiology of the primary underlying disease process must be determined before specific therapy for malassimilation syndrome can be initiated. Specific therapy for most causes of malassimilation is not available, except for lesions due to parasite damage. Anticoccidial and larvacidal dewormings may improve the condition; however, a complete healing and return to full absorption capacity is not always achievable depending on the damage. Anti-inflammatory agents (eg, NSAIDs, corticosteroids) may also help decrease the inflammatory response within the affected bowel. Supportive care and facilitation of nutrient absorption from more caudal parts of the intestine must be encouraged until the intestinal epithelium recovers and new villous cells are produced. Maturation and healing of the intestinal absorptive surfaces may take weeks to months in severe cases.

Calves and foals with acquired lactase deficiency after diarrheal disease (viral, bacterial, protozoal) often respond well to supportive care (correction of acid-base, electrolyte, and glucose abnormalities) and feeding of enzymatically treated milk until the small-intestinal mucosa has regenerated. Foals and calves should be fed small amounts of high-quality roughage or grain (if they are able to tolerate it) to help meet their energy needs, although enteral feeding should be continued whenever possible. Young foals and calves that do not tolerate feedings of milk or enzymatically treated milk may benefit from short-term (<24 hr) withdrawal of milk. These animals need alternative sources of energy and nutrients such as short-term feeding (≤24 hr) of glucose-containing electrolyte solutions or, in more severe cases, partial or total parenteral nutrition. Dietary change to a soy-based, non-lactose-containing milk replacer and early weaning are advised for animals with nonresponsive lactose intolerance.

Treatment of inflammatory bowel disease in horses has been attempted but is often unsuccessful even with aggressive corticosteroid administration. Sulfasalazine and isoniazid have been recommended, but their usefulness is unproved. Similarly, the usefulness of dimethyl sulfoxide in the treatment of intestinal amyloidosis is unknown. Animals with anaerobic or aerobic bacterial overgrowth may respond to antimicrobial administration. Adequate penetration of antimicrobials into inflammatory bowel lesions (*Rhodococcus equi* in foals) is doubtful. Successful treatment of *Lawsonia intracellularis* in foals has been achieved with longterm administration of antimicrobials (erythromycin, azithromycin, clarithromycin, chloramphenicol, oxytetracycline, doxycycline) and aggressive supportive care (fluids, plasma) as dictated by the animal's clinical condition. Any treatment attempt of cattle with clinical signs of Johne's disease have proved to be unsuccessful; slaughter or euthanasia is recommended. *Eimeria macusaniensis* infections in affected camelids may successfully be treated if diagnosed early. Treatment currently involves administration of amprolium, sulfonamides, ponazuril, or toltrazuril with appropriate supportive care.

Horses with malabsorption due to a disease process or after small-bowel resection must be fed a diet that optimizes digestion of feeds in the large intestine. The diet should provide easily absorbed protein, carbohydrates, fat, and water-soluble vitamins and maintain mineral balance. Increased concentrate-to-forage ratios decrease digestion of feeds in the large intestine and should be avoided. Horses benefit from a fiber-based diet. To enhance digestion in the large intestine, easily fermentable roughages (eg, alfalfa) should be fed. High-quality fiber, metabolized in the cecum and colon to volatile fatty acids, may partially compensate for small-intestinal losses. In young animals, the diet may be supplemented with milk protein if lactase deficiency is not present. Fat may be added to the diet to enhance caloric intake. Calcium, magnesium, phosphate, zinc, copper, and iron may need to be supplemented, because they are absorbed in horses in the small intestine only. Water-soluble (especially vitamin B_{12}) and fat-soluble vitamins should be supplemented parenterally as needed. Excessive supplementation, which could lead to toxicosis, should be avoided.

Horses that will not eat may have to be force-fed via nasogastric tube. The horse should be fed small, frequent meals to take advantage of the limited remaining absorptive ability of the small intestine without overloading it. Preruminant calves that are repeatedly tube-fed may develop ruminal acidosis due to deposition of fermentable feed material into the rumen (rumen drinker) rather than the abomasum. Partial or total parenteral nutrition may be necessary for animals that refuse to eat or that cannot tolerate force-feeding. However, total parenteral nutrition is expensive and difficult to continue on a long-term basis in horses or even impossible in ruminants.

Prognosis: Efforts should be made to determine an etiologic diagnosis once malassimilation has been confirmed so that an accurate prognosis can be given and appropriate therapy prescribed. Most conditions causing malassimilation in adult large animals warrant a poor prognosis, and treatment is commonly unsuccessful.

However, parasitic infection of the bowel or its blood supply can respond to anthelmintic therapy. Occasionally, a non-neoplastic infiltration of the bowel may respond to corticosteroids, but the response may be transient in some cases. Calves, foals, and kids with lactase deficiency may respond well to supportive care and dietary management. Prognosis for horses with malabsorption due to inflammatory bowel disease is poor; most reported cases have been fatal.

ABDOMINAL FAT NECROSIS

Hard masses of necrotic fat are occasionally identified in the peritoneal cavity of mature cattle, especially the Channel Island breeds, Japanese Black cattle, and beef cattle grazing fescue for long periods. The disease has also been seen in goats and some species of deer maintained on pastures consisting primarily of tall fescue. The masses are commonly mistaken for a developing fetus on palpation per rectum because they feel like "floating corks" similar to cotyledons. The masses of necrotic fat usually do not cause clinical signs but in advanced cases can create an extraluminal obstruction that results in episodes of moderate abdominal pain, distention of intestine proximal to the fat, and the passage of small amounts of feces.

The composition of the deposits in cattle with fat necrosis is identical to that of fat in healthy cows. The abnormal fat deposition is confined to abdominal fat and is consistent with current understanding that abdominal fat is controlled in a different manner than fat deposits elsewhere in the body. Fat necrosis has historically been termed lipomatosis, but this term is now considered inappropriate because the masses are not neoplastic or hyperplastic.

The etiology is unknown, but one proposed cause is consumption of feeds containing high concentrations of long-chain, saturated fatty acids. Fat necrosis is most commonly seen in beef cattle ≥2 yr old after prolonged grazing of tall fescue infected with the endophyte *Neotyphodium (Acremonium) coenophialum* (*see also* FESCUE POISONING, p 3016); fat necrosis is associated with endophyte infection rates of ≥65%. Fat necrosis is seen throughout the southeastern USA where tall fescue is the primary pasture plant for grazing.

Hard masses of necrotic fat form in the omentum, mesentery, and perirenal fat. The masses may cause clinical disease when they compress the abomasum, small intestine, and spiral colon; obstruct the birth canal; or more rarely compress the ureters. Palpation per rectum is useful in diagnosis and in determining prevalence in a cattle herd. Advanced cases in aged dairy cows may be detected by abdominal ballottement with the identification of large firm masses in the abdomen. Ultrasonographic examination of the abdomen reveals the presence of hyperechoic masses of variable size in the omentum, with localized masses appearing to float in an excess of peritoneal fluid. Hyperechoic masses adjacent to intestine may be associated with luminal constriction. A presumptive diagnosis of abdominal fat necrosis can be made using ultrasound-guided biopsy of the echogenic masses or by direct biopsy during right flank exploratory laparotomy. Less commonly, isolated fat masses may be found freely floating in the peritoneal fluid at surgery. The size of the masses usually slowly increases, but spontaneous resolution can occur. Removal of cattle from fescue pastures or dilution of fescue intake by supplying legume or other grass pasture can promote the slow reduction in the size of masses. Isoprothiolone (50 mg/kg/day, PO, for 8 wk) effectively decreases the size of fat necrosis lesions in Japanese Black cattle.

In affected deer herds, 90% of the females may be affected with fat necrosis. Clinical signs include slow development of anorexia, depression, and uremia associated with large masses of necrotic abdominal fat constricting the ureters, causing hydroureter and hydronephrosis.

A second form of abdominal fat necrosis in domestic animals, less well defined, appears to be related to pancreatitis. Although not associated with a clinical syndrome, the lesions (discrete or confluent masses of necrotic adipose tissue) are usually confined to peripancreatic fat. However, fat necrosis lesions may also be found throughout the abdomen.

A third form, a focal necrosis of abdominal and retroperitoneal fat (steatitis or yellow-fat disease) is seen most often in sheep but also in pigs, horses, cats, and other species. Little information is available about the condition in these species, but abdominal radiography or ultrasonography may help identify focal necrosis in cats.

DISEASES OF THE MOUTH IN SMALL ANIMALS

For a discussion of developmental diseases of the mouth, *see* p 162. For EOSINOPHILIC GRANULOMA COMPLEX, *see* p 971.

The primary function of the mouth is to introduce food into the digestive tract. Additional functions include communication and social interaction, grooming, protection, heat regulation (particularly in dogs), and grasping objects. The latter is very important for performance animals (eg, retrievers, military and police dogs). Similar to other areas of the alimentary tract, the mouth in the normal, healthy state supports a large and diverse population of bacteria that lives primarily in biofilm communities. Unlike other areas of the body, the mouth also contains nonvital surfaces (enamel of teeth) that have neither local immune system defenses nor the ability to regenerate through cellular replacement. The oral mucosal tissues have an excellent vascular supply, and the tightly adherent gingiva protects the underlying alveolar bone from trauma, thermal injury, and bacterial invasion.

Food prehension requires a complex interaction of the muscles of mastication, the teeth, the tongue, and the pharyngeal muscles. When any of these become compromised through disease or trauma, malnutrition and dehydration may result.

A complete oral examination should be included in every physical examination, because oral diseases are most effectively treated when diagnosed early. Unfortunately, many problems remain hidden in the mouth until they have progressed to an advanced stage.

ORAL INFLAMMATORY AND ULCERATIVE DISEASE

Inflammation of the oral tissues can be either primary or secondary. Inflammation in the oral cavity may affect the gingiva (gingivitis), nongingival tissues of the periodontium (periodontitis), alveolar mucosa (alveolar mucositis), sublingual mucosa (sublingual mucositis), lip and cheek mucosa (labial and buccal mucositis), lip (cheilitis), oral mucosa (stomatitis), mucosa of the dorsal or ventral tongue surface (glossitis), mucosa of the caudal oral cavity (caudal mucositis), mucosa forming the lateral walls of the pharynx (faucitis), mucosa of the palate (palatitis), palatine tonsil (tonsillitis), or mucosa of the pharynx (pharyngitis). The nature and severity of the lesions vary greatly depending on the etiology and duration of the disease. Contact mucositis and contact mucosal ulceration represent lesions in susceptible animals that are secondary to mucosal contact, with a tooth surface bearing the responsible irritant, allergen, or antigen. They have also been called "contact ulcers" and "kissing ulcers." Stomatitis is inflammation of the mucous lining of any of the structures in the mouth; in clinical use, the term should be reserved to describe widespread oral inflammation (beyond gingivitis and periodontitis) that may also extend into submucosal tissues (eg, marked caudal mucositis extending into submucosal tissues may be termed caudal stomatitis).

Periodontal disease, including gingivitis and periodontitis, is the most common oral problem in small animals. Gingivitis is a gingival inflammatory response to the presence of bacterial plaque on an adjacent tooth surface. Periodontitis is inflammation of nongingival tissues of the periodontium (namely periodontal ligament and alveolar bone); it results from the combination of bacterial periodontopathogens and the host's immune response that together destroy the tooth-supporting tissues. (*See also* PERIODONTAL DISEASE, p 178.)

Periapical disease (granuloma, abscess, or cyst) is usually caused by endodontic disease (spread of infection and inflammation from within the tooth through the apical foramina into the periapical tissues). Clinically, a sinus tract may develop that manifests as a circular raised area of inflamed granulation tissue with a central draining fistula that opens near the mucogingival junction. The tract can be followed to the primary periodontal or periapical lesion, and the etiology resolved. (*See also* ENDODONTIC DISEASE, p 180.) A parulis is a true periodontal abscess (eg, an encapsulated mucopurulent lesion within a periodontal pocket).

Other causes of oral inflammatory conditions include immunopathy (eg, autoimmune disease, immune deficiency), chemical agents, infectious disease, trauma, metabolic disease, developmental anomalies or conformational anatomy that predisposes to irritation or inflammation, burns, radiation therapy, or neoplasia. Infectious agents that have been associated with oral inflammation, glossitis, stomatitis, and oral ulcerations include feline herpesvirus, feline calicivirus, feline leukemia virus, feline immunodeficiency virus, canine distemper virus, *Bartonella henselae*, and certain *Leptospira* serovars. Traumatic stomatitis may be seen after oral exposure to plant material (embedded plant awns) or fiberglass insulation. When chewed, plants of the species *Dieffenbachia* may also cause oral inflammation and ulcers. Contact with processionary caterpillars may also cause severe glossitis. Thallium is the major heavy metal responsible for oral lesions; incidence of this toxicity is low. Uremia can cause stomatitis and oral ulcers. Recurrent oral ulcerations are also seen in gray Collies with cyclic hematopoiesis.

Signs vary widely with the cause and extent of inflammation. Anorexia may be seen, especially in cats. Halitosis and drooling are common with caudal stomatitis or glossitis, and saliva may be blood tinged. The animal may paw at its mouth and resent any attempt to examine the oral cavity because of pain. Regional lymph nodes may be enlarged.

Feline Stomatitis

(Gingivostomatitis, Caudal stomatitis, Lymphocytic-plasmacytic stomatitis)

Feline stomatitis (FS) is a relatively uncommon (3% of feline oral problems) but serious condition. Affected cats present with progressively worsening inflammation of oral mucosal tissues (particularly the gingiva, alveolar mucosa, labial and buccal mucosa, sublingual mucosa, and mucosa of the caudal oral cavity) and increasing levels of discomfort. More significantly, the mucosa of the caudal oral cavity and the area at and lateral to the palatoglossal folds are often severely ulcerated, friable, inflamed, and proliferative. Severe ulceroproliferative inflammation that involves this area bilaterally in the back of the mouth is pathognomonic for FS. The cause is unproved, but it is suspected to result from an inappropriate inflammatory response in affected cats to one or more antigens. A high percentage of affected cats (100% in some studies) are chronic carriers of feline calicivirus. FS may be caused by the sum of multiple sensitivities in an individual, with antigen on the tooth surfaces, including the root surfaces and periodontal ligament, exceeding a threshold.

The most immediate sign is severe pain when opening the mouth. Cats vocalize and jump when they yawn or open their mouth to eat. Halitosis, ptyalism, and dysphagia may be seen. Cats often show an "approach-avoidance" behavior as they approach their food in hunger, then hiss and run off in anticipation of discomfort. If the condition is severe and of long duration, weight loss may be evident. The disease is slowly progressive and may not be recognized until lesions have become severe. Mandibular lymphadenopathy is sometimes present. Pain often prevents adequate examination of the oral cavity without sedation or anesthesia.

Diagnosis: Diagnosis is made by visual identification of bilateral inflammation of the mucosa of the caudal oral cavity and the tissues at or lateral to the palatoglossal folds during oral examination. In advanced cases, the cat will strongly object to opening the mouth. Additional tests include virus isolation (eg, calicivirus and herpesvirus), retroviral tests, and evaluation for systemic disease (eg, renal failure). Although a definitive association with *Bartonella* infection has not been shown, testing has been recommended. In atypical cases (unilateral involvement, usually proliferative focal lesion), biopsy and histopathologic evaluation is required to exclude oral neoplasia or other specific oral disorders. Most biopsy samples collected from chronic inflammatory or ulcerated lesions reveal a predominance of lymphocytes and plasma cells, which indicate the chronic inflammatory nature of the lesion without elucidating the primary etiology.

Treatment: Partial-mouth extraction (removal of all premolars and molars) or full-mouth extraction (removal of all teeth) and debridement of the associated soft and hard tissues is the only treatment to provide lasting improvement and aid in overall longterm control. Partial- or full-mouth extractions provide significant improvement in 60%–80% of affected cats when done early in the disease course and when no root tips or fragments are left behind. Chronically affected cats treated medically for many months have a poorer prognosis after surgery. Dental radiographs of areas with missing teeth are required to check for retained roots. Any retained root fragments must be removed, because they will prevent improvement. Postoperatively, medical therapy focuses on controlling inflammation, infection, and pain. Oral administration of corticosteroids such as prednisolone is less effective than SC or IM injection of methylprednisolone. An alternative is transdermal administration of prednisolone. In refractory cases, use of interferon omega may be considered, injected intralesionally before the start of oral administration. Commonly used antibiotics include amoxicillin-clavulanic acid or clindamycin, but the response to treatment may be lacking or only transient. Culturing the lesions and performing susceptibility tests are rarely indicated, even in chronic or recurrent infections. Nutritional support is required in chronic cases with severe weight loss and dehydration. Pain control with sublingual buprenorphine or a transdermal fentanyl patch should also be considered, along with dietary changes (nonallergenic, soft palatable foods) and administration of topical antiseptics (eg, dilute chlorhexidine or zinc ascorbate). Placement of a feeding tube should be considered in debilitated cats that do not respond to therapy.

Many other treatments for FS have been reported, including good home oral hygiene, periodontal therapy, frequent dental cleanings, cyclosporine therapy, laser therapy, and bovine lactoferrin. Perhaps with the exception of cyclosporine, none of these provide longterm resolution. Corticosteroid administration alone usually results in significant and immediate clinical improvement from modulation of the excessive inflammatory response, but it is not recommended except as a last resort. Without surgery (ie, partial- or full-mouth extractions), repeated use of corticosteroids is frequently required. This treatment becomes progressively less effective and eventually completely ineffective. In addition, cats that have received repeated corticosteroid treatments have a poorer prognosis once the teeth are extracted. Partial- or full-mouth extractions often result in significant improvement or complete resolution of the inflammation if performed early in the course of the disease and before multiple corticosteroid treatments.

Canine Stomatitis

Characteristics of canine stomatitis that often manifest as contact mucositis and contact mucosal ulceration (also called chronic ulcerative paradental syndrome or CUPS) include severe gingivitis, multiple sites of gingival recession and dehiscence, and large areas of ulcerated labial and buccal mucosa adjacent to the surfaces of large teeth. The problem commonly affects Greyhounds, and it has also been seen in Maltese, Miniature Schnauzers, Labrador Retrievers, and other breeds.

Diagnosis: Diagnosis of canine stomatitis is by clinical observation of the typical oral lesions after excluding other etiologies such as uremic stomatitis, caustic stomatitis, or specific infectious agents. The characteristic lesion is the contact ulcer that develops where the lip or cheek mucosa contacts the tooth surface, most commonly on the inner surface of the upper lip adjacent to the upper canine and carnassial teeth. These lesions have also been termed "kissing ulcers" or "kissing lesions," because they are found where the lips "kiss" the teeth. An immune profile should be done, and a biopsy considered for histopathology.

Treatment: The underlying pathology of canine stomatitis is an immunopathy that results in an excessive local inflammatory response to the antigens in dental plaque. Eliminating, or at least minimizing, plaque through professional dental cleaning and meticulous home oral hygiene (twice daily tooth brushing) may resolve the problem. However, even slight residual plaque on the tooth surfaces will perpetuate the inflammation and ulcerations. Supplemental antimicrobial measures with topical chlorhexidine gluconate rinses or gels and possibly oral antibiotic treatment with metronidazole should also be used. In severe cases, topical anti-inflammatory preparations to modulate the inflammatory response may provide comfort. Discomfort caused by the ulcers complicates efforts to brush the teeth and administer oral medications. In cases in which discomfort is severe and the owners are unable or unwilling to brush the teeth, extraction of all teeth associated with ulcers may be necessary to remove the contact surfaces on which plaque accumulates. Although this may help control the lesions, it is not curative, because plaque forms on mucosal surfaces in the mouth, including the tongue. In some cases with complete extractions, dogs continue to develop lesions due to a hyperimmune response to the plaque.

Lip Fold Dermatitis and Cheilitis

Lip fold dermatitis is a chronic, moist dermatitis seen most commonly in breeds that have pendulous lips and lower lateral lip folds (eg, spaniels, English Bulldogs, Saint Bernards) that have prolonged contact with saliva. The lesions may be exacerbated when poor oral hygiene results in increased salivary bacterial levels. The lower lip folds can become very malodorous, inflamed, uncomfortable, and swollen.

Lip wounds, resulting from fights or chewing on sharp objects, are common and vary widely in severity. Thorns, grass awns, plant burrs, and fishhooks may embed in the lips and cause marked irritation or severe wounds. Irritants such as plastic or plant material can produce inflammation of the lips. Lip infections may develop secondary to wounds or foreign bodies or can be associated with inflammation of adjacent areas. Direct extension of severe periodontal disease or stomatitis can produce cheilitis. Licking areas of bacterial dermatitis or infected wounds can spread the infection to the lips and lip folds. Other causes of inflammation of the lips include parasitic infections, autoimmune skin diseases, and neoplasia.

Clinical Findings and Diagnosis: Inflammation of the lips and lip folds can be acute or chronic. Animals with cheilitis may paw, scratch, or rub at their mouth or lip; have a foul odor on the breath; and occasionally salivate excessively or be anorectic. With chronic infection of the lip margins or folds, the hair in these areas is discolored, moist, and matted with a thick, yellowish or brown, malodorous discharge overlying hyperemic and sometimes ulcerated skin.

Cheilitis due to extension of infection from the mouth or another area of the body usually is detected easily because of the primary lesion.

Treatment: Medical management of lip fold dermatitis includes clipping the hair, cleaning the folds 1–2 times/day with benzoyl peroxide or a mild skin cleanser, and keeping the area dry. Topical diaper rash cream applied daily may be helpful. Surgical correction (cheiloplasty) of deep lip folds is a more longlasting remedy.

Cheilitis that is unrelated to lip folds usually resolves with minimal cleansing, appropriate antibiotics if a bacterial infection is present, and specific treatment of primary etiologies (eg, autoimmune skin disease). Wounds of the lips should be cleaned and sutured if necessary. Treatment of periodontal disease or stomatitis is necessary to prevent recurrence.

Infectious cheilitis that has spread from a lesion elsewhere usually improves with treatment of the primary lesion, but local treatment also is necessary. With severe infection, hair should be clipped from the lesion and the area gently cleaned and dried. Antibiotics are indicated if the infection is severe or systemic.

Mycotic Stomatitis

Mycotic stomatitis caused by overgrowth of the opportunistic yeast *Candida albicans* is an uncommon cause of stomatitis in dogs and cats. It is characterized by stomatitis, halitosis, ptyalism, anorexia, oral ulceration, and bleeding from the oral tissues. It is usually thought to be associated with other oral diseases, longterm antibiotic therapy, or immunosuppression. Diagnosis is confirmed by culture of the organism from the lesion or by histologic evidence of tissue invasion.

Any existing underlying local or systemic diseases affecting the oral cavity should be treated. Ketoconazole or a related benzimidazole should be administered until the lesions resolve, after which antibiotic therapy should be discontinued. An adequate level of nutrition should be maintained. The prognosis is guarded if predisposing diseases cannot be adequately treated or controlled.

Acute Necrotizing Ulcerative Gingivitis

(Necrotizing ulcerative gingivostomatitis, Ulceromembranous stomatitis, Necrotizing ulcerative stomatitis, Vincent stomatitis, Trench mouth)

Acute necrotizing ulcerative gingivitis (ANUG) is a relatively uncommon disease of dogs characterized by severe gingivitis, ulceration, and necrosis of the oral mucosa. *Fusobacterium* spp and spirochete organisms (*Borrelia vincenti*), normal inhabitants of the mouth, have been suggested as a cause of this disease after some predisposing factor increases their numbers or decreases the local resistance of the oral mucosa. The role, if any, of these organisms in causing disease is unknown. In people, *Bacteroides melaninogenicus intermedius* may play a more important role. Other potential factors are stress, excess glucocorticoid administration in susceptible dogs, and poor nutrition.

The disease appears first as reddening and swelling of the gingival margins and interdental papillae, which are painful, bleed easily, and may progress to gingival recession. Extension to other areas of the oral mucosa is common, resulting in ulcerated, necrotic mucous membranes and exposed bone in severe cases, leading to osteomyelitis and osteonecrosis. Halitosis is severe, and the animal may be anorectic because of pain. Ptyalism sometimes occurs, and the saliva may be blood tinged. Differential diagnoses include severe periodontal disease, autoimmune skin disease, uremia, neoplasia, and other systemic disease associated with oral lesions.

Diagnosis is made by exclusion of other etiologies.

Treatment of periodontal disease, partial- or full-mouth extractions, debridement of lesions, oral hygiene, antibiotics (amoxicillin-clavulanate, ampicillin, clindamycin, metronidazole, tetracyclines), and oral antiseptics (dilute chlorhexidine solution or gel) are indicated.

Glossitis

Glossitis, an acute or chronic inflammation of the tongue, may be due to infectious (calicivirus, herpesvirus, rhinotracheitis virus, leptospirosis), physical (irritation from excess calculus and periodontal disease, foreign bodies that penetrate or become lodged under the tongue, traumatic wounds), or chemical agents; metabolic disease (uremia, hypoparathyoidism, diabetes); or other causes such as electric or thermal burns and insect stings. Foreign body glossitis is especially a problem in longhaired dogs that attempt to remove plant burrs from their coats.

Drooling and a reluctance to eat are common signs, but the cause may go undiscovered unless the mouth is carefully examined. Periodontitis may result in reddening, swelling, and occasionally ulceration of the lateral edges and the tip of the tongue. A thread, string, or other linear foreign body may get caught under the tongue. There may be no inflammation of the dorsal surface of the tongue, but the ventral surface is painful, shows acute or chronic irritation, and frequently is lacerated by the foreign body. Porcupine quills, plant material, and other foreign materials may become embedded so deeply they are not palpable. Insect stings cause acute swelling of the tongue.

In chronic cases of ulcerative glossitis, a thick, brown, foul-smelling discharge (occasionally with bleeding) may be present. Frequently, the animal is reluctant to allow oral examination.

Fissured, or plicated, tongue (lingua dissecta) describes a textural variation of the dorsum of the tongue with deep central or lateral longitudinal grooves. The fissure deepens with age and is therefore thought to be acquired from some extrinsic factor. However, it may also represent a developmental anomaly. The groove often becomes deeply filled with hairs that act as a local irritant, causing inflammation and discomfort.

Any foreign bodies or hairs should be removed, and broken or diseased teeth removed or treated. Bacterial infectious glossitis should be treated with an appropriate systemic antibiotic. Debridement and dilute chlorhexidine mouthwashes are beneficial in some cases. Lingual curettage is sometimes required if foreign material is embedded in the tongue. A soft diet and parenteral fluids are administered as needed. If the animal is debilitated and unable to eat well for a prolonged period, a feeding tube to allow for nutritional support should be considered. Acute glossitis due to insect stings may require emergency treatment.

If the glossitis is secondary to another condition, the primary disease should be treated. Tongue tissues heal rapidly after irritation and infection have been eliminated.

SOFT-TISSUE TRAUMA

Chewing Lesions

A proliferative, verrucous lesion along the bite-plane of the cheek or sublingual region may result from self-trauma when the tissue becomes entrapped between the teeth during chewing. Surgical removal of the excess tissue prevents further trauma.

Mouth Burns

Thermal, chemical, or electric burns involving the mouth are not uncommon.

The animal should be evaluated and treated for systemic involvement, which may be life-threatening (neurogenic pulmonary edema). The tongue, lips, cheeks, labial and buccal mucosa, and palate are frequently involved with electric burns. The injuries may be mild with only temporary discomfort, or they may be destructive with loss of tissue, scar formation, and subsequent deformity or tissue deficits. Chewing on an electric cord is most frequently a problem in kittens, puppies, and pet rabbits. These animals often have a linear scar across the dorsum of the tongue, outlining the path of the electric cord. One or both lip commisures may have a scar or wound, and the adjacent carnassial teeth may be discolored and eventually require endodontic treatment.

The owner may have observed the incident, but more commonly it occurs in the owner's absence. The animal hesitates to eat or drink, drools, and resents handling of its mouth or face. If tissue destruction is marked, ulcerative or gangrenous stomatitis can develop, with secondary bacterial infections. If recent contact with a corrosive alkaline chemical has occurred, the mouth should be flushed with mild solutions of vinegar or citrus juice; if the chemical was acidic, a solution of sodium bicarbonate should be used. Copious flushing of the mouth with water helps remove some of the chemical substances. More commonly, the animal is seen too long after the exposure for neutralization to be effective. The hair should be clipped and/or washed if it is suspected to be a continued source of a chemical that caused the caustic mucosal lesions.

Animals that have inflamed oral mucosa without tissue defects require no specific supportive treatment other than a soft or liquid diet until the lesion has healed. If tissue damage is extensive, treatment includes lavage with dilute chlorhexidine solution and conservative tissue debridement. The risk of secondary infection should be minimized with systemic antibiotic therapy for several days.

PAPILLOMAS

Papillomas are benign growths caused by the canine papillomavirus (*see* p 952). The oral mucosa and commissures of the lip are most frequently involved, but the growths (usually *multiple but sometimes single*) can involve the palate and oropharynx. Papillomas are most common in young dogs and appear suddenly, with rapid growth and spread. Signs are seen when the growths interfere with prehension, mastication, or swallowing. Occasionally, if the growths are numerous, the dog may bite them when chewing, causing them to bleed and become infected. They may regress spontaneously within a few weeks to months, and removal is generally not necessary. If necessary, the exophytic lesion can be debulked with electro- or radiosurgery or by sharp resection. Surgical removal of one or more of the papillomas may initiate regression. The use of commercial or autogenous vaccines should be considered in very severe cases in which the dog cannot swallow or breathe normally. The self-limiting character of the disease makes evaluation of any treatment difficult. Severe oral papillomatosis may be seen in immunocompromised dogs with lymphoma.

Other wart-like lesions are benign exophytic proliferations of squamous epithelium. They are clinically indistinguishable from virus-induced papillomas but are generally slow growing and solitary. They most commonly remain benign, and surgical removal is curative.

ORAL TUMORS

Benign Oral Tumors

Peripheral odontogenic fibromas (previously called fibromatous epulis or ossifying epulis) are the most common benign oral tumors. These firm masses involve the gingival tissue adjacent to a tooth. They affect dogs of any age but are most common in dogs >6 yr old. Some develop centers of ossification, visible as distinct alveolar bone proliferation extending into the soft-tissue mass. They are generally solitary, although multiple lesions may be present. The tumors do not metastasize but may become quite extensive. They arise from the periodontal ligament of the affected tooth, and complete surgical removal must include tissues up to and including the periodontal ligament. This usually necessitates conservative resection of the neoplastic lesion, extraction of the affected tooth or teeth, and curettage of the extraction sites (ie, removal of remaining periodontal ligament). Complete excision is curative.

The canine acanthomatous ameloblastoma (previously called acanthomatous epulis) is much more locally aggressive, quickly invading the local tissues including bone. This tumor does not metastasize, but because of its locally aggressive nature, surgical excision should include a 1-cm margin of clinically normal tissue (including bony margins) to prevent recurrence. Radiation therapy may minimize disfigurement when treating large tumors. Adequate surgical removal is curative.

Malignant Oral Tumors

In dogs, the three most common malignant oral tumors are malignant melanoma, squamous cell carcinoma, and fibrosarcoma. The incidence of malignant oral tumors is higher in dogs >8 yr old.

Squamous cell carcinomas are by far the most common malignant oral neoplasms in cats; they commonly involve the gingiva and tongue and are locally highly invasive. Fibrosarcomas are the next most common. In cats, these tumors are locally invasive and, if extensive, carry a poor prognosis.

Clinical Findings: Signs of malignant oral tumors vary depending on the location and extent of the neoplasm. Halitosis, reluctance to eat, and hypersalivation are common. If the oropharynx is involved, dysphagia may be present. The tumors frequently ulcerate and bleed. The face may become swollen as the tumor enlarges and invades surrounding tissue. Regional lymph nodes often become swollen before oral and pharyngeal tumors are seen.

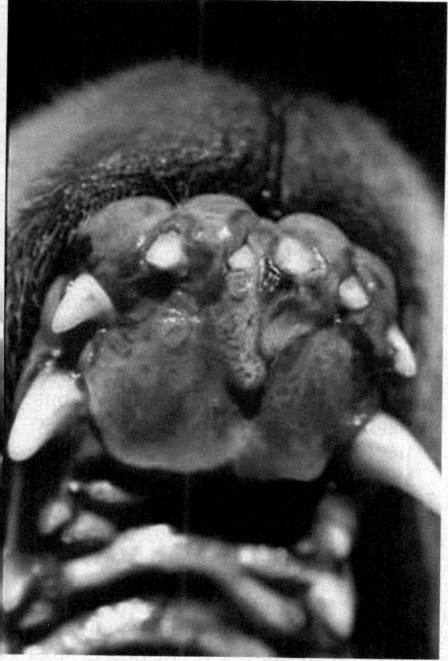

Oral mast cell tumor in a dog. *Courtesy of Dr. Ben Colmery III.*

Diagnosis: Because of the varied behavior of oral and maxillofacial tumors, presurgical characterization is valuable to plan the extent of the required surgery. Biopsy is the most reliable method to obtain a definitive diagnosis; however, a cytologic diagnosis from impression smears of a fine-needle aspirate is possible in many cases. Therefore, a histologic diagnosis is typically necessary to plan for accurate treatment. Malignant melanomas are variable in appearance, pigmented or nonpigmented, and should be considered in the diagnosis of any oral tumor. Squamous cell carcinomas commonly involve the gingiva or palatine tonsils (unilateral), and lymphosarcoma should be a differential diagnosis for bilaterally enlarged tonsils. Lymph nodes and the lungs should be evaluated for regional and distant metastasis.

Treatment: Malignant melanomas are highly invasive and metastasize readily; consequently, the prognosis is guarded to poor. Surgical resection can extend survival and may be curative, particularly with masses in the rostral areas of the mouth. However, local recurrence is common. Immunotherapy is available as an adjunct treatment to radical surgery and chemotherapy. Nontonsillar squamous cell carcinomas are locally invasive with a low rate of metastasis, and the prognosis in dogs is good with aggressive and complete surgical resection, radiation therapy, or both. Tonsillar squamous cell carcinomas are aggressive and have a poor prognosis. Fibrosarcomas have a guarded prognosis because of their locally aggressive nature. Recurrence of tumor growth after resection is common.

In cats, squamous cell carcinoma has a poor prognosis unless the entire tumor can be removed, and longterm survival is usually seen only if diagnosed and treated early.

SALIVARY DISORDERS

Ptyalism

Ptyalism is drooling of saliva. This may be caused by hypersialosis (hypersecretion of saliva) or pseudoptyalism (secondary to conformational abnormalities or swallowing disorders in animals producing a normal quantity of saliva). Both are discussed together as ptyalism.

Ptyalism may result from the following: 1) drugs, toxins, or poisons, eg, organophosphates; 2) local irritation or inflammation associated with stomatitis, glossitis (especially in cats), oral foreign bodies, neoplasms, injuries, or other mucosal defects; 3) infectious diseases (eg, rabies), the nervous form of distemper, or other convulsive disorders; 4) motion sickness, fear, nervousness, or excitement; 5) reluctance to swallow or interference with swallowing (from irritation of the esophagus, esophageal obstruction by regional pathology, or from stimulation of GI receptors caused by gastritis or enteritis); 6) sublingual lesions (eg, linear foreign body, tumor); 7) tonsillitis; 8) administration of medicine (particularly in cats); 9) conformational defects (eg, heavy, pendulous lower lips); 10) metabolic disorders (eg, hepatic encephalopathy [especially in cats]) or uremia; 11) abscess or other inflammatory blockage or condition of the salivary gland.

The possibility of rabies should be eliminated before oral examination. The underlying cause, local or systemic, should be determined and treated. Acute moist dermatitis of the lips and face may develop if the skin is not kept as dry as possible. Cleansing with a dilute chlorhexidine solution or benzoyl peroxide may be helpful.

Salivary Mucocele

A salivary mucocele (or sialocele) is an accumulation of saliva in the submucosal or subcutaneous tissues after damage to the salivary duct or gland capsule. This is the most common salivary gland disorder of dogs. Although any of the salivary glands may be affected, the ducts of the sublingual and mandibular glands are involved most commonly. Saliva often collects in the intermandibular or cranial cervical area (cervical mucocele). It can also collect in the sublingual tissues on the floor of the mouth (sublingual mucocele or ranula). A less common site is in the pharyngeal wall (pharyngeal mucocele) or lower eyelid (zygomatic mucocele).

The cause may be traumatic or inflammatory blockage or rupture of the duct or capsule (with damage of parenchyma) of the sublingual, mandibular, parotid, or zygomatic salivary gland. Usually, the exact cause is not determined, but a developmental predisposition in dogs has been suggested.

Signs depend on the site of saliva accumulation. In the acute phase of saliva accumulation, the inflammatory response results in the area being swollen and painful. Frequently, this stage is not seen by the owner, and the first noticed sign may be a nonpainful, slowly enlarging, fluctuant mass, frequently in the cervical region. A ranula may not be seen until it is traumatized and bleeds. A pharyngeal mucocele can obstruct the airways and result in moderate to severe respiratory distress. A zygomatic mucocele may result in exophthalmos or enophthalmos, depending on its size and location.

A mucocele is detectable as a soft, fluctuant, painless mass that must be differentiated from abscesses, tumors, and other retention cysts of the neck. Pain or fever may be present if the mucocele becomes infected. A salivary mucocele usually can be diagnosed by palpation and aspiration of light brown or blood-tinged, viscous saliva. Usually, careful palpation with the animal in dorsal recumbency can determine the affected side; if not, sialography may be helpful.

Surgery is recommended to remove the damaged salivary gland and duct. Periodic drainage if surgery is not an option is usually only a temporary measure and has the potential for iatrogenic infection. Marsupialization is often ineffective. Gland-duct removal has been recommended for curative treatment of salivary mucoceles.

Salivary Fistula

Salivary fistula is an uncommon problem that can result from trauma to the mandibular, zygomatic, or sublingual salivary glands. Wounds of the parotid gland are most likely to develop a fistula. Parotid duct injury may be the result of a traumatic wound (eg, bite wound), abscess drainage, or prior surgery in the area with iatrogenic rupture. The constant flow of saliva prevents healing, and a fistula develops.

History of injury in the gland area, location of the fistula, and nature of the discharge are characteristic. A salivary fistula must be differentiated from a draining sinus (due to a penetrating foreign body or endodontic disease of a mandibular tooth) in the neck or from sinuses arising from congenital defects. Surgical ligation of the duct usually results in resolution, but excision of the associated gland may also be necessary.

Salivary Gland Tumors

Salivary gland tumors are rare in dogs and cats, although cats are affected twice as frequently as dogs. Most are seen in dogs and cats >10 yr old. There is no clear breed or sex predilection, although Poodles and Spaniel breeds may be predisposed. Most salivary gland tumors are malignant, with carcinomas and adenocarcinomas the most common. Local infiltration and metastasis to regional lymph nodes and lungs are common, as is local recurrence after surgical excision. Radiotherapy, with or without surgery, offers the best prognosis.

Sialadenitis

Sialadenitis, or inflammation of the salivary gland, is rarely a clinical problem in dogs and cats. However, it is frequently an incidental finding on histopathology at necropsy.

The cause may be trauma from penetrating wounds or systemic infection affecting the salivary gland or surrounding tissue. Sialadenitis as a component of systemic disease has been reported with rabies, distemper, and the paramyxovirus that causes mumps in people.

Signs include fever, depression, and painful, swollen salivary glands. Rupture of an abscessed gland discharges pus into the surrounding tissue or the mouth. Rupture through the skin may cause a salivary fistula to form. Swelling of the parotid gland is most prominent below the ear, swelling of the mandibular gland at the angle of the jaw, and swelling of the zygomatic gland just caudal to the eye. Zygomatic gland involvement may result in retrobulbar swelling, divergent strabismus of the affected eye, exophthalmos, excess tearing, and reluctance to open the mouth or eat. Abscesses of the zygomatic and parotid glands are acutely painful; the animal may hold its head rigidly and resent any manipulation involving the head or neck.

Radiographs and laboratory tests are usually not helpful, although evaluation of fluid in an abscess can lead to a diagnosis. Histopathology of salivary gland tissue can reveal acute or chronic inflammatory changes or necrosis.

Mild sialadenitis requires no treatment, and recovery is usually rapid and complete. A developed abscess should be drained through the overlying skin or, if involving the zygomatic gland, behind the last upper molar on the affected side. Systemic antibiotics should be administered.

Lack of resolution or recurrence necessitates cytology of aspirated material, biopsy, or surgical removal of the affected gland.

Sialadenosis in Dogs

Sialadenosis is a non-inflammatory, non-neoplastic, usually bilateral enlargement of the mandibular salivary glands, associated with regional swelling (dependent on location) and exophthalmos but no apparent pain. The dog may retch and gulp, which is elicited by mild excitement and occurs several times a day. There may be weight loss, reluctance to exercise, snorting, lip smacking, nasal discharge, hypersalivation, inappetence, and depression. Histologically, there are no obvious abnormalities. Excessive saliva production may be associated with increased parasympathetic activity or changes in sympathetic innervation. Phenobarbital administration usually results in lasting improvement, providing support for a neurogenic pathogenesis.

Necrotizing Sialometaplasia in Dogs

Necrotizing sialometaplasia has also been termed salivary gland necrosis or infarction. There is squamous metaplasia of the salivary gland ducts and lobules, with ischemic necrosis of the salivary gland lobules. It can be seen in dogs (mostly small breeds such as terriers) of all ages, most often 3–8 yr old. Affected dogs usually are depressed, nauseous, and anorectic. Clinical signs include salivary gland enlargement that may be painful on palpation, weight loss, ptyalism, retching, gagging, regurgitation, and vomiting. Other signs include persistent swallowing, lip smacking, coughing, tachypnea, dyspnea, and abdominal respiration. Examination of samples from fine-needle aspirates or biopsies often reveal no abnormalities. Diagnosis requires excluding other causes of enlargement. Surgical removal of the affected salivary gland produces minimal if any improvement. Pain management, antibiotics (based on culture and sensitivity of the fluid/tissue aspirate), NSAIDs, antiinflammatory doses of glucocorticoids, and control of internal parasites have resulted in favorable responses in some cases. Phenobarbital administration (1–2 mg/kg, PO, bid, or higher initial doses) has resulted in dramatic improvement in several cases, providing more support for a neurogenic pathogenesis..

Xerostomia

Hypoptyalism is a decreased secretion of saliva that can result in a dry mouth (xerostomia). It can cause significant discomfort and difficulty during eating. It is uncommon in dogs and cats but is very common in people who have undergone radiation therapy for tumors of the head and neck that resulted in collateral radiation injury to the salivary glands. As radiation treatment is used more commonly in veterinary medicine, xerostomia may become more frequent in animals. Decreased salivary secretion may also result from use of certain drugs (eg, atropine), extreme dehydration, pyrexia, or anesthesia. It is seen in some dogs with keratoconjunctivitis sicca and can be immune-mediated. Occasionally, it is due to disease of the salivary gland. Determination and treatment of the underlying cause is of primary importance. Physiologically balanced mouthwashes relieve the discomfort that results from xerostomia. Fluids should be administered if the animal is dehydrated. Immunosuppressive therapy is indicated if immune-mediated disease is suspected.

DISEASES OF THE ESOPHAGUS IN SMALL ANIMALS

CRICOPHARYNGEAL ACHALASIA

Cricopharyngeal achalasia is characterized by inadequate relaxation of the cricopharyngeal muscle, which leads to a relative inability to swallow food or liquids. It is seen primarily as a congenital defect but is occasionally seen in adult dogs. The cause is generally unknown, but in adult animals it may be associated with acquired neuromuscular disorders. Repeated attempts to swallow are followed by gagging and regurgitation. Aspiration pneumonia is a common complication. An accurate diagnosis requires fluoroscopic evaluation of swallowing after oral administration of contrast material alone and mixed with food. Abnormal function (lack of relaxation) of the cricopharyngeal muscle results in retention of barium in the posterior pharynx.

Treatment consists of cricopharyngeal myotomy or cricopharyngeal and thyropharyngeal myectomy, which usually results in normal swallowing immediately after surgery. The success rate of surgery approaches 65%. Dogs with acquired neuromuscular disorders are less likely to respond to surgery but may respond to treatment of the underlying disease. Aspiration pneumonia should be treated aggressively if present.

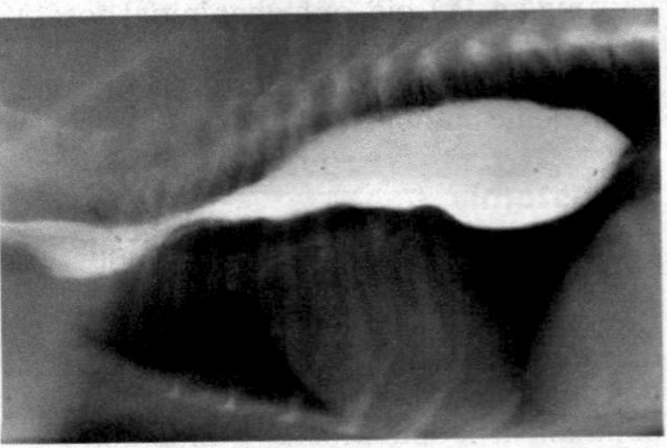

Esophagram demonstrating dilatation of the esophagus (megaesophagus), lateral projection. *Courtesy of Dr. Ronald Green.*

DILATATION OF THE ESOPHAGUS

(Megaesophagus)

Megaesophagus may be due to a congenital defect or may be an adult-onset, acquired disorder. Congenital defects that may result in megaesophagus include vascular ring anomalies, esophageal diverticula, congenital myasthenia gravis, and an idiopathic form. (*See also* CONGENITAL AND INHERITED ANOMALIES OF THE ESOPHAGUS, p 166.) Adult-onset megaesophagus may be primary (idiopathic) or secondary to systemic disease. Secondary megaesophagus may be due to myasthenia gravis, systemic lupus erythematosus, polymyositis, hypoadrenocorticism, heavy metal (lead) toxicity, thallium toxicity, glycogen storage disease, neurotoxin-induced cholinesterase inhibition, dysautonomia, CNS disorders including neoplasia, and possibly hypothyroidism. Esophageal dilatation may also develop cranial to an esophageal lesion such as an esophageal stricture, foreign body, neoplasia, or extraesophageal compression.

The cardinal sign is regurgitation. A puppy with congenital megaesophagus characteristically begins to regurgitate at weaning when it starts to eat solid food. Affected pups are generally unthrifty and smaller than their littermates. Pressure applied to the abdomen may cause ballooning of the esophagus at the thoracic inlet. Aspiration pneumonia is a complication with associated signs of cough, fever, and sometimes nasal discharge. Adult animals that develop megaesophagus also start to regurgitate and ultimately lose weight. Respiratory signs may predominate, with little or no apparent regurgitation. Thoracic radiographs reveal air, fluid, or food in a dilated esophagus. The esophagus is usually uniformly dilated. A large ventral deviation may be present cranial to the heart. Megaesophagus secondary to a stricture, foreign body, neoplasia, or vascular ring anomaly is visualized as a dilatation of the esophagus cranial to the defect only. Strictures, foreign bodies, or vascular ring anomalies can be excluded with an esophagram and/or esophagoscopy.

In adult dogs, associated diseases (eg, myasthenia gravis) should be excluded or, if found, treated. Surgery is indicated for a vascular ring anomaly. Surgery may not successfully resolve the clinical signs in longstanding cases with severe esophageal dilatation cranial to the anomaly. Medical management is indicated for congenital or acquired idiopathic megaesophagus. Congenital megaesophagus may resolve as the animal ages, usually by 6 mo of age. The consistency of the diet that best prevents regurgitation varies from dog to dog; a soft gruel works for some, while dry food works for others. Another possibility is canned food formed into a meatball shape. Frequent, small meals work best for most dogs. Feeding from an elevated position with the forelimbs higher than the hindlimbs and holding that position for at least 10–15 min after eating allows gravity to assist food passage into the stomach. Neither surgery nor medications improve esophageal function. Ultimately, most animals succumb to aspiration pneumonia.

ESOPHAGEAL DYSMOTILITY

Young dogs may have a disorder of esophageal dysmotility without overt megaesophagus. Clinical signs can be similar to those of megaesophagus, although some dogs without clinical signs have abnormal motility during an esophagram. In one study in more than half the cases, the condition improved or resolved with age. Terrier breeds were overrepresented. Cats can also have esophageal dysfunction, which can be idiopathic; congenital; or secondary to myasthenia gravis, mediastinal masses, vascular ring anomalies, dysautonomia, and strictures. Many cats improve with medical management such as the use of sucralfate, H_2-blockers, and metoclopramide.

ESOPHAGEAL STRICTURES

(Esophageal stenosis)

Esophageal stricture is a pathologic narrowing of the lumen that may develop after anesthesia, trauma (eg, foreign body), ingestion of caustic substances, exposure to certain drugs (such as doxycycline or clindamycin), esophagitis, gastroesophageal reflux, or tumor invasion. Most strictures develop in the thoracic portion of the esophagus. Esophageal tumors are rare, but esophageal sarcomas may be associated with *Spirocerca lupi* infection (*see* p 412), requiring consideration in areas where this parasite is prevalent. Esophageal compression by vascular ring anomalies or extramural tumors may mimic the signs of strictures.

Clinical signs are similar to those associated with foreign bodies and include regurgitation, ptyalism, dysphagia, and pain. An esophagram under fluoroscopy is the preferred tool for diagnosis, because it allows visualization of the number, length, location, and severity of strictures. Esophagoscopy can also be diagnostic but does not allow visualization beyond the stricture unless esophageal balloon dilation is also performed.

Treatment with balloon catheter dilation has been the most successful. Bougienage is another, less available, technique. It theoretically causes more shear stress on the esophagus but has not been shown to have a significantly different complication rate than balloon dilation. Some cases can require multiple dilation procedures. Esophageal stents have been used in strictures that have been refractory to dilation procedures. However, this method has been limited by a high rate of complications, including stent migration, stent shortening, stent breakage, recurrence of stricture, infection, megaesophagus, overgrowth of tissue into the stent, ptyalism, apparent nausea, gagging, vomiting, regurgitation, and tracheal-esophageal fistula. Surgical resection of a single stricture is another option; however, it is less successful. These treatments are likely to induce some degree of esophagitis, which must be treated to decrease the chance of stricture reformation. The use of corticosteroids, either systemically or intralesionally, to help prevent stricture reformation is controversial. No data exist regarding the success of this adjunct therapy for esophageal strictures in dogs and cats, but intralesional use has been helpful in reducing recurrence in people.

ESOPHAGITIS

Inflammation of the esophagus is usually caused by foreign bodies, gastroesophageal reflux, and occasionally certain drugs (eg, doxycycline). Gastroesophageal reflux is usually associated with anesthesia, drugs that decrease lower esophageal sphincter tone (eg, atropine, acepromazine), and acute or chronic vomiting. Other causes of esophagitis include ingestion of an irritating or caustic substance, neoplasia, and *Spirocerca lupi* infection (*see* p 412). Feeding tubes that traverse the gastroesophageal junction may result in gastroesophageal reflux. Calicivirus in cats may also cause esophagitis.

Regurgitation is the classic sign of esophagitis; others include ptyalism, repeated swallowing attempts, pain, depression, anorexia, dysphagia, and extension of the head and neck. Mild esophagitis may have no associated clinical signs.

Endoscopy is the diagnostic tool of choice. It allows visualization of any associated problems (eg, foreign body) and direct assessment of esophageal damage. Plain radiographs are of little or no benefit in the diagnosis of esophagitis. An esophagram under fluoroscopy demonstrates any associated esophageal motility defects secondary to the esophagitis and may demonstrate esophageal wall defects if severe.

Mild esophagitis may require no treatment. If clinical signs are present, medical therapy should be instituted. Esophagitis secondary to gastroesophageal reflux is treated by decreasing gastric acidity, increasing lower esophageal sphincter tone, increasing the rate of gastric emptying, and providing pain control. In most cases, H_2-receptor antagonists (eg, ranitidine, famotidine) are sufficient to decrease gastric acid production; however, in severe cases of esophagitis, a proton pump inhibitor (eg, omeprazole) is preferred. Cisapride and metoclopramide increase lower esophageal tone and the rate of gastric emptying. Cisapride is more potent than metoclopramide. A sucralfate slurry may also be administered orally for esophageal cytoprotection. Soft food, low in fat and fiber, should be fed in small, frequent meals. Systemic analgesics may be used for pain relief.

If esophagitis is severe, a gastrostomy tube may be used to completely rest the esophagus. The administration of corticosteroids to prevent esophageal stricture formation is controversial. Broad-spectrum antibiotics should be used for concurrent aspiration pneumonia and may be useful in severe esophagitis as an attempt to prevent bacterial invasion and infection.

ESOPHAGEAL FOREIGN BODIES

Esophageal foreign bodies are more common in dogs than cats. Bones are the most common foreign body, but needles, fishhooks, wood, rawhide, and dental chew treats may also become lodged in the esophagus. Objects usually lodge in the areas of the esophagus with the least distensibility: the thoracic inlet, over the heart base, or the caudal esophagus just cranial to the diaphragm. Occasionally, an object may lodge in other locations such as the upper esophageal sphincter.

Ptyalism, gagging, dysphagia, regurgitation, and repeated attempts to swallow are signs of an esophageal foreign body. Often, the owner may see the animal eat the foreign body. The signs depend on the location of the foreign body and on the degree and duration of obstruction. A partial obstruction may allow fluids but not food to pass. With a chronic obstruction, anorexia, weight loss, and lethargy are common.

Perforation of the cervical esophagus may result in local abscessation or subcutaneous emphysema; perforation of the thoracic esophagus may result in pleuritis, mediastinitis, pyothorax, pneumothorax, bronchoesophageal fistula formation, or fatal aortic esophageal fistula formation. Esophagitis, mucosal laceration, esophageal stricture, and esophageal diverticulum formation are also potential complications. Esophageal stricture formation is the most common complication associated with an esophageal foreign body. Aspiration pneumonia may also be seen secondary to the regurgitation.

Many esophageal foreign bodies are radiopaque and can be seen on plain radiographs. A contrast esophagram or esophagoscopy is often required to identify radiolucent foreign bodies. If a perforation is suspected, an iodinated contrast medium should be used instead of barium suspensions. Esophagoscopy permits evaluation of both the foreign body and the esophageal wall and often allows therapeutic intervention.

Esophageal foreign bodies, once diagnosed, should be removed immediately. Most often, a foreign body can be removed per os with a flexible endoscope and forceps. A rigid endoscope can also be used if a flexible scope is not available, but care must be taken when manipulating the scope in the esophagus to prevent lacerations or perforations. If the foreign body is smooth, a Foley catheter can be inserted distal to the foreign body, inflated, then removed orally, bringing the foreign body with it. A large endotracheal tube can be placed over the endoscope to remove sharp foreign bodies such as fish hooks, which can be drawn up into the endotracheal tube and removed without damaging the esophagus on the way out. If a foreign body cannot be removed per os, it may be pushed into the stomach where it can either be digested (eg, bones), passed, or removed via a gastrotomy. Surgery is indicated if a perforation has occurred or the foreign body cannot be removed via endoscopy; in one study, the recovery rate was 93% after surgery. However, there is potential for stricture formation and complications secondary to the poor wound-healing ability of the esophagus. Esophagitis, if present, should be treated appropriately (*see* above).

ESOPHAGEAL DIVERTICULA

Diverticula are pouch-like dilatations of the esophageal wall and may be congenital or acquired. They are rare in dogs and cats. Acquired diverticula are of two types: pulsion or traction. **Pulsion diverticula** are caused by increased intraluminal pressure or deep esophageal inflammation, which can lead to mucosal herniation. Predisposing conditions include esophagitis, esophageal stricture, foreign bodies, vascular ring anomalies, megaesophagus, and hiatal hernia. This type of diverticulum involves the esophageal epithelium and connective tissue. **Traction diverticula** result from inflammation in the chest cavity in close proximity to the esophagus. Fibrous tissue is produced, which then contracts, pulling the esophageal wall outward. This diverticulum involves all layers of the esophagus.

Small diverticula may be subclinical. Large diverticula allow food to become trapped in the pouch, leading to postprandial dyspnea, regurgitation, and anorexia. Survey radiographs may show the diverticulum if it is full of ingesta or air, but contrast radiographs are best to demonstrate the pouch. Endoscopy will also allow visualization and can identify ulceration and scarring.

Small diverticula may be treated with a bland, soft diet fed with the animal in an upright position. Large diverticula require surgical excision and reconstruction of the esophageal wall. The prognosis after surgery is fair to good.

BRONCHOESOPHAGEAL FISTULA

Bronchoesophageal fistulas are rarely seen in dogs and cats. They most commonly develop secondary to foreign body penetration of the esophagus. Fistulas may develop between the esophagus and any part of the respiratory tree. A congenital form has been described, and Cairn Terriers may be predisposed. The most common clinical sign is coughing after eating or drinking. Regurgitation may also be seen, and anorexia, fever, and lethargy may be related to pneumonia.

Survey radiographs may reveal a radiopaque foreign body and pneumonia. Contrast esophagrams will show the communication between the esophagus and airways. Use of a small amount of barium is recommended—iodinated contrast agents are hyperosmolar and can cause pulmonary edema.

Surgical correction consisting of a lung lobectomy and repair of the defect in the esophagus is required. The prognosis after surgery is good.

DISEASES OF THE STOMACH AND INTESTINES IN SMALL ANIMALS

CANINE PARVOVIRUS

Etiology and Pathophysiology:

Canine parvovirus (CPV) is a highly contagious and relatively common cause of acute, infectious GI illness in young dogs. Although its exact origin is unknown, it is believed to have arisen from feline panleukopenia virus or a related parvovirus of nondomestic animals. It is a nonenveloped, single-stranded DNA virus, resistant to many common detergents and disinfectants, as well as to changes in temperature and pH. Infectious CPV can persist indoors at room temperature for at least 2 mo; outdoors, if protected from sunlight and desiccation, it can persist for many months and possibly years. In North America, clinical disease is largely attributed to CPV-2b; however, infection with a newer and equally virulent strain, CPV-2c, is increasingly common, having been identified in at least 15 states. To date, no association has been identified between CPV strain and severity of clinical disease.

Young (6 wk to 6 mo), unvaccinated or incompletely vaccinated dogs are most susceptible. Rottweilers, Doberman Pinschers, American Pit Bull Terriers, English Springer Spaniels, and German Shepherds have been described to be at increased risk of disease. Assuming sufficient colostrum ingestion, puppies born to a dam with CPV antibodies are protected from infection for the first few weeks of life; however, susceptibility to infection increases as maternally acquired antibody wanes. Stress (eg, from weaning, overcrowding, malnutrition, etc), concurrent intestinal parasitism, or enteric pathogen infection (eg, *Clostridium* spp, *Campylobacter* spp, *Salmonella* spp, *Giardia* spp, coronavirus) have been associated with more severe clinical illness. Among dogs >6 mo old, intact male dogs are more likely than intact female dogs to develop CPV enteritis.

Virus is shed in the feces of infected dogs within 4–5 days of exposure (often before clinical signs develop), throughout the period of illness, and for ~10 days after clinical recovery. Infection is acquired through direct oral or nasal contact with virus-containing feces or indirectly through contact with virus-contaminated fomites (eg, environment, personnel, equipment). Viral replication occurs initially in the lymphoid tissue of the oropharynx, with systemic illness resulting for subsequent hematogenous dissemination. CPV preferentially infects and destroys rapidly dividing cells of the small-intestinal crypt epithelium, lymphopoietic tissue, and bone marrow. Destruction of the intestinal crypt epithelium results in epithelial necrosis, villous atrophy, impaired absorptive capacity, and disrupted gut barrier function, with the potential for bacterial translocation and bacteremia.

Lymphopenia and neutropenia develop secondary to destruction of hematopoietic progenitor cells in the bone marrow and lymphopoietic tissues (eg, thymus, lymph nodes, etc) and are further exacerbated by an increased systemic demand for leukocytes. Infection in utero or in pups <8 wk old or born to unvaccinated dams without naturally occurring antibodies can result in myocardial infection, necrosis, and myocarditis. Myocarditis, presenting as acute cardiopulmonary failure or delayed, progressive cardiac failure, can be seen with or without signs of enteritis. However, CPV-2 myocarditis is infrequent, because most bitches have CPV antibodies from immunization or natural exposure.

Clinical Findings: Clinical signs of parvoviral enteritis generally develop within 5–7 days of infection but can range from 2–14 days. Initial clinical signs may be nonspecific (eg, lethargy, anorexia, fever) with progression to vomiting and hemorrhagic small-bowel diarrhea within 24–48 hr. Physical examination findings can include depression, fever, dehydration, and intestinal loops that are dilated and fluid filled. Abdominal pain warrants further investigation to exclude the potential complication of intussusception. Severely affected animals may present collapsed with prolonged capillary refill time, poor pulse quality, tachycardia, and hypothermia—signs potentially consistent with septic shock. Although CPV-associated leukoencephalomalacia has been reported, CNS signs are more commonly attributable to hypoglycemia, sepsis, or acid-base and electrolyte abnormalities. Inapparent or subclinical infection is common.

Lesions: Gross necropsy lesions can include a thickened and discolored intestinal wall; watery, mucoid, or hemorrhagic intestinal contents; edema and congestion of abdominal and thoracic lymph nodes; thymic atrophy; and, in the case of CPV myocarditis, pale streaks in the myocardium. Histologically, intestinal lesions are characterized by multifocal necrosis of the crypt epithelium, loss of crypt architecture, and villous blunting and sloughing. Depletion of lymphoid tissue and cortical lymphocytes (Peyer's patches, peripheral lymph nodes, mesenteric lymph nodes, thymus, spleen) and bone marrow hypoplasia are also seen. Pulmonary edema, alveolitis, and bacterial colonization of the lungs and liver may be seen in dogs that died of complicating acute respiratory distress syndrome, systemic inflammatory response syndrome, endotoxemia, or septicemia.

Diagnosis: CPV enteritis should be suspected in any young, unvaccinated, or incompletely vaccinated dog with relevant clinical signs, especially those living in or newly acquired from a shelter or breeding kennel. During the course of the illness, most dogs develop a moderate to severe leukopenia characterized by lymphopenia and neutropenia. Leukopenia, lymphopenia, and the absence of a band neutrophil response within 24 hr of starting treatment has been associated with a poor prognosis. Prerenal azotemia, hypoalbuminemia (GI protein loss), hyponatremia, hypokalemia, hypochloremia, and hypoglycemia (due to inadequate glycogen stores in young puppies and/or sepsis, potentially a poor prognostic indicator), and increased liver enzyme activities may be noted on the serum biochemical profile. Commercial ELISAs for detection of antigen in feces are widely available and have good to excellent sensitivity and specificity, even for the more recently evolved CPV-2c strain. All animals with relevant clinical signs should be immediately tested, so appropriate isolation procedures can be initiated. Most clinically ill dogs shed large quantities of virus in the feces. However, false-negative results can be seen early in the course of the disease (before peak viral shedding), because of the dilutional effect of large volume diarrhea, or after the rapid decline in viral shedding that tends to occur within 10–12 days of infection. False-positive results can be seen within 4–10 days of vaccination with modified-live CPV vaccine. Alternative ways to detect CPV antigen in feces include PCR testing, electron microscopy, and virus isolation. Serodiagnosis of CPV infection requires demonstration of a 4-fold increase in serum IgG titer throughout a 14-day period or detection of IgM antibodies in the absence of recent (within 4 wk) vaccination.

Treatment and Prognosis: The main goals of treatment for CPV enteritis include restoration of fluid, electrolyte, and metabolic abnormalities and prevention of secondary bacterial infection. In the absence of significant vomiting, oral electrolyte solutions can be offered. Administration SC of an isotonic balanced electrolyte solution may be sufficient to correct mild fluid deficits (<5%) but is insufficient for dogs with moderate to severe dehydration. Most dogs will benefit from IV fluid therapy with a balanced electrolyte solution. Correcting dehydration, replacing ongoing fluid losses, and providing maintenance fluid needs are essential for effective treatment. Dogs must be monitored for development of hypokalemia and hypoglycemia. If electrolytes and serum blood glucose concentration cannot be routinely monitored, empirical supplementation of IV fluids with potassium (potassium chloride 20–40 mEq/L) and dextrose (2.5%–5%) is appropriate.

If GI protein loss is severe (albumin <20 g/L, total protein <40 g/L, evidence of peripheral edema, ascites, pleural effusion, etc), colloid therapy should be considered. Nonprotein colloids (eg, pentastarch, hetastarch) can be administered in boluses (5 mL/kg, maximum of 20 mL/kg) throughout at least 15 min. The remainder of the maximal dosage of 20 mL/kg can be administered as a constant-rate infusion throughout 24 hr, and the volume of crystalloids administered decreased by 40%–60%. Alternatively, transfusion of fresh frozen plasma may partially replace serum albumin while providing serum protease inhibitors to counter the systemic inflammatory response. There is no evidence to support the use of serum from dogs recovered from CPV-enteritis (convalescent or hyperimmune serum) as a means of passive immunization.

Antibiotics are indicated because of the risk of bacterial translocation across the disrupted intestinal epithelium and the likelihood of concurrent neutropenia. A β-lactam antibiotic (eg, ampicillin or cefazolin [22 mg/kg, IV, tid]) will provide appropriate gram-positive and anaerobic coverage. For severe clinical signs and/or marked neutropenia, additional gram-negative coverage (eg, enrofloxacin [5 mg/kg/day, IM or IV] or gentamicin [6 mg/kg/day, IV]) is indicated. Aminoglycoside antibiotics must not be administered until dehydration has been corrected and fluid therapy established. Enrofloxacin has been associated with articular cartilage damage in rapidly growing dogs 2–8 mo old and should be discontinued if joint pain or swelling develops. Second- or third-generation cephalosporins (eg, cefoxitin, ceftazidime, cefovecin, others) can also be considered for their relatively wide spectrum of activity against gram-positive and gram-negative bacteria.

Antiemetic therapy is indicated if vomiting is protracted, perpetuates dehydration and electrolyte abnormalities, or limits oral administration of medications and nutritional support. α-Adrenergic antagonists (eg, prochlorperazine, 0.1–0.5 mg/kg, SC, tid) can worsen hypotension in hypovolemic animals, whereas prokinetic agents (eg, metoclopramide, 0.3 mg/kg, PO or SC, tid, or 1–2 mg/kg/day as a constant-rate infusion) may increase the risk of intussusception; use of either agent should be restricted to dogs that are rehydrated and being appropriately monitored. In dogs with CPV enteritis, maropitant (1 mg/kg/day, IV) and ondansetron (0.5 mg/kg, IV, tid) appear to be equally effective at controlling vomiting, although maropitant may be associated with an improved ability to maintain body weight during illness. Vomiting may persist despite antiemetic administration. Antidiarrheals are not recommended, because retention of intestinal contents within a compromised gut increases the risk of bacterial translocation and systemic complications. A successful protocol for outpatient treatment of dogs with parvoviral enteritits, consisting of maropitant (1 mg/kg/day, SC), cefovecin (8 mg/kg, SC, every 14 days), and SC crystalloid fluids (tid), has been described.

Previous anecdotal recommendations for nutritional management of CPV enteritis included withholding food and water until cessation of vomiting. However, evidence suggests early enteral nutrition is associated with earlier clinical improvement, weight gain, and improved gut barrier function. For anorectic dogs, placement of a nasoesophageal or nasogastric tube for continual feeding of a prepared liquid diet (eg, Clinicare®, or dilute, blended canned diet) should be instituted within 12 hr of hospital admission. Once vomiting has subsided for 12–24 hr, gradual reintroduction of water and a bland, low-fat, easily digestible commercial or homemade (eg, boiled chicken or low-fat cottage cheese and rice) diet is recommended. Partial or total parenteral nutrition is reserved for dogs with anorexia >3 days that cannot tolerate enteral feeding.

Oseltamivir is an antiviral agent, usually used to treat influenza virus infections in people. In a single published study of naturally occurring CPV enteritis in dogs, treatment with oseltamivir (2 mg/kg, PO, bid for 5 days) did not decrease duration of hospitalization, clinical disease severity, or mortality. However, treated dogs did not experience weight loss or a decrease in WBC count, as were observed in untreated control dogs. The potential for induction of drug resistance to human or avian influenza viruses has led some to question the appropriateness of oseltamivir administration to animals. Other adjunctive treatments such as recombinant human granulocyte colony-stimulating factor, recombinant bactericidal/permeability-increasing protein, and feline interferon-ω have not been shown to be beneficial.

Intussusception, bacterial colonization of IV catheters, thrombosis, urinary tract infection, septicemia, endotoxemia, acute respiratory distress syndrome, and sudden death are potential complications of CPV enteritis. Most puppies that survive the first 3–4 days of illness make a full recovery, usually within 1 wk. With appropriate supportive care, 68%–92% of dogs with CPV enteritis will survive. Dogs that recover develop longterm, possibly lifelong immunity.

Prevention and Control: To limit environmental contamination and spread to other susceptible animals, dogs with confirmed or suspected CPV enteritis must be handled with strict isolation procedures (eg, isolation housing, gowning and gloving of personnel, frequent and thorough cleaning, footbaths, etc). All surfaces should be cleaned of gross organic matter and then disinfected with a solution of dilute bleach (1:30) or a peroxygen, potassium peroxymonosulfate, or accelerated hydrogen peroxide disinfectant. The same solutions may be used as footbaths to disinfect footwear.

To prevent and control CPV, vaccination with a modified-live vaccine is recommended at 6–8, 10–12, and 14–16 wk of age, followed by a booster administered 1 yr later and then every 3 yr. Because of potential damage by CPV to myocardial or cerebellar cells, inactivated rather than modified-live vaccines are indicated in pregnant dogs or colostrum-deprived puppies vaccinated before 6–8 wk of age. It has been suggested that the presence of maternally acquired CPV antibodies may interfere with the effectiveness of vaccination in puppies <8–10 wk old. However, current modified-live CPV vaccines are sufficiently immunogenic to protect puppies from infection in the presence of low levels of interfering maternal antibody, and vaccination of 4-wk-old puppies with a high antigen titer vaccine results in seroconversion and may decrease the window of susceptibility to infection. Current vaccine products protect similarly well against CPV-2 as against other strains of the virus.

As described above, CPV can remain viable in the environment for an extended period. In a kennel, shelter, or hospital situation, cages and equipment should be cleaned, disinfected, and dried twice before reuse. The same concepts can be applied to a home situation. Removal of contaminated organic material is important in outdoor situations where complete disinfection is not practical. Disinfectants can be applied outdoors with spray hoses, but disinfection will be less effective than when applied to clean, indoor surfaces. In a home situation, only fully vaccinated puppies (at 6, 8, and 12 wk) or fully vaccinated adult dogs should be introduced into the home of a dog recently diagnosed with CPV enteritis. Booster vaccination of in-contact healthy dogs that are up-to-date on parvovirus vaccination is reasonable but potentially unnecessary given the extended duration of immunity to CPV.

COLITIS

The colon helps maintain fluid and electrolyte balance and absorb nutrients; it is also the major site of fecal storage until expulsion and provides an environment for microorganisms. Disruptions to normal colonic function lead to changes in both absorption and motility; clinically, this often manifests as large-bowel diarrhea. Approximately one-third of dogs with a history of chronic diarrhea have colitis. Chronic colitis is defined as inflammation of the colon that is present for ≥2 wk. Inflammation of the colon reduces the amount of water and electrolytes absorbed and changes colonic motility by suppressing the normal colonic contractions that mix and knead and by stimulating giant migrating contractions (ie, more powerful contractions that rapidly propel intestinal contents). Colitis has been classified into four forms: lymphocytic-plasmacytic, eosinophilic, neutrophilic, and granulomatous. Lymphocytic-plasmacytic is the most common form in both dogs and cats. Most dogs are middle-aged, and there is no sex predilection. There may be an association between colitis and perianal fistula, especially in German Shepherds. Cats with chronic colitis tend to be middle-aged and more commonly purebred. Typically, there is an increased number of lymphocytes and plasmocytes in the lamina propria (less frequently in the submucosa and muscularis).

Eosinophilic colitis is characterized by an increased number of eosinophils in the lamina propria. It is less common than lymphocytic-plasmacytic colitis, the animals tend to be younger, and it is more difficult to treat. Infectious agents, parasites, and food allergies may be inciting factors, but none has been proved. The CBC may reveal eosinophilia. Hypereosinophilic syndrome in cats is a variant of eosinophilic enteritis with eosinophilic involvement not only of the bowel but also of the liver, spleen, mesenteric lymph nodes, kidney, adrenal glands, and heart.

Granulomatous colitis (GC) is a rare, breed-specific inflammatory bowel disease of young Boxer dogs. It is seen as a segmental, thickened, partially obstructed segment of bowel (ileum and colon most commonly), characterized by the presence of macrophages and other inflammatory cells within the lamina propria. These macrophages are not periodic acid-schiff positive. Because of the histologic characteristics, it is important to exclude inflammation secondary to fungal disease, intestinal parasites, feline infectious peritonitis, and foreign material. Treatment remains controversial. Although surgery was previously recommended because GC was refractory to medical treatment and associated with high mortality rates, recent research using culture-independent molecular analysis has shown a correlation between GC and *Escherichia coli* invasion within colonic mucosal macrophages. Current treatment recommendations for GC require antimicrobials effective against *E coli* and that penetrate intracellularly, such as enrofloxacin.

Etiology and Pathophysiology:

Inflammation of the colon may be acute or chronic. In most cases, the inciting factors are unknown. Bacterial, parasitic, fungal, traumatic, uremic, and allergic causes have been postulated. Inflammation may be the result of a defect in mucosal immunoregulation. After initial mucosal injury, submucosal lymphocytes and macrophages become exposed to luminal antigens and subsequently trigger inflammation. An exaggerated reaction to dietary or bacterial factors within the lumen of the bowel, genetic predisposition, psychologic pathology affecting the neurologic or vascular supply to the colon, or sequelae of previous infectious or parasitic disease have also been implicated.

In acute colitis, there is mucosal infiltration with neutrophils and epithelial disruption and ulceration. Chronic colitis is most often characterized by mucosal infiltration of plasma cells and lymphocytes, fibrosis, and sometimes ulceration. Goblet cells are stimulated to secrete excessive quantities of mucus. Absorption of water and electrolytes is impaired, and motility is reduced. Inflammation disrupts intracellular tight junctions and reduces the transmucosal electrical potential difference, interrupting the ability of the colon to absorb sodium. Normal segmentation is inhibited; giant migrating muscular contractions proceed down the length of the colon and rapidly expel luminal contents. The inflamed bowel is more sensitive to stretch, and contents entering the colon stimulate strong migrating muscular contractions, an urge to defecate, and abdominal discomfort.

Fructooligosaccharides (FOSs) enhance colonic microflora and assist in the prevention and treatment of colonic disease. These complex carbohydrates are not digested in the small intestine. They are fermented by specific colonic bacteria that use them as an energy source. FOSs promote the growth of beneficial bacteria and inhibit growth of potentially harmful bacteria. They are responsible for the production of short-chain fatty acids (SCFAs).

SCFAs (acetate, propionate, butyrate) are an important energy source essential for maintenance of normal mucosal health. They help maintain intestinal motility and ameliorate intestinal inflammation. Alteration of fatty acids leads to mucosal atrophy and injury.

Clinical Findings: The most common clinical sign of chronic colitis is large-bowel diarrhea, characterized by mucus, hematochezia, tenesmus, and occasionally pain when defecating. There is often an increased urgency and frequency of defecation, with decreased fecal volume per bowel movement. Weight loss and vomiting can occur but are uncommon; they are seen more often when small intestine is involved. Clinical signs may wax and wane. Initially, the clinical signs may be sporadic, but progression usually occurs. Physical examination is unremarkable in most cases. A thorough rectal examination may reveal rectal polyps or malignant neoplasms that can mimic signs of chronic colitis.

Diagnosis: The initial approach should include a complete history and physical examination, including rectal palpation and evaluation of feces. Fecal smears for *Giardia* and fungal elements (*Histoplasma capsulatum*, *Pythium insidiosum*), fecal flotation for parasite identification (*Trichuris vulpis* in dogs, *Tritrichomonas foetus* in cats), and culture for bacteria (*Campylobacter*, *Salmonella*, *Clostridium*) are suggested in cases of chronic colitis. Rectal cytology is an important tool to exclude other causes of large-bowel diarrhea. It can reveal inflammatory cells, neoplastic cells, and certain infectious agents (eg, *H capsulatum*). Cases of suspected clostridial colitis (>5 endospores per field) should be confirmed by identifying *Clostridium perfringens* enterotoxin A and B in feces using a commercially available ELISA after a fecal bacterial culture is performed.

A dietary trial is recommended before pursuing more advanced diagnostics. If clinical signs persist, a CBC, biochemical profile, and urinalysis should be performed to exclude other diseases; however, in most cases of chronic colitis, the results are normal. For cats, feline leukemia virus/feline immunodeficiency virus testing is also recommended as well as a thyroid level if age appropriate. Routine abdominal radiographs are also usually normal. Contrast radiographs may occasionally demonstrate intraluminal narrowing, which could indicate an infiltrative disease process. Ultrasonography allows the visualization of colonic mucosa, localized lesions, and the size and echogenicity of lymph nodes.

Colonoscopy is indicated to visually inspect the mucosal surface of the colon and to obtain biopsy specimens. Preparation of the colon is essential to avoid missing small or subtle lesions because of residual fecal material on the mucosal surface. Food should be withheld for 24–48 hr before the procedure, followed by a combination of enemas and an oral colonic lavage solution. Several agents can be used to clean the bowel, such as sodium picosulfate and bisacodyl. Multiple samples from the cecum and ascending, transverse, and descending colon should be obtained, regardless of gross morphologic appearance. Because of poor correlation between gross appearance and histopathologic results, results should be interpreted in light of the physical examination and history. A normal mucosal biopsy or one with evidence of a hyperplastic mucosa, in conjunction with clinical signs supportive of large-intestinal diarrhea, is compatible with irritable bowel syndrome. Peripheral eosinophilia is invariably present in cats with hypereosinophilic syndrome.

Treatment and Control: If possible, the inciting cause should be identified and eliminated. Food should be withheld for an initial 24–48 hr in animals with acute colitis in an effort to "rest" the bowel.

Because shedding of ova by whipworms is intermittent, therapeutic deworming (eg, fenbendazole 50 mg/kg/day, for 3 days, repeated in 3 wk and again in 3 mo if there is a positive response) should be done even if results of fecal examinations are negative.

Supplementing the diet with fiber (1–6 tsp of psyllium hydrophilic mucilloid or 1–4 tbsp of coarse wheat bran/feeding) improves diarrhea in many animals. Dietary fiber reduces free fecal water, prolongs luminal transit time (increasing the opportunity to absorb water), absorbs toxins, increases fecal bulk and stretches the colonic smooth muscle, and improves contractility. However, the addition of fiber alone rarely results in complete resolution of clinical signs of large-intestinal diarrhea in dogs, and beneficial effects may take as long as 6 wk to become evident. Over time, the fiber dose can be reduced or eliminated in some dogs and a standard dog food substituted without causing a return of the diarrhea.

Novel protein diets have effectively controlled clinical signs of colitis in both dogs and cats. The protein source used should be one to which the animal has not previously been exposed. In one study, clinical signs associated with lymphocytic-plasmacytic colitis resolved in all dogs within ~2 wk after feeding a low-residue, digestible, hypoallergenic diet (1 part low-fat cottage cheese and 2 parts boiled white rice). Thereafter, most dogs were maintained without recurrence of clinical signs on commercially available prescription diets they had not been previously fed. Currently, a number of commercially available diets contain rice with mutton or lamb, venison, or rabbit.

Hydrolyzed diets have also been effective in treatment of colitis. These specialized diets disrupt the protein structure sufficiently to remove any allergens and allergenic epitopes and, therefore, prevent immune recognition.

If feeding a high-fiber or novel protein diet is not beneficial, a commercial, low-residue diet may be tried, especially one that contains FOSs.

Cats with lymphocytic-plasmacytic colitis may respond to dietary management alone (eg, lamb and rice, horsemeat, or a commercially available diet). In one study, cats were initially treated with dietary fiber or with dietary fiber and pharmacologic intervention (prednisone, tylosin, or sulfasalazine). Most cats were eventually maintained on high-fiber diets or a highly digestible diet.

Metronidazole is considered one of the primary pharmacologic agents in chronic colitis in cats. Its therapeutic effects include antiprotozoal and antimicrobial activity and inhibition of some aspects of cell-mediated immunity. It is not usually used as a sole agent but rather in combination with either dietary management or another drug. Although metronidazole is well tolerated in both dogs and cats, adverse effects can occur (mostly neurologic, eg, nystagmus, ataxia, vestibular signs, seizures), either with chronic therapy or at high dosages. However, neurotoxicoses should be reversible within 5–7 days after treatment is discontinued.

Tylosin, a macrolide antibiotic used primarily in food animals, is useful in chronic enteropathies, because it interferes with bacterial adhesion to the mucosa and has some antibacterial and immunomodulating effects. It targets mainly facultative and obligate anaerobic gram-positive bacteria and some gram-negative bacteria. However, *E coli* and *Salmonella* are resistant to tylosin. Tylosin is well tolerated in both dogs and cats with minimal effects.

Clinical signs resolve more rapidly when anti-inflammatory medication is given, along with the change in diet. Sulfasalazine, prednisone or prednisolone, and azathioprine are used most commonly. Sulfasalazine is often used to treat lymphocytic-plasmacytic colitis in dogs (12.5 mg/kg, qid for 14 days, then 12.5 mg/kg, bid for 28 days). Longterm use is discouraged, because it predisposes to keratoconjunctivitis sicca. Sulfasalazine is a prostaglandin synthetase inhibitor and has antileukotriene activity. It consists of mesalamine linked to sulfapyridine in an azochemical bond; this linkage prevents absorption in the upper GI tract and allows most of the drugs to be transported to the large intestine. Once it has reached the large intestine, it is metabolized by cecal and colonic bacteria, releasing both components. Mesalamine acts locally to reduce colonic mucosal inflammation. Sulfapyridine is believed to be systemically absorbed and therefore does not have any local therapeutic effect in colitis but is blamed for the adverse effects of sulfasalazine. Salicylates are metabolized in the liver by hepatic enzymatic processes involving glucuronyl transferase. Because cats are deficient in this enzymatic pathway, salicylates have prolonged half-lives in this species. Therefore, sulfasalazine is not used as the drug of choice in colitis in cats because of the risk of salicylate toxicity.

Glucocorticoids, in combination with dietary management and metronidazole, are the treatment of choice for chronic colitis in cats. They may be introduced into the therapeutic plan for dogs when the previously discussed therapies are not successful or if the 5-aminosalicylates result in adverse effects. If used in combination with sulfasalazine or metronidazole, prednisone may be given at a reduced dosage. Prednisone should be started at 2 mg/kg/day, PO; for 2 wk after clinical signs resolve, the dosage should be reduced by 25% every 2–4 wk, which can usually maintain remission.

Cats usually tolerate glucocorticoids very well; adverse effects are common in dogs and include polyuria, polydipsia, polyphagia, GI bleeding, increased susceptibility to infection, iatrogenic hyperadrenocorticism, and pituitary-adrenocortical suppression.

Budesonide is a nonhalogenated glucocorticoid used in treatment of Crohn's disease in people. Budesonide undergoes significant first-pass metabolism in the liver; theoretically, this should reduce the adverse effects often seen with traditional glucocorticoids, because little of the active drug is systemically available. In one study of 10 healthy dogs, the pituitary-adrenocortical axis was suppressed, but no other adverse effects were seen.

Immunosuppressive drugs are mostly used in combination with glucocorticoids when the response is not satisfactory with the latter alone. The most commonly used are azathioprine and chlorambucil in dogs and cats. Azathioprine (2 mg/kg/day, and then tapered), alone or in combination with prednisone, has been used to control clinical signs associated with lymphocytic-plasmacytic colitis. Azathioprine may be considered in cases that are poorly responsive to prednisone or to prednisone with sulfasalazine. The serious adverse effects of azathioprine in cats (myelosuppression and hepatotoxicity) limit its use in feline colitis. Instead, chlorambucil (0.1–0.2 mg/kg or 1 mg/cat, daily initially until clinical signs are markedly improved, which may require 4–8 wk) is used in cats in combination with prednisone if needed.

Cyclosporine has been effective in steroid-refractory cases of colitis, but it has not been evaluated in cats. Adverse effects include GI disturbances, gingival disease, and alopecia.

Some animals also require short-term use of motility modifiers until inflammation is controlled. Loperamide (0.1–0.2 mg/kg, bid-qid) stimulates segmental activity and slows passage of fecal contents. It also decreases colonic secretion, enhances salt and water absorption, and increases anal sphincter tone. It is contraindicated in cases of infectious colitis (eg, caused by *Salmonella, Campylobacter*, or *Clostridium*).

Prognosis: The short-term prognosis for chronic colitis is good for both dogs and cats. However, longterm prognosis for complete resolution without relapses appears poor. Most cases of inflammatory bowel disease are not curable, and some form of treatment will likely be necessary longterm. For some animals, especially cats, longterm management of chronic colitis may be possible with diet alone.

Most cases of idiopathic lymphocytic-plasmacytic colitis respond to appropriate dietary and medical changes. Stricture formation and extensive fibrosis warrant a more guarded prognosis. Eosinophilic colitis in dogs responds favorably to controlled diets and glucocorticoid therapy. In cats, the prognosis is more guarded, and more aggressive treatment with immunosuppressive agents is required. Hypereosinophilic syndrome is a progressive, fatal disease that has no effective treatment in animals.

Histiocytic colitis of Boxers carries a grave prognosis unless treatment is started early in the course of the disease. The immunoproliferative enteropathy of Basenjis also carries a poor prognosis; most dogs die within 2 yr of diagnosis, although some have been reported to live as long as 5 yr. Similarly, the prognosis for the diarrheal syndrome reported in Lundehunds is also poor.

CONSTIPATION AND OBSTIPATION

Constipation is the infrequent or difficult evacuation of feces, which are typically dry and hard. Constipation is a common clinical problem in small animals. In most instances, the problem is easily rectified; however, in more debilitated animals, accompanying clinical signs can be severe. As feces remain in the colon longer, they become drier, harder, and more difficult to pass. Obstipation is intractable constipation characterized by an inability to evacuate the mass of dry, hard feces; impaction extending from the rectum to the ileocolic valve can result. Megacolon is a pathologic condition of hypomotility and dilation of the large intestine that results in constipation and obstipation.

Etiology and Pathophysiology: Peristaltic waves are responsible for the aboral movement of fecal material in the colon. Giant migrating waves that occur intermittently throughout the day move this matter farther and more rapidly. These waves constitute the "gastrocolic reflex" and are common after ingestion of a meal. A reduction or loss of these waves may contribute to constipation. Similarly, an increase in segmentation wave activity may predispose to constipation. However, diet is the most important local factor affecting colonic function.

Chronic constipation may be due to intraluminal, extraluminal, or intrinsic (ie, neuromuscular) factors. Intraluminal obstruction is most common and is due to the inability to pass poorly digested, often firm matter (eg, hair, bones, litter) mixed with fecal material. The lack of water intake or the reluctance to defecate on a regular basis because of environmental (eg, stress) or behavioral (eg, dirty litter box) factors or painful anorectal disease predisposes to formation of hard, dry feces. Intraluminal tumors may also impede the passage of feces. Extraluminal obstruction may be caused by compression of the colon or rectum from a narrowed pelvic inlet after suboptimal healing of pelvic fractures or from enlarged sublumbar lymph nodes or prostate gland. Colonic stricture due to trauma or neoplasia should also be considered. Finally, some animals (usually cats) with chronic constipation or obstipation may have megacolon, likely caused by a lesion of the neuromuscular bed of the colon. The etiology of megacolon often remains undiagnosed. Other diseases that affect neuromuscular control of the colon and rectum include hypothyroidism, dysautonomia, and lesions of the spinal cord (eg, Manx sacral spinal cord deformity) or pelvic nerves. Hypokalemia and hypercalcemia also adversely affect muscular control. Some drugs (eg, opioids, diuretics, antihistamines, anticholinergic agents, sucralfate, aluminum hydroxide, potassium bromide, and calcium channel-blocking agents) promote constipation via differing mechanisms.

Clinical Findings: The classic clinical signs of constipation are tenesmus and the passage of firm, dry feces. If the passage of feces is hindered by an enlarged prostate or sublumbar lymph nodes, the feces may appear thin or "ribbon-like" in appearance. Abdominal palpation and rectal examination can confirm the presence of large volumes of retained fecal matter. Passed feces are often putrid. Some animals are quite ill and also have lethargy, depression, anorexia, vomiting (especially cats), and abdominal discomfort.

Diagnosis: A history of dietary indiscretion and physical evidence of retained feces confirms the diagnosis. Detailed information regarding the duration of constipation and influencing factors may help determine the cause, as will a history of ingestion of indigestible material that may increase fecal bulk or cause pain that can terminate the defecation reflex. Other historical factors that may be relevant include recent surgery, previous pelvic trauma, and possibly radiation therapy. A complete neurologic examination with special emphasis on caudal spinal cord function should be performed to identify neurologic causes of constipation, eg, spinal cord injury, pelvic nerve trauma, and Manx sacral spinal cord deformity.

Abdominal palpation and rectal examination, including evaluation of the prostate and sublumbar lymph nodes, should be performed to determine the presence of perineal hernia, foreign material, pain, or masses. Plain abdominal radiographs may help establish the inciting factor(s) of fecal retention and give some indication of what the feces contain (eg, bones). A barium enema, ultrasonography, or colonoscopy may facilitate demonstration of obstructive lesions or predisposing causes of chronic constipation.

A CBC, biochemical profile including a serum T_4 level, urinalysis, and detailed neurologic examination should be completed in cases of chronic or recurring constipation.

Treatment and Control: Affected animals should be adequately hydrated. Mild constipation can often be treated by dietary adjustment consisting of avoidance of dietary indiscretion, ready access to water and high-fiber diets, and use of suppository laxatives. Continued or longterm use of laxatives should be discouraged unless absolutely necessary to avoid constipation.

A number of pediatric rectal suppositories are available for management of mild constipation. They include dioctyl sodium sulfosuccinate (DSS; emollient laxative), glycerin (lubricant laxative), and bisacodyl (stimulant laxative). The use of suppositories requires a compliant pet and a willing owner. Suppositories can be used alone or in conjunction with oral laxative therapy.

Mild to moderate or recurrent episodes of constipation may require administration of enemas or manual extraction of impacted feces, or both. Types of enemas include warm tap water (5–10 mL/kg), warm isotonic saline (5–10 mL/kg) with or without a mild soap to act as an irritant, DSS (5–10 mL/cat), mineral oil (5–10 mL/cat), or lactulose (5–10 mL/cat). Enema solutions should be administered slowly with a 10–12 French rubber catheter or feeding tube.

Phosphate-containing enemas must be avoided in cats.

If enemas are unsuccessful, manual extraction of impacted feces may be needed. After adequate rehydration, the animal should be anesthetized with an endotracheal tube in place to prevent aspiration in case the colonic manipulation induces vomiting. Complete removal of all feces may require 2–3 attempts over as many days. Concurrent fluid and electrolyte abnormalities should also be corrected.

Laxatives are classified as bulk-forming, lubricant, emollient, osmotic, or stimulant types. Most act on fluid transport mechanisms and colonic motor stimulation. They should be avoided in the presence of dehydration. Bulk-forming laxatives are added to the diet. These products are dietary fiber supplements of poorly digestible polysaccharides and celluloses derived principally from cereal grains, wheat bran, and psyllium. They absorb water, soften feces, add bulk, stretch the colonic smooth muscle, and improve contractility. Many constipated cats respond to dietary supplementation with one of these products. Dietary fiber is preferable because it is well tolerated, more effective, and more physiologic than other laxatives. Commercial fiber-supplemented diets are available, or the pet owner may add psyllium (1–4 tsp/meal), wheat bran (1–2 tbsp/meal), or pumpkin (1–4 tbsp/meal) to canned food. Animals should be well hydrated before starting fiber supplementation to minimize the potential for impaction of fiber in the constipated colon.

Emollient laxatives are anionic detergents that increase the miscibility of water and lipids in digesta, thereby enhancing lipid absorption and impairing water absorption. DSS and disoctyl calcium sulfosuccinate are emollient laxatives available in oral and enema form. Docusate sodium (cats: 50-mg capsule/day; dogs: 50-mg capsule, 1–4/day) and docusate calcium (cats: 50-mg capsule, 1–2/day; dogs: 50-mg capsule, 2–3/day) are other examples of emollient laxatives.

Mineral oil and white petroleum are lubricant laxatives that impede colonic water absorption and permit greater ease of fecal passage. These effects are moderate, and lubricant laxatives are beneficial only in mild cases of constipation. Mineral oil use should be limited to rectal administration because of the risk of aspiration pneumonia with oral administration.

Hyperosmotic laxatives consist of poorly absorbed polysaccharides (eg, lactulose, 0.5 mL/kg, PO, bid-tid), magnesium salts (eg, magnesium citrate, magnesium hydroxide, magnesium sulfate), and the polyethylene glycols. Lactulose is the most effective agent of this group. The organic acids produced from lactulose fermentation stimulate colonic fluid secretion and propulsive motility. Lactulose osmotically retains water in the bowel to soften fecal material. It is also useful in management of hepatic encephalopathy because it decreases luminal pH, reduces bacterial production of ammonia, and favors formation of ammonium ions that are poorly absorbed. Stimulant laxative products (eg, bisacodyl [cats and small dogs: 5 mg; medium-sized dogs: 10 mg; large dogs: 15–20 mg]) increase the propulsive activity of the bowel. They are contraindicated in the presence of bowel obstruction.

Colonic prokinetic agents (eg, cisapride) enhance colonic propulsive motility by activating colonic smooth muscle 5-hydroxytryptamine-2A receptors in a number of species. Anecdotal experience suggest that cisapride (0.1–0.5 mg/kg, PO, bid-tid) effectively stimulates colonic propulsive motility in cats with mild to moderate idiopathic constipation. Higher dosages (up to 1 mg/kg) may be necessary in cats with moderate to severe constipation. No significant adverse effects have been reported in cats treated with cisapride at dosages of 0.1–1 mg/kg, PO, bid-tid). Cats with longstanding obstipation and megacolon are not likely to improve with cisapride therapy.

Ranitidine and nizatidine, H_2-receptor antagonists, are reported to stimulate colonic motility by inhibiting acetylcholinesterase. They stimulate motility by increasing the amount of acetylcholine available to bind smooth muscle muscarinic cholinergic receptors.

To prevent recurrence, high-fiber diets are recommended, ready access to water should be maintained, and frequent opportunities to defecate allowed.

Cases of simple intraluminal obstruction due to dietary indiscretion respond well to bowel evacuation and prevention of this habit in the future. Chronic constipation unresponsive to medical management (eg, some cats with megacolon) may respond to subtotal or total colectomy. Colectomy with colocolonic, ileocolonic, or jejunocolonic anastomosis may be performed depending on the extent of the disease. Mild to moderate diarrhea may occasionally persist for weeks to months after surgery, and some cats may have recurrent constipation. Pelvic osteotomy without colectomy has been recommended for cats with pelvic fracture malunion and hypertrophic megacolon of <6 mo duration. In such cases, pathologic hypertrophy may be reversible with early pelvic osteotomy. Subtotal colectomy is recommended in cats with pelvic fractures if hypertrophy and clinical signs have persisted for >6 mo. In these cases, hypertrophy is followed by muscular degeneration and pathologic dilatation, and pelvic osteotomy alone will not provide relief from obstipation.

FELINE ENTERIC CORONAVIRUS

Feline enteric coronavirus (FECV) is an enveloped, single-stranded RNA virus that is highly prevalent in domestic cat populations worldwide. Infection is often subclinical or characterized by transient, mild GI illness in kittens. Mutation of FECV to a biotype capable of infection and replication within macrophages is responsible for development of feline infectious peritonitis (FIP), a highly fatal, multisystemic disease (*see* p 780).

Etiology and Pathophysiology: Fecal shedding of FECV begins within 1 wk of initial infection and persists at high levels for 2–10 mo, followed by an extended period (up to 24 mo) of lower level, potentially intermittent, viral shedding. At least 13% of infected cats shed the virus indefinitely.

Cats become infected through ingestion or inhalation of virus-containing feces or through contact with contaminated fomites (eg, litter boxes, mutual grooming, housing, personnel). FECV is relatively fragile but can survive in dry environments for up to 7 wk. Close contact between cats (eg, catteries and multicat households) facilitates transmission. Vertical transmission from infected queens to kittens does occur. Kittens generally do not begin to shed virus before 9–10 wk of age, although viral shedding as early as 4 wk of age has been reported. Soon after infection, virus may replicate in oropharyngeal tissue, resulting in transient (hours to days) salivary shedding. FECV infects and replicates in mature apical epithelial cells of the intestinal villi, causing brush border shortening and destruction.

Clinical Findings: Most FECV infections are clinically inapparent or characterized by mild, self-limiting gastroenteritis. Occasionally, vomiting and diarrhea can be acute and severe or chronic and unresponsive to treatment. Although diarrhea is the most common clinical sign of infection in kittens, upper respiratory tract signs have also been reported.

Diagnosis: The viral DNA can be detected in feces by reverse transcriptase PCR (RT-PCR). Because chronic carriers of FECV tend to be asymptomatic, FECV can be assumed to be the cause of the diarrhea only after other causes (eg, infectious, dietary, inflammatory bowel disease, neoplasia, etc) have been excluded. The clinical utility of serologic evaluation for antibodies to FECV is questionable. Positive coronavirus antibody titers are detected in up to 40% of pet cats and in up to 90% of cats in catteries or multicat households. Positive FECV antibody titers are indicative only of exposure to the virus and are not suggestive of the etiology of the current disease, do not correlate with the risk of developing FIP, and are not diagnostic for FIP. Histologic lesions suggestive of FECV enteritis include intestinal villous fusion, atrophy, or sloughing. Because these lesions are nonspecific, definitive diagnosis requires immunohistochemical or immunofluorescent detection of viral antigen in intestinal epithelial cells.

Treatment, Control, and Prevention: The mild, transient clinical signs are unlikely to require therapy. Treatment, if required, is symptomatic and supportive (ie, fluid therapy, oral electrolyte solutions, antiemetics). There is no specific antiviral therapy. Death due to the FECV-associated gastroenteritis is uncommon.

Control and prevention of FECV are usually a concern only in breeding catteries and rescue shelters. Ingestion of virus-contaminated fecal particles should be prevented as much as possible. Fecal contamination of the environment can be minimized with sufficient litter box numbers, daily litter box cleaning, weekly litter box disinfection, and clipping/cleaning fur from the hind end of long-haired cats. FECV can survive indoors for up to 7 wk under dry conditions but is readily inactivated by most commercial disinfectants.

Ideally, cats should be housed in small (three or four cats), closed groups. The room, cages, bedding, and litter boxes should be disinfected between groups. Although impractical in a shelter situation, cats should be housed in groups according to their antibody (immunofluorescent antibody test seropositive or seronegative) and virus shedding (based on fecal PCR) status. Seropositive cats can be retested every 3–6 mo and moved into seronegative groups as their antibody titer decreases. In a rescue or shelter situation, cats should be housed singly. Identification of FECV carrier cats requires nine monthly, consecutive positive fecal RT-PCR tests, whereas identification of a cat that has eliminated FECV infection requires five consecutive negative fecal RT-PCR tests.

Seropositive cats should be mated only to other seropositive cats, and seronegative cats to other seronegative cats. Kittens born of seropositive matings or to a seropositive queen are protected from infection by maternally derived immunity until ~6 wk of age. Kittens weaned from seropositive queens by 6 wk of age are unlikely to acquire infection from the queen. Serologic testing of kittens should be delayed until 10–11 wk of age, by which time seroconversion is likely.

New cats should be serologically tested before introduction into a cattery or breeding program. Only seronegative and virus-free (fecal PCR) cats should be introduced into an FECV-free cattery or a cattery attempting to eliminate the virus. Seropositive cats are less likely to develop FIP than seronegative cats when introduced to an FECV-endemic environment. Vaccination with an intranasal, temperature-sensitive FECV mutant is not generally recommended but can be considered in seronegative cats >16 wk old introduced into an FECV-endemic environment. Vaccination will lead to seroconversion and does not completely protect cats previously exposed to FECV from developing FIP.

GASTRIC DILATION AND VOLVULUS

(Bloat)

Gastric dilation and volvulus (GDV) is an acute, life-threatening condition that primarily affects large- and giant-breed dogs. Immediate medical and surgical intervention is required to optimize chance of survival.

Etiology and Pathophysiology: The etiology of GDV is unknown, but several phenotypic and environmental risk factors have been identified for developing GDV. Breeds at risk of GDV include the Great Dane, German Shepherd, Irish Setter, Gordon Setter, Weimaraner, Saint Bernard, *Standard Poodle*, and Bassett Hound. No sex predisposition exists, and dogs appear to be at increased risk with advancing age. Other reported predisposing factors include lean body condition, deep/narrow thoracic conformation, a first-degree relative with a history of GDV, stress, aggressive or fearful behavior, once daily feeding, dry food, rapid consumption of food, previous splenic disease, and increased gastric ligament laxity.

It is unclear whether dilation or volvulus occurs first during the development of GDV, although it is postulated that volvulus occurs first. Dilation of the stomach results from accumulation of gas and/or fluid, and volvulus prevents the normal release of these contents. During volvulus, the pylorus and duodenum first migrate ventrally and cranially. Viewed from a caudal to cranial direction, the stomach may rotate from 90° to 360° in a clockwise fashion about the distal esophagus. This rotation displaces the pylorus to the left of midline, entrapping the duodenum between the distal esophagus and the stomach. Depending on the degree of volvulus, the spleen may vary in position from the left caudodorsal to the right craniodorsal abdomen. A volvulus of >180° causes occlusion of the distal esophagus.

After volvulus of the stomach, gas is trapped within this compartment and intragastric pressure rises. Gastric outflow obstruction may be caused by compression of the duodenum by the distending stomach against the body wall, or it may be due to the presence of neoplasia, a gastric foreign body, or pyloric stenosis. Splenic entrapment often accompanies GDV. The progressively distending stomach compromises venous return by compression of the caudal vena cava. Sequestration of blood in the dilated splanchnic, renal, and posterior muscular capillary beds results in portal hypotension, GI tract ischemia, hypovolemia, and systemic hypotension. These factors combine with the loss of fluid in the obstructed stomach and a lack of water intake to produce signs of hypovolemic shock. Dogs are at risk of endotoxemia, hypoxemia, metabolic acidosis, and disseminated intravascular coagulation.

Clinical Findings: Dogs may present with a history of nonproductive retching, hypersalivation, and restlessness. Acute or progressive abdominal distention may be noted, or the affected dog may be found recumbent and depressed with an enlarged abdomen.

Physical examination findings include an enlarged or tympanic abdomen. Abdominal pain and/or splenomegaly may be appreciated on abdominal palpation. Progression from gastric dilation to volvulus predisposes to hypovolemic shock. Signs of shock are common and can include weak peripheral pulses, tachycardia, prolonged capillary refill time, pale mucous membranes, and dyspnea. An irregular heart rate and pulse deficits indicate the presence of a cardiac arrhythmia. Additionally, the expanding stomach may compress the thoracic cavity and inhibit diaphragmatic movement, leading to respiratory distress.

Diagnosis: Suspicion of GDV is usually high after considering the history, signalment, and clinical signs. Radiographs help distinguish simple gastric dilation from GDV. The preferred radiographic views for identification of GDV are right lateral and dorsoventral recumbency. Ventrodorsal positioning must be avoided because of the potential for aspiration of gastric contents.

The right lateral radiograph usually reveals a large, distended, gas-filled gastric shadow with the pylorus located dorsal and slightly cranial to the fundus. The gastric shadow is frequently compartmentalized or divided by a soft-tissue "shelf" between the pylorus and fundus. This shelf, or reverse "C" sign, is created by the folding of the pyloric antral wall onto the fundic wall. Splenic enlargement or malposition may be noted on radiographs. Gas within the gastric wall is suggestive of tissue compromise, whereas free gas within the abdomen indicates gastric rupture.

PCV, total solids, electrolytes, blood glucose, and serum lactate levels should be evaluated, and blood drawn for a CBC, serum biochemical profile, and coagulation assays. Continuous ECG and blood pressure monitoring are recommended.

Prerenal azotemia is a common finding in animals with GDV and is secondary to systemic hypotension. Increased CK levels may be present due to striated muscle damage, and serum potassium levels may increase subsequent to cell membrane damage. Serum ALT and AST levels may increase secondary to hypoxic damage. Increased lactate is a common finding and is secondary to systemic hypotension and inflammation. Hyperlactatemia (>6 mmol/L) is associated with an increased likelihood of gastric necrosis and the need for partial gastric resection.

Treatment: Immediate goals in treatment of GDV include restoring circulating volume and gastric decompression. Rapid surgical correction of the volvulus follows initial patient stabilization. Because duration of clinical signs is one of the risk factors of GDV-associated death, it is imperative to recognize and correct this condition immediately.

Correction of hypovolemia is the first treatment priority and is achieved by rapid fluid replacement with one or more large bore (16- to 18-gauge) IV catheters placed in cranial (jugular, cephalic) veins. Shock rate (90 mL/kg/hr) fluid therapy with crystalloids should begin immediately. Fluid therapy with combinations of crystalloids, colloids (eg, hetastarch at a rate of 10–20 mL/kg, IV), or hypertonic saline (eg, 7% hypertonic saline solution with dextran 70 at a rate of 5 mL/kg over 15 min) can be considered for animals in severe shock, and the rate of crystalloid fluid infusion reduced by as much as 40% if these products are used. These fluid rates are guidelines only, and fluid resuscitation choices must be tailored to the individual patient's needs. Flow-by oxygen should be provided during stabilization. Electrolyte and acid-base disturbances are usually corrected by adequate fluid therapy and gastric decompression. Because of the potential risk of endotoxemia and GI translocation of bacteria, antibiotics (eg, ampicillin 22 mg/kg, tid-qid, and continued for 2–3 days after surgery) are often given.

Gastric decompression occurs concurrently with fluid resuscitation. Initial decompression attempts should be made with an orogastric tube, which can be performed after sedation with fentanyl (2–5 mcg/kg, IV) or hydromorphone (0.05–0.1 mg/kg, IV), with or without diazepam (0.25–0.5 mg/kg, IV). Agents that cause vasodilation (eg, phenothiazines) should be avoided. A stomach tube is measured from the incisors to the last rib and marked. The tube must not be placed beyond this marking. The lubricated tube is introduced into the mouth (often held open with a roll of tape or bandage material) while the dog is in a sitting position. Some resistance is typically encountered at the esophageal-gastric sphincter. Gentle manipulation and counterclockwise movement of the tube may be necessary to allow passage of the tube into the stomach, but caution must be exercised because it is possible to perforate the esophagus with the tube. Once the tube enters the stomach, gastric gas rapidly escapes. Successful passage of a stomach tube does not exclude the presence of volvulus. After gas and stomach contents are released from the stomach via the tube, the stomach should be lavaged with warm water to decrease the rate of redilation with gas.

If an orogastric tube cannot be readily passed, percutaneous gastrocentesis may be performed to release excess gastric gas.

An area (10 cm × 10 cm) over the right abdominal wall caudal to the last rib and ventral to the transverse vertebral process is clipped and aseptically prepared. Percussion of the area should reveal tympany; this helps avoid accidental puncture of an overlying spleen. If a tympanic structure is not appreciated, the left paracostal region should be assessed. A large-bore needle or over-the-needle catheter is introduced through the skin and body wall into the stomach at the site of greatest tympany. Decompression usually allows for subsequent passage of an orogastric tube and lavage of the stomach.

Surgical correction of GDV rapidly follows the initial stabilization. Aseptic preparation of the abdomen is performed before surgery, and a cranioventral midline approach is performed. Before correcting the gastric torsion, the stomach should be decompressed with the help of an assistant placing an orogastric tube or via gastrocentesis intraoperatively. The stomach is then returned to its normal position, and the stomach and spleen are evaluated for ischemia. Any areas of ischemic gastric wall are removed, and a splenectomy is performed if necessary. Extensive gastric necrosis and necrosis of the gastric cardia are considered poor prognostic indicators. The stomach is emptied of contents, and a gastropexy is performed to decrease risk of recurrence. Several gastropexy techniques have been described and include a simple incisional pexy, a circumcostal (belt-loop) pexy, and a tube gastrotomy and pexy.

Pre-, intra-, and postoperative monitoring should include continuous ECG, intermittent blood pressure measurement, and frequent assessment of vital parameters, PCV, total solids, electrolytes, blood glucose, and serum lactate.

Postoperative medical management includes IV fluid therapy and analgesia. Food should be withheld for 48 hr after surgery. Antiemetic agents (metoclopramide at 0.2–0.5 mg/kg, SC, or 1–2 mg/kg/day, constant-rate IV infusion; maropitant at 1 mg/kg/day, SC) may be administered in cases of continued vomiting. Postoperative cardiac arrhythmias are common, but treatment is often not indicated. Criteria to initiate antiarrhythmic therapy include signs of persistent tachycardia (>140 bpm), hypotension (systolic blood pressure <90 mmHg), hypoperfusion (prolonged capillary refill time, weak pulses), "R on T wave" pattern (a phenomenon that predisposes to ventricular fibrillation), or multifocal ventricular premature contractions. A bolus of 2% lidocaine (2–4 mg/kg, slowly IV) can be administered and repeated twice in a 30-min period if necessary; a continuous IV infusion (30–80 mcg/kg/min) may be indicated to control arrhythmias. Cardiac arrhythmias associated with GDV are often difficult to control. If the arrhythmia is poorly responsive to this therapy, procainamide (6–10 mg/kg, IV over 15 min) should be given. Life-threatening arrhythmias may respond to 20% magnesium sulfate (0.15–0.3 mEq/kg, or 12.5–35 mg/kg, IV over 15–60 min).

Less common postoperative complications can include life-threatening conditions such as sepsis, peritonitis, and disseminated intravascular coagulation.

Overall mortality rate associated with GDV is ~25%–30%. Risk factors associated with short-term death from GDV include duration of clinical signs >6 hr before examination, performing splenectomy and a partial gastrectomy, hypotension at any time during hospitalization, peritonitis, sepsis, and disseminated intravascular coagulation. Preoperative plasma lactate concentration has been shown to be a good predictor of gastric necrosis and a negative prognostic indicator for outcome for dogs with GDV.

Prophylactic gastropexy is currently being recommended by many veterinary surgeons for breeds at risk or for dogs with relatives that have been affected by GDV. Prophylactic gastropexy can be performed at the time of sterilization surgeries (spay/neuter). Minimally invasive techniques such as laparoscopic-assisted gastropexy are gaining favor. Prophylactic gastropexy has not been shown to prevent development of GDV if performed at the time of neuter but has been shown to help prevent recurrence if performed at the time of the first GDV correction. However, in one study of five large dog breeds predisposed to GDV, mortality was reduced (versus no gastropexy) ranging from 2.2-fold (Rottweiler) to 29.6-fold (Great Dane). A prospective study reported a median survival time of 547 days in dogs that underwent gastropexy versus 188 days for dogs that did not. Owners of breeds at high risk of GDV should be educated about the risk factors for and signs of GDV, and advised to seek immediate veterinary care if clinical signs are apparent. Additional precautions include avoiding stress, feeding multiple rather than single daily meals, avoiding exercise immediately after feeding, and not using elevated food dishes.

GASTRITIS

Gastritis is a general term used to describe a syndrome of acute or chronic vomiting secondary to inflammation of the gastric mucosa. Irritation, infection, antigenic stimulation, or injury (eg, chemical, erosion, ulceration) of the gastric mucosa stimulates the release of inflammatory and vasoactive mediators with subsequent disruption of gastric epithelial cells, increased gastric acid secretion, and impaired gastric barrier function. Visceral receptors sensitive to gastric distention, gastric inflammation, and tonicity of gastric contents send impulses via vagal and sympathetic nerves to the vomiting center of the medulla oblongata, thereby stimulating the vomiting reflex.

Acute Gastritis: In acute gastritis, vomiting of sudden onset is presumed or confirmed to be secondary to inflammation of the gastric mucosa. Causes include dietary indiscretion or intolerance (eg, ingestion of novel, spoiled, or contaminated foods, or of foreign material), drug or toxin ingestion (eg, antibiotics, NSAIDs, corticosteroids, plants, chemicals), systemic illness (eg, pancreatitis, uremic gastropathy, hypoadrenocorticism), endoparasitism (eg, *Physaloptera* sp [dog], *Ollulanus* sp [cat]), or bacterial (eg, *Helicobacter*-associated disease) or viral (eg, canine parvovirus gastroenteritis, feline panleukopenia) infection. Vomiting of sudden onset is characteristic. The vomitus may contain bile, food, froth, blood (frank or digested), or evidence of an ingested substance (eg, grass, bones, foreign material, etc). Additional clinical signs depend on the severity and frequency of vomiting as well as on the underlying cause.

Diagnosis is usually based on a thorough history, clinical findings, and response to symptomatic treatment. A specific diagnosis should be sought if the animal has had access to foreign objects or toxins, if clinical signs do not resolve within 2 days of symptomatic therapy, if hematemesis or melena are present, if the animal is systemically unwell, or if abnormalities are noted on abdominal palpation. Dogs may signal the presence of cranial abdominal discomfort by adopting a "praying" posture (hindquarters raised and chest and forelegs held close to floor), which seems to provide some sense of relief. A CBC, serum biochemical profile, and urinalysis may be followed by more specific clinicopathologic testing (eg, basal serum cortisol concentration, adrenocorticotropic hormone [ACTH] stimulation test, evaluation of vomitus for specific toxins). Diagnostic imaging, including plain and/or barium contrast abdominal radiographs and abdominal ultrasound, may be indicated.

Treatment of acute gastritis is generally symptomatic and supportive. Small amounts of oral fluids can be given frequently, with the volume increasing as vomiting subsides. Ice (crushed or cubes) can be provided as the only source of water initially. Subcutaneous administration of an isotonic balanced electrolyte solution may be sufficient to correct mild fluid deficits (<5%). If dehydration is moderate to severe or the clinical condition of the animal warrants IV fluid therapy, a more extensive diagnostic evaluation is indicated. If vomiting is acute, oral intake should be discontinued for ≥24 hr. Small amounts of a bland, low-fat, easily digestible diet (eg, boiled lean beef, chicken, or cottage cheese and rice, or a commercially available prescription diet) fed frequently can be introduced, with gradual transition to the usual diet over 3–5 days.

Antiemetic drugs should be used to control vomiting only after an etiologic diagnosis has been made or if vomiting is protracted or severe enough to cause dehydration or electrolyte imbalances. Metoclopramide (0.3 mg/kg, PO or SC, tid, or 1–2 mg/kg/day as a constant-rate infusion) increases gastric contractions; relaxes the pyloric sphincter; and increases gastric, duodenal, and proximal jejunal peristalsis. It is contraindicated in confirmed or suspected GI obstructions. Alternative antiemetics include maropitant (1 mg/kg/day, SC, or 2 mg/kg/day, PO, for 5 days) and ondansetron (0.1–1 mg/kg, PO, once to twice daily). Gastroprotectants such as H_2-receptor antagonists (eg, famotidine 0.5–1 mg/kg, PO, SC, or IV, bid) or proton pump inhibitors (eg, omeprazole 0.7–2 mg/kg/day, PO, or pantoprazole 1 mg/kg/day, IV) may also be indicated. In dogs, omeprazole may provide better gastric acid suppression and better prevention of exercise-induced gastritis than famotidine.

Chronic Gastritis: Chronic gastritis should be considered in animals with intermittent or persistent vomiting that lasts >7 days and that cannot be attributed to dietary indiscretion or intolerance; drug, toxin, or foreign body ingestion; systemic illness; endoparasitism; infection (bacterial or viral); or neoplasia. The most common clinical sign is intermittent vomiting of food or bile. Systemic illness, weight loss, and GI ulceration are infrequent and should raise suspicion of a more serious condition or diffuse GI inflammation (eg, inflammatory bowel disease, pythiosis, etc).

Histologic evaluation of endoscopic or surgical gastric biopsies is required for definitive diagnosis and classification of chronic gastritis. A CBC, serum biochemical profile, urinalysis, total thyroid hormone concentration (cats), basal serum cortisol concentration possibly with an ACTH-stimulation test (to exclude canine hypoadrenocorticism), and fecal evaluation for endoparasitism are indicated but are frequently unremarkable in animals with chronic gastritis. Diagnostic imaging (plain and/or barium contrast abdominal radiographs, abdominal ultrasound) can identify foreign objects, neoplasia, pyloric stenosis, gastric antral mucosal hypertrophy, discrete or multifocal mucosal or mural abnormalities, intra-abdominal lymphadenomegaly, or other intra-abdominal pathology, and is indicated before gastric biopsy.

Lymphocytic-plasmacytic gastritis and **eosinophilic gastritis** are characterized by diffuse infiltration of the gastric mucosa and lamina propria with lymphocytes and plasma cells, or eosinophils, respectively. Similar cellular infiltrates may be seen in the small intestine. Concomitant lymphoid hyperplasia, mucosal atrophy, or mucosal fibrosis is infrequently seen. Dietary allergy or intolerance, occult parasitism, or hyperimmune response to normal antigens have been proposed as possible causes. Eosinophilic gastritis with eosinophilia and/or skin lesions should raise suspicion for dietary sensitivity or hypereosinophilic syndrome (cats).

Animals with mild clinical signs and mild histologic lesions may respond to symptomatic care (*see* p 387), empirical deworming, and exclusive feeding of a hypoallergenic or novel protein diet (eg, balanced homemade diet or many commercially available options). In addition to symptomatic care, empirical deworming, and dietary modification, animals with moderate to severe, histologically confirmed disease generally require immunosuppressive therapy. Prednisone (or prednisolone in cats) is started at 2 mg/kg/day, PO (dogs), or 2–4 mg/kg/day, PO (cats), and tapered to the lowest dosage that controls clinical signs. Assuming continued clinical remission, prednisone therapy is ultimately discontinued and strict adherence to dietary therapy maintained. If clinical signs persist despite gastroprotectant therapy, dietary modification, and prednisone therapy, treatment with an additional immunosuppressive agent (dogs: azathioprine 2 mg/kg, PO, every 24–48 hr; cats >4 kg: chlorambucil 2 mg [total dose], PO, every 48 hr for 2–4 wk then tapered to 2 mg every 72–96 hr; cats <4 kg: chlorambucil 2 mg [total dose] every 72 hr; dogs and cats: cyclosporine 3–5 mg/kg/day, PO) can be considered.

Chronic atrophic gastritis is often characterized by marked mononuclear cell infiltration, thinning of the gastric mucosa, and atrophy of the gastric glands. A unique, breed-associated form of atrophic gastritis in Norwegian Lundehunds has not been associated with *Helicobacter* spp infection but has been associated with gastric adenocarcinoma. The role, if any, of *Helicobacter* spp infection in the development of atrophic gastritis is unknown. However, if *Helicobacter* spp organisms are identified in gastric biopsy specimens, treatment is indicated (*see* p 394). Additional treatment options include dietary management and immunosuppression as for lymphocytic-plasmacytic and eosinophilic gastritis (*see* above); however, data with respect to treatment efficacy and prognosis are lacking.

Chronic hypertrophic gastropathy is characterized by diffuse or focal hypertrophy of the gastric mucosa, muscularis, or both, with variable inflammatory infiltrates. The lesion is often most pronounced in the pyloric region, with resultant gastric outflow obstruction. Projectile vomiting of food within hours of eating may be described. Older, male, small-breed dogs are overrepresented (eg, Lhasa Apso, Shih Tzu, Maltese, Miniature Poodle). Hypergastrinemia due to exaggerated secretion (eg, gastrin-secreting neoplasia, Basenji gastroenteropathy) or inadequate clearance (eg, hepatic or renal disease, achlorhydria) may initiate mucosal hypertrophy. Surgical correction via pyloroplasty and/or removal of hypertrophied tissue may be required to alleviate clinical signs.

GASTROINTESTINAL NEOPLASIA

GI neoplasia is uncommon in dogs and cats, with gastric tumors representing <1% and intestinal tumors <10% of overall neoplasia in these species. GI neoplasms tend to be malignant. The average age of dogs with GI neoplasia is 6–9 yr and of cats 10–12 yr.

Etiology and Pathophysiology: Specific etiologic agents for GI neoplasia have not been identified. The increased risk of Belgian Shepherds for gastric carcinoma, and of Siamese cats for intestinal adenocarcinoma and lymphoma may reflect genetic predispositions. Feline leukemia has been suggested to be an underlying factor in development of feline GI lymphoma, even in cats with a negative retroviral status.

Helicobacter infections are associated with gastric neoplasia in people, but similar direct links have not been established in dogs or cats.

Adenocarcinomas are the most common GI neoplasia in dogs and are typically found in the duodenum, colon, and rectum. Gastric adenocarcinomas are common in dogs and frequently affect the lower 1/3 of the stomach (eg, lesser curvature and pyloric region). Adenocarcinoma is commonly identified in the feline intestinal tract, especially in the jejunum and ileum. Adenocarcinomas are very aggressive and frequently metastasize to regional lymph nodes, liver, and lung. At the time of diagnosis in dogs, as many as 44% of intestinal and as many as 95% of gastric adenocarcinomas have metastasized. Adenomas and carcinomas in situ are uncommonly found in the GI tract of dogs or cats. These polyp-like masses are usually solitary and located in the colon or rectum in dogs.

Lymphoma is the most common feline GI neoplasia, and it is also common in dogs. GI lymphoma most commonly affects the small intestine as well as extra-gastrointestinal organs such as the liver. Two subtypes of feline GI lymphoma have been reported: a low-grade, small-cell lymphocytic lymphoma and a more aggressive, poorly differentiated, large-cell, lymphoblastic lymphoma. Canine GI lymphoma is usually poorly differentiated and aggressive, similar to lymphoblastic lymphoma in cats.

GI stromal tumors (GISTs) are mesenchymal in origin in dogs; they are rarely seen in cats. One of the major diagnostic criteria for GISTs include positive c-kit (CD117) reaction on immunohistochemistry. Before the recognition of GISTs, many of these tumors were likely classified as leiomyosarcomas. GISTs typically are found in the cecum and large intestine. In contrast, leiomyosarcomas are most common in the stomach and small intestine. The metastatic rate is as high as 30% with leiomyosarcomas and likely lower with GISTs. Uncommon GI tumors of dogs and cats include mast cell tumors, leiomyomas and leiomyosarcomas, fibrosarcomas, and plasmacytomas.

Clinical Findings: Clinical signs of GI neoplasia depend on the location and extent of the tumor and its possible metastases or paraneoplastic syndromes (eg, hypercalcemia, hypoglycemia). The most common clinical signs associated with GI neoplasia include vomiting (with or without blood), anorexia, weight loss, diarrhea, and lethargy. Signs of constipation or tenesmus may accompany colonic and rectal tumors. An abdominal mass or organomegaly may be palpable on physical examination. Abdominal pain and ascites may reflect peritonitis secondary to a ruptured portion of neoplastic bowel.

Diagnosis: Routine laboratory studies and plain radiographs do not show specific changes associated with GI neoplasia. Hypoglycemia is often associated with leiomyomas/leiomyosarcomas. Hypercholesterolemia and increased alkaline phosphatase activity has been seen in some nonlymphomatous neoplasia. Microcytic anemia with or without hypoproteinemia is a common finding with ulcerated masses and chronic blood loss. Electrolyte and acid-base disturbances may reflect ongoing vomiting and can include hypochloremia, hypokalemia, and metabolic alkalosis or acidosis. Paraneoplastic hypercalcemia has been associated with lymphoma and intestinal adenocarcinoma.

Contrast abdominal radiographs may reveal mass lesions in the GI tract or areas of ulceration. Abdominal ultrasonography may reveal focal or diffuse thickening of the GI tract and loss of normal layering. Regional lymph nodes may be enlarged, and splenomegaly and/or hepatomegaly may accompany some cases of GI lymphoma. Ultrasound can facilitate fine-needle aspirates or needle biopsy sample collection for cytologic or histologic analysis.

Endoscopy of the upper and lower GI tract can facilitate identification and partial-thickness biopsy of GI neoplasia. However, endoscopic biopsy collection is limited by the small size and superficial nature of the biopsy, because some GI tumors are submucosal and this technique may only collect superficial mucosa. A false diagnosis of gastritis or enteritis may reflect inflammation of the mucosa overlying a neoplastic process. In one study, endoscopic biopsies were adequate to detect feline gastric lymphoma but not adequate to differentiate inflammatory bowel disease from lymphoma in the GI tract. Recent studies suggest that endoscopic ileal biopsies aid in the diagnosis of lymphoma and other GI diseases, compared with endoscopic duodenal biopsies. Full-thickness surgical biopsies collected via laparoscopy or laparotomy may more suitably establish a diagnosis and will allow for biopsy of regional lymph nodes and liver to evaluate for metastasis. Immunohistochemistry may be required to differentiate between types of neoplasia for GI biopsies.

PCR for antigen receptor rearrangement detects clonality of a population of lymphocytes and can aid in the diagnosis of GI lymphoma when performed on inconclusive biopsy sections, especially in cats.

Treatment and Prognosis: Surgical excision of the tumor is recommended for nonmetastatic, nonlymphomatous neoplasia. Curative resection, with margins of ≥4 cm, should be attempted.

The median survival time for GI adenocarcinoma in dogs is 10–15 mo if the tumor was focal and completely resected but only 3 mo if metastasis is present at diagnosis. Adjuvant chemotherapy (eg, carboplatin) may be prescribed; optimized chemotherapy protocols for treatment of GI adenocarcinoma have not been reported. GI lymphoma is typically treated with chemotherapy. Phenotypic variations of feline GI lymphoma warrant different treatment strategies.

Small-cell (well-differentiated, low-grade) lymphoma is treated with prednisone (2 mg/kg/day, PO) and chlorambucil (either 2 mg PO every other day or 15 mg/m^2 daily for 4 days, every 3 wk). The prognosis associated with small-cell GI lymphoma is good, with a median survival time of 765 days. Poorly differentiated GI lymphoma in dogs and cats is poorly responsive to chemotherapy. If treatment is attempted, a multidrug chemotherapy protocol (eg, Wisconsin-Madison) is recommended, but complete remission rates are low, and median survival times are usually <3 mo. Focal lymphoma may be surgically excised, and follow-up chemotherapy may be recommended. GISTs and leiomyosarcomas are slow-growing and slow to metastasize. In a study of dogs with a diagnosis of either leiomyosarcoma or GIST, median survival time was 37 mo after complete resection, although another report suggests that GISTs are associated with a better survival rate than leiomyosarcomas. Malignant GI neoplasia usually has a poor prognosis (survival <6 mo), even with surgical and medical therapy. Benign lesions, such as leiomyomas and colorectal adenomas, have a good prognosis with surgical excision.

GASTROINTESTINAL OBSTRUCTION

GI obstruction often leads to intractable vomiting, the consequences of which can be life-threatening and include possible aspiration, electrolyte and acid-base disturbances, and dehydration. Depending on the underlying cause of the obstruction, the site can undergo tissue damage resulting in perforation, endotoxemia, and hypovolemic shock. Therefore, GI obstruction should be treated as an emergency.

Etiology and Pathophysiology: GI obstruction can be secondary to extraluminal, intramural, or intraluminal causes. The most common extraluminal cause of GI obstruction is intussusception, in which an invaginated segment of the GI tract becomes enveloped by an antegrade or retrograde segment. Intussusception can be secondary to endoparasitic infection, parvoviral infection, foreign body ingestion, or neoplasia, but is often idiopathic. Intestinal intussusception occurs most commonly at the ileocecocolic junction. Gastroesophageal and pylorogastric intussusceptions are uncommon, acute, severe forms of intussusception associated with a high mortality rate. German Shepherds may be predisposed to gastroesophageal intussusception. Intestinal entrapment in hernias or mesenteric rents can result in strangulation of bowel and rapid development of hypovolemic shock.

Intramural obstruction can be caused by infiltrative disease such as neoplasia, fungal infection (eg, pythiosis), and granulomas (eg, secondary to feline infectious peritonitis). Pyloric stenosis can cause gastric outflow obstruction and has been reported as a congenital condition in brachycephalic breeds. Intraluminal obstruction commonly occurs in dogs and cats secondary to ingestion of a foreign body.

Most cases of acute vomiting are not a result of GI obstruction and are self-limiting. Vomiting may be a result of dietary indiscretion, parasitic infection, bacterial or viral gastroenteritis, anxiety, or motion sickness. In these cases, treatment usually involves withholding food for a short period, feeding an easily digested diet, and offering small amounts of water frequently. Careful monitoring for persistent vomiting, depression, abdominal discomfort, and/or fever is critical. If vomiting persists, reevaluation is warranted. Abdominal palpation should be performed, looking for signs of a foreign body or abdominal discomfort. Careful examination of the oral cavity in cats, looking for evidence of yarn, thread, or needles, is important. Abdominal radiographs should be performed, looking for radiopaque foreign objects or signs of intestinal distention, indicating possible obstruction.

Obstruction secondary to foreign body ingestion can be partial or complete if the foreign body is unable to pass through the GI tract. Linear or small foreign bodies are more likely to cause partial obstruction, whereas large, round objects often result in complete obstruction. Foreign bodies are usually objects that cannot be digested (eg, plastic, rocks), are slowly digested (eg, bones), or are too large to pass through the GI tract. Some dogs are indiscriminate eaters and will consume such objects, whereas cats more typically ingest linear foreign bodies (eg, string, yarn, dental floss) while playing with them.

GI obstruction may be due to one or more foreign bodies. The decision to treat medically or proceed with surgery can be a challenge. Some small objects identified radiographically will pass through the GI tract. Passage of these objects can be monitored with serial radiographs if the animal is clinically stable. Failure of these objects to pass within 48 hr, serial radiographic evidence that the objects are not moving, or a deterioration of clinical signs necessitate surgical removal. Presence of uncooked bone matter in the stomach should be monitored but is usually resolved by normal digestive processes in the stomach.

Regardless of underlying etiology, unresolved GI obstruction leads to distention of the more proximal GI tract with fluid and gas. If entrapment of GI loops results secondary to hernias or mesenteric rents, strangulation and bowel incarceration occurs. Venous return is impaired but arterial flow maintained, leading to congestion, anoxia, and necrosis. Obstruction or strangulation of bowel can result in devitalization of the GI tissue and translocation of bacteria such as *Escherichia coli* and *Clostridium* spp from the GI lumen to the tissue. If not corrected, edema, hemorrhage, mucosal sloughing, and eventually bowel necrosis occur.

Clinical Findings: Intussusception occurs most commonly in young dogs. Intestinal intussusception typically causes signs of abdominal pain, vomiting, and diarrhea with or without blood. More proximal intussusceptions (ie, gastroesophageal, pylorogastric) result in vomiting and regurgitation.

Young cats and young, large-breed dogs are more likely to present with signs of foreign body obstruction than older animals. Clinical signs are variable, depending on duration, degree, and location of the foreign body but often include vomiting and anorexia. Vomiting is less common with distal, small-intestinal obstruction. Diarrhea, weight loss, lethargy, and signs of septic shock are less common. Physical examination may be unremarkable or may reveal signs of abdominal pain or a palpable intestinal mass. Physical examination must be thorough and include inspection of the oral cavity, because linear foreign bodies in cats may be anchored to the base of the tongue. If a linear foreign body is present in the oral cavity, it must be cut immediately and never pulled in hopes of retrieving the foreign body.

Signs of hypovolemic shock and abdominal pain usually accompany cases of intestinal incarceration.

Diagnosis: Laboratory findings associated with GI foreign bodies include leukocytosis with a mild left shift. Marked leukocytosis or leukopenia with a degenerative left shift can be present in cases of GI perforation and secondary bacterial peritonitis or sepsis. A wide variety of electrolyte and acid-base changes have been described. Proximal GI obstruction has typically been associated with hypochloremia, hypokalemia, and metabolic alkalosis, whereas more distal GI obstruction is associated with metabolic acidosis. In a study in dogs, hypochloremia and metabolic alkalosis were the two most common changes regardless of the site of GI obstruction. Hyperlactatemia and hemoconcentration (increased PCV and total solids) are also frequently identified.

Plain radiographs may assist in diagnosis of GI obstruction in cases of radiopaque foreign bodies. Complete obstruction may result in radiographic findings such as ileus and intestinal loop dilation with fluid and/or gas, whereas linear foreign bodies can create intestinal plication. These findings are not specific for GI foreign bodies, however, and can be seen with other causes of GI obstruction, including intestinal stricture, adhesions, intussusception, and neoplasia. Contrast abdominal radiographs may be useful in detection of radiolucent foreign bodies that create filling defects and in cases of intussusception. Barium is commonly used for contrast radiographs, but if GI perforation is suspected, aqueous iodine or iohexol should be used instead.

Abdominal ultrasonography can help identify the presence of GI foreign bodies and dilation of intestinal loops with fluid. Transverse sonographic views of intestinal intussusceptions often show a "target-like" lesion with concentric hyperechoic and hypoechoic rings. Large amounts of intestinal gas may obscure the ultrasound view. Signs of peritonitis and GI perforation detectable with radiographs or ultrasound include abdominal effusion or free gas. Abdominal effusion, if present, should be cytologically examined to evaluate for septic peritonitis. Endoscopic examination may help identify foreign bodies and mass lesions.

Treatment: Small, smooth foreign bodies may pass uneventfully through the GI tract. If this approach is taken, monitoring with abdominal radiographs to track the movement of the foreign body is recommended. If the foreign body is not moving, and if obstruction or worsening of clinical signs is apparent, intervention is required.

In most cases, removal of detected foreign bodies via endoscopic or surgical retrieval is recommended because of the potential for obstruction or perforation. Detection of colonic foreign bodies is often incidental, and these usually do not require removal. If a colonic foreign body is causing clinical signs, endoscopic removal is preferred over surgically opening the colon. Fluid, electrolyte, and acid-base disturbances should be corrected before anesthesia if possible.

Endoscopic or surgical retrieval of foreign bodies causing GI obstruction is associated with a high survival rate. The utility of endoscopy is typically limited to the retrieval of gastric foreign bodies. Endoscopy cannot assess the GI tract distal to the pyloric or proximal duodenal region. If endoscopy is used to retrieve a proximal GI foreign body, the scope should be passed into the small intestine as distally as possible for evaluation, with radiographs taken before recovery from anesthesia to exclude the presence of multiple foreign bodies.

An exploratory laparotomy is indicated if a foreign body distal to the pyloric region is present, if there are foreign bodies at multiple locations, if there are signs of septic peritonitis, or if endoscopy is not available. Exploratory laparotomy is also indicated over endoscopy in cases of suspected intussusception and obstruction secondary to a mass lesion. The entire GI tract must be inspected for objects that could cause obstruction. Vitality of the GI tract must also be assessed, and areas of perforation or ischemia resected. If a linear foreign body is present in the stomach and extends into the small intestine, gentle manipulation may easily free the foreign body from its distal attachments, allowing removal through the gastrotomy incision. Otherwise, multiple enterotomies may be indicated. The minimal number of enterotomies possible to remove the foreign body or bodies is recommended to help decrease the risk of postoperative dehiscence. Linear foreign bodies in cats can be particularly challenging, because the foreign material may be a single piece of thread, yarn, or dental floss that is not palpable, which makes assessment of its length difficult. Multiple solid, smooth intestinal foreign bodies can often be "milked" through the intestine and removed through one incision. Linear foreign bodies are more likely to cause GI mucosal damage and devitalization and can affect a large section of the GI tract. Devitalized or perforated areas of the GI tract must be resected, and the remaining GI tract anastomosed. Intussusceptions are manually reduced or resected, and the remaining bowel anastomosed if reduction is not possible or the bowel loop appears compromised. Laparoscopic-assisted exploration and foreign body retrieval is gaining popularity among veterinary surgeons with suitable expertise and equipment.

After foreign body retrieval, correction of fluid, electrolyte, and acid-base disturbances should continue. Peritonitis is treated with antibiotics and closed suction drains. If the animal is not vomiting, water may be offered 12 hr after anesthetic recovery. Food may be introduced 12–24 hr after recovery if there is no vomiting.

Prognosis and Prevention: Outcome for animals with GI foreign body obstruction is good if the condition is recognized and treated quickly. Animals with severe clinical signs resulting from systemic factors such as concurrent infection or debilitation, hypovolemia, and shock are at higher risk of delayed healing and incisional breakdown. Marked preoperative hypoalbuminemia (<2–2.5 g/dL) is associated with a higher rate of postoperative dehiscence. Animals presenting with signs of peritonitis or sepsis have more postoperative complications and are at higher risk of enterotomy dehiscence. Animals with signs of peritonitis, or those requiring resection of a large amount of intestine leading to short-bowel syndrome, have a guarded prognosis. Dehiscence of the intestinal surgical site most commonly occurs 3–5 days after surgery at the end of the lag phase of healing. Until this point, most tensile strength has been provided by formation of a fibrin seal that is debrided by macrophages 3–5 days after surgery. Postoperative dehiscence usually requires a second surgery and is associated with a high mortality rate.

Gastroesophageal and pylorogastric intussusceptions are associated with a high mortality rate, and rapid diagnosis and surgical intervention are essential to maximize chance of survival in these cases. GI obstruction secondary to neoplasia is uncommon, and prognosis depends on the type of neoplasia.

GASTROINTESTINAL ULCERS

Ulceration and disruption of the GI mucosal barrier can be a consequence of several drugs and diseases in small animals. As a result, gastroprotectant therapies are widely used in veterinary patients.

Etiology and Pathophysiology: The gastric mucosal barrier is a complex defense mechanism that protects the normal mucosa from the harsh chemical environment of the gastric luminal contents. The acids, pepsin, and proteolytic enzymes normally present in the gastric lumen have a pH of 2. The mucous layer provides a weak buffer, maintaining a pH of 4–6 and neutralizing the acidic luminal contents. The GI barrier is maintained by a protective layer that includes mucosal cells, tight junctions, and a thick layer of mucus. High blood flow to this area supports cellular metabolism and rapid renewal of injured cells. Prostaglandins (mainly E and I) help maintain the GI mucosal blood flow and integrity, increase secretion of mucus and bicarbonate, decrease acid secretion, and stimulate epithelial cell turnover. Tight junctions seal the cellular layers of the gastric mucosa, ensuring that the luminal contents do not leak into or around these cells. The small amount of gastric acid that diffuses into the epithelial cells is quickly cleared by the high blood flow to this area.

A defect in the GI mucosal barrier leads to a self-perpetuating cycle of mucosal damage. Injury to this barrier allows hydrochloric acid, bile acids, and proteolytic enzymes to degrade the epithelial cells, disrupt lipid membranes, and induce inflammation and apoptosis. Back diffusion of luminal contents through the tight junctions leads to inflammation and hemorrhage of the GI cells, with further acid secretion mediated by inflammatory cells and their products. Mast cell degranulation occurs, causing histamine release that perpetuates further gastric acid secretion. The inflammatory environment also causes decreases in blood flow (resulting in ischemia), ability for cellular repair, and secretion of mucus and cytoprotective prostaglandins. Mucosal ulceration can result, exposing the submucosa or deeper layers of the GI tissue to the luminal contents.

In the normal GI tract, the potential disruptive properties of the luminal contents are balanced by the defense mechanisms of the GI mucosal barrier. However, many drugs and disease have the potential to upset the balance between the harsh luminal contents and the GI protective barrier.

The incidence of GI ulceration in dogs and cats is unknown. NSAID administration, neoplasia, and hepatic disease are the most common causes in dogs. NSAIDs can cause direct topical damage to the GI mucosa, and inhibition of cyclooxygenase (COX)-1 decreases production of protective prostaglandins. The use of COX-2-specific NSAIDs is thought to decrease GI ulceration, but ulceration and perforation still occur with use of these medications. Corticosteroids potentiate the effects of mucosal damage by decreasing cell turnover and mucus production and by stimulating gastrin (and acid) production.

Hepatic disease is associated with increased gastric acid secretion and alterations in mucosal blood flow, potentially leading to ulcer formation. Primary GI neoplasia such as lymphoma, adenocarcinoma, leiomyoma, and leiomyosarcoma can result in ulceration. Additionally, paraneoplastic syndromes secondary to mast cell tumors and gastrinomas (Zollinger-Ellison syndrome) have been associated with increased gastric hydrochloric acid production and ulceration in dogs.

Other drugs and diseases associated with GI ulceration in dogs include corticosteroid use in dogs with spinal disease, renal disease, hypoadrenocorticism, stress, primary GI disease (eg, inflammatory bowel disease), extreme exercise (eg, sled dog racing), shock, and sepsis. The role of *Helicobacter* infection in GI ulceration is unknown, because *Helicobacter* organisms have been found in healthy dogs and cats.

GI ulceration is uncommonly reported in cats. Neoplasia (eg, lymphoma, adenocarcinoma) has been associated with GI ulceration in cats, but the cause is often unknown.

Clinical Findings: Specific clinical signs of GI ulceration include melena, hematemesis, and hematochezia. Abdominal pain, anorexia, and signs of underlying disease may be present. Cats with GI ulceration rarely show specific signs such as melena or hematemesis but frequently show signs of life-threatening hemorrhage. Animals with severe ulceration and/or GI perforation may present with signs of pain, weakness, pallor, and shock. Clinical signs of a causative factor may be seen. Some dogs and cats with GI ulceration do not show any clinical signs.

Diagnosis: A CBC, serum biochemistry profile, and urinalysis can help differentiate primary GI disease from non-GI disease and can identify metabolic derangements resulting from GI disease. Additional testing, such as liver function tests or an adrenocorticotropic hormone stimulation test, may be warranted depending on the clinical findings and initial test results.

Abdominal radiographs generally do not help diagnose GI ulceration, but they can help exclude GI obstruction, intussusceptions, and peritonitis. Abdominal ultrasonography may show abnormalities in GI wall thickness or presence of a mass, but its primary utility is the identification of non-GI lesions. Endoscopy allows visualization of the esophagus, stomach, duodenum, and colon and identification of mucosal lesions and ulcers. Endoscopy also allows for fine-needle aspirates of lesions or collection of biopsy samples, although full-thickness surgical biopsies may be required to identify infiltrative disease and tumors. Ulcerated areas should be biopsied only on the periphery to avoid perforation. Gastric fluid can be tested for pH to help diagnose hypersecretory states.

Treatment and Control: Primary treatment of GI ulceration is directed at the underlying cause. Supportive care may be required to correct metabolic derangements and can include fluid therapy. Medication directed at the ulcer itself reduces gastric acidity, prevents further destruction of GI mucosa, and promotes ulcer healing. In general, antiulcerative therapy should be continued for 6–8 wk.

Gastric acid production is stimulated by histamine (most potent), gastrin, and acetylcholine. Drugs that decrease acid secretion help protect damaged GI mucosa. H_2- receptor blockers (eg, cimetidine, famotidine) help promote mucosal healing, and some agents also act as prokinetics (eg, ranitidine). Famotidine (0.5–1 mg/kg, bid, PO, SC, or IV) has been shown to be more potent in reducing gastric pH than other H_2-blockers such as cimetidine or ranitidine. Proton pump inhibitors (eg, omeprazole 0.5–1 mg/kg/day, PO, or pantoprazole 0.5–1 mg/kg/day, IV) offer more complete inhibition of gastric acid secretion and are therefore useful for more severe ulcers. Prophylactic use of H_2-blockers and proton pump inhibitors to prevent GI ulceration is controversial but may be considered in animals receiving NSAIDs or that have other risk factors.

Cytoprotective agents include antacids and sucralfate. Antacids are weak bases that help neutralize gastric acid within the stomach lumen. These drugs may also promote gastric prostaglandin production. Aluminum or magnesium-containing antacids are considered the most effective agents with the fewest adverse effects, although these drugs can lead to constipation. Because of their short half-life (2–3 hr), animals may experience a rebound gastric acidity between doses, and the drugs must be given frequently. Sucralfate (dogs: 0.5–1 g, PO, bid-tid; cats: 0.25 g, PO, bid-tid) is a polyaluminum sucrose sulfate that binds to areas of eroded or ulcerated GI mucosa. Because this drug inhibits absorption, it should not be given within 1–2 hr of food or other drugs.

The prostaglandin E_2 analogue misoprostol is used to help prevent NSAID-associated ulcer formation but does not assist in mucosal healing or decrease acid secretion.

Prophylactic use of antibiotics can be considered in cases of major GI mucosal barrier disruption or shock, or in other cases when clinicopathologic signs (eg, fever, hematochezia, leukopenia, neutrophilia) suggest that bacterial translocation is of concern. First-line antibiotic therapy includes the β-lactams, with additional gram-negative coverage if necessary.

Prognosis: The prognosis for GI ulceration in dogs is favorable when the underlying cause can be treated or removed, ulceration is mild, or the condition is rapidly diagnosed and treated. Ulceration associated with severe or end-stage conditions (eg, hepatic insufficiency) is difficult to control. Mortality rates associated with GI perforation range as high as 70%.

GI ulceration in cats is often related to neoplasia. Intensive care frequently is needed because of the high prevalence of marked hemorrhage. In one report, median survival of cats with gastric ulceration treated with surgery and palliative care ranged from 12–15 mo. Cats with GI ulceration secondary to a non-neoplastic disease have less severe clinical disease and a good prognosis.

HELICOBACTER INFECTION

Helicobacter spp are commonly found in the stomachs of both healthy and vomiting dogs and cats, but their significance is not well defined. Although *H pylori* infections in people have been linked to gastritis, peptic ulcers, and a higher rate of gastric neoplasia, similar direct casual relationships between *Helicobacter* infections and GI disease have not been established in dogs and cats.

Etiology and Pathophysiology: *Helicobacter* organisms are spiral or curved, gram-negative, motile, flagellated organisms. *H pylori* is the most commonly reported species in human GI infections, but non-*H pylori* organisms (such as *H felis*, *H heilmannii*, and *H bizzozeronii*) are more common in dogs and cats. At least 38 different *Helicobacter* species have been identified in animals, and infected animals can harbor multiple species.

Helicobacter organisms have been identified most commonly in the gastric tissue of dogs and cats, especially in the fundus and cardia of the stomach, but they are also found in the intestinal tract. Colonization of gastric mucosa appears to be most prevalent in the surface mucus layer, as well as within the gastric glands and parietal cells. There have been sporadic reports of *Helicobacter* organisms identified in the hepatic tissue of a dog with multifocal necrotizing hepatitis, as well as in healthy cats and in cats with cholangiohepatitis.

Transmission of *Helicobacter* infections between groups of dogs or cats is unclear, and reservoir hosts have not been defined. Because of the increased rate of morbidity and mortality associated with *Helicobacter* infections in people, concern of zoonotic transmission has been raised (*see* below).

Clinical Findings and Diagnosis: Studies report as many as 100% of healthy dogs and cats are positive for *Helicobacter* infections; similar infection rates are reported in vomiting dogs and cats. In people, *H pylori* infection is associated with gastritis, peptic ulcers, and an increased risk of gastric neoplasia. Gastritis, vomiting, and diarrhea have been associated with *Helicobacter* infection, although a direct causal relationship has not been identified. Peptic ulceration is rarely associated with *Helicobacter* infections in dogs and cats.

Diagnosis involves upper GI endoscopy or exploratory laparotomy. Surface mucus from a large area of the stomach can be obtained by taking brush samples via endoscopy. If organisms are present, they are readily identified under 100× oil-immersion magnification. Because brush cytology samples a large area of the stomach, the sensitivity of this test is high.

Gastric biopsies should be obtained from multiple areas in the stomach, because organism distribution can be patchy. Routine H&E staining is usually sufficient to identify organisms, although special silver stains may be required if the organisms have a glandular location. Mucosal inflammation, glandular degeneration, and lymphoid follicle hyperplasia accompany some infections. Cytology and histopathology is not sufficient to identify specific species. A commercially available rapid urease test to detect production of bacterial urease in gastric biopsies can identify the presence of *Helicobacter* organisms. However, because cytology and histopathology are highly sensitive and specific for detection of *Helicobacter* infections, urease testing may not add further diagnostic information in some cases.

Noninvasive tests for *Helicobacter* infection available in the research setting include urea breath testing, fecal antigen detection, and serology.

Treatment: The lack of knowledge regarding the pathogenicity of *Helicobacter* infections in dogs and cats makes treatment decisions difficult. *H pylori* infections in people are treated with double or triple antimicrobial agent therapy plus an acid secretory inhibitor (eg, clarithromycin, amoxicillin, bismuth, and ranitidine) for 2 wk, and similar therapeutic approaches have been used in veterinary medicine.

Currently, the role of *Helicobacter* as a causative agent of gastritis in dogs and cats is unclear. Treatment decisions for dogs and cats should be based on presence of *Helicobacter*, in combination with appropriate clinical signs and/or gastric lesions. In many veterinary studies, *Helicobacter* infections have been difficult to eradicate. Recommended treatment regimens include amoxicillin or tetracycline, metronidazole, bismuth subsalicylate, and a proton pump inhibitor (eg, omeprazole) or H_2-receptor blocker (eg, famotidine) for 2–3 wk. Other treatment combinations of omeprazole and azithromycin or clarithromycin have been described. Although many dogs and cats treated with the above combinations did not experience longterm eradication of *Helicobacter* infection, when retested, the frequency of vomiting and gastric lesions did improve with therapy for many patients.

Zoonotic Risk: Zoonotic transmission of *Helicobacter* infections from dogs and cats to people is possible. *H canis*, *H felis*, *H heilmannii*, and other species naturally colonize the stomachs of dogs and cats, and these strains of *Helicobacter* have been linked to gastritis, ulcers, and lymphoma in people. Whereas many strains of *Helicobacter* in dogs and cats are genetically distinct from those implicated in human infections, at least one case report documents a genetically identical strain of *H heilmannii* infecting pet dogs and a child in the same house. Although some studies have suggested a higher risk of *Helicobacter* infection in people in contact with dogs and cats, other research refutes this. Given the unknown risk of transmission, proper hygiene practices are encouraged, and identification of infections in dogs and cats with chronic gastritis and vomiting is likely prudent.

HEMORRHAGIC GASTROENTERITIS

Hemorrhagic gastroenteritis (HGE) is a syndrome of dogs characterized by acute vomiting and hemorrhagic diarrhea, often accompanied by hemoconcentration. Young (median age 5 yr), small and toy breed dogs (Yorkshire Terrier, Miniature Pinscher, Miniature Schnauzer, Miniature Poodle, Maltese) are overrepresented. No sex predisposition has been identified.

Etiology and Pathophysiology: The precise etiology and pathogenesis are unclear, but suspicion that HGE is the result of infection with or hypersensitivity to *Clostridium perfringens* seems reasonable. *Clostridium* spp has been identified by bacterial culture or immunohistopathology in small-intestinal biopsies from dogs with HGE, suggesting an association with clostridial overgrowth. Acute intestinal mucosal hemorrhagic necrosis and neutrophilic inflammation are the predominant histologic lesions, with the most severe lesions occurring in the large intestine. Histologic mucosal lesions are not generally identified in the stomach, leading some to suggest "acute hemorrhagic diarrhea syndrome" may be a more appropriate descriptor. Leakage of fluid, plasma proteins, and RBCs into the intestinal lumen occur secondary to increased intestinal permeability.

Clinical Findings: An acute onset of profuse hemorrhagic diarrhea (often said to resemble raspberry jam) in a small or toy breed dog is characteristic of HGE. Vomiting, anorexia, lethargy, and abdominal pain are common. Vomiting may precede the onset of bloody diarrhea. Marked, peracute fluid loss can result in hypovolemic shock before clinically recognizable dehydration. Other historical findings (eg, dietary indiscretion, vaccination status, etc) are unremarkable. HGE is not considered contagious.

Diagnosis: The diagnosis is typically based on signalment and acute onset of clinical signs with hemoconcentration (PCV 55%) and normal to slightly decreased total plasma protein concentration. Selective culture for fecal pathogens (eg, *Clostridium* spp, *Salmonella* spp, *Yersinia* spp, *Clostridium* spp, *Campylobacter* spp, enterotoxigenic *Escherichia coli*, etc) and evaluation for *Clostridium* spp enterotoxin by fecal ELISA can be considered. Abnormalities on CBC are usually limited to hemoconcentration and neutrophilic leukocytosis. If neutropenia is present, sepsis and/or parvovirus enteritis may be a concern. Serum biochemical profile may be unremarkable or show mild panhypoproteinemia, hypoglycemia (sepsis, decreased intake with limited hepatic glycogen stores), and electrolyte abnormalities consistent with GI loss and decreased intake (ie, hypokalemia, hyponatremia, hypochloremia). There have been anecdotal reports of mildly prolonged (<10%) coagulation times (activated clotting time, prothrombin time, partial thromboplastin time), potentially attributable to inflammation or interference due to hemoconcentration. If coagulation times are moderately or markedly prolonged, coagulopathy or disseminated intravascular coagulation (DIC) should be investigated. Basal serum cortisol concentration should be normal to increased and is an appropriate screening test for hypoadrenocorticism. Radiographic and ultrasound abnormalities should be limited to diffuse ileus and fluid-filled loops of bowel. Differential diagnoses include bacterial, viral (eg, parvovirus, coronavirus), and parasitic (eg, *Trichuris vulpis*, *Ancylostoma* spp, *Uncinaria* spp) gastroenteritis; systemic disturbances with secondary GI involvement (eg, hypoadrenocorticism, pancreatitis, renal failure, hepatic disease, etc); coagulopathy (eg, rodenticide toxicosis, thrombocytopenia, thrombocytopathia, etc); severe GI ulceration; neoplasia; and GI perforation of any etiology.

Treatment and Prognosis: Aggressive IV fluid therapy is the mainstay of treatment. The rate of isotonic fluid administration is based on patient perfusion, degree of dehydration, and ongoing losses. Dogs markedly hypoproteinemic or in shock may benefit from synthetic or natural colloid (stored or fresh frozen plasma) therapy. Parenteral antibiotics effective against *Clostridium* spp (eg, ampicillin 22 mg/kg, IV, tid-qid, or metronidazole 7.5 mg/kg, IV, bid) and to decrease the potential for sepsis secondary to intestinal bacterial translocation are indicated. Additional antibiotic coverage for gram-negative bacteria (eg, enrofloxacin 5–10 mg/kg/day, IV) is indicated in animals with sepsis or neutropenia. In a prospective study of dogs with HGE and no clinical indices of sepsis, treatment with amoxicillin-clavulanic acid did not affect mortality rate, duration of hospitalization, or severity of clinical signs. This might suggest not all cases of HGE are due to primary bacterial infection or that the bacteria involved may not be susceptible to amoxicillin-clavulanic acid. Depending on serum potassium concentration, maintenance fluids should be supplemented with potassium chloride at 20–40 mEq/L to prevent development of hypokalemia. Hypoglycemic dogs require dextrose supplementation (2.5%–5%) of maintenance IV fluids. Additional supportive care, including antiemetic therapy and dietary management, are as described above (*see* CANINE PARVOVIRUS, p 373, and ACUTE GASTRITIS, p 387). Rehydration with a balanced oral electrolyte solution (an initial volume of 7% dehydration [to be replaced over 12 hr] should be offered every 4 hr, along with volumes to account for maintenance fluid requirements and ongoing losses) may be appropriate for dogs with mild dehydration and mild clinical signs.

Prognosis is good with appropriate treatment. However, serious complications, including marked hypoproteinemia, DIC, sepsis, hypovolemic shock, and death, can occur.

INFLAMMATORY BOWEL DISEASE

Idiopathic inflammatory bowel disease (IBD) constitutes a group of GI diseases characterized by persistent clinical signs and histologic evidence of inflammatory cell infiltrate of unknown etiology. The various forms of IBD are classified by anatomic location and the predominant cell type involved. Lymphocytic-plasmacytic enteritis is the most common form in dogs and cats, followed by eosinophilic inflammation. There are occasional reports of inflammation with a granulomatous pattern (regional enteritis). A neutrophilic predominance in the inflammatory infiltrate is rare. A mixed pattern of cellular infiltrate is described on many occasions. Certain unique IBD syndromes occur more often in some breeds, such as the protein-losing enteropathy/nephropathy complex in Soft-coated Wheaten Terriers, immunoproliferative enteropathy of Basenjis, IBD in Norwegian Lundehunds, and histiocytic ulcerative colitis in Boxers.

Etiology and Pathophysiology: The etiology of IBD is unknown. Several factors may be involved, such as GI lymphoid tissue (GALT); permeability defects; genetic, ischemic, biochemical, and psychosomatic disorders; infectious and parasitic agents; dietary allergens; and adverse drug reactions. IBD may also be immune mediated. The intestinal mucosa has a barrier function and controls exposure of antigens to GALT. The latter can stimulate protective immune responses against pathogens, while remaining tolerant of harmless environmental antigens (eg, commensal bacteria, food). Defective immunoregulation of GALT results in exposure and adverse reaction to antigens that normally would not evoke such a response. Although dietary allergy is an unlikely cause of IBD (except in eosinophilic gastroenteritis), it may contribute to increased mucosal permeability and food sensitivity.

Current evidence supports the likely involvement of hypersensitivity reactions to antigens (eg, food, bacteria, mucus, epithelial cells) in the intestinal lumen or mucosa. More than one type of hypersensitivity reaction is involved in IBD. For example, type I hypersensitivity is involved in eosinophilic gastroenteritis, whereas type IV hypersensitivity is likely involved in granulomatous enteritis. The hypersensitivity reaction incites the involvement of inflammatory cells, resulting in mucosal inflammation that impairs the mucosal barrier, in turn facilitating increased intestinal permeability to additional antigens. Persistent inflammation may result in fibrosis.

Clinical Findings: There is no apparent age, sex, or breed predisposition associated with IBD; however, it may be more common in German Shepherds, Yorkshire Terriers, Cocker Spaniels, and purebred cats. The mean age reported for development of clinical disease is 6.3 yr in dogs and 6.9 yr in cats, but IBD has been documented in dogs <2 yr old. Clinical signs are often chronic and sometimes cyclic or intermittent. Vomiting, diarrhea, changes in appetite, and weight loss may be seen. In a retrospective study of cats with lymphocytic-plasmacytic enterocolitis, weight loss, intermittent vomiting progressing to more frequent vomiting on a daily basis, diarrhea, and anorexia were seen most often. Vomiting, melena, and cranial abdominal pain are often seen with gastroduodenal ulceration and erosion. Weight loss, vomiting, diarrhea, ascites, and peripheral edema can be seen in the cases of protein-losing enteropathy. Pulmonary thromboembolism is a rare complication; however, it can occur if there is severe intestinal protein loss (loss of antithrombin III). Clinical signs of large-intestinal diarrhea, including anorexia and watery diarrhea, are not uncommon.

An association between gastric dilation and volvulus (*see* p 384) and IBD in dogs has also been postulated. In this case, inflammation of the bowel may cause alterations in gastric motility and emptying and in GI transit time, thus predisposing to dilation and volvulus.

An association between inflammatory hepatic disease, pancreatitis, and IBD has been reported in cats, although an etiology for this triad of diseases has not been established. However, cats with cholangiohepatitis should also be evaluated for IBD and pancreatitis. Although unproved, it has been suggested that severe IBD in cats may progress to lymphosarcoma.

Diagnosis: There are no specific abnormalities on CBC, biochemical evaluations, or radiographs.

Hypoproteinemia due to reduced dietary intake and malabsorption or increased loss via the GI tract may be seen. Hypocalcemia and hypocholesterolemia may be attributed to malabsorption. Increases in serum amylase as a consequence of bowel inflammation have been reported. Hypokalemia secondary to anorexia, potassium loss from vomiting and diarrhea, and mild increases in serum levels of liver enzymes can be expected. Low serum levels of folate and cobalamin because of malabsorption are also documented.

Eosinophilia may be associated with eosinophilic enteritis; however, this is not a sensitive parameter. Microcytic anemia may be present with loss of iron, associated with chronic loss of blood. Nonresponsive anemia, if present, likely reflects anemia of chronic or inflammatory disease.

Erythrocytosis, associated with fluid loss from vomiting and diarrhea, and a stress leukogram may be seen. Radiographic changes may include gas or fluid distention of the stomach and increased total diameter of small-intestinal loops. Contrast films may show diffuse or focal mucosal irregularities suggestive of infiltrative disease. Loss of contrast can be related to ascites.

Fecal examination is important to exclude other causes of mucosal inflammation, such as nematodes, *Giardia* infection, and bacterial infection. *Giardia* may be difficult to detect because of intermittent shedding, and empirical treatment with fenbendazole is recommended in all cases.

Abdominal ultrasonography can be used to assess all abdominal organs, examine the entire intestinal tract, and measure wall thickness (although the latter measurement is of no significant value in IBD diagnosis). Small-intestinal hyperechoic mucosal striations are frequently associated with mucosal inflammation and protein-losing enteropathy. Ultrasonography also helps eliminate the possibility of disease in other organs, localize the disease, and determine whether endoscopy would allow biopsy of the site.

Endoscopy allows examination of the esophagus, stomach, duodenum, and sometimes the jejunum, depending on the size of the animal. Colonoscopy allows exploration of the colon. In some cases, gross mucosal lesions may be seen endoscopically, including erythema, friability, enhanced granularity, erosion, and ulceration. In many cases, the endoscopic appearance is normal. However, biopsy samples should always be taken, because the macroscopic and microscopic appearance of the intestinal mucosa are poorly correlated. At least six biopsies of each segment of the GI tract are recommended. Endoscopy is the easiest way to collect biopsy samples, but such samples are superficial and usually can be collected only from the proximal small intestine. One study suggested that ileal biopsies can reveal lesions not apparent in the duodenum and, therefore, should be performed routinely. More specifically, feline lymphoma was much more likely to be found in the ileum than the duodenum. In some cases, exploratory celiotomy and full-thickness biopsy are necessary to reveal histopathologic changes at the level of the mucosa (eg, dilation of the lacteals in lymphangiectasia). However, wound healing can be compromised if there is severe hypoproteinemia or if urgent steroid treatment is needed. For this reason, most clinicians choose to perform endoscopic biopsies unless biopsies of other abdominal organs are required.

Small populations of lymphocytes, plasma cells, macrophages, eosinophils, and neutrophils are normal components of intestinal mucosal tissue. Increased numbers of plasma cells, lymphocytes, eosinophils, and neutrophils in the lamina propria are seen in IBD. However, these morphologic features may also be seen with other causes of GI disease (eg, *Giardia*, *Campylobacter*, *Salmonella*, lymphangiectasia, lymphosarcoma). Although histopathologic assessment of intestinal biopsy material remains the gold standard for diagnosis of many IBDs, it has marked limitations. Specimen quality can vary, pathologic diagnoses are inconsistent, and differentiation between normal specimens and those showing IBD and even lymphoma can be difficult. Biopsy must always be considered in relation to clinical signs, and the animal treated accordingly.

Treatment and Control: The goals of therapy are to reduce diarrhea and vomiting, promote appetite and weight gain, and decrease intestinal inflammation. If a cause can be identified (eg, dietary, parasitic, bacterial overgrowth, drug reaction, etc), it should be eliminated.

Dietary manipulation by itself may be effective in some cases (eg, in chronic colitis); in other cases, it can enhance the efficacy of concurrent medical therapy, allowing for the drug dosage to be reduced or for drug therapy to be discontinued once clinical signs are in remission. Corticosteroids, azathioprine, sulfasalazine, tylosin, and metronidazole are among the drugs most often used in management of IBD.

Unless the animal is debilitated, it is better to institute therapeutic modalities sequentially. The frequency and nature of clinical signs should be monitored, and therapy adjusted as needed. Treatment should begin with anthelmintic/antiparasitic medication (eg, fenbendazole at 50 mg/kg/day, PO, for 3–5 days). This is followed by dietary modification (preferably with an antigen-limited or hydrolyzed protein diet) for 3–4 wk, then a 3- to 4-wk antibacterial trial (usually tylosin 10 mg/kg, PO, tid, or metronidazole 10 mg/kg, PO, bid), and finally trial immunosuppressive therapy (initially prednisolone, 1 mg/kg, PO, bid).

Dietary modification generally involves feeding a hypoallergenic or elimination diet with a source of protein to which the animal has not been previously exposed (eg, homemade diets of lamb and rice or venison and rice, commercial diets). This diet should be the sole source of food for a minimum of 4–6 wk; no treats of any kind should be fed. Dogs with large-intestinal diarrhea may benefit from diets high in insoluble fiber content (*see* p 379). Supplementation of dietary fiber alone is rarely effective in animals with severe inflammatory cell infiltrate.

Sulfasalazine (and related drugs) are often used in dogs when IBD is limited to the large intestine. In the colon, this drug is split to release 5-aminosalicylic acid, which exerts its anti-inflammatory activity in the mucosa. The principal adverse effects in dogs are keratoconjunctivitis sicca and vasculitis. Because of the risk of salicylate toxicity in cats (*see* p 379), sulfasalazine is not routinely used in feline colitis. Newer aminosalicylic drugs without some of sulfasalazine's adverse effects are available, eg, olsalazine (dogs: 10–20 mg/kg, PO, tid) and mesalamine (dogs: 10 mg/kg, PO, tid).

The use of antibiotics can be justified in part by the potential to treat any undiagnosed enteropathogens. Metronidazole (10–20 mg/kg, PO, bid) is the preferred antibacterial for most forms of IBD in small animals. It may have immunomodulatory effects. Tylosin (10 mg/kg, PO, tid) may also have immunomodulatory effects and may have some efficacy in canine IBD. Histiocytic ulcerative colitis of Boxers is responsive to enrofloxacin, which supports the hypothesis that this particular form of IBD is the consequence of an infection with a specific organism.

Corticosteroids may be useful for both small- and large-intestinal disease. Initial dosages are 2 mg/kg/day for prednisone or prednisolone and 0.25 mg/kg/day for dexamethasone. Adverse effects include polyuria, polydipsia, polyphagia, and GI disturbances (eg, vomiting, melena, diarrhea). Dosages should be tapered every 7–10 days to the lowest possible dose required to control clinical signs and, if possible, discontinued altogether. An enteric-coated formulation of the glucocorticoid budesonide has successfully maintained remission in human IBD. A preliminary study has shown apparent efficacy in dogs and cats, but information on use of this drug is limited. It undergoes substantial first-pass elimination via rapid inactivation in the liver; the result is lower systemic bioavailability and reduced effects on the hypothalamic-pituitary-adrenal axis, making iatrogenic hyperadrenocorticism less common than with other glucocorticoids. The optimal dosage in dogs is unknown. Anecdotally, a dosage of 1 mg/m^2/day, PO, in dogs, and 1 mg/cat/day, PO, in cats, has been recommended.

In refractory cases, adding an immunosuppressive drug to corticosteroid therapy may be beneficial. Azathioprine (for dogs) and chlorambucil (for cats) can be used. The dosage of azathioprine is 2.2 mg/kg/day, PO. Adverse effects include myelosuppression, pancreatitis, and hepatotoxicity. The dosage of azathioprine can be tapered after several weeks. Typically, the prednisone is tapered first (by 25% every 2–3 wk). After prednisone has been tapered to 0.5 mg/kg every other day without a relapse, then azathioprine is given every other day. If response to steroids is poor, even if combined with azathioprine, cyclosporine can be added at 5–10 mg/kg/day, PO, for at least 8–10 wk. No study has been done to compare cyclosporine and azathioprine. However, one recent study suggested that the combination of chlorambucil-prednisolone was more efficient to treat chronic enteropathy with concurrent protein-losing enteropathy in dogs than the azathioprine-prednisolone protocol.

Azathioprine is not recommended in cats because of sensitivity to adverse effects. Instead, cats are treated with a combination of prednisone and chlorambucil (0.1–0.2 mg/kg or 1 mg/cat). Clinical signs typically improve in 3–5 wk, although 4–8 wk of treatment may be needed. A CBC should be done every 2 wk to monitor for evidence of myelosuppression.

Adjunctive treatment may include ursodeoxycholic acid in cats (10–15 mg/kg/day, PO), cobalamine supplementation (20 mg/kg, SC, every 7 days for 4 wk and then every 28 days for a further 3 mo) in dogs and cats, and other supportive therapy as needed.

The response rate to treatment of IBD is variable. Quality of life tends to be poor, and prognosis is guarded. Hypoalbuminemia is a negative prognostic sign. Prognosis is worse in cases with severe histologic lesions, mucosal fibrosis, eosinophilic enteritis, protein-losing enteropathy, or hypereosinophilic syndrome. Relapses occur and are most often precipitated by dietary indiscretion.

MALABSORPTION SYNDROMES

Malabsorption is the defective uptake of a dietary constituent resulting from interference with its digestion or absorption, due to either exocrine pancreatic insufficiency (EPI) or small-intestinal disease. Malabsorption typically results in diarrhea, altered appetite, and weight loss, but a number of animals (especially cats) will not have overt diarrhea because of the ability of the colon to conserve water.

The primary function of the small intestine is digestion and absorption of nutrients, and it occurs in sequential phases: intraluminal digestion, mucosal digestion and absorption, and delivery of nutrients to the body. Many chronic, small-intestinal diseases cause malabsorption by interfering with one or several of these processes. Malabsorptive syndromes have been studied in most detail in dogs, but basic diagnostic and therapeutic principles are relevant to other species.

Physiology: The normal digestive processes convert polymeric dietary nutrients into forms (mainly monomers) that can cross the luminal surface (brush border) of intestinal absorptive epithelial cells (ie, enterocytes). Most digestive enzymes are secreted by the pancreas; EPI is thus a major cause of malabsorption. Terminal digestion before absorption is performed by brush border enzymes, either at the brush border surface of the enterocyte in association with transport proteins for the specific products, or when released into the intestinal lumen through cleavage by pancreatic peptidases or through loss of senescent enterocytes.

The main dietary carbohydrates are starch, glycogen, sucrose, and lactose. Starch and glycogen are first hydrolyzed by pancreatic amylase to the oligosaccharides maltose, maltotriose, and α-limit dextrins. These oligosaccharides and ingested disaccharides (sucrose, lactose) are further hydrolyzed to monosaccharides by enzymes located on the brush border of the enterocytes. Brush border lactase activity declines after weaning, especially in cats, and animals may become lactose intolerant, especially if the brush border has been damaged by another disease. The final products of mucosal hydrolysis (glucose, galactose, and fructose) are actively transported into the enterocyte by sodium-linked carrier-mediated processes, driven by a sodium-potassium ATPase. Once in the cell, glucose is not used by the glycolytic pathway but is passed by facilitated diffusion via a transport protein on the basolateral enterocyte membrane down a concentration gradient into the extracellular space, and then by diffusion into the portal venous circulation.

Protein digestion and absorption follow a similar pattern. Proteolytic enzymes from the stomach and pancreas degrade protein into a mixture of short-chain oligopeptides, dipeptides, and amino acids. Oligopeptides are further hydrolyzed by brush-border peptidases to dipeptides and amino acids that cross the brush-border membrane on specific carrier proteins.

Fat-soluble molecules do not need specific carriers to cross the phospholipid barrier of the brush border. However, intraluminal degradation of large lipids is essential. Fat in the duodenum stimulates release of cholecystokinin, which, in turn, stimulates secretion of pancreatic lipase. After solubilization by bile salt micelles, triglycerides are digested by pancreatic lipase to monoglycerides and free fatty acids. At the enterocyte membrane, the monoglycerides and free fatty acids disaggregate from the micelle and are passively absorbed into the cell. Released bile acids remain within the lumen and are ultimately reabsorbed by the ileum and undergo enterohepatic recycling. Once inside the cell, the monoglycerides and free fatty acids are reesterified to triglycerides and incorporated into chylomicrons, which subsequently enter the central lacteal of the villus, being delivered to the venous circulation via the thoracic duct. Medium-chain triglycerides (C_8–C_{10}) may be absorbed directly into the portal blood, providing an alternative route for fat uptake in case of lymphatic obstruction, but some do normally enter the circulation via the thoracic duct. Consequently, they are no longer recommended in management of lymphangiectasia.

Etiology and Pathophysiology: Malabsorption is a consequence of interference with mechanisms responsible for either the degradation or absorption of dietary constituents (*see* TABLE 7).

Diseases that disrupt the synthesis or secretion of digestive pancreatic enzymes cause maldigestion with subsequent malabsorption, so that the end result is the same. An important syndrome is EPI (*see* p 409), which occurs if there is a loss of ~85%–90% of exocrine pancreatic mass. EPI is characterized by severe maldigestion-malabsorption of starch, protein, and most notably, fat. In dogs, EPI is most commonly due to acinar atrophy; chronic pancreatitis is less common and is seen in older animals, and pancreatic hypoplasia is a rare congenital cause. EPI in dogs is often complicated by secondary antibiotic-responsive diarrhea, which further disrupts nutrient digestion and absorption. EPI is relatively uncommon in cats and is most frequently due to chronic pancreatitis.

Intraluminal effects of bacteria can also have important consequences. Bacterial deconjugation of bile salts interferes with micelle formation, which results in malabsorption of lipid. Deconjugated bile salts and hydroxy fatty acids exacerbate diarrhea by stimulating colonic secretion.

TABLE 7 MECHANISMS OF MALABSORPTION

Location	Disease	Mechanism
Luminal	Exocrine pancreatic insufficiency	Lack of pancreatic enzymes (maldigestion)
	Antibiotic-responsive diarrhea, secondary small-intestinal bacterial overgrowth	Bacterial activity: bile salt deconjugation, fatty acid hydroxylation, competition for cobalamin and nutrients
Mucosal	Inflammatory bowel disease, infectious enteropathies, dietary sensitivities, neoplastic infiltration	Mucosal damage: inflammation, brush border defects, disturbed enterocyte function, reduction of surface area
	Villous atrophy	Reduction in surface area, immature enterocytes due to increased cell turnover
	Brush border enzyme deficiencies	Lactase deficiency, diffuse small-intestinal disease
Postmucosal	Lymphangiectasia	Lymphatic obstruction impairs delivery of chylomicrons
	Vasculitis, portal hypertension	Impaired delivery

True small-intestinal bacterial overgrowth (SIBO) can be secondary to defective gastric acid secretion, interference with normal motility or mechanical obstruction of the intestine, interference with the function of the ileocecal valve, and local immunodeficiency. In other cases, there is no evidence of overgrowth and no defined cause but a lack of overt mucosal damage. However, a positive response to antibiotic therapy indicates that the malabsorption is related to bacteria, perhaps in how the innate immune system (toll-like receptors) respond to bacterial components. Originally called idiopathic SIBO, this syndrome is better termed antibiotic-responsive diarrhea (ARD).

Fat malabsorption may also be seen with a deficiency of intraluminal bile salts due to cholestatic liver disease, biliary obstruction, or ileal disease resulting in defective absorption of conjugated bile salts.

Small-intestinal disease can cause malabsorption by reduction of the number or function of individual enterocytes. Diffuse diseases of the mucosa can result in reduced activities of brush border enzymes, decreased carrier-protein function, decreased mucosal absorptive surface area, and interference with final transport of nutrients into the circulation. Weight loss may be compounded by reduced nutrient intake due to inappetence. In addition, malabsorbed nutrients exert strong intraluminal osmotic effects that diminish intestinal and colonic absorption of water and electrolytes, resulting in diarrhea. This may be exacerbated if mucosal damage is accompanied by intestinal inflammation, which can cause secretory and permeability diarrhea.

Potential causes of mucosal damage include idiopathic inflammatory bowel disease (IBD), enteric pathogens (eg, enteric viruses, pathogenic bacteria, *Giardia*, *Histoplasma*, *Pythium*), dietary sensitivity, ARD, and intestinal neoplasia (eg, lymphosarcoma). Histologic changes such as villous atrophy and infiltration with inflammatory cells indicate intestinal disease but do not identify the underlying cause. For example, lymphocytic-plasmacytic enteritis may be a common response pattern of the intestinal mucosa to more than one provocative agent, particularly microbial and dietary antigens. Definite associations with parasites, pathogenic bacteria, and dietary sensitivity have been demonstrated in dogs, but often the underlying cause cannot be identified.

Mucosal damage may also occur without obvious changes under light microscopy. This is typified by infection with enteropathogenic *Escherichia coli* (which specifically cause ultrastructural damage to microvilli in an attaching-effacing lesion) and by ARD in dogs, which can cause biochemical damage to the intestinal brush border, interfering with enterocyte function.

The main brush border enzyme deficiency reported is a relative lactase deficiency, leading to milk intolerance in adult dogs and cats. Acquired brush border defects also may be seen in the course of generalized small-intestinal disease.

Postmucosal obstruction may be seen with lymphatic obstruction (especially lymphangiectasia) and vascular compromise (portal hypertension, vasculitis). Intestinal lymphangiectasia causes intestinal protein loss as well as severe fat malabsorption.

Usually, in malabsorption a number of nutrients are affected and consequently diarrhea occurs; malabsorption of a single ingredient without any GI signs is rare (eg, selective cobalamin malabsorption in Giant Schnauzers, Australian Shepherds, and Border Collies). Again, it should be noted that the large absorptive capacity of the colon may prevent overt diarrhea in some animals (especially cats) despite significant malabsorption and weight loss.

Clinical Findings: Clinical signs of malabsorption are mainly the result of lack of nutrient uptake and losses in the feces. The duration, severity, and primary cause determine the severity of signs, which typically include chronic diarrhea, weight loss, and altered appetite (anorexia or polyphagia). The absence of diarrhea does not exclude the possibility of severe GI disease. Weight loss may be substantial despite a ravenous appetite, sometimes characterized by coprophagia and pica. Typically, animals with malabsorption are systemically well unless there is severe inflammation or neoplasia. Nonspecific signs may include dehydration, anemia, and ascites or edema in cases of hypoproteinemia. Thickened bowel loops or enlarged mesenteric lymph nodes may be palpable, especially in cats.

Diagnosis: Chronic diarrhea and weight loss are nonspecific signs common to a variety of systemic and metabolic diseases, as well as malabsorption, although, typically, systemic diseases cause anorexia. A thorough diagnostic approach in dogs and cats with signs suggestive of malabsorption is therefore needed to help exclude association with possible underlying systemic or metabolic disease. A precise diagnosis is also important to determine treatment and prognosis.

The history is particularly important, because it may suggest specific dietary intolerance, indiscretion, or sensitivity. Weight loss may indicate malabsorption or protein-losing enteropathy (PLE) but may also be due to anorexia, vomiting, or extraintestinal disease. Small- and large-intestinal diarrhea may be distinguished by a number of features (*see* TABLE 1, p 157). This distinction is more helpful in dogs than in cats, which rarely have exclusively large-intestinal disease. Suspected large-intestinal disease in dogs may be further evaluated by colonoscopic biopsy of the large intestine. However, if signs of large-intestinal disease are accompanied by weight loss or large volumes of feces, then there is probably also concurrent small-intestinal disease.

A thorough physical examination should be performed. Abdominal palpation is essential to identify abnormalities, and rectal examination is required even when no large-intestinal disease is suspected, both to provide a fecal sample and possibly to identify previously unreported melena. In older cats, the thyroid should be palpated carefully and serum T_4 assayed, because signs of hyperthyroidism can closely mimic those of malabsorption.

Initial evaluation should include a CBC, biochemical profile, urinalysis, fecal examination, abdominal ultrasonography and, when indicated by clinical signs or abnormal abdominal palpation, plain radiography. Hematologic correlates in small-intestinal diseases sometimes include anemia of chronic blood loss (microcytic, hypochromic) or chronic inflammation (normocytic, normochromic); neutrophilia and/or monocytosis associated with intestinal inflammation, infectious enteropathies, or neoplasia; eosinophilia associated with parasitism and eosinophilic enteritis; and lymphopenia that may be associated with intestinal lymphangiectasia in dogs. Lymphocytosis in a dog with diarrhea raises the suspicion of hypoadrenocorticism.

Biochemical tests and urinalysis help to exclude systemic diseases that cause chronic diarrhea, most notably hypoadrenocorticism, protein-losing nephropathies, renal failure, and liver disease. Hypoproteinemia frequently is secondary to PLE and is seen more commonly in dogs than cats. In most cases of PLE, serum albumin and globulin are both low, but a low albumin alone does not exclude it; inflammatory bowel disease (IBD) and neoplasia are rarely associated with hyperglobulinemia as well as hypoalbuminemia. Liver enzymes (ALT, AST) may be increased as a consequence of increased intestinal permeability, allowing more antigens to reach the liver; in such cases, a bile acid stimulation test as well as ultrasonography should be performed to exclude primary liver disease. However, in cats there may be concurrent IBD and cholangitis. Hypocholesterolemia may develop with fat malabsorption and is most notable in lymphangiectasia. Urinalysis is important to exclude renal causes of hypoalbuminemia and/or renal disease. However, sometimes both may be seen together (eg, the familial PLE and nephropathy of Soft-coated Wheaten Terriers). Hyperthyroidism in cats should be excluded by measuring serum T_4 concentrations. Serologic tests for feline leukemia and feline immunodeficiency viruses should also be performed, not only because both may be associated with secondary, chronic diarrhea but also because they are important prognostic factors. Feline infectious peritonitis and toxoplasmosis have also been described as occasional causes of chronic diarrhea in cats.

The presence of fat, undigested muscle fibers, or starch in feces may provide indirect evidence for malabsorption, but these are unreliable. Feces should be examined for parasites (especially hookworms and *Giardia* in dogs and *Tritrichomonas* and *Giardia* in cats) and potentially pathogenic bacteria (including *Salmonella* and *Campylobacter*). Speciation of *Campylobacter* isolates by PCR allows distinction of the pathogenic *C jejuni* from the more common and probable commensal *C upsaliensis*. Pathogenic *Escherichia coli* are emerging as a potentially important problem in dogs, but molecular techniques to identify genes encoding pathogenicity determinants are required for diagnosis. *Giardia* can be detected using serial zinc sulfate fecal flotations or a commercially available ELISA; the latter is easier to perform, and its sensitivity is better than fecal flotation performed by inexperienced personnel. *Tritrichomonas* typically causes colitis in cats rather than malabsorption and is best diagnosed by pouch culture or PCR. Detection of excessive leukocytes on fecal cytology may indicate chronic intestinal inflammation or the presence of enteric pathogens. Cytology of rectal scrapings may reveal *Histoplasma* organisms.

Abdominal radiography is more useful when vomiting is present or palpable abnormalities are detected, but ultrasonography is an important part of the investigation of most small-intestinal diseases. It can be used to measure intestinal wall thickness, layering, and luminal diameter and to detect other intestinal lesions (eg, masses, intussusception), mesenteric lymphadenopathy (in neoplasia and inflammatory bowel disease), and abnormalities in other organs. Mucosal striations have been associated with lymphatic dilatation.

Once obvious dietary, systemic, parasitic, and infectious causes of chronic small-intestinal diarrhea have been eliminated, the next step is differentiation of EPI from intestinal malabsorption; the diagnosis of EPI is relatively straightforward, whereas that of small-intestinal disease is more complex. Numerous tests have been used for dogs and cats with suspected EPI, but they are too inaccurate or impractical to be recommended. Assay of serum trypsin-like immunoreactivity (TLI) is a highly sensitive and specific test and should be used for diagnosis of EPI. This assay measures trypsinogen, some of which normally leaks from the pancreas into the blood, thereby providing an indirect assessment of functional pancreatic tissue. In EPI, functional exocrine tissue is severely depleted and serum TLI concentrations are extremely low, clearly distinguishing EPI from other causes of malabsorption. This test requires a fasted serum sample. Species-specific canine and feline TLI tests are available.

The diagnosis of small-intestinal disease is difficult because of limitations of routine screening procedures, the need for biopsy, and frequently the absence of diagnostic histologic changes. Bacteriologic culture of duodenal fluid obtained endoscopically or at laparotomy has been used to confirm a diagnosis of ARD. However, the exact cut-off point at which small-intestinal bacterial numbers are considered excessive is a matter of debate, because numbers $>10^5$ total or $>10^4$ obligate anaerobic colony-forming units (CFU)/mL may be found in apparently clinically healthy dogs, depending on circumstances, including *environment, diet, scavenging,* and coprophagia.

The assay of serum folate and cobalamin (vitamin B_{12}) concentrations can be a helpful initial test in assessment of small-intestinal disease. Folate is absorbed primarily by the proximal small intestine (jejunum), whereas cobalamin is absorbed by the distal small intestine (ileum). As a result, serum folate concentrations can be decreased in proximal small-intestinal diseases, serum cobalamin concentrations can be decreased in distal diseases, and both can be decreased in diffuse enteropathies. Other factors such as the severity, extent, and duration of a mucosal abnormality; dietary intake; and vitamin supplementation also influence these concentrations. In addition, EPI can affect serum folate and cobalamin concentrations, and changes in serum folate and cobalamin concentrations are unreliable for the diagnosis of ARD and secondary antibiotic-responsive diarrhea. The validity of serum folate and cobalamin concentrations as markers of small-intestinal disease in cats is less clear, but low serum cobalamin concentrations may be found with both small-intestinal disease and EPI. Hypocobalaminemia is particularly associated with IBD and alimentary lymphoma and results in metabolic changes, including methylmalonic acidemia, that can lead to anorexia; low cobalamin concentrations are an indication for parenteral supplementation.

A further indirect approach to detect small-intestinal disease is assessment of intestinal function and permeability by oral administration of test substances that are subsequently measured in blood or urine samples. Historically, the xylose absorption test was used to assess intestinal function, but it was insensitive, especially in cats, and is no longer used. Measurements of the differential absorption of D-xylose/3-O-methyl-D-glucose and of intestinal permeability have not been shown to be clinically useful. Hydrogen breath testing after oral administration of individual sugars was considered a simple test to detect malabsorption and to assess transit time, but it has also fallen out of favor. Attempts to diagnose ARD by breath hydrogen or measurement of serum unconjugated bile acids were unreliable, because bacterial numbers may not actually be increased in ARD.

IV administration of ^{51}Cr-labeled albumin (or $^{51}CrCl_3$ to label endogenous albumin) has been used historically to document PLE in dogs. Measurement of 3-day fecal excretion of this radioactive marker provides an estimation of labeled albumin and hence protein loss into the intestinal lumen. However, its use is very limited because of the use of radioactive markers. An alternative approach is the measurement of α-1 protease inhibitor in the feces. This plasma protein is lost into the intestinal lumen together with albumin, but unlike albumin it is an antiprotease and is excreted in the feces essentially intact. Species-specific assays have been developed. Three fresh fecal samples passed by spontaneous evacuation are required; any GI bleeding invalidates the result.

Definitive diagnosis of chronic small-intestinal disease typically includes histologic examination of intestinal biopsies taken by endoscopy or at laparotomy. Endoscopy is minimally invasive and allows visualization of the mucosa and targeted biopsy sampling. However, endoscopic mucosal biopsies may not always give an adequate representation of deeper disease and are limited to the parts of the small intestine (duodenum and sometimes proximal jejunum and ileum) that can be visualized via colonoscopy. Endoscopic biopsy is preferred initially because the risk of intestinal surgical wound dehiscence can exceed 10% in debilitated, malnourished, or hypoproteinemic animals. However, surgery is the preferred option when there is a concern about deeper or extraintestinal disease or a focal lesion. If a laparotomy is performed, multiple elliptical, longitudinal biopsy samples should be collected from the duodenum, jejunum, and ileum; mesenteric lymph nodes should be biopsied and other organs examined.

Histologic examination of intestinal biopsy specimens can identify morphologic changes in intestinal inflammation (including lymphocytic-plasmacytic enteritis and eosinophilic enteritis), intestinal lymphangiectasia, villous atrophy, and intestinal neoplasia. The description of morphologic abnormalities can provide a baseline to evaluate response to treatment if sequential small-intestinal biopsies are possible. Morphologic abnormalities may also provide prognostic information, because more severe enteropathies tend to be more difficult to manage. However, there may be minimal or no obvious abnormalities in certain disorders (eg, ARD) despite considerable interference with intestinal function. Histologic descriptions alone provide little information on possible etiology or underlying mechanisms of damage, which would clearly assist effective management. Furthermore, inconsistencies in histologic descriptions between pathologists is a recognized problem. However, the World Small Animal Veterinary Association GI Standardization Group has published a descriptive template as a basis for concordance.

Treatment: Treatment of malabsorption involves treatment of the primary cause (if identified), dietary therapy, and management of complications. Management of EPI in dogs is relatively straightforward (*see* p 409) and includes feeding a low-fiber diet that contains moderate levels of fat or highly digestible fat, very digestible carbohydrate, and high-quality protein. Specific treatment involves lifelong supplementation of each meal with pancreatic extract. Powdered extracts (1 tsp/10 kg body wt) are preferable to tablets, capsules, and most enteric-coated preparations. Fresh or frozen pancreas can be used as an alternative (100 g/meal for an adult German Shepherd). If the response to pancreatic replacement therapy is poor, secondary antibiotic-responsive diarrhea may be suspected, and the animal should be treated concurrently with oral antibiotics for ≥1 mo (*see* below). Acid suppressants (eg, H_2-receptor blockers, such as cimetidine or ranitidine; proton pump inhibitors, such as omeprazole) may be given 20 min before a meal to inhibit acid secretion and to minimize acid degradation of enzymes in the pancreatic extract, but they are expensive and their value is questionable. Oral multivitamin supplementation should be considered as supportive therapy, but cobalamin (500–1,000 mcg/wk until normalized) should be given parenterally. Dietary requirements of cats with EPI can generally be met by conventional commercial diets, but pancreatic replacement therapy is still needed, as well as parenteral cobalamin supplementation in cats with low serum cobalamin concentrations.

Effective treatment of **small-intestinal disease** depends on the nature of the disorder, but therapy may be empirical when a specific diagnosis cannot be made. In dogs with ARD, a low-fat diet may help by minimizing secretory diarrhea due to bacterial metabolism of fatty acids and bile salts. Oral broad-spectrum antibiotic therapy with oxytetracycline (10–20 mg/kg, tid for 28 days) has been successful. Metronidazole (10–20 mg/kg, bid) and tylosin (20 mg/kg, tid) are effective alternatives; there is rarely a need to use other antibiotics, and the nontargeted use of fluoroquinolones should be avoided. Repeated or longterm treatment may be necessary in dogs with **idiopathic ARD**. Vitamin supplementation may be helpful, particularly for animals with cobalamin deficiency. Secondary antibiotic-responsive diarrhea usually resolves with appropriate management of the underlying disease, but idiopathic ARD can be difficult to control, especially in young German Shepherds, which are predisposed to developing the condition.

Dietary modification is an important aspect of the management of small-intestinal disease in both dogs and cats. Diets generally contain moderate levels of limited protein sources and highly digestible carbohydrates (to reduce protein antigenicity, reduce osmolar effects, and improve nutrient availability) and low to moderate levels of fat. In addition, they are lactose and gluten free; may be fiber-restricted; and may contain increased levels of antioxidants, prebiotics (eg, fructo-oligosaccharides), or omega-3 fatty acids. These additives are thought to modulate the inflammatory response and increase the health of the bacterial gut flora and enterocytes. Treatment with an exclusion diet consisting of a single novel protein source or a hydrolyzed protein should be used as trial therapy when dietary sensitivity is suspected. Intestinal inflammation is sometimes a manifestation of dietary sensitivity, and an initial exclusion food trial is indicated in mild cases of IBD before other treatments. Boiled white rice and potato are suitable carbohydrate sources, while fish, lamb, or chicken are often used as a protein source, depending on the dietary history. Cottage cheese, horsemeat, rabbit, or venison may be acceptable alternatives. Commercial exclusion diets are not necessary to diagnose food hypersensitivity; however, they are preferred for maintenance to reduce potential dietary imbalances. Protein hydrolysates may be the most effective diets to detect dietary sensitivity. The response to an exclusion diet is often rapid, but the diet must be fed for at least 3 and, in a few cases, up to 10 wk before being considered a failure. Oral prednisolone (1 mg/kg, bid for 2–4 wk, followed by a reducing dose) in combination with an exclusion diet may be useful in animals in which idiopathic IBD is suspected but dietary sensitivity has not yet been excluded.

Treatment of **idiopathic inflammatory bowel disease** should initially attempt to eliminate or control an underlying antigenic stimulus that may be playing a primary or secondary role in the damage. Treatment should first involve the use of a protein hydrolysate diet. The diet should comprise digestible carbohydrate (preferably rice, which is most digestible) and high-quality protein. Restriction of fat content may also be valuable and can minimize the secretory diarrhea that is a consequence of bacterial metabolism of fatty acids and bile salts. Oral prednisolone (1 mg/kg, bid for 1 mo, followed by a reducing dose) is indicated in cases of intestinal disease with an obvious inflammatory component, such as lymphocytic-plasmacytic enteritis and eosinophilic enteritis. In more severe cases, it may be necessary to add chlorambucil (2–6 mg/m^2/day, PO, until remission, followed by drug tapering) in cats or azathioprine (2–2.5 mg/kg/day) in dogs.

Cats are often given adjunctive metronidazole (10 mg/kg, bid); the beneficial effect of metronidazole may be a result of an inhibition of cell-mediated immune responses as well as anaerobic antibacterial activity. However, the value of metronidazole in combination with prednisolone in the treatment of IBD in dogs has been questioned.

In **lymphangiectasia**, a severely fat-restricted, calorie-dense, highly digestible diet reduces diarrhea but tends to exacerbate weight loss. Supplementation with fat-soluble vitamins is advised, and additional medium-chain triglycerides have been recommended as an easily absorbable fat source that bypasses the lymphatics, although this mechanism is now doubted. Prednisone/prednisolone therapy may be beneficial for its anti-inflammatory and immunosuppressive effects, especially if there is associated lipogranulomatous lymphangitis. The response to treatment is variable; clinical signs may sometimes abate for months or even years, but the longterm prognosis is grave.

Giardiasis can be treated with metronidazole or fenbendazole, and **histoplasmosis** with itraconazole (cats) or ketoconazole (dogs), with or without amphotericin B. In cases of **lymphosarcoma**, treatment involves an appropriate chemotherapy regimen, but response is poor in dogs and in cats with lymphoblastic forms. In cats, treatment of **small-cell villous lymphoma** with oral prednisone and chlorambucil is associated with prolonged remission.

Prognosis: The prognosis in cases of malabsorption is good if there is a simple solution, eg, 85% of cases of EPI respond well to enzyme replacement therapy. The prognosis is worse the more severe the small-intestinal pathology. A poorer prognosis has been associated with severe intestinal inflammation, neoplastic disease, severe weight loss, hypoalbuminemia and ascites (PLE), anorexia, and hypocobalaminemia.

THE EXOCRINE PANCREAS

The pancreas has both endocrine and exocrine functions. The exocrine pancreas is made up of pancreatic acinar cells and a duct system that opens into the proximal duodenum. Pancreatic acinar cells synthesize and secrete digestive enzymes (eg, amylase, lipase, and others) or inactive proenzymes, and zymogens (eg, trypsinogen, chymotrypsinogen, proelastase, prophospholipase, and others) of digestive enzymes, which are essential for the digestion of dietary components such as proteins, triglycerides, and complex carbohydrates. The exocrine pancreas also secretes other essential substances, such as large amounts of bicarbonate, which buffers gastric acid, intrinsic factor, which is needed for cobalamin absorption, and colipase, which is an essential cofactor for pancreatic lipase.

PANCREATITIS

Pancreatitis is the most common exocrine pancreatic disease in both dogs and cats. It can be acute or chronic, depending on whether the disease has led to permanent changes of the pancreatic parenchyma, mainly atrophy and/or fibrosis. Both acute and chronic pancreatitis can be subclinical, mild and associated with vague clinical signs, or severe and associated with pancreatic necrosis and systemic complications. Thus a distinction between the two is clinically of little significance.

Etiology and Pathogenesis: Most cases of pancreatitis in dogs and cats are idiopathic. However, several risk factors have been described. Miniature Schnauzers have been identified to be dramatically overrepresented in some studies, and it has been speculated that they may have a genetic predisposition similar to that in families of human patients with hereditary pancreatitis. Other studies have reported an increased prevalence in Yorkshire Terriers, Cocker Spaniels, Dachshunds, Poodles, sled dogs, or other breeds. Dietary indiscretion is believed to be a common risk factor in dogs. Also, hypertriglyceridemia in dogs, if severe (ie, generally serum concentrations ≥500 mg/dL), is considered a risk factor for pancreatitis. Hyperadrenocorticism has been cited in some studies as a risk factor for pancreatitis in dogs. Severe blunt trauma, such as can be sustained during a traffic accident or in cats with high-rise syndrome, can also cause pancreatitis. Surgery has been considered another risk factor; however, most postsurgical cases of pancreatitis are now believed to be due to pancreatic hypoperfusion during anesthesia. Infectious diseases have been implicated, but the evidence for a cause and effect relationship is weak in most cases. In dogs, pancreatitis has been reported with *Babesia canis* or *Leishmania* infection. In cats, *Toxoplasma gondii*, *Amphimerus pseudofelineus*, and feline infectious peritonitis are considered most important.

Many drugs have been implicated in causing pancreatitis in people, but very few have been confirmed in dogs and cats. In general, most drugs should be viewed as potential causes of pancreatitis; cholinesterase inhibitors, calcium, potassium bromide, phenobarbital, L-asparaginase, estrogen, salicylates, azathioprine, thiazide diuretics, and vinca alkaloids are probably the most important.

Many different insults may ultimately lead to pancreatitis through a common pathway. Secretion of pancreatic juice decreases during the initial stages of pancreatitis. This is followed by co-localization of zymogen granules and lysosomes, leading to activation of trypsinogen to trypsin within the co-localized organelles. Trypsin, in turn, activates more trypsinogen and also other zymogens. Prematurely activated digestive enzymes lead to local damage of the exocrine pancreas with pancreatic edema, bleeding, inflammation, necrosis, and peripancreatic fat necrosis. The ensuing inflammatory process leads to recruitment of WBCs and cytokine production. The activated enzymes, and more importantly, the cytokines circulate in the bloodstream and lead to distant complications such as generalized inflammation, disseminated intravascular coagulation, disseminated lipodystrophy, pancreatic encephalopathy, hypotension, renal failure, pulmonary failure, myocarditis, or even multiorgan failure.

Clinical Findings: Anorexia (91%), vomiting (90%), weakness (79%), abdominal pain (58%), dehydration (46%), and diarrhea (33%) have been reported as the most common clinical signs in dogs with severe pancreatitis. Clinical signs in cats with severe pancreatitis are even less specific, with anorexia (87%), lethargy (81%), dehydration (54%), weight loss (47%), hypothermia (46%), vomiting (46%), icterus (37%), fever (19%), and abdominal pain (19%) most commonly reported. Dogs and cats with milder forms of pancreatitis may be subclinical or may have only vague clinical signs, such as anorexia, lethargy, or diarrhea. The low rate of abdominal pain reported is remarkable given that >90% of human patients with pancreatitis report abdominal pain, so it is most likely due to lack of recognition in veterinary patients.

Diagnosis: A history of dietary indiscretion combined with vomiting and abdominal pain may suggest pancreatitis in dogs, but most cats present with nonspecific histories and clinical signs. Findings on CBCs and serum biochemistry profiles may suggest an inflammatory disease process but are nonspecific. In dogs, thrombocytopenia and neutrophilia with a left shift are common. Azotemia and increases in liver enzymes and bilirubin are common, nonspecific findings in both dogs and cats. Thus, while basic blood work is not useful for the diagnosis of pancreatitis, it is crucial to systematically evaluate the animal and diagnose systemic complications. Abdominal radiographs may show decreased detail in the proximal abdominal cavity and displacement of abdominal organs, but these findings are also nonspecific and a diagnosis based on radiographic findings alone is not reliable. However, abdominal radiographs are valuable in animals suspected of having pancreatitis to exclude other differential diagnoses. Abdominal ultrasonography, if stringent criteria are applied, is highly specific for pancreatitis, but pancreatic enlargement and fluid accumulation around the pancreas alone are not sufficient for diagnosis. A combination of pancreatic enlargement, fluid accumulation around the pancreas, changes in echogenicity (ie, decreased echogenicity suggesting pancreatic necrosis, increased echogenicity around the pancreas suggesting peripancreatic fat necrosis, increased echogenicity suggesting pancreatic fibrosis), and/or a pancreatic mass effect are suggestive of pancreatitis. Care should be taken not to overinterpret findings, because modern ultrasonographic equipment has a very high resolution, and pancreatic nodular hyperplasia may lead to changes in echogenicity, falsely suggesting the presence of pancreatitis. Also, the sensitivity of abdominal ultrasonography is highly operator-dependent, with sensitivities as high as 35% in cats and 68% in dogs in the most experienced hands.

Several diagnostic markers for pancreatitis have been evaluated in dogs and cats. In general, the clinical usefulness of serum lipase and amylase activity is limited in dogs and even more so in cats. In-clinic tests for the semiquantitative evaluation of serum pancreatic lipase immunoreactivity are available. A negative semiquantitative test suggests that pancreatitis is very unlikely, whereas a positive test suggests pancreatitis. In the latter case, pancreatic lipase immunoreactivity (PLI) concentration should be measured in a serum sample and evaluated to confirm the diagnosis and to determine a baseline concentration. This allows use of serum PLI concentration as a monitoring tool for the disease. In both dogs and cats, serum PLI concentration is highly specific for exocrine pancreatic function and is also the most sensitive diagnostic test for pancreatitis currently available (sensitivity >80%). However, as for any disease, no test should be used in isolation for diagnosis, and all clinical findings should be used in conjunction to arrive at the most appropriate diagnosis.

Pancreatic cytology or histopathology can also be used to definitively diagnose pancreatitis. Fine-needle aspiration of the pancreas is safe and can show acinar cells and inflammatory cells, allowing a definitive diagnosis of pancreatitis. However, lack of inflammatory cells does not exclude pancreatitis, because the inflammatory infiltrate can be highly localized. Pancreatic biopsy for histopathologic evaluation may be associated with a higher risk of pancreatitis than fine-needle aspiration (due to more aggressive pancreatic handling and longer anesthesia). Also, even if the presence of pancreatitis seems obvious on macroscopic examination of the pancreas, a biopsy specimen should be collected because the definitive diagnosis of pancreatitis requires the identification of an inflammatory infiltrate during histopathology. Finally, animals with severe pancreatitis are often poor anesthetic risks, and exploratory laparotomy or even fine-needle aspiration may not be justified.

Treatment: The mainstay of therapy of severe pancreatitis is supportive care with fluid therapy, vigorous monitoring, and early intervention to prevent systemic complications. Fluid therapy should be based on calculation of degree of dehydration (to be replaced over 4–8 hr if there is no contraindication), maintenance, and ongoing losses (eg, due to vomiting or diarrhea). In those few cases in which the cause is known, specific therapy against the inciting cause may be initiated. Antibiotics are of questionable value and should not be used routinely. Resting the pancreas is suggested only if the animal vomits uncontrollably (ie, the animal vomits frequently and violently despite appropriate antiemetic therapy). In fact, early nutritional support is considered a key component of successful treatment of human patients with severe pancreatitis. Also, enteral nutritional support is considered superior to parenteral nutrition. Animals that vomit should be treated with an entiemetic, such as maropitant (NK1 antagonist), ondansetron or dolasetron (HT3 antagonists), or in most animals a combination of both. Even animals that do not actively vomit may benefit from such antiemetic support, because they may be nauseated, leading to hyporexia or even anorexia. Metoclopramide is not considered effective as an antiemetic agent and should not be used in these animals. Abdominal pain should be assumed to be present and treated until contrary evidence is available. Intermittent meperidine, butorphanol, or buprenorphine may be used in animals with mild or moderate abdominal pain. Animals with severe pain are often treated with a constant-rate infusion of an opioid, such as morphine, fentanyl, or methadone, or with a combination therapy of fentanyl, ketamine, and lidocaine. Plasma appears to be helpful in severe cases of canine pancreatitis. It should be given daily until improvement is significant or adverse effects are identified. Many other treatments have been investigated in dogs, cats, and people, but unfortunately none has been shown to be useful.

Animals with mild forms of pancreatitis should be carefully assessed for the presence of risk factors (eg, hypertriglyceridemia, hypercalcemia, history of medications that can cause pancreatitis) and concurrent diseases (eg, cholangitis, hepatitis, inflammatory bowel disease, diabetes mellitus). In dogs, feeding an ultra-low-fat diet is crucial for treatment success. In cats, a moderately fat-restricted diet is recommended. Antiemetic drugs are helpful for animals that may not eat due to nausea.

If animals do not respond to therapy, a trial with prednisone (dogs), prednisolone (dogs and cats), or cyclosporine (dogs or cats) may be attempted. Cyclosporine is advantageous in animals with concurrent diabetes mellitus, because it has a smaller impact on insulin resistance than glucocorticoids. However, data are limited to date, and indiscriminate use of glucocorticoids or cyclosporine in dogs and cats with chronic pancreatitis should be discouraged.

The prognosis in mild cases is good, but prognosis in severe cases of pancreatitis is guarded in both dogs and cats. Systemic complications such as hypothermia, acidosis, hypocalcemia, and single- or multiple-organ failure are considered risk factors for a poor outcome. It can be challenging to identify severe cases early during the disease process and prevent complications in those animals.

EXOCRINE PANCREATIC INSUFFICIENCY

Exocrine pancreatic insufficiency (EPI) is a syndrome caused by insufficient synthesis and secretion of digestive enzymes by the exocrine portion of the pancreas. EPI is less common than pancreatitis in both dogs and cats, but it is the second most common exocrine pancreatic disorder in both species.

Etiology and Pathogenesis: Pancreatic acinar atrophy is the most common cause of EPI in German Shepherds, Rough Collies, and Eurasians, whereas chronic pancreatitis is the most common cause in dogs of other breeds and cats. Less common causes of EPI in dogs and cats are pancreatic or extrapancreatic masses that lead to obstruction of the pancreatic duct. The exocrine pancreas has a remarkable functional reserve, ~90% of which must be lost before clinical signs of EPI develop. Pancreatic acinar enzymes play an integral role in the assimilation of all major macronutrients, and a lack of pancreatic digestive enzymes leads primarily to maldigestion. However, animals with EPI also show evidence of malabsorption, the pathogenetic basis of which is less well understood (*see also* MALABSORPTION SYNDROMES, p 400). The nutrients remaining in the intestinal lumen lead to loose, voluminous feces and steatorrhea. The lack of nutrients also causes weight loss and may lead to vitamin deficiencies. In animals with EPI caused by chronic pancreatitis, destruction of pancreatic tissue may not be limited to the acinar cells, and concurrent diabetes mellitus may develop.

Clinical Findings: EPI due to pancreatic acinar atrophy is most frequent in young adult German Shepherds but has also been described in Rough Collies and Eurasians. Dogs and cats with EPI due to other causes are usually middle-aged to older and can be of any breed. Clinical signs most commonly reported are polyphagia, weight loss, and diarrhea. Vomiting and anorexia are observed in some animals and may be a sign of concurrent conditions rather than EPI. The feces are most commonly pale, loose, and voluminous and may be malodorous. In rare cases, watery diarrhea may be seen. In a small portion of cats with EPI, the high fat content of the feces can lead to a greasy appearance of the hair coat, especially in the perianal and tail region.

Diagnosis: A serum trypsin-like immunoreactivity (TLI) concentration of ≤2.5 mcg/L in dogs or ≤8.0 mcg/L in cats is diagnostic for EPI. Because digestion of a macronutrient can often be accomplished by more than one enzyme, lack of exocrine pancreatic secretions does not necessarily lead to clinical signs. For example, several German Shepherds with subclinical EPI have been reported. These dogs had severely decreased serum TLI concentrations and a lack of exocrine pancreatic tissue, but no or only intermittent clinical signs of EPI.

An assay that measures fecal elastase in dogs has been validated. Unfortunately, some healthy dogs or dogs with chronic small-intestinal disease may have a severely decreased fecal elastase concentration, making this test much less reliable than serum TLI concentration.

Treatment: Most dogs and cats with EPI can be successfully treated by supplementation with pancreatic enzymes. Powder is more effective than tablets, capsules, and especially enteric-coated products. Initially, 1 teaspoon/10 kg should be given with each meal for dogs and 1 teaspoon/cat with each meal for cats. Once the clinical signs have completely resolved, the dose can be slowly decreased until the lowest effective dose has been reached. However, it should be noted that the lowest effective dose can vary between enzyme batches. Oral bleeding has been reported in 3 of 25 dogs with EPI treated with pancreatic enzyme supplements; the bleeding stopped in all three dogs after a dose reduction. Moistening the food and pancreatic powder mix may also decrease the frequency of this adverse effect.

Fresh pancreas may be a viable alternative to the use of powder; 1–3 oz (30–90 g) of raw chopped pancreas can replace 1 teaspoon of pancreatic extract. Raw pancreas can be kept frozen for several months without loss of enzymatic activity. Preincubation of the food with pancreatic enzymes or supplementation with bile salts is not necessary.

Even though pancreatic enzyme supplementation decreases the clinical signs in almost all animals, nutrient absorption, especially that of fats, is not normalized. Feeding low-fat diets to accommodate impaired fat digestion has been suggested, but this may further decrease fat assimilation and lead to deficiencies of fat-soluble vitamins and/or essential fatty acids. Some types of dietary fiber interfere with pancreatic enzyme activity, and a diet low in insoluble or nonfermentable fiber should be fed.

Enzyme supplementation alone may not lead to complete resolution of clinical signs; cobalamin deficiency should be considered as a possible cause. Cobalamin absorption depends on adequate synthesis and secretion of intrinsic factor. In both dogs and cats, the majority of intrinsic factor is synthesized and secreted by the exocrine pancreas, and >80% of dogs and almost all cats with EPI are cobalamin deficient. Also, cobalamin deficiency was the only independent risk factor for poor outcome in a study of dogs with EPI. Thus, serum cobalamin and folate concentrations should be routinely evaluated in small animals with suspected EPI. Dogs and cats with cobalamin deficiency, suggested by a severely decreased serum cobalamin concentration, should be parenterally supplemented with cobalamin. Other hypovitaminoses have also been reported in animals with EPI. For example, vitamin K deficiency leading to a coagulopathy has been reported in some cats with EPI.

Some animals may not respond to enzyme supplementation and cobalamin therapy and likely have concurrent small-intestinal disease. Animals with EPI commonly have concurrent small-intestinal dysbiosis and may need antibiotic therapy. Inflammatory bowel disease also occurs in some animals with EPI. In those that do not respond to therapy, a proton pump inhibitor can also be tried.

Prognosis: EPI results from an irreversible loss of pancreatic acinar tissue in most cases, and recovery is rare. However, with appropriate management and monitoring, these animals usually gain weight quickly, pass normal feces, and can live a normal life for a normal life span.

PANCREATIC NEOPLASMS

Neoplasias of the exocrine pancreas can be primary or secondary and can be classified as benign or malignant. Most exocrine pancreatic neoplasias in dogs and cats are secondary.

Pancreatic adenomas are benign tumors that are usually singular and can be differentiated from pancreatic nodular hyperplasia by the presence of a capsule. Pancreatic adenocarcinoma is the most common primary neoplastic condition of the exocrine pancreas in dogs and cats but is rare overall in both species.

Pathogenesis: Benign neoplasms of the exocrine pancreas can lead to transposition of organs of the cranial abdominal cavity. However, these changes are subclinical in most cases, and the diagnosis is often made as an incidental finding during necropsy. In rare cases, the neoplastic growth can obstruct the pancreatic duct and cause secondary atrophy of the remaining exocrine pancreas, leading to exocrine pancreatic insufficiency. Adenocarcinomas may lead to tumor necrosis if the tumor outgrows its blood supply. Tumor necrosis causes local inflammation, which can lead to clinical signs of pancreatitis. Malignant neoplasms may also spread to neighboring or distant organs.

Clinical Findings: The presentation of dogs and cats with exocrine pancreatic neoplasia is nonspecific, and many cases remain subclinical until late in the disease process. Some animals show clinical signs suggestive of pancreatitis. Obstructive jaundice may be seen if bile duct obstruction develops. Clinical signs related to metastatic lesions have also been reported in some cases of pancreatic adenocarcinoma and may present as lameness, bone pain, or dyspnea. Finally, paraneoplastic alopecia has been reported in cats with pancreatic adenocarcinoma.

Diagnosis: Several nonspecific findings, such as neutrophilia, anemia, hypokalemia, bilirubinemia, azotemia, hyperglycemia, and increased hepatic enzyme activities, have been reported in dogs and cats with pancreatic adenocarcinoma. However, results of routine blood tests may be unremarkable. Increased serum lipase and amylase activities and trypsin-like immunoreactivity and pancreatic lipase immunoreactivity concentrations have not been commonly reported in either dogs or cats with pancreatic adenocarcinoma but may be seen in either species.

Radiographic findings are also nonspecific in most cases. Abnormal findings include decreased contrast in the cranial abdomen suggesting peritoneal effusion, transposition of the spleen caudally, and shadowing in the pyloric region. In some cases, abdominal radiographs suggest a cranial abdominal mass. Abdominal ultrasonography generally shows a soft-tissue mass near the pancreas, but in many cases, continuation of the mass with pancreatic tissue cannot be conclusively demonstrated. Also, neoplastic lesions of neighboring organs may be falsely presumed to be of pancreatic origin. Finally, animals with severe pancreatitis may show a mass effect in the area of the pancreas on abdominal ultrasonography that must not be confused with a pancreatic neoplasia.

If peritoneal effusion is present, a sample should be aspirated and evaluated cytologically. However, in most cases neoplastic cells do not readily exfoliate into the peritoneal effusion, and no neoplastic cells are identified on cytology. Fine-needle aspiration or transcutaneous biopsy under ultrasonographic guidance can be attempted when suspicious masses are identified. However, in many cases, the diagnosis is made at exploratory laparotomy or necropsy.

Treatment and Prognosis: Pancreatic adenomas are benign and theoretically do not require therapy unless they cause clinical signs due to the effects of an intra-abdominal space-occupying lesion. However, because the final diagnosis of pancreatic adenocarcinoma is often made at exploratory laparotomy, a partial pancreatectomy should be performed even in cases of suspected pancreatic adenoma. The prognosis in these cases is excellent. Animals with pancreatic adenocarcinomas often present at a late stage of the disease, and metastatic disease at the time of diagnosis is quite common in both dogs and cats. Common sites for metastasis are the liver, abdominal and thoracic lymph nodes, mesentery, intestines, and the lungs, but other metastatic sites have also been reported. In those few cases when gross metastatic lesions are not identified at the time of diagnosis, surgical resection of the tumor may be attempted, but clean surgical margins can almost never be achieved, and owners should be forewarned. Both chemotherapy and radiation therapy have shown little success in human or veterinary patients with pancreatic adenocarcinomas.

Thus, the prognosis for dogs and cats with pancreatic adenocarcinoma is grave.

PANCREATIC ABSCESSES

By definition, a pancreatic abscess is a collection of pus, usually in proximity to the pancreas, containing little or no pancreatic necrosis. Pancreatic abscesses are considered a complication of pancreatitis, and thus their clinical presentation is similar to that of pancreatitis, although most cases are associated with mild chronic pancreatitis, and clinical signs may be more vague. A bacterial infection may or may not be present, but almost all cases reported in small animals have been sterile. Increased serum trypsin-like immunoreactivity and pancreatic lipase immunoreactivity concentrations have not been reported in dogs or cats with a pancreatic abscess, but anecdotal reports suggest that both serum parameters are increased in these animals. Surgical drainage and aggressive antimicrobial therapy are the treatments of choice in human patients with an infected pancreatic abscess. Dogs and cats may also respond favorably to surgical drainage. However, in one report, only slightly more than 50% of animals survived the immediate postsurgical period. Thus, given the mixed results and risks, difficulties, and expenses associated with anesthesia, surgery, and postoperative care, surgery may not be warranted unless there is clear evidence of an enlarging mass and/or sepsis in a medically managed animal.

PANCREATIC PSEUDOCYST

A pancreatic pseudocyst is a collection of sterile pancreatic fluid enclosed by a wall of fibrous or granulation tissue; these structures are also considered a complication of pancreatitis. Several cases of pancreatic pseudocysts in dogs and cats have been described. Clinical signs are usually nonspecific and mimic those of pancreatitis. On abdominal ultrasonography, a cystic structure in close proximity to the pancreas can be identified. Aspiration of the pseudocyst is relatively safe and should be attempted for diagnostic and therapeutic purposes. Fluid from a pancreatic pseudocyst should have few cells and should not contain any evidence of inflammation. Pancreatic pseudocysts can be treated medically or surgically. Medical management involves ultrasonographic-guided percutaneous aspiration and close monitoring of the size of the pseudocyst. Surgery may be indicated in animals with persistent clinical signs or when the pseudocyst fails to regress over time.

GASTROINTESTINAL PARASITES OF SMALL ANIMALS

SPIROCERCA LUPI

(Esophageal worm)

Adult *Spirocerca lupi* are bright red worms, 40 mm (male) to 70 mm (female) long, generally located within nodules in the esophageal, gastric, or aortic walls. Infections are seen in southern areas of the USA as well as in many tropical and subtropical regions worldwide (eg, Greece, India, Israel, Japan, South Africa). Dogs are infected by eating an intermediate host (usually dung beetle) or a transport host (eg, chickens, reptiles, or rodents). The larvae migrate via the wall of the celiac artery to the thoracic aorta, where they usually remain for ~3 mo. Eggs are passed in feces ~5–6 mo after infection.

Clinical Findings: Most dogs with *S lupi* infection show no clinical signs, but when signs are present, they most commonly include weight loss, coughing, and dyspnea. When the esophageal lesion is very large (usually when it has become neoplastic), the dog has difficulty swallowing and may vomit repeatedly after trying to eat. Such dogs salivate profusely and eventually become emaciated. In addition, dogs may develop thickening of the long bones characteristic of hypertrophic osteopathy. These clinical signs are suggestive of spirocercosis with associated neoplasia in regions where the parasite is prevalent. Occasionally, a dog dies suddenly as the result of massive hemorrhage into the thorax after rupture of the aorta damaged by the developing worms.

Lesions: The characteristic lesions are aneurysm of the thoracic aorta, reactive granulomas of variable size around worms in the esophagus, and exostoses that bridge between ventral aspects of thoracic vertebrae. Esophageal sarcoma, often with metastases, is sometimes associated (apparently causally) with *S lupi* infection, particularly in hound breeds. Dogs with *Spirocerca*-related sarcoma often develop hypertrophic osteopathy (*see* p 1205).

Diagnosis: Diagnosis can be made by demonstrating the characteristic small (11–15 × 30–38 μm), elongated eggs (by $NaNO_3$ [specific gravity 1.36] or sugar flotation) that contain larvae in the feces. However, eggs are sporadically voided in feces and can be difficult to find. Gastroscopy occasionally reveals a nodule or an adult worm. A presumptive diagnosis can be made by radiographic examination when it reveals dense masses in the esophagus; a positive-contrast barium study may help define the lesion. CT is an additional useful diagnostic tool, with a higher level of sensitivity than thoracic radiography for *S lupi*. However, while CT generally provides more information on the location and severity of the infection than radiographs, the specificity of the findings for *S lupi* is currently unclear.

Many infections are not diagnosed until necropsy. The granulomas vary greatly in size and location in the esophagus but usually are sufficiently characteristic to be diagnostic, even if the worms are no longer present. Worms and granulomas may be present in the lungs, trachea, mediastinum, stomach wall, or other abnormal locations. Healed aneurysms of the aorta persist for the life of the dog and are diagnostic of previous infection. When sarcomas are associated with the infection, the esophageal lesion usually is larger and often contains cartilage or bone; metastases frequently are present in the lungs, lymph nodes, heart, liver, or kidneys.

Treatment and Control: In endemic areas, dogs should be prevented from eating dung beetles, frogs, mice, lizards, etc, and not fed raw chicken scraps. In Europe, monthly treatment with topical moxidectin/imidacloprid is approved for use in dogs as a preventive for *S lupi* infection. Treatment of clinical cases is often not practical. However, efficacy has been demonstrated with doramectin (0.2 mg/kg, SC, three doses at 2-wk intervals; 0.4 mg/kg, SC, six doses at 2-wk intervals; 0.5 mg/kg, SC, two doses 2 wk apart; 0.5 mg/kg/day, PO, for 42 days; 0.8 mg/kg, SC, two doses 1 wk apart; additional treatments may be required), and with ivermectin (0.6 mg/kg, SC, two doses 2 wk apart) combined with prednisolone (0.5 mg/kg, PO, bid for 2 wk and then tapered), although none of these treatments is approved. The specific breed toxicity associated with ivermectin in Collies and other herding dog breeds also occurs with doramectin. Surgical removal usually is unsuccessful because of the large areas of the esophagus involved.

PHYSALOPTERA SPP

(Stomach worm)

Several species of these stomach nematodes of dogs and cats are seen throughout the world. They are usually firmly attached to the gastric mucosa. The males are ~30 mm long, and the females ~40 mm. The eggs are oval, 42–53 × 29–35 μm, thick-shelled, and larvated.

Encysted infective larvae of *Physaloptera* spp have been found in several species of insects, including beetles, cockroaches, and crickets. Mice and frogs may be paratenic hosts. After the dog or cat ingests the intermediate or paratenic host, development of larvae to adults is direct. Although infections are often subclinical, these parasites may cause gastritis that can result in vomiting, anorexia, and dark feces. Bleeding, ulcerated areas remain on the gastric mucosa when the parasites move to other locations; in heavy infections, anemia and weight loss may develop. Gastroscopy is the most efficient means of diagnosis, and immature worms are often found in the vomitus of puppies or kittens. The eggs are difficult to find in feces, because they do not readily float; eggs are best detected by fecal sedimentation. In cats, pyrantel pamoate (5 mg/kg, PO, two doses 2–3 wk apart; 20 mg/kg, PO, once) and ivermectin (0.2 mg/kg, SC or PO, two doses 2 wk apart) can be used for *Physaloptera* infections. In dogs, fenbendazole (50 mg/kg/day, PO, for 3 days), pyrantel pamoate (5 mg/kg, PO, two doses 2–3 wk apart; 15 mg/kg, PO, two doses 2–3 wk apart; 20 mg/kg, PO, once), and ivermectin (0.2 mg/kg, SC or PO, two doses 2 wk apart) can be used. None of these drug regimens is approved for treatment of *Physaloptera* in either dogs or cats.

OLLULANUS SP

Ollulanus tricuspis is a small worm, ≤1 mm long, that infects several animal species, typically cats and other felids, and occasionally induces a mild erosive or catarrhal gastritis. Vomiting minutes to a few hours after eating is a common sign. The female worms are viviparous, so massive infections can build up endogenously. Transmission is via vomitus. Diagnosis is by microscopic demonstration of larvae (~500 μm) or adult worms in vomitus or stomach contents. The use of a Baermann apparatus enables the separation of the worms from ingesta, after which they are easier to observe. Parasites are rarely seen in feces, because they are usually digested before being passed. Therapeutic efficacy in cats has been demonstrated with fenbendazole (20–50 mg/kg/day, PO, for 3 days) and levamisole (5 mg/kg, SC, once), although these are not approved treatments.

STRONGYLOIDES SP

Strongyloides stercoralis is a small, slender nematode that when fully mature is ~2 mm long, located at the base of the villi in the anterior half of the small intestine of dogs and cats. The worms are almost transparent and all but impossible to see grossly at necropsy. Usually, infections are associated with warm, wet, crowded, unsanitary housing. The species found most often in dogs is identical to that found in people.

The parasitic worms are all females. The eggs embryonate rapidly, and most larvae hatch before being passed in the feces. Under appropriate conditions of warmth and moisture, development in the environment is rapid; the third larval stage may be reached in little more than a day. Some of these larvae develop into infective filariform larvae; others develop into free-living worms that mate and produce progeny similar to that of the parasitic female. The filariform larvae penetrate the skin but also may infect a host via ingestion. Transmammary transmission is possible. Progeny may be shed in the feces 7–10 days after infection. Autoinfection caused by larvae that developed to the infective stage within the GI tract can result in infections in which dogs shed larvae for lengthy periods.

Clinical Findings: The presence of clinical signs indicates that a heavy infection has been building up for some weeks. A blood-streaked, mucoid diarrhea, usually seen in young animals during hot humid weather, is characteristic. Emaciation is often prominent, and reduced growth rate may be one of the first signs. Appetite usually is good, and the dog is normally active in the earlier stages of the disease. In the absence of concurrent secondary infections, there is little or no fever. Usually in advanced stages, there is shallow, rapid breathing and fever, and the prognosis is grave. Autoinfection may be induced by the use of corticosteroids or other factors that affect immunocompetence. There may be larvae in tissues, and these dogs are more likely to die. At necropsy, there can be evidence of verminous pneumonia with large areas of consolidation in the lungs as well as marked enteritis with hemorrhage, mucosal exfoliation, and much secretion of mucus.

Diagnosis: First-stage larvae (~380 μm long) are identified by direct microscopic evaluation of a small quantity of feces. Usually, the Baermann technique is used to separate larvae from fecal material. It is important to use fresh fecal material obtained from an infected dog so the larvae can be easily differentiated from hookworm larvae or free-living soil nematodes. Occasionally, eggs (50–60 × 30–35 μm) may be identified by flotation of fresh feces. Adult female worms can be identified by scraping the mucosa of the small intestine. They are only ~2 mm long, but the presence of eggs in the uterus easily differentiates them from larvae of other nematodes.

Treatment and Control: Poor sanitation and mixing of susceptible with infected dogs can lead to a rapid buildup of the infection in all dogs in a kennel or pen. Dogs with diarrhea should be promptly isolated from dogs that appear healthy. Direct sunlight, increased soil or surface temperatures, and desiccation are deleterious to all free larval stages. Thorough washing of wooden and impervious surfaces with steam or concentrated salt or lime solutions, followed by rinsing with hot water, effectively destroys the parasite. Because the disease in people can be serious, caution should be exercised when handling infected dogs. The disease in people (as in dogs) is much more likely to be severe if the person is immunosuppressed.

Infections in dogs can be treated with ivermectin (0.2 mg/kg, SC or PO, once, with a second dose 4 wk later; 0.8 mg/kg, PO, once), fenbendazole (50 mg/kg/day, PO, for 5 days, repeated 4 wk later), or thiabendazole (100–150 mg/kg/day, PO, for 3 days, repeated weekly until larvae are not detected in feces—toxicity may be seen with this regimen). In cats, fenbendazole (50 mg/kg/day, PO, for 3 days) can be used. These are not approved regimens in either cats or dogs. In all animals, feces should be examined regularly for at least 6 mo after treatment to confirm efficacy.

ROUNDWORMS

The large roundworms (ascaridoid nematodes) of dogs and cats are common, especially in puppies and kittens. Of the three species *Toxocara canis*, *Toxascaris leonina*, and *Toxocara cati*, the most important is *T canis*, not only because its larvae may migrate in people (as do larvae of *T cati*), but also because infections are generally common and may impact puppy health. Also, fatal infections may occasionally be seen in young pups. *T leonina* is seen in adolescent/adult dogs and cats. These species also infect wild carnivores, especially those in zoos or other captive settings.

In puppies, the usual mode of infection with *T canis* is transplacental transfer. If pups <3 mo old ingest embryonated infective eggs, the hatched larvae penetrate the intestinal mucosa, reach the lungs via the liver and bloodstream, are coughed up, swallowed, and mature to egg-producing adults in the small intestine. However, when infective eggs of *T canis* are swallowed by older dogs, the larvae hatch, penetrate the intestinal mucosa, and migrate to the liver, lungs, muscles, connective tissue, kidneys, and many other tissues, where development is arrested. In pregnant bitches, these dormant larvae mobilize and migrate into the developing fetus; they can be found in the intestine of puppies as early as 1 wk after birth. Some larvae migrate to the mammary gland, so pups may also be infected via the milk. During this perinatal period, the immunity of the bitch to ascarid infection is partially suppressed, and substantial numbers of eggs may be passed in the feces of the bitch. Development of these patent infections appears to be associated with maturation of arrested larvae in the bitch, which migrate to the intestine via the lungs. Patency may also occur as a result of ingestion and maturation of larvae that are passed in the feces of puppies.

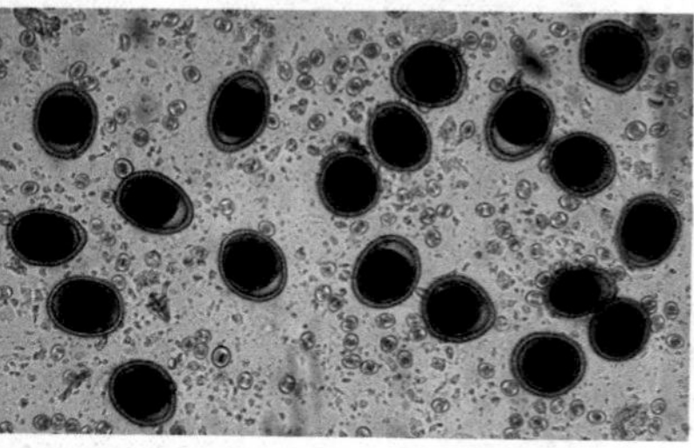

Toxocara canis ova (larger structures) and *Cystoisospora* oocysts (smaller structures). *Courtesy of Dr. Andrew Peregrine and Ontario Veterinary College.*

After ingestion of infective eggs, larvae of ascaridoid nematodes may migrate into the tissues of many animals and thus provide an alternative source of infection, particularly for cats and wild carnivores. Such migration also occurs if larvated eggs of *Toxocara* spp are swallowed by people. Most human infections are asymptomatic, but fever, persistent eosinophilia, and hepatomegaly (sometimes with pulmonary involvement) may occur, resulting in a condition known as **visceral larva migrans**. Rarely, a larva may settle in the retina and impair vision, resulting in a condition known as **ocular larva migrans**.

The life cycle of *T cati* is similar to that of *T canis*, except that no prenatal infection occurs. Furthermore, transmammary transmission appears to occur only when queens acquire infection during late gestation. Thus, overall, this route of infection appears to play a minor role in transmission. With *T leonina*, migration is restricted to the intestinal wall so that neither prenatal nor transmammary transmission occurs.

Clinical Findings and Lesions: The first indication of infection in young animals is lack of growth and loss of condition. Infected animals have a dull coat and often are "potbellied." Worms may be vomited and are often voided in the feces. In the early stages, migrating larvae may cause an eosinophilic pneumonia, which can be associated with coughing. Diarrhea with mucus may be evident.

In puppies with severe infections, verminous pneumonia, ascites, fatty liver, and mucoid enteritis are common. Cortical kidney granulomas containing larvae may be seen.

Diagnosis: Infection in dogs and cats is diagnosed by detection of eggs in feces. Distinguishing the spherical, pitted-shelled eggs of *Toxocara* spp (*T canis* 80–90 × 75 μm; *T cati* 65 × 75 μm) from the oval, smooth-shelled eggs of *Toxascaris leonina* (75–85 × 60–75 μm) is important because of the public health significance of the former.

Treatment and Control: In dogs, compounds approved for treatment of roundworm infections include fenbendazole, milbemycin, moxidectin, piperazine, and pyrantel (*see* TABLE 8). In Europe, selamectin is approved to treat *T canis* infections with a single dose, whereas in Canada approved treatment requires two doses 1 mo apart. Preventive programs for heartworm infection using milbemycin, milbemycin/lufenuron, milbemycin/praziquantel, milbemycin/spinosad, moxidectin/imidacloprid, ivermectin/pyrantel, or ivermectin/pyrantel/praziquantel also control intestinal ascarid infections. In addition, selamectin is approved for this indication in some countries but not in the USA (*see* TABLE 8).

Drugs approved for treatment of ascarid infections in cats include emodepside, fenbendazole, milbemycin, moxidectin, piperazine, pyrantel, and selamectin (*see* TABLE 9). Heartworm-preventive programs that use milbemycin, milbemycin/praziquantel, moxidectin/imidacloprid, or selamectin also control ascarid infections in cats (*see* TABLE 9).

Environmentally resistant larvated eggs on the ground and somatic larvae in the bitch are the main reservoirs of infection. Perinatal transmission of infection can be greatly reduced by treating bitches with 1) daily doses of fenbendazole (25 mg/kg, PO) from day 40 of gestation to day 2 after whelping (approved in the UK), 2) ivermectin (0.3 mg/kg, SC) on days 0, 30, and 60 of gestation, and 10 days after whelping, 3) ivermectin (0.5 mg/kg) on days 38, 41, 44, and 47 of gestation, or 4) ivermectin (1 mg/kg) on days 20 and 42 of gestation; these uses of ivermectin are extra-label. Otherwise, to minimize egg output, pups should be treated as early as possible; ideally, treatment should be given 2 wk after birth and repeated at 2-wk intervals to 2 mo of age, and then monthly to 6 mo of age. Nursing bitches should be treated at the same times as puppies. In cats, perinatal transmission can be greatly reduced by treating queens with a single dose of emodepside/praziquantel spot-on in the last week of pregnancy. Kittens should be treated with an appropriate anthelmintic at 3, 5, 7, and 9 wk of age, and then monthly to 6 mo of age. Nursing queens should be treated at the same time as kittens. In other animals, the appropriate frequency of preventive treatment for roundworms should be based on a risk assessment of the animal's environment.

Because the eggs adhere to many surfaces and become mixed in soil and dust, strict hygiene should be observed by people, particularly children, exposed to potentially contaminated animals or areas.

Baylisascaris in Dogs

The raccoon roundworm, *Baylisascaris procyonis*, is a common infection of raccoons in parts of North America and Europe. Adult parasites reside within the small intestine of raccoons and occasionally in the small intestine of dogs. It is thought that dogs become infected via ingestion of infective eggs or paratenic hosts (eg, rodents, rabbits, birds).

Ingestion of infective eggs results in visceral and neural larva migrans in many species, including people. As a result, the parasite is a significant zoonotic concern.

Clinical disease has not been reported in dogs with intestinal infections. However, signs are likely to be similar to those of *T canis* infections. In contrast, severe or fatal neural larva migrans has occasionally been reported in dogs.

Patent intestinal infections appear to occur uncommonly in dogs. However, it is likely that such infections are underdiagnosed; the eggs of *B procyonis* are similar in appearance to those of *T canis*, except they are slightly smaller (63–75 × 53–60 μm) and darker in color. Eggs of *B procyonis* may be found in dog feces as a result of ingestion of raccoon feces; shedding of such eggs should cease within 1–2 days.

Adult *B procyonis* and *T canis* passed in feces can be difficult to differentiate; female parasites should be dissected, and the eggs examined for identification.

Because of the zoonotic potential of *B procyonis* eggs, it is important that patent infections in dogs are diagnosed promptly and that appropriate treatment administered immediately. Ivermectin/pyrantel and milbemycin oxime/lufenuron at approved dosages have been shown to exhibit significant activity against intestinal infections in dogs with cure rates of 100% and 75%, respectively, after treatment with a single dose. However, these are not approved treatment protocols. Dogs should be confined and feces/parasites collected and disposed of for at least 3 days after treatment.

HOOKWORMS

Ancylostoma caninum is the principal cause of canine hookworm disease in most tropical and subtropical areas of the world. *A tubaeforme* of cats has a similar but more sparse distribution. *A braziliense* of dogs and cats is sparsely distributed from Florida to North Carolina in the USA. It is also found throughout Central and South America and Africa. *A ceylanicum* of dogs, cats, and people is widely distributed throughout Asia, the Middle East, and parts of South America. *Uncinaria stenocephala* is the principal canine hookworm in cooler regions; it appears to be the predominant canine hookworm in Canada and the northern fringe of the USA, where it is primarily a fox parasite. *U stenocephala* also is seen in cats. *A caninum* males are ~12 mm long, females, ~15 mm; the other species are somewhat smaller. The infective larvae of canine hookworms, particularly those of *A braziliense*, may penetrate and wander under the skin of people and cause **cutaneous larva migrans**.

The elongate (>65 µm), thin-walled, hookworm eggs in the early cleavage stages (2–8 cells) are first passed in the feces 15–20 days after infection; they complete embryonation and hatch in 24–72 hr on warm, moist soil. Transmission may result from ingestion of infective larvae from the environment and additionally, in the case of *A caninum*, via the colostrum or milk of infected bitches. Infections with *A caninum*, *A braziliense*, *A tubaeforme*, or *A ceylanicum* can also result from larval invasion through the skin, but this route is of little significance for *U stenocephala*. Skin penetration in young pups is followed by migration of the larvae through the blood to the lungs, where they are coughed up and swallowed to mature in the small intestine. However, in animals >3 mo old, *A caninum* larvae, after migration through the lungs, are arrested in the somatic tissues. These arrested larvae are activated during pregnancy, then accumulate in the mammary glands. Arrested development may also occur in the mucosa of the small intestine; activation may occur after removal of adult worms from the intestine.

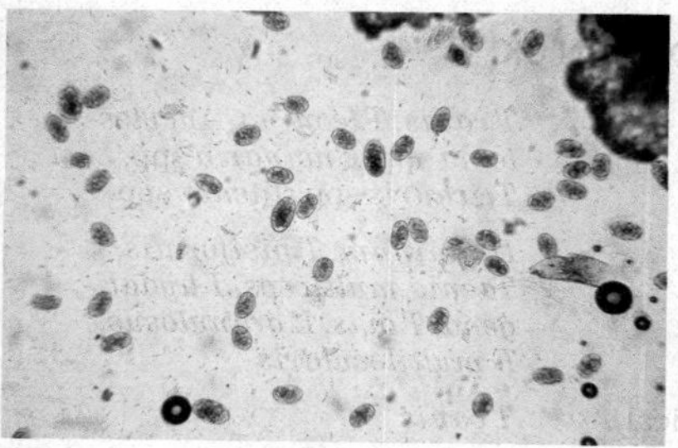

Hookworm eggs of *Ancylostoma* (smaller) and *Uncinaria* (larger) spp. *Courtesy of Dr. Andrew Peregrine and Ontario Veterinary College.*

Clinical Findings: An acute normocytic, normochromic anemia followed by hypochromic, microcytic anemia in young puppies is the characteristic, and often fatal, clinical manifestation of *A caninum* infection. Surviving puppies develop some immunity and show less severe clinical signs. Nevertheless, debilitated and malnourished animals may continue to be unthrifty and suffer from chronic anemia. Mature, well-nourished dogs may harbor a few worms without showing signs; they are of primary concern as the direct or indirect source of infection for pups. Diarrhea with dark, tarry feces accompanies severe infections. Anemia, anorexia, emaciation, and weakness develop in chronic disease.

Lesions: Anemia results directly from the bloodsucking and the bleeding ulcerations that result when *A caninum* shift feeding sites. The amount of blood loss due to a single worm in 24 hr has been estimated to be up to 0.1 mL. There is no interference with erythropoiesis in uncomplicated hookworm disease. The liver and other organs may appear ischemic, and some fatty infiltration of the liver may occur. Hemorrhagic enteritis with a swollen intestinal mucosa that shows red, small ulcers and attached worms is usually seen in acute, fatal cases. *A braziliense*, *A tubaeforme*, *A ceylanicum*, and *U stenocephala* are not avid blood feeders, and anemia rarely develops. However, hypoproteinemia is characteristic, and serum seepage around the site of attachment in the intestine may reduce blood protein by >10%.

In dogs, dermatitis due to larval invasion of the skin may be seen with any of the hookworms but has been seen most frequently in the interdigital spaces with *U stenocephala*; skin infections with *U stenocephala* rarely mature. Pneumonia and lung consolidation may result from overwhelming infections in pups.

Diagnosis: The characteristic thin-shelled, oval eggs are easily seen on flotation of fresh feces from infected dogs and cats (*Ancylostoma* spp 52–79 × 28–58 µm; *Uncinaria* sp 71–92 × 35–58 µm). Acute anemia and death from infections acquired via milk may be seen in young pups before eggs are passed in their feces, ie, as early as 1–2 wk of age.

Treatment and Control: Bitches should be free of hookworms before breeding and

TABLE 8 DRUGS FOR INTESTINAL HELMINTHS OF DOGS APPROVED IN THE USA AND UK

Drug or Drug Combination	Dosage (mg/kg)	Route of Administration	Helminths Active Against[a]
APPROVED ONLY IN USA			
Fenbendazole	50, daily for 3 days	PO	*Toxocara canis, Toxascaris leonina, Ancylostoma caninum, Uncinaria stenocephala, Trichuris vulpis, Trichuris pisiformis*
Epsiprantel	5.5	PO	*D caninum, T pisiformis*
Milbemycin oxime	0.5	PO	*T canis, T leonina, A caninum, T vulpis*
Milbemycin oxime + spinosad	0.5/30	PO	*T canis, T leonina, A caninum, T vulpis*
Moxidectin	0.17	SC	*A caninum, U stenocephala*
Piperazine (various salts)	48–66[b, d]	PO	*T canis, T leonina*
Praziquantel	5–12.5	PO	*D caninum, T pisiformis, Echinococcus granulosus*[c], *E multilocularis*[c]
	5–11.4	SC, IM	*D caninum, T pisiformis, E granulosus, E multilocularis*
Pyrantel pamoate	5 (10 for dogs ≤2.3 kg)	PO	*T canis, T leonina, A caninum, U stenocephala*
Ivermectin + pyrantel pamoate	0.006/5	PO	*T canis, T leonina, A caninum, A braziliense, U stenocephala*
Praziquantel + pyrantel pamoate	5/5	PO	*T canis, T leonina, A caninum, A braziliense, U stenocephala, D caninum, T pisiformis*
Praziquantel + pyrantel pamoate + febantel	5/5/25	PO	*T canis, T leonina, A caninum, U stenocephala, T vulpis, D caninum, T pisiformis, E granulosus, E multilocularis*
Praziquantel + pyrantel pamoate + ivermectin	5/5/0.006	PO	*T canis, T leonina, A caninum, A braziliense, U stenocephala, D caninum, T pisiformis*
APPROVED ONLY IN UK			
Fenbendazole	100; 50, daily for 3 days	PO	*T canis, T leonina, Ancylostoma* spp, *Uncinaria* spp, *Trichuris* spp, *Taenia* spp
Praziquantel	5	PO	*D caninum, T pisiformis, Taenia multiceps, T hydatigena, T ovis, E granulosus, E multilocularis*
Selamectin	6	Topical	*T canis*
Febantel + pyrantel embonate	15/14.4	PO	*T canis, T leonina, A caninum, U stenocephala, T vulpis*

TABLE 8 DRUGS FOR INTESTINAL HELMINTHS OF DOGS APPROVED IN THE USA AND UK *(continued)*

Drug or Drug Combination	Dosage (mg/kg)	Route of Administration	Helminths Active Against[a]
Milbemycin oxime + praziquantel	0.5/5	PO	*T canis, T leonina, A caninum, T vulpis, D caninum, Taenia* spp, *Echinococcus* spp, *Mesocestoides* spp
Praziquantel + pyrantel embonate + febantel	5/14.4/15	PO	*T canis, T leonina, A caninum, U stenocephala, T vulpis*[c], *D caninum*[c], *Taenia* spp (*T hydatigena*[c], *T pisiformis*[c]), *Echinococcus* spp[c] (*E granulosus*[c], *E multilocularis*[c])
Praziquantel + pyrantel embonate + oxantel embonate	5/5/20	PO	*T canis, T leonina, A caninum, U stenocephala, T vulpis, D caninum, Taenia* spp[c] (*Taenia ovis*[c], *T pisiformis*[c], *T hydatigena*[c], *T multiceps*[c]), *Echinococcus* spp[c] (*E granulosus*[c], *E multilocularis*[c]), *Mesocestoides* spp[c]
APPROVED IN BOTH USA AND UK			
Milbemycin oxime + lufenuron	0.5/10	PO	*T canis, T leonina*[d], *A caninum, T vulpis*
Moxidectin + imidacloprid	2.5/10	Topical	*T canis, T leonina, A caninum, U stenocephala, T vulpis, Spirocerca lupi*[e]

[a] Many of these drugs are also approved for use against other types of parasites (eg, fleas, heartworm) not listed here.

[b] Repeat in 10–20 days

[c] Only some products

[d] Only in the USA

[e] Only in the UK

kept out of contaminated areas during pregnancy. Sanitary quarters should be provided for whelping and nursing. Concrete runways that can be washed at least twice a week in warm weather are best. Sunlit clay or sandy runways can be decontaminated with sodium borate (1 kg/2 m^2).

In dogs, fenbendazole, moxidectin, and pyrantel are approved for treatment of *A caninum* and *U stenocephala* infections. Milbemycin is also approved for treatment of *A caninum* infections (*see* TABLE 8). Nitroscanate is also approved for both hookworms at 50 mg/kg in some countries (eg, Canada). When anemia is severe, chemotherapy may have to be supported by blood transfusion or supplemental iron, followed by a high-protein diet until the Hgb level is normal. Heartworm prevention with products containing milbemycin control *A caninum*, whereas ivermectin/pyrantel, ivermectin/pyrantel/praziquantel, moxidectin, and moxidectin/imidacloprid control *A caninum* and *U stenocephala*. Heartworm preventives containing pyrantel also have activity against *A braziliense* (*see* TABLE 8) and are approved for this purpose. Finally, the injectable formulation of moxidectin for heartworm prevention in dogs also has significant efficacy against infection with *A caninum* and *U stenocephala* for at least 3 mo. For *A ceylanicum*, the combination product containing pyrantel embonate/febantel/praziquantel is approved for treatment in Australia.

TABLE 9 DRUGS FOR INTESTINAL HELMINTHS OF CATS APPROVED IN THE USA AND UK

Drug or Drug Combination	Dosage (mg/kg)	Route of Administration	Helminths Active Against[a]
APPROVED ONLY IN USA			
Epsiprantel	2.75	PO	*Dipylidium caninum*, *Taenia taeniaeformis*
Ivermectin	0.024	PO	*Ancylostoma tubaeforme*, *A braziliense*
Milbemycin oxime	2	PO	*Toxocara cati*, *A tubaeforme*
Piperazine (various salts)	48–88[b, d]	PO	*T cati*[c], *Toxascaris leonina*
Praziquantel	4.6–10	PO	*D caninum*, *T taeniaeformis*
	5–10	SC, IM	*D caninum*, *T taeniaeformis*
Praziquantel + pyrantel pamoate	5/20	PO	*T cati*, *A tubaeforme*, *D caninum*, *T taeniaeformis*
APPROVED ONLY IN UK			
Fenbendazole	50, daily for 3 days; 100	PO	*T cati*, *T leonina*, *Ancylostoma* spp, *Uncinaria* spp, *Taenia* spp
Praziquantel	5	PO	*D caninum*, *T taeniaeformis*, *Echinococcus multilocularis*[c]
	8	Topical	*D caninum*, *Taenia* spp, *E multilocularis*
Milbemycin oxime + praziquantel	2/5	PO	*T cati*, *A tubaeforme*, *D caninum*, *Taenia* spp, *E multilocularis*
Praziquantel + pyrantel embonate	5/57.5	PO	*T cati*, *T leonina*, *D caninum*, *T taeniaeformis*
APPROVED IN BOTH USA AND UK			
Emodepside + praziquantel	3/12	Topical	*T cati*, *A tubaeforme*, *D caninum*, *T taeniaeformis*, *T leonina*[d], *E multilocularis*[d]
Moxidectin + imidacloprid	1/10	Topical	*T cati*, *A tubaeforme*
Selamectin	6	Topical	*T cati*, A tubaeforme

[a] Many of these drugs are also approved for use against other types of parasites (eg, fleas, heartworms) not listed here.

[b] Repeat in 10–14 days for most products

[c] Only some products

[d] Only in the USA

In cats, drugs approved for treatment of *A tubaeforme* include emodepside, fenbendazole, ivermectin, milbemycin, moxidectin, pyrantel, and selamectin (*see* TABLE 9). Heartworm prevention with ivermectin, milbemycin, milbemycin/praziquantel, moxidectin/imidacloprid, or selamectin controls *A tubaeforme*, whereas ivermectin also controls *A braziliense* (*see* TABLE 9).

When neonatal pups die due to hookworm infection, subsequent litters from the bitch should be treated weekly for *A caninum* for ~12 wk beginning at 2 wk of age. In addition, fenbendazole (25 mg/kg, PO) given daily to pregnant bitches from day 40 of pregnancy to day 2 after whelping greatly reduces transmammary transmission to the pups (approved in the UK). Likewise, treatment of the bitch with ivermectin (0.5 mg/kg) on two occasions (4–9 days before whelping and 10 days later), or with moxidectin/imidacloprid spot-on on day 56 of pregnancy, has the same effect (extra-label use).

Resistance of *A caninum* to pyrantel has been reported in parts of Australia.

WHIPWORMS

Adult *Trichuris vulpis* are 45–75 mm long and consist of a long, slender anterior portion and a thick posterior third. They commonly inhabit the cecum and colon of dogs, where they are firmly attached to the wall with their anterior end embedded in the mucosa. Thick-shelled eggs with bipolar plugs are passed in the feces and become infective in 1–2 mo in a warm, moist environment. Although eggs may remain viable in a suitable environment for up to 5 yr, they are susceptible to desiccation. The life cycle is direct. After infective eggs are ingested, the larvae hatch and develop in the wall of the distal ileum, cecum, and colon, and the adults mature in ~11 wk. They may remain for up to 16 mo.

No signs are seen in light infections, but as the worm burden increases and the inflammatory (and occasionally hemorrhagic) reaction in the cecum and colon becomes more pronounced, weight loss and diarrhea become evident. Fresh blood may be seen in the feces of heavily infected dogs, and anemia occasionally follows.

Trichuris infections are rarely seen in cats in North and South America and the Caribbean but may occasionally be associated with clinical signs similar to those described for dogs.

Treatment and Control: The eggs are susceptible to desiccation; therefore, by maintaining cleanliness and eliminating moist areas, the risk of infection in dogs can be reduced considerably, although *T vulpis* infections can be difficult to control. For anthelmintic treatment of dogs, approved compounds include febantel, fenbendazole, milbemycin, moxidectin (topical), and oxantel (*see* TABLE 8). Treatment should be repeated three times at monthly intervals because of the long prepatent period. Finally, milbemycin, milbemycin/lufenuron, milbemycin/spinosad, milbemycin/praziquantel, and moxidectin/imidacloprid, when administered for heartworm prevention, are also approved for control of *T vulpis* infections.

Effective therapy has yet to be described for *Trichuris* infections in cats. If required, treatment should be attempted on an experimental basis using a compound with approved activity against *T vulpis*.

ACANTHOCEPHALANS

(Thorny-headed worms)

Oncicola spp

Oncicola canis and other species are rarely found in the small intestine of dogs and cats. They are white and ~8–15 mm long, and their thorny heads are embedded in the mucosa. The females lay brown, thick-shelled, embryonated, wide oval eggs (43–50 × 67–72 μm). The life cycle is not completely known, but it is thought to include an arthropod intermediate host and paratenic hosts such as lizards, birds, or armadillos. Most infections cause no clinical signs.

Macracanthorhynchus sp

Macracanthorhynchus ingens, naturally a parasite of raccoons, is occasionally found in dogs. The usual observation is of a large (8–12 cm), white, wrinkled worm passed in the feces. No clinical signs have been definitively associated with the infection. The life cycle requires a millipede as an intermediate host, but other animals may serve as paratenic hosts. The eggs look similar to those of *Oncicola canis* but are larger (~50 × 100 μm). Diagnosis of patent infections is unlikely, because experimentally induced infections did not persist after 1–12 days of patency. No treatment is necessary.

TAPEWORMS

(Cestodes)

Most urban dogs and cats eat prepared foods and have restricted access to natural

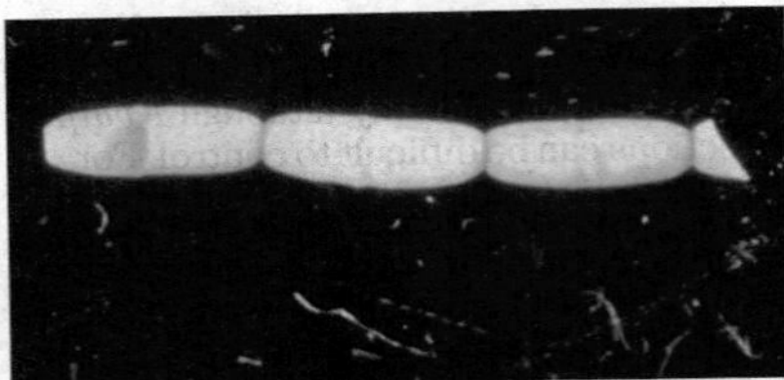

Dipylidium caninum segments. *Courtesy of Dr. Andrew Peregrine and Ontario Veterinary College.*

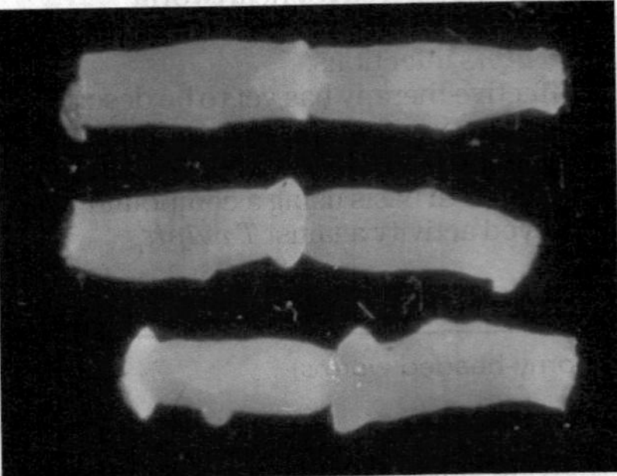

Taenia sp segments. *Courtesy of Dr. Andrew Peregrine and Ontario Veterinary College.*

prey. Such animals may acquire *Dipylidium caninum* (the double-pored dog tapeworm) by ingesting fleas. Cats with access to infected house (or outdoor) mice and rats also can acquire *Taenia taeniaeformis*. In certain parts of the world (eg, India, the Middle East, North Africa, southeast Asia, southern Europe), dogs and cats with access to reptiles may acquire *Joyeuxiella pasqualei*. Suburban, rural, and hunting dogs have more access to various small mammals, in addition to raw meat and offal from domestic and wild ungulates. A number of cestodes can be expected in such dogs (*see* TABLE 10). On sheep ranges and wherever wild ungulates and wild canids are common, dogs may acquire *Echinococcus granulosus* (the hydatid tapeworm). Sylvatic *Echinococcus multilocularis* (the alveolar hydatid tapeworm), previously known only from arctic North America, has been found in wildlife in midwestern and western USA and Canada. The parasite is also endemic in many parts of central and eastern Europe, particularly France, Germany, and Switzerland. Thus far, infections in cats or dogs are generally rare. However, in addition to multiple reports from dogs and cats in central Europe, the parasite has recently been identified in a few dogs

TABLE 10 CESTODES OF DOGS AND CATS IN NORTH AMERICA

Cestode	Definitive Host	Intermediate Host and Organs Invaded[a]
Dipylidium caninum	Dog, cat, coyote, wolf, fox, other wild canids and felids	Fleas and more rarely lice; free in body cavity
Taenia taeniaeformis	Cat, dog, lynx, fox, other animals	Various rats, mice, other rodents; in large cysts in liver
Taenia pisiformis	Dog, fox, wolf, coyote, other animals	Rabbits and hares, rarely squirrels and other rodents; in pelvic or peritoneal cavity attached to viscera
Taenia hydatigena	Dog, wolf, coyote, weasel, fox	Domestic and wild cloven-hoofed animals, rarely hares and rodents; in liver and abdominal cavity

across Canada. *Spirometra mansonoides* is an uncommon (but not rare) parasite of cats and occasionally of dogs along the eastern and Gulf Coast areas of North America.

Association with infected dogs may result in human infection with metacestodes of *E granulosus*, *E multilocularis*, *T multiceps*, *T serialis*, or *T crassiceps* in various tissues (by ingestion of eggs passed in dog feces), or adult *D caninum* in the intestine (by ingestion of infected fleas). The presence of metacestodes in livestock may limit commercial use of such carcasses or offal meats. Thus, cestodes of dogs and cats may be of both economic and public health importance (*see* TABLE 11).

Adult cestodes in the intestine of dogs and cats rarely cause serious disease, and clinical signs, if present, may depend on the degree of infection, age, condition, and breed of host. Clinical signs vary from unthriftiness, malaise, irritability, capricious appetite, and shaggy coat to colic and mild diarrhea; rarely, intussusception or blockage of the intestine, emaciation, and seizures are seen.

Diagnosis is based on finding proglottids or eggs in the feces. The eggs of *Taenia* spp and *Echinococcus* spp cannot be differentiated by microscopic examination; PCR methods are required. Direct microscopic examination of fecal samples or fecal flotation may reveal the eggs of *Spirometra mansonoides*, which are sometimes mistaken for trematode eggs, although they are larger and possess an operculum that is often difficult to see.

Control of tapeworms of dogs and cats requires therapy and prevention. Animals that roam freely often become reinfected by ingestion of metacestodes in carrion or prey animals. *Dipylidium caninum* is different, because it can cycle through fleas that may be associated with confined infected animals. An accurate diagnosis is necessary for effective advice on preventing reinfection.

Effective treatment should remove the attached scolices from the small intestine of infected animals. (*See* TABLE 10 for specific approved treatments.) For dogs, fenbendazole and praziquantel are approved for treatment of *Taenia* spp (ie, more than just *T pisiformis*, for which epsiprantel is approved); epsiprantel, nitroscanate, and praziquantel are approved for *D caninum*; and praziquantel is approved for treatment of *Echinococcus* spp (*see* TABLE 8). For cats, fenbendazole and praziquantel are approved for treatment of *Taenia* spp (ie, more than just *T taeniaeformis*, for which epsiprantel is approved); epsiprantel and

TABLE 10 CESTODES OF DOGS AND CATS IN NORTH AMERICA *(continued)*

Diagnostic Features of Adult Worm	Comments	Approved Treatment[b]
Strobila 15–70 cm long and up to 3 mm in maximum width, 30–150 rostellar hooks of rose-thorn shape in 3 or 4 circles; large hooks 12–15 µm, smallest 5–6 µm long. Segments shaped like cucumber seeds, with pore near middle of each lateral margin.	Probably most common tapeworm of dogs and cats; cosmopolitan. Occasionally infects people, particularly infants.	Dogs and cats: epsiprantel, praziquantel
Strobila 15–60 cm long, 5–6 mm in maximum width, 26–52 rostellar hooks in double row; large hooks 380–420 µm, small hooks 250–270 µm long. No neck. Sacculate lateral branches of uterus difficult to count.	Common cestode of cats, rare in dogs; cosmopolitan	Cats: epsiprantel, praziquantel, fenbendazole
Strobila 60 cm to 2 m long, 5 mm in maximum width, ~34–48 rostellar hooks in double row; large hooks 225–290 µm, small hooks 132–177 µm long. Each side of gravid uterus has 5–10 lateral branches.	Particularly common in suburban, farm, and hunting dogs that eat rabbits and rabbit viscera.	Dogs: epsiprantel, fenbendazole, praziquantel
Strobila to 5 m long and 7 mm in maximum width; ~26–44 rostellar hooks in double row; large hooks 170–220 µm, small hooks 110–160 µm long. Each side of gravid uterus 5–10 lateral branches.	In farm dogs, more rarely hunting dogs; cosmopolitan	Dogs: praziquantel, fenbendazole

TABLE 10 CESTODES OF DOGS AND CATS IN NORTH AMERICA *(continued)*

Cestode	Definitive Host	Intermediate Host and Organs Invaded[a]
Spirometra mansonoides	Cat, dog, raccoon, bobcat	Copepods, frogs, rodents, snakes; connective tissue
Diphyllobothrium spp	People, dog, cat, other fish-eating animals	Encysted in various organs, or free in body cavity of various fish
Echinococcus granulosus	Dog, wolf, coyote, fox, and several other wild carnivores	Sheep, goats, cattle, pigs, horses, deer, moose, some rodents, occasionally people and other animals; commonly in liver and lungs, occasionally in other organs and tissues
Echinococcus multilocularis	Arctic, red, and gray foxes; coyote, cat, dog	Microtine rodents, occasionally in people; in the liver and other organs
Mesocestoides spp	Many wild canids, felids, mustelids; other animals, including dog and cat	Complete life cycle unknown; arthropod intermediate hosts suspected; juvenile tetrathyridia in abdominal cavity and elsewhere of various mammals, birds, and reptiles; tetrathyridia in intestine of dogs may enter abdomen through intestinal wall.
Taenia multiceps	Dog, coyote, fox, wolf	Sheep, goats, and other domestic or wild ruminants, rarely people; usually in brain or spinal cord
Taenia serialis	Dog, coyote, fox, wolf	Rabbit, hare, squirrel, rarely people; in subcutaneous connective tissue or retroperitoneally
Taenia crassiceps	Dog, coyote, fox, wolf	Various rodents, a few records in people; subcutaneous and in body cavities

TABLE 10 CESTODES OF DOGS AND CATS IN NORTH AMERICA *(continued)*

Diagnostic Features of Adult Worm	Comments	Approved Treatment[b]
Strobila 0.5 m long, 8 mm in maximum width. Scolex with 2 grooves and no hooks. Genital pores ventral midline of segment.	Eastern and Gulf Coast, North America	*See* text for extra-label treatment
Strobila to 10 m long, 20 mm in maximum width but usually smaller. Scolex with 2 grooves (bothria) and no hooks. Genital pores ventral midline of segment.	Canada, Alaska and various other states of the USA, Siberia, and other areas	*See* text for extra-label treatment
Strobila 2–6 mm long with 3–5 segments; 28–50 (usually 30–36) rostellar hooks in double row; large hooks 27–40 µm, small hooks 21–25 µm long.	Foci among North American range sheep and dogs associating with them; sylvatic moose-wolf cycle where these animals are found; probably cosmopolitan	Dogs: praziquantel
Strobila 1.2–2.7 mm long with 2–4 segments; 26–36 rostellar hooks in double row; large hooks 23–29 µm, small hooks 19–26 µm long.	Central and eastern Europe, former USSR, Alaska, and midwestern USA and Canada; thus far, significant cycle in cats and dogs in North America not recognized. However, multiple cases of alveolar echinococcosis have been diagnosed in dogs across Canada.	Dogs and cats: praziquantel
Strobila 10 cm long and 2–5 mm wide. Scolex with 4 suckers but no rostellum or hooks. Genital pore ventral in midline of worm. Gravid segments with parauterine organ.	Reported in dogs and cats in midwest and west; in wild animals elsewhere in USA and Canada	Dogs: praziquantel
Strobila 40–100 cm long and up to 5 mm wide. Scolex with 4 suckers and 22–32 hooks in double row; large hooks 150–170 µm, small hooks 90–130 µm long. Vagina with reflexed curve near lateral excretory canal; 9–26 lateral branches on gravid uterus.	Rare in domestic carnivores in western North America; more common in wild animals	Dogs: praziquantel, fenbendazole
Strobila 20–72 cm long and 3–5 mm wide; 26–32 hooks in double row; large hooks 110–175 µm, small hooks 68–120 µm long. Vagina with reflexed curve near lateral excretory canal; 20–25 lateral branches on gravid uterus.	Primarily in wild canids; considered by some authorities as not distinct from *T multiceps*	Same as for *T multiceps*
Strobila 70–170 mm long and 1–2 mm wide. Scolex with 30–36 hooks in double row; large hooks 158–187 µm, small hooks 119–141 µm long. Uterus has 16–21 lateral branches, sometimes becoming diffuse.	Reported from Canada and northern USA, including Alaska	Same as for *T multiceps*

TABLE 10 CESTODES OF DOGS AND CATS IN NORTH AMERICA *(continued)*

Cestode	Definitive Host	Intermediate Host and Organs Invaded[a]
Taenia krabbei	Dog, coyote, wolf, bobcat	Moose, deer, reindeer; in striated muscle
Taenia ovis	Dog, wild canids	Sheep and goat; in skeletal and cardiac muscle, rarely elsewhere

praziquantel are approved for treatment of *D caninum*, and praziquantel is approved for treatment of *E multilocularis* (*see* TABLE 9). Outside the USA and UK, praziquantel is approved for use in multiple countries at 5 mg/kg for treatment of *J pasqualei* in dogs (as praziquantel/pyrantel/febantel) and cats (as praziquantel/pyrantel).

Praziquantel at 7.5 mg/kg, PO, for 2 consecutive days is effective against *Diphyllobothrium* sp in dogs. Furthermore, a single dose of 35 mg/kg, PO, eliminates *D latum* from infected cats. Both treatments are extra-label.

Infections with *Spirometra* sp in dogs and cats can be treated with praziquantel at 7.5 mg/kg, PO, for 2 consecutive days. *Spirometra* sp infections in cats can also be treated with a single dose of praziquantel at 30 mg/kg, SC, IM, or PO. Mebendazole at 11 mg/kg, PO, has also been successful. All these treatments are extra-label.

FLUKES

Intestinal Flukes

Nanophyetus salmincola, the "salmon poisoning" fluke, is a small (~0.5 × 0.3 mm), oval fluke found in the small intestine of dogs, cats, and many wild fish-eating mammals in the northwestern USA, southwestern Canada, and Siberia. The eggs, which pass in the feces of infected hosts, are light brown, 72–97 × 35–55 µm, and indistinctly operculated with a small knob at one pole. The life cycle includes an extended period (3 mo) of embryonation. The first intermediate hosts are snails found in endemic locations (eg, *Oxytrema silicula* in the USA). The cercariae from these snails penetrate the skin of young salmonid fishes and encyst as metacercariae in their muscles and organs. Dogs and other animals become infected by eating raw or improperly prepared infected fish.

Because these flukes embed deeply between the villi of the intestine, infection with a large number may cause enteritis. Most infections, however, are complicated through development of the salmon poisoning complex caused by rickettsial organisms, which the fluke transmits (*see* p 808). Praziquantel (20–30 mg/kg, PO or SC, once) and fenbendazole (50 mg/kg/day, PO, for 10–14 days) are both effective, but not approved, treatments for dogs.

Alaria alata, *A canis*, and other *Alaria* spp are small (2–6 mm) flukes usually found in the small intestine of dogs, cats, foxes, mink, and wild carnivores in the western hemisphere, as well as in Europe, Australia, and Japan. The anterior part of the body is flat, and the posterior part is conical. The eggs are oval, light brown, and fairly large (98–134 × 62–68 µm). The life cycle includes freshwater snails (eg, *Helisoma* spp) as first intermediate hosts. Cercariae emerge from the snails, penetrate tadpoles, and develop into mesocercariae. Frogs, snakes, and mice then acquire infection by eating tadpoles; the mesocercariae transfer to their tissues and remain as this life-cycle stage. Dogs and other definitive hosts become infected by feeding on these animals. The young flukes migrate through various organs of the definitive host, including the diaphragm and

TABLE 10 CESTODES OF DOGS AND CATS IN NORTH AMERICA *(continued)*

Diagnostic Features of Adult Worm	Comments	Approved Treatment[b]
Strobila ~20 cm long and up to 9 mm wide. Scolex small with 26–36 hooks in double row; large hooks 146–195 µm, small hooks 85–141 µm long. Gravid uterus has 18–24 straight and narrow lateral branches.	Reported from Canada and northern USA, including Alaska; considered by some a subspecies of *T ovis*	Same as for *T multiceps*
Strobila 45–110 cm long and up to 4–8.5 mm wide. Scolex with 32–38 hooks in double row; large hooks 170–191 µm, small hooks 111–127 µm long. Gravid uterus has 20–25 lateral branches. Vagina crosses ovary on poral side of segment.	Reported from western and central Canada and the southern USA	Same as for *T multiceps*

[a] In all cases in which the life cycle is known, cats and dogs become infected by eating animals (or parts) that contain the infective metacestode. These intermediate hosts become infected by ingesting tapeworm eggs (except in *Mesocestoides*, *Spirometra*, and *Diphyllobothrium* spp, which have an extra stage in the life cycle), which are passed in the feces of the definitive host.

[b] *See* TABLE 8 and TABLE 9 for drug dosages.

lungs, before reaching the small intestine. Although the flukes are generally considered to be nonpathogenic, large numbers may cause pulmonary hemorrhages during migration or enteritis when they mature in the small intestine. These flukes may infect people. Infections can be treated with praziquantel using the approved cestocidal dosage (*see* TABLE 8 and TABLE 9 for drug dosages.). However, such treatment is extra-label.

Other species of flukes, usually not pathogenic, have been found occasionally in the intestine of dogs, cats, and other carnivores; these include *Heterophyes heterophyes* in some north African and Asian countries; *Metagonimus yokogawai* in Asia; *Cryptocotyle lingua* in the USA, Canada, Japan, Siberia, and Europe; and *Apophallus donicum* in North America and eastern Europe. Their life cycles include snails as first intermediate hosts and fish as second intermediate hosts, in which metacercariae become encysted.

Heterobilharzia americana is found in the mesenteric veins of dogs and wild animals, especially raccoons, in the southeastern USA. The eggs pass through the tissues of the intestine to the lumen and then are voided in the feces. From the snail intermediate host, cercariae escape into water and penetrate the skin of dogs and other definitive hosts, migrate to the liver, mature, and move to the mesenteric vessels. Granulomas form around the eggs in the wall of the intestine, the liver, and other parts of the body. Lethargy, weight loss, vomiting, and/or diarrhea may develop in heavy infections. "Water dermatitis" is sometimes seen when cercariae penetrate the skin. The eggs do not readily float and, if placed in water, hatch within minutes; therefore, a sedimentation method using 0.85% saline is useful in separating eggs from ingesta. In infected dogs, eggs are passed intermittently, so on a given day eggs may not be found in feces. Fenbendazole at 50 mg/kg/day, PO, for 10 days, is an effective treatment. Praziquantel at 25 mg/kg, tid, for 2 days is also effective. Both are extra-label uses.

Hepatic Flukes

Flukes in the bile ducts and gallbladder cause mild to severe fibrosis. Many species of distome trematodes have been reported from the liver of dogs and cats in most parts of the world. Mild infections may pass unnoticed; however, in severe infection, dogs may develop progressive weakness, ending in complete exhaustion, coma, and death. The following are some of the most commonly encountered trematodes.

Opisthorchis felineus is parasitic in the bile duct, pancreatic duct, and small intestine of dogs and cats in Italy, eastern Europe, and parts of Asia. *O viverrini* is seen in dogs as well as in domestic and wild cats in southeast Asia. They are small

TABLE 11 CESTODES OF PUBLIC HEALTH IMPORTANCE

Cestode[a]	Host of Adult Worm	Name of Metacestode (Intermediate) Stage	Measurements of Metacestode	Principal Intermediate Hosts	Site of Metacestode
Taenia saginata	People only	Cysticercus "beef measles"	9 × 5 mm	Cattle	Skeletal and cardiac muscle
Taenia solium	People only	Cysticercus "pork measles"	6–10 × 5–10 mm	Pigs, rarely dogs (people may be both definitive and intermediate hosts)	Skeletal and cardiac muscle, occasionally nervous system
Diphyllobothrium spp	People, dogs, cats, and other fish-eating mammals	Procercoid in copepod, plerocercoid in fish	2–25 × 2.5 mm for plerocercoid	Copepod, then fish	Mesenteric tissues, testes, ovary, muscles of fish
Echinococcus granulosus	Dogs, wolves, foxes, and several other wild carnivores	Hydatid cyst	Diameter 50–100 mm, sometimes ≥150 mm	Sheep, cattle, pigs, horses, moose, deer; occasionally people	Commonly in liver and lungs, occasionally in other organs and tissues
Echinococcus multilocularis	Canids and domestic cats	Alveolar hydatid cyst	Variable, penetrates like neoplastic tissue	Field mice, voles, lemmings, sometimes domestic mammals and people	Usually liver, various other organs and tissues

[a] Human infections with the metacestodes of *Taenia crassiceps*, *T multiceps*, *Mesocestoides* spp, and other cestodes not listed here occur rarely. Children occasionally become infected with adult *Dipylidium caninum*, which appears to have no medical significance but important aesthetic aspects.

(9 × 2 mm) and elongate. Their life cycle includes certain snails (*Bithynia* sp) and cyprinid fishes as intermediate hosts. A related species, *Clonorchis sinensis*, the Oriental liver fluke of people, also has been found in the bile ducts and pancreatic ducts of dogs, cats, and other animals. It is larger than *Opisthorchis* spp. The operculated eggs of these parasites may be identified in the feces of infected animals.

Longterm presence of these flukes in the bile duct causes epithelial hyperplasia and fibrosis of the duct wall. Carcinomas in the liver or pancreas have been seen in chronic and severe cases. Treatment of *Opisthorchis* spp infections in dogs may be attempted with fenbendazole (200 mg/kg/day, PO, for 3 days) or praziquantel (20 mg/kg, PO, once). Treatment of *C sinensis* infections in dogs may be attempted with praziquantel (30 mg/kg/day, PO, for 3 days). All these treatments are extra-label.

Platynosomum concinnum is a small fluke (6 × 2 mm) found in the bile and pancreatic ducts of Felidae in southeastern USA, Puerto Rico and other Caribbean Islands, South America, some of the Pacific islands, and parts of Africa. Its life cycle includes the snail *Sublima octona* and a crustacean (wood louse) as intermediate hosts and certain lizards as paratenic hosts. Cats acquire the parasite by feeding on infected lizards. In mild cases, nonspecific chronic signs of unthriftiness may be seen. Severe infections, however, may cause the "lizard poisoning" syndrome, which is characterized by anorexia, lethargy, depression, persistent vomiting, diarrhea, jaundice, and an enlarged abdomen, leading to death. Treatment with praziquantel (20 mg/kg/day, PO, for 3–5 days, ideally, repeated 12 wk later), or nitroscanate (100 mg/kg, PO, once) has been successful, although these drugs are not approved for this use. Praziquantel appears to be the most effective agent. Bile duct surgery may also be required.

Metorchis albidus and *M conjunctus* are two small flukes (5 × 1.5 mm) that have been found in the bile ducts and gallbladder of dogs, cats, and other carnivores in North America, Europe, and the former USSR. They seldom cause any recognizable clinical signs. Their eggs are small (24–30 × 13–16 μm), and the life cycle includes certain freshwater snails and fish as intermediate hosts. Treatment of *Metorchis* spp infections in dogs may be attempted with praziquantel (20 mg/kg, PO, once), although this is an extra-label use.

Eurytrema procyonis is a small fluke (2.1 × 1 mm) commonly seen in the pancreatic duct of raccoons in the eastern USA and occasionally found in the pancreatic duct, bile duct, and gallbladder of domestic cats. Infection may be associated with weight loss and intermittent vomiting. The eggs are medium sized (45–53 × 29–36 μm), and the life cycle involves a land snail and a second intermediate host thought to be an arthropod. Treatment may be attempted with fenbendazole (30 mg/kg/day, PO, for 6 days) or praziquantel/pyrantel/febantel (praziquantel and pyrantel each at 5.8 mg/kg/day and febantel at 28.8 mg/kg/day, PO, for 5 days), although these drugs are not approved for this use.

HEPATIC DISEASE IN SMALL ANIMALS

The liver performs numerous functions, including but not limited to lipid, carbohydrate, and protein metabolism; storage, metabolism, and activation of vitamins; storage of minerals, glycogen, and triglycerides; extramedullary hematopoiesis; and synthesis of coagulant, anticoagulant, and several acute phase proteins. It also influences immunologic responses and contributes to digestion through synthesis and enterohepatic circulation of bile acids and detoxification of many endogenous and exogenous compounds, toxins, and xenobiotics. Because the liver has a large functional reserve and the ability to regenerate, hepatic injury must be considerable or chronic and recurrent to cause overt hepatic dysfunction or failure.

Active liver injury is accompanied by increased liver enzyme activity, with cytosolic transaminases (ALT, AST) acutely reflecting altered membrane permeability or viability or the phenomenon of membrane blebbing, and membrane-affiliated enzyme induction (alkaline phosphatase [ALP], γ-glutamyl transferase [GGT]) reflecting cholestasis and increased protein transcription (enzyme induction). The liver is predisposed to secondary injury owing to its sentinel position between the systemic circulation and GI tract and because it contains the largest population of fixed macrophages (Kupffer cells) in the body. Macrophage phagocytosis can initiate release of a cascade of inflammatory cytokines, leading to local cellular damage and recruitment of inflammatory infiltrates. The considerable metabolic activity of the liver exaggerates its exposure to noxious products, particularly in the centrilobular region, where high cytochrome p450 activity produces noxious products and adducts. Hepatocytes in this region also are more easily injured by hypoxia. The accumulation of hepatic copper and/or iron can initiate and augment liver injury through oxidative mechanisms.

Clinical signs of liver injury vary depending on the type, mechanism, and chronicity of the insult. Common clinical features may include anorexia, vomiting, diarrhea, weight loss, and fever. With severe, diffuse liver injury, animals may become jaundiced and demonstrate polyuria and polydipsia (PU/PD), coagulation abnormalities, and ascites. Ascites indicates development of portal hypertension and is typically associated with formation of acquired portosystemic shunts (APSSs) and concurrent hypoalbuminemia. Hepatic encephalopathy (HE) develops in acquired liver disease only when diffuse fibrosis and APSSs have developed, in acute fulminant liver failure, or secondary to congenital portosystemic shunts (congenital malformations of the portal vein that shunt portal blood directly to the systemic circulation). Fecal color may change with complete occlusion of bile ducts (acholic or pale-colored feces) or because of increased enteric bilirubin elimination (green fecal color). Hepatomegaly is found with diffuse infiltrative or storage disorders, acute extrahepatic bile duct obstruction (EHBDO), congenital biliary cystic malformations, or passive congestion, whereas microhepatica (small liver) usually reflects portal venous hypoperfusion, diversion of enteric hepatotrophic factors normally delivered in the portal circulation, or the presence of chronic hepatic fibrosis in dogs.

LABORATORY ANALYSES AND IMAGING

HEMATOLOGY

Depending on the severity and underlying cause of liver disease, a nonregenerative or regenerative anemia may develop. Severe or acute anemia can impact the liver as a result of hypoxia, causing alterations in hepatocyte membranes, leading to release of transaminases and induction of ALP. Altered RBC morphology (poikilocytes, irregularly irregular RBCs) is common in cats with cholangiohepatitis and hepatic lipidosis (HL). Cats with HL, severe cholangiohepatitis, and EHBDO also may develop Heinz bodies, reflecting oxidative injury that may lead to hemolysis. Severe hypophosphatemia in HL may develop secondary to a re-feeding syndrome and cause hemolysis severe enough to require a blood transfusion; this can be avoided by providing fluid therapy supplemented with potassium phosphate when nutritional support is implemented. In dogs with diffuse necroinflammatory liver disease (altered sinusoidal perfusion), RBCs with microvascular shearing (eg, schistocytes, acanthocytes) may be seen. RBC microcytosis is common in congenital or acquired portosystemic shunting, although the pathologic mechanism remains unclear.

Change in WBC count or distribution are variable. Leukocytosis may reflect inflammatory, infectious, necrolytic, or diffuse infiltrative hepatic disorders, or release of endogenous glucocorticoids or administration of glucocorticoids. Leukopenia can reflect sepsis or toxicosis. In severe diffuse necroinflammatory liver injury, damaged sinusoidal microvasculature can provoke platelet aggregation, contributing to thrombocytopenia and disseminated intravascular coagulation.

COAGULATION TESTS

Coagulation abnormalities can develop as a result of decreased synthesis or activation of coagulation factors and anticoagulant proteins produced in the liver (ie, factors V, VII, IX, X, XI, XII, fibrinogen, prothrombin, antithrombin, protein C, plasminogen, α_2-macroglobulin, and α_1-antitrypsin). Decreased enteric absorption of fat-soluble vitamins can lead to vitamin K–responsive bleeding in animals with EHBDO or bile duct immunoinjury (feline sclerosing cholangitis), or in cats with HL. Cats with liver disease appear predisposed to vitamin K–responsive coagulopathies. Conventional coagulation assessments may not reflect impending coagulopathies that remain unsuspected after physical examination, analysis of urine or feces, or mucosal bleeding time test. Dogs with congenital or acquired portosystemic shunting usually develop low protein C activity (<70% activity) that seemingly reflects the severity of portosystemic shunting. Although coagulation factors may be significantly lower in some of these dogs than in age-matched control groups, symptomatic coagulopathy is rare.

ENZYME ACTIVITY

Liver disease is often first suspected based on increased liver enzyme activity. However, abnormally increased liver enzyme activity is considerably more common than the prevalence of liver disease. A wide spectrum of nonhepatic disorders may influence liver enzyme activity. It is important to recognize that liver enzyme measurements are not liver function tests but rather reflect hepatocyte membrane integrity, hepatocyte or biliary epithelial necrosis, cholestasis, or induction phenomenon.

The pattern of liver enzyme abnormalities in relation to the signalment, history, total bilirubin concentration, serum bile acid values, and comorbid conditions/medications provides the first indication of a liver-specific disorder. A full assessment of liver enzyme aberration considers: 1) the predominant pattern of enzyme change (hepatocellular leakage enzymes vs cholestatic enzymes), 2) the magnitude of increase of enzyme activity above the normal reference range (mild is <3 times the upper reference range, moderate is 3–9 times, marked is >10 times), 3) the rate of change (increase or resolution) with sequential sampling, and 4) the nature of the course of change (fluctuation vs progressive increase or decrement). Up to 2.5% of clinically "normal" animals can have borderline abnormal enzyme values.

Recognizing whether enzyme abnormalities are persistent or cyclic helps categorize likely causes. Investigating liver function with paired fasting and postprandial total serum bile acids (TSBAs) or urine bile acid/creatinine measurements (urine collected 4–8 hr after meal ingestion) may expedite a decision to pursue liver biopsy when clinical signs remain vague and enzymes are only mildly increased. Imaging studies help detect primary underlying disorders that have secondarily influenced the liver, causing increased enzyme activity. Ultrasonographic assessment may help determine the method of liver biopsy; needle biopsies are ill advised in animals with microhepatica, ascites, or difficult-to-sample focal liver lesions.

Age-appropriate reference ranges for serum liver enzyme activity are essential to interpret laboratory values in puppies and kittens. Plasma enzyme activities of ALP and GGT in neonatal dogs and cats are remarkably higher than those of adults. Differences reflect physiologic adaptations during the transition from fetal and neonatal life stages, colostrum ingestion, maturation of metabolic pathways, growth effects, differences in volume of distribution and body composition, and nutritional intake. Serum activities of ALP, AST, CK, and LDH in neonates usually increase greatly during the first 24 hr of life. In kittens, serum activities of ALP, CK, and LDH exceed adult values through 8 wk of age. Serum ALP increases remarkably in day-old puppies and kittens after colostrum ingestion, as also observed in neonatal calves, lambs, pigs, and foals.

Aminotransferases: AST and ALT are commonly measured to detect liver injury; however, both enzymes are present in high concentrations in liver and several other tissues. AST activity is higher in kidney, heart, and skeletal muscle than liver, whereas ALT activity is highest in liver. Because hepatic ALT activity is 10,000-fold greater than plasma enzyme activity in healthy animals, it has high diagnostic utility to detect "liver lesions." The cytosolic location of transaminases allows their immediate release with even minor change in hepatocellular membrane integrity. Unfortunately, indiscriminate leakage limits their diagnostic utility. Nonetheless, duration and magnitude of transaminase activities measured sequentially can predict disease activity and severity and roughly estimate the number of involved cells.

Hepatic transaminases increase with muscle injury as well as vigorous physical activity in dogs. Persistence of transaminases in plasma contributes to their sustained high activities in certain disorders. Because transaminase catabolism occurs by absorptive endocytosis at the hepatocyte sinusoidal border, slow enzyme clearance may sustain plasma enzyme activity in hepatic insufficiency associated with liver fibrosis, nodular regeneration, and development of APSSs.

Alanine Aminotransferase: The largest increases in ALT develop with hepatocellular necrosis and inflammation. After acute severe hepatocyte necrosis, serum ALT activity increases sharply within 24–48 hr to values often >100-fold normal, peaking during the first 5 days of injury. If the injurious event resolves, ALT activity gradually declines to normal over 2–3 wk. Although this pattern is considered classic, some severe hepatotoxins are not associated with increased ALT activity, because they inhibit gene transcription or interfere with ALT biosynthesis (eg, aflatoxin B1 hepatotoxicity, microcystin hepatotoxicity). A declining ALT also may represent a paucity of viable hepatocytes in end-stage chronic hepatitis or severe acute liver disease.

Examples of classic necrotizing hepatotoxins are carbon tetrachloride, acetaminophen, and nitrosamine. A single exposure to carbon tetrachloride causes an acute sharp increase in ALT that resolves over the ensuing week. Hepatotoxicity induced by acetaminophen causes a marked increase in ALT and AST within 24 hr that may decline within 72 hr to near normal values. This toxin is highly dose dependent in dogs and cats. Cats are exceedingly susceptible, with hematologic signs dominating after ingestion of as little as 125 mg. However, in dogs, a dosage of 200 mg/kg may be life-threatening, with susceptibility heightened by antecedent exposure to phenobarbital. Hepatocellular necrosis induced by nitrosamines increases plasma ALT activity, but not significantly, until after 1 wk of intermittent chronic exposure. The ALT activity persists for weeks until necrosis resolves. Low-grade hepatocellular degeneration, observed in some dogs with congenital portosystemic shunts, reflects delayed enzyme clearance and low-grade hepatocyte dropout; most of these dogs have small lipogranulomas reflecting single hepatocyte dropout/necrosis in the absence of an inflammatory response.

Acute hepatic necrosis caused by infectious canine hepatitis increases plasma ALT activity by 30-fold, peaking within 4 days. Thereafter, chronic sustained ALT activity persists as chronic hepatitis develops in dogs unable to clear the virus. Hepatic injury induced by toxins usually causes plasma ALT activity to increase, peak, and return to normal sooner than it does in infectious viral hepatitis. Chronic hepatitis, an idiopathic or copper-associated persistent or cyclic necroinflammatory liver injury in dogs is associated with varying severities of necrosis and fibrosis. Cyclic disease activity is reflected by plasma enzyme "flares." At times, plasma ALT activity is >10-fold normal. Enzyme fluctuations contrast with profiles associated with single injurious events. In dogs with hepatitis, serum ALT activity declines as injury resolves, but serum ALP activity may increase as a result of regenerative responses (progenitor cell proliferation, ductal or oval cell response). Dogs treated with glucocorticoids may develop mildly increased ALT activity that resolves within several weeks of glucocorticoid withdrawal.

Despite high sensitivity of ALT to identify liver disorders, its lack of specificity to differentiate clinically significant liver disease, specific histologic abnormalities, or hepatic dysfunction requires that it be interpreted in conjunction with other diagnostic tests.

Aspartate Aminotransferase: AST is present in substantial concentrations in a wide variety of tissues, especially muscle. Increased AST activity can reflect reversible or irreversible changes in hepatocellular membrane permeability, cell necrosis, hepatic inflammation, and in dogs, microsomal enzyme induction. After acute diffuse severe hepatic necrosis, serum AST sharply increases during the first 3 days to values 10- to 30-fold above normal in dogs and up to 50-fold above normal in cats. If necrosis resolves, AST activity gradually declines over 2–3 wk. In most cases, AST parallels changes in ALT activity.

Although increased AST activity in the absence of abnormal ALT activity implicates an extrahepatic enzyme source (notably in muscle injury), there are clinical exceptions that may relate to severity and zonal location of hepatic damage. In some cats with liver disease, AST is a more sensitive marker of liver injury than ALT (eg, hepatic necrosis, cholangiohepatitis, myeloproliferative disease, hepatic infiltrative lymphoma, and EHBDO). A similar trend is evident in some dogs. Because AST is located within the mitochondria and free within the cytosol of hepatocytes, AST in fold increases greater than those of ALT may reflect mitochondrial injury. Dogs treated with glucocorticoids may develop mildly increased AST activity that resolves within several weeks of glucocorticoid withdrawal.

Alkaline Phosphatase: Increased ALP activity in dogs is the most common abnormality on routine biochemical testing; its high sensitivity and low specificity can defy diagnostic interpretation without a liver biopsy. ALP activity in dogs has the lowest specificity of routinely used liver enzymes as a result of its complexity associated with induction of different isozymes.

In dogs and cats, tissues containing highest ALP activity (in descending order) are intestine, kidney (cortex), placenta (dogs only), liver, and bone. Distinct serum ALP isozymes can be extracted from some of these tissues in each species; eg, bone (B-ALP), liver (L-ALP), and glucocorticoid-induced (G-ALP) isoenzymes in canine serum. In dogs, L-ALP and G-ALP are primarily responsible for high serum ALP activity, whereas L-ALP is primarily responsible in cats. Increased ALP activity develops in up to 75% of hyperthyroid cats, depending on the chronicity of the condition, with B-ALP substantially contributing.

The comparably small magnitudes of ALP activity in cats with liver disease (2- to 3-fold normal) relative to dogs (usually >4- to 5-fold) reflect the lower specific activity of ALP in feline liver and its shorter half-life. Nevertheless, ALP activity remains clinically useful in the diagnosis of feline liver disease when the species-appropriate perspective is maintained.

The utility of serum ALP activity as a diagnostic indicator in dogs is complicated by the common accumulation of L-ALP and G-ALP isozymes, which can both be induced by steroidogenic hormones.

Because the B-ALP isozyme increases secondary to osteoblast activity, it is detected in young growing animals and in animals with bone tumors, secondary renal hyperparathyroidism, and osteomyelitis. However, the minor contribution of B-ALP to total serum ALP activity usually does not lead to an erroneous diagnosis of cholestatic liver disease. Bone remodeling secondary to neoplasia may not substantially affect serum ALP activity or may cause only a trivial increase (2- to 3-fold) in dogs. In young growing cats, increased B-ALP activity may simulate enzyme activity seen in hepatobiliary disease.

Although ALT is immediately released from the hepatocellular cytosol in acute hepatic necrosis, the small quantities of membrane-bound ALP are not. It takes several days for induction of membrane-associated enzyme to "gear up" and spill into the systemic circulation. Increased serum ALP reflects enhanced *de novo* hepatic synthesis, canalicular injury, cholestasis, and solubilization of its membrane anchor (by bile salts). The largest increases in serum ALP activity (L-ALP and/or G-ALP ≥100-fold normal) develop in dogs with diffuse or focal cholestatic disorders, massive hepatocellular carcinoma, bile duct carcinoma, and those exposed to steroidogenic hormones.

Although serum activity of ALP may be normal or only modestly increased in dogs with metastatic neoplasia involving the liver, it may also increase dramatically in dogs with mammary neoplasia. High serum ALP activity develops in ~55% of dogs with malignant and 47% with benign mammary tumors, with highest ALP activity seen in dogs with malignant mixed tumors. Nevertheless, serum ALP has no value as a diagnostic or prognostic marker in mammary cancer; it remains unclear whether disease remission (surgical, chemotherapy) is followed by a regression in serum ALP activity or whether serum ALP activity functions as a paraneoplastic marker.

After acute severe hepatic necrosis, ALP activity increases 2- to 5-fold in dogs and cats, stabilizes, and then gradually declines over 2–3 wk. Sustained ALP activity usually correlates with a reparative ductal response (progenitor or oval cell hyperplasia). In cats, EHBDO results in a 2-fold increase in ALP within 2 days, as much as a 4-fold increase within 1 wk, and up to a 9-fold increase within 2–3 wk. Thereafter, activity stabilizes and gradually declines but usually not into the normal range; the declining enzyme activity coordinates with developing biliary cirrhosis (*see* EXTRAHEPATIC BILE DUCT OBSTRUCTION, p 478). Inflammatory disorders involving biliary or canalicular structures or disorders compromising bile flow increase serum ALP activity secondary to membrane inflammation/disruption and local bile acid accumulation. In both dogs and cats, similar increases in serum ALP activity develop in intrahepatic (metabolic, biochemical, sepsis) associated cholestasis or obstruction involving the extrahepatic biliary structures. Consequently, ALP activity cannot differentiate between intra- and extrahepatic cholestatic disorders.

Many extrahepatic and primary hepatic conditions are associated with increased L-ALP. In cats, HL (*see* p 456) is associated with marked increase in ALP activity and jaundice. The increased ALP seemingly reflects canalicular dysfunction or compression. Although ALP in cats is rarely affected by anticonvulsants or glucocorticoids, it can increase with diabetes mellitus, hyperthyroidism, and pancreatitis.

In dogs, primary hepatic inflammation as well as systemic infection or inflammation and exposure to steroidogenic hormones may induce a glycogen-associated vacuolar hepatopathy (VH). When severe, VH has a cholestatic effect that seemingly causes canalicular compression. Although glycogen-associated VH was initially characterized as a glucocorticoid-initiated lesion, it is now established that nearly 50% of dogs with glycogen-associated VH lack overt exposure to steroidogenic substances. Chronically ill dogs may produce the G-ALP isozymes secondary to stress-induced glucocorticoid release. Such dogs with glycogen-associated VH (lacking exogenous glucocorticoid exposure) may demonstrate normal dexamethasone suppression and adrenocorticotropic hormone (ACTH) response tests. However, in some dogs, high ALP with a glycogen-associated VH signals the presence of atypical adrenal hyperplasia associated with abnormal sex hormone production. There is no consistent relationship between the magnitude of serum ALP activity, the presence of high G-ALP activity, or histologic lesions. Unfortunately, G-ALP is not useful for syndrome characterization because it can become the predominant ALP isoenzyme in dogs treated with glucocorticoids and in dogs with spontaneous or iatrogenic hyperadrenocorticism, hepatic or nonhepatic neoplasia, hepatic inflammation, or numerous diverse chronic illnesses, including primary liver disease.

The magnitude of ALP activity induced by glucocorticoid administration depends on the type of drug and dose given, as well as the individual's response. The production of G-ALP does not imply that a dog treated with cortisone has iatrogenic hyperadrenocorticism, a suppressed pituitary-adrenal axis, or a clinically important glycogen-associated VH. By comparison, the feline liver is relatively insensitive to glucocorticoids, with rare development of a glycogen-associated VH or acceleration of hepatocyte lipid vacuole accumulation.

In dogs, serum total ALP activity and L-ALP isozyme also may be induced by administration of certain anticonvulsants (phenobarbital, primidone, and phenytoin) and other drugs; in this circumstance, the ALP activity usually increases 2- to 6-fold normal. In contrast, serum ALP and L-ALP did not increase in cats after administration of phenobarbital (0.25 grain, bid) for 30 days.

Gamma-Glutamyl Transferase: Gamma-glutamyl transferase (GGT) is a membrane-bound glycoprotein that plays a critical role in cellular detoxification (involved with glutathione availability), conferring resistance against a number of toxins and drugs. Tissue concentrations of GGT in dogs and cats are highest in the kidney and pancreas, with lesser amounts in the liver, gallbladder, intestines, spleen, heart, lungs, skeletal muscle, and erythrocytes. However, serum GGT activity is largely derived from the liver, although there is considerable species variation in its localization within this organ.

Acute, severe, diffuse necrosis is associated with either no change or only mild increases (1- to 3-fold normal) in GGT activity that resolve in ~10 days. In dogs with EHBDO, serum GGT activity increases 1- to 4-fold above normal within 4 days, and 10- to 50-fold within 1–2 wk. Thereafter, values may plateau or continue to increase as high as 100-fold. In cats with EHBDO, serum GGT activity may increase up to 2-fold within 3 days, 2- to 6-fold within 5 days, 3- to 12-fold within 1 wk, and 4- to 16-fold within 2 wk. Glucocorticoids and certain other microsomal enzyme inducers may stimulate GGT production in dogs, similar to their influence on ALP. Administration of dexamethasone (3 mg/kg/day) or prednisone (4.4 mg/kg/day, IM) may increase GGT activity within 1 wk to 4- to 7-fold above normal and up to 10-fold within 2 wk. Dogs treated with phenytoin or primidone develop only a modest increase in serum GGT activity (up to 2- to 3-fold), unless they develop anticonvulsant hepatotoxicosis that is often associated with marked enzyme activity.

Cats with advanced necroinflammatory liver disease, EHBDO, or inflammatory intrahepatic cholestasis can develop a larger increase in GGT activity relative to ALP. Glucocorticoids and other enzyme inducers in dogs do not clinically influence serum GGT in cats. The normal range for serum GGT activity in cats is much narrower and lower than that in dogs; therefore, assays must be sensitive enough to detect low GGT activity.

GGT values can be markedly increased in dogs and cats with primary hepatic or pancreatic neoplasia. However, GGT does not appear to be suitable for surveillance of hepatic metastasis in either species.

Like ALP, GGT lacks specificity in differentiating between parenchymal hepatic disease and obstructive biliary disease. It is not as sensitive in dogs as ALP but does have higher specificity. In cats with inflammatory liver disease, it is more sensitive but less specific than ALP; these two enzymes should be interpreted simultaneously. The likelihood that HL has developed secondary to necroinflammatory liver disease, EHBDO, or pancreatic disease can be predicted by examining the relative increases in GGT and ALP. Necroinflammatory disorders involving biliary structures, the portal triad, or pancreas are often associated with a greater fold increase in GGT than in ALP. With the exclusion of these underlying disorders, cats with HL usually have a higher fold increase in ALP relative to GGT; this has important diagnostic utility in discerning the underlying cause of HL.

Neonatal animals of several species, including dogs but not cats, develop high serum GGT activity secondary to colostrum ingestion.

OTHER SERUM BIOCHEMICAL MEASURES

Albumin: Albumin is produced exclusively by the liver and has a half-life in healthy dogs estimated at ~8 days. Because the healthy liver is estimated to maintain albumin synthesis at 33% maximal capacity, it has a large reserve capability for albumin synthesis. Albumin functions as an essential transport molecule, maintaining normal drug-receptor interactions. In liver disease, decline in albumin concentration compromises its transport functions, increasing risk of adverse drug reactions (more free or unbound drug). Albumin's large role in maintaining colloid osmotic pressure reflects its lower molecular weight compared with other plasma proteins and its higher intravascular concentration. In inflammatory disease or during malnutrition, albumin may increase its transcapillary escape rate, augmenting distribution into the interstitial space. This phenomenon hastens onset of hypoalbuminemia in animals with necroinflammatory liver disease, long before development of ascites. Concurrent hypoalbuminemia and development of hepatic presinusoidal, sinusoidal, or postsinusoidal portal hypertension is commonly associated with ascites in animals with chronic severe liver disease.

Albumin also functions as a scavenger of oxygen radicals and other oxidizing agents. These antioxidant effects may be compromised in necroinflammatory liver disease and fulminant hepatic failure. Any disease processes promoting an oxidative environment (eg, diabetes mellitus, renal disease, hepatic insufficiency, hyperthyroidism) can irreparably damage the albumin molecule, accelerating its turnover (synthesis and catabolism).

In many animals with liver disease, an early trend toward hypoalbuminemia often reflects systemic inflammation (negative acute phase effect). Only in severe hepatic insufficiency (eg, chronic progressive hepatitis) is synthetic failure a driving cause of hypoalbuminemia. Protein-losing nephropathy (glomerular disease) or protein-losing enteropathy must be excluded as underlying causes of hypoalbuminemia. Glomerular causes are associated with a urine protein:creatinine ratio >3 and hypercholesterolemia, whereas protein-losing enteropathy is associated with panhypoproteinemia and hypocholesterolemia.

Bilirubin: Total bilirubin >2.5–3 mg/dL results in clinical icterus. Hyperbilirubinemia can reflect prehepatic (eg, hemolysis), hepatic (impaired uptake, intracellular transport, glucuronide conjugation, or canalicular elimination), or posthepatic/extrahepatic causes (EHBDO, biliary tree rupture). Total bilirubin concentrations vary markedly with different disease processes. Concentrations are highest in dogs with hemolytic disorders and in cats with HL and EHBDO. Bilirubinuria can be detected in healthy dogs because of their ability to conjugate bilirubin in renal tubules (low renal threshold). However, bilirubinuria in cats is always abnormal and should be investigated. Fractionation of total bilirubin into direct (conjugated) and indirect (unconjugated) moieties offers little diagnostic utility. Bilirubin covalently bound to albumin (biliprotein complexes) remains in the circulation and is not excreted in urine. Chronic retention can impart tissue jaundice in the absence of bilirubinuria long after a cholestatic disorder has resolved.

Common causes of hyperbilirubinemia include increased hemoprotein liberation (eg, hemolytic anemia, ineffective erythropoiesis, body cavity hemorrhage), bile duct occlusion, ruptured biliary tract, intrahepatic cholestasis, impaired hepatobiliary bilirubin processing, and sepsis. Jaundiced dogs and cats presenting with regenerative anemia should be tested for hemolytic disorders, including immune-mediated hemolytic anemia, Heinz body hemolysis, zinc toxicity, and erythroparasites (including hemotropic *Mycoplasma* [cats, dogs] and *Babesia* [dogs]).

BUN and Creatinine: There are no characteristic changes in BUN or creatinine concentrations with liver disorders except that low values are associated with portosystemic shunting and feeding of a restricted protein diet (only BUN, not creatinine) formulated to reduce signs of HE. The concentration of BUN reflects numerous variables, including hydration status, nutritional support, enteric bleeding, tissue catabolism, and the hepatic capacity to detoxify ammonia. Anorexia, feeding a low-protein diet, or hepatic insufficiency can result in low normal to subnormal concentration of BUN, whereas increased values relative to creatinine (discordant BUN:creatinine ratio) may reflect dehydration, enteric bleeding, or consumption of a high-protein diet. Compared with BUN, serum creatinine concentrations are less affected by dietary protein intake. The low BUN and low normal or low creatinine concentration often seen in animals with portosystemic shunting reflect increased water turnover that increases glomerular filtration rate (up to 2-fold), contributing to PU/PD. Reduced hepatic synthesis of creatinine also contributes to low creatinine concentrations in animals with hepatic insufficiency, considering that creatinine depends on hepatic synthesis of creatine in the transmethylation pathway.

Glucose: Hypoglycemia is uncommon in acquired liver disease except end-stage cirrhosis or fulminant liver failure. The inability to store hepatic glycogen or convert glycogen to glucose is more common in neonates and juvenile small-breed dogs with congenital portosystemic shunts. Other causes of hypoglycemia, including sepsis, insulinoma, iatrogenic insulin overdose, rare glycogen storage disorders, or paraneoplastic effects of large primary hepatic neoplasia (canine hepatocellular carcinoma or adenoma) or other tumors should be considered in an animal with suspected liver disease.

Cholesterol: All cells in the body except RBCs synthesize cholesterol for intracellular use. Cholesterol incorporated in plasma lipoproteins is synthesized only in the liver and distal small intestine. Bile provides the major excretory pathway for cholesterol. Hypocholesterolemia may reflect endocrine, metabolic, and nutritional factors as well as hepatic insufficiency and portosystemic shunting. Nonhepatic disorders associated with hypocholesterolemia include hypoadrenocorticism, maldigestion/malabsorption, pancreatic exocrine insufficiency, severe starvation, cachexia, sepsis, and hyperthyroidism (cats); hepatic causes include portosystemic shunting (congenital or acquired) and severe hepatic insufficiency (eg, end-stage cirrhosis, fulminant hepatic failure). Hypercholesterolemia is more common in ill animals and requires careful consideration of potential nonhepatic disorders, including hypothyroidism, diabetes mellitus, pancreatitis, nephrotic syndrome, hyperadrenocorticism or treatment with glucocorticoids, idiopathic dyslipidemias, and rarely a postprandial effect. Hypercholesterolemia is usually seen in EHBDO and in some animals with diffuse intrahepatic cholestasis, destructive cholangitis, and marked hepatic regeneration.

HEPATIC FUNCTION TESTS

Total Serum Bile Acids: TSBA concentrations sensitively detect cholestatic disorders and conditions associated with portosystemic shunting. TSBA concentration should be measured before and 2 hr after meal ingestion; fasting is not required. Insufficient hepatic mass or deviated portal circulation to the systemic circulation via extrahepatic portosystemic shunts (congenital or acquired) or microscopic shunts within the liver (congenital microvascular dysplasia) cause high TSBA concentrations, particularly in postprandial samples. TSBA concentrations are usually lower before a meal than 2 hr after a meal. However, ~15%–20% of dogs and 5% of cats have higher TSBA concentrations before a meal than after, likely reflecting physiologic variables influencing the enterohepatic circulation of bile acids (ie, the rate of gallbladder contraction, gastric emptying, and intestinal transit of bile acids to the ileum where they are actively resorbed). TSBA concentrations in dogs >25 μM/L or in cats >20 μM/L are abnormal either before or after a meal (fasting ranges should not be applied because of the variables influencing the TSBA enterohepatic circulation). Collecting a single sample for TSBA measurement (random fasting or a single postprandial sample) can miss detection of abnormal values. Because TSBA concentrations are a more sensitive indicator of cholestasis than total bilirubin, measuring TSBA concentration is redundant in animals with nonhemolytic jaundice. Use of TSBAs as a liver function test can indicate need for a liver biopsy. TSBA concentrations should be routinely measured in all young (6 mo), small, "terrier-like breeds" to detect dogs with microvascular dysplasia (MVD). Finding increased TSBA concentrations in apparently healthy, young, terrier-like breeds, including but not restricted to Yorkshire Terriers, Maltese, Shih Tzus, Miniature Schnauzers, Cairn Terriers, Norfolk Terriers, Havanese, Papillons, Tibetan Spaniels, and Pugs, allows detection of dogs in which TSBA concentration will be misleading if discovered in later life during evaluation of illness.

Ammonia: Measurement of blood ammonia can detect hepatic disorders associated with HE. Ammonia is derived predominantly from protein degradation, with most generated in the intestines from consumed food and enteric bacterial ureases that catabolize urea into ammonia and carbon dioxide. Portal transport of ammonia from the intestines to the liver results in a direct 85% detoxification to urea. Ammonia intolerance (impaired clearance) occurs in any disorder associated with portosystemic shunting and in acute fulminant hepatic failure. Ammonia is not influenced by cholestasis or liver disorders that do not deviate the portosystemic circulation or extensively reduce hepatic parenchymal mass.

Although ammonia is regarded as a pivotal cause of HE, animals with overt HE may have normal blood ammonia concentrations owing to complicated pathologic mechanisms driving HE. A single normal ammonia value cannot discount HE in an animal with suspected chronic liver disease, and serial ammonia measurements may not correlate with an evolving clinical scenario of HE. Thus, ammonia measurements cannot reliably diagnose HE.

Measurement of blood ammonia is complicated. Spurious hyperammonemia can reflect slow blood collection, tight tourniquet technique, conditions promoting ammonia liberation from muscle (seizures, crush injuries), sample contamination (human sweat, cigarette smoke, open urine vials), and spontaneous generation in samples not immediately cooled on collection or not promptly analyzed. Ammonia is highly volatile, and samples cannot be mailed for analyses. Blood samples should be collected into pre-cooled tubes and transported on melting ice to the laboratory for analysis within 20 min. Enzymatic-based methodologies are difficult to standardize. Nonhepatic causes of hyperammonemia also exist, with the most common disorders involving bacterial infection of the urinary tract with a urease-producing organism associated either with uroabdomen or obstructive uropathy.

If a random blood ammonia concentration is within normal limits but hepatic insufficiency and portosystemic shunting suspected, an ammonia tolerance test can be conducted. Ammonium chloride is given at 100 mg/kg in a 5% solution orally (can induce vomiting) or at 2 mL/kg of a 5% solution administered rectally (instilled 30 cm deep) after a cleansing enema, with blood ammonia measured at baseline and then at 20, 30, 40, or 60 min later. Unfortunately, an ammonia tolerance test may induce iatrogenic HE in susceptible animals.

The presence of ammonium biurate crystalluria in an animal with high TSBAs is pathognomonic for hyperammonemia and portosystemic shunting. A minimum of three urine samples collected at separate daily intervals should be inspected to optimize surveillance for crystal discovery. In animals on restricted protein intake using diets specifically formulated for hepatic insufficiency, finding ammonium biurates may be difficult because of the high efficacy of such diets to control hyperammonemia.

IMAGING

Radiography: Routine abdominal radiographs are useful to determine liver size and may detect irregular liver borders. Mineralized densities that involve parenchyma or the biliary tree can reflect stasis of bile flow, dystrophic mineralization associated with congenital malformations, acquired duct "sacculation," chronic duct inflammation, or choleliths. Choleliths that contain enough calcium bilirubinate or calcium carbonate are radiographically visible. A mass effect in the right cranial quadrant in suspected EHBDO may represent an engorged gallbladder, pancreatitis, neoplasia, or focal bile peritonitis. Radiographic suspicion of abdominal effusion (poor abdominal detail) may prompt diagnosis of bile peritonitis and ascitic effusion. Gas within hepatic parenchyma or biliary structures indicates an emphysematous process (eg, cholecystitis, choledochitis, infected biliary cyst, hepatic abscess, necrotic tumor mass) and warrants prompt antimicrobial therapy and either surgical intervention or percutaneous, ultrasound-guided aspiration/lavage. Thoracic radiography can indicate signs of systemic disease (eg, metastatic lesions, pleural fluid). Finding sternal lymphadenopathy is common in cats with the cholangitis/cholangiohepatitis syndrome, in which it reflects hepatic inflammation.

Although cholecystography can be accomplished with iodinated contrast given PO or IV, contrast radiographic imaging of the biliary system is rarely pursued. Distribution and concentration of contrast agents within biliary structures is influenced by numerous variables, including hyperbilirubinemia and major duct occlusion. At best, these agents may disclose choleliths, polyps, or sludged bile but are insufficient to confirm bile peritonitis or to localize the site of leakage. Multisector CT and/or hepatic ultrasonography are more useful to discern these processes.

Contrast studies of the portal vasculature are the gold standard for confirmation of a congenital portosystemic shunt. Radiographs should be taken in right and left lateral and ventrodorsal positions for best test sensitivity. Multisector CT imaging produces exceptional images and has replaced radiographic portography for diagnosis of congenital portosystemic shunts because it allows contrast injection into a peripheral vessel, can capture numerous images per second, and allows three-dimensional anatomic reconstruction.

Ultrasonography: There are many diagnostic applications of hepatic ultrasonography: 1) identify distention and determine thickness of biliary structures; 2) verify common bile duct obstruction; 3) detect gallbladder mucoceles and cholelithiasis; 4) differentiate between diffuse and focal hepatic abnormalities; 5) identify and determine dimensions of "mass lesions"; 6) identify pancreatic, mesenteric, and perihepatic lymphadenomegaly; 7) in conjunction with vascular studies, identify congenital intrahepatic and extrahepatic portosystemic vascular anomalies (PSVAs), APSSs, arteriovenous malformations, and hepatic venule distention reflecting passive congestion; and 8) detect small volume abdominal effusion and small volume of fluid surrounding the gallbladder. However, although abdominal ultrasonography has become an indispensable diagnostic tool to assess the liver and biliary system, its use is highly operator dependent, and findings must always be reconciled with the history, physical examination findings, and clinicopathologic data. Reconciliation of data is best done by the principal clinician managing the case, who has the most knowledge of the animal's management and prognosis.

Computed Tomography: Multisector CT imaging, available in specialty referral practices and university teaching hospitals, can distinguish mass lesions, detect changes in structure of hepatic parenchyma and the biliary system, identify choleliths, detect abnormal hepatic perfusion (involving the portal vein, hepatic artery, or hepatic vein), and portal thrombi, and can detail the extent of traumatic hepatobiliary injuries.

CHOLECYSTOCENTESIS

Cholecystocentesis is the aspiration sampling of gallbladder bile; this can be completed using a percutaneous transhepatic ultrasound-guided approach, by laparoscopic assistance, or during exploratory abdominal surgery. Samples of bile are collected for cytologic investigation and culture of aerobic and anaerobic bacteria and fungi; collection of bile that contains particulate debris or sediment has the highest yield to find microorganisms (cytologically, by culture). Complications of cholecystocentesis may include intraperitoneal bile leakage (reduced by using a transhepatic approach), hemorrhage, hemobilia, bacteremia, and vasovagal reaction, especially in cats, that may result in ventilatory arrest, severe bradycardia, and death. If a gallbladder mucocele or EHBDO is suspected, cholecystocentesis is contraindicated. It is better to perform a cholecystectomy for gallbladder mucocele and surgically decompress EHBDO (relieve or bypass the obstruction).

LIVER CYTOLOGY

Ultrasonographic-guided fine-needle aspirates are routinely used to confirm a diagnosis of HL in cats and to identify suppurative septic inflammation, neoplasia, and glycogen-like VH. However, definitive diagnosis of hepatic disease is otherwise impossible with liver aspirates because the absence of acinar architecture compromises anatomic orientation and correct interpretation. Cytologic interpretation of liver aspirates are notoriously discordant with histologic findings on biopsy specimens. Neither neoplasia nor sepsis can be definitively excluded using cytology, and inflammatory disease is too often suspected. Cytology should not be the basis to recommend immunomodulatory or antifibrotic medications or longterm chelation therapy for copper-associated hepatopathy. Rather, liver biopsy remains the standard for diagnoses of most hepatic disorders.

LIVER BIOPSY

Hepatic needle true-cut biopsies (especially 18-gauge) collected under ultrasonographic guidance may yield samples too small and fragmented for accurate diagnosis because of a lack of representative acinar units (at least 15 portal triads should be sampled). Furthermore, needle biopsies are usually only collected from the more safely sampled left-side lobes, which may miss lesions differentially affecting liver lobes (eg, cholangiohepatitis in cats). Blind-needle biopsies done without ultrasonographic guidance are hazardous and ill advised in animals with suspected hepatic hilar or mesenteric lymphadenomegaly; involvement of the common bile duct, gallbladder, intestines (eg, inflammatory bowel disease, infiltrative disease), or pancreas; or multiple organ abnormalities. An exploratory laparotomy is more appropriate. When possible, wedge biopsies or laparoscopic cup forcep biopsies are preferred, because samples of adequate size can be easily and safely acquired from multiple liver lobes, ensuring accurate disease representation.

These methods also permit assessment of the gross appearance of the liver. Notably, laparoscopic methods are not recommended when disease of the common bile duct or gallbladder is suspected that may necessitate a decompressive biliary procedure, cholecystectomy, or cholestotomy. Liver biopsy should always be done even if an obvious biliary abnormality is the predominant disease process, because underlying histologic liver lesions may indicate another primary disease process. It is also important to biopsy grossly normal liver when focal lesions are identified. This practice ensures 1) characterization of "normal" liver histology, 2) determines whether an underlying liver disease coexists, 3) investigates histology of liver distant to the gallbladder in animals undergoing cholecystectomy, and 4) provides multiple liver lobe samples needed to confirm suspected MVD (because this lesion is variable among liver lobes).

Routine biopsy evaluation should include examination of a cytologic imprint, Gram stain (if suppurative or pyogranulomatous inflammation is cytologically detected), routine H&E staining and interpretation, as well as staining with a reticulin stain (discloses sinusoidal collapse of the supporting scaffolding of the liver), Masson's trichrome (to confirm presence and severity of fibrillar connective tissue deposition), Prussian blue to identify iron retention in Kupffer cells (fixed macrophages) and hepatocytes (helps confirm lobular involvement in inflammation, Kupffer cell activation, presence of rare hemochromatosis), rhodanine stain for copper (confirms and can be used to quantify copper with digital scanning of the rhodanine-stained section), aerobic and anaerobic bacterial cultures of liver and bile, and quantification of liver metals (copper, iron, and zinc concentrations because these values can help evaluate risk of oxidative injury and need for zinc supplementation). A tissue sample (formalin fixed) should also be reserved for other special case-specific studies such as special immunohistochemical stains or for PCR testing for infectious agents.

Before biopsy, bleeding tendencies should be evaluated by careful review of the history, physical examination, blood smear (to confirm platelets ≥100,000/μL), routine coagulation profile (prothrombin time [PT], activated partial thromboplastin time [APTT]), von Willebrand factor (vWF) activity in high-risk breeds, and a buccal mucosal bleeding time. Routine coagulation assessments have low reliability to detect bleeding risk. The buccal mucosal bleeding time is more relevant when performed immediately before the procedure. Animals suspected to have bleeding tendencies should be treated with vitamin K_1 (0.5–1 mg/kg, SC or IM) at 0, 12, and 24 hr before tissue sampling. If buccal mucosal bleeding time is >5 min, a fresh frozen plasma transfusion is indicated, as is administration of desmopressin acetate (DDAVP, 0.3–1 mcg/kg diluted in saline), which increases plasma vWF 2-fold over baseline within 1 hr as well as plasma activity of Factor VIII. DDAVP can initiate a hemostatic effect in dogs with type 1 vWF (partial quantitative deficiency) but not in dogs with qualitative defects or complete vWF deficiency. In many people with liver disease, DDAVP has improved coagulation ability, although the exact mechanisms remain incompletely clarified.

PATHOLOGIC CHANGES IN BILE

(White bile syndrome, Inspissated bile syndrome, Bilirubin deconjugation)

In animals with bile stasis, nonabsorbable bile constituents (bile salts, phospholipids, glycoproteins, and cholesterol) are subject to concentration or dilution when water and inorganic electrolytes (sodium, chloride, bicarbonate) are resorbed or added by the biliary epithelium. EHBDO can produce a "white bile" syndrome reflecting the absence of bilirubin pigments; this usually is found in animals with an obstructed gallbladder at the level of the cystic duct or in animals with obstruction of the hepatic ducts. Stasis of bile flow also may cause bile dehydration, promoting a pathologically thickened or sludged bile typically dark green to black in color. Formation of a gallbladder mucocele involves the entrapment, retention, dehydration, and local overproduction of mucin that lends a rubbery viscosity to bile. Bile stasis in obstructed ducts can lead to bilirubin deconjugation, which reduces bilirubin solubility and favors cholelith precipitation. Choleresis (enhanced bile flow) produces "watery," dilute bile and is a therapeutic goal in disorders associated with bile stasis.

NUTRITION

Nutritional support has a pivotal influence in cats with HL and is an important component of at-home treatment in animals with slowly progressive hepatobiliary disorders. Proper nutritional support improves quality of life in animals with hepatic insufficiency prone to HE. Diets for animals with hepatobiliary disease should be easily digestible, highly palatable, calorically dense, easy for the owner to prepare and feed, and fed frequently as small meals. Objectives are to optimize food digestion and assimilation and to achieve voluntary food consumption.

If animals are anorectic, tube feeding should be considered. Nasogastric tubes are inexpensive, easily placed, and recommended as a short-term solution. Esophagostomy tubes are preferred in cats with HL for longer dietary support. Use of appetite stimulants remains controversial, because they may delay institution of regimented nutritional support. In addition, some commonly used drugs are metabolized in the liver. Diazepam and oxazepam may rarely lead to idiopathic fulminant hepatic failure in cats.

Dietary modification for animals with liver disease depends on their clinical status, the definitive diagnosis, and assessment of liver function. Diets should be balanced and supplemented with water-soluble vitamins. In severe cholestatic disorders that impede enteric access of bile (eg, EHBDO, advanced sclerosing cholangitis in cats), fat-soluble vitamins may become depleted. Vitamin K_1 can be supplemented via parenteral injection of 0.5–1.5 mg/kg every week (titrated against a thrombotest [PIVKA assay] or PT). If vitamin K_1 depletion is confirmed, vitamin E also likely needs supplementation. Because vitamin E is a fat-soluble vitamin, a unique, water-soluble form may be necessary for oral administration: polyethylene glycol α-tocopherol succinate (10 IU/kg/day, PO). It is important to follow dosing recommendations, because excessive vitamin K can lead to hemolytic anemia (in cats), and excessive vitamin E can interfere with vitamin K function.

Liver function also has considerable influence on glucose homeostasis (glycogenolysis or gluconeogenesis from amino acids and lactate), detoxification of nitrogen (urea cycle), and ketogenesis (from fatty acids). In rare circumstances, in animals prone to hypoglycemia, low-dose IV glucose may be transiently needed. Protein modification and restriction is used to address insufficient nitrogen detoxification (*see* below).

Energy Allowance: Energy allocation should be estimated based on ideal body weight, with modified diets gradually introduced. Initial intake should be no greater than 50% of the calculated daily energy requirement on day 1, increased to 75% on day 2, and then to 100% by day 3–5. Energy allowances may require adjustment after the diet is accepted, the animal is stable, and weight and body condition reassessments confirm a need for higher or lower intake. Estimation of initial energy intake is calculated using formulas that predict resting energy requirements in healthy animals. Formulas for estimation of initial energy allocations for dogs are $30 \times$ body wt (kg) + 70 (for dogs 2–16 kg); $70 \times$ body wt (kg)$^{0.75}$ (for dogs <2 or >16 kg); or $99 \times$ body wt (kg)$^{0.67}$ (safe initial intake for a healthy dog).

For cats, $60 \times$ body wt (kg) is often used, unless the cat is markedly overconditioned or has a subnormal metabolic rate or activity level. Frequent reassessment is necessary with energy allowances tailored to response.

Dietary Protein Allowance: A diagnosis of liver disease should not automatically dictate a need for protein restriction. In fact, protein restriction can be detrimental in some animals, eg, cats with HL or animals with chronic but stable necroinflammatory liver disease that do not have APSSs or HE. Unfortunately, altering nutritional support can be difficult and challenging in animals that reject novel diet modifications. Protein restriction is appropriate when HE is suspected, ammonium biurate crystalluria is observed in an animal with suspected hepatic insufficiency, or portosystemic shunting (congenital or acquired) is either confirmed by imaging studies or suggested by protein C assessments.

The protein allowance for an animal with HE should maintain a positive nitrogen balance, avoiding tissue catabolism. Because maintenance of lean body mass (muscle) provides a temporary respite from ammonia toxicity, body condition should be monitored regularly for comparative estimates, with the goal being to maintain muscle mass.

When protein restriction is deemed necessary, initial restriction to 2.5 g protein/kg body wt (<5 g protein/100 kcal diet) for dogs and 3.5 g protein/kg body wt (<7 g protein/100 kcal) for cats is advised. Sequential historical, physical, and clinicopathologic assessments judge treatment response and guide further tailoring of these recommendations.

Most protein-restricted diets are used in dogs with chronic, severe liver disease or that have PSVA. If a dog responds well to an initial protein restriction, ~0.25–0.5 g/kg/day can be added, using a tofu or dairy-based protein source. Animals should be monitored every 1–2 wk for signs of HE and alterations in albumin, BUN, and appearance of ammonium biurate crystalluria during dietary protein titration. Three urine samples should be collected: first thing in the morning, 4–8 hr after feeding, and late in the evening to optimize scrutiny for ammonium biurate crystalluria.

Dietary protein should not be restricted in cats with HL, because protein restriction compromises survival. Protein should not be restricted in most dogs and cats with chronic necroinflammatory liver disorders at the time of diagnosis, because many of these animals may have higher protein requirements than a comparably sized, healthy, age-matched control for tissue repair and cell replication. In people with similar health status, nitrogen requirements increase as needed for increased nitrogen utilization (tissue repair and regeneration).

Modified Protein Quality/Source: Altering the type and quality of protein intake for dogs with HE can help achieve good life quality. A high energy:nitrogen ratio should be maintained, because this optimizes use of dietary protein. In dogs, dairy and vegetable quality protein (soy) sources work best. Dairy quality protein (amount per 8 oz) can be found in the following products: whole milk (8 g in 157 cal), yogurt (8 g in 139 cal), cottage cheese (28–31 g in 200–250 cal), and cheddar cheese (57 g in 800–900 cal). Alternatively, in dogs, calcium caseinate can provide 88 g protein, 2 g fat, and 370 kcal/100 g portion. Using dairy quality and vegetable-derived protein can be estimated using the Nutritional Analysis Tool 2.0 (human nutrition). In cats, which are pure carnivores, a meat-based protein source is recommended in a balanced diet that contains adequate arginine (~250 mg/100 kcal diet) and taurine for feline metabolism (several commercial prescription foods meet these requirements).

Dietary Fat: There is no need to restrict dietary fat in most animals with hepatobiliary disease, because these animals typically have no problems with fat digestion or assimilation. Fat ingestion is important to provide essential fatty acids and fat-soluble vitamins. One exception is animals with chronic EHBDO or cats with sclerosing cholangitis (destructive cholangitis) with symptomatic "ductopenia" (pale acholic feces, bleeding tendencies, marked jaundice). These animals have reduced entry of bile into the alimentary canal and impaired enterohepatic circulation of bile acids, limiting emulsification, digestion, and assimilation of ingested fat. Another exception is dogs with gallbladder mucoceles, some of which have idiopathic hyperlipidemia; in these, feeding a high-fat diet can facilitate rapid maturation of the gallbladder mucocele.

Micronutrients and Vitamins: Water-soluble vitamins should be supplemented (via IV fluids) in animals with chronic liver disease and cats with HL (*see* TABLE 12). Cats are especially susceptible to thiamine (B_1), cobalamin (B_{12}), and vitamin K_1 deficiency when they are chronically inappetent, treated with antimicrobials, have severe intestinal or pancreatic disease, or demonstrate chronic cholestasis. Hyperthyroid cats may develop malabsorptive problems and may be more prone to these complications when also affected with cholangiohepatitis or HL. Vitamin C is not recognized as a commonly depleted micronutrient in either dogs or cats. Dogs with copper storage hepatopathy and animals with large hepatic iron stores should probably not receive vitamin C supplements, because this may augment oxidative injury associated with transition metal accumulation.

Supplementation of **fat-soluble vitamins** is important in animals with fat malabsorption and obstructed bile flow. Vitamin K_1 depletion develops when the enterohepatic bile acid cycle is interrupted in animals demonstrating acholic feces (eg, EHBDO, severe destructive [sclerosing ductopenic] cholangiohepatitis in cats), HL (cats), exocrine pancreatic insufficiency, severe malabsorptive intestinal disease, after feeding a vitamin K–deficient diet, animals chronically treated with oral antimicrobials, and in animals with severe liver disease causing insufficiency. Vitamin K should be administered to any jaundiced animal with suspected liver disease as early as possible (0.5–1.5 mg/kg, SC or IM, three times at 12-hr intervals) before invasive procedures (insertion of catheters in large veins, cystocentesis, insertion of feeding tubes, hepatic aspiration sampling, or liver biopsy). In ductopenic feline sclerosing cholangitis or chronic EHBDO, animals require intermittent vitamin K_1 injections (eg, every 7–21 days), monitored by PIVKA or PT clotting tests. Overdosing with vitamin K_1 can lead to symptomatic Heinz body hemolytic anemia in cats.

Vitamin E is an important antioxidant, antiinflammatory, and antifibrotic used in necroinflammatory and cholestatic liver disorders. Oral D-α-tocopherol acetate is given at 10 IU/kg/day. Higher dosages (100 IU/kg/day) are needed in animals with

TABLE 12 FORMULATION OF A FORTIFIED, WATER-SOLUBLE VITAMIN SUPPLEMENT[a] FOR DOGS AND CATS WITH LIVER DISEASE

Vitamin Supplement	Concentration per mL
Thiamine hydrochloride (vitamin B_1)	50 mg
Riboflavin 5′ phosphate sodium (vitamin B_2)	2–2.5 mg
Niacinamide (vitamin B_3)	50–100 mg
D-Panthenol (vitamin B_5)	5–10 mg
Pyridoxine HCl (vitamin B_6)	2–5 mg
Cyanocobalamin (vitamin B_{12})	Variable; 0.4–50 mcg (low B_{12} values necessitate additional supplementation in deficient cats, SC or IM)
Benzyl alcohol (preservative)	1.5%

[a] 2 mL/L of IV fluid

chronic EHBDO or feline destructive cholangitis (ductopenic sclerosing cholangitis). Alternatively, α-tocopherol polyethylene glycol succinate (water-soluble vitamin E) can be used at 10 IU/kg/day. Dosing of vitamin E should not exceed recommended amounts, because too much vitamin E can interfere with vitamin K activity, provoking coagulopathies. Too much vitamin E also can impart oxidant injury secondary to accumulation of the tocopheroxy radical.

DISEASES OF THE LIVER

FULMINANT HEPATIC FAILURE

Fulminant hepatic failure is a syndrome defined by the abrupt loss of liver function, associated with hepatic encephalopathy (HE) and coagulopathy. Early, appropriate therapy is critical. In chronic or end-stage liver disease with an acute or chronic insult and in acute liver injury with no apparent underlying cause, treatment provides supportive care to allow time for hepatic regeneration and compensation.

Specific treatment should be administered if an underlying cause is determined. Decontamination of oral, dermal, and enteric surfaces is mandatory if toxin exposure has occurred within 36 hr. If an adverse drug reaction is implicated, the drug in question must be discontinued and antidotes investigated. Life-threatening infection, cerebral edema, and coagulopathies are major complications.

Attention to fluid, electrolyte, and acid-base balance, glycemic status, and nutritional support optimizes chance of survival. Restoration of intravascular volume and systemic perfusion may prevent or mitigate the severity of organ failure that often accompanies fulminant hepatic failure (eg, renal, cardiac, adrenal, pancreatic dysfunction). Lactated Ringer's solution should be avoided in animals with compromised lactate metabolism, leading to lactic acidosis. Chronic vomiting and diarrhea often accompany fulminant hepatic failure and can lead to dehydration, hypokalemia, hypochloremia, and metabolic alkalosis. Alkalosis and hypokalemia can each escalate renal ammonia production, contributing to hyperammonemia and HE. Neuroglycopenia can induce neurologic signs that can be confused with and augment HE. Administration of 0.9% NaCl with supplemental vitamins and glucose is usually a safe first option unless portal hypertension and ascites complicate the syndrome. Dextrose (2.5%) and potassium (sliding scale) should be judiciously added to IV fluids, as well as water-soluble vitamins (fortified B-soluble vitamins at 2 ml/L of fluid). Ascites may develop in animals with an acute sinusoidal collapse or acute or chronic fibrosing hepatic injury.

In cats, a B_{12} injection (250–1,000 mcg total dose, IM or SC) should be considered if severe gut disease, pancreatic disease, or starvation are suspected; a plasma sample for assessment of B_{12} should be collected before treatment. Definitive assessment of methylmalonic acidemia defines B_{12} adequacy but cannot be completed in a timely manner for clinical application in emergent liver failure. Thiamine deficiency (B_1) can also complicate clinical status, producing neurobehavioral signs overlapping with HE. Although hyperglycemia must be avoided because it can worsen cerebral edema, euglycemia must be established before thiamine administration; otherwise, thiamine-provoked neuroglycopenia may aggravate neurologic injury and clinical signs. Thiamine is especially important in cats and can be supplemented PO or slowly with IV fluids (fortified B-soluble vitamin solution); 25–100 mg/day is recommended.

Animals with acute liver failure have high energy expenditure and protein catabolism. Nutritional support should be attempted enterically with protein intake initially restricted to 2.5 g/kg body wt in dogs and 3.5 g/kg body wt in cats, with overt HE. If neurologic signs are inapparent, protein restriction is not advised.

Broad-spectrum antibiotics should be given empirically if HE, renal failure, or components of the systemic inflammatory response syndrome (SIRS) are identified. As for other suspected bacterial infections involving the liver, a combination of ticarcillin, metronidazole (7.5 mg/kg, bid, PO or IV), and enrofloxacin are advised.

In most cases, N-acetylcysteine is administered for the first 2 days to provide cysteine for glutathione synthesis, to improve microcirculatory perfusion, and to protect against development of SIRS. A loading dose (140 mg/kg) is initially administered through a 0.25 μM filter and given over 20 min; prolonged infusion can precipitate hyperammonemia. Thereafter, 70 mg/kg is given IV at intervals of 6–8 hr for 2 days. Rarely, an adverse reaction develops, manifesting as urticaria, pruritic rash, vomiting, and most severely as angioneurotic edema.

When oral medications can be tolerated, biologically available S-adenosylmethionine (SAMe) is recommended at 20–40 mg/kg/day, PO, given on an empty stomach to sustain hepatic glutathione adequacy.

Initially, vitamin K_1 (0.5–1.5 mg/kg, IM or SC) is given in three doses at 12-hr intervals. Repeated dosing may be necessary in animals with overt coagulopathies. However, a balanced hemostatic defect with loss of hepatic procoagulant synthesis paralleled by the loss of hepatically derived anticoagulants results in the lack of an overt coagulopathy. Inhibition of gastric acid secretion with an H_2-receptor antagonist (eg, famotidine, faster onset) or HCl pump inhibitor (eg omeprazole, slower onset) is advised. Omeperazole inhibits certain p450 cytochromes and may result in polypharmacy drug interactions. If overt hemorrhagic tendencies are seen, fresh frozen plasma or cryoprecipitate (for vWF and fibrinogen) may be needed. Desmopressin acetate (DDAVP, 0.3 mcg/kg, IV, diluted to 10% in saline) can sometimes arrest serious clinical hemorrhage by improving primary hemostasis. With acute portal hypertension, diapedesis of blood into the enteric lumen may develop before opening of APSSs; this can lead to lethal blood loss and/or aggravate HE. In this scenario, only a whole blood transfusion or administration of packed RBCs and species-specific plasma can replace extracorporeal losses. Concurrent propranolol administration may reduce portal hypertension, which may lessen the rate of blood loss.

The goal of therapeutic strategies in fulminant hepatic failure is to prevent the onset of encephalopathy, limit its severity, and reduce the risk of cerebral edema. Development of cerebral edema is multifactorial, complex, and incompletely understood. Mediators of systemic and local inflammation and circulating neurotoxins (especially ammonia) contribute to its development. HE also can be precipitated by systemic infection, hypotension, and systemic vasodilatation. Altered cerebral endothelial permeability in response to neurotoxins (eg, ammonia) and inflammatory mediators, inflammatory responses, and altered cerebral blood flow are also recognized to trigger or worsen HE.

The head and neck should be maintained in a neutral position, avoiding compression of jugular blood flow; elevation of the head and neck can reduce intracranial pressure and decrease CSF hydrostatic pressure. Central venous lines increase risk of serious iatrogenic hemorrhage, which may require use of compression bandaging. Spontaneous hyperventilation sustains a mild respiratory alkalosis that promotes cerebral arterial vasoconstriction, which tends to reduce intracerebral pressure. Hypoxia must be avoided because of its associated cerebral vasodilatory effect. Mannitol (0.25–0.5 g/kg, given as an IV bolus) can help reduce cerebral edema; boluses can be repeated if serum osmolality has not increased. Furosemide (0.5–1 mg/kg, every 6–8 hr) has been used to increase renal elimination of sodium and water. Use of hypothermia, barbiturate coma, hypertonic saline, or flumazenil infusions are not recommended.

HEPATIC ENCEPHALOPATHY

Hepatic encephalopathy (HE) develops in liver disorders associated with portosystemic shunting, fulminant hepatic failure, or cirrhosis (acquired portosystemic shunts, reduced functional hepatic mass, intrahepatic shunting of blood around regenerative nodules). Clinical signs vary but involve disturbed sensorium ranging from mild dullness and an inability to respond to basic commands to overt abnormalities, including propulsive circling, head pressing, aimless wandering, weakness, ataxia, amaurosis (unexplained blindness), ptyalism, dementia, behavior change (eg, aggression), collapse, seizures, and coma. Although the pathophysiologic mechanisms of HE are not completely known, synergistic effects between the failure of the liver to detoxify ammonia and other endogenous substances, increased cerebral inflammatory cytokines, impaired brain perfusion, development of neuronal edema, hypoxia, mitochondrial dysfunction, neuroglycopenia, and oxidative injury are important interdependent mechanisms. Increased production of reactive oxygen and nitrogen oxide species are thought to trigger protein and RNA modifications that deleteriously influence brain function. The integrated concept of HE explains episodic variability and heterogeneous precipitating factors that correlate with diverse clinical scenarios.

Ammonia plays a key role in HE and is thought to sensitize the brain to numerous other precipitating factors/mediators. However, blood and cerebral ammonia concentrations are often discordant, disqualifying blood ammonia as a simplistic measure of HE. In healthy animals, most ammonia is removed by hepatocytes, converted into amino acids or urea, and excreted via kidneys in urine. In liver failure or portosystemic shunting, blood ammonia concentrations increase because of inadequate hepatic detoxification. In the circulation, ammonia can also be excreted by the kidneys (tubular secretion) and used for glutamine synthesis in skeletal muscle (temporary ammonia detoxification). This latter mechanism is why maintenance of lean body mass (muscle) is essential in animals with hepatic insufficiency that are susceptible to hyperammonemia and HE. A number of clinical scenarios and mechanisms can augment blood ammonia concentrations and precipitate HE, including dehydration (prerenal/renal azotemia), alkalemia, hypokalemia, hypoglycemia, catabolism, infection, PU/PD, anorexia, constipation, hemolysis, blood transfusion, GI hemorrhage, high dietary protein, and various drugs (eg, benzodiazepines, tetracyclines, antihistamines, methionine, barbiturates, organophosphates, phenothiazines, diuretics [overdosage], metronidazole (overdosage), and certain anesthetics).

Ammonia can influence multiple neurotransmitter systems directly (chemical influence) and indirectly (altered substrate availability for transmitters). There is substantial evidence that astrocytes play an important role in the pathogenesis of HE. Ammonia and other endogenous products, inflammatory cytokines, and hyponatremia (associated with portal hypertension) induce astrocyte swelling that can lead to brain edema and herniation most common in acute liver failure and acute severe HE.

Treatment of acute HE is aimed at providing supportive care and rapidly reducing neurotoxins produced in the GI tract. Severely encephalopathic animals may be semicomatose or comatose. Benzodiazepines and other sedatives should not be administered. Food should be withheld until neurologic status improves. Fluids (2.5% dextrose and 0.45% saline with potassium chloride and vitamin B complex added) should be administered to correct dehydration, electrolyte, and acid-base imbalances, but monitoring of plasma osmolality is essential to avoid hypoosmolality. Lactated Ringer's solution should be avoided, because hepatic failure may thwart lactose metabolism and cause lactic acidosis. Cleansing enemas of warm soapy water are followed by retention enemas of either lactulose or lactitol (3 parts lactulose or lactitol to 7 parts water at 20 mL/kg), 10% povidone-iodine solution (20 mL/kg, rinsed well after 10–15 min dwell), neomycin (22 mg/kg mixed with water), or diluted metronidazole (7.5 mg/kg suspended in water at 10–20 mL/kg) given every 8 hr until the animal is neurologically responsive. Retention enemas should be maintained for 15–20 min by use of a Foley catheter. Administration (oral or rectal) of live *Lactobacillus* and *Bifidobacillus* organisms (live yogurt cultures or probiotic products) also can assist in displacing ammonia-producing microbes but remains a controversial intervention. Metronidazole, neomycin, and povidone-iodine solutions can directly alter colonic bacterial flora, decreasing populations of ammonia-producing organisms. However, care is warranted in using neomycin with concurrent inflammatory bowel disease because increased systemic uptake can increase potential for renal and otic (cochlear) toxicity. Metronidazole must be restricted to ≤7.5 mg/kg every 8 hr (combined oral and rectal dosing); higher dosages confer risk of iatrogenic neurotoxicity (vestibular signs initially).

Once the animal is stabilized, treatment is aimed at preventing recurrence. Protein-modified restricted diets should be fed (*see* p 439). Oral probiotic yogurt and lactulose (0.1–0.5 mL/kg, PO, bid-tid, initial dose) can be used, with initial dose titrated to achieve several soft, pudding-like stools per day. Feeding milk may achieve a similar effect in some animals. The goal of administration of nondigestible carbohydrate is to promote fermentation in the gut. Concentrated probiotic organisms can prevent other bacteria from growing and replicating through substrate competition and pH-related (acid) growth inhibition or mechanical cleansing (catharsis) induced by fermentation products. These effects diminish uptake of ammonia, inflammatory and oxidative substrates, lipopolysaccharide, and other toxic enteric products contributing to HE. Unfortunately, the efficacy of probiotics remains unestablished for this purpose.

In recalcitrant HE, antibiotic therapy, preferably metronidazole (7.5 mg/kg, PO, bid) or amoxicillin (13–15 mg/kg, PO, bid) rather than neomycin, is recommended. Antibiotic therapy works synergistically to reduce enteric toxins along with indigestible carbohydrates. Rifaximin (approved for treatment of HE in people in 2010 because of its few adverse effects and pharmacologic benefits) is a semisynthetic, gut-selective, nonabsorbable oral antibiotic derived from rifamycin and a structural analogue of rifampin. It acts locally in the GI tract, with systemic adverse effects similar to those of placebo in people. It is active against a variety of aerobic and anaerobic gram-positive and gram-negative organisms, as well as protozoal infections. In vitro data indicate that the susceptibility of gram-positive organisms to rifaximin is greater than that of gram-negative organisms. Dosing at 5 mg/kg, once to twice daily, has been used in a small number of dogs and cats with recalcitrant HE with apparent positive response. Optimal dosing has not been determined.

Clinical signs of HE can be exacerbated by GI bleeding, infection, glucocorticoid use (enhanced catabolism of tissue protein), hypoglycemia, neoplasia, fever, azotemia or dehydration (increased BUN increases enteric ammonia production), constipation (increased generation and absorption of colonic neurotoxins), metabolic alkalosis (favoring both production of ammonia by the kidneys and uptake of ammonia across the blood-brain barrier), and use of diazepam and barbiturates (synergetic neuroinhibitors). Use of H_2-receptor antagonists and sucralfate, control of fever and infection, proper hydration, and minimal (if any) use of anticonvulsant medications can help alleviate HE complications. For additional considerations, *see* p 442.)

PORTAL HYPERTENSION AND ASCITES

Ascites develops secondary to portal hypertension and low albumin concentrations. Physiologic responses triggered to maintain euvolemia and splanchnic perfusion pressure signal systemic conservation of sodium and water.

Portal hypertension represents circulatory dynamics thwarting craniad flow of blood through the liver. Prehepatic causes include stenosis, stricture, or thrombi involving the extrahepatic portal vein. Intrahepatic causes include the sequela of chronic hepatitis resulting in collagenization and capillarization of hepatic sinusoids, accumulation of connective tissue encircling portal triads or the hepatic venule (centrilobular area), architectural remodeling of the liver by formation of regenerative nodules (cirrhosis), vascular occlusion of hepatic or portal veins (eg, thrombi, neoplasia, vasculitis), or diffuse dissemination of neoplastic cells within sinusoids or storage materials (amyloid within the space of Disse, fat or glycogen within hepatocytes). Rarely, arterialization of the hepatic parenchyma by an intrahepatic arteriovenous malformation leads to arterialization of the intrahepatic circulation and causes portal hypertension and ascites. Intrahepatic causes of portal hypertension are categorized as presinusoidal, sinusoidal, and postsinusoidal. Post-hepatic causes of portal hypertension include obstruction of blood flow from the liver through the hepatic vein; this can begin at the level of the heart (eg, right heart failure, cor triatriatum dexter, hemangiosarcoma involving the right atrium), pericardium (eg, restrictive pericarditis, pericardial tamponade), or vena cava (eg, thrombi, congenital or acquired "kink," heartworm-associated vena caval syndrome).

In all cases of hepatic portal hypertension, intrahepatic portal hypoperfusion (portal perfusion pressure is ~5–8 mmHg) is compensated by an increase in hepatic arterial perfusion that maintains organ circulation. This causes hepatofugal (backward) flow of blood into the valveless portal system and formation of acquired portosystemic shunts (APSSs).

Compensatory imbalance of sodium and water homeostasis becomes clinically apparent at the onset of portal hypertension and is typically associated with a subnormal albumin concentration. Ascitic effusion associated with hepatic disease is usually a modified or pure transudate (serum albumin <1.8 g/dL). Consequences of portal hypertension include development of ascitic effusion, splanchnic vasodilation, risk of bleeding from APSSs, development of a portal-enteric vascuolopathy, and increased risk of septic abdominal effusion.

The standard treatment to reduce splanchnic portal hypertension in people is nonselective β-blockade using propranolol, administered to control or reduce risk of spontaneous bleeding from APSSs. Other pharmacologic interventions remain controversial and have not been shown in placebo-controlled trials to provide greater benefit. Therapeutic strategies for control of ascites include dietary sodium restriction, administration of diuretics to increase urinary sodium elimination, and therapeutic abdominocentesis (when necessary). The first step is dietary sodium restriction to an intake of ≤100 mg sodium/100 kcal diet (25 mg/kg/day; <0.1% dry-matter basis in food). However, sodium-restriction alone is often insufficient and too slow in onset for efficient management. Thus, diuretics are usually also recommended. Diuretic therapy should slowly reduce ascites without causing dehydration, metabolic alkalosis, or hypokalemia. Reducing ascites by ≤1%–1.5% of total body wt/day is recommended by initially using combined treatment with furosemide (1–2 mg/kg, PO, bid) and spironolactone (loading dosage 2–4 mg/kg × 2–3 doses, then 1–2 mg/kg, PO, bid). Reevaluation every 7–10 days allows for careful upward titration of diuretic dosages. Combining a loop diuretic (furosemide) with spironolactone (aldosterone antagonist) reduces risk of iatrogenic hypokalemia.

If ascites is slow to mobilize, measuring the urinary fractional excretion of sodium can help determine whether dietary restriction and diuretic dosing are adequate. If ascites causes tense abdominal distention compromising ventilation, appetite, or patient comfort, therapeutic abdominocentesis may be undertaken. In people, 8 g of human albumin is administered for every 5 L of effusion removed to offset the development of postdiuresis circulatory dysfunction developing ~12 hr after effusion removal. Postdiuresis circulatory dysfunction reflects reequilibration of body fluids and worsened hypoalbuminemia (removed by abdominocentesis), leading to systemic hypotension (response to redistribution of removed ascitic fluid) and splanchnic and renal vasoconstriction. The latter responses increase risk of development of the hepatorenal syndrome (reversible renal vasoconstriction associated with liver failure complicated by ascites). Because there is no access to species-specific albumin for dogs and cats, polyionic fluids may be used when therapeutic abdominocentesis to remove large amounts of ascitic fluid is performed. Large-volume abdominocentesis should never be performed without concurrent diuretic administration. In removing ascitic effusion, the goal is to remove enough volume to improve patient comfort. Rational use of therapeutic abdominocentesis reduces abdominal pressure, improves renal perfusion and cardiac output, and improves response to diuretic therapy. Once ascitic effusion is mobilized, diuretics can often be used intermittently with concurrent dietary sodium restriction.

PORTOSYSTEMIC VASCULAR MALFORMATIONS

The most common circulatory anomalies of the liver in dogs are microvascular dysplasia (MVD) and portosystemic vascular anomalies (PSVAs, also referred to as portosystemic shunts or portocaval shunts). Cats also are affected with PSVAs but less commonly than dogs. MVD and PSVAs are related polygenic disorders affecting small-breed dogs. PSVAs may be extrahepatic (more common in small-breed dogs) or intrahepatic (more common in large-breed dogs). MVD has not been characterized in large-breed dogs or in cats.

Microvascular Dysplasia

MVD is far more common than PSVAs in affected kindreds of small "terrier" type dogs. A diagnosis of MVD denotes abnormal development of the fine (tertiary) branches of the intrahepatic portal veins and is associated with lobular atrophy and a compensatory increase in arterial perfusion (hepatic arterial buffer response), which manifests as coiling of hepatic arteriole branches and development of arterial twigs. The arteriolar response results in increased numbers of thick-walled arterial cross-sections in portal tracts and orphaned random arterioles within the hepatic parenchyma. Other additional MVD microanatomic abnormalities variably include large numbers of binucleate hepatocytes (especially adjacent to the portal tract), merging of hepatic venules with portal tracts, abnormal sinusoidal organization and expansion, thickening of the throttling muscle of the hepatic venule in dogs, and formation of random foci of lipogranulomas. A diagnosis of "portal hypoplasia" cannot be made on the basis of a liver biopsy, because any reduction in hepatic portal venous perfusion causes identical microanatomic changes. Rather, this histologic pattern is better termed "portal hypoperfusion." Dogs with MVD have high TSBA concentrations but do not demonstrate clinical illness or other laboratory abnormalities found in dogs with PSVAs. They do not demonstrate HE, do not develop ammonium biurate crystalluria, and typically have a normal protein C activity. A normal lifespan should be expected in dogs with MVD. This diagnosis does not warrant feeding a special diet or liver-specific medications (eg, lactulose, SAMe, milk thistle). However, because dogs with MVD may have trouble metabolizing drugs that require rapid hepatic delivery and extraction, care is necessary when prescribing certain medications. Because MVD is genetically linked with PSVAs, TSBAs should be measured in all young puppies of predisposed breeds for future health care considerations; discovery of high TSBA concentrations during an illness may lead to inappropriate, invasive, and expensive diagnostic testing. Selection of breeding stock in affected kindreds should target dogs with normal TSBA concentrations. However, because the trait is polygenic, breeding dogs with normal TSBAs may result in puppies affected with MVD and PSVAs. Once high TSBA concentrations are detected in young (<6 mo) small terrier-type breeds lacking clinical signs of PSVA, repeated bile acid measurements are not warranted; TSBA concentrations will remain variably increased for the animal's life. Knowing that a dog has high bile acids likely caused by MVD will define utility of the TSBA test for future health care assessments.

Definitive diagnosis of MVD is possible only by consideration of the liver biopsy and vascular imaging studies. Liver biopsy demonstrates lesions identical to those of PSVAs. The severity of MVD lesions varies among liver lobes, necessitating collection of samples from three different lobes for definitive characterization. Liver biopsy by the tru-cut method is strongly discouraged for diagnosis of portal hypoperfusion (PSVAs, MVD) because this diagnosis is based on examination of multiple acinar units to detect lobular atrophy, portal triad arteriolarization, and other characteristic features. Needle biopsies restrict the number of acinar units sampled. However, steps to pursue a definitive diagnosis *are not* recommended in most dogs with suspected MVD (no clinical signs, no hematologic or biochemical markers typical of PSVA). Instead, it is prudent to consider that a dog at risk of hepatic vascular malformations has MVD as the underlying cause of high TSBAs unless it exhibits clinical (HE) or clinicopathologic features (RBC microcytosis, low BUN, creatinine, and cholesterol concentrations, low protein C activity) associated with PSVAs.

Portosystemic Vascular Anomalies

A portosystemic vascular anomaly (PSVA) is a grossly apparent aberrant connection between the extrahepatic portal vasculature and the systemic circulation (connecting a branch of the portal vein to the vena cava or azygous vein) that diverts blood to the systemic circulation, bypassing the liver. Reduced portal flow to the liver causes hepatic lobular atrophy. Because the portal circulation transports microorganisms, toxins, nutrients, and other materials from the intestines to the liver, detoured blood is not cleansed or processed before circulation to the brain and systemic circulation. Consequently, neurotoxic substances that can provoke encephalopathic effects can be circulated directly to the brain, causing HE. Other noxious products and infectious agents inefficiently removed by the liver in animals with PSVAs result in a more severe clinical challenge to what should be mild health concerns (eg, infectious diarrhea, infected wounds, dermatitis, tick bites, other).

Congenital PSVAs are seen primarily in purebred dogs with extrahepatic PSVAs, predominantly in small purebred terrier-type dogs (eg, Yorkshire Terriers, Maltese, Shih Tzu, Havanese, Papillon, Miniature Schnauzers, Pugs, Cairn Terriers, Norfolk Terriers, Tibetan Spaniels, and others). Intrahepatic PSVAs predominate in large-breed dogs, including (but not exclusively) Irish Wolfhounds, Old English Sheepdogs, Labrador Retrievers, and Golden Retrievers. Extrahepatic PSVAs usually arise from the portal vein, left gastric vein, or splenic vein and connect to the caudal vena cava (most common), the azygous vein, or rarely another systemic vessel. An intrahepatic PSVA represents the retention of an embryonic vessel that carries fetal blood from the placenta to the heart, through the middle of the liver but bypassing the hepatic circulation (ductus venosus). This malformation is only occassionally seen in small-breed dogs and cats.

Congenital PSVAs in cats are seen more frequently in mixed breeds, but the prevalence may be increased in purebred Himalayans and Persians. However, the higher prevalence of polycystic liver disease and associated portal hypertension and acquired portosystemic shunts in these breeds complicates diagnosis of PSVAs. In cats, extrahepatic PSVAs involving the left gastric vein are most common.

Animals with PSVAs are often smaller than littermates, fail to thrive, and can have other congenital abnormalities (eg, cryptorchidism in dogs and cats, heart murmurs in cats). Clinical signs are highly variable, and 10%–20% of affected animals may be asymptomatic. The presence of clinical signs depends on the severity of portosystemic shunting. In symptomatic animals, clinical signs are usually evident by 6 mo of age in cats and before 1 yr in dogs. Clinical signs include nausea, ptyalism (especially cats), vomiting, diarrhea, pica, intermittent anorexia, PU/PD, amaurosis (unexplained blindness), excessive vocalization, hallucinations, apparent neck or spinal pain, hematuria, pollakiuria, stranguria, urethral obstruction associated with formation of ammonia biurate uroliths, and additional neurobehavioral signs reflecting HE. Signs referable to urinary tract calculi may be the only presenting complaint. Cats with PSVAs have a unique, homogenous, copper-colored iris that appears to be genetically linked with the disorder; the exception is blue-eyed cats. However, because a copper-colored iris is typical for Persians and Russian blue cats that do not have a PSVA, it is important to consider this observation in perspective of clinical signs and finding high TSBA concentrations.

Laboratory abnormalities may include microcytic RBCs (low MCV), mild nonregenerative anemia, poikilocytosis (cats), target cells (dogs), mild hypoproteinemia and hypoalbuminemia, hypoglycemia (rare, primarily young toy-breed dogs), low BUN and creatinine, hypocholesterolemia, normal to mildly increased liver enzyme activity (ALT, AST, and ALP), normal bilirubin, dilute urine (hyposthenuria or isothenuria), and ammonia biurate crystalluria. Fasting and postprandial TSBA *concentrations* are usually markedly increased; however, measurement of TSBAs or ammonia after a prolonged fast may yield normal values. Postprandial TSBAs and ammonia (after NH_4Cl administration) are markedly abnormal. Routine coagulation assessments are usually within normal limits, but protein C activity is usually <70%. The protein C test is valid for use in dogs. This test reflects the severity of shunting; the lower the value, seemingly the more severe the shunt. In asymptomatic PSVA dogs with a protein C >70%, surgical ligation has been very successful. Those with a protein C <70% may not tolerate complete shunt attenuation.

Abdominal radiographs reveal microhepatica and "plump" kidneys. Ammonium biurate uroliths are radiolucent and thus not detected with radiographic imaging. Ultrasonography can noninvasively identify a PSVA if done by an experienced operator using color-flow Doppler in a fasted, cooperative patient. However, extrahepatic PSVAs can be missed on ultrasonographic imaging and even falsely identified in animals with MVD. Although discovery of intrahepatic PSVAs is relatively easy using ultrasonography, identification of extrahepatic PSVAs can be challenging because bowel gas and animal cooperation may limit imaging in critical regions. Ultrasonographic examination can identify radiolucent uroliths in the renal pelvis or urinary bladder. Colorectal portal scintigraphy or splenoportal scintigraphy, available in specialty clinics or teaching hospitals, can clearly determine the presence of portosystemic shunting. However, scintigraphy is unable to identify the anatomic location of involved shunting vasculature with certainty. Splenoportal scintigraphy requires percutaneous injection of isotope into the spleen, is considered an invasive test, and does not provide better resolution, specificity, or sensitivity over routine colorectal scintigraphy to determine the presence of portosystemic shunting or definitively identify the involved vasculature. Contrast radiographic portography, the traditional gold standard test to confirm PSVAs, requires catheterization of a branch of the portal vein and injection of radiodense iodinated contrast to illustrate portal vascular anatomy. Noninvasive multisector CT has replaced simple contrast radiographic portography, providing better anatomic mapping of portal vasculature. This imaging modality requires short-term anesthesia with contrast injected into a peripheral vessel and permits 3-dimensional anatomic reconstruction of the splanchnic circulation, vascular anomaly, and adjacent viscera. A liver biopsy is always indicated in PSVA patients during surgical shunt ligation, or if multiple shunts are noted, to determine primary underlying disorders or acquired liver diseases that may coexist and require specific intervention.

Although the treatment of choice for symptomatic PSVAs is surgical attenuation or ligation, not all dogs can tolerate shunt attenuation, and a subset of dogs (asymptomatic, minimally symptomatic) survive with good quality of life with medical management only. Surgical management of PSVAs may include direct shunt ligation at surgery to the animal's tolerance (judged by measurements of portal pressure, vital signs, local visceral response) or application of an ameroid ring (inner lining gradually expands over a few days to slowly occlude the shunting vasculature). The most common postsurgical complication of PSVA attenuation is short-term benign abdominal effusion that typically resolves within a few days. The most serious postsurgical complication is acute portal hypertension, characterized by development of abdominal effusion, bloody diarrhea, abdominal pain, ileus, endotoxic shock, and cardiovascular collapse. This complication requires immediate removal of the shunt ligature. Other complications include seizures (rare) and formation of blood clots within the portal vein. Unfortunately, in some dogs, acquired portosystemic shunts silently develop at varying intervals after surgery for a PSVA. The ligation site also may be circumvented by formation of a medusa of vessels around the ligated site or recanalization of the PSVA that reestablishes portosystemic shunting several years after initial surgery. The greatest risk of insidious postoperative complications is associated with ameroid constrictors, because the extent of vessel occlusion remains ill defined unless repeat imaging studies are undertaken. In rare cases, ameroids have eroded through the shunting vasculature, causing acute collapse, hemoabdomen, and death that may occur months after their application. Excellent outcomes have been observed with careful intraoperative graded ligation of extrahepatic PSVAs (observing portal pressure and visceral response, systemic blood pressure, and heart rate) as well as with application of ameroid rings. Surgical intervention for intrahepatic shunts is more complicated and less successful. Coil embolization of intrahepatic shunting vessels by interventional radiographic technique is an alternative procedure but can be associated with adverse effects (portal hypertension, portal or vena caval clot formation) and can be prohibitively expensive; in addition, more than a single intervention may be needed to substantially reduce portosystemic shunting. Survival analyses of >450 dogs with PSVAs managed with surgical versus longterm medical management estimated a median survival time of 11 yr for dogs with extrahepatic PSVAs treated surgically, with no significant difference for dogs treated solely by medical management. However, this result is biased, because owners of the population of dogs optimally responding to medical management were more inclined to decline surgical intervention. Median survival time in dogs with intrahepatic PSVAs (n=34) treated surgically was estimated as 5 yr and was not significantly different from a larger population of dogs treated by medical management alone. In a report of 96 dogs with intrahepatic shunts treated by one or more coil embolization procedures, the estimated median survival time was 6 yr.

Male dogs with repeated bouts of ammonium biurate urolithiasis requiring medical or surgical resolution (those undergoing surgical correction of PSVAs in which the shunt could not be fully attenuated as in those on medical management) should have a permanent prescrotal urethrostomy created to allow passage of small calculi. This will avert subsequent development of an obstructive uropathy.

Overall, prognosis after surgical ligation of a single extrahepatic PSVA is usually good. Prognosis is less favorable in dogs with multiple acquired shunts secondary to severe intrahepatic portal vein atresia and in those with intrahepatic shunts. Surgery is less successful in cats than in dogs, with cats more likely to develop multiple acquired portosystemic shunts after PSVA ligation. Staging surgeries to gradually attenuate PSVAs in dogs or cats has not improved outcomes.

Dogs with relatively asymptomatic PSVAs can often be managed with special diets indicated for hepatic insufficiency. Lifelong dietary support is required, but good health and normal lifespan can be achieved. However, dogs managed medically are always at risk of more severe effects from health issues involving other organ systems, infections, or GI signs. The best protein sources for dogs are soy and dairy quality protein with a protein intake starting at 2.5 g/kg/day. Red meat, fish, and organ meats must be avoided. Additional dairy quality protein is usually easily tolerated and can be used to increase protein, phosphate, and fermentable carbohydrate intake. Treats of raw vegetables (eg, broccoli, carrots), cheese, probiotic yogurt, popcorn, modest numbers of dog biscuits, animal crackers, and limited supervised activity with rawhide bones can be offered without adverse consequences. If rawhide chews result in oral hemorrhage, they should be avoided because swallowed blood can provoke encephalopathic signs. Variation in the need for daily lactulose and metronidazole administration (*see* p 443) is broad, such that individualization of treatments is advised. Medically managed dogs remain at risk of developing HE. Owners should be educated to recognize early signs of HE and complicating health issues, how to administer cleansing and retention enemas, and how to administer subcutaneous fluids. This training allows early intervention of HE episodes and reduces the number of emergency veterinary visits.

ACQUIRED PORTOSYSTEMIC SHUNTS

Acquired portosystemic shunts (APSSs) form secondary to portal hypertension caused by 1) chronic liver disease (fibrosis, regenerative nodules), 2) congenital severe portal vein atresia, 3) acquired damage to the fine branches of the intrahepatic portal vein (noncirrhotic portal hypertension), 4) hepatic arteriovenous malformations, 5) congenital hepatic fibrosis associated with polycystic liver malformations (ductal plate malformations), 6) portal vein thrombosis or stricture, or 7) outflow obstruction through the hepatic vein/venules (thrombosis [Budd-Chiari syndrome], hepatic vein injury [veno-occlusive syndrome]). The main body of the portal vein lacks valves and maintains a blood pressure of <8 mmHg. Any disorder diminishing hepatic portal perfusion results in a hepatic arterial buffer response that increases hepatic arterial perfusion. High-pressure retrograde arterial flow into portal vasculature leads to formation of APSSs as blood follows the path of least resistance to the vena cava. In animals with extrahepatic portal atresia or portal thrombi, splanchnic circulatory hypertension leads to an APSS. In animals with occluded hepatic venular outflow or fibrotic hepatic remodeling, sinusoidal and postsinusoidal hypertension also results in retrograde flow of blood into the valveless portal system. APSSs represent nests of tortuous veins uniting portal vasculature with the abdominal vena cava.

The most common sites of APSSs are caudal to the left kidney, in the region of the colorectal vasculature, and associated with vessels of the spleen. Nests of small tortuous vessels can usually be identified during ultrasound examination using Doppler color flow. Although esophageal varicoceles are most common in people, this location does not predominate in animals. Surgical exploration for shunt ligation should not be done in animals with suspected PSVAs associated with APSSs, because finding an APSS confirms the presence of portal hypertension. Liver biopsies are needed to determine the underlying cause of portal hypertension.

Clinical signs of APSSs include episodic HE, PU/PD, vomiting, diarrhea (sometimes bloody), and abdominal effusion. Laboratory abnormalities consistent with a primary underlying hepatic disease can be seen in addition to markers of shunting (RBC microcytosis, low BUN and creatinine, hypocholesterolemia, ammonium biurate crystalluria, and subnormal protein C activity). Hyperbilirubinemia may be present, depending on the underlying cause. Ligation of multiple APSSs is contraindicated, because this is a compensatory response to portal hypertension. Banding of the vena cava to reduce the extent of shunting is ill advised. Medical treatment to minimize signs of HE along with sodium restriction and combination diuretic therapy are used to control abdominal effusion. Dogs and cats with APSSs can live several years without clinical signs, some having a normal lifespan uneventfully when provided with appropriate medical and nutritional support.

OTHER HEPATIC VASCULAR DISORDERS

Other vascular abnormalities seen in dogs and cats include hepatic arteriovenous "fistulas," hepatic venous outflow obstruction, (veno-occlusive disease, Budd-Chiari syndrome), and portal venous thromboembolism. These are relatively uncommon compared with PSVAs and MVD and other acquired hepatic disorders.

Hepatic Arteriovenous Malformation

A hepatic arteriovenous (AV) malformation is a direct intrahepatic connection between the high-pressure hepatic arterial system and the low-pressure portal venous system. High-pressure arterialized blood flows retrograde into the portal vasculature, causing intrahepatic and extrahepatic portal hypertension, ascites, and APSS formation. These may be congenital or, less commonly, acquired from trauma, biopsy lesions, or neoplasia. Clinical signs of a congenital AV malformation initially manifest in young animals and include HE, abdominal effusion, inappetence, vomiting, and diarrhea (often bloody). A murmur or bruit associated with turbulent blood flow may be audible over the affected liver lobe. Rarely, an intrahepatic AV malformation represents a variant of an intrahepatic PSVA.

Laboratory abnormalities are identical to those associated with more common PSVAs (*see* p 447) and additionally may disclose erythrocyte changes reflecting turbulence or a shearing effect (ie, schistocytes). Although ascites is a feature distinguishing an AV malformation from a PSVA, dogs with severe congenital portal atresia also may develop abdominal effusion (if they do not manifest a PSVA). Abdominal ultrasonography can easily identify an intrahepatic AV malformation (pulsing flow) and the associated APSS on color-flow Doppler interrogation. Definitive imaging requires contrast angiography via the celiac or anterior mesenteric artery (former "gold standard") or multisector contrast angiographic CT (current "gold standard").

Multiple AV connections are often evident within an affected liver lobe. Although surgical lobectomy or ligation of the nutrient artery is the conventional treatment, many affected dogs have other microvascular malformations causing intrahepatic shunting along with APSSs thwarting efficacy of lesion ablation. Biopsy of the liver from sites distant to the AV malformation (other liver lobes) is imperative to detect other intrahepatic vascular malformations. Surgical management has a dismal prognosis for cure because of the widespread intrahepatic distribution of microscopic vascular malformations and the presence of functional APSSs. Intravascular acrylamide injection using an interventional radiographic approach is an alternative salvage procedure. Unfortunately, this also cannot guarantee clinical cure because of the complex effect of this malformation on hepatic microvasculature. Limited outcome data for this approach describes treatment failures, some procedural complications (unintended embolization of nontargeted vasculature), and need for chronic medical management of HE.

Hepatic Vein Outflow Obstruction

Hepatic venous outflow obstruction can result from cardiac or pericardial disorders causing passive congestion of the caudal vena cava (eg, right heart failure, pericardial disease causing tamponade, congenital defects [cor triatriatum dexter], cardiac tumors), obstruction of the caudal vena cava (eg, postcaval syndrome associated with heartworm disease, congenital "kinking" of the caudal vena cava, vascular or neoplastic thrombosis of the caudal vena cava, diaphragmatic hernia compressing the caudal vena cava), or obstruction of the efferent hepatic venous system (eg, liver lobe torsion, compression by a hepatic mass, idiopathic postsinusoidal venous obstruction secondary to acquired fibrosis or hepatic venular destruction, severe occlusive or obstructive extramedullary hematopoiesis, or hepatic venule obstruction by occlusive lipogranulomas (subset of dogs with extrahepatic PSVAs or MVD).

Clinical features of occlusive disorders include hepatomegaly (unless cause is associated with PSVAs or MVD), ascites, formation of APSSs, and signs suggestive of the underlying primary disorders. Simple passive congestion leads to hepatomegaly, modest increases in liver enzymes, normal bile acid concentrations, and an abdominal effusion characterized as a modified transudate. Laboratory abnormalities of veno-occlusive disease (hepatic venule occlusion) or a Budd-Chiari syndrome (thrombosis of the hepatic vein or vena cava) reflect portosystemic shunting (eg, high TSBA concentrations, hypocholesterolemia, and usually low protein C activity), mild to moderate increases in hepatic transaminases, and variable total bilirubin and albumin concentrations. A modified transudative abdominal effusion is common.

Thoracic and abdominal radiographs help distinguish cardiac from other causal disorders; these may disclose kinking or impingement of the caudal diaphragmatic region of the vena cava. Cardiac ultrasonography helps identify causes of passive congestion (eg, differentiate between pericardial disease, cardiac tumors, congenital malformations, or intrathoracic masses compressing the caudal vena cava). Abdominal ultrasonography discloses hepatic venular distention in passive congestion and diminished hepatic venule size in veno-occlusive or Budd-Chiari syndromes associated with hepatic dysfunction and APSSs. Treatment and prognosis depend on the underlying disease.

HEPATOTOXINS

Although many drugs have been associated with hepatic dysfunction, their influence on liver pathology varies depending on the pathomechanism of liver injury and the acinar zone of metabolic or circulatory disturbance.

Primidone, phenytoin, and phenobarbital can cause acute fulminant liver failure, chronic cholestatic liver disease, or a diffuse progressive degenerative vacuolar hepatopathy (VH) leading to metabolic epidermal necrosis (also known as necrolytic migratory erythema or hepatocutaneous syndrome). Although a diffuse glycogen-like VH (steroid hepatopathy) is usually a benign, reversible change associated with high-dose, longterm glucocorticoid administration, longer-term administration of high doses can cause a diffuse, severe degenerative VH leading to jaundice (in dogs) and hepatic lipidosis (in cats). Increases in ALP and, to a lesser extent, ALT are seen as early as 2 days after glucocorticoid administration in dogs.

Lomustine, a chemotherapeutic agent used mostly in dogs, causes an idiosyncratic unpredictable and progressive hepatitis culminating in cirrhosis. Oxidative injury secondary to drug metabolite accumulation is a suspected pathomechanism of liver injury, because treatment with biologically available SAMe before lomustine administration is seemingly protective.

Danazol, an impeded androgen, can cause idiosyncratic reversible jaundice in dogs.

Androgenic anabolics can induce hepatic lipidosis in inappetent cats or in cats fed a protein-restricted diet. Androgenic anabolics also increase risk of hepatocellular carcinoma.

Thiacetarsamide, previously used to treat dirofilariasis, causes hepatotoxicity owing to its arsenical content.

Toxicity is associated with increased ALT activity and, in some dogs, jaundice. High liver enzymes were used as an indication to suspend therapy; thereafter, hepatic injury resolved. Mebendazole-associated idiosyncratic hepatotoxicity caused fatal acute hepatic necrosis or chronic hepatitis in some dogs. Chronic oxibendazole-diethylcarbamazine administration in dogs was shown to cause increased ALT and ALP activity, hyperbilirubinemia, periportal hepatitis, and fibrosis. Progressive injury and clinical signs resolved in many but not all dogs after drug discontinuation.

Many NSAIDs are mitochondrial toxins, and some are associated with idiosyncratic acute hepatocellular toxicity. In particular, carprofen was shown to cause idiosyncratic hepatic necrosis in some dogs, particularly Labrador Retrievers. Dogs may recover fully if toxicity is recognized early and drug administration suspended. Based on retrospective liver biopsy inspection, the concurrent presence of excessive hepatocellular copper seemingly augmented NSAID toxicity in Labrador Retrievers. In dogs, trimethoprim-sulfadiazine also can cause idiosyncratic hepatotoxicity that may involve an immune-mediated component. A reversible cholestatic hepatopathy or acute/subacute massive fatal hepatic necrosis has been observed, sometimes after only a few treatments using a conventional dose. Halothane and methoxyflurane can be associated with a sensitization reaction leading to hepatic necrosis in dogs. Xylitol, a commonly used artificial sweetener in human foods, may be an intrinsic hepatotoxin for dogs, with ingestion of small doses leading to intractable hypoglycemia and lethal hepatic failure. Toxicity may lead to death before liver enzyme activity increases. However, there is some evidence suggesting a breadth of individual responses to this toxin.

Tetracyclines can rarely lead to idiosyncratic necrosis in dogs and cats and have been shown to augment hepatocellular lipid accumulation in many species. Itraconazole and ketoconazole in dogs and cats can cause idiosyncratic hepatotoxicity associated with high liver enzyme activity and jaundice. Clinical signs resolve with drug withdrawal.

Acetaminophen predictably causes centrilobular hepatic necrosis in dogs at dosages >200 mg/kg. Methemoglobinemia is also seen. Toxicity in cats is seen acutely at a much lower dosage (56 mg/kg), with hematologic signs predominating (eg, methemoglobinemia and Heinz body hemolysis). (*See also* p 3029.)

Methimazole hepatotoxicity in cats causing hepatic degeneration and necrosis appears to be idiosyncratic but also may involve immune-mediated mechanisms. Clinical features include inappetence, jaundice, and increased liver enzyme (ALT, AST) activity that resolve after drug discontinuation.

In cats, griseofulvin-associated hyperbilirubinemia with increased ALT appears to be idiosyncratic. Clinical signs and liver injury are reversible upon drug discontinuation. Idiopathic diazepam toxicity in cats causes fulminant hepatic failure associated with panlobular necrosis; signs of toxicity are evident within several days of initial drug administration. Toxicity has mainly been seen with medication given PO for behavior modification or to treat feline lower urinary tract disease. Unfortunately, idiosyncratic diazepam hepatotoxicity is usually fatal in cats. Proactive monitoring of liver enzymes can identify adverse reactions early in their course, allowing for prompt drug discontinuation. Similar toxicity has also been seen with oxazepam.

Other specific hepatotoxins include aflatoxins, toxins derived from amanita mushroom (amanitin), blue-green algae (microcystin), cycad-associated (Sago palm) cycasin, and β-methylamino L-alanine, a neurotoxic amino acid. There are many plants in the Sago palm family, which are used as yard ornamentals in temperate climates in North America and also are commonly sold as bonsai plants in large retail stores.) Each of these toxins can cause lethal hepatic necrosis. Other chemicals reported to be hepatotoxic include heavy metals, certain herbicides, fungicides, insecticides, and rodenticides. (*See also* TOXICOLOGY, p 2948, et seq.)

Important steps to minimize absorption of ingested toxins or overdose of oral drugs include vigorous decontamination of the stomach and intestines by gastric lavage, induced vomiting, and decreasing enteric toxin absorption. Vomiting can be induced within 30 min up to 2 hr after ingestion by oral administration of 3% hydrogen peroxide (2.2 mL/kg [1 mL/lb] to a maximum of 45 mL/dog, repeated once after 10–15 min if vomiting does not occur) or administration of apomorphine hydrochloride (0.03 mg/kg [0.014 mL/lb], IV, once; or a crushed tablet dissolved in saline [0.9% NaCl] solution instilled into the conjunctival sac and rinsed away with water or saline solution after emesis) or syrup of ipecac given orally (1–2 mL/kg).

Activated charcoal without sorbitol (2 g/kg, PO, repeated every 6–8 hr) may be administered to reduce absorption of toxins if the animal is conscious. Activated charcoal may also be administered as a high-retention enema. Gastric lavage is important to prevent absorption in unconscious animals. High-cleansing colonic enemas should also be given, using polyionic warmed fluids in dehydrated animals. Clinical observation suggests that cholestyramine might provide benefit for dogs after acute cycad ingestion if given after initial enteric decontamination steps (induced vomiting, gastric lavage). If there is no specific treatment for a hepatotoxin, judicious, supportive care should be provided.

INFECTIOUS DISEASES OF THE LIVER

Viral Diseases

Viral diseases associated with liver dysfunction include infectious canine hepatitis, canine herpesvirus, inadvertent parenteral injection of an intranasal *Bordetella bronchiseptica* vaccine in dogs, feline infectious peritonitis, and virulent systemic calicivirus infection in cats. Rarely, canine parvovirus can lead to hepatic injury as a result of portal systemic sepsis.

Infectious canine hepatitis is caused by canine adenovirus 1. In addition to acute hepatic necrosis, chronic hepatitis and hepatic fibrosis can be sequelae if neutralizing antibody is inadequate to eliminate the infection during the active phase. *See* p 798 for clinical findings, diagnosis, treatment, and control.

Canine herpesvirus affects neonatal puppies, causing hepatic necrosis as well as other systemic changes. It is usually fatal in puppies.

Accidental parenteral injection of intranasal *B bronchiseptica* vaccine in dogs can cause both a local inflammatory reaction at the injection site and acute, nonseptic hepatocellular degeneration and necrosis that evolves into chronic hepatitis. There is no known treatment other than symptomatic therapy for chronic inflammatory liver disease.

Feline infectious peritonitis virus is a coronavirus that causes diffuse pyogranulomatous inflammation and vasculitis. Icterus, abdominal effusion, vomiting, diarrhea, and fever are common clinical signs. *See* p 780 for clinical findings, diagnosis, treatment, and control.

Virulent systemic calicivirus, a recently emerged variant of feline calicivirus, can have mortality rates of 33%–60% in adult cats. Primarily identified in shelter or cattery populations, this virus causes profound fever, anorexia, marked subcutaneous edema (limbs and face especially), jaundice, alopecia, and crusting and ulceration of the nose, lips, ears, and feet. Adult cats are most severely affected. Individual hepatocyte necrosis ranging to centrilobular or more extensive necrosis is associated with neutrophilic inflammatory foci and intrasinusoidal fibrin deposits.

Bacterial Diseases

Leptospirosis: Infections with *Leptospira interrogans* serovars Icterohemorrhagiae and Pomona and chronic infections with Grippotyphosa have been associated with liver disease in dogs. Other serotypes may also involve the liver. No specific histologic lesions are pathognomonic. Markedly increased liver enzyme activity and hyperbilirubinemia indicate hepatic involvement. However, these parameters may reflect hepatic response to a sepsis syndrome rather than specific organ invasion in acutely ill dogs. Clinical and clinicopathologic features of liver involvement may worsen initially with treatment (fever, liver enzymes, hyperbilirubinemia), a Jarisch-Herxheimer reaction. Diagnosis depends on demonstrating a rise in convalescent titer or PCR detection of leptospiral DNA in blood or urine. Identification of organisms in stained liver specimens is difficult. Treatment includes supportive care and specific antimicrobial therapy. Penicillins are used initially for the acute phase, (eg, ampicillin [22 mg/kg, IV, qid] or amoxicillin [22 mg/kg, PO, bid]). Aminoglycosides (dose depends on drug used; streptomycin was historically used to clear leptospirosis) or doxycycline (5 mg/kg, PO, bid for 4 wk) are recommended to treat the carrier phase. Aminoglycosides are currently not recommended for treatment of leptospirosis owing to the high risk of causing nephrotoxicity. Special precautions are recommended when handling animals suspected of having leptospirosis (and their urine specimens) because of the zoonotic potential. (*See also* LEPTOSPIROSIS, p 646.)

Tyzzer Disease: Tyzzer disease (*see* p 199) is a rare but fatal condition caused by *Clostridium piliforme*. Infections in dogs or cats most commonly occur in immunocompromised hosts, either neonatal animals or adults affected with other conditions. Because *C piliforme* is a commensal organism in the intestines of laboratory rodents, infection is acquired by contact with or ingestion of rodent feces transporting bacterial spores. Clinical signs (lethargy, anorexia, abdominal discomfort) are acute in onset, and illness rapidly progresses to death within 24–48 hr. Marked increase in ALT activity immediately precedes death. Special stains are needed to identify organisms in liver tissue because organisms do not grow in routine bacterial culture media. Although there is no effective treatment, a vaccine has been developed for research colony animals.

***Mycobacterium avium* Infection:** Hepatic infection with disseminated *M avium* has been described in young Abyssinian and Somali cats that had an apparent innate immunodeficiency (unknown cause). The clinical course included vague illness characterized by a several month history of weight loss in the face of polyphagia. Marked diffuse interstitial pulmonary infiltrates developed in cats with and without respiratory signs. Hepatomegaly and increased ALT and AST activities were notable. Liver samples revealed granulomatous inflammation. Treatment with clarithromycin (62.4 mg/cat, PO) combined with either clofazimine (25 mg/cat/day, PO, or 50 mg/cat, PO, every other day) or rifampicin (5–10 mg/kg, bid, PO) and a fluoroquinolone or doxycycline (5–10 mg/kg, bid, PO) achieved remission in affected cats. Relapse should be expected because of the immunocompromised status of these cats.

Systemic infections, including granulomatous hepatitis due to *Mycobacterium* spp has been reported by several investigators in Basset Hounds, Miniature Schnauzers, and additional dogs. Affected dogs are suspected to have some form of cell-mediated immunodeficiency (Basset Hounds) or unique exposure to another infected animal or person. Susceptibility to various *Mycobacterium* spp vary among mammals. *M tuberculosis* can induce progressive disease in people, nonhuman primates, dogs, and swine. Clinical signs in animals infected with *M tuberculosis* depend on the route of exposure and degree of localization of the infection or its systemic dissemination. Early infection is subclinical, leading to cachexia, weakness, anorexia, dyspnea, and a low-grade, fluctuating fever. Hepatic involvement caused increased transaminase activity, reflecting pyogranulomatous hepatitis. Many animals infected with *Mycobacterium* spp are euthanized because of the severity of organ involvement at the time of diagnosis and because of zoonotic concerns. Diagnosis of *M tuberculosis* in an animal should be reported to local health officials. At least 6–9 mo of treatment using a multidrug regimen is advised; single-agent treatment is not advised owing to concern for emergence of resistant strains. Treatment recommendations include combined administration of isoniazid, ethambutol, and rifampin, with pyrazinamide sometimes substituted for ethambutol. However, experience in longterm treatment of dogs is lacking.

Diagnosis of *Mycobacterium* can be difficult because many of these organisms are slow growing (requires >1 mo), acid-fast organisms may not be found in tissue sections, and PCR from formalin-fixed tissue may be falsely negative. However, *Mycobacterium* sp have also been detected by both histologic staining and by PCR from formalin-fixed liver specimens from dogs with pyograulomatous hepatitis.

Extrahepatic and Intrahepatic Bacterial Infections and Sepsis: Extrahepatic infection and sepsis can cause cholestasis and hyperbilirubinemia. Increases in serum bilirubin may range from moderate to marked, while increases in liver enzyme activity remain modest. This type of jaundice has been seen in dogs with leptospirosis and in dogs and cats with ill-defined sepsis syndromes. Appropriate treatment targets the underlying organism causing infection. Increased liver enzyme activity in septicemia/sepsis also can reflect bacterial invasion of the liver or hepatocellular damage by associated cytokine release or hypoxia.

Animals with acute hepatic failure, chronic hepatobiliary disease, and cholestatic disorders are predisposed to systemic bacterial infection and endotoxemia due to diminished function of hepatic reticuloendothelial cells (hepatic Kupffer cells comprise the largest fixed macrophage population in the body) and reduced biliary elimination of bacteria derived from the enterohepatic circulation in bile. In acute fulminant hepatic failure, sepsis or septicemia may be masked by fever, hypoglycemia, and leukocytosis that might also represent clinical manifestations of hepatic injury.

Animals with chronic disorders causing stasis of bile flow or with chronic hepatic neoplasia are more likely to develop intrahepatic infections. Risk factors associated with biliary tract infection include advanced age, recent episodes of cholangitis, acute cholecystitis, choledocholithiasis, and obstructive jaundice.

Treatments that reduce susceptibility to infection and liver injury during fulminant hepatic failure and extrahepatic bile duct occlusion include administration of N-acetylcysteine, α-tocopherol, glutamine, oral bile acids, and enteric and systemic antibiotics. These strategies increase microvascular perfusion, reduce enteric bacterial translocation, augment innate immunity, and protect against oxidant injury. While awaiting results of culture and sensitivity (tissue, abdominal effusion, bile), antibiotics against enteric opportunists should be administered empirically, avoiding drugs extensively metabolized in the liver. Combination of a β-lactamase–resistant penicillin, metronidazole (7.5 mg/kg, PO, bid), and enrofloxacin (2.5–5 mg/kg, PO, IM, or IV, bid), may be beneficial during initial treatment when the underlying infectious cause remains unclear.

Mycotic Diseases

The most common mycotic infections associated with liver dysfunction are coccidioidomycosis (*see* p 637) and histoplasmosis (*see* p 639). In severely affected animals, clinical signs include ascites, jaundice, and hepatomegaly, in addition to signs associated with other involved organ systems. Antifungal treatment is variable, determined by the severity of infection, organ involvement, and individual clinical response. Because liver involvement in histoplasmosis is seen with disseminated disease, aggressive chemotherapy (including combinations of either itraconazole or ketoconazole and amphotericin B) are recommended. Debilitated animals have a poor prognosis. Coccidioidomycosis can be treated successfully with several antifungal medications (itraconazole and fluconazole are preferred to ketoconazole). Chronic treatment (6–12 mo) is required, and relapses may occur. Treatment efficacy is determined based on resolution of clinical signs and radiographic lesions and reduction in serologic titers. Termination of treatment should not be based on serologic titers alone, because these stabilize and persist in many dogs after clinical recovery. Owners must be informed that discontinuing medication may result in relapse. Animals recovering from CNS infection should receive lifelong treatment. Similarly, animals with disseminated disease suffering infection relapse after treatment discontinuation should continue on longterm or lifetime treatment with an azole antifungal. For chronic treatment, drug doses that effectively maintain remission may be lower than those needed to induce remission.

Protozoal Diseases

Toxoplasmosis: Toxoplasmosis (*see* p 685) can cause acute hepatic failure associated with hepatic necrosis. *Toxoplasma gondii* is more commonly seen in cats positive for feline immunodeficiency virus and feline leukemia virus. Icterus, abdominal effusion, fever, lethargy, vomiting, and diarrhea are seen in addition to clinical signs consistent with CNS, ocular, or pulmonary involvement. Liver disease in dogs is rare but when seen is either in an immunocompromised host or in young dogs and also involves systemic infection. Young dogs may be concurrently infected with canine distemper virus; in these, illness is acute in onset and rapidly fatal. Diagnosis of toxoplasmosis can be difficult; while a positive IgM titer indicates active clinical disease, IgG titers may be found in chronic infections and in animals lacking clinical disease. Clindamycin (12.5 mg/kg, PO or IM, bid for 4 wk) is the drug of choice. Because clindamycin is metabolized in the liver, dosage reduction may be necessary in severe hepatic insufficiency. Oral clindamycin should be followed by a bolus of water or food to prevent esophageal irritation. In some cases, initial treatment is combined with anti-inflammatory glucocorticoids to protect against tissue injury caused by inflammatory responses initiated by protozoal death. Prognosis depends on the degree of debilitation and stage of disease at initial diagnosis and the associated disorder causing immunosuppression. Despite improvement with treatment, animals should be considered chronically infected and thus must undergo surveillance for recrudescent disease.

Leishmaniosis: Canine leishmaniosis (*see* p 589) is a multisystemic disease caused by protozoan parasites of the genus *Leishmania*, most commonly encountered in animals that have lived in Mediterranean countries, Portugal, the Middle East, and some parts of Africa, India, and Central and South America. It also is occasionally encountered in dogs in the USA (especially Foxhounds). A serosurvey of >12,000 dogs (Foxhounds, other breeds, wild canids) and 185 people in 35 states and 4 Canadian provinces was done to assess geographic distribution prevalence, host range, and modes of transmission within North America and to assess possible infection in people. Findings identified *Leishmania* spp–infected Foxhounds in 18 states and 2 Canadian provinces but no evidence of human infection. North America leishmaniosis appears widespread in Foxhounds and is limited to dog-to-dog transmission. However, if the organism becomes adapted for vector transmission by indigenous phlebotomines, the probability of human exposure may greatly increase.

Clinical features in dogs with naturally occurring leishmaniosis include nonregenerative anemia, increased enzyme (ALP, ALT, and AST) activity, hypoalbuminemia, and variable bilirubinemia. Histologic response is characterized by a multifocal pyogranulomatous hepatitis associated with hepatocyte vacuolar degeneration with phagocytized organisms seen within macrophages. Severity of liver lesions represents sequential stages of hepatic infection in chronic visceral leishmaniosis. However, no correlation has been shown between histologic features and breed, sex, age, clinical features, or hepatic parasite load.

Treatment is rarely curative, and prognosis for debilitated animals is poor. Owing to the zoonotic potential of the organism, owners must be informed that their pet will never be completely free of the disease and that relapses may require repeated treatment. This is particularly important if an owner is immunocompromised. In the absence of renal insufficiency, a high-protein diet is recommended. The most common specific treatment recommended in the USA is allopurinol (7–20 mg/kg, PO, once to three times daily) given for 3–24 mo or indefinitely lifelong; other first-line treatments include meglumine antimony (100 mg/kg/day, IV or SC), sodium stibogluconate (30–50 mg/kg/day, IV or SC), or liposomal amphotericin B (0.25–0.5 mg/kg, IV, every other day until a total dose of 5–10 mg/kg is achieved). Numerous other second-line drugs have also helped control infections.

FELINE HEPATIC LIPIDOSIS

Hepatic lipidosis (HL), the most common acquired and potentially lethal feline liver disease, is a multifactorial syndrome. In most cases, a primary disease process causing anorexia sets the stage for HL in overconditioned cats. Peripheral fat mobilization exceeding the hepatic capacity to either redistribute or use fat for β-oxidation (producing energy) leads to profound hepatocyte cytosolic expansion with triglyceride (fat) stores. In fewer cases, inappetence is caused by environmental stresses (eg, forced weight loss with unacceptable food substitutions, moving to a new household, newly introduced or loss of pets or family members, boarding, accidental confinement [eg, locked in a garage, basement, or attic], or an inside-only cat being lost outside). The term "idiopathic HL" is appropriate only when an underlying disease condition or event leading to inappetence cannot be identified.

HL has no necroinflammatory component, and the severe cholestasis is caused by canalicular compression secondary to hepatocyte triglyceride vacuolar distention. The syndrome is associated with a number of metabolic deficits, including low hepatic and RBC glutathione, low plasma taurine, low vitamin K_1 causing coagulopathies in some cats, thiamine and/or cobalamin deficiency and likely other B vitamin depletions, and electrolyte aberrations (especially low potassium and low phosphorus).

Clinical signs vary but usually include dramatic weight loss (>25%, may include dehydration deficits), lethargy, vomiting, ptyalism, pallor, neck ventroflexion, hepatomegaly, jaundice, gastroparesis and intestinal ileus (due to electrolyte aberrations), and retention of omental and falciform fat despite diminished peripheral fat stores. Diarrhea is common in HL cats with inflammatory bowel disease or enteric lymphoma as primary disease processes. Classic signs of HE are not seen, and ammonium biurate crystalluria is unusual, although bleeding tendencies may develop. Vitamin K_1 deficiency has been confirmed in numerous HL cats by observation that bleeding tendencies and coagulation test abnormalities resolve with vitamin K_1 therapy.

Laboratory results reflect the HL syndrome as well as the primary underlying disease. A nonregenerative anemia, poikilocytosis, increased RBC Heinz bodies, variable WBC count, hyperbilirubinemia and bilirubinuria, mild to marked increases in ALT and AST, and marked increases in ALP are common. In cats with a primary necroinflammatory process involving the pancreas, liver, bile ducts, or gallbladder, GGT activity will be increased, usually exceeding the fold increase in ALP. In all other conditions causing HL, GGT activity is normal or only modestly increased. The GGT:ALP relationship is useful in discerning underlying cholangitis/cholangiohepatitis and other diseases involving biliary structures (including pancreatitis). Finding a high GGT also predicts whether a liver or pancreatic biopsy is indicated. Depending on underlying disorders, hypoalbuminemia and hyperglobulinemia may be found. Prolonged PT or APTT may develop; the PIVKA clotting time is more sensitive for detection of vitamin K_1 sufficiency. In the earliest stages of the HL syndrome, TSBAs are abnormal before onset of jaundice (this circumstance is rarely encountered). Peritoneal effusion is rare but when found represents the primary disease process or iatrogenic fluid overload.

Ultrasonographic evaluation reveals homogeneous hyperechoic hepatic parenchyma and subjective hepatomegaly. Hyperechogenicity is determined by comparing hepatic parenchyma to falciform fat and the spleen (liver is normally hypoechoic vs spleen). Kidneys also may appear hyperechoic because of increased renal tubular fatty vacuolation. Ultrasonographic examination should carefully assess the entire abdomen for evidence of an underlying disease process and include evaluation of the biliary tree, gallbladder, pancreas, intestinal wall thickness, hepatic and mesenteric lymph nodes, kidneys, and urinary bladder, and scrutiny for uroliths in the kidneys, ureters, or bladder.

Definitive diagnosis is based on the history, physical examination findings, laboratory features, ultrasonographic appearance of the liver, and ultrasound-guided hepatic aspiration cytology. Liver biopsy is not necessary to diagnose HL; however, underlying cholangitis/cholangiohepatitis or hepatic lymphoma may eventually require biopsy for definitive diagnosis. Cytology preparations show profound vacuolar distention of hepatocytes involving >80% of hepatocytes aspirated. Canalicular cholestasis is commonly seen. Mistaken aspiration of omental fat rather than liver is easily deduced by the absence of hepatocytes.

Treatment of HL is aimed at correcting fluid, electrolyte, and metabolic deficits and initiating food intake. Because cats with HL may have high lactate concentrations and may not be able to metabolize acetate, 0.9% NaCl is the fluid of choice. Fluids should not be supplemented with dextrose, because this will reduce utilization of intrahepatic fatty acids for β-oxidation. Because affected cats are usually overconditioned, fluid therapy must be based on ideal body weight. Overhydration is common when fluid dosage is based on total overconditioned body weight and can lead to pleural and abdominal effusion and pulmonary edema.

Fluids should be appropriately supplemented with potassium (using the sliding scale) based on electrolyte status. If initial serum phosphate concentration is low (<2 mg/dL), potassium phosphate should be added at a rate of 0.01–0.03 mmol/kg/hr. Potassium chloride supplementation must be judiciously adjusted, considering concurrent potassium phosphate supplements to avoid iatrogenic hyperkalemia. Potassium phosphate supplements (up to 0.06 mmol/kg/hr) are commonly initiated when feeding is started to guard against development of severe hypophosphatemia associated with the "refeeding syndrome."

A fortified water-soluble vitamin solution (2 mL/L of fluids, *see* TABLE 12, p 442) should be added to the IV fluids. Thiamine supplements (50–100 mg/day) are specifically indicated in HL and provided in water-soluble fluid supplements or by the oral route. Rare anaphylactoid reactions and neuromuscular paralysis have been seen in a few cats treated with thiamine by SC or IM injection.

A diagnostic blood sample should be collected for B_{12} determination followed by empirical B_{12} administration (250–1,000 mcg/cat, SC). Cobalamin deficiency is seemingly common in HL cats and may predispose individuals to this syndrome. When present, B_{12} deficiency confounds intermediary metabolism; however, this is confirmed only by assessment of methylmalonic acid, which confirms functional B_{12} insufficiency. Unfortunately, this assessment cannot be promptly completed. Consequently, B_{12} supplementation (which has no adverse effects) is routinely supplemented with the less exacting measurement of plasma B_{12} used to determine propriety of longterm supplementation. Treatment with N-acetylcysteine is initiated during the first 2–3 days (140 mg/kg, IV, administered through a 0.25-μm filter over 20 min, then 70 mg/kg, IV, tid-qid; diluted to a 10% solution). N-acetylcysteine should not be given as a prolonged (>1 hr) constant-rate infusion, because it may induce hyperammonemia by deviating substrates from the urea cycle.

Vitamin K_1 is given with a small needle (0.5–1.5 mg/kg, SC or IM, three doses given at 12-hr intervals) before procedures that might provoke bleeding (eg, insertion of a jugular catheter, esophageal feeding tube, cystocentesis, or hepatic aspiration sampling).

Some cats may develop renal potassium wasting as a result of underlying renal disease or lipid accumulation in their renal tubules. The fractional excretion of potassium can be estimated by measuring potassium and creatinine in simultaneously collected baseline serum and urine samples: fractional potassium excretion = ([urine potassium/urine creatinine] × [serum creatinine/serum potassium]) × 100%. In a hypokalemic cat, a value <1% is expected. Values >20% represent marked renal potassium wasting and indicate the need for aggressive potassium supplementation. Cats with prodigious potassium needs should have potassium gluconate added to their food as soon as oral intake is established. This will reduce the concentrations of potassium needed in the IV fluids and associated risk of iatrogenic hyperkalemia.

Nutritional support is the cornerstone of recovery (*see* p 439). Feeding is initiated after the cat is rehydrated and has reasonable electrolyte balance, because these are requisite factors enabling normal enteric motility. Because cats with HL are in metabolic liver failure, appetite stimulants are inappropriate; diazepam, oxazepam, cyproheptidine, and mirtazepine should not be used and will not recover an affected cat. Occasionally, an appetite stimulant may help initiate feeding early in syndrome development.

A palatable odiferous food should be offered initially. If the cat salivates or objects, all food should be removed because of the risk of inducing a "food aversion syndrome." If oral feeding is not tolerated, feeding a liquid diet (eg, CliniCare®) with supplements via a nasoesophageal tube is cautiously initiated as a first step. A 5–10 mL volume of tepid water is administered first to assess the cat's tolerance and response. If no vomiting or signs of discomfort are noted, the process is repeated with liquefied food. After a few days of nasoesophageal feeding, if the cat is judged to be a reasonable anesthetic risk, an esophagostomy tube (E-tube) is placed with the distal tip 2–4 cm craniad to the esophageal-gastric junction. This should be documented with a lateral thoracic radiograph.

A high-protein, calorie-dense, balanced feline diet is recommended for E-tube feeding. Only rarely should a protein-restricted diet be used, because protein restriction can aggravate hepatic lipid accumulation. Rather, use of lactulose and oral amoxicillin or low-dose metronidazole (7.5 mg/kg, bid) can optimize nitrogen tolerance to allow feeding of a normal feline diet (these measures modify enteric flora, substrate utilization, and increase colonic catharsis or cleansing). A number of metabolic supplements have improved recovery of affected cats: taurine (250–500 mg/cat/day), medical grade liquid oral L-carnitine (250–500 mg/cat/day), vitamin E (10 IU/kg/day), and potassium gluconate (if hypokalemia is persistent).

Initial feedings are small and given frequently or by constant-rate infusion. On the first day, one-third to one-half of the cat's energy requirements are fed; the amount fed is then gradually increased over the next 2–4 days to the ideal intake. If vomiting occurs, electrolytes must be rechecked, feeding tube position verified, and factors relevant to the underlying disease process considered. Metoclopramide (0.05–0.1 mg/kg, IM, up to tid, or 0.25–0.5 mg/kg divided per day as a constant-rate infusion), ondansetron (0.025 mg/kg, IV, up to bid), or maropitant (1 mg/kg/day, no more than 5 days) may be used as antiemetics. Enteric motility may be stimulated by exercise during owner visits.

To avert development of hypophosphatemia induced by re-feeding, which can cause weakness, hemolysis, encephalopathy, and other adverse effects, serum phosphorus concentrations should be serially monitored and supplemental potassium phosphate judiciously provided. Routine IV potassium phosphate supplementation is administered when feeding is initiated to obviate persistent or feeding-induced hypophosphatemia. If gastritis is suspected, an H_2-blocker (eg, famotidine or ranitidine) may be used, and carafate administered PO (but not via E-tube). If the cat tolerates oral medications, SAMe at 40 mg/kg/day is given between meals once N-acetylcysteine treatment is completed. SAMe supplementation must be accompanied by sufficient B_{12}, folate, and other water-soluble vitamins to ensure optimal metabolic benefit (metabolism to glutathione and methyl group donation for transmethylation reactions). Use of ursodeoxycholate in HL may be detrimental because TSBAs are extraordinarily high in these cats and because bile acid profiles resemble those associated with EHBDO (increased secondary bile acids). All bile acids are toxic to cells in high concentrations and, in HL, bile acids are seemingly trapped by canalicular compression.

In the rare circumstance that signs of HE are encountered, lactulose, amoxicillin, or low-dose metronidazole (≤7.5 mg/kg, PO, bid) may be useful. In symptomatic pancreatitis, feeding distal to the pancreas is done using a constant-rate infusion of CliniCare® mixed with supplemental pancreatic enzymes through a jejunostomy tube. Alternatively, parenteral nutrition can be provided, although this may delay recovery and provoke hepatic triglyceride retention.

Prognosis for cats with HL is good with early diagnosis, full treatment support, and control of underlying disease. Monitoring liver enzymes has no value in predicting recovery. However, a decline in total bilirubin by 50% within the first 7–10 days portends an excellent chance of full recovery. Concurrent pancreatitis is a poor prognostic indicator. Monitoring ALP of obese cats undergoing weight reduction may identify emerging HL that will allow suspension of the weight loss program and early treatment intervention. Recurrence of HL is rare in recovered cats.

BILIARY CIRRHOSIS

Biliary cirrhosis refers to periportal bridging fibrosis associated with marked hepatic architectural remodeling and biliary hyperplasia subsequent to chronic (months) of EHBDO or years of nonsuppurative cholangiohepatitis. However, it is uncommon in cats with cholangitis/cholangiohepatitis, because these animals usually succumb before biliary cirrhosis develops. Biliary cirrhosis is misidentified in cats with ductal plate malformations (a form of polycystic liver disease). Clinical features of biliary cirrhosis include variable inappetence, cachexia, jaundice, variable liver size, and ascites. Liver enzymes may be normal. Hypoalbuminemia, hyperglobulinemia, hyperbilirubinemia, and coagulopathies are common. The liver may be considered large on abdominal radiographs and appears nodular on ultrasonographic evaluation. Biopsies are needed for definitive diagnosis. Coagulation deficits complicate tissue sampling and necessitate vitamin K_1 supplementation and fresh frozen plasma transfusions before procedures. Treatment is symptomatic, requiring management of HE, hypoalbuminemia, EHBDO, and ascites. Prognosis is generally poor. Biliary cirrhosis is most commonly seen in animals with chronic EHBDO caused by obstructive neoplasia. Although cholecystoenterostomy or choledochoenterostomy can avert progression of EHBDO to biliary cirrhosis, it introduces recurrent retrograde infection through biliary structures causing chronic or recurrent septic cholangitis.

CANINE CHOLANGIOHEPATITIS

Cholangiohepatitis in dogs is rare and usually associated with suppurative inflammation and ascending biliary tree infection with a wide variety of bacterial organisms (both gram-negative and gram-positive enteric bacteria, *Salmonella*, *Campylobacter jejuni*, coccidiosis). Canine cholangiohepatitis is most commonly associated with disorders causing stasis of bile flow, biliary mucocele formation, cholelithiasis, and surgical manipulations of the biliary tree. Clinical signs include anorexia, vomiting, diarrhea, lethargy, PU/PD, fever, and abdominal pain.

Laboratory abnormalities are consistent with hepatic cholestasis and include hyperbilirubinemia and increased activities of ALP, GGT, and transaminases. Ultrasonography may or may not reveal abnormalities involving the biliary tree or gallbladder. In some cases, a coarse hepatic echogenicity is identified, reflecting portal tract inflammatory infiltrates and connective tissue. In some cases, ultrasonographic findings may indicate need for emergency surgical intervention (eg, mature gallbladder mucocele, cholelithiasis associated with EHBDO). Aspirates or impression smears of liver or bile may reveal suppurative septic inflammation. Samples collected from liver, bile, and sections of the biliary tree should be submitted for aerobic and anaerobic culture and sensitivity. Antibiotic treatment should be based on cultured organisms, and other treatments should target underlying disease processes. Initial treatment with combination of ticarcillin, metronidazole, and enrofloxicin is commonly used before culture and biopsy results are available. For best outcome in animals undergoing surgery, antimicrobials should be started before the surgical procedure.

CANINE CHRONIC HEPATITIS

Chronic hepatitis that does not focus on biliary structures is more common in dogs than cats. Several breeds are predisposed, including Bedlington Terriers, Labrador Retrievers, Cocker Spaniels, Doberman Pinschers, Skye Terriers, Standard Poodles, West Highland White Terriers, Springer Spaniels, Chihuahuas, and Maltese. Although there is an identifiable etiology for some categories of chronic hepatitis, in most cases the cause remains unidentified. Increased hepatocellular copper and Kupffer cell iron stores are common in dogs with chronic hepatitis. The degree of metal accumulation and its acinar location help determine its relevance to tissue injury.

Other associated conditions include infectious canine hepatitis, chronic hepatitis secondary to infectious processes, and chronic exposure to xenobiotics (including certain drugs, biologic toxins, and chemicals). Terminology that reflects specific etiology or breed predilection, such as drug-associated chronic hepatitis, infectious chronic hepatitis, copper-associated hepatitis, etc, is preferred. The term idiopathic chronic hepatitis indicates that an etiology has not been determined.

Histopathologic changes are generally similar in all cases of chronic hepatitis, regardless of the underlying cause, and include a lymphocytic-plasmacytic inflammation with infiltrates extending into hepatic parenchyma, variable single cell or piecemeal necrosis, and in advanced disease, development of bridging fibrosis and nodular regeneration. The acinar zone of involvement varies with the underlying cause.

Copper-associated Hepatopathy

Copper-associated hepatopathy is a leading cause of chronic hepatitis in dogs, increasing in prevalence since 1997 when copper supplements in commercial dog foods were modified to a more bioavailable form. Retrospective evaluation of liver biopsies from Labrador Retrievers and Doberman Pinschers from 1980 to 2013 indicated that dogs of these breeds, with and without chronic hepatitis, had significantly higher hepatic copper concentrations in the last 10 yr of the study. Management of body copper homeostasis relies on numerous copper transporters, chaperones, and binding proteins, as well as biliary canalicular egress. Copper-associated hepatopathy is best characterized in Bedlington Terriers, which have a mutation (deletion of exon 2) of the COMMD1 copper transporter protein. Careful breeding programs guided by liver biopsy and genetic testing (PCR gene mutation test) have remarkably reduced disease frequency in Bedlington Terriers. However, some Bedlington Terriers with biopsy-confirmed copper-associated hepatopathy lack this specific gene mutation.

Failure to excrete copper into bile leads to chronic hepatitis and, eventually, cirrhosis and liver failure. Affected dogs develop high liver copper concentrations by 1 yr of age (normal: <400 mcg/g dry liver or 400 ppm), which progressively increase during the first 6 yr of life (values may be >12,000 ppm). Liver injury is reflected by increased ALT activity and has been shown in dogs with hepatic copper as low as 600 ppm.

Three disease phases were historically characterized in Bedlington Terriers. Acute hepatic necrosis occurred in dogs <6 yr old, presenting with hepatomegaly, vomiting, lethargy, anorexia, jaundice, copper-induced hemolytic anemia, and hemoglobinuria. Copper-associated hemolytic anemia occurs only with massive hepatic necrosis, which releases large amounts of copper into the systemic circulation. Death usually occurs within 48–72 hr of onset of clinical signs. In this group of dogs, untreated survivors suffered recurrent bouts of critical illness induced by stress (eg, whelping, attending dog shows, traveling). Another clinical presentation involves chronic hepatitis associated with clinical features, including chronic weight loss, HE, ascites, and jaundice. Some dogs develop an acquired Fanconi syndrome (glucosuria, aminoaciduria, metabolic acidosis, inappropriately alkaline urine pH), signaling renal tubular copper toxicity. The last clinical presentation was recognized in young, clinically healthy dogs, simply demonstrating increased ALT activity and increased hepatic copper concentrations (on liver biopsy). This presentation progresses to acute hepatic necrosis or chronic hepatitis. Rarely, an affected dog remained asymptomatic until another disease process caused liver injury augmented by excessive hepatic copper stores.

Genetic testing is recommended for selection of Bedlington Terrier breeding stock. However, definitive diagnosis of copper-associated hepatopathy requires liver biopsy in adult dogs with qualitative copper stains reconciled with quantitative copper measurements.

Many other purebred and mixed-breed dogs of all ages also may develop copper-associated hepatopathy. More commonly and perhaps more severely affected are Labrador Retrievers; whether the high breed popularity influences this observation remains unclear. Doberman Pinschers, West Highland White Terriers, and some dogs related to Dalmatians also may develop profoundly increased hepatic copper concentrations accompanied by severe liver injury. A genetic cause has not been identified in any of these breeds. It is important to emphasize that copper-associated hepatopathy can be the primary cause of hepatitis in any dog (purebred or mixed breed) and can be definitively diagnosed only by liver biopsy. There is no recognized gender predisposition.

Histologic features of copper-associated hepatopathy include a focus on the centrilobular region (zone 3), finding eosinophilic granules within the cytosolic compartment of hepatocytes and within macrophages in areas of single cell necrosis. Small granulomas develop subsequent to hepatocyte necrosis and release of copper granules into the surrounding parenchyma. Zone 3 lesional–associated parenchymal collapse is verified with reticulin staining (centrilobular collapse) and fibrillar collagen deposition with Masson trichrome staining (centrilobular connective tissue deposition). With advanced injury, regenerative nodules and regions of parenchymal extinction are seen. The prominent role of copper in driving tissue injury is verified by finding copper granules (rhodanine staining) in nearly every hepatocyte within regenerative nodules.

Treatment of copper-associated hepatopathy requires copper chelation with concurrent restriction of copper intake from dietary and water sources. Dietary copper restriction can be achieved by feeding a prescription diet formulated for dogs with HE (delivering 2.2–2.5 g of protein/kg body wt). These low-protein formulas can be supplemented with protein sources low in copper to raise the dietary protein intake to 3.5 g of protein/kg body wt. Supplementary protein sources are selected using the USDA food tables (sort based on copper concentration), with feeding amounts of selected foods calculated using the Nutritional Analysis Tool 2.0 (human nutrition). Copper in water should contain <0.1 ppm (0.1 mcg copper/L); if copper pipes transport water, flushing the system for 5 min will eliminate any leached copper.

Administration of antioxidants is important, because copper induces liver damage through oxidative injury. Chelation therapy with D-penicillamine (15 mg/kg, PO, bid, given 30 min before feeding, for ≥4–6 mo) is the gold standard treatment. Thereafter, chronic therapy may be instituted by reducing the D-penicillamine dosage by half and administering the drug every other day while maintaining dietary copper restriction. Alternatively, the dog may be treated with zinc acetate (*see* below). Concurrent administration of pyridoxine (25 mg/day) is advised during D-penicillamine treatment, because this drug has antipyridoxine (vitamin B_6) effects. If D-penicillamine chelation is not tolerated, trientene hydrochloride can be used (5–7 mg/kg, PO, bid, given 30 min before feeding). Caution is warranted with trientine used at the originally higher recommended dose, because this has induced acute renal failure in dogs with severe copper storage hepatopathy.

An alternative approach to manage copper storage hepatopathy is daily administration of oral zinc (acetate, gluconate, sulfate) to inhibit copper uptake from the GI tract (zinc induces enterocyte metallotheinine, which irreversibly binds copper and prohibits its absorption; copper is subsequently eliminated with effete enterocytes in feces). Although zinc treatment theoretically increases dietary options, study of the efficacy of zinc treatment in people with Wilson disease confirms unreliable control of dietary copper uptake. Zinc therapy must not be given concurrent with chelation therapy, because this will thwart efficacy of each treatment. Oral zinc is not well tolerated by some dogs, commonly causing vomiting, nausea, and inappetence. If zinc therapy seems more suitable for chronic treatment in a specific dog, a loading phase of elemental zinc at 5–10 mg/kg/day is given in two divided doses, 30 min before meals. Plasma zinc concentrations are monitored to ensure that circulating zinc is not nearing toxic values (>800 ppm). After several months, the dosage can be reduced to 2–3 mg/kg/day divided bid, but without study of radiolabelled copper uptake the efficacy of treatment in an individual dog remains unknown.

Vitamin E (10 IU/kg/day, PO) and biologically available SAMe (20 mg/kg/day, PO, on an empty stomach) are recommended antioxidants that also have anti-inflammatory and potentially antifibrotic effects. Vitamin C is contraindicated in copper storage hepatopathy, because it may foster injurious transition metal effects.

After chelation therapy, it is essential to continue to limit copper ingestion in food and water lifelong. Adherence to a copper-restricted diet and water source may obviate the need for continual chelation or zinc therapy.

Chronic Hepatitis with or without Increased Hepatic Copper in West Highland White Terriers: Although West Highland White Terriers have been shown to accumulate excessive hepatic copper, not all dogs with high hepatic copper concentrations develop hepatitis. Some dogs with severely increased hepatic copper concentrations die of old age without necroinflammatory liver lesions. Although West Highland White Terriers with chronic hepatitis usually do have high tissue copper concentrations, they differ from Bedlington Terriers with copper storage hepatopathy in that: 1) the mode of inheritance has not been determined, 2) maximal copper accumulation occurs by 6 mo of age and may then decline, 3) overall hepatic copper concentrations are lower than in Bedlington Terriers, and 4) hemolytic anemia has not been reported.

Focal hepatitis may be seen in asymptomatic young adult dogs. Chronic hepatitis is associated with anorexia, nausea, vomiting, diarrhea, jaundice, and later ascites. Increased liver enzymes develop first with focal disease, followed by increased TSBA concentrations and then hyperbilirubinemia as the severity of liver injury advances. Histopathologic changes include multifocal necroinflammatory hepatitis with typical copper-affiliated granulomas and single cell necrosis, with advanced disease culminating in cirrhosis. Treatments target copper primarily if an association between inflammation and copper accumulation is histologically verified. (For treatment recommendations, *see* COPPER-ASSOCIATED HEPATITIS, p 460, and CANINE CHRONIC HEPATITIS, p 460.)

Idiopathic Chronic Hepatitis

Idiopathic chronic hepatitis is defined as chronic necroinflammatory self-perpetuating liver disease associated with a nonsuppurative inflammatory infiltrate. To qualify as an idiopathic syndrome, an underlying cause should have been rigorously pursued yet not discovered. Autoimmune hepatitis is included in this classification. An antinuclear antibody test, testing for endemic infectious diseases (titer or antigen tests), and investigation of drug and toxin exposure, along with dietary, environmental, and family history, must be undertaken. Middle-aged to older adult dogs are more commonly affected; there are no breed or gender predilections.

Clinical features include variable anorexia or hyporexia, lethargy, weakness, vomiting, diarrhea, weight loss, jaundice, PU/PD, and in severe or advanced disease, coagulopathies, ascites, and HE. Earliest laboratory findings are persistent or cyclic increases in activity of ALT, AST, ALP, and GGT. With advancing disease, increased TSBA concentrations are followed by hyperbilirubinemia. Other findings may include a nonregenerative anemia, leukocytosis, and hyperglobulinemia. In late-stage disease, portal hypertension causes development of APSSs and the associated laboratory markers of RBC microcytosis, hypocholesterolemia, hypoalbuminemia, prolonged APTT and/or PT, and ammonium biurate crystalluria. At this stage, overt signs of HE may manifest. In early disease, liver size is normal and there may be no demonstrable ultrasonographic lesions. In late-stage disease, radiographs may demonstrate a small liver with nodular lesions detected on ultrasound examination. Ultrasonographic evaluations also may disclose ascites and APSSs in dogs with advanced liver injury.

Definitive diagnosis requires liver biopsy to detail acinal distribution of liver injury, the type of inflammatory infiltrates, the presence of lobular remodeling and fibrosis, and accumulation of copper and/or iron. Chronic, sustained, unexplained increases in liver enzymes usually indicate liver biopsy. Biopsy specimens should be submitted for both aerobic and anaerobic bacterial cultures and quantification of copper, iron, and zinc. Copper stains must be reconciled with quantitative copper measurements to avoid erroneous interpretations. Liver biopsies must be large enough to detail at least 15 contiguous portal triads, and biopsies must be taken from several different liver lobes. Samples collected only from apparent "mass lesions" can lead to erroneous diagnoses. Application of special stains will disclose the acinar location of liver injury (reticulin staining); presence of collagen deposition of fibrosis (Masson's trichrome staining); extent of iron accumulation in macrophages, Kupffer cells, and hepatocytes (Prussian blue staining); and the extent and location of hepatocellular copper accumulation (rhodanine staining).

Supportive care (nutritional, vitamin supplementation) and use of specific therapies to slow inflammation and fibroplasia and to restore liver antioxidant status are recommended. Antibiotics are initially prescribed empirically until results of the biopsy and tissue cultures become available, and then adjusted or discontinued based on culture results. Additional treatments include ursodeoxycholic acid as a hepatoprotectant and anti-inflammatory choleretic (15–20 mg/kg, PO, divided bid, given with food), polyunsaturated phosphatidylcholine as an antifibrotic (PhosChol® [the specific source used containing 52% of the active antifibrotic component dilinoleoylphosphatidylcholine] 25–50 mg/kg/day, given PO with food), vitamin E as an antifibrotic and antioxidant (10 IU/kg/day, given with food), and bioavailable SAMe as an antioxidant (20–40 mg/kg/day, PO, on an empty stomach).

Immunosuppressive drugs are used only after careful consideration and exclusion of infectious or toxic causes and when an active disease process (nonsuppurative or pyogranulomatous inflammation) is characterized on liver biopsy. Prednisolone or prednisone is usually started at a dosage of 2–4 mg/kg/day, for 7–10 days and titrated downward to a maintenance level of 0.5–1 mg/kg, given every 24 hr or on alternate days, depending on patient response. In the presence of ascites or APSSs, dexamethasone is used instead of prednisone or prednisolone, because it is a synthetic glucocorticoid lacking mineralocorticoid effects. The dose is adjusted considering its longer biologic half-life (72–96 hrs) and higher potency (7–10 fold more than prednisolone or prednisone) such that dexamethasone is used at 0.1–0.2 mg/kg, PO, given every 3 days after a daily loading dose for 3 days. An immunomodulatory agent additional to the glucocorticoid is used to enable titration of the glucocorticoid dosage to the lowest effective dose. This reduces the dose of each immunosuppressive drug, reducing their adverse effects and achieving a multimodal immunosuppressive effect. Adverse effects of glucocorticoids in chronic hepatobiliary disease include sodium and water retention (which can exacerbate or promote ascites), catabolic effects (which can promote HE), GI ulceration and enteric bleeding (which can precipitate HE), pancreatitis, predisposition to secondary infections, glucose intolerance, and iatrogenic hyperadrenocorticism (glycogen-like VH).

Azathioprine is most commonly used at a dosage of 1–2 mg/kg/day for 3–5 days, then every other day. Beneficial effects may not be seen for up to 8 wk. Because azathioprine can cause bone marrow suppression and gastroenteric, pancreatic, and rarely liver toxicity, frequent follow-up assessments are imperative. If azathioprine causes acute bone marrow suppression (within 1 mo), treatment is discontinued until recovery, then restarted with a 25%–50% reduction in dosage. If bone marrow toxicity is identified only after chronic administration (months), azathioprine should be permanently discontinued. Pancreatitis and idiopathic hepatotoxicity are rare adverse effects that also mandate drug discontinuation. Mycophenolate mofetil is used in dogs that cannot tolerate azathioprine or, alternatively, as an initial immunosuppressant. Recommended dosing is 10–20 mg/kg, PO, bid for 7–10 days, then every 24 hr, followed by dosage titration based on patient response. Cyclosporin is another alternative immunosuppressant used in combination therapy. Some dogs previously managed well on azathioprine have lost remission on conversion to cyclosporin. Other dogs started on cyclosporin as their primary immunosuppressant have responded well. In the absence of placebo-controlled clinical trials for treatment of canine immune-mediated hepatitis, treatment is individualized to each dog based on sequential monitoring and, sometimes, follow-up liver biopsy. Discontinuation of immunosuppressive therapy is not recommended in dogs with chronic hepatitis; if drugs are discontinued, they should be withdrawn gradually, with close monitoring (serum biochemical profiles).

Because complete remission is difficult to evaluate clinically, a follow-up biopsy may be required. In most cases, serum ALT activity serves as a surrogate marker of disease activity. Prognosis is widely variable. Some dogs live ≥5 yr after initial diagnosis. Dogs with ascites require dietary sodium restriction and treatment with furosemide and spironolactone (*see* p 445). Dogs with HE require dietary protein modification and may benefit from lactulose and administration of low-dose metronidazole.

If immune-mediated hepatitis is considered the definitive diagnosis, careful consideration should be given before administration of routine vaccinations. Nonspecific immune stimulation may adversely stimulate hepatitis and cause disease flare.

Breed-specific Chronic Hepatitis

Labrador Retrievers: This popular breed is predisposed to chronic hepatitis that is commonly associated with pathologic accumulation of hepatocellular copper (*see* COPPER-ASSOCIATED HEPATITIS, p 460). However, this breed also can develop a primary lymphoplasmacytic hepatitis that appears to involve immune-mediated mechanisms. Clinical features at diagnosis (in order of highest frequency) include jaundice, inappetence, vomiting, lethargy, and weight loss, with some dogs demonstrating abdominal discomfort, PU/PD, or no signs relevant to hepatitis. Common laboratory features include a normal PCV, leukocytosis, increased ALT (10-fold), increased ALP (5-fold), modest or no increases in AST and GGT, hyperbilirubinemia, prolonged APTT, and transient glucosuria if severe copper-associated hepatopathy is a concurrent problem. Ultrasonographic imaging often demonstrates hypoechoic and hyperechoic parenchymal nodules, subjective microhepatica, and less frequently, irregular liver margins and ascites. A lymphocytic-plasmacytic hepatitis with single cell necrosis and remodeling may focus on the portal tract or be diffusely disseminated. If pathologic copper accumulation is a leading cause of the liver injury, inflammatory responses are focused in the centrilobular region. When both disorders coexist, marked lymphoplasmacytic infiltrates are seen within sinusoids of all acinar zones. Copper-associated hepatopathy is not typically associated with a marked lymphoplasmacytic infiltrate. In dogs with coexistent lesions, it remains unclear whether sensitization to epitopes on hepatocytes damaged from copper toxicity is the primary underlying etiopathogenesis of the immune-mediated response.

Treatment decisions are based on liver biopsy findings with routine and special liver stains and tissue copper quantification. Copper chelation and restricted copper intake (food and water) establishes complete remission in dogs with overt copper overload (>800 mcg/g dry weight tissue but lacking a nonsuppurative inflammatory reaction). Response to treatment is rapid and dramatic if diagnosed early but lifelong management of copper-associated hepatopathy (*see* p 460) is required. Labrador Retrievers with chronic nonsuppurative immune-mediated hepatitis not associated with hepatic copper retention are treated lifelong as for idiopathic chronic hepatitis (*see* above). Response to treatment can be dramatic and is especially effective when diagnosis is made early in the disease process.

Doberman Pinschers: An idiopathic, chronic, immune-mediated hepatitis recognized in Doberman Pinschers in the mid 1980s predominantly involved middle-aged adult female dogs. Copper retention appears to play a role in some dogs, which currently contributes to hepatitis seen in this breed.

In dogs with advanced disease, clinical features include cyclic illness involving anorexia, weight loss, vomiting, diarrhea, PU/PD, jaundice, coagulopathies (melena, epistaxis), splenomegaly, microhepatica, ascites, and HE. Laboratory features may include a nonregenerative anemia, leukocytosis, thrombocytopenia, increased ALP and ALT activities, hyperbilirubinemia, hypoalbuminemia, prolonged APTT, and a pure or modified transudative abdominal effusion. Ultrasonography may identify nodular liver lesions.

Liver biopsy is necessary for definitive diagnosis and treatment recommendations.

Treatment in dogs with immune-mediated nonsuppurative hepatitis includes immunomodulation with prednisone (1–2 mg/kg/day for several weeks, slowly titrated to 0.5 mg/kg/day and if possible, to every other day) and antioxidants, with or without azathioprine. In dogs with developing fibrosis, PhosChol® polyunsaturated phosphatidylcholine is also recommended (25–50 mg/kg, PO, with food). Nutritional support depends on the presence of HE and the need for copper restriction. Prognosis is poor for dogs diagnosed with advanced nonsuppurative hepatitis. Dogs diagnosed early can achieve remission for several years with prednisone, vitamin E, antioxidants, and ursodeoxycholic acid. Prognosis for dogs with apparent copper-associated hepatopathy can be good if diagnosed early in the disease process (*see* COPPER-ASSOCIATED HEPATITIS, p 460).

Cocker Spaniel Hepatopathy: Chronic Cocker Spaniel hepatopathy is associated with a degenerative vacuolar hepatopathy (glycogen, lipid, and hydropic degeneration) associated with low-grade nonsuppurative inflammation and sinusoidal myofibrocyte activation that leads to sinusoidal deposition of fine tendrils of fibrillar collagen. Disease is typically advanced at initial presentation. Definitive diagnosis by liver biopsy demonstrates regenerative nodules and marked distortion of the hepatic architecture consistent with micronodular and macronodular cirrhosis. There is no gender predisposition, and most dogs are diagnosed as young adults (4–4.6 yr, range 2–11 yr). Most dogs lack signs of liver disease antecedent to development of portal hypertension, ascites (pure or modified transudate), hypoalbuminemia, abrupt onset of HE, and APSSs. Clinical signs at presentation may include (in declining frequency) inappetence, lethargy, diarrhea, weight loss, melena, vomiting, and amaurosis. In some dogs, hepatopathy is discovered during abdominal ultrasonography for another health problem. Clinicopathologic features include modestly increased to normal liver enzyme activity, hypoalbuminemia, hypocholesterolemia, and increased TSBAs in the absence of hyperbilirubinemia. Normal fibrinogen, clotting times, normal or increased C-reactive protein, and subnormal antithrombin activity argue for a lack of acute phase marker induction and an inflammatory phenotype. Some dogs have moderate to abundant copper (on copper-specific staining), which may represent copper retention secondary to cholestasis (mild copper retention) or a more primary copper-associated injury (copper >800 ppm). In the latter dogs, foci of hepatocellular damage coordinate with regions of dense copper retention.

Strong sinusoidal staining with alpha-smooth muscle actin confirms transformation of resting stellate cells (Ito cells) that normally store retinoic acid (vitamin A) into activated myofibrocytes. Although the lesion has been labeled "lobular dissecting hepatitis" and Cocker Spaniel "hepatitis," the minimal inflammation and necrosis and lack of clinicopathologic markers of inflammation suggest that "hepatopathy" is better terminology. Chronic Cocker Spaniel hepatopathy studied in Sweden nearly 20 yr ago investigated whether a genetic abnormality causing alpha$_1$-antitrypsin (AAT) deficiency was involved. AAT is an important serum protease inhibitor synthesized in the liver and exported to the systemic circulation. Study of plasma AAT protein configuration and immunohistochemistry of AAT in canine liver biopsies implicated a unique enzyme phenotype associated with AAT globules evident in hepatocytes of some but not all Cocker Spaniels. Unfortunately, retention of AAT in damaged or dysfunctional hepatocytes may also occur as an epiphenomenon of compromised protein transcription consequent to hepatocellular injury (but usually not retention of globules) as demonstrated in affected dogs. Yet it remains unknown whether AAT plays a role in this breed-related syndrome. In people, treatment for AAT deficiency is liver transplant.

Treatment is supportive and symptomatic using a balanced protocol as described for chronic hepatitis. Early glucocorticoid immunomodulation (eg, before the diagnosis of liver disease, glucocorticoids prescribed for ear or skin disorders) has seemingly prolonged survival in affected dogs. However, in dogs with hypoalbuminemia or ascites, glucocorticoids are poorly tolerated and may cause melena, ascites, HE, etc. If a glucocorticoid trial is undertaken, dexamethasone should be used instead of prednisone to avoid mineralocorticoid effects. Ursodeoxycholic acid, vitamin E, SAMe, polyunsaturated phosphatidylcholine (PhosChol®), and individually tailored nutritional support are recommended. A permanent urethrostomy may be necessary in male dogs that develop ammonium biurate calculi. Successful treatment of severely affected dogs has been possible for several years. Need for copper chelation is based on specific stains and copper quantification. Management of HE (dietary modification, lactulose, low-dose metronidazole, or nonabsorbable orally administered antimicrobials), and management of ascites (sodium restriction, diuretics, judicious therapeutic abdominocentesis) as described previously are recommended. Dogs receiving glucocorticoids as treatment for antecedent health issues before hepatopathy diagnosis and dogs treated with glucocorticoids with or without azathioprine after diagnosis may have improved survival. Additional supportive treatments reported include ursodeoxycholic acid, antioxidants, and antifibrotics. Although there was no correction of hypoalbuminemia in most dogs, survival beyond 3 yr of diagnosis was documented.

Skye Terriers: Three reports of hepatitis in Skye Terriers, one characterizing disease in nine related dogs, described no age or gender predilection and clinical signs ranging from asymptomatic to end-stage liver failure at time of initial diagnosis.

Three separate liver disorders were described: mild inflammation with no evidence of cirrhosis or copper accumulation, advanced macronodular cirrhosis with cholestasis, and marked copper accumulation. Treatment is based on liver biopsy, as described previously for these disorders.

Maltese Dog Zone 3 (Centrilobular) Hepatopathy: Maltese dogs have a high prevalence of congenital hepatic vascular malformations (MVD, PSVAs). Dogs with MVD vastly outnumber those with PSVAs. Within kindreds, finding high TSBAs in 60%–90% of dogs confirms high trait prevalence. Clinicians and breed enthusiasts have been confused by a published article proposing that TSBA quantification in Maltese dogs is confounded by interfering analytes. Liver biopsies from Maltese dogs with increased TSBA concentrations strongly refute that supposition, with >250 studied cases (60% lacking PSVAs) demonstrating lesions of portal hypoperfusion. An inflammatory and degenerative zone 3 (centrilobular) hepatic lesion develops in a subset of dogs with the MVD/PSVA trait; the lesion often coexists with marked persistent or cyclic increases of serum ALT activity. Histologic lesions vary in severity and may be progressive, eventually culminating in cirrhosis. This hepatopathy is often associated with concurrent inflammatory bowel disease and may derive from splanchnic delivery of inflammatory cytokines and inflammatory cells. Histologic lesions in dogs with increased serum ALT and high TSBA concentrations typically consist of a lymphoplasmacytic infiltrate with or without eosinophils adjacent to and sheathing hepatic venules (centrilobular, zone 3). Dogs develop a degenerative hepatopathy with lipogranulomas (foamy macrophage aggregates) located adjacent to hepatic venules that appear to partially or completely obscure vascular lumen. A spectrum of histologic severities exists within biopsy sections from an individual dog. Severe lesions provoke postsinusoidal intrahepatic portal hypertension and development of APSSs. Although cirrhosis has been confirmed in a small subset of dogs, ascites is detected clinically in nearly 75% of those affected. In dogs with ascites, ultrasonography usually discloses hepatic parenchymal nodules, a nodular liver surface contour consistent with hepatic remodeling, and narrowing of hepatic venules on color-flow vascular interrogation. A small subset of dogs may have copper-associated hepatopathy (rhodanine staining and quantified tissue copper >1,200 ppm). Dogs with zone 3 degenerative hepatopathy concurrent with a PSVA usually respond poorly to surgical or ameroid shunt attenuation.

Treatment focuses on management of associated inflammatory bowel disease (hypoallergenic diets, home-cooked nutritionist-formulated or commercially available diets), metronidazole (7.5 mg/kg, PO, bid [low dose because of portal hypoperfusion]), and glucocorticoids avoiding use of drugs with mineralocorticoid effects (eg, dexamethasone, every 3 days, anti-inflammatory dose). Vitamin E (10 IU/kg/day) and SAMe (20 mg/kg/day) are recommended for antioxidant and antifibrotic benefits. Because a subset of severely affected dogs have developed thromboemboli involving hepatic venules and/or portal veins, minidose aspirin (0.5 mg/kg, PO, once to twice daily) has been prescribed for some dogs until inflammation abates (assumed based on decline in liver enzyme activity with maintained synthetic markers). Inflammation also has been successfully managed with budesonide in some dogs. In dogs treated with glucocorticoids, dosage is titrated to response (enzymes, clinical features) to minimize undesirable adverse effects. Some dogs require combined immunomodulation to achieve control of inflammation or because of unacceptable glucocorticoid effects. In these, azathioprine or cyclosporine are used in combination with or to replace glucocorticoids. Ascites is managed with sodium restriction and combined furosemide and spironolactone administration. A loading dose of spironolactone (2–4 mg/kg, PO, given once) followed by 1–2 mg/kg, PO, bid. Furosemide is dosed at 1 mg/kg, PO, once to twice daily. Diuretic treatment is suspended when ascites is in remission and reinstituted on recurrence, with continued sodium restriction.

LOBULAR DISSECTING HEPATITIS

Lobular dissecting hepatitis is a unique hepatic reaction pattern rather than a unique hepatic syndrome. The histologic features are typified by liver injury associated with intrasinusoidal nonsuppurative inflammatory infiltrates leading to panlobular sinusoidal fibrosis. Although more commonly described in juvenile to young adult dogs and in a small group of related Standard Poodles, this disorder seemingly has no breed, gender, or age predilection. Weight loss and ascites, with or without jaundice, are common clinical features. Laboratory abnormalities include hypoalbuminemia, hypocholesterolemia, low BUN, and increased TSBA concentrations in nonjaundiced dogs. Liver enzymes may be normal or mildly or markedly increased. APSSs develop due to acquired intrahepatic sinusoidal portal hypertension. Hepatic copper concentrations are not consistently increased. The syndrome commonly progresses to cirrhosis. Supportive treatment is recommended for HE, ascites, and control of fibroplasia and inflammation as described previously. Colchicine (0.03 mg/kg, PO, daily to every other day) has been used to control fibrosis and sinusoidal inflammation in some dogs. Other dogs have been managed with more conventional immunomodulatory protocols with PhosChol® (polyunsaturated phosphatidylcholine with 52% dilinoleoyl-phosphatidylcholine, 25–50 mg/kg/day), used as an antifibrotic with fewer adverse affects. This is a poorly understood and characterized syndrome and in some cases may reflect hepatotoxin exposure.

CANINE VACUOLAR HEPATOPATHY

Vacuolar hepatopathy (VH) is a commonly diagnosed canine liver syndrome in which hepatocytes become markedly distended with cytosolic glycogen with or without discrete membrane-bound lipid inclusions. Glycogen-like VH is associated with typical or atypical hyperadrenocorticism or endogenous release of corticosteroids in response to chronic stress, illness, inflammation, or neoplasia. Liver biopsy is often pursued because of unexplained increases in serum ALP activity. Transaminase activity may be only modestly increased; GGT may or may not be increased.

Abdominal radiography may reveal hepatomegaly or changes associated with an underlying disease process. Metastatic disease or mineralized airways (chronic hyperadrenocorticism) may be seen on thoracic radiography. Ultrasonography reveals subjective hepatomegaly and hypoechoic hepatic nodules against a hyperechoic parenchymal background, the so-called "Swiss cheese pattern" that cannot be differentiated from infiltrative mass lesions, hepatic fibrosis, nodular hyperplasia, regenerative nodules, or cirrhosis. In some cases, grossly evident hepatic nodules cannot be discerned by ultrasound examination. VH usually is the underlying hepatic lesion in dogs with idiopathic nodular hyperplasia and also is common in dogs with hepatic adenomas, hepatocellular carcinoma, and gallbladder mucoceles. Progressive VH merges into the classic hepatic syndrome associated with the hepatocutaneous lesion (*see* below). Hepatic biopsy is needed for definitive diagnosis, because glycogen-vacuolated hepatocytes are also seen in necroinflammatory liver disorders. Intrahepatic extramedullary hematopoiesis is common.

It is critical to determine and treat any underlying disease process. Careful scrutiny for adverse drug reactions is also necessary, with a focus on drugs associated with "induction phenomenon." These should be discontinued and replaced with an alternative therapy. Clinicians should investigate any use of holistic or herbal remedies that may have systemic glucocorticoid or adrenocorticotropic hormone (ACTH) effects.

Nutritional support is important and must be individualized. In most cases, a normal protein intake is appropriate. VH in dogs with hyperlipidemia requires treatment with a fat-restricted diet (<2 g fat/100 kcal of diet). A protein-restricted diet should not be fed, unless indicated (eg, demonstration of HE or ammonium biurate crystalluria). In fact, protein restriction may augment development of this liver lesion, especially if it is associated with hypoaminoacidemia as in the hepatocutaneous syndrome. A supplemental water-soluble vitamin is recommended for all dogs. Antioxidants should be provided, because some experimental evidence implicates oxidative injury in degenerative VH. Ursodeoxycholic acid is recommended if TSBA concentrations are increased.

Vacuolar Hepatopathy in Scottish Terriers: VH associated with a progressive increase in ALP activity is common in Scottish Terriers. Studies suggest this syndrome is linked with a breed-related abnormality involving adrenal steroidogenesis, leading to overproduction of progestins and androgens. Severe progressive VH is first noted in middle-aged dogs and can be either slowly progressive or progress rapidly over a few years to liver failure, cirrhosis, APSSs, ascites, and hyperbilirubinemia. Ultrasonographic imaging discloses the typical "Swiss cheese" pattern of VH (described above). High risk of hepatocellular carcinoma is recognized in dogs demonstrating progressive hepatic remodeling. Liver biopsy often discloses dysplastic proliferative lesions antecedent to formation of hepatocellular carcinoma. Adrenomegaly is common and may be bilateral or unilateral. Treatment with adrenal-modulating drugs can be hazardous and appears ineffective. Supportive care as for dogs with declining hepatic function, monitoring both sequential biochemical profiles for sudden marked increases in ALP or ALT activity that may signal tumor formation, and serial ultrasonographic evaluations for enlarging hepatic mass lesions are recommended. Early surgical excision of enlarging hepatic mass lesions that likely represent hepatocellular carcinomas is recommended to allow complete excision. A subset of dogs studied also have copper-associated liver injury that cannot be inferred on the basis of biochemical assessments but rather require liver biopsy for definitive diagnosis.

METABOLIC DISEASES AFFECTING THE LIVER

Diabetes mellitus, hyperadrenocorticism, hypothyroidism, and hyperthyroidism can cause changes in the liver.

HL can develop secondary to diabetes mellitus because of increased lipid metabolism and mobilization; notable are hepatomegaly and increased liver enzyme activities. Dogs with diabetes mellitus rarely manifest liver dysfunction unless they develop severe progressive VH associated with the hepatocutaneous syndrome (*see* below). Most of these dogs have markedly increased ALP with lesser increases in transaminase activity. Diabetic cats also may develop increased ALT and ALP activities and may become hyperbilirubinemic with onset of HL. Diabetic animals have increased risk of pancreatitis that may progressively lead to EHBDO and cholangitis. These animals have increased risk of bacterial infections involving biliary structures (emphysematous cholecystitis, cholangitis).

Cats with hyperthyroidism usually develop increases in ALP and ALT activities and are rarely hyperbilirubinemic. Liver function is usually normal. The underlying cause of altered enzyme activity is not fully understood but postulated to involve toxic effects of excessive thyroxine, malnutrition, cardiac dysfunction, induction phenomenon, and increased bone turnover (causing increase in the bone isoenzyme of ALP). Liver enzymes return to normal with successful treatment; however, methimazole also can lead to a drug-associated hepatopathy that resolves only after drug discontinuation.

HEPATOCUTANEOUS SYNDROME

(Superficial necrolytic dermatitis, Necrolytic migratory erythema, Glucagonoma syndrome)

Hepatocutaneous syndrome is a rare, chronic, progressive, and usually fatal disorder. Although typically associated with diabetes mellitus, the liver lesion is a severe, degenerative, glycogen-like VH that also can accompany pancreatic or neuroendocrine tumors and severe VH secondary to endogenous steroidogenic hormone release or chronic phenobarbital therapy.

Bilaterally symmetric crusting and ulcerative lesions are found on mucocutaneous junctions and cutaneous regions susceptible to pressure injury (eg, footpads, ears, periorbital regions, and limb pressure points). Skin lesions are characterized by a marked parakeratotic epidermis. Edematous spaces between cells are filled with neutrophils, necrotic cells, and debris that create an "eosinophilic" layer. Mild neutrophilic perivascular inflammation is also seen. Lesions are commonly referred to as "red, white, and blue" on H&E staining (red for parakeratosis, white for edema, and blue for hyperplasia). Skin lesions are seen initially in most affected dogs, but liver lesions may precede cutaneous changes.

Clinical features include anorexia, weight loss, lethargy, PU/PD, mild nonregenerative anemia, marked increases in ALP and moderate increases in ALT and AST, hyperglycemia, decreased plasma amino acid concentrations (by 50% of normal), hypoalbuminemia, and increased TSBA concentrations. High plasma glucagon levels are inconsistent. Liver size is variable. On ultrasound, multiple hypoechoic nodules surrounded by hyperechoic parenchyma are diffusely scattered throughout the liver, described as a "Swiss cheese" pattern. The association between the cutaneous and hepatic lesions is not understood but is speculated to involve hypoaminoacidemia or abnormal zinc metabolism. Liver lesions are not necroinflammatory and are not associated with fibrosis or cirrhosis. The prognosis for recovery from hepatocutaneous syndrome in dogs is poor.

Treatment focuses on correcting amino acid deficiencies and providing symptomatic care for cutaneous lesions and VH. In general, corticosteroids are contraindicated for the skin lesions. A commercial diet high in protein or formulated for dogs with hepatic insufficiency with an added "body-building" amino acid concentrate can be used. Administration of IV amino acids requires delivery through a catheterized jugular vein. Aminosyn 10% crystalline amino acid solution (100 mL contains 10 g of amino acids) can be given IV, 500 mL/dog, over 8–12 hr. Symptoms from hyperammonemia may develop in susceptible dogs (previously demonstrating HE) but should resolve within 12 hr after completion of the infusion. The IV amino acid infusion is repeated 7–10 days later if skin lesions persist; four cycles can be given. If no response is seen, further amino acid infusions are futile. Amino acid treatment results in regression of skin lesions and hepatopathy in some dogs.

Control of concurrent diabetes mellitus can be challenging, because insulin resistance suggests involvement of counter-regulatory hormones (glucagon, glucocorticoids, others). Supportive care requires use of appropriate broad-spectrum antifungals or antibiotics for superficial secondary bacterial and fungal invaders, zinc methionine supplementation (1.5–2 mg/kg/day, PO), water-soluble vitamins (doubled daily dose), essential fatty acid supplements, and topical lesion cleansing. Some dermatologists also recommend treatment with niacinamide (250–300 mg/dog, PO, bid). Ursodeoxycholic acid (15–20 mg/kg, divided and given bid with food) and antioxidants (vitamin E and SAMe) are recommended. Identification and treatment of underlying metabolic conditions is essential for control. Chronic phenobarbital therapy has been an underlying cause in some dogs. Successful treatment with long-acting somatostatin (octreatide; prohibitively expensive) has been described in a single dog with hepatocutaenous syndrome secondary to metastatic glucagonoma.

NODULAR HYPERPLASIA

Nodular hyperplasia (proliferative hepatocytes maintaining single-celled hepatic cord architecture with normal reticulin support) occurs as a benign, age-related microscopic or grossly apparent small mass lesion in dogs. It is often associated with a VH, lacks a defining remodeled border (as characterizes regenerative nodules), and may be confused histologically with adenomatous hyperplasia or hepatic adenoma (demonstrating proliferative disorganized hepatocytes forming thick hepatic cords with diminished reticulin support). Although nodular hyperplasia does not cause clinical disease, it can be accompanied by increased liver enzyme activity, particularly ALP. Unless the liver is diffusely remodeled with nodular lesions (secondary to degenerative VH), TSBA concentrations remain normal. Ultrasonographically, nodular hyperplasia is associated with hypoechoic hepatic nodules set against a hyperechoic background (if associated with glycogen-like VH). Cytology of an aspirate may discriminate dysplastic, neoplastic, or inflammatory cells but cannot exclude any of these disorders. Biopsy is necessary to differentiate between nodular hyperplasia, dysplastic microscopic nodules, regenerative nodules, cirrhosis, and neoplasia.

HEPATIC NEOPLASIA

Primary hepatic neoplasms are less common than metastatic neoplasms in the liver and are either carcinomas, carcinoids, sarcomas, or of hemolymphatic origin. Metastatic neoplasia of the liver can originate from multiple visceral organs and can include lymphosarcoma. There may be no clinicopathologic features indicating the presence of metastatic neoplasia within the liver.

Primary tumors are most often found in older animals (>9 yr) and can be malignant or benign. The most common primary hepatic neoplasm in dogs is hepatocellular carcinoma, whereas the most common primary hepatic neoplasms in cats include biliary adenomas and carcinomas and cystadenomas (not considered a neoplasm) most common in older cats. Additional tumor types include hemangiosarcomas, carcinoids, and sarcomas in dogs; lymphomas and myeloproliferative disease in cats; and less frequently, leiomyosarcomas, GI stromal tumors, and myelolipomas.

Hepatocellular Carcinomas: Hepatocellular carcinoma is most common in dogs but also may occur rarely in cats. Diagnosis may be initially pursued because of palpation of an abdominal mass or recognition of serially increasing ALT, ALP, or GGT activities. Less commonly, mass lesions are discovered as the cause of critical abdominal hemorrhage. Radiography may disclose a large mass lesion or emphysematous abscess within a necrotic tumor core. Ultrasonography is more sensitive for detection of mass lesions and can discriminate single from multiple lobe involvement. Small hepatocellular carcinomas may appear hypoechoic, hyperechoic, or heteroechoic. However, the large size of some masses precludes clear differentiation of tumor impingement on or invasion into adjacent viscera and vasculature. Hepatocellular carcinomas can occur as a single large mass in one liver lobe with or without smaller masses in other lobes (massive), as discrete nodules located in multiple lobes (nodular), or as infiltrative disease throughout the liver without obvious discrete nodularity (diffuse). Nodular and diffuse hepatocellular carcinomas, which account for 29% and 10%, respectively, of all hepatocellular carcinomas, involve multiple liver lobes and are not usually amenable to surgical removal. Single massive hepatocellular carcinomas represent 61% of all canine hepatocellular carcinomas and are potentially resectable with good outcome. Tumors involving the left liver lobes carry the best prognosis. Hepatocellular carcinomas are locally invasive and may spread to local lymph nodes but are slow to metastasize elsewhere. Multiple histologic patterns have been characterized for canine hepatocellular carcinoma, including (but not limited to) solid, clear cell, trabecular, peliod, pseudoglandular, scirrhous, and anaplastic.

Common clinical signs in dogs include weight loss, inappetence, fever, and lethargy; less common signs include vomiting, PU/PD, and seizures (hypoglycemia). However, dogs may be asymptomatic until the tumor reaches massive size or develops a necrotic core leading to critical abdominal hemorrhage. On abdominal palpation, a mass may be detected, and pain notable. Abdominal effusion is uncommon. Laboratory tests may indicate nonregenerative anemia, RBC microcytosis, thrombocytosis, increased serum activity of ALP and AST, and hypercholesterolemia. High ALT and AST concentrations may reflect invasion of adjacent normal tissue or central tumor necrosis and may indicate a poor prognosis. Increased ALP may reflect association with increased steroidogenesis (particularly androgens and progestins). Hypoglycemia may develop either due to large tumor mass or a paraneoplastic effect. Pulmonary metastases are uncommon. Tumor margins should be demarcated on submitted specimens to judge adequacy of mass resection (tumor-free margin). Mass excision with wide margins can be curative in both dogs and cats. Liver biopsies from regions distal to the tumor are recommended in dogs, because antecedent dysplastic foci may portend possible tumor recurrence. Finding dysplastic foci should increase ultrasonographic and clinicopathologic (a sudden peak in ALP or transaminase activity) surveillance for tumor recurrence.

Hepatocellular Adenomas and Adenomatous Hyperplasia or Dysplastic Foci: Differentiation of hepatocellular carcinoma from hepatocellular adenoma can be difficult, involving judgement of the degree of dysplasia and characterization of the histologic features. Like hepatocellular carcinomas, adenomas also may be accompanied by microscopic dysplastic foci in unaffected liver lobes. Hepatocellular adenomas and dysplastic foci are more common in dogs with atypical adrenal hyperplasia associated with increased androgen or progesterone concentrations. Both lesions are often associated with increased liver enzyme activity (ALP primarily, with more modest change in transaminases). Rather than single mass lesions, multiple dysplastic foci are commonly identified within a single biopsy sample and among multiple biopsies from the same animal. Neoplastic transformation of dysplastic foci is suspected.

Similar to hepatocellular carcinomas, hepatocellular adenomas may outgrow their central blood supply, developing a necrotic core that may serve as a nidus for abscess formation. Mass lesions also may rupture and cause critical abdominal hemorrhage. Hepatocellular adenoma is curable by wide resection, although recurrence is possible in dogs with dysplastic foci. Tumor margins should be demarcated on submitted specimens to enable microscopic assessment of the adequacy of mass resection (tumor-free margin).

Biliary Adenocarcinomas: Variably classified as cholangiocellular carcinoma or adenocarcinomas and hepatocellular adenocarcinomas, these tumors are the most common primary malignant hepatic neoplasm in cats and may derive from intrahepatic or extrahepatic bile ducts, pancreas, or gallbladder. Pancreatic adenocarcinomas, invasive into hepatic structures, are also common in cats. Immunohistochemical staining may be necessary to definitively characterize the tissue of origin (biliary epithelium vs hepatocellular). Biliary cysts can be mistaken on gross inspection for primary biliary adenocarcinomas.

Clinical signs usually include anorexia, lethargy, and vomiting, and some cats are jaundiced. Many cats have a history of antecedent liver disease based on historical biochemical profiles; histologically, the chronic liver disease is a nonsuppurative cholangiohepatitis. A mass or large liver may be palpable. Increased ALT, AST, ALP, and GGT activities and increased cholesterol and bilirubin concentrations are common. However, some cats with biliary adenocarcinomas have no clinical signs or laboratory abnormalities. Biliary tree obstruction is identified in some but not all cats with neoplasia associated with the common bile duct and gallbladder. Abdominal radiographs may disclose mass lesions disrupting the hepatic silhouette. Ultrasonography usually delineates mass lesions, their dimensions, and lobe location and documents the presence or absence of biliary tree and/or gallbladder obstruction. Some cats develop abdominal effusion and carcinomatosis.

Surgical resection of neoplastic lesions associated with biliary structures distal to the porta hepatis and lesions associated with the gallbladder is possible. Neoplasia involving the common duct may be palliated with stent placement through the sphincter of Oddi into the duodenum (poorly tolerated by cats) or surgical creation of a biliary diversion. Some cats survive for months with palliative supportive care (without surgery) despite total bile duct obstruction. However, the longterm prognosis is poor. Metastatic lesions are often found in the local lymph nodes, peritoneum, and lungs.

Lymphoma: The most common hemolymphatic tumor found in the liver in both dogs and cats is lymphoma; this may be primary or metastatic (from primary enteric or multifocal disease). Other myeloproliferative diseases and mast cell neoplasia also can involve the liver, especially in cats. Animals with infiltrative hepatic lymphoma may remain asymptomatic in regard to clinicopathologic features except for hyperbilirubinemia and hepatomegaly. Ultrasonographic imaging may not recognize architectural changes or discover nodules or mass lesions. Abdominal effusion may develop secondary to compressive presinusoidal and sinusoidal intrahepatic portal hypertension. Sampling of the effusion and hepatic aspiration may allow cytologic diagnosis of lymphoma. Circulating blood should first be reviewed for presence of neoplastic lymphocytes.

Myelolipomas: These benign tumors are composed of adipose cells and hematopoietic elements. The cellular composition closely resembles cellular elements found in bone marrow. These tumors are usually serendipitously discovered during abdominal ultrasonography, appear densely hyperechoic, have a clearly demarcated border, and are usually small. Aspiration cytology can easily characterize the cellular features. Unless large vessels and biliary structures are compressed, these lesions do not require surgical removal.

Metastatic Neoplasia: The most common tumors metastasizing to the liver in dogs include lymphoma, pancreatic carcinoma, mammary carcinoma, pheochromocytoma, intestinal carcinoma, thyroid carcinoma, fibrosarcoma, osteosarcoma, hemangiosarcoma, mast cell tumors, and transitional cell carcinoma. Metastatic tumors of the liver are less common in cats but include pancreatic, intestinal, and renal cell carcinomas; mast cell tumors; and lymphoma. Metastatic tumors are often multifocal but may initially exist only within vascular and lymphatic elements.

Clinical signs can be nonspecific or specific to the liver and resemble features associated with primary hepatobiliary neoplasia, including anorexia, weight loss, vomiting, PU/PD, and variable hyperbilirubinemia. Metastatic hepatic neoplasia is more likely to be associated with a malignant abdominal effusion. Neurologic signs may indicate metastatic lesions within the brain, with associated clinical signs mistaken for HE. Abnormalities on baseline hematologic or chemistry profiles may be minimal. Although a nonregenerative anemia may develop, there are no consistent changes in WBC count or distribution. Schistocytes may be seen when neoplasia invades hepatic sinusoids, creating a shearing effect on RBCs. Eosinophilia can develop with mast cell tumors and lymphoma, especially in cats. Liver enzymes may be normal or variably increased. Hypoglycemia due to large tumor mass (enhanced glucose utilization) or a paraneoplastic effect (insulin-like effect) is sometimes identified. Hyperbilirubinemia and increased AST are more frequent in canine metastatic disease than in primary hepatic neoplasia. Although radiographic findings are variable, ultrasonography can discriminate single vs multiple lobe involvement from diffuse infiltrative disease. However, aspirates of mass lesions or biopsy is needed for definitive diagnosis. If one liver lobe is involved, surgical removal is recommended. If lymphoma or mastocytosis is diagnosed, appropriate chemotherapy may prolong life.

Hepatic hemangiosarcoma is treated by surgical resection as primary therapy if a defined mass lesion is characterized, with follow-up chemotherapy. There is no specific study of survival expectations of dogs with hepatic hemangiosarcoma, with or without surgical debulking or chemotherapy. Surgery is palliative to arrest active hemorrhage but does not provide longterm survival benefit for most dogs with liver involvement. Survival in dogs with grossly evident metastatic disease have the worst prognosis, with median survival ranging from 68–136 days. A number of combination chemotherapy protocols have been investigated in dogs with hemangiosarcoma, providing median survival ranging from 145 to 250 days in dogs with incisional or excisional biopsies (all sites of tumor not limited to the liver). In a chemotherapy study with doxorubin (free or pegylated liposome-encapsulated drug) compared with a random prospective clinical trial (n=17 for each group), there was no survival difference between treatments in dogs with splenic hemangiosarcoma. Pegylated liposome-encapsulated doxorubicin was associated with more adverse effects. Another combination protocol for dogs with advanced-stage noncutaneous hemangiosarcoma (doxorubicin, dacarbazine, and vincristine) with nonresectable stage II and stage III hemangiosarcoma (doxorubicin and dacarbazine day 1, vincristine days 8 and 15, protocol repeated every 21 days for a maximum of six cycles or until disease progression) was studied. In this study of 24 dogs, a 47.4% response rate (five complete responses, four partial responses) was realized; median time to tumor progression was 101 days with a median survival of 125 days. Significant toxicities included hematologic and GI adverse effects.

MISCELLANEOUS LIVER DISEASES

Glycogen Storage Disease: Of the four glycogen storage diseases reported in dogs, types I and III directly affect the liver, causing massive hepatomegaly in young puppies. These disorders are characterized by excessive accumulation of glycogen in the liver and other organs. Accumulated glycogen is unavailable for conversion to glucose as a result of defective glycolytic enzyme activity.

Type Ia glycogen storage disease, caused by deficiency of glucose-6-*phosphatase-α*, has been reported in toy-breed dogs, particularly Maltese. There is no gender predilection, and disease transmission is autosomal recessive. Clinical signs include emaciation, stunted growth, abdominal distention due to massive hepatomegaly (glycogen and lipid vacuolation of hepatocytes), and lethargy and weakness associated with severe hypoglycemia. Histologic lesions are also seen in renal tubular epithelium. Affected dogs develop lactic acidemia, hypercholesterolemia, hypertriglyceridemia, and hyperuricemia. Clinical signs progress to death or euthanasia by 60 days of age. A genetic test is available for type 1 disease in Maltese dogs.

Type III glycogen storage disease, caused by a deficiency in glycogen debranching enzymes, has been reported in German Shepherds and Curly Coated Retrievers. There is no gender predilection, and an autosomal recessive transmission has been confirmed. Clinical signs include abdominal distention due to hepatomegaly and mild hypoglycemia. Glycogen stores are notable in both liver and skeletal muscle. In Curly Coated Retrievers, the mutation leads to profound hepatocyte glycogen vacuolation, resulting in progressive hepatic fibrosis and liver failure. Affected dogs also develop a progressive degenerative myopathy. A genetic test is available for type III disease in Curly Coated Retrievers.

Diagnosis of these disorders is based on a high index of suspicion considering breed affiliation and symptomatic hypoglycemia. Abdominal radiography reveals hepatomegaly, and ultrasonography reveals hyperechoic hepatic parenchyma consistent with hepatic glycogen or lipid accumulation. Differential diagnoses include other causes of juvenile hypoglycemia (including malnutrition, endoparasitism, transient fasting hypoglycemia in toy breeds, and PSVAs) and other causes of muscular weakness (including endocrinopathies, immune-mediated disorders, infectious diseases, hypokalemia, and neuromyopathies). Supportive care consists of fluid support, IV dextrose to achieve euglycemia, and frequent feedings of a high-carbohydrate and protein diet. Diagnosis is confirmed by tissue enzyme analyses, confirmation of excess glycogen stores in liver tissue, or genetic testing. Prognosis is poor. Affected dogs and their parents should be eliminated from breeding programs.

Hepatic Amyloidosis: Amyloidosis is a familial disease of Abyssinian, Siamese, and Oriental short-hair cats and Chinese Shar-Pei dogs. Affected Shar-Pei are more likely to demonstrate episodic fever and swollen hocks (Shar-Pei fever) with or without renal failure, but the liver may also be affected by diffuse amyloid deposition. Affected Abyssinian cats often present with clinical signs related to the kidneys or with complications associated with diffuse hepatic amyloidosis or amyloid deposition in other organs. Oriental short-hair and Siamese cats generally present with amyloid-related hepatic complications. Other conditions associated with hepatic amyloidosis include a diversity of chronic infections or antigen exposures (eg, coccidioidomycosis in dogs, cyclic hematopoiesis in Gray Collies, infusion of porcine insulin in dogs) and hypervitaminosis A in cats.

Although animals may be asymptomatic for long intervals, clinical signs may include fever, lymphadenopathy, vomiting, inappetence, weight loss, PU/PD, jaundice, and hepatomegaly. Acute presentation for severe abdominal hemorrhage subsequent to liver lobe rupture usually leads to the diagnosis in Oriental short-hair and Siamese cats. Ultrasonography can often identify a developing hematoma at the site of liver lobe rupture. Aspiration of abdominal effusion confirms active hemorrhage. Diagnosis can be made by aspiration cytology if amyloid fibrils are retrieved. Otherwise, diagnosis is made by identifying amyloid deposits in a liver biopsy; amyloid is confirmed by tissue staining with Congo red and examination under polarized light.

Because familial amyloidosis is a progressive systemic disorder, prognosis is poor. Cats surviving acute, severe hepatic hemorrhage by aggressive administration of blood component therapy subsequently succumb to renal amyloidosis. (*See also* AMYLOIDOSES, p 592.) Colchicine and dimethyl sulfoxide have been used to slow progression of systemic amyloidosis in Shar-Pei dogs and in cats, with limited success. Anecdotally, hepatic amyloid has regressed in Shar Pei treated with colchicine (0.03 mg/kg/day, daily to every other day). Longterm survival in Shar Pei demonstrating systemic signs of Shar-Pei fever is possible with early institution of colchicine therapy. In predisposed Shar Pei, a duplication mutation upstream of the hyaluronic acid synthase 2 (HAS2) gene amplifies production of hyaluronic acid, which initiates chronic inflammation and amyloid formation. Additional genetic studies have identified complex polygenic modifier genes.

DISEASES OF THE GALLBLADDER AND EXTRAHEPATIC BILIARY SYSTEM

Jaundice is often the primary presenting sign in animals with disorders involving the gallbladder or extrahepatic biliary structures; abdominal effusion may reflect bile peritonitis. Finding a higher bilirubin concentration in an effusion relative to serum (>10-fold difference) confirms leakage of bile into the abdominal cavity and constitutes a surgical emergency.

CHOLECYSTITIS

In **non-necrotizing cholecystitis**, inflammation of the gallbladder may involve nonsuppurative or suppurative inflammation; may be associated with infectious agents, systemic disease, or neoplasia; or may reflect blunt abdominal trauma or gallbladder obstruction by occlusion of the cystic duct (eg, cholelithiasis, neoplasia, or choledochitis). Cystic duct occlusion incites gallbladder inflammation secondary to bile stasis; this process is augmented by mechanical irritation of a cholelith. The gallbladder wall thickens, and the lumen distends with a white, viscid, mucin-laden bile (white bile).

Necrotizing cholecystitis more commonly affects middle-aged to older adult dogs and may develop secondary to thromboembolism, blunt abdominal trauma, bacterial infection, EHBDO (cystic duct obstruction or distal duct obstruction by choleliths, stricture, or neoplasia), or a mature gallbladder mucocele (causing tense gallbladder distention). Extension of an inflammatory or neoplastic process from adjacent hepatic tissue also may be an underlying cause. Necrotizing cholecystitis can present with or without gallbladder rupture, or as a chronic syndrome associated with adhesions between the gallbladder, omentum, and adjacent viscera. Bacteria are commonly cultured from the gallbladder wall.

Necrotizing cholecystitis requires prompt surgical intervention (cholecystectomy and potential biliary diversion). Clinical signs usually develop acutely and include abdominal pain, fever, and increased liver enzyme activity. However, signs may remain vague and episodic, and hyperbilirubinemia is inconsistent.

Clinical Findings and Diagnosis: Signs of acute cholecystitis include abdominal pain (may only be postprandial), fever, vomiting, ileus, and mild to moderate jaundice. Some animals present in endotoxic shock. The hemogram discloses variable leukocytosis, with or without toxic neutrophils or a left shift. Hyperbilirubinemia and development of jaundice depend on chronicity, involvement of extrahepatic biliary structures, presence or extent of biliary tree occlusion, bile peritonitis, and endotoxemia. Liver enzyme activity is variable, but ALP and GGT are usually moderately to markedly increased. Gallbladder rupture leads to pericholecystic abscess formation (localized by the omentum) or focal or generalized bile peritonitis. Abdominal radiography may reveal indistinct detail in the cranial abdomen consistent with focal peritonitis; a sentinel intestinal loop may implicate focal ileus. Rarely, the gallbladder wall may become radiodense due to dystrophic mineralization secondary to chronic inflammation. Choleliths may be found on ultrasonography. Detection of gas within the biliary tree or gallbladder heralds an emphysematous process associated with sepsis and should prompt antibiotic administration before surgical intervention. Consideration of triage for emergency cholecystectomy is appropriate in some cases. Pericholecystic fluid can be sampled using ultrasonographic guidance to confirm bile leakage and infection. Comparison of total bilirubin concentration in effusion versus serum helps confirm bile leakage.

Diagnosis is based on clinical signs, clinicopathologic features, and ultrasonographic imaging. Ultrasonographic detection of a thickened gallbladder wall or cystic bile duct and tenderness during the imaging procedure or on deep abdominal palpation may be the only evidence of illness. Because necrotizing cholecystitis is often associated with gallbladder mucocele in dogs, early intervention by prophylactic cholecystectomy may reduce need for emergency surgery.

Treatment and Prognosis: Management of cholecystitis focuses on restoration of fluid and electrolyte status, treatment with broad-spectrum antibiotics effective against enteric opportunists, and prompt surgical intervention. In some cases, colloids and plasma transfusion are necessary (plasma preferred to colloids). Because EHBDO is a differential diagnosis, vitamin K_1 should be administered (0.5–1.5 mg/kg, IM or SC, three doses at 12-hr intervals) before surgery to avert hemorrhagic complications. If emergency surgery is necessary, fresh frozen plasma should be given judiciously based on coagulation tests and a buccal mucosal bleeding time. Careful exploration of all biliary structures is warranted during surgery. Patency of the cystic and common bile ducts must be determined, and viability of the gallbladder ascertained as surgical assessments are made.

Cholecystectomy is the treatment of choice in most cases. However, some animals benefit from a cholecystoenterostomy or choledochoenterostomy to circumvent a permanently occluded distal common bile duct. Placement of a temporary biliary stent may be appropriate but should be carefully considered because of the high rate of complications, especially in cats. Cats with EHBDO secondary to pancreatitis demonstrate greater morbidity associated with this technique than dogs. In one case series of seven cats with EHBDO secondary to pancreatitis, after stent insertion, two cats reobstructed within 1 wk, one cat developed ascending cholangitis, two cats suffered chronic intermittent vomiting, and two cats died during the perioperative period.

Samples of bile, gallbladder wall, choleliths, and liver tissue should be submitted for aerobic and anaerobic culture. Cytologic evaluations of tissue imprints and bile help initial selection of antimicrobials (based on bacterial morphology and Gram staining). A combination of metronidazole, ampicillin-clavulanate, and enrofloxacin provides broad protection against commonly encountered enteric opportunists. If only the gallbladder is involved, simple cholecystectomy may be curative. If the common bile, cystic, or hepatic ducts are involved, a more guarded prognosis is warranted, and longterm antibiotic therapy recommended.

There are few adverse consequences of cholecystectomy, although episodic abdominal pain and diarrhea associated with fat malabsorption have been described. Cholecystectomy results in loss of the absorptive and pressure-regulating function of the gallbladder and the fasting reservoir where bile is concentrated. After cholecystectomy, the volume of bile increases because of reduced sodium and water resorption that normally occurs in the gallbladder, the size of the bile acid pool diminishes, and the enterohepatic circulation of bile becomes continuous. Bile composition shifts because of the increased exposure of bile acids to enteric flora with increased formation of secondary bile acids.

Animals undergoing biliary tree decompression by biliary enteric anastomo ses are thereafter susceptible to retrograde septic cholangitis and choledochitis. Dogs tolerate this procedure with fewer clinical signs than cats. Animals should be monitored for fever, inappetence, vomiting, and signs of cyclic illness. A hemogram and liver enzymes should be monitored quarterly. Chronic or intermittent antimicrobial administration may be needed to control ascending cholangitis. Fortunately, illness is usually transient and responsive to antibiotics. Longterm survival with good quality of life is expected in the absence of neoplasia. Owners should be instructed to monitor the rectal temperature of animals with cyclic illness to detect episodes of septic cholangitis to enable institution of at-home antimicrobial therapy.

Emphysematous Cholecystitis/ Choledochitis

Emphysematous cholecystitis/choledochitis is an uncommon condition associated with gas within the wall or lumen of the gallbladder or segments of the biliary tree. In dogs, it has been associated with diabetes mellitus, acute cholecystitis with or without cholecystolithiasis, traumatic ischemia, mature gallbladder mucocele formation, and neoplasia. Gas within the biliary structure indicates serious septic inflammation associated with a gas-forming bacteria such as *Escherichia coli* or *Clostridium* spp. Treatment requires cholecystectomy and antimicrobial therapy based on culture and sensitivity of bile and involved biliary tissues. Broad-spectrum antibiotic coverage should be initiated before surgical exploration. Use of a β-lactamase–resistant penicillin, with enrofloxacin and metronidazole, is initially indicated until culture and sensitivity results are available.

CANINE GALLBLADDER MUCOCELE

Canine gallbladder mucocele (GBM) is characterized by progressive accumulation of tenacious, pale yellow to dark green, mucin-laden bile, which may extend into the cystic, hepatic, and common bile ducts, resulting in variable degrees of bile duct obstruction. Progressive expansion of a GBM leads to gallbladder ischemia and necrosis, bile peritonitis, and sometimes opportunistic infection. Gallbladder stasis, perhaps reflecting dysmotility, and distention predispose to cholecystitis. A GBM should be considered when sequential ultrasonographic examinations fail to indicate a reduction in gallbladder volume after feeding, confirming lack of movement of luminal "sludge." Feeding a dog (100 g of food) and recording gallbladder dimensions at 0, 15, 30, 45, 60, 90, and 120 min, recorded in cm ([width × height × length] × 0.52) yields the gallbladder volume in mL. Failure to reduce baseline gallbladder volume by at least 25% suggests dysmotility. Erythromycin (0.5–1 mg/kg, PO, one dose) combined with a small meal also may stimulate initiation of gallbladder motility; however, in healthy dogs studied, neither feeding with or without erythromycin was consistently superior to initiate contraction.

Dogs with GBM range in age from 3–14 yr old with no gender predisposition. Incidence is increased in Shetland Sheepdogs, Miniature Schnauzers, and Cocker Spaniels. A genetic mutation in the ABCB4 (MDR3) phospholipase flippase transporter was demonstrated in Shetland Sheepdogs and other dogs with GBM. All affected dogs were heterozygous for this mutation.

Factors predisposing to GBM formation include middle to older age, endocrinopathies (typical and atypical hyperadrenocorticism, hypothyroidism, diabetes mellitus), hyperlipidemia or hypercholesterolemia (idiopathic, nephrotic syndrome, feeding of a high-fat diet, pancreatitis), gallbladder dysmotility, and cystic hyperplasia of the gallbladder mucosa (shown to be inducible by progestins in dogs). The inciting cause of mucus hypersecretion or accumulation is unproved and may be multifactorial. Nevertheless, mucin imparts important viscoelastic properties to bile and likely importantly contributes to GBM formation. Decreased gallbladder motility leads to luminal bile stasis and enhanced absorption of electrolytes and fluid, promoting biliary sludge formation. Dogs with risk factors may rapidly mature a developing mucocele after beginning glucocorticoid therapy or a high-fat diet (eg, some diets for renal disease or hepatic insufficiency). Because concurrent VH is common, associated underlying disorders should be investigated.

Clinical Findings and Diagnosis: Symptomatic illness averages ~5 days, although some dogs have vague episodic signs (ie, inappetence, vomiting, vague abdominal pain) for months. In decreasing order of frequency, clinical signs include vomiting, abdominal discomfort, anorexia or hyporexia, jaundice, tachypnea, tachycardia, PU/PD, fever, diarrhea, and abdominal distention. Dogs progressing to gallbladder rupture usually demonstrate abdominal pain, jaundice, tachycardia, tachypnea, and fever. However, occasionally, ruptured

GBMs asymptomatic with a free-moving congealed mucocele have been imaged in the peritoneal cavity. Typical clinicopathologic indicators include leukocytosis with a mature neutrophilia and monocytosis and sometimes a left shift, high liver enzyme activities (ALP, GGT, ALT, and AST), hyperbilirubinemia, and inconsistent hypercholesterolemia. Aerobic bacteria may be cultured from bile or the gallbladder wall, with a number of enteric organisms identified, including *Escherichia coli*, *Enterobacter* spp, *Enterococcus* spp, *Staphylococcus* spp, *Micrococcus* spp, and *Streptococcus* spp. Transhepatic ultrasound–guided cholecystocentesis should not be performed if a GBM is suspected. Ultrasonography may detect hepatomegaly and either a heterogeneous or hyperechoic hepatic parenchyma. Hypoechoic "nodules" correspond to a severe VH with formation of reticulin-defined nodules and regenerative repair. After gallbladder removal, sequential hepatic ultrasonographic evaluations are necessary to determine whether parenchymal lesions resolve. A liver biopsy should be collected from a liver lobe distant to the gallbladder to evaluate for underlying or coexisting disorders; sections collected adjacent to the gallbladder contain peribiliary glands and numerous ductal elements that may result in erroneous assessments.

Histologically, cystic mucosal hyperplasia of the gallbladder wall is common. All dogs have thick biliary debris; some components may be profoundly viscous and mucin laden, others more liquid, some dark green to black, some with white bile, some contain gritty black material, and some contain a firm, organized gelatinous matrix. Transmural ischemic necrosis may develop and lead to necrotizing cholecystitis and gallbladder rupture. Liver biopsies may disclose a VH or mild to moderate portal hepatitis or periductal fibrosis; the later changes reflect associated cholangitis or transient biliary tree occlusion. Some dogs lack concurrent hepatic lesions, especially when cholecystectomy is done preemptively (before GBM maturation).

Treatment: Dogs without signs of mucocele leakage or biliary tree obstruction at the time of initial diagnosis may benefit from hydrocholeresis induced by administration of ursodeoxycholic acid (15–25 mg/kg, PO, divided bid and given with food), SAMe (20–40 mg/kg/day, PO, after an overnight fast; food should also be withheld for 2 hr after dosing), and antimicrobial coverage. Biochemical and ultrasonographic evaluations every 6 wk are useful to monitor treatment response or syndrome progression. Rarely, an evolving GBM may resolve with medical treatment. However, progression in any clinical, clinicopathologic, or imaging parameter indicates poor control and need for surgical intervention.

Cholecystectomy is the best course of treatment and is essential for most dogs with clinical signs and clinicopathologic findings consistent with biliary tree inflammation, obstruction, or rupture. Because bile stasis predisposes to infection, broad-spectrum antimicrobials should be initiated before surgical intervention. Examination and staining of cytologic preparations of bile and imprints of liver and biliary tree biopsies may be invaluable if antibiotic coverage interferes with submitted cultures. Evidence of bacteria in cytologic samples or histologic confirmation of suppurative cholecystitis or cholangitis indicates a need for chronic postoperative antimicrobial administration. The resected gallbladder should be submitted for histopathology (sectioned before fixation to allow formalin penetration), and a liver biopsy collected distant to the site of surgery. Perioperative mortality is high for symptomatic dogs with a ruptured gallbladder complicated by sepsis. If bile peritonitis is present, the peritoneal cavity must be extensively cleansed with sterile, warm, polyionic fluids to remove debris, bacteria, and injurious bile salts. Abdominal drains may be necessary. Antibiotics should be administered for 4–6 wk after surgery.

Cholecystotomy for removal of gallbladder contents without cholecystectomy is not advised, because GBMs usually recur. Furthermore, necrosis of the gallbladder wall may not be grossly evident at surgery, leading to postoperative gallbladder rupture. After gallbladder resection, chronic choleretic therapy is recommended, especially for Shetland Sheepdogs in which a genetic risk is surmised for sludged bile. Underlying causes of hyperlipidemia or endocrine disorders should be identified and managed appropriately. Clinicopathologic abnormalities (high ALP usually) normalize after gallbladder removal in most dogs, except those with associated suppurative cholangiohepatitis, unresolved endocrinopathies, persistent hyperlipidemia, or surgical complications of cholecystectomy. Feeding a protein-restricted, high-fat diet to hyperlipidemic animals may be detrimental and is not recommended.

OTHER DISORDERS OF THE GALLBLADDER

Gallbladder agenesis describes the congenital absence of the gallbladder. In the absence of congenital malformations of the intrahepatic biliary structures, this is an inconsequential abnormality.

Biliary atresia describes the congenital maldevelopment of intrahepatic biliary structures and is uncommonly encountered. Affected individuals are jaundiced and unthrifty at a young age. Prognosis is poor.

A bilobed gallbladder is occasionally identified in cats during ultrasonography or at surgery as an inconsequential abnormality.

Cystic mucosal hyperplasia of the gallbladder is also known as cystic mucinous hypertrophy, cystic mucinous hyperplasia, and mucinous cholecystitis (although it is not an inflammatory lesion). The role of steroid hormones in lesion induction remains unclear but is suspected. There is no associated inflammation, and the serosal surface of the gallbladder remains intact. These hyperplastic lesions are routinely identified in dogs with gallbladder mucocele, in which "cystic" structures are filled with tenacious viscoelastic mucin.

Gallbladder dysmotility is proposed as an emerging syndrome in dogs and may precede GBM development. The syndrome may be linked to steroid hormones, based on early observations of an apparent link between mucocele development and treatment with progestational compounds. Sex hormones (progestins, androgens) have been shown experimentally (in vitro) to reduce contractility of gallbladder smooth muscle in experimental animal models.

OTHER DISORDERS OF THE BILE DUCTS

Benign Hepatic or Biliary Cysts: These single cysts are often limited to one liver lobe, usually cause no substantial compressive injury, and are occasionally discovered serendipitously during ultrasonographic examinations for other disorders, at surgery, or at necropsy. They do not expand to damage adjacent tissues, are not associated with increased liver enzyme activity, and are considered inconsequential. However, they may be problematic if they enlarge or interfere with bile flow at the porta hepatis.

Hepatic Fibropolycystic Disorders: Hepatic fibropolycystic disorders are congenital disorders that have been identified in dogs and cats and reflect embryologic malformations involving the ductal plate (portal triad). Ductal plate malformations (DPMs) reflect embryogenic malformations due to dysfunction of primary cilia causing defective tubulogenesis, affecting formation of bile ducts and renal tubules. Either or both organs may be affected. Fibropolycystic syndromes are divided into six categories in people, and this divisional classification also appears relevant to animals: 1) diffuse DPMs associated with increased deposition of extracellular matrix (congenital hepatic fibrosis) causing intrahepatic presinusoidal portal hypertension, 2) Caroli malformation causing sacculation of large intrahepatic or interlobular bile duct (may be associated with increased deposition of extracellular matrix), 3) von Meyenburg complexes representing microscopic isolated DPMs, 4) simple hepatic cysts, 5) choledochal cysts representing an appendix-like diverticulum from the extrahepatic bile duct that can act as an infection sump, and 6) biliary cystadenomas that likely represent expanding cystic malformations involving large biliary ducts usually located adjacent to the gallbladder and cystic duct. Different malformations can predispose to cholangitis, lead to prehepatic portal hypertension, or evolve into space-occupying cystic lesions. A single genetic mutation in cats (autosomal onset dominant polycystic kidney disease) can lead to biliary ductule malformations and hepatic fibrosis, which are commonly misidentified as advanced biliary cirrhosis subsequent to the feline cholangitis/cholangiohepatitis syndrome. Most cats with this mutation demonstrate polycystic renal malformations rather than biliary malformations, although a small subset of cats develop diffuse fibropolycystic liver lesions. Multiple mutations have been identified to cause fibropolycystic malformations in people, and it is suspected that a similar spectrum of gene mutations also may underlie similar syndromes in dogs and cats. In some cats, many large hepatic cysts cause profound hepatomegaly, requiring repeated drainage, fenestration, marsupialization, or surgical resection. Uncommonly, cystic structures may become mineralized or complicated by formation of mineralized choleliths.

Cats with diffuse DPMs have islands of normal hepatic parenchyma segregated by bridging portal tracts that represent proliferative malformed bile ductules embedded in a complex of extracellular matrix (dense fibrillar collagen). Extensive connective tissue causes intrahepatic portal hypertension, a firm large liver, development of APSSs, signs of HE, and ascites. Affected cats may present with increased liver enzyme activity (ALT, AST, ALP) due to low-grade inflammation or development of septic cholangitis or cholelithiasis. Most are not hyperbilirubinemic or jaundiced. Liver enzymes may be within the normal range, with diagnostic biopsy initiated by ultrasonographic findings.

Biliary dysplastic syndromes rarely occur in dogs concurrent with renal cystic malformations. However, DPMs are as commonly identified in dogs as in cats. Affected dogs may develop increased ALP activity and increased TSBA concentrations. As in cats, extensive connective tissue deposition in the portal tract can cause portal-to-portal bridging fibrosis, intrahepatic presinusoidal portal hypertension, APSSs, HE, and ascites.

The only treatment for DPM associated with bridging portal fibrosis is to palliate HE with protein-modified diets and efforts to alter the enteric microbial flora and pH (lactulose, milk, or low-dose metronidazole). Diuretics and dietary sodium restriction are used to control ascites. Similar syndromes in people are managed by liver transplantation.

Choledochal Cyst: Congenital, appendix-like cystic dilation of the extrahepatic bile duct is recognized uncommonly in cats. Clinical signs include fever, abdominal pain, and jaundice, associated with cyst infection, with the amotile cyst functioning as an infected sump. Surgical exploration is usually required for definitive diagnosis. Extirpation of the cystic malformation or its marsupialization into the common bile duct has been a successful treatment. Postoperative longterm antimicrobial therapy is guided by bile culture, cytology, and repeated ultrasonographic imaging.

Biliary Cystadenoma: These lesions, also termed cystadenomas, bile-duct adenomas, cholangiocellular adenomas, cystic cholangiomas, and hepatobiliary cystadenomas, are benign lesions most commonly encountered in older cats. Well-demarcated, single lesions often have a complex internal structure and may invade or compress adjacent hepatic parenchyma, causing compressive atrophy. Cyst contents range from clear, watery fluid to viscous or solid material; typically there are no bile acids or bilirubin. Cyst sizes vary, ranging from 1 mm to 8 cm, with masses ranging from 5 mm to 12.5 cm. Imaging studies (ultrasonography or CT) are key to diagnosis.

Although surgical excision is the treatment of choice, this may not be possible if the structure integrates into the porta hepatis. However, because these lesions are often discovered serendipitously, surgical excision is commonly not indicated. Prognosis after complete cystadenoma excision is good; however, if surgical intervention is necessary and complete excision is not possible, partial resection may delay complications from mechanical invasion of normal tissue. Repeated aspiration, catheter drainage, marsupialization, and partial excision have been used for palliative management but carry risk of infections. Neoplastic transformation is also possible. Cystadenomas are usually difficult to aspirate owing to their complex internal structure.

EXTRAHEPATIC BILE DUCT OBSTRUCTION

Obstruction of the common bile duct is associated with a number of diverse primary conditions, including inflammation (eg, pancreatitis, duodenitis, duodenal foreign body, etc), cholelithiasis, gallbladder mucocele, choledochitis/cholecystitis, neoplasia, bile duct malformations, parasitic infection, extrinsic compression, fibrosis, and bile duct stricture. Hepatomegaly and distention of intrahepatic bile ducts promptly follow EHBDO. If obstruction resolves within a few weeks, resolution of fibrosis and bile duct distention can follow. However, obstruction for >6 wk results in persistent peribiliary fibrosis, connective tissue bridging between portal tracts, remodeling of the liver consistent with biliary cirrhosis, portal hypertension, and formation of APSSs.

Complete EHBDO may result in development of white bile within the bile duct or gallbladder, reflecting the absence of bilirubin pigments in bile; ie, bile cannot enter the distal "stagnant loop" of the ductal system or gallbladder (cystic duct occlusion). Increased ductal mucin contributes to duct distention and the color of luminal contents. In some cases, the biliary tree becomes colonized by bacteria, which are not cleared because of failed mechanical expulsion of bile and inadequate antibiotic penetration into bile.

Clinical Findings and Diagnosis: Acute complete EHBDO leads to lethargy, cyclic fever, and prompt development of jaundice; total bilirubin concentration increases within 4 hr. Vomiting may be episodic. Some animals are intermittently inappetent, whereas others become polyphagic, reflecting fat maldigestion due to the lack of enteric bile acids and consequent fat malabsorption. Hepatomegaly, acholic feces, and the absence of urine urobilinogen (inconsistent) usually develop within the first week. Bleeding tendencies may be notable within 2–3 wk and are more common in cats and develop earlier. GI ulceration at the pyloric-duodenal junction is common and can lead to considerable blood loss. Even with miniscule enteric bleeding, bilirubin pigments gain access to the bowel, allowing feces to become brown (stercobilin formation) and urine to test positive for urobilinogen, negating the reliability of finding acholic feces and negative urine urobilinogen for EHBDO diagnosis.

The hemogram may reveal a nonregenerative anemia with chronic obstruction or a strongly regenerative anemia in animals with substantive enteric bleeding. A neutrophilic leukocytosis with or without a left shift is common. As bile stagnates in the biliary tree, serum ALT and AST activities increase. Serum ALP and GGT activities increase within 8–12 hr of obstruction and are substantial within a few days. Parenchymal necrosis, periductal inflammation, and cholestasis sustain serum transaminase and cholestatic enzyme activity. In cats, the magnitude of ALP and GGT are less dramatic than in dogs but nevertheless are useful indicators of biliary tree obstruction, injury, and inflammation. Hypercholesterolemia develops within 10–14 days of complete obstruction, reflecting impaired cholesterol elimination and possibly increased hepatic cholesterol biosynthesis. With chronic obstruction and development of biliary cirrhosis, serum cholesterol declines, reflecting impaired cholesterol synthesis and APSSs. Coagulopathies associated with vitamin K deficiency may develop within 2–3 wk in dogs and earlier (within 1 wk) in cats. Response to vitamin K_1 administration is usually dramatic. EHBDO is confirmed with ultrasonographic imaging and exploratory laparotomy.

Treatment: Surgical inspection of the liver and biliary structures and appropriate biliary decompression are requisites for optimal therapy. Gross inspection of the gallbladder and common bile duct usually reveals the site and cause of obstruction; duct palpation is essential to identify intramural mass lesions. A grossly distended, tortuous common bile duct makes the diagnosis apparent. Gentle gallbladder compression is used to verify obstruction and the site of restricted bile flow. The most difficult obstructions to confirm and resolve involve hepatic ducts. A duodenotomy, cholecystotomy, or choledochotomy may be necessary for passage of a flexible catheter into the common bile duct to verify the site of obstruction and to allow removal of inspissated biliary sludge or choleliths. Successful treatment of biliary tract sepsis requires mechanical removal of biliary debris and infectious material and a decompressive maneuver often involving a surgical correction. Animals with biliary tree infections tend to become hypotensive and are susceptible to endotoxic shock during surgery and anesthesia, especially cats. Liver biopsy by percutaneous needle or laparoscopic methods does not allow safe biliary decompression and may lacerate distended bile ducts, leading to bile peritonitis; thus, laparotomy is the optimal managerial and assessment approach.

Controversy exists regarding the need for biliary tree decompression in animals with EHBDO secondary to pancreatitis. In most dogs, obstruction resolves spontaneously over several weeks as the inflammation resolves. In animals with obstruction persisting beyond 2–3 wk, temporary (stenting of the bile duct at the sphincter of Oddi) or permanent decompression of the biliary tree is usually considered. The risk of mortality in dogs with pancreatitis undergoing extrahepatic biliary surgery may be as high as 50%. Transhepatic ultrasound-guided aspiration of the gallbladder as a decompressive approach has been successfully completed in some affected animals but has high risk of focal or more generalized bile peritonitis.

CHOLELITHIASIS

Most choleliths in dogs and cats are clinically silent. Diagnosis of this disorder has increased subsequent to routine use of abdominal ultrasound as a diagnostic modality. Choleliths are more common in middle-aged to older animals, and incidence may be higher in small-breed dogs. Most choleliths in dogs and cats contain calcium carbonate and calcium-bilirubinate pigments and are considered "pigment stones." However, many stones do not contain enough mineral for detection on survey radiographs. Pigment gallstones are divided into two categories: "black-pigment" stones composed primarily of bilirubin polymers, reflecting prolonged hyperbilirubinemia, and "brown-pigment" stones composed predominantly of calcium bilirubinate, which are associated with bacterial infections and biliary stasis. Mucin production, enhanced by local inflammation and prostaglandins, entangles calcium bilirubinate and bilirubin polymers into cholelith aggregates. This process is augmented by gallbladder dysmotility and bile stasis.

Clinical Findings and Diagnosis: Cholelithiasis may be associated with vomiting, anorexia, jaundice, fever, and abdominal pain. However, many animals remain asymptomatic or display postprandial discomfort (eg, stretching, position of relief, changing postures, wandering, pacing). Laboratory features of cholelithiasis most commonly reflect related cholecystitis or choledochitis, or cholangitis (intrahepatic choleliths or hepatolithiasis). In animals with small duct lithiasis, clinicopathologic features reflect involvement of biliary structures (high ALP and GGT activities). Jaundice is only directly related to cholelithiasis associated with EHBDO or sepsis; thus, many animals with cholelithiasis are not hyperbilirubinemic. Cholelithiasis may develop secondary to infection, or stones may promote infection secondary to amechanical trauma derived from choleliths. Animals with DPMs, especially Caroli malformation (sacculation of large intrahepatic bile ducts) are predisposed to intrahepatic cholelithiasis and infection. High vigilance for signs of sepsis is warranted in any animal with cholelithiasis.

The hemogram may be normal or reflect inflammation or infection. A serum biochemical profile may be normal or reveal high cholestatic enzyme activity or evidence of obstructive jaundice. Ultrasonography can detect stones >2 mm in diameter in the gallbladder; however, both skill and luck are needed to recognize stones lodged in segments of the common bile duct or in the hepatic bile ducts. For animals with small duct cholelithiasis, biopsy and culture of liver tissue is necessary to identify underlying disease processes and associated bacterial infections.

Treatment: Medical treatment of cholelithiasis includes broad-spectrum *antibiotics* and a choleretic regimen of ursodeoxycholic acid at 15–25 mg/kg, PO, divided bid and given with food, and SAMe at 20–40 mg/kg/day, PO, on an empty stomach. Liver biopsy determines whether immunomodulatory therapy is appropriate. Vitamin E at 10 U/kg/day can be used for its antioxidant and anti-inflammatory effects.

Surgical intervention is necessary if choleliths are associated with cholecystitis, are causing cystic duct obstruction, or are occluding the common bile duct. Successful treatment of cholecystitis and cystic duct occlusion requires cholecystectomy and lavage of the common bile duct. The causal factors of cholelith formation must be carefully considered; retaining a diseased or dysmotile gallbladder imposes risk of recurrent lithiasis or necrotizing cholecystitis. In cases in which obstruction of the common bile duct is irresolvable, a cholecystoenterostomy is necessary, followed by longterm monitoring for septic cholangitis. Chronic pulsatile antimicrobial administration may be needed to control retrograde infections of the biliary tree thereafter. Biopsy of involved biliary structures and liver is essential to determine whether an underlying primary inflammatory, septic, or neoplastic disease is present and predisposing to cholelith formation. Tissue (liver, bile duct, gallbladder), bile, and cholelith nidus should be submitted for aerobic and anaerobic bacterial cultures.

Cholecystoduodenostomy and cholecystojejunostomy are the most common surgical procedures for biliary bypass in small animals. Cystoenteric anastomosis to the proximal duodenum is most physiologic, because it allows bile to enter the duodenum in a position that closely maintains normal physiologic responses in the proximal bowel to allow coordinated mixing of bile acids and pancreatic enzymes necessary for digestion and assimilation.

BILIARY TREE RUPTURE AND BILE PERITONITIS

Rupture of the common bile duct, cystic duct, hepatic ducts, or gallbladder is most often associated with cholelithiasis, necrotizing choledochitis or cholecystitis, blunt abdominal trauma, or neoplasia. In dogs, necrotizing cholecystitis most often occurs as a result of a mature gallbladder mucocele that stretches the gallbladder wall to the extent of causing ischemic necrosis. Regardless of cause, rupture of any portion of the biliary tree can lead to bile peritonitis. Clinical signs may be minimal early in the disease process, consisting only of inappetence and vague abdominal discomfort. With chronicity, free bile initiates an inflammatory reaction (chemical peritonitis), an abdominal effusion accumulates, and vivid jaundice develops.

Ultrasonography should guide collection of abdominal effusion as close to the biliary tree as possible, because this will increase detection of free and phagocytized bilirubin crystals and bacterial organisms. Abdominal adhesions develop with delay in diagnosis and complicate surgical remediation.

Surgical interventions are specific to the causal lesions and may involve biliary tree decompression, cholecystectomy, cholecystotomy, choledochotomy, biliary-enteric anastomosis, or bile duct stent insertion. A liver biopsy should be collected to identify antecedent or coexistent hepatobiliary disease. Portions of the ruptured structure, bile, and abdominal effusion should be sampled and cultured for aerobic and anaerobic bacteria. Affected tissue and adjacent and nonadjacent liver tissue should be biopsied. The abdominal cavity must be thoroughly lavaged with sterile warm saline to remove bile contamination. Antibiotic coverage against likely enteric opportunists (gram-negative bacteria) and anaerobic flora is recommended, eg, ticarcillin, piperacillin, third-generation cephalosporins, or enrofloxacin combined with metronidazole. Antimicrobial therapy should begin before surgery and, if sepsis is confirmed, continued for 4–8 wk. Antimicrobial selection should be guided initially by results of cytology and Gram staining, and adjusted based on results of culture and sensitivity. Animals with chronic jaundice should receive vitamin K_1 (0.5–1.5 mg/kg, IM or SC, bid for up to three doses) before surgical intervention. Fresh frozen plasma may be necessary to abate bleeding tendencies during emergency surgery. Antiemetics are recommended if the animal is vomiting; H_2-receptor antagonists are used if enteric bleeding is identified, because these act quickly. In animals with cholelithiasis and in dogs with gallbladder mucocele, hydrocholeresis (ursodeoxycholic acid and SAMe) and antioxidants (vitamin E and SAMe) are recommended postoperatively.

FELINE CHOLANGITIS/ CHOLANGIOHEPATITIS SYNDROME

Feline cholangitis/cholangiohepatitis syndrome (CCHS) is the most common acquired inflammatory liver disease in domestic cats. Both cholangitis and cholangiohepatitis are more common in cats than dogs. The anatomic difference between the biliary and pancreatic ducts in cats compared with dogs has long been considered an underlying risk factor. Feline CCHS coexists with inflammatory processes in the duodenum, pancreas, and kidneys (chronic interstitial nephritis). Numerous concurrent conditions have been identified in cats with CCHS, whether the inflammatory infiltrate is predominantly neutrophilic (suppurative), lymphocytic or lymphoplasmacytic (nonsuppurative), or whether it actively involves bile duct destruction. Disorders associated with feline CCHS include bacterial infections (primary or chronic), septicemia, cholecystitis, cholelithiasis, EHBDO, trematode infestation, toxoplasmosis, inflammatory bowel disease, primary cholangitis, pancreatitis, neoplasia (eg, pancreatic or gallbladder or bile duct adenocarcinoma), biliary cystadenoma, and various ductal malformations (eg, choledochal cyst, diffuse ductal plate malformation [congenital hepatic fibrosis associated with polycystic liver malformation], Caroli malformation).

Liver lobe involvement in feline CCHS is variable, and the extent and severity of histologic lesions may not be fully ascertained on a single liver biopsy or with small tru-cut biopsies (eg, 18 gauge). Some biopsy sections may show modest or moderate periductal inflammation and hepatitis, whereas other liver lobes reveal complete elimination of bile ducts and lack active inflammation owing to loss of bile duct epitopes that may drive the inflammation. Cats with disease in multiple organ systems have significantly shorter survival times if untreated. However, because CCHS is slowly progressive, cats can survive several years beyond initial diagnosis without therapeutic interventions.

Suppurative CCHS causes the most overt clinical illness. These cats have a shorter duration of illness before presentation (<5 days), with young or middle-aged adults predominating (range 3 mo to 16 yr). Clinical signs include pyrexia, lethargy, dehydration, inappetence, vomiting, and variable jaundice. Many cats manifest abdominal pain, and some have palpable hepatomegaly. Clinicopathologic features are similar to those of other forms of CCHS, with moderate to marked increases in transaminases (ALT, AST) and more modest increases in ALP and GGT activities. Surprisingly, some cats lack cholestatic enzyme abnormalities. Most cats are hyperbilirubinemic, some have concurrent renal azotemia, and many demonstrate a left shift and toxic neutrophils on their leukogram. Concurrent HL may confuse initial assessments. Abdominal ultrasonography may reveal EHBDO; abnormalities consistent with cholecystitis, choledochitis, pancreatitis, or inflammatory bowel disease; diffuse hepatic parenchymal hyperechogenicity consistent with HL; coarse parenchymal echogenicity; or no abnormalities. A coarse or heterogeneous hepatic parenchymal pattern sometimes recognized may reflect parenchymal inflammation and/or periductule or portal tract fibrosis and inflammation. Thoracic radiography often reveals a large sternal lymph node reflecting abdominal inflammation/sepsis.

Medical treatment is usually provided before surgical intervention (biliary decompression surgery for EHBDO, cholecystectomy for cholecystitis, cholecystotomy for cholelithiasis) and liver biopsy. Disorders causing stasis of bile flow must be rectified, because they increase risk of opportunistic infection involving the biliary system. Aspiration or biopsy imprint cytology of liver and bile usually reveal bacterial organisms and suppurative inflammation. Gram-stain characterization of bacteria on cytologic specimens assists in selection of antimicrobial agents and may provide the only confirmation of bacterial infection. Cultures may be negative because of prior antibiotic administration or failure to culture for anaerobic bacteria. Commonly isolated bacteria include *Escherichia coli*, *Streptococcus*, *Clostridium*, *Bacteroides*, and *Actinomyces*.

Treatment involves broad-spectrum antimicrobials effective against anaerobic and gram-negative enteric opportunists, ursodeoxycholic acid, SAMe, vitamin E, water-soluble vitamins, enteral alimentation with a maximum-calorie diet formulated for cats, and judicious administration of fluids and electrolyte supplements to correct and maintain hydration and electrolyte status. Antioxidants are provided during critical illness by administration of N-acetylcysteine (140 mg/kg initial dose [10% solution in NaC1], 70 mg/kg thereafter, bid-tid, infused IV over 20 min through a 0.25-μm filter); when oral administration is possible, SAMe is given by mouth. A combination of enrofloxacin, metronidazole, and ampicillin/sulbactam is often initially administered and adjusted based on culture and sensitivity reports from hepatobiliary or bile aspirates or tissue samples. Antimicrobial treatment should begin before surgical intervention (because sepsis compromises postoperative survival) and continue for 8–12 wk or until liver enzymes normalize. If liver enzymes remain increased, repeat ultrasonographic assessment is warranted to check for abnormalities involving biliary structures, pancreas, or gut, or development of lymphadenopathy. Repeat aspiration cytology or liver biopsy may be necessary.

Feline lymphocytic portal hepatitis is a diagnosis demonstrating inflammatory infiltrates without tropism for bile ducts but showing single cell hepatocyte necrosis. It is presumed that many of these cats are responding to antigens or debris from the alimentary canal or reflect inflammatory cells delivered in the portal circulation. Otherwise, this diagnosis may represent mild lesions in cats with CCHS when only a few portal triads are sampled from a relatively uninvolved liver lobe. Low-yield needle biopsies from cats with nonsuppurative CCHS may generate this diagnosis. In some cats, however, an inflammatory portal tract infiltrate is associated with single cell hepatocyte necrosis, qualifying as a true portal hepatitis.

Nonsuppurative CCHS without destructive cholangitis is usually a T-cell or mixed T-cell with B-cell mediated inflammatory syndrome affecting middle-aged or older cats. Concurrent infection with feline leukemia virus or feline immunodeficiency virus is uncommon, and there is no gender or breed predisposition. Duration of illness ranges from 2 wk to several years, with most cats demonstrating signs of illness for several months before initial presentation. Clinical signs include intermittent vomiting and diarrhea and episodic illness characterized by anorexia or hyporexia, reclusiveness, or self-resolving jaundice. Hepatomegaly is common. It is uncommon for nonsuppurative CCHS to cause portal hypertension, APSSs, and abdominal effusion, because cats usually succumb to the effects of this syndrome before diffuse fibrosis evolves. Rather, cats with these features more likely have fibropolycystic biliary malformations (*see* p 477).

The hemogram is variable, commonly demonstrating poikilocytosis and Heinz bodies. The leukogram is variable but typically does not display a left shift or toxic neutrophils. Hyperglobulinemia develops with chronicity; most cats have moderate to marked increases in ALT and AST activities with widely variable ALP and GGT activities depending on cyclic activity of the disease process. Hyperbilirubinemia is inconsistent and also appears cyclic. Some cats are persistently jaundiced secondary to inflammatory obstruction or destruction of small and medium-sized bile ducts (nonsuppurative CCHS with destructive cholangitis); these often develop symptomatic coagulopathies responsive to vitamin

K administration. Abdominal ultrasonographic findings overlap with those of suppurative CCHS; a nonuniform or coarse parenchymal pattern may be identified. However, cats with marked nonsuppurative CCHS may lack ultrasonographic hepatic or biliary abnormalities. Severity of histologic lesions is highly variable within and between liver lobes and between cats.

Initial treatment consists of appropriate antimicrobials (*see* above), SAMe, vitamin E, supplementation of B vitamins, enteral alimentation with a maximum-calorie diet formulated for cats, and fluids and electrolyte supplements to correct and maintain hydration and electrolyte abnormalities. Broad-spectrum antimicrobial coverage (against anaerobic and gram-negative enteric opportunists) is recommended pending liver biopsy and culture results. Longterm treatment requires immunomodulation. Ursodeoxycholic acid is used in cats lacking evidence of destructive cholangitis. However, ursodeoxycholic acid is no longer recommended for cats with destructive cholangitis based on evidence (experimental animal models, people with sclerosing cholangitis) that it may provoke small duct injury in destructive cholangiopathies. First-line immunosuppressive therapy is prednisolone, initially administered at 2–4 mg/kg ideal body weight, PO, daily, with the dose titrated to 5–10 mg/day, administered daily to every other day. Glucocorticoid dosing is titrated based on clinical assessments. Metronidazole (7.5 mg/kg, PO, bid) s also recommended to assist with immunomodulation and control of associated nflammatory bowel disease; adding this drug may allow reduction of the glucocorticoid dose. Continued administration of SAMe (40–50 mg/kg/day, PO) and vitamin E (10 U/kg/day) is recommended.

As a single agent, SAMe has reduced nonsuppurative CCHS-associated inflammaion in a few studied cats. Chlorambucil 2 mg/cat/day, titrated to every other or every hird day) is used in cats that do not respond o anti-inflammatory glucocorticoid and metronidazole therapy. Treatment usually eturns bilirubin concentrations to normal, but cyclic increases in enzyme activity emain although at lower magnitudes.

Cats with **nonsuppurative CCHS with destructive cholangitis (sclerosing cholangitis)** can eventually develop widespread small duct destruction causing permanent hyperbilirubinemia and ntermittent acholic feces due to a histoogic progressive "ductopenia." This subset f CCHS is confirmed by finding defining histologic features that include the following: 1) infiltration of bile ductules with lymphocytes, 2) peripheralization of bile ductules to the margin of portal tracts, 3) evidence of involuting bile ducts, 4) lipogranulomas (when ducts have been eliminated), 5) scant lymphoid nodules (B cells) consistent with an inflammation, and 6) periductular sclerosing fibrosis without other features suggesting EHBDO. In some cases, confirmation of bile duct involution and peripheralization to the edge of portal tracts requires immunohistochemistry using a cytokeratin antibody. Marked differences between liver lobes in status of portal tract inflammation may be seen; in lobes with elimination of biliary ductules, inflammation can be mild or inapparent. Approximately 30% of cats with destructive cholangitis treated with glucocorticoids develop diabetes mellitus. Involvement of pancreatic ducts with the T-cell ductal targeting inflammation may influence this outcome.

Symptomatic ductopenic cats require once or twice weekly vitamin K_1 injections (*see* p 439) and water-soluble vitamin E (polyethylene glycol α-tocopherol succinate, 10 U/kg/day, PO). Overdosing vitamin K_1 can cause serious hemolytic anemia, and overdosing vitamin E can lead to insufficient vitamin K activity. Affected cats should be investigated for severe inflammatory bowel disease and B_{12} adequacy. Hematology and serum biochemistry features are similar to those of cats with non-duct destructive CCHS. Immunomodulation with prednisolone does little to moderate enzyme activity or hyperbilirubinemia in destructive CCHS when used as monotherapy immunosuppression. Instead, methotrexate or chlorambucil are used initially with glucocorticoids. Pulsatile methotrexate is given at a total daily dose of 0.4 mg/cat divided into three treatments given on a single day (0.13 mg per dose, PO) once every 7–10 days. Alternatively, methotrexate may be given IV or IM with a 50% dose reduction. Folic acid, 0.25 mg/day, PO, is concurrently administered to prevent methotrexate-associated hepatotoxicity, GI toxicity, or hematopoietic effects. The dosage of methotrexate must be reduced in cats with renal azotemia. Methotrexate imposes profound immunosuppression at the recommended dosage, and careful monitoring for complicating infections is essential. Alternatively, treatment with chlorambucil, as described above, can be used instead of methotrexate. Concurrent treatment with SAMe is recommended, along with low-dose prednisolone and metronidazole. Treatment for concurrent inflammatory bowel disease with a hypoallergenic diet also may be beneficial. Cobalamin deficiency must be corrected, with cats chronically supplemented if deficiency is proved through laboratory testing. Low cobalamin concentrations should raise concern for severe small-bowel malabsorption (especially small-cell lymphoma) or severe pancreatic disease.

In **lymphoproliferative disease masquerading as lymphocytic CCHS**, lesions are characterized by dense portal lymphocyte infiltrates that penetrate hepatic sinusoids. However, involved lymphocytes lack convincing morphology for classification as a neoplastic population; this syndrome may represent a transition phase between conventional inflammatory disease and overt neoplasia. Treatment with chlorambucil has proved beneficial in some cats (2 mg/cat, given every other or every third day), combined with treatments previously described for CCHS. Affected cats may survive for several years with minimal clinical signs. Immunohistochemical staining and other molecular tests (investigation of clonality) may help differentiate this syndrome from lymphoma.

In **small-cell lymphoma masquerading as lymphocytic CCHS**, dense lymphocytic portal infiltrates penetrate hepatic sinusoids. However, this population of cells has morphology consistent with a diagnosis of small-cell lymphoma. Treatment with chemotherapy protocols for feline lymphoma is recommended, along with judicious administration of nutritional, vitamin, and antioxidant support. Many of these cats respond to chlorambucil, as described above, for several years. Affected cats may have concurrent intestinal involvement, although some cats with overt hepatic lymphosarcoma have inflammatory bowel disease, and some cats with overt enteric lymphosarcoma have non-neoplastic nonsuppurative CCHS. Evolution of chronic inflammation to a neoplastic process is suspected in each organ system.

HEPATOBILIARY FLUKE INFECTION

Infection with liver flukes in endemic regions can cause acute and chronic cholangitis in cats and less frequently in dogs. The most common fluke infecting cats is *Platynosomum concinnum* in Florida, Hawaii, and other tropical areas. Infestation is acquired by ingesting an infected intermediate host, usually a lizard or frog; ~15%–85% of cats with access to intermediate hosts are infected in endemic areas. After infection, young flukes emerge in the intestines and migrate into the common bile duct, gallbladder, or hepatic ducts, where they mature within 8–12 wk. Embryonated eggs thereafter pass from bile into the alimentary canal, where they may be detected in feces as early as 12 wk after infection (sedimentation, Baermann test).

Clinical signs depend on severity of infection (parasite burden); however, most infested cats remain asymptomatic. Symptomatic cats demonstrate progressive illness characterized by progressive lethargy, fever, hepatomegaly, and abdominal distention. These cats may become jaundiced and emaciated secondary to anorexia, vomiting, and mucoid diarrhea. Chronic fluke infestation can be fatal in severely affected cats. First clinical signs develop between 7 and 16 wk of infection. In some cases, clinical signs resolve by 24 wk after infection without treatment. A circulating eosinophilia may develop 3–14 wk after infection and may persist. In heavily infected cats, ALT and AST activities may increase, while ALP activity may remain normal or only increase mildly. Hyperbilirubinemia may develop within 7–16 wk after infection.

Hepatic histologic lesions develop after 3 wk and are progressive in persistent infections. Inflammation and distention of large bile ducts is associated with mixed neutrophilic and eosinophilic inflammatory infiltrates. By 4 mo, severe adenomatous biliary hyperplasia and peribiliary inflammation are well established. By 6 mo, progressive fibrosis is obvious and evolves into biliary cirrhosis. Regional lymphadenopathy may be notable. Bile duct distention increases with growth of adult flukes, and when flukes become sexually mature, bile ducts become fibrotic. During this time, serum transaminase activities decline and may normalize. Abdominal ultrasonography may reveal apparent biliary obstruction involving the gallbladder, common bile duct, and/or intrahepatic ducts. Gallbladder debris associated with flukes may appear as oval hypoechoic structures having echoic centers. A thickened gallbladder wall associated with a double-rim sign may reflect cholecystitis. Hypoechoic hepatic parenchyma with prominent hyperechoic portal regions (ducts) reflects cholangitis and cholangiohepatitis.

Canine infection with *Heterobilharzia americana*, a schistisomal fluke, has also been characterized in dogs from Texas,

North Carolina, Louisiana, and Florida. Infection is acquired through skin penetration by cercariae released from snails. These forms migrate through the host as schistosomula, reaching the lungs within 5–9 days and liver within 7–45 days. Schistosomes grow and mature in liver, with adults migrating to mesenteric veins, where they release eggs and also proteolytic enzymes upon migration to the bowel lumen. Eggs provoke a granulomatous reaction. Healing of the host leads to scar formation and organ injury that can result in liver failure and GI malabsorption.

Clinical signs of illness in dogs with schistosomiasis may manifest as early as a few days to months after infection. Young adult dogs are more commonly affected. Common clinical features (in descending order) include lethargy, weight loss, vomiting, diarrhea, inappetence, hypercalcemia, PU/PD, and more rarely, melena. The most common hematologic findings are lymphopenia and mild to marked thrombocytopenia, with eosinophilia being uncommon. Schistocytes have been seen in some dogs, reflecting intravascular shearing injury of RBCs. Common serum biochemical features include modest azotemia (BUN and creatinine), hyperglobulinemia, total and ionized hypercalcemia, and hyperglobulinemia. Liver enzyme activity is variable. Hypercalcemia is thought to reflect granulomatous inflammation. Acquired immunodeficiency (neoplasia, drug therapy) may increase susceptibility to infection.

Because fluke-infected cats may remain asymptomatic, diagnosis can be difficult. Eggs may not be detected on fecal examination, because they are only sporadically passed and demonstrate variable morphology (immature and embryonated forms). Furthermore, fluke eggs are small, and routinely used fecal methods are relatively insensitive for fluke egg detection. In addition, development of bile duct obstruction and fibrosis may impede passage of fluke eggs into bile and feces.

Suspected fluke infestation is treated with praziquantel (based on dosing extrapolated from experimentally infected animals and proved to control schistosome infection in dogs). Praziquantel at 20–25 mg/kg body wt, tid for 3 days, has been effective in some but not all treated animals. Eggs may continue to be passed in feces for up to 2 mo after successful treatment in cats, and reinfection may complicate assessment of treatment response. Some infected dogs have been treated with fenbendazole (50 mg/kg body wt/day, PO, for 10 days) with or without concurrent praziquantel administration. Prednisolone is used to reduce fluke-associated inflammation (2 mg/kg/day for 2–4 wk, tapered in 50% decrements every 2 wk). Ursodeoxycholic acid is recommended for bile duct–associated lesions given at 15–20 mg/kg, PO, divided bid and administered with food to initiate hydrocholeresis. Broad-spectrum antibiotic coverage is recommended to protect against secondary bacterial infections associated with migrating or dying flukes. Vitamin E (10 IU/kg/day, PO) and SAMe (20–40 mg/kg/day, PO) are given until liver enzymes normalize. If necessary, an antiemetic can be administered, eg, metoclopramide (0.2–0.5 mg/kg, PO or SC, every 6–8 hr) or maropitant (1 mg/kg/day for no more than 5 consecutive days).

Treatment results are variable, but prognosis is favorable in mild fluke infestation. Other rare parasites of the biliary tract include *Amphimerus pseudofelineus*, *Metorchis conjunctus*, and *Eurytrema procyonis*. (*See also* HEPATIC FLUKES, p 427.) Similar assessment and treatment strategies are warranted.

EYE AND EAR

THE EYE

THE EAR

OPHTHALMOLOGY

PHYSICAL EXAMINATION OF THE EYE

The initial examination of the eye should assess symmetry, conformation, and gross lesions; the eye should be viewed from 2–3 ft (~1 m) away, in good light, and with minimal restraint of the head. The anterior ocular segment and pupillary light reflexes are examined in detail with a strong light and under magnification in a darkened room. Baseline tests like the Schirmer tear test, fluorescein staining, and tonometry (intraocular pressure measurement) may be followed by ancillary tests such as taking corneal and conjunctival cytology and cultures, everting the eyelids for examination, and flushing the nasolacrimal system to evaluate the external parts of the eye, including the anterior segment. Diseases of the vitreous and ocular fundus are evaluated by direct and indirect ophthalmoscopy (usually performed after inducing mydriasis) and vision testing (menace reflex, obstacle course, dazzle reflex, etc).

Schirmer tear tests and cultures should be performed before topical anesthetic is instilled. Fluorescein staining and eversion of the eyelids do not require topical anesthesia, but tonometry, examination of the bulbar surface of the nictitating membrane, conjunctival and corneal cytology, gonioscopy, and lavage of the nasolacrimal system usually do. To avoid false-positives, samples for corneal and conjunctival cytology that will be analyzed by fluorescent antibody procedures should be collected before topical fluorescein staining.

Special examinations such as slit-lamp biomicroscopy, ultrasonography, fluorescein angiography, and electroretinography may require sedation or local, regional, or general anesthesia, depending on the species.

EYELIDS

The eyelids consist of four parts: 1) the outer very thin and mobile skin; 2) the strong and encircling orbicularis oculi muscle anchored at the medial canthus; 3) the thin and poorly developed fibrous tarsus, which contains the sebaceous Meibomian glands and attaches the lid to the bony orbital rim; and 4) the thin and flexible palpebral conjunctiva, which continues to the conjunctival fornix or conjunctival cul-de-sac. Eyelid disorders may be associated with facial and orbital abnormalities, specific breeds, and adjunct skin diseases, as well as with many systemic diseases.

Conformational Abnormalities

Entropion is an inversion of all or part of the lid margins that may involve one or both

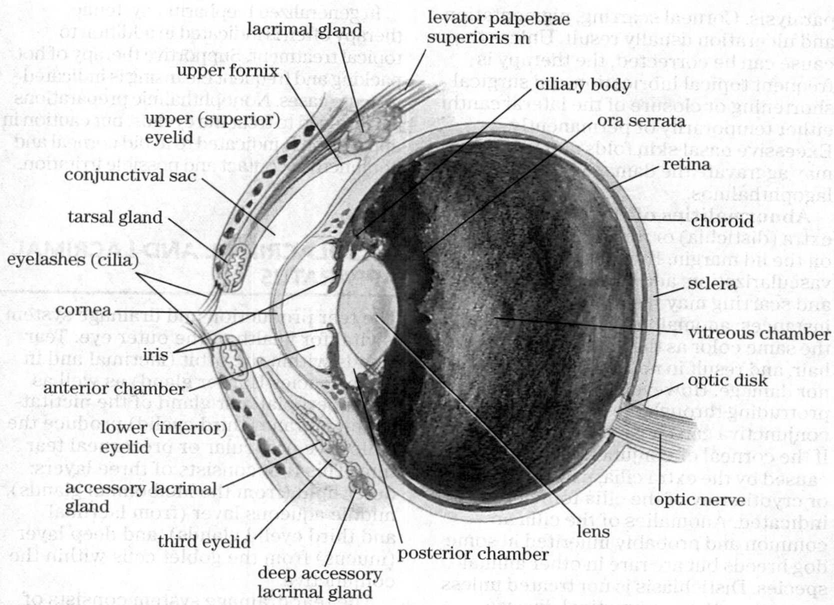

The eye and eyelids, median section. *Illustration by Dr. Gheorghe Constantinescu.*

eyelids and the canthi. It is the most frequent inherited eyelid defect in many canine and ovine breeds and may also follow cicatrix formation and severe blepharospasm due to ocular or periocular pain. Inversion of the cilia (or eyelashes) or facial hairs causes further discomfort, conjunctival and corneal irritation, and if protracted, corneal scarring, pigmentation, and possibly ulceration. Early spastic entropion may be reversed if the inciting cause is quickly removed or if pain is alleviated by everting the lid hairs away from the eye with mattress sutures in the lid, by subcutaneous injections (eg, of procaine penicillin) into the lid adjacent to the entropion, or by palpebral nerve blocks. Temporary stay sutures or surgical staples left in place for 2–3 wk may be used to treat entropion in very young puppies. Established entropion usually requires surgical correction.

Ectropion is a slack, everted lid margin, usually with a large palpebral fissure and elongated eyelids. It is a common bilateral conformational abnormality in a number of dog breeds, including the Bloodhound, Bull Mastiff, Great Dane, Newfoundland, St. Bernard, and several Spaniel breeds. Contracting scars in the lid or facial nerve paralysis may produce unilateral ectropion in any species. Conjunctival exposure to environmental irritants and secondary bacterial infection can result in chronic or recurrent conjunctivitis. Topical antibiotic-corticosteroid preparations may temporarily control intermittent infections, but surgical lid-shortening procedures are often indicated. Mild cases can be controlled by repeated, periodic lavage with mild decongestant solutions.

Lagophthalmos is an inability to fully close the lids and protect the cornea from drying and trauma. It may result from extremely shallow orbits (in brachycephalic breeds), exophthalmia due to a space-occupying orbital lesion, or facial nerve

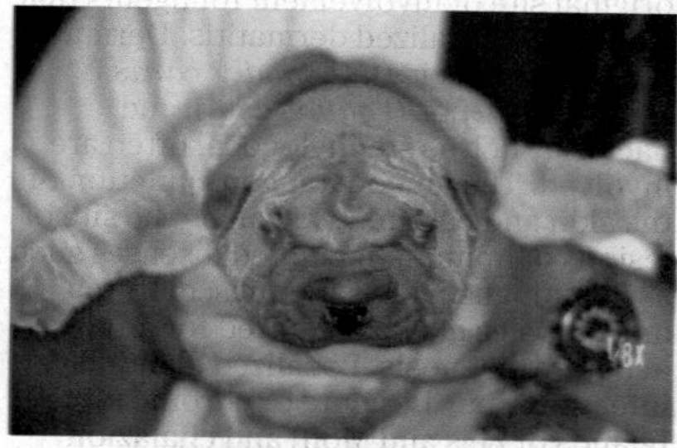

Bilateral entropion, Shar Pei puppy. *Courtesy of K. Gelatt.*

paralysis. Corneal scarring, pigmentation, and ulceration usually result. Unless the cause can be corrected, the therapy is frequent topical lubrication and surgical shortening or closure of the lateral canthi either temporarily or permanently. Excessive nasal skin folds and facial hair may aggravate the damage caused by lagophthalmos.

Abnormalities of the cilia include extra (distichia) or misdirected eyelashes on the lid margin. Epiphora, corneal vascularization, and corneal ulceration and scarring may result. In many instances, anomalous cilia are very fine, the same color as the surrounding eyelid hair, and result in neither clinical signs nor damage. However, ectopic cilia protruding through the dorsal palpebral conjunctiva can cause profound pain. If the corneal or conjunctival damage is caused by the extra cilia, excision, cautery, or cryothermy of the cilia follicles is indicated. Anomalies of the cilia are common and probably inherited in some dog breeds but are rare in other animal species. Distichiasis is not treated unless corneal and/or conjunctival disease results. Successful removal of distichia requires destruction of the follicular base of the eyelids while not injuring the eyelid margin. The most popular method is cryotherapy applied at the base of the cilia beneath the palpebral conjunctiva at the eyelid margin. Depigmentation of the eyelid margin may result after cryotherapy but usually re-pigments in the subsequent months. Inadequate cryotherapy can result in distichia recurrence.

Inflammation

Blepharitis (inflammation of the eyelids) can result from extension of a generalized dermatitis, conjunctivitis, local glandular infections, or irritants such as plant oils or solar exposure. The lids can be the original site of involvement for agents that lead to a generalized dermatitis. Dermatophytes (all species), *Demodex canis* (dogs), *D cati* or *D gatoi* (cats), and bacteria such as staphylococci often are involved. The mucocutaneous junction of the skin and conjunctiva can be the site of lesions of immune-mediated diseases such as pemphigus. Skin scrapings, cultures, and biopsies may be required for an accurate diagnosis. Localized glandular infections may be acute or chronic (stye [glands of Zeis and Moll] and chalazion [Meibomian glands]).

In generalized blepharitis, systemic therapy often is indicated in addition to topical treatment. Supportive therapy of hot packing and frequent cleansing is indicated in acute cases. Nonophthalmic preparations can be used to treat the eyelids, but caution in application is indicated to avoid corneal and conjunctival contact and possible irritation.

NASOLACRIMAL AND LACRIMAL APPARATUS

The tear production and drainage system is vital for health of the outer eye. Tear glands within the orbit (lacrimal and in some species Harder gland) as well as the superficial tear gland of the nictitating membrane (third eyelid) produce the collective preocular or precorneal tear film. This film consists of three layers: outer lipid (from the Meibomian glands), middle aqueous layer (from lacrimal and third eyelid glands), and deep layer (mucus) from the goblet cells within the conjunctiva.

The tear drainage system consists of two lacrimal puncta (except in the rabbit and pig, which have only one punctum), two canaliculi, the lacrimal sac (within the bony lacrimal fossa), and the long and often tortuous lacrimal duct (to empty tears within the forward nasal cavity).

Hypertrophy, inflammation, and prolapse of the gland of the nictitating membrane (**cherry eye**) is common in young dogs and certain breeds (eg, American Cocker Spaniel, Beagle, Lhasa Apso, Pekingese, English Bulldog). In the acute stage, the red glandular mass swells and protrudes over the leading margin of the nictitans, and there is a mucopurulent discharge. Although the swelling may recede for short periods, the gland eventually often remains prolapsed. Because it is a major tear gland, it should be preserved if possible; the gland should be replaced and anchored with sutures to the orbital rim, periorbital fascia, or nictitans cartilage, or covered with adjacent mucosa (envelope or pocket techniques). Partial excision should be avoided. Complete excision may predispose to keratoconjunctivitis sicca (*see* p 492) in 30%–40% of dogs in later life. Surgical or medical resolution of cherry eye still predisposes ~20% of these dogs to future keratoconjunctivitis sicca. Therefore, these dogs should be monitored for several years after undergoing surgery.

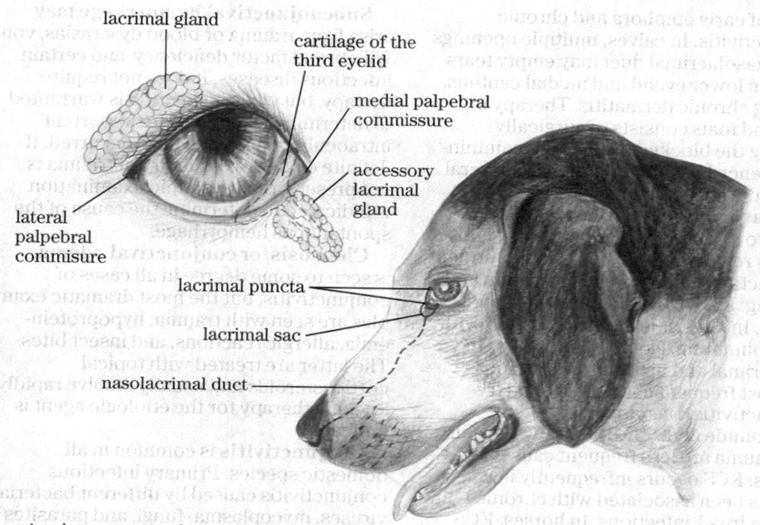

Lacrimal apparatus, dog. *Illustration by Dr. Gheorghe Constantinescu.*

Dacryocystitis (inflammation of the lacrimal sac) usually is caused by obstruction of the nasolacrimal sac and proximal nasolacrimal duct by inflammatory debris, foreign bodies, or masses pressing on the duct. It results in epiphora, secondary conjunctivitis refractory to treatment, and occasionally a draining fistula in the medial lower eyelid. Irrigation of the nasolacrimal duct reveals an obstruction of the duct, reflux of mucopurulent discharge from the lacrimal puncta, or both. Radiographs of the skull after injection of contrast material into the duct (dacryocystorhinography) may be necessary to establish the site, cause, and prognosis of chronic obstructions. Therapy consists of maintaining patency of the duct and instilling topical antibiotic solutions. Tubing (polyethylene or silicone) or 2-0 monofilament nylon suture temporarily catheterized in the duct may be necessary to maintain patency during healing. When the nasolacrimal apparatus has been irreversibly damaged, a new drainage pathway can be constructed surgically (conjunctivorhinostomy or conjunctivoralostomy) to empty tears into the nasal cavity, sinus, or mouth.

Imperforate lacrimal puncta are an infrequent cause of epiphora in young dogs. In foals, atresia of the nasal (distal) end of the nasolacrimal duct is a common

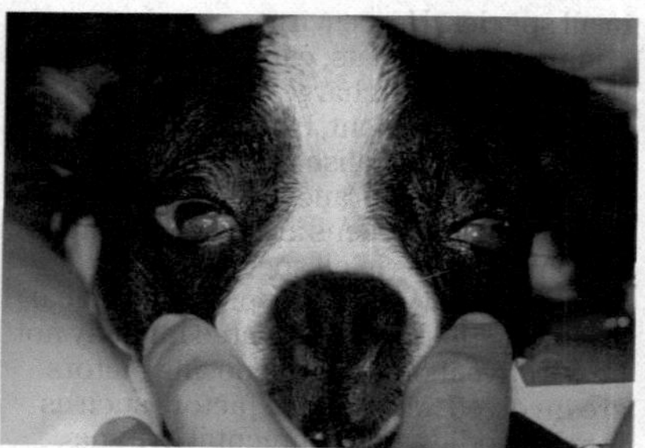

Bilateral inflammation and prolapse of the nictitating membrane (cherry eye), young Boston Terrier. *Courtesy of K. Gelatt.*

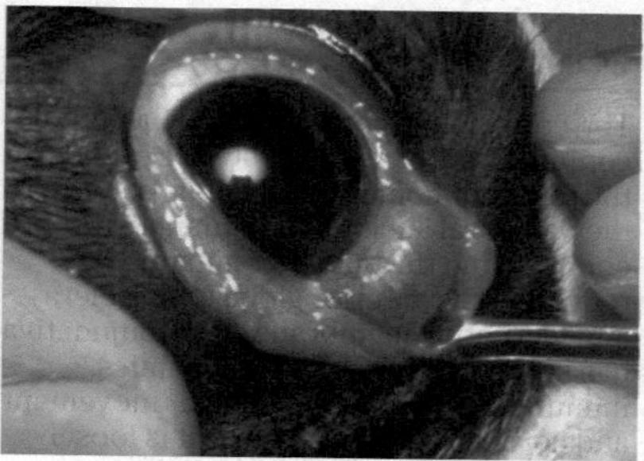

Exposure of inflamed, prolapsed nictitating membrane using thumb forceps, Boston Terrier. *Courtesy of K. Gelatt.*

cause of early epiphora and chronic conjunctivitis. In calves, multiple openings of the nasolacrimal duct may empty tears onto the lower eyelid and medial canthus, causing chronic dermatitis. Therapy in dogs and foals consists of surgically opening the blocked orifice and maintaining patency by catheterization for several weeks during healing.

Keratoconjunctivitis sicca (KCS) is due to an aqueous tear deficiency and usually results in persistent, mucopurulent conjunctivitis and corneal ulceration and scarring. KCS occurs in dogs, cats, and horses. In dogs, it is often associated with an autoimmune dacryoadenitis of both the lacrimal and nictitans glands and is the most frequent cause of secondary conjunctivitis. Distemper, systemic sulfonamide and NSAID therapy, heredity, and trauma are less frequent causes of KCS in dogs. KCS occurs infrequently in cats and has been associated with chronic feline herpesvirus 1 infections. In horses, KCS may follow head trauma.

Topical therapy consists of artificial tear solutions, ointments, and, if there is no corneal ulceration, antibiotic-corticosteroid combinations. Lacrimogenics such as topical cyclosporin A (0.2%–2%, bid), tacrolimus (0.02%, bid), or pimecrolimus (1%) may increase tear production; cyclosporine increases tear formation in ~80% of dogs with Schirmer tear test values ≥2 mm wetting/min. Ophthalmic pilocarpine mixed in food may be useful for neurogenic KCS (dogs 20–30 lb [10–15 kg] should be started on 2–4 drops of 2% pilocarpine, bid). Mucolytic agents (eg, 10% acetylcysteine) lyse excess mucus and restore the spreading ability of other topical agents. In chronic KCS refractory to medical therapy, parotid duct transplantation is indicated. In general, canine KCS requires longterm (often for life) topical lacrimogenic therapy.

CONJUNCTIVA

The conjunctiva consists of the palpebral conjunctiva (lining the posterior eyelids), the fornix or conjunctival cul-de-sac where the palpebral and bulbar conjunctiva connect, and the bulbar conjunctiva (covering the anterior globe or episclera) and nictitating membrane. The conjunctiva has important roles in tear dynamics, immunologic protection, ocular movement, and corneal healing. Because it is loosely attached to the episclera, the bulbar conjunctiva is a useful tissue to graft to weakened, ulcerated corneas.

Subconjunctival hemorrhage may arise from trauma or blood dyscrasias, von Willebrand factor deficiency, and certain infectious diseases. It does not require therapy, but close inspection is warranted to determine whether more important intraocular alterations have occurred. If definite evidence or history of trauma is not present, then systemic examination is indicated to determine the cause of the spontaneous hemorrhage.

Chemosis, or **conjunctival edema**, is seen to some degree in all cases of conjunctivitis, but the most dramatic examples are seen with trauma, hypoproteinemia, allergic reactions, and insect bites. The latter are treated with topical corticosteroids and usually resolve rapidly. Specific therapy for the etiologic agent is indicated.

Conjunctivitis is common in all domestic species. Primary infectious conjunctivitis caused by different bacteria, viruses, mycoplasma, fungi, and parasites affect several species. The etiologic agents vary from infectious to environmental irritants. The signs are hyperemia, chemosis, ocular discharge, follicular hyperplasia, and mild ocular discomfort. The appearance of the conjunctiva usually is not sufficiently distinctive to suggest the etiologic agent, and specific diagnosis depends on history, physical examination, conjunctival scrapings and culture, Schirmer tear test, and occasionally biopsy. Unilateral conjunctivitis may result from a foreign body, dacryocystitis, or keratoconjunctivitis sicca (*see* above). In cats, feline herpesvirus 1 (FHV-1), *Mycoplasma*, or *Chlamydia psittaci* may produce conjunctivitis that begins in one eye and becomes bilateral after ~1 wk. Specific diagnosis is made most rapidly by demonstrating the inclusions or the agent in conjunctival scrapings. Bilateral conjunctivitis is common in viral infections in all species. Herpesviruses produce conjunctivitis in cats, cattle, horses, and pigs. Purulent discharge indicates a bacterial component, but this may be opportunistic because of debilitation of the mucous membrane. Environmental irritants and allergens are common causes of conjunctivitis in all species. If a mucopurulent exudate is present, topical antibiotic therapy is indicated but may not be curative if other predisposing factors are involved. Mechanical factors such as foreign bodies, environmental irritants, parasites, and eyelid conformational defects should be removed or corrected. Selected antibiotics are indicated for chlamydial and mycoplasmal infections; topical antiviral preparations (eg, 1% idoxuridine, 3% adenine arabinoside, or 1% trifluorothymidine (often instilled tid–qid and administered for 7–14 days) are indicated for herpesvirus infections when both the cornea and conjunctiva are involved. Oral supplementation in cats with 250–500 mg of L-lysine daily (often placed in the treats) may reduce the severity and frequency of recurrence of FHV-1 conjunctivitis and keratitis.

CORNEA

The size of the nearly round to oval cornea (vertical/horizontal) varies by animal species: dog (8.5 × 9.5 mm), cat (8.4 × 8.9 mm), horse (16.6 × 17.9 mm), and cow (15.2 × 16.4 mm). The animal cornea consists of the superficial epithelium and basement membrane, large and relatively acellular stroma, deeper Descemet membrane, and deep single layer endothelium. The cornea maintains a strong and durable barrier between the eye and environment, as well as a transparent medium to permit passage of light and images into the posterior segment. Corneal diseases are common in most animal species and fortunately can be treated successfully by medical, surgical, or a combination of these methods. The accessibility of the cornea permits several detailed and noninvasive diagnostic techniques.

Superficial keratitis is common in all species and is characterized by corneal vascularization and opacification, which may be due to edema, cellular infiltrates, pigmentation, or fibroplasia. If ulceration is present, pain—manifest by epiphora and blepharospasm—is an outstanding sign. Unilateral keratitis frequently is traumatic in origin. Mechanical factors, such as lid conformational defects and foreign bodies, should always be eliminated as possible causes, because improvement will not occur until they are resolved. Ulcerative keratitis may be complicated by secondary invasion by bacteria and, in horses, by saprophytic fungi. Bilateral superficial keratitis may be immune-mediated or associated with a lack of tears, eyelid conformational defects, or infectious agents.

Pannus, or Uberreiter disease, is a specific, bilateral, progressive, proliferative, chronic, superficial keratitis that begins laterally and/or medially at the limbus and eventually extends from all quadrants to cover the cornea. Inflammatory cells (lymphocytes and plasma cells) infiltrate the cornea from the limbus, accompanied

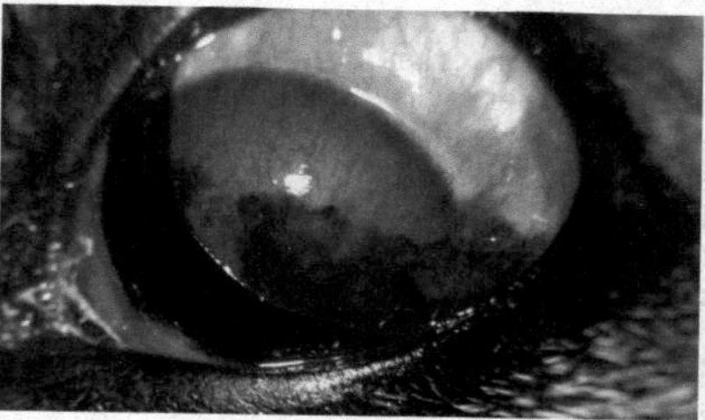

Chronic superficial keratitis, early, German Shepherd. The cornea is progressively infiltrated with superficial blood vessels, followed by inflammation (lymphocytes and plasma cells), and lastly pigmentation.
Courtesy of K. Gelatt.

by superficial blood vessels. This immune-mediated keratitis is common in German Shepherds, Belgian Tervurens, Border Collies, Greyhounds, Siberian Huskies, and Australian Shepherds. Specific therapy consists of topical antibiotics, antiviral or antimycotic agents when appropriate, removal of any mechanical irritants, tear replacement when deficient, and corticosteroids or cyclosporin A (or both) when immune-mediated. The latter may need to be continued indefinitely and the frequency varied depending on the response. Chronic superficial keratitis when immune-mediated is a lifelong disease, requiring lifelong topical anti-inflammatory therapy. The disease appears more aggressive in young dogs and in dogs that live outside in higher altitudes. Generally, topical 1% prednisolone, 0.1% dexamethasone, or 0.2%–1% cyclosporine instilled in both eyes bid-qid is sufficient to control the disease and prolong vision. The intensity of the inflammatory response in both eyes is quite variable and may change by age, season, amount of time the dog spends outside, and other factors. To minimize costs and adverse effects, but control the disease, topical therapy is adjusted to the individual animal (topical therapy ranges from one drop in the affected eye every other day to as frequent as one drop in the affected eyes qid).

Interstitial keratitis is a deep involvement of the corneal stroma that represents one of the clinical signs associated with all chronic and many acute cases of anterior uveitis. The corneal vascularization is less branching, finer, and deeper than in superficial keratitis; if the endothelium has been disrupted, corneal edema is often marked. Systemic diseases, such as infectious canine hepatitis, bovine malignant catarrhal fever, systemic mycoses in many species, and neonatal septicemias that localize in the eye, can cause bilateral or unilateral interstitial keratitis. Therapy is directed at the anterior uveitis, the systemic infection, or both. A specific, nonulcerative, peripheral, stromal keratitis and persistent anterior uveitis (keratouveitis) occurs in horses; prognosis and response to treatment are poor.

Ulcerative keratitis may be divided based on onset, depth, and position within the cornea. Ulcerative keratitis (based on depth) may be superficial, deep, deep with descemetocele, or perforating. Progression of the corneal ulcer is based on the microbes involved and on the release of microbe and tissue enzymes that digest the corneal stroma. Pain, corneal irregularity, edema, and eventually vascularization are signs of ulceration. A dense, white infiltrate at the ulcer margin indicates strong leukotaxis and bacterial involvement. To detect small ulcers, topical fluorescein may be required. In dogs and horses, most ulcers are mechanical in origin; in cattle, sheep, goats, cats, and reindeer, infectious agents and mechanical causes are important; in cats and horses, herpesvirus infection is a frequent cause. All ulcers have the potential for secondary bacterial contamination as well as endogenous proteinase "melting" of the stroma. Therapy for superficial ulcers is usually medical and consists of topical broad-spectrum antibiotic(s) administered 3–6 times daily, correction of any mechanical factors, and limited 1% topical atropine to maintain iridocycloplegia and reduction of ocular pain. Adverse effects of atropine-induced reduced tear production in all species and colic in horses must be considered. Antiproteinase therapy for melting stromal ulcers includes topical serum and other drugs, and for acute ulcerations they may be instilled 4–6 times daily for the first several days. Corneal healing is monitored by frequent clinical examinations and gradual reduction in the size of the fluorescein retention by the nonepithelialized ulcer.

Syndromes of very slow-healing and recurrent superficial ulcers occur in dogs, cats, and horses; in dogs, they may be due to basement membrane disease causing faulty attachment of the corneal epithelium, whereas in cats and horses, and recently in dogs, herpesvirus should be suspected. Initial therapy is ulcer debridement followed by topical antibiotics and atropine. For refractory cases in dogs, multiple punctures or cross-hatching (punctate and grid keratotomies) of affected corneas with a 22-gauge needle stimulates most indolent ulcers to heal within 7–10 days. Early reports suggest these keratotomies in cats may predispose to corneal sequestration and should be used with great care. Nictitating membrane flaps (or soft contact lenses or collagen shields) act as a pressure bandage and often are therapeutic for shallow ulcers. Medical treatment of deep ulcers is similar to that of superficial ulcers, but many deep ulcers also require conjunctival grafts to strengthen and maintain the integrity of the cornea.

Corneal sequestration and keratitis appear to be unique to the cat. It occurs in all breeds of cats but may be more frequent in the Siamese, Persian, and Himalayan breeds. Initially, a very small dark area develops within the anterior stroma and under intact corneal epithelium (that stains with rose Bengel and occasionally very faintly with topical fluorescein). Eventually, the stromal spot becomes larger and either dark brown or black, and is not covered by epithelium. There is variable pain and a central to paracentral, brown to black opacity composed of necrotic stroma, vascularization, and surrounding inflammation. Spontaneous extrusion may occur, especially with superficial sequestra. Treatment consists of superficial keratectomy of the entire sequestrum, that, with deeper lesions, is covered with conjunctival grafts.

Corneal stromal abscesses in horses may be sequelae of healing corneal ulcers or defects and the trapping of bacteria or fungal organisms (or both) within the stroma after reepithelialization. Recently, fungi (both *Candida* and *Aspergillus*) have been demonstrated in horses' subepithelial cornea devoid of iridocyclitis, suggesting another mode of entry. A variable, white to yellow, stromal infiltrate is surrounded by

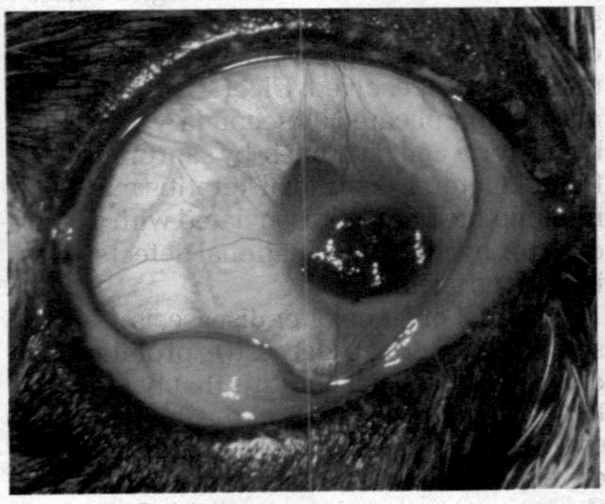

Corneal sequestrum, domestic cat. *Courtesy of K. Gelatt.*

an intense stromal keratitis and vascularization and a variable but sometimes intense anterior uveitis. At least seven to nine different species of fungi have been isolated in corneal ulcers and stromal abscesses in horses, but *Aspergillus* and *Fusarium* spp are the most frequent isolates. Treatment consists of intensive topical and occasional systemic antibiotics (and if indicated, antifungals), iridocycloplegics, NSAIDs, and often surgical removal of the abscess with conjunctival and tectonic corneal grafts.

Corneal dystrophies and degenerations occur frequently in dogs, infrequently in cats, and rarely in horses. Corneal dystrophies are bilateral and often thought inherited in dogs. The appearance of these two diseases may be divided into the following categories: 1) part of cornea affected (epithelium, stroma [anterior, middle, and deep], and endothelium), 2) area of the involved cornea (central, paracentral, and limbal), and 3) possible cause (primary/inherited or secondary). Corneal dystrophies may affect the epithelium and endothelium but appear clinically to involve the stroma most frequently. The corneal degenerations are secondary to other ocular disease or systemic conditions.

Corneal dystrophies affecting the epithelium are associated with recurrent corneal erosions in dogs. The defective corneal epithelium fails to normally adhere to its defective basement membrane and results in recurrent superficial erosions (more frequent in the Boxer breed) and prolonged healing.

The stromal dystrophies appear as white, irregular deposits within the different depths of the stroma and are sometimes labeled corneal lipidosis. Corneal dystrophies are most frequent in dogs, appear inherited in ~20 breeds, affect mostly the corneal stroma, and are usually bilateral. Of the breeds affected, the Siberian Husky corneal stromal dystrophy has been investigated in the greatest detail. Most often, the corneal opacities consist of triglycerides and both intracellular and extracellular cholesterol. Treatment is not usually necessary unless vision is impaired or the deposits become irritating. For these lipid deposits to be viewed histologically, the corneas must be processed as frozen sections and alcohol dehydration processing avoided.

The corneal endothelial dystrophies occur in dogs and rarely in cats (Manx breed). In dogs, it primarily affects older Boston Terriers, Chihuahuas, and Dachshunds.

Female Boston Terriers are affected more frequently than males (with a mean age of ~7.5 yr), and this breed's disease has both clinical and histopathology similarities to those of Fuch corneal endothelial dystrophy in people. With the dystrophic and degenerating endothelium, progressive but painless bilateral corneal edema develops starting centrally. With extensive and full-thickness corneal edema, corneal epithelial bullae may develop and are quite painful. Treatment of early cases before complete corneal involvement consists of topical hyperosmotics (2%–5% sodium chloride or 40% glucose) applied frequently and, for advanced cases, thermokeratoplasty (Salaras procedure) or full-thickness (penetrating) keratoplasty.

Corneal degenerations are often unilateral and usually secondary to ocular or systemic diseases. Deposits of triglycerides, cholesterol, and also calcium are present in corneal degenerations. Corneal degeneration may be associated with other ocular diseases, such as corneal ulcerations, phthisis bulbus, lagophthalmos, and prolonged NSAID therapy. If associated with hyperlipoproteinemias or hypercholesterolemia and high-fat diets, corneal degenerations can affect both eyes, and these deposits are usually associated with corneal vascularization. They also can be altered by significant changes in diet. Baby rabbits or puppies fed whole cow milk may develop extensive lipid deposits in the corneal stroma sufficient to impair vision. Treatment for most corneal degenerations is not usually necessary, unless related to dietary or systemic diseases.

ANTERIOR UVEA

The anterior uvea consists of the iris, ciliary body, and anterior chamber (or iridocorneal) angle. The iris provides most of the eye color as well as an aperture (pupil) to regulate the amount of light that enters the eye and posterior segment. Pupil shape varies widely among animal species, including circle, vertical slit, horizontal oval, square, or even multiple pupils. The ciliary body processes provide most of the aqueous humor to nourish the anterior segment and remove its metabolic wastes, as well as the outflow channels (anterior chamber angle) for aqueous humor to reenter the venous system. The ciliary body musculature also regulates lens curvature (accommodation), which is more limited in domesticated animals than in people. The ciliary body continues posteriorly as the choroid, and diseases of the iris and ciliary body also often involve the choroid. Diseases of the anterior uvea are common in domestic animals.

Persistent pupillary membranes are remnants of the normal prenatal vascular network that fills the pupillary region. Persistence of pigmented strands across the pupil from one area of the iris to another, or to the lens or cornea, is not uncommon in dogs and occurs occasionally in other species. In Basenjis, the condition is inherited.

Atrophy of the iris is common in older dogs and may involve the pupillary margin or the stroma. Atrophy of the pupillary margin creates a scalloped border and a weakening of the sphincter muscle, which is manifest as a moderately dilated pupil(s) or by sluggish pupillary light reflexes and increased sensitivity to bright illumination. Stromal atrophy results in dramatic holes in the iris and, often, displacement of the pupil. Neither form of atrophy appears to affect vision. Animals lacking a functional iridal sphincter may show increased sensitivity to bright light.

Iridic cysts are seen in dogs, cats, and horses. In dogs, they usually are free-floating, pigmented spheres in the aqueous humor within the pupil and anterior and posterior chambers. Although innocuous in most breeds of dogs, anterior uveal cysts (iris and ciliary body) in Golden Retrievers and Great Danes are associated with exfoliation of pigmented cells, chronic uveitis, glaucoma, and cataract formation. In cats, the cysts frequently are not usually free-floating but attached at the pupillary margin. In horses, they are present in the stroma of the iris and more frequently involve blue irides. Because vision is infrequently impaired, therapy is rarely necessary, but aspiration or noninvasive laser-induced deflation can be performed. Transillumination will usually demonstrate their cystic nature and differentiate them from neoplasms. Enlarged and cystic dorsal corpora nigra may impair vision and mimic iridic melanomas in horses. Surgical excision or aspiration may be indicated.

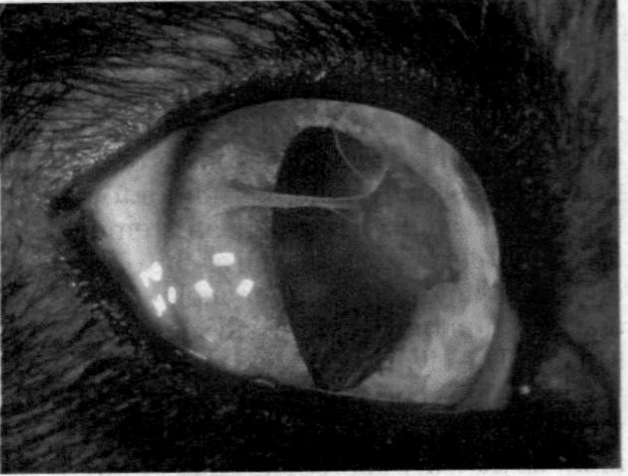

Persistent pupillary membranes, cat. *Courtesy of K. Gelatt.*

Iris colobomas are rare in animals but occur occasionally in Australian Shepherds. They are usually in the upper iris, mainly in heterochromic irides, and cause an irregularity to the pupil. Viewed closely, the defect involves the iridal anterior stroma and apparently the sphincter muscle, but the pigment layer is present.

Anterior uveitis, or **iridocyclitis**, when acute, is manifest by miosis, increased protein and cells in the anterior chamber (aqueous flare), low intraocular pressure, bulbar conjunctival hyperemia, iridal swelling, photophobia, and blepharospasm. Secondary glaucoma, cataract, and corneal opacification may be complications. Concurrent posterior uveitis or choroiditis is frequent. Causes of anterior uveitis can be separated into exogenous and endogenous. Penetrating and nonpenetrating trauma and, rarely, intraocular neoplasms or intraocular helminths are causes of unilateral uveitis. Common causes of bilateral uveitis include immune-mediated diseases and infectious diseases such as infectious canine hepatitis, feline infectious peritonitis, feline leukemia, feline immunodeficiency, feline toxoplasmosis, systemic mycoses in dogs and cats, canine brucellosis, leptospirosis in horses, bovine malignant catarrhal fever, infectious bovine rhinotracheitis, equine viral arteritis, classical swine fever, canine ehrlichiosis, and neonatal bacterial infections (joint, navel, and gut) of calves, lambs, kids, and foals. Recurrent uveitis that is at least in part immune-mediated affects horses (periodic ophthalmia or recurrent uveitis) and dogs (panuveitis with dermal depigmentation or uveodermal syndrome). Recurrent and chronic anterior uveitis are most often associated with complications and can produce secondary cataract formation with posterior synechiae, and glaucoma. A thorough history; examination of the cornea for injuries; physical examination; serum serology; and centesis of the aqueous for culture, serology, and cytology aid in diagnosis.

Nonspecific therapy consists of topical mydriatics to maintain pupillary dilation and movement, topical corticosteroids (if nonbacterial), a darkened environment, and prostaglandin inhibitors (such as aspirin, flunixin meglumine, or phenylbutazone). If bacterial in origin, topical, systemic, and perhaps intraocular antibiotics are indicated. Treatment of immune-mediated processes may require systemic or subconjunctival as well as topical corticosteroids and oral azathioprine.

Hyphema or hemorrhage in the anterior chamber has several clinical appearances, including the following: 1) small, focal blood clots suspended within the anterior chamber or adhered to the posterior cornea, iris, or anterior lens capsule; 2) diffuse, unclotted hemorrhage throughout the entire anterior chamber, occluding deeper eye examination and vision; and 3) multiple layers of recurrent or chronic unclotted hemorrhage (the oldest is a purple or black layer in the bottom of the anterior chamber and the most recent hemorrhage is the dorsal bright red layer). Causes of hyphema include uveitis, trauma, intraocular neoplasia, retinal detachments and retinal tears, systemic hypertension, coagulation factor abnormalities, platelet disorders, hyperviscosity, congenital ocular anomalies, anterior segment neovascularization, and glaucoma. Resolution of hyphema requires exit of intact RBCs through the aqueous humor outflow channels.

Acute hyphema generally has a good prognosis provided the cause is identified and treated. Recurrent and/or chronic hyphema has a poor to guarded prognosis, because secondary glaucoma or phthisis bulbus is likely. No drugs have been proved to facilitate resolution of hyphema, but intracameral tissue-plasminogen activator (TPA) can dissolve fibrin that is <10–14 days old and release the entrapped RBCs within the anterior chamber. TPA does not prevent future fibrin formation, but topical and systemic corticosteroids may.

GLAUCOMA

The glaucomas are generally related to reduced outflow of aqueous humor through the trabecular meshwork of the anterior chamber or iridocorneal angle (conventional outflow, ~85%), and through the uveoscleral network (through the ciliary body and subscleral space, ~15%). Excessive production of aqueous humor in people appears to be rare as a cause of glaucoma and has not been reported in animals. Changes in the composition of aqueous humor have been reported recently in human and animal glaucomas and appear important in the disease genesis and progression.

The glaucomas represent a group of diseases characterized by increased intraocular pressure with resultant retinal and optic disk destruction. Low-tension glaucoma, characterized in people by normal levels of intraocular pressure and progressive optic disk damage, has not been documented in domestic animals. In dogs, the primary (inherited) and secondary glaucomas occur in ~1.7% of the canine population in North America. The frequency of bilateral primary breed-predisposed glaucomas in purebred dogs is the highest of any animal species, except people (0.9%). Primary open-angle glaucoma in Beagles has been associated with the ADAMTS10 mutation. In cats, the glaucomas are predominately secondary to anterior uveitis and neoplasms; however, primary open-angle glaucoma occurs in the Siamese breed. In horses, the glaucomas appear underdiagnosed, because applanation tonometry is not routinely done; they appear most frequently in older animals, Appaloosas, and with concurrent anterior uveitis. In cattle, the glaucomas have been associated with congenital iridocorneal anomalies and anterior uveitis.

Diagnostic procedures essential to manage the glaucomas include tonometry, ophthalmoscopy (direct and indirect), and gonioscopy (visualization of the iridocorneal angle and anterior ciliary cleft). Newer electrophysiologic techniques, such as pattern electroretinograms and visual evoked potentials, estimate damage to the retinal ganglion cells and their axons and appear to be sensitive indicators of glaucoma-related destruction of these cells. New, clinical high-resolution imaging techniques, including ultrasound biomicroscopy for anterior segment changes and optical coherence tomography for retinal and optic nerve head changes, permit noninvasive detailed intraocular examinations. In small animals, the Schiotz indentation tonometer has been replaced by newer and more accurate applanation tonometers used to estimate intraocular pressure; in horses and cattle, only applanation-type tonometers can be used.

Intraocular pressure is reasonably consistent in most species (*see* TABLE 1), and diurnal variations have been documented in dogs, cats, rabbits, and nonhuman primates. Ophthalmoscopy permits detection of the intraocular pressure-related damage to the retina and optic disk. Gonioscopy is the basis for classification of all glaucomas; it detects iridocorneal and sclerociliary cleft opening outflow changes as the glaucoma progresses and helps determine the most appropriate medical and surgical treatments. Ultrasound biomicroscopy

TABLE 1 INTRAOCULAR PRESSURE (IOP) BY APPLANATION TONOMETRY

Species	Tonometer	IOP (mmHg) Mean ± SD[a]
Dog	MacKay-Marg	15.7 ± 4.2
	Tono-Pen™	18.7 ± 5.5 12.9 ± 2.7
	Tono-Vet®	10.8 ± 3.1
Cat	Tono-Pen	19.7 ± 5.6
Rabbit	Pneumatonograph	19.5 ± 1.8 17.9 ± 2.1
Horse	Tono-Pen	29.6 ± 6.2 23.3 ± 6.9
Cow	Tono-Pen	26.9 ± 6.7
Llama/alpaca	Tono-Pen	16.6 ± 3.6
Monkey (ketamine)	Tono-Pen	13.6 ± 3.7
Alligator	Tono-Pen	23.7 ± 2.1
Ferret	Tono-Pen	22.8 ± 5.5
Rat	Tono-Pen	17.3 ± 5.3
Hawk	Tono-Pen	20.6 ± 3.4
Owl	Tono-Pen	10.8 ± 3.6

[a] Duplicate figures represent different reports for that species.

(50–100 MHz) permits further examination of the anterior chamber angle and the entire sclerociliary cleft.

Clinical signs are traditionally divided into acute and chronic; in reality, most cases of acute high-pressure glaucoma are superimposed on chronic glaucoma rather than occurring as singular events. Most dogs with early to moderate chronic glaucoma are not taken to the veterinarian because the early clinical signs—sluggish to slightly dilated pupils, mild bulbar conjunctival venous congestion, and early enlargement of the eye (buphthalmia or megaloglobus)—are so subtle. To detect early glaucoma, repeated tonometry should be routinely performed on high-risk breeds of dogs as part of the annual, general physical examination. The clinical signs of acute and often markedly increased levels of intraocular pressure are a dilated, fixed, or sluggish pupil; bulbar conjunctival venous congestion; corneal edema; and a firm globe. With prolonged increases of intraocular pressure, secondary enlargement of the globe, lens displacement, and breaks in Descemet membrane (corneal striae) result. Pain usually is manifest by behavioral changes and occasional periorbital pain, rather than by blepharospasm.

Classification of the glaucomas assists in the optimal plan for clinical management and preservation of vision. The choice of medical or surgical treatment, or most frequently a combination of both, is based on the progressive iridocorneal angle closure that occurs in most of the glaucomas. As the glaucoma progresses and aqueous humor outflow continues to reduce, the need for a combination of medical therapies increases. For open-angle glaucoma in dogs, short- and longterm management is by treatment with miotics, topical and systemic carbonic anhydrase inhibitors, prostaglandins, osmotics, and β-blocking adrenergics. These same treatments are used for initial control of narrow and closed-angle glaucoma, but short- and longterm management often requires supplemental surgery, eg, filtering procedures, anterior chamber shunts, cyclocryotherapy, or laser transscleral cyclophotocoagulation. Short- and longterm management of end-stage glaucoma with buphthalmia and blindness in dogs also requires surgery, eg, intrascleral prosthesis, enucleation, cyclocryothermy, or intravitreal gentamycin (10–25 mg) combined with 1 mg dexamethasone. Surgical procedures in dogs have traditionally provided only short-term resolution, because the filtering fistulas eventually scar over and fail. More recently, anterior chamber shunts, with and without valves, offer improved results. Antifibrotic drugs, such as mitomycin C and 5-fluorouracil, may delay or prevent scarring of the alternative aqueous outflow channels and prolong their function. In cats, medical therapy is usually the mainstay and consists of topical β-blocking adrenergics (caution in small cats), topical carbonic anhydrase inhibitors, and for those glaucomas associated with anterior uveitis, topical and/or systemic corticosteroids. In horses, single and/or repeated laser transscleral cyclophotocoagulation is most effective.

LENS

The optically clear and avascular lens consists of (from anterior to posterior) the anterior lens capsule, anterior cortex, nucleus, posterior cortex, and very thin posterior lens capsule. The lens is formed early in the development of the eye and coated with its basement membranes (anterior and posterior lens capsules), which insulate the lens proteins from the later-developing immune system. Hence in later life, if the lens capsule barrier is compromised by trauma or surgery, the immune system "attacks" the foreign lens material. The sole function of the lens is to allow unaltered passage of light and images to the retina. Diseases of the lens involve changes in its transparency.

Cataracts are an opacity of the lens or its capsule and should be differentiated from the minor lens imperfections in young dogs (seen on slit-lamp biomicroscopy) and the normal increase in nuclear density (nuclear sclerosis) that occurs in older animals. Cataract formation and cataract surgery in people and dogs have many similarities, but dogs experience more postoperative anterior uveitis. Cataract surgery is highly effective (95%) in people and is performed with advanced nuclear sclerosis and the failure of missing two lines on the Snellen eye acuity test. Cataracts usually are classified by their age of onset (congenital, juvenile, senile), anatomic location, cause, degree of opacification (incipient, immature, mature, hypermature), and shape. Most cataracts can be detected by dilating the pupil and examining the pupillary region against the retroillumination of the tapetal fundus. Slit-lamp biomicroscopy permits optimal direct examination of the lens. Cataracts (often inherited) are more common in dogs than in other species (*see* TABLE 2), and vary by age of onset, rate of progression, and original site of cataract formation. Other causes include diabetes mellitus (the second most frequent group of cataract surgeries in the dog), malnutrition, radiation, inflammation, and trauma. In cats and horses, most cataracts are secondary to anterior uveal inflammation. Most reported inherited cataracts in cats are in young animals. Population studies on cataracts in cattle, rabbits (laboratory and pet), and guinea pigs suggest spontaneous cataracts occur not infrequently, but these species infrequently become blind.

In dogs, cataracts that are secondary related to diabetes mellitus are increasingly common; these cataracts represent the second largest group of cataracts operated on in dogs in the USA. The increased blood glucose causes intralenticular sorbitol to accumulate, which increases the osmotic forces of the lens, causing the lens to imbibe water and result in fiber swelling, rupture, and death. Typically, these cataracts develop rapidly and can occasionally rupture the equatorial or posterior lens capsule. Cataract surgery appears to yield the same success rate as for inherited cataracts in dogs. Other ocular sequelae of diabetes mellitus in dogs are occasional small retinal hemorrhages, presumed corneal neuropathy, and reduced corneal sensitivity. Cats seem quite resistant to diabetic cataract formation, perhaps associated with lower aldose reductase activity than in dogs.

Sight may be regained in some young dogs, cats, and horses when cataracts undergo sufficient spontaneous resorption; congenital nuclear cataracts in young animals may reduce in size with growth of the lens to permit restoration of vision as the animal matures. Animals with immature and incomplete cataracts may benefit from topical ophthalmic atropine 2–3 times/wk, which allows vision around a central or nuclear cataract. However, the only definitive therapy for cataracts is surgical removal of the lens. In dogs and horses, cataract extraction, often by phacoemulsification and with intraocular lens implantation, yields best results when performed before cataract maturation is complete and lens-induced uveitis (due to leakage of lens

TABLE 2 INHERITED CATARACTS IN DOMESTIC ANIMALS

Breed	Age of Onset	Initial Localization	Mode of Inheritance
		DOGS	
Afghan Hound	6–12 mo	Equatorial/posterior cortex	Autosomal recessive
American Cocker Spaniel	1–6 yr	Posterior/anterior cortex	Autosomal recessive polygenetic
Australian Shepherd	2–4 yr	Posterior cortex	Autosomal dominant[a]
Bichon Frise	2–6 yr	Posterior/anterior cortex	Autosomal recessive
Boston Terrier	Congenital or juvenile	Posterior sutures/ nuclear	Autosomal recessive[a]
	Late onset	Equatorial/anterior cortex	Autosomal recessive
Chesapeake Bay Retriever	≥1 yr	Nuclear/cortex	Incomplete dominant
Entelbucher Mountain Dog	1–2 yr	Posterior cortex	Autosomal recessive
German Shepherd	≥8 wk	Posterior sutures/ cortex	Incomplete dominant
Golden Retriever	≥6 mo	Posterior subcapsular (triangular)	Incomplete dominant
Labrador Retriever	≥6 mo	Posterior subcapsular (triangular)	Incomplete dominant
Havanese	2–6 yr	Posterior/anterior cortex	Possible autosomal recessive
Miniature Schnauzer	Congenital	Nuclear/posterior cortex	Autosomal recessive
	≥6 mo	Posterior cortex	Autosomal recessive
Norwegian Buhund	≥1 yr	Nuclear/cortex	Autosomal dominant
Old English Sheepdog	Congenital	Nuclear/cortex	Autosomal recessive
Rottweiler	≥10 mo	Posterior polar/ complete	Unknown
Siberian Husky	≥6 mo	Posterior subcapsular/ posterior sutures	Autosomal recessive
Staffordshire Bull Terrier	≥6 mo	Posterior sutures/cortex	Autosomal recessive[a]
Standard Poodle	≥1 yr	Equatorial cortex	Autosomal recessive
Welsh Springer Spaniel	Congenital	Nuclear/posterior cortex	Autosomal recessive
West Highland White Terrier	Congenital	Posterior sutures	Autosomal recessive

(continued)

TABLE 2 INHERITED CATARACTS IN DOMESTIC ANIMALS *(continued)*

Breed	Age of Onset	Initial Localization	Mode of Inheritance
		HORSES	
Belgian	Congenital	Nuclear/cortex	Autosomal dominant
Morgan	Congenital	Nuclear	Autosomal dominant
		CATTLE	
Holstein-Friesian	Congenital	Nuclear/cortex	Autosomal recessive
Jersey	Congenital	Nuclear	Autosomal recessive
		SHEEP	
New Zealand Romney	Congenital	Anterior/posterior cortex	Autosomal dominant

[a] Associated with mutations in HSF4 gene.

material) is established. Lens-induced uveitis is intensified by cataract surgery and contributes substantially to postoperative complications. In animals in which cataract surgery is not performed, continued clinical monitoring is important. The secondary lens-induced anterior uveitis often requires longterm monitoring and repeated tonometry, with occasional corticosteroid and mydriatic therapy. Secondary glaucoma and phthisis bulbus formation are possible complications.

Lens displacement (subluxation, anterior or posterior luxation) occurs in all species but is common as a primary inherited defect associated with the ADAMTS17 mutation in several terrier breeds. Complete displacement into the anterior chamber produces acute signs and frequently is accompanied by glaucoma and corneal edema. Treatment is surgical removal by phacoemulsification or intracapsular lens extraction. Posterior displacement into the vitreous cavity is asymptomatic or associated with ocular inflammation or glaucoma. Subluxated lenses are recognized by an aphakic crescent and trembling or instability of the iris (iridodonesis) and lens (phacodonesis). The decision to remove subluxated lenses is based on the severity of ocular disease that can be attributed to the lens displacement. Lens displacements also can be produced by trauma, enlargement of the globe with glaucoma, and degenerative zonular changes with hypermature cataracts. Procedures to remove the lens for lens displacement are associated with higher levels of postoperative complications of glaucoma and retinal detachment.

OCULAR FUNDUS

The ocular fundus consists of the upper tapetal fundus, ventral and surrounding nontapetal fundus, retinal vasculature, and optic disk (optic nerve head or optic papilla). Histologically, the posterior segment consists, from superficial to deep, of the following structures: 1) posterior sclera; 2) choroid, which contains pigmented cells, blood vessels to support the high metabolic needs of the outer retina, and the tapetum lucidum to enhance vision in dim light (tapetum cellulosum in carnivores and tapetum fibrosum in herbivores); 3) retina, which consists of the nine layers of neurosensory retina and the outer retinal pigment epithelium; and 4) the optic disk, where the retinal ganglion axons leave the eye through a weak and fenestrated scleral lamina cribrosa to synapse in the lateral geniculate body (vision) or middle brain (pupillary light reflex [Edinger-Westphal nucleus] or dazzle reflex [midbrain and rostral colliculi]). Whereas dogs, cats, horses, cattle, sheep, goats, and many other species have an upper tapetal fundus, pigs and rabbits are typically atapetal.

Diseases of the ocular fundus may be primary or may be manifestations of systemic diseases. Inherited abnormalities may be congenital or appear later and are important in the pathogenesis of retinopathies in dogs and cats. Trauma, metabolic disturbances, systemic infections, neoplasms, blood dyscrasias, hypertension, and nutritional deficiencies are possible underlying causes for retinopathies in all species.

Inherited Retinopathies

Collie eye anomaly is a congenital, recessively inherited (CEA-CH mutation), ocular defect with variable expression in rough- and smooth-coated Collies. It also is seen in Shetland Sheepdogs, Border Collies, Australian Shepherds, Lancashire Heelers, Long-haired Whippets, Boykin Spaniels, and Nova Scotia Duck Tolling Retrievers. The basic lesion is an area of choroidal or chorioretinal hypoplasia that on ophthalmoscopy appears as a focal, variable-sized, pale area lateral to the optic disk. More severely affected dogs (10%–20%) can have additional colobomatous lesions of the optic papilla or peripapillary region and occasional retinal detachments (2%–5%). Intraocular hemorrhage may occur. Vision is not appreciably affected unless retinal detachment develops. With recent availability of the CEA-CH DNA test, additional breeds of dogs diagnosed ophthalmoscopically with Collie eye anomaly can be confirmed having the same mutation as well as potential carrier dogs within affected breeds before breeding.

Retinal dysplasia is a congenital, focal, geographic, or generalized maldevelopment of the retina that may arise from trauma, genetic defect, or intrauterine damage such as viral infections. Most forms of retinal dysplasia in dogs are inherited, and many DNA mutations have been reported. Maternal viral infections, especially during early fetal development, can result in multiple ocular anomalies with retinal dysplasia in kittens (panleukopenia virus), lambs (bluetongue disease), puppies (herpesvirus), and calves (bovine viral diarrhea). Breeds of dogs with focal, geographic, and generalized retinal dysplasia thought to be inherited as an autosomal recessive trait include American Cocker Spaniels, Beagles, Labrador Retrievers, Rottweilers, and Yorkshire Terriers. Focal areas of retinal maldevelopment may be asymptomatic or interfere with central vision. Generalized retinal dysplasia with retinal detachment, visual impairment, or blindness is inherited in English Springer Spaniels, Bedlington Terriers, Sealyham *Terriers, Labrador Retrievers*, Doberman Pinschers, and Australian Shepherds. Other ocular anomalies, including microphthalmia and congenital cataracts, often accompany the generalized forms. In Labrador Retrievers and Samoyeds, retinal dysplasia may be associated with skeletal dysplasia (shortening) of the forelegs.

Progressive retinal atrophy (PRA) is a group of degenerative retinopathies consisting of inherited photoreceptor dysplasia and degenerations that have a similar clinical appearance. A large number of mutations and DNA tests have been reported for these diseases that vary by breed of dog. The photoreceptor dysplasias inherited as autosomal recessive traits in which clinical signs develop in the first year are seen in Irish Setters, Collies, Norwegian Elkhounds, Miniature Schnauzers, and Belgian Sheepdogs. The photoreceptor degenerations inherited as autosomal recessive traits in which clinical signs develop at 3–5 yr are seen in Miniature and Toy Poodles, English and American Cocker Spaniels, Labrador Retrievers, Tibetan Terriers, Tibetan Spaniels, Papillons, English Springer Spaniels, Miniature Longhaired Dachshunds, Akitas, and Samoyeds. In Siberian Huskies, PRA is inherited as an X-linked trait, whereas in Old English Mastiffs and Bull Mastiffs, PRA is inherited as an autosomal dominant. Many other breeds of dogs are also suspected of having inherited PRA. In Abyssinian cats, PRA occurs as both photoreceptor dysplasia and degeneration. Night blindness is noted early and progresses to total blindness over months to years. Ophthalmoscopic lesions are a bilateral symmetric increase in reflectivity

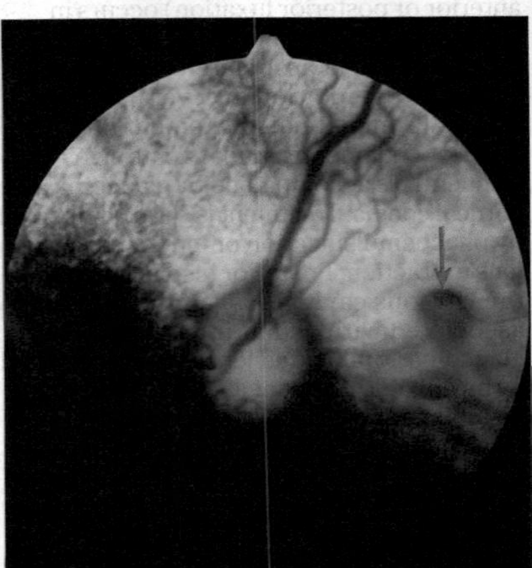

Choroidal hypoplasia and peripapillary coloboma (arrow), Collie. Both ocular defects support the diagnosis of Collie eye anomaly. *Courtesy of K. Gelatt.*

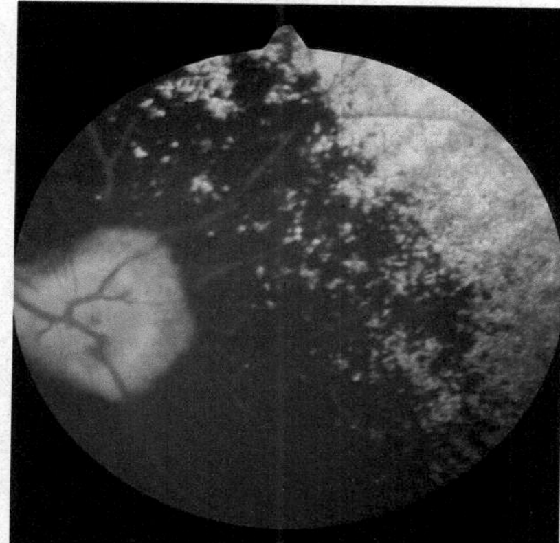

Progressive retinal atrophy, Miniature Poodle. Changes in tapetal reflectivity, reduced retinal vascularity, and early optic nerve atrophy are consistent with the diagnosis of progressive retinal atrophy. *Courtesy of K. Gelatt.*

of the tapetal fundus, decreased pigmentation of the nontapetal fundus, attenuation and a decrease in the number of retinal vessels, and eventual atrophy of the optic papilla. Electroretinography is often used to investigate and diagnose the condition. Cortical cataracts are common late in the course of PRA in many breeds and may mask the underlying retinopathy. No effective therapy is available. Blood and buccal mucosa-based DNA marker and specific gene tests have been developed to detect carrier and affected dogs before clinical signs develop in many breeds. The list of breeds affected with inherited retinal degenerations and causative genes continues to increase; for current information consult the recent literature.

Retinal pigment epithelial dystrophy (central progressive retinal atrophy) is seen in Labrador Retrievers, smooth and rough Collies, Border Collies, Shetland Sheepdogs, and Briards. The condition may be inherited in Labrador Retrievers as a dominant trait with variable penetrance. Early ophthalmoscopic findings (often before clinical signs are apparent) are small foci of irregular pigmentation in the tapetal fundus, which eventually coalesce and fade as reflectivity of the tapetal fundus increases. The pigmented nontapetal fundus becomes mottled, the retinal vasculature gradually decreases, and the optic disk atrophies. Progressive visual impairment occurs gradually over several years. Cataract formation occurs late in the disease. There is no treatment. Studies in English Cocker Spaniels suggest vitamin E disorders may also be important in the pathogenesis of this disease complex. A similar condition in horses, equine motor neuron disease (*see* p 1248), has similar focal yellow-brown areas scattered throughout the tapetal fundus and has also been associated with vitamin E deficiency.

Chorioretinitis

Chorioretinitis frequently is a manifestation of systemic infectious disease; it is important as both a convenient diagnostic clue and a prognosticator of visual function. Unless the lesions are generalized or involve the optic nerve, they often are "silent." Scars may be differentiated from active lesions by the haze and ill-defined borders of the latter. Routine ophthalmoscopic examinations of all animals with systemic diseases often permit rapid diagnosis of many specific diseases. Chorioretinitis may be present with canine distemper, systemic mycoses in dogs and cats, protothecosis, feline toxoplasmosis, tuberculosis, bacterial septicemias in young animals, feline infectious peritonitis, thromboembolic meningoencephalitis in cattle, bovine malignant catarrhal fever, classical swine fever, and leptospirosis and onchocerciasis in horses. Therapy is directed at the systemic disease.

Retinal Detachments

Retinal detachments occur in most species. In dogs, retinal detachment or separation of the neurosensory retina from the retinal pigment epithelium is associated with congenital retinal disorders (retinal dysplasia and Collie eye anomaly), chorioretinitis, trauma, intraocular surgery, and posterior segment neoplasia. In cats, retinal detachments occur with chorioretinitis associated with feline infectious peritonitis, feline viral leukemia, and systemic hypertension. In horses, the most frequent causes are trauma, intraocular surgery, and recurrent uveitis.

Retinal detachments are divided clinically into nonrhegmatogenous (serous, exudative, hemorrhagic, secondary to vitreal syneresis) and rhegmatogenous (with retinal breaks [hole or tear]). Clinical signs include mydriasis, anisocoria, vision impairment, and intraocular hemorrhage. Diagnosis is by ophthalmoscopy and, in eyes with an opaque cornea or lens, ocular ultrasonography.

Nonrhegmatogenous serous retinal detachments are usually treated medically, with therapy directed at the primary

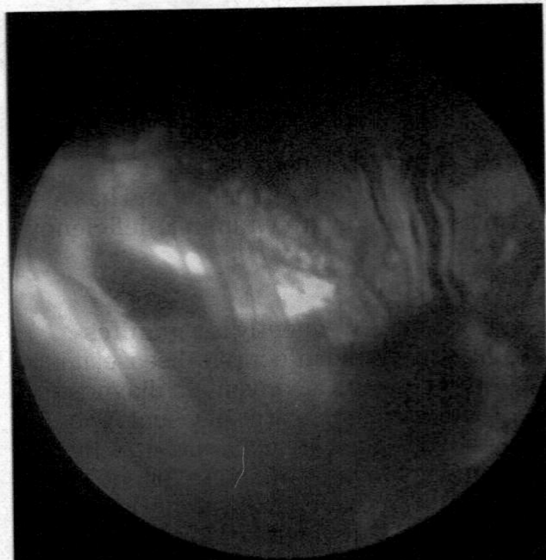

Early retinal detachment and hemorrhage developing lateral to the optic disc in a Collie puppy with Collie eye anomaly.
Courtesy of K. Gelatt.

disease. Retinal reattachment occurs with resolution of the subretinal exudates and hemorrhage. Variable retinal degeneration may follow in the detached areas. Rhegmatogenous retinal detachments with retinal breaks generally require surgical correction.

OPTIC NERVE

Optic nerve diseases are often difficult to detect and diagnose. Of the optic nerve diseases, inflammation of the optic nerve (optic neuritis) is most frequent.

Optic nerve hypoplasia may be inherited in Miniature Poodles; in kittens and calves, it may result from in utero infections with panleukopenia and bovine viral diarrhea, respectively. In calves, the cause may be maternal avitaminosis A. The condition may be unilateral or bilateral, and it can occur with or without other ocular anomalies. Bilateral involvement is manifest as blindness in the neonate; unilateral involvement is often an incidental finding later in life or becomes manifest if the other eye acquires a blinding disease.

Bilateral optic neuritis produces acute blindness and dilated and fixed pupils. On ophthalmoscopy, the optic nerve head or optic disc is raised, edematous with blurred margins and peripapillary hemorrhages, venous congestion, and often inflammatory cells in the adjacent retina and vitreous. Causes of optic neuritis may vary by species affected and include viral, mycotic, protozoan and parasitic infections, trauma, reticulosis, toxins, and other causes. Complete physical and medical evaluations are usually necessary to establish the possible diagnoses. Specific therapies are directed toward the cause, and systemic corticosteroids are important to reduce inflammation of and damage to the optic nerve.

Papilledema is rare in animals and often associated with orbital masses in most domestic species. Increased intracranial pressure does not usually result in papilledema in animals, except in calves with avitaminosis A. The optic disk appears raised above the surface of the adjacent retina, and venous congestion is present. Vision and the light pupillary reflexes are not usually affected unless optic atrophy develops.

Optic atrophy may develop after glaucoma, trauma, advanced retinal degeneration, prolonged ocular hypotension, or inflammation. The optic disk appears depressed and smaller than normal; it is often pigmented, with marked reduction in the optic nerve and retinal vasculature. Both direct pupillary reflex and vision are absent. There is no treatment.

ORBIT

Signs of **orbital cellulitis** are acute pain on opening the mouth, eyelid swelling, unilateral prolapse of the nictitating membrane, forward displacement of the globe, and conjunctivitis. Keratitis may develop from lagophthalmos. The condition is seen predominantly in large and hunting breeds of dogs and is rare in other species. Foreign bodies (eg, migrating grass awns) and zygomatic sialadenitis are additional causes. Orbital hemorrhage and neoplasia may mimic inflammation, except there is usually no pain on opening the mouth. In acute cases, systemic broad-spectrum antibiotics are usually curative, but if swelling behind the last molar is present, drainage of this area is indicated. Warm compresses and topical lubricants to protect the cornea are also indicated. Relapses may occur, and radiographs and ultrasonography of the adjacent teeth, sinuses, and nasal cavity are recommended.

PROLAPSE OF THE EYE

Acute prolapse or proptosis of the eye occurs as a result of trauma. It is common in dogs and infrequent in cats. Prognosis depends on the extent of the trauma, the breed of dog, depth of the orbit, duration of the proptosis, resting pupil size, condition of the exposure keratitis, and other periocular damage. In cats, proptosis usually results from severe trauma to the head; often, other facial bones are fractured. The globe should be replaced as soon as possible if the animal's physical condition will permit induction of general anesthesia (*see* p 1696). Treatment consists of systemic antibiotics and occasionally corticosteroids, combined with topical antibiotics and mydriatics. Although the prognosis for retention of vision is guarded, the globe is usually saved. Return of vision occurs in ~50% of dogs but is rare in cats.

OPHTHALMIC MANIFESTATIONS OF SYSTEMIC DISEASES

Ophthalmic manifestations of systemic diseases are not uncommon with inherited, infectious, degenerative, and neoplastic disorders in animals. Often, ophthalmic examinations can assist in timely identification of the systemic disorder. Diseases affecting the vascular and nervous systems are likely to show ocular manifestations. Animals with bilateral ocular disease should be carefully evaluated for systemic diseases.

In dogs, ophthalmic diseases, such as retinal dysplasia, microphthalmia, and cataracts, have been associated with dwarfism, albinism, and merling. Infectious diseases often involve the uveal tract and present as iridocyclitis, choroiditis, and panuveitis. They may be caused by viruses (distemper, infectious hepatitis), rickettsial diseases (ehrlichiosis and Rocky Mountain spotted fever), bacteria (*Brucella canis* and *Borrelia burgdorferi*), fungi (*Blastomyces*, *Coccidioides*, *Histoplasma*, *Cryptococcus*, and *Aspergillus*), protozoa (*Toxoplasma*, *Neospora*, *Leishmania*, and *Hepatozoon*), algae (*Prototheca*), or parasites (*Dirofilaria*, *Toxocara*, and *Diptera* spp). Metabolic diseases associated with eye diseases in the dog include diabetes mellitus (cataract formation), hypocalcemia (cataracts), hyperadrenocorticism (corneal disease, cataracts, and lipemia retinalis), and hypothyroidism (keratoconjunctivitis sicca, intraocular hemorrhages from increased systemic blood pressure, and lipemia retinalis [hyperlipidemia]). Blood and vascular disorders may present as intraocular hemorrhage, retinal detachment, secondary glaucoma, and papilledema. Metastatic neoplasms, such as lymphosarcoma, most often affect the uvea, presenting as persistent uveitis, overt intraocular masses, intraocular hemorrhage, secondary glaucoma, or retinal detachment.

In cats, systemic diseases frequently affect the eye and associated structures. Eyelid inflammations are often associated with systemic *Demodex cati* and *D gatoi*, *Notoedres cati* (scabies), ringworm, and immune-mediated skin diseases. The pathogens that commonly cause infectious diseases of cats, eg, feline herpesvirus 1, *Chlamydia*, and *Mycoplasma*, frequently present as acute and recurrent conjunctivitis. Feline herpesvirus 1 is also associated with ulcerative and stromal keratitis, proliferative keratoconjunctivitis, corneal sequestrum, corneal symblepharon, and keratoconjunctivitis sicca. Feline infectious peritonitis, toxoplasmosis, feline immunodeficiency virus, and feline leukemia virus often present as anterior and posterior uveitis, chronic uveitis, retinal detachment, and secondary glaucoma. Acute vision loss with intraocular hemorrhage and retinal detachment in older cats may be secondary to systemic hypertension and is often associated with chronic renal failure or hyperthyroidism. Resolution of intraocular hemorrhages, repair of the retinal detachment, and possible restoration of vision depends on the successful lowering of blood pressure to normal levels, often using amlodipine, an oral calcium channel blocker.

In horses, systemic infectious diseases, such as adenovirus in immunodeficient Arabian foals, equine influenza, strangles (*Streptococcus equi*), *Rhodococcus equi* infection, leptospirosis, Lyme disease (*Borrelia burgdorferi*), and salmonellosis, may present as conjunctivitis, anterior uveitis, or posterior uveitis. Ophthalmic onchocerciasis can be markedly reduced by frequent administration of ivermectin but can present with anterior and posterior uveitis, peripapillary chorioretinitis, keratitis, keratoconjunctivitis, or lateral conjunctival vitiligo. Habronemiasis presents with inflammatory conjunctival masses of the periocular area (especially the medial canthus) associated with the aberrant migration of larvae of *Habronema muscae*, *H microstoma*, and *Draschia megastoma*. Therapy is usually systemic ivermectin.

In cattle, microphthalmia, cataracts, retinal dysplasia, and retinal detachments are associated with hydrocephalus and in utero infection of calves with bovine viral diarrhea. The same ophthalmic defects occur in lambs affected in utero with bluetongue virus. Vitamin A deficiency in

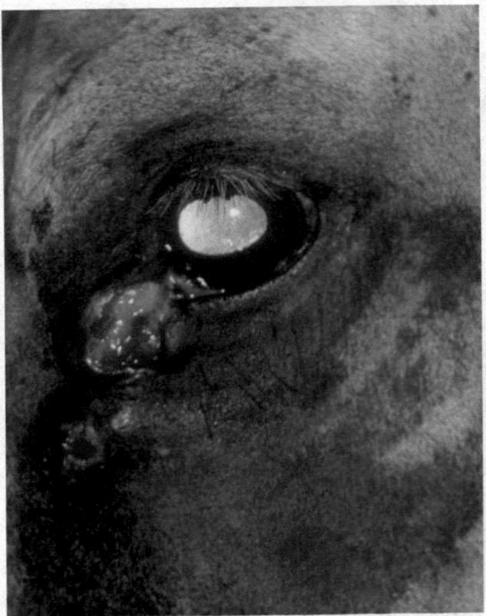

Conjunctival habronemiasis may be concurrent with "summer sores" in horses. *Courtesy of K. Gelatt.*

piglets causes microphthalmia, and in calves blindness and optic nerve hypoplasia. Vitamin A deficiency in adult or growing cattle results in night blindness, mydriasis, and eventually total blindness. Ophthalmoscopic abnormalities include papilledema, retinal degeneration, and optic nerve atrophy. Vitamin A supplementation may restore vision in animals with night blindness only. Lymphosarcoma in cattle may present as bilateral progressive exophthalmia. Many infectious diseases, such as rhinotracheitis, malignant catarrhal fever, thromboembolic meningoencephalitis, and neonatal septicemia, may present with conjunctivitis or anterior or posterior uveitis. Intoxications such as male fern poisoning (*Dryopteris filix*), bracken fern poisoning (*Pteridium aquilinum*) in sheep, coumarin poisoning (sweet clover poisoning) in cattle, and phenothiazine toxicity in cattle present with clinical signs of blindness from retinal degeneration, intraocular hemorrhage, or corneal edema. (*See also* TOXICOLOGY, p 2948.)

CHLAMYDIAL CONJUNCTIVITIS

Etiology and Epidemiology: Chlamydiae are obligate intracellular bacteria that form inclusions within the cytoplasm of epithelial cells. The life cycle of chlamydiae involves an alternation between the intracellular reticulate body and the extracellular elementary body, which is the infectious form of the organism. Several members of the family Chlamydiaceae have been associated with conjunctivitis in the host species they infect, including *Chlamydia caviae* (guinea pigs), *C suis* (pigs), *C psittaci* (birds), and *C pecorum* (cattle and sheep). Although chlamydial infection has been associated with keratoconjunctivitis in sheep and goats, a study that used molecular techniques to detect chlamydiae in sheep did not find a clear association between infection and disease. Chlamydial conjunctivitis in cats is caused by *C felis* (formerly *Chlamydophila felis*). *C pneumoniae* has also been detected in cats with conjunctivitis using molecular methods. *C psittaci* has been isolated from dogs with keratoconjunctivitis and respiratory signs in a dog breeding facility. Trachoma and inclusion conjunctivitis in people are caused by *C trachomatis*. Chlamydia-like organisms (*Parachlamydia acanthamoebae*) that reside and proliferate within free-living amoeba have been detected in the eyes of cats, guinea pigs, pigs, and sheep with conjunctivitis. The pathogenic role of these organisms and their amoebic hosts is unclear.

Although the disease in cats has been referred to as feline pneumonitis, chlamydiae rarely cause pneumonia in cats. The infection always involves the eye, occasionally causing signs of rhinitis, with sneezing and nasal discharge. Although antibody titers to *C felis* are common in some cat populations, the organism is rarely isolated from clinically healthy cats. Cats with chlamydial conjunctivitis are generally <1 yr old, and cats 2–6 mo old appear to be at highest risk of infection. Cats with conjunctivitis that are >5 yr old are very unlikely to be infected, and cats <8 wk old may be less at risk because of the presence of maternal antibody. Transmission occurs as a result of direct, close contact between cats, because the organism survives poorly in the environment. Infected cats also shed chlamydiae from their rectum and vagina, although whether venereal transmission may occur has not been confirmed. There is weak evidence that chlamydiae may be capable of causing reproductive disease and lameness in cats, although these associations have not been definitively documented.

Chlamydial infection is one of the most common causes of conjunctivitis in guinea pig populations, in which it is also known as guinea pig inclusion conjunctivitis (*see* p 2017). As with cats, young guinea pigs, especially those 1–2 mo old, are predisposed. Subclinical disease may also occur. Rhinitis, lower respiratory tract disease, and genital infections, causing salpingitis and cystitis in female guinea pigs and urethritis in males, may also occur.

Clinical Findings: In cats, the incubation period after exposure to an infected cat ranges from 3 to 10 days. Signs can include serous to mucopurulent conjunctivitis, nasal discharge, and sneezing. Cats with signs of rhinitis in the absence of conjunctivitis are unlikely to be infected with *C felis*. Early signs include unilateral or bilateral conjunctival hyperemia, chemosis, and serous ocular discharge, with prominent follicles on the inside of the third eyelid in more severe cases. Keratitis is rare, and if present, may be the result of coinfection with organisms such as feline herpesvirus 1. The signs are most severe 9–13 days after onset and then become mild over a 2- to 3-wk period. In some cats, clinical signs can last for weeks despite treatment, and recurrence of signs is not uncommon. Untreated cats may harbor the organism for months after infection.

Guinea pigs may develop mild to severe conjunctivitis, with conjunctival hyperemia, chemosis, and mucopurulent ocular discharge.

Diagnosis: Chlamydial conjunctivitis in cats should be differentiated from conjunctivitis caused by feline herpesvirus 1 and feline calicivirus, and in guinea pigs from mycoplasmal and other bacterial infections (eg, "pinkeye"). Diagnosis is best confirmed using PCR for chlamydial DNA on conjunctival swabs. Cell culture for *Chlamydia* is sensitive and specific but not widely available or practical for routine diagnostic purposes. Special chlamydial transport media is required for transport of specimens for culture.

A diagnosis of ocular chlamydiosis can also be made by demonstration of intracytoplasmic chlamydial inclusions in exfoliative cytologic preparations. Scrapings for cytologic examination are prepared by lightly but firmly moving a spatula over the conjunctiva and smearing the scraped material onto a glass slide; the preparation is air-dried and stained. Chlamydial inclusions, which contain reticulate bodies, are round and generally stain purple with Romanowsky stains. Conjunctival cytology from guinea pigs generally reveals a neutrophilic inflammatory response. Inclusions are generally visible only early in the course of infection and sometimes not at all. Melanin granules and remnants of some ophthalmic preparations may be mistaken for inclusions, leading to false-positives, so other diagnostic tests are recommended to confirm the diagnosis.

Prevention and Treatment: Vaccines are available for chlamydiosis in cats but not for other species. Feline chlamydial vaccines do not provide complete protection from infection but may reduce disease severity and infection rates. Their use may be considered in catteries where chlamydiosis is endemic.

All *Chlamydia* isolates are susceptible to tetracyclines. The treatment of choice is doxycycline (10 mg/kg/day) for at least 4 wk. Systemic therapy is superior to topical therapy and is logical given that organisms are shed from sites other than the conjunctiva. Treatment for up to 6 wk has been required to eliminate infection in some cats. All cats in the household must be treated. Fluoroquinolones, such as enrofloxacin and pradofloxacin, and amoxicillin-clavulanic acid, also have been used to successfully treat feline chlamydiosis, although their efficacy may be less than that of doxycycline. Azithromycin does not appear to be effective.

Zoonotic Risk: On rare occasions, *C felis* and *C caviae* have been isolated from people living with infected cats and guinea pigs. Follicular conjunctivitis was described in a single immunocompromised person who was found to be infected with *C felis*. There was one report of detection of *C caviae* in a person with serous ocular discharge who worked with ~200 diseased guinea pigs. *C caviae* was also detected in conjunctival swabs of this person's cat and rabbit, the latter of which had signs of mild conjunctivitis. Routine hygiene practices, such as hand washing before and after handling sick pets, may reduce the potential for transmission of these organisms from affected animals to people.

EQUINE RECURRENT UVEITIS

(Periodic ophthalmia, Moon blindness, Equine uveitis)

Equine recurrent uveitis (ERU) is an important ophthalmic condition with a reported prevalence of 2%–25% worldwide. The classic form of ERU is characterized by episodes of active intraocular inflammation followed by variable quiescent periods. However, some horses experience insidious ERU in which subclinical ocular inflammation persists without obvious signs of discomfort. With chronicity, the inflammatory bouts cause secondary ocular changes such as cataracts, lens luxation, glaucoma, phthisis bulbi, and retinal degeneration. As a result, ERU is the most common cause of blindness in horses in the world.

Etiology and Pathogenesis: ERU is an autoimmune syndrome that ensues after an initial episode of acute uveitis. Although not every horse with a single bout of uveitis will develop ERU, horses that have experienced acute uveitis are at risk of developing ERU for several years after the primary episode. While numerous bacterial, viral, protozoan, parasitic, and noninfectious causes, including ocular trauma, have been linked to the initiation of ERU, the pathophysiology of ERU is complex and multifactorial. Of the infectious causes investigated, *Leptospira* spp, especially *L interrogans* serogroup Pomona, have been most studied with regard to their role in the initiation of ERU. The precise mechanisms by which *Leptospira* spp initiate ERU remain unknown, but it is likely that loss of ocular immune tolerance, cross-reaction between *Leptospira* organisms and self-antigen, and intra- and intermolecular epitope spreading all play a critical role. There is no gender or age predisposition for ERU. However, Appaloosas, warmbloods, and draft breeds are overrepresented among horses diagnosed with ERU, which suggests a heritable component. Genes of the major histocompatibility complex (MHC) have been most widely investigated and likely play a role in susceptibility to ERU and/or to leptospirosis as an inciting trigger for ERU. The prevalence of ERU varies with geographic region, with higher rates reported in tropical and temperate climates than in arid, dry climates, an observation that may be partially attributable to differences in persistence of pathogenic *Leptospira* spp within the environment. Thus, the underlying cause of the primary uveitis, genetic composition of the horse, and environmental factors are all integral to the development of ERU.

Clinical Findings and Lesions: Clinical findings associated with ERU include acute signs of active inflammation as well as chronic secondary complications. Changes in ocular immunity allow leukocytes to invade the uvea and release proinflammatory cytokines such as prostaglandins and leukotrienes. These inflammatory mediators cause increased vascular permeability within the uvea, breakdown of the blood-ocular barrier, iris sphincter muscle spasm, decreased aqueous humor production, and ciliary body muscle spasm. These changes are responsible for the classic signs of acute uveitis: epiphora, blepharospasm, corneal edema, episcleral congestion, aqueous flare and cell, and fibrin in the anterior chamber. These anterior segment signs often reduce visualization of the posterior segment. Active posterior segment inflammation can result in vitreous haze secondary to cellular infiltrate, fibrinous traction bands, focal or diffuse retinal detachment, or chorioretinitis. Chronic sequelae of ERU include corneal scarring, iridal fibrosis, corpora nigra atrophy, posterior synechia, cataract, lens dislocation, glaucoma, phthisis bulbi, and chorioretinal scarring. ERU can be unilateral or bilateral and can affect the eyes asymmetrically.

Horses with primary ocular disease, especially corneal disease, experience many clinical signs typical of ERU, especially epiphora, blepharospasm, miosis, and corneal edema. It is critical to differentiate primary corneal disease from ERU considering the marked differences in treatment. A complete ophthalmic examination and fluorescein stain are essential. A thorough ophthalmic examination, including fundoscopy, is also critical during prepurchase or soundness examinations. Horses with chronic ERU may exhibit subtle or no anterior segment signs but have significant retinal degeneration and thus potential for vision compromise.

Diagnosis: Diagnosis is based on characteristic clinical signs combined with a history of recurrent or persistent episodes of uveitis. A thorough ophthalmic examination of the anterior and posterior segment is critical to observing signs consistent with ERU and to excluding other primary ocular diseases. Tonometry should be performed in all cases to exclude glaucoma and document hypotony that is common with ERU. Application of fluorescein stain is important to assess corneal epithelial integrity and exclude reflex uveitis from ulcerative keratitis. In cases of acute uveitis, a physical examination is performed to exclude systemic disease. A CBC and serum biochemistry panel are often warranted as part of the minimum database. Specific tests may assist in determining the underlying cause of a primary bout of uveitis. Serologic testing for *Leptospira* spp may confirm exposure to this common risk factor but is not helpful in determining treatment. Anterior chamber or vitreous cavity paracentesis may aid in identifying a causative organism, but this procedure may cause severe intraocular damage and is not recommended.

Treatment, Prevention, and Control: The primary goals of therapy are to reduce inflammation, relieve discomfort, and prevent vision loss. If possible, the specific underlying cause should be diagnosed and addressed as part of the initial treatment regimen. Regardless of whether the underlying cause is identified, aggressive treatment with systemic and topical anti-inflammatory medications is initiated immediately to minimize damage from intraocular inflammation. Flunixin meglumine administered systemically (especially IV) is critical to the initial management of acute uveitis in horses. The typical initial IV dosage is 1.1 mg/kg, administered at the time of diagnosis, followed by a 5- to 7-day course at a dosage of 0.5–1.1 mg/kg, PO, bid. As inflammation resolves, the dosage can be reduced to 0.25–0.5 mg/kg once daily or every other day throughout a 1- to 3-mo treatment period. Because of the potential for renal toxicity, serum creatinine is intermittently monitored if flunixin meglumine is used for >1 mo. Horses treated with flunixin meglumine should also be observed for signs of GI ulceration, and concurrent prophylactic administration of omeprazole (2 mg/kg/day, PO) may be indicated. If flunixin meglumine is not tolerated, phenylbutazone (2–4 mg/kg, PO, once to twice daily) or aspirin (10–25 mg/kg, PO, once to twice daily) can be used alternatively, but neither is as potent or effective. Historically, horses with frequent recurrences or chronic, low-grade uveitis were managed medically with daily (or every other day) doses of oral phenylbutazone or aspirin. Although most horses tolerate this regimen well, these medications can have adverse GI, hematologic, or renal effects, and these regimens frequently do not eliminate recurrence. Systemic steroids, specifically prednisolone (100–300 mg/day) and dexamethasone (5–10 mg/day) have also been successfully used to treat acute uveitis episodes, but their longterm use has been associated with laminitis. Except in cases when bacterial infection is present, systemic antibiotics are not indicated.

Topical steroidal medications, including dexamethasone (0.1% suspension or ointment) and prednisolone acetate (1% suspension), are very effective at decreasing inflammation. Topical acetate and suspension preparations of steroids are designed to penetrate the cornea and achieve adequate uveal concentrations and are thus preferred to sodium phosphate formulations. Topical hydrocortisone should be avoided, because it lacks adequate corneal penetration and is not sufficiently potent to treat anterior uveitis. A fluorescein stain is warranted before initiation of topical steroids, because these medications are contraindicated with corneal ulceration and/or infection. Topical nonsteroidal medications include flurbiprofen (0.03% solution) and diclofenac (0.1% solution); they are less potent than topical steroids but offer a wider safety margin in cases of concurrent corneal disease. Frequency of administration depends on inflammation severity; initially, administration may be 4–6 times daily. With improvement in clinical signs, frequency of administration of topical steroidal or nonsteroidal medications can be gradually decreased. However, therapy should continue for 1 mo after complete resolution of active inflammation. Topical atropine (1% solution or ointment) causes mydriasis (which decreases the likelihood of posterior synechia formation) and cycloplegia (which decreases pain associated with ciliary body muscle spasm) and stabilizes the blood-aqueous barrier. Atropine is applied topically 2–3 times daily until the pupil is widely dilated; the frequency can then be adjusted to maintain mydriasis. Because atropine decreases GI motility, horses treated with topical atropine should be monitored for signs of ileus. If frequent topical medication is not possible, subconjunctival injections of triamcinolone acetamide (1–2 mg) provide adequate intraocular anti-inflammatory concentrations for 7–10 days and are less likely to cause abscess or granuloma formation than other steroids, including methylprednisolone acetate (10–40 mg).

However, all subconjunctival steroids should be used with caution, because they cannot be easily removed once injected and can have devastating consequences if an infectious component is present or a corneal ulcer develops.

Two surgical procedures are commonly used in longterm management. A suprachoroidal cyclosporine implant is a sustained-release medication device that provides therapeutic concentrations of cyclosporine A, an immunosuppressive T-cell inhibitor, for ~3 yr after implantation. During this procedure, a cyclosporine A disk (~5 mm in diameter) is implanted under a scleral flap created ~8 mm posterior to the dorsolateral aspect of the limbus. Horses with implants have markedly fewer uveitic episodes than they did before surgery, and this device results in effective longterm control of ERU. Core vitrectomy removes virtually all of the vitreous through an incision posterior to the dorsolateral aspect of the limbus. The vitreous is then replaced with either balanced salt solution or saline. The theorized benefit of this procedure is that organisms, especially *Leptospira* spp, and/or inflammatory cells in the vitreous significantly contribute to the chronic inflammation of ERU. By removing these factors, the frequency and severity of uveitic episodes are minimized.

Good husbandry practices to manage ERU ensure proper health maintenance, prevent ocular trauma, and reduce environmental triggers. Specific management recommendations include routine deworming and vaccinations, proper nutrition and dental care, a quality fly mask, minimizing contact with cattle or wildlife, draining stagnant ponds or restricting access to swampy pastures, effective fly control, and frequent bedding changes. Although such measures benefit individual horses, the extent to which they impact the clinical course of ERU has not been evaluated.

EYEWORM DISEASE

(Thelaziasis)

LARGE ANIMALS

Etiology and Epidemiology: Eyeworms (*Thelazia* spp) are common parasites of horses and cattle in many countries, including those of North America. Horses are infected primarily by *T lacrymalis*, whereas cattle are mainly infected by *T gulosa*, *T skrjabini*, and *T rhodesii*. The latter is the most common and harmful to cattle in the Old World, but it has not been recently reported in North America. The prevalence of *Thelazia* spp in livestock has declined in at least some areas where macrocyclic lactone endectocides such as ivermectin and doramectin are in common use. *Thelazia* spp are also found in pigs, sheep, goats, deer, water buffalo, dromedaries, hares, dogs and cats (*see* p 512), birds, and people.

The face fly, *Musca autumnalis*, is the vector of *T lacrymalis*, *T gulosa*, and *T skrjabini* in North America. Feeding habits of this fly include a preference for ocular secretions, which are ideal for transmission. The life cycle of *Thelazia* is as follows: female worms are ovoviviparous and discharge larvae into the ocular secretions; the larvae are ingested by the fly and become infective in 2–4 wk. Infective third-stage larvae emerge from the labellae of infected flies and are mechanically deposited in the host's eye by the fly during feeding. Development of sexually mature worms takes 1–4 wk in cattle, depending on worm species, and 10–11 wk for *T lacrymalis* in horses. Infections may be found year-round, but clinical disease outbreaks, particularly in cattle, usually are associated with warm season activities of the flies. *Thelazia* sp larvae may overwinter in face flies. Infection rates generally tend to increase with advancing host age, although some studies report maximal levels in hosts 2–3 yr old.

Pathogenesis: The lacrimal gland and its ducts are common sites for *T lacrymalis* and *T gulosa*, with the glands of the nictitating membrane and the nasolacrimal ducts less so. *T skrjabini* is normally found within the lacrimal ducts of the nictitating membrane. Superficial locations on the cornea, in the conjunctival sac, and under the eyelids and nictitating membrane are more typical for *T rhodesii*, but *T lacryma-*

lis, *T skrjabini*, and *T gulosa* may be found in these sites, too. Worms may also be found on the periorbital hair or skin during anesthesia or following migration after death of the host. Localized irritation and inflammation is likely due to the serrated cuticle of the worms, especially for *T rhodesii*. Invasion of the lacrimal gland and excretory ducts may cause inflammation and necrotic exudation. Inflammation of the lacrimal ducts and sac has also been reported in horses. Mild to severe conjunctivitis and blepharitis are common. Also, keratitis, including opacity, ulceration, perforation, and permanent fibrosis, may develop in severe cases, particularly with *T rhodesii* infection in cattle.

Clinical Findings and Diagnosis: Asymptomatic infections in horses and cattle appear to be typical of thelaziasis in North America. Infection may be encountered incidentally during surgery or at necropsy. However, *Thelazia* infections in cattle in North America may not always be innocuous. They may produce mild conjunctivitis, excessive lacrimation, localized edema, corneal clouding, and occasionally, subconjunctival cysts. In Europe and Asia, thelaziasis is commonly associated with severe clinical manifestations, including conjunctivitis, photophobia, and keratitis. Characteristically, there is chronic conjunctivitis with lymphoid hyperplasia and a seromucoid exudate.

A clinically feasible technique for reliable detection of adult eyeworms is lacking. Gross inspection of the eyes may reveal the worms and is generally recommended for *T rhodesii*, commonly found in the conjunctival sac. However, *T gulosa* and *T skrjabini* in cattle, and *T lacrymalis* in horses, tend to be more invasive and are less apt to be seen. Topical anesthetics allow for tissue manipulation and are useful for detection and recovery of worms. Microscopic examination of lacrimal fluids for embryonated eggs or larvae may be attempted.

Clinical signs may be helpful in differential diagnosis. Thelaziasis tends to cause a chronic conjunctivitis. In cattle, infectious keratoconjunctivitis (*see* below) is an acute, rapidly spreading infection of the cornea. In horses, infective larvae of the stomach worms *Draschia* and *Habronema* sp may also produce ophthalmic lesions. These tend to occur near the medial canthus of the eyelid and are raised, ulcerative granulomas, often containing characteristic yellow, plaque-like "sulfur granules" 1–2 mm in diameter. Likewise, microfilariae of *Onchocerca* sp invade the eye and may result in ophthalmic manifestations. Small (<1 mm), raised, white nodules in the pigmented conjunctiva adjacent to the temporal limbus are pathognomonic of *Onchocerca* infection. Depigmentation of the bulbar conjunctiva in this area is also common. Other lesions of onchocerciasis involve the cornea and include edema and punctate or streaking opacities of the stroma, superficial erosions, and a wedge-shaped sclerosing keratitis emanating from the temporal limbus. Intraocular structures also may be affected by microfilariae of *Onchocerca* sp (*see* p 905). Worms may be identified morphologically. In addition, PCR and sequencing assays have been developed to confirm the identity of some species, but these are not used routinely.

Treatment and Control: Mechanical removal with forceps after instillation of a local anesthetic is useful for *T rhodesii* in cattle. This also may be feasible for the more invasive *T gulosa* or *T skrjabini* in cattle or for *T lacrymalis* in horses. Irrigation of the eyes with 50–75 mL aqueous solution of 0.5% iodine and 0.75% potassium iodide has been recommended for *T gulosa* and *T skrjabini*. This also may be effective for *T lacrymalis* in horses. Topical application of 0.03% echothiophate iodide or 0.025% isofluorophate (both organophosphates) has been successful for *T lacrymalis* in horses. Concurrent use of antibiotic-steroid ointment for the inflammation and secondary invaders is recommended. These topical agents should also be useful for *T gulosa* and *T skrjabini* in cattle. Certain systemic anthelmintics have exhibited activity against eyeworms. In cattle, levamisole at 5 mg/kg, SC, and ivermectin and doramectin, both at 0.2 mg/kg, SC or IM, have shown activity against *Thelazia* spp. Pour-on formulations of ivermectin or doramectin, delivered to achieve a dosage of 0.5 mg/kg, are also effective. Doramectin has been approved in the USA for treatment of adult eyeworms in cattle. For *T lacrymalis* in horses, single doses of the commonly used anthelmintics, including ivermectin, administered via stomach tube at 0.2 mg/kg, have had limited, if any, effect on eyeworms. In contrast, the multidose regimen of fenbendazole (10 mg/kg/day for 5 days) is efficacious against *T lacrymalis*.

Fly control measures, directed especially against the face fly, aid in the control of thelaziasis in cattle and horses. Cattle on dry, open pastures have fewer face flies than those on pastures where shade and water are present.

SMALL ANIMALS

Thelazia californiensis is found in dogs, cats, and deer in western USA; *T callipaeda* is found in dogs, cats, foxes, wolves, martens, and rabbits in Europe and Asia. *T callipaeda* appears to be spreading in some regions of Europe. Both species are zoonotic. The worms are whitish, 7–19 mm long, and move in a rapid serpentine motion across the eye. Up to 100 eyeworms may be seen in the conjunctival sac, tear ducts, and on the conjunctiva under the nictitating membrane and eyelids. Filth flies (*Musca* spp, *Fannia* spp) serve as intermediate hosts and deposit infective larvae on the eye while feeding on ocular secretions. Zoophilic fruit flies have emerged as potential intermediate hosts of *T callipaeda*. These include *Phortica variegata* in Europe and *Amiota* spp in Asia.

Clinical signs include excessive lacrimation and epiphora, ocular pruritus, conjunctivitis, keratitis with corneal opacity and ulceration, hyperemia, and rarely, blindness. After local anesthetic, diagnosis and treatment are readily accomplished by observing and removing the parasites with forceps. *Thelazia* spp infections have been successfully eliminated from dogs with ivermectin SC at 0.2 mg/kg, milbemycin oxime PO at a minimum dosage of 0.5 mg/kg (two treatments 1 wk apart improved efficacy), or spot-on treatment with moxidectin 2.5%. Ocular solutions (1% moxidectin or 2% levamisole) or ointments (1% levamisole or 4% morantel) also may be effective. Infection with *T callipaeda* has been prevented for the full season in dogs with sustained-release moxidectin at 0.17 mg/kg, SC, with milbemycin oxime PO at the dosage recommended for heartworm prevention, and with ivermectin PO at 0.2 mg/kg. Milbemycin oxime at the minimum oral dosage of 2 mg/kg showed high therapeutic efficacy in cats infected with *T callipaeda*.

INFECTIOUS KERATOCONJUNCTIVITIS

(Pinkeye, Infectious ophthalmia)

Infectious keratoconjunctivitis of cattle, sheep, and goats is characterized by blepharospasm, conjunctivitis, lacrimation, and varying degrees of corneal opacity and ulceration.

Infectious bovine keratoconjunctivitis (IBK) is the most common ocular disease of cattle and is seen worldwide. The gram-negative rod *Moraxella bovis* is the only organism demonstrated to cause IBK in cattle. Seven different serogroups of *M bovis* are currently recognized. Most other ocular infections of cattle are characterized by conjunctivitis with minimal or no keratitis. The primary differential diagnosis is infectious bovine rhinotracheitis (IBR), which causes severe conjunctivitis and edema of the cornea that originates near the limbus; however, corneal ulceration is uncommon. *Mycoplasma* spp may cause conjunctivitis of cattle, either alone or in conjunction with *M bovis*. Infection with IBR virus or other microbes may increase the severity of infection with *M bovis*. Another *Moraxella* species that has been frequently isolated from eyes of cattle with IBK is *Moraxella bovoculi* (not to be confused with *Mycoplasma bovoculi*). Recent studies do not support a role for *Moraxella bovoculi* as a primary pathogen in causing corneal ulceration associated with IBK. It is likely that *Moraxella bovoculi* may act as a risk factor for IBK by causing conjunctivities similar to other risk factors for infectious agents such as *Mycoplasma* spp and IBR virus. *Moraxella bovoculi* has also been reported in cases of infectious keratoconjunctivitis in reindeer. Plant awns, face flies, ultraviolet radiation from bright

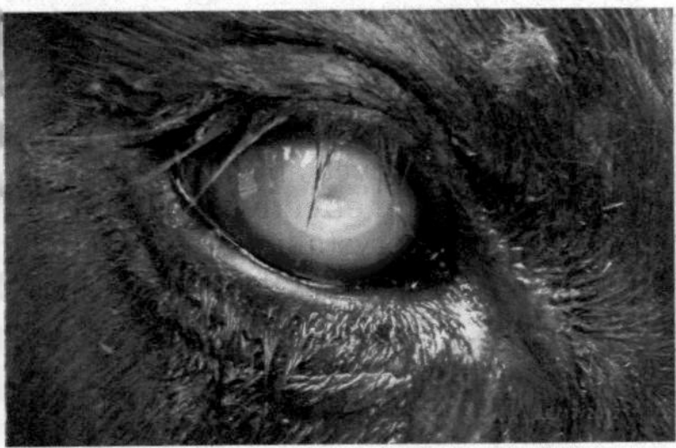

Infectious bovine keratoconjunctivitis with corneal ulceration in a calf. Note severe corneal edema (opacity), corneal neovascularization, and epiphora. *Courtesy of Dr. John A. Angelos.*

sunlight, dry and dusty environmental conditions, and shipping stress are all risk factors associated with IBK in cattle. In cattle, additional risk factors that should be considered when making herd management decisions include trace mineral deficiencies such as selenium and copper deficiency. Flies can also serve as vectors for *M bovis*.

In sheep and goats, naturally occurring conjunctivitis or keratoconjunctivitis can be associated with *Chlamydia pecorum*, *Mycoplasma* spp (notably *M conjunctivae*), *Moraxella ovis*, *Colesiota conjunctivae*, *Listeria monocytogenes*, *Acholeplasma oculi*, and *Thelazia* spp.

Clinical Findings: The disease usually is acute and tends to spread rapidly. In all species, young animals are affected most frequently, but animals of any age are susceptible. One or both eyes may be affected. The earliest clinical signs are photophobia, blepharospasm, and epiphora; later, the ocular discharge may become mucopurulent. Conjunctivitis, with or without varying degrees of keratitis, is usually present. In sheep and goats, concurrent polyarthritis may be present in association with *C pecorum* infections. Appetite may be depressed because of ocular discomfort or visual disturbance that results in inability to locate food. The usual clinical course varies from a few days to several weeks. Most corneal ulcers in cattle with IBK heal without loss of vision; however, corneal rupture and permanent blindness can occur in the most severe cases.

Lesions: Lesions vary in severity. In cattle, one or more small ulcers typically develop near the center of the cornea. Initially, the cornea around the ulcer is clear, but within a few hours a faint haze appears that subsequently increases in opacity. Lesions may regress in the early stages or may continue to progress. After 48–72 hr in severe cases, the entire cornea may become opaque, blinding the animal in that eye. Blood vessels may invade the cornea from the limbus and move toward the ulcer at ~1 mm/day. Corneal opacity may result from edema (hazy white to blue corneas), which is a part of the inflammatory process, or leukocyte infiltration (milky white to yellow corneas), which indicates severe infection. Continued active ulceration may cause corneal rupture. Relapse may occur at any stage of recovery.

Diagnosis: In all species, presumptive diagnosis is based on ocular signs and concurrent systemic disease. It is important to distinguish that the lesions are not due to foreign bodies or parasites (*see* p 510). In IBR, upper respiratory signs and conjunctivitis predominate, while keratitis accompanied by ulceration is rare. In bovine malignant catarrhal fever, respiratory signs are prominent with primary uveitis and associated keratitis. Microbial culture may be beneficial in confirming the causative organisms. *Chlamydia* and *Mycoplasma* spp require special media; the diagnostic laboratory should be consulted before sample collection. Cytologic evaluation of stained slides prepared from conjunctival scrapings of sheep and goats may reveal *Chlamydia* organisms; however, intracytoplasmic inclusion bodies can be difficult to recognize. PCR analysis can be used to detect *Chlamydia* and *Mycoplasma* spp.

Prevention and Treatment: Good management practices are of paramount importance to reduce or prevent spread of infection in cattle, sheep, and goats. Separation of infected animals is beneficial when possible. Gloves and protective clothing should be worn and then disinfected between animals when affected individuals are being handled. Temporary isolation and preventive treatment of animals newly introduced to the herd may be helpful, because some of these animals may be asymptomatic carriers. Ultraviolet radiation from sunlight may enhance disease (particularly in cattle); therefore, affected animals should be provided with shade. Dust bags or insecticide-impregnated ear tags can be used to reduce the number of face flies (*Musca autumnalis*), an important vector for *M bovis*.

M bovis bacterins are available and can be administered before the beginning of fly season. Cattle should be started on *M bovis* vaccine series 6–8 wk before the anticipated first cases of IBK to allow time for adequate immune responses to develop. The efficacy of current commercially available *M bovis* bacterins is controversial and likely varies because of vaccinal versus outbreak strains of *M bovis* and varying degrees of cross-protection afforded by vaccination. Vaccination may reduce the severity and duration of infection in affected animals. IBR may predispose cattle to infection with *M bovis*; thus, vaccination of herds against IBR may reduce outbreaks of *M bovis*. The use of modified-live IBR vaccines has been associated with outbreaks of IBK in cattle; IBR vaccination must be appropriately timed with cattle shipments so that these events do not coincide. Vaccination of cattle with a modified-live IBR vaccine could likely exacerbate an outbreak of IBK associated with *M bovis* and/or *Moraxella bovoculi* because of increased ocular and nasal secretions spreading bacteria between herdmates as well as corneal epithelial damage. In recent studies, the efficacy of autogenous *Moraxella* spp bacterins to prevent IBK has not been demonstrated in randomized controlled field trials. Nevertheless, anecdotal evidence has suggested that, for some herds, *M bovis* and/or *Moraxella bovoculi* autogenous bacterins have provided benefit in reducing IBK problems. It is unlikely that any *Moraxella* spp vaccine will ever completely control IBK in the face of overwhelming challenge from and exposure to other risk factors such as flies, dust, other infectious agents, and trace mineral deficiencies. As such, planning and implementing a successful IBK control program should address multiple issues that may potentially reduce susceptibility of cattle to IBK beyond just vaccines against *Moraxella* spp.

M bovis is susceptible to many antibiotics. Because antibiotic susceptibility may vary in different geographic locations, bacterial culture and susceptibility testing is advised. One common treatment is bulbar conjunctival injection with penicillin. In the USA, long-acting oxytetracycline (two injections of 20 mg/kg, IM or SC, at a 48- to 72-hr interval) and tulathromycin (2.5 mg/kg, SC, given once) are currently approved antibiotics to treat IBK in cattle. Other effective antibiotics include ceftiofur crystalline free acid (6.6 mg/kg, SC, at the base of the ear) and florfenicol (20 mg/kg, IM, two doses at a 2-day interval). A single injection of long-acting oxytetracycline (20 mg/kg, IM) along with oral oxytetracycline (2 g/calf/day for 10 days) fed in alfalfa pellets has also been shown to be effective at reducing severity of IBK during a herd outbreak. Topical applications of ophthalmic preparations should be applied at least three times a day to be effective, and thus are often not cost-effective or practical in herd settings. Effective antibiotics for topical ophthalmic use include triple antibiotic, gentamicin, and a combination oxytetracycline/polymyxin B ointment. A third-eyelid flap or partial tarsorrhaphy, which will shade the cornea from sunlight, together with subconjunctival injection, may reduce morbidity in severely affected animals. A temporary eye patch glued to the hair surrounding the eye is an inexpensive and easily applied treatment. The eye patch provides shade, prevents exposure to flies, and may help to decrease spread of organisms.

For sheep and goats in which chlamydial and mycoplasmal infections are suspected, respectively, topical tetracycline, oxytetracycline/polymyxin B, or erythromycin ointments are treatments of choice. These preparations are all effective against *Chlamydia* or *Mycoplasma* and should be applied 3–4 times daily. If topical therapy is not practical, long-acting oxytetracycline (20 mg/kg, IM) or the addition of oxytetracycline to the feed (80 mg/animal/day) may be beneficial.

Animals with substantial uveitis secondary to keratoconjunctivitis that is particularly painful may benefit from topical ophthalmic application of 1% atropine ointment 1–3 times daily. This will prevent painful ciliary body spasms and reduce the likelihood of posterior synechia formation that occurs with miosis. Because of mydriasis caused by atropine, treated animals should be provided with shade. Systemic NSAID treatment may be used to provide relief from secondary uveitis.

NEOPLASIA OF THE EYE AND ASSOCIATED STRUCTURES

The different tissues of the eye and associated structures can be the site of primary or metastatic neoplasms. Ophthalmic neoplasms vary in histologic type, frequency, and importance in different species and are a significant group of diseases in veterinary ophthalmology.

CATTLE

The most frequent ophthalmic neoplasms in cattle are the squamous cell carcinoma complex and the orbital infiltration associated with lymphosarcoma (*see* p 743). The latter, with extensive invasion of the orbital structures, results in progressive bilateral exophthalmia, reduced ocular mobility, exposure keratitis, and corneal ulcerations that can lead to perforation.

Ocular squamous cell carcinoma (cancer eye) is the most common neoplasm of cattle. It results in significant economic loss due to condemnation at slaughter and a shortened productive life. It occurs more frequently in the *Bos taurus* than the *Bos indicus* breeds, and it is seen most often in Herefords, less often in Simmentals and Holstein-Friesians, and rarely in other breeds. The peak age of incidence is 8 yr; actual incidence varies from 0.8% to 5.0% among herds. The cause is multifactorial, with heritability, sunlight, nutrition, eyelid pigmentation, and perhaps viral involvement playing roles. The medial and lateral limbal regions (corneoscleral junction) are affected most frequently, but the eyelids, conjunctivae, and nictitating membrane may be affected. Bilateral involvement varies but can be as high as 35%. Eyelid and conjunctival pigmentation are highly heritable and can reduce the frequency of lid squamous cell carcinomas, but they have limited effect on the development of tumors of the conjunctiva and nictitating membrane. The cancerous or precancerous lesions are bilateral or multiple in the same eye in ~28% of cases. Ultraviolet radiation and a high plane of nutrition are contributing factors. The viruses of infectious bovine rhinotracheitis and papilloma have been isolated from the neoplasms, but their significance is unknown.

The lesions usually begin as benign, smooth, white plaques on the conjunctival surfaces; they may progress to a papilloma and then to a squamous cell carcinoma or go directly to the malignant stage. Lid lesions usually begin as either an ulcerative or a hyperkeratotic lesion (cutaneous horn). While in this benign stage, ~30% may spontaneously regress. The tumor may become quite large without invading the globe, but invasion into the eye and orbit and metastasis to parotid and submandibular lymph nodes occur in late stages of the disease. Diagnosis usually is made by the typical clinical appearance but can be confirmed rapidly by cytologic examination of impression smears. The intraocular tumor invasion must be differentiated from severely damaged and disorganized eyes after trauma or advanced infectious keratoconjunctivitis (*see* p 512).

Squamous cell carcinomas may respond to excision, cryotherapy, hyperthermia, radiation therapy, local chemotherapy using 5-fluorouracil, immunotherapy, or often a combination of these therapies. Surgical excision is indicated for small lesions or for debulking the larger lesions before cryotherapy or hyperthermia. Superficial keratectomy can be used to excise the limbal plaques, papillomas, and squamous cell carcinomas. After superficial keratectomy and tumor removal, cryotherapy, hyperthermia, or a permanent bulbar conjunctival graft have yielded excellent short-term results, but recurrence at the same or a different site is ~25%.

For advanced lesions confined to the globe, enucleation is recommended. When adjacent tissues are affected, removal of the globe and all orbital contents (exenteration) should be performed. Immunotherapy is

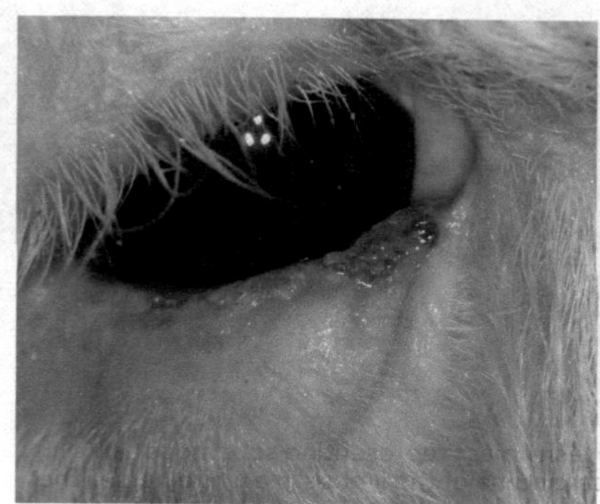

Squamous cell carcinoma, eyelid, cow. *Courtesy of K. Gelatt.*

still experimental, and the resulting tumor regression may be temporary. Radiation therapy is not practical in the field but may be an option for valuable animals.

Owners of problem herds should be advised of the heritability factor, with affected animals and their offspring culled to decrease the incidence of tumors. Active breeding bulls with ocular squamous cell carcinoma should be culled.

HORSES

In horses, tumors of the skin, eye, and genital system are the most frequent, and ~80% of eye neoplasms are malignant. Neoplasms of the eyelids and conjunctivae are the most frequent ophthalmic tumors in horses; most are either squamous cell carcinoma or sarcoid. Orbital neoplasms are rare and are usually local extensions of eyelid, conjunctiva, or sinus tumors or systemic neoplasms, including lymphosarcoma. Intraocular neoplasms, usually malignant melanomas, are rare.

Squamous cell carcinoma occurs most frequently in horses 8–10 yr old and may occur more frequently in those with non- or lightly pigmented eyelids. The Appaloosa and draft breeds are affected most frequently. Ultraviolet radiation may be important, because the incidence in North America is higher in southern and western mountainous areas and in areas of increased altitude or mean solar radiation. The eyelids (~15%), conjunctivae and limbus (~25%), and nictitating membrane (~30%) can be affected with ulcerative or proliferative masses. Bilateral involvement is infrequent (~15%). Squamous cell carcinoma of the nictitans is more likely to invade the orbit than are those from other sites. Treatment of ocular squamous cell carcinoma in horses is similar to that in cattle, although presentation for treatment is usually earlier, and greater emphasis is placed on cosmetic appearance after therapy. Surgical excision for equine squamous cell carcinoma yields ~50% success when used alone. When surgery is combined with cryotherapy, hyperthermia, or local chemotherapy, the success rate is markedly increased. As expected, small squamous cell carcinomas can be excised more widely, and the need for later reconstructive blepharoplasties or corneoconjunctival surgeries is more limited. Often, referral to specialty services that routinely treat these types of neoplasms can yield the best possible outcomes. The preventive role of face shields or masks with the goal of reduced ultraviolet exposure to the external eye is unknown, but their use should start at a very young age.

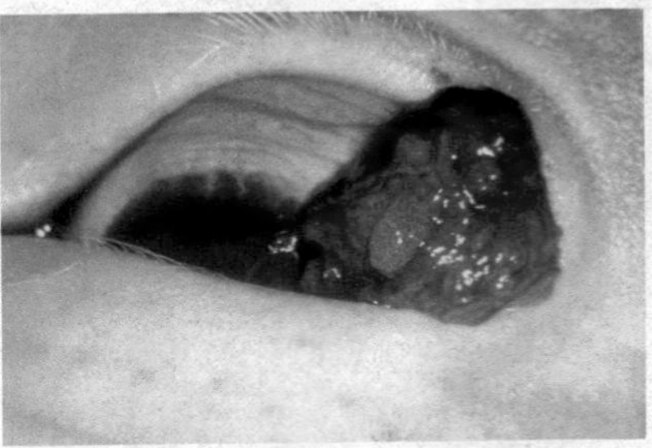

Fleshy mass representing squamous cell carcinoma of the limbus in a white horse. The area should be closely examined, because this mass often can be removed by keratectomy and covered by a permanent advancing bulbar conjunctival graft. *Courtesy of K. Gelatt.*

The equine sarcoid (*see* p 954) generally affects young horses (average 3.8 yr old) and represents ~40% of all neoplasms in horses. Because sarcoids are locally destructive and have a high recurrence rate after surgery, effective treatment when the periocular tissues are involved presents cosmetic and functional problems. Sarcoids are grouped into occult, verrucose, nodular, fibroblastic, mixed, and malignant types, and they are divided histologically into neurofibroma, neurofibrosarcoma, myxosarcoma, and fibromyxosarcoma. They appear initially as subcutaneous masses in the eyelids or canthi; they usually enlarge rapidly and may invade the skin, appearing as red, fleshy masses. Treatment is surgery, hyperthermia, cryotherapy, chemotherapy, radiation, or a combination of these therapies. After attempts to surgically remove the sarcoid, recurrence may be rapid and precede wound healing. Immunotherapy using BCG (bacille Calmette-Guérin) as a potentiator of the cellular immune system is often successful (~70%). Injections should be repeated at 2- to 4-wk intervals until the mass disappears. Systemic corticosteroids and antiprostaglandins before and after treatment may decrease the likelihood of systemic anaphylactic reactions. Gamma radiation therapy using platinum-sheathed iridium^{192} is highly successful (~95%) but less convenient and available and usually requires a total dose of 7,000–9,000 rads.

DOGS

Eyelid neoplasms are the most frequent group of ophthalmic neoplasms in dogs. Adenoma and adenocarcinoma of the meibomian gland are the most common lid neoplasms (~60%) in older dogs; local disfigurement and irritation necessitate excision, which is usually successful. Meibomian (sebaceous) adenocarcinomas are locally invasive and histologically malignant but are not known to metastasize. Lid melanomas, exhibited as spreading pigmented masses on the eyelid margin or a mass within the lid, should be widely excised. Other frequent eyelid neoplasms include histiocytoma, mastocytoma, and papilloma and may require biopsy to determine the best mode of therapy and prognosis. The vast majority of canine eyelid neoplasms are treated successfully by only surgical excision.

Canine conjunctival neoplasms have a greater propensity for maligancy and local infiltration than eyelid neoplasms and require more extensive surgical excision. Because recurrence may occur, periodic reexaminations are recommended.

Orbital neoplasms in dogs produce exophthalmia, conjunctival and eyelid swelling, strabismus, and exposure keratitis. The globe cannot be retropulsed. Usually, there is no pain. Because ~90% of the neoplasms are malignant and ~75% arise within the orbit, the prognosis for longterm survival is often poor. The most frequently diagnosed tumors include osteosarcomas, fibrosarcomas, and nasal adenocarcinomas. The neoplasm type should be determined histologically, and the extent of the mass determined by physical examination, skull radiographs (including special contrast procedures, CT, and MRI), and ultrasonography before treatment by surgical excision or radiation. Excision of the orbital mass with the globe and all orbital tissues (including adjacent bone) may decrease the possibility of recurrence but is more disfiguring, especially in shorthaired dogs. Prognosis is guarded or poor; 25%–40% of affected dogs are euthanized on diagnosis. Surgery, sometimes combined with chemotherapy, can often prolong life for ≥6 mo.

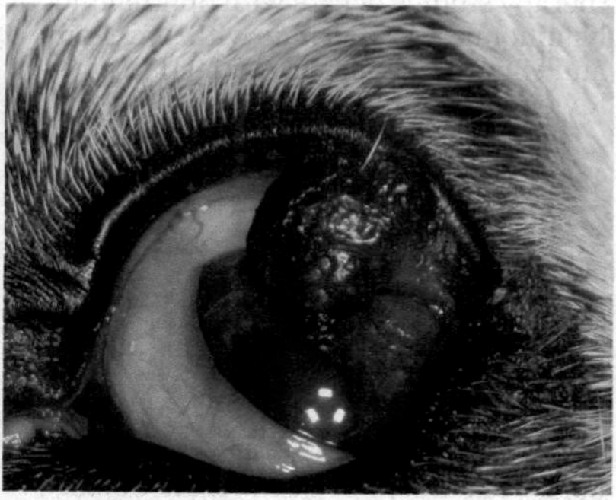

Lid masses in dogs are mostly adenomas or adencarcinomas that arise from the meibomian glands. Surgical excision is usually effective, with infrequent recurrence. *Courtesy of K. Gelatt.*

Corneal and limbal neoplasms are uncommon in dogs and can be confused with nodular fasciitis and proliferative keratoconjunctivitis in Collies. Biopsy is often necessary to establish the diagnosis and the specific plan for the best therapy. Limbal or epibulbar malignant melanomas are focal, usually superficial, pigmented masses that extend both onto the cornea and caudally toward the globe's equator. After close intraocular examination (including gonioscopy and B-scan ultrasonography) to detect possible penetration of the sclera, partial to full-thickness surgical excision with scleral grafts, cryotherapy, or laser photocoagulation is usually successful. If intraocular extension occurs, enucleation is performed.

Melanomas are the most common uveal neoplasm, are usually pigmented, and most frequently involve the iris and ciliary body, with the latter being the site of origin. Choroidal melanomas, common in people, are rare in dogs. Clinical signs of anterior uveal melanomas may include an obvious mass, persistent iridocyclitis, hyphema, glaucoma, and pain. These melanomas are divided into melanocytic melanomas (80%–90%) and malignant melanomas (10%–15%). Metastasis is infrequent (<5%). Ciliary body adenoma and adenocarcinoma are the most frequent epithelial neoplasms of the anterior uvea. Signs may include hyphema, glaucoma, and usually a nonpigmented mass behind the iris and in the pupil. Neoplasms of neuroectodermal origin are rare. Treatment is usually enucleation. Recent studies in iridal melanomas, especially in young Labrador Retrievers, suggest that noninvasive diode laser photocoagulation may be effective and can be repeated if necessary, thereby avoiding enucleation.

Secondary uveal adenocarcinomas are relatively infrequent and originate from a number of distant sites. Other neoplasms, such as transmissible venereal tumor and hemangiosarcoma, may metastasize to the anterior uvea. Lymphosarcoma frequently involves the anterior uvea and other ocular structures and may present as bilateral disease. Systemic therapy with topical and/or systemic anti-inflammatory treatment for intraocular lymphoma may be attempted using one of several available lymphoma protocols (eg, combination of cyclophosphamide, prednisolone, vincristine, and/or doxorubicin), but dogs with both intraocular and systemic lymphoma have shorter survival times.

CATS

Ocular neoplasms are less frequent in cats than in dogs and tend to be more malignant. Approximately 2% of feline patients present with neoplasia, and of these, 2% are affected with ophthalmic tumors. Eyelid and conjunctival tumors are the most frequent primary ophthalmic neoplasms. These neoplasms are usually malignant and more difficult to treat in cats than in dogs. Squamous cell carcinomas, which are more common in white cats with nonpigmented eyelid margins, can involve the eyelids, conjunctivae, and the nictitating membrane; they are pink, roughened, irregular masses or thickened ulcerations. Other less frequent neoplasms include adenocarcinomas, fibrosarcomas, neurofibrosarcomas, and basal cell carcinomas. Treatment varies with the tumor type, location, and size and includes surgical excision, radiation therapy, and cryotherapy. Prognosis for these malignant tumors is poor, with survival of only 1–2 mo.

The most common primary intraocular neoplasm in cats is diffuse iridal melanoma, which presents as progressive hyperpigmentation of the iris with an expanding irregular surface. Pupillary abnormalities, secondary glaucoma due to iridocorneal angle obstruction, and buphthalmia occur late in the disease. Enucleation is recommended for masses that are fast-growing or produce pupillary abnormalities, iridocorneal angle involvement, and/or glaucoma, because metastasis is frequent in advanced cases.

Post-traumatic intraocular sarcoma occurs in older cats with a history of chronic uveitis, previous intraocular damage, or intraocular injections of gentamicin. Clinical signs are either glaucoma, phthisis bulbi, or chronic uveitis. Intraocular cartilage and osteoid production is common. Early enucleation is recommended.

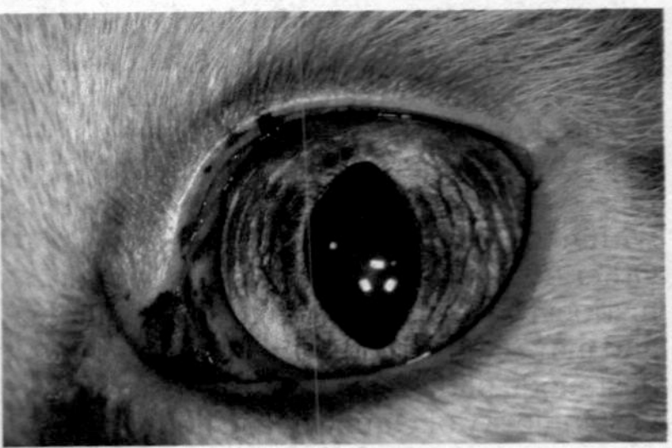

Diffuse iridal melanoma in a cat, with progressive pigmentation of the anterior surface of the iris. *Courtesy of K. Gelatt.*

Feline lymphosarcoma-leukemia complex (FeLLC) is the most common secondary ocular neoplasm. Cats with ocular FeLLC have clinical signs ranging from isolated ocular lesions (affecting one or both eyes) to severe systemic illness. Corneal abnormalities may include keratitis, edema, neovascularization, corneal infiltrates, and hemorrhages within the stroma. Ulcerative keratitis may result. Masses can be found in the orbit, globe, conjunctivae, and eyelids. Pupillary abnormalities, including mydriasis, anisocoria, spastic pupil syndrome, "D" or reverse "D" pupil shape, and lack of light-induced pupillary reflexes, may develop months before other clinical signs. Anterior uveitis is the most common clinical finding in FeLLC. Other findings include ocular hypotension, changes in iridal pigmentation and color, keratic precipitates, hyphema, anterior and posterior synechiae, miosis, and aqueous flare. Posterior segment changes include retinal hemorrhages, tortuous dilated vessels, perivascular cuffing, and detachment and degeneration of the retina. Few therapy studies of cats with ophthalmic lymphoma exist, but cats with lymphoma and feline leukemia virus infection have lower overall survival times.

DEAFNESS

Deafness—the absence of perception of sound—and reduced hearing are common in dogs and cats, and to a lesser extent in other species. Deafness can be hereditary or acquired, and sensorineural or conductive.

Hereditary deafness can be cochleosaccular or neuroepithelial in origin. Cochleosaccular deafness is usually seen in dogs with the piebald or merle genes and in cats with white coat color. It produces deafness in one or both ears and is often associated with blue eyes and white pigmentation. Pigment-associated deafness also occurs in equine, bovine, porcine, and other species. This is the most common cause of deafness in dogs and cats and should be the first differential diagnosis considered in an animal with any white pigmentation. The condition develops within 1–3 wk after birth secondary to stria vascularis degeneration that results from the suppression of melanocytes by the pigment gene, leading to cochleosaccular neuronal degeneration. Unilaterally deaf animals may go undetected without brain stem auditory evoked response (BAER) testing but will pass on an increased deafness risk to offspring if bred; inheritance does not appear to be simple autosomal. Neuroepithelial deafness is not associated with pigment patterns, is usually bilateral, and results from primary hair cell loss over the same time course as cochleosaccular deafness; vestibular signs may also be present (eg, in Doberman Pinschers).

Congenital deafness (usually hereditary) has been reported in ~100 dog breeds and is especially prevalent in the piebald-carrying breeds of Dalmatian, Bull Terrier, Australian Cattle Dog, English Setter, English Cocker Spaniel, Boston Terrier, and Parson Russell Terrier, and in the different merle-carrying breeds. The prevalence of deafness in white cats (dominant white gene), especially those with blue eyes, is high, but blue-eyed cats from Siamese breeds do not appear to be affected. No DNA testing is currently available to identify carriers of genetic deafness in dogs or cats, so BAER testing and selective breeding are the only available options to reduce prevalence within breeds. A late-onset form of genetic neuroepithelial deafness may exist in Rhodesian Ridgebacks.

Conduction deafness results from obstruction or reduction of sound reaching the cochlea, usually from otitis media (*see* p 531), chronic otitis externa (*see* p 527), or excess cerumen, and less commonly from tympanum rupture or ossicle damage. Resolution of the obstruction or tissue damage usually restores hearing. Recovery after otitis media may require weeks while the body phagocytizes the infection residue, accompanied by progressive recovery of hearing. Primary secretory otitis media (glue ear), especially in Cavalier King Charles Spaniels, produces a persistent conductive deafness that may be treated by myringotomy, bulla osteotomy, or tympanostomy tubes.

Sensorineural deafness results from loss of cochlear nerve cells and is not reversible in mammalian species. Acquired sensorineural deafness may result from intrauterine infection or toxins, otitis interna or meningitis, mechanical or noise trauma, ototoxicity, anesthesia, neoplasms, or aging (presbycusis). Loss can be bilateral or unilateral, and partial or complete. Otitis interna (*see* p 531) will frequently be accompanied by vestibular signs such as head tilt and circling. Hunting or military dogs exposed to loud percussive sounds such as gunfire experience cumulative losses that may initially go unnoticed. This is often observed in hunting dogs, in which the distance at which a trained dog responds to commands shrinks by half or more.

A variety of drugs and chemicals are ototoxic and vestibulotoxic, especially the aminoglycoside antibiotics (gentamicin, amikacin), antineoplastic drugs (cisplatin), salicylates, diuretics (ethacrynic acid, furosemide), and antiseptics (chlorhexidine). The toxicity is permanent. Aminoglycoside toxicity, the most common, functions through reactive oxygen species, and human studies have shown that coadministration with aspirin or N-acetylcysteine ameliorates the toxicity; it is unknown if postexposure treatment is of value. High frequencies are affected first, slowing recognition of the toxicity, which may appear at a delay of weeks after treatment has been discontinued. Dogs or cats undergoing general anesthesia for teeth or ear cleaning occasionally awaken bilaterally deaf, but the mechanisms, which can be conductive or sensorineural, are unknown. Few reports have been seen for procedures on body regions other than mouth and ear, and no unilateral deafness from anesthetic procedures has been reported.

Many geriatric animals develop **presbycusis**. Mid to high frequencies are affected first, followed by progressive loss at all frequencies. The loss may appear to be acute in onset but reflects the animal's eventual inability to compensate for the progressive loss that had been developing for some time. There does not appear to be a gender difference in prevalence. Onset is typically in the last third of a breed's typical lifespan and will progress to complete deafness if the animal lives long enough.

Unilaterally deaf animals show negligible signs, primarily an inability to localize sound origins and orienting toward the good ear, but many compensate and show no signs. Bilateral orienting pinnae movements persist in unilaterally deaf animals. Bilaterally deaf animals do not respond to sound stimuli but become adept at increased attention to other sensations such as vision and vibration. Affected animals "key" off the behavior of littermates or other household pets. Breeders of breeds with high prevalence often choose to euthanize bilaterally deaf (and spay/neuter unilaterally deaf) animals because of a frequent outcome of poor quality of life and liabilities from owning a deaf dog, such as startle biting. Bilaterally deaf dogs can be successfully raised, but more dedication than normal is required. Owners of deaf dogs should be counseled to protect their pets against undetected dangers such as motor vehicles.

Dogs that lose hearing later in life appear to cope well but on occasion exhibit transient behavior suggestive of auditory sensations similar to subjective tinnitus in people. There is no evidence that deaf animals otherwise experience pain or discomfort from the condition.

Identification of deafness is most accurate with BAER testing at referral centers, but behavioral testing is typically used in the clinic. Observations are made for a response to a sound stimulus outside the animal's visual field. Limitations include the inability to identify unilateral deafness, stimulus detection through other senses, blunted responses in stressed animals, and failed responses from expired novelty of a repeated stimulus. Failure of a sleeping animal to waken to an auditory stimulus that does not activate other senses is a reliable indicator of bilateral deafness in the home environment.

Otoscopic examination of the external ear and tympanum, radiography of the tympanic bullae, and neurologic examination may reveal the cause, especially in conduction deafness, which usually responds to appropriate medical or surgical treatment. Early intervention in ototoxicity may reduce or reverse loss but usually is not successful. Once developed, sensorineural deafness cannot be reversed, and its cause cannot be determined. Congenital deafness in breeds with white pigmentation is nearly always of genetic origin.

DISEASES OF THE PINNA

A variety of dermatologic conditions affect the pinna. Rarely, a disease affects the pinna alone or the pinna is the initial site affected. As with all dermatologic conditions, a diagnosis is best made with the results of a thorough history, a complete physical and dermatologic examination, and with careful selection and evaluation of specific diagnostic tests. This overview is not all inclusive but discusses diseases that solely or commonly affect the pinna of domestic animals.

ARTHROPOD BITE PINNAL DERMATITIS

Arthropods commonly cause dermatitis of the pinnae either through direct damage from the bite of the parasite or as a result of hypersensitivity. Ticks can cause irritation at the site of attachment and may be found on the pinna or in the ear canal. The spinous ear tick (*Otobius megnini*), found in the southwestern USA, south and central Americas, southern Africa, and India, is a soft-shelled tick, the larval and nymphal forms of which parasitize the external ear canal of horses, cattle, sheep, goats, deer, rabbits, cats, and dogs. Clinical signs include head shaking, head rubbing, or drooped pinnae. Both the animal and the environment should be treated. Treatment involves mechanical removal of as many ticks as possible with a forceps and spraying or dipping the coat with pyrethrin/pyrethroid products or malathion. Treatment of secondary bacterial or yeast otitis externa is also important. Precautions to prevent reinfestations should be instituted.

Gotch ear is a condition described in cattle, and also in a goat, that results from infestation of the pinna with the Gulf Coast tick, *Amblyomma maculatum*. Adult ticks prefer feeding on animal ears, and when ticks are present in sufficient numbers the pinna becomes edematous, erythematous, and crusting at the tick-attachment sites. Curling of the tip of the ear and excoriations may also be seen. Spotted fever group rickettsiae, such as *Rickettsia parkeri*, have been suggested to cause the skin lesions, because ticks removed from the pinna of animals with gotch have been, in some cases, positive for *Rickettsia* spp by PCR. However, efforts to find the organisms in skin samples from affected areas have failed. Removal of ticks and treatment of any secondary infection are curative.

INSECT BITE DERMATITIS

This worldwide problem is caused by inflammatory mediators or toxic substances present in the saliva of various hematophagous insects. It typically affects dogs, cats, and horses. Clinical signs are characterized by small papules and wheals with central hemorrhagic crusts that can progress to multiple small ulcers. Lesions are found on the apexes of the pinnae of cats and dogs with erect ears or on the folded surfaces of the pinnae of dogs with flopped ears. The causative insect can vary with the season and environment and include, among others, mosquitoes (*Aedes* spp, *Culex* spp), the stable fly (*Stomoxys calcitrans*), and black flies (*Simulium* spp). Mosquitoes can also cause a hypersensitivity reaction in cats characterized by inflammatory lesions on the pinnae, face, and feet (*see* below). The rabbit flea (*Spilopsyllus cuniculi*) is found mainly in Europe and Australia and can be transmitted to dogs and cats. It adheres tightly to the skin of the host and typically affects the tip of the pinna, where it may cause dermatitis. In horses, bites of the stable fly, black flies, and *Culicoides* spp can cause a hypersensitivity reaction or severe dermatitis that results in lesions on the dorsal and/or ventral trunk and face in addition to the pinna. Treatment includes fly repellents, controlling the fly population with environmental clean up (manure, compost, etc), and insecticides. Topical or oral short-acting glucocorticoids may be necessary to reduce the inflammation and pruritus in severe cases.

MITE INFESTATIONS

Sarcoptes scabiei is a common mange mite in pigs and dogs, and *Notoedres cati* is common in cats throughout the world (*see also* MANGE, p 914). In the USA, sarcoptic mange is rare in horses and sheep and is considered a reportable disease. Papular eruptions progress to scaling, crusting, and excoriations of the ear margins and other parts of the body. Pruritus is severe. Transmission is by direct contact with infected animals or contaminated fomites. Diagnosis is based on clinical signs, history, and discovery of mites from multiple skin scrapings. Negative scrapings do not exclude the diagnosis, however, because mites are often difficult to find. If the diagnosis is suspected, treatment should be instituted. Mites are much easier to find on skin scrapings of cats with notoedric acariasis. Treatment options include 2%–4% lime sulfur dips (safe in all species) every 5 days for 4–6 treatments, amitraz dips at a strength of 250 ppm (in dogs only) applied weekly for 4 to 6 treatments, and ivermectin at 200–300 mcg/kg, PO or SC, every 1–2 wk for 3–4 treatments. Treatment response is not consistent when using lime sulfur dips or amitraz in small animals; therefore, these topicals are not good options for a treatment trial (ie, mites are not found on skin scrapings). Oral milbemycin oxime has been reported to be safe and effective in the treatment of sarcoptic mange in dogs but is not FDA approved for this purpose. The recommended treatment protocol is 2 mg/kg once weekly for 4 to 6 treatments or twice weekly for 3 wk. Selamectin, also extra-label, has also shown efficacy; the recommended protocol is four applications at 2-wk intervals. Moreover, imidacloprid 10%/moxidectin 2.5% spot-on applied twice at a 30-day interval or every 3 wk for three treatments has been shown to be efficacious. There are also anecdotal reports of efficacy of these treatment modalities for treatment of notoedric mange in cats. Because mites can survive off the host for a variable amount of time, all bedding, brushes, tack, and fomites should be treated as well. All in-contact animals also should be treated because of the contagious nature of these acarioses.

Ivermectin is widely used to treat sarcoptic mange in dogs and has been used to treat notoedric mange in cats, but it is not approved by the FDA for these indications. Therefore, every caution should be taken, and clients specifically informed of inherent risks with this drug. Dog breeds susceptible to ivermectin toxicity include Collies, Shetland Sheepdogs, Australian Shepherds, English Shepherds, Longhaired Whippets, McNabs, Silken Windhounds, and Old English Sheepdogs. Before using ivermectin in any of these breeds, a genetic test for the mutation of the ABCB1 (formerly MDR1) gene, which encodes for the multidrug transporter P-glycoprotein, should be performed. (This test is available at the University of Washington.)

Nonburrowing psoroptic mites cause otitis externa in horses and goats. Animals may be asymptomatic or present with pruritus, head shaking, and a drooping ear. Crusted papules, alopecia, and/or scaling are typically present on the pinnae. Diagnosis is confirmed by finding the mites on skin scraping or in otic exudate, but mites may be difficult to find in the ear canal. Ivermectin at 200 mcg/kg, PO, every 2 wk for two treatments has been shown to be effective.

ALLERGY

Environmental-induced (eg, house dust, house dust mites, pollens of trees, grasses and weeds, molds) or food-induced **atopic dermatitis** are common allergic disorders of dogs and cats and frequently cause erythema and pruritus of the pinnae and external ear canals. The allergic condition predisposes to develop secondary bacterial or yeast otitis externa, which can extend to the pinna. In these cases, papules, crusts, and lichenification may develop in addition to the erythema. Other body sites such as the face (ie, periocular region, muzzle, chin), axilla, groin, and feet are also often affected. Diagnosis is based on a characteristic history, clinical signs, and the elimination of other pruritic skin diseases. A strict food elimination trial is important for animals with year-round clinical signs to determine whether food allergens are triggering the atopic signs. If food allergy is excluded or is only part of the allergic condition, intradermal or serologic allergy tests can be performed to support a presumptive diagnosis of environmental-induced atopic dermatitis and, more importantly, to institute allergen-specific immunotherapy. It is very important to identify and treat any secondary ear and skin bacterial or yeast infections, because they aggravate the allergic dermatitis. Treatment of food-induced atopic dermatitis consists of solely feeding the diet used during the food trial or avoiding food ingredients known to trigger the allergic reaction. Treatment of atopic dermatitis consists of using anti-inflammatory/immunomodulatory drugs, including oral short-acting glucocorticoids such as prednisone or prednisolone at 1 mg/kg/day and tapering to the lowest possible dosage administered every other day. Cyclosporine at 5 mg/kg/day can also be used in animals that cannot tolerate or do not respond well to glucocorticoid therapy. Omega-3 and/or omega-6 fatty acids can be used as adjunctive therapy. H_1-receptor antihistamines typically are not very efficacious to control the pruritus or inflammation associated with atopic dermatitis, but their safety profile and relatively low cost make them worthwhile to try. Allergen-specific immunotherapy based on intradermal or serologic test results is currently the only specific therapy for atopic dermatitis and should be considered as a treatment option.

Feline mosquito hypersensitivity is an allergic reaction to mosquito bites that can cause an ulcerative and crusted dermatitis of the pinnae, nose, and less commonly the footpads, eyelids, chin, and lips of cats. Lesions progress from wheals to papules to plaques to crusted ulcers that coalesce to affect extensive areas. Pruritus is a consistent sign, and regional lymphadenopathy may occur. In severe cases, fever or other systemic signs may develop. Histologically, the lesions are characterized by severe superficial and deep perivascular to interstitial eosinophilic dermatitis, often associated with flame figures, folliculitis, and furunculosis. Differential diagnoses include pemphigus foliaceus, herpesvirus ulcerative dermatitis, other causes of eosinophilic dermatitis (food allergy, atopy, idiopathic), notoedric mange, and dermatophytosis. Treatment includes keeping the cat inside and using a pyrethrin repellent (avoid permethrin-containing products in cats) when exposure to mosquitoes is anticipated. Systemic glucocorticoids may be necessary in severe cases. (*See also* MOSQUITOES, p 888.)

AURAL CONTACT DERMATITIS

Aural contact dermatitis commonly affects the concave aspect of the pinna, likely because it lacks hair. Topical ear medications, particularly those containing aminoglycosides and/or propylene glycol, are common causes in animals being treated for otitis externa. Lesions may develop 1–7 days after starting therapy. Contact dermatitis can also result from ointments applied transdermally to the concave aspect of the pinnae. Clinical signs include erythema, edema, papules that may coalesce and form plaques, erosions, and/or ulcerations. Pruritus and pain are variable. A definitive diagnosis can rarely be made, because drug challenge is not recommended. Discontinuation of all topical medications is the indicated treatment. Changing to a different topical drug is not recommended because most products have identical vehicles, which are the offending cause in most cases.

PINNAL ALOPECIA

Symmetrical noninflammatory alopecic disorders affecting the pinna, such as periodic pinnal alopecia, pattern baldness, and alopecia associated with melanoderma, may affect dogs and cats and are typically idiopathic.

Periodic pinnal alopecia in Miniature Poodles is characterized by progressive bilateral alopecia of the convex surfaces of the ear. The hair loss is acute in onset and progresses throughout several months, but hair may spontaneously regrow. There are no other clinical signs. A similar condition was reported in Siamese cats in which complete or patchy alopecia of the convex aspect of both pinna develops. Treatment is unnecessary.

Pattern baldness affecting only the pinna has been reported in Dachshunds, Chihuahuas, Italian Greyhounds, and Whippets and is thought to have a hereditary predisposition. The age of onset is ≤1 yr of age. Lesions start as thinning of the hair coat, and complete pinnal alopecia may occur by 8–9 yr of age. Other commonly affected areas are the ventral neck and thorax and the caudal medial thighs. The hair loss is asymptomatic. Histologically, the skin is normal, and hair follicles are diminished in size but normal in appearance. No effective treatment has been reported, but pentoxifylline (15–20 mg/kg, bid-tid), melatonin (3 mg for small breeds and 6 mg for large breeds, bid-tid), and topical minoxidil have anecdotally been described as helpful. Pattern baldness restricted to the pinna has also been reported in cats; however, use of minoxidil in cats should be avoided, because it has been associated with death in two cases.

Alopecia associated with melanoderma has been described mostly in Yorkshire Terriers and occasionally in Doberman Pinchers. Alopecia and marked hyperpigmentation (melanoderma) are first noticed between 6 mo and 3 yr of age and affect both pinna and the bridge of the nose. Other areas such as the tail and feet may also be affected. The alopecic and hyperpigmented skin has a smooth, shiny, and leathery appearance. The condition tends to worsen as the dog ages, and it typically does not spontaneously resolve. There is no treatment.

EAR MARGIN SEBORRHEA

This condition is common in Dachshunds, although other breeds with pendulous pinnae may be affected. Lesions usually affect the apex of the pinnae on both sides but can progress to involve the whole ear margin. The cause is unknown. Lesions appear as waxy, gray to yellow scales adherent to the base of hair shafts. Plugs of hair can be easily epilated, leaving behind a shiny surface to the skin. In severe cases, the ear margins are edematous and fissured. Histologic findings include severe hyperkeratosis and follicular keratosis with dilated follicles filled with keratin debris. Differential diagnoses include sarcoptic mange, pinnal alopecia, proliferative thrombovascular necrosis, dermatophytosis, and frostbite. Dermatophytosis, in particular, can cause a scaling pinnal dermatitis in dogs, cats, and horses, but the ear margin is not typically involved and other areas of the body are generally affected as well. Treatment includes antiseborrheic shampoos (eg, sulfur, salicylic acid, benzoyl peroxide), keratolytic products, dioctyl sodium sulfosuccinate (DSS), and systemic medications that may help normalize the abnormal keratinization process (eg, vitamin A and synthetic retinoids, essential fatty acids). Topical or oral glucocorticoids and pentoxifylline (10–15 mg/kg, bid-tid) may be beneficial when severe inflammation and fissures develop.

SEBACEOUS ADENITIS

Sebaceous adenitis is uncommon in dogs and rare in cats. The cause is unknown, but the strong predisposition of certain canine breeds suggests that genetics plays a role. The proposed pathogenesis includes cell-mediated immunologic destruction of the sebaceous gland; a primary cornification disorder of the glandular duct, resulting in obstruction and secondary inflammation of the gland; an anatomic defect of the sebaceous gland, leading to lipid leakage and a foreign body reaction; or an abnormal lipid metabolism, leading to glandular destruction. Predisposed breeds include Standard Poodles, Akitas, Samoyeds, Vizslas, Havanese, Springer Spaniels, and Lhasa Apsos; however, various other breeds can be affected. Lesions typically affect the pinnae, forehead, face, tail, and dorsal trunk and are characterized by alopecia and adherent scales that cast hair shafts. The severity and characteristics of clinical signs vary among breeds. Pruritus is variable and mostly associated with secondary bacterial infection. Histopathologic findings include diffuse absence of sebaceous glands, granulomatous to pyogranulomatous inflammation at the site of previous glands, and follicular keratosis. Currently, the most efficacious therapy for sebaceous adenitis is oral cyclosporine (5 mg/kg/day) in association with topical therapy. Oral vitamin A (1,000 IU/kg/day) or synthetic retinoids (eg, isotretinoin or acitretin) may be efficacious in some cases. The combination of tetracycline (250 mg, tid, for dogs <10 kg; 500 mg, tid, for dogs >10 kg) or doxycycline (5 mg/kg, bid) and niacinamine

(250 mg, tid, for dogs <10 kg; 500 mg, tid, for dogs >10 kg) is an option for milder cases or when owners are concerned about costs and/or adverse effects associated with cyclosporine or retinoids. Topical therapy in the form of medicated shampoos and emollient rinses or sprays should be used in conjunction with systemic therapy. Omega-3 and omega-6 fatty acids can also be used as adjunctive therapy. To help soften the adherent scales, a mixture of 70%–75% propylene glycol in water can be sprayed or used as a rinse on the animal's coat and allowed to act for 2–3 hr before bathing with a medicated shampoo. Another option is to apply baby oil soaks (undiluted or diluted with water 1:1) for 1–6 hr before bathing with a medicated shampoo.

AURICULAR HEMATOMAS

Auricular hematomas are small-to-large, fluid-filled swellings that develop on the concave surface of the pinnae in dogs, cats, and pigs. The pathogenesis for the development of the lesions is unknown, but head shaking or ear scratching due to pruritus is almost always involved. In dogs, the condition is seen with atopic dermatitis and food allergy in which the ear canals are the primary sites of allergic inflammation, pruritus, and secondary infection. In pigs, sarcoptic mange, pediculosis, and meal in the ears (from overhead feeders) have been implicated as a cause of head-shaking that has led to auricular hematomas. Bites from other pigs also may be at fault (*see* below). Treatment is surgical to allow drainage. After draining and flushing, several mattress sutures can be placed to eliminate the "pocket." The addition of a drain made out of a teat tube, piece of soft urinary catheter, or IV catheter increases the success rate of surgery. Drainage and glucocorticoid instillation are successful in ~50% of cases. Drainage is best obtained with a butterfly connection or an IV catheter. Glucocorticoids are instilled to fill the cavity without causing skin distention. A short course of a low anti-inflammatory dosage of oral glucocorticoids is commonly added to this treatment.

EQUINE AURAL PLAQUES

Equine aural plaques, also known as papillary acanthoma or ear papillomas, are caused by papillomavirus. Currently, four papillomaviruses have been isolated from aural plaques. Black flies (*Simulium* spp) are likely the mechanical vector. The flies are active at dawn and dusk, when they attack the head, ears, and ventral abdomen of horses. Clinically, the lesions are characterized by depigmented, hyperkeratotic, coalescing papules and plaques localized to the concave aspect of the pinna. Often, both pinnae are affected. Lesions are usually asymptomatic, but in some cases the fly bite itself causes dermatitis and discomfort. Histologically, the lesions are characterized by mild papillated epidermal hyperplasia and marked hyperkeratosis. Increased size of keratohyalin granules, koilocytosis, and hypomelanosis may also be present in the epidermis. Intranuclear viral particles have been seen in electron microscope studies. Various treatments have been anecdotally tried, with minimal to no response. A recent, open-label pilot study showed that imiquimod cream is effective in the treatment of aural plaques; however, the severe inflammation induced by the drug makes this treatment difficult to use, with most horses requiring sedation. The recommended protocol consists of applying imiquimod 2–3 times weekly (nonconsecutive days) every other week. Frequent applications of fly repellent and stabling the horse during the fly's feeding times are important measures to reduce discomfort and prevent recurrence. Lesions typically do not regress spontaneously.

NECROTIC EAR SYNDROME IN SWINE

(Ear necrosis, Necrotic auricular dermatitis)

Pigs with necrotic ear syndrome have unilateral or bilateral necrosis of the pinnae, are unthrifty, and commonly develop septic arthritis or die from secondary bacterial septicemia. The condition occurs sporadically in weaned and growing pigs under all management systems, particularly when challenged with endemic diseases that may influence feed intake.

Etiology, Transmission, and Pathogenesis: The causes have not been determined conclusively. Circumstantial evidence strongly suggests that necrotic ear syndrome is due to trauma (fighting) and subsequent bacterial invasion of the damaged tissue. Another potential factor that may contribute to the problem is inadequate dietary lysine levels in the feed, although no scientific data exist to prove this assumption.

Histologic and microbiologic findings suggest that the aggressive, erosive to ulcerative lesion is due to secondary bacterial infection. In the early phases of the disease, large numbers of *Staphylococcus hyicus* and low to moderate numbers of β-hemolytic streptococci are found in the surface exudate; later, during the ulcerative and necrotic stage, large numbers of the streptococci are found deep in the lesion. It is hypothesized that *S hyicus* colonizes the traumatized tissue, which prepares the way for the highly invasive streptococci that induce the changes that lead to ulceration and necrosis. Efforts to reproduce the disease by experimental inoculation of the two organisms have been unsuccessful. Spirochetes have also been found in skin samples from ear lesions using silver stain, and *Treponema* spp were amplified and sequenced from DNA prepared from ear lesion scrapings and broth cultures. However, the primary role of spirochetes in causing ear necrosis in pigs is unknown at this time. Moreover, porcine circovirus type 2 infection may contribute to ear necrosis, because controlling the infection through systematic vaccination has been reported to reduce the frequency of ear necrosis on farms.

Clinical Findings, Lesions, and Diagnosis: The nature and extent of clinical signs depend on the severity of the local lesion and development of secondary bacterial septicemia. Thus, a spectrum of signs, including unthriftiness, anorexia, fever, septic arthritis, collapse, and death, may be seen.

Mild lesions consist of superficial scratches covered with thin, dry, brown crusts. Mild edema or erythema may be present near the scratches. In more severe cases, thick, brown, moist crusts cover deep ulcers. In the most severe cases, there is extensive necrosis. The lesions evolve from mild, superficial dermatitis to severe, deep inflammation with exudation, ulceration, thrombosis, and necrosis. In mild cases, resolution occurs with no loss of ear tissue; in severe cases, the margins, tips, or even the entire pinna may be lost.

Diagnosis is made based on the appearance of the affected ears.

Management and Control: Tincture of iodine, applied topically bid for 1 wk, has reduced the incidence and severity of the disease. Antibacterial drugs administered in the feed are effective in some herds but not in others. Lack of effectiveness could be due to drug resistance. In cases of antibacterial ineffectiveness, specimens should be collected aseptically from the deep aspect of the ulcerative lesions for culture and sensitivity testing. Traumatizing events should be minimized. Management practices (ventilation, location and functioning of waterers, pen design, group size, mixing) and proper levels of dietary lysine should be checked and corrected if deficiencies are detected. Proper immunization against porcine circovirus type 2 is important to reduce the frequency of ear necrosis on farms.

MISCELLANEOUS DISEASES OF THE PINNA

Several immune-mediated diseases such as **pemphigus foliaceus, pemphigus erythematosus, drug eruption, toxic epidermal necrolysis**, and **immune-mediated vasculitis** may affect the pinna and the ear canal. (*See also* AUTOIMMUNE SKIN DISORDERS, p 827.) Other areas of the body are typically affected and may include footpads, mucous membranes, mucocutaneous junctions, nails and nail beds, and the tip of the tail. Immune-mediated diseases are confirmed with biopsy of primary lesions (papules, vesicles, pustules, erythematous margins of secondary lesions) and histologic evaluation by a dermatohistopathologist.

Folded ear tips in cats are most often associated with longterm glucocorticoid therapy (eg, daily eye or otic preparations). They may also be caused by solar radiation damage. Ear folding may not be reversible.

Feline solar dermatitis or actinic dermatitis is seen most commonly in white cats or cats with white pinnae that have been chronically exposed to sun. Lesions first appear as erythema and scaling on the sparsely haired tips of the ears. Crusting, exudation, and ulceration may develop as the actinic keratosis undergoes transformation into a squamous cell carcinoma. During early stages of the disease, treatment consists of limiting exposure to ultraviolet light through confinement indoors between the hours of 10 AM and 4 PM and the use of topical sunscreens. Squamous cell carcinoma of the pinnae is treated with surgical excision followed by radiation therapy. If surgery and radiation therapy are not an option, topical treatment with imiquimod cream 2–3 times weekly has shown promising results.

Feline proliferative and necrotizing otitis externa is a rare disease of unknown cause. It can affect cats from 2 mo to 12 yr of age, with most cases occurring at 4 yr of age. No breed predilection has been reported, but males appear to be overrepresented. It most commonly affects the concave aspect of the pinna and external aural orifice, but it can extend into the ear canal. The preauricular, periocular, and perioral regions may also be affected. Lesions are characterized by thick hyperkeratotic crusts covering erythematous plaques that may erode or ulcerate. Secondary bacterial and yeast infections may aggravate the condition. Most cats appear indifferent to the lesions, but mild pruritus and discomfort may be present when ulceration develops. Diagnosis is confirmed by the histopathologic findings, which are characterized by epidermal hyperplasia associated with scattered apoptotic-appearing keratinocytes that extend to the superficial follicular epithelium. Parakeratotic hyperkeratosis is also a feature. Spontaneous resolution has been reported to occur in some cases but only after 12–24 mo. Therapy with topical tacrolimus or oral cyclosporine at 5 mg/kg/day is reported to be efficacious.

Proliferative thrombovascular necrosis of the pinnae is rare in dogs. There are no known breed, sex, or age predilections, and the cause is unknown. Lesions, which consist of scaly, thickened, hyperpigmented skin surrounding a necrotic ulcer, begin at the apex of the ear and spread along the concave surface. Eventually, necrosis may deform the margin of the pinna. Pentoxifylline (15–20 mg/kg, bid-tid) and/or the combination of tetracycline (250 mg tid for dogs <10 kg; 500 mg tid for dogs >10 kg) or doxycycline (5 mg/kg bid) and niacinamine (250 mg tid for dogs <10 kg; 500 mg tid for dogs >10 kg) have been anecdotally reported to be efficacious in some cases. Topical glucocorticoids are also an option but must be used carefully because of their atrophogenic effects. If medical therapy has failed, surgical removal of diseased tissue should be considered.

Auricular chondritis has been reported rarely in cats and dogs. Clinical signs include pain, swelling, erythema, and deformation of the pinnae. Both ears are typically affected. Systemic signs may accompany some cases, and involvement of other organs such as the joints, eyes, and heart has been reported. Histologically, lesions consist of lymphoplasmacytic infiltrates, basophilia, and loss or necrosis of cartilage. Treatment may not be required if the condition is nonpainful and no systemic signs are present. Oral glucocorticoids have been reported to be ineffective, but dapsone (1 mg/kg/day) has induced remission in some cases. Permanent deformity of the pinnae is to be expected whether or not treatment has been instituted.

Vasculitis is an uncommon disorder of dogs and cats. Lesions consist of purpura, erythema, well-demarcated ulcers, crusts, and sloughing of necrotic tissue. The pinnae, tail, and footpads are typically affected. It is usually difficult to determine the triggering cause, which may be immune-mediated, drug-induced, a concurrent infection, neoplasia, or idiopathic. Differential diagnoses include fight wounds, cold agglutinin diseases, frostbite, and coagulopathies. Treatment involves identifying and eliminating the inciting cause and administering oral, short-acting glucocorticoids (such as prednisone/prednisolone at 1–2 mg/kg/day, then tapering to the lowest possible dose administered every other day), tetracycline (250 mg tid for dogs <10 kg; 500 mg tid for dogs >10 kg) or doxycycline (5 mg/kg bid) and niacinamine (250 mg tid for dogs <10 kg; 500 mg tid for dogs >10 kg), pentoxifylline (15–20 mg/kg, bid-tid), and cyclosporine (5 mg/kg/day) or other immunomodulating drugs.

Frostbite may occur in animals poorly adapted to cold climates and is more likely in wet or windy conditions. It typically affects poorly insulated body regions, including the tips of the ears, feet, and tail. The skin may be pale or erythematous, edematous, and painful. In severe cases, necrosis and sloughing of the ear tips may follow. Treatment consists of rapid, gentle warming and supportive care. Amputation of affected regions may be required but should be delayed until the extent of viable tissue is determined, which may take some time.

Canine juvenile cellulitis is an uncommon disorder of puppies and is characterized by sterile papules, nodules, and pustules on the face and pinnae, in addition to submandibular lymphadenopathy. It is seen in puppies 3 wk to 4 mo old and rarely in older animals. Golden Retrievers, Gordon Setters, and Dachshunds appear to be at greater risk than other breeds. A purulent otitis externa is common, along with edematous, thickened pinnae. Systemic signs such as anorexia, lethargy, and fever may be present in some cases. The diagnosis can be confirmed by biopsy, which shows a pyogranulomatous inflammatory infiltrate with no microorganisms, and by negative bacteriologic culture. Early treatment is recommended to avoid scarring. Prednisone or prednisolone (2 mg/kg, PO, divided bid) should be tapered slowly throughout 4–6 wk or until the disease is inactive. Antibiotics may be needed to treat secondary bacterial infection. Cyclosporine at 10 mg/kg/day has been reported to be effective in a case refractory to glucocorticoid therapy.

Canine sterile nodular granulomatous dermatitis of the pinna is a rare condition reported only anecdotally to date. Currently, existence of an age predilection is unknown, and Great Danes and Rottweilers appear to be overrepresented. Clinical signs are characterized by multiple nodules that tend to coalesce and are primarily localized to the ear margin. Loose to adhered scales typically cover the nodules. Histopathology shows multiple dermal nodules composed primarily of histiocytes. Leishmaniasis (*see* p 800) is an important differential diagnosis in endemic areas. Other sterile nodular diseases that need to be excluded are sterile granuloma and pyogranuloma disease and cutaneous reactive histiocytosis; however, other body sites are commonly affected in these diseases. Cases typically respond to oral glucocorticoids (eg, prednisone/prednisolone 1–2 mg/kg/day until remission then tapered) or cyclosporine (5 mg/kg/day); however, more conservative treatments, such as topical glucocorticoid (0.01% flucinolone acetonide plus 60% DMSO) and tetracycline (250 mg tid for dogs <10 kg; 500 mg tid for dogs >10 kg) or doxycycline (5 mg/kg bid) combined with niacinamine (250 mg tid for dogs <10 kg; 500 mg tid for dogs >10 kg), have been efficacious in some cases. Once the disease is in remission, a maintenance treatment regimen must be instituted.

OTITIS EXTERNA

Otitis externa is inflammation of the external ear canal distal to the tympanic membrane; the ear pinna may or may not be involved. It may be acute or chronic and unilateral or bilateral. It is one of the most common reasons for small animals to be presented to the veterinarian. Clinical signs can include any combination of headshaking, odor, pain on manipulation of the ear, exudate, and erythema. It can be seen in rabbits (in which it is usually due to the mite *Psoroptes cuniculi*) and is uncommon in large animals.

Etiology and Classification System:

Causes of otitis externa are now defined as primary or secondary, with factors that contribute to or promote disease. It is also standard of care to determine whether the cause is curable or lifelong management is required. **Primary causes** of otitis externa are those that create disease in a normal ear. They can cause otitis without any other cause or factor and can be subtle; they often go unrecognized by owners and veterinarians until secondary causes develop. Primary factors alter the ear environment, which allows secondary infections to develop. The major primary causes of otitis externa are allergy, autoimmune (eg, pemphigus), endocrine, epithelialization disorders, foreign bodies, glandular disorders, immune-mediated (eg, drug reactions), fungal (eg, aspergillosis), parasites, viral (eg, canine distemper), and miscellaneous (auricular chondritis, eosinophilic diseases, juvenile cellulitis, proliferating necrotitizing otitis of cats). **Secondary causes** are those that cause disease in an abnormal ear. These causes are relatively easy to eliminate and include bacteria, fungi, medication reactions, overcleaning, and yeast overgrowth.

Factors are elements related to the disease or pet that contribute to or promote the otitis externa by altering the structure, function, or physiology of the ear canal. Factors are subdivided into predisposing factors, which are present before the development of the ear disease, and perpetuating factors, which occur as a result of the inflammation. **Predisposing factors** include conformation of the ear, excessive moisture, obstruction of the ear canal (eg, polyp, feline apocrine cystadenomatosis), primary otitis media (eg, primary secretory otitis media, otitis media due to neoplasia or respiratory disease), systemic diseases (eg, catabolic states), and treatment effects (eg, alterations of normal microflora, trauma from cleaning). **Perpetuating factors** include changes in the ear epithelium (eg, failure of migration), ear canal (eg, edema, stenosis, proliferation), tympanic membrane (eg, dilated, ruptured), glandular (eg, sebaceous hyperplasia), pericartilaginous fibrosis (eg, calcification), and middle ear (eg, filled with debris, otitis media). This system is currently referred to as the PSPP classification system. A prognosis should be given for otitis externa. Curable means that the component of the problem is readily resolved with treatment (for weeks) or via surgery. Longterm management indicates that the component of the ear problem may be resolvable, but it can take months of treatment. Lifelong treatment indicates that the owner will need to play an active role in management for the life of the pet.

Clinical Findings and Diagnosis: There is no recognized sex distribution for otitis externa. Young animals may be more commonly affected. There are clear breed predispositions for otitis, which directly reflect the breed predispositions for skin disease (eg, allergies in retrievers and terriers). The most common historical findings are headshaking and aural pruritus.

The first step in physical examination is determination of the severity of pain. This can be done by gentle palpation or petting of the animal. If the ear is painful or the degree of discomfort is high, the animal should be sedated before performing any further diagnostic testing. The second step is gentle palpation and manipulation of the ear canal and pinna to determine the presence of swelling, pruritus, fibrosis, or calcification. The presence or absence of these findings will help determine whether advanced diagnostics are needed, specifically imaging of the ear canal. Next, the outside of the ear should be examined, noting erythema, edema, crusts, scale, ulcers, lichenification, hyperpigmentation, or exudate. The pinnae and periauricular regions should be examined for evidence of self-trauma, erythema, and primary and secondary skin lesions. Pinnal deformities, hyperplastic tissue in the canal, and headshaking suggest chronic otic discomfort. If the otitis is unilateral, the unaffected ear should be examined first to prevent iatrogenic contamination of the unaffected ear with organisms (eg, *Pseudomonas aeruginosa* or *Proteus mirabilis*) that may be present in the diseased ear. The unaffected ear may, in fact, be diseased, meaning that the differential diagnosis list should also include causes of bilateral otitis.

Otoscopic examination is often not possible because the ear is painful, *swollen, or filled* with exudate; sedation is usually required. Swelling of the ear canal often makes it impossible to see the tympanic membrane. A handheld otoscope must have enough light and magnification to clearly visualize the external canal to the level of the tympanic membrane. Disposable otoscopic ear cones are recommended, because studies have demonstrated contamination of cones. Handheld otoscopes are available with a variety of heads, including magnification options and surgical operating heads, that allow for visualization of the ear canal while inserting another instrument. The surgical head is used when biopsies, foreign body removal, or deep flush of the canal is anticipated.

A video otoscope provides magnifcation of the ear canal and tympanic membrane. Most have a working channel through which biopsy instruments, catheters for flushing debris from the canal, and laser tips can be passed. Video otoscopes allow visualization through water and saline to determine the integrity of the tympanic membrane and to facilitate sampling and culture of the middle ear.

During an otoscopic examination, the ear canal should be inspected for changes in diameter, pathologic changes in the skin, quantity and type of exudate, parasites, foreign bodies, neoplasms, and changes in the tympanic membrane. The tympanic membrane should be examined for evidence of disease or rupture. However, in many cases of otitis, the character of the ear canal and tympanic membrane cannot be visualized at all until the exudate is gently flushed from the canal. Samples for cytologic evaluation and culture should be obtained before the ear is flushed. Examination is attempted again after the ear is dried. In chronic cases, the canal may be too stenotic, either from hyperplasia or edema, to be examined. Systemic glucocorticoids given daily for 1 wk may reduce swelling enough to allow examination.

If sedation is not needed, samples for ear diagnostic tests should be collected: skin cytology from the external and inner pinnae, cytology of any exudates present, hair trichograms and skin scrapings for *Demodex*, and ear swab cytology with mineral oil in young and adult animals (especially cats, because feline demodicosis can present as pruritic otitis). Wood's lamp examinations need to be done with care, keeping in mind that the key color is apple-green fluorescense and that sebum can glow yellow. Dermatophytosis affects the hair of the pinnae and hairs in the concave surface of the ear canal.

Cytologic evaluation of exudate or cerumen taken from the horizontal ear canal may provide immediate diagnostic information. The external ear canals of most dogs and cats harbor small numbers of commensal gram-positive cocci. These organisms may become pathogenic if the microenvironment is changed and encourages their overgrowth. Exudate obtained with a cotton-tipped applicator can be rolled onto a glass slide, stained with a 3-step quick stain or modified Wright's stain, and examined under a microscope. (A study has shown that heat fixing is not necessary for ear swab cytology.) Smears should be examined microscopically under 4×, 10×, and oil immersion to look for numbers and morphology of keratinocytes, bacteria, yeasts, and WBCs; evidence of phagocytosis of microorganisms; fungal hyphae; and acantholytic or neoplastic cells.

A stained smear can quickly determine whether microbial overgrowth is present. Coccal organisms are usually staphylococci or streptococci. Rod-shaped organisms are usually *Pseudomonas aeruginosa*, *Escherichia coli*, or *Proteus mirabilis*; their appearance in large numbers indicates that a bacterial culture with antibiotic sensitivity should be performed because of their known resistance to many antimicrobial agents. The presence of many neutrophils phagocytizing bacteria confirms the pathogenic nature of the organisms.

The yeast *Malassezia pachydermatis* is found in low numbers in the ear canals of many healthy dogs and cats. Because yeasts colonize the surface of the ear canal, they are most easily found adhered to clumps of exfoliated squamous epithelial cells. *M pachydermatis* is identified readily on microscopic examination and its numbers easily assessed. There is no specific number that indicates yeast overgrowth. The key determining factor is whether the ears are pruritic. In addition, if previous treatment did not include antifungal therapy and if otitis externa is recurrent, antifungal therapy is warranted.

A dark exudate in the canal usually signals the presence of either *Malassezia* spp or a parasite but may also be seen with a bacterial or mixed infection. In addition to stained cytology, otic exudate should be examined for eggs, larvae, or adults of the ear mite *Otodectes cynotis* and for *Demodex* mites in dogs and cats, and *Psoroptes cuniculi* in rabbits and goats. Smears are made by combining cerumen and otic discharge with a small quantity of mineral oil on a glass slide. A coverglass should be used, with the smear examined under low-power magnification. Rarely, refractory ceruminous otitis externa may be associated with localized proliferation of *Demodex* sp in the external ear canals of dogs and cats and may be the only area on the body affected.

Microbial cultures are taken before otoscopy is completed and before any cleaning is done. Samples for culture should be taken with a sterile culturette from the horizontal canal (the region where most infections arise) or from the middle ear in cases of tympanic rupture. A bacterial culture and antibiotic sensitivity and an antibiotic mean inhibitory concentration should be done.

Histopathologic changes associated with chronic otitis externa are often nonspecific. Histopathologic evidence of a hypersensitivity response may support a recommendation for intradermal allergy testing or for a hypoallergenic diet trial. In addition, biopsies from animals with chronic, obstructive, unilateral otitis externa may reveal whether neoplastic changes are present.

Radiography of the osseous bullae is indicated when proliferative tissues prevent adequate visualization of the tympanic membrane, when otitis media is suspected as a cause of relapsing bacterial otitis externa, and when neurologic signs accompany otitis externa. Fluid densities and proliferative or lytic osseous changes provide evidence of middle ear involvement. Unfortunately, radiographs are normal in many otitis media cases. CT or MRI, if available, should be performed for cases of severe, chronic otitis.

Treatment: Key to treatment is a discussion with the owner regarding the suspected or known cause of the otitis externa, whether the otitis is curable, and whether treatment must be longterm for resolution or lifelong management will be required. All primary and secondary causes and predisposing factors need to be identified, managed, and treated. Management of pain or pruritus must be included in the initial treatment protocol. Tramadol for the first 5–7 days at 5 mg/kg, PO, tid, may be especially beneficial. In addition, otitis externa is one of the few dermatologic conditions in which glucocorticoids are beneficial in the face of concurrent antimicrobial use or sepsis. Glucocorticoids decrease swelling of the ear canal and may be key to successful treatment. Prednisone or triamcinolone is used most commonly. Duration depends on the severity. Ear hygiene is important; in particular, the hair from the pre- and periauricular area should be clipped, as well as hair from the surface of the inner pinnae and ends of the ears. This facilitates cleaning and treatment of the ears. Plucking of hair from the ear canal is controversial but may be needed to adequately resolve the ear infection. Hair plucking is painful and should be done under anesthesia.

The first ear cleaning should be done in the veterinary clinic, and owners should be instructed not to clean the ears until recheck in 5–7 days. Owners are often unable to clean the ears and/or are too aggressive, causing further damage. Owners should initally focus on administration of topical and/or systemic drugs and can begin to clean the ears after the first recheck and if the otitis is resolving. It is important to remember that topical medications are inactivated by exudates, and excessive cerumen may prevent medications from reaching the epithelium. The ears should be gently cleaned with an ear cleaner that will remove the debris in the canal. Thick, dry, or waxy material requires a ceruminolytic solution such as carbamide peroxide or dioctyl sodium sulfosuccinate (DSS). If rods are seen, the ear cleaner should contain squalene, because one possible cause is *Pseudomonas*, which can produce a biofilm that protects bacteria from antibiotics. The ears should be thoroughly rinsed with warm water to remove residual ear cleaner. If the tympanic membrane is ruptured, detergents and DSS are contraindicated; milder cleansers (eg, saline, saline plus povidone iodine, Tris EDTA) should be used to flush the ear.

Effective treatment may require both topical and systemic antimicrobial therapy, along with pain medications and glucocorticoids.The duration of treatment may vary from 7–10 days to >30 days, depending on the diagnosis. In treatment of acute bacterial otitis externa, antibacterial agents in combination with corticosteroids reduce exudation, pain, swelling, and glandular secretions. The least potent corticosteroid that will reduce the inflammation should be used (*see* p 2710).

Most commercial topical products contain a combination of antibiotic/antifungal and glucocorticoids. The volume of the ear canal in most dogs is 1 mL, and adequate treatment requires instillation of at least this volume twice daily. Products with an aqueous base or those that have a thin film should be used; ointments are to be avoided.

Irritating medications (eg, home remedies and vinegar dilutions) should be avoided. They cause swelling of the lining of the ear canal and an increase in glandular secretions, which predispose to opportunistic infections. Substances that are usually not irritating in normal ear canals may cause irritation in an ear that is already inflamed. This is particularly true of propylene glycol. Powders, such as those used after plucking hair from the canal, can form irritating concretions within the ear canal and should not be used.

Systemic therapy should be incorporated into the treatment regimen in most cases of chronic otitis and in any case in which otitis media is suspected. The most common cause of recurrent otitis externa is undiagnosed otitis media. Failure to use systemic antimicrobial therapy is an important cause of chronic ear disease in dogs. Systemic antibiotics should be used when neutrophils or rod-type bacteria are found on cytology, in cases of therapeutic failure with topical antimicrobial agents, in chronic recurring ear infections, and in all cases of otitis media. (*See also* SYSTEMIC PHARMACOTHERAPEUTICS OF THE INTEGUMENTARY SYSTEM, p 2571.) Yeast infections in dogs can be treated with oral ketoconazole 5 mg/kg/day, PO, for 15–30 days. Ketoconazole should not be used in cats; itraconazole 2–3 mg/kg/day for 15–30 days or one week on/one week off is recommended.

Duration of treatment will vary depending on the individual case but should continue until the infection is resolved based on reexamination and repeat cytology and culture. Animals with bacterial and yeast infections should be physically examined, with cytologies evaluated weekly to every other week until there is no evidence of infection. For most acute cases, this takes 2–4 wk. Chronic cases may take months to resolve, and in some instances, a therapeutic regimen must be continued indefinitely.

Methicillin-resistant *Staphylococcus intermedius* and *Pseudomonas* otitis (caused by *Pseudomonas aeruginosa*) have emerged as frustrating and difficult perpetuating causes of otitis because of the development of resistance to most common antibiotics. These infections are often chronic in course (>2 mo) and associated with marked suppurative exudation, severe epithelial ulceration, pain, and edema of the canal. Successful treatment is multifaceted and should include the following steps: 1) identify the primary cause of the otitis and manage it, 2) remove the exudate via irrigation of the ear canal, 3) identify and treat concurrent otitis media, 4) select an appropriate antibiotic from the results of culture and mean inhibitory concentration on the organism and use it at an effective dosage for an appropriate duration, and 5) treat topically and systemically until the infection resolves (weeks to months).

The best treatment of chronic otitis is prevention. In addition to identifying the cause of acute otitis, topical and/or systemic medications should be chosen based on cytology or culture; they should have a narrow spectrum and be specific for the current condition. Aminoglycosides and fluoroquinolone antibiotics should not be used unless absolutely required for successful treatment but are the most common ingredients in topical otic medications. Because many topical products contain a combination of glucocorticoid, antibiotic, and antifungal medications, it is imperative to educate the owner on proper use (frequency and duration). Many owners discontinue treatment when the ear "looks better" before the infection is resolved. Polymyxin B and fluoroquinolone antibiotics have shown the best success in controlling *Pseudomonas* infections in cases in which resistance has been identified through culture. However, resistance is developing to fluoroquinolones.

Maintenance Care: Owners should be shown how to properly clean the ears. The frequency of cleaning usually decreases over time from daily to once or twice weekly as a preventive maintenance procedure. The ear canals should be kept dry and well ventilated. Using topical astringents in dogs that swim frequently and preventing water from entering the ear canals during bathing should minimize maceration of the ear canal. Chronic maceration impairs the barrier function of the skin, which predisposes to opportunistic infection. Preventive otic astringents may decrease the frequency of bacterial or fungal infections in moist ear canals. Clipping hair from the inside of the pinna and around the external auditory meatus, and plucking it from hirsute ear canals, improves ventilation and decreases humidity in the ears. However, hair should not routinely be removed from the ear canal if it is not causing a problem, because doing so can induce an acute inflammatory reaction.

OTITIS MEDIA AND INTERNA

Otitis media, inflammation of the middle ear structures, is seen in small and large domestic animals, including dogs, cats, rabbits, ruminants, horses, pigs, and camelids. It can be unilateral or bilateral and can affect animals of all ages. Although typically sporadic, outbreaks are possible in herds. Otitis media usually results from extension of infection from the external ear canal through the tympanic membrane or from migration of pharyngeal microorganisms through the auditory tube. Occasionally, infection extends from the inner ear to the middle ear, or reaches the middle ear by the hematogenous route. Primary otitis media has been reported in certain breeds of dogs, particularly Cavalier King Charles Spaniels. Untreated otitis media can lead to **otitis interna** (inflammation of the inner ear structures) or to rupture of an intact tympanic membrane with subsequent otorrhea or otitis externa.

Clinical Findings and Diagnosis: Signs of otitis media include head shaking, rubbing or scratching the affected ear, and tilting or rotating the head toward the affected side; self-trauma can lead to aural hematoma. The most common cause of recurrent otitis externa is undiagnosed otitis media. When otitis externa (*see* p 527) accompanies otitis media, the external ear canal may look inflamed and contain an abnormal discharge. The pinna or ear canal may be painful and malodorous, and the hair surrounding the base of the ear may be wet or matted. Because the facial (cranial nerve VII) and sympathetic nerves course through the middle ear, animals with otitis media may exhibit signs of facial nerve paralysis (eg, ear droop, lip droop, ptosis, collapse of the nostril) and/or Horner syndrome (eg, miosis, ptosis, enophthalmos, protrusion of the nictitating membrane) on the same side as the affected ear. Exposure keratitis and corneal ulceration may develop. With facial paralysis, the nasal philtrum or lip may deviate away from the affected side. These signs help to distinguish otitis media from simple otitis externa.

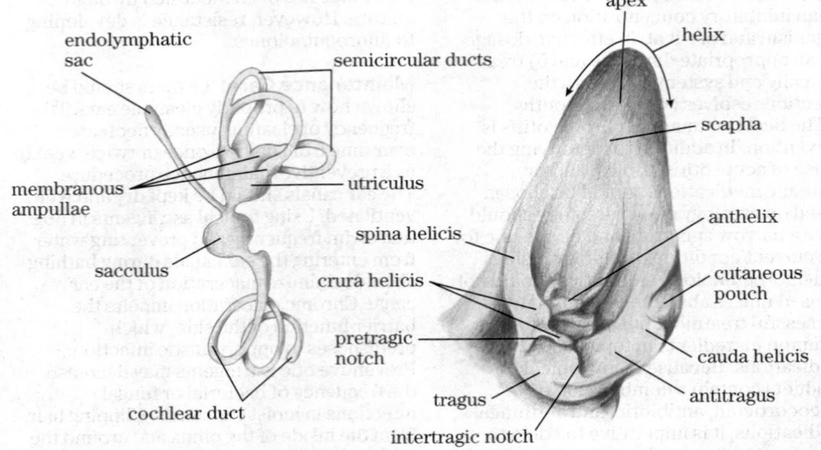

Left: Membranous labyrinth, internal ear, dog. Right: External ear, dog. *Illustration by Dr. Gheorghe Constantinescu.*

With otitis interna, inflammation impairs function of the vestibulocochlear nerve (cranial nerve VIII), resulting in hearing loss and signs of peripheral vestibular disease such as head tilt, circling, leaning or falling toward the affected side, general incoordination, or spontaneous horizontal nystagmus with the fast phase away from the affected side. Extension of infection from the inner ear to the brain leads to meningitis, meningoencephalitis, or abscesses, with signs referable to those conditions. In horses, severe otitis media/interna can result in fusion and fracture of the tympanohyoid joint; extension of the fracture line to the calvarium can lead to intracranial spread of infection or cause hematoma and death.

Whereas animals with otitis media/interna are usually alert, nonfebrile, and have a good appetite, those with meningitis

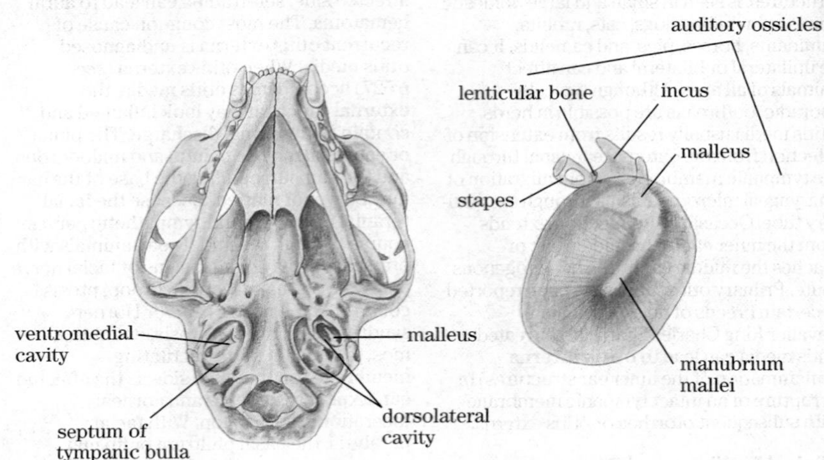

Deep structures of tympanic bulla and tympanic membrane, cat. *Illustration by Dr. Gheorghe Constantinescu.*

or meningoencephalitis are usually depressed, febrile, and inappetent. A major differential diagnosis for otitis media/interna in ruminants is listeriosis. However, in listeriosis, cranial nerves other than VII and VIII may be affected, causing signs such as dysphagia or loss of facial sensation, and affected animals are usually depressed.

In large animals, otitis media and interna are presumptively diagnosed based on history and clinical signs. A history of bottle feeding or feeding of contaminated milk to neonates, concurrent or previous respiratory disease, chronic ear infection, or aural foreign body, in conjunction with typical signs of otitis media/interna, should prompt examination of the ear canal. Otitis media is confirmed by visualizing a bulging, discolored, or ruptured tympanic membrane. Although the tympanic membrane may be visualized using a simple otoscope in many cases, the anatomy of the ear canal hinders visualization in some species, such as horses and llamas; endoscopy, or video otoscopy, is an alternative approach. Imaging methods assist in diagnosis and assessment of lesion severity. Radiography can detect osseous changes in the tympanic bulla and fluid in the tympanic cavity if appropriate positioning and techniques are used. However, CT and MRI are more sensitive and are the preferred methods when feasible. In some cases, diagnosis is made only at necropsy, using special techniques to expose the tympanic region. Diagnosis of clinical otitis media/interna in one ear should always prompt examination of the other ear to determine whether subclinical otitis is present.

Otitis media has been reported to be present in 16% of dogs with otitis externa and in >50% of dogs with chronic otitis externa. The tympanic membrane has also been reported to be intact in >70% of cases, and the disease is usually bilateral in dogs. Primary and secondary causes and factors of otitis externa can lead to otitis media. Diagnosis can be challenging, because the tympanic membrane can be intact. Palpation of the tympanic membrane with a blunt instrument is not an accurate method of determining the patency of the tympanic membrane. Advanced imaging techniques (CT or MRI) are more sensitive than routine radiographs but are not 100% sensitive and specific. In some cases, exploratory (and therapeutic) bulla osteotomy may be necessary.

Treatment and Prognosis: Treatment of otitis media/interna is most successful when started early in the course of the disease. Chronic cases are often refractory to treatment or recur after apparent remission. When otitis externa accompanies otitis media/interna, the ear should be examined closely for mites and foreign bodies, such as plant awns, and the discharge cultured for bacteria. Many aerobic and anaerobic bacteria have been cultured from the ears of animals with otitis media/interna, and mixed infections are common. Pathogens that warrant mentioning because of their frequency of isolation include *Malassezia* spp and *Pseudomonas* spp in small animals; *Streptococcus suis* in pigs; *Streptococcus* spp in horses; *Mycoplasma* spp in goats; and *Mannheimia haemolytica*, *Pasteurella multocida*, *Histophilus somni*, and *Mycoplasma bovis* in cattle. *M bovis* is particularly problematic in dairy calves fed unpasteurized waste milk from cows with intramammary infection. However, other pathogens, such as coliform bacteria, *Staphylococcus* spp, *Neisseria* spp, corynebacteria, and *Trueperella pyogenes* are frequently isolated from the ears of affected animals. Isolation of a bacterial pathogen(s) or mites from the ear helps direct initial treatment but does not necessarily imply causation of otitis media/interna, because the same organisms can be isolated from the external ear canals of apparently healthy animals.

Ear mites, when present, should be treated with an appropriate systemic antiparasitic agent (*see* p 2576). Topical acaricides can be instilled into the external ear canal once it is cleaned. Bacterial infection should be treated with appropriate systemic antimicrobial agents (*see* p 2571), based on culture and susceptibility test results. If the tympanic membrane is intact, a culture can be obtained via a myringotomy incision with a tom cat catheter. It may be possible to aspirate fluid. If not, 0.5 mL of sterile water can be instilled into the bulla and the fluid aspirated for culture. No antimicrobial agents are labeled for treatment of otitis media/interna in food-producing animals in the USA, so extra-label drug use guidelines must be followed and prohibited drugs avoided.

In addition to antimicrobial and/or anthelmintic therapy, the external ear canal should be cleaned and flushed if otorrhea or otitis externa is present; physiologic saline or dilute antiseptic solutions, such as iodine, chlorhexidine, or hydrogen peroxide, are commonly used for flushing. Steroids or NSAIDs can help reduce inflammation and pain associated with otitis media/interna. Corneal ulceration, aural hematomas, and concurrent infections should be treated appropriately, if present, and the animal protected from further self-injury.

If the tympanic membrane is intact and otitis media/interna does not respond sufficiently to systemic antimicrobial and anti-inflammatory therapy, myringotomy (perforation of the tympanic membrane) can be performed to relieve pressure and enable culture and drainage of fluid from the tympanic cavity. In chronic, nonresponsive or recurrent cases of otitis media/interna, it may be necessary to perform bulla osteotomy or total ear canal ablation to establish sufficient drainage and enable effective lavage. Tympanostomy tubes can be implanted into the tympanic membrane after myringotomy to allow continuous drainage in Cavalier King Charles Spaniels with primary secretory otitis, but such tubes are not useful to drain more purulent exudate.

Early diagnosis and treatment of otitis media/interna can result in complete resolution of infection and clinical signs. However, with severe, chronic, or nonresponsive cases, owners should be advised that neurologic deficits and hearing loss may persist even if infection is resolved. In small animals, otitis media may be resolved only by surgery (total ear canal abalation), particularly if multidrug-resistant bacteria are present.

TUMORS OF THE EAR CANAL

Ear canal tumors may arise from any of the tissues lining or supporting the ear canal, including the squamous epithelium, the ceruminous or sebaceous glands, or the mesenchymal tissues. Malignant tumors arising from the external ear canal and pinna are more common in cats than in dogs.

True neoplasia in the ear is often misdiagnosed during physical examination, because hyperplastic epithelial tissue and glands can appear as growths along the canal. Treatment of the infection and inflammation over time can change the appearance of these growths and, in some cases, they will actually disappear. In contrast, neoplastic growths will not resolve with topical otic therapy.

Although the precise cause of ear canal tumors is unknown, several theories have been postulated. Chronic inflammation of the ear canal may lead to hyperplasia, followed by dysplasia and finally neoplasia. Bacterial degradation of the fatty acids and other products produced in inspissated apocrine secretions from hyperplastic ceruminous glands during otitis externa episodes may also stimulate carcinogenesis in the ear canal. Middle-aged dogs and cats are more likely to have benign otic tumors, whereas dogs and cats >11 yr old seem to have more malignant tumors. This seems to be attributed to chronicity of ear disease rather than simply age. Tumors in the ear canal decrease the lumen volume, which leads to decreased drying of the canal and impaired drainage of inflammatory exudates and volatile fatty acids. Chronic infection and inflammation do not subside, allowing neoplastic changes to continue to develop.

Incidence of benign and malignant ear tumors is higher in American Cocker Spaniels than in other breeds. The density of glandular tissue in the ear canal of this breed may be the reason. Middle-aged to older cats are predisposed to benign and malignant ear canal tumors, whereas young cats (3 mo to 5 yr) are more likely to develop nasopharyngeal polyps. Clinical signs of an ear canal tumor include unilateral chronic otic discharge (ceruminous, purulent, mucoid, or hemorrhagic) and necrotic odor, head shaking, and ear scratching. Often, aural hematomas result from the head shaking associated with ear canal tumors. Draining abscesses in the parotid region below the affected ear may result. If there is middle or inner ear involvement, neurologic signs may be present, including deafness, vestibular signs (eg, head tilt, ataxia, nystagmus), facial nerve palsy or paralysis (facial drooping, salivation, and dropping food from the lips), Horner syndrome (eyelid droop, pinpoint pupil, and inward rolling of the globe), and occasional protrusion of the third eyelid. In any case of medically refractory unilateral otitis, a neoplasm of the ear canal or middle ear should be suspected.

Ear canal tumors in dogs are more likely to be benign than malignant. Malignant otic neoplasms are locally invasive, with <10% showing any lymph node involvement. Invasion of tumor into the bulla or surrounding tissue indicates a poorer prognosis. Cats have a higher incidence of malignant otic tumors. The most common pinnal neoplasms in dogs are sebaceous gland tumors, histiocytoma, and mast cell tumors. In cats, common pinnal neoplasms include squamous cell carcinoma, basal cell tumors, hemangiosarcoma, and melanocytic tumors. The most common external ear canal tumors reported in dogs are ceruminous gland adenomas and adenocarcinomas. Other tumors reported in the external ear canal of dogs include inflammatory polyps, papillomas, sebaceous gland adenomas, histiocytomas, plasmacytomas, melanomas, fibromas, squamous cell carcinomas, and hemangiosarcomas. The most common external ear canal masses reported in cats are nasopharyngeal polyps, squamous cell carcinomas, and ceruminous gland adenocarcinomas. Lymphoma, fibrosarcoma, and squamous cell carcinomas are occasionally seen in the middle or inner ear of dogs and cats. (*See also* TUMORS OF THE SKIN AND SOFT TISSUES, p 942.)

CERUMINOUS GLAND TUMORS

(Ceruminous gland adenoma or adenocarcinoma)

Ceruminous gland tumors are best visualized in a degreased, clean ear using a video otoscope. These tumors may be pedunculated or broad based but rise above the level of the epithelium. They may be smooth or multilobulated in appearance. In breeds other than the American Cocker Spaniel, these tumors are often primarily in the vertical ear canal. In the American Cocker, these tumors can be found in the horizontal ear canal as well. Properly taken, ear canal biopsies can give useful information. However, superficial ear canal biopsies are often reported as polyps with granulation tissue covered by epithelium. Deep en-bloc biopsies of the same tissue are often reported correctly as tumors. CT or MRI may be very useful in assessing the tympanic bulla more completely and in determining the extent of tumor invasion, especially in malignant tumors.

Surgical removal of benign ear canal tumors may be accomplished via lateral ear canal resection for access to the tumor mass. Laser surgery, especially when used in conjunction with a video otoscope, has made intraotic removal of these tumors relatively easy without having to open the canal surgically. More aggressive surgeries, such as total ear canal ablation and bulla osteotomy, are recommended for malignant tumors of the middle ear. Lateral ear canal resection for malignancies results in a >75% recurrence rate. Median survival time for animals with malignant ear canal tumors has been reported to be >58 mo in dogs and >11.7 mo in cats. Dogs with extensive tumor involvement had a less favorable prognosis. Radiation therapy can be used to treat excised ceruminous gland adenocarcinomas in dogs and cats, with a 56% 1-yr survival rate reported. No data are available on the efficacy of chemotherapy for otic tumors of dogs and cats.

Prognosis of animals with otic neoplasms can best be determined by histopathologic examination of removed tissues.

NASOPHARYNGEAL POLYPS

Nasopharyngeal polyps are uncommon, benign, smooth, pink, fleshy, pedunculated, inflammatory growths of connective tissue found in the external ear canals of young cats. They arise from the mucosal lining of the tympanic bulla, the pharyngeal mucosa, or the auditory tube. These polyps may be congenital, or they may result from chronic bacterial otitis media, commonly found in cats with upper respiratory diseases. They are rarely found in dogs. They are not neoplastic, and viruses have not been identified in polyp tissue.

Diagnosis involves sedation and deep otoscopic examination of the horizontal canal. Purulent discharge from the bulla may need to be flushed and suctioned from the ear canal to visualize the polyp. Use of a video otoscope greatly facilitates visualization and treatment of polyps. Polyps originating from the eustachian tube may be seen by retracting the soft palate rostrally. Radiography of the bullae may reveal an opacity in the affected bulla. CT or MRI may be helpful if a mass is suspected in the tympanic bulla that cannot be seen otoscopically. Definitive diagnosis is made via histopathology.

Surgical removal is curative as long as the entire polyp and stalk are removed. This often involves performing a bulla osteotomy, because the base of the polyp is often in the tympanic bulla. Incomplete removal of the base of the polyp by traction avulsion alone leads to rapid regrowth and return of clinical signs in 15%–50% of cats. Topical steroids in the bulla for 30–45 days seems to retard this regrowth. Systemic antibiotic therapy for the bacterial otitis media is also indicated.

ENDOCRINE SYSTEM

ENDOCRINE SYSTEM INTRODUCTION

The endocrine system encompasses a group of tissues that release hormones into circulation for travel to distant targets. An endocrine tissue is typically a ductless gland (eg, pituitary, thyroid) that releases its hormones into capillaries permeating the tissue. These glands are richly supplied with blood. However, nontypical endocrine tissues also contribute important hormones to circulation, eg, secretion of atrial natriuretic peptide from the heart, erythropoietin from the kidney, insulin-like growth factor from the liver, and leptin from fat. New hormones continue to be discovered. Some act only on a single tissue, whereas others have effects on virtually all cells of the body. The effects of hormones on their targets are varied—from enhancement of nutrient uptake to altering cell division and differentiation, among many others.

GENERAL CHEMICAL STRUCTURE AND FUNCTION

There are three main chemical categories of hormones: protein/polypeptides, steroids, and those made from modified amino acids.

Protein/Polypeptide Hormones:

Examples of protein/polypeptide hormones include adrenocorticotropin (ACTH) from the pituitary, insulin from the pancreas, and parathyroid hormone (PTH). These hormones range in size from three amino acids (thyrotropin-releasing hormone) to *considerably larger proteins* with subunit structure (eg, luteinizing hormone). They are produced in their endocrine tissue of origin by transcription/translation of the gene coding for the hormone and synthesized initially as larger products (prepro- or pre-forms) that undergo processing to authentic hormone inside the cell before secretion. Embedded in the gene coding for protein structure are amino acid sequences (signal peptides) that communicate to the cell that these molecules are destined for the regulated secretory pathway. Other post-translational modifications may occur during processing, including folding, glycosylation, disulfide bond formation, and subunit assembly. The folded and processed hormone is then stored in secretory granules or vesicles in preparation for release by the exocytotic process. Release of hormone is triggered by unique signals; eg, secretion of PTH is stimulated by a decline in the concentration of ionic or free calcium present in the extracellular fluid bathing the parathyroid chief cells. In most cases, cells producing protein/polypeptide hormones store significant amounts of these substances intracellularly; therefore, they can respond quickly when increased amounts are needed in circulation. Generally, protein/polypeptide hormones have relatively short half-lives in blood (minutes) and do not travel in blood-bound carrier proteins (exceptions exist, eg, insulin-like growth factor 1 is highly protein bound).

Protein/polypeptide hormones act on their target cells by binding to receptors located on the cell surface. These receptors are proteins and glycoproteins embedded in the cell membrane that traverse the membrane at least once so that the receptor is exposed to both the extracellular and intracellular environments. There are several classes or types of cell surface hormone receptors that translate the hormonal message to the cell interior by different means. Some are the G-protein (guanosine) coupled type, with seven transmembrane spanning domains. After hormone binding, these receptors activate a G-protein that is also located in the membrane. One or more of the G-protein subunits affects other downstream molecules (known as effectors) such as enzymes (eg, adenylate cyclase or phospholipase C) or ion channels. Activation may result in production of a second messenger, such as cyclic AMP, that can then bind to protein kinase A, causing its activation and subsequent phosphorylation of other proteins. Thus, signal transduction is a cascading and often amplifying series of events triggered when a hormone binds to its receptor. The ultimate effects in target cells are multiple and include such things as triggering secretion, increasing uptake of a molecule, or activating mitosis. Other receptors, such as the one for insulin, not only bind hormone but also act as enzymes, with the ability to phosphorylate tyrosine residues. The phosphorylated tyrosines in turn serve as docking sites for downstream signaing proteins.

Cell surface receptors are dynamic; their numbers and/or activity change with physiologic conditions. In some cases, such as exposure to excessive amounts of hormone, receptor down-regulation can occur. Down-regulation and a decline in target tissue responsiveness may be due to internalization of receptors after ligand binding or to desensitization whereby the receptor is chemically modified and becomes less active. Conversely, a lack of hormonal exposure can lead to an increase in receptor numbers on target cells (up-regulation). Diseases have been linked to mutations in hormone receptors, which can result in inactivation or constitutive or nonhormonal activation of the pathway. In some instances, a single amino acid substitution is responsible.

Steroid Hormones: Steroid hormones are derivatives of cholesterol and include products of the adrenal cortex, ovaries, and testes as well as the related molecule, vitamin D. Unlike protein/polypeptide hormones, steroid hormones are not stored in large amounts. When needed, they are rapidly synthesized from cholesterol by a series of enzymatic reactions. Most of the cholesterol needed for rapid steroid hormone synthesis is stored intracellularly in the tissue of origin. In response to appropriate signals, the precursor is moved to organelles (mitochondria and smooth endoplasmic reticulum), where a series of enzymes (eg, isomerases, dehydrogenases) rapidly convert the molecule to the appropriate steroid hormone. The identity of the final steroidal product is thus dictated by the set of enzymes expressed in that tissue.

Steroid hormones are hydrophobic and pass through cell membranes easily. In the blood, they are bound to a great extent to carrier proteins. Albumin binds many steroids fairly loosely; in addition, specific binding globulins exist for many steroid hormones. Most of the steroid hormone in circulation is bound to carrier proteins, and a small fraction circulates free or unbound. This latter fraction is thought to be available for target cell entry, ie, the biologically active portion. A rapid equilibrium exists between protein-bound and unbound steroid in extracellular fluid. Possible roles for steroid hormone–binding proteins include aiding in tissue delivery of steroids by providing an even distribution to all cells within a target tissue, buffering against large fluctuations in free hormone, and prolonging the half-life of steroids in blood. Relative to protein/polypeptide hormones, steroids usually have longer half-lives, often in the range of many minutes to hours.

Steroid hormones act on target cells via receptors located in the cell interior. These receptors are generally found in the nucleus, although some appear to reside, when unoccupied, in the cytoplasm. There are several classes of steroid receptors—those for glucocorticoids, mineralocorticoids, progestins, etc. Steroid receptors comprise a family of related proteins that also show homology to receptors for the thyroid hormones and vitamin D. The receptor has regions or domains that carry out specific tasks: one for recognition and binding of the steroid, another for binding to a specific region on chromosomal DNA, and a third for helping regulate the transcriptional complex. Steroid hormones enter targets by diffusing through the cell membrane and then binding to the receptor, causing a conformational change in the new complex. This, in turn, leads to release of associated proteins (eg, heat-shock proteins) and movement to the nucleus (if necessary), followed by binding of the complex to regions of DNA located near specific steroid-regulated genes. The result is a change in the rate of transcription of specific genes, either increasing or decreasing their expression. Thus, steroid hormones primarily function by affecting the production rates of specific messenger RNA and proteins in targets. Steroid action is relatively slow in onset (hours) but may be long lasting because of the duration of production and half-lives of the messenger

RNA and proteins induced in target cells. It is increasingly clear that some steroids also act via nongenomic mechanisms. For example, many of the anti-inflammatory effects of glucocorticoids are thought to be due to the glucocorticoid-receptor complex binding to, and inhibiting the action of, pro-inflammatory transcription factors inside cells.

Steroids in the blood are eliminated by metabolism in the liver. Reduced forms are produced and subsequently conjugated to glucuronic acid and sulfate. These metabolites are freely soluble in blood and are eliminated from the body by renal excretion and through the GI tract. Small amounts of free steroid hormone are also directly excreted by the kidneys.

Modified Amino Acid Hormones: This class of hormones is made by chemical modification of amino acids, mainly tyrosine. They include thyroid hormones and the catecholamines epinephrine and norepinephrine. Thyroxine (T_4) and triiodothyronine (T_3) are stored in the thyroid as a part of thyroglobulin; secretion of these hormones involves thyroidal cell uptake and breakdown of this large molecule liberating T_4 and T_3. Thyroid hormones act on targets much like steroids; they are relatively water insoluble, transported by carrier proteins in blood, and act on targets via intracellular receptors. Catecholamines are manufactured by hydroxylation, decarboxylation, and methylation of tyrosine and are secreted into the blood from the adrenal medulla. They have exceedingly short half-lives (<5 min), are not protein bound, and act on targets via cell surface receptors (α- and β-adrenergic receptors).

MEASUREMENT OF HORMONES

Because hormones circulate in low quantities in blood, accurate measurement of these substances requires sensitive assays, usually in the form of a competitive immunoassay. The original method (still widely used) is radioimmunoassay employing an antibody directed against the hormone and a radio-labeled form of the hormone. The labeled hormone competes with unlabeled hormone for antibody-binding sites. A standard curve containing known amounts of hormone is used for comparison to calculate the concentration of hormone in patient samples. The use of radioactive tags permits detection of low concentrations of hormone, which typically circulate in the pico- (10^{-12}) or nanomolar (10^{-9}) range. In recent years, nonradioactive tags, "sandwich-type" assays, and ELISA methods have been developed for hormone measurement.

Accurate measurement in veterinary species presents some challenges, because normal concentrations of a given hormone can vary significantly between species. For example, normal total T_4 concentrations in dogs and cats are ~4 times lower than those in people. Concern about cross-reactivity is important; protein/polypeptide hormones vary in amino acid composition and in other structural ways (eg, patterns of glycosylation) across species. As a consequence, antibodies made against a particular hormone may not recognize that material from another species. Finally, while steroid hormones are structurally identical across species (cortisol in dogs is identical to that in people), substances present in the serum of a given species can sometimes interfere in an assay, leading to inaccurate results. Overall, it is important that a laboratory providing measurement of a particular hormone in a species demonstrate that the assay is valid in that species and that the laboratory has established normal ranges.

REGULATION OF ENDOCRINE SYSTEMS

Secretion of hormones is regulated by a system of sensing elements possessing the means to detect need for both increased and decreased secretion. The particular sensing network, feedback elements, and network of control responses are unique for each hormone. Hormonal pathways maintain homeostasis, and adjustments in secretion usually result in changes that will help maintain the status quo. In addition, secretion and activity of a particular hormone may be adjusted upward or downward in response to challenges such as chronic stress, disease, or change in nutritional status. The concept of negative feedback and its relationship to control of hormonal pathways is important in understanding pathway regulation and evaluation of endocrine function tests. For example, insulin is released in response to an increase in glucose concentration bathing the β-cells in the pancreatic islets of Langerhans. One of insulin's actions is to lower glucose concentrations in extracellular fluid by enhancing its uptake in target tissues. This decline in glucose leads to reductions in insulin secretion. In patients suspected of having an insulin-secreting tumor, the finding of a low blood glucose concentration (hypoglycemia) together with an increased insulin concentration demonstrates inappropriate feedback, characteristic of such a tumor. In another example, patients showing increased blood calcium concentrations should have low levels of PTH in circulation. Measurement of high PTH levels in such patients indicates a malfunction at the level of the parathyroid, most often associated with parathyroid adenoma.

Secretory patterns of hormones vary tremendously. The thyroid hormones tend to have less variability than the steroid hormones and show only moderate daily or weekly variation. In contrast, blood levels of the adrenal steroid cortisol show much more fluctuation, with occasional bursts of secretion followed by periods of low activity (low blood levels) occurring throughout the day.

PATHOGENESIS OF ENDOCRINE DISEASE

Endocrine diseases can arise from many causes. Hormones can be over- or underproduced, receptors can malfunction, and normal pathways for hormone removal may be disrupted. Clinical signs consistent with malfunction in an endocrine tissue may develop because of a problem originating in the source of the hormone itself or may be due to disruption in another location that is secondarily affecting hormone secretion or action.

In veterinary medicine, the most common types of endocrine disease are hormonal overproduction associated with either a tumor or hyperplastic tissue manufacturing excessive amounts of hormone, and hormonal deficiency due to destruction of the endocrine tissue source. Common diseases associated with hormonal overproduction are hyperthyroidism in cats and hyperadrenocorticism (Cushing disease) in dogs. Often, the abnormal endocrine tissue not only overproduces hormone but also fails to respond normally to feedback signals, contributing to inappropriate release of hormone. Hormonal overproduction from an endocrine tissue can also result from stimulation arising from a secondary source; eg, renal disease can result in parathyroid hyperplasia and oversecretion of PTH. Hyperphosphatemia occurs as a consequence of some types of renal disease. This leads to decreased formation of the active form of vitamin D, 1,25-dihydroxycholecalciferol (calcitriol). In turn, low calcitriol concentrations contribute to low calcium levels in extracellular fluid, which act as a stimulus for PTH secretion. Nonendocrine tissues can produce and secrete hormones in sufficient amounts to cause clinical signs; eg, certain tumors (apocrine gland tumors of the anal sac in dogs, lymphoma) can manufacture PTH-related protein that can mimic PTH action, resulting in hypercalcemia.

Syndromes associated with deficient or absent hormone secretion also have multiple causes. Endocrine tissue destruction secondary to cell-mediated autoimmune attack is often believed to be the cause. Examples of endocrine hypofunction resulting from primary tissue loss include canine hypothyroidism, type 1 diabetes mellitus, primary hypoparathyroidism, and primary hypoadrenocorticism. In early stages of tissue loss, compensatory mechanisms involving feedback pathways stimulate activity (hormone production) from the remaining tissue. For example, in primary hypoadrenocorticism (Addison disease), secretion of pituitary ACTH increases as the adrenal cortex disappears. The increased trophic support results in full activation of the remaining tissue and often provides sufficient hormone secretion to delay signs of deficiency until tissue loss simply eliminates the hormonal source. Disorders resulting in clinical signs of endocrine hypoactivity may also occur due to disruption in tissues distant from the hormone source. Secondary hypothyroidism results from pituitary thyroid-stimulating hormone insufficiency that reduces the stimulus needed at the thyroid for T_4 and T_3 production and secretion. Patients receiving glucocorticoid therapy may experience atrophy of the cortisol-producing zones in the adrenal cortex. The exogenous steroid initiates negative feedback on the pituitary gland, suppressing ACTH secretion and leading to adrenal cortical atrophy. Another potential cause of endocrine hypofunction relates to tissue loss secondary to compressive and/or destructive growth of nonfunctional tumors.

Endocrine disease and related maladies also result from alterations in tissue responsiveness to hormones. An important example is type 2 or non-insulin-dependent diabetes mellitus, in which relative insensitivity to insulin is observed, often associated with obesity. Nephrogenic diabetes insipidus is due to renal insensitivity to the actions of vasopressin (antidiuretic hormone). The renal insensitivity to vasopressin in this syndrome may relate to congenital abnormalities in the vasopressin receptor but more often is secondary to other diseases (eg, pyometra, hyperadrenocorticism) or abnormalities in ion concentrations (eg, hypokalemia, hypercalcemia).

PRINCIPLES OF THERAPY

Endocrine diseases involving hyperactivity may be treated surgically (tumor removal), by radiotherapy (eg, ^{131}I for hyperthyroidism), or medically (eg, methimazole as an antithyroid drug). Syndromes of hormone deficiency are often successfully managed by simply replacing the missing hormone(s), such as insulin treatment in diabetes mellitus or thyroid hormone replacement therapy in hypothyroidism. Replacement therapy for deficiencies related to protein/polypeptide hormones can present a challenge. Often, the species-specific version of the hormone is not available, the drug may need to be injected several times per day, or the possibility of antibody formation and anaphylaxis must be considered. Steroid and thyroid hormones can usually be administered orally. Some protein/polypeptide hormones or analogues are effective when given by routes other than injection (eg, the antidiuretic hormone analogue desmopressin acetate is effective when administered by a variety of routes).

Hormonal replacement therapy should be monitored by assessment of clinical response and other suitable measures such as therapeutic blood monitoring (eg, post-pill measurement of T_4 concentrations, measurement of sodium and potassium in serum in patients with primary hypoadrenocorticism). Replacement therapy is often required for a time after surgical removal of an endocrine tumor. However, remaining normal tissue that was atrophied as a consequence of the disease often recovers activity in a fairly short period of time, obviating need for lifelong replacement therapy. Animals show significant variation in drug bioavailability; thus, a proper dosing schedule should be tailored to each patient.

Glucocorticoids are commonly used therapeutic drugs, particularly because of their anti-inflammatory and anti-allergic activity. Proper use requires an understanding of their adverse effects, including the potential appearance of signs of hyperadrenocorticism resulting from longterm therapy or from use of potent derivatives. Such adverse effects can be minimized by use of orally administered glucocorticoids given on alternate days.

THE PITUITARY GLAND

The pituitary gland (hypophysis) is composed of the adenohypophysis (anterior lobe) and the neurohypophysis (posterior lobe).

Adenohypophysis: The adenohypophysis, which surrounds the pars nervosa of the neurohypophyseal system to varying degrees in different species, consists of the pars distalis, the pars tuberalis, and the pars intermedia. The pars distalis is the largest part and contains multiple populations of endocrine cells. The pars tuberalis functions primarily as a scaffold for the capillary network of the hypophyseal portal system. The pars intermedia forms the junction between the pars distalis and pars nervosa. It contains two populations of cells in dogs, one of which synthesizes adrenocorticotropic hormone (ACTH).

A specific population of endocrine cells in the pars distalis (and in the pars intermedia for ACTH in dogs) synthesizes and secretes each of the pituitary trophic hormones. Pituitary cells have a secretory cycle and enter an actively synthesizing phase in response to increased demand for a particular hormone. Secretory cells in the adenohypophysis are often subdivided into chromophils (acidophils, basophils) and chromophobes based on interaction of the secretory granules with pH-dependent histochemical stains.

Acidophils are further subdivided into somatotrophs that secrete growth hormone (GH, somatotropin) and lactotrophs that secrete prolactin. Basophils include gonadotrophs that secrete both luteinizing hormone (LH) and follicle-stimulating hormone (FSH), and thyrotrophs that secrete thyrotropic hormone (thyroid-stimulating hormone [TSH]). Chromophobes include the endocrine cells involved in the synthesis of ACTH and melanocyte-stimulating hormone (MSH), nonsecretory follicular cells, and undifferentiated stem cells.

Endocrine cells in the adenohypophysis are under the control of corresponding hypothalamic-releasing hormones. These releasing hormones are conveyed by the hypophyseal portal system to specific cells in the adenohypophysis, where they stimulate the rapid release of preformed trophic hormones.

Separate hypothalamic-releasing hormones regulate the rate of secretion of each trophic hormone from the adenohypophysis. For most pituitary trophic hormones, negative feedback control is accomplished by a feedback loop involving the blood concentration of the hormone produced by the target endocrine gland (eg, thyroid gland, adrenal cortex, ovary, and testis). Hormones such as prolactin, GH, and MSH have more complex feedback mechanisms. For example, prolactin affects primarily the mammary gland, and GH has its principal effect on the liver—both nonendocrine tissues. The negative feedback in such cases includes metabolites and other messengers (eg, insulin-like growth factor I produced by the liver). In the case of GH, there is an inhibitory (somatostatin) as well as stimulatory (GH-releasing hormone) hypothalamic regulator.

Neurohypophysis: The neurohypophysis (pars nervosa, posterior lobe) has three anatomic subdivisions. Secretion granules that contain the neurohypophyseal hormones, ie, antidiuretic hormone (ADH, vasopressin) and oxytocin, are synthesized in the hypothalamus but are released into the bloodstream in the pars nervosa. The infundibular stalk joins the pars nervosa to the overlying hypothalamus.

ADH, an octapeptide synthesized in the hypothalamus, is packaged into membrane-limited granules with a corresponding binding protein (neurophysin) and transported to the pars nervosa, where it is released into the circulation. ADH binds to specific receptors in the distal part of the nephron and collecting duct of the kidney; it increases the renal tubular reabsorption of water from the glomerular filtrate.

The output of ADH is directly related to the degree of hydration of the body. Hydration of the body inhibits release of ADH, whereas dehydration or injection of hypertonic electrolyte solutions favors release of ADH, which in turn causes increased water resorption from the glomerular filtrate, resulting in dilution and decreased osmolarity of body fluids. Barbiturates, ether, chloroform, morphine, acetylcholine, nicotine, and pain increase ADH release, which leads to less urine formation. Ethanol inhibits ADH release, which leads to diuresis.

The pressor effect of ADH is less prominent than the antidiuretic effect. At a dosage several hundred times larger than the antidiuretic dosage, ADH has a pronounced pressor effect, which may also lead to coronary constriction. The contractile mechanism of the capillaries, as well as GI and uterine muscle, is stimulated, and a prolonged increase in blood pressure follows.

Oxytocin has specific effects on the smooth muscle of the uterus and the myoepithelial cells of the mammary gland. It has no established physiologic function in the male, although an effect on sperm transport has been suggested.

HYPERADRENOCORTICISM

(Cushing disease)

Hyperadrenocorticism may be divided into two broad categories. One category, pituitary-dependent hyperadrenocorticism, arises from adenomatous enlargement of the pituitary gland, resulting in excessive ACTH production. The other category, adrenal-dependent disease, is associated with functional adenomas or adenocarcinomas of the adrenal gland. Ectopic ACTH secretion has not been reported in dogs; however, in people, ectopic ACTH secretion is associated with certain lung tumors. Iatrogenic hyperadrenocorticism results from chronic excessive exogenous steroid administration.

Clinical Findings: Hyperadrenocorticism is seen in middle-aged to older dogs (7–12 yr old); ~85% have pituitary-dependent hyperadrenocorticism (PDH), and ~15% have adrenal tumors. Breeds in which PDH is commonly seen include Miniature Poodles, Dachshunds, Boxers, Boston Terriers, and Beagles. Large-breed dogs often have adrenal tumors, and there is a distinct predilection in females (3:1). In cats, hyperadrenocorticism is found in middle-aged to older cats, with a slight predilection in females (60%).

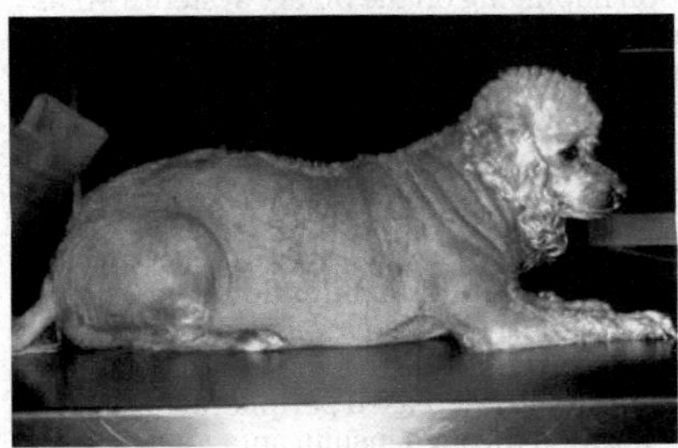

Hyperadrenocorticism in a 7-yr-old intact, female Miniature Poodle. *Courtesy of Dr. Stephen White.*

The most common clinical signs in dogs and cats are polydipsia, polyuria, polyphagia, heat intolerance, lethargy, abdominal enlargement or "potbelly," panting, obesity, muscle weakness, and recurrent urinary tract infections. The panting and increased respiratory rate may be a result of the enlarged liver pushing against the diaphragm and limiting the depth of respiration. Dermatologic manifestations of hyperadrenocorticism in dogs can include alopecia (especially truncal), thin skin, phlebectasias, comedones, bruising, cutaneous hyperpigmentation, calcinosis cutis, pyoderma, dermal atrophy (especially around scars), secondary demodicosis, and seborrhea. In cats, the most striking dermatologic sign is increased skin fragility; many cats present with self-inflicted cutaneous wounds. Secondary infections (especially respiratory) are also common in cats.

Uncommon clinical manifestations include hypertension, pulmonary thromboembolism, bronchial calcification, congestive heart failure, and neurologic signs, such as polyneuropathy or myopathy, behavior changes, blindness, or pseudomyotonia. Hypercortisolemia may be evident as weakening of collagen manifesting as cranial cruciate rupture (small dog) or a nonhealing corneal ulceration. Reproductive signs of hyperadrenocorticism can include perianal adenoma in a female or castrated male, clitoral hypertrophy in females, testicular atrophy in intact males, or prostatomegaly in castrated male dogs.

In dogs, serum chemistry abnormalities associated with hypercortisolemia include increased serum alkaline phosphatase (SAP), increased ALT, hypercholesterolemia, hyperglycemia, and decreased BUN. Hypercholesterolemia is due to steroid stimulation of lipolysis. SAP is increased primarily from induction of a specific hepatic isoenzyme; some also comes from hepatic glycogen deposition and vacuolization impinging on the biliary system. SAP is seldom increased in cats (<20%), because they lack the specific hepatic isoenzyme for it. Increased serum ALT and AST are caused by hepatocellular necrosis, glycogen accumulation, and swollen hepatocytes. Decreased serum phosphorus may be a result of increased urinary excretion due to polyuria. Abnormalities noted on the biochemical profile may also include hyperglycemia due to increased gluconeogenesis and decreased peripheral tissue *utilization* through insulin antagonists. Approximately 10% of Cushingoid dogs are diabetic; however, in cats with hyperadrenocorticism, almost 80% present with overt diabetes mellitus and insulin resistance. The hemogram is characterized by evidence of regeneration (erythrocytosis, nucleated RBCs) and a classic stress leukogram (eosinopenia, lymphopenia, and mature leukocytosis). Basophilia is occasionally seen. Many dogs with hyperadrenocorticism show evidence of urinary tract infection without pyuria (positive culture), bacteriuria, and proteinuria resulting from glomerulosclerosis. In cats, polydipsia and polyuria are a result of concurrent diabetes mellitus, and urine specific gravity is usually high. In dogs, cortisol-induced interference with ADH binding results in hyposthenuria, and central diabetes insipidus may occur as a result of pituitary tumor enlargement.

Diagnosis: There is no single test or combination of tests that is 100% accurate for diagnosing hyperadrenocorticism. The sensitivity and specificity of individual tests or combinations of tests are increased when they are applied to a patient population likely to have hyperadrenocorticism. The diagnosis should be based on appropriate clinical signs followed by supporting minimum database abnormalities (eg, high cholesterol, SAP), and confirmed via an appropriate screening test for hyperadrenocorticism. If screening test results are inconclusive, or if laboratory abnormalities associated with hyperadrenocorticism (eg, increased SAP) are noted in a dog without clinical signs, the dog should be retested 3–6 mo later rather than treated without a definitive diagnosis. In particular, the diagnosis of sex steroid–induced Cushing disease may be especially difficult.

The urine cortisol to creatinine ratio (UCCR) is a highly sensitive test to differentiate healthy dogs from those with hyperadrenocorticism, but it is not highly specific because dogs with moderate to severe nonadrenal illness also exhibit increased ratios. UCCR should be determined based on free-catch urine collected at home by the owner. The stress of transporting the dog to the veterinary hospital, the stress of cystocentesis, or both, can be enough to cause a falsely increased UCCR. An increased UCCR should be confirmed with an ACTH stimulation test, an IV low-dose dexamethasone suppression (LDDS) test, or an oral LDDS test.

The LDDS test is the screening test of choice for canine hyperadrenocorticism when properly used. Only 5%–8% of dogs with PDH exhibit suppressed cortisol concentrations at 8 hr (ie, are false-negatives). In addition, 30% of dogs with PDH exhibit suppression at 3 or 4 hr followed by "escape" of suppression at 8 hr;

this pattern is diagnostic for PDH, making further testing unnecessary. The major disadvantage of the LDDS test is the lack of specificity in dogs with nonadrenal illness: >50% of dogs with nonadrenal illness have a positive LDDS test. In such cases, the dog should be allowed to recover from the nonadrenal illness before testing for hyperadrenocorticism with an LDDS test. Another option, particularly in cats, is to perform an oral LDDS test using the UCCR as the discriminator. In this test, morning urine is collected for a baseline on days 1 and 2. On the second day after urine collection, three doses of dexamethasone at 0.1 mg/kg (cats) or 0.01 mg/kg (dogs) is administered every 6 hr and a urine sample is collected for UCCR measurement the next morning. The first two samples can be combined into a single "pre" or baseline sample. If the UCCR does not decrease into the normal range after oral dexamethasone, the diagnosis of hyperadrenocorticism can be confirmed.

The ACTH stimulation test is used to diagnose various adrenopathic disorders, including endogenous or iatrogenic hyperadrenocorticism and spontaneous hyperadrenocorticism. As a screening test for the diagnosis of naturally occurring hyperadrenocorticism, it has a diagnostic sensitivity of ~80%–85% and a higher specificity than the LDDS test. In one study, only 15% of dogs with nonadrenal disease had an exaggerated response to ACTH stimulation. Adrenal tumors may be particularly difficult to diagnose using an ACTH stimulation test; however, an ACTH stimulation test is the test of choice for iatrogenic hyperadrenocorticism.

Dogs with adrenal sex steroid excess may have negative ACTH stimulation and LDDS tests, because serum cortisol concentrations are normal. This may be due to excess cortisol precursors. Increases in progesterone, 17-OH-progesterone, androstenedione, testosterone, and estrogens may require dynamic adrenal testing using the ACTH stimulation test and measurement of sex steroids in addition to cortisol.

After the diagnosis of hyperadrenocorticism has been confirmed, differentiation of pituitary- versus adrenal-dependent disease may be necessary. Although most dogs with hyperadrenocorticism have PDH, in atypical cases (eg, anorectic dogs with hyperadrenocorticism), a differentiation test is appropriate. In particular, differentiation of PDH (often macroadenomas) from adrenal tumors is often necessary in large breeds.

The high-dose dexamethasone suppression (HDDS) test works on the principle that autonomous ACTH hypersecretion by the pituitary can be suppressed by supraphysiologic concentrations of steroid. Dogs with autonomous cortisol-producing adrenal tumors have maximally suppressed ACTH production via the normal feedback mechanism; therefore, administration of dexamethasone, no matter how high the dose, cannot suppress serum cortisol concentrations. In dogs with PDH, however, the high dose of dexamethasone is able to suppress ACTH and, hence, cortisol secretion. One important caveat is that dogs with pituitary macroadenomas (15%–50% of dogs with PDH) do not suppress on the HDDS test.

Measurement of endogenous plasma ACTH concentrations is the most reliable way to discriminate between PDH and adrenal tumors. Dogs with adrenal tumors have low to undetectable ACTH concentrations; in contrast, dogs with PDH have normal to increased ACTH concentrations. Recently, researchers have found that the addition of the protease inhibitor, aprotinin, to whole blood in EDTA tubes inhibits the degradation of ACTH. Samples may be collected, spun in a nonrefrigerated centrifuge, and kept for as long as 4 days at <4°C.

Diagnostic imaging of the pituitary and the adrenal glands can be accomplished via abdominal radiography, ultrasonography, CT, or MRI. Abdominal radiographs should be performed in all dogs that do not suppress on an HDDS; ~30%–50% of dogs with adrenal tumors have a mineralized mass in the area of the adrenal glands. Abdominal ultrasonography is a more sensitive way to identify adrenal tumors. In addition, liver metastasis or invasion into the vena cava may be demonstrated in dogs with adrenal carcinomas. CT or MRI of the brain or abdominal cavity in dogs that do not suppress on the HDDS may demonstrate unilateral adrenal enlargement (50%), pituitary macroadenoma (25%), or pituitary microadenoma (25%).

Treatment and Prognosis: Three treatment options are available for hyperadrenocorticism in dogs. Medical, surgical, and radiation therapy have all been used with varying degrees of success.

Dogs with PDH may be treated using the adrenolytic agent mitotane (o,p′-DDD), beginning with an induction dosage of 25–50 mg/kg/day for 7–10 days. Dogs should be monitored for signs of hypoadrenocorticism, such as anorexia, vomiting, and diarrhea; if such signs occur, mitotane therapy should be discontinued and glucocorticoids administered. Water consumption or appetite may be measured to provide an endpoint for therapy; water consumption should decrease to <60 mL/kg/day (dogs). After 7–10 days of therapy with mitotane or a reduction in water or food consumption, an ACTH response test should be performed to determine whether cortisol suppression is adequate. Cortisol levels measured both before and after the ACTH response test should be in the normal range. To maintain suppression of cortisol secretion, mitotane is administered at a dosage of 50 mg/kg/wk. Dogs on longterm treatment with mitotane should have an examination and ACTH response test every 3–4 mo. Gradually increasing dosages of the drug are often required to maintain adequate clinical remission.

Adverse effects of mitotane at the recommended dosage include GI irritation (vomiting and anorexia), CNS disturbances (ataxia, weakness, seizures), mild hypoglycemia, and a moderate increase in SAP. Signs such as depression or ataxia can be alleviated by dividing the daily dose into two equal parts administered at 8- to 12-hr intervals. Persistence of CNS signs after mitotane is discontinued suggests an expanding pituitary macroadenoma.

Reports have demonstrated the efficacy of the adrenal enzyme inhibitor trilostane in the treatment of PDH in dogs. Studies in dogs with hyperadrenocorticism have shown that trilostane is an effective steroid inhibitor with minimal adverse effects. Trilostane must be administered daily and often twice daily to achieve a decrease in glucocorticoid secretion from the adrenal glands. Mineralocorticoid insufficiency, which is reversible, can also be seen in animals receiving trilostane; a few cases of adrenal necrosis with permanent adrenal insufficiency have been seen after trilostane administration. Trilostane may prove to be a reasonable alternative to mitotane therapy for PDH in dogs. Dogs with sex steroid imbalance also may benefit from trilostane therapy, because the enzyme inhibitor affects precursors of cortisol synthesis in addition to inhibiting cortisol synthesis itself.

Radiation therapy of pituitary tumors is associated with a high rate of response; however, most dogs and cats require ancillary trilostane or mitotane therapy for several months after radiation treatment because of residual ACTH secretion. In dogs with PDH undergoing hypophysectomy, 80% achieved remission, with an 11% recurrence; thyroid and glucocorticoid support may be needed after surgery, and animals may lose the ability to secrete vasopressin, leading to diabetes insipidus as well. Selegiline is an irreversible monoamine oxidase (type B) inhibitor that increases dopamine levels. Dopamine inhibits ACTH release from the pituitary gland. However, only ~20% of cases with PDH can be expected to respond; no significant changes in serum cortisol or creatinine, ACTH stimulation, or LDDS have been noted with selegiline therapy.

Treatment of iatrogenic hyperadrenocorticism should include a change to an oral, short-acting steroid such as prednisone or prednisolone. Gradually, the steroid dose is decreased from ~1 mg/kg to 0.5 mg/kg throughout several weeks and then tapered to an alternate-day schedule until the adrenal glands can respond to ACTH stimulation. Monthly ACTH stimulation tests may be performed to determine when steroid treatment can be discontinued.

Surgical removal of unilateral adrenal adenomas or adenocarcinomas may be indicated in some cases; however, surgical and anesthetic complications (eg, hypotension) may develop secondary to hypoadrenocorticism, which occurs immediately after surgical removal of the tumor. Median survival for dogs with carcinomas treated with surgical excision was 778 days. The metastatic rate was 5% at time of surgery and 14% longterm. With unilateral adrenalectomies, mortality within 1 mo after surgery was 14%–60%; overall rate for cure for adrenal tumors was ~50%. Medical treatment of adrenal tumors is difficult, because they tend to be resistant to the effects of mitotane. Adrenal tumors are relatively resistant to mitotane; dogs require as much as four times the dose of mitotane to respond, and clinical response tends to be less favorable. Finally, if the dog is showing neurologic signs (eg, anorexia, stupor, or seizures) and a large pituitary tumor (macroadenoma) is identified, radiation therapy of the pituitary gland is indicated. Newer types of radiation therapy (cyberknife, gamma knife) may prove to be superior to previously available modalities and can treat pituitary tumors in <3 days with minimal adverse effects. Results of radiation therapy in dogs show that this is an effective method of treatment with low morbidity; however, it may take several months for the signs of PDH to subside. These dogs do well longterm, however, because the primary disease process (pituitary tumor) has been addressed.

Prognosis of dogs with PDH has been estimated to be ~2 yr with or without medical therapy. Radiation treatment of pituitary tumors causing PDH or hypophysectomies is associated with a relatively good longterm prognosis (2–5 yr). Prognosis of dogs with unilateral adrenalectomy was 18 mo.

NONFUNCTIONAL PITUITARY TUMORS

Nonfunctional pituitary tumors are uncommon in most species. Chromophobe adenomas appear to be endocrinologically inactive, but they may cause compression atrophy of adjacent portions of the pituitary gland and extend into the overlying brain. Clinical disturbances occur because of either a lack of secretion of pituitary trophic hormones and diminished target organ function (eg, adrenal cortex) or dysfunction of the CNS. Affected animals often are depressed, incoordinated, and weak and may collapse with exercise. (*See also* ADULT-ONSET PANHYPOPITUITARISM, below.)

Endocrinologically inactive pituitary adenomas often attain considerable size before they cause obvious signs (or death). The proliferating tumor cells incorporate the remaining structures of the adenohypophysis and infundibular stalk. The entire hypothalamus may become compressed and replaced by the tumor.

HIRSUTISM ASSOCIATED WITH ADENOMAS OF THE PARS INTERMEDIA

(Hypertrichosis)

Hirsutism is the long, nonshedding hair coat that develops in older horses (typically ≥18 yr old) and is associated with pituitary pars intermedia dysfunction (PPID) caused by an adenoma of the cells of the pars intermedia of the pituitary gland. Such adenomas often severely compress the overlying hypothalamus, which is the primary center for homeostatic regulation of body temperature, appetite, and cyclic shedding of hair. In addition, pars intermedia adenomas secrete increased amounts of alpha melanocyte-stimulating hormone (MSH), a factor in the growth of a long hair coat in winter.

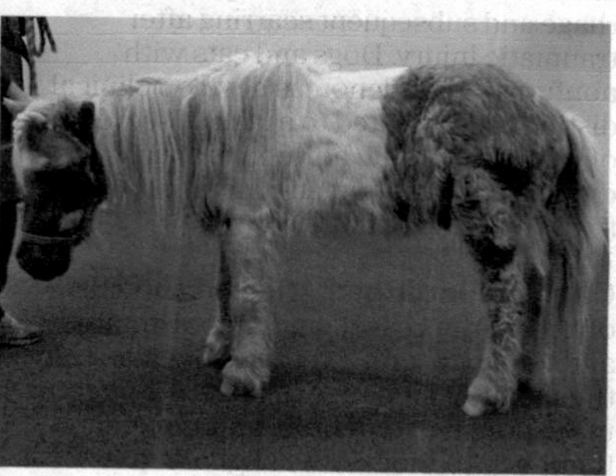

Hirsutism in a pony, associated with advanced pituitary pars intermedia dysfunction. *Courtesy of Dr. Janice Kritchevsky.*

Clinical Findings and Lesions: Signs of PPID include polyuria and polydipsia (PU/PD), poor muscle tone, weakness, somnolence, abnormal distribution of adipose tissue, swelling of the periorbital fossa, laminitis, increased susceptibility to infections, intermittent hyperpyrexia, and generalized hyperhidrosis. Hirsutism often becomes evident because of failure of the cyclic seasonal shedding of hair. Before generalized hirsutism is observed, horses may have longer hair on the legs, ventral abdomen, and throat latch. Eventually, the hair over most of the trunk and extremities becomes long (up to 4–5 in. [10–12 cm]), abnormally thick, wavy, and often matted.

Pars intermedia adenomas are the most common pituitary tumors in horses. They are yellow to white, multinodular, and compress the pars nervosa. Horses with PPID may have hyperglycemia (insulin-resistant) and glycosuria. It is not known why some horses with PPID become insulin resistant and others do not. However, cortisol and other hormones that may be present in increased concentrations in horses with PPID are insulin antagonists.

Plasma immunoreactive adrenocorticotropin and alpha-MSH levels may range from modestly to extremely increased. Blood cortisol concentrations generally remain in the normal range but lack normal diurnal rhythm and escape suppression by administration of dexamethasone much more quickly than in healthy animals.

Diagnosis: Hyperglycemia and insulin insensitivity are suggestive of pituitary adenoma in horses, but because they occur in horses with equine metabolic syndrome (*see* p 1006) or other insulin dysregulation syndromes, they are not diagnostic of PPID. Other nonspecific findings include an absolute or relative neutrophilia, eosinopenia, and lymphopenia; lipemia; hypercholesterolemia; and a mild, normochromic, normocytic anemia. Liver enzymes may be increased. Electrolytes are usually normal. Urinalysis is normal except for occasional glycosuria and a low to normal specific gravity.

Definitive diagnosis is based on evocative testing or measurement of resting endogenous ACTH concentrations. Dexamethasone (40 mcg/kg, IM) often will not suppress cortisol levels to at least 30% of baseline or to <1 mcg/dL, as it does in healthy horses 6–15 hr after administration. In addition, cortisol concentrations return to within 80% or greater of baseline values 24 hr after dexamethasone administration in horses with PPID. Healthy horses have suppressed cortisol levels 24 hr after dexamethasone administration. Horses with PPID react with an exaggerated response to domperidone administration. Increase in plasma endogenous ACTH to ≥100% of baseline levels 2–4 hr after administration of domperidone at 5 mg/kg, PO, is consistent with PPID. Horses with PPID have an increase in plasma endogenous ACTH concentration 10 min after administration of 1 mg thyroid-releasing hormone (TRH), and the TRH stimulation test is believed to be the most sensitive means to detect a pituitary tumor. Horses experience a seasonal rise in endogenous ACTH in the autumn (August through November in the northern hemisphere). Healthy horses are less likely to have a decreased cortisol concentration in response to dexamethasone administration and may demonstrate an exaggerated response to domperidone or TRH in the autumn as well. For this reason, unless there are season-specific normal values available for the testing being performed, it is recommended to perform diagnostic testing for PPID from January through July.

Differential diagnoses include syndromes resulting in chronic debilitation, eg, poor management and nutrition, parasitism, and chronic systemic diseases. The PU/PD must be differentiated from that due to chronic renal disease or diabetes insipidus. The hyperglycemia, glycosuria, and PU/PD must be differentiated from that caused by primary diabetes mellitus. High insulin concentrations or an increased glucose to insulin ratio must be differentiated from primary hyperinsulinemia (equine metabolic syndrome). Pheochromocytomas (*see* p 576) may cause hyperhidrosis, hyperglycemia, and tachypnea, although they usually are nonfunctional and found only incidentally at necropsy. Differential diagnosis for hirsutism includes being of the Bashkir Curly breed or having a congenital curly coat abnormality. There is no other recognized condition in which adult horses acquire a long, curly hair coat. For this reason, hirsutism can be considered a *positive* diagnostic test for PPID.

Treatment: Horses with PPID are relatively fragile, with poor immune function. Thus, most require diligent attention to good husbandry. Pergolide, a dopaminergic agonist, is currently the only agent demonstrated to decrease endogenous ACTH concentrations in horses with PPID. Starting dosages are 0.006–0.01 mg/kg/day, PO. This typically results in a dose of 0.5–1 mg/day. If this amount does not result in improvement in clinical signs and endocrinologic testing, it may be increased gradually. Reported adverse effects of pergolide therapy include depression and anorexia. Often, these signs are transitory and resolve over time. If they do not, the dose may be decreased temporarily or split and given twice daily. Although its use has not been documented to result in improvement in clinical signs when given alone, cyproheptadine at a dosage of 0.6–1.2 mg/kg/day, PO, may exert synergistic effects when combined with pergolide, and the combination may result in outcomes better than those achieved with pergolide alone. Trilostane, a competitive 3-β hydroxysteroid dehydrogenase inhibitor, has not been investigated adequately in the horse, although its use has improved clinical results.

ADULT-ONSET PANHYPOPITUITARISM

Endocrinologically inactive, nonfunctional pituitary tumors develop most commonly in adult to aged animals; there is no apparent breed predisposition. The most common cause is a chromophobe adenoma arising in the pars distalis. Other infrequent causes include extensive inflammatory destruction of pituitary tissue, ischemic necrosis of the pituitary due to infarction from invasion of tumor cells, parasitic or septic emboli, diffuse necrosis associated with toxemia, invasion by neoplasms arising in adjacent structures (eg, meninges, sphenoid bone, nasal cavity, etc), and widespread hemorrhage and subsequent scarring after traumatic injury. Dogs and cats with nonfunctional adenomas develop clinical disturbances related to a lack of secretion of pituitary trophic hormones and diminished target organ function or to dysfunction of the CNS.

Clinical Findings: Affected animals often are depressed and incoordinated and collapse with exercise. Occasionally, they exhibit a change in attitude, become unresponsive to people, and develop a tendency to hide at the slightest provocation. In chronic cases, there may be evidence of blindness, with dilated and fixed pupils due to compression and disruption of optic nerves by dorsal extension of the pituitary tumor. Affected dogs often show a progressive weight loss with muscle atrophy due to loss of the protein anabolic effect of growth hormone. Compression of the cells that secrete gonadotropic hormones or the corresponding releasing hormone from the hypothalamus results in atrophy of the gonads. Disturbances of water balance result from interference with the synthesis of antidiuretic hormone (ADH) or its release into capillaries of the pars nervosa. The posterior lobe, infundibular stalk, and hypothalamus are compressed or disrupted by neoplastic cells.

Animals with panhypopituitarism appear dehydrated despite increased water consumption. Dogs and cats with large nonfunctional pituitary tumors usually excrete large volumes of dilute urine with a low specific gravity (≤1.007) and may break housetraining. Clinical signs are not highly specific and can be confused with those of other CNS disorders (eg, brain tumors or encephalitis) or chronic renal disease.

Hypopituitarism caused by pituitary tumors should be included in the differential diagnosis of diseases characterized by incoordination, depression, polyuria, blindness, and sudden behavioral changes in adult or aged animals. Because the blindness is central in origin, ophthalmoscopic examination usually does not reveal significant lesions. There is no effect on body stature associated with compression of the pars distalis and probable interference of growth hormone secretion, because these tumors usually arise in dogs that have already completed their growth. Parakeets with chromophobe adenomas often develop exophthalmos due to extension of neoplastic cells along the optic nerve.

Lesions: Endocrinologically inactive pituitary adenomas usually reach considerable size before they cause obvious signs or death. The proliferating tumor cells incorporate the remaining structures of the adenohypophysis and infundibular stalk. The entire hypothalamus may be compressed and replaced by tumor.

Thyroid glands in dogs and cats with large pituitary adenomas often are smaller than normal, although to a much lesser degree than the adrenal cortex. The adrenal glands are small and consist primarily of medullary tissue surrounded by a narrow zone of cortex. Seminiferous tubules are small and show little evidence of active spermatogenesis.

Skin atrophy and loss of muscle mass may be related to a lack of protein anabolic effects of growth hormone in an adult dog or cat. Interference with the secretion of pituitary trophic hormones often results in gonadal atrophy resulting in either decreased libido or anestrus.

JUVENILE-ONSET PANHYPOPITUITARISM

(Pituitary dwarfism)

Pituitary dwarfism occurs most frequently in German Shepherds but has been reported in other breeds such as the Spitz, Miniature Pinscher, and Karelian Bear Dog. It is inherited as a simple autosomal recessive trait.

Pituitary dwarfism is usually associated with a failure of the oropharyngeal ectoderm of the cranial pharyngeal duct (Rathke's pouch) to differentiate into trophic-hormone-secreting cells of the pars distalis. Consequently, the adenohypophysis is not completely developed. The second most common cause is craniopharyngioma, a benign tumor derived from the oropharyngeal ectoderm of Rathke's pouch. Compared with other types of pituitary neoplasms, these tumors tend to develop in younger dogs. Craniopharyngiomas cause subnormal secretion of growth hormone, which results in dwarfism.

Clinical Findings: Dwarf pups are indistinguishable from normal littermates up to 2 mo old. Subsequently, the slower growth rate compared with littermates, retention of puppy coat, and lack of primary guard hairs gradually become evident. German Shepherds with pituitary dwarfism appear coyote- or fox-like, owing to their small size and soft, woolly coat. Bilaterally symmetric alopecia develops gradually and often becomes complete except for the head and tufts of hair on the legs. Permanent dentition is delayed or completely absent. Closure of the epiphyses is delayed as long as 4 yr depending on the severity of the hormonal insufficiency and is caused by deficiencies of both thyroid-stimulating hormone and growth hormone. The testes and penis are small, calcification of the os penis is delayed or incomplete, and the penile sheath is flaccid. The ovarian cortex is hypoplastic, and estrus is irregular or absent. Lifespan is shortened because of the resulting secondary endocrine dysfunction, such as hypothyroidism and hypoadrenocorticism. Puppies with panhypopituitarism often have a shrill bark.

Lesions: Pituitary cysts fill with mucus and eventually occupy the entire pituitary area, resulting in severe compression of the pars nervosa and infundibular stalk. Craniopharyngiomas are large, solid, cystic areas that extend into the overlying hypothalamus. They may also grow along the ventral aspect of the brain, where incorporation of several cranial nerves results in specific nerve function deficits.

Diagnosis: Levels of thyroxine, triiodothyronine, and cortisol are reduced or in the low-normal range. In those animals with an equivocal change in basal hormone level, the responses to challenge by exogenous thyrotropin or adrenocorticotropin are subnormal, owing to the hypoplasia or atrophy of the thyroid gland and adrenal cortex. Other useful diagnostic aids include comparison of height with that of littermates, evidence of delayed epiphyseal closure or dysgenesis on skeletal radiographs, and skin biopsy. Cutaneous lesions include hyperkeratosis, follicular keratosis, hyperpigmentation, adnexal atrophy, loss of elastin fibers, and a loose network of collagen fibers in the dermis. Hair shafts are absent, and hair follicles are primarily in the telogen stage of the growth cycle.

The activity of somatomedin C (insulin-like growth factor 1) is low in dwarf dogs. Intermediate somatomedin C activity is present in phenotypically normal ancestors suspected to be heterozygous carriers. Assays for somatomedin C provide an indirect measurement of circulating growth hormone activity in dogs with suspected pituitary dwarfism. Basal levels of circulating canine growth hormone are reported to be detectable but low (normal range: 1.75 ± 0.17 mg/mL) in pituitary dwarfs and do not increase after a provocative test for secretion via clonidine injection (30 mcg/kg, IV) as they do in healthy dogs. Insulin hypersensitivity has been demonstrated in pituitary dwarf dogs, probably due to a change in insulin receptor numbers or affinity of binding in response to the low level of growth hormone.

DIABETES INSIPIDUS

Central diabetes insipidus is caused by reduced secretion of antidiuretic hormone (ADH). When target cells in the kidney lack the biochemical machinery necessary to respond to the *secretion* of normal or increased circulating levels of ADH, nephrogenic diabetes insipidus results. It occurs infrequently in dogs, cats, and laboratory rats, and rarely in other animals.

Etiology: The hypophyseal form develops as a result of compression and destruction of the pars nervosa, infundibular stalk, or supraoptic nucleus in the hypothalamus. The lesions responsible for the disruption of ADH synthesis or secretion in hypophyseal diabetes insipidus include large pituitary neoplasms (endocrinologically active or inactive), a dorsally expanding cyst or inflammatory granuloma, and traumatic injury to the skull with hemorrhage and glial proliferation in the neurohypophyseal system.

Clinical Findings: Affected animals excrete large volumes of hypotonic urine and drink equally large amounts of water. Urine osmolality is decreased below normal plasma osmolality (~300 mOsm/kg) in both hypophyseal and nephrogenic forms, even if the animal is deprived of water. The increase of urine osmolality above that of plasma in response to exogenous ADH in the hypophyseal form, but not in the nephrogenic form, is useful in the clinical differentiation of the two forms of the disease.

Lesions: The posterior lobe, infundibular stalk, and hypothalamus are compressed or disrupted by neoplastic cells. This interrupts the nonmyelinated axons that transport ADH from its site of production (hypothalamus) to its site of release (pars nervosa).

Diagnosis: This is based on chronic polyuria that does not respond to dehydration and is not due to primary renal disease. To evaluate the ability to concentrate urine, a water deprivation test should be done if the animal is not dehydrated and does not have renal disease. The bladder is emptied, and water and food are withheld (usually 3–8 hr) to provide a maximum stimulus for ADH secretion. The animal should be monitored carefully to prevent a loss of >5% body wt and severe dehydration. Urine and plasma osmolality should be determined; however, because these tests are not readily available to most practitioners, urine specific gravity is frequently used instead. At the end of the test, urine specific gravity is >1.025 in those animals with only a partial ADH deficiency or with antagonism to ADH action caused by hypercortisolism. There is little change in specific gravity in those animals with a complete lack of ADH activity, whether due to a primary loss of ADH or to unresponsiveness of the kidneys.

An ADH response test should follow to differentiate among conditions that may result in large volumes of urine that is chronically low in specific gravity but otherwise normal. These include nephrogenic diabetes insipidus (an inability of the kidneys to respond to ADH), psychogenic diabetes insipidus (a polydipsia in response to some psychological disturbance but a normal response to ADH), and hypercortisolism (which results in a partial deficiency of ADH activity due to the antagonistic effect of cortisol on ADH activity in the kidneys). This test also can be used to evaluate animals in which a water deprivation test could not be performed. Urine specific gravity is determined at the start of the test, desmopressin acetate is administered (2–4 drops in the conjunctival sac), the bladder is emptied at 2 hr, and urine specific gravity is measured at set intervals (4, 8, 12, 18, and 24 hr) after ADH administration. Specific gravity peaks at >1.026 in animals with a primary ADH deficiency, is significantly increased above the level induced with water deprivation in those with a partial deficiency in ADH activity, and shows little change in those with nephrogenic diabetes insipidus.

If osmolality is measured, the ratio of urine to plasma osmolality after water deprivation is >3 in healthy animals, 1.8–3 in those with moderate ADH deficiency, and <1.8 in those with severe deficiency. The ratio of urine osmolality after ADH administration as compared with water deprivation is >2 in animals with primary ADH deficiency, between 1.1 and 2 in those with inhibitors to ADH action, and <1.1 in those unresponsive to ADH.

As an alternative to the water deprivation test, or in cases in which this test does not establish a definitive diagnosis, a closely monitored therapeutic trial with desmopressin (*see* below) can be performed. Again, all other causes of polyuria and polydipsia should initially be excluded, limiting the differential diagnosis to central diabetes insipidus, nephrogenic diabetes insipidus, and psychogenic polydipsia. For cats, the owner should measure the animal's 24-hr water intake 2–3 days before the therapeutic trial with desmopressin, allowing free-choice water intake. The intranasal preparation of desmopressin is administered in the conjunctival sac (1–4 drops, bid) for 3–5 days. A dramatic reduction in water intake (>50%) during the first treatment day strongly suggests an ADH deficiency and a diagnosis of central diabetes insipidus or partial nephrogenic diabetes insipidus.

Diabetes insipidus also needs to be distinguished from other diseases with polyuria. The most common are diabetes mellitus with glycosuria and high urine specific gravity, and chronic nephritis with a urine specific gravity that is usually low and shows evidence of renal failure (protein, casts, etc).

Treatment: Polyuria may be controlled using desmopressin acetate, a synthetic analogue of ADH. The initial dose is 2 drops applied to the nasal mucosae or conjunctivae; this is gradually increased until the minimal effective dose is determined. Maximal effect usually occurs in 2–6 hr and lasts for 10–12 hr. Water should not be restricted. Treatment should be continued once or twice daily for the life of the animal.

FELINE ACROMEGALY

Acromegaly, or hypersomatotropism, results from chronic, excessive secretion of growth hormone in the adult animal. Acromegaly in cats is caused by a growth hormone–secreting tumor of the anterior pituitary. In cats, these tumors grow slowly and may be present for a long time before clinical signs appear.

Clinical Findings: Feline acromegaly occurs in older (8–14 yr) cats and appears to be more common in males. Clinical signs of uncontrolled diabetes mellitus are often the first sign of acromegaly in cats; therefore, polydipsia, polyuria, and polyphagia are the most common presenting signs. Net weight gain of lean body mass in cats with uncontrolled diabetes mellitus is a key sign of acromegaly. Organomegaly, including renomegaly, hepatomegaly, and enlargement of endocrine organs, is also seen. Some, but not all, cats show the classic enlargement of extremities, body size, jaw, tongue, and forehead that is characteristic of acromegaly in people. Some of the most striking manifestations are seen in the musculoskeletal system and include an increase in muscle mass and growth of the acral segments of the body, including the paws, chin, and skull. Stridor may be detected as a result of increased soft-tissue enlargement of the epiglottis and surrounding tissues. Cardiovascular abnormalities such as cardiomegaly (radiographic and echocardiographic), systolic murmurs, and congestive heart failure develop late in the disease course. Azotemia also develops late in the course of the disease in ~50% of acromegalic cats. Neurologic signs of acromegaly in people, such as peripheral neuropathies (paresthesias, carpal tunnel syndrome, sensory and motor defects) and parasellar manifestations (headache and visual field defects), are not generally detected in acromegalic cats.

Impaired glucose tolerance and insulin resistance resulting in diabetes mellitus are seen in all cats with acromegaly. Measurement of endogenous insulin reveals dramatically increased serum insulin concentrations. Despite severe insulin resistance and hyperglycemia, ketosis is rare. Hypercholesterolemia and mild increases in liver enzymes are attributed to the diabetic state. Hyperphosphatemia without azotemia is also a common clinicopathologic finding. Urinalysis is unremarkable except for persistent proteinuria. In a recent study, acromegaly was the most common (25%) underlying cause of non-insulin–dependent diabetes mellitus in cats, and it should be suspected in any cat that does not respond to standard therapy for type 2 diabetes mellitus (high-protein, low-carbohydrate diet and glargine insulin) within 4 mo of initiating therapy.

Lesions: Gross necropsy findings in acromegalic cats may include a large expansile pituitary mass, hypertrophic cardiomyopathy with marked left ventricular and septal hypertrophy (early) or dilated cardiomyopathy (late), hepatomegaly, renomegaly, degenerative joint disease, lumbar vertebral spondylosis, moderate enlargement of the parathyroid glands, adrenocortical hyperplasia, and diffuse enlargement of the pancreas with multifocal nodular hyperplasia. Histopathologic examination of the endocrine glands reveals acidophil adenoma of the pituitary; adenomatous hyperplasia of the thyroid gland; and nodular hyperplasia of the adrenal cortices, parathyroid glands, and pancreas.

Diagnosis: A definitive diagnosis requires measurement of increased plasma growth hormone or insulin-like growth factor 1 (IGF-1) concentrations in suspected cases. Unfortunately, feline growth hormone assays are no longer available. Serum IGF-1 concentrations are often dramatically increased in acromegalic cats (as in affected people). Currently, the most definitive diagnostic test is CT of the pituitary region. Results of CT, coupled with the exclusion of other disorders that cause insulin resistance (hyperthyroidism, hyperadrenocorticism) and clinical signs and laboratory abnormalities, support a diagnosis of acromegaly.

Treatment and Prognosis: Medical therapy in people includes the use of dopamine agonists, such as bromocriptine, and somatostatin analogues (octreotide). Treatment with octreotide has been unsuccessful in acromegalic cats. The lack of efficacy of the long-acting somatostatin analogues may result from species-specific tissue binding. Radiation therapy probably offers the greatest chance for success with low rates of morbidity and mortality. The disadvantages include the slow rate of tumor shrinkage (>3 yr) and the occurrence of hypopituitarism, cranial and optic nerve damage, and radiation injury to the hypothalamus.

The short-term prognosis in cats with untreated acromegaly is fair to good. Insulin resistance is generally controlled satisfactorily by using large doses of insulin divided into several daily doses. Mild cardiac disease can be managed with diuretics and vasodilators. The longterm prognosis is relatively poor, however, and most cats die of congestive heart failure, chronic renal failure, or signs of an expanding pituitary mass. The longterm prognosis may improve with early diagnosis and treatment.

THE THYROID GLAND

All vertebrates have a thyroid gland. In mammals, it is usually bilobed and located just caudal to the larynx, adjacent to the lateral surface of the trachea. The two lobes may be connected by a fibrous isthmus (eg, ruminants, *horses*), or a connecting isthmus may be indistinct (eg, dogs, cats). The gland is extremely vascular. In birds, it is found within the thoracic cavity; both lobes are located near the syrinx, adjacent to the carotid artery near the origin of the vertebral artery.

Ectopic or accessory thyroid tissue is relatively common in most species, especially dogs and cats. It may be located anywhere from the larynx to the diaphragm and may be responsible for maintaining normal thyroid function after surgical thyroidectomy. In addition, ectopic thyroid tissue occasionally is the site of hyperplasia or neoplasia.

Physiology: Thyroid hormones are the only iodinated organic compounds in the body. Thyroxine (T_4) is the main secretory product of the normal thyroid gland. However, the gland also secretes 3,5,3′-triiodothyronine (T_3), reverse T_3, and other deiodinated metabolites. T_3 is ~3–5 times more potent than T_4, whereas reverse T_3 is thyromimetically inactive.

Although all T_4 is secreted by the thyroid, a considerable amount of T_3 is derived from T_4; therefore, T_4 has been called a prohormone. Its activation to the more potent T_3 is a step regulated individually by peripheral tissues.

Thyroid hormone secretion is regulated primarily via negative-feedback control through the coordinated response of the hypothalamic-pituitary-thyroid axis: thyrotropin-releasing hormone (TRH) binds to the thyrotroph cell in the pituitary and stimulates secretion of thyrotropin (thyroid-stimulating hormone, TSH), which binds to the follicular cell membrane and stimulates thyroid hormone synthesis and secretion.

Thyroid hormones are water-insoluble lipophilic compounds that are bound to plasma proteins (thyroxine-binding protein, thyroxine-binding prealbumin [transthyretin], and albumin). The major function of the thyroid hormone–binding proteins is probably to provide a hormone reservoir in the plasma and to "buffer" hormone delivery into tissue. In healthy euthyroid animals, 0.1% of total serum T_4 is free (not bound to thyroid hormone–binding proteins), whereas ~1% of circulating T_3 is free. Evidence suggests that the fractions of circulating free T_4 and free T_3 determine the amount of hormone available for uptake by tissues.

Action of Thyroid Hormones: Thyroid hormones act on many different cellular processes; however, no single reaction or metabolic event can be equated with their action. Although both T_4 and T_3 have intrinsic metabolic activity, T_3 is 3–5 times more potent in binding to the nuclear receptors and similarly more potent in stimulating oxygen consumption.

Effects of thyroid hormones generally are divided into two categories: those that manifest within minutes to hours after hormone receptor binding and do not require protein synthesis, and those that manifest later (usually >6 hr) and require synthesis of new proteins. About half the increase in oxygen consumption produced by thyroid hormones is related to activation of the plasma membrane–bound Na^+/K^+ ATPase; thyroid hormones also stimulate mitochondrial oxygen consumption. These changes are linked directly to the calorigenic effect of thyroid hormones. More chronic effects invariably are related to the cellular actions that require interaction with nuclear T_3 receptors, followed by an increase in protein synthesis crucial to physiologic processes such as growth, differentiation, proliferation, and maturation.

Thyroid hormones, in physiologic quantities, are anabolic. In conjunction with growth hormone and insulin, protein synthesis is stimulated and nitrogen excretion is reduced. However, in excess (hyperthyroidism), they can be catabolic, with increased gluconeogenesis, protein breakdown, and nitrogen wasting.

HYPOTHYROIDISM

In hypothyroidism, impaired production and secretion of the thyroid hormones result in a decreased metabolic rate. This disorder is most common in dogs but also develops rarely in other species, including cats, horses, and other large, domestic animals.

Etiology: Although dysfunction anywhere in the hypothalamic-pituitary-thyroid axis may result in thyroid hormone deficiency, >95% of clinical cases of hypothyroidism in dogs appear to result from destruction of the thyroid gland itself (primary hypothyroidism). The two most common causes of adult-onset primary hypothyroidism in dogs include lymphocytic thyroiditis and idiopathic atrophy of the thyroid gland. Lymphocytic thyroiditis, probably immune-mediated, is characterized histologically by a diffuse infiltration of the gland by lymphocytes, plasma cells, and macrophages and results in progressive destruction of follicles and secondary fibrosis. Idiopathic atrophy of the thyroid gland is characterized histologically by loss of thyroid parenchyma and replacement by adipose tissue. (*See also* AUTOIMMUNE THYROIDITIS, p 831.)

In dogs, the most common cause of secondary hypothyroidism is destruction of pituitary thyrotrophs by an expanding, space-occupying tumor. Because of the nonselective nature of the resulting compressive atrophy and replacement of pituitary tissue by such large tumors, deficiencies of other (one or more) pituitary hormones also usually occur.

Other rare forms of hypothyroidism in dogs include neoplastic destruction of thyroid tissue and congenital (or juvenile-onset) hypothyroidism. Congenital primary hypothyroidism may result from one of various forms of thyroid dysgenesis (eg, athyreosis, thyroid hypoplasia) or from dyshormonogenesis (usually an inherited inability to organify iodide). Congenital secondary hypothyroidism (associated with clinical signs of disproportionate dwarfism, lethargy, gait abnormalities, and constipation) has been reported in Giant Schnauzers, Toy Fox Terriers, and Scottish Deerhounds. Congenital secondary hypothyroidism also has been reported in German Shepherds with pituitary dwarfism associated with a cystic Rathke's pouch. However, the degree of TSH deficiency in these dogs is variable, and clinical signs are usually caused primarily by deficiency of growth hormone (rather than thyroid hormone).

In cats, iatrogenic hypothyroidism is the most common form. Hypothyroidism develops in these cats after treatment for hyperthyroidism with radioiodine, surgical thyroidectomy, or use of an antithyroid drug. Although naturally occurring hypothyroidism is an extremely rare disorder in adult cats, congenital or juvenile-onset hypothyroidism does also occur. Recognized causes of congenital hypothyroidism in cats include intrathyroidal defects in thyroid hormone biosynthesis (dyshormonogenesis), an inability of the thyroid gland to respond to TSH, and thyroid dysgenesis. All reported cats with hypothyroidism have had the primary (thyroidal) disorder. Secondary (pituitary) or tertiary (hypothalamic) hypothyroidism has not been well described in either juvenile or adult cats but has been reported after severe head trauma.

In foals, congenital hypothyroidism may develop when pregnant mares graze plants that contain goitrogens, or are fed diets either deficient in or containing excessive amounts of iodine. Most commonly, congenital hypothyroidism develops in association with a specific syndrome of neonatal foals characterized by thyroid gland hyperplasia together with multiple congenital musculoskeletal anomalies. This syndrome, reported most commonly in western Canada, has been referred to as either thyroid hyperplasia and musculoskeletal deformities syndrome or as congenital hypothyroidism and dysmaturity syndrome and may be related to feeding a high nitrate diet to pregnant mares. In adult horses, hypothyroidism appears to be very rare but, as in other species, is commonly misdiagnosed.

Clinical Findings: Although onset is variable, hypothyroidism is most common in dogs 4–10 yr old. It usually affects mid- to large-size breeds and is rare in toy and miniature breeds. Breeds reported to be predisposed include the Golden Retriever, Doberman Pinscher, Irish Setter, Miniature Schnauzer, Dachshund, Cocker Spaniel, and Airedale Terrier. There does not appear to be a sex predilection, but spayed females appear to have a higher risk of developing hypothyroidism than intact females.

A deficiency of thyroid hormone affects the function of all organ systems; as a result, clinical signs are diffuse, variable, often nonspecific, and rarely pathognomonic. Although the disorder should be highly suspect, overdiagnosis should be avoided, because many diseases, especially those of the skin, can easily be misdiagnosed as hypothyroidism.

Many of the clinical signs associated with canine hypothyroidism are directly related to slowing of cellular metabolism, which results in development of mental dullness, lethargy, exercise intolerance, and weight gain without a corresponding increase in appetite. Mild to marked obesity develops in some dogs. Difficulty maintaining body temperature may lead to frank hypothermia; the classic hypothyroid dog is a heat-seeker. Alterations in the skin and coat are common. Dryness, excessive shedding, and retarded regrowth of hair are usually the earliest dermatologic changes. Nonpruritic hair thinning or alopecia (usually bilaterally symmetric) that may involve the ventral and lateral trunk, the caudal surfaces of the thighs, dorsum of the tail, ventral neck, and the dorsum of the nose is seen in about two-thirds of dogs with hypothyroidism. Alopecia, sometimes associated with hyperpigmentation, often starts over points of wear. Occasionally, secondary pyoderma (which may produce pruritus) is seen.

In moderate to severe cases, thickening of the skin occurs secondary to accumulation of glycosaminoglycans (mostly hyaluronic acid) in the dermis. In such cases, myxedema is most common on the forehead and face, resulting in a puffy appearance and thickened skin folds above the eyes. This puffiness, together with slight drooping of the upper eyelid, gives some dogs a "tragic" facial expression. These changes also have been described in the GI tract, heart, and skeletal muscles.

In intact dogs, hypothyroidism may cause various reproductive disturbances: in females, failure to cycle (anestrus) or sporadic cycling, infertility, abortion, or poor litter survival; and in males, lack of libido, testicular atrophy, hypospermia, or infertility.

A variety of neurologic disorders, including megaesophagus, laryngeal paralysis, facial nerve paralysis, and vestibular disease, have been related to hypothyroidism. However, all such peripheral and central nervous disease is uncommon, at least compared with the metabolic and dermatologic changes commonly seen in hypothyroid dogs. In addition, such neurologic signs do not always resolve after thyroid hormone replacement therapy.

Myxedema coma, a rare syndrome, is the extreme expression of severe hypothyroidism. The course can develop rapidly; lethargy progresses to stupor and then coma. The common signs of hypothyroidism (eg, hair loss) are usually present, but other signs, such as hypoventilation, hypotension, bradycardia, and profound hypothermia, are usually seen as well.

During the fetal period and in the first few months of postnatal life, thyroid hormones are crucial for growth and development of the skeleton and CNS. Therefore, in addition to the well-recognized signs of adult-onset hypothyroidism, disproportionate dwarfism and impaired mental development (cretinism) are prominent signs of congenital and juvenile-onset hypothyroidism. In primary congenital hypothyroidism, enlargement of the thyroid gland (goiter) also may be detected, depending on the cause of the hypothyroidism. Radiographic signs of epiphyseal dysgenesis (underdeveloped epiphyses throughout the long bones), shortened vertebral bodies, and delayed epiphyseal closure are common.

In dogs with congenital hypopituitarism (pituitary dwarfism, *see* p 549), there may be variable degrees of thyroidal, adrenocortical, and gonadal deficiency, but clinical signs are primarily related to growth hormone deficiency. Signs include proportionate dwarfism (rather than the disproportionate form of dwarfism characteristic of congenital hypothyroidism), loss of primary guard hairs with retention of the puppy coat, hyperpigmentation of the skin, and bilaterally symmetric alopecia of the trunk.

In adult cats, clinical signs associated with advanced or severe hypothyroidism include lethargy, dullness, nonpruritic seborrhea sicca, hypothermia, decreased appetite, and occasionally bradycardia. Obesity may develop, especially in cats with iatrogenic hypothyroidism, but it is not a consistent sign. Bilaterally symmetric alopecia, except for pinnal involvement, does not appear to develop, but focal areas of alopecia over the craniolateral carpi, caudal hocks, and dorsal and lateral tailbase have occasionally been seen. However, in many cats with mild iatrogenic hypothyroidism, very mild or no obvious clinical signs are seen. In young cats with congenital or juvenile-onset hypothyroidism, the clinical signs are more obvious and include disproportionate dwarfism, severe lethargy, mental dullness, constipation, inappetence, and bradycardia.

Diagnosis of Hypothyroidism:

Hypothyroidism is probably one of the most overdiagnosed diseases in dogs. Many diseases and conditions can mimic hypothyroidism, and some of the clinical signs, even in dogs with normal thyroid function, can improve after administration of exogenous thyroid hormone. In addition, a variety of nonthyroidal factors (eg, nonthyroidal illness and prior administration of certain drugs) can lead to low serum thyroid hormone measurements in euthyroid dogs, cats, and other species. Definitive diagnosis of canine hypothyroidism requires careful attention to clinical signs and results of routine laboratory testing. Tests that may confirm the diagnosis include measurement of the serum concentrations of total T_4, free T_4, and TSH; provocative thyroid function tests (eg, TSH stimulation test); thyroid gland imaging; and response to thyroid hormone supplementation. Choice and interpretation of diagnostic tests is based heavily on the index of suspicion for hypothyroidism.

There are well-recognized clinicopathologic abnormalities associated with hypothyroidism, the severity of which usually correlates with the severity and chronicity of the hypothyroid state. These changes are nonspecific and may be associated with many other diseases in dogs. Their presence, however, adds supportive evidence for a diagnosis of hypothyroidism in a dog with relevant clinical signs. The classic hematologic finding associated with hypothyroidism, found in 40%–50% of cases, is a normocytic, normochromic, nonregenerative anemia. The classic serum biochemical abnormality is hypercholesterolemia, which occurs in ~80% of dogs with hypothyroidism. The value of serum cholesterol determination as a screening test for hypothyroidism cannot be overemphasized, because cholesterol concentrations are a sensitive and inexpensive biochemical marker for this disease in dogs. Other clinicopathologic abnormalities may include high serum concentrations of triglycerides, alkaline phosphatase, and CK.

Total T_4 concentration is the most commonly performed static thyroid hormone measurement and is a good initial screening test for hypothyroidism, with a diagnostic sensitivity of ~90%. A dog or cat with a T_4 concentration well within reference range limits may be assumed to have normal thyroid function. However, a subnormal basal T_4 concentration alone is not diagnostic; it may indicate an animal that is normal, hypothyroid, or suffering from a nonthyroidal illness with a secondary decrease in the basal T_4 concentration (sick euthyroid syndrome; *see* below).

Because only the unbound fraction of serum T_4 is biologically active, measurement of free T_4 has been hypothesized to be more useful to differentiate euthyroid dogs from hypothyroid dogs than total T_4 concentrations. However, most single-stage solid phase (analogue) commercial assays for free T_4 do not appear to be superior to measurement of total T_4 in dogs, probably because of differences in serum binding proteins. A free T_4 assay that uses an equilibrium dialysis step (direct dialysis) has better accuracy than the analogue methods. Compared with the total T_4 assay, the free T_4 assay by dialysis has greater diagnostic sensitivity and specificity.

Because T_3 is the most potent thyroid hormone at the cellular level, it would seem logical to measure its concentration for diagnostic purposes. However, serum T_3 concentrations may be low, normal, or (occasionally) high in dogs with documented hypothyroidism. The diagnostic value of a serum T_3 determination is particularly weak during early thyroid failure because the "failing" thyroid tends to increase the relative synthesis and secretion of T_3 versus T_4. In hypothyroid dogs in which values for serum T_3 are high, anti-T_3 antibodies, which produce spurious results in most T_3 radioimmunoassays, should be suspected.

Determination of serum TSH concentrations by use of a valid species-specific TSH assay can be a useful adjunctive test for hypothyroidism in dogs, cats, and horses. Animals with primary hypothyroidism (by far the most common type) would be expected to have low serum T_4 and/or free T_4 concentrations with high endogenous TSH concentrations. Unfortunately, serum TSH concentrations remain within the reference range in 20%–40% of dogs with confirmed hypothyroidism. Although a few dogs with normal serum TSH concentrations have secondary hypothyroidism, pituitary TSH deficiency is extremely rare, and most dogs with normal TSH concentrations (ie, a false-negative result) have primary hypothyroidism. In contrast, falsely high serum TSH concentrations (ie, a false-positive result) are occasionally found in euthyroid dogs with nonthyroidal illness. Thus, serum TSH determinations should never be evaluated alone but always in conjunction with the dog's history, routine laboratory abnormalities, and total or free T_4 concentrations.

The TSH stimulation test evaluates the response of the thyroid gland to exogenously administered TSH and is a test of thyroid reserve. It is an accurate test of thyroid function in dogs but its use is limited by the expense and limited availability of TSH. The protocol requires collection of a serum sample for measurement of a basal T_4, followed by administration of bovine TSH given IV at a dosage of 0.1 U/kg (maximum dose 5 units). A second sample for measurement of T_4 is collected 6 hr later. Human recombinant TSH is available, although expensive, and may be frozen for at least 8 wk with no loss of potency. The recommended dose is 75 mcg, IV, with collection of 0- and 6-hr samples. Results are similar to those obtained using the bovine product. Results may reveal a normal response, a blunted response (sick euthyroid syndrome), or no response (hypothyroidism).

Both ultrasonography and scintigraphy of the thyroid gland have been evaluated as diagnostic tests for hypothyroidism in dogs. With an experienced radiologist, use of thyroid sonography (ie, decreased echogenicity and decreased thyroid volume) can be an effective ancillary diagnostic tool to differentiate between canine hypothyroidism and euthyroid sick syndrome. The best imaging technique may be the use of technetium 99m (^{99m}Tc) uptake and imaging of the thyroid gland. With quantitative measurement of thyroidal ^{99m}Tc uptake, there is little to no overlap between dogs with primary hypothyroidism and dogs with nonthyroidal illness.

In some cases, the most practical approach to confirming the diagnosis of hypothyroidism is a therapeutic trial using appropriate guidelines. Every attempt should be made to exclude nonthyroidal illness before starting a therapeutic trial. There is no evidence that thyroid hormone supplementation is beneficial in dogs with sick euthyroid syndrome, and it may be detrimental. Thyroxine supplementation should be started at a dosage of 20 mcg/kg (administered without food, on an empty stomach), once to twice daily. Objective criteria should be used to assess the response to treatment. If response to treatment is positive, the clinician should be prepared to withdraw therapy to confirm that clinical signs return. This will ensure that dogs with thyroid-responsive diseases (ie, those in which the clinical signs improve because of the nonspecific effects of thyroid hormone or unrelated to therapy) do not remain on thyroid supplementation for life. If therapy is unsuccessful, therapeutic monitoring should be performed to identify the cause of treatment failure. Because an incorrect diagnosis is the most common cause of treatment failure, the clinician should be prepared to withdraw therapy and pursue other diagnoses.

In cats, hypothyroidism can also be diagnosed on the basis of finding low to low-normal serum concentrations of total T_4, free T_4, and T_3, with high serum TSH concentrations. A feline-specific TSH assay is not available, but the canine TSH assay can be used as a test for feline hypothyroidism.

Diagnosis of Thyroiditis: Circulating antithyroglobulin antibodies can be detected in as many as half of dogs with hypothyroidism and are believed to reflect a state of autoimmune thyroiditis. Measurement of these antibodies in breeding studs and bitches has been proposed as a method to identify dogs with autoimmune thyroid disease. Serum thyroglobulin autoantibody determinations may be a useful adjunctive diagnostic aid for hypothyroidism. However, the test can never be used alone to confirm a diagnosis of hypothyroidism, because a positive antithyroglobulin antibody titer may occur in euthyroid dogs with early stages of lymphocytic thyroiditis. Identification of these autoantibodies supports the diagnosis if the dog has clinical signs and other laboratory data consistent with the disorder.

Although extremely rare in dogs, circulating thyroid hormone autoantibodies (anti-T_3 or anti-T_4 antibodies) are occasionally detected and also are believed to reflect a state of autoimmune thyroiditis. These antibodies, which can be formed against either T_3 or T_4 (or both), produce a spurious increase in the apparent T_3 or T_4 concentrations, into the hyperthyroid range in most dogs. Of all the thyroid hormones, only measurement of free T_4 (by dialysis) is not affected by autoantibodies directed at T_4 or T_3, because the serum autoantibodies are removed in the dialysis step. Therefore, if hypothyroidism is suspected in a dog with circulating thyroid hormone autoantibodies, serum free T_4 concentration should be determined to help confirm the diagnosis.

Nonthyroidal Factors That Affect Interpretation of Thyroid Function Tests: Certain breeds have normal thyroid hormone ranges that differ from most other breeds. Few have been evaluated, but Greyhounds have serum total T_4 and free T_4 concentrations that are considerably lower than those of most other breeds. Scottish Deerhounds also have total T_4 concentrations that are well below the mean concentration of dogs in general, and other sight hounds may have similar findings. Alaskan sled dogs have serum total T_4, T_3, and free T_4 concentrations that are below the reference range of most pet dogs, particularly during periods of intense training or racing.

Illness not involving the thyroid gland can alter thyroid function tests and has been labeled "nonthyroidal illness" or "euthyroid sick syndrome." Any illness can alter thyroid function tests, causing a fairly consistent decrease in total T_4 and T_3 concentrations in proportion to the severity of illness. Serum TSH concentration is increased in 8%–10% of dogs with nonthyroidal illness. Serum free T_4 measured by equilibrium dialysis is less likely to be affected but can be increased or decreased. However, in dogs with substantial nonthyroidal illness, the free T_4 is likely to be decreased. Testing of thyroid function should be postponed until the nonthyroidal illness is resolved. If this is not possible, measurement of T_4, TSH, and free T_4 are indicated.

Glucocorticoids, phenobarbital, sulfonamides, clomipramine, and aspirin are known to commonly alter thyroid function tests. Glucocorticoids suppress total T_4 and sometimes free T_4 concentrations. Phenobarbital causes decreased total T_4 and mildly increased TSH. Sulfonamides can induce overt primary hypothyroidism with clinical signs and thyroid function tests that support the diagnosis. All changes are reversible when the medication is discontinued. Dozens of drugs affect thyroid function and thyroid function tests in people, so many others likely affect animals as well.

Treatment: Thyroxine (T_4) is the thyroid hormone replacement compound of choice in dogs and cats. With few exceptions, replacement therapy is necessary for the remainder of the animal's life; careful initial diagnosis and tailoring of treatment is essential. The reported replacement dosages for T_4 in dogs and cats range from a total dosage of 0.01–0.02 mg/lb (0.02–0.04 mg/kg), daily, given once or divided bid without food (on an empty stomach).

The most important indicator of the success of therapy is clinical improvement. Reversal of changes in coat and body weight should be assessed only after 1–2 mo of therapy. When clinical improvement is marginal or signs of thyrotoxicosis are seen, the clinical observations can be supported by therapeutic monitoring of serum thyroid hormone concentrations ("post-pill testing"). With once-daily administration of T_4, the peak serum concentration of T_4 generally should be slightly high to high-normal 4–6 hr after dosing and should be low-normal to normal 24 hr after dosing. Animals on bid administration probably can be checked at any time, but peak concentrations can be expected at the middle of the dosing interval (4–6 hr) and the nadir just before the next dose. After the dosage is stabilized, serum T_4 (with or without T_3) concentrations should be checked 1–2 times per year.

If clinical signs of hypothyroidism remain despite the use of reasonable doses of thyroid hormone, the following must be considered: 1) the dosage or frequency of administration is improper; 2) the owner is not complying with instructions or is not successfully administering the medication; 3) the animal is not absorbing the medication well, or is metabolizing and/or excreting it too rapidly; 4) the medication is outdated; or 5) the diagnosis is incorrect.

NON-NEOPLASTIC ENLARGEMENT OF THE THYROID GLAND

(Goiter)

An enlarged thyroid gland is, by definition, a goiter. Non-neoplastic and noninflammatory enlargements of the thyroid gland develop in all domestic mammals as well as birds. The major causes of goiter include iodine deficiency, ingestion of goitrogenic substances, dietary iodine excess, and inherited enzyme defects in the biosynthesis of thyroid hormones. Many animals with goiter appear to remain euthyroid, but clinical *signs of hypothyroidism* may develop in some, especially in newborns.

Iodine Deficiency: Thyroid hyperplasia due to iodine deficiency was common in many goitrogenic areas throughout the world before the widespread supplementation of iodized salt to animal diets. Although outbreaks of iodine-deficient goiter are now sporadic and fewer animals are affected, iodine deficiency is still responsible for most non-neoplastic goiters seen in large domestic animals.

Iodine atoms are a part of the thyroid hormones thyroxine and triiodothyronine; thus, insufficient iodine reduces the ability of the thyroid to make these hormones. With reduced circulating thyroid hormone levels, the pituitary secretes more thyroid-stimulating hormone (TSH), which acts as a stimulus for hyperplasia of the thyroid gland and subsequent development of a goiter. The hyperplastic gland may, and usually does, compensate for the reduced availability of iodine; therefore, goiter is in no way synonymous with hypothyroidism. Fetal thyroid glands are more susceptible to the effects of high or low iodine intake; animals born to females on iodine-deficient diets are more likely to develop severe thyroid enlargement and have clinical signs of hypothyroidism.

Goiter caused by iodine deficiency is most common in newborn pigs, lambs, and calves in iodine-deficient areas. The thyroid lobes of the young animal usually are at least twice normal size, soft, and dark red. In severe cases, there is an accompanying lack of hair (especially in pigs) or wool (lambs). The neck is usually grossly enlarged, and the skin and other tissue may be thickened, flabby, and edematous. In mildly affected animals, treatment with iodized salt (containing >0.007% iodine) may resolve the goiter and associated clinical signs, but many die before or soon after birth. Prophylaxis is more effective than treatment. Using stabilized iodized salt or ensuring that the ration is balanced for iodine content is recommended in all areas known or suspected to be iodine deficient.

Iodine Toxicity: Goiter and hypothyroidism occur in foals of dams fed excess iodine during gestation. Mares supplemented with iodine at ≥35 mg/day may produce affected foals. Foals receive the excess iodine both in utero and via the milk, because mares on high-iodine diets secrete higher than normal amounts of iodine in their milk. Clinical signs vary and may include goiter, weakness, and musculoskeletal abnormalities. Mares are invariably asymptomatic. Foals may improve or recover once the excess iodine is removed.

Goitrogenic Substances: Certain plants may produce goiter when ingested in sufficient amounts, especially in the absence of adequate iodine intake. Soybeans are most notable, but cabbage, rape, kale, and turnips all contain less potent goitrogens. Cooking or heating (and the usual processing of soybean meal) destroys the goitrogenic substance in these plants. All of the goitrogenic substances act by interfering with production of thyroid hormone. As with iodine deficiency, the pituitary responds to the reduced circulating thyroid hormone levels by increasing its secretion of TSH, which results in thyroid gland enlargement. In adult animals the disease is usually not significant, but severe thyroid enlargement and hypothyroidism may develop in newborns.

Congenital Hypothyroidism and Dysmaturity Syndrome of Foals: Congenital hypothyroidism and dysmaturity syndrome of neonatal foals was first recognized in the early 1980s and is characterized by hyperplasia of the thyroid gland, goiter, and multiple congenital musculoskeletal anomalies. It is most common in western Canada but has been seen in the Pacific Northwest and sporadically in other areas of the USA. There is no sex or breed predilection. Foals with this syndrome are born after a prolonged gestation (340–400 days) but appear dysmature with pliable ears, muscle weakness, and incomplete skeletal development. Common musculoskeletal defects include flexural deformities of the forelimbs, ruptured tendons of the common digital extensor muscles, mandibular prognathia, and immature carpal and tarsal bones. Multiple cases may appear on a farm, with no recurrence in subsequent years. The underlying etiology is unknown but may be the result of diets that contain high levels of nitrate (eg, greenfeed) combined with low iodine intake or ingestion of an unidentified goitrogen. Most affected foals either die or are euthanized within the first week of life.

Familial Dyshormonogenetic Goiter: Familial dyshormonogenetic goiter has been reported in sheep, cattle, goats, and pigs and appears to be inherited as an autosomal recessive trait. Essentially, it is a genetic enzyme defect in the biosynthesis of thyroid hormones. As with iodine deficiency, reduced thyroid hormone production leads to secretion of increased levels of TSH and subsequent goiter. Clinical signs may include subnormal growth rate, absence of normal wool development or a sparse coat, myxedematous swelling of subcutaneous tissues, and weakness. Many affected animals die shortly after birth or are very sensitive to adverse environmental conditions.

HYPERTHYROIDISM

Excessive secretion of the thyroid hormones, T_4 and T_3, results in signs that reflect an increased metabolic rate and produces clinical hyperthyroidism. It is most common in middle-aged to old cats but also develops rarely in dogs.

Functional thyroid adenoma (adenomatous hyperplasia) is the most common cause of feline hyperthyroidism; in ~70% of cases, both thyroid lobes are enlarged. Thyroid carcinoma, the primary cause of hyperthyroidism in dogs, is rare in cats (1%–2% of hyperthyroidism cases).

Clinical Findings and Diagnosis: The most common signs include weight loss, increased appetite, hyperexcitability, polydipsia, polyuria, and palpable enlargement of the thyroid gland. GI signs are also common and may include vomiting, diarrhea, and increased fecal volume. Cardiovascular signs include tachycardia, systolic murmurs, dyspnea, cardiomegaly, and congestive heart failure. Rarely, hyperthyroid cats exhibit apathetic signs (eg, anorexia, lethargy, and depression); weight loss remains a common sign in these cats.

High basal serum total thyroid hormone concentration is the hallmark of hyperthyroidism and confirms the diagnosis. Although serum total T_4 concentrations are high in most cats with hyperthyroidism, ~5%–10% of cats have normal T_4 values. Most cats with normal serum T_4 values have either mild or early hyperthyroidism or hyperthyroidism with concurrent nonthyroidal illness, which has caused suppression of a high total T_4 concentration to within reference range limits. In these cats, a high free T_4 concentration along with consistent history and physical examination findings is diagnostic of hyperthyroidism.

Treatment: Cats with hyperthyroidism can be treated by radioiodine therapy, thyroidectomy, chronic administration of an antithyroid drug, or lifelong nutritional therapy (iodine-deficient diet). Radioactive iodine provides a simple, effective, and safe treatment and is considered the treatment of choice. The radioiodine is concentrated within the thyroid tumor, where it selectively irradiates and destroys hyperfunctioning thyroid tissue.

Surgical thyroidectomy is also an effective treatment for hyperthyroidism in cats. With unilateral thyroid tumors, hemithyroidectomy corrects the hyperthyroid state, and thyroxine supplementation usually is not necessary. For bilateral thyroid tumors, complete thyroidectomy is indicated, but parathyroid function must be preserved to avoid postoperative hypocalcemia. Thyroxine supplementation should be started 1–2 days after complete thyroidectomy. If iatrogenic hypoparathyroidism develops, treatment with vitamin D and calcium is also indicated.

Treatment with methimazole, an antithyroid drug, controls hyperthyroidism by blocking thyroid hormone synthesis. Carbimazole is a similar antithyroid drug available in many European countries, Australia, and Japan; it exerts its effects through immediate conversion to methimazole after administration. Propylthiouracil, another antithyroid drug, is not recommended for use in cats because of the high incidence of serious adverse effects (especially hemolytic anemia and thrombocytopenia). The recommended initial daily dose of methimazole is 2.5–5 mg in two divided doses. The dosage is adjusted to maintain circulating thyroid hormone concentrations within the mid-normal range and is given daily. Adverse effects, the more serious of which are agranulocytosis and thrombocytopenia, develop in <5% of treated cats. If this occurs, methimazole should be discontinued and supportive therapy instituted; these adverse reactions should resolve within 2 wk. To maintain normal levels of thyroid hormone and to monitor for adverse reactions during the first 3 mo of treatment (when the most serious adverse effects associated with methimazole therapy develop), CBCs and serum thyroid hormone determinations should be repeated at 2- to 4-wk intervals, with the drug dosage adjusted as necessary. Subsequently, serum T_4 concentrations should be measured at 3- to 6-mo intervals to monitor dosage requirements and response to treatment.

The use of medical therapy other than methimazole may be required if adverse effects develop. For the most part, these alternative medical therapies are for short-term use and are only recommended before use of a more permanent treatment option.

Propranolol and *atenolol* are the most frequently used β-adrenoceptor blocking agents in hyperthyroid cats. These drugs do not lower the circulating T_4 concentration but are used to symptomatically control the tachycardia, tachypnea, hypertension, and hyperexcitability associated with hyperthyroidism.

Oral cholecystographic agents (eg, ipodate, iopanoic acid, or diatrizoate meglumine) acutely inhibit conversion of peripheral T_4 to T_3. In one study of hyperthyroid cats, administration of calcium ipodate normalized serum total T_3 concentrations and produced clinical improvement in >60% of cats treated. Ipodate (308 mg iodine/500 mg calcium ipodate) is no longer marketed in the USA, but iopanoic acid (333 mg iodine/500 mg iopanoic acid) and diatrizoate meglumine (370 mg iodine/mL) have been used anecdotally in hyperthyroid cats at comparable dosages. None of these drugs provides complete resolution of clinical signs or biochemical features associated with hyperthyroidism. In addition, waning of the thyroid-lowering effect is common after 3 mo of therapy with any of these drugs.

A fouth treatment option for cats with hyperthyroidism is the use of a prescription diet with severely restricted iodine levels (Hill's® y/d Feline Thyroid Health™). The basis for using this diet is that iodine is an essential component of both T_4 and T_3; without sufficient iodine, the thyroid cannot produce excess thyroid hormones. This is an iodine-deficient diet, containing iodine levels below the minimum daily requirement for adult cats. A major indication for use of this diet for management of feline hyperthyroidism is in cats that are not candidates for definitive treatment of the underlying thyroid tumor(s) with surgery or radioiodine, which remain the treatments of choice. In addition, nutritional management could be considered in cats whose owners are not able to give oral medication or in cats that develop adverse effects from methimazole or carbimazole.

Most hyperthyroid cats exclusively fed this iodine-restricted diet become euthyroid in 8–12 wk. This therapy appears to be more effective in cats with only moderate increases of T_4 than in cats with severe hyperthyroidism. Despite some advantages, nutritional management has disadvantages: 1) feeding this diet can only control (by withholding "fuel" for the thyroid tumor) but not cure hyperthyroidism; 2) cats fed this diet must not eat any other cat diet, table food, or treats, because even tiny amounts of iodine can render the diet ineffective in controlling hyperthyroidism; and 3) relapse will occur if the diet is stopped, so the cat must eat only this diet for the rest of its life.

In dogs, a thyroid tumor causing hyperthyroidism should always be presumed to be a carcinoma until proved otherwise. This is in contrast to the case in hyperthyroid cats, in which thyroid carcinoma is present in <5%.

Treatment of thyroid neoplasia and hyperthyroidism in dogs is dictated by the size of the primary tumor, extent of local tissue invasion, presence of detectable metastasis, and available treatment options. Surgery, chemotherapy, cobalt irradiation, and use of radioactive iodine therapy, alone or in combination, may be indicated depending on the individual. The hyperthyroid state can be medically controlled by daily administration of an antithyroid drug such as methimazole or carbimazole (5–15 mg/dog, bid), but such treatment will not prevent tumor growth or metastasis. Because canine hyperthyroidism is almost always associated with thyroid carcinoma, the longterm prognosis in these dogs is poor to grave.

THE PARATHYROID GLANDS AND DISORDERS OF CALCIUM METABOLISM

The physiology and disorders of calcium and phosphate metabolism, the function of vitamin D (which acts more like a hormone than a vitamin), and the formation of bone are all tied together in a common system along with two other regulatory hormones—parathyroid hormone (PTH) and calcitonin. Therefore, PTH, calcitonin, and vitamin D are discussed in this chapter together with the associated disorders of calcium homeostasis.

Because aberrant calcium and phosphorus metabolism is reflected in the skeletal system, specific syndromes are presented in that section. (*See also* DYSTROPHIES ASSOCIATED WITH CALCIUM, PHOSPHORUS, AND VITAMIN D, p 1050.)

CALCIUM PHYSIOLOGY AND CALCIUM-REGULATING HORMONES

The concentration of calcium in the blood of mammals is ~10 mg/dL, with some variation due to species (eg, as much as 13 mg/dL is normal in horses and rabbits), age, dietary intake, and analytic method. Calcium in plasma or serum exists in three forms or fractions: 1) Protein-bound calcium accounts for approximately one-third of the total serum calcium concentration. Protein-bound calcium cannot diffuse through membranes and thus is not usable by tissues. 2) Ionized or free calcium is the physiologically active form that accounts for 50%–60% of total calcium concentration. 3) Complexed or chelated calcium is bound to phosphate, bicarbonate, sulfate, citrate, and lactate and accounts for ~10% of the total calcium concentration.

The calcium ion is an essential structural component of the skeleton and plays a key role in muscle contraction, blood coagulation, enzyme activity, neural excitability, secondary messengers, hormone release, and membrane permeability. Precise control of calcium ion in extracellular fluids is vital to health. Three major hormones (PTH, vitamin D, and calcitonin) interact to maintain a constant concentration of calcium, despite variations in intake and excretion. Other hormones, such as adrenal corticosteroids, estrogens, thyroxine, somatotropin, and glucagon, may also contribute to the maintenance of calcium homeostasis.

Parathyroid Hormone: PTH is synthesized and stored in the chief cells of the parathyroid glands. Synthesis is regulated by a feedback mechanism involving the level of blood calcium (and, to a lesser degree, that of magnesium). In addition, biological amines, peptides, steroids, and several classes of drugs can influence PTH secretion.

The primary function of PTH is to control calcium concentration in the extracellular fluid, which it does by affecting the rate of transfer of calcium into and out of bone, resorption in the kidneys, and absorption from the GI tract. The effect on the kidneys is the most rapid, causing reabsorption of calcium and excretion of phosphorus. The major initial effect on bone is to mobilize calcium from the bone to the extracellular fluid; later, bone formation may be enhanced. PTH does not directly affect calcium absorption from the gut. Its effect is mediated indirectly by regulation of synthesis of the active metabolite of vitamin D.

Vitamin D: The second major hormone involved in the regulation of calcium metabolism and skeletal remodeling is vitamin D, which includes cholecalciferol (vitamin D_3) of animal origin, as well as ergocalciferol (vitamin D_2) of plant origin. Vitamin D has long been considered an essential dietary ingredient, but in several species, including sheep, cattle, horses, pigs, and people, vitamin D can be formed in the skin from a cholesterol metabolite (7-dehydrocholesterol) after exposure to ultraviolet light. In contrast, dogs and cats are not able to synthesize vitamin D_3 adequately in the skin and mainly depend on dietary intake.

Vitamin D must be metabolically activated before it can function physiologically. The biologic actions of vitamin D depend on hydroxylation in the liver and kidneys to form the biologically active 1,25-dihydroxyvitamin D (calcitriol). This conversion in the kidneys is the rate-limiting step in vitamin D metabolism, and it is partly responsible for the delay between vitamin D administration and expression of its biologic effects. PTH and conditions that stimulate its secretion, as well as hypophosphatemia, increase the formation of the active vitamin D metabolite. High circulating phosphorus concentrations have the opposite effect. Under certain conditions, prolactin, estradiol, placental lactogen, and possibly somatotropin have a similar enhancing effect. Increased secretion of these hormones, either alone or in combination, appears to be important in the efficient adaptation to the major calcium demands of pregnancy, lactation, and growth.

Calcitonin: Calcitonin is a 32-amino acid polypeptide hormone secreted by the parafollicular cells (C-cells) of the thyroid gland in mammals and by ultimobranchial tissue in avian and other nonmammalian species. The concentration of calcium ion in extracellular fluids is the principal stimulus for the secretion of calcitonin by C-cells. In hypercalcemia, the rate of secretion of calcitonin is increased greatly by rapid discharge of stored hormone from C-cells into interfollicular capillaries. Hyperplasia of C-cells occurs in response to longterm hypercalcemia. When blood calcium is lowered, the stimulus for calcitonin secretion is diminished. The storage of large amounts of preformed hormone in C-cells and rapid release in response to a moderate rise in circulating calcium probably reflect the physiologic role of calcitonin as an "emergency" hormone to protect against development of hypercalcemia.

Calcitonin exerts its effects by interacting with target cells, primarily in bone and kidney. The actions of PTH and calcitonin are antagonistic on bone resorption but synergistic on decreasing the renal tubular reabsorption of phosphorus. The hypocalcemic effects of calcitonin are primarily the result of decreased entry of calcium from the skeleton into plasma, resulting from a temporary inhibition of PTH-stimulated bone resorption. The hypophosphatemia develops from a direct action of calcitonin, which increases the rate of movement of phosphorus out of plasma into soft tissue and bone and inhibits the bone resorption stimulated by PTH and other factors. Although many effects have been attributed to calcitonin at pharmacologic doses, their physiologic relevance is suspect. Physiologically, calcitonin has at best a minor role in regulating blood concentrations of calcium. Neither chronically high (eg, as in animals with medullary thyroid cancer) nor chronically low (eg, as in animals after surgical removal of the thyroid gland) circulating calcitonin concentrations result in any changes in the serum calcium concentration.

HYPERCALCEMIA IN DOGS AND CATS

Hypercalcemia can be toxic to all body tissues, but major deleterious effects occur in the kidneys, nervous system, and cardiovascular system. The development of clinical signs from hypercalcemia depends on the magnitude of the calcium increase, how quickly it develops, and its duration. Serum total calcium concentrations of ≤15 mg/dL may not be associated with systemic signs, but serum concentrations of >18 mg/dL are often associated with severe, life-threatening signs. Polydipsia and polyuria are the most common signs of hypercalcemia and result from an impaired ability to concentrate urine and a direct stimulation of the thirst center. Anorexia, vomiting, and constipation can also develop as a result of decreased excitability of GI smooth muscle. Decreased neuromuscular excitability may lead to signs of generalized weakness, depression, muscle twitching, and seizures.

There are many potential causes of hypercalcemia (*see* TABLE 1). In hypercalcemic dogs, neoplasia (lymphosarcoma) is

TABLE 1 CAUSES OF HYPERCALCEMIA IN DOGS AND CATS

Acromegaly
Apocrine gland adenocarcinoma
Carcinoma (squamous cell, mammary, bronchogenic, prostate, thyroid, nasal cavity)
Chronic and acute renal failure
Factitious: lipemia, postprandial, young dog (<6 mo old)
Granulomatous disease
Hematologic malignancies (bone marrow osteolysis)
Humoral hypercalcemia
Hypercalcemia of malignancy
Hyperthyroidism
Hypervitaminosis D: iatrogenic, plants (eg, day-blooming jessamine), rodenticides, antipsoriatic cream
Hypoadrenocorticism (Addison disease)
Iatrogenic disorders: excess calcium or oral phosphate binders
Idiopathic hypercalcemia of cats
Laboratory error
Lymphoma (lymphosarcoma)
Metastatic or primary bone neoplasia
Multiple myeloma
Myeloproliferative disease (rare)
Primary hyperparathyroidism
Skeletal lesions: osteomyelitis, hypertrophic osteodystrophy

the most common cause, followed by hypoadrenocorticism, primary hyperparathyroidism, and chronic renal failure. Other causes of hypercalcemia in dogs, in an approximate incidence order as seen in practice, include vitamin D toxicosis, apocrine gland carcinoma of the anal sac, multiple myeloma, carcinomas (lung, mammary, nasal, pancreas, thymus, thyroid, vaginal, and testicular), and finally, certain granulomatous diseases (blastomycosis, histoplasmosis, schistosomiasis). Approximately 70% of hypercalcemic dogs are also azotemic. However, azotemia is uncommon in dogs with hyperparathyroidism.

In cats, idiopathic hypercalcemia appears to be the most frequent cause of a high total calcium concentration, followed by renal failure and malignancy. Ionized hypercalcemia in conjunction with chronic renal failure is more common in cats than dogs. The most common tumor types associated with hypercalcemia of malignancy in cats are lymphoma and squamous cell carcinoma. Primary hyperparathyroidism occurs in cats but not as frequently as in dogs. Rarely, hypercalcemia is seen in cats with hyperthyroidism.

Hypercalcemia of Malignancy

Malignancy is the most common cause of persistent hypercalcemia in dogs and is a common cause in cats. In hypercalcemia of malignancy, the hypercalcemia primarily results from increased osteoclastic bone resorption, but increased renal tubular resorption and increased intestinal absorption may also play a role. Factors that may be produced by tumors and result in humoral hypercalcemia of malignancy include PTH, PTH-related protein (PTHrP), transforming growth factor, 1,25-dihydroxyvitamin D, prostaglandin E_2, osteoclast-activating factor, and other cytokines (interleukin-1, interleukin-2, and γ-interferon). Although many tumors have been associated with hypercalcemia in people, malignancy-associated hypercalcemia in dogs has been most commonly linked to lymphoma, adenocarcinoma of the apocrine glands of the anal sac, and multiple myeloma. Other tumors (thymoma, squamous cell carcinoma, nasal carcinoma, hemangiosarcoma, and undifferentiated adenocarcinoma) have also been associated with hypercalcemia in dogs. In cats, humoral hypercalcemia of malignancy occurs less frequently than in dogs but has been reported with squamous cell carcinoma, multiple myeloma, and lymphoproliferative diseases.

Lymphoma (Lymphosarcoma): The most common tumor associated with hypercalcemia in dogs, lymphoma is also one of the tumors associated with hypercalcemia in cats. The pathogenesis of the hypercalcemia may involve two general mechanisms. One is local elaboration of an osteolytic factor that induces resorption of bone and mobilization of calcium when the bone marrow is infiltrated by tumor cells. The other, probably more important, is humoral hypercalcemia in which neoplastic cells produce a humoral factor that acts at a distance from the tumor. As evidence for secretion of a humoral substance by tumor cells, increased bone resorption, phosphaturia, and urinary excretion of cyclic adenosine monophosphate (cAMP) have been documented in dogs with lymphoma. Serum concentrations of both PTH and 1,25-dihydroxyvitamin D are generally low in these dogs, but PTHrP has been detected in dogs with lymphoma (*see* TABLE 2).

Of dogs with lymphoma, 10%–40% have concurrent hypercalcemia, and a large number of these cases also have the mediastinal form of lymphoma. Although detectable lymphadenopathy is usually present, hypercalcemia may be the first abnormality noted. A thorough physical examination, together with thoracic and abdominal radiographs, abdominal ultrasonography, multiple lymph node aspirates or biopsies, and multiple bone marrow aspirates may be necessary to make the diagnosis. Treatment with glucocorticoids (eg, prednisone) lowers serum calcium concentrations; however, steroids are lympholytic and make identification of lymphoma difficult.

Although remission rates in dogs with lymphoma and hypercalcemia are not statistically different from those without hypercalcemia, survival times are considerably less, indicating that hypercalcemic lymphomas have a poorer prognosis. (*See also* CANINE MALIGNANT LYMPHOMA, p 40, and FELINE LEUKEMIA VIRUS AND RELATED DISEASES, p 790.)

Adenocarcinoma of the Apocrine Glands of the Anal Sac: This tumor usually occurs in older dogs of either sex, with hypercalcemia developing in ~90% of cases. Humoral mechanisms are most likely responsible for the hypercalcemia, because a PTH-like protein has been identified from tumor tissue in dogs. This tumor is usually malignant and has metastasized to regional lymph nodes by the time of diagnosis. Surgical resection is associated with reduction of serum calcium. Failure to remove all of the tumor or recurrence of the tumor usually results in recurrence of hypercalcemia. Despite surgical excision, radiation, and various chemotherapy protocols, the tumor usually recurs within a few months, and prognosis is poor.

Multiple Myeloma: This malignancy in dogs and cats has been associated with hypercalcemia in 10%–15% of cases. The pathogenesis of the hypercalcemia is most likely multifactorial. Myeloma cells are known to produce osteoclast-activating factor in people, which may partially account for the hypercalcemia. The presence of extensive bony lysis may also contribute to the increased serum calcium. Although serum protein concentration is usually increased in multiple myeloma, increased protein binding of calcium rarely accounts for the hypercalcemia. Treatment of multiple myeloma with chemotherapy has been associated with longterm survival, but the presence of associated hypercalcemia, light chain proteinuria, and extensive bony lesions is associated with a shorter survival time.

Primary Hyperparathyroidism

Primary hyperparathyroidism results from excessive secretion of PTH by one or more abnormal (usually neoplastic) parathyroid glands. It is relatively rare in dogs and cats. Persistent hypercalcemia is characteristic. Solitary adenoma of the external or internal parathyroid gland is the most common cause of primary hyperparathyroidism, whereas parathyroid carcinoma has been infrequently reported. Hyperplasia of one or all four parathyroid glands has been described but is very rare.

Clinical Findings: Polydipsia, polyuria, anorexia, lethargy, and depression are the most common signs, but many animals with milder degrees of hypercalcemia may be asymptomatic. Constipation, weakness, shivering, twitching, vomiting, stiff gait, and facial swelling are less often reported.

Diagnosis: Hypercalcemia, normal to low serum phosphorus, and low urine specific gravity are the most consistent findings. Azotemia commonly develops as a consequence of moderate to severe hypercalcemia. In hypercalcemic animals that still have relatively normal renal function (normal serum creatinine and urea nitrogen concentrations), determination of serum PTH is helpful in diagnosis. The finding of high-normal to high serum PTH concentrations in hypercalcemic animals with normal renal function is consistent with primary hyperparathyroidism, whereas the finding of low PTH concentrations is consistent with hypercalcemia of malignancy. Ultrasonography of the parathyroid glands is a useful diagnostic technique but requires an ultrasound unit with a high frequency transducer in the 7.5- to 10-MHz range to achieve the necessary resolution. Normal parathyroid glands are not always visualized on ultrasonographic examination, but enlarged parathyroid glands appear as rounded hypoechoic or anechoic structures associated with the thyroid gland. Finding a solitary parathyroid gland in a hypercalcemic animal supports a diagnosis of primary hyperparathyroidism, whereas finding multiple enlarged parathyroid glands is compatible with secondary hyperparathyroidism. Ultrasound cannot distinguish a parathyroid adenoma from an adenocarcinoma. Exploratory surgery of the cervical region is a diagnostic alternative if no other cause of hypercalcemia can be determined.

Treatment: The most cost-effective and expedient approach to management is surgical exploration of the neck and removal of the abnormal parathyroid tissue. Percutaneous ultrasound-guided chemical (ethanol) or heat ablation of the parathyroid has been used and may be a feasible alternative to surgery in some cases. Attempts to lower the serum calcium concentration with IV fluids (saline) and furosemide before surgery or ablation may be beneficial (*see* p 568). No medical treatment exists for primary hyperparathyroidism, although treatment for hypercalcemia can be done if surgery is declined.

Hypercalcemia Associated with Hypoadrenocorticism

Mild hypercalcemia (≤15 mg/dL) has been reported in as many as 30% of dogs with hypoadrenocorticism (Addison disease). Multiple factors may result in the hypercalcemia, including increased calcium citrate (complexed calcium), hemoconcentration (relative increase), increased renal resorption of calcium, and increased affinity of serum proteins for calcium. Although total serum calcium concentrations may be increased, the ionized fraction usually is normal. The hypercalcemia resolves quickly with successful treatment for hypoadrenocorticism.

Renal Failure

In cats, chronic renal failure (usually associated with chronic interstitial nephritis) appears to be the most common cause of hypercalcemia. The pathogenesis of the hypercalcemia is not known, but the ionized calcium concentrations remain normal. In dogs, renal failure caused by familial renal disease is more often associated with hypercalcemia than are other forms of chronic renal failure. Hypercalcemia may also be present in acute renal failure during the polyuric phase, but this is rare.

Idiopathic Hypercalcemia of Cats

A syndrome in young to middle-aged cats, first described in the early 1990s, involves hypercalcemia that occurs without obvious explanation. It has been suggested that the feeding of acidifying, magnesium-restricted diets predisposes cats to idiopathic hypercalcemia. Another plausible hypothesis is that excessive dietary vitamin D content in some cat foods may contribute to this condition. Total serum calcium is increased for months to years, often without obvious clinical signs in the early stages. Ionized calcium is increased, sometimes out of proportion to the increase in total serum calcium. Longhaired cats may be over-represented; most are not azotemic at initial diagnosis but may later develop azotemia. PTH levels are either low or remain within the reference range, PTHrP is not detectable, and 25-hydroxyvitamin D and calcitriol levels are within normal limits.

Intensive treatment for idiopathic hypercalcemia is rarely indicated, because hypercalcemia has developed gradually and is relatively longstanding, and dramatic clinical signs are usually absent. Most cats can be treated as outpatients with dietary change either alone or in combination with drug therapy.

Diet modification is recommended as a first-line treatment. If an acidifying diet is being fed, it should be discontinued. A number of different diets have been recommended, including high-fiber diets, kidney diets, or diets developed to prevent calcium oxalate urolithiasis. Others recommend feeding canned diets with a composition similar to what cats would eat in the wild (ie, 40%–60% of calories as protein, 30%–50% fat, and <15% carbohydrates). No matter what type of diet is chosen, it is best to feed a wet-only diet to promote urinary dilution and lessen the chance of calcium oxalate stone formation. Administration of prednisone results in longterm decreases in ionized and total calcium concentrations in some cats.

If normocalcemia has not been restored after a dietary feeding trial of 6–8 wk, treatment with glucocorticosteroids or bisphosphonates should be considered. Prednisone is given orally at 5 mg/cat/day for 1 mo before reevaluation. If the serum ionized calcium concentration is normal, this dose is continued for several months. If the ionized calcium value is still increased, the dosage is gradually increased to 10–20 mg/cat/day as needed to restore normocalcemia. Alternatively, treatment with the bisphosphonate alendronate can be instituted, starting at 10 mg orally once weekly; the dosage can be increased to 20–30 mg per week, as needed. It is extremely important to administer alendronate after a 12-hour fast, because food significantly reduces drug absorption; the fast should also be continued for at least 2 hr after alendronate administration. Erosive esophagitis is a known adverse effect of oral bisphosphonates in human patients. Although the risk of development of esophagitis in cats is unknown, the owner can give 5–6 mL of water to the cat with a dosing syringe immediately after administration of the alendronate; a small amount of butter applied to the cat's lips may increase licking and salivation and promote the transit of the pill to the stomach. The longterm safety and efficacy of oral bisphosphonates in cats are currently unknown, but alendronate appears to be relatively safe for use in cats.

Osteolytic Lesions

Hypercalcemia resulting from tumor invasion or metastasis to bone develops very rarely in animals. Primary bone tumors (eg, osteosarcoma) and neoplastic cells within the bone marrow (eg, multiple myeloma) may occasionally produce hypercalcemia. The mechanisms whereby bony neoplasia may produce hypercalcemia include mechanical destruction by the infiltrating cells (as occurs with metastatic tumors and osteosarcoma) and local production of osteoclast-activating factor (as occurs with multiple myeloma). Bacterial and mycotic osteomyelitis can also occasionally produce hypercalcemia. The hypercalcemia may result from direct bone lysis or may be mediated by bone-resorbing factors (eg, prostaglandins, osteoclast-activating factor).

Other Causes of Hypercalcemia

Hypervitaminosis D: Vitamin D toxicity refers to the effects of excessive intake of bioactive metabolites of vitamin D. Toxicity caused by ergocalciferol (vitamin D_2) or cholecalciferol (vitamin D_3) can occur from excessive dietary supplementation (most common in young growing dogs) for treatment of primary hypoparathyroidism. Both of these forms of vitamin D have a slow onset of action and prolonged duration, making correct dosing difficult. Treatment is directed at discontinuing the supplement or decreasing the dose of vitamin D. Toxicity caused by calcitriol (1,25-dihydroxyvitamin D), the most active form of vitamin D, most commonly occurs after treatment of primary hypoparathyroidism. Calcitriol is also the active ingredient in some rodenticides, but these products are no longer widely available in the USA.

In dogs, a newly emerging cause of vitamin D toxicity is ingestion of the calcitriol analogue, calcipotriene (also called tacalcitol), which is a topical preparation used to treat psoriasis in people. Calcipotriene toxicity in dogs can result in severe metastatic calcification in the GI tract, kidney, and other tissues; the condition is commonly fatal.

Houseplants: Certain house plants (eg, *Cestrum diurnum* [the day-blooming jessamine], *Solanum malacoxylon*, *Trisetum flavescens*) may contain a substance similar to vitamin D that may cause hypercalcemia when ingested.

Granulomatous Disease: Hypercalcemia associated with granulomatous disease arises from an alteration of endogenous vitamin D metabolism. Macrophages activated in response to granulomatous inflammation can develop the capability to convert vitamin D precursors to the active form of vitamin D (ie, calcitriol) in an unregulated manner. A similar alteration of vitamin D metabolism in people may explain hypercalcemia in non-Hodgkin lymphoma, Hodgkin lymphoma, and lymphomatoid granulomatosis.

In companion animals, hypercalcemia related to granulomatous disease has been reported in disseminated histoplasmosis, blastomycosis, coccidiomycosis, tuberculosis, and schistosomiasis. Animals with hypercalcemia related to granulomatous disease are expected to have high serum concentrations of ionized calcium and low values for PTH. Serum calcium concentrations return to normal with treatment (ie, antifungal drugs and surgical removal).

Diagnostic Tests for Hypercalcemia

The first step in investigating hypercalcemia is to exclude the possibility of spurious test results. Ideally, a fasting sample should be resubmitted, because sample conditions (lipemia or hemolysis) can artifactually increase total serum calcium values reported by colorimetric analyzers.

If the hypercalcemia is repeatable, ionized calcium should be measured, because it is a better reflection of the biologically active form of calcium. Total or adjusted total calcium are not reliable measurements of calcium status.

In some animals with persistent ionized hypercalcemia, identification of the cause will be obvious after analysis of history (vitamin D exposure, drugs, ingestion of houseplants) and physical examination findings (masses, organomegaly, cancer, or granulomatous disease). In other animals, the cause will not be obvious, and hematology, serum biochemistry, body cavity imaging, cytology, and histopathology may be required. In many animals, use of specialized assays, including measurement of PTH, PTHrP, and/or vitamin D is necessary to confirm a diagnosis.

If lymphadenopathy is present, a lymph node aspirate or biopsy should be performed to check for lymphosarcoma. If a tumor of the anal sac is found, surgical removal should be attempted. Any other neoplasm should be treated by surgical removal, chemotherapy, or radiation therapy. Problems may arise when hypercalcemia is complicated by renal failure, or when primary hyperparathyroidism or occult malignancy is suspected. In these cases, the cause of hypercalcemia may not be obvious, and additional steps must be taken to differentiate primary hyperparathyroidism from occult tumors causing hypercalcemia.

Ionized Calcium: Because the ionized calcium fraction is the biologically active form and the component that regulates production of PTH, measurement of the ionized calcium concentration is the first step in evaluation of calcium abnormalities. If ionized calcium is normal, even if total calcium is increased, no further diagnostics are warranted. If ionized calcium is increased, then PTH and PTHrP determinations should be considered if there are no obvious causes of the hypercalcemia.

In many cases of hyper- or hypocalcemia, the total calcium and ionized calcium concentrations are highly correlated (*see* TABLE 2). However, in some instances the concentration of total calcium does not reflect the status of ionized calcium. In dogs with renal failure, total calcium is high, but ionized calcium is normal or surprisingly low. In this situation, the total calcium increase seems to reflect increased amounts of calcium complexed to anions, an effect that would not be identified in albumin-adjusted calcium concentrations.

Ionized calcium is measured in serum or heparinized plasma by an instrument using a calcium-specific electrode. Serum ionized calcium may be falsely high when collected in serum separator tubes. There is simultaneous measurement of pH, which affects the binding of calcium to protein in an inverse manner. An increase in pH is accompanied by a decrease in ionized calcium. Serum samples collected and handled in anaerobic conditions provide the best results with ionized calcium assays. Samples collected in EDTA tubes are unsuitable, because EDTA binds available ionized calcium.

Parathyroid Hormone: Assay of PTH is the next step in evaluation of calcium abnormalities, once hypercalcemia has been confirmed by measurement of the ionized calcium concentration. Evaluation of PTH can reveal whether the parathyroid glands are responding appropriately to the change in calcium concentration or whether inappropriate production of PTH is the cause of the disorder. If calcium metabolism is normal, small increases of ionized calcium inhibit secretion of PTH and small decreases of ionized calcium prompt release of PTH.

Serum or plasma PTH determinations are very useful in evaluation of hypercalcemic dogs and cats. Animals with primary hyperparathyroidism should have mid-normal to high concentrations of PTH, whereas those with most other forms of hypercalcemia have low PTH concentrations (*see* TABLE 2).

Parathyroid Hormone-related Protein (PTHrP): Hypercalcemia associated with nonparathyroid neoplasia is often caused by production of a humoral factor, PTHrP, that has parathyroid hormone–like bioactivity. Since its discovery in the 1980s, PTHrP has been found to be associated with a variety of tumors that cause hypercalcemia of malignancy in people.

Assay of PTHrP can be used to confirm hypercalcemia of malignancy (*see* TABLE 2). There is a relatively high prevalence of positive results in dogs with apocrine gland adenocarcinoma of the anal sac, lymphoma, or other miscellaneous tumors. However, humoral hypercalcemia of malignancy always remains a differential diagnosis in a hypercalcemic dog with a low PTH and a normal or negative PTHrP. In cats, high PTHrP is also consistent with humoral hypercalcemia of malignancy, especially in cats with carcinoma.

Vitamin D Metabolites (Calcidiol and Calcitriol): Because metabolites of vitamin D are chemically identical in all species, radioimmunoassays developed for use in people are satisfactory for measurement in animals. Calcidiol (25-hydroxyvitamin D) concentration is a good indicator of vitamin D ingestion and can be used to diagnose hypervitaminosis D.

Vitamin D metabolites resulting from the ingestion of cholecalciferol present in rodenticides can be measured with the calcidiol assay. Toxicity from ingestion of cholecalciferol or ergocalciferol would be detected by an increase of calcidiol that may persist for weeks after exposure. Assay of calcidiol also may be used to confirm toxicity from ingestion of rodenticides that contain vitamin D_3 as the active ingredient.

Calcipotriene, the vitamin D analogue *found in antipsoriasis creams*, is not measured with the assay for calcidiol but would be detected in the assay for calcitriol. Unfortunately, the calcitriol assay is not widely available for clinical use.

See TABLE 2 for a summary of the anticipated PTH, ionized calcium, and PTHrP values in the various disorders causing hypercalcemia. Generally, the PTH level is normal to high with primary, secondary, or tertiary hyperparathyroidism. The PTH level is low with other causes of hypercalcemia (eg, hypervitaminosis D, malignancy associated, renal failure, hypoadrenocorticism).

Treatment of Hypercalcemia

A mild degree of hypercalcemia may not be immediately dangerous; there is time to establish a definitive diagnosis before starting treatment. In animals with severe clinical signs associated with hypercalcemia, diagnostic and therapeutic efforts may proceed concurrently. No single treatment protocol is consistently effective for all causes of hypercalcemia; each animal must be approached individually, and the cause of the hypercalcemia must be determined. The definitive treatment of hypercalcemia is treating or removing the underlying cause. Unfortunately, the cause may not be apparent, and supportive measures must be taken to decrease the serum calcium concentration. The goal of all supportive treatment is to enhance urinary excretion of calcium and to prevent calcium resorption from bone.

Fluid Therapy: Volume expansion with 0.9% saline, ~100–125 mL/kg/day, IV, decreases hemoconcentration and increases renal calcium loss by improving glomerular filtration rate and sodium excretion, which results in less calcium reabsorption.

Diuretics: Loop diuretics such as furosemide (2–4 mg/kg, bid-tid) increase calcium excretion by the kidneys; however, higher dosages may be needed. If dehydration is present, fluid therapy should be instituted first because volume contraction and further hemoconcentration may worsen the hypercalcemia. Thiazide diuretics are contraindicated in hypercalcemia, because these agents decrease calcium excretion by the kidneys and worsen the hypercalcemia.

Glucocorticoids: Glucocorticoids such as prednisone (1–2 mg/kg, bid) or dexamethasone (0.1–0.2 mg, bid) provide a second tier of treatment for hypercalcemic cases that do not respond adequately to IV fluids and furosemide. They reduce bone resorption of calcium, reduce

TABLE 2 CHARACTERISTIC LABORATORY ABNORMALITIES ASSOCIATED WITH COMMON CAUSES OF HYPERCALCEMIA

Diagnosis	Total Calcium	Ionized Calcium	Intact PTH	1,25-Dihydroxy-vitamin D	Phosphorus	PTHrP
Primary hyperthyroidism	High	High	Normal to high	Normal	Normal to low	Negative
Malignant hypercalcemia	High	High	Low to low-normal	Low to normal	Normal to low	Positive (sometimes)
Hypoadrenocorticism (Addison disease)	Low, normal, or high	Normal	Normal	Normal	Normal to high	Negative
Chronic renal failure	Low, normal, or high	Normal to low	Normal to high	Low to normal	High	Negative
Hypervitaminosis D (calcitriol or calcitriol analogue)	High	High	Low to low-normal	Low to normal	Normal to high	Negative
Hypervitaminosis D (D_2 or D_3 toxicity)	High	High	Low to low-normal	High	Normal to high	Negative
Granulomatous disease	High	High	Low to low-normal	Low to normal	Normal to high	Negative
Idiopathic hypercalcemia of cats	High	High	Normal	Normal	Normal	Negative

intestinal calcium absorption, increase renal calcium excretion, and are cytotoxic to malignant lymphocytes, leading to substantial reduction in serum calcium concentration in animals with hypercalcemia secondary to lymphoma, myeloma, hypervitaminosis D, granulomatous disease, and hypoadrencorticism. However, use of glucocorticoids may make definitive diagnosis of the underlying cause of the hypercalcemia difficult. This is especially true with lymphosarcoma, because steroids are lymphocytolytic and may alter lymph node architecture and patterns of lymphocyte infiltration in bone marrow.

Miscellaneous Agents: The third tier of treatment is to add a bisphosphonate, mithramycin, or calcitonin for more longterm control of hypercalcemia. Bisphosphonates assist in lowering serum calcium by reducing the number and action of osteoclasts. Pamidronate is the most commonly used parenteral drug; the recommended dosage in dogs is 1–2 mg/kg, IV, mixed in 0.9% saline given throughout 2 hr. In cats, alendronate is the most common oral preparation used to control idiopathic hypercalcemia. Adequate hydration is essential when treating with bisphosphonates, because these drugs may cause nephrotoxicity, especially at higher doses. The drug can be repeated in 3–4 wk if needed.

Mithramycin, an inhibitor of RNA synthesis in osteoclasts, is an effective treatment for hypercalcemia; the dosage is 25 mcg/kg, IV, given throughout 4–6 hr. A single dose is usually successful in normalizing the serum calcium concentration; effects last from a few days to several weeks. Adverse effects may include thrombocytopenia, nephrotoxicity, and hepatotoxicity but are unlikely after a single dose. However, this drug must be used with extreme caution.

Calcitonin inhibits bone resorption by inhibiting the activity and formation of bone osteoclasts. The dose of calcitonin is 4–8 U/kg, SC, bid-tid. Calcitonin is the most rapidly acting hypocalcemia agent, causing serum calcium to decrease within a few hours after administration. Its effect is rather transient, however, and the maximal reduction in calcium is not as great as that seen with bisphosphonates or mithramycin.

Calcimimetics, a new class of drugs, are calcium-sensing receptor agonists. The mostly commonly used drug of this class is cinacalcet. By interacting with the calcium-sensing receptors in the parathyroid glands, these drugs reduce the secretion of PTH and can effectively suppress circulating PTH in all forms of hyperparathyroidism. They have become a major therapy for secondary hyperparathyroidism associated with renal failure as well as for treatment of primary hyperparathyroidism.

HYPERCALCEMIA IN HORSES

Like dogs and cats, horses can develop hypercalcemia due to several disorders, including chronic renal failure, vitamin D toxicosis, and primary hyperparathyroidism. The most common cause of hypercalcemia in horses is chronic renal failure. The equine kidney is important in the excretion of calcium; therefore, impaired renal calcium excretion associated with normal intestinal calcium absorption may explain the hypercalcemia found in these horses.

Humoral hypercalcemia of malignancy has been reported to be associated with gastric squamous cell carcinoma, adrenocortical carcinoma, squamous cell carcinoma of the vulva, lymphosarcoma, and ameloblastoma. These horses have hypercalcemia, hypophosphatemia, increased serum concentrations of PTHrP, and decreased serum concentrations of PTH.

Intoxication with ergocalciferol or cholecalciferol has been reported in horses. Ingestion of plants containing 1,25-dihydroxyvitamin D–like compounds (*Solanum malacoxylon*, *S sodomaeum*, *Cestrum diurnum*, *Trisetum flavescens*) causes typical clinical signs of vitamin D intoxication, including hypercalcemia.

Primary hyperparathyroidism is a rare disorder in ponies and horses. As in dogs and cats, hypercalcemia, hypophosphatemia, and high serum PTH concentrations are reported in horses with the disorder. Additional tests to exclude other conditions associated with hypercalcemia may include measurement of PTHrP and vitamin D metabolite concentrations.

As in other species, the definitive treatment of equine hypercalcemia is treating or removing the underlying cause. Unfortunately, the cause may not be readily apparent, and supportive measures (eg, fluid therapy, diuretics, and/or glucocorticoids) must sometimes be used to enhance urinary excretion of calcium and to decrease the serum calcium concentration.

HYPOCALCEMIA IN DOGS AND CATS

Hypocalcemia causes the major clinical manifestations of hypoparathyroidism by increasing the excitability of both the central and peripheral nervous systems. Peripheral neuromuscular signs classically include muscle tremors, twitches, and tetany. Generalized convulsions, resembling those of an idiopathic seizure disorder, are the predominant CNS manifestation of hypoparathyroidism.

Hypoparathyroidism

Hypoparathyroidism is a metabolic disorder characterized by hypocalcemia and hyperphosphatemia and either transient or permanent PTH insufficiency. The spontaneous disorder is uncommon in dogs and rarely reported in cats. Iatrogenic injury or removal of the parathyroid glands during thyroidectomy for treatment of hyperthyroidism is the most common cause in cats. Postoperative hypoparathyroidism secondary to parathyroidectomy for parathyroid tumor may occur because of atrophy of the remaining glands in either dogs or cats.

Diagnosis: Diagnosis is based on history, clinical signs, laboratory evidence of hypocalcemia and hyperphosphatemia, and exclusion of other causes of hypocalcemia (eg, hypoproteinemia, malabsorption, pancreatitis, renal failure). If idiopathic hypoparathyroidism is suspected, it should be confirmed by histologic examination of the parathyroid glands and documentation of parathyroid atrophy or destruction. Because the parathyroid glands are not grossly evident in animals with hypoparathyroidism, a unilateral thyroidectomy should be performed to ensure that adequate parathyroid tissue is available for examination. Determination of serum PTH concentrations might be helpful in the diagnosis of idiopathic hypoparathyroidism and may thereby eliminate the need for cervical exploratory surgery and histologic verification.

Treatment: Treatment is directed at restoring the serum calcium concentration to the low end of the normal range. This should include use of calcium supplements and vitamin D for either iatrogenic or idiopathic forms of hypoparathyroidism. If hypocalcemic tetany or seizures are present, calcium should be administered IV immediately. For maintenance of normocalcemia, oral calcium should be administered together with a vitamin D preparation.

The major complication associated with treatment of hypoparathyroidism is hypercalcemia, which develops as a consequence of overtreatment with calcium and vitamin D. If this occurs, calcium and vitamin D therapy should be temporarily discontinued; saline and furosemide should be administered if hypercalcemia is severe (*see* p 568). With idiopathic hypoparathyroidism, longterm management with vitamin D (with or without calcium supplementation) is necessary. In contrast, with iatrogenic hypoparathyroidism, spontaneous recovery of parathyroid function or accommodation of calcium-regulating mechanisms to the absence of PTH may occur weeks to months after surgery.

Other Causes of Hypocalcemia

Renal Disease: Chronic renal failure is probably the most frequently encountered cause of hypocalcemia. Azotemia and hyperphosphatemia result from decreased glomerular filtration rates. Mechanisms of hypocalcemia include decreased renal tubular calcium resorption, hyperphosphatemia, decreased formation of 1,25-dihydroxyvitamin D, hypoalbuminemia, and chelation of calcium with oxalate. Parathyroid gland hyperplasia occurs to maintain serum calcium in normal ranges. High PTH concentrations result in increased bone resorption. The hypocalcemia associated with renal failure, however, is rarely clinically significant (ie, muscle tremors, twitches, tetany, or convulsions do not develop). In addition, most animals with chronic renal failure have normal serum calcium concentrations. Treatment should be directed at lowering the serum phosphate concentrations by dietary restriction of phosphorus and intestinal phosphate binders. (*See also* RENAL DYSFUNCTION IN SMALL ANIMALS, p 1512.)

Hypoproteinemia: Animals with hypoalbuminemia may be hypocalcemic because of a decrease in the protein-bound fraction of calcium, but the ionized calcium fraction may remain normal. Clinical signs of hypocalcemia do not usually develop. The magnitude of hypocalcemia is usually mild.

Pancreatitis: When hypocalcemia occurs in animals with pancreatitis (*see* p 407), it is usually mild and subclinical. The exact mechanism is unknown, but a commonly accepted theory is that calcium is precipitated in the form of insoluble soaps through saponification of peripancreatic fatty acids formed subsequent to release of the pancreatic enzyme lipase. More recent work suggests that hypocalcemia may result from a shift of calcium into soft tissues, especially muscle.

Puerperal Tetany: Puerperal tetany (eclampsia, *see* p 992) is an acute, life-threatening disease caused by an extreme fall in circulating calcium concentrations in the lactating bitch or queen. Severe hypocalcemia associated with eclampsia develops during the nursing period (several days to several weeks postpartum). The pathophysiology remains poorly understood but appears to result from an imbalance between the rate of inflow (eg, bone resorption, GI absorption) and outflow (eg, mammary gland) from the extracellular calcium pool. Treatment consists of slow IV administration of calcium (*see* below) and weaning of the litter, if possible.

Phosphate Enema Toxicity: Hypertonic sodium phosphate (eg, Fleet®) enemas may result in severe biochemical abnormalities, especially when administered to dehydrated cats with colonic atony and mucosal disruption. Hypernatremia and hyperphosphatemia result from the colonic absorption of sodium and phosphate from the enema solution, as well as transfer of intravascular water to the colonic lumen (because of the hypertonic enema). Hyperphosphatemia leads to precipitation of serum calcium with resultant hypocalcemia. Clinical signs of phosphate enema toxicosis, which result from these electrolyte and fluid alterations, include shock and neuromuscular irritability. Treatment consists of IV volume expansion with an electrolyte-poor solution (eg, 5% dextrose in water), as well as treatment of hypocalcemia (*see* below).

Chelating Agents: EDTA (ethylenediaminetetraacetic acid), citrated blood, and oxalic acid (a metabolite of the ethylene glycol in antifreeze) all complex calcium and can cause hypocalcemia. Animals with ethylene glycol intoxication (*see* p 3046) also have severe metabolic acidosis, azotemia, and hyperphosphatemia from the oliguric renal failure, which results from calcium oxalate crystal precipitation in the renal tubules.

Treatment of Hypocalcemia

The definitive treatment for hypocalcemia is to eliminate the underlying cause. Supportive measures, including the following, to restore normocalcemia can be administered pending the diagnosis.

Parenteral Calcium: Hypocalcemic tetany or convulsions are indications for the immediate IV administration of 10% calcium gluconate (1–1.5 mL/kg), which should be slowly infused throughout a 10-min period. Close monitoring is mandatory; if bradycardia or shortening of the QT interval occurs, the IV infusion should be slowed or temporarily discontinued.

Once the life-threatening signs of hypocalcemia have been controlled, calcium can be added to the IV fluids and administered as a slow continuous infusion (eg, 10% calcium gluconate, 2.5 mL/kg every 6–8 hr). The rate of calcium administration should be adjusted as necessary to maintain a normal serum calcium concentration, and the infusion should be continued for as long as necessary to prevent recurrence of hypocalcemia. Although this continuous calcium infusion will maintain normocalcemia, its effects are short-lived; hypocalcemia will recur within hours of stopping the infusion unless other treatment is given.

Oral Calcium: Oral calcium supplementation may be beneficial in some conditions (eg, hypoparathyroidism, puerperal tetany). The daily requirements are 1–4 g for dogs and 0.5–1 g for cats. The daily dose of calcium should be based on the amount of elemental calcium in the product, rather than on the weight of the calcium salt.

Vitamin D: In some conditions, vitamin D supplementation is necessary to increase calcium absorption from the intestines. There are three main preparations of vitamin D available, including vitamin D_2 (ergocalciferol), dihydrotachysterol, and 1,25-dihydroxyvitamin D (calcitriol). The dosage and duration of response of these drugs depends on the form used. For vitamin D_2, the initial required dosages are generally 4,000–6,000 IU/kg/day, whereas the final dosages required to maintain normocalcemia range from 1,000–2,000 IU/kg, once daily to once weekly. For dihydrotachysterol, initial loading dosages of 0.02–0.03 mg/kg/day are usually administered, with maintenance dosages of 0.01–0.02 mg/kg given every 24–48 hr. For 1,25-dihydroxyvitamin D, a daily dosage of 0.025–0.06 mcg/kg (25–60 ng/kg/day) is generally required. Because the available capsule sizes (250 and 500 ng) are not well formulated for the small body size of most dogs and cats, and these capsules cannot be readily divided, it may be desirable to contact a pharmacist who can reformulate these products to a size that is appropriate for the individual pet. With all vitamin D preparations and dosage regimens, the development of iatrogenic hypercalcemia is a common complication of treatment.

HYPOCALCEMIC DISORDERS OF HORSES

Primary hypoparathyroidism is a rare but well documented disorder in horses. Affected horses have clinical signs consistent with hypocalcemia (ataxia, seizures, hyperexcitability, synchronous diaphragmatic flutter, tachycardia, tachypnea, muscle fasciculation, and ileus). As in other species, the diagnosis is based on the finding of low serum concentrations of calcium and PTH with high levels of phosphorus. As described above, treatment with intravenous and subsequently oral calcium combined with large doses of vitamin D should result in the remission of clinical signs associated with hypoparathyroidism.

Sepsis is one of the most common causes of hypocalcemia in horses admitted to veterinary hospitals. Total and ionized hypocalcemia are common in horses with severe GI disease and sepsis. Hypocalcemia with inappropriately low serum PTH concentrations also has been reported in foals. The underlying cause of hypocalcemia in foals remains to be determined. However, these foals may possibly have some form of hypoparathyroidism associated with sepsis.

THE ADRENAL GLANDS

The adrenal glands of mammals are located near the cranial pole of the kidneys. They consist of two distinct parts, the outer cortex and inner medulla, that differ in morphology, function, and origin.

ADRENAL CORTEX

The adrenal cortex is subdivided into three layers, or zones, although the demarcation between zones often is indistinct. The zona glomerulosa, the outer zone, is responsible for the secretion of mineralocorticoid hormones. The zona fasciculata, the middle zone, comprises ~70% of the cortex and is composed of cells that contain abundant cytoplasmic lipid and the glucocorticoid hormones. The zona reticularis, the inner zone, is responsible for the secretion of sex steroids.

Mineralocorticoids, of which the most potent naturally occurring one is aldosterone, are adrenal steroids that have their principal effects on ion transport by epithelial cells, resulting in a loss of potassium and retention of sodium. Sweat glands and the electrolyte "pumps" in epithelial cells of the renal tubule respond similarly. In the distal convoluted tubule of the mammalian nephron, a cation-exchange mechanism resorbs sodium from the glomerular filtrate and secretes potassium into the lumen. These reactions are accelerated by mineralocorticoids and proceed more slowly in their absence. A lack of secretion of mineralocorticoids (Addison disease) may result in a lethal retention of potassium and loss of sodium.

Cortisol and lesser amounts of corticosterone are the most important glucocorticoid hormones secreted by the adrenal gland in many species. In general, the actions of glucocorticoids on carbohydrate, protein, and lipid metabolism result in sparing of glucose and a tendency to result in hyperglycemia and increased glucose production. In addition, they decrease lipogenesis and increase lipolysis in adipose tissue, which results in release of glycerol and free fatty acids.

Glucocorticoids also suppress inflammatory and immunologic responses, thereby attenuating associated tissue destruction and fibroplasia. However, high levels of glucocorticoids reduce resistance to bacteria, viruses, and fungi, which favors the spread of infection. Glucocorticoids may impair the immunologic response at any stage, from the initial interaction and processing of antigens by cells of the reticuloendothelial system, through the induction and proliferation of immunocompetent lymphocytes and subsequent antibody production. Inhibition of a number of lymphocyte functions forms part of the basis for immunosuppression.

Glucocorticoids may have a profound negative effect on wound healing. High therapeutic doses of adrenal corticosteroids or the syndrome of hyperadrenocorticism may cause wound dehiscence after surgery. The inhibition of fibroblast proliferation and collagen synthesis leads to a decrease in scar tissue formation.

Progesterone, estrogens, and androgens are adrenal sex hormones. Excess secretion may be associated with a neoplasm of the zona reticularis. The manifestation of virilism, precocious sexual development, or feminization depends on which steroid is secreted in excess, sex of the individual, and age of onset. In addition, a syndrome termed atypical hyperadrenocorticism has been reported in association with excessive production of adrenal sex steroids. The symptoms mirror those of Cushing syndrome (*see* p 543), despite normal or low levels of cortisol concentrations after provocative testing. Dogs with this syndrome have increased concentrations of one of several adrenal steroids, which lead to the clinical signs. Treatment options are similar to those used in the management of Cushing syndrome.

HYPERADRENOCORTICISM

(Cushing syndrome)

Hyperadrenocorticism may be the most frequent endocrinopathy in adult to aged dogs but is infrequent in other domestic animals. The clinical signs and biochemical abnormalities result primarily from chronic excess production of cortisol. Increased cortisol levels in dogs may result from one of several mechanisms. The most common is an adenoma or hyperplasia of the adrenocorticotropic hormone (ACTH)–containing cells of the pituitary gland (pars distalis or pars intermedia), which results in bilateral adrenal cortical hypertrophy and hyperplasia. This form of the disease is referred to as pituitary-dependent hyperadrenocorticism (Cushing disease) and is seen in ~90% of cases. Functional adrenal tumors, a far less frequent cause of hyperadrenocorticism in dogs, may secrete cortisol or sex steroids, resulting in a variety of clinical signs. Many of the clinical signs and biochemical abnormalities seen with naturally occurring hyperadrenocorticism can be induced by longterm, daily administration of large doses of corticosteroids. Dogs develop a spectrum of clinical signs and laboratory abnormalities as a result of the combined gluconeogenic, lipolytic, protein catabolic, and anti-inflammatory effects of the glucocorticoid hormones on many organ systems. The disease is insidious and slowly progressive. (For discussion of the clinical signs, laboratory abnormalities, diagnosis, and treatment of hyperadrenocorticism, *see* p 543.)

HYPOADRENOCORTICISM

(Addison disease)

A deficiency in adrenocortical hormones is seen most commonly in young to middle-aged dogs and occasionally in horses. The disease may be familial in Standard Poodles, West Highland White Terriers, Great Danes, Bearded Collies, Portuguese Water Dogs, and a variety of other breeds. The cause of primary adrenocortical failure usually is unknown, although most cases probably result from an autoimmune process. Other causes include destruction of the adrenal gland by granulomatous disease, metastatic tumor, hemorrhage, infarction, adrenolytic agents (mitotane), or adrenal enzyme inhibitors (trilostane).

Clinical Findings: Many of the functional disturbances of chronic adrenal insufficiency are not highly specific; they include recurrent episodes of gastroenteritis, a slowly progressive loss of body condition, and failure to respond appropriately to stress. Although hypoadrenocorticism is seen in dogs of any breed, sex, or age, idiopathic adrenocortical insufficiency is most common in young female adult dogs. This may be related to its suspected immune-mediated pathogenesis.

A reduction in secretion of aldosterone, the principal mineralocorticoid, results in marked alterations of serum levels of potassium, sodium, and chloride. Potassium excretion by the kidneys is reduced and results in a progressive increase in serum potassium levels. Hyponatremia and hypochloremia result from renal tubular loss. Severe hyperkalemia may result in bradycardia and an irregular heart rate with changes in the ECG. Some dogs develop a pronounced bradycardia (heart rate ≤50 bpm) that predisposes to weakness or circulatory collapse after minimal exertion.

Although the development of clinical signs is often unnoticed, acute circulatory collapse and evidence of renal failure frequently occur. A progressive decrease in blood volume contributes to hypotension, weakness, and microcardia. Increased excretion of water by the kidneys, because of decreased reabsorption of sodium and chloride, results in progressive dehydration and hemoconcentration. Emesis, diarrhea, and anorexia are common and contribute to the animal's deterioration. Weight loss is frequently severe. Similar clinical signs are seen in cats with hypoadrenocorticism.

Decreased production of glucocorticoids results in several characteristic functional disturbances. Decreased gluconeogenesis and increased sensitivity to insulin contribute to the development of moderate hypoglycemia. In some dogs, hyperpigmentation of the skin is seen because of the lack of negative feedback on the pituitary gland and increased ACTH release. Atypical Addison disease has been reported in dogs and is associated with hypocortisolemia with normal electrolytes. Clinical signs are similar to those seen in dogs with both glucocorticoid and mineralocorticoid insufficiency.

Lesions: The most common abnormality in dogs is bilateral idiopathic adrenocortical atrophy, in which all layers of the cortex are markedly reduced in thickness. The adrenal cortex is reduced to one-tenth or less of its normal thickness and consists primarily of the adrenal capsule. The adrenal medulla is relatively more prominent and, with the capsule, makes up the bulk of the remaining adrenal glands.

All three zones of the adrenal cortex are involved, including the zona glomerulosa, which is not under ACTH control; however, no obvious pituitary lesions have been seen in dogs with idiopathic adrenal cortical atrophy.

A destructive pituitary lesion that decreases ACTH secretion is characterized by severe atrophy of the inner two cortical zones of the adrenal gland; the zona glomerulosa remains intact.

Diagnosis: A presumptive diagnosis is based on the history and supportive (although not specific) laboratory abnormalities, including hyponatremia, hyperkalemia, a sodium:potassium ratio of <25:1, azotemia, mild acidosis, and a normocytic, normochromic anemia. Severe GI blood loss has also been reported. Occasionally, mild hypoglycemia is present. The hyperkalemia results in ECG changes: an elevation (spiking) of the T wave, a flattening or absence of the P wave, a prolonged PR interval, and a widening of the QRS complex. Ventricular fibrillation or asystole may occur with potassium levels >11 mEq/L.

Differential diagnoses include primary GI disease (especially whipworm infection), renal failure, acute pancreatitis, and toxin ingestion. For definitive diagnosis, evaluation of adrenal function is required. After obtaining a baseline blood sample, ACTH (gel or synthetic) is administered. Gel preparations are administered IM, and a second blood sample is obtained 2 hr later. Synthetic preparations are administered IM or IV with a second blood sample 1 hr later. Baseline (resting) cortisol concentrations >2.5 mcg/dL effectively exclude the diagnosis of hypoadrenocorticism, whereas values <2.5 mcg/dL require the use of ACTH stimulation testing to confirm the diagnosis. Affected dogs have low baseline cortisol levels, and there is little response to ACTH administration in classic and atypical cases. This test can be completed in most animals before replacement hormone therapy is started.

Treatment: An adrenal crisis is an acute medical emergency. An IV catheter should be inserted, and an infusion of 0.9% saline begun. If the dog is hypoglycemic, the saline should include 2.5%–5% dextrose. The hypovolemia is corrected rapidly by administering 0.9% saline (60–70 mL/kg over the first 1–2 hr). Urine output should be assessed to determine whether the dog is becoming anuric. Fluids should be continued, at a rate appropriate to match ongoing losses, until the clinical signs and laboratory abnormalities have resolved.

Prednisolone sodium succinate (22–30 mg/kg) or dexamethasone sodium phosphate (0.2–1 mg/kg) may be used in the initial management of shock. Dexamethasone will not interfere with cortisol measurements during the ACTH stimulation test. Prednisolone or prednisone should be given at 1 mg/kg, bid, for the first few days of therapy and then at 0.25–0.5 mg/kg/day. Mineralocorticoid replacement therapy (*see* below) is also begun to help with electrolyte imbalances and hypovolemia. Electrolytes, renal function, and glucose should be monitored regularly to assess response to therapy.

In cases of severe, nonresponsive hyperkalemia, 10% glucose in 0.9% saline can be given for 30–60 min to increase potassium movement into the cells. Regular insulin (0.25–1 U/kg) administered IM will enhance glucose and potassium uptake, but 10% glucose (20 mL per unit of insulin) should be administered IV concurrently to avoid hypoglycemia.

For longterm maintenance therapy, the mineralocorticoid desoxycorticosterone pivalate (DOCP) is administered at 2.2 mg/kg, IM or SC, every 25–28 days. Electrolytes should be measured at 3 and 4 wk after the first few injections to determine the duration of action. Alternatively, fludrocortisone acetate is administered PO at 10–30 mcg/kg/day. Serum electrolytes should be monitored weekly until the proper dose is determined. Some dogs (especially dogs on DOCP) also require daily oral glucocorticoid therapy to adequately control clinical signs. Replacement doses of prednisone (0.2–0.4 mg/kg/day) are required in ~50% of dogs. Additional glucocorticoid supplementation may be required (2–5 times maintenance) during times of illness or stress. Dogs with atypical Addison disease require only replacement doses of prednisone, although it is recommended that electrolytes be monitored every 3 mo for the first year after diagnosis. Dogs with chronic hypoadrenocorticism should be reexamined every 3–6 mo.

Treatment of horses with hypoadrenocorticism is similar—aggressive replacement of fluids, steroids, and glucose if needed in an adrenal crisis. Supportive therapy and rest are indicated in cases of chronic Addison disease.

ADRENAL MEDULLA

The adrenal medulla, although apparently not essential to life, plays an important role in response to stress or hypoglycemia. It secretes epinephrine and norepinephrine, which increase cardiac output, blood pressure, and blood glucose, and decrease GI activity.

Pheochromocytomas (*see* below) may develop in domestic animals, most often in cattle and dogs. These secrete epinephrine, norepinephrine, or both. Clinical signs are often absent, and tumors may be incidental findings during evaluation for other conditions or at necropsy.

Other adrenal tumors, such as neuroblastomas and ganglioneuromas, may arise in the chromaffin cells of the sympathetic nervous system.

NEUROENDOCRINE TISSUE TUMORS

Neuroendocrine cells are characterized by their ability to produce and secrete a neuromodulator, transmitter, or hormone. In addition, these cells contain dense core secretory granules, the storage site for the secreted product(s). Neuroendocrine cells are capable of releasing this product in a regulated manner by classic exocytosis. Neuroendocrine cells differ from classic neurons in that they lack axons and synapses. Certain molecules, particularly those of the granin family (eg, chromogranin) are synthesized and stored in neuroendocrine cells and serve as immunohistologic markers.

Previously, neuroendocrine cells were classified as amine precursor uptake and decarboxylation (APUD) cells and were believed to be solely derived from neuroectoderm. However, more recent evidence supports a more diverse embryologic origin.

Tumors that arise from this cell type comprise a family of neuroendocrine tumors, or NETs. Because of the diffuse distribution of cells, particularly within the GI tract, NETs are found in a wide variety of locations. Overall, NETs are rare tumors in people and animals. Some NETs oversecrete their normal product, and the excessive levels result in the observed signs. Other NETs are nonfunctional, and clinical signs instead result from physical forces associated with expansion and/or metastasis.

Examples of NETs include carcinoids, gastroenterohepatic tumors (gastrinoma, insulinoma, glucagonoma), pheochromocytoma of the adrenal gland, medullary carcinoma of the thyroid gland, some pituitary tumors, small-cell lung cancer, multiple endocrine neoplasia (MEN types 1 and 2), and tumors of the chemoreceptor organs. Interestingly, devil facial tumor disease, a devastating transmissible cancer affecting Tasmanian devils (*see* p 2044), appears to be an NET. NETs are identified and classified by their microscopic appearance, the immunohistologic identification of classic neuroendocrine cell markers (such as chromogranin A), and staining for their characteristic transmitter or hormonal product.

Insulinoma and Gastrinoma: Insulinoma (functional islet cell tumor) is the most common NET in domestic species. For discussions of insulinoma and gastrinoma, *see* p 582 and p 583.

Carcinoids: Carcinoids are a heterologous group of NETs that occur in various regions of the GI tract. In dogs and cats, carcinoids have been reported to occur in the stomach. The most common sign reported in affected animals is chronic vomiting. In people (but not yet documented in companion animals), carcinoids serve as a source of serotonin or histamine. Excessive release of these transmitters can cause a syndrome of flushing, hypotension, wheezing, and diarrhea.

Glucagonoma: Glucagonomas have been found in a small number of dogs. Interestingly, affected animals show cutaneous lesions characterized by a superficial necrolytic dermatitis affecting mucocutaneous junctions, footpads, elbows, or the abdomen.

TUMORS OF THE ADRENAL MEDULLA

Pheochromocytomas: Pheochromocytomas occur in domestic species, including dogs and cats. Incidental masses in the area of the adrenal glands are being discovered with greater frequency because of the increased use of abdominal ultrasound and other imaging techniques. Pheochromocytoma, although rare, should be a differential diagnosis whenever such a mass is identified. Pheochromocytomas arise from the adrenal medullary chromaffin cells that normally synthesize and secrete the catecholamines epinephrine and norepinephrine. These tumors have been identified more often in dogs than in cats, usually affect only one gland, and tend to occur in older animals. They are often locally invasive (may result in thrombus formation in the adjacent vena cava) and metastasize in ~25% of cases. Diagnosis of pheochromocytoma is challenging. Clinical signs are nonspecific and may appear sporadically, possibly related to periodic or intermittent release of catecholamines. In addition, signs may vary depending on which catecholamine predominates. Signs reported in most dogs include weight loss, anorexia, depression, weakness, and occasional collapse. Dyspnea and tachycardia may be seen, and hypertension is common; indirect blood pressure measurement can help establish the diagnosis. Imaging, such as ultrasonography or CT scans, is very useful in confirmation of a suspected adrenal mass. Although surgical removal is the treatment of choice, animals with pheochromocytoma present an anesthetic risk secondary to the cardiovascular effects of the catecholamines. Surgery is additionally complicated by the tendency toward local invasion of these tumors and their proximity to large vessels.

Adrenal Medullary Hyperplasia: Diffuse or nodular adrenal medullary hyperplasia appears to precede the development of pheochromocytomas in bulls with C-cell tumors of the thyroid gland. This diffuse proliferation of chromaffin cells is nonencapsulated but compresses the surrounding adrenal cortex. In bulls with prominent diffuse medullary hyperplasia, there are often a few small foci of intense nodular proliferation of medullary cells.

THYROID C-CELL TUMORS

Tumors derived from C-cells (parafollicular, ultimobranchial cells) of the thyroid gland are most common in adult to aged bulls and horses and in certain strains of laboratory rats. A high percentage of aged bulls has been reported to develop C-cell tumors (≥30%) or hyperplasia of C-cells and ultimobranchial derivatives (≥15%–20%). These have not been seen in cows fed similar diets. The incidence in bulls increases with advancing age and is often associated with development of increased vertebral density. Multiple endocrine tumors, especially bilateral pheochromocytomas and occasionally pituitary adenomas, are detected coincidentally in bulls with C-cell tumors. A high frequency of thyroid C-cell tumors and pheochromocytomas has been reported in a family of Guernsey bulls, which suggests an autosomal dominant pattern of inheritance. A diffuse or nodular hyperplasia of secretory cells in the adrenal medulla often precedes the development of pheochromocytoma.

In dogs, C-cell tumors of the thyroid occur as a small percentage of all thyroid tumors (estimates range from 0.1%–12%), but the incidence may be higher. Distinguishing these tumors from other thyroid carcinomas is challenging with light microscopy alone, and confirmation requires immunohistologic staining. These tumors are usually well encapsulated and do not show the tendency for metastasis other thyroid carcinomas exhibit. Oversecretion of calcitonin has not been clearly documented in affected animals. Perhaps related to excessive release of prostaglandins or serotonin, diarrhea is a common clinical sign in dogs with C-cell tumors of the thyroid.

Adenomas: C-cell adenomas appear in one or both thyroid lobes as discrete, single or multiple, gray to tan nodules. Adenomas are smaller (~1–3 cm in diameter) than carcinomas and are separated from the thyroid parenchyma by a thin, fibrous connective tissue capsule. The adjacent thyroid is compressed but not invaded by the tumor. In horses, C-cell adenomas may result in a palpable enlargement in the anterior cervical region. Larger C-cell adenomas incorporate most of the thyroid lobe, but a rim of dark brown-red thyroid often is present on one side.

Carcinomas: Thyroid C-cell carcinomas cause extensive multinodular enlargements of one or both thyroid lobes and may incorporate the entire thyroid gland. If present, metastases in anterior cervical lymph nodes usually are large and have areas of necrosis and hemorrhage. Pulmonary metastases are infrequent and appear as discrete tan nodules throughout all lobes of the lung.

The chronic stimulation of C-cells by longterm dietary intake of excess calcium may be related to the high incidence of these tumors in bulls; adult bulls frequently were fed diets with 3.5–6 times the amount of calcium normally recommended for maintenance, and incidence of the tumors declined significantly when calcium intake was reduced.

Syndromes associated with abnormalities in the secretion of calcitonin are recognized much less frequently than disorders involving parathyroid hormone (PTH). Hypersecretion of calcitonin has been reported in people, bulls, and laboratory rats with medullary (ultimobranchial) thyroid neoplasms derived from C-cells. Osteosclerotic changes have been reported in bulls with this syndrome, but the relationship of longterm excess calcitonin secretion to the pathogenesis of the skeletal lesions and their occurrence in other species is unclear.

In dogs, the histologic grading of thyroid carcinoma has been important in prognosis, although histologic type has not. Of greater importance is the volume of tumor and its relation to the potential for metastasis; also, the more deeply fixed the tumor is to underlying structures, the less likely surgical resection will be complete. Surgery is the primary therapy, but some form of adjuvant therapy is reasonable because of the potential for metastatic spread and residual nonresectable tissue. A combination of radiotherapy and chemotherapy would be ideal in theory, and there is increasing interest in such combined therapy. For the rather rare functional thyroid carcinoma in dogs, treatment with ^{131}I would be a reasonable choice.

CHEMORECEPTOR ORGANS

Chemoreceptor organs are sensitive barometers of changes in the carbon dioxide and oxygen content and pH of the blood and aid in the regulation of respiration and circulation. Although chemoreceptor tissue appears to be widely distributed in the body, tumors (chemodectomas) develop principally in the aortic (more frequent in animals) and carotid (more frequent in people) bodies. These tumors are found primarily in dogs and rarely in cats and cattle. Brachycephalic breeds of dogs, such as the Boxer and Boston Terrier, are predisposed to tumors of the aortic and carotid bodies.

Aortic body tumors appear most frequently as single masses or as multiple nodules within the pericardial sac near the base of the heart. They vary considerably in size (0.5–12.5 cm), with carcinomas generally larger than adenomas. Solitary, small adenomas either are attached to the adventitia of the pulmonary artery and ascending aorta or are embedded in the adipose connective tissue between these major vascular trunks. Larger adenomas may indent the atria or displace the trachea, are multilobular, and partially surround the major arterial trunks at the base of the heart.

In dogs, malignant aortic body tumors occur less frequently than adenomas. Carcinomas may infiltrate the wall of the pulmonary artery to form papillary projections into the lumen or invade through the wall into the lumen of the atria. Although tumor cells often invade blood vessels, metastases to the lungs and liver are infrequent in dogs with aortic body carcinomas. Nonetheless, the local and physiologic effects are important, including those of adenomas.

Aortic body tumors in animals are not functional (ie, they do not secrete excess hormone into the circulation) but, as space-occupying lesions, may result in various functional disturbances. These include manifestations of cardiac decompensation due to pressure on the atria or vena cava (or both) associated with larger aortic body adenomas and carcinomas. Aortic body tumors tend to be more benign than carotid body tumors. They grow slowly by expansion and exert pressure on the vena cava and atria. Aortic body carcinomas may invade locally into the atria, pericardium, and adjacent large, thin-walled vessels.

Carotid body tumors arise near the bifurcation of the common carotid artery, usually as a unilateral, slow-growing mass. Adenomas are usually 1–4 cm in diameter. The bifurcation of the carotid artery is incorporated in the mass, and tumor cells are firmly adherent to the tunica adventitia. Complete excision or biopsy often is difficult because of the high degree of vascularity and intimate relationship with major arterial trunks in the neck.

Malignant carotid body tumors are larger and more coarsely multinodular than adenomas. Although carcinomas appear to be encapsulated, tumor cells invade the capsule and penetrate into the walls of adjacent vessels and lymphatics. The external jugular vein and several cranial nerves may be incorporated by the neoplasm. Metastases of carotid body tumors occur in ~30% of cases and have been found in the lung, bronchial and mediastinal lymph nodes, liver, pancreas, and kidneys. Multicentric neoplastic transformation of chemoreceptor tissue occurs frequently in brachycephalic breeds of dogs.

The histologic characteristics of chemodectomas are essentially similar whether derived from the carotid or aortic body.

Although the etiology of carotid and aortic body tumors is unknown, it has been suggested that a genetic predisposition aggravated by chronic hypoxia may account for the higher risk in certain brachycephalic breeds. Carotid bodies of several mammalian species, including dogs, have undergone hyperplasia when subjected to chronic hypoxia by living in a high-altitude environment.

THE PANCREAS

The endocrine function of the pancreas is performed by small groups of cells, the islets of Langerhans, that are completely surrounded by acinar (exocrine) cells that produce digestive enzymes. The endocrine and exocrine portions of the pancreas are closely related during development, and evidence suggests that islet, acinar, and ductal cells arise from a common multipotential precursor cell.

Pancreatic islets contain α, β, and δ cells, each of which synthesize a unique polypeptide hormone. β cells account for 60%–70% of the islet-cell population and secrete insulin, α cells secrete glucagon, and δ cells secrete somatostatin.

The pancreatic islets function as discrete microendocrine organs. They are distributed throughout the pancreas with a characteristic pattern of cellular interrelationships to assure an appropriate balance of hormones. Afferent vessels and nerves enter the islet in the peripheral tricellular region. The close anatomic relationship of α, β, and δ cells in this heterogeneous cortical region allow it to function as a local glucose sensor, permitting a coordinated output of insulin and glucagon in response to fluctuations in blood glucose. Specialized tight junctions between membranes of adjacent endocrine cells tend to partition the intercellular space and may permit somatostatin to exert a direct local (paracrine) inhibitory effect on glucagon and insulin release.

Insulin is formed initially as a single polypeptide chain of 81–86 amino acid residues. This prohormone (proinsulin) contains the A and B chains of the insulin molecule, plus a connecting peptide. Proinsulin is converted enzymatically to insulin before storage in membrane-limited secretory granules.

The major physiologic stimulus for the release of insulin from β cells is an increase in the concentration of glucose in the extracellular fluid. Specific glucoreceptors that bind with glucose exist on the plasma membrane of β cells. An appropriate level of extracellular calcium is required for insulin secretion. Other sugars (fructose, mannose, ribose), amino acids (leucine, arginine), hormones (glucagon, secretin), drugs (sulfonylurea, theophylline), short-chain fatty acids, and ketone bodies may also stimulate insulin secretion under certain conditions. Pancreatic β cells are able to respond to a specific physiologic stimulus with release of stored hormone in a modulated fashion, rather than releasing all of the stored hormone at once.

Insulin affects, either directly or indirectly, the function of every organ in the body. Tissues that are especially responsive to insulin include skeletal and cardiac muscle, adipose tissue, fibroblasts, liver, WBCs, mammary glands, cartilage, bone, skin, aorta, pituitary gland, and peripheral nerves. The main function of insulin is to stimulate anabolic reactions involving carbohydrates, fats, proteins, and nucleic acids. Liver, adipose cells, and muscle are three principal target sites for insulin. Insulin catalyzes the formation of macromolecules used in cell structure and energy stores, and it regulates many cell functions. In general, insulin increases the transfer of glucose and certain other monosaccharides, some amino acids and fatty acids, and potassium and magnesium ions across the plasma membrane of target cells. It also decreases the rate of lipolysis, proteolysis, ketogenesis, and gluconeogenesis.

Glucagon is secreted in response to a reduction in blood glucose. It promotes mobilization of stores of energy-yielding nutrients by increasing glycogenolysis, gluconeogenesis, and lipolysis. At physiologic concentrations, glucagon increases both hepatic glycogenolysis and gluconeogenesis, thereby increasing blood glucose.

Insulin and glucagon act in concert to maintain the concentration of glucose in extracellular fluids within relatively narrow limits. A glucose sensor in the pancreatic islets controls the relative amounts of insulin and glucagon secreted. Glucagon controls glucose release from the liver into the extracellular space, and insulin controls glucose transport from the extracellular space into insulin-sensitive tissues such as fat, muscle, and liver.

DIABETES MELLITUS

Diabetes mellitus is a chronic disorder of carbohydrate metabolism due to relative or absolute insulin deficiency. Most cases of spontaneous diabetes occur in middle-aged dogs and middle-aged to older cats. In dogs, females are affected twice as often as males, and incidence appears to be increased in certain small breeds such as Miniature Poodles, Dachshunds, Schnauzers, Cairn Terriers, and Beagles, but any breed can be affected. In one study, obese male cats were more commonly affected than females; no breed predilection is seen in cats.

Etiology and Pathogenesis: The pathogenic mechanisms responsible for decreased insulin production and secretion are multiple, but usually they are related to destruction of islet cells, secondary to either immune destruction or severe pancreatitis (dogs) or amyloidosis (cats). Chronic relapsing pancreatitis with progressive loss of both exocrine and endocrine cells and their replacement by fibrous connective tissue results in diabetes mellitus. The pancreas becomes firm and multinodular and often contains scattered areas of hemorrhage and necrosis. Later in the course of disease, a thin, fibrous band of tissue near the duodenum and stomach may be all that remains of the pancreas. In other cases, the numbers of β cells are decreased, and the cells become vacuolated; in chronic cases, the islets are difficult to find. Insulin resistance and secondary diabetes mellitus are also seen in many dogs with spontaneous hyperadrenocorticism and after chronic administration of glucocorticoids or progestins. Pregnancy and diestrus also can predispose to diabetes mellitus. In dogs, but not cats, progesterone leads to release of growth hormone from mammary tissue, resulting in hyperglycemia and insulin resistance. Obesity also predisposes to insulin resistance in both dogs and cats.

Cats with diabetes mellitus usually have specific degenerative lesions localized selectively in the islets of Langerhans, whereas the remainder of the pancreas appears to be normal. The selective deposition of amyloid in islets, with degenerative changes in β cells, is the most common pancreatic lesion in many cats with diabetes. The amyloid appears to arise from islet-associated polypeptide (IAPP), which is secreted together with insulin from the β cells. Cats are unable to process IAPP normally, which leads to excessive accumulation and conversion into amyloid. As cats age, a greater percentage of their islets contain amyloid. Cats with diabetes have a greater percentage of their islets affected with larger amounts of amyloid than age-matched cats without diabetes. The amyloid or IAPP (or both) lead to physical disruption of the β cell and insulin resistance, resulting in diabetes.

Infection with certain viruses in people may cause selective islet damage or pancreatitis and has been suggested to be responsible for certain cases of rapidly developing diabetes mellitus. This has yet to be documented in dogs or cats. The selective degeneration and necrosis of β cells is accompanied by infiltration of the islets by lymphocytes and macrophages. Stress, obesity, and administration of corticosteroids or progestogens may increase the severity of clinical signs.

Complete expression of the complex metabolic disturbances in diabetes mellitus appears to be the result of a bihormonal abnormality. Although a relative or absolute deficiency of insulin action in response to a rising extracellular glucose concentration has long been recognized as the major hormonal abnormality, the importance of an absolute or relative increase of glucagon secretion has been appreciated more recently. Hyperglucagonemia in diabetes may be the result of increased secretion of pancreatic glucagon, enteroglucagon, or both. Increased glucagon appears to contribute to development of severe hyperglycemia by mobilizing hepatic stores of glucose and to development of ketoacidosis by increasing the oxidation of fatty acids in the liver.

Clinical Findings: The onset of diabetes is often insidious, and the clinical course chronic. Common signs in dogs include polydipsia, polyuria, polyphagia with weight loss, bilateral cataracts, and weakness. The disturbances in water metabolism develop primarily because of an osmotic diuresis. The renal threshold for glucose is ~180 mg/dL in dogs and ~280 mg/dL in cats.

Diabetic animals have decreased resistance to bacterial and fungal infections and often develop chronic or recurrent infections such as cystitis, prostatitis, bronchopneumonia, and dermatitis. This increased susceptibility to infection may be related in part to impaired chemotactic, phagocytic, and antimicrobial activity associated with decreased neutrophil function. Radiographic evidence of emphysematous cystitis (rare) due to infections with glucose-fermenting organisms (such as *Proteus* sp, *Aerobacter aerogenes*, and *Escherichia coli*), which results in gas formation in the wall and lumen of the bladder, is suggestive of diabetes mellitus. Emphysema also may develop in the wall of the gallbladder in diabetic dogs.

Hepatomegaly due to lipid accumulation is common in diabetic dogs and cats. The fatty liver results from increased fat mobilization from adipose tissue. Individual liver cells are greatly enlarged by the accumulation of multiple droplets of neutral lipid. In cats, hepatic lipidosis may occur in conjunction with diabetes mellitus.

Cataracts develop frequently in dogs (not cats) with poorly controlled diabetes mellitus. The lenticular opacities appear initially along the suture lines of lens fibers and are stellate ("asteroid") in shape. Cataract formation in dogs is related to the unique sorbitol pathway by which glucose is metabolized in the lens, which leads to edema of the lens and disruption of normal light transmission. Although the same sorbitol pathway seems to be present in cats, the development of cataracts is rare. Other extrapancreatic lesions associated with diabetes mellitus in people, such as nephropathy, retinopathy, and micro- and macrovascular angiopathy, are rare in dogs and cats.

Diagnosis: A diagnosis of diabetes mellitus is based on persistent fasting hyperglycemia and glycosuria. The normal fasting value for blood glucose in dogs and cats is 75–120 mg/dL. In cats, stress-induced hyperglycemia is a frequent problem, and multiple blood and urine samples may be required to confirm the diagnosis. Measurement of serum fructosamine can assist in differentiating between stress-induced hyperglycemia and diabetes mellitus. In cases of stress-induced hyperglycemia, the fructosamine concentrations are normal. In all cases, a search should be made for drugs or diseases that predispose to diabetes.

Treatment: Longterm success depends on the understanding and cooperation of the owner. Treatment involves a combination of weight reduction, diet, insulin, and possibly oral hypoglycemics. Intact females should be neutered. In cats, recent evidence has supported the use of high-protein, low-carbohydrate diets. In dogs, diets that are high in fiber and complex carbohydrates are preferred. Diet and weight reduction alone will not control the disease, so initial therapy with insulin is required. Most dogs require two doses of insulin a day. In general, NPH or lente is the initial insulin of choice at a dose of 0.5 U/kg, bid. With twice daily injections, two meals of equal calories are given at the time of insulin administration. Diets high in simple sugars (semimoist foods) should be avoided. Clinical signs and serial blood glucose determinations are used to monitor therapy after initial stabilization at home for 5–7 days.

In dogs with poor glycemic control on NPH or lente insulin, use of the basal insulin detemir should be considered. Because of its potency, the starting dosage of detemir is 0.1 U/kg, bid, with reassessment of clinical signs and glycemic control in 1 wk.

It is usually preferable to have blood glucose testing performed at home to avoid changes in the pet's routine and the stress of in-hospital testing. Studies in both dogs and cats have shown that at-home monitoring improves glycemic control and increases the likelihood of obtaining remission in diabetic cats. In cats, high-protein diets along with insulin therapy are initiated, with reevaluation in 5–7 days. In newly diagnosed cats, insulin glargine is the insulin of choice. Glargine is a long-acting basal insulin. Used in conjunction with high-protein, low-carbohydrate diets, it is associated with remission of diabetes and discontinuation of insulin therapy in 80%–90% of cases within the first 3–4 mo of treatment. NPH, lente, or PZI insulins may also be used in cats, with starting dosages ranging from 1 to 3 units, bid. However, these insulins are not associated with high rates of diabetic remission.

The use of oral hypoglycemic agents (glipizide) has been evaluated in diabetic cats. Glipizide is a sulfonylurea that stimulates the release of insulin from functional β cells. Glipizide should not be used in thin or ketonuric cats when absolute insulin deficiency is likely and exogenous insulin administration is required. Glipizide is administered at an initial dose of 2.5 mg, bid, PO, in conjunction with dietary management. Clinical response is seen at 3–4 wk. Short-term success is seen in 50% of treated cats, with longterm success rates (>1 yr) of ~15%. Alternatively, glimepiride and glyburide (other sulfonylureas) may be administered to cats at 2 mg/day (glimepiride) or 0.625 mg/day (glyburide). Acarbose, an oral α-glucosidase inhibitor, has also been used in cats at a dose of 12.5–25 mg, bid-tid, in conjunction with diet and/or insulin to control hyperglycemia.

Ketoacidosis is a serious complication of diabetes mellitus and should be regarded as a medical emergency. Therapy includes correcting dehydration by administration of IV fluids, such as 0.9% NaCl or lactated Ringer's solution; reducing hyperglycemia and ketosis by administration of crystalline zinc (regular) insulin; maintaining serum electrolyte levels, especially potassium, through supplemental administration of appropriate electrolyte solutions; and identifying and treating underlying and complicating diseases, such as acute pancreatitis or infections.

Numerous insulin regimens have been used in treatment of ketoacidotic diabetes mellitus. In the intermittent insulin regimen, regular insulin at 0.2 U/kg, IM, is the initial dosage, followed by hourly administration of 0.1 U/kg. Once the serum glucose is <250 mg/dL, the insulin is administered SC at 0.25–0.5 U/kg, every 4–6 hr, with careful monitoring of the serum glucose at 1- to 2-hr intervals. During aggressive treatment with insulin, blood glucose levels may fall rapidly, and the addition of 2.5%–5% dextrose to the IV fluids may be required.

When insulin therapy has been instituted, the blood glucose should be checked frequently until an adequate maintenance dose has been determined. Once the animal is on maintenance therapy and its condition is stable, it should be reassessed every 4–6 mo.

FUNCTIONAL ISLET CELL TUMORS

The most frequent pancreatic islet tumor is an islet cell carcinoma derived from insulin-secreting β cells. These neoplasms frequently are hormonally active and secrete excessive amounts of insulin, which causes hypoglycemia. Endocrine pancreatic tissue appears to be derived from multipotential ductal epithelial cells, which differentiate into one of the several cell types present within the islets. Gastrin, somatostatin, pancreatic polypeptide, and vasoactive intestinal peptide may also be produced in excess in islet cell tumors. β-cell neoplasms of the pancreatic islets (insulinomas) are seen most frequently in dogs 5–12 yr old. They are common in ferrets and have also been less frequently reported in cats and in older cattle.

Clinical Findings: The clinical signs seen with insulinomas result from excessive insulin secretion, which leads to an increased rate of transfer of glucose from the extracellular fluid to body tissues and thus to severe hypoglycemia. The clinical signs are a reflection of the hypoglycemia and are not specific for hyperinsulinism associated with β-cell neoplasms. Initial signs include posterior weakness, fatigue after exercise, generalized muscular twitching and weakness, ataxia, mental confusion, and changes of temperament. Dogs are easily agitated, and there are intermittent periods of excitability and restlessness. Periodic seizures may occur, and episodes of collapse resembling syncope have also been reported.

Clinical signs are characteristically episodic and occur initially at widely spaced intervals but become more frequent and prolonged as the disease progresses. Hypoglycemic attacks may be precipitated by physical exercise (increased use of glucose) or fasting (decreased availability of glucose), as well as by ingestion of food (stimulation of insulin release). Administration of glucose rapidly alleviates the signs.

The predominance of clinical signs relating to the CNS demonstrates the primary dependence of the brain on the metabolism of glucose for energy. When the brain is not supplied with glucose, cerebral oxidation decreases and manifestations of anoxia appear. Because clinical signs are compatible with primary disease of the CNS, functional islet cell tumors may be misdiagnosed as idiopathic epilepsy, brain tumors, or other organic neurologic disease. Repeated episodes of prolonged and severe hypoglycemia may result in irreversible neuronal degeneration throughout the brain. Permanent neurologic disability probably accounts for the terminal coma, unresponsiveness to glucose, and eventual death of some dogs.

Lesions: Insulinomas usually appear as single, yellow to dark red, spherical, small (1–3 cm) nodules visible from the serosal surface. They occur as single or occasionally multiple nodules in the same or different lobes of the pancreas. They are of similar consistency to or slightly firmer than the surrounding pancreatic parenchyma. A thin layer of fibrous connective tissue separates the neoplasm from the adjacent parenchyma. Insulinomas frequently metastasize to regional lymph nodes or the liver (or both) before diagnosis. True benign adenomas of islet cells are rare.

Diagnosis: A blood glucose determination should be done on all older dogs with a history of periodic weakness, collapse, or seizures. Fasting hypoglycemia (≤60 mg/dL) in a middle-aged to older dog is strong support for an insulinoma. Serum insulin concentrations taken at the time of hypoglycemia are normal to increased in animals with an insulinoma. Differential diagnoses for hypoglycemia include hypoadrenocorticism, hepatic failure, large extrapancreatic neoplasms, sepsis, polycythemia, insulin overdosage, and laboratory error.

Treatment: Although insulinomas are usually solitary in dogs, the entire pancreas should be examined carefully for multiple tumors. Complete excision of the tumor ameliorates the hypoglycemia and associated neurologic signs, unless there have been irreversible changes in the CNS. If there are nonvisible metastases, hypoglycemia may persist after surgery. Even though the potential for malignancy of insulinomas is high, many dogs live >1 yr with acceptable quality of life if all visible tumors are debulked at surgery. Dogs with inoperable tumors may be managed fairly well with multiple feedings per day and glucocorticoid administration (0.5–1 mg/kg/day). Diazoxide (20–80 mg/kg/day, divided into three equal doses) may also alleviate clinical signs in some dogs, although problems with availability have limited its use. The chemotherapeutic agent streptozotocin has been investigated for the treatment of islet cell tumors in dogs and may be considered after surgical resection.

GASTRIN-SECRETING ISLET CELL TUMORS

Gastrinomas of the pancreas have been reported in people, dogs, and a cat. Hypersecretion of gastrin in people results in the Zollinger-Ellison syndrome, consisting of hypersecretion of gastric acid and recurrent peptic ulceration in the GI tract. The tumors, derived from ectopic amine precursor uptake decarboxylase (APUD) cells in the pancreas, produce an excess of the hormone gastrin, which normally is secreted by cells of the antral and duodenal mucosa.

Clinical Findings: These tumors are rare; they occur less frequently than the insulin-secreting β-cell neoplasms. The few documented cases have had anorexia, hematemesis, intermittent diarrhea (usually with dark blood present), progressive weight loss, and dehydration. The prominent functional disturbances appear to result from multiple ulcerations of the GI mucosa that develop from gastrin hypersecretion.

Lesions: Animals studied with the Zollinger-Ellison-like syndrome have had single or multiple tumors of varying size in the pancreas. The tumors were firm on palpation because of an increase of fibrous connective tissue in the stroma, and all had evidence of metastasis before diagnosis.

Diagnosis: Serum gastrin levels have been evaluated in a limited number of dogs with gastrinomas. Gastrin levels in a dog with a Zollinger-Ellison–like syndrome varied from 155 to 2,780 pg/mL, whereas the mean serum gastrin in clinically normal (control) dogs was 70.9 pg/mL. Recurrent gastric or duodenal ulcers in dogs with no identified cause warrants exploratory surgery and careful inspection of the pancreas.

Treatment: Excision of the gastrin-secreting mass in the pancreas can be attempted. However, all such tumors that have been studied in dogs have had evidence of local invasion into adjacent parenchyma and had metastasized to regional lymph nodes and liver. The dogs had either single or multiple ulcerations in the gastric or duodenal mucosa associated with free blood in the lumen. Medical management with H_2-receptor antagonists (famotidine or ranitidine) or the proton-pump inhibitor omeprazole may temporarily alleviate clinical signs in animals with inoperable disease.

GENERALIZED CONDITIONS

MORE THAN ONE SPECIES

HORSES

PIGS

RUMINANTS

SMALL ANIMALS

ACTINOBACILLOSIS

Actinobacillosis refers to a group of diseases caused by gram-negative coccobacilli in the genus *Actinobacillus*. Although there are >22 different bacterial species in this genus, only four (*A pleuropneumoniae*, *A suis*, *A equuli*, and *A lignieresii*) are frequently associated with disease in animals.

A pleuropneumoniae causes contagious pleuropneumonia in pigs (*see* p 1469). Disease ranges from acute, severe fibrinous pleuropneumonia to subacute or chronic infection with pleuritis and pulmonary abscessation. Immune complexes formed as a result of host response may damage endothelial cells, resulting in vasculitis and thrombosis, with edema, necrosis, infarction, and hemorrhage. Infection is usually restricted to pigs <5 mo old. *A pleuropneumoniae* may be normal mucosal flora in pigs, cattle, and sheep. Diagnosis is by culture of the organism from nasal swabs or lung tissue at necropsy. Molecular techniques such as PCR have also been developed to detect the presence of *A pleuropneumoniae* in tissue samples. Treatment involves use of antibiotics, including penicillin, tetracycline, spectinomycin, cephalosporins, or fluoroquinolones. Control focuses on good management combined with the use of vaccines or eradication of the infection from the herd by depopulation.

A suis is part of the normal flora of the oral cavity of pigs. It causes septicemia in young pigs and arthritis, pneumonia, and pericarditis in older pigs. It may also cause septicemia, arthritis, pneumonia, and purulent nephritis in neonatal and postnatal foals. Disease follows a break in the integrity of the oral mucosa or may be associated with immunosuppression. The organism is typically susceptible to sulfonamides and cephalosporins.

The natural host of *A equuli* is the horse, and infections are seen in both foals and adult horses. Disease in foals may manifest as diarrhea, followed by meningitis, pneumonia, purulent nephritis, or septic polyarthritis (sleepy foal disease or joint-ill). Infection may be acquired through a contaminated umbilicus or by inhalation or ingestion. The incidence of foal infection is reduced with greater attention to sanitation in the foaling environment, and maternal antibodies in colostrum are often protective. Abortions, septicemia, nephritis, peritonitis, and endocarditis may result from *A equuli* infection in adult horses. A syndrome of acute peritonitis in adult horses associated with *A equuli* has been described in Australia as well as sporadically in other parts of the world. *A equuli* isolates have also been recovered from fetuses of mares affected with mare reproductive loss syndrome; however, it is not clear whether the bacteria is directly associated with the pregnancy loss. In both foals and adult horses, several other bacteria can cause the same clinical disease syndromes as *A equuli*. Therefore, definitive diagnosis of *A equuli* relies on isolating the bacteria by culture. Infected horses may be treated with chloramphenicol, gentamicin, or third-generation cephalosporins, depending on the nature of the Infection and the ability to achieve therapeutic concentrations at the site of infection. β-Lactam antibiotics and potentiated sulfonamides have been recommended; however, resistance to both of these types of antibiotics is occasionally reported.

A arthritidis, previously classified as Bisgaard taxon 9, has been isolated from horses with arthritis and septicemia.

A lignieresii causes tumorous abscesses of the tongue, usually referred to as wooden tongue. It is seen primarily in cattle but also

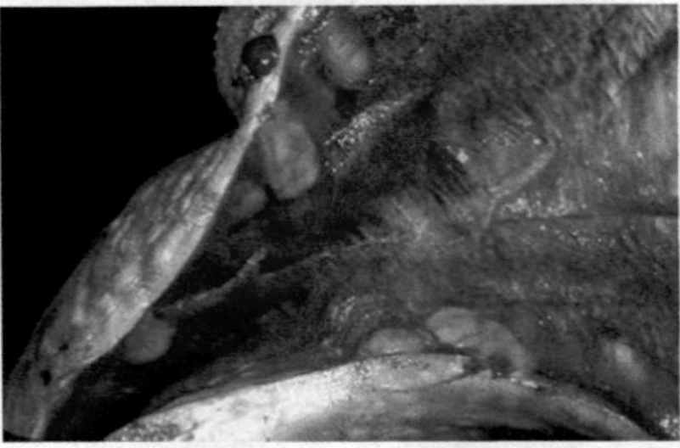

Actinobacillosis in a cow. Note the characteristic large granulomas in the substance of the tongue. *Courtesy of Dr. John Prescott.*

in sheep, horses, pigs, and dogs. It is a rare cause of disease in chickens. The organism may also cause pyogranulomatous lesions in soft tissues associated with the head, neck, limbs, and occasionally the lungs, pleura, udder, and subcutaneous tissue. *A lignieresii* is part of the normal mucosal flora of the upper GI tract and causes disease when it gains access to adjacent soft tissue via penetrating wounds. It causes localized infections and can spread via the lymphatics to other tissues. The primary lesion associated with *A lignieresii* infection in cattle is a very hard, diffusely swollen, painful tongue. This leads to excessive salivation, the inability to prehend food normally, and sometimes a visibly enlarged tongue that protrudes from the mouth. On palpation, the tongue will feel very hard. Diagnosis requires culture and biopsy of the lesion. Pus from an abscess crushed between two glass slides may show club-like spicules of calcium phosphate, giving the appearance of sulfur granules <1 mm diameter. No reliable serologic tests are available for actinobacillosis, and the hematologic and clinical chemistry findings are generally normal. Gross pathology generally reveals a firm, pale tongue containing multifocal nodules. These nodules are often filled with thick yellow-white pus. Histologically, the primary lesion is a granulomatous abscess.

This form of actinobacillosis is found worldwide but is sporadic and thus difficult to prevent. Herd outbreaks are possible and are generally associated with consumption of coarse, abrasive feeds that encourage formation of lesions in the mouth. Sodium iodide is the treatment of choice in actinobacillosis in ruminants. IV sodium iodide (70 mg/kg of a 10%–20% solution) is given once and then repeated once or twice at 7- to 10-day intervals. If clinical signs of iodine toxicity develop (including dandruff, diarrhea, anorexia, coughing, and excessive lacrimation), iodine administration should be discontinued. Clinical improvement is often seen within 48 hr of therapy, and treatment is usually successful when only the tongue is involved. Systemic antibacterial agents, such as ceftiofur, penicillin, ampicillin, florfenicol, and tetracyclines may be effective and are primarily recommended in severe cases of actinobacillosis or in cases refractory to sodium iodide therapy. Surgical debulking of lesions, especially if they interfere with breathing, may be useful. This is particularly true when large granulomatous masses that do not respond to medical therapy are present. Prevention of actinobacillosis in ruminants primarily relies on avoidance of coarse, stemmy feedstuffs and pastures full of hard, penetrating plant awns (ie, foxtails or thistles).

A ureae has caused upper respiratory tract infections in people and abortions in pigs. In addition, *A actinoides* has occasionally been associated with suppurative pneumonia in calves and seminal vesiculitis in bulls.

ACTINOMYCOSIS

Members of the genus *Actinomyces* are gram-positive, anaerobic, non-acid-fast rods, many of which are filamentous or branching. Branches are <1 μm in diameter, as opposed to fungal filaments, which are >1 μm in diameter. Although they are normal flora of the oral and nasopharyngeal membranes, several species are associated with diseases in animals.

A bovis is the etiologic agent of lumpy jaw in cattle. It has also been isolated from nodular abscesses in the lungs of cattle and infrequently from infections in sheep, pigs, dogs, and other mammals, including chronic fistulous withers and chronic poll evil in horses. Lumpy jaw is a localized, chronic, progressive, granulomatous abscess that most frequently involves the mandible, the maxillae, or other bony tissues in the head. Disease is seen when *A bovis* is introduced to underlying soft tissue via penetrating wounds of the oral mucosa from wire or coarse hay or sticks. Involvement of adjacent bone frequently results in facial distortion, loose teeth (making chewing difficult), and dyspnea from swelling into the nasal cavity. Any part of the head can be affected; however, the alveoli around the roots of the cheek teeth are frequently involved. The primary lesion appears as a slow-growing, firm mass that is attached to or part of the mandible. Ulceration forms in some cases, with or without fistulous tracts, and drainage of purulent exudate may occur. Presumptive diagnosis is often based on clinical signs. The diagnosis can be confirmed by culture of the organism from the lesion; however, this requires anaerobic conditions and is frequently negative. A Gram stain of purulent material will reveal gram-positive, club-shaped rods and filaments (sulfur granules). Radiology of the head is also useful; the primary radiographic lesion consists of multiple, centrally radiolucent areas of osteomyelitis surrounded by periosteal new bone and fibrous tissue. As a last resort, a biopsy sample can be taken with a trephine and submitted for histopathology.

The goal of treatment is to kill the bacteria and stop the spread of the lesion. However, the hard mass will usually not regress significantly. Sodium iodide is the treatment of choice in ruminant actinomycosis. Sodium iodide (70 mg/kg of a 10%–20% solution, IV) is given once and repeated several times at 7- to 10-day intervals. If signs of iodine toxicity develop (eg, dandruff, diarrhea, anorexia, coughing, and excessive lacrimation), iodine administration should be discontinued or treatments given at longer intervals. Sodium iodide has been shown to be safe for use in pregnant cows and presents little risk of causing abortion. Concurrent administration of antimicrobials, including penicillin, florfenicol, or oxytetracycline, is recommended. Surgery to debride large mandibular lesions has also been described in conjunction with iodine and antimicrobial therapy. Because *A bovis* is part of the normal oral flora in ruminants, control focuses on avoiding coarse, stemmy feeds or feeds with plant awns that might damage the mucosal epithelium. When multiple cases are seen in a herd, it is not from the contagious nature of the pathogen but the widespread exposure to a risk factor (eg, coarse feed).

A actinoides is occasionally found as a secondary invader in enzootic pneumonia of calves and seminal vasculitis in bulls.

A israelii is primarily associated with chronic granulomatous infections in people but has also been isolated rarely from pyogranulomatous lesions in pigs and cattle. Treatment involves surgical debridement and administration of penicillin.

A naeslundii has been isolated from suppurative infections in several animal species, the most common being aborted porcine fetuses.

A suis causes pyogranulomatous porcine mastitis, characterized by small abscesses containing thick, yellow pus surrounded by a wide zone of dense connective tissue. Yellow "sulfur granules" may be scattered throughout the pus, as in *A bovis* in cattle. Chronic, deep-seated abscesses may fistulate. Sows may also develop ventral subcutaneous granulomatous lesions, and occasional pyogranulomatous infections develop in lungs, spleen, kidneys, and other organs. Diagnosis is based on clinical signs and on isolation and identification of the etiologic agent. Treatment is rarely successful, primarily due to the inability of an antibacterial agent to penetrate the infected tissue. Infected tissue may be surgically removed to salvage sows for slaughter.

A hordeovulneris is a rare cause of canine actinomycosis, which can present with either localized abscesses or systemic infections such as pyogranulomatous pleuritis, peritonitis, visceral abscesses, or septic arthritis. A common predisposing factor is the presence of tissue-migrating foxtail grass (*Hordeum* spp) particles, and the primary route of infection appears to be via inhalation of the bacteria. History and clinical signs may contribute to the diagnosis, but demonstration of the causative agent by Gram stain and bacteriologic culture is necessary for confirmation. Treatment includes surgical debridement and/or longterm treatment with penicillin, cephalosporins, or sulfonamides. Pyothorax is frequently seen in canine actinomycosis and requires repeated drainage of the chest in addition to antimicrobial therapy.

A viscosus causes cutaneous actinomycosis in dogs, which appears as localized subcutaneous abscesses. These usually occur secondary to perforating injuries caused by bite wounds or foreign bodies. The most common sites for abscesses are the head, neck, thorax, and abdomen. *A viscosus* can also cause pneumonia, pyothorax, and rarely pyogranulomatous meningoencephalitis. Diagnosis may be based on history and clinical signs, including the presence of soft, grayish white granules in the pus or exudate. Cytology (of pus or pleural fluid) is useful and will reveal gram-positive, filamentous organisms. Definitive diagnosis is based on isolation and identification of *A viscosus*. Treatment of pyothorax with penicillin, sulfonamides, or cephalosporins may be successful if begun early in the clinical course. A successful outcome is more likely with cutaneous infections, which should also be treated with the same antimicrobials.

AMYLOIDOSES

The amyloidoses are diseases that result from errors in protein folding. When new proteins are made, their peptide chains normally fold into the correct shape. Sometimes, however, the peptide chains fold incorrectly and form highly stable β-sheets that are insoluble and resistant to proteolytic digestion. When this insoluble protein is deposited in tissues, it is called amyloid. Amyloid proteins may be deposited in a localized fashion or widely distributed throughout the body. They cause damage by displacing normal cells. If critical organs such as the kidneys, liver, or heart are extensively disrupted, the disease may be fatal. Amyloidosis can affect all domestic mammals, and minor, asymptomatic deposition of amyloid proteins is common in aged animals.

The most common form of amyloid is generated by misfolding of the major acute-phase protein, serum amyloid A (SAA). Levels of SAA in the blood climb significantly in animals with severe inflammation. If SAA fails to fold correctly, it forms a very stable protein called AA amyloid. Amyloidosis thus develops as a result of chronic inflammatory diseases, chronic bacterial infections, and malignant tumors. It is a common cause of death in horses aggressively immunized for antiserum production. AA amyloid is usually deposited in parenchymal organs, such as the spleen, where it may not cause clinical signs. If the kidneys are involved, the presence of amyloid in glomeruli may lead to severe proteinuria, eventually resulting in renal failure and death. There is no practical treatment for this form of amyloidosis, although removal of the source of inflammation may slow amyloid deposition and hence progression of the disease.

Misfolding of immunoglobulin light chains generates a second form of amyloid, AL amyloid. This commonly results from the overproduction of monoclonal light chains in animals with plasma cell tumors (myelomas). AL amyloid tends to be deposited in mesenchymal tissues, especially nervous tissues and joints. It is rare in domestic animals.

At least 20 other proteins have been shown to misfold, form β-sheets, and become deposited in the tissues as amyloid. There are also hereditary amyloidoses, such as those described in Abyssinian cats and Chinese Shar-Pei dogs, in which mutations result in protein misfolding. Some amyloid is formed in all aged animals (senile systemic amyloidosis); eg, in aged dogs, amyloid is commonly deposited in the media of meningeal and cortical arteries. Tumor-like amyloid nodules and subcutaneous amyloid have been reported in horses.

Some forms of amyloid may be transmitted between animals. The most important of these are the transmissible spongiform encephalopathies, such as bovine spongiform encephalopathy (*see* p 1284) and scrapie (*see* p 1288). These are caused by the production of misfolded prion proteins. Indeed, even AA amyloid is somewhat transmissible, because experimental administration of small amounts of amyloid protein to an animal can accelerate its development. Cheetahs are especially prone to amyloidosis and shed an infectious form of amyloid protein in their feces.

Because of its diffuse distribution and insidious onset, amyloidosis is difficult to diagnose clinically. However, amyloidosis should be suspected if progressive renal or hepatic failure develops in animals subsequent to chronic infections or inflammation. There is no specific therapy that can prevent the development of amyloidosis or promote the resorption of fibrils. Animals with persistent inflammation should be treated to reduce the severity of their inflammatory response and hence the availability of SAA. Amyloidosis is readily recognized at necropsy and in histologic sections by its affinity for dyes such as Congo red.

ANTHRAX

(Splenic fever, Siberian ulcer, Charbon, Milzbrand)

Anthrax is a zoonotic disease caused by the sporeforming bacterium *Bacillus anthracis*. Anthrax is most common in wild and domestic herbivores (eg, cattle, sheep, goats, camels, antelopes) but can also be seen in people exposed to tissue from infected animals, to contaminated animal products, or directly to *B anthracis* spores under certain conditions. Depending on the route of infection, host factors, and potentially strain-specific factors, anthrax can have several different clinical presentations. In herbivores, anthrax commonly presents as an acute septicemia with a high fatality rate, often accompanied by hemorrhagic lymphadenitis. In dogs, people, horses, and pigs, it is usually less acute although still potentially fatal.

B anthracis spores can remain viable in soil for many years. During this time, they are a potential source of infection for grazing livestock but generally do not represent a direct risk of infection for people. Grazing animals may become infected when they ingest sufficient quantities of these spores from the soil. In addition to direct transmission, biting flies may mechanically transmit *B anthracis* spores from one animal to another. The latter follows when there have been rains encouraging a high fly hatch and reporting has been delayed on the index ranch, such that there are 4–6 moribund or dead cattle for the flies to feed on. Feed contaminated with bone or other meal from infected animals can serve as a source of infection for livestock, as can hay muddy with contaminated soil. Raw or poorly cooked contaminated meat is a source of infection for zoo carnivores and omnivores; anthrax resulting from contaminated meat consumption has been reported in pigs, dogs, cats, mink, wild carnivores, and people.

Epidemiology: Underdiagnosis and unreliable reporting make it difficult to estimate the true incidence of anthrax worldwide. However, anthrax has been reported from nearly every continent and is most common in agricultural regions with neutral or alkaline, calcareous soils. In these regions, anthrax periodically emerges as epizootics among susceptible domesticated and wild animals. These epizootics are usually associated with drought, flooding, or soil disturbance, and many years may pass between outbreaks. During interepidemic periods, sporadic cases may help maintain soil contamination. But it is now absent from some countries in western Europe, north Africa, and east of the Mississippi in the USA.

Human cases may follow contact with contaminated carcasses or animal products. The risk of human disease in these settings is comparatively small in developed countries, partly because people are relatively resistant to infection. However, in developing countries, each affected cow can result in up to 10 human cases because of home slaughter and sanitation issues. In cases of natural transmission, people exhibit primarily cutaneous disease (>95% of all cases). GI anthrax (including pharyngeal anthrax) may be seen among human populations after consumption of contaminated raw or undercooked meat. Under certain artificial conditions (eg, laboratories, animal hair processing facilities, exposure to weaponized spore products), people may develop a highly fatal form of disease known as inhalational anthrax or woolsorter's disease. Inhalational anthrax is an acute hemorrhagic lymphadenitis of the mediastinal lymph nodes, often accompanied by hemorrhagic pleural effusions, severe septicemia, meningitis, and a high mortality rate. Of late, injection anthrax has emerged in conjunction with contaminated heroin.

The precise incidence of anthrax among animals in the USA is unknown. Throughout the past hundred years, animal infections have been seen in nearly all states, with highest frequency from the Midwest and West. Presently, anthrax is enzootic in west Texas and northwest Minnesota; sporadic in south Texas, Montana, eastern North and South Dakota; and only occasionally seen elsewhere. The annual incidence of human anthrax in the USA has declined from ~130 cases annually in the beginning of the last century to no reported cases in 2004–2005.

In addition to causing naturally occurring anthrax, *B anthracis* has been manufactured as a biologic warfare agent. *B anthracis* was used successfully as a weapon of terrorism in 2001, killing 5 people and causing disease in 22. Probably because of the method of delivery (via mail), no known animal disease resulted from this attack. Weaponized spores represent a threat to both human and animal populations. The World Health Organization has estimated that 50 kg of *B anthracis* released upwind of a population center of 500,000 could result in 95,000 deaths and 125,000 hospitalizations. The effect on animal populations has not been estimated, but because livestock are more susceptible to *B anthracis* infection than primates, the outcome of an aerosol attack with *B anthracis* spores against livestock would result in higher and earlier mortality and morbidity rates than among a human population. Subsequent to the 1979 Severdlovsk incident, human cases were seen up to 4 km from the source, but dead sheep were noted 64 km downwind, and in villages between.

Pathogenesis: After wound inoculation, ingestion, or inhalation, spores infect macrophages, germinate, and proliferate. In cutaneous and GI infection, proliferation can occur at the site of infection and in the lymph nodes draining the site of infection. Lethal toxin and edema toxin are produced by *B anthracis* and respectively cause local necrosis and extensive edema, which are frequent characteristics of the disease. As the bacteria multiply in the lymph nodes, toxemia progresses and bacteremia may ensue. With the increase in toxin production, the potential for disseminated tissue destruction and organ failure increases. After vegetative bacilli are discharged from an animal after death (by carcass bloating, scavengers, or postmortem examination), the oxygen content of air induces sporulation. Spores are relatively resistant to extremes of temperature, chemical disinfection, and dessication. Necropsy is discouraged because of the potential for blood spillage and vegetative cells to be exposed to air, resulting in large numbers of spores being produced. Because of the rapid pH change after death and decomposition, vegetative cells in an unopened carcass quickly die without sporulating.

Clinical Findings: Typically, the incubation period is 3–7 days (range 1–14 days). The clinical course ranges from peracute to chronic. The peracute form (common in cattle and sheep) is characterized by sudden onset and a rapidly fatal course. Staggering, dyspnea, trembling, collapse, a few convulsive movements, and death may occur in cattle, sheep, or goats with only a brief evidence of illness.

In acute anthrax of cattle and sheep, there is an abrupt fever and a period of excitement followed by depression, stupor, respiratory or cardiac distress, staggering, convulsions, and death. Often, the course of disease is so rapid that illness is not observed and animals are found dead. Body temperature may reach 107°F (41.5°C), rumination ceases, milk production is materially reduced, and pregnant animals may abort. There may be bloody discharges from the natural body openings. Some infections are characterized by localized, subcutaneous, edematous swelling that can be quite extensive. Areas most frequently involved are the ventral neck, thorax, and shoulders.

The disease in horses may be acute. Signs may include fever, chills, severe colic, anorexia, depression, weakness, bloody diarrhea, and swellings of the neck, sternum, lower abdomen, and external genitalia. Death usually occurs within 2–3 days of onset.

Although relatively resistant, pigs may develop an acute septicemia after ingestion of *B anthracis*, characterized by sudden death, oropharyngitis, or more usually a mild chronic form. Oropharyngeal anthrax is characterized by rapidly progressive swelling of the throat, which may cause death by suffocation. In the chronic form, pigs show systemic signs of illness and gradually recover with treatment. Some later show evidence of anthrax infection in the cervical lymph nodes and tonsils when slaughtered (as apparently healthy animals). Intestinal involvement is seldom recognized and has nonspecific clinical characteristics of anorexia, vomiting, diarrhea (sometimes bloody), or constipation.

In dogs, cats, and wild carnivores, the disease resembles that seen in pigs. In wild herbivorous animals, the expected course of illness and lesions varies by species but resembles, for the most part, anthrax in cattle.

Lesions: Rigor mortis is frequently absent or incomplete. Dark blood may ooze from the mouth, nostrils, and anus with marked bloating and rapid body decomposition. If the carcass is inadvertently opened, septicemic lesions are seen. The blood is dark and thickened and fails to clot readily. Hemorrhages of various sizes are common on the serosal surfaces of the abdomen and thorax as well as on the epicardium and endocardium. Edematous, red-tinged effusions commonly are present under the serosa of various organs, between skeletal muscle groups, and in the subcutis.

Hemorrhages frequently occur along the GI tract mucosa, and ulcers, particularly over Peyer's patches, may be present. An enlarged, dark red or black, soft, semifluid spleen is common. The liver, kidneys, and lymph nodes usually are congested and enlarged. Meningitis may be found if the skull is opened.

In pigs with chronic anthrax, the lesions usually are restricted to the tonsils, cervical lymph nodes, and surrounding tissues. The lymphatic tissues of the area are enlarged and are a mottled salmon to brick-red color on cut surface. Diphtheritic membranes or ulcers may be present over the surface of the tonsils. The area around involved lymphatic tissues generally is gelatinous and edematous. A chronic intestinal form involving the mesenteric lymph nodes is also recognized.

Diagnosis: A diagnosis based on clinical signs alone is difficult. Confirmatory laboratory examination should be attempted if anthrax is suspected. Because the vegetative cell is not robust and will not survive 3 days in transit, the optimal sample is a cotton swab dipped in the blood and allowed to dry. This results in sporulation and the death of other bacteria and contaminants. For carcasses dead >3 days, either the nasal turbinates should be swabbed or turbinate samples removed. Pigs with localized disease are rarely bacteremic, so a small piece of affected lymphatic tissue that has been collected aseptically should be submitted. Before submission, the receiving reference laboratory should be contacted regarding appropriate specimen labelling, handling, and shipping procedures.

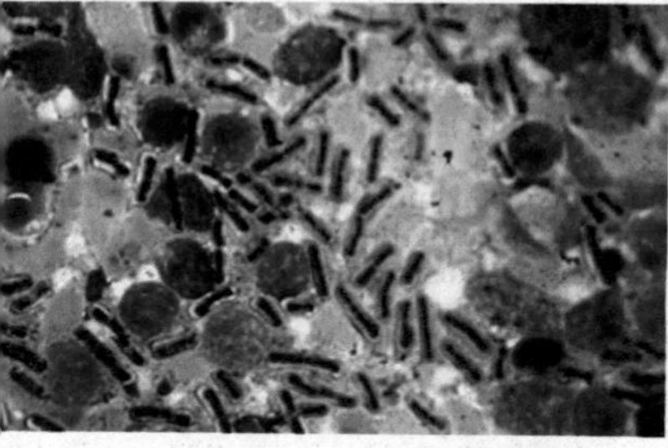

Bacillus anthracis, methylene blue stain of tissue smear, high power. Note the intense red stain of the large capsule of this organism. *Courtesy of the Department of Pathobiology, University of Guelph.*

Specific diagnostic tests include bacterial culture, PCR tests, and fluorescent antibody stains to demonstrate the agent in blood films or tissues. Western blot and ELISA tests for antibody detection are available in some reference laboratories. Lacking other tests, fixed blood smears stained with Loeffler's or MacFadean stains can be used and the capsule visualized; however, this can result in ~20% false positives.

In livestock, anthrax must be differentiated from other conditions that cause sudden death. In cattle and sheep, clostridial infections, bloat, and lightning strike (or any cause of sudden death) may be confused with anthrax. Also, acute leptospirosis, bacillary hemoglobinuria, anaplasmosis, and acute poisonings by bracken fern, sweet clover, and lead must be considered in cattle. In horses, acute infectious anemia, purpura, colic, lead poisoning, lightning strike, and sunstroke may resemble anthrax. In pigs, acute classical swine fever, African swine fever, and pharyngeal malignant edema are diagnostic considerations. In dogs, acute systemic infections and pharyngeal swellings due to other causes must be considered.

Treatment, Control, and Prevention: Anthrax is controlled through vaccination programs, rapid detection and reporting, quarantine, treatment of asymptomatic animals (postexposure prophylaxis), and burning or burial of suspect and confirmed cases. In livestock, anthrax can be controlled largely by annual vaccination of all grazing animals in the endemic area and by implementation of control measures during epizootics. The nonencapsulated Sterne-strain vaccine is used almost universally for livestock immunization. Vaccination should be done at least 2–4 wk before the season when outbreaks may be expected. Because this is a live vaccine, antibiotics should not be administered within 1 wk of vaccination. Before vaccination of dairy cattle during an outbreak, all of the procedures required by local laws should be reviewed and followed. Human anthrax vaccines currently licensed and used in the USA and Europe are based on filtrates of artificially cultivated *B anthracis*.

Early treatment and vigorous implementation of a preventive program are essential to reduce losses among livestock. Livestock at risk should be immediately treated with a long-acting antibiotic to stop all potential incubating infections. This is followed by vaccination ~7–10 days after antibiotic treatment. Any animals becoming sick after initial treatment and/or vaccination should be retreated immediately and revaccinated a month later. Simultaneous use of antibiotics and vaccine is inappropriate, because available commercial vaccines for animals in the USA are live vaccines. Animals should be moved to another pasture away from where the bodies had lain and any possible soil contamination. Suspected contaminated feed should be immediately removed. Domestic livestock respond well to penicillin if treated in the early stages of the disease. Oxytetracycline given daily in divided doses also is effective. Other antibacterials, including amoxicillin, chloramphenicol, ciprofloxacin, doxycycline, erythromycin, gentamicin, streptomycin, and sulfonamides also can be used, but their effectiveness in comparison with penicillin and the tetracyclines has not been evaluated under field conditions.

In addition to therapy and immunization, specific control procedures are necessary to contain the disease and prevent its spread. These include the following: 1) notification of the appropriate regulatory officials; 2) rigid enforcement of quarantine (after vaccination, 2 wk before movement off the farm, 6 wk if going to slaughter); 3) prompt disposal of dead animals, manure, bedding, or other contaminated material by cremation (preferable) or deep burial; 4) isolation of sick animals and removal of well animals from the contaminated areas; 5) cleaning and disinfection of stables, pens, milking barns, and equipment used on livestock; 6) use of insect repellents; 7) control of scavengers that feed on animals dead from the disease; and 8) observation of general sanitary procedures by people who handle diseased animals, both for their own safety and to prevent spread of disease. Contaminated soils are very difficult to completely decontaminate, but formaldehyde will be successful if the level is not excessive. The process generally requires removal of soil.

Human infection is controlled through reducing infection in livestock, veterinary supervision of animal production and slaughter to reduce human contact with potentially infected livestock or animal products, and in some settings either pre- or postexposure prophylaxis. In countries where anthrax is common and vaccination coverage in livestock is low, people should avoid contact with livestock and animal products that were not inspected before and after slaughter. In general, consumption of meat from animals that have exhibited sudden death, meat obtained via emergency slaughter, and meat of uncertain origin should be avoided. Routine vaccination against anthrax is indicated for individuals engaged in work involving large quantities or concentrations of *B anthracis* cultures or activities with a high potential for aerosol production. Laboratory workers using standard Biosafety Level 2 practices in the routine processing of clinical samples are not at increased risk of exposure to *B anthracis* spores. The risk for workers who come into contact with imported animal hides, furs, bone meal, wool, animal hair, or bristles has been reduced by improvements in industry standards and import restrictions. Routine preexposure vaccination is recommended for people in this group only when these standards and restrictions are insufficient to prevent exposure to anthrax spores. Routine vaccination of veterinarians in the USA is not recommended because of the low incidence of animal cases. However, vaccination may be indicated for veterinarians and other high-risk individuals handling potentially infected animals in areas where there is a high incidence of anthrax cases.

The CDC has recommended that those at risk of repeated exposure to *B anthracis* spores in response to a bioterrorism attack should be vaccinated. Those groups include some emergency first responders, federal responders, and laboratory workers. Vaccination in anticipation of a terrorist attack is not recommended for other populations.

For people, postexposure prophylaxis against *B anthracis* is recommended after an aerosol exposure to *B anthracis* spores. Prophylaxis may consist of antibiotic therapy alone or the combination of antibiotic therapy and vaccination, if vaccine is available (most human vaccines are not live). Although there is no approved regimen, the CDC has suggested that antibiotics may be discontinued after three doses of vaccine have been administered according to the standard schedule (0, 2, and 4 wk). Because of availability and ease of dosing, doxycycline or ciprofloxacin may be chosen initially for antibiotic chemoprophylaxis until the susceptibility of the infecting organism is determined. Penicillin and doxycycline are approved by the FDA for treatment of anthrax in people and have traditionally been considered the drugs of choice. Both ciprofloxacin and ofloxacin have demonstrated in vitro activity against *B anthracis*. Although naturally occurring *B anthracis* resistance to penicillin is infrequent, it is reported; resistance to other antibiotics has been noted. Antibiotics are effective against the germinated form of *B anthracis* but are not effective against the spore form of the organism. Spores may survive in the mediastinal lymph nodes in the lungs for months without germination in nonhuman primates.

There are currently no approved vaccination regimens for postexposure prophylaxis after *B anthracis* exposures. Although postexposure chemoprophylaxis using antibiotics alone has been effective in animal models, the definitive length of treatment remains unclear. Antibiotic chemoprophylaxis may be switched to penicillin VK or amoxicillin in children or pregnant women once antibiotic susceptibilities are known and the organism is found to be susceptible to penicillin. The safety and efficacy of anthrax vaccine in children or pregnant women has not been studied; therefore, a recommendation for use of vaccine in these groups cannot be made. Although the shortened vaccine regimen has been effective when used in a postexposure regimen that includes antibiotics, the duration of protection from vaccination is not known. The existing evidence suggests that vaccine protection is adequate for 12 mo. If subsequent exposures occur, additional vaccinations may be required.

There are no definitive recommendations for postexposure prophylaxis after cutaneous or GI exposures of people to *B anthracis*. Based on the slow progression of disease, low fatality rate, and ease of antibiotic treatment of cutaneous anthrax, and the general low risk of cutaneous disease after natural exposure, postexposure prophylaxis is not recommended after direct cutaneous exposure to contaminated animals or animal products. However, immediate washing of the exposed areas is advised. Those exposed should be advised of the signs of cutaneous anthrax (ie, an inflamed but painless area with or without circumferential small vesicles, enlargement of the regional lymph nodes) and should seek medical assistance if illness develops. Because of the high fatality rate and rapid progression of GI anthrax, serious consideration should be given to initiating postexposure antibiotic prophylaxis for those who consume contaminated undercooked or raw meat. There is no current indication for vaccination after either cutaneous exposure or ingestion.

BESNOITIOSIS

Besnoitiosis (originally named globidiosis) is a cyst-forming, usually nonfatal disease caused by a number of different species of the apicomplexan protozoa *Besnoitia*. Lesions are commonly seen in the dermis and in mucous and serous membranes, as well as in other tissues. These *Besnoitia* species tend to be confined to specific animal hosts that include large and small mammals, as well as reptiles.

Etiology and Transmission: The most significant condition in domestic animals is that of cattle, in which *B besnoiti* causes economic loss through reduced milk production, infertility and sterility, skin lesions, and increased mortality; similar effects are likely with *B caprae* in goats in Africa, southern Europe, and New Zealand. Recent studies indicate that infection is being detected more commonly in cattle in Europe (ie, Spain, Portugal, Italy, Germany, Switzerland, Hungary, and Greece). *B bennetti* has been reported to be present in donkeys in Africa, southern France, Mexico, and in a number of locations in the USA. *B bennetti* is also found in horses, especially, but not only, those living in the tropics. *B jellisoni* and *B wallacei* have been described from rodents; *B tarandi* from reindeer or caribou; *B darlingi* from lizards, opossums, and snakes; and *B sauriana* from lizards. Viscerotropic strains of *B besnoiti* have been isolated from African antelopes; and serologic evidence of infection was detected in red and roe deer. Wildlife in Australia and blue duiker, impala, and blue wildebeest in Africa have been affected; to date it has not been reported in cattle in North America. A recent addition to these species and their hosts is *B oryctofelisi* in Argentinian rabbits.

It is thought that these parasites may have both definitive and intermediate hosts, and although the cat is often named as the likely candidate for the role of definitive host, this has not yet been clearly defined for most *Besnoitia* sp. Various animals, usually rodents or small mammals, such as woodrats and opossums, have been suggested as intermediate hosts.

These *Toxoplasma/Neospora*-like organisms multiply in endothelial, macrophage, and other cells and produce characteristic large, thick-walled cysts filled with bradyzoites. These, along with the oocyte stage in cats and the tachyzoite stage in other animals, are the infectious forms.

The true route(s) of transmission remains unclear despite many experimental and epidemiologic attempts. Experimental cyclic transmission with intestinal sexual stages in a definitive host—the cat—has been reported for *B besnoiti*, *B wallacei*, and *B darlingi*, and experimental transmission using genetically modified mice and tissue culture has been achieved with *B oryctofelisi*. Transmission of *B besnoiti* from cattle to cats has not been substantiated by subsequent studies. The suggestion that biting insects may transmit *B besnoiti* mechanically remains a possibility but has not been substantiated; *Besnoitia* spp can be transmitted artificially to suitable hosts by needle inoculation of tissues that contain cysts. Water or feed contaminated by infected cat feces are other possible routes of transmission.

Clinical Findings: Infected cattle often show no clinical signs other than a few cysts in the scleral conjunctiva or a localized, scaly, papular dermal change. Illness begins with fever followed by warm, painful swellings ventrally (anasarca). Swollen lymph nodes, diarrhea, anorexia, photophobia, rhinitis, and orchitis also are seen. Anasarca gives way to sclerodermatitis. The skin becomes hard, thick, and wrinkled and develops cracks that allow secondary bacterial infection and myiasis to develop; movement is painful. There is loss of hair and epidermis. In addition to the skin lesions, there may be focal, disseminated myositis, keratitis, periostitis, endostitis, lymphadenitis, pneumonia, periorchitis, orchitis, epididymitis, arteritis, and perineuritis. Severely affected animals become emaciated. Although mortality is low, convalescence is slow in severe cases. Severely affected bulls can become permanently sterile. Affected animals remain carriers for life. The disease in goats is similar to that in cattle. In horses, the clinical signs are similar but tend to be less severe or invasive. Infected donkeys, which are most commonly young (<2 yr old), also present with similar signs and symptoms, which are often more severe than those seen in horses.

The appearance of cysts in the scleral conjunctiva and nasal mucosa are useful diagnostic indicators. Parasitologic diagnosis is made by finding the crescent-shaped bradyzoites in biopsies or skin/conjunctival scrapings.

Prevention and Treatment: *B besnoiti* infections are economically important to cattle owners in endemic areas because of mortality (although usually <10%), sterility (which may be temporary or permanent), loss of condition, lower market value, and damage to the hide.

Although the route of transmission remains unclear, cattle are usually isolated and protected from biting insects and ticks to reduce transmission, and then treated symptomatically. In some countries, cattle are immunized with a live, tissue culture–adapted vaccine. Chemotherapy remains very limited and only minimally effective. Both antimony and sulfanilamide complex prevented cyst development by *B besnoiti* in rabbits, and oxytetracycline may have some therapeutic value if given early in the disease course. Clindamycin has been used to treat cats, but this has no positive effect on the stages present in other animals. Ponazuril has been found to be generally ineffective in infected donkeys.

CHLAMYDIOSIS

Bacteria of the order Chlamydiales are ubiquitous, obligate intracellular gram-negative bacteria. Within the host cell, they replicate via a unique developmental cycle competing with the host for intracellular nutrient pools. Virtually any chlamydial organism can infect any eukaryotic host cell, resulting in various infections.

Chlamydial taxonomy with two genera, *Chlamydia* and *Chlamydophila*, was proposed in 1999 but is no longer valid. A single genus, *Chlamydia*, is now used, as well as nine species (*abortus*, *caviae*, *felis*, *muridarum*, *pecorum*, *pneumoniae*, *psittaci*, *suis*, and *trachomatis*). Genome comparison revealed a high level of sequence conservation and synteny across taxa with the major exception of the human pathogen *C trachomatis*. Two additional new species have been discovered recently, ie, *C avium* and *C gallinacea*.

Etiology and Epidemiology: Traditional classification of chlamydiae was based on host and/or disease association, without a high degree of consistency. Different efficiencies in infectivity and replication determine consistent, but not absolute, associations between chlamydial strain, host, and disease manifestation. The *Chlamydia* species known so far were traditionally attributed to their main hosts.

C abortus (formerly *C psittaci* serotype 1) is an agent causing primarily abortion in small ruminants, mainly sheep (ovine enzootic abortion, now ovine chlamydiosis; *see* p 1338) and goats (*see* p 1340). *C caviae* was found in guinea pigs and was related to ocular and urogenital infections. *C felis* is associated with acute or chronic conjunctivitis (*see* p 506), rhinitis, and bronchopneumonia in both stray and domestic cats. *C muridarum* was isolated from a mouse colony with pneumonia. Infections with *C pecorum* are ubiquitous in cattle herds with multiple organ manifestations (*see also* ABORTION IN LARGE ANIMALS, p 1332). *C pneumoniae* is a respiratory pathogen in people and is involved in community-acquired respiratory tract infections as well as exacerbations of chronic obstructive airway diseases. *C psittaci* is the causative agent of avian chlamydiosis (*see* p 2808), formerly called psittacosis or ornithosis in psittacine birds or poultry/fowl, respectively. In swine, *C suis* (former porcine serovar of *C trachomatis*) is the most prevalent chlamydial agent that might be involved in multiple infection sites of the body. *C trachomatis* causes a variety of diseases in people, such as trachoma, urogenital infection, and lymphogranuloma venereum. With respect to the two new species, *C avium* has already been identified as a pathogen in pigeons and in psittacines, whereas the role of *C gallinacea* in poultry has yet to be defined.

With the availability of molecular diagnostic tools, the presence of chlamydiae has been frequently noticed in clinically inconspicuous animals (pets and farm animals). Epidemiologic data indicate that chlamydial infections are disseminated worldwide, but the epidemiologic importance of these findings is still unknown.

Transmission and Zoonotic Risk: Recent studies indicate that host specificity of different species is not as clear as previously thought. Most members of the genus *Chlamydia* have shown to be transmissible among species, including people. Zoonotic transmission from animals to people is well known for *C psittaci*, *C abortus*, and *C felis*. Conversely, chlamydial species of people have been detected in numerous animal species.

Transmission of avian *C psittaci* strains to people may result in atypical pneumonia or even life-threatening acute illness (ie, psittacosis in people). Transmission between companion parrots and dogs or cats, respectively, has also been associated with clinical cases. Furthermore, *C psittaci* has been found in numerous other mammalian species (eg, cattle, swine, horses, small ruminants, rodents, wildlife). An association between *C psittaci* genotypes with host species has recently been detected, but the pathogenetic relevance as well as the zoonotic potential of non-avian *C psittaci* strains have yet to be defined.

C abortus may cause abortion and fetal death in pregnant women after transmission from goats or sheep. It has also been found in other animals (cattle, swine, wild suidae, horses, and birds). Zoonotic risks resulting from these hosts and the role of this pathogen in these hosts are unknown.

Natural transmission of *C felis* mostly occurs through close contact with other infected cats, their aerosol, and fomites, but the pathogen has also been found in dogs. With respect to people, there is clear evidence that *C felis* acquired from cats may occasionally cause keratoconjunctivitis. Reports are rare, attributing this pathogen to serious systemic disease or atypical pneumonia.

The known human pathogen *C pneumoniae* was detected in cats with conjunctivitis and also infects koalas, horses, and frogs. *C trachomatis*, the other human pathogen, was found in pigs and birds so far.

The risk of zoonotic transmission of other chlamydial species found in numerous animal species beside their main hosts, including the two new species *C avium* and *C gallinacea*, has yet to be defined.

Clinical Findings: Chlamydial infections do not present a typical clinical picture. In general, they affect multiple organs and can generate a variety of clinical manifestations, ranging from acute to chronic inflammation and from a severe to a mild or even subclinical course. Because aerosol transmission of the pathogen is one of the main infection routes, the respiratory system is often involved.

In birds, avian chlamydiosis is accompanied by conjunctivitis, serositis, fibrinopericarditis, hepato- or splenomegaly, anemia, and leukocytosis or monocytosis. Dogs infected by *C psittaci* (most likely transmitted from birds) present a clinical picture of bronchopneumonia that may include fever and dry cough, but also keratoconjunctivitis, GI signs (vomiting, diarrhea), and even neurologic signs. In cats, infections with *C felis* clinically result in rhinitis, conjunctivitis, and/or bronchopneumonia, but seropositive cats are often asymptomatic. Lambs delivered by ewes with *C abortus* infection may develop acute chlamydial pneumonia. They become febrile, lethargic, and dyspneic and develop a serous and later mucopurulent nasal discharge.

In cattle and pigs, chlamydial infections must be regarded as widespread but often underdiagnosed. Chlamydiae detected so far in cattle herds include mainly *C pecorum*, but also *C abortus*, *C psittaci*, and *C suis*. In pig herds, *C suis* dominates, but *C psittaci*, *C abortus*, *C perorum*, and even *C trachomatis* have been found in parallel. Mixed infections are common in herds and even in individual animals. Clinical pictures of bovine and porcine chlamydioses are highly variable, although most infections remain clinically inapparent. Current knowledge suggests these infections manifest clinically when they coincide with additional risk factors. In acute infection, clinical symptoms include fever and depression. Respiratory disorders may affect upper airways as well as the lower respiratory tract and result in pneumonia with the typical signs (nasal secretions, dry hacking cough, and dyspnea). In reproducing cows and sows, chlamydial infections might be associated with abortion, disorders in fertility, and mastitis. Other disease manifestations of acute chlamydiosis include enteritis and diarrhea, polyarthritis (*see* p 1065), keratoconjunctivitis, encephalomyelitis (*see* p 1308), pericarditis, or hepatitis. In chlamydia-positive herds, newborns are free of chlamydiae but start to acquire chlamydial infections within 2 wk of birth. Thus, young animals develop more clinical signs than older ones.

Equine chlamydiosis has been described as variable. Bronchopneumonia may be accompanied by abortions in mares, polyarthritis in foals, hepatitis, and fatal cases of encephalomyelitis. Recent data indicate a role of *C psittaci* and/or *C abortus* in equine recurrent airway obstruction as trigger factors of inflammation or indicators of severe disease.

Based on serologic data, most chlamydial infections in farm animals do not necessarily result in clinical illness. However, they may lead to chronic-persistent or recurrent chlamydial infections on a subclinical level. Because of the potential role of chlamydiae as bystanders, copathogens, or etiologic agents of latent persisting infections, clinically inapparent chlamydial infections are probably economically more important than rare outbreaks of severe chlamydial disease.

Lesions: Acute pulmonary lesions include bronchiolitis, severe focal pneumonia, and dystelectases. Dissemination of chlamydial bodies in lung tissue is usually accompanied by an influx of macrophages, granulocytes, and activated T cells. Pulmonary edema may occur. Disturbances in gas exchange and acid-base status (hypoxemia and/or respiratory acidosis) or even acute respiratory distress are attributed to multiple disorders in pulmonary functions.

Bronchointerstitial pneumonia and alveolitis may be accompanied by progression to type II pneumocyte hyperplasia and interstitial thickening due to ingress of mixed inflammatory cells. Lymphocytic aggregates are frequently seen around airways and pulmonary vessels.

In chronic (often subclinical) chlamydial infections, macroscopic examination of the respiratory tract reveals only mild lesions or a few foci of atelectasis, predominantly affecting the apical lobes. Histologic lesions may include neutrophil inflammation, follicular bronchiolitis, and active lymphoid tissues (tonsils, tracheobronchial and pulmonary lymph nodes, etc). Both activated bronchus-associated lymphoid tissue of bronchioles (bronchiolar cuffing) and hyperplastic bronchial and bronchiolar epithelium contribute to chronic small airway obstruction and persistent airflow limitation.

Diagnosis: Neither clinical signs nor lesions allow a definitive diagnosis of chlamydiosis. Detection of *Chlamydia* species is not part of routine veterinary bacteriologic diagnosis, and infections caused by these intracellular pathogens have long been underestimated because of the requirement for special laboratory facilities. Isolation of the pathogen strictly depends on cell culture techniques.

Confirmation of chlamydial infection requires collection of an appropriate clinical sample from the animal, followed by direct detection of the organism using a suitable diagnostic test. In vivo, swabs (nasal, ocular, rectal, vaginal), tracheal washing, or bronchoalveolar lavage fluid are useful. Chlamydial inclusion bodies may be detected in affected tissues. Appropriate tests include direct impression smears and cytologic staining, cell culture isolation of the agent, immunofluorescence tests, and nucleic acid amplification–based tests (PCR and microarray techniques).

Because most chlamydial infections do not elicit sufficiently high changes in antibody levels, serologic detection is generally more suitable for prevalence surveys than for the retrospective diagnosis of chlamydial infection. Species-specific serologic tests are still lacking. Most commercially available ELISA methods may detect infections caused by the family Chlamydiaceae but do not differentiate between chlamydial species. Sensitivity and specificity of these serologic tests are much lower than direct detection of the antigen by PCR.

Prevention and Treatment: The classic concept of prophylactic immunization that elicits sterilizing immunity and virtually 100% protection from disease does not apply to chlamydiae. However, therapeutic vaccination may nevertheless provide substantial health and economic benefits. To prevent abortion in small ruminants, *C abortus* live vaccines are available. There is, however, an ongoing and controversial discussion whether the vaccine strain might even be involved in enzootic abortion. Vaccines against *C felis* are available for pet cats, but little has been reported about their efficacy.

Several antimicrobials (eg, tetracyclines, quinolones, macrolides, lincosamides, rifamycins) can interfere with chlamydial replication. Tretracyclines or fluoroquinolones (eg, enrofloxacin) are generally the drugs of choice. Treatment must start as early as possible and continue for at least 7 days.

No antibiotic treatment for chlamydiae is bactericidal. It is suspected that antibiotics frequently induce persistent chlamydial infections by reducing antichlamydial immunity due to suppression of antigen production while not completely eliminating chlamydiae.

CLOSTRIDIAL DISEASES

Clostridia are relatively large, anaerobic, sporeforming, rod-shaped, gram-positive organisms. They are found either as living cells (vegetative forms) or as dormant spores. Their natural habitats are soils and intestinal tracts of animals, including people. Dormant spores of several clostridial species have been found in healthy muscular tissue of horses and cows. The endospores are oval, sometimes spherical, and are located centrally, subterminally, or terminally. The vegetative forms of clostridia in tissue fluids of infected animals occur singly, in pairs, or rarely in chains. Differentiation of the various pathogenic and related species is based on cultural characteristics, spore shape and position, biochemical reactions, and the antigenic specificity of toxins or surface antigens. The genomes of many clostridia have been sequenced and are available online. Pathogenic strains or their toxins may be acquired by susceptible animals by either wound contamination or ingestion. Diseases thus produced are a constant threat to successful livestock production in many parts of the world.

Clostridial diseases can be divided into two categories: 1) those in which the organisms actively invade or when locally dormant spores are activated and reproduce in the tissues of the host, with the production of toxins that enhance the spread of infection (the gas-gangrene group, the clostridial cellulitides group); and 2) those characterized by toxemia resulting from the absorption of toxins produced by organisms within the digestive system (the enterotoxemias), in devitalized tissue (tetanus), or in food or carrion outside the body (botulism). Clostridial diseases are not spread from animal to animal.

BACILLARY HEMOGLOBINURIA

(Red water disease)

Bacillary hemoglobinuria is an acute, infectious, toxemic disease caused by *Clostridium haemolyticum*. It affects primarily cattle but has also been found in sheep and rarely in dogs. It occurs in the western part of the USA, along the Gulf of Mexico, in South America, Great Britain, the Middle East, India, Japan, and other parts of the world.

Etiology: *C haemolyticum* is a soilborne organism naturally found in the GI tract of some cattle. It can survive for long periods in contaminated soil or in bones from carcasses of infected animals. After ingestion, latent spores ultimately become lodged in the liver. The incubation period is extremely variable, and onset depends on the presence of a locus of anaerobiosis in the liver. Such a nidus for germination is most often caused by liver fluke (*Fasciola hepatica*) infection, rarely by high nitrate content of the diet, accidental liver puncture, liver biopsy, or any other cause of localized necrosis. When conditions for anaerobiosis are favorable, the spores germinate, and the resulting vegetative cells multiply and produce β toxin (phospholipase C). This causes intravascular hemolysis, resulting in hemolytic anemia and hemoglobinuria.

Clinical Findings: Cattle may be found dead without premonitory signs. Usually, there is a sudden onset of severe depression, fever, abdominal pain, dyspnea, dysentery, and hemoglobinuria. Anemia and jaundice are present in varying degrees. Edema of the brisket may occur. Hgb and RBC levels are quite low. The duration of clinical signs varies from ~12 hr in pregnant cows to ~3–4 days in other cattle. Mortality in untreated animals is ~95%. Some cattle suffer from subclinical attacks of the disease and thereafter act as immune carriers.

Lesions: Dehydration, anemia, and sometimes subcutaneous edema are seen. There is bloody fluid in the abdominal and thoracic cavities. The lungs are not grossly affected, and the trachea contains bloody froth with hemorrhages in the mucosa. The small intestine and occasionally the large intestine are hemorrhagic; their contents often contain free or clotted blood. An ischemic infarct in the liver is characteristic; it is slightly elevated, lighter in color than the surrounding tissue, and outlined by a bluish red zone of congestion. The kidneys are dark, friable, and usually studded with petechiae. The bladder contains purplish red urine. After death, rigor mortis sets in quickly.

Diagnosis: The general clinical picture and postmortem findings usually permit a tentative diagnosis. The most striking sign is the typical port-wine-colored urine, which foams freely when voided or on agitation. The presence of the typical liver infarct is sufficient for a presumptive diagnosis. The normal size and consistency of the spleen serve to exclude anthrax and anaplasmosis. Bracken fern poisoning and leptospirosis also should be considered. Diagnosis can be confirmed by isolating *C haemolyticum* from the liver infarct, but the organism is difficult to culture. Rapid and accurate diagnosis can be made by demonstrating the organism in the liver tissue by a fluorescent antibody or immunohistochemical test or by demonstrating the toxin in the fluid in the peritoneal cavity or in a saline extract of the infarct. PCR has also been used to diagnose clinical bacillary hemoglobinuria in a cow in Japan.

Control: Early treatment with penicillin or tetracyclines at high doses is essential. Whole blood transfusions and fluid therapy also are helpful early in the disease. *C haemolyticum* bacterin prepared from whole cultures confers immunity for ~6 mo. In areas where the disease is seasonal, one preseasonal dose is usually adequate; where the disease occurs throughout the year, semiannual vaccination is necessary. Cattle in contact with animals from areas where this disease is endemic should be vaccinated, because the latter may be carriers.

BIG HEAD

(Swollen head)

Big head is an acute, infectious disease, caused by *Clostridium novyi*, *C sordellii*, or rarely *C chauvoei*, characterized by a nongaseous, nonhemorrhagic, edematous swelling of the head, face, and neck of young rams. This infection is initiated in young rams by fighting or continual butting of one another. It has also been associated with the practice of dipping immediately after shearing. The bruised and battered subcutaneous tissues provide conditions suitable for growth of pathogenic clostridia, and the breaks in the skin offer an opportunity for their entrance. Treatment is with broad-spectrum antibiotics or penicillin.

BLACKLEG

Blackleg is an acute, febrile, highly fatal disease of cattle and sheep caused by *Clostridium chauvoei* and characterized by emphysematous swelling, commonly affecting heavy muscles (clostridial myositis). It is found worldwide.

Etiology: *C chauvoei* is found naturally in the intestinal tract of animals. Spores remain viable in the soil for years and are purported to be a source of infection. Outbreaks of blackleg have occurred in cattle on farms in which recent excavations have occurred or after flooding. The organisms probably are ingested, pass through the wall of the GI tract, and after gaining access to the bloodstream, are deposited in muscle and other tissues (spleen, liver, and alimentary tract) and may remain dormant indefinitely.

In cattle, blackleg infection is endogenous. Lesions develop without any history of wounds, although bruising or excessive exercise may precipitate disease in some cases. Commonly, the animals that contract blackleg are of the beef breeds, in excellent health, and gaining weight. Outbreaks occur in which a few new cases are found each day, sometimes for several days. Most cases are seen in cattle from 6–24 mo old, but thrifty calves as young as 6 wk and cattle as old as 10–12 yr may be affected. The disease usually occurs in summer and fall and is uncommon during the winter. Interestingly, in sheep, the disease is almost always the result of a wound infection and often follows some form of injury such as shearing cuts, docking, crutching, or castration. The case fatality rate approaches 100%. In New Zealand, blackleg is seen more frequently in sheep.

Clinical Findings and Lesions: Usually, onset is sudden, and a few cattle may be found dead without premonitory signs. Acute, severe lameness and marked depression are common. Initially, there is a fever but, by the time clinical signs are obvious, body temperature may be normal or subnormal. Characteristic edematous and crepitant swellings develop in the hip, shoulder, chest, back, neck, or elsewhere. At first, the swelling is small, hot, and painful. As the disease rapidly progresses, the swelling enlarges, there is crepitation on palpation, and the skin becomes cold and insensitive with decreased blood supply to affected areas. General signs include prostration and tremors. Death occurs within 12–48 hr. In some cattle, the lesions are restricted to the myocardium and the diaphragm.

Diagnosis: A rapidly fatal, febrile disease in well-nourished young cattle, particularly of the beef breeds, with crepitant swellings of the heavy muscles suggests blackleg. The affected muscles are dark red to black and dry and spongy, have a sweetish odor, and are infiltrated with small bubbles but little edema. The lesions may be seen in any muscle, even in the tongue or diaphragm. In sheep, because the lesions of the spontaneously occurring type are often small and deep, they may be overlooked. Occasionally, the tissue changes caused by *C septicum*, *C novyi*, *C sordellii*, and *C perfringens* may resemble those of blackleg. At times, both *C septicum* and *C chauvoei* may be isolated from blackleg lesions, particularly when the carcass is examined ≥24 hr after death, which allows time for postmortem invasion of the tissues by *C sordellii*. Field diagnoses are confirmed by laboratory demonstration of *C chauvoei* in affected muscle (standard methods: culture and biochemical identification). The samples of muscle should be taken as soon after death as possible. The fluorescent antibody test for *C chauvoei* is rapid and reliable. A PCR is available and reported to be very good for clinical samples but not for environmental samples.

Control: A multivalent vaccine containing *C chauvoei*, *C septicum* and, where needed, *C novyi* antigens is safe and reliable for cattle and sheep. Calves 3–6 mo of age should be vaccinated twice, 4 wk apart, followed by annual boosters before the anticipated danger period (usually spring or early summer). In an outbreak, all susceptible cattle should be vaccinated and treated prophylactically with penicillin (10,000 IU/kg, IM) to prevent new cases for as long as 14 days. Cattle should be moved from affected pastures. Vaccine failure has been observed locally and attributed to a deficient spectrum of antigens in the vaccine. In such instances, a bacterin vaccine is produced with local, previously identified clostridial strains of *C chauvoei*.

Naive ewes should be vaccinated twice 1 mo before lambing and then with yearly boosters. In outbreaks in flocks of ewes, prophylactic penicillin and antiserum treatments are recommended. Young sheep should be vaccinated before going to pasture. Immunity in young sheep is relatively short. Clostridial vaccines are reported to create a weaker immune response in sheep and goats than in cattle. Carcasses should be destroyed by burning or buried deeply in a fenced-off area to limit heavy spore contamination of the soil.

INFECTIOUS NECROTIC HEPATITIS

(*Clostridium novyi* infection, Black disease)

Infectious necrotic hepatitis is an acute toxemia of sheep that is sometimes seen in cattle and is rare in pigs and horses.

Etiology and Pathogenesis: The etiologic agent, *Clostridium novyi* type B, is soilborne and present in the intestines and livers of herbivores; it may be present on skin surfaces and dormant in muscles and is a potential source of wound infections. Fecal contamination of pasture by carrier animals is the most important source of infection. The organism multiplies in areas of liver necrosis caused by migration of liver flukes and produces a powerful necrotizing toxin (α toxin). The disease is distributed worldwide, wherever sheep and liver flukes are both found, and is increasing in cattle where liver flukes are accidentally introduced.

C novyi has been suspected but not yet confirmed as a cause of sudden death in cattle and pigs fed high-level grain diets, and in which preexisting lesions of the liver were not detectable. The lethal and necrotizing toxins damage hepatic parenchyma, thereby permitting the bacteria to multiply and produce a lethal amount of toxin.

Clinical Findings: Usually, death is sudden with no well-defined signs. Affected animals often are 2–4 yr old, tend to lag behind the flock, assume sternal recumbency, and die within a few hours. Most cases occur in the summer and early fall when liver fluke infection is at its peak. The disease is most prevalent in well-nourished adult sheep and seems to be limited to animals infected with liver flukes. Differentiation from acute fascioliasis may be difficult, but peracute deaths of animals that show typical lesions on necropsy should arouse suspicion of infectious necrotic hepatitis.

Lesions: The most characteristic gross lesions are grayish yellow, necrotic foci in the liver along migratory tracks of the young flukes. Histologically, the liver lesions include central eosinophilic inflammation (fluke induced) surrounded by coagulation necrosis with an outer rim of neutrophils. The lesion is positive for gram-positive rods. Other common findings are an enlarged pericardial sac filled with straw-colored fluid and excess fluid in the peritoneal and thoracic cavities. Usually, there is extensive rupture of the capillaries in the subcutaneous tissue, which causes the adjacent skin to turn black (hence the common name, black disease).

Control: The incidence may be lowered by reducing the numbers of *Lymnaea* spp snails, the intermediate hosts for the liver flukes, or by otherwise reducing the fluke infection of sheep. However, these procedures are not always practical, and active immunization with *C novyi* aluminum-precipitated toxoid seems more effective and can be also performed during outbreaks. Longterm immunity is produced by one vaccination. After this, only new introductions to the flock (lambs and sheep brought in from other areas) need to be vaccinated. This is best done in early summer. Pasture contamination can be minimized by proper disposal of carcasses (burning).

MALIGNANT EDEMA

Malignant edema is an acute, generally fatal toxemia affecting all species and ages of animals and is usually caused by *Clostridium septicum*. Other clostridial species have been isolated, indicating mixed infections. Additional clostridia implicated in wound infections include *C chauvoei*, *C perfringens*, *C novyi*, and *C sordellii*. The disease occurs worldwide.

Etiology and Pathogenesis: *C septicum* is found in soil and intestinal contents of animals throughout the world. Infection ordinarily occurs through contamination of wounds containing devitalized tissue, soil, or some other tissue debilitant or through activation of dormant spores. Wounds caused by accident, castration, docking, insanitary vaccination, and parturition may become infected. Potent clostridial toxins cause local and systemic signs, often resulting in death. Local exotoxins cause excessive inflammation, resulting in severe edema, necrosis, and gangrene. Risk factors include IM injections in horses; shearing, docking, and lambing in sheep; and traumatic parturition and castration in cattle. Horses and probably cows have dormant spores present in muscle tissues.

Clinical Findings: General signs, such as anorexia, intoxication, and high fever, as well as local lesions, develop within 6–48 hr after predisposing injury or activation of dormant spores. The local lesions are soft swellings that pit on pressure and extend rapidly because of the formation of large quantities of exudate that infiltrate the subcutaneous and intramuscular connective tissue of the affected areas. The muscle in such areas is dark brown to black. Accumulations of gas in subcutaneous tissue and along muscle fascias may or may not be present. These muscle infections are extremely painful, and systemic toxemia may evolve. Extensive local sloughing of

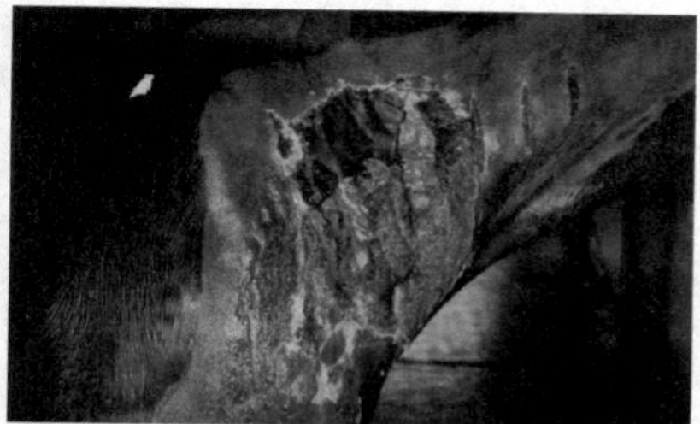

Clostridial myonecrosis due to *C perfringens* type A in a horse. *Courtesy of Dr. Henry Stämpfli.*

skin and tissues is often seen in progressed states of malignant edema. Severe edema of the head of rams develops after infection of wounds inflicted by fighting. Malignant edema associated with lacerations of the vulva at parturition is characterized by marked edema of the vulva, severe toxemia, and death in 24–48 hr.

Diagnosis: Similarity to blackleg (*see* p 602) is marked, and differentiation made on necropsy is unreliable; laboratory confirmation is the only certain procedure. Horses and pigs are susceptible to malignant edema but not to blackleg. An important differential diagnosis in these species is anthrax (*see* p 593).

C septicum also causes **braxy** in sheep, a highly fatal infection characterized by toxemia and inflammation of the abomasal wall. This disease seems to be confined mostly to European sheep fed on "frosted" pasture.

Diagnosis can be confirmed rapidly on the basis of fluorescent-antibody staining of *C septicum* from a tissue smear. However, *C septicum* is an extremely active postmortem invader from the intestine, and its presence in a specimen taken from an animal that has been dead for ≥24 hr is not significant. PCR can be used for direct identification and differentiation of clostridia associated with malignant edema. The presence of type III echinocytes or spheroechinocytes in blood smears may help diagnose immune-mediated hemolytic anemia associated with clostridial infections in horses. Fine-needle aspirates and Gram stain may confirm the presence of gram-positive rods before confirmation by anaerobic culture.

Control: Bacterins are used for immunization. *C septicum* usually is combined with *C chauvoei* in a blackleg/malignant edema vaccine and is available in multivalent vaccines. In endemic areas, animals should be vaccinated before they are castrated, dehorned, or docked. Calves should be vaccinated at ~2 mo of age. Two doses 2–3 wk apart generally give protection. In high-risk areas, annual vaccination is indicated, as is revaccination after severe trauma.

Treatment with high doses of parenteral penicillin, tetracyclines, or broad-spectrum antibiotics is indicated early in the disease. Although injection of penicillin directly into the periphery of the lesion may minimize spread of the lesion, the affected tissues usually slough. Supportive therapy with NSAIDs (flunixin meglumine for cattle and horses) is recommended. Local treatment includes surgical incision of skin and fascia to allow drainage. Animals with systemic toxic signs will need supportive treatments such as IV perfusion.

BOTULISM

(Lamziekte)

Botulism is a rapidly fatal motor paralysis caused by ingestion of the toxin produced by *Clostridium botulinum* types A-G. The spore-forming anaerobic organism proliferates in decomposing animal tissue and sometimes in plant material.

Etiology: Botulism is in most cases an intoxication, not an infection, and results from ingestion of toxin in food. There are seven types of *C botulinum*, differentiated on the antigenic specificity of the toxins: A, B, C_1, D, E, F, and G. Types A, B, and E are most important in people; C_1 in most animal species, notably wild ducks, pheasants, chickens, mink, cattle, and horses; and D in cattle. In horses, the most common type in North America and Europe is type B (>85% of USA cases), and in the western USA type A has been reported in only two outbreaks, both in people, known to have been caused by type F. Type G, isolated from soil in Argentina, is not known to have been involved in any outbreak of botulism. The usual source of the toxin is decaying carcasses or vegetable materials such as decaying grass, hay, grain, or spoiled silage. Toxins of all types have the same pharmacologic action. Like tetanus toxin, botulinum toxin is a zinc-binding metalloprotease that cleaves specific proteins in synaptic vesicles. Motor neuron surface receptors vary for the different botulinum toxins, explaining some of the species differences in susceptibility to the different toxins.

The exact incidence of botulism in animals is not known, but it is relatively low in cattle and horses, probably more frequent in chickens, and high in wild waterfowl. Probably 10,000–50,000 birds are lost in most years, with losses reaching 1 million or more during the great outbreaks in the western USA. Most affected birds are ducks, although loons, mergansers, geese, and gulls also are susceptible. (*See also* BOTULISM IN POULTRY, p 2889.) Dogs, cats, and pigs are comparatively resistant to all types of botulinum toxin when challenged orally; however, there are recent individual case reports mentioning botulism in dogs.

Most botulism in cattle occurs in South Africa and South America, where a combination of extensive agriculture, phosphorus deficiency in soil, and *C botulinum* type D in animals creates conditions ideal for the disease. The phosphorus-deficient cattle chew any bones with accompanying bits of flesh they find on the range; if these came from an animal carrying type D strains of *C botulinum*, intoxication is likely to result. Any animal eating such material also ingests spores, which germinate in the intestine and, after death of the host, invade the musculature, which in turn becomes toxic for other cattle. Type C strains also cause botulism in cattle in a similar fashion. This type of botulism in cattle is rare in the USA, although a few cases have been reported from Texas under the name of **loin disease**, and a few cases have occurred in Montana. Hay or silage contaminated with toxin-containing carcasses of birds or mammals and poultry litter fed to cattle have also been sources of type C or type D toxin for cattle ("forage botulism"). Big bale silage and haylage seem to be a particular risk and result in botulism problems if fermentation fails to produce a low and stable pH (<4.5). Botulism in sheep has been encountered in Australia, associated not with phosphorus deficiency as in cattle, but with protein and carbohydrate deficiency, which results in sheep eating carcasses of rabbits and other small animals found on the range. Botulism in horses often results from forage contaminated with type C or D toxin. In six out of eight outbreaks of equine botulism associated with type A, the source of infection was confirmed to be hay or silage.

Toxicoinfectious botulism is the name given the disease in which *C botulinum grows in tissues of a living animal and* produces toxins there. The toxins are liberated from the lesions and cause typical botulism. This has been suggested as a means of producing the **shaker foal syndrome**. Gastric ulcers, foci of necrosis in the liver, abscesses in the navel and lungs, wounds of the skin and muscle, and necrotic lesions of the GI tract are predisposing sites for development of toxicoinfectious botulism. This disease of foals and adult horses appears to resemble "wound botulism" in people. Type B toxin is often implicated in botulism in horses and foals in the eastern USA. Toxicoinfection is also suggested as a cause of equine grass sickness (equine dysautonomia, *see* p 1257).

Botulism in mink usually is caused by type C strains that have produced toxin in chopped raw meat or fish. Type A and E strains are occasionally involved. Botulism has not been reported in cats but occurs sporadically in dogs. Type C toxin is usually responsible, but there have been reports in which type D was incriminated.

Clinical Findings and Lesions: The signs of botulism are caused by flaccid muscle paralysis and include progressive motor paralysis, disturbed vision, difficulty in chewing and swallowing, and generalized progressive paresis. Death is usually due to respiratory or cardiac paralysis. The toxin prevents release of acetylcholine at motor endplates (neuromuscular junction). Passage of impulses down the motor nerves and contractility of muscles are not hindered. No characteristic gross and histologic lesions develop, and pathologic changes may be ascribed to the general paralytic action of toxin, particularly in the muscles of the respiratory system, rather than to the specific effect of toxin on any particular organ.

Epidemics have occurred in dairy herds in which up to 65% of adult cows developed clinical botulism and died 6–72 hr after the onset of recumbency. Major clinical findings included drooling, decreased tongue tone, dysphagia, inability to urinate, and sternal recumbency that progressed to lateral recumbency just before death. Skin sensation is usually normal, and withdrawal reflexes of the limbs are weak. Initially, clinical signs resemble second-stage parturient paresis (*see* p 988), but the cows do not respond to parenteral calcium therapy.

Reported clinical signs in horses are very similar, with progressive muscle paresis, recumbency, dysphagia, and decreased muscle tone (tail, tongue, jaw), respiratory distress, and death.

In the shaker foal syndrome, foals are usually <4 wk old. They may be found dead without premonitory signs; most often, they exhibit signs of progressive symmetric motor paralysis. Stilted gait, muscular tremors, and the inability to stand for >4–5 min are salient features. Other clinical signs include dysphagia, constipation, mydriasis, and frequent urination. As the disease progresses, dyspnea with extension of the head and neck, tachycardia, and respiratory arrest occur. Death ensues most often 24–72 hr after the onset of clinical signs due to respiratory failure. The most consistent necropsy findings are pulmonary edema and congestion and excessive pericardial fluid, which contains free-floating strands of fibrin.

Diagnosis: Although sporadic cases of botulism often are suspected because of the characteristic motor paralysis, it is difficult to establish the diagnosis by demonstrating the toxin in animal tissues or sera or in the suspect feed. Commonly, the diagnosis is made by eliminating other causes of motor paralysis (flaccid paralysis). Filtrates of the stomach and intestinal contents should be tested for toxicity in mice, but a negative answer is unreliable. Primary supportive evidence is provided by feeding suspect material to susceptible animals. In peracute cases, the toxin may be detectable in the blood by mouse inoculation tests but usually is not detectable in the average field case in farm animals. Use of ELISA methodology for detection of the toxin makes it feasible to test large numbers of samples, increasing the chances of diagnosis confirmation. In toxicoinfectious botulism, the organism may be cultured from tissues of affected animals.

Treatment and Control: Any dietary deficiencies in range animals should be corrected and carcasses disposed of, if possible. Decaying grass or spoiled silage should be removed from the diet. Immunization of cattle with types C and D toxoid has proved successful in South Africa and Australia. Toxoid is also effective in immunizing mink and has been used in pheasants.

Botulinum antitoxin has been used for treatment with varying degrees of success, depending on the type of toxin involved and the species of host. Treatment of ducks and mink with type C antitoxin is often successful; however, such treatment is rarely used in cattle. Early administration of antitoxin (type B) specific or polyvalent to foals before recumbency (30,000 IU, IV) is reported to be successful. Supportive care in valuable animals is essential; prognosis is poor in recumbent animals. In endemic areas (eg, Kentucky), vaccination with type B toxoid appears to be effective.

CLOSTRIDIUM DIFFICILE AND *C PERFRINGENS* INFECTIONS

Clostridium difficile is a large, gram-positive, anaerobic, spore-forming motile rod and is the major cause of antibiotic-associated colitis in people. *C difficile*–associated diarrhea and disease develops spontaneously in a variety of other species including horses, pigs, calves, dogs, cats, hamsters, guinea pigs, rats, and rabbits. *C difficile* produces protein toxins A, B, and/or the binary toxin CDT in the intestine. Toxin A is an enterotoxin that causes hypersecretion of fluid into the intestinal lumen and also causes tissue damage. Toxin B is a potent cytotoxin that induces inflammation and necrosis. The mechanism of action of CDT is not known. Disruption of colonic microflora together with the presence of toxigenic *C difficile* strains that overgrow in the intestines are the prerequisites for disease. Diagnostic tests for *C difficile* toxins include cell cytoxicity assays and ELISA on fecal samples, anaerobic culture, and PCR to discriminate between toxigenic and nontoxigenic strains. *C perfringens* is widely distributed in the soil and the GI tract of animals and is characterized by its ability to produce potent exotoxins, some of which are responsible for specific enterotoxemias. Five types (A, B, C, D, and E) have been identified and produce one or more of four major toxins (alpha, beta, epsilon, and iota). *C perfringens* type A is most common and the most variable strain in toxigenic properties. Alpha toxin production is associated with gas gangrene, traumatic infections, avian and canine necrotic enteritis, colitis in horses, and diarrhea in pigs. *C perfringens* types B and C cause severe enteritides, dysentery, toxemia, and high mortality in young lambs, calves, pigs, and foals (beta toxin). Type C causes enterotoxemia in adult cattle, sheep, and goats. The diseases are listed below, categorized as to cause and host.

Clostridia-associated Enterocolitides in Horses

Clostridium difficile and *C perfringens* have been implicated in this acute, sporadic disease of horses characterized by diarrhea and colic. Because of uncertainty about the etiology, the condition has also been referred to as idiopathic colitis, but there is now good evidence that these organisms are responsible for enterocolitis in horses in approximately 20%–30% of cases of acute diarrhea. (*See also* p 285.)

Etiology: *C difficile* may be found in low concentrations in the feces of as many as 10% of healthy horses. *C difficile* and *C perfringens* organisms may be present in soil or the environment and be ingested by horses. The factors that trigger disease are not well known, but it is presumed that some alteration in the normal flora permits excessive multiplication of the bacteria, which produce toxins capable of causing intestinal damage and systemic effects.

Predisposing factors that have been suggested include change in diet and antibiotic therapy. Other host factors that may determine whether disease develops include age, immunity, and presence or absence of intestinal receptors for the clostridial toxins. Recent antibiotic therapy is a common feature of the history of horses with *C difficile*–induced diarrhea. Certain antibiotics, notably macrolides and especially erythromycin ethylsuccinate, β-lactam antibiotics, and trimethoprim/sulfonamide, are more likely than others to be associated with *C difficile* colitis. Mares with foals that are being treated with erythromycin ethylsuccinate appear to be at high risk. Elimination of roughage from the diet before surgery is also reported to predispose to *C difficile* colitis. Acute diarrhea has been reproduced in healthy neonatal foals using *C difficile* spores and vegetative cell forms. Acute anterior enteritis (duodenitis-jejunitis, *see* p 285) has also been associated with *C difficile* in a case-control study.

C perfringens type A is believed to cause diarrhea by elaboration of an enterotoxin (CPE), which is released during sporulation and stimulates intestinal epithelial cells to secrete excess fluid into the lumen. A novel necrotizing toxin, called β2, produced by some strains of *C perfringens*, has recently been strongly associated with colitis in horses.

Clinical Findings: Foals and adult horses may be affected. Typically, there are signs of abdominal pain and diarrhea with or without blood. There may be abdominal distention, especially in cases of *C difficile*–induced diarrhea. Dehydration, toxemia, and shock may develop, and the mortality rate is variable. One or several animals on a farm may be affected. Horses with anterior enteritis have associated severe recurrent nasogastric reflux, fever, and malaise.

Lesions: The characteristic lesion is a necrotizing enterocolitis-typhlitis. There is severe loss of colonic and cecal mucosal epithelial cells, hemorrhagic colitis and typhlitis, and thrombosis in capillaries of the intestinal mucosa. Horses with anterior enteritis will mostly have hemorrhagic duodenitis.

Diagnosis: Clinical features of the disease are similar to those of acute salmonellosis (*see* p 195), Potomac horse fever (*see* p 283), or monocytic ehrlichiosis. The identification of *C perfringens* as the cause of diarrhea in horses depends on demonstration of the presence of enterotoxin or the gene for CPE in the feces or intestinal fluid and the absence of other likely etiologic agents. Most *C perfringens* found in the intestine of horses lack the gene for CPE expression. Large numbers of *C perfringens* in anaerobic fecal culture of horses with diarrhea is not diagnostically significant. The diagnosis of *C difficile* diarrhea is suggested by a history of recent treatment with antibiotics and is supported by demonstration of the presence of *C difficile* toxin A and/or B in a freshly passed or frozen fecal sample submitted to a laboratory using a human ELISA validated in horses, with good sensitivity and specificity. The toxin gene may be identified by PCR ribotyping.

Control: Steps may be taken to reduce the opportunity for *C difficile* infections in horses. Proper isolation procedures and infectious disease control should be applied to high-risk horses receiving antibiotics. The environmental load of *C difficile* spores may be reduced by surface disinfection with sporicidal disinfectants, and the spread may be reduced by hand washing and by isolation of infectious horses and foals. There are no control measures available for prevention of *C perfringens*–induced diarrhea. Oral metronidazole (15 mg/kg, tid) is recommended for treatment of either of these clostridial infections. Metronidazole might be teratogenic, so its use should be avoided if possible in pregnant mares.

Clostridium difficile in Swine

Clostridium difficile has emerged as an important cause of diarrhea in neonatal swine. In some studies, it has been identified as the second most frequent cause of diarrhea in 1- to 7-day-old pigs. Mesocolonic edema is a characteristic feature of the disease seen in almost all affected pigs, but this lesion is not pathognomonic. Diagnosis of the disease depends on detection of toxins as described for the disease in horses. Porcine, equine, bovine, and canine *C difficile* isolates may show an antimicrobial susceptibility profile overlapping that of isolates from human patients, raising the possibility for interspecies transmission of *C difficile*. Dormant *C difficile* spores have been found in meat of pigs and beef cattle. Some of the ribotypes isolated were similar or identical to human pathogenic strains.

Clostridium difficile in Dogs

Clostridium difficile has not been established as a primary pathogen in dogs. However, human toxigenic *C difficile* strains have been frequently isolated from rectal swabs of dogs visiting human patients in hospitals. Human ELISA for *C difficile* toxins does not perform well in dogs with diarrhea and has poor sensitivity and specificity. Approximately 10% of asymptomatic dogs shed toxigenic *C difficile* in feces.

Clostridium difficile in Calves

Clostridium difficile has been identified as a potential cause of diarrhea in young calves. The disease could not be reproduced in colostrum-deprived neonatal calves with spores or vegetative cells. *C difficile* has been found in high prevalence in veal calves early in the veal production process.

Clostridium perfringens in Adult Cattle

In the past few years, hemorrhagic bowel, bloody gut, or jejunal hemorrhage syndrome has emerged sporadically in individual, high-producing dairy cows in early lactation. Although no specific etiology has been established, it is assumed that *Clostridium perfringens* type A is involved, because large numbers of this clostridia may be recovered in most cases. The clinical course is peracute, with anorexia, colic, drop in milk yield, hemorrhage into the intestine, and sudden death despite aggressive supportive and surgical treatment. Gross postmortem findings include severe hemorrhage and necrosis in the intestines. Prevention consists of optimizing nutritional management and avoiding sudden feed changes. Autogenous vaccines in affected dairy herds have been tried with anecdotal success.

ENTEROTOXEMIAS

(*Clostridium perfringens* infections)

Enterotoxemia Caused by *Clostridium perfringens* Type A

Type A strains of *C perfringens* are commonly found as part of the normal intestinal microflora of animals and lack some of the powerful toxins produced by strains of other types. *C perfringens* enterotoxin (CPE) is the principal toxin involved in *C perfringens* foodborne illness and is associated with nonfoodborne diarrheal disease in different animals. *C perfringens* also produces a necrotizing toxin associated with necrotic enteritis in poultry (*see* p 2802) and dogs, colitis in horses, and diarrhea in pigs. *C perfringens* type A is implicated in a rarely occurring hemorrhagic diarrhea in dogs and has been associated with nosocomial and acquired acute and chronic diarrhea in dogs. The acute form is characterized by a necrotic enteritis in which there is massive destruction of the villi and coagulation necrosis of the small intestine. Many large, gram-positive rods are visible in fecal smears, and large numbers of *C perfringens* type A are recovered on anaerobic culture of feces of dogs with acute diarrhea. Fecal tests are not useful in determining the cause of diarrhea, however, because of a high number of false-positive results. A commercial ELISA for CPE in dogs is quite specific. PCR for CPE gene expression in dogs is being evaluated. Type A strains from pigs with diarrhea have produced enterotoxin in vitro, and anti-enterotoxin antibodies in sows indicate that enterotoxin is produced in vivo. Enterotoxin has also been demonstrated in the feces of pigs with diarrhea but not in feces of healthy animals. *C perfringens* isolated from pigs with diarrhea are typically nonenterotoxigenic but produce the cytotoxic β2 toxin, which possibly plays a role in disease. Experimental disease has been produced in pigs challenged orally with *C perfringens* type A.

Enterotoxemia Caused by *Clostridium perfringens* Types B and C

Infection with *C perfringens* types B and C causes severe enteritis, dysentery, toxemia, and high mortality in young lambs, calves, pigs, and foals (*see* TABLE 1). Types B and C both produce the highly necrotizing and lethal beta toxin responsible for severe intestinal damage. This toxin is sensitive to proteolytic enzymes, and disease is associated with inhibition of proteolysis in the intestine. Sow colostrum, which contains a trypsin inhibitor, has been suggested as a factor increasing the susceptibility of young piglets. Type C also causes enterotoxemia in adult cattle, sheep, and goats.

Clinical Findings: Lamb dysentery is an acute disease of lambs <3 wk old. Many may die before clinical signs are seen, but some newborn lambs stop nursing, become

TABLE 1 ENTEROTOXEMIA CAUSED BY *CLOSTRIDIUM PERFRINGENS* TYPES B AND C

Disease	*C perfringens* Type	Host
Lamb dysentery	Type B	Lambs ≤3 wk old
Calf enterotoxemia	Types B and C	Well-fed calves ≤1 mo old
Pig enterotoxemia	Type C	Piglets in first few days of life
Foal enterotoxemia	Type B	Foals in first week of life
Struck	Type C	Adult sheep
Goat enterotoxemia	Type C	Adult goats

listless, and remain recumbent. A fetid, blood-tinged diarrhea is common, and death usually occurs within a few days. In calves, there is acute diarrhea, dysentery, abdominal pain, convulsions, and opisthotonos. Death may occur in a few hours, but less severe cases survive for a few days, and recovery is possible. Pigs become acutely ill within a few days of birth and there is diarrhea, dysentery, reddening of the anus, and a high fatality rate; most affected piglets die within 12 hr. In foals, there is acute dysentery, toxemia, and rapid death. Struck in adult sheep is characterized by death without premonitory signs.

Lesions: Hemorrhagic enteritis with ulceration of the mucosa is the major lesion in all species. Grossly, the affected portion of the intestine is deep blue-purple and appears at first glance to be an infarction associated with mesenteric torsion. Smears of intestinal contents can be examined for large numbers of gram-positive, rod-shaped bacteria, and filtrates can be made for detection of toxin and subsequent identification by neutralization with specific antisera.

Treatment and Control: Treatment is usually ineffective because of the severity of the disease but, if attempted, includes specific hyperimmune sera and oral antibiotics. The disease is best controlled by vaccination of the pregnant dam during the last third of pregnancy, initially with two vaccinations 1 mo apart and annually thereafter. When outbreaks occur in newborn animals from unvaccinated dams, antiserum should be administered immediately after birth.

Type D Enterotoxemia

(Pulpy kidney disease, Overeating disease)

This classic enterotoxemia of sheep is seen less frequently in goats and rarely in cattle. It has a worldwide distribution and affects animals of any age. It is most common in lambs either <2 wk old or weaned in feedlots and on a high-carbohydrate diet or, less often, on lush green pastures. The disease has been suspected in well-nourished beef calves nursing high-producing cows grazing lush pasture and in sudden death syndrome in feedlot cattle; however, supportive laboratory evidence in the latter is lacking.

Etiology: The causative agent is *C perfringens* type D. Predisposing factors are essential, the most common being the ingestion of excessive amounts of feed or milk in the very young and of grain in feedlot lambs. In young lambs, the disease usually is restricted to ewes with single lambs, because ewes with twins seldom give enough milk to allow enterotoxemia to develop. In the feedlot, the disease usually is seen in lambs switched rapidly to high-grain diets. As starch intake increases, it provides a suitable medium for overgrowth of *C perfringens*, producing epsilon toxin. The toxin causes vascular damage, particularly in capillaries of the brain. Many adult sheep carry strains of *C perfringens* type D as part of their normal intestinal microflora, which is the source of organisms that infect the newborn. Most such carriers have nonvaccinal antitoxin serum titers.

Clinical Findings: Usually, sudden deaths in the best-conditioned lambs are the first indication of enterotoxemia. In some cases, excitement, incoordination, and convulsions occur before death. Opisthotonos, circling, and pushing the head against fixed objects are common neurologic signs; frequently, hyperglycemia or glycosuria is present. Diarrhea may or may not develop. Occasionally, adult sheep are affected too, showing weakness, incoordination, convulsions, and death within 24 hr. In goats, the course of disease ranges from peracute to chronic, with signs that vary from watery diarrhea with or without blood to sudden death. Affected calves not found dead show mania, convulsions, blindness, and death within a few hours. Subacutely affected calves are stuporous for a few days and may recover. In goats, diarrhea and nervous signs are seen, and death may occur over several weeks. Type D enterotoxemia occasionally is seen in young horses that have overeaten.

Lesions: Necropsy may reveal only a few hyperemic areas on the intestine and a fluid-filled pericardial sac. This is particularly the case in young lambs. In older animals, hemorrhagic areas on the myocardium may be found as well as petechiae and ecchymoses of the abdominal muscles and serosa of the intestine. Bilateral pulmonary edema and congestion frequently occur but usually not in young lambs. The rumen and abomasum contain an abundance of feed, and undigested feed often is found in the ileum. Edema and malacia can be detected microscopically in the basal ganglia and cerebellum of lambs. Rapid postmortem autolysis of the kidneys has led to the popular name of pulpy kidney disease; however, pulpy kidneys are by no means always found in affected young lambs and are seldom found in affected goats or cattle. Hemorrhagic or necrotic enterocolitis may be seen in goats.

Diagnosis: A presumptive diagnosis of enterotoxemia is based on sudden, convulsive deaths in lambs on carbohydrate-rich feed. Smears of intestinal contents reveal many short, thick, gram-positive rods. Confirmation requires demonstration of epsilon toxin in the small-intestinal fluid. Fluid, not ingesta, should be collected in a sterile vial within a few hours after death and sent under refrigeration to a laboratory for toxin identification. Chloroform, added at 1 drop for each 10 mL of intestinal fluid, will stabilize any toxin present. Although immunologic tests have been developed to replace the traditional mouse assay for detection of toxin, they are less sensitive. A PCR for detection of epsilon toxin gene is available for identification of the isolates as either type B or D.

Control: The method of control depends on the age of the lambs, the frequency with which the disease appears on a particular property, and the method of husbandry. If the disease is seen consistently in young lambs, ewe immunization probably is the most satisfactory method of control. Breeding ewes should be given two injections of type D toxoid in their first year, a booster injection 4–6 wk before lambing, and each year thereafter.

Enterotoxemia in feedlot lambs can be controlled by reducing the amount of concentrate in the diet. However, this may not be economical, and immunization of all lambs with toxoid on entering the feedlot likely will reduce losses to an acceptable level. Two injections, 2 wk apart, will protect lambs through the feeding period. When aluminum-precipitated toxoids or bacterins are used, the injection should be given at such a site that the local cold abscesses, which commonly develop, can be removed easily during normal dressing and will not blemish the carcass.

TETANUS

(Lockjaw)

Tetanus toxemia is caused by a specific neurotoxin produced by *Clostridium tetani* in necrotic tissue. Almost all mammals are susceptible, although dogs and cats are relatively more resistant than any other domestic or laboratory mammal. Birds are quite resistant; the lethal dose for pigeons and chickens is 10,000–300,000 times greater (on a body wt basis) than that for horses. Horses and lambs seem to be the most sensitive of all species, with the possible exception of people. Although tetanus is worldwide in distribution, there are some areas, such as the northern Rocky Mountain section of the USA, where the organism is rarely found in the soil and where tetanus is almost unknown. In general, the occurrence of *C tetani* in the soil, especially in cultivated soil, and the incidence of tetanus in people, horses, and lambs is higher in the warmer parts of the various continents.

Etiology and Pathogenesis: *C tetani*, an anaerobe with terminal, spherical spores, is found in soil, especially cultivated soil, and intestinal tracts. In most cases, it is introduced into the tissues through wounds, particularly deep puncture wounds, that provide a suitable anaerobic environment. In lambs, however, and sometimes in other species, tetanus often follows docking or castration. Sometimes, the point of entry cannot be found because the wound itself may be minor or healed.

The spores of *C tetani* are unable to grow in normal tissue or even in wounds if the tissue remains at the normal oxidation-reduction potential of the circulating blood. Suitable conditions for multiplication occur when a small amount of soil or a foreign object causes tissue necrosis. The bacteria remain localized in the necrotic tissue at the original site of infection and multiply. As bacterial cells undergo autolysis, the potent neurotoxin is released. The neurotoxin is a zinc-binding protease that cleaves synaptobrevin, a vesicle-associated membrane protein. Usually, toxin is absorbed by the motor nerves in the area and travels retrograde up the nerve tract to the spinal cord, where it causes ascending tetanus.

The toxin causes spasmodic, tonic contractions of the voluntary muscles by interfering with the release of inhibitory neurotransmitters from presynaptic nerve endings. If more toxin is released at the site of the infection than the surrounding nerves can take up, the excess is carried off by the lymph to the bloodstream and thus to the CNS, where it causes descending tetanus. Even minor stimulation of the affected animal may trigger the characteristic tetanic muscular spasms. The spasms may be severe enough to cause bone fractures. Spasms affecting the larynx, diaphragm, and intercostal muscles lead to respiratory failure. Involvement of the autonomic nervous system results in cardiac arrhythmias, tachycardia, and hypertension.

Clinical Findings: The incubation period varies from one to several weeks but usually averages 10–14 days. Localized stiffness, often involving the masseter muscles and muscles of the neck, the hindlimbs, and the region of the infected wound, is seen first; general stiffness becomes pronounced ~1 day later, and tonic spasms and hyperesthesia become evident. Because of their high resistance to tetanus toxin, dogs and cats often have a long incubation period and frequently develop localized tetanus; however, generalized tetanus does develop in these species.

The reflexes increase in intensity, and the animal is easily excited into more violent, general spasms by sudden movement or noise. Spasms of head muscles cause difficulty in prehension and mastication of food, hence the common name, **lockjaw**. In horses, the ears are erect, the tail stiff and extended, the anterior nares dilated, and the third eyelid prolapsed. Walking, turning, and *backing are difficult*. Spasms of the neck and back muscles cause extension of the head and neck, while stiffness of the leg muscles causes the animal to assume a "sawhorse" stance. Sweating is common. General spasms disturb circulation and respiration, which results in increased heart rate, rapid breathing, and congestion of mucous membranes. Sheep, goats, and pigs often fall to the ground and exhibit opisthotonos when startled. Consciousness is not affected. In dogs and cats, localized tetanus often presents as stiffness and rigidity in a limb with a wound. The stiffness progresses to involve the opposing limb and may advance anteriorly. The appearance in generalized tetanus is similar to that described for horses except that the partially open mouth with the lips drawn back (as seen in people) is usually evident. Young, large-breed dogs seem to be most commonly affected.

Usually, the temperature remains slightly above normal, but it may rise to 108°–110°F (42°–43°C) toward the end of a fatal attack. In mild attacks, the pulse and temperature remain nearly normal. Mortality averages ~80% (~50% in dogs in one study). In animals that recover, there is a convalescent period of 2–6 wk; protective immunity usually does not develop after recovery.

Diagnosis: The clinical signs and history of recent trauma are usually adequate for a clinical diagnosis of tetanus. It may be possible to confirm the diagnosis by demonstrating the presence of tetanus toxin in serum from the affected animal. In cases in which the wound is apparent, demonstration of the bacterium in gram-stained smears and by anaerobic culture may be attempted.

Treatment and Control: When administered in the early stages of the disease, curariform agents, tranquilizers, or barbiturate sedatives, in conjunction with 300,000 IU of tetanus antitoxin IV, bid, have been effective in the treatment of horses. Good results have been obtained in horses by injecting 50,000 IU of tetanus antitoxin directly into the subarachnoid space through the cisterna magna. Such therapy should be supported by draining and cleaning the wounds and administering penicillin or broad-spectrum antibiotics. Good nursing is invaluable during the acute period of spasms. The horse should be placed in a quiet, darkened box stall with feeding and watering devices high enough to allow use without lowering the head. Slings may be useful for horses having difficulty standing or rising.

The same approach as described for horses is used in treatment of dogs and cats, except that caution must be exercised in the IV administration of antitoxin, because the equine antitoxin may induce anaphylaxis. In one study, antitoxin was given to dogs with tetanus only after an intradermal test to detect hypersensitivity reactions. In addition, all dogs received IV penicillin and some also received metronidazole orally. A combination of chlorpromazine and phenobarbital or diazepam may be used to reduce hyperesthetic reactions and convulsions.

Active immunization can be accomplished with tetanus toxoid. If a dangerous wound occurs after immunization, another injection of toxoid to increase the circulating antibody should be given. If the animal has not been immunized previously, it should be treated with 1,500–3,000 IU or more of tetanus antitoxin, which usually provides passive protection for as long as 2 wk. Toxoid should be given simultaneously with the antitoxin and repeated in 30 days. Even though it is not scientifically based, yearly booster injections of toxoid in animals are advised; in people the toxoid is given every 10 yr. The toxoid vaccination interval is currently debated among vaccine recommendations for sport horses. Mares should be vaccinated during the last 6 wk of pregnancy and foals vaccinated at 5–8 wk of age. In high-risk areas, foals may be given tetanus antitoxin immediately after birth and every 2–3 wk until they are 3 mo old, at which time they can be given toxoid. The decision to vaccinate lambs or calves depends on the prevalence of the disease in the area. All animals that have recovered from tetanus should be regularly vaccinated. Animals surviving tetanus do not build a good immunity and should be vaccinated with tetanus toxoid.

All surgical procedures should be conducted with the best possible aseptic techniques. After surgery, animals should be turned out on clean ground, preferably grass pastures. Only oxidizing disinfectants such as iodine or chlorine dependably kill the spores.

CLOSTRIDIAL VACCINES

Vaccination is frequently practiced for protection of animals against clostridial diseases. A wide variety of vaccines is available, singly or in combinations that consist of bacterins, toxoids, or mixtures of bacterins and toxoids. Single vaccination with most clostridial vaccines does not provide adequate levels of protection and must be followed by a booster dose within 3–6 wk. Vaccination of young animals does not yield adequate protective immunity until they are at least 1–2 mo old. Therefore, most vaccination strategies target the pregnant dam so that maximal immunity is transferred to the neonate in colostrum. Most commercial vaccines are inactivated and usually contain 2-, 4-, 7-, or 8-way combinations of clostridial organisms/toxoids. These should be optimally timed for provision of maximal protection at the most likely age of susceptibility.

Tetanus toxoid is commonly used as a single vaccine in horses but is often used in combination in sheep, goats, and cattle. In sheep and goats, a common combination is tetanus toxoid plus *Clostridium perfringens* types C and D. In cattle, a combination frequently used in feedlots is a 4-way vaccine that consists of killed cultures of *C chauvoei*, *C septicum*, *C novyi*, and *C sordellii* to protect against blackleg and malignant edema. A more complex clostridial vaccine that contains *C perfringens* types C and D in addition to the components of the 4-way vaccine may be used to protect cattle against enterotoxemias as well. The addition of *C haemolyticum* extends the protection to include infectious bacillary hemoglobinuria. The clostridial vaccines often cause tissue reactions and swelling and should therefore be administered to cattle in the neck and by the SC rather than the IM route.

CONGENITAL AND INHERITED ANOMALIES

Embryonic and fetal development are the result of a complex series of well orchestrated events. When properly accomplished, the outcome is a healthy neonate. Errors in the sequential steps of development may be followed by embryonic loss, fetal death, fetal mummification, abortion, stillbirth, birth of nonviable neonates, or birth of viable offspring with defects. When a developmental disruption results in a deviation from normal that is present or apparent at birth, the defect is said to be congenital. Other developmental defects may not become apparent until later in life, and although the disruptive event occurred before birth, the defect is not strictly classified as congenital. Although the event or agent resulting in disrupted development remains undefined for many recognizable congenital conditions, technologic advances in the field of teratology have identified an increasing number of specific genetic, environmental, and infectious agents as etiologic determinants of certain cases of defective fetal development.

Teratogens are agents or factors that cause development of physical defects in the embryo or fetus. The timing of teratogenic exposure influences the eventual outcome. Although zygotes, the cells resulting from the union of gametes, are relatively resistant to the effects of most teratogens, they may be affected by chromosomal alterations or aberrations that occur during the process of gametogenesis or fertilization, as well as by genetic mutations that may be passed from one or both parents. As the zygote develops into the embryo and organogenesis progresses, susceptibility to environmental teratogens and teratogenic infectious agents increases. As the conceptus ages further, the fetus becomes increasingly resistant to environmental teratogens. Late-differentiating structures such as the palate, cerebellum, and urogenital system remain at risk well into the fetal period.

Similar, and perhaps indistinguishable, defects may be induced by more than one agent. Exposure to toxic or infectious agents at critical phases of embryonic or fetal development may induce congenital anomalies that closely resemble heritable conditions. With increased awareness of the importance of inherited anomalies by breeders and breed associations, practitioners and diagnosticians must be thorough in investigating cases, to avoid failing to recognize conditions that may be heritable and to avert improperly implicating breeding lines as a cause.

Structural and functional congenital defects have been described in all domestic species. Although congenital defects are often classified or described by the body system or part primarily involved, such classification systems are complicated by frequent simultaneous involvement of multiple body systems. Even so, descriptive classifications provide a basis for comparison and allow for estimation of the time of the disruptive event relative to fetal development, and sometimes etiology (*see* TABLE 2).

Etiology

Identification of molecular signals that guide sequential development of organs and organ systems, coupled with molecular diagnostic tools and genomic testing, allow a more detailed understanding of many observed congenital anomalies. It is likely that as these technologies improve, the etiology of other conditions will be clarified.

Chromosomal abnormalities occurring during gametogenesis or fertilization may result in embryo lethal anomalies or occasionally in abnormal but viable offspring. Errors in oogenesis can be associated with increased maternal age in several species and may result in failure of fertilization, reduced embryo viability, or in deficiencies expressed during fetal development. Chromosomal errors such as trisomy, in which there are three instances of a particular chromosome instead of the normal two, have been reported in veterinary medicine, and increasing availability of karyotyping and ancillary chromosomal analysis have increased recognition of these defects. Aging of gametes after suboptimal timing of insemination represents another source of chromosomal abnormality leading to errors in embryonic and fetal development. All cells of the defective embryo may be aneuploid (the presence of an abnormal number of chromosomes in a cell) or various degrees of mosaicism (the presence of two or more populations of cells with different genotypes in one individual who has developed from a single fertilized egg) may exist.

Chromosomal and epigenetic abnormalities may occur during assisted reproductive techniques that involve oocyte collection, culture, and fertilization. Bovine pregnancies resulting from somatic cell nuclear transfer or, to a lesser extent, from in vitro fertilization, are at increased risk of development of abnormal offspring syndrome due to failures in physiologic mechanisms necessary for proper fetal and placental development. These errors in development and placentation can result in fetal death, abortion, abnormally large or small birth weights, or birth of defective neonates, and are often associated with dystocia.

Inherited Defects

Inherited defects resulting from mutant genes present in breeding lines or families have been seen in all breeds. They may be expressed in typical patterns of inheritance such as the common simple autosomal recessive pattern typified by the recently described arthrogryposis multiplex anomaly of Angus cattle. Dominant defect traits are inherited as well and are sometimes selected for.

TABLE 2 SOME COMMON CONGENITAL DEFECTS OF DOMESTICATED ANIMALS

Amelia	Absence of a limb or limbs
Arthrogryposis	Persistent flexure or contracture of a joint or joints
Atresia	Absence or closure of a normal body opening or passage
Brachygnathia	Abnormally short lower jaw
Campylognathia	Curved jaw
Cheiloschisis	Abnormal division of the lip (harelip)
Cryptorchidism	Failure of the testis to descend into the scrotum
Hemimelia	Absence of all or part of the distal half of a limb
Hernia	Abnormal protrusion of an organ or portion of an organ through a defect or natural opening
Hydranencephaly	Virtual absence of cerebral hemispheres and replacement by CSF
Hydrocephalus	Abnormal fluid in the cranial vault accompanied by enlargement of the head
Kyphosis	Abnormally increased convexity of the thoracic spine
Microophthalmia	Abnormally small eye
Palatoschisis	Fissure of the palate (cleft palate)
Perosomus	Developmental anomaly characterized by a greatly deformed body or trunk
Polydactyly	Supernumerary digits
Porencephaly	The presence of cavities in the brain developed during fetal life
Prognathia	Marked projection of the lower jaw
Schistosomia	Developmental anomaly characterized by fissure of the abdominal wall
Scoliosis	Lateral deviation of the spinal axis
Syndactyly	Fusion of the digits
Thoracoschisis	Fissure of the thoracic wall, which may result in herniation of lung tissue

Some polygenetic defects require inclusion of more than one interacting gene. Rat tail syndrome, a congenital form of hypotrichosis in cattle, is controlled by genes at two interacting loci.

Because animals heterozygous for undesirable or lethal recessive traits often cannot be detected by visual examination, and sometimes exhibit a phenotype that is thought to be desirable, inadvertent selection may help spread genetic defects in a particular breed. For example, cattle heterozygous for tibial hemimelia reportedly have rear limb conformation and hair coat characteristics preferred by some breeders, and phenotypic selection of certain sires may have increased the allele frequency in the population. Similarly, while the Overo color pattern is attractive to some horse breeders, animals homozygous for this color pattern are often affected with a lethal congenital anomaly due to failure of intestinal tract innervation secondary to ileocolonic agangliosis. It is recommended to include only one Overo parent in a mating. The dominant inheritance of polledness in dairy goats is associated with coinheritance of a recessive allele that results in masculinization of homozygous females (the so-called polled intersex goat). Restrictive breeding programs that ensure at least one member of the breeding pair has horns are recommended to avoid this defect.

Heritable defects in metabolic function may result in embryonic or fetal death, birth of nonviable neonates, or birth of compromised offspring that survive. Such defects may be lethal in utero or early in the postnatal period, or animals may survive in a compromised form. Careful observation and diagnostic evaluation are required to properly identify these conditions and link them to pedigree information.

Deficiency of monophosphate synthase (DUMPS) is a lethal autosomal recessive trait formerly widely dispersed in Holstein cattle. When breeding of two DUMPS carriers results in a homozygous embryo, apparently normal fertilization and embryonic development is followed by death of the fetus in early gestation. Screening of sires destined for use in artificial insemination has successfully reduced the incidence of DUMPS.

Citrullinemia in cattle results in disruption of the urea cycle due to arginosuccinate synthetase deficiency and is lethal in the homozygous state. Affected calves appear healthy at birth but develop increased blood ammonia concentrations and die within a few days.

Defects found on the X chromosome, such as the one responsible for canine X-linked muscular dystrophy in Golden Retrievers, Labrador Retrievers, and other breeds, are expressed in males carrying only a single copy of a defective allele. Both parents are unaffected, with the dam carrying a single copy of the defective gene on an X chromosome.

For a partial list of inherited disorders with a known molecular basis, *see* TABLE 3.

Use of elite genetic lines in domestic species increased with the rapid and widespread adoption of reproductive technologies, particularly artificial insemination, embryo transfer, and in vitro fertilization. Dissemination of undetected genetic recessives to a large portion of the population domestically and internationally has been an inadvertent and unintended consequence. As the percentage of animals carrying undesirable recessive traits grows, an increased opportunity for breeding genetically related individuals is followed by the expression of the undesirable phenotype. Complex vertebral malformation in Holstein-Friesian dairy cattle was spread internationally primarily due to the influence of a single Holstein sire from the USA *and his offspring*. Similarly, arthrogryposis multiplex in Angus cattle received international attention due to the influence of a popular bull, his offspring, and descendants. In both cases, genetic testing developed after description of the condition provided breed associations and breeders opportunities to minimize the effects or eliminate the conditions.

By the time detrimental genetic conditions are recognized in a population or breed, the abnormal allele is often widely distributed. Early recognition and detection are desirable to minimize this possibility. All congenital anomalies should be investigated, and when a condition appears to have an underlying genetic component, appropriate techniques to assess pedigree information and identify the mutated homozygous phenotype should be explored. A structured system of reporting and recording, beginning with accurate clinical and pathologic descriptions, is necessary to centralize data and focus attention on physical and physiologic abnormalities that may be genetic in origin. Pedigree analysis and test mating of closely related animals coupled with recently developed DNA-based testing have the potential to identify specific genetic aberrations, in some cases relatively rapidly after recognition of the defect. Most breed associations have procedures to report congenital anomalies and work with pathologists, geneticists, and molecular biologists to identify emerging genetic defects.

Once known genetic recessive conditions are identified, several options exist to minimize their occurrence. For complex vertebral malformation, testing of all Holstein sires entering artificial insemination programs was chosen. Bulls were identified as being either carriers or free of the defect. The resulting decline in use of semen from carrier bulls led to a decrease in the occurrence of the condition and the allelic frequency within the breed. Other genetic recessive conditions in the same breed, including bovine leukocyte adhesion deficiency and DUMPS were handled similarly, and the recently identified brachyspina syndrome will likely be managed in the same manner. The extensive use of artificial insemination in dairy cattle allows this strategy to have a rapid impact.

In breeds or species with less use of artificial insemination, a more aggressive approach may be required. After recognition of arthrogryposis multiplex, the American Angus Association mandated testing and identification of all sires in active artificial insemination programs. They also required genetic testing to determine carrier status of all animals with suspect pedigrees submitted for registration. No certificate of registration will be issued to carrier animals born after a specified date. Similar requirements for

TABLE 3 CONGENITAL DISORDERS WITH A KNOWN MOLECULAR BASIS

Species	Disorder
Cat	Gangliosidosis (GM1, GM2) Mucopolysaccharidosis (I, VI, VII) Muscular dystrophy (Duchenne, Becker) α-Mannosidosis
Dog	C3 deficiency α-Fucosidosis Glycogen storage disease (I, VII) Hemophilia B Krabbe disease Leukocyte adhesion deficiency Mucopolysaccharidosis (I, VII) Muscular dystrophy (Becker, Duchenne [X-linked]) Myotonia Narcolepsy Nephritis, X-linked Pyruvate kinase deficiency of RBCs Rod-cone dysplasia Severe combined immunodeficiency Tremor, X-linked von Willebrand disease III
Cattle	Arthrogryposis multiplex (Angus, Angus-influenced breeds) Brachyspina syndrome (Holstein) Chédiak-Higashi syndrome Complex vertebral malformation (Holstein) Citrullinemia Deficiency of uridine monophosphate synthetase (Holstein) Ehlers-Danlos syndrome (II, V) Glycogen storage disease Goiter, familial (Holstein) Leukocyte adhesion deficiency α-Mannosidosis β-Mannosidosis Maple syrup urine disease Muscular hypertrophy (Shorthorn, Maine-Anjou) Pulmonary hypoplasia with anasarca (Shorthorn) Progressive degenerative myeloencephalopathy (Brown Swiss) Protoporphyria Spinal muscular atrophy (Brown Swiss) Syndactyly (Holstein, Angus) Tibial hemimelia (Shorthorn, Maine-Anjou)
Sheep	Ceroid lipofuscinosis Chondrodysplasia Glycogen storage disease IV
Goat	Goiter, familial β-Mannosidosis Mucopolysaccharidosis III Reduced casein concentration Polled intersex syndrome
Horse	Hyperkalemic periodic paralysis (Quarter horse, Paint, others) Megacolon Severe combined immunodeficiency (Arabians)
Pig	Hypercholesterolemia Malignant hyperthermia

animals with pedigrees tracing to carriers of neurogenic hydrocephalus have been put in place by this breed association. Extensive testing and identification of carrier individuals is used by the American Quarter Horse Association to minimize the incidence of hyperkalemic periodic paralysis.

As new genetic recessive abnormalities are identified and characterized, genetic tests to determine carrier status can be developed. Breed associations and breeders will adopt testing and identification strategies similar to those mentioned above. However, implementation of testing strategies will be more complicated for nonlethal defects and for conditions in which heterozygotes have a phenotype perceived as desirable.

Environmental Teratogens

Environmental teratogens include plant toxins, viruses, drugs, trace elements, nutritional deficiencies, and physical agents such as irradiation, hyperthermia, uterine positioning, and perhaps pressure during rectal examination for pregnancy. Although the defects produced in the neonate may resemble or mimic heritable defects, they do not follow a familial pattern. Specific causes may be difficult to identify but often follow seasonal patterns associated with growth characteristics of toxic plants or availability of suitable vectors of arthropodborne viruses. Although congenital anomalies may follow maternal disease due to plant intoxication or viral infection, teratogenic effects sometimes occur in the absence of observed clinical signs in the dam.

Biologically active products produced by many plants are known to be teratogens. (*See also* POISONOUS PLANTS, p 3103.) Ingestion may result in abortion, birth of nonviable neonates, or production of neonates that are abnormal at birth. Production losses can be significant if large numbers of animals gain access to affected plants at critical times in embryonic or fetal development. *Veratrum californicum* (skunk cabbage) has been implicated as a cause of fetal gigantism, prolonged gestation, and craniofacial deformities in sheep grazing rangelands containing the plant. Cyclopamine, a steroidal alkaloidal compound produced by the plant, is the teratogenic agent. Experimental dosing with this toxin in ewes on day 13–15 of pregnancy can cause a variety of congenital anomalies. Ingestion on day 14 specifically induces synophthalmia or cyclopean defect. Ewes exposed later in gestation may deliver healthy lambs, illustrating the critical interaction of time of exposure and gestational age.

In cattle, ingestion of several species of lupines (*Lupinus laxiflorus, L caudatus, L sericeus*, or *L nootkatensis*) has resulted in "crooked calf disease," characterized by joint contractures, torticollis, scoliosis or kyphosis, cleft palate, or combinations of these defects. The quinolizidine alkaloid anagyrine is identified as the teratogen, and the critical window for exposure is 40–70 days gestational age. Ingestion of *L formosus* causes similar skeletal defects and cleft palate in cattle and goats; the teratogen is the alkaloid piperidine. With either toxin, defects are thought to be related to an alkaloidal toxin–induced inhibition of fetal movement during critical gestational periods. Periodic losses due to lupine-induced crooked calf disease occur in the western USA after ingestion by cattle on rangeland.

Conium maculatum (poison hemlock) causes contracture defects and occasionally cleft palate in cattle, goats, sheep, and pigs. Both the plant and seed contain the teratogenic alkaloidal toxin coniine.

Ingestion of *Nicotiana tabacum* (cultivated tobacco) produces skeletal defects in pigs similar to those induced in cattle and pigs by *Lupinus* spp and *C maculatum*. Congenital amelia and hemimelia in piglets that occurred when pregnant sows were allowed access to tobacco stalks are seldom seen today due to changes in swine management. *Nicotiana glauca* (tree tobacco) also induces contracture defects and cleft palate in cattle, sheep, and goats.

Other plants suspected of causing similar defects in calves include *Senecio* spp, *Cycadales, Blighia, Papaveraceae, Colchicum, Vinca* spp, and *Indigofera spicata* and related plants. Sudan grass (*Sorghum vulgare*) has been incriminated as a cause of congenital joint contracture in horses, and *S sudanense* may cause arthrogryposis in calves.

Pregnant mares consuming fescue pasture or fescue hay infected with the fungal endophyte *Neotyphodium coenophialum* are at risk of abortion, prolonged gestation, hypogalactia, and delivery of weak or dysmature foals (*see* p 3016). Ergovaline and other ergot alkaloids produced by the endophyte are the cause of fescue toxicosis. Endophyte-free fescue and fescue infected by nontoxic strains of endophyte reportedly can be grazed safely by pregnant mares.

Congenital hypothyroidism in foals has been linked to increases of dietary nitrate concentrations in pregnant mares in western Canada and to dietary exposure of late gestation mares to *N coenophialum*–infected fescue.

Pesticides, herbicides, pharmaceutical agents, and other chemicals have been incriminated as teratogenic agents. Currently, drugs and chemicals undergoing approval processes in the USA, Canada, and many other countries must be tested for teratogenic potential before commercial licensing. Products may be labeled with instructions to specifically avoid use in animals that are pregnant or may be pregnant. Other products may be labeled as safe for pregnant animals once the fetus exceeds a specified gestational age. When using some herbicides, it may be necessary to withhold animals from pasture for specified periods after application. Extra-label use of pharmaceutical agents in pregnant animals and inadvertent exposure to pesticides and other chemicals carries inherent risks, including adverse effects on the developing fetus. Practitioners and producers should be aware of the potential for pregnancy loss or development of congenital anomalies after administration of therapeutic agents or exposure to pesticides and chemicals and should exercise appropriate caution when using such products.

Infectious Agents

Prenatal viral infections may be teratogenic in cattle, sheep, goats, pigs, dogs, and cats but have rarely been incriminated in congenital defects in horses. The stage of fetal or embryonic development at the time of exposure determines the type and extent of the anomalies observed. Viral infection in late gestation may result in fetal infection and seroconversion without observed clinical signs, while exposure during earlier stages may induce pregnancy loss or induce congenital defects.

Production of neonates with congenital anomalies after in utero infection may follow observable clinical disease in the dam; however, anomalies are also seen without history of disease during pregnancy. On occasion, use of modified-live virus vaccines in pregnant animals has produced congenital defects; such use is discouraged.

Pestivirus infections are teratogenic in many species. Bovine viral diarrhea virus (BVDV) is among the most economically significant infectious agents affecting cattle worldwide, and prenatal infection can cause a variety of congenital defects in survivors, including cerebellar hypoplasia, brachygnathia, alopecia, ocular defects, internal hydrocephalus, and impaired immunocompetence. Immunotolerant, persistently infected animals may result from fetal infection with noncytopathic BVDV before gestational day 120. These animals serve as a major reservoir of infection.

Pestivirus infections in other species also result in congenital defects. Infection of pregnant ewes with border disease virus (*see* p 622) may manifest as embryonic and fetal death or congenital defects involving the integumentary, nervous, skeletal, endocrine, and immune systems. Defects include tremors, ataxia, abnormal hair coat, low birth weight, facial and ocular abnormalities, depressed immune response, and birth of small, weak lambs with poor growth and viability. Infection of pregnant ewes with BVDV from cattle has produced identical congenital anomalies in sheep.

Classical swine fever (*see* p 713), a pestivirus infection of swine, was once known as hog cholera. The virus has been eradicated in the USA but remains a major cause of swine disease in some areas. Prenatal infection can result in congenital defects similar to those seen in cattle infected with BVDV.

Cache Valley virus infection of pregnant ewes may result in anomalies in their lambs, including arthrogryposis, torticollis, scoliosis, lordosis, hydranencephaly, microcephaly, porencephaly, and cerebellar and muscular hypoplasia. This bunyavirus is spread by mosquitoes and is found in the USA, Canada, and Mexico. Other ruminant species may be affected, and other bunyaviruses have been reported to cause similar congenital defects.

Bluetongue virus, an orbivirus endemic in many areas of North America, South America, Africa, and parts of Asia, has recently expanded its range in Europe. In utero exposure may induce hydranencephaly, porencephaly, and arthrogryposis in sheep, and it can result in abortion, stillbirths, arthrogryposis, campylognathia, prognathia, hydranencephaly, and "dummy calf" syndrome in cattle. Other orbiviruses such as Chuzan virus and perhaps epizootic hemorrhagic disease may cause abortion, congenital defects, and neonatal losses similar to bluetongue virus.

Akabane virus (*see* below), an orbivirus present in many tropical and subtropical areas, is spread by *Culicoides* spp (biting midges). Infection of naive animals can be followed by transplacental infection of the fetus and may produce deformities similar to those seen with viruses such as bluetongue and Cache Valley virus.

Congenital cerebellar hypoplasia in kittens has long been recognized as a result of infection of pregnant queens with feline panleukopenia virus. Infection of pregnant ferrets with feline panleukopenia virus also can result in congenital cerebellar hypoplasia.

Nutritional Factors

Deficiency of one or more nutrients during pregnancy may result in congenital defects in the newborn. Microminerals and vitamins are implicated in a variety of developmental defects. Severe deficiencies may interrupt pregnancy or result in weak or nonviable young.

Iodine deficiency may cause congenital goiter or cretinism in all species. Copper deficiency is a cause of enzootic ataxia in lambs. Manganese deficiency can result in congenital limb deformities in calves. Vitamin D deficiency may cause neonatal rickets, and vitamin A deficiency may cause eye defects or harelip. Experimentally, teratogenic effects have been induced by deficiencies of choline, riboflavin, pantothenic acid, cobalamin, and folic acid, and by hypervitaminosis A.

Physical Agents

Congenital joint contracture after birth of relatively large calves or foals, or associated with cases of twin pregnancy in these normally monotocous species, is a result of restricted motion due to uterine crowding. Many cases are mild and potentially self-correcting after birth.

Torticollis, scoliosis, and limb abnormalities in foals have been associated with intrauterine fetal positioning after transverse or caudal presentation. Pervious urachus in foals is reportedly associated with umbilical cord twisting.

In cattle, aggressive transrectal palpation of the amnionic vesicle before day 42 of gestation (eg, during pregnancy diagnosis) may disrupt vascular supply to the intestinal tract and induce atresia coli. Most cases of this malformation are seen in Holstein cattle, and a genetic predisposition may exist. At least one report suggests an autosomal recessive inheritance pattern for atresia coli.

Gestational Accidents of Unknown Etiology

In many cases of congenital anomalies, the etiology or predisposing factors remain unknown. Some specific anomalies of unknown etiology occur frequently enough to be readily recognized by veterinarians in the field.

Perosomus elumbis is a congenital anomaly that occurs primarily in cattle but also in small ruminants and swine. Affected calves have agenesis of segments of the lumbosacral spinal cord and vertebral column, with secondary hypoplasia, arthrogryposis, and ankylosis of the pelvic limbs. Other anomalies associated with development of the GI and urogenital systems accompany this condition. The body, limbs, and organs cranial to the developmental defect in the spinal cord appear normal. The condition is fatal, resulting in stillbirth or requiring euthanasia on humane grounds. Dystocia is a frequent complication. Although there are suggestions of inheritance, no definitive cause is recognized. Aberrations in the homeobox gene family, responsible for cranial to caudal patterning, may be involved.

Schistosomus reflexus, a fatal congenital disorder seen in ruminants, is characterized by severe retroflexion of the spinal column, resulting in positioning of the hindlimbs adjacent to the skull, ankylosis of appendicular joints, and failure of closure of the abdominal wall with consequential presence of abdominal viscera outside the body. Other anomalies, including thoracoschisis, may accompany the condition. The presence of an affected fetus results in dystocia, frequently requiring surgical intervention or fetotomy. Some reports utilizing pedigree analysis suggest a genetic etiology, but no specific defect or mode of inheritance has been found. Interestingly, cases involving one affected calf and a healthy co-twin have been reported.

Fetal anasarca is a fatal anomaly seen in several breeds of dogs. The cause remains unknown and may vary from breed to breed. This condition frequently results in dystocia due to the disproportionately large fetus at term. Single or multiple pups within a litter may be affected.

AKABANE VIRUS INFECTION

Akabane is an insect-transmitted virus that causes congenital abnormalities of the CNS in ruminants. Disease due to Akabane virus has been recognized in Australia, Israel, Japan, and Korea; antibodies to it have been found in a number of countries in southeast Asia, the Middle East, and Africa. The disease affects fetuses of cattle, sheep, and goats. Asymptomatic infection has been demonstrated serologically in horses, buffalo, deer, and pigs (but not in people) in endemic areas.

Etiology, Epidemiology, and Transmission: The causal agent, Akabane virus, is an orthobunyavirus and member of the Simbu serogroup of the family Bunyaviridae. It is spread by biting midges (*Culicoides* spp) in Australia, Japan, and Kenya.

Akabane virus is common in many tropical and subtropical areas between ~35°N and 35°S. In these endemic areas, herbivores are bitten by the vectors, become infected at an early age, and develop a long-lasting immunity by the time of breeding; thus, congenital abnormalities are seldom seen. However, under favorable environmental conditions such as an extended humid summer, the vector (and hence the virus) may spread beyond its usual range into new areas, and outbreaks of congenital infection may be expected. These outbreaks usually occur at the northern or southern limits of the vector distribution or in areas of higher altitude. Similarly, pregnant ruminants from virus- and vector-free areas moved to virus-infected areas are at risk.

The incidence of Akabane virus–induced disease is influenced by the time of gestation at which infection occurs and by the strain of virus. Infections in cattle during the last 3 mo of pregnancy result in a relatively low incidence of disease (5%–10% of calves are affected). The peak incidence is seen after infection in the third and fourth months, when up to 40% of calves may be born with defects. Some strains of Akabane virus produce a very low incidence of abnormalities (<20%) even at the most susceptible stages of gestation, whereas the most severe can cause disease in up to 80% of infected animals.

In sheep and goats, disease is seen but the distinct sequential manifestation of different abnormalities seen in cattle does not occur because of the shorter period of gestation and the shorter period of susceptibility. Most abnormalities develop after infection between days 28–56 of gestation. Few, if any, abnormalities are seen after infection at other times. However, it is not known whether infection in large or small ruminants very early in gestation results in lethal infection, with abortion of the fetus.

Clinical Findings and Lesions: The clinical signs and pathology of Akabane virus infection depend on the species of animal and time of infection. In a herd of cattle with an extended or year-round calving period, the full range of abnormalities may be seen. The most severe defects are seen after susceptible cows have been infected between ~80–150 days of gestation; however, calves can be affected at most times after the first 2 mo of gestation. Calves infected late in pregnancy may be born alive but unable to stand and may have a flaccid paralysis of the limbs, or may be incoordinated and on necropsy show a disseminated encephalomyelitis. Those infected earlier (120–180 days of gestation) have rigid fixation of limbs, usually in flexion (arthrogryposis), and sometimes also torticollis, kyphosis, and scoliosis with associated neurogenic muscle atrophy due to loss of spinal motor neurons. These abnormalities usually cause dystocia and can result in severe obstetric complications, sometimes resulting in infertility and even death of cows. The first calves born with arthrogryposis are less severely affected than those born during the next 4–6 wk. Initially, only one or two joints may be affected on a single limb, but later cases can have severe fixation of multiple joints on several or all limbs. Calves infected at 80–120 days of gestation are usually born alive and, if able to stand, walk poorly and are depressed and blind. These calves have varying degrees of cavitation of cerebral hemispheres, ranging from porencephaly to severe hydranencephaly. The latter is common, especially among those infected in the earlier stages of pregnancy. Some calves may be affected with both arthrogryposis and hydranencephaly. Calves with severe hydranencephaly may be aborted in midgestation. A useful differential diagnostic feature is the virtual absence of either gross or histologic lesions in the cerebellum, distinguishing Akabane virus infection from other teratogenic viruses such as bovine viral diarrhea virus (BVDV, *see* p 267). Infrequently, strains of Akabane virus are encountered that cause disease when calves are infected in the first few weeks of life. A range of neurologic signs and pathology consistent with an acute viral encephalitis may be seen. In Japan, strains of Akabane virus that cause disease in adult cattle have also been described.

In small ruminants, the lesions of arthrogryposis and hydranencephaly are often seen concurrently and are common in the same animals. In lambs and kids, a range of other defects may occur, including pulmonary hypoplasia and hypoplasia of the spinal cord. Most Akabane-infected lambs or kids are stillborn or die soon after birth. Abortions are also seen.

Akabane virus–induced congenital abnormalities (especially arthrogryposis and hydranencephaly) have been suspected in horses, but laboratory confirmation has been inconclusive.

Diagnosis: A presumptive diagnosis can be made on the gross CNS lesions, but the disease must be differentiated from other infectious and genetic conditions. Infection can be confirmed by testing sera or body fluids (eg, pericardial or pleural fluid) from unsuckled, affected offspring and their dams for antibodies against Akabane virus. While the detection of antibody in maternal serum does not confirm Akabane as an etiologic agent, its absence is definitive for exclusion.

Other vectorborne viruses (and also non-vectorborne viruses such as BVDV) can cause congenital defects identical to those of Akabane virus. Aino virus, a relative of Akabane, is found in Australia, Japan, and several other countries where Akabane virus is found and has been an infrequent cause of disease in cattle. In late 2011, Schmallenberg, a newly recognized orthobunyavirus, spread throughout most of western Europe and extended to the UK and also north to Scandinavian countries. This Simbu virus caused disease indistinguishable from Akabane infection in sheep, although the incidence of congenital defects was generally low compared with that caused by Akabane virus. Disease was occasionally seen in cattle but at a very low prevalence. In Japan, Chuzan virus, a reovirus, is transmitted by *Culicoides oxystoma* and causes congenital infection in calves similar to Akabane virus. In the USA, Cache Valley virus, another vectorborne bunyavirus unrelated to Akabane virus, has been associated with congenital defects in sheep and perhaps cattle in some states.

Treatment and Control: There is no specific treatment for animals affected by Akabane virus infection. Measures should be directed at the prevention of infection of susceptible animals with Akabane virus during pregnancy. Introduction of stock from nonendemic to endemic areas should be done well before first breeding. Effective vaccines are available in Japan.

BORDER DISEASE

(Hairy shaker disease)

Border disease (Britain) or hairy shaker disease (Australia and New Zealand) is a congenital disorder of lambs characterized by low birth weight and viability, poor conformation, tremor, and an excessively hairy birth coat in normally smooth-coated breeds. Goat kids may also be affected, and a similar condition occasionally occurs in calves. The disease has been recognized in most sheep-rearing areas of the world, including the western USA. There are currently seven recognized genotypes (BDV-1 to BDV-7) for the border disease virus.

Etiology, Pathogenesis, and Epidemiology: Border disease is caused by infection of the fetus in early pregnancy with a pestivirus (Flaviviridae) closely related to the viruses of classical swine fever (*see* p 713) and bovine viral diarrhea/mucosal disease (*see* p 267). Surviving lambs are persistently viremic, and the virus is present in their excretions and secretions, including semen. Cattle, goats, and pigs are also susceptible to infection with border disease virus. Persistently infected individuals have been demonstrated in all of the aforementioned species from natural in-utero infection. Transmission of border disease virus to cattle can occur from commingled grazing with persistent or acutely infected sheep. Acute infections in immunocompetent animals are usually transient and subclinical and result in immunity to challenge with homologous but not heterologous strains of virus.

Virus acquired in early pregnancy by previously unexposed animals crosses the placenta and invades the fetus. Placentitis occurs 10–30 days after infection and may cause fetal death with expulsion, resorption, or mummification. Abortion may occur at any stage of pregnancy and may pass unnoticed because there is little maternal malaise.

In sustained pregnancies, the virus becomes widely distributed in fetal tissues, but pathologic changes are most obvious in the skin, skeleton, and CNS. Affected lambs may be born 2–3 days early, and many die before or at weaning. In survivors, the clinical signs gradually regress, but such animals remain persistently infected and excrete virus for the remainder of their lives, exposing their progeny and flockmates. Death from a syndrome similar to bovine mucosal disease may occur in these clinically "recovered" hairy-shaker sheep at any time.

In naive flocks exposed to bovine viral diarrhea virus (BVDV), up to 50% or more of lambs born may be affected with border disease. Thereafter, the prevalence declines, although the disease may become endemic when "recovered" lambs are retained for breeding. The virus is most commonly introduced into susceptible flocks by the addition of persistently infected sheep or pregnant ewes carrying an infected fetus. However, sheep can also acquire infection from transiently or persistently infected cattle. For practical purposes, it should be assumed that sheep and cattle are equally susceptible to all strains of border disease virus and BVDV, even though at least four phylogenetic groups of pestiviruses have been identified in domestic ruminants.

Clinical Findings: Affected flocks probably are recognized first at lambing time by an increase in the number of barren ewes and in the birth of undersized lambs with excessively hairy and sometimes excessively pigmented fleece. Skeletal abnormalities that may be seen in newborn lambs include a decreased crown-rump length, shortened tibia and radius, and a shortened longitudinal axis of the cranium. Some lambs exhibit involuntary muscular tremors, particularly of the trunk and hindlegs. The tremors are reduced at rest and exacerbated by purposeful movement. In others, skeletal defects such as dropped pasterns and mandibular brachygnathia may predominate. Affected lambs have a poor survival rate. In survivors, nervous signs gradually disappear within 3–4 mo. Even in the absence of typical hairy-shaker lambs, outbreaks of low fertility in ewes and poor viability and ill-thrift in lambs may be associated with border disease virus infection.

Lesions: In severe cases, abnormal development of the cerebrum may be seen at necropsy, resulting in hydrocephalus, hydranencephaly, porencephaly, or microcephaly. Cerebellar hypoplasia or cerebellar dysplasia may also occur. Otherwise, the characteristic lesions are microscopic and involve the white matter of the CNS. There is a deficiency of myelin and an increase in interfascicular glial cells, in which myelin-like lipid droplets may accumulate. These changes are most obvious in the newborn and gradually resolve.

Diagnosis: Clinical findings usually allow a diagnosis, although abnormal hairiness of the birth coat may not be apparent in rough-coated breeds of sheep. The diagnosis can be confirmed by histologic demonstration of the pathognomonic lesions in the CNS and with immunocytochemical staining of the virus. In typical hairy-shaker lambs, the virus or viral antigen may be demonstrated readily in blood and tissues by virus isolation, fluorescent antibody tests, immunohistochemistry, or PCR. When testing blood in newborn lambs, precolostral blood is ideal because colostral antibody can mask virus for up to 2 mo. Virus can be isolated from serum or buffy coat cells in cell cultures, but a viral antigen detection ELISA using heparinized or EDTA blood is available. Reverse transcriptase-PCR can also be used to detect viral RNA in clinical specimens and to type ruminant pestiviruses.

Other causes of ovine abortion (eg, bluetongue, *Chlamydia*, listeriosis, *Salmonella*, *Campylobacter*, *Rickettsia* spp, *Toxoplasma gondii*, and Akabane virus) should be considered in the differential diagnosis. In live-born lambs, border disease must be differentiated from swayback (enzootic ataxia), bacterial meningoencephalitis, focal symmetric encephalomalacia, and "daft lamb" disease.

Control: There is no effective treatment for persistently infected lambs. Bulk tank milk samples can be tested for antibodies to BVDV to screen for the presence of virus within dairy sheep flocks. Serology should be performed on the dams of affected lambs. Most should have high levels of antibody and be immune to further challenge with the same strain of virus in subsequent pregnancies. Those that do not have antibody titers should be screened for virus to identify any that are persistently infected. Recovered lambs should not be retained for breeding but can be mixed with replacement stock well before breeding season to maximize opportunities for the latter to become infected and develop immunity before subsequent matings. There is no effective vaccine. BVDV vaccines for cattle cannot be recommended for use in sheep, because border disease viruses most commonly isolated from sheep are antigenically distinct from BVDV most common in cattle.

COXIELLOSIS

Coxiellosis is a zoonotic bacterial infection associated primarily with parturient ruminants, although domestic animals such as cats and a variety of wild animals have been identified as sources of human infection. The zoonotic infection in people associated with *Coxiella burnetii* is widely known as Q fever. Coxiella is considered a potential agent of bioterrorism because of its low infectious dose, stability in the environment, and capability for aerosol dispersion.

Etiology, Epidemiology, and Transmission: Coxiellosis is caused by the gram-negative coccobacillus *C burnetii*. Although classically considered a rickettsial agent, recent phylogenetic analyses suggest that *C burnetii* is more closely related to *Legionella* and *Francisella* than to the genus *Rickettsia*. It resides and reproduces in the acidified phagolysosomes of host monocytes and macrophages. Two forms exist: the large cell variant is a vegetative form found in infected cells, and the small cell variant is the extracellular infectious form shed in milk, urine, and feces and found in high concentration (10^9 ID_{50}/g) in placental tissue and amniotic fluid. The small cell variant is resistant to heat, drying, and many common disinfectants and remains viable for weeks to years in the environment. Once a domestic ruminant is infected, *C burnetii* can localize in mammary glands, supramammary lymph nodes, placenta, and uterus, from which it may be shed in subsequent parturitions and lactations.

The epidemiology of *C burnetii* is complex because there are two major patterns of transmission. In one, the organism circulates between wild animals and their ectoparasites, mainly ticks; the other occurs in domestic ruminants, independent of the wild animal cycle. Ixodid and argasid ticks can act as reservoirs of the organism. Distribution is worldwide (except New Zealand), and the host range includes various wild and domestic mammals, arthropods, and birds. The disease is enzootic in most areas where cattle, sheep, and goats are kept. In the USA, seroprevalence studies have shown significant variability in prevalence of antibodies to *C burnetii* based on difference in test population, test used, and time of year. Evaluation of bulk tank milk sampling of USA cattle dairies has demonstrated prevalence of the organism at the farm level of 77% to >90%. In a comprehensive seroprevalence study conducted in Canada, 48.6% of sheep operations and 63.2% of goat operations had at least one positive animal. Not surprisingly, seroprevalence in veterinarians and small ruminant farmers is also high.

The greatest risk of transmission occurs at parturition by inhalation, ingestion, or direct contact with birth fluids or placenta. The organism is also shed in milk, urine, and feces. High-temperature pasteurization effectively kills the organism. Ticks may transmit the disease among domestic ruminants but are not thought to play an epidemiologically important role in transmission of disease to people.

Clinical Findings and Diagnosis: Infection in ruminants is usually subclinical but can cause anorexia and late abortion. When infection is subclinical, animals shed much lower bacterial loads of the organism than when abortion occurs. Reports have implicated *C burnetii* as a cause of infertility and sporadic abortion with a necrotizing placentitis in ruminants. New evidence has shown an association of *C burnetii* with subclinical mastitis among dairy cows, although additional work regarding causality is required before this can be considered clinically valid. Experimental infection in cats causes transient fever, dullness, and anorexia lasting several days.

In domestic ruminants, gross lesions are nonspecific, and differential diagnosis should include infectious and noninfectious agents that cause abortion. Immunofluorescence test on paired sera taken ≥2 wk apart can be used to detect recent infection; however, shedding of *C burnetii* may occur in the absence of a measurable serum antibody titer in up to 20% of infected animals. Culture, immunohistochemical, and PCR tests may be used to identify *C burnetii* in tissues. Studies conducted in veterinary diagnostic laboratories suggest that *C burnetii* is often found concurrently with other organisms isolated in cases of infectious abortions, so mixed infections may be important. Seasonal variability in shedding of the organism hinders interpretation of a single PCR test. Shedding is highest in the periparturient period and may drop below detectable levels for a significant period during the year despite persistent infection.

Treatment and Control: Q fever in people is a notifiable disease in the USA, primarily because of its status as a possible bioterrorism agent; reporting requirements for animals vary by state. Vaccines for people and animals have been developed but are not commercially available in the USA. Vaccination has prevented infection when administered to uninfected calves and has improved fertility and reduced shedding in previously infected animals.

There is little evidence-based data to suggest that antibiotic treatment in animals provides significant benefit. Human clinical disease is typically treated with tetracyclines, but significant benefit from tetracycline treatment has not been demonstrated in controlled studies in abortion outbreaks of sheep in Europe. Despite the lack of evidence, some practitioners still advocate the use of parenteral tetracyclines during abortion storms. In known infected herds, the periparturient period represents a significant risk period for transmission because of the large amount of environmental contamination associated with abortion. Standard abortion control measures, including prompt removal of aborted materials (using zoonotic precautions), segregation of animals by pregnancy status, and diagnostic evaluation of abortions, are all warranted.

Zoonotic Risk: Q fever occurs more frequently in persons who have occupational contact with high-risk species. The clinical presentation in people is highly variable clinically, ranging from a self-limiting, influenza-like illness to pneumonia, hepatitis, and endocarditis. *C burnetii* is highly infectious, and a single organism can reportedly cause infection via the aerosol route in people. Individuals who have artificial heart valves are at particular risk, as well as anyone who is significantly immunocompromised. *C burnetii* has been associated with human abortions, and pregnant women should take precautions to prevent exposure.

The majority of outbreaks in people have been associated with wind dispersion of desiccated reproductive products, contaminated with *C burnetii*, from sites where sheep, goats, or cattle are kept. Farmers and veterinarians are at risk while assisting birthing. Slaughterhouse workers are at risk from contact with infected carcasses, hair, and wool. Transmission may also occur by consumption of unpasteurized milk. Handling of infected tissue poses a threat to laboratory personnel. Q fever has been seen in personnel and human patients in medical institutions where latently infected sheep were used for research. Medical facilities using ruminants in research should attempt to purchase animals from flocks free of coxiellosis or use male animals when possible. In addition, workers should use adequate personal protective equipment to protect against small droplet and aerosol exposure during high-risk medical procedures.

ERYSIPELOTHRIX RHUSIOPATHIAE INFECTION

(Erysipelas, Nonsuppurative polyarthritis, Postdipping lameness)

Erysipelothrix rhusiopathiae is a significant bacterial pathogen of swine, turkeys, and sheep. It is distributed worldwide and has also been isolated from cattle, horses, dogs, cats, mice, rats, fresh and saltwater fish, domestic poultry, and a variety of wild birds and mammals. Erysipeloid, a condition characterized by localized skin infections and cellulitis, may develop in people who work with infected animals, infected carcasses, or infected animal byproducts.

The bacterium can survive in the soil for up to 5 wk; however, soil is not an effective growth medium, and the organism is unable to survive for extended periods of time in the environment. Soil and surface water contamination represent routes of exposure. Asymptomatic carriers are the usual source of infectious organisms, but the bacteria may also be introduced to animal production units by surface water runoff, wild mammals, wild birds, pets, and biting insects. *E rhusiopathiae* has food safety implications, because it can survive for several months in animal tissues such as frozen or chilled pork, cured and smoked ham, and feed byproducts such as dried blood.

E rhusiopathiae is a nonmotile, gram-positive, facultative anaerobic bacillus. It is catalase negative, coagulase positive, oxidase negative, resistant to high salt concentrations, and produces H_2S on triple sugar iron media. Colonies of *E rhusiopathiae* are either smooth or rough, with rough colonies being slightly larger, with irregular edges. On agar media, colonies are clear, circular, and very small (0.1–1.5 mm in diameter) after 24 hr of incubation, but they increase in size after 48 hr.

The organism is very hardy and can survive and grow in a wide range of pH and environmental temperatures. *E rhusiopathiae* has demonstrated the ability to resist the action of several classes of disinfectants used in animal production units, including alcohols, aldehydes, oxidizing agents, and phenols. Classes of disinfectants and/or compounds considered to effectively inactivate *E rhusiopathiae* include hypochlorites (bleach) and caustic soda (lye; NaOH). The organism is sensitive to the β-lactam (penicillin, ampicillin), cephalosporin (ceftiofur), and tetracycline classes of antibiotics and is resistant to sulfonamides.

SWINE ERYSIPELAS

Infectious disease caused by *Erysipelothrix rhusiopathiae* in pigs is known as erysipelas and is one of the oldest recognized diseases that affect growing and adult swine. Up to 50% of pigs in intensive swine production areas are considered to be colonized with *E rhusiopathiae*. The organism commonly resides in the tonsillar tissue. These typical healthy carriers can shed the organism in their feces or oronasal secretions and are an important source of infection for other pigs.

Disease outbreaks may be acute or chronic, and clinically inapparent infections also occur. Acute outbreaks are characterized by sudden and unexpected deaths, febrile episodes, painful joints, and skin lesions that vary from generalized cyanosis to the often-described diamond skin (rhomboid urticaria) lesions. Chronic erysipelas tends to follow acute outbreaks and is characterized by enlarged joints and lameness. A second form of chronic erysipelas is vegetative valvular endocarditis. Pigs with valvular lesions may exhibit few clinical signs; however, when exerted physically they may show signs of respiratory distress, lethargy, and cyanosis, and possibly suddenly succumb to the infection.

Etiology: Growth of *E rhusiopathiae* on nonenriched media produces pinpoint, nonhemolytic colonies after incubation for 24 hr. After 48 hr of incubation, a zone of incomplete hemolysis becomes evident around colonies. The genus of *Erysipelothrix* is subdivided into two major species: *E rhusiopathiae* and *E tonsillarum*. In addition, there are other strains that constitute one or more additional species known as *E* species 1, *E* species 2, *E* species 3, and *E inopinata*. At least 28 different serotypes of *Erysipelothrix* spp are recognized, and pigs are considered to be susceptible to at least 15. Field cases of swine erysipelas are predominately caused by *E rhusiopathiae* serotypes 1a, 1b, or 2.

On farms where the organism is endemic, pigs are exposed naturally to *E rhusiopathiae* when they are young. Maternal-derived antibodies provide passive immunity and suppress clinical disease. Older pigs tend to develop protective active immunity as a result of exposure to the organism, which does not necessarily lead to clinical disease. *E rhusiopathiae* is excreted by infected pigs in feces and oronasal secretions, effectively contaminating the environment. When ingested, the organism can survive passage through the hostile environment of the stomach and intestines and may remain viable in the feces for several months. Recovered pigs and chronically infected pigs may become carriers of *E rhusiopathiae*. Healthy swine also may be asymptomatic carriers. Infection is by ingestion of contaminated feed, water, or feces and through skin abrasions.

Clinical Findings: The acute and chronic forms of swine erysipelas may occur in sequence or separately. Pigs that succumb to the acute septicemic form may die suddenly without previous clinical signs. This form occurs most frequently in growing and finishing pigs. Acutely infected pigs are depressed, febrile (104°–108°F [40°–42°C]), and reluctant to stand and move. Affected pigs squeal excessively when handled, require assistance to stand, and prefer to lie down soon after being forced to stand. Affected pigs may also walk stiffly on their toes and shift weight from limb to limb when standing. Anorexia and thirst are common, and febrile pigs will often seek wet, cool areas to lie down. Skin discoloration may vary from widespread erythema and purplish discoloration of the ears, snout, and abdomen, to diamond-shaped skin lesions almost anywhere on the body, but particularly on the lateral and dorsal regions. The lesions may occur as discrete, pink or purple areas of varying size that become raised and firm to the touch within 2–3 days of illness. They may disappear over the course of a week or progress to a more chronic type of lesion, commonly referred to as diamond skin disease. If untreated, necrosis and separation of large areas of skin can occur, and the tips of the ears and tail may become necrotic and slough.

Clinical disease is usually sporadic and affects individuals or small groups, but sometimes larger outbreaks occur. Mortality is variable (0–100%), and death may occur up to 6 days after the first signs of illness. Acutely affected pregnant sows may abort, probably due to the fever, and lactating sows may show agalactia. Untreated pigs may develop the chronic form of the disease, usually characterized by chronic arthritis, vegetative valvular endocarditis, or both. Such lesions may also be seen in pigs with no previous signs of septicemia. Valvular endocarditis is most common in mature or young adult pigs and is frequently manifest by death, usually from embolism or cardiac insufficiency. Chronic arthritis, the most common form of chronic infection, produces mild to severe lameness. Affected joints may be difficult to detect initially but eventually become hot and painful to the touch and later visibly enlarged. Dark purple, necrotic skin lesions that commonly slough may be seen. Mortality in chronic cases is low, but growth rate is retarded.

Lesions: At necropsy, acutely infected pigs may exhibit skin lesions, enlarged and congested lymph nodes, edematous and congested lungs, splenomegaly, and hepatomegaly. Petechial hemorrhages may be seen on the kidneys and heart.

In chronic erysipelas, valvular endocarditis is seen as proliferative, granular growths on the heart valves, and embolisms and infarctions may develop. Arthritis may involve joints of one or more legs, and the intervertebral articulations may be involved. Affected joints may be enlarged, with proliferative, villous synovitis and increased viscosity of synovial fluid, inflammatory exudates, and thickening of the joint capsule. Proliferation and erosion of articular cartilage may result in fibrosis and ankylosis of the joint.

Diagnosis: Diagnosis of erysipelas is based on clinical signs, gross lesions, response to antimicrobial therapy, and demonstration of the bacterium or DNA in tissues from affected animals. Acute erysipelas can be difficult to diagnose in individual pigs showing only fever, poor appetite, and listlessness. However, in outbreaks involving several animals, the presence of skin lesions and lameness is likely to be seen in at least some cases and would support a clinical diagnosis. Rhomboid urticaria or diamond skin lesions are almost diagnostic when present; however, similar lesions can also be seen with classical swine fever virus infection (*see* p 713), *Actinobacillus suis* septicemia, or the porcine dermatitis and nephropathy syndrome. Isolation of *E rhusiopathiae* from blood of affected pigs, especially after enrichment, is possible in acute cases and helps establish a diagnosis. In addition, molecular methods capable of detecting *E rhusiopathiae* DNA in affected tissues or blood (ie, PCR assays) can also be used. Recently, immunohistochemical methods to demonstrate the organisms in formalin-fixed paraffin-embedded tissues have become available and are useful in cases when pigs have been treated with antimicrobials before sample submission. A rapid, positive response to penicillin therapy in affected pigs supports a diagnosis of acute erysipelas because of the sensitivity of the organism to penicillin.

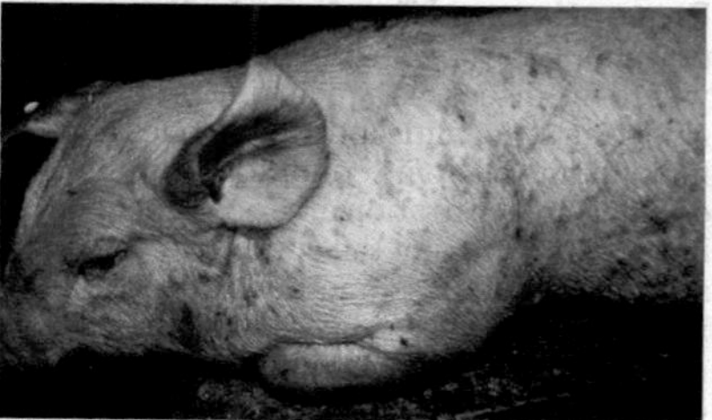

Acute, severe skin form of swine erysipelas with extensive small, raised, pink/red lesions and some developing dark scabs. *Courtesy of Dr. Ranald D. A. Cameron.*

Chronic erysipelas can be difficult to definitively diagnose. Arthritis and lameness, coupled with the presence of vegetative valvular endocarditis postmortem, may support a presumptive diagnosis of chronic erysipelas. However, these lesions can be caused by other infectious agents. A positive culture of valvular vegetations or demonstration of *E rhusiopathiae* DNA in the lesions by PCR is definitive for diagnosing chronic erysipelas.

Serologic tests cannot reliably diagnose erysipelas but can be useful to determine previous exposure or success of vaccination protocols, because antibody titers should increase after vaccination. For this purpose, ELISAs and complement fixation tests are available in selected laboratories.

Differential diagnoses to consider include conditions that can precipitate gross lesions suggestive of acute septicemia. Septicemic salmonellosis due to *Salmonella* Choleraesuis infection, classical swine fever due to pestivirus infection, and septicemia and endocarditis due to *Streptococcus suis* infection should be considered, based on similarity of lesions. Glasser's disease (*see* p 720) due to *Haemophilus parasuis* infection and *Mycoplasma hyosynoviae* infection can precipitate similar changes in synovial tissues and joints of affected pigs.

Treatment: *E rhusiopathiae* is sensitive to penicillin. Ideally, affected pigs should be treated at 12-hr intervals for a minimum of 3 days, although longer durations of therapy may be necessary to resolve severe infections. On an economic basis, penicillin is the best choice for antibiotic therapy, but ampicillin and ceftiofur also yield satisfactory results in acute cases. When injecting large numbers of affected pigs is impractical, tetracyclines delivered in the feed or water may be useful. Fever associated with acute infections can be managed by administration of NSAIDs such as flunixin meglumine or by delivery of aspirin in the water. Erysipelas antiserum is described as an effective adjunct to antibiotic therapy in treating acute outbreaks but is not commonly available. Treatment of chronic infections is usually ineffective and not cost effective.

Prevention: Vaccination against *E rhusiopathiae* is very effective in controlling disease outbreaks on swine farms and should be encouraged. Cessation of vaccination on some farms has been linked to disease outbreaks. Injectable bacterins and attenuated, live vaccines delivered via the water are available and provide extended duration of immunity. Optimal timing of vaccination may vary from farm to farm. When *E rhusiopathiae* is endemic in the production environment, vaccination should precede anticipated outbreaks. Susceptible pigs may be vaccinated before weaning, at weaning, or several weeks after weaning. Male and female swine selected for addition to the breeding herd should be vaccinated with a booster 3–5 wk later. Thereafter, breeding stock should be vaccinated twice yearly. Vaccines should not be administered to animals undergoing antibiotic therapy, because antibiotics can interfere with the subsequent immune response to the vaccine.

Vaccination failures may occur in some herds due to management stresses that compromise the immune system of vaccinated pigs. Antigenic differences between serotypes in vaccines and serotypes circulating on farms can also result in incomplete immunity and disease outbreaks, but this is a rare event because there is good cross-protection among the major *E rhusiopathiae* strains infecting pigs.

In addition to vaccination, attention to sanitation and hygiene and elimination of pigs with clinical signs suggestive of erysipelas infection represent other viable methods that may help control the disease on swine farms.

NONSUPPURATIVE POLYARTHRITIS IN LAMBS

Nonsuppurative polyarthritis is an infectious condition of older, growing lambs (6–16 wk old) characterized by high morbidity and moderate to severe lameness with enlargement of affected joints.

Etiology: The infectious agent of nonsuppurative polyarthritis, *Erysipelothrix rhusiopathiae*, is thought to infect the animal through wounds created as a result of tail docking and castration procedures. However, outbreaks may also occur after "bloodless" procedures, particularly during extended periods of wet weather, which increases the level of stress and appears to enhance the survivability of the organism in the environment. *E rhusiopathiae* localizes in joints via hematogenous dissemination and infects the synovial membrane. Progression of the synovial infection results in synovitis and damage to articular cartilage and underlying subchondral bone.

Clinical Findings and Lesions: Sudden onset of moderate to severe lameness in a high number of growing lambs is suggestive of nonsuppurative polyarthritis. Lameness typically occurs in two or more limbs, and the joints most often affected are the carpus and hock. Affected lambs are reluctant to move and spend extended periods of time in sternal recumbency. Growth is often severely depressed. Progression of the condition results in proliferation of the synovial membrane, thickening of the joint capsule without significant joint effusion, and eventual erosion of articular cartilage.

Diagnosis: Sudden onset of lameness in a large number of growing-age lambs is suggestive of polyarthritis due to *E rhusiopathiae*. Because joint effusions are minimal, attempts to obtain a sample from affected joints for culture and other diagnostics may be unsuccessful.

Prevention and Treatment: Vaccination should be considered on premises where the disease is a recurring problem. Adopting strict antiseptic techniques and maintaining hygienic conditions for tail docking and castration are recommended but may not prevent the condition. The so-called "bloodless" methods of performing both procedures may reduce the chances of wound contamination, but outbreaks are still possible. Administration of penicillin for 5 days is recommended for effective treatment of the nonsuppurative polyarthritis. Administration of NSAIDs helps improve lameness.

POSTDIPPING LAMENESS IN SHEEP

Postdipping lameness affects lambs and adult sheep. It is characterized by severe lameness that results from infection caused by the penetration of *Erysipelothrix rhusiopathiae* through skin abrasions in the hoof. Postdipping lameness, which normally occurs in outbreaks, has been described in most sheep-raising countries. Because of the reduced usage of sheep dips in recent years, this manifestation is seen less frequently now.

Etiology: With time and repeated use, dipping solutions, which have little or no bacteriostatic activity, become heavily contaminated with various species of bacteria. *E rhusiopathiae* is a common contaminant, and its presence in the dipping vat, sometimes in enormous numbers, leads to infection of skin wounds during dipping. Small skin abrasions in the region of the hoof and fetlock joint are a common portal of entry. Lesions extending from these wounds to the laminae of the hoof cause acute postdipping lameness. Outbreaks may also occur when sheep must walk through wet and muddy areas that are heavily contaminated with the organism.

Clinical Findings: Two to 4 days after dipping, a variable number (up to 90%, but usually ~25%) of sheep in the flock may be lame in one or more limbs. Affected limbs appear normal except for the hoof and pastern regions, where the coronary band may be swollen, hot, and painful. Most sheep recover spontaneously in 2–4 wk with nothing more serious than a slight loss of body weight. In some outbreaks, however, administration of penicillin for 5 days may be necessary to salvage affected sheep. Septicemia and polyarthritis are not common with this condition.

Prevention and Treatment: Discarding heavily contaminated dips is the best way to prevent infection with *E rhusiopathiae* and the lameness associated with this condition. Using an appropriate bacteriostat in dip solutions may reduce the incidence of the condition.

FOOT-AND-MOUTH DISEASE

Foot-and-mouth disease (FMD) is a highly communicable viral disease caused by an *Aphthovirus* of the family Picornaviridae. There are 7 serotypes: A, O, C, Asia 1, and SAT (Southern African Territories) 1, 2, and 3. Further diversity is found in strains within each serotype. It primarily affects cloven-hooved animals of the order Artiodactyla. Livestock hosts include cattle, pigs, sheep, goats, and experimental infections in alpacas and llamas. FMD virus has also been reported in >70 species of wild artiodactyls, including bison, giraffes, Indian elephants, and several species of deer and antelope. The disease is characterized by fever and vesicles in the mouth and on the muzzle, teats, and feet and is spread through direct contact or aerosolized virus via respiratory secretions, milk, semen, and ingestion of feed from infected animals (meat, offal, milk). In a susceptible population, morbidity reaches 100% with rare fatalities except in young animals. FMD was once distributed worldwide but has been eradicated in some regions, including North America and Western Europe. In endemic countries, FMD places economic constraints on the international livestock trade and can be easily reintroduced into disease-free areas unless strict precautions are in place. Outbreaks can severely disrupt livestock production and require significant resources to control, as in the 2001 UK outbreak.

Epidemiology and Transmission: FMD is endemic in many countries of the Middle East, Africa, Asia, and in parts of South America. Where FMD still occurs, serotypes are not uniformly distributed. Six of the 7 serotypes have occurred in Africa (O, A, C, SAT-1, SAT-2, SAT-3), 4 in Asia (O, A, C, Asia-1), and 3 in South America (O, A, C). North and Central America, Australia, New Zealand, Greenland, Iceland, and Western Europe are free of FMD. In 2001, FMD was introduced into the UK, where it spread to Ireland, the Netherlands, and France. The highly virulent pan-Asiatic serotype O causing the outbreak was the same found throughout Asia.

The virus is transmitted via direct or indirect contact with infected secretions and excretions (including semen and milk), mechanical vectors (people, horses, dogs, cats, birds, vehicles), and air currents over land or water. The virus can enter the body via inhalation, ingestion, or through skin wounds and mucous membranes. Breeding is a possible route of transmission for the SAT viruses in African buffalo populations. An example scenario for introduction into a previously FMD-free area is for a susceptible population, such as pigs, given imported food derived from an infected animal (meat, offal, milk). Virus then spreads from pigs, which can expire up to 3,000 times more virus than cattle, to more susceptible cattle hosts via aerosol. Virus was reported to travel over water >250 km (155 miles) from Brittany, France, to the Isle of Wight, UK, in 1981, but it usually travels no more than 10 km (~6 miles) over land. FMD has high agroterrorism potential because of its infectivity, high transmissibility through wind and inanimate objects, and potential for large economic losses.

People can act as mechanical vectors of FMD by carrying virus on clothing or skin. FMD is not considered a public health problem, but there are reports of people who work in FMD vaccine laboratories who have developed antibodies to the virus. There are few reports of people with laboratory-confirmed cases of clinical illness between 1921 and 1969. The disease in people is usually short-lived and mild, with symptoms including vesicular lesions and influenza-like illness.

Pathogenesis: The primary site of infection and replication of FMD is in the mucosa of the pharynx. The virus may also enter through skin lesions or the GI tract. Once distributed throughout the lymphatic system, the virus replicates in the epithelium of the mouth, muzzle, teats, feet, and areas of damaged skin (eg, knees and hocks of pigs). Vesicles then develop at the organs and rupture within 48 hr. More than 50% of ruminants that recover from illness and those that are vaccinated and have been exposed to virus can carry virus particles in the pharyngeal region—up to 3.5 yr in cattle, 9 mo in sheep, and >5 yr in African buffalo.

FMD virus is environmentally resistant and inactivates outside the pH range 6–9 and desiccation and at temperatures >56°C (132.8°F). It is resistant to lipid solvents such as ether and chloroform, but sodium hydroxide (lye), sodium carbonate (soda ash), citric acid, and acetic acid (vinegar) are effective disinfectants. Iodophores, quaternary ammonium compounds, hypochlorite, and phenols are less effective disinfectants, especially in the presence of organic matter.

FMD is shed into milk in dairy cows before clinical signs develop, so there is opportunity for virus to spread farm to farm and from cow to calf via raw milk. FMD may survive pasteurization depending on the method (high temperature short time, ultra high temperature, laboratory pasteurization); the lipid component of milk protects virus during heating. FMD virus survives up to 20 wk on hay or straw bedding, in dry fecal matter for up to 14 days in summer, in a fecal slurry for up to 6 mo in winter, in urine for 39 days, and in soil for 3 (summer) to 28 (winter) days.

The incubation period of FMD is variable and depends on the host, environment, route of exposure, and virus strain. After infection with FMD virus, the average incubation period for sheep and goats is 3–8 days, ≥2 days for pigs, and 2–14 days in cattle. The incubation period can be as short as 18 hr for host-adapted strains in pigs, especially under intense direct contact.

Clinical Findings: Clinical signs in cattle include pyrexia of ~104° F, followed by vesicular development on the tongue, hard palate, dental pad, lips, gums, muzzle, coronary band, interdigital cleft, and teats in lactating cows. Acutely affected individuals may salivate profusely, stamp their feet, and prefer to lie down. Ruptured oral vesicles can coalesce and form erosions but heal rapidly, roughly 11 days after vesicle formation. Feet vesicles take longer to heal and are susceptible to bacterial infection leading to chronic lameness. Secondary bacterial mastitis is common due to infected teat vesicles and resistance to milking. After vesicular disease develops, cattle quickly lose condition and milk yield, which can persist chronically.

Infected pigs show mild lameness and blanching around the coronary band and may develop a fever of up to 107°F. Affected pigs become lethargic, huddle among other pigs, and have little interest in feed. Vesicles develop on the coronary band, heel of the foot including accessory digits, snout, mandible, and tongue. Additional vesicles may form on the hocks and knees of pigs housed on rough surfaces. Depending on the severity of vesicles, the horn of the foot may completely slough off and cause chronic lameness in recovered pigs. Young pigs <14 wk old may die without clinical signs of illness because of viral damage to the developing myocardium.

Lameness is usually the first clinical sign of FMD infection in sheep and goats. This is followed by fever and vesicular development on the interdigital cleft, heel bulbs, coronary band, and mouth. Vesicles may also form on the teats of lactating animals and rarely on the vulva and prepuce. Secondary infections result in reduced milk yield, chronic lameness, and predisposition to other viral infections, including sheep/goat pox (*see* p 869) and peste des petits ruminants (*see* p 766). Similarly to young pigs, infection in immature sheep and goats results in death without clinical signs due to heart failure.

Experimentally infected camelids are commonly reported to have mild clinical illness, if at all, but can have severe infections resulting in salivation and mouth lesions and sloughing of the footpad and skin of the tarsal and carpal joints. Water buffalo can have mouth and foot lesions, which heal faster and are less severe than those in cattle. FMD infections in wildlife resemble clinical illness in their domestic counterparts, but more severe lesions such as sloughing of antlers or toe horn are reported.

Diagnosis: In cattle and pigs, the clinical signs of FMD are indistinguishable from those of vesicular stomatitis (*see* p 694), and in pigs from those of swine vesicular disease (*see* p 735) and vesicular exanthema (*see* p 738). Therefore, laboratory confirmation is essential for diagnosis of FMD and should be performed in specialized laboratories that meet OIE requirements for Containment Group 4 pathogens. Countries lacking access to a national or regional laboratory meeting these guidelines should send specimens to an OIE FMD reference laboratory. The tissue of choice for sampling is vesicular epithelium or fluid. At least 1 g of epithelium should be placed in a transport medium of phosphate-buffered saline (PBS) or equal parts glycerol and phosphate buffer with pH 7.2–7.6. Samples should be kept refrigerated or transported on ice. If vesicles are not present, oropharyngeal fluid can be collected via probang cup or pharyngeal swabbing for virus isolation or reverse transcription PCR (RT-PCR). Serum (blood) samples may also be tested by these means (OIE *Terrestrial Manual* 2012). Repeated sampling may be necessary to identify a carrier, because virus presence may be low and fluctuate.

Laboratory diagnosis is usually performed via antigen capture–ELISA or serotyping ELISA. This is the preferred method for countries with endemic FMD for viral antigen detection and serotyping (OIE *Terrestrial Manual* 2012). Concurrent virus isolation may be performed, preferably in primary bovine thyroid cell culture. Detecting nucleic acids via RT combined with real-time PCR is more sensitive and rapid than conventional methods and may be more useful when samples contain low concentrations of virus. ELISA is preferred over complement fixation tests because of its increased sensitivity and specificity, but complement fixation may be performed if ELISA reagents are not available. Commercially available lateral flow devices have not yet been validated by the OIE.

Serologic tests for FMD are used to certify animals for import/export (ie, trade), confirm suspected cases of FMD, test efficacy of vaccination, and provide evidence for absence of infection. Testing cut-offs may be set at different levels for herd-based surveillance versus certifying freedom of infection for trade purposes. The choice of serologic test depends on the vaccination status of the animals. Serologic tests for antibodies to the viral structural (capsid) proteins cannot be used in vaccinated animals, because FMD vaccines induce antibodies to these proteins. Detection of antibodies to nonstructural proteins, which are expressed only during virus replication, can be used to determine past or present infection with any of the 7 serotypes, whether or not the animal has been vaccinated. However, they are less sensitive and may result in false-negatives in cases with limited virus replication such as vaccinated animals that become infected, because the vaccine suppresses viral replication (OIE *Terrestrial Manual* 2012).

Treatment, Control, and Prevention: The OIE classifies countries and regions as FMD-free without vaccination, FMD-free with vaccination, suspended FMD-free status with or without vaccination, and unrecognized (World Organization for Animal Health, 2013). The current global status of FMD distribution shows geographic areas of viral "hotspots" where FMD prevalence indices are highest over long periods of time. They are commonly located in poor countries where veterinary services and resources are inadequate to control or eradicate FMD. Combined use of trade and movement restrictions of animals and animal products has not completely prevented introductions of FMD into FMD-free areas. These viral incursions into countries or regions where FMD is not enzootic are usually controlled by slaughter of all infected and susceptible animals, strict restriction of animal and vehicle movement around infected premises, proper carcass disposal, and environmental disinfection, without the use of vaccines. Inactivated virus vaccines are limited in their use, because they protect for only 4–6 mo against the specific serotype(s) contained in the vaccine and protect animals from clinical illness but not viral persistence in the pharyngeal region; therefore, they can induce a carrier state. Additionally, it is difficult to distinguish infected animals from vaccinated animals unless purified killed vaccines are used. Therefore, vaccination is used more in enzootic countries to protect producing animals, particularly high-yielding dairy cattle, from clinical illness because slaughter of all at-risk individuals may be economically unfeasible and can cause food shortages.

Rapid disease reporting is essential to control an FMD outbreak in nonendemic countries. Veterinarians who encounter any vesicular disease in the USA should immediately inform their state or federal veterinary authorities. After an outbreak, tracing is done through epidemiologic inquiries to help identify the source of disease introduction. In countries where mass slaughter is not possible, strict quarantining and movement restriction should be enforced. However, quarantine may not be long enough to prevent carrier animal movement after an outbreak. When mass euthanasia is performed, infected carcasses must be disposed of via incineration, burial, or rendering on or close to the infected premises. Scavengers and rodents should be prevented or killed to prevent mechanical dissemination of virus. Buildings should be cleaned with a mild acid or alkali disinfectant and fumigation, and people that have come into contact with virus may be asked to decontaminate their clothing and avoid contact with susceptible animals for a period of time.

In some regions, FMD persistence in wildlife populations, such as the wild African buffalo, can make FMD eradication unrealistic. Control measures, such as fencing of wildlife reserves to prevent contact with domestic livestock, have helped limit the spread of virus in certain areas. A twice-yearly vaccination buffer zone in livestock proximal to endemic wildlife reserves may additionally help decrease outbreak occurrence.

There is no specific treatment for FMD, but supportive care may be allowed in countries where FMD is endemic.

FUNGAL INFECTIONS

(Mycoses)

Systemic mycoses are infections with fungal organisms that exist in the environment, enter the host from a single portal of entry, and disseminate within the host usually to multiple organ systems. The soil reservoir is the primary source of most infections, which can be acquired by inhalation, ingestion, or traumatic introduction of fungal elements. (*See also* DERMATOPHILOSIS, p 858.)

Pathogenic fungi establish infection in apparently normal hosts, and such diseases as histoplasmosis, coccidioidomycosis, blastomycosis, and cryptococcosis are regarded as primary systemic mycoses. Opportunistic fungi usually require a host that is debilitated or immunosuppressed to establish infection. Prolonged administration of antimicrobials or immunosuppressive agents appears to increase the likelihood of infection by the opportunistic fungi that cause diseases such as aspergillosis and candidiasis, which may be focal or systemic.

Clinical findings and gross lesions are often suggestive of systemic mycoses, but definitive diagnosis requires microscopic identification, culture of the organism, or PCR. Identification of the fungus and the tissue reaction via microscopic examination of exudates and biopsy material is adequate for diagnosis of histoplasmosis, cryptococcosis, blastomycosis, coccidioidomycosis, and rhinosporidiosis. Other diseases, such as candidiasis, aspergillosis, zygomycosis, phaeohyphomycosis, hyalohyphomycosis, and oomycosis (pythiosis and lagenidiosis), usually require more than microscopic evaluation for a definitive diagnosis. Some of these fungi are also common contaminants of cultures; thus, tissue invasion and reaction must be demonstrated for the culture isolation to be considered significant. Serology may be useful for diagnosis (and prognosis) of some mycotic diseases such as coccidioidomycosis, pythiosis, and lagenidiosis. Antigen titers have proved useful for cryptococcosis, histoplasmosis, and blastomycosis.

For treatment, *see* discussions of specific systemic mycoses (below) and *see* SYSTEMIC PHARMACOTHERAPEUTICS OF THE INTEGUMENTARY SYSTEM, p 2571.

ASPERGILLOSIS

Aspergillosis is caused by several *Aspergillus* spp, especially *A fumigatus* and *A terreus*. *A niger*, *A nidulans*, *A viridinutans*, *A flavus*, and *A felis* are being recognized more commonly with increasing use of molecular techniques for identification. *Aspergillus* infection is found worldwide and in almost all domestic animals and birds as well as in many wild species. It is primarily a respiratory infection that may become generalized; however, tissue predilection varies among species. The most common forms are pulmonary infections in poultry and other birds; mycotic abortion in cattle; guttural pouch mycosis in horses; infections of the nasal and paranasal tissues, intervertebral sites, and kidneys of dogs; and sinonasal, sino-orbital, and pulmonary infection in domestic cats.

Clinical Findings and Lesions: In **birds**, aspergillosis (*see* p 2901) is primarily bronchopulmonary, with dyspnea, gasping, and polypnea accompanied by somnolence, anorexia, and emaciation. Mycotic tracheitis has also been described. Torticollis and disturbances of equilibrium are seen when infection disseminates to the brain. Yellow nodules of varying size and consistency or plaque lesions are found in the respiratory passages, lungs, air sacs, or membranes of body cavities. Fur-like growth of fungus may be found on the thickened walls of air sacs. Other species with bronchopulmonary aspergillosis may have nodular lesions in the lungs or an acute pneumonia accompanied by serosanguineous fluid in the pleural cavity and a fibrinous pleuritis.

In **ruminants**, aspergillosis may be asymptomatic, appear in a bronchopulmonary form, cause mastitis, or cause placentitis and abortion. Mycotic pneumonia may be rapidly fatal. Signs include pyrexia; rapid, shallow, stertorous respiration; nasal discharge; and a moist cough. The lungs are firm, heavy, and mottled and do not collapse. In subacute to chronic mycotic pneumonia, the lungs contain multiple discrete granulomas, and the disease grossly resembles tuberculosis (*see* p 687).

In the absence of pneumonia, infected cows generally have no signs except for abortion; a dead fetus is aborted at 6–9 mo gestation, and the fetal membranes are retained. Lesions are found in the uterus, fetal membranes, and often the fetal skin. In the uterus, the intercaruncular areas are grossly thickened, leathery, dark red to tan, and contain elevated or eroded foci covered by a yellow-gray adherent pseudomembrane. Maternal caruncles are dark red to brown, and the adherent fetal cotyledons are markedly thickened. Cutaneous lesions in aborted fetuses consist of soft, red to gray, elevated, discrete foci that resemble ringworm.

In **horses**, epistaxis and dysphagia are common complications of gutturomycosis (*see* p 1463). The infected guttural pouch is characterized by a necrotizing inflammation and is thickened, hemorrhagic, and covered by a friable pseudomembrane. Mycotic rhinitis characterized by dyspnea and nasal discharge has also been described. Aspergillosis can be a rapidly fatal disease associated with diffuse pulmonary invasion. In these cases, acute enteritis is often a predisposing factor. The colitis is thought to result in a profound neutropenia that decreases the immunocompetence of the host, followed by the invasion of *Aspergillus* from disrupted intestinal mucosa. Locomotor and visual disturbances, including blindness, may occur when the infection spreads to the brain and optic nerve.

In **dogs**, aspergillosis is typically localized to the nasal cavity or paranasal sinuses and is usually caused by infection with *A fumigatus*. Nasal aspergillosis is seen mainly in dolichocephalic breeds; it begins in the posterior region of the ventral maxilloturbinate with signs of lethargy,

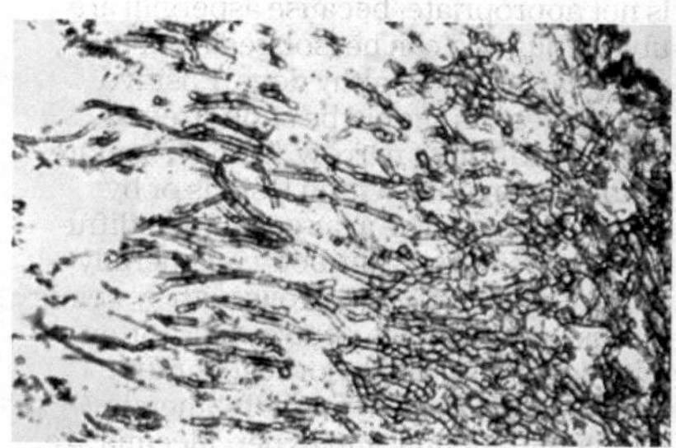

Aspergillus fumigatus from canine nasal infection. *Courtesy of Ontario Veterinary College.*

nasal pain, ulceration of the nares, sneezing, unilateral or bilateral sanguinopurulent nasal discharge, frontal sinus osteomyelitis, and epistaxis. Gross lesions vary considerably with site of infection, but the mucosa of the nasal and paranasal sinuses may be covered by a layer of necrotic material and white to gray-white fungal growth. The mucosa and the underlying bone may be necrotic with loss of bone definition on radiographs or CT.

Disseminated disease in dogs is seen most often in middle-age, female German Shepherds and usually involves *A terreus*, *A deflectus*, and *A niger*. The clinical signs of disseminated aspergillosis may include lethargy, lameness, anorexia, weight loss, muscle wasting, pyrexia, hematuria, urinary incontinence, generalized lymphadenopathy, and neurologic deficits. Lesions are frequently found in the abdominal and thoracic lymph nodes, kidneys, spleen, and vertebrae. Discospondylitis is common.

In **cats**, sinonasal and sino-orbital disease is seen most often. Aspergillosis is rare in cats compared with dogs. Sinonasal disease can present similarly to the disease in dogs, but sino-orbital disease can be very aggressive, often causing severe facial swelling. In some cases, a mass in the pterygopalatine fossa or ulceration of the hard palate may be seen. The CNS may be invaded, causing neurologic signs.

Diagnosis: Radiographs in dogs with nasal aspergillosis may show generalized radiolucence of the nasal cavity secondary to turbinate tissue destruction. Frontal sinus osteomyelitis is seen in as many as 80% of dogs. Cross-sectional imaging via CT is more sensitive than plain radiographs in demonstrating consistent changes. Visualization of fungal plaques by rhinoscopy together with serologic and either mycologic or radiographic evidence of disease is often how a diagnosis is made. A diagnosis based on culture results alone is not appropriate, because aspergilli are ubiquitous and can be isolated from the nasal cavities of healthy dogs. Positive culture results should be supported by demonstration of narrow, hyaline, septate, branching hyphae within lesions or by serologic tests. The agar-gel double-diffusion test for serum antibody is generally considered unreliable. Dogs with systemic disease usually have neutrophilia, often with a left shift, and a nonregenerative anemia. Azotemia, hyperglobulinemia, hypoalbuminemia, and hypercalcemia are common. Ultrasound usually reveals abdominal lymphadenopathy and renal lesions. Systemic disease is usually diagnosed by culture of the organism, often from urine. A blood and urine galactomannan antigen assay for diagnosis of systemic aspergillosis in dogs has been described to have moderate sensitivity and specificity.

Treatment: In dogs, topical treatment is considered the treatment of choice for nasal and paranasal aspergillosis. Several surgical techniques and drug regimens have been used with varying success. Clotrimazole formulated in a polyethylene glycol base is generally considered the first-line treatment. It can be administered through indwelling tubes trephined into the frontal sinuses or via the nares as a single infusion. If infusion is via the nares, Foley catheters are used to instill 0.5 g in each side of the nasal cavity. The infused solution is left in place for 1 hr, during which the dog's position is changed periodically to maximize penetration. There is an ~80% success rate using local infusions in this manner. Enilconazole, 10 mg/kg, instilled bid for 7–14 days, via tubes implanted surgically into the frontal sinuses, has also been used with a similar success rate. Drugs given systemically have included ketoconazole, itraconazole, fluconazole, voriconazole, and posaconazole. Fluconazole (2.5–10 mg/kg, divided bid) and itraconazole (5–10 mg/kg/day) are cost-effective options. Ketoconazole (5–10 mg/kg, bid for 6–8 wk), although cost-effective, is not as effective clinically. Voriconazole (3–6 mg/kg/day) is probably the most effective of the azole antifungals for treating aspergillosis, but the cost is much higher than that of the other choices.

In horses, surgical exposure and curettage have been used to treat gutturomycosis. Topical natamycin and oral potassium iodide have been reported effective in cases of *Aspergillus* infection. Itraconazole (3 mg/kg, bid for 84–120 days) has been reported effective in *Aspergillus* rhinitis in horses.

Bovine mastitis has been treated successfully with combined intra-arterial and intramammary injection with miconazole.

BLASTOMYCOSIS

Blastomycosis, caused by the dimorphic fungus *Blastomyces dermatitidis*, is characterized by pyogranulomatous lesions in various tissues. It is most common in people, dogs, and cats but has also been described in such widely divergent species as horses, ferrets, deer, wolves, African lions, bottlenosed dolphins, and sea lions. It appears not to be a disease of cattle, sheep, or pigs. Blastomycosis is generally limited to North America, and most cases have occurred in the Mississippi, Missouri, Tennessee, and Ohio River basins and along the Great Lakes and the St. Lawrence Seaway. There is an endemic area in the Pacific northwest. Even within these river basins, the organism is found in geographically restricted areas. Beaver dams and other habitats where soil is moist, acidic, and rich in decaying vegetation may serve as the ecologic niche for the organism, but it is often difficult to find in the environment. The organism has also been recovered from pigeon and bat feces. Rain, dew, or fog may play a critical role in liberating the infective conidia, which then are aerosolized and inhaled. When respiratory defenses are overwhelmed or immunosuppressed, disseminated disease occurs via hematogenous spread from the lungs. Cutaneous lesions may result from a primary entry through the skin or, more commonly, by dissemination from a pulmonary focus. Needle-stick injuries to veterinary personnel after aspiration of cutaneous lesions from infected animals have resulted in primary cutaneous infection. Ocular lesions tend to develop first in the posterior segment, resulting in granulomatous chorioretinitis and retinal detachment. Anterior segment involvement often follows, resulting in anterior uveitis and panophthalmitis.

Clinical Findings: The signs vary with organ involvement and are not specific. Weight loss may be accompanied by coughing, anorexia, lymphadenopathy, dyspnea, ocular disease, lameness, skin lesions, and fever. Dry, harsh lung sounds from lung lesions are common in dogs with blastomycosis. Signs of pulmonary involvement are seen in as many as 85% of affected dogs. Severe pulmonary involvement results in hypoxemia, which indicates a poor prognosis. Lymph node involvement is seen in approximately half of affected dogs, which is about the same proportion of dogs that have cutaneous involvement. Skin lesions may include proliferative granulomas and subcutaneous abscesses that ulcerate and drain a serosanguineous discharge. The skin lesions are often very small and multifocal in dogs, but large abscesses are occasionally seen, especially in cats. The planum nasale, face, and nail beds are most often involved. Signs of ocular blastomycosis are seen in 30%–50% of affected dogs and include blindness, uveitis, glaucoma, and retinal detachment. Lameness associated with fungal osteomyelitis or severe paronychia occurs in approximately one quarter of affected dogs. CNS signs are uncommon, occurring in <5% of dogs, but they may be more common in cats. The pattern of systemic involvement is similar in cats, but cats are affected far less commonly than dogs. Hematuria and dysuria may be seen with urogenital blastomycosis.

Lesions: Gross lesions consist of few to numerous, variable-sized, irregular, firm, gray to yellow areas of pulmonary consolidation and nodules in the lungs and thoracic lymph nodes. Dissemination may result in nodular lesions in various organs but especially the skin, eyes, and bone. Cutaneous lesions are single or multiple papules, or chronic, draining, nodular pyogranulomas.

Diagnosis: Blastomycosis should be considered in dogs with draining cutaneous nodules and signs of respiratory disease. In cats, respiratory tract involvement is seen most frequently, followed by involvement of the CNS, regional lymph nodes, skin, eyes, and GI and urinary tracts. Radiographic findings in the lungs include noncalcified nodules or consolidation, with enlargement of the bronchial and mediastinal lymph nodes. The predominant patterns on thoracic radiographs are those of diffuse nodular interstitial and peribronchial densities. Commonly, the bronchial lymph nodes are greatly enlarged and appear in radiographs as dense masses. Diagnosis can be made from biopsy of tissue or aspirated specimens taken from cutaneous lesions or other involved organs by the presence of thick-walled yeast that often have daughter cells budding from a broad base. These round to ovoid, pale pink (H&E) blastospores measure 8–25 µm and have a refractile, double-contoured wall. They may be empty or contain basophilic nuclear material and have single, broad-based buds. An antibody response, detected by agar gel immunodiffusion, usually occurs, but this response is neither sensitive nor specific when attempting to make a definitive diagnosis. An enzyme immunoassay for antibodies to rBAD-1 repeat has shown improved sensitivity. A recently developed antigen enzyme immunoassay has been used in both serum and urine to detect cell-wall galactomannan that is immunologically indistinguishable in histoplasmosis and blastomycosis. Although the titer is not useful in differentiating between the two infections, it helps diagnose the presence of one of these two systemic mycoses.

Treatment: Itraconazole (5 mg/kg/day) is the treatment of choice for dogs and cats with blastomycosis. A minimum of 2 mo of treatment is necessary, and the drug should be continued until active disease is not apparent. Clinical cure can be expected in ~70% of dogs, with recurrence months or years after treatment noted in ~20% of treated dogs. Most dogs will respond to retreatment with itraconazole. Other azoles such as fluconazole and ketoconazole are not as effective as itraconazole, but a study evaluating cost-effectiveness of fluconazole showed it to be a less expensive alternative, despite longer treatment times. In fulminating cases of blastomycosis, especially those with evidence of hypoxemia, combination therapy with amphotericin B and itraconazole is recommended. Short courses of anti-inflammatory dosages of glucocorticoids have been advocated during the first few days of treatment by some, but steroid use is controversial and may actually worsen the prognosis. The prognosis is best for dogs with only mild lung disease, is more guarded for dogs with moderate to severe lung disease, and is poorest for dogs with CNS involvement.

CANDIDIASIS

Candidiasis is a localized mucocutaneous disease caused by species of the yeast-like fungus *Candida*, most commonly *C albicans*. It is distributed worldwide in a variety of animals. *C albicans* is a normal inhabitant of the nasopharynx, GI tract, and external genitalia of many species of animals and is opportunistic in causing disease. Factors associated with candidal infections are disruption of mucosal integrity; indwelling, intravenous, or urinary catheters; administration of antibiotics; and immunosuppressive drugs or diseases. The organism most frequently infects birds (*see* p 2791), in which it involves the oral mucosa, esophagus, and crop. Superficial infections limited to the mucous membranes of the intestinal tract have been described in pigs and foals. Systemic candidiasis has also been described in cattle, calves, sheep, and foals secondary to prolonged antibiotic or corticosteroid therapy. In cats, candidiasis is rare but has been associated with oral and upper respiratory disease, pyothorax, ocular lesions, intestinal disease, and urocystitis. Infections are rare in dogs and horses. However, *Candida* spp have been considered a cause of arthritis in horses and mastitis and abortion in cattle. Fungemia and *Candida* peritonitis have been noted in dogs with perforating intestinal lesions after surgery, and mucosal and cutaneous candidiasis has been noted in immunosuppressed dogs and in dogs with diabetes mellitus.

Clinical Findings and Lesions: Signs are variable and nonspecific and may be associated more with the primary or predisposing conditions than with the candidiasis itself. Calves with forestomach candidiasis have watery diarrhea, anorexia, and dehydration, with gradual progression to prostration and death. Affected chicks are listless and have reduced feed intake and growth rate. Porcine candidiasis affects the oral, esophageal, and gastric mucosa, with diarrhea and emaciation the most consistent signs.

Gross lesions of the skin and mucosae are generally single or multiple, raised, circular, white masses covered with scabs. The organism can penetrate keratinized epithelium and cause marked keratinous thickening of the mucosae of the tongue, esophagus, and rumen. In birds, the crop and esophageal lesions are white, circular ulcers with raised surface scabs that produce thickening of the mucosa; an easily removed pseudomembrane is common.

Diagnosis: Fungal organisms are numerous in proliferating epithelial tissue, and diagnosis can be made by examination of scrapings or biopsy specimens from mucocutaneous lesions. *C albicans* are ovoid, budding yeast cells (2–4 μm in diameter) with thin walls, or they occur in chains that produce pseudohyphae when the blastospores remain attached after budding division. Filamentous, regular, true hyphae also may be visible. The fungal cells generally are limited to epithelial tissue and rarely extend deeper.

Treatment: Nystatin ointment or topical application of amphotericin B or 1% iodine solution may be useful in the treatment of oral or cutaneous candidiasis. Amphotericin B, 500 g in 1 L of 5% dextrose, was administered IV, every 48 hr for 24 days and then every 72 hr for 15 days, to successfully resolve arthritis induced by *C fumata* in a horse. Fluconazole (5 mg/kg/day, PO, for 4–6 wk) was also used to successfully treat disseminated candidiasis in foals. Itraconazole and amphotericin B lipid complex are considered the treatments of choice in dogs, but few cases have been treated.

COCCIDIOIDOMYCOSIS

(Valley Fever)

Coccidioidomycosis (Valley Fever) is a dustborne, noncontagious infection caused by the dimorphic fungus *Coccidioides immitis*. Infections are limited to arid and semiarid regions of the southwestern USA and to similar areas of Mexico and Central and South America. Although many species of animals, including people, are susceptible, only dogs are affected significantly. Placental infection leading to abortion and osteomyelitis have been described in horses. Ruminants and pigs may have subclinical infections with lesions restricted to foci in the lungs and to thoracic lymph nodes. Inhalation of fungal spores is the only established mode of infection, and spores may be carried on dust particles. Epidemics may occur when rainy periods are followed by drought, resulting in dust storms. Most bovine infections are contracted in dusty feedlots.

Clinical Findings and Lesions: The disease varies from inapparent (cattle, sheep, pigs, dogs, cats) to progressive, disseminated, and fatal (dogs, nonhuman primates, cats, and people). Coccidioidomycosis is primarily a respiratory disease that ranges from self-limiting to chronic. Dissemination occurs in ~20% of canine infections, with many tissues, especially eyes, joints, and bone, affected. Clinical signs can vary greatly, depending on organ involvement and severity of infection. Dogs with disseminated disease may have chronic cough, anorexia, cachexia, lameness, enlarged joints, fever, and intermittent diarrhea. Dissemination to the skin with draining ulceration may occur, but primary infection through the skin is rare. Cats infected with *C immitis* most often present with dermatologic signs (draining skin lesions, subcutaneous granulomatous masses, abscesses), fever, inappetence, and weight loss. Less common clinical signs in cats include respiratory (dypsnea), musculoskeletal (lameness), neurologic, and ophthalmologic abnormalities. Approximately 50% of infected cats appear to have disseminated disease.

Gross lesions may be limited to the lungs, mediastinum, and thoracic lymph nodes, or may be disseminated to various organs. Lesions are discrete, variable-sized nodules with a firm, gray-white cut surface, and resemble those of tuberculosis (*see* p 687). The nodules are pyogranulomas composed of epithelioid and giant cells, and the center of some foci may contain purulent exudate and fungal organisms. Some lesions may have mineralized foci.

Diagnosis: In endemic areas, coccidioidomycosis should be considered in dogs with chronic bronchopulmonary disease and when pulmonary nodules and enlarged lymph nodes are found on thoracic radiographs. The lesions are pyogranulomas that contain *C immitis* free in the exudate and in epithelioid and multinucleate giant cells. The organisms vary in size and appear as relatively large (20–80 µm, up to 200 µm) spherules with a double-contoured wall. The mature spherules (sporangia) contain endospores (sporangiospores) 2–5 µm in diameter. Diagnosis is established by demonstrating the spherules in tissues. Serum can also be tested by agar gel immunodiffusion (AGID) assays for detection of precipitin and complement-fixing antibodies. Currently, most commercial laboratories run AGID assays for IgG and IgM antibodies; results of these assays are specific but relatively insensitive. An enzyme immunoassay for *Coccidioides* galactomannan antigen useful in human infections has proved insensitive in dogs. A presumptive diagnosis can be made when serology is positive in an animal with consistent clinical signs. Attempts to culture the fungus should be restricted to those laboratories equipped to handle such dangerously infective cultures.

Treatment: Disease is often self-limiting, but if chronic respiratory signs or multisystemic disease are present, longterm antifungal therapy is needed; with disseminated infection, treatment of at least 6–12 mo is typical. Fluconazole (2.5–10 mg/kg/day) is the most commonly used drug to treat disseminated or chronic respiratory infections. Ketoconazole (10–30 mg/kg/day) and itraconazole (10 mg/kg/day) are also commonly used to treat dogs with coccidioidomycosis but are more expensive and have a higher incidence of adverse effects. Amphotericin B may be the most effective antifungal drug, but it is highly nephrotoxic. It may be indicated in animals that either do not improve or are unable to tolerate the azole antifungals.

CRYPTOCOCCOSIS

Cryptococcosis is a systemic fungal disease that may affect the respiratory tract (especially the nasal cavity), CNS, eyes, and skin (particularly of the face and neck of cats). The causal fungi, *Cryptococcus neoformans* and *C gattii*, exist in the environment and in tissues in a yeast form. Infection occurs worldwide. The fungi are found in soil and fowl manure, especially in pigeon droppings. Transmission is by inhalation of spores or contamination of wounds. In avian droppings, it may occur in a noncapsulated form as small as 1 μm, which can be inhaled into the deeper portions of the lungs. Cryptococcosis is most common in cats but also is seen in dogs, cattle, horses, sheep, goats, birds, and wild animals. In people, many cases are associated with a defective cell-mediated immune response.

Clinical Findings and Lesions: Bovine cryptococcosis has been associated only with cases of mastitis, and many cows in a herd may be infected. Affected cows have anorexia, decreased milk flow, swelling and firmness of affected quarters, and enlarged supramammary lymph nodes. The milk becomes viscid, mucoid, and gray-white, or it may be watery with flakes. The disease in horses almost invariably is a respiratory ailment with obstructive growths in the nasal cavities.

In cats, upper respiratory signs secondary to nasal cavity infection are most common and include sneezing; mucopurulent, serous, or hemorrhagic unilateral or bilateral chronic nasal discharge; polyp-like mass(es) in the nostril; and/or a firm, subcutaneous swelling over the bridge of the nose. Cutaneous lesions are also common and are characterized by papules and nodules that are fluctuant to firm. Larger lesions tend to ulcerate, leaving a raw surface with a serous exudate. Neurologic signs associated with cryptococcosis of the CNS may include depression, changes in temperament, seizures, circling, paresis, and blindness. Ocular abnormalities may also develop, including dilated unresponsive pupils and blindness due to exudative retinal detachment, granulomatous chorioretinitis, panophthalmitis, and optic neuritis.

In contrast to cats, dogs often have disseminated disease with CNS or ocular involvement. Clinical signs are often related to meningoencephalitis, optic neuritis, and granulomatous chorioretinitis. Lesions in the nasal cavity of many dogs have been reported, but they are usually not the primary finding or reason for presentation. Approximately 50% of dogs have lesions in the respiratory tract, usually the lungs, and most have granulomas present in multiple systems. Structures often involved in order of decreasing frequency are kidneys, lymph nodes, spleen, liver, thyroid, adrenals, pancreas, bone, GI tract, muscle, myocardium, prostate, heart valves, and tonsils.

Lesions associated with cryptococcosis vary from a gelatinous mass, consisting of numerous organisms with minimal inflammation, to granuloma formation. The lesion is usually composed of aggregates of encapsulated organisms within a connective tissue reticulum. The cellular response is primarily macrophages and giant cells with a few plasma cells and lymphocytes. Epithelioid giant cells and areas of caseous necrosis are less common than with the other systemic mycoses.

Diagnosis: The most rapid method of diagnosis is cytologic evaluation of nasal exudate, skin exudate, CSF, or samples obtained by paracentesis of the aqueous or vitreous chambers of the eye or by impression smears of nasal or cutaneous masses. Gram stain is most useful; the organism retains the crystal violet, whereas the capsule stains lightly red with safranin. India ink is also used to visualize the organism, which appears unstained and silhouetted against a black background. It is not as definitive as Gram stain unless budding is seen, because lymphocytes, fat droplets, and aggregated India ink particles may be confused with the organism. Wright stain has been used most often in diagnosing canine and feline cases, but this stain can cause the organism to shrink and the capsule to become distorted. New methylene blue and periodic acid-Schiff (PAS) stains are better than Wright stain for this reason. Because cytologic evaluation is rapid, impression smears or potassium hydroxide preparations should always be made of suspected cryptococcal lesions.

If no organisms are seen, a biopsy of the lesion can be taken; part of the sample can be used for culture and the rest processed for routine histology. The organism can be stained with H&E, but the capsule does not stain. The organism is more easily visualized with PAS and Gomori methenamine silver stains, but the capsule does not stain with these, either. The best stain for *Cryptococcus* is Mayer mucicarmine because of its ability to stain the capsule. Immunofluorescent staining can also be used. The large capsule and thin cell wall of *Cryptococcus* differentiate it from *Blastomyces*. *Cryptococcus*, by its budding and lack of endospores, can be distinguished from *Coccidioides immitis*.

Detection of cryptococcal capsular antigen in serum, urine, or CSF is a useful, rapid method of diagnosis in those suspected cases in which the organism is not identified. A latex agglutination test is commercially available in kit form. The antigen titer can also be used to help determine response to therapy.

The organism can be cultured from exudate, CSF, urine, joint fluid, and tissue samples if a large enough sample volume is available. Sabouraud agar with antibiotics is used if bacterial contamination is likely.

Treatment: Fluconazole (2.5–10 mg/kg/day) or itraconazole (10 mg/kg/day) are considered the treatments of choice. Amphotericin B can be given SC (0.5–0.8 mg/kg diluted in 0.45% saline containing 2.5% dextrose; 400 mL for cats, 500 mL for dogs <20 kg, 1,000 mL for dogs >20 kg), 2–3 times per wk. Amphotericin B lipid complex (1–2 mg/kg for cats or 2–3 mg/kg for dogs) can also be given 3 times/wk for 12–15 treatments. Flucytosine can be used alone; however, drug resistance may develop, so combination therapy with amphotericin is recommended.

EPIZOOTIC LYMPHANGITIS

Epizootic lymphangitis is a chronic granulomatous disease of the skin, lymph vessels, and lymph nodes of the limbs and neck of Equidae caused by the dimorphic fungus *Histoplasma farciminosum*. The disease is seen in Asian and Mediterranean areas but is unknown in the USA. The fungus forms mycelia in nature and yeast forms in tissues and has a saprophytic phase in soil. Infection probably is acquired by wound infection or transmission by bloodsucking insects.

Clinical Findings and Lesions: The disease is characterized by freely movable cutaneous nodules, which originate from infected superficial lymph vessels and nodes and tend to ulcerate and undergo alternating periods of discharge and closure. Affected lymph nodes are enlarged and hard. The skin covering the nodules may become thick, indurated, and fused to the underlying tissues. Lesions also may be present in the lungs, conjunctiva, cornea, nasal mucosa, and other organs. The nodules are pyogranulomas with a thick, fibrous capsule and contain thick, creamy exudate and the causative organisms.

Diagnosis: The clinical features are highly suggestive. Diagnosis can be confirmed by microscopic examination of exudates and biopsy specimens. The yeast forms of the organisms distend the cytoplasm of macrophages and appear in H&E sections as globose or oval bodies (3–4 μm) with a central basophilic body surrounded by an unstained zone. The organism closely resembles *H capsulatum*. Serologic testing is available with serum agglutination titers of 1:80 or higher reported to be positive. Positive titers may be reflective of past exposure, with specificity for current infection being low.

Treatment: No completely satisfactory treatment is known. Surgical excision of lesions combined with antifungal drugs (amphotericin B) could be used.

HISTOPLASMOSIS

Histoplasmosis is a chronic, noncontagious, disseminated, granulomatous disease of people and other animals caused by the dimorphic fungus *Histoplasma capsulatum*. The organism is commonly found in soil that contains bird and bat manure. It produces mycelial growth in the soil and in culture at room temperature and grows in a yeast form in tissues and in cultures at 37°C.

Histoplasmosis is found worldwide. Endemic areas in the USA include the Mississippi and Ohio River valleys. Infection has been described in many animal species, but disease is uncommon to rare in all but dogs and cats. Infection is commonly via aerosol contamination of the respiratory tract, and the lungs and thoracic lymph nodes are the sites of primary infection, although the GI tract may be a primary site of infection, especially in dogs. The organisms enter the bloodstream from a primary focus and become disseminated throughout the body; they may localize in bone marrow or the eyes, where they produce chorioretinitis or endophthalmitis.

Clinical Findings: The signs vary and are nonspecific, reflecting the various organs involved. Chronic GI signs, especially large intestinal diarrhea, are usually most obvious in dogs, but cats tend to have respiratory and nonspecific clinical signs. Many dogs have a protracted course of weight loss to emaciation, chronic cough, persistent diarrhea, fever, anemia, hepatomegaly, splenomegaly, lymphadenopathy, and nasopharyngeal and GI ulceration. Obstructive respiratory difficulty due to tracheobronchial lymphadenopathy also has been seen in dogs. Dissemination may involve the skin, in which weeping, ulcerated, nodular lesions develop. Polyarthropathy, chorioretinitis, and retinal detachment have also been reported in a dog with disseminated histoplasmosis. Acute histoplasmosis may be fatal after 2–5 wk. In cats, disseminated infection is common. Clinical signs may be nonspecific but often include respiratory difficulty, fever, depression, anorexia, and weight loss. Lymphadenopathy, hepatomegaly, ocular disease (conjunctivitis, granulomatous chorioretinitis, retinal detachment, optic neuritis), lameness, and cutaneous nodules or ulcers may also be seen.

Lesions: Gross lesions include enlargement of the liver, spleen, and mesenteric lymph nodes; ascites; yellow-white, variable-sized nodules in the lungs; and enlargement of bronchial lymph nodes. The enlarged liver may have multiple, scattered, irregular-shaped, pale yellow foci of granulomatous inflammation. Pale foci may be present in the myocardium, and the small intestine may have thickened, gray walls and ulceration of the mucosa.

Diagnosis: Histoplasmosis should be considered when the clinical signs include weight loss, chronic diarrhea, respiratory distress, enlarged bronchial lymph nodes, and pulmonary nodules. *Histoplasma* organisms are usually numerous in affected tissues, and a definitive diagnosis can often be made by fine-needle aspiration and exfoliative cytology. Cytology of bone marrow may be diagnostic in cats. Tissue biopsy may be required if cytology is not diagnostic. *Histoplasma* organisms are difficult to detect with routine H&E stain but stain well with PAS, Gomori methenamine silver, and Gridley fungal stains. Yeast forms in macrophages and giant cells are round to ovoid (1–4 µm) structures with a thin cell wall and a thin, clear zone between the cell wall and cellular cytoplasm. *H capsulatum* can also be cultured from tissue specimens, fine-needle aspirates, and body fluids. Antigen testing using a quantitative antigen ELISA can be performed on urine, serum, and CSF. Cross-reactivity occurs with blastomycosis.

Treatment: Itraconazole (10 mg/kg/day) is the treatment of choice for disseminated histoplasmosis in dogs and cats, although fluconazole is probably also effective. Ketoconazole, 10–15 mg/kg, bid for 4–6 mo, may be effective in early or mild cases of histoplasmosis in dogs. For severe cases, concurrent treatment with amphotericin B or amphotericin B lipid complex is suggested.

HYALOHYPHOMYCOSIS

Hyalohyphomycosis is infection caused by nonpigmented fungi (other than the genera *Aspergillus* or *Penicillium* or the class Zygomycetes) that in tissue form hyphal elements with hyaline or clear walls. Examples of genera causing hyalohyphomycosis in people and other animals include *Acremonium*, *Fusarium*, *Geotrichum*, *Paecilomyces*, *Pseudallescheria*, *Sagenomella*, *Phialosimplex*, *Geosmithia*, *Geomyces*, and *Scedosporium*. Hyalohyphomycosis is far less common than phaeohyphomycosis.

Clinical Findings: Lesions range from local cutaneous, subcutaneous, corneal, or nasal mucosal disease to disseminated disease involving the lungs and multiple other organ systems. Disseminated and corneal forms have been reported most commonly. Animals presenting with cutaneous lesions should be evaluated for systemic disease. Animals being treated with immunosuppressive drugs for immune-mediated disease may develop cutaneous hyalohyphomycosis and not have lesions at other sites, whereas immunocompetent animals that develop hyalohyphomycosis most often do have disseminated disease, or at least disease that is not confined to the skin.

Diagnosis: The several causative fungi cannot be identified by their histologic features in tissues; culture isolation and/or PCR are required.

Treatment: Surgical removal with or without azole antifungal therapy is the treatment of choice for local disease. Disseminated disease typically carries a grave prognosis. Treatment with newer azole antifungals and/or amphotericin B lipid complex may be attempted and is most likely to be effective if immunosuppressive drugs can be tapered.

MYCETOMAS

Mycetomas are granulomatous nodules of the subcutaneous tissues that contain tissue grains or granules. Within the grains are dense colonies of the organism. When such lesions are caused by fungi, they are known as eumycotic mycetomas. The causal agents of eumycotic mycetomas include a variety of saprophytic geophilic fungi. Eumycotic mycetomas caused by pigmented fungi such as *Curvularia* spp and *Madurella* spp are called black- or dark-grain mycetomas. White-grained mycetomas are caused by unpigmented fungi such as *Acremonium* spp and *Scedosporium apiospermum* (the asexual state of *Pseudallescheria boydii*).

Clinical Findings and Lesions: Most eumycotic mycetomas are confined to the subcutaneous tissue, but white-grain mycetomas may be extensions of abdominal cavity disease. Peritonitis or abdominal masses are typically seen in white-grain mycetomas. Black-grain mycetomas are usually characterized by relatively poorly circumscribed cutaneous nodules on the extremities or face. The lesions may ulcerate or form fistulas. When the feet or limbs are involved, the infection may extend to the underlying bone.

The fungal mycelia proliferate in the lesions and organize into aggregates known as granules or grains. In these granules, the mycelium is compact and frequently bizarre and distorted in form. Chlamydospores are frequent, especially at the periphery, and the mycelium may or may not be embedded in an amorphous, cement-like substance. Histologically, the granules are frequently surrounded by eosinophilic deposits. Granules may be of various colors and sizes, depending on the species of fungus involved.

Diagnosis: A presumptive diagnosis can be made if there are grains within the exudate of draining tracts. For cytology, the grains should be examined for the presence of fungal elements. If no tissue grains are found in the exudate, a biopsy of the lesion should be taken for histopathologic examination. Cultures should be performed to confirm cytologic findings and to identify the causative agent. Either tissue grains or biopsy specimens should be cultured.

Treatment: The prognosis for abdominal mycetomas is guarded, because tissue involvement is usually extensive. Cutaneous mycetomas, while not life-threatening, are often difficult to resolve. Radical surgical excision, including limb amputation, may be effective for some cases of cutaneous mycetomas. Effectiveness of antifungal chemotherapy has been reported in only a few cases. In one report, fluconazole, 50 mg/day for 6 wk, was used to successfully treat a dog with intra-abdominal maduromycosis. In another report, longterm treatment with itraconazole, 5–10 mg/kg/day, failed to resolve a disseminated *Acremonium* infection in a dog.

OOMYCOSIS

(Pythiosis, Lagenidiosis)

Oomycosis is caused by pathogens in the class Oomycetes. These organisms are not true fungi but are aquatic pathogens in the kingdom Stramenopila. They are more closely related to algae than fungi but cause disease that closely resembles zygomycosis (*see* p 645). Organisms of significance in veterinary medicine include various species of *Saprolegnia* and *Achyla* (eg, *S diclina*), which are the common agents of cutaneous disease in fishes; *Pythium insidiosum*, the cause of a cutaneous and subcutaneous mycosis in horses (bursatti, swamp cancer, leeches), a cutaneous, subcutaneous, and GI disease in dogs, and a cutaneous and paranasal disease of cats; and *Lagenidium* spp, the cause of cutaneous and systemic lesions and large-vessel aneurysms in dogs. Pythiosis is a common disease of domestic animals in some tropical and subtropical areas of the world. In dogs, pythiosis is most often encountered in southeast Asia, eastern coastal Australia, South America, and in the USA, especially along the Gulf coast. In the USA, the disease most often is seen in fall and winter months.

Clinical Findings and Lesions: In horses, lesions are large, roughly circular, granulomatous, ulcerated, fistulated nodules, or subcutaneous swellings with yellow-gray necrotic masses or cores. The lesions are most common on the legs (especially the lower limbs), abdomen, chest, and genitalia. Distribution of lesions is attributable to the aquatic nature of the

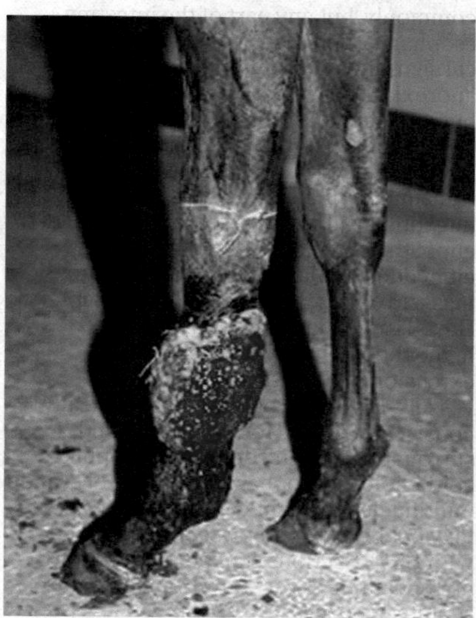

Prominent granulation tissue and inflammation due to *Pythium insidiosum* in a horse. *Courtesy of Dr. Corrie Brown.*

organism. The lesions are pruritic, discharge a mucosanguineous exudate, and often are self-traumatized. The granulomas contain firm, yellowish, coralliform masses of necrotic tissue known as "kunkers," which may be removed intact. Kunkers are foci of coagulative necrosis in vessels that have become sequestered from the surrounding tissue; they contain broad, branching aseptate hyphae and are 1–10 μm in diameter. Bone involvement may be a feature of chronic pythiosis. Enteric pythiosis in horses is characterized by fibrosing and stenotic GI lesions containing intralesional foci of caseous material and fungal hyphae.

Specimens removed at surgery or necropsy consist of fibrous tissue with irregularly spaced, firm, focal areas of necrosis that vary in size and color. Microscopically, alterations vary from foci of acute exudative inflammation with numerous eosinophils to a granulomatous reaction with sequestered areas of necrosis and a framework of hyphae that are thick-walled, branching, and slightly irregular in width.

GI and cutaneous forms of pythiosis are seen and are characterized by severe granulomatous and eosinophilic inflammation. *P insidiosum* infection is seen most often in the GI tract of young adult dogs, especially Labrador Retrievers. The stomach, proximal small intestine, and ileocolic junction are affected most commonly, but any part of the intestine, esophagus, and colon can be diseased. Clinical signs include vomiting, weight loss, and anorexia. The weight loss can be severe, but affected dogs usually do not appear systemically ill until late in the disease. The lesions are typically characterized by severe transmural thickening of the gastric or intestinal wall, with mesenteric lymphadenopathy in which the lymph nodes are embedded in a large, firm granulomatous mass involving the surrounding mesentery. Bowel ischemia, infarction, or acute hemoabdomen may develop due to extension of disease into mesenteric vessels. Enteric pyogranulomas typically consist of necrotic foci infiltrated and surrounded by neutrophils, eosinophils, epithelioid macrophages, plasma cells, and multinucleated giant cells. Etiologic agents may not be apparent on sections stained with H&E. Sections stained with Gomori methenamine silver show branching, rarely septate hyphae.

Cutaneous pythiosis is typified by nonhealing wounds, invasive masses, and ulcerated nodules with draining tracts. The extremities, tail head, ventral neck, or perineum are affected most commonly. Pythiosis in cats is rare and typified by either cutaneous or nasopharyngeal lesions.

Lagenidiosis is an oomycotic infection of dogs characterized by progressive, multifocal cutaneous and subcutaneous lesions, most often affecting the extremities, mammary region, perineum, or trunk. Regional lymphadenopathy is common. At least two species of *Lagenidium* have been shown to affect dogs. One of the *Lagenidium* spp causes more aggressive cutaneous infection with systemic involvement, whereas a less aggressive *Lagenidium* spp tends to cause more slowly progressive cutaneous disease. Cutaneous lesions are characterized as firm dermal or subcutaneous nodules, or as ulcerated, thickened, edematous areas of deep cellulitis with regions of necrosis and numerous draining tracts. In contrast to the clinical course of cutaneous pythiosis, in dogs with aggressive *Lagenidium* spp, involvement at distant sites is often seen. Thoracic and abdominal lymph nodes, lungs, and especially great vessels may be affected. Animals with great vessel or sublumbar lymph node involvement typically have cutaneous or subcutaneous lesions on the hindlimbs and often develop hindlimb edema. Great vessel aneurysms may acutely rupture, resulting in hemoabdomen and sudden death.

Diagnosis: In horses, lesions of pythiosis are similar to those of zygomycosis (*see* p 645) and may be confused with cutaneous habronemiasis (*see* p 904), excessive granulation tissue, and certain equine neoplasms. In pythiosis, the necrotic cores are distinct from the surrounding tissue, and a seropurulent discharge from the sinus tracts is prominent. The lesions contain irregular, branching (at right angles), rarely septate hyphae, 4–8 μm in diameter.

In dogs, diagnosis can be made by isolation of *P insidiosum* from infected tissues. Culture identification or PCR has been used. Immunoblot serology for detection of anti-*P insidiosum* antibodies is available and appears to be both sensitive and specific. Immunoblot serology for detection of anti-*Lagenidium* antibodies in canine serum can provide a presumptive diagnosis of lagenidiosis but must be interpreted in conjunction with results of serologic testing for *P insidiosum* infection because of the potential for cross-reactivity in serum from dogs with pythiosis. The histologic features of lagenidiosis are similar to those of pythiosis and zygomycosis. However, *Lagenidium* hyphae are usually much larger and visible on H&E-stained tissues. Definitive diagnosis of lagenidiosis and pythiosis is best made by culture and PCR identification.

Treatment: The prognosis for pythiosis or lagenidiosis is poor if surgical excision cannot be done. Complete surgical excision is the treatment of choice, but the disease is often too extensive at the time of diagnosis to allow complete resection. In animals with lesions limited to a single distal extremity, amputation is recommended. Medical therapy for pythiosis should include itraconazole (10 mg/kg/day) and terbinafine (5–10 mg/kg/day). Steroids may decrease inflammation and improve clinical signs in the short term. Treatment with amphotericin B lipid complex can also be attempted. Approximately 20% of dogs with pythiosis respond to longterm antifungal therapy. Lagenidiosis appears to be poorly responsive to medical therapy. In horses, the prognosis is guarded, and timely recognition and treatment are essential for successful management. Factors that influence prognosis include size and site of lesion and duration of infection. Small lesions of short duration that have not invaded critical structures usually respond best to treatment. Surgical excision, immunotherapy, or a combination of both may be effective. Immunotherapy consists of a series of intradermal or SC injections of killed, sonicated, whole-cell hyphal antigens or precipitated soluble antigens of the causative fungus. Subcutaneous abscesses at the sites of injection, osteitis, or deep-seated laminitis may be a complication of such therapy. Surgical removal plus systemic or local administration of amphotericin B may be a satisfactory treatment if the disease is localized.

PENICILLIOSIS

Infections with *Penicillium* spp are rare in domestic animals. In dogs, infections of the nasal cavity, lungs, lymph nodes, and bones have been reported. Nasal disease is most common and behaves similar to nasal aspergillosis. In cats, the fungus has been isolated from the nasal cavity, orbital cellulitis and sinusitis, and lungs. It has also been reported to cause systemic disease in captive toucanets (*P griseofulvum*) and bamboo rats (*P marneffei*) in southeast Asia. *Penicillium* spp are widely distributed in nature and are found in soils, grains, and various foods and feeds.

Clinical Findings and Lesions: Dogs with nasal penicilliosis have chronic sneezing and an acute to chronic nasal discharge that varies from intermittent hemorrhagic to intermittent or continuous mucoid or mucopurulent. Radiographic findings include areas of turbinate destruction with increased radiolucency. Grossly, the nasal mucosa has foci of necrosis and ulceration; microscopically, fungal hyphae may form a thick mat over an intact mucosa adjacent to these foci. Systemic disease often affects long bones, resulting in lameness.

Diagnosis: Diagnosis is based on fungal culture, character of the lesions, presence of fungal hyphae, and a positive agar-gel double-diffusion test. Cultural isolation of a *Penicillium* sp must be accompanied by demonstration of tissue invasion by the fungus for confirmation. In tissues, *P marneffei* closely resemble the yeast phase of *Histoplasma capsulatum*.

Treatment: Very little has been reported concerning treatment of penicilliosis. Surgical turbinectomy with curettage has been combined with flushing of the nasal cavity with 1% tincture of iodine or povidone-iodine (10:1) and oral thiabendazole. Fluconazole, 2.5–5 mg/kg/day for 2 mo, has been used to successfully treat some dogs with nasal penicilliosis.

PHAEOHYPHOMYCOSIS

Phaeohyphomycosis refers to chronic cutaneous, subcutaneous, mucosal, cerebral, or systemic infection caused by one of several genera and species of pigmented fungi of the family Dematiaceae. Several fungal genera have been reported to affect people and other animals, including *Alternaria*, *Bipolaris*, *Cladophialophora* (*Xylohypha*, *Cladosporium*), *Curvularia*, *Exophiala*, *Fonsecaea*, *Moniliella*, *Phialophora*, *Ramichloridium*, and *Scolecobasidium*. Fungi in this category are saprophytic, widely distributed organisms found in soil, water, and decaying vegetable matter. Infection may result from fungal implantation into tissue at the site of an injury.

Clinical Findings and Lesions: Phaeohyphomycosis has been described in cows, cats, horses, and dogs. The most common clinical presentations include ulcerated cutaneous nodules of the digits, pinnae, nasal planum, and nasal/paranasal tissues in cats. The nodules may ulcerate and have draining fistulous tracts. These pyogranulomas contain pigmented, septate hyphae with irregular enlargements and thin-walled, budding, yeast-like forms. Granulomatous meningoencephalitis caused by pigmented fungi has been reported in dogs and cats. Dogs treated with multiple immunosuppressive agents, especially cyclosporine, appear to be predisposed to developing multifocal cutaneous lesions. Systemic dissemination is most likely in animals treated with immunosuppressive drugs.

Diagnosis: Phaeohyphomycosis can be diagnosed by microscopic examination of exudate and biopsy specimens, which reveals pigmented, dark-walled, irregularly septate filamentous hyphae (2–6 μm in diameter) or yeast-like cells. Infected tissues may be grossly pigmented, giving an appearance of melanoma. The several causative fungi cannot be identified by their histologic features in tissues; cultural isolation and/or PCR are required. The differential diagnosis should include neoplasia, other granulomas, and epidermoid cysts.

Treatment: Phaeohyphomycosis is generally poorly responsive to treatment. Wide excision of cutaneous or subcutaneous lesions is recommended, followed by 6–12 mo of treatment with itraconazole (10 mg/kg/day). Nonresectable disease should be treated with itraconazole. Voriconazole or posaconazole may be more effective, but voriconazole is not recommended in cats. In dogs being treated with immunosuppressive therapy, the prognosis may be better if the immunosuppressive drugs (especially cyclosporine) can be discontinued.

RHINOSPORIDIOSIS

Rhinosporidiosis is a chronic, nonfatal, pyogranulomatous infection, primarily of the nasal mucosa and occasionally of the skin of horses, cattle, dogs, cats, and aquatic birds, caused by the fungus *Rhinosporidium seeberi*. Uncommon in North America, it is seen most often in India, Africa, and South America. The organism has not been cultured, and its natural habitat is unknown. Trauma may predispose to infection, which is not considered transmissible.

Clinical Findings and Lesions: Infection of the nasal mucosa is characterized by polypoid growths that may be soft, pink, friable, lobulated with roughened surfaces, and large enough to occlude the nasal passages. The cutaneous lesions may be single or multiple, sessile or pedunculated. The nasal polyps and cutaneous lesions have a granulomatous, fibromyxoid inflammatory component and contain the fungal organism.

Diagnosis: Rhinosporidiosis may be confused with other granulomatous lesions of the nasal mucosa and skin, including aspergillosis, entomophthoromycosis, "nasal granuloma," and cryptococcosis. Microscopic demonstration of spherules (sporangia) of *R seeberi* in biopsy specimens confirms the diagnosis. The spherules may be numerous, vary in size (up to 300 μm), have thick walls that stain periodic acid-Schiff positive, and contain endospores 4–19 μm in diameter. Developing stages of varying size without spores are distributed throughout the lesion.

Treatment: Surgical excision of the lesions is considered standard, but recurrence is common. Amphotericin B and itraconazole have been described for medical treatment but are generally not as effective as surgery.

SPOROTRICHOSIS

Sporotrichosis is a sporadic, chronic, granulomatous disease of people and various domestic and laboratory animals caused by *Sporothrix schenckii*. The organism is dimorphic and forms mycelia on vegetation and in Sabouraud dextrose agar at 25°–30°C (77°–86°F) but is yeast-like in tissue and media at 37°C (98.6°F). It is ubiquitous in soil, vegetation, and timber; is distributed worldwide; and in the USA is most commonly found in coastal regions and river valleys. Infection usually results from direct inoculation of the organism into skin wounds via contact with plants or soil or penetrating foreign bodies. Disseminated disease caused by inhalation of spores is rare.

Sporotrichosis has been reported in dogs, cats, horses, cows, camels, dolphins, goats, mules, birds, pigs, rats, armadillos, and people. Zoonotic infections can occur. The cat may be the species with the greatest zoonotic potential, and transmission from cats to people has been reported without evidence of trauma. In contrast, transmission from other infected species appears to require inoculation of previously traumatized skin. The large number of organisms shed from the wound and in the feces of infected cats is believed to be responsible for the increased zoonotic potential of feline sporotrichosis. Epidemics of sporotrichosis have been reported in Brazil. Data from these studies support the importance of cats in the zoonotic transmission of the organism. Caretakers of infected cats were four times more likely to become infected than others living in the same household.

Clinical Findings and Lesions: Sporotrichosis may be grouped into three forms: lymphocutaneous, cutaneous, and disseminated. The lymphocutaneous form is the most common. Small, firm dermal to subcutaneous nodules, 1–3 cm in diameter, develop at the site of inoculation. As infection ascends along the lymphatic vessels, cording and new nodules develop. Lesions ulcerate and discharge a serohemorrhagic exudate. In cats, lesions are most often seen on the head, especially on the bridge of the nose and pinnae. Although systemic illness is not seen initially, chronic illness may result in fever, listlessness, and depression. Respiratory signs may be apparent. The cutaneous form tends to remain localized to the site of inoculation, although lesions may be multicentric. Disseminated sporotrichosis is rare but potentially fatal and may develop with neglect of cutaneous and lymphocutaneous forms or if the animal is inappropriately treated with corticosteroids. Infection develops via hematogenous or tissue spread from the initial site of inoculation to the bone, lungs, liver, spleen, testes, GI tract, or CNS.

Diagnosis: Diagnosis can be made by culture (samples obtained from unopened lesions) or microscopic examination of the exudate or biopsy specimens. In tissues and exudate, the organism is present as few to numerous, cigar-shaped, single cells within macrophages. The fungal cells are pleomorphic and small (2–10 × 1–3 μm); buds may be present and give the appearance of a ping-pong paddle. A fluorescent antibody technique has been used to identify the yeast-like cells in tissues. In species other than cats, *Sporothrix* organisms are often sparse in exudate and infected tissue, so that diagnosis usually requires culture. In cultures, a true mycelium is produced, with fine, branching, septate hyphae bearing pear-shaped conidia on slender conidiophores.

Treatment: Itraconazole (10 mg/kg/day) is considered the treatment of choice for sporotrichosis. Treatment should be continued 3–4 wk beyond apparent clinical cure. Terbinafine has also been used successfully. Alternatively, a supersaturated solution of potassium iodide, administered PO, has been used with some success; therapy is continued 30 days beyond apparent clinical cure. During treatment, the animal should be monitored for signs of iodide toxicity: anorexia, vomiting, depression, muscle twitching, hypothermia, cardiomyopathy, cardiovascular collapse, and death. Cats are especially sensitive to iodides and the development of iodism.

Zoonotic Risk: Sporotrichosis is an important zoonosis, with animal-to-human transmission well documented. Strict hygiene must be observed when handling animals (especially cats) with suspected or diagnosed sporotrichosis. People in contact with infected animals should be informed of the contagious nature of the disease when therapeutic options are discussed.

ZYGOMYCOSIS

(Basidiobolomycosis, Conidiobolomycosis, Entomophthoromycosis)

Zygomycosis is used to describe infection with fungi in the class Zygomycetes and two genera in the order Entomophthorales, *Basidiobolus* and *Conidiobolus*. True zygomycete infections are rare, but conidiobolomycosis and basidiobolomycosis are more common and cause pyogranulomatous lesions grossly and histologically similar to those caused by pythiosis and lagenidiosis. This is primarily an infection of the nasopharyngeal mucosa and subcutaneous tissue of horses and rarely other animals (llamas, sheep) by *C coronatus*, *C incongruus*, *C lamprauges*, or *B ranarum*. These ubiquitous fungi are present in soil and decaying vegetation and, in the case of basidioboli, the GI tracts of amphibians, reptiles, and macropods. *C coronatus* affects almost exclusively the mucosa of the nose and mouth. *Basidiobolus* infects the lateral aspects of the head, neck, and body. *C coronatus* is also an important insect pathogen.

Clinical Findings: Ulcerative pyogranulomas of the mucous membrane of the nasopharyngeal tissue, mouth, or nodular growths of the nasal mucosa and the lips may be seen with conidiobolomycosis, resulting in mechanical obstruction of the nasal cavity, dyspnea, and nasal discharge. Local dissemination into the retropharyngeal, retrobulbar, or other tissues of the face may be noted. Lesions in basidiobolomycosis are usually single, circular, ulcerative, pruritic nodules of the skin of the upper body. Fistulous tracts discharge a serosanguineous fluid from the lesions, which frequently are traumatized. Extension to regional lymph nodes results in swelling of the nodes and development of yellow necrotic foci. Lesions may contain a creamy, yellow central core of necrotic tissue. Disseminated basidiobolomycosis is rare but has been described in dogs and a mandrill.

Lesions: In excised tissues or necropsy specimens, a thickened fibrotic dermis has scattered, red or creamy white areas. The lesions, which contain hyphal forms, a heavy infiltrate of eosinophils, and sequestered areas of necrosis, have histologic features of infectious granulomas.

Diagnosis: Clinically, zygomycosis may be confused with cutaneous habronemiasis (*see* p 904) and oomycosis (*see* p 641) but can be differentiated by microscopic examination of tissues. In H&E sections, the fungus appears as holes and elongated channels, and many hyphae have a wide eosinophilic cuff; in sections stained for fungi, the organism consists of large, branching, sometimes septate, 2.5–25 µm hyphae. Cultural examination is required to identify the causative fungus.

Treatment: Longterm itraconazole administration is recommended for treatment of nasopharyngeal infection. Although lesions often regress, recurrence is common after treatment is discontinued. Cutaneous zygomycete infections should be treated with wide surgical resection followed by longterm itraconazole.

LEPTOSPIROSIS

Leptospirosis is a zoonotic disease with a worldwide distribution caused by infection with any of several pathogenic serovars of *Leptospira*. The disease affects virtually all mammals and has a broad range of clinical effects, from mild, subclinical infection to multiple-organ failure and death.

Etiology: *Leptospira* are aerobic, gram-negative spirochetes that are fastidious, slow growing, and have characteristic corkscrew-like motility. The taxonomy of *Leptospira* is complex and can be confusing. Traditionally, *Leptospira* were divided into two groups; the pathogenic *Leptospira* were all classified as members of *L interrogans*, and the saprophytic *Leptospira* were classified as *L biflexa*. Within each of these species, leptospiral serovars were recognized, with >250 different serovars of pathogenic *Leptospira* identified (based on surface antigens) throughout the world. The serovars are often grouped into antigenically related serogroups. With the increased use of genomic information for the classification of bacteria, the genus *Leptospira* was reorganized. There are currently 21 recognized genomospecies of leptospires, including both pathogenic, intermediate, and nonpathogenic organisms. Pathogenic leptospires are now identified in 9 species of *Leptospira*, with 6 species being regarded as intermediate in pathogenicity, and 6 being nonpathogenic. Some of the common leptospiral pathogens of domestic animals now have different species names. For example, *L interrogans* serovar Grippotyphosa is now *L kirschneri* serovar Grippotyphosa. The two types of serovar Hardjo have been formally split into two species: serovar Hardjo type hardjobovis (found in the USA and much of the world) is now *L borgpetersenii* serovar Hardjo and the less common serovar Hardjo type hardjo-prajitno (found primarily in the UK) is now *L interrogans* serovar Hardjo. The revised nomenclature is now reflected in the scientific literature but not on labels for vaccines and pharmaceutical products. Fortunately for clinicians, the serovar and serogroup names remain in common use and are useful when discussing the epidemiology, serology, clinical features, treatment, and prevention of leptospirosis.

Host Susceptibility, Epidemiology, and Transmission: Essentially all mammals are susceptible to infection with pathogenic *Leptospira*, although some species are more resistant to disease. Among common companion animals and livestock, leptospirosis is most frequently recognized in cattle, swine, dogs, and horses. Cats have historically been considered to be resistant to disease but have been shown to seroconvert on exposure to leptospires. Recent evidence suggests that the role of leptospires in the pathogenesis of feline renal disease should be reexamined. Leptospirosis in wildlife is common, although the disease is most often noticed only when the wildlife serve as a source of infection for domestic animals or people.

Leptospirosis is found throughout the world. The infection (and disease) is more prevalent in warm, moist climates and is endemic in much of the tropics. In temperate climates, the disease is more seasonal, with the highest incidence after periods of rainfall.

Although >250 serovars of pathogenic *Leptospira* are recognized, a subset of leptospiral serovars are prevalent within a particular region or ecosystem and are associated with one or more maintenance hosts, which serve as reservoirs of infection (*see* TABLE 4). Maintenance hosts are often wildlife species and, sometimes, domestic animals and livestock. Each serovar behaves differently within its maintenance host species than it does in other, incidental host species. In maintenance hosts, leptospirosis is generally characterized by a high prevalence of infection, relatively mild acute clinical signs, and persistent infection in the kidneys and sometimes the genital tract.

Diagnosis of maintenance host infections is difficult because of relatively low antibody responses and the presence of few organisms in the tissues of infected animals. Examples of this type of infection are serovar Bratislava infection in swine and serovar Hardjo infection in cattle. In incidental hosts, leptospirosis is characterized by a low prevalence of infection, severe clinical signs, and a short renal phase of infection. Diagnosis of incidental host infections is less problematic because of a marked antibody response to infection and the presence of large numbers of organisms in tissues of infected animals. Examples of this type of infection are serovar Grippotyphosa infection in dogs or serovar Icterohaemorrhagiae infection in cattle and swine.

Characterization of a host/serovar interaction as a maintenance or incidental host infection is not absolute. For example, swine and cattle infected with serovar Pomona behave as a host intermediate between the two forms, with the organism persisting in the kidneys but the host showing a marked antibody response to infection.

Transmission among maintenance hosts is often direct and involves contact with infected urine, placental fluids, or milk. In addition, the infection can be transmitted venereally or transplacentally with some host/serovar combinations. Infection of incidental hosts is more commonly indirect, by contact with areas contaminated with urine of asymptomatic maintenance hosts that shed leptospires in their urine. Environmental conditions are critical in determining the frequency of indirect transmission. Survival of leptospires is favored by moisture and moderately warm temperatures; survival is brief in dry soil or at temperatures <10°C or >34°C. The organisms are killed by freezing, dehydration, or direct sunlight.

Pathogenesis: Despite the many serovars of *Leptospira* and host species, the key steps in pathogenesis of the disease are similar in all host/serovar combinations. Leptospires invade the body after penetrating exposed mucous membranes or

TABLE 4 COMMON MAINTENANCE HOSTS OF THE PATHOGENIC LEPTOSPIRES ASSOCIATED WITH DISEASE IN DOMESTIC ANIMALS IN THE USA AND CANADA

Leptospiral Serovar	Maintenance Hosts
Canicola	Dogs
Pomona	Pigs, cattle, opossums, skunks
Grippotyphosa	Raccoons, muskrats, skunks, voles
Hardjo	Cattle
Icterohaemorrhagiae	Rats
Bratislava	Pigs, mice (?), horses (?)

damaged skin. After a variable incubation period (4–20 days), leptospires circulate in the blood and replicate in many tissues including the liver, kidneys, lungs, genital tract, and CNS for 7–10 days. During the period of bacteremia and tissue colonization, the clinical signs of acute leptospirosis, which vary by serovar and host, occur. Agglutinating antibodies can be detected in serum soon after leptospiremia occurs and coincide with clearance of the leptospires from blood and most organs. As the organisms are cleared, the clinical signs of acute leptospirosis begin to resolve, although damaged organs may take some time to return to normal function. In some cases, severely damaged organs may not recover, leading to chronic disease or death.

At this point, the disease in incidental and maintenance hosts diverges. Leptospires remain in the tubules of the kidneys of incidental hosts for a short period of time and are shed in the urine for a few days to several weeks. In maintenance hosts, however, leptospires often remain in the renal tubules, genital tract, and less commonly, the eyes, despite the presence of high levels of serum antibody. Leptospires are shed in the urine and genital secretions of persistently infected animals for months to years after initial infection, and these animals become an important reservoir of infection, with the potential to transmit infection to other reservoir hosts or to incidental hosts at risk of developing clinical disease.

Clinical Findings: The clinical signs of leptospirosis depend on the host species, the pathogenicity of the strain and serovar of *Leptospira*, and the age and physiologic state of the animal. Subclinical infections are common, particularly in the maintenance host. In incidental hosts, leptospirosis is an acute, systemic, often febrile illness characterized by renal and/or hepatic damage. In addition, there may be effects on other body systems resulting in clinical problems such as uveitis, pancreatitis, bleeding, hemolytic anemia, muscle pain, or respiratory disease.

In both incidental and maintenance hosts that are pregnant at the time of infection, localization and persistence of the organism in the uterus may result in fetal infection, with subsequent abortion, stillbirth, birth of weak neonates, or birth of healthy but infected offspring. In general, incidental hosts abort acutely, whereas in maintenance hosts, abortions or other reproductive sequelae may be delayed by several weeks or months.

Diagnosis: Diagnosis of leptospirosis depends on a good clinical and vaccination history and laboratory testing. Diagnostic tests for leptospirosis include those designed to detect antibodies against the organism and those designed to detect the organism in tissues or body fluids. Serologic testing is recommended in each case, combined with one or more techniques to identify the organism in tissue or body fluids.

Serologic assays are the most commonly used technique to diagnose leptospirosis in animals. The microscopic agglutination test (MAT) is most frequently used. It involves mixing appropriate dilutions of serum with live leptospires of serovars prevalent within the region. The presence of antibodies is indicated by the agglutination of the leptospires, with the reported titer being the highest dilution of serum that results in 50% agglutination. The MAT is a complex test to perform and interpret, and it requires the maintenance of live leptospiral cultures. An ELISA test to diagnose canine leptospirosis is offered by a commercial laboratory in the USA. This test detects antibodies to LipL32, a membrane protein found on pathogenic leptospires. The currently available assay provides a qualitative negative or positive result and will also detect antibodies induced by vaccination. A comparison of this test to the MAT has not been reported, and it is likely that the numerical titers provided by the MAT will provide more diagnostically useful information than a qualitative ELISA.

Interpretation of serologic results from the MAT is complicated by a number of factors, including cross-reactivity of antibodies, antibody titers induced by vaccination, and lack of consensus about the level of antibody titer that indicates infection. Antibodies produced in an animal in response to infection with a given serovar of *Leptospira* often cross-react with other serovars. In some cases, these patterns of cross-reactivity are predictable based on the antigenic relatedness of the various serovars of *Leptospira*, but the patterns of cross-reactive antibodies vary between host species. Paradoxical reactions may occur with the MAT early in the course of an acute infection, with a marked agglutinating antibody response to a serovar other than the infecting serovar. In addition, there is evidence of lack of consistency between diagnostic laboratories. For these reasons, the infecting serovar in an individual animal cannot be reliably identified as the serovar to which the animal develops the highest titer. The real value of the MAT is in providing a numerical titer to allow comparison of acute and convalescent values.

Widespread vaccination of dogs and livestock with leptospiral vaccines also complicates interpretation of leptospiral serology. In general, vaccinated animals develop relatively low agglutinating antibody titers (1:100 to 1:400) in response to vaccination, and these titers persist for 1–4 mo after vaccination. However, some animals develop high titers after vaccination which persist for ≥6 mo.

Consensus is lacking as to what constitutes a diagnostic titer for leptospiral infection. A low antibody titer does not necessarily exclude a diagnosis of leptospirosis, because titers are often low in acute disease and in maintenance host infections. In cases of acute leptospirosis, a 4-fold rise in antibody titer is often observed in paired serum samples collected 7–10 days apart. Diagnosis of leptospirosis based on a single serum sample should be made with caution and with full consideration of the clinical picture and vaccination history of the animal. In general, with a compatible clinical history and vaccination >3 mo ago, a titer of 1:800 to 1:1,600 is good presumptive evidence of leptospiral infection. The use of paired acute and convalescent titers is strongly recommended whenever possible. Antibody titers can persist for several months after infection and recovery, although there is usually a gradual decline with time.

Immunofluorescence can be used to identify leptospires in tissues, blood, or urine sediment. The test is rapid and has reasonable sensitivity, but interpretation requires a skilled laboratory technician. Immunohistochemistry is useful to identify leptospires in formalin-fixed tissue but, because there may be small numbers of organisms present in some tissues, the sensitivity of this technique is variable. A number of PCR procedures are available, and each laboratory may select a slightly different procedure. Unfortunately, few publications have confirmed the validity of all the commercially available PCRs, which likely vary considerably in their performance. PCR techniques allow detection of pathogenic leptospires in blood, urine, or tissue samples but do not determine the infecting serovar. Culture of blood, urine, or tissue specimens is the only method to definitively identify the infecting serovar. Blood may be cultured early in the clinical course; urine is more likely to be positive 7–10 days after clinical signs appear. Culture is rarely positive after antibiotic therapy has begun. Culture of leptospires requires specialized culture medium, the organisms are fastidious and slow-growing, and diagnostic laboratories rarely culture specimens for the presence of leptospires. Thus, culture is of little value to clinicians.

Prevention: Avoidance of exposure to free-ranging wildlife and domestic animals that may be maintenance hosts for *Leptospira* is difficult because rodents, raccoons, opossums, and skunks are frequently found in rural and urban environments. The cornerstone of leptospirosis prevention is vaccination with polyvalent inactivated vaccines. Immunity to leptospirosis is believed to be serovar specific and, therefore, vaccines are formulated for various species to include the relevant serovars. There are currently no leptospiral vaccines for horses. Leptospiral vaccines are generally designed and evaluated for the ability to prevent clinical signs of disease, although some vaccines have also been shown to significantly reduce renal colonization and urine shedding.

Zoonotic Risk: People are susceptible to infection with most of the pathogenic serovars of *Leptospira* but are incidental hosts and, therefore, not important reservoirs of infection. Occupational exposure is a rick factor, and veterinarians, veterinary staff, livestock producers, and dairy workers are at increased risk. In addition, recreational exposure to waters contaminated with urine of domestic animals or wildlife presents a risk. Animal owners have contracted leptospirosis via contact with infected companion animals and livestock.

The principal route of infection is contact with infectious body fluids (blood in acute cases or urine) via mucous membranes. In people, the disease varies from subclinical to severe and can be fatal when renal or hepatic failure occurs. The most common signs are fever, headaches, rash, ocular pain, myalgia, and malaise. Transplacental infection, abortion, and infection of infants via breast feeding have been described, making exposure of pregnant women of particular concern. Laboratory techniques are necessary for a definitive diagnosis. Because diagnosis of leptospirosis in animals is difficult based on clinical signs, veterinarians may wish to implement an infection control program in which animal body fluids are handled only with gloved hands and hand washing is routine. It is also essential for staff to take precautions when handling or nursing animals suspected or confirmed to have leptospirosis. Appropriate precautions include wearing gowns, shoe covers, and gloves to avoid contaminating exposed skin or spreading organisms. Face shields should be worn when handling wet bedding or cleaning cages, stalls, or runs to avoid contact of aerosolized organisms with mucous membranes.

LEPTOSPIROSIS IN DOGS

Dogs are the maintenance host for *Leptospira interrogans* serovar Canicola, and before widespread vaccination programs, serovars Canicola and Icterohaemorrhagiae were the most common serovars in dogs in the USA. The prevalence of canine serovars has shifted significantly in the last 20 years; currently the most prevalent serovars are believed to be Grippotyphosa, Pomona, and Bratislava; however, this belief is largely based on serologic results that are now known to be inaccurate in predicting the infecting serovar in dogs with leptospirosis. The serovars that cause disease in dogs are likely to vary with geographic region and the presence of reservoir hosts. Unfortunately, current understanding of the serovars that cause natural disease in dogs is limited by the fact that isolation of leptospires is rarely performed; thus, studies to date have relied on serologic data. As noted above, it is now accepted that the results of the MAT do not reliably predict the infecting serovar in dogs (or people) with leptospirosis; thus, the true infecting serovar is unknown in most cases. However, it is likely that the serovars that cause disease in dogs are those circulating in local wildlife. Experimental infections and isolation of organisms from a small number of sick dogs have shown that serovars Icterohaemorrhagiae, Canicola, Autumnalis, Pomona, Bratislava, Sejroe, and Ballum are capable of causing disease in dogs. Knowledge of the infecting serovar in dogs is essential for epidemiologic studies and vaccine development; it is less important for clinicians managing individual cases. It is currently not known whether specific serovars are associated with specific clinical signs in dogs, and there is no published evidence to guide therapy based on serovar identification. It is, however, extremely important for veterinarians to maintain a high index of suspicion for leptospirosis, because this is a zoonotic disease and has a wide range of clinical presentations in dogs. Any age, breed, or sex of dog is susceptible to leptospirosis, and the diagnosis should not be excluded on the basis of signalment or lifestyle. Canine leptospirosis is not restricted to large-breed dogs, male dogs, or dogs with a predominantly outdoor lifestyle.

Acute kidney injury has been the most common presentation for canine leptospirosis in recent years. Affected dogs may present with lethargy, anorexia, vomiting, abdominal pain, and history of polyuria, oliguria, or anuria. Dogs that survive acute renal failure may return to baseline or progress to chronic kidney disease. Leptospirosis should also be considered in any dog with previously diagnosed chronic kidney disease that develops “acute-on-chronic” kidney injury. Renal tubular damage in leptospirosis may manifest as cylindruria, proteinuria, or glycosuria. In people, acute kidney injury due to leptospirosis is often nonoliguric and can be associated with hyponatremia and hypokalemia. These electrolyte changes have also been noted in canine leptospirosis, along with the expected changes of azotemia, hyperphosphatemia, and acidosis of renal failure. Hyperkalemia is also possible. Polyuria and polydipsia (PU/PD) in the absence of azotemia is a less common manifestation of the renal effects of leptospirosis. PU/PD may be due to a decrease in glomerular filtration rate that is sufficient to cause loss of renal concentrating ability without azotemia. However, PU/PD can also be due to nephrogenic diabetes insipidus.

Acute liver disease may accompany acute renal failure in dogs with leptospirosis, or it may occur alone. Affected dogs may be icteric, and serum biochemistry analysis reveals increased bilirubin and alkaline phosphatase. ALT is typically less markedly increased than alkaline phosphatase. In people and dogs, the jaundice of acute leptospirosis appears to be associated with minimal histopathologic changes in the liver, suggesting that it is due to the “cholestasis of sepsis” rather than to hepatocellular damage.

Muscle pain, stiffness, weakness, trembling, or reluctance to move can be seen in dogs with leptospirosis. These may be the result of vasculitis, myositis, or nephritis. Myalgia is commonly reported in human leptospirosis and is associated with the septicemic phase of the disease.

Less common manifestations of canine leptospirosis include bleeding disorders characterized by petechial hemorrhages, epistaxis, melena, and hematemesis. These findings are most likely due to vasculitis.

Affected dogs may also be thrombocytopenic; however, platelet counts are rarely low enough to be responsible for spontaneous bleeding. The causes and mechanisms of bleeding disorders in leptospirosis are poorly understood, but they have been suggested to be associated with endothelial cell damage. Pulmonary hemorrhage is now one of the most common clinical signs in outbreaks of human leptospirosis. This is a less common finding in canine leptospirosis; however, cough or dyspnea, or radiographic abnormalities have been noted in a number of affected dogs. Uveitis is an uncommon manifestation of leptospirosis in dogs. It appears to be infrequently associated with experimental canine leptospirosis, but rare case reports exist. Additional clinical signs reported in dogs with leptospirosis include vomiting, diarrhea, weight loss, fever, hypothermia, oculonasal discharge, lymphadenopathy, effusions, and edema.

CBC changes may include neutrophilia, lymphopenia, monocytosis, and mild anemia. These changes are nonspecific; however, mild to moderate thrombocytopenia is seen in >50% of cases and, if detected in combination with azotemia or evidence of cholestasis, should prompt diagnostic testing for leptospirosis. Coagulation abnormalities may include increased fibrin degradation products and prolonged prothrombin time (PT) or activated partial thromboplastin time (APTT). Urinalysis may reveal hyposthenuria, isosthenuria, or hypersthenuria, depending on the degree of renal involvement. Other changes may include proteinuria, glucosuria, cylindruria, hematuria, and pyuria. Leptospirosis could also potentially be associated with renal tubular acidosis.

Reticulonodular pulmonary opacities have been described in the thoracic radiographs of dogs with leptospirosis and attributed to pulmonary hemorrhage. These changes may be diffuse or predominantly involve the caudodorsal lung fields. Abdominal radiographs may be unremarkable or may show renomegaly or hepatomegaly. Changes noted on ultrasonography include renomegaly, pyelectasia, increased cortical echogenicity, perinephric effusion, and a hyperechoic medullary band. However, these changes are not specific for leptospirosis, and absence of these findings does not exclude the diagnosis.

Gross necropsy findings can include jaundice, effusions, and petechial or ecchymotic hemorrhages on any organ, pleural, or peritoneal surface. The kidneys and liver may be enlarged, and lungs may be wet, heavy, and discolored. The liver is often friable with an accentuated lobular pattern and may have a yellowish brown discoloration. The kidneys may have white foci on the subcapsular surface. Microscopic findings in the liver may include mild random hepatocytic necrosis, nonsuppurative hepatitis, and intrahepatic bile stasis, while swollen tubular epithelial cells, tubular necrosis, and a mixed inflammatory reaction may be seen in the kidneys.

Ideally, a combination of serology and organism detection should be used for diagnosis of canine leptospirosis. Serology is the most frequently used diagnostic test for dogs. Acute and convalescent titers may be necessary to confirm a diagnosis; hence, the use of the MAT is preferred over the ELISA. PCR-based tests are widely available, and collection of both blood and urine samples before administration of antibiotics should be considered for maximal sensitivity. The results of all diagnostic tests should be interpreted in light of the animal's vaccination history, clinical signs, and clinicopathologic findings.

Renal failure and liver disease are treated with fluid therapy and other supportive measures to maintain normal fluid, electrolyte, and acid-base balance. Supportive measures may include antiemetics, GI protectants, phosphate binders, and hepatic support medications. Renal replacement therapy with intermittent hemodialysis or continuous renal replacement therapy should be considered for dogs that are anuric or oliguric despite appropriate supportive therapy. Antibiotic therapy is indicated whenever leptospirosis is suspected and should be instituted before confirmatory test results are available. There are no experimental studies in dogs to guide selection of antibiotic protocols for this species. Current recommendations are to treat with doxycycline (5 mg/kg, PO, every 12 hours) for 2 wk. For dogs that cannot tolerate doxycycline, initial therapy with a penicillin is appropriate, but this should be followed by a 2-wk course of doxycycline to eliminate the renal carrier phase of infection. Dogs recently exposed to leptospirosis may be treated prophylactically with oral doxycycline for 14 days.

Commercial bacterins for dogs are available for serovars Canicola, Icterohaemorrhagiae, Grippotyphosa, and Pomona. Vaccinated dogs may potentially be susceptible to infection with other serovars, although this has not been tested in an experimental setting. In general, currently available vaccines provide good protection from clinical disease and also appear to reduce renal colonization and urine shedding. Concerns exist regarding hypersensitivity reactions after leptospiral vaccination in dogs, but these appear to be unjustified based on more recent studies and perhaps associated with the use of more highly purified vaccines. Canine challenge studies have demonstrated duration of immunity of at least 1 yr; thus, prior recommendations for vaccinating every 6 mo are no longer justified.

Because leptospirosis is a zoonotic disease, all veterinary personnel should take appropriate precautions when handling known or suspected infected animals. Such dogs do not need to be placed in isolation but should be nursed with barrier precautions, paying particular attention to avoiding exposure of skin or mucous membranes to urine or blood. Infected dogs should be allowed to urinate in designated areas that can subsequently be cleaned and disinfected. The organisms are killed by all commonly used disinfectants. Owners of dogs recently diagnosed with leptospirosis should be advised of the zoonotic nature of the disease and contact their physicians with any health concerns. Owners should wear gloves when cleaning up urine and should wash their hands after handling the dog, at least until the course of antibiotic therapy is completed.

LEPTOSPIROSIS IN HORSES

In the USA and Canada, *Leptospira interrogans* serovar Pomona type kennewicki and serovar Grippotyphosa are the most common causes of equine leptospirosis. The prevalence of leptospirosis in horses is unknown, but serologic evidence indicates a higher incidence than is apparent clinically. Antibodies to serovar Bratislava are reported frequently in horses in the USA and in Europe; horses are thought to be a maintenance host for this organism, and clinical disease has not been confirmed with Bratislava infections. Acute Pomona infections also commonly cause cross-reacting antibodies for Bratislava and Icterohaemorrhagiae on the MAT, which may explain some of the commonly observed high titers to Bratislava. Clinical leptospirosis in horses is most commonly associated with abortions, acute renal failure, rarely pulmonary or systemic illness in foals, and most importantly recurrent uveitis.

Leptospira interrogans serovar Pomona abortions may account for ~13% of bacterial abortions in mares in endemic regions, although incidence varies considerably between years. The reason for the yearly variation in incidence of abortions is not clear. Serovar Pomona type kennewicki is responsible for most of the leptospiral abortions in North America, but serovars Grippotyphosa and Hardjo have also been reported. Skunks, raccoons, and red foxes are known to harbor Pomona type kennewicki. Most abortions occur after 9 mo of gestation, and rarely a live foal may be born ill from leptospirosis. Macroscopic lesions are edema, areas of necrosis in the chorion, and placentitis that does not involve the cervical star. Microscopic lesions include necrosis and calcification of the placenta. Placental disease may result in the mare developing hydroallantois. Macroscopically, the fetal liver may have yellow discoloration. Liver disease in the fetus is a multifocal necrosis and giant cell hepatopathy. Tubulonephrosis and interstitial nephritis may be detected in the kidneys of the aborted fetus. Inflammation of the umbilical cord (funisitis) may be recognized by diffuse yellowish discoloration. Aborting mares typically have very high leptospiral antibody titers at the time of abortion and, although quite variable, the time of urine shedding of leptospires after an abortion is often 2–3 mo.

Occasionally, *Leptospira interrogans* serovar Pomona causes fever and acute renal failure in horses. The kidneys become swollen as a result of tubulointerstitial nephritis, and urinalysis may reveal hematuria and pyuria without visible bacteria. On rare occasions, multiple weanling or yearling horses may be affected with fever and acute renal failure after infection.

The most important clinical disease associated with *L interrogans* serovar Pomona infection in adult horses in North America and *L kirschneri* serovar Grippotyphosa in Europe is equine recurrent uveitis (ERU). ERU is believed to be an immune-mediated disease sometimes involving antibody against certain *Leptospira* antigens, specifically the LruC outer membrane protein, which cross-reacts with tissues of the lens, cornea, and possibly retina. Live *Leptospira* organisms can be found in the aqueous or vitreous fluid of horses with ERU. High concentration of antibody against *L interrogans* serovar Pomona in the aqueous humor, compared with serum titers, also suggests persistent local antigenic stimulation. Survival of the organism in the face of high ocular antibody indicates an absence of cells or molecules (eg, complement) involved in bacterial clearance, suggesting an ocular immune privilege similar to that of the CNS. Recurrent episodes of the disease may be related to a Th17 response of autoreactivity following mimicry and inter- or intramolecular epitope spreading, or both.

Genetic factors are likely involved in the disease process, helping to explain why only some horses infected with *Leptospira* develop uveitis. Appaloosas are thought to be genetically predisposed, and specific MHC markers on ECA1, ELA class 1, and an ELA class II microsatellite are strongly associated with the disease. The prevalence of ERU is unknown, but reports suggest that ≥1% of horses will develop the disease during their lifetime. It is probable that some cases of ERU are not associated with *Leptospira* infection, and this may vary by geographic region. In some regions, more than 50% of ERU cases are associated with persistent ocular infections with *Leptospira*. *Leptospira*-associated uveitis may cause corneal, anterior chamber, and posterior chamber disease. Therefore, clinical findings may vary from corneal edema, clinically quiet retinal lesions observed on funduscopic examination, and most dramatically recurrent and progressive painful uveitis. The chronic disease of the globe may cause cataracts, retinal degeneration, or even glaucoma.

Diagnosis of *Leptospira* abortion is best accomplished by fluorescent antibody testing (FAT) or immunohistochemical evaluation of the placenta, umbilical cord, fetal liver, or fetal kidney. The sensitivity and specificity of the FAT in these tissues (but not urine) are nearly 100%. Examination of silver-stained kidney samples in horses with renal disease does not yield high accuracy, because there may be false-negative and false-positive findings, likely a result of nonpathogenic serovars. PCR testing is preferred for evaluation of fluids, such as urine, ocular fluids, and blood. Marked increases in serum antibody titers often accompany *Leptospira* abortions or acute renal failure, but serum titers may be low in horses with recurrent uveitis because of the chronic and localized nature of infection. Acute *L interrogans* serovar Pomona infections often cause marked increases in antibody titers to several serovars (especially Icterohemorrhagiae and Bratislava, but the noninfecting serovar titers usually decline much more quickly over several weeks than the titers to the actual infecting serovar. Collection of a voided urine sample after furosemide administration may improve sensitivity of PCR, darkfield staining, or culture testing. A combination of serology, culture, and PCR testing of aqueous fluid may be the only way to confirm *Leptospira*-associated uveitis. In ERU, the organism is most commonly found in the vitreous rather than aqueous fluid, which limits the practical application of ocular fluid PCR testing.

In acute disease, systemic antibiotics such as enrofloxacin, penicillin, tetracyclines, or aminoglycosides are useful, but this has not been proved to be the case with recurrent uveitis. There are no leptospiral vaccines approved for horses, although many veterinarians have used vaccines approved for cattle on horse farms that have endemic *Leptospira* abortions or uveitis.

LEPTOSPIROSIS IN RUMINANTS

Leptospiral serovars of major importance in cattle are Hardjo and Pomona in North America, with serovars Grippotyphosa, Bratislava, Icterohaemorrhagiae, and Canicola occasionally implicated. The most commonly documented cause of leptospirosis among cattle in the USA and throughout much of the world is serovar Hardjo, for which cattle are the maintenance host. Risk factors for Hardjo infection in cattle have been reported to include open herds, access to contaminated water sources, co-grazing with sheep, and use of natural breeding. Serovar hardjo has the ability to colonize and persist in the genital tract of infected cows and bulls.

Many leptospiral infections in cattle are subclinical, particularly in nonpregnant and nonlactating animals. Acute or subacute leptospirosis is most commonly associated with incidental host infections and occurs during the leptospiremic phase of infection. Clinical signs associated with chronic infections are usually associated with reproductive loss through abortion and stillbirth. Persistent colonization by serovar Hardjo of the uterus and oviducts may be associated with infertility characterized by increased services per conception and prolonged calving intervals.

Uncommonly, severe acute disease occurs in young stock infected with incidental serovars, particularly serovar Pomona and less commonly Icterohemorrhagiae. Clinical signs include high fever, hemolytic anemia, hemoglobinuria, jaundice, pulmonary congestion, occasionally meningitis, and death. In lactating cows, incidental infections may be associated with agalactia with small quantities of blood-tinged milk. A less severe form of this "milk drop syndrome" may occur in Hardjo-infected lactating cows in the absence of other clinical evidence of infection. In lactating cows, incidental infections have been reported to cause blood-tinged milk.

The chronic phase of disease is associated with fetal infection in pregnant cows presenting as abortion, stillbirth, or birth of premature and weak infected calves. Infected but healthy calves also may be born. Abortion or stillbirth is commonly the only manifestation of infection but may sometimes be related to an episode of illness up to 6 wk (Pomona) or 12 wk (Hardjo) earlier. Abortions associated with incidental host infection tend to occur late term and in groups or so-called "abortion storms." In contrast, abortions occurring after infection with serovar Hardjo tend to be more sporadic and can occur mid- to late pregnancy and several months after initial infection.

Diagnosis of incidental host infections in cattle is relatively straightforward. In general, infected animals develop high titers to the infecting serovar; an antibody titer >1:800 at the time of abortion is considered evidence of leptospirosis. Leptospires can be demonstrated in placenta and the fetus in some cases by immunofluorescence, PCR, and immunohistochemistry. Diagnosis of serovar Hardjo infection is more difficult and requires a combination of approaches. Serology alone often fails to identify animals infected with serovar Hardjo, because seronegative shedders are common in infected cattle herds. The recommended diagnostic testing strategy includes the primary use of a test (immunofluorescence or PCR) to detect the organism in the urine from a sample of cattle in the herd followed by serologic testing to provide insight into the likely infecting serovar of *Leptospira*.

Cattle with acute leptospirosis can be treated with the label dosage of tetracycline, oxytetracycline, penicillin, ceftiofur, tilmicosin, or tulathromycin. Leptospires also are highly susceptible to erythromycin, tiamulin, and tylosin, although these antibiotics cannot be relied on to remove the renal carrier state. Injectable, long-acting oxytetracycline (20 mg/kg) and sustained-release ceftiofur have been shown to effectively eliminate shedding in cattle infected with serovar Hardjo. Vaccination can be combined with antibiotic treatment in the face of an outbreak of leptospirosis, but vaccination alone will not reduce urinary shedding. All appropriate withdrawal times should be observed.

Bovine leptospirosis vaccines available in the USA and Canada are pentavalent and contain leptospiral serovars Pomona, Grippotyphosa, Canicola, Icterohaemorrhagiae, and Hardjo. These vaccines provide good protection against disease caused by each of these serovars, with the possible exception of serovar Hardjo. Experimental and field evidence indicates that some traditional five-way leptospirosis vaccines do not provide good protection from serovar Hardjo infection. New vaccines have been introduced to address this issue. If a primary goal of a vaccination program is protection of cattle against Hardjo, care should be taken in selection of a vaccine product. In general, annual vaccination of all cattle in a closed herd or low incidence area, or twice-yearly vaccination in an open herd or high incidence area, is the most effective approach to control.

Relative to cattle and pigs, sheep and goats have been considered resistant to leptospiral infection, with low seroprevalences and only a small number of serogroups being implicated in clinical disease. Sheep can serve as a maintenance host for serovar Hardjo and therefore spread infection to cattle. Incidental infections may cause sporadic outbreaks of acute disease characterized by hematuria, hemoglobinuria, jaundice, and death (usually in lambs), and occasional abortions.

LEPTOSPIROSIS IN SWINE

Leptospira interrogans (serovars Pomona, Icterohaemorrhagiae, Canicola, Hardjo, and Bratislava), *L borgpetersenii* (serovars Sejroe and Tarassovi), and *L kirschneri* (serovar Grippotyphosa) are all reported to infect pigs. Serovars Pomona and Bratislava are uniquely adapted to swine; others are maintained in other species but sometimes infect swine. Swine are maintenance hosts for serovar Bratislava, and infected pigs rarely develop signs typical of acute leptospirosis—rather, reproductive failure as evidenced by infertility and sporadic abortion is the most common clinical sign, and venereal transmission may occur. Serovar Pomona, in contrast, is of intermediate pathogenicity for swine, with acute clinical signs seen in young pigs and abortions (often in groups) occurring in pregnant swine. Although Pomona infections are associated with acute, sometimes severe clinical signs suggestive of an incidental host infection, pigs often remain infected and shed serovar Pomona for weeks to a few months after infection. This feature of Pomona infection can be associated with high rates of pig-to-pig transmission among swine reared in confinement. Incidental infections may occur from strains belonging to the Grippotyphosa, Icterohaemorrhagiae, and Canicola serogroups.

Abortions occurring 2–4 wk before term are the most common manifestation of leptospirosis in pigs. Piglets produced at term may be dead or weak and may die soon after birth. The principal differential diagnosis is porcine reproductive and respiratory syndrome (*see* p 729), although brucellosis, parvovirus, and SMEDI (stillbirth, mummification, embryonic death, and infertility) share some features with leptospirosis. Acute leptospirosis, as described in calves, has been described in piglets but is rare. Treatment and control are similar to those described for cattle, using a combination of medication either to prevent infection or to decrease shedding, vaccination, rodent and small mammal control, and feed and water free of *Leptospira* organisms. Immunization through use of bacterins is widely practiced in breeding herds and will reduce the prevalence of infection and abortions. The bacterin must be serovar specific for protection. Bacterins should not be expected to eliminate infection in carriers.

LIGHTNING STROKE AND ELECTROCUTION

Injury or death of an animal due to high-voltage electrical currents may be the result of lightning, fallen transmission wires, faulty electrical circuits, or chewing on an electrical cord. Electrocution due to lightning stroke is seasonal and tends to be geographically restricted. Investigation of possible electrocution should always proceed with caution, because the electrification resulting from broken transmission wires, for example, may still be present. Once the site is clearly safe, the investigation should include the location of the dead animals, examination of all affected animals, and necropsy of those that died.

Certain types of trees, especially hardwoods such as oaks and those that are tall and have spreading root systems just beneath the ground surface, tend to be struck by lightning more often than others. Electrification of such roots charges a wide surface area, particularly when the ground is already damp; passage of charged roots beneath a shallow pool of water causes it to become electrified. A tile drain may spread an electric charge throughout its course. Fallen or sagging transmission wires also may electrify a pool of water, fence, or building, and an animal may also directly contact such wires. Differences exist in conductivity of soil; loam, sand, clay, marble, and chalk are good conductors (in decreasing order), whereas rocky soil is not.

Accidental electrocution of farm animals in a barn or adjacent confinement pen usually occurs as a result of faulty wiring. Electrification of a water or milk line stanchion or a metal creep or guard rail can result in widespread distribution of an electric current throughout the stable (*see also* STRAY VOLTAGE IN ANIMAL HOUSING, p 2113) that may result in signs of water deprivation or feed refusal.

Death from electric shock usually results from cardiac or respiratory arrest. Passage of current through the heart usually produces ventricular fibrillation, and involvement of the CNS may affect the respiratory or other vital centers.

Clinical Findings: Varying degrees of electric shock may occur. In most instances of electrocution by lightning stroke, death is instantaneous and the animal falls without a struggle. Occasionally, the animal becomes unconscious but may recover in a few minutes to several hours; residual nervous signs (eg, depression, paraplegia, cutaneous hyperesthesia, blindness) may persist for days or weeks or be permanent. Singe marks on or damage to the carcass, damage to the immediate environment, or both, occur in ~90% of cases of lightning stroke but are less likely to be found if the animal is electrocuted by standing on electrified earth. Singe marks tend to be linear and are more commonly found on the medial sides of the legs, although rarely much of the body may be affected. Beneath the singe marks, capillary congestion is common; the arboreal pattern characteristic of lightning stroke can be visualized best from the dermal side of the skin by subcutaneous extravasations of blood. Singe marks are rarely found on recovered animals. Smaller animals such as pigs that contact electrified water bowls or creeps may be killed instantly or be thrown some distance by the strength of the shock. Electrocuted pigs are often recumbent and may have sustained spinal, pelvic, or limb fractures, resulting from severe muscular contractions.

Diagnosis: The diagnosis is almost always made on circumstantial evidence, ie, location of the carcass(es) and absence of any disease processes when examined by necropsy. The presence of dead animals under a tree, hanging through or near a wire fence, or clustered around a light pole is strong evidence of electrocution by lightning stroke even in the absence of physical evidence like recent burning of tree bark or splitting of poles or boards in a fence.

Rigor mortis develops and passes quickly. Postmortem distention of the rumen occurs rapidly and must be differentiated from antemortem ruminal tympany (*see* p 227); in both conditions, the blood tends to clot slowly or not at all. The mucosae of the upper respiratory tract, including the turbinates and sinuses, are congested and hemorrhagic; linear tracheal hemorrhages are common, and large blood clots are occasionally found in the trachea, but the lungs are not compressed as in bloat. All other viscera are congested, and petechiae and ecchymoses may be found in many organs. Due to postmortem ruminal distention, the poorly clotted blood is passively moved to the periphery of the body, resulting in postmortem extravasation of blood in muscles and superficial lymph nodes of the head, neck, and thoracic limbs, and to a lesser extent in the hindquarters. Probably the best indication of instantaneous death is the presence of hay or other feed in the animal's mouth; supportive evidence includes the presence of normal ingesta (especially in the rumen), lack of frothy ingesta (frothy bloat), and presence of normal feces in the lower tract and occasionally on the ground behind the animal. Few conditions affecting livestock cause such peracute death clustered in a small area.

Farm animals often are insured against lightning stroke, and the insurance claims agent or the veterinarian requested to sign an insurance form should closely observe the situation that initiated the claim. The investigator should ascertain that the animal actually died in the high-risk location rather than having been moved after death. This could be done to merely clean up or to deliberately confuse the investigation. Similarly, examination of recent weather information confirming thunderstorms is an important part of the process to substantiate an insurance claim. A well-documented description of where the animal(s) died and the results of a necropsy examination are usually acceptable to support an insurance claim of lightning stroke.

Treatment: Those animals that survive may require supportive and symptomatic therapy. Euthanasia is warranted for those animals recumbent with fractures or severe muscle injuries.

LISTERIOSIS

(Listerellosis, Circling disease)

Listeriosis is a sporadic bacterial infection that affects a wide range of animals, including people and birds. It is seen worldwide, more frequently in temperate and colder climates. There is a high incidence of intestinal carriers. Encephalitis or meningoencephalitis in adult ruminants is the most frequently recognized form.

Etiology and Epidemiology: *Listeria monocytogenes* is a small, motile, gram-positive, nonsporeforming, extremely resistant, diphtheroid coccobacillus that grows under a wide temperature range 4°–44°C (39°–111°F). Its ability to grow at 4°C is an important diagnostic aid (the "cold enrichment" method) for isolation of the organism from brain tissue but not from placental or fetal tissues. Primary isolation is enhanced under microaerophilic conditions. It is a ubiquitous saprophyte that lives in a plant-soil environment and has been isolated from ~42 species of domestic and wild mammals and 22 species of birds, as well as fish, crustaceans, insects, sewage, water, silage and other feedstuffs, milk, cheese, meconium, feces, and soil.

The natural reservoirs of *L monocytogenes* appear to be soil and mammalian GI tracts, both of which contaminate vegetation. Grazing animals ingest the organism and further contaminate vegetation and soil. Animal-to-animal transmission occurs via the fecal-oral route.

Listeriosis is primarily a winter-spring disease of feedlot or housed ruminants. The less acidic pH of spoiled silage enhances multiplication of *L monocytogenes*. Outbreaks typically occur ≥10 days after feeding poor-quality silage. Removal or change of silage in the ration often stops the spread of listeriosis; feeding the same silage months later may result in new cases.

Pathogenesis: *Listeria* organisms that are ingested or inhaled tend to cause septicemia, abortion, and latent infection. Those that gain entry to tissues have a predilection to localize in the intestinal wall, medulla oblongata, and placenta or to cause encephalitis via minute wounds in buccal mucosa.

The various manifestations of infection occur in all susceptible species and are associated with characteristic clinical syndromes: abortion and perinatal mortality in all species, encephalitis or meningoencephalitis in adult ruminants, septicemia in neonatal ruminants and monogastric animals, and septicemia with myocardial or hepatic necrosis (or both) in poultry (*see* p 2839).

Listeric encephalitis affects sheep, cattle, goats, and occasionally pigs. It is essentially a localized infection of the brain stem that develops when *L monocytogenes* ascends the trigeminal nerve. Clinical signs vary according to the function of damaged neurons but often are unilateral and include depression (ascending reticular activating system), ipsilateral weakness (long tracts), trigeminal and facial nerve paralysis, and less commonly, circling (vestibulocochlear nucleus). Neurologic signs indicating bilateral cranial nerve deficits are occasionally seen in lambs <4 mo old.

Septicemic or visceral listeriosis is most common in monogastric animals, including pigs, dogs, cats, domestic and wild rabbits, and many other small mammals. These animals may play a role in transmission of *L monocytogenes*. This form is also found in young ruminants before the rumen is functional. Although rare, septicemia has been reported in older domestic ruminants and deer. The septicemic form affects organs other than the brain, the principal lesion being focal hepatic necrosis.

The uterus of all domestic animals, especially ruminants, is susceptible to infection with *L monocytogenes* at all stages of pregnancy, which can result in placentitis, fetal infection and death, abortion, stillbirths, neonatal deaths, metritis, and possibly viable carriers. The metritis has little or no effect on subsequent reproduction; however, *Listeria* may be shed for ≥1 mo via the vagina and milk.

Infections acquired via ingestion tend to localize in the intestinal wall and result in prolonged fecal excretion. It has been postulated that contaminated silage results in latent infections, often approaching 100% of the exposed herd or flock, but clinical listeriosis in only a few animals.

Clinical Findings: Encephalitis is the most readily recognized form of listeriosis in ruminants. It affects all ages and both sexes, sometimes as an epidemic in feedlot cattle or sheep. The course in sheep and goats is rapid, and death may occur 24–48 hr after onset of signs; however, the recovery rate can be up to 30% with prompt, aggressive therapy. In cattle, the course is less acute, and the recovery rate approaches 50%. Lesions are localized in the brain stem, and the signs indicate dysfunction of nerve nuclei, including those of the third to seventh cranial nerves.

Initially, affected animals are anorectic, depressed, and disoriented. They may propel themselves into corners, lean against stationary objects, or circle toward the affected side. Facial paralysis with a drooping ear, deviated muzzle, flaccid lip, and lowered eyelid often develops on the affected side, as well as lack of a menace

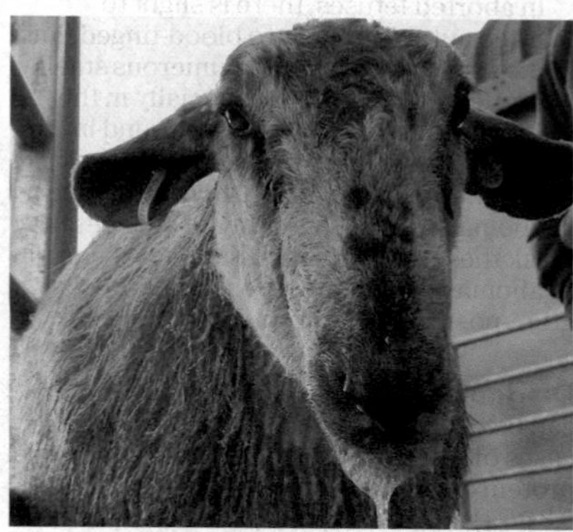

Right-sided facial and trigeminal nerve paralysis with profuse salivation caused by listeriosis in a goat. *Courtesy of Dr. Philip Scott.*

response and profuse, almost continuous, salivation; food material often becomes impacted in the cheek due to paralysis of the masticatory muscles. Terminally affected animals fall and, unable to rise, lie on the same side; involuntary running movements are common.

Listeric encephalitis may recur on the same premises in successive years. The number of animals clinically involved in an outbreak usually is <2% but in exceptional circumstances may reach 10%–30% in a flock of sheep.

Listeric abortion usually occurs in the last trimester without premonitory signs. Fetuses usually die in utero, but stillbirths and neonatal deaths occur. The abortion rate varies and may reach 20% in sheep flocks. Fatal septicemia of the dam secondary to metritis is rare. Encephalitis and abortion usually do not occur simultaneously in the same herd or flock. However, the clinical pattern in sheep in the UK has been changing; abortions, encephalitis, and diarrhea are increasing, and outbreaks of abortions and encephalitis occur together in the same flock.

Listeriosis is relatively uncommon in pigs, with septicemia occurring in those <1 mo old and encephalitis in older pigs; it has a rapid, fatal course of 3–4 days.

Lesions: In listeric encephalitis, there are few gross lesions except for some congestion of meninges. Microscopic lesions are confined primarily to the pons, medulla oblongata, and anterior spinal cord.

In septicemic listeriosis, small necrotic foci may be found in any organ, especially the liver. In calves that die when <3 wk old, in addition to focal hepatic necrosis, there is frequently marked hemorrhagic gastroenteritis.

In aborted fetuses, there is slight to marked autolysis, clear to blood-tinged fluid in the serous cavities, and numerous small necrotic foci in the liver, especially in the right half. Necrotic foci may be found in other viscera such as lung and spleen. Shallow erosions, 1–3 mm, may be present in abomasal mucosa. Autolytic changes may mask these lesions. Gram-stained smears of abomasal contents reveal numerous gram-positive, pleomorphic coccobacilli.

Diagnosis: Samples of lumbosacral CSF can be collected under local anesthesia. In cases of listeriosis, the CSF has an increased protein concentration (0.6–2 g/L [normal 0.3 g/L]) and a mild pleocytosis composed of large mononuclear cells.

Listeriosis is confirmed only by isolation and identification of *L monocytogenes*. Specimens of choice are brain from animals with CNS involvement and aborted placenta and fetus. If primary isolation attempts fail, ground brain tissue should be held at 4°C (39°F) for several weeks and recultured weekly. Occasionally, *L monocytogenes* has been isolated from spinal fluid, nasal discharge, urine, feces, and milk of clinically ill ruminants. Serology is not used routinely for diagnosis, because many healthy animals have high *Listeria* titers. Immunofluorescence is effective for rapidly identifying *L monocytogenes* in smears from animals dead or aborted from listeriosis and from milk, meat, and other sources.

Listeriosis can be differentiated from pregnancy toxemia in ewes (*see* p 1021) or ketosis in cattle (*see* p 1024) by careful clinical examination, CSF changes, and 3-OH butyrate concentrations well below 3 mmol/L. Furthermore, facial and ear paralysis are absent in pregnancy toxemia or ketosis. In cattle, the unilateral signs of trigeminal and facial paralysis (often subtle) help differentiate listeriosis from bovine spongiform encephalopathy (*see* p 1284), thromboembolic meningoencephalitis (*see* p 754), polioencephalomalacia (*see* p 1281), sporadic bovine encephalomyelitis (*see* p 1308), and lead poisoning (*see* p 3078). Rabies (*see* p 1302) must always be considered in the differential diagnosis of listeriosis. Animals with brain abscesses and coenurosis (*see* p 1311) present with circling, contralateral blindness, and proprioceptive deficits, but show no cranial nerve deficits. Vestibular disease is common in growing ruminants; these animals typically show ipsilateral spontaneous nystagmus or strabismus, and remain bright and alert without trigeminal nerve dysfunction.

Treatment and Control: Recovery depends on early, aggressive antibiotic treatment. If signs of encephalitis are severe, death usually occurs despite treatment. *L monocytogenes* is susceptible to penicillin (the drug of choice), ceftiofur, erythromycin, and trimethoprim/sulfonamide. High doses are required because of the difficulty in achieving minimum bactericidal concentrations in the brain.

Penicillin G should be given at 44,000 U/kg body wt, IM, daily for 1–2 wk; the first injection should be accompanied by the same dose given IV. Supportive therapy, including fluids and electrolytes, is required for animals having difficulty eating and drinking. High-dose dexamethasone (1 mg/kg, IV) at first examination is considered beneficial by some but is controversial and will cause abortion during the last two trimesters in cattle and after day 135 in sheep.

Results with vaccines have been equivocal, which together with the sporadic nature of the disease, lead to questions about the cost-benefit of vaccination. In an outbreak, affected animals should be segregated. If silage is being fed, use of the particular silage should be discontinued on a trial basis. Spoiled silage should be avoided. Corn ensiled before being too mature and grass silage containing additives are likely to have a more acid pH, which discourages multiplication of *L monocytogenes*.

Zoonotic Risk: Whether animals serve as a reservoir of infection for people may be questioned, because *Listeria* organisms have been isolated from feces of a significant number of apparently healthy people as well as other animals. However, despite this and the apparently low invasiveness of *L monocytogenes*, all suspected material should be handled with caution. Aborted fetuses and necropsy of septicemic animals present the greatest hazard. In cases with encephalitis, *L monocytogenes* is usually confined to the brain and presents little risk of transmission unless the brain is removed. People have developed fatal meningitis, septicemia, and papular exanthema on the arms after handling aborted material. Pregnant animals (including women) should be protected from infection because of danger to the fetus, with possible abortion, stillbirth, and infection of neonates. Although human listeriosis is rare (upper estimate of 12 cases per million population per yr), mortality can reach 50%. Most cases involve older patients, pregnant women, or immunocompromised people.

L monocytogenes can be isolated from milk of mastitic, aborting, and apparently healthy cows. Excretion in milk is usually intermittent but may persist for many months. Infected milk is a hazard, because the organism may survive certain forms of pasteurization. *Listeria* also have been isolated from milk of sheep, goats, and women.

LYME BORRELIOSIS

(Lyme disease)

Lyme borreliosis is a bacterial, tick-transmitted disease of animals (dogs, horses, probably cats) and people. Many additional mammalian and avian species become infected but do not develop overt clinical signs. Areas of greatest incidence in the USA are regions in the northeast (particularly the New England states), the upper Midwest, and the Pacific coast. Lyme borreliosis also occurs in moderate climatic regions of Europe and Asia.

Etiology and Transmission: On the basis of DNA analysis, 19 different genospecies fall within the *Borrelia burgdorferi* sensu lato complex. Within this complex, the most important spirochete species are *B burgdorferi* sensu stricto (North America, Europe), *B afzelii* (Europe, Asia), *B bavariensis*, and *B garinii* (Europe, Asia), all of which are pathogenic for people. Only *B burgdorferi* sensu stricto has been shown so far to be pathogenic for domestic animals under experimental conditions. Tick vectors of *B burgdorferi* sensu lato are hard-shelled *Ixodes* ticks. In the USA, these are primarily *I scapularis* in the northeast and Midwest and *I pacificus* on the Pacific coast. *I ricinus* and *I persulcatus* are the primary vectors in Europe and Asia. *B miyamotoi* is another member of the genus *Borrelia*. Although this spirochete is transmitted by ixodid ticks and may cause infections in mammals characterized by clinical signs such as fever, headache, fatigue, and muscle aches, the bacterium is a relapsing, fever-causing organism.

Ixodid ticks hatch from eggs as uninfected larvae. Both larvae and nymphs may acquire spirochetes from *Borrelia*-carrying hosts. Small mammals, especially rodents, play a major role as reservoir hosts. Birds and lizards may also harbor certain *Borrelia* species and serve as reservoir hosts. Infection rates of the vectors vary according to region and season and can be as high as 50% in adult ticks. After tick attachment,

>24 hr elapse before the first *B burgdorferi* sensu lato organisms are transmitted into the host's skin. Stable infection of the host occurs at >53 hr into the blood meal. Therefore, early removal of attached ticks reduces the potential for spirochete transmission. *B burgdorferi* sensu lato organisms are not transmitted by insects, body fluids (urine, saliva, semen), or bite wounds. Experimental studies have shown that dams infected before gestation may transmit spirochetes to their pups in utero.

Clinical Findings: Numerous clinical syndromes have been attributed to Lyme borreliosis in domestic animals, including limb and joint disease and renal, neurologic, and cardiac abnormalities. In dogs, intermittent, recurrent lameness; fever; anorexia; lethargy; and lymphadenopathy with or without swollen, painful joints are the most common clinical signs. The second most common syndrome associated with Lyme borreliosis is renal failure, which is generally fatal. It is characterized by uremia, hyperphosphatemia, and severe protein-losing nephropathy, often accompanied by peripheral edema. Bernese Mountain Dogs and Labrador Retrievers in particular often show high *Borrelia*-specific antibody levels; immune complexes in kidney tissues lead to severe inflammation. In human medicine, single case reports have described abnormalities with bradycardia with the cardiac form of Lyme borreliosis, whereas facial paralysis and seizure disorders are thought to be expressions of the neurologic form.

Diagnosis: Diagnosis is based on history, clinical signs, elimination of other diagnoses, laboratory data, epidemiologic considerations, and response to antibiotic therapy. Autoimmune panels, CBC, blood chemistry, radiographs, and other laboratory data are generally normal, except for results pertaining directly to the affected system (eg, soft-tissue swelling in limbs, neutrophil accumulation in synovial fluids of affected joints, uremia in renal disease).

Serologic testing for antibodies specific for *B burgdorferi* sensu lato is an adjunct to clinical diagnosis. Antibodies can be detected with ELISA (including rapid test systems), Western blots, line immunoassays (LIA), and with fluorescent bead-based multiplex assays. Because of their low specificity, indirect immunofluorescent antibody assays are no longer recommended. The standard procedure for antibody detection is a two-tiered approach in which samples are screened with a sensitive ELISA, and only positively reacting samples are rechecked with specific confirmatory tests. Western blot or LIA testing helps to differentiate the immune response elicited by infection from that induced by vaccination.

Alternatively, blood or serum samples can be tested with peptide-based assays (C6 peptide), which is specific for infection-induced antibodies. However, demonstration of specific antibodies indicates exposure to bacterial antigen only and does not equate to clinical disease. Approximately 5%–10% of dogs in central Europe carry *Borrelia*-specific antibodies with no clinical signs. Additionally, false-negative results can occur with the C6 peptide assays shortly after infection. Long incubation periods, persistence of antibodies for months to years, and the disassociation of the antibody response from the clinical stage of disease make diagnosis by blood testing alone impossible.

Lymphocyte stimulation tests are available that measure the cellular immune response to *Borrelia*. In culture, *Borrelia* antigens are processed by antigen-presenting cells with which specific lymphocytes interact. Released cytokines (eg, interleukin-1 beta) in the culture supernatant are correlates for preceding *Borrelia* infections of the host. Scant information is available in terms of the test's sensitivity and specificity.

Isolation of *B burgdorferi* sensu lato by culture or detection of specific DNA by PCR from joints, skin tissue samples, or other sources may also help in diagnosis. However, direct detection of the organism is difficult, time consuming (up to 6 wk for culture), and in most cases produces negative results. Only a positive result is meaningful. Blood samples are generally negative, because the organism resides in tissue and not in the circulation.

Clinical signs of Lyme borreliosis are nonspecific. In addition to other orthopedic disorders (eg, trauma, osteochondritis dissecans, immune-mediated diseases), other infections should be considered. *Anaplasma phagocytophilum* can also induce intermittent, recurrent lameness. *A phagocytophilum* is transmitted by the same tick genus, and epidemiologic studies have revealed that up to 30% of all dogs in central Europe carry antibodies specific for this agent. Mixed infections should be considered when clinical signs are apparent.

Treatment: Antibiotic therapy is indicated in all cases with clinical signs attributed to Lyme borreliosis. Antimicrobials in the tetracycline (eg, doxycycline 10 mg/kg, PO, bid) and penicillin (eg, amoxicillin 20 mg/kg, PO, tid) groups are effective, and rapid response is seen in limb and joint disease in most cases, although incomplete or transient resolution of signs occurs in a significant number of affected animals. Doxycycline is preferred over penicillins, because mixed infections with other tickborne pathogens are often found in animals with clinical signs. Clinical and research data indicate that low-level infection in animals, including people, may persist despite antibiotic therapy. In dogs, standard antibiotic doses and treatment for 4 wk have been demonstrated to be effective. If clinical signs recur, the antibiotics mentioned above can be used again, because persistent infection is not the result of acquired antibiotic resistance. Prolonged antibiotic therapy (>4 wk) may be beneficial for animals with continuing disease signs.

Symptomatic therapy directed toward the affected organ system and clinicopathologic abnormalities is also important, especially in renal disease. In limb and joint disease, the use of NSAIDs concurrent with antibiotic therapy may lead to confusion over the source of clinical improvement and make diagnosis based on therapeutic response difficult.

Control and Prevention: Tick avoidance plays an important role in disease control. Although highly effective repellents and acaricides in collars, sprays, and spot-ons are available for use on dogs, lack of owner compliance in application may often be a barrier to effective, longterm tick avoidance.

Killed, whole-cell bacterins to prevent Lyme borreliosis in dogs have been in use since the early 1990s. Vaccines that contain only recombinant outer surface protein A (rOspA) have since been licensed for use in dogs. Vaccines are available in Europe that contain antigens from different species of the *B burgdorferi* sensu lato complex. All current vaccines induce a strong antibody response predominately to OspA (lysate vaccines) or only against OspA (recombinant vaccines). During the tick's blood meal, antibodies against OspA bind to *Borrelia* organisms residing in the tick. Bound antibodies prevent spirochete migration within the tick and consequently *Borrelia* transmission from ticks to hosts. Later, during the blood meal, *B burgdorferi* sensu lato organisms in the engorging tick stop producing OspA and begin expressing new proteins, OspC and others, before transmission. Development of vaccines that contain multiple *B burgdorferi* antigens that may contribute to enhanced protection is being pursued.

In endemic areas, dogs should be vaccinated before natural exposure to ticks to attain the highest degree of protection. Dogs that have been exposed to ticks should be tested serologically for established infection before vaccination. Postinfection vaccination has little to no therapeutic effect on established infections. Two doses of vaccine should be administered SC to dogs ≥9–12 wk old at 3-wk intervals, or according to label directions. Because antibody levels often drop quickly after the initial two immunizations, additional booster vaccinations should be administered twice within the next year, preferably at 6-mo intervals (suggested schedule: spring, fall, spring) with annual vaccinations thereafter.

Zoonotic Risk: Lyme borreliosis is an important zoonotic disease. Animals and people are infected during the blood meal of hard-shelled ticks (*Ixodes* spp). Companion and farm animals are not the source of infection in people. Pets may bring unattached infected ticks into the household and subsequently the vectors may be passed on to other animals or people during close contact.

MELIOIDOSIS

(Pseudoglanders, Whitmore disease)

Melioidosis is a bacterial infection of animals and people. It is often associated with suppurative or caseous lesions, comprising a mixed purulent and granulomatous response that can occupy any body organ.

Etiology and Epidemiology: The etiologic agent is *Burkholderia pseudomallei*, an oval, motile, gram-negative, facultative anaerobic bacillus with bipolar staining. The organism is ubiquitous throughout southeast Asia, northern

Australia, and the South Pacific. Its distribution is predominantly tropical and subtropical with "hyperendemicity" in the top end of the Northern Territory of Australia and northeast Thailand. The true boundaries of its endemicity are ambiguous because of movement of the organism and its ability to travel to and exist in temperate regions (eg, southwest Australia, France), where it may cause sporadic disease and outbreaks. *B pseudomallei* has been introduced to new environments with the export of animals, and shipments of contaminated soil and water could potentially produce the same results. Reports of possible autochthonous melioidosis have also come from India, Pacific islands, Central and South America, the Caribbean, Africa, and the Middle East.

B pseudomallei is a widespread saprophyte and has been isolated from various soil types and surface water of varying depths. Melioidosis outbreaks have coincided with heavy rainfall and flooding associated with high humidity or temperature. Major excavations and disturbances in plumbing resulting in contamination of water supplies have also resulted in outbreaks.

Melioidosis is most commonly seen in sheep, goats, and pigs; other affected species include cattle, buffalo, horses, mules, deer, camels, alpacas, dogs, cats, dolphins, wallabies, koala, primates, birds, tropical fish, reptiles, and people. Laboratory animals affected by melioidosis include hamsters, guinea pigs, rabbits, mice, and rats. Host susceptibility and disease manifestations vary between species. The introduction of naive livestock to endemic regions may predispose them to disease, as seen with sheep, goats, pigs, and camelids. Other species (eg, dogs and cats) may succumb to infection due to immunocompromising conditions.

Transmission: Infection is thought to be opportunistic and primarily a result of transmission from the environment (eg, contaminated soil and surface waters) rather than from animal to animal. The most common routes of infection are via percutaneous inoculation, contamination of wounds, ingestion of soil or contaminated carcasses, or inhalation. Transplacental infection resulting in abortion has been reported in goats. Transmission during breeding and other means of host-to-host transmission may occur. Laboratory-acquired infection and iatrogenic infection via contaminated antiseptics, injections, or other hospital or surgical equipment have been reported.

Pathogenesis: The virulence of *B pseudomallei* appears to vary among isolates, but these virulence factors are not well understood. Molecular-typed clonal outbreaks have produced a range of different clinical presentations, which indicate that host factors and infecting dose may be just as important in determining the severity of disease. The incubation period ranges from a few days to months or even years. *B pseudomallei* is a facultative intracellular pathogen that can remain dormant for many years before emerging as an active infection.

Clinical Findings: Signs can vary widely within a species, depending on the site of infection, and range from acute to chronic. Fever, anorexia, or swollen glands may be noted. Subclinical infection is common. Infection may be associated with single or multiple suppurative or caseous nodules/abscesses, which can be located in any organ tissue with variable effects. Disease most likely due to percutaneous inoculation often develops at distant sites without evidence of active infection at the inoculation site. The organs most commonly affected include the lungs, spleen, liver, and associated lymph nodes.

Goats often develop mastitis, and aortic aneurysms have been reported. The respiratory system is involved preferentially in sheep; signs can include fever, severe coughing, respiratory distress, and mucopurulent nasal and ocular discharge. CNS disease, with signs that include circling, incoordination, blindness, nystagmus, and spasms, has been seen in cattle, horses, sheep, and goats. Pigs often have asymptomatic lesions on the spleen that are incidental findings at slaughter. Lameness due to septic arthritis and osteomyelitis can occur. Fatalities often occur in association with acute fulminating infections or when vital organs are affected. Various forms of melioidosis have been reported in horses; signs may include weakness, edema and lymphangitis of the limbs, mild colic, diarrhea, coughing, or nasal discharge. Skin infections may resemble fungal eczema initially, progressing to become papular. In dogs, disease may be acute, subacute, or chronic. In acute cases, septicemia with fever, severe diarrhea, and fulminant pneumonia are common. Subacute cases may present as a skin lesion with lymphangitis and lymphadenitis; untreated cases may progress to septicemia. Chronic disease can occur in any organ with clinical signs that include anorexia, myalgia, edema of the limbs, and skin abscesses.

Lesions: Multiple abscesses that contain thick, caseous greenish yellow to off-white material are noted at necropsy. The organs most commonly involved are the lungs, spleen, lymph nodes, liver, and subcutaneous tissues. Exudative bronchopneumonia, consolidation, and abscesses may be found in the lungs of animals with respiratory disease. Nodules and ulcers may be found on the nasal mucosa and septum and on the turbinates; these may coalesce into irregular plaques. Meningoencephalitis, severe enteritis, suppurative polyarthritis, and other syndromes also have been reported.

Diagnosis: The clinical signs of melioidosis are not diagnostic because of the protean nature of the disease. For a definitive diagnosis, isolation and identification of the organism are required. The organism can be isolated from lesions and discharges. It is possible to culture the organism on routine diagnostic media; however, Ashdown's media is preferred because of a consistently distinctive colony morphology and odor. Gram-stained smears of exudate or pus can sometimes identify bipolar "safety pin"–shaped, gram-negative rods. Serologic tests such as complement fixation and indirect hemagglutination are effective herd surveillance tools. More recently, DNA probes and PCR tests have been developed.

Treatment and Prevention: Treatment with the appropriate antibiotics should be based on culture and sensitivity results. Treatment may be expensive, prolonged, and possibly unsuccessful, with the risk of recrudescence once treatment is discontinued. The possibility of underlying immunosuppressive conditions should be investigated in less susceptible species. With severe disease, treatment regimens can follow guidelines for human melioidosis with initial intensive therapy using the newer β-lactams (ceftazidime and the carbepenems), possibly in combination with cotrimoxazole for up to 2 mo. This should be followed by subsequent eradication therapy for a minimum of 3 mo with high-dose cotrimoxazole or conventional combination therapy using chloramphenicol, cotrimoxazole, and doxycycline or amoxicillin/clavulanate. Preventive measures are more practical and economical in intensive farming environments and involve raising the animals off the soil, especially avoiding exposing animals to muddy or water-inundated regions and providing clean drinking water via chlorination and filtration. Minimization of environmental contamination by diseased animals is also an important control measure. There is no effective vaccine.

Zoonotic Risk: Melioidosis has zoonotic potential. Infected animals can shed the organism in wound exudates and, depending on the site of infection, from other sources, including nasal secretions, milk, feces, and urine. Mastitis in goats is a common manifestation, and *B pseudomallei* has been isolated from milk, resulting in the requirement for pasteurization of commercial goats' milk in the tropics. Infected animal carcasses are condemned at the abattoir.

NEOSPOROSIS

Neospora caninum is a microscopic protozoan parasite with worldwide distribution. Many domestic (eg, dogs, cattle, sheep, goats, water buffalo, horses, chickens) and wild and captive animals (eg, deer, rhinoceros, rodents, rabbits, coyotes, wolves, foxes) can be infected. Neosporosis is one of the most common causes of bovine abortion, especially in intensively farmed cows. Neosporosis abortion also occurs in sheep, goats, water buffalo, and camelids, although they may be less susceptible than cattle.

A second *Neospora* species, *N hughesi*, is a cause of myelitis in horses and shares clinical features with equine protozoal myelitis, which in North and South America is usually caused by *Sarcocystis neurona* (*see* p 1309). The life cycle of *N hughesi* is unknown. Discussion in this chapter deals only with *N caninum* infection.

Epidemiology: Neosporosis in cattle herds manifests in both endemic and epidemic abortion patterns, but it is also possible for a herd to have a high infection prevalence without a noticeable abortion problem. Both endemic and epidemic transmission patterns in cattle are positively associated with the presence and number of dogs in and around farms. Endemic abortion is mainly associated with recrudescence of latent organisms during pregnancy followed by transplacental transmission to the fetus, although occasional transmission from dogs or other canids may compound the problem. Epidemic abortion is a possible consequence of sudden large-scale transmission to pregnant cattle, presumably by ingestion of a mixed ration or water that has been contaminated with infected canine feces. The use of mixed rations in dairy herds probably accounts for the greater prevalence of neosporosis in dairy cattle than in extensively grazed beef cattle.

Transmission: Dogs are definitive hosts of *N caninum* and are capable of shedding oocysts in feces after eating tissues of infected animals. Gray wolves, coyotes, and dingoes are also definitive hosts, and many other wild canids are suspected. *Neospora* oocysts have an impervious shell that enables survival in soil and water for prolonged periods after canine feces have decomposed. Intermediate hosts such as cattle become infected by ingesting oocysts. Cattle do not produce oocysts and thus do not transmit infections horizontally to other cattle, but latent infection may endure permanently in their tissues and is transmitted to canids by carnivorism.

In cattle, *N caninum* can be transmitted transplacentally from an infected cow to the developing fetus, an event that may occur in multiple pregnancies of the same cow. Because most congenital infections are subclinical, congenitally infected heifer calves may be retained and added to the breeding herd and, in turn, may pass infections transplacentally to their own offspring. This endogenous transplacental transmission may enable transgenerational maintenance of the parasite even if the herd does not have frequent transmission from dogs. Exogenous transplacental transmission may occur when a previously uninfected cow ingests *Neospora* oocysts during pregnancy and the fetus becomes infected.

Dogs have been shown to become infected by eating infected cattle (including placentas) and deer and are presumed to become infected by consuming raw meat diets, barnyard chickens, and a variety of wild animals.

Clinical Findings: Most neosporosis abortions occur in mid to late gestation. Congenitally infected calves may be born weak or with neurologic deficits. However, most congenital infections are subclinical.

In dogs, subclinical infection is the rule, although there are a greater variety of exceptions. Litters or individual puppies may develop progressive hindlimb paresis associated with polyradiculoneuritis, myositis, and muscle atrophy. Adult dogs may have encephalomyelitis, focal cutaneous nodules or ulcers, pneumonia, peritonitis, hepatitis, or myocarditis with use of immunosuppressive drugs.

Diagnosis of Bovine Abortion: Because neosporosis is only one of many causes of abortion, diagnostic efforts should focus on an array of possible causes. Aborted fetuses should be submitted to a veterinary diagnostic laboratory, together with placenta and a serum sample from the aborting dam. Examination of multiple fetuses increases the odds of accurate diagnosis. If it is impractical to submit an entire fetus, as many of the following specimens as possible should be submitted to exclude other causes of abortion: aseptically collected and chilled lung, liver, spleen, and abomasal fluid; an eyeball for nitrate testing; formalin-fixed specimens of brain (even if soft), lung, thymus, liver, kidney, spleen, adrenal gland, skeletal muscle (eg, tongue and diaphragm), and placental cotyledon; serum from the aborting dam; and thoracoabdominal fluid from the fetus for serology.

A diagnosis of neosporosis abortion can be made with great confidence from the following constellation of findings: 1) lack of other etiologic agents; 2) nonsuppurative inflammation in multiple fetal organs, especially including the brain, heart, and skeletal muscle; 3) immunohistochemical or PCR detection of *Neospora* in fetal tissues; and 4) *Neospora* seropositivity of the dam or fetus. However, such unequivocal findings are not always present. A lesion that is nearly specific for neosporosis abortion in cattle is multifocal cerebral necrosis surrounded by nonsuppurative leukocytic reaction. Confidence in the diagnosis increases with the strength of the *Neospora* antibody level in the aborting dam, with high seropositive reactions at the time of abortion having greater predictive value than low seropositive reactions. Neosporosis is generally excluded in seronegative dams.

Toxoplasmosis is a more common cause of abortion in sheep and goats and has lesions similar to those of neosporosis, but toxoplasmosis abortion in cattle is rare or nonexistent.

Serologic testing of multiple cows or heifers can be used as an alternative or complementary method to determine whether neosporosis is a major reproductive problem in a herd. This strategy can be helpful when investigating herds with endemic abortion problems. Serum samples should be collected from aborting dams and from an equal number of matched herdmates with normal gestation (generally ≥10 per group). Sera should be tested and classified for *Neospora* antibodies. If most cows in the aborting group are seropositive and few are seropositive in the normal group, then neosporosis should be suspected as a cause of abortion in the herd; this may be confirmed by statistical comparison. If most aborting cattle are seronegative, then neosporosis is unlikely to be a major problem.

Diagnosis of Canine Neosporosis: Clinically affected dogs often have *Neospora* antibody levels much higher than levels seen in subclinically infected individuals. Biopsy of clinically affected tissues demonstrates nonsuppurative inflammation and may reveal the presence of protozoal organisms, but immunohistochemistry or PCR may be required to detect the organisms or to differentiate them from other protozoa.

Dogs with symptomatic neosporosis usually do not shed oocysts in feces. The finding of *Neospora* in routine fecal floats is serendipitous, because dogs typically shed oocysts for only a period of days or weeks after ingesting tissue of an infected animal. The tiny oocysts are round to slightly oval and 10–11 microns in diameter; in comparison, *Giardia* cysts are oblong and approximately 9 × 13 microns, and coccidia are 2–4 times the diameter of *Neospora*. A smooth outer contour helps to differentiate *Neospora* oocysts from pitted pollen grains of similar size. The oocysts are nearly identical to those of *Hammondia heydorni*, a closely related parasite that has not been associated with systemic disease in dogs or with abortion in ruminants. PCR may be necessary to distinguish between oocysts of *N caninum* and *H heydorni*.

Treatment: There is no approved treatment for neosporosis in cattle. Clinical neosporosis in dogs is treated with prolonged administration of clindamycin or potentiated sulfa drugs. The prognosis is negatively associated with the severity of presenting clinical signs and with delayed treatment. The prognosis is poor in puppies if disease has progressed to hindlimb paresis with atrophied, rigid limbs.

Control: Currently, there are no available *Neospora* vaccines for cattle or dogs.

It is common for dairy and beef herds to have at least a small percentage of *Neospora*-infected cattle. Although reducing the risk of *Neospora* transmission is a useful goal, complete eradication from a herd is usually impractical. Contamination of feedstuffs used in mixed rations by canine feces should be avoided. Large dairies can consider erecting dog-proof fences around the area in which feedstuffs are stored outdoors, and automatic gates can be installed to facilitate the daily traffic of heavy machinery. Smaller dairy farms may be able to protect feedstuffs within traditional buildings such as barns, grain bins, and silos.

In addition to protecting feedstuffs, herds with endemic neosporosis abortions may consider not retaining heifer calves born to seropositive cows, thereby reducing the number of congenitally infected replacement heifers that enter the breeding herd. If this technique is used, seropositive dairy cows could be bred using beef semen. For seropositive cows with valuable genetics, the use of embryo transfer to *Neospora*-seronegative surrogates, a technique that blocks endogenous transmission, can be considered.

Dead stock, offal from home slaughter, and placentas should be discarded in a manner that prevents ingestion by dogs to reduce the risk that dogs will become infected and shed *Neospora* oocysts on the farm. Dogs seropositive for *Neospora* have reduced likelihood for future shedding of oocysts than do seronegative dogs; therefore, serologic testing of farm dogs is seldom useful.

Zoonotic Risk: Despite its similarity to *Toxoplasma*, *Neospora* infection has not been clearly associated with any human disease. Laboratory workers should guard against inoculation, which caused fetal lesions in parenterally inoculated primates.

NOCARDIOSIS

Nocardiosis is an opportunistic, noncontagious, pyogranulomatous to suppurative disease of domestic animals, wildlife, and people.

Mastitis, pneumonia, abscesses, and cutaneous/subcutaneous lesions are the major clinical manifestations of nocardiosis in livestock and companion animals.

Nocardia species are aerobic actinomycetes that belong to the order Actinomycetales, which comprises a complex group of pathogens, including the genera *Rhodococcus*, *Mycobacterium*, and *Corynebacterium*, which are related to severe infectious diseases and usually refractory to conventional therapy.

Etiology: *Nocardia* is a pleomorphic, gram-positive, facultative intracellular bacterium, nonmotile and non-spore-forming. In Gram smears, it appears as rods, cocci, or coccobacilli forms with characteristic long or branching filaments and a tendency to fragment into rods and cocci. When cultured, some species of *Nocardia* produce aerial filaments. Components of the cell wall, particularly mycolic acids, render *Nocardia* spp partially acid-fast. Pathogenic *Nocardia* spp are strictly aerobic, growing over a wide temperature range (10°–50°C [50°–122°F]).

In past decades, *Nocardia* species identification has been traditionally based on phenotypic methods, including hydrolysis of different substrates (casein, xanthine, hypoxanthine, and tyrosine), carbohydrate assimilation (glucose, glycerol, galactose, glucosamine, inositol, adonitol, and trehalose), and antimicrobial susceptibility profile. Based on this former classification, the most important pathogenic species for animals and people were represented by the *Nocardia asteroides* complex (*N asteroides*, *N nova*, *N farcinica*), *N brasiliensis*, *N pseudobrasiliensis*, *N otitidiscaviarum*, and *N transvalensis*. However, diagnosis based exclusively on phenotypic assays leads to misidentification or is insufficient to distinguish some species of *Nocardia*. More recently, studies in domestic animals and people have revealed that speciation of *Nocardia* requires confirmation by molecular methods. However, most of the literature about nocardiosis in animals and people was published before this new molecular speciation. Thus, because of the taxonomic transition of *Nocardia* speciation, for purposes of this chapter, the remaining text will use the former *Nocardia* spp (in reference to the old classification) or molecular species detection of *Nocardia* (in reference to the new taxonomy).

To date, >90 valid species of *Nocardia* are recognized. Of these, >30 have been described as causes of opportunistic human infections, and at least 30 as responsible for animal diseases. Recent use of molecular techniques has led to large taxonomic changes in the *Nocardia* classification, and new species continue to be described.

Epidemiology: *Nocardia* spp are ubiquitous organisms, a component of normal soil microflora; they are commonly found in soil, organic material, freshwater and saltwater, dust, compost vegetation, and other environmental sources.

Nocardiosis is considered an uncommon disease in animals and people. However, reports of animal nocardiosis have increased worldwide.

Infections in livestock and companion animals caused by *Nocardia* spp are acquired by inhalation, traumatic percutaneous introduction of the microorganism, ingestion, or by the intramammary route. The occurrence of disease and infective *Nocardia* spp may vary geographically, influenced by animal management strategies as well as environmental factors, such as dry, dusty, or windy conditions.

Nocardia spp is considered an agent of mastitis of environmental origin in cattle and small ruminants. Nocardial mastitis usually affects herds with a history of inadequate milking management and/or poor hygiene conditions before and after milking. Mammary infections are predominantly caused by soil contamination of teat dips, udders, and milking equipment during washing procedures and by intramammary infusion therapy. Dairy herds affected by nocardial mastitis also have a history of inadequate concentrations of antiseptics in teat dips. Outbreaks of nocardial mastitis have been reported associated with dry-cow therapy (eg, neomycin) or improper intramammary therapy.

In companion animals, disease transmission is related to the inoculation of organisms through puncture wounds or foreign bodies, or secondary to bites, wounds, or scratches after cat fights. Canine infections have rarely been related to inhalation of the bacterium. The occurrence of nocardiosis in dogs and cats is intimately associated with underlying immunosuppressive disorders, particularly dogs infected by distemper virus and cats affected by leukemia or immunodeficiency virus. Canine nocardiosis occurs at any age group and in both sexes, although it appears to affect mainly males, particularly between 1–2 yr old.

Nocardiosis in horses is recognized as an opportunistic infection and is usually related to immune disorders. In most reported cases of equine clinical nocardiosis, there were underlying immunosuppressive problems, particularly pituitary pars intermedia dysfunction (*see* p 547) or severe combined immunodeficiency in Arabian foals (*see* p 818).

Pathogenesis: Pathogenicity of *Nocardia* in domestic animals is attributed to the virulence of the strain, the structure of the bacterial cell wall, host susceptibility, route of transmission, coinfection with immunosuppressive diseases, and development of pyogranulomatous lesions. However, the outcome of *Nocardia* infections is intimately linked to the ability of the strain to resist the initial neutrophil and activated macrophage attack and the cell-mediated immune response.

Immune response against nocardial infections is primarily cell-mediated. These intracellular organisms are able to inhibit phagosome-lysosome fusion in neutrophils and macrophages because of the presence of mycolic acids in their bacterial cell wall. *Nocardia* is also resistant to acids, oxidative enzymes (catalase and superoxide dismutase), and other enzymatic mechanisms of phagocytic cells. In addition, some toxins have been identified in *Nocardia* spp that appear to contribute to the virulence of pathogenic strains.

Nocardia does not induce an effective humoral immune response mediated by the action of B lymphocytes.

Clinical Findings: Mastitis, cutaneous/subcutaneous lesions, abscesses in organs, and pneumonia are the most common clinical signs of nocardiosis in livestock and companion animals.

Mastitis in Ruminants: Former *N asteroides*, *N nova*, *N otitidiscaviarum*, and *N farcinica* are the most common species described in mammary nocardiosis of domestic ruminants. More recently, based on 16S rRNA sequencing, *N nova* and *N farcinica* were the most frequent species detected in 80 different cases of bovine mastitis in Brazil and, unexpectedly, *N puris*, *N veterana*, *N cyriacigeorgica*, *N arthritidis*, and *N africana* were identified as well.

Nocardial mastitis is generally characterized by a history of chronic evolution and is usually refractory to antimicrobial therapy. Classically, clinical cases of mammary nocardiosis were predominantly seen in one or two animals in the herd, during lactation or the dry period. Clinical examination of the udder shows enlargement, edema, fibrosis, either diffuse or multifocal nodules, and occasionally draining tracts. Strip cup testing reveals serous to purulent milk secretion, showing white to yellow particles ("sulfur granules"). Infected cows have high somatic cell counts. Less frequently, the organism may disseminate from the mammary gland to other organs, causing regional lymphadenitis and pyogranulomatous lesions.

Bovine Farcy: This particular manifestation of bovine nocardiosis is usually limited to the tropics. Bovine farcy is caused by former *N farcinica*. Occasionally, *Mycobacterium farcinogenes* and *M senegalense* are also identified in similar lesions. Bovine farcy is an uncommon cause of chronic lymphangitis, lymphadenitis, and cutaneous nodules. Initially, the lesions consist of cutaneous nodules, particularly in the leg and neck regions. These nodules may slowly enlarge and coalesce to lesions of up to 10 cm in diameter, which rarely ulcerate. The lymphatic vessels appear cord-like.

Horses: Nocardiosis is an uncommon disease in horses. Most nocardial infections in horses were described involving former *N asteroides* and occasionally *N brasiliensis*. More recently, based on molecular assays, *N nova* was described causing recurrent airway obstruction in a horse. Severe pneumonia, pleuritis, disseminated (systemic) abscesses in organs, cutaneous lesions, mycetomas, and rarely, abortion represent the main clinical signs of equine nocardiosis.

Systemic nocardiosis occurs by hematogenous dissemination of bacteria causing abscesses in various organs. Pulmonary nocardiosis is characterized by increased respiratory rate, cough, labored breathing, and nasal secretion. Cutaneous and subcutaneous lesions are generally secondary to traumatic introduction of

Nocardia into the skin, leading to pyodermatitis, cellulitis, and cutaneous nodules located anywhere in the body. The lesions may ulcerate and have an odorless, gray to white discharge. Mycetomas are another type of cutaneous infection and consist of chronic and progressive skin lesions caused after transcutaneous inoculation of *Nocardia* spp. Painless nodules, purulent to necrotic, commonly form, usually limited to the site of injury, and occasionally show purulent discharge through the sinus tract.

Abortion rarely occurs in mares. Two cases were reported in Arabian and Thoroughbred mares at ~6 mo of gestation, both with history of failure to maintain gestation to term. Fetal necropsies showed lesions in lung and liver. *N asteroides* was cultured from the uterus of the Arabian mare.

Companion Animals: In dogs and cats, former *N asteroides*, *N brasiliensis*, *N otitidiscaviarum*, and *N nova* are the most frequent species identified. Recently, based on molecular methods, *N africana*, *N elegans*, and *N tenerifensis* were reported in cats, and *N abscessus* in a dog.

Superficial skin, lymphocutaneous, and thoracic infections, as well as disseminated forms, are the major clinical pictures of nocardiosis in dogs and cats. Cutaneous/subcutaneous abscesses with fistulous tracts, ulcers, mycetomas, and regional lymphadenitis are frequent clinical manifestations of the disease, associated with local skin or lymphocutaneous lesions in cats and resembling human nocardiosis. Skin lesions are seen mainly in the extremities, flank, nose, and neck areas. Canine and feline pulmonary nocardiosis are characterized by mucopurulent oculonasal discharge, anorexia, hyperthermia, weight loss, cough, dyspnea, and hemoptysis. Other systemic or disseminated forms of the disease in companion animals are represented by the presence of abscesses or lesions in two or more sites, including liver, kidneys, spleen, eyes, bones, joints, and abdominal lymph nodes, as well as development of peritonitis, pleuritis, and pyothorax. GI infection can lead to gingivitis, halitosis, and ulceration of the oral cavity. Rarely, the organism affects the urinary tract and heart. Nocardial infection in the CNS is associated with seizures, alertness, and deficits in proprioception.

Miscellaneous: Bovine or equine oral infection secondary to ingestion of fibrous foods can lead to development of pyogranulomatous lesions in the jaw. Abortion may also occur in sows and cows. Submandibular and mesenteric lymphadenitis was reported in pigs. Nocardiosis in wildlife and fishes generally causes organ abscesses and pneumonia.

Diagnosis: Routine diagnosis is based on epidemiologic findings, clinical signs, and microbiologic examination. Samples of abscesses, skin, tracheobronchial lavage fluid, milk, aspirates, organs, or other tissues should be cultured on sheep blood and/or Sabouraud agar and incubated aerobically for 2–7 days at 37°C and 25°C [98.6°F and 77°F], respectively. However, growth of some *Nocardia* spp in culture media is slow, and incubation should be extended for at least 2 wk. Colonies are circular, convex, smooth or rough, firmly adherent to agar surface, odorless, with various carotenoid-like pigments (cream, white, orange, pink, or red), and present aerial hyphae and typical powdery and dry surface, like fungal organisms. Because *Nocardia* spp are ubiquitous in the environment, microbiologic isolation of a small number of organisms from clinical specimens must be evaluated together with clinical signs and other diagnostic methods.

Microscopically, gram-positive, typically filamentous organisms are seen, with a tendency to fragmentation. Modified Ziehl-Neelsen stain shows partially acid-fast organisms. Fine-needle aspiration has been used in the diagnosis of skin nocardiosis in companion animals. Gram, Giemsa, and panoptic stains show filamentous organisms in aspirated specimens. The leukogram reveals mainly leukocytosis with neutrophilia and monocytosis, whereas the erythrogram shows moderate anemia.

Radiographic images of dogs with pulmonary nocardiosis show diffuse inflammation, nodules, abscesses, and lobar consolidation. Differential diagnoses in domestic animals include infections with *Actinomyces* or *Streptomyces* spp because of the similarities in microbiologic appearance and clinical signs. Face and jaw enlargement in cattle and horses caused by oral nocardiosis should be differentiated from *Actinomyces bovis* (actinomycosis, *see* p 590), *Actinobacillus lignieresii* (actinobacillosis, *see* p 589), and *Staphylococcus aureus* (botryomycosis).

Postmortem examination of internal organs and tissues reveals abscesses and/or numerous small to large nodules, discrete to coalescing, of white to gray color. Histologic findings of nocardiosis are characterized by pyogranulomatous to suppurative lesions with areas of necrosis. The lesions or nodules show a suppurative, necrotic center containing filamentous organisms surrounded by macrophages, lymphocytes, and plasma cells. Occasionally, epithelioid and multinucleated giant cells are found. Histolopathology sometimes reveals small, soft granules in discharges of lesions, formed by microcolonies of the organism. Lymph nodes are enlarged.

Different serologic (immunodifusion, complement fixation, and ELISA) and cutaneous hypersensitivity tests have been proposed to diagnose nocardiosis in animals. However, host animals commonly develop a nonspecific antibody response against *Nocardia*, limiting the use of serologic tests in routine diagnosis.

Currently, phenotypic diagnoses of *Nocardia* spp have been confirmed using molecular methods, including PCR, restriction endonuclease analysis of amplified 65-kDa heat shock protein gene (hsp65), 16S rRNA gene sequence, essential secretory protein A (secA1), gyrase B (gyrB), and DNA-DNA hybridization. These molecular techniques offer a timesaving and reliable means of speciation and have led to a number of taxonomic changes and the identification of new species of *Nocardia*.

Treatment: Animal and human nocardiosis is usually refractory to conventional therapy because of the intracellular location of the bacterium, development of pyogranulomatous lesions, and antimicrobial resistance patterns.

The antimicrobial susceptibility profile varies dramatically between *Nocardia* spp and geographic areas. The National Committee for Clinical Laboratory Standards approved an in vitro standardized susceptibility test for *Nocardia* by broth microdilution. The modified disc diffusion method has been used as well.

Trimethoprim-sulfonamides, aminoglycosides (amikacin, gentamicin), linezolid, amoxicillin-clavulanate, imipenem, and some cephalosporins (cefotaxime, ceftriaxone) are considered drugs of choice for nocardiosis therapy in animals and people. Ampicillin, clarithromycin, doxycycline, erythromycin, and minocycline are described as treatment alternatives for animals. Combined therapy using amikacin with sulfonamides, and amikacin with imipenem or cephalosporins (cefotaxime, ceftriaxone) also have been proposed. Intramammary infusions of trimethoprim-sulfonamides, cephalosporins or aminoglycosides (gentamicin) have been used for 5–7 days to treat clinical mastitis in cattle and goats.

Long-term therapy (1–6 mo in domestic animals and 6–12 mo in people) is required because of clinical relapses after short-term protocols. In companion animals, surgical procedures (debridement, drainage, extirpation of foreign bodies, and washing of lesions with antiseptic solutions) are indicated in cutaneous/subcutaneous lesions and osteomyelitis. However, antimicrobial therapy is successful in only 30%–50% of cases of mastitis in cattle and goats, as well as in pulmonary or extrapulmonary (disseminated or systemic) infections in companion animals and horses. The mortality of animal nocardiosis is attributed mainly to underlying conditions, delayed diagnosis, and improper therapy.

Control and Prevention: There are no specific or effective measures to control animal and human nocardiosis, probably because of the wide distribution of the microorganism in the environment.

In companion animals, immunosuppressive pathogens or debilitating conditions should be investigated as predisposing factors to development of nocardiosis.

Control and prevention of nocardial mastitis is based on measures recommended for environmental agents. Thus, the best measures to control and/or prevent nocardial mastitis remain the early microbiologic diagnosis of mastitis, proper hygiene conditions, cleaning the environment during milking, correct antiseptic concentrations in post- and mainly in pre-dipping solutions, high-quality water to wash the animals and milking equipment, removal of organic material from the milking area, and appropriate intramammary therapy procedures. Because of poor success rates in treatment of mammary infections, segregation of infected animals, chemical drying of affected quarters, or culling of animals are also recommended in control of nocardial mastitis in dairy herds.

Public Health Considerations: Human nocardiosis is an opportunistic disease. In some countries, the clinical impact of nocardiosis is fragmentary, indicating that diagnosis of disease may be neglected or underestimated. Curiously, reports of human nocardiosis have recently increased all over the world. Although the disease typically occurs in immunocompromised patients, nocardiosis has been described in immunocompetent people as well. Former *N asteroides* complex is the main species described in human nocardiosis. Currently, based on molecular methodologies and rearranged taxonomy, *N cyriacigeorgica*, *N brasiliensis*, *N asteroides*, *N nova*, *N farcinica*, *N transvalensis*, *N pseudobrasiliensis*, and *N otitidiscaviarum* have most frequently been detected in human patients.

Pneumonia, cutaneous-subcutaneous lesions, mycetoma, and neurologic manifestations are the most common clinical signs. However, clinical cases of human nocardiosis are intimately associated with immunosuppressive or debilitating disorders, such as AIDS, organ transplants, cirrhosis, diabetes, alcoholism, rheumatic and malignancy diseases (lymphosarcoma, lymphoma), or prolonged use of corticosteroids.

The environment is the natural reservoir of *Nocardia* spp for human and animal infections. Most cases of transmission to people probably occur by inhalation of the organism in dry and warm climate regions (aerosolization). Trauma with skin inoculation is another form of transmission of the bacterium to people. Cases of cutaneous/subcutaneous nocardiosis have been reported in some patients, secondary to bites or scratches of clinically ill dogs and cats. However, human nocardiosis is apparently not directly transmitted person-to-person or by nosocomial infections. Interestingly, studies have shown great similarity between *Nocardia* spp involved in human and animal infections. Experimental studies regarding temperature resistance using former *N asteroides* and *N brasiliensis* isolated from bovine milk and submitted to time/temperature conditions used in usual pasteurization procedures indicated a potential risk of *Nocardia* transmission by milk.

Precautions should be taken among human patients who have immune dysfunctions or debilitating diseases, with special reference to contact with soil or organic material from environments contaminated by domestic animals, contamination of traumatic cutaneous lesions, or close contact with animals suspected of having nocardiosis.

PERITONITIS

Peritonitis is an inflammation of the serous membranes of the peritoneal cavity. It may be a primary disease or secondary to other pathologic conditions. Different infectious and noninfectious agents may cause peritonitis, which may result in a variety of clinical manifestations, disease progression, and outcome. Peritonitis may be acute or chronic, septic or nonseptic, local or diffuse, or adhesive or exudative. The term "tertiary peritonitis," used in human medicine for particular cases of chronic peritonitis with a small number of bacteria or fungi, is not used in veterinary medicine.

Etiology: Primary peritonitis is less common than secondary peritonitis and may be infectious or idiopathic. In infectious primary peritonitis, infectious agents spread via the bloodstream into the peritoneal cavity of animals that are often immunocompromised. Such infectious agents include feline coronavirus (FCoV), which causes feline infectious peritonitis (FIP); *Nocardia* spp; *Mycobacterium* spp; *Haemophilus parasuis*; and other infectious agents. Progression of primary peritonitis tends to be chronic.

Peritonitis occurs secondary to another disease as the result of exposure of the peritoneal cavity to nonspecific infectious or noninfectious agents. It is often acute and frequently results in a progressive, systemic disease. Secondary septic peritonitis is commonly associated with perforation of and leakage from GI organs (eg, traumatic reticuloperitonitis in cattle), with subsequent processes allowing transmural migration of bacteria (eg, neoplasia, intestinal ischemia), or with perforation/rupture of or leakage from other infected viscera (eg, abscesses in liver, spleen, omentum, cystitis, endometritis, pyometra). Furthermore, migration of parasites through the abdominal cavity may also result in leakage of chyme with subsequent septic peritonitis. Perforating wounds of the abdominal wall (eg, dog bites) or dehiscence of abdominal wound closure may result in laceration of viscera and inoculation of foreign material and microorganisms into the peritoneal cavity.

Microorganisms associated with septic peritonitis usually reflect the source of contamination. A mixed bacterial population is seen in GI tract perforation, whereas perforation of nongastrointestinal viscera (eg, urinary or gall bladder, uterus, prostate) or hematogeous infection of the peritoneal cavity may be more typically associated with aerobic organisms, including *Escherichia coli*, *Streptococcus equi zooepidemicus*, *Staphylococcus*, *Proteus*, *Rhodococcus*, *Klebsiella*, *Salmonella*, *Enterobacter*, *Pseudomonas*, or *Corynebacterium*.

Secondary aseptic peritonitis occurs after contamination of the abdominal cavity with chemical irritants (eg, bile, urine, drugs) or intestinal ischemia. Common conditions are urolithiasis and rupture of the urinary or gall bladder; however, these conditions are not always aseptic. The originally aseptic peritoneal inflammations may later become septic. In addition, intraperitoneal administration of drugs or fluids may result in temporary inflammatory reactions of the peritoneum. Because New World camelids show severe inflammatory reactions to infections with *Dicrocoelium dentriticum*, peritonitis may develop subsequent to the severe hepatitis. In large animals, peritonitis is most commonly seen in cattle, less often in horses, and rarely diagnosed in pigs, sheep, and goats. It is a serious and often fatal condition in cats (FIP). For common causes of peritonitis in various species, *see* TABLE 5.

TABLE 5 COMMON CAUSES OF PERITONITIS

Species	Cause
Cattle	Traumatic reticuloperitonitis; rumenitis; abomasal ulcer (perforation); abomasal volvulus; cecal torsion; dystocia (uterine torsion, cesarean section); metritis or pyometra; abdominal surgery; intestinal, rectal, or uterine rupture; liver or abdominal abscess rupture; omphalitis (calves); fat necrosis/pancreatitis; neoplasia (eg, mesothelioma, ileal adenocarcinoma); iatrogenic (eg, rectal perforation, liver biopsy, intraperitoneal injection, rumenocentesis); green algae infection (rare); *Setaria* infection (rare)
Horses	Parasitic (larval) migration; intestinal injury and ischemia (colic); abdominal abscess rupture (*Rhodococcus*, *Streptococcus*); abdominal surgery (colic surgery, castration); gastric, intestinal, or uterine rupture; gastroduodenoenteritis, colitis; omphalitis, persistent urachus, or bladder rupture (foals); gastric ulcer (perforation); fat necrosis/pancreatitis; neoplasia (eg, cholangiocellular carcinoma); penetrating trauma to abdominal wall; iatrogenic (rectal perforation, intraperitoneal injection)
Small ruminants	Primary peritonitis (*Mycoplasma* spp); parasitic (larval) migration (eg, liver fluke, lungworm, *Setaria* sp); traumatic reticuloperitonitis (less common than in cattle); abdominal abscess rupture; neoplasia (eg, mesothelioma, cholangiocellular carcinoma); iatrogenic (eg, liver biopsy, intraperitoneal injection)
New World camelids	Sequela of parasitic migration/acute hepatitis (dicrocoeliosis of special importance); perforating third-compartment or duodenal ulcers; sequela of urolithiasis/ruptured urinary bladder; traumatic reticuloperitonitis (rare)
Pigs	Glässer's disease (*Haemophilus parasuis*); intestinal (ileal) perforation; dystocia; sequela of septicemic infections (*Salmonella* Choleraesuis, *Streptococcus suis*); polyserositis (*Mycoplasma hyorhinis*)
Dogs and cats	Feline infectious peritonitis (FCoV); ingested intestinal foreign bodies; gastric, intestinal, rectal, bladder, or uterine rupture; abdominal or intestinal surgery; gastric and duodenal ulcers/perforation; abdominal neoplasia (eg, mesothelioma); hepatitis, gallbladder diseases/rupture; pancreatitis/fat necrosis; gastric dilatation volvulus (dog); penetrating trauma to abdominal wall; *Candida albicans* (rare); *Neospora caninum* (rare)

Pathogenesis: Inflammation of the peritoneum is the result of a variety of possible pathogenetic pathways that are species-dependent (eg, peritoneal inflammatory response in cattle is characterized by extensive fibrin formation, horses tend to develop exudative peritonitis) and mainly influenced by etiology (eg, primary or secondary, septic or nonseptic). Because of the release of inflammatory mediators after contact with mechanical, chemical, or infectious agents, serosal capillary permeability is increased and results in leakage of plasma proteins, solutes, and water into the peritoneal cavity. Exudation of protein-rich fluid may result in hypoproteinemia and facilitates bacterial proliferation. The combined effect of large fluid losses into the peritoneal cavity and vasodilatory effects of absorbed toxins may produce profound hypotension and hypovolemia. The inflammation may decrease the animal's antioxidative capacity and result in oxidative stress.

Rupture or perforation of the forestomach, stomach, or intestine with spillage of large volumes of gastric or intestinal contents and rupture or perforation of the contaminated uterus leads to an acute septic peritonitis. Toxins produced by bacteria and tissue breakdown are readily absorbed through the peritoneum and have severe systemic effects leading to hypotension, shock, systemic inflammatory response syndrome (SIRS), and disseminated intravascular coagulation (DIC). Endotoxins and acid-base and electrolyte disturbances directly affect cardiac function, leading to reduced cardiac output and circulatory failure. Paralytic ileus is considered to be a frequent result of acute peritonitis, causing functional obstruction and an increased mortality rate. Large volumes of inflammatory exudates may be secreted into the peritoneal cavity during peritonitis and may lead to impaired respiration by impinging on the diaphragm. Spillage of small amounts of gastric or intestinal content (eg, after transcutaneous rumenocentesis, bar suture techniques for left displaced abomasum surgery) normally result in local peritonitis.

Chronic peritonitis is often characterized by extensive secretion of fibrinogen and subsequent formation of fibrinous/fibrous adhesions. Such adhesions help localize the inflammatory process (eg, traumatic *reticuloperitonitis in cattle*, type 3 abomasal ulcers in cattle) but may cause mechanical or functional obstruction of the GI tract. Chronic peritonitis in horses often results in recurrent colic episodes.

Clinical Findings: Clinical signs vary depending on the type and etiology of peritonitis. Affected animals may develop toxemia and septicemia, shock, hemorrhage, abdominal pain, paralytic ileus, fluid accumulation, and adhesions in varying degrees. However, there are reports of apparently clinically healthy animals having chronic bacterial peritonitis.

Shock, hypotension, acid-base disturbances, and circulatory collapse after acute septic peritonitis associated with rupture of intestines or uterus often lead to sudden death. These animals normally show only limited clinical signs of peritonitis. In less severe cases, abdominal pain and fever are common. Hypothermia can also be seen as a result of dehydration, hypovolemia, and sepsis. Abdominal pain may be permanent and severe, characterized by guarding the abdomen, stiff gait, or recumbency. In all species, pain responses are most evident in the early stages. Abdominal distention, which may be inapparent, usually is due to accumulation of peritoneal exudates, paralytic ileus, or peritoneal adhesions. Fecal output is often decreased, although frequency of defecation may be increased in the early stages of peritonitis. Animals with secondary peritonitis may also show clinical signs associated with the primary disease.

Rectal palpation is a useful diagnostic technique to evaluate the peritoneum and accessible abdominal organs in large animals; however, local peritonitic processes in the cranial abdomen (eg, traumatic reticuloperitonitis in cattle) do not result in clinical signs that can be diagnosed by rectal examination. Abdominal radiography may be used in small animals. In horses and cattle, radiography can be also used as a diagnostic tool, but high-power x-ray machines are required; therefore, this technique is limited to stationary units in veterinary clinics. Generally, ultrasonography is the most valuable diagnostic tool to examine the abdominal cavity and assess the extent, localization, and character of peritonitis. Additionally, ultrasonography allows a guided abdominocentesis, which can be used (in both large and small animals) to obtain fluid for cytologic and biochemical examination and bacteriologic culture. Diagnostic peritoneal lavage can be used if peritoneal fluid cannot be obtained by abdominocentesis. Diagnostic laparoscopy or laparotomy can be considered to verify the diagnosis. Diagnostic laparotomy is frequently used in cattle because it is inexpensive, can be performed in standing position, and is associated with few or minor complications; it also makes additional diagnostic procedures unnecessary and can often be combined with therapeutic measures.

Cattle: Clinical signs of peritonitis in cattle are often nonspecific and characterized by reduced feed intake, drop in milk production, and decreased rumination activity. In chronic cases, ruminal contractions may be present but reduced in intensity. Abdominal percussion may reveal ruminal tympany or pneumoperitoneum. Moderate fever is typical during the first 24–36 hr in cattle with acute, local peritonitis. High fever suggests acute, diffuse peritonitis. Cattle with peritonitis often have a shuffling, cautious gait with a rigid arched back, and grunt when walking or passing urine or feces. Deep palpation of the abdominal wall and pain provocation tests result in pain response. Chronic peritonitis is associated with development of fibrous adhesions. Depending on localization, rectal palpation may reveal adhesions between intestinal loops and peritoneum. Cattle may suffer from chronic indigestion (Hoflund syndrome, abomasal impaction) or toxemia, with periods of acute, severe illness caused by partial intestinal obstruction. The majority of cattle develop a localized peritonitis by extensive fibrin formation; however, in a few cases the abdominal cavity contains large volumes of turbid, infected peritoneal fluid.

Small Ruminants, New World Camelids, and Pigs: Generally, the clinical signs in small ruminants, New World camelids, and pigs are similar to those in other animals. However, peritonitis is rarely diagnosed clinically in pigs, sheep, or goats, although it is not an uncommon finding on routine meat inspection after slaughter of pigs. It is more common in llamas and alpacas.

Horses: Clinical signs include colic, distended intestines on rectal examination, gastric reflux, and occasionally diarrhea. Rectal palpation may reveal tacky, dry mucosa and in some cases fibrinous or fibrous adhesions between intestinal loops and other abdominal organs. Intestinal peristaltic sounds are reduced. Tachycardia, weak pulses, poor peripheral perfusion, and fever are common. Weight loss and intermittent abdominal pain (colic) may be seen in horses with chronic peritonitis.

Dogs and Cats: In small animals, anorexia and depression are nonspecific signs of peritonitis, often accompanied by vomiting and decreased defecation. The abdomen may be distended. Abdominal palpation may be painful, and abdominal masses may be detected. Icterus may be present in generalized biliary peritonitis in small animals. Abdominal radiographs may reveal GI obstruction, bowel dilatation, free abdominal air, ascites, or radiodense foreign material. Loss of serosal details in radiographs indicates abdominal fluid.

Diagnosis: Laboratory analyses are helpful to confirm the clinical diagnosis and determine the severity of peritonitis, and should include a CBC and several biochemical parameters in blood and peritoneal fluid.

Acute, diffuse peritonitis with toxemia is usually accompanied by leukopenia, neutropenia, and a marked increase in immature neutrophils (degenerative left shift). In less severe acute peritonitis, leukocytosis may occur as a result of increased neutrophil production. Acute, localized peritonitis may reveal a normal WBC count with a regenerative left shift. The total WBC count in chronic peritonitis may be normal, with an occasional increase in lymphocytes and monocytes. Anemia may occur due to hemorrhage into the peritoneal cavity but is also commonly associated with chronic inflammatory processes. A number of abnormalities of serum biochemical parameters (eg, total protein, albumin, fibrinogen, bilirubin, LDH, alkaline phosphatase, CK) may accompany peritonitis. Hypoalbuminemia, hyperglobulinemia, and hyperbilirubinemia are frequently present. Generally, the changes in hematologic and biochemical parameters indicate inflammatory processes and tissue damage, but they are not pathognomonic for peritonitis.

The peritoneal fluid is a plasma dialysate with specific physical and chemical properties that depend on membrane permeability, concentrations and electrical charges of ions, and osmotic pressure. The fluid contains cells deriving from the mesothelium and the blood or lymphatic vessels. Under physiologic conditions, peritoneal fluid is a transudate, whereas peritonitis results in a fluid that is typically characterized as an exudate. Analysis of peritoneal fluid is a useful diagnostic method in gastroenterology, because the fluid generally reflects abdominal conditions. The volume of peritoneal fluid is frequently increased in peritonitis. In cases of septic peritonitis, samples of peritoneal fluid should be examined microbiologically to characterize infectious pathogens.

The parameters of the classic transudate-exudate categorization system are shown in TABLE 6. A peritoneal fluid showing properties of both a transudate and an exudate is commonly called a modified transudate. Use of a scoring system allows further classification as mild, moderate, or severe peritonitis. In practice, however, analysis of peritoneal fluid may be inconsistent, leading to inconclusive results. Therefore, the diagnostic value of this traditional concept is limited. To improve the sensitivity of the distinction between an exudate and transudate of pleural and peritoneal effusions in human medicine, Light's criteria (fluid to serum protein ratio >0.5, fluid to serum LDH ratio >0.6, or fluid LDH activity >200 U/L), cutoff values for ratios between peritoneal fluid and plasma or serum of various parameters (eg, lactate, glucose, enzymes), and the serum-ascites albumin gradient (SAAG) have been established. These concepts have been applied to some animal species (ie, horses, cattle, small animals).

Under physiologic conditions, the ratio between lymphocytes and neutrophils is close to 1:1. Acute peritonitis usually results in an increased number of leukocytes, and the percentage of neutrophils can be 60%–90%. However, in cases of peracute septic inflammation, the number of leukocytes may decrease due to necrosis and cell damage. Histologically, a high rate of degenerative leukocytes (cytolysis, karyorrhexis, or karyolysis) can be found. In chronic peritoneal inflammation, the proportion of neutrophils decreases and the proportion of monocytes increases. The presence of intra- or extracellular bacteria confirms septic peritonitis. Gram-staining enables differentiation between gram-positive and gram-negative bacteria and facilitates early antibiotic treatment.

The physiologic total protein concentration in peritoneal fluid is 20–25 g/L. The normal protein ratio between peritoneal fluid and serum is lower than 1:2. The SAAG is calculated by subtracting the peritoneal fluid albumin concentration from the serum concentration. The cutoff value of 11 g/L for people seems suitable for monogastric animals. However, the reference values for protein ratio and SAAG are not applicable to dairy cattle, mainly because of their higher serum protein and albumin concentrations than those of monogastric animals and people. In addition, in cattle, the protein ratio and SAAG did not show higher diagnostic values than the total protein concentration in peritoneal fluid alone.

In healthy animals, glucose concentration is the same in both serum and peritoneal fluid. Bacterial infection of the peritoneal cavity results in a major decrease of peritoneal glucose concentration. A peritoneal fluid:serum ratio of glucose concentrations <0.5 is highly sensitive and specific for septic peritonitis. Because in animals with septic peritonitis the glucose concentration in peritoneal fluid frequently falls below the detection limit, it is often not even necessary to measure the glucose concentration in serum.

Intestinal ischemia results in an increase of L-lactate concentration in plasma and peritoneal fluid. Although an association exists between L-lactate concentration in peritoneal fluid and plasma, L-lactate in peritoneal fluid is considered to be more closely correlated to the severity of intestinal ischemia. Physiologically, L-lactate concentration in peritoneal fluid is lower than that in plasma (in healthy horses, the ratio is ~1:2). This ratio is reversed in colicky horses with intestinal ischemia, cows with abomasal volvulus, and dogs with gastric dilatation volvulus. Similar to that in horses, an increased L-lactate concentration in

TABLE 6 CHARACTERISTICS OF TRANSUDATES AND EXUDATES IN CATTLE, HORSES, DOGS, AND CATS

Parameter	Species	Transudate	Exudate
Total protein (g/dL)	All	<2.5	>3
Specific gravity	All	<1.020	>1.025
Cell count (10^9/L)	Cattle	0.5–5	>8
	Horses	0.5–5	>8
	Dogs, cats	<3	>5
Color	All	Colorless to yellow	Variable
Turbidity	All	Clear to moderate	Moderate to opaque
Bacteria	All	Absent	May be present

peritoneal fluid has been found in cattle with abomasal volvulus and dogs with gastric dilatation volvulus. In addition, lactate is also a bacterial metabolite (predominately D-lactate); therefore, increased lactate concentration in peritoneal fluid may also indicate septic peritonitis. The accuracy of peritoneal lactate concentration in differentiating septic and nonseptic peritonitis varies between species (eg, 90%–95% in dogs but 65%–70% in cats).

Inflammation can be monitored using acute phase proteins such as C-reactive protein or haptoglobin (in cattle) as markers. Acute phase protein concentrations are increased in peripheral blood and in peritoneal fluid in animals with peritonitis; however, these parameters are general indicators for inflammation and not specific for peritonitis.

Fibrinogen concentration in peritoneal fluid may be increased in animals with peritonitis. However, fibrinogen concentration has limited diagnostic value, because there is only a weak association between peritoneal and blood fibrinogen concentration. An increased concentration of the fibrin degradation product D-dimer indicates intestinal ischemia and inflammation with high sensitivity and specificity. Normal values for human plasma are <0.3 mg/L. Reference values for small animals and horses seem to be similar to those in people. The peritoneal fluid D-dimer concentration in healthy cows is <0.6 mg/L; increased values indicate peritonitis with high sensitivity and specificity.

Inflammation, intestinal ischemia, and reperfusion affect the activities of several enzymes (alkaline phosphatase [ALP], AST, CK, LDH) in peritoneal fluid and peripheral blood. CK activity is primarily increased in serum and peritoneal fluid in cases of intestinal ischemia. The origin of CK is thought to be the muscular layer of the strangulated, ischemic intestines. However, other tissues (eg, striated muscle after colic episodes in horses) may be sources of higher CK activities; therefore, the sensitivity and specificity of CK are low.

LDH activity is a measure of inflammatory response and has been used to differentiate exudate from transudate (peritoneal fluid:serum LDH ratio >0.6; LDH activity of peritoneal fluid >200 U/L). The reference values for monogastric animals, but not those for cattle, are similar to those for people. For cattle, a cut-off value of 960 U/L has been identified.

An increase of ALP during intestinal ischemia and reperfusion has been found in peritoneal fluid of horses with colic and cows with displaced abomasum. However, the origin of the ALP was not exclusively the damaged stomach or intestine. Other sources of the increased ALP activity in these cases include hepatocytes and granulocytes. Normally, serum ALP activity does not show major changes during intestinal ischemia.

Increased concentrations of protein and globulin in serum and peritoneal fluid are often seen in cats with FIP. However, neither parameter is accurate enough for diagnosis, especially if measured in serum. Calculation of the albumin:globulin ratio may improve the diagnostic value. The traditional Rivalta's test simply differentiates transudates from exudates. Although it produces false-positive results in cats with septic bacterial peritonitis, it still seems useful for FIP diagnosis. The widely used parameter α-1-acid glycoprotein indicates inflammation but is not specific for FIP. Serum anti-feline coronavirus (FCoV) antibody titers must be interpreted critically, because many healthy cats are anti-FCoV-antibody positive. The diagnostic value of anti-FCoV antibody titers in peritoneal fluid is still under discussion. A number of advanced diagnostic methods (eg, immunofluorescent staining of FCoV antigen in peritoneal macrophages, ELISA to detect antigen-antibody complexes in serum, reverse transcriptase-PCR) have been introduced as diagnostic measures to improve accuracy of FIP diagnosis. Generally, the laboratory tests performed on peritoneal fluid are superior to those that use serum. Further immunohistochemistry for intracellular FCoV antigen in macrophages derived from ocular or dermal lesions of FIP cats may aid the diagnosis. (*See also* FELINE INFECTIOUS PERITONITIS, p 780.)

Prognosis: Although the mesothelium of the peritoneum is able to regenerate rapidly, peritonitis must be considered a severe, life-threatening disease with a guarded prognosis. Prognosis strongly depends on the character and severity of the disease and, therefore, must be determined individually. General survival rates of 50%–70% have been reported, with much lower rates for return of productivity in farm animals. In horses, the prognosis for further use in equestrian sport is guarded. Furthermore, horses that survive peritonitis frequently suffer from recurrent colic episodes. Despite new developments in therapy, the prognosis for cats with FIP remains poor. It is still a lethal disease with no effective long-term treatment.

Treatment: Adequate therapy depends on the diagnosis and the results of physical examination and laboratory analyses. In severe cases of septic peritonitis, the initial treatment must be directed toward saving the life of the animal and stabilizing cardiovascular and other organ functions. In severe cases, euthanasia is a consideration. Therapy should include treatment of hypovolemic/toxemic shock, aggressive anti-inflammatory therapy, and treatment of the metabolic and rheologic disturbances (eg, electrolyte and acid-base disorders, disseminated intravascular coagulation). Replacement fluids, electrolytes, plasma, or whole blood may be necessary to maintain cardiac output and improve circulation. It is of major importance to prevent circulatory failure from complications of disseminated intravascular coagulation. Antioxidative treatment using vitamins C and E or short-acting glucocorticoids might be useful. Additional prokinetic drugs might be necessary to increase and coordinate the motility of the GI tract.

Appropriate antimicrobial therapy should be started once septic peritonitis is suspected or confirmed. Peritoneal fluid samples should be obtained for culture and sensitivity testing. Parenteral broad-spectrum antimicrobial therapy must be applied initially. Aminoglycoside or fluoroquinolone antibiotics are effective against gram-negative organisms, and penicillins or cephalosporins are effective against gram-positive bacteria. The antimicrobial drug may be changed later according to the results of cytology and culture and sensitivity testing. Antimicrobial and anti-inflammatory treatment should continue through the healing period.

If possible, therapy should be initiated to eliminate the cause of peritonitis. In animals with suspected leakage of abdominal organs, surgery should be performed immediately to explore the abdomen and repair the defects, followed by peritoneal lavage with an isothermic, isotonic, balanced electrolyte solution before the abdominal cavity is closed. Although frequently performed, there is no proven clinical benefit in adding antimicrobial drugs to the lavage solution. Solutions containing antiseptics (eg, povidone-iodine) also have no proven clinical benefit and may even function as chemical irritants and exacerbate the inflammation. Heparin treatment may be considered in cases of DIC and may prevent extensive fibrin formation within the peritoneal cavity.

The application of abdominal drains and subsequent lavage is possible in small and large animals to treat severe peritonitis, removing septic and proinflammatory material from the abdominal cavity. Whereas the removal of septic peritoneal fluid is generally accepted as beneficial, the efficacy of repeated peritoneal lavage is under debate. Whereas some reports describe positive effects, others claim that intensive lavage may disturb healing of the epithelium and result in further spread of the inflammation. The composition of the lavage solution is also under debate; there are no or very few advantages to adding antibiotics or antiseptics. The decision to manage peritoneal drainage is based on the severity of the case, experience level, intensive care possibility, and equipment. Maintenance of drain patency can be difficult, especially in cattle, caused by the extensive fibrin formation in the abdominal cavity. In animals treated by peritoneal drainage or lavage, serum protein and electrolyte levels should be monitored periodically, because both are lost with drainage of exudate.

Nutritional support should be anticipated, because many animals with peritonitis will not eat. Enteral nutrition helps to maintain the health of the intestinal mucosa; however, vomiting (dogs and cats) or anorexia may force the consideration of alternatives. In ruminants and New World camelids, transfaunation using rumen fluid obtained from other animals or commercially available products has proved beneficial. In certain animals, total or partial parenteral nutrition may be necessary to provide a portion of the nutritional requirements while enteral nutrition is being initiated. Administration of antioxidants and vitamins should be considered. Vomiting is sometimes a sequela of peritonitis in small animals; antiemetic treatment is indicated in such cases.

Feline coronaviral infection may cause a primary feline infectious peritonitis (FIP). Therapy is palliative (eg, interferon therapy, glucocorticoids, supportive therapy) and directed toward slowing down the inflammation. However, no effective long-term therapy is available. Commercial vaccines for prophylaxis are available in some countries; however, there are conflicting reports on their efficacy and safety. The vaccine is not effective when administered to animals already exposed to FCoV; however, it may offer some protection when administered to seronegative animals.

In chronic adhesive peritonitis, laparoscopy or laparotomy may be considered to cut adhesions that prevent intestinal motility or to remove/drain intestinal abscesses. However, the success of such interventions might be limited.

PLAGUE

Plague, caused by *Yersinia pestis*, is an acute and sometimes fatal bacterial zoonosis transmitted primarily by the fleas of rats and other rodents. Enzootic foci of sylvatic plague exist in the western USA and throughout the world, including Eurasia, Africa, and North and South America. In addition to rodents, other mammalian species that have been naturally infected with *Y pestis* include lagomorphs, felids, canids, mustelids, and some ungulates. Domestic cats and dogs have been known to develop plague from oral mucous membrane exposure to infected rodent tissues, typically when they are allowed to roam and hunt in enzootic areas. Birds and other nonmammalian vertebrates appear to be resistant to plague. On average, 10 human plague cases are reported each year in the USA; most are from New Mexico, California, Colorado, and Arizona. Most human cases result from the bite of an infected flea, although direct contact with infected wild rabbits, rodents, and occasionally other wildlife and exposure to infected domestic cats are also risk factors.

Etiology: *Y pestis* is a gram-negative, nonmotile, coccobacillus belonging to the Enterobacteriaceae family. It exhibits a bipolar staining, "safety pin" appearance when stained with Wright, Giemsa, or Wayson stains. *Y pestis* grows slowly even at optimal temperatures (28°C [82.4°F]) and can require ≥48 hr to produce colonies. Several types of media can be used to grow *Y pestis*, including blood agar, nutrient broth, and unenriched agar. Colonies are small (1–2 mm), gray, nonmucoid, and have a characteristic "hammered copper" appearance. Different virulence factors are expressed by the organism at different temperatures and environments, allowing the organism to survive in flea vectors and then be transmitted to and multiply in mammalian hosts. The organism does not survive for long at high temperatures or in dry environments.

Epidemiology and Transmission: *Y pestis* is maintained in the environment in a natural cycle between susceptible rodent species and their associated fleas. Commonly affected rodent species include ground squirrels (*Spermophilus* spp) and wood rats (*Neotoma* spp). Cats and dogs are usually exposed to *Y pestis* by mucous membrane contact with secretions or tissues of an infected rodent or rabbit or by the bite of an infected flea. People are usually exposed by an infected flea bite but are sometimes exposed due to contact with infected animals or via respiratory droplet transmission from pneumonic cases. Risk factors for cats acquiring plague include hunting and eating rodents and rabbits, visiting an enzootic plague area, finding dead rodents around the yard or areas that the animal frequents, and exposure to infected fleas. Plague epizootics cause nearly 100% mortality in affected wild rodent and rabbit populations. Once their host has died, *Y pestis*–infected rodent and rabbit fleas will seek other hosts, including cats and dogs, and potentially be transported into homes. Rodent and rabbit flea species are different from dog and cat fleas (*Ctenocephalides* spp), although most veterinarians and pet owners will not be able to visually distinguish flea species. Dog and cat fleas are rare in most plague-enzootic areas of the western USA; therefore, fleas on pets in these areas may be more likely to be fleas from wildlife, including rodents or rabbits.

Pathogenesis: Fleas become infected with *Y pestis* when feeding on a bacteremic mammal. It has been thought that most flea transmission of plague occurs when the bacteria multiply and block the flea's digestive tract, preventing it from digesting subsequent blood meals; the flea then regurgitates the plague bacteria and inoculates the host on which it is attempting to feed. Recent experiments have shown that some species of unblocked fleas are better transmitters of plague. These fleas became infectious within a day of feeding and remained infectious for ≥4 days, also inoculating the host on which they are feeding with plague bacteria that have been multiplying within the flea's upper GI tract. In mammalian hosts, plague presents clinically in one of three forms: bubonic, septicemic, or pneumonic. After inoculation into the skin by a flea bite or into mucous membranes by contact with infectious secretions or tissues, the bacteria travel via lymphatic vessels to regional lymph nodes. These infected lymph nodes are called buboes, the typical lesion of bubonic plague.

Secondary septicemic plague can develop when the organism spreads from the affected lymph nodes via the bloodstream but can also occur without prior lymphadenopathy (primary septicemic plague) and affect numerous organs, including the spleen, liver, heart, and lungs. Pneumonic plague can develop from inadequately treated septicemic plague (secondary pneumonic plague) or from infectious respiratory droplets (primary pneumonic plague), typically from a coughing pneumonic plague patient (animal or human).

Clinical Findings and Lesions: The clinical presentation of plague in cats is most commonly bubonic plague. The incubation period ranges from 1–4 days. Cats with bubonic plague typically present with fever, anorexia, lethargy, and an enlarged lymph node that may be abscessed and draining. Oral and lingual ulcers, skin abscesses, ocular discharge, diarrhea, vomiting, and cellulitis have also been documented. A retrospective review of 119 naturally infected cats found that 53% of cats had bubonic plague; of those, 75% had submandibular lymphadenopathy, with bilateral enlargement in ~1/3 of cases. Affected lymph nodes show necrosuppurative inflammation, edema, and hemorrhages and contain numerous *Y pestis* organisms. In experimentally infected cats, fever was as high as 106°F (41°C), peaking ~3 days after exposure; mortality was as high as 60% in untreated cats. Ten of 16 (62.5%) cats exposed orally developed enlarged lymph nodes in the medial retropharyngeal, submandibular, sublingual, and tonsillar regions, palpable 4–6 days after exposure. *Y pestis* was isolated from the throats of 15 of these cats. In 6 subcutaneously exposed cats (mimicking a flea bite), none had palpably enlarged lymph nodes in the head or neck region, but four had subcutaneous abscesses at the inoculation site.

Cats with primary septicemic plague have no obvious lymphadenopathy but present with fever, lethargy, and anorexia. Septic signs may also include diarrhea, vomiting, tachycardia, weak pulse, prolonged capillary refill time, disseminated intravascular coagulopathy, and respiratory distress. Primary pneumonic plague has not been documented in cats. Cats with secondary pneumonic plague may present with all the signs of septicemic plague along with a cough and other abnormal lung sounds. Characteristic necropsy findings can include livers that are pale with light-colored necrotic nodules, enlarged spleens with necrotic nodules, and lungs with diffuse interstitial pneumonia, focal congestion, hemorrhages, and necrotic foci.

Dogs infected with plague are less likely to develop clinical illness than cats, although cases have been seen in enzootic areas. Symptomatic plague infection has been documented in three naturally infected dogs; clinical signs included fever, lethargy, submandibular lymphadenopathy, a purulent intermandibular lesion, oral cavity lesions, and cough.

Cattle, horses, sheep, and pigs are not known to develop symptomatic illness from plague, whereas clinical illness has been documented in goats, camels, mule deer, pronghorn antelope, nonhuman primates, and a llama. Infected mountain lions and bobcats have shown clinical signs and mortality similar to those of domestic cats.

Diagnosis: Plague must be differentiated from other bacterial infections, including tularemia (*see* p 692), abscesses due to wounds (cat fight bites), and staphylococcal and streptococcal infections. During acute illness, preferred antemortem samples for culture include whole blood, lymph node aspirates, swabs from draining lesions, and oropharyngeal swabs from cats with oral lesions or pneumonia. Diagnostic samples should be taken before antibiotics are administered. *Y pestis* cultures can take 48 hr for visible growth to develop. An air-dried glass slide smear of a bubo aspirate can be used for a fluorescent antibody test that detects the F1 antigen on *Y pestis* cells. This test can be performed in a matter of hours in an experienced laboratory and is both sensitive and specific.

Postmortem specimens should include samples of liver, spleen, and lung (for pneumonic cases) and affected lymph nodes. In areas where tularemia is also present, samples should be collected under a biosafety hood, or the entire animal submitted to a veterinary diagnostic laboratory where aerosol precautions can be implemented. Serologic antibody tests can be confirmatory but require acute and convalescent samples taken 2–3 wk apart, demonstrating a 4-fold rise in antibody titer. Single acute sera are often negative if taken early in the course of illness or can be problematic in an enzootic area where animals may retain antibody titers from previous exposures.

Treatment: Because of the rapid progression of this disease, treatment for suspected plague (and infection control practices) should be started before a definitive diagnosis is obtained. Streptomycin has been considered the drug of choice in human cases but is difficult to obtain and rarely used today. Gentamicin is currently used to treat most human plague cases and should be considered a suitable alternative choice in veterinary medicine for seriously ill animals, although it is not approved for this purpose. Animals with renal failure require adjusted dosages.

Doxycycline is appropriate for treatment of less complicated cases and to complete treatment of seriously ill animals after clinical improvement. Tetracycline and chloramphenicol are also options. Penicillins are not effective in treating plague. In treatment studies with experimentally infected mice, the fluoroquinolones performed as well as streptomycin. Fluoroquinolones have not been studied in any veterinary clinical trials, but there is growing evidence from their use in enzootic areas that they are effective in the treatment of plague in dogs and cats. The recommended duration of treatment is 10–21 days, with clinical improvement (including defervescence) expected within a few days of treatment initiation.

The duration of infectivity in treated cats is not definitively known, but cats are thought to be noninfectious after 72 hr of appropriate antibiotic therapy with indications of clinical improvement. During this infectious period, cats should remain hospitalized, especially if there are signs of pneumonia. Human cases have occurred in cat owners trying to give oral medications at home, exposing them to contact with the oral cavity and associated infectious secretions.

Prevention and Zoonotic Risk: Along with treatment and diagnostic considerations, protection of people and other animals and initiation of public health interventions are critical when an animal is suspected to have plague. Animals with signs suggestive of plague should be placed in isolation, with infection control measures implemented for the protection of staff and other animal patients without waiting for a definitive diagnosis. The use of gloves, surgical masks, eye protection (if splashes or sprays are anticipated), patient isolation (animal or human), and standard hygiene and disinfection procedures for protection from potentially contaminated respiratory droplets, body fluids, and secretions from the patient (animal or human) are essential. Of the 23 human patients who developed cat-associated plague in the USA between 1977 and 1998, 6 were veterinary staff; the rest were cat owners or others handling a sick cat. After pneumonia has been excluded, or once there is evidence of clinical improvement after 72 hr of appropriate therapy, isolation procedures may be relaxed, but standard disinfection and hygiene procedures should continue.

Local or state public health officials should be notified promptly when plague is suspected to help conduct appropriate diagnostic tests, initiate an environmental investigation, and assess the need for fever watch or prophylactic antibiotics in potentially exposed people. To decrease the risk of pets and people being exposed to plague, pet owners in enzootic areas should keep their pets from roaming and hunting, limit their contact with rodent or rabbit carcasses, and use appropriate flea control. Epidemiologic data, fact sheets, public education brochures, and other information on plague is available on the Web sites of the CDC and the New Mexico Department of Health.

RHODOCOCCOSIS

Rhodococcosis is a pyogranulomatous disease of domestic animals, wildlife, and people. It is caused by *Rhodococcus equi* (formerly *Corynebacterium equi*), the pathogenicity of which has been mainly attributed to the presence of virulence-associated antigens and plasmids.

Etiology: *Rhodococcus* spp belong to the aerobic actinomycetes in the order Actinomycetales, which is taxonomically related to the genera *Mycobacterium*, *Corynebacterium*, and *Nocardia*. *R equi* is a facultative intracellular opportunistic pathogen. In Gram smears, the bacteria appear as gram-positive rods, cocci, or rod-shaped (pleomorphic) organisms.

The virulence of *R equi* is intimately associated with its ability to survive and multiply inside macrophages, mainly the presence of a large plasmid that contains genes encoding a number of proteins associated with virulence (*Vap*). Seven genes have been classically associated with *R equi* virulence, the most important being the *VapA* plasmid because of its probable regulatory action over other genes. This gene regulation of *R equi* is a complex mechanism, influenced by various factors, including iron and magnesium availability, as well as environmental conditions such as temperature and pH.

Epidemiology: *R equi* has been isolated from a wide variety of species, including horses, cattle, swine, sheep, goats, dogs, cats, camelids, birds, and wild animals.

R equi is distributed worldwide. It is widespread in surface soil, particularly in feces of foals and other herbivores, and in their environment. *R equi* may survive up to 12 mo in soil and can multiply in a wide temperature range (15°–40°C) and neutral pH (6.5–7.3).

Inhalation of soil dust particles is considered the main route of infection for domestic animals. Contaminated water and food is a less frequent route of infection, except for swine. Infected sputum may be swallowed by foals with pneumonia, causing ulcerative colitis and mesenteric lymphadenitis. Foals showing clinical and subclinical disease may spread *R equi* via aerosol.

Risk factors associated with a higher prevalence of disease in horses include large numbers of foals and mares, transient equine population, high foal density, foals born to mares that shed high numbers of the microorganism in the feces, and inadequate transfer of maternal antibodies. Poor animal management, housing, seasonal effect on foals' birth, and environmental conditions (eg, dry, dusty, windy) have also been reported as predisposing conditions.

VapA plasmid is usually found in foal and bovine rhodococcosis cases, indicating a major risk of infection to companion animals by contact with livestock or their environment.

Pathogenesis: The outcome of exposure to *R equi* is strongly influenced by the virulence, infective dose, and age and immune response of the host. Virtually all foals are exposed to *R equi* shortly after birth, although most do not develop clinical signs. Adult horses are commonly resistant to the clinical disease, because they have developed effective immune responses against *R equi*.

R equi may invade the animal via the respiratory or digestive tracts or the skin. It then spreads through hemolymphatic vessels, reaching different tissues and organs and developing pyogenic reactions in the liver, spleen, kidneys, bones, brain, and lymph nodes.

The basis of pathogenicity is attributed to the ability of the organism to survive and multiply inside macrophages, subsequently destroying these phagocytic cells. Other factors that contribute to the pathogenesis include the iron acquisition mechanism and the presence of phospholipase C and cholesterol oxidase (so called "equi factors"). In nonequine species, immunosuppressive conditions of the host may enable avirulent or less virulent strains to persist inside phagocytes.

Passive humoral immunity generated by ingestion of mare colostrum contributes to the control of *R equi* infection in foals. However, humoral response by itself does not confer complete protection. Consistent evidence supports the essential role of cellular immune response in control of *R equi* infections.

Clinical Findings: Suppurative bronchopneumonia and ulcerative colitis in foals, lymphadenitis in cattle and swine, and cutaneous or organ abscesses are the major clinical manifestations of rhodococcosis in domestic animals. *R equi* infections are frequently found only in foals and swine, whereas they are rare or uncommon in small ruminants, companion animals, birds, and wildlife.

In **horses**, *R equi* is a commensal intestinal organism; it can actively multiply in the intestines of foals up to ~3 mo old and can also be isolated from the feces of adult horses. Suppurative bronchopneumonia is the primary clinical sign in foals. Foals are affected between 2 wk and 6 mo of age, although foals 1–3 mo old are most commonly affected, possibly because of the decline in maternal antibodies at ~6 wk of age. On endemic farms, it is estimated that 5%–40% of foals may develop clinical signs, and up to 50% of cases may be fatal. Foals >6 mo old appear to be refractory to development of clinical signs. (*See also* RHODOCOCCUS EQUI PNEUMONIA IN FOALS, p 1451.)

Initially, foals show nonspecific signs, including fever, lack of appetite, and reluctance to move and suckle. Most foals with lung infections show respiratory distress, with tachycardia, tachypnea, and a strong inspiratory effort manifested by abdominal movement and nostril flaring. On auscultation, inspiratory and expiratory wheezes and crackles are possibly audible, predominantly in the cranioventral region. Decreased airway sounds suggest consolidation, extensive abscess formation, or occasional pleural effusion. Mucous membranes may be pale or cyanotic. Weight loss, cough, and serous to mucopurulent nasal secretion are not consistent signs. Typically, the disease is insidious in foals because of the ability of horses to compensate for respiratory lesions, making early diagnosis difficult.

Abdominal *R equi* infections in foals are clinically manifest by diarrhea, ulcerative colitis, mesenteric lymphadenitis, abdominal abscesses, typhlitis, and peritonitis. Foals rarely develop intestinal signs without pulmonary signs, but intestinal lesions are found in ~30%–50% of foals with pulmonary rhodococcosis. Colic, diarrhea, and weight loss are the major clinical signs of the intestinal form.

Immune-mediated polysynovitis affects ~20%–30% of foals, caused by immune complex deposition in joints. Any joint may be involved, although the tibiotarsal and stifle joints are most commonly affected. Synovial fluid aspiration reveals nonseptic mononuclear pleocytosis, without isolation of *R equi*. Septic arthritis of foals is another joint lesion caused by *R equi*. Different from immune-mediated polysynovitis, the septic lesion is usually combined with lameness signs.

A variety of other *R equi* infections are sporadically seen in horses, including cellulitis, ulceration, subcutaneous abscesses, lymphangitis, lymphadenitis, renal abscesses, pleuritis, hepatitis, and hepatoencephalopathy. Ocular signs, such as hypopyon and immune-mediated uveitis, may be seen. Osteomyelitis causing ataxia, decubitus, and limb paralysis is uncommon. Rarely, *R equi* is associated with abortion, placentitis, and infertility in mares, and it has been occasionally isolated from equine semen.

Clinical manifestations in adult horses are uncommon. The disease probably affects immunocompromised horses, or animals coinfected with immunosuppressive agents, infected by plasmid strains expressing *VapA*. The predominant clinical signs in adult horses are similar to those in foals, with suppurative bronchopneumonia, pleuritis, enteritis, lymphadenitis, and osteomyelitis.

In **swine**, *R equi* infections are basically restricted to the lymphatic tract. Usually, pyogranulomatous cervical lymphadenitis is seen, although mesenteric, bronchial, and other lymph nodes may be involved. *R equi* has also been isolated from apparently normal lymph nodes. Occasionally, pneumonia may be seen. Gross lesions in lymph nodes caused by *R equi* observed in slaughterhouses resemble those caused by *Mycobacterium* spp, a major cause of swine lymphadenitis (*see* p 690).

Rhodococcosis is rare in **dogs and cats**, although it is more commonly reported in cats than in dogs. The most common routes of infection in dogs and cats are traumatic percutaneous introduction of microorganisms, primary contamination of wounds, or secondary to scratches in cat fights. Most cats present with cutaneous lesions on one extremity, along with localized swelling, ulcers, and fistulas with purulent drainage. The lesions are commonly painful, and usually no systemic signs are seen. Regional lymph nodes may be enlarged. Respiratory and visceral involvement represents the systemic or disseminated form of disease. Pyothorax is usually caused by dissemination of the organism from mediastinal lymph nodes. These animals present with fever, anorexia, dyspnea, and weight loss. In visceral infections, there is abdominal distention with palpable fluid, splenomegaly, hepatomegaly, and mesenteric lymphadenomegaly. Underlying conditions, including immunosuppressive viral infections, should be investigated in cats with rhodococcosis.

In **ruminants**, lymphadenitis (mesenteric, submaxillary, and bronchial), pneumonia, pyometra, ulcerative lymphangitis, and occasionally mastitis have been reported in cattle and buffalo. Pneumonia is the most common clinical picture in goats. Sporadic abortion and organ abscesses have been reported in sheep and goats.

Diagnosis: Periodic clinical examinations, WBC counts, serum fibrinogen levels, serologic tests, and diagnostic imaging have been proposed as measures for early diagnosis, mainly because of the insidious and precocious characteristic of foal rhodococcosis. Weekly physical examination, including thoracic auscultation, is an effective clinical practice for early diagnosis. Monthly or more frequent monitoring of increased WBC counts (>13,000 cells/μL), serum fibrinogen concentration (>400 mg/dL), and thoracic ultrasonography are also valuable procedures for early diagnosis. Efficacy of periodic immunodiffusion testing in predicting individual cases in affected foals is controversial.

Supportive clinical and epidemiologic findings are important in presumptive diagnosis, but diagnosis by isolation, microbiologic culture, and phenotypic characterization of *R equi* is considered the "gold standard." Tracheobronchial lavage, skin, synovial and peritoneal fluid, organs, and abscesses are the main clinical specimens used. On staining, the presence of gram-positive pleomorphic organisms supports a presumptive diagnosis, although this preliminary identification of the organism should be carefully evaluated, because few bacteria may be present in some clinical samples. Tracheobronchial lavage is the main clinical specimen for isolation of *R equi* in foals. However, the organism may occasionally be isolated from the trachea of foals without signs of pneumonia. Nasal swabs of foals are not indicated as evidence of rhodococcosis because of contamination with local microflora. Likewise, the presence of *R equi* in the nasal region is not predictive of pulmonary infection.

R equi is naturally isolated from feces of most livestock species, especially foals. Despite the fact that foals often swallow sputum containing *R equi*, <20% of foals confirmed with pulmonary rhodococcosis show positive fecal isolation of bacterium.

R equi can be isolated from feces, soil, or other contaminated samples. Potentially contaminated material, including feces, soil, and sand of parks and yards, should be submitted to selective culture media.

Neutrophilic leukocytosis, hyperfibrinogenemia, and hyperglobulinemia are the most consistent hematologic findings in foals with rhodococcosis. Thrombocytosis and monocytosis are variable findings. Serum amyloid A (SAA), an acute-phase protein, has been proposed as an inflammatory marker of rhodococcosis because of increased SAA levels in foals with *R equi* infections. Abdominal and thoracic effusions are usually exudates and reveal increased protein levels and nucleated cell counts.

Thoracic, abdominal, and joint radiography have also been used in diagnosis. Initial pneumonia is characterized by a mild to moderate, diffuse bronchointerstitial pattern, revealing small nodules and possibly cavitary masses, which can be multiple and large in severe cases. Occasionally, mediastinal lymphadenomegaly is seen. Thoracic ultrasonography is valuable to evaluate mainly peripheral lung lesions.

Serologic assays (eg, agar-gel immunodiffusion, ELISA, synergistic hemolysis inhibition) have been proposed for use in diagnosis, particularly of horses. However, titer results have varied greatly, probably because of differences in antigen preparation, interference of maternal antibodies, and continuous exposure to *R equi* in the environment. In addition, these tests have failed to differentiate between healthy and sick foals and, therefore, are inappropriate for diagnosis of individual cases.

Detection of *R equi*-specific DNA by PCR is also available for rapid and reliable diagnosis. However, because *R equi* can be found in the trachea of foals without pulmonary signs, PCR may be positive in healthy animals. Thus, epidemiologic aspects, clinical signs, hematologic tests, imaging findings, microbiologic culture, and/or molecular assays must all be considered in making a diagnosis.

Lesions: Suppurative abscesses with necrotic areas and regional lymphadenitis are the major gross lesions seen at necropsy. Typically, pulmonary lesions reveal multiple firm nodules, atelectasis, congestion, and cavitary lesions. Multiple miliary lesions may be seen as well. Multifocal enteritis, typhlitis, mesenteric lymphadenitis, and Peyer's patches reaction are seen in cases of intestinal involvement. Abdominal dissemination is characterized by peritonitis and organ abscesses. Septic arthritis, hypopyon, and vertebral osteomyelitis are signs indicative of hematogenous dissemination. Abortion, placentitis, and fetal infection are uncommon.

Histologically, the tissue and organ lesions are characterized as pyogranulomatous lesions containing foci of necrosis. The lesions reveal numerous gram-positive pleomorphic organisms phagocytized by macrophages, multinucleate giant cells, and fewer neutrophils. Moderate infiltrate of plasma cells and lymphocytes are also found.

The primary pathogens that should be differentiated from *R equi* as causal agents of foal respiratory diseases are *Salmonella* spp, *Streptococcus equi*, influenza virus, herpesvirus, and migrating stages of *Parascaris equorum*. Differential diagnosis of *R equi* causing intestinal manifestations should be performed with *Clostridium* spp, *Salmonella* spp, *Escherichia coli*, *Strongyloides westeri*, rotavirus, and coronavirus. Septic arthritis caused by *R equi* should be differentiated, especially from *Salmonella* spp and *Streptococcus equi*. Swine lymphadenitis caused by *Mycobacterium* spp should be differentiated from *R equi* because of similar appearance of lymph nodes at the slaughterhouse.

Treatment: Treatment involves appropriate antimicrobial therapy, surgical drainage, debridement, and supportive care.

R equi is typically refractory to conventional antimicrobial therapy. Successful therapy varies dramatically between animal species, probably because of the intracellular location of the pathogen, development of pyogranulomatous lesions, and antimicrobial resistance patterns of the isolates. Antimicrobial susceptibility profile of animal and human strains usually shows in vitro sensitivity to rifampin, erythromycin, aminoglycosides (lincomycin, gentamicin), and imipenem. However, lipid-soluble drugs are the antimicrobials of choice because of the need for adequate tissue and cellular penetration, particularly into macrophages.

Since 1980, the standard effective chemotherapy protocol for foals is based on administration of rifampin (5 mg/kg, PO, bid, or 10 mg/kg/day, PO) and erythromycin (25 mg/kg, PO, tid, or 37.5 mg/kg, PO, bid). These drugs have a synergic effect, and their combined use decreases resistance rates. Throughout the past decade, the macrolides clarithromycin (7.5 mg/kg, PO, bid) and azithromycin (10 mg/kg/day, PO) have been investigated as treatment alternatives because of their bioavailability, stability, and higher concentration in the cells than erythromycin. The combination of rifampin and clarithromycin has shown better efficacy than rifampin-erythromycin or azithromycin-rifampin.

The duration of treatment is variable, although 4–8 wk is frequently recommended. Therapy may be extended in complicated cases in foals. However, after a longer course of therapy, some foals may develop antibiotic-associated colitis. Recent resistance of *R equi* isolates to rifampin and erythromycin have been described, especially with use of these drugs as monotherapy.

Azithromycin has been used as an alternative to erythromycin in foals with adverse signs after the use of erythromycin, including respiratory distress and diarrhea. However, there is a paucity of information regarding prolonged use (≥4 wk) and adverse effects of this drug.

In companion animals, combined therapy using rifampin (10 mg/kg/day, PO) and clarithromycin (7.5–12.5 mg/kg, PO, bid) for 2–5 wk may be recommended. Combined treatment using lincomycin (20 mg/kg, PO, bid, for 7–10 days) and gentamicin (5–8 mg/kg/day, SC, IM, or IV, for 5 days) has been effective in some cats, although longterm therapy or a second course of antimicrobials may be necessary. Erythromycin (15 mg/kg, PO, bid, for 14 days) may be combined with rifampin or other drugs in treatment of dogs and cats.

Surgical drainage of abscesses and debridement are indicated in some cutaneous lesions. Hydration and adequate nutrition are recommended as supportive care. NSAIDs may be used to control fever and in animals with arthritis.

Despite appropriate antimicrobial therapy and supportive care, domestic animals with respiratory distress, tachycardia, severe thoracic imaging abnormalities, and osteomyelitis have a poor prognosis.

Control and Prevention: Control procedures are recommended to maximize the resistance of foals to infection and to reduce infection pressure in their environment. Adequate transfer of colostral immunoglobulins to foals is essential. Different measures have been proposed to prevent and control animal rhodococcosis, particularly in foals, including decrease in environmental exposure to *R equi*, passive immunization (hyperimmune plasma), active immunization (vaccination), and early diagnosis of disease.

The exposure of domestic animals, particularly foals, to *R equi* in the environment is theoretically the main risk factor for transmission. A high number of mares and foals on farms, and high density, leading to higher levels of *R equi* in manure, appear to be predominant risk factors for equine rhodococcosis. Thus, decreasing the number of mares and foals and reducing foal density have been recommended on farms with endemic rhodococcosis.

Removal of excess manure from livestock paddocks, stalls, and pastures could theoretically decrease growth of *R equi*, and consequently, the risk of infection. However, high concentrations of pathogenic *R equi* are usually found in the feces of foals, because they commonly swallow sputum containing virulent strains and excrete the pathogen in their feces. Infected foals should be isolated and their manure removed immediately to help control the disease.

Direct involvement of dust as the major risk factor for livestock rhodococcosis is controversial. Nevertheless, irrigation of paddocks and stalls, as well as growing grass in foal environments that are excessively dusty, may decrease aerosolization.

The use of hyperimmune plasma as an alternative prophylactic measure for equine passive immunization against *R equi* is based on the protective action of plasma components (immunoglobulin, interferon, complement factors, cytokines, and fibronectin). Hyperimmune plasma decreases the severity of clinical signs in foals, although it does not seem to have a curative effect or to shorten the course of disease. Protocols for administration are variable, but hyperimmune plasma is most effective when used before exposure to *R equi*. Most commonly, 1 L of hyperimmune plasma (or 20 mL/kg of foal), IV, is used for foals 1–60 days old. The initial dose for foals is variable, given at 1–10 days of age, and followed by a second dose at 30–50 days of age. However, because foals are challenged early (in the first days of life), the first dose is probably the most effective for protection.

Different vaccines have been developed to induce active immunity in foals. Most foals challenged with virulent *R equi* strains develop a protective and prolonged immune response. However, insufficient neonatal response or relative immunologic immaturity, interference with maternal antibodies, and the intracellular location of *R equi* limit the active immunization of foals in field conditions.

Killed vaccines have shown ineffective or controversial results in inducing a cellular immune response against *R equi*.

Infection with *R equi* strains without *VapA* and *VapB* genes does not induce protection of foals, indicating that virulent strains are essential for composition of effective vaccines. Studies in experimental and field conditions using *VapA* vaccines have shown enhanced clearance of *R equi*. Administration of oral live *VapA* vaccines has induced high concentrations of *VapA*-specific antibodies, despite being considered impractical for vaccination of a large number of animals. Efforts are ongoing to develop vaccines using modern concepts, such as transposons, and recombinant and DNA vaccines containing *VapA* antigen, which induces humoral and especially cellular immune response.

Zoonotic Risk: Traditionally, contact with soil or manure, or inhalation of aerosols contaminated by livestock, represents the major routes of transmission of *R equi* to people. Alternatively, human infection may occur by transcutaneous trauma, ingestion, or wound contamination. Recent evidence supports that consumption of pork products or undercooked pork may be a probable route of infection to people because of contamination of the meat with lymph node content or feces.

R equi has emerged as a pulmonary pathogen among immunocompromised people. Therefore, it is recommended that immunocompromised people avoid contact with livestock and their environment, as well as consumption of undercooked pork products.

SWEATING SICKNESS

Sweating sickness is an acute, febrile, tickborne toxicosis characterized mainly by a profuse, moist eczema and hyperemia of the skin and visible mucous membranes. It is essentially a disease of young calves, although adult cattle are also susceptible. Sheep, pigs, goats, and a dog have been infected experimentally. It occurs in eastern, central, and southern Africa and probably in Sri Lanka and southern India.

Etiology: The cause of sweating sickness is an epitheliotropic toxin produced by females of certain strains of *Hyalomma truncatum*. The toxin develops in the tick, not in the vertebrate host. Four tick salivary gland proteins with molecular mass ranging from 27–33 kDA have been proposed to be associated with sweating sickness immunodominance, whereas a 32 kDA band salivary gland protein was found to be unique to a sweating sickness–positive strain. The potential to produce toxin is retained by ticks for as long as 20 generations, and possibly longer. Attempted experimental transmissions between affected and healthy animals by contact or inoculations of blood have been unsuccessful.

Graded periods of infestation of a susceptible host by "infected" ticks have different effects on the host. A very short period has no effect; the animal remains susceptible. A period just long enough to produce a reaction may confer immunity, but if the exposure is >5 days, severe clinical signs and death may result. Recovery confers a durable immunity, which may last ≥4 yr. Other closely related forms of *H truncatum* toxicoses have been described.

Clinical Findings: After an incubation period of 4–11 days, signs appear suddenly and include hyperthermia, anorexia, listlessness, watering of the eyes and nose, hyperemia of the visible mucous membranes, salivation, necrosis of the oral mucosa, and hyperesthesia. Later, the eyelids stick together. The skin feels hot, and a moist dermatitis soon develops, starting from the base of the ears, the axillae, groin, and perineum and extending over the entire body. The hair becomes matted, and beads of moisture may be seen on it. The skin becomes extremely sensitive and emits a sour odor. Later, the hair and epidermis can be readily pulled off, exposing red, raw wounds. The tips of the ears and the tail may slough. Eventually, the skin becomes hard and cracked and predisposed to secondary infection or screwworm infestation. Affected animals are sensitive to handling, show pain when moving, and seek shade.

Often, the course is rapid, and death may occur within a few days. In less acute cases, the course is more protracted and recovery may occur. Mortality in affected calves is 30%–70% under natural conditions. Morbidity in endemic areas is ~10%. The severity of infection is influenced by the number of ticks as well as by the length of time they remain on the host.

Lesions: Emaciation, dehydration, diphtheroid stomatitis, pharyngitis, laryngitis, esophagitis, vaginitis or posthitis, edema and hyperemia of the lungs, atrophy of the spleen, and congestion of the liver, kidneys, and meninges are found, in addition to the skin lesions. Experimentally infected adult cattle showed typical lesions of moist eczema, and mucous membrane changes were accompanied by a marked decrease in circulating leukocytes with severe neutropenia.

Diagnosis: For diagnosis, it is essential to determine the presence of the vector. Typically, there is a generalized hyperemia with subsequent desquamation of the superficial layers of the mucous membranes of the upper respiratory, GI, and external genital tracts, and profuse moist dermatitis followed by superficial desquamation of the skin.

Prevention and Treatment: Control of tick infestation is the only effective preventive measure. Adult ticks show a predilection to attach in the tail switch. Removal of ticks, symptomatic treatment, and good nursing care are indicated. Non-nephrotoxic antibiotics and anti-inflammatory agents are useful to combat secondary infection. Immune serum can be an effective specific treatment, although associated with problems of donor availability, possible serum contamination, and IV administration of a relatively large volume. A refined precipitated immunoglobulin suspension proved ineffective as a specific treatment, probably because of low concentrations of effective immunoglobulins.

TOXOPLASMOSIS

Toxoplasma gondii is a protozoan parasite that infects people and other warm-blooded animals, including birds and marine mammals (*see* p 1865). It has been found worldwide from Alaska to Australia.

Etiology and Pathogenesis: Felids are the only definitive hosts of *T gondii*; both wild and domestic cats therefore serve as the main reservoir of infection. There are three infectious stages of *T gondii*: tachyzoites (rapidly multiplying form), bradyzoites (tissue cyst form), and sporozoites (in oocysts).

T gondii is transmitted by consumption of infectious oocysts in cat feces, consumption of tissue cysts in infected meat, and by transplacental transfer of tachyzoites from mother to fetus. *T gondii* initiates enteroepithelial replication in unexposed cats after ingestion of uncooked meat containing tissue cysts. Bradyzoites are released from tissue cysts by digestion in the stomach and small intestine, invade intestinal epithelium, and undergo sexual replication, culminating in the release of oocysts (10 μm diameter) in the feces. Oocysts are first seen in the feces at 3 days after infection and may be released for as long as 20 days. Oocysts sporulate (become infectious) outside the cat within 1–5 days, depending on aeration and temperature, and remain viable in the environment for several months. Cats generally develop immunity to *T gondii* after the initial infection and therefore shed oocysts only once in their lifetime.

After being consumed in uncooked meat containing tissue cysts (carnivores) or in feed or drink contaminated with cat feces containing oocysts (all warm-blooded animals), *T gondii* initiates extraintestinal replication. Bradyzoites and sporozoites, respectively, are released and infect intestinal epithelium. After several rounds of epithelial replication, tachyzoites emerge and disseminate via the bloodstream and lymph. Tachyzoites infect tissues throughout the body and replicate intracellularly until the cells burst, causing tissue necrosis. Tachyzoites measure 4–6 × 2–4 µm in diameter. Young and immunocompromised animals may succumb to generalized toxoplasmosis at this stage. Older animals mount a powerful, cell-mediated immune response to the tachyzoites (mediated by cytokines) and control infection, driving the tachyzoites into the tissue cyst or bradyzoite stage. Tissue cysts are usually seen in neurons but also seen in other tissues. Individual cysts are microscopic, up to 70 µm in diameter, and may enclose hundreds of bradyzoites in a thin, resilient cyst wall. Tissue cysts in the host remain viable for many years, and possibly for the life of the host.

Clinical Findings: The tachyzoite is the stage responsible for tissue damage; therefore, clinical signs depend on the number of tachyzoites released, the ability of the host immune system to limit tachyzoite spread, and the organs damaged by the tachyzoites. Because adult immunocompetent animals control tachyzoite spread efficiently, toxoplasmosis is usually a subclinical illness. However, in young animals, particularly puppies, kittens, and piglets, tachyzoites spread systemically and cause interstitial pneumonia, myocarditis, hepatic necrosis, meningoencephalomyelitis, chorioretinitis, lymphadenopathy, and myositis. The corresponding clinical signs include fever, diarrhea, cough, dyspnea, icterus, seizures, and death. *T gondii* is also an important cause of abortion and stillbirth in sheep and goats and sometimes in pigs. After infection of a pregnant ewe, tachyzoites spread via the bloodstream to placental cotyledons, causing necrosis. Tachyzoites may also spread to the fetus, causing necrosis in multiple organs. Finally, immunocompromised adult animals (eg, cats infected with feline immunodeficiency virus) are extremely susceptible to developing acute generalized toxoplasmosis.

Diagnosis: Diagnosis is made by biologic, serologic, or histologic methods, or by some combination of these. Clinical signs of toxoplasmosis are nonspecific and are not sufficiently characteristic for a definite diagnosis. Antemortem diagnosis may be accomplished by indirect hemagglutination assay, indirect fluorescent antibody assay, latex agglutination test, or ELISA. IgM antibodies appear sooner after infection than IgG antibodies but generally do not persist past 3 mo after infection. Increased IgM titers (>1:256) are consistent with recent infection. In contrast, IgG antibodies appear by the fourth week after infection and may remain increased for years during subclinical infection. To be useful, IgG titers must be measured in paired sera from the acute and convalescent stages (3–4 wk apart) and must show at least a 4-fold increase in titer. Additionally, CSF and aqueous humor may be analyzed for the presence of tachyzoites or anti-*T gondii* antibodies. Postmortem, tachyzoites may be seen in tissue impression smears. Additionally, microscopic examination of tissue sections may reveal the presence of tachyzoites or bradyzoites. *T gondii* is morphologically similar to other protozoan parasites and must be differentiated from *Sarcocystis* species and *Neospora caninum*.

Treatment: For animals other than people, treatment is seldom warranted. Sulfadiazine (15–25 mg/kg) and pyrimethamine (0.44 mg/kg) act synergistically and are widely used for treatment of toxoplasmosis. Although these drugs are beneficial if given in the acute stage of the disease when there is active multiplication of the parasite, they will not usually eradicate infection. These drugs are believed to have little effect on the bradyzoite stage. Certain other drugs, including diaminodiphenylsulfone, atovaquone, and spiramycin are also used to treat toxoplasmosis in difficult cases. Clindamycin is the treatment of choice for dogs and cats, at 10–40 mg/kg and 25–50 mg/kg, respectively, for 14–21 days.

Prevention and Zoonotic Risk: *T gondii* is an important zoonotic agent. In some areas of the world, as much as 60% of the human population has serum IgG titers to *T gondii* and are likely to be persistently infected. Toxoplasmosis is a major concern for people with immune system dysfunction. In these individuals, toxoplasmosis usually presents as meningoencephalitis and results from the emergence of *T gondii* from tissue cysts located in the brain as immunity wanes rather than from primary *T gondii* infection. Toxoplasmosis is also a concern for pregnant women because tachyzoites can migrate transplacentally and cause birth defects in human fetuses. Infection with *T gondii* may occur after ingestion of undercooked meat or accidental ingestion of oocysts from cat feces. To prevent infection, the hands of people handling meat should be washed thoroughly with soap and water after contact, as should all cutting boards, sink tops, knives, and other materials. The stages of *T gondii* in meat are killed by contact with soap and water. *T gondii* organisms in meat can also be killed by exposure to extreme cold or heat. Tissue cysts in meat are killed by heating the meat throughout to 67°C (152.6°F) or by cooling to −13°C (8.6°F). *Toxoplasma* in tissue cysts are also killed by exposure to 0.5 kilorads of gamma irradiation. Meat of any animal should be cooked to 67°C (152.6°F) before consumption, and tasting meat while cooking or while seasoning should be avoided. Pregnant women should avoid contact with cat litter, soil, and raw meat. Pet cats should be fed only dry, canned, or cooked food. The cat litter box should be emptied daily, preferably not by a pregnant woman. Gloves should be worn while gardening. Vegetables should be washed thoroughly before eating, because they may have been contaminated with cat feces.

There is currently no vaccine to prevent toxoplasmosis in people.

TUBERCULOSIS AND OTHER MYCOBACTERIAL INFECTIONS

Tuberculosis (TB) is considered a reemerging, infectious granulomatous disease in animals and people caused by acid-fast bacilli of the genus *Mycobacterium*. Although commonly defined as a chronic, debilitating disease, TB occasionally assumes an acute, rapidly progressive course. The disease affects practically all species of vertebrates. The widespread occurrence of multidrug-resistant (MDR) strains and extensively drug-resistant (XDR) strains of *M tuberculosis* is of concern to clinicians and public health and regulatory officials involved in the control of disease. Bovine TB is still a significant zoonosis in nonindustrialized countries of the world. Signs and lesions are generally similar in the various species.

Etiology: The main types of *M tuberculosis* complex (mammalian tubercle bacilli) recognized are *M tuberculosis*, *M canettii*, *M bovis*, *M caprae*, *M pinnipedii*, *M microti*, *M mungi*, and *M africanum*. The *M avium* complex includes *M avium avium* (avian tubercle bacilli), *M avium hominissuis* (isolated from people, swine, and other mammals), and *M intracellulare*. The types differ in cultural characteristics and pathogenicity. Several serovars of *M avium avium* are recognized; however, only serovars 1, 2, and 3 are pathogenic for birds. *M bovis* may survive on pasture for ≥2 mo, and *M avium* may survive in soil for ≥4 yr.

All types may produce infection in host species other than their own. *M tuberculosis* is most specific; it rarely produces progressive disease in animals other than people and nonhuman primates, infrequently in dogs and pigs, and has very rarely been isolated from skin lesions in exotic birds. *M bovis* can cause progressive disease in most warm-blooded vertebrates, including people. *M caprae*, an organism closely related to *M bovis*, has been isolated from people, goats, cattle, and several other species in Europe. *M avium avium* is the species of most importance in birds, but it has a wide host range and is also pathogenic for pigs, cattle, sheep, deer, mink, dogs, cats, certain exotic hoofed animals, and some cold-blooded animals. *M avium hominissuis* is the cause of tuberculosis in people, swine, and other animals. *M genavense* and other pathogenic mycobacteria are infrequently isolated from exotic and free-living wild and domestic birds (*see* p 692). *M intracellulare* causes disease in cold-blooded animals and has been isolated from many other species.

Pathogenesis: Inhalation of infected droplets expelled from the lungs is the usual route of TB infection, although ingestion, particularly via contaminated milk or water, also occurs. Intrauterine and coital methods of infection are recognized less commonly. Inhaled bacilli are phagocytosed by alveolar macrophages that may either clear the infection or allow the mycobacteria to proliferate. In the latter instance, a primary focus may form, mediated by cytokines associated with a hypersensitivity reaction that consists of dead and degenerate macrophages surrounded by epithelioid cells, granulocytes, lymphocytes, and later, multinucleated giant cells. The purulent to caseous, necrotic center may calcify, and the lesion may become surrounded by granulation tissue and a fibrous capsule to form the classic "tubercle." The primary focus plus similar lesions formed in the regional lymph node is known as the "primary complex." In alimentary forms of disease, the primary focus may be found in the pharynx or mesenteric lymph nodes or, less commonly, in the tonsils or intestines. The cellular composition of and presence of acid-fast bacilli in tuberculous lesions differ between and within host species.

The primary complex seldom heals in animals and may progress slowly or rapidly. Dissemination through vascular and lymphatic channels may be generalized and rapidly fatal, as in acute miliary TB. Nodular lesions may form in many organs, including the pleura, peritoneum, liver, kidney, spleen, skeleton, mammary glands, reproductive tract, and CNS. A prolonged, chronic course may also ensue, with lesions usually having a more localized pattern of distribution.

Clinical Findings: The clinical signs of TB reflect the extent and location of lesions. Generalized signs include progressive emaciation, lethargy, weakness, anorexia, and a low-grade, fluctuating fever. The bronchopneumonia of the respiratory form of the disease causes a chronic, intermittent, moist cough with later signs of dyspnea and tachypnea. The destructive lesions of the granulomatous bronchopneumonia may be detected on auscultation and percussion. Superficial lymph node enlargement may be a useful diagnostic sign when present. Affected deeper lymph nodes cannot always be palpated, but they may cause obstruction of the airways, pharynx, and gut, leading to dyspnea and ruminal tympany.

In pigs, lesions caused by *M avium hominissuis* or *M avium avium* are most often seen in lymph nodes associated with the GI tract, although generalized disease involving the liver, lung, and spleen does occur.

Diagnosis: The single most important diagnostic test for TB is the intradermal tuberculin test. Old tuberculin prepared from the culture filtrate of *M tuberculosis* is used to detect disease in nonhuman primates exposed to *M tuberculosis* or *M bovis*. In other animals, purified protein derivatives (PPDs) prepared from the culture filtrate of *M bovis* or *M avium* can be used. Diagnosis based on clinical signs alone is very difficult, even in advanced cases. Radiography is useful in nonhuman primates and small animals. Microscopic examination of sputum and other discharges is sometimes used. Necropsy findings of the classic "tuberculous" granulomas are often very suggestive of the disease. Confirmation of diagnosis is by isolation and identification of the organism, with culture usually taking 4–8 wk, or by PCR, which requires only a few days. Molecular techniques, such as restriction fragment length polymorphism (RFLP) or variable number tandem repeat (VNTR) provide definitive information useful in conducting epidemiologic investigations.

The delayed-type hypersensitivity response of the host, responsible for much of the pathology of TB, is fundamental to the tuberculin skin test widely used for diagnosis in large animals. The single intradermal (SID) test involves inoculation of PPD prepared by precipitation of protein from the culture filtrate of *M bovis*. PPD preparations improve specificity. In a reactor, the antigen stimulates a local infiltrate of inflammatory cells and causes skin swelling that can be detected by palpation and measured by calipers. The reaction is read at 48–72 hr for maximum sensitivity and at 96 hr for maximum specificity. Test sites used vary in sensitivity and between countries/areas and include the neck region, caudal fold at the tail base, and vulval lip. One disadvantage of the *M bovis* SID test is that cross-reactions may occur in animals infected with *M kansasii*, *M avium*, *M tuberculosis*, *M avium paratuberculosis*, or other mycobacteria that share some antigenic determinants with *M bovis*.

In areas with a high incidence of avian TB or other mycobacterial infections such as paratuberculosis, the comparative tuberculin skin test can be used, with biologically balanced *M bovis* and *M avium* PPD tuberculins inoculated simultaneously but at separate sites in the neck. The agent causing sensitization provokes the greater skin reaction. Other diagnostic tests used for TB include the thermal test, which may detect a pyrexic peak (104°F [>40°C]) at 6–8 hr after SC inoculation with tuberculin. The Stormont test uses an intradermal inoculation of PPD followed by a second inoculum at the same site 7 days later. The test is read for swelling 24 hr later.

False-negative results may occur in animals with poor immune response such as those in the early stages of infection, nonresponsive cases in advanced disease, or old animals. Cattle that have recently calved may also have false-negative results. Current research is focused on the identification of antigens such as secretory proteins and genetically engineered proteins of *M bovis* for use in improved in vitro diagnostic tests. Serologic tests such as ELISA appear to be of limited diagnostic use, consistent with the lesser role of antibody compared with the cellular immune response in TB. In vitro cellular assays have been developed (ie, interferon-γ assay) using WBCs stimulated with *M bovis* antigen and may be used as a supplemental test to the widely used SID test; however, they have not come into widespread use in many nonindustrialized countries because of cost and the necessity to conduct cellular assays in the laboratory within 24 hr after collection of blood specimens.

Control: The main reservoir of *M bovis* infection is cattle. However, other animals have been found to be reservoirs in some countries, including badgers and red deer (England, Ireland); red deer, possums, and ferrets (New Zealand); mule deer, white-tailed deer, elk, and American bison (North America); African buffalo (South Africa); and water buffalo (Australia). The prevalence of disease in such reservoirs influences the incidence of disease in other species. Carnivores and scavengers can acquire *M bovis* by consumption of infected carcasses. These species include lion, coyote, wolf, hyena, cheetah, black bear, bobcat, and leopard. Warthogs, ferrets, raccoon, European wild boar, opossums, and feral pigs have also been found to be infected with *M bovis*.

The three principal approaches to the control of TB are test and slaughter, test and segregation, and chemotherapy. The test and slaughter policy is the only one assured of eradicating TB and relies on the slaughter of reactors to the tuberculin test. In an affected herd, testing every 2 mo is recommended to rid the herd of individuals that can disseminate infection. Routine hygienic measures aimed at cleaning and disinfecting contaminated food, water troughs, etc, are also useful. Test and slaughter has been used widely in the UK, USA, Canada, Germany, New Zealand, and Australia. In some European countries, where test and slaughter would have been impractical, varying forms of test and segregation have been used, with test and slaughter used only in the final stages of eradication.

The BCG (bacille Calmette-Guérin) vaccine, sometimes used to control TB in people, has proved to provide little protection against virulent *M bovis* in most animal species, and inoculation often provokes a severe local granulomatous reaction. Moreover, BCG-vaccinated animals usually respond on the tuberculin skin test.

CATTLE

Most of the general discussion above applies to bovine TB. The introduction of milk pasteurization was a major step in the fight against *Mycobacterium bovis* TB and continues to be an important control procedure in many nonindustrialized countries.

SHEEP AND GOATS

Lesions caused by *Mycobacterium bovis* in the lungs and lymph nodes of sheep and goats are similar to those seen in cattle, and the organism may sometimes disseminate to other organs. Sheep and goats are quite resistant to *M tuberculosis* infection. The intradermal skin test is commonly used for diagnosis. The comparative tuberculin skin test conducted in the cervical region using biologically balanced purified protein derivative tuberculins of *M bovis* and *M avium* can be used to differentiate sensitization to other mycobacteria. The responses should be observed at 48 and 72 hr for induration and swelling.

DEER AND ELK

Tuberculosis due to *Mycobacterium bovis* is an important problem in most species of farmed and wild cervids, including axis deer, fallow deer, roe deer, mule deer, sika deer, as well as red deer/elk/wapati. Deer appear to be unusually susceptible to *M bovis* infections. *M avium* infections may produce similar lesions. *M tuberculosis* infection is uncommon. Tuberculous lesions may be confined to isolated lymph nodes of the head, or they may be found extensively in lymph nodes and organs after a rapid, fulminating disease course. Abscessation in deer should always raise suspicions of tuberculosis. A presumptive diagnosis may be made using the tuberculin skin test and/or by in vitro cellular assays (blood lymphocyte immune-stimulation test or γ interferon assay), or a combination of these tests. Infection should be confirmed by an organism-based test.

HORSES

Horses are relatively resistant to tuberculosis caused by *Mycobacterium tuberculosis*; however, they are susceptible to *M bovis*. When tuberculosis does develop, tuberculous, noncalcified lesions are often found in the liver, mesenteric lymph nodes, lungs, and other sites. Tuberculin test results are rather erratic.

ELEPHANTS

Tuberculosis due to *Mycobacterium tuberculosis* has been reported in captive elephants. Lesions most often involve the lung and associated lymph nodes. Nonspecific responses are observed on tuberculin skin tests and on some in vitro immunologic tests; therefore, diagnosis should be made on an organism-based test of trunk washes. Multidrug regimens, including isoniazid and rifampin, have been developed that eliminate shedding of *M tuberculosis* in discharges and minimize development of drug-resistant strains. It is important to emphasize that drug sensitivity tests should be conducted to determine the susceptibility of the organism. Also, blood concentrations should be monitored periodically to confirm they are high enough to kill the bacteria.

PIGS

Pigs are susceptible to *M tuberculosis*, *M bovis*, and *M avium* complex. *M avium avium* and *M avium hominissuis* are most frequently isolated; serologic identification of isolates is useful in epidemiologic investigations. Granulomatous lesions are most often found in the cervical, submandibular, and mesenteric lymph nodes, but in advanced disease lesions may also be found in the liver and spleen. Typically, enlarged nodes contain small, white or yellow, caseous foci, usually without any evidence of mineralization. Pigs with disease due to *M tuberculosis* may have similar regionalized lesions. Pigs are particularly susceptible to *M bovis*, which is usually acquired from shared grazing or ingestion of contaminated dairy products. This can cause a rapidly progressive, disseminated disease with caseation and liquefaction of lesions. The single intradermal test conducted on the dorsal surface of the ear or in skin of the vulva is often useful for diagnosis. Test responses should be observed at 48 hr after injection of tuberculin.

DOGS

Dogs may be infected with *Mycobacterium tuberculosis*, *M bovis*, and occasionally with *M avium* complex or *M fortuitum*, commonly from a human or bovine source. Tuberculous lesions are usually found in the lungs, liver, kidney, pleura, and peritoneum; they have a gray appearance, usually with a noncalcified, necrotic center. Lesions are often exudative and can produce a large quantity of straw-colored fluid in the thorax. False-negative tuberculin tests are often seen in dogs. Radiographs and a thorough history are useful in diagnosis. Treatment is not often recommended. Affected dogs in close contact with people should be euthanized because of public health concerns.

CATS

Cats are quite resistant to infection with *Mycobacterium tuberculosis* but are susceptible to *M bovis*, *M avium* complex, or *M microti*. *M lepraemurium* has been isolated from granulomatous lesions in the skin. Some unclassified acid-fast bacilli have also been isolated. Contaminated milk causing GI tract lesions, typically in the mesenteric lymph nodes, is the most common circumstance, and historically this was responsible for a very high percentage of tuberculous cats in Europe. Rapid, hematogenous dissemination to other organs, including the lungs and regional lymph nodes, can occur. Infected skin or deeper wounds sometimes give rise to tuberculous sinuses. Lesions have a central area of necrosis, usually without calcification. The tuberculin skin test is considered unreliable in cats. Diagnosis may be assisted by radiography and ELISA. Identification of the organism is necessary to confirm a diagnosis. Efficacious treatment protocols are not available. Therefore, it is recommended that cats infected with *M bovis* be euthanized because of public health concerns.

RABBITS

Naturally occurring, or so-called spontaneous tuberculosis in rabbits is an uncommon finding; most cases are caused by *Mycobacterium bovis* or *M avium*. Rabbits apparently become infected when exposed to other tuberculous animals or by ingesting milk from tuberculous cattle. *M avium* has been reported in rabbits that are housed in close contact with domestic or exotic birds infected with *M avium*. Rabbits are relatively resistant to *M tuberculosis*; such infections are seldom reported. Rabbits infected with *M avium* complex may develop miliary lesions involving the lung and liver. Tuberculin skin tests may be conducted on the skin of the abdomen. Test sites should be observed for induration and swelling at 24 and 48 hr after injection of *M bovis* purified protein derivative.

GUINEA PIGS

Guinea pigs are quite susceptible to infection with either *Mycobacterium tuberculosis* or *M bovis*. Lesions are most often seen in the parenchyma of the lung and adjacent lymph nodes. Also, guinea pigs are susceptible to certain serovars of *M avium* complex with lesions seen in lymph nodes associated with the GI tract. Tuberculin skin tests can be conducted by injection of purified protein derivative of *M bovis* and of *M avium* (1:100 dilution containing 5,000 tuberculin units) at separate sites in the skin of the abdomen. The preferred injection site is 2 cm posterior to the xyphoid cartilage and 2 cm lateral on each side of the linea alba. The injection sites should be observed at 24 and 48 hr for induration and swelling. The presence of erythema at the injection site is of little or no significance.

NONHUMAN PRIMATES

In monkeys and large apes, *Mycobacterium tuberculosis*, *M bovis*, and *M avium* complex can cause severe disease of the lungs and other organs. Epidemics in primate colonies may be caused by contact with infected human caregivers. Transmission is usually by aerosol with respiratory infection, but the oral route is also possible. Bacilli may also be shed in urine. Old tuberculin is used in skin tests in preference to purified protein derivative (PPD), because it provides greater sensitivity in detecting animals infected with *M tuberculosis* or *M bovis*. Biologically balanced PPDs prepared from *M bovis* or *M avium* can be injected intradermally at separate sites on the abdomen to conduct a comparative test. Skin tests are observed at 24, 48, and 72 hr for induration and swelling. Tuberculins prepared for use in people are not of sufficient potency to elicit a response in nonhuman primates. Treatment of cases of tuberculosis in nonhuman primates has been attempted using drugs that have had success in people, eg, isoniazid, ethambutol, and rifampin. Drug sensitivity tests should be conducted to determine sensitivity of isolates. Efficacy is limited, and there are overriding arguments against therapy, based on the removal of infected animals, zoonotic risks, and the danger of developing drug resistance. Exacerbations may occur.

FREE-RANGING AND CAPTIVE HOOFED ANIMALS

The major wildlife reservoirs of *Mycobacterium bovis* infection in addition to cervids are African buffalo, wood bison, North American bison, white-tailed and mule deer, lechwe, and elk. Also, brushtail possums and European badgers are considered reservoirs of *M bovis* infection. Other species in which *M bovis* infection has been reported but not implicated as reservoirs and are considered spillover hosts include fennic fox, coyote, Arabian oryx, muntjac, impala, sitatunga, springbok, moles, voles, hares, eland, yak, bactrian camel, wildebeest, European wild goat, large spotted genet, tapir, moose, otters, feral water buffalo, hedgehogs, European wild boar, greater kudu, tiger, white and black rhinoceros, and giraffe. *M tuberculosis* has been isolated from oryx, black rhinoceros, Asian elephant, addax, and Rocky Mountain goats. Tuberculous lesions vary in consistency from purulent to caseous and often involve the lungs and regional lymph nodes, with liver, spleen, and serosal surfaces as other potential sites. Tuberculin skin tests are conducted in the cervical region using *M bovis* purified protein derivative (PPD) containing 5,000 tuberculin units prepared for veterinary use. Nonspecific responses may occur in some species with no history of tuberculosis. Therefore, it may be necessary to use biologically balanced PPDs prepared from *M avium* and *M bovis* injected at separate injection sites. Skin tests are observed for swelling and induration at 48 and 72 hr.

MARINE MAMMALS

Mycobacterium pinnipedii (a seal-adapted variant of *M bovis*) causes tuberculous lesions in fur seals and sea lions. The organism has been isolated from four species of fur seals and two species of sea lions in several countries as well as from some other animals. In seals, the organism causes lesions in the peripheral lymph nodes, spleen, peritoneum, and lungs. The presence of acid-fast organisms in the granulomatous lesions varies. Aerosols are considered the main route of transmission. Because of the zoonotic risk, precautions should be taken when handling these animals. (*See also* MYCOBACTERIOSIS IN MARINE MAMMALS, p 1863.)

MYCOBACTERIAL INFECTIONS OTHER THAN TUBERCULOSIS

Mycobacteria found in soil and water have been isolated from tissues of animals. *Mycobacterium fortuitum*, a rapidly growing organism highly resistant to penicillin G, streptomycin, ampicillin, sulfamethoxazole, and chloramphenicol, has been associated with mastitis in cows, pulmonary infections in dogs, lymph node lesions in pigs and certain exotic animals, and cutaneous lesions in cats and dogs. Drug susceptibility tests indicate the organism is inhibited by capreomycin and by ethionamide. *M chelonae*, another rapidly growing *Mycobacterium* similar to *M fortuitum* in biochemical reactions, has been isolated from contaminated wounds and injection abscesses. These organisms must be distinguished from *M phlei*, *M smegmatis*, and *M vaccae*, which are rarely if ever pathogenic.

Fish and other cold-blooded animals may be infected with *M marinum*, certain serovars of *M avium* complex, or *M intracellulare*, which have been recognized as human pathogens. A photochromogenic organism, *M kansasii*, has been isolated from pigs, cattle, and nonhuman primates. These organisms can be differentiated by biochemical and seroagglutination tests.

M avium paratuberculosis, the cause of Johne's disease, has been isolated from domestic and wild ruminants (*see also* PARATUBERCULOSIS, p 762). It is a slowly progressive diarrheal disease resulting in weight loss and emaciation. Lesions are most often seen in the ileocecal valve and associated lymph nodes. Diagnosis should be based on an organism-based test. No treatment is available.

M scrofulaceum, a scotochromogen, has been isolated from lymph node lesions in pigs, cattle, and certain nonhuman primates. *M xenopi*, a slowly growing scotochromogen, has been isolated from pigs, seafowl, and amphibians. These organisms should be differentiated from *M gordonae* and *M flavescens* and from other slowly growing scotochromogenic mycobacteria that are common contaminants of water.

Numerous nonpathogenic, nonphotochromogenic mycobacteria that closely resemble potential pathogens can be isolated from water and soil; *M nonchromogenicum*, *M gastri*, *M triviale*, and *M terrae*, which closely resemble strains of the *M avium* complex, may be differentiated by in vitro laboratory examinations, including molecular techniques.

Although opportunistic mycobacteria usually do not produce progressive disease, they may be important in inducing transient tuberculin skin sensitivity in animals. The application of comparative skin tests, using biologically balanced purified protein derivative tuberculins prepared from culture filtrates of *M bovis* and *M avium*, provides useful information on the possible cause of tuberculin skin sensitivity. Tuberculins prepared for veterinary use, containing ~5,000 tuberculin units per test dose, should be used for skin tests in free-ranging, captive, wild, and exotic animals.

M lepraemurium, a nonphotochromogenic, slow-growing, acid-fast bacillus, causes a disease in cats and rats similar in some respects to leprosy in people. It can be grown on media containing cytochrome C and α-ketoglutarate. *M leprae*, the cause of leprosy in people, has been found in spontaneously occurring disease in armadillos. This organism has not been grown on artificial culture medium; however, *M leprae* DNA can be identified by molecular techniques.

TULAREMIA

Tularemia is a bacterial septicemia that affects >250 species of wild and domestic mammals, birds, reptiles, fish, and people. It is listed as a category A bioterrorism agent because of the potential for fatality, airborne dissemination, and societal disruption if released.

Etiology: The causative bacterium, *Francisella tularensis*, is a nonspore-forming, gram-negative coccobacillus antigenically related to *Brucella* spp. It is a facultative intracellular parasite that is killed by heat and proper disinfection but survives for weeks or months in a moist environment. It can be cultured readily on blood supplemented with cysteine but must be differentiated from other gram-negative bacteria on blood agar. The taxonomic status of *Francisella* has been revised and debated, but recent consensus establishes the subspecies *F tularensis tularensis*, associated with type A tularemia; *F tularensis holarctica*, which causes type B tularemia; and a third type, C, associated with *F novicida*, which has low virulence and is less common than the other two. Type A has been found predominantly in North America and is more virulent; in people, the mortality rate may be as high as 30% if untreated. Type B is less virulent and occurs in both the Old and New Worlds.

Epidemiology and Transmission: Among domestic animals, sheep are the most common host, but clinical infection has also been reported in cats, dogs, pigs, and horses. Cats are at increased risk because of predatory behavior and appear to have an increased susceptibility, whereas cattle appear to be resistant. Little is known of the true incidence and spectrum of clinical disease in domesticated animals. Important wild animal hosts for *F tularensis tularensis* include cottontail and jackrabbits, whereas the most common vectors are the ticks *Dermacentor andersoni* (the wood tick), *Amblyomma americanum* (the lone star tick), *D variabilis* (the American dog tick), and *Chrysops discalis* (the deer fly). Animal hosts of *F tularensis holarctica* are lagomorphs, beaver, muskrat, voles, and sheep. Ticks, flies, fleas, and exposure to contaminated water sources are all associated with transmission of this subspecies, which has also been found to persist naturally in a water-associated amoeba.

Natural foci of infection exist in North America and Eurasia. Although found in every state except Hawaii, tularemia is most often reported in the southcentral and western USA (eg, California, Missouri, Oklahoma, South Dakota, and Montana).

Tularemia can be transmitted by aerosol, direct contact, ingestion, or arthropods. Inhalation of aerosolized organisms (in the laboratory or as an airborne agent in an act of bioterrorism) can produce a pneumonic form. Direct contact with, or ingestion of, infected carcasses of wild animals (eg, cottontail rabbit) can produce the ulceroglandular, oculoglandular, oropharyngeal (local lesion with regional lymphadenitis), or typhoidal form. Immersion in or ingestion of contaminated water can result in infection in aquatic animals. Ticks can maintain infection transstadially and transovarially, making them efficient reservoirs and vectors.

The most common source of infection for people and herbivores is the bite of an infected tick, but people who prepare or eat improperly cooked wild game are also at increased risk. Dogs, cats, and other carnivores may acquire infection from ingestion of an infected carcass. Case reports have implicated cats as a source of infection in people.

Clinical Findings: The incubation period is 1–10 days. The most severely and commonly affected livestock species are sheep; Type A tularemia is particularly pathogenic for lagomorphs, and cats and nonhuman primates have been reported to be infected. The clinical presentation depends on host species, subspecies of the bacteria, and route of infection. Sheep and cats may be subclinically infected or develop bacteremia, fever, and respiratory infection. Cats may also develop ulceroglandular or oropharyngeal disease, presumably through exposure to infected prey items. Clinical signs include increased pulse and respiratory rates, coughing, diarrhea, and pollakiuria with lymphadenopathy and hepatosplenomegaly. Prostration and death may occur in a few hours or days. Sporadic cases are best recognized by signs of septicemia. Outbreaks in untreated lambs may have up to 15% mortality.

Lesions: The most consistent lesions are miliary, white to off-white foci of necrosis in the liver and sometimes in the spleen, lung, and lymph nodes. Organisms can be readily isolated from necropsy specimens by use of special media. The infective dose required to transmit this pathogen is extremely low; thus, risk of infection during necropsy or to laboratory personnel is significant, and special procedures and facilities are essential.

Diagnosis: Tularemia must be differentiated from other septicemic diseases (especially plague and pseudotuberculosis) or acute pneumonia. When large numbers of sheep show typical signs during periods of heavy tick infestation, tularemia or tick paralysis (*see* p 1314) should be suspected. Tularemia should be considered in cats with signs of acute lymphadenopathy, malaise, oral ulcers, and history of recent ingestion of wild prey.

Diagnosis of acute infection is confirmed by culture and identification of the bacterium, direct or indirect fluorescent antibody test, or a 4-fold increase in antibody titer between acute and convalescent serum specimens. A single titer of ≥1:80 by the tube agglutination test is presumptive evidence of prior infection. When tularemia is suspected, laboratory personnel should be alerted as a precaution to reduce the risk of laboratory-acquired infection. In some jurisdictions, tularemia in animals is reportable to public health authorities.

Treatment and Control: Streptomycin, gentamicin, and tetracyclines are effective at recommended dose levels. Gentamicin should be continued for 10 days. Because tetracycline and chloramphenicol are bacteriostatic, they should be continued for 14 days to minimize the risk of relapse. Early treatment is important to minimize risk of fatality. Because of the substantial sylvatic (wildlife and tick) component of the *Francisella* life cycle, control is limited to reducing arthropod infestation and to rapid diagnosis and treatment.

VESICULAR STOMATITIS

Vesicular stomatitis is a viral disease caused by two distinct serotypes of vesicular stomatitis virus—New Jersey and Indiana. Vesiculation, ulceration, and erosion of the oral and nasal mucosa and epithelial surface of the tongue, coronary bands, and teats are typically seen in clinical cases, along with crusting lesions of the muzzle, ventral abdomen, and sheath. Clinical disease has been seen in cattle, horses, and pigs and very rarely in sheep, goats, and llamas. Serologic evidence of exposure has been found in many species, including cervids, nonhuman primates, rodents, birds, dogs, antelope, and bats.

Etiology: The viruses are members of the family Rhabdoviridae and genus *Vesiculovirus*. Vesicular stomatitis viruses are the prototypes of the *Vesiculovirus* genus. They are bullet shaped and generally 180 nm long and 75 nm wide. The genomic structure is a single strand of negative-sense RNA composed of five genes (N, P, M, G, and L, representing the nucleocapsid protein, phosphoprotein, matrix protein, glycoprotein, and the large protein, which is a component of the viral RNA polymerase). Although there are many members of the *Vesiculovirus* genus, the New Jersey and Indiana serotypes are of particular interest in the Western hemisphere. These two viruses are similar in size and morphology but generate distinct neutralizing antibodies in infected animals. They have both been isolated in recent outbreaks in the USA.

Epidemiology and Transmission: Vesicular stomatitis is seen sporadically in the USA. Outbreaks historically occurred in all regions of the country but since the 1980s have been limited to western states and occur seasonally, usually May through October. Outbreaks occurred in the USA in 1995, 1997, 1998, 2004, 2005, 2006, 2009, 2010, and 2012. The largest outbreak in the past decade occurred in 2005 and affected nine states. Vesicular stomatitis viruses are endemic in South America, Central America, and parts of Mexico but have not been seen naturally outside the Western hemisphere. The virus can be transmitted through direct contact with infected animals with clinical disease (those with lesions) or by blood-feeding insects. In the southwestern USA, black flies (Simulidae) are the most likely biologic insect vector. In endemic areas, sand flies (*Lutzomyia*) are proven biologic vectors. Other insects may act as mechanical vectors. Exposure to insects that carry the virus is often associated with nearby moving water sources such as creeks or rivers or irrigation of pastures. Experimental studies have shown that feeding of infected insects on mucosal surfaces and nonhaired areas of the body were more often associated with development of lesions at those sites than if insects fed on haired areas of the body. The prevalence of clinical cases in a herd is generally low (10%–20%), but seroprevalence within the herd may approach 100%. Viremia has not been detected in livestock species that exhibit clinical signs of vesicular stomatitis, although experimental studies have shown transmission of virus, presumably via lymphatics, between co-feeding black flies on cattle. Virus is routinely isolated from active lesions in affected animals, and these lesions serve as a source of virus spread by direct contact and contamination of shared feed and water stations. Many vertebrate species have serologic evidence of exposure and may serve as reservoirs of infection. No definitive reservoir or amplifying host of vesicular stomatitis viruses in the USA has been identified.

Clinical Findings: The incubation period is 2–8 days and is typically followed by a fever. By the time animals develop other signs and are examined, however, they are rarely febrile. Ptyalism is often the first sign of disease. Vesicles in the oral cavity are rarely seen in naturally occurring cases because of rupture soon after formation; therefore, ulcers are the most common lesion seen during initial examination. Ulcers and erosions of the oral mucosa, sloughing of the epithelium of the tongue, and lesions at the mucocutaneous junctions of the lips are commonly seen in both cattle and horses. Ulcers and erosions on the teats are not uncommon in cattle and may result in secondary cases of mastitis in dairy cows. Coronitis with erosions at the coronary band are seen in some cattle, horses, and pigs, with subsequent development of lameness. Crusting lesions of the muzzle, ventral abdomen, sheath, and udder of horses are typical during outbreaks in the western USA. Loss of appetite due to oral lesions, and lameness due to foot lesions, are normally of short duration, because the disease is generally self-limiting and resolves completely within 10–14 days. Virus-neutralizing antibodies to either serotype persist and have been documented in individual horses that had previous clinical disease for >8 yr after an outbreak, but reinfection can occur after a second exposure.

Diagnosis: In most areas, including the USA, vesicular stomatitis is a reportable disease. Samples for diagnostic purposes are generally taken by a foreign animal disease diagnostician or other regulatory veterinarians and are tested by officially designated government laboratories. Diagnosis is based on the presence of typical signs and either antibody detection through serologic tests, viral detection through isolation, or detection of viral genetic material by molecular techniques. Samples for viral isolation may include vesicular fluid, epithelial tags from lesions, or swabs of lesions. Vesicular stomatitis viruses are easily propagated in cell culture. Three commonly used serologic tests are competitive ELISA, virus neutralization, and complement fixation. PCR tests may also be used to identify the virus. Of primary concern in diagnosis is differentiation of vesicular stomatitis from clinically indistinguishable but much more devastating viral diseases, including foot-and-mouth disease in ruminants and swine (*see* p 629), swine vesicular disease (*see* p 735), and vesicular exanthema of swine (*see* p 738). Horses are not susceptible to foot-and-mouth disease. Both noninfectious and infectious causes of oral lesions must be considered.

Treatment, Control, and Prevention: No specific treatment is available or warranted. Cachexia can be avoided by providing softened feeds. Cleansing lesions with mild antiseptics may help avoid secondary bacterial infections. Management factors suggested to reduce risk of exposure to the virus include limiting time on pasture during insect season, providing shelters or barns during insect feeding times, and implementing other procedures that reduce animal contact with insects, such as application of insecticides. This should include application to the inner surface of the pinna, where black flies feed. If livestock need to be kept on pasture during outbreaks of vesicular stomatitis, then keeping them pastured away from moving surface water (such as streams, irrigation canals, or rivers) may reduce the risk of exposure to *Vesiculovirus*. Affected animals should be isolated, and movement of other animals from the affected premises restricted. Vesicular stomatitis is a reportable disease in most areas, including the USA, so state and federal animal health officials must be notified when it is suspected. Commercially produced vaccines are not available in the USA, but vaccines for livestock are available in some Latin American countries.

Veterinarians act as a part of the surveillance network as they examine animals involved in shows, exhibitions, races, and interstate or international movement in order to write a health certificate (ie, certificate of veterinary inspection). When practitioners observe suspect cases of vesicular stomatitis, they should report to both their state and federal animal health officials. Reporting will prompt a regulatory investigation. Mucosal swab and serum samples from suspected animals are submitted for testing to veterinary diagnostic laboratories. During outbreak years, data regarding laboratory-confirmed cases of vesicular stomatitis, along with the number of premises with cases, are posted on the Web site of the Animal and Plant Health Inspection Service of the USDA.

Zoonotic Risk: The vesicular stomatitis viruses are zoonotic and may cause self-limiting influenza-like disease (headache, fever, myalgia, and weakness) lasting 3–5 days in people working in close contact with the virus (eg, laboratory exposure, direct contact with lesions in infected animals). Rarely, people can develop vesicles on the buccal and pharyngeal mucosa, lips, and nose. More severe signs, including encephalitis, are rare.

AFRICAN HORSE SICKNESS

African horse sickness (AHS) is an insect-borne, viral disease of equids that is endemic to sub-Saharan Africa. It can be acute, subacute, or subclinical and is characterized by clinical signs and lesions associated with respiratory and circulatory impairment.

Etiology and Epidemiology: AHS is caused by African horse sickness virus (AHSV), which is 55–70 nm in diameter and of the genus *Orbivirus* in the family Reoviridae. There are nine immunologically distinct serotypes of AHSV. The virus is inactivated at a pH of <6 (but is stable at higher pH), or by formalin, β-propiolactone, acetylethyleneimine derivatives, or radiation.

In endemic regions of Africa, the appearance of AHS may be preceded by seasons of heavy rain that alternate with hot and dry climatic conditions, which favor transmission by the insect (biting midge) vector. Outbreaks in central and east Africa have occasionally extended to Egypt, the Middle East, and southern Arabia. In 1959–1961, a major epidemic, caused by AHSV serotype 9, extended from Africa through the Near East and Arabia as far as Pakistan and India, causing the deaths of an estimated 300,000 equids. A further epidemic of the same serotype in 1965–1966 centered on northwest Africa (Morocco, Algeria, and Tunisia) but also extended briefly into southern Spain. This outbreak in Spain was eliminated by a vigorous vaccination and slaughter campaign. In July 1987, AHS caused by AHSV serotype 4 was reported in central Spain, due to the importation of infected zebra from Namibia. The outbreak lasted until the cold weather started in October 1987; however, the virus survived the winter and caused disease in southern Spain, Portugal, and Morocco in subsequent years before its elimination in 1991. AHS outbreaks continue to occur in endemic regions of southern and eastern Africa, and in 2007, AHS serotype 2 was reported in West Africa (Nigeria and Senegal), and serotype 7 in Senegal. Outbreaks of AHS caused by any one of several serotypes have recently been reported in Ethiopia.

Transmission: *Culicoides* spp are the principal vectors of all nine serotypes of AHSV, with *C imicola* usually considered to be the most important. Consequently, AHS is seen during warm, rainy seasons, which favor propagation of the vectors, and disappears when cold weather stops or significantly reduces vector activity. The virus also has been isolated from the dog tick *Rhipicephalus sanguineus sanguineus*, and the camel tick *Hyalomma dromedarii* during the winter in southern Egypt, where the disease is endemic. AHSV has apparently been transmitted between dogs by infected mosquitoes. Furthermore, dogs, and possibly large African carnivores such as lions and leopards, can be infected by ingestion of meat from AHSV-infected equids. However, it is generally considered that dogs and other large carnivores, ticks, and mosquitoes play little part in the epidemiology of AHS.

Clinical Findings and Lesions: Mortality depends on the virulence of the particular AHSV strain and susceptibility of the host. In naive populations of horses, which are the most susceptible equids, mortality may reach 90% in epidemics. The acute respiratory form is characterized by an incubation period of 3–5 days, interlobular edema, and hydropericardium. Death occurs in ~1 wk. A fever of 40°–40.5°C (104°–105°F) for 1–2 days is followed by dyspnea, spasmodic coughing, and dilated nostrils. The animal stands with its legs apart and head extended. The conjunctivae are congested, and the supraorbital fossae may be edematous. Recovery is rare, and the animal dies of anoxia, congestive heart failure, or both. At necropsy, pulmonary edema is especially visible in the intralobular spaces. The lungs are distended and heavy, and frothy fluid may be found in the trachea, bronchi, and bronchioles. There may be pleural effusion. Thoracic lymph nodes may be edematous, and the gastric fundus may be congested. Petechiae are found in the pericardium, and there is an increase in pericardial fluid; however, cardiac lesions usually are not outstanding. The abdominal viscera may be congested. A frothy exudate may ooze from the nostrils. The pulmonary form is the predominant form in dogs, which are usually infected by ingesting virus-contaminated meat.

The cardiac form of AHS is subacute with an incubation period of 1–2 wk. A fever of <1 wk is followed by edema of the supraorbital fossae. Swelling may extend to the eyelids, facial tissues, neck, thorax, brisket, and shoulders. Death usually occurs within 1 wk and may be preceded by colic. The mortality rate is ~50%. Petechiae and ecchymoses on the epicardium and endocardium are prominent. The lungs are usually flaccid or slightly edematous. There are yellow, gelatinous infiltrations of the subcutaneous and intramuscular tissues, especially along the jugular veins and ligamentum nuchae. Other lesions include hydropericardium, myocarditis, hemorrhagic gastritis, and petechiae on the ventral surface of the tongue and peritoneum.

A mixed pulmonary and cardiac form is most commonly seen in outbreaks, with a mortality rate in horses of ~80%.

Subclinical AHSV infection occurs in partially immune equids, such as those previously vaccinated against the disease, or in equids naturally infected with live-attenuated vaccine strains of AHSV. Subclinical infections are also characteristic in zebras and certain other equids.

Diagnosis: In endemic areas, clinical signs and lesions may lead to a presumptive diagnosis. However, laboratory confirmation is essential for definitive diagnosis and determination of the serotype; the latter is important for control measures. Anticoagulated blood should be obtained at the peak of fever and transported (at 4°C) to the laboratory. Spleen samples collected from freshly dead animals should be kept on ice. Presence of virus is best detected by group-specific reverse-transcriptase polymerase chain reaction (RT-PCR). AHSV also can be isolated by intracerebral inoculation of suckling mice or in mammalian or insect cell cultures. Although not widely available, indirect sandwich ELISA is also useful for rapid identification of AHSV antigen in tissues from animals that have died from acute infection.

Serotyping of AHSV previously relied on virus neutralization tests using type-specific antisera, which take ≥5 days. The recent development of type-specific RT-PCR can now confirm the serotype of an AHSV within 24 hr.

Prevention and Control: There is no specific treatment for animals with AHS apart from rest and good husbandry. Complicating and secondary infections should be treated appropriately during recovery. AHSV is typically noncontagious and spread exclusively via the bites of infected *Culicoides* spp or by the direct inoculation of infectious material (via blood-feeding insects, needles, etc). Various methods of control may be attempted, such as introducing animal movement restrictions to prevent infected animals initiating new foci of infection, and husbandry modification to deny or reduce vector access to susceptible or infected animals (eg, stabling in vector-proof housing). It is rarely possible to completely eliminate populations of vector *Culicoides*, especially in extensive pasture systems.

Live-attenuated virus vaccines are available for immunization of equids against AHS. These are typically based on cell culture–attenuated viruses and generally provide good, but not absolute, protection. Annual revaccination is recommended in regions where these vaccines are used. However, there are increasing concerns regarding use of live-attenuated AHSV vaccines because of their potential reversion to virulence, capacity for transmission by vector *Culicoides* midges, and reassortment of their gene segments with other vaccine and field strains of virus, leading to the creation of novel virus progeny. Inactivated and subunit vaccines avoid these potential drawbacks and, assuming they are commercially available, would likely be used after incursion of AHSV into previously unaffected regions.

Transport of equids from countries where AHSV occurs to virus-free areas is subject to strict regimens of testing and quarantine, although the precise requirements may vary from country to country. The presence of antibodies alone should not preclude such movements as long as AHSV is not present.

EQUINE GRANULOCYTIC EHRLICHIOSIS

Equine granulocytic ehrlichiosis is an infectious, noncontagious, seasonal disease, originally seen in the USA in northern California but now recognized in many states where the tick vector occurs; it is also seen in Europe, Africa, and South America. (*See also* POTOMAC HORSE FEVER, p 283.)

Etiology, Epidemiology, and Transmission: The causal rickettsial agent was initially termed *Ehrlichia equi*, but based on DNA sequence relationships, the organism is now referred to as *Anaplasma phagocytophilum*. It is not similar or clinically related to anaplasmosis in cattle. The organism has a wide host range; naturally occurring infections have been seen in horses, burros, dogs, llamas, and rodents. A rickettsia infection in people, the human granulocytic anaplasmosis (HGA) agent, caused by a similar strain as the equine infection, has been identified in cases of human illness in the upper midwestern and northeastern states in the USA and many other countries worldwide.

A phagocytophilum frequently infects horses wherever the tick vector (*Ixodes* sp) is present. States in which clinical infection has been confirmed include Connecticut, Illinois, Arkansas, Washington, Pennsylvania, Colorado, Minnesota, New York, Massachusetts, and Florida. It has also been confirmed in British Columbia, Sweden, Great Britain, and South America.

A phagocytophilum resembles the etiologic agents of tickborne fever (*see* p 772), bovine petechial fever (*see* p 745), and the HGA agent based on morphology, cell tropism, and 16S rRNA gene sequence data. It is present in cytoplasmic vacuoles of neutrophils and occasionally eosinophils during the acute phase. Blood smears stained with Giemsa or Wright-Leishman stains reveal one or more loose aggregates (morulae or inclusion bodies, 1.5–5 μm in diameter) of blue-gray to dark blue coccoid, coccobacillary, or pleomorphic organisms within the cytoplasm of neutrophils.

The infection can be transmitted experimentally to susceptible horses by whole blood from infected horses or from people with HGA. The incubation period is 1–3 wk. *I pacificus* (the western blacklegged tick) and *I scapularis* can transmit *A phagocytophilum* to horses.

The zoonotic risk of infection to people via horses has not been observed to occur. Although horses and people appear to be infected with strains of the same agent, it is believed that human exposure occurs through tick bites, and not by direct transmission from horses to people.

Clinical Findings: Severity of signs varies with age of the horse and duration of the illness. Signs may be mild. Horses <1 yr old may have a fever only; horses 1–3 yr old develop fever, depression, mild *limb edema, and ataxia.* Adults exhibit the characteristic signs of fever, partial anorexia, depression, reluctance to move, limb edema, petechiation, and icterus. The fever, which is highest during the first 1–3 days of infection at 103°–104°F (39.5°–40°C), persists at 102°–104°F (39°–40°C) for 6–12 days. Signs become more severe over several days. Rarely, myocardial vasculitis may cause transient ventricular arrhythmias. Other clinical presentations for acute infection have included recumbency and severe myopathy. Any concurrent infection (eg, a leg wound or respiratory infection) can be exacerbated. Cytoplasmic inclusion bodies are few during the first 48 hr and increase to 30%–40% of circulating neutrophils at days 3–5 of infection. The disease is seasonal in California, occurring in the late fall, winter, and spring.

Lesions: Gross petechiation, ecchymoses, and edema develop in the subcutis and fascia. Vasculitis is regional, with the subcutis and fascia of the legs predominantly affected.

Diagnosis: Demonstration of the characteristic cytoplasmic inclusion bodies in a standard blood smear is diagnostic. However, inclusion bodies are difficult to see in the first day or two of fever. PCR can detect *A phagocytophilum* DNA in unclotted blood or buffy coat smears. An indirect fluorescent antibody test can detect rising antibody titers to *A phagocytophilum*. Differential diagnoses include viral encephalitis, primary liver disease, equine infectious anemia, purpura hemorrhagica, and viral arteritis.

Treatment and Control: Oxytetracycline is extremely effective against *A phagocytophilum*, and systemic treatment with tetracycline, 7 mg/kg/day, IV, for 8 days, has eliminated the infection. Penicillin, chloramphenicol, and streptomycin have no inhibitory effect. Horses treated early in infection for shorter durations may relapse within the following few weeks. Horses with severe ataxia and edema may benefit from short-term corticosteroid treatment (dexamethasone, 20 mg/day, for 2–3 days). The risk of laminitis appears to be very low; no laminitis has occurred in clinical cases or experimental infections. Recovered horses are solidly immune for ≥2 yr and are not believed to be carriers. Persistence of infection has been suggested with some European strains, but further verification is required. Tick control measures are mandatory for control of disease. There is no vaccine.

EQUINE INFECTIOUS ANEMIA

Equine infectious anemia (EIA) is a noncontagious, infectious disease of horses and other Equidae. It is caused by an RNA virus classified in the *Lentivirus* genus, family Retroviridae. EIA can present as an acute, subacute, or chronic infection. On occasion, the virus can be a cause of significant morbidity and mortality. The most frequently encountered form of the disease is the inapparent, chronically infected carrier.

Transmission and Pathogenesis: Under natural conditions, the most important mode of transmission of EIA is by the transfer of virus-infective blood by blood-feeding insects between horses in close proximity. Virus is found free in the plasma or cell associated, principally in monocytes and macrophages of infected animals. Although infection is considered primarily blood borne, all tissues and body fluids are potentially infectious, especially during episodes of clinical disease when viral burdens are high. Transmission of EIA by biting flies is purely mechanical; the virus does not replicate in the vector. The chance of transmission of EIA is directly proportional to the volume of blood retained on the mouthparts of the insect after feeding. In that respect, horse flies, deer flies, and to a lesser extent, stable flies are likely the most efficient vectors. It is also because they are capable of triggering host defensive behavior that interrupts feeding and results in their seeking a new susceptible host to complete their blood meal.

Additionally, EIA can be readily transmitted iatrogenically through use of blood-contaminated syringes, needles, or surgical equipment, or by transfusion of infective blood or blood products. Infrequently, transplacental transmission can occur in infected mares that experience one or more clinical episodes during pregnancy. There is evidence, although circumstantial, from a significant outbreak of EIA in an equine hospital in Ireland, of probable spread of the virus by direct or indirect transfer between horses in stalls sharing the same barn.

A very close relationship exists between presence and severity of clinical signs of EIA and the amount of virus present in infected animals. Viral burdens are highest during febrile episodes of the disease. Many of the clinical signs associated with the acute form of EIA result from infection of macrophages and the release of pro-inflammatory mediators or cytokines, specifically tumor necrosis factor α, IL-1, IL-6, and transforming growth factor ß. This response together with suppression of platelet production are believed to be the factors responsible for the thrombocytopenia that is a characteristic feature of EIA. In addition, immune responses play a major role in the pathogenesis of EIA. Platelets from infected horses have significant amounts of bound IgG or IgM, which leads to their immune-mediated destruction, contributing to both splenomegaly and hepatomegaly.

Clinical Findings: The clinical findings and course of EIA are variable, depending on the virulence of the virus strain, viral dose, and susceptibility of the horse. After an incubation period of 15–45 days or longer in naturally acquired cases of infection, classic cases of the disease progress through three clinical phases. An initial or acute episode lasting 1–3 days is characterized by fever, depression, and thrombocytopenia. Because these signs can be mild and transitory, they are often overlooked. Typically, this initial phase is followed by a prolonged period associated with recurring episodes of fever, thrombocytopenia, anemia, petechiation on mucous membranes, dependent edema, muscle weakness, and loss of condition. The interval between episodes can range from days to weeks or months. In most cases, the episodes of clinical disease subside within a year, and infected horses become inapparent carriers and reservoirs of EIA virus. Many of these horses remain clinically normal.

Although the foregoing represents the most commonly described clinical course of the disease, some outbreaks of EIA can be associated with peracute infection in which the primary viral infection is uncontrolled; this can result in a very high fever, severely reduced platelet counts, and acute depression, leading to death. In view of the wide variation in response seen in natural cases of infection, it is not possible to confirm a diagnosis of EIA based solely on clinical grounds.

Lesions: Gross lesions frequently seen in acute cases of EIA include enlargement of the spleen, liver, and abdominal lymph nodes; dependent edema; and mucosal hemorrhages. Chronic cases of infection are characterized by emaciation, pale mucous membranes, petechial hemorrhages, enlargement of the spleen and abdominal lymph nodes, and dependent edema. Histopathologically, there is a nonsuppurative hepatitis and, in some cases, a glomerulonephritis, periventricular leukoencephalitis, meningitis, or encephalitis. Proliferation of reticuloenthelial cells is evident in many organs, especially in the liver, where there is also accumulation of hemosiderin in Küpffer cells. Perivascular accumulation of lymphocytes can be found in various organs.

Diagnosis: A provisional clinical diagnosis of EIA must be confirmed by demonstration of antibodies to the virus in blood. Although the internationally accepted serologic test is the agar gel immunodiffusion or Coggins test, there is increasing acceptance of a variety of ELISA tests, either competitive or synthetic antigen–based, because they can provide rapid results. Because ELISA tests can give a higher rate of false positives, all ELISA positive results must be confirmed by the Coggins test. When used in combination, ELISA and agar gel immunodiffusion tests provide the highest level of sensitivity combined with specificity. The Western blot is a supplemental test that can be resorted to in cases of conflicting results with other diagnostic tests. A problem with available serologic tests is that they can give negative results when testing sera collected within the first 10–14 days of infection. Whereas the vast majority of horses infected with EIA virus will have seroconverted by 45 days, there have been exceptional cases in which the interval has been ≥90 days. Virus detection assays such as the reverse transcription PCR assay are not routinely used to diagnose EIA. Notwithstanding their sensitivity, they may not detect virus in carrier horses with very low viral loads. Although the animal inoculation test is highly sensitive for detection of EIA virus, for logistical and economic reasons, it is no longer in vogue as a means of diagnosis of EIA.

Treatment and Control: No specific treatment or safe and effective vaccine is *available*. Because equids infected with EIA virus present the only known source of infection, antibody-positive animals should be kept at a safe distance (~200 m) from other equids. The only recognized exception to this rule is the progeny of seropositive mares, which may possess maternal antibodies to the virus after ingesting colostrum. In most cases, passive antibody against EIA virus wanes and is no longer detectable in the Coggins test by 6–8 mo of age; detectable antibody may persist up to 12 mo, however, if ELISA testing is used.

The risk associated with maintaining infected breeding stock varies. Field studies have indicated excellent success in raising test-negative foals from inapparent carriers of EIA virus. The risks of infection in utero increase dramatically if clinical signs of EIA are seen in the mare before parturition. Unfortunately, it is not possible to accurately determine the risk posed by any equid infected by EIA virus. Inapparent carrier horses maintain low-level viremias that may increase under stressful circumstances. As compared with seronegative healthy horses, inapparent carriers have increased serum globulin concentrations and lymphocyte subset changes that are consistent with immune activation or chronic inflammation. Because EIA virus persists in infected equids for life, most regulatory agencies assume all equids seropositive for EIA virus pose the same high risk.

In the USA, seropositive horses must be placed under quarantine within 24 hr after the positive test results are known. The quarantine area must provide separation of at least 200 yd from all other equids. After a confirmatory test is performed, seropositive horses must be permanently identified using the National Uniform Tag code number assigned by the USDA to the state in which the reactor was tested, followed by the letter "A." This identification may take the form of a hot brand, chemical brand, freezemark, or lip tattoo, and it must be applied by a USDA representative. Reactor horses must be removed from the herd by euthanasia, slaughter, or quarantine at the premises of origin. They may move interstate only under official permit to a federally inspected slaughter facility or a federally approved diagnostic or research facility, or to return to the premises of origin. After a reactor is detected in a herd, testing for EIA must be performed on all horses on the premises and repeated until all remaining equids on the premises test negative. These horses must be retested at 30- to 60-day intervals until no new cases are found. Quarantine on the premises is released when tests on the entire herd have been negative for at least 60 days after the reactor equids have been removed.

All equids shipped across state lines in the USA must be tested for EIA with a negative result within 12 mo before transport. All equids sold, traded, or donated within a state must have tested negative for EIA no more than 12 mo before change in ownership and, preferably, no more than 60–90 days. All equids entering horse auctions or sales markets are required to have a negative test before sale, or the horse must be held in quarantine within the state until the test results are known.

It is recommended that horse owners implement an EIA control plan for their premises. All horses should be tested every 12 mo as part of a routine health program. More frequent testing may be indicated in areas that perennially have a high incidence of EIA. Owners of equids entering shows or competitive events should present proof to event officials of a negative EIA test. All new equids introduced to a herd should have a negative EIA test before entry or be isolated while tests are pending. Vector control practices, including application of insecticides and repellents and environmental insect control, should be implemented. Good hygiene and disinfection principles should be maintained to prevent iatrogenic infection of horses with contaminated needles, syringes, or equipment.

EQUINE VIRAL ARTERITIS

(Epizootic cellulitis-pinkeye, Equine typhoid, Rotlaufseuche)

Equine viral arteritis (EVA) is an acute, contagious, viral disease of equids caused by equine arteritis virus (EAV). Typical cases are characterized by fever, depression, anorexia, leukopenia, dependent edema (especially of the lower hind extremities, scrotum, and prepuce in the stallion), conjunctivitis, supra- or periorbital edema, nasal discharge, respiratory distress, skin rash, temporary subfertility in affected stallions, abortion, and infrequently, illness and death in young foals. A variable percentage of postpubertal colts and stallions become carriers and semen shedders after infection with EAV.

Etiology and Pathogenesis: EAV is a small, enveloped single-stranded positive-sense RNA virus and the prototype virus of the genus *Arterivirus*, family Arteriviridae, order Nidovirales. It has 10 open reading frames (ORFs), of which ORFs 2a, 2b, 3, 4, 5, 5a, 6, and 7 encode the viral structural proteins. EAV is one of the three most important equine viral respiratory pathogens. The virus is not especially resistant outside the body, and survival ≥37°C can be short-lived. In contrast, EAV can maintain infectivity in tissues or bodily fluids for extended periods at storage temperatures equal to or below freezing. It can remain viable in frozen semen for many years.

Although only one major serotype of EAV has so far been identified, the prototype Bucyrus strain, genomic and antigenic variation exists among temporally and geographically different isolates. Pathogenicity also varies among viral strains, with some capable of causing moderate to severe signs of disease whereas others only induce a fever.

After respiratory exposure, EAV invades the upper and lower respiratory tract and multiplies in nasopharyngeal epithelium and tonsillar tissue and in bronchial and alveolar macrophages. Infected cells of the monocytic lineage and CD3$^+$ T lymphocytes transport the virus to the regional lymph nodes, where it undergoes a further cycle of replication before being released into the bloodstream. The cell-associated viremia that follows ensures dissemination of EAV throughout the body. By day 6–8, the virus localizes in the vascular endothelium and medial myocytes of the smaller blood vessels, especially the arterioles, and causes a panvasculitis. It can also be found in the epithelium of certain tissues, particularly the adrenals, seminiferous tubules, thyroid, and liver. Vascular lesions include endothelial swelling and degeneration, neutrophilic infiltration, and necrosis of the tunica media of affected vessels. These lesions give rise to edema and hemorrhage, which are believed to result from activation of the proinflammatory cytokines IL-1 beta, IL-6, IL-8, and possibly TNF-α. Maximal vascular injury occurs by about day 10, after which lesions begin to resolve.

Based on experimental infection of pregnant mares with the experimentally derived highly virulent Bucyrus strain of

EAV, abortion is believed to result from a myometritis that gives rise to impairment of the placental circulation and death of the fetus. However, this is unlikely to represent the pathogenesis of abortion in naturally acquired cases of EAV infection, which has yet to be determined.

Except in certain infected stallions that become carriers of the virus, EAV is no longer detectable in tissues and body fluids beyond day 28 after primary infection. However, stallions that remain persistently infected harbor the virus principally in certain accessory sex glands, especially the ampulla of the vas deferens, where it can remain for many years. Some carrier stallions may shed EAV from their reproductive tracts for an extended period.

Epidemiology and Transmission: While the natural and experimental host range of EAV is restricted principally to equids, there are very limited data to suggest the virus may also infect alpacas and llamas. There is no evidence that EAV is transmissible to people. Based on serologic surveys and reported outbreaks of equine viral arteritis, EAV is present in equine populations in many countries worldwide, with the notable exceptions of Japan and Iceland. The prevalence of infection varies widely both between countries and among breeds in the same country. It is frequently highest in Standardbreds and Warmbloods. Despite the widespread global distribution of EAV, laboratory-confirmed outbreaks of EVA are relatively uncommon. However, this situation appears to be changing in more recent years, with an increase in the number of verified occurrences of the disease being reported. A major factor contributing to this change is the continued growth in the volume of international trade in horses and equine semen.

The epidemiology of EVA involves virus-, host-, and environment-related factors, including variability in pathogenicity among naturally occurring strains of the virus, modes of transmission, occurrence of the carrier state in stallions, and the nature of acquired immunity to infection. Outbreaks of EVA are most often linked to the movement of infected animals or the shipment of virus-contaminated semen. Frequently, viral transmission occurs with minimal if any detectable clinical signs in acutely infected equids.

Transmission of EAV can occur by respiratory, venereal, and congenital routes or by indirect means. Spread by the respiratory route is the principal mode of dissemination of the virus during the acute phase of infection. It is primarily responsible for transmission of EAV among naive equids kept in close contact (eg, at racetracks, shows, sales, veterinary hospitals, and under conditions of intensive management on breeding farms). EAV can also be transmitted venereally by the acutely infected mare and by the acutely or chronically infected stallion. Mares can be readily infected by the venereal route after breeding to a carrier stallion either by live cover or artificial insemination with fresh-cooled or cryopreserved semen. There is evidence that EAV can be spread through embryo transfer. Infection can also be spread through indirect contact with virus-contaminated fomites (eg, breeding shed equipment, shanks, or twitches) or on the hands or apparel of animal handlers.

The carrier state has been confirmed in sexually mature intact males, specifically postpubertal colts and stallions, but not in mares, geldings, sexually immature colts, or fillies. Establishment and persistence of EAV in the reproductive tract of stallions is testosterone-dependent. The carrier stallion is the natural reservoir of EAV and is responsible for its dissemination and persistence in equine populations. Frequency of the carrier state can vary from <10% to >70%. There is evidence that stallions with $CD3^+$ T lymphocytes that are susceptible to EAV infection are at higher risk of becoming carriers than stallions with the $CD3^+$ T lymphocyte–resistant phenotype. Persistently infected stallions shed EAV constantly in the sperm-rich fraction of the semen but not in any other secretions or excretions. Duration of the carrier state can range from weeks to many years. Persistent EAV infection clears spontaneously in a variable percentage of stallions, with no evidence of subsequent reversion to a shedding state. Existence of the carrier state does not appear to impair the fertility of infected stallions nor otherwise adversely affect their clinical condition. Carrier stallions also serve as the principal means by which genetic diversification of EAV can occur, with potential emergence of novel viral variants.

Compared with other equine respiratory viruses, EAV stimulates a stronger, longer-lasting immunity that is protective against development of clinical disease, including abortion and establishment of the carrier state in stallions. High levels of neutralizing antibodies that frequently persist for at least 2–3 yr can be stimulated by natural exposure to the virus and by vaccination.

Clinical Findings: Exposure to EAV may result in clinical or asymptomatic infection, depending on the relative pathogenicity of the virus strain involved, viral dose, age and physical condition of the animal, and various environmental factors. Most cases of primary infection are asymptomatic. Onset of the acute phase of EAV infection, whether associated with clinical signs or not, is preceded by an incubation period of 3–14 days, which varies mainly with the route of exposure. The interval is usually 6–8 days after venereal transmission of the virus. Clinical signs can differ in range and severity between disease outbreaks and between affected individuals in the same outbreak. Any combination of the following may be seen: fever lasting 2–9 days, leukopenia, depression, anorexia, limb edema (especially of the lower hindlimbs), and edema of the scrotum and prepuce. Less frequently encountered signs include conjunctivitis, lacrimation and photophobia, periorbital or supraorbital edema, rhinitis and nasal discharge, edema of the ventral body wall (including the mammary glands of mares), an urticarial-type skin reaction (often localized to the sides of the face, neck, or over the pectoral region, although it can be generalized), stiffness of gait, dyspnea, petechiation of mucous membranes, diarrhea, icterus, and ataxia.

Strains of EAV can cause abortion throughout much of pregnancy (3 mo to more than 10 mo). Abortion may occur late in the acute phase or early in the convalescent phase of the infection, with or without prior clinical signs of EVA. In natural outbreaks, abortion rates can vary from <10% to as high as 60%. There is no evidence confirming that mares bred with EAV-infective semen will abort later in gestation. Mares that abort from the virus are already pregnant at time of exposure; this occurs primarily by the respiratory route through direct proximity with an acutely infected animal. Abortion occurs 1–4 wk later. Mares exposed very late in gestation may not abort but give birth to a foal congenitally infected with the virus. Mares that abort from EAV infection have not been proved to be less fertile.

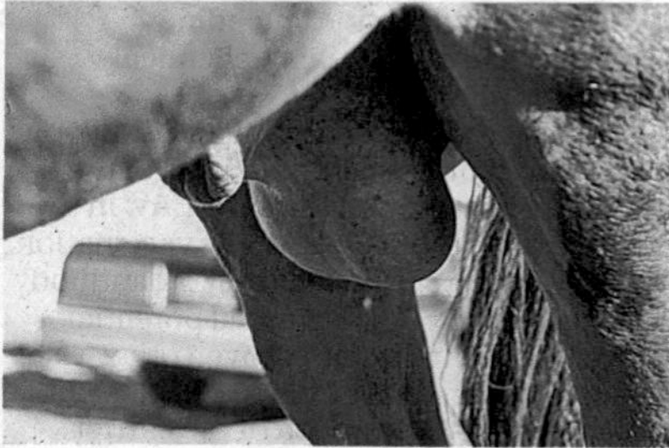

Equine viral arteritis, scrotal edema. *Courtesy of Dr. Peter J. Timoney.*

Stallions with EVA may undergo a period of short-term subfertility. This has been observed in individuals that develop a high and prolonged fever and extensive scrotal edema. Affected stallions may exhibit reduced libido associated with decreases in total and progressively motile sperm, curvilinear velocity, percentage of live spermatozoa, and percentage of morphologically normal spermatozoa. The changes in semen quality are believed to result from increased intratesticular temperature and not from the direct effect of EAV on spermatogenesis and testicular function. There is strong evidence that fever and scrotal edema exert independent effects on semen quality. Semen changes can last for 14–16 wk before returning to normal. No longterm adverse effects on fertility have been seen in fully recovered stallions.

The frequency and severity of clinical illness associated with EAV infection tend to be greater in very young, old, or debilitated individuals and under adverse climatic conditions. Regardless of severity of clinical signs, affected horses invariably make complete recoveries, even in the absence of symptomatic treatment. Mortality in older horses is very rarely encountered in natural outbreaks. However, it can occur in neonatal and in young foals up to a few months of age that succumb from a fulminating pneumonia or pneumoenteritis.

Lesions: The gross and microscopic lesions in fatal cases of EVA reflect the extensive and considerable vascular damage caused by the virus; these descriptions are primarily based on experimental infection with the highly pathogenic Bucyrus strain of EAV. The most significant gross findings include edema, congestion, and hemorrhages, especially in the subcutis of the limbs and abdomen; excess peritoneal, pleural, and pericardial fluid; and edema and hemorrhage of the intra-abdominal and thoracic lymph nodes and of the small and large intestine, especially the cecum and colon. Pulmonary edema, emphysema and interstitial pneumonia, enteritis, and infarcts in the spleen have been reported in naturally acquired fatal cases of the disease in foals.

Aborted fetuses are often partly autolyzed. Gross lesions are usually absent; if present, they are limited to an excess of fluid in body cavities and a variable degree of interlobular pulmonary edema. The vascular damage and immune-mediated lesions seen in older animals are seldom found in infected fetuses.

The characteristic microscopic lesion seen in cases of EAV infection is a vasculitis, involving primarily smaller arterioles and venules. Histologically, changes can range from vascular and perivascular edema, with occasional lymphocytic infiltration and endothelial cell hypertrophy in mild cases, to fibrinoid necrosis of the tunica media, extensive lymphocytic infiltration, necrosis and loss of endothelium, and thrombus formation in severe cases. Microscopic lesions are frequently not seen in cases of abortion. If present, vasculitis has been seen in the placenta and the brain, liver, spleen, and lungs of the fetus.

Fatal cases of EAV infection in young foals are characterized by interlobular edema, congestion and mononuclear cell infiltration in the lungs, and lymphoid depletion and hemorrhage in lymphoreticular tissues. Focal hemorrhages and necrosis of the intestinal mucosa have been described when there is an associated enteritis.

Diagnosis: The symptomatology of EVA can mimic that of a range of other respiratory and nonrespiratory equine diseases. Accordingly, laboratory examination of appropriate specimens is essential to confirm diagnosis. Equine influenza, equine herpesvirus 1 and 4–related diseases, infection with equine rhinitis A and B viruses or equine adenoviruses, and purpura hemorrhagica are among the more common equine illnesses that clinically resemble EVA. The latter must also be differentiated from equine infectious anemia, toxicosis caused by hoary alyssum (*Berteroa incana*), and allergy-induced urticaria. Several foreign diseases that should be considered in a differential diagnosis of EVA include Getah virus infection, dourine, and African horse sickness (*see* p 696).

Abortion caused by EAV must be differentiated from that due to equine herpesvirus 1 or 4. A helpful but not always reliable distinguishing feature is that mares that abort because of EAV may display prior clinical signs of EVA, whereas mares that abort because of equine herpesvirus seldom exhibit any premonitory clinical evidence of infection. Furthermore, EAV-infected fetuses not infrequently are somewhat autolyzed at time of expulsion and very often are devoid of any gross and even microscopic lesions. In contrast, herpesvirus-infected fetuses are invariably fresh and usually display characteristic gross and microscopic lesions.

Laboratory confirmation of a provisional clinical diagnosis of EVA should be pursued without delay in suspected outbreaks. This can be based on virus isolation, detection of viral nucleic acid, visualization of viral antigen by immunohistochemical examination, or demonstration of a recent humoral antibody response by testing paired (acute and convalescent) sera collected 3–4 wk apart.

The most appropriate samples for virus isolation and/or detection of viral nucleic acid by reverse transcriptase-PCR (RT-PCR) are nasopharyngeal swabs or washings and unclotted (citrated or EDTA) blood samples. To optimize the chances of isolation or detection, samples should be collected as early as possible after the onset of clinical signs or suspicion of EAV infection. After collection, swabs should be transferred directly into viral transport medium and shipped refrigerated or frozen in an insulated container via an overnight delivery service to a laboratory capable of testing for this infection. Unclotted blood samples should be transported refrigerated but not frozen.

In suspect cases of EAV-related abortion, virus detection should be attempted from placental tissues and fluids and from fetal lung, liver, lymphoreticular tissues (especially thymus), and peritoneal or pleural fluid. Chorioallantoic membrane and fetal lung are the tissues of choice for recovery of virus. When EAV is suspected in deaths of young foals or older horses, a wide range of tissue specimens, especially the lymphatic glands in the thoracic and abdominal cavities and related organs, should be collected and submitted for laboratory examination, including histologic and immunohistochemical testing.

Detection of the carrier state in a stallion is based initially on determination of the individual's serologic status for EAV. In the absence of a certified history of vaccination, stallions with a serum neutralizing antibody titer ≥1:4 should be considered potential carriers of the virus until proven otherwise, based on an absence of detectable EAV in their semen. Confirmation of the carrier state is based on demonstration of virus in a semen sample containing the sperm-rich fraction of the ejaculate either by isolation of virus in cell culture or its detection by RT-PCR. Under controlled laboratory conditions, sensitivity of virus isolation and real-time RT-PCR are essentially equivalent for detection of EAV in stallion semen; however, the RT-PCR assay has the advantage of providing a more rapid result. The carrier state can also be determined by test breeding a stallion to two seronegative mares and checking the mares for seroconversion 28 days after breeding.

Of the serologic assays evaluated for detection of antibodies to EAV, the complement-enhanced virus neutralization test continues to be the most reliable for the diagnosis of acute EAV infection and for seroprevalence studies. A number of ELISA tests have been developed, only a few of which offer comparable but not equivalent sensitivity and specificity. None of the available serologic tests can differentiate antibody titers resulting from natural infection from those due to vaccination.

Treatment, Prevention, and Control: There is no specific antiviral treatment currently available for EVA. Aside from young foals, virtually all naturally affected horses make complete clinical recoveries. Symptomatic treatment (eg, antipyretic, anti-inflammatory, and diuretic drugs) is indicated only in severe cases, especially in stallions. Prompt symptomatic treatment of stallions with a high or prolonged fever and significant scrotal and preputial edema can reduce the likelihood of short-term subfertility. Good nursing care, adequate rest, and a gradual return to normal activity are indicated. There is no effective treatment for EVA-related cases of pneumonia or pneumoenteritis in foals. Because congenitally infected foals are very productive sources of EAV and their chances of survival are essentially nil, early euthanasia should be considered to minimize the risk of further spread of the virus to any susceptible contacts, especially pregnant mares and young foals. Although there is some evidence that temporary down-regulation of circulating testosterone by GnRH immunization or through the use of a GnRH antagonist promotes clearance of EAV from the reproductive tract of carrier stallions, neither strategy has yet been adequately validated.

EVA is a manageable and preventable disease that can be controlled by observance of sound management practices together with a targeted vaccination program. Only one commercial vaccine, a modified-live virus product, is currently available in North America. The vaccine protects against development of EVA, including abortion, and establishment of the carrier state in stallions. Although the vaccine is safe and immunogenic for stallions and nonpregnant mares, the manufacturers do not recommend its use in pregnant mares, especially in the final 2 mo of gestation or in foals <6 wk of age, unless under circumstances of high risk of exposure to natural infection. Experimental and field studies have shown that there are no adverse consequences to vaccinating pregnant mares up to 3 mo before foaling and during the immediate postpartum period. However, there is a low risk of abortion in mares vaccinated during the last 2–3 mo of pregnancy. Minimizing or eliminating direct or indirect contact of unprotected horses with infected animals or with virus-infective semen is critical to the success of any prevention program.

The primary focus of current control programs is to restrict the spread of EAV in breeding populations and to reduce the risk of outbreaks of virus-related abortion, death in young foals, and establishment of the carrier state in stallions and postpubertal colts. Although EAV has occasionally been responsible for extensive outbreaks of disease at racetracks, shows, sales, and veterinary hospitals, these have been so sporadic that no specific control programs have been developed to prevent such occurrences.

Effective control programs are predicated on observance of sound management practices similar to those recommended for other respiratory infections. These include isolation of new arrivals on a premises for 3–4 wk before allowing them to co-mingle with the resident equine population, maintenance of pregnant mares in small isolated groups, identification of carrier stallions, annual immunization of noncarrier breeding stallion populations, and vaccination of colts at 6–12 mo of age to minimize their risk of becoming carriers later in life. Carrier stallions should be managed separately and bred only to naturally seropositive mares or mares vaccinated against EVA. Because fresh-cooled or frozen semen can be an important source of EAV, it should be tested by a laboratory with appropriate diagnostic expertise to confirm its negative EAV status, especially if imported. When breeding a mare artificially with virus-infective semen, the same precautions apply as if breeding by live cover to a carrier stallion.

In the event of a suspected outbreak of EVA, relevant animal health authorities should be promptly notified, with affected and in-contact horses isolated, and restrictions immediately imposed on movement of horses onto and off the affected premises. Appropriate specimens should be collected as soon as possible after onset of clinical signs and submitted for laboratory confirmation of a diagnosis of EVA. Breeding activity should be suspended on breeding farms to minimize risk of further spread of the infection. Stalls and equipment that might have come in contact with infected animals should be thoroughly sanitized. Vaccination of the at-risk equine population on a premises should be seriously considered as a means of restricting further transmission of EAV and of expediting control and resolution of an outbreak. Movement restrictions should not be lifted until at least 3 wk after the last clinical or suspected case of EVA or laboratory-confirmed case of EAV infection.

GLANDERS

(Farcy)

Glanders is a contagious, acute or chronic, usually fatal disease of Equidae caused by *Burkholderia mallei* and characterized by serial development of ulcerating nodules that are most commonly found in the upper respiratory tract, lungs, and skin. Felidae and other species are susceptible, and infections are usually fatal. The organism is infectious for people, with a 95% fatality rate in untreated septicemia cases, and is considered a potential bioterrorism agent. Glanders is one of the oldest diseases known and once was prevalent worldwide. It has now been eradicated or effectively controlled in many countries, including the USA. In recent years, the disease has been reported in the Middle East, Pakistan, India, Mongolia, China, Brazil, and Africa.

Etiology: *Burkholderia mallei*, a clonal gram-negative facultative intracellular obligate pathogen, is present in nasal exudates and discharges from ulcerated skin of infected animals. Glanders is commonly contracted by ingesting food or water contaminated with nasal discharges of carrier animals, by contact with harness components, and by ingestion of meat from affected horses. The organism is susceptible to heat, light, and disinfectants; survival in a contaminated area is limited to 1–2 mo. Humid, wet conditions favor survival. A polysaccharide capsule is an important virulence factor and enhances survival in the environment.

Clinical Findings: After an incubation period of 3 days to 2 wk, acutely affected animals usually have septicemia, high fever (as high as 106°F [41°C]), weight loss, and subsequently, a thick, mucopurulent nasal discharge and respiratory signs. Death occurs within a few days. The chronic disease is common in horses and is seen as a debilitating condition with nodular or ulcerative lesions of the skin and internal nares. Infected animals may live for years and continue to disseminate the organism. In some, the infection may be latent and persist for long periods.

Nasal, pulmonary, and cutaneous forms of glanders are recognized, and an animal may be affected by more than one form at a time. In the **nasal form**, nodules develop in the mucosa of the nasal septum and lower parts of the turbinates. The nodules degenerate into deep ulcers with raised irregular borders. Characteristic star-shaped cicatrices remain after the ulcers heal. In the early stage, the submaxillary lymph nodes are enlarged and edematous and later become adherent to the skin or deeper tissues.

In the **pulmonary form**, small, tubercle-like nodules, which have caseous or calcified centers surrounded by inflammatory zones, are found in the lungs. If the disease process is extensive, consolidation of the lung tissue and pneumonia may be present. The nodules tend to break down and may discharge their contents into the bronchioles, resulting in extension of the infection to the upper respiratory tract.

In the **cutaneous form** ("farcy"), nodules appear along the course of the lymph vessels, particularly of the extremities. These nodules degenerate and form ulcers that discharge a highly infectious, sticky pus. The liver and spleen also may show typical nodular lesions. Histologically, there may be vasculitis, thrombosis, and infiltration of degenerating inflammatory cells.

Diagnosis: The typical nodules, ulcers, scar formation, and debilitated condition may provide sufficient evidence for a clinical diagnosis. However, because these signs usually do not develop until the disease is well advanced, specific diagnostic tests should be used as early as possible. Culture of *B mallei* from lesions confirms the diagnosis. A test for delayed hypersensitivity is performed by intrapalpebral inoculation of mallein, a secreted glycoprotein of *B mallei* found in culture supernatant. Infected hypersensitive horses develop a purulent conjunctivitis within 24 hr and swelling of the eyelid. Complement fixation is also used to screen for infection. Competitive ELISA is more sensitive than complement fixation and may become positive as early as 3 days after infection. PCR based on 16S and 23S rRNA gene sequences may be used for specific identification.

Prevention and Treatment: There is no vaccine. Protective immunity involves T cell responses elicited by live attenuated bacteria. Prevention and control depend on early detection and elimination of affected animals, as well as complete quarantine and rigorous disinfection of the area involved. Treatment is given only in endemic areas but does not reliably produce a bacteriologic cure. Doxycycline, ceftrazidime, gentamicin, streptomycin, and combinations of sulfazine or sulfamonomethoxine with trimethoprim were effective in the prevention and treatment of experimental glanders.

HENDRA VIRUS INFECTION

Hendra virus was first described in 1994 after an outbreak of acute respiratory disease in a Thoroughbred training stable in Australia in which horses and one person were fatally infected. Sporadic cases continue to occur in eastern Australia, typically presenting as an acute febrile illness and rapidly progressing with variable system involvement, notably acute respiratory and/or severe neurologic disease. Fruit bats (suborder Megachiroptera) are the natural reservoir of the virus. Hendra virus is classified as a biosafety Level 4 agent (defined as posing a high risk of life-threatening disease in people), and the use of safe work practices and personal protective equipment is essential to manage the risk of human exposure. The earlier names of equine morbillivirus and acute equine respiratory syndrome are no longer appropriate.

Etiology and Pathogenesis: Hendra virus is a large, pleomorphic enveloped RNA virus. Although initially considered to be more closely related to members of the genus *Morbillivirus* than to other genera in the family Paramyxoviridae, subsequent studies showed limited sequence homology with respiroviruses, morbilliviruses, and rubulovirus and negligible immunologic cross-reactivity with other paramyxoviruses. Hendra virus is genetically and antigenically closely related to Nipah virus (*see* p 721), with which it shares >90% amino acid homology. Both viruses have been classified in a new genus, *Henipavirus*, in the subfamily Paramyxovirinae.

It is increasingly evident that Hendra virus strain variation is minimal and that clinical presentation and pathology more likely vary with the route of infection. Historically, interstitial pneumonia of variable severity was the principal finding in naturally infected horses and in experimentally infected horses exposed by the respiratory or parenteral routes. Hendra virus has a specific tropism for vascular tissues, regardless of route of challenge. In early infection, the vascular lesions may include edema and hemorrhage of vessel walls, fibrinoid degeneration with pyknotic nuclei in endothelial and tunica media cells, and numerous giant cells (syncytia) in the endothelium and sometimes the tunica media of affected vessels (both venules and arterioles). The virus becomes more widely distributed in various tissues throughout the body as infection progresses, presumably as a result of a leukocyte-associated viremia. Virus has been demonstrated in the vascular endothelium of subarachnoid and cerebral vessels and in the vasculature of the renal glomerulus and pelvis, lamina propria of the stomach, spleen, various lymph nodes, and myocardium. When respiratory disease is present, there is progressive destruction of alveolar walls, with the appearance of alveolar and intravascular macrophages. In addition to its vascular tropism, Hendra virus can also be neurotropic, causing neuronal necrosis and focal gliosis. A feature of one outbreak at an equine veterinary clinic in Australia in 2008 was severe neurologic disease and an absence of respiratory disease. Thus, Hendra virus should no longer be regarded as causing predominantly respiratory disease in horses.

Epidemiology and Transmission: Naturally occurring disease caused by Hendra virus has been reported only in horses and people. Experimentally, disease has been produced in cats, hamsters, ferrets, monkeys, pigs, and guinea pigs, but not in mice, rats, rabbits, chickens, or dogs. The clinical response and pathologic findings in cats are very similar to those seen in horses. Hendra virus infection and disease in horses has only been reported in Australia, and events are sporadic and infrequent, with 14 events recorded between 1994 and 2010. Most of these were single horse events. Thus, Hendra virus appears to have limited infectivity, and under field conditions, transmission between infected and noninfected horses occurs infrequently. However, the frequency of Hendra virus infection in horses has increased since 2011, with 18 incidents in 2011, 8 in 2012, 8 in 2013, and 3 in 2014 (up to October), with extended geographic locations (between far north Queensland to north New South Wales, Australia). In July 2011, a dog on a property with horses infected with Hendra virus (in Queensland) was identified as seropositive without any clinical signs. In July 2013, a dog on a property (in New South Wales) with Hendra virus infection in a horse was confirmed to be infected with the same virus. Further research is underway to investigate whether these increased incidents in horses were because of greater public awareness in reporting the disease or whether environmental or ecologic factors triggered this increased number of cases and extended geographic occurrence.

Experimentally, attempted transmission from virus-infected horses to in-contact horses or cats has been unsuccessful. Nonetheless, the possibility of respiratory transmission cannot be excluded. The frothy nasal discharge (originating from the lungs) sometimes observed terminally in naturally affected horses could plausibly provide a source of virus for aerosol transmission. Hendra virus has been found in the urine, blood, and nasal and oral secretions of naturally infected horses and cats. Based on available field and laboratory data, infection of people or animals appears to require direct contact with virus-infective secretions (lung exudates), excretions (urine), body fluids, or tissues. Although Hendra virus appears to have limited infectivity, the case fatality rate in individuals that become infected is high: 75% in horses, 57% in people.

Available epidemiologic, serologic, and virologic evidence implicates fruit bats as the natural reservoir of Hendra virus. Serologic surveys have revealed a high prevalence of neutralizing antibodies in wild-caught fruit bats (*Pteropus* spp) in Australia and Papua New Guinea. The geographic distribution of the virus in fruit bats appears to be limited to Australia and Papua New Guinea, although a transition of Hendra-like to Nipah-like viruses may occur beyond Australia. Infection in fruit bats (either natural or experimental) causes no evident disease. There is field and experimental evidence of vertical transmission, with isolates recovered from the uterine fluid and fetal tissues of a grey-headed flying fox (*P poliocephalus*) and a black flying fox (*P alecto*). The infrequent occurrence and sporadic nature of equine cases suggest that exposure of horses to Hendra virus is, at least in part, a chance event. The modes of transmission between bats, and from bats to horses, are uncertain, as are factors that may facilitate spillover. Hendra virus has been identified in the birthing fluids, placental material, aborted pups, and urine of naturally infected fruit bats and in the urine of experimentally infected fruit bats. The related Nipah virus has been detected in bat urine and on fruit partially eaten by bats. Horses are hypothesized to be infected through contact with food or water contaminated with material from infected fruit bats, but the definitive mechanism remains to be determined.

Clinical Findings: Because of its affinity for endothelial cells, Hendra virus can cause a range of clinical signs in horses. The predominant clinical presentation may depend on which organ system sustains the most severe or compromising endothelial damage.

Hendra virus infection should be considered when there is acute-onset fever and rapid progression to death, possibly associated with either severe respiratory or neurologic signs; however, the absence of these should not preclude consideration of Hendra virus. Infection is not always fatal, with 25% of known cases having recovered from clinical disease.

Clinical signs that should prompt a veterinarian to consider Hendra virus infection include acute onset of illness, fever, and rapid deterioration. Respiratory signs can include pulmonary edema and congestion, respiratory distress (increased respiratory rate), and terminal nasal discharge, which may be clear initially and progress to stable white or blood-stained froth. Neurologic signs can include “wobbly gait” progressing to ataxia, altered consciousness (apparent loss of vision in one or both eyes, aimless walking in a dazed state), head tilt, circling, muscle twitching (myoclonic spasms have been seen in acutely ill and recovered horses), urinary incontinence, recumbency with inability to rise, terminal weakness, ataxia, and collapse. Other clinical signs may include depression, highly increased heart rate, facial edema, muscle trembling, anorexia, congestion of oral mucous membranes, colic-like symptoms (generally quiet abdominal sounds on auscultation of the abdomen in preterminal cases), and stranguria in both males and females. Proximity to fruit bat roosts or feeding sites should increase the index of suspicion.

Where horses are paddocked, Hendra virus infection is more likely to manifest as a single sick or dead horse than as multiple cases. Most paddock infections have involved a single fatally infected horse with no transmission to in-contact companion horses. However, on several occasions, one or more companion horses have become infected after close contact with the index case before or at the time of death. Where horses are stabled, it appears that Hendra virus has the potential to spread either through close direct contact with infectious body fluids, or through indirect transmission via contaminated fomites, including inadvertent human-assisted transfer. Hendra virus infections in horse stables to date have resulted in multiple horses becoming infected, which appear to have arisen from a horse infected in a paddock or outside yard being brought into the stable.

Lesions: The presence of large endothelial syncytial cells on histopathology is characteristic of Hendra virus infection. Although most prominent in pulmonary capillaries and arterioles, these cells are also seen in other organs (lymph nodes, spleen, heart, stomach, kidneys, and brain). Widespread fibrinoid degeneration of small blood vessels is seen in many organs, including the lungs, heart, kidneys, spleen, lymph nodes, meninges, GI tract, skeletal muscle, and bladder. Antigen specific for Hendra virus can be demonstrated by immunohistochemical staining in the vascular lesions and along alveolar walls. Intracytoplasmic viral inclusion bodies can be seen in infected endothelial cells by electron (but not light) microscopy. When respiratory disease is predominant, the principal gross lesions are severe edema and congestion of the lungs and marked dilatation of the subpleural lymphatics. The airways are filled with thick froth, which is often blood-tinged. Additional lesions seen in some affected horses include increased pleural and pericardial fluids, congestion of lymph nodes, hemorrhages in various organs, and slight jaundice.

Microscopically, the primary lesions are those of an acute interstitial pneumonia. Severe vascular damage, with serofibrinous alveolar edema, hemorrhage, thrombosis of capillaries, necrosis of alveolar walls, and alveolar macrophages are evident in the lungs.

If neurologic disease is predominant, lesions of nonsuppurative meningitis or meningoencephalitis, including perivascular cuffing, neuronal degeneration, and focal gliosis, have been seen.

Diagnosis: Hendra virus infection should be considered when there is acute onset fever and rapid progression to death, but a nonfatal outcome should not preclude consideration of Hendra virus. Confirmation of the diagnosis is based on laboratory examination of appropriate specimens to detect virus, viral antigen, viral nucleic acid, or specific antibodies. The approach to specimen collection should reflect the serious zoonotic potential of Hendra virus and should incorporate appropriate measures to avoid human exposure. Minimum recommended samples include a blood sample (whole and/or EDTA) and nasal, oral , and/or rectal swabs. These can be taken from both live and dead horses. Necropsy specimens, both fresh and fixed in 10% formalin, of lung, kidney, spleen, liver, lymph nodes, and brain will increase the likelihood of reaching a conclusive diagnosis but also potentially increase the risk of human exposure. The number and type of specimens collected should follow a careful risk analysis by the veterinarian to prevent human exposure and consider many factors, including personal protective equipment available, training, and prior experience. If there are personal safety concerns, only a minimal set of samples (blood, swabs) should be collected. Submitting a combination of EDTA blood, serum, nasal, oral, and rectal swabs should be sufficient to detect Hendra virus infection in a horse highly suspected to be infected. Recommended procedures for safe handling of suspect Hendra cases are available at the Biosecurity Queensland Web site (www.daff.qld.gov.au).

The virus can be isolated in a range of cell lines; Vero cells are the cell line of choice. Viral cytopathic effect, which typically develops after 3 days, is characterized by syncytia formation in infected cells. Virus isolation and other diagnostic tests involving live virus should only be attempted under biosecurity Level 4 conditions. Serologic confirmation of infection is based on testing acute and convalescent sera collected 2–4 wk apart in a virus neutralization test. Presence of the characteristic vascular lesions on histopathology is highly suggestive of the infection; specificity of the lesions can be confirmed by immunochemical labeling with Hendra virus reference antiserum.

African horse sickness can clinically mimic Hendra virus infection and should be considered in the differential diagnosis. Other causes of sudden death that must be excluded include anthrax, botulism, certain bacterial infections (eg, pasteurellosis, equine influenza, peracute equine herpesvirus 1 infection), snake bite, and plant or chemical poisoning.

Treatment, Prevention, and Control: There is no specific antiviral treatment for Hendra virus infection. A vaccine, containing a noninfectious protein component (G protein) of the virus, has been developed; it was introduced in November 2012 and is available through accredited veterinarians in Australia. Healthy horses can be vaccinated from 4 mo of age with two doses at a 21-day interval, followed by boosters every 6 mo. Studies are being conducted to determine whether the period of booster vaccination can be extended to 1 yr.

Confirmed cases should be euthanized on humane grounds and to limit risk of human exposure. In Australia, euthanasia of recovered seropositive horses is also recommended, because the currently available evidence cannot exclude the possibility of recrudescence in these animals.

Prevention focuses on minimizing contact with fruit bat body fluids/contaminants and includes simple, practical measures such as placing feed and water containers under cover and minimizing the number of bat food trees/shrubs (fruiting and/or flowering) in horse paddocks or excluding horses from the vicinity of such trees/shrubs. Control is based on euthanasia and deep burial of cases; monitoring, isolating, and restricting movement of in-contact animals; and disinfection of potentially contaminated surfaces.

Zoonotic Risk: Human infection with Hendra virus has a 57% case fatality rate. All human infections have occurred from handling infected horses (both live horses and dead horses at necropsy), so great care should be taken to ensure the personal safety of all people in contact with suspect or confirmed equine cases. Neither bat-to-human nor human-to-human transmission has been recorded.

Protocols to minimize risk of human exposure should be implemented on suspicion of Hendra virus infection in a horse, not on confirmation. An outline of the approach developed by Biosecurity Queensland includes the following steps to minimize risk. First, a plan should be made in advance that outlines how Hendra virus risks will be managed by the practice and individual veterinarians in that practice. This includes 1) taking precautions based on suspicion of Hendra virus and not waiting for confirmation of infection; 2) isolating sick or dead horse(s) from people and all other animals, including pets; 3) limiting human contact with in-contact horses to only essential people; 4) promoting personal hygiene (especially hand washing, showering) for in-contact staff; 5) identifying hazards and taking steps to minimize the risks associated with these (eg, if decontaminating an area, avoid generating splashes and aerosols by not using a high-pressure hose); 6) informing people who may be potentially exposed such as owners, handlers, and others (including other veterinarians and veterinary assistants) of the risk and the appropriate procedures to be followed; and 7) referring to relevant animal health and public health authorities.

Second, adequate personal protective equipment should be used: 1) all exposed skin, mucous membranes and eyes should be protected from direct contact; 2) inhalation of airborne particulates should be prevented; 3) regular hand washing and washing of exposed skin with soap should be promoted; and 4) cuts and abrasions should be covered by water-resistant occlusive dressings that are changed as necessary.

In particular, blood and other body fluids (especially respiratory and nasal secretions, saliva, and urine) and tissues from sick or dead horses should be treated as potentially infectious and appropriate precautions taken to prevent any direct contact with, splashback of, or accidental inoculation with these body fluids.

AFRICAN SWINE FEVER

African swine fever (ASF) is a highly contagious hemorrhagic disease of pigs that produces a wide range of clinical signs and lesions that closely resemble those of classical swine fever (*see* p 713). It is an economically important disease that is enzootic in many African countries and the Mediterranean island, Sardinia. In June 2007, ASF was confirmed for the first time in Georgia in the Caucasus region. Since its introduction into Georgia, African swine fever virus (ASFV) has spread rapidly into vast areas of western and southern Russia, where it is currently (2013) circulating out of control in domestic and wild pig populations. The virus has spread to the edges of Europe, with outbreaks reported in both the Ukraine and Belarus in 2013, putting at risk the very large pig populations present in Eastern Europe.

Etiology and Epidemiology: ASFV is a large, enveloped, double-stranded DNA virus that replicates primarily in cells of the mononuclear phagocytic system. It is currently classified as the only member of a family called African swine fever–like viruses (Asfarviridae). The prolonged period during which ASF has been an enzootic disease in Africa is likely to have led to the selection of viruses of varying virulence. Distinct genotypes of ASFV have been differentiated by sequence analysis of the genomes of viruses obtained from different geographic areas over a long time. The virus is highly resistant to a wide pH range and to a freeze/thaw cycle and can remain infectious for many months at room temperature or when stored at 4°C. Virus in body fluids and serum is inactivated in 30 min at 60°C, but virus in unprocessed pig meat, in which it can remain viable for several weeks, can be inactivated only by heating to 70°C for 30 min. Although ASFV can be adapted to grow in cells from different species, it does not replicate readily in any species other than swine.

The disease is limited to all breeds and types of domestic pigs and European wild boar. All age groups are equally susceptible. In Africa, the virus produces inapparent infection in two species of wild swine—warthog (*Phacochoerus aethiopicus*) and bushpig (*Potamochoerus porcus*)—and in the soft tick *Ornithodoros moubata*. When the disease was endemic in southern Spain and Portugal, a different species of soft tick, *O erraticus*, became infected with the virus. Several other *Ornithodoros* spp that are not usually associated with pigs or wild swine have been infected experimentally. ASF has been reported in a large number of countries in Africa south of the Sahara, either as an enzootic disease or as sporadic epidemics in domestic pigs. The first spread of the disease outside Africa was into Europe (Portugal) in 1957 as a result of waste from airline flights being fed to pigs near Lisbon airport. Although this incursion of disease was almost certainly eradicated, a further outbreak occurred in 1960 in Lisbon, and ASF then remained endemic in the Iberian peninsula until the mid-1990s. Outbreaks of ASF were reported in a number of other European countries during the 20th century, including Malta (1978), Italy (1967, 1980), France (1964, 1967, 1977), Belgium (1985), and the Netherlands (1986). The disease was eradicated from each of these countries but has remained endemic in Sardinia since its introduction in 1978. During the 1970s, ASFV spread to the Caribbean and South America. An outbreak in south Brazil in 1978–1979 was eradicated by stamping out, and Brazil regained its ASF-free status in December 1984.

The spread of ASF out of Africa has been a relatively rare event, but in June 2007 ASF was confirmed in pigs in the former Soviet republic of Georgia in the Caucasus region. Genetic analysis revealed the genotype of the Georgia isolate to be closely related to isolates in circulation in Mozambique, Madagascar, and Zambia. It is therefore likely that pigs were fed ASFV-contaminated pig meat transported by ship from the southeastern part of Africa. By July 2007, the outbreak had spread to 56 of 61 districts in Georgia; soon after, outbreaks of ASF were reported in neighboring regions, including the autonomous republic of Abkhazia, Armenia, and Nagorno-Karabakh. Later in the year, infection of wild boar was confirmed in the Russian republic of Chechnya. In 2008, the spread of ASF continued into North Ossetia; it then jumped over 1,000 km into Orenburg, illustrating its potential for rapid spread over long distances. By October 2008, a total of 21 outbreaks of ASF had been officially reported in five Russian administrative divisions. From 2009–2013, the virus has continued to spread within the Russian Federation, and there are currently (Oct 2013) two main expanding hotbeds of infection in Russia, one in the southern part of the center of the Rostov region (Oblast) and the other in the Tver region (Oblast) and the adjoining areas. In 2013, outbreaks of ASF were reported in both the Ukraine and Belarus, putting at risk large pig populations in eastern Europe.

Transmission and Pathogenesis: ASFV is maintained in Africa by a natural cycle of transmission between warthogs and the soft tick vector *O moubata*, which inhabits warthog burrows and from which it is unlikely ever to be eliminated. The spread of virus from the wildlife reservoirs to domestic pigs can be by the bite of an infected soft tick or by ingestion of warthog tissues. Virulent viruses produce acute disease, and all body fluids and tissues contain large amounts of infectious virus from the onset of clinical disease until death. Pigs infected with less virulent isolates can transmit virus to susceptible pigs as long as 1 mo after infection; blood is infectious for as long as 6 wk, and transmission can occur if blood is shed. Pigs usually become infected via the oronasal route by direct contact with infected pigs or by ingestion of waste food containing unprocessed pig meat or pig meat products. The primary route of infection is the upper respiratory tract, and virus replicates in the tonsil and lymph nodes draining the head and neck, with generalized infection rapidly following via the bloodstream. High concentrations of virus are then present in all tissues. The factors that produce the hemorrhagic lesions are not fully defined, but severe disruption to the blood clotting mechanism plays a major role. Virus is excreted mainly from the upper respiratory tract and is also present in secretions and excretions containing blood.

Pigs that survive infection with the less virulent isolates may be persistently infected and have circulating antibody, although they do not excrete virus or transmit virus to their offspring in utero. Their role in the epidemiology of the disease is not fully understood; however, they are resistant to disease when challenged with related highly virulent isolates, indicating some level of cross-protective immunity between strains.

Clinical Findings and Lesions: Peracute, acute, subacute, and chronic forms of ASF occur, and mortality rates vary from 0 to 100%, depending on the virulence of the virus with which pigs are infected. Acute disease is characterized by a short incubation period of 3–7 days, followed by high fever (up to 42°C) and death in 5–10 days. The least variable clinical signs are loss of appetite, depression, and recumbency; other signs include hyperemia of the skin of the ears, abdomen, and legs; respiratory distress; vomiting; bleeding from the nose or rectum; and sometimes diarrhea. Abortion is sometimes the first event seen in an outbreak. The severity and distribution of the lesions also vary according to virulence of the virus. Hemorrhages occur predominantly in lymph nodes, kidneys (almost invariably as petechiae), and heart; hemorrhages in other organs are variable in incidence and distribution. Some isolates produce an enlarged and friable spleen; straw-colored or blood-stained fluid in pleural, pericardial, and peritoneal cavities; or edema and congestion of the lungs. Some viruses of low virulence have been isolated in Europe and produce nonspecific clinical signs and lesions. Chronic disease is characterized by emaciation, swollen joints, and respiratory problems. This form of the disease is rarely seen in outbreaks.

Diagnosis: ASF cannot be differentiated from classical swine fever (hog cholera) by either clinical or postmortem examination. Samples of blood, serum, spleen, tonsil, and gastrohepatic lymph nodes from suspected cases should be submitted to the laboratory for confirmation. Virus can be isolated by inoculation of primary cultures of pig monocytes, in which it produces hemadsorption of pig red cells to the surface of infected cells. Classical swine fever virus does not replicate in these cells. There are nonhemadsorbing viral isolates, some of which produce virulent disease. These isolates produce only a cytopathic effect in pig leukocytes. Confirmation of ASF in these cases has to be performed by either PCR or an antigen-detection ELISA. Viral antigen can be detected in infected tissue smears or sections by staining with labeled antibodies (several enzyme-labeled tests are available, eg, immunofluorescence), and viral DNA by PCR or hybridization of nucleic acid probes to tissue sections. The most appropriate tests to detect antibody in serum or tissue fluids are the ELISA and indirect immunofluorescence.

Other differential diagnoses include hemorrhagic bacterial infections and certain types of poisons.

Control: There is no treatment for ASF, and all attempts to develop a vaccine have so far been unsuccessful. Prevention depends on ensuring that neither infected live pigs nor pig meat products are introduced into areas free of ASF. All successful eradication programs have involved the rapid diagnosis, slaughter, and disposal of all animals on infected premises. Sanitary measures must also be applied and include control of movement and treatment of waste food. Subsequently, a serologic survey of all pig farms within a specific control zone must be conducted to ensure that all infected pigs have been identified.

CLASSICAL SWINE FEVER

(Hog cholera, Swine fever)

Classical swine fever is a contagious, often fatal, disease of pigs clinically characterized by high body temperature, lethargy, yellowish diarrhea, vomiting, and a purple skin discoloration of the ears, lower abdomen, and legs. It was first described in the early 19th century in the USA. Later, a condition in Europe termed "swine fever" was recognized to be the same disease. Both names continue to be used, although in most of the world the disease is now called classical swine fever (CSF) to distinguish it from African swine fever (*see* p 711), which is a clinically indistinguishable disease but caused by an unrelated DNA virus. Because of the severe economic impact of CSF, outbreaks are notifiable to the OIE. CSF has the potential to cause devastating epidemics, particularly in countries free of the disease. In these countries, vaccination is allowed only under emergency circumstances. In case of a new outbreak, strict measures are enforced to control spread, eg, culling of infected and disease suspect herds and strict movement restrictions. This can have severe consequences for the swine industry, especially in densely populated livestock areas. Awareness and vigilance are essential, so that outbreaks are detected early and control measures instituted rapidly to prevent further spread of CSF. The "high risk period," ie, the time between introduction of the virus and detection of the outbreak, must be kept as short as possible.

Etiology and Epidemiology: CSF is caused by a small, enveloped RNA virus in the genus *Pestivirus* of the family Flaviviridae. Classical swine fever virus (CSFV) is antigenically related to the other pestiviruses, mainly to bovine viral diarrhea virus (BVDV, *see* p 1436) of cattle and to border disease virus (BDV, *see* p 622) of sheep. These viruses are highly prevalent in bovine and ovine populations and can infect pigs. Although infections of pigs with ruminant pestiviruses in most cases do not lead to clinical disease and are rapidly cleared, infections with both BVDV and BVD induce an antibody response in swine. Therefore, antibody discrimination tests must be applied to differentiate CSF infections from infections caused by ruminant pestiviruses. Transmission of ruminant pestiviruses to pigs usually requires direct contact with cattle, sheep, or goats. CSFV naturally infects members of the Suidae family, ie, domestic and wild pigs.

In the laboratory, CSFV is cultured in cells of porcine origin, notably in the PK-15 cell line (porcine kidney), but does not generally cause a visible cytopathic effect. The virus has only one serotype, although some minor antigenic variability between strains is seen. Strains can be typed for epidemiologic mapping purposes by sequencing the entire viral genome or specific regions of the viral genome (ie, 5′UTR, E2, and NS5B regions) combined with phylogenetic analysis.

CSFV is moderately fragile and does not persist in the environment or spread long distances by the airborne route. However, it can survive for prolonged periods in a moist, protein-rich environment such as pork tissues or body fluids, particularly if kept cold or frozen. Virus survival times up to several years have been observed in frozen pork meat. CSFV may also survive months in chilled or cured cuts.

CSF has a worldwide distribution. It is considered endemic in certain countries of Central and South America, in the Caribbean basin, and in many pork-producing countries in Asia. Australia, New Zealand, Canada, and the USA are free of the disease, as well as most countries of western and central Europe, although sporadic outbreaks occur in Europe. CSF is considered endemic in several countries in eastern Europe. The main source of CSFV infection is the pig, either via infected live animals or via uncooked pork products. In areas where CSF is endemic, the major concern relates to the spread of disease through movement of infected animals, which may lead to widespread outbreaks, particularly in areas where there is large-scale transport of pigs among farms or to slaughter houses. In Europe, CSFV is considered endemic in wild boar populations, and infected wild boars are a source for CSF outbreaks among domestic pigs. However, the most probable source of CSFV infection for wild boars is contaminated garbage or even "spillover" from infected domestic pigs. The outcome of such infections mainly depends on the size and density of the wild boar populations affected. Outbreaks in small populations of wild boars living within natural confines, such as valleys, tend to be self-limiting, and the disease fades away over time. In contrast, infections leading to outbreaks in large areas densely populated with wild boars often become endemic.

Another major risk for CSF outbreaks is the accidental introduction of CSFV into herds through illegally imported pork meat or pork products that often find their way into the porcine food chain via swill feeding. However, CSFV is readily inactivated by heat (ie, cooking), which emphasizes the importance of enforcing regulations for heat treatment of swill feed. In addition, many countries have completely banned swill feeding practices.

Mechanical transmission by vehicles and equipment, as well as by personnel (notably veterinarians) travelling between pig farms, are also significant means of spread of CSF within infected areas. The persistence of CSFV within herds for long periods has been observed. Infections of sows during pregnancy with low to moderately virulent strains of CSFV may lead to in utero infections of fetuses. These infections lead to litters born persistently infected with CSFV that are carriers of the virus and source for new infections. Persistently infected carrier pigs usually do not show clinical signs but constantly shed CSFV into the environment. Therefore, it is particularly important to consider CSFV infections while investigating herds presenting with unexplained reproductive failures that include clinical manifestations in piglets such as congenital tremor or congenital abnormalities.

Clinical Findings and Lesions: CSF is characterized by fever, hemorrhages, ataxia, and purple discoloration of the skin; however, the clinical presentation varies, depending on host characteristics and the particular virus strain causing the infection. CSF occurs in several forms, including highly lethal, acute, chronic, or subclinical. Acute forms of CSF, associated with highly virulent CSFV strains, are characterized by an incubation period that is typically 3–7 days, with death occurring within 10 days after infection. Fever >41°C (105.8°F) is usually seen and persists until terminal stages of the disease when body temperature drops and becomes subnormal. Constipation followed by diarrhea and vomiting is common.

The principal lesion produced by CSFV infection is a generalized vasculitis, clinically manifested as hemorrhages and cyanosis of the skin, notably at the ears, lower abdomen, and extremities. There may also be a generalized erythema of the skin. Vasculitis in the CNS leads to incoordination (ie, staggering gait) or even convulsions. Histologically, nonsuppurative encephalitis with a characteristic vascular cuffing is common. At necropsy, the principal findings are widespread petechial and ecchymotic hemorrhages, especially in lymph nodes (eg, mandibular and retropharyngeal), tonsils, larynx, kidneys, spleen, urinary bladder, and ileum. Infarction may be seen, particularly in the periphery of the spleen. Subacute and chronic forms of the disease are also characterized by high fever, staggering gait, cough, diarrhea, purple discoloration of the skin, and death. In the subacute form, death generally happens within 20–30 days after infection; in the chronic form, death may occur much later. Subacute and chronic forms of the disease are associated with

CSFV strains of moderate to low virulence, respectively. Low virulence strains can be difficult to detect; the only clinical expression may be poor reproductive performance of sows and the birth of piglets with neurologic defects (eg, congenital tremor). In chronic forms of CSF after an initial acute febrile phase, infected animals may show an apparent recovery but then relapse, with anorexia, depression, fever, and progressive loss of condition (ie, marked weight loss). Macroscopically, in addition to the lesions described above, "button" ulcers may develop in the intestine, particularly near the ileocecal junction. Histologically, atrophy of the thymus and depletion of lymphoid follicles in lymph nodes are seen.

Diagnosis: CSF is first detected by veterinarians in the field. Because clinical signs manifested by CSFV-infected pigs are also seen with other diseases of swine, laboratory confirmation is always required. Clinically, the differential diagnosis varies according to the course of the disease, and primarily includes African swine fever. Hemorrhagic lesions must also be distinguished from those seen in porcine dermatitis and nephropathy syndrome and postweaning multisystemic wasting syndrome. Hemolytic disease of the newborn, porcine reproductive and respiratory syndrome, Aujeszky disease, parvovirus, thrombocytopenic purpura, anticoagulant poisoning (eg, warfarin), and salt poisoning should also be considered as possible differential diagnoses. Septicemic diseases, including salmonellosis, erysipelas, pasteurellosis, actinobacillosis, *Haemophilus suis* infections, and eperythrozoonosis may resemble CSF. Congenital infections with ruminant pestiviruses can resemble CSF reproductive failures caused by low virulence strains of CSFV. Poor reproductive performance in sows can also be associated with pseudorabies, parvovirus, and other noninfectious causes.

Virologic tests are essential to confirm the diagnosis of CSF. Advice on sample submission should be sought from the laboratory. Suitable tissues to detect the presence of the virus are tonsils, lymph nodes (mandibular, retropharyngeal, gastrohepatic, and mesenteric), spleen, kidney, and ileum. Whole blood collected with EDTA as anticoagulant can be used for virus isolation or virus detection, particularly during the viremic phase of the infection. Clotted blood samples (serum) are taken when serologic tests for detection of CSFV antibodies are pursued. Nasal swabs and/or tonsil scrapings are commonly collected clinical samples used to detect the virus (ie, viral RNA).

Significant amounts of CSFV are shed from infected animals into the environment via the oronasal route, particularly early during infection. Detection of CSFV antigen can be performed using direct immunofluorescence on frozen tissue sections, particularly in tonsil samples using specific antibodies. Antigen detection can also be done using ELISA; however, this assay has low sensitivity and is only useful for screening for the presence of CSFV at the herd level. More commonly, viral nucleic acid detection is done using reverse transcriptase (RT)-PCR. The assay is highly specific and can differentiate CSFV from BVDV and BDV. Standardized methods such as RT-PCR can be scaled up to screen large numbers of samples, giving rapid results while retaining high sensitivity. This is particularly useful to screen herds during an outbreak of CSF.

For virus isolation, cell cultures are inoculated with tissue suspensions or WBCs, fixed after 2–3 days, and the virus is detected using specific antibodies directed against CSFV (eg, fluorescent or enzymatic methods). Final results may not be available for 4–7 days. This method is labor intensive and time consuming. Virus characterization using virus-specific monoclonal antibodies or RT-PCR is performed to differentiate CSFV from the other pestiviruses. Positive results of antigen detection or virus isolation are not confirmed until virus identification is completed. Virus neutralization tests and ELISA tests are available to detect antibodies against CSFV. Because the virus is noncytopathogenic in culture, the neutralization test requires an additional immunostaining step to reveal the presence of neutralizing antibodies. ELISA tests are suitable for large-scale serology when large number of samples are processed, ie, for surveillance purposes. Cross-reactions between pestivirus antibodies are seen in diagnostic tests. The presence of antibodies against ruminant pestiviruses in pigs may hamper the serologic diagnosis of CSF. BVDV or BDV-specific antibodies are sporadically detected in pig populations. Risk factors related with ruminant pestivirus antibodies in pigs are associated with the presence of cattle on the same farm and high density of sheep and/or goats in the area. Some commercial ELISAs can distinguish CSF from BVDV or BDV antibodies, although confirmatory testing is advised usually via neutralizing peroxidase-linked assays.

New generations of CSFV marker vaccines have been developed to make emergency vaccination compatible with control of CSF. The application of a marker vaccine is possible if tests such as ELISA can distinguish between antibodies produced in response to a natural infection and those produced by vaccination. This is the DIVA principle (differentiation of infected from vaccinated animals) that is based on detection of CSFV-specific antibodies that develop in the host only with CSFV infection but not on vaccination with a marker vaccine. These assays have been developed as necessary companion tests for CSF marker vaccines.

Control: CSF is a notifiable disease. Control is usually strictly regulated by local laws that establish strict sanitary measures. No treatment is available. Outbreaks in countries free of CSF are controlled rapidly via culling of infected animals and preemptive slaughter of susceptible animals within determined distances from the focus. Restriction of movement within a well-defined radius from the outbreak is applied to contain spread of the infection. Eventually, emergency vaccination can be authorized to control the further spread of CSFV. Countries will regain their CSF-free status (no antibodies or virus detected) after establishing that CSFV is no longer present in the national pig herd.

Countries free of CSF usually implement preventive measures to avoid outbreaks of CSF by controlling movement of live animals and pork products at borders. Countries free of CSF forbid the use of prophylactic vaccination. In countries where CSF is endemic, prophylactic vaccination is regularly practiced and is mandatory in some cases. Prophylactic vaccination has been used worldwide as a tool to control and eradicate CSF. In these countries, herds affected by an outbreak are quarantined and if possible eliminated. Emergency ring vaccination around the outbreak is done to prevent further spread of CSFV. CSF live attenuated vaccines are safe and highly efficient, being able to induce protection shortly after vaccination (within 3 days after vaccination). Several live attenuated vaccines, such as the Chinese lapinized vaccine (C-strain), the Japanese GPE-strain, and the French Thiverval strain, have been developed and used in different countries. More recently, subunit CSFV vaccines containing only the major viral surface glycoprotein of the virus have been licensed. Although these vaccines have DIVA capabilities, they lack the efficiency of live attenuated vaccines. Oral vaccination of wild boars has been used successfully within the European Union using a live attenuated vaccine delivered via baits. Oral vaccination has been a key strategy to control CSF, particularly where parenteral vaccine delivery is not feasible.

EDEMA DISEASE

(*Escherichia coli* enterotoxemia)

Edema disease is a peracute toxemia caused by specific pathotypes of *Escherichia coli* that affect primarily healthy, rapidly growing nursery pigs. Other names for edema disease include "gut edema" or "bowel edema" because of the prominent edema of the submucosa of the stomach and mesocolon.

Etiology and Pathogenesis: Edema disease is caused by hemolytic *E coli* that produce F18 pili and Shiga toxin 2e (Stx2e, also known as verotoxin 2e or VT2e). The F18 pili have two major antigenic variants, F18ab and F18ac; F18ab is characteristic of edema disease strains, and F18ac is associated primarily with enterotoxigenic *E coli*. A new variant of F18 has been identified on strains of *E coli* that carry the Stx2e gene, but the role of these strains in edema disease is not known. The Shiga toxin–producing *E coli* implicated in edema disease most commonly belong to four specific serotypes: O138:K81:NM, O139:K12:H1, O141:K85ab:H4, and O141:K85ac:H4. However, other serotypes of *E coli* may be implicated, and strains of serogroup O147 have been dominant in parts of the USA. These O147 strains typically carry the H17 flagella, but some have H14 or H4. Some of these O147 strains are not typeable with O147 specific antiserum but can be identified by their O antigen genes.

Pigs become infected initially by a contaminated environment or the sow. Spread of infection among penmates is facilitated by the large numbers of edema disease–producing *E coli* that are shed by colonized pigs. Some strains of *E coli* that cause edema disease also carry genes for enterotoxins and can cause diarrhea as well as edema disease. Ingestion of edema disease strains of *E coli* is followed by colonization of the intestine in pigs in which intestinal epithelial cells carry receptors for the F18 pili. Expression of the receptors is age-related, so younger pigs are less susceptible to colonization than older pigs. Some pigs carry a specific mutation in a gene required for expression of the receptors and are thereby resistant to infection.

Resistance/susceptibility is determined by a single locus with a dominant susceptibility allele and a recessive resistant allele; it is possible to select resistant pigs, which can be identified by a simple PCR test that identifies presence or absence of the specific mutation. Some concern about selection for resistance to F18+ *E coli* has been expressed, because a very high association between presence of the marker for resistance to F18+ *E coli* and presence of the marker for stress susceptibility was shown in Swiss Landrace pigs. However, this association does not exist in Belgian pigs.

Stx2e produced in the intestine of colonized pigs is responsible for the major clinical signs and pathology seen. This cytotoxin inhibits protein synthesis, leading to cell death. The toxin is absorbed from the intestine and targets vascular endothelium in specific sites believed to have high concentrations of the toxin receptors globotriaosyl ceramide and globotetraosyl ceramide. A study showed that edema disease strains of *E coli* may colonize the mesenteric lymph nodes and produce Stx2e there. This may be an additional site from which the toxin is absorbed into the bloodstream. The Stx2e toxin binds readily to pig RBCs, which may transport the toxin to various sites in the body. Sites highly susceptible to the toxin include the submucosa of the stomach, the colonic mesentery, the subcutaneous tissues of the forehead and eyelids, the larynx, and the brain. Damage to vascular endothelium results in edema, hemorrhage, intravascular coagulation, and microthrombosis.

High-protein diets increase the susceptibility of pigs to the disease. Factors associated with weaning, including the stresses of mixing pigs, changes in diet, and the loss of milk antibodies from the intestine, appear to be important elements in enhancing the susceptibility of weaned pigs to the disease.

Clinical Findings: Clinical signs range from peracute death with no signs of illness to CNS involvement with ataxia, paralysis, and recumbency. Edema disease usually occurs 1–2 wk after weaning and typically involves the healthiest animals in a group. The disease is seen occasionally in nursing pigs or in adult pigs. The average morbidity is 30%–40%, and the mortality among affected pigs is often as high as 90%. Periocular edema, swelling of the forehead and submandibular regions, dyspnea, and anorexia are common.

Lesions: Edema disease is primarily a disease of the vasculature, and gross lesions consist of subcutaneous edema and edema in the submucosa of the stomach, particularly in the glandular cardiac region. The edema fluid is usually gelatinous and may extend into the mesocolon. The edema may be accompanied by hemorrhage. Fibrin strands may be found in the peritoneal cavity, and serous fluid may be found in both the pleural and peritoneal cavities. Microscopically, a degenerative angiopathy affecting arteries and arterioles and necrosis of the smooth muscle cells in the tunica media are present. Lesions of focal encephalomalacia in the brain stem are characteristic and thought to result from vascular damage, leading to edema and ischemia.

Diagnosis: A clinical history of peracute death in healthy, well-conditioned, recently weaned pigs, along with observation of periocular edema and extensive edema of the stomach and mesocolon, are helpful in diagnosis. There may be a characteristic squeal due to edema of the larynx. Diarrhea may precede the signs of edema disease if the *E coli* responsible also possesses genes for enterotoxins. Characteristically, the stomach is full of dry feed. Diagnosis is easily made in an outbreak in which the full range of clinical signs and pathologic features are likely to occur. It is more difficult when only a few animals are affected or when the disease occurs in an atypical age group. Isolation and characterization of the *E coli* are required for a definitive diagnosis. Culture of the small intestine and colon typically yields a heavy growth of hemolytic *E coli*, but in some cases the organism may no longer be present in the intestine at the time of death. Demonstration that the hemolytic *E coli* isolated is an edema disease strain may be done by PCR amplification of the genes for the F18 pili and Stx2e. Recently, quantitative PCR for several pig bacterial enteropathogens, including edema disease strains of *E coli*, was shown to be a rapid and sensitive method for detection and quantification of these bacteria in pig feces. Serotyping of the isolate is useful to track the persistence of a particular type of the organism on a farm. The F18 pili are not readily expressed on organisms that are cultured, but the genes that encode them are easily detected by PCR.

Treatment and Control: Because the onset of disease is often sudden and the course rapid, treatment is often ineffective. Oral medication with antibiotics via the drinking water may be used to protect clinically unaffected pigs in a herd in which cases of the disease have been detected. Antibiotic sensitivity should be determined on the isolate from an affected pig; medication should be changed if the initial choice was ineffective. Control is also difficult. Several experimental approaches have been shown to be effective, but none are economical to date. These methods include feeding a high-fiber and low-protein diet, reducing the amount of feed given to weaned pigs, vaccinating by a systemic route with Stx2e toxoid, oral vaccination with an F18+ nontoxigenic *E coli*, passive systemic immunization with antitoxin, and passive oral immunization with anti-F18 antibodies. Mucosal immunization with purified F18 fimbriae has proved to be ineffective, possibly because the portion of the F18 fimbria that binds to the intestine is a small fraction of the total fimbrial structure. Incomplete protection was reported after vaccination of pigs with the receptor portion of the F18 fimbriae conjugated with F4 fimbriae. Two important developments are the rapid and inexpensive methods for purification of Stx2e toxin or toxoid and the demonstration that immunization of pregnant sows with Stx2e toxoid resulted in protection of their weaned offspring against a challenge with a lethal dose of Stx2e toxin. The flagella of F18ab edema disease *E coli* has been shown to be involved in adherence to pig intestinal epithelial cells in vitro and could be a new target for vaccines against edema disease.

ENCEPHALOMYOCARDITIS VIRUS INFECTION

Encephalomyocarditis (EMC) is a significant viral infection of swine and zoologic mammals. It is caused by members of the genus *Cardiovirus* in the family Picornaviridae and recognized in many parts of the world. Although EMC virus (EMCV) isolates from various regions and countries have differed in pathogenicity and virulence, until recently all EMC viruses were considered to exist as a single serotype (EMCV-1). A cardiovirus isolated from a wood mouse in Germany in 2012 was distinguished from EMCV-1 by serologic and molecular means and has been designated EMCV-2. Although EMCV-1 infects a wide variety of hosts, the host range and pathogenicity of EMCV-2 remains to be determined.

Swine may die acutely at any age due to associated myocardial failure or may be affected with near-term abortions, fetal mummification, and apparent reproductive failure. Type A strains cause porcine reproductive problems, whereas type B strains cause heart failure. With the recognition of porcine reproductive and respiratory syndrome (PRRS) in 1987, however, the overall significance of EMCV-1 as a cause of reproductive disease in swine has been questioned. The high mutation rate of the PRRS arterivirus complicates the maintenance of reliable diagnostic PCR assays for that virus, while a concurrent EMCV infection may be easily detected by virus isolation. Most outbreaks of EMCV infection have been associated with captive animals in swine production units, primate research centers, and zoos. Sudden death is often the first indication of infection. A variety of exotic mammals have been fatally afflicted with EMC in zoologic parks in the USA, Australia, and other parts of the world and have included African elephants, rhinoceroses, hippopotamuses, sloths, llamas, various antelope species, and many types of nonhuman primates (chimpanzees, orangutans, baboons, monkeys, lemurs, etc). An episode of lion deaths at a zoo in the USA was associated with the feeding of the carcass of an African elephant that had died of EMC, and a spontaneous outbreak of fatal EMC was reported in free-ranging African elephants at Kruger National Park in South Africa in 1995. Reports of outbreaks of EMCV-associated disease are solicited and recorded at the Pirbright Institute in the UK.

Epidemiology: Cardioviruses are small, nonenveloped viruses that are almost always associated with rodents, and the disease in other mammalian species has often been attributed to spillover from populations of wild mice and rats. These, and presumably other rodent species, shed the viruses in feces and urine, which may contaminate food and water supplies of large mammals. Ingestion of rodents dead or dying of EMC may be another means of infection. Pigs shed virus in nasal secretions and feces during the first 3 days of experimental infection. During this short period, the virus may be transmitted to other pigs by contact. Cardioviruses are resistant to adverse environmental influences and may remain infective for weeks to months under favorable conditions.

Clinical Findings and Lesions: The disease is named for its predilection for the CNS and cardiovascular systems of experimental mice, and both encephalotropic and cardiotropic strains have been defined. In swine and zoologic species, however, acute and subacute deaths are almost always attributed to the destructive effects of the virus on the myocardium, with resultant cardiac insufficiency, pulmonary edema, and frothy transudation into the respiratory tract. Affected animals often appear to have asphyxiated in their own respiratory fluids. Other clinical signs may include fever, anorexia, listlessness, trembling, staggering, dyspnea, and paralysis. Mortality approaching 100% has been described in suckling swine but becomes successively lower in older age groups. Strains of EMC viruses that target the pancreas and are diabetogenic in experimental mice have been recognized, but the significance of this finding for other mammals has not been established.

EMC viruses are known to cross the placenta in swine and have been recovered from conceptuses in cases of reproductive failure due to near-term abortions (107–111 days of gestation), stillbirths, and mummifications. Reproductive problems have been reported to involve sows of all parities, often persisting in affected herds for 2–3 mo, but the possibly more significant contribution of PRRS should be investigated.

Diagnosis: Because the pale necrotic heart muscle lesions that may be seen in fatal EMC infections are also seen in septic infarction or vitamin E/selenium deficiency, a definitive diagnosis requires virus recovery and identification. Heart, liver, kidney, and spleen collected from acutely dead animals or abortuses are the specimens of choice for virus isolation. Because EMC viruses are very stable, they may be recovered from frozen tissues.

Serologic diagnosis via virus neutralization, hemagglutination-inhibition, or ELISA is possible if acute and convalescent sera are collected, but the frequency of subclinical EMC infections makes single serum determinations of little value in aborting sows. Detection of antibody against EMC viruses in stillborn or large mummified fetuses is significant for fetal infection, however, because maternal immunoglobulins are not passed across the placenta in swine.

Treatment, Control, and Prevention: There is no specific treatment for EMC, but mortality may be minimized by avoiding stress or excitement in animals at risk. EMC viruses appear to cycle in rodents and are most likely to affect swine and zoo animals when rodent populations are high. Rodent control is thus critical to minimize exposure of susceptible species. Prompt and proper disposal of animals that have died of the disease is also recommended. EMC viruses are inactivated by the judicious use of many disinfectants labeled for livestock use.

Killed vaccines for the prevention of myocarditis in weaned swine have been patented but are no longer commercially available in the USA except as autogenous products. The current impetus for vaccine development has come largely from zoos and amusement parks where EMC has been problematic. Success with a genetically engineered attenuated virus vaccine has been reported in primates, pigs, and various zoologic hoofstock species. Commercial EMCV vaccine production has been limited by the apparent lack of need in most domestic livestock situations.

Zoonotic Risk: EMC viruses have rarely been recognized as the cause of human illness, and the severe myocarditis and acute fatal infections seen in many other species have not been reported in people. Nevertheless, serologic surveys have revealed human EMCV infections are common in many parts of the world; most are asymptomatic or not recognized. Human disease has been characterized by fever, chills, nausea, headache, nuchal rigidity, delirium, delusions, vomiting, photophobia, and pleocytosis.

GLÄSSER'S DISEASE

(Porcine polyserositis, Infectious polyarthritis)

Pigs can be colonized by different microorganisms before weaning, but some of those early colonizing agents are potentially pathogenic. This is the case with *Haemophilus parasuis*, a commensal organism of the upper respiratory tract of swine that causes severe systemic disease characterized by fibrinous polyserositis, arthritis, and meningitis. Disease has a sudden onset, short course, and high morbidity and mortality. Young animals (4–8 wk old) are primarily affected, although sporadic disease can be seen in adults (eg, introduction of a naive adult to a healthy herd). Survivors can develop severe fibrosis in the abdominal and thoracic cavities, which can result in reduced growth rate and carcass condemnation at slaughter. Glässer's disease is seen worldwide, and its incidence appears to have increased since the introduction of porcine reproductive and respiratory syndrome (*see* p 729).

Etiology: The causal agent, *H parasuis*, is a small, gram-negative pleomorphic bacterium of the family Pasteurellaceae that requires V factor (NAD) supplementation but not X factor (hemin) for growth. In the laboratory, *H parasuis* grows on enriched chocolate agar; it can also be cultured in blood agar with a staphylococcal nurse streak. However, *H parasuis* is fastidious, and its isolation in pure culture from diseased animals is usually difficult and frequently complicated because of antibiotic treatments. Fifteen serovars of *H parasuis* have been reported, but a high percentage of the evaluated isolates cannot be typed. Wide differences in serovar virulence have been described. Serovars 1, 2, 4, 5, 12, 13, 14, and some isolates that cannot be typed are usually isolated from systemic disease cases, while serovars 3, 6, 7, 9, and other nontyped isolates are frequently isolated from the upper respiratory tract. The factors involved in systemic invasion by *H parasuis* are still unknown. Moreover, the correlation between serovar and virulence is not clear, and strains belonging to the same serovar may vary in virulence. Serotyping also has been used as the basis to establish vaccination criteria, but the cross-protection between different serovars is variable and difficult to predict. Therefore, current methods of *H parasuis* identification and characterization are primarily genotyping (fingerprinting or sequencing methods). The identification of virulence genes has received increased attention because of the possibility of differentiating strains with pathogenic potential as well as of developing vaccines.

Clinical Findings: Clinical signs are seen mainly in pigs 4–8 wk old, although the age of affected animals may vary, depending on the level of acquired maternal immunity.

Peracute disease has a short course and may result in sudden death without the presence of characteristic gross lesions; petechiae may be seen in some organs in these cases, indicating septicemia.

The typical clinical signs of acute Glässer's disease include high fever (41.5°C [106.7°F]), severe coughing, abdominal breathing, swollen joints, and CNS signs such as lateral decubitus, paddling, and trembling. These signs may be seen jointly or independently. Chronically affected animals may have a reduced growth rate as a result of severe fibrosis in the thoracic and peritoneal cavities.

Dyspnea and coughing not usually associated with Glässer's disease have been described, together with *H parasuis* isolation from the lungs of pigs with catarrhal purulent bronchopneumonia and even fibrinohemorrhagic pneumonia. However, *H parasuis* is not considered a significant cause of coughing.

Disease prevalence is modulated by concomitant environmental stressors as well as by viral infections affecting the immune system, mainly porcine reproductive and respiratory syndrome and porcine circovirus type 2 systemic disease.

Lesions: Peracute disease may cause petechiae in some tissues, with no gross lesions observed. Histologically, these pigs show septicemia-like microscopic lesions such as DIC and microhemorrhages. Increased fluid in the thoracic and abdominal cavities, without the presence of fibrin, can also be seen in peracute cases.

Acute systemic infection is characterized by development of fibrinous polyserositis, arthritis, and meningitis. The fibrinous exudate can be seen on the pleura, pericardium, peritoneum, synovia, and meninges and is usually accompanied by an increased amount of fluid. Fibrinous pleuritis may be accompanied by cranioventral consolidation (catarrhal-purulent bronchopneumonia). Lack of characteristic gross lesions is also common in swine showing CNS signs. Chronically affected pigs usually have severe fibrosis of the pericardium and pleura, which may or may not be present in the peritoneal cavity.

Diagnosis: Diagnosis is based on observation of characteristic clinical signs and lesions, in association with detection of *H parasuis* in affected swine by isolation or by molecular methods such as PCR.

Most current diagnostic methods do not differentiate virulent from nonvirulent isolates, so it is important to sample only from systemic sites such as pleura, pericardium, peritoneum, joints, and brain. Isolation of *H parasuis* from the upper respiratory tract has no relevance in the diagnosis of systemic infection. Samples collected from clinically affected animals that were euthanized increase the chances of isolation. Recently, a multiplex PCR technique able to differentiate between virulent and nonvirulent isolates has been developed. This technique might be used to prevent introduction of pigs carrying potentially virulent strains onto farms that are free of clinical Glässer's disease.

Differential diagnoses of Glässer's disease include infections by *Streptococcus suis*, *Mycoplasma hyorhinis*, septicemic *Escherichia coli*, *Actinobacillus suis*, *Erysipelothrix rhusiopathiae*, and *Salmonella* Choleraesuis.

Treatment and Control: *H parasuis* is one of the few gram-negative organisms that can be successfully treated with synthetic penicillin. Other antimicrobials used include ceftiofur, ampicillin, enrofloxacin, erythromycin, tiamulin, tilmicosin, florfenicol, and potentiated sulfonamides. Individual treatments must be given parenterally to see a significant effect, and all pigs in the affected group (not just those showing clinical signs) should be treated. Preventive treatments can be given via water or feed medication. Either commercial or autogenous vaccines can be used to control *H parasuis* infection, although their efficacy has been variable. The broad range of potentially pathogenic serovars and genotypes has impaired the development of a universal vaccine for *H parasuis*. Homologous protection between isolates from the same serovar group is relatively satisfactory, whereas heterologous protection is restricted to a few serovars. So far, several "universal" (independent of serovar) vaccine prototypes have been experimentally developed but are not yet commercially available.

NIPAH VIRUS INFECTION

(Porcine respiratory and neurologic syndrome, Barking pig syndrome)

Nipah virus disease is a relatively newly discovered disease of swine and people associated with infection with a novel paramyxovirus named Nipah virus. This disease emerged in Malaysia in 1998 and 1999. It was linked to severe encephalitis among people occupationally exposed to infected pigs in Malaysia and Singapore. The disease was eradicated from the national commercial swine population by control efforts. Fruit bats of the genus *Pteropus* appear to be reservoirs of the virus.

Etiology and Epidemiology: The etiologic agent, Nipah virus (genus *Henipavirus*, family Paramyxoviridae), is an enveloped, negative-sense, single-stranded RNA virus. The virus is closely related to Hendra virus (*see* p 707), the only other member of the genus. The human outbreak in Malaysia and Singapore followed contact with infected swine and resulted in encephalitis with ~40% case mortality. The virus is assumed to have been introduced into the swine population from one of the two species of *Pteropus* found with antibodies during investigation of the outbreak. *Pteropus* spp range from the Western Pacific through southeast Asia, and south Asia down through coastal African islands, including Madagascar. Several species of *Pteropus* have been found with antibodies, suggesting that the virus or closely related viruses occur in other areas within the range of this genus of bats. In Malaysia, genetic analysis of virus from human and swine clinical materials strongly supported a single introduction of the virus with spread through the commercial swine population. There was evidence of infection among several other species of domestic animals, including dogs, cats, and horses. Human encephalitis caused by Nipah viruses in south Asia has been a regular occurrence since 2001 in Bangladesh and more recently in adjacent areas of India. In these areas, epidemiology has not supported the role of intermediary domestic species but rather more direct transmission from the flying fox reservoir of the virus. More recently, fruit bats belonging to the family Pteropidae, but not the genus *Pteropus*, were found to harbor related viruses in Africa.

Transmission and Pathogenesis: Infection in pigs is assumed to have been a transfer from the reservoir bat species to pigs. Once the virus was introduced into an intensive swine husbandry setting, infection of animals within premises was rapid, and serologic tests suggested that nearly all pigs on an affected premise were infected. Transmission between premises was thought to be by poor biosecurity procedures and movement of infected animals. Experimental infection of swine with Nipah virus in a high biosecurity facility in Geelong supported that transmission between swine in close contact occurred readily. In south Asia, infection of people appears to occur by indirect means from the reservoir fruit bats; contamination of sap collected in pots on palm trees is a recurring means of infection in regular cases occurring in Bangladesh. Other similar circumstances, such as contact with trees contaminated by bats or consumption of fruit partially eaten by bats, are other documented means of infection in Bangladesh. Person-to-person transmission, although not evident in Malaysia, has also occurred in south Asia.

Clinical Findings: Because of the danger of human infection from infected pigs and the emergency setting, clinical observations were not detailed in the field during the original epidemic. Most pigs developed a febrile respiratory disease with a severe cough that led to the local names for the disease—"barking pig syndrome" and "one-mile cough." Encephalitis was also noted, particularly in the sows and boars in affected facilities. The proportion of animals with each form of the disease is uncertain, although the respiratory form predominated. Overall mortality within affected facilities was also not well documented but probably was not >5% among all age groups.

Diagnosis: Laboratory diagnosis can be made by isolation of the virus, identification of the RNA by use of reverse transcriptase-PCR, detection of antigens in tissues by immunohistochemical staining with specific antibodies, or serologic tests such as indirect ELISA and virus neutralization tests. The virus is considered biosafety level 4 in the USA and Australia, and stringent laboratory containment at limited laboratories is a special consideration.

Treatment: Treatment of affected swine was not attempted during the Malaysian emergency. Human patients required intensive care with ventilation support to manage the encephalitis; no specific treatment is available. Ribavirin was administered to some patients, but subsequent studies in laboratory animals suggest that it is ineffective.

Control and Prevention: Control of the epidemic/epizootic in Malaysia was dependent on the initiation of strict quarantine procedures and the slaughter of all swine from affected facilities. Adherence to appropriate biosecurity and quarantine procedures within facilities, as with other contagious diseases, is of paramount importance in preventing spread of the infection. An active surveillance and slaughter program successfully eliminated the virus from the national commercial swine population, which has remained free of infection. Presence of the virus in reservoir species of bats in a wide geographic range emphasizes the importance of good disease surveillance and biosecurity practices to promote early detection and confine the disease to initial premises should reintroduction occur.

Zoonotic Risk: Transmission of the virus from infected pigs to people was largely in an occupational setting, and a study of risk factors associated with human infection suggests that close contact with live infected swine was the means of infection of nearly all human Nipah virus infections in Malaysia.

Continued sporadic clusters in horses and subsequent human cases with Hendra virus in Australia, with serious disease in some of these clusters, emphasize the importance of use of appropriate personal protective equipment in veterinary clinical examinations or postmortem procedures when Hendra or Nipah virus infection is suspected.

PORCINE CIRCOVIRUS DISEASES

(Postweaning multisystemic wasting syndrome, Porcine dermatitis and nephropathy syndrome)

A novel, noncytopathogenic, picornavirus-like contaminant in the porcine kidney cell line PK-15 (ATCC-CCL33) was described in 1974. This agent was later shown to be a small, nonenveloped virus containing a single-stranded, circular DNA genome; it was named porcine circovirus (PCV). PCV antibodies in swine were found to be widespread, and experimental infections with this virus in pigs did not result in clinical disease, suggesting that PCV was nonpathogenic.

A new disease was described in Western Canada during the early and mid 1990s. The etiology was unknown, and the condition was named postweaning multisystemic wasting syndrome (PMWS). Affected pigs, mainly nursery pigs, showed primarily poor growth rate, ill thrift, and/or wasting, and they were histopathologically characterized by systemic inflammatory lesions. In the late 1990s, an apparently novel PCV-like virus was isolated from PMWS-affected pigs. The new virus was antigenically and genetically distinct from the PCV contaminant of PK-15 cell cultures. Subsequently, PCV isolates from diseased pigs were designated as porcine circovirus type 2 viruses (PCV2) and the original PCV from PK-15 cell cultures as porcine circovirus type 1.

PCV2 has been further associated with a number of disease syndromes in pigs, so the term porcine circovirus disease (PCVD) was proposed as a collective name. Recently, the terms PCV2-systemic disease (PCV2-SD) and PCV2-reproductive disease (PCV2-RD) have been proposed to replace PMWS and PCV2-associated reproductive failure, respectively. Moreover, it is currently thought that the most important PCVD is the PCV2-subclinical infection (PCV2-SI), which is linked with growth retardation without overt clinical signs. Porcine dermatitis and nephropathy syndrome (PDNS) is also included as a PCVD, although there is still no proof of PCV2 as the antigen linked with this immunocomplex disease. PCV2 has also been associated with porcine respiratory disease complex, although its impact is probably linked to the occurrence of PCV2-SD. PCV2-SD and PCV2-SI are the PCVDs considered to severely impact swine production worldwide, but the introduction of efficacious vaccines to the market has largely ameliorated their effects.

Etiology and Pathogenesis: Circoviruses are small (17–22 nm in diameter), nonenveloped viruses that contain a single strand of circular DNA. There are two types of porcine circovirus, although only PCV2 is considered pathogenic. Phylogenetic studies have shown that at least three genotypes of PCV2 exist (PCV2 a, b, and c). Recent studies suggested a genotype shift (from a to b; PCV2c has been retrospectively detected in Denmark during the 1980s) coincidental with major outbreaks of PCV2-SD in North America, Japan, and some European countries. It is not clear whether differences in virulence exist among or within PCV2 genotypes.

Serologic surveys show that PCV2 is widespread in swine, independent of the PCV2-SD status of the farm. Results from retrospective serologic studies indicate that PCV2 has been infecting pigs for >50 years so far, and phylogenetic studies indicate that PCV2 has probably circulated in pigs during the past 100 years.

Initially, PCV2-SD was identified in high health herds that were free of most common swine pathogens. However, under field conditions, swine that show signs of PCV2-SD usually are infected with multiple agents, including porcine parvovirus, porcine reproductive and respiratory syndrome virus, *Mycoplasma hyopneumoniae*, *Actinobacillus pleuropneumoniae*, *Pasteurella multocida*, *Haemophilus parasuis*, *Staphylococcus* spp, and *Streptococcus* spp.

Accounts of multiple attempts to experimentally reproduce PCV2-SD have been published. Some early trials (using tissue homogenates from pigs affected with PCV2-SD or a PCV2 isolate) reproduced PCV2-SD–like histologic lesions but not the wasting condition. However, occasional studies subsequently reproduced clinical disease and lesions consistent with PCV2-SD using only PCV2, presumably, as inoculum. Consequently, it was suggested that PCV2 infection, linked to other cofactors, was necessary for the consistent development of full clinical disease. It appears that a number of factors, such as age and source of pigs, environmental conditions, genetics, the nature of the PCV2 inoculum used, and the immunologic status of the pig at PCV2 infection, play a significant role in the consistent experimental reproducibility of the disease. In fact, the more consistent and repeatable PCV2-SD disease models have been obtained using infectious and noninfectious cofactors as triggers. Also, the coinfection of PCV2a and b genotypes has been linked to reproduction of clinical disease under experimental conditions. The mechanisms by which other viruses or immunostimulation may trigger the development of wasting in PCV2-infected pigs is still unknown. High loads of PCV2 in blood, lymphoid, and other tissues and in potential excretion routes are associated with the expression of disease.

When multisystemic disease and wasting is apparent, damage to the immune system is the main feature suggesting that affected pigs have an acquired immunodeficiency. Lymphocyte depletion of lymphoid tissues, changes in peripheral blood mononuclear cell subpopulations, and altered cytokine expression patterns have all been demonstrated in pigs naturally and experimentally affected with PCV2-SD.

The identification of cells that support PCV2 replication has been a matter of controversy. The large amount of PCV2 virus antigen found in the macrophages and dendritic cells of diseased pigs appears to be the result of accumulation of viral particles. However, epithelial and endothelial cells seem to be the main target for PCV2 replication, as well as a small proportion of macrophages and lymphocytes.

Much less is known regarding the pathogenesis of other PCVDs. PCV2 is able to replicate in fetuses as well as in zona pellucida–free embryos. Moreover, an experiment with embryos exposed to PCV2 and then transferred to receptor sows suggested that infection can lead to embryonic death. Therefore, it is believed that one of the potential outcomes of PCV2 infection in sows could be return to estrus. Transplacental transmission of PCV2 has been demonstrated. However, experiments using pregnant sows inoculated intranasally have yielded variable results. When successful, those studies have shown that PCV2 may cause fetal death, similar to that of porcine parvovirosis, with live pigs together with dead piglets and mummies of different sizes.

PDNS is considered a type III hypersensitivity reaction in which the antigen present in the immune complexes is unknown. It has been speculated that PCV2 could be the antigen, but there is no definitive proof that PCV2 causes PDNS lesions. Indirect evidence exists, such as significantly higher serum antibody titers to PCV2 in affected pigs compared with healthy or PCV2-SD-affected pigs.

Epidemiology and Transmission: PCV2 is considered a ubiquitous virus in countries with and without PCVDs, including PCV2-SD. PCV2 infection and PCV2-SD have also been described in wild boars. The disease has been reported worldwide.

Transmission may be by direct contact with infected pigs. PCV2 has been detected in almost all potential excretion routes such as nasal, ocular, and bronchial secretions; saliva; urine; and feces. The virus can be found in semen, but the practical importance of this is probably negligible. Artificial insemination (AI) of sows with PCV2-infected semen from experimentally inoculated boars did not result in sow infection or fetal infection. However, when such AI was performed with PCV2-spiked semen, reproductive problems were developed. Therefore, it seems that reproductive disease linked to AI is possible, but only when semen has a high virus load, which is unlikely under natural conditions. Although not demonstrated, it is assumed that contact with contaminated fomites, exposure to contaminated feeds or biologic products, multiple use of hypodermic needles, or biting insects may play a role in transmission.

PCV2 may persist in swine for several months under either experimental or field conditions. Convalescent swine may carry virus for extended periods and be important in disease transmission. PCV2 is fairly resistant to commonly used disinfectants and to irradiation, probably allowing it to accumulate in the environment and be infective for new groups of susceptible pigs if rigorous sanitary measures are not followed. The decline of colostral antibody titer in pigs is associated with onset of PCV2-SD in late nursery or finishing pigs. Transplacental infection with PCV2 has been documented, but it is not known whether pigs infected in utero are able to subsequently develop clinical PCV2-SD.

Some reports have suggested that animals other than swine may be infected with PCV2 or PCV-like viruses. However, results of serologic studies for antibody against PCV in cattle and other livestock have been contradictory, and experimental induction of disease using PCV1 or PCV2 in species of livestock other than swine has not been successful. Mice may be able to replicate and harbor the virus.

Clinical Findings: PCV2-SD is characterized by overt weight loss. Disease often occurs in the fattening units in pigs 8–18 wk old, although the disease can be also seen in older or younger pigs. Morbidity is typically 5%–20% among cohorts in the late nursery or finishing stages. Mortality in swine with signs of PCV2-SD can occasionally be >50%. In addition to death loss, PCV2-SD in finishing pigs may cause a substantial increase in time to reach market weight, resulting in economic loss. Growth retardation, wasting, and dyspnea are the clinical signs seen most frequently in outbreaks. Pallor, anemia, jaundice, diarrhea, and palpable inguinal lymphadenopathy also are seen in some affected pigs. A low-grade fever (104°–106°F [40°–41°C]) that lasts several days may be seen as well. Overcrowding, poor air quality, insufficient air exchange, and commingled age groups seem to exacerbate the course of the disease. Usually, only a few pigs in a group show wasting. The onset of disease may be acute, leading to death within a few days in some pigs. Other pigs show a more chronic disease and fail to gain weight or thrive.

PCV2-SI is believed to occur in pigs that become infected with the virus and suffer from growth retardation (significantly lower average daily weight gain [ADWG]) but not overt clinical signs. In fact, in a farm affected by PCV2-SD, a variable proportion of pigs developed the systemic disease, while most had only subclinical infection. PCV2-SI had been unnoticed for many years until the advent of vaccines drew attention to this condition. Vaccinated pigs have an increased ADWG compared with nonvaccinated, apparently healthy counterparts. Such difference has been demonstrated to vary between 10–40 g/d, depending on the farm.

PCV2-RD characterized by late-term abortions and stillbirths in the absence or presence of other well-known reproductive pathogens seems to be the hallmark of clinical PCV2 infection in sows. Most of these descriptions come from North America and usually occur in start-up herds. Return to estrus due to embryonic death as a potential outcome of intrauterine PCV2 infection has been suggested based on experimental data. However, there are no field data unequivocally supporting this effect.

PDNS may affect nursery and growing pigs and, sporadically, adult animals. The prevalence of the syndrome in affected herds is relatively low (<1%), although higher prevalences (>20%) have been described occasionally. Pigs with severe acute disease die within a few days after the onset of clinical signs, due to acute renal failure with a significant increase in serum levels of creatinine and urea. Surviving pigs tend to recover and gain weight 7–10 days after the beginning of the syndrome. Affected pigs have anorexia, depression, prostration, stiff gait and/or reluctance to move, and normal temperatures or mild fever. The most obvious sign in the acute phase is the presence of irregular, red-to-purple macules and papules on the skin of the hindlimbs and perineal area, although distribution may be generalized in severely affected animals. With time, the lesions become covered by dark crusts and fade gradually (usually in 2–3 wk), sometimes leaving scars.

Lesions: PCV2-SD is diagnosed by characteristic histopathologic findings in affected pigs. Grossly, lymph nodes may be substantially enlarged and pale on cut surface, the thymus atrophied, and the tonsils thinner than normal. Splenic infarcts also may be present in a low proportion of pigs affected with PCV2-SD. Histopathologic lymphoid lesions are characteristic, showing lymphocytic depletion and granulomatous inflammation, sometimes with the presence of multinucleate giant cells and amphophilic botryoid intracytoplasmic inclusion bodies of different sizes caused by accumulation of PCV2 particles.

Lesions in the lung are common in affected pigs; their severity is influenced by duration of disease and presence of concurrent infections. Gross lung lesions may include failure to collapse, firmness, diffuse pulmonary edema, mottling, and consolidation. Microscopically, a variable degree of lymphohistiocytic interstitial pneumonia to granulomatous bronchointerstitial pneumonia with bronchiolitis and bronchiolar fibrosis can be seen.

Grossly, the liver may appear icteric and/or atrophic in a low proportion of affected pigs. Interlobular connective tissue may be prominent. Microscopic lesions range from single cell necrosis (apoptosis) with mild lymphocytic infiltration of portal zones to extensive lymphohistiocytic periportal hepatitis with diffuse necrosis of hepatocytes. The kidneys may be enlarged and show scattered to diffuse white foci on the cortical surface. Microscopic lesions include interstitial lymphohistiocytic infiltration. Other lesions seen in affected pigs include gastric ulceration (probably due in part to a prolonged fattening period in chronically affected pigs) and occasional multifocal lymphohistiocytic myocarditis. In severely affected pigs, lymphohistiocytic infiltrates can be seen in virtually all tissues.

PCV2-SI pigs do not show gross lesions attributable to PCV2 infection. These animals may show microscopic lymphoid lesions similar to those seen in pigs with PCV2-SD, although only to a mild degree.

In PCV2-RD, stillborn and nonviable neonatal piglets show chronic passive congestion of the liver and cardiac hypertrophy with multifocal areas of myocardial discoloration. The key histopathologic feature is fibrosing and/or necrotizing myocarditis in fetuses.

PDNS is easy to detect from a clinical point of view because of the red-to-dark macules and papules, which correspond microscopically to necrosis and hemorrhage secondary to necrotizing vasculitis of dermal and hypodermal capillaries and arterioles. Necrotizing vasculitis is a systemic feature, but it is more prominent in the skin, renal pelvis, mesentery, and spleen (splenic infarcts may also be present as a result of necrotizing vasculitis of splenic arteries or arterioles). Apart from skin lesions, pigs that die acutely with PDNS have firm, bilaterally enlarged kidneys, with a fine granular cortical surface and edema of the renal pelvis. The renal cortex displays multiple, small, reddish pinpoint lesions, similar to petechial hemorrhages, which microscopically correspond to enlarged and inflamed glomeruli (fibrinonecrotizing glomerulitis). Histologically, a moderate to severe nonpurulent interstitial nephritis with dilation of renal tubules is also seen. Usually, both skin and renal lesions are present, but in some cases, skin or renal lesions may occur alone. Lymph nodes may be enlarged and red due to blood drainage from affected zones with hemorrhages (mainly skin). Histopathologically, PCV2-SD–like lesions such as lymphocyte depletion and histiocytic and/or multinucleate giant cell infiltration (although less severe) are usually found in lymphoid tissues of affected pigs, although to a milder degree.

Diagnosis: The PCV2-SD case definition includes three main diagnostic criteria: 1) clinical signs of wasting or ill thrift, 2) presence of gross and microscopic (moderate and severe) lesions characteristic of the disease, and 3) presence of viral antigen or DNA (moderate to high amount) in the microscopic lymphoid lesions. Visualization of viral DNA or antigen in lesions is usually done using in situ hybridization or immunohistochemistry, respectively, and moderate to high amounts of virus are linked to the disease. A herd case definition has been proposed, which includes two main criteria: 1) significant increase of mortality and number of runt pigs or pigs failing to gain weight or thrive in comparison to previous values for the farm, and 2) fulfillment of the three individual criteria listed above in at least one of five examined pigs. Differential diagnoses include conditions causing increased mortality and growth retardation, such as PRRS, chronic respiratory disease, Glässer's disease, salmonellosis, porcine intestinal adenomatosis, and many others.

Because PCV2 is ubiquitous and the virus replicates in individual pigs for weeks to months, isolation of virus, detection of PCV2 DNA in serum or tissues, or detection of PCV2 antibodies in serum is not sufficient to establish a diagnosis of PCV2-SD. Antibodies against PCV2 may be detected by ELISA, indirect fluorescent antibody, or immunoperoxidase staining of infected cell cultures. Viral isolation can be done on several porcine cell lines (mainly porcine kidney cells) using serum, bronchiolar lavage fluid, or tissue homogenates. Viral DNA can be detected using PCR in most tissues or in serum from affected pigs. Several tissue samples from multiple pigs may be required for detection of virus in cases of chronic disease. Virus quantification in serum by real time quantitative PCR (qRT-PCR) has been suggested as a potential diagnostic method in live pigs. Values of

>107 PCV2 genome copies/mL of serum usually have been linked with PCV2-SD occurrence. However, PCV2 infection is extremely common in clinically healthy pigs, and interpretation of positive qRT-PCR results is not always straightforward.

The diagnostic approach of PCV2-SI is of less interest for clinicians, because lack of overt clinical signs plus demonstration of infection by PCR would be enough to establish such a diagnosis. Values of >105 or 106 PCV2 genome copies/mL of serum usually have been linked with the subclinical infection.

The diagnosis of PCV2-RD should include the following criteria: 1) late-term abortions and stillbirths, sometimes with hypertrophy of the fetal heart, 2) extensive fibrosing and/or necrotizing myocarditis, and 3) high concentrations of PCV2 in the myocardial lesions and other fetal tissues. Differential diagnoses for PCV2-RD include PRRS, porcine parvovirus, pseudorabies (Aujeszky disease), leptospirosis, and other diseases that cause late abortions, stillbirths, and weak piglets. So far, there are no formal criteria to diagnose a putative return to estrus associated with PCV2 infection. However, the occurrence of such signs together with evidence of viral circulation during the clinical episode should be demonstrated.

The case definition for PDNS is relatively simple and includes two main criteria: 1) presence of hemorrhagic and necrotizing skin lesions, mainly located on the hindlimbs and perineal area, and/or swollen and pale kidneys with generalized cortical petechiae, and 2) presence of systemic necrotizing vasculitis as well as necrotizing and fibrinous glomerulonephritis. From a diagnostic point of view, detection of PCV2 is not included in the diagnostic criteria.

Differential diagnosis of PDNS depends on the most significant pathologic outcome. Cutaneous manifestations may be confused with classical and African swine fever, swine erysipelas, septicemic salmonellosis, infection with *Actinobacillus suis*, porcine stress syndrome, transit erythema (urine-soaked floors, chemical burns, etc), and other bacterial septicemias. Differential diagnoses for kidney lesions include classical and African swine fever, swine erysipelas, and septicemic salmonellosis. Serum biochemical analyses may help differentiate PDNS from other diseases; urea and creatinine concentrations are markedly increased.

Treatment and Control: Because PCV2-SD is a multifactorial disease, effective control measures before the advent of PCV2 vaccines were focused on control or eradication of these triggers. The most widely used control measures were the use of antibiotics to prevent concurrent bacterial infections, improvement of biosecurity and sanitary measures such as isolation of affected pigs and disinfection of pens after their use, decreasing stressors (eg, high stocking density, inadequate ventilation, inadequate temperature control), and control of concomitant viral infections, especially PRRS. Other prevention and control measures used on young pigs before the anticipated time of onset include injection of vitamins, IP injection of serum harvested from finishing pigs, and vaccination against common pathogens.

Currently, control of PCV2-SD as well as PCV2-SI is based on use of PCV2 vaccines. There are four major commercial vaccines worldwide (plus a higher number with regional availability, mainly in southeast Asia). The first commercial vaccine was based on an inactivated PCV2 isolate and was licensed for use in sows and gilts. The same vaccine was later licensed for use in piglets. Subsequently, three more vaccines have been developed, all for use in piglets ~2–3 wk old or older. Two of these are subunit vaccines (PCV2 capsid protein produced in a baculovirus system), and the third is an inactivated virus constructed by replacing the capsid gene of the nonpathogenic PCV1 with that of PCV2. In addition to significantly reducing mortality and runting percentages, these vaccines seem to improve ADWG, batch uniformity, slaughter weight uniformity, and feed conversion rate.

All commercial PCV2 vaccines are based on PCV2a isolates, but cross-protection has been demonstrated against PCV2b. All PCV2 vaccines are able to generate both cellular and humoral immune responses, which are believed to be the key features to control the subsequent PCV2 infection that occurs under field conditions.

No treatment has proved successful for PDNS. Only those epizootic cases with moderate to high morbidity and mortality rates may be important in terms of economic losses. Treatment using a wide range of antimicrobial agents has been unsuccessful. Because the antigen responsible for triggering PDNS is not known, no preventive recommendations are indicated. Importantly, the use of PCV2 vaccines worldwide has significantly reduced occurrence of this condition, emphasizing the putative implication of PCV2 in its pathogenesis.

PORCINE HEMAGGLUTINATING ENCEPHALOMYELITIS

(Vomiting and wasting disease, Coronaviral encephalomyelitis)

Porcine hemagglutinating encephalomyelitis, a viral disease of young pigs, is characterized by vomiting, constipation, and anorexia and results either in rapid death or chronic emaciation (vomiting and wasting). Also, motor disorders due to acute encephalomyelitis (hemagglutinating encephalomyelitis) are often seen during field outbreaks.

Etiology, Epidemiology, and Pathogenesis: The causal coronavirus, porcine hemagglutinating encephalomyelitis virus (PHEV), is of a single antigenic type, and it grows in several types of porcine cell cultures, in which it causes syncytia. It agglutinates RBCs of several animal species. Pigs are the only natural host. The virus is spread via aerosol. It has no public health significance.

Based on virus detection and/or serology, PHEV Infection has been reported from several countries in Europe and from North and South America (Argentina), Australia, and Asia (Mainland China, Taiwan,PRC, South Korea); thus, it appears to be widespread. The virus is endemic in most breeding herds, and a herd immunity exists. The infection usually remains subclinical. Immune sows transfer maternal antibodies to their piglets, which are protected until they have developed an age resistance; thus, clinical outbreaks are rare. However, if the virus enters a susceptible herd with neonatal piglets, morbidity and mortality may be high.

The virus first replicates in the nasal mucosa, tonsils, lungs, and to a very limited extent, in the small intestine. From these sites of entry, the virus invades defined nuclei of the medulla oblongata via the peripheral nervous system and subsequently spreads to the entire brain stem, and possibly to the cerebrum and cerebellum. Vomiting is thought to be caused by viral replication in the vagal sensory ganglion. Wasting is due to vomiting and delayed emptying of the stomach, which is the result of virus-induced lesions in the intramural plexus. Infection of cerebral and cerebellar neurons may cause motor disorders.

Clinical Findings: Both clinical syndromes, the vomiting and wasting disease (VWD) and the encephalitic forms, are confined almost exclusively to pigs <4 wk old. The "VWD form" has an incubation period of 4–7 days. Repeated retching and vomiting are seen. Pigs start suckling but soon stop, withdraw from the sow, and vomit the milk they have ingested. They dip their mouths into water bowls but drink little, possibly indicative of pharyngeal paralysis. The persistent vomiting results in a rapid decline of condition. Neonatal pigs become dehydrated, cyanotic, and comatose and die. Older pigs continue to vomit, although less frequently than in the early stage of the disease. They lose appetite and become emaciated. A large distention of the cranial abdomen can develop. This "wasting" state may persist for 1–6 wk until the pigs die of starvation. Mortality approaches 100% within the litter, and survivors remain permanently stunted.

The "encephalomyelitic form" also starts with vomiting, usually 4–7 days after birth. Vomiting continues intermittently for 1–2 days, but it is rarely severe and does not result in dehydration. After 1–3 days, generalized muscle tremors and hyperesthesia are seen. The pigs tend to walk backward, often ending in a dog-sitting position. They soon become weak, are unable to rise, and paddle their limbs. Blindness, opisthotonos, and nystagmus also occur. After a few days, they become dyspneic, comatose, and die. More recently, some outbreaks have been reported from Taiwan,PRC and South Korea in which pigs 30–50 days old showed motor disorders. Morbidity and mortality of the encephalomyelitic form are high (as much as 100%) in neonatal pigs but both decrease with increasing age. Both clinical forms of PHEV infection may be seen during an outbreak on the same farm.

From onset to disappearance, an outbreak on a farm lasts 2–3 wk. Disappearance of disease coincides with the development of immunity in sows in late pregnancy, which subsequently protects piglets via maternal antibodies.

Lesions: Cachexia and abdominal distention are seen in chronically affected pigs. Their stomachs are dilated and filled with gas. Microscopically, perivascular cuffing, gliosis, and neuronal degeneration are found in the medulla in 70%–100% of pigs with nervous signs and in 20%–60% of pigs with VWD. Neuritis of peripheral sensory ganglia, particularly the trigeminal ganglia, is seen regularly. Degeneration of the ganglia of the stomach wall and perivascular cuffing are found in 15%–85% of pigs with VWD. The lesions are most pronounced in the pyloric gland area.

Diagnosis: A laboratory diagnosis can be made routinely by virus isolation from the brain stem and, to be successful, the pigs are preferably euthanized within 2 days after signs appear. It is difficult to isolate the virus from pigs that have been affected for >2–3 days. Other diagnostic techniques, based on antigen or nucleic acid (RT-PCR) detection, have been developed and applied recently.

A significant rise in antibody titer can be demonstrated in paired serum samples. Because of the rather long incubation period, pigs may start to build up a low antibody titer 2–3 days after the first signs appear. Therefore, the acute serum must be collected immediately after disease starts.

Differential diagnoses include pseudorabies (*see* p 1300) and teschovirus encephalomyelitis (*see* p 1307). Respiratory signs in older pigs and abortions in sows are part of a pseudorabies outbreak. In teschovirus encephalomyelitis, older pigs are usually involved.

Control: There is no treatment. Once signs are evident, the disease runs its course. Spontaneous recoveries are rare. Piglets born from nonimmune sows during the outbreak can be protected by being injected, at birth, either with hyperimmune serum or, if this is not available, with pooled serum collected from older sows at a slaughterhouse. However, the time lapse between diagnosis and cessation of the disease is usually too short for this procedure to be effective. Maintaining the virus on the farm (thus retaining naturally induced immunity in the sows) avoids outbreaks in piglets.

PORCINE REPRODUCTIVE AND RESPIRATORY SYNDROME

Porcine reproductive and respiratory syndrome (PRRS) was first reported in the USA in 1987. Since then, outbreaks of PRRS and successful isolation of the virus have been confirmed throughout North America and Europe.

Etiology and Epidemiology: The etiologic agent is a virus in the group Arteriviridae. The virus is enveloped and ranges in size from 45 to 80 mm. Inactivation is possible after treatment with ether or chloroform; however, the virus is very stable under freezing conditions, retaining its infectivity for 4 mo at –70°C (–94°F). As the temperature rises, infectivity is reduced (15–20 min at 56°C [132.8°F]).

After infection of a naive herd, exposure of all members of the breeding population is inconsistent, leading to development of naive, exposed, and persistently infected subpopulations of sows. This situation is exacerbated over time through the addition of improperly acclimated replacement gilts and leads to shedding of the virus from carrier animals to those that have not been previously exposed.

The primary vector for transmission of the virus is the infected pig. Contact transmission has been demonstrated experimentally, and spread of virus from infected seedstock originating from a single source has been described. Introduction of infected seedstock can lead to the introduction and coexistence of genetically diverse isolates of PRRS virus on the same farm. Controlled studies have indicated that infected swine may be longterm carriers, with adults able to shed PRRS virus for up to 86 days after infection, and weaned pigs able to harbor virus for 157 days. Experimentally infected boars can shed virus in the semen up to 93 days after infection.

Aerosol transmission of the virus has been confirmed as an indirect route of transmission and may depend on isolate pathogenicity. Highly virulent isolates that produce high titers of virus in blood and tissues have been shown to be spread via aerosols at a significantly higher frequency than less pathogenic isolates. Environmental factors, such as wind direction and velocity, significantly impact spread via this route as well. PRRS virus can also be transmitted by fomites, such as contaminated needles, boots, coveralls, transport vehicles, and shipping containers. Farm personnel are not a risk, unless hands are contaminated with blood from viremic pigs. Finally, transmission via certain species of insects (mosquitoes [*Aedes vexans*] and house flies [*Musca domestica*]) has been reported.

Clinical Findings: PRRS appears to have two distinct clinical phases: reproductive failure and postweaning respiratory diseases. The reproductive phase of the disease includes increases in the number of stillborn piglets, mummified fetuses, premature farrowings, and weak-born pigs. Stillbirths and mummies may increase up to 25%–35%, and abortions can be >10%. Anorexia and agalactia are evident in lactating sows and result in increased (30%–50%) preweaning mortality. Suckling piglets develop a characteristic thumping respiratory pattern, and histopathologic examination of lung tissue reveals a severe, necrotizing, interstitial pneumonia. PRRS is capable of crossing the placenta in the third and possibly second trimester of gestation. Piglets may also be born viremic and transmit the virus for 112 days after infection. Performance after weaning is also affected. Infection with PRRS virus results in destruction of mature alveolar macrophages, which has led to the hypothesis that infection results in immune suppression; however, controlled studies indicate that the virus may actually enhance specific parameters of the immune response.

Outbreaks of the reproductive form of PRRS have been reported to last 1–4 mo, depending on the facilities and initial health status of the pigs. In contrast, the postweaning pneumonic phase can become chronic, reducing daily gain by 85% and increasing mortality to 10%–25%. Numerous other pathogens are commonly isolated along with PRRS virus from affected nursery or finishing pigs. Other bacteria such as *Streptococcus suis*, *Escherichia coli*, *Salmonella* Choleraesuis, *Haemophilus parasuis*, and *Mycoplasma hyopneumoniae* have been reported, as well as viruses such as porcine respiratory coronavirus and *swine influenza virus*. Finally, differences in the clinical response to PRRS virus may also be due to strain variation. Studies have demonstrated the ability of different isolates to induce varying degrees of interstitial pneumonia in cesarean-derived/colostrum-deprived (CD/CD) piglets after intranasal inoculation.

Diagnosis: The most commonly used serologic assay is the ELISA. It measures IgG antibodies to PRRS virus. It cannot measure the level of immunity in an animal or predict whether the animal is a carrier. Titers are detected within 7–10 days after infection and can persist for up to 144 days. Tests for PRRS virus include PCR, virus isolation, and immunohistochemistry. Nucleic acid sequencing of the open reading frame 5 region of the virus is an excellent tool for epidemiologic investigations in the field to confirm similarity between isolates recovered from different sites. Recently, oral fluid sampling has been widely applied as a means to sample a population of pigs. This method is cost effective and convenient and can be used for both virus and antibody detection at the pen level.

Treatment and Control: Currently, there are no effective treatment programs for acute PRRS. Attempts to reduce fever using NSAIDs (aspirin) or appetite stimulants (B vitamins) appear to have minimal benefit. The use of antibiotics or autogenous bacterins to reduce the effects of opportunistic bacterial pathogens has also been reported; however, results have been mixed.

Prevention of infection appears to be the primary means of control. Understanding the PRRS status of replacement gilts and boars, as well as proper isolation and acclimatization of incoming stock, are critical measures to prevent viral introduction. Pigs should be retested on arrival at the isolation facility and 45–60 days later, before entry to the herd. Elimination of existing infection by multisite production and segregated early weaning has also been described. Although these strategies have had some success, the longterm risks of reinfection appear high. Prevention of viral spread by nursery depopulation has been described. This is successful when virus transmission is not occurring in the sow herd (usually 12–18 mo after initial outbreak), but the nurseries and growing/finishing pigs are still infected. All nursery pigs are removed from the farm to be finished elsewhere. The nurseries are then aggressively washed and disinfected and left empty for 7–14 days, after which they can be used normally. The technique has successfully eliminated PRRS virus from several herds, and pigs have remained seronegative (for >1 yr) to market age; production in the nurseries has improved, both in growth rate and mortality.

Commercial modified-live vaccines have been licensed and have been effective in controlling outbreaks, reducing shedding, and preventing economic losses.

Elimination of PRRS virus has been demonstrated to be possible on an individual farm basis. Methods such as whole herd depopulation-repopulation, test and removal, and herd closure have been documented as effective methods to eliminate PRRS virus from endemically infected herds. Unfortunately, a number of eradication efforts have failed because of introduction of new isolates through unidentifiable routes. This has resulted in an increased level of biosecurity on farms. Strict quarantine and testing programs, the purchase of PRRS virus-naive breeding stock and semen, sanitation of transport vehicles, and strict protocols of fomite and personnel movement between farms are critical components of an effective program. Recent advances in monitoring the status of artificial insemination centers include PCR analysis of blood samples collected from the auricular vein (blood swab). In addition, the application of air filtration to artificial insemination centers and breeding herds has been shown to significantly reduce the risk of airborne entry of the virus.

STREPTOCOCCAL INFECTIONS IN PIGS

Of the bacterial group of gram-positive cocci comprising the genera *Streptococcus*, *Enterococcus*, and *Peptostreptococcus*, streptococci constitute the most significant pathogens of swine. Streptococci are also associated with infectious conditions of people, cattle, sheep, goats, and horses. Relative to pigs, *S suis* (an α-hemolytic *Streptococcus*) is by far the most important agent of infectious diseases in this group, affecting mainly nursing and recently weaned pigs. Septicemia, meningitis, polyserositis, polyarthritis, and bronchopneumonia are associated with *S suis* infections. *Streptococcus dysgalactiae equisimilis* is considered the most important β-hemolytic *Streptococcus* involved in lesions in pigs, and it has been judged to be of etiologic significance in autopsy reports. *S porcinus*, another β-hemolytic *Streptococcus*, has been associated particularly in the USA with a contagious clinical entity in growing pigs known as streptococcal lymphadenitis, jowl abscesses, or cervical abscesses. Enterococci reside in the intestinal tract and may cause disease in multiple species. In pigs, the *E faecium* species group, mainly *E durans* and *E hirae*, are especially associated with enteritis and diarrhea.

STREPTOCOCCUS SUIS INFECTION

S suis is a significant pathogen of swine and one of the most important causes of bacterial mortality in piglets after weaning. It is considered a normal inhabitant of the upper respiratory tract (especially nonvirulent strains) and can be easily found in tonsils, which are considered a natural niche. It can also be isolated from the reproductive and GI tracts of clinically healthy pigs.

Etiology and Pathogenesis: *S suis* possesses antigens somehow related to Lancefield group D streptococcus , but it is taxonomically far from other members of this group. It is considered a facultatively anaerobic, gram-positive, nonmotile coccus, oriented in chains of varying lengths. *S suis* produces α-hemolysis (incomplete hemolysis) on blood agar and is catalase negative. It has a worldwide distribution, and originally 35 serotypes based on capsular antigens had been described (serotypes 1 to 34 and serotype 1/2). However, there is still some controversy, because serotypes 20, 22, 26, 32, 33, and 34 have been suggested as not being part of the *S suis* species. Nonetheless, the number of serotypes considered as highly virulent is relatively small and depends mainly on geographic location.

Most studies on virulence factors of *S suis* have been performed with serotype 2 only. Type 2 virulent and nonvirulent strains exist, but characterization of virulence factors is still incomplete. Capsular polysaccharide is so far the most important critical virulence factor. However, well encapsulated nonvirulent serotype 2 strains do exist. Some proteins, such as the muramidase-released protein, the extracellular factor, and the hemolysin (suilysin), constitute virulence-related proteins for serotype 2 strains isolated in Europe and Asia but not for North American strains. So far, there is no single true predictor of pathogenicity. In fact, serotype 2 strains from different continents are phenotypically and genotypically very different. Most strains from Asia and Europe belong mainly to the sequence type or ST1, as characterized by multilocus sequence typing, and are highly virulent. Serotype 2 strains from North America belong to ST25 and ST28, presenting lower virulence capacities, which may explain the importance of other serotypes in this continent, such as serotypes 3 and 1/2.

The mechanisms that enable *S suis* to disseminate throughout the animal are not well understood. The bacterium is able to spread systemically from the nasopharynx, occasionally resulting in septicemia and death. The palatine and pharyngeal tonsils are both potential portals of entry for *S suis*, leading to subsequent hematogenous or lymphogenous dissemination. Survival of the organism once in the bloodstream may be facilitated by the capsular polysaccharide as well as cell wall components, which efficiently hamper phagocytosis. If *S suis* does not cause acute fatal septicemia, bacteria are able to reach the CNS via mechanisms that are only partially elucidated, such as invasion of brain microvascular endothelial cells or through the choroid plexus epithelial cells. In both septicemic and CNS cases, excessive host inflammation seems to play an important role in the pathogenesis of infection.

Epidemiology and Transmission: *S suis* is present in all parts of the world in swine intensive areas. Serotypes 1–9 (including serotype 1/2 that shares antigens with serotypes 1 and 2) represent >70% of *S suis* isolates recovered from diseased pigs, mainly in North America where most studies have been done. Serotype 2 is, in general, the most prevalent worldwide, but its importance is lower in North America and higher in Asia and some countries in Europe, such as France. Serotype 9 is the most frequently isolated type in other European countries, such as Spain, Germany, and the Netherlands.

Most clinically healthy pigs are carriers of multiple serotypes of *S suis*, although a few are colonized by virulent strains. Piglets become colonized with *S suis* from vaginal secretions during parturition and while nursing. Asymptomatic carriers serve as a source of infection for their pen mates after they are mixed and commingled in the nursery, when maternal antibodies are no longer present. Clinical infections are seen mainly in weaned pigs (2–5 wk after weaning), growing pigs, and less frequently, suckling piglets and adult animals. Transmission between herds occurs by the movement and mixing of healthy carrier pigs. The introduction of a highly virulent strain into a naive herd may result in subsequent onset of disease in weaned and/or growing pigs. However, some herds with animals harboring virulent strains but not showing illness may suddenly develop serious clinical disease in the presence of other predisposing factors such as overcrowding, poor ventilation, excessive temperature fluctuations, mixing of pigs with an age spread of >2 wk, and coinfections with other pathogens. Disease outbreaks due to *S suis* infection have been frequently reported with coinfections of porcine reproductive and respiratory syndrome virus (*see* p 729). *S suis* might also be transmitted via fomites and flies, although probabilities are low. Although *S suis* has been isolated from different mammal species and birds, the importance of such reservoirs is unknown.

Clinical Findings: Even when the carrier rate in pigs is near 100%, the incidence of the disease varies from period to period and is usually <5%. However, in the absence of treatment, mortality rates can reach 20%. The earliest sign is usually fever, which may occur initially without other obvious signs. It is accompanied by a pronounced septicemia that may persist for several days if untreated. During this period, there is usually a fluctuating fever and variable degrees of inappetence, depression, and shifting lameness. In peracute cases, pigs may be found dead with no premonitory signs. Meningitis is the most striking feature and the one on which a presumptive diagnosis is usually based. Pigs in the early stages of meningitis may hold their ears back and squint their eyes. Other early nervous signs include depression, incoordination, and adoption of unusual stances (eg, dog-sitting), which soon progress to inability to stand, paddling, opisthotonos, convulsions, and nystagmus. Swollen joints and lameness are indicative of polyarthritis, which is common in North America. Endocarditis is also a frequent finding in older piglets, with affected pigs dying suddenly or showing signs of dyspnea, cyanosis, and wasting. Signs of respiratory disease may be seen in some outbreaks, although the role of *S suis* as a primary agent of pneumonia, in the absence of other pathogens, remains controversial.

Lesions: Lesions are mainly seen in weaned and growing pigs and are associated with lymphadenopathy, meningitis, arthritis, and endocarditis. Polyserositis similar to that seen in Glässer's disease is sometimes seen. Lesions may include fibrinopurulent exudates in the brain, swollen joints, fibrinous serositis, and cardiac valvular vegetations. Splenomegaly and petechial hemorrhages indicating septicemia are common. Significant microscopic lesions are usually limited to the brain, heart, and joints. The predominant lesions are neutrophilic meningitis and chorioiditis, with hyperemic meningeal blood vessels, and fibrinopurulent or suppurative epicarditis. Evidence of encephalitis, edema, and congestion of the brain may be present. The choroid plexus may have disruption of the plexus brush border, and fibrin and inflammatory cell exudates may be present in the ventricles. Microscopic lesions do not seem to be associated with a given serotype.

Diagnosis: Presumptive diagnosis is generally based on history, clinical signs, age of animals, and gross lesions. Isolation and serotyping of the infectious agent and evaluation of microscopic lesions in affected tissues confirm the diagnosis. After isolation, biochemical identification of *S suis* isolates recovered from diseased animals is possible with a minimum of biochemical tests. Serotyping is important to confirm and implement preventive measures, and several multiplex PCR tests to easily serotype *S suis* strains have been reported (and can be used by any laboratory). Validated and specific serologic tests to detect antibodies are not available for *S suis*. Genetic characterization, including multilocus sequence typing, is done in some laboratories and is particularly useful for epidemiologic studies. For European and Asian strains of serotype 2, detection of the muramidase-released protein, the extracellular factor, and the hemolysin (suilysin) by PCR as an indication of virulence can also be done.

Detection of virulent strains of *S suis* from tonsils or nasal cavities cannot be done, because universal virulence factors are unknown. These sites are highly contaminated, and traditional bacterial isolation has a low sensitivity. Strains isolated from tonsils must be confirmed by PCR as being *S suis*, because biochemical tests are not able to correctly differentiate this bacterial species from other streptococci normally present in the upper respiratory tract of swine.

Differential diagnoses include polyserositis caused by *Haemophilus parasuis* or *Mycoplasma hyorhinis*; meningitis caused by *H parasuis*; endocarditis caused by *Erysipelothrix rhusiopathiae*; septicemia caused by *H parasuis*, *Actinobacillus suis*, *Escherichia coli*, *Erysipelothrix rhusiopathiae*, or *Salmonella* Choleraesuis; and polyarthritis caused by other streptococci, staphylococci, *E coli*, or *A suis*.

Treatment, Control, and Prevention: Prompt recognition of the early clinical signs of streptococcal meningitis, followed by immediate parenteral treatment of affected pigs with an appropriate antibiotic, is currently the best method to maximize survival. The early stages of meningitis may be difficult to detect, so weaned pigs should be observed 2–3 times daily on farms where *S suis* infections are a problem. Resistance of isolates to penicillin has been reported and varies among countries, but extended spectrum β-lactams such as ampicillin and amoxicillin appear to retain some good effectiveness. Treatment can also be administrated via the drinking water or in amoxicillin-medicated feed. However, because of the method of spread of the disease, treatment needs to be started quickly. Whichever method of medication is used, treatment should be continued for at least 5 days. Administration of an anti-inflammatory preparation is sometimes recommended to reduce inflammation of affected tissues and improve the overall condition of pigs with *S suis* meningitis. Treatment of sows with antibiotics before farrowing may reduce pathogen transmission to piglets, although results are controversial.

Vaccines available in the field are bacterins (inactivated whole cells), and they have proved to be relatively ineffective in preventing outbreaks. If somehow useful, the protection would be serotype-specific. Because affected animals are in general 6–10 wk old, interference with maternal antibodies should be considered. In addition, the adjuvant used seems to play an important role; a bacterin with a water-in-oil emulsion as an adjuvant provided better results than the same bacterin with an aluminum hydroxide–based adjuvant. Sow vaccination also had poor results.

One main problem is that *S suis* is one of several bacterial pathogens that have been able to defeat eradication efforts in nursing or early weaned pigs, because animals are already colonized immediately after or even during farrowing.

Streptococci are susceptible to the action of aldehyde, biguanide, hypochlorite, iodine, and quaternary ammonium disinfectants.

Zoonotic Risk: Human infections with *S suis* can result in septicemia, meningitis, permanent hearing loss, endocarditis, and arthritis. In Western countries, mortality has been reported to approach 7%, and most cases are related to employment in the swine industry (ie, pig farmers, abattoir workers, persons transporting pork, meat inspectors, butchers, and veterinarians). In Asia, the general population is at risk, and mortality rates can be >20%. *S suis* is considered one of the most common causes of adult meningitis in Thailand, Vietnam, and Hong Kong SAR,PRC. Serotype 2 and, to a lesser extent, serotype 14 are mainly involved in human cases. Transmission to people occurs via contamination of skin wounds or mucous membranes by blood or secretions from infected pigs or by consuming raw meat or blood (as is the case in Asia). The disease is considered to be underdiagnosed and underreported in several countries.

STREPTOCOCCUS DYSGALACTIAE EQUISIMILIS INFECTION

Alpha- and nonhemolytic streptococci of Lancefield group C are defined as *S dysgalactiae dysgalactiae*, whereas β-hemolytic streptococci belonging to groups C, G, or L are named *S dysgalactiae equisimilis*.

In swine, β-hemolytic *S dysgalactiae equisimilis* usually belong to Lancefield group C. Although members of the normal flora, they are considered the most important β-hemolytic streptococci involved in lesions in pigs, and these agents were judged to be of etiologic significance in autopsy reports. These streptococci are common in nasal and throat secretions, tonsils, and vaginal and preputial secretions. Vaginal secretions and milk from postparturient sows are the most likely sources of infection for the piglets.

Streptococci enter the bloodstream via skin wounds, the navel, and tonsils. A bacteremia or septicemia occurs, and the organisms then settle in one or more tissues, giving rise to arthritis, endocarditis, or meningitis.

Clinical Findings and Lesions: Infection is usually first seen in pigs 1–3 wk old. Joint swelling and lameness are the most obvious and persistent clinical signs. Increased temperatures, lassitude, roughened hair coat, and inappetence may also be noted. Early lesions consist of periarticular edema; swollen, hyperemic synovial membranes; and turbid synovial fluid. Necrosis of articular cartilage may be seen 15–30 days after onset and may become more severe. Fibrosis and multiple focal abscessation of periarticular tissues and hypertrophy of synovial villi also occur. Endocarditis occurs but is difficult to diagnose antemortem. Lesions consist of yellow or white vegetations of different sizes, often covering the entire surface of the affected valve.

Diagnosis: Diagnosis of streptococcal septicemia, arthritis, or endocarditis is best accomplished by necropsy and bacteriologic examination of affected pigs. Only small numbers of organisms or no organisms may be isolated from affected joints, especially when inflammation is advanced.

Treatment and Prevention: β-hemolytic streptococci are sensitive to β-lactam antibiotics. Long-acting antibacterial agents may be beneficial, and treatment should be given before inflammation is well advanced. There are no recent reports about vaccination against these streptococci. Autogenous bacterins are sometimes used, and there were reports of a reduced incidence of arthritis when sows were vaccinated before farrowing. However, no recent data have confirmed such information.

Adequate intake of colostrum may ensure that piglets receive protective antibodies. Traumatic injuries to the feet and legs should be minimized by reducing the abrasiveness of the floor surface in the farrowing area.

S dysgalactiae is not recognized as a zoonotic pathogen.

STREPTOCOCCUS PORCINUS INFECTION

(Streptococcal lymphadenitis, Jowl abscess, Cervical abscess)

S porcinus Lancefield group E has been associated in the USA with a contagious clinical entity in growing pigs known as streptococcal lymphadenitis, jowl abscesses, or cervical abscesses. Losses due to this disease in the USA were important in the 1960s, but its incidence has since declined, and the disease is not recognized as an important economic entity in other countries, where the bacterium represents only a few percent of the microorganisms isolated from abscesses in swine. Interestingly, it was recently reported that almost 20% of tonsils from a slaughterhouse were positive for *S porcinus*. Although pathology is not frequently seen, the pathogen is still prevalent in swine.

Transmission is possible by contact or ingestion of food or water contaminated by purulent material from abscesses or feces containing the organism. Organisms infect the pig through the mucosa of the pharyngeal or tonsillar surfaces and are carried to the lymph nodes, primarily of the head and neck region, where abscesses are formed. Abscesses may be seen at slaughter, and enlargement of lymph nodes in the throat region may be evident. *S porcinus* is also occasionally found in the vaginal mucus of sows and the semen and prepuce of boars. It is generally considered to be a secondary invader.

Scattered miliary abscesses develop in the mandibular, parotid, or retropharyngeal lymph nodes within 7 days after infection. By 21 days, abscesses measuring 5–8 cm in diameter are common; they destroy the internal structure of affected nodes and may extend into adjacent tissues. Developing abscesses may reach the skin, rupture, and drain in 7–10 wk. The drained lesions heal by granulation, leaving a dense, fibrous, subcutaneous tract that resolves after several weeks. Deep-seated abscesses may remain undetected until slaughter and tend not to drain into the pharynx.

S porcinus is sensitive to penicillins, and antibiotic therapy will usually resolve acute infections if detected. However, antibiotic treatment is not usually successful in treating swine with established abscesses or in eliminating carriers. Resistance to tetracycline has been reported, but pulsing tetracyclines in the feed at the therapeutic level of 400 g/ton is commonly used in an attempt to control this condition. Vaccination (autogenous) is possible but has not been widely used, because cervical abscesses are not a widespread problem.

S porcinus Lancefield groups P, U, and V have been isolated from lungs, genital organs, and brains of pigs. However, no histologic lesions could be associated with their presence. *S porcinus* groups P and V have also been associated with abortions in pigs.

Many strains of *S porcinus* have been recovered from the human female genitourinary tract. However, it has been reported later that these strains belong to a different and new species, *Streptococcus pseudoporcinus* sp nov (novel species).

OTHER STREPTOCOCCAL AND ENTEROCOCCAL INFECTIONS

Bacterial streptococcal strains were isolated from the lungs and kidney of two pigs with lesions associated with pneumonia and septicemia, respectively. The two isolates were recovered from different animals, on different farms located in difference provinces of Spain, and in different years. The isolates were classified as a new species, *Streptococcus plurextorum* sp nov (novel species). Other isolates associated with pneumonia were also defined as a new species, *Streptococcus porci* sp nov. So far, there are no data about the habitat and/or virulence properties of these two species.

Enterococci are known as part of the intestinal flora, but some strains can extensively colonize the mucosal surface of the small intestine. Some enterococcal species that show typical adhesion to the apical surface of the enterocytes of the small intestine of young animals have been described as associated with diarrhea in different species, including piglets 2–20 days old. Taxonomic studies have shown that most of these enterococci are members of the *E faecium* species group, mainly *E durans* and *E hirae*.

SWINE VESICULAR DISEASE

Swine vesicular disease (SVD) is typically a transient disease of pigs in which vesicular lesions appear on the feet and snout and in the mouth. SVD is usually mild in nature and may infect pigs subclinically. However, the disease is of major economic importance, because it must be differentiated from foot-and-mouth disease, eradication is costly, and embargoes on export of pigs and pork products are often imposed on nations not free of SVD.

Pigs are considered the only natural host of the virus, although it can infect sheep in close contact with infected pigs and infection of one laboratory worker was reported. SVD has been reported only in Europe and Asia, having been first identified in Italy in 1966 and subsequently in Hong Kong SAR,PRC, Japan, Taiwan,PRC and 16 other countries in Europe. Although SVD virus was eradicated from Japan in the mid-1970s and most European countries by the mid-1980s, it has remained endemic in Italy and caused sporadic outbreaks of disease in other European countries during the 1990s and in Portugal in 2003, 2004, and 2007.

Etiology: The causal agent is an enterovirus of the family Picornaviridae. It belongs to the species Human enterovirus B and is thought to have evolved from the human pathogen coxsackievirus B5, with which it shares a close antigenic and genetic relationship. There is only one serotype of SVD virus, although isolates may be differentiated by antigenic or genetic typing and may differ in virulence. SVD virus is transmitted by direct or indirect contact or by feeding infected pork or pork products. Infection is via the oral route or through skin abrasions and can give rise to viremia, fecal viral shedding, and generalized vesicles that rupture to release large amounts of virus.

Clinical Findings and Lesions: The primary signs are fresh or healing vesicular lesions on the feet, especially the coronary band, and less often other areas such as the mouth, lips, teats, or snout. The lesions may be mild or inapparent, especially when pigs are kept on soft bedding. The lesions are similar to those of foot-and-mouth disease (*see* p 629), vesicular exanthema of swine (*see* p 738), and vesicular stomatitis (*see* p 694); however, affected pigs usually do not lose condition, and the lesions heal rapidly. Nervous signs have been described but are rarely seen in the field. The OIE recommends that any outbreaks of vesicular disease in pigs should be assumed to be foot-and-mouth disease until proved otherwise by laboratory testing.

Diagnosis: Diagnosis is confirmed by laboratory tests on epithelial samples, feces, or serum. Virus detection is by antigen-detection ELISA, virus isolation, or reverse-transcriptase PCR. Serology is by antibody-detection ELISA or virus neutralization test, but low specificity may be a concern, particularly in older animals. In clinical cases, the preferred specimens are lesion material collected in phosphate-buffered saline. Subclinical infection may be detected by testing of pen-floor feces using reverse-transcriptase PCR or virus isolation.

Control: Countries free of the disease can remain so by controlling the import of pigs and pork products or by ensuring that pork products are treated (heat or otherwise) to kill the virus. Feeding of garbage to pigs may be banned or regulated to ensure thorough cooking. Any suspected outbreak should be reported to the appropriate authorities. If SVD does occur, control is by zoosanitary measures, including restrictions on pig movement. There are no commercially available vaccines. Extensive serosurveillance is necessary to detect subclinically infected herds, and seroreactor herds must be followed up by clinical inspection and fecal virus testing. The virus is extremely resistant in the environment and is stable over a wide pH range (2.5–12); thus, disinfection of premises, trucks, and equipment must be thorough. The most effective disinfectants are strong alkalis, although hypochlorites or acid-containing iodophors can be used when organic material is not present.

TRICHINELLOSIS

(Trichinosis)

Trichinellosis is a parasitic disease of public health importance caused by the nematode *Trichinella spiralis*. Human infections are established by consumption of insufficiently cooked infected meat, usually pork or bear, although other species have been implicated. Natural infections are found in wild carnivores; trichinellosis has also been found in horses, rats, beavers, opossums, walruses, whales, and meat-eating birds. Most mammals are susceptible. The number of human cases has declined in the past 50 years due in part to the move to modern production facilities (confinement) that reduces or eliminates exposure to rodents and other wildlife.

Etiology and Epidemiology: The genus *Trichinella* is currently considered a complex of nine species and three additional genotypes (T6, T8, and T9) of undetermined taxonomic status. Other than for the existence of two clades defined by the presence or absence of a collagen capsule (cyst) surrounding the parasite in the muscle, there are few distinct morphologic differences. Taxon identification is based on characteristics such as reproductive isolation, infectivity to certain hosts, resistance to freezing, geographic cruising range, PCR and DNA sequencing, and isoenzyme analysis. *T spiralis* (T1) is the most common and widely distributed of the encapsulated species affecting people and domestic animals in temperate regions; it has high infectivity for pigs and rodents, exhibits low resistance to freezing, and is broadly infective for most sylvatic hosts. The other cyst-forming species include *T nativa* (T2), found in arctic carnivores; *T britovi* (T3), found throughout the entire European continent, northwest Africa, and southwest Asia; *T murrelli* (T5), restricted to North America; *T nelsoni* (T7), found only in eastern Africa; and the most recently named *T patagoniensis* (T12), found in Argentina. There are three other encapsulated genotypes: *Trichinella* T6, which is very similar to *T nativa* and is found in carnivores of North America; T8, which shows similarities to *T britovi* and is present in carnivores of Africa; and T9, which has been identified only in sylvatic hosts from Japan but is genetically more similar to *T murrelli* of the USA. There are three additional species—*T pseudospiralis* (T4), *T papuae* (T10), and *T zimbabwensis* (T11), which constitute the nonencapsulated clade (lack a cyst in the muscle). *T pseudospiralis* has a cosmopolitan distribution and is the only species capable of infecting mammals and birds. *T papuae* was first identified in pigs from Papua New Guinea, but its presence is suspected to extend into Australasia and southeast Asia. *T zimbabwensis* is present in sub-Saharan Africa. Both *T papuae* and *T zimbabwensis* are capable of infecting crocodiles.

Infection generally occurs by ingestion of larvae encysted in muscle. The cyst wall is digested in the stomach, and the liberated larvae penetrate into the duodenal and jejunal mucosa. Within ~4 days, the larvae develop into sexually mature adults. After mating, the females (3–4 mm) penetrate deeper into the mucosa and discharge living larvae (up to 1,500) throughout 4–16 wk. After reproduction, the adult worms die and usually are digested. The young larvae (0.1 mm) migrate into the lymphatics, are carried via the portal system to the peripheral circulation, and reach striated muscle, where they penetrate individual muscle cells. They grow rapidly (to 1 mm) and begin to coil within the cell, usually 1 per cell. Capsule formation begins ~15 days after infection and is completed by 4–8 wk, at which time the larvae are infective. The cell degenerates as the larva grows, and then calcification occurs (at different rates in various hosts). Larvae may remain viable in the cysts for years, and their development continues only if ingested by another suitable host. The diaphragm, tongue, masseter, and intercostal muscles are among those most heavily involved in pigs.

If larvae pass through the intestine and are eliminated in the feces before maturation, they are infective to other animals.

Clinical Findings and Diagnosis: Most infections in domestic and wild animals go undiagnosed. In people, heavy infections may produce serious illness with three clinical phases (intestinal, muscle invasion, and convalescent) and occasionally death.

Although antemortem diagnosis in animals other than people is rare, trichinellosis may be suspected if there is a history of eating rodents, wildlife carcasses, or raw, infected meat. Microscopic examination of a muscle biopsy sample (usually tongue) may confirm but not necessarily exclude trichinellosis. ELISA is a reliable test to detect anti-*Trichinella* antibodies. Seroconversion may not occur for weeks after infection, although as little as 0.01 larvae per gram of meat can be detected.

Control: Treatment is generally impractical in animals. The objective is to prevent ingestion by any animal, including people, of viable *Trichinella* cysts in muscle (trichinae). In pigs, this may be accomplished with good management that includes controlling rodents, cooking garbage (fed to the pigs) for 30 min at 212°F (100°C), and preventing cannibalism (ie, tail biting) and access to wildlife carcasses.

Inspection of meat for viable trichinae at the time of slaughter (by trichinoscopic or digestion methods) is effective to prevent human infection in many countries. In North America, the assumption is that pork may be infected; therefore, those products that appear as "ready to eat" must be processed by adequate heating, freezing, or curing to kill trichinae before marketing. Other pork should be cooked to assure that all tissue is heated to an internal temperature of 145°F (63°C) for roasts or 160°F (71°C) for ground meats. Freezing pork at an appropriate temperature for an appropriate time is also effective (5°F [−15°C] for 20 days, −9.4°F [−23°C] for 10 days, or −22°F [−30°C] for 6 days). Freezing cannot be relied on to kill trichinae in meat other than pork.

VESICULAR EXANTHEMA OF SWINE

(San Miguel sea lion virus disease)

Vesicular exanthema of swine (VES) is an acute, highly infectious disease characterized by fever and formation of vesicles on the snout, oral mucosa, soles of the feet, coronary band, and between the toes.

VES has been reported only in the USA, and not since 1959, but it remains of historic importance because of its clinical similarity to foot-and-mouth disease. Since 1972, San Miguel sea lion virus (SMSV), a virus indistinguishable from VES virus (VESV), and related caliciviruses have been isolated from marine mammals on the west coast of the USA.

VESV, SMSV, and related viruses are members of the genus *Vesivirus* in the family Caliciviridae. Many immunologically distinct serotypes have been demonstrated (13 types of VESV from pigs and at least 16 types of SMSV from marine sources). In addition, a number of serotypes have been isolated from other host species and named accordingly: bovine, primate, cetacean, walrus, skunk, mink, rabbit, and reptile caliciviruses. In some cases, serotypes initially isolated in terrestrial animals (eg, reptile calicivirus) have subsequently been found in marine mammals. All of these viruses (except for SMSV-8, SMSV-12, and mink calicivirus) form a single virus species, vesicular exanthema of swine virus.

SMSV has also been isolated from vesicular lesions on marine mammals, seal meat, and perch-like fish in California. SMSV can produce lesions indistinguishable from those of VES in pigs, and the diverse pool of marine caliciviruses on the west coast of the USA are a reservoir of potential swine pathogens. Two marine caliciviruses, serotype SMSV-5 and an unknown virus, have been isolated from vesicular lesions or throat washings of two people with vesicular lesions, but the viruses are considered of minimal significance to public health.

In pigs, the clinical disease is indistinguishable from foot-and-mouth disease (*see* p 629), vesicular stomatitis (*see* p 694), and swine vesicular disease (*see* p 735).

Presumptive diagnosis in pigs is based on fever and the presence of typical vesicles, which break within 24–48 hr to form erosions. Diagnosis can be confirmed by ELISA, reverse-transcriptase PCR, complement-fixation tests, and electron microscopy on epithelial tissue, or after passage in swine tissue cultures. Serum neutralization tests and electron microscopy are also used.

Suspected cases of vesicular exanthema should be reported immediately to the appropriate authorities. Feeding of food scraps (garbage, swill) to pigs is illegal in many countries and can be done only under license and after cooking in the USA.

BLUETONGUE

Bluetongue is an infectious arthropod-borne viral disease primarily of domestic and wild ruminants. Infection with bluetongue virus (BTV) is common in a broad band across the world, which until recently stretched from ~35°S to 40°–50°N. Since the 1990s, BTV has extended considerably north of the 40th and even the 50th parallel in some parts of the world (eg, Europe). The geographic *restriction is in* part related to the climatic and environmental conditions necessary to support the *Culicoides* vectors. Most infections with BTV in wild ruminants and cattle are subclinical. Bluetongue (the disease caused by BTV) is usually considered to be a disease of improved breeds of sheep, particularly the fine-wool and mutton breeds, although it has also been recorded in cattle and some wild ruminant species, including white-tailed deer (*Odocoileus virginianus*), pronghorn antelope (*Antilocapra americana*), and desert bighorn sheep (*Ovis canadensis*) in North America, and European bison (*Bison bonasus*) and captive yak (*Bos grunniens grunniens*) in Europe.

Etiology and Transmission: Bluetongue virus is the type-species of the genus *Orbivirus* in the family Reoviridae. There are at least 24 serotypes worldwide, although not all serotypes exist in any one geographic area; eg, 13 serotypes (1, 2, 3, 5, 6, 10, 11, 13, 14, 17, 19, 22, and 24) have been reported in the USA and 8 serotypes (1, 2, 4, 6, 8, 9, 11, and 16) in Europe. Distribution of BTV throughout the world parallels the spatial and temporal distribution of vector species of *Culicoides* biting midges, which are the only significant natural transmitters of the virus, as well as the temperatures at which BTV will replicate in and be transmitted by these vectors. Of more than 1,400 *Culicoides* species worldwide, fewer than 30 have been identified as actual or potential vectors of BTV to date. Continued cycling of the virus among competent *Culicoides* vectors and susceptible ruminants is critical to viral ecology. In the USA, the principal vectors are *C sonorensis* and *C insignis*, which limit the distribution of BTV to southern and western regions. In northern and eastern Australia the principal vector is *C brevitarsis*, whereas in Africa, southern Europe, and the Middle East it is *C imicola*. In northern Europe, the major vectors are species within the *C obsoletus-dewulfi* complex. In each geographic region, secondary vector species may attain local importance.

Vectors become infected with BTV by imbibing blood from infected vertebrates; transovarial transmission has not been reported. High affinity of the virus to blood cells, especially the sequestering of viral particles in invaginations of RBC membranes, contributes to prolonged viremia in the presence of neutralizing antibody. The extended viremia in cattle (occasionally up to 11 wk), and the host preference of some vector species of *Culicoides* for cattle, provide a mechanism for year-round transmission in domestic ruminants in locations where the vector-free (winter) period is relatively short. Mechanical transmission by other bloodsucking insects is of minor significance.

Vector-borne transmission through *Culicoides* spp is the primary way BTV spreads. Virus concentrations in secretions and excretions are minimal, making direct, indirect, or aerosol transmission unlikely. However, in-contact transmission of BTV serotype 26 has been demonstrated in goats. The significance of this form of transmission in the ecology of this serotype is not known. Semen from viremic bulls can serve as a source of infection for cows through natural service or artificial insemination. Embryo transfer is regarded as safe, provided that donors are not viremic and an appropriate washing procedure for embryos is used. Transplacental transmission of field strains of BTV from dam to fetus, leading to the birth of viremic calves, is reported in cattle, but the epidemiologic significance of this mechanism is unclear. Accidental infection has been reported in dogs in the USA after administration of a modified-live canine virus vaccine that was contaminated with BTV. Serologic evidence of infection with BTV has been found in wild and captive carnivores in Africa and Europe, perhaps as a result of ingesting virus-infected viscera. The epidemiologic importance of this oral infection mechanism is at present uncertain. Serologic evidence of BTV exposure has been demonstrated in domestic dogs fed commercial diets.

Clinical Findings: The course of the disease in sheep can vary from peracute to chronic, with a mortality rate of 2%–90%. Peracute cases die within 7–9 days of infection, mostly as a result of severe pulmonary edema leading to dyspnea, frothing from the nostrils, and death by asphyxiation. In chronic cases, sheep may die 3–5 wk after infection, mainly as a result of bacterial complications, especially pasteurellosis, and exhaustion. Mild cases usually recover rapidly and completely. The major production losses include deaths, unthriftiness during prolonged convalescence, wool breaks, and reproductive losses.

In sheep, BTV causes vascular endothelial damage, resulting in changes to capillary permeability and subsequent intravascular coagulation. This results in edema, congestion, hemorrhage, inflammation, and necrosis. The clinical signs in sheep are typical. After an incubation period of 4–6 days, a fever of 105°–107.5°F (40.5°–42°C) develops. The animals are listless and reluctant to move. Clinical signs in young lambs are more apparent, and the mortality rate can be high (up to 30%). Approximately 2 days after onset of fever, additional clinical signs may be seen, such as edema of lips, nose, face, submandibular area, eyelids, and sometimes ears; congestion of mouth, nose, nasal cavities, conjunctiva, and coronary bands; and lameness and depression. A serous nasal discharge is common, later becoming mucopurulent. The congestion of nose and nasal cavities produces a "sore muzzle" effect, the term used to describe the disease in sheep in the USA. Sheep eat less because of oral soreness and will hold food in their mouths to soften before chewing. They may champ to produce a frothy oral discharge at the corners of the lips. On close examination, small hemorrhages can be seen on the mucous membranes of the nose and mouth. Ulceration develops where the teeth come in contact with lips and tongue, especially in areas of most friction. Some affected sheep have severe swelling of the tongue, which may become cyanotic ('blue tongue") and even protrude from the mouth. Animals walk with difficulty as a result of inflammation of the hoof coronets. A purple-red color is easily seen as a band at the junction of the skin and the hoof. Later in the course of disease, lameness or torticollis is due to skeletal muscle damage. In most affected animals, abnormal wool growth resulting from dermatitis may be seen.

Clinical signs in cattle are rare but may be similar to those seen in sheep. They are usually limited to fever, increased respiratory rate, lacrimation, salivation, stiffness, oral vesicles and ulcers, hyperesthesia, and a vesicular and ulcerative dermatitis. Susceptible cattle and sheep infected during pregnancy may abort or deliver malformed calves or lambs. The malformations include hydranencephaly or porencephaly, which results in ataxia and blindness at birth. White-tailed deer and pronghorn antelope develop severe hemorrhagic disease leading to sudden death. Pregnant dogs abort or give birth to stillborn pups and then die in 3–7 days.

Diagnosis and Lesions: The typical clinical signs of bluetongue enable a presumptive diagnosis, especially in areas where the disease is endemic. Suspicion is confirmed by the presence of petechiae, ecchymoses, or hemorrhages in the wall of the base of the pulmonary artery and focal necrosis of the papillary muscle of the left ventricle. These highly characteristic lesions are usually obvious in severe clinical infections but may be barely visible in mild or convalescent cases. These lesions are often described as pathognomonic for bluetongue, but they have also been seen occasionally in other ovine diseases such as heartwater, pulpy kidney disease, and Rift Valley fever. Hemorrhages and necrosis are usually found where mechanical abrasion damages fragile capillaries, such as on the buccal surface of the cheek opposite the molar teeth and the mucosa of the esophageal groove and omasal folds. Other autopsy findings include subcutaneous and intermuscular edema and hemorrhages, skeletal myonecrosis, myocardial and intestinal hemorrhages, hydrothorax, hydropericardium, pericarditis, and pneumonia.

In many areas of the world, BTV infection in sheep, and especially in other ruminants, is subclinical. Laboratory confirmation is based on virus isolation in embryonated chicken eggs or mammalian and insect cell cultures, or on identification of viral RNA by PCR. The identity of isolates may be confirmed by the group-specific antigen-capture ELISA, group-specific PCR, immunofluorescence, immunoperoxidase, serotype-specific virus neutralization tests, serotype-specific PCR, or hybridization with complementary gene sequences of group- or serotype-specific genes. For virus isolation, blood (10–20 mL) is collected as early as possible from febrile animals into an anticoagulant such as heparin, sodium citrate, or EDTA and transported at 4°C (39.2°F) to the laboratory. For longterm storage when refrigeration is not possible, blood is collected in oxalate-phenolglycerin (OPG). Blood to be frozen should be collected in buffered lactose peptone and stored at or below −70°C (−94°F). Blood collected at later times during the viremic period should not be frozen, because lysing of the RBCs on thawing releases the cell-associated virus, which may then be neutralized by early humoral antibody. The virus does not remain stable for long at −20°C (−4°F). In fatal cases, specimens of spleen, lymph nodes, or red bone marrow are collected and transported to the laboratory at 4°C (39.2°F) as soon as possible after death.

A serologic response in ruminants can be detected 7–14 days after infection and is generally lifelong after a field infection. Current recommended serologic techniques for detection of BTV antibody include agar gel immunodiffusion and competitive ELISA. The latter is the test of choice and does not detect cross-reacting antibody to other orbiviruses, especially anti-EHDV (epizootic hemorrhagic disease virus) antibody. Various forms of the serum neutralization test, including plaque reduction, plaque inhibition, and microtiter neutralization, can be used to detect type-specific antibody.

Prevention and Control: There is no specific treatment for animals with bluetongue apart from rest, provision of soft food, and good husbandry. Complicating and secondary infections should be treated appropriately during the recovery period.

Prophylactic immunization of sheep remains the most effective and practical control measure against bluetongue in endemic regions. Attenuated and inactivated vaccines against BTV are commercially available in some countries. Three polyvalent vaccines, each comprising five different BTV serotypes attenuated by serial passage in embryonated hens' eggs followed by growth and plaque selection in cell culture, are widely used in southern Africa and elsewhere, should epizootics of bluetongue occur. A monovalent (BTV type 10) modified-live virus vaccine propagated in cell culture is available for use in sheep in the USA. Use of vaccines with different serotypes does not provide consistent cross-protection. Live-attenuated vaccines should not be used during *Culicoides* vector seasons, because these insects may transmit the vaccine virus(es) from vaccinated to nonvaccinated animals, eg, other ruminant species. This may result in reassortment of genetic material and give rise to new viral strains. Abortion or malformation, particularly of the CNS, of fetuses may follow vaccination of ewes and cows with attenuated live vaccines during the first half and the first trimester of pregnancy, respectively. Passive immunity in lambs usually lasts 2–4 mo.

The control of bluetongue is different in areas where the disease is not endemic. During an outbreak, when one or a limited number of serotypes may be involved, vaccination strategy depends on the serotype(s) causing infection. Use of vaccine strains other than the one(s) causing infection affords little or no protection and is not recommended. The potential risk from vaccine virus reassortment with wild-type viral strains, virus spread by the vectors to other susceptible ruminants, and reversion to virulence of vaccine virus strains or even the production of new BTV strains of uncertain virulence should also be considered. The use of inactivated vaccines in BTV incursions into northern Europe has played a major part in controlling virus spread in those regions where significant cover (>80%) has been achieved.

Control of vectors by using insecticides or protection from vectors may lower the number of *Culicoides* bites and subsequently the risk of exposure to BTV infection. However, these measures alone are unlikely to effectively halt a bluetongue epidemic and should be regarded as mitigation measures to be used alongside a comprehensive and vigorous vaccination program.

BOVINE EPHEMERAL FEVER

(Three-day sickness)

Bovine ephemeral fever is an insect-transmitted, noncontagious, viral disease of cattle and water buffalo that is seen in Africa, the Middle East, Australia, and Asia. Inapparent infections can develop in Cape buffalo, hartebeest, waterbuck, wildebeest, deer, and possibly goats. Low levels of antibody have been recorded in several other antelope species and giraffe, but the specificity has not been confirmed.

Etiology and Epidemiology: Bovine ephemeral fever virus (BEFV) is classified as a member of the genus *Ephemerovirus* in the family Rhabdoviridae (single-stranded, negative sense RNA). The virus is ether-sensitive and readily inactivated at pH levels below 5 and above 10. Although no evidence of immunogenic diversity is reported, antigenic variation has been demonstrated using panels of monoclonal antibodies and by epitope mapping. Several closely related ephemeroviruses (including Berrimah virus, Kimberley virus, Malakal virus, Adelaide River virus, Obodhiang virus, Puchong virus, kotonkan virus, and Koolpinyah virus) have been identified. However, of these, only kotonkan virus (isolated in Nigeria) has been associated with clinical ephemeral fever in cattle.

BEFV can be transmitted from infected to susceptible cattle by IV inoculation; as little as 0.005 mL of blood collected during the febrile stage is infective. Although the virus has been recovered from several *Culicoides* species and from Anopheline and Culicine mosquito species collected in the field, the identity of the major vectors has not been proved. Transmission by contact or fomites does not occur. The virus does not appear to persist in recovered cattle, which often have a lifelong immunity.

The prevalence, geographic range, and severity of the disease vary from year to year, and epidemics occur periodically. During epidemics, onset is rapid; many animals are affected within days or 2–3 wk. Bovine ephemeral fever is most prevalent in the wet season in the tropics and in summer to early autumn in the subtropics or temperate regions (when conditions favor multiplication of biting insects); it disappears abruptly in winter. Virus spread appears to be limited by latitude rather than topography or availability of susceptible hosts. Morbidity may be as high as 80%; overall mortality is usually 1%–2%, although it can be higher in lactating cows, bulls in good condition, and fat steers (10%–30%). However, reported overall mortality rates have exceeded 10% in outbreaks in several countries in recent years.

Clinical Findings: Signs, which occur suddenly and vary in severity, can include biphasic to polyphasic fever (40°–42°C [104°–107.6°F]), shivering, inappetence, lacrimation, serous nasal discharge, drooling, increased heart rate, tachypnea or dyspnea, atony of forestomachs, depression, stiffness and lameness, and a sudden decrease in milk yield. Clinical signs are generally milder in water buffalo. Affected cattle may become recumbent and paralyzed for 8 hr to >1 wk. After recovery, milk production often fails to return to normal levels until the next lactation. Abortion, with total loss of the season's lactation, occurs in ~5% of cows pregnant for 8–9 mo. The virus does not appear to cross the placenta or affect the fertility of the cow. Bulls, heavy cattle, and high-lactating dairy cows are the most severely affected, but spontaneous recovery usually occurs within a few days. More insidious losses may result from decreased muscle mass and lowered fertility in bulls.

Lesions: Bovine ephemeral fever is an inflammatory disease. The most common lesions include polyserositis affecting pleural, pericardial, and peritoneal surfaces; serofibrinous polysynovitis, polyarthritis, polytendinitis, and cellulitis; and focal necrosis of skeletal muscles. Generalized edema of lymph nodes and lungs, as well as atelectasis, also may be present.

Diagnosis: Diagnosis is based almost entirely on clinical signs in an epidemic. All clinical cases have a neutrophilia with the presence of many immature forms, although this is not pathognomonic. Serofibrinous inflammation in the tendon sheaths, fascia, and joints, together with pulmonary lesions, may substantiate a presumptive diagnosis.

Laboratory confirmation is by serology, rarely by virus isolation. Whole blood should be collected from sick and apparently healthy cattle in affected herds and must be sufficient to provide two air-dried blood smears, 5 mL of whole blood in anticoagulant (not EDTA), and ~10 mL of serum. A differential WBC count on blood smears can either support or refute a presumptive field diagnosis.

Virus is best isolated by inoculation of mosquito (*Aedes albopictus*) cell cultures with defibrinated blood, followed by transfer to baby hamster kidney (BHK-21 or BHK-BSR) or monkey kidney (Vero) cell cultures after 15 days. Suckling mice may also be used for primary isolation by intracerebral inoculation. Isolated viruses are identified by PCR, neutralization tests using specific BEFV antisera, and ELISA using specific monoclonal antibodies. The neutralization test and the blocking ELISA are recommended for antibody detection and give similar results. A 4-fold rise in antibody titer between paired sera collected 2–3 wk apart confirms infection.

Treatment and Control: Complete rest is the most effective treatment, and recovering animals should not be stressed or worked because relapse is likely. Anti-inflammatory drugs given early and in repeated doses for 2–3 days are effective. Oral dosing should be avoided unless the swallowing reflex is functional. Signs of hypocalcemia are treated as for milk fever (*see* p 988). Antibiotic treatment to control secondary infection and rehydration with isotonic fluids may be warranted.

Attenuated virus vaccines appear to be effective but should be used only in endemic areas. Inactivated virus vaccines have not produced longterm protection against experimental challenge with virulent virus and cannot guarantee lasting immunity, but they may boost the immunity produced by live virus vaccine. Although a subunit vaccine that protects against field and laboratory challenge has been described, it is not commercially available. The efficacy of vector control remains uncertain, because the insect vectors have not been fully identified. There is no evidence that people can be infected.

BOVINE LEUKOSIS

(Bovine lymphosarcoma, Leukemia, Malignant lymphoma)

Lymphosarcoma in cattle may be sporadic or result from infection with bovine leukemia virus (BLV); the latter is often referred to as an enzootic bovine leukosis. Sporadic lymphosarcoma in cattle is unrelated to infection with BLV. Despite the lack of association, animals with sporadic lymphosarcoma may possibly be infected with the virus. Sporadic lymphosarcoma manifests in three main forms: juvenile, thymic, and cutaneous. Juvenile lymphosarcoma occurs most often in animals <6 mo old, thymic lymphosarcoma affects cattle 6–24 mo old, and cutaneous lymphosarcoma is most common in cattle 1–3 yr old.

Etiology, Transmission, and Epidemiology: Enzootic bovine leukosis is caused by BLV, an exogenous C-type oncogenic retrovirus of the BLV-human T-lymphotropic virus group. BLV has a stable genome, does not cause chronic viremia, and has no preferred site of proviral integration. Despite the lack of preferred proviral integration sites, the tumors generated by the virus in a single individual are typically monoclonal and have a single integration site. The virus escapes the immune response by low levels of viral replication. It appears that replication is blocked at the transcriptional level, but the mechanism is not completely understood.

The prevalence of BLV infection varies from country to country. Many European countries, Australia, and New Zealand have eradication programs in place that have led to negligible rates of BLV infection. Although voluntary control programs are in place in the USA, prevalence is high compared with much of the rest of the world. The most recent surveys in the USA estimate that 44% of dairy and 10% of beef cattle are infected with the virus. Prevalence tends to increase on dairies with increasing herd size, while the converse is true in beef cattle. In general, the prevalence of viral infection increases with age.

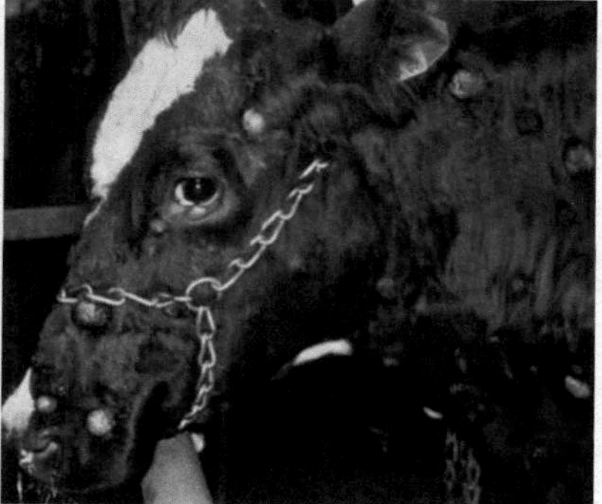

Cutaneous lymphosarcoma. *Courtesy of Dr. Peter Constable.*

Cattle are infected with BLV through the transfer of blood and blood products that contain infected lymphocytes. Once infected, cattle develop a lifelong antibody response, primarily to the gp51 envelope protein and the p24 capsid protein. B lymphocytes harbor the integrated provirus but rarely express viral proteins on their cell surface. The exact site of viral replication and expression that drives the immune response remains elusive.

Under experimental conditions, most routes of viral exposure can successfully transmit infection. However, many of these settings are unlikely to be encountered naturally. Many bodily fluids, including urine, feces, saliva, respiratory secretions, semen, uterine fluids, and embryos, have been examined for their ability to transmit BLV and are considered to be noninfectious. Only on rare occasion has virus been found in these fluids. Colostrum from BLV-positive cows contains virus and has been found to be infectious experimentally. However, colostrum also contains large amounts of antibody, and it is believed that the protective effects of colostral antibody outweigh the infectious potential when colostrum is administered in a normal fashion.

Most BLV transmission is horizontal. Close contact between BLV-negative and BLV-positive cattle is thought to be a risk factor. Many common farm practices have been implicated in viral transmission, including tattooing, dehorning, rectal palpation, injections, and blood collection. Vectors such as tabanids and other large biting flies also may transmit the virus. Vertical transmission may occur transplacentally from an infected dam to the fetus, intrapartum by contact with infected blood, or postpartum from the dam to the calf through ingestion of infected colostrum.

Any material that is blood contaminated or lymphocyte rich has the potential to infect animals with BLV.

Pathogenesis: There are three main outcomes in cattle infected with BLV. Most animals remain persistently infected with no outward signs of infection. Approximately 29% of BLV-infected cattle develop persistent lymphocytosis, while <5% of BLV-infected cattle develop lymphosarcoma.

Persistent lymphocytosis is sometimes referred to as a preneoplastic syndrome, but there is no convincing evidence that affected cattle have an increased risk of developing lymphosarcoma. The lymphocytes present in persistent lymphocytosis are not neoplastic, although they may have mild reactive changes consistent with normal blood smears in cattle. Persistent lymphocytosis is considered a benign condition associated with BLV infection. For this reason, it is often overlooked. However, these cows may serve as a reservoir of infection. The increased lymphocyte count is attributed to a 45-fold increase of infected $CD5^+$ and a 99-fold increase in infected $CD5^-$ B cells. It has been suggested that cows with persistent lymphocytosis may be at greater risk of passing BLV infection on to their calves in utero and may show decreased milk production and alteration of milk components.

Lymphosarcoma is rarely seen in animals <2 yr old and is most common in the 4- to 8-yr-old age group. Less than 5% of BLV-infected cattle develop lymphosarcoma. Lymphosarcoma, including both sporadic and enzootic forms, is one of the main causes of condemnation of adult dairy cows at slaughter.

Clinical Findings: Clinical signs associated with development of lymphosarcoma are highly variable, because the affected organ(s) will dictate the predominant clinical signs.

Juvenile lymphosarcoma is often characterized by a sudden onset of diffuse lymphoid hyperplasia with or without visceral organ involvement. Weight loss, fever, tachycardia, dyspnea, bloat, and posterior paresis have all been described with this form of lymphosarcoma. Profound lymphocytosis (>50,000/μL) often accompanies this fatal form of bovine lymphosarcoma. Thymic lymphosarcoma may involve the cervical or intrathoracic thymus, or both. Clinical signs associated with this form of lymphosarcoma depend heavily on the location and size of the tumor. A cervical swelling may be evident. Dyspnea, bloat, jugular distention, tachycardia, anterior edema, and fever have been documented. The affected cell population is an immature, poorly differentiated lymphocyte. Cutaneous lymphosarcoma presents as cutaneous plaques, 1–5 cm in diameter, on the neck, back, rump, and thighs. Regional lymph nodes may also be enlarged. This form of lymphosarcoma may undergo spontaneous remission; however, relapses may occur.

Lesions: Animals with BLV-associated lymphosarcoma commonly show lesions in the central or peripheral lymph nodes, leading to lymphadenopathy. Lesions of the abomasum may lead to signs of cranial abdominal pain, melena, or abomasal outflow obstruction. Pelvic limb paresis progressing to paralysis can occur in animals with extradural spinal lesions. Retrobulbar lesions cause protrusion of the globe, resulting in exposure keratitis and eventually proptosis. Lesions of the right atrium may be mild and undetectable clinically, or may cause arrhythmias, murmurs, or heart failure. Uterine lesions may lead to reproductive failure or abortion. Lesions of the internal organs typically involve the spleen, liver, or kidneys and ureters. Lesions of the spleen are often initially asymptomatic but may result in rupture of the spleen and exsanguination into the peritoneal cavity. Lymphosarcoma of the liver is often asymptomatic but may lead to jaundice and liver failure. Disease of the kidney and ureter can lead to abdominal pain and the subsequent development of hydroureter or hydronephrosis and clinical signs associated with renal failure.

Lymphosarcoma may appear as yellow-tan, discrete nodular masses or a diffuse tissue infiltrate. The latter pattern results in an enlarged, pale organ and can be easily misinterpreted as a degenerative change rather than neoplasia. Histologically, the tumor masses are composed of densely packed, monomorphic lymphocytic cells.

Diagnosis: Lymphosarcoma is often included on the differential diagnosis list for many diseases because of the wide range of clinical findings. Viral infection is diagnosed by serology or virology, persistent lymphocytosis is identified by hematology, and neoplastic tumors are identified by histologic examination of biopsies. Positive serology or virology for BLV confirms viral infection but not the presence of lymphosarcoma.

Serology is the most common and reliable way to diagnose infection with BLV. Agar gel immunodiffusion is still recognized by most countries as the official import/export test, but ELISA is the most common test for routine diagnostic use. Serology is unreliable in calves that have ingested colostrum from BLV-positive cows because of the passive acquisition of maternal antibodies that typically wane by 4–6 mo of age. PCR is a sensitive and specific assay for diagnosis of BLV infection in peripheral blood lymphocytes. This test can identify proviral DNA of BLV in the lymphocytes of infected animals and differentiate positive from negative calves in the presence of maternal antibodies.

The diagnosis of lymphosarcoma must be made by cytology or histopathology. Cytologic diagnosis is sometimes difficult because of the frequency of blood contamination of the aspirates.

Treatment and Control: There is no treatment for viral infection or for lymphosarcoma in cattle, although parenteral corticosteroids can transiently decrease the severity of clinical signs. Eradication programs have been developed but success has been variable, primarily because of the expense and high prevalence of infection among cattle in the USA relative to the economic cost of disease. The most commonly recommended eradication protocol is as follows: 1) identify infected animals using a serologic test, 2) cull seropositive animals immediately, 3) retest the herd in 30–60 days, 4) use PCR to test young calves and as a complementary test to clarify test results in herds with a low prevalence of infection, and 5) repeat testing and cull until the entire herd tests negative. Testing is then repeated every 6 mo. The herd is declared free when there have been no positive tests for 2 yr. Additions to the herd should have two negative tests 30 and 60 days before arrival.

When test and cull programs are economically untenable, test and segregation programs have been recommended but are rarely implemented. These programs necessitate running two completely separate operations and require additional resources, including money, time, and available workforce.

Prevention: Eliminating the movement of blood from infected animals to naive animals is the cornerstone of prevention protocols. In calves, feeding colostrum from seronegative cows is often advocated. However, most epidemiologic evidence suggests that the protective effect of colostral antibody outweighs the risk of infections, particularly in high prevalence herds. The replacement of whole milk feeding with high-quality milk replacer may also be considered. Bloody milk should never be fed to calves.

Cautery or other bloodless methods of dehorning should be used. Equipment used for castration, tattooing, ear tagging, or implanting should be adequately cleaned and disinfected between animals.

Transmission can be decreased in adult cattle by changing rectal sleeves in between cows. Artificial insemination or embryo transfer (using negative recipients) may limit transmission. In beef herds, the use of a negative bull may limit transmission, but natural service is an uncommon method of viral transmission unless breeding is traumatic.

Additional recommendations include disinfection of equipment that has come in contact with blood or body tissue. Single use, disposable needles should always be used for blood collection and IM injections. It is preferable to use single-use disposable needles for vaccination, but the risk of transmitting BLV virus via SC vaccination is low. Handling facilities that become contaminated with blood should be cleaned between animals. Fly control helps minimize the potential for tabanid-associated transmission. Blood transfusions and vaccines containing blood, such as those used for babesiosis and anaplasmosis, are particularly potent ways to spread the disease, and donors must be carefully screened.

BOVINE PETECHIAL FEVER

(Ondiri disease)

Bovine petechial fever is a rickettsiosis of cattle characterized by high fever, hemorrhages, and edema. Its occurrence has been confirmed in the highlands of Kenya and Tanzania at altitudes >5,000 ft (1,500 m), although it is considered likely to occur in neighboring countries with similar topography. The importance of bovine petechial fever lies in its threat to dairy development in the highlands of eastern Africa, but no outbreak has been reported for more than a decade.

Etiology and Epidemiology: The disease is caused by *Ehrlichia ondiri*, an intracellular rickettsia that resides in cytoplasmic vacuoles of circulating leukocytes. The organism can multiply after experimental infection in cattle, sheep, goats, bushbuck, duiker, impala, Thomson's gazelles, and wildebeest, and hence, probably in most domestic and wild ruminants. *E ondiri* is believed to be endemic in wild ruminants, particularly bushbuck, and it sporadically overspills into domestic cattle grazing forest edges or scrubs.

The disease is restricted to scrub or forest edge areas that have heavy shade, a thick litter layer that provides high relative humidity, and a residual population of bushbuck and duiker, the two wild ruminants believed to be the main amplifying and reservoir hosts. It is seen sporadically throughout the year in imported breeds of cattle. It is not known how the disease is transmitted. As in other rickettsial infections, an arthropod vector is suspected, but extensive attempts to incriminate ticks, biting insects, and mites have failed.

Pathogenesis: The route of infection is not known, but *E ondiri* can be seen in circulating granulocytes (neutrophils and eosinophils) and monocytes while cattle are ill, and in the spleen at necropsy. Electron microscopic studies have shown that *E ondiri* can also infect endothelial and Kupffer cells, and it may be free in capillary lumens in the heart. It is believed that *E ondiri* initially multiplies in the spleen, with subsequent spread to other areas. Damage to the vascular endothelium would explain the hemorrhages and edema, as in many other rickettsial infections.

Clinical Findings: The disease is characterized by a high, fluctuating fever, apathy, lowered milk yield, and widespread petechiation of mucous membranes. After an incubation period of 4–14 days, animals develop a high fever; 2–3 days later, most animals appear dull, and petechiae may be seen on mucous membranes, particularly the lower surface of the tongue and the vaginal mucosa. These hemorrhages enlarge over several days and then regress as the animal begins to recover. Marked conjunctival edema and hemorrhage ("poached egg eye") are characteristic in some severe cases. The conjunctival sacs are swollen and everted around a tense and protruding eyeball, and there may be blood in the aqueous humor. Pregnant cows may abort, most likely from the high fever. Other clinical signs are absent. The case mortality rate in untreated cases can be as high as 50% in imported animals or in animals newly introduced to the area. Latent infections develop after recovery in some animals, especially in indigenous stock and in bushbuck. After recovery from the disease, affected cattle are immune against experimental challenge for ~2 yr.

Lesions: Typically, eosinopenia and lymphopenia are marked, followed by an equally pronounced neutropenia. Anemia is characteristically a sequela, and organisms can be demonstrated in Giemsa-stained smears of blood or spleen. At necropsy, widespread serosal and mucosal hemorrhages and edema are accompanied by lymphoid hyperplasia. Organs frequently affected include the heart, GI tract from the forestomach to the colon, liver, gallbladder, kidneys, and urinary bladder. The edema is characterized by gelatinous fluid in the intermuscular connective tissue, lymph nodes, and abomasum. No characteristic histologic abnormalities have been described, but there is vascular proliferation with prominent endothelial swelling and mild mononuclear infiltration.

Diagnosis: In areas where the disease is endemic, a history of movement to forest edge areas, coupled with clinical signs and postmortem lesions, allows for a presumptive diagnosis. Definitive diagnosis requires demonstration of the causal organism in Giemsa-stained smears of blood or spleen or by electron microscopy. *E ondiri* stains blue with Giemsa and can be seen as small bodies (0.4 µm), larger bodies (1–2 µm), groups of small and large bodies, and groups or morulae of small bodies. They are seen in cytoplasmic vacuoles and are most commonly seen in neutrophils. Tissue suspensions (spleen) can also be inoculated into susceptible cattle or sheep. Blood smears from the recipient animal should be made daily for as long as 10 days, by which time *E ondiri* should be detectable in neutrophils. The disease is difficult to differentiate from other hemorrhagic diseases of cattle such as Rift Valley fever, acute trypanosomosis (hemorrhagic *Trypanosoma vivax*), acute theileriasis, heartwater, hemorrhagic septicemia, and bracken fern poisoning.

Treatment and Control: Dithiosemicarbazone and tetracyclines have been used successfully to treat early experimental cases but are ineffective in advanced cases. The former is said to be more effective. In endemic areas, the disease can be prevented by avoiding areas associated with previous cases. However, this may not always be practical.

CAPRINE ARTHRITIS AND ENCEPHALITIS

Caprine arthritis and encephalitis (CAE) virus infection is manifested clinically as polysynovitis-arthritis in adult goats and less commonly as progressive paresis (leukoencephalomyelitis) in kids. Subclinical or clinical interstitial pneumonia, indurative mastitis ("hard udder"), and chronic wasting have also been attributed to infection with this virus. Most CAE virus infections, however, are subclinical. Infection with the CAE virus decreases the lifetime productivity of dairy goats and is a barrier to exportation of goats from North America.

CAE virus infection is widespread among dairy goats in most industrialized countries but rare among indigenous goat breeds of developing countries unless they have been in contact with imported goats. In countries such as Canada, Norway, Switzerland, France, and the USA, seroprevalence of CAE virus is >65%.

Etiology, Epidemiology, and Pathogenesis: The CAE virus is an enveloped, single-stranded RNA lentivirus in the family Retroviridae. There are several, genetically distinct isolates of the virus that differ in virulence.

The CAE virus of goats is closely related to the ovine lentiviruses causing ovine progressive pneumonia and maedi-visna in North America and Europe, respectively. Cross-species transmission is possible through feeding of infected milk and colostrum. Therefore, the ovine and caprine lentiviruses are now commonly referred to as small ruminant lentiviruses.

CAE virus infection is widespread in dairy goat breeds but uncommon in meat- and fiber-producing goats. This has been attributed to genetics, management practices such as feeding colostrum and milk from a single dam to multiple kids, and industrialized farming practices (eg, frequent introductions of new animals into a herd). Prevalence of infection increases with age but is not influenced by sex. Most goats are infected at an early age, remain virus positive for life, and develop disease months to years later.

The chief mode of spread of CAE is through ingestion of virus-infected goat colostrum or milk by kids. The feeding of pooled colostrum or milk to kids is a particularly risky practice, because a few infected does will spread the virus to a large number of kids. Horizontal transmission also contributes to disease spread within herds and may occur through direct contact, exposure to fomites at feed bunks and waterers, ingestion of contaminated milk in milking parlors, or serial use of needles or equipment contaminated with blood. Unlikely methods of transmission, as indicated by experimental studies, include in utero transmission to the fetus, infection of the kid during parturition, and infection through breeding or embryo transfer.

The pathogenesis of CAE is not fully understood. Virus-infected macrophages in colostrum and milk are absorbed intact through the gut mucosa. Infection is subsequently spread throughout the body via infected mononuclear cells. Periodic viral replication and macrophage maturation induces the characteristic lymphoproliferative lesions in target tissues such as the lungs, synovium, choroid plexus, and udder. Persistence of the CAE virus in the host is facilitated by its ability to become sequestered as provirus in host cells. Infection induces a strong humoral and cell-mediated immune response, but neither is protective.

Clinical Findings: Clinical signs are seen in ~20% of CAE virus–infected goats during their lifetime. The most common manifestation of infection is polysynovitis-arthritis, which is primarily seen in adult goats but can occur in kids as young as 6 mo old. Signs of polysynovitis-arthritis include joint capsule distention and varying degrees of lameness. The carpal joints are most frequently involved. The onset of arthritis may be sudden or insidious, but the clinical course is always progressive. Affected goats lose condition and usually have poor hair coats. Encephalomyelitis is generally seen in kids 2–4 mo old but has been described in older kids and adult goats. Affected kids initially exhibit weakness, ataxia, and hindlimb placing deficits. Hypertonia and hyperreflexia are also common. Over time, signs progress to paraparesis or tetraparesis and paralysis. Depression, head tilt, circling, opisthotonos, torticollis, and paddling have also been described. The interstitial pneumonia component of CAE virus infection rarely produces clinical signs in kids. However, in adult goats with serologic evidence of CAE virus infection, chronic interstitial pneumonia that leads to progressive dyspnea has been documented. The "hard udder" syndrome attributed to CAE virus infection is characterized by a firm, swollen mammary gland and agalactia at the time of parturition. Milk quality is usually unaffected. Although the mammary gland may soften and produce close to normal amounts of milk, production remains low in many goats with indurative mastitis.

Lesions: Pathologic lesions of CAE virus infection are generally described as lymphoproliferative with degenerative mononuclear cell infiltration. Lesions in joints are characterized by thickening of the joint capsule and marked proliferation of synovial villi. In chronic cases, soft-tissue calcification involving joint capsules, tendon sheaths, and bursae is not uncommon. Severe cartilage destruction, rupture of ligaments and tendons, and periarticular osteophyte formation have also been described in advanced cases. Microscopic features of articular lesions include synovial cell hyperplasia, subsynovial mononuclear cell infiltration, villous hypertrophy, synovial edema, and synovial necrosis. Gross lesions associated with the neurologic form of CAE include asymmetric, brownish pink, swollen areas, most commonly in the cervical and lumbosacral spinal cord segments. Histopathologically, these lesions are characterized by multifocal, mononuclear cell inflammatory infiltrates and varying degrees of demyelination. On gross examination, lungs of affected goats are firm and gray-pink with multiple, small, white foci, and do not collapse. The bronchial lymph nodes are invariably enlarged. Histologic findings include chronic interstitial pneumonia with mononuclear cell infiltration in alveolar septae and in perivascular and peribronchial regions. In does with udder induration, mononuclear infiltration of periductular stroma obliterates normal mammary tissue.

Diagnosis: A presumptive diagnosis can be based on clinical signs and history. Infectious arthritis caused by *Mycoplasma* spp and traumatic arthritis are differential diagnoses for arthritis induced by CAE virus. Differential diagnoses for the progressive paresis and paralysis exhibited by young kids should include enzootic ataxia, spinal cord abscess, cerebrospinal nematodiasis, spinal cord trauma, and congenital anomalies of the spinal cord and vertebral column. If the neurologic examination indicates brain involvement, polioencephalomalacia, listeriosis, and rabies should be considered as possible causes. The pulmonary form of caseous lymphadenitis may have a similar clinical presentation to the pulmonary form of CAE in adult goats.

Both an agar gel immunodiffusion test and ELISA for CAE virus are considered sufficiently reliable for use in control programs. The agar gel immunodiffusion test is reported to be more specific but less sensitive than the ELISA. A positive test result in an adult goat implies infection but does not confirm that the clinical signs are caused by CAE virus. Kids infected at birth develop a measurable antibody response 4–10 wk after infection. However, positive test results in kids <90 days old usually reflect colostral antibody transfer. Negative test results do not reliably exclude CAE virus infection, because the time for postinfection seroconversion is variable and occasional goats have a very low titer that may not be detectable. Low antibody titers are common in late pregnancy. Because of the limitations of serologic testing, definitive diagnosis of clinical CAE requires demonstration of characteristic lesions in biopsy specimens or at necropsy. Virus isolation or PCR to demonstrate presence of viral antigen in tissues may be used to further substantiate the diagnosis.

Treatment and Control: There are no specific treatments for any of the clinical syndromes associated with CAE virus infection. However, supportive treatments may benefit individual goats. The condition of goats with the polysynovitis-arthritis may be improved with regular foot trimming, use of additional bedding, and administration of NSAIDs such as phenylbutazone or aspirin. Goats with encephalomyelitis can be maintained for weeks with good nursing care. Antimicrobial therapy is indicated to treat secondary bacterial infections that may complicate the interstitial pneumonia or indurative mastitis components of CAE virus infection. Providing high-quality, readily digestible feed to goats positive for CAE virus may delay the onset of the wasting syndrome.

In commercial herds, one or more of the following have been recommended for control of CAE: 1) permanent isolation of kids beginning at birth; 2) feeding of heat-treated colostrum (45°C [113°F] for 60 min) and pasteurized milk; 3) frequent serologic testing of the herd (semiannually), with identification and segregation of seronegative and seropositive goats; and 4) eventual culling of seropositive goats. If the control program includes segregation of herds into seropositive and seronegative groups, groups should be separated by a minimum of 6 ft (1.8 m), and shared equipment should be disinfected using phenolic or quaternary ammonium compounds.

COLISEPTICEMIA

(Septicemic colibacillosis, Septicemic disease)

Septicemia caused by *Escherichia coli* is a common disease of neonatal calves, and to a lesser extent lambs. It may present with signs of acute septicemia or as a chronic bacteremia with localization.

Etiology and Epidemiology: The disease is caused by specific invasive serotypes of *E coli* that possess virulence factors enabling them to cross mucosal surfaces, overcome the bactericidal plasma factors, and produce bacteremia and septicemia. The main determinant of the disease is deficiency of circulating immunoglobulins as the result of a failure in passive transfer of colostral immunoglobulin.

Colisepticemia is seen during the first weeks of life, with the highest incidence in animals 2–5 days old. Bacteremia and septicemia in calves and lambs are most commonly associated with *E coli* and to a lesser extent *Salmonella* spp. Approximately 30% of diarrheic calves with severe systemic clinical signs were found to be bacteremic or septicemic, with *E coli* the most commonly isolated pathogen from blood cultures.

Transmission and Pathogenesis: It is assumed that the primary source of the infection is the feces of infected animals, including the healthy dams and neonates, and diarrheic newborn animals, which act as multipliers of the organisms. Invasion occurs primarily through the nasal and oropharyngeal mucosa but can also occur across the intestine or via the umbilicus and umbilical veins. Septicemic strains of *E coli* produce endotoxin, which results in shock and rapid death. There is a period of subclinical bacteremia that, with virulent strains, is followed by rapid development of septicemia and death from endotoxemic shock. A more prolonged course, with localization of infection, polyarthritis, meningitis, and less commonly uveitis and nephritis, is seen with less virulent strains. Chronic disease also develops in calves that have acquired marginal levels of circulating immunoglobulin. The organism is excreted in nasal and oral secretions, urine, and feces; excretion begins during the preclinical bacteremic stage. Initial infection can be acquired from a contaminated environment. In groups of calves, transmission is by direct nose-to-nose contact, urinary and respiratory aerosols, or as the result of navel sucking or fecal-oral contact.

Clinical Findings and Diagnosis: In the peracute and acute disease, the clinical course is short (3–8 hr), and signs are related to development of septic shock. Fever is not prominent, and the rectal temperature may even be subnormal. Listlessness and an early loss of interest in sucking are followed by depression, poor response to external stimuli, collapse, recumbency, cold extremities, and coma.

Tachycardia, a weak pulse, and prolonged capillary refill time are seen. The feces are loose and mucoid, but severe diarrhea is not seen in uncomplicated cases. Tremor, hyperesthesia, opisthotonos, and convulsions are seen occasionally, but stupor and coma are more common. Mortality approaches 100%. With a more prolonged clinical course, the infection may localize. Polyarthritis, ophthalmitis, omphalophlebitis, and meningitis may occur within the first week of the initial bacteremic phase.

No single laboratory parameter is considered reliable for early diagnosis of septicemia. A moderate but significant leukocytosis and neutrophilia are seen early, but leukopenia is more common in severe and advanced cases. A left shift of neutrophils and signs of toxicity of neutrophils as well as hypoglycemia are common findings. Because failure of transfer of passive immunity is the single most important predisposing factor, subnormal serum IgG and total protein concentrations are common. Subnormal platelet counts are the result of a consumptive coagulopathy. In cases of arthritis, the joint fluid has an increased inflammatory cell count and protein concentration. With meningitis, the CSF shows pleocytosis and an increased protein concentration; organisms may be evident on microscopic examination. Less commonly, other bacteria, including other Enterobacteriaceae, *Streptococcus* spp, and *Pasteurella* spp, produce septicemic disease in young calves. These organisms are more common in sporadic cases than as causes of outbreaks. They produce similar clinical disease but can be differentiated by culture. As with colisepticemia, the primary determinant of these infections is a failure of passive transfer of colostral immunoglobulins.

The diagnosis is based on history and clinical findings, demonstration of a severe deficiency of circulating IgG, and ultimately, demonstration of the organism in blood or tissues.

Treatment: Treatment requires aggressive antimicrobial, fluid, and anti-inflammatory therapy. Although blood cultures are recommended to retrospectively confirm the diagnosis, antimicrobial therapy must be initiated immediately in any animal suspected of being septic. Because there is no time for sensitivity testing, the initial choice should be a bactericidal drug that has a high probability of efficacy against gram-negative organisms. Administration IV of large volumes of balanced electrolyte solutions over several hours is essential to correct hypovolemia and assure adequate peripheral tissue perfusion; fluids should include glucose to correct hypoglycemia. The beneficial effect of NSAIDs has been attributed to their anti-inflammatory, antipyretic, and analgesic properties. Glucocorticoids have also been proposed to treat septicemia, although their benefits for treatment of sepsis are less well established.

Control and Prevention: Calves that acquire adequate concentrations of immunoglobulin from colostrum are resistant to colisepticemia. Therefore, prevention depends primarily on management practices that ensure an adequate and early intake of colostrum. The adequacy of the farm's practice of feeding colostrum should be monitored, and corrective strategies applied as required. In North American Holstein dairy herds, natural sucking does not guarantee adequate concentrations of circulating immunoglobulins, and calves should be fed 2–4 L of first-milking colostrum containing a minimal total mass of 100 g of IgG, using a nipple bottle or an esophageal feeder, within 2 hr of birth; this is followed by a second feeding at 12 hr. A cow-side immunoassay test can assist in selection of colostrum with adequate immunoglobulin concentration. Although the circulating concentration of immunoglobulin required to protect against colisepticemia is low, high concentrations are desirable to decrease susceptibility to other neonatal infectious diseases.

When natural colostrum is not available for a newborn calf, commercial colostrum substitutes containing 25 g of IgG will provide sufficient immunoglobulin for protection against colisepticemia if fed early in the absorptive period. Plasma containing at least 4 g and preferably 8 g of IgG, administered parenterally, will provide some protection for older calves that have not been fed colostrum and are unable to absorb immunoglobulins from the intestine. Small-volume hyperimmune serum is of benefit only when it contains antibody specific to the particular serotype associated with an outbreak. The risk of early infection should be minimized by hygiene in the calving area and disinfection of the navel at birth. To minimize transmission, calves reared indoors should be in separate pens (without contact) or reared in calf hutches.

CRIMEAN-CONGO HEMORRHAGIC FEVER

Crimean-Congo hemorrhagic fever (CCHF) is a severe hemorrhagic viral disease of people acquired from infected ticks, tissues of infected wild or domestic animals, and from human patients with the disease.

Etiology and Epidemiology: The etiologic agent, CCHF virus (genus *Nairovirus*, family Bunyaviridae), is an enveloped negative-sense, trisegmented, single-stranded RNA virus. The virus has been reported in a wide area from South Africa through southern Europe, Eurasia, and into parts of western China. The virus is principally associated with ticks of the genus *Hyalomma*, although it has also been isolated from other genera of ixodid ticks. The global distribution of the virus roughly approximates that of *Hyalomma* spp ticks. Recent analyses of the genome of the virus suggest that there is significant genetic diversity somewhat correlated with geographic origin of the virus. However, anomalies to this pattern suggest that dispersal of host ticks by migratory wildlife such as birds or the movement of livestock (by people) may act to perturb the "normal" geographic distribution of CCHF virus subpopulations.

Transmission and Pathogenesis: The virus replicates in the host tick as it passes from larval through adult stages (transstadial transmission), and it can also be transmitted from one generation to the next (transovarial transmission). Thus, the tick not only is a vector but also can be a reservoir of the virus via vertical transmission. Small rodents, lagomorphs, and birds have all been incriminated as sources of infection of immature stages of the tick, while most *Hyalomma* spp ticks are multihost and use larger vertebrates as the host for the adult stage of their life cycle.

Clinical Findings and Diagnosis: In experimental inoculations, sheep and cattle become infected but develop only transient and mild increases of body temperature with little evidence of clinical disease. Viremia levels and duration are relatively low and short, and antibodies are detectable shortly after cessation of viremia. Reverse transcriptase-PCR assays can detect the virus, but primer design should match the viruses found in the region in which human patients, or other materials, have originated. Some tests (principally IgG ELISA) can detect antibodies for the remainder of the life of the animal, while other tests, such as complement fixation and indirect fluorescent antibody, can detect antibodies for shorter periods after infection. Antibody prevalence in adult livestock species in endemic regions can be >50%.

Treatment: The antiviral drug ribavirin has been used in treatment of human disease in South Africa, although placebo-controlled trials have not been completed. Lack of significant clinical disease in livestock warrants no treatment considerations.

Control and Prevention: Control strategies for human infection include the avoidance of tick bites through the use of repellents and appropriate protection when slaughtering or grooming animals. Movement of naive animals into endemic areas provides opportunity for vertebrate amplification of the virus and increasing occupational risk to butchers and hide preparers; tick control when naive animals and endemic stock are mixed is paramount. Medical personnel should use appropriate barrier nursing techniques and universal (standard) precautions when handling suspect patients.

HEARTWATER

(Cowdriosis)

Heartwater is an infectious, noncontagious, tickborne rickettsial disease of ruminants. The disease is seen only in areas infested by ticks of the genus *Amblyomma*. These include regions of Africa south of the Sahara and the islands of the Comores, Zanzibar, Madagascar, Sao Tomé, Réunion, and Mauritius. Heartwater was introduced to the Caribbean, and it and its vector (*A variegatum*) are endemic on the islands of

Guadeloupe and Antigua. *A variegatum*, but not the rickettsia, has since spread to several other islands despite attempts at eradication. Possible spread to the mainland threatens the livestock industry of regions from northern South America to Central America and the southern USA. In heartwater endemic areas in southern Africa, it is estimated that mortalities due to the disease are more than double those due to bacillary hemoglobinuria (red water, *see* p 601) and anaplasmosis (*see* p 18) combined. Cattle, sheep, goats, and some antelope species are susceptible to heartwater. In endemic areas, some animals and tortoises may become subclinically infected and act as reservoirs. Indigenous African cattle breeds (*Bos indicus*), especially those with years of natural selection, appear more resistant to clinical heartwater than *B taurus* breeds.

Etiology and Transmission: The causative organism is an obligate intracellular parasite, previously known as *Cowdria ruminantium*. Molecular evidence led to reclassification of several organisms in the order Rickettsiales, and it is now classified as *Ehrlichia ruminantium*. Under natural conditions, *E ruminantium* is transmitted by *Amblyomma* ticks. These three-host ticks become infected during either the larval or nymphal stages and transmit the infection during one of the subsequent stages (transstadial transmission). The progeny of an infected female tick are most probably not infective (ie, there is no epidemiologically significant transovarial transmission). This and the fact that ticks are indiscriminate feeders probably play a role in the low infection rate in tick populations.

E ruminantium can be propagated experimentally by serial passage, either by inoculating infective blood into, or by feeding infected nymphal or adult stages of a vector tick on, susceptible animals. The organism can also be propagated in tissue culture, most reliably in endothelial cells, but also in primary neutrophil cultures and macrophage cell lines. At room temperature, infective material loses its infectivity within a few hours, but the organism, together with suitable cryoprotectants, may be viably preserved in liquid nitrogen for years.

Immunity to heartwater appears to be *chiefly, if not exclusively*, cell mediated, because spleen cells from an immune donor inoculated into susceptible recipients protects, whereas serum from an immune donor fails to protect recipients when challenged. There is no, or only partial, cross-protection between different stocks (strains) of *E ruminantium*. Most of these stocks are infective for, but cannot be serially passaged in, mice; however, a few are pathogenic to mice infected by the IV route.

Pathogenesis: The pathogenesis of heartwater has not been elucidated; however, the tick probably infects the host via organisms in the saliva or regurgitated gut content while feeding. Replication of the *E ruminantium* organisms in the tick probably occurs in the intestinal epithelium and is significantly amplified. Once in the host, the organisms may replicate first within the regional lymph nodes with subsequent dissemination via the bloodstream to invade endothelial cells of blood vessels elsewhere in the body. In domestic ruminants, there does seem to be a predilection for endothelial cells of the brain. Organisms can often be found in colonies (commonly but mistakenly referred to as morulas) within the cytoplasm of endothelial cells. Colonies can vary in size, as can the organisms that reside in them. Generally, small-sized organisms are found in larger colonies and vice versa. The smaller organisms are usually referred to as elementary bodies and represent the infective stage, the larger organisms as reticulated bodies and the proliferative stage, and those in between as intermediate bodies.

During the febrile stage, and for a short while thereafter, the blood of infected animals is infective to susceptible animals if subinoculated. Signs and lesions are associated with functional injury to the vascular endothelium, resulting in increased vascular permeability without recognizable histopathologic or even ultrastructural pathology. The concomitant fluid effusion into tissues and body cavities precipitates a fall in arterial pressure and general circulatory failure. The lesions in peracute and acute cases are hydrothorax, hydropericardium, edema and congestion of the lungs and brain, splenomegaly, petechiae and ecchymoses on mucosal and serosal surfaces, and occasionally hemorrhage into the GI tract, particularly the abomasum. The typically straw-colored effusions are high in large-molecular-weight proteins, including fibrinogen; hence, this fluid readily clots on exposure to air. The amount of effusion seen, particularly in body cavities, is not necessarily proportionate to the concentration of parasitic colonies detected in endothelial cells.

Clinical Findings: The clinical signs are dramatic in the peracute and acute forms. In peracute cases, animals may drop dead within a few hours of developing a fever, sometimes without any apparent clinical signs; others display an exaggerated respiratory distress and/or paroxysmal convulsions. In the acute form, animals often show anorexia and depression along with congested and friable mucous membranes. Respiratory distress slowly develops along with nervous signs such as a hyperaesthesia, a high-stepping stiff gait, exaggerated blinking, and chewing movements. Terminally, prostration with bouts of opisthotonus; "pedaling," "thrashing," or stiffening of the limbs; and convulsions are seen. Diarrhea is seen occasionally. In subacute cases, the signs are less marked and CNS involvement is inconsistent.

Diagnosis: In clinical cases, heartwater must be differentiated from a wide range of infectious and noninfectious diseases, especially plant poisonings, that manifest with CNS signs. In acute clinical cases in endemic areas, clinical signs alone may suggest the etiology, but demonstration of colonies of organisms in the cytoplasm of capillary endothelial cells is necessary for a definitive diagnosis. Traditionally, this is done with "squash" smears of cerebral or cerebellar gray matter stained with Romanowsky-type stains. Low concentration Giemsa stain developed for 30 min gives the best color differentiation and batch-to-batch consistency. Organisms in autolyzed material lose their stainability, and diagnosis then becomes difficult.

For the "brain squash smear," a piece of gray matter (~3 × 3 mm) is macerated between two microscope slides; the softened material is then spread like a blood smear with the material pushed rather than pulled along. A slight lifting of the spreader slide about every 5–10 mm creates several thick ridges across the slide, from which capillaries are arranged straight and parallel in the thin sections of the smear for easier examination. The endothelial cells of all the capillaries on a smear should be carefully scrutinized for presence of the dark purple colonies made up of clusters of individual organisms (granules) of *E ruminantium*. The size of the granules can vary between animals, or smears from the same animal, or even between colonies on the same smear, but is usually uniform within a particular colony.

Using immunoperoxidase staining methods, a definitive diagnosis can be made on any formalin-fixed tissue samples, even from autolyzed carcasses. The contrasting color makes the search for and identification of the rickettsial colonies much quicker, although the substructure of the colonies should be identified before the diagnosis is confirmed. Because of the nature of the test, false-positive reactions may arise with some closely related organisms. On brain squash smears, *Chlamydia pecorum* can be confused with *E ruminantium*, but histopathology or the immunoperoxidase technique allow differentiation. Serodiagnosis of animals previously exposed to the disease, ie, recovered from subclinical or clinical infection, still poses problems. Several tests are in use, including several indirect fluorescent antibody and ELISA tests. All serologic tests, including an ELISA that uses recombinant antigen, are plagued by cross-reactions with sera from animals infected with one of several *Ehrlichia* or *Anaplasma* organisms (false positive) and the fact that immune cattle on repeated exposure may become seronegative (false negative). DNA probes, available at research institutions, can be used together with PCR technology. A combination of a pCS20 probe and probes to 16S ribosomal RNA of several of the stocks are used routinely to examine samples from animals when permits for movement of animals from endemic to nonendemic areas are required. Real-time PCR has also come into use.

Treatment, Control, and Prevention: Oxytetracycline at 10 mg/kg/day, IM, or doxycycline at 2 mg/kg/day will usually effect a cure if administered early in the course of heartwater infection. A higher dosage of oxytetracycline (20 mg/kg) is usually required if treatment begins late during the febrile reaction or when clinical signs are evident. In such cases, the first treatment should preferably be given slowly IV. A minimum of three daily doses should be given regardless of temperature; if fever persists, oxytetracycline treatment should continue for a fourth and fifth day. If the fever still does not abate, a potentiated sulfonamide at 15 mg/kg/day, IM, has been successful. The withdrawal times for milk and meat after treatment with doxycycline, short- or long-acting oxytetracycline, and sulfonamides must be observed based on local regulations.

Corticosteroids have been used as supportive therapy (prednisolone

1 mg/kg, IM), although there is debate as to the effectiveness and rationale for their use.

Diazepam may be required to control convulsions.

Affected animals must be kept quiet in a cool area with soft bedding and be totally undisturbed; any stimulation can preempt a convulsive episode and subsequent death.

Vaccination can help with the control of heartwater; however, it is neither easily administered nor monitored and gives variable to no cross-protection to the various *E ruminantium* stocks. The "infection and treatment method" for immunization is in use in southern Africa, where infected sheep blood containing fully virulent organisms of the Ball 3 stock is used for infection, followed by monitoring of rectal temperature and antibiotic therapy after a fever develops. In certain circumstances, the "controlled" infection is followed by preventive "block treatment" without temperature recording (cattle on day 14 [susceptible *B taurus* breeds] or day 16 [for the more resistant *B indicus* breeds], sheep and Angora goats on day 11, and Boer and crossbreed goats on day 12). Young calves (<4 wk old), lambs, and kids (<1 wk old) have an innate age-related resistance to heartwater, so if challenged by natural or induced infections within this time period, most recover spontaneously and develop a reasonable immunity.

Control of tick infestation is a useful preventive measure in some instances but may be difficult and expensive to maintain in others. Excessive reduction of tick numbers, however, interferes with the maintenance of adequate immunity through regular field challenge in endemic areas and may periodically result in heavy losses.

Chemoprophylaxis involves a series of oxytetracycline injections to protect susceptible animals from contracting heartwater when introduced into endemic areas while also allowing them to develop a natural immunity.

HISTOPHILOSIS

Histophilosis, or *Histophilus somni*–associated disease, is a common disease in North American cattle. It also has been reported to occur sporadically in beef and dairy cattle worldwide. *H somni* predominantly causes an acute, often fatal, septicemic disease that can involve the respiratory, cardiovascular, musculoskeletal, or nervous systems, either singly or together in confined cattle. The reproductive system is often affected without clinical signs or other systemic involvement; however, herd infertility has been reported to occur more frequently.

Etiology and Transmission: *H somni* is a gram-negative, nonmotile, nonspore-forming, nonencapsulated, pleomorphic coccobacillus that requires an enriched medium and a microaerophilic atmosphere for culture. Hemolysis on blood agar occurs within 48 hr due to an exotoxin produced by most disease-causing isolates. Pathogenic and nonpathogenic strains have been differentiated. The virulence of the organism may vary by region and age group.

H somni is considered a commensal of bovine mucous membranes. Pathogenic and nonpathogenic strains of *H somni* are found in the sheath and prepuce of males, the vagina of females, and in the nasal passages of both sexes. Nasal and urogenital secretions are believed to be sources of the organism. The organism may colonize the respiratory tract, presumably after inhalation, and gain access to the bloodstream via that route. Colonization of the male and female reproductive tracts may involve venereal spread.

Epidemiology: Recently weaned calves are at higher risk of infection and death from histophilosis than are previously weaned older calves, yearlings, or mature animals. The risk of infection with *H somni* is highest early in the feeding period, with "high-risk" calves in confinement establishing peak titers to *H somni* at ~21–23 days after arrival. Although calves are generally exposed to *H somni* earlier in the feeding period, the average time on feed for calves that die of histophilosis has been reported to be 30–60 days. Sudden death due to peracute septicemia usually occurs within 21 days after arrival, although it may occur throughout the feeding period. Reproductive disease manifestations, including granular vulvovaginitis, abortion, and mastitis, can affect individual beef and dairy cattle or more of the herd.

Pathogenesis: Septicemia is likely required for most forms of histophilosis. Strains of *H somni* that cause disease adhere to the endothelium of vessels, resulting in contraction, exposure of collagen, platelet adhesion, and thrombus formation. The primary disease mechanism likely involves a thrombus, rather than a thromboembolism as once thought. Some bacterial strains may adhere to the endothelium in vessels of the pleura, myocardium, pericardium, synovium, or a variety of other tissues (eg, brain, larynx). Interruption of the blood supply in those areas results in the formation of an infarction with destruction of tissue and the formation of a necrotic sequestrum. The development of clinical signs is associated with the extent of organ system involvement. The susceptibility of individual animals and variations in the preference of strains of the organism for vessels in different tissues may be important in the development of the different forms of the disease, but these have not been extensively studied.

The apparent preference of *H somni* for different organ systems has defined the changing character of histophilosis. Initially, the disease presented primarily as an encephalitic syndrome that changed to one in which pleuritic and myocardial forms predominated. Anecdotal observations suggest that the organism may be changing again (eg, from a focal to a more generalized myocarditis). Recent microbiologic examinations of the organism have identified a variety of mechanisms that contribute to its diverse virulence and ability to withstand treatment.

Reproductive disease has not been associated with systemic infection; the inflammation appears to be more local, even though the pathogenesis in these situations is not well understood.

Clinical Findings: Sudden death is usually the first indication of *H somni* infection in a group of confined animals and is often mistaken by the stock attendants as evidence of a digestive tract upset such as bloat. A profound depression has been described as the most noticeable clinical sign of encephalitic histophilosis. Other findings are determined by the system(s) involved and may include rapid respiration, stiffness, muscle weakness, ataxia, lameness, and severe behavioral changes. Animals affected with pleuritic histophilosis are usually found dead without any treatment history; if alive, they may exhibit extreme dyspnea. Animals with myocarditis display very poor exercise tolerance and may collapse and die when movement to a handling facility is attempted. Animals with the encephalitic form and early depression rapidly proceed to recumbency, with occasional signs of hyperesthesia before death. Animals found dead and confirmed with *H somni* infection often have a history of treatment for undifferentiated fever or depression in the previous 14 days.

Closer individual examination usually reveals a febrile animal. Polypnea and/or dyspnea may be evident overtly and are easily confirmed by auscultation. Hypoxemia associated with a malfunctioning pulmonary or cardiovascular system can be easily confused with other clinical signs such as depression or even blindness. A sterile blood sample obtained from an untreated animal at this time tests positive for *H somni* in a high percentage of cases.

Lesions: Feedlot cattle that die of possible histophilosis should be examined at necropsy. These animals may exhibit an array of postmortem findings, including fibrinous pleuritis without bronchopneumonia, a focal myocardial lesion (often in the papillary muscle of the left ventricle), fibrinous pericarditis, bronchopneumonia, polyarthritis, and a fibrinous laryngitis. Less common gross postmortem lesions include polyserositis, fibrinous gonitis, and a fibrinopurulent meningitis. Probably the most common lesion seen in the feedyard is that of “left heart failure” associated with a marked necrotic sequestrum in the myocardial wall.

In animals that survive long enough to allow the pathology to progress, the fibrinous portion of the lesions becomes fibrotic, and the infarctions or sequestrae in the heart or larynx liquefy and wall off to become an abscess. Lesions of the reproductive tract may include suppurative vaginitis, cervicitis, and endometritis.

Diagnosis: A definitive diagnosis is based on sampling and examination of affected tissues collected during a necropsy or clinical examination. A diagnosis at necropsy of “left heart failure” with a concomitant myocardial lesion or a carcass in which the thoracic space is filled with fluid and fibrin with little pneumonia is considered definitive for histophilosis. Historically, isolation of the organism from CSF, brain, blood, urine, joint fluid, or other sterile, internal organs or fluids has been used to confirm the diagnosis. Because *H somni* is a commensal of the mucous membranes of cattle, the bacterium should be isolated in predominant or pure culture from the respiratory or urogenital tract to be considered a significant etiologic agent. This may be difficult, because antimicrobial treatment often interferes with recovery of the organism. The characteristic histologic lesion is suppurative with heavy infiltrations of neutrophils in all tissues where localization of the bacteria occurs. Currently, the diagnosis is usually confirmed with molecular techniques such as immunohistochemical staining of H&E-stained tissues or a fresh lesion swab subjected to a specific PCR test.

Treatment and Prevention: A major hindrance to successful treatment of individual histophilosis cases is the difficulty in identifying affected animals early in the course of disease because of its often rapidly fatal nature. Antimicrobial treatment is most effective in the early stages of disease. Florfenicol (20 mg/kg, IM, repeated in 48 hr, or 40 mg/kg, SC, once) may be the antimicrobial of choice if histophilosis is the tentative diagnosis in an individual animal.

Evidence supporting the use of prophylactic or metaphylactic treatment with a sustained-action antimicrobial or an oral antimicrobial supplement in the feed on arrival at the feedlot or in the face of occurring cases to reduce histophilosis mortality is scant. This contrasts with the evidence that *H somni* is susceptible in vitro to a wide range of antimicrobials, including florfenicol, tilmicosin, tulathromycin, tetracyclines, trimethoprim-sulfadoxine, fluoroquinolones, and ceftiofur. Historically, the precise mechanism by which the organism is able to avoid systemic antimicrobial blood levels has not been well understood. Recently, it has been postulated that as *H somni* proliferates, it forms biofilms that allow it to adhere to the endothelium and to withstand an otherwise adequate level of an antimicrobial.

Bacterins containing different strains of the organism have been used to immunize cattle against *H somni*. A favorable humoral response generated by a single immunization with a commercial vaccine has been shown to be improved when boosted with a second immunization. Calves initially immunized before "turn out" (estimated age to be 2 mo) will respond to a second immunization anamnestically on their arrival at the feedlot after weaning. Although protection with current bacterins and immunogens against histophilosis morbidity and mortality has been reported, the ability of immunization to consistently spare cattle from the disease is compromised when immunization and challenge occur at the same time (ie, arrival at the feedlot).

HEMORRHAGIC SEPTICEMIA

Hemorrhagic septicemia (HS) is an acute, highly fatal form of pasteurellosis that affects mainly water buffalo, cattle, and bison. It is considered the most economically important bacterial disease of water buffalo and cattle in tropical areas of Asia, particularly in southeast Asia, where water buffalo populations are high. Disease is most devastating to smallholder farmers where husbandry and preventive practices are poor and free-range management is common. HS is also an important disease in Africa and the Middle East, with sporadic outbreaks occurring in southern Europe. The only confirmed outbreaks of HS in the Americas occurred in bison in Yellowstone National Park, most recently from 1965–1967. Natural disease occurs infrequently in pigs, sheep, and goats and has been reported in camels, elephants, horses, donkeys, yaks, and various species of deer and other wild ruminants.

Etiology: Classical HS as defined by the OIE is caused by *Pasteurella multocida* serotypes B:2 and E:2 (Carter and Heddleston classification system). Serotype B:2 has been identified in most areas where the disease is endemic, whereas serotype E:2 has been found only in Africa. Septicemic pasteurellosis that is clinically similar to HS can be caused by a wide variety of other *P multocida* serotypes and has been reported worldwide.

Transmission, Epidemiology, and Pathogenesis: The tonsils of up to 5% of healthy water buffalo and cattle are colonized by small numbers of *P multocida* serotype B:2 or E:2, which can be shed during periods of stress. Common stressors associated with outbreaks include high temperature and humidity, concurrent infection (blood parasites or foot and mouth disease), poor nutrition, or work stress. Although outbreaks can occur at any time, disease is most prevalent during the rainy season. Increased outbreaks associated with high rainfall are most likely due to the multiple stressors present during this time and the moist conditions, which prolong the survival time of the organism in the environment. Infection occurs by contact with infected oral or nasal secretions from either healthy carrier animals or animals with clinical disease, or by ingestion of contaminated feed or water. Infection begins in the tonsil and adjacent nasopharyngeal tissues. Subsequently, bacteremia leads to dissemination and rapid growth of bacteria in various locations, tissue injury, a host cytokine response, and release of lipopolysaccharides that results in a rapidly progressing endotoxemia. Clinical signs can appear 1–3 days after infection, and death can occur within 8–24 hr after the first signs develop. In endemic areas, HS affects older calves and young adults, and morbidity and mortality are variable. In nonendemic areas, epizootics can occur with high morbidity and mortality that can reach 100%. Water buffalo tend to be more susceptible and have more severe clinical disease than cattle. Recovery can stimulate acquired immunity to homologous and often heterologous strains of *P multocida*, and some of these animals become healthy carriers that can provide a source of infection for future outbreaks.

Clinical Findings: Many cases of HS are peracute and result in death within 8–24 hr. These animals often have fever, hypersalivation, nasal discharge, and difficult respiration, but because of the short duration of disease these signs may easily be overlooked. Acute disease can persist up to 3 days, and less often 5 days, and is characterized by fever of 104°–106°F (40°–41.1°C), apathy or restlessness and reluctance to move, hypersalivation, lacrimation, nasal discharge that begins as serous and progresses to mucopurulent, subcutaneous swelling in the pharyngeal region that extends to the ventral neck and brisket (and sometimes the forelegs), progressive respiratory difficulty, cyanosis, terminal recumbency, and possibly abdominal pain with diarrhea.

Lesions: The characteristic lesion of HS is swelling of the subcutis and muscle of the submandibular region, neck, and brisket by clear to blood-tinged edema fluid. Serous to serofibrinous fluid may also be present in the thorax, pericardium, and abdominal cavity. There is typically widespread congestion with petechiae and ecchymoses in tissues and on serosal surfaces. Hemorrhages are often most prominent in the pharyngeal and cervical lymph nodes. Pulmonary congestion and edema, sometimes with interstitial pneumonia, and gastroenteritis may occur in some cases.

Diagnosis: Clinical diagnosis of HS in endemic areas is based on history, lapses in vaccination, environmental conditions, and the characteristic clinical signs and lesions of disease. Although typical outbreaks of HS are not difficult to recognize in endemic regions, acute salmonellosis, anthrax, and noninfectious toxicities should also be considered. Sporadic cases are more difficult to diagnose clinically and could be confused with blackleg, lightning strike, or snakebite. A definitive diagnosis of HS is based on isolation of *P multocida* serotype B:2 or E:2 (or other less common serotypes recognized by the OIE as causing HS) from the blood and tissues of an animal with typical signs. Various other *P multocida* serotypes can cause HS-like disease in cattle and water buffalo, which must be differentiated from classical HS. The passive mouse protection test using specific B:2 and E:2 immune rabbit sera has been used in Asia and Africa to identify these serotypes. More precise tests, such as indirect hemagglutination, coagglutination, counter immunoelectrophoresis, and immunodiffusion tests have also been used in some laboratories. More recently, molecular techniques, including pulsed field gel electrophoresis, southern blots, and

PCR-based protocols, have been used to differentiate between capsular and somatic serotypes. The PCR techniques are most feasible for use in endemic areas and can be used with various samples, including blood, tissues, or bacteria from broth or plate cultures.

Treatment and Prevention: Antimicrobials are effective against HS if administered very early in the disease. However, because HS progresses rapidly, therapy is often unsuccessful. During outbreaks, any animal with a fever should be treated with IV antimicrobials as soon as possible to quickly obtain systemic bactericidal antimicrobial concentrations. Various sulfonamides, tetracyclines, penicillin, gentamicin, kanamycin, ceftiofur, enrofloxacin, tilmicosin, and chloramphenicol have been used effectively to treat HS. However, plasmid- and chromosomal-mediated multidrug resistance seems to be increasing for some strains of *P multocida*, and resistance to tetracyclines and penicillin has been reported for serotype B:2.

Killed vaccines are most commonly used for prevention and include bacterins, alum-precipitated and aluminum hydroxide gel vaccines, and oil-adjuvant vaccines. In animals >3 yr old, an initial two doses, 1–3 mo apart, is recommended, followed by booster vaccinations once or twice yearly. The oil-adjuvant vaccine provides protection for 9–12 mo and is given annually. Although it provides the best immunity, it is unpopular in the field because of its viscosity and difficulty of administration. Oil-based vaccines combined with tween 80 or saponin have also been used in attempts to increase the ease of administration or immune protection. The commonly used alum-precipitated and aluminum hydroxide gel vaccines have shorter durations of immunity, and twice yearly booster vaccinations are recommended. It is important that the vaccines are made from the strains of *P multocida* circulating in the regions of intended use to obtain maximal effectiveness. Attenuated or modified-live vaccines have been used with some success. A live avirulent vaccine prepared from a *P multocida* serotype B:3(4) of fallow deer origin seems effective and is recommended for use by the Food and Agricultural Organization of the United Nations (FAO) in southeast Asia. Various modified-live and subunit vaccines made from either purified or recombinant bacterial components have also been investigated experimentally.

Zoonotic Risk: The *P multocida* serotypes that cause HS have not been recovered from human infections. However, because many serotypes of *P multocida* have the potential to infect people, appropriate precautions should be taken when dealing with suspected cases of HS or HS-like disease.

MALIGNANT CATARRHAL FEVER

(Malignant head catarrh, Snotsiekte, Catarrhal fever, Gangrenous coryza)

Malignant catarrhal fever (MCF) is an infectious systemic disease that presents as a variable complex of lesions affecting mainly ruminants and rarely swine. It is principally a disease of domestic cattle, water buffalo, Bali cattle (banteng), American bison, and deer. In addition to these farmed animals, MCF has been described in a variety of captive ruminants in mixed zoologic collections. In some species, such as bison and some deer, MCF is acute and highly lethal, capable of affecting large numbers of animals. With occasional exceptions, the disease in cattle normally is seen sporadically and affects single animals. MCF is typically fatal; however, there are outbreaks in which several animals are affected, with evidence of recovery and mild or inapparent infections in some cases. It also occasionally presents as chronic alopecia and weight loss. Its distribution is essentially worldwide, mirroring that of the principal carriers, domestic sheep and wildebeest. MCF has long been a major problem in farmed deer operations, and in recent years has emerged as a severe threat to the commercial bison industry.

Etiology: MCF results from infection by one of several members of a group of closely related ruminant gammaherpesviruses of the *Rhadinovirus* genus. Although the MCF group of ruminant rhadinoviruses currently comprises approximately 10 known members, only a few are known to be pathogenic under natural conditions. The principal carriers and their viruses are sheep (ovine herpesvirus-2), wildebeest (alcelaphine herpesvirus-1), and goats (caprine herpesvirus-2). Another strain of unidentified origin has caused MCF in white-tailed deer. Virtually all clinical cases are caused by the sheep or wildebeest viruses.

The viruses are maintained within the sheep and wildebeest populations in similar but not identical patterns. Lambs are infected usually at 3–6 mo of age by aerosol transmission from other individuals within the flock and begin to actively shed virus at ~6–9 mo of age. Shedding decreases at ~10 mo, with adults shedding at a much lower rate than adolescents. Wildebeest calves, in contrast, are infected in the perinatal period by horizontal and occasional intrauterine transmission, and actively shed virus until 4–6 mo of age. Transmission is by transfer of virus-laden nasal secretions by direct contact or poorly defined airborne routes. Transmission from sheep to cattle has been demonstrated at distances of at least 70 m in cattle and at distances of up to 5.1 km in bison. In Africa, most wildebeest-associated MCF is seen around the time of wildebeest calving; however, sheep-associated MCF (SA-MCF) does not follow the same pattern. Ewes do not shed virus in placental tissues or secretions and do not experience more frequent shedding episodes around lambing time. The only rational and established factors contributing to seasonality of SA-MCF are climatic influences on virus survival and the age-related shedding patterns in lambs. The epidemiology of the caprine MCF virus appears similar to that of sheep.

The severity of SA-MCF outbreaks depends on factors such as the total numbers, population density, and species of susceptible hosts involved; the closeness of contact; and the amount of shed virus available for transmission. Cases usually are seen sporadically in European breeds of cattle (*Bos taurus*), because they are a relatively resistant species. By contrast, Bali cattle, bison, and some but not all cervid species (eg, white-tailed deer, Pere David's deer) are highly susceptible. Infectious dose of virus is a primary determinant of infection and clinical disease, with bison being >1,000 times more susceptible to infection than cattle. As agricultural systems involving bison and deer production have developed, MCF has become more troublesome. It is a leading cause of infectious disease losses on New Zealand deer farms. In bison exposed to large numbers of adolescent sheep, losses can be devastating. Approximately 800 head died in one outbreak in the USA in 2003. The incubation period is variable and ranges from 14 to >200 days from initial exposure.

Among animals that survive, infection is lifelong. Some susceptible species, including cattle and bison, may be latently infected. Recrudescence of latent infections is possible and must be considered for cases with no known history of contact with carriers.

MCF is transmitted only between carriers and clinically susceptible animals. Affected animals do not transmit MCF to their cohorts.

Clinical Findings: Acute MCF cases caused by ovine herpesvirus-2 and alcelaphine herpesvirus-1 are similar clinically and pathologically. Disease course may range from peracute to chronic. Cases in deer and bison are often peracute with sudden death. Deer that survive for a few days and bison usually develop hemorrhagic diarrhea, bloody urine, and corneal opacity before expiring. High fever (106°–107°F [41°–41.5°C]) and depression are common. Other possible signs include catarrhal inflammation; erosions and mucopurulent exudation affecting the upper respiratory, ocular, and oral mucosa; swollen lymph nodes; lameness; and CNS signs (depression, trembling, hyporesponsiveness, stupor, aggressiveness, convulsions). Historically, MCF has been described as having several "forms"—mild, peracute, head and eye, intestinal, etc. There is little basis for this division and it is of little utility. Variation in organ system involvement sometimes can be seen in the same outbreak and is at least partially related to survival time after disease onset. On average, the time to death in European cattle breeds is somewhat longer than in deer, bison, water buffalo, and Bali cattle. In cattle, swollen lymph nodes and severe eye lesions (panophthalmitis, hypopyon, corneal opacity) are more frequent, and hemorrhagic enteritis and cystitis less frequent, than in deer and bison. Peripheral (centripetal) corneal opacity is an important clinical sign suggestive of MCF in cattle. Skin lesions (erythema, exudation, cracking, crust formation) are common in animals that do not succumb quickly.

Hematologic changes are variable, and an inflammatory leukogram may not be present, even in febrile animals with severe lesions. As many as 25% of cattle experience chronic disease, and sometimes the disease waxes and wanes. Mortality rates in clinically affected animals generally approach 95%. However, in limited circumstances, survival in cattle can be higher, although survivors can rarely return to normal production.

In a few outbreaks, the goat MCF virus (caprine herpesvirus-2) induced disease in white-tailed and Sika deer. These cases were subacute to chronic, with weight loss, dermal inflammation, and alopecia as the primary signs. Whether this strain of virus causes disease in species other than deer is not known.

Lesions: The disease is systemic, and lesions may be found in any organ, although severity and frequency varies greatly. The principal lesions are inflammation and necrosis of respiratory, alimentary, or urinary mucosal epithelium; subepithelial lymphoid infiltration; generalized lymphoid proliferation and necrosis; and widespread vasculitis. Mucosal ulcerations and hemorrhage are common. Hemorrhages may be present in many parenchymatous organs, particularly lymph nodes. A classic but not pathognomonic histologic lesion is fibrinoid necrosis of small muscular arteries, but vessels of all types may be inflamed, including those in the brain. Prominent white nodules representing intramural and perivascular proliferation may be apparent, particularly in the kidneys.

Diagnosis: Diagnosis of MCF is based on clinical signs, gross and histologic lesions, and laboratory confirmation. Primary differential diagnoses include bovine viral diarrhea/mucosal disease, rinderpest, infectious bovine rhinotracheitis, and East Coast fever (theileriosis). When CNS involvement is prominent, MCF can resemble rabies and the tickborne encephalitides. A history of contact with a carrier species (sheep, goats, or wildebeest) can be helpful, although recrudescent cases can be seen without such a history. Reliable and specific laboratory assays for antibody and for viral DNA are available. The test of choice for clinical diagnosis is PCR to detect viral DNA. Preferred tissues for testing are anticoagulated blood, kidney, intestinal wall, lymph node, and brain.

Serology is used to survey healthy animals and is indicative only of infection—latent infection among susceptible animals may render serology alone inconclusive evidence of current disease. Several seroassays are available, including viral neutralization, immunoperoxidase, immunofluorescence, and ELISA. The polyclonal assays are hampered by cross-reactivity. The monoclonal-based competitive ELISA is currently the most specific and detects antibody against all of the known MCF group viruses. Only PCR can discriminate between the different viruses.

Treatment and Control: The prognosis is grave. No treatment has been found to provide any consistent benefit. Stress reduction of subclinical or mildly affected animals is indicated. No vaccine is currently available. Sheep can be produced that are free of virus by early weaning and isolation. The only other effective control strategy is separation of carriers from susceptible species. When large numbers of potent shedders are present, such as in lamb feedlots, distances >1 km may be necessary to protect highly susceptible species such as bison.

NAIROBI SHEEP DISEASE

Nairobi sheep disease (NSD) is a tickborne viral disease of sheep and goats characterized by fever and hemorrhagic gastroenteritis, abortion, and high mortality. The disease was first identified near Nairobi, Kenya, in 1910, and NSD virus was shown to be the causative agent in 1917. The disease is endemic in Kenya, Uganda, Tanzania, Somalia, Ethiopia, Botswana, Mozambique, and Republic of Congo. Human infections are rare; however, accidental infections have been reported among laboratory workers, resulting in fever, joint aches, and general malaise. The African field rat (*Arvicathus abysinicus nubilans*) is a potential reservoir host. NSD is a reportable disease in the USA and is one of the OIE listed diseases.

Etiology and Transmission: NSD virus is classified in the genus *Nairovirus*, family Bunyaviridae, and is possibly the most pathogenic virus known for sheep and goats. It is identical to or closely related to Ganjam virus, a tickborne infection of sheep, goats, and people in India. Genetic and serologic data demonstrate that Ganjam virus is an Asian variant of NSD virus. Both Ganjam and NSD viruses are phylogenetically more closely related to Hazara virus than Dugbe virus. In addition, the NSD virus is serologically related to Dugbe virus, another tickborne infection in cattle, and to Crimean-Congo hemorrhagic fever virus (*see* p 751). It is transmitted transovarially and transstadially by the brown ear tick, *Rhipicephalus appendiculatus*, in which it can survive up to 800 days. The unfed adult ticks can transmit NSD virus for >2 yr after infection. Other *Rhipicephalus* spp and *Amblyomma variegatum* ticks also may transmit the disease. The virus is shed in urine and feces, but the disease is not spread by contact.

Clinical Findings: In natural outbreaks, disease usually occurs 5–6 days after susceptible animals move to areas infested with *R appendiculatus*. Clinical signs begin with a steep rise in body temperature (41°–42°C [105.8°–107.6°F) that persists for 1–7 days. Leukopenia and viremia usually coincide with the febrile phase. Diarrhea usually appears 1–3 days after the onset of fever and worsens as infection progresses. Illness is manifest by depression; anorexia; mucopurulent, blood-stained, nasal discharge; occasional conjunctivitis; and fetid dysentery that causes painful straining. Pregnant animals frequently abort. In peracute and acute cases, the time between the appearance of disease and death is usually 2–7 days but may be as long as 11 days in less acute cases. Experimental infection has shown that indigenous Persian fat-tailed and European breeds of sheep are equally susceptible; however, mortality rate in the field is as high as 70%–90% for indigenous breeds of sheep and 30% for exotic and cross-breeds. The clinical signs in goats are similar to those in sheep but less severe, although 80% mortality has been reported. The presence of colostral immunity not only protects lambs and kids from early exposure to infection but also allows development of active immunity, enabling survival in tick-infested areas.

Lesions: The most striking features on external examination of the carcass are the hindquarters soiled with feces (or a mixture of blood and feces) and dehydration, especially in animals with prolonged scouring. Also common are conjunctivitis and dried crusts around the nostrils as a result of nasal discharge. Necropsy findings include enlarged and edematous lymph nodes; mild splenomegaly; and hemorrhages in the GI (particularly the abomasum), respiratory, and female genital tracts, as well as in the gallbladder, spleen, and heart. Petechial and ecchymotic hemorrhages in the mucosa of the cecum and colon frequently appear as longitudinal striations and are sometimes the only lesion evident. Subserosal hemorrhages may be seen in the cecum, colon, gallbladder, and kidneys. Conjunctivitis with dried crusts around the nostrils is often noted. Common histopathologic lesions are hyperplasia of lymphoid tissues, myocardial degeneration, nephrosis, and coagulative necrosis of the gallbladder.

Diagnosis: The occurrence of a disease in sheep or goats with high mortality accompanied by a tick infestation is suggestive, especially if it follows movements into endemic areas or changes in tick populations that have been induced by heavy and prolonged rainfall. Confirmation of suggestive signs and lesions requires detection of virus or viral antigen and antibodies. The preferred specimens are plasma from febrile animals, mesenteric lymph nodes, spleen, and serum. Personal protective equipment should be used when conducting a necropsy and handling the agent in the laboratory. Mouse inoculation and cell cultures can be used for primary isolation of virus. Sheep are the most sensitive animals for isolation, whereas a baby hamster kidney cell line and lamb or hamster kidney cell cultures are the most sensitive cells. Agar gel immunodiffusion, complement fixation, and ELISA can be valuable for detection of antigen in the infected tissues or tissue culture. New probes have been developed targeting the S and L segments of Dugbe virus and can potentially be used as a rapid diagnostic tool for NSD. Antibodies in infected or recovered animals can be detected by immunodiffusion, complement fixation, indirect fluorescent antibody tests, hemagglutination, and ELISA.

Differential diagnoses include peste des petits ruminants (*see* p 766), Rift Valley fever (*see* p 768), heartwater (*see* p 751), and salmonellosis (*see* p 195).

Treatment and Control: No specific antiviral agent is available for treatment. Unaffected animals in the flock may be treated with acaricides (eg, pyrethroids in a grease, cypermethrin "pour-on" products, various dip preparations). Longterm tick control is not cost-effective in endemic areas.

In endemic areas, clinical signs are not seen unless susceptible animals are introduced. Such animals should be vaccinated, as should those exposed when the range of the tick vector extends. Two types of experimental vaccines have been developed—a modified-live virus vaccine attenuated in mouse brain and an inactivated oil adjuvant vaccine. A single dose of the modified-live vaccine produces rapid immunity; however, revaccination is necessary to maintain full protection. Two doses of the inactivated vaccine are required to elicit good protection. Neither of these vaccines is produced commercially.

PARATUBERCULOSIS

(Johne's disease)

Paratuberculosis is a chronic, contagious granulomatous enteritis characterized in cattle by persistent diarrhea, progressive weight loss, debilitation, and eventually death. It is considered a listed disease by the OIE, meaning it is a priority disease for international trade. The etiologic agent, *Mycobacterium paratuberculosis*, also known as *Mycobacterium avium* subsp *paratuberculosis*, is believed capable of infecting and causing disease in all other ruminants (eg, sheep, goats, llamas, deer) and in captive and free-ranging wildlife. The infection has also been recognized in omnivores and carnivores such as wild rabbits, foxes, weasels, pigs, and nonhuman primates. Distribution is worldwide. National control programs include those established in Australia, Norway, Iceland, Japan, The Netherlands, Denmark, Ontario, Canada, and the USA. The highest published prevalence is in dairy cattle, with 20%–80% of herds infected in many of the major dairy-producing countries. Limited information is available about the prevalence in other species. The disease is of economic importance for the goat industry in Spain and the sheep industry in Australia.

Etiology and Pathogenesis: *M paratuberculosis* is excreted in large numbers in feces of infected animals and in lower numbers in their colostrum and milk. It is resistant to environmental factors and can survive on pasture for >1 yr; survival in water is longer than in soil. The infection is usually acquired through the fecal-oral route; the dose needed to infect an animal is not known. Introduction of the disease into a noninfected herd is usually through herd expansion or replacement purchases; the infection is introduced via subclinically infected carriers.

Infection is acquired early in life—often soon after birth—but clinical signs rarely develop in cattle <2 yr old, because progression to clinical disease occurs slowly. Resistance to infection increases with age, and cattle exposed as adults are much less likely to become infected. Infection is acquired by ingestion of the organism when nursing on contaminated teats; consumption of milk, solid feed, or water contaminated by the organism; or licking and grooming behavior in a contaminated environment. In the later, bacteremic stages of infection, intrauterine infections can be seen. After ingestion and uptake in the Peyer's patches of the lower small intestine, this intracellular pathogen infects macrophages in the GI tract and associated lymph nodes. It is possible that some animals may eliminate infection through a cell-mediated immune response that encourages microbiocidal activity in macrophages, but the frequency with which this occurs is unknown. In most cases, the organisms multiply and eventually provoke a chronic granulomatous enteritis that interferes with nutrient uptake and processing, leading to the cachexia typical of advanced infections. This may take months to years to develop and is usually paralleled by a decline in cell-mediated immunity, a rise in serum antibody, and bacteremia with dissemination of the infection beyond the GI tract. Fecal shedding begins before clinical signs are apparent, and animals in this "silent" stage of infection are important sources of transmission.

Clinical Findings: Paratuberculosis in cattle is characterized by weight loss and diarrhea in the late phases of infection, but infected animals can appear healthy for months to years. In cattle, diarrhea may be constant or intermittent; in sheep, goats, and other ruminants, diarrhea may not be seen. It typically does not contain blood, mucus, or epithelial debris and is passed without tenesmus. Throughout weeks or months, the diarrhea becomes more severe, further weight loss occurs, coat color may fade, and ventral and intermandibular edema may develop due to a protein-losing enteropathy. This leads to low concentrations of total protein and albumin in plasma, although gamma globulin levels are normal. In dairy cattle and goats, milk yield may drop or fail to reach expected levels. Animals are alert, and temperature and appetite are usually normal, although thirst may be increased. The disease is progressive and ultimately terminates in emaciation and death. In infected herds, the mortality rate may be low for a number of years, but as many as 50% of animals may be infected subclinically with associated production losses. The disease in sheep and goats is similar, but diarrhea is not a common feature, and advanced cases may shed wool easily. In cervids (deer and elk), the course of the disease may be more rapid.

Lesions: A diverse array of pathology may be seen in infected animals, ranging from a complete lack of gross lesions to a thickened and corrugated intestine with enlarged and edematous neighboring lymph nodes. Often, there is no correlation between clinical signs and the severity of lesions. Carcasses may be emaciated, with loss of pericardial and perirenal fat in more advanced, cachectic cases. Intestinal lesions can be mild, but typically the distal small-intestinal wall is diffusely thickened with a nonulcerated mucosa thrown into prominent transverse folds. Lesions may extend proximally and distally to the jejunum and colon. Serosal lymphangitis and enlargement of mesenteric and other regional lymph nodes are usually apparent. Histologically, there is a diffuse granulomatous enteritis characterized by the progressive accumulation of epithelioid macrophages and giant cells in the mucosa and submucosa of the gut. Sparse to myriad acid-fast organisms may be seen within the macrophages. Often, there is no correlation between clinical signs and the severity of lesions. Sheep, goats, and deer sometimes develop foci of caseation with calcification in the intestinal wall and lymph nodes.

Diagnosis: There are many commercially available tests for paratuberculosis, each with their own advantages, disadvantages, and appropriate application. The assays focus on detecting the organism in feces or tissue (culture, PCR), on finding evidence of cellular immune response to infection (skin testing, interferon-γ), or on detecting antibody to *M paratuberculosis* antigens (ELISA). Use of different tests in combination can increase diagnostic sensitivity. Given the biology of the infection and the need to manage it on a herd basis, diagnostic information should be gathered for a group of animals rather than for an individual case. An animal showing signs of disease is more likely to provide diagnostic evidence of the infection (shedding, antibody production) than an animal at the preclinical stage of infection. Necropsy with culture and histopathology on multiple tissues is the gold standard for definitive diagnosis. Ziehl-Neelsen stains of tissue samples for acid-fast bacteria usually reveal abundant mycobacteria in lesions; however, in some cases, a careful search still may not reveal their presence. Acid-fast staining of an impression smear made from the ileum of a cow with typical pathology is a quick, low-cost (albeit insensitive) method to arrive at a preliminary diagnosis. Biopsy of full-thickness sections of ileum and regional lymph nodes for culture and histopathology may provide a definitive diagnosis; however, this approach is usually restricted to particularly valuable animals. *M paratuberculosis* has been isolated from a wide variety of tissue sites, but the mesenteric and ileocecal lymph nodes, ileum, and liver are most frequently recommended for diagnostic sampling.

Serologic tests are rapid, low-cost methods for antemortem confirmation of a clinical diagnosis; sensitivity is >85% in clinically affected animals. They are also useful to detect infection in clinically normal cattle in the later stages of infection that are shedding large numbers of *M paratuberculosis*; sensitivity is ~45%. Of the serologic tests, those based on ELISA technology offer the highest sensitivity and specificity and are best used to determine the infection prevalence in a herd. Quantitative use of ELISA to identify animals for selective culling or isolation in herds may be a cost-effective strategy for disease control; higher ELISA values are associated with higher probabilities of infection and higher rates of fecal shedding. Fecal culture is more sensitive and more specific than serology, but the organism grows very slowly (2–4 mo) and the assay is more costly than serology. Pooling of fecal samples (eg, five samples per pool) or culture of manure from farm sites where cattle commingle (environmental sampling) can establish a herd's infection status at a lower cost, despite some reduction in test sensitivity. Proficiency at isolation of this pathogen varies significantly among laboratories. Use of a laboratory that has passed a proficiency test is recommended. Most strains infecting sheep will not grow on solid media but may be isolated using liquid culture media systems. Genetic probes for an element specific for *M paratuberculosis* DNA, such as IS900, can be used in conjunction with culture or directly on fecal samples. Commercial PCR kits are as sensitive and specific as fecal culture and much more rapid. Cost of culture and PCR is comparable.

Tests of cell-mediated immunity, such as the intradermal Johnin test, lymphocyte transformation test, and interferon-γ, are used more on a research basis and may be negative in advanced clinical cases. The genome of *M paratuberculosis* has been described and may provide the basis for new diagnostic approaches.

Tests that have fallen out of favor because of reports of low sensitivity and/or specificity are microscopic examination of Ziehl-Neelsen–stained fecal samples and the IV Johnin test. The complement fixation (CF) test also reportedly is less accurate than other serologic tests. The CF test is still required by many countries for importation of animals, although many of the reagents used in the CF test are made to different specifications in different countries, resulting in a lack of standardization.

Control: No satisfactory treatment is known. Control requires good sanitation and management practices aimed at limiting the exposure of young animals to the organism. Calves, kids, or lambs should be birthed in areas free of manure, removed from the dam immediately after birth in the case of dairy cattle, bottle-fed colostrum that has been pasteurized or obtained from dams that test negative, and then reared segregated as much as possible from adults and their manure until >1 yr old. Use of milk replacer is recommended instead of waste milk unless the milk has been pasteurized. A routine testing program for adults can help focus efforts in controlling the disease. Low-cost tests (eg, ELISA) have the greatest cost benefit for commercial dairy herds that are confirmed infected by culture or PCR. Animals testing positive, particularly heavy shedders or that have strong-positive ELISA results, should be sent to slaughter as soon as economically feasible. Retesting at least annually should be continued until herd tests indicate a low (<5%) infection prevalence. Because intrauterine infection can occur, more aggressive control programs include culling of calves from dams that have or develop signs of the disease. Herd replacements should be obtained from herds believed to be free of the disease, and the replacements themselves should be tested before introduction to the new herd. More general procedures to minimize fecal contamination on the farm can also help, eg, elevating food and water troughs, providing piped water in preference to ponds, and harrowing frequently to disperse feces on pasture. Herd owners should be advised that paratuberculosis control takes at least 5 yr.

The formulation of *M paratuberculosis* vaccines varies by manufacturer. In many countries, their use is subject to approval by regulatory agencies and may be restricted to heavily infected herds. Vaccination of calves <1 mo old can reduce disease incidence but does not prevent shedding or new cases of infection in the herd. Vaccination thus does not eliminate the need for good management and sanitation. In the goat industry in Spain and Australia, vaccination has increased productive herd life. Cattle inoculated with an inactivated whole-cell, mineral-oil vaccine develop granulomas, one to several inches in diameter, at the site of inoculation (brisket) and may react positively on subsequent tuberculin tests. Accidental self-inoculation can result in severe acute reactions with sloughing and chronic synovitis and tendinitis.

Zoonotic Risk: There are conflicting data on the involvement of the causative organism in Crohn disease, a chronic granulomatous enteritis of unknown cause in people. However, *M paratuberculosis* is consistently detected by PCR in people with Crohn disease. This fact, coupled with its broad host range, including nonhuman primates, indicates that paratuberculosis should be considered a zoonotic risk until the situation is clarified.

PASTEURELLOSIS OF SHEEP AND GOATS

Pasteurella and *Mannheimia* organisms are β-hemolytic, gram-negative, aerobic, nonmotile, nonsporeforming coccobacilli in the family Pasteurellaceae. This family tends to inhabit the mucosal surfaces of the GI, respiratory, and genital tract of mammals. Many are known as opportunistic secondary invaders. Some species show preferences for specific surfaces and hosts. Updating of phylogenetic data has resulted in renaming based on gene sequence analysis. As a result, *P haemolytica* biotypes A and T were reclassified as *M haemolytica* (biotype A) and *P trehalosi* (biotype T). More recently, *P trehalosi* has been reclassified as *Bibersteinia trehalosi*. Each isolate of *M haemolytica* and *B trehalosi* is designated with a biotype and serotype. *M haemolytica* A2 is the most common strain isolated from sheep and goat respiratory pasteurellosis, although A6, A13, and Ant have been reported in sheep and Ant in goats. *M haemolytica* A2 is routinely reported from cases of mastitis in sheep. *B trehalosi* T3, T4, T10, and T15 have been most often associated with the systemic or septicemic form of pasteurellosis affecting lambs. These serotypes have been regrouped to *B trehalosi* biotype 2, and a new biotype 4 has been added. *B trehalosi* is often isolated from the lungs of sheep, goats, and cattle, but pathogenicity is variable and may be incidental. *P multocida* has also been reported as a cause of pneumonic pasteurellosis in sheep and goats and has been isolated in herd outbreaks of septic arthritis. *M haemolytica* is the most commonly isolated bacteria in clinical cases, followed closely by *B trehalosi*, with *P multocida* seen less frequently.

Etiology and Pathogenesis: *M haemolytica* and *B trehalosi* are distributed worldwide, and diseases caused by them are common in sheep and goats of all ages, although the prevalence of serotypes may vary by region and flock. *M haemolytica*, *B trehalosi*, and *P multocida* are common commensal organisms of the tonsils and nasopharynx of healthy sheep and goats. The presence of multiple *Pasteurella* spp may serve to keep the bacterial populations in check, because there appears to be some interference with growth when multiple species are present. For these organisms to cause infection, a combination of stressors, including heat, overcrowding, exposure to inclement weather, poor ventilation, handling, and transportation, leaves sheep and goats susceptible to respiratory viral infections. Parainfluenza 3, adenovirus type 6, respiratory syncytial virus, possibly bovine adenovirus type 2, ovine adenovirus types 1 and 5, and reovirus type 1 cause primary respiratory infections that are rarely life threatening but predispose to secondary *M haemolytica* infections. Respiratory infections with *Mycoplasma ovipneumoniae* and *Bordetella parapertussis* have also been reported to be associated with secondary *M haemolytica* infections. The combination of stressors and primary infections are thought to break down the mucosal barrier integrity of the lower respiratory tract, allowing *M haemolytica* to colonize, proliferate, and induce significant tissue damage.

The virulence of *M haemolytica* and *B trehalosi* is mediated by the action of several factors, including endotoxin, leukotoxin, and capsular polysaccharide, that afford the bacteria advantages over host immunity. The leukotoxin is particularly important in the pathogenesis, because it is specifically toxic to ruminant leukocytes, resulting in fibrin deposition in lungs and on pleural surfaces. The lipopolysaccharide endotoxin contributes to adverse reactions in the lungs and also leads to systemic circulatory failure and shock. The capsular polysaccharide prevents the phagocytosis of the bacteria and assists in attachment to the alveolar epithelial surface. Survival of the acute phase of pneumonic pasteurellosis depends on the extent of lung involvement and damage in the lower respiratory tract. Sheep and goats that recover may have chronic respiratory problems, including reduced lung capacity and weight gain efficiency if ≥20% of the lung was damaged. In one review, there was no association between virulence and the presence of hemolysis on blood agar culture plates.

Clinical Findings and Lesions: *B trehalosi* mainly causes septicemia and systemic pasteurellosis in sheep <2 mo old. The systemic form of pasteurellosis caused by *B trehalosi* is characterized by fever, listlessness, poor appetite, and sudden death in young sheep. The organism is thought to move from the tonsils to the lungs and pass into the blood. This results in septicemia and localization of the infection in one or more tissues such as the joints, udder, meninges, or lungs. *P multocida* has been reported to be isolated from polyarthritis in young lambs. *M haemolytica* has been reported from cases of mastitis, especially in sheep. All of these bacteria can cause a severe fibrinonecrotic pneumonia in sheep and goats. The disease is characterized by acute onset of illness, very high fevers, dyspnea, anorexia, and often death.

Diagnosis: The differentiation of pasteurellosis from other causes of respiratory disease is based on the high mortality and rapid progression to death. Diagnosis of pneumonic and septicemic forms of pasteurellosis is based on necropsy examination, gross and histopathologic findings, and isolation of organisms from a range of tissues. Lesions include subcutaneous hemorrhage; epithelial necrosis of the tongue, pharynx, esophagus, or occasionally the abomasum and intestine; enlargement of tonsils and retropharyngeal lymph nodes; and peracute, multifocal, embolic, necrotizing lesions in the lung and liver. There is better correlation with PCR analysis of lung tissue than with microbial culture in identifying the presence of *M haemolytica*, *B trehalosi*, and *P multicoda*.

Treatment: Early identification of respiratory disease and introduction of effective antibiotic therapy is necessary. Death losses are high in severely affected animals. Antimicrobial susceptibility patterns of *M haemolytica*, *B trehalosi*, and *P multicoda* have shown resistance to penicillins (all three organisms), sulfadimethoxine (*P multocida*), and tetracyclines (*B trehalosi*). Ampicillin, ceftiofur, danofloxacin, enrofloxacin, florfenicol, trimethoprim-sulfamethoxazole, and tulathromycin would be expected to have good efficacy, although extra-label use of fluoroquinolones is prohibited in the USA. Treatment is frequently unrewarding unless begun very early in the disease process because of rapid progression of lung damage and endotoxin release. Parenteral fluids and anti-inflammatory agents are important adjuncts to antibiotic therapy. Although septicemic pasteurellosis has favorable antimicrobial susceptibility, response to therapy is often disappointing. Administering prophylactic antibiotics to at-risk lambs may be beneficial.

Prevention: Pasteurellosis prevention would be desirable given the economic costs of treatment, losses, and reduction of weight gains in survivors. Commercial vaccines are available for cattle but unfortunately are specific for *M haemolytica* A1, and there is little or no cross-protection against *M haemolytica* A2 experimentally. Commercial vaccines for *M haemolytica* A2 are available in the UK and have been reported to be beneficial in reducing death losses and decreased weight gains from both septicemic and pneumonic forms of pasteurellosis. An intranasal recombinant vaccine has protected lambs challenged with *P multocida*, but this vaccine is not commercially available. There are no commercial vaccines in the USA, but producers can get autogenous bacterins for their flocks; however, evidence that these are efficacious is anecdotal. Prevention of respiratory viruses by using a vaccination program would be expected to decrease respiratory pasteurellosis by preventing the initial insult that allows colonization. Inclusion of prophylactic antibiotics, mainly tetracycline, in the feed during the months of the year with the highest incidence is a common management practice. Avoidance or reduction of known stressors such as heat, overcrowding, exposure to inclement weather, poor ventilation, handling, and transportation should also be considered.

PESTE DES PETITS RUMINANTS

Peste des petits ruminants (PPR) is an acute or subacute viral disease of goats and sheep characterized by fever, necrotic stomatitis, gastroenteritis, pneumonia, and sometimes death. It was first reported in Cote d'Ivoire (the Ivory Coast) in 1942 and subsequently in other parts of West Africa. Goats and sheep appear to be equally susceptible to the virus, but goats exhibit more severe clinical disease. The virus also affects several wild small ruminant species. Cattle, buffalo, and pigs are only subclinically infected. People are not at risk.

Etiology and Epidemiology: The causal virus, a member of the *Morbillivirus* genus in the family Paramyxoviridae, preferentially replicates in lymphoid tissues and epithelial tissue of the GI and respiratory tracts, where it produces characteristic lesions.

PPR has been reported in virtually all parts of the African continent, except for the southern tip; the Middle East; and the entire Indian subcontinent. In the last 15 yr, PPR has rapidly expanded within Africa and to large parts of Central Asia, South Asia, and East Asia (including China).

Because PPR virus and the now-eradicated rinderpest virus (*see* p 771) are cross-protective, it is possible that the recent rapid expansion of the PPR virus within endemic zones and into new regions may be because of disappearance of the cross-protection previously afforded by natural rinderpest infection of small ruminants and/or the hitherto use of rinderpest vaccine to prevent small ruminant infection with PPR virus in certain endemic areas. Based on this theory, PPR virus has the potential to cause severe epidemics, or even pandemics, in more small ruminant populations in an increasingly expanding area of the developing world.

At a local level, such epidemics may eliminate the entire goat or sheep population of an affected village. Between epidemics, PPR can assume an endemic profile. Mortality and morbidity rates vary within an infected country, presumably due to two factors: the varying immune status of the affected populations and varying levels of viral virulence.

Transmission: Transmission is by close contact, and confinement seems to favor outbreaks. Secretions and excretions of sick animals are the sources of infection. Transmission can occur during the incubation period. It is generally accepted that there is no carrier state. The common husbandry system whereby goats roam freely in urban areas contributes to spread and maintenance of the virus. There are also numerous instances of livestock dealers being associated with the spread of infection, especially during religious festivals when the high demand for animals increases the trade in infected stock.

Several species of gazelle, oryx, and white-tailed deer are fully susceptible; these and other wild small ruminants may play a role in the epidemiology of the disease, but few epidemiologic data are available for PPR in wild small ruminants. Cattle, buffalo, and pigs can become naturally or experimentally infected with PPR virus, but these species are dead-end hosts, because they do not exhibit any clinical disease and do not transmit the virus to other in-contact animals of any species.

Clinical Findings: The acute form of PPR is accompanied by a sudden rise in body temperature to 40°–41.3°C (104°–106°F). Affected animals appear ill and restless and have a dull coat, dry muzzle, congested mucous membranes, and depressed appetite. Early, the nasal discharge is serous; later, it becomes mucopurulent and gives a putrid odor to the breath. The incubation period is usually 4–5 days. Small areas of necrosis may be observed on the mucous membrane on the floor of the nasal cavity. The conjunctivae are frequently congested, and the medial canthus may exhibit a small degree of crusting. Some affected animals develop a profuse catarrhal conjunctivitis with matting of the eyelids. Necrotic stomatitis affects the lower lip and gum and the gumline of the incisor teeth; in more severe cases, it may involve the dental pad, palate, cheeks and their papillae, and the tongue. Diarrhea may be profuse and accompanied by dehydration and emaciation; hypothermia and death follow, usually after 5–10 days. Bronchopneumonia, characterized by coughing, may develop at late stages of the disease. Pregnant animals may abort. Morbidity and mortality rates are higher in young animals than in adults.

Lesions: Emaciation, conjunctivitis, and stomatitis are seen; necrotic lesions are observed inside the lower lip and on the adjacent gum, the cheeks near the commissures, and on the ventral surface of the tongue. In severe cases, the lesions may extend to the hard palate and pharynx. The erosions are shallow, with a red, raw base and later become pinkish white; they are bounded by healthy epithelium that provides a sharply demarcated margin. The rumen, reticulum, and omasum are rarely involved. The abomasum exhibits regularly outlined erosions that have red, raw floors and ooze blood.

Severe lesions are less common in the small intestines than in the mouth, abomasum, or large intestines. Streaks of hemorrhages, and less frequently erosions, may be present in the first portion of the duodenum and terminal ileum. Peyer's patches are severely affected; entire patches of lymphoid tissue may be sloughed. The large intestine is usually more severely affected, with lesions developing around the ileocecal valve and at the cecocolic junction and rectum. The latter exhibits streaks of congestion along the folds of the mucosa, resulting in the characteristic "zebra-striped" appearance.

Petechiae may appear in the turbinates, larynx, and trachea. Patches of bronchopneumonia may be present.

Diagnosis: A presumptive diagnosis is based on clinical, pathologic, and epidemiologic findings and may be confirmed by viral isolation and identification. Historically, simple techniques such as agar-gel immunodiffusion have been used in developing countries for confirmation and reporting purposes. However, PPR virus cross-reacts with rinderpest virus in these tests. Virus isolation is a definitive test but is labor intensive, cumbersome, and takes a long time to complete. Currently, antigen capture ELISA and reverse transcription-PCR are the preferred laboratory tests for confirmation of the virus. For antibody detection (such as might be needed for epidemiologic surveillance, confirmation of vaccine efficacy, or confirmation of absence of the disease in a population), competitive ELISA and virus neutralization are the OIE-recommended tests. The specimens required are lymph nodes, tonsils, spleen, and whole lung for antigen or nucleic acid detection, and serum for antibody detection. The virus neutralization test may also be used to confirm an infection if paired serum samples from a surviving animal yield rising titers of ≥4-fold. PPR must be differentiated from other GI infections (eg, GI parasites), respiratory infections (eg, contagious caprine pleuropneumonia), and such other diseases as contagious ecthyma, heartwater, coccidiosis, and mineral poisoning.

Control: Local and federal authorities should be notified when PPR is suspected. PPR is also an OIE-reportable disease worldwide. Eradication is recommended when the disease appears in previously PPR-free countries. There is no specific treatment, but treatment for bacterial and parasitic complications decreases mortality in affected flocks or herds. An attenuated PPR vaccine prepared in Vero cell culture is available and affords protection from natural disease for >1 yr. Encouraged by the successful global eradication of rinderpest, international organizations such as OIE, Food and Agriculture Organization of the United Nations (FAO), and International Atomic Energy Agency (IAEA) are making plans (2015) for global eradication of PPR. The available homologous PPR vaccine would play an important role in that effort.

RIFT VALLEY FEVER

Rift Valley fever (RVF) is a peracute or acute, mosquito-borne, zoonotic disease of domestic and wild ruminants in Africa, Madagascar, and the Arabian Peninsula. Large outbreaks of clinical disease are usually associated with heavy rainfall and localized flooding. During epidemics, the occurrence of abortions in livestock and deaths among young animals, particularly lambs, together with an influenza-like disease in people, is characteristic. However, infections are frequently subclinical or mild.

Etiology and Epidemiology: RVF virus belongs to the genus *Phlebovirus* and is a typical Bunyavirus. An enveloped spherical particle of 80–100 nm in diameter, it has a three-segmented, single-stranded, negative-sense RNA genome with a total length of ~11.9 kb. Each of the segments, L (large: 6.4 kb), M (medium: 3.9 kb), and S (small: 1.7 kb), is contained in a separate nucleocapsid within the virion. Remarkably little genetic diversity has been found between RVF virus isolates from many countries, and no significant antigenic differences have been demonstrated, but differences in pathogenicity are seen. The disease is endemic in many tropical and subtropical regions of Africa, Madagascar, and the Arabian Peninsula. Thought to have been originally confined to the Rift Valley region of eastern and southern Africa, the virus has recently expanded its range, with major outbreaks having occurred in Egypt since 1977, West Africa since 1987, Madagascar since 1990, and the Arabian Peninsula in 2000. Particularly large epidemics with large numbers of human cases occurred in Egypt in 1977–1978 and in Kenya in 2006–2007. It is considered a threat to regions further afield, where competent mosquito vectors are present. Sporadic, large epidemics have occurred at 5–10 yr intervals in drier areas of eastern Africa, and less frequently in southern Africa. Outbreaks are usually associated with periods of abnormally heavy rainfall or, in some cases, with localized flooding due to dam building or flood irrigation. During interepidemic periods, the virus may remain dormant in eggs of floodwater-breeding aedine mosquitoes in the dry soil of small, ephemeral wetlands (dambos or pans). In some areas, this transovarial transmission is believed to be the most important interepidemic survival strategy of the virus; however, inapparent cycling of the virus between vectors and wild or domestic mammalian hosts has been shown to occur in many areas. RVF virus may also spread by movement of viremic animals and possibly by wind-borne mosquitoes. When emergence of infected mosquitoes, or introduction of virus to an area, coincides with abnormally wet conditions and the presence of a highly susceptible host population, a large epidemic may ensue when the virus is amplified in ruminants and spread locally by many species of mosquitoes or mechanically by other insects. The incidence of RVF peaks during the late rainy season. In areas with cold winters, both the disease and vectors may disappear after the first frost. In warmer climates where insect vectors are present continuously, seasonality is not seen.

People are readily infected through blood aerosols from infected animals during slaughter, or by exposure to infected animal tissues, aborted fetuses, mosquito bites, and laboratory procedures. Therefore, veterinarians, farm laborers, and abattoir workers are particularly at risk. People can also act as amplifying hosts and introduce the disease (via mosquitoes) to animals in uninfected areas.

Clinical Findings: Clinical signs of RVF tend to be nonspecific, rendering it difficult to recognize individual cases. The incubation period is 12–36 hr in lambs, and a biphasic fever of up to 108°F (42°C) may develop. Affected animals are listless and reluctant to move or feed and may show signs of abdominal pain. Mortality in young lambs is high (90%–100%), and animals usually die within 2–3 days. Adult sheep are less susceptible, with 10%–30% mortality; the incubation period is 24–72 hr, and animals show a generalized febrile response, lethargy, hematemesis, hematochezia, and nasal discharge, although infection may also be inapparent. Calves are less susceptible than lambs, but mortality may still be as high as 70%; clinical signs are similar to those in sheep, but icterus is more common. Disease in adult cattle is often inapparent, but they may show anorexia, lacrimation, salivation, nasal discharge, dysgalactia, and a bloody or fetid diarrhea, with a mortality of 5%–10%. Sometimes, abortion may be the only sign of infection; the aborted fetus is usually autolyzed. In pregnant ewes, abortion rates vary from 5% to almost 100% in different outbreaks and on different farms; abortion rates in cattle are usually <10%. Vaccination of ewes with live Smithburn strain vaccine may result in early embryonic death, congenital CNS anomalies and arthrogryposis, or abortion or stillbirth. Clinical signs and abortions have also been reported in goats, and occasionally in camels, water buffalo, and some wild ungulate species. In people, RVF is usually inapparent or associated with a self-limiting febrile illness characterized by abrupt onset of malaise, myalgia, and arthralgia. A minority (1%–2%) may develop severe disease with ocular lesions, encephalitis, or severe hepatic lesions with hemorrhages; in such cases, the fatality rate may be 10%–20%.

Lesions: The hepatic lesions are similar in all species and vary mainly with the age of the affected individual. The most severe lesions, seen in aborted fetuses and newborn lambs, are moderately to greatly enlarged, soft, friable livers with irregular congested patches. Numerous grayish white necrotic foci are invariably present but may not be clearly visible. Hemorrhage and edema of the wall of the gallbladder and mucosa of the abomasum are common. Intestinal contents are dark chocolate-brown. In all animals, the spleen and peripheral lymph nodes are enlarged and edematous and may show petechiae. Histopathologically, the liver lesions are severe and extensive, with hepatic necrosis being the most striking microscopic lesion of RVF in all domestic animals and people.

Diagnosis: RVF should be suspected when abnormally heavy rains and flooding are followed by widespread occurrence of abortions and mortality among newborn animals characterized by necrotic hepatitis, concurrent with influenza-like disease in people handling animals or their products.

The necropsy of infected animals poses considerable risk to the operator and should be performed only by trained personnel, using appropriate personal protective equipment. The virus can readily be isolated from tissues of aborted fetuses and the blood of infected animals. The viral titer in these tissues is often high enough to use organ suspensions as antigen for a rapid diagnosis in neutralization, complement fixation, ELISA, agar gel diffusion tests, or staining of organ impression smears; however, these tests should be supplemented by isolation in suckling mice or hamsters injected intracerebrally or in cell cultures such as baby hamster kidney (BHK21), monkey kidney (Vero), chicken embryo–related (CER) and mosquito cells, or primary kidney and testis cell cultures of lambs. Detection of viral nucleic acid by PCR is possible, and reverse transcriptase-PCR tests have been described. Virus can be demonstrated in organ sections using immunohistochemical stains.

All conventional serologic tests can be used to detect antibody against RVF virus and are helpful in epidemiologic studies. In some areas, however, serologic surveys may be complicated by cross-reactivity between RVF virus and other phleboviruses; virus neutralization tests are the most specific in this situation. An IgM ELISA can demonstrate recent infection using a single serum sample.

Wesselsbron disease (*see* p 775) and other insect-borne viral diseases tend to occur under the same climactic conditions. RVF mortality associated with hepatic lesions should be distinguished from hepatotoxic plant and algal intoxications; bacterial septicemias such as pasteurellosis, salmonellosis, and anthrax; and other viral infections such as Nairobi sheep disease and peste des petits ruminants. When abortion is the only finding, other important diseases such as brucellosis, leptospirosis, chlamydiosis, campylobacteriosis, *Coxiella burnetii* infection, and salmonellosis should be eliminated.

Control and Prevention: Immunization remains the only effective way to protect livestock from RVF. The mouse neuro-adapted Smithburn strain of RVF virus can readily be produced in large quantities, is inexpensive, and induces a durable immunity 6–7 days after inoculation. It should normally not be used for protection of pregnant animals, because it may cause abortion, congenital defects, and hydrops amnii in the ewe; however, its use may be contemplated during an outbreak when possible adverse effects may be outweighed by the dangers of natural infection. Although not proved, it is theoretically possible for the attenuated virus to revert to virulence. A small-plaque variant and a mutagen-induced strain have been investigated as potential vaccine candidates but have not been accepted as replacements for the Smithburn strain. More recently, a naturally attenuated avirulent isolate of Rift Valley fever, clone 13, has been used in a commercially available vaccine. It is not advisable to use live attenuated vaccines in nonendemic countries. Possible future recombinant DNA vaccines and viral strains with deletions of the major virulence genes should offer a better alternative. Control of vectors, movement of stock to high-lying areas, and confinement of stock in insect-proof stables are usually impractical, instituted too late, and of little value.

Much work has gone into attempts to predict RVF outbreaks using meteorologic and remote-sensing data to identify high-risk areas and time periods; this has been somewhat successful in predicting outbreaks in eastern Africa but less so in southern Africa. However, outbreaks cannot yet reliably be predicted and are usually of sudden onset. Therefore, routinely immunizing lambs at 6 mo of age, which should afford lifelong protection, is advisable. The offspring of susceptible e wes can be immunized at any age. Pregnant ewes and cattle can be vaccinated with a formalin-inactivated vaccine, which elicits a better immunity in cattle and is safe in pregnancy. Revaccination after 3 mo is advisable to induce an immunity that will last >1 yr and to confer colostral immunity to the offspring.

Zoonotic Risk: Because RVF virus can cause a severe and potentially fatal disease in people, those involved in the livestock industry should be made aware of the potential dangers of exposure to RVF-infected animals and tissues. Appropriate protective measures should be taken when investigating cases of abortion, handling potentially infected animals, and collecting diagnostic samples.

RINDERPEST

(Cattle plague)

Historically, rinderpest virus was a scourge that wrought economic havoc throughout Africa, Asia, and Europe. The need to combat rinderpest provided the impetus for the establishment of the first modern veterinary school in Lyon (France) in 1762. After several decades of success in eradicating rinderpest from Europe, the disease recurred unexpectedly in Belgium in 1920, and renewed efforts to eradicate it resulted in the creation of the World Organization for Animal Health (OIE) in 1924. Shortly after the creation of the Food and Agriculture Organization (FAO) of the United Nations in 1946, the OIE and FAO signed a cooperation agreement in 1952. Since then, the two organizations (FAO and OIE) have been major participants in several global campaigns to combat rinderpest, which culminated in global eradication of the disease in 2011. In fact, the last reported rinderpest outbreak occurred in Kenya in 2001, but a 10-yr active surveillance period was necessary before global eradication could be declared. Rinderpest is only the second viral disease, after smallpox, to have been successfully eradicated worldwide.

The successful eradication of rinderpest shows that smallpox eradication in 1980 was not an unrepeatable feat and should provide a certain degree of confidence to the international community that concerted, science-based efforts can result in future successes. Rinderpest virus is biologically similar to the virus of peste des petits ruminants (*see* p 766), which has been targeted by the OIE and FAO as the next animal disease for global eradication.

Rinderpest was a disease of cloven-hoofed animals characterized by fever, necrotic stomatitis, gastroenteritis, lymphoid necrosis, and high mortality. In epidemic form, it was the most lethal plague known in cattle. All wild and domesticated species of the order Artiodactyla were variably susceptible to rinderpest, although dissemination of the virus largely depended on continual transmission among domesticated cattle, domesticated buffalo, and yaks. The virus also infected goats and sheep, leading to under-diagnosis of the clinically similar peste des petits ruminants in regions where the two diseases coexisted.

Etiology, Epidemiology, and Transmission: Rinderpest virus is a *Morbillivirus*, closely related to the viruses causing peste des petits ruminants, canine distemper (*see* p 777), and measles. Strains of varying virulence for cattle occurred and could be differentiated genetically. However, a single serotype of the virus existed, and a vaccine prepared from any strain could protect against all strains.

Rinderpest virus is shed in nasal and ocular secretions and can be transmitted during the incubation period (1–2 days before onset of fever). Transmission required direct or close indirect contact between susceptible animals and sick animals shedding the virus. The role of fomites in transmission was negligible, because the virus is fragile, being inactivated within 12 hr of exposure to atmospheric heat and light. There was no carrier state, and recovered animals acquired lifelong immunity. In endemic areas, young cattle became infected after maternal immunity disappeared and before vaccinal immunity began, with possible auxiliary cycles in wild ungulates.

Clinical Findings: After an incubation period of 3–15 days, fever, anorexia, depression, and oculonasal discharges developed, followed by necrotic lesions on the gums, buccal mucosa, and tongue. The hard and soft palates were often affected. The oculonasal discharge became mucopurulent, and the muzzle appeared dry and cracked. Diarrhea, the final clinical sign, could be watery and bloody. Convalescence was prolonged and could be complicated by concurrent infections due to immunosuppression. Morbidity was often 100% and mortality was up to 90% in epidemic areas, but in endemic areas morbidity was low and clinical signs were often mild.

Lesions: Gross pathologic lesions occurred throughout the GI and upper respiratory tracts, either as areas of necrosis and erosion, or congestion and hemorrhage, the latter creating classic "zebra-striping" in the rectum. Lymph nodes could be enlarged and edematous, with white necrotic foci in the Peyer's patches. Histologic lesions included lymphoid and epithelial necrosis with viral-induced syncytia, and intracytoplasmic and intranuclear inclusions were often seen.

Diagnosis: Clinical and pathologic findings were sufficient for diagnosis in endemic areas and after initial laboratory confirmation of an outbreak. In areas where rinderpest was uncommon or absent, laboratory tests had to be used to differentiate it from bovine viral diarrhea in particular, as well as East Coast fever, foot-and-mouth disease, infectious bovine rhinotracheitis, and malignant catarrhal fever. Viral isolation and detection of specific viral antigens in affected tissues using an immunodiffusion test was the standard, but simpler, more rapid and more discriminating tests, such as immune capture ELISA and reverse transcription-PCR (RT-PCR), were favored toward the end of the eradication campaign. The RT-PCR technique allowed phylogenetic characterization of the virus and helped trace the origin of strains in new outbreaks. A simple lateral flow penside test for field use also proved useful in the final stages of the eradication campaign. In the 10-yr period between occurrence of the last outbreak and the official declaration of eradication, active rinderpest surveillance in recent endemic areas included the testing of all susceptible cloven-hoofed animals presenting with erosive stomatitis.

Control: Active immunity was lifelong, whereas maternal immunity lasted 6–11 mo. Control in endemic areas was by immunization of all cattle and domestic buffalo >1 yr old with an attenuated cell culture vaccine. In these areas, outbreaks were controlled by quarantine and "ring vaccination" and sometimes by slaughtering. In epidemics, the disease was best eliminated by imposing quarantine and by slaughtering affected and exposed animals. Control of animal movements was paramount to control rinderpest; many outbreaks were due to the introduction of infected cattle to hitherto uninfected herds. The lessons learned from this huge success will be instrumental in the fight against peste des petits ruminants.

TICKBORNE FEVER

(Pasture fever)

Tickborne fever is a febrile disease of domestic and free-living ruminants in the temperate regions of Europe. It is prevalent in sheep and cattle in the UK, Ireland, Norway, Finland, The Netherlands, Austria, and Spain. Disease is transmitted by the hard tick *Ixodes ricinus*. A similar disease transmitted by other ticks has been described in India and South Africa. The main hosts are sheep and cattle, but goats and deer are also susceptible.

Etiology: The causative agent is now classified as a member of the order Rickettsiales, family Anaplasmataceae, as *Anaplasma phagocytophilum*, which includes the granulocytic agents formerly known as *Ehrlichia phagocytophila*, *Ehrlichia equi*, and the agent of human granulocytic ehrlichiosis.

The organism infects eosinophils, neutrophils, and monocytes, in that order. Cytoplasmic inclusions are visible as grayish blue bodies in Giemsa-stained blood smears and may contain one or more rickettsial particles of variable size and shape. The varied morphologic types in the cytoplasmic inclusions do not represent stages of development, as in chlamydiae, but rather are rickettsial colonies within cytoplasmic vacuoles.

The disease is transmitted by the hard tick *I ricinus*. Adult ticks infected as larvae or nymphs can transmit the disease as can nymphs infected as larvae, but infections do not appear to pass from the adult female to the larva via the egg. The rickettsiae can survive in infected ticks for long periods and, because *I ricinus* can survive unfed for >1 yr awaiting a new host, ticks infected in their previous instar can still be infective after long periods of hibernation. The ready transmission of infection by injecting infected blood suggests that the organism could be transmitted mechanically by biting insects. In addition, if the organisms reported to cause a similar disease in ruminants in India and South Africa are indeed *A phagocytophilum*, it is most likely that ticks other than *I ricinus* are involved.

Clinical Findings: After infestation with infected ticks, the incubation period may be 5–14 days, but after injection with infected blood, the incubation period is 2–6 days. In sheep, the main clinical sign is a sudden fever (105°–108°F [40.5°–42.0°C]) for 4–10 days. Other signs are either absent or mild, but the animals generally appear dull and may lose weight. Respiratory and pulse rates are usually increased, and a cough often develops.

In cattle, the disease is known as pasture fever in many parts of Europe, including Finland, Norway, Austria, Spain, and Switzerland. The disease occurs as an annual minor epidemic when dairy heifers and cows are turned out to pasture in the spring and early summer. Within days, the cows are dull and depressed, with a marked loss of appetite and milk yield. Affected cows usually suffer from respiratory distress and coughing. Clinical signs are more obvious and last longer in newly purchased animals than in home-bred animals. Often, veterinary advice is sought after a sudden drop in milk yield.

Abortions affect susceptible ewes and cows newly introduced onto tick-infested pastures during the last stages of gestation, with abortions occurring 2–8 days after the onset of fever. Except for aborting ewes, death due to tickborne fever is rare. The semen quality of infected rams and bulls may be greatly reduced. Variations in severity of the clinical effects may be related to differences between strains of *A phagocytophilum* or in host susceptibility.

Perhaps the most significant effect of infection is its serious impairment of humoral and cellular defense mechanisms, which results in increased susceptibility to secondary infections such as tick pyemia, pneumonic pasteurellosis, louping ill, and listeriosis.

Lesions: Tickborne fever is characterized by transient but distinct hematologic changes. A modest neutrophilia develops 2–4 days after natural or experimental infection and is followed by a severe leukopenia due to lymphocytopenia and neutropenia. The lymphocytopenia lasts 4–6 days, whereas the neutropenia develops progressively and becomes more marked ~10 days after infection. Studies with monoclonal antibodies that recognize surface markers for lymphocyte subsets have shown that both T and B lymphocytes are reduced. The number of circulating eosinophils is also depressed for as long as 2 wk. After the febrile period has subsided, the number of monocytes may increase. At the peak of reaction, >90% of circulating neutrophils and eosinophils may be infected. The monocytes are predominantly infected during the later stages of bacteremia, whereas the granulocytes are usually infected throughout the period of bacteremia. The number of circulating thrombocytes is also reported to be depressed during the febrile period, and the occasional hemorrhagic syndromes associated with tickborne fever are probably related to the reduction in circulating thrombocytes.

Diagnosis: In sheep, the onset of high fever in tick-infested areas during the spring and summer in association with hematologic changes and the presence of inclusions within granulocytes or the detection of specific DNA by PCR is diagnostic. PCR and other molecular methods are particularly useful during the late stages of primary bacteremia and during persistent infection when it is difficult to detect inclusion bodies in blood smears. Clinical disease usually is seen only in young lambs born in tick-infested areas or in older animals newly introduced to such areas. Demonstration of typical inclusion bodies in blood smears or specific DNA by PCR should indicate the association of tickborne fever and cases of tick pyemias and abortions, particularly when abortions occur after pregnant animals are moved from tick-free to tick-infested pastures. Infection could be established retrospectively by demonstrating a rise in antibody titers by indirect immunofluorescence or ELISA.

In affected dairy cattle, the main signs are abortions and a sudden drop in milk yield. The other common clinical sign in infected cattle is respiratory illness after a herd is introduced to tick-infested pastures. Tickborne fever must also be considered when abortions and stillbirths, particularly in heifers, occur soon after their introduction to tick-infested pastures. Therefore, in areas where the disease is enzootic, blood smears must be examined for the presence of organisms in all cases of abortion in sheep and cattle and when milk yield drops suddenly soon after the animals have returned to pasture.

Treatment and Control: The short-acting oxytetracyclines are regarded as the most effective treatment, because other antibiotics such as penicillin, streptomycin, and ampicillin do not prevent relapses. Sulfamethazine has also proved useful. If dairy cattle are treated with oxytetracyclines within a few days of infection, the pyrexia is reduced quickly and milk yield restored.

There are three important aspects of control: vector control, chemotherapy, and immunity. Effective control can be achieved by eliminating or markedly reducing contact with the tick vector either by grazing sheep and cattle on tick-free pastures in lowland areas or by use of acaricides. In sheep practice, this commonly involves keeping ewes and lambs in a fenced, relatively tick-free pasture until the lambs are ~6 wk old. Lambs also benefit from improved nutrition of the ewes. Dipping lambs within 1–2 wk of birth is not commonly practiced because of difficulties of gathering the lambs on widely dispersed hill farms, the risks of mismothering, and the relatively short duration of protection provided by acaricides, possibly because of the short fleece and rapid growth rate of lambs. However, dipping twice with a 2- to 3-wk interval or use of pour-on preparations or smears applied before lambs are moved from lambing fields to hill pastures reportedly controls ticks effectively. Pregnant animals should not be moved from tick-free to tick-infested pastures.

In enzootic areas, treatment with long-acting tetracyclines may be used as a prophylactic measure. When susceptible animals, particularly pregnant ewes and cows and newborn lambs, are to be moved from tick-free to tick-infested areas, it may be necessary to combine dipping with prophylactic use of long-acting tetracyclines. Such treatment of lambs in the first 2–3 wk of life can be protective for as long as 3 wk and helps reduce secondary infections such as tick pyemia, pasteurellosis, and colibacillosis. It may also improve growth rate.

Several aspects of immunity remain controversial, but it is generally accepted that sheep and cattle are immune to challenge after recovery from one or two bouts of clinical disease caused by tickborne fever. The immunity may last for several months but wanes rapidly if the animals are removed from tick-infested areas. Secondary infections are usually milder as residual immunity persists. There is a variable degree of cross-protection among strains of *A phagocytophilum*. No effective vaccines are available to protect ruminants from clinical tickborne fever. However, if susceptible animals are being brought into tick-infested pastures, it may be sensible to deliberately infect them before introduction and treat them with oxytetracyclines before or immediately after the onset of fever. This allows multiplication of the organism and therefore stimulation of immune responses without uncontrolled clinical disease; a minimum duration of bacteremia may be required for protective immunity to develop. Because not all strains of *A phagocytophilum* are cross-protective, strains specific to the area must be used.

TICK PYEMIA

Tick pyemia affects lambs 2–12 wk old and is characterized by debility, crippling lameness, and paralysis. Pyemic abscesses are common in joints but may be found in virtually any organ. The disease causes significant economic loss through debilitation and death. The disease is enzootic in many regions of the UK and Ireland where the tick *Ixodes ricinus* is common, and it is likely to be present in other parts of Europe where the same tick is found.

Etiology: *Staphylococcus aureus* is regarded as the main cause of the pyemic abscesses, because it has been isolated consistently from superficial and deep-seated lesions and it is rare to find other bacteria. The bacteria are believed to gain entry into the bloodstream either by direct inoculation during tick feeding, from local superficial wounds, or through the infected umbilicus. However, there is clinical and experimental evidence that *I ricinus* does not simply act as a vector directly injecting staphylococci into the bloodstream. The main role of *I ricinus* is as a vector of the rickettsial agent *Anaplasma phagocytophilum*, which causes tickborne fever (*see* p 772), which in turn creates factors favorable to development of pyemia. Lambs affected with tickborne fever have severe leukopenia, and their peripheral blood neutrophils are less capable of phagocytizing and killing *S aureus*. Experimental studies have shown that lambs with tickborne fever were more susceptible to experimental infections with *S aureus* during the period of neutropenia and that as many as 30% of lambs with tickborne fever may develop staphylococcal infections.

The epidemiology of the disease is closely related to the biology of *I ricinus*. The disease is limited to areas populated by *I ricinus* and to seasons of the year climatically favoring high tick population and activity.

Clinical Findings: Abscesses form in various parts of the body, mainly in the joints, tendon sheaths, and muscles, resulting in lameness—hence the common use of the term "crippled lambs." In some outbreaks, >30% of lambs may be affected; they are usually dull and lame and often suffer from loss of body condition. Internal abscesses without joint lesions may result in no clinical signs other than the loss of condition, but when lesions are present in the CNS, there may be ataxia, paraplegia, or other nervous signs. The crippling disease lasts for days or weeks, but the disease may also appear as an acute septicemia. On occasion, there may be sudden deaths resulting from multiple internal abscesses without other visible signs. As many as 50% of affected lambs may die, and the survivors recover slowly.

Lesions: Apart from the joints and other superficial structures, abscesses are commonly found in the liver, lungs, and kidneys. They may also be present in the meninges of the spinal cord and in the pericardium and myocardium. The diaphragm, thymus, and adrenal glands are less commonly affected. Ticks are often found attached to an inflamed area.

Diagnosis: History and clinical signs are valuable indicators. The restriction of the disease to tick-infested areas, its occurrence during seasons of tick activity, and demonstration of *A phagocytophilum* or specific DNA by PCR in the blood of affected lambs or other sheep in the flock are diagnostic features. Isolation of *S aureus* from lesions and the absence of other bacteria will help to confirm tick pyemia. The loss of condition and ill-thrift without lameness may be difficult to recognize as tick pyemia, and the acute condition can be confused with other septicemic diseases. Tick pyemia may also resemble other suppurative infections of the newborn, including navel ill and joint ill due to infections by other bacteria such as streptococci and *Trueperella pyogenes*.

Treatment and Control: Treatment of clinical cases of tick pyemia with penicillin or tetracycline can be effective, provided the lesions are not too advanced.

Control of tick infestation is the most effective prevention. This can be achieved either by restricting lambs and ewes to low-ground, tick-free pastures for the first few weeks of life or by dipping ewes before lambing and administering acaricides as dips or smears on lambs. In young lambs, pour-on preparations of cypermethrin or smears applied before lambs are moved from lambing fields to hill pastures reportedly control ticks effectively.

Administration of long-acting oxytetracycline at the time of risk can help prevent both tickborne fever and tick pyemia during the first weeks of life. A single injection at double the standard dose given at 3 wk of age can significantly reduce mortality and morbidity in young hill lambs on tick-infested pasture and improve weight gains and condition in the remainder. Prophylactic treatment with a long-acting antibiotic may prevent development of tickborne fever for as long as 3 wk, without pyrexia and immunosuppression, so that the incidence of tick pyemia and other infections such as pasteurellosis and colibacillosis are reduced. Although treatment with oxytetracycline may inhibit the development of immunity, if the lambs eventually develop tickborne fever, they are several weeks older and apparently less susceptible to tick pyemia. Deliberate exposure of lambs by injections, followed by treatment with oxytetracycline, could provide some immunity before the lambs enter tick-infested areas; however, strains specific to the area must be used because some strains of *A phagocytophilum* have no cross-immunity.

WESSELSBRON DISEASE

Wesselsbron disease is an acute, arthropod-borne flavivirus infection of mainly sheep, cattle, and goats in sub-Saharan Africa. Infection is common, but clinical disease is infrequent although likely under-reported. Newborn lambs and goat kids are most susceptible, and mortality may occur. Infection in adult sheep, cattle, and goats is usually subclinical, but disease may be severe in sheep with preexisting liver pathology. Occasional abortion in ewes, together with congenital malformation of the CNS with arthrogryposis of the ovine (and also the bovine) fetus and hydrops amnii in ewes, is seen. Incidental spillover occurs to people, causing a nonfatal, influenza-like disease.

Etiology and Epidemiology: Wesselsbron disease is caused by a flavivirus, which is an enveloped, positive-sense RNA virus. It has not been well characterized but has properties typical of a hemagglutinating flavivirus. It has been isolated from vertebrates and arthropods from many sub-Saharan African countries, and serologic surveys provide evidence of its occurrence in other countries. Evidence of infection has been reported in cattle, sheep, goats, camels, pigs, donkeys, horses, ostriches, and wild ruminants. Based on the distribution of aedine mosquitoes associated with Wesselsbron disease, the incidence of infection is likely greater than is generally realized. The high prevalence of antibodies in warmer and moister coastal areas of southern and eastern Africa suggests that domestic herbivores may play a significant role in maintenance of the virus, and activity appears to occur year round. In drier areas, however, seroprevalence is generally lower, with irregular disease outbreaks occurring, usually in conjunction with Rift Valley fever (*see* p 768) when abnormally heavy rains lead to an abundance of floodwater-breeding mosquitoes. People may become infected by mosquitoes or by handling organs from infected animals.

Clinical Findings: After an incubation period of 1–3 days in newborn lambs, nonspecific signs of illness, including fever, anorexia, listlessness, weakness, and increased respiration, become evident. Death may occur within 72 hr. In calves and adult sheep, goats, and cattle, nonfatal febrile or inapparent infection occurs. Occasional abortion, congenital CNS malformations with arthrogryposis, and hydrops amnii are seen in ewes. Wesselsbron disease and Rift Valley fever share many clinical and pathologic features. However, Wesselsbron disease is usually milder, producing much lower mortality, fewer abortions, and less destructive liver lesions. The virus appears to be more neurotropic than that of Rift Valley fever, and severe fetal teratology of the CNS is seen after experimental infection. Use of the attenuated vaccine in pregnant ewes may result in early embryonic death, severe teratology of the CNS, arthrogryposis, hydrops amnii, abortion, or fetal mummification. In people, mild to severe, nonfatal influenza-like symptoms are seen.

Lesions: In newborn and young animals, a moderate to severe icterus and hepatomegaly are seen with Wesselsbron disease; the liver is yellowish to orange brown. Petechiae and ecchymoses are commonly found in the mucosa of the abomasum, the contents of which are chocolate-brown in color. Histopathology reveals mild to extensive necrosis of the parenchyma as well as individual or small, scattered groups of necrotic hepatocytes. Lesions in adult animals are usually much milder.

Diagnosis: The clinical signs and epidemiology, together with a relatively high mortality in lambs, are an indication of Wesselsbron disease. It should, however, be distinguished from Rift Valley fever, and the two diseases may occur together. The virus can be isolated from almost all organs of lambs that have died during the clinical stage of the disease. Intracerebral inoculation of newborn mice is the best method of isolation. The virus can be distinguished from that of Rift Valley fever by intraperitoneal inoculation of weaned mice; Wesselsbron disease virus will not kill such mice, whereas Rift Valley fever virus will. Confirmation of the viral identity can be accomplished by virus neutralization.

Serodiagnosis has been based on hemagglutination-inhibition, complement fixation, and virus neutralization. Flavivirus cross-reactivity is marked in hemagglutination-inhibition tests but less so in complement fixation, a test that is specific in cattle sera. Nevertheless, homologous Wesselsbron titers greatly exceed heterologous flavivirus titers.

Control: Production of an attenuated vaccine was discontinued shortly before 2000. Incidence of disease is low in sheep, but injudicious use of the vaccine in pregnant ewes resulted in severe economic losses in the past due to abortion and fetal malformations. Attempts to control mosquito vectors are of little value as a preventive measure.

CANINE DISTEMPER

Canine distemper is a highly contagious, systemic, viral disease of dogs seen worldwide. Clinically, it is characterized by a diphasic fever, leukopenia, GI and respiratory catarrh, and frequently pneumonic and neurologic complications. Its epidemiology is complicated by the large number of species susceptible to infection. The disease is seen in Canidae (dog, fox, wolf, raccoon dog), Mustelidae (ferret, mink, skunk, wolverine, marten, badger, otter), most Procyonidae (raccoon, coatimundi), some Viveridae (binturong, palm civet), Ailuridae (red panda), Ursidae (bear), Elephantidae (Asian elephant), primates (Japanese monkey), and large Felidae. Domestic dogs (including feral populations) are considered to be the reservoir species in most, if not all, locations. Antigenic drift and strain diversity is increasingly documented in association with outbreaks in wild species, domestic dogs, and exotic animals held in zoos and parks.

Etiology and Pathogenesis: Canine distemper is caused by a paramyxovirus closely related to the viruses of measles and rinderpest. The fragile, enveloped, single-strand RNA virus is sensitive to lipid solvents, such as ether, and most disinfectants, including phenols and quaternary ammonium compounds. It is relatively unstable outside the host. The main route of infection is via aerosol droplet secretions from infected animals. Some infected dogs may shed virus for several months.

Virus initially replicates in the lymphatic tissue of the respiratory tract. A cell-associated viremia results in infection of all lymphatic tissues, which is followed by infection of respiratory, GI, and urogenital epithelium, as well as the CNS and optic nerves. Disease follows virus replication in these tissues. The degree of viremia and extent of viral spread to various tissues is moderated by the level of specific humoral immunity in the host during the viremic period.

Clinical Findings: A transient fever usually occurs 3–6 days after infection, and there may be a leukopenia (especially lymphopenia) at this time; these signs may go unnoticed or be accompanied by anorexia. The fever subsides for several days before a second fever occurs, which may be accompanied by serous nasal discharge, mucopurulent ocular discharge, lethargy, and anorexia. GI and respiratory signs, typically complicated by secondary bacterial infections, may follow; rarely, pustular dermatitis may be seen. Encephalomyelitis may occur in association with these signs, follow the systemic disease, or occur in the absence of systemic manifestations. Dogs surviving the acute phase may have hyperkeratosis of the footpads and epithelium of the nasal planum, as well as enamel hypoplasia in incompletely erupted teeth.

Overall, a longer course of illness is associated with the presence of neurologic signs; however, there is no way to anticipate whether an infected dog will develop neurologic manifestations. CNS signs include circling, head tilt, nystagmus, paresis to paralysis, and focal to generalized seizures. Localized involuntary twitching of a muscle or group of muscles (myoclonus, chorea, flexor spasm, hyperkinesia) and convulsions characterized by salivation and, often, chewing movements of the jaw ("chewing-gum fits") are considered classic neurologic signs. Emerging viral strains may be associated with greater neurotropism; increased morbidity and mortality from neurologic complications has been observed.

A dog may exhibit any or all of these multisystemic signs during the course of the disease. Infection may be mild and inapparent or lead to severe disease with most of the described signs. The course of the systemic disease may be as short as 10 days, but the onset of neurologic signs may be delayed for several weeks or months as a result of chronic progressive demyelination within the CNS.

Clinicopathologic findings are nonspecific and include lymphopenia, with the possible finding of viral inclusion bodies in circulating leukocytes very early in the course of the disease. Thoracic radiographs may reveal an interstitial pattern typical of viral pneumonia.

Chronic distemper encephalitis (old dog encephalitis, [ODE]), a condition often marked by ataxia, compulsive movements such as head pressing or continual pacing, and incoordinated hypermetria, may be seen in fully vaccinated adult dogs without a history suggestive of systemic canine distemper infection. Although canine distemper antigen has been detected in the brains of some dogs with ODE by fluorescent antibody staining or genetic methods, dogs with ODE are not infectious, and replication-competent virus has not been isolated. The disease is caused by an inflammatory reaction associated with persistent canine distemper virus infection in the CNS, but mechanisms that trigger this syndrome are unknown.

Lesions: Thymic atrophy is a consistent postmortem finding in infected young puppies. Hyperkeratosis of the nose and footpads is often found in dogs with neurologic manifestations. Depending on the degree of secondary bacterial infection, bronchopneumonia, enteritis, and skin pustules also may be present. In cases of acute to peracute death, exclusively respiratory abnormalities may be found. Histologically, canine distemper virus produces necrosis of lymphatic tissues, interstitial pneumonia, and cytoplasmic and intranuclear inclusion bodies in respiratory, urinary, and GI epithelium. Lesions found in the brains of dogs with neurologic complications include neuronal degeneration, gliosis, noninflammatory demyelination, perivascular cuffing, nonsuppurative leptomeningitis, and intranuclear inclusion bodies predominately within glial cells.

Diagnosis: Distemper should be considered in the diagnosis of any febrile condition in dogs with multisystemic manifestations. Characteristic signs sometimes do not appear until late in the disease, and the clinical picture may be modified by concurrent parasitism and numerous viral or bacterial infections. Distemper is sometimes confused with other systemic infections such as leptospirosis (*see* p 650), infectious canine hepatitis (*see* p 798), or Rocky Mountain spotted fever (*see* p 806). Intoxicants such as lead or organophosphates can cause simultaneous GI and neurologic signs. A febrile catarrhal illness with neurologic sequelae justifies a clinical diagnosis of distemper.

In dogs with multisystemic signs, the following can be examined by immunofluorescent assay or reverse transcriptase (RT) PCR: smears of conjunctival, tracheal, vaginal, or other epithelium; the buffy coat of the blood; urine sediment; or bone marrow aspirates. Commercially available quantitative RT-PCR can usually distinguish natural infection from vaccinal virus. A combined two-step RT-PCR to distinguish vaccinal strains from emerging wild-type strains has also been described; this assay would be of particular value in epidemiologic investigations or in outbreaks in non-canine species. Antibody titers or ELISA can be performed on CSF and compared with peripheral blood; a relatively higher level in the CSF is typical of natural infection versus vaccination. Viral antigen immunofluorescent assay (IFA) or fluorescent in situ hybridization for viral DNA can be performed on biopsies from the footpads or from the haired skin of the dorsal neck.

At necropsy, diagnosis is usually confirmed by histologic lesions, IFA, or both. These samples are often negative when the dog is showing only neurologic manifestations or when circulating antibody is present (or both), requiring that the diagnosis be made by CSF evaluation or RT-PCR as described above.

Treatment: Treatments are symptomatic and supportive, aimed at limiting secondary bacterial invasion, supporting fluid balance, and controlling neurologic manifestations. Broad-spectrum antibiotics, balanced electrolyte solutions, parenteral nutrition, antipyretics, analgesics, and anticonvulsants are used, and good nursing care is essential. No single treatment is specific or uniformly successful. Experimental in vitro work with antiviral agents shows promise, but these agents have not yet been widely used.

Unfortunately, treatment for acute neurologic manifestations of distemper is frequently unsuccessful. If the neurologic signs are progressive or severe, the owner should be appropriately advised. With prompt, aggressive care, dogs may recover completely from multisystemic manifestations, but in other cases, neurologic signs may persist after GI and respiratory signs have resolved. Some dogs with chronic progressive or vaccine-induced forms of neurologic disease may respond to immunosuppressive therapy with anti-inflammatory or greater dosages of glucocorticoids.

Prevention: With the potential increasing virulence of emerging strains and the wide host range of canine distemper virus, widespread vaccination of domestic dogs is essential. Successful immunization of pups with canine distemper modified-live virus (MLV) vaccines depends on the lack of interference by maternal antibody. To overcome this barrier, pups are vaccinated with MLV vaccine when 6 wk old and at 3- to 4-wk intervals until 16 wk old. Alternatively, measles virus vaccine induces immunity to canine distemper virus in the presence of relatively greater levels of maternal distemper antibody. MLV measles vaccine is administered IM to pups 6–7 wk old and is followed with at least two more doses of MLV distemper vaccine when 12–16 wk old.

Many varieties of attenuated distemper vaccine are available and should be used according to manufacturers' directions. MLV vaccines should not be used in late-pregnant or early-lactation bitches. MLV vaccines can produce postvaccinal illness in some immunosuppressed dogs. A recombinant canarypox vector vaccine expressing distemper virus proteins is licensed for use in ferrets; the American Assocation of Zoo Veterinarians recommends its extra-label use in many at-risk species held in zoos and parks. Historically, annual revaccination has been standard because of the breaks in protection that can occur in stressed, diseased, or immunosuppressed dogs, and because vaccines have been labeled for annual use. Substantial evidence supports the finding that immunity induced by MLV distemper vaccines lasts ≥3 yr. However, in most cases, this remains an extra-label use of the vaccine; thus, decisions to revaccinate less often than annually should be considered in light of local prevalence of the disease and other potential risk factors, as well as industry and professional organization recommendations.

CANINE HERPESVIRAL INFECTION

Canine herpesvirus is best known as a severe viral infection of puppies worldwide, which often has a 100% mortality rate in affected litters. Increasingly sensitive molecular diagnostics have enabled its recognition in adult dogs with upper respiratory infection, ocular disease, vesicular vaginitis or posthitis, and in dogs with no clinical signs. As is typical of herpesviruses, recovery from clinical disease is associated with lifelong latent infection. Only canids (dogs, wolves, coyotes) are known to be susceptible. The seroprevalence in dog populations worldwide ranges from 20% to 98% depending on the region. Because latently infected animals may transiently convert to seronegative status, any seroprevalence study likely underestimates the true rate of exposure and carriage.

Etiology and Pathogenesis: The disease is caused by an enveloped DNA canine herpesvirus (CHV) that is sensitive to lipid solvents (such as ether and chloroform) and most disinfectants. CHV is relatively unstable outside the host, so close contact is required for transmission.

Transmission usually occurs by contact between susceptible individuals and the infected oral, nasal, or vaginal secretions of shedding dogs. Many dogs shedding virus exhibit no clinical signs. Immunologically naive pregnant bitches are at risk of acute infection, which may be transmitted to fetuses or neonatal pups; previously infected bitches are unlikely to transmit infection. The most significant systemic disease occurs in fetal or neonatal puppies from in utero infection, or infection in the first 3 wk of life. After this time, natural resistance to infection improves as puppies mature and maintain a higher body temperature.

Infection of susceptible animals results in replication of CHV in the surface cells of the nasal mucosa, pharynx, and tonsils. In the case of newborn susceptible pups or other dogs with compromised immune response, viremia and invasion of diverse visceral organs occur. Primary systemic infection is associated with a high degree of viral shedding; shedding by latently infected animals after clinical or subclinical recrudescence is of lesser severity and duration.

Clinical Findings: Deaths due to CHV infection usually occur in puppies 1–3 wk old, occasionally in puppies up to 1 mo old, and rarely in pups as old as 6 mo. Typically, onset is sudden, and death occurs after an illness of ≤24 hr. If clinical signs are observed, they may include lethargy, decreased suckling, diarrhea, nasal discharge, conjunctivitis, corneal edema, erythematous rash, rarely oral or genital vesicles, and the notable absence of fever. Thoracic radiographs show a diffuse unstructured interstitial pattern that is typical of viral pneumonia, but, in contrast to other viral diseases of puppies, leukocytosis may be present.

Older dogs exposed to or experimentally inoculated with CHV may develop a mild rhinitis, which may be part of the "kennel cough" syndrome (infectious tracheobronchitis, *see* p 1490) or a vesicular vaginitis or posthitis. There are also reports of conjunctivitis and dendritic corneal ulcers in the absence of other upper respiratory signs. Acutely infected pregnant bitches may abort a litter, or deliver a partially stillborn litter; however, they seldom exhibit other clinical signs, and future breedings are likely to be successful.

Lesions: The characteristic gross lesions at necropsy consist of disseminated focal necrosis and hemorrhages. The most pronounced lesions are seen in the lungs, cortical portion of the kidneys, adrenal glands, liver, and GI tract. All lymph nodes are enlarged and hyperemic, and the spleen is swollen. Lesions may also be found in the eyes and CNS. The basic histologic lesion is necrosis with hemorrhage in the adjacent parenchyma. The inflammatory reaction in many organs may be limited, but marked neutrophilic and mononuclear infiltration is seen in ocular lesions. Single, small, basophilic, intranuclear inclusion bodies are most common in areas of necrosis in the lung, liver, and kidneys; occasionally, they are seen as faintly acidophilic bodies located within the nuclear space.

Diagnosis: In systemically affected puppies, CHV infection may be confused with infectious canine hepatitis (*see* p 798), but it is not accompanied by the thickened, edematous gallbladder often associated with the latter. The focal areas of necrosis and hemorrhage, especially those that are seen in the kidneys, distinguish it from hepatitis and neosporosis (*see* p 663). CHV causes serious disease only in very young puppies. The rapid death and characteristic lesions distinguish it from canine distemper (*see* p 777).

Hemagglutination, ELISA, and immunofluorescence antibody tests are available, and PCR is highly sensitive and specific when used on fresh tissue and fluid samples. In cases of neonatal mortality, the diagnosis typically is made postmortem with virus isolation from fresh lung, liver, kidney, and spleen by cell culture techniques and subsequent identification by PCR and sequencing, transmission electron microscopy, immunofluorescence, or fluorescence in situ hybridization. The tissues should be submitted to the laboratory refrigerated but not frozen.

Treatment: Therapy is typically unrewarding in systemically affected puppies, and the prognosis for puppies that do survive is guarded because damage to lymphoid organs, brain, kidneys, and liver may be irreparable. Before onset of clinical signs in littermates or other nearby puppies, rearing in incubators at an increased temperature (95°F [35°C], 50% relative humidity), and/or passive immunization with intraperitoneal serum may reduce losses within an exposed litter. Limited studies with antiviral agents such as vidarabine are inconclusive, but immediate recognition and treatment would be needed to have any possibility of success.

Adult dogs with ocular, respiratory, or genital disease often experience mild and self-limiting signs. Ophthalmic antiviral cidofovir (0.5% bid) has been used successfully in one reported case of primary ocular infection in an adult dog and may be useful for persistent or painful ocular lesions.

Prevention: No vaccine is available in the USA. Infected bitches develop antibodies, and litters subsequent to the first infected litter receive maternal antibodies in the colostrum. Puppies that receive maternal antibodies may be infected with the virus, but disease does not result. Isolation of pregnant bitches from other dogs during the last 3 wk of gestation and first 3 wk postpartum, with excellent hygiene by human handlers, is the most effective way to minimize risk to puppies. Because of the high seroprevalence among adult dogs and because virus may be shed by asymptomatic individuals, complete avoidance of exposure is not a reasonable management strategy for most dogs.

FELINE INFECTIOUS PERITONITIS

Feline infectious peritonitis (FIP) is an immune-mediated disease triggered by infection with a feline coronavirus (FCoV). FCoV belongs to the family Coronaviridae, a group of enveloped, positive-stranded RNA viruses frequently found in cats.

Coronavirus-specific antibodies are present in as many as 90% of cats in catteries and in as many as 50% of those in single-cat households. However, <5% of FCoV-infected cats develop FIP in multicat households.

Geographic Distribution: FCoV infection and FIP occur worldwide with similar prevalence and are found in domestic and wild cats. FCoV strains can be classified into serotypes I and II, depending on their antigenetic relationship to canine coronavirus (CCV), and these subtypes vary in proportion among different countries. Among FCoV strains isolated in the field in the USA and Europe, 70%–95% are serotype I. In contrast, in Japan serotype II predominates. Most cats with FIP are infected with FCoV serotype I. However, both serotypes can cause FIP and both can cause clinically inapparent FCoV infections.

FCoV belongs to the same taxonomic cluster of coronaviruses as transmissible gastroenteritis virus, porcine respiratory coronavirus, CCV, and some human coronaviruses. In many species, coronaviruses have a relatively restricted organ tropism, mainly infecting the respiratory and/or GI tracts. In cats and mice, however, coronavirus infections can, in certain circumstances, involve multiple organs.

In addition to cats, other felid species are susceptible, and FCoV is also an important pathogen in nondomestic felids. There was evidence of FCoV infection in 195 of 342 nondomestic felids in southern Africa, which included both wild and captive animals. There is also a high incidence of FIP in nondomestic felids in captivity in the USA and Europe. Cheetahs in captivity seem to be highly prone to developing FIP; loss of genetic diversity and a genetic deficiency in their cellular immunity is thought to predispose them to the disease. Although FIP can only occur in felids, a clinically similar condition in ferrets is associated with ferret systemic coronavirus.

Etiology and Pathogenesis: FIP is a sporadic disease thought to be caused by viral variants that develop within each specific cat. The pathogenesis of FIP is unclear, but there are two main hypotheses. The "internal mutation theory" states that cats are infected with the primarily avirulent FCoV that replicates in enterocytes; in some cats, a mutation occurs in a certain region of the FCoV genome that creates a new phenotype with the ability to replicate within macrophages. The presence of highly virulent strains of FCoV capable of consistently inducing FIP support this theory, albeit under experimental conditions. Several researchers speculate that some circulating feline enteric coronaviruses are closer to making critical mutations necessary for development of FIP, possibly explaining FIP outbreaks. No consistent mutation has yet been identified, although studies have suggested sequence differences in the spike protein, membrane protein, or NSP3c correlate with disease manifestation. Recent studies have found feline coronaviruses to have intact NSP3c genes, whereas most isolates from diseased tissues of FIP cases had disrupted NSP3c genes. Findings suggested that 3c-inactivated viruses only rarely replicate in the intestine, which possibly explains the rare incidence of FIP outbreaks. In additional work, it was concluded that mutation of the S1/S2 locus and modulation of a furin recognition site normally present in the S gene of enteric coronaviruses is a critical contributing factor for development of FIP.

The second hypothesis for the development of FIP is the existence of distinct circulating virulent and avirulent strains in a population, and exposure to the pathogenic strain, the viral load, and the cat's immune response determine whether FIP will develop. It is likely both viral genetics and host immunity play a role. In both hypotheses, the key pathogenic event in the development of FIP is the massive replication of FCoV in macrophages. If the cat does not eliminate macrophages infected with replication-competent virus early in infection, the presence of the virus within circulating macrophages initiates an ultimately fatal arthus-type immune-mediated reaction, which defines FIP.

Factors that increase FCoV replication in the intestines (and increase the probability of the mutation) include young age, breed predisposition, immune status, stress, corticosteroid treatment, and surgery, as well as dosage and virulence of the virus and reinfection rate in multicat households. Crowded environments, such as catteries or shelters, also may increase stress and exposure to FCoV. Whenever FCoV infection exists, so does the potential for development of FIP.

After a cat becomes infected with FCoV via fecal-oral transmission (or less commonly, inhalation), the main site of viral replication is the intestinal epithelium. Replication of FCoV in the cytoplasm can destroy intestinal epithelial cells, leading to diarrhea in some cats. In many cats, infection persists for weeks to months in the absence of clinical signs. These cats shed FCoV either intermittently or continually and act as a source of infection for other cats. Previously, it was believed that avirulent FCoV remained confined to the digestive tract, did not cross the gut mucosa, and did not spread beyond the intestinal epithelium and regional lymph nodes. However, PCR can detect FCoV in the circulating macrophages of healthy cats from households with endemic FCoV, indicating that avirulent FCoV may also cause viremia.

FIP is an immune complex disease involving viral antigen, antiviral antibodies, and complement. Within weeks after macrophage invasion and replication, virions are found in the cecum, colon, intestinal lymph nodes, spleen, and liver after distribution by macrophages in the whole body, including the CNS. There are two possible explanations for the events that follow viral dissemination from the intestines. The first proposed mechanism is that FCoV-infected macrophages leave the bloodstream and carry virus into the tissues. The virus attracts antibodies, complement is fixed, and more macrophages and neutrophils are attracted to the lesion; as a consequence, typical pyogranulomatous changes develop. The alternative explanation is that FIP occurs as a result of circulating immune complexes lodging in blood vessel walls, fixing complement, and leading to development of the pyogranulomatous changes. It is assumed that these antigen–antibody complexes are recognized by macrophages but are not, as they should be, presented to killer cells, and thus are not destroyed.

In addition to virus, chemotactic substances, including complement and inflammatory mediators, are released from infected macrophages. Complement fixation leads to the release of vasoactive amines, which cause endothelial cell retraction and thus increased vascular permeability. Retraction of capillary endothelial cells allows exudation of plasma proteins and, hence, development of characteristic protein-rich exudates. Inflammatory mediators activate proteolytic enzymes that cause tissue damage.

Epidemiology and Transmission:

FCoV and FIP are a major problem in multicat households. The virus is endemic in environments in which many cats are kept together in a confined space (eg, catteries, shelters, pet stores). FCoV is found less commonly in free-roaming community cats, because they do not typically use the same locations to bury their feces; shared litter boxes are a major source of transmission in multicat households.

Although the prevalence of FCoV infection is very high in multicat households, <5% of cats in these situations develop FIP; the number is even lower in a single cat environment. The risk of developing FIP is higher for young and immunocompromised cats because the replication of FCoV in these animals is less controlled and, thus, the critical mutation is more likely to occur. More than half of the cats with FIP are <12 mo old. Sexually intact cats, males, and purebred cats have a higher incidence of FIP. Epidemiologic data suggest that the cat's genetic background contributes to the manifestation of FIP. Investigators have described variation in breed resistance and susceptibility to FIP. Susceptibility to FIP is a polygenic inherited trait in Persians and Birmans. Breeds with higher prevalence of FIP include Abyssinian, Bengal, Birman, Himalayan, Ragdoll, and Rex.

FCoV is shed mainly in the feces. Infection is generally via the oronasal route. After natural infection, cats begin to shed virus in feces within 1 wk. In very early infection, it may be found in saliva, respiratory secretions, and urine. When naive cats in multicat households first encounter FCoV, it is likely that all will become infected (and develop antibodies); most will shed virus intermittently for a period of weeks or months. Some cats become chronic FCoV shedders, providing a continual source for reinfection of other cats. Cats that are antibody-negative are very unlikely to shed, whereas approximately one-third of all FCoV antibody-positive cats shed virus. Cats with high antibody titers are more likely to shed FCoV. They also are more likely to shed consistently and higher amounts of the virus. Most cats with FIP also shed non-mutated FCoV; however, the virus load in feces seems to decrease after a cat has developed FIP.

The major sources of FCoV for naive cats are litter boxes shared with shedding cats. Also, continuous reinfection through the contaminated litter box of a cat already infected seems to play an important role in the endemic survival of the virus. Rarely, virus can be transmitted through saliva, by mutual grooming, sharing the same food bowl, and through close contact. Sneezed droplet transmission is also rare but possible. It is uncertain whether FCoV transmission occurs to a significant degree at cat shows. Transmission by lice or fleas is considered unlikely. Transplacental transmission can occur but is very uncommon under natural circumstances. Most kittens that are removed from contact with virus-shedding adult cats at 5–6 wk of age do not become infected. Most commonly, kittens are infected at the age of

6–8 wk at a time when their maternal antibodies wane, mostly through contact with feces from their mothers or other FCoV-excreting cats.

FCoV is a relatively fragile virus that is destroyed by most household disinfectants and detergents. However, it may survive in cold or dry conditions (eg, in carpet) for as long as 7 wk outside the cat. Indirect fomite transmission is possible, and the virus can be transmitted for a short time via clothes, toys, and grooming tools.

Clinical Findings:

Feline Coronavirus Infection: FCoV infection can cause a transient and clinically mild diarrhea and/or vomiting due to replication of FCoV in enterocytes. Kittens infected with FCoV may have a history of stunted growth or upper respiratory tract signs. Occasionally, the virus may cause severe diarrhea with weight loss, which may be unresponsive to treatment and continue for months. However, most FCoV-infected cats do not show clinical signs.

Feline Infectious Peritonitis: Clinical signs of FIP vary depending on organ involvement. Many organs, including the liver, kidneys, pancreas, CNS, and eyes, can be involved. The clinical signs and pathologic findings are a consequence of the vasculitis and, less commonly, organ failure resultant from damage to the blood vessels that supply them. In all cats with nonspecific clinical signs, such as chronic weight loss or fever of unknown origin resistant to antibiotic treatment or recurrent in nature, FIP should be on the list of differential diagnoses.

The length of time between infection and development of clinical signs is unknown and depends on the immune response of the individual cat. Disease generally becomes apparent from a few weeks to 2 yr after the mutation has occurred. Cats are at greatest risk of developing FIP in the first 6–18 mo after infection with FCoV; the risk decreases to ~4% at 36 mo after infection.

Previously, three different forms of FIP were distinguished: 1) an effusive, exudative, "wet form"; 2) a noneffusive, nonexudative, granulomatous, parenchymatous "dry form"; and 3) a mixed form. The first form was characterized by a fibrinous peritonitis, pleuritis, and/or pericarditis with effusion in the abdomen, thorax, and/or pericardium, respectively. The second form was characterized by granulomatous changes in different organs that may include the eyes and CNS. Differentiation between these forms is not useful and is of value only for the diagnostic approach, because there is nearly always effusion to a greater or lesser degree in combination with more or less granulomatous changes present in cats with FIP. In addition, the forms can transform into each other. Cats with FIP may be alert or depressed. Some eat with a normal or even increased appetite; others are anorectic. Fever, weight loss, and/or icterus may be noted.

In cats with ascites, an abdominal swelling is commonly noticed. Fluctuation and a fluid wave may be present; in less severe cases, fluid can be palpated between the intestinal loops. Abdominal masses can sometimes be palpated, reflecting omental and visceral adhesions or enlarged mesenteric lymph nodes. Thoracic effusions may cause dyspnea, tachypnea, open-mouth breathing, or cyanotic mucous membranes. Auscultation reveals muffled heart sounds. In cats with pericardial effusions, heart sounds are muffled and typical changes can be seen on ECG and echocardiography. Effusions can be visualized by diagnostic imaging (eg, radiographs, ultrasound) and verified by a fluid centesis.

In cats without obvious effusion, in which mainly granulomatous changes are present, signs are often vague and include fever, weight loss, lethargy, and decreased appetite. If the lungs are involved, cats can be dyspneic, and thoracic radiographs may reveal patchy densities in the lungs. Abdominal palpation may reveal enlarged mesenteric lymph nodes and irregular kidneys or nodular irregularities in other viscera. Presenting clinical signs sometimes can be unusual. In some cats, abdominal tumors are suspected, but FIP is finally diagnosed at surgery or necropsy.

Cats with FIP frequently have ocular lesions. The most common ocular lesions are retinal changes, and a retinal examination should be performed in all cats with suspected FIP. FIP can cause cuffing of the retinal vasculature, which appears as fuzzy grayish lines on either side of the blood vessels. Occasionally, granulomatous changes are seen on the retina. Retinal hemorrhage or detachment may also occur. These changes, however, are not pathognomonic; similar changes can be seen in other systemic infectious diseases, including toxoplasmosis, systemic fungal infections, and feline immunodeficiency virus or feline leukemia virus infection. Uveitis is another common manifestation. Mild uveitis can manifest by color change of the iris. Uveitis may also manifest as aqueous flare, with cloudiness of the anterior chamber, which can be detected in a darkened room using focal illumination. Large numbers of inflammatory cells in the anterior chamber settle on the back of the cornea and cause keratic precipitates, which may be hidden by the nictitating membrane. Hemorrhage into the anterior chamber can occur. If aqueous humor is sampled, it may reveal increased protein and pleocytosis.

Neurologic signs are common in cats with FIP. These are variable and reflect the area of CNS involvement. The lesions are usually multifocal. The most common clinical sign is ataxia followed by nystagmus and seizures. In addition, incoordination, intention tremors, hyperesthesia, behavioral changes, and cranial nerve involvement can be seen. If cranial nerves are involved, neurologic signs such as visual deficits and loss of menace reflex may be present. When FIP lesions are located on a peripheral nerve or the spinal column, lameness, progressive ataxia, or paresis may be seen. Finding hydrocephalus on a CT scan is suggestive of neurologic FIP. In a study of 24 cats with FIP with neurologic involvement, 75% were found to have hydrocephalus on postmortem examination.

Solitary mural intestinal lesions have been described in cats with a histologic diagnosis of FIP. Diarrhea, vomiting, or obstruction can occur, and a suspected neoplastic mass can be found in the colon or ileocecocolic junction, with associated lymphadenopathy, and a markedly thickened and firm segment of bowel with multifocal pyogranulomas extending through the intestinal wall on histology.

Skin fragility syndrome was described in a cat with FIP, and other skin lesions (eg, nodular skin lesions, papular skin lesions, pododermatitis) may be present as well. Reproductive disorders, neonatal deaths, and fading kittens are not usually associated with FIP.

Lesions: Histology of lesions is usually pathognomonic and is traditionally considered the gold standard for diagnosis of FIP. H&E-stained samples typically contain localized perivascular mixed inflammation with macrophages, neutrophils, lymphocytes, and plasma cells. FCoV can be identified by immunohistochemistry in the macrophages within the lesions. Pyogranulomas may be large and consolidated, sometimes with focal tissue necrosis, or numerous and small. Lymphoid tissues in cats with FIP often show lymphoid depletion caused by apoptosis.

Diagnosis: Reliable and rapid diagnosis of FIP is important but can be challenging. Difficulties arise from the lack of noninvasive confirmatory tests in cats without obvious effusion. Obtaining and analyzing effusion is minimally invasive and much more sensitive than diagnostic tests in blood. In cats with no effusion, several parameters including history, clinical signs, laboratory changes, and level of antibody titers should be considered to determine whether to use invasive confirmative diagnostic methods.

Hematology and Serum Biochemistry: WBC counts can be decreased or increased. Lymphopenia is commonly present, mainly caused by apoptosis of uninfected T cells, primarily $CD8^+$ T cells, as a result of high TNF-α concentrations produced by virus-infected macrophages. However, lymphopenia in combination with neutrophilia can occur in many severe diseases in cats. A mild to moderate nonregenerative anemia is another nonspecific finding that may be seen in almost any chronic disease in cats.

The most common laboratory abnormality in cats with FIP is an increase in total serum protein concentration caused by increased globulins, mainly γ-globulins, which occurs in >70% of cats with FIP. Total protein in cats with FIP can reach very high concentrations of ≥12 g/dL. The albumin to globulin ratio, however, has a significantly higher diagnostic value to distinguish FIP from other diseases than total serum protein or γ-globulin concentrations, because serum albumin also may decrease. Albumin loss in cats with FIP may be caused by glomerulonephritis secondary to immune complex deposition, by loss of protein due to exudative enteropathy in cases of granulomatous changes in the intestines, or by extravasation of protein-rich fluid during vasculitis. An optimal cut-off value of 0.8 was determined for the albumin to globulin ratio (specificity 82%, sensitivity 80%). If the serum albumin to globulin ratio is <0.8, the probability that the cat has FIP is high (92% positive predictive value [PPV]); if the albumin to globulin ratio is >0.8, the cat likely does not have FIP (61% negative predictive value [NPV]). Reference laboratories have variation in techniques for measurement of serum proteins. Serum protein electrophoresis may be performed in cats with suspected FIP to distinguish a polyclonal from a monoclonal hypergammaglobulinemia to differentiate FIP (and other chronic infection) from tumors such as multiple myelomas or other plasma cell tumors. However, hyperglobulinemia is generally nonspecific and reflects active inflammation.

Other laboratory parameters, including liver enzymes, bilirubin, urea (or BUN), and creatinine, can be variably increased depending on the degree and localization of organ damage but are not helpful in establishing an etiologic diagnosis. Hyperbilirubinemia and icterus are often seen in cats with FIP. High bilirubin (in the absence of hemolysis) and increased liver enzyme activity should raise the suspicion of FIP.

High serum levels (>3 mg/mL) of α-1-acid glycoprotein (AGP), a serum acute phase protein that is increased in cats with FIP, can support diagnosis, but levels also are increased in other inflammatory conditions; thus, these changes are not specific. Additionally, AGP may also be high in asymptomatic cats infected with FCoV, especially in households where FCoV is endemic. However, the most prominent increases in serum AGP concentration have been recorded in cats with FIP. Levels of AGP in serum and effusions increased 2- to 5-fold in cats with FIP, more than in diseases such as neoplasia and cardiomyopathy. In a study with a small number of cases, measurement of serum AGP concentrations was demonstrated to be most helpful, because it was the only diagnostic test in complete concordance with immunohistochemistry. Two factors must be considered when evaluating AGP concentration to support a clinical diagnosis of FIP: the magnitude of the increase in concentration and the pretest probability of FIP (compatible history and clinical findings). Serum amyloid A (SAA), another acute phase protein, increases 10-fold in the serum of cats with FIP compared with asymptomatic cats exposed to feline enteric coronaviruses. SAA may be a useful biomarker in the future.

Diagnostic Imaging: A recent study highlighted specific concurrent ultrasonographic findings that should increase the index of suspicion for FIP, including abdominal lymphadenopathy, peritoneal or retroperitoneal effusion, renomegaly, irregular renal contour, hypoechoic subcapsular echogenicity, and diffuse changes within the intestines. In most cats in the study population, the liver and spleen were normal in echogenicity. A normal abdominal ultrasound does not exclude the possibility of FIP infection.

Effusion Fluid: Tests on effusion have a much higher diagnostic value than tests performed on blood. Fluid can be obtained through ultrasound-guided fine-needle aspiration or by using the “flying cat technique” in case of ascites. Although clear yellow effusions of sticky consistency are considered typical, the presence of this type of fluid in body cavities alone is not diagnostic. Cases with pure chylous effusion have been reported. Usually, the protein content is very high (>3.5 g/dL), consistent with an exudate, whereas the cellular content is low (<5,000 nucleated cells/mL), resembling a modified transudate or even pure transudate. Major differential diagnoses for these effusions include inflammatory liver disease, lymphoma, heart failure, and bacterial peritonitis or pleuritis. LDH activity typically is high (>300 IU/L). Cytology is variable but often consists predominantly of macrophages and nondegenerate neutrophils (in much lower numbers than seen with bacterial infection). These effusions can usually be differentiated from bacterial infection or lymphoma by the presence of malignant cells, degenerate neutrophils, or intracellular bacteria on cytology and bacterial growth on culture, respectively. The albumin to globulin ratio of the effusion can be measured: a ratio of <0.5 is strongly correlated with FIP, with a PPV between 66% and 95%, depending on the prevalence of FIP in the cat’s environment. An albumin to globulin ratio >0.81 has a 100% NPV, essentially excluding FIP.

Rivalta’s test is a simple, inexpensive method that does not require special laboratory equipment and can be performed easily in private practice. It is very useful in cats to differentiate between effusions caused by FIP and effusions caused by other diseases. The high protein content and high concentrations of fibrin and inflammatory mediators lead to a positive reaction. To perform the test, a transparent reagent tube (10 mL) is filled with ~8 mL distilled water, to which 1 drop of acetic acid (highly concentrated vinegar, 98%) is added and mixed thoroughly. On the surface of this solution, 1 drop of the effusion fluid is carefully layered. If the drop disappears and the solution remains clear, the Rivalta’s test is defined as negative. If the drop retains its shape, stays attached to the surface, or slowly floats down to the bottom of the tube (drop- or jelly-fish-like), the test is defined as positive. Rivalta’s test has a high PPV (86%) and a very high NPV (96%) for FIP. Positive results can sometimes be seen in cats with bacterial peritonitis or lymphoma. Those effusions, however, are usually easy to differentiate through macroscopic examination, cytology, and bacterial culture.

Cerebrospinal Fluid: Analysis of cerebrospinal fluid (CSF) from cats with neurologic signs due to FIP lesions may reveal increased protein (50–350 mg/dL with a normal value of <25 mg/dL) and pleocytosis (100–10,000 nucleated cells/mL) containing mainly neutrophils, lymphocytes, and macrophages (a relatively nonspecific finding). Many cats with neurologic signs caused by FIP have normal CSF. In one study, typical CSF findings in cats with FIP were a protein concentration >200 mg/dL and a WBC count of >100 cells/µL, which consisted predominantly of neutrophils.

Measurement of Antibodies: There is no FIP-specific antibody test; all that can be measured is antibodies against FCoV. Antibody titers measured in serum are extensively used as a diagnostic tool. However, most FCoV antibody-positive cats never develop FIP. Thus, antibody titers must be interpreted extremely cautiously and should never be used as the sole test to diagnose FIP. Antibody testing still has a certain role in the diagnosis and, more importantly, in the management of multicat households, when done by appropriate methodologies and when results are properly interpreted. However, antibody testing can only be useful if the laboratory is reliable and consistent. Low or medium titers have no diagnostic value. If interpreted carefully, however, very high titers can be of certain diagnostic value. A very high titer in a cat with compatible clinical signs (1:1,600) has a 94% PPV for FIP; a negative titer has a 90% NPV for FIP. Cats with high antibody titers are more likely to shed FCoV and to shed more consistently higher amounts of the virus. Thus, the titer is directly correlated with virus replication rate and the amount of virus in the intestines. Screening a cattery for the presence of FCoV or screening a cat before introduction into an FCoV-free cattery are additional indications.

Measuring antibodies in fluids (eg, effusion, CSF) other than blood has been investigated. Detection of anticoronavirus antibodies in effusion fluid has a PPV of 90% and a NPV of 29% for diagnosis of FIP. Presence of antibodies in effusion is correlated with the presence of antibodies in blood; thus, antibody titers in effusions are not very helpful. One study investigating the diagnostic value of antibody detection in CSF reported a very good correlation to the presence of FIP when compared with histopathology; however, two studies investigating a large number of cats presented to veterinary teaching hospitals revealed no significant difference in antibody titers in CSF from cats with neurologic signs due to FIP compared with cats with other neurologic diseases confirmed by histopathology.

Feline Coronavirus Reverse Transcriptase PCR: FCoV reverse transcriptase PCR in blood is used with increasing frequency as a diagnostic tool for FIP. However, so far, no PCR has been developed that can definitively diagnose FIP. PCR can be false-negative (eg, because the assay requires reverse transcription of viral RNA to DNA before amplification of DNA, and degradation of RNA can occur due to contamination with ubiquitous RNAases) or false-positive (eg, the assay does not distinguish between virulent and avirulent FCoV strains and will not discriminate FCoV from coronaviruses of other species). Furthermore, viremia appears to occur not only in cats with FIP but also in healthy carriers. FCoV RNA has been detected in the blood of cats with FIP but also in healthy cats that did not develop FIP for as long as 70 mo. Therefore, the results of PCR tests in general must be interpreted carefully, and PCR cannot be used as a tool to definitively diagnose FIP.

PCR has been used to detect FCoV in fecal samples, and it is sensitive and useful to document that a cat is shedding FCoV in feces. The strength of the PCR signal in feces correlates with the amount of virus present in the intestines. These results can be useful to detect cats that chronically shed high virus loads and that pose a high risk in multicat households.

Immunostaining of Feline Coronavirus Antigen: Direct staining of FCoVs within macrophages by immunofluorescence in cytocentrifuged effusions or immunohistochemistry in tissue is considered the most specific test to confirm FIP. Immunostaining cannot differentiate between the "harmless" FCoV and FIP-causing FCoV, but finding infected macrophages in characteristic pyogranulomatous lesions or in inflammatory effusions is highly associated with FIP. In a recent study in which a large number of cats with confirmed FIP and controls with other confirmed diseases were investigated, positive immunofluorescence staining of intracellular FCoV antigen in macrophages of the effusion was 100% predictive of FIP. Unfortunately, the NPV of the test is not very high (57%), which can be explained by low numbers of macrophages on effusion smears resulting in negative staining. Immunohistochemistry can be used to detect the expression of FCoV antigen in tissue and is also 100% predictive of FIP if positive. However, invasive methods (eg, laparotomy or laparoscopy) are usually necessary to obtain appropriate tissue samples. Either histology itself is confirmative, or immunohistochemistry staining of

FCoV antigen in tissue macrophages can be used to diagnose FIP.

Treatment, Control, and Prevention: Because of the high prevalence of FCoV antibodies in healthy cats, widespread antibody testing of healthy cats is not an appropriate screening test for FIP in pet cats. Nor should cats in shelters be screened for antibodies before adoption. No treatment of healthy antibody-positive cats has been shown to prevent development of FIP.

Treatment of cats with FIP remains frustrating and is limited to the cases that respond favorably within the first few days. The prognosis for a cat with FIP is very poor. In a prospective study including 43 cats with confirmed FIP, the median survival after the definitive diagnosis was 9 days. Some cats, however, may live for several months. Factors that indicate a poor prognosis and a short survival time are low Karnofsky score (index for quality of life), low platelet count, low lymphocyte count, high bilirubin concentration, and a large amount of effusion. Seizures are an unfavorable prognostic sign; they are significantly more frequent in cats with marked extension of the inflammatory lesions to the forebrain. Cats that show no improvement within 3 days after treatment initiation are unlikely to show any benefit from therapy, and euthanasia should be considered. Longer survival or remission from clinical signs is rare.

Supportive treatment is aimed at suppressing the immune overreaction, usually using corticosteroids. However, there are no controlled studies that indicate whether corticosteroids have any beneficial effect. Cats treated with corticosteroids have shown anecdotal improvement for as long as several months. Immunosuppressive drugs such as prednisolone (2–4 mg/kg/day, PO) are commonly used. More potent cytotoxic drugs such as cyclophosphamide (4 mg/kg/day) have also been suggested. Cats with large effusions benefit from removal of the fluid; injection of dexamethasone into the abdominal or thoracic cavity may follow (1 mg/kg/day until no effusion is present).

Cats with FIP should receive supportive therapy, including fluids and nutritional support, and their quality of life should be monitored. Anecdotal reports suggest that ozagrel hydrochloride, a thromboxane synthetase inhibitor that inhibits platelet aggregation, and pentoxifylline, a drug that decreases vasculitis and inhibits several cytokines (such as interleukins and TNF-α), may be beneficial in some cats.

Immune modulators (eg, *Propionibacterium acnes*, acemannan, tylosin, promodulin, interferon-α) have been used to treat cats with FIP. However, controlled trials are lacking, and anecdotal reports often lack definitive diagnosis. It has been suggested that these agents may benefit infected animals by restoring compromised immune function. However, a nonspecific stimulation of the immune system would seem to be contraindicated in FIP, because clinical signs develop and progress as a result of an immune-mediated response.

A number of studies have investigated effectiveness of various antiviral treatments in cats with FIP, including interferons and ribavirin. To date, none have proved to be very successful. *See* TABLE 7.

Interferons have been used frequently in cats with FIP. Human interferon-α has a direct antiviral effect, and in vitro antiviral efficacy against an FIP-causing FCoV strain has been demonstrated. In a controlled study, cats with confirmed FIP treated with interferon-α at 106 IU/kg in combination with *Propionibacterium acnes* survived for ~3 wk. Feline interferon-ω is available in some European countries and Japan. FCoV replication is inhibited by feline interferon-ω in vitro, but there was no statistically significant difference in the mean survival time of cats enrolled in a randomized placebo-controlled double-blind treatment trial. Cats survived for 3–200 days, regardless of whether they received the drug or placebo.

Management of Exposed Cats: When a cat in a household develops FIP, all in-contact cats will have already been exposed to the same FCoV. Under natural circumstances, it appears that the FIP-causing virus strain is not excreted in such cases, and FIP is not transmitted from cat to cat. However, under experimental conditions it has been possible to transmit FIP-causing virus from a cat with FIP to in-contact cats. Still, it appears to be relatively safe for a cat with FIP to remain in the same household with cats that have already been in contact to the FCoV strain. However, it is not recommended to allow contact between a cat with FIP and any new "naive" cat. Kittens, which are more susceptible to FIP than adults, should not be introduced to households with a recent history of FIP.

If a cat has been euthanized or has died due to FIP, the owner should wait 2 mo before obtaining another cat. FCoV can remain infectious for at least 7 wk in the environment, particularly where litter boxes are in use. Other cats currently in the household are most likely infected with and shedding FCoV. Cats are commonly presented to the veterinarian for evaluation after contact with a cat with FIP or a suspected or known virus excretor. The owner may want to know the prognosis for the exposed cat or whether it is shedding FCoV. Such cats will likely be antibody positive, because 95%–100% of cats exposed to FCoV become infected and develop antibodies ~2–3 wk after exposure. A few cats may be resistant to FCoV infection. Some cats in FCoV-endemic multicat households continuously remain antibody negative. The mechanism of action for this resistance is unknown.

Although exposed cats will most likely have antibodies, this is not necessarily associated with a poor prognosis. Most cats infected with FCoV will not develop FIP, and many cats in single- or two-cat households will eventually clear the infection and become antibody negative in a few months to years (usually ~6 mo). If titers are monitored, cats should be retested (using the same laboratory) every 6–12 mo until the antibody test is negative. Some cats will remain antibody positive for years. The value of serial antibody or PCR testing is mostly limited to protocols aimed at creating FCoV-free closed catteries.

Management of Multicat Households: In most multicat households with unusually high cat numbers, FCoV is endemic and FIP is almost inevitable. Households of <5 cats may spontaneously and naturally become FCoV-free, but in households of >10 cats per group, this is almost impossible because the virus passes from one cat to another, maintaining the infection. In these FCoV-endemic environments, such as breeding catteries, shelters, foster homes, and other multicat homes, there is virtually nothing to prevent FIP.

Various tactics have been used to eliminate FCoV from an endemic cattery. Reducing the number of cats (especially of kittens <12 mo old) and keeping suspected FCoV-contaminated surfaces clean can minimize population loads of the virus. Antibody or fecal PCR testing and removal of positive cats should be performed to stop exposure and reinfection of recovered cats. Approximately ⅓ of antibody-positive cats excrete virus; thus, every antibody-positive cat should be considered infectious. After 3–6 mo, antibody titers can be retested. Alternatively, PCR testing of (several) fecal samples can be performed to detect chronic FCoV carriers; these cats should be removed. In large, multicat environments, 40%–60% of cats shed virus in their feces at any given time. Approximately 20% will shed virus persistently. If a cat remains persistently PCR-positive for >6 wk, it should be placed in a single-cat environment or with other chronic shedders.

Kittens of FCoV-shedding queens are often protected from infection by maternally derived antibodies until they are 5–6 wk old. An early weaning protocol for prevention of FCoV infection in kittens has been proposed and consists of isolation of queens 2 wk before parturition, strict quarantine of queen and kittens, and early weaning at 5 wk of age. Early removal of kittens from the queen and prevention of infection from other cats may succeed in keeping kittens free of infection. Kittens should be taken to a new home (with no FCoV-infected cats) at 5 wk of age. Although straightforward in concept, the protocol requires quarantine rooms and procedures to ensure that new virus does not enter. Special care must be taken during this

TABLE 7 DRUGS THAT HAVE BEEN SUGGESTED FOR USE IN FELINE INFECTIOUS PERITONITIS CASES

Drug[a]	Comment	ABCD Recommendation (EBM Level[b])
	ANTIVIRALS	
Ribavirin	Active in vitro but toxic in cats	Not recommended (2)
Vidarabin	Active in vitro but toxic in cats	Likely ineffective (4)
Human interferon-α, SC, high dose	Although effective in vitro against FCoV, SC treatment did not work in an experimental trial	Ineffective (2)

TABLE 7 DRUGS THAT HAVE BEEN SUGGESTED FOR USE IN FELINE INFECTIOUS PERITONITIS CASES *(continued)*

Drug[a]	Comment	ABCD Recommendation (EBM Level[b])
Human interferon-α, PO, low dose	No trials. Only acts as immunostimulant if given orally; immune stimulation should be avoided in cats with FIP	Contraindicated (4)
Feline interferon-ω	Single placebo-controlled study of naturally occurring cases and one uncontrolled study	No benefit was observed (level 1 study); may require further studies in view of anecdotal clinical evidence (4)
Polyprenyl immunostimulant (investigational drug)	Upregulation biosynthesis of mRNA of TH1 cytokines, uncontrolled study treating three noneffusive cases, long survival	May have some beneficial effect in noneffusive FIP (3); controlled studies required
IMMUNOSUPPRESSANTS		
Prednisolone/ dexamethasone (immunosuppressive doses)	No controlled studies; some cats improved during treatment and survived for several months; does not cure FIP	Currently supportive treatment of choice (3); if effusion is present, dexamethasone intrathoracic or intraperitoneal may be helpful
Pentoxyfylline	Aimed at treating vasculitis	Ineffective in one case study (4)
Ozagrel hydrochloride	Thromboxane synthesis inhibitor aimed at treating inflammatory response; only used in two cases with beneficial effect	Controlled studies needed (3)
Cyclosporin A	Immunosuppressive; no published studies	Not recommended; more directed against cellular immunity than humoral (lack of data) (4)
Cyclophosphamide	Immunosuppressive; no published studies	Might be considered in combination with glucocorticoids (4)
Chlorambucil	Immunosuppressive; no published studies	Might be considered in combination with glucocorticoids (4)
Azathioprine	Toxic in cats; immunosuppressive; no published studies	Not recommended (4)
Acetylsalicylic acid (aspirin), platelet inhibitory dosage	To treat inflammatory response as well as vasculitis; no published studies	May have some beneficial effect, but adverse effects possible if used in combination with high-dose glucocorticoids

[a] Many of the treatments listed represent extra-label use for treatment of FIP.

[b] Evidence-based medicine (EBM) level 1 = confirmed by randomized controlled clinical trials in target species; EBM level 2 = confirmed by randomized controlled experimental studies in target species; EBM level 3 = supported by case series, other experimental studies, nonrandomized clinical trials; EBM level 4 = based on expert opinion, case reports, studies in other species. Modified, with permission, from Feline infectious peritonitis. Guidelines of The European Advisory Board on Cat Diseases (ABCD), © 2012 Advisory Board on Cat Diseases.

period to socialize the kittens. The success of early weaning and isolation depends on effective quarantine and low numbers of cats (<5) in the household.

Another possible approach is to maximize heritable resistance to FIP in breeding catteries. Genetic predisposition plays a role in the disease but is not completely understood. Full-sibling littermates of kittens with FIP have a higher likelihood of developing FIP than other cats in the same environment. A cat that has two or more litters in which kittens develop FIP should not be bred again. Particular attention should be paid to pedigrees of toms in which FIP is overrepresented. Because line breeding often uses valuable tomcats extensively, eliminating such animals may have an effect on improving overall resistance.

In shelters, prevention of FIP is virtually impossible unless cats are strictly separated and handled only through sterile handling devices (comparable to isolation units). Isolation is often not effective because FCoV is easily transported on clothes, shoes, dust, and cats. There appears to be significant correlation between the number of handling events outside the cages and stress and the percentage of antibody-positive cats. Studies have shown dramatic increases in fecal shedding of FCoV in infected cats after entering an animal shelter. Half of the cats that were originally FCoV-negative were shedding FCoV within 1 wk of entering the shelter environment. Shelters should have written information sheets or contracts informing adopters about FCoV and FIP. Personnel should understand that FCoV is an unavoidable consequence of endemic FCoV in multicat environments. Good husbandry practices and facilities that can be cleaned easily may minimize virus spread.

Vaccination: A vaccine developed with a temperature-sensitive mutant of the FCoV strain DF2-FIPV, which is reported to replicate in the cool lining of the upper respiratory tract but not at higher internal body temperature, is available in the USA, Canada, and Europe. This vaccine is administered intranasally and produces local immunity (IgA antibodies) at the site where FCoV first enters the body (the oropharynx), as well as cell-mediated immunity. Vaccination in an FCoV-endemic environment or in a household with known cases of FIP is not effective, probably because most cats are already seropositive for FCoV. The vaccine is labeled for use beginning at 16 wk of age, which may be too late to protect kittens against FCoV in endemic populations. Most cats develop systemic antibodies after vaccination, thus making the establishment and control of an FCoV-free household difficult. The American Association of Feline Practitioners lists the FIP vaccine as "not recommended."

Zoonotic Risk: Although coronaviruses shared with animals, such as severe acute respiratory syndrome (SARS) and Middle East respiratory syndrome (MERS), are responsible for severe respiratory disease outbreaks in people, there is no indication that FCoV is infectious to people.

FELINE LEUKEMIA VIRUS AND RELATED DISEASES

(Feline lymphoma and leukemia, Lymphosarcoma)

Feline leukemia virus (FeLV) remains one of the most important infectious diseases of cats globally. It manifests primarily through profound anemia, malignancies, and immunosuppression and infects domestic cats and other species of Felidae. In the laboratory, cells from a much wider range of species can be infected by some strains of the virus.

The Feline Retrovirus Management Guidelines published by the American Association of Feline Practitioners is a key resource for expert consensus on prevention, diagnosis, and management of FeLV for veterinary practitioners in private practice, animal shelters, and catteries (*see* TABLE 8).

Etiology and Epidemiology: FeLV is a retrovirus in the family Oncovirinae. Other oncoviruses include feline sarcoma virus, mouse leukemia viruses, and two human T-lymphotropic viruses. Although oncogenesis is one of their more dramatic effects, oncoviruses cause many other conditions, including degenerative, proliferative, and immunologic disorders.

TABLE 8 SUMMARY OF CLINICAL MANAGEMENT OF FELINE RETROVIRUS

Test cats that are:	Sick regardless of age and previous test status Entering a new household 30 days since last high potential for exposure At risk with unknown infection status Receiving routine veterinary care and have outdoor access or live in a home with FeLV-positive cats Candidates for blood donation
Vaccinate cats that are:	Kittens, as part of the initial vaccination series Often outdoors In transient group situations such as foster homes or temporary colony housing Living with known FeLV-positive cats *Note:* All cats should be tested for FeLV before vaccination.
Diagnostic considerations	Antigen tests do not detect previous vaccination. Positive results on immunofluorescent assay or PCR confirm positive infection status, but a negative result creates a discordant situation that clouds confirmation of true infection status. Current test modalities cannot exclude the potential of a regressive infection with subsequent negative tests after any initial positive result.
Management of infected cats	Infected cats may have a good quality of life. Although many cats succumb within 3 yr of diagnosis, others remain clinically healthy for multiple years. Preventive veterinary care, including frequent physical examination, laboratory monitoring, core vaccination, spay/neuter surgery, dental prophylaxis, and parasite control, is essential. Avoid transmission to other cats by preventing access to outdoors and other uninfected cats in household. Many antiviral and immunotherapeutic treatments are described in early trials or anecdotal use, but none has both wide availability and demonstrated clinical efficacy in controlled field studies.

Adapted from the Feline Retrovirus Management Guidelines, American Association of Feline Practitioners, 2008.

There are four FeLV subgroups of clinical importance. Almost all naturally infected cats are originally infected by FeLV-A, the original, archetypical form of the virus. Additional mutated forms of the original FeLV-A subtype as well as FeLV-B, FeLV-C, or FeLV-T may develop in infected cats. FeLV-B increases the frequency of neoplastic diseases; FeLV-C is strongly associated with development of erythroid hypoplasia and consequent severe anemia; and FeLV-T has the propensity to infect and destroy T lymphocytes, leading to lymphoid depletion and immunodeficiency. Viruses of all four subgroups are detected (but cannot be distinguished) by commonly used FeLV diagnostic test kits.

The prevalence of FeLV infection documented in cross-sectional surveys in North America has been declining throughout the past three decades and is attributed to testing and vaccination efforts. In the USA, 3.1% of cats in a large, nationwide data set tested positive for FeLV in 2010, with increased risk among outdoor cats, unneutered males, and cats with other disease conditions (particularly respiratory disease, oral disease, and abscessation). Prevalence was highest in the midwestern and western regions of the USA and lowest in the northeast. Seroprevalence surveys of varying statistical power have found rates of positive test results to range from 3.6% in Germany and Canada to 4.6% in Egypt and 24.5% in Thailand.

Persistently infected, healthy cats serve as reservoirs of FeLV for both vertical and horizontal viral transmission. Oronasal contact with infectious saliva or urine represents the most likely mode of horizontal transmission; vertical transmission in utero or through nursing is also common. Tears and feces may contain virus but are not considered to be clinically significant in disease transmission or diagnostic detection. Although direct contact, mutual grooming, and shared litter trays and food dishes are the primary methods of horizontal transmission, infection through bite wounds is possible. In a national (USA) study, FeLV infection was diagnosed in 9% of cats undergoing treatment for bite wounds, approximately three times the rate for cats in general. Because FeLV is a fragile, enveloped virus, horizontal transmission between adults usually requires prolonged, intimate contact. In addition, the dose required for oronasal transmission of the virus is relatively high.

FeLV is considered to be an age-dependent disease; young kittens are at higher risk of progressive infection and more rapid disease progression, whereas adults display some degree of age resistance. However, transmission can occur at any age, and factors affecting clinical course of disease are complex and incompletely understood.

Pathogenesis: After oronasal inoculation, the virus first replicates in oropharyngeal lymphoid tissue. From there, virus is carried in blood mononuclear cells to spleen, lymph nodes, epithelial cells of the intestine and bladder, salivary glands, and bone marrow. Virus also appears in secretions and excretions of these tissues and in peripheral blood leukocytes and platelets. Viremia is usually evident 2–4 wk after infection. The acute stage of FeLV infection occurring 2–6 wk after infection is rarely detected but typically characterized by mild fever, malaise, lymphadenopathy, and blood cytopenias. Cats unable to mount an adequate immune response become persistently viremic and develop a progressive infection, often leading to fatal disease. Oncogenesis occurs when FeLV virus inserts into the host cellular genome, either in proximity to an oncogene resulting in activation or directly into the oncogene itself to form a recombinant subgroup virus such as FeLV-B that can induce new neoplastic activity in any cell the recombinant virus enters.

The most recent classification system for FeLV labels infections as progressive, abortive, regressive, and focal. Progressive infections are defined by uninhibited viral replication with subsequent persistent viremia and probable eventual manifestation of clinical disease. Previously, most adult cats were thought to have abortive infections in which transient viremia was followed by complete clearance of viral infection. However, improved sensitivity of PCR testing has revealed that antigen-negative cats may still harbor FeLV provirus in tissues; this is termed regressive infection. It is believed that cats with regressive infections generally are aviremic, do not shed infectious virus, and do not develop FeLV-associated diseases; however, they are considered carriers with the potential for reactivation and future shedding. It is likely that FeLV can be transmitted by blood transfusion from cats with regressive infection, so feline blood donors should have PCR testing performed as a screening test before donating. The incidence of regressive infections and the causes and frequency of reactivation of viral shedding among these cats are incompletely understood. Focal infections, rare in natural infections, involve viral replication in specific tissues, such as the eyes or bladder, releasing low levels of viral antigen and, therefore, variable results on diagnostic testing.

Disorders Caused by FeLV: FeLV-related disorders are numerous and include anemia, neoplasia, immunosuppression, immune-mediated diseases, reproductive problems, enteritis, neurologic dysfunction, and stomatitis.

The anemia caused by FeLV is typically nonregenerative and normochromic. Less commonly, macrocytosis or regenerative hemolytic anemia is seen in only 10% of FeLV-induced anemia cases. The cause of nonregenerative anemia is usually bone marrow suppression due to viral infection of the hematopoietic stem cells and the supporting stromal cells. Platelet dysfunction, thrombocytopenia, and neutropenia are all possible sequelae as well.

Lymphoma is the most frequently diagnosed malignancy of cats. Tumors such as lymphoma and lymphoid leukemia develop in as many as 30% of cats with progressive FeLV infections. Regressive infections are also implicated in the occurrence of these tumors in the absence of viremia, but cats with progressive infections may face an increased risk of lymphoma development as high as 60-fold. Most American cats with mediastinal, multicentric, or spinal forms of lymphoma are FeLV-positive. However, these forms of lymphoma are becoming less common as the prevalence of FeLV decreases. Diffuse GI lymphoma is now more likely to be found in FeLV-negative cats of middle or older age and can be difficult to differentiate from inflammatory bowel disease. Fibrosarcomas and quasi-neoplastic disorders such as multiple cartilaginous exostoses (osteochondromatosis) can be FeLV-associated. Other types of tumors share a suspected but not yet clearly defined link with the FeLV virus.

Leukemia is characterized by the neoplastic proliferation of hematopoietic cells originating in the bone marrow, including neutrophils, basophils, eosinophils, monocytes, lymphocytes, megakaryocytes, and erythrocytes. Feline leukemias are strongly associated with FeLV infection and typically involve neoplastic cells circulating in the blood. Lymphoid leukemias are further classified as acute and chronic. Acute lymphocytic leukemia is characterized by lymphoblasts circulating in the blood, whereas chronic lymphocytic leukemias have an increased number of circulating lymphocytes with mature morphology.

The immunosuppression caused by FeLV creates increased susceptibility to bacterial, fungal, protozoal, and viral infections. Numbers of neutrophils and lymphocytes in the peripheral blood of affected cats may be reduced, and those cells that are present may be dysfunctional. Many FeLV-positive cats have low blood concentrations of complement; this contributes to FeLV-associated immunodeficiency and oncogenicity, because complement is vital for some forms of antibody-mediated tumor cell lysis.

Immune complexes formed in the presence of moderate antigen excess can cause systemic vasculitis, glomerulonephritis, polyarthritis, and a variety of other immune disorders. In FeLV-infected cats, immune complexes form under conditions in which FeLV antigens are abundant and anti-FeLV IgG antibodies are sparse, a situation ideal for the development of immune-mediated disease.

Reproductive problems are commonly associated with FeLV infection. Fetal death, resorption, and placental involution may occur in the middle trimester of pregnancy, presumably as a result of in utero infection of fetuses by virus transported across the placenta in maternal leukocytes. Abortion typically occurs in late gestation accompanied by risk of bacterial endometritis, especially in neutropenic queens. Transmission during birth and nursing constitutes the greatest risk of producing live, viremic kittens. There is some evidence that regressively infected queens may pass virus on to their kittens either in utero or in milk. Neonatal kittens are at risk of rapidly progressive infection with clinical manifestations of hypothermia, dehydration, failure to nurse, and early mortality collectively termed "fading kitten syndrome." It is likely that transmission from infected queens to their kittens is the single greatest source of FeLV infections.

Coinfection with FeLV and feline panleukopenia virus (FPV) has been implicated in feline panleukopenia-like syndrome (FPLS), which is also termed FeLV-associated enteritis. FPLS resembles feline panleukopenia both clinically and histopathologically and is characterized clinically by progressive anorexia, depression, vomiting, hemorrhagic diarrhea, weight loss, gingivitis, oral ulceration, severe neutropenia, and septicemia. FPV antigen is inconsistently present on diagnostic testing in these cases, and the pathogenesis and exact role of each virus in the development of this syndrome are incompletely understood.

Although neurologic disorders associated with FeLV are most often caused by compression of the brain and spinal cord by lymphoma tumor tissue, a mechanism for neuropathology is also suspected to result in peripheral neuropathies, urinary incontinence, and ocular pathology, including anisocoria, mydriasis, Horner syndrome, and central blindness even in the absence of visible compressive lesions on diagnostic imaging. If antineoplastic therapy is planned, it is important to distinguish neoplasia from neuropathy.

Stomatitis is more classically associated with FIV infection, but FeLV infection can also predispose cats to chronic ulcerative proliferative gingivostomatitis. Clinical sequelae include pain, anorexia, and tooth loss. An immune-mediated mechanism is likely, particularly in combination with coinfections such as feline calicivirus.

Diagnosis: Testing for FeLV infection is recommended when cats are first acquired, before vaccination against FeLV, if there has been potential exposure or bite wound from a cat of unknown or positive retroviral status; annually if they live in a household with FeLV-positive cats; before blood donation; and regularly if they have outdoor access. For cats entering a new home or known to be at high risk of exposure, testing should be repeated 30 days after the first test in case of recent infection that has not yet resulted in detectable circulating antigen. Documentation of a previous negative test does not negate the need for repeat testing in the above situations. Prior vaccination does not interfere with diagnostic testing unless performed immediately before blood collection for antigen testing.

Three types of tests are now readily available for clinical use: immunochromatography (such as ELISA), immunofluorescent assay (IFA), and PCR. Virus isolation is considered the gold standard diagnostic test but is not generally available to private practitioners. ELISA or other point-of care antigen test kits can be used in the veterinary clinic to detect the presence of soluble FeLV p27 antigen in whole blood or serum using a lateral flow test kit or a multi-well plate. Saliva and tears are not considered to be reliable samples for testing purposes. Several different test kits are available; most have sensitivities and specificities of ~98%.

IFA tests for the presence of FeLV p27 and other structural core antigens in the cytoplasm of cells. In clinical practice, peripheral blood smears are usually used for IFA, but cytologic preparations of bone marrow or other tissues can also be used. IFA requires submission to a diagnostic laboratory and cannot detect infection until bone marrow involvement occurs. False-negative test results may occur because of leukopenia or lack of bone marrow involvement, whereas technical error is most often the cause of false-positive results. Like ELISA, IFA cannot detect regressive infection because of the lack of sufficient viral antigen production. Historically, cats with nonregenerative anemia or other cytopenias and negative FeLV antigen tests on blood samples were subjected to bone marrow testing in search of occult FeLV infections. Several recent studies have indicated this is unnecessary, because cats with FeLV-associated bone marrow suppression invariably have positive results on blood tests.

Discordant results between tests, often a positive initial ELISA followed by negative results on either repeat ELISA or IFA, may reflect the inconsistent antigen circulation during various stages of FeLV infection, technical error, or possibly regressive infection status. These cats are generally considered presumptively infected and potential sources of infection until further clarification is possible. Standard recommendations to resolve discordant testing dictate repeating both tests in 30–60 days using serum instead of whole blood. It is not uncommon for cats, especially kittens, to test negative on a subsequent test. This could indicate a false-positive on the first test, a false-negative on the second test, or development of a regressive or abortive infection status. Once a single positive test result has been obtained, it can be difficult to ever know the true status of the cat, even if subsequent tests are negative.

PCR testing on whole blood, bone marrow, and other tissues is increasingly available through diagnostic laboratories, although validated sensitivity and specificity studies are often lacking. Real-time PCR offers great potential to provide extremely sensitive detection of FeLV rapidly after infection and can be useful to detect regressive infections and resolve conflicting test results if a positive result is obtained.

Diagnosis of FeLV-induced neoplasia is similar to that of other tumors. Cytologic examination of fine-needle aspirates of masses, lymph nodes, body cavity fluids (eg, pleural effusion), and affected organs may reveal malignant lymphocytes. Bone marrow examination may reveal leukemic involvement, even when the peripheral blood appears normal. Biopsy with histopathologic examination of abnormal tissues is often necessary for diagnostic confirmation. Cellular phenotyping via flow cytometry, immunocytochemistry, or other techniques can provide additional diagnostic information.

Treatment and Prognosis: Unfortunately, no curative treatment currently exists to eradicate retroviral infection.

In vitro studies have yielded cautiously promising results suggesting virus-suppressing activity of FDA-approved drugs used to treat HIV and other myelodysplastic syndromes against FeLV virus (eg, raltegravir, tenofovir, gemcitabine, decitabine). Further research is needed to demonstrate efficacy and safety in vivo and in field trials, as well as to address affordability of these drugs for most cat owners. Feline interferon omega and human interferon alpha have been associated with improved survival, but concerns surrounding availability, cost, and absence of strong evidence in controlled field studies have limited their widespread integration into standard treatment protocols for FeLV.

Anecdotal reports of various antiviral and immunotherapeutic agents to reverse viremia, improve clinical signs, and prolong survival are abundant. Controlled studies using naturally infected cats have either not been performed or have not confirmed anecdotal observations. Treatment efficacy must be demonstrated in controlled clinical trials, because spontaneous reversion to seronegative status or prolonged survival is not uncommon, even in the absence of medical treatment.

Some FeLV-positive cats can live without major disease complications for years with routine prophylactic care, good husbandry, minimal stress, and avoidance of secondary infections. Infected cats should be kept strictly indoors to reduce the risk of exposure to infectious agents and to prevent transmission of the virus to other cats. Routine vaccinations should be administered based on individual risk assessment and in compliance with local laws. Use of inactivated vaccines could be considered because of concerns regarding use of live vaccines reverting to virulence in immunocompromised animals, although this does not appear to be common. FeLV vaccinations should not be administered, because there is no evidence to suggest a benefit after infection. Physical examinations focusing on external parasites, skin infections, dental disease, lymph node size, and body weight should be performed semiannually, along with a routine program for parasite control and annual fecal, CBC, chemistry panel, and urinalysis testing. All infected cats should be neutered. Owners should be advised to watch for signs of FeLV-related disease, particularly secondary infections. Although FeLV-positive cats often respond well to treatment, therapy for such infections or other illnesses should be early and aggressive because of immunocompromise.

Because FeLV is historically associated with rapid and grave disease, the modern prognosis varies considerably depending on husbandry, veterinary care, and individual immune system variation. Large-scale studies have demonstrated an average survival of 2.4 yr after diagnosis among positive cats (versus 6 yr after testing for negative control cats), with 50% mortality in 2 yr and 80% mortality by 3 yr after diagnosis. Progression of disease is much more rapid in kittens, whereas some adult cats remain healthy for many years and may succumb to conditions unrelated to their retroviral status.

Lymphoma Treatment: Feline lymphoma can be treated with cytotoxic drugs. These drugs may cause significant toxicities if not dosed and administered properly. Most cytotoxic drugs are also carcinogens and must be handled properly. Before administering these drugs, veterinarians should familiarize themselves with proper dosing and administration procedures, appropriate monitoring of the patient, toxicities and complications, and safe handling to prevent exposure of veterinary personnel and owners to the agents and their metabolites.

Approximately 50% of cats with lymphoma that are treated obtain a complete remission, defined as no clinical evidence of disease. FeLV-negative cats that attain a complete remission live an average of 9 mo, whereas survival among FeLV-positive cats averages 6 mo. Cats not treated or those not responding to treatment survive an average of 2–6 wk.

Many protocols for treatment of feline lymphoma have been published; most use similar drugs with differing schedules of administration. One widely used protocol consists of an intensive induction phase (vincristine weekly for 4 wk, cyclophosphamide every 3 wk on the same day as vincristine, and prednisolone daily), followed by a less intensive maintenance phase (vincristine and cyclophosphamide given every 3 wk on the same day, and prednisolone continued daily). Treatment is continued for 1 yr or until relapse. With this protocol, 79% of cats attained remission, and average survival was 150 days. Changing the maintenance protocol to doxorubicin every 3 wk provided an average remission of 281 days. When relapse occurs, the drug regimen can be changed and a second remission achieved; however, second remissions seldom last as long as the first.

Another popular chemotherapy protocol involves an initial treatment with L-asparaginase and vincristine. Treatment is continued with daily prednisolone and alternating doses of cyclophosphamide, vincristine, and doxorubicin for a total of three cycles. When relapse occurs, the protocol is started again. Using this protocol, the median survival has been reported to be 210 days. Other protocols incorporating alkylating agents such as mustargen and procarbazine have demonstrated efficacy as well, sometimes even after other combination therapies have not achieved remission.

Most lymphomas have an intermediate or high histopathologic grade and are clinically aggressive, except for a subset identified as small-cell lymphoma or lymphocytic lymphoma. Small-cell lymphomas are characterized by a diffuse infiltration of malignant lymphocytes throughout affected organs, typically intestines, and can often be successfully treated with less aggressive chemotherapy. Administration of prednisolone and chlorambucil orally daily for 4 consecutive days every 3 wk has been used. Using these drugs in clinical trials to treat small-cell lymphoma involving the GI tract produced a median survival of 963 days. If other sites were involved, with or without GI disease, the median survival was 636 days.

In addition to small-cell lymphoma, large granular lymphocyte lymphoma also affects the intestinal tract. This is an extremely aggressive disease, with a response to chemotherapy of ~30% and a median survival of 57 days. An intestinal mass is usually present and may cause intestinal obstruction.

Acute lymphocytic leukemia is treated with the same protocol as lymphoma, but only ~25% of cats obtain remission for an average of 7 mo. Chronic lymphocytic leukemia typically carries a much better prognosis than the acute form and is best treated with chlorambucil and prednisolone given every other day on alternating days. Leukemias other than lymphocytic are rarely treated because of severity of illness at diagnosis and poor response to therapy.

Prevention and Control: FeLV virus is unstable in the environment and is susceptible to all common detergents and disinfectants. In a hospital or boarding setting, infected cats may be kept in the general population as long as they are housed in separate cages. Medical and surgical equipment contaminated with body fluids, even when dried, can be fomites for infection. Thorough cleaning and sterilization of equipment, strict attention to washing contaminated hands, and avoiding reuse and sharing of single use and consumable supplies between patients are critical practices to prevent iatrogenic transmission.

FeLV vaccines are non-core and are intended to protect cats against FeLV infection or to reduce the likelihood of persistent viremia. Types of vaccines include killed whole virus, subunit, and genetically engineered. Vaccines may vary in protective effect, and manufacturers' claims and independent comparative studies should be carefully noted. Vaccines are indicated only for uninfected cats, because there is no benefit in vaccinating an FeLV-positive cat.

The American Association of Feline Practitioners (AAFP) Feline Retrovirus Management Guidelines include the recommendation that all kittens should receive the two-dose FeLV vaccination as a component of the routine initial vaccination series and should also receive a booster vaccination 1 yr later. This is prudent, because rehoming and lifestyle changes such as outdoor access frequently occur as cats mature. Annual revaccination after maturity would depend on the cat's risk of FeLV exposure.

The adult cat's risk of exposure to FeLV-positive cats should be assessed, and vaccines used only for those cats at risk. FeLV vaccines have been associated with development of sarcomas at the vaccination site, although the risk of tumor development is very low. Uninfected cats in a household with infected cats should be vaccinated; however, vaccination is not universally protective, and other means of reducing transmission to uninfected cats, such as physical separation, should also be used.

While testing of cats in an animal shelter environment is considered optional for individual housing, FeLV status should be determined before placement in group housing and is recommended at the time of adoption or foster home placement. Because tests are not 100% accurate, shelter cats placed in group housing should be vaccinated against FeLV, especially in longterm conditions such as sanctuaries. Because of the equivalent prevalence of FeLV among feral and free-roaming pet cats and the role of neutering in decreasing the spread of infection, expending resources on FeLV testing is not considered a mandatory component of community trap-neuter-return programs.

Zoonotic Risk: Some strains of FeLV can be experimentally grown in human tissue cultures, leading to concerns of potential for transmission to people. Studies addressing this concern have shown no evidence that any zoonotic risk exists, and there are no known cases of zoonotic transmission.

FELINE PANLEUKOPENIA

(Feline infectious enteritis, Feline parvoviral enteritis)

Feline panleukopenia is a highly contagious, often fatal, viral disease of cats that is seen worldwide. Kittens are affected most severely. The causative parvovirus is very resistant; it can persist for 1 yr at room temperature in the environment, if protected in organic material. Feline panleukopenia is now diagnosed infrequently by veterinarians, presumably as a consequence of widespread vaccine use.

However, infection rates remain high in some unvaccinated cat populations, and the disease occasionally is seen in vaccinated, pedigreed kittens that have been exposed to a high virus challenge.

Etiology, Transmission, and Pathogenesis: Feline panleukopenia virus (FPV) is closely related to mink enteritis virus and the type 2 canine parvoviruses (CPV) that cause canine parvoviral enteritis. FPV can cause disease in all felids and in some members of related families (eg, raccoon, mink), but it does not harm canids. Conversely, some currently circulating CPV strains (CPV-2a, -2b, and -2c) have been shown to cause a panleukopenia-like illness in domestic cats and larger felids. In some parts of Asia, CPV strains are reported to rival FPV as the major cause of feline panleukopenia, although FPV still dominates worldwide. Vaccines that contain FPV only provide some protection to cats against disease caused by CPV, but it has been suggested by some authorities that inclusion of CPV-2c in feline vaccines would broaden and improve the degree of protection provided.

Virus particles are abundant in all secretions and excretions during the acute phase of illness and can be shed in the feces of survivors for as long as 6 wk after recovery. Being highly resistant to inactivation, parvoviruses can be transported long distances via fomites (eg, shoes, clothing). However, FPV can be destroyed by exposure to a 1:32 dilution of household bleach (6% aqueous sodium hypochlorite), 4% formaldehyde, and 1% glutaraldehyde for 10 min at room temperature. Peroxygen disinfectants are also highly effective.

Cats are infected oronasally by exposure to infected animals, their feces, secretions, or contaminated fomites. Most free-roaming cats are thought to be exposed to the virus during their first year of life. Those that develop subclinical infection or survive acute illness mount a robust, long-lasting, protective immune response.

FPV infects and destroys actively dividing cells in bone marrow, lymphoid tissues, intestinal epithelium, and—in very young animals—cerebellum and retina. In pregnant queens, the virus may spread transplacentally to cause embryonic resorption, fetal mummification, abortion, or stillbirth. Alternatively, infection of kittens in the perinatal period may destroy the germinal epithelium of the cerebellum, leading to cerebellar hypoplasia, incoordination, and tremor. FPV-induced cerebellar ataxia has become a relatively rare diagnosis, because most queens passively transfer sufficient antibodies to their kittens to protect them during the period of susceptibility.

Clinical Findings: Most infections are subclinical, as evidenced by the high seroprevalence of anti-FPV antibodies among unvaccinated, healthy cats. Those cats that become ill are usually <1 yr old. Peracute cases may die suddenly with little or no warning (fading kittens). Acute cases show fever (104°–107°F [40°–41.7°C]), depression, and anorexia after an incubation period of 2–7 days. Vomiting usually develops 1–2 days after the onset of fever; it is typically bilious and unrelated to eating. Diarrhea may begin a little later but is not always present. Extreme dehydration develops rapidly. Affected cats may sit for hours at their water bowl, although they may not drink much. Terminal cases are hypothermic and may develop septic shock and disseminated intravascular coagulation.

Physical examination typically reveals profound depression, dehydration, and sometimes abdominal pain. Abdominal palpation—which can induce immediate vomiting—may reveal thickened intestinal loops and enlarged mesenteric lymph nodes. In cases of cerebellar hypoplasia, ataxia and tremors with normal mentation are seen. Retinal lesions, if present, appear as discrete gray foci.

The duration of this self-limiting illness is seldom >5–7 days. Mortality is highest in young kittens <5 mo old.

Lesions: There are typically few gross lesions, although dehydration is usually marked. Bowel loops are usually dilated and may have thickened, hyperemic walls. There may be petechiae or ecchymoses on the intestinal serosal surfaces. Perinatally infected kittens may have a noticeably small cerebellum. Histologically, the intestinal crypts are usually dilated and contain debris consisting of sloughed necrotic epithelial cells. Blunting and fusion of villi may be present. Eosinophilic intranuclear inclusion bodies are seen only occasionally in formalin-fixed specimens; use of Bouin's or Zenker's fixative will increase the likelihood of seeing these.

Diagnosis: A presumptive diagnosis is usually based on compatible clinical signs in an inadequately vaccinated cat and the presence of leukopenia (nadir 50–3,000 WBC/µL). Neutropenia is a more consistent finding than lymphopenia. Total WBC counts <2,000 cells/µL are associated with a poorer prognosis. During recovery from infection, there is typically a rebound neutrophilia with a marked left shift. Diagnosis can sometimes be confirmed using an in-office immunochromatographic test kit intended for detection of fecal CPV antigen. However, fecal antigen is detectable only for a short time after infection. False-negative results are common.

Differential diagnoses include other causes of profound depression, leukopenia, and GI signs. Salmonellosis (*see* p 195) and infections with feline leukemia virus (FeLV, *see* p 790) and feline immunodeficiency virus (*see* p 821) should be considered. Concurrent infection with FeLV and FPV can cause a panleukopenia-like syndrome in adult cats.

Treatment and Prevention: Successful treatment of acute cases requires vigorous fluid therapy and supportive nursing care in the isolation unit. Electrolyte disturbances (eg, hypokalemia), hypoglycemia, hypoproteinemia, anemia, and opportunistic secondary infections often develop in severely affected cats. Anticipation of these possibilities, close monitoring, and prompt intervention are likely to improve outcome. IV fluid replacement and maintenance with a balanced isotonic crystalloid solution (eg, lactated Ringer's solution with calculated potassium supplementation) is the foundation of therapy. B vitamins should be added to the infusion, together with 5% glucose if hypoglycemia is suspected or proved. In addition to crystalloid infusion, transfusion of fresh-frozen plasma helps support plasma oncotic pressure and provides clotting factors to severely ill, hypoproteinemic kittens. Whole blood is preferable for the occasional cat that is severely anemic. Parenteral, broad-spectrum antibiotic therapy is indicated; however, nephrotoxic drugs (eg, gentamicin, amikacin) should be avoided until dehydration has been corrected. Antiemetic therapy (eg, metoclopramide, ondansetron, maropitant) may provide some relief and allow earlier enteral feeding of soft, easily digested food. Parenteral nutrition is indicated for severely affected cases. Recombinant feline interferon omega (rFeIFN; 1 MU/kg/day SC for 3 days) should be considered for use in the treatment of feline panleukopenia. Although rFeIFN is not approved by the FDA for this purpose, it is approved and effective in the treatment of canine parvoviral enteritis.

Excellent inactivated and modified-live virus vaccines that provide solid, long-lasting immunity are available for prevention of feline panleukopenia. Live vaccines should not be given to cats that are pregnant, immunosuppressed, or sick, or to kittens <4 wk old. Most authorities recommend that kittens receive two or three modified-live vaccine doses SC, 3–4 wk apart. The first vaccination is usually given at 6–9 wk of age. The last dose of the initial vaccination series should not be administered before the kitten is 16 wk old, to ensure that interfering maternal antibodies do not inactivate the modified-live virus. Exposure to virus should be avoided until 1 wk after the initial vaccination series has been completed. Cats should be revaccinated 1 yr later, and triennially or less frequently thereafter, although some manufacturers continue to recommend annual revaccination.

INFECTIOUS CANINE HEPATITIS

Infectious canine hepatitis (ICH) is a worldwide, contagious disease of dogs with signs that vary from a slight fever and congestion of the mucous membranes to severe depression, marked leukopenia, and coagulation disorders. It also is seen in foxes, wolves, coyotes, bears, lynx, and some pinnipeds; other carnivores may become infected without developing clinical illness. In recent years, the disease has become uncommon in areas where routine immunization is done, but periodic outbreaks, which may reflect maintenance of the disease in wild and feral hosts, reinforce the need for continued vaccination.

Etiology and Pathogenesis: ICH is caused by a nonenveloped DNA virus, canine adenovirus 1 (CAV-1), which is antigenically related only to CAV-2 (one of the causes of infectious canine tracheobronchitis, *see* p 1491). CAV-1 is resistant to lipid solvents (such as ether), as well as to acid and formalin. It survives outside the host for weeks or months, but a 1%–3%

solution of sodium hypochlorite (household bleach) is an effective disinfectant.

Ingestion of urine, feces, or saliva of infected dogs is the main route of infection. Recovered dogs shed virus in their urine for ≥6 mo. Initial infection occurs in the tonsillar crypts and Peyer patches, followed by viremia and disseminated infection. Vascular endothelial cells are the primary target, with hepatic and renal parenchyma, spleen, and lungs becoming infected as well. Chronic kidney lesions and corneal clouding ("blue eye") result from immune-complex reactions after recovery from acute or subclinical disease.

Clinical Findings: Signs vary from a slight fever to death. The mortality rate ranges from 10%–30% and is typically highest in very young dogs. Concurrent parvoviral or distemper infection worsens the prognosis. The incubation period is 4–9 days. The first sign is a fever of >104°F (40°C), which lasts 1–6 days and is usually biphasic. If the fever is of short duration, leukopenia may be the only other sign, but if it persists for >1 day, acute illness develops.

Signs are apathy, anorexia, thirst, conjunctivitis, serous discharge from the eyes and nose, and occasionally abdominal pain and vomiting. Intense hyperemia or petechiae of the oral mucosa, as well as enlarged tonsils, may be seen. Tachycardia out of proportion to the fever may occur. There may be subcutaneous edema of the head, neck, and trunk. Despite hepatic involvement, there is a notable absence of icterus in most acute clinical cases.

Clotting time is directly correlated with the severity of illness and is the result of disseminated intravascular coagulation induced by vascular endothelial compromise, coupled with failure of the liver to rapidly replace consumed clotting factors. It may be difficult to control hemorrhage, which is manifest by bleeding around deciduous teeth and by spontaneous hematomas. CNS involvement is unusual and is typically the result of vascular injury. Severely infected dogs may develop convulsions from forebrain damage. Paresis may result from brain stem hemorrhages, and ataxia and central blindness have also been described. Foxes more consistently have CNS signs and intermittent convulsions during the course of illness, and paralysis may involve one or more limbs or the entire body. Respiratory signs usually are not seen in dogs with ICH; however, CAV-1 has been recovered from dogs with signs of infectious tracheobronchitis despite high serologic titers against parenteral disease.

Clinicopathologic findings reflect the coagulopathy (prolonged prothrombin time, thrombocytopenia, and increased fibrin degradation products). Severely affected dogs show acute hepatocellular injury (increased ALT and AST). Proteinuria is common. Leukopenia typically persists throughout the febrile period. The degree of leukopenia varies and seems to be correlated with the severity of illness.

On recovery, dogs eat well but regain weight slowly. Hepatic transaminase activities peak around day 14 of infection and then decline slowly. In ~25% of recovered dogs, bilateral corneal opacity develops 7–10 days after acute signs disappear and usually resolves spontaneously. In mild cases, transient corneal opacity may be the only sign of disease.

It has long been thought that chronic hepatitis may develop in dogs that have low levels of passive antibody when exposed, although a recent PCR-based study did not confirm this theory.

Lesions: Endothelial damage results in "paint-brush" hemorrhages on the gastric serosa, lymph nodes, thymus, pancreas, and subcutaneous tissues. Hepatic cell necrosis produces a variegated color change in the liver, which may be normal in size or swollen. Histologically, there is centrilobular necrosis, with neutrophilic and monocytic infiltration, and hepatocellular intranuclear inclusions. The gallbladder wall is typically edematous and thickened; edema of the thymus may be found. Grayish white foci may be seen in the kidney cortex.

Diagnosis: Usually, the abrupt onset of illness and bleeding suggest ICH, although clinical evidence is not always sufficient to differentiate ICH from distemper (*see* p 777). Definitive antemortem diagnosis is not required before institution of supportive care but can be pursued with commercially available ELISA, serologic, and PCR testing. PCR or restriction fragment length polymorphism is required to definitively distinguish CAV-1 from CAV-2, if clinically necessary. Postmortem gross changes in the liver and gallbladder are more conclusive, and diagnosis is confirmed by virus isolation, immunofluorescence, characteristic intranuclear inclusion bodies in the liver, or PCR or fluorescence in situ hybridization studies of infected tissue.

Treatment: Treatment is symptomatic and supportive. The goals of therapy are to limit secondary bacterial invasion, support fluid balance, and control hemorrhagic tendencies. Broad-spectrum antibiotics and intravenously administered balanced electrolyte solutions with 5% dextrose supplementation are indicated. Plasma or whole blood transfusions may be necessary in severely ill dogs.

Although the transient corneal opacity (which may be seen during the course of ICH or associated with vaccination with attenuated CAV-1 vaccines) usually requires no treatment, atropine ophthalmic ointment may alleviate the painful ciliary spasm sometimes associated with it. Dogs with corneal clouding should be protected against bright light. Systemic corticosteroids are contraindicated for treatment of corneal opacity associated with ICH.

Prevention: Modified-live virus (MLV) injectable vaccines are available and are often combined with other vaccines. Vaccination against ICH is recommended at the time of canine distemper vaccinations. Maternal antibody from immune bitches interferes with active immunization in puppies until they are 9–12 wk old. Attenuated CAV-1 vaccines have produced transient unilateral or bilateral opacities of the cornea, and the virus may be shed in urine. For these reasons, CAV-2 attenuated live virus strains, which provide cross-protection against CAV-1, are preferentially used because they have very little tendency to produce corneal opacities or uveitis, and the virus is not shed in urine. Historically, annual revaccination against ICH was standard, and vaccines are labeled for annual use. Increasing evidence suggests that immunity induced by MLV CAV-1 injectable vaccines lasts ≥3 yr, although this remains an extra-label use of commercially available vaccines.

LEISHMANIOSIS

(Visceral leishmaniasis)

Leishmaniosis is a disease caused by protozoan parasites of the genus *Leishmania* and transmitted through the bites of female phlebotomine sand flies. More than 23 species of *Leishmania* have been described, most of which are zoonotic. The most important *Leishmania* parasite to affect domestic animals is *L infantum*, also known as *L chagasi* in Latin America. Dogs are the main reservoir host for human visceral leishmaniosis caused by *L infantum*, and the disease is potentially fatal in dogs and people. Because the internal organs and skin of the dog are affected, the canine disease is termed viscerocutaneous or canine leishmaniosis. Cats, horses, and other mammals can be infected by *L infantum* or other *Leishmania* species. The disease in cats is rarer than in dogs and may manifest in cutaneous or visceral organs. *L braziliensis*, the cause of tegumentary canine leishmaniosis, is widespread in regions of South America and may geographically overlap with *L chagasi*.

Canine leishmaniosis is a major zoonosis endemic in >70 countries. It is prevalent in southern Europe, Africa, Asia, South and Central America, and sporadically in the USA. It is also of concern in nonendemic countries where imported disease constitutes a veterinary and public health problem.

Transmission: *Leishmania* is a diphasic parasite that completes its life cycle in two hosts: a sand fly that harbors the flagellated extracellular promastigote form and a mammal in which the intracellular amastigote parasite form develops.

Transmission is a complex process that requires special adaptation between the sand fly host and the particular *Leishmania* species transmitted. There are numerous species of sand flies, only a minority of which are competent vectors of *Leishmania*. Dogs with or without clinical signs are infectious to sand flies and may transmit leishmaniosis. Congenital vertical transmission of canine leishmaniosis from an infected dam to its offspring has been reported but appears to be uncommon. Transmission by transfusion of blood products from infected dogs has been shown to cause infection in recipients. Direct dog-to-dog transmission by contact has been suggested as a mode of disease transmission in an effort to explain the spread of infection among kenneled Foxhounds in the USA in the absence of proven sand fly vectors. At present, the validity of direct transmission is unknown.

Clinical Findings: Dogs are infected by *L infantum* promastigotes deposited into the skin via the bites of infected sandflies. The promastigotes invade host macrophages and replicate as intracellular amastigotes. The immune responses mounted at the time of infection and thereafter appear to be the most important factor in determining whether a persistent infection will develop and progress from subclinical to clinical disease. The incubation period may last months to years, during which the parasite disseminates from the skin throughout the host's body (primarily to the hemolymphatic system organs). Age, breed, host genetics, nutrition, concurrent diseases, and other factors may also influence the progression from infection to clinical disease.

Canine leishmaniosis is a multisystemic disease with a highly variable spectrum of immune responses and clinical manifestations. In endemic areas, the prevalence of dogs carrying infection is much higher than those demonstrating clinical disease. Clinical disease is associated with a marked antibody response that does not confer protection. In fact, immune-mediated mechanisms are responsible for much of the pathology in canine leishmaniosis.

The typical history reported by owners of dogs with clinical disease due to *L infantum* includes the appearance of skin lesions, ocular abnormalities, or epistaxis. These are frequently accompanied by weight loss, exercise intolerance, and lethargy. The main physical examination findings are dermal lesions in 80%–90% of the dogs, lymphadenomegaly in 62%–90%, ocular disease in 16%–81%, splenomegaly in 10%–53%, and abnormal nail growth (onychogryphosis) in 20%–31%. Other clinical findings may include polyuria and polydipsia due to kidney disease, vomiting, colitis, melena, and lameness due to joint, muscle, or bone lesions. The sole presenting signs of disease could be epistaxis, ocular abnormalities, or manifestations of kidney disease without dermal abnormalities. The dermal lesions associated with canine leishmaniosis include exfoliative dermatitis, which can be generalized or localized over the face, ears, and limbs. Ulcerative, nodular, or mucocutaneous dermatitis are also seen. Cutaneous ulcers over the ears or other locations may be associated with considerable bleeding. A mild form of papular dermatitis has been reported in dogs with no other signs of disease. Ocular or periocular lesions include keratoconjunctivitis and uveitis.

Clinical laboratory findings include mild to moderate nonregenerative or more rarely regenerative anemia in 60%–73% of the dogs; thromobocytopenia is less common. The most consistent serum biochemistry findings in dogs with clinical canine leishmaniosis are serum hyperproteinemia with hyperglobulinemia and hypoalbuminemia, frequently expressed by a decreased albumin:globulin ratio. Marked hyperglobulinemia with no apparent cause in dogs from *Leishmania*-endemic regions should suggest possible canine leishmaniosis. Grossly increased activities of liver enzymes or azotemia are found in only a minority of infected dogs. Some degree of renal pathology is present in most dogs with canine leishmaniosis. Subsequent renal failure due to immune-complex glomerulonephritis may eventually develop and is believed to be the main natural cause of death. The presence of proteinuria should be evaluated and kidney disease staged with measurement of the urine protein:creatinine ratio.

Lesions: The typical histopathologic finding in canine leishmaniosis is granulomatous inflammation associated with a variable number of *Leishmania* amastigotes with macrophages. Protective immunity against *Leishmania* parasites is mediated through CD4+T_H cells and the activation of a complex cascade of cytokine mediators. Circulating immune complexes and antinuclear antibodies can be detected in animals with canine leishmaniosis, and deposition of immune complexes in the kidneys, blood vessels, and joints occurs as infection progresses. Glomerulonephritis associated with the renal immune complexes is a hallmark of this disease. Renal pathology, including glomerulonephritis and interstitial nephritis, is evident by histopathology, even if not manifested clinically in most dogs infected with *L infantum*.

Diagnosis: Diagnostic tests include a CBC, biochemical profile, urinalysis, and one or more specific tests to confirm infection. Quantitative serology is useful, especially when compatible clinical signs are present. High antibody titers are found in 80%–100% of dogs with clinical disease and could be conclusive of a diagnosis. Various quantitative serologic methods to detect anti-*Leishmania* antibodies have been developed, including indirect immunofluorescence assays, ELISA, and direct agglutination assays. Purified recombinant antigens such as rK39 are also used to detect leishmaniosis in dogs and people. Serologic cross-reactivity with trypanosomes may be found in regions where *Trypanosoma* infection is prevalent, particularly with *T cruzi* in Latin America.

Detection of parasite-specific DNA by PCR allows sensitive and specific diagnosis of infection. Several different assays with various target sequences using genomic or kinetoplast DNA (kDNA) have been developed for canine leishmaniosis. PCR can be performed on DNA extracted from tissues, blood, or even from histopathologic specimens. Assays based on kDNA are the most sensitive for direct detection in infected tissues. Bone marrow, lymph node, conjunctival swabs, or spleen samples are superior to blood with most of the current PCR techniques.

Leishmania amastigotes can be demonstrated by cytology from lymph nodes, spleen, skin impressions, bone marrow, or joint fluids stained with Giemsa stain or a quick commercial stain. Detection of amastigotes by cytology is sometimes unrewarding because of a low number of detectable parasites, even in dogs with full-blown clinical disease. *Leishmania* parasites may also be viewed in histopathologic formalin-fixed, paraffin-embedded biopsy sections of the skin or other infected organs. Identification of parasites within tissue macrophages may be difficult; immunolabeling with immunohistochemical staining can verify the presence of *Leishmania* in the tissue.

Detection of infection in dogs with no clinical disease for purposes such as importation to nonendemic countries or use as blood donors may require PCR, which is the most sensitive diagnostic technique. Cross-sectional studies of dog populations in highly endemic areas have shown that infection rates can reach 65%–80%. Typically, only approximately 10%–13% manifest clinical signs of disease, 26% are seropositive and include sick and subclinically infected dogs, and an additional 40%–60% are carriers positive only by tissue PCR.

Treatment: The main protocol used for treatment of canine leishmaniosis includes N-methylglucamine antimoniate (not approved for use in dogs in the USA) at 75–100 mg/kg, SC, for 4–8 wk combined with allopurinol (10 mg/kg, PO, bid, for 6–12 mo or longer as needed). Allopurinol may also be used as a single therapeutic agent at the same dose. Miltefosine (not approved for use in dogs in the USA) at 2 mg/kg/day, PO, for 4 wk can also be combined with allopurinol (10 mg/kg, PO, bid) as an alternative to N-methylglucamine antimoniate. Treatment frequently achieves only temporary clinical improvement in dogs and often does not eliminate the parasites. Treated dogs can remain carriers of infection and may relapse. They may remain infectious to sand flies. Stopping treatment with allopurinol is recommended only when clinical signs disappear, hematologic and serum biochemistry abnormalities return to normal, and the animal becomes seronegative by a quantitative laboratory serologic test.

Specific repellent topical insecticides effectively reduce sand fly bites and disease transmission. A deltamethrin-impregnated collar and a spot-on formulation of permethrin and imidacloprid have been shown to confer protection against sand fly bites. The application of protective insecticides is recommended for dogs in *Leishmania*-endemic areas, dogs traveling to sites of infection, and infected dogs (to reduce potential transmission). Purified-fraction commercial vaccines against canine leishmaniosis are marketed in Europe and Brazil, and other vaccines are under development.

Zoonotic Risk: Human visceral leishmaniosis caused by *L infantum* is a serious public health problem in areas where canine leishmaniosis is endemic and dogs are the main reservoir of infection. It is mostly a disease of young children. Malnutrition has been recognized as a risk factor and may explain why this disease is more prevalent among children in poor countries than among those in affluent ones, despite high prevalence rates in the canine populations. Human disease is also prevalent in immunosuppressed individuals; HIV patients are the predominant risk group for human leishmaniosis in southern Europe. HIV and leishmaniosis coinfection has been reported from >33 countries worldwide and does not respond well to therapy. Efforts to control canine leishmaniosis and the human disease in endemic areas focus on disrupting the transmission of infection and preventing canine infection at the population level.

RICKETTSIAL DISEASES

EHRLICHIOSIS AND RELATED INFECTIONS

In the past, a number of obligate intracellular organisms that infect eukaryotic cells were classified in the genus *Ehrlichia* on morphologic and ecologic grounds. With newer genetic analyses, these agents have been reclassified into the genera of *Ehrlichia*, *Anaplasma*, and *Neorickettsia*, all of which are in the family Anaplasmataceae. However, usage of the term "ehrlichiosis" to broadly describe these infections may still persist.

Etiology: Canine ehrlichiosis is primarily caused by *Ehrlichia canis*, which predominantly involves monocytes; although it is not considered a primary zoonosis, human infection with this agent has been occasionally reported. Another common ehrlichial pathogen of dogs is *E chaffeensis*, which causes a monocytic form of illness and is the primary species causing human ehrlichiosis infection in the USA. Human cases are reported throughout the mid to southeastern and central USA. Several published reports of monocytic ehrlichiosis in cats suggest that feline infection may occur, albeit uncommonly. *E ewingii*, which primarily infects the granulocytes of susceptible hosts, has been isolated from dogs and people in the southern, western, and midwestern USA. In 2009, an organism either identical or related to *E muris* was identified as a cause of human illness in the upper Midwest; the role of this *E muris*–like (EML) agent as a possible pathogen of dogs or cats is currently unknown.

A phagocytophilum, formerly known as both *E equi* and the agent of human granulocytic ehrlichiosis, has been reported as a cause of illness in dogs. It is known to cause human illness in the USA, primarily in northeastern, upper midwestern, and western states. Infection with this agent is most appropriately referred to as anaplasmosis, and the pathogen is found predominantly in granulocytes.

A platys, which infects platelets, is the cause of infectious cyclic thrombocytopenia of dogs.

Epidemiology: *E canis* is transmitted by the brown dog tick, *Rhipicephalus sanguineus*, which is found worldwide; accordingly, canine monocytic ehrlichiosis also has a worldwide enzootic distribution. Acute *E canis* cases may resemble infection with *Rickettsia rickettsii* (the agent of Rocky Mountain spotted fever, which can also be transmitted by the brown dog tick). *Rhipicephalus* ticks become infected with *E canis* after feeding on infected dogs, and ticks transmit infection to other dogs during blood meals taken in successive life stages. Blood transfusions, or other means by which infected WBCs can be transferred, may also transmit the pathogen. *E chaffeensis* and *E ewingii* have sylvan cycles in the environment that involve tick species and wildlife reservoir hosts. In the USA, *E chaffeensis* and *E ewingii* are transmitted by *Amblyomma americanum*, the lone star tick, and white-tailed deer are thought to play an important role as reservoir hosts. Dogs are also considered a possible reservoir for *E ewingii*. A case of human *E ewingii* contracted via blood infusion has been reported, and organ transplantation of *E chaffeensis* infection has been suspected. The ecologic cycle for the EML agent has not yet been elucidated but is suspected to involve *Ixodes scapularis*, the black-legged tick.

A phagocytophilum is transmitted by *Ixodes* species of ticks; in the northeastern USA, infection is transmitted by *I scapularis*, whereas infection in western states is primarily associated with *I pacificus*, the Western black-legged tick. In nature, the enzootic cycle is most likely associated with small rodents. People and domestic animals are incidental hosts of these pathogens. Human-to-human transmission via transfusion of packed RBCs has been reported; the risk of canine-associated infections after blood transfusion is unknown.

A platys is transmitted by *R sanguineus* and is enzootic in many parts of the USA and worldwide. Coinfection with *E canis* may occur, because the same tick vector is responsible for transmission of both pathogens.

Clinical Findings: In dogs, *E canis* causes the most potentially severe clinical presentation of the *Ehrlichia* spp. Signs arise from involvement of the hemic and lymphoreticular systems and commonly progress from acute to chronic, depending on the strain of organism and immune status of the host. In acute cases, there is reticuloendothelial hyperplasia, fever, generalized lymphadenopathy, splenomegaly, and thrombocytopenia. Variable signs of anorexia, depression, loss of stamina, stiffness and reluctance to walk, edema of the limbs or scrotum, and coughing or dyspnea may be seen. Most acute cases are seen in the warmer months, coincident with the greatest activity of the tick vector. Chronic cases may present at any time of year.

During the acute phase of *E canis* infection in dogs, the hemogram is usually normal but may reflect a mild normocytic, normochromic anemia; leukopenia; or mild leukocytosis. Thrombocytopenia is common, but petechiae may not be evident, and platelet decreases may be mild in some animals. Vasculitis and immune-mediated mechanisms induce a thrombocytopenia and hemorrhagic tendencies. Lymph node aspiration reveals hyperplasia. Death is rare during this phase; spontaneous recovery may occur, the dog may remain asymptomatic, or chronic disease may ensue.

Chronic ehrlichiosis caused by *E canis* may develop in any breed, but certain breeds, eg, German Shepherds, may be predisposed. Seasonality is not a specific hallmark of chronic infection, because appearance of chronic signs may be variably delayed after acute infection. In chronic cases, the bone marrow becomes hypoplastic, and lymphocytes and plasmacytes infiltrate various organs. Clinical findings vary based on the predominant organs affected and may include marked splenomegaly, glomerulonephritis, renal failure, interstitial pneumonitis, anterior uveitis, and meningitis with associated cerebellar ataxia, depression, paresis, and hyperesthesia. Severe weight loss is a prominent finding.

The hemogram is usually markedly abnormal in chronic cases. Severe thrombocytopenia may cause epistaxis, hematuria, melena, and petechiae and ecchymoses of the skin. Variably severe pancytopenia (mature leukopenia, nonregenerative anemia, thrombocytopenia, or any combination thereof) may be seen. Aspiration cytology reveals reactive lymph nodes and, usually, marked plasmacytosis. Frequently, polyclonal, or occasionally monoclonal, hypergammaglobulinemia develops.

Other ehrlichial infections caused by *E chaffeensis*, *E ewingii*, or *A phagocytophilum* appear clinically similar to acute *E canis* infection, but the clinical course is usually more self-limiting. Shifting leg lameness and fever of unknown origin may be present. Thrombocytopenia and mild leukopenia or leukocytosis may occur during the acute course of infection, which is clinically more discrete. Chronic canine disease, as seen with *E canis* infection, is not typically seen with other infections.

Dogs infected with *A platys* generally show minimal to no signs of infection despite the presence of the organism in platelets. The primary finding is cyclic thrombocytopenia, recurring at 10-day intervals. Generally, the cyclic nature diminishes, and the thrombocytopenia becomes mild and slowly resolves.

Lesions: During the acute or self-limiting phase of *E canis* infections, lesions generally are nonspecific, but splenomegaly is common. Histologically, there is lymphoreticular hyperplasia and lymphocytic and plasmacytic perivascular cuffing. In chronic cases, these lesions may be accompanied by widespread hemorrhage and increased mononuclear cell infiltration in perivascular regions of many organs.

Diagnosis: Because thrombocytopenia is a relatively consistent finding with these infections, a platelet count is an important screening test. Clinical diagnosis may be confirmed by demonstrating the organisms within WBCs or platelets, seen in intracytoplasmic inclusion bodies called morulae. This method of diagnosis lacks sensitivity, because low numbers of organisms make demonstration difficult. More commonly, a diagnosis is made by a combination of clinical signs, positive serum indirect fluorescent antibody (IFA) titer, and response to treatment. In-house tests for *E canis*, *A phagocytophilum*, *A platys*, and *E ewingii* based on enzyme immunoassay methods are also available. The antibody response may be delayed for several weeks; thus, serologic testing may not be a reliable diagnostic tool early in the course of the disease. Furthermore, antibodies can persist for months or years after infection, making in-house tests for the organisms problematic for confirmation of acute infection, particularly in highly enzootic areas where many dogs may have antibodies to these agents because of previous infections. Testing of paired sera and demonstration of increased antibody titers is recommended to confirm infection when possible, although treatment of suspected cases should never be delayed or withheld on the basis of test results, either positive or negative. Serologic cross-reactivity is strong between *E canis*, *E chaffeensis*, and *E ewingii*; some cross-reactivity to *A phagocytophilum* is also seen. In people, the EML agent shows cross-reactivity to *E chaffeensis*. In some areas, ~50% of dogs infected with *E canis* also have a titer to *A platys*, which likely reflects coinfection; cross-reactivity between these agents is not seen.

PCR has been used to detect and identify specific *Ehrlichia* and *Anaplasma* species in infected people and animals. Samples appropriate for PCR include blood, tissue aspirates, or biopsy specimens of reticuloendothelial organs, such as lymph nodes, spleen, liver, or bone marrow. PCR can also be used to detect the effectiveness of treatment in clearing infection. PCR is not routinely available through commercial veterinary laboratories, although some veterinary schools and research institutions offer it. PCR is available through several commercial human laboratories.

During the acute stage, differential diagnoses include other causes of fever and lymphadenomegaly (eg, Rocky Mountain spotted fever, brucellosis, blastomycosis, endocarditis), immune-mediated diseases (eg, systemic lupus erythematosus), and lymphosarcoma. During the chronic stage of *E canis* infection, differential diagnoses include estrogen toxicity, myelophthisis, immune-mediated pancytopenia, and other multisystemic diseases associated with specific organ dysfunction (eg, glomerulonephritis).

Treatment: The drug of choice for infection with *Ehrlichia* and *Anaplasma* spp is doxycycline because of its superior intracellular penetration and bacteriostatic properties against rickettsiae. Doxycycline is recommended for dogs of all ages. If infection is suspected, dogs should be treated empirically; treatment should not be withheld or delayed pending laboratory results. Early seronegative tests should not be considered a reason to stop therapy, because antibodies may take ≥1 wk to develop in acute cases. The recommended dosage of doxycycline in dogs is 5–10 mg/kg/day, PO or IV, for 10–21 days. Tetracycline (22 mg/kg, PO, tid) can also be used for ≥2 wk in acute cases and 1–2 mo in chronic cases. Two doses of imidocarb dipropionate (5–7 mg/kg, IM), 2 wk apart, are variably effective against both ehrlichiosis and some strains of babesiosis. In acute cases receiving appropriate antibiotic therapy, body temperature is expected to return to normal within 24–48 hr after treatment. In chronic cases associated with *E canis* infection, the hematologic abnormalities may persist for 3–6 mo, although clinical response to treatment often occurs much sooner. Supportive therapy may be necessary to combat wasting and specific organ dysfunction; platelet or whole-blood transfusions may be required if hemorrhage is extensive. Concurrent broad-spectrum antibiotics may be needed if the dog has severe leukopenia. The *E canis* antibody titer should be measured again within 6 mo of illness to confirm a low or seronegative status indicative of successful therapy. Serum titers that persist at lower but positive levels should be rechecked in another 6 mo to ensure that they are not increasing.

Prevention: Prevention is enhanced by controlling ticks on dogs, through use of reliable methods. In particular, medications and products with proven efficacy against *R sanguineus* are important to use. Because *R sanguineus* infestations can be problematic in kennels and around homes, and longterm tick control is needed for management, use of effective long-acting collars on all susceptible dogs might be considered; collars containing propoxur, amitraz, or flumethrin have proven activity against *R sanguineus*. Prevention of transfusion-associated transmission can be reduced by using seronegative screened blood donors, although new donors with a negative screen cannot be presumed free of infection for several weeks because they may be incubating infection. Prophylactic administration of tetracycline at a lower dosage (6.6 mg/kg/day, PO) is effective in preventing *E canis* infection in kennels where disease is endemic. Treatment must be extended for many months through at least one tick season if the endemic cycle is to be successfully eliminated, and tick control should be implemented as well.

Zoonotic Risk: *E chaffeensis*, *E ewingii*, and *A phagocytophilum* are considered zoonoses. Despite the occurrence of disease in both animals and people, the involvement of a required intermediate tick vector for transmission means dogs and other infected animals do not pose a direct transmission risk in normal circumstances. Infection in dogs may indicate a heightened risk of human infections related to tick exposure in a given area.

ROCKY MOUNTAIN SPOTTED FEVER

(*Rickettsia rickettsii* infection)

Etiology: Rocky Mountain spotted fever (RMSF) is a disease of people and dogs caused by *Rickettsia rickettsii*. *R rickettsii* and closely related members of the spotted fever group of rickettsiae are considered endemic throughout much of North, South, and Central America. These pathogens are transmitted primarily through the bites of infected ticks. The ability of genetically similar rickettsial organisms, such as *R parkeri*, to cause clinically similar disease in dogs is unknown. Because of their susceptibility to *R rickettsii* and relatively higher rates of tick exposure, dogs may serve as excellent sentinels of risk for *R rickettsii* infection in people. Clusters of disease are frequently reported in defined geographic areas, and temporally associated infections may be seen in both dogs and their owners.

Epidemiology: In the USA, *Dermacentor variabilis* (the American dog tick) and *D andersoni* (the Rocky Mountain wood tick) are considered the primary vectors for *R rickettsii*. In South America, several *Amblyomma* spp of ticks have been implicated in transmission. The organism has also been isolated from *Rhipicephalus sanguineus* ticks (the brown dog tick), which appear to be the primary vector in some focal areas of Arizona, particularly on American Indian tribal lands, and may also play an as-yet unappreciated role in outbreaks elsewhere in the USA. *R sanguineus* ticks are also associated with transmission of *R rickettsii* in Central America and with large city-based outbreaks in Mexico. The pathogen is acquired by larval and nymph stages of ticks while feeding on infected vertebrate hosts and is also passed from female ticks to progeny through transovarial transmission. An estimated <1% of *Dermacentor* spp ticks carry *R rickettsii*, even in areas considered highly endemic. In highly enzootic regions of Arizona where *R rickettsii* is transmitted by the brown dog tick, as many as 5% of ticks may be infected.

Seroprevalence in dogs from endemic areas ranges from 4.3%–77%, but these values do not accurately reflect infection rates because of the detection of cross-reacting antibodies to other genetically similar rickettsiae. RMSF transmission through blood transfusion has been documented in a single human case and should be considered when selecting canine blood donors. Direct transmission from dogs to people has not been reported, although human infection may occur after contact of abraded skin or conjunctiva with tick hemolymph or excreta during removal of engorged ticks from pets.

Clinical Findings: Dogs are highly susceptible to clinical infection with *R rickettsii*; in contrast, it is rarely diagnosed in cats. Early signs in dogs may include fever (up to 105°F [40.5°C]), anorexia, lymphadenopathy, polyarthritis, coughing or dyspnea, abdominal pain, vomiting and diarrhea, and edema of the face or extremities. Petechial hemorrhages of the conjunctiva and oral mucosa may be seen in severe cases. Focal retinal hemorrhage may be seen during the early course of disease. Neurologic manifestations such as altered mental states, vestibular dysfunction, and paraspinal hyperesthesia may occur.

Thrombocytopenia is common. Leukopenia develops during the early stages of infection and, in untreated cases, is followed by progressive leukocytosis. Serum biochemical abnormalities may include hypoproteinemia, hypoalbuminemia, azotemia, hyponatremia, hypocalcemia, and increased liver enzyme activities. Case fatality rates of ~1%–10% are expected.

Lesions: Vascular endothelial damage is due to direct cytopathic effects of the rickettsiae. Severity of the necrotizing vasculitis can be directly correlated to the infective dose. Vascular endothelial damage and thrombocytopenia contribute to development of petechiae and ecchymoses. Necrosis of the extremities (acryl gangrene) or disseminated intravascular coagulation can develop in severely affected dogs.

Diagnosis: Currently, there are no in-house diagnostic tests available for diagnosis of acute RMSF in dogs. Indirect fluorescent antibody titer (IFA) is preferred for serologic testing. However, because of the high incidence of cross-reacting antibodies to a variety of nonpathogenic spotted fever group rickettsiae, as well as longterm persistence of antibodies after acute RMSF infection, demonstration of a 4-fold rise in titer should be documented in conjunction with a compatible clinical syndrome. Differential diagnoses include other causes of fever of unknown origin. The therapeutic response is usually dramatic, as it is in other canine rickettsial diseases. Animals with neurologic dysfunction may have residual deficits. Immunity appears to be lifelong after natural infection; therefore, recurrent episodes should not be attributed to RMSF.

Treatment: Antibiotic treatment should be administered based on clinical suspicion without waiting for results of serologic tests, because delayed administration of antibiotics may result in higher rates of severe or fatal outcome. Doxycycline is the treatment of choice, regardless of age of the dog, and should be administered at a dosage of 5–10 mg/kg/day, PO or IV, for 10–21 days. Tetracycline at 22 mg/kg, PO, tid for 2 wk is also effective. Chloramphenicol has been used to treat RMSF in the past, but its use is associated with higher rates of fatal outcome in human patients, and it is not recommended. Other broad-spectrum antibiotics are ineffective against *R rickettsii* infection, and there is some evidence in human cases that use of fluoroquinolones may actually worsen infection. Early seronegative tests should not be considered a reason to stop therapy, because antibodies may take ≥1 wk to develop in acute cases. Supportive care for dehydration and hemorrhagic diathesis may be necessary. Because of alterations in vascular integrity, conservative rates of fluid administration are advised. Precautions should be taken for the safe removal and control of ticks. In settings in which *R rickettsii* transmission from *R sanguineus* is suspected, medications and products with proven efficacy against this tick species are important to use. Because *R sanguineus* infestations can be problematic in kennels and around homes, and longterm tick control is needed for outbreak control, use of effective long-acting tick collars on all susceptible dogs might be considered; collars containing propoxur, amitraz, or flumethrin have proven activity against *R sanguineus*.

Zoonotic Risk: *R rickettsii* is considered a zoonotic pathogen. The potential for household clustering and large urban outbreaks, particularly in areas with transmission by brown dog ticks, makes RMSF a disease of significant public health concern. Although clinical disease occurs in both animals and people, the involvement of a required intermediate tick vector for transmission means dogs and other infected animals do not pose a direct transmission risk in normal circumstances. Infection in dogs indicates a heightened risk of human infections related to tick exposure in a given area, and serologic studies of dogs in emerging areas may help predict human risk of infection. Particularly in areas where transmission occurs via *R sanguineus*, close cooperation between veterinary, medical, and public health officials is important to achieve control.

MURINE TYPHUS

(*Rickettsia typhi* infection, *R felis* infection)

Rickettsia typhi, the causative agent of murine typhus, and *R felis* are zoonotic pathogens maintained primarily in rodent reservoirs (rats, mice) that may also be associated with enzootic cycles involving opossums and domestic cats. Infection is transmitted to people and other animals through contact with infected fleas.

Epidemiology: Infection in people is primarily thought to occur through exposure of abraded skin with infectious flea feces; aerosolization of infectious materials may occur in limited settings. Dogs and cats are presumably exposed in a similar fashion. Although known to occur worldwide, currently fewer than several hundred human cases of murine typhus are reported in the USA each year. Enzootic infection is the most commonly reported from southern Texas, California, and Hawaii, although the disease is believed to be underreported.

Clinical Findings: Clinical illness associated with canine and feline infection with *R typhi* and *R felis* is not well documented, but evidence of exposure based on presence of antirickettsial antibodies has been noted, particularly in association with outbreaks of human disease. Although a role as a possible reservoir for infection has been suggested, particularly for cats, the importance of domestic animals in maintenance of enzootic cycles has not been well elucidated. Nonetheless, dogs and cats may, at a minimum, serve as a source of fleas that may pose a transmission risk to people. Regular flea control is recommended to reduce risk of flea-associated transmission to people.

Diagnosis: An indirect fluorescent antibody (IFA) titer assessed in paired sera is preferred for serologic testing and is most commonly used in conjunction with environmental assessments around a human outbreak. There is some degree of antibody cross-reactivity with antibodies from other rickettsial infections, including *R rickettsii*, so assessments should ideally be made with paired sera. PCR of whole blood may also be used, but its utility in assessing canine and feline infection is unknown because the animals may not exhibit clinical signs during periods of rickettsemia, making it difficult to determine the optimal time for assessment.

Treatment: In the absence of clinical signs, specific treatment is not recommended. If clinical illness associated with *R typhi* or *R felis* infection is suspected in a dog or cat, doxycycline may be administered at a dosage of 5–10 mg/kg/day, PO or IV, for 10–21 days. Animals should be provided with routine preventive treatments to control fleas. Control programs involving animal removal from an area of enzootic activity should be accompanied by pesticide treatment of the environment to prevent fleas feeding on people after the removal of preferred blood-meal hosts.

Zoonotic Risk: *R typhi* is considered a zoonotic pathogen. Serologic evidence of exposure or past infection in dogs or cats indicates a heightened risk of human infections in a given area, and flea control for pets is an essential component of disease control.

SALMON POISONING DISEASE AND ELOKOMIN FLUKE FEVER

(*Neorickettsia* spp infection)

Salmon poisoning disease (SPD) is an acute, infectious disease of canids, in which the infective agent is transmitted through the various stages of a fluke in a snail-fish-dog life cycle. The name of the disease is misleading, because no toxin is involved. Elokomin fluke fever (EFF) is an acute infectious disease of canids, ferrets, bears, and raccoons that resembles SPD but has a wider host range. In people, *Neorickettsia sennetsu* causes a disease known as Sennetsu ehrlichiosis, and in horses *N risticii* causes a disease known as Potomac horse fever; these have not been reported as a cause of illness in dogs except for one report of *N risticii* in Illinois.

Etiology: SPD is caused by *N helminthoeca* and is sometimes complicated by a second agent, *N elokominica*, which causes EFF. The vector for these *Neorickettsia* agents is a small fluke, *Nanophyetus salmincola*. Dogs and other animals become infected by ingesting trout, salmon, or Pacific giant salamanders that contain the encysted metacercaria stage of the rickettsia-infected fluke. In the dog's intestine, the metacercarial flukes excyst, embed in the duodenal mucosa, become gravid adults, and transmit the rickettsiae to monocytes-macrophages. The fluke infection itself produces little or no clinical disease. A recent report of SPD in two captive Malayan sun bears underscores the need to consider this etiology in non-native exotic species with compatible exposure and clinical histories.

Epidemiology: The life cycle of *Neorickettsia helminthoeca* is maintained by the release of infected fluke ova in the feces of the mammalian host. Infected miracidia develop from these ova and infect the snails *Juga plicifera* and *Juga silicula* to form infected rediae. Rediae develop into infected cercariae that are released from the snail, penetrate the salmon or trout, and develop into encysted metacercariae infected with *Neorickettsia*. The cycle is completed when mammals eat the fish, and infected metacercariae become infected gravid adults and pass *Neorickettsia* to fluke eggs. Although *Neorickettsia* infection of dogs is not required for the life cycle of *Neorickettsia*, mammalian infection is required to maintain the trematode life cycle. Transmission by cage-to-cage contact, rectal thermometers, or aerosols is rare.

There are no age, sex, or breed predilections; however, the disease prevalence is higher when the availability of trematode-infected fish is greater. Infected fish are found in the Pacific Ocean from San Francisco to the coast of Alaska, but SPD is more prevalent from northern California to Puget Sound. It is also seen inland along the rivers of fish migration. SPD also has been reported in southern California and Brazil. The snail is the primary factor for geographic limitation, but dogs fed undercooked or raw fish from the supermarket may have developed SPD.

Clinical Findings: In SPD, signs appear suddenly, usually 5–7 days after eating infected fish, but may be delayed as long as 33 days, and persist for 7–10 days before culminating in death in up to 90% of untreated animals. Body temperature peaks at 104°–107.6°F (40°–42°C) 1–2 days later, then gradually declines for 4–8 days and returns to normal. Frequently, animals are hypothermic before death. Fever is accompanied by depression and complete anorexia in virtually all cases. Persistent vomiting usually occurs by day 4 or 5. Vomiting occurs in most cases, and diarrhea, which develops by day 5–7, often contains blood and may be severe. Dehydration and extreme weight loss occur. When severe, the GI signs are clinically indistinguishable from those of canine parvoviral infection. Generalized lymphadenopathy develops in ~60% of cases. Nasal or conjunctival exudate may be present and mimic signs of distemper. Neutrophilia is common, but a marked, absolute leukopenia with a degenerative left shift may occur. Thrombocytopenia is reported in 94% of the cases. Serum chemistry values are normal.

Clinically, EFF is a milder infection than SPD. Severe GI signs are less commonly seen in EFF infections, and lymphadenopathy may be a more pronounced finding. Case fatality rates with EFF are lower, at ~10% of untreated cases.

Lesions: Infection appears to chiefly affect the lymphoid tissues and intestines. There is enlargement of the GI lymph follicles, lymph nodes, tonsils, thymus, and to some extent, the spleen, with microscopic necrosis, hemorrhage, and hyperplasia. Remarkable abdominal or mesenteric lymphadenomegaly may be seen. A variable but often severe nonhemorrhagic enteritis is seen throughout the intestine with SPD but is less commonly seen with EFF. Microscopic foci of necrosis also appear apart from the follicles. Nonsuppurative meningitis or meningoencephalitis has been identified in some dogs.

Diagnosis: Fluke ova are found on fecal examination in ~92% of cases, which supports the diagnosis. The ova are oval, yellowish brown, rough-surfaced, and ~87–97 × 35–55 μm, with an indistinct operculum and a small, blunt point on the opposite end. During the first day or two, few ova may be passed. Intracellular organisms have been demonstrated by Romanowsky staining on lymph node aspirates in ~70% of cases. PCR testing to detect DNA-specific *N helminthoeca* (or *Neorickettsia* genus) is recommended for accurate diagnosis. Serologic testing using the *N helminthoeca* organism has been developed. Other causes of fever of unknown origin, generalized lymphadenopathy, vomiting, and diarrhea are differential diagnoses. When diarrhea and exudative conjunctivitis occur, distemper should be considered.

Prevention and Treatment: Currently, the only means of prevention is to restrict the ingestion of uncooked salmon, trout, steelhead, and similar freshwater fish. In animals that recover, a profound humoral immune response persists, but there is no cross-resistance between *N helminthoeca* and *N elokominica*. Sulfonamides are not effective and may exacerbate the clinical disease. Recommended treatment is parenteral oxytetracycline (7 mg/kg, IV, tid for 5 days) or doxycycline (10 mg/kg, bid for 7 days). Oral tetracycline or doxycycline is contraindicated because of impinging GI signs. Animals usually succumb because of dehydration, electrolyte and acid-base imbalances, and anemia. Therefore, general supportive therapy to maintain hydration and acid-base balance, while meeting nutritional requirements and controlling diarrhea, is often essential. Judicious use of whole blood transfusions may be helpful.

IMMUNE SYSTEM

THE BIOLOGY OF THE IMMUNE SYSTEM

Animals are under constant threat of invasion by a diverse range of microorganisms that seek to enter the body and exploit its resources for shelter and food. To ensure survival and prevent such exploitation, the body combats the most dangerous of these invaders with an equally complex set of defensive mechanisms that can be thought of as a series of barriers. These mechanisms include physical barriers to invasion such as a tough, thick skin or the ability to cough and sneeze. The second line of defense is a “hard wired” system of innate immunity that depends on a rapid, stereotyped response to stop and kill both bacterial and viral invaders. This is typified by the process of acute inflammation and by the classic sickness responses such as a fever. The third line of defense is the highly complex, adaptable, and incredibly effective adaptive immune system.

Innate immune responses are highly effective against opportunistic organisms or those of low virulence, but by their very nature cannot do more than delay highly pathogenic microbial invaders. Longterm resistance and survival depends on adaptive immunity. The adaptive immune system is effective against a wide variety of pathogens. Its effectiveness improves each time it is activated in response to microbial invasion. Because the body accumulates immune memory cells as it ages, adaptive immunity provides an almost insurmountable barrier to most potential invaders. In its absence, the animal dies.

The adaptive immune system faces complex challenges. Many different microorganisms, including bacteria, viruses, protozoa, and helminths, may attempt invasion. The optimal immune responses to this diversity of invaders must also be very diverse. For example, invaders such as bacteria that live outside body cells are best attacked by an antibody-mediated (or humoral) immune response, whereas viruses living within cells are best destroyed by the killing of infected cells through cell-mediated mechanisms.

PHYSICAL BARRIERS

The physical barriers on the surface of the body play a significant role in slowing or blocking microbial invasion. Very few microorganisms can penetrate intact skin; instead, invaders usually enter through wounds or by being injected, such as by mosquito bites. Skin wounds heal rapidly to reestablish the protective barrier. A complex population of normal skin bacteria tends to exclude new invaders, while antimicrobial molecules in sweat can kill many would-be invaders. In the airways, the structure of the upper respiratory tract serves as an effective filter of small particles. The airways themselves are lined with a layer of adhesive mucus that can entrap microbes. The mucus contains multiple antimicrobial proteins such as defensins, lysozyme, and surfactants. "Dirty" mucus is constantly being replaced by clean material as ciliary action carries it to the pharynx where it is swallowed. Coughing and sneezing remove larger irritants from the airways and nasal passages and are essential defensive reactions. The defense of the intestine centers largely on the presence of the huge and immensely complex normal commensal microbiota. Potential invaders may be unable to colonize the intestine in the presence of a well-adapted population of commensal microbes. If all else fails, invaders may be rapidly removed from the GI tract by vomiting and diarrhea.

The intestinal microbiota plays a critical role in maintaining animal health. First, it is a source of nutrients, especially in herbivores, in which it provides a means of exploiting a cellulose-rich diet and a source of essential vitamins. This microbiota also plays a critical role in the defense of the body. The large, well-adapted microbial population excludes many potential pathogens through competition. More importantly, the constant stimulus provided by the presence of the microbiota effectively stimulates the correct development of the adaptive immune system and regulates the level of inflammation mediated by innate immune systems.

INNATE IMMUNITY

Microbes that succeed in penetrating the physical barriers of the body are rapidly detected, and the innate defenses are activated. Although multiple innate mechanisms exist, acute inflammation is the central feature of innate immunity. The first step in the inflammatory process is the early detection of either invading organisms or damaged tissues. Most invaders are recognized by pattern-recognition receptors that bind and recognize conserved molecules expressed on microbial surfaces. There are many different pattern-recognition receptors, but the most important are the toll-like receptors (TLRs). TLRs are a family of at least 10 different receptors found on the surface or in the cytoplasm of cells such as macrophages, intestinal epithelial cells, and mast cells. The TLRs on cell surfaces bind to molecules commonly expressed by extracellular bacteria such as lipopolysaccharides or lipoproteins. The cytoplasmic TLRs, in contrast, bind to the nucleic acids of intracellular viruses. Once they bind their ligands, the TLRs trigger the production of proteins such as interleukin 1 (IL-1) or interferon α (IFN-α).

IL-1 and the other cytokines produced in response to TLR stimulation then trigger acute inflammation. They initiate the adherence of circulating leukocytes to blood vessel walls close to sites of invasion. These leukocytes, especially neutrophils, then leave the blood vessels and migrate to invasion sites, attracted by microbial products, small proteins called chemokines, and molecules from damaged cells. Once they arrive at the invasion site, the neutrophils bind invading bacteria, ingest them through the process of phagocytosis, and kill the ingested organisms. This killing is largely mediated by a metabolic pathway called the respiratory burst that generates potent oxidants such as hydrogen peroxide and hypochloride ions. Neutrophils, however, have minimal energy reserves and can undertake only few phagocytic events before they are depleted.

Even if the initial inflammatory response is successful in killing all invaders, the body must still remove cell debris, eliminate any surviving microbes and dying neutrophils, and repair the damage. This is the task of macrophages. Tissue macrophages originate as blood monocytes. They, like neutrophils, are attracted to sites of microbial invasion and tissue damage by chemokines and damaged tissues, where they finish off any surviving invaders. They also ingest and destroy any remaining neutrophils, thus ensuring that the neutrophil oxidants are removed without toxic spills occurring in the tissues. Finally, another population of these macrophages begins the process of tissue repair. Macrophages that complete the destructive process are optimized for microbial destruction and are called M1 cells. Macrophages optimized for tissue repair and removal of damaged tissues are called M2 cells.

Many of the molecules produced as a result of inflammation and tissue damage, such as IL-1 and tumor necrosis factor, can reach the bloodstream where they circulate. They enter the brain and trigger sickness behavior; for example, they alter the thermoregulatory centers to cause a fever, act on appetite-controlling centers to suppress appetite, and act on sleep centers to produce sleepiness and depression. They also mobilize energy reserves from adipose tissue and muscle. This sickness behavior is believed to enhance the defense of the body by redirecting energy toward fighting off invaders.

Circulating cytokines from inflammatory sites also act on liver cells, causing the cells to secrete a mixture of "acute-phase proteins," so-called because their blood levels climb steeply when acute inflammation develops. Different species have different acute-phase proteins, including serum amyloid A, C-reactive protein, and many different iron-binding proteins. Acute-phase proteins also serve to promote innate immunity.

Complement

Although acute inflammation is central to the processes of innate immunity, the body possesses other innate defenses. Tissues contain antimicrobial peptides that can bind and kill invading bacteria. These include detergent-like molecules such as the defensins or cathelicidins that can lyse bacterial cell walls, enzymes such as lysozyme that kill many gram-positive bacteria, and iron-binding proteins such as hepcidin or haptoglobin that prevent bacterial growth by depriving them of essential iron supplies. Perhaps the most important of these innate defenses is the complement system, which consists of a complex group of ~30 proteins that act collectively to kill invading microbes. The primary function of the complement system is to bind two proteins called C3 and C4 irreversibly to microbial surfaces. Once bound, these complement components may either kill microbes by rupturing them using another protein called C9 or simply coat them so that they are rapidly and effectively phagocytized by leukocytes.

The complement system can be activated in three ways. One way, called the alternative pathway, is triggered by the presence of bacterial surfaces that consist largely of carbohydrates and can bind the complement protein C3. Once bound, the C3 acts as an enzyme to activate and bind more C3. These C3-coated bacteria are rapidly and effectively phagocytized and destroyed. Alternatively, surface-bound C3 can activate additional complement components that eventually cause a protein called C9 to insert itself within bacterial cell walls, where it causes bacterial rupture. A second complement-activating pathway is triggered when bacterial surface carbohydrates bind to a mannose-binding protein in serum. This binding activates an enzyme pathway that leads to activation of C3 or C9. The third, or classic, pathway of complement activation is triggered when antibodies bind to microbial surfaces. It is thus triggered by adaptive immune responses. As with the mannose pathway, this eventually leads to activation of C3 and C9. Because of its potential ability to cause severe tissue damage, the complement system is carefully regulated through multiple complex regulatory pathways.

Cells of Innate Immunity

The key to an effective innate immune response is prompt recognition of invasion and a rapid cellular response. Several cell types function as sentinel cells; three of the most important are macrophages, dendritic cells, and mast cells. These cell types express pattern recognition receptors such as TLRs and can sense the presence of microbial invaders. They also express multiple other receptors that can detect microbes and tissue damage. When these receptors are engaged, they signal through a molecule called NF-κB to turn on the production of cytokines such as IL-1, IFN-α, and TNF-α. They also release vasoactive and pain molecules such as histamine, leukotrienes, prostaglandin, and specialized peptides that initiate the vascular events in inflammation.

The purpose of inflammation is to ensure that leukocytes are delivered as promptly as possible to sites of microbial invasion. This involves attracting these cells from the bloodstream where they circulate and inducing them to migrate through the tissues to the invasion sites where they engulf and kill invaders. There are three major leukocyte populations that can kill invaders. Granulocytes are especially effective at killing invading bacteria. They engulf the invaders, activate a metabolic pathway called the respiratory burst, and generate lethal oxidizing molecules such as hydrogen peroxide and hypochloride ions that kill most ingested bacteria. Eosinophils are specialized killers of invading parasites. They contain enzymes that are optimized to kill migrating helminth larvae. The third major killing cell population are M1 macrophages. These cells migrate into areas of microbial invasion more slowly than granulocytes. However, they are capable of sustained and effective phagocytosis. They contain the highly lethal antimicrobial factor nitric oxide and thus can kill organisms resistant to neutrophil killing.

When inflammation leads to activation of macrophages, they secrete a cytokine called IL-23. This, in turn, acts on a population of T cells (called Thl7 cells), causing them to secrete IL-17. IL-17 recruits granulocytes to sites of inflammation, infection, and tissue damage.

While many leukocytes are optimized to kill invading bacteria, viruses also present a potent threat. Natural killer (NK) cells are a population of innate cells optimized to kill virus-infected cells. NK cells, a form of lymphocyte, can kill virus-infected or other "abnormal" cells that fail to express major histocompatibility complex (MHC) class I molecules. MHC class I molecules bind to *NK cell receptors* and switch off their killing abilities. In the absence of this signal, the NK cells bind to target cells, inject them with apoptosis-inducing proteins, and kill them.

ADAPTIVE IMMUNITY

Innate immunity, although critical to the defense of the body, is insufficient to guarantee protection. It lacks the flexibility to respond optimally to a diversity of microorganisms and by its very nature may cause significant tissue damage. A third layer of defense is required that can act automatically in response to microbial invasion, generate resistance proportional to the threat, and improve with experience. These are the key features of the adaptive immune system. Adaptive immune responses are of two major types: antibody (humoral) immunity directed against extracellular invaders, and cell-mediated immunity directed against intracellular invaders.

Adaptive immune responses are complex and must be very carefully regulated. The immune defenses of the body constitute a potent system of protection that must be carefully controlled to minimize damage to normal tissues. As a result, a major portion of the immune system is devoted to the production of regulatory cells that function to ensure that adaptive immune responses occur only under appropriate circumstances. If these regulatory pathways fail, disease or death may result.

The adaptive immune system functions through a series of steps that must occur sequentially for either an antibody-mediated or cell-mediated immune response to occur. The first step involves the capture and processing of foreign antigens. Once processed, these antigens are transported to cell surfaces, where they can be recognized by lymphocytes carrying receptors for specific antigens. Each antigen receptor is highly specific, and each lymphocyte expresses only a single form of antigen receptor. Thus, millions of cells have the potential to recognize millions of antigens. To ensure that only foreign antigens trigger adaptive immunity, cells with receptors that bind and respond to normal body antigens are selectively killed early in their development. The surviving cells are located within lymphoid organs at sites where they can most effectively encounter antigens on microbial invaders, triggering them to respond by mounting immune responses. There are three major populations of lymphocytes: **B cells** that are responsible for antibody responses, **effector T cells** that are responsible for cell-mediated immune responses, and **regulatory T cells** that control these responses and minimize inappropriate responses.

Antibody Responses (Humoral Immunity)

Antibodies are protein molecules that serve as B-cell antigen receptors that can be synthesized in large quantities and secreted by the cell into the bloodstream where they circulate. These proteins are produced by B cells and from B cell–derived plasma cells. Antibodies bind to foreign molecules and mark them for destruction by phagocytic cells or complement-mediated lysis. Plasma cells are differentiated B cells optimized to synthesize and secrete enormous quantities of antibodies. Antibodies are critical to host defense against extracellular invaders such as most bacteria, some blood parasites, and viruses traveling between cells.

B cells originate in the bone marrow and reside in lymphoid tissues such as lymph nodes, bone marrow, Peyer's patches, and the spleen. Each B cell is covered by several thousand identical antigen receptors and can bind and respond to only a single antigenic molecule. When a microbe enters the body, it will inevitably encounter B cells that can bind to some of its surface antigens. As a result of antigen binding, and under suitable circumstances, these B cells divide repeatedly and differentiate into two subpopulations. One subpopulation is composed of antibody-producing plasma cells, which are capable of enormously increased protein synthesis and are the major sources of antibodies. The other subpopulation is composed of B cells that develop into memory B cells and persist in lymphoid tissues for months or years. When an animal encounters an antigen for a second time, these memory B cells respond rapidly, producing large numbers of plasma cells (and more memory cells). As a result, the animal mounts a vastly improved antibody response and the invader is rapidly eliminated. Subsequent exposure to a microbe leads in turn to the accumulation of more memory cells, resulting in better protection and virtually guaranteeing that the organism will never be able to cause disease in that animal. This response is the basis of all vaccination programs.

Although simple in concept, B cell responses and antibody production are made more complex by the need to ensure their careful regulation. Thus, a B cell is not usually able to respond to a bound foreign antigen unless it also receives "permission" in the form of a second signal from cells called helper T cells. These T cells in turn can only be activated if they are presented with antigen under carefully controlled circumstances.

Antibodies: Antibodies are composed of proteins called immunoglobulins. Mammals use five different classes of antibodies: immunoglobulin G (IgG), IgM, IgA, IgE, and IgD. The class of immunoglobulin secreted by B cells and plasma cells depends on their location. Cells located in lymphoid organs within the body secrete IgM and IgG, whereas cells located on body surfaces secrete IgM, IgA, and IgE.

IgG is the most abundant immunoglobulin found in the bloodstream and plays the major role in eliminating organisms that succeed in penetrating deep into the body. IgM serves as a "back-up" for IgG and is usually confined to the bloodstream. IgM is produced early in the antibody response, when its high effectiveness compensates for its low quantity.

IgA is produced by B cells and plasma cells located on mucosal surfaces. As a result, IgA is produced and secreted in large amounts into the upper respiratory tract, the GI tract, tears, sweat, etc. In these locations, it complements the physical barriers of the body and prevents microbial invasion. IgE serves as a "back-up" for IgA and is also mainly produced on body surfaces. IgE is optimized to control invasion by parasites such as helminths or arthropods. However, it also mediates a rapid acute inflammation in allergic states and hence may mediate life-threatening anaphylaxis. The function of IgD is unclear, but it is believed to be of minimal significance.

T Cell Help: Most antibody responses are regulated by the need to receive prior approval from T cells. The T cells in turn are activated only when they bind antigen fragments presented by specialized antigen-presenting cells called dendritic cells.

Dendritic cells are macrophage-like cells that capture and process foreign antigens. Their name derives from their many long, thin, filamentous processes or dendrites that extend through tissues to form an effective antigen-trapping web. For example, a subpopulation of dendritic cells (Langerhans cells) is found in the dermis, where its web of dendrites traps microorganisms seeking to enter the body through damaged skin. Dendritic cells capture and phagocytize invading microorganisms. Fragments of these foreign antigens persist within the dendritic cells, where they become attached to receptor molecules (major histocompatibility complex [MHC] molecules). Once formed, these antigen-receptor complexes move to the cell surface where they can be recognized by T cells.

The receptors in dendritic cells that bind and present antigen fragments are specialized proteins encoded by genes clustered together in the MHC (originally identified as the antigens that cause graft rejection, hence their unusual name). There are many thousands of different MHC molecules expressed within an animal population but relatively few (3–6) different molecules expressed in any individual animal. Because they play a critical role in binding antigen fragments and activating T cells, MHC molecules effectively determine whether an individual can respond to a foreign antigen. An individual animal possesses MHC molecules that can bind many, perhaps most, foreign antigens, but not all of them. If an animal lacks MHC molecules that can bind an antigen, it will be unable to respond to that specific antigen. The set of antigens to which an individual can respond (and against which it is protected) are determined by its MHC haplotype. All domestic animal species possess their own unique MHC. The receptors coded for these genes are named after the specific species; thus, BoLA is the name of these molecules in cattle, ELA in horses, SLA in swine, etc.

As with B cells, T cells possess specific antigen receptors on their surface that are generated randomly when the cells are first produced. As T cells mature within the thymus, cells with receptors that can bind normal body components are killed. Surviving T cells can respond only to foreign antigens. The antigen receptors on T cells, like those on B cells, are identical on any single cell. Unlike those on B cells, however, the receptors can recognize antigen only when it is bound to an MHC molecule. Thus, when a dendritic cell presents MHC-associated antigen to T cells, only those T cells with appropriate receptors will bind to the dendritic cells. Once in contact, the cells exchange signals that confirm that the T cell is responding to a correctly processed antigen. After T cells receive all the necessary signals, they secrete a mixture of cytokines that permit their attached B cells to respond to antigens and allow antibody production to proceed.

Antibodies are produced in response to, and directed against, extracellular bacteria. Cell-mediated responses, in contrast, are directed against viruses and intracellular bacteria. The determination as to the appropriate form of the immune response is made at an early stage in the immune response. Thus, there are two populations of dendritic cells that can trap and process antigens. One population (DC1 cells) triggers cell-mediated immunity, whereas the other (DC2 cells) triggers antibody formation. These dendritic cell populations send different messages to T cells, because they use different cytokines for signaling; DC1 cells secrete IL-12, whereas DC2 cells secrete IL-1. In turn, these different cytokines stimulate two different T cell populations: Th1, which promotes cell-mediated immunity, and Th2, which promotes B cell responses and antibody production. Th1 cells secrete a mixture of cytokines typified by interferon-γ (IFN-γ). Th2 cells secrete a mixture of cytokines typified by IL-4. B cells will usually respond optimally to a foreign antigen only if they are stimulated by the presence of IL-4 from Th2 cells.

Cell-mediated Immunity

As described above, cell-mediated immune responses are required to combat intracellular invaders such as viruses and some intracellular bacteria. The immune system blocks virus infections by killing the cells that they infect. The cells responsible are called effector, or cytotoxic, T cells. Like T cells, effector T cells undergo development and selection within the thymus, so any T cells capable of killing normal healthy cells are eliminated. The surviving T cells are released into the body, where they circulate continuously through the tissues seeking out abnormal cells.

All nucleated cells produce many different proteins when functioning normally. Virus-infected cells, however, are forced by the virus to produce viral proteins. The body therefore requires that all nucleated cells send a sample of their newly synthesized proteins to the cell surface. This involves the cell diverting a small sample of each newly formed protein and fragmenting it in a complex enzyme system called a proteasome. The resulting protein fragments are then attached to MHC molecules and carried to the cell surface, where they are available for inspection by effector T cells. If the cell's receptors do not engage a protein fragment, nothing happens. If, however, their antigen receptors bind to a foreign antigen fragment in an MHC-protein complex, the T cell will be signaled to kill the offending cell. Like B cells, effector T cells function only if they receive permission from a helper T cell, specifically a Th1 cell. The cytokines from Th1 cells, especially IFN-γ, must be present if an effector T cell is to kill its target.

Effector T cells bind tightly to target cells expressing foreign antigens and then signal them to destroy themselves through apoptosis. The T cells inject their targets with enzymes called granzymes that trigger this process. As a result, effector T cells eliminate virus-infected cells but not normal, healthy cells. Most effector T cells die within a few days once they are no longer needed, but a few survive to become long-lived memory cells that respond rapidly should the animal encounter the virus again.

Effector T cells are especially effective at killing target cells that produce foreign antigens. However, some intracellular organisms, especially intracellular bacteria, are best destroyed by other cell-mediated mechanisms. In these cases, IFN-γ from Th1 cells activates M1 macrophages. As a result, bacteria that can survive within normal macrophages are rapidly destroyed by activated macrophages.

Immunologic Memory

The effectiveness of adaptive immunity is largely a result of its ability to recognize antigens encountered previously and to mount an enhanced and accelerated response against them. The more an animal encounters an antigen, the greater will be its immune response. Immunologic memory depends on the presence of persistent populations of memory cells that accumulate as an animal ages. These memory cells may be very long-lived or, more likely, turn over very slowly. As a result, animals may make small amounts of antibodies to vaccine antigens for many years after vaccination. Cell-mediated memory may also be due to the development of very long-lived populations of memory T cells. The effectiveness of vaccines in inducing long-lasting immunity depends in large part on their ability to induce memory cell populations.

Cytokines

The cells of the adaptive immune system communicate in several ways. They can come into physical contact and exchange signals through receptors within the contact area or immunologic synapse. Examples include the contact between T cells and dendritic cells or between effector T cells and their targets. Immune cells can also signal nearby cells by secreting small signaling proteins called cytokines. Several hundred different cytokines have been identified. Signaling cells secrete a mixture of cytokines that then bind to receptors on nearby cells. The target cell receives multiple signals that it must integrate to respond appropriately. Cytokines, acting through their specific receptors, can turn the synthesis of specific proteins on or off. They can cause the target cell to divide or differentiate, and they may trigger apoptosis. With hundreds of different cytokines acting in complex mixtures it is sometimes difficult to predict exactly how a specific target cell will respond. Major families of cytokines include the interleukins that mediate signaling between leukocytes, interferons that mediate interactions between cells and have significant antiviral activity, growth factors that regulate growth and differentiation of many different cell types, and tumor necrosis factors that modulate inflammatory responses.

Regulatory Cells

The adaptive immune system is carefully regulated by several different cell populations. The most important are T_{reg} cells, which secrete a mixture of cytokines that inhibit conventional immune responses. They serve to turn off an immune response once it has completed its task and the invading microorganism is eliminated. T_{reg} cells also play a central role in preventing the development of autoimmunity. Another important population of regulatory T cells are called Th17 cells. These cells, so called because they secrete IL-17, regulate the innate immune system and the development of inflammation.

IMMUNOLOGIC DISEASES

The primary role of the immune system is the detection and destruction of invading microorganisms. Because of the great diversity of microbial invaders, the immune system has evolved an equally complex mixture of protective mechanisms. These may be simply classified as innate immunity (*see* p 812) and adaptive immunity (*see* p 814). Protection within the first few days of microbial invasion is the responsibility of the "hard-wired" innate immune system. Longterm protection is the responsibility of the adaptive immune system.

In general, disease associated with the immune system takes two forms: insufficient immune function causing immunodeficiencies, manifested as increased susceptibility to infections, and diseases resulting from excessive immune function, resulting in hypersensitivities and autoimmunity.

Under certain circumstances, normally protective immune responses can cause significant tissue damage. In general, excessive innate immune responses do this by triggering inappropriate inflammation leading to collateral damage to nearby tissues, or by producing vastly excessive amounts of inflammatory cytokines. Excessive adaptive immune responses, in contrast, can cause damage by multiple mechanisms. One simple classification divides diseases due to excessive adaptive immune responses into four distinct types. Each involves the activities of different cell populations or complement. Type I is mediated by mast cells and eosinophils, Type II by complement and some macrophages, Type III by neutrophils, and Type IV is T cell–mediated.

Inflammation and limited tissue destruction are features of the normal innate and adaptive immune responses. Clinical disease occurs when this inflammation is excessive or in an inappropriate location. This may be due to external environmental factors, such as the composition of the intestinal microflora, together with genetic and hormonal influences.

IMMUNODEFICIENCY DISEASES

Immunodeficiency diseases manifest clinically as a predisposition to infections. They are usually recognized when an animal makes multiple visits to a veterinarian for infections that would normally be relatively easy to control. Two major groups of immunodeficiency disease occur. One group is inherited as a result of mutations or other genetic disease. These primary or congenital immunodeficiency diseases usually develop in very young animals (<6 mo old). The second group of immunodeficiency diseases are secondary to some other stimulus such as a viral infection or tumor. These secondary or adaptive diseases tend to occur in adult animals. One other general rule in diagnosing immunodeficiencies is that defects in the innate and antibody-mediated immune systems tend to result in uncontrollable bacterial infections, whereas defects in the cell-mediated immune system tend to result in overwhelming viral and fungal infections.

PRIMARY IMMUNODEFICIENCIES

Defects in Innate Immunity

Phagocytosis is a central feature of innate immunity. Phagocytic cells are found underlying the mucous membranes and skin and in the bloodstream, spleen, lymph nodes, meninges, synovial membrane, bone marrow, and around blood vessels throughout the body. Phagocytes are either in the tissue (histiocytes, synovial macrophages, Kupffer cells, etc) or in the blood (neutrophils and monocytes). Phagocytes have receptors for immunoglobulins and complement on their surfaces that assist in the engulfment (opsonization) of foreign material coated with specific antibody (opsonins) or complement, or both. Phagocytosis involves chemotaxis of the phagocyte toward foreign, noxious, or damaged tissues; adherence of microorganisms to the plasma membrane of the phagocyte; incorporation of the organisms into a phagosome; and activation of the respiratory burst and lysosomal enzymes in the phagosome, leading to microbial death and destruction.

Deficiencies in Phagocytosis:

Deficiencies in phagocytic activity can be due to acquired or congenital defects in any of these steps, or simply to a deficiency of phagocytic cells themselves. They often manifest as an increased susceptibility to bacterial infections of the skin, respiratory system, and GI tract. These infections respond poorly to antibiotics. Secondary phagocytic deficiencies include disorders that lead to profound and chronic depressions of WBCs. Feline leukemia virus infection, feline panleukopenia virus infection, feline immunodeficiency virus infection, tropical canine pancytopenia, idiopathic granulocytopenias, drug-induced granulocytopenias (antineoplastic drugs, estrogens, anticonvulsants, sulfonamides, etc), and myeloproliferative disorders are some of the conditions in which secondary infections can develop as life-threatening complications.

A cyclic decrease of all cellular elements, most notably neutrophils, occurs in the peripheral blood and lowers the resistance to infection of certain lines of gray Collies and Collie crosses.

Congenital abnormalities that lead to impaired phagocytosis are well documented in people. Deficiencies of opsonins, complement factors, chemotactic abilities, and myeloperoxidase have been recognized in people but not in other animals. Chediak-Higashi syndrome results from a defect in phagosomal function and has been recorded in cats, mink, cattle, and orcas. Chronic granulomatous disease has been recognized as an X-linked defect in some Irish Setters (canine granulocytopathy syndrome). Some lines of Weimaraners develop bacterial septicemias (usually manifested by bone and joint infections) as puppies. The underlying causes of these defects are unknown; some of the affected dogs have lower than normal levels of IgM and IgG, and their WBCs have a bactericidal defect.

Leukocyte Adhesion Deficiency: Leukocyte adhesion deficiency is an autosomal recessive primary immunodeficiency. It has been described in people, Irish Setters, and Holstein cows. The deficiency results from the absence of an integrin, an essential surface glycoprotein expressed on leukocytes. Clinically, it is characterized by recurrent severe bacterial infections, impaired pus formation, and delayed wound healing. Infected animals usually have severe pyrexia, anorexia, and weight loss. Response to antibiotic therapy is usually poor. Extreme, persistent leukocytosis may occur (>100,000 WBCs/mL) and consists predominantly of mature neutrophils. The integrin deficiency prevents blood leukocytes from leaving blood vessels and entering the tissues, so they cannot contribute to the defense of tissues against infections.

Complement Deficiencies: A congenital deficiency of C3 has been described in Brittany Spaniels. These dogs developed recurrent bacterial infections, especially skin diseases and pneumonias. Although complement is necessary for opsonization and neutrophil chemotaxis, bacterial infections do not always develop in people or laboratory animals with complement deficiencies, because the existence of multiple pathways provides a way to activate the system even if one pathway is blocked. Diagnosis is based on a blood test showing reduced C3 levels.

A congenital deficiency in the C1 inhibitor has been recognized in people and occurs rarely in dogs. This can lead to uncontrolled complement activation and inflammation. Affected animals have recurrent bouts of facial edema.

There is no specific treatment for complement deficiencies. Vaccination and antibiotics are used to prevent and treat infection. As with all inherited diseases, subsequent breeding programs must be carefully assessed to prevent the reappearance of the disease in future generations.

Deficiencies in Adaptive Immunity

Humoral Immunodeficiencies: These deficiencies may be acquired or congenital. Acquired deficiencies are seen in neonates that do not receive adequate maternal antibodies (failure of passive transfer) or in older animals due to conditions that decrease active immunoglobulin synthesis. Failure of passive transfer occurs in species that use colostrum as the major source of maternal antibodies. It is commonly associated with recurrent infections in calves, lambs, and foals. Failure of passive transfer can occur when the young animal fails to nurse properly during the first several days of life or when the dam's colostrum contains low levels of specific antibodies. Defects in the absorption of immunoglobulin from ingested milk may also occur. Immunoglobulin levels <400 mg/dL in a postnursing serum sample indicate a failure of passive transfer in foals. Premature weaning of calves is a problem in dairy herds and is a leading cause of failure of passive transfer in dairy calves. Newborn animals that do not receive sufficient maternal antibodies often succumb to fatal bacterial or viral infections of the GI and respiratory tracts.

Hypogammaglobulinemia of clinical significance can be associated with any disorder that interferes with antibody synthesis. Tumors, such as plasma cell myelomas or lymphosarcomas that secrete large amounts of monoclonal antibody, can be associated with profound antibody deficiencies. This is because the tumor cells outcompete normal immunoglobulin-producing cells, or because regulatory pathways inhibit immunoglobulin production. Animals with tumors that produce monoclonal antibodies may have severe secondary infections. Some viral infections, eg, canine distemper and canine parvovirus, may damage the immune system so severely that antibody production is virtually stopped.

Congenital hypogammaglobulinemia has been recognized either alone or in combination with defects in cell-mediated immunity (combined immunodeficiency, *see* p 816). Deficiencies in IgG subclasses have been seen in some breeds of cattle; IgM deficiency has been described in horses; and IgA deficiencies have been described in Beagles, German Shepherds, and Chinese Shar-Pei. Cattle with IgG subclass deficiency are usually asymptomatic. Older foals with IgM deficiencies develop respiratory infections. Dogs with IgA deficiency, like their human counterparts, are prone to chronic skin infections, chronic respiratory infections, and possibly allergies. IgA deficiency of Beagles appears to be due to a defect in the secretion of IgA, because IgA-positive cells are present in normal numbers. Some German Shepherds have lower IgA levels than other breeds and a higher incidence of intestinal infections. IgA deficiency in Shar-Pei is highly variable; some have negligible serum and secretory levels, and some have normal serum levels and low or negligible secretory levels. Like German Shepherds, affected Shar-Pei have more problems than expected with allergies. Dogs with these immunodeficiency syndromes may have a higher than usual incidence of autoimmune diseases and autoantibodies, such as autoimmune hemolytic anemia, thrombocytopenia, and systemic lupus erythematosus. Longterm treatment with broad-spectrum antibiotics is required and is often unsatisfactory.

Transient hypogammaglobulinemia has been recognized most frequently in foals and puppies. It may be more common in Spitz-type puppies than in other breeds. It results from a delayed onset of immunoglobulin production in the newborn and is associated with defects in both T_H function and the B cell response to foreign antigens. Puppies with this condition develop recurrent respiratory infections at 1–6 mo of age but recover by 8 mo. Affected foals frequently develop clinical signs of hypogammaglobulinemia (usually respiratory infections) at ~6 mo of age when their maternal antibody reaches a very low level. After another 3–5 mo they begin to produce immunoglobulin. Appropriate antibiotic treatment and supportive therapy is often sufficient.

Deficiencies in Cell-mediated Immunity: Deficiencies in cell-mediated immune responses are associated with **thymic aplasia**, an absent or very small thymus. This has been seen in some inbred lines of dogs, cats, and cattle; these animals were deficient in cell-mediated immune functions, as well as having pituitary dysfunction.

Combined Immunodeficiency Diseases: If both humoral and cell-mediated immune responses are deficient, they are classified as combined immunodeficiencies (CID). These result from inherited defects in the earliest lymphocyte progenitors. An autosomal recessive CID has been identified in Arabian foals and Basset Hounds. It results from a defect in DNA repair enzymes and prevents the production of functional antigen receptors. Sporadic cases of CID have also been seen in Toy Poodle, Rottweiler, and mixed-breed puppies. Affected dogs are frequently asymptomatic during the first several months of life but become progressively more susceptible to microbial infections as maternal antibody wanes. Puppies with CID are clinically normal until 6–12 wk of age. The most common cause of death from CID is canine distemper as a consequence of routine immunization with modified-live virus distemper vaccine. Arabian foals with CID frequently succumb to adenovirus pneumonia or other infections when ~2 mo old. The foals are persistently lymphopenic. Precolostral serum samples have no detectable IgM antibody. Immunoglobulin levels are normal initially but then progressively decrease compared with levels in normal foals. At necropsy, the thymus is difficult to identify and is architecturally abnormal. Lymphocyte numbers are depleted in the lymph nodes, Peyer's patches, and spleen. A PCR test can confirm CID in foals and the presence of the gene in heterozygote animals. As a result of such testing, the prevalence of equine CID has declined significantly.

Selective Immunodeficiencies: A large number of immunodeficiency diseases have yet to be fully analyzed, so their precise mechanisms remain unknown. For example, Rottweiler puppies have a breed predilection for severe and often fatal canine parvovirus infections (*see* p 373). Their resistance to other infections is essentially normal, and the basis of this selective immunodeficiency is unknown.

Persian cats have a predilection toward severe, and sometimes protracted, dermatophyte infections (*see* p 874). In some Persian cats, the fungal infections invade the dermis and cause granulomatous disease (mycetomas).

Mink with the Aleutian coat color mutation are susceptible to chronic parvovirus infection and so develop Aleutian disease (*see* p 1872). Other strains of mink are susceptible to infection with this virus but do not develop clinical disease. This is due to inherited Chediak-Higashi syndrome.

Focal and systemic aspergillosis (*see* p 633), and mycoses due to related fungi, affect certain types of dogs. Long-nosed breeds, in particular German Shepherds and Shepherd-crosses, are prone to develop focal aspergillosis in the nasal passages. Systemic aspergillosis is seen almost exclusively in German Shepherds. It is characterized by fungal pyelonephritis, osteomyelitis, and discospondylitis. The organism can be isolated readily from blood and urine.

Diagnosis of Primary Immunodeficiencies

Recurrent persistent infections in young animals suggest some form of immunodeficiency. A complete differential leukocyte count will reveal whether all leukocyte types are present in appropriate numbers. Immunoglobulin deficiencies can only be detected by means of a quantitative immunoassay such as radial immunodiffusion, although turbidity tests such as those used for the diagnosis of failure of passive transfer are relatively easy to perform and may provide useful diagnostic information.

Primary immunodeficiencies as genetic diseases are generally not treatable and, if diagnosed, steps should be taken to ensure that parent animals that carry defective traits are no longer used for breeding.

SECONDARY IMMUNODEFICIENCIES

In adult animals, immunodeficiencies often occur as a consequence of virus infections, malnutrition, stress, or toxins. These are called secondary immunodeficiencies. Virus-induced secondary immunodeficiencies are the most important of these.

Virus-induced Immunodeficiencies

One way in which viruses survive in infected animals is by immunosuppression. For example, canine distemper virus infects and kills lymphocytes, causing a profound combined immunodeficiency in affected puppies. This infection is associated with a progressive decline in immunoglobulin levels and increased susceptibility to organisms normally controlled by cellular immunity such as *Pneumocystis* and *Toxoplasma*. Parvoviral infection in both dogs and cats also causes a profound depression in the resistance to fungal infections such as aspergillosis, mucormycosis, or candidiasis in the immediate postrecovery period.

Feline Leukemia Virus (FeLV): FeLV is associated with an increased susceptibility to secondary and opportunistic infections. Acquired immunodeficiency in FeLV infection is multifactorial. Infected cats can have deficiencies of neutrophils, decreased synthesis of antibodies (especially to bacterial antigens), decreased cellular immunity, and reduced complement levels. Immune responses to FeLV infection also appear to suppress immunity to the feline infectious peritonitis (FIP) coronavirus and may lead to reactivation of quiescent FIP. (*See also* p 790.)

Simian Type D Retrovirus: This viral infection of macaques has a similar pathogenesis to that of FeLV infection of cats but can induce even more severe immunodeficiency. Type D retrovirus infection of macaques can cause severe disease in adolescent animals. Affected macaques may either die within several months with fever, lymphadenopathy, and opportunistic infections of the CNS, respiratory tract, and intestines; become lifelong asymptomatic carriers; or sometimes recover fully.

Simian Immunodeficiency Virus (SIV): This lentivirus is closely related to human immunodeficiency virus. Many strains of SIV exist in nature. The common hosts are African primates such as African green monkeys, sooty mangabeys, mandrills, baboons, and other guenons. Transmission between infected and noninfected monkeys is probably a result of bites or in utero exposure. SIV is not present in native populations of Asian primates. It rarely causes disease in the host African species. If infected animals are under heavy stress, as in captivity, some may develop AIDS-like disease. SIV, especially of sooty mangabey origin, causes severe disease in macaques (rhesus, stump-tail, pig-tail, bonnet, etc). The immunosuppression associated with SIV can last for weeks or years. Encephalitis (usually asymptomatic except for wasting) and lymphomas are frequent consequences of SIV infection in macaques.

Feline Immunodeficiency Virus (FIV): FIV has been identified in domestic and wild felids. The infection is endemic in cats throughout the world. Virus is shed in the saliva, and biting is the principal mode of transmission. As a result, free-roaming, male, and aged cats are at greatest risk of infection. FIV infection is uncommon in closed purebred catteries. After infection, there is a transient fever, lymphadenopathy, and neutropenia. Most cats then recover and appear to be clinically normal for many months or years before progressive immunodeficiency develops. Cats with acquired immunodeficiency induced by FIV then develop chronic secondary and opportunistic infections of the respiratory, GI (including mouth), and urinary tracts, as well as the skin. FIV-infected cats have a higher than expected incidence of FeLV-negative lymphomas, usually of the B-cell type, and myeloproliferative disorders (neoplasia and dysplasias).

Bovine Immunodeficiency-like Virus: This lentivirus has been isolated from cattle with persistent lymphocytosis, hemolymphadenopathy, and BLV-negative lymphosarcomas. The overall prevalence in North American cattle appears to be ~1%, although in some herds it may be as much as 15%. The virus does not appear to be pathogenic.

EXCESSIVE IMMUNE FUNCTION

There are many different ways by which excessive immune function can cause disease or death. These include excessive innate responses, excessive adaptive responses, and tumors of the immune system.

EXCESSIVE INNATE RESPONSES

While acute inflammation is a defensive process and central to innate immunity, it may occur without appropriate provocation and in locations where it causes discomfort, tissue damage, or systemic disease. This results in significant morbidity and resulting disability.

Canine Rheumatoid Arthritis: This disease results from excessive, uncontrolled inflammation around joints. It manifests initially as a shifting lameness with soft-tissue swelling around involved joints. Within weeks or months, the disease localizes in individual joints, and characteristic radiographic changes develop. The earliest radiographic changes consist of soft-tissue swelling and a loss of trabecular bone density in the area of the joint. Lucent cyst-like areas frequently are seen in the subchondral bone. The most prominent lesion is a progressive erosion of cartilage and subchondral bone in the area of synovial attachments, resulting in loss of articular cartilage and collapse of the joint space. Angular deformities often occur, and luxation of the joint is a frequent sequela. *Deformities are most* frequent in the carpal, tarsal, and phalangeal joints and less frequent in the elbow and stifle. Synovial fluid examination shows a sterile, inflammatory synovitis, with increased cell count and a high proportion of neutrophils in the synovial fluid cell population. The excessive inflammation is believed to be due to the deposition of immune complexes in the synovia with subsequent complement activation.

An erosive arthritis has also been recognized in cats. It tends to occur in older male cats and frequently is associated with feline syncytia-forming virus infection. The development of disease in cats is much more insidious than in dogs.

Canine rheumatoid arthritis responds poorly to systemic glucocorticoids alone. Immunosuppressive agents with anti-inflammatory activity such as cyclophosphamide and azathioprine are used with glucocorticoids to treat these disorders; NSAIDs (eg, aspirin, carprofen, etodolac, meloxicam) may bring relief.

Plasmacytic-Lymphocytic Synovitis: Possibly a variant of rheumatoid arthritis, this synovitis occurs in medium-sized and large breeds of dogs. Although multiple joints often are involved, the disease has a predisposition for the stifle. The most common clinical sign is hindlimb lameness and anterior drawer motion of the stifles. Lymphocytes, plasma cells, and neutrophils predominate in the synovial fluid, although in some cases the fluid is essentially normal. Gross inspection of the joint shows proliferation of the synovial membrane and stretching or rupture of the cruciate ligaments. Treatment is as for canine rheumatoid arthritis, above.

Idiopathic Polyarthritis: Arthritis of unknown etiology is most common in large dogs, particularly German Shepherds, Doberman Pinschers, retrievers, spaniels, and pointers. In toy breeds, it is most frequent in Toy Poodles, Yorkshire Terriers, and Chihuahuas, or mixes of these breeds. There is no evidence of a primary chronic infectious disease process or of systemic lupus erythematosus. Arthritis is often the sole manifestation.

Diagnosis is based on the history of cyclic antibiotic-unresponsive fever, malaise, and anorexia, with stiffness or lameness. Bony changes are not seen on radiographs until the disease is well established. Even then, radiographic changes are mild and can mimic degenerative joint disease. Synovial fluid contains leukocytes but is sterile.

The disease may be controlled with daily high-dose glucocorticoids followed by low-dose, alternate-day therapy. Treatment usually can be discontinued after 3–5 mo. Dogs with poor response to such therapy (>50%) may be treated with more potent immunosuppressive drugs such as azathioprine or cyclophosphamide in addition to glucocorticoids. Gold salts help augment glucocorticoid therapy in some animals.

Immune-mediated Meningitis: This disease occurs in adolescent or young adult Beagles, Boxers, German Shorthaired Pointers, and Akitas but is very rare in other pure and mixed breeds. The clinical signs consist of cyclic episodes of fever, severe neck pain and rigidity, reluctance to move, and depression. Each attack lasts 5–10 days, with intervening periods of complete or partial normality lasting approximately a week. During attacks, protein and neutrophils in the CSF are increased. The lesion is an arteritis, primarily of the meningeal vessels, but occasionally of other organs as well. The disease is often self-limiting over several months; attacks become milder and less frequent. Glucocorticoid therapy reduces the severity of attacks. In some animals, the disease becomes chronic and only partially amenable to therapy.

A more severe form of this meningitis has been reported in young Bernese Mountain Dogs. The disease in this breed is somewhat cyclical, but the resolution in intervening periods is less than in other species. CSF abnormalities resemble those seen in other breeds. The condition requires longterm, high-dose glucocorticoid therapy.

A syndrome of meningitis, often associated with polyarthritis, is seen in young Akitas. The dogs show severe episodes of fever, depression, cervical pain and rigidity, and generalized stiffness. Affected dogs grow slowly and often appear unthrifty. The condition responds poorly to glucocorticoid and combination immunosuppressive therapy, and most affected dogs are euthanized as young adults. In older Akitas, a milder and more drug-responsive form of the disease is seen, which may be associated with pemphigus foliaceus, uveitis, and plasmacytic-lymphocytic thyroiditis.

Systemic Inflammatory Response Syndrome

In severe infections or after massive tissue damage, large amounts of cytokines and reactive oxygen and radicals enter the bloodstream and cause a form of shock known as systemic inflammatory response syndrome.

Septic shock is the name given to the systemic inflammatory response syndrome specifically caused by severe infections and associated with trauma, ischemia, and tissue injury. Animals with severe infections may generate vastly excessive cytokine production, most notably IL-1, TNF-α, IL-8, and IL-6. This massive cytokine release has been called "a cytokine storm." High doses of cytokines are toxic and induce severe acidosis, fever, lactate release in tissues, an uncontrollable drop in blood pressure, increased plasma catecholamines, and eventually renal, hepatic, and lung injury and death. The procoagulant-anticoagulant balance is upset so that endothelial procoagulant activity is enhanced, while many anticoagulant pathways are inhibited, leading to disseminated intravascular coagulation and capillary thrombosis.

All these effects are initiated by excessive triggering of toll-like receptors leading to a massive and uncontrolled release of cytokines. The cytokines damage vascular endothelial cells, activating them so that procoagulant activity is enhanced, which leads to blood clotting. The nitric oxide causes vasodilation and a drop in blood pressure. The widespread damage to vascular endothelium eventually causes organ failure. Multiple organ dysfunction syndrome is the end stage of severe septic shock. It is characterized by hypotension, insufficient tissue perfusion, uncontrollable bleeding, and organ failure caused by hypoxia, tissue acidosis, tissue necrosis, and severe local metabolic disturbances. The severe bleeding is due to disseminated intravascular coagulation. The sensitivity of mammals to septic shock varies greatly. Species with pulmonary intravascular macrophages (cat, horse, sheep, and pig) tend to be more susceptible than dogs.

EXCESSIVE ADAPTIVE RESPONSES

Excessive activity of the adaptive immune system can lead to inflammation and tissue damage, autoimmunity, or amyloidosis. For many years it has been customary to classify excessive adaptive immune system function into four types on the basis of the mechanisms involved.

Type I Reactions

(Atopic disease, Anaphylactic reactions)

Type I, or immediate hypersensitivity, encompasses these IgE-mediated reactions to other, nonparasitic antigens. This inflammation may be minor or local, or severe and generalized. In its most extreme form, it causes a potentially lethal shock syndrome called anaphylaxis. Anaphylaxis is an acute systemic manifestation of the interaction of an antigen (allergen) binding to IgE antibodies attached to mast cells and basophils. This binding of antigens to cell-bound IgE antibodies triggers the release of biologically active inflammatory mediators, including histamine, leukotrienes, eosinophilic chemotactic factors, platelet activating factor, kinins, serotonin, proteases, and cytokines. These molecules directly affect both the vascular system, causing vasodilation and increased vascular permeability, and smooth muscles, causing contraction. Additionally, they attract pro-inflammatory eosinophils to the triggering site.

The severity of anaphylaxis depends on the type of antigen, the amount of IgE produced, and the amount of antigen and route of exposure. If the animal has been previously sensitized by exposure to an allergen (antigen) and produces IgE antibodies, then injection of the sensitizing antigens directly into the bloodstream can result in anaphylactic shock and related reactions (eg, hives, urticaria, facial-conjunctival edema). If the sensitizing allergen enters through the mucous membranes or the skin, allergic reactions tend to be more localized. Agents that can trigger anaphylactic and allergic reactions are numerous and include the venom of stinging and biting insects, vaccines, drugs, foods, and blood products.

Systemic Anaphylaxis (Generalized Anaphylactic Reactions): Anaphylactic shock occurs in sensitized animals after exposure to antigens in sensitizing vaccines or drugs, ingestion of foods, or insect bites. Clinical signs occur within seconds to minutes after exposure to the allergen. In most domestic animals, the lungs are the primary target organs, and the portal-mesenteric vasculature is a secondary target; this is reversed in dogs. Mast cell degranulation in the pulmonary vasculature causes constriction of bronchial airways or pulmonary veins and pooling of blood and edema in the pulmonary vascular bed, which results in severe respiratory distress. Mast cell degranulation in the portosystemic vasculature causes venous dilatation and pooling of blood in the intestines and liver.

Clinical signs can be localized or generalized and include restlessness and excitement, pruritus around the head or site of exposure, facial edema, salivation, lacrimation, vomiting, abdominal pain, diarrhea, dyspnea, cyanosis, shock, incoordination, collapse, convulsions, and death. In dogs, the major organ affected by anaphylactic shock is the liver, and signs are associated with constriction of hepatic veins, which results in portal hypertension and visceral pooling of blood. GI signs rather than respiratory signs are more apt to be seen in dogs. Supportive therapy, in addition to treating respiratory distress, consists of the administration of epinephrine (both locally and systemically as needed). IV fluids for the treatment of shock, antihistamines (systemically for severe acute anaphylaxis or orally as a means to control chronic signs of allergy or milder allergic signs), and corticosteroids if needed. Ancillary support of blood pressure and respiration may be necessary.

Urticarial reactions (hives or angioedematous plaques) of the skin and subcutaneous tissue and acute edema of the lips, conjunctiva, and skin of the face (facial-conjunctival angioedema) are less severe forms of Type I hypersensitivity. Hives are the least severe reaction and may not be associated with other clinical abnormalities. Facial-conjunctival edema is more severe and can be associated with mild to moderately severe systemic anaphylaxis. These reactions usually follow administration of vaccines or drugs, ingestion of certain foods, or insect bites. Urticarial reactions and facial-conjunctival edema occur in most species and usually resolve spontaneously within 24 hr. Not all urticarial reactions are mediated by Type I hypersensitivity. (*See also* URTICARIA, p 857.)

Milk allergy occurs occasionally in cows and less frequently in mares. This occurs when a cow makes IgE autoantibodies to its own milk components, notably casein. When intramammary pressure rises, these milk proteins gain access to the circulation and induce a Type I hypersensitivity. The reaction can be localized or systemic. Recovery occurs once the animal is milked.

Localized Anaphylactic Reactions: Allergic rhinitis, manifest by serous nasal discharge and sneezing, is less common in domestic animals than in people. Often, it is seasonal, correlating with pollen exposure. Nonseasonal rhinitis may be associated with exposure to ubiquitous allergens, such as molds, danders, bedding, and feeds. Recurrent airway obstruction in horses (*see* p 1455) is probably a reaction to chronic exposure to molds present in moldy hay and poorly ventilated stables. Summer snuffles is a seasonal allergic rhinitis occurring commonly in Guernsey or Jersey cattle placed on certain types of flowering pastures in late summer and early autumn. Allergic rhinitis can be diagnosed tentatively by the following: 1) identification of eosinophils in the nasal exudate, 2) demonstration of a favorable response to antihistamines, 3) disappearance of signs when the offending allergen is removed, or 4) occasionally, its seasonal nature. Skin testing is not an accurate means to diagnose nasal allergies in animals.

Chronic allergic bronchitis has been characterized in dogs. A dry, harsh, hacking cough that is easily precipitated by exertion or by pressure on the trachea is a characteristic clinical sign. The disease may be seasonal or occur year-round. Usually, it is not associated with other signs of illness. The bronchial exudate is rich in eosinophils and free of bacteria. Chest radiographs are normal, and there may or may not be a low-grade peripheral eosinophilia. The condition is treated with bronchodilators and expectorants (aminophylline and potassium iodide or guaifenesin). Glucocorticoids will alleviate clinical signs, especially when their use can be limited to certain seasons or to low-dose, alternate-day therapy. Avoidance of the offending allergen(s) usually is not possible.

Allergic bronchiolitis is most common in cats. It is manifest by a low-grade cough, wheezing, some dyspnea, and increased peribronchiolar density on radiographs, and it may be mistaken for other conditions (allergic asthma or lungworm disease). Early in the course of the disease, clinical signs can be modified by antihistamine therapy, but if the disease increases in severity, moderate to high dosages of corticosteroids may be necessary. The offending allergen usually is not identified.

Eosinophilic bronchopneumopathy occurs most frequently in dogs but has been recognized in all species. It is associated with diffuse inflammatory infiltrates in the lungs and a pronounced peripheral eosinophilia; frequently, the serum globulins are increased. Unlike in allergic bronchitis, affected animals are often dyspneic or tire easily with exercise. Diffuse bronchial exudate contains numerous eosinophils. The specific offending allergen is rarely identified. Glucocorticoids are the treatment of choice. A similar syndrome is also associated with resident or migratory parasitic infections of the lungs in young animals.

Allergic asthma occurs most frequently in cats, in which the signs are similar to those in people. It occurs more frequently in summer and after going outdoors; individual attacks can be transient and mild, or protracted and severe (status asthmaticus). Mild attacks may manifest as wheezing and coughing; in severe attacks, there may be expiratory dyspnea, hyperinflation of the lungs, aerophagia, cyanosis, and frantic attempts to obtain air.

Intestinal allergies (food allergies) are principally seen in dogs and cats, particularly kittens. (*See also* p 855 and p 2379.) Allergic gastritis is manifest by vomiting, which occurs 1 to >12 times weekly, within 1–2 hr of eating. The vomitus may be tinged with bile. In cats, vomiting may be the sole sign; dogs may also have intermittent loose feces. Cats and dogs with allergic gastritis are usually healthy except for vomiting, although there can be loss of weight and coat condition in severe cases. Allergic enteritis is associated with a mild inflammation of the small intestine but with little or no eosinophilia. Feces usually are normal in volume and frequency but vary from semiformed to watery. They may be extremely odorous, especially in cats. Affected animals may be excessively thin despite good appetite. Skin lesions and poor coat are commonly associated with food allergies in cats but less commonly in dogs. The allergy often develops after episodes of viral, bacterial, or protozoal enteritis (a phenomenon known as allergic breakthrough). Eosinophilic enteritis, the most severe form of allergic intestinal disease, manifests by moderate to severe inflammation of the intestines and a pronounced eosinophilia. Diarrhea, weight loss, and poor coat condition are usually evident. The prevalence of allergic colitis is greater in cats than in dogs, although in general it is not common. In dogs, it is often associated with frequent defecation and soft, mucus-laden and sometimes bloody feces; in cats, it most frequently manifests by more normal feces coated or spotted with fresh blood. (For diagnosis and treatment of food allergies, *see* p 855.)

Atopic dermatitis (*see* p 853) is a complex pruritic, chronic skin disorder that occurs in many species but has been studied mostly in dogs. Some animals with atopic dermatitis may have a genetic predisposition that leads to excessive production of reaginic (IgE) antibodies. It has been estimated that ~10% of all dogs suffer from atopy, with a breed predisposition in terriers, Dalmatians, and retrievers. Atopic dermatitis of dogs often is triggered by inhaled allergens, eg, house dust mites, pollens, molds, and danders. Atopic dogs often chew at their feet and axillae. Excessive sweating is especially noticeable in hairless areas. The severity of the skin lesions are greatly increased by licking, scratching, flea infestation, and secondary bacterial or yeast infection. Atopic skin lesions in cats are either miliary (small scabs) and widespread, or larger and more localized. Localized lesions are often pruritic.

In cats, food allergens probably are a more common cause of skin lesions than are inhaled allergens. Sweet itch (*see* p 887) is a seasonal allergic dermatitis of horses associated with certain insect bites, especially night-feeding *Culicoides*. Intensely pruritic lesions appear along the dorsum from the ears to tail head and perianal area. Similar allergic skin reactions to insect bites can be seen around the ears and face of cats and dogs. (For diagnosis and treatment, *see* p 853.)

Type II Reactions

(Antibody-mediated cytotoxic reactions)

Type II reactions occur when an antibody binds to an antigen present on the surface of cells. This bound antibody can then activate the classical complement pathway, resulting in cell lysis, phagocytosis, or antibody-mediated cytotoxicity. Many different antigens may trigger this cell destruction, but an infection in a genetically predisposed animal appears to be a major triggering pathway. Cross-reactive antibodies can develop during infections. These cross-reactive antibodies directed toward an infectious agent may bind to normal tissue antigens and trigger antibody-mediated cytotoxicity. For example, in streptococcal infection in horses, a cross-reaction between *Streptococcus equi* antigen and vascular basement membranes can occur, leading to purpura hemorrhagica. Pathogens such as *Babesia* or *Mycoplasma haemofelis*, which parasitize cells, trigger an immune response that destroys those cells as part of the protective mechanism. The most common manifestations of Type II hypersensitivity involve blood cells. These include hemolytic anemia if RBCs are involved, leukopenia involving WBCs, or thrombocytopenia involving platelets. Under some circumstances, a cytotoxic attack on vascular epithelial cells will cause a vasculitis with local vascular leakage.

Immune-mediated Hemolytic Anemia (IMHA) and Thrombocytopenia:

The production of autoantibodies against erythrocyte or platelet antigens leads to anemia and thrombocytopenia, the most common Type II reactions. Antibody and complement attach to RBCs either directly or indirectly via an absorbed antigen and then mediate RBC destruction, resulting in a severe, life-threatening anemia. Concurrent thrombocytopenia is found in 60% of cases. IMHA can be associated with systemic lupus erythematosus or with lymphoreticular malignancies. Drugs or infections may trigger episodes of hemolytic anemia or thrombocytopenia in many species. More often than not, the initiating cause is unknown.

IMHA occurs in several clinical forms: peracute, acute or subacute, chronic, cold agglutinin disease, and red cell aplasia. Most cases are treatable, but relapses are common. (*See also* p 10.)

Peracute IMHA is seen mainly in middle-aged, larger breeds of dogs. Affected dogs are acutely depressed and have a rapid decrease in PCV within 24–48 hr with bilirubinemia, variable icterus, and sometimes hemoglobinuria. Initially, the anemia is nonresponsive, but it may respond within 3–5 days. Thrombocytopenia may also be present. Antiglobulin tests are often negative, and spherocytes may or may not be present, but tube or slide agglutination of RBCs is marked. The autoagglutination is not dispersed by saline dilution, hence the term hemolytic anemia with in-saline agglutinins. The serum usually contains autoantibodies that cause agglutination of most donor RBCs. The prognosis of peracute IMHA is poor even with prompt and vigorous therapy. The most effective therapy involves immediate use of high dosages of glucocorticoids plus cyclophosphamide, together with a compatible blood transfusion. If incompatible blood must be used, the animal should first be heparinized and maintained on heparin for 10 days. Even without transfusion, heparinization may be beneficial for the first 2 wk or more. Bovine hemoglobin blood substitute and human immunoglobulins can be used as supportive therapy until immunosuppressive treatment reduces the destruction of RBCs.

Acute IMHA is the most common form of the disease, with a breed predilection in Cocker Spaniels. Initial signs are pallor, fatigue, and less commonly, icterus. Hepatosplenomegaly is a prominent sign. The WBC count may be increased due to bone marrow hyperplasia. Autoagglutination of RBCs is uncommon, and the antiglobulin test is generally positive. These animals usually respond well to glucocorticoid therapy. If a favorable response is not seen within 7–10 days, cytotoxic drugs (cyclophosphamide or azathioprine) should be added to the regimen.

Chronic IMHA differs from the acute form in that the PCV falls to a constant level and remains there for weeks or months. The bone marrow is either normal or hyperresponsive, and the antiglobulin test is often negative. Chronic IMHA is relatively more common in cats than in dogs. Usually, the anemia is responsive early in the course of disease but responds minimally or not at all by the time it becomes severe. Initial treatment is with glucocorticoids; if there is no response within 2 wk, cytotoxic drugs may be added to the regimen.

Cold agglutinin disease is an IMHA of dogs and horses. Its cause is usually unknown but may be secondary to infection, other autoimmune diseases, or neoplasia. The IgM autoantibodies can be agglutinating or nonagglutinating. Complete agglutination does not occur at body temperature but only when the blood is chilled; thus, it is more frequent in colder climates and seasons. Initial signs may be of a hemolytic disease; in the agglutinating type, vascular blockage may lead to necrosis of the nose, tips of the ears and tail, digits, scrotum, and prepuce. Diagnosis is based on a reversible autoagglutination that occurs only at 4°C. The direct antiglobulin reaction is usually negative for IgG, frequently positive for C3, and usually positive for IgM if the reaction is performed in the cold. Mortality is high. In the absence of an obvious initiating cause such as infection or neoplasia, the disease is best controlled with high doses of glucocorticoids in combination with cyclophosphamide.

Red cell aplasia (*see* p 13) is most common in dogs. It occurs in two forms, one in postweanling to adolescent puppies and the other in adults. Unlike in IMHA, the bone marrow shows a selective depression of erythroid elements; granulocytes and platelets are unaffected. Therefore, the peripheral anemia is unresponsive. The immune attack is directed against erythroid stem cells, and the antiglobulin test is usually negative. Treatment is usually as for chronic IMHA, but recovery may be very slow.

Immune-mediated thrombocytopenia is common in dogs. It occurs more often in females than males. The most frequent clinical signs are hemorrhages of the skin and mucous membranes. Melena, epistaxis, and hematuria may be accompanying features and can cause profound anemia. Hemolytic anemia and thrombocytopenia sometimes occur together. Immune-mediated thrombocytopenia usually is diagnosed on the basis of low peripheral platelet counts despite a pronounced megakaryocytosis in the marrow. Occasionally, megakaryocytes may be selectively absent from the marrow. Tests for antiplatelet antibodies are difficult to conduct, so diagnosis is usually made on clinical presentation and response to therapy. (*See also* p 46.)

Animals with immune-mediated thrombocytopenia that show only petechial and ecchymotic hemorrhages, with no significant blood loss and megakaryocytes in the marrow, may be treated initially with glucocorticoids. The clinical signs should abate and the platelet count begin to rise after 5–7 days. If the platelet count has not increased significantly by 7–10 days, cyclophosphamide, azathioprine, or vincristine can be added to the glucocorticoid regimen. In animals with megakaryocytes in the marrow and severe blood loss, a more rapid response to therapy is desirable. Such animals are treated with a single injection of vincristine combined with daily glucocorticoids; a favorable response usually occurs after 3–5 days. If the blood loss is life-threatening, platelet-rich whole blood should be administered. If the platelet count has risen by day 7, remission is maintained on glucocorticoids alone. If there is no response after 7 days, a second dose of vincristine is given. If the platelet count is still low after 2 wk, vincristine is discontinued and either cyclophosphamide or azathioprine is added. Animals with thrombocytopenia and no megakaryocytes respond much more slowly to glucocorticoids, or to glucocorticoids and vincristine. Preferred treatment for these animals is with prednisolone and cyclophosphamide, and a response should not be expected earlier than 1–2 wk after beginning therapy. Therapy may be discontinued in most animals with immune-mediated thrombocytopenia 1–3 mo after the platelet count returns to normal. Some animals have a persistent thrombocytopenia despite drug therapy, or they can be maintained in remission only with chronic high-dose treatment. The alternatives are to allow the animal to live with the thrombocytopenia if signs are minimal or to use longterm combination drug therapy with glucocorticoids and either vincristine, azathioprine, or cyclophosphamide. Splenectomy is seldom curative by itself but may allow use of lower and safer dosages of immunosuppressive drugs.

Autoimmune Skin Disorders: In these diseases, affected animals make autoantibodies against the intracellular cement proteins in the epidermis. This promotes local proteolysis, leading to separation of the epidermal cells (acantholysis) and development of vesicles within the skin. Although not strictly a Type II disease, it is best considered here.

Pemphigus foliaceus is the most common of these diseases, occurring more often in dogs than in cats and horses.

It is characterized by the development of erosions, ulcerations, and thick encrustations of the skin and mucocutaneous junctions. The absence of lesions in the mouth, and the widespread thick, crusty nature of the skin lesions, tend to differentiate pemphigus foliaceus from the much rarer pemphigus vulgaris. Autoantibodies in the skin react with intracellular cement (desmoglein), resulting in its degradation and separation of the cornified and uncornified cell layers. Immunosuppression is required to treat the disease. High doses of glucocorticoids are used initially, but low-dose, alternate-day therapy is used once the disease is under control. More potent immunosuppressive drugs such as cyclophosphamide or azathioprine may be used with glucocorticoids in cases unresponsive to steroids. Animals that respond poorly to initial therapy, or require high dosages of drugs to control lesions, have a poor longterm prognosis.

Pemphigus vulgaris is a much less common autoimmune skin disease than pemphigus foliaceus. It is characterized by vesicle formation along the mucocutaneous junctions of the mouth, anus, prepuce, and vulva, and in the oral cavity. Other areas of the skin are only mildly involved. Because the epidermis of animals is relatively thin (compared with human skin), these blisters rupture rapidly and form erosions; consequently, characteristic bullae are seldom seen. The vesicles develop as a result of suprabasilar acantholysis. Secondary bacterial infection often complicates the lesions, and if untreated, the disease is often fatal. It is treated with high doses of glucocorticoids alone or in combination with other drugs such as cyclophosphamide, azathioprine, or gold salts. Pemphigus vulgaris is difficult to maintain in remission, and the longterm prognosis of affected animals is fair to poor.

Bullous pemphigoid is a rare canine skin disease recognized most often in Collies and Doberman Pinschers. Lesions are often widespread but tend to be concentrated in the groin. The involved skin resembles a severe scald. Bullae also develop; they are subepidermal and may be full of eosinophils. Autoantibodies to the basal lamina can be detected in immunohistopathologic sections. The treatment of choice is prednisolone and azathioprine used in combination; remission is frequent, but continual drug therapy at relatively high dosages may be required to keep the disease under control. The longterm prognosis is poor.

Myasthenia Gravis: Myasthenia gravis is an autoimmune disease in which autoantibodies directed against the acetylcholine receptors on muscle cells cause receptor degradation or blockage and so block neuromuscular transmission. The disease is characterized by extreme generalized muscle weakness, which is accentuated by mild exercise. Megaesophagus due to paralysis of esophageal muscles is a frequent primary or accompanying complaint in dogs. Thymomas are often associated with myasthenia gravis in people but are uncommon in domestic species. Administration of a short-acting anticholinesterase (edrophonium chloride) produces a dramatic increase in muscle strength. Treatment is with a long-acting anticholinesterase. Chronic immunosuppressive drug therapy for this disease is logical. Autoantibodies to the acetylcholine receptors can be detected in the serum of affected animals by an indirect immunohistopathologic assay using normal muscle as a substrate.

Type III Reactions

(Immune complex disease)

Antigen-antibody complexes (immune complexes) deposited in tissues may cause acute inflammation. By activating the classical complement pathway, the complexes produce potent chemoattractants that attract large numbers of neutrophils. These cells, especially if they release their enzymes and oxidants, cause acute inflammation and tissue damage. The most frequently affected sites include the joints, skin, kidneys, lungs, and brain.

The prerequisite for the development of immune complex disease is the persistent presence of soluble antigen and antibody. These form insoluble immune complexes that become trapped on the basement membrane of small blood vessels. The deposited immune complexes then activate the classical complement pathway. Complement fragments attract neutrophils and are also directly vasoactive, triggering a vasculitis. Antigens persist for a number of reasons, including chronic infections and certain neoplastic conditions, particularly lymphoreticular neoplasms. Chronic antigen exposure also occurs with inhaled antigens and, in such cases, immune complexes form in the alveolar walls. Lastly, some animals respond to self-antigens, which then act as a source of chronic antigen exposure. In many cases, the origin of the antigen within these immune complexes cannot be determined.

The location of the immune complexes is largely determined by the route by which antigen enters the body. Inhaled antigens give rise to a pneumonitis, antigens that enter through the skin cause local skin lesions, and antigens that access the bloodstream form immune complexes that are deposited in renal glomeruli or joints. Clinical signs are therefore variable but may include fever, cutaneous signs (such as erythema multiforme), and polyarthritis (shifting-leg lameness or painful, swollen joints). Other signs include ataxia, behavior change, proteinuria, isosthenuria, polydipsia, polyuria, or nonspecific signs such as vomiting, diarrhea, or abdominal pain. Diagnosis is based on the elimination of more common causes of clinical signs. Supporting evidence to confirm the diagnosis includes establishing a temporal relationship if a drug or infectious agent is suspected as the cause, identifying chronic infections or malignancies, and performing histopathology and immunohistochemistry on biopsies to identify immune-mediated vasculitides or nephritis.

Therapy should include supportive treatment, removal of the causative agent, or treatment of the underlying disorder (eg, appropriate antibiotic therapy for bacterial infections, surgical drainage of abscesses or infected tissue, therapy for heartworm disease, the withdrawal of drugs). Immunosuppressive therapy may be needed to prevent the continued deposition of immune complexes.

Membranoproliferative Glomerulonephritis: This lesion is caused by immune complexes that form within the bloodstream and are filtered out in the glomeruli (*see* p 1517). In effect, the insoluble complexes collect on the glomerular basement membrane. Depending on their size, they may be deposited on the subendothelial or subepithelial surface of the membrane. Secondary glomerulonephritis occurs as a sequela of chronic infectious, neoplastic, or immunologic disorders. Animals with idiopathic glomerulonephritis (>50% of cases) usually have signs of renal disease, whereas secondary glomerulonephritis is often a relatively minor part of a more serious disease.

Hypersensitivity Pneumonitis: When inhaled antigens meet circulating antibodies in the walls of the alveoli, immune complexes form in the alveolar walls and trigger acute inflammation. Hypersensitivity pneumonitis is most common in large animals exposed over a long time to antigenic dusts. The most potent antigens of this type are those contained in the spores of thermophilic actinomycetes from moldy hay. Inhalation of these spores causes farmer's lung disease in people and a similar condition in cattle (*see* p 1441). Hypersensitivity pneumonitis is characterized by the onset of respiratory distress 4–6 hr after exposure to moldy hay. The most effective treatment is removal of the source of the antigen; otherwise, corticosteroid therapy may help.

Systemic Lupus Erythematosus (SLE): This complex autoimmune disease occurs in dogs, is rare in cats, and has been reported in large animals. It has two consistent immunologic features: immune complex disease and a tendency to produce multiple autoantibodies. Clinically, it reflects a combination of Type II and III mechanisms. Antibodies to nucleic acids are the diagnostic hallmark of SLE, but in many individuals, antibodies to RBCs, platelets, lymphocytes, clotting factors, immunoglobulin (rheumatoid factors), and thyroglobulin are also present. The presence of autoantibodies to nucleic acids, antinuclear antibodies (ANA), can be diagnostic of the disease. Either the immune complex or the autoantibody component of the disease tends to predominate in a given animal. Immune complex deposition around small blood vessels may lead to synovitis, dermal reactions, oral erosions and ulcers, myositis, neuritis, meningitis, arteritis, myelopathy, glomerulonephritis, or pleuritis. Glomerulonephritis is one of the major life-threatening complications of SLE in cats but not in dogs. Psychosis, a major sign of SLE in people, is also seen in animals with SLE. Autoimmune hemolytic anemia or thrombocytopenia, or both, are the most common presentations of SLE in animals.

SLE is characterized by the presence of ANA, and tests for these or the associated lupus cells may help in diagnosis. However, some healthy animals may have ANA, and not all animals with SLE have detectable ANA in their blood. Diagnosis of SLE must therefore be based on the entire clinical syndrome—not just on the presence or absence of ANA.

SLE usually can be treated with glucocorticoids. Initially, they are used in high daily doses, and when remission occurs, alternate-day, low-dose therapy is used. Drug treatment should be continued for 2–3 mo after all clinical signs have resolved. Cyclophosphamide or azathioprine, or both, are used in combination with glucocorticoids in animals with SLE that is difficult to control with glucocorticoids alone.

Vasculitis: Vasculitis mediated by immune complexes occurs in animals, especially dogs and horses. Lesions are most prevalent in the dermis of the distal limbs and mucous membranes of the mouth, particularly the palate and tongue (dogs) and lips (horses). Involvement of the nose, ears, eyelids, cornea, and anus is less common. Early lesions develop as reddened areas that rapidly form shallow erosions. A scab quickly forms over dermal erosions. Limb edema is common in horses and a less frequent but equally striking sign in dogs. Vasculitis is a feature of SLE in some animals but most often is idiopathic. Drug-induced vasculitis has been well recognized in dogs. The vasculitis is detected on histopathologic and immunohistopathologic examination of superficial and deep biopsies taken from the margins of lesions.

Vasculitis is treated by withdrawal of offending drugs and, if necessary, by immunosuppressive drug therapy. Glucocorticoids used alone or in combination with other agents such as azathioprine or cyclophosphamide are usually used to treat non-drug-induced cases.

Periarteritis Nodosa (Polyarteritis Nodosa, Necrotizing Polyarteritis): This rare disease of domestic animals is caused by deposition of immune complexes and inflammation in walls of small and medium-sized arteries. Among farm animals, it is most common in pigs, usually associated with erysipelas and streptococcal infections, and is attributed to a Type III reaction to these bacteria or to their vaccines. It has been reported in cats, although it may be mistaken for the noneffusive form of feline infectious peritonitis.

Other Type III Reactions: **Purpura hemorrhagica** of horses is a severe nonthrombocytopenic purpura (*see* p 47) that often follows a *Streptococcus equi* respiratory infection; it is mediated by immune complexes of antibody and streptococcal antigen deposited in vascular basement membranes.

Anterior uveitis ("blue-eye," *see* p 495) is an immune complex–mediated reaction that frequently occurs in the recovery stage of infectious canine hepatitis (*see* p 798). It results from the reaction of serum antibodies with uveal endothelial cells infected with canine adenovirus 1. Similarly, severe **equine recurrent uveitis** (*see* p 508) is associated with immunologic reactions to *Leptospira* or *Onchocerca* spp. This periodic ophthalmia results from autoimmune attack. Antibodies against some serovars of *Leptospira* can cross-react with retinal antigens and so trigger severe ophthalmia. Uveitis caused by *Toxoplasma* and feline infectious peritonitis virus infections of cats may also have an immunologic basis.

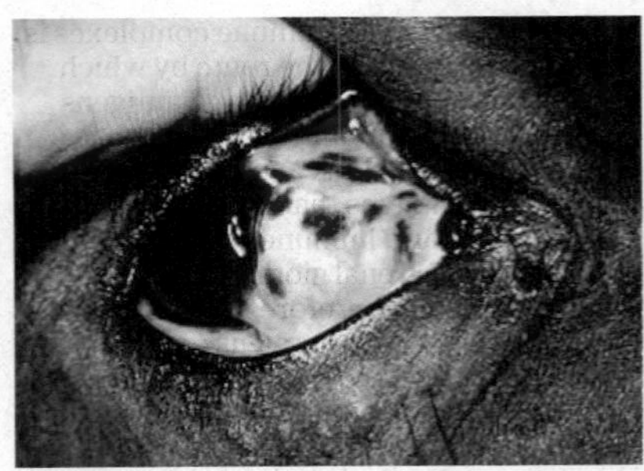

Purpura hemorrhagica, ocular lesions, in a horse. *Courtesy of Dr. Thomas Lane.*

Type IV Reactions

(Cell-mediated immune reactions)

Cell-mediated immune reactions occur when antigen triggers T_H1 responses. Multiple cytokines as well as activated macrophages and cytotoxic T cells are produced. The infiltration of mononuclear cells and the elaboration of a variety of inflammatory molecules from these cells in tissues result in the pathologic processes of cell-mediated immune reactions. The antigens usually responsible for the development of Type IV reactions include intercellular bacteria or parasites, some viruses, chemicals, and (in certain situations) cellular antigens. The lesions commonly occur in the skin (allergic contact dermatitis) when the antigen comes into contact with the skin. The diagnosis is based on eliminating other causes of disease and on histology. The goals of treatment are to identify and eliminate the source of antigen responsible for the reaction and to provide anti-inflammatory or immunosuppressive therapy as required.

Granulomatous Reactions: T cell–mediated granulomatous reactions may also occur around persistent infectious foci. These reactions to microorganisms such as mycobacteria, *Coccidioides* spp, *Blastomyces* spp, and *Histoplasma* spp, and possibly feline infectious peritonitis virus, may be a result of chronic cell-mediated immune reactions and localized macrophage activation. Although cell-mediated immunity effectively controls these types of infections in most animals, for poorly understood reasons, these same mechanisms are only partially effective in others. These granulomatous reactions are characterized by the development of a fibrous stroma and an infiltration of macrophages, giant cells, and lymphocytes around the persistent antigen.

Lymphocytic Choriomeningitis: Lymphocytic choriomeningitis, a viral infection of mice (*see* p 2025), results from the destruction of virus-infected cells by T cells, leading to CNS damage and a choriomeningitis.

Old-dog Encephalitis: Old-dog encephalitis (*see* p 777) may also result from cell-mediated immune mechanisms directed against cells persistently infected with canine distemper virus. The initiating canine distemper virus infection is usually clinically inapparent and may precede the development of encephalitis by many years.

Allergic Contact Hypersensitivity: Allergic contact hypersensitivity results from chemicals reacting with and modifying normal dermal proteins. The modified proteins trigger a cell-mediated immune response, which causes inflammation and damages the skin (eg, poison oak and poison ivy reactions in people). This reaction has been described in dogs, cattle, and horses and usually occurs as a result of contact with sensitizing chemicals incorporated in plastic food dishes, plastic collars, and drugs placed on the skin.

Autoimmune Thyroiditis: Autoimmune thyroiditis in dogs is characterized by destruction of the thyroid gland by an autoimmune process that has both humoral (Type II) and cell-mediated (Type IV) components. It is particularly prevalent in Doberman Pinschers, Beagles, Golden Retrievers, and Akitas. Hypothyroidism (*see* p 553) may be the sole manifestation of the disease or may be a clinical or subclinical component of a broader autoimmune disorder such as systemic lupus erythematosus or panendocrinopathy.

Autoimmune Adrenalitis: Autoimmune adrenalitis has been reported in dogs. The adrenal glands are slowly destroyed by a plasmacytic-lymphocytic infiltrate. When sufficient glandular tissue is destroyed, the dogs develop Addison syndrome (adrenocortical insufficiency, *see* p 574). The condition is sometimes associated with autoimmune thyroiditis (*see* above).

Keratitis Sicca: Keratitis sicca is a "dry eye" syndrome that occurs in dogs. It can occur in either a primary form or secondary to chronic use of sulfonamides. It results from immune-mediated destruction of the lacrimal glands and is similar to Sjögren syndrome of people. Affected dogs may respond favorably to cyclosporine eye drops.

TUMORS OF THE IMMUNE SYSTEM

The cells of the immune system may become neoplastic. This may result in the production of tumor cells that are nonfunctional and hence lead to immunodeficiencies. Alternatively, they may be functional, and some cancerous B cells may produce large quantities of immunoglobulins.

Tumor cells escape from the immune attack by relying on both immunosuppression and tumor cell modification. The demonstration that even bulky, invasive tumors can undergo complete remission under appropriate stimulation (eg, IL-2) has shown that it is indeed possible to treat some cancers successfully by immune manipulation.

Lymphomas are common tumors in dogs and cats. The normal adaptive response requires a burst of rapid proliferation of lymphocytes. On occasion, however, this proliferation may be uncontrolled, and lymphoid neoplasms result. Because lymphocytes are present in all organs, lymphoid tumor development can occur in any organ. Lymphomas can be multicentric, mediastinal, GI, renal, nervous, or leukemic. Less commonly, they occur in the eyes, skin, or nose. To determine the stage of the disease, CBC, serum chemistry profiles, abdominal ultrasound, abdominal radiographs, and bone marrow analyses are useful. Immunofluorescent staining and immunophenotyping can be performed in dogs and cats to characterize lymphomas. They may be either T cell or B cell in origin.

Most cases of canine lymphosarcoma, Marek's disease, calf leukosis, and feline leukemia are of T-cell origin, as are thymomas. Many T-cell lymphomas are associated with a simultaneous immunosuppression manifest by a predisposition to recurrent infections.

Adult bovine and ovine leukosis, alimentary feline leukemia, and avian leukosis are usually of B-cell origin. Under some circumstances, neoplastic B cells may develop into plasma cells. Plasma-cell tumors are known as myelomas. Because neoplastic plasma cells can secrete immunoglobulins, they give rise to gammopathies (*see* below).

GAMMOPATHIES

Gammopathies are conditions in which serum immunoglobulin levels are greatly increased. They can be classified either as polyclonal (increases in all major immunoglobulin classes) or monoclonal (increases in a single homogeneous immunoglobulin).

Polyclonal gammopathies result from chronic stimulation of the immune system. They can therefore be caused by chronic pyodermas; chronic viral, bacterial, or fungal infections; granulomatous bacterial diseases; abscesses; chronic parasitic infections; chronic rickettsial diseases, such as tropical canine pancytopenia; chronic immunologic diseases, such as systemic lupus erythematosus, rheumatoid arthritis, and myositis; or by some neoplasia. In many cases, there is no obvious predisposing cause. In some animals, the gammopathy may initially be monoclonal because of the predominance of a single immunoglobulin class (usually IgG). This has been seen in cats with noneffusive feline infectious peritonitis and in dogs with chronic tropical canine pancytopenia.

Monoclonal gammopathies are characterized by the production of large amounts of a single immunoglobulin protein. Monoclonal gammopathies are either benign (ie, associated with no underlying disease), or more commonly, associated with immunoglobulin-secreting tumors.

Tumors that secrete monoclonal antibodies originate from plasma cells (myelomas). Myelomas can secrete intact proteins of any immunoglobulin class or immunoglobulin subunits (light chains or heavy chains). Myeloma proteins in dogs are commonly IgG or IgA and less commonly IgM. Myelomas of the IgA type are particularly common in Doberman Pinschers. Myeloma proteins in cats and horses usually are IgG and, uncommonly, IgM, IgG3 (horses), or IgA.

Clinical signs depend on the location and severity of the primary neoplasm and on the amount and type of immunoglobulin secreted. Plasma-cell myelomas frequently develop in marrow cavities of flat bones of the skull, ribs, and pelvis, and in the vertebrae and cause severe bone erosion. Pathologic fractures of diseased bone can lead to spinal pain and lameness.

Disease can result from the presence of the monoclonal protein itself. For example, some forms of amyloidosis (*see* p 592) are due to deposition of immunoglobulin light chains in tissues (SAA amyloid). Hyperviscosity syndrome occurs in 20% of dogs with IgM or IgA monoclonal proteins if the protein levels in blood are high. In this syndrome, plasma viscosity can be many times normal, resulting in profound vascular disturbances, thrombosis, and bleeding. Depression, blindness, and neurologic manifestations can be due to hemorrhage in the nervous system and retina. Some IgM monoclonal proteins are cryoglobulins and aggregate in vitro and in vivo when the plasma is cooled. Animals with cryoglobulinemia often develop gangrenous sloughs of the ear tips, eyelids, digits, and tip of the tail, especially during cold weather. Animals with monoclonal gammopathies may have depressed levels of normal immunoglobulins and are therefore immunodeficient.

Immunoglobulin-secreting tumors usually are treated with appropriate chemotherapy. Plasmapheresis may be required to lower serum viscosity in animals with clinical signs of hyperviscosity syndrome.

INTEGUMENTARY SYSTEM

NEOPLASTIC SKIN DISEASES

MISCELLANEOUS SKIN DISEASES

INTEGUMENTARY SYSTEM INTRODUCTION

The skin is the largest organ of the body and, depending on the species and age, may represent 12%–24% of an animal's body weight. The skin has many functions, including serving as an enclosing barrier and providing environmental protection, regulating temperature, producing pigment and vitamin D, and sensory perception. Anatomically, the skin consists of the following structures: epidermis, basement membrane zone, dermis, appendageal system, and subcutaneous muscles and fat.

Epidermis: The epidermis is composed of multiple layers of cells consisting of keratinocytes, melanocytes, Langerhans cells, and Merkel cells.

Keratinocytes function to produce a protective barrier. They are produced from columnar basal cells attached to a basement membrane. The rate of cell mitosis and subsequent keratinization are controlled by a variety of factors, including nutrition, hormones, tissue factors, immune cells in the skin, and genetics. The dermis may also exert significant control over the growth of the epidermis. It has been hypothesized that photoperiod and reproduction cycles may affect the epidermis in animals. Glucocorticoids decrease mitotic activity; disease and inflammation also alter normal epidermal growth and keratinization. As keratinocytes migrate upward, they undergo a complex process of programmed cell death or keratinization. The goal of this process is to produce a compact layer of dead cells called the stratum corneum, which functions as an impermeable barrier to the loss of fluids, electrolytes, minerals, nutrients, and water, while preventing the penetration of infectious or noxious agents into the skin. The structural arrangement of keratin and the lipid content of the skin are critical to this function. The vitamin D precursor, 7-dehydrocholesterol, is formed in the epidermis. The epidermis is thickest in large animals. The stratum corneum is continuously shed or desquamated.

Melanocytes are located in the basal cell layer, outer root sheath, and ducts of sebaceous and sweat glands. They are responsible for the production of skin and hair pigment (melanin). Production of pigment is under hormonal and genetic control.

Langerhans cells are mononuclear dendritic cells that are intimately involved in regulating the immune system of the skin. They are damaged by excessive UV light exposure and glucocorticoids. Antigenic and allergenic material is processed by these cells and transported to local and nodal T cells to induce hypersensitivity reactions. Epidermal proteins may also conjugate with exogenous haptens, rendering them antigenic.

Merkel cells are specialized sensory cells associated with skin sensory organs, eg, whiskers and tylotrich pads.

Basement Membrane Zone: This area serves as a site for attachment of basal epidermal cells and as a protective barrier between the epidermis and dermis. A variety of skin diseases, including several autoimmune conditions, can cause damage to this zone. Vesicles are an example of a damaged basement membrane zone.

Dermis: The dermis is a mesenchymal structure that supports, nourishes, and to some degree, regulates the epidermis and appendages. The dermis consists of ground substance, dermal collagen fibers, and cells (fibroblasts, melanocytes, mast cells, and occasionally eosinophils, neutrophils, lymphocytes, histiocytes, and plasma cells). Blood vessels responsible for thermoregulation, nerve plexuses associated with cutaneous sensation, and both myelinated and unmyelinated nerves are present in the dermis. Motor nerves are primarily adrenergic and innervate blood vessels and arrector pili muscles. Except in horses, apocrine glands do not appear to be innervated. Sensory nerves are distributed in the dermis, hair follicles, and specialized tactile structures. The skin responds to the sensations of touch, pain, itch, heat, and cold.

Appendageal System: These structures grow out of (and are continuous with) the epidermis and consist of hair follicles, sebaceous and sweat glands, and specialized structures (eg, claw, hoof). The hair follicles of horses and cattle are simple, ie, the follicles have one hair emerging from each pore. The hair follicles of dogs, cats, sheep, and goats are compound, ie, the follicles have a central hair surrounded by 3–15 smaller hairs all exiting from a common pore. Animals with compound hair follicles are born with simple hair follicles that develop into compound hair follicles.

The growth of hair is controlled by a number of factors, including nutrition, hormones, and photoperiod. The growing stage of the hair is referred to as anagen, and the resting stage (mature hair) is referred to as telogen. The transitional stage between anagen and telogen is catagen. Animals normally shed their hair coat in response to changes in temperature and photoperiod; most animals undergo a shed in the early spring and early fall. The size, shape, and length of hair is controlled by genetic factors but may be influenced by disease, exogenous drugs, nutritional deficiencies, and environment. Hormones have a significant effect on hair growth. Thyroxine initiates hair growth, and glucocorticoids inhibit hair growth. The primary functions of the hair coat are to provide a mechanical barrier, to protect the host from actinic damage, and to provide thermoregulation. In most species, trapping dead air space between secondary hairs conserves heat. This requires that the hairs be dry and waterproof; the cold-weather coat of many animals is often longer and finer to facilitate heat conservation. The hair coat can also help cool the skin. The warm-weather coat of animals, particularly large animals, consists of shorter thicker hairs and fewer secondary hairs. This anatomic change allows air to move easily through the coat, which facilitates cooling. The hair coat also helps conceal or camouflage the animal.

Sebaceous glands are simple or branched alveolar, holocrine glands that secrete sebum into the hair follicles and onto the epidermal surface. They are present in large numbers near the mucocutaneous junction, interdigital spaces, dorsal neck area, rump, chin, and tail area; in some species, they are part of the scent-marking system. For example, in cats, sebaceous glands are present on the face, dorsum, and tail in high concentration; cats mark territories by rubbing their face on objects and depositing a layer of sebum laced with feline facial pheromones. Sebum is a complex lipid material containing cholesterol, cholesterol esters, triglycerides, diester waxes, and fatty acids. Sebum is important to keep the skin soft and pliable and to maintain proper hydration; it gives the hair coat sheen and has antimicrobial properties.

Sweat glands (epitrichial [formerly apocrine] and atrichial [formerly eccrine]) are part of the thermoregulatory system. The evaporation of sweat from the skin is the primary body cooling mechanism for horses and primates and, to a lesser degree, pigs, sheep, and goats. There is some clinical evidence to suggest that limited sweating occurs in dogs and cats, and that it may have a minor role in cooling the body. Dogs and cats thermoregulate primarily by panting, drooling, and spreading saliva on their coats (cats). Cats also sweat through their paws, especially when excited; this is most commonly seen as wet paw prints on surfaces, eg, examination tables.

Subcutaneous Muscles and Fat: The "twitch muscle" (panniculus carnosus) is the major subcutaneous muscle. The subcutaneous fat (panniculus adiposus) serves many functions, including insulation; reservoir for fluids, electrolytes, and energy; and shock absorber.

DERMATITIS

Inflammation of the skin can be produced by numerous agents, including external irritants, burns, allergens, trauma, and infection (bacterial, viral, parasitic, or fungal). It can be associated with concurrent internal or systemic disease; hereditary factors also may be involved. Allergies form an important group of etiologic factors, especially in small animals.

The skin's response to insult is generically called dermatitis and manifests as any combination of pruritus, scaling, erythema, thickening or lichenification of the skin, hyperpigmentation, oily seborrhea, odor, and hair loss. The usual progression of a skin disease involves an underlying trigger (disease syndrome) that causes primary lesions such as papules, pustules, and vesicles. Pruritus is a common clinical sign in many diseases, and in conditions that are not inherently pruritic, it is often present because of secondary infections or as a result of production of inflammatory mediators. As the inflammatory changes progress, crusting and scaling develop. If the process involves the deeper dermis, exudation, pain, and sloughing of the skin may occur. Secondary bacterial and yeast infections commonly develop as a result of skin inflammation. As dermatitis becomes chronic, acute signs of inflammation (eg, erythema) subside and primary lesions become obscured by signs of chronic inflammation (thickening of the skin, hyperpigmentation, scaling, seborrhea). Often, the skin becomes drier; if pruritus is not a component of the underlying trigger, it will often develop at this stage. Resolution of dermatitis requires identification of the underlying cause and treatment of secondary infections or other complications.

DERMATOLOGIC PROBLEMS

Dermatitis is a nonspecific term usually used until the dermatologic history, clinical signs, and physical examination can more precisely define the problem. Dermatologic problems are a major category of clinical findings that can be caused by a number of skin diseases; many skin diseases look alike and are differentiated by working through diagnostic flow charts and a process of elimination. The most common dermatologic problems include pruritus, alopecia, crusting and scaling, otitis, nonhealing wounds, nodules and tumors, and ulcerative disorders. In some species, such as cats, there may be well-recognized subcategories of dermatologic problems (eg, head and neck pruritus, symmetric alopecia, eosinophilic exudation/dermatitis, etc). Defining the major dermatologic problem will help create a specific differential diagnosis list and aid selection of appropriate diagnostic tests. The animal's dermatologic problem may or may not be the owner's chief complaint. It is important to be sensitive to owners' perceptions of problems or complaints, especially if odor or aesthetics are involved, and to address them (eg, bathing to minimize odor while the key problem is being evaluated).

DIAGNOSIS OF SKIN DISEASES

Definitive diagnosis of the causes of various skin diseases requires a detailed history, physical examination, and appropriate diagnostic tests. Many skin diseases look alike, and a definitive diagnosis is made over time by including or excluding possible causes, evaluating responses to therapy, and/or process of elimination.

History

A careful dermatologic history is critical to interpret the physical examination findings and choose appropriate diagnostic tests. A complete general history should be obtained, including information about prior illnesses, vaccinations, husbandry (housing, feeding practices, etc), changes in attitude and food consumption, elimination practices, exposure to other animals, and travel within the past 6–12 mo. This should be followed by a detailed dermatologic history. Use of a preprinted history form can be very useful for chronic or complicated cases. A good history is important, because many skin diseases that look similar are differentiated based on interpreting clinical signs and historical patterns.

The following information should be obtained: 1) the primary complaint; 2) length of time the problem has been present; 3) age at which the skin disease started (distinct age predilections are seen in many diseases, eg, demodicosis and dermatophytosis in pediatric animals and signs of atopic dermatitis in animals 1–3 yr old); 4) breed (breed predilections include a predisposition of Cocker Spaniels to primary disorders of keratinization, and of terriers to atopic dermatitis); 5) presence and severity of pruritus (including licking, rubbing, scratching, or chewing behaviors—owners often do not realize licking may be a sign of pruritus); 6) how the disease started and its progression (diseases that begin with pruritus may lead to self-trauma and subsequent development of secondary skin lesions [alopecia, seborrhea] or infections [bacterial or yeast pyoderma]); 7) type and progression of lesions noted by the owner; 8) evidence of seasonality (suggesting fleas, allergic skin disease, or weather-related diseases); 9) area on the body the problem was first noticed (ie, regional patterns seen in atopic dermatitis [typically the face and feet], cheyletiellosis [primarily dorsal], scabies [primarily ventral], and endocrine hair loss [usually involves the trunk and spares the head and legs]); 10) any previous treatments and the responses to such (ie, antibiotic-responsive skin diseases suggest a bacterial cause; pruritus that responds to small doses of glucocorticoids, antihistamines, or essential fatty acids suggests allergic dermatitis); 11) frequency of bathing and when the last bath was given (recent bathing may obscure or change important clinical lesions, excessive bathing and wetting of the skin can predispose to skin disease); 12) presence of fleas, ticks, or mites; 13) other contact animals (ie, evidence of contagion, which suggests fleas, scabies, cheyletiellosis, or dermatophytosis); 14) the environment of the animal (housing changes can influence the development of certain skin diseases, eg, contact dermatitis, contagious diseases); and 15) signs or reports of systemic illness (endocrine [eg, hypothyroidism and hyperadrenocorticism] disorders and metabolic diseases [eg, diabetes mellitus, renal disease, liver disease] should be noted, because the skin can be the first place signs of systemic illness are noted).

Physical Examination

A complete physical examination should always be performed. Many skin diseases are manifestations of systemic diseases, eg, hypothyroidism, hyperadrenocorticism, hepatocutaneous syndrome, systemic lupus erythematosus. (*See also* MISCELLANEOUS SYSTEMIC DERMATOSES, p 973.) A good dermatologic examination requires very close inspection of the entire hair coat and skin under strong lighting; flashlights may be necessary to examine the skin of large animals. It is important to examine the ventrum of the animal, where many primary lesions and cutaneous parasites are found.

Clinical lesions are described in a variety of ways. Gross lesions can be described as focal, multifocal, or diffuse in distribution, followed by a description of the affected region (eg, mucocutaneous, truncal). On closer inspection, lesions may be further described as primary or secondary. Primary lesions include macules or patches (non-elevated areas of discoloration); papules or plaques (elevated lesions, the latter coalescing); pustules, vesicles, or bullae (fluid-filled lesions); wheals (flat-topped, steep-walled, solid elevations of the skin arising from histamine release); or nodules or tumors (large solid elevations of the skin). Secondary lesions include epidermal collarettes (late stage of a pustule), scars, excoriation (areas of self-trauma), erosions or ulcers (loss of the epidermis), fissures, lichenification (increased thickening and hyperpigmentation of the skin), and calluses. Some lesions may be either primary or secondary, depending on the cause of the disease. These include alopecia, scale, crusts, follicular casts (plugging of hair follicles with visible keratin), comedones (blackheads), and pigmentary changes.

Laboratory Procedures for Skin Diseases

Skin Scrapings: Skin scrapings are part of the basic database for all skin diseases. There are two types of skin scrapings, superficial and deep. Superficial scrapings do not cause capillary bleeding and provide information from the surface of the epidermis. Deep skin scrapings collect material from within the hair follicle; capillary bleeding indicates that the sampling was deep enough. Skin scrapings are used primarily to determine the presence or absence of mites. Skin scrapings are best performed using a skin-scraping spatula, which is a thin metal weighing spatula commonly found in pharmacy or chemical supply catalogs. These spatulas are reusable and do not cause injury.

Combing of the Hair Coat: This technique, commonly referred to as "flea combing," is useful to collect large amounts of skin debris and trap cutaneous parasites. Combings are particularly useful to find fleas, ticks, lice, and some mites. A clean scrub brush or curry comb can be used to collect material into a flat container (eg, pie plate) in large animals.

Examination of Hairs: Microscopic examination of hair shafts can be used to look for evidence of self-trauma, dermatophyte infections (requires clearing agents and special staining), dysplastic hairs, and sometimes, genetic diseases of the hair coat.

Cytology: Cutaneous and auricular cytology is helpful to identify bacterial, fungal, and, possibly, neoplastic skin diseases. At least 4–6 impression smears should be made; several slides should be saved for examination at a reference laboratory if necessary. When performing impression smears of the skin, the glass slide should be placed directly over the site to be sampled. An index finger or thumb should be placed directly over the slide and very firm pressure exerted. Alternatively, clear acetate tape can be used to sample the skin. Adequate sampling will produce a "thumb print" from the surface. At least one slide should be heat fixed with a match or lighter before staining. In most cases, a

Romanowsky-type stain is adequate. In pruritic animals, material should be scraped from beneath nail beds and smeared onto glass slides for heat fixing, staining, and cytologic examination. Specimens should be examined under 4×, 10×, and oil immersion magnification.

Fungal Cultures: Dermatophyte infections are best identified with a fungal culture on either dermatophyte test medium or on plain Sabouraud agar. Plates that are easily inoculated are preferred; glass, screw-topped jars are difficult to inoculate and obtain samples from and are best avoided. Cats are best sampled using a new toothbrush aggressively combed over the affected lesions. Dogs can be sampled with either a toothbrush or via a hair plucking technique. In large animals, hairs should be gently wiped with alcohol before collecting to minimize contaminant growth. Intermediate and deep fungal organisms are best cultured at a reference laboratory using a skin biopsy specimen (6–8 mm in size).

Bacterial Cultures: Intact pustules can be cultured by rupturing the pustule with a sterile needle and swabbing the lesion with a sterile culture swab. Lesions should not be scrubbed before sampling. Deep pyodermas are best cultured from a skin biopsy (6–8 mm). The reference laboratory should be informed as to what pathogens are suspected, because this may affect how the exudate is cultured. Systemic and topical agents should be withheld for at least 72 hr before sampling.

Biopsy: Skin biopsies are indicated in any case that appears severe, unusual, or does not respond to appropriate therapy. Lesions should not be scrubbed before biopsy, because surface pathology is important in the diagnosis of many skin diseases. Several samples from a variety of lesions should be submitted for examination. Primary lesions should be sampled whenever possible; otherwise, the report is often not very helpful in making a diagnosis or narrowing a list of differential diagnoses. Biopsy specimens require examination by a pathologist familiar with skin diseases of animals. Direct immunofluorescence is not necessary to diagnose autoimmune skin diseases; routine histopathology is the test of choice.

Routine Blood and Urine Tests: In most dermatologic cases, these tests do not help to make a definitive diagnosis. If systemic signs of illness are present, then a CBC, serum chemistry panel, and urinalysis may be helpful to identify the cause. In dogs with recurrent infections, these tests may identify an underlying subclinical disease.

Intradermal Skin Testing: This test is not necessarily required to make a diagnosis of atopic dermatitis. A positive intradermal skin test reaction indicates past exposure to a particular allergen. Inhalant allergies are best diagnosed based on a compatible history, physical examination findings, and judicious use of intradermal skin testing or in vitro testing for allergies. Intradermal skin testing is recommended for animals in which immunotherapy is indicated because of the severity or duration of allergic signs. Potential drug interactions that can interfere with testing should be considered before intradermal skin testing is performed.

In Vitro Diagnostic Tests: In vitro diagnostic tests (ELISA or RAST tests) are an alternative to intradermal skin testing. Although in vitro tests are considered less reliable because of the large number of false-positive reactions, most complications in interpretation are the result of poor patient selection. Like intradermal skin tests, in vitro tests reflect exposure and must be interpreted in light of the animal's clinical signs and history.

COMMON DERMATOLOGIC PROBLEMS

The two most common dermatologic problems are alopecia and pruritus.

ALOPECIA

(Hair loss)

Alopecia is the partial or complete lack of hairs in areas where they are normally present. If an animal is presented for the problem of hair loss and pruritus is present, the problem of pruritus should be investigated first (*see* p 843).

Etiology: There are many causes of alopecia; any disease that can affect hair follicles can cause hair loss. There are two broad etiologic categories of alopecia: 1) congenital or hereditary and 2) acquired. Acquired alopecia is further divided into two categories: inflammatory and noninflammatory.

Congenital or hereditary alopecia (*see* p 846) has been described in cows, horses, dogs, cats, and pigs. Hairless breeds of mice, rats, cats, and dogs have been bred and developed for personal and research interests. Congenital alopecia may or may not be hereditary; it is caused by a lack of development of hair follicles and is apparent at, or shortly after, birth. Animals with tardive alopecias are born with normal coats, and focal or generalized hair loss occurs when the animal sheds its juvenile coat or when it becomes a young adult. Examples of this include pattern baldness of Dachshunds, color dilution alopecia (most commonly seen in Doberman Pinschers), and certain types of follicular dysplasias.

Acquired alopecia encompasses all other causes of hair loss. In this type of alopecia, the animal is born with a normal hair coat, has or had normal hair follicles at one time, and is or was capable of producing structurally normal hairs. Acquired alopecia may be noninflammatory, as is seen in endocrine alopecia or some types of immune-mediated alopecia, or inflammatory. Inflammatory acquired alopecia is the most common cause of alopecia. Acquired alopecia develops because a disease destroys the hair follicle or shaft, interferes with the growth of hair or wool, or causes the animal discomfort (eg, pain, pruritus), leading to self-trauma and loss of hair.

Diseases that can directly cause destruction or damage to the hair shaft or follicle include bacterial skin diseases, dermatophytosis, demodicosis, severe inflammatory diseases of the dermis (eg, juvenile cellulitis, deep pyoderma), traumatic episodes (eg, burns, radiation), and rarely, poisonings caused by mercury, thallium, and iodine. These diseases tend to be inflammatory.

Diseases that can directly inhibit or slow hair follicle growth include nutritional deficiencies (particularly protein deficiencies), hypothyroidism, hyperadrenocorticism, and excessive estrogen production or administration (hyperestrogenism, Sertoli cell tumors, estrogen injections for mismating). Temporary alopecia in horses, sheep, and dogs can occur during pregnancy, lactation, or several weeks after a severe illness or fever. Marked hair loss (effluvium) is common in cats after respiratory infection. These types of alopecia tend to be noninflammatory unless a secondary skin infection develops.

Pruritus or pain is a common cause of acquired inflammatory alopecia in animals. Diseases that commonly cause pruritus or pain include infectious skin diseases (eg, *bacterial pyoderma* and dermatophytosis), ectoparasites, allergic skin diseases (eg, atopic dermatitis, food allergy, contact, insect hypersensitivity), and less commonly, neoplastic skin diseases. Friction may cause local hair loss, eg, poorly fitted halters or collars. Rarely, excessive grooming may be the cause of hair loss in some animals, particularly cats.

Feline endocrine alopecia is no longer recognized as a bona fide syndrome; the current name is feline acquired symmetric alopecia. To date, there is no documented evidence of an endocrine disease in these cats, and the symmetric alopecia seen is a clinical sign of an underlying disease, most commonly a pruritic disease. The most common cause of feline symmetric alopecia is flea allergy dermatitis. In cats that do not have an obvious flea infestation, a CBC with differential is recommended; many cats that have flea allergy dermatitis have an eosinophilia. This finding may help convince owners to pursue flea control as a first diagnostic step.

Clinical Findings and Lesions: The clinical signs of hair loss may be obvious or subtle, depending on the disease. Congenital or hereditary hair loss is commonly symmetric and not accompanied by many inflammatory changes; in some cases, the areas of hair loss are localized to one region (eg, ear flaps) or to well-demarcated areas.

The clinical signs of acquired hair loss are varied and often influenced by the underlying cause(s); the pattern of hair loss may be focal, multifocal, symmetric, or generalized. Inflammatory changes such as hyperpigmentation, lichenification, erythema, scaling, excessive shedding, and pruritus are common. Some causes of acquired alopecia may predispose the animal to development of secondary skin diseases, such as a bacterial pyoderma or seborrhea. Pruritus is variable, depending on the primary cause. In endocrine alopecias, the hair loss usually develops in a symmetric pattern, often in wear areas first; pruritus is uncommon unless there is a secondary infection. Contrary to previous thought, hair loss is not generally an early clinical sign of an endocrine alopecia.

Many owners seek veterinary assistance because of perceived excessive shedding. Shedding may be abnormal (excessive) if it results in obvious loss of the hair coat and areas of alopecia. A common cause of abnormal shedding is bacterial pyoderma. If, however, the shedding is not accompanied by development of patchy or symmetric hair loss, it is likely that it is just a stage in the natural replacement of the hair coat.

Diagnosis: An accurate diagnosis of the cause of alopecia requires a careful history and physical examination. Key points in the history include recognition of breed predispositions for congenital or hereditary alopecias; the duration and progression of lesions; and the presence or absence of pruritus, evidence of contagion, or nondermatologic problems, eg, polyuria and polydipsia. On physical examination, the distribution of lesions should be noted (focal, multifocal, symmetric, generalized), and the hairs examined to determine whether they are being shed from the hair follicle or broken off—the latter suggesting pruritus. Signs of secondary skin infections or ectoparasites should be noted, and a careful nondermatologic examination should be performed.

Initial diagnostic tests include skin scrapings for ectoparasites (particularly *Demodex* mites); combing of the hair coat for fleas, mites, and lice; impression smears of the skin for evidence of bacterial or yeast infections; fungal cultures for identification of dermatophytosis; and examination of plucked hairs, looking at both the shaft and the ends for evidence of dermatophytosis or that the hairs were chewed off. In many cases of bacterial pyoderma, impression smears of the skin do not show neutrophils and/or cocci, but they may show large numbers of shed keratinocytes. Neutrophils and cocci are seen if pustules or recently ruptured pustules are sampled.

If these tests do not identify or suggest an underlying cause, a skin biopsy may be indicated to evaluate hair follicle structures, numbers, and anagen/telogen ratios and to look for evidence of bacterial, fungal, or parasitic skin infections. In addition, skin biopsies are often needed to confirm congenital or tardive causes of hair loss and to identify inflammatory or neoplastic causes of hair loss. Skin biopsies from normal and abnormal sites should be submitted for evaluation. CBC, serum chemistry panels, and urinalyses are generally only helpful when an endocrinopathy is suspected. Specific endocrine function tests can be performed based on findings of routine laboratory work or clinical signs.

Treatment: Successful therapy depends on the underlying cause and specific diagnosis.

PRURITUS

(Itching)

Pruritus is defined as an unpleasant sensation within the skin that provokes the desire to scratch.

Pathophysiology: Pruritus may be well or poorly localized. It may manifest as a sharp or diffuse, burning sensation. Although the skin is richly innervated, there are no known specialized pruritus receptors. The sensation of itch is transmitted via a specialized set of afferent fibers. Myelinated fibers that conduct sensations at 10–20 m/sec carry the well-localized pricking itch sensation. In contrast, the sensation of burning itch is transmitted via nonmyelinated fibers that conduct sensations at 2 m/sec. Both of these fibers enter the dorsal root of the spinal cord, ascend through the dorsal column, and cross into the lateral spinothalamic tract. From there they go to the thalamus and on to the sensory cortex.

The mediators of pruritus are controversial and may vary depending on the species. These putative mediators include histamines (released from mast cell degranulation), proteolytic enzymes (proteases), and leukotrienes. Proteases are released by fungi, bacteria, and mast cell degranulation, and during antigen-antibody reactions. Leukotrienes, prostaglandins, and thromboxane A_2, which are broken down from arachidonic acid, are pro-inflammatory. Essential fatty acids, particularly glinolenic acid, have been used to counter the inflammation mediated by leukotrienes and thromboxane A_2. The sensation of pruritus may be affected by a variety of factors, including boredom, competing sensations, and anxiety. Stress may potentiate pruritus via the release of opioid peptides.

Etiology: Pruritus is a clinical sign and not a diagnosis or specific disease. In general, the most common causes of pruritus are parasites, infections, allergic skin diseases, and miscellaneous causes (eg, cutaneous neoplasia). Many diseases that are nonpruritic (eg, endocrinopathies) become pruritic when the animal develops secondary bacterial or yeast infections.

Diagnosis: A thorough dermatologic history and physical examination should be performed. Parasitic causes of pruritus, including *Demodex*, fleas and ticks, contagious mites, and lice, should be excluded, because they are most common. Skin scrapings can exclude (or include) various mite infestations, including *Demodex*. However, some mite infestations (eg, *Sarcoptes*, *Cheyletiella*, *Psoroptes*, *Chorioptes*) might be missed on skin scrapings. If a mite infestation is suspected, a response to therapy trial should be undertaken. The most commonly used drug in these cases is ivermectin. Fleas can be excluded or included based on a history of flea control, response to flea control, or finding evidence of flea infestation via a flea combing. Flea control practices can also exclude louse infestations.

The next most important group of pruritic diseases to exclude is infectious causes of skin disease. These include bacterial infections (primarily staphylococcal infections, *Malassezia* overgrowth, and dermatophytosis). A fungal culture should be performed in any cat presented for pruritus. It is also highly recommended in dogs that are newly acquired, any animal with a possible history of exposure and/or compatible clinical signs, or when there is a history of people with skin disease. Concurrent bacterial and yeast infections are increasingly recognized as a common cause of pruritus in dogs, cats, and large animals. Bacterial pyoderma is underdiagnosed in cats, and a response to therapy trial may be needed to exclude or include it.

Infectious causes of pruritus commonly induce clinical signs of hair loss, scaling, scales piercing hairs, odor, and/or greasy seborrhea. Marked pedal pruritus and facial rubbing are common in animals with concurrent yeast and bacterial infections. Before pursuing allergies as a cause of pruritus or performing skin biopsies or other more expensive and/or invasive diagnostic testing, a concurrent bacterial and yeast infection should be excluded. A 21–30 day concurrent course of an antibiotic effective against *Staphylococcus* spp (eg, cephalexin 30 mg/kg, PO, bid) and a systemic antifungal (eg, ketoconazole, itraconazole, or fluconazole 5–10 mg/kg/day, PO) should be prescribed. If the pruritus resolves, then existing pruritus was due to a microbial infection.

It is possible that the initial trigger has long passed or is seasonal. However, if the animal's pruritus is unchanged or only somewhat better, the most likely underlying cause is allergic (assuming parasitic causes have been excluded). The most common causes of allergic pruritus are insect bite hypersensitivity (eg, flea allergy, mosquito bite allergy, fly bite), food allergy, and atopic dermatitis. Flea allergy dermatitis and insect bite hypersensitivity are excluded based on response to insect control. Animals that do not have insect bite hypersensitivity but are seasonally pruritic most likely have atopic dermatitis. Animals with year-round allergic pruritus have atopic dermatitis and/or food allergy. Food allergy is excluded or included based on response to a diet trial and provocative challenge. Atopic dermatitis is a clinical diagnosis; in vitro allergy testing and intradermal skin testing show only antigen exposure patterns. These tests are used to determine the contents of an immunotherapy vaccine.

Treatment: Successful therapy depends on identification of the underlying cause. Animals with idiopathic pruritus or those in which treatment of the underlying disease does not eliminate the pruritus (eg, atopic animals) require medical management of pruritus. Currently, evidence-based reviews of antipruritic do not support the use of antihistamines to control pruritus.

Essential Fatty Acids: Essential fatty acids are rarely effective as sole antipruritic agents and are not suitable for acute flares of pruritus. If they are beneficial, it is a longterm therapy.

Glucocorticoids: Glucocorticoids are the most effective drugs in the management of pruritus. However, they cannot be used safely for longterm management because of adverse effects (eg, suppression of adrenal function, risk of development of diabetes mellitus, risk of secondary urinary tract infections). In addition, owners can rarely tolerate the common adverse effects (polydipsia, polyuria, polyphagia, and panting) for long periods. Anti-inflammatory dosages range from 0.5–1 mg/kg/day, PO, for 5–10 days and then every other day. Topical spray formulations of triamcinolone acetate are highly effective and good alternatives to oral steroids.

Other Systemic Antipruritic Agents: Cyclosporine modified is a highly effective nonsteroidal drug for control of pruritus. The only formulation that can be used is modified cyclosporine. The dosage is 5 mg/kg for dogs and 7 mg/kg for cats. Maximal benefit can take as long as 30 days to observe. Once efficacy is established, dose tapering to every other day can be attempted. Common adverse effects include vomiting and diarrhea (common) and gingival hyperplasia (less common). Another drug for control of pruritus in dogs is oclacitinib, a Janus kinase inhibitor that provides rapid relief from pruritus and inflammation in dogs with short- and longterm allergic skin disease.

PRINCIPLES OF TOPICAL THERAPY

See also SYSTEMIC PHARMACOTHERAPEUTICS OF THE INTEGUMENTARY SYSTEM, p 2571.

Topical therapy is an important part of veterinary dermatology. It is often beneficial in improving the cosmetic appearance or odor of the animal, pending the final diagnosis. It can be beneficial as an adjunct to systemic therapy. Finally, it may be the preferred method of treatment for some diseases, eg, flea infestations.

The following are some basic guidelines to consider when prescribing topical therapy:

1) As much of the hair coat as possible should be removed when treating skin diseases. Good grooming practices facilitate topical therapy and can significantly help shorten the course of disease. 2) The cooperation of the owner (and animal) should be evaluated before any topical therapy is prescribed. 3) Animals tend to groom off topical products and may vomit after ingestion. The risk of toxicity is a constant worry for owners. Local ointments, gels, and sprays are best used sparingly, under occlusion, and for specific diseases. Such medications often sting when applied to the skin, especially many of those instilled into the ears. Many agents also may mat the hair. 4) Tepid water is the temperature of choice for bathing animals. 5) The old adage, "If it's wet, dry it and if it's dry, wet it," has some truth to it; however, this advice should not be carried to extremes. Exudative lesions, eg, areas of pyotraumatic dermatitis, heal faster if they are kept clean and covered with an antibiotic ointment or gel (previous recommendations suggested aggressive astringent use). Dry, lichenified skin is often pruritic, and the judicious use of emollients may be beneficial. 6) The animal should be monitored closely for possible development of irritant or allergic contact dermatitis from topical agents. Many topical agents have very similar bases or ingredients, and changing from one to another may only exacerbate the problem. 7) Owners should be given careful and thorough instructions on how to administer the therapy.

Shampoo Therapy: Shampoos are the most commonly used topical treatments. There are three broad classes of shampoos: cleansing, antiparasitic, and medicated. **Cleansing shampoos** remove dirt and excess oils from the coat. These products include over-the-counter dog grooming shampoos, flea shampoos, and many mild human products. These products lather well and must be rinsed from the coat. **Antiparasitic shampoos** are "flea shampoos." In most cases, the amount of insecticide in these products is not adequate to kill all the fleas in a severe infestation. However, these products are excellent routine cleansing products. **Medicated shampoos** include antimicrobial and antiseborrheic products. The most widely used antibacterial shampoos contain chlorhexidine or benzoyl peroxide. Antiseborrheic shampoos contain some combination of tar, sulfur, and salicylic acid—ingredients that are keratoplastic and keratolytic. Tar is recommended for oily seborrhea, and sulfur and salicylic acid are recommended for scaly seborrhea. Most animals benefit from products that contain all three agents; however, tar products are contraindicated in cats.

When a medicated shampoo is used, the animal should be washed in a cleansing shampoo before the medicated shampoo and rinsed well. Medicated shampoos often are not good cleansing agents, do not lather well, or do not work well in the presence of organic debris. The medicated shampoo should be applied evenly to the hair coat after being prediluted in water. Prediluting the shampoo will facilitate it being rinsed from the coat and minimize the potential for irritant or allergic contact dermatitis. Depending on the shampoo, the concentration of shampoo to water will vary between 1:3 and 1:4. If possible, the medicated shampoo should be allowed to have a contact time of 10 min with the skin and then rinsed thoroughly from the coat. Shampoo residue is a common cause of irritant reactions. Finally, the medicated shampoo should be used often, usually 2–3 times/wk during the early stages of therapy.

The use of medicated antimicrobial shampoo therapy is increasing because of concerns over development of methicillin-resistant staphylococcal infections.

CONGENITAL AND INHERITED ANOMALIES OF THE INTEGUMENTARY SYSTEM

Congenital dermatoses of the skin may be genetic or arise during embryogenesis because of nongenetic factors. Genetic mutations that cause skin anomalies may be present at birth or become apparent weeks to months later. These late-onset manifestations are referred to as tardive developmental defects. Both congenital and tardive developmental dermatoses are fairly common in domestic animals of all species, with the greatest number of well-defined defects described in cattle and dogs.

CONGENITAL ANOMALIES OF THE SKIN

Epitheliogenesis imperfecta (aplasia cutis) is a congenital discontinuity of squamous epithelium. It is seen in cattle (autosomal recessive trait), horses, swine, sheep, cats, and dogs, although it is rare in the latter three species. In cattle, affected breeds include Holstein-Friesian, Hereford, Ayrshire, Jersey, Shorthorn, Angus, Dutch Black Pied, Swedish Red Pied, and German Yellow Pied. It is common in swine, in which large lesions are obvious at birth as glistening red, well-demarcated discontinuities in the skin or mucous membranes. Infection and ulceration are early consequences. One or more hooves or claws may be deformed or absent; in some affected animals, there are other associated congenital anomalies. The condition is fatal when extensive, but small defects can be surgically corrected. Ultrastructural evaluation of this condition in American Saddlebred foals has demonstrated a relationship with junctional epidermolysis bullosa (*see* p 850).

Focal cutaneous hypoplasia and **subcutaneous hypoplasia** are congenital, circumscribed hypoplastic defects of multiple or deeper skin layers in swine. The lesions manifest as skin depressions in which all skin layers or the subcutaneous fat layers fail to develop normally.

A **nevus** is a circumscribed developmental defect of the skin, whereas a **hamartoma** is a hyperplastic mass formed as a result of a developmental defect in any organ. Both nevi and hamartomas have been described as congenital skin defects, but the problem may not become obvious until later in life. In dogs, sebaceous nevi, pigmented epidermal nevi, inflammatory linear verrucous epidermal nevi, nevi comedonicus, linear organoid nevi, and follicular hamartomas are known to occur. In horses, cannon keratosis and linear epidermal nevi have been described. Doubtless, similar defects occur in all species. Mixed, or organoid, nevi consist of circumscribed collections of densely packed adnexal structures (pilosebaceous nevus and pilosebaceosudoriferous nevus). Collagenous nevi are nodules composed of focal collagen hyperplasia that displace the normal structures of the skin. Most lesions are alopecic, with pigmented, pitted surfaces. When not extensive, nevi can be excised; otherwise there is no known effective treatment.

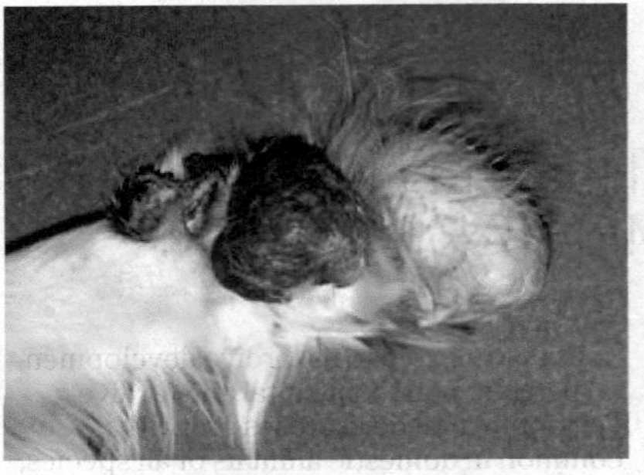

Collagenous nevus in a dog. *Courtesy of Dr. Robert Dunstan.*

Dermoid sinuses or **cysts** are seen in Thoroughbred horses and Rhodesian Ridgebacks (in which they are inherited) and occasionally other breeds of dogs. These are cystic structures lined with skin in which exfoliated skin, hair, and glandular debris accumulate. They are caused by failure of complete separation of the neural tube from the epidermis during embryogenesis; cysts are found on the dorsal midline and are rarely associated with spinal cord neural deficits. They can be removed by surgical excision.

Follicular cysts develop by abnormal hair follicle morphogenesis and by retention of follicular or glandular products. They may be congenital when caused by the failure of the follicular orifice to develop normally. Congenital cysts are most commonly identified in Merino and Suffolk sheep. Periauricular (dentigerous) cysts are seen in horses and, although present at birth, may not be recognized until adulthood. Wattle cysts are seen in Nubian goats; these arise from the bronchial cleft. Porcine wattles are seen fairly frequently in all breeds of swine. These are teat-like growths on the lower jaw.

HEREDITARY ALOPECIA AND HYPOTRICHOSIS

Alopecia is the absence of hair; hypotrichosis, which is much more common, is the presence of less hair than normal. Although these defects can be generalized, they commonly develop in patterns that spare the extremities or correlate with hair color. These ectodermal defects can be congenital or tardive and can be associated with abnormal or absent adnexa, with defects in other ectodermal structures (such as teeth, claws, and eyes), or with skeletal and other developmental defects. There are various modes of inheritance in those instances in which familial occurrence has been studied.

X-linked ectodermal dysplasia has been reported in German Shepherds. Hairless breeds of dogs (eg, Mexican Hairless, Chinese Crested, American Hairless Terrier) and cats (Sphinx) have been bred for these ectodermal defects. Many sporadic cases of ectodermal defects are described in dogs, most often in males. Affected dogs, including most of the hairless breeds, often have patchy or pattern hypotrichosis as well as associated dental anomalies. All animals with abnormal follicular development are prone to comedone formation, hair follicle infections, and hair foreign-body granulomas.

At least 13 types of **hypotrichosis** have been described in cattle, affecting Angus, Ayrshire, Brangus, Holstein-Friesian, Hereford, polled Hereford, Guernsey, Gelbvieh, Jersey, as well as Normandy-Maine, Anjou-Charolais, and Simmental crosses. Most have autosomal recessive or sex-linked modes of inheritance. Associated defects include failure of horn development, hypophyseal hypoplasia, macroglossia, dental anomalies, abnormal coat coloration, and death (lethal hypotrichosis). Viable hypotrichosis, hypotrichosis with anodontia, semihairlessness, streaked hairlessness, black hair follicle dysplasia (Holstein), and cross-related hypotrichosis (rat tail) are specific types described in cattle.

In sheep, hypotrichosis is rarely reported, with the best known syndrome affecting the Polled Dorset. This involves the hair of the face most severely, but the wool is also of poor quality. In goats, hypotrichosis is associated with congenital goiter. In swine, two forms of hypotrichosis are known (Mexican Hairless, German), one of which is associated with goiter and death in the homozygote.

In dogs, there are several tardive **follicle dysplasias**, including color dilution alopecia. This is found in some dogs bearing the coat color genotype dd, which renders black genotypes blue and liver genotypes beige or fawn. This syndrome is best known in Doberman Pinschers but is also commonly seen in color dilute Dachshunds, Italian Greyhounds, Greyhounds, Whippets, Yorkshire Terriers, and tricolor hounds and has been reported in a German Shepherd. Recently, "silver Labrador Retrievers" with color dilution alopecia have been reported. Affected dogs are born with normal hair coats but before 1 yr of age begin to develop folliculitis and hypotrichosis that is progressive and confined to the blue- or fawn-colored areas. Black hair follicle dysplasia, a similar but earlier developing and more complete hypotrichosis, is seen in black and white piebald dogs. The hypotrichosis develops shortly after birth and affects only the black-colored areas. This syndrome is best known in the Papillon and Bearded Collie. Recent genetic analysis in Large Munsterlanders has indicated an autosomal recessive inheritance in this breed. A similar follicular dysplasia is reported in nonpiebald breeds. Other types of follicular dysplasias of uncertain cause include seasonal flank alopecia of Boxers and Airedale Terriers and various woolly syndromes and post-clipping alopecia in Spitz-type breeds. Familial hypotrichosis of Irish Water Spaniels develops at 2–4 yr of age, and a dominant mode of inheritance has been suggested. The condition formerly known as growth hormone-responsive alopecia in Pomeranians and other breeds is now called alopecia X, reflecting the complexity of factors, hereditary and otherwise, influencing these syndromes.

In cats, follicular dysplasia is seen in the Devon Rex. In horses, both color dilution alopecia and black hair follicle dysplasias are occasionally reported, especially in Appaloosas. Congenital progressive hypotrichosis has been reported in a blue roan Percheron. Reported hair shaft structural abnormalities of dogs and cats include pili torti (American Wirehaired Cat), trichorrhexis nodosa, and spiculosis (Kerry Blue Terrier).

HYPERPLASTIC AND SEBORRHEIC SYNDROMES

Many anomalies affect keratinization; some are associated with hereditary hypotrichoses (*see* p 846), whereas others are associated with systemic metabolic derangements. Those for which none of these associations has yet been made are a diverse group of syndromes that may affect localized parts of the epithelium or that may be generalized. Among the latter are the poorly characterized congenital or familial seborrheic syndromes, the best known of which is idiopathic seborrhea of Spaniels and idiopathic facial dermatitis of Persian cats. **Hereditary congenital follicular parakeratosis** is a syndrome of female Rottweilers and Siberian Huskies. It is a severe keratinization defect associated with various noncutaneous abnormalities.

Cutaneous ichthyoses are characterized by abnormal and hypertrophic epithelial proliferation, with accumulation of extensive scale and hyperkeratosis on the skin surface. Cases have been described mostly in cattle and dogs, but chicken and several mouse models are also known, and there is one report in a llama. In cattle, the severity varies; some forms are lethal shortly after birth. Affected breeds include Red Poll, Friesian, Holstein, Brown Swiss, Pinzgauer, and Chianina.

Canine ichthyosiform dermatoses are also heterogeneous and occur sporadically in a number of breeds, including Doberman Pinschers, Rottweilers, Irish Setters, Collies, English Springer Spaniels, Cavalier King Charles Spaniels, Golden Retrievers, Labrador Retrievers, and terriers (including Parson Russell Terriers). There is some evidence of a familial inheritance pattern in Parson Russell Terriers and Golden Retrievers. In dogs, the body is covered with large adherent scales that may flake off in large sheets. The planum nasale and digital pads may be markedly thickened in some forms; the latter usually is associated with apparent discomfort. Clinical management is difficult, but signs may be ameliorated with keratinolytic shampoos or solutions (eg, selenium disulfides, lactic acid, benzoyl peroxide) and with humectants (eg, lactic acid, urea, propylene glycol, and essential fatty acid preparations). Experimental use of synthetic retinoids has been helpful. Control of secondary pyoderma is frequently required.

Psoriasiform-lichenoid dermatosis affects young English Springer Spaniels and is presumed to be genetic. The erythematous, symmetric lesions, which consist of papules and plaques on the pinnae and inguinal region, are covered with scales and become increasingly hyperkeratotic if left untreated. In some affected dogs, the lesions may eventually spread, and the skin is severely greasy. Spontaneous remissions and a waxing and waning course are recorded. Some dogs respond to antibiotic treatment or to synthetic retinoids, but most are refractory to therapy. Cyclosporine therapy has been used with mixed results in some dogs.

Pityriasis rosea of pigs is a familial disease in which the mode of inheritance is not known. (*See* p 979 for clinical findings, diagnosis, and treatment.) **Dermatosis vegetans** of Landrace pigs is a hereditary, possibly congenital, disorder with an autosomal recessive mode of inheritance. It must be differentiated in the early stages from pityriasis rosea. This is a more serious disease and affects the hooves as well as the skin. Lesions begin as macules and papules and are scaly as in pityriasis rosea. They later become covered with brown-black crusts and are associated with coronitis and hoof deformity. Piglets fail to thrive and eventually develop pneumonia; the disease is not uniformly fatal, but affected survivors are stunted. There is no effective treatment.

Familial footpad hyperkeratosis is reported in Irish Terriers and Dogues de Bordeaux. All pads of all feet are involved from a young age, although the disease is not usually congenital. When hyperkeratosis is severe, horns, fissures, and secondary infection cause pain and lameness. No other skin lesions are present. Treatment is symptomatic, with soaking, keratolytic and emollient treatments, with treatment of bacterial pyoderma. No reports of the use of synthetic retinoids are available. Major differential diagnoses for footpad hyperkeratosis include hepatocutaneous syndrome, a disorder of keratinization, and pemphigus.

Granulomatous sebaceous adenitis is an idiopathic disease that destroys the sebaceous glands and, in some breeds of dogs, is associated with a severe seborrheic and alopecic dermatosis. It is hereditary in Standard Poodles and suspected to be familial in Akitas. It first manifests itself in young adults, but inapparent carriers are known in Poodles. Marked hyperkeratosis precedes development of hair coat abnormalities, which begin as loss of normal hair kinkiness and progress to patchy alopecia. Akitas tend to have more seborrhea oleosa and less alopecia than Poodles. Response to treatment is inconsistent and incomplete. Mildly affected dogs are treated with antiseborrheic shampoos and treatment of pyoderma as needed. Severely affected dogs have benefited from propylene glycol or hot oil treatments. Some dogs respond to oral supplementation with omega-3 fatty acids, and some respond to synthetic retinoids. Spontaneous remission has been recorded. Recently, modified cyclosporine A (5 mg/kg/day, PO) has been very effective in the treatment of many dogs.

PIGMENTARY ABNORMALITIES

Many associations between skin and coat color and developmental anomalies have been recorded in domestic animals. Some of the associations with hypotrichosis are discussed under hereditary alopecia (*see* p 846).

Albinism appears to be rare in domestic animals. True albinism is always associated with pink or pale irises and with visual defects and increased risk of solar radiation–induced neoplasms of the skin. It has been noted in Icelandic sheep and in Guernsey, Austrian Murboden, Shorthorn,

Brown Swiss, and Charolais cattle. Albinism must be differentiated from extreme white spotting or piebaldism and dominant white. Some animals with extreme piebaldism or dominant white have associated neurologic anomalies or deafness, or suffer death in utero. Lethal white foal syndrome is one that results from breeding two Overo Paints. In dogs and cats, dominant white or extreme piebaldism can be associated with unilateral or bilateral deafness and sometimes with blue irides or iris heterochromia. White cats with bilateral blue eyes have a 75% chance of deafness. In dogs, deafness may also be associated with merle hair coats and is found in Dalmatians, Sealyham Terriers, harlequin Great Danes, Collies, and white Bull Terriers. Cyclic neutropenia may be found in gray or pale merle Collies. In Rhodesian Ridgebacks, pale coat color is associated with cerebellar degeneration. In Chédiak-Higashi syndrome (*see* p 50) of cats and cattle (Herefords, Japanese Black, Brangus), coat color dilution (blue smoke in cats) is associated with neutrophil and platelet abnormalities and shortened life span. This is inherited as an autosomal recessive trait. Male tricolor cats (calico and tortoiseshell) are sterile because the gene for orange is X-linked and recessive, and males have the abnormal XXY genotype.

Pigmentary abnormalities may be acquired, and some of these may be hereditary or familial, as in **vitiligo**. As a familial disease, vitiligo is best recognized in Arabian horses (Arabian fading syndrome, pinky syndrome); it may also be familial in cattle (Holstein-Friesian), Siamese cats, and in some breeds of dogs (Belgian Tervuren, Rottweiler). Affected animals develop somewhat symmetric macular depigmentation of the skin that occasionally also affects the hair coat and claws or hooves. The onset is usually in young adulthood. Most lesions are on the face, especially the muzzle or planum nasale or around the eyes. Depigmentation may wax and wane. Complete remission may occur but is rare. There is no accompanying systemic or cutaneous pathology. No treatment is available; treatments used in people with vitiligo are unlikely to provide significant cosmetic results in animals.

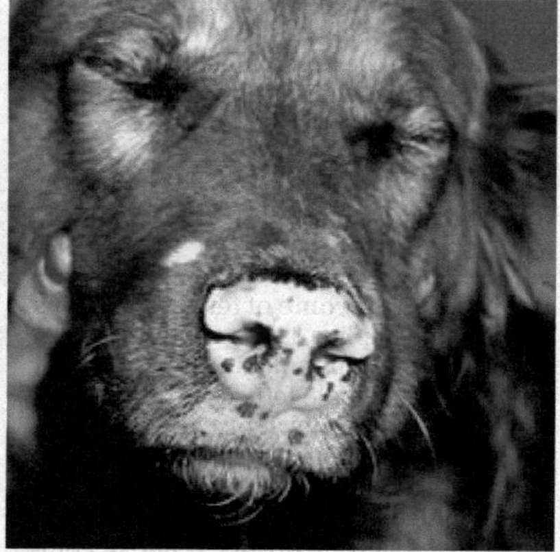

Vitiligo in an adult Golden Retriever. *Courtesy of Dr. Stephen White.*

Lentigo in orange and orange-faced male cats is marked by the development of asymptomatic, pigmented macules. Lesions are first seen on the lips and eyelids at <1 yr of age. Other sites include the planum nasale and gingivae. Lentigines are not precancerous and have no medical consequence.

Acquired aurotrichia of Miniature Schnauzers is a familial syndrome in which hair along the dorsal midline changes to golden from the normal black or gray of this breed. The onset is usually in young adulthood. The change may be associated with thinning in the hair coat but no other cutaneous or systemic signs. In most dogs, coat color reverts to normal within 1–2 yr.

DEFECTS OF STRUCTURAL INTEGRITY

This category includes genetic defects in structural elements responsible for the integrity of the epidermis and dermal-epidermal junction, as well as some dermal structural anomalies.

Cutaneous asthenia (dermatosparaxis, Ehlers-Danlos syndrome) is a group of syndromes characterized by defects in collagen production. This results in a variety of clinical signs including loose, hyperextensible, fragile skin; joint laxity; and other connective tissue dysfunctions. These collagen defects have been described in cattle (Belgian Blue and White, Charolais, Hereford, Holstein-Freisian, Simmental), a goat, sheep (Norwegian Dala, Border Leicester-Southdown, Finnish-Merino cross, Romney, White Dorper), pigs (Large White-Essex cross), horses (Quarter horse, Arabian cross), rabbits (New Zealand white), cats (Himalayan and domestic shorthair), mink, and dogs (a litter of Garafiano Shepherds, sporadically in several breeds). The mode of inheritance has been demonstrated for Himalayan cats (recessive) and domestic shorthair cats (dominant).

Clinical features include fragile skin from the time of birth, wounds that heal with thin scars, delayed wound healing, pendulous skin, and hematoma and hygroma formation. In lambs, rupture of the GI tract and arterial aneurysms are features, and the disease is fatal in lambs and calves. In horses, the onset is later and the lesions are well circumscribed, consisting of hyperextensible and somewhat fragile skin. In dogs and cats, the disease is not fatal, and older animals develop hanging folds of skin and exhibit extensive scarring; some have joint laxity or ocular anomalies.

Diagnosis is based on clinical signs and histopathologic studies of the collagen structure, which require age and breed-matched controls. For diagnosis in cats and dogs, a skin extensibility index has been developed. There are anecdotal reports of improvement of affected dogs with vitamin C supplementation. The major differential diagnosis in adult cats is feline hyperadrenocorticism with acquired skin fragility.

The **epidermolysis bullosa syndromes** are a group of congenital and hereditary diseases that result from defects in the dermal-epidermal attachment structures. These are known as mechanobullous diseases, because minor cutaneous trauma results in dermal-epidermal separation with formation of flaccid bullae that soon rupture, leaving glistening, flat erosions. Syndromes are classified according to the ultrastructural location of the epidermal-dermal defect: simplex, in the epidermal basal cell layer; junctional, within the basement membrane; and dystrophic, below the basement membrane in the subepidermal anchoring fibrils.

In large animals, lesions are most common on the gingivae, palate, lips, tongue, and feet. Some forms of epidermolysis bullosa are scarring, and most are fatal. In large animals, epidermolysis bullosa syndromes are known in calves (Simmental, Brangus), domestic buffalo, lambs (Suffolk, South Dorset Down, Scottish Blackface, Weisses Alpenschaf, Welsh Mountain), and Belgian foals. All three forms of epidermolysis bullosa have been characterized in dogs and cats. Epidermolysis bullosa simplex has been described in Collies and Shetland Sheepdogs. Junctional epidermolysis bullosa has been reported in a Toy Poodle, German Shorthaired Pointers, mixed-breed dogs, and Siamese cats and tentatively identified in Beaucerons. Dystrophic epidermolysis bullosa has been reported in a domestic shorthair cat and a Persian and in Golden Retrievers and Akitas. Lesions may be present at birth or develop within the first weeks of life. The most severe lesions are on the feet, with sloughing of hooves, claws, or footpads, and oral mucous membrane and facial and perigenital skin (erosions). Except for epidermolysis bullosa simplex, these diseases are fatal.

Canine benign familial chronic pemphigus is a mechanobullous disorder that is caused by a defect in cell-to-cell adhesion in the epidermis. This disorder has been described in a family of English Setters. It develops within a few weeks of birth and causes crusting alopecic lesions on the pressure points of the skin that slowly enlarge as the puppies grow. The disease is benign, and no treatment is reported. **Familial acantholysis**, reported in New Zealand Angus calves, is a similar syndrome. This fatal syndrome is reported to be an autosomal recessive trait. Affected calves develop erosions, with collarettes and crusts, in areas subjected to trauma. Some show partial separation of the hooves. Diagnosis in both puppies and calves is established by skin biopsy of newly forming lesions.

Cutaneous mucinosis is thought to be a familial problem in some lines of Chinese Shar-Pei. Normal Shar-Pei have more cutaneous mucin than other dogs, but in some young dogs, cutaneous mucin formation in the dermis is so excessive that the skin exhibits pronounced folding and mucinous vesiculation. Diagnosis is by skin prick of the vesicles and observation of the strings of mucus that have the same appearance as normal joint fluid or, alternatively, by skin biopsy. The syndrome is partially responsive to corticosteroids, but they are contraindicated because of the young age of the affected dogs. As these dogs mature, the severity of the syndrome may abate, but it can be exaggerated by the development of allergic skin disease, which is common in the breed. The major differential diagnosis is hypothyroidism.

CUTANEOUS MANIFESTATIONS OF MULTISYSTEMIC AND METABOLIC DEFECTS

Baldy calf syndrome of female Holsteins, as the name implies, is associated with hypotrichosis. This autosomal recessive trait is lethal to male fetuses. Affected calves appear normal at birth but lose condition and patches of hair beginning 1–2 mo later. The skin then becomes thickened and wrinkled, and the tips of the ears may curl. Calves salivate profusely and become emaciated, and affected female calves die by 6–8 mo of age. The underlying metabolic defect is not known. A similar appearing syndrome, known as **congenital anemia, dyskeratosis, and progressive alopecia**, is described in polled Hereford calves of either sex. Anemia and small size are noted at birth and become progressively more severe. Alopecia, abnormal curly hair, and hyperkeratosis begin around the muzzle and ear margins and become more extensive as the calves mature. Later, the skin becomes markedly wrinkled, and neurologic abnormalities develop. Calves have diarrhea and die before 6 mo of age.

Familial vasculopathy has been described in German Shepherds and Parson Russell Terriers. In these dogs, the skin lesions develop shortly after the first set of puppy vaccinations and seem to be exacerbated after subsequent vaccinations. The main cutaneous signs are footpad swelling and depigmentation that may progress to ulceration; all footpads are typically affected. Crusting and ulceration of the ear and tail tips and depigmentation of the planum nasale are also features. As the dogs mature, the disease may resolve, but pad lesions may be so severe that euthanasia is warranted. No known treatment is uniformly effective, although some dogs appear to respond to high dosages of corticosteroids. A severe form of **neutrophilic vasculitis** recently described in young Chinese Shar-Pei may be familial.

Familial dermatomyositis is an idiopathic inflammatory disease of the skin and muscles of young Collies and Shetland Sheepdogs. The mode of inheritance is reported to be autosomal dominant in Collies, but there is some evidence of a role for an unidentified infectious agent in the pathogenesis. A vasculopathy is associated with the early inflammatory stages of the disease in the skin and muscle; in both tissues, the eventual sequela is atrophy. The onset is typically at <6 mo of age, although onset in adulthood has been recorded. Progression of lesions is variable, and individual pups within a litter may be affected mildly to severely. Skin lesions appear in areas of increased trauma and are seen on the face, ear tips, tail tips, and lateral surfaces of the extremities. Skin lesions, which consist of erosion, crusting, and alopecia, are exacerbated by heat and sun exposure. The muscles affected most severely are on the head and extremities. Diagnosis is established by evaluation of littermates and family history, skin biopsy, electromyography, and muscle biopsy, which must be performed early in the course of the disease. There are reports of disease amelioration with dosages of corticosteroids, vitamin E, and omega-3 fatty acids, but severely affected dogs rarely respond satisfactorily to treatment. Pentoxifylline (10 mg/kg, PO, bid) has been helpful in many dogs.

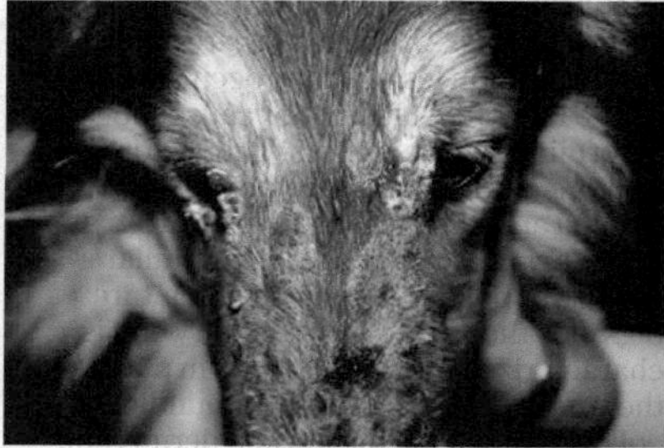
Familial dermatomyositis in a Collie. *Courtesy of Dr. Robert Dunstan.*

Hereditary lupoid dermatosis of German Shorthaired Pointers is first noted when the dog is ~6 mo old. It begins with scaling and crusting on the head and dorsum and quickly progresses to generalized scaling with erythema. The dermatopathy appears to be either painful or pruritic. Affected dogs become pyrexic and develop lymphadenopathy. Some develop a poorly characterized enteropathy; most lose condition. As the name implies, skin biopsy specimens reveal features of a lupus-like dermatitis. The disease is progressive and ultimately fatal. No successful treatment has been reported.

Hereditary zinc deficiency syndromes are best known in cattle and have also been described in dogs. In cattle, these syndromes include hereditary parakeratosis, lethal trait A46, edema disease, and hereditary thymic hypoplasia. Affected breeds include Friesian, Shorthorn, Angus, and Black Pied. These syndromes all become apparent within days to weeks of birth and are characterized by symmetric, mostly acral, hyperkeratosis; crusting and unthriftiness; susceptibility to infection; and early death. Affected calves exhibit conjunctivitis, ptyalism, rhinitis, and diarrhea and often succumb to pneumonia. In most breeds of cattle, the trait appears to be autosomal recessive and associated with intestinal malabsorption of dietary zinc, which is more or less responsive to dietary zinc supplementation. In some breeds, the defect in absorption is absolute, and parenteral administration of zinc is needed to achieve remission. Because such treatment is rarely feasible in production animals, these are lethal traits. Diagnosis is established by excluding dermatophilosis (*see* p 858) and by skin biopsy (showing mostly parakeratosis), by measuring serum zinc levels, and by necropsy findings that include hypoplasia of thymus and lymph nodes.

In dogs, there are two familial zinc deficiency syndromes. In white Bull Terriers, **lethal acrodermatitis** is characterized by retarded growth; progressive, acral, hyperkeratotic dermatitis; and pustular dermatitis around mucocutaneous junctions. These signs are apparent by 10 wk of age and are later accompanied by diarrhea, pneumonia, and death before 2 yr of age. In older dogs, footpad hyperkeratosis and paronychia contribute significantly to morbidity. The severity of the cutaneous disease can be ameliorated somewhat by control of secondary bacterial and *Malassezia* infections and, with aggressive medical treatment, the lives of affected dogs can be prolonged. These dogs do not respond to oral zinc therapy. A **familial zinc-responsive dermatopathy** that is manifest mostly by cutaneous lesions and is responsive to supplemental oral zinc is seen in Alaskan Malamutes, Huskies, and German Shorthaired Pointers. Signs develop at weaning or later in life and consist of crusting and hyperkeratosis of the extremities and mucocutaneous junctions. Often, bitches will develop signs associated with estrus or whelping and lactation. Secondary *Malassezia* infections are common. Diagnosis is established by skin biopsy and response to oral zinc supplementation.

Tyrosinemia has been described in a German Shepherd puppy. It was compared to a type of tyrosinemia in people and thus thought to be hereditary. Clinical manifestations included erosions and ulcerations of the footpads and nose and bullous lesions and depigmentation of the skin, loss of claws, and eye lesions. It must be differentiated from the familial vasculopathy of German Shepherds described above. In the puppy, serum tyrosine levels were 20–30 times above normal levels, and urine specimens contained similar high concentrations.

Porphyria is an inherited defect in the metabolism of hemoglobin and its byproducts. In cattle, accumulation of aberrant porphyrins in the skin increases sensitivity to ultraviolet light. (Porphyria has been described in cats and swine but does not result in photosensitivity.) In cattle, there are two types of inherited porphyries. Bovine protoporphyria has been reported in crossbred Limousin cattle and is inherited as an autosomal recessive trait. Signs include photodermatitis and photophobia. Affected calves may die, but mature animals may be less severely affected. Bovine erythropoietic porphyria (*see* p 986) is more common and more severe. It is reported in several breeds (including Shorthorn, Holstein-Friesian, and Hereford) as an autosomal recessive trait. In addition to severe photosensitivity, signs include red-brown discoloration of teeth, bones, and urine; regenerative anemia; and stunted growth. Teeth and urine from affected animals fluoresce orange under a Wood's lamp. Skin biopsy is also useful in diagnosis.

Leukocyte adhesion deficiency in Holstein cattle is an inherited disease (autosomal recessive) with many manifestations. It is fatal before adulthood. Skin lesions are frequently seen in affected calves and include dermatitis and vasculitis. This disease can be diagnosed by molecular methods with PCR analysis of fresh or fixed tissue providing identification of affected, carrier, and normal cattle.

CONGENITAL AND HEREDITARY NEOPLASMS AND HAMARTOMAS

Congenital neoplasms are common in large animals. **Mastocytosis**, **melanocytosis**, **cutaneous lymphosarcoma**, and **vascular hamartomas** are found in calves. Melanocytomas may also arise shortly after birth in calves and may be hereditary. These are thought to be benign.

Melanomas are seen in Duroc-Jersey and Sinclair miniature pigs as familial traits. These may undergo spontaneous remission or may behave as malignant tumors. Piglets have also been described with vascular hamartomas and with congenital **fibropapillomatosis**, which is likely infectious.

Congenital tumors are rare in dogs and cats. One dog with a giant congenital pigmented nevus had a malignant melanoma develop within the lesion. In cats, familial benign mastocytosis is described in young Siamese cats.

A syndrome of multiple collagenous nevi is seen in some families of German Shepherds and is called **nodular dermatofibrosis**. Affected dogs are adults. Dozens of skin lesions may occur, and those on the feet often ulcerate or cause foot deformities and lameness. This syndrome is a cutaneous marker for renal cystadenocarcinoma and uterine leiomyoma. **Progressive dermal collagenosis** is a similar disease of postpubertal male miniature pigs. It is thought to be hereditary and is characterized by symmetric, firm plaques on the trunk that consist of thick bundles of collagen replacing the normal dermis and panniculus. A connection with internal malignancy has not been reported.

Urticaria pigmentosa is caused by mast cell hyperplasia and has been described in cats. Affected cats have multifocal, partially coalescing macular and crusted papular eruption on the head, neck, and legs. Diagnosis is made by skin biopsy. There is evidence of a familial history.

ATOPIC DERMATITIS

Atopic dermatitis (AD) is a genetically predisposed inflammatory and pruritic allergic skin disease with characteristic clinical features. It is most commonly associated with IgE antibodies to environmental allergens. The atopic phenotype (*see* clinical signs, below) can be seen in animals with IgE-mediated skin disease, food allergy, or a condition called "atopic-like dermatitis" (ALD). ALD is defined as a pruritic skin disease in dogs with characteristic features of AD but negative tests for IgE antibodies. Feline atopic dermatitis has many similarities to canine atopic dermatitis.

Etiology and Pathogenesis: The etiology and pathogenesis of AD is complex and involves a genetic predisposition, impairment of the normal barrier function of the skin, and immunologic aberrations. Animals with AD are thought to be genetically predisposed to become sensitized to allergens in the environment. Allergens are proteins that, when inhaled or absorbed through the skin, respiratory tract, or GI tract, evoke allergen-specific IgE production. These allergen-specific IgE molecules affix themselves to tissue mast cells or basophils. When these primed cells come in contact with the specific allergen again, mast cell degranulation results in the release of proteolytic enzymes, histamine, bradykinins, and other vasoactive amines, leading to inflammation (erythema, edema, and pruritus). The skin is the primary target organ in dogs and cats, but rhinitis and asthma can also occur in ~15% of affected animals.

CANINE ATOPIC DERMATITIS

Clinical Findings: There is no sex predilection in canine AD. There are breed predilections, but the prevalence within a breed largely depends on the genetic pool and region. Breeds predisposed to development of AD include Chinese Shar-Pei, Wirehaired Fox Terrier, Golden Retriever, Dalmatian, Boxer, Boston Terrier, Labrador Retriever, Lhasa Apso, Scottish Terrier, Shih Tzu, and West Highland White Terrier. The age of onset is generally between 6 mo and 3 yr. Clinical signs usually occur on a seasonal basis but may be seen year-round with time. Pruritus is the characteristic sign of AD. The feet, face, ears, flexural surfaces of the front legs, axillae, and abdomen are the most frequently affected areas. Primary lesions consist of erythematous macules, patches, and small papules. Lesions that develop secondary to self-trauma include alopecia, erythema, scaling, salivary staining, hemorrhagic crusts, excoriations, lichenification, hyperpigmentation, superficial staphylococcal pyoderma, *Malassezia* and bacterial overgrowth, and allergic otitis externa. Chronic or recurrent otitis is the only complaint in a small number of animals.

Diagnosis: The diagnosis is challenging and is based on signalment, clinical signs, and disease history and not on laboratory tests. Prospective studies have revealed the following clinical features compatible with a diagnosis of AD: onset of clinical signs before 3 yr of age, dogs that live mostly indoors, glucocorticoid-responsive pruritus, pruritus without skin lesions, affected front feet, affected ear pinnae, nonaffected ear margins, and nonaffected dorsolumbosacral areas. These clinical signs can overlap with other diseases, so parasites, pruritic microbial overgrowth, food allergy, and flea allergy need to be excluded. Allergy testing (intradermal or serologic) is a diagnostic aid that measures increased levels of tissue-bound or circulating IgE; alone, it is not diagnostic but rather reflects exposure. The primary reason to pursue intradermal or serologic allergy testing is to identify the offending allergens in an individual animal and to formulate specific immunotherapy. Test results are significant only if the offending allergens identified are compatible with the history or seasonality of pruritus. Animals with classic clinical signs but negative allergy tests are given the diagnosis of ALD. Immunotherapy would be difficult if not impossible in these animals.

Treatment: AD and ALD cannot be cured. Client education is important, because this is a lifelong disease that requires lifelong management and regular progress checks. Management options depend on the severity of the clinical signs and whether the pruritus is seasonal or year round.

Avoidance of allergens: This may be the best choice, but it is difficult, if not impossible, to do unless a specific allergen can be identified.

Relief from pruritus: By definition, this is a pruritic skin disease; itching may be relieved via antipruritic drugs alone or in combination with allergen-specific immunotherapy (ASIT [*see* below]).

Bathing and coat hygiene: Bathing dogs with AD may decrease pruritus. In dogs with a history of flares due to microbial overgrowth, routine use of antimicrobial shampoos can be of benefit. Except for the use of lipid-containing shampoos, there is no evidence of benefit from shampoos or conditioners that contain oatmeal, pramoxine, antihistamines, or corticosteroids.

Recognition and control of flare factors: A relapse of clinical signs in a dog that is otherwise well controlled should prompt an investigation into what caused the exacerbation of pruritus. Recognized flare factors include, but are not limited to, fleas, food and environmental allergens, secondary microbial overgrowth, and poor coat hygiene. These need to be investigated before using systemic antipruritic drugs.

Antipruritic drugs for acute flares: In many dogs, the flare may present as allergic otitis, and topical use of otic corticosteroids may be adequate. There is good evidence for a short course of a topical triamcinolone or hydrocortisone aceponate spray for local pruritus. If the pruritus is too severe or extensive to be controlled with topical formulations, then oral steroids may be needed. Options include prednisone, prednisolone, or methylprednisone administered PO at 0.5 mg/kg, once to twice daily, until clinical signs are in remission. Tacrolimus, cyclosporine, or essential fatty acids are unlikely to be beneficial for acute flares.

Antipruritic drugs for chronic AD: Systemic reviews of clinical trials have not shown conclusively that omega-3 and omega-6 essential fatty acids alone are likely to reduce pruritus. Use may help improve coat quality. Cyclosporine can provide relief similar to that seen with glucocorticoids. A reported 50% reduction in pruritus in 70% of dogs with AD given cyclosporine A parallels the response seen with glucocorticoids but with fewer adverse effects. Some animals can be maintained comfortably with this drug alone. Tacrolimus ointment provides a benefit in animals with more localized lesions. However, drugs in this category tend to be more expensive than other symptomatic treatments. Another option is oclacitinib (a Janus kinase inhibitor), which has been shown to be safe and effective in control of pruritus.

Immunotherapy: Immunotherapy or ASIT is arguably the best treatment option for AD, because it is the only therapy that potentially leads to remission of signs without addition of other medications. It remains the treatment of choice of most dermatologists and allergists. ASIT attempts to increase an animal's tolerance to environmental allergens (subjectively measured when an individual is exposed to an identified allergen without developing clinical signs). Although the mode of action is not completely understood, the primary theory states that IgG increases during the first few months of hyposensitization and exerts a blocking effect on circulating allergens by binding them and preventing mast cell degranulation. Another theory states that immunotherapy causes a shift away from TH_2 toward TH_1 by enhancing γ-interferon expression. After an injection, however, allergen-specific IgE levels may also increase when immunotherapy is initiated due to a response to the additional allergen load from the immunotherapy injections. This may result in increased pruritus in some animals. Reducing the amount of allergen given often alleviates this reaction, and with time, allergen-specific IgE levels decrease. However, decreased IgE levels and clinical improvement are not always directly correlated.

ASIT can be administered via injections or allergy drops, which are equally effective. Immunotherapy is best considered for animals with problematic clinical signs that occur for several months during the year. For injections, the animal must also be cooperative enough to receive allergy injections. For allergy drops, the owner must be able to handle the animal's mouth and be able and willing to administer the drops twice a day every day. The criteria for successful hyposensitization include appropriate interpretation of test results, careful selection of allergens, adequate control of secondary infections, control of other allergies (food or flea), systematic administration of immunotherapy injections, and periodic communications between the owner and veterinarian. The longterm commitment needed from both the owner and the veterinarian for successful immunotherapy cannot be overemphasized. The owner must be willing to follow instructions accurately, be patient, and communicate effectively with the veterinarian. The veterinarian must recognize and treat other primary or secondary causes of pruritus and manage flare factors (eg, otitis, pyoderma, *Malassezia* dermatitis, insect hypersensitivity) as they occur and guide the owner through these challenges until improvement is seen. Symptomatic therapy is required in almost every case during the induction period and at various times of the year (*see* above).

Allergen selection is determined by correlating the positive allergens on the test results with the prominent allergens during the time of year when the animal is symptomatic. If the test shows positive results for pollens that have no clinical relevance (eg, high pollen count during a period when the animal is not pruritic, positive reaction to an allergen not in the geographic area), then either the allergic reaction is mild (subthreshold) or it is a false-positive reaction. Either way, the allergen is not included in the allergen mixture.

Allergen protocols vary but usually have induction and maintenance periods. During the induction period, the dosage of allergen gradually increases until an arbitrary maintenance dosage is reached. Once the maximal dosage is given, this maintenance level is continued. The interval between maintenance dosages may vary from 3–4 days to 3 wk. Adjustments in the interval are based on the animal's response. Owners are advised not to expect much response for 6 mo and are asked to commit to at least 1 yr of therapy before deciding the usefulness of immunotherapy. The best assessment of response is to compare the degree of disease or discomfort between similar seasons.

FELINE ATOPIC DERMATITIS

Feline AD is similar to canine AD. It is a pruritic disease in which affected cats have a hypersensitivity reaction to inhaled or contacted environmental allergens. The age of onset is variable but generally is <5 yr. The signs may be seasonal or nonseasonal. Purebred cats may have a higher risk than domestic shorthaired cats. As in dogs, pruritic cats may have several clinical presentations (eg, miliary dermatitis, symmetric alopecia, eosinophilic granuloma complex, head and neck pruritus) that are consistent with a diagnosis of AD but that must be differentiated from other diseases with similar clinical signs. Differential diagnoses include flea allergy, various mite infestations (eg, *Cheyletiella*, *Demodex*, *Notoedres*, *Sarcoptes*, *Otodectes*), mosquito bite hypersensitivity, food allergy, autoimmune disease (eg, pemphigus foliaceus), dermatophytosis, and cutaneous neoplasia. A thorough review of the cat's history and complete dermatologic and physical examination, along with the standard flea combing, skin scrapings, and fungal cultures, are mandatory first steps. The diagnosis of AD is made when the other differential diagnoses have been eliminated. Response to glucocorticoids is excellent initially but decreases over time.

Intradermal allergy testing and hyposensitization procedures in cats are similar to those used in dogs, but the intradermal test results are more difficult to read because the reactions are less dramatic and dissipate more rapidly in cats. The same avoidance recommendations made for dogs apply to cats. Symptomatic therapy includes control of secondary infections and use of antipruritic drugs. The approved formulation of cyclosporine for use in cats is liquid; the dosage is 7 mg/kg, and it can be administered PO or in food. After 30 days, the dosage can be tapered to every other day in ~70% of cats and to twice a week in ~50% of cats. Response to immunotherapy is similar to that in dogs (*see* above); owners are advised to commit to 1 yr of therapy before deciding its usefulness.

FOOD ALLERGY

(Adverse food reactions)

Adverse food reactions comprise allergic reactions termed food allergy as well as nonallergic reactions termed food intolerance. On a practical level, these terms are frequently interchanged, because the precise immunologic processes of most adverse food reactions are usually not known. Immunologic reactions types I, III, and IV are thought to be the most likely causes, but this is conjectural for most reported cases in small animals. Food allergies are very rare in herbivores. In this chapter, the more commonly used term food allergy will be used for all adverse food reactions.

Food allergy is ~10% as common as atopic dermatitis in dogs and perhaps as common as atopic dermatitis in cats. The history is that of a nonseasonal pruritus, with little variation in the intensity of pruritus from one season to another in most cases. Most reports do not suggest a breed predilection; however, one report indicated an increased relative risk in Labrador Retrievers, West Highland White Terriers, and Cocker Spaniels. Food hypersensitivities have been reported in Soft-coated Wheaten Terriers in association with protein-losing enteropathy and nephropathy. The age of onset is variable, from 2 mo to 14 yr old. One report indicated that most food allergies begin at <12 mo of age. In adult-onset food allergy, most dogs have been fed the offending allergen for >2 yr.

The distribution of pruritus and lesions varies markedly between animals. Ear canal disease that manifests as pruritus and secondary infection with bacteria (usually *Staphylococcus pseudintermedius*, *Pseudomonas* spp) or yeast (*Malassezia pachydermatis*) is common and may be the only presenting complaint. Other patterns seen include blepharitis, generalized pruritus, generalized seborrhea (scaling), a papular eruption, or a distribution pattern that may mimic that of atopic dermatitis (feet, face, and ventrum) or flea allergy dermatitis (dorsal lumbosacrum and hindlegs). The most common areas of involvement include the ears, feet, inguinal region, axillary area, proximal anterior forelegs, periorbital region, and muzzle. The degree of pruritus is usually moderate to severe. Response to glucocorticoids varies from poor to excellent.

There is no reliable diagnostic test other than a strict food elimination diet. Serologic testing and intradermal testing for food allergens have proved unreliable. The ideal food elimination diet should be balanced and nutritionally complete and not contain any ingredients that have been previously fed. Many diets contain novel protein or carbohydrate sources (eg, venison and rice). However, if a previously fed ingredient is present in the elimination diet, and the animal is allergic to that ingredient, the diet trial will be a failure. Another option is the use of hydrolyzed protein diets, in which the protein source is hydrolyzed to small molecular weights that are not allergenic. It is estimated that hydrolyzation of the protein may still trigger an allergic response in ~10% of animals allergic to the unhydrolyzed form.

The trial diet should be fed for up to 3 mo. The key point in any food elimination diet trial is that *only* the designated food ingredients can be fed. Thus, no treats, flavored toys, medications, or toothpaste are allowed. If marked or complete resolution in the pruritus and clinical signs occurs during the elimination diet trial, food allergy can be suspected. To confirm that a food allergy exists and that the clinical improvement was not just coincidental, the animal must be challenged with the previously fed food ingredients and a relapse of clinical signs must occur. The return of clinical signs after challenge is usually between 1 hr and 14 days. Once a food allergy is confirmed, the elimination diet should be reinstituted until clinical signs resolve, which usually takes <14 days. At this point, previously fed individual ingredients should be added to the elimination diet for up to 14 days. If pruritus recurs, the individual ingredient is considered positive for having a causative role in the food allergy. If pruritus does not recur, the individual ingredient is not considered important in causing the clinical signs.

The number of offending food allergens varies from one to five ingredients. The most frequently identified causative allergens in canine food allergy include beef, chicken, eggs, corn, wheat, soy, and milk. Once the offending allergens are identified, control of the food allergy is by strict avoidance. Concurrent diseases (such as atopic dermatitis or flea allergy) may complicate the identification of underlying food allergies. Infrequently, a dog will react to new food allergens over time.

Clinical presentations of food allergy in cats include miliary dermatitis, feline symmetric alopecia, eosinophilic granuloma complex (primarily the eosinophilic plaque), and severe head and neck pruritus. No breed, sex, or age predilection is seen. Age of onset varies from 3 mo to 11 yr. In one study, however, 46% of affected cats became symptomatic at ≤2 yr of age, and Siamese cats represented 30% of the cases.

Response to glucocorticoids is variable, but about two-thirds of cats show excellent response initially. In many cats, response to glucocorticoids becomes poor with repeated treatments. As with food allergy in dogs, an elimination diet should be fed for up to

3 mo. The elimination diet should not contain any previously fed ingredients. Food elimination diets can be difficult in cats, because many cats are reluctant to change diets. Cats should not be starved or forced into eating a new elimination diet because of the serious nature of hepatic lipidosis that may be induced by prolonged anorexia.

Time until relapse of pruritus after challenge with the offending food varies from 15 min to 10 days. The most frequently identified food allergens in cats include fish, beef, milk, and chicken. Avoidance of the offending allergens will control the clinical signs associated with the food allergy.

URTICARIA

(Hives, Nettle rash)

Urticaria is characterized by multiple plaque-like eruptions that are formed by localized edema in the dermis and that often develop and disappear suddenly. It occurs in all domestic animals but most often in horses. Allergic urticaria may be exogenous or endogenous. Exogenous hives may be produced by toxic irritating products of the stinging nettle, the stings or bites of insects, topical medications, or exposure to chemicals (eg, carbolic acid, turpentine, carbon disulfide, or crude oil). Nonimmunologic factors such as pressure, sunlight, heat, exercise, psychologic stress, and genetic abnormalities may precipitate or intensify urticaria. Pruritus is not always present, particularly in horses.

Sensitive animals, particularly short-haired dogs and purebred horses, also rarely may exhibit **dermographism**, a phenomenon wherein pressure applied to the skin produces linear urticarial lesions. The clinical significance is unknown.

Endogenous urticaria may develop after exposure to topical, inhaled, or ingested allergens or administration of medications; it has been seen mostly in horses and dogs. In horses, it has been noted in the course of GI conditions, particularly severe constipation or inflammation of the intestinal mucosa. A unique form of urticaria in cattle has been described chiefly in the Channel Island breeds (Jersey, Guernsey), which become sensitized to the casein in their own milk ("milk allergy"); it occurs in cases of milk retention or unusual engorgement of the udder with milk. Urticaria has been seen in bitches during estrus. In young horses, dogs, and pigs, urticaria may be associated with intestinal parasites. **Angioneurotic edema** is a life-threatening variant of urticaria in which there is diffuse subcutaneous edema, often localized to the head, limbs, or perineum. In horses, dermatophytosis (ringworm) and pemphigus foliaceus may present as urticaria early in the disease. In horses, vasculitis may also present with urticaria.

Clinical Findings: The wheals or plaques appear within a few minutes or hours of exposure to the causative agent. In severe cases, the cutaneous eruptions are preceded by fever, anorexia, or dullness. Horses often become excited and restless. The skin lesions are elevated, round, flat-topped, and 0.5–8 in. (1–20 cm) in diameter; they may be slightly depressed in the center. They can develop on any part of the body but are seen mainly on the back, flanks, neck, eyelids, and legs. In advanced cases, they may be found on the mucous membranes of the mouth, nose, conjunctiva, rectum, and vagina. In general, the lesions disappear as rapidly as they arise, usually within a few hours.

In sheep, lesions usually are seen only on the udder and hairless parts of the abdomen. In pigs, eruptions have been seen around the eyes, between the hindlegs, and on the snout, abdomen, and back.

In general, the prognosis is favorable. Fatalities are rare and are probably due to anaphylaxis or associated angioedema involving the respiratory passages.

Chronic urticaria is a diagnostic challenge. All allergens in an environment should be considered potential causes, and elimination of exposure instituted, if possible. Persistent urticarial lesions, particularly those that progress to thickened crusts, should be biopsied.

Treatment: Acute urticaria usually disappears spontaneously. The rapid-acting glucocorticoids, eg, hydrocortisone sodium succinate or prednisolone sodium succinate or hemisuccinate are reported to be useful. Dexamethasone (0.1 mg/kg) has been useful in dogs, cats, and horses. Antihistamines are of questionable value and may induce urticaria if given IV. Epinephrine may be given in life-threatening situations. The lesions promptly disappear but return rapidly if the allergen is not eliminated. Usually, local treatment of the lesions is not necessary. In chronic urticaria in horses, the antihistamine hydroxyzine at 0.4–0.8 mg/kg, bid, or the tricyclic antidepressant doxepin (which has antihistaminic properties) at 0.6 mg/kg, bid, may be useful.

DERMATOPHILOSIS

(Dermatophilus infection, Cutaneous streptothricosis, Lumpy wool, Strawberry footrot)

This infection of the epidermis, seen worldwide but more prevalent in the tropics, is also erroneously called mycotic dermatitis. The lesions are characterized by exudative dermatitis with scab formation. *Dermatophilus congolensis* has a wide host range. Among domestic animals, cattle, sheep, goats, and horses are affected most frequently, and pigs, dogs, and cats rarely. It is commonly called cutaneous streptothricosis in cattle, goats, and horses; in sheep, it is termed lumpy wool when the wooled areas of the body are affected. Infection in camel herds has been related to drought and poverty. Recent isolates from chelonids may represent a new species of *Dermatophilus*. It is also a common disease in farmed crocodiles. The few human cases reported usually have been associated with handling diseased animals.

Etiology, Transmission, and Epidemiology: *D congolensis* is a gram-positive, non-acid-fast, facultative anaerobic actinomycete. It is the only currently accepted species in the genus, but a variety of strains can be present within a group of animals during an outbreak. It has two characteristic morphologic forms: filamentous hyphae and motile zoospores. The hyphae are characterized by branching filaments (1–5 µm in diameter) that ultimately fragment by both transverse and longitudinal septation into packets of coccoid cells. The coccoid cells mature into flagellated ovoid zoospores (0.6–1 µm in diameter).

The natural habitat of *D congolensis* is unknown. Attempts to isolate it from soil have been unsuccessful, although it is probably a saprophyte in the soil. It is believed to be spread by direct contact between animals, through contaminated environments, or possibly via biting insects. It has been isolated only from the integument of various animals and is restricted to the living layers of the epidermis. Asymptomatic chronically infected animals are considered the primary reservoir.

Factors such as prolonged wetting by rain, high humidity, high temperature, and various ectoparasites that reduce or permeate the natural barriers of the integument influence the development, prevalence, seasonal incidence, and transmission of dermatophilosis. Ticks and lice are major predisposing factors in cattle and sheep, respectively.

The organism can exist in a quiescent form within the epidermis until infection is exacerbated by climatic conditions. Epidemics usually occur during the rainy season. Moisture facilitates release of zoospores from preexisting lesions and their subsequent penetration of the epidermis and establishment of new foci of infection. High humidity also contributes indirectly to the spread of lesions by allowing increases in the number of biting insects, particularly flies and ticks, that act as mechanical vectors. Shearing, dipping, or introducing an infected animal into a herd or flock can spread infection.

Dermatophilosis is contagious only in that any reduction in systemic or local skin resistance favors establishment of infection and subsequent disease.

Pathogenesis: To establish infection, the infective zoospores must reach a skin site where the normal protective barriers are reduced or deficient. The respiratory efflux of low concentrations of carbon dioxide from the skin attracts the motile zoospores to susceptible areas on the skin surface. Zoospores germinate to produce hyphae, which penetrate into the living epidermis and subsequently spread in all directions from the initial focus. Hyphal penetration causes an acute inflammatory reaction. Natural resistance to the acute infection is due to phagocytosis of the infective zoospores, but once infection is established, there is little or no immunity. In most acute infections, the filamentous invasion of the epidermis ceases in 2–3 wk, and the lesions heal spontaneously. In chronic infections, the affected hair follicles and scabs are sites from which intermittent invasions of noninfected hair follicles and epidermis occur. The invaded epithelium cornifies and separates in the form of a scab. In wet scabs, moisture enhances the proliferation and release of zoospores from hyphae. The high carbon dioxide concentration produced by the dense population of zoospores accelerates their escape to the skin surface, thus completing the unique life cycle.

Clinical Findings: Dermatophilosis is seen in animals at all ages but is most prevalent in the young, in animals chronically exposed to moisture, and in immunosuppressed hosts. Lesions on a host can vary from acute to chronic. Age, sex, and breed do not seem to affect host susceptibility. Pruritus is variable. Most affected animals recover spontaneously within 3 wk of the initial infection (provided chronic maceration of the skin does not occur). In general, the onset of dry weather speeds healing. Uncomplicated skin lesions heal without scar formation. These infections usually have little effect on general health. Animals with severe generalized infections often lose condition, and movement and prehension are difficult if the feet, lips, and muzzle are severely affected; these animals are often sent to slaughter as incurable. Deaths occasionally occur, particularly in calves and lambs, because of generalized disease with or without secondary bacterial infection and secondary fly or screwworm infestation. The primary economic consequences are damaged hides in cattle, wool loss in sheep, and lameness and loss of performance in horses when severely affected around the pastern area. Cattle with lesions covering >50% of the body are likely to become seriously ill.

Lesions: Distribution of the gross lesions on cattle, sheep, and horses usually correlates with the predisposing factors that reduce or permeate the natural barriers of the integument. In cattle, the lesions can be observed in three stages: 1) hairs matted together as paint-brush lesions, 2) crust or scab formation as the initial lesions coalesce, and 3) accumulations of cutaneous keratinized material forming wart-like lesions that are 0.5–2 cm in diameter. Typical lesions consist of raised, matted tufts of hair. Most lesions associated with prolonged wetting of the skin are distributed over the head, dorsal surfaces of the neck and body, and upper lateral surfaces of the neck and chest. Cattle that stand for long periods in deep water and mud develop lesions in areas such as skin folds of the flexor surfaces of the joints. Dairy cows may present with papular crusted lesions on the udder. Lesions initiated by biting flies (mechanical vectors) are found primarily on the back, whereas lesions induced by ticks are primarily on the head, ears, axillae, groin, and scrotum.

Chronic lumpy wool infections are characterized by pyramid-shaped masses of scab material bound to wool fibers. The crusts are primarily on the dorsal areas of the body and prevent the shearing of sheep; spiny plants often predispose to lesions on the lips, legs, and feet. Strawberry footrot is a proliferative dermatitis affecting the skin from the coronet to the carpus or hock.

Lesions on horses with long winter hair coats are similar to those of cattle, developing with matted hair and paint-brush lesions leading to crust or scab formation with yellow-green pus present under larger scabs. With short summer hair, matting and scab formation is uncommon; loss of hair with a fine paint-brush effect can be extensive. Persistent wetting of pasterns in wet yards, stables, or at pasture leads to lower limb infection; white legs and the white-skinned areas of the lips and nose are more severely affected. Generalized disease is also associated with prolonged wet weather. Outbreaks occur on farms with previously affected horses.

Histopathologic examination reveals the characteristic branching hyphae with multidimensional septations, coccoidal cells, and zoospores in the epidermis. The organisms are usually abundant in active lesions but can be sparse or absent in chronic lesions.

Diagnosis: Presumptive diagnosis depends largely on the appearance of lesions in clinically diseased animals and demonstration of *D congolensis* in stained smears or histologic sections from scabs. A definitive diagnosis is made by demonstrating the organism in cytologic preparations, isolation via culture, and/or via skin biopsy.

An indirect fluorescent antibody technique and a single dilution ELISA test have been developed for large serologic and epidemiologic surveys. The most practical diagnostic test is cytologic examination of fresh crusts and/or impression smears of the underside of freshly avulsed lesions. Fresh crusts are minced on a glass microscope slide with a sterile scalpel blade in several drops of sterile saline. The slide is allowed to air dry and is then stained with a fast Giemsa or Romanowski stain. The organisms are seen under oil immersion as 2–6 parallel rows of gram-positive cocci that look like railroad tracks. Differential diagnoses include dermatomycoses in most species, warts and lumpy skin disease (*see* p 868) in cattle, contagious ecthyma (*see* p 866) and ulcerative dermatosis (*see* p 872) in sheep, and dermatophytosis (*see* p 872) and immune-mediated scaling diseases of horses (eg, pemphigus foliaceus).

Treatment and Control: It was previously thought that because acutely infected animals usually heal rapidly and spontaneously, treatment was indicated only for cosmetic reasons in food-producing animals. However, in certain parts of the world, the disease is associated with significant morbidity and mortality, loss of body condition, decreased milk production, and increased somatic cell counts in milk. Treatment is recommended in horses because the lesions interfere with use and are painful. Organisms are susceptible to a wide range of antimicrobials: erythromycin, spiramycin, penicillin G, ampicillin, chloramphenicol, streptomycin, amoxicillin, tetracyclines, and novobiocin. Two doses of long-acting oxytetracycline (20 mg/kg) 1 day apart have shown to be curative in 85% of cattle and 100% of sheep, compared with cure rates of 71% in cattle and 80% in sheep for a single dose. In food-producing animals, topical applications of lime sulfur are a cost-effective adjuvant to antibacterial therapy. Insecticides applied externally are frequently used to control biting insects.

In horses, the lesions should be gently soaked and removed. Topical antibacterial shampoo therapy is effective as adjuvant therapy. Chlorhexidine is recommended. Topical treatment with povidone-iodine is superior to parenteral oxytetracycline alone (100% and 66% effective, respectively).

Isolating clinically affected animals, culling affected animals, and controlling ectoparasites are methods used to break the infective cycle. Preventing chronic maceration of the skin and keeping the animals dry are important. Zinc levels should be checked in the feed of cattle, because outbreaks have been associated with zinc deficiencies.

Zoonotic Risk: Dermatophilosis can be transmitted to people. Direct contact with an infected animal can lead to infections on the hands and arms. Affected animals should be handled with gloves, and thorough handwashing with an antibacterial soap is recommended after contact with an infected animal.

EXUDATIVE EPIDERMITIS

(Greasy pig disease)

Exudative epidermitis is a generalized dermatitis that occurs in 5- to 60-day-old pigs and is characterized by sudden onset, with morbidity of 10%–90% and mortality of 5%–90%. The acute form usually affects suckling piglets, whereas a chronic form is more commonly seen in weaned pigs. It has been reported from most swine-producing areas of the world.

Lesions are caused by *Staphylococcus hyicus*, which can produce an exfoliative toxin but seems unable to penetrate intact skin. Both virulent and avirulent strains exist. Abrasions on the face, feet, and legs or lacerations on the body precede infection. Such injuries are usually caused by fighting or by abrasive surfaces such as new concrete. Other predisposing factors that may affect the severity and progress of the disease include immunity, hygiene, nutrition, and the presence of mange mites or anything that damages the skin. Mature sows that have acquired a high level of immunity from previous exposure will provide protection to piglets via their colostrum. The incidence is often higher in

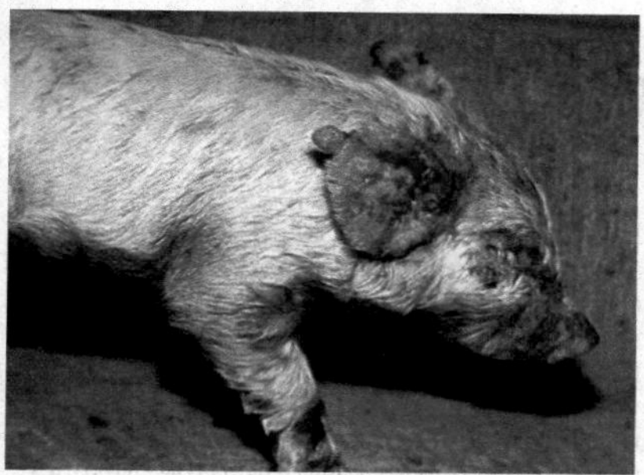

Chronic exudative epidermitis over the entire body in a 5-wk-old weaner pig. *Courtesy of Dr. Ranald D. A. Cameron.*

gilt litters and in newly established SPF herds in which most breeders are gilts.

Pigs develop resistance with age, but *S hyicus* may be recovered from the skin of older pigs, the vagina of sows, and the preputial diverticulum of boars. These inapparent carriers serve as a source of contamination for naive herds. Suckling pigs are usually infected by their dams, in some cases during birth from sows with vaginal infections, or from contamination in the farrowing unit. Suckling piglets are the most commonly and severely affected, but cross-infection occurs after mixing at weaning with a morbidity of as much as 80%. However, mortality is usually low in this age group. The incidence appears to have increased because of pig production units with high stocking densities and possibly earlier weaning. There are recent reports of exudative epidermitis associated with ST398 methicillin-resistant *S aureus* (MRSA) infections, but a causal role has not been clearly demonstrated.

Clinical Findings and Lesions: The first signs are listlessness and reddening of the skin in one or more piglets in the litter. Affected pigs rapidly become depressed and refuse to eat. Body temperature may increase early in the disease but thereafter is near normal. The skin thickens, and reddish brown spots (macules) appear around the eyes, nose, lips, and ears from which serum and sebum exude. The lesions increase in size and develop a vesicular or pustular appearance.

The body is rapidly covered with a moist, greasy exudate of sebum and serum that becomes crusty. Accumulation of dirt gives the affected area a black color. Vesicles and ulcers may also develop on the nasal disk and tongue. The feet are nearly always involved, with erosions at the coronary band and heel; the hoof may be shed in rare cases. In the acute disease, death occurs within 3–5 days. In older animals, the chronic form of the disease is seen as thick, crusty lesions over the entire body or as discrete circumscribed lesions that do not coalesce. Mortality is low except in very young suckling piglets. However, recovery is slow and growth is retarded and often associated with diarrhea, emaciation, and dehydration.

Necropsy of severely affected pigs reveals marked dehydration, congestion of the lungs, and inflammation of the peripheral lymph nodes. Distention of the kidneys and ureters with mucus, cellular casts, and debris is common in peracute and acute forms of the disease. Differential diagnoses include sarcoptic mange (*see* p 919), nutritional deficiencies including zinc (parakeratosis, *see* p 975), ringworm (*see* p 872), and pityriasis rosea (*see* p 979).

Treatment: The causative organism is inhibited by many antibiotics, including amoxicillin, ampicillin, erythromycin, lincomycin, penicillin, tylosin, trimethoprim-sulfonamide, the aminoglycosides, and cephalosporins. Successful treatment requires that the antimicrobial be given in high dosages early in the disease and for 7–10 days. Success is greatest when antimicrobial therapy is combined with daily applications of antiseptics to the entire body surface. Treatment is less effective in very young pigs and ineffective in advanced cases. In severe outbreaks, in-contact pigs should also be given antibiotics for several days. Sows due to farrow, and their housing, should be thoroughly disinfected to prevent outbreaks. Hygiene in the weaner accommodation and strategic in-water or in-feed medication for 3–5 days will help control outbreaks after weaning. Other procedures that may decrease the severity of an outbreak include clipping the needle teeth of newborn pigs, providing soft bedding, segregating infected animals, and avoiding mixing of animals to decrease the possibility of skin lesions due to fighting. Autogenous bacterins have been used with some success to reduce the incidence of disease in chronically infected herds.

INTERDIGITAL FURUNCULOSIS

Interdigital furuncles, often incorrectly referred to as interdigital cysts, are painful nodular lesions located in the interdigital webs of dogs. Histologically, these lesions represent areas of nodular pyogranulomatous inflammation—they are almost never cystic. Canine interdigital palmar and plantar comedones and follicular cysts is a recognized syndrome that may be a subtype of interdigital furuncles or a separate disease.

Etiology: The most common cause is a deep bacterial infection. Many dog breeds (eg, Chinese Shar-Pei, Labrador Retriever, English Bulldog) are predisposed to bacterial interdigital furunculosis because of the short bristly hairs located on the webbing between the toes, prominent interdigital webbing, or both. The short shafts of hairs are easily forced backward into the hair follicles during locomotion (traumatic implantation). Hair, ie, keratin, is very inflammatory in the skin, and secondary bacterial infections are common. Less commonly, foreign material is traumatically embedded in the skin. Demodicosis (*see* p 920) may be a primary cause of interdigital furunculosis. Canine atopic dermatitis (*see* p 853) is also a common cause of recurrent interdigital furunculosis.

The cause of canine interdigital palmar and plantar comedones and follicular cysts is unknown but most likely involves trauma, resulting in epidermal and follicular infundibular hyperkeratosis, acanthosis, plugging or narrowing of the follicular opening, and retention of the follicular contents.

Clinical Findings and Lesions: Early lesions of interdigital furunculosis may appear as focal or generalized areas of erythema and papules in the webbing of the feet that, if left untreated, rapidly develop into single or multiple nodules. The latter usually are 1–2 cm in diameter, reddish purple, shiny, and fluctuant; they may rupture when palpated and exude a bloody material. Interdigital furuncles are most commonly found on the dorsal aspect of the paw but may also be found ventrally. Furuncles are usually painful, and the dog may be obviously lame on the affected foot (or feet) and lick and bite at the lesions. Lesions caused by a foreign body, eg, a grass awn, are usually solitary and are often found on a front foot; recurrence is not common in these cases. If bacteria cause the interdigital furunculosis, there may be several nodules with new lesions developing as others resolve. A common cause of recurrence is the granulomatous reaction to the presence of free keratin in the tissues.

Dogs with interdigital comedones and follicular cysts typically present with lameness and draining tracts. Skin lesions are not often seen unless the hair coat is clipped. Areas of alopecia and thickened, firm, callus-like skin with multiple comedones are typical.

Diagnosis: For furunculosis, the diagnosis is often based on clinical signs alone. The major differential diagnoses are traumatic lesions, foreign bodies, follicular comedone cysts, and neoplasia, although the latter is rare. The most useful diagnostic tests include skin scrapings for *Demodex* mites, impression smears, or fine-needle aspirates to confirm the presence of an inflammatory infiltrate. Unusual or recurrent lesions should be excised for histopathologic examination. Solitary lesions may require surgical exploration to find and remove foreign bodies such as grass awns.

Definitive diagnosis of palmar and plantar follicular cysts requires a skin biopsy. However, these cysts are suspected when clinical examination reveals draining tracts associated with callus-like lesions or obvious comedone formation. Moderate to extensive compact hyperkeratosis and acanthosis of the epidermal and follicular infundibulum is found. Follicular cysts consisting of keratin are common. Often, lesions are complicated by secondary infection and concurrent bacterial furunculosis.

Treatment: Bacterial interdigital furuncles respond best to a combination of topical and systemic therapy. Treatment is best based on culture and susceptibility, because these are deep infections and may require longterm therapy, particularly if multifocal. Pending culture, application of warm water compresses and topical triple antibiotic ointment or mupirocin antibiotic ointment are recommended. Foot soaks in chlorhexidine solution are also helpful. Because the lesions are pyogranulomatous, it may be difficult for antibiotics to penetrate them; therefore, >8 wk of systemic antibiotic therapy may be required for lesions to completely resolve. These lesions are often complicated by concurrent *Malassezia* spp infections. Oral ketoconazole or itraconazole (5–10 mg/kg) for 30 days may be indicated. The presence of *Malassezia* can be documented by cytologic examination of nail bed debris and/or impression smears of the skin.

Chronic, recurrent interdigital furunculosis is most often caused by inappropriate antibiotic therapy (too short a course, wrong dosage, wrong drug), concurrent corticosteroid administration, demodicosis, an anatomic predisposition, or a foreign body reaction to keratin. Lesions that recur despite therapy can also be a sign of an underlying disease, eg, atopy, hypothyroidism, or concurrent *Malassezia* infection. Lesions in confined dogs are likely to recur unless the dog is removed from wire or concrete surfaces. In some chronic cases, surgical excision or surgical correction of the webbing via fusion podoplasty may be needed. Alternatively, pulse antibiotic therapy (full dosage therapy 2–3 times/wk) or chronic low dosage antibiotic therapy (eg, 500 mg/day/dog, PO) may help maintain clinical remission and provide pain relief in dogs with chronic lesions. This therapy is recommended only when the inciting cause cannot be identified (eg, idiopathic pyoderma), treated (eg, anatomic predisposition), or resolved (eg, chronic infection caused by foreign body material or keratin).

Treatment of interdigital palmar and plantar comedones and follicular cysts can be successfully accomplished by laser therapy. Postoperative care is time intensive, with hydrotherapy and bandage changes once or twice daily.

PYODERMA

Pyoderma literally means "pus in the skin" and can be caused by infectious, inflammatory, and/or neoplastic etiologies; any condition that results in the accumulation of neutrophilic exudate can be termed a pyoderma. Most commonly, however, pyoderma refers to bacterial infections of the skin. Pyodermas are common in dogs and less common in cats.

Bacterial pyodermas are either simple infections or complex infections. Simple infections are those occurring in young animals that are triggered by one-time or simple events, eg, flea infestation. Complex infections are recurrent and are associated with underlying diseases, such as allergies (flea allergy, atopic dermatitis, food allergy), internal diseases (particularly endocrinopathies such as hypothyroidism or hyperadrenocorticism), seborrheic conditions (including follicular or sebaceous gland diseases), parasitic diseases (eg, *Demodex canis*), or anatomic predispositions (eg, skin folds). Either simple or complex infections can be superficial or deep. Bacterial pyodermas limited to the epidermis and hair follicles are referred to as superficial, whereas those that involve the dermis, deep dermis, or cause furunculosis are referred to as deep. Etiologic classification refers to the pathogenic organism involved in the infection (eg, staphylococci, streptococci, etc). Infections are superficial and secondary to a variety of other conditions.

Etiology: Bacterial pyoderma is usually triggered by an overgrowth/overcolonization of normal resident or transient flora. The primary pathogen of dogs is *Staphylococcus pseudintermedius*.

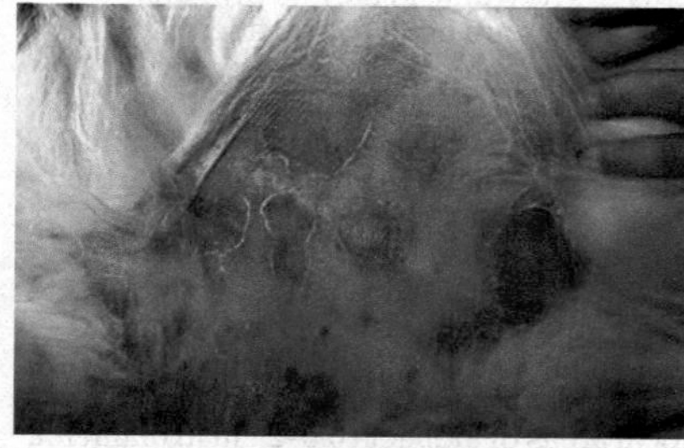

Superficial pyoderma in a dog. *Courtesy of Dr. Stephen White.*

Normal resident bacteria in canine skin also include coagulase-negative staphylococci, streptococci, *Micrococcus* sp, and *Acinetobacter*. Transient bacteria in canine skin include *Bacillus* sp, *Corynebacterium* sp, *Escherichia coli*, *Proteus mirabilis*, and *Pseudomonas* sp. These organisms may play a role as secondary pathogens, but often *S pseudintermedius* is required for a pathologic process to ensue. Normal resident bacteria in feline skin include *Acinetobacter* sp, *Micrococcus* sp, coagulase-negative staphylococci, and α-hemolytic streptococci. Transient bacteria in feline skin include *Alcaligenes* sp, *Bacillus* sp, *Escherichia coli*, *Proteus mirabilis*, *Pseudomonas* sp, coagulase-positive and coagulase-negative staphylococci, and α-hemolytic streptococci.

The most important factor in superficial pyodermas that allows a bacteria to colonize the skin surface is bacterial adherence, or "stickiness," to the keratinocytes. Warm, moist areas on the skin, such as lip folds, facial folds, neck folds, axillary areas, dorsal or plantar interdigital areas, vulvar folds, and tail folds, often have higher bacterial counts than other areas of skin and are at an increased risk of infection. Pressure points, such as elbows and hocks, are prone to infections, possibly because of follicular irritation and rupture due to chronic repeated pressure. Any skin disease that changes the normally dry, desert-like environment to a more humid environment can predispose the host to overcolonization of the skin with resident and transient bacteria.

Clinical Findings and Lesions: The most common clinical sign of bacterial pyoderma in both dogs and cats is excessive scaling; scales are often pierced by hairs. Pruritus is variable. In dogs, superficial pyoderma commonly appears as multifocal areas of alopecia, follicular papules or pustules, epidermal collarettes, and serous crusts. The trunk, head, and proximal extremities are most often affected. Shorthaired breeds often present with multiple superficial papules that look similar to urticaria because the inflammation in and around the follicles causes the hairs to stand more erect. These hairs are often easily epilated, an important feature that helps to distinguish superficial pyoderma from true urticaria, in which hairs do not epilate. In bacterial pyoderma, affected hairs epilate and progress to form focal areas of alopecia 0.5–2 cm in diameter. At the margins of the hair loss, mild epidermal collarette formation may be present, but follicular pustules and erythema are often absent in shorthaired breeds, making diagnosis difficult. Collies and Shetland Sheepdogs often have diffuse areas of widespread alopecia with mild erythema and epidermal collarette formation at the leading edge of the expanding area, often mimicking an endocrinopathy. Pustules and crusts are infrequently found.

The hallmarks of deep pyoderma in dogs are pain, crusting, odor, and exudation of blood and pus. Erythema, swelling, ulcerations, hemorrhagic crusts and bullae, hair loss, and draining tracts with serohemorrhagic or purulent exudate may also be seen. The bridge of the muzzle, chin, elbows, hocks, interdigital areas, and lateral stifles are more prone to deep infections, but any area may be involved. Acral lick granulomas and areas of pyotraumatic dermatitis are also clinical manifestations of deep pyoderma. Interdigital furunculosis (*see* p 862) is another manifestation of deep pyoderma. Plant awns, naked keratin from hair shafts or ruptured hair follicles, and other foreign bodies play a significant role in the inflammatory process associated with deep pyodermas.

Superficial pyoderma in cats is usually due to *Staphylococcus* spp. It is often overlooked and underdiagnosed. The most common clinical finding is scaling, particularly over the lumbosacral area; scales pierced by hairs are a common finding. Intact pustules are almost never found. Feline pyoderma is most common in allergic skin diseases, parasitic diseases, and feline chin acne.

Miliary dermatitis can be a clinical manifestation of superficial pyoderma. Cats with deep pyodermas often present with alopecia, ulcerations, hemorrhagic crusts, and draining tracts. Eosinophilic plaques are a common clinical presentation of deep pyoderma secondary to an allergic disease. Recurrent nonhealing deep pyoderma in cats can be associated with systemic disease, such as feline immunodeficiency virus or feline leukemia virus, or atypical mycobacteria.

Diagnosis: The diagnosis of superficial pyoderma is usually based on clinical signs—hair loss, scaling, erythema, papules, pustules, and epidermal collarettes. Differential diagnoses for superficial pyoderma include demodicosis (*see* p 920), *Malassezia* dermatitis, dermatophytosis (*see* p 872), other causes of folliculitis, and uncommon crusting diseases such as pemphigus foliaceus. Diagnosis of pyoderma should also include steps to identify any predisposing causes.

Identification of the dermatologic lesions described above allows a tentative diagnosis of superficial pyoderma. Direct impression smears of intact pustules, areas underlying crusts or epidermal collarettes, or moist erythematous areas may reveal cocci, rods, or inflammatory cell infiltrates. Impression smears of areas of hair loss and scaling may only reveal large numbers of exfoliative keratinocytes. One of the most important reasons to do impressions is to determine whether a concurrent *Malassezia* infection or overcolonization is present; there is a symbiotic relationship between *Staphylococcus* and *Malassezia*, and both are found in ~50% of cases. The infection will not resolve without concurrent systemic antimicrobial therapy. Multiple deep skin scrapings are needed to exclude parasitic infections, particularly *Demodex canis*. Dermatophyte cultures should be done to exclude dermatophytosis. Bacterial culture and susceptiblity testing is highly recommended because of the increased prevalence of methicillin-resistant *Staphylococci*.

Accurate test results are most likely obtained from intact pustules or induced rupture of deep lesions. Caution should be exercised in interpreting culture results from samples submitted from crusted lesions, papules, epidermal collarettes, and fistulous tracts, because contamination of the sample is more likely than with samples obtained from a closed lesion. Pending culture and susceptibility, topical antimicrobial therapy is recommended, using chlorhexidine-based baths or solutions.

The most common underlying triggers of superficial pyoderma include fleas, flea allergy dermatitis, atopic dermatitis, food allergy, hypothyroidism, hyperadrenocorticism, and poor grooming. Appropriate diagnostic testing and treatment of underlying triggers is mandatory. The most common causes of recurrent bacterial pyoderma include failure to identify an underlying trigger, antibiotic undertreatment (dosage too low or duration of therapy too short), concurrent use of glucocorticoids, wrong antibiotic, or wrong dose.

Treatment: The primary treatment of superficial pyoderma is with appropriate antibiotics for ≥21, and preferably 30, days. All clinical lesions (except for complete regrowth of alopecic areas and resolution of hyperpigmented areas) should be resolved for at least 7 days before antibiotics are discontinued. Chronic, recurrent, or deep pyodermas typically require 8–12 wk or longer to resolve completely.

Amoxicillin, penicillin, and tetracycline are inappropriate choices to treat superficial or deep pyodermas, because they are ineffective in 90% of these cases. Fluoroquinolones should be used only if based on culture and susceptibility.

Topical antibiotics may be helpful in focal superficial pyoderma. A 2% mupirocin ointment penetrates skin well and is helpful in deep pyoderma, is not systemically absorbed, has no known contact sensitization, and is not used as a systemic antibiotic that would increase the likelihood of cross-resistance. It is not very effective against gram-negative bacteria. This ointment should not be used in cats with any known or suspected history of renal disease, because the preparation contains propylene glycol. Neomycin is more likely to cause a contact allergy than other topicals and has variable efficacy against gram-negative bacteria. Bacitracin and polymyxin B are more effective against gram-negative bacteria than other topical antibiotics but are inactivated in purulent exudates.

Attention to grooming is often overlooked in the treatment of both superficial and deep pyoderma. The hair coat should be clipped in animals with deep pyoderma, and a professional grooming is recommended in medium- to longhaired dogs with generalized superficial pyoderma. Clipping will remove excessive hair that can trap debris and bacteria and will facilitate grooming. Longhaired cats usually benefit most from having the hair coat clipped.

Dogs with superficial pyoderma should be bathed 2–3 times/wk during the first 2 wk of therapy and then 1–2 times until the infection has resolved. Dogs with deep pyoderma may require daily hydrotherapy. Medicated shampoos should be prediluted 1:2 to 1:4 before application to facilitate lathering, dispersal, and rinsing. Appropriate antibacterial shampoos include benzoyl peroxide, chlorhexidine, chlorhexidine-ketoconazole, ethyl lactate, and triclosan. Shampooing will remove bacteria, crusts, and scales, as well as reduce the pruritus, odor, and oiliness associated with the pyoderma. Clinical improvement in superficial pyodermas may not be evident for at least 14–21 days, and recovery may not be as rapid as expected.

Of increasing concern is the development of methicillin-resistant staphylococci, and narrow-spectrum antibiotics should be used in treatment of pyoderma to minimize development of resistance. Recurrent bacterial pyoderma, deep pyoderma, and/or animals with a history of extensive antibiotic use are best treated based on culture and sensitivity. Concurrent aggressive topical antimicrobial therapy is helpful. Avoidance of fluoroquinolones and second- and third-generation cephalosporins as empirical therapy is important to minimize the development of multistrain-resistant staphylococci.

CONTAGIOUS ECTHYMA

(Orf, Contagious pustular dermatitis, Sore mouth)

Contagious ecthyma is an infectious dermatitis of sheep and goats that affects primarily the lips of young animals. The disease is usually more severe in goats than in sheep. People are occasionally affected through direct contact.

Etiology and Epidemiology: The causal parapoxvirus is related to pseudocowpox (*see* p 868) and bovine papillar stomatitis (*see* p 215). Infection occurs by contact. The virus is highly resistant to desiccation in the environment, having been recovered from dried crusts after 12 yr. In the laboratory, it is also resistant to glycerol and to ether.

Contagious ecthyma is found worldwide and is common in young lambs reared artificially and in older lambs during late summer, fall, and winter on pasture, and during winter in feedlots.

Clinical Findings and Diagnosis: The primary lesion develops at the mucocutaneous junction of the lips and around erupting incisor teeth and may extend to the mucosa of the buccal cavity. Occasionally, lesions are found on the feet and around the coronet, where secondary bacterial infection with *Dermatophilus congolensis* commonly causes "strawberry footrot." Ewes nursing infected lambs may develop lesions on the teats extending onto the udder skin. The lesions develop as papules and progress through vesicular and pustular stages before encrusting. Coalescence of numerous discrete lesions often leads to the formation of large scabs, and the proliferation of dermal tissue produces a verrucose mass under them. When the lesion extends to the oral mucosa, secondary necrobacillosis (*see* p 1429) frequently develops.

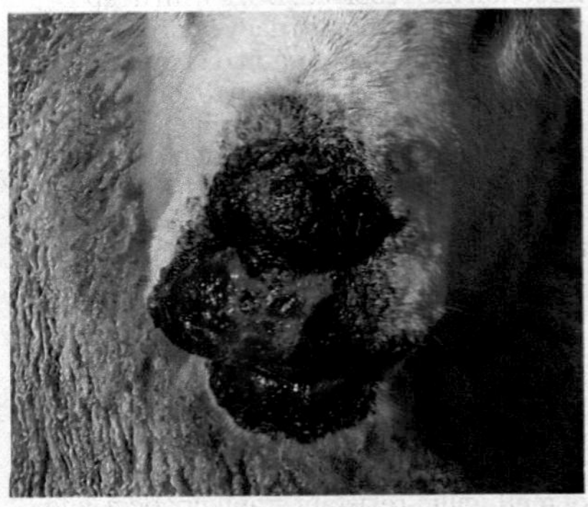

Proliferative contagious ecthyma (orf) lesion extends from the mucocutaneous junction of the lips in a sheep. *Courtesy of Dr. Philip Scott.*

During the course of the disease (1–4 wk), the scabs drop off and the tissues heal without scarring. During active stages of infection, more severely affected lambs do not eat normally and lose condition. Extensive lesions on the feet cause lameness. Mastitis, sometimes gangrenous, may occur in ewes with lesions on the teats.

The lesion is characteristic. The disease must be differentiated from ulcerative dermatosis (*see* p 872), which produces tissue destruction and crateriform ulcers. Ecthyma usually affects younger animals than does ulcerative dermatosis, although this criterion can only be used presumptively. Foot-and-mouth disease (*see* p 629) and bluetongue (*see* p 738) infection should be considered if morbidity is high and clinical signs include salivation, lameness, and fever. Staphyloccocal folliculitis affects the skin of the muzzle and surrounding the eyes. Direct demonstration of virus in scab material by electron microscopy has now been replaced by PCR as the diagnostic method of choice for ecthyma. Historically, positive differentiation could be obtained by inoculating susceptible and ecthyma-immunized sheep.

Treatment and Control: Both parenteral and topical antibiotics may help combat secondary bacterial infection of the skin lesions. In endemic areas, appropriate repellents and larvicides should be applied to the lesions to prevent myiasis. The virus is transmissible to people, and the lesions, usually confined to the hands and face, are more proliferative and occasionally very distressing. Veterinarians and sheep handlers should exercise reasonable protective precautions and wear disposable gloves. Diagnosis in people is established by transmitting the virus to sheep; a complement-fixation test may be of value.

Sheep that have recovered from natural infection are highly resistant to reinfection. Despite a multiplicity of immunogenic virus strains, the presently used commercial single-strain live vaccines have produced fair immunity in all parts of the USA (with an occasional exception more usually seen in goats). Vaccine breaks appear to be due to the virulence of the infecting strain rather than to differences in antigenicity of the vaccine. Sheep immunized against contagious ecthyma remain susceptible to ulcerative dermatosis.

Live vaccines should be used cautiously to avoid contaminating uninfected premises, and vaccinated animals should be segregated from unprotected stock until the scabs have fallen off. A small amount of the live vaccine is brushed over light scarifications of the skin, usually on the inside of the thigh or behind the elbow or caudal fold. Lambs should be vaccinated when ~1 mo old. For best results, a second vaccination ~2–3 mo later is suggested. Nonimmunized lambs should be vaccinated ~1–2 mo before entering infected feedlots.

POX DISEASES

Pox diseases are acute viral diseases that affect many animals, including people and birds. Some poxviruses also cause zoonoses. Typically, lesions of the skin and mucosae are widespread and progress from macules to papules, vesicles, and pustules before encrusting and healing. Most lesions contain multiple intracytoplasmic inclusions, which represent sites of virus replication in infected cells. In some poxvirus infections, vesiculation is not clinically evident, but microvesicles can be seen on histologic examination and, in some, proliferative lesions are characteristic.

Infection is acquired either by inhalation or through the skin (eg, sheeppox). In certain instances (eg, fowlpox, swinepox), the virus is transmitted mechanically by biting arthropods. Infection may be followed by generalized lesions (eg, sheeppox) or remain localized (eg, pseudocowpox). Strains of poxvirus with reduced virulence are used to immunize against some infections, the classic example being the global eradication of smallpox in people by immunization with strains of live vaccinia virus.

Poxviruses can be classified according to their physicochemical and biologic properties. Immunologically, the viruses of smallpox, cowpox, monkeypox, etc, are closely related to vaccinia virus and are classified within the genus *Orthopox*. The avian poxviruses, the myxoma viruses, and some of the other poxviruses (eg, swinepox) are species-specific. The viruses of orf, pseudocowpox, and bovine papular stomatitis are parapoxviruses. It has been recognized that several orthopoxvirus infections of domestic animals and people, notably cowpox and monkeypox, are acquired from rodent reservoir hosts. Many of these rodent hosts have not been unequivocally identified. Thus, although the use of adjectives such as "cowpox" and "monkeypox" to describe these viruses may be epidemiologically inaccurate and misnomers, their retained use reflects both historical association and, until a better nomenclature evolves, pragmatism (*see* p 870).

Poxvirus infections can be confirmed in the laboratory using several diagnostic techniques. The orthopoxviruses can usually be isolated in cell culture and by inoculation of embryonated eggs. Examination of clinical samples by negative-staining electron microscopy is frequently used to visualize virus particles. PCR is widely used to further characterize virus isolates.

COWPOX

In this mild, eruptive disease of dairy cows, lesions are seen on the udder and teats. Although once common, cowpox is now extremely rare and reported only in western Europe (*see also* p 870).

The virus of cowpox is closely related antigenically to vaccinia and smallpox viruses. Indeed, the first two can be differentiated only by sophisticated laboratory techniques. Before vaccination of the general population against smallpox was discontinued, some outbreaks of cowpox in cows in North America and Europe were due to infection with vaccinia from recently vaccinated persons. Vaccinia-related viruses continue to cause occasional outbreaks of teat infections in dairy cattle in South America and buffalo in the Indian subcontinent. These viruses often spread to people in contact with cattle. The epidemiology of these viruses is unknown, but it has been suggested that they are vaccine viruses that spread to animals during the smallpox vaccination campaigns.

The disease spreads by contact during milking. After an incubation period of 3–7 days, during which cows may be mildly febrile, papules appear on the teats and udder. Vesicles may not be evident or may rupture readily, leaving raw, ulcerated areas that form scabs. Lesions heal within 1 mo. Most cows in a milking herd may become affected. Milkers may develop fever and have lesions on the hands, arms, or face. Occasionally, cowpox in people can cause generalized disease, and fatalities have been recorded.

Cowpox or vaccinia infection may be confused with bovine herpes mammillitis (*see* p 1385); because the lesions of these two conditions are superficially similar, laboratory confirmation is required. The viruses of cowpox and vaccinia can be easily visualized by electron microscopy. Although they cannot be distinguished from each other, their morphology by electron microscopy is distinct from that of pseudocowpox virus and bovine herpes mammillitis virus. Both vaccinia and cowpox viruses grow readily in cell cultures.

Measures to prevent spread of cowpox within a herd must be based on segregation and hygiene. Cowpox and vaccinia viruses are important causes of zoonoses.

PSEUDOCOWPOX

(Milker's nodes, Paravaccinia)

Pseudocowpox, a common, mild infection of the udder and teats of cows, is caused by a parapoxvirus and is widespread worldwide. The virus of pseudocowpox is related to those of contagious ecthyma (*see* p 866) and bovine papillar stomatitis (*see* p 215). These parapoxviruses differ morphologically from vaccinia virus and other poxviruses. They have a limited host range and cannot be propagated in fertile eggs, and they will grow in some cell cultures, although relatively poorly.

Lesions begin as small, red papules on the teats or udder. These may be followed rapidly by scabbing, or small vesicles or pustules may develop before scabs form. Scabs may be abundant but can be removed without causing pain. Granulation occurs beneath the scabs, resulting in a raised lesion that heals from the center and leaves a characteristic horseshoe or circular ring of small scabs. This stage is reached in ~7–12 days. Some lesions persist for several months, giving the affected teats a rough feel and appearance, and more scabs may form. The infection spreads slowly throughout milking herds, and a variable percentage of cows shows lesions at any time. Cattle may become reinfected in subsequent lactations.

The scabbed lesions may be confused with mild traumatic injuries to the teats and udder. Scabs examined with an electron microscope frequently show characteristic virus particles.

Control of infection within a herd is difficult and depends essentially on hygienic measures, such as teat dipping, to destroy the virus and prevent transmission. Little immunity appears to develop.

People may become infected with painless but itchy purplish red nodules that are generally present on the fingers or hands. These lesions cause little disturbance and disappear after several weeks.

LUMPY SKIN DISEASE

Lumpy skin disease is an infectious, eruptive, occasionally fatal disease of cattle characterized by nodules on the skin and other parts of the body. Secondary bacterial infection often aggravates the condition. Traditionally, lumpy skin disease is found in southern and eastern Africa, but in the 1970s it extended northwest through the continent into sub-Saharan west Africa. Since 2000, it has spread to several countries of the Middle East and in 2013 was confirmed in Turkey.

Etiology and Epidemiology: The causal virus is related to that of sheeppox. The prototype strain is known as the

Neethling poxvirus. Lumpy skin disease appears epidemically or sporadically. Frequently, new foci of infection appear in areas far removed from the initial outbreak. Its incidence is highest in wet summer weather, but it may occur in winter. It is most prevalent along water courses and on low ground. Because quarantine restrictions designed to limit the spread of infection have failed, biting insects have been suspected as vectors; however, outbreaks have occurred under conditions in which insects practically could be excluded. Experimentally, three species of hard ticks found in Africa have been shown to biologically transmit the virus. Because the disease can be experimentally transmitted by infected saliva, contact infection is considered as another route of infection. African buffalo are suspected as maintenance hosts in Kenya.

Clinical Findings: A subcutaneous injection of infected material produces a painful swelling and then fever, lacrimation, nasal discharge, and hypersalivation, followed by the characteristic eruptions on the skin and other parts of the body in ~50% of susceptible cattle. The incubation period is 4–14 days.

The nodules are well circumscribed, round, slightly raised, firm, and painful and involve the entire cutis and the mucosa of the GI, respiratory, and genital tracts. Nodules may develop on the muzzle and within the nasal and buccal mucous membranes. The skin nodules contain a firm, creamy-gray or yellow mass of tissue. Regional lymph nodes are swollen, and edema develops in the udder, brisket, and legs. Secondary infection sometimes occurs and causes extensive suppuration and sloughing; as a result, the animal may become extremely emaciated, and euthanasia may be warranted. In time, the nodules either regress, or necrosis of the skin results in hard, raised areas ("sit-fasts") clearly separated from the surrounding skin. These areas slough to leave ulcers, which heal and scar.

Morbidity is 5%–50%; mortality is usually low. The greatest loss is due to reduced milk yield, loss of condition, and rejection or reduced value of the hide.

Diagnosis: The disease may be confused with **pseudo-lumpy skin disease**, which is caused by a herpesvirus (bovine herpesvirus 2). These diseases can be similar clinically, although in some parts of the world the herpesvirus lesions seem confined to the teats and udder of cows, and the disease is called bovine herpes mammillitis (*see* p 1385).

Pseudo-lumpy skin disease is a milder disease than true lumpy skin disease, but differentiation depends essentially on isolation and identification of the virus. Histologic and ultrastructural examination of nodules may be helpful. Poxlike intracytoplasmic inclusion bodies or eosinophilic intranuclear herpesvirus inclusions may be seen in the nodules.

Dermatophilus congolensis also causes skin nodules in cattle (*see* p 858).

Prevention and Treatment: Quarantine restrictions are of limited use. Vaccination with attenuated virus offers the most promising method of control. The viruses of goatpox and sheeppox passed in tissue culture also have been used.

Administration of antibiotics to control secondary infection and good nursing care are recommended.

SHEEPPOX AND GOATPOX

Sheeppox and goatpox are serious, often fatal, diseases characterized by widespread skin eruption. Both diseases are confined to parts of southeastern Europe, Africa, and Asia. The poxviruses of sheep and goats (capripoxviruses) are closely related, both antigenically and physicochemically. They are also related to the virus of lumpy skin disease (*see* above). Reports on the natural susceptibility of sheep to the virus of goatpox and vice versa are conflicting; at least some strains seem capable of infecting both species.

The incubation period of sheeppox is 4–8 days and that of goatpox 5–14 days. The clinical picture is similar in the two diseases but is generally less severe in goats. Fever and a variable degree of systemic disturbance develop. Eyelids become swollen, and mucopurulent discharge crusts the nostrils. Widespread skin lesions develop and are most readily seen on the muzzle, ears, and areas free of wool or long hair. Palpation can detect lesions not readily seen. Lesions start as erythematous areas on the skin and progress rapidly to raised, circular plaques with congested borders caused by local inflammation, edema, and epithelial hyperplasia. Although microvesicles are present histologically, vesicles and pustules are not evident clinically. Virus is abundant in skin lesions at this stage. As lesions start to regress, necrosis of the dermis occurs and dark, hard scabs form, which are sharply separated from the surrounding skin. Regeneration of the epithelium beneath the scabs takes several weeks. When scabs are removed, a star-shaped scar, free of hair or wool, remains. In severe cases, lesions can develop in the lungs. In some sheep and in certain breeds, the disease may be mild or the infection inapparent.

It has been suggested that transmission may be airborne, may occur by direct contact with lesions, or mechanically by biting insects.

The disease in either species must be differentiated from the milder infection, contagious ecthyma (orf, *see* p 866), which mainly causes crusty, proliferative lesions around the mouth.

Infection results in solid and enduring immunity. Live, attenuated virus vaccines induce longer immunity than inactivated virus vaccines. Live, attenuated, lumpy skin disease virus also can be used as a vaccine against sheeppox and goatpox.

SWINEPOX

Swinepox is an acute, often mild, infectious disease characterized by skin eruptions that affects only pigs. It is present in the USA, particularly in the Midwest, and has been reported from all continents, although the incidence is generally low.

Historically, vaccinia virus was involved in some outbreaks; currently, swinepox virus appears to be the only cause. The disease described here is that caused by the latter. Swinepox virus is distinct from other poxviruses and does not protect against infection with vaccinia virus. It will grow on pig cell cultures but not embryonating eggs. It is relatively heat stable and survives for ~10 days at 37°C (98.6°F).

The disease is most frequently seen in young pigs, 3–6 wk old, but all ages may be affected. After an incubation period of ~1 wk, small red areas may be seen most frequently on the face, ears, inside the legs, and abdomen. These develop into papules and, within a few days, pustules or small vesicles may be seen. The centers of the pustules become dry and scabbed and are surrounded by a raised, inflamed zone so that the lesions appear umbilicated. Later, dark scabs (1–2 cm in diameter) form, giving affected piglets a spotted appearance. These eventually drop or are rubbed off without leaving a scar. Successive crops of lesions can occur so that all are not at the same stage. The early stage of the disease may be accompanied by mild fever, inappetence, and dullness. Few pigs die of uncomplicated swinepox.

Virus is abundant in the lesions and can be transferred from pig to pig by the biting louse (*Haematopinus suis*). The disease also may be transmitted, possibly between farms, by other insects acting as mechanical carriers.

Recovered pigs are immune. There is no specific treatment. Eradication of lice is important.

COWPOX VIRUS INFECTIONS IN CATS AND OTHER SPECIES

Many orthopoxvirus infections of domestic animals and people result from "spill over" from rodent reservoir hosts. Although traditionally described as infecting cattle, infections of cattle with cowpox virus are now very rare. Domestic cats in Europe are now the most commonly recognized species clinically affected by cowpox virus. Cowpox infections are apparently restricted to Europe. The virus has not been isolated in the Americas, but there is a single report of raccoonpox virus (a related orthopoxvirus) causing a paw lesion in a cat in Canada.

Etiology and Epidemiology: All orthopox isolates from domestic cats in Europe are currently considered to be cowpox virus, although molecular characterization indicates significant heterogeneity in isolates that may be indicative of different rodent hosts. Infection due to cowpox virus has also been recorded in other domestic species (dogs, horses, and llamas) and in a wide range of captive species in various European zoos. Cowpox virus is also infectious to people, and cat-to-human transmission has been recorded. Owners should be advised accordingly.

It is assumed that because of a domestic case of raccoonpox infection in a cat in Canada with a localized infection of a paw, cats may become infected when hunting. Most affected cats come from rural environments and are known to hunt rodents; the initial lesion is often described as having originated as a small bite-like wound. Infection in cats has a marked seasonal incidence, with most cases occurring between September and November. Cat-to-cat transmission can also occur but usually results in only subclinical infection.

The significance of the disease and its relatively recent recognition in cats is an enigma. It may have always been present in the feline population but not recognized. Alternatively, the disease may be increasing in importance as a result of a change either in the epidemiology of the disease, in the reservoir host, or in the nature of the dominant biotype of the virus itself.

Pathogenesis: The most common route of entry appears to be through the skin, but oronasal infection is also possible. After local replication and development of a primary skin lesion, the virus spreads to local lymph nodes, and a leukocyte-associated viremia develops. The viremic phase may be associated with pyrexia and depression and, during this period, virus can be isolated from various tissues, including the skin, turbinates (and sometimes lungs), and lymphoid organs. Widespread secondary skin lesions appear a few days after the onset of viremia, and new lesions continue to appear for 2–3 days, at which time the viremia subsides.

Clinical Findings: Most affected cats have a history of a single primary skin lesion, usually on the head, neck, or a forelimb. The primary lesion can vary from a small, scabbed wound to a large abscess. Approximately 7–10 days after the primary lesion appears, widespread secondary lesions begin to appear. Throughout 2–4 days, these develop into discrete, circular, ulcerated papules ~0.5–1 cm in diameter. The ulcers soon become covered by scabs, and healing is usually complete by ~6 wk. Many cats show no signs other than skin lesions, but ~20% may develop mild coryza or conjunctivitis. Some cats may also be pyrexic, depressed, and inappetent during the viremic phase just before and during the early development of secondary lesions. Concurrent bacterial infection, particularly of the primary lesions, may give rise to systemic signs. However, most domestic cats recover uneventfully. More severe pulmonary disease is uncommon in domestic cats but frequently occurs in cheetahs and is often fatal in both species. More severe disease in domestic cats is often associated with immunosuppression, either after treatment with corticosteroids or associated with infection with feline leukemia or immunodeficiency viruses.

Lesions: Because most cats survive, skin biopsies generally are the only tissue available for histologic examination. Early lesions consist of areas of epidermal hyperplasia and hypertrophy with vesiculation of the prickle cell layer. Many of the epidermal cells bordering such vesicles contain characteristic eosinophilic cytoplasmic inclusions. Later, there is ulceration and necrosis of the epidermis and replacement by an eosinophilic coagulum of necrotic cells and fibrin. A heavy, mixed inflammatory cell exudate is present in the dermis surrounding the lesion. As healing ensues, a thin layer of epidermis covers the skin beneath the scabs, early scar tissue is present, and there is a moderate, mainly mononuclear cell infiltrate.

In rarer cases, in which the disease has generalized, lesions may also be present in the liver, lungs, trachea, bronchi, oral mucosa, and small intestine.

Diagnosis: If multiple, well-circumscribed skin lesions are present, and especially if there is a history of hunting or exposure to a rural environment, a presumptive diagnosis may be based on clinical signs. Cowpox virus infection also should be suspected when skin lesions do not respond to antibiotics. Differential diagnoses include miliary dermatitis, feline herpesvirus or calicivirus infection, eosinophilic granuloma, bite wounds, ringworm, and other chronic bacterial or fungal conditions.

Presumptive and rapid diagnosis can be made in most cases from unfixed scab, exudate, or biopsy material examined for characteristic brick-shaped orthopox virions by electron microscopy. A more accurate and sensitive method of diagnosis is by PCR, or isolation of virus in cell culture or on the chick chorioallantois. Fixed biopsy material for histologic examination and serum for antibody determination also can be sent to the laboratory.

Treatment and Control: In both domestic cats and cheetahs, it is important that cowpox be diagnosed promptly, because steroid treatment, which is often used in therapy of other skin conditions, is contraindicated. Although the disease is often severe in cheetahs, in domestic cats supportive treatment (broad-spectrum antibiotics, fluid therapy) is generally successful, and mortality is low.

Because it seems that infection in domestic cats is mainly sporadic and acquired from chance contact with an infected wildlife reservoir, it is difficult to control the exposure of outdoor cats to this virus. In wildlife parks, where big cats are at risk from contact with small wild rodents, and especially where the disease has already occurred, vaccination may be helpful. Vaccinia virus appears to be of low pathogenicity in domestic cats, and cheetahs appear to be refractive. Currently, management of outbreaks among large cats depends on prompt diagnosis and segregation of affected animals to reduce the possibility of cat-to-cat spread. Rodent control should be evaluated and premises disinfected. At ambient temperatures, poxviruses are relatively resistant and may remain infective in dried crusts for months.

ULCERATIVE DERMATOSIS OF SHEEP

(Lip and leg ulceration, Venereal balanoposthitis and vulvitis)

Ulcerative dermatosis is an infectious disease of sheep caused by a virus similar to the ecthyma virus. It manifests in two somewhat distinct forms, one characterized by formation of ulcers around the mouth and nose or on the legs (lip and leg ulceration), and the other as a venereally transmitted ulceration of the prepuce and penis or vulva.

Clinical Findings: The lesion, regardless of location, is an ulcer with a raw crater that bleeds easily, varies in depth and extent, and contains an odorless, creamy pus; it is covered from the beginning with a scab.

Face lesions occur on the upper lip, between the border of the lip and the nasal orifice, on the chin, and on the nose. In severe cases, the ulcers may perforate the lip. Foot lesions are seen anywhere between the coronet and the carpus or tarsus.

Venereal lesions partially or completely surround the preputial orifice and may become so extensive as to cause phimosis. Rarely, the ulcers may extend to the glans penis so that the ram becomes unfit for natural breeding. In ewes, edema, ulceration, and scabbing of the vulva have less serious consequences.

There are no noticeable early systemic reactions. Morbidity rates of 15%–20% are usual, although up to 60% of a flock may be infected. Often, the disease remains unrecognized until the lesions are so advanced that signs of lameness or disturbed urination become apparent.

Diagnosis: Diagnosis depends entirely on recognition of the characteristic ulcerative lesion. Differentiation between this lesion and that of contagious ecthyma (*see* p 866), which is essentially proliferative in character, is fundamental. In most cases, on removal of the scabs, the lesions of ulcerative dermatosis are crateriform or ulcerative, whereas lesions of contagious ecthyma are proliferative. The question of the similarity of the agents of these two conditions is not clearly defined, but inoculation of sheep previously immunized against contagious ecthyma helps in making a diagnosis. It is also difficult, and in some instances impossible, to differentiate between ulcerative posthitis and vulvitis (*see* p 1372) and ulcerative dermatosis without resorting to sheep inoculation.

Prevention and Treatment: Infected sheep should be isolated, and those with genital lesions should not be bred. Recovery takes 2–8 wk and is not greatly influenced by treatment. Therapy is usually not attempted unless the animals are to be bred soon, lip lesions interfere with eating, foot lesions make the animals so lame that they are losing condition, or secondary bacterial infections become severe.

Treatment consists of removing the scabs and all necrotic tissue from the ulcers and applying any one of the following preparations: silver nitrate (styptic pencil), strong tincture of iodine, 30% copper sulfate solution, 4% formaldehyde, 5% cresol (sheep dip), or sulfa-urea powder. Foot and lower leg lesions can be treated with copper sulfate or formaldehyde solutions in footbath troughs.

DERMATOPHYTOSIS

(Ringworm)

Dermatophytosis is an infection of keratinized tissue (skin, hair, and claws) by one of the three genera of fungi collectively called dermatophytes—*Epidermophyton*, *Microsporum*, and *Trichophyton*. (*See also* FUNGAL INFECTIONS, p 632.) These pathogenic fungi are found worldwide, and all domestic animals are susceptible. In developed countries, the greatest economic and human health consequences come from dermatophytosis of domestic cats and cattle. A few dermatophyte species are soil inhabitants (geophilic), eg, *M gypseum* and *T terrestre*, and cause disease in animals that are exposed while digging or rooting. Other species are host-adapted to people (anthropophilic), eg, *M audouinii* and *T rubrum*, and infect other animals rarely. The most important animal pathogens worldwide are *M canis*, *M gypseum*, *T mentagrophytes*, *T equinum*, *T verrucosum*, and *M nanum*. These species are zoonotic, especially *M canis* infections of domestic cats and *T verrucosum* of cattle and lambs. The zoophilic species are transmitted primarily by contact with infected individuals and contaminated fomites such as furniture, grooming tools, or tack. Exposure to a dermatophyte does not always result in infection. The likelihood of infection depends on several factors, including the fungal species, host age, immunocompetence, condition of exposed skin surfaces, host grooming behavior, and nutritional status. Infection elicits specific immunity, both humoral and cellular, that confers incomplete and short-lived resistance to subsequent infection or disease. New information concerning dermatophytic virulence factors, notably secreted proteases involved in the invasion of keratin, aspects of host immune response against dermatophytes, and new molecular tools available for studying dermatophytes should hasten development of safe and effective vaccines against dermatophytosis in species without vaccination options.

Under most circumstances, dermatophytes grow only in keratinized tissue, and advancing infection stops when reaching living cells or inflamed tissue. Infection begins in a growing hair or in the stratum corneum, where threadlike hyphae develop from the infective arthrospores or fungal hyphal elements. Hyphae can penetrate the hair shaft and weaken it, which, together with follicular inflammation, leads to a common clinical sign of patchy hair loss. As the infection matures, clusters of arthrospores develop on the outer surface of infected hair shafts. Broken hairs infected with spores are important sources for spread of the disease. Under experimental conditions, the housefly, *Musca domestica*, can transmit *M canis* mechanically with its outer body surface for as long as 5 days. The clinical relevance is yet to be determined. As inflammation and host immunity develop, further spread of infection is inhibited, although this process may take several weeks. Thus, for most healthy adult hosts, dermatophyte infections are self-limiting. In young or debilitated animals and, to some extent, in Yorkshire Terriers and longhaired breeds of domestic cats, infection may be persistent and widespread.

Dermatophytosis is diagnosed by fungal culture, examination with a Wood's lamp, and direct microscopic examination of hair or skin scale. Fungal culture is the most accurate means of diagnosis. Dermatophyte test medium (DTM) may be used in a clinical setting. Selected lesions should have the hair clipped to a length of ~0.3 cm. The area should be gently patted with an alcohol-moistened sponge and then patted dry to reduce contamination with saprophytic fungi. Hair stubble and skin scale are collected for placement on the growth agar. The container is then loosely capped to prevent drying. Incubation at room temperature is sufficient except when culturing for *T verrucosum* from food and fiber animals, in which case incubation at 37°C is necessary. *T equinum* requires nicotinic acid if subcultured from primary growth, and some *T verrucosum* isolates require thiamine or thiamine and inositol.

Dermatophyte growth is usually apparent within 3–7 days but may require up to 3 wk on any type of DTM. Dermatophytes growing on DTM cause the medium to change to red at the time of first visible colony formation. Dermatophyte fungi have white to buff-colored, fluffy to granular mycelia. Saprophytic contaminant colonies are white or pigmented and almost never produce an initial color change on DTM. Definitive diagnosis and species identification require removal of hyphae and macroconidia from the surface of the colony with acetate tape and microscopic examination with lactophenol cotton blue stain. Dysgonic strains do exist, but lack of growth of suspected ringworm is most likely due to lack of expertise in culture technique and fungal identification or to disease processes other than ringworm that cause clinical signs.

The Wood's lamp is useful as a screening tool for *M canis* infections in cats and dogs. Infected hairs fluoresce yellow-green; however, only ≤50% of *M canis* infections fluoresce, and other fungal species in animals do not. Therefore, negative Wood's lamp examinations are not meaningful. False-positive examinations may occur and are especially likely in oily, seborrheic skin conditions. Fluorescing hairs should always be cultured to confirm the diagnosis.

Direct microscopic examination of hairs or skin scrapings may enhance clinical suspicion by demonstrating characteristic hyphae or arthrospores in the specimen. The technique is more useful in diagnosing dermatophytosis in large animals than in small animals. Hairs (preferably white ones) and scrapings from the periphery of lesions are examined for fungal elements in a wet preparation of 20% potassium hydroxide that has been gently warmed or incubated in a humidity chamber overnight.

An ELISA for the serodiagnosis of canine dermatophytosis has been researched but is not commercially available. The sensitivity and specificity is high and similar to that of fungal culture with DTM, but positive results can be seen after elimination of the dermatophyte infection. Cross-reactivity between the various dermatophytes would not allow for species identification, which is important for identification of the source of infection.

CATTLE

Trichophyton verrucosum is the usual cause of ringworm in cattle, but *T mentagrophytes*, *T equinum*, *Microsporum gypseum*, *M nanum*, *M canis*, and others have been isolated. Dermatophytosis is most commonly recognized in calves, in which nonpruritic periocular lesions are most characteristic, although generalized skin disease may develop. Cows and heifers are reported to develop lesions on the chest and limbs most often, and bulls in the dewlap and intermaxillary skin. Lesions are characteristically discrete, scaling patches of hair loss with gray-white crust formation, but some become thickly crusted with suppuration. Ringworm as a herd health problem is more common in the winter and is more commonly recognized in temperate climates and in English rather than Zebu breeds of cattle.

Many topical treatments have been reported to be successful in cattle, but because spontaneous recovery is common, claims of efficacy are difficult to substantiate. Valuable individual animals should still be treated, because this may well limit both progression of existing lesions and spread to others in the herd. Thick crusts should be removed gently with a brush, and the material burned or disinfected with hypochlorite solution. Treatment options depend on allowed usage of some agents in animals destined for slaughter. Agents reported to be of use include washes or sprays of 4% lime sulfur, 0.5% sodium hypochlorite (1:10 household bleach), 0.5% chlorhexidine, 1% povidone-iodine, natamycin, and enilconazole. Individual lesions can be treated with miconazole or *clotrimazole* lotions.

A live attenuated fungal vaccine is in use in some countries other than the USA. The vaccine has been used in control and eradication programs to successfully decrease the number of new infected herds. The duration of immunity is long lasting. The vaccine prevents development of clinical lesions, transmission to other animals, and contamination of the environment. A vaccination program combined with a cleaning and disinfection protocol can help eliminate signs of ringworm and eradicate it from the herd. Vaccination has greatly reduced the incidence of zoonotic disease in farmers, their households, veterinarians, and people working in abattoirs and tanneries. No live attenuated vaccine is available in North America.

DOGS AND CATS

In dogs, ~70% of cases are caused by *Microsporum canis*, 20% by *M gypseum*, and 10% by *Trichophyton mentagrophytes*; in cats, 98% are caused by *M canis*. The Wood's lamp is useful in establishing a tentative diagnosis of dermatophytosis in dogs and cats but cannot be used to exclude this type of infection. Definitive diagnosis is established by DTM culture (*see* p 872). Detection of infection in asymptomatic carrier animals is facilitated by brushing the coat with a new toothbrush and then inoculating a culture plate with the collected hair and scale by pressing the bristles to the surface of the medium.

The clinical appearance of ringworm in cats is quite variable. Kittens are affected most commonly. Typical lesions consist of focal alopecia, scaling, and crusting; most are located around the ears and face or on the extremities. Cats with clinically inapparent infections can serve as a source of infection to other cats or people. Occasionally, dermatophytosis in cats causes feline miliary dermatitis and is pruritic. Cats with generalized dermatophytosis occasionally develop cutaneous ulcerated nodules, known as dermatophyte granulomas or pseudomycetomas. Devon Rex cats can have a maculopapular hyperpigmented, crusted disease that histopathologically is an eosinophilic/mastocytic dermatitis.

Lesions in dogs are classically alopecic, scaly patches with broken hairs. Dogs may also develop regional or generalized folliculitis and furunculosis with papules and pustules. A focal nodular form of dermatophytosis in dogs is the kerion reaction. Generalized ringworm in adult dogs is uncommon and is usually accompanied by immunodeficiency, especially endogenous or iatrogenic hyperadrenocorticism. Differential diagnoses for classic ringworm lesions in dogs include demodicosis, bacterial folliculitis, and seborrheic dermatitis.

Dermatophytosis in dogs and shorthaired cats may be self-limiting, but resolution can be hastened by treatment. Another primary objective of therapy is to decrease environmental contamination and prevent spread of infection to other animals and people. Although no controlled studies exist that prove clipping of the hair coat shortens the duration of infection, clinical studies support this recommendation, at least for cats with long hair and/or generalized dermatophytosis, even if it initially worsens or spreads the lesions. Environmental decontamination with bleach (1:10 dilution) or enilconazole solution (0.2%) is effective.

Whole-body topical therapy may hasten a clinical cure (if not a mycologic cure) and decrease environmental contamination. Based on in vitro and in vivo studies, whole-body lime sulfur dips (1:16), 0.2% enilconazole rinses, 2% miconazole, and a combined 2% miconazole/chlorhexidine shampoo were found to be antifungal. These may be appropriate for adjunctive therapy. Enilconazole rinse is not currently available in the USA in a formulation approved for dogs and cats. Topical use of enilconazole may have been the cause of hypersalivation, idiopathic muscle weakness, and slightly increased serum ALT concentration in one study. Local lesions can be treated effectively with topical miconazole or clotrimazole.

For chronic or severe cases and for ringworm in longhaired breeds of cats and Yorkshire Terriers, systemic treatment is indicated. Itraconazole, fluconazole, terbinafine, ketoconazole, and griseofulvin have all been used successfully. The microsized formulation of griseofulvin can be used in dogs (25–100 mg/kg, daily or in divided doses) and in cats (25–50 mg/kg, daily in divided doses) and is best absorbed when given with a fatty meal. The ultramicrosized formulations should be used at lower dosages (10–15 mg/kg/day). There is no veterinary-labeled griseofulvin currently approved for use in dogs and cats in the USA. Cats may develop bone marrow suppression, especially neutropenia, at higher doses as idiosyncratic reactions. This is more common in feline immunodeficiency virus–positive cats. In both dogs and cats, GI upset is a fairly common sequela of griseofulvin administration.

Other effective treatments include itraconazole (5–10 mg/kg/day, or pulse therapy 5–10 mg/kg/day for 28 days then on an alternate-week regimen [1 week on, 1 week off]), ketoconazole (5–10 mg/kg/day), terbinafine (30–40 mg/kg/day), and fluconazole (5–10 mg/kg/day). Fluconazole may be the least effective of these drugs. Terbinafine was found to be at levels higher than the minimum inhibitory concentration on the hair of treated animals for 5.3 wk after 2 wk of daily therapy. This may indicate its potential for use as a pulse therapy drug after 2 wk of daily administration. None of these drugs is approved for use in domestic animals in the USA. In addition, ketoconazole is often a cause of anorexia in cats and is not used as often in this species. Systemic and topical treatments for dermatophytosis should be continued until a negative brush culture is obtained. A brush culture is usually submitted after a minimum of 1 mo of therapy or when clinical lesions are minimal to resolved. In chronic disease and/or challenging environments, the endpoint of treatment may more appropriately be two or three consecutive negative fungal cultures obtained at weekly or biweekly intervals. Efficacy of lufenuron either to treat or prevent *M canis* infection has not been confirmed in controlled studies.

HORSES

Trichophyton equinum and *T mentagrophytes* are the primary causes of ringworm in horses, although *Microsporum gypseum*, *M canis*, and *T verrucosum* have also been isolated. Clinical signs consist of one or more patches of alopecia and erythema, scaling, and crusting, which are present to varying degrees. Early lesions may resemble papular urticaria but progress with crusting and hair loss within a few days. Diagnosis is confirmed by culture. Differential diagnoses include dermatophilosis, pemphigus foliaceus, and bacterial folliculitis. Transmission is by direct contact or by grooming implements and tack. Most lesions are seen in the saddle and girth areas ("girth itch").

Treatment is generally topical because systemic therapy is expensive and of unproven efficacy. Whole-body rinses as described earlier for cattle may be recommended, and individual lesions treated with clotrimazole or miconazole preparations. Grooming implements and tack should be disinfected, and affected horses should be isolated.

PIGS, SHEEP, AND GOATS

Dermatophytosis in pigs is usually caused by *Microsporum nanum*. Lesions are rings of inflammation or brown discoloration that spread centrifugally up to a diameter of 6 cm. Lesions are fairly asymptomatic in adults, and ringworm in swine is generally of little economic consequence. Zoonotic infections in farm workers are not common.

Ringworm is a common, troublesome problem in show lambs but is otherwise uncommon in production flocks of sheep and goats. The infecting species include *M canis*, *M gypseum*, and *Trichophyton verrucosum*. Lesions in lambs are most often noticed on the head, but widespread lesions under the wool may be apparent when lambs are sheared for show, or may develop later as a consequence of contamination from clippers at shearing. Infected lambs should not be issued certificates for transport to show until the infection is cleared. Because there is little evidence that lambs with a functional rumen absorb griseofulvin to effective levels, treatment is best accomplished with sodium hypochlorite solutions or enilconazole rinses (where available). In healthy lambs, as in other species, these infections are self-limiting, but resolution may not be evident in time for show purposes.

CATTLE GRUBS

Hypodermosis of cattle in the northern hemisphere is caused by bot fly larvae (cattle grubs or ox warbles) of *Hypoderma* spp (order Diptera, family Oestridae). In Central and South America, larvae (tropical warbles) of *Dermatobia hominis* (order Diptera, family Cuterebridae) are important pests of cattle.

HYPODERMA SPP

Two species of *Hypoderma*, *H bovis* (common cattle grub) and *H lineatum* (northern cattle grub), are economically important and primary pests of cattle. They are found between 25° and 60° latitude in the northern hemisphere in >50 countries of North America, Europe, Africa, and Asia. In North America, *H lineatum* is found in Canada, the USA, and northern Mexico, whereas *H bovis* is generally found north of the 35th parallel. Occurrence in cattle and American bison was historically common. However, widespread use of macrocyclic lactones have decreased the prevalences of *H lineatum* and *H bovis* in cattle in North America. *H tarandi* parasitizes native Cervidae and reindeer in arctic and subarctic regions. Larvae of *Hypoderma* spp also have been reported in horses, sheep, goats, and people.

Life Cycle: Adult *Hypoderma*, known *also as heel flies* or gad flies, are ~15 mm long, hairy, and bee-like in appearance. In late spring or early summer, they attach their eggs on the hair of cattle, particularly on the legs and lower body regions. The eggs hatch in 3–7 days, and first-stage larvae travel to the base of the hair shaft and penetrate the skin. Normally, the first-stage larvae travel through the fascial planes between muscles, along connective tissue, or along nerve pathways. They secrete proteolytic enzymes that facilitate their movement. During fall and winter, larvae migrate toward two different regions, depending on the species. *H lineatum* larvae migrate to the submucosal connective tissue of the esophageal wall, where they accumulate for 2–4 mo. *H bovis* larvae migrate to the region of the spinal canal, where they are found in the epidural fat between the dura mater and the periosteum for a similar period.

Beginning in early winter, the larvae arrive in the subdermal tissue of the back of the host, where they make breathing holes (central punctum) through the skin. Cysts or warbles form around the larvae, which undergo two molts (second and third stage). The warble stage lasts 4–8 wk. Finally, third-stage larvae emerge through the breathing holes, drop to the ground, and pupate. Flies emerge from the pupae in 1–3 mo, depending on weather conditions. Adult flies, which do not feed, live <1 wk. The life cycle is complete in 1 yr.

For the two species, seasonal events are similar except that those for *H lineatum* occur ~6–8 wk earlier than those of *H bovis*. These events vary from year to year but correlate with local and regional climatic conditions. Larvae first appear in backs of cattle about mid September in southern USA but not until late January or later in northern USA. Grubs first emerge from the back during the last half of November in Texas and during the first half of March in Montana. When both species are present, third-stage larvae may appear in the back for ~5–6 mo; when only one species is present, the larvae may appear for ~3–4 mo. The activity of ovipositing (by female flies) is at its height from January to March in southern USA and from May to July in northern USA.

Clinical Findings and Pathogenesis: During periods of sunshine on warm days, cattle may run with their tails high in the air when chased by female heel flies, particularly *H bovis*. This behavior in cattle is referred to as "gadding" and is a strategy to avoid female flies and their attempt to deposit eggs. Not all stampeding or gadding of this kind is the result of heel fly attacks, because this activity has been seen in the absence of heel flies. Gadding in cattle may result in loss of production, altered reproduction, self-injury, or death.

In otherwise healthy cattle, *H bovis* larvae and their secretions in the epidural fat of the spinal canal are associated with dissolved connective tissue, fat necrosis, and inflammation. Sometimes, the inflammation extends to the periosteum and bone, producing a localized area of periostitis and osteomyelitis. Occasionally, the epineurium and perineurium may become involved. In rare severe cases, paralysis or other nervous disorders may occur. Similarly, *H lineatum* in the submucosa of the esophagus may cause sufficient inflammation and edema in the surrounding tissues to hinder swallowing or eructation. It is unusual, however, for clinical signs of parasitism to be evident during the migratory phase.

Penetration of the skin by newly hatched larvae may produce a hypodermal rash, most often in older, previously infested cattle. The points of penetration are painful and inflamed and usually exude a yellowish serum. Warbles may be found in the back from tailhead to shoulders, and from topline to about one-third the distance down the sides. Usually, the warbles are firm and raised considerably above the normal contour of the skin. In each warble, there is a breathing hole, ranging in size from a small slit to a round hole (3–4 mm in diameter) for more mature larvae. Generally, secondary infection is depressed; however, warbles may occasionally develop in large, suppurating abscesses. The emergence of the third-stage larvae, their forced expulsion, or their death within the cysts usually results in healing of the lesions without complications. Carcasses and hides of cattle infested with cattle grubs show marked evidence of the infestation and are reduced in value.

An infested animal may have 1 to ≥300 warbles but generally <100; infested herds often have individual animals with no larvae. Young animals are most heavily infested.

If migrating *Hypoderma* die in esophageal tissue (*H lineatum*) or near the spinal cord (*H bovis*), they can cause severe, sometimes fatal, reactions. These reactions appear to be related to the numbers of larvae but are rare in any case.

Death of first-stage larvae of *H lineatum* in the submucosal connective tissue of the esophagus causes inflammation of the esophageal wall, dysphagia, drooling, and bloat. Again, recovery is usually rapid and complete (48–72 hr after treatment), but in severe cases, the bloat may be fatal. Rupture of the esophagus may be caused by attempted passage of a stomach tube in an affected animal.

Death of first-stage larvae of *H bovis* in the spinal canal of cattle after systemic insecticide treatment has resulted in stiffness, ataxia, muscular weakness, and paralysis of hindlimbs. Recovery is usually rapid and complete, but occasionally, paralysis may be permanent.

Concurrent with the decrease in the prevalences of *H lineatum* and *H bovis* in cattle, widespread use of macrocyclic lactones has also led to a decline in the clinical relevances of these parasites in North America. However, serologic surveys have demonstrated that cattle are still exposed to *Hypoderma* spp. Should treatment programs stop or move away from products that have efficacy against *Hypoderma* spp, clinical signs due to infestation will likely reappear.

Diagnosis: Third-stage larvae of *Hypoderma* spp are found in warbles, the furuncle-like nodules or cysts along the back of cattle. On recovery from a warble, third-stage larvae can be easily differentiated. *H bovis* is longer (27–28 mm) and has no spines on the tenth segment and a funnel-shaped spiracular plate. *H lineatum* is slightly shorter (25 mm) and has spines on the tenth segment and typically a flat spiracular plate. In cases of bloat or paralysis, the presence of disintegrating grubs and the associated hemorrhage and tissue damage distinguishes animals that are parasitized from those that are not. ELISA-based tests have been developed to

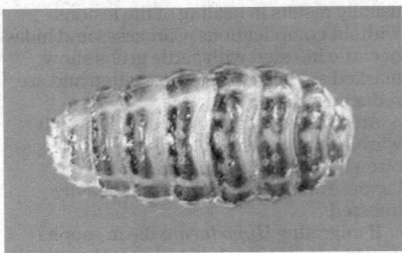

Hypoderma spp, third-stage larva. *Courtesy of Dr. Raffaele Roncalli.*

detect anti-*Hypoderma* antibodies in sera and milk. These ELISA tests are often used to measure risk of exposure and do not correlate well with observation of clinical hypodermosis in cattle.

Treatment and Control: Systemic insecticides in various formulations are available for treatment. Pour-on products containing macrocyclic lactones (doramectin, eprinomectin, ivermectin, or moxidectin) are poured evenly along the midline of the back. Some products must not be applied when the skin or hair coat are wet or when rain is expected to wet cattle within 6 hr. The application site should be free of skin lesions, mud, or manure. Cattle stressed by castration, overheating, vaccination, or shipping should not be treated.

In the USA, registrations of most, if not all, systemic organophosphate insecticides for cattle grub control have been cancelled, and the practices of dipping or spraying cattle for cattle grub control have been replaced by pour-on and/or injectable treatments.

Doramectin and ivermectin are systemically active against *Hypoderma* larvae when injected SC. Ivermectin is also available as an oral paste. The injectable and pour-on systemic treatments are approved for control of *Hypoderma* and other myiasis-causing flies in many countries.

Eprinomectin and moxidectin pour-on formulations are approved for treatment of both beef and dairy cattle. Otherwise, use of drugs for cattle grub control is prohibited in dairy animals of breeding age. Because residues may be present in cattle for varying *periods after* treatment, withdrawal times for all treatments must be observed.

In areas where *Hypoderma* spp are prevalent, cattle, especially calves, should be treated as soon as possible after the end of the heel fly season. They should not be treated later than 8–12 wk before the anticipated first appearance of grubs in the backs, because adverse reactions may occur when migrating larvae are killed.

Where systemic insecticides cannot be used, *Hypoderma* spp larvae can be controlled by applying tetrachlorvinphos dust to the warbles in the back. The dust should be applied to the animal's back and worked into the grub holes. Because new grubs continue to appear in the back, treatment must be repeated every 30–45 days during the warble season.

On small groups of tractable animals, mechanical extraction by instrument or hand expulsion (ie, squeezing) of the individual larva is effective. Larvae can also be removed by carefully injecting 1 mL of 3% hydrogen peroxide with a blunt cannula through the central punctum. However, care must be used to not rupture or pierce the larvae during removal. Rarely, when these procedures are performed carelessly, larvae are crushed or pierced, inducing an anaphylaxis-type reaction. This anaphlyaxis is believed to result from the overwhelming and sudden release of *Hypoderma* spp antigens. Experimental studies have also demonstrated that this anaphylaxis-type reaction is due to the release of toxins from *Hypoderma* larvae.

Research to develop vaccines against *Hypoderma* spp infestations was conducted as early as the 1950s. Even though some natural and recombinant antigens were demonstrated to have efficacy against *Hypoderma* spp infestations, the high efficacy and ease of use of macrocyclic lactones have precluded modern vaccine development.

DERMATOBIA HOMINIS

The tropical warble fly or torsalo, one of the most important parasites of cattle in Latin America, is distributed between southern Mexico and northern Argentina. Larval stages are found in many hosts, including cattle, sheep, goats, pigs, buffalo, dogs, cats, rabbits, and people. Cattle and dogs are infected most commonly. *D hominis* is thought to initiate the lesion that gives rise to lechiguana, a disease of cattle (*see* below).

Life Cycle: The adult fly is 12–15 mm long and has a short life span (1–9 days). The adult fly fastens its eggs to different types of insects (49 have been described as vectors of *D hominis* in Latin America; most are mosquitoes or muscoid flies) that then transport them to warm-blooded hosts, where they hatch as the insects feed. The larvae penetrate the skin of the animal within a few minutes of hatching and remain in the subcutaneous tissue for 4–18 wk. During this period, the larvae grow within warbles with breathing holes. When mature, the larvae leave the host and drop to the ground, burrow, and pupate. After the pupal period, which lasts 4–11 wk, the flies emerge as adults. The complete life cycle takes 11–17 wk.

Clinical Findings and Pathogenesis: Larval penetration of the skin is accompanied by pain and local inflammation, and pus gradually forms. Infested hides are condemned at slaughter, and production of milk and meat is reduced. In 1982, it was estimated that cattle infested with *D hominis* resulted in a yearly reduction in weight of 40.6 g/larva. In 2014, combining losses due to reduced weight gain and hide damage, infestation by *D hominis* in cattle raised in Brazil was estimated to cost producers $383 million USD annually. Efforts to characterize and produce antigenic proteins that confer immunity against *D hominis* have resulted in identification of a candidate vaccine, with 90% efficacy in immunized cattle.

Treatment and Control: Different contact and systemic insecticides in various formulations are available for treatment. Generally, *D hominis* infestations in cattle are susceptible to systemic organophosphates and macrocyclic lactone endectocides, which may be approved and available locally.

Lechiguana

Lechiguana is a sporadic, chronic disease of cattle that, thus far, has been reported only from southern and southeastern Brazil, in areas where infection by *Dermatobia hominis* is common. It is characterized by large, hard, subcutaneous swellings that develop rapidly, mainly in the scapular and adjacent areas (chest, neck, shoulders, and ribs). Most cattle affected have only one swelling, but two swellings are occasionally seen. The regional lymph nodes are enlarged and without treatment may become enormous.

Mannheimia granulomatis has been recovered from lesions and is considered causal. The lesion that gives rise to lechiguana is initiated by *D hominis* larvae. *M granulomatis* is consistently recovered from lesions of the clinical disease, and it is thought to be mainly responsible for the characteristic tissue changes. The involvement of a myofibroblast-like cell population that expresses mRNA for type I collagen is suggested to be associated with the increase of collagen deposition. It has also been demonstrated that macrophages activated by *M granulomatis* induce fibroblast proliferation. The habitat or source of *M granulomatis* is not known. It has not been recovered from cattle without lechiguana.

Histologically, lesions consist of focal proliferation of fibrous tissue infiltrated by plasma cells, eosinophils, lymphocytes, and sometimes neutrophils. The primary lesion is an eosinophilic lymphangitis, which results in eosinophilic abscesses, with occasional rosettes containing bacteria in their centers. The subcutaneous, tumorous mass produced may attain a size as large as 40 × 50 cm in 2 mo. Without treatment, death occurs after 3–11 mo, probably due to inanition resulting from the enormous swellings.

When well established, the disease is clinically obvious. Diagnosis is confirmed by recovery of *M granulomatis* and observation of the characteristic histopathologic lesions.

Treatment with chloramphenicol (3 g/day for 5 days) or danofloxacin mesylate (1.25 mg/kg/day for 3 days) results in rapid reduction of swellings, with almost complete regression in 30 days. Conducting susceptibility tests is advisable before using other antimicrobials.

CUTEREBRA INFESTATION IN SMALL ANIMALS

This opportunistic, parasitic infestation of dogs, cats, and ferrets is caused by the rodent or rabbit bot fly, *Cuterebra* spp (order Diptera, family Cuterebridae). Flies are usually host- and site-specific relative to their life cycle. However, rabbit *Cuterebra* are less host-specific and are usually associated with dog and cat infestations. Rarely, cats and dogs may be infested with *Hypoderma* spp or *Dermatobia hominis*. Ferrets housed outside may be infested by *Hypoderma* or *Cuterebra* spp.

Etiology: Adult *Cuterebra* flies are large and bee-like and do not feed or bite. Females deposit eggs around the openings of animal nests, burrows, along runways of the normal hosts, or on stones or vegetation in these areas. A female fly may deposit 5–15 eggs per site and >2,000 eggs in her lifetime. Animals become infested as they pass through contaminated areas; the eggs hatch in response to heat from a nearby host. In the target host, the larvae enter the body through the mouth or nares during grooming or, less commonly, through open wounds. After penetration, the larvae migrate to various species-specific subcutaneous locations on the body, where they develop and communicate with the air through a breathing pore. After ~30 days, the larvae exit the skin, fall to the soil, and pupate. The duration of pupation varies depending on the environmental factors and winter diapause.

Clinical Findings and Diagnosis: *Cuterebra* lesions are most common in the summer and fall when the larvae enlarge and produce a fistulous swelling ~1 cm in diameter. Dogs, cats, and ferrets are abnormal hosts for this parasite; aberrant migrations can involve the head, brain, nasal passages, pharynx, and eyelids. In the skin, typical lesions are seen around the head, neck, and trunk. The hair is often matted, and a subcutaneous swelling is present beneath the lesions. Cats often groom the area aggressively. Pain at the site is variable and usually associated with secondary infections. Purulent material may exude from the lesion; the most common differential diagnosis is an abscess or foreign body.

Free-roaming cats are more likely to develop lesions than indoor cats. Clinical signs are often associated with the CNS and typically occur between July and September. Cats may have depression, lethargy, or seizures; upper respiratory infections; or abnormal body temperatures (either hyperthermia or hypothermia). One key historical finding in cats with neurologic signs caused by *Cuterebra* infestations is an acute episode of violent sneezing weeks to months before clinical presentation. Common neurologic findings include blindness, abnormal mentation, and signs of unilateral prosencephalic disease. Idiopathic vestibular signs in cats may be due to aberrant migration of the parasite.

Definitive diagnosis is made by finding and identifying a larva. In cats, CT scans may help identify larvae. Second instar larvae are 5–10 mm long and are gray to cream in color. Third instar larvae are dark, thick, heavily spined and are the stage most commonly seen by veterinarians.

Treatment: Suspect lesions should be explored by carefully enlarging and probing the breathing pore or fistula with mosquito forceps. It is not unusual for the parasite to retreat into the opened pore, making it difficult to grasp. Covering the breathing pore with white petroleum jelly for 10–15 minutes before grasping the parasite can make it easier to remove. The lesion should not be squeezed, because this may rupture the larva and lead to a chronic foreign body reaction and secondary infection. There are anecdotal reports of larval rupture causing anaphylaxis. If possible, the larva should be removed in one piece; recurrent abscesses at the site of previous *Cuterebra* infestation suggest residual infection or remaining pieces of larva. The area should be thoroughly flushed with sterile saline, debrided (if necessary), and allowed to heal by granulation. Healing may be slow. Ivermectin has been described as a treatment for cats with CNS cuterebriasis. Diphenhydramine (4 mg/kg, IM) is administered 1–2 hr before ivermectin (400 mcg/kg, SC) and dexamethasone (0.1 mg/kg, IV). Ivermectin is not approved for use in cats.

FLEAS AND FLEA ALLERGY DERMATITIS

There are >2,200 species of fleas recognized worldwide. In North America, only a few species commonly infest dogs and cats: *Ctenocephalides felis* (the cat flea), *Ctenocephalides canis* (the dog flea), *Pulex simulans* (a flea of small mammals), and *Echidnophaga gallinacea* (the poultry sticktight flea). However, by far the most prevalent flea on dogs and cats is *C felis*. Cat fleas cause severe irritation in animals and people and are responsible for flea allergy dermatitis. They also serve as the vector of typhus-like rickettsiae and *Bartonella* sp and are the intermediate host for filarid and cestode parasites. Cat fleas have been found to infest >50 different mammalian and avian hosts throughout the world. In North America, the most commonly infested hosts are domestic and wild canids, domestic and wild felids, raccoons, opossums, ferrets, and domestic rabbits.

Transmission, Epidemiology, and Pathogenesis: Cat fleas deposit their eggs in the pelage of their host. The eggs are pearly white, oval with rounded ends, and 0.5 mm long. They readily fall from the pelage and drop onto bedding, carpet, or soil, where hatching occurs in ~1–6 days. Newly hatched flea larvae are 1–5 mm long, slender, white, segmented, and sparsely covered with short hairs. Larvae are free-living, feeding on organic debris found in their environment and on adult flea feces, which are essential for successful development. Flea larvae avoid direct light and actively move deep in carpet fibers or under organic debris (grass, branches, leaves, or soil).

Larvae are susceptible to desiccation, with prolonged exposures to relative humidity <50% being lethal. The areas within a home with the necessary humidity are limited, and suitable outdoor sites are even rarer. Flea development occurs outdoors only where the ground is shaded and moist (1%–20% soil moisture content) and where the flea-infested animal spends a significant amount of time so that adult flea feces will be deposited into the larval environment. In the indoor environment, flea larvae probably survive only in the protected microenvironment deep within carpet fibers, in cracks between hardwood floors in humid climates, and on unfinished concrete floors in damp basements. The larval stage usually lasts 5–11 days but may be prolonged for 2–3 wk, depending on availability of food and climatic conditions.

After completing its development, the mature larva produces a silk-like cocoon in which it pupates. The cocoon is ovoid, ~0.5 cm long, whitish, and loosely spun. Flea cocoons can be found in soil, under vegetation, in carpets, under furniture, and on animal bedding. Once the pupa has fully developed (1–2 wk), the adult flea can emerge from the cocoon when properly stimulated by physical pressure, carbon dioxide, substrate movement, or heat.

The preemerged adult (which is a fully formed adult flea) residing in the cocoon is the stage that can extend the longevity of the flea. If the preemerged adult does not receive the proper stimulus to emerge, it can remain quiescent in the cocoon for several weeks until a suitable host arrives. Emergence can be delayed up to 350 days if preemerged adults are protected from desiccation. Newly emerging fleas move to the top of the carpet pile or vegetation, where they are more likely to encounter a passing host. Under ideal conditions of temperature (27°C [80.6°F]) and relative humidity (90%), a newly emerged cat flea can survive ~12 days before requiring a blood meal; at 50% relative humidity, this interval drops to ~3 days. It is these newly emerged unfed fleas that infest animals and bite people. There is generally minimal inter-host movement of cat fleas. However, it has been documented that before *C felis* reaches reproductive status, there can be some limited movement on and off hosts. Cat fleas that have found a preferred host (eg, dog, cat, opossum, etc) and have initiated reproduction generally do not leave their host unless forced off by grooming or insecticides.

Depending on temperature and humidity, the entire life cycle of the cat flea can be completed in as little as 12–14 days or can be prolonged for up to 350 days. However, under typical household conditions with normal pet and human activity, cat fleas complete their life cycle in 3–8 wk.

Adults begin feeding almost immediately once they find a host. Female cat fleas can consume 13.6 µL of blood daily, which is 15 times their body weight. After rapid transit through the flea, the excreted blood dries within minutes into reddish black fecal pellets or long tubular coils (flea dirt). Fleas mate after feeding, and egg production begins within 24–48 hr of females taking their first blood meal. Female cat fleas can produce up to 40–50 eggs/day during peak egg production, averaging 27 eggs/day through 50 days. Individual females may continue to produce eggs for >100 days.

Cat fleas are susceptible to cold. No stage of the life cycle (egg, larva, pupa, or adult) can survive exposure to <3°C (37.4°F) for several days. Therefore, cat fleas survive winters in north temperate climates as adults on untreated dogs and cats or on small wild mammals (eg, raccoons or opossums) in the urban environment. As these animals pass through yards in the spring or set up nesting sites in crawl spaces or attics, the eggs laid by surviving female fleas drop off and subsequently develop to adults. Cat fleas may also survive the winter as preemerged adults in microenvironments protected from the cold.

Fleas can cause iron-deficiency anemia in heavily infested hosts, particularly in young animals. Fleas in the genus *Ctenocephalides* have been reported to produce anemia in poultry, dogs, cats, goats, calves, and sheep.

Cat fleas are also involved in disease transmission. Murine typhus, caused by *Rickettsia typhi* and *Rickettsia felis*, is a mild to severe febrile disease of people characterized by headaches, chills, and skin rashes, with infrequent involvement of the kidneys and CNS. The disease is seen in people and many small mammals along the southeastern, southwestern, and Gulf coasts. In the USA, the principal transmission cycle involves opossums and cat fleas. Cat fleas also serve as the intermediate host of the nonpathogenic subcutaneous filarid nematode of dogs, *Dipetalonema reconditum*. *Dipylidium caninum*, the common intestinal cestode of dogs and cats (and rarely children), develops as a cysticercoid in *C felis*, *C canis*, and *Trichodectes canis*. Flea larvae ingest the eggs of the tapeworm, which develop into cysticercoids in the body of the flea. When grooming themselves, dogs and cats may ingest infected fleas, and the cysticercoids are released.

FLEA ALLERGY DERMATITIS

Flea allergy dermatitis (FAD) or flea bite hypersensitivity is the most common dermatologic disease of domestic dogs in the USA. Cats also develop FAD, which is one of the major causes of feline miliary dermatitis. FAD is most prevalent in the summer, although in warm climates flea infestations may persist throughout the year. In north temperate regions, the close association of pets and their fleas with human dwellings creates conditions that permit a year-round problem. Temperature extremes and low humidity tend to inhibit flea development.

When feeding, fleas inject saliva that contains a variety of histamine-like compounds, enzymes, polypeptides, and amino acids that span a wide range of sizes (40–60 kD) and induce Type I, Type IV, and basophil hypersensitivity. Flea-naive dogs exposed intermittently to flea bites develop either immediate (15 min) or delayed (24–48 hr) reactions, or both, and detectable levels of both circulating IgE and IgG antiflea antibodies. Dogs exposed continuously to flea bites have low levels of these circulating antibodies and either do not develop skin reactions or develop them later and to a considerably reduced degree. This could indicate that immunologic tolerance may develop naturally in dogs continually exposed to flea bites. Although the pathophysiology of FAD in cats is poorly understood, similar mechanisms may exist.

Clinical Findings: Clinical signs associated with FAD are variable and depend on frequency of flea exposure, duration of disease, presence of secondary or other concurrent skin disease, degree of hypersensitivity, and effects of previous or current treatment. Nonallergic animals may have few clinical signs other than occasional scratching due to annoyance of flea bites. Those that are allergic will typically have a dermatitis characterized by pruritus.

In dogs, the pruritus associated with FAD can be intense and may manifest over the entire body. Classic clinical signs are papulocrustous lesions distributed on the lower back, tailhead, and posterior and inner thighs. Dogs may be particularly sensitive in the flanks, caudal and medial thighs, ventral abdomen, lower back, neck, and ears. Affected dogs are likely to be restless and uncomfortable, spending much time scratching, licking, rubbing, chewing, and even nibbling at the skin. Hair may be stained brown from the licking and is often broken off. Common secondary lesions include areas of alopecia, erythema, hyperpigmented skin, scaling, papules, and broken papules covered with reddish brown crusts. The rump and tailhead areas are typically the first, most evident, areas affected. As FAD progresses and becomes chronic, the areas become alopecic, lichenified, and hyperpigmented, and the dog develops secondary bacterial and yeast infections.

In extremely hypersensitive dogs, extensive areas of alopecia, erythema, and self-trauma are evident. Traumatic moist dermatitis (hot spots) can also occur. As the disease becomes chronic, generalized alopecia, severe seborrhea, hyperkeratosis, and hyperpigmentation may develop.

In cats, clinical signs vary from minimal to severe, depending on the degree of sensitivity. The primary dermatitis is a papule, which often becomes crusted. This miliary dermatitis is typically found on the back, neck, and face. The miliary lesions are not actual flea bites but a manifestation of a systemic allergic reaction that leads to generalized pruritus and an eczematous rash. Pruritus may be severe, evidenced by repeated licking, scratching, and chewing. Cats with FAD can have alopecia, facial dermatitis, exfoliative dermatitis, and "racing stripe" or dorsal dermatitis.

Diagnosis: A number of factors must be considered in the diagnosis of FAD, including history, clinical signs, presence of fleas or flea excrement, results of intradermal testing, and exclusion of other causes of dermatologic disease.

Most cases are seen in the late summer, corresponding to the peak of flea populations. In these cases, history can be highly suggestive. Age of onset is also important, because FAD does not ordinarily occur before 1 yr of age. Usually, diagnosis is made by visual observation of fleas on the infested pet. Demonstration to the owner of the presence of fleas or flea excrement is helpful. Slowly parting the hair against the normal lay often reveals flea excrement or the rapidly moving fleas. Flea excrement is reddish black, cylindrical, and pellet- or comma-shaped. Placed in water or on a damp paper towel and crushed, the excrement dissolves, producing a reddish brown color.

Extremely hypersensitive animals are likely to be virtually free of fleas because of excessive self-grooming. In these cases, it is usually difficult to find evidence of fleas, thus making it harder to convince owners of the problem. Use of a fine-toothed flea comb (32 teeth/in.) facilitates finding of fleas and their excrement. Examination of the pet's bedding for eggs, larvae, and excrement is also useful.

Intradermal skin testing may be used to support a presumptive diagnosis of FAD. Positive immediate reactions are characterized by a wheal 3–5 mm larger in diameter than the negative control. Alternatively, a positive wheal measurement can be defined as a response that is at least equal to the halfway point between the size of positive and negative control reactions. Observations for an immediate reaction (15–20 min) and, if negative, a 24-hr delayed reaction are recommended. The delayed reaction may not be seen as a discrete wheal but rather as a diffuse erythematous reaction. A positive reaction does not conclusively indicate that the clinical condition is FAD—it indicates only that the animal is allergic to the flea antigen, either from present or past exposure. The reliability of intradermal skin testing in cats to diagnose FAD is variable.

Serologic testing of IgE directed against flea-specific salivary antigens can be used to aid in the diagnosis of FAD.

FAD must be differentiated from other causes of dermatologic disease. The presence of fleas or a positive reaction to an intradermal test does not exclude the presence of another dermatologic disease responsible for the clinical signs. In dogs, differential diagnoses include atopic dermatitis, food allergy dermatitis, sarcoptic or demodectic mange, other ectoparasites, and bacterial folliculitis. In cats, other conditions that can result in miliary dermatitis include external parasites (cheyletiellosis, trombiculosis, notoedric mange, and pediculosis), dermatophytosis, drug hypersensitivity, food allergy, atopic dermatitis, bacterial folliculitis, and idiopathic miliary dermatitis.

Treatment and Control: *See also* ECTOPARASITICIDES USED IN SMALL ANIMALS, p 2754.

Flea control measures have changed dramatically over the years. The development of insecticides and insect growth regulators (IGRs) with convenient dosage formulations and prolonged residual activity has dramatically improved owner compliance and helped eliminate recurrent infestations. The goals of flea control are elimination of fleas on pet(s), elimination of existing environmental infestation, and prevention of subsequent reinfestation. The first step is still the elimination of existing pet flea infestations. Elimination of those fleas currently established on the dog or cat is necessary to eliminate pet discomfort. One common consideration is termed rate or speed of flea kill on a pet. However, it is important to differentiate between speed of elimination of established infestations and speed of elimination of newly acquired fleas after a product has been applied. When treating a dog or cat with a topically applied formulation, it could take several hours (12–36 hr) until the compound has spread sufficiently or reached sufficient systemic concentrations to eliminate all existing fleas. If a more rapid rate of kill is needed, a flea spray or oral product such as nitenpyram, afoxolaner, fluralaner, or spinosad may be desirable.

Several available insecticides provide excellent elimination of established flea infestations on both dogs and cats, including afoxolaner (dogs only), dinotefuran, fipronil, fluralaner (dogs only), imidacloprid, indoxacarb, metaflumizone, nitenpyram, selamectin, spinosad, and pyrethroids.

The second step is to eliminate the existing infestation in the pet's environment. This can be accomplished in several ways: 1) topical application of residual insecticides that kill newly acquired fleas (within 24 hr) before they can initiate reproduction; 2) administration of topical, injectable, or oral IGRs to stop flea reproduction; 3) repeated application of insecticides and/or IGRs to the premises; or 4) combinations of the above.

Administration of topical or systemic residual insecticides and administration of topical, injectable, or oral IGRs have become the preferred methods to eliminate flea infestations. Several of these insecticides and IGRs have very effectively controlled fleas on pets living in infested premises. Field studies have shown that afoxolaner, fipronil with or without the addition of (S)-methoprene, imidacloprid, indoxacarb, fluralaner, lufenuron (with an adulticide), selamectin, and spinosad can effectively control flea infestations, without the need for premise treatment. Flea infestations can be eliminated via regular monthly use of topical and systemic approaches, because most fleas are killed before and/or directly inhibited from reproducing. However, even if the systemic or topical insecticide used is 100% effective, control of an existing infestation will typically take 2–3 mo because of the existing flea life stages in the environment.

If residual flea products are applied at the appropriate dose and treatment intervals, residual activity between applications may be adequate to kill many newly acquired fleas before egg production is initiated. However, flea survival and reproduction may occur before the next application for a variety of reasons: 1) residual activity <100% within the labeled time frame, 2) rate of flea kill slows during the third or fourth week, 3) delayed or infrequent product reapplication, 4) simple under-dosing, and 5) mechanical removal of water-soluble insecticides during bathing or swimming. These problems may result in delays in control or outright treatment failures.

Some of the currently available residual flea products may not be 100% effective against all cat flea strains between labeled reapplication periods because of genetic variability of different flea populations. Many of the factors that allow flea infestations to persist could possibly lead to genetic selection of resistant flea populations. Surviving fleas may be capable of producing viable eggs. Continued reproduction must be halted to prevent persistent flea infestations and selection for resistant fleas. Reproduction can be prevented by administration of topical or systemic IGRs, which provide prolonged residual ovicidal activity, interrupting future flea development even after residual activity of an insecticide is diminished. Application of methoprene or pyriproxyfen to the hair coat of dogs and cats rapidly kills developing flea eggs in addition to residual ovicidal activity. The combination of fipronil/(S)-methoprene or other adulticidal/ovicidal products has demonstrated activity against adult fleas and provides prolonged residual ovicidal activity, thus reducing the potential for genetic selection. Not only have topically applied IGRs been shown to be ovicidal, but orally administered or injectable (cats only) lufenuron also provides ovicidal activity. Although not an IGR, selamectin also demonstrates ovicidal activity in cats.

Many pet owners mistakenly think that flea products either kill all newly acquired fleas within seconds to minutes or completely repel them. But repellency may sometimes be nonexistent, and residual products do not kill most fleas within minutes. Often fleas may live for 6–24 hr and consume blood before being killed. Therefore, close scrutiny of treated pets in an infested environment occasionally results in a few flea sightings on pets for up to 8 wk and occasionally longer until the infestation is eliminated.

An additional complication for pet owners is infestation of the yard by wildlife, feral cats and dogs, or other infested pets. Often owners will treat their pets, but do not realize the environment their pet frequents may be constantly infested with fleas by wildlife or feral animals (especially cats). Even when pets go outdoors for only brief periods, they are susceptible to becoming infested. Additionally, people can act as carriers, bringing fleas into the household and infesting unprotected pets.

In cases of severe, massive flea infestations or severe pet or human flea allergy, treatment of the premises may be necessary. Pet owners should begin by conducting a mechanical control program. Helpful procedures include washing pet blankets, throw rugs, and pet carriers; in addition, pet sleeping and resting areas should be vacuumed thoroughly to help remove flea eggs and larvae. Seat cushions and pillows on sofas and chairs should be removed and vacuumed, and special attention given to crevices in sofas and chairs and to areas beneath sofas or beds where flea eggs and feces may drop from the pet and accumulate. Intermittent-light flea traps can also be beneficial. The overall goal of mechanical intervention is to reduce preexisting biomass of immature and adult life stages in the premises. In addition, treatment of the premises with adulticides and IGRs may still be necessary in some infestations. Control may be achieved by using insecticides with residual activity (or by repeated application of short-acting insecticides) in combination with an IGR to prevent development of flea eggs and larvae. Methoprene and pyriproxyfen are the currently available

IGRs for premise application. Insecticides and IGRs can be applied by broadcast treatment (hand pump sprayers or pressurized aerosols) or with total release aerosols or "foggers." During application, the surface of all rugs and carpets must be treated adequately. Efforts should be directed to areas where flea eggs and larvae accumulate, such as carpets, cracks, grooves in hardwood floors, behind baseboards, under the edge of rugs, beneath furniture (beds, tables, and sofas), and within closets. In severe infestations, a second treatment may be necessary 7–10 days later because of continued emergence of adult fleas from cocoons hidden deep within carpets.

Elimination of fleas in the yard can be an important aspect of flea control. Outdoor treatments (eg, imidacloprid, cyfluthrin, fenvalerate) should concentrate on primary areas of flea development, including protected microhabitats such as dog houses, within garages, under porches, and in animal lounging areas beneath shrubs or other shaded areas. Spraying flea control products over the large expanse of a shade-free lawn generally is not beneficial in control efforts and is poor environmental practice.

Despite the efforts of pet owners, the total elimination of fleas may not be feasible in some situations or may not occur rapidly enough to control clinical signs of FAD. Supportive medical therapy must be instituted to control pruritus and secondary skin disease in hypersensitive animals. Systemic glucocorticoids are often needed to control inflammation and associated pruritus. Short-acting prednisone or prednisolone can be administered initially at a dosage of 0.5–1 mg/kg/day, tapering the dosage and using alternate-day therapy until the lowest dose possible that still controls the pruritus is given. As soon as flea control is accomplished, the glucocorticoid can be discontinued. Anti-inflammatory therapy should never be used as a substitute for flea control.

Secondary bacterial skin infection can be associated with FAD. Systemic antibiotics are commonly used to control the pyoderma and thus reduce the associated inflammation and pruritus. Selection of an appropriate antibiotic should be based on bacterial cultures and results of antibiotic sensitivity tests.

Hyposensitization consists of administering allergens to a hypersensitive animal on a regular basis in an attempt to obtain a state of clinical nonreactivity to flea bites. The effectiveness of currently available whole flea extracts is controversial.

FLIES

Flies belong to the order Diptera, a large, complex order of insects. Most members of this order have two wings (one pair) as adults. However, there are a few wingless dipterans. Dipterans vary greatly in size, food source preference, and in the developmental stage that parasitizes the animal or produces pathology. As adults, dipterans may intermittently feed on vertebrate blood or on saliva, tears, or mucus. These dipterans are referred to as periodic parasites and may serve as intermediate hosts for helminth parasites or for protozoan parasites. They may also alternately feed both on feces and on food and may possibly serve as vectors for bacteria, viruses, spirochetes, chlamydiae, etc. As larvae (maggots), dipterans may develop in the subcutaneous tissues of the skin, respiratory passages, or GI tract of vertebrate hosts and produce a condition known as myiasis.

DIPTERANS WITH BITING MOUTHPARTS

Blood-feeding dipterans can be classified based on which sexes feed on vertebrate blood and on food preference. In certain species of dipterans, only the females feed on vertebrate blood, which is required for egg laying; these species include black flies, sand flies, biting midges, mosquitoes, horse flies, and deer flies. In other species of blood-feeding dipterans, both male and female flies feed on vertebrate blood; these species include stable flies, horn flies, buffalo flies, tsetse flies, sheep keds, and hippoboscid or louse flies.

BLACK FLIES

Members of the family Simulidae are commonly called black flies (although their coloration may vary from black to gray to yellow to olive) or buffalo gnats (because their thorax is humped over the head, giving the appearance of a buffalo's hump). Black flies are the tiniest of the blood-feeding dipterans, 1–6 mm long. They have broad, unspotted wings with thick, prominent veins along the anterior margins. Black flies have compound eyes; eyes of females are distinctly separated, whereas those of the males are contiguous above the antennae. The palps have five segments. Female black flies have scissor-like mouthparts with tiny, sharp, serrated edges. The female flies require a blood meal to lay eggs. Males are never bloodfeeders but instead feed on nectar from flowers.

Although there are >1,000 species of black flies, only a few are considered important as pests. Black flies feed on all classes of livestock, wildlife, birds, and people.

Black flies are distributed throughout the world in areas where conditions permit development of the immature forms. Larvae nearly always are found in swiftly flowing, well-aerated water; shallow mountain torrents are favored breeding places. Some species breed in larger rivers; others live in temporary or semipermanent streams. Black flies are particularly abundant in the north temperate and subarctic zones, but many species are found in the subtropics and tropics where factors other than seasonal temperatures affect their developmental and abundance patterns.

Larval black flies are cylindrical and attach themselves by a large posterior sucker. On the anterior end are the mouthparts and a pair of brush-like organs. The larvae are carnivorous. Just below the mouthparts is an arm-like appendage called the proleg. Larvae attach to rocks or other solid objects in the stream, sometimes clinging to aquatic or emergent vegetation. The mature larva spins a triangular cocoon on the floor of the stream. The oblong pupa has one dorsal and one ventral respiratory tube, the branches of which float out of the cocoon.

Black flies produce one to six generations per year, depending on the species and climatic conditions. Adult female feeding activity may last from 2–3 wk to 3 mo. Adult black flies may fly 8–11 miles (12–18 km) from swiftly flowing streams; migrating windborne swarms have been known to travel ≥250 km.

Pathology: Because of their tiny, serrated mouthparts, female black flies inflict painful bites. The ears, neck, head, and abdomen of cattle are favorite feeding sites. In addition to local reactions (redness, itching, wheals) at the bite site, there may be general conditions that vary in intensity with the sensitivity of the animal and the number of bites. Attacks by large numbers of black flies can cause severe damage and high mortality in livestock. People may be similarly attacked.

Death from black fly attack apparently results from a toxin in the saliva, which increases capillary permeability and permits the fluid from the circulatory system to ooze into the body cavity and tissue spaces. The animal rapidly succumbs to a mass attack but can recover quickly if protected from further attacks. Reduced milk, meat, and egg production may result from less extensive attacks. Certain species of black flies sometimes cause losses in poultry, either by direct attack or through transmission of *Leucocytozoon* spp. In Africa, *Simulium damnosum* and *S neavei* are important as vectors of *Onchocerca* spp. *S neavei* is an important vector of *O volvulus*. In Central America, *S ochraceum*, *S metallicum*, *S callidum*, and *S exiguum* are important vectors of *Onchocerca* spp. *S ochraceum* and *S metallicum* also are vicious biters.

Diagnosis: Black flies are most often collected in the field and not found on the animals. Adult flies can be identified by their small size, humped back, prominent venation in the anterior region of the wings, and tiny, serrated mouthparts. Identification of black flies to genus and species is probably best left to an entomologist.

Treatment and Control: If public funds and trained supervisory personnel are available, large-scale control of black flies is possible by treating breeding streams with an approved larvicide. However, black fly control is difficult because of the large number of flowing water breeding sites. Streams can be treated using the natural product, *Bacillus thuringiensis* var *israelensis*, a product with no mammalian toxicity.

Treatment of streams and rivers involves techniques similar to those used by mosquito abatement programs. As a rule, pesticides should not be used owing to their potential negative effects on the environment. Pesticide treatments involving water surfaces or large land areas are subject to governmental regulation and must be performed with due regard for possible deleterious environmental effects and residues in food products.

Adult black flies are small enough to pass through window screens or may come indoors on or within a pet's hair coat. More often, the adult female flies prefer to feed outdoors and during the daylight hours. Because black flies feed predominantly during the daylight hours, it is wise to limit exposure of pets to swiftly flowing streams. Pet owners concerned about black fly bites may use over-the-counter insect repellents. Aerosols containing pyrethrins may provide only temporary relief.

Because area-wide control of black flies is difficult and expensive, livestock producers frequently resort to the daily use of repellents to protect their animals. Extension entomology personnel should be contacted for the latest approved recommendations and withdrawal times.

SAND FLIES

The phlebotomine sand flies, *Phlebotomus* spp (Old World sand flies) and *Lutzomyia* spp (New World sand flies), are members of the family Psychodidae. These flies are confined primarily to the tropical and subtropical regions of the world. Members of these genera are tiny, moth-like flies, ~1.5–4 mm long. The legs are as long as the antennae, comprising 16 segments that often have a beaded, hairy appearance. They are commonly known as sand flies, moth flies, or owl midges. The key morphologic feature for identification is that the body of the sand fly is covered with fine hairs. The females have piercing mouthparts and feed on blood of a variety of warm-blooded animals, including people. Many species feed on reptiles. Male sand flies suck moisture from any available source and are even said to suck perspiration from people. Sand flies tend to be active only at night and are weak fliers; their flying is deterred by air currents, even slight ones. During the day, sand flies seek protection in crevices and caves, among vegetation, and within dark buildings. They often seek protection within rodent and armadillo burrows; these mammals can serve as reservoir hosts for *Leishmania* spp. Sand flies breed in dark, humid environments that have a supply of organic matter that serves as food for the larvae. They do not breed in aquatic environments.

Pathology: These tiny flies serve as an intermediate host for *Leishmania* spp, a protozoan parasite that infects the reticuloendothelial cells of capillaries, the spleen, and other organs but may be seen in monocytes, polymorphonuclear leukocytes, and macrophages of people, dogs, cats, horses, and sheep (*see* p 800).

Diagnosis: Like black flies, sand flies can most often be collected in the field and are not found on animals. They can be identified by their small size and hairy wings and bodies. Identification of genus and species is probably best left to an entomologist.

Treatment and Control: Insecticide spraying of larval habitat is usually not possible because of the difficulty of accessing breeding sites. Removal of dense vegetation discourages breeding. Spraying of residual insecticides on surfaces in the home is the main way to control sand flies; however, this is ineffective for species that bite away from the home. In general, populations of sand flies have been reduced as a result of intense mosquito control programs. Deltamethrin-impregnated collars may be recommended to dog owners to protect their pets from sand fly bites.

BITING MIDGES

The biting midges, "no-see-ums," or punkies belong to the family Ceratopogondiae. The most common biting midges are *Culicoides* spp. They are associated with aquatic or semiaquatic habitats, eg, mud or moist soil around streams, ponds, and marshes. Biting midges are tiny gnats (1–3 mm long) and, like black flies, inflict painful bites and suck the blood of their hosts, both people and livestock.

Pathology: *Culicoides* spp are vicious biters and can cause intense irritation and annoyance. In large numbers, they can cause livestock to be nervous and interrupt their feeding patterns. These gnats tend to feed on the dorsal or ventral areas of the host; feeding site preference depends on the species of biting gnat. They fly only in the warm months of the year and are most active before and during dusk. They feed often on the mane, tail, and belly of horses. Horses often become allergic to the bites, scratching and rubbing these areas, causing alopecia, excoriations, and thickening of the skin. This condition has several names, including culicoid hypersensitivity in Canada, Queensland itch in Australia, Kasen in Japan, sweat itch, and sweet itch. Because it is often seen during the warmer months of the year, it is also referred to as summer dermatitis. These flies also serve as the intermediate host for *Onchocerca cervicalis*; the microfilariae of this nematode are found in the skin of horses. Onchocerciasis (*see* p 905) is a nonseasonal dermatosis that is similar to sweet itch but usually is less pruritic and affects the head, neck, and belly. These flies also transmit the bluetongue virus (*see* p 738) in sheep and cattle.

Diagnosis: Like black flies and sand flies, biting midges are most often collected in the field and not found on the animals. In contrast to the clear, heavily veined wings of black flies, the wings of *Culicoides* spp are mottled. Identification is probably best left to an entomologist.

Treatment and Control: Larvae may be attacked in their breeding grounds. Extension entomology personnel should be contacted for the latest approved recommendations.

Bio Kill Stable Spray™, a modified permethrin, is approved for the spraying of stables and horseboxes to aid in the control of biting midges. A backpack or handheld bulk pesticide spray pack, turbo-blower, or fogger should be used. A fine spray should be produced under pressure, in the amount of 500–750 mL per stable (stable size: 3 m × 3.5 m to 4 m × 4 m). All surfaces in the stable should be sprayed. A reapplication 7–10 days later is needed. Thereafter, application every 3–4 wk should provide ample product buildup on the walls.

Because *Culicoides* spp are poor flyers, an electric fan may be used in the stable to create air movement around the horses. Fly repellent ear tags attached to the horse's mane and tail (not approved in the USA); pyrethrum synergized with piperonyl butoxide, applied weekly; butoxypolypropylene glycol 800, applied daily; stable blankets; and fine screens on stable doors and windows have been used with mixed success. Topical insecticides such as pyrethrins (eg, cypermethrin or cyfluthrin), especially in pour-on formulations, may also be used to control these adult pests in large animals.

MOSQUITOES

Mosquitoes are members of the family Culicidae. Important genera include *Aedes*, *Anopheles*, *Culex*, *Culiseta*, and *Psorophora*. Although they are tiny, fragile dipterans, mosquitoes are perhaps some of the most voracious of the blood-feeding arthropods. Approximately 300 species have been described worldwide, with ~150 species found in the temperate regions of North America. Mosquitoes are found in such diverse areas as salt marshes of the coastal plains to snow pools above 14,000 ft (4,300 m) to the gold mines of India 3,600 ft (1,100 m) below sea level. The volume of water in which mosquitoes will breed varies from that within an empty can or tree hole to large shallow pools of accumulated, standing water from either rain or snow melt.

Mosquitoes lay their eggs either on the surface of standing water (eg, *Aedes* and *Psorophora* spp) or on a substrate (such as damp soil) where the eggs hatch after inundation from rainfall, irrigation, snow melt, etc. Larval mosquitoes are known as wrigglers, whereas pupal mosquitoes are known as tumblers. These stages are always aquatic and are found in a wide variety of habitats. Large numbers of mosquitoes can be produced from eggs laid in relatively small bodies of water. Some species have several generations per year. The flight habits of adult mosquitoes vary with the species; some *Aedes* sp migrate many miles for their aquatic, larval habitat. In strong winds, mosquitoes may be carried great distances. Some species overwinter as eggs, while others overwinter as adults.

Pathology: Only female mosquitoes actively take a blood meal so that they can lay eggs. Males feed on nectar, plant juices, and other liquids. Mosquitoes annoy livestock, cause blood loss, and transmit disease. Also, the toxins injected at the time of biting may cause systemic effects. The feeding of large numbers of swarming mosquitoes can cause significant anemia in domestic animals. Although they are known for spreading malaria, yellow fever, dengue, and elephantiasis in people, mosquitoes are probably best known in veterinary medicine as the intermediate host for the canine heartworm, *Dirofilaria immitis*, and as the vectors of the equine viral encephalitides, including West Nile virus.

Anopheles quadrimaculatus is the intermediate host for malaria (*Plasmodium* spp) in people and other primates. *Aedes aegypti* is the yellow fever mosquito, transmitting this virus among people. *Psorophora columbiae* is a severe pest of both livestock and people in the rice fields of Louisiana and Arkansas. *Culex tarsalis* is an important vector of Western equine encephalitis and is found in the western, central, and southern USA. *Aedes vexans* is an important nuisance species found in the Midwest. *Aedes albopictus* is a recently introduced Asian species that also spreads yellow fever, dengue, and equine encephalitis. Certain *Mansonia* spp are severe pests of livestock in Florida. In Central and South America, the adult female bot fly *Dermatobia hominis* fastens her eggs to a species of *Psorophora* mosquito, which then transmits them to the mammalian host during feeding.

Diagnosis: Adult mosquitoes are most often collected in the field and are not found on animals. Adults are 3–6 mm long and slender, with small, spherical heads and long legs. The wing veins, body, head, and legs are covered with tiny, leaf-shaped scales. The long, filamentous antennae have 14–15 segments and are plumose in the males of most species. They also have proboscides designed for lacerating tiny blood vessels and sucking up pooled blood. Identification of the plethora of mosquito species (adult, larval, and pupal stages) is probably best left to an entomologist.

Treatment and Control: Area control of mosquitoes usually involves the cooperation of many individuals and can be accomplished successfully by experienced personnel with proper equipment. Areas that can serve as breeding sites for mosquito larvae should be eliminated or reduced. In addition, area programs generally include extensive use of larvicides; however, mosquito larvicides can disrupt the normal ecologic balance within an ecosystem. Recently, the use of various species of fish as biologic controls has been successful. In massive emergence of adult mosquitoes, particularly when disease transmission is a concern, application of an insecticide active against the adult may be necessary.

Caution is advised with area treatment programs, because many nontarget organisms (eg, fish, shrimp, bees) may be exposed to insecticides. A local extension entomologist should be consulted regarding appropriate materials for use on animals or within premises. Large-scale programs usually are coordinated by mosquito abatement district or other government agencies.

It is difficult for individual producers to protect their animals; residual sprays on the animals do not prevent feeding females from landing, and currently available repellents do not confer adequate protection during massive emergence. Protection from adult mosquitoes may be provided by ground and, in some cases, aerial application of an insecticide at the time of emergence. Depending on local conditions, this protection may be of short duration. Valuable animals should be housed in closed or screened buildings and the mosquitoes inside killed with a fog or aerosol formulation of an approved insecticide. Temporary relief may be afforded by a spray or "wipe on" of materials commercially available.

Walking pets or allowing pets free range, outdoor access in the early morning or early evening hours when adult mosquitoes are most abundant should be avoided to reduce exposure to mosquito bites. Imidacloprid has been used as a topical prevention and treatment of ticks, fleas, and mosquitoes on dogs and puppies ≥7 wk old, weighing >2 lb (0.91 kg). It has been shown to repel adult female mosquitoes for as long as 4 wk. Unfortunately, it cannot be used on cats. Mosquitoes are not attracted to light; thus, electrocution devices are not helpful in mosquito control and may actually be detrimental, because they may destroy beneficial insects that prey on mosquitoes.

A combination of two compounds, imidacloprid and permethrin, works to repel and kill the many species of blood-feeding mosquitoes that often feed on dogs. Monthly application of this product repels and kills mosquitoes, preventing their blood-feeding activity and ostensibly helping to prevent transmission of organisms such as *Dirofilaria immitis* from dog to dog. This product may not be used on cats.

HORSE FLIES AND DEER FLIES

Tabanus spp (horse flies) and *Chrysops* spp (deer flies) are large (up to 3.5 cm long), heavy bodied, robust dipterans with powerful wings and very large eyes. They are swift fliers. These flies are the largest in the dipteran group, in which only the females feed on vertebrate blood. Horse flies are larger than deer flies; many horse flies are highly colored. Deer flies are medium sized; they have a dark band passing from the anterior to the posterior margin of the wings and a yellow to brown abdomen with black patches and longitudinal bands.

Adult horse flies and deer flies lay eggs in the vicinity of open water. Larval stages are found in aquatic to semiaquatic environments, often buried deep in mud at the bottom of lakes and ponds. The developing larval stages have sharp mandibles and are predatory on smaller vetebrates and invertebrates; they will even lightly nip at the toes of people wading in shallow water. This is an unusual dipteran fly in that both larval stages and adult flies are capable of inflicting pain as they bite.

Pathology: Adults are seen in summer, particularly in sunlight. Adult females of both species feed in the vicinity of open water and have reciprocating, scissor-like mouthparts, which they use to lacerate tissues and lap up the oozing blood. They consume 0.1–0.3 mL of blood at a single feeding. Bites are painful and irritating. These flies feed primarily on large animals, such as cattle and horses, which become restless when the flies are present. Site preferences include the underside of the abdomen around the navel, the legs, or the neck and withers. Horse flies and deer flies feed a number of times in multiple feeding sites before they become replete. When disturbed by the animal's swatting tail or by the panniculus reflex, the flies leave the host, yet blood continues to ooze from the open wound. These flies may act as mechanical transmitters of anthrax, anaplasmosis, tularemia, and the virus of equine infectious anemia.

Diagnosis: These flies can be identified by their large size, powerful wings, compound eyes, and lacerating scissor-like mouthparts. Species identification of intact adult and larval horse and deer flies is probably best left to an entomologist.

Treatment and Control: Horse flies and deer flies are the most difficult to control of all of the bloodsucking flies. Many of the adulticide compounds used for other biting flies can kill both horse and deer flies. However, because these flies are intermittent feeders that alight on the host for only a short time, they may not be exposed to these compounds long enough to be affected. Thus, larger doses of the compounds may be required.

Horse fly traps have been effective when used around cattle confined to manageable areas. For livestock, pyrethroid pourons function as limited repellents. Self-application techniques are usually not effective for horse and deer flies.

Manipulation of these flies' aquatic habitat has been attempted by removing unnecessary woody plants from residential areas or draining wet areas. Application of insecticides in the water may have detrimental environmental effects.

STABLE FLIES

The stable fly, *Stomoxys calcitrans*, is often called the biting house fly. It is about the same in size and general appearance as *Musca domestica*, the house fly. It is brownish gray, the outer of four thoracic stripes is broken, and the abdomen has a checkered appearance. It has a bayonet-like, needle-sharp proboscis that, when at rest, protrudes forward from the head. The wings, when at rest, are widely spread at the tips. These flies are found throughout the world. In the USA, they are found in the midwestern and southeastern states.

The larval and pupal forms develop in decaying organic matter, including grass clippings and seaweed along beaches. In the midwestern USA, larvae can be found in wet areas around the edges of hay stacks and silage pits. Where cattle are fed hay, breeding can occur at the edge of the feeding area where hay has become mixed with urine and feces. The life cycle in the field can be completed in 2–3 wk, and adults may live ≥3–4 wk.

Pathology: Both male and female stable flies are avid blood feeders, feeding on any warm-blooded animal. Stable flies stay on the host for short periods of time, during which they obtain blood meals. This is an outdoor fly; however, in the late fall and during rainy weather, it may enter barns.

Horses are the preferred hosts. The fly usually lands on the host with its head and proboscis pointed upward and inflicts painful bites that puncture the skin and bleed freely. It is a sedentary fly, not moving on the host. Stable flies usually attack the legs and ventral abdomen and may also bite the ears. They can be a problem in cattle feedlots in the Midwestern USA. The damage inflicted to cattle is caused by the painful bite and blood loss, and the irritation results in a reduced efficiency in converting feed to meat or milk. In pets, stable flies prefer to feed on the tips of the ears of dogs with pointed ears, especially German Shepherds.

Stable flies are mechanical vectors of anthrax, surra, and equine infectious anemia. They are the intermediate host for *Habronema muscae*, a nematode found in the stomach of horses.

Diagnosis: Stable flies are easily identified by their size (about the same as that of the house fly), coloration, and bayonet-like proboscis that protrudes forward from the head.

Treatment and Control: The main consideration in stable fly control is sanitation, which can effect up to 90% control. Areas along fence rows, under feed bunks, or wherever manure and straw or decaying matter can accumulate should be kept clean, because these substrates provide the medium in which the larval flies develop. If good sanitation procedures are practiced, chemical control is less likely to be needed. Various insecticides can be sprayed where flies may be resting in barns or on fence rows.

Stable flies feed on the lower portions of cattle, around the legs and belly, including the udder. They usually feed only once or twice daily for short periods, thus minimizing exposure to compounds applied to these areas. Often, insecticides applied to these body regions are rubbed off by contact with dense vegetation and mud or rinsed off when dairy cattle are rinsed before milking. Direct animal application of sprays and dusts may be used in some instances to protect large animals. Insecticides used for direct animal application usually have short residual activity. This type of application is quite labor intensive.

A combination of two compounds, imidacloprid and permethrin, works to repel *S calcitrans*. Monthly application repels these flies and prevents their blood feeding on dogs, but the product does not kill this type of biting fly.

HORN FLIES

The common name of *Haematobia irritans* comes from the fact that these flies often cluster in the hundreds around the base of the horns of cattle. This major pest of cattle is found in most cattle-producing areas of the world. Populations are common in Europe, North Africa, Asia Minor, and the Americas. Throughout North America, horn flies are found almost exclusively on cattle, but they will feed on horses, sheep, goats, and wildlife. Horn flies are found in much larger numbers and for longer periods of time in the southern and southwestern USA.

Adult horn flies spend their entire life on their host, and females leave only to oviposit eggs on fresh cow feces, where larval and pupal development occurs. In the southern USA, the life cycle can be as short as 1 wk, but in cooler climates and in the spring or fall, development can take 2–3 wk. In some warmer areas (south Florida and southernmost Texas), horn flies reproduce throughout the year.

When the air temperature is <70°F (21°C), horn flies cluster around the base of the horns of cattle. In warmer climates, the flies often cluster in large numbers on the shoulders, back, and sides; these areas are least disturbed by tail switching. On hot, sunny days, horn flies accumulate on the ventral abdomen.

Newly emerged flies seeking their host may travel 7–10 miles (11–15 km) but usually find a host in much shorter distances. Migration seldom occurs over any great distance. In the southern USA, fly populations on individual animals may be in the thousands, especially on bulls not receiving chemical treatment; in the north, they may not exceed 100, although the damage inflicted is similar.

Pathology: Horn flies feed frequently (as many as 20 times/day), sucking blood and other fluids; female flies are more aggressive than males. Feeding causes pain, annoyance, and blood loss in cattle. Irritated animals also lose weight because of their less efficient use of feed. Heavy infestations cause lesions along the ventral midline of the animal. Horn flies cause great economic losses annually in the USA; 14% reductions in weight gains on range cattle and losses of 12–14 lb (5–6 kg/head) in weaned calves are common. In dairy cattle, milk production may be reduced 10%–20%. These flies also serve as the intermediate host for *Stephanofilaria stilesi* (*see* p 907), a filarial parasite that produces plaquelike lesions on the ventral abdomen of cattle.

Diagnosis: Horn flies can be easily identified by their dark color, size (~3–6 mm long, approximately half the size of a stable fly), and bayonet-like proboscis that protrudes forward from the head.

Treatment and Control: Horn flies are relatively easy to control with whole-animal chemical sprays and with self-treating devices (eg, dust bags or back rubbers) in a forced-use manner. Dust bags are most effective when cattle are required to pass under them daily to reach water or mineral supplements. Dust bags leave a deposit of insecticides along the dorsum, the areas where horn flies spend most of their time. Back rubbers allow cattle to treat themselves as they scratch. The insecticide should be diluted with a good grade of mineral oil according to label instructions. Feed additives pass through the animal to kill larval stages that develop in fresh cow feces. All animals must consume a minimum dose of a feed additive regularly. Insect growth regulators also prevent development of larvae in cow feces. When used according to label directions, insecticide-impregnated cattle ear tags (eg, pyrethroids) release small amounts of insecticides that are distributed over the animal during grooming or rubbing. Animals should be tagged at or near the beginning of fly season, the tags removed at or near the end of fly season, and alternative methods with nonpyrethroid insecticides used near the end of fly season. Pour-on insecticide formulations are also effective against horn flies. These compounds are applied to cattle in measured doses based on body weight. Most of these pour-ons function as contact insecticides.

BUFFALO FLIES

Buffalo flies, *Haematobia irritans exigua*, are similar to horn flies in size and appearance and in feeding and breeding habits. The buffalo fly is a primary pest of cattle and water buffalo but occasionally feeds on horses, sheep, or wildlife. It is distributed throughout northern Australia and New Guinea and is found in parts of southern, southeastern, and eastern Asia as well as Oceania; it is not found in New Zealand. Its life cycle is similar to that of the horn fly; the adult leaves the host long enough to oviposit on fresh manure, where development occurs. The life cycle may take as few as 7–10 days, depending on weather conditions.

Pathology: Buffalo flies irritate and annoy animals, usually biting about the shoulders and withers. Bite wounds may provide a site for screwworm (*Chrysomya bezziana*) infection. During hot weather, the flies move to shaded parts of the body. Affected animals suffer blood loss and are irritated by the flies; feed efficiency and production may be affected adversely.

Diagnosis: Buffalo flies can be identified by their dark color, size (approximately half that of a stable fly), and bayonet-like proboscis that protrudes forward from the head.

Treatment and Control: Insecticides should be avoided in the treatment of buffalo fly populations. Many of the chemicals used to treat these flies result in meat residues. Buffalo flies have developed resistance to the synthetic pyrethroids and to some of the organophosphates. Buffalo fly traps have been developed in Australia. The trap consists of a rounded, clear plastic tent through which the cattle walk. The flies are brushed off the cattle within the tent and are then trapped inside where they die of desiccation. These traps remove ~80% of the buffalo flies each time the cattle pass through. When cattle pass through the trap every day or every second day, sufficient fly control is usually achieved.

TSETSE FLIES

The tsetse flies, *Glossina* spp, are important blood-feeding flies found in Africa (latitude 5°N to 20°S). Tsetse flies are narrow bodied, yellow to dark brown, and 6–13.5 mm long. When resting, their wings are held over the back in a scissor-like configuration. The thorax has a dull greenish color with inconspicuous spots or stripes. The abdomen is light to dark brown.

Both sexes are avid blood feeders. One copulation renders a female fly fertile for her lifetime, during which she can produce as many as 12 larvae. She produces one larva at a time, retaining it within her uterus; after ~10 days, the larva is deposited on loose, sandy soil, where it digs in and begins pupation within 60–90 min. This pupation period averages ~35 days, after which the adult emerges. Adult flies feed avidly on vertebrate blood approximately every 3 days.

Pathology: Tsetse flies serve as the intermediate hosts for several species of trypanosomes that cause fatal diseases of both domestic animals (nagana) and people (African sleeping sickness). Trypanosomes invade the blood, lymph, CSF, and various organs of the body, such as the liver and spleen. Nagana, a related complex in cattle caused by *Trypanosoma brucei*, has occurred throughout enormous areas estimated to be as great as one quarter of the African continent. The disease is fatal to horses, mules, camels, and dogs. Cattle, sheep, and goats usually survive, except when parasitized by certain strains. Many wild ungulates native to Africa show no evidence of harm. (*See also* TRYPANOSOMIASIS, p 35.)

Diagnosis: Tsetse flies can be identified by their honeybee-like appearance, the long proboscis with its onion-shaped bulb at the base, and the unique wing venation with the characteristic cleaver- or hatchet-shaped cell in the center of the wing.

Treatment and Control: Tsetse flies can be controlled by catching and trapping (tsetse traps), bush clearing, fly screens, repellents, insecticides, and sterile male release techniques.

SHEEP KEDS

The sheep ked, *Melophagus ovinus*, is one of the most widely distributed and important external parasites of sheep. There are also keds that parasitize deer in North America (*Lipoptena depressa* and *Neolipoptena ferrisi*).

Keds are wingless dipterans. The adult is ~7 mm long, brown or reddish in color, and covered with short, bristly hairs. The head is short and broad, and the legs are strong and armed with stout claws.

The female gives birth to a single, fully developed larva, which is cemented to the wool and pupates within 12 hr. A young ked emerges after ~22 days. Females live 100–120 days and produce ~10 larvae during this time; males live ~80 days. The entire life cycle is spent on the host. Keds that fall off the host usually survive <1 wk and present little danger of infestation to a flock. Ked numbers increase during the winter and early spring when they spread rapidly through a flock, particularly when sheep are assembled in close quarters for feeding or shelter.

Pathology: To feed, sheep keds pierce the skin with their mouthparts and suck blood. They usually feed on the neck, breast, shoulder, flanks, and rump but not on the back where dust and other debris collect in the wool. Ked bites cause pruritus over much of the host's body; sheep often bite, scratch, and rub themselves, thus damaging the wool. The fleece becomes thin, ragged, and dirty. The excrement of the keds causes a permanent brown discoloration, which is likely to reduce the value of the wool. Keds also cause a defect in hides called a cockle, which affects the grade and value of the sheep skin. Infested sheep, particularly lambs and pregnant ewes, may lose vitality and become unthrifty. Heavy infestations can considerably reduce the condition of the host and even cause anemia. Keds also transmit *Trypanosoma melophagium*, a nonpathogenic protozoan parasite of sheep.

Diagnosis: Close inspection of the damaged, dirty wool and underlying skin reveals infestation by the unique appearance of these wingless, hairy flies.

Treatment and Control: Shearing removes many pupae and adults. Thus, shearing before lambing and subsequent treatment of the ewes with insecticides to control the remaining keds can greatly reduce the possibility of lambs becoming heavily infested. Sheep are usually treated after shearing, and best results are obtained if an insecticide that has a residual activity of ≥3–4 wk is used. By this means, the keds that emerge from the pupae are also killed. Modern treatments to control lice also control keds.

Dipping is an effective method of treatment. Completely submerging the sheep in vats ensures the destruction of all keds present but, in most instances, does not kill the pupated larvae; a long-acting insecticide is required to kill newly emerging keds. Large flocks of range sheep should be treated in a permanently constructed dipping vat. Smaller flocks and farm flocks may be successfully treated in portable, galvanized-iron dipping vats or in smaller tanks, tubs, or canvas dipping bags.

Spraying may be as effective as dipping and is more convenient in some areas. Pressures of 100–200 lb/sq in. (7–14 kg/cm^2) for short wool and 300–350 lb/sq in. (21–28 kg/cm^2) for long wool are commonly used.

Shower dipping is also sometimes used; the sheep are held in a special pen and showered from above and below until the fleece is saturated. The run-off is returned for recirculation, and the concentration of insecticide used is the same as for dipping. The concentration of the insecticide can drop rapidly and become ineffective if the instructions for replenishment are not followed explicitly.

Jetting involves the forceful application of the insecticide by means of a hand-held, multiple-jet comb drawn through the short fleece. Although a little slower and less effective than dips or sprays, jetting may be advantageous for smaller flocks because it is economical and does not require a permanent installation.

Spot-on or pour-on formulations of the newer pyrethroids are easy to apply and very effective.

Powder dusting fits well into management practices at shearing time. It is rapid, economical, and avoids wetting the animals. Various types of equipment for dusting are available commercially.

SPIDER FLIES/NEW FOREST FLIES

The spider or new forest fly, *Hippobosca equina*, is widely distributed throughout Europe, Asia, and Africa. These winged keds parasitize horses and rarely cattle throughout the UK. Its bite is characterized as a nuisance and disturbance to large domestic animals. It has a predilection for feeding sites in the perineal region and between the hind legs.

The winged adult is ~10 mm long with a flattened, shriveled body. The life cycle is similar to that of *Melophagus ovinus*, in that the female produces one larva at a time, and at the time of maturity the larva falls away from the female fly and pupates in the soil.

Treatment is rarely indicated, but many of the repellents used for other blood-feeding periodic parasites may be used.

HIPPOBOSCID OR LOUSE FLIES

The hippoboscid or louse flies, *Pseudolynchia* and *Lynchia* spp, are winged versions of the keds. They infest many song birds, raptors, and pigeons. The pigeon fly, *P canariensis*, is an important parasite of domestic pigeons throughout the tropical and subtropical regions of the world. It is found throughout the southern USA and northward along the Atlantic coast to New England. These dark brown flies have long wings (6.5–7.5 mm) and are able to fly swiftly from the host.

Pathology: Hippoboscid flies move about quickly on their avian hosts and bite and suck blood from parts that are not well feathered. They may serve as intermediate hosts for many avian blood protozoans of the genus *Haemoproteus*. Pigeon flies readily attack people who handle adult birds; the bite is said to be as painful as a bee sting, and its effects may persist for ≥5 days.

Diagnosis: Close inspection of the ruffled feathers and underlying skin reveals infestation by the unique appearance of these winged, swiftly flying flies.

Treatment and Control: Any flies on the birds can be killed by spraying the birds with permethrin. Thorough cleaning of the premises and destruction of the debris are essential for control. Spraying the loft with permethrin, when coupled with cleaning, will alleviate the infestation.

DIPTERANS WITH NONBITING MOUTHPARTS

FACE FLIES

Face flies, *Musca autumnalis*, are so named because they gather around the eyes and muzzles of livestock, particularly cattle. They may also be found on the withers, neck, brisket, and sides. Their mouthparts are adapted for sponging up saliva, tears, and mucus. Face flies are usually not considered blood feeders because their mouthparts are a sponging type and not piercing or bayonet-like, as are those of *Stomoxys calcitrans*. However, they follow blood-feeding flies, disturb them during the feeding process, and then lap up the blood and body fluids that accumulate on the host's skin. Face flies are found on animals that are outdoors and usually do not follow animals into barns.

Face flies are found on range cattle throughout southern Canada and most of the USA. The mouthparts consist of sponging labellae, and there are four longitudinal stripes on the abdomen. Although similar in appearance to the common house fly, face flies can be differentiated by the closeness and angles of the interior margins of the eyes and by the distinctive coloration of the face and abdomen. Speciation requires the skills of a trained entomologist.

Cattle are the principal host of the face fly in the USA, but face flies will also feed on horses and probably sheep and goats. The face fly is a pest of range cattle; it is not seen in feedlot situations and thus is not a parasite of confined cattle. The eggs are laid in fresh cattle feces in rangeland situations and hatch in ~1 day. The yellowish larvae develop in 2–4 days and, when mature, leave the manure to pupate in the surrounding soil. The complete life cycle from egg to adult requires 12–20 days, depending on climatic conditions. The diapausing adult overwinters within buildings and other protective places.

Pathology: Face flies annoy the host and ultimately interfere with the host's productivity. Females feed on facial secretions, such as tear fluid, nasal mucus, and saliva, to obtain protein for egg development. The irritation around the host's eyes stimulates the flow of tears, which attracts even more flies.

Face flies also feed on other fluid sources, such as blood from wounds and milk on calves' faces. Because face flies have small, rough spines (prestomal teeth) on their sponging mouthparts, they can cause irritation and mechanical damage to the eye tissue of the host. The feeding activity of face flies enhances transmission of *Moraxella bovis* (*see* p 512). Face flies can also serve as intermediate hosts for *Thelazia* spp (*see* p 510) and for *Parafilaria bovicola* (*see* p 906).

Diagnosis: Adult face flies are morphologically similar to house flies. These two species can be differentiated only by minor differences in eye position and color of the abdomen. Speciation requires the skills of a trained entomologist. In general, if a medium-sized fly is seen feeding around the eyes and nostrils of a cow or horse, it is most probably a face fly.

Treatment and Control: Control of face flies is difficult. Much effort has been made using various insecticides and application techniques, such as dust bags, mist sprays, and wipe-on formulations. Also, insecticides and insect growth regulators are used as feed additives. However, results are usually less than satisfactory. The introduction of insecticide-impregnated ear tags has provided somewhat better control, but generally, seasonal face fly reduction of only 70%–80% has been achieved, even with two tags (one in each ear) per animal.

HEAD FLIES

(Plantation flies)

Head flies or plantation flies, *Hydrotaea irritans*, are nonbiting flies found in large numbers in northern European countries, especially Denmark and Great Britain, where they are pests of cattle, sheep, and other livestock. This fly resembles the house fly and is ~4–7 mm long. The thorax is black with gray patches, the abdomen is olive green, and the wing bases are orange yellow.

Head flies are a nuisance to domestic animals and people because they are attracted to the mouth, nose, ears, eyes, and wounds to feed on secretions. Unlike other *Hydrotaea* spp, *H irritans* produces one generation per year, with three larval instar stages. Eggs deposited in late summer hatch out larvae within a few days. The saprophagous stage is brief, before development to the stage that is predatory on other insect larvae. Overwintering occurs as late-stage larvae. Adults are most active from early June until late September and are common in the vicinity of thickets or woodlands in which they shelter between periods of feeding.

Pathology: In Great Britain, sheep are mainly affected. Large swarms of flies, attracted by the movement of animals, congregate to feed on secretions from the eyes and nose and on the cellular debris at the grown horn base. To alleviate the persistent irritation, sheep scratch and rub their heads, resulting in raw wounds or "broken heads," especially on the poll. Flies, attracted by the blood, settle on these self-inflicted lesions and extend the margins by their feeding activity. Sheep of all ages are involved, but breeds with horns and without wool on the head are most severely affected.

Head flies also attack people, deer, horses, cattle, and rabbits. Although no corresponding broken head lesions develop in cattle, the occurrence of summer mastitis (due to *Trueperella pyogenes*) and the seasonal activity of head flies are closely associated, especially in Denmark. Head flies may also be involved in the spread of myxomatosis in rabbits (*see* p 1950).

Treatment and Control: The development, emergence, and congregation of head flies, which occur away from farm areas, preclude the traditional methods of insecticide spraying of generalized breeding sites and resting habitats. Control at the point of contact between the feeding adult insects and the mammalian hosts is also limited in value. With sheep, the retention of organophosphate compounds or pyrethrin derivatives on the susceptible head areas is of short duration, which necessitates impractical reapplications in free-ranging animals. Use of insecticide-impregnated ear tags in cattle decreases the incidence of summer mastitis, presumably by reducing transmission by head flies.

Removal of livestock from infested locations during the fly season is the only completely effective way to prevent damage. Once broken heads have occurred, the housing of sheep is the only successful method to stop further fly damage.

FILTH-BREEDING FLIES

The following adult dipterans are often referred to as filth-breeding flies: *Musca domestica* (the house fly); *Calliphora*, *Phaenicia*, *Lucilia*, and *Phormia* spp (the blow flies or bottle flies); *Sarcophaga* spp (the flesh flies); *Fannia* spp (the little house flies); *Muscina* spp (the false stable flies); and *Hermetia illucens* (the black soldier flies). Large populations of these adult flies are often found around facilities associated with animal feces. Larval stages may be associated with skin wounds contaminated with bacteria or with a matted hair coat contaminated with feces (*see* p 897). The life cycle of *M domestica* will be used as a representative example of the life cycles of the assorted filth-breeding flies.

The house fly is commonly found around livestock and poultry operations, where it readily breeds in accumulating manure sources. It is a medium-sized (as large as 9 mm), grayish fly with four dark thoracic stripes and sponging, nonbiting mouthparts designed for sucking semiliquid food (there are no mandibles or maxillae). The labium is expanded into two labellae that can transfer fluids and semifluids.

After oviposition, the creamy-white, banana-shaped egg (~1 mm long) hatches in 6–12 hr in optimal conditions. The eggs are not resistant to drying, and few appear to survive temperatures >40°C or <15°C. Larvae may develop in a few days to 3 wk, depending on the temperature and availability of food. When temperature for larval development is optimal (~36°C), the larvae develop to pupae in ~6 hr. Pupae persist 4–5 days in warm weather. After the adults emerge, the flies search for food and copulate after a few days. The life cycle is usually completed in ~3 wk, although it can be completed in as little as 10–14 days under favorable conditions. In temperate climates, it is thought that house flies overwinter as pupae.

Pathology: Even though these flies do not feed on blood, annoyance caused by their movement on and off animals can lead to reduced performance. In addition, they have been implicated in the transmission of numerous pathogens (helminth, protozoan, bacterial, and viral) of people and other animals. Large populations of these adult flies often are found around poorly managed livestock or poultry facilities and become a public annoyance. These are synanthropic flies, ie, they are often associated with human dwellings. The flies are "vomit drop" feeders and fly from feces to food, spreading bacteria on their feet and within their disgorged stomach contents.

Diagnosis: All adult filth-breeding flies have similar sponging, nonbiting mouthparts, designed for sucking semiliquid food. The identification of adult flies is probably best left to a specialist. House flies are medium-sized, grayish flies with four dark thoracic stripes. A preliminary identification of blow flies or bottle flies may be made on the basis of the metallic coloring of the adults. Flesh flies are medium-sized, grayish flies with a checkerboard abdominal pattern.

Treatment and Control: A thorough sanitation program is necessary to control fly populations in and around livestock and poultry facilities. All manure accumulations should be removed at least twice a week or handled properly, if stored on the premises, to minimize fly breeding. If solid manure management practices are applied, efforts should be made to reduce manure moisture. If a liquid manure pit is used, manure should not be allowed to accumulate above the waterline, either floating or sticking to the sides, because this is an ideal site for fly reproduction. Insecticides should be considered as supplementary to sanitation and management measures aimed at preventing fly breeding. Residual sprays providing 2–4 wk control with one treatment may be applied to fly-resting surfaces. Space sprays, mists, or fogs with quick knockdown but no residual action can be used for immediate reduction of high numbers of adult flies. Other measures for control of adult flies include use of insecticide resin strips or various fly baits. These measures also can be applied directly to fly-breeding sources; however, this should be considered only for fly-breeding spots that cannot be eliminated by normal sanitation practices.

EYE GNATS

The eye gnats or the eye flies (*Hippelates* spp) are very small (1.5–2.5 mm long) flies that frequently congregate around the eyes as well as mucous and sebaceous secretions, pus, and blood.

In the desert and foothill regions of southern California, adult Hippelates flies are present throughout the year; they are annoying from April through November. During the peak months, they are noticeable in the early morning and late afternoon. They gather in deep shade, such as among densely planted shrubs or in the shade of a dwelling. The eggs are ~0.5 mm long, fluted, and distinctly curved. They are deposited on or below the surface of the soil. The larvae hatch and feed on decaying organic matter, including excrement. The larval stage lasts 7–11 days. During the winter months, the larval and pupal stages may persist for many weeks. Pupation occurs close to the surface of the soil and lasts ~6 days. The entire life cycle lasts ~21 days. The adults are generally strong flyers, flying both with and against the wind.

Pathology: Some species are attracted to the genital organs of mammals; for example, *H pallipes* clusters around a dog's penis. These gnats quietly approach their mammalian hosts. They usually alight some distance from their feeding site and then crawl over the skin, or fly intermittently and alight, thus avoiding annoyance to the host. They are persistent and, if brushed away, quickly return to continue engorging themselves. They are nonbiting flies; however, the labellae have spines that scarify host tissue and allow entrance of pathogenic organisms. *Hippelates* flies often hover around the body orifices of calves, yearlings, pregnant heifers, and lactating cows. They feed on lacrimal fluid, fatty body secretions, milk droplets, and on secretions at the tips of the teats of animals. *Hippelates* flies also serve as vectors for *Trueperella pyogenes* (summer mastitis) and *Moraxella bovis* (pinkeye, *see* p 512).

Diagnosis: These small flies have sponging type mouthparts. Although eye gnats have much smaller mouthparts, they closely resemble house flies in form and structure and have short aristate antennae.

Treatment and Control: Repellents, such as those recommended for mosquitoes, provide temporary relief from eye gnats. Applications of insecticides on a community-wide basis (as would take place with mosquito abatement) may provide temporary control of adults, but more adults invade the treated area after the insecticide has dissipated.

DIPTERANS THAT PRODUCE MYIASIS

Larval dipterans may develop in the subcutaneous tissues of the skin or organs of many domestic animals, producing a condition known as **myiasis**. There are two types of myiases based on degree of host dependence. In **facultative myiasis**, the fly larvae are usually free-living; however, in certain circumstances, these larvae can adapt themselves to a parasitic dependence on a host. In **obligatory myiasis**, the fly larvae are completely parasitic, ie, they depend on the host to complete the life cycle. Without the host, obligatory parasites will die.

FACULTATIVE MYIASIS-PRODUCING FLIES

Facultative myiasis-producing flies of veterinary importance covered in other chapters include *Gasterophilus* spp in horses (*see* p 315), *Oestrus ovis* in sheep (*see* p 1473), and *Cuterebra* spp in dogs and cats (*see* p 879). The following larval dipterans are often referred to as facultative myiasis-producing flies: *Musca domestica* (the house flies); *Calliphora, Phaenicia, Lucilia,* and *Phormia* spp (the blow flies or bottle flies); and *Sarcophaga* spp (the flesh flies). Their adult stages are synanthropic flies, ie, they are often associated with human dwellings and readily fly from feces to food. Larval stages are usually associated with skin wounds of any domestic animal that have become contaminated with bacteria or with a matted hair coat contaminated with feces. In the larval stages, the characteristics of the distinctive posterior spiracular plates and the cephalopharyngeal skeleton are unique for each species and are used for identification.

The life cycle of *M domestica* is a representative example of that of the filth-breeding flies (*see* p 895). Several species of blow flies cause myiasis in sheep. Primary flies in the USA and Canada are *Phormia regina* and *Protophormia terraenovae* (the black blow flies) and *Lucilia sericata* (the green bottle fly). *L illustris, Cochliomyia macellaria* (secondary screwworm), and some others are usually secondary invaders. *L cuprina* is the most important primary fly in Australia and South Africa; *L sericata* in Great Britain; and *L cuprina, L sericata,* and *Calliphora stygia* in New Zealand.

Pathology: In normal conditions, adult flies of these genera lay their eggs in feces or in decaying animal carcasses. In facultative myiasis, the adult flies are attracted to a moist wound, skin lesion, or soiled hair coat. A common site is the breech, where flies may be attracted to wool soaked with urine or feces. As adult female flies feed in these sites, they lay eggs, which hatch within 24 hr if conditions are moist. Larvae (maggots) move independently about the wound surface, ingesting dead cells, exudate, secretions, and debris, but not live tissue. This condition is known as strike or fly strike. The larvae irritate, injure, and kill successive layers of skin and produce exudates. Maggots can tunnel through the thinned epidermis into the subcutis. This process produces tissue cavities in the skin that measure up to several centimeters in diameter. Once established, strikes can spread rapidly and attract more blow flies, secondary as well as primary. Mild strikes can cause rapid loss of condition, and bad strikes can be fatal. Unless the process is halted by appropriate therapy, the infested animal may die from shock, intoxication, histolysis, or infection. A peculiar, distinct, pungent odor permeates the infested tissue and the affected animal. Advanced lesions may contain thousands of maggots.

The body of the sheep also may be struck. This is usually associated with soaking rains that cause the development of fleece rot, often characterized by discoloration due to *Pseudomonas* spp or dermatophilosis. Other sites are the horns of rams, wool around the prepuce, sides where feet with footrot come in contact with fleece, and wounds.

As adults, these flies can be pestiferous in veterinary clinics, farms, or poultry operations. The flies are vomit drop feeders and fly from feces to food, spreading bacteria on their feet and from their disgorged stomach contents.

These fly larvae have also been associated with toxic effects in chickens. Botulism (*see* p 2889), also known as limberneck in chickens, has been associated with ingestion of large numbers of larvae of *Lucilia caesar*, *Phaenicia sericata*, and other species of flies. *Clostridium botulinum* multiplies in carrion, where it may be picked up by fly larvae breeding in that medium and then passed on to chickens that eat the maggots. Dead animals should be quickly and safely disposed of, preferably by incineration.

Diagnosis: Strikes should be diagnosed early; behavior of sheep is a good indicator of myiasis. Affected animals become depressed, stand with their heads down, do not feed, and attempt to bite the infested areas. Screwworm may be suspected if the larvae are associated with wounds.

The species of myiasis-producing flies can be definitively identified by closely examining the larvae. The extreme caudal ends of several third-stage larvae infesting the wound should be sliced using a scalpel blade held perpendicularly to the larval body. When the sliced caudal ends are placed cut surface down on a glass slide, covered with a coverglass, and examined under a compound microscope, a dichotomous key can be used to identify the genus or genera of flies within the wound. The unique spiracular plates are distinct for a particular genus, much like a human fingerprint. Several specimens should be examined because more than one genus may be present within the lesion. The first larvae to hatch in the lesion often create a favorable medium attractive to flies of other genera. Also, the possibility of obligatory myiasis caused by *Cochliomyia hominivorax* (*see* below) or *Chrysomya bezziana* (*see* p 900) should be considered, depending on geographic locale.

Treatment and Control: Blow fly infestation of the breech can be effectively controlled for ~6–8 wk by tagging or crutching (ie, wool is shorn between the legs and around the tail). Complete shearing controls outbreaks involving other parts of the body. Wool removed from around the head and the prepuce can prevent strike in these areas. Urine staining of the crutch of Merino ewes can be virtually eliminated by removal of breech wrinkles (Mules operation), and fecal contamination can be greatly reduced by docking tails at the third joint. Scouring should be controlled. Odors and associated moisture attract flies and stimulate oviposition, particularly during hot, humid weather.

Chemoprophylaxis consists of wetting to complete saturation of susceptible areas with suitable insecticidal and larvicidal preparations, such as the organophosphate insecticides or cyromazine, a specific larvicide in dips and sprays. Jetting is the most efficient procedure—insecticide is forced into the fleece, usually locally to the breech and along the back and head, under high pressure. Protection can last 6–8 wk, but where the primary fly is resistant (eg, *L cuprina* in Australia), it may last only 2–3 wk. Weekly application of agents such as ronnel (2.5%) under pressure to wounds until healed can be highly beneficial, particularly for screwworm infestation. Before suitable agents are applied, all wool should be removed from the struck area and around it.

Burning or deep burying of the carcass may be a valuable general hygienic measure but may have little effect on primary strikes. The main source of primary flies is the struck sheep. A genetic manipulation approach has been used to control a strain of blow fly in Australia; male flies are partially sterile but transmit a gene that causes blindness in female offspring.

Treatment and control measures for myiasis in dogs and cats are limited. If these larvae are detected in small animals, immediate therapy is necessary. The hair coat should be clipped to determine the extent of the lesion and to remove many of the larvae present in the hair. Removing maggots from existing deep tissue pockets may be difficult, and sedating or even anesthetizing the animal may be necessary. The lesion should be examined on successive days; adult flies lay eggs in the wound at different times, and hatching of larvae may not be synchronous.

Depressed, febrile, and prostrate animals should be treated according to their clinical signs. Ideally, culture and sensitivity studies should be performed on samples or scrapings of the wounds. If secondary bacterial or fungal infections are present, administration of broad-spectrum antibiotics is advisable.

With respect to prevention, owners should be educated about the effectiveness of treating all skin wounds. Animals with skin wounds should be confined to fly-free areas. The hair coat should be kept clean of urine or feces and should not be permitted to become matted. Contaminated wounds and matted hair coats soaked in urine or feces rapidly attract adult myiasis-producing flies. The control of adult flies in the field and the destruction of their breeding places are excellent preventive measures. All areas should be free of opened garbage cans and decaying carcasses or carrion.

OBLIGATORY MYIASIS-PRODUCING FLIES

Many dipteran flies produce larvae that must lead a parasitic existence and result in obligatory myiasis. Only one fly in North America, *Cochliomyia hominivorax*, is a primary invader of fresh, uncontaminated skin wounds of domestic animals. Another species of screwworm, *Chrysomya bezziana*, is found in Africa and southern Asia, including Papua New Guinea.

Cochliomyia hominivorax

(Primary screwworm, New World screwworm)

Cochliomyia hominivorax is distributed throughout the neoarctic and neotropical regions of the western hemisphere. As a result of massive state, federal, and international eradication programs, extant populations of *C hominivorax* are no longer found in the USA or Mexico; isolated reports are often traced to importation of infested animals from locations where the screwworm is still prevalent. Extant populations are found in Central and South America and in certain Caribbean Islands.

Adult female flies lay batches of 200–400 eggs in rows that overlap like shingles in a mass on the edge of a fresh wound. After 12–21 hr, larvae hatch, crawl into the wound, and burrow into the flesh. The larvae feed on wound fluids and live tissue. After 5–7 days, grown larvae exit from the wound, fall to the ground, and burrow in the soil to pupate. The pupal period varies from 7 days to 2 mo, depending on the temperature. Freezing or sustained soil temperatures <46°F (8°C) kill the pupae. Adults breed only once during their lifetime, a fact that can be used as an advantage in biologic control. Adult flies usually mate when 3–4 days old, and gravid females are ready to oviposit when ~6 days old. In warm weather, the life cycle may be completed in 21 days. Only female flies feed and oviposit on wounds; males and younger, virgin females gather to mate in vegetation, especially flowering vegetation.

Pathology: Newly infested wounds contain screwworm larvae of a single age; older, larger wounds may contain larvae of various ages and of different species of flies. The malodorous, reddish brown fluid produced in the wound usually drains and may stain the hair or wool around or below the wound. As annoyance increases, the infested animal seeks protection by retreating to the densest available shade. Even a small and relatively inconspicuous wound infested with screwworm larvae attracts not only more screwworm flies but also facultative myiasis-producing flies. Necrotic tissues attract even more flies. The wound can become greatly enlarged due to multiple infestation and, unless treated, usually results in death of the animal.

Diagnosis: The parasitic larvae are tapered and have mouth hooks at the narrow end and breathing spiracles at the wide end. Body segments are ringed with spines. Fully grown larvae can be as long as 1.5 cm. Larvae are often identified by their "wood screw" shape and appearance and can be distinguished from the larvae of the facultative myiasis-producing flies by the darkly pigmented tracheal tubes on the dorsal aspect of the posterior end of third-stage larvae. These tubes can be easily visualized through the larval cuticle.

Adult screwworm flies are similar in appearance to other blow flies. The adult stage is never recovered in a veterinary case scenario. They are bluish to bluish green, have a reddish orange head and eyes, and are slightly larger than a house fly. If collected, they are difficult to distinguish from other blow flies or bottle flies. Identification of adult screwworms is probably best left to an entomologist.

Treatment and Control: Screwworm infestation must be reported to both state and federal authorities. *C hominivorax* has been eradicated from the USA but occasionally enters the country surreptitiously on imported animals. In the USA, if a wound is thought to be infested with screwworm larvae, the USDA can be contacted.

Screwworms in wounds can be killed by direct application of a wound dressing, called a smear. Such smears, which contain lindane or ronnel, may be difficult to find in the USA because of the eradication program. Smears are best applied with a 1-in. (2.5-cm) paint brush and should reach all of the many pockets formed by the burrowing larvae in deep wounds. A thin layer should also be applied to the skin surrounding the wound to protect it from reinfestation. Wounds may also be treated with aerosol, dust, or foam formulations of coumaphos, lindane, or ronnel. To protect animals from infestation and also to kill larvae in small wounds that are difficult to detect, animals can be sprayed thoroughly with ronnel or sprayed with or dipped in coumaphos.

Sterile Male Release Eradication Program: In 1958, the USDA initiated a program in the southeastern states to eliminate screwworms by the sterile male release technique. When reared artificially and exposed to irradiation shortly before they emerge from the pupae, male flies are able to mate but sterile. The female mates only once and, when mated with a sterile male, lays eggs that do not hatch. Therefore, release of sufficient numbers of sterile males in an area throughout a period of time leads to eradication. By 1959, screwworms had been eliminated from Florida.

This program was expanded to cover the rest of the area involved in the USA and then, via a joint Mexico—USA agreement, to include most of Mexico. This, along with the use of screwworm attractant and an insecticide system that attracted and killed adults, led to eradication of screwworms from Mexico. There is interest in expanding this area throughout Central America and the Caribbean. However, until this has been achieved, constant vigilance by all who deal with animals in the southern USA and Mexico is necessary to detect an infestation quickly and to eradicate it before the flies reproduce and spread.

Chrysomya bezziana

(Old World screwworm, Oriental fly, Bezzi's blow fly)

Chrysomya bezziana is found in Africa, the Indian subcontinent, and southeast Asia *from Taiwan,PRC in the north to* Papua New Guinea in the south. This fly is not indigenous to Australia. Owing to its geography, the most likely potential port of entry for *C bezziana* to the USA is Hawaii.

Adult screwworms are usually not seen in the field. The adult fly has a dark metallic green body with abdominal segments with narrow bands along the posterior margins. The legs are black or partially brown. The face is orange/yellow. The first larval stage probably goes unnoticed because of its small size, as long as 3 mm at the time of its molt to the second stage. The second stage is quite similar to the third but is 4–9 mm long. The third-stage larvae are large, as long as 18 mm. The body is composed of 12 segments that have broad encircling bands of spinules. All three stages are maggot-like in their appearance and have posterior spiracles that are unique to the species. The posterior end of the larva has its spiracular plate located in a deep cleft at the end of the eighth abdominal segment. The spiracular plates are large and well separated. The peritreme and the three breathing slits are wide.

C bezziana produce a particularly vile myiasis. Female flies are attracted to open wounds of people and domestic and wild animals, laying their eggs in masses of 150–500 at the edge of wounds or near body orifices. Larvae develop to the third stage ~2 days after hatching. They burrow deep into the wound such that only their posterior ends are visible. The entire larval stage lasts 5–6 days. The pupal stage lasts 7–9 days in tropical conditions and longer in cooler environments. The adult flies emerge later to mate, locate a new host, and continue the cycle. Female flies mate only once during their lifetime—a fact paramount in prevention and control. Under favorable conditions, there may be ≥8 generations per year.

Pathology: The larvae of *C bezziana* are obligatory wound parasites, never developing in carcasses or decomposing organic material. Although female flies are attracted to open wounds, occasionally eggs are deposited on the unbroken, soft skin of various parts of the body, especially if contaminated by blood or mucous discharge. When the larvae hatch, they burrow into the flesh of the host, using their hooked mouthparts to scrape away at the tissues and lacerate the fine blood vessels. Larvae are voracious blood feeders. During the bloodsucking phase, only the caudal ends of the maggots with their blackish peritremes remain visible at the surface of the lesion, enabling the larvae to breathe. As many as 300 maggots have been seen in some wounds. In untreated wounds, the destructive activity of the larvae may lead to the death of the animal within a very short time.

Secondary infestation with the facultative myiasis-producing flies (*see* p 897) may complicate treatment and control.

Diagnosis: The identification of the rarely observed adult flies and their associated larval stages is best left to an entomologist. A definitive diagnosis can be made only after observation, extraction, and identification of typical larvae. Diagnosis may often be made by residence in or history of travel to an area endemic for *C bezziana*. If a wound is thought to be infested with larvae of *C bezziana*, samples should be collected and sent to appropriate eradication officials.

Treatment and Control: Treatment of screwworm infestation involves killing the larvae in the lesions, promoting healing, and preventing secondary reinfestation with larvae of the facultative myiasis-producing flies. The extent of the lesions is determined by clipping the hair coat and removing as many larvae as possible. The larvae that are removed should be killed to prevent them from pupating and developing into adults. Larvae located deep within tissues must be extracted.

Ivermectin at dosages of 50, 100, and 300 mcg/kg administered to infested cattle resulted in 100% larval mortality for at least 6, 12, and 14 days, respectively. Depending on their age, larvae survived in established strikes after treatment at 200 mcg/kg. Mortality was 100% in larvae up to 2 days old but less in older larvae. However, many of the larvae that survived ivermectin therapy failed to develop to the adult stage. After treatment with 200 mcg/kg, residual protection lasted 16–20 days, 2–3 times that of most insecticide smears.

All wounds on domestic animals should be properly dressed, and all elective surgical procedures avoided during the fly season.

The fact that the female flies mate only once during their lifetime is an important fact to consider in the control of *C bezziana*. Pupal flies exposed to irradiation lead to sterile adults that can be released to mate with wild male and female flies. As a result, no viable offspring are produced in the wild.

Wolves (Warbles) of Small Animals

Larvae of the genus *Cuterebra* are often referred to as wolves, warbles, rabbit bots, or rodent bots. These fly larvae infest the skin of rabbits, squirrels, mice, rats, chipmunks, and occasionally dogs and cats. (For clinical findings, diagnosis, and treatment, *see* p 879.)

Gray Flesh Flies

The gray flesh fly, *Wohlfahrtia vigil*, is responsible for cutaneous myiasis in North America, particularly in southern Canada and the northern part of the USA. The adult flies have been recorded from the New England states to Alaska, but most reports are from eastern sections of Canada and the neighboring northeastern parts of the USA. All reports of infestation are in the skin of healthy animals, particularly the unbroken skin of the young.

All three larval stages are maggot-like in their appearance and have posterior spiracles unique to the species. The first larval stage is 1.5 mm at hatching and grows to 3.5 mm at the time of its molt to the second stage. The third stage is 7–18.5 mm long. Its posterior end is narrow, and it is covered with many irregular rows of small spines that have dark points and are directed posteriorly. This larva is better adapted to maintain an attachment to living tissues. The oral hooks are strongly developed. The posterior end of the larva has its spiracular plate located in a deep pit formed by the margins of the segment. The posterior spiracles have wide slits and a strong peritreme.

The gray flesh fly is larviparous—it deposits larvae instead of eggs on healthy, uninjured skin of suitable hosts, particularly young animals. Larvae penetrate the unbroken skin and form a boil-like (furuncular) swelling. Development to the infective third-larval stage is usually completed in 9–14 days. The parasites then drop to the ground and pupate for ~11–18 days, varying with the season of the year and the temperature. When cold weather approaches, the pupation period is greatly prolonged. Under laboratory conditions, it has been observed to last 7 mo. Parasites survive the winter in pupal form. Adults emerge and mate after ~3–4 days. Female flies begin larviposition ~1 wk later, depositing 6–16 larvae at a time. Female flies live for 35–40 days; males seldom survive >3 wk.

Pathology: Female *W vigil* deposit active larvae near or directly on the host. Although larvae usually penetrate unbroken skin, in small animals, penetration may go deeper than the dermal tissue, even into the coelomic cavity.

The first indication that an animal is infected is exudation of serum and matting of the hair coat over the site of penetration. In light-skinned animals, a small inflammatory area, with a tiny hole visible in the center or to one side, is noticeable. These lesions may be palpated as they develop. On the third or fourth day, the larvae are 1.5–2 cm long and produce abscess-like lesions resembling those of *Hypoderma* spp in cattle. These lesions vary in size, shape, position, and the number of larvae they contain. The hair coat often becomes parted over the summit of the lesions and reveals an opening 2–3 mm in diameter. The posterior aspect of the larva is visible in these openings, through which it breathes. Openings are generally circular and well-defined; however, if several larvae are present in a single lesion, the shape of the opening is quite variable. Small animals infected with ≥5 larvae for several days become emaciated, and the skin becomes dry and loses its luster.

The penetration of the skin by the larvae, their development in the subcutaneous tissues, and secondary bacterial infection produce intense irritation and inflammation. Attempts by the animal to remove the larvae or relieve the irritation tend to aggravate the condition. Young animals may die from exhaustion. It has also been suggested that the larvae may produce toxic secretions. *W vigil* has been isolated from the skin of young children, particularly infants.

Diagnosis: Adult gray flesh flies are nonparasitic and as a result will probably not be seen by owners or veterinarians. They are large grayish flies (~13 mm long), about twice the size of a house fly. The dorsal surface of the thorax is marked with three longitudinal bands, and the dorsal surface of the abdomen has three well-defined rows of oval black spots that are confluent with one another.

The identification of adult flies and their associated larval stages should be left to an entomologist. The presence of a dermal swelling with a central opening may lead to a tentative diagnosis of myiasis due to *W vigil*. A definitive diagnosis can be made only after extraction and identification of a typical larva. Extensive descriptions and dichotomous keys for the three larval stages are available. A tentative diagnosis may often be made by a history of either residence in or travel to a geographic area endemic for *W vigil*.

Treatment and Control: Larvae must be extracted from the skin. Applying heavy oil, liquid paraffin, or petrolatum jelly to the opening of the lesions will occlude the airway of the larvae. Applying a small amount of chloroform or ether to the opening may be helpful before removing larvae with forceps. Lidocaine hydrochloride can also be injected into the furuncular lesion to facilitate extraction. Great care should be taken during the extraction process to avoid rupturing larvae in situ, although anaphylaxis has not been reported. Antibiotics should be prescribed.

W vigil often infects young mink. A teaspoon of ronnel can be placed in the bedding of mink nest boxes as a control measure; however, ronnel should not be used in the bedding of kits <3 days old. Protection can be provided by using wire gauze to keep flies out of cages.

African Tumbu Flies

(Mango fly, Skin maggot fly, Ver du Cayor, Worms of Cayor)

The African tumbu fly, *Cordylobia anthropophaga*, is responsible for another boil-like (furuncular) myiasis in both people and animals in Africa, particularly in the sub-Saharan regions.

The adult flies are nonparasitic and as a result are not seen by owners or veterinarians. They are stout, compact flies, 6–12 mm long. They are light brown, with diffuse blue-gray patches on the thorax and dark gray on the posterior part of the abdomen. The face and legs are yellow. The second- and third-stage larvae are the stages usually seen in the animal's skin.

Second-stage larvae are slightly club-shaped and exhibit large, black cuticular spines directed posteriorly and distributed irregularly over segments 3–8. Segments 9–11 are almost bare when compared with the preceding segments. The segments have a few rows of small, pale spines posteriorly. Segment 12 is densely covered with these spines. Segment 13 is indistinctly demarcated, lacking spines but possessing two pair of short processes. Each tracheal tube opens through two slightly bent slits. The second-stage larvae are 2.5–4 mm long. The size of advanced second-stage larvae varies greatly, as does the size of third-stage larvae. Fully mature larvae are 1.3–1.5 cm long. The body is cylindrical with 12 identifiable segments. Curved spines that are directed posteriorly are densely arranged at least up to segment 7; the last 5 segments may be either partially or densely covered with spines.

After fertilization, female flies produce 100–500 banana-shaped eggs, usually depositing them in dry, shady, sandy soil that has often been contaminated by urine or feces. Eggs are never deposited on the skin of the host. Eggs hatch after 1–3 days, and the larvae are initially 0.5–1 mm long. Larvae can survive as long as 15 days while waiting for a host and can penetrate the host in as little as 25 sec. After penetration, larvae reside in a cavity in the dermis and hypodermis. This cavity communicates to the external environment by means of a central breathing pore, which corresponds to the caudal end of the larva with its spiracles. A single larva is found in each cavity, within which the larva develops to the second and third stages. Larvae require 7–15 days to mature and then emerge through the breathing pore and drop to the ground, where they pupate. Adult flies emerge 10–20 days later, and the cycle begins again.

Rats and dogs are the usual definitive host; however, people, mice, monkeys, mongooses, squirrels, leopards, boars, antelopes, cats, goats, pigs, rabbits, guinea pigs, and chickens can be infested.

Pathology: Clinically, the infestation is characterized by a small erythematous papule that appears 2–3 days after larval penetration. Within days, the papule enlarges until it becomes a nodule that resembles a boil (furuncle); hence, the description furunculoid myiasis. At the center of the nodule is a pore through which serous fluid oozes. This fluid can be hemorrhagic or purulent and contains larval feces.

Dogs with thin, soft skin seem to be more suitable hosts for larval development than dogs with thick skin. Preferential sites of infestation are the feet, genitals, tail, and axillae. In endemic areas, mild infestations in dogs do not produce clinical distress. Massive infestation may induce marked swelling and edema, especially if larvae are in close proximity to each other. Larvae can penetrate deep into tissues and cause considerable damage and even death.

Diagnosis: The presence of a dermal swelling with a central opening may lead to a tentative diagnosis of myiasis due to *C anthropophaga*. A definitive diagnosis can be made only after extraction and identification of typical larvae. The identification of adult flies and their associated larval stages should be left to an entomologist.

A tentative diagnosis may often be made by a history of either residence in or travel to a geographic area endemic for *C anthropophaga*. However, the parasite has also been diagnosed in travelers and their accompanying pets from geographic areas where the parasite is not found.

Treatment and Control: Larvae can be removed by coating the breathing pore with a thick, viscous compound, such as heavy oil, liquid paraffin, sticking plaster, or petrolatum jelly. Clogging the pore causes the larva to become hypoxic and leave the cavity in search of oxygen. Light pressure at the edge of the lesion also aids in larval removal.

Lidocaine hydrochloride can be injected into the furuncular lesion to facilitate larval extraction with thumb forceps. Surgical excision is usually unnecessary and unwarranted while the larvae are alive but is used to remove dead or decaying larvae. Great care should be taken during the extraction process to avoid rupturing larvae in situ, although anaphylaxis has not been reported. Antibiotics should be prescribed.

Adult flies should be killed if seen indoors. Larvae should be removed from animals entering the house and destroyed. All rats should be killed and burned. Prevention of an infestation depends on cleanliness and regular disinfection of the animal's sleeping quarters. In the case of valuable animals (eg, Angora rabbits), flies may be kept out of rabbit pens using wire gauze.

Because the adult female flies lay eggs in sandy soil contaminated by feces or urine, the parasite can be controlled in the pet's environment by prompt removal of the pet's feces and by covering urination sites on the premises with a layer of dirt.

PSEUDOMYIASIS

In pseudomyiasis, dipteran larvae have been accidentally ingested and are found within an animal's GI tract, where they are not able to continue their development. Dogs or cats infested with larvae of the facultative myiasis-producing flies in wounds or in the hair coat often ingest larvae while licking or grooming. These larvae pass through the GI tract and appear in the feces undigested. Dipteran larvae may also be passed in the feces when a roaming dog or cat ingests carrion that contains maggots; these maggots pass to the external environment undigested.

Pseudomyiasis can also occur if feces submitted for parasitologic examination are not fresh. Adult facultative-myiasis flies may have laid their eggs in these feces, and larval development may have begun.

Eristalis tenax, the rat-tailed maggot, may be seen in the gutter behind cows in dairy barns. These maggots are associated with liquid feces and with feces that have not been removed from the environment. The larvae are known as rat-tailed maggots because their breathing pores are found at the tip of a long, siphon-like breathing tube on their posterior end. Many farmers erroneously assume that the cows defecated these maggots. The adults are nonparasitic, free-living flies.

HELMINTHS OF THE SKIN

CUTANEOUS HABRONEMIASIS

(Summer sores, Jack sores, Bursatti)

Cutaneous habronemiasis is a skin disease of Equidae caused in part by the larvae of the spirurid stomach worms (*see* p 315). When the larvae emerge from flies feeding on preexisting wounds or on moisture of the genitalia or eyes, they migrate into and irritate the tissue, which causes a granulomatous reaction. The lesion becomes chronic, and healing is protracted. Diagnosis is based on finding nonhealing, reddish brown, greasy skin granulomas that contain yellow, calcified material the size of rice grains. Larvae, recognized by spiny knobs on their tails, can sometimes be demonstrated in scrapings of the lesions. Many different treatments have been tried, most with poor results. Symptomatic treatment, including use of insect repellents, may be of benefit, and organophosphates applied topically to the abraded surface may kill the larvae. Surgical removal or cauterization of the excessive granulation tissue may be necessary. Treatment with ivermectin (200 mcg/kg) has been effective, and although there may be temporary exacerbation of the lesions (presumably in reaction to the dying larvae), spontaneous healing may be expected. Moxidectin at 400 mcg/kg also appears to be active against *Habronema* spp in the stomach. Control of the fly hosts and regular collection and stacking of manure, together with anthelmintic therapy, may reduce the incidence.

DRACUNCULUS INFECTIONS

Dracunculus insignis is found mainly in the subcutaneous connective tissues of the legs of raccoons, mink, and other animals, including dogs and cats, in North America and possibly other parts of the world. The females (≥300 mm long) are much longer than the males (~20 mm). They produce ulcers in the skin of their host, through which their anterior end is protruded on contact with water. Females produce characteristic long, thin-tailed larvae. Water fleas (*Cyclops* sp) are the intermediate host in which infective larvae develop. Dogs become infected through ingestion of contaminated water or a paratenic host (frogs).

Subcutaneous, serpentine, inflammatory tracts and nonhealing, crater-like, edematous skin ulcers are seen. Infections are rare but are occasionally found in animals that have been around small lakes and bodies of shallow, stagnant water. Treatment is by careful, slow extraction of the parasite. Administration of miridazole or benzimidazole compounds may be useful.

D medinensis, the guinea worm of parts of Africa, Asia, and the Middle East, although primarily a parasite of people, is also found in dogs and other animals.

ELAEOPHOROSIS

(Filarial dermatosis, "Clear-eyed" blindness, Sorehead)

Elaeophora schneideri is a parasite of mule deer and black-tailed deer found in the mountains of western and southwestern USA and in Nebraska; it also has been found in white-tailed deer in southern and southeastern regions in the USA. Adult parasites are 60–120 mm long and usually are found in the common carotid or internal maxillary arteries. The microfilariae, which are ~275 μm long and 15–17 μm thick, normally are found in skin capillaries on the forehead and face. Development in the intermediate hosts, horse flies of the genera *Tabanus* and *Hybomitra*, requires ~2 wk. Infective larvae invade the host as the horse fly feeds, migrate to the leptomeningeal arteries, and develop to immature adults in ~3 wk. These young adults migrate against the blood flow and establish in the common carotid arteries, where they continue to grow. The parasites reach sexual maturity ~6 mo later and begin producing microfilariae. The life span of adults is 3–4 yr.

Clinical Findings: Clinical disease has not been reported in mule deer and black-tailed deer; therefore, they are considered to be the normal definitive hosts. When horse flies transmit the infective larvae to elk, moose, domestic sheep and goats, sika deer, and possibly white-tailed deer, the larvae develop in the leptomeningeal arteries and cause ischemic necrosis of brain tissue, resulting in blindness, brain damage, and sudden death. Blindness in these animals is characterized by absence of opacities in the refractive media of the eye ("clear-eyed" blindness).

Domestic sheep and goats, especially lambs, kids, and yearlings, may die suddenly 3–5 wk after infection. Death is usually preceded by incoordination and circling and often by convulsions and opisthotonos. Numerous thrombi occur in the cerebral and leptomeningeal arteries. One or more young adult *E schneideri* accompany each thrombus. If sheep or goats survive the early infection, a raw bloody dermatitis on the poll, forehead, or face ("sorehead") develops 6–10 mo later. Lesions occasionally develop on the legs, abdomen, and feet. These lesions are an allergic dermatitis in response to the microfilariae lodged in capillaries. Lesions persist, with periods of intermittent and incomplete healing for ~3 yr, followed by spontaneous recovery. Hyperplasia and hyperkeratosis develop in the epidermis of the parasitized area.

Diagnosis: Differential diagnoses include coenurosis (*Taenia*, *see* p 1311), cerebrocortical necrosis (*see* p 1281), and enterotoxemia (*see* p 609). Elaeophorosis should not be considered unless sheep have been in endemic areas during the summer. Diagnosis in lambs, kids, or elk yearlings or calves usually is made at necropsy; numerous thrombi and parasites are found in the common carotid, internal maxillary, cerebral, and leptomeningeal arteries. Presumptive diagnosis in mature sheep is based on history and location and type of lesion. The skin lesion must be differentiated from that of ulcerative dermatosis (*see* p 872). Confirmation is by recovery of microfilariae from the lesion or by postmortem recovery of the adult parasites. A skin biopsy of the lesion is macerated in isotonic saline solution and allowed to stand ≥6 hr at room temperature. The skin is strained off and the fluid examined for the typical microfilariae.

Treatment: Piperazine salts (220 mg/kg, PO) are effective. Complete recovery occurs in 18–20 days. No treatment is available for the cerebral form of the disease.

ONCHOCERCIASIS

The taxonomic status of the three species of *Onchocerca* currently recognized in the USA, and other previously recognized species, is under debate. *O cervicalis* is found in the ligamentum nuchae and possibly other sites in Equidae. In cattle, *O gutturosa* locates in the ligamentum nuchae, and *O lienalis* in the gastrosplenic ligament. Adults are associated with connective tissues; they are very thin and 3–60 cm long. Microfilariae are found in the dermis and on rare occasions circulating in peripheral blood. The microfilariae lack a sheath and are 200–250 μm long with a short, sharply pointed tail. *Culicoides* spp (*see* p 887) are the intermediate hosts for *O cervicalis*, and *Simulium* spp for *O gutturosa* and *O lienalis*.

Clinical Findings: *O cervicalis* has been associated with fistulous withers, poll evil, dermatitis, and uveitis in horses. However, because *O cervicalis* in large numbers is common in horses without these diseases, there is some debate about its role in the pathogenesis of these conditions.

Adults in the ligamentum nuchae induce inflammatory reactions ranging from acute edematous necrosis to chronic granulomatous changes, resulting in marked fibrosis and mineralization. Mineralized nodules are more common in older horses. Although lesions are found in these areas, presumably associated with dead parasites, it is generally agreed that fistulous withers and poll evil are not caused by *O cervicalis* infections.

Microfilariae concentrate in the skin of the ventral midline. Large numbers can be found in horses without dermatitis as well as in horses with dermatitis of the face, neck, chest, withers, forelegs, and abdomen. These lesions may be pruritic and often include areas of scale, crusts, ulceration, alopecia, and depigmentation. The dermatitis may be associated with an immunologic reaction to dead and dying microfilariae. Although the pathogenesis of these lesions is unclear, treatment with microfilaricidal drugs may result in dramatic improvement. Allergic reactions to the bites of small flies may produce similar lesions or exacerbate microfilaria-associated dermatitis. Thus, diagnosis of *Onchocerca*-associated dermatitis may be based on responsiveness to microfilaricidal treatment.

Microfilariae also accumulate in the eyes of horses, but not all agree that a clear association has been made between microfilariae and equine uveitis (*see* p 508) or other ocular lesions in horses.

Diagnosis: The most effective method of diagnosis is by skin biopsy, preferably a full-thickness biopsy ≥6 mm. The tissue is minced and macerated in isotonic saline for several hours. Microfilariae are concentrated and stained with new methylene blue after removal of skin pieces. The microfilariae can be differentiated microscopically from *Setaria* spp, found in the blood of cattle, and Equidae by the presence of a sheath around *Setaria*.

Treatment: No treatment is effective against the adults. Ivermectin (200 mcg/kg) and moxidectin (400 mcg/kg) are efficacious (>99%) against microfilariae and produce marked clinical improvement in horses with onchocercal dermatitis. A small portion of horses infected with *O cervicalis* react to the treatment with a marked, edematous ventral midline swelling 1–3 days after treatment. Ocular lesions have also been reported. These reactions usually resolve spontaneously, but symptomatic treatment may be necessary.

PARAFILARIA INFECTION

Parafilaria bovicola

This filarial parasite of cattle causes subcutaneous lesions that resemble bruising. It also has been reported from water buffalo (*Bubalus bubalis*). The worm is whitish; adult females are 50–65 mm long, and males 30–35 mm. It is found in Asia (Philippines, Japan, Russia, Pakistan, India), Europe (Bulgaria, Romania, France, Sweden), and Africa (Morocco, Tunisia, Rwanda, Burundi, South Africa, Namibia, Botswana, Zimbabwe). A specimen was recovered in Canada from a bull imported from France, but *P bovicola* does not appear to have established itself on the American continents and has not been reported from Australia.

Parafilaria infection has been identified as a source of considerable economic loss to the beef industries of South Africa and Sweden, despite their climatic differences. It is found primarily in range cattle in the savanna areas of southern Africa, whereas in Sweden it has emerged as a problem in cattle following spring turnout to pasture after winter housing.

Clinical Findings: The only external signs of infection in cattle are focal cutaneous hemorrhages ("bleeding spots") that may ooze for some hours before clotting and drying in the matted hair of the coat. Bleeding spots are induced by the female worm, which causes the formation of a small nodule, perforates the skin, and oviposits in the blood dripping from the central wound. The tiny eggs contain the first larval stage (microfilariae) of the parasite. In both the northern and southern hemispheres, bleeding spots are markedly seasonal, being most common in spring and early summer. Most bleeding spots occur along the dorsum of the animal, particularly in the forequarters.

The invertebrate hosts are face flies of the genus *Musca* (subgenus *Eumusca*), which ingest the eggs when feeding at the bleeding spots. *M autumnalis* has been identified as a host in Sweden, *M lusoria* and *M xanthomelas* in South Africa, and *M vitripennis* in Asia. Development to infective third-stage larvae in the fly takes 10–12 days. Transmission to cattle probably occurs when the flies feed on wounds, *Parafilaria* bleeding spots, or ocular secretions.

Because of seasonal bleeding and the cutaneous nodules, severe infections of *P bovicola* have been reported to impair the productivity of working bullocks in India; however, the major importance of *Parafilaria* in beef-producing countries is damage to the subcutaneous tissues. Carcasses of infected animals display irregular, edematous, greenish yellow lesions that resemble bruising. These are usually superficial but occasionally underlying muscles are extensively involved. Lesions are most severe during the spring and summer.

Trimmed carcasses are often seriously disfigured and consequently downgraded. In severe cases, the carcass may be condemned. Lesions are more common and severe in bulls than in steers, which in turn are less severely affected than female animals.

Diagnosis: The seasonal bleeding spots are sometimes confused with those caused by thorns, wire, ticks, or biting insects. For differentiation, either fresh or dried blood should be mixed with water in a test tube and centrifuged. The characteristic eggs are found on microscopic examination of the sediment.

Carcass lesions can be differentiated from bruising by the presence of numerous eosinophils in Giemsa-stained impression smears made from the lesions. In addition, affected tissue has a characteristic, disagreeable, metallic smell.

Usually, only small numbers of worms are present in affected carcasses and are often difficult to find because of their color and the accompanying inflammatory reaction. Affected tissues can be incubated in warm saline to facilitate the recovery of parasites. An ELISA for the detection of antibodies against *P bovicola* is available.

Treatment and Prevention: Ivermectin (200 mcg/kg) or nitroxynil (20 mg/kg) given SC reduces the number and surface area of *Parafilaria* lesions. Animals should be treated at least 70–90 days before slaughter to provide sufficient time for lesions to resolve. The treatment-to-slaughter interval should not be >120 days, because unaffected larval forms of the parasite may induce fresh lesions as they mature.

In trials in Sweden, use of pyrethroid-impregnated ear tags gave good control of flies and reduced parafilarial lesions at slaughter by 75%. Ear tagging all cattle in an area resulted in total control of the parasite. The use of residually active, synthetic pyrethroid dips has also effectively reduced transmission.

It may be possible to screen imported animals with an ELISA to prevent spread of the disease to unaffected countries or, in conjunction with residual insecticides and effective anthelmintics, to eradicate new foci of infection.

Parafilaria multipapillosa

P multipapillosa is found in the subcutaneous tissues of horses in various parts of the world; it is especially common in the Russian steppes and eastern Europe. It is similar in size, appearance, life cycle, and development to *P bovicola*. Bloodsucking *Haematobia* spp are thought to be the invertebrate hosts.

In spring and summer, the parasite causes skin nodules, particularly on the head and upper forequarters. These bleed transiently but often profusely ("summer bleeding") and then resolve; other hemorrhaging nodules develop as the parasite moves to a different site. Occasionally, the nodules suppurate. The nodules and bleeding are unsightly and interfere with harnesses of working horses but generally are of little consequence. The clinical signs are pathognomonic.

No satisfactory treatment has been reported, but fly control may reduce the incidence.

PELODERA DERMATITIS

(Rhabditic dermatitis)

This rare, nonseasonal, acute dermatosis results from invasion of the skin by larvae of the free-living saprophytic nematode *Pelodera strongyloides*. The larvae are ubiquitous in decaying organic matter and on or near the surface of moist soil but are only occasionally parasitic. Exposure to the larvae occurs through direct contact with infested material such as damp, filthy bedding. The larvae may not be able to invade healthy skin; preexisting dermatoses or environmental conditions favoring maceration of the skin, eg, constant exposure to mud or damp bedding, may facilitate invasion. *Pelodera* dermatitis has been reported in dogs, cows, horses, sheep, guinea pigs, and people.

Typically, lesions are confined to body areas in contact with the infested material, such as the extremities, ventral abdomen and thorax, and perineum. Affected skin is erythematous and partially to completely alopecic, with papules, pustules, crusts, erosions, or ulcerations. Pruritus is usually intense but can be moderate or even absent. Differential diagnoses include demodicosis, canine scabies, dermatophytosis, pyoderma, and other rare cutaneous larval infestations such as hookworm dermatitis, dirofilariasis, dipetalonemiasis, and strongyloidiasis.

Diagnosis is confirmed easily by finding live, motile *P strongyloides* larvae in skin scrapings of affected areas. The larvae are cylindrical and ~600 × 38 μm. Histologic examination of skin biopsy specimens reveals larvae in the hair follicles and superficial dermis and usually an inflammatory dermal infiltrate. The larvae are readily cultivated on blood agar plates at 77°F (25°C).

Effective treatment consists primarily of removing and destroying moist, infested bedding material and moving the animal to a clean, dry environment. Usually, spontaneous recovery ensues. It may be desirable to dip or spray the affected animals with an insecticidal preparation at least twice at weekly intervals. Short-term use of corticosteroids may be indicated if pruritus is severe.

STEPHANOFILARIASIS

(Filarial dermatitis of cattle)

Stephanofilaria stilesi is a small, filarial parasite that causes a circumscribed dermatitis along the ventral midline of cattle. It has been reported throughout the USA but is more common in the west and southwest. Adult worms are 3–6 mm long and usually are found in the dermis, just beneath the epidermal layer. Microfilariae are 50 µm long and are enclosed in a spherical, semirigid vitelline membrane. The intermediate host for *S stilesi* is the female horn fly, *Haematobia irritans* (*see* p 892). Horn flies feeding on the lesion ingest microfilariae that develop to third-stage infective larvae in 2–3 wk. The infective larvae are introduced into the skin as the horn fly feeds.

The dermatitis develops along the ventral midline, usually between the brisket and navel. With repeated exposure, the lesion spreads and often involves the skin posterior to the navel. Active lesions are covered with blood or serous exudate, while chronic lesions are smooth, dry, and devoid of hair. Hyperkeratosis and parakeratosis develop in the epidermis of the parasitized area.

Deep skin scrapings are macerated in isotonic saline solution and examined microscopically for adults or microfilariae. The microfilariae must be differentiated from microfilariae of *Onchocerca lienalis*, *O gutturosa*, and *Setaria* spp, which are much larger (200–250 µm), and *Pelodera strongyloides* (*see* above), a small free-living nematode occasionally responsible for a moist, superficial dermatitis. The rhabditiform esophagus of *P strongyloides* is not found in filarial nematodes.

No approved treatment is available for *S stilesi*, but topically applied organophosphates (trichlorfon 6%–10%, daily or on alternate days for 7 days) have proved effective against other species of *Stephanofilaria*. Ivermectin is reported to be effective against microfilariae of *S zaheeri*.

LICE

(Pediculosis)

Numerous species of lice parasitize domestic animals. Lice are largely host specific, living on one species or several closely related species. Lice are obligate ectoparasites and depend on the host to complete their life cycle. Recent taxonomic changes have complicated the orders and suborders of lice. In general, lice are divided into two categories: bloodsucking (or sucking) lice (order Anoplura) and chewing (or biting) lice (formerly the order Mallophaga, now composed of three suborders). Bloodsucking lice are parasites of mammals, whereas chewing lice infest both mammals and birds. Lice live within the microenvironment provided by the skin and its hair or feathers, and are transmitted primarily by contact between hosts. All life stages occur on the host, although lice may survive off the host for a period of time. In temperate regions, lice are most abundant during the colder months and often are difficult to find in the summer. Infestations are most often seen on stressed animals, and husbandry and individual health are important in treatment and management of these parasites. (*See also* p 2875.)

Etiology and Pathogenesis: Lice are wingless, flattened insects, usually 2–4 mm long, although the species infesting animals may range from 1–8 mm long. The claws of the legs are adapted for clinging to and moving among hairs or feathers; the size and shape of the claws tend to be specialized for the average width of a hair shaft of the host species. This characteristic plays an important role in host specificity. The mouthparts also aid in attachment to the host. Chewing lice have ventral chewing mandibles; they feed on epidermal debris, primarily skin scales, sebaceous secretions, and feathers, if applicable. The heads of chewing lice have a blunted appearance, with the head being wider than the thorax. As the name implies, bloodsucking lice have piercing mouthparts that allow them to feed on the blood of their host. In contrast to the heads of chewing lice, those of bloodsucking lice have a pointed appearance, and the heads are narrower than the thorax. When not in use, their mouthpart stylets are retracted within the head. The distinction between chewing lice and bloodsucking lice is important when choosing an effective therapy for treatment of pediculosis.

On mammalian hosts, louse eggs, sometimes called "nits," are glued to hairs near the skin surface and are pale, translucent, and suboval. The three nymphal stages, of increasing size, are smaller than adults but otherwise resemble adults in habits and appearance. Approximately 3–4 wk are required to complete one generation, but this varies by species. Adult lice are visible to the naked eye, but magnification is often required to identify the species.

Pediculosis can result in dermatologic disease, production loss, and occassionally anemia due to blood loss. Additionally, lice may be vectors of more arthropod-borne infections than previously believed. Lice have been shown to transmit viruses, bacteria, fungi, and protozoa. Most of the research has focused on agents transmitted by human lice species that are known to transmit a variety of pathogens to their hosts, including the causative agents of epidemic typhus (*Rickettsia prowazekii*), louse-borne relapsing fever (*Borrelia recurrentis*), and trench fever (*Bartonella recurrentis*), among others. Until recently, relatively few diseases were known to be vectored by domestic animal lice. A number of agents are now known or suspected to be vectored by lice.

Clinical Findings and Diagnosis: Pediculosis is manifested by pruritus and dermal irritation, with resultant scratching, rubbing, and biting of infested areas. A generally unthrifty appearance, rough coat, and lowered production in farm animals is common. In severe infestations, there may be loss of hair and local scarification. Extreme infestation with bloodsucking lice can cause anemia. In sheep and goats, rubbing and scratching often results in broken fibers, which gives the fleece a "pulled" appearance. In dogs, the coat becomes rough and dry and, if lice are numerous, the hair may be matted. Sucking lice cause small wounds that may become infected. The constant crawling and piercing or biting of the skin may cause restless behavior in hosts.

Diagnosis is based on the presence of lice. The hair should be parted, and the skin and proximal portion of the coat examined under good lighting conditions. The hair of large animals should be parted on the face, neck, ears, topline, dewlap, escutcheon, tail base, and tail switch. The head, legs, feet, and scrotum should not be overlooked, particularly in sheep. On small animals, the ova are more readily seen. Occasionally, when the coat is matted, the lice can be seen when the mass is broken apart. Biting lice are active and can be seen moving through the hair. Sucking lice usually move more slowly and are often found with mouthparts embedded in the skin. Diagnosis may be aided by use of a magnification device. An otoscope, without the otoscopy cone, may be useful for this purpose.

Pediculosis of livestock is most prevalent during the winter; severity is greatly reduced with the approach of summer. Infestations of both chewing and sucking lice may become severe. In dairy herds, the young stock, dry cows, and bulls may escape early diagnosis and suffer more severely. Young calves may die, and pregnant cows may abort.

Transmission usually occurs by host contact. Lice dropped or pulled from the host die in a few days, but disengaged ova may continue to hatch over 2–3 wk in warm weather. Therefore, premises recently vacated by infested stock should be disinfected before being used for clean stock.

Treatment: Successful louse control is a multifactorial process. Factors to address include treatment of the affected animal(s), treatment of contact animals, environmental control, and properly addressing the stressors that either permitted initial infestation or exacerbated infestation. Effective treatment results in prompt improvement of clinical signs. Specific pediculosis treatments are discussed below.

It is the practitioner's duty to recommend a safe and effective treatment regimen. In the USA, ectoparasiticides are regulated by the Environmental Protection Agency (EPA) or the FDA Center for Veterinary Medicine. As a general rule, if a product is applied topically to an animal to treat ectoparasites, and the compound is not absorbed systemically, it likely falls under the jurisdiction of the EPA. If a product is administered parenterally, or if it is applied topically for systemic absorption, it likely falls under the jurisdiction of the FDA. This distinction is important for practitioners to recognize, because there is no legal extra-label use of products regulated by the EPA. Label directions must be followed regarding species treated, product concentration, product dosage, individuals allowed to administer application, and re-treatment interval. Because products regulated by the FDA are approved animal drugs, extra-label use may be allowed under the Animal Medicinal Drug Use and Clarification Act (AMDUCA) (*see* p 2748 and *see* p 2637). The Food Animal Residue Avoidance Databank (FARAD) can be consulted for extra-label drug use recommendations and calculated meat and milk withdrawal times.

Treatment of individual animals may be aided by debulking the infested coat if weather and coat type permit. Clipping an infested animal's long, heavily soiled, or matted coat can immediately reduce the parasite burden on an affected animal, allow topical products to be distributed evenly, and allow for treatment of secondary infections if present. Many compounds effectively kill adult and nymphal life stages, but few have been tested for ovicidal capabilities. Therefore, many sources recommend re-treatment at intervals of 7–10 days until the infestation has been controlled. Contact animals should also be treated to prevent spread of infestation within a herd, flock, or household. Animal equipment or bedding should be washed frequently with hot, soapy water until infestation is controlled. Finally, addressing animal overcrowding, poor feed quality, and underlying health issues are the final steps to manage pediculosis and prevent recurrence. New animals should be quarantined and inspected for infestation before herd or flock integration.

CATTLE

In temperate climates, domestic cattle may be infested with one species of chewing louse (*Damalinia bovis*, formerly *Bovicola bovis*) and four species of bloodsucking lice (*Linognathus vituli*, *Solenopotes capillatus*, *Haematopinus eurysternus*, and *H quadripertuses*). Except for *H quadripertuses*, these lice have a cosmopolitan distribution, ie, they are found throughout most of the world. *H quadripertuses*, the cattle tail louse, is a tropical louse that has extended its distribution into subtropical areas. In the USA, *H quadripertuses* has been reported in California, Florida, and in other Gulf Coast states. The cattle tail louse is known to parasitize both European and Zebu breeds of cattle.

Cattle, especially young animals, may be infested with multiple species of lice simultaneously. *S capillatus* and *H eurysternus* infestations are more often recognized on mature animals, whereas *L vituli* is more commonly seen on calves and on dairy stock. For all age classes of cattle, stressors such as high stocking density, poor feed quality, gestational status, and underlying health issues are often contributing factors to susceptibility and degree of infestation. For site predilection on the host, *see* TABLE 1.

Pathogenesis and Disease Transmission: Pediculosis in cattle can decrease weight gain and milk production, result in weight loss, and cause hide and hair damage. Some sources have reported up to 9% reduced gain in cattle moderately to heavily infested with lice.

L vituli can serve as a mechanical vector for *Anaplasma marginale*, the causative

TABLE 1 SITE PREDILECTION OF CATTLE LICE

	Site Predilection
	CHEWING LICE
Damalinia bovis (cattle biting louse, red louse)	Most commonly found on dorsum Infestation may extend cranially to head and caudally to tailhead
	BLOODSUCKING LICE
Linognathus vituli (long-nosed cattle louse)	Most commonly found over withers, lateral shoulders, and dewlap May have generalized distribution over animal In early infestations, may be found in clusters In heavy infestations, may be found over most of body
Haematopinus eurysternus (short-nosed cattle louse)	Often found on front half of host from ears to dewlap Infestations tend to be heavier in anterior portions of the body, including the ears, during warm weather
Solenopotes capillatus (little blue cattle louse)	Found in distinct clusters, mainly on head and face Heavy infestations may extend to dewlap or surround eyes
Haematopinus quadripertuses (cattle tail louse)	Adults often confined to the tail, eggs commonly noted on tail switch

agent of bovine anaplasmosis (*see* p 18). Outside the USA, *H eurysternus* populations have been found to contain multiple *Rickettsia* spp, but the role lice play in transmitting rickettsial agents is not well understood.

Treatment: A variety of compounds effectively control lice in cattle, including synergized pyrethrins; the synthetic pyrethroids cyfluthrin, permethrin, zetacypermethrin, and cyhalothrin (including gamma- and lambda-cyhalothrin) (beef cattle only); the organophosphates phosmet, chlorpyrifos (beef and nonlactating dairy cattle only), tetrachlorvinphos, coumaphos, and diazinon (beef and nonlactating dairy cattle only); and the macrocyclic lactones ivermectin, eprinomectin, and doramectin. Pour-on formulations are effective against biting and bloodsucking lice, whereas injectable formulations are primarily effective against bloodsucking lice.

Multiple pour-on formulations of 5% permethrin/5% piperonyl butoxide, 5% diflubenzuron/5% permethrin, and gamma-cyhalothrin are labeled for season-long control (~3–4 mo) of lice on beef and dairy cattle. Although both amitraz and spinosad are effective against lice, the last cattle products containing amitraz were removed from the USA market in 2014. Spinosad formulations for use on cattle were officially discontinued in the USA in 2010.

Certain Brahman and Brahman-cross cattle have organophosphate hypersensitivity, which should be considered when selecting a treatment compound.

Because of ease of application and reduced stress to the treated animal, the pour-on method has become a popular way to apply insecticides. Self-treatment devices also can be used, such as back rubbers, oilers, dust bags, and ear tags. Cattle dips have fallen out of favor in the USA because of the labor-intensive nature of the process and amount of chemical needed to keep vats charged with active compound. The compound chosen must be appropriate for the animal's age, reproductive status, and production system. The treatment of meat and dairy animals must be restricted to uses specified on the product label, and all label precautions should be carefully observed. Appropriate meat and milk withdrawal times must be observed. In most countries, regulatory agencies specify tissue residue limits of insecticides and carefully regulate insecticide use on livestock. All regulations are subject to change, and pertinent current local laws and requirements should be determined before treatment.

Husbandry issues (overcrowding, poor feed quality, etc) and underlying health conditions in animals should be addressed. Treatment will be most effective if stock trailers, chutes, and other areas cattle have contacted are cleaned and treated with an appropriate premise spray.

SHEEP AND GOATS

Sheep may become infested with one species of chewing louse, *Damalinia ovis* (formerly *Bovicola ovis*), and three species of bloodsucking lice: *Linognathus pedalis*, *L ovillus*, and *L africanus* (*see* TABLE 2). Outside the USA, *D ovis* is also referred to as the sheep

TABLE 2 SITE PREDILECTION OF SHEEP LICE

	Site Predilection
CHEWING LICE	
Damalinia ovis (sheep biting louse)	Most commonly found on the dorsum Infestation may extend cranially to head and caudally to tailhead
BLOODSUCKING LICE	
Linognathus pedalis (sheep foot louse)	Confined to hairy parts of the foot, except in very heavy infestations
Linognathus ovillus (sheep face and body louse)	Usually found on hairy parts of the sheep's skin As populations increase, lice spread to other parts of body
Linognathus africanus (African blue louse)	Often found on flanks of sheep Forms clusters Slippage of wool is common

body louse. Despite its name, *L africanus* is found outside Africa, including in the USA, Central America, and India. *L africanus* has also been reported from a variety of hosts, including goats and several species of deer.

Goats can be parasitized by three types of chewing lice, namely *Damalinia caprae* (formerly *Bovicola caprae*), *D limbata* (formerly *B limbata*), and *D crassipes* (formerly *Holokartikos crassipes*); and two types of bloodsucking lice, namely *Linognathus stenopsis* and *L africanus*. *L stenopsis* is found on both short-haired and Angora breeds of goats. *L stenopsis* has occasionally been reported from sheep in various parts of the world. It is found mostly on the long-haired parts of the hindlegs and back. Severe infestations are rare. *D caprae*, the goat biting louse, is most frequently found on short-haired goats. Both *D crassipes* and *D limbata* (the Angora goat biting louse) are serious pests of Angora breeds.

Pathogenesis and Disease Transmission: Affected animals often rub vigorously on fencing and pens, damaging the coat and causing excoriations. Pediculosis is one cause of "wool slip" in sheep.

Sheep and goat lice are not known to vector any disease agents within the USA.

Treatment: Pyrethrins and pyrethroids are labeled for control of lice in sheep and goats. Shearing may be necessary to achieve effective louse control on sheep and goats. Re-treatment is often necessary. Husbandry issues and individual health issues within the flock or herd should be addressed. Shearing must be done carefully, because clippers may carry lice from animal to animal.

Treatment of meat and dairy animals must be restricted to uses specified on the product label, and all label precautions should be carefully observed. Appropriate meat and milk withdrawal times must be observed.

HORSES AND DONKEYS

Horses and donkeys may be infested by two species of lice, *Haematopinus asini*, the horse bloodsucking louse, and *Damalinia equi*, the horse biting louse. *D equi* is also called *Werneckiella equi* and was formerly known as *Bovicola equi*, *Trichodectes equi*, and *T parumpilosus*. Both species are distributed worldwide. *D equi* is a small louse, 1–2 mm long, and *H asini* is 3–3.5 mm long. There have been reports of poultry chewing lice (*see* p 2876) infesting horses when poultry and horses are housed in the same facilities. This problem is exacerbated when the poultry are removed without concurrent animal or premise treatments, leaving horses as the only host available.

Stressors such as high stocking density, poor feed quality, gestational status, and underlying health issues are often contributing factors to susceptibility and degree of infestation. Longer body hair, whether a winter coat or feathering, appears to allow for higher densities of lice to be sustained, because they have greater surface area to infest. Infestations are most common in winter and early spring. For site predilection on host by species of louse, *see* TABLE 3.

Pathogenesis and Disease Transmission: *D equi* and *H asini* are not known to vector any disease agents in the USA.

Treatment: A variety of compounds effectively control lice on horses, including synergized pyrethrins, synthetic pyrethroids, and the organophosphate coumaphos. Diazinon is no longer labeled for use on horses in the USA.

Pyrethrin and pyrethroid sprays are the most popular method for lice control on horses in the USA. Pyrethrin or pyrethroid formulations also are available

TABLE 3 SITE PREDILECTION OF EQUINE LICE

	Site Predilection
CHEWING LICE	
Damalinia equi (also called *Werneckiella equi*)	Found most commonly on the finer hairs of the body Found on lateral aspects of the neck, flanks, and base of the tail
BLOODSUCKING LICE	
Haematopinus asini	Found most commonly at roots of the forelock and mane, around base of the tail, and on hairs just above the hoof (especially in breeds with feathering)

in wipe-on, pour-on, and powder applications. Coumaphos is available as a powder or spray. Caution is warranted in mares with foals at their side, because the foals may be exposed to larger amounts of the compound than intended, especially with powdered formulations. When using sprays, certain formulations require soaking the hair to the skin, including mane and tail, whereas others may require only a light, misting application. Label instructions should be read carefully, and the manufacturer consulted if necessary.

Depending on the severity of infestation, the coat may be clipped. Long hair such as feathers on certain breeds, winter coats, or resultant from endocrine disorder (eg, pituitary pars intermedia dysfunction, *see* p 547) may make treatment more difficult.

Husbandry issues (overcrowding, poor feed quality, etc) and underlying health conditions should be addressed. Treatment will be most effective if trailers, stalls, wash racks, and other areas where horses have contacted are cleaned and treated with an appropriate premise spray.

PIGS

Domestic pigs are infested with only one species of louse, *Haematopinus suis*, the hog louse. This very large (5–6 mm) sucking louse is common on domestic swine worldwide. Swine pediculosis is more common in smaller or backyard populations than in large, commercial operations. Nymphal lice are normally found on the inside of the ears (often in the ear canal), on the skin behind the ears, in the folds of the neck, and on the medial aspects of the legs. In severe infestations, *H suis* may be found elsewhere on the body.

H suis can cause severe anemia, especially in piglets, because of the amount of blood imbibed by this large louse species. Extreme pruritus and subsequent self-trauma (alopecia, erythema, excoriations, and crusting) can be seen as hogs alleviate the irritation associated with the lice feeding.

Pathogenesis and Disease Transmission: *H suis* is a vector of swine pox virus, and it has also been implicated as a vector of *Eperythrozoon suis* and *E parvum*, the causative agents of swine eperythrozoonosis and of African swine fever virus in regions where these agents are endemic. Except for swine pox virus, transmission of these agents by *H suis* is considered rare.

Treatment: A variety of compounds effectively control lice on swine, including synergized pyrethrins; pyrethroids; the organophosphates phosmet, coumaphos, and tetrachlorvinphos; and the macrocyclic lactones ivermectin and doramectin.

Amitraz is no longer available for use on swine in the USA. Although eprinomectin is used in cattle, this compound should not be used in unapproved animal species, because severe adverse reactions, including fatalities, may result.

For severe infestations in swine, dust formulations can be used to treat bedding. Husbandry and underlying health issues should be addressed.

DOGS AND CATS

Dogs can be infested with one species of bloodsucking lice, *Linognathus setosus*, and two species of chewing lice, *Trichodectes canis* and *Heterodoxus spiniger*. *H spiniger* is considered rare in North America. It is distributed worldwide but appears to be more common in warmer environments; infestations are heavier on animals in poor physical condition. *H spiniger* exhibits atypical behavior for a chewing louse—it is a blood-feeder. Dogs neglected or in poor health may become heavily infested with *L setosus*, which tends to prefer longhaired breeds. *T canis* prefers the head, neck, and tail of the host, and it may be found around wounds and body openings. Infestations may be heavy on very young and very old animals. Infested dogs rub, bite, and scratch the affected area and have a rough, matted coat.

Cats can be infested with one species of chewing lice, *Felicola subrostratus*, although there are rare reports of *H spiniger* on feral cats in other regions of the world. The louse may be seen more frequently on older, longhaired cats that are unable to groom themselves.

Practitioners should be able to distinguish *Phthirus pubis*, the human crab louse, from the lice of dogs and cats. This species may be presented for identification by owners who claim to have found them on an animal. *P pubis* does not typically infest dogs or cats; there have been only two reports of dogs infested with *P pubis*, both of which occurred from sharing bedding with a person who was severely infested.

With widespread use of monthly flea and tick preventives, pediculosis in dogs and cats has become rare in the USA. Infestation is usually seen on debilitated, feral, stray, or shelter animals.

Pathogenesis and Disease Transmission: *T canis* can serve as an intermediate host to the double-pored tapeworm, *Dipylidium caninum*. This parasite of dogs and cats can occasionally infect people. *H spiniger* has been found to contain the filarial nematode *Acanthocheilonema reconditum* (formerly *Dipetalonema reconditum*), but its competence as a vector has not been demonstrated.

Treatment: A variety of compounds effectively control lice on dogs and cats, including many of the topical, monthly flea and tick control products. Pyrethrins and pyrethroids are very effective pediculicides. However, caution must be exercised when using these products on cats, because this species is highly sensitive to pyrethrins and pyrethroids, lacking the ability to metabolize high doses. Limited pyrethrin or pyrethrin products are labeled for use on cats; the products either contain very low concentrations of the active compound or are available in a slow-release formulation (eg, flumethrin/imidacloprid collar). Selamectin, imidacloprid, and fipronil have all been used successfully to treat lice on dogs and cats.

Although carbamates are effective against lice, carbaryl-containing collars were removed from the USA market in 2010, and propoxur-containing collars will no longer be available for sale in the USA after April 1, 2016. Extra-label use of eprinomectin or doramectin may result in fatalities.

Currently, spot-on products are the most popular way to treat lice in dogs and cats. However, other formulations, such as collars, shampoos, sprays, or dusts, are available for insect control on pets.

If the animal is heavily matted or long-haired, treatment may be facilitated by clipping the coat. Bedding should be washed frequently in hot, soapy water or treated with an approved bedding or premise spray until the infestation is controlled. Certain fipronil products are labeled for this use. Nutritional deficiencies or concurrent health conditions should be addressed.

MANGE

(Cutaneous acariasis, Mite infestation)

Mange is a contagious disease characterized by crusty or scaly skin, pruritus, and alopecia. Mange is a general term for cutaneous acariasis and is the result of infestation with one of several genera of parasitic mites, including *Chorioptes*, *Demodex*, *Psorobia* (formerly *Psorergates*), *Psoroptes*, *Sarcoptes*, and others. The term "scabies" most appropriately refers to infestation with *Sarcoptes* sp mites (ie, sarcoptic mange); however, this term is commonly misused to refer to any type of mange.

Historically, mange in large animals was a reportable disease because of the severity of clinical signs and contagiousness. However, widespread use of macrocyclic lactones beginning in the 1990s has provided effective treatment and decreased the prevalence. As a result, mange is no *longer a federally reportable* disease in the USA. However, some types of mange in large animals remain reportable to certain state agencies, although this may change as the lists are revised.

Successful mange treatment is a multifactorial process, including treatment of the affected animal(s), treatment of contact animals, and environmental control. Isolation of affected animals for 2 wk is often recommended to prevent or limit spread of contagious mites. Care should be taken to prevent contact of naive animals with potentially infested fomites (eg, animal bedding, feed and water buckets, tack and other equipment). Specific treatments are discussed for each species below.

CATTLE

Sarcoptic Mange (Scabies): *Sarcoptes scabiei* var *bovis* is a highly contagious disease spread by direct contact between infested and naive animals or by contaminated fomites. Lesions caused by this burrowing mite start on the head, neck, and shoulders and can spread to other parts of the body. The whole body may be involved in 6 wk. Pruritus is intense, and papules develop into crusts; the skin thickens and forms large folds. Diagnosis is made by deep skin scrapings, skin biopsy, or response to therapy. *S scabiei* var *bovis* can be transmitted to people and result in a transient, self-limiting dermatitis.

The following compounds are approved for use against sarcoptic mange mites in cattle at the labeled injectable and pour-on dosages: doramectin, eprinomectin, and ivermectin. Hot lime sulfur dips or sprays may be used, following the label instructions for species-specific dilution, with treatment repeated at 12-day intervals as needed, usually for a maximum of three treatments. Phosmet is also labeled for use against sarcoptic mange mites in cattle; two treatments may be required. Label instructions for dilution (multiple dilutions are listed) should be followed as appropriate. Certain spray formulations of permethrin are labeled for use against sarcoptic mange mites, but it is generally not considered the compound of choice. If permethrin is used, the animals should be wet thoroughly with the product and re-treated in 10–14 days.

Practitioners and producers should take care to note whether the compound, dose, and formulation are appropriate for the age of the animal and the production system in use. Eprinomectin and moxidectin pour-on formulations, as well as hot lime sulfur, are approved for use on dairy animals in the USA.

Psoroptic Mange: Psoroptic mange in cattle is caused by infestation with *Psoroptes ovis*. Current taxonomic and systematic classification of *Psoroptes* spp indicates that *P ovis* and *P cuniculi* (ear canker in rabbits, ear mange in sheep and goats) are strains or variants of the same species, with *P ovis* being found primarily on the backs and flanks of infested animals and *P cuniculi* in the ears. *P ovis* is not zoonotic.

P ovis is a nonburrowing mite that lives on the skin surface. All stages of the mite are found on the host, and transmission is through direct contact of infested and susceptible hosts. Transmission is also possible through contact with contaminated environments or fomites, because *P ovis* can survive off the host for ≥2 wk under the right conditions.

P ovis is a common parasite of cattle with a distribution limited to continental Europe and parts of the USA. It can be found in range and feedlot beef cattle from the central and western states, with the largest numbers of outbreaks historically reported from Texas, New Mexico, Oklahoma, Kansas, Colorado, and Nebraska. Clinical signs of *P ovis* infestation are rare in dairy cattle. These mites pierce host tissue and feed on serum and other fluid secretions from the bite wound. Exudates coagulate to form thick, scabby crusts. Alopecia is common with exudative dermatitis. Infestations are intensely pruritic, with papules, crusts, excoriation, and lichenification on the shoulders and rump initially, spreading to cover almost the entire body. Secondary bacterial infections are common in severe cases. Death in untreated calves, weight loss, decreased milk production, and increased susceptibility to other diseases can occur.

Treatment can be done by spray dipping or vat dipping; topical application of nonsystemic acaricides; and oral, topical, or injectable formulations of systemic drugs. Spray dipping is time consuming but useful for small herds, whereas vat dipping has fallen out of favor in the USA because of expense and the difficulty in managing proper concentrations of therapeutic compounds and proper cleanup. Toxaphene spray (0.5%–0.6%) was used historically; however, all uses of toxaphene were banned in the USA in 2001 and prohibited internationally through the Stockholm Convention on Persistent Organic Pollutants, effective 2004.

In the USA, the following treatments are labeled for use against *P ovis* in cattle at the labeled dosages: injectable doramectin, injectable ivermectin, and moxidectin (pour-on and injectable formulations). Hot lime sulfur dips or sprays may be used, following the species-specific dilution labeled on the package, with treatment repeated at 12-day intervals as needed, usually for a maximum of three treatments. Of these, only pour-on moxidectin and hot lime sulfur are approved for use on dairy animals. Certain spray formulations of permethrin are labeled for use against mange mites in cattle, but it is generally not considered the compound of choice. If permethrin is used, the animals should be thoroughly wet with the product and re-treated in 10–14 days. Outside the USA, other treatments are available and labeled for the control of mange, including flumethrin pour-on (2 mg/kg, repeated 10 days later), 0.3% coumaphos, 0.1% phoxim, 0.075% diazinon, and 0.025–0.05% amitraz. There are currently no amitraz products labeled for use on cattle in the USA. Diazinon is available for use on cattle only in an ear tag formulation in the USA; it is not labeled for treatment or prevention of mange. Products labeled for treatment and control of sarcoptic mange in cattle are considered effective against *P ovis*.

Chorioptic Mange (Leg Mange, Foot and Tail Mange, Symbiotic Mange, Barn Itch): Chorioptic mange in cattle is caused by infestation with *Chorioptes bovis* or *C texanus*. Species of *Chorioptes* are not host specific, and *C bovis* can be found on domestic ruminants and horses throughout the world. Chorioptic mange caused by infestation with *C bovis* is the most common type of mange in cattle in the USA. *C texanus* has been reported on cattle from Brazil, China, Germany, Israel, Japan, Malaysia, South Korea, and USA. *C bovis* and *C texanus* are not zoonotic.

C bovis live on the skin surface and do not burrow. Life cycle stages include egg, larval, two nymphal, two female, and one male stage. Eggs are deposited on the skin, and secretions from female mites help secure eggs to the surface of their hosts. Eggs require 5–6 days to hatch, whereas each larval and nymphal stage requires 3–5 days for development. The entire life cycle may be completed in 21–26 days and depends on temperature and humidity. Transmission is by direct contact of infested and naive hosts. *C bovis* can live off their host for up to 3 wk and can be transmitted to cattle through contact with contaminated fomites and housing.

C bovis likely feeds on sloughed skin cells and other surface debris. While feeding, *C bovis* irritates the host skin, causing abrasions that become contaminated with secretions and feces from the mites. Most cattle are subclinically infested with *C bovis*. However, *C bovis* may cause an allergic, exudative, mildly pruritic, flaky dermatitis. Lesions include nodules, papules, crusts, and ulcers that typically begin at the pastern and spread up the legs to the udder, scrotum, tail, and perineum. Self-trauma and alopecia may be evident. Lesions and clinical signs appear in late winter and spontaneously regress during summer months. Chorioptic mange is less pathogenic than sarcoptic or psoroptic mange in cattle. Diagnosis is by observation of mites in skin scrapings.

In the USA, the following treatments are approved for use against *C bovis* at the labeled dosages: pour-on doramectin, eprinomectin (both pour-on and injectable formulations), and pour-on moxidectin. Hot lime sulfur dips or sprays are labeled for use against chorioptic mites and may be used following the label directions for species-specific dilution. Lime sulfur treatment should be repeated at 12-day intervals if needed. Of these, the pour-on formulations of eprinomectin and moxidectin as well as hot lime sulfur are approved for use on dairy animals in the USA.

Demodectic Mange (Follicular Mange, Bovine Demodicosis): Three species of *Demodex* are known to infest cattle: *D bovis*, *D ghanensis*, and *D tauri*. *D bovis* is the most common and infests hair follicles of cattle worldwide. *D ghanensis* infests meibomian glands of cattle from Ghana, and *D tauri* has been recovered from hair follicles and sebaceous glands of cattle from Czechoslovakia. Species of *Demodex* are host specific and not zoonotic.

Demodex spp are unique among parasitic mites, because they are elongated with short, stumpy legs. Their distinct morphology is a presumed adaptation to living in hair follicles and sebaceous glands of their hosts. All life cycle stages are found on the host and include egg, larvae, two nymphs, and adults. These mites feed on sebum, protoplasm, and epidermal debris. Transmission of *D bovis* occurs through close contact of infested and naive hosts, with the transfer of mites from infested dams to neonates being the primary route.

Lesions consist of follicular papules and nodules, especially over the withers, neck, back, and flanks. Invasion by *D bovis* results in chronic inflammation, with formation of ulcers, abscesses, and fistulae due to follicular rupture or secondary staphylococcal infection. Pruritus is absent. Infestation of *D bovis* may result in considerable damage to hides. Cattle of any age are susceptible to demodectic mange, although disease is more evident in the young. Most cases are seen in dairy cattle in late winter or early spring. Infestation with *D bovis* is usually subclinical, and infestation may

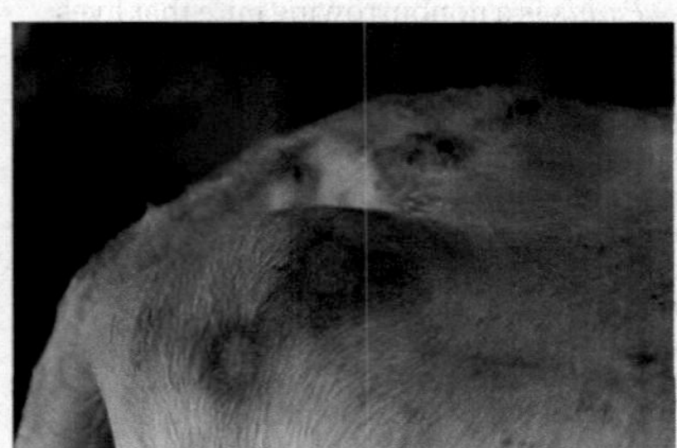

Demodex bovis, skin lesions. Courtesy of Dr. Raffaele Roncalli.

extend for many months. Diagnosis is by observation of mites in deep skin scrapings. Recovery is usually spontaneous; consequently, treatment is rarely performed. If therapy is instituted, the macrocyclic lactones listed for treatment of *Sarcoptes scabiei* var *bovis* or *Chorioptes ovis* should be considered.

Psorergatic Mange (Itch Mite): *Psorobia bos* (formerly *Psorergates bos*) is a small mite that lives in the superficial layers of cattle skin. In most instances, *P bos* is nonpathogenic, and few cattle exhibit clinical signs of infestation. On rare occasions, mild pruritus, alopecia, and increased licking and rubbing have been attributed to infestation with *P bos*. This mite has been reported from cattle in the USA, Canada, the UK, and South Africa. *P bos* is not zoonotic. The disease does not cause significant economic losses; therefore, animals are usually not treated. The macrocyclic lactone products labeled for use for sarcoptic, chorioptic, and psoroptic mange likely control this infestation effectively.

SHEEP AND GOATS

It is the practitioner's duty to recommend a safe and effective treatment regimen, but this proves difficult when treating mange in sheep and goats. In the USA, ectoparasiticides are regulated by the Environmental Protection Agency (EPA) or the FDA Center for Veterinary Medicine. As a general rule, if a product is applied topically to an animal to treat ectoparasites, it likely falls under the jurisdiction of the EPA. If a topical product is used to treat both external and internal parasites, it likely falls under jurisdiction of the FDA. This distinction is important for practitioners to recognize, because there is no legal extra-label use of products regulated by the EPA. Label directions must be followed regarding species treated, product concentration, product dosage, individuals allowed to administer application, and re-treatment interval. Because products regulated by the FDA are approved animal drugs, extra-label drug use may be allowed under the Animal Medicinal and Drug Use and Clarification Act (AMDUCA). (*See* also p 2748 and *see* p 2637.) The Food Animal Residue Avoidance Databank (FARAD) can be consulted for extra-label drug use recommendations and calculated meat and milk withdrawal times.

Hot lime sulfur spray or dip is labeled for use against sarcoptic, psoroptic, and chorioptic mites in sheep. Treatment should be repeated every 12 days if needed. Certain formulations of permethrin sprays are labeled for mange in sheep and goats. As with cattle, permethrin is generally not considered the compound of choice, but if used, the animals should be thoroughly wet with the product and re-treated in 10–14 days. Topical treatments are more likely to be effective if sheep are freshly shorn. Oral ivermectin sheep drench is not labeled for treatment or control of mange. Although single doses of oral ivermectin have been shown to reduce the number of *Psoroptes ovis* mites within 24 hr, a single oral dose is not considered curative. For these reasons, extra-label drug use of macrocyclic lactones in sheep and goats is common. However, practitioners should consider compounds labeled for a large range of species, the production system of the animals treated, and any warnings against use in species not listed on the label. Outside the USA, injectable ivermectin is approved to treat *P ovis* in sheep at the labeled dosage of 200 mcg/kg, two doses given 7 days apart.

Sarcoptic Mange: *Sarcoptes scabiei* var *ovis* infests sheep, and *S scabiei* var *caprae* infests goats, throughout the world. However, *S scabiei* var *ovis* is rare in the USA. This mite infests nonwooly skin, usually on the head and face. Typical of scabies, lesions manifest with formation of crusts and intense pruritus. Affected animals have decreased reproduction, meat gain, and milk yield. In goats, *S scabiei* var *caprae* is responsible for a generalized skin condition characterized by marked hyperkeratosis. Lesions start usually on the head and neck and can extend to the inner thighs, hocks, brisket, ventral abdomen, and axillary region. Both *S scabiei* var *ovis* and *S scabiei* var *caprae* are zoonotic. Consistent with other animal variants of *Sarcoptes*, zoonoses are initiated from direct contact with infested animals but are self-limiting infestations.

Chorioptic Mange: *Chorioptes bovis* infests sheep and goats worldwide. Prevalence of *C bovis* is more common in rams than ewes or lambs. Infestation of *C bovis* on goats is fairly common, with most of a herd infested. Distribution of lesions is the same as that in cattle, with papules and crusts seen on the feet and legs. Most sheep are subclinically infested with *C bovis*. However, *C bovis* can cause exudative dermatitis on the lower legs and scrota of rams (scrotal mange). Semen quality may be affected, presumably due to increased temperature of infested scrota.

Psoroptic Mange (Sheep Scab, Ear Mange): *Psoroptes ovis* is a highly contagious and severe infestation of sheep. This mite has been eradicated from sheep in Canada, New Zealand, and the USA. However, sheep scab persists in many countries, including some in Europe. Intense pruritus leads to large, scaly, crusted lesions that develop in more densely haired or woolly parts of the body. Lesions begin on the back and side but may become generalized and cover a large portion of the body. Animals bite, lick, and scratch in response to the pruritus, which results in wool loss and secondary bacterial infection. If affected sheep are not treated, infested animals may become emaciated and anemic and possibly die.

Psoroptic mange (ear mange) in goats and sheep is caused by *P cuniculi*, which is likely a variant of *P ovis*. *P cuniculi* typically infests the ears of goats but can spread to the head, neck, and body. Infestation of *P cuniculi* in goats can be common, with 80%–90% of a herd infested. Disease can range from subclinical to scaling, crusting, inflammation, alopecia, ear scratching, head shaking, and rubbing of ears and head to alleviate irritation. Although the course is chronic, the prognosis is good with appropriate treatment.

Demodectic Mange (Ovine Demodicosis, Caprine Demodicosis): *Demodex ovis* infests sheep, and *D caprae* infests goats. Demodectic mange in sheep is not common, whereas *D caprae* are relatively common in goats. Lesions are similar to those in cattle. In goats, nonpruritic papules and nodules develop, especially over the face, neck, shoulders, and sides or udder. Demodectic mange in goats occurs most commonly in kids, pregnant does, and dairy goats. The nodules contain a thick, waxy, grayish material that can be easily expressed; mites can be found in this exudate. The disease can become chronic. Historically, in some cases, localized lesions in goats have been managed by incision, expression, and infusion with Lugol's iodine or rotenone in alcohol (1:3). This practice should not be continued or condoned. Rotenone, a plant-derived ketone once a popular pesticide and ectoparasiticide approved for use in organic farming, is now available only as a piscicide in the USA and Canada.

Psorergatic Mange (Itch Mite, Australian Itch): *Psorobia ovis* (formerly *Psorergates ovis*) is a common skin mite of sheep in Africa, Australia, New Zealand, and South America. Most infested sheep are not affected. However, intense generalized pruritus and scaliness, with matting and loss of wool can result from infestation with *P ovis*. All breeds of domestic sheep are susceptible. Because of their small size, the mites are difficult to find in skin scrapings. This disease can cause significant economic losses through weight loss and wool damage. Treatments effective against sarcoptic, chorioptic, and psoroptic mange in sheep are expected to be efficacious for psorergatic mange.

HORSES

The last large animal mange reportable to the OIE was horse mange, but this was removed in 2006. Mange in horses was removed from the list of federally reportable diseases in the USA prior to this date, although it remains reportable to some state veterinary agencies.

Sarcoptic Mange: *Sarcoptes scabiei* var *equi* is rare but is the most severe type of mange in horses. The first sign of infestation is intense pruritus due to hypersensitivity to mite products. Early lesions appear on the head, neck, and shoulders. Regions protected by long hair and lower parts of the extremities are usually not involved. Lesions start as small papules and vesicles that later develop into crusts. Alopecia and crusting spread, and the skin becomes lichenified, forming folds. If infestations are not treated, lesions may extend over the whole body, leading to emaciation, general weakness, and anorexia. Negative skin scrapings do not exclude the disease; biopsy may establish a diagnosis.

Hot lime sulfur spray or dip is labeled for use against sarcoptic, psoroptic, and chorioptic mites in horses. Treatment should be repeated every 12 days if needed, following the species-specific dilution on the label. Although certain spray formulations of permethrin are labeled for use against mange in horses, it is generally not considered the compound of choice. If permethrin is used, the animals should be thoroughly wet with the product and re-treated in 10–14 days. Although not labeled for treatment of mange in horses, two doses of oral ivermectin at 200 mcg/kg given 14 days apart (field studies), or a single treatment of oral moxidectin at 400 mcg/kg, have effectively treated psoroptic, chorioptic, and sarcoptic mange in horses.

Psoroptic Mange: *Psoroptes ovis* (formerly *P equi*) and *P cuniculi* (likely a variant of *P ovis*) both infest horses. *P ovis* is rare in horses. However, infestations can produce lesions on thickly haired regions of the body, such as under the forelock and mane, at the base of the tail, under the chin, between the hindlegs, on the udder, and in the axillae. *P cuniculi* can sometimes cause otitis externa in horses and may cause head shaking. Pruritus is characteristic. Lesions start as papules and alopecia and develop into thick, hemorrhagic crusts. Psoroptic mites are more easily recovered from skin scrapings than are sarcoptic mites. Topical and oral treatments recommended for other types of mange are effective. Hot lime sulfur is labeled for use against *Psoroptes* in horses (*see* above). Although not labeled for treatment of mange in horses, oral ivermectin at 200 mcg/kg given for two doses 14 days apart (field studies), or a single treatment with oral moxidectin at 400 mcg/kg, has effectively treated psoroptic, chorioptic, and sarcoptic mange in horses.

Chorioptic Mange (Leg Mange): Chorioptic mange is caused by infestation with *Chorioptes bovis* (formerly *C equi*) and is the most common form of mange in horses. Draft horses are commonly infested, although all breeds are susceptible. Lesions caused by *C bovis* start as a pruritic dermatitis affecting the distal limbs around the foot and fetlock. Papules are seen first, followed by alopecia, crusting, and thickening of the skin. A moist dermatitis of the fetlock develops in chronic cases. Infested horses may stamp their feet or rub one foot against the opposite leg or object. Chorioptic mange is a differential diagnosis for "greasy heel" in draft horses. The signs subside in summer but recur with the return of cold weather. The disease course is usually chronic without treatment, but the prognosis is favorable when treated. Topical and oral treatments recommended for other types of mange are effective. Hot lime sulfur is labeled for use against *Chorioptes* in horses (*see* above). Treatment is aided by clipping long hair from infested areas. Although not labeled for treatment of mange in horses, oral ivermectin at 200 mcg/kg given for two doses 14 days apart (field studies), or a single treatment with oral moxidectin at 400 mcg/kg, has effectively treated psoroptic, chorioptic, and sarcoptic mange in horses.

Demodectic Mange (Equine Demodicosis): Demodectic mange in horses is caused by infestation with *Demodex equi* or *D caballi*. *Demodex* mites infest hair follicles and sebaceous glands. *D equi* lives on the body, and *D caballi* on the eyelids and muzzle. Demodectic mange is rare in horses but can manifest as patchy alopecia and scaling or as nodules. Lesions appear on the face, neck, shoulders, and forelimbs. It has been reported in association with pituitary pars intermedia dysfunction (*see* p 547) and chronic corticosteroid treatment. Pruritus is absent; therefore, secondary infections due to excoriation are rare. Therapy is rarely done, although there is limited evidence that the macrocyclic lactones may be effective. Lesions have also been reported to resolve without treatment.

Trombiculidiasis (Chiggers, Harvest Mite): Trombiculid mites can parasitize the skin of horses, especially during the late summer and fall. The adult mites live on invertebrates and plants; the larvae normally feed on small rodents, but they can opportunistically feed on people and domestic animals, including horses. Lesions consist of severely pruritic papules and wheals on the face, lips, and feet. At the time of diagnosis, a topical pyrethrin or pyrethroid labeled for horses can be used to kill any remaining larvae still feeding. Symptomatic treatment with a glucocorticoid for pruritus can be added to minimize further self-trauma and associated secondary infections. Any secondary infections should be treated. Repellents may help prevent infestation.

Straw Itch Mite (Forage Mite): These mites usually feed on organic material in straw and grain and can opportunistically infest the skin of horses. Papules and wheals appear on the face and neck if horses are fed from a hay rack, and on the muzzle and legs if fed from the ground. Pruritus is variable. Treatment for trombiculidiasis may be used for straw itch mite infestations.

PIGS

Mange in pigs is principally due to infestation with *Sarcoptes scabiei* var *suis*. Rarely, infestation with *Demodex phylloides* has been reported to cause clinical disease in pigs.

Sarcoptic Mange: Sarcoptic mange, caused by infestation with *Sarcoptes scabiei* var *suis*, is of primary importance in pigs worldwide. *S scabiei* var *suis* in a herd typically becomes established after introduction of infested breeding stock.

Transmission of *S scabiei* var *suis* can occur rapidly through direct contact of infested and naive pigs. However, transmission to naive pigs is also possible through contact with fomites contaminated with *S scabiei* var *suis*. Survival of the mite eggs away from the host is limited. However, exposure for as little as 24 hr to contaminated pens that were recently vacated by infested pigs resulted in transmission of the mite. Laboratory experiments indicated that *S scabiei* var *suis* did not survive >96 hr at temperatures <25°C or >24 hr at 20°–30°C. Survival was <1 hr at temperatures >30°C. Unless pigs originated from SPF colonies or after mange eradication programs, all pig herds must be considered potentially infested even if acaricides are used routinely.

Lesions due to infestation with *S scabiei* var *suis* usually start on the head, especially the ears, then spread over the body, tail, and legs. Itching can be intense and associated with a hypersensitivity reaction to the mites. As the hypersensitivity subsides, typically after several months, the thickened, rough, dry skin is covered with grayish crusts. Infestations are negatively correlated with daily weight gains and feed conversion in pigs.

Experimental studies of *S scabiei* var *suis* in pigs have demonstrated that infestation alters the microbial community on the skin. Comparing the microbiome of bacteria on pigs without *S scabiei* var *suis* versus that of infested pigs showed that noninfested pigs had low relative abundances of *Staphylococcus*, whereas the relative abundance of *Staphylococcus* increased significantly on pigs with *S scabiei* var *suis* during the course of infestations. Specifically, the staphylococci population shifted from *S hominis* to that of the more pathogenic *S chromogenes* as scabies progressed.

Diagnosis is best performed by combining different approaches: dermatitis score recorded at slaughter, scratching index, observation of clinical signs of mange, ear or skin scrapings for microscopic examination, and ELISA for detection of specific antibodies. The usefulness of each criterion may vary according to the group age. This global approach is particularly useful during an eradication campaign.

Injectable doramectin and ivermectin are labeled for use against *S scabiei* var *suis* and are considered highly effective treatments. In some instances, a second dose of macrocyclic lactone 14 days later may be necessary for complete resolution. Hot lime sulfur is labeled for use against mange in swine. In swine, lime sulfur dips are repeated at intervals of 3–7 days to treat mange, unlike in other species in which they are repeated every 12 days. Label instructions must be followed closely, because there are three possible lime sulfur dilutions for use on swine. Unlike phosmet, lime sulfur spray can be applied to suckling pigs. Certain spray formulations of permethrin are labeled for use against mites on swine, but it is generally not considered the compound of choice. If permethrin is used, animals should be wet thoroughly with the product and re-treated in 14 days. Phosmet spray is approved for sarcoptic mange in swine at the species-specific dilution instructions on the label. A single treatment is usually effective, but a second treatment can be applied 14 days later if necessary. Phosmet should not be applied directly to suckling pigs. Coumaphos sprays are available for use on swine in the USA, but they are labeled only for control of lice.

Demodectic Mange (Swine Demodicosis): Demodectic mange caused by infestation with *Demodex phylloides* is possible in pigs. Clinical signs of *D phylloides* infestation include reddening of the skin, pustules, and alopecia. Although rare in domestic pigs, *D phylloides* infestation can be common in wild boars without overt signs of clinical disease. In wild boars, the highest prevalence and greatest numbers of *D phylloides* were found in sebaceous glands in eyelids and cheeks. *D phylloides* can also be found around the eyes, mouth, snout, ventral neck, ventrum, and thighs. There is no reliable treatment.

DOGS AND CATS

Sarcoptic Mange (Canine Scabies): *Sarcoptes scabiei* var *canis* infestation is a highly contagious disease of dogs found worldwide. The mites are fairly host specific, but animals (including people) that come in contact with infested dogs can also be affected. Adult mites are 0.2–0.6 mm long and roughly circular in shape; their surface is covered with small triangular spines, and they have four pairs of short legs. Females are almost twice as large as males. The entire life cycle (17–21 days) is spent on the dog. Females burrow tunnels in the stratum corneum to lay eggs. Sarcoptic mange is readily transmitted between dogs by direct contact; transmission by indirect contact may also occur. Clinical signs may develop anytime from 10 days to 8 wk after contact with an infected animal. Asymptomatic carriers may exist. Intense pruritus is characteristic and probably due to hypersensitivity to mite products. Primary lesions consist of papulocrustous eruptions with thick, yellow crusts, excoriation, erythema, and alopecia. Secondary bacterial and yeast infections may develop. Typically, lesions start on the ventral abdomen, chest, ears, elbows, and hocks and, if untreated, become generalized. Dogs with chronic, generalized disease develop seborrhea, severe thickening of the skin with fold formation and crust buildup, peripheral lymphadenopathy, and emaciation; dogs so affected may even die. "Scabies incognito" has been described in well-groomed dogs; these dogs, infested with sarcoptic mites, are pruritic, but demonstrating the mites on skin scrapings is difficult because the crusts and scales have been removed by regular bathing. Atypical, including localized, clinical forms that are probably linked to extensive use of insecticides or acaricides are being increasingly seen.

Diagnosis is based on the history of severe pruritus of sudden onset, possible exposure, and involvement of other animals, including people. Making a definitive diagnosis is sometimes difficult because of negative skin scrapings. Concentration and flotation of several scrapings may increase chances of finding the mites, eggs, or feces. Several extensive superficial scrapings should be done of the ears, elbows, and hocks; nonexcoriated areas should be chosen. A centrifugation fecal flotation using sugar solutions may reveal mites or eggs. A specific and sensitive commercially available ELISA to detect specific antibodies has been developed and may be useful. Because mites can be difficult to detect, if *Sarcoptes* is on the differential diagnosis list but no mites are found, a therapeutic trial is warranted.

Systemic treatments of scabies are based on administration of macrocyclic lactones, some of which are FDA approved for this purpose. Among them, selamectin is given as a spot-on formulation at 6 mg/kg. This drug appears to be safe, even in ivermectin-sensitive breeds. Another is the imidacloprid-moxidectin formulation, which may be used on dogs as young as 7 wk of age. In some countries, moxidectin is also registered for treatment of scabies. It is available as a spot-on formulation in combination with imidacloprid and should be given in two doses of 2.5 mg/kg, 4 wk apart; additionally, oral uptake should be prevented in breeds at risk of avermectin sensitivity. Other endectocides, such as milbemycin oxime and ivermectin, which are not registered for treatment of sarcoptic mange in dogs, have been reported to be effective depending on the dosage and route of administration. The recommended dosage for milbemycin oxime is 2 mg/kg, PO, weekly for 3–4 wk; potential toxicity should be considered in dogs with avermectin sensitivity. Ivermectin (200 mcg/kg, PO or SC, 2–4 treatments 2 wk apart) is very effective and usually curative. Ivermectin at this dosage is contraindicated in avermectin-sensitive breeds. Additionally, the microfilaremic (*Dirofilaria immitis*) status of the dog should be evaluated before treatment with a macrocyclic lactone. For topical treatment, hair can be clipped, the crusts and dirt removed by soaking with an antiseborrheic shampoo, and an acaricidal dip applied. Lime sulfur is highly effective and safe for use in young animals; several dips 7 days apart are recommended. Amitraz is an effective scabicide, although it is not approved for this use. It should be applied as a 0.025% solution at 1- or 2-wk intervals for 2–6 wk. In addition, the owner must observe certain precautions to avoid self-contamination. Fipronil spray was reported to be effective but should be considered an aid in control rather than a primary therapy. Treatment can be topical or systemic, and should include all dogs in contact.

Notoedric Mange (Feline Scabies): This rare, highly contagious disease of cats and kittens is caused by *Notoedres cati*, which can opportunistically infest other animals, including people. The mite and its life cycle are similar to the sarcoptic mite. Pruritus is severe. Crusts and alopecia are seen, particularly on the ears, head, and neck, and can become generalized. Mites can be found quite easily in skin scrapings. Treatment consists of both topical and systemic therapies. Nonapproved but effective and safe treatments include selamectin (6 mg/kg, spot-on) and moxidectin (1 mg/kg, spot-on, in the imidacloprid-moxidectin formulation). Ivermectin (200 mcg/kg, SC) has also been used. Another effective topical therapy is lime sulfur dips at 7-day intervals.

Otodectic Mange: *Otodectes cynotis* mites are a common cause of otitis externa, especially in cats but also in dogs. Mites that belong to the family Psoroptidae are usually found in both the vertical and horizontal ear canals but are occasionally seen on the body. Clinical signs include head shaking, continual ear scratching, and ear droop.

Pruritus is variable but may be severe. Dark brown cerumen accumulation in the ear and suppurative otitis externa with possible perforation of the tympanic membrane may be seen in severe cases. Affected and in-contact animals should receive appropriate parasiticide treatment in the ears. Systemic therapies have been approved and include topically applied selamectin and moxidectin. Direct applications to the external ear canal of cats using approved ivermectin and milbemycin formulations are also effective. As a general rule, ear cleansing with an appropriate ceruminolytic agent is indicated with any therapy.

Cheyletiellosis (Walking Dandruff): *Cheyletiella blakei* infests cats, *C yasguri* infests dogs, and *C parasitovorax* infests rabbits, although cross-infestations are possible. This disease is very contagious, especially in animal communities. Human infestation is frequent. Mite infestations are rare in flea-endemic areas, probably because of the regular use of insecticides. These mites have four pairs of legs and prominent hook-like mouthparts. They live on the surface of the epidermis, and their entire life cycle (3 wk) is spent on the host. Female mites can, however, survive for as long as 10 days off the host. Clinical disease is characterized by scaling, a dorsal distribution, and pruritus, which varies from none to severe. Cats can develop dorsal crusting or generalized miliary dermatitis. Asymptomatic carriers may exist. The mites and eggs may not be easy to find, especially in animals that are bathed often. Acetate tape preparations, superficial skin scrapings, and flea combing can be used to make the diagnosis.

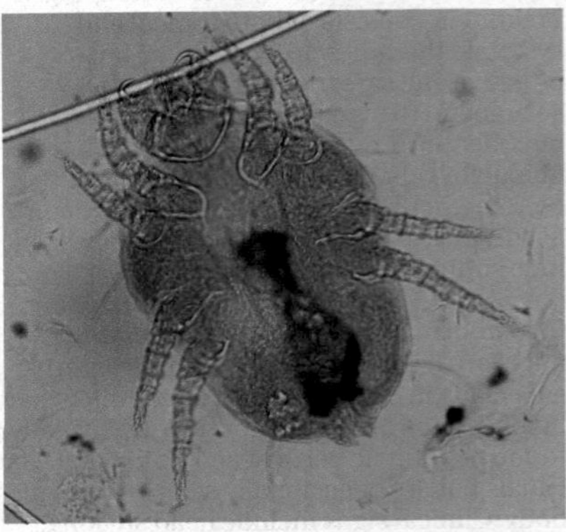

Cheyletiella sp. Courtesy of Dr. Michael W. Dryden.

Both topical and systemic acaricides are effective against cheyletiellosis, although no drugs are currently licensed for this indication. In addition to treatment of the affected animals, it is necessary to treat all in-contact animals. Topical drugs include lime sulfur, fipronil spot-on and spray, permethrin, and amitraz (the latter two drugs are contraindicated in cats). Extra-label systemic drugs include selamectin spot-on, milbemycin oxime (PO), and ivermectin (SC). Care must be taken to avoid or minimize the risks of adverse reactions as described above (*see* p 920). The treatment period depends on the selected drug but must be long enough to eradicate the mites from both the animals and their environment, which can be difficult in animal communities (eg, breeding colonies, kennels). In practice, treatment lasts 6–8 wk and should continue for a few weeks beyond clinical cure until parasitologic cure is achieved.

Canine Demodicosis: Canine demodicosis occurs when large numbers of *Demodex canis* mites inhabit hair follicles and sebaceous glands. In small numbers, these mites are part of the normal flora of canine skin and usually cause no clinical disease. The mites are transmitted from dam to puppies during nursing within the first 72 hr after birth. The mites spend their entire life cycle on the host, and the disease is not considered to be contagious. The pathogenesis of demodicosis is complex and not completely understood; evidence of hereditary predisposition for generalized disease is strong. Immunosuppression, natural or iatrogenic, can precipitate the disease in some cases. Secondary bacterial deep folliculitis, furunculosis, or cellulitis may occur, leading to a guarded prognosis.

Three forms of demodicosis are seen in dogs: localized demodectic mange, juvenile-onset generalized demodicosis, and adult-onset generalized demodicosis. Localized demodicosis is seen in dogs usually <1 yr old, and most of these cases resolve spontaneously. Lesions often consist of one to five well-demarcated small areas of alopecia, erythema, and scaling. Lesions are usually confined to areas around the lips, periorbital area, and forelimbs but may be found in other locations. Pruritus is usually absent or mild. A small percentage of these cases, especially the diffuse localized forms, progress to a more severe generalized form. Juvenile-onset generalized demodicosis is the result of an inherited immunologic defect with functional abnormality associated with the cell-mediated immune system. It is a severe disease of young dogs with generalized lesions (erythema, papules, alopecia, oily seborrhea, edema, hyperpigmentation, and crusts) that are usually aggravated by secondary bacterial infections (pyodemodicosis). Accompanying pododermatitis is common. Dogs can have systemic illness with generalized lymphadenopathy, lethargy, and fever when deep pyoderma, furunculosis, or cellulitis is seen. Diagnosis is not difficult; deep skin scrapings or hair plucking typically reveal mites, eggs, and larval forms in high numbers. The third form is adult-onset generalized demodicosis and clinically appears similar to juvenile-onset generalized demodicosis but is seen in adult dogs. It is typically associated with or triggered by some neoplastic process or debilitating disease that may be producing immunosuppression, such as malignant lymphosarcoma, malignant melanoma, hyperadrenocorticism, hypothyroidism, diabetes mellitus, etc. However, in many cases an underlying immunosuppressive condition may not be found.

Localized demodicosis can generally be left untreated. The prognosis for this form is usually good, and spontaneous recovery is frequent. In contrast, treatment is required in cases of generalized demodicosis, for which prognosis is guarded. Hair clipping and body cleansing, especially with benzoyl peroxide shampoo used for its follicular flushing activity, may be required. Whole-body amitraz dips (0.025%) applied every 2 wk remains the only approved treatment in the USA for generalized demodicosis. Higher concentrations (0.05%) and shorter treatment intervals (1 wk) may be more efficient.

A number of other protocols are commonly used for refractory generalized demodicosis. Among macrocyclic lactones, milbemycin oxime (0.5–1 mg/kg/day, PO), moxidectin, and ivermectin have all demonstrated varying degrees of effectiveness. Moxidectin is available as a spot-on formulation in combination with a flea product (imidacloprid) and should be given at 2.5 mg/kg at 1–4 wk intervals. More frequent applications are associated with higher degrees of success. Other reportedly successful but unapproved systemic treatments include moxidectin (400 mcg/kg/day, PO) and ivermectin (300–600 mcg/kg/day, PO). For the latter, different therapeutic protocols have been proposed with a gradually increased dosage and thorough monitoring of treated animals to detect any potentially toxic effect. Ivermectin is contraindicated in Collies and Collie crosses. However, idiosyncratic toxicity may be seen in any breed. Testing for mutation in the MDR1 allele (ABCB1) may be required before initiating therapy. Local and systemic corticosteroids are contraindicated in any animal diagnosed with demodicosis. Secondary bacterial infections must be treated aggressively with an appropriate antibiotic. Antiparasitic therapy must be continued not only until clinical signs abate but also until at least two consecutive negative skin scrapings are obtained at 1-mo intervals. Although some dogs respond rapidly, others may need several months of treatment. Recurrence within the first year of treatment is not uncommon. As the sole prophylactic measure, dogs developing juvenile-onset generalized demodicosis should not be used for breeding.

Feline Demodicosis: Feline demodicosis is an uncommon to rare skin disease caused by at least two species of demodectic mites. *Demodex cati* is thought to be a normal inhabitant of feline skin. It is a follicular mite, similar to but narrower than the canine mite, that can cause either localized or generalized demodicosis. One other species of *Demodex* (named *D gatoi*) is shorter, with a broad abdomen, and is found only in the stratum corneum. It causes a contagious, transmissible, superficial demodicosis that is frequently pruritic and can be generalized. In follicular localized demodicosis, there are one or several areas of focal alopecia most commonly on the head and neck. In generalized disease, alopecia, crusting, and potential secondary pyoderma of the whole body are seen. The generalized form is often associated with an underlying immunosuppressive or metabolic disease such as feline leukemia virus infection, feline immunodeficiency virus infection, diabetes mellitus, or neoplasia. In some cases, ceruminous otitis externa is the only clinical sign.

Diagnosis is made by superficial (*D gatoi*) and deep (*D cati*) skin scrapings, although mite numbers are often small, especially with *D gatoi*. Medical evaluation is indicated in cats with generalized disease. Dermatophyte cultures are essential, because dermatophytosis and demodicosis can be concomitant conditions. Prognosis of generalized demodicosis is unpredictable because of its potential relationship with systemic disease. Some cases spontaneously resolve. Weekly lime sulfur dips (2%) are safe and usually effective; amitraz (0.0125%–0.025%) has been used but is not approved for use in cats and can cause anorexia, depression, and diarrhea. The use of antiparasitic macrocyclic lactones has been reported but their efficacy is unclear.

Trombiculosis: Trombiculosis is a common, seasonal, noncontagious acariasis caused by the parasitic larval stage of free-living mites of the family Trombiculidae (chiggers). It can affect domestic carnivores, other domestic or wild mammals, birds, reptiles, and people. Two common species found in cats and dogs, *Neotrombicula autumnalis* and *Eutrombicula alfreddugesi*, are reported in Europe and in America, respectively. Adults (harvest mites) and nymphs look like small spiders and live on rotting detritus. In temperate areas from summer to fall, dogs and cats can acquire the larvae as parasites when lying on the ground or walking in suitable habitat. In warmer regions, infestation occurs throughout the year. The larvae (0.25 mm long) attach to the host, feed for a few days, and leave when engorged. At that time, they are easily identified as ovoid, 0.7 mm long, orange to red, immobile dots, usually found clustering on the head, ears, feet, or ventrum. Pathogenicity is through traumatic and proteolytic activities. Hypersensitivity reactions are suspected in some animals, because pruritus may vary from none to severe. Lesions include erythema, papules, excoriations, hair loss, and crusts. When present, intense pruritus can persist for hours to several days even after the larvae have left the animal.

Diagnosis is based on history and clinical signs. The infestation is a seasonal threat to free-ranging dogs and cats. Differential diagnoses include other pruritic dermatoses. Diagnosis is confirmed by careful examination of the affected areas. Microscopic examination of samples obtained from skin scrapings may help to identify the larvae, which have an oval-shaped body densely covered with setae, six long legs, and curved pedipalps terminating in claws.

Management is difficult. The most useful approach, if feasible, consists of keeping pets away from areas known to harbor large numbers of mites to prevent reinfestation during periods of risk. The application of pyrethroids (dogs only) with repellent-like activity to prevent infestation has yielded variable results. Fipronil and permethrin (dogs only) can be used, both for prevention and treatment of infested animals. Symptomatic treatment may be required in cases of severe pruritus.

Straelensiosis: Canine straelensiosis is a rare, noncontagious, sporadic, but potentially emerging parasitic dermatitis caused by the temporary encystment in the epidermis of the parasitic larval stage of *Straelensia cynotis*. This mite belongs to a family close to the family Trombiculidae. To date, the life cycle is largely unknown, and the disease has been reported only in France, Portugal, Spain, and Italy. Transmission occurs mainly in rural and small-sized hunting dogs, probably through contact with contaminated soil, litter, and other terrestrial habitat of foxes. No contagion has been reported to congeners and people. *S cynotis* has distinct differences from other trombidioid mites, especially in clinical presentation, histopathologic features, and response to treatment.

Straelensiosis is sudden in onset and may be accompanied by systemic signs such as anorexia and prostration. Lesions are painful, variably pruritic, and either generalized or multifocal, most often affecting the dorsal regions of the head and trunk. The characteristic erythematous papules and nodules resemble small craters. Scaling, pustules, and crusts can be seen.

Differential diagnoses include bacterial folliculitis, sarcoptic mange, and gunshot. Microscopic examination of samples obtained from deep skin scrapings may help identify the larvae (0.7 mm long, 0.45 mm wide), each in a thick-walled cyst. The larvae, which resemble *Neotrombicula*, are more easily visualized by histopathology.

The prognosis is favorable; a self-cure generally occurs after several months if reinfestation is prevented. However, management of clinical signs is difficult. Amitraz may be somewhat effective.

Lynxacariasis: Feline lynxacariasis is a quite common but to date geographically restricted (Australia, Brazil, Hawaii, Florida, North Carolina, Texas) parasitic dermatitis caused by the fur mite *Lynxacarus radovskyi*, which belongs to the family Listrophoridae. The life cycle remains poorly described, and this species has not been reported from hosts other than cats. Infestation typically occurs by direct contact, but fomites may be important for transmission. Clinical signs include a salt-and-pepper appearance of the hair coat, variable pruritus, and alopecia. Diagnosis is based on visualization of mites (0.5 mm long) using a magnifying glass or on isolation of any parasitic stage in skin scrapings or acetate tape preparations. Treatment with acaricidal sprays, weekly lime sulfur dips, and ivermectin (300 mcg/kg, SC) are effective. The only case of contagion to people that has been reported involved a transient rash in an owner with a heavily infested cat.

TICKS

Ticks are obligate ectoparasites of most types of terrestrial vertebrates virtually wherever these animals are found. Ticks are large mites and thus are arachnids, members of the subclass Acari. They are more closely related to spiders than to insects. The ~850 described species are exclusively bloodsucking in all feeding stages. Ticks transmit a greater variety of infectious organisms than any other group of arthropods and, worldwide, are second only to mosquitoes in terms of their public health and veterinary importance. Some of these agents are only slightly pathogenic to livestock but may cause disease in people; others cause diseases in livestock that are of tremendous economic importance. In addition, ticks can harm their hosts directly by inducing toxicosis (eg, sweating sickness [*see* p 684], tick paralysis [*see* p 1314] caused by salivary fluids containing toxins), skin wounds susceptible to secondary bacterial infections and screwworm infestations, and anemia and death. International movement of animals infected with the tick-transmitted blood parasites *Theileria*, *Babesia*, and *Anaplasma* spp and *Ehrlichia (Cowdria) ruminantium* is widely restricted.

Movement of tick-infested livestock over great distances is an important factor in the extensive distribution and prevalence of many tick species and tickborne disease agents. A number of introduced tick species thrive in the vast grazing and browsing environments established during recent centuries of human and livestock population explosions. Conversely, introduction of livestock into areas with exotic tick species and tickborne agents to which they have no immunity or innate resistance often results in significant losses.

Two of the three families of ticks parasitize livestock: the Argasidae (argasids, "soft ticks") and the Ixodidae (ixodids, "hard ticks"). Although they share certain basic properties, argasids and ixodids differ in many structural, behavioral, physiologic, ecologic, feeding, and reproductive patterns. Tropical and subtropical species may undergo one, two, or rarely three complete life cycles annually. In temperate zones, there is often one annual cycle; in northern regions and at higher elevations in temperate regions, at least 2–4 yr are required by most species.

There are four developmental stages: egg, larva, nymph, and adult. All larvae have three pairs of legs; all nymphs and adults have four. Adults have a distinctive genital and anal area on the ventral body surface. The foreleg tarsi of all ticks bear a unique sensory apparatus—Haller's organ—to sense carbon dioxide, chemical stimuli (odor), temperature, humidity, etc. Pheromones stimulate group assembly, species recognition, mating, and host selection.

Certain tick species that parasitize livestock can survive several months, and occasionally a few years, without food if environmental conditions permit. Tick host preferences are usually limited to a particular genus, family, or order of vertebrates; however, certain ticks are exceptionally adaptable to a variety of hosts, so each species must be evaluated separately. The larvae and nymphs of most ixodids that parasitize livestock feed on small wildlife such as birds, rodents, small carnivores, or even lizards.

In the Argasidae, the leathery dorsal surface lacks a hard plate (scutum). Male and female argasids appear to be much alike, except for the larger size of the female and differences in external genitalia. The argasid capitulum (mouthparts) arises from the anterior of the body in larvae but from the ventral body surface in nymphs and adults.

In the Ixodidae, the male dorsal surface is covered by a scutum. The scutum of the ixodid female, nymph, and larva covers only the anterior half of the dorsal surface. The ixodid capitulum arises from the anterior end of the body in each developmental stage.

Argasid Parasitism

The world's argasid tick fauna comprises 185 species in four genera, namely *Argas*, *Carios*, *Ornithodoros*, and *Otobius*, in the family Argasidae. The Argasidae are highly specialized for sheltering in protected niches or crevices in wood or rocks, or in host nests or roosts in burrows and caves. Some argasid species are known to survive for several years between feedings. Most of these leathery parasites inhabit tropical or warm, temperate environments with long dry seasons. Hosts are those that either rest in large numbers near the argasid microhabitat or return from time to time to rest or breed there. Soft ticks can be a serious pest in poultry and pig operations in tropical and subtropical countries. Blood loss and subsequent anemia can be significant and substantially affect weight gains and egg-laying performance. Massive infestations can cause numerous fatalities.

An argasid population typically parasitizes only a single kind of vertebrate and inhabits its shelter area. Argasids use multiple hosts, ie, the larvae feed on one host and drop to the substrate to molt; the several nymphal instars each feed separately, drop, and molt; adults feed several times (but do not molt). Argasid nymphs and adults feed rapidly (usually 30–60 min). Larvae of some argasids also feed rapidly; others require several days to engorge fully. Adult argasids mate off the host several times; afterward, females deposit a few hundred eggs in several batches and feed between ovipositions.

Most of the 57 described *Argas* spp parasitize birds that breed in colonies in trees or against rock ledges; others parasitize cave-dwelling bats. Few feed on reptiles or wild mammals, and none on livestock. Several species have become important pests of domestic fowl and pigeons; among these are the vectors of *Borrelia anserina* (avian spirochetosis) and the rickettsia *Anaplasma (Aegyptianella) pullorum* (aegyptianellosis). *Argas* spp also cause tick paralysis and transmit *Pasteurella multocida* (agent of fowl cholera), and many are vectors of a variety of arboviruses, some of which infect people.

Genus *Carios* includes 88 species, most of which are parasites of mammals, especially bats and rodents. Depending on the species, they inhabit dens or roosts of bats located in caves or tree holes or rodent burrows. Several species parasitize colonial nesting birds and dwell in the substrate or under stones and debris in ground-level bird colonies. Many of these ticks parasitize only a single host species or a group of closely related hosts. However, some *Carios* ticks will feed on people and domestic animals if the primary host is not available. *C kelleyi*, a tick associated with bats and bat habitats, has been reported to carry a novel spotted fever group *Rickettsia* and a relapsing fever spirochete closely related to *Borrelia turicatae*. The seabird tick *C capensis* has been shown to transmit West Nile virus to ducklings. The American *C puertoricensis* and *C talaje* are potential vectors of African swine fever virus.

The majority of nearly 37 species belonging to the genus *Ornithodoros* inhabit animal burrows and lairs in hot, arid climates and feed on most any potential hosts that enter their habitat. Larvae in this nidicolous genus do not feed, which may be related to the fact that these ticks dwell in burrows that may house hosts irregularly. A few species have adapted to living in crevices of walls and under fences where livestock are confined and also are pests of people. Certain species are vectors of relapsing fever spirochetes (*Borrelia* spp) and African swine fever virus; some species cause toxicosis, and one species (*O coriaceus*) transmits a spirochete causing epizootic bovine abortion in the western USA. Numerous *Ornithodoros*-transmitted salivary toxins or arboviruses cause irritation or febrile illnesses in people.

The unique argasid genus *Otobius* (*see* p 939) has three species, which do not feed in the adult stage. *O megnini* (spinose ear tick) is exceedingly specialized biologically and structurally. It infests the ear canals of pronghorn antelope, mountain sheep, and Virginia and mule deer in low rainfall biotopes of the western USA, Mexico, and western Canada. Cattle, horses, goats, sheep, dogs, various zoo animals, and people are similarly infested. This well-concealed parasite has been transported with livestock to western South America, Galapagos, Cuba, Hawaii, India, Madagascar, and southeastern Africa. Notably, adults have nonfunctional mouthparts and remain nonfeeding on the ground but may survive for almost 2 yr. Females can deposit as many as 1,500 eggs in a 2-wk period. Larvae and two nymphal instars feed for 2–4 mo, mostly in winter and spring. There can be two or more generations per year. People and other animals may have severe irritation from ear canal infestations, and heavily infested livestock lose condition during winter. Tick paralysis of hosts and secondary infections by larval screwworms are reported. *O megnini* is infected by the agents of coxiellosis/Q fever, tularemia, Colorado tick fever, and Rocky Mountain spotted fever. Another species, *O lagophilus*, feeds on the heads of jackrabbits (hares) and rabbits in western USA.

Ixodid Parasitism

The Ixodidae number >600 species, occupy many more habitats and niches than do argasids, and parasitize a greater number of vertebrates in a wider variety of environments. Most ixodid species have a three-host life cycle, others have a two-host cycle, and a few have a one-host cycle. Each ixodid postembryonic developmental stage (larva, nymph, adult) feeds only once but for a period of several days. Males and females of most species that parasitize livestock mate while on the host, although some mate off the host on the ground or in burrows. Males take less food than females but remain longer on the host and can mate with several females. During inactive seasons, few or no females are found feeding, even though males may remain attached to the hosts. Such males may contribute to transmission of pathogens to new susceptible animals by serial interhost transfer. Larval and nymphal population activity generally peaks during the "off seasons" of adults, although in some species there is overlap in the seasonal dynamics of immatures and adults.

The ixodid males, except those in the genus *Ixodes*, become sexually mature only after beginning to feed, after which they mate with a feeding female. Only after mating does the female become replete and proceed to develop eggs. She then detaches, drops from the host, and over a period of several days deposits a single batch of many eggs on or near the ground, usually in crevices or under stones, leaf litter, or debris. Depending on species and quantity of female nourishment, the egg batch usually numbers 1,000–4,000 but may be >12,000. The female dies after ovipositing. Notably, ixodids (except one- and two-host species, which use vertebrate host animals as habitat for much of their life cycle) spend >90% of their lifetime off the host, a fact of utmost significance in planning control measures. The several-day feeding process progresses slowly; the balloon shape characteristic of engorged larvae, nymphs, and females develops only during the final half day of feeding and is followed by detaching. The dropping time at certain hours of the day or night is governed by a circadian rhythm closely associated with the activity cycle of the principal host.

It is also important, especially in understanding the epidemiology of tickborne pathogens, to know whether immatures of an ixodid species feed on the same host species as do the adults, or on smaller vertebrates. Where acceptable smaller-sized hosts are scarce, immatures of some ixodid species can feed on the same livestock hosts as adults; immatures of other species seldom or never do so.

The proximity of acceptable hosts, air temperature gradients, and atmospheric humidity during resting and questing periods are among the factors that regulate the development of each stage and, in the case of females, oviposition.

Three-host Ixodids: Most ixodids have a three-host cycle. The recently hatched larvae quest for a suitable host, usually from vegetation, feed for several days, drop, and molt to nymphs, which repeat these activities and molt to adults. Of the three-host species that parasitize livestock or dogs, a few have immatures and adults that parasitize the same kind of host; these often develop tremendous population densities. The success of ixodid species that require smaller-size hosts for immatures depends on the availability of those hosts in the livestock browsing and grazing grounds. The natural hazards inherent in the three-host cycle have been compensated for by the benefits afforded adaptable tick species by animal husbandry practices. Only certain ixodids specific for herbivores have adapted to coexistence with livestock, and therein lies the answer to numerous livestock tick problems in Africa, where hosts for adults and immatures are abundant.

Two-host Ixodids: Some ixodids, especially those that parasitize wandering mammals (and also birds in certain cases) in inclement environments of the Old World, have developed a two-host cycle in which larvae and nymphs feed on one host, and adults on another. As in three-host species, both hosts may be different or may be the same species. Two-host parasites of livestock thrive in both inclement and clement environments and are difficult to control. This is especially true of two-host species that feed in the ears and anal areas of livestock.

One-host Ixodids: Among the most economically important ticks are several one-host species. These parasites evolved together with herbivores that wandered in extensive ranges in the tropics (*Rhipicephalus* [*Boophilus*] spp, *Dermacentor nitens*, etc) or in temperate zones (*D albipictus*, *Hyalomma scupense*). Larvae, nymphs, and adults feed on a single animal until the mated, replete females drop to the ground to oviposit.

Feeding Sites: Each species has one or more favored feeding sites on the host, although in dense infestations, other areas of the host may be used. Some feed chiefly on the head, neck, shoulders, and escutcheon; others in the ears; others around the anus and under the tail; and some in the nasal passages. Other common feeding sites are the axillae, udder, male genitalia, and tail brush. Immatures and adults often have different preferred feeding sites. Attachment of the large, irritating *Amblyomma* spp is regulated by a male-produced aggregation-attachment pheromone, which ensures that the ticks attach at sites least vulnerable to grooming.

IMPORTANT IXODID TICKS

The important ixodid ticks include *Amblyomma* spp, *Anomalohimalaya* spp, *Bothriocroton* spp, *Cosmiomma* sp, *Dermacentor* spp, *Haemaphysalis* spp, *Hyalomma* spp, *Ixodes* spp, *Margaropus* spp, *Nosomma* sp, *Rhipicentor* spp, and *Rhipicephalus* spp.

AMBLYOMMA SPP

More than half of the ~140 known *Amblyomma* species are endemic to the New World. *Amblyomma* ticks are large, three-host parasites. They have eyes and long, robust mouthparts. They are more or less brightly ornamented and generally confined to the tropics and subtropics. Adults and immatures of 37 species in this genus parasitize reptiles, which together with ground-feeding birds, are often hosts of immature *Amblyomma* ticks that have adapted, in the adult stage, to parasitizing mammals. Their long mouthparts make *Amblyomma* ticks especially difficult to remove manually and frequently cause serious wounds that may become secondarily infected by bacteria or screwworms and other myiasis flies.

Several African *Amblyomma* that infest livestock are vectors of *Ehrlichia (Cowdria) ruminantium*, the rickettsial agent that causes heartwater (*see* p 751), whereas New World *Amblyomma* spp carry agents of monocytic and granulocytic ehrlichioses as well as several *Rickettsia* spp, including *R rickettsii*, the agent of Rocky Mountain spotted fever.

A americanum, the lone-star tick, is abundant in the southern USA from Texas and Missouri to the Atlantic Coast and ranges northward into Maine. Southward, its distribution extends into northern Mexico. Because of the changing climate, the geographic range of this species continues to expand.

The scutum is distinctive because of pale ornamentation in males and a conspicuous, silvery spot ("star") near the posterior margin in females. Larvae, nymphs, and adults are indiscriminate in host choice and parasitize a variety of livestock, pets, and wildlife as well as people. Activity in the USA continues from early spring to late fall. Feeding sites on domestic and wild mammals are usually skin areas with sparse hair; wounds at these sites predispose livestock to attack by the screwworm fly *Cochliomyia hominivorax*.

A americanum is a vector of *Francisella tularensis*, the etiologic agent of tularemia; *Ehrlichia chaffeensis*, which causes monocytic ehrlichiosis in people; *E ewingii*, which causes granulocytic ehrlichiosis in dogs and people; and a recently described Panola Mountain *Ehrlichia* closely related to the agent of heartwater, which is pathogenic to at least goats and people. This tick also transmits *Rickettsia amblyommii*, *Borrelia lonestari*, and the Heartland virus pathogenic to people. A *Coxiella* sp symbiontic bacteria, closely related to the agent of Q fever, can be present in the majority of ticks in a population but is unknown to cause infections in people or other animals. *A americanum* may cause tick paralysis in people and dogs. In addition, Lone star virus (Bunyaviridae) has been isolated from a single *A americanum* nymphal tick that had been removed from a woodchuck (*Marmota monax*) in Kentucky.

A cajennense, the Cayenne tick, ranges from South America into southern Texas. This species is found most commonly in dry tropical habitats and lower elevations of subtropical highlands. As with *A americanum*, each active stage is indiscriminate in host choice: livestock and a large variety of avian and mammalian wildlife serve as hosts. People are severely irritated by clusters of *A cajennense* larvae ("seed ticks") in wooded and high-grass areas. Most adults attach on the lower body surface, especially between the legs; some feed elsewhere on the body. Activity continues throughout the year. *A cajennense* is a vector of *R rickettsii* in Central and South America from Panama to Argentina and has been experimentally shown to transmit *Ehrlichia ruminantium*. Wad Medani virus (an Orbivirus, Reoviridae), an African virus transported to Caribbean islands by *A variegatum*–infested cattle from Senegal, has been isolated from *A cajennense* in Jamaica.

A maculatum, the Gulf Coast tick, is an important pest of livestock, particularly cattle, from South America to southern USA. Optimal habitats are warm areas with high rainfall, near seacoasts. Immatures usually parasitize birds and small mammals; adults parasitize deer, cattle, horses, sheep, pigs, and dogs. Adult feeding activity is chiefly in late summer and early fall but may begin later after a dry summer. Most adults infest the ears, where the feeding wounds are initial sites of screwworm infestations. Clustered feeding adults also cause much irritation to the upper parts of the neck of cattle and to the humps of Brahman cattle. *A maculatum* is the primary vector of *R parkeri*, and in some tick populations as many as 50% of individual ticks may be infected with this pathogen.

A imitator parasitizes livestock from Central America to southern Texas; it has been shown to transmit *R rickettsii* in Mexico. Occasional pests of livestock in tropical America are *A neumanni* (Argentina), *A ovale* and *A parvum* (Argentina to Mexico), *A tigrinum* (much of South America), and *A tapirellum* (Colombia to Mexico).

A testudinarium inhabits Asian tropical wooded environments from Sri Lanka and India to Malaysia and Vietnam, Indonesia, Borneo, Philippines, Taiwan, PRC and southern Japan. Adults are particularly abundant on wild and domestic pigs and also infest deer, cattle, other livestock, and people. Immatures parasitize birds and small mammals as well as people. In India and Sri Lanka, adult *A integrum* and *A mudlairi* also parasitize livestock, wild ungulates, and people.

A hebraeum, the southern Africa bont tick, inhabits warm, moderately humid savannas of South Africa, Namibia, Botswana, Zimbabwe, Malawi, Mozambique, and Angola. Immatures feed on various small mammals, ground-feeding birds, and reptiles. Adults infest livestock, antelope, and other wildlife. Adults, attached chiefly to body areas with relatively little hair, cause serious wounds that become secondarily infected by bacteria and the screwworm *Chrysomya bezziana*. Like other African *Amblyomma* ticks (bont ticks) that parasitize livestock, *A hebraeum* is an important vector of *Ehrlichia ruminantium* and the principal vector of *Rickettsia africae*, the agent of African tick bite fever, in southern Africa.

A variegatum, the tropical African bont tick, is an easily visible, brightly colored parasite found throughout sub-Saharan savannas southward to the range of *A hebraeum*, and also in southern Arabia and several islands in the Indian and Atlantic Oceans and the Caribbean. An eradication program is in progress in the Caribbean; St. Kitts, St. Lucia, Montserrat, Anguilla, Barbados, and Dominica qualified for "provisionally free" certification by 2002, although St. Kitts was reinfested in 2004. Host preferences are similar to those of *A hebraeum* but also include camels. The bites of the tropical bont tick are severe. They may result in septic wounds and abscesses, inflammation of the teats of cows, and considerable damage to hides and skins. Adults feed chiefly during rainy seasons, immatures during dry seasons. Most adults attach to the underside of the host body, on the genitalia, and under the tail.

A variegatum injuries to hosts and transmission of *E ruminantium* are similar to those of *A hebraeum* but also include the spread of acute bovine dermatophilosis (*see* p 858). This tick is not considered to be an effective vector of Nairobi sheep disease virus but is a secondary vector of Crimean-Congo hemorrhagic fever virus. Dugbe virus has been isolated from *A variegatum* in six countries north of the equator; the Thogoto and Bhanja viruses are also associated with this tick in various areas north of the equator. Notably, yellow fever virus has been isolated from *A variegatum* collected from cattle in the Central African Republic and has been demonstrated to be transovarially transmitted to the progeny of infected females. Jos virus infects *A variegatum* from Ethiopia to Senegal and has been transported in this tick to Jamaica.

A lepidum, the East African bont tick, inhabits xeric savanna environments from northern Tanzania to central Sudan. *A gemma*, the gem-like bont tick, occurs in similar environments of Tanzania, Somalia, Kenya, and Ethiopia. A small variety of the buffalo bont tick, *A cohaerens*, is abundant on cattle in Ethiopian highlands, but from Zaire to Tanzania the larger variety of *A cohaerens* parasitizes chiefly Cape buffalo. Other African *Amblyomma* ticks of Cape buffalo and various other large mammals, including livestock, are *A pomposum* of humid highland forests in Angola, Zaire, Uganda, southern Sudan, Kenya, and Zimbabwe, and *A astrion* of West Africa and Zaire.

In Central and South America, numerous *Amblyomma* spp parasitize livestock and dogs, often in large numbers. Among those, *Amblyomma* and *A ovale* adults feed primarily on carnivores and *A parvum* on carnivores and armadillos. *A auricularium* has been found on wild hosts of the families Myrmecophagidae and occasionally Didelphidae, Caviidae, Chinchillidae, Hydrochaeridae, Muridae, Canidae, Mustelidae, and Procyonidae; it transmits *R rickettsii* in Brazil. *A pseudoconcolor* has been found occasionally on wild hosts of the family Didelphidae. *A naponense* is common on peccaries, and *A oblongoguttatum* has been found on a variety of hosts in several South and Central American countries. The South American tapir (*Tapirus terrestris*) seems to be the primary host for the adult stage of *A latepunctatum*, *A scalpturatum*, and *A incisum*. *A dissimile* is a common parasite of reptiles and true toads of the genus *Bufo*, from Argentina northward to southern Mexico, the Caribbean islands, and southern Florida.

ANOMALOHIMALAYA SPP

The three *Anomalohimalaya* spp are found in mountains of Central Asia—Pamir, Tian Shan, Tibet, and Himalayas. All stages of these three-host ticks parasitize rodents, shrews, and less frequently hares.

BOTHRIOCROTON SPP

Genus *Bothriocroton* (formerly *Aponomma*) includes seven species of ticks indigenous to Australia and Papua New Guinea (*B oudemansi*). *Bothriocroton* spp resemble *Amblyomma* spp except they have no eyes. In this group, *B aruginans* is a parasite of wombats; *B concolor* and *B oudemansi* are ectoparasites of echidnas in Australia and Papua New Guinea, respectively. The other four species in this genus parasitize reptiles almost exclusively. *B hydrosauri*, the blue-tongued lizard tick, is the reservoir of *Rickettsia honei* on Flinders Island, Australia.

COSMIOMMA SP

Genus *Cosmiomma* contains a single species, *C hippopotamensis*, which is found in southwestern and eastern Africa. It feeds primarily on white and black rhinoceroses and less frequently on antelopes.

DERMACENTOR SPP

Of the 36 *Dermacentor* spp, 19 inhabit temperate zones. Of the tropical species, *D (Anocenter) nitens* is of major veterinary importance, although others may transmit zoonotic infections, and adults may be common on wildlife such as pigs, deer, and antelope. Immatures infest chiefly rodents and lagomorphs. *Dermacentor* spp in cold areas and *D nitens* in tropical America have specialized life cycles and seasonal dynamics of activity, each of which must be considered separately. Except for *D nitens*, *D albipictus*, and *D dissimilis*, the *Dermacentor* life cycle is of the typical three-host pattern.

D nitens, the one-host tropical horse tick, is of considerable veterinary importance. It originally parasitized deer (*Mazama*) in the forests of northern South America. With the introduction of Equidae and other livestock into its habitat, it adapted to these animals. Spending its entire parasitic life deep in the hosts' ears, this parasite was easily spread by human activities to other areas of the Americas, including Florida and Texas. In addition to ear cavities, each active stage may infest nasal passages and the mane, ventral abdomen, and perianal area. *D nitens* transmits *Babesia caballi* transovarially to successive generations and is important in the horse-racing industry. It also is an experimental vector of *Anaplasma marginale* to cattle.

Another American one-host species, *D albipictus*, the winter or moose tick, ranges from Canada and northern USA into western USA and Mexico. A brownish form, sometimes called *D nigrolineatus*, is distributed from New Mexico to southern and eastern USA and may merit subspecies, if not full-species, rank. The larval-nymphal-adult feeding period on a single host (moose, deer, elk, or domestic cattle or horses) extends from fall to spring. Heavily infested hosts may die. *D albipictus* causes the often fatal "phantom moose disease" of Canada, is a secondary vector of Colorado tick fever virus, and is an experimental vector of *B caballi*; it is a natural vector of *A marginale* in Oklahoma.

In Mexico and central America, *D dissimilis* parasitizes a variety of equine and ruminant hosts and may be a one-host tick on horses.

The Rocky Mountain wood tick, *D andersoni*, is found from Nebraska westward to the western mountains (Cascades and Sierra Nevadas), in northern New Mexico and Arizona, and in western Canada.

The American dog tick, *D variabilis*, is found west of the Cascades and Sierra Nevadas, in Mexico, from Montana to Texas and east to the Atlantic, and in eastern Canada. Both species may cause tick paralysis in livestock, wildlife, and people. They are the primary vectors of *Rickettsia rickettsii*, the agent of Rocky Mountain spotted fever (*see* p 806). *D andersoni* is also the chief vector of Colorado tick fever virus and transmits Powassan virus, *A marginale*, *A ovis*, and the agents of tularemia and coxiellosis/Q fever. *D variabilis* is an experimental vector of *A marginale*, *B caballi*, and *B equi*. In addition, sawgrass virus, *Ehrlichia chaffeensis*, and *E ewingii* have been detected in questing *D variabilis* adults. Adults of both species parasitize livestock and wildlife, including deer, bison, and elk, but those of *D variabilis* prefer skunk, raccoon, puma, etc, and domestic dogs. Immatures feed on rodents and other small wild mammals. A related, biologically similar species, *D occidentalis*, is restricted to the Pacific lowlands and foothills from Oregon to Baja California and is a natural vector of *A marginale*.

In western USA and Mexico, *D parumapterus*, *D hunteri*, and *D halli* parasitize various hares and rabbits, mountain sheep, and peccaries, respectively. These ticks seldom make contact with livestock. *D hunteri* is an experimental vector of *A marginale* and *A ovis*. In Costa Rica and Panama, *D latus* infests tapirs.

In Eurasian steppes, forests, and mountains, *D marginatus*, *D reticulatus*, and *D silvarum*, collectively, are vectors of *Rickettsia slovaca* and *R raoultii* (the causative agents of tickborne lymphadenopathy), *R sibirica* (the agent of Siberian tick typhus), *Babesia bovis*, *B caballi*, *B equi*, *B canis*, *Theileria ovis*, and *A ovis*, together with the agents of tularemia and coxiellosis/Q fever, and Russian spring-summer encephalitis. *D marginatus* is found in forests, marshes, semideserts, and alpine zones from France to southwestern Siberia, Kazakhstan, Xinjiang Uygur Autonomous Region of China, Iran, and northern Afghanistan. *D reticulatus* ranges from Ireland and Britain to northwestern Siberia and Xinjiang, China, in meadows, floodplains, and deciduous and deciduous-conifer forests. *D silvarum* ranges from central Siberia and northeastern China to Japan in marshes, meadows, shrubby and secondary forests, and farmlands in taiga forest areas. Some males in populations of each of these three species remain attached to the host during winter. Adults and immatures may overwinter on the ground. Greatest adult activity is from early spring to summer with a lower peak in fall. Larvae and nymphs are active from spring through fall. The life cycle may be completed in 1 yr or extended by one or more summer or winter diapauses to 2–4 yr.

About 12 other *Dermacentor* spp inhabit certain lowland, mountain steppe, and semidesert areas of temperate Asia. Their adults are commonly taken from camels, cattle, horses, sheep, and goats. In tropical Asia, the several species of the *Dermacentor* subgenus *Indocentor* are parasites of wild pigs; they also infest larger wildlife but seldom if ever feed on livestock.

HAEMAPHYSALIS SPP

Few of the 166 species of *Haemaphysalis* parasitize livestock, but those that do are economically important in Eurasia, Africa, Australia, and New Zealand. Some haemaphysaline parasites of wild deer, antelope, and cattle have adapted to domestic cattle and, to a lesser extent, to sheep and goats. Others, originally specific for various wild sheep and goats, have adapted chiefly to the domestic breeds of these animals. A few African species that evolved together with carnivores now parasitize domestic dogs. Immatures of species that parasitize livestock generally feed on small vertebrates, but there are a few notable exceptions. All *Haemaphysalis* spp have a three-host life cycle. They are small (unfed adults <4.5 mm long), brownish or reddish, and eyeless. Most have very short mouthparts. Different species cause tick paralysis and are vectors of the agents that cause coxiellosis/Q fever, tularemia, and brucellosis, and of *Theileria orientalis*, *T ovis*, *Babesia major*, *B motasi*, *B canis*, *Anaplasma mesaeterum*, etc.

H punctata, the red sheep tick, is widely distributed where sheep, goats, and cattle feed in certain open forests and shrubby pastures from southwestern Asia (Iran and former USSR) to much of Europe, including southern Scandinavia and Britain. It usually does not appear in large numbers. Immatures infest birds, hedgehogs, rodents, and reptiles. *H punctata* can cause tick paralysis. In addition to transmitting *Anaplasma*, *Brucella*, *Theileria*, *Babesia* spp , and tularemia, different *H punctata* populations are infected by Russian spring-summer encephalitis virus, Tribec virus, Bhanja virus, and Crimean-Congo hemorrhagic fever virus. *H concinna* is found in Central Europe, East and Southeast Asia, China, and Japan. It is found in humid scrubby forests as well as in meadows and peat-lands but avoids dense forests. *H concinna* can transmit tularemia, several *Rickettsia* spp, including mildly pathogenic *R heilongjiangensis*, and several encephalitis viruses.

H sulcata adults parasitize livestock (chiefly sheep and goats) from northwestern India and southern former USSR to Arabia, Sinai, and southern Europe. *H parva* adults parasitize these hosts from southwestern former USSR and the Near East to the Mediterranean area (but not Egypt). Immature *H sulcata* are especially common on lizards, but the range of hosts of larvae and nymphs of both species is similar to that of *H punctata*.

H longicornis is a parasite of deer and livestock in Japan and northeast Asia; there is a bisexual form (race) in southern areas and a parthenogenetic race in northern areas. The latter has been introduced into Australia, New Zealand, and the Pacific islands, where it preserves this unusual reproductive ability. Immatures usually parasitize small mammals and birds but may also feed on livestock; heavy population densities may become serious pests of deer and livestock. This tick is the chief vector of *Theileria orientalis* and also transmits *Babesia ovata*, *B gibsoni*, and the agents of coxiellosis/Q fever, Powassan encephalitis, and Russian spring-summer encephalitis. Larval feeding causes acute dermatitis in people.

H inermis is found in lowlands from northern Iran and southwestern former USSR to central and southeastern Europe to Italy, where it prefers deciduous and mixed forests as well as grasslands. It can cause tick paralysis. Other Eurasian haemaphysalines of livestock are *H pospelovashtromae* (mountains of southern former USSR and Mongolia), *H kopetdaghicus* (Caspian Sea area, mountains of former USSR, and Iran), and *H tibetensis*, *H xinjiangensis*, and *H moschisuga* (China).

Of the several *Haemaphysalis* spp parasitizing livestock in southeast Asia, three are especially noteworthy: *H bispinosa* ranges to Pakistan, Bangladesh, Nepal, Bhutan, Sri Lanka, and Malaysia, and transmits *Babesia* spp to cattle, sheep, and dogs; *H spinigera* is the chief vector of Kyasanur Forest disease virus in people in Karnataka state, India; and *H anomala* ranges from the Nepal lowlands to Sri Lanka and the mountains of northwestern Thailand.

In temperate Asia, 18 other haemaphysalines parasitize livestock: 9 high in the Himalayas and outlying mountains, and 9 in northeastern Russia, Korea, and Japan. Yak and yak-cattle hybrids are among the livestock hosts of Himalayan haemaphysalines. Several Himalayan species appear to prefer sheep and goats.

H leachi, the yellow or African dog tick, is found in tropical and southern Africa. It can transmit canine and feline babesiosis, Mediterranean spotted fever, coxiellosis/Q fever, and Boutonneuse fever. Other haemaphysalines that infest livestock in highland forests or lowland, humid, secondary or riparian forests in sub-Saharan Africa are *H parmata* (Ethiopia and Kenya, Central and West Africa, to Angola), *H aciculifer* (Ethiopia to Cameroon and Zimbabwe, introduced into South Africa), *H rugosa* (southern Sudan and Uganda to Ghana and Senegal), and *H silacea* (Zululand and eastern South Africa).

HYALOMMA SPP

Hyalomma ticks are often the most abundant tick parasites of livestock, including camels, in warm, arid, and semiarid, generally harsh lowland and middle altitude biotopes, and those with long dry seasons, from central and southwest Asia to southern Europe and southern Africa. Of the ~30 known *Hyalomma* spp, at least half are important vectors of infectious agents to livestock and people. The three-host life cycle predominates in this genus, but some species have either a one- or two-host cycle. Some three-host species can develop in one- or two-host cycles, a facultative ability unique to this ixodid genus. *Hyalomma* spp are mostly moderately large to large ticks with long mouthparts.

In the subgenus *Hyalommasta*, immatures of the single species, *H aegyptium*, parasitize tortoises and small wildlife and livestock from Pakistan to both sides of the Mediterranean basin. Adults are specific for tortoises.

The subgenus *Hyalommina* is found on the Indian subcontinent and in Somalia. Each of the six species has a three-host cycle. Immatures parasitize small mammals, especially rodents. Adult host preferences among livestock reflect the wild gazelle, bovine, caprine, or ovine group with which each species evolved. Two species infest chiefly cattle and the domestic buffalo: *H brevipunctata* (India and Pakistan) and *H kumari* (India, Pakistan, Afghanistan, northwestern Iran, and Tadzhikistan). Three usually parasitize sheep and goats: *H hussaini* (India, Pakistan, Burma), *H rhipicephaloides* (Dead Sea and Red Sea areas), and *H arabica* (Yemen and Saudi Arabia). *H punt* (Somalia and Ethiopia) feeds on antelope, camels, cattle, sheep, and goats.

The subgenus *Hyalomma* contains ticks of veterinary and public health importance that affect cattle, sheep, goats, horses, camels, dromedaries, dogs, cats, and people. Chief among these is the two-host *H anatolicum anatolicum*, which ranks high among the world's most damaging ticks and has been widely distributed by camels, cattle, and horses in steppe and semidesert environments from central Asia to Bangladesh, the Middle and Near East, Arabia, southeastern Europe, and Africa north of the equator. Immatures and adults generally infest the same kinds of hosts. Nymphs and unfed adults spend the dry and winter season in crevices in stone walls, stables, and weedy or fallow fields. When immatures infest smaller mammals, birds, or reptiles, the life cycle type is three-host. In addition to significantly weakening affected animals, causing weight loss, reduced fertility, and decreased milk production, *H anatolicum anatolicum* transmits *Theileria annulata*, *Babesia equi*, *B caballi*, *Anaplasma marginale*, *Trypanosoma theileri*, and at least five arboviruses; it is a significant vector of Crimean-Congo hemorrhagic fever virus to people.

Immatures of the subspecies *H anatolicum excavatum* (a three-host parasite) infest chiefly burrowing rodents in somewhat different biotopes in the same environments as *H anatolicum anatolicum*. Adults of both species may infest the same animal. Distribution of *H anatolicum excavatum* is somewhat more limited than that of *H anatolicum anatolicum*, but its winter season population densities are often greater. A closely related species, *H lusitanicum*, replaces *H anatolicum anatolicum* from central Italy to Portugal, Morocco, and the Canary Islands; it is associated with equine and bovine babesiosis. In addition to livestock, deer and rabbits serve as hosts.

The *H marginatum* complex consists of four species, each apparently invariably two-host. Adults parasitize livestock and wild herbivores. Immatures primarily parasitize birds. Rodents are rarely, if ever, parasitized. Hares and hedgehogs are secondary hosts. This group includes *H marginatum marginatum* (Caspian area of Iran and former USSR to Portugal and northwestern Africa), *H marginatum rufipes* (south of the Sahara to South Africa, also Nile Valley and southern Arabia), *H marginatum turanicum* (Pakistan, Iran, southern former USSR, Arabia, parts of northeastern Africa—introduced with sheep from Iran to Karoo), and *H marginatum isaaci* (Sri Lanka to southern Nepal, Pakistan, northern Afghanistan). Ticks belonging to the *H marginatum* complex are major vectors of the Crimean-Congo hemorrhagic fever virus. They also transmit *Rickettsia aeschlimannii* and several *Babesia*, *Anaplasma*, *Theileria*, and *Trypanosoma* spp that infect wildlife, livestock, and people. *H truncatum* can cause paralysis in livestock, pets, and people.

The *H asiaticum* complex includes three species with three-host life cycles and inhabits deserts, semideserts, and steppes from southwestern China, Mongolia, and the southern former USSR into the Middle East as far as Iraq. Rodents are the chief hosts of immatures; hares also may be infested. Adults parasitize livestock, particularly camels. The subspecies from east to west, *H asiaticum kozlovi*, *H asiaticum asiaticum*, and *H asiaticum caucasicum*, are of veterinary and medical importance.

Three additional three-host *Hyalomma* spp that parasitize camels and other livestock are *H dromedarii* (India to Africa north of the equator), *H schulzei* (eastern Iran to Arabia and northern Egypt), and *H franchinii* (Syria to Tunisia). Immatures parasitize rodents and other small mammals, birds, and reptiles; those of *H dromedarii* also infest livestock. *H dromedarii* is of veterinary and medical importance; the other two species have been little investigated.

H detritum, an important vector of *Theileria annulata*, is a three-host species; both adults and immatures parasitize livestock. Its biotopes are humid areas in steppes, deserts, and semideserts from southern China, Mongolia, and Nepal lowlands to southern Europe and northern Africa. *H impeltatum* ranges from Iran and Arabia to northern Tanzania and Chad. Adults parasitize livestock; immatures feed on rodents and other small mammals, birds, and reptiles.

H scupense, a one-host parasite of cattle and horses in southwestern former USSR and southeastern Europe, is unusual (like Canadian strains of *Dermacentor albipictus*) in that it overwinters on the host, which often suffers greatly from the long feeding period of numerous larvae (late fall), nymphs (winter), and adults (spring). *H scupense* is a vector of *T annulata* and *B equi*.

In addition to the several species already mentioned, the African savannas harbor five other *Hyalomma* spp of livestock and wildlife: *H (Euhyalomma) glabrum truncatum* (southeastern Egypt to southern Africa), *H albiparmatum* (southern Kenya, northern Tanzania), *H erythraeum* (eastern Somalia and Ethiopia, Yemen), *H impressum* (western Sudan, West Africa), and *H nitidum* (Central African Republic, West Africa). The preferred hosts of its adults are large herbivores such as zebras, gemsbok, and eland. Immatures of these three-host species generally infest small mammals, less often ground-frequenting birds and reptiles. *H truncatum glabrum*, which causes bovine sweating sickness and lameness and also human and ovine tick paralysis, is a vector of Crimean-Congo hemorrhagic fever virus, *Coxiella burnetii* (Q fever), and *Rickettsia conorii* (African tick typhus, Boutonneuse fever).

IXODES SPP

Ixodes spp, the largest genus of the family Ixodidae, contains 249 species and is highly specialized both structurally and biologically. So far as is known, all *Ixodes* spp have a three-host life cycle. Almost all inhabit temperate or tropical forest zones or wooded or shrubby grasslands; fewer are adapted to humid areas in semideserts or to arctic or sub-Antarctic nesting colonies of marine birds. Hosts are a wide variety of birds and mammals and a few reptiles. Most species parasitize burrowing hosts or those that return regularly to caves, dens, or terrestrial or arboreal nesting colonies. The few *Ixodes* spp that parasitize wandering artiodactyls or perissodactyls are exceptionally adaptable; they also parasitize livestock and are important pests or vectors of agents that infect livestock and people.

The *I ricinus* group of Eurasia, northwestern Africa, and North and South America is especially important. *I ricinus*, the so-called sheep tick and prototype of this group, inhabits relatively humid, cool, shrubby and wooded pastures, gardens, windbreaks, floodplains, and forest through much of Europe to the Caspian Sea and northern Iran, and also northwestern Africa. Its life cycle is 2–4 yr, depending on environmental temperature. (In drier, warmer, eastern Mediterranean biotopes, *I ricinus* is replaced by *I gibbosus*, which completes its life cycle in 1 yr.) *I ricinus* larvae feed on small reptiles, birds, and mammals. Nymphs feed on small and medium-sized vertebrates, and adults feed chiefly on herbivores and livestock. All stages, especially nymphs and adults, parasitize people. Male *I ricinus* take little or no food and can mate either on or off the host. Unfed adults often mate while on vegetation. Adult activity peaks in spring; in some populations, there is a lower peak of adult activity in the fall. Chief among the numerous arboviral diseases transmitted by *I ricinus* are louping ill, tickborne encephalitis, and Crimean-Congo hemorrhagic fever. Other agents transmitted to livestock are *Coxiella burnetii*, *Anaplasma marginale*, *Babesia divergens*, and *A phagocytophilum*, various strains of which cause bovine, ovine, and human granulocytic anaplasmoses.

I persulcatus, the taiga tick, is closely related to *I ricinus* and has similar host preferences. It ranges from the central and eastern mountains of Europe through the lowland forests from the Baltic Sea and Karelia eastward through the Siberian taiga to the Seas of Japan and Okhotsk and the northern islands of Japan. The life cycle can be completed in 3–4 yr but can last up to 7 yr in regions with a short summer season. It is one of the main vectors of Russian spring-summer encephalitis virus and *Borrelia burgdorferi*. In addition, it transmits *Babesia* spp, *Ehrlichia muris*, and the agents of human and ovine anaplasmoses and tularemia.

Other Asian representatives of the *I ricinus* group are *I sinensis* of China; *I kashmiricus* of mountainous northern India, Pakistan, and Kyrgyzstan; *I pavlovskyi* of the southern Siberian mountains of Russia; and *I kazakstani* of mountain taiga and deciduous forest in Kazakhstan, Kyrgyzstan, and Turkmenistan.

In the Americas, representatives of the *I ricinus* group include *I scapularis*, *I pacificus*, *I affinus*, *I jellisoni*, *I minor*, and *I muris*. *I scapularis* is distributed throughout the eastern and northcentral USA and southern Canada. It is a vector of *Borrelia burgdorferi*, the agent of Lyme disease, and *A phagocytophilum*, which causes granulocytic anaplasmosis in people, horses, and dogs. It also transmits *Babesia microti*, the agent of human babesiosis in coastal areas from Rhode Island to Virginia, and an *E muris*–like agent causing granulocytic ehrlichiosis in people and rodents in the midwestern USA. The chief hosts of adult *I scapularis* are deer; livestock seldom graze in the wooded zones inhabited by this tick. Adults of *I pacificus* parasitize livestock from Baja California to British Columbia and in inland pockets of Idaho, Nevada, and Oregon. *I pacificus* and *I neotomae* transmit the agents of Lyme disease, tularemia, and a rickettsia of the Rocky Mountain spotted fever group; *I pacificus* also transmits *A phagocytophilum*. The tick bites cause slowly healing ulcers. A related species, *I affinis*, ranges from South Carolina and Florida to Argentina. It is recorded chiefly from wildlife and has not been shown to be a vector.

In Africa, only four *Ixodes* spp have adapted to livestock. Chief among these is the South African paralysis tick, *I rubicundus*, of humid hill and mountain karoo vegetation in South Africa. Its salivary toxins cause a flaccid tetraplegia in livestock, people, dogs, and jackals. Immatures parasitize the rock hare, other hares, and elephant shrews. Other parasites of livestock in African highlands are *I drakenbergensis* (Natal), *I lewisi* (Kenya), and *I cavipalpus* (southern Sudan to Zimbabwe and Angola).

I holocyclus, the Australian paralysis tick, is considered the most medically important of the Australian tick fauna. Although most cases of tick bite are uneventful, some can result in life-threatening illnesses, including paralysis, tick typhus, and severe allergic reactions. The species is found throughout the year in a variety of habitats, particularly wet sclerophyll forests and temperate rainforest areas, across the humid coastal regions of eastern Australia. Adults are more abundant in the spring and early summer, larvae in mid to late summer, and nymphs during winter. Natural hosts include bandicoots, kangaroos, possums, birds, and sometimes even reptiles, but it regularly attaches to domestic animals, including dogs, cats, cattle, and horses, and occasionally people. The tick injects a neurotoxin that causes progressive motor paralysis, respiratory depression, and death in animals that have no immunity to the toxin. Most cases of tick paralysis seen by veterinarians are in dogs and cats, but other species can be affected. The condition has been recorded in sheep, cattle, goats, llamas, and Muscovy ducks. Fatal cases have occurred in people. In the larger species, the younger and smaller animals are likely to be affected.

I rubicundus, the karoo paralysis tick, may cause paralysis in sheep and goats in southern Africa. The immature stages of *I rubicundus* can be found on scrub hares and elephant shrews. The life cycle of the tick is ~2 yr. The ticks can often be found along the lower line of the neck, chest, and belly. The active period for adult ticks begins usually late in summer and reaches peak levels in autumn and early winter (April/May) and declines thereafter. The paralysis commonly occurs from February and reaches a peak in April and May.

MARGAROPUS SPP

Ticks of the genus *Margaropus* resemble *Rhipicephalus (Boophilus)* ticks but do not have festoons or ornamentations. They are characterized by greatly enlarged posterior legs and a prolonged median plate. The three highly specialized beady-legged, one-host *Margaropus* spp are restricted to limited areas of Africa. *M reidi* and *M wileyi* are recorded from giraffes in the Sudan and in Kenya and Tanzania, respectively. *M wileyi* is also known to parasitize zebras and gnu. *M winthemi*, a winter-feeding parasite of zebras, horses, and less often other livestock and antelope, is confined to mountains of South Africa and may contribute to loss of condition during winter.

NOSOMMA SP

Adults of the single species in this genus, *N monstrosum*, particularly parasitize wild and domestic buffalo, and also people, livestock, and wildlife, through much of India, Nepalese lowlands, Bangladesh, Thailand, and Laos. Immatures parasitize chiefly murid rodents.

RHIPICENTOR SPP

The genus *Rhipicentor* is composed of two species, namely *R bicornis* and *R nuttalli*, and both are found only in Africa south of the Sahara. *R bicornis* feeds on goats, cattle, horses, dogs, and carnivores in southern and central Africa. *R nuttalli* has a widespread distribution in South Africa. Immature stages feed on elephant shrews. The preferred hosts of the adults are domestic dogs, leopards, and South African hedgehogs. The life cycle of these ticks probably takes a year to complete in the field.

RHIPICEPHALUS SPP

Approximately 60 of the 81 rhipicephalid species are found in sub-Saharan Africa. The other rhipicephalid species have their origins in Eurasia and northern Africa, with *R sanguineus* and *R (Boophilus) microplus* being spread by human activities into Asia, Australia, and the Americas. Adults of most species parasitize wild and domestic artiodactyls, perissodactyls, or carnivores. Immatures feed mostly on smaller mammals; however, of those that parasitize rodents or hyraxes, and of those that parasitize artiodactyls, a few feed on the same host as the adults. The rhipicephalid life cycle is typically three-host, but in the Mediterranean climatic zone (long, warm summer with low rainfall) *R bursa* has a two-host cycle. In sub-Saharan Africa with long dry seasons, *R evertsi* and *R glabroscutatum* also have two-host cycles. In contrast, each of the five species in subgenus *Boophilus* has a one-host life cycle that may be completed in 3–4 wk (*see* below).

A number of *Rhipicephalus* spp have long been difficult to identify or have been incorrectly identified. Current concepts of tick phylogeny, taxonomy, and nomenclature are based on molecular analyses.

Subgenus *Boophilus* spp

Each of the five *Rhipicephalus (Boophilus)* spp has a one-host life cycle that may be completed in 3–4 wk and results in a heavy tick burden. Under these conditions, acaricide resistance becomes a major problem in control efforts. Zebu cattle, which have served for centuries as hosts of *R (B) microplus* in the Indian region, have developed resistance to feeding by large numbers of ticks and are used (purebred or crossbred) in integrated control programs. *R (B) microplus*, considered the world's most important tick parasite of livestock, has been introduced from the bovid- and cervid-inhabited forests of the Indian region to many areas of tropical and subtropical Asia, northeastern Australia, Madagascar, the coastal lowlands of southeastern Africa to the equator, and much of South and Central America, Mexico, and the Caribbean. *R (B) microplus* and *R (B) annulatus* were eradicated from the USA after a long, costly control program. Constant surveillance is maintained to prevent their reintroduction. *R (B) annulatus* of southern former USSR, the Middle East, and the Mediterranean area, was introduced with livestock of the early Spanish colonialists into northeastern Mexico but has not spread into Central America. In Africa, south of the Sahara and north of the equator, cattle movements probably account for the many *R (B) annulatus* populations.

R (B) decoloratus, which ranges from southern Africa to the Sahara, is being replaced in the southeastern part of this area by *R (B) microplus*. In more humid West African zones, *R (B) annulatus* mixes with or is totally replaced by *R (B) geigyi*. Scattered *R (B) geigyi* populations are found as far east as southern and central Sudan. The only boophilid restricted to sheep and goats (and occasionally horses) is *R (B) kohlsi* of Syria, Iraq, Israel, Jordan, western Saudi Arabia, and Yemen. *R (B) microplus* is an experimental vector of *Babesia equi* and has been collected from the nasal passages of equids in Panama. This tick and *R (B) annulatus* are major vectors of *Babesia bigemina*, *B bovis*, and *Anaplasma marginale*. *R (B) decoloratus* is an efficient vector of *B bigemina* and *A marginale* but does not transmit *B bovis* or *B equi*.

Subgenus *Rhipicephalus* spp

Tropical Asia is the home of five *Rhipicephalus (Rhipicephalus)* spp; adults of two species parasitize domestic animals. *R haemaphysaloides* infests all types of livestock, and wild antelope, deer, carnivores, and hares in continental southeast Asia (and Taiwan,PRC and the Philippines) westward to India, Sri Lanka, Nepal, Pakistan, and western Afghanistan. *R pilans* infests livestock and wildlife in Indonesia and Borneo. Immatures of both species feed chiefly on rodents, also on shrews, hares, and smaller carnivores.

From central Europe to Kazakhstan, *R rossicus*, *R schulzei*, and *R pumilio* are of medical and veterinary importance. In southwestern Europe, *R pusillus* infests dogs as well as European rabbits, foxes, and wild pigs. *R turanicus*, as presently recognized, ranges from China, southern former USSR, India into southern Europe, and Africa as far south as South Africa. A member of the taxonomically difficult *R sanguineus* group, "*R turanicus*" and its various populations, which may represent separate species, requires further studies of its abilities as a vector.

An easily recognized two-host species, *R bursa*, ranges from the western Mediterranean area of Europe to Iran and Kazakhstan. Adults and immatures parasitize livestock, hares, deer, wild sheep and goats, people, and infrequently dogs. It causes ovine paralysis and transmits Crimean-Congo hemorrhagic fever virus and other viruses to people, and numerous microbial diseases of livestock such as various species of *Babesia*, *Anaplasma*, and *Theileria* (notably *Theileria parva*, the agent of East Coast Fever, often fatal for cattle), *Ehrlichia (Cowdria) ruminantium* (the agent of heartwater), and *Trypanosoma vivax* (an agent of sleeping sickness).

The best known African rhipicephalid, *R sanguineus*, the kennel tick or brown dog tick, has spread worldwide with domestic dogs. It is now established in buildings as far north as Canada and Scandinavia and as far south as Australia. In Africa, the Near East, and parts of southern Europe, adults parasitize wild and domestic carnivores, sheep, goats, camels, other livestock, and various wild mammals, especially hares and hedgehogs. Immatures in nature in this area feed on small mammals. However, in urban situations everywhere, dogs are virtually the only hosts of immatures and adults. People are attacked infrequently, more often in situations when children play and sleep in close contact with heavily infested dogs. Strains of adult *R sanguineus* that feed on cattle are recorded in parts of Mexico and in Tahiti. This tick is active throughout the year in the tropics and subtropics but only from spring to fall in temperate zones. Newly active adults and nymphs are frequently seen climbing walls from floor-level cracks. *R sanguineus* is a vector of *Babesia canis*, *Ehrlichia canis*, *Rickettsia conorii*,

R massiliae, *R rickettsii*, and *R rhipicephali*, Crimean-Congo hemorrhagic fever virus, and Thogoto virus. In southcentral USA, *R sanguineus* is associated with scattered foci of *Leishmania mexicana*. Certain American populations have become resistant to insecticides. The hymenopteran (chalcid) parasite of ticks, *Hunterellus hookeri*, frequently infests nymphal *R sanguineus* in East Africa.

R appendiculatus, the brown ear tick, is a major pest in cool, shaded, woody and shrubby savannas from southern Sudan and eastern Zaire to Kenya and South Africa. Adults and immatures feed in the ears of cattle, other livestock, and antelope, but also on other areas when the infestation is massive. Immatures may infest small antelope and carnivores, and occasionally rodents. Engorged females lay as many as 5,000 eggs. The life cycle lasts 3–9 mo. Seasonal activity is closely associated with temperature and rain periods. As many as three generations a year can follow in regions with two rainy seasons. *R appendiculatus* is the major vector of the *Theileria parva* group of diseases (East Coast fever, Corridor disease, Zimbabwe malignant theileriosis) and Nairobi sheep disease virus, and is also a vector of *T taurotragi*, *Ehrlichia bovis*, *R conorii*, and Thogoto virus. Heavy infestations on susceptible *Bos taurus* cattle cause a sometimes fatal toxemia, loss of resistance to various infections, and severe damage to the host's ears.

The closely related *R zambeziensis*, with similar host preferences, is found in drier lowland savannas in Tanzania, Zimbabwe, Zambia, Botswana, and Transvaal; it also is a vector of East Coast fever. Other species closely related to *R appendiculatus* include *R nitens* in the Cape Province of South Africa and *R duttoni* in Angola and Zaire.

The ivory-ornamented *R pulchellus*, a parasite of zebras, also infests livestock and game animals in savanna habitats east of the Rift Valley from southern Ethiopia to Somalia and northeastern Tanzania. Adults and immatures generally infest the same host; however, immatures also feed on hares, and larvae ("seed ticks") are notoriously annoying pests of people. *R pulchellus* feeds in the ears and on the lower abdomen, chiefly during wet seasons. This tick is a vector of *Babesia equi* (among zebra), *Theileria* spp, *Trypanosoma theileri*, *Rickettsia conorii*, several Bunyaviridae (Crimean-Congo hemorrhagic fever virus; Nairobi sheep disease; and Kajiado, Kismayo, and Dugbe viruses), and Barur virus.

The two-host African rhipicephalids are *R evertsi* subspecies and *R glabroscutatum*. *R evertsi evertsi*, a large, beady-eyed, red-legged tick, a parasite of the East African zebra, parasitizes all types of herbivorous wildlife and livestock (but seldom pigs). Immatures and adults infest the same hosts; immatures are also recorded from hares. It ranges from South Africa through eastern Africa east of the Nile to southern Sudan and is established in the mountains of Yemen. Scattered foci, introduced by domestic animals, are found west of the Nile. Immatures feed in the ear canal; adults feed mostly around the anus and under the tail but also in the axillae and groin and on the sternum. Large numbers on a single host are common on Equidae and are difficult to control because of their concentrations in difficult-to-reach feeding sites. Adult females lay as many as 7,000 eggs. The life cycle takes 36 mo to complete, depending on weather conditions. *R evertsi evertsi* transmits *Babesia equi*, *Theileria parva* (secondary vector), *Borrelia theileri*, *Rickettsia conorii*, and Kerai, Wad Medani, and Thogoto viruses. The banded-legged (*Hyalomma*-like) western subspecies, *R evertsi mimeticus*, found from western Botswana to Namibia, Angola, and Zaire, is like the nominate subspecies in host preferences, feeding sites, and life cycle.

The tiny *R glabroscutatum* has become a common pest of sheep, goats, and other livestock in the arid, small-shrub savanna of southeastern Cape Province, South Africa. Kudu and other small antelope are also infested. The few records of immatures are from rodents.

The *R pravus* group, currently under taxonomic study, consists of four or more species of which the adults feed on livestock and herbivorous wildlife (including hares); immatures feed on elephant shrews (insectivores), hares, and other small mammals. *R pravus*, a brown, convex-eyed tick, is found in shrubby and wooded savannas in east Africa. It is infected by *Kadam virus*. The closely related *R occulatus*, a parasite of hares, and another related, unnamed parasite of livestock are found in southern Africa.

The difficult-to-classify *R punctatus* group of parasites of livestock and wild artiodactyls consists of *R punctatus* (Angola, Mozambique, Tanzania), *R kochi (neavi)* (Botswana to Kenya and Zaire), and an as yet unnamed species from Zimbabwe and South Africa.

The *R capensis* group is also under study. Originally parasites of the Cape buffalo, these species now parasitize livestock and wildlife in Namibia and South Africa (*R capensis* and *R gertrudae*), East Africa (*R compositus* and *R longus*), and West Africa to southwestern Sudan (*R pseudolongus*).

Above 5,900 ft (1,800 m) altitude in East African forest and shrub zones, *R hurti* and *R jeanelli* infest livestock and Cape buffalo and other large game animals. *R hurti* also inhabits mountains in Zaire. Both species feed chiefly in the hosts' ears; *R jeanelli* also feeds in the tailbrush.

R simus, the prototype of the *R simus* group and long considered to be a well-established species, is divided into several species. *R simus sensu stricto* is found through central and southern Africa, roughly south of latitude 8°S, where it is a competent experimental vector of *Anaplasma marginale* and *A centrale*. In eastern and northern Africa, *R simus* is replaced by a less punctate species, *R praetextatus*, which ranges from central Tanzania to Egypt. Adults of both species parasitize livestock, dogs, wild carnivores, large and medium-sized game animals, and people. Occurrence and densities on livestock are inexplicably erratic. Immature stages feed on the common burrowing rodents in savannas. Both species cause tick paralysis of people and transmit *Rickettsia conorii* and *Coxiella burnetii*. In Kenya, *R praetextatus* is a vector of Thogoto virus and may be a secondary vector of Nairobi sheep disease virus. West of the Nile, these species are replaced by *R senegalensis* and *R muhsamae*.

Much literature regarding *R tricuspis* (Tanzania to South Africa) and *R lunulatus* (West Africa to Ethiopia and Tanzania) has been incorrect. The chief feeding site of both on livestock and wildlife is the tailbrush, but other parts of the host may also be feeding sites.

R sanguineus and *R turanicus* of the *R sanguineus* group are described above. Related species are *R camicasi* and *R bergeoni* of northeastern Africa, *R guilhoni* and *R moucheti* of West Africa, and two widely distributed "forms" of *R sulcatus*, which are under study.

Two quite distinctive species often confused with *R appendiculatus* are *R supertritus* (Natal to southern Sudan) and *R muhlensi* (Kenya and southern Sudan to Central Africa). Adults of both species parasitize cattle, Cape buffalo, antelope, and big game animals; *R supertritus* also is found on carnivores.

IMPORTANT ARGASID TICKS

The important argasid ticks include *Argas* spp, *Carios* spp, *Ornithodoros* spp, and *Otobius* spp.

ARGAS SPP

Most of the 57 known *Argas* spp are specific for birds or bats; a few parasitize wild terrestrial mammals or Galapagos giant tortoises. *A persicus* (the fowl or poultry tick) is an important poultry pest worldwide in warm climates. *A miniatus* (the South American chicken tick) and *A radiatus* (the North American bird tick) can present a problem for traditional or outdoor poultry operations from Caribbean to Central America and from Caribbean to North America, respectively. The species of importance in transmitting *Aegyptianella pullorum* and *Borrelia anserina* to poultry are *A persicus* (many tropical and subtropical areas of the world), *A arboreus* (much of Africa, including Egypt), *A africolumbae* (tropical Africa), *A walkerae* (southern Africa), and *A miniatus* (South and Central America). Other species that infest poultry appear to transmit both *A pullorum* and *B anserina*. (*See also* p 2876.) Tick paralysis is caused by feeding *A persicus*, *A arboreus*, *A walkerae*, *A miniatus*, *A radiatus*, and *A sanchezi* (USA). These and other *Argas* spp can cause great irritation when feeding on people.

CARIOS SPP

Most of the 88 *Carios* spp are species-specific parasites of bats and rodents. Several species infest birds nesting in rocks and caves. These ticks normally live alongside their hosts in caves, hollow trees, and rock crevices, and therefore rarely come in contact with domestic animals. However, in locations where bats occupy roof cavities, their parasites may present a problem for people and their pets. Ticks *C kelleyi* in North America and *C vespertilionis* in Europe, which in nature feed almost exclusively on rock- and tree-roosting bats, have been found in massive numbers in homes with associated bat colonies and have been reported to attach to people. Nest parasites of colonial birds such as *C amblus*, *C capensis*, and *C denmarki* may pose a distinct threat to breeding colonies and are known to cause the death of chicks.

ORNITHODOROS SPP

Most of the 37 *Ornithodoros* spp inhabit protected niches in burrows, caves, dens, cliffsides, and bird colonies. Among the few that parasitize livestock, *O savignyi* and *O coriaceus* are exceptional, because they have eyes and because they rest just below or above ground level under the shade of trees and rocks where livestock and game animals rest and sleep. *O savignyi*, the sand tampan, lives in semiarid areas from Namibia to India and Sri Lanka and is often tremendously abundant. It can cause fatal tick paralysis in calves. People and tethered livestock suffer severe irritation, allergy, and toxicosis from sand tampan bites, and paralysis and death of animals are recorded. *O coriaceus*, the "pajaroello" of hillside scrub oak habitats from northern California and Nevada to Chiapias, Mexico, occupies deer beds under trees and near large rocks. It is well known for irritating deer and cattle, and in people, its bite causes a severe skin reaction. Epizootic bovine abortion, caused by an unnamed bacterum (in the order Myxococcales), is transmitted by *O coriaceus*. *O gurneyi* shelters in tree-shaded soil in arid zones of Australia where kangaroos and people rest; livestock are rare or absent in these habitats.

Among the numerous *Ornithodoros* spp that inhabit burrows, several species are either naturally infected with African swine fever (ASF) virus in Africa or have the laboratory-confirmed ability to harbor and transmit the agent in Europe and the Americas. The natural reservoir and vector of ASF virus is *O porcinus*, which is abundant in burrows of tropical African pigs and also of antbears and porcupines. It has secondarily adapted to human dwellings and domestic animal shelters, where it lives in the cracks of walls and floors. Domestic pig populations in the vicinity of infected wild pigs can be decimated by ASF. Wild and domestic pigs are not involved in the epidemiology of *Borrelia duttoni*, the agent of human African relapsing fever, which is transmitted by *O moubata*. ASF virus has been transported in infected meat to Spain where *O marocanus*, an inhabitant of rodent burrows and pig sties, is an efficient vector. *O marocanus* is also a reservoir and vector of *Borrelia hispanica*, the agent of Spanish-northwest African human relapsing fever. ASF has likewise been introduced in Brazil, Haiti, the Dominican Republic, and Cuba. The American *O turicata*, *O dugesi*, and *O coriaceus* are potential vectors of ASF virus.

O tholozani (*O papillipes*, also *O crossi*) infests burrows, caves, stables, stone and clay fences, and human habitations in semidesert, steppe, and long dry-season environments from China, southern former USSR, northwestern India, and Afghanistan to Greece, northeastern Libya, and eastern Mediterranean islands. Numerous rodents, hedgehogs, porcupines, and domestic animals support *O tholozani* populations. People develop severe, sometimes fatal, Persian relapsing fever when bitten by *O tholozani* infected with *Borrelia persica*.

O lahorensis, originally a parasite of wild sheep resting in the lee of cliffsides, is an important pest of stabled livestock in lowlands and mountains of Tibet Autonomous Region, Kashmir, and southern former USSR to Saudi Arabia and Turkey, Greece, Bulgaria, and Yugoslavia. The two-host life cycle and long wintertime attachment of *O lahorensis* is biologically remarkable. It is deleterious to livestock held for much of the winter in heavily infested stables; it may cause paralysis, anemia, and toxicosis, and it transmits the agents of piroplasmosis, brucellosis, coxiellosis/Q fever, tularemia, and possibly *Borrelia persica*, the agent of Persian relapsing fever.

O turicata parasitizes rodents that live in burrows, crevices, or caves; owls; snakes; tortoises; and also domestic pigs and other livestock in southern USA and Mexico. Contrary to most *Ornithodoros* feeding patterns, immature *O turicata* engorge in <30 min, but adults may attach for as long as 2 days. *O turicata* has been associated with diseases of pigs, and serious toxic reactions and secondary infections can result when people are bitten.

O furucosus parasitizes people and livestock in houses and stables in northwestern South America. Other South American pests of livestock and people, probably originally parasites of the peccary, are *O braziliensis* and *O rostratus*.

OTOBIUS SPP

Otobius megnini, which is exceedingly specialized biologically and structurally, infests the ear canals of pronghorn antelope, mountain sheep, and Virginia and mule deer in low rainfall biotopes of western USA and in Mexico and western Canada. Cattle, horses, goats, sheep, dogs, and people are similarly infested. This well-concealed parasite has been transported with livestock to western South America, Galapagos, Cuba, Hawaii, India, Madagascar, and southeastern Africa. Notably, adults have nonfunctional mouthparts and remain nonfeeding on the ground but may survive for almost 2 yr. Females can deposit as many as 1,500 eggs in a 2-wk period. Larvae and two nymphal instars feed for 2–4 mo, mostly in winter and spring. There can be two or more generations per year. In contrast with most other ticks, the bites of *O megnini* are painful for the hosts. People and other animals may suffer severe irritation from ear canal infestations, and heavily infested livestock lose condition during winter. Tick paralysis of hosts and secondary infections by larval screwworms are reported. *O megnini* is infected by the agents of coxiellosis/Q fever, tularemia, Colorado tick fever, and Rocky Mountain spotted fever, although its ability to transmit these pathogens to the hosts is uncertain. The second *Otobius* sp, *O lagophilus*, feeds on the heads of jackrabbits (hares) and rabbits in western USA.

TICK REMOVAL

Ticks found attached to people or domestic animals should be removed immediately. The longer a tick remains attached to the skin, the more pathogen- and/or toxin-containing saliva is being injected into the host. Therefore, prompt removal is imperative. Several tick removal devices are on the market, but ticks are most effectively removed by a plain set of fine-tipped tweezers.

The CDC recommends the following method of tick removal: 1) Use tweezers to grasp the tick as close to the skin surface as possible. 2) Pull upward with steady, even pressure. 3) Do not twist the tick, because this will cause the mouthparts to break off and remain in the skin. If this happens and the mouthparts cannot easily be removed with clean tweezers, leave it alone and let the skin heal. Chances of a local infection being caused by remaining tick mouthparts are insignificant compared with the risk of pathogen transmission by an attached tick. 4) Avoid crushing the tick. Do *not* squash the tick with your fingers; the contents of the tick can transmit disease through skin abrasions. 5) After removing the tick, thoroughly clean the bite area and your hands with rubbing alcohol, an iodine scrub, or soap and water.

Avoid folklore remedies such as "painting" the tick with nail polish or petroleum jelly or using a hot match to make the tick detach from the skin. The goal is to remove the tick as quickly as possible, not to wait for it to detach. Using irritants such as petroleum jelly, a hot match, or alcohol will *not* cause the tick to "back out" and in fact, may cause more disease-carrying tick saliva to be deposited in the wound.

TICK CONTROL

The main reasons for tick control are to protect hosts from irritation and production losses, formation of lesions that can become secondarily infested, damage to hides and udders, toxicosis, paralysis, and of greatest importance, infection with a wide variety of disease agents. Control also prevents the spread of tick species and the diseases they transmit to unaffected areas, regions, or continents.

Cultural and Biologic Control: These measures can be directed against both the free-living and parasitic stages of ticks. The free-living stages of most tick species, both ixodid and argasid, have specific requirements in terms of microclimate and are restricted to particular microhabitats within the ecosystems inhabited by their hosts. Destruction of these microhabitats reduces the abundance of ticks. Alteration of the environment by removal of certain types of vegetation has been used in the control of *Amblyomma americanum* in recreational areas in southeastern USA and in the control of *Ixodes rubicundus* in South Africa. Control of argasid ticks such as *Argas persicus* and *A walkerae* in poultry can be achieved by eliminating cracks in walls and perches, which provide shelter to the free-living stages.

The abundance of tick species can also be reduced by removal of alternative hosts or hosts of a particular stage of the life cycle. This approach has occasionally been advocated for control of three-host ixodid ticks such as *Rhipicephalus appendiculatus*, *Amblyomma hebraeum*, and *Ixodes rubicundus* in Africa, and *Hyalomma* spp in southeastern Europe and Asia.

Rotation of pastures or pasture spelling has been used in control of the one-host ixodid tick *Rhipicephalus (Boophilus) microplus* in Australia. The method could also be applied to other one-host ticks, in which the duration of the spelling period is determined by the relatively short life span of the free-living larvae. However, it has minimal application to multihost ixodid ticks or argasid ticks because of the long survival periods of the unfed nymphs and adults.

Predators, including birds, rodents, shrews, ants, and spiders, play a role in some areas in reducing the numbers of free-living ticks. In the New World, fire ants

(*Pheidole megacephala*) are noteworthy tick predators. Engorged ticks may also become parasitized by the larvae of some wasps (Hymenoptera), but these have not significantly reduced tick populations.

Zebu (*Bos indicus*) and Sanga (a *B taurus*, *B indicus* crossbreed) cattle, the indigenous breeds of Asia and Africa, usually become very resistant to ixodid ticks after initial exposure. In contrast, European (*B taurus*) breeds usually remain fairly susceptible. The tick resistance of Zebu breeds and their crosses is being increasingly exploited as a means of control of the parasitic stages. The introduction of Zebu cattle to Australia has revolutionized the control of *R microplus* on that continent. Use of resistant cattle as a means of tick control is also becoming important in Africa and the Americas. In Africa, infestations of ixodid ticks on livestock and wild ungulates may also be reduced by oxpeckers (*Buphagus* spp), which are birds that feed on attached ticks.

Chemical Control: *See also* ECTOPARASITICIDES, p 2748.

Control of ticks with acaricides may be directed against the free-living stages in the environment or against the parasitic stages on hosts. Control of ixodid ticks by acaricide treatment of vegetation has been done in specific sites (eg, along trails) in recreational areas in the USA and elsewhere, to reduce the risk of tick attachment to people. This method has not been recommended for wider use because of environmental pollution and the cost of treatment of large areas. Dog kennels, barns, and human dwellings may also require periodic treatment with acaricides to control the free-living stages of ixodid ticks such as the kennel tick, *Rhipicephalus sanguineus*.

The free-living stages of argasid ticks, which infest specific foci such as fowl runs, pigeon lofts, pig sties, and human dwellings, are more frequently and more effectively treated with acaricides.

Treatment of hosts with acaricides to kill attached larvae, nymphs, and adults of ixodid ticks and larvae of argasid ticks has been the most widely used control method. In the first half of the century, the main acaricide was arsenic trioxide. Subsequently, organochlorines, organophosphates, carbamates, amidines, pyrethroids, and avermectins have been used in different parts of the world. The introduction of new compounds, such as the phenylpyrazoles, has been necessary because of the development of resistance in tick populations.

Acaricides are most commonly applied to livestock by use of dips or sprays, with dips being considered the more effective. In recent years, several other means of acaricide application have been developed, including slow release of systemics from implants and boluses, slow release of conventional acaricides from impregnated ear tags, pour-ons (which are applied on the back and spread rapidly over the entire body surface), and spot-ons (which are similar but have less ability to spread). Acaricides are usually applied as dusts or washes on cats, and as dusts on dogs and fowl.

For many years, pyrethroids and organophosphates formulated as dusts, dips, or collars were used on dogs and cats to control ticks. With the advent of the phenylpyrazoles, long-lasting spray and convenient spot-on formulations were introduced. Pyrethroids are available as highly concentrated spot-on products that are labeled only for dogs because of their toxicity in cats. Use of these concentrated pyrethroids is not advised on dogs if a cat is even in the same household.

Vaccines: An advance of potentially great importance has been the production, using biotechnology, of a promising vaccine against *R microplus*. The immunizing agent is a concealed tick antigen, not normally encountered by the host. The immune mechanism it stimulates is different from that stimulated by exposure to ticks (ie, tick feeding). The antigen was derived from a crude extract of partially engorged adult female ticks. It stimulates the production of an antibody that damages tick gut cells and kills the ticks or drastically reduces their reproductive potential.

Prospects of developing similar vaccines against other ixodid tick vectors of cattle diseases of major veterinary importance are not clear. *Rhipicephalus* ticks are good candidates for such vaccines in that they are one-host ticks and show a marked preference for bovine hosts, which act as the principal reservoir of perhaps the most important group of disease agents (*Babesia* spp) these ticks transmit. By contrast, most other tick vector species of agents that cause important cattle diseases (eg, anaplasmosis, heartwater, theileriosis) are three-host ticks, which infest not only cattle but also wild ungulate species, for which vaccination is not feasible. Moreover, many wild ungulate hosts of the vector ticks serve as reservoirs of these disease agents. For these reasons, vaccines against nonboophilid vector ticks may be unable either to eradicate the ticks or to eliminate important sources of the disease agents they transmit.

Control Strategies: Initially, the main uses of acaricides were for tick eradication, prevention of spread of ticks and tickborne diseases (quarantine), and eradication and control of tickborne diseases. The eradication programs were successful in some ecologically marginal subtropical areas, such as southern USA and central Argentina where *Rhipicephalus* spp and babesiosis were eradicated, and southern Africa where East Coast fever (caused by *Theileria parva parva*) was eradicated. The programs were less successful in the ecologically more favorable tropical areas of northeastern Australia, Central America, the Caribbean Islands, and East Africa.

In the areas where eradication was not achieved, costs of maintaining intensive tick control programs often have become prohibitive. For this reason, integrated biologic and chemical control strategies are being adopted. The effectiveness of these cost-containment strategies requires better knowledge of the dynamic associations among the disease agents, their vertebrate hosts, the tick vectors, and the environment. Strict quarantine measures to prevent reintroductions are enforced in countries from which ticks and tickborne diseases have been eradicated. Climate-matching models, geographic information systems, and expert systems (models based on expert knowledge and artificial intelligence) are being used to identify unaffected areas in which tick pests could become established if introduced.

Control of these diseases will require use of the principles of endemic stability and development of improved recombinant vaccines. A current, promising strategy is the identification of receptor sites on the midgut of vector ticks and the development of antibodies that bind with these sites, thereby blocking tick-ingested tickborne pathogens from infecting the tick. Cattle injected with receptor-site antigens may produce antibodies that feeding ticks ingest.

TUMORS OF THE SKIN AND SOFT TISSUES

Cutaneous tumors are the most frequently diagnosed neoplastic disorders in domestic animals, in part because they can be identified easily and in part because the constant exposure of the skin to the external environment predisposes this organ to neoplastic transformation. Chemical carcinogens, ionizing radiation, and viruses all have been implicated, but hormonal and genetic factors may also play a role in development of cutaneous neoplasms.

The skin is a complex structure composed of various epithelial (epidermis, adnexa), mesenchymal (fibrous connective tissues, blood vessels, adipose tissue), and neural and neuroectodermal tissues (peripheral nerve, Merkel cells, melanocytes), all with the potential to develop distinctive tumors. Because cutaneous tumors are so diverse, their classification is difficult and often controversial. There is also controversy regarding the criteria used to define whether a lesion that arises in the skin or soft tissues is neoplastic and, if so, whether it is benign or malignant. To avoid confusion, the following terms are used in this discussion: A **hamartoma (nevus)** is a localized developmental defect associated with enlargement of one or more elements of the skin. A sebaceous hamartoma, for example, refers to a localized region of the skin where sebaceous glands are extremely prominent and sometimes malformed. Although by strict definition hamartomas are present at birth, they may occasionally take a long time to reach a clinically apparent size and may not be diagnosed until an animal is mature. To confuse matters further, some lesions with clinical and histologic features of congenital hamartomas may develop in adult animals. Such "acquired" hamartomas are difficult to separate from benign epithelial and mesenchymal neoplasms. In human medical literature and some veterinary texts, the term "nevus" is used synonymously with hamartoma. A **benign neoplasm** is localized, noninfiltrative, and because it is surrounded by a capsule, easily excisable. A **neoplasm of intermediate malignancy** is locally infiltrative and difficult to excise but does not metastasize. A **malignant neoplasm** is infiltrative with metastatic potential.

Although cutaneous neoplasms characteristically are nodular or papular, they also can occur as localized or generalized alopecic plaques, erythematous and pigmented patches and plaques, wheals, or nonhealing ulcers. The variability in clinical presentation can make distinguishing a neoplasm from an inflammatory disease difficult; furthermore, distinguishing a benign tumor from a malignant tumor is even more subjective because sarcomas or carcinomas early in their development may palpate as discrete, encapsulated masses. To establish a definitive diagnosis, histopathology is generally required. Cytologic evaluation is very useful and should be used to exclude mast cell tumor before surgery so that wide adequate margins are planned as appropriate. For some neoplasms (eg, round cell tumors), cytology can rival or even surpass the value of histologic examination.

Therapy depends largely on the type of tumor, its location and size, and signalment of the animal. For benign neoplasms associated with neither ulceration nor clinical dysfunction, no therapy may be the most prudent option, especially in aged companion animals.

Fine-needle aspiration cytology should be performed initially on all tumors to determine the type of tumor and treatment planning. For more aggressive neoplastic diseases or for benign tumors that inhibit normal function or are cosmetically unpleasant, there are several therapeutic options. For most, surgical intervention with complete excision provides the best chance of a cure with the least cost and often with the fewest adverse events.

Histologic assessment of margin status is useful to predict local recurrence of cutaneous malignant tumors in dogs and cats treated by means of excision alone. However, method accuracy varies among tumor types and grades. Recurrence times suggest postsurgical follow-up should continue for ≥2 yr. Careful postsurgical management is recommended for animals with both infiltrated and close tumor margins.

Lumpectomy is adequate for benign lesions, but if a malignancy is suspected, the lesion should be removed with wide (3 cm) surgical margins. For tumors that cannot be completely excised, partial removal or debulking may prolong the life of the animal and increase the effectiveness of radiation or chemotherapy. Cryosurgery is also an option, although it is more effective for benign, superficial lesions than for malignant cutaneous neoplasms. Radiation therapy is of most value for infiltrative neoplasms not surgically resectable, or when surgical intervention would cause unacceptable physical impairment. Chemotherapy can be used either systemically (and if appropriate, intralesionally) as a primary method for treatment of malignant neoplasms or as an adjunct to surgery or radiation therapy. In the skin, radiation is most commonly used to treat round cell tumors (eg, lymphosarcomas, mast cell tumors, transmissible venereal tumors, etc) or solid tumors that cannot be excised completely. Although generally palliative, long remissions may sometimes be obtained with radiation therapy. Other forms of therapy include hyperthermia, laser therapy, photodynamic therapy, antiangiogenic therapy, metronomic therapy, gene therapy, immunotherapy, and multimodal therapy using a combination or sequencing of various therapies.

EPIDERMAL AND HAIR FOLLICLE TUMORS

Ceruminous gland tumors are discussed in TUMORS OF THE EAR CANAL (*see* p 535).

Benign, Nonvirus-associated Papillomatous Lesions

For a discussion of papillomas (viral warts), the most common, viral-induced neoplasms of the skin, *see* p 952. Benign, proliferative lesions not associated with papilloma virus infection can have a gross morphology similar to that of papillomas.

Epidermal hamartomas (nevi) are rare proliferations identified only in dogs, most often in the young. The disease may be heritable in Cocker Spaniels. Grossly, epidermal nevi appear as pigmented, hyperkeratotic, vaguely papillated papules and plaques that are occasionally arranged in a linear pattern. Some forms are associated with pustules and acantholytic cells. They are benign, but their appearance is unpleasant, and the extensive hyperkeratosis is prone to secondary bacterial infection. Localized lesions can be excised; dogs with multiple lesions or lesions too large to be surgically removed may be responsive to isotretinoin or etretinate. Hyperkeratosis may be transiently controlled by use of topical keratolytic shampoos and emollients.

Congenital papillomas of foals are rare and probably a developmental defect rather than a result of papilloma virus infection. They are found anywhere on the body but most commonly on the head. Thoroughbreds may be predisposed. Present at birth, the lesions are often several centimeters in diameter, hairless, pedunculated, and exophytic, with a papillated surface reminiscent of a cauliflower. They are benign, and excision is curative.

Canine warty dyskeratomas are rare, benign neoplasms of uncertain derivation but with histologic features of follicular or apocrine neoplasms (or both). They appear grossly as verrucous papules or nodules with a keratotic, umbilicated center. Excision is curative.

Basal Cell Tumors and Basal Cell Carcinomas

(Basal cell epitheliomas, Basaliomas, Trichoblastomas, Basosquamous cell carcinomas)

Basal cell tumors represent a heterogeneous group of cutaneous epithelial neoplasms recognized most commonly in cats, less commonly in dogs, occasionally in horses and sheep, and seldom in other domestic animals. These neoplasms are composed of a proliferation of small basophilic cells that exhibit morphology reminiscent of the progenitor cells of the epidermis and adnexa. As these tumors have been examined more closely, evidence of differentiation (follicular, sebaceous, etc) has been discovered, giving justification for reclassification. For example, in dogs, what in the past was called a basal cell tumor is best characterized as a **trichoblastoma**, a tumor of hair bulb (the site of the follicle that produces the hair shaft) origin.

Some reclassification schemes have suggested that the use of the term basal cell tumor be restricted to a benign neoplasm in cats (the derivation of which has yet to be defined). Because this revised terminology is being adopted slowly, traditional terminology will be used herein. That is, a benign proliferation of basal cells will be called a basal cell tumor; a malignant proliferation will be called a basal cell carcinoma. In domestic animals, most basal cell tumors are benign and originate in the mid to deep dermis, indicating probable adnexal derivation. These features distinguish basal cell tumors in domestic animals from those in people, the latter being locally invasive (ie, they are true carcinomas) and originating in the epidermis. In addition, solar injury is a common cause of neoplasms derived from basal cells in people, but its role in inducing basal cell tumors of other animals is unknown.

Canine basal cell tumors generally develop in middle-aged to older dogs of predisposed breeds such as Wirehaired Pointing Griffons, Kerry Blue Terriers, and Wheaten Terriers. These tumors are found most commonly on the head (especially the ears), the neck, and forelimbs. Older domestic longhair, Himalayan, and Persian cats are the breeds most at risk. Feline basal cell tumors may develop almost anywhere on the body. In both dogs and cats, these tumors generally appear as firm, solitary, encapsulated, and often hairless or ulcerated nodules that may be pedunculated; they vary in size from <1 cm to >10 cm in diameter. In cats more often than dogs, these tumors are often densely pigmented, and on cut section, they can be difficult to distinguish from dermal melanocytomas. Cystic variants are also more common in cats. Although basal cell tumors are benign, they are expansive neoplasms and may be associated with extensive ulceration and secondary inflammation. Complete excision is curative.

Basal cell carcinomas are more frequently recognized in aged cats than in dogs. Persian-type breeds are predisposed. They often appear as ulcerated plaques on the head, extremities, or neck. Unlike benign basal cell tumors, these carcinomas generally have continuity with the epidermis, are locally invasive, and may be multicentric. Although evidence of vascular invasion may be identified on histologic sections, local or systemic metastasis rarely occurs. Consequently, surgical excision is the treatment of choice.

In dogs, most basal cell carcinomas have histologic evidence of cornification, a feature they have in common with squamous cell carcinomas. Therefore, they are generally called **basosquamous cell carcinomas**. These tumors are generally recognized in older dogs. Saint Bernards, Scottish Terriers, and Norwegian Elkhounds are most at risk. Unlike canine basal cell tumors, basosquamous cell carcinomas do not tend to develop on the head and can be found almost anywhere on the body where they have continuity with the epidermis and appear as exoendophytic nodules or plaques. These tumors are locally invasive but seldom metastasize. Surgical excision is the treatment of choice.

Intracutaneous Cornifying Epitheliomas

(Keratoacanthoma, Infundibular keratinizing acanthoma)

Intracutaneous cornifying epitheliomas are benign neoplasms of dogs and possibly cats. As in human keratoacanthomas, these lesions most likely arise from the hair follicle and not from the interfollicular epidermis. They can develop anywhere on the body, with the back, tail, and extremities the most common sites affecting middle-aged dogs. Norwegian Elkhounds, Belgian Sheepdogs, Lhasa Apsos, and Bearded Collies are most likely to develop these tumors, with Norwegian Elkhounds and Lhasa Apsos at risk of developing generalized lesions. The most characteristic presentation is a papule or nodule with a central cornified pore that may protrude above the epidermal surface, giving the appearance of a horn; however, many of these tumors never have continuity with the epidermis and may appear solely as cornified cysts. These tumors are benign and treatment is optional, provided a definitive diagnosis has been established and there is no self-trauma, ulceration, or secondary infection. Tumor wall rupture releases keratin into surrounding tissues, evoking a pyogranulomatous and granulomatous inflammatory response. Excision is curative; however, dogs are prone to develop additional tumors over time. For animals with a generalized form of the disease, oral retinoids (eg, isotretinoin or etretinate) may be of therapeutic benefit.

Squamous Cell Carcinomas

(Epidermoid carcinomas, Prickle cell carcinomas)

Thought to arise from either the epidermis or the epithelium of the superficial (infundibular) regions of the outer root sheath of the hair follicle, squamous cell carcinomas have been recognized in all domestic animals. Although most arise without prior cause, in many species, especially in the face and ear tips of white cats and in the ventral nonpigmented skin of dogs, prolonged exposure to sunlight on sparsely haired, minimally pigmented areas of the body is a major predisposing factor. The grooming habits of cats also expose them to particulate carcinogens from cigarette smoke and flea collars. In addition, a unique form of feline squamous cell carcinoma associated with papilloma virus infection has been described (*see* below).

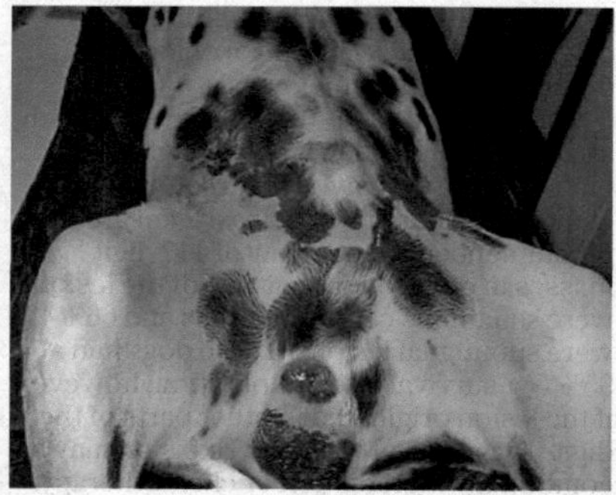

Solar-induced squamous cell carcinoma in the white skin of a Dalmation dog. *Courtesy of Dr. Alice Villalobos.*

In dogs, squamous cell carcinomas are the most frequently diagnosed carcinomas arising in the skin. Two forms are recognized: cutaneous and subungual. **Cutaneous squamous cell carcinomas** are tumors of older dogs, with Bloodhounds, Basset Hounds, and Standard Poodles at greatest risk. Lesions commonly arise on the head, distal extremities, ventral abdomen, and perineum. Most cutaneous squamous cell carcinomas appear as firm, raised, frequently ulcerated plaques and nodules; sometimes they can be extremely exophytic and have a wart-like surface. The etiology of most of these tumors is undefined; however, some are induced by prolonged solar injury. These usually develop on ventral abdominal, preputial, scrotal, and inguinal skin in white-skinned, shorthaired breeds such as Dalmatians, Bull Terriers, Pit Bulls, and Beagles. Lesions develop in a ventral location because the poorly haired skin has minimal shielding from ultraviolet radiation, many animals sun themselves lying on their backs, and perhaps because solar radiation reflects from the ground. Before a carcinoma develops, animals acquire focal zones of lichenification, hyperkeratosis, and erythema known as **solar keratosis** (solar dermatosis, actinic keratosis, senile keratosis).

Subungual squamous cell carcinomas are most commonly found in older Giant and Standard Schnauzers, Gordon Setters, Briards, Kerry Blue Terriers, Standard Poodles, and Scottish Terriers. Generally, all are darkhaired breeds, and a dark coat color has been associated with development of subungual squamous cell carcinomas that arise from the nailbed epithelium and invade the medullary and cortical bone of P3. They may arise on multiple digits, often appear on different extremities, and may metastasize via lymphatics to regional lymph nodes and lungs in as many as 13% of cases. Females have a slight predilection, and both fore- and hindlimbs are equally predisposed to tumor development.

In cats, cutaneous squamous cell carcinomas most commonly develop in conjunction with chronic solar injury.

Consequently, they usually develop on the pinnae, frontal ridges, eyelids, nose, or lips of cats that have white skin in these regions. There is no breed or sex predilection. As in dogs, solar keratosis or carcinoma in situ (early superficial stage) often precedes development of a malignant tumor. Recently, coat-associated particulate carcinogens from exposure to cigarette smoke and flea collars have been identified as risk factors for cats with oral squamous cell carcinoma. Lesions not caused by sun exposure may develop on the digits and are presumed to be metastatic from primary squamous cell carcinomas of the lung, but primary subungual forms are uncommon in cats.

Cutaneous squamous cell carcinomas are the most common malignant neoplasm in horses. They generally develop in adult or aged horses with white or part-white coats; breeds at risk include Appaloosa, Belgian, American Paint, and Pinto. Although they can arise anywhere on the body, these tumors most commonly arise in nonpigmented, poorly haired areas near mucous membranes. Thus, the periorbital regions, lips, nose, anus, and external genitalia (especially the penile sheath) are sites most likely to be affected.

In cattle, these tumors are most common in breeds with white hair and poorly pigmented skin (especially Holsteins and Ayrshires) and, as in horses, develop around the mucous membranes, usually at the mucocutaneous junctions, particularly the periocular and vulvar regions. In India, squamous cell carcinomas of the horn core are common in aged bullocks. The most common cause is actinic injury. Solar keratoses often precede development of an invasive tumor; genetic factors, immunodeficiency, and viruses may also play a role.

In sheep, squamous cell carcinomas are of economic significance in some parts of the world. In a study in Australia, they were responsible for more than one-third of all condemnations before slaughter. The Merino breed is most at risk, and females more so than males. The most common sites are the poorly haired skin of the ears, lips, muzzle, and the vulvar lips after they have been externalized by a Mules operation to prevent fly strike. Tumors at these sites develop in conjunction with solar injury, which is heightened when animals ingest photosensitizing plants. Tumors of the ears also develop more frequently after a procedure such as ear tagging. Squamous cell carcinomas can develop from follicular cysts on sites not commonly exposed to sunlight.

In goats, squamous cell carcinomas develop most frequently in females, in which tumors develop on the perineal and vulvar regions and on the skin of the teats and udders. Both males and females can develop sun-induced tumors on the ears. Although Angoras are most at risk, Saanan goats occasionally develop squamous cell carcinomas on the udder in association with papillomas. The role papilloma viruses play in tumor progression is considered contributory.

Squamous cell carcinomas are extremely uncommon in swine.

Most squamous cell carcinomas are solitary lesions; however, multiple tumors may develop in conjunction with solar injury in the "field cancerization" model. They appear as endophytic or exoendophytic lesions, the former as raised, irregular dermal masses with an ulcerated surface, and the latter as raised, irregular dermal masses covered by a papillated epidermis. Cats initially exhibit small crusting facial sores that do not heal. The lesions often persist for months before defects appear on the ear tips, nares, and eyelids. Subungual squamous cell carcinomas of dogs are first identified by lameness or nail malformation, an infection that mimics chronic osteomyelitis, or loss of the claw of the affected digit. In cattle with involvement of the horn, the first sign is distorted growth.

Squamous cell carcinomas are characteristically invasive into adjacent soft and bony tissues. Infrequently, in cattle, they regress spontaneously. In small animals, longterm survival and the likelihood of metastasis are correlated with histologic differentiation. Well-differentiated tumors are slowly progressive or remain localized; undifferentiated tumors are more likely to metastasize or recur within 20 wk of excision. In general, failure of treatment is due to late diagnosis and lack of control of local disease rather than metastasis.

For dogs and cats, surgical excision, such as amputation of the involved digit or pinnae or nosectomy, is the treatment of choice, and margins of at least 2 cm are recommended. One review of 117 digit masses in dogs found that 25% of the lesions were squamous cell carcinomas and 66% were subungual lesions. These dogs had a 95% 1-yr survival after amputation; however, if the lesion originated in other parts of the digit, 1-yr survival was 60%. Excision may be combined with radiation or chemotherapy. Feline squamous cell carcinomas are more radiosensitive than their canine counterparts. Still, the 1-yr survival rate is <10%

for invasive neoplasms. Cryosurgery and hyperthermia can be very helpful for local therapy especially in early (carcinoma in situ) lesions, but controlled studies have not been done to determine their effectiveness. Intralesional implant chemotherapy with 5-fluorouracil (dogs only), cisplatin (dogs only), or carboplatin along with retinoids and photodynamic therapy has been used with variable success. Intratumoral injection of nasal planum squamous cell carcinomas in cats using carboplatin in a water-sesame seed oil emulsion resulted in a 70% general response with 1-yr progression-free survival rate of ~50%. In dogs with multiple ventral actinic keratoses, topical dinitrochlorbenzene or 5-fluorouracil (5%) may be of benefit. Cats should not be given any form of 5-fluorouracil therapy. More recently, the use of topical immunomodulating antineoplastics such as imiquimod cream applied topically on lesions twice daily for 2 wk creates a local application site inflammatory reaction and often resolves lesions. Imiquimod stimulates Toll-like receptor 7 and dendritic cells, modifying immune responses to destroy the targeted carcinoma cells. The response may be enhanced by the application of 6 joules of cold laser therapy to the lesions every 2 wk until regression. Limiting exposure to ultraviolet radiation may help prevent solar-induced squamous cell carcinomas in dogs and cats. This may be accomplished by using UV window screens, sunscreen, and keeping companion animals indoors during hours of peak sunlight between 10 AM and 2 PM. Tattoos, magic markers, and sunscreen are used with variable success.

In horses, radiotherapy using surface or interstitial brachytherapy is the treatment of choice for squamous cell carcinomas. Other options include ^{90}Sr or ^{192}Ir implants, wide surgical excision (especially for neoplasms of the third eyelid, penis, and prepuce), and cryosurgery. Immunotherapy, with either an autogenous vaccine made from the tumor tissue suspended in Freund's adjuvant, or nonspecific immunomodulation using *Corynebacterium parvum*, has had some success in treating ocular or horn core squamous cell carcinomas in cattle.

Feline multicentric squamous cell carcinoma in situ (feline Bowen disease) is a disease of aged (>10 yr old) cats and may be associated with immunosuppression. There is no defined breed or sex predilection. Clinically, lesions appear as multiple discrete, erythematous, black or brown hyperkeratotic plaques and papules. Lesions are nonpruritic, and ulceration is uncommon. Their development is associated with the presence of a papilloma virus. The term in situ refers to a malignant proliferation of epidermal and follicular outer sheath cells that are not invasive into the underlying dermis. Unfortunately, lesions may progress over time into an invasive carcinoma. Metastasis is extremely uncommon. These lesions usually develop in systemically ill or immunosuppressed cats and are believed to be virally induced. They have not been amenable to therapy; however, cryotherapy of local lesions and topical imiquimod as described above may increase time to progression.

Keratinized Cutaneous Cysts

Most keratinized cutaneous cysts are malformations of the hair follicle. They are common in dogs; occasionally identified in cats, horses, goats, and sheep; and rare in cattle and pigs. Excision is the treatment of choice. Vigorous squeezing of these lesions is contraindicated, because it often incites a severe foreign body inflammatory response due to the release of keratin into surrounding tissues.

Infundibular follicular cysts (epidermoid cysts, epidermal inclusion cysts, erroneously called sebaceous cysts) are the most common. They are a cystic dilatation of the upper portion of the outer sheath of the hair follicle (the infundibulum) lined by a layer of stratified cornifying epithelial cells indistinguishable from the epidermis. These cysts vary in size from 2 mm to >5 cm (lesions <5 mm in diameter are often called milia). The only domestic animals identified at risk are Merino sheep, in which these cysts are often multiple and may progress to squamous cell carcinomas. As with all follicular cysts, these are usually solitary, papular to nodular lesions that are freely movable. They are generally partially compressible on palpation and occasionally have a small opening through the epidermis from which the cystic contents can be extruded. On cut surface, they are filled with a gray, brown, or yellowish, granular, "cheesy" material that is lumenal keratin.

Isthmus catagen cysts (trichilemmal cysts, pilar cysts, cystic intracutaneous cornifying epithelioma) are follicular cysts that have the keratinization pattern of the lower portion of the outer root sheath. They have been definitively identified only in dogs and (rarely) in cats.

Matrix cysts are follicular cysts in which the wall resembles the epithelium of the hair bulb (the matrix portion of the hair follicle) and the inner root sheath. They occur predominantly in dogs and cats. Many progress to pilomatricomas (*see* p 948).

Hybrid cysts (panfollicular cysts) are follicular cysts that have a combination of the characteristics of epidermal inclusion, trichilemmal, and matrix cysts and that are found predominantly in dogs and cats. Many progress to trichoepitheliomas (*see* below).

Dermoid cysts are congenital malformations found most commonly on the dorsal midline of the head or along the vertebral column. They are most commonly identified in Boxers, Kerry Blue Terriers, and Rhodesian Ridgeback dogs; Thoroughbred horses; and possibly Suffolk sheep. Typically multiple, they differ from other follicular cysts in that on cut surface they contain fully formed hair shafts. They are arguably the only true epidermal inclusion cysts, because they most likely represent an embryonal invagination of the epidermis with associated adnexa. These adnexa are responsible for the hair shafts within the cyst lumens.

Keratomas are cystic lesions in the hoof wall of the toe or, less frequently, the quarter or heel in simple or cloven-hoofed animals. They often develop secondary to a traumatic injury. Although often asymptomatic, they commonly induce lameness and deformity of the hoof wall or sole and may be associated with distal phalangeal lysis. Keratomas are seldom >5 cm in diameter and contain white to brown laminated keratin, often with a necrotic center associated with secondary inflammation. When lameness is present, surgical excision and curettage of the underlying bone, if affected, is the treatment of choice.

Dilated pores of Winer are rare, hair-follicle neoplasms recognized only in aged cats. Males may be predisposed. These lesions most often develop on the head. Clinically, they appear as solitary, dome-shaped lesions with the appearance of a giant comedo. Compact keratin may protrude through (above) the surface, giving them the appearance of a cutaneous horn. These lesions are benign, and complete excision is curative.

Tumors of the Hair Follicle

The hair follicle is a complex structure composed of eight different epithelial layers. Hair-follicle tumors display a similar complexity, and much work needs to be done to characterize them further. They are most common in dogs, less frequent in cats, and rare in other domestic animals.

Tricholemmomas are rare, benign, hair-follicle neoplasms of dogs, most commonly found on the head. Poodles may be predisposed. These tumors are derived from the lower portion of the outer root sheath and often have areas of transition into basal cell tumors. They have little in common with a tumor of the same name in people that represents an old wart. They appear as firm, ovoid masses, 1–7 cm in diameter, that are encapsulated but expand over time. Excision is curative.

Trichofolliculomas are extremely rare follicular tumors of dogs composed of the inferior and isthmic regions of multiple abortive follicles that extrude their lumenal contents into a dilated abnormal cystic infundibulum. Too few have been recognized to determine age, breed, or sex predilection. Considered by some to be more a hamartoma than a true neoplasm, these tumors are benign, and complete surgical excision is curative.

Trichoepitheliomas are cystic hair follicle neoplasms of dogs and, less commonly, cats, in which all elements of the hair follicle (infundibulum, isthmus, and inferior portions) and the patterns of cornification they produce are represented. The epithelium and cornification of the infundibular and isthmic portions predominate. Benign and malignant forms are recognized. In dogs, these lesions can be seen at any age but are found most commonly during late middle age. Many breeds are predisposed, including Basset Hounds, Bull Mastiffs, Irish Setters, Standard Poodles, English Springer Spaniels, and Golden Retrievers. There is no defined sex predilection. Tumors can develop anywhere on the body but are most common on the trunk in dogs and on the head, tail, and extremities in cats. Benign forms appear as palpably encapsulated cystic nodules (1–5 cm in diameter) in the dermis and subcutaneous fat. Expansion of cysts or self-trauma may induce ulceration associated with extrusion of lumenal keratin that appears as a condensed, yellow, granular, "cheesy" material. Excision is curative; however, animals that develop one such tumor are prone to develop additional lesions at other sites. This is especially true for Basset Hounds and English Springer Spaniels.

Malignant trichoepitheliomas are much less common than benign trichoepitheliomas and are differentiated by their local invasiveness; continuity with the epidermis; and association with extensive inflammation, necrosis, and fibrosis. Metastasis is uncommon. Wide surgical excision is the treatment of choice and is often curative in those tumors that are invasive but have minimal metastatic potential.

Pilomatricomas (hair matrix tumors, calcifying epitheliomas of Malherbe) are cystic hair-follicle neoplasms recognized almost exclusively in dogs. Unlike trichoepitheliomas, in which all elements of the follicle are represented, in pilomatricomas only the cells of the matrix region of the inferior part of the hair follicle and the cornification patterns they produce (hair shaft and inner root sheath) are present. Benign and malignant forms are recognized. Benign tumors are most common on the trunk of middle-aged dogs. Kerry Blue and Wheaten Terriers, Bouviers des Flandres, Bichons Frises, and Standard Poodles are most at risk. Grossly, these tumors are indistinguishable from trichoepitheliomas, but their cystic contents are often gritty because of mineralization. Excision is the treatment of choice. As in trichoepitheliomas, when one such lesion develops, additional lesions often develop over time.

Malignant pilomatricomas (malignant hair matrix tumor, matrical carcinoma) are rare and have been identified most often in dogs. They are a tumor of old dogs and grossly characterized as solitary or multinodular, variably cystic tumors that are often firmly attached to subjacent soft tissues. Because they are invasive, they are difficult to excise, and recurrence is common after attempts at surgical excision. They often metastasize to draining lymph nodes and internal organs, especially the lungs. Aggressive surgery is recommended. It is unknown whether they respond to radiation or chemotherapy.

Cutaneous Apocrine Gland Tumors

Sweat glands are of two types: apocrine and eccrine. Apocrine glands are tubular glands with a coiled secretory portion and a long, straight duct that flows into the follicular infundibulum. In domestic animals, all hair follicles have apocrine glands. Apocrine glands in dogs and cats are also present in association with the anal sac, and modified apocrine glands, known as ceruminous glands, are present in the external auditory meatus. In most mammals, apocrine glands produce an odiferous, oily compound that is a sexual attractant, a territorial marker, and a warning signal. In horses and cattle, these glands play a role in thermoregulation by producing sweat.

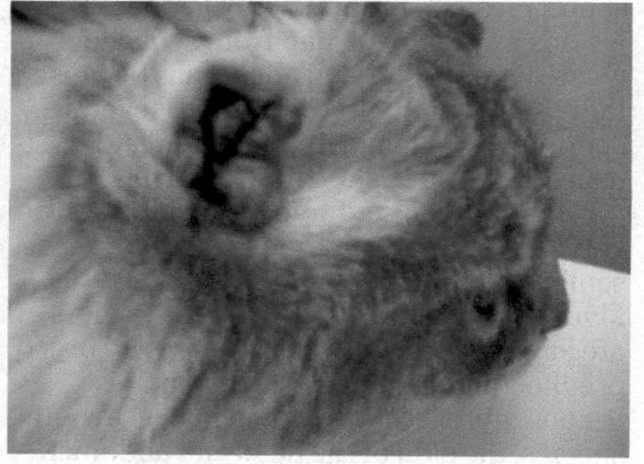

Ceruminous gland carcinoma, right ear of a cat. *Courtesy of Dr. Alice Villalobos.*

Apocrine gland tumors and malformations are most common in dogs and cats. Three diseases of apocrine glands of haired skin have been characterized.

Cystic apocrine gland dilations (apocrine gland cysts, cystic apocrine gland hyperplasia, apocrine cystomatosis) are best characterized as hamartomas. Two forms exist: a cystic form in which one or more cysts develop in the mid to upper dermis with a poor association with hair follicles, and a more diffuse form characterized by cystically dilated apocrine glands associated with multiple hair follicles in nontraumatized skin. Both are found in middle-age or older dogs and, less commonly, cats. The head and neck are the most common sites where these lesions develop. In both species, lesions appear as fluctuant dermal cysts or as translucent bullae. Complete excision is curative; however, this may be difficult to accomplish in the more diffuse form.

Apocrine gland adenomas are diagnosed almost exclusively in dogs, cats, and rarely horses. Two types are recognized based on whether their histologic appearance primarily resembles the secretory or ductular portion of the apocrine gland. **Apocrine adenomas** resemble the secretory region of the apocrine glands. They are found in older dogs and cats. Great Pyrenees, Chow Chows, and Alaskan Malamutes are the most commonly affected breeds. The head, neck, and extremities are the most frequent sites of development. In cats, apocrine adenomas are more likely to be seen in males, and no breed appears at greater risk than any other. The vast majority of apocrine adenomas occur on the head, especially the pinnae. In horses, no age, sex, or breed association is known. The pinnae and vulva are the most likely regions to develop these tumors. In all species, these tumors appear as firm to fluctuant cysts, seldom >4 cm in diameter. They contain varying amounts of clear to brownish fluid. In cats, the luminal fluid may be darkly pigmented, and apocrine cysts can be confused clinically with melanocytomas, especially when present on the inner aspect of the ears. **Apocrine ductular adenomas** are less common. They are found in older dogs and cats and are putatively derived from or show differentiation toward apocrine ducts. In dogs, these tumors are most commonly recognized in Peekapoos, Old English Sheepdogs, and English Springer Spaniels. They are often smaller, firmer, and less cystic than apocrine adenomas. Because they often consist of a large population of basal cells and because evidence of ductular differentiation can be extremely subtle, these tumors are often diagnosed histologically as basal cell tumors (*see* p 944). Apocrine adenomas and apocrine ductular adenomas are benign, and complete surgical excision is curative.

Apocrine gland adenocarcinomas of haired skin are rare in all domestic animals but most frequently identified in older dogs and cats. In dogs, Treeing Walker Coonhounds, Norwegian Elkhounds, German Shepherds, and mixed-breed dogs are most at risk; in cats, Siamese may be predisposed. In both species, this tumor most commonly arises in axillary and inguinal regions—sites that allow it to be easily confused clinically and histologically with mammary gland ductular adenocarcinomas. Apocrine gland adenocarcinomas generally are larger than adenomas and have a variable clinical appearance ranging from fibrotic dermal nodules to ulcerated plaques. They are locally invasive and frequently metastasize to draining lymph nodes. Less commonly, skin and lung metastasis may occur. Complete surgical excision is the treatment of choice. Little is known about response to adjunct chemotherapy.

Apocrine Gland Tumors of Anal Sac Origin

Apocrine gland tumors of anal sac origin have been definitively identified only in dogs, although anecdotal reports suggest they may also be seen in cats. Older English Cocker and Springer Spaniels, Dachshunds, Alaskan Malamutes, German Shepherds, and mixed-breed dogs are most at risk. Unlike hepatoid gland tumors (*see* p 951), these apocrine gland tumors have no sex predilection. They most commonly appear as deep, firm, nodular masses near the anal sac. As these lesions grow, they may *compress the rectum* and induce constipation. Some of these tumors are associated with paraneoplastic hypercalcemia, which causes anorexia, weight loss, polyuria and polydipsia, and mineralization of renal tissue with increased BUN and creatinine values. These tumors are often highly infiltrative into the pelvic canal and commonly (90%) metastasize to the sublumbar lymph nodes or to distant internal organs (40%). Wide surgical excision, including involved lymph nodes, is the treatment of choice. Even if the tumor cannot be totally resected, debulking can be of value in dogs with pseudohyperparathyroidism, because the hypercalcemia is related to the production of parathormone-like hormone from the total tumor volume. Adjunct chemotherapy along with tyrosine kinase inhibitors, metronomic chemotherapy, and radiation therapy may also be of benefit to increase time to progression, but few dogs are reported to live >1 yr after the tumor has been recognized.

Eccrine Gland Tumors

Eccrine glands are the coiled, tubular, sweat glands present on the footpads of carnivores, the frog of ungulates, the carpus of pigs, and the nasolabial region of ruminants. Tumors derived from these glands are extremely rare and have been identified only on the footpads of dogs and cats. Most are malignant and invasive. These tumors are reported to have a high potential to metastasize to draining lymph nodes.

Sebaceous Gland Tumors

Tumors and tumor-like conditions of sebaceous glands are common in dogs, infrequent in cats, and rare in other domestic animals. Based on morphologic more than on behavioral features, four categories of benign sebaceous gland proliferations have been described. In people, in which a roughly similar classification scheme is traditionally used, it has been proposed that all benign sebaceous gland tumors be called sebaceomas.

Sebaceous gland hamartomas are solitary lesions reported only in dogs. These lesions are distinguished from sebaceous gland hyperplasias and adenomas because they are linear or circumscribed, several centimeters in length or diameter, and usually identified shortly after birth.

Sebaceous gland hyperplasias (senile sebaceous hyperplasias) represent a senile change in dogs and cats. In dogs, Manchester, Wheaten, and Welsh Terriers are at greatest risk. In cats, there is no breed predilection, but females develop these lesions more frequently than males. In both species, the skin of the head and abdomen are affected most commonly. Sebaceous hyperplasias commonly appear as papillated masses seldom >1 cm in diameter, often with a shiny, keratotic surface.

Sebaceous gland adenomas are seen in all domestic animals but are so common in older dogs and cats they can be considered primarily a small animal neoplasm. Coonhounds, English Cocker Spaniels, Cocker Spaniels, Huskies, Samoyeds, and Alaskan Malamutes are the canine breeds most likely to develop these tumors; Persians are the feline breed most predisposed. In dogs, these tumors frequently are clinically indistinguishable from sebaceous hyperplasias, but they tend to be larger (typically >1 cm). They are often multiple and may develop anywhere on the body but are commonly found on the head. Sebaceous adenomas may be covered with a serocellular crust and exhibit pleocellular inflammation and superficial pyoderma. **Sebaceous gland epitheliomas** are a variant of sebaceous adenoma distinguished by lobules composed primarily of basal progenitor cells rather than mature sebocytes. Because they often have irregular lobules that extend into the deep dermis, they can occasionally be confused with sebaceous carcinomas. These tumors are found in older dogs and rarely in cats. They appear as ulcerated nodules that may be several centimeters in diameter. A papillated epidermal surface and pigmentation are variable findings.

Sebaceous gland adenocarcinomas are rare in domestic animals. They are recognized almost exclusively in dogs and cats, generally in middle-aged or older animals. Cavalier King Charles Spaniels; Cocker Spaniels; and Scottish, Cairn, and West Highland White Terriers are most at risk. Male dogs and female cats may be predisposed. These lesions are often ulcerated and may be indistinguishable from sebaceous epitheliomas or other cutaneous carcinomas. They are locally infiltrative and may metastasize to regional lymph nodes late in the disease.

Once a diagnosis is established, treatment is optional for benign sebaceous gland tumors unless they are secondarily inflamed and infected. For malignant adenocarcinomas, excision is the treatment of choice, but complete removal can be difficult because of the infiltrative nature of this tumor; adjunct radiotherapy may be required. Even benign sebaceous gland growths recur if remnants are left at the surgical site. In addition, animals that develop one sebaceous gland hyperplasia or adenoma often develop new lesions at other sites over time. No established protocol of chemotherapy for any of these lesions has been defined. Oral retinoids may prevent recurrence of sebaceous hyperplasia, but their use remains poorly defined, and consultation with a veterinary oncologist or dermatologist is strongly recommended.

Hepatoid Gland Tumors

(Perianal gland tumors, Circumanal gland tumors)

These common neoplasms arise from modified sebaceous glands that are most abundant in the cutaneous tissues around the anus but may also be present along the ventral midline from the perineum to the base of the skull, the dorsal and ventral tail, and in the skin of the lumbar and sacral regions. Because androgens stimulate the development of hepatoid glands, the incidence of proliferative lesions of hepatoid glands in intact, male dogs is three times that in females.

Benign hepatoid gland tumors are divided into hepatoid gland hyperplasias and adenomas; however, as with benign sebaceous gland tumors, there is a continuum from hyperplasia to adenoma. Here, they will be considered as a single entity. Hepatoid gland adenomas are most common in aged dogs. Siberian Huskies, Samoyeds, Pekingese, and Cocker Spaniels are most commonly affected. Tumors may develop at any site where hepatoid glands are present, but 90% are found in the perianal region. Grossly, they appear as one or (more commonly) multiple intradermal nodules 0.5–10 cm in diameter. Larger lesions commonly ulcerate, and hemorrhagic, proteinacious material can often be extruded with local pressure. Large tumors can compress the anal canal and make defecation difficult. Up to 95% of male dogs respond completely to castration; in those that do not, the pituitary-adrenal axis should be evaluated and, if no abnormality is detected, the dog should be reevaluated for the presence of a low-grade hepatoid gland adenocarcinoma. Excision may be used concurrently to remove extremely large or ulcerated tumors that have become secondarily infected. Surgery is the treatment of choice for females with hepatoid gland adenomas but may need to be repeated, because recurrence is common. Radiation therapy is also an option and has a 2-yr cure rate of 69% for benign tumors. Cryosurgery is another therapeutic alternative, but because of the complication of fecal incontinence, should be used only when tumors are not amenable to surgical intervention. Diethylstilbestrol has been used in the past as an alternative to castration, but because of severe adverse effects, including aplastic anemia and cystic prostatic hyperplasia, it should be used with extreme caution, if at all. Antiandrogens may have a role as an alternative to castration.

Hepatoid gland adenocarcinomas are uncommon canine neoplasms that generally appear as nodular lesions affecting the perianal region. These tumors are found in male dogs 10 times more commonly than in females. Siberian Huskies, Alaskan Malamutes, and Bulldogs are most likely to develop this tumor. Histologic evaluation is the best means of diagnosis; however, there is debate about how to distinguish low-grade malignant tumors from hepatoid adenomas, because well-differentiated forms can be confused with adenomas, and anaplastic forms can be confused with apocrine gland adenocarcinomas of anal sac origin. These tumors have metastatic potential and often spread to regional lymph nodes. Treatment consists of wide surgical excision including involved lymph nodes and, possibly, subsequent radiation. These tumors are generally not responsive to castration or to estrogen therapy; however, some studies show that the use of masitinib and other tyrosine kinase inhibitors may overcome chemoresistance, inhibit the proliferation of tumor cells, and prevent the emergence of metastasis. These findings may increase the benefit of combining targeted agents with various forms of chemotherapy such as oral piroxicam and capecitabine or with metronomic chemotherapy to prevent or treat local recurrence and metastatic disease. The overall prognosis is guarded.

Primary Cutaneous Neuroendocrine Tumors

(Merkel cell tumors, Atypical histiocytomas, Trabecular carcinomas, Extramedullary plasmacytomas)

In veterinary medicine, the diagnosis of tumors derived from Merkel cells (tactile, neurosecretory cells of epithelial derivation present in the basal cell layer of the epidermis) has fallen in disfavor, and most pathologists consider this tumor to be an extramedullary plasmacytoma. Merkel cell tumors most likely develop in animals but are not recognized as such.

Papillomas

(Warts)

Papilloma viruses are small, double-stranded DNA viruses of the Papovaviridae family. Some mammals have several distinct papilloma viruses: people have >20; cattle, 6; dogs, 3; and rabbits, 2. Different papilloma viruses often have considerable species, site, and histologic specificity. The virus is transmitted by direct contact, fomites, and possibly by insects. Papillomas have been reported in all domestic animals, birds, and fish. Multiple papillomas (**papillomatosis**) of skin or mucosal surfaces generally are seen in younger animals and are usually caused by viruses. Papillomatosis is most common in cattle, horses, and dogs. Single papillomas are more frequent in older animals, but they may not always be caused by viral infection.

When lesions are multiple, they may be sufficiently characteristic to confirm the diagnosis; however, there are many simulants of warts, and a definitive diagnosis requires identification of the virus or its cytopathic effects on individual cells—a change known as koilocytic atypia or koilocytosis.

In cattle, warts commonly are found on the head, neck, and shoulders, and occasionally on the back and abdomen. The extent and duration of the lesions depend on the type of virus, area affected, and degree of susceptibility. Warts appear ~2 mo after exposure and may last ≥1 yr. Papillomatosis becomes a herd problem when a large group of young, susceptible cattle becomes infected. Immunity usually develops 3–4 wk after initial infection, but papillomatosis occasionally recurs, probably due to loss of immunity.

Although most warts appear as epidermal proliferations that have a keratotic surface resembling a cauliflower (verruca vulgaris), some bovine papilloma viruses (bovine papilloma types 1 and 2) involve dermal fibroblasts and keratinocytes and appear as a papulonodule with a warty surface. Such fibropapillomas may involve the venereal regions, where they can cause pain, disfigurement, infection of the penis of young bulls, and dystocia when the vaginal mucosa of heifers is affected.

A form of persistent cutaneous papillomatosis with smaller numbers of papillomas may be seen in herds of older cattle. A bovine papilloma virus has been demonstrated in bladder tumors associated with bracken fern ingestion (*see* p 3089) and in upper GI tract papillomas of cattle in Scotland. It is believed that the papilloma virus acts as a co-carcinogen. When bovine papilloma virus type 1 or 2 is injected into the skin of horses, a dermal tumor similar to equine sarcoid develops.

In horses, small, scattered papillomas develop on the nose, lips, eyelids, distal legs, penis, vulva, mammary glands, and inner surfaces of the pinnae, often secondary to mild abrasions. They can be a herd problem, especially when young horses are kept together, but regress in a few months, as a foal's immune system matures. When they develop in older horses, they often persist for >1 yr. So-called aural plaques are also thought to be a flat form of papilloma (verruca planum). Equine papillomas are disfiguring but benign. They should be distinguished from verrucous equine sarcoid (*see* p 954).

In dogs, three clinical presentations of canine papilloma virus infection have been described. The first is **canine mucous membrane papillomatosis**, which primarily affects young dogs. It is characterized by the presence of multiple warts on oral mucous membranes from lips to (occasionally) the esophagus and on the conjunctival mucous membranes and adjacent haired skin. When the oral cavity is severely affected, there is interference with mastication and swallowing. A viral etiology has been clearly established for these lesions. Azithromycin therapy has been shown to speed up regression in dogs. The second presentation is **cutaneous papillomas**, which are indistinguishable from the warts that develop on or around mucous membranes. However, they are more frequently solitary and develop on older dogs. Cocker Spaniels and Kerry Blue Terriers may be predisposed. A definitive viral etiology has not been established, and lesions may be confused with cutaneous tags. A syndrome characterized by papillomatosis of one or more footpads has also been described. Clinically, lesions appear as multiple, raised keratin horns. A viral etiology has been suggested but not proved. The third presentation is **cutaneous inverted papillomas**, which have more in common clinically with intracutaneous cornifying epitheliomas. In this disease of young, mature dogs, lesions most commonly develop on the ventral abdomen, where they appear as raised papulonodules with a keratotic center. Infrequently, viral papillomas in dogs may progress to invasive squamous cell carcinomas.

In cats, papilloma virus infection appears most commonly as a multicentric squamous cell carcinoma (*see* p 945). The typical warty lesions associated with papilloma virus infection in most species are not present. Papillomas may affect the skin of goats, and infection on the teats has been reported to induce malignant transformation. In sheep, papillomas are rare and most commonly appear as fibropapillomas. In pigs, they are very rare and when present are identified as solitary or multiple lesions on the face or genitalia. (For discussion of papillomatosis in rabbits, *see* p 1950.)

A cutaneous fibroma occurs in white-tailed, black-tailed, and mule deer, and in antelope, moose, and caribou. It is caused by a papilloma virus that resembles a bovine papilloma virus and is found only in the epithelium that covers the tumors.

Infectious papillomatosis is a self-limiting disease, although the duration of warts varies considerably. A variety of treatments have been advocated without agreement on efficacy. Surgical removal is recommended if the warts are sufficiently objectionable. However, because surgery in the early growing stage of warts may lead to recurrence and stimulation of growth, the warts should be removed when near their maximum size or when regressing. Affected animals may be isolated from susceptible ones, but with the long incubation period, many are likely to have been exposed before the problem is recognized.

Vaccines are of some value as a preventive but are of little value in treating cattle that already have lesions. Because wart viruses are mostly species-specific, there is no merit in using a vaccine derived from one species in another. An intralesional lymphocyte T-cell immunomodulator, which stimulates T cells and endogenous interleukin 2 levels, may benefit individual animals that develop multiple or persistent warts. In addition to azithromycin, topical imiquimod cream may also help the immune system to resolve these warts in dogs.

When the disease is a herd problem, it can be controlled by vaccination with a suspension of ground wart tissue in which the virus has been killed with formalin. Autogenous vaccines may be more effective than those commercially available. It may be necessary to begin vaccination in calves as early as 4–6 wk of age with a dose of ~0.4 mL intradermally given at two sites. The vaccination is repeated in 4–6 wk and at 1 yr of age. Immunity develops in a few weeks but is unrelated to whatever mechanism is involved in spontaneous regression. If the animal was exposed to the virus before vaccination, immunity may develop too late to prevent warts. A vaccination program must be in effect for ~3–6 mo before its preventive value will be evident. Vaccination should be continued for ≥1 yr after the last wart disappears, because the premises may still be contaminated. Stalls, stanchions, and other inert materials can be disinfected by fumigating with formaldehyde.

EQUINE SARCOIDS

Equine sarcoids are the most commonly diagnosed tumor of equids, representing 20% of all equine neoplasms and 36% of all skin tumors in horses. Studies suggest there is no significant gender or age predisposition.

Equine sarcoids are rarely life threatening but can compromise function and be a major economic concern. Sarcoids may also cause significant welfare dilemmas, particularly in developing countries where equids, principally donkeys, are widely used as work animals (eg, brick-carrying donkeys in India).

Sarcoids can occur as single or multiple lesions in different forms, ranging from small, wart-like lesions to large, ulcerated, fibrous growths. Six distinct clinical entities are recognized: 1) Occult—flat, gray, hairless, and persistent; often circular or roughly circular. 2) Verrucose—gray, scabby, or warty in appearance and may contain small, solid nodules; possible surface ulceration; well-defined or cover large, ill-defined areas. 3) Nodular—multiple, discrete, solid nodules of variable size; may ulcerate and bleed. 4) Fibroblastic—fleshy masses, either with a thin pedicle or a wide, flat base that commonly bleed easily; may have a wet, hemorrhagic surface. 5) Mixed—variable mixtures of two or more types. 6) Malevolent—an extremely rare, aggressive tumor that spreads extensively through the skin; cords of tumor tissue intersperse with nodules and ulcerating fibroblastic lesions.

Lesions can develop anywhere on the body but are most common in the paragenital region, the ventral thorax and abdomen, and the head. They frequently are seen at sites of previous injury and scarring. Equine sarcoids can resemble other skin tumors such as benign fibropapillomas and also other cutaneous conditions such as exuberant granulation tissue (proud flesh). An individual lesion on a horse can be difficult to diagnose, but multiple tumors (often of more than one type) with characteristic features on an individual horse make the clinical diagnosis reasonably straightforward. A definitive diagnosis can be made by biopsy; however, acquiring the sample carries the risk of triggering a considerable and uncontrollable expansion of the lesion.

Bovine papillomavirus (BPV), primarily types 1 and 2, is now considered the main etiologic agent of equine sarcoids. There may also be a genetic predisposition associated with equine leukocyte antigens; particular breeds and bloodlines appear to be more susceptible to the disease.

The mode of transmission has not been confirmed. BPV-1 has recently been detected in several common fly species (eg, house fly and stable fly), and because there is an apparent predilection for sarcoid development at wound sites, it has been proposed that flies may act as vectors as they move between wound sites on different horses. Alternatively, BPV infection may be transmitted via stable management practices, such as the sharing of contaminated tack, or be passed into existing wounds from contaminated pasture.

There is a wide range of therapies for sarcoids, and many tumors recur. Pedunculated sarcoids with a discernible neck are ideally suited to ligation with rubber bands or elasticized suture material, usually in combination with a topical preparation once the tumor is detached. Other commonly used treatments include cryotherapy, surgical or laser excision, and local immune modulation (Bacillus Calmette-Guérin [BCG] therapy). Surgical excision with margins of at least 0.5–1 cm is recommended. Preplaced sutures or releasing incisions are often needed for primary closure. Local radiotherapy (interstitial brachytherapy), using permanently implanted radon-222 or gold-198 seeds or removable needles of radium-226, cobalt-60 or, more often, iridium-192 (^{192}Ir) implants, is a highly effective treatment for tumors less amenable to traditional therapy (eg, those on the limbs or around the eye). However, ^{192}Ir implants and other radioisotopes are expensive and not widely available but may be the best option for recurrent aggressive lesions. Sarcoids have a 15%–82% recurrence rate if treated by surgical excision alone. Excised sarcoids often regrow more aggressively within 6 mo, which may be due to activation of latent BPV in apparently normal tissue surrounding the lesion. Larger tumors may require a combination of therapies (eg, surgical debulking or CO_2 laser vaporization followed by topical or intracavitary chemotherapy or local electrochemotherapy).

Several promising treatments now available or in the final stages of clinical trials include the use of intra-tumoral bioabsorbable cisplatin beads/emulsion (9% recurrence rate), the application of topical imiquimod every other day for 32 wk or until resolution (60%), autologous implantation, and topical acyclovir creams for treatment of flat, occult sarcoids (68% response rate) or applied to the wound bed of larger tumors removed by surgical excision. Acyclovir is relatively inexpensive and has a wide safety margin, but its method of action is unknown. Other products used to treat sarcoids are topical ointments that contain heavy metals, thiouracils, and 5-fluorouracil; an escharotic salve containing bloodroot powder extract and zinc chloride; and an IV immunostimulant of nonviable *Propionibacterium acnes* and BCG. The development of preventive and/or therapeutic vaccines may form a significant part of disease control strategies in the future, but trials so far have shown limited success.

A novel therapeutic approach using small interfering RNA molecules to target viral gene expression is being investigated. This technique has been shown to selectively destroy BPV-1–infected equine skin cells in vitro.

CONNECTIVE TISSUE TUMORS

Benign Fibroblastic Tumors

Collagenous nevi are benign, focal, developmental defects associated with increased deposition of dermal collagen. They are common in dogs, uncommon in cats, and rare in large animals. They generally are found in middle-aged or older animals, most frequently on the proximal and distal extremities, head, neck, and areas prone to trauma. They are sessile to raised, dermal nodules, often with a papillated surface. Two forms are seen: one develops in the interfollicular dermis or subcutaneous fat that is not accompanied by adnexal involvement, and one incorporates adnexa and induces enlarged, often malformed follicles, sebaceous glands, and apocrine glands. This latter form has been called **focal adnexal dysplasia**. Excision of both forms is generally curative although, infrequently, expansive forms have been identified that may grow too large to be surgically removed.

Generalized nodular dermatofibrosis (dermatofibromas), recognized rarely in German Shepherds (believed to be an inherited, autosomal dominant trait) and even less commonly in other canine breeds, is a syndrome in which multiple collagenous nevi are associated with renal cystadenocarcinomas and, in females, multiple uterine leiomyomas. Skin lesions, first recognized when animals are 3–5 yr old, are characterized by the development of multiple collagenous nevi varying from barely palpable to large and nodular, generally on the limbs, feet, head, and trunk. They may be symmetrically distributed. Renal disease develops ~3–5 yr after the skin lesions are recognized. No known therapy can prevent development of the renal and uterine neoplasms.

Acrochordons (cutaneous tags, soft fibromas, fibrovascular papillomas) are distinctive, benign, cutaneous lesions of older dogs. These lesions are common, may be single or multiple, and can develop in any breed, although large breeds may be at increased risk. Most commonly, they appear as pedunculated exophytic growths, often covered by a verrucous epidermal surface. Treatment is optional, but a biopsy is recommended to confirm the diagnosis. Acrochordons are amenable to excision, electrosurgery, and cryosurgery, but dogs that develop one are prone to develop others over time.

Fibromas are discrete, generally cellular proliferations of dermal fibroblasts. Histologically, they resemble collagenous nevi or cutaneous tags. Fibromas occur in all domestic species but are primarily a tumor of aged dogs. Doberman Pinschers, Boxers (predisposed to developing multiple tumors), and Golden Retrievers are most at risk. The head and extremities are the most likely sites. Clinically, the lesions appear as discrete, generally raised, often hairless nodules originating in the dermis or subcutaneous fat. They palpate as either firm and rubbery (**fibroma durum**) or soft and fluctuant (**fibroma molle**). These lesions are benign, but complete excision is recommended if they change appearance or grow large.

Soft-tissue Sarcomas

This group of malignancies includes equine sarcoids, fibromatoses, fibrosarcomas, malignant fibrous histiocytomas, neurofibrosarcomas, leiomyosarcomas, rhabdomyosarcomas, and variants of liposarcomas, angiosarcomas, synovial cell sarcomas, mesotheliomas, and meningiomas. As a group, sarcomas are widely recognized, yet poorly characterized neoplasms. The confusion stems in part from the fact that spindle-cell sarcomas demonstrate much greater morphologic heterogeneity than carcinomas; often, features of one sarcoma are intermixed with features of another. Consequently, it is widely accepted that the cell of origin of all soft-tissue sarcomas is a primitive mesenchymal cell that can differentiate in many different directions. This makes it difficult to define histopathologic criteria necessary for making an unequivocal diagnosis of specific spindle-cell sarcomas.

In addition, comparing neoplastic mesenchymal cells with the normal cell they most closely resemble does not imply origin from those cells.

A second cause for the confusion stems from the difficulty in determining whether these are benign or malignant or what their biologic behavior will be in certain locations or breeds. Most spindle-cell sarcomas of domestic animals are locally infiltrative, difficult to excise, and yet seldom metastasize. Because, by definition, only malignant tumors have metastatic potential, these tumors should be considered benign; however, again by definition, benign neoplasms are not infiltrative, and those tumors should be considered malignant and treated aggressively from the start. In human pathology, infiltrative but nonmetastasizing mesenchymal spindle-cell tumors have been defined as sarcomas of intermediate malignancy, a concept used below.

Clinically, four general principles relate to spindle-cell sarcomas and soft-tissue sarcomas: The more superficial the location, the more likely the tumor is to be benign (deep tumors tend to be malignant). The larger the tumor, the more likely it is to be malignant. A rapidly growing tumor is more likely to be malignant than one that develops slowly. Benign tumors are relatively avascular, whereas most malignancies are hypervascular. The type of sarcoma, its size, location, stage and histologic grade (low, intermediate, high [or I, II, III]), which depends on the degree of differentiation, the number of mitotic figures per 10 high-power fields, and percent that is necrotic, will help guide treatment planning.

Surgical excision is the treatment of choice. Wide excision or amputation should be performed when anatomically feasible because spindle-cell sarcomas often infiltrate along fascial planes, making it difficult to determine from gross examination the peripheral margins of the tumor. The best, if not only, opportunity to completely remove a spindle-cell sarcoma is during the first surgical attempt. A presurgical biopsy should be performed and, if possible, tumor imaging with CT or MRI or ultrasound to provide a clear surgical plan that includes the intention of complete removal, with biopsy samples submitted for margin determinations. Those sarcomas that recur have a greater potential for metastasis, and the time to recurrence often shortens with each subsequent attempt at excision. In addition, many soft-tissue tumors have a pseudocapsule, which on gross examination gives the impression of complete encapsulation; these tumors should not be "shelled out," because neoplastic cells are usually present in the pericapsular connective tissues. Many sarcomas are shaped like an octopus, with tentacles that extend deeply into the tumor bed. Except for equine sarcoids, cryosurgery is usually not used for these tumors because some types, most notably fibrosarcomas, are resistant to freezing. Spindle-cell sarcomas generally do not respond well to conventional doses of radiation; however, higher doses have been reported to control ~50% of them for 1 yr. Surgical debulking followed by intraoperative placement of carboplatinum-containing biodegradable beads, intracavitary chemotherapy with follow-up intratumor bed chemotherapy, and/or follow-up radiation therapy are options to enhance local control.

Chemotherapeutic protocols for sarcomas that include targeted therapy agents such as tyrosine kinase (T-K) inhibitors have become more accepted as a means of treatment. Most older protocols involve the use of adriamycin often in combination with other agents, including cyclophosphamide, vincristine, dacarbazine, and methotrexate. Some clinicians prefer to use a combination of carboplatin, T-K inhibitors, and metronomic chemotherapy, whereas others rotate carboplatin with adriamycin. Although chemotherapy may cause temporary adverse events, it can improve the length and overall quality of life; it is seldom curative.

Fibromatosis (aggressive fibromatosis, extra-abdominal desmoids, desmoid tumors, low-grade fibrosarcomas, nodular fasciitis) is a sclerosing and infiltrative proliferation of well-differentiated fibroblasts derived from aponeuroses and tendon sheaths. They are generally seen on the heads of dogs, especially Doberman Pinschers and Golden Retrievers, where they are commonly diagnosed as nodular fasciitis. In veterinary medicine, the term nodular fasciitis is applied to two different diseases: one that behaves as a fibromatosis and one that commonly affects the periocular tissues (known as canine fibrous histiocytoma [*see* p 957]). Fibromatoses are infrequently diagnosed in cats and horses. Grossly, fibromatoses are generally indistinguishable from infiltrative fibrosarcomas; however, they can be differentiated on histologic examination. Focal lymphoid nodules are scattered throughout the tissues. The fibromatoses are locally infiltrative, with essentially no metastatic potential. If feasible, wide, complete excision with local control techniques as described above is the treatment of choice at diagnosis. Recurrence is common, and radiation therapy may be of value for local control.

Fibrosarcomas are aggressive mesenchymal tumors in which fibroblasts are the predominant cell type. They are the most common soft-tissue tumors in cats and are also common in dogs but rare in other domestic animals. In dogs, these tumors are most common on the trunk and extremities. Gordon Setters, Irish Wolfhounds, Brittany Spaniels, Golden Retrievers, and Doberman Pinschers may be predisposed. Fibrosarcomas vary markedly in their appearance and size. Neoplasms arising in the dermis may appear nodular. Those arising in the subcutaneous fat or subjacent soft tissues may require palpation to identify. They appear as firm, fleshy lesions involving the dermis and subcutaneous fat and often invade musculature along fascial planes. When tumors are multiple, they are usually found within the same anatomic region. Fibrosarcomas with abundant interstitial proteoglycans (connective tissue mucins) are called **myxosarcomas** or **myxofibrosarcomas**. Myxosarcomas remain poorly defined in veterinary medicine, and many of them could be characterized as variants of liposarcomas or malignant fibrous histiocytomas. Fibrosarcomas in dogs are invasive tumors; ~10% metastasize. Factors that affect whether a fibrosarcoma can be completely excised include the skill of the surgeon; rate of growth (as defined by the mitotic index and quantity of necrosis); degree of cellular atypia; and the tumor's infiltrative nature, size, and location (which may require imaging to define properly).

Three forms of fibrosarcoma are recognized in cats: a multicentric form in the young (generally <4 yr old) caused by the feline sarcoma virus (FSV); a solitary form in the young or old, in which FSV has not been implicated; and a fibrosarcoma that develops in the soft tissues where cats are commonly vaccinated (*see* p 2169). An association with rabies and feline leukemia virus vaccinations is better defined than with vaccinations for other viral or bacterial diseases. Aluminum hydroxide (commonly used in adjuvants) has been identified in vaccine-induced fibrosarcomas, and a prolonged proliferation of fibroblasts in response to the adjuvant may predispose these cells to undergo neoplastic transformation. These tumors appear as nodules or plaques between the shoulder blades, in the soft tissues of the proximal hindlimbs, or less commonly, over the lumbar areas. Although commonly classified as fibrosarcomas, vaccination-site sarcomas are extremely heterogeneous and may be appropriately called malignant fibrous histiocytomas (giant cell tumors), liposarcomas, osteosarcomas, or chondrosarcomas.

Wide and deep surgical excision is the treatment of choice for fibrosarcomas, but because the necessary margin extent is commonly underestimated, recurrence is common (>70% within 1 yr of the initial surgery). The rate of recurrence is >90% for vaccine-associated sarcomas. Even when surgical excision is clinically and histologically complete, recurrence is still the rule. Therefore, multimodal therapy combining presurgical imaging, aggressive surgery, intracavitary chemotherapy with carboplatin, followed by radiation therapy and IV carboplatin every 21 days for 4–6 treatments with tyrosine kinase (T-K) inhibitors as adjunctive therapy may yield the best results. Chemotherapy with carboplatin, doxorubicin and cyclophosphamide, or dacarbazine, along with T-K inhibitors, has been recommended for nonresectable tumors. Initial results using a biologic response modifier (used intratumorally before excision and followed by radiation therapy) appear promising. Further work suggests that its effectiveness as an adjunct to surgery and radiation may increase tumor-free intervals up to 20% compared with historical controls.

Fibrohistiocytic Tumors

These pleomorphic, mesenchymal tumors composed of fibroblasts and histiocytic cells (often present as multinucleated giant cells) remain poorly defined in veterinary medicine. A lesion called **canine fibrous histiocytoma** (nodular granulomatous episclerokeratitis, nodular fasciitis, proliferative keratoconjunctivitis, conjunctival granuloma, Collie granuloma) is recognized at the episcleral junction and cornea primarily in young to middle-aged (2–4 yr old) Collies, but the histologic features are more suggestive of a granulomatous inflammatory response than a neoplasm. As might be expected for a noninfectious inflammatory process, these are generally responsive to sublesional injections of 10–40 mg of methylprednisolone.

Malignant fibrous histiocytomas (extraskeletal giant cell tumors, giant cell tumors of soft parts, dermatofibrosarcomas) are most frequently found in the skin and soft tissues of cats, occasionally found in horses and mules, and rarely in the skin of other domestic species, including dogs. In cats, malignant fibrous histiocytomas are most common on the distal extremities or ventral cervical regions of the aged but may also be diagnosed at vaccination sites. In horses and mules, these have been described as giant cell tumors of soft parts. Seen in young adult to middle-aged Equidae, they are firm, nodular to diffuse swellings that are white on cut surface, with variable hemorrhage. Malignant fibrous histiocytomas are sarcomas of intermediate malignancy. They are locally invasive and tend to recur after attempts at complete excision but seldom metastasize. Radical excision is recommended.

Peripheral Nerve Sheath Tumors

Amputation neuromas (traumatic neuromas) are non-neoplastic, disorganized proliferations of peripheral nerve parenchyma and stroma that form in response to amputation or traumatic injury. They are most commonly identified after tail docking in dogs or neurectomy in the distal extremities of horses. The most common clinical presentation is a young dog that continuously traumatizes its docked tail. In horses, such a lesion appears as a firm, often painful swelling at a neurectomy surgery site. Excision is curative.

Neurofibromas and **neurofibrosarcomas** (perineuromas, neurilemmomas, nerve sheath tumors, hemangiopericytomas, neurothekomas, schwannomas) are spindle-cell tumors that arise from the connective tissue components of the peripheral nerve. They are believed to arise from Schwann cells, but they could also arise from mesenchymal cells, which produce the nonmyelinated connective tissues that surround the myelinated nerve fiber. In dogs, forms of this tumor can be virtually indistinguishable from hemangiopericytomas and may be the same tumor.

In dogs and cats, peripheral nerve sheath tumors of the skin are found in older animals. In cattle, they have a suspected genetic basis, may be multiple, can develop in both the young and old, and are generally an incidental finding at slaughter; they arise from the deep nerves of the thoracic wall and viscera, and cutaneous involvement is rare. Regardless of the species, these tumors appear as white, firm, nodules. *Attachment to* a peripheral nerve may occasionally be noted. Both benign and intermediate-grade malignant variants are recognized. Benign tumors are most common in cattle in which, because of their indolent nature, treatment is optional; also, additional tumors often develop spontaneously at other sites over time. In dogs, cats, and horses, most are locally infiltrative but do not metastasize. Complete excision is the treatment of choice. When margins are narrow or insufficient, followup radiation therapy, postoperative intralesional tumor bed chemotherapy (using the patient's serum mixed with the chemotherapy agent), electrochemotherapy, or systemic chemotherapy with carboplatin or metronomic chemotherapy may increase the tumor-free interval.

Adipose Tissue Tumors

Lipomas are benign tumors of adipose tissue, perhaps more accurately characterized as hamartomas. They are common in dogs, occasionally identified in cats and horses, and rare in other domestic species. In dogs, they generally develop in older, obese females, most commonly on the trunk and proximal limbs. The breeds most at risk are Doberman Pinschers, Labrador Retrievers, Miniature Schnauzers, and mixed-breed dogs. Older, neutered male Siamese cats are predisposed, and tumors are most commonly found on the ventral abdomen. Obesity does not appear to be a factor in the development of lipomas in cats. Affected horses are generally <2 yr old. Lipomas typically appear as soft, occasionally pedunculated, discrete nodular masses, and most are freely movable. In dogs and cats, >5% are multiple. In general, these tumors float when placed in formalin.

A rare variant of this tumor, **diffuse lipomatosis**, has been identified in Dachshunds. Virtually the entire skin is affected, resulting in prominent folds on the neck and truncal skin. Many lipomas merge imperceptibly with the adjacent non-neoplastic adipose tissue, making it difficult to determine when the entire lesion is excised. Lipomas with an abundant connective tissue stroma (fibrolipomas), cartilaginous stroma (chondrolipomas), or a prominent vascular component (angiolipomas) are also recognized. Despite their benign nature, lipomas should not be ignored because they tend to enlarge over time, and their gross presentation may be indistinguishable from that of infiltrative lipomas or liposarcomas (*see* below). Excision is curative. In dogs, dietary restriction to 70% of normal intake for several weeks before surgery may allow for better definition of the surgical margins of the tumor.

Infiltrative lipomas (intra- and intermuscular lipomas) are rare in dogs and even less common in cats and horses. In dogs, they are most common in middle-aged females, usually on the thorax and limbs. The breeds (dogs) most at risk are the same as those for lipomas. These tumors are poorly confined, soft, nodular to diffuse swellings that typically involve the subcutaneous fat and underlying muscle and connective tissue stroma. Infiltrative lipomas, which dissect along fascial planes and between skeletal muscle bundles, are considered sarcomas of intermediate malignancy. They rarely metastasize. Aggressive excision is recommended, and amputation may be necessary.

Liposarcomas are rare neoplasms in all domestic animals. Most are recognized in older male dogs in which they usually develop on the trunk and extremities; Shetland Sheepdogs and Beagles may be predisposed. In cats, feline leukemia virus infection has been infrequently associated with their development; whether this is a coincidence or such infections play a causative role remains unclear. Liposarcomas are nodular and soft to firm. They may exude a mucinous fluid when sectioned. Many have palpable, partially encapsulated areas, but these zones should not be construed as evidence of a benign tumor. Liposarcomas are malignant neoplasms that have a low metastatic potential but are frequently pseudoencapsulated. Wide excision is recommended. Recurrence is common, so followup radiation therapy is indicated in cases with insufficient margins.

Vascular Tumors

Hemangiomas of the skin and soft tissues are benign proliferations that closely resemble blood vessels. Whether these are neoplasms, hamartomas, or vascular malformations remains undefined, and no clear criteria exist that allow for their separation. They are most commonly identified in dogs, occasionally in cats and horses, and rarely in cattle and pigs; they are an exceptional finding in other domestic animals. In dogs, they are tumors of adult dogs and most commonly develop on the trunk and extremities. Many canine breeds (including Gordon Setters; Boxers; and Airedale, Scottish, and Kerry Blue Terriers) are considered to be at risk. Cats most frequently develop hemangiomas when they are adults. Lesions are most common on the head, extremities, and abdomen. In horses, they are most common on the distal extremities of young (<1 yr old) animals. In cattle, they may be seen as congenital lesions or in older animals. Dairy cattle are predisposed to developing disseminated hemangiomas (angiomatosis) in the skin and internal organs. In pigs, these lesions generally develop in the scrotal or perineal skin of Yorkshire, Berkshire, and less commonly Chester White boars. In the first two breeds, the disease is believed to be genetically transmitted. Hemangiomas are single to multiple, circumscribed, often compressible, red to black nodules. The lining epidermis may be unaffected or ulcerated or papillated. Small, superficial hemangiomas that often appear as a "blood blister" are known as angiokeratomas. When erythrocytes are sparse or absent within vascular lumens, the term lymphangioma is applied. Hemangiomas are benign, but their tendency to ulcerate and grow quite large, along with the importance of confirming the diagnosis to make a prognosis, indicate removal. Excision is the treatment of choice; however, in large animals in which the lesions may be large and involve the distal extremities, this may be difficult. In these cases, cryosurgery or radiation therapy may be necessary. Except in dairy cattle with angiomatosis, development of additional tumors at new sites after complete excision is uncommon.

Hemangiopericytomas (canine spindle-cell sarcoma, canine malignant fibrous histiocytoma, canine neurofibrosarcoma, canine perineuroma) are common in dogs and rare in cats (if they occur at all). This tumor was initially named because it was thought to be derived from fibroblastic cells that surround small vessels; however, the appropriateness of the name remains a topic of debate. These tumors develop most commonly on the distal extremities and thorax of older dogs. Females appear to be predisposed, and Siberian Huskies, mixed-breed dogs, Irish Setters, and German Shepherds are most at risk. Hemangiopericytomas typically present as firm, multilobulated, solitary lesions with irregular borders, most commonly in the subcutaneous fat but sometimes in the dermis. They are of intermediate malignancy and have limited metastatic potential. Complete excision with adequate margins is the treatment of choice but, because of the infiltrative nature of these tumors, excisions are incomplete or margins are narrow in most surgeries; therefore, ~30% recur. If the first excision of any sarcoma does not have adequate margins, ie, clean, wide surgical margins ("complete" may include narrow margins not considered adequate for local tumor control), followup surgery to remove the tumor bed and increase the margins is indicated. At surgery, intracavitary chemotherapy with carboplatin or 5-fluorouracil mixed with the patient's serum, and/or intraoperative radiation therapy with followup intratumor bed chemotherapy, and/or followup radiation therapy may increase the tumor-free interval.

Angiosarcomas, arguably the most aggressive of all soft-tissue tumors, are composed of cells that have many functional and morphologic features of normal endothelium. Although these tumors are often divided into hemangiosarcomas (of purported blood vessel origin) and lymphangiosarcomas (of lymphatic vessel origin), such a distinction is arbitrary. The term **angioendothelioma** is also used. These tumors generally arise spontaneously. In the nonpigmented skin of dogs with short, often white coats, chronic solar injury may induce transformation in the superficial vascular plexus, which initially appears as a hemangioma and then progresses to a malignant vascular tumor. The light-skinned breeds prone to actinically induced dermal angiosarcomas are Whippets, Italian Greyhounds, White Boxers, and Pit Bulls. Pathologists often diagnose these lesions as cutaneous hemangiosarcomas. Because histogenesis of dermal hemangiosarcoma is often related to that of chronic solar irritation, predisposed breeds should be protected from sun exposure. Dermal hemangiosarcomas have a moderately high potential for malignancy; therefore, wide surgical excision is the treatment of choice for tumors >0.5 cm. Cryosurgery or laser surgery can effectively control multifocal, small, early lesions. When metastasis occurs, it is by the hematogenous route to the lungs and spleen. Up to one-third of splenic hemangiosarcomas arise in the skin or peripheral tissue and end up in the spleen because of splenic filtering of cells in the bloodstream.

Angiosarcomas of the skin and soft tissues are seen in all domestic animals but are most common in dogs, generally in adult or aged animals. In dogs, they most frequently develop on the trunk, hip, thigh, and distal extremities. In addition to the breeds prone to actinically induced angiosarcomas, Irish Wolfhounds, Vizslas, Golden Retrievers, and German Shepherds are also at risk. In cats, this tumor is seen most commonly in older, neutered males, on the extremities and trunk. Cats with skin, *subcutaneous, or visceral* involvement develop distant metastasis. Angiosarcomas can vary markedly in appearance. Most commonly, they appear as one or more erythematous nodules present anywhere in the skin or underlying soft tissues. Less frequently, they appear as a poorly defined bruise. All grow rapidly, often are associated with large zones of necrosis and thrombosis, and typically are red to black on cut section. Tumors often diagnosed as lymphangiosarcomas may have much less lumenal blood, and the vascular spaces are typically filled with serum. Characteristically, angiosarcomas create their own vascular space by dissecting through soft tissues. Distant metastasis, especially to the lungs and liver, is common. In other domestic animals, these tumors do not appear to behave as aggressively, and postexcisional recurrence rather than metastasis is more common.

For all species, because of the aggressiveness of these nodules, wide excision with intraoperative placement of carboplatin beads or intracavitary carboplatin mixed with the patient's serum may be the treatment of choice. Solar-induced canine cutaneous hemangiosarcomas generally do not have an aggressive biologic behavior, although numerous lesions may continue to appear over a period of several years. Superficial lesions are easily destroyed with topical cryotherapy, which may control the disease for years; however, if lesions become large (>1 cm) or cystic, they are best controlled with excision. If multiple cystic lesions appear, the animal may benefit from a combination of local control and antiangiogenic therapy. Avoidance of further sun irradiation injury may reduce the development of new lesions; however, previously exposed skin may continue to develop lesions as a result of "field cancerization." Adjuvant chemotherapy consisting of vincristine, doxorubicin, and cyclophosphamide (the VAC protocol) has been reported to shrink angiosarcomas;

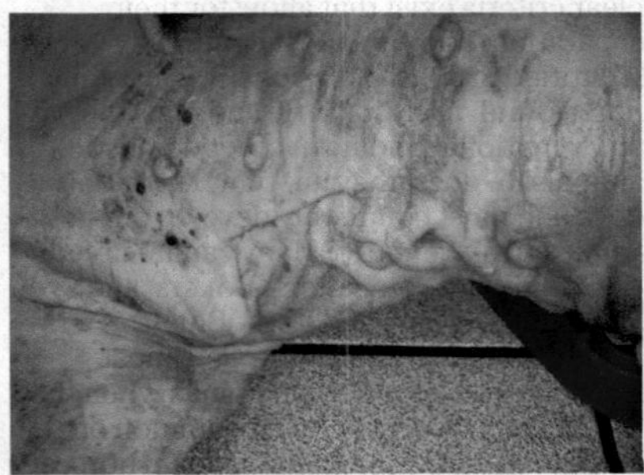

Solar-induced cutaneous hemangiosarcoma, older Bulldog. Lesions appear as multiple, red, flat or blood-filled cysts in sun-exposed nonpigmented skin. *Courtesy of Dr. Alice Villalobos.*

carboplatin is also helpful. However, the effects of chemotherapy for systemic control or radiation therapy for local control and longterm survival remain to be defined. Electrochemotherapy delivering bleomycin and platinum-containing drugs into tumors has shown cytotoxic efficacy leading to endothelial cell death in 1 to 3 treatment sessions under heavy sedation. These agents may also be administered intraoperatively. The role of NSAIDs such as piroxicam, meloxicam, etc, is still not completely understood and may vary from drug to drug. Antiangiogenic or angiostatic compounds such as canine recombinant canstatin that attack the blood supply of tumors may control and prevent metastases; however, results of clinical trials remain elusive.

Cutaneous Smooth Muscle Tumors

Because they either are not recognized or do not develop with any regularity in domestic animals, cutaneous smooth muscle tumors (leiomyomas or leiomyosarcomas) are diagnosed rarely. Those reported generally have been malignant and found in dogs and cats. Usually, they are firm cutaneous masses. Leiomyomas are small and tend to be limited to the dermis, whereas leiomyosarcomas are larger and most arise from (or extend into) the subcutaneous fat. The behavior of malignant smooth muscle tumors remains poorly defined. Complete excision is the treatment of choice for both leiomyomas and leiomyosarcomas. They have been responsive to vincristine chemotherapy given IV weekly for 6 wk then tapered; they may also respond to oral masitinib therapy and other tyrosine-kinase inhibitors.

UNDIFFERENTIATED AND ANAPLASTIC SARCOMAS

These malignant mesenchymal tumors are difficult to characterize microscopically. Undifferentiated sarcomas lack distinctive features (eg, architectural patterns, cytoplasmic and nuclear features, cell products). Anaplastic sarcomas have most of the following features: variations in size and shape of nuclei, nuclear hyperchromasia, striking irregularity of chromatin pattern, abnormal mitotic figures, and large numbers of mitotic figures. As such, anaplastic sarcomas are generally undifferentiated, but undifferentiated sarcomas do not have to be anaplastic. In both cases, excision should be deep and wide, with 3-cm margins along with a combination of the intraoperative and followup oncologic therapy techniques described above, because the first surgery with immediate followup is most important in determining outcome. The prognosis is generally poorer for anaplastic sarcomas than for undifferentiated sarcomas.

LYMPHOCYTIC, HISTIOCYTIC, AND RELATED CUTANEOUS TUMORS

Lymphoid Tumors of the Skin

Canine extramedullary plasmacytomas (atypical histiocytomas, cutaneous neuroendocrine tumors [*see* p 952], reticulum cell sarcomas, cutaneous nodular amyloidosis) are relatively common cutaneous tumors. Although their derivation was long debated, neoplastic cells characteristically express cytoplasmic immunoglobulin and may produce primary amyloid, leaving little doubt as to their lymphoplasmacytic origin. These tumors of dogs and, rarely, cats are most frequently identified on the head (including ears, lips, and oral cavity) and extremities of mature to aged animals. Cocker Spaniels, Airedales, Scottish Terriers, and Standard Poodles are most at risk. The tumors are generally small (<5 cm) and sometimes pedunculated. Most of these tumors are locally confined, and complete but conservative surgical excision is the treatment of choice. Infrequently, extracutaneous plasmacytomas may be locally invasive or multiple (or both), especially when they occur in the oral cavity. Recurrence has also been correlated with the presence of amyloid (*see* p 592). Treatment for these tumors targets local control using localized techniques described above. For recurrent, invasive tumors, more aggressive attempts at excision may be required. When tumors are multiple or when surgical excision is not feasible, radiation therapy appears to be the best secondary treatment. For tumors resistant to radiation and for those animals unable to receive radiation therapy, systemic treatment with chemotherapeutic agents, including melphalan, chlorambucil, cyclophosphamide, and glucocorticoids, have been recommended and have yielded longterm survival.

Cutaneous lymphosarcoma may occur as a disease in which the skin is the initial and primary site of involvement, or it may be secondary to systemic, internal disease. (*See also* CANINE MALIGNANT LYMPHOMA, p 40; BOVINE LEUKOSIS, p 743; and FELINE LEUKEMIA VIRUS AND RELATED DISEASES, p 790.)

Cutaneous lymphosarcoma is uncommon but has been identified in all domestic species. In general, two distinct forms are recognized—an epitheliotropic form (in which there is infiltration by malignant lymphocytes into the epidermis and adnexa) and a nodular, nonepitheliotropic form. Both usually express surface and cytoplasmic antigens characteristic of T cells; this, along with the frequent identification of at least small foci of epitheliotropism in many cases of "nonepitheliotropic" forms in dogs and cats, suggest they may be different variants of the same tumor.

Epitheliotropic cutaneous lymphosarcoma (ECL, mycosis fungoides) is the most frequently recognized form of cutaneous lymphosarcoma in dogs and arguably cats. It is a disease of middle-aged and older dogs, and Poodles and Cocker Spaniels may be predisposed. Classically, the lesions progress from patch to plaque to tumor; however, one or any combination of these three primary lesions may be present. For example, a form of ECL known as Pagetoid reticulosis has minimal to no dermal involvement, and cutaneous lesions always appear as erythematous patches. Another common feature of the disease in dogs is the presence of areas of alopecia due to follicular atrophy caused by infiltration of neoplastic cells into the outer sheath and lumen of hair follicles. Although most cases are associated with diffuse cutaneous involvement, forms limited primarily to mucous membranes or the footpads have been identified. Because of the variable clinical appearance of this tumor, diagnosis based on clinical features can be very difficult, and early stages can be confused with allergic, autoimmune, endocrine, infectious, or seborrheic diseases. Most cases are limited to the cutis until late in the course of the disease. ECL with concurrent leukemia is known as Sézary syndrome.

In dogs, ECL is a slow to moderately progressive disease for which a number of therapies have been attempted. To date, all appear more effective in improving the clinical features of the disease than in prolonging an affected dog's life. Methchlorethamine (nitrogen mustard) has been used in the past as a topical therapy, but because large areas of a dog's body may be affected (including the mucous membranes) and because of its sensitizing potential in people, it is infrequently used. The disease is often transiently responsive to steroids. Chemotherapeutic agents, such as combinations of adriamycin, chlorambucil, cyclophosphamide, doxorubicin, and vincristine, are variably effective. Lomustine (an alkylating nitrosourea), retinoids with and without glucocorticoids, and high-dose linoleic acid supplementation (safflower oil at 3 mL/kg, 3 consecutive days/wk) may occasionally achieve partial or complete remission. Studies show that a lymphocyte T-cell immunomodulator, which signals the differentiation of late stage CD_4 lymphocytes and causes apoptosis of malignant T cells, is a reasonable adjunctive therapeutic agent to use and may improve the clinical course in some cases.

ECL is rare in cats and tends to develop in older animals. Lesions often follow a defined progression, appearing initially as a crusty plaque that is variably pruritic. Biopsies of early lesions are often diagnosed as lymphocytic mural folliculitis. In many cases in which this diagnosis is applied, the lesions evolve into unequivocal cutaneous lymphosarcoma. In contrast to ECL in dogs, epitheliotropism is often extremely subtle in cats. Little is known about therapy or whether therapy used in dogs would be effective if used in cats; however, since the availability of a lymphocyte T-cell immunomodulator for use in cats with feline leukemia virus, it can be offered as a viable option.

Nonepitheliotropic cutaneous lymphosarcoma (NECL) is the most recognized form of cutaneous lymphosarcoma in all domestic animals but dogs and cats. In dogs, NECL is most common in middle-aged or older animals. Lesions are nodules or plaques that most commonly develop on the trunk. They generally are multiple, although solitary lesions may be noted, especially in cats. In many cases, NECL is grossly indistinguishable from the tumor stage of ECL. A definitive diagnosis is important because NECL in dogs is generally more aggressive than ECL, and systemic involvement occurs commonly and early in the course of the disease. Various modes of therapy, including excision, chemotherapy, and less frequently radiotherapy, have been used as monotherapy and in combination. Excision is the choice when the disease is limited to a solitary tumor, and complete cures have occasionally been obtained. Excision or cryosurgery in more diffuse forms infrequently elicit longterm remissions. Chemotherapy or chemoimmunologic protocols used for other forms of canine lymphosarcoma should be considered as palliative. The average remission time is ~8 mo.

In cats, NECL is a rare disease of middle-aged or older animals. The role of feline leukemia virus remains undefined. The lesions are plaques or nodules that may be solitary or multiple, alopecic or haired, and ulcerated or lined by an intact epidermis. Feline NECL is aggressive; even when complete excision of a solitary nodule is attempted, recurrence is common. No definitive therapy is known; however, using a combination of lomustine, steroids, linolenic acid (oil of evening primrose), and injections of a lymphocyte T-cell immunomodulator may be of some value.

In horses, NECL (nodular lymphosarcoma, subcutaneous lymphosarcoma, lymphohistiocytic lymphosarcoma) may be recognized at any age but is most common in young and middle-aged animals. Firm, nonulcerated nodules are most common in the subcutaneous fat of the ventral body surface. Microscopically, two types of nodular lymphosarcoma are recognized in horses. The most common consists of a mixture of histiocytes and small, well-differentiated lymphocytes, occasionally with plasmacytoid features; the second consists of a monomorphic population of large atypical lymphocytes, with only occasional histiocytic cells. Differentiation between these two forms is important because most cases of cutaneous lymphosarcoma in horses with a monomorphic pattern of cells have internal involvement, and the disease progresses rapidly. In contrast, the lymphohistiocytic form seldom is associated with internal involvement, and affected horses may live for years. As the lymphohistiocytic form progresses, the nodules tend to become more frequent on the ventral cervical regions. In many cases, euthanasia may be warranted when pharyngeal involvement induces dyspnea. Because of the expense of cytotoxic drugs, therapy is generally limited to glucocorticoids administered orally or intralesionally; remission, if induced, is usually short term.

In cattle, cutaneous lymphosarcoma is a disease of young animals (generally <4 yr old). It is one of the sporadic bovine leukosis syndromes that is not transmissible. The term sporadic bovine leukosis is usually reserved for calf, cutaneous, and thymic types of lymphoma, which are defined by the young age of occurrence and the distribution of tumors. The cause or causes are not known. Only lymphomas caused by bovine leukemia virus infection should be termed leukosis or enzootic bovine leukosis. There may also be lymphosarcomatous conditions that do not fall into either the sporadic or enzootic bovine leukosis categories, ie, adult multicentric lymphoma with sporadic occurrence of unknown etiology. Cutaneous lymphosarcoma of young cattle is presumed not to be associated with bovine leukemia virus infection (*see* p 743) and presently has an unknown etiology. The lesions are typically nodular, involve the dermis or subcutaneous fat, and are often ulcerated. There is no known therapy.

Cutaneous Mast Cell Tumors

(Mastocytomas, Mast cell sarcomas)

These tumors are the most frequently recognized malignant or potentially malignant neoplasms of dogs. In addition, visceral and leukemic forms can occur. A viral etiology has been speculated but remains controversial. Tumors may be seen in dogs of any age (average 8–10 yr). They may develop anywhere on the body surface as well as in internal organs, but the limbs (especially the posterior upper thigh), ventral abdomen, and thorax are the most common sites; ~10% are multicentric. However, studies suggest that multiple tumors do not carry a worse prognosis when they are all adequately excised if grade 1 or low grade. Initial size at the time of surgery is highly predictive of outcome; tumors >3 cm correlate with decreased survival time. Tumors that are incompletely excised, grow rapidly, or arise from mucocutaneous junctions, muzzle, ventrum, prepuce, or subungual areas or in animals with clinical signs at diagnosis are associated with more aggressive biologic behavior.

Many breeds appear to be predisposed, especially Boxers and Pugs (in which tumors are often multiple), Rhodesian Ridgebacks, and Boston Terriers. The tumors vary markedly in size, and clinical appearance alone cannot establish a diagnosis. Most commonly, they appear as raised, nodular masses that may be soft to solid on palpation. Although they often seem encapsulated, mast cell tumors in dogs are seldom discrete. Rather, they consist of a highly cellular center surrounded peripherally by a halo of smaller numbers of mast cells that palpate as normal skin. Dogs can also develop clinical signs associated with the release of vasoactive products from the malignant mast cells. Most common is gastroduodenal ulceration that may be present in up to 25% of cases. Cytologic evaluation of Wright-stained, fine-needle aspirates or impression smears can be used to establish the diagnosis of mast cell tumors in dogs. All skin tumors should be examined by fine-needle aspiration cytology before excision to exclude mast cell tumor. If the surgeon is aware that the tumor is of mast cell origin, a surgical plan for wide and deep excision will yield the best results. All mast cell tumors should be submitted for biopsy to determine margins and grade, because cytology is not a substitute for histopathology—only the latter has been well correlated with prognosis. However, certain cytologic features can be used to identify high-grade tumors. Two systems of histopathologic grading have been defined, the Bostock system of 1973 and the Patnaik et al system of 1984. To avoid confusion, it is essential to know which system is being used. The commonly used Patnaik grading system has the following designations: grade 1 = low grade, grade II = intermediate grade, grade III = high grade. Up to 80% of canine mast cell tumors are classified as grade II and are further divided into subgroups of low grade II (mitotic index ≤5) and high grade II (mitotic index >5) along with characteristics that may predict clinical behavior in this large category.

Although there is believed to be a benign variant of canine mast cell tumor, there is no clinical or microscopic means of identifying it. In addition, small mast cell tumors may remain quiescent for long periods before becoming aggressive. A subcutaneous variant of canine mast cell tumor, which does not have a primary infiltrative dermal involvement, occurred in ~10% of biopsied tissues in one study. This variant appeared most frequently in the hindlimb, with 66% having incomplete excision, most commonly at the deep margin. These tumors have intermediate histologic grade, a lower rate of recurrence (only 9%), and extended mean survival times, with only a 6% rate of metastases.

Up to 65% of incompletely excised mast cell tumors do not recur. This suggests that their biologic behavior is not always aggressive and that aggressive treatment may not always be warranted. Specialized stains can be used to distinguish tumor grades more adequately. Proliferation marker expression can help determine the likelihood that an incompletely removed mast cell tumor will recur or metastasize. The combination of Ki-67 >23/grid; proliferating cell nuclear antigen, Agnor count >54; mutations in exon 8 and exon 11 of c-Kit gene; and increased PCNA levels are prognostic for local recurrence and a poor prognosis. Correlation of test results with *survival times can be useful* but is not always a reliable predictor of the outcome. There is agreement on cytologic features for high-grade mast cell tumors: seven or more mitotic figures/10 high-power fields (hpf), three multinucleated cells/10 hpf, three bizarre nuclei/10 hpf, and karyomegaly in 10% of the cells. These high-grade features confer a prognosis of a 4-mo survival time vs >2 yr for low-grade mast cell tumors. Because of the difficulty of subcategorizing canine mast cell tumors, all should be treated as at least potential malignancies. The Mast Cell Tumor Panel to determine prognosis and treatment guidance can be requested for grade II tumors at the Diagnostic Center for Population and Animal Health at Michigan State University.

Treatment depends on the clinical stage of the disease and the predicted aggressive biologic behavior. For Stage I tumors (a solitary tumor confined to the dermis without nodal involvement), the preferred treatment is complete excision with a wide margin; at least 3 cm of healthy tissue surrounding all palpable borders should be removed in an attempt to excise both the nodule and its surrounding halo of neoplastic cells. Intraoperative cytology (examination of impression smears at the excised tissue margins) can guide the surgeon, who should continue to remove tissue until the margins are adequate and free of mast cells. If histologic evaluation suggests that the tumor extends beyond the surgical margins, reexcision or tumor bed excision should be attempted. Because mast cells are sensitive to radiation, intraoperative radiation therapy is an option along with followup external beam radiation therapy, which may be curative if the remaining tumor is small or microscopic. Combination or multimodal treatments using radiation therapy (if affordable), with intralesional chemotherapy and or local hyperthermia or electrochemotherapy along with systemic chemotherapy including tyrosine-kinase inhibitors, may be more effective than radiation alone to control biologically and locally aggressive mast cell tumors.

There is no agreed upon mode of therapy for Stage II-IV mast cell tumors; however, the advent of multikinase inhibitors represents a new option, which when used in combination with cytotoxic chemotherapy, requires dose reduction to avoid adverse events. Standard care options for Stage II tumors (a solitary tumor with regional lymph node involvement) include excision of the mass and the affected regional node (if feasible), prednisolone, and radiotherapy, used either singly or in combination. Triamcinolone or dexamethasone sodium phosphate, mixed with the patient's serum and injected evenly into the tissues of the tumor bed at the time of surgery or postoperatively as a followup series, may also help reduce recurrence. Intraoperative radiation therapy and/or followup external beam therapy is still considered the highest standard of care but is often declined because of cost. Injections into the tumor bed after incomplete excision using hypotonic, deionized, or distilled water has been debated. Treatment of Stage III (multiple dermal tumors with or without lymph node involvement) or Stage IV (any tumor with distant metastasis or recurrence with metastasis) tumors is generally considered palliative. One recommended therapy is prednisolone (2 mg/kg, PO, for 5 days, followed by a maintenance dose of 0.5 mg/kg/day) or intralesional injections of triamcinolone (1 mg/cm diameter of tumor, every 2 wk). Treatment with H_1- and H_2-receptor antagonists for the peripheral and gastric effects of histamine, respectively, may be indicated for animals with systemic disease or clinical signs referable to histamine release. Chemotherapy with vinca alkaloids (vincristine, vinblastine), L-asparaginase, and cyclophosphamide has also been used with some effectiveness. Prednisone and vinblastine used as adjuvant chemotherapy to incomplete surgical resection conferred an apparent improvement over historical survival data using surgery alone, yielding a 57% 1- and 2-yr disease-free state and a 45% survival at 1 and 2 yr for dogs with grade III tumors. In 19 dogs on a high dose of lomustine given every 21 days, 42% of mast cell tumors showed measurable responses, ranging from stable to partial with one complete response. Neutropenia appears 7 days after treatment, with neutrophil counts of 1,500 cells/μL. Vincristine doses must be lowered if used in combination with multikinase inhibitors. Lomustine at metronomic doses given daily along with multikinase inhibitors may be helpful and may avoid the adverse events associated with high-dose lomustine.

Novel small molecule multikinase inhibitors such as masitinib mesylate and toceranib phosphate are available to treat mast cell tumors and have been shown to be very helpful in management of difficult cases. They inhibit the c-Kit tyrosine kinase receptor, an activated or mutated proto-oncogene associated with the development of mast cell tumors. Tissue sampling to determine the biologic aggressiveness of mast cell tumors and to look for the presence of the mutated tyrosine kinase c-Kit receptor has been recommended before starting treatment, although evidence shows that many mast cell tumors respond regardless of their c-Kit status. A study of 202 client-owned dogs with or without prior treatment, having measurable cutaneous grade II or III mast cell tumors without nodal or visceral metastasis, found that masitinib (12.5 mg/kg/day, PO) was a relatively safe and beneficial treatment option. Another clinical trial found that toceranib (3.25 mg/kg, PO, every 48 hr), a receptor tyrosine kinase inhibitor, results in inhibition of Kit phosphorylation in canine mast cell tumors and was of clinical benefit with continued use. Note that the toceranib dosage stated on the package insert may lead to unacceptable toxicity. Veterinary oncologists are the most informed sources for clinical application using these novel tyrosine kinase inhibitor drugs against mast cell tumors, which may also benefit other malignancies.

In cats, cutaneous mast cell tumors are the second most common skin tumor; however, the disease is seen only occasionally in practice. In addition to cutaneous tumors, primary splenic, systemic, leukemic, and GI forms have been recognized. Two distinct variants of the cutaneous form occur—a mast cell type analogous to, but not identical with, cutaneous mast cell tumors in dogs, and a histiocytic type unique to cats. Feline cutaneous mast cell tumors may be either solitary or multiple. Primary splenic, systemic, recurrent, and multiple tumors (five or more) are associated with a guarded prognosis.

The mast cell type is most common. It is found primarily in cats >4 yr old and may develop anywhere on the body but most commonly on the head and neck. The tumors are single, alopecic nodules, generally 2–3 cm in diameter, that occasionally extend into the subcutaneous fat. Lymphoid nodules are common; eosinophils are rare. Unlike mast cell tumors in dogs, those in cats are generally benign; atypia and clinical behavior are poorly correlated. Surgical excision is the treatment of choice; 30% of tumors recur after surgery and some metastasize. Cryotherapy may be a good option to treat multiple recurrent small lesions to avoid anesthesia. Recurrent tumors may respond to chemotherapy, radiation therapy, and novel small molecule targeted therapy (*see* above).

The histiocytic type of cutaneous mast cell tumor in cats is recognized primarily in Siamese cats <4 yr old. Lesions may develop anywhere on the body and appear as multiple (miliary), small (generally 0.5–1 cm in diameter), firm, subcutaneous papulonodules. Usually, the older the cat, the fewer the lesions. This variant may be difficult to distinguish morphologically from a granulomatous inflammatory response. Because some of these tumors are reported to resolve spontaneously, treatment may not be necessary.

In horses, mast cell tumors are uncommon and generally benign, although metastasis has been reported and should be considered. There has been debate as to whether mast cell tumors are actually a neoplastic process or an unusual inflammatory response; however, they are currently considered a neoplastic process caused by a gain of function mutation of the Kit proto-oncogene. Lesions may develop anywhere on the body but are most common on the head and legs. Typically, there is a single, solitary mass in the dermis or subcutaneous fat that rarely expands to involve the underlying musculature. Erythema and wheal formation (Darrier sign) is not a clinical feature of equine mastocytoma. Most affected horses are male, with an average age of 7 yr (range 1–18 yr). The tumor begins as a nodule composed of a generally monomorphic proliferation of mast cells. As the lesion evolves, the mast cells are limited to aggregates in a fibrous stroma that surrounds large foci of liquefactive necrosis containing numerous eosinophils. In the late stages, the necrotic foci undergo dystrophic mineralization, and mast cells may be very difficult to identify. Once mineralization occurs, the lesion is gritty on sectioning. The classification system used to grade mast cell tumors in dogs is unreliable in horses because of the variable histologic appearance of tumors in this species. Alopecia and ulceration are variable features.

A variant of cutaneous mast cell tumor is seen in newborn foals, in which the lesions may become generalized but regress over time, suggesting an equine equivalent of urticaria pigmentosa in people.

Conventional therapy for equine metastatic mast cell cancer is suboptimal. Excision is the treatment of choice; however, lesions have been reported to metastasize occasionally. Affordable protein tyrosine kinase inhibitors or "small molecule" drugs such as masitinib mesylate and toceranib phosphate that selectively target mutated forms of the c-Kit tyrosine kinase receptors may become available in the future.

In pigs and cattle, mast cell tumors are rare. In pigs, most appear as discrete, solitary, cutaneous nodules. Most are benign but disseminated, and leukemic variants do occur. In cattle, most are malignant and characterized by multiple cutaneous nodules often accompanied by systemic involvement; purely cutaneous forms have been recognized occasionally.

Tumors with Histiocytic Differentiation

Tumors with histiocytic differentiation comprise a group of poorly defined skin diseases all characterized by a proliferation of histiocytes (tissue macrophages) in the absence of any known stimulus.

Cutaneous histiocytomas are common in dogs and rare in goats and cattle; it is debatable whether they are found in cats. Strong immunohistochemical evidence suggests that in dogs they are derived from Langerhans (intraepidermal antigen processing) cells. These tumors are typically seen in dogs <3.5 yr old but can be seen at any age. English Bulldogs, Scottish Terriers, Greyhounds, Boxers, and Boston Terriers are most at risk. The head (including the pinnae) and limbs are the most common sites of involvement. These classic "button tumors" appear as solitary, smooth, pink, raised nodules that are generally covered by alopecic skin, or they may be ulcerated. They are freely movable. Although a common neoplasm, histiocytomas are not always easy to diagnose histologically and can be confused with granulomatous inflammation, mast cell tumors, plasmacytomas, and cutaneous lymphosarcomas. Canine histiocytomas should be considered benign, and most resolve spontaneously within 2–3 mo without treatment. Surgical excision is optional once the diagnosis is established (which can often be made via cytology).

In goats and cattle, histiocytomas are extremely rare and behave the same as those in dogs. Histiocytomas have also been reported in young cats; however, they most likely represent the histiocytic form of mast cell tumor in cats.

Cutaneous histiocytosis is associated with development of numerous plaques and nodules involving the dermis or subcutaneous fat. It is rare in dogs and can develop at any age but is most common in young adults. Chinese Shar Pei, Collies, Border Collies, Shetland Sheepdogs, Briards, Bernese Mountain Dogs, Golden Retrievers, and German Shepherds may be predisposed. Shar-Pei have excessive skin folding and severe cutaneous mucinosis due to an accumulation of dermal hyaluronan, a protein associated with angiogenesis and tumor cell motility. The nodules and plaques tend to wax and wane, and the extremities and trunk are involved most commonly. Lesions also occur on the face and nasal planum, and swelling of the nares may cause difficulty breathing. Lesions are nonpruritic, and larger lesions may ulcerate. Cutaneous histiocytosis seldom involves internal organs, but its diffuse nature and the unsightly appearance often force the owner to consider euthanasia. Various forms of therapy have been tried, including systemic glucocorticoids and a combination of glucocorticoids and chemotherapy and more recently in combination with masitinib and other tyrosine kinase inhibitors. Leflunomide without steroids has been used as well as azathioprine and cyclosporine. Response is variable; the lesions in some dogs respond rapidly and permanently, whereas in others, lesions are either transiently improved or unchanged.

The **histiocytoses of Bernese Mountain Dogs** are systemic, familial disorders of unknown etiology with two manifestations: a more indolent and generally cutaneous form known as systemic histiocytosis and a more aggressive form in which skin lesions are rare, known as malignant histiocytosis. Malignant histiocytosis has been infrequently identified in other canine breeds. In systemic histiocytosis, males (mean age at onset 4 yr) are affected more often than females. There are multiple cutaneous nodules, papules, and plaques involving the skin (especially of the scrotum), nasal mucosa, and eyelids. The lesions are poorly circumscribed and variably alopecic and may be ulcerated; they develop in waves and slowly regress, only to recur several months later. The clinical disease tends to become more severe with each new wave of eruptions. Although the skin is the primary target organ, lesions may also develop in other organs, including lymph nodes, spleen, and bone marrow. The disease may be episodic in its clinical presentation, but it is progressive and eventually fatal.

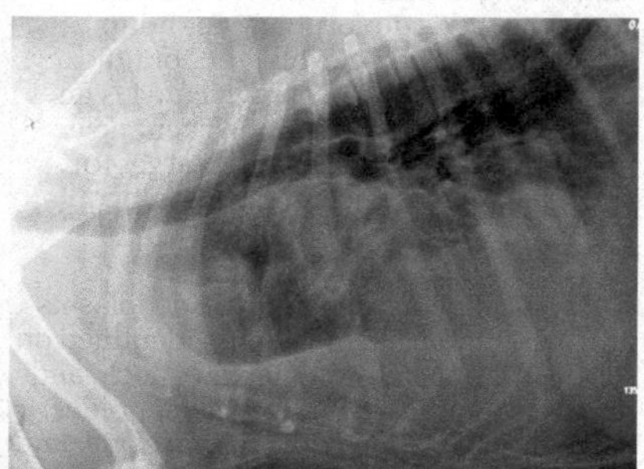

Malignant histiocytosis and pleural effusion in thorax of a dog. *Courtesy of Dr. Alice Villalobos.*

Malignant histiocytosis is seen in male Bernese Mountain Dogs (mean age at onset 7 yr) and, less frequently, in other canine breeds. The lungs, lymph nodes, and liver are the most common organs affected, and the disease tends to spare the skin. Grossly, the lesions appear as large, solitary, firm masses that may cause pleural effusion or efface large portions of affected internal organs. The disorder is rapidly progressive and does not wax and wane as does systemic histiocytosis. Few dogs survive >6 mo.

Various chemotherapeutic regimens mentioned above have been used to treat both forms; hopefully, masitinib and other tyrosine kinase inhibitors used in combination with vincristine or other combinations of antineoplastic drugs will be of benefit. Bovine thymosin fraction 5 may help induce remissions, especially in the systemic form. However, both forms of the disease are ultimately fatal.

Transmissible Venereal Tumors

See also CANINE TRANSMISSIBLE VENEREAL TUMOR, p 1408. These can also develop initially on haired skin due to inoculation via cutaneous injuries.

TUMORS OF MELANOCYTIC ORIGIN

These tumors are most common in dogs, gray horses, and miniature pigs; uncommon in goats and cattle; and rare in cats and sheep. The terminology used to describe melanocytic lesions in veterinary medicine is different from that used in human dermatology. In animals, the terms melanocytoma and malignant melanoma are used to describe benign and malignant melanocytic proliferations, respectively. In people, a benign melanocytic proliferation (whether congenital or acquired) is called a nevus, and the term melanoma by definition refers to a malignancy (ie, in people, there are no benign melanomas). In addition, although solar injury is a common cause of melanocytic tumors in people, actinic damage is seldom associated with development of analogous tumors in domestic animals.

Dogs: Melanocytomas of the skin are diagnosed much more frequently than malignant melanomas. They most commonly develop on the head and forelimbs in middle-aged or older dogs. There may be a predilection for males. Miniature and Standard Schnauzers, Doberman Pinschers, Golden Retrievers, Irish Setters, and Vizslas are the breeds in which these tumors are most commonly recognized. They can appear as macules or patches; as papules or plaques; or as elevated, occasionally pedunculated masses. Most have a pigmented surface. Although generally solitary, lesions may be multiple, especially in the breeds at risk. These tumors are benign, and complete excision is curative.

Malignant melanomas most commonly develop in dogs somewhat older than those that develop melanocytomas. Miniature and Standard Schnauzers and Scottish Terriers are most at risk. The mucocutaneous junctions of the lips, in the oral cavity (*see* p 366), and in the nail beds are the most common sites of development. Malignant melanomas of haired skin are rare, and most arise on the ventral abdomen and the scrotum. Males are affected more commonly than females. Most malignant melanomas appear as raised, generally ulcerated nodules that are variably pigmented depending on the melanin content; some malignant melanomas are amelanotic. When present on the mucocutaneous regions of the lip, the tumors may be pedunculated with a papillated surface; when present in the nail bed, they appear as swellings of the digit, often with loss of the nail and destruction of underlying bone, mimicking osteomyelitis. Whenever a toe is festering in an older dog, radiographs and a deep punch biopsy that includes bone are indicated for diagnosis. Canine malignant melanomas are locally aggressive and have a high potential for metastasis; however, there is considerable variability in reported survival times. Reported median survival times for dogs with oral malignant melanomas treated with definitive surgery alone are 511 days for WHO stage I disease, 324 days for stage II, and 336 days for stage III disease. A comprehensive study found that up to 32% of oral melanocytic tumors in dogs exhibited less aggressive biologic behavior, which emphasizes the need to accurately classify them in clinical trials.

Treatment generally consists of complete excision; however, the infiltrative nature of the tumor may make achieving adequate margins difficult. When present on the digits, amputation is indicated; when present on the mandible, a hemimandibulectomy may allow for complete excision with adequate margins and an acceptable postsurgical cosmetic appearance and survival. Lesions at rostral locations on the maxilla or mandible allowed the best survival times of 10.9 mo in one study. Melanomas are generally considered insensitive to radiation therapy, and there is no established chemotherapeutic protocol shown to be highly effective. Survival times range from 1–36 mo, indicating that individual variations in host defense mechanisms and aggressiveness of the tumor may play a role in establishing a prognosis. The nuclear protein Ki67 has been established as a highly sensitive and specific immunohistochemical marker for predicting the outcome of oral malignant melanoma, with indices >19.5 corresponding to lower survival times. A mitotic index of >4/10 high-power field and a nuclear atypia score of >30% also indicate poor survival times. In one study of 117 dogs with digit masses, 24 had melanoma and a median survival time of 12 mo, with 42% alive at 1 yr and 13% alive at 2 yr.

A series of novel xenogeneic gene therapy vaccinations using plasmid DNA encoding human tyrosinase can induce an immune response in dogs, resulting in antibody and cytotoxic T-cell responses that may shrink their melanomas. A canine melanoma vaccine was shown to have potential therapeutic value for dogs as an adjuvant therapy for completely removed oral melanoma and for some advanced malignant melanoma cases in clinical trials in the New York area. It was conditionally licensed in the USA in 2007; however, no benefit was found in a study that followed 23 vaccinated dogs and 17 nonvaccinated dogs in Michigan. A clinical trial using masitinib in combination with the canine melanoma vaccine in dogs with melanomas expressing mutated c-Kit and another study that adds doxorubicin for nonmutated c-Kit are being evaluated for efficacy. Chondroitin sulfate proteoglycan-4 is an immunohistochemical biomarker and a potential immunotherapeutic target for canine malignant melanoma, as in people.

Cats: Cutaneous melanocytic neoplasms are uncommon and most often identified on the head (especially the pinnae), neck, and distal extremities in middle-aged or older cats. An association with the oral cavity and subungual regions is less well defined than in dogs, and a higher percentage are malignant. Excision is the treatment of choice.

Horses: Most melanocytic neoplasms are in gray horses, in which the coat turns gray (or white) with age. They are especially common in Lipizzaners, Arabians, and Percherons, and 80% of gray or white horses of these breeds may be affected. They are generally recognized in older horses but usually begin their development when animals are 3–4 yr old. The perineum and the base of the tail are the most common sites of development, but these tumors may develop in any location, including the parotid area. The tumors are often multiple and may appear as coalescent, frequently pedunculated nodules that often extend in a linear arrangement up the tail base. They increase in size and number over time. Although most are benign, invasive variants, some with metastatic potential, can develop. Most are black on cross-section. Many gray horses have evidence of lymph node involvement; however, there is debate as to whether this represents metastasis or whether the intranodal melanocytes and melanophages represent a stimulation of extracutaneous melanocytes that are normally present in the lymph node. Treatment consists of surgical or cryosurgical removal; however, affected horses are predisposed to develop additional tumors over time. Little is known about the use of radiation or chemotherapy for the treatment of equine melanocytoma or malignant melanoma. Cimetidine was reported to be of value in controlling recurrence, but followup studies did not find benefit. Electrochemotherapy or intralesional chemotherapy with cisplatin or carboplatin after surgical debulking may be of benefit in the treatment of large or inoperable masses. Recurrent tumors do not develop resistance to cisplatin, and they can be treated a second time, sometimes with good results.

Melanocytic neoplasms of nongray horses are rare tumors usually found on the trunk and extremities of young (often <2 yr old) horses. They may represent expansion of a congenital lesion. Masses characteristically appear as solitary nodules. Most are benign; however, congenital malignant melanomas may infrequently develop. Such tumors are invasive, with little metastatic potential. Surgical excision or cryosurgery is the treatment of choice. If the tumors are benign and surgically extirpated, the prognosis is excellent. For invasive tumors, the prognosis is guarded.

Pigs: Melanocytic neoplasms of pigs are seen as congenital lesions and sporadically in adults of the Sinclair (Hormel) miniature pigs and Duroc and Duroc crosses. Selective breeding in these strains has increased the prevalence of tumors. These tumors develop both pre- and postnatally, anywhere on the body. Generally multiple, they can appear as pigmented macules or patches with smooth borders; as raised, often ulcerated pigmented lesions; or as deeper, slightly raised, blue masses. Deeply invasive melanomas are often associated with metastatic disease. The lymph nodes and lungs are the most common sites of metastasis. Not all of these tumors become invasive, and many undergo spontaneous regression associated with an intense lymphocytic infiltrate. Melanocytic lesions in pigs are not treated; because of the heritable nature of the disease, prevention by selective breeding is recommended if lesions are frequently recognized in a herd.

Cattle: Melanocytic neoplasms in cattle develop infrequently anywhere on the body. They can be found at any age but are most commonly recognized in young animals; congenital forms have been recognized. Angus cattle appear to be predisposed. Most commonly, the tumors are large nodular masses, densely pigmented on cut surface, and benign. Excision is curative for most; however, rare malignant variants have been recognized with distant metastasis.

Sheep: Melanocytic neoplasms in sheep are most common in middle-aged or older animals but have been recognized in neonates. They are most common in Suffolks and Angoras, in which they appear as multiple, densely pigmented dermal or subcutaneous masses. They should be considered malignant; metastasis is common.

Goats: Melanocytic tumors in goats are rare. They are most common in middle-aged or older animals and possibly in Angoras. There may be a site predilection for the coronary band and udder. Lesions are seen as solitary or multiple masses with variable pigmentation on cut surface. Most tend to grow rapidly, and metastasis is common.

METASTATIC TUMORS

The spread of a primary neoplasm to the skin is unusual in domestic animals. It is occasionally identified in dogs; less commonly in cats; and rarely in horses, cows, sheep, goats, and pigs. Although all malignant neoplasms are capable of secondary cutaneous involvement, metastatic potential is greatest in mammary gland adenocarcinomas, squamous cell carcinomas, transitional cell carcinomas, transmissible venereal tumors, pulmonary adenocarcinomas, and angiosarcomas. Although appearance is variable, the lesions most commonly are multiple, ulcerated papulonodules. Early cutaneous metastasis is characterized by aggregates of neoplastic cells within superficial and deep dermal vessels. As these lesions evolve, they extend into the dermis and are associated with effacement of adnexa. Generally, it is difficult to distinguish the primary neoplasm based on the morphologic features of a metastatic site. This is because only a small population of cells in the primary tumor have the potential for metastasis, and these cells may have different microscopic features. In cats, pulmonary adenocarcinomas appear to preferentially metastasize to the distal extremities, and when carcinomas are diagnosed on multiple feet, radiographic examination for a primary lung tumor should be performed. Cutaneous metastasis is usually a feature of aggressive tumors and is associated with a guarded to poor prognosis.

ACANTHOSIS NIGRICANS

Acanthosis nigricans is a clinical reaction in dogs characterized by axillary and inguinal hyperpigmentation, lichenification, and alopecia.

Etiology and Clinical Findings: Acanthosis nigricans is a disorder of hyperpigmentation. There is no sex predilection. Primary acanthosis nigricans is a genodermatosis that can occur in many breeds but particularly Dachshunds. Clinical signs are usually present by 1 yr of age in this breed. Secondary acanthosis nigricans or postinflammatory hyperpigmentation can occur in any breed of dog and at any age; it is most common in breeds predisposed to conditions that result in inflammation of the axillary or inguinal region due to conformational abnormalities, obesity, endocrinopathies (eg, hypothyroidism, hyperadrenocorticism, sex hormone abnormalities), axillary and inguinal pruritus associated with atopic dermatitis, food allergy, contact dermatitis, primary disorders of keratinization, and skin infections (eg, staphylococcal pyoderma, *Malassezia* dermatitis).

Clinical signs start with increased pigmentation in the axillary and/or inguinal region. In primary acanthosis nigricans, the hyperpigmentation is initially diffuse and noninflammatory. It tends to develop uniformly in the affected areas. In secondary acanthosis nigricans, the distribution is patchy and often starts with a lacey appearance. It may not develop in all areas at the same time. Inflammation is mild but becomes more severe with time. Lesions of postsecondary inflammation are not necessarily present in both the axillary and inguinal region, nor are they necessarily symmetric. In primary acanthosis nigricans, secondary inflammatory lesions (ie, lichenification) most commonly develop as a result of conformational friction. Postinflammatory hyperpigmentation is triggered by inflammation and/or friction. Lesions can develop into severe areas of hyperpigmentation, with marked lichenification, hair loss, and seborrhea. Often, these areas are odiferous and may be painful. The edges of these lesions are often erythematous; this is a sign of secondary bacterial and/or yeast pyoderma. With time, lesions may spread to the ventral neck, groin, abdomen, perineum, hocks, periocular area, and pinnae. Pruritus is variable and is usually the result of secondary microbial overgrowth (staphylococcal or *Malassezia* dermatitis) or pruritus from the underlying disease.

Diagnosis: The physical findings compatible with a clinical diagnosis of primary acanthosis nigricans are not difficult to recognize. Postinflammatory hyperpigmentation is a clinical sign of an underlying disease and should be aggressively evaluated through a careful history and physical examination to identify the underlying trigger. Skin scrapings should be performed to exclude demodicosis, and impression smears should be performed to confirm suspected bacterial and *Malassezia* infections. Postinflammatory inflammation associated with endocrinopathies is not pruritic, and testing for thyroid and adrenal disease may be useful in older dogs; endocrine skin diseases are not pruritic unless accompanied by secondary skin infections. Intradermal skin testing and/or a food trial may be necessary. Skin biopsies are usually not necessary to confirm primary disease and are usually not helpful in identification of underlying disease associated with secondary disease, with the possible exception of primary seborrhea. In some cases, skin biopsy can identify secondary bacterial infections not previously recognized. The presence of such infections is common; secondary infections are underdiagnosed in this condition. In most cases, it is useful to treat the secondary bacterial and/or *Malassezia* infections before proceeding with other diagnostic tests.

Treatment: Primary acanthosis nigricans in Dachshunds is not curable. In some dogs, lesions do not progress beyond a cosmetic problem. If inflammation is present, early cases may respond to antimicrobial shampoo therapy and local topical glucocorticoids, eg, triamcinolone acetate spray or betamethasone valerate ointment. As lesions progress, more aggressive systemic therapy may be useful. The following systemic therapies have been used, alone or in combination, with varying degrees of success: vitamin E, 200 IU, PO, bid, for 2–3 mo; systemic glucocorticoids, 1 mg/kg/day, PO, for 7–10 days, then on alternate days; melatonin, 2 mg/day/dog, SC, for 3–5 days, then weekly or monthly as needed. The concurrent treatment of secondary bacterial or *Malassezia* infections is helpful and is required before systemic glucocorticoids are administered; antimicrobial therapy is compatible with the other therapies. Antiseborrheic shampoos are often beneficial for removing excess oil and odor but must be used frequently (ie, 2–3 times/wk).

In postinflammatory hyperpigmentation, most of the lesions will resolve after identification and correction of the underlying cause. Some residual lacey hyperpigmentation may remain. Treatment of secondary bacterial and yeast overgrowth is critical. If the dog has not been previously treated for a staphylococcal bacterial infection of the skin, therapy with narrow-spectrum drugs based on culture and susceptibility and/or use of topical chlorhexidine spray or baths is recommended. Culture is recommended to minimize development of methicillin-resistant staphylococci. Yeast infections may be successfully treated with concurrent oral itraconazole or ketoconazole (5–10 mg/kg). Affected dogs benefit greatly from appropriate antimicrobial therapy and antiseborrheic shampoos (2–3 times/wk). If the lesions are caused by friction, emollients may be beneficial.

Clinical signs resolve slowly, possibly over months.

EOSINOPHILIC GRANULOMA COMPLEX

The cause of this group of diseases that affects cats, dogs, and horses is primarily an underlying hypersensitivity reaction. This is particularly true in cats and horses. Insect, environmental, and dietary hypersensitivities have been documented in cats, while insect hypersensitivity has been seen in some equine cases and in a smaller number of canine cases. Genetic predisposition and bacterial infections have also been noted as causes in cats. In all species, idiopathic cases exist.

CATS

In cats, three disease entities have been grouped in the complex.

Eosinophilic Ulcer: This well-circumscribed, erythematous, ulcerative lesion, often neither painful nor pruritic, is usually found on the upper lip. Some are associated with a hypersensitivity to flea bites. Although reported to occur, progression to squamous cell carcinoma is extremely rare. Histology shows an ulcerative dermatitis, with a cellular infiltrate of eosinophils, neutrophils, plasma cells, and mononuclear cells predominating. Mild to moderate fibroplasia is common. Peripheral eosinophilia is not as common as in the eosinophilic plaque or the linear granuloma. Occasional cases due to pyoderma or dermatophytes have been reported; thus, a fungal culture of the surrounding hairs is recommended.

Eosinophilic Plaque: This well-circumscribed, erythematous, raised lesion is most commonly found in the medial thigh and abdominal regions; it is extremely pruritic. Regional lymphadenopathy can be seen. Histology shows a diffuse eosinophilic dermatitis with marked epidermal inter- and intracellular edema and vesicles containing eosinophils. Mast cells may also be present in the dermis. Peripheral eosinophilia is common.

Eosinophilic Granuloma: These typically raised, well-circumscribed, yellowish to pink lesions may be found anywhere on the body but are most common on the caudal thighs and in the oral cavity. When these lesions develop on the head, face, bridge of the nose, pinnae, or pads of the feet, mosquito bites may be the inciting cause. The caudal thigh lesions are usually distinctly linear. Histologically, a granulomatous inflammatory response surrounds collagen fibers. Tissue and peripheral eosinophilia are marked when the lesions are in the mouth but vary when lesions are on the skin.

Treatment: Hypersensitivity disorders (allergy to fleas, food, or inhalants) should be investigated by instituting strict flea control, testing for environmental allergens (intradermal or in vitro), and conducting dietary elimination trials. Hyposensitization, continued insect control, and dietary management should be used when appropriate. Antibiotic therapy (amoxicillin-clavulanate, cephalosporins, or fluoroquinolones) should be tried empirically, especially in refractory cases. If no underlying cause can be determined and the condition is refractory, corticosteroids, such as methylprednisolone acetate (4 mg/kg, IM, once every 2 wk for 2–3 injections), oral prednisolone (2–4 mg/kg/day), or oral triamcinolone (0.8 mg/kg/day), can be tried. Oral corticosteroids should be tapered to alternate days (or to every third day in the case of triamcinolone) and dosages reduced when used for long-term management. Long-acting injectable methylprednisolone acetate should not be used more often than every 12 wk because of the potential to induce hyperadrenocorticism and/or diabetes mellitus. Cyclosporine (7 mg/kg/day) has been used successfully in the eosinophilic granuloma and plaque, less so in the lip ulcer. This may require laboratory monitoring (at least twice yearly) for metabolic (eg, renal) changes, although internal organ dysfunction is relatively rare. Progestational drugs, such as megestrol acetate or medroxyprogesterone acetate, have also been effective; however, they are not recommended because of their potential adverse effects.

DOGS

In dogs, the lesions reported as eosinophilic granulomas histologically resemble the eosinophilic granuloma of cats, with marked collagen degeneration surrounded by a granulomatous and eosinophilic infiltrate. These lesions may be seen as ulcerated or vegetative masses in the oral cavity or, less commonly, as plaques, nodules, or papules on the lips and other areas of the body. Any breed may be affected, but Siberian Huskies and Cavalier King Charles Spaniels may be at greater risk.

Most lesions respond to corticosteroids, and therapy is usually oral prednisone or prednisolone (0.5–2 mg/kg/day initially, tapering the dosage throughout 20–30 days). Lesions recur in some dogs, in which case low-dose, every-other-day corticosteroid therapy is indicated.

Canine eosinophilic furunculosis is a closely related disease. It has been reported in many breeds but typically is seen in long-nosed large breeds or curious small breeds (eg, terriers) with potential access to wasps, bees, ants, spiders, etc. It is thus felt to be due to arthropod bites or stings. Consistent with this, the disease may be very rapid in onset, leading to nasal/muzzle swelling, exudation, and pain. Large, swollen erythematous lesions on the muzzle are the most common lesions, but in some dogs similar lesions may be seen on the head, periocularly and around the pinna. Impression smears often show eosinophils. Although diagnosis is usually done on a clinical basis, histologic confirmation will show lesions similar to that of the canine eosinophilic granuloma but with more eosinophilic infiltration into the epidermis and follicular wall, a furunculosis, and fewer areas of eosinophilic debris-coated collagen. Treatment is as described for feline eosinophilic granuloma.

HORSES

In horses, the disease also has been termed equine eosinophilic granuloma with collagen degeneration, nodular necrobiosis of collagen, and collagenolytic granuloma. The lesions are nodular, nonulcerative, and nonpruritic. They often are found in the saddle, central truncal, and lateral cervical areas and may have a gray-white central core. Older lesions may become mineralized. Both insect bites and trauma have been suggested as causes, although the occasional onset during winter in cold climates and in noncontact saddle or tack areas suggests multifactorial causes. Histology reveals multifocal areas of collagen fibers surrounded by granulomatous inflammation containing eosinophils. Thus, histologically, this lesion is similar to eosinophilic granuloma of cats and dogs.

Solitary lesions may be treated with surgical excision or sublesional corticosteroid injections. Mineralized lesions often require excision. Triamcinolone acetonide (3–5 mg/lesion) or methylprednisolone acetate (5–10 mg/lesion) is effective. No more than a total of 20 mg triamcinolone acetonide should be administered sublesionally at any one time because of the potential to induce laminitis. Horses with multiple lesions may be treated with oral prednisone or prednisolone at 1.1 mg/kg/day, for 2–3 wk. In horses with recurrent lesions, intradermal allergy testing, particularly with insect antigens, is recommended. Hyposensitization and insect control can be palliative in some cases.

HYGROMA

A hygroma is a false bursa that develops over bony prominences and pressure points, especially in large breeds of dogs. Repeated trauma from lying on hard surfaces produces an inflammatory response, which results in a dense-walled, fluid-filled cavity. A soft, fluctuant, fluid-filled, painless swelling develops over pressure points, especially the olecranon. If longstanding, severe inflammation may develop, and ulceration, infection, abscesses, granulomas, and fistulas may occur. The bursa contains a clear, yellow to red fluid.

If diagnosed early and if still small, hygromas can be managed medically via aseptic needle aspiration, followed by corrective housing. Soft bedding or padding over pressure points is imperative to prevent further trauma. Surgical drainage, flushing, and placement of Penrose drains are indicated for chronic hygromas. Small lesions can be treated with laser therapy. Areas with severe ulceration may require extensive drainage, extirpation, or skin grafting procedures. Use of intrahygromal corticosteroids is not recommended. Severe lesions can develop into decubital ulcers.

Hygromas can become complicated with comedones and furunculosis. Furthermore, some dogs develop follicular cysts or calcinosis cutis circumscripta at these sites. A skin biopsy of atypical lesions or lesions that do not respond to conservative medical therapy is recommended.

MISCELLANEOUS SYSTEMIC DERMATOSES

A number of systemic diseases produce various lesions in the skin. Usually, the lesions are noninflammatory, and alopecia is common. In some instances, the cutaneous changes are characteristic of the particular disease. Often, however, the dermatosis is not obviously associated with the underlying condition and must be carefully differentiated from primary skin disorders. Some of these secondary dermatoses are mentioned briefly below and are also described in the chapters on the specific disorders.

Dermatosis may be associated with nutritional deficiency, especially of proteins, fats, minerals, some vitamins, and trace elements. However, this is uncommon in dogs and cats fed modern, balanced diets. Siberian Huskies, and occasionally other breeds, may develop a disease similar to parakeratosis in pigs and require additional zinc in their diet (elemental zinc at 2–3 mg/kg/day). Zinc-responsive dermatoses also have been reported in cattle, sheep, goats, and llamas and may be associated with either a higher individual requirement or a dietary deficiency. The latter may be precipitated by oversupplementation of calcium. A zinc-responsive dermatosis has also been reported in a dingo and a red wolf.

Dermatitis is sometimes seen in association with disorders of internal organs, such as the liver, kidneys, or pancreas. Hepatic parenchymal dysfunction has been associated with superficial necrolytic dermatitis (hepatocutaneous syndrome, diabetic dermatosis) in old dogs and rarely in cats. This has been associated with hypoaminoacidemia. The cutaneous lesions include erythema, crusting, oozing, and alopecia of the face, genitals, and distal extremities, as well as hyperkeratosis and ulceration of the footpads. The skin disease may precede the onset of signs of the internal disease. Histopathologic findings are diagnostic and include superficial perivascular to lichenoid dermatitis, with marked diffuse parakeratotic hyperkeratosis and striking inter- and intracellular edema limited to the upper half of the epidermis. Hyperglucagonemia has also been documented in dogs with this syndrome; however, dogs tend to have hepatic parenchymal dysfunction more commonly than glucagonomas. In dogs, therapy relies on IV or oral amino acid treatment or surgical removal of the glucagonoma. Skin fragility syndrome (excessive skin friability) in cats has been seen in association with pancreatic or hepatic neoplasia, hepatic lipidosis, or adrenal dysfunction. Pancreatic neoplasia has also been associated with crusting of the footpads and alopecia in cats. A generalized nodular dermatofibrosis syndrome in German Shepherds, and occasionally other breeds, associated with renal cystadenomas, cystadenocarcinomas, or renal epithelial cysts, has been reported. Histopathologic examination of the skin nodules reveals dense collagen fibrosis.

Poisoning by thallium sulfate (rat poisons, *see* p 3165), ergot (*see* p 3012), mercury (*see* p 3080), and iodides may cause various skin changes. Hyperkeratosis in cattle can be caused by chlorinated naphthalene toxicity.

In dogs, dermatosis can develop as a result of endocrine dysfunction (*see* THE ENDOCRINE SYSTEM, p 538 et seq). In males with Sertoli cell tumors, bilateral alopecia and occasional pruritus with a papular eruption may be seen. Intact female dogs with hormonal imbalances are usually pruritic and have a papular eruption, mammary tissue enlargement, and frequent estrous cycles. The skin lesions of both disorders may begin in the inguinal or flank region and progress cranially. Dermatosis due to neutering is not common in dogs and cats; when it does occur, it is generally nonpruritic, with mild alopecia in the perineal or inguinal areas.

Dermatoses have been seen in hypothyroidism (*see* p 553). The skin lesions are characterized by diminished hair growth and bilaterally symmetric alopecia. The skin is dry, scaly, thickened, and sometimes cool to the touch. Pyoderma and seborrhea may occur. The margins of the pinna may develop excess scale. In rare cases, cutaneous myxedema develops.

Faulty production of hypophyseal hormones may rarely cause dermatoses. Hypopituitarism is characterized by alopecia, especially in the axillary regions and on the lateral thorax and abdomen. Hyperadrenocorticism also is manifest by skin changes such as hyperpigmentation, alopecia, seborrhea, calcinosis cutis, and secondary pyoderma. In cats, the skin becomes extremely friable. In diabetes mellitus, pruritus and secondary infection sometimes occur, especially in cats with generalized *Malassezia* sp infection.

The canine nasal mite (*Pneumonyssoides caninum*, *see* p 1480) is a parasite found in the nasal cavity and sinuses of the dog. *P caninum* infection in dogs causes nonspecific clinical signs of the upper respiratory tract, such as sneezing, reverse sneezing, rhinitis, impaired scenting ability, and pawing at the muzzle.

Rarely, underlying neurologic disorders, especially in dogs, may manifest as cutaneous lesions. These include sensory neuropathies in English Pointers and Longhaired Dachshunds, cauda equina syndrome, pseudorabies, neoplasia of peripheral nerves, and syringomyelia and/or Chiari-like malformation of Cavalier King Charles Spaniels. Clinical signs generally include pruritus and/or scratching (sometimes "air scratching" in some cases of syringomelia/Chiari-like malformation) but also manifest as pain in the cauda equina syndrome and self-mutilation in the sensory neuropathies.

Treatment of all the above conditions depends on a specific etiologic diagnosis. Once this is established and managed, the skin lesions usually need only symptomatic care (eg, control of scratching) until they resolve with resolution of the primary disease.

NASAL DERMATOSES OF DOGS

(Collie nose, Nasal solar dermatitis)

Nasal dermatoses of dogs may be caused by many diseases. Lesions may affect the haired bridge of the muzzle, the planum nasale, or both. In pyoderma, dermatophytosis, and demodicosis, the haired portions of the muzzle are affected. In systemic lupus erythematosus or pemphigus, the whole muzzle is often crusted (with occasional exudation of serum) or ulcerated. In systemic and discoid lupus, and occasionally in pemphigus and cutaneous lymphoma, the planum nasale is depigmented, erythematous, and eventually may ulcerate. The normal "cobblestone" appearance of the nasal planum is effaced.

Nasal dermatosis due to solar radiation probably is not as common as previously thought and may often be a misdiagnosis for the lupus variants. In true nasal solar dermatitis, the nonpigmented areas of the planum nasale are affected first, and occasionally the bridge of the nose may become inflamed and sometimes ulcerated. The lesions are worse in the summer, although lupus and pemphigus may also show this seasonal variation.

Any of the diseases listed above may affect the periocular areas. (*See also* SYSTEMIC LUPUS ERYTHEMATOSUS, p 829, and AUTOIMMUNE SKIN DISORDERS, p 827.) A sudden onset of nasal swelling, erythema, and exudation is often eosinophilic furunculosis; this is thought to be caused by an arthropod sting or bite. The protozoal disease leishmaniasis may cause depigmentation of the nasal planum.

Treatment depends on the cause. Diagnostic tests should include skin scrapings, bacterial and fungal cultures, and biopsies for both histopathology and immunologic testing, although such testing is not used as often as in the past because of the increase in veterinary dermatopathologists who may be able to make the diagnosis based on histopathology alone. If systemic lupus erythematosus is considered, blood for an antinuclear antibody test should be obtained.

If the diagnosis is nasal solar dermatitis, a topical corticosteroid lotion (betamethasone valerate, 0.1%) may help relieve inflammation. Exposure to sunlight must be severely curtailed. Topical sunscreens may be effective but need to be applied at least twice daily. Treatment for eosinophilic furunculosis is systemic corticosteroids, prednisone or prednisolone at 1 mg/kg, bid, for 1 wk, after which the dosage should be gradually decreased over the course of 1 mo.

PARAKERATOSIS

Parakeratosis is a nutritional deficiency disease of 6- to 16-wk-old pigs characterized by lesions of the superficial layers of the epidermis. It is a metabolic disturbance resulting from a deficiency of zinc (*see also* p 2337) or inadequate absorption of zinc due to an excess of calcium, phytates, or other chelating agents in the diet. Predisposing factors include rapid growth, deficiency of essential fatty acids, or malabsorption due to GI diseases. Parakeratosis is unlikely in commercial swine unless errors have been made in diet formulation, but it may be seen in backyard pigs. The widespread use of high zinc levels in feed to prevent enteric disease in weaned pigs has further reduced the likelihood of the disease.

Signs are limited to the skin, although mild lethargy, anorexia, and growth depression may be seen in severe cases; there is little if any pruritus. The outstanding lesions are symmetrically distributed areas of excessive and abnormal keratinization of the epidermis with the formation of horny scale and fissures. Brown spots or papules are first seen on the ventrolateral areas of the abdomen and inner thigh, pastern, fetlock, hock, and tail regions. These lesions coalesce to involve larger areas until the entire body may be covered. The scale is horny, dry, and usually easily removed. Occasionally, secondary infection of the cracks and fissures causes them to fill with dark, sticky exudate and debris, which may resemble exudative epidermitis (*see* p 860); however, this usually occurs in younger piglets. Chronic sarcoptic mange and deficiencies of B vitamins or iodine must also be considered in the differential diagnosis. Clinical signs, skin biopsy, and low serum levels of zinc and alkaline phosphatase help confirm the diagnosis.

Highly satisfactory results can be obtained by adjusting the intake of calcium or zinc, or both. Nursery pig diets should contain 0.8%–0.85% calcium (with standardized total tract digestible phosphorus of 0.4%–0.45%) and 100 mg/kg of zinc, assuming daily feed intake of 280–500 g. Grower diets should contain 0.6%–0.65% calcium and 60 ppm zinc, whereas finisher diets should contain 0.45%–0.5% calcium and 50 ppm zinc. Sow and boar diets should contain 0.9% calcium and 150 ppm zinc. Correction of the deficiency results in rapid recovery.

PHOTOSENSITIZATION

Photosensitization occurs when skin (especially areas exposed to light and lacking significant protective hair, wool, or pigmentation) becomes more susceptible to ultraviolet light because of the presence of photodynamic agents. Photosensitization differs from sunburn and photodermatitis, because both of these conditions result in pathologic skin changes without the presence of a photodynamic agent.

In photosensitization, unstable, high-energy molecules are formed when photons react with a photodynamic agent. These high-energy molecules initiate reactions with substrate molecules of the skin, causing the release of free radicals that in turn result in increased permeability of outer cell and lysosomal membranes. Damage to outer cell membranes allows for leakage of cellular potassium and cytoplasmic extrusion. Lysosomal membrane damage releases lytic enzymes into the cell. This can lead to skin ulceration, necrosis, and edema. The time interval between exposure to the photodynamic agent and the onset of clinical signs depends on the type of agent, its dose, and the exposure to sunlight.

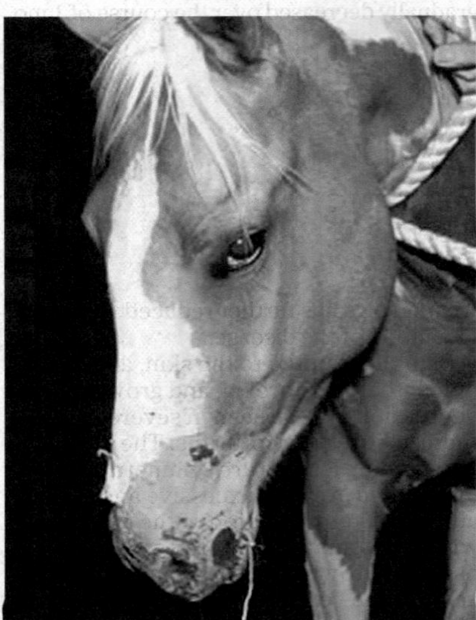

Photosensitization, causing cracking and peeling of the skin, in an adult horse. *Courtesy of Dr. Stephen White.*

Photosensitization is typically classified according to the source of the photodynamic agent. These categories include primary (type I) photosensitivity, aberrant endogenous pigment synthesis (type II) photosensitivity, and hepatogenous (secondary, type III) photosensitivity. A fourth category termed idiopathic (type IV) photosensitivity has been described.

A wide range of chemicals, including some that are fungal and bacterial in origin, may act as photosensitizing agents. However, most compounds that are important causes of photosensitivity in veterinary medicine are plant-derived. Photosensitization occurs worldwide and can affect any species but is most commonly seen in cattle, sheep, goats, and horses.

Primary Photosensitization: Primary photosensitization occurs when the photodynamic agent is either ingested, injected, or absorbed through the skin. The agent enters the systemic circulation in its native form, where it results in skin cell membrane damage after the animal is exposed to ultraviolet light. Examples of primary photosensitizing agents include hypericin (from *Hypericum perforatum* [St. John's wort]) and fagopyrin (from *Fagopyrum esculentum* [buckwheat]). Plants in the families Umbelliferae and Rutaceae contain photoactive furocoumarins (psoralens), which cause photosensitization in livestock and poultry. *Ammi majus* (bishop's weed) and *Cymopterus watsonii* (spring parsley) have produced photosensitization in cattle and sheep, respectively. Ingestion of *A majus* and *A visnaga* seeds has produced severe photosensitization in poultry. Species of *Trifolium*, *Medicago* (clovers and alfalfa), *Erodium*, *Polygonum*, and *Brassica* have been incriminated as primary photosensitizing agents. Many other plants have been suspected, but the toxins responsible have not been identified (eg, *Cynodon dactylon* [Bermudagrass]). Additionally, coal tar derivatives such as polycyclic aromatic hydrocarbons, tetracyclines, and some sulfonamides have been reported to cause primary photosensitization. Phenothiazine anthelmintics have been reported to cause primary photosensitivity in cattle, sheep, goats, and swine.

Aberrant Pigment Metabolism: Type II photosensitivity due to aberrant pigment metabolism is known to occur in both cattle and cats. In this syndrome, the photosensitizing porphyrin agents are endogenous pigments that arise from inherited or acquired defective functions of enzymes involved in heme synthesis. Bovine congenital erythropoietic porphyria (*see* p 986) and bovine erythropoietic protoporphyria (*see* p 852) are the most commonly reported diseases in this category.

Secondary (Hepatogenous) Photosensitization: Secondary or type III photosensitization is by far the most frequent type of photosensitivity observed in livestock. The photosensitizing agent, phylloerythrin (a porphyrin), accumulates in plasma because of impaired hepatobiliary excretion. Phylloerythrin is derived from the breakdown of chlorophyll by microorganisms present in the GI tract. Phylloerythrin, but not chlorophyll, is normally absorbed into the circulation and is effectively excreted by the liver into the bile. Failure to excrete phylloerythrin due to hepatic dysfunction or bile duct lesions increases the amount in the circulation. Thus, when it reaches the skin, it can absorb and release light energy, initiating a phototoxic reaction.

Phylloerythrin has been incriminated as the phototoxic agent in the following conditions: common bile duct occlusion; facial eczema (*see* p 3015); lupinosis (*see* p 3018); congenital photosensitivity of Southdown and Corriedale sheep (*see* p 978); and poisoning by numerous plants, including *Tribulis terrestris* (puncture vine), *Lippia rehmanni*, *Lantana camara*, several *Panicum* spp (kleingrass, broomcorn millet, witch grass), *Cynodon dactylon*, *Myoporum laetum* (ngaio), and *Narthecium ossifragum* (bog asphodel).

Photosensitization also has been reported in animals that have liver damage associated with various poisonings: pyrrolizidine alkaloid (eg, *Senecio* spp, *Cynoglossum* spp, *Heliotropium* spp, *Echium* spp [*see* p 978]), cyanobacteria (*Microcystis* spp, *Oscillatoria* spp), *Nolina* spp (bunch grass), *Agave lechuguilla* (lechuguilla), *Holocalyx glaziovii*, *Kochia scoparia*, *Tetradymia* spp (horse brush or rabbit brush), *Brachiaria brizantha*, *Brassica napus*, *Trifolium pratense* and *T hybridum* (red and alsike clover), *Medicago sativa*, *Ranunculus* spp, phosphorus, and carbon tetrachloride. Phylloerythrin is likely the phototoxic agent in many of these poisonings.

Type IV Photosensitivity: Photosensitivity in which the pathogenesis is unknown or the photodynamic agent is not identified is classified as type IV. One such example involved a case of primary photosensitivity in cattle presumed to be caused by *Thlaspi arvense* (field pennycress), even though field pennycress has not been reported to cause photosensitization. Outbreaks of photosensitization have been reported in cattle exposed to water-damaged alfalfa hay, moldy straw, and foxtail-orchardgrass hay. These cases were suspected to be hepatogenous in origin. *Ranunculus bulbosus* (buttercup) has also been presumed to be a cause of hepatogenous photosensitization. Other plants associated with photosensitization include winter wheat (cattle), *Medicago* spp (alfalfa), *Brassica* spp (mustards), and *Kochia scoparia* (fireweed). Many of these plants are believed to be type I photosensitizers. Forages such as oats, wheat, and red clover have been suspected in cases of photosensitization and may be associated with specific environmental conditions such as heavy rainfall.

Clinical Findings and Lesions: Dermatologic signs associated with photosensitivity are similar regardless of the cause. Photosensitive animals are photophobic immediately when exposed to sunlight and appear agitated and uncomfortable. They may scratch or rub lightly pigmented, exposed areas of skin (eg, ears, eyelids, muzzle). Lesions initially appear in white-haired, nonpigmented, or hairless areas such as the nose and udder. However, severe phylloerythrinemia and bright sunlight can induce typical skin lesions, even in black-coated animals. Erythema develops rapidly and is soon followed by edema. If exposure to light stops at this stage, the lesions soon resolve. When exposure is prolonged, lesions may progress to include vesicle and bulla formation, serum exudation, ulceration, scab formation, and skin necrosis. The final stage involves skin sloughing. In cattle, and especially in deer, exposure of the tongue while licking may result in glossitis, characterized by ulceration and deep necrosis. Irrespective of coat color, cattle may develop epiphora, corneal edema, and blindness.

Depending on the initial cause of the accumulation of the photosensitizing agent, other clinical signs may be seen. For example, if the photosensitivity is hepatogenous, icterus may be present. In bovine congenital erythropoietic porphyria, discoloration of dentin, bone (and other tissues), and urine often accompanies the skin lesions. Photodermatitis is the sole manifestation seen in bovine erythropoietic protoporphyria.

Diagnosis: Diagnosis of photosensitization is based on clinical signs, evidence or history of exposure to photosensitizing agents or hepatotoxins, and characteristic lesions. Photophobia in combination with erythema and edema of hairless, nonpigmented areas of skin is strongly suggestive of the disease. The period from exposure to photodynamic or hepatotoxic agents to the onset of clinical signs can vary from several hours up to 10 days. Clinical signs; increased serum biochemical measurements, including sorbitol dehydrogenase, gamma glutamyltransferase, alkaline phosphatase, and direct bilirubin; and gross or histologic signs of liver disease help support a diagnosis of hepatogenous photosensitization. A presumptive diagnosis of *porphyria is based on signalment* (sex, breed, age) combined with clinical signs, and a definitive diagnosis can be made by measuring porphyrin levels in blood, feces, and urine.

Treatment: The prognosis for animals with hepatogenous photosensitization and porphyria is poor; however, the prognosis for animals with primary photosensitization is generally good. Treatment involves mostly palliative measures. While photosensitivity continues, animals should be shaded fully or, preferably, housed and allowed to graze only during darkness. The severe stress of photosensitization and extensive skin necrosis can be highly debilitating and increase mortality. Corticosteroids, given parenterally in the early stages, may be helpful. Secondary skin infections and suppurations should be treated with basic wound management techniques, and fly strike prevented. The skin lesions heal remarkably well, even after extensive necrosis.

CONGENITAL PHOTOSENSITIZATION IN SHEEP

Southdown and Corriedale sheep may inherit a hepatobiliary incompetence that results in photosensitization.

In mutant Southdown sheep, the inherited defect involves hepatic uptake of unconjugated bilirubin and organic anions. Plasma levels of unconjugated bilirubin are consistently increased and, because bilirubin is partially excreted, icterus is not a clinical feature. Phylloerythrin is less effectively excreted, and affected lambs become photosensitized when they first begin grazing green plant material. Unless chlorophyll is excluded from the diet, or exposure to sunlight is prevented, lesions and stress of photosensitization result in death within weeks. Mutant sheep so protected develop progressive renal lesions in which radial, fibrous bands form in the medulla, along with increasing numbers of cystic tubules. The changes ultimately result in renal insufficiency and death. The liver is small, with pericanalicular deposits of lipofuscin. This semilethal trait appears to be inherited as a simple recessive trait. Elimination of carriers is the only feasible control.

In mutant Corriedale sheep, the hepatocellular incompetence involves excretion of conjugated bilirubin and other conjugated metabolites. There is no obvious icterus, but phylloerythrin excretion is sufficiently impaired to produce photosensitization. Hepatic pigmentation is obvious grossly. Brown-black, melanin-like pigment is confined to centrilobular parenchymal cells. This condition is transmitted as an autosomal recessive trait. Control is by detection and removal of carriers.

PITYRIASIS ROSEA IN PIGS

(Porcine juvenile pustular psoriasiform dermatitis)

Pityriasis rosea is a sporadic disease of unknown etiology of pigs, usually 8–14 wk old, but occasionally as young as 2 wk and very rarely in pigs as old as 10 mo. One or more pigs in a litter may be affected. The disease is mild, but transient anorexia and diarrhea have been reported. The initial skin lesions are characterized by small erythematous papules, which rapidly expand to form a ring (collarette) with distinct raised and reddened borders. The lesions enlarge at their periphery, and adjacent lesions may coalesce. The center of the lesion is flat and covered with a bran-like scale overlaying normal skin. The lesions are found predominantly on the ventral abdomen and inner thighs but occasionally may be seen over the back, neck, and legs. Characteristically, there is no pruritus, and recovery is spontaneous in 6–8 wk. Treatment is generally considered unnecessary. Diagnosis can usually be made from the characteristic lesions, but laboratory tests, culture, and biopsy may be used to differentiate it from dermatomycosis, exudative epidermitis, dermatosis vegetans, and swinepox.

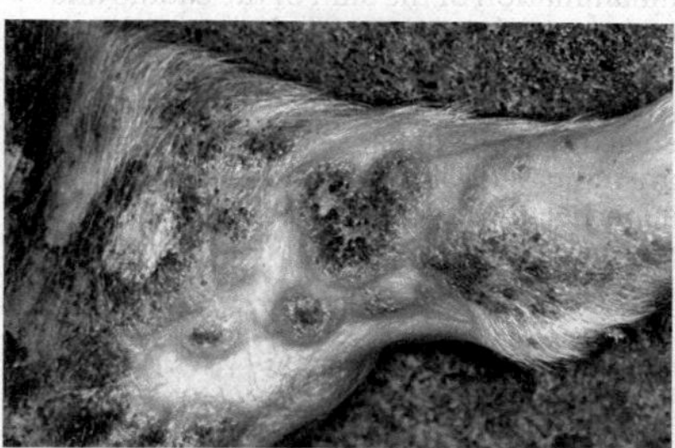

Pityriasis rosea lesions, hindlimb, pig. Note the small, ring-like early stage lesions and the older, expanding larger rings healing centrally as they expand. *Courtesy of Dr. Ranald D. A. Cameron.*

The disease is considered to be partially hereditary, pigs of the Landrace breed being most commonly affected, but the mode of inheritance is uncertain. The disease does not resemble pityriasis rosea in people clinically or pathologically.

Lesions appear to be more extensive in pigs reared in high stocking densities with high ambient temperatures and high humidity. Under these conditions, secondary bacterial infection (eg, *Staphylococcus hyicus*) is common. Treatment is of little value and does not affect the course of the disease; however, treatment aimed at controlling secondary infections may be warranted.

SADDLE SORES

(Collar galls)

The area of riding horses that is under saddle, or the shoulder area of those driven in harness, is frequently the site of injuries to the skin and deeper soft and bony tissues. Clinical signs vary according to the depth of injury and the complications caused by secondary infection. Emaciated horses are at increased risk. Sores affecting only the skin are characterized by inflammatory changes that range from erythematous to papular, vesicular, pustular, and finally necrotic. Frequently, the condition starts as an acute inflammation of the hair follicles and progresses to a purulent folliculitis. Affected areas show hair loss and are swollen, warm, and painful. The serous or purulent exudate dries and forms crusts. Advanced lesions are termed "galls." When the skin and underlying tissues are more severely damaged, abscesses may develop. These are characterized as warm, fluctuating, painful swellings from which purulent and serosanguineous fluid can be aspirated. Severe damage to the skin and subcutis or deeper tissues results in dry or moist necrosis. Chronic saddle sores are characterized by a deep folliculitis/ furunculosis (boils) with fibrosis or a localized indurative and proliferative dermatitis. Lesions are usually caused by poorly fitting tack.

Identification and elimination of the offending portion of tack is more important than any other treatment. Excoriations and inflammation of the skin of the saddle and harness regions are treated as any other dermatosis. Absolute rest of the affected parts is necessary. During the early or acute stages, astringent packs (Burow solution) are indicated. Chronic lesions and those superficially infected may be treated by warm applications and topical or systemic antibiotics. Hematomas should be aspirated or incised. Necrotic tissue should be removed surgically. In severe folliculitis and furunculosis, antibiotics, ideally chosen on the basis of culture and sensitivity, are always indicated. Scars and/or leukotrichia (white hairs) are common sequelae of healed areas. Recurrence of hematomas, seromas, and/or sloughing skin upon initial saddlings of a young Quarter horse or Paint horse should elicit suspicion of the genetic disease hereditary equine dermal asthenia. A simple DNA test, performed on the hair bulbs of the tail, will confirm this diagnosis.

SEBORRHEA

Primary idiopathic seborrhea is a skin disease seen in dogs and rarely in cats. It is characterized by a defect in keratinization or cornification that results in increased scale formation, occasionally excessive greasiness of the skin and hair coat, and often secondary inflammation and infection. Secondary seborrhea, in which a primary underlying disease causes similar clinical signs, is more common than primary seborrhea. Seborrhea in horses is usually secondary to either pemphigus foliaceus or equine sarcoidosis (chronic granulomatous disease).

Etiology, Clinical Findings, and Diagnosis: Primary seborrhea is an inherited skin disorder characterized by faulty keratinization or cornification of the epidermis, hair follicle epithelium, or claws. It is seen more frequently in American Cocker Spaniels, English Springer Spaniels, Basset Hounds, West Highland White Terriers, Dachshunds, Labrador and Golden Retrievers, and German Shepherds. There is usually a familial history of seborrhea, suggesting genetic factors. The disease begins at a young age (usually <18–24 mo) and typically progresses throughout the animal's life. A diagnosis of generalized primary idiopathic seborrhea should be reserved for cases in which all possible underlying causes have been excluded.

Most seborrheic animals have secondary *seborrhea, in which* a primary underlying disease predisposes to excessive scaling, crusting, or oiliness, often accompanied by superficial pyoderma, *Malassezia* (yeast) infection, and alopecia. The most common underlying causes are endocrinopathies and allergies. The goal is to identify and treat any underlying cause of the seborrhea. Palliative therapies that do not compromise the diagnostic evaluation should be instituted concurrently to provide as much immediate relief as possible.

Underlying diseases may present with seborrhea as the primary clinical problem. The signalment (age, breed, sex) and history may provide clues in diagnosing the underlying cause. Environmental allergies (atopic dermatitis) are more likely to be the underlying cause if age at onset is <5 yr, whereas an endocrinopathy or neoplasia (especially cutaneous lymphoma) is more likely if the seborrhea begins in middle-aged or older animals.

The degree of pruritus should also be noted. If pruritus is minimal, endocrinopathies, other internal diseases, or certain diseases limited to the skin (eg, demodicosis or sebaceous adenitis) should be excluded. If pruritus is significant, allergies and pruritic ectoparasitic diseases (eg, scabies, fleas) should be considered. The presence of pruritus does not exclude nonpruritic disease as the underlying cause, because the presence of a pyoderma, *Malassezia* infection, or inflammation from the excess scale can cause significant pruritus. However, a lack of pruritus helps to exclude allergies, scabies, and other pruritic diseases as the underlying cause.

Other important considerations include the presence of polyuria, polydipsia, or polyphagia; heat-seeking behavior; abnormal estrous cycles; occurrence of pyoderma; the influence of seasonality; diet;

response to previous medications (including corticosteroids, antibiotics, antifungals, antihistamines, or topical treatments); zoonosis or contagion; and the environment. The duration and severity of disease as well as level of owner frustration are important factors in determining the aggressiveness of the diagnostic plan.

A thorough physical examination, including internal organ systems and a comprehensive dermatologic examination, is the first step in identifying the underlying cause. The dermatologic examination should document the type and distribution of the lesions; the presence of alopecia; and the degree of odor, scale, oiliness, and texture of the skin and hair coat. The presence of follicular papules, pustules, crusts, and epidermal collarettes usually indicates the existence of a superficial pyoderma. Hyperpigmentation indicates a chronic skin irritation (such as pruritus, infection, or inflammation), and lichenification indicates chronic pruritus. Yeast (*Malassezia* spp) infection should always be considered when evaluating a seborrheic animal.

Secondary infection plays a significant role in most cases of seborrhea. The sebum and keratinization abnormalities that are common in seborrhea frequently provide ideal conditions for bacterial and yeast infections. The self-trauma that occurs in pruritic animals increases the likelihood of a secondary infection. Often, coagulase-positive *Staphylococcus* spp or *Malassezia* spp are present. The infections add to the pruritus and are usually responsible for a significant amount of the inflammation, papules, crusts, alopecia, and scales.

One of the first diagnostic steps is to obtain superficial cytology of the affected areas to identify the quantity and type of bacteria or yeast present. If numerous cocci and neutrophils are present, pyoderma is likely. In addition to systemic therapy, topical shampoos will aid in the treatment of secondary infections. In a seborrheic dog with pruritus, the infection may cause all or most of the pruritus. Instead of considering allergies as the underlying disease in these dogs, nonpruritic diseases (eg, endocrinopathies) may be uncovered by addressing the infections.

After the infections have been addressed, other diagnostic tests that should be considered include multiple deep skin scrapings, dermatophyte culture, impression smears, trichograms, and flea combing. If these are negative or normal, a skin biopsy, CBC, serum biochemical profile, and complete urinalysis will complete the minimum database. Examples of diagnostic clues include increased serum alkaline phosphatase (which may suggest hyperadrenocorticism or previous steroid therapy), cholesterol (which may suggest hypothyroidism), blood glucose (which suggests diabetes mellitus), and BUN or creatinine (which may suggest renal disease).

Treatment: Palliative therapy is needed to keep the animal comfortable while the underlying cause is identified and secondary skin diseases are corrected. For treatment of pyoderma, an antibiotic with known sensitivity against *Staphylococcus pseudintermedius* should be appropriate. Examples of such antibiotics are amoxicillin-clavulanate 13.75 mg/kg bid, cephalexin 20–30 mg/kg bid-tid, cefpodoxime 5–10 mg/kg/day, lincomycin 20 mg/kg bid, ciprofloxacin 30 mg/kg/day, enrofloxacin 5–10 mg/kg/day, marbofloxacin 3–6 mg/kg/day, azithromycin 10 mg/kg/day, 4 days/wk, doxycycline 5 mg/kg bid, trimethoprim-sulfa 30 mg/kg bid, clindamycin 11 mg/kg bid, and chloramphenicol 50 mg/kg tid in dogs and 12.5–20 mg/kg bid in cats. Because most staphylococcal infections in seborrhea cases are superficial pyodermas, they should be treated for a minimum of 4 wk.

With the increase in methicillin-resistant *S pseudintermedius*, *S aureus*, and *S schleiferi*, it is now strongly recommended to perform a bacterial culture of any animal with pyoderma that does not begin to respond to an antibiotic after 3–4 wk. Epidermal collarettes may be cultured using a dry sterile culturette rolled across the collarettes. Although methicillin-resistant *S pseudintermedius* infections are more difficult to treat, they are not more virulent or visually striking than those due to methicillin-susceptible *S pseudintermedius*. Previous (ie, within the past year) hospitalization, surgery, or previous antibiotic treatment are all possible risk factors for development of methicillin-resistant *S pseudintermedius* infections.

Malassezia may be treated systemically with an azole such as ketoconazole or fluconazole (5 mg/kg/day, for 4 wk). In addition to addressing any secondary infections, antipruritic therapy and shampoo therapy are usually needed to help control the seborrhea and speed the return of the skin to a normal state. Shampoo therapy can decrease the number of bacteria and yeast on the skin surface, the amount of scale and sebum present, and the level of pruritus; it also helps normalize the epidermal turnover rate.

In the past, seborrhea has been classified as seborrhea sicca (dry seborrhea), seborrhea oleosa (oily seborrhea), or seborrheic dermatitis (inflammatory seborrhea). Most seborrheic animals have varying degrees of all three of these classifications of seborrhea.

Most products contained in shampoos can be classified based on their effects as keratolytic, keratoplastic, emollient, antipruritic, or antimicrobial. **Keratolytic products** include sulfur, salicylic acid, tar, selenium sulfide, propylene glycol, fatty acids, and benzoyl peroxide. They remove stratum corneum cells by causing cellular damage that results in ballooning and sloughing of the surface keratinocytes. This reduces the scale and makes the skin feel softer. Shampoos containing keratolytic products frequently exacerbate scaling during the first 14 days of treatment because the sloughed scales get caught in the hair coat. The scales will be removed by continued bathing, but owners should be warned that the scaling often worsens initially. **Keratoplastic products** help normalize keratinization and reduce scale formation by slowing down epidermal basal cell mitosis. Tar, sulfur, salicylic acid, and selenium sulfide are examples of keratoplastic agents. **Emollients** (eg, lactic acid, sodium lactate, lanolin, and numerous oils, such as corn, coconut, peanut, and cottonseed) are indicated for any scaling dermatosis, because they reduce transepidermal water loss. They are most effective after the skin has been rehydrated and are excellent adjunct products after shampooing. **Antibacterial agents** include benzoyl peroxide, chlorhexidine, ethyl lactate, tris-EDTA, and triclosan. **Antifungal ingredients** include chlorhexidine, sulfur, ketoconazole, and miconazole. Boric and acetic acids are also used as topical antimicrobials.

It is important to know how individual shampoo ingredients act, as well as any additive or synergistic effects they have, because most shampoos are a combination of products. The selection of appropriate antiseborrheic shampoo therapy is based on hair coat and skin scaling and oiliness, of which there are four general presentations: 1) mild scaling and no oiliness, 2) moderate to marked scaling and mild oiliness (the most common), 3) moderate to marked scaling and moderate oiliness, 4) mild scaling and marked oiliness. These categories are intended to guide the type of shampoo therapy necessary; however, all factors for each individual animal should be considered.

Animals with mild scaling and no oiliness need mild shampoos that are gentle, cleansing, hypoallergenic, or moisturizing. These shampoos are indicated for animals that have mild seborrheic changes, are irritated by medicated shampoos, or bathed too often. These products often contain emollient oils, lanolin, lactic acid, urea, glycerin, or fatty acids. Emollient sprays or rinses are often used in conjunction with these shampoos.

Animals with moderate to marked scaling and mild to marked oiliness should be bathed with shampoos that contain sulfur and salicylic acid. Both agents are keratolytic, keratoplastic, antibacterial, and antipruritic. In addition, sulfur is antiparasitic and antifungal. Some of these shampoos also contain ingredients that are antibacterial, antifungal, and moisturizing, which can help control secondary pyoderma, *Malassezia* spp, and excessive scaling. Shampoos that contain ethyl lactate lower the cutaneous pH (which has a bacteriostatic or bactericidal action by inhibiting bacterial lipases), normalize keratinization, solubilize fats, and decrease sebaceous secretions. These actions also result in potent antibacterial activity.

In the past, dogs with moderate to severe scaling and moderate oiliness were often treated with tar-containing shampoos. However, because tar shampoos usually have an unpleasant odor and can be irritating, along with poor owner compliance, they usually are no longer recommended.

In animals with severe oiliness and minimal scaling, profound odor, erythema, inflammation, and a secondary generalized pyoderma or *Malassezia* dermatitis are often present. Shampoos that contain benzoyl peroxide provide strong degreasing actions along with potent antibacterial and follicular flushing activities. Because benzoyl peroxide shampoos are such strong degreasing agents, they can be irritating and drying. Other antibacterial shampoos are better suited in animals that have superficial pyoderma without significant oiliness. These shampoos usually contain 2%–4% chlorhexidine (often in assoication with tris-EDTA) or ethyl lactate. The follicular flushing action of benzoyl peroxide makes it helpful for animals with numerous comedones or with demodicosis. Benzoyl peroxide gels (5%) are good choices when antibacterial, degreasing, or follicular flushing actions are desired for focal areas, such as in localized demodicosis, canine acne, or Schnauzer comedone syndrome. However, these gels also may be irritating.

METABOLIC DISORDERS

METABOLIC DISORDERS INTRODUCTION

Metabolic diseases may be inherited or acquired, the latter being more common and significant. Metabolic diseases are clinically important because they affect energy production or damage tissues critical for survival.

METABOLIC STORAGE DISORDERS AND INBORN ERRORS OF METABOLISM

Storage diseases and inborn errors of metabolism are classified as either genetic or acquired. These diseases are characterized by the accumulation or storage of specific lysosomal enzyme substrates or byproducts within cells because of partial or complete deficiency of those enzymes. Although lysosomal storage diseases are often widespread throughout the body, the majority of clinical signs are due to the effects on the CNS.

Genetic storage diseases are named according to the specific metabolic byproduct that accumulates in the lysosomes. Animals are typically normal at birth, then manifest clinical signs within the first weeks to months of life. These diseases are progressive and usually fatal, because specific treatments do not exist. In small animals, the gangliosidoses (GM_1 and GM_2) are seen in Siamese, Korat, and domestic cats, and in Beagle crosses, German Shorthaired Pointers, and Japanese Spaniels. Sphingomyelinosis is seen in German Shepherds and Poodles and in Siamese and domestic shorthaired cats. Glucocerebrosidosis is seen in Australian Silky Terriers and Dalmatians. Ceroid lipofuscinosis is seen in English Setters, Cocker Spaniels, Dachshunds, Chihuahuas, Salukis, Border Collies, and domestic cats. Mannosidosis is seen in Persian and domestic cats. Glycogenosis is seen in Silky Terriers and in domestic shorthaired and Norwegian forest cats. Globoid cell leukodystrophy (Krabbe disease) is seen in Cairn Terriers, West Highland White Terriers, Beagles, Bluetick Hounds, Poodles, and domestic shorthaired cats. Mucopolysaccharidosis type I is seen in Siamese, Korat, and domestic shorthaired cats; type IV is seen in Siamese cats. In dogs, mucopolysaccharidosis is seen in Miniature Pinschers, Plott Hounds, and mixed-breed dogs and is associated with lameness. Diseases associated with decreased RBC survival and anemia include pyruvate kinase deficiency in Basenjis, Beagles, and West Highland White and Cairn Terriers; phosphofructokinase deficiency in English Springer and American Cocker Spaniels; and porphyria in Siamese and domestic shorthaired cats.

In large animals, α-mannosidosis occurs in Angus, Murray Grey, Simmental, Galloway, and Holstein cattle. β-Mannosidosis is seen in Saler cattle and Nubian and Nubian-cross goats. Generalized glycogenosis (GM_1) is seen in Holstein cattle and Suffolk sheep. Generalized glycogenosis (GM_2) is seen in Shorthorn and Brahman cattle, and in pigs. Globoid cell leukodystrophy is seen in polled Dorset sheep. Other identified diseases that are manifest by neurologic signs and appear to be inherited include neuronal lipodystrophy in Angus and Beefmaster cattle, shaker calf syndrome of horned Hereford cattle, maple syrup urine disease of Hereford and polled Shorthorn cattle, and hereditary neuraxial edema of polled and horned Hereford and Hereford-Friesian cross cattle. There have been no reports of lysosomal storage diseases in horses; however, inherited diseases manifest by neurologic signs include inherited myoclonus of Peruvian Paso foals and congenital encephalomyelopathy in Quarter horses.

Other inherited diseases that involve basic errors of metabolism in various tissues include goiter of sheep and goats, inherited parakeratosis (edema disease) of cattle, osteogenesis imperfecta of sheep and cattle, and possibly cardiomyopathy of cattle, the hypotrichoses, baldy calves, photosensitization of sheep (*see* p 978), dermatosis vegetans and porcine stress syndrome (*see* p 1027) of pigs, dermatosparaxia and Ehlers-Danlos syndrome of cattle, hemochromatosis of cattle (*see* p 349), and Marfan syndrome in cattle. Many other inherited defects, especially those based on abnormal growth of collagen, cartilage, and bone, also are likely to have basic errors of metabolism of structural tissues. Many disorders of metabolism have been described involving dysfunctions of the immune system.

Acquired storage diseases are caused by ingestion of plants that contain inhibitors of specific lysosomal catabolic enzymes. Chronic ingestion of locoweed plants (*Astragalus* or *Oxytropis* spp) results in an acquired neurologic storage disease. Several toxic components, including locoine, swainsonine n-oxide, and indolizidine alkaloids, interfere with α-mannosidase activity. Horses are most susceptible to intoxication; however, cattle, sheep, and goats can also be affected. (*See also* p 3103.)

PRODUCTION-RELATED METABOLIC DISORDERS

Although the development of the following diseases is largely related to production or management factors, the pathogenesis of each disease is primarily related to alterations in metabolism. In most cases, the basis of disease is not a congenital or inherited error in metabolism, but rather an increased demand for a specific nutrient that has become deficient under certain conditions. Diseases such as hypocalcemia, hypomagnesemia, and hypoglycemia are augmented by management practices directed toward improving and increasing production. They are therefore correctly considered production diseases. However, they are also metabolic diseases because management of the animal is directed at production, which at its peak is beyond the capacity of that animal's metabolic reserves to sustain a particular nutrient at physiologic concentrations. For example, parturient paresis of cows (*see* p 988) occurs when the mass of calcium in the mammary secretion is greater than the cow's diet or its skeletal reserves can supply. Comparable situations occur with magnesium and glucose metabolism, and with phosphorus in relation to postparturient hemoglobinuria (*see* p 1002).

Most production-induced metabolic diseases result from a negative balance of a particular nutrient. In some cases, dietary intake of the nutrient is rapidly reduced because of an ongoing, high metabolic requirement for that nutrient. Examples include pregnancy toxemia in ewes (*see* p 1021), protein-energy malnutrition in beef cattle (*see* p 2248), fat cow syndrome in dairy cattle (*see* p 1018), and hyperlipemia in ponies (*see* p 346). Furthermore, some diseases may be precipitated when producers, primarily because of economic concerns, are compelled to not supplement the diet of animals that already have a substandard nutritional plane.

Exertional rhabdomyolysis of horses (*see* p 1178) is another production-induced metabolic disease. In this case, the production activity (draft or racing) is maintained by and matched to a level of caloric intake. Management decisions not to work or race these horses without a concomitant decrease in caloric intake may result in accumulation of muscle glycogen to dangerous levels. Disease results when work is resumed and the production of lactate exceeds its metabolism.

The difference between production-related metabolic diseases and nutritional deficiencies is often subtle. Typically, nutritional deficiencies are longterm, steady-state conditions that can be corrected through dietary supplementation. Metabolic diseases are generally acute states that dramatically respond to the systemic administration of the deficient nutrient or metabolite, although affected animals may require subsequent dietary supplementation to avoid recurrence. An important aspect of dealing with production-induced metabolic diseases is accurate and rapid diagnosis. Ideally, diagnostic tests can be used to predict the occurrence of disease before its clinical onset.

CONGENITAL ERYTHROPOIETIC PORPHYRIA

(Porphyrinuria, Pink tooth, Osteohemochromatosis)

Congenital erythropoietic porphyria (CEP) is a rare hereditary disease of cattle, pigs, cats, and people that results from a significant yet variable decrease in uroporphyrinogen III synthase (URO-synthase) activity. URO-synthetase is the fourth enzyme in the heme biosynthesis pathway, and it normally converts hydroxymethylbilane to uroporphyrinogen III. With decreased URO-synthase activity, hydroxymethylbilane accumulates primarily in erythrons and is nonenzymatically converted to uroporphyrinogen I. Further decarboxylation of uroporphyrinogen I leads to the formation of various porphyrinogen I isomers, with coproporphyrinogen I occurring as the final product. Coproporphyrinogen l cannot be further metabolized to heme and is thus nonphysiologic. Porphyrinogen l isomers are pathogenic when they accumulate in large amounts and are oxidized to their corresponding porphyrins. Accumulation of porphyrinogen isomers in bone marrow erythroid precursors results in cell damage and hemolysis. Porphyrin I isomers are also released into circulation and deposited in skin, bone, and other tissues. Cutaneous photosensitivity occurs, because porphyrins deposited in skin are photocatalytic and cytotoxic. Presumably, exposure of skin to sunlight (and other sources of long-wave ultraviolet light) leads to phototoxic excitation of isomers, formation of oxygen radicals, and subsequent tissue and vessel damage. Urinary porphyrin excretion is greatly increased (100–1,000 times normal) and primarily consists of uroporphyrin l and coproporphyrin I with lesser amounts of other isomers. Although isomer l porphyrins predominate, isomer lll porphyrins are also increased.

CEP was first reported in South African Shorthorn cattle; however, most cases have since been reported in the Holstein breed. It is inherited as a simple autosomal recessive and is usually confined to herds in which inbreeding or close line-breeding is practiced. It has been recognized in the USA, Canada, Denmark, Jamaica, England, South Africa, Australia, and Argentina. This broad geographic distribution suggests that the disease likely is found worldwide and probably affects all meat-producing animals, especially cattle, swine, and sheep.

Heterozygous animals seem to be normal, but homozygous recessive animals are affected at birth with reddish brown discoloration of the teeth, bones, and urine that persists for life. The excess coproporphyrin I and uroporphyrin I in the urine colors it an amber or reddish brown. Bones, urine, and teeth (especially the deciduous teeth) fluoresce pink when irradiated with near-ultraviolet light. Prolonged exposure to sunlight causes typical lesions of photosensitization with hyperemia, vesicle formation, and superficial necrosis of unpigmented portions of the skin. Severity of the skin lesions depends on the intensity of the solar radiation and the extent of cutaneous pigmentation found in specific families of animals. A normochromic, hemolytic anemia with macrocytes and microcytes and marked basophilic stippling develops. Splenomegaly eventually develops. The texture of bones is not altered except in cases in which bones have increased fragility because of a diminished cortex. Affected animals are generally of medium to good condition unless solar injury has occurred. Some animals become progressively unthrifty unless protected from sunlight. A similar disease, bovine protoporphyria (*see* p 852), causes photosensitivity only in Limousin cattle and people. A recent molecular study of CEP in cattle supports the hypothesis that CEP is caused by a mutation affecting the URO-synthetase gene; however, additional functional studies are needed to identify the exact causative mutation.

In people, a series of porphyrias caused by defective functions of enzymes in porphyrin-heme biosynthesis have been described and grouped according to their presenting signs. These vary broadly and may include severe cutaneous lesions on exposed areas of the body, acute photosensitivity reactions, serious liver damage, and acute attacks of neurologic dysfunction. In animals, the recognized diseases are commonly classified as CEP, congenital erythropoietic protoporphyria, or porphyria. It is likely that all of the syndromes described in people also occur in animals and that a broader classification could be used.

Porphyria in swine is rare and incompletely described. Affected pigs have discoloration of teeth and excessive uroporphyrin in urine. In contrast to CEP in cattle and people, affected swine are not anemic and do not present with signs of photosensitization. The specific genetic defect is unknown; therefore, its relevance to CEP in other animals is also unknown. Nonetheless, the disorder is inherited as an autosomal dominant trait.

Recently, the first feline model of human CEP due to deficient URO-synthase activity was identified by characteristic clinical phenotype and confirmed by biochemical and molecular genetic studies. In this case, sequencing of the cat's URO-synthetase gene revealed two homozygous, missense mutations in exons 3 and 6. This synergistic interaction of two rare amino acid substitutions in the URO-synthase polypeptide resulted in the feline model of human CEP. Previously, cats presenting with brownish discolored teeth that fluoresced pink under UV light and increased URO and coproporphyrinogen concentrations were believed to have CEP. The disease was also observed to be inherited as an autosomal dominant trait (as in some pig models), whereas in people and cattle, the disease is inherited as an autosomal recessive trait. It is now understood that cats with the CEP-like phenotype and autosomal dominant inheritance actually have feline acute intermittent porphyria and not CEP.

Diagnosis should be based on the excretion of abnormal uroporphyrins, the brown discoloration of the teeth (which fluoresce when irradiated with near-ultraviolet light), the appearance of discolored urine, and hemolytic anemia.

The recessive genetic character is widely distributed in cattle, but the clinical condition is comparatively rare. Clinically normal heterozygotes have lower levels of uroporphyrinogen III cosynthetase than do normal animals, but laboratory identification of the carrier state is impractical because of the low incidence of the disease and is not widely used. Morbidity can be controlled by keeping affected animals indoors and out of direct sunlight.

DISORDERS OF CALCIUM METABOLISM

HYPOCALCEMIC TETANY IN HORSES

(Transport tetany, Lactation tetany, Eclampsia)

Hypocalcemic tetany in horses is an uncommon condition associated with acute depletion of serum ionized calcium and sometimes with alterations in serum concentrations of magnesium and phosphate. It occurs after prolonged physical exertion or transport (transport tetany) and in lactating mares (lactation tetany). Signs are variable and relate to neuromuscular hyperirritability.

Etiology: Mechanisms of hypocalcemia include decreased absorption from the intestines; increased loss of calcium from the kidneys, sweat, or milk; or inhibition of osteolysis due to alterations in parathyroid hormone, calcitonin, or vitamin D. In lactating mares, high milk production and grazing of lush pastures appear to be predisposing factors. Hypocalcemia after prolonged physical activity (eg, endurance rides) results from sweat loss of calcium, increased calcium binding during hypochloremic alkalosis, and stress-induced high corticosteroid levels. Corticosteroids inhibit vitamin D activity, which leads to decreased intestinal absorption and skeletal mobilization of calcium. Stress and lack of calcium intake have been associated with transport tetany. Occasionally, hypocalcemic tetany may be precipitated by hypocalcemia after blister beetle ingestion (*see* p 3157).

Clinical Findings: The severity of clinical signs corresponds with the serum concentration of ionized calcium. Increased excitability may be the only sign in mild cases. Severely affected horses may show synchronous diaphragmatic flutter (*see* p 1183), anxious appearance, and signs of tetany, including increased muscle tone, stiffness of gait, muscle tremors, prolapse of the third eyelid, inability to chew, trismus, salivation, recumbency, convulsions, and cardiac arrhythmias. In lactating mares, if not treated, the disease may take a progressive and sometimes fatal course over 24–48 hr.

Differential diagnoses include tetanus, endotoxemia, colic, exertional rhabdomyolysis or other muscle disorder, seizure disorder, laminitis, and botulism.

Diagnosis: A tentative diagnosis is based on clinical signs, history, and response to treatment. Definitive diagnosis requires demonstration of low serum levels of ionized calcium. Most laboratories measure only total (protein-bound and free) serum calcium, which is an acceptable diagnostic test in most cases. However, discrepancies may arise in alkalotic and hypoalbuminemic horses. Alkalosis increases albumin binding of calcium, which results in a decreased concentration of ionized calcium. Thus, alkalotic horses may have normal total serum calcium while exhibiting signs of hypocalcemia. Likewise, hypoalbuminemic or acidotic horses may have decreased total serum calcium without developing signs of hypocalcemia. Total serum calcium can be adjusted for albumin concentration by the following formula:

adjusted Ca^{2+} = measured Ca^{2+} – serum albumin concentration + 3.5

Treatment: IV administration of calcium solutions, such as 20% calcium borogluconate or solutions recommended for treatment of periparturient paresis in cattle, usually results in full recovery. These solutions should be administered slowly (over 20 min) at 250–500 mL/500 kg, diluted at least 1:4 in saline or dextrose, and the cardiovascular response should be closely monitored. An increased intensity of heart sounds is expected. If arrhythmias or bradycardia develop, the IV treatment should be discontinued immediately. Once the heart rate has returned to normal, the infusion may be resumed at a slower rate. If the horse does not improve within 1–2 hr of the initial infusion, a second dose may be given, although laboratory verification of hypocalcemia is indicated. Some horses require repeated treatments over several days to recover from hypocalcemic tetany. Mildly affected horses may recover without specific treatment. If the tetany is associated with physical exertion, incorporating magnesium into the solution may be advisable.

Prevention: A balanced feed ration should be provided to supply adequate amounts and ratios of calcium and phosphorus throughout gestation. In times of increased calcium demand such as lactation, fasting should be avoided and high-quality forage such as alfalfa or calcium-containing mineral mixes should be provided. Stress and fasting during transport should be minimized. In endurance horses, water and electrolyte deficits associated with prolonged exercise and sweating may be prevented by provision of a sufficient water supply and electrolyte supplementation.

PARTURIENT PARESIS IN COWS

(Milk fever, Hypocalcemia)

Parturient paresis is an acute to peracute, afebrile, flaccid paralysis of mature dairy cows that occurs most commonly at or soon after parturition. It is manifest by changes in mentation, generalized paresis, and circulatory collapse.

Etiology: Dairy cows will secrete 20–30 g of calcium in the production of colostrum and milk in the early stages of lactation. This secretion of calcium causes serum calcium levels to decline from a normal of 8.5–10 mg/dL to <7.5 mg/dL. The sudden decrease in serum calcium levels causes hyperexcitability of the nervous system and reduced strength of muscle contractions, resulting in both tetany and paresis. Parturient paresis may be seen in cows of any age but is most common in high-producing dairy cows entering their third or later lactations. Incidence is higher in Channel Island breeds.

Clinical Findings and Diagnosis: Parturient paresis usually occurs within 72 hr of parturition. It can contribute to dystocia, uterine prolapse, retained fetal membranes, metritis, abomasal displacement, and mastitis.

Parturient paresis has three discernible stages. During stage 1, animals are ambulatory but show signs of hypersensitivity and excitability. Cows may be mildly ataxic, have fine tremors over the flanks and triceps, and display ear twitching and head bobbing. Cows may appear restless, shuffling their rear feet and bellowing. If calcium therapy is not instituted, cows will likely progress to the second, more severe stage.

Cows in stage 2 are unable to stand but can maintain sternal recumbency. Cows are obtunded, anorectic, and have a dry muzzle, subnormal body temperature, and cold extremities. Auscultation reveals tachycardia and decreased intensity of heart sounds. Peripheral pulses are weak. Smooth muscle paralysis leads to GI stasis, which can manifest as bloat, failure to defecate, and loss of anal sphincter tone. An inability to urinate may manifest as a distended bladder on rectal examination. Cows often tuck their heads into their flanks, or if the head is extended, an S-shaped curve to the neck may be noted.

In stage 3, cows lose consciousness progressively to the point of coma. They are unable to maintain sternal recumbency, have complete muscle flaccidity, are unresponsive to stimuli, and can suffer severe bloat. As cardiac output worsens, heart rate can approach 120 bpm, and peripheral pulses may be undetectable. If untreated, cows in stage 3 may survive only a few hours.

Differential diagnoses include toxic mastitis, toxic metritis, other systemic toxic conditions, traumatic injury (eg, stifle injury, coxofemoral luxation, fractured pelvis, spinal compression), calving paralysis syndrome (damage to the L6 lumbar roots of sciatic and obturator nerves), or compartment syndrome. Some of these diseases, in addition to aspiration pneumonia, may also occur concurrently with parturient paresis or as complications. (*See also* p 1188.)

Treatment: Treatment is directed toward restoring normal serum calcium levels as soon as possible to avoid muscle and nerve damage and recumbency. Recommended treatment is IV injection of a calcium gluconate salt, although SC and IP routes are also used. A general rule for dosing is 1 g calcium/45 kg (100 lb) body wt. Most solutions are available in single-dose, 500-mL bottles that contain 8–11 g of calcium. In large, heavily lactating cows, a second bottle given SC may be helpful, because it is thought to provide a prolonged release of calcium into the circulation. SC calcium alone may not be adequately absorbed because of poor peripheral perfusion and should not be the sole route of therapy. No matter what route is used, strict asepsis should be used to lessen the chance of infection at the injection site. Solutions containing formaldehyde or >25 g dextrose/500 mL are irritating if given SC. Many solutions contain phosphorus and magnesium in addition to calcium. Although administration of phosphorus and magnesium is not usually necessary in uncomplicated parturient paresis, detrimental effects of their use have not been reported. Magnesium may protect against myocardial irritation caused by the administration of calcium. Magnesium is also necessary for appropriate parathyroid hormone (PTH) secretion and activity in response to hypocalcemia. Most products available to veterinarians contain phosphite salts as the source of phosphorus. However, phosphorus found in blood and tissues of cattle is primarily in the form of the phosphate anion. Because no pathway exists for the conversion of phosphite to the usable phosphate form, it is unlikely these solutions are of any benefit in addressing hypophosphatemia.

Calcium is cardiotoxic; therefore, calcium-containing solutions should be administered slowly (10–20 min) while cardiac auscultation is performed. If severe dysrhythmias or bradycardia develop, administration should be stopped until the heart rhythm has returned to normal. Endotoxic animals are especially prone to dysrhythmias caused by IV calcium therapy.

Administration of oral calcium avoids the risks of cardiotoxic adverse effects and may be useful in mild cases of parturient paresis; however, it is not recommended as the sole approach for clinical milk fever cases. Products containing calcium chloride are effective but can be caustic to oral and pharyngeal tissues, especially if used repeatedly. Calcium propionate in propylene glycol gel or powdered calcium propionate (0.5 kg dissolved in 8–16 L water administered as a drench) is effective, less injurious to tissues, avoids the potential for metabolic acidosis caused by calcium chloride, and supplies the gluconeogenic precursor propionate. Oral administration of 50 g of soluble calcium results in ~4 g of calcium being absorbed into the circulation.

Regardless of the source of oral calcium, it is important to note that cows with hypocalcemia often have poor swallowing and gag reflexes. Care must be exercised during administration of calcium-containing solutions to avoid aspiration pneumonia. Gels containing calcium chloride should not be administered to cows unable to swallow.

Hypocalcemic cows typically respond to IV calcium therapy immediately. Tremors are seen as neuromuscular function returns. Improved cardiac output results in stronger heart sounds and decreased heart rate. Return of smooth muscle function results in eructation, defecation, and urination once the cow rises. Approximately 75% of cows stand within 2 hr of treatment. Animals not responding by 4–8 hr should be reevaluated and retreated if necessary. Of cows that respond initially, 25%–30% relapse within 24–48 hr and require additional therapy. Incomplete milking has been advised to reduce the incidence of relapse. Historically, udder inflation has been used to reduce the secretion of milk and loss of calcium; however, the risk of introducing bacteria into the mammary gland is high.

Prevention: Historically, prevention of parturient paresis has been approached by feeding low-calcium diets during the dry period. The negative calcium balance results in a minor decline in blood calcium concentrations. This stimulates PTH secretion, which in turn stimulates bone resorption and renal production of 1,25 dihydroxyvitamin D. Increased 1,25 dihydroxyvitamin D increases bone calcium release and increases the efficiency of intestinal calcium absorption. Although mobilization of calcium is enhanced, it is now known that feeding low-calcium diets is not as effective as initially believed. Furthermore, on most dairy farms today, it is difficult to formulate diets low enough in calcium (<20 g absorbed calcium/cow/day), although the use of dietary straw and calcium-binding agents such as zeolite or vegetable oil may make this approach more useful.

Alternative methods to prevent hypocalcemia include delayed or incomplete milking after calving, which maintains pressure within the udder and decreases milk production; however, this practice may aggravate latent mammary infections and increase incidence of mastitis. Prophylactic treatment of susceptible cows at calving may help reduce parturient paresis. Cows are administered either SC calcium on the day of calving or oral calcium gels at calving and 12 hr later.

Most recently, the prevention of parturient paresis has been revolutionized by use of the dietary cation-anion difference (DCAD), a method that decreases the blood pH of cows during the late prepartum and early postpartum period. This method is more effective and more practical than lowering prepartum calcium in the diet. The DCAD approach is based on the finding that most dairy cows are in a state of metabolic alkalosis due to the high potassium content of their diets. This state of metabolic alkalosis with increased blood pH predisposes cows to hypocalcemia by altering the conformation of the PTH receptor, resulting in tissues less sensitive to PTH. Lack of PTH responsiveness prevents effective use of bone calcium, prevents activation of osteoclastic bone resorption, reduces renal reabsorption of calcium from the glomerulus, and inhibits renal conversion to its active form.

An important strategy to decrease blood pH in periparturient cattle is to reduce the potassium content of the diet. It is essential to include corn silage as a major portion of the dry cow's diet, because it tends to have the lowest content potassium of available forages. Alfalfa is another forage source that may prove beneficial in maintaining proper blood pH. In the past, including alfalfa in a dry cow ration was not considered ideal because of the high calcium content. However, it has since been determined that calcium has little effect on the alkalinity of cow's blood. Withholding potassium fertilizers on fields used to grow dry cow forages is another way to decrease potassium levels in hay fed to dry cows. Alternatively, readily absorbable anions can be added to the diet to increase the total negative charges in the blood, allowing more H^+ to exist, decreasing the pH of the blood. Anionic salts to consider include calcium chloride, magnesium chloride, magnesium sulfate, calcium sulfate, ammonium sulfate, and ammonium chloride. Research evaluating the acidifying activity of different anionic salts has resulted in the following equation that describes the ion balance in rations:

$$DCAD = (Na^+ + K^+) - (Cl^- + S^{-2})$$

The target value for close-up dry cow rations is −15 to +15 mEq/100 g dry matter. Sodium and potassium should be provided as close to the required levels as possible (0.1% dietary dry matter sodium, and 1% dietary dry matter potassium). Chloride should be added to the ration to offset the effects of low levels of potassium on blood alkalinity. In general, providing ~0.5% less dietary chloride than the concentration of potassium being fed will result in appropriate acidification. Urine pH provides an inexpensive and relatively accurate estimate of blood pH in dairy cattle. Mean urine pH ranges from ~6–6.5 are optimal to manage DCAD and prevent milk fever. Urine should be measured >24 hr after addition of an anionic diet in pre-fresh cows.

An important drawback to feeding anionic salts is poor palatability, which can be overcome by using a mixture of anionic salts within a moist, palatable ration such as corn silage, brewer's grain, distiller's grain, or molasses. Although sulfate salts are more palatable than chloride salts, they are less effective in acidifying the blood. Dietary sulfur should be >0.22% dry matter to support rumen microbial amino acid synthesis but <0.4% dry matter to avoid neurologic signs associated with sulfur toxicity. If dry matter intake drops >1 kg/day in a group of pre-fresh dry cows fed an acidifying diet, the dose of anions should be decreased to the point that dry matter intake is restored.

Administration of vitamin D_3 and its metabolites effectively prevents parturient paresis. Large doses of vitamin D (20–30 million U/day), given in the feed for 5–7 days before parturition, reduces the incidence. However, if administration is stopped >4 days before calving, the cow is more susceptible. Dosing for periods longer than those recommended should be avoided because of potential toxicity. A single injection (IV or SC) of 10 million IU of crystalline vitamin D given 8 days before calving is an effective preventive. The dose is repeated if the cow does not calve on the due date. Newer compounds used (where available and approved) in lieu of vitamin D and less likely to cause hypervitaminosis include 25-hydroxycholecalciferol, 1,25-dihydroxycholecalciferol, and 1α-hydroxycholecalciferol. After calving, a diet high in calcium is required. Administering large doses of calcium in gel form (PO) is commonly practiced. Doses of 150 g of calcium gel are given 1 day before, the day of, and 1 day after calving.

Use of synthetic bovine PTH may prove to be superior to administration of vitamin D metabolites. Vitamin D metabolites enhance GI calcium absorption, whereas PTH enhances GI calcium absorption and stimulates bone resorption. PTH is administered either IV 60 hr before parturition, or IM 6 days before parturition. Drawbacks to the use of PTH include increased labor requirements for administration, as well as the availability of such compounds.

PARTURIENT PARESIS IN SHEEP AND GOATS

(Milk fever, Hypocalcemia)

Parturient paresis in pregnant and lactating ewes and does is a disturbance of metabolism characterized by acute-onset hypocalcemia and rapid development of hyperexcitability and ataxia, progressing to depression, recumbency, coma, and death. Unlike parturient paresis in dairy cattle, which primarily occurs within a few days of calving, the condition in ewes and does usually occurs before and less commonly after parturition. This condition may be underdiagnosed in some situations.

Etiology: Parturient paresis is caused by a decrease in calcium intake under conditions of increased calcium requirements, usually during late gestation. This results in a low serum calcium concentration, particularly in animals pregnant with multiple fetuses. Some cases are complicated by concurrent pregnancy toxemia. Ewes that are both hypocalcemic and hyperketonemic may not be able to produce endogenous glucose as readily as ewes that are only hyperketonemic, leading to the risk of more severe disease developing when both conditions are present. Parturient paresis can occur at any time from 6 wk before to 10 wk after parturition; however, the greatest demand for calcium because of mineralization of the fetal skeleton occurs 1–3 wk prepartum, particularly when multiple fetuses are present in utero. Whenever an abrupt decrease in calcium intake occurs, the body requires 24–72 hr to activate the metabolic machinery necessary to mobilize stored calcium. Mobilization of stored calcium can be inadequate to meet the animal's needs in older ewes and does, in animals with chronic calcium deficiency, and when diets are calcium deficient. Examples of forages with low calcium levels include cereal hays or pasture, poor-quality grassy hays and pasture, and corn silage. Most grains also contain little calcium but additionally have high levels of phosphorus, causing an inverse calcium:phosphorus ratio, increasing dietary risk. Vitamin D deficiency, which occurs in housed ruminants during winter months, also depresses calcium absorption from the GI tract.

Clinical Findings and Diagnosis: Characteristically, parturient paresis occurs in outbreaks, with most cases occurring in the last few weeks of gestation, although it is not uncommon for individual animals to be affected. Usually, <5% of animals are affected, but severe outbreaks may involve up to 30% of the flock. The onset is sudden and often follows—within 24 hr—an abrupt change of feed, a sudden change in weather, or short periods of fasting imposed by circumstances such as shearing or transportation (*see also* p 1030). In early hypocalcemia in sheep, the most commonly noted signs are stiff gait, ataxia, salivation, constipation, and depressed rumen motility, progressing to hyposensitivity, bloat, recumbency, loss of anal reflex and, if untreated, death. Tachycardia may be present; heart sounds are quieter than normal. Often when recumbent, ewes are in a sternal frog-lying position, with the hindlegs extended behind. Goats have a similar presentation, although muscle tremors are more commonly seen than in sheep.

A working diagnosis is based on the history and clinical signs. In outbreaks occurring before parturition, pregnancy toxemia (*see* p 1021) is the main differential diagnosis. These diseases also occur concurrently. A tentative diagnosis of acute hypocalcemia is supported by a dramatic and usually lasting response to slow IV administration of calcium. Diagnosis can be confirmed by testing serum calcium levels before treatment. Urine ketone or serum β-hydroxybutyrate levels should always be evaluated at the same time. Hypocalcemia is often classified as total serum calcium levels <2 mmol/L or, if expressed as ionized calcium, <1.1 mmol/L. Normal values are reported as 2.8–3.2 mmol/L for sheep and 2.2–3.05 mmol/L for goats. (To convert from mmol/L to mg/dL, divide the value by 0.25.) Animals with low serum albumin, such as occurs with Johne's disease and clinical GI parasitism, may have low total serum calcium and normal ionized calcium.

Treatment and Prevention: Treatment should be initiated immediately, usually administered as calcium borogluconate IV (50–150 mL of a 23% solution). Calcium-containing products that also contain phosphorus and magnesium, as well as dextrose, likely have additional therapeutic value. Oral or SC administration of a calcium solution helps to prevent relapse. During treatment, the heart should be monitored, and therapy slowed or stopped if arrhythmias occur. For ease of IV administration, it may be preferred to increase the volume of the product by adding 50–150 mL of a 23% calcium borogluconate or gluconate solution to 1 L of a 5% dextrose solution and administering this volume over 10 min. Dietary modifications to increase the calcium:phosphorus ratio (>1.5:1) and ensure total calcium in the diet meets NRC requirements (*see* TABLE 1), as well as vitamin D levels, may help to prevent further cases in pregnant animals. Sudden dietary changes or other stressors should be avoided during late gestation, and risk factors for pregnancy toxemia investigated.

PUERPERAL HYPOCALCEMIA IN SMALL ANIMALS

(Postpartum hypocalcemia, Periparturient hypocalcemia, Puerperal tetany, Eclampsia)

Puerperal hypocalcemia is an acute, life-threatening condition usually seen at peak lactation, 2–3 wk after whelping. Small-breed bitches with large litters are most often affected. Hypocalcemia may also occur during parturition and may precipitate dystocia.

Etiology and Pathogenesis: Hypocalcemia most likely results from loss of calcium into the milk and from inadequate dietary calcium intake. This imbalance in calcium metabolism occurs because calcium mobilization from bone into the serum pool is insufficient to maintain the efflux of calcium leaving through the mammary glands. Heavy lactational demands from large puppies or a large litter are often noted. The incidence is increased in small breeds of dogs, although puerperal hypocalcemia can occur in any breed, with any size litter, and at any time during lactation. Rarely, it occurs during late gestation in bitches. Although uncommon in queens, it may occur during early lactation. In dogs, supplementation with oral calcium during pregnancy may predispose to eclampsia during peak lactation, because excessive calcium intake during pregnancy causes downregulation of the calcium regulatory system and subsequent clinical hypocalcemia when calcium demand is high.

TABLE 1 CALCIUM REQUIREMENTS OF A MEAT EWE AND DAIRY DOE DURING GESTATION AND LACTATION

70-kg adult with twins	Calcium Requirements (g/day)			
	Early gestation	Late gestation	Early lactation	Mid lactation
Ewe (meat)	6.5	8.8	7.9	6.5
Doe (parlour milked)	6.6	6.6	20.7	21.4

Adapted, with permission, from *Nutrient Requirements of Small Ruminants*, Animal Nutrition Series, 2007. National Academy of Sciences, National Academy Press, Washington DC.

Inadequate production of parathyroid hormone (PTH) during the hypocalcemic crisis is not responsible for eclampsia in dogs. In dairy cows with a similar condition (*see* p 988), production of PTH is adequate, but the pool of osteoclasts for PTH to stimulate is not. The small osteoclast pool results from feeding a high level of dietary calcium during the nonlactating period, which suppresses parathyroid gland secretion of PTH and stimulates parafollicular C-cell secretion of calcitonin. Hypocalcemia at parturition interferes with the release of acetylcholine at the neuromuscular junction, which is normally mediated by extracellular calcium entering presynaptic nerve terminals through voltage-gated calcium channels and triggering the fusion of acetylcholine-filled synaptic vesicles with the presynaptic nerve terminus. The paresis seen in cattle, rather than the tetany seen in dogs, is probably the result of a combination of factors. Cows often have concurrent mild hypermagnesemia. Magnesium is a calcium-channel antagonist and plays a key role in modulating any activity governed by intracellular calcium fluxes. Cows also have increased volatile fatty acids (which are inhibitory at neuromuscular synapses), and cows have a higher threshold potential at neuromuscular junctions than do dogs.

In dogs with hypocalcemia, unlike cows, excitation-secretion coupling is maintained at the neuromuscular junction. The low concentration of calcium in the extracellular fluid has an excitatory effect on nerve and muscle cells, because it lowers the threshold potential (voltage level at which sodium channels become activated) so it is closer to the resting membrane potential. With hypocalcemia, sodium channels become activated (opened) by very little increase in membrane potential from their normal, negative level. Therefore, the nerve fiber becomes highly excitable, sometimes discharging repetitively without provocation rather than remaining in the resting state. The probable way that calcium ions affect the sodium channels are that calcium ions bind to the exterior surfaces of sodium channels. The positive charge of these calcium ions alters the electrical state of the sodium channel protein, thus altering the voltage level required to open the sodium channel. Because of the loss of stabilizing membrane-bound calcium ions, nerve membranes become more permeable to sodium ions and require a stimulus of lesser magnitude to depolarize. Tetany occurs as a result of spontaneous repetitive firing of motor nerve fibers. Hypoglycemia can occur concurrently.

Clinical Findings: Panting and restlessness are early clinical signs. Mild tremors, twitching, muscle spasms, and gait changes (stiffness and ataxia) result from increased neuromuscular excitability. Behavioral changes such as aggression, whining, salivation, pacing, hypersensitivity to stimuli, and disorientation are frequent. Severe tremors, tetany, generalized seizure activity, and finally coma and death may be seen. Hyperthermia may occur in severe cases. Prolonged seizure activity may cause cerebral edema. Tachycardia, hyperthermia, polyuria, polydipsia, and vomiting are sometimes seen. Historically, the bitch has been otherwise healthy and the neonates have been thriving.

Although hypocalcemia usually occurs postpartum, clinical signs can appear prepartum or at parturition. Mild hypocalcemia (serum calcium concentration >7 mg/dL but below the normal reference range) may contribute to ineffective myometrial contractions and slow the progression of labor without causing any other clinical signs.

Heavy panting may produce a respiratory alkalosis. Ionized calcium is the physiologically available fraction; it is affected by protein concentration, acid-base status (alkalosis favors protein binding of serum calcium and will decrease blood levels of the biologically important ionized calcium, thus exacerbating hypocalcemia), and other electrolyte imbalances. Thus, the severity of clinical signs may not correlate with total calcium concentration.

Diagnosis: Diagnosis is often made from the signalment, history, clinical signs, and response to treatment. A pretreatment total serum calcium concentration <7 mg/dL (<6 mg/dL in cats) confirms the diagnosis. (IV therapy with calcium is often started, however, before serum calcium concentration is determined.) A serum chemistry profile is useful to exclude concurrent hypoglycemia and other electrolyte imbalances. Prolongation of the QT interval and ventricular premature contractions may be seen on the ECG.

Differential diagnoses include other causes of seizures such as hypoglycemia, toxicoses, and primary neurologic disorders such as idiopathic epilepsy or meningoencephalitis. Other causes of irritability and hyperthermia such as metritis and mastitis should also be excluded. If the parathyroid glands are functioning normally, serum PTH will be increased in the face of hypocalcemia. Low or undetectable serum PTH in a hypocalcemic animal is strongly suggestive of primary hypoparathyroidism (*see* p 1057). A commercially available human intact-PTH assay has been validated in both cats and dogs; PTH-calcium curves are also similar in cats and dogs.

Treatment and Prevention: Slow IV administration of 10% calcium gluconate is given to effect (0.5–1.5 mL/kg over 10–30 min; 5–20 mL is the usual dose). This usually results in rapid clinical improvement within 15 min. Muscle relaxation should be immediate.

During administration of calcium, heart rate should be carefully monitored by auscultation or by ECG for bradycardia or arrhythmias. Signs of toxicity from too rapid administration of calcium include bradycardia, shortening of the QT interval, and premature ventricular complexes. If an arrhythmia develops, calcium administration should be discontinued until the heart rate and rhythm are normal; then administration is resumed at half the original infusion rate.

It is important to calculate the dosage of calcium based on elemental (available) calcium, because different products vary in the amount of calcium available. The dosage of elemental calcium for hypocalcemia is 5–15 mg/kg/hr. Calcium gluconate, 10%, contains 9.3 mg of elemental calcium/mL. Calcium chloride, 27%, contains 27.2 mg of elemental calcium/mL. Thus, for 10% calcium gluconate the dosage is 0.5–1.5 mL/kg/hr, IV, and for 27% calcium chloride the dosage is 0.22–0.66 mL/kg/hr, IV. Calcium gluconate, as a 10% solution, is recommended because, unlike calcium chloride, calcium gluconate extravasation is not caustic.

Once the animal is stable, the dose of calcium gluconate needed for initial control of tetany may be diluted in an equal volume of normal (0.9%) saline and given SC, tid, to control clinical signs. (Calcium chloride cannot be given SC.) Alternatively, 5–15 mg of elemental calcium/kg/hr can be continued IV. This protocol effectively supports serum calcium concentrations while waiting for oral vitamin D and calcium therapy to have effect. Ideally, serum calcium concentration should be maintained >8 mg/dL. Serum calcium concentrations <8 mg/dL indicate the need to increase the dosage of parenteral calcium, whereas concentrations >9 mg/dL suggest that it be reduced. The aim of longterm therapy is to maintain the serum calcium concentration at mildly low to low-normal concentrations (8–9.5 mg/dL).

The bitch may remain nonresponsive after correction of hypocalcemia if cerebral edema has developed. Cerebral edema, hyperthermia, and hypoglycemia should be treated if present. Fever usually resolves rapidly with control of tetany, and specific treatment for fever may result in hypothermia.

It is best not to let the puppies or kittens nurse for 12–24 hr. During this period, they should be fed a milk substitute or other appropriate diet; if mature enough, they should be weaned. If tetany recurs in the same lactation, the litter should be removed from the bitch and either hand raised (<4 wk old) or weaned (>4 wk old).

After the acute crisis, elemental calcium at 25–50 mg/kg/day in three or four divided doses is given PO for the remainder of the lactation. Again, the dose of calcium is based on the amount of elemental calcium in the product (ie, calcium carbonate tablets contain 295 mg elemental calcium/1 g tablet). In dogs, the dosage is usually 1–4 g/day, in divided doses. In cats, the dosage of calcium is ~0.5–1 g/day, in divided doses. Longterm maintenance therapy with oral vitamin D and oral calcium supplementation usually requires a minimum of 24–96 hr before an effect is achieved. Hypocalcemic animals should, therefore, receive parenteral calcium support during the initial posttetany period. Calcium carbonate is a good choice because of its high percentage of elemental calcium, general availability in drugstores in the form of antacids, low cost, and lack of gastric irritation. The dosage of calcium can be gradually tapered to avoid unnecessary therapy; there is usually sufficient calcium in commercial pet food to meet the needs of dogs and cats. However, to avoid acute problems of hypocalcemic tetany, oral calcium supplementation should continue throughout lactation.

Vitamin D supplementation is used to increase calcium absorption from the intestines. The concentration of serum calcium should be monitored weekly. The dosage of 1,25-dihydroxyvitamin D (calcitriol) is 0.03–0.06 mcg/kg/day. Calcitriol has a rapid onset of action (1–4 days) and short half-life (<1 day). Iatrogenic hypercalcemia is a common complication of this therapy. If hypercalcemia results from overdosage, it can be rapidly corrected by discontinuing calcitriol. The toxic effects resolve in 1–14 days. This is a much briefer period than that seen with dihydrotachysterol (1–3 wk) or ergocalciferol (vitamin D_2; 1–18 wk) therapy.

Corticosteroids lower serum calcium and, therefore, are contraindicated. They may interfere with intestinal calcium transport and increase urinary loss of calcium.

Owners should be warned that puerperal hypocalcemia is likely to recur with future pregnancies. Preventive steps to consider in the bitch include feeding a high-quality, nutritionally balanced, and appropriate diet during pregnancy and lactation, providing food and water ad lib during lactation, and supplemental feeding of the puppies with milk replacer early in lactation and with solid food after 3–4 wk of age. Oral calcium supplementation during gestation is not indicated and may cause rather than prevent postpartum hypocalcemia. Calcium administration during peak milk production may be helpful in bitches with a history of puerperal hypocalcemia.

HYPOCALCEMIA AS AN ELECTROLYTE DISTURBANCE IN SMALL ANIMALS

Hypocalcemia is also an important electrolyte disturbance in critically ill dogs and cats. The incidence of hypocalcemia is 16% in critically ill dogs and 24% in dogs with sepsis. Hypocalcemia is best detected by measuring ionized calcium (<2.5 mEq/L), which is the biologically active form, rather than total or corrected calcium. Hypocalcemia, hypovitaminosis D, and metabolic acidosis occur in dogs with induced endotoxemia. LPS may mediate a decrease in vitamin D–binding protein, with subsequent loss of vitamin D in the urine. Also, dogs with blunt and penetrating traumatic injuries, particularly abdominal trauma, are significantly more likely to have ionized hypocalcemia (16% incidence). These dogs spend longer time in the hospital and ICU, require more intensive therapies, and are less likely to survive (57% survival rate) than dogs with normocalcemia (89% survival rate). Hypocalcemia from critical illness or traumatic injury can cause clinical signs similar to those of puerperal hypocalcemia (hyperexcitability, including tremors, twitching, spasms, or seizures, or more subtle signs related to cardiovascular collapse).

DISORDERS OF MAGNESIUM METABOLISM

Magnesium (Mg) homeostasis is not under direct hormonal control but is mainly determined by absorption from the GI tract; excretion by the kidneys; and the varying requirements of the body for pregnancy, lactation, and growth. Magnesium is the second most common intracellular cation after potassium, with 50%–60% of total body Mg distributed in bone, 40%–50% in soft tissues, and <1% in the extracellular fluid. Therefore, plasma Mg does not provide an indication of intracellular or bone Mg stores. Intracellular Mg is required for activation of enzymes involving phosphate compounds such as ATPases, kinases, and phosphatases; and for synthesis of RNA, DNA, and protein. Magnesium is a cofactor for >300 enzymatic reactions involving ATP, including glycolysis and oxidative phosphorylation. It is also important in the function of the Na^+/K^+-ATPase pump, membrane stabilization, nerve conduction, ion transportation, and calcium channel activity. Magnesium also regulates the movement of calcium into smooth muscle cells, giving it a pivotal role in cardiac contractile strength and peripheral vascular tone. Low ionized Mg concentrations accelerate the transmission of nerve impulses. Clinical manifestations of severe hypomagnesemia include muscle weakness, muscle fasciculations, ventricular arrhythmias, seizures, ataxia, and coma.

Similar to calcium, serum total magnesium (tMg) can be divided into three forms. The physiologically active (free) fraction is ionized magnesium (iMg^{2+}), whereas the protein-bound and chelated fractions are unavailable for biochemical processes. Serum iMg^{2+} cannot be accurately calculated from serum tMg and albumin concentrations; therefore, serum iMg^{2+} concentration must be determined by direct measurement. Because iMg^{2+} concentrations represent the functional pool of serum Mg, determination of iMg^{2+} may provide a better physiologic assessment of Mg status than does tMg. A commercially available ion-selective electrode for Mg allows routine measurement of iMg^{2+} concentrations.

Magnesium is cleared by glomerular filtration and, in the absence of renal disease, renal homeostatic mechanisms will attempt to maintain Mg balance. When the diet contains excessive Mg, renal tubular resorption decreases, maintaining serum concentrations of Mg within narrow physiologic limits. Renal excretion of Mg may be used to evaluate Mg balance.

IV administration of large doses of Mg is safely used to concurrently diagnose and treat hypomagnesemia. The IV Mg retention test, which involves the determination of urinary Mg retention, has become the gold standard to determine Mg status in human medicine and has been validated in horses, dogs, and cattle. Animals deficient in Mg will retain a large proportion of the administered Mg, whereas animals with sufficient Mg will excrete most of it.

Fractional clearance relates the amount of substance excreted to the amount filtered by the glomerulus without the need for volumetric urine collection. Fractional clearance can be calculated by using concurrently collected spot samples of urine and serum and by measuring the concentrations of creatinine and the electrolyte of interest. This allows assessment of urinary electrolyte excretion without the need for timed urine collections and takes into account variability in urine concentration due to hydration status.

Ruminants are more prone to hypomagnesemia than monogastric animals. The variation in Mg metabolism among species is mainly because of anatomic and physiologic differences in digestive tracts. Ruminants absorb Mg less efficiently than nonruminants (35% vs 70% of intake). The rumen is the main site of absorption, and there are active transport mechanisms. Absorption from the large intestine occurs with high Mg intakes. In nonruminants, the small intestine is the main site of absorption. Species differences in Mg metabolism are attributable to variation in both absorption efficiency of Mg from the gut and reabsorption of Mg by the kidney tubules.

HYPERMAGNESEMIA

Hypermagnesemia (plasma Mg concentration >2 mg/dL [1.1 mmol/L]) is a rare condition reported only in monogastric animals. Horses show signs of sweating and muscle weakness within 4 hr of receiving excessive oral doses of magnesium sulfate administered as a cathartic for treatment of large-intestinal impactions. This is followed by recumbency, tachycardia (120 bpm), and tachypnea (60 breaths/min). Signs subside after treatment with slow IV infusion of calcium gluconate (23% solution). Hypermagnesemia has been reported in cats with renal failure that were receiving IV fluid therapy. As plasma Mg concentrations exceed 2.5 mmol/L, there may be ECG changes with prolongation of the PR interval; at 5 mmol/L, deep tendon reflexes disappear, followed by hypotension and respiratory depression. Cardiac arrest may occur with blood Mg levels >6.0–7.5 mmol/L.

HYPOMAGNESEMIC TETANY IN CATTLE AND SHEEP

(Grass tetany, Grass staggers)

Hypomagnesemic tetany is a complex metabolic disturbance characterized by hypomagnesemia (plasma tMg <1.5 mg/dL [<0.65 mmol/L]) and a reduced concentration of tMg in the CSF (<1.0 mg/dL [0.4 mmol/L]), which lead to hyperexcitability, muscular spasms, convulsions, respiratory distress, collapse, and death. Adult lactating animals are most susceptible because of the loss of Mg in milk. Hypomagnesemic tetany occurs mainly when animals are grazed on lush grass pastures or green cereal crops but can occur in lactating beef cows fed silage indoors. It is rare in nonlactating cattle but has occurred when undernourished cattle were introduced to green cereal crops.

Etiology: The disorder occurs after a decrease in plasma Mg concentration when absorption of dietary Mg is unable to meet the requirements for maintenance (3 mg/kg body wt) and lactation (120 mg/kg milk). This can arise after a reduction in food intake during inclement weather, transport, or when cows graze short-grass dominant pastures containing <0.2% Mg on a dry-matter basis. Low herbage availability (<1,000 kg dry matter/hectare) results in liveweight losses during lactation, and plasma Mg decreases because insufficient Mg is obtained from body tissues mobilized during loss of liveweight to support lactation.

Mg absorption from the rumen may be reduced when potassium and nitrogen intakes are high and sodium and phosphorus intakes are low. Soils naturally high in potassium and those fertilized with potash and nitrogen are high-risk areas for hypomagnesemic tetany. The more complex mineral interactions are likely to be involved in herds in which hypomagnesemic tetany occurs in first- and second-calving cows as well as in older cows.

Cows often do not develop signs of hypomagnesemic tetany until blood calcium concentrations are <0.8 mg/dL (0.35 mmol/L), which commonly occurs in cattle grazing green cereal crops. The hypocalcemia arises from either a reduction in calcium intake or absorption, or both. Lush grass pastures and green cereal crops may predispose cattle to metabolic alkalosis (urine pH >8.5) with a reduced available pool of ionized calcium and magnesium, thereby increasing the risk of hypocalcemia and hypomagnesemia. Urine Mg concentrations are a useful guide to Mg status and are undetectable in cows with hypomagnesemia.

Clinical Findings: In the most acute form, affected cows, which may appear to be grazing normally, suddenly throw up their heads, bellow, gallop in a blind frenzy, fall, and exhibit severe paddling convulsions. These convulsive episodes may be repeated at short intervals, and death usually occurs within a few hours. In many instances, animals at pasture are found dead without observed illness, but an indication that the animal had convulsions before death may be seen from marks on the ground. In less severe cases, the cow is obviously ill at ease, walks stiffly, is hypersensitive to touch and sound, urinates frequently, and may progress to the acute convulsive stage after a period as long as 2–3 days. This period may be shortened if the cow is transported or driven to a fresh pasture. When animals have hypocalcemia and hypomagnesemia, the signs shown depend on which predominates. With hypomagnesemia, tachycardia and loud heart sounds are characteristic signs.

Clinical signs of hypomagnesemic tetany in sheep occur when hypomagnesemia (plasma tMg <0.5 mg/dL [0.2 mmol/L]) occurs concomitantly with hypocalcemia (plasma tCa <8 mg/dL [2.0 mmol/L]). The disease in lactating ewes occurs under essentially the same conditions and has the same clinical signs as in cattle.

Diagnosis: Diagnosis is usually confirmed by response to treatment, followed by confirmation of hypomagnesemia in samples taken before treatment. Tetany usually occurs when plasma tMg is <1.2 mg/dL (0.5 mmol/L) in cattle and <0.5 mg/dL (0.2 mmol/L) in sheep. Urine Mg is usually undetectable in cows with hypomagnesemic tetany. Mg concentrations <1.8 mg/dL (0.75 mmol/L) in the vitreous humour of the eye removed from animals within 24 hr after death are indicative of hypomagnesemic tetany.

Treatment: Animals showing clinical signs require treatment immediately with combined solutions of calcium and Mg, preferably given slowly IV while monitoring the heart (*see* p 988). The response to treatment is slower in animals with hypomagnesemic tetany than in animals with hypocalcemia alone, because of the time it takes to restore Mg in the CSF. The animal should not be stimulated during treatment, because this could trigger fatal convulsions. Additional Mg sulfate (200 mL of a 50% solution/cow) can be given SC. After treatment, cows should be left to respond without stimulation and then moved off the tetany-prone pasture, if possible. Animals must be provided with hay treated with 2 oz (60 g) of Mg oxide daily; if this is not done, the condition can recur within 36 hr after initial therapy.

Prevention: Mg must be given daily to animals at risk, because the body has no readily available stores. Daily oral supplements of Mg oxide (2 oz [60 g] to cattle and ⅓ oz [10 g] to sheep) should be given in the danger period. Most Mg salts are unpalatable and must be combined with other palatable ingredients such as molasses, concentrates, or hay. Feeding hay alone may be all that is required to prevent hypomagnesemic tetany in herds in which only old cows (>6 yr) are affected. If slow-release intraruminal Mg devices are administered, the animals also should be provided with hay. Fertilizers containing Mg effectively increase herbage Mg only on certain soil types. Herbage may be dusted with powdered Mg oxide (500 g/cow) or sprayed with a 2% solution of Mg sulfate at intervals of 1–2 wk. If rainfall exceeds 40–50 mm within 2–3 days of dusting, the herbage will require another dusting.

Out-wintered stock should be protected from wind and cold and provided with supplementary food. Sheep and cattle should have access to hay, particularly when grazing either green cereal crops or pastures fertilized with potassium or nitrogen (or both).

Hypomagnesemic Tetany in Calves

Magnesium absorption efficiency in calves fed milk falls from 87% at 2–3 wk to 32% at

7–8 wk of age. Hypomagnesemic tetany occurs in 2- to 4-mo-old calves being fed milk only, or in younger calves with chronic scours while being fed milk replacer.

Clinical signs are similar to those of hypomagnesemic tetany in adult cattle (*see* above) and include hyperexcitability, muscular spasms, convulsions, and death.

Hypomagnesemic tetany in calves must be differentiated from acute lead poisoning (*see* p 3078), tetanus (*see* p 611), strychnine poisoning (*see* p 3170), polioencephalomalacia (*see* p 1281), and enterotoxemia caused by the toxin of *Clostridium perfringens* (*see* p 609). Analysis of bone aids diagnosis—normal bone has a Ca:Mg ratio of 70:1; in hypomagnesemic calves, the ratio may be ≥90:1.

Affected calves require prompt treatment with a 10% solution of Mg sulfate (100 mL, SC) followed by Mg oxide at 10 g/day, PO. Provision of good-quality legume hay and a starter ration from 2 wk of age prevents the disorder.

MAGNESIUM AS AN EQUINE DIETARY SUPPLEMENT

Dietary Mg deficiency in horses is very rare, unless extreme conditions combine to result in decreased consumption and increased demand, eg, long-distance transportation of unfed lactating mares or prolonged administration of enteral or parenteral fluid or nutrition solutions deficient in Mg. Despite this, Mg supplements have been advocated by laymen as a calming agent or as an adjunctive therapy for equine metabolic syndrome, and even to prevent laminitis. There is no evidence that these uses are beneficial or effective, and such practices should be discouraged. One randomized placebo controlled study showed no difference in either insulin sensitivity or morphometric variables in horses supplemented with Mg (8.8 g/d) and chromium. Although sedation can be seen in horses administered >500 g of $MgSO_4$ as a cathartic via stomach tube, low level Mg supplements are unlikely to influence behavior, and larger amounts would be unpalatable in the feed or even dangerous if administered as repeated dosages via nasogastric tube (*see* p 996). Recommended doses of 3–10 g are unlikely to have a clinical benefit. However, low-level supplementation is considered relatively safe even if not efficacious, because excess Mg will be readily excreted by the kidneys in animals with normal renal function.

The maintenance Mg requirement for horses has been estimated at 13 mg/kg body wt/day and can be provided by a diet containing 0.16% Mg (1,600 ppm of feed) or by adding Mg oxide at 31 mg/kg/day, $MgCO_3$ at 64 mg/kg/day, or $MgSO_4$ at 93 mg/kg/day. This may be important when formulating oral replacement fluids for inappetent horses. For a 500-kg horse, this would equate to Mg oxide at ~16 g/day, $MgCO_3$ at 32 g/d, or $MgSO_4$ at 47 g/day. Growing, lactating, and exercising animals may require double these amounts. Horses that are obtaining adequate feed by grazing, with hay or grain, are unlikely to be Mg deficient. Horses are able to absorb 30%–60% of the Mg provided in their feed, which is higher than the absorption rate in ruminants.

If a pasture is considered Mg deficient (winter pastures with little herbage that have been fertilized with potash and /or nitrogen), then renal excretion of Mg may be used to evaluate Mg balance. With low dietary Mg intake, urinary Mg excretion falls to negligible levels. Renal Mg excretion is measured in urine collected throughout 24 hr (mg/kg/day). The fractional clearance of Mg can be determined by expressing the renal Mg clearance relative to the creatinine clearance and requires only a single sample each of urine and serum. Fractional clearance of Mg in healthy horses fed grass hay ranges from 15% to 35%, and values <6% indicate inadequate dietary Mg intake. A Mg retention test to assess total body status has been evaluated in horses receiving Mg-deficient diets, but this test offered no benefit over performing fractional clearances and requires 48 hr of volumetric urine collection.

SUBCLINICAL HYPOMAGNESEMIA IN CRITICALLY ILL ANIMALS

Subclinical hypomagnesemia is common in critically ill horses and small animals and can increase the severity of the systemic inflammatory response syndrome; worsen the systemic response to endotoxin; and lead to ileus, cardiac arrhythmias, refractory hypokalemia, and hypocalcemia.

Low serum Mg concentrations have been reported to occur in 65% of critically ill people, 39%–46% of dogs and cats in the intensive care unit (ICU), 49% of hospitalized horses, 54% of equine surgical colic patients, and 78% of horses with enterocolitis. In human and canine ICU populations, hypomagnesemic patients had higher rates of concurrent hypokalemia and hyponatremia and a longer length of hospitalization. In another study, 54% of equine surgical colic patients had low iMg levels, and these horses had a significantly greater prevalence of postoperative ileus.

Although diets for horses and small animals are rarely deficient in Mg, subclinical acute hypomagnesemia is very common in critically ill animals. Serum Mg concentration may be low as a result of altered Mg homeostasis, cellular or third-space redistribution, GI loss of Mg, or diuresis secondary to aggressive fluid therapy with IV fluids unsupplemented with Mg.

Hypocalcemia is also frequently seen in the equine ICU. Although the mechanism of action is unknown, serum Mg may influence serum calcium concentrations; human hypocalcemic patients with concurrent hypomagnesemia are often refractory to calcium therapy unless the low serum Mg levels are identified and corrected. Despite the precise regulation of serum Mg concentration by the kidney, Mg does not have a complex homeostatic endocrine regulating mechanism. This is in contrast to calcium, which is tightly regulated by parathyroid hormone (PTH), calcitonin, and calcitriol. However, PTH, vitamin D, calcitonin, arginine vasopressin, glucagons, and calcium concentrations do influence Mg absorption and excretion to some degree.

Mild hypocalcemia and hypomagnesemia stimulate PTH release, but severe Mg depletion and acute hypermagnesemia decrease PTH release. Consequently, parallel determination of calcium and PTH concentrations is important in the investigation of Mg homeostasis.

If longterm fluid therapy is required to support an inappetent animal in the ICU, Mg should be supplemented. A constant rate infusion of Mg sulfate at 50–150 mg/kg/day, IV (0.1–0.3 mL/kg/day of the 50% solution), provides daily requirements.

DISORDERS OF PHOSPHORUS METABOLISM

Phosphorus (P) is a macromineral with a plethora of important biologic functions. In addition to being essential for the structural stability of bones and teeth, cell membranes (phospholipids), and nucleic acid molecules, phosphorus plays an important role in metabolic activity such as carbohydrate and energy metabolism that inherently depends on the capacity to phosphorylate intermediate metabolites and to store energy released during oxidation in high-energy phosphate bonds such as ATP or phosphocreatine. Phosphorus is an integral component of 2,3-DPG, a compound that regulates oxygen release from hemoglobin and therefore is critical for oxygen delivery to tissues. Inorganic phosphorus (phosphate, PO_4, or Pi) is also an important buffer in the body.

In the body, phosphorus is present as a stable inorganic phosphate (Pi), an organic phosphate ester, or a phospholipid. By far the largest fraction of the body phosphorus (~85% of total body phosphorus) is incorporated into bone in an insoluble inorganic phosphate form (dihydroxyapatite). The remainder is largely located in the intracellular space (ICS, ~14%), while <1% of the total body phosphorus is found in the extracellular space (ECS), which includes blood serum or plasma. In the ECS, phosphorus is present either as Pi, forming the metabolically relevant fraction, or as phospholipids. The extracellular Pi fraction is largely (~85%) ionized (either $H_2PO_4^-$ or HPO_4^{2-}), while ~10% is protein bound and 5% is complexed with other minerals such as calcium or magnesium.

The concentration of Pi in the ECS and thus in serum is dictated by the equilibrium between Pi uptake from the digestive tract; Pi excretion in urine (monogastric species), saliva (ruminants), and milk; the uptake or release of Pi from bone; and compartmental Pi shifts between the ECS and ICS. Accordingly, hypophosphatemia that is defined as subnormal serum or plasma Pi concentration can be caused by decreased oral phosphorus uptake, increased phosphorus loss, increased cellular phosphorus uptake, or a combination of these factors. Because only increased phosphorus loss and decreased phosphorus uptake are associated with phosphorus depletion of the body but compartmental shifts of phosphorus between the ICS and ECS can strongly affect the extracellular Pi concentration, the serum Pi concentration is an unreliable parameter to assess the phosphorus status of an animal. Despite the difficult interpretation of the serum Pi concentration, it is still the most commonly used measurement of phosphorus status in veterinary medicine.

HYPOPHOSPHATEMIA

Etiology and Pathogenesis: Chronic phosphorus deficiency is commonly caused by inadequate feed intake or inadequate phosphorus content in the ration over an extended time. This can be seen in grazing animals in arid regions with low phosphorus content in soil. Phosphorus depletion can also result from chronic renal tubular disease due to impaired renal reabsorption of phosphorus (eg, Fanconi syndrome) or primary hyperparathyroidism causing increased renal phosphorus excretion. Hypophosphatemia is a common finding in horses with chronic renal failure.

Acute phosphorus losses associated with hypophosphatemia are a well-recognized problem in high-yielding dairy cows at the onset of lactation. The sudden onset of phosphorus losses through the mammary gland at the onset of lactation and the decreased feed intake around parturition are believed to be the major contributors to periparturient hypophosphatemia of dairy cows. Nonetheless, periparturient hypophosphatemia has also been documented in mastectomized cows, indicating that other mechanisms, such as compartmental shifts, impaired intestinal absorption, or increased losses through the digestive or urinary tracts, must contribute to this phenomenon.

Hypophosphatemia without phosphorus depletion may occur after oral or parenteral carbohydrate administration and after parenteral insulin administration as a result of increased cellular phosphorus uptake in combination with glucose. Alkalemia and respiratory alkalosis enhance cellular phosphorus uptake and therefore also have a hypophosphatemic effect.

Clinical Findings and Lesions: Signs of chronic phosphorus depletion are most commonly seen in cattle fed a phosphorus-deficient diet over several months. Young animals grow slowly, develop rickets, and tend to have a rough hair coat, whereas adult animals in early stages may become lethargic, anorectic, and lose weight. Decreased milk production and fertility have erroneously been attributed to phosphorus depletion. These signs appear to be the result of decreased energy and protein intake in animals that are anorectic due to phosphorus depletion. In later stages, animals may develop pica, osteomalacia, abnormal gait, and lameness, and eventually become recumbent.

Acute hypophosphatemia has been associated with anorexia, muscle weakness, muscle and bone pain, rhabdomyolysis, increased fragility of RBCs, and ensuing intravascular hemolysis. Other potential effects of hypophoshatemia are neurologic signs presumably related to the altered energy metabolism, impaired cardiac and respiratory function (decreased contractility of striated and heart muscle), and dysfunction of WBCs and platelets that are believed to be caused by ATP depletion.

In cattle, hypophosphatemia occurring at the onset of lactation is widely believed to be associated with periparturient recumbency and the downer cow syndrome (*see* p 1188). However, this association is based on empirical observation and is not supported by unequivocal evidence. Postparturient hemoglobinuria is another but rare condition seen in high-yielding dairy cows in the first days of lactation. It is characterized by acute intravascular hemolysis and hemoglobinuria, frequently with fatal outcome.

It is currently not well understood whether the above-mentioned clinical signs and conditions are caused by low levels of phosphorus in the blood or by overall depletion of phosphorus in the body.

Necropsy findings in cases of chronic phosphorus depletion are those specific to rickets or osteomalacia. Carcasses appear emaciated with a dull hair coat. Fractures of ribs, vertebrae, or the pelvis, as well as widened growth plates and costochondral junctions, angular deformities, and shortened long bones are common.

Diagnosis: Phosphorus depletion is not readily diagnosed in living animals. Because chronically phosphorus-depleted animals can maintain the serum Pi concentration within normal limits by mobilizing Pi from bone, and because the serum Pi concentration can be decreased even in the absence of phosphorus depletion, the Pi concentration in serum is an unreliable proxy to diagnose chronic phosphorus depletion. Although acute phosphorus depletion can reflect accurately in the serum Pi concentration, the considerable diurnal variation, effects of physical activity, and feed intake complicate the interpretation of results from a single blood sample. Dextrose administered parenterally shortly before blood sampling can decrease the serum Pi concentration by >30%; 4–6 hr should elapse between the end of dextrose infusion and blood sampling to allow the serum Pi concentration to return to baseline. Other factors that can affect the serum Pi concentration include physical exercise shortly before blood sampling or the site of blood collection. Vigorous physical activity can result in markedly decreased serum or plasma Pi concentrations for >1 hr.

Determination of the bone density or bone phosphorus content in a rib biopsy has been proposed as a reliable parameter to diagnose chronic phosphorus depletion in cattle. Nonetheless, the bone phosphorus content is slow to respond to changes in dietary phosphorus supply, which means the nutritional history has a strong impact on the mineral content of fresh bone. The phosphorus content in fresh bone is therefore a good indicator of body phosphorus reserves but not of current dietary phosphorus supply. Furthermore, obtaining bone biopsies is impractical under field conditions, and determination of bone phosphorus content is generally restricted to postmortem examination or research activities. Alternatively, the extent of bone resorption activity can be determined by measuring the urinary hydroxyproline concentration, an amino acid liberated from collagen as bone is demineralized. Radiographic examination of bone will reveal reduced radiopacity of the bones in chronically phosphorus-depleted animals.

Feed samples can be submitted to determine the phosphorus content in the ration, allowing an estimate of phosphorus intake if the daily feed intake is known. In grazing animals, the phosphorus concentration in either soil or in a fecal sample can be determined and used as an indirect and crude parameter to assess adequacy of the dietary phosphorus content.

Treatment and Prevention: Chronic phosphorus depletion and hypophosphatemia is most effectively treated by providing sufficient amounts of feed with adequate phosphorus content; however, the most appropriate treatment approach for acute phosphorus depletion and hypophosphatemia is controversial. IV administration of phosphorus-containing solutions is often recommended as the most appropriate approach. In small animals, this is achieved by slow IV infusion of sodium phosphate salt solutions, or in case of concomitant hypokalemia of potassium phosphate solutions. In cattle, rapid administration of sodium phosphate salt solutions is commonly practiced. Mono- or dibasic phosphate salts (either Na_2HPO_4 or NaH_2PO_4) infused IV rapidly increase the serum Pi concentration. Tribasic phosphate (Na_3PO_4) is a caustic detergent that cannot be used under any circumstances for PO or IV phosphorus supplementation. An issue with the IV infusion of phosphorus salt solutions is that unbound Pi in plasma reaching the kidney is filtered by the renal glomeruli and must then be reabsorbed in the renal tubules. Because tubular reabsorption is a saturable process, infusing Pi at a rate that increases plasma Pi concentration above the renal threshold disproportionally increases renal Pi excretion and therefore only transiently increases the plasma Pi concentration. This explains the short-lived effect (<2 hr) of sodium phosphate solutions when administered as an IV bolus as recommended for cattle. Rapid administration of sodium phosphate salts causes transient but severe hyperphosphatemia and therefore bears the risk of causing hypocalcemia due to precipitation of calcium phosphate salts. This risk of calcium phosphate precipitation also precludes the parenteral administration of phosphate salts in combination with parenteral calcium or magnesium infusions. Infusing phosphorus salts slowly over several hours results in a more sustained effect and reduces the risk of hypocalcemia. Currently, no sodium phosphate salt–containing solutions are approved by the FDA for IV administration in cattle; therefore, any effective IV phosphate administration is off-label.

In cattle, solutions containing not phosphate but phosphite (PO_3), hypophosphite, or organic phosphorus compounds such as butaphosphan or toldimphos are often used to supplement phosphorus IV, frequently in combination with calcium, magnesium, and other minerals. However, these phosphorus compounds are not suitable to correct hypophosphatemia, because mammals are unable to convert phosphite or the above-mentioned organic compounds into phosphate (PO_4) and so do not contribute to the biologically active plasma Pi pool. Even when organic phosphorus compounds are usable metabolically, pharmaceutical products containing organic phosphorus compounds administered at label dose do not provide nearly enough phosphorus to correct severe phosphorus depletion, which would be the primary indication for IV treatment.

Mild to moderate phosphorus depletion can be treated effectively by oral Pi supplementation either by adding dairy products to the diet (monogastric species) or by providing solutions of sodium phosphate salts for oral consumption. Oral Pi administration rapidly increases plasma Pi concentration and is safe and effective, but it may not be appropriate in vomiting and possibly in diarrheic animals. In cattle, oral sodium phosphate salts increase the plasma Pi concentration within 3–4 hr and exert a sustained effect lasting >12 hr. Other phosphate salts that have been proposed for rapid correction of hypophosphatemia in cattle include monopotassium phosphate and monocalcium phosphate. Dicalcium phosphate is commonly used for longterm supplementation of phosphorus-deficient diets but because of its poor solubility characteristics is unsuitable for rapid correction of hypophosphatemia.

Phosphorus depletion in healthy grazing animals is prevented by assuring sufficient feed intake with adequate phosphorus content. In animals grazing on phosphorus-deficient soils, depletion may be prevented by fertilizing the soils with phosphorus or by supplementing feeds or the water supply with phosphate salts. In the dairy industry, overfeeding phosphorus is more common because of the widely held but incorrect assumption that feeding phosphorus in excess of the daily requirements improves fertility and milk production. Research consistently confirms that phosphorus concentration of 0.42% in dry matter is adequate for high-yielding dairy cows.

Currently, no effective approach to prevent hypophosphatemia and phosphorus depletion at the onset of lactation is known. Feeding higher amounts of dietary phosphorus during the last weeks of gestation is contraindicated, because it decreases the intestinal absorption rate of phosphorus and increases the risk of periparturient hypocalcemia. The dietary Ca:P ratio that appears to be essential in horses and other species to prevent secondary hypo- or hyperparathyroidism is not important in ruminants. Cattle tolerate Ca:P ratios between 1:1 and 8:1, provided the ration meets minimal requirements for both minerals. This peculiarity in ruminants can be explained by the high *salivary phosphorus* concentration (5- to 10-fold the concentration in serum) and the large amounts of saliva produced that alter the Ca:P ratio of the rumen content considerably.

HYPERPHOSPHATEMIA

Physiologically increased serum and plasma Pi concentrations are seen in young and growing animals due to enhanced intestinal phosphorus uptake and decreased renal phosphorus excretion, presumably to facilitate bone mineralization. Pathologically increased extracellular phosphorus concentrations can be the result of hemoconcentration, decreased renal excretion, decreased intracellular uptake, or cellular release of phosphorus after cell lysis. Decreased urinary phosphorus excretion in association with chronic renal failure is the most common cause of hyperphosphatemia in many monogastric species except horses. In ruminants, hyperphosphatemia is commonly seen in dehydrated animals and is most likely due to hemoconcentration and a concomitant reduction in saliva production. Massive tissue injury with rhabdomyolysis results in damaged cell membrane integrity, which leads to release of phosphorus together with other predominantly intracellular compounds such as potassium into the extracellular space. Hypoparathyroidism may result in hyperphosphatemia due to increased renal phosphorus reabsorption in the absence of PTH. Incidental cases of severe acute hyperphosphatemia were reported after repeated treatment with enemas containing hypertonic sodium phosphate solutions in people and small ruminants.

Hemolysis occurring during or after blood sample collection results in release of intracellular phosphorus from RBCs and therefore gives erroneously high serum Pi concentrations. Therefore, hemolytic blood samples should not be used to determine the serum or plasma Pi concentration.

Hyperphosphatemia as it occurs during hemoconcentration or decreased glomerular filtration is unlikely to be of any clinical relevance. In more severe cases, concomitant hypocalcemia may result from precipitation of excessive phosphorus with calcium and cause muscle fasciculations and tetanic muscle contractions. In sustained cases, precipitation of calcium-phosphate salts results in extraskeletal tissue mineralization with a potentially fatal outcome.

POSTPARTURIENT HEMOGLOBINURIA

Postparturient hemoglobinuria is a sporadic condition seen worldwide that most commonly affects individual high-yielding dairy cows at the onset of lactation. It is characterized by development of peracute intravascular hemolysis and anemia with potentially fatal outcome. Beef and nonlactating cattle are rarely affected. The exact cause is unknown, but phosphorus depletion or hypophosphatemia has been incriminated as a major predisposing factor. Severe intracellular phosphorus depletion of RBCs is known to increase osmotic fragility of the RBCs, possibly predisposing to intravascular hemolysis. Although marked hypophosphatemia is commonly diagnosed in affected animals, most cases of severe hypophosphatemia are not associated with intravascular hemolysis, suggesting that hypophosphatemia is not the sole causative factor responsible for postparturient hemoglobinuria. A similar condition reported in New Zealand was associated with copper deficiency, potentially making RBCs more susceptible to oxidative stress. Other potential causes are hemolytic or oxidative plant toxins (often from *Brassica* spp, sugar beets, or green forage).

Clinical cases are rare, but when they occur the case fatality rate is high (10%–30%). With clinical disease, rapid intravascular hemolysis leads to severe anemia, tachycardia, weakness, hemoglobinuria with dark brown or red urine, and pallor over several days. Milk production drops rapidly. Affected cows also may have fever, diarrhea, and tachypnea. Cows that survive the hemolytic crisis may take several months to recover completely. Convalescent cows and cows with subclinical disease develop icterus and evidence of increased erythropoiesis.

Diagnosis is usually made by recognition of clinical signs, particularly dark urine and anemia during the characteristic stage of lactation. Hemoglobinuria may best be diagnosed by noting failure of the urine to clear with centrifugation (excluding hematuria) and presence of concurrent severe anemia. Intravascular hemolysis caused by *Babesia* (*see* p 21) or *Theileria* (*see* p 33) may be excluded by blood smear analysis, and standard laboratory methods can be used to exclude leptospirosis (*see* p 646) or bacillary hemoglobinuria (*see* p 601). Diagnostic testing and feed or pasture analysis can be performed to identify toxic plants and deficiency of phosphorus, copper, and other antioxidants.

Transfusion of large quantities of whole blood is the best treatment for severely affected cows. Crystalloid fluids may be beneficial if blood is not available and may protect the kidneys against toxic and anoxic damage, but monitoring the PCV and the total protein concentration is required to prevent third spacing due to the decreased intravascular oncotic pressure. Parenteral treatment with monosodium dihydrogen phosphate (60 g in 300 mL of sterile water) IV followed by oral treatment with 200–300 g of sodium phosphate salts every 12 hr is suitable to rapidly correct hypophosphatemia. Copper glycinate (120 mg available copper) has been recommended in cases in which copper deficiency is suspected as the underlying cause. The efficacy of these treatments to prevent further hemolysis is not documented. No sodium phosphate or copper glycinate solution approved for parenteral administration by the FDA is currently available for use in ruminants. The use of these compounds in dairy cows is therefore extra-label. Correction of mineral deficiencies and elimination of plant toxins from the diet may help prevent recurrence.

DISORDERS OF POTASSIUM METABOLISM

Potassium homeostasis is mainly determined by the balance between absorption of potassium from the GI tract and subsequent excretion by the kidneys (all animals) and saliva (in adult ruminants). Transport of potassium is passive in the small intestine and active in the colon under the influence of aldosterone. The most important hormone affecting renal and salivary potassium excretion is aldosterone, which is released from the zona glomerulosa of the adrenal gland in response to hyperkalemia and other factors. One of aldosterone's primary actions is to enhance the secretion of potassium ions in the distal renal tubules and collecting ducts. At least 95% of whole body potassium is intracellular, with skeletal muscle containing 60%–75% of the intracellular potassium. Marked changes in serum or plasma potassium concentrations alter the resting membrane potential of cells, because the potassium gradient generated by Na^+/K^+-ATPase is the main cause for the negative electric potential across cell membranes. Therefore, hypokalemia or hyperkalemia alters the resting membrane potential, resulting in clinically significant changes in cellular and organ function. Hypokalemia usually indicates whole body depletion of potassium, whereas in hyperkalemia, whole body potassium status cannot be inferred because many animals with hyperkalemia have concurrent acidemia and whole body potassium depletion.

Hypokalemia can occur in any animal receiving large volumes of IV fluid or having a marked and sustained reduction in feed intake. The clinical signs in most animals with mild to moderate hypokalemia are mild and nonspecific. Severe hypokalemia is associated with ventroflexion of the head or recumbency due to generalized muscle weakness and cardiac arrhythmias, including both atrial and ventricular premature complexes that may lead to more complex cardiac arrhythmias. Prolonged and profound hypokalemia can result in a myopathy that is difficult to treat. Cats can be affected by a hypokalemic polymyopathy (*see* p 1201), and Burmese cats have an autosomal recessive disorder that leads to hypokalemic myopathy (*see* p 1232).

Hyperkalemia usually results from inadequate urinary excretion of ingested potassium and is common in monogastric animals with urinary tract obstruction and bladder rupture. Hyperkalemia in horses and ruminants can also result from exertional rhabdomyolysis, because skeletal muscle contains a large percentage of whole body potassium. Hyperkalemia also occurs in heavily muscled Quarter horses and related breeds as a genetic disorder (hyperkalemic periodic paralysis, *see* p 1047). Hyperkalemia is frequently present in dogs with hypoadrenocorticism (*see* p 574). Severe hyperkalemia is associated with generalized muscle weakness, depression, and cardiac conduction disturbances that may lead to lethal cardiac arrhythmias. Pseudohyperkalemia in serum can occur in animals with thrombocytosis as a result of the excessive release of intracellular potassium stores from platelets during clotting. Pseudohyperkalemia in serum and plasma occurs when extensive hemolysis is present due to the high potassium concentration in RBCs.

HYPOKALEMIA IN ADULT CATTLE

Hypokalemia occurs commonly in inappetant adult cattle, particularly in lactating dairy cows because of the additional loss of potassium in the milk.

Etiology: Hypokalemia is common in adult cattle with prolonged inappetence (>2 days), or in those receiving more than one injection of corticosteroids that have mineralocorticoid activity, eg, isoflupredone acetate. This is because mineralocorticoid activity enhances renal and GI losses of potassium. Hypokalemia is extremely rare in adult ruminants with adequate dry matter intake.

Clinical Findings and Diagnosis: Animals with hypokalemia have generalized muscle weakness, depression, and muscle fasciculations. Severely affected animals are unable to stand or lift their head from the ground.

Serum biochemical analysis is required to confirm a suspected diagnosis of hypokalemia. A serum potassium concentration <2.5 mEq/L reflects severe hypokalemia; most animals will be weak, and some will be recumbent. A serum potassium concentration of 2.5–3.5 mEq/L reflects moderate hypokalemia, and some cattle will be recumbent or appear weak with depressed GI motility. In addition to measurement of serum potassium concentration, measurement of serum concentrations of sodium, chloride, calcium, and phosphorus, and serum activities of CK and AST can be very helpful in guiding treatment. Aciduria may be present in response to a marked decrease in urine potassium concentration.

Treatment: Oral potassium administration is the treatment of choice for hypokalemia. Inappetant lactating dairy cattle should be treated with 60–120 g of feed grade KCl twice at a 12-hr interval, with the KCl placed in gelatin boluses or administered by ororuminal intubation. Adult cattle with severe hypokalemia (<2.5 mEq/L) should initially be treated with 120 g of KCl PO, followed by a second 120-g dose of KCl 12 hr later, for a total 24-hr treatment of 240 g KCl. Higher oral doses are not recommended, because they can lead to diarrhea, excessive salivation, muscular tremors of the legs, and excitability.

Potassium is rarely administered IV; the IV route is used only for initial treatment of recumbent ruminants with severe hypokalemia and rumen atony, because it is much more dangerous and expensive than oral treatment. The most aggressive IV treatment protocol is an isotonic solution of KCl (1.15%), which should be administered at <3.2 mL/kg/hr, equivalent to a maximal delivery rate of K^+ at 0.5 mEq/kg/hr. Higher rates of potassium administration run the risk of inducing hemodynamically important arrhythmias, including premature ventricular complexes that can lead to ventricular fibrillation and death.

Prevention: Oral administration of potassium is a mandatory component of fluid and electrolyte administration to inappetant cattle. Ensuring adequate dry-matter intake is the best method to prevent hypokalemia in adult cattle.

HYPERKALEMIA

Etiology: Hyperkalemia is common in neonatal ruminants with diarrhea, dehydration, acidemia, and strong ion (metabolic) acidosis. Hyperkalemia often accompanies acidemia, because low blood pH results in intracellular acidosis and leakage of potassium from the intracellular compartment to the extracellular space. Hyperkalemia is common in neonatal foals with uroabdomen secondary to ruptured bladder associated with parturition, and in male cats with uroabdomen secondary to obstructive urolithiasis and bladder rupture. Hyperkalemia is rare in steers, wethers, and bucks with obstructive urolithiasis and bladder or urethral rupture, because excess potassium is secreted in adult ruminant saliva and affected animals have a decrease in potassium intake due to illness. Hyperkalemia can be present in horses and ruminants with exertional rhabdomyolysis due to damage to skeletal muscle cells.

Clinical Findings and Diagnosis: Severe hyperkalemia is usually associated with depression, weakness, lethargy, cardiac arrhythmias, and ECG abnormalities, particularly when the serum potassium concentration is >7 mEq/L. Severe cardiotoxic effects are evident when the serum potassium concentration is 8–11 mEq/L.

Serum biochemical analysis is required to confirm a suspected diagnosis of hyperkalemia. In addition to measurement of serum potassium concentration, measurement of serum concentrations of sodium, calcium, phosphorus, urea, and creatinine; the serum activities of CK and AST; and blood gas analysis can be helpful in guiding treatment. ECG may reveal bradyarrhythmias, suppression in P wave amplitude or loss of the P wave, widened QRS complexes, and symmetric T waves (narrowing of T wave duration and "tenting" of the T wave). The ECG effects of hyperkalemia are exacerbated by the presence of hyponatremia, acidemia, and hypocalcemia. The ratio of serum sodium to potassium concentration is important in development of cardiac arrhythmias; hyperkalemia in the presence of hyponatremia (sodium:potassium ratio <25:1) is commonly associated with the occurrence of cardiac arrhythmias and ECG abnormalities.

Treatment: Hyperkalemia should initially be treated by IV administration of 0.9% NaCl to increase the rate of urine production in dehydrated animals with a patent urinary system, and in selected cases by IV administration of sodium bicarbonate, glucose, insulin, and sometimes calcium. Urine should be removed from the abdomen of animals with obstructive urolithiasis and ruptured bladder, and urethral patency established. Sodium bicarbonate is administered to correct systemic and intracellular acidosis. The rationale for IV glucose and insulin administration is that insulin-mediated glucose entry into cells is accompanied by movement of potassium from the extracellular space to the intracellular compartment. The rationale for calcium administration is that calcium counteracts many of the deleterious effects of hyperkalemia on arrhythmogenesis, and the IV administration of calcium may therefore improve cardiac output. However, hypertonic saline (2,400 mOsm/L) is just as effective as hypertonic sodium bicarbonate in decreasing hyperkalemia and hyperkalemia-associated bradyarrhythmias, probably because of hypernatremia-mediated intracellular movement of potassium, extracellular volume expansion, and increased rate of urine production. The focus of treatment in hyperkalemia should therefore be identification and correction of acidemia, plasma volume expansion to assist in renal excretion of potassium, and increasing the serum sodium concentration. Glucose and insulin do not appear to be routinely needed to correct hyperkalemia.

Prevention: Hyperkalemia can be prevented by early diagnosis and treatment of its most common causes. Hyperkalemic periodic paralysis can be prevented in horses by feeding a low-potassium diet or the oral administration of acetazolamide.

EQUINE METABOLIC SYNDROME

(Insulin dysregulation syndrome, Equine syndrome X, Peripheral Cushing disease)

Equine metabolic syndrome (EMS) describes a characteristic collection of clinical signs and clinicopathologic changes in equids. It is found in both horses and ponies and has also been recognized in donkeys. Affected animals typically are obese, with increased condition score overall and increased adiposity in the neck and tailhead regions. Laminitis, both chronic and acute, is common. Hyperinsulinemia with normal blood glucose concentrations (insulin resistance) is the primary clinical pathologic finding. Other associated signs include infertility, altered ovarian activity, and increased appetite. Other laboratory findings include hypertriglyceridemia, increased serum concentrations of leptin, and arterial hypertension. Previously, this cluster of clinical signs in horses was referred to as hypothyroidism, peripheral Cushing disease, prelaminitic syndrome, or Syndrome X. EMS replaces these earlier terms. EMS may be the end result of an inability to properly metabolize dietary carbohydrate, and many horses exhibit exaggerated glucose and insulin responses to an oral hexose load before developing true insulin resistance. Any abnormality in carbohydrate metabolism in horses has been termed insulin dysregulation.

EMS first develops in horses 5–16 yr old. Breeds most commonly affected include ponies, Saddlebred, Tennessee Walking, Paso Fino, Morgan, Mustang, and Quarter horses. Thoroughbreds and Standardbreds infrequently develop EMS. There is no recognized sex predilection.

Etiology and Pathogenesis: The underlying reason why some horses develop EMS and others do not is not known. There appears to be a genetic disposition, both within and between breeds. Affected horses may possess a "thrifty" gene that enabled their ancestors to survive in harsh environments. This increased efficiency of energy metabolism became maladaptive in modern environments with plentiful, nutrient-dense feedstuffs.

The common denominators behind many of the signs associated with EMS appear to be increased adiposity, insulin resistance, and hyperinsulemia. When obesity develops, adipose tissues elaborate leptin and other adipokines as well as tumor necrosis factor and other inflammatory mediators. Increased fat stores in the liver may also predispose to insulin resistance due to down-regulation of insulin receptors.

Experimentally, high blood insulin levels lead to laminitis in horses and ponies. Insulin has vasoregulatory actions. Insulin resistance can decrease nitric oxide production and promote vasoconstriction. Altered glucose and insulin levels may also lead to altered epidermal cell function and glucose uptake by epidermal laminar cells. These effects predispose horses with EMS to develop laminitis.

Horses with EMS respond to high carbohydrate meals with an exaggerated increase in insulin, a higher than expected blood glucose level, and a very slow return of blood glucose concentrations to baseline values. This indicates a resistance to the peripheral effects of insulin (EMS) and/or an inability to metabolize oral carbohydrate normally (insulin dysregulation).

EMS may be a predisposing factor for pituitary pars intermedia dysfunction (PPID; also called equine Cushing disease). Both endocrine disorders can occur concurrently in middle-aged and older horses. Horses with EMS should therefore be monitored to detect the onset of PPID. (*See also* p 547.)

Clinical Findings: There is no clinical picture that is pathognomonic for insulin resistance. Horses may exhibit all the phenotypic characteristics of EMS with normal responses to evocative testing. In most instances, the animals in question are obese because of excess calorie intake rather than any underlying metabolic alteration.

Affected horses typically are obese with a body condition score >6 out of 9. Even if the overall condition score is not extremely high, there is increased fat deposition in the neck, leading to a "cresty" appearance. Fat deposition over the ribs and over the top line to the tail head is also common. Geldings may have increased fat deposition in the prepuce, whereas mares may have increased fat deposition around the mammary gland. Laminitis is a common finding. Horses brought in for evaluation with no previous history of laminitis often show evidence of prior episodes such as abnormal hoof growth rings and radiographic evidence of third phalanx rotation or pedal osteitis. Laminitis may occur secondary to ingestion of feeds high in soluble carbohydrates, either in the form of lush pasture or high-carbohydrate hays and supplements. This can result in bouts of laminitis developing in the spring, when new pasture growth appears, and in the fall, when night temperatures are below freezing.

Horses with EMS may not lose weight without extreme feed restriction; owners commonly report that affected horses remain obese even when fed minimal amounts. Obesity may be exacerbated by laminitis, which may limit exercise. Horses appear to have increased appetites and often will eat continually as long as feed is available. Infertility and abnormal reproductive cycles occur in mares affected with EMS.

Lesions: Increased general adiposity and laminitis are often documented. The pituitary gland is normal in younger horses with EMS, but lesions consistent with PPID may be found in older horses with EMS that are concurrently affected by EMS and PPID.

Diagnosis: Diagnostic testing for EMS should concentrate on documenting insulin resistance while excluding PPID. The presence of obesity and the cresty neck phenotype is not sufficient to make a diagnosis. A careful dietary history and physical examination are essential. Establishing baseline body condition score and neck circumference will enable assessment of the horse's response to treatment. Even if there is no history of laminitis, careful examination of the feet, including lateral images of P3, are indicated.

Because many conditions, including diet, pain, and stress, can affect blood glucose and insulin levels, diagnostic testing should be performed in a controlled manner in a low-stress environment. If the horse has laminitis, diagnostic testing should be delayed until the feet have stabilized and are relatively pain free.

Blood glucose concentrations are in the normal range or only slightly increased with EMS. If persistent hyperglycemia is documented, concurrent PPID should be strongly suspected. Because many factors influence blood glucose and insulin levels, a one-time blood insulin measurement should be used only as a screening test for insulin resistance. Insulin should be determined after the horse has been fasted for 6–8 hr. This can be done by leaving only one flake of hay with the horse after 10 PM the night before and then collecting the blood sample the next morning. If those conditions are met, a blood insulin concentration >20 μU/mL is suggestive of insulin resistance.

To document insulin resistance, the horse's ability to handle glucose should be evaluated. Because a subset of horses are normal in all respects except for their ability to handle an oral carbohydrate load, an oral sugar test (OST) or oral glucose test (OGT) should be performed. The OST is easy to perform in North America, where corn syrup is readily available, whereas the OGT can be performed in other parts of the world. The OST is performed by fasting the horse for 6–8 hr and then giving an oral dose of corn syrup at 0.15 mL/kg. Blood should be collected at 60 or 90 min after administration of the corn syrup for insulin determination. An insulin concentration >60 mU/L is abnormal. The OGT is performed by giving a fasted horse 0.5 kg of chaff-based feed to which dextrose powder at 1 g/kg has been added. An insulin concentration >87 mU/L in a blood sample collected 2 hr later is abnormal. To determine whether insulin can stimulate normal glucose uptake by peripheral tissues, an insulin tolerance test can be performed. This is accomplished by collecting a baseline blood sample for glucose concentration, giving regular human recombinant insulin at 0.1 IU/kg, IV, and then collecting a second blood sample for glucose concentration 30 min later. A second blood glucose concentration that does not decrease to 50% or less of the baseline value indicates insulin resistance. Other diagnostic testing that has been described includes the IV glucose tolerance test or a combined glucose-insulin response test. The oral glucose tolerance test can be altered by delayed gastric emptying or poor GI absorption and is less desirable. Because of the large number of blood samples required and the fact that change from baseline—not absolute glucose values—is of interest, a hand-held glucometer to determine blood glucose concentration may be used when performing these tests.

Tests for PPID such as measuring endogenous ACTH concentration, the dexamethasone suppression test, domperidone response test,or thyroid releasing hormone response test are normal in horses with EMS. Positive results indicate that the horse is concurrently affected by EMS and PPID, which can occur in older horses. Detection of PPID is important, because it is thought that PPID exacerbates insulin resistance in horses previously affected by EMS.

Treatment and Prevention: Treatment for EMS involves dietary management and, if diet and exercise is not sufficient to treat the condition, medical therapy. Correction of the diet may be all that is needed to return the horse to normal body weight. Dietary carbohydrate restriction is essential to decrease glycemic and insulinemic response; total calorie intake is restricted to reduce body weight. Pasture access should be eliminated or severely restricted. Use of a grazing muzzle may aid in decreasing pasture ingestion.

The nonstructural carbohydrate (NSC) content of forage should be determined by feed analysis. This can be calculated by adding starch and water-soluble carbohydrate percentages. Ideally, NSC should comprise <10% of the hay dry matter, and it should never exceed 16%. Soaking hay in water for 60 min has been recommended to lower water-soluble carbohydrate concentrations, but the actual amount reduced is extremely variable; hence, this is not a reliable method to produce a low-NSC forage. Supplements should be given to add needed vitamins and minerals but not additional calories. Complete feeds that are formulated to be low in digestible energy and carbohydrate specifically designed for horses with insulin resistance may be used in place of forage and supplements. Numerous dietary supplements have been suggested to increase insulin sensitivity, including cinnamon, chromium, and magnesium. None has been shown to improve insulin sensitivity in horses in experimental situations.

Horses should initially be fed 1.5% of their ideal body weight in forage per day. This amount can be lowered to 1.25% and then to 1% of ideal body weight after 30 days, if necessary. Sudden feed restriction should be avoided, because it may lead to hyperlipemia and further exacerbate insulin resistance. Increasing the amount and level of exercise will increase the rate of weight loss. The amount of exercise necessary to provide maximal benefits has not been established, but five sessions per week that include at least 30 min of trotting and lunging is a realistic goal. In horses with laminitis, walking as pain allows may be of some benefit.

Weight reduction should be documented by scale weight or weight tapes. In addition, neck thickness and diameter can be monitored over time. If increased exercise and dietary modification is not sufficient to decrease body weight, medical therapy may be of benefit.

The thyroid hormone thyroxine, in the form of levothyroxine sodium, will accelerate weight loss and thereby improve insulin sensitivity when combined with dietary interventions in horses. Horses weighing >350 kg can be given 48 mg/day, PO; smaller horses and ponies should receive 24 mg/day, PO. Treatment periods of 3–6 mo are often needed to achieve desirable weight loss. At that time, the horse should be weaned off the medication over 3–4 wk. If feed intake is not limited concurrently, treatment with levothyroxine is unlikely to resolve clinical signs.

Metformin is poorly absorbed in equids but may decrease postprandial glucose and insulin levels.. It may lead to improvement in hyperinsulinemic horses at a dosage of 30 mg/kg, PO, tid or bid. It should be given 30 min before a meal if possible. However, the longterm efficacy and safety of metformin has not been established in horses. If it is used, blood glucose should be carefully monitored. Use of metformin should be discontinued if hypoglycemia is documented.

Prevention of EMS should focus on maintaining normal weight in horses, particularly in high-risk breeds. Because these horses may be more efficient users of ingested calories than others, it is imperative to feed appropriately to maintain an ideal condition score and not to use arbitrary feeding guidelines. Particular care should be exercised when turning horses on pasture during times of high-soluble carbohydrate content, eg, spring and autumn.

FATIGUE AND EXERCISE

Muscular fatigue during exercise is the inability to continue to perform at the same *level of intensity, resulting from the inability* of the muscles to produce force. Fatigue may occur during both aerobic and anaerobic exercise, and at submaximal effort depending on the ambient temperature, hydration status, electrolyte concentrations, external motivation, and the animal's desire to work. As effort increases, glycogen depletion, intracellular acidosis, and accumulation of metabolic by-products will contribute to the onset of fatigue. Fatigue during exercise can also be the result of pathologic conditions, including diseases that affect oxygen uptake, energy metabolism, or neuromuscular function. This chapter will focus on muscular fatigue in normal, healthy animals.

Fatigue is considered a normal consequence of exercise of prolonged duration or high intensity, and is regarded as an intrinsic safety mechanism. Without the onset of fatigue, or if fatigue is delayed for a time, structural damage to the myocytes and supportive tissues may occur. Most knowledge of fatigue has been described in horses using high-speed treadmill exercise, to allow for investigation of the respiratory, cardiovascular, and metabolic responses during exertion. Tests involved include spirometry, arterial blood gases, hematologic analysis, kinematics, electromyography, and muscle biopsies. Fatigue in these studies has been defined as the inability or unwillingness of the horse to maintain the same velocity as the treadmill at a determined speed despite minimal encouragement. Horses run to the point of fatigue on a treadmill exhibit characteristic changes in gait, including decreased stride frequency and a longer stride length.

Fatigue has been classified into two types: peripheral and central. Peripheral fatigue is described as fatigue secondary to altered muscle function. The primary cause is failure of ATP to resynthesize with accumulation of ADP and inorganic phosphate ions. Studies of muscle metabolism after exercise to identify peripheral fatigue have relied mainly on muscle biopsies and direct measurement of muscle glycogen, creatine phosphate, ATP, ADP, inosine monophosphate, inorganic phosphate, glycolytic intermediary products, pH, and other metabolites. Other studies have investigated the expression of mRNA in muscle tissue to monitor adaptations in gene expression of proteins that regulate oxygen-dependent metabolism, glucose metabolism, and fatty acid utilization. Indirect serum biomarkers associated with fatigue may include lactate, ammonia, hypoxanthine and xanthine, ammonia, markers of oxidative damage (thiobarbituric acid reactive substances, glutathione, and glutathione peroxidase), inflammatory mediators, and lymphocytes.

Central fatigue is defined as an alteration in the signals arising from the CNS, directly decreasing performance by modifying the frequency of the action potential in the motor neurons. Central fatigue may occur secondary to pain, dyspnea, perceptions of exertion, hypoglycemia, hyperthermia, ammonia accumulation, increases in serotonin, altered amino acid metabolism, and changes in extracellular ions. Central fatigue is associated with decreased motivation, lethargy, tiredness, and loss of muscle coordination. However, the cause of central fatigue is multifactorial, and the response to these stimuli is highly variable. For example, some horses can continue endurance exercise at speed despite severe hyperthermia, dehydration, and plasma electrolyte disturbances.

FATIGUE DURING HIGH-INTENSITY EXERCISE

For all intensities of exercise, there is a degree of anaerobic metabolism, but for brief, high-intensity exercise, anaerobic metabolism predominates. Catabolism of creatine phosphate and glycogen is the anaerobic source of energy during high-intensity exercise. This type of exercise at an individual animal's highest attainable speed cannot be maintained for >30–40 seconds. Thereafter, fatigue occurs and the animal slows down.

Energetics of Exercise and Fatigue:

The contribution of aerobic or anaerobic energy pathways during exercise depends on the duration and energy demands of the event. In short, intense exercise lasting 20–30 seconds (eg, Quarter horse races [400 m], some Greyhound races), 60% of energy demands is supplied by anaerobic sources. For intense exercise at maximal speeds for a longer duration (eg, Standardbred or Thoroughbred races [1,600–2,100 m] lasting 1–3 min), it has been estimated that the energy supply is 20%–30% anaerobic. In contrast, events lasting many hours (eg, endurance races for horses, camels, and dogs) have >90% of energy demands met by aerobic sources.

During brief, high-intensity exercise, fatigue is secondary to engagement of muscle fibers that heavily rely on anaerobic metabolism. The higher the intensity, the greater the anaerobic demand. Fatigue is the result of an increase in hydrogen ions, lactate, inorganic phosphate, ammonia, and ADP, and a decrease in ATP, phosphocreatine, and pH in active muscle cells. Clinically, fatigue is initially identified by a decrease in exercise intensity or a drop in the maximal speed.

As anaerobic metabolism increases, lactate production is directly correlated to the percentage of type IIB muscle fibers present and corresponds to the accumulation of protons in the muscle tissue. Intracellular acidosis caused by lactate accumulation has a negative feedback effect on the glycolytic enzymes required for energy production and mitochondrial respiration, resulting in a decline in ATP concentrations. Lack of ATP prevents calcium recycling through the sarcoplasmic reticulum, resulting in accumulation of calcium in the sarcoplasm and slowing of the relaxation phase of muscle contraction. Acidosis also interferes with excitation-contraction coupling by interfering with calcium binding to troponin C, reducing the ability of the muscles to contract. Unfortunately, there is no correlation between muscle lactate concentration and placement in a race, or plasma lactate concentrations and performance indexes.

A decrease in muscle ATP after maximal exercise has been noted in conjunction with high muscle lactate concentrations. For high-intensity exercise, eg, a Thoroughbred race lasting 2 min, intramuscular stores of ATP can decrease from 14% to 50%. Depletion of ATP varies by muscle fiber type. In type I fibers, depletion is negligible, whereas in type IIB fibers, ATP loss is significant. Low levels of ATP impair optimal functioning for muscle contraction, reuptake of calcium by the sarcoplasmic reticulum, and the sodium potassium exchange. Fatigue is associated with depletion of phosphocreatine stores and accumulation of ADP and inorganic phosphate. A correlation between stride length and muscle ADP accumulation has been seen at the time of fatigue.

Muscular Fatigue: Increased ADP concentration results in accumulation of AMP, inosine monophosphate, allantoin, ammonia, and uric acid in horses. In treadmill studies, the decrease in muscle ATP during intense exercise is correlated with an increase in plasma uric acid concentration 30 min after exercise. Running time during treadmill tests is correlated with uric acid concentrations after exercise. Significant but low correlations have also been found between racing performance of Standardbred pacers and uric acid concentrations after a race.

Ammonia accumulation in plasma is correlated to decreased ATP and increased muscle lactate. It has been postulated that ammonia accumulation in the plasma may contribute to fatigue. However, infusion with ammonium acetate during treadmill exercise until fatigue did not significantly affect time to fatigue, suggesting plasma ammonia levels do not have a role in fatigue during intense exercise.

Similar to ATP depletion, muscle glycogen concentration decreases up to 30% after a single exercise bout and by as much as 50% with repeated bouts of intense exercise. Again, depletion varies between muscle fiber types, with greater depletion seen in type IIB muscle fibers. Glycogen depletion may play a role in fatigue, in that horses that perform repeated bouts of exercise before an anaerobic exercise session may be at increased risk of fatigue because of the slow rate of glycogen repletion in this species.

During high-intensity exercise, the normal equilibrium between release of potassium from recruited muscle and uptake by inactive muscle fibers is lost, resulting in a continual increase of extracellular potassium until the onset of fatigue. Changes in the ratio of intracellular to extracellular potassium across the sarcolemma alter the resting membrane potential and decrease sarcolemma excitability and the ability to generate an action potential. Reduced excitability contributes to reduced calcium release by the sarcoplasmic reticulum (a process that requires ATP) and a consequent reduction in the force of muscle contraction. This loss of force may relate to the idea of an inherent safety mechanism, in that plasma potassium rapidly declines after cessation of exercise by reuptake into the now inactive muscle.

Intracellular acidosis as a result of lactate accumulation has been blamed for the decrease in efficiency or force of muscle contractions. However, in vitro research has demonstrated a protective effect of lactic acidosis or hydrogen ions in maintaining sarcolemma function and muscle force production in the face of potassium shifts within the cell and plasma associated with intense exercise.

Thermoregulation and Fatigue: Fatigue during high-intensity exercise is also influenced by environmental conditions. Intense exercise in hot conditions is associated with earlier onset of fatigue, due to increased blood flow to the skin for thermoregulation at the expense of cardiac output and oxygen delivery to the exercising muscle. Attenuation of normal increases in muscle blood flow during exercise in hot environments has been suggested as a contributor to the onset of fatigue. There is also a central effect of high temperatures, resulting from increased blood temperature at the hypothalamus. Early onset of fatigue in hot conditions is thought to be a protective response to avoid heat stroke.

FATIGUE DURING PROLONGED EXERCISE

Fatigue as a result of prolonged exercise depends on the duration and intensity of the activity, liver glycogen stores, the ambient temperature, and mechanisms of central fatigue. Prolonged exercise mainly depends on aerobic metabolism. Fatigue during prolonged exercise has been associated with depletion of glycogen stores in muscle and liver, and with hypoglycemia. Intramuscular glycogen provides 50% of the energy during the first 30 min of submaximal exercise but drops to <20% after 1 hr. Blood glucose makes a smaller contribution, providing only 10% of total energy utilized. Although circulating fatty acids may provide an energy source during prolonged exercise, fatigue will set in before these fat stores are completely exhausted.

In prolonged exercise, the heat generated during aerobic ATP resynthesis imposes a high thermoregulatory demand on the animal. Only 25% of the total energy produced by the muscles is converted to mechanical energy, leaving 75%–80% of that energy that must be removed as heat. Physiologic responses to heat production include sweating and/or panting to remove excess heat from the body. Complications from these compensatory mechanisms include dehydration, acid base and electrolyte disturbances (which are implicated as causes of fatigue), exhaustion, and even death (which can occur after prolonged exercise).

Exhausted Horse Syndrome: Horses occasionally develop severe clinical signs of fatigue at endurance events, despite current preventive practices, including evaluation of recovery at rest stops. Horses that compete in sports that include 3-day eventing, endurance rides, or combined driving are at risk of presenting with life-threatening exhaustion. In hot conditions, horses may lose body fluids at a rate of 10–15 L/hr through sweat during prolonged exercise. Urgent treatment of fluid and electrolyte deficits and hyperthermia (rectal temperatures >40.5°C [104.9°F]) may be required. Exhausted horses may lose up to 10% of their body weight in water, with some having body fluid deficits of up to 40 L, depending on their size. Water lost as sweat is mainly lost from the extracellular fluid and circulating plasma. Decreased blood volume reduces perfusion to vital organs and hampers thermoregulation. In severe cases, cardiovascular compromise may result in multiorgan failure, including damage to the kidneys, GI mucosa, and lamina of the hoof.

Sweating is associated with the loss of electrolytes, mainly sodium, potassium and chloride, as well as calcium and magnesium. Alterations in muscle electrolytes can contribute directly to signs of fatigue. The most common acid-base alteration resulting from electrolyte imbalances is metabolic alkalosis. Aerobic energy metabolism of endurance events produces minimal amounts of lactic acid; therefore, alkalosis caused by alterations in strong ions (hypochloremia and hypokalemia) predominates. Depletion of magnesium and calcium may contribute further to neuromuscular dysfunction, causing ileus, cardiac arrhythmias, and synchronous diaphragmatic flutter. Unlike endurance riding, anaerobic metabolism predominates in 3-day eventing and combined driving, resulting in metabolic acidosis during the event. After recovery, which can range from 30 min to 2 hr after the event, lactate is oxidized and the acidosis resolves. Metabolic alkalosis will then predominate.

Horses affected by exhausted horse syndrome demonstrate a range of symptoms, from changes in attitude and gait inconsistencies to colic, laminitis, clinical signs of myopathies (hard muscle bellies, pain on palpation), depression, ataxia, and eventually recumbency. Persistent tachycardia and tachypnea are noted despite rest, and rectal temperature may be ≥42°C (107.6° F). Perfusion abnormalities and signs of dehydration may be seen. Sweating may be inappropriate or absent.

Treatment involves cooling the horse and providing fluid therapy to restore circulating volumes. Hyperthermic horses should be moved to shade and treated with cool or cold water sponge baths, cold hosing, or misting fans. Water should be scraped off the haircoat and reapplied repeatedly, to prevent an insulating layer of water from forming. Application of ice water should be avoided, as well as alcohol baths or direct ice application, to prevent tissue damage. Cool-water enemas, or peritoneal and gastric lavage, may help to reduce body temperature in severe cases.

Isotonic balanced electrolyte solutions may be provided for dehydration by nasogastric intubation if the horse has normal borborygmi. Horses may be given up to 8 L initially, with subsequent administration of 4–8 L every 1–2 hr, as needed. Commercial electrolyte mixtures for horses are suitable, but hypertonic, hypotonic, and alkaline solutions should not be used. In severe cases, IV fluid therapy is preferred.

A shock dose of a balanced electrolyte solution should be provided initially (20–40 mL/kg bolus) with addition of 100 mL 23% calcium gluconate per 5 L, and 5% dextrose. Additional fluids and additives should be based on reevaluation of serum chemistries and hydration status.

Additional treatments may include NSAIDs for muscle pain and colic, administered simultaneously with fluid therapy to prevent renal injury, and phenothiazines for anxiety caused by myopathies. Anticonvulsant medications may be required, and dexamethasone may help reduce cerebral edema. DMSO may be useful to further reduce inflammation, and low-molecular-weight heparin can be administered to treat coagulopathies.

Environmental temperature and humidity have a major impact on the severity of disturbance of the horse's fluid balance during prolonged exercise. It is important to ensure adequate hydration before an event, especially after long trailer rides to the competition, and to provide access to fluids during and after exercise to reduce the likelihood of dehydration. Administration of supplementary fluids, electrolytes, and glucose before and during competition, when allowed by doping regulations, may reduce the incidence of exhausted horse syndrome.

Overtraining Syndrome: Highly intense exercise training over many weeks can result in a form of chronic fatigue referred to as overtraining syndrome. Racehorse trainers have long used the terms "overtraining," "staleness," or "sourness" to describe a syndrome of poor performance, failure to recover from exercise, and prolonged fatigue that does not resolve for weeks or months. By definition, signs of overtraining syndrome should persist after >2 wk of rest or reduced physical activity. A less severe form of overtraining syndrome is termed "overreaching," which is also a syndrome of poor performance and fatigue, but athletic recovery in overreaching typically occurs from a few days to 2 wk after a reduced workload.

Overtraining syndrome was first reported in Swedish Standardbred trotters based on observations of horses with signs of fatigue and poor performance combined with weight loss, inappetence, and signs of stress, including tachycardia, nervousness, muscle tremors, sweating, and diarrhea. The severity of clinical signs of overtraining was associated with the degree of red cell hypervolemia, and horses exhibited adrenal exhaustion that may be similar to parasympathetic overtraining reported in people.

In experimental studies, a milder form of overtraining has been reproduced, without any evidence of red cell hypervolemia, inappetance, or adrenal gland exhaustion. However, this syndrome was associated with a decrease in the plasma cortisol response to intense exercise, suggesting that overtraining is associated with dysfunction of the hypothalamic-pituitary-adrenal axis. Recent research has shown that overtrained horses have altered growth hormone activities, with an increase in the normal pulsatile growth hormone activity overnight, in addition to altered glucose metabolism. Biomarkers of skeletal muscle metabolism are currently being investigated as a means to identify overtraining syndrome but require invasive muscle biopsies for measurement.

Overtraining syndrome should be suspected in horses with evidence of sustained decreased performance in association with one or more physiologic or behavioral signs. While no single physiologic marker is able to identify the syndrome, clinical signs in horses may include decreased body weight, increased heart rate during exercise, decreased plasma cortisol response to exercise, and increased plasma concentrations of muscle enzymes or gamma glutamyl transferase. Behavioral signs are a consistent and early marker of overtraining syndrome, and development of a behavioral score to assist in early detection of overtraining syndrome in horses is warranted.

PREVENTION OF FATIGUE

Physical Training: Physical training is the most effective way to reduce fatigue and increase capacity for exercise. Physiologic responses to training that contribute to increased exercise capacity include increases in the maximal rate of oxygen transport, cardiac stroke volume, muscle capillary density, circulating blood volume, and total hemoglobin content. Hypertrophy of muscle cells occurs, coupled with increases in concentrations of mitochondria, glycogen, and enzymes concerned with cellular energy production.

Sport-specific training can result in specific adaptions. For example, sprint training can result in decreased proportions of slow-twitch muscle fibers, whereas endurance training can result in increased oxidative capacity of fast-twitch muscle fibers. Sprint training also modulates the ionic changes associated with intense exercise, including decreased potassium efflux from working muscles, resulting in a smaller increase in plasma potassium and delayed onset of fatigue. Training also modulates the exercise-induced decline in both calcium reuptake by the sarcoplasmic reticulum and calcium-ATPase activity associated with fatigue.

Adaptations to training in skeletal muscle depend on the training intensity. Horses trained at intensities >80% of their maximal oxygen uptake (VO_{2max}) had an increase in their percentage of fast-twitch muscle fibers and an 8% increase in the buffering capacity of exercised muscle. These responses did not occur in horses trained at 40% of VO_{2max}.

Heart rate meters can be used to guide the intensity of training to improve the adaptive response to training. Heart rates that result in 80% of VO_{2max} are ~90% of maximal heart rate, which typically ranges from 210 to 240 bpm in horses. Heart rate meters can be used to measure an individual horse's heart rates during slow and fast exercise and to calculate the exercise velocities that result in heart rates of 90% of maximal heart rate. Blood lactate after exercise can also be used to measure the appropriate training intensity. At an exercise intensity of 80% VO_{2max}, plasma lactate concentrations during treadmill exercise are in the range of 4–10 mmol/L.

Warm-up: Warm-up before exercise significantly increases the time to fatigue during intense exercise. Warm-up increases muscle temperature before exercise, increases the rate at which oxygen uptake increases, and reduces lactate accumulation by enhancing aerobic metabolism. The effect is similar whether the warm-up is low intensity (5–10 min at 50% VO_{2max}), moderate intensity (1 min at 70% VO_{2max}), high intensity (1 min at 115% $VO_{2\,max}$), or a combination of low- and high-intensity. The practical importance of this finding is that a warm-up before competition involving intense exercise is likely to increase the time to fatigue during Quarter horse, Thoroughbred, and Standardbred races.

Manipulation of Acid-Base Balance, Diet, and Hydration: It has been suggested that fatigue during intense exercise may be delayed by manipulation of acid-base status before exercise to increase the plasma-buffering capacity. Although some trainers have administered sodium bicarbonate before races, this practice is now banned by many racing administrations. The treatment does alter blood pH and lactate concentrations during exercise; however, the effect of alkalinizing solutions on equine performance is equivocal. Studies using bicarbonate at a dosage of 0.6 g/kg have not shown an effect on the time at which fatigue occurs. Although a metabolic alkalosis could be induced, administration of sodium bicarbonate before intense treadmill exercise did not have any significant effect on metabolic response to exercise. In Greyhounds, a dose of sodium bicarbonate at 0.4 g/kg did not have a significant effect on race time in races >400 m long. However, there may be an ergogenic effect when sodium bicarbonate is administered at high dosages. Sodium bicarbonate at a dosage rate of 1 g/kg (by nasogastric tube) increased the time to fatigue in horses running on a treadmill, and it was concluded that treatment at this dose affected performance.

Energy supply and hydration are frequently manipulated in human athletes to limit fatigue during endurance exercise. Dehydration before exercise results in higher core temperatures during exercise in horses. It would be inappropriate for an animal to begin an endurance exercise with suboptimal hydration. Horses are more susceptible to hyperthermia during prolonged exercise than people because of their high body mass to surface area ratio, which inhibits heat loss. Equine thermoregulation also results in extreme changes to total body fluid status, and there is increasing interest in the way of limiting these excessive responses to exercise by preexercise fluid administration.

Hyperhydration by administration of electrolytes or saline solutions orally before exercise will result in expansion of the blood volume during the event. Studies suggest that hyperhydration before prolonged exercise helps conserve plasma volume during exercise but does not lower body temperature or improve arterial hypoxemia. Maintenance of euhydration with water or a carbohydrate-electrolyte solution during exercise improves perfusion parameters and sweating rates and reduces heat storage. Horses should be acclimated to hot environments before competition.

Horses should not be given large meals (equal to half the ration) 1–2 hr before intense exercise, because plasma volume is decreased for at least 1 hr after a large meal. Large meals may also shift fluid to the GI tract, reducing cardiovascular and thermoregulatory function during exercise. Feeding smaller rations every 4 hr does not result in changes in plasma volume. A short-term reduction in fiber intake before high-intensity racing (fed as ~1% of body wt in hay for 3 days before high-intensity exercise) is a strategy to reduce GI water volume and, hence, body weight. For endurance exercise, feeding before exercise, especially high-fiber feeds, is likely to be beneficial, because the increased water in the GI tract can be an important reservoir for water and electrolytes to replace sweat losses. Feeding high-fiber feeds also increases voluntary water intake.

Glucose supplementation may be important in limiting fatigue in endurance exercise in horses. Endurance time during treadmill running was prolonged by the IV infusion of a glucose solution during exercise. Plasma glucose was higher than controls, and plasma lactate and body temperature were lower at the point of fatigue. These results suggest that supplemental glucose during exercise prolongs performance time in horses. This increase may be due to increased glucose availability, reduced reliance on anaerobic energy production, lower core temperature, and better maintenance of plasma volume. In endurance horses, hydrolyzable starches and sugars fed within 3 hr of a race may increase glucose utilization in the short term but inhibit lipid oxidation, which could be detrimental for energy production.

Glycogen concentration in skeletal muscle before performance is relevant to fatigue during both short-term/intense and prolonged endurance exercise. Depletion of muscle glycogen before exercise causes a decrease in anaerobic power generation and capacity for high-intensity work. Intense or prolonged exercise depletes the muscle glycogen stores, and it may take 48 hr for glycogen to be replenished in the horse. Although modest increases in glycogen stores may be obtained using high-starch diets in the horse, no benefit on performance has been shown. On the contrary, high-carbohydrate diets have increased heart rates and blood lactate concentrations during intense exercise. Use of glucose or other carbohydrate solutions before racing to promote performance in Standardbred and Thoroughbred racehorses has no scientific basis.

Fat supplementation is now a widespread practice in diets for athletic horses and can increase performance during endurance exercise. Increased free fatty acid concentrations in the bloodstream before prolonged exercise results in an increased use of fat as an energy source and in higher blood glucose and muscle glycogen concentrations during exercise. The shift to increased use of fat as a fuel results in lower respiratory demands for exercise, because less carbon dioxide must be expired when more fat is used for energy. Fat adaptation appears to facilitate the metabolic regulation of glycolysis by sparing glucose and glycogen at low-intensity work and by promoting glycolysis when power is needed for high-intensity exercise. Adding fat to the diet also affects the metabolic and thermoregulatory response to exercise. Feeding vegetable oil at a rate of 10%–12% of the total diet on a dry-matter basis has been suggested, but horses must be acclimated to high-fat diets. In horses not acclimated, fat supplementation can slow the rate of muscle glycogen repletion.

Creatine has been used in horses as an ergogenic aid, but there is no evidence of its efficacy. Horses receiving 25 g of creatine monohydrate bid for 6.5 days did not have significantly different run times until fatigue on a treadmill than control horses. Supplementation with creatine also had no significant effect on muscle or blood creatine concentrations at rest or after exercise until fatigue.

An association between plasma vitamin E concentration and performance has been described in sled dogs. Dogs with a higher prerace vitamin E concentration were more likely to finish the race and were less likely to be withdrawn during the race for poor health, fatigue, or other reasons. Vitamin E concentrations for the dog team overall were not associated with speed during the race. Additional studies are needed to investigate whether the reduced signs of fatigue are directly linked to higher vitamin E concentrations in the bloodstream.

Recovery: Recovery of horses after endurance exercise is influenced by the rehydration strategy used. After prolonged treadmill exercise and furosemide-induced dehydration, horses offered a saline solution (0.9% NaCl) as the initial rehydration fluid maintained a plasma sodium concentration higher than that of control horses. The recovery of body weight was more rapid than in horses offered plain water. A similar study noted ambient temperature fluids were more palatable (20°C [68°F]) and increased voluntary intake. Water intake can also be increased by providing a saline solution (0.9% NaCl) both during and after endurance exercise. Sodium chloride solutions may increase plasma chloride and accentuate a metabolic acidosis; as a result, isotonic polyionic electrolyte solutions formulated specifically for horses should be selected. When providing electrolyte solutions, horses may need to be trained to drink these fluids, and plain water should always be available. However, use of electrolyte solutions should be encouraged, especially in horses required to compete on consecutive days, such as in endurance rides and 3-day events.

FEVER OF UNKNOWN ORIGIN

In both veterinary and human patients, fever may indicate infectious, inflammatory, immune-mediated, or neoplastic disease. In most cases, the history and physical examination reveal the cause of the fever, or the fever resolves spontaneously or in response to antibiotic therapy. However, in a small percentage of patients, the cause of fever is not readily apparent, and the problem becomes persistent or recurrent. These patients are said to have fever of unknown origin (FUO).

In human medicine, classic FUO is defined as fever >101°F (38.3°C) on several occasions over a period >2–3 wk with no diagnosis established after 3 outpatient visits or 3 days in the hospital. There is no recognized definition of this syndrome in veterinary medicine, making it difficult to determine its true prevalence. FUO is probably less prevalent now than in the past because of improved diagnostic technology (eg, imaging, molecular diagnostic tests).

Body Temperature Regulation: Body temperature is regulated by the hypothalamus. This area of the brain acts as a thermostat to maintain temperature as close as possible to a normal set-point. The hypothalamus receives input from internal and external thermoreceptors, and it activates physiologic and behavioral activities that influence heat production, heat loss, and heat gain.

Hyperthermia refers to any increase in body temperature above the normal range. Fever is a particular form of hyperthermia in which the heat loss and heat gain mechanisms are adjusted to maintain body temperature at a higher hypothalamic set-point; thus, fever is essentially a regulated hyperthermia. In nonfebrile cases of hyperthermia (eg, heat stroke, exercise-induced hyperthermia, malignant hyperthermia, seizure), body temperature is increased by abnormal and unregulated heat loss, heat gain, or heat production, and the hypothalamic set-point is not altered. Depending on their severity, these conditions can potentially result in body temperatures ≥106°F (41.1°C). In comparison, most patients with true fever have body temperatures in the range of 103°–106°F (39.5°–41.1°C).

An increase in the hypothalamic set-point may be initiated by exogenous pyrogens, which include drugs, toxins, and viral or bacterial products (eg, endotoxin). These pyrogenic stimuli lead to the release of cytokines, termed endogenous pyrogens, from inflammatory cells. Ultimately, locally synthesized prostaglandin E_2 in the hypothalamus is responsible for increasing the set-point, resulting in fever.

Etiology and Pathogenesis: FUO may be defined as fever that does not resolve spontaneously in the period expected for self-limited infection and for which a cause cannot be found despite considerable diagnostic effort. This excludes patients that respond to antibiotic therapy (and do not relapse) and patients in which the cause of fever is determined from initial history, physical examination, or laboratory tests, or in which fever resolves spontaneously.

Infectious, immune-mediated, and neoplastic disease are the most common causes of FUO in dogs. In a study of 101 dogs with fever, 22% had immune-mediated diseases, 22% primary bone marrow abnormalities, 16% infectious diseases, 11.5% miscellaneous conditions, 9.5% neoplasia, and 19% genuine FUO. In cats, the cause is more likely to be infectious, but there are fewer published data on feline cases than on canine cases. In a case series of horses with FUO, 43% had infectious disease, 22% neoplasia, 6.5% immune-mediated disease, 19% miscellaneous causes, and in 9.5% the cause was not determined. In farm animals, the most likely causes of FUO are infectious or inflammatory diseases such as pneumonia, peritonitis, abscesses, endocarditis, metritis, mastitis, polyarthritis, and pyelonephritis.

Diagnosis: The key to diagnosis of FUO is to develop and follow a systematic plan that allows for the detection of both common and uncommon causes of fever. The plan should always include repetition of relevant tests, because findings can change over time. Owners should be informed that diagnosis of FUO may require considerable time and patience and may demand more advanced or expensive diagnostic tests. Nevertheless, simple and inexpensive tests may also reveal diagnostic clues that eventually point to the cause of the fever. In one retrospective study of fever in dogs, radiography, cytology, and bacterial or fungal cultures of tissues or fluids were found to be the most useful diagnostic tests.

A staged or tiered approach to diagnosis can assist in choosing appropriate tests. The first stage should include history, physical examination, ophthalmic and neurologic examinations, CBC, fibrinogen, serum chemistry profile, urinalysis and urine culture, feline leukemia virus and feline immunodeficiency virus tests (cats), and usually thoracic and abdominal radiographs in small animals. Any medications that could induce fever should be discontinued. In the second stage, some first-stage tests may be repeated (particularly the physical examination), and additional specialized tests are performed. These may be dictated by abnormal findings in the first stage of testing or may be determined by consideration of the most common known causes of FUO. Tests included in this stage include blood cultures, arthrocentesis, abdominal ultrasonography, lymph node aspiration, aspiration of other organs or masses, analysis of body fluids (eg, fluid from body cavities, milk samples, reproductive tract secretions), rectal cytology, fecal culture, echocardiography (in the presence of a murmur), long-bone and joint radiographs, contrast radiographs, serology, and molecular diagnostic tests. In the third stage, earlier tests may be repeated again, as well as additional specialized procedures. These procedures are most likely to be chosen on the basis of previous findings but may also be considered when all previous testing has been unrewarding. Examples include echocardiography (in the absence of a murmur), dental radiographs, bone marrow aspiration, bronchoscopy and bronchoalveolar lavage, CSF analysis, CT, MRI, laparoscopy, thoracoscopy, biopsies, exploratory surgery, or trial therapy.

History and Physical Examination: Epidemiologic characteristics such as vaccination, parasite control, exposure to vectors, and travel history should always be reviewed. The response to previous medications should be determined, as well as the presence of illness in other animals or people. Owners should be questioned carefully about specific clinical signs, because these may help localize the source of the fever. The physical examination should be detailed; always include fundic, neurologic, and rectal examinations; and repeated frequently.

CBC and Serum Chemistry Profile: The CBC and chemistry changes in animals with FUO are often nonspecific but may suggest further diagnostic tests. For example, bile acids assay may be indicated in an animal with changes suggestive of hepatic dysfunction. The CBC should always be accompanied by blood smear evaluation to detect parasites or morphologic changes.

Urine Culture: This test is always indicated to evaluate FUO in small animals, regardless of the appearance of the urine sediment.

Radiography and Advanced Imaging: Thoracic and abdominal radiographs are useful screening tools for the early localization of fever. Skeletal radiographs and contrast radiographs may subsequently be considered, depending on initial findings. For example, myelography may be used to investigate back pain. The use of techniques such as CT or MRI is determined by the results of initial diagnostic testing or by consideration of the body system of interest, eg, MRI is particularly useful to evaluate the CNS. Advanced imaging with nuclear scintigraphy or positron emission tomography is used in human patients with FUO but is not yet widely reported in veterinary medicine.

Ultrasonography and Echocardiography: Abdominal ultrasonography may reveal a source of fever in the abdomen, such as neoplasia, peritonitis, pancreatitis, or abscesses. The thoracic cavity, limbs, and retrobulbar areas may also be examined by ultrasound. Echocardiography is indicated at the early stages of evaluation of the FUO patient with a murmur. This may aid in the detection of endocarditis, although this diagnosis should also be based on signalment, characteristics of the heart murmur, and blood culture results.

Bone Marrow Evaluation: Bone marrow cytology and histology should be evaluated in any animal with unexplained CBC abnormalities. Bone marrow disease is a common cause of FUO in small animals; therefore, bone marrow aspiration and biopsy, if possible, should also be included in the second stage of diagnostic testing in these patients. When obtaining bone marrow aspirates from cats, a sample should be saved for possible molecular diagnostic testing for feline leukemia virus.

Arthrocentesis: Because immune-mediated polyarthritis is a common cause of FUO in dogs, arthrocentesis of multiple joints is included in the second stage of diagnostic testing in this species, even if the joints are normal on palpation. Some dogs with steroid-responsive meningitis-arteritis also have concurrent immune-mediated polyarthritis; therefore, arthrocentesis should be performed in dogs with spinal pain. Infectious polyarthritis is more commonly recognized in large animals, in which arthrocentesis is an important diagnostic test.

CSF Analysis: CSF sampling is recommended for dogs with FUO if less invasive tests do not reveal the cause of the fever. Fluid should be submitted for cytology, protein measurement, and culture.

Blood Culture: Blood cultures are recommended in all animals with unexplained fever. The techniques used should allow the collection of adequately large volumes of blood under aseptic conditions. If the size of the animal allows collecting more than one set of samples for blood culture, using appropriately sized aerobic and anaerobic bottles increases the sensitivity and specificity of the test. Special enrichment culture methods may be considered for certain organisms, eg, *Bartonella* spp.

Infectious Disease Testing: Tests available for the diagnosis of infectious diseases include assays for detection of antibodies or antigen in blood, body fluids, or tissues. Molecular diagnostic tests detect nucleic acid, with PCR being the most common in this category. Selection of these tests should be based on the signalment, clinical signs, and epidemiologic characteristics of the animal. Interpretation of test results requires an understanding of disease prevalence, vaccination history, and sensitivity and specificity of the test. When requesting PCR-based assays, it is important to use laboratories that have quality management programs that address test performance and consistency, and control for sample contamination.

Other Serologic Tests: The value of immune panels or autoantibody screens in small animal patients with FUO is unclear. Neither antinuclear antibody nor rheumatoid factor titers alone should be used to diagnose systemic lupus erythematosus or rheumatoid arthritis, respectively.

Microbiology, Cytology, and Histology: Fine-needle aspirates are safe and simple to obtain from effusions, masses, nodules, organs, tissues, and body fluids. Fluids should be examined cytologically and also submitted for microbiologic or molecular diagnostic testing. Tissue biopsies are generally obtained in the second or third stages of diagnostic testing, after clinical signs or initial diagnostic tests have localized the fever. When biopsies are obtained, sufficient samples should be submitted for histopathology, appropriate culture (aerobic and anaerobic, fungal, mycoplasmal, mycobacterial, etc), molecular diagnostics, and special stains. If exploratory surgery is performed, biopsies should be obtained from several sites.

Treatment: In some FUO cases a specific diagnosis is not reached, or diagnostic testing is discontinued, leading to consideration of therapy in the absence of a diagnosis. Options include antibiotics, antifungal agents, and anti-inflammatory or immunosuppressive therapy (usually with corticosteroids). Trial therapy may resolve the clinical signs or confirm a presumptive diagnosis, but it is also associated with significant risk. Before pursuing a therapeutic trial, the owner should be informed of the potential risks and should be committed to careful monitoring of the animal for an appropriate length of time. The therapeutic trial should be based on a tentative diagnosis and should define the parameters to be followed and the criteria used to determine treatment success or failure. If an animal is likely to be referred for in-depth investigation of FUO, trial therapy should not be started because it may affect the results of further testing.

In true fever, the increase in body temperature is regulated; therefore, cooling methods such as water baths work against the body's own regulatory mechanisms. It is also likely that fever itself has some beneficial effects, particularly in infectious diseases. However, fever can lead to anorexia, lethargy, and dehydration. Thus, animals with FUO may benefit from IV fluid therapy or antipyretic medications. Examples include NSAIDs such as aspirin, carprofen, ketoprofen, and meloxicam in small animals, and flunixin meglumine or phenylbutazone in large animals.

HEPATIC LIPIDOSIS

FATTY LIVER DISEASE OF CATTLE

Fatty liver results from a state of negative energy balance and is one of the important metabolic diseases of postparturient dairy cows. Although often considered a postpartum disorder, it usually develops before and during parturition. Periparturient depression of feed intake, and endocrine changes associated with parturition and lactogenesis contribute to development of fatty liver. Cows that are overconditioned at calving are at highest risk. Fatty liver can develop whenever there is a decrease in feed intake and may occur secondary to the onset of another disorder. Fatty liver at calving is commonly associated with ketosis (*see* p 1024).

Etiology: Mobilization of body fat reserves that is triggered by hormonal cues in states of negative energy balance results in the release of nonesterified fatty acids (NEFAs) from adipose tissue. The liver retains ~15%–20% of the NEFAs circulating in blood and thus accumulates increased amounts during periods when blood NEFA concentrations are increased. The most dramatic increase occurs at calving, when plasma concentrations are often >1,000 μEq/L. Concentrations can reach that level if the animal goes off feed. NEFAs taken up by the liver can either be oxidized or esterified. The primary esterification product is triglyceride, which can either be exported as part of a very low density lipoprotein (VLDL) or be stored in liver cells. In ruminants, export occurs at a very slow rate relative to many other species because of impaired VLDL synthesis. Therefore, under conditions of increased hepatic NEFA uptake and esterification, triglycerides accumulate. Oxidation of NEFAs leads either to the production of ATP in the tricarboxylic acid cycle or to the formation of ketones through peroxisomal or β-oxidation. Ketone formation is favored when blood glucose concentrations are low. Conditions that lead to low blood glucose and insulin concentrations also contribute to fatty liver, because insulin suppresses fat mobilization from adipose tissue.

The greatest increase in liver triglyceride typically occurs at calving. The extent of feed intake depression before and after calving or during disease in combination with the amount of available body fat reserves moderates the degree of triglyceride accumulation. Excessive intracellular triglyceride accumulation in liver cells results in disturbed liver function and cell damage. Fatty liver can develop within 24 hr of an animal going off feed. Although lipid accumulation in the liver is a reversible process, the slow rate of triglyceride export as lipoprotein causes the disorder to persist for an extended period. Depletion of the liver lipid content usually begins when the cow reaches positive energy balance and may take several weeks to fully subside.

Fatty liver is not a consequence of positive energy balance or overfeeding. Energy consumption above requirements for maintenance and productive purposes will not directly result in deposition of triglyceride in hepatic tissue. Triglyceride deposition will occur only if the animal becomes overconditioned and consequently reduces feed intake.

Clinical Findings: There are no pathognomonic clinical signs of fatty liver disease in cattle. The condition is often associated with feed intake depression, decreased milk production, and ketosis. Increased blood NEFA concentration has been associated with impaired immune function and a proinflammatory effect, presumably reflecting in increased incidence of clinical mastitis, metritis, and other periparturient infectious diseases. However, cause and effect has not been established. Metabolic consequences of triglyceride accumulation in the liver include reduced gluconeogenesis, ureagenesis, hormone clearance, and hormone responsiveness. Consequently, hypoglycemia, hyperammonemia, and altered endocrine profiles may accompany fatty liver.

Fatty liver is likely to develop concurrently with another disease, typically disorders that are seen at or shortly after calving. These include metritis, mastitis, abomasal displacement, or hypocalcemia. Field observations suggest that response to treatment of concurrent disorders is poor if cows have extensive triglyceride infiltration of the liver. Cows slow to increase in milk production and feed intake after calving are likely to have fatty liver. However, fatty liver is probably the result rather than the cause of poor feed intake. Fatty liver is often associated with obese cows and downner cows (*see* p 1188) but is unlikely to be a direct cause of the downer cow syndrome. Overconditioned cows exhibit more pronounced feed intake depression before and after calving than nonobese cows and, therefore, are susceptible to fatty liver. Although obesity predisposes to fatty liver disease, it is not restricted to obese cows. Similarly, obese cows do not necessarily have fatty liver.

Diagnosis: Diagnostic tools for fatty liver are of limited value. Fatty liver is usually diagnosed after the animal has been off feed or has died because of another disease. A positive diagnosis does not mean that clinical signs of illness are the result of fatty liver, and misinterpretation of a positive diagnosis is common.

Liver biopsy is a minimally invasive procedure that is the only direct and most reliable method to determine severity of fatty liver in dairy cattle. Measurement of total lipid or triglyceride content by gravimetric or chemical methods after extraction from tissue by organic solvents is necessary for quantitative assessment; however, these assays are not routinely conducted in commercial laboratories. Estimation of triglyceride content by flotation characteristics of the tissue in copper sulfate solutions of varying specific gravity is rapid, easy, and available for use under field conditions.

Blood and urine metabolites or blood enzyme activity have been proposed as indirect diagnostic parameters. Blood glucose concentrations are low and blood NEFA and β-hydroxybutyrate concentrations are high when conditions are conducive to the development of fatty liver. Blood cholesterol concentration is usually low when fatty liver occurs, which may reflect an impaired ability of the liver to secrete lipoproteins. AST, ornithine decarboxylase, and sorbitol dehydrogenase are hepatic enzymes that may be positively associated with liver triglyceride and liver damage. The total bilirubin concentration in blood is often positively associated with the NEFA concentration in blood. Blood metabolites or enzymes are unreliable indices of the degree of fatty liver, because normal concentrations vary widely among animals. The same problem exists when attempting to determine liver function by measuring sulfobromophthalein clearance from blood.

With the availability of handheld devices allowing cowside testing, measuring β-hydroxybutyrate concentration in blood has become a popular way to identify herds that may be at risk of developing fatty liver. Measurement of plasma NEFA concentration is more expensive and requires submission of blood samples to a diagnostic laboratory. In addition to extreme variations in plasma NEFA concentrations among animals, there is extreme variation in a single individual, because concentrations increase dramatically immediately before and after calving. Therefore, a large number of animals must be sampled at a consistent time relative to calving. Care must be taken not to excite animals before sampling blood, because NEFAs increase rapidly in response to stress; samples should be drawn at standardized times using standardized procedures. The plasma NEFA concentrations at which triglyceride accumulates in the liver have not been established but are probably ~600 μEq/L and higher. These concentrations are common within 24–48 hr of parturition. However, prolonged exposure of the liver to concentrations >600 μEq/L will likely lead to fatty liver. Primiparous cows are less susceptible to fatty liver during periods of increased plasma NEFAs. Therefore, mature animals should be sampled when using plasma NEFAs as a predictor of fatty liver. To screen a herd for the prevalence and severity of hepatic lipidosis, determination of plasma NEFAs not earlier than 1 wk antepartum is recommended. Even though plasma NEFA concentration is a direct parameter for the lipid mobilization and thus the liver lipid accumulation, after parturition the plasma β-hydroxybutyrate concentration has been found to more accurately reflect the severity of hepatic lipidosis.

Microscopic evaluation can be used to estimate the volume of the tissue occupied by fat. Estimates obtained by this method agree fairly well with chemical determination of triglyceride when expressed as a percentage of tissue dry weight. Mild, moderate, and severe fatty liver are often defined as <20%, 20%–40%, and >40% fat (percentage of cell volume), respectively, but these values have little meaning relative to impact on physiologic function or clinical signs of the animal. However, clinical signs potentially associated with fatty liver disease are rarely seen in animals with <10% fat in wet liver tissue. Use of ultrasonography as an alternative noninvasive procedure is being developed to determine the severity of fatty liver but is not yet routinely available.

Prevention and Treatment: Reducing severity and duration of negative energy balance is crucial to prevent fatty liver. This can be achieved by avoiding overconditioning cattle, rapid diet changes, unpalatable feeds, periparturient diseases, and environmental stress. Cows within a herd should enter the dry period with an average body condition score (BCS) of 3–3.5 (scale: 1 = thin, 5 = obese). Thin cows (BCS ≤2.5) can be fed additional energy during the dry period to replenish condition without fear of causing fatty liver. Overconditioned cattle (BCS ≥4) should not be feed restricted, because this will promote fat mobilization from adipose tissue and increase blood NEFAs and liver triglyceride.

The critical time for prevention of fatty liver is ~1 wk before through 1 wk after parturition, when cows are most susceptible. Cows that are candidates for preventive measures are those that are overconditioned or starting to go off feed. Propylene glycol, 300–600 mL/day, given as an oral drench during the final week prepartum has effectively reduced plasma NEFAs and the severity of fatty liver at calving. Propylene glycol can be fed, but feeding may not be as effective if the full dose is not consumed in a short period of time. Glycerin may be a less expensive alternative to propylene glycol.

Glucose or glucose precursors are effective, because they may cause an insulin response. Insulin is antilipolytic, ie, it decreases lipid mobilization from adipose tissue. Slow-release insulin compounds are available but are not approved for use in food-producing animals. A single 100 IU IM dose of a 24-hr slow-release insulin immediately after calving may be prophylactic. Higher doses may cause severe hypoglycemia and should not be used without concurrent glucose administration. Glucagon stimulates glycogenolysis, gluconeogenesis, and insulin production. In contrast to that in nonruminants, the lipolytic effect of glucagon in ruminants is negligible. Glucagon (10 mg/day, IV, for 14 days) is effective at reducing liver triglyceride. A more practical protocol for use of glucagon to prevent fatty liver has not been established. Niacin is an antilipolytic agent that may have potential for prevention of fatty liver, but unequivocal evidence supporting niacin supplementation of animals at risk is not available.

Minimizing stress is important for prevention of fatty liver. Sudden changes in environment should be avoided. For example, changes in ration, housing, temperature, herdmates, etc, may cause a reduction in feed intake and trigger catecholamine-mediated increases in fat mobilization.

Other than longterm IV infusion of glucagon, there is no proven treatment for fatty liver. Repeated IV bolus administration of 500 mL of 50% dextrose solution is commonly used in dairy practice and can be combined with administration of propylene glycol 250 mL, PO, bid. Dextrose administration at a continuous infusion rate of up to 40 g/hr, IV, suitable to increase the plasma glucose concentration to 100–150 mg/dL without surpassing the renal threshold for glucose, can be used in a clinical setting. Although this treatment effectively suppresses lipolysis and ketogenesis, treatment-induced hyperglycemia is likely to negatively affect feed intake. It is therefore advisable to reduce the infusion rate after 2–3 days and to determine whether the animal is able to maintain normoglycemia as the parenteral glucose supply decreases.

Use of glucocorticoids in cows with fatty liver is controversial because of their potential lipolytic effect. Recent literature suggests that short-term treatment with dexamethasone does not induce lipolysis in dairy cows. The gluconeogenic effect of glucocorticoids that is well documented in several monogastric species has thus far not been confirmed in cattle. The well-established hyperglycemic effect of glucocorticoids in cattle has primarily been attributed to an impaired glucose uptake by the mammary gland in treated cows. In addition, glucocorticoids are thought to have a positive effect on feed intake. In theory, effective treatments would be those that enhance lipoprotein triglyceride export from the liver. However, compounds that are known lipotropic agents in nonruminants have not been proved to be effective in ruminants. IV administration of choline, inositol, methionine, and vitamin B_{12} are often suggested as treatments, but scientific data are insufficient to support their use. Oral administration of these compounds is not effective, because they are degraded in the rumen. In essence, treatment is the same as prevention; attempts should be made to avoid negative energy balance and to minimize fatty acid mobilization from adipose tissue. Once positive energy balance is attained, liver triglyceride can be reduced significantly in 7–10 days.

PREGNANCY TOXEMIA IN COWS

Pregnancy toxemia in cows is similar to the condition in small ruminants and is the result of fetal carbohydrate or energy demand exceeding maternal supply during the last trimester of pregnancy. It is precipitated by large or multiple fetuses, feed low in energy or protein or high in poorly digestible fiber, and health conditions that increase energy demand or decrease ability to take in nourishment (eg, lameness and oral diseases). Cold, snowy weather may contribute by increasing the animal's energy requirement and by covering available forage. Inflammation is also increasingly being associated with disorders of energy metabolism; inflammatory mediators tend to promote mobilization of lipid stores and antagonize the actions of insulin. The fetoplacental unit uses carbohydrate for energy and removes these compounds from the blood in an insulin-independent fashion. When this demand exceeds maternal supply, adipose tissue is mobilized to supply energy as acetate or ketone bodies, sparing carbohydrate consumption by other maternal tissues. However, only a small amount of new carbohydrate is generated from fat metabolism (from glycerol). This condition is more severe than ketosis (*see* p 1024) because fetal demand increases during pregnancy, while milk demand can decline in response to negative energy balance.

Although the mechanism is unknown, clinical disease develops in some cows with negative energy or carbohydrate balance. Proposed mediators of clinical disease include glucose deficiency with intermittent hypoglycemia, ketone body accumulation with metabolic acidosis or appetite suppression, and death of the fetus with secondary infection and toxemia. Individual cows of any breed can be affected, but herd problems are most common in beef cattle, which frequently are managed so that late pregnancy coincides with the poorest availability of feed. Both thin and fat cows can be affected, but the first noted abnormality often is loss of body condition over 1–2 wk. Decreased appetite, rumination, fecal production, and nose-licking are general signs of illness. With time, affected cows become markedly depressed, weak, ataxic, and recumbent. Opisthotonos, seizures, or coma may be seen terminally. Ketonuria is present from the early stage of disease and is the most specific finding; even mild ketonuria should not be found in healthy pregnant cows until a few days before calving. Inexpensive ketone meters are now available and augment the older techniques of nitroprusside tablets or strips. Hypoglycemia is also common, but excited or seizuring cows may have hyperglycemia. With more advanced disease, there may be variable increases in serum activities of muscle or liver enzymes, as well as clinicopathologic evidence of infection, metabolic acidosis, internal organ dysfunction or failure, and circulatory collapse. Hepatic lipidosis in conjunction with large or multiple fetuses is a common necropsy finding; evidence of muscle pressure necrosis and toxemia may also be found.

Successful treatment requires early identification of the disease. There are few differential diagnoses, and pregnancy toxemia must be considered a factor in any disease that affects cattle in late gestation. Cattle that have lost weight but are still eating may be managed by feeding concentrate or propylene glycol (0.5–1 g/kg/day for up to 5 days). Anorectic cattle must be treated aggressively, because the decrease in energy intake causes the disease to progress rapidly. Propylene glycol can be force-fed, or dextrose given IV (0.5 g/kg at least once a day). Cattle with dehydration, organ dysfunction, or metabolic acidosis should be treated with large volumes (20–60 L/day, PO or IV) of electrolyte fluids; if IV fluid administration is practical, continuous dextrose infusion (5%) is recommended. Protamine zinc insulin (200 U, SC, every 48 hr) may be given after dextrose administration to suppress ketogenesis. However, insulin is not approved for use in cattle in the USA. Recumbent cattle may benefit from good nursing care (*see* p 1188) but rarely respond to treatment. To decrease the energy drain of any cow with pregnancy toxemia, induction of parturition or removal of the fetus by cesarean section should be considered.

On the herd level, the disease can be prevented by adequate attention to nutrition and health care of cattle in late gestation. For the individual cow, recognition of the precarious state of energy and carbohydrate balance during late gestation dictates careful monitoring of energy intake, attitude, and fat mobilization, especially during times of illness or other stress.

PREGNANCY TOXEMIA IN EWES AND DOES

(Twin lamb disease, Pregnancy ketosis)

Pregnancy toxemia affects ewes and does during late gestation and is characterized by partial anorexia and depression, often with neurologic signs, progressing to recumbency and death. It is seen more often in animals carrying multiple fetuses. Generally, clinically affected animals have other risk factors, at either the individual or flock/herd level.

Epidemiology and Pathogenesis: The primary predisposing cause of pregnancy toxemia is inadequate nutrition during late gestation, usually because of insufficient energy density of the ration and decreased rumen capacity as a result of fetal growth. In the last 4 wk of gestation, metabolizable energy requirements rise dramatically. For example, the energy requirement of a 70-kg ewe carrying a single lamb is 2.8 Mcal/day in early gestation compared with 3.45 Mcal/day in late gestation, or an increase of 23%. This change is more dramatic in ewes bearing twins, with an energy requirement of 3.22 Mcal/day in early and 4.37 Mcal/day in late gestation (36% increase), and in ewes bearing triplets, with an energy requirement of 3.49 Mcal/day in early and 4.95 Mcal/day in late gestation (42% increase). Dairy goats have similar changes in needs.

In late gestation, the liver increases gluconeogenesis to facilitate glucose availability to the fetuses. Each fetus requires 30–40 g of glucose/day in late gestation, which represents a significant percentage of the ewe's glucose production and which is preferentially directed to supporting the fetuses rather than the ewe. Mobilization of fat stores is increased in late gestation as a way to assure adequate energy for the increased demands of the developing fetus(es) and impending lactation. However, in a negative energy balance, this increased mobilization may overwhelm the liver's capacity and result in hepatic lipidosis, with subsequent impairment of function. Additionally, twin-bearing ewes appear to have more difficulty producing glucose and clearing ketone bodies, thus increasing their susceptibility to pregnancy toxemia.

Females with a poor body condition score (BCS ≤2) or that are overconditioned (BCS ≥4) and carrying more than one fetus are most at risk of developing pregnancy toxemia, although the condition can occur even in ideally conditioned ewes on an adequate ration. Susceptible, thin ewes or does develop ketosis because a chronically inadequate ration is offered or because other diseases limit intake (eg, lameness, dental disease) and, with increasingly insufficient energy to meet increasing fetal demands, the ewe or doe mobilizes more body fat, with resultant ketone body production and hepatic lipidosis. Overconditioned animals may have depressed appetites, and adipose mobilization quickly overwhelms the liver's capacity, resulting again in hepatic lipidosis. In addition, there may be a population of animals less responsive to insulin production when nutritional intake is inadequate. Ewes fitting these criteria may quickly shift from subclinical ketosis to clinical pregnancy toxemia if feed intake is acutely curtailed by such events as adverse weather, transport, handling for shearing or preventive medication, or other concomitant disease (footrot, pneumonia, etc). These variants of pregnancy toxemia have been termed primary pregnancy toxemia (thin ewes and inadequate nutrition), estate ketosis (fat ewes), and secondary pregnancy toxemia (ewes suffering from other disease). Dairy does often experience ketosis after kidding (serum β-hydroxybutyrate [BHB] >1.7 mmol/L), which may or may not be connected with pregnancy ketosis before kidding. Ketosis after kidding appears to be more common in herds using a complete pelleted ration.

Clinical Findings: Early clinical signs can be detected by an observant producer. Most cases develop 1–3 wk before parturition. Onset earlier than day 140 of gestation is associated with more severe disease and increased risk of mortality. Decreased aggressiveness at feeding, particularly with grain consumption, indicates a problem. Animals will spend more time lying and have more frequent bouts of lying than their healthy herdmates. As the disease advances, ewes or does may also show signs of listlessness, aimless walking, muscle twitching or fine muscle tremors, opisthotonos, and grinding of the teeth. This progresses (generally over 2–4 days) to blindness, ataxia, and finally sternal recumbency, coma, and death. Cerebral hypoglycemia coupled with ketosis, ketoacidosis, and reduced hepatic and renal function lead to the clinical signs and fetal death. Blood glucose levels may return to normal or even become high terminally, possibly indicating death of the fetus(es). Septicemia develops in the ewe or doe after fetal death.

Lesions: Postmortem changes demonstrate varying degrees of fatty liver, enlarged adrenal glands, and often include multiple fetuses in a state of decomposition indicating premortem death. Very thin animals may appear starved (eg, serous atrophy of the kidney and heart fat). However, these signs alone are not pathognomonic for death due to pregnancy toxemia. Postmortem samples of aqueous humor or CSF can be analyzed for BHB. Levels >2.5 and 0.5 mmol/L, respectively, are consistent with a diagnosis of pregnancy toxemia.

Diagnosis: Laboratory findings in individual animals may include hypoglycemia (often <2 mmol/L), increased urine ketone levels (evaluated by commercial qualitative test strips), increased serum BHB levels (normal <0.8 mmol/L, subclinical ketosis ≥0.8 mmol/L, and clinical disease >3 mmol/L), and occasionally hypocalcemia. Hypoglycemia is not a consistent finding, with up to 40% of cases having normal glucose levels and up to 20% having hyperglycemia. If the diagnosis needs further confirmation, CSF glucose levels may be more accurate than blood; they remain low even when serum glucose rebounds in advanced cases after fetal death. BHB is a more reliable indicator of disease severity than are blood glucose levels. Nonesterified fatty acids can also be increased above 0.4 mmol/L, indicating likely hepatic lipidosis, resulting in impaired hepatic function.

Although hypocalcemia is often found in cases of pregnancy toxemia, it should also be considered when formulating hypotheses regarding recumbent late gestational sheep and goats (*see* p 991). This is similarly true with hypomagnesemia, which is a common finding in cases of pregnancy toxemia but should also be considered as a differential diagnosis for periparturient CNS disease. Other CNS diseases to be considered include polioencephalomalacia, pulpy kidney disease (enterotoxemia), rabies, scrapie, maedi visna/ovine progressive pneumonia, lead poisoning, chronic copper toxicity, and listeriosis. These can be differentiated based on clinical and laboratory findings or during necropsy.

Treatment: Ewes or does in the early stages (ie, are ambulatory, have a decreased appetite for grain, and are showing few nervous signs) can often be treated successfully with oral propylene glycol (60 mL, bid, for 3 days, or 100 mL/day). Adding oral calcium (12.5 g calcium lactate), oral potassium (7.5 g KCl), and insulin (0.4 IU/kg/day, SC) has increased survival rates. Oral commercial calf electrolyte solutions containing glucose may also be given by stomach tube at a dose of 3–4 L, qid, or drenched as a concentrated solution. It may also be prudent to induce parturition/abortion if the ewe or doe is also thin or fat and cannot manage fetal demands that late in pregnancy. This can be done by administering dexamethasone (20 mg, IV or IM). Parturition is expected within 24–72 hr, with most animals giving birth within 36 hr. Does may also benefit by the addition of prostaglandin $F_2\alpha$ (dinoprost [10 mg, IM] or cloprostenol [75 mcg/45 kg body wt]). Contributing factors (eg, nutrition, housing, illness, other stressors) should be corrected for the group, and feeding management assessed (eg, adequate feeder space, feeding frequency, protection from adverse weather).

Treatment of advanced cases of pregnancy toxemia is frequently unrewarding. If a ewe or doe is already comatose, humane euthanasia is warranted, and treatment should focus on the rest of the flock. However, if the female is valuable and the owner wishes to pursue treatment despite the poor prognosis, then aggressive therapy should be directed against the ketoacidosis and hypoglycemia. Before starting this therapy, it should be determined whether the fetuses are alive (eg, real-time or Doppler ultrasonography). If the fetuses are alive and within 3 days of a calculated due date (gestation length 147 days), then an emergency cesarean section may be considered if economically viable. If the fetuses are dead or too premature to survive a cesarean section, it is less stressful to the ewe or doe to induce early parturition with dexamethasone (as above). Prophylactic antibiotics (usually procaine penicillin G at 20,000 IU/kg/day) are appropriate if the fetuses are thought to be dead.

Hypoglycemia can be treated by a single injection of 50% dextrose, 60–100 mL, IV, followed by balanced electrolyte solution with 5% dextrose. IV drips and lower dextrose levels in solution might cause less of a diuretic effect; however, this is often impractical in a field setting. Repeated boluses of IV glucose should be avoided, because they may result in a refractory insulin response. Insulin can be administered (20–40 IU protamine zinc insulin, IM, every other day). Calcium (50–100 mL of a commercial calcium gluconate or borogluconate solution, SC) can be given safely without serum biochemistry data. If serum biochemistry demonstrates hypocalcemia, ~50 mL of a commercial calcium solution can be given by slow IV injection while monitoring the heart. Oral potassium chloride (KCl) can be given as well, because serum potassium levels are often depressed. Use of flunixin meglumine at 2.5 mg/kg improved survival rate of ewes and their lambs, although the mechanism is unknown. Although aggressive therapy and intensive nursing care may be successful, it is not unusual to see case fatality rates >40%. Given the cost, it is prudent to share the guarded prognosis with owners before undertaking treatment.

A sample of late-gestation ewes or does can be tested for serum BHB levels to determine the extent of the risk in the rest of the flock. Generally, 10–20 animals in late gestation should be sampled (3%–20% of the pregnant flock). The risk of the flock can be determined based on the mean value of these results: normal (low risk) 0–0.7 mmol/L, moderate underfeeding (moderate risk) 0.8–1.6 mmol/L, and severe underfeeding (high risk) 1.7–3.0 mmol/L. Other diseases should be treated (eg, footrot). Females off feed should be separated from the group and hand fed, keeping in mind they should be able to see the group to feel comfortable.

Prevention: Ewes or does should not enter the last 6 wk of gestation with a BCS <2.5; this can be prevented by good feeding management, eg, adequate feeder space for pregnant animals, sorting (based on BCS, fetal numbers, and animal size), forage analysis (for energy, digestible fiber, and protein levels), and ration formulation. During the last 6 wk of gestation, grain is required as a source of carbohydrates in the ration to maintain the health of multiple-bearing females. Amount varies depending on forage quality, adult body weight and condition score, and number of fetuses, but protein must also be balanced for rumen microbes to make optimal use of available carbohydrates.

Producers should ideally assess BCS at breeding and midgestation, usually at the time of pregnancy scanning, so that thin animals can be fed as a separate group. It takes ~6 wk to raise BCS by 1 point, so early intervention is important to avoid late-gestation problems. If real-time ultrasound scanning allows for fetal number determination, then animals should also be managed based on fetal numbers. Producers may find it convenient to feed pregnant ewe-lambs or doelings with twin-bearing females and thin, single-bearing females because of the added energy young animals need for growth. With prolific breeds, triplet-bearing ewes and thin, twin-bearing ewes can be fed together. Overconditioned females (ie, BCS ≥4) are not as common but may be seen in small hobby flocks. Fat females are much less responsive to therapy, and owners should be advised on how to avoid the problem through proper feeding management. However, late pregnancy is not the time to reduce BCS in overconditioned females. BHB serum levels can be used as a flock screening test to detect flocks at risk of pregnancy toxemia. In flocks with values ranging from >0.8–3 mmol/L, feeding management should be corrected quickly to avoid clinical disease.

Research has supported the use of ionophores, particularly monensin, in transition dairy cows to prevent subclinical ketosis and other early postpartum diseases. Ionophores improve feed efficiency by changing microflora populations in the rumen, resulting in increased feed efficiency and production of propionic acid, followed by improved gluconeogenesis. There is some evidence that monensin may be beneficial for late-gestation ewes (although not for dairy goats); it improved feed efficiency by lowering feed intake. Treated ewes also showed lower serum BHB levels in late gestation, with no adverse effects on lamb birth weights. It may help prevent ketosis in postpartum dairy goats. Lasalocid has been similarly studied. Again, feed intake was suppressed, but lamb survival was better in the treatment group. More work needs to be done with both drugs to assess their use in preventing pregnancy toxemia in prolific ewes.

KETOSIS IN CATTLE

(Acetonemia, Ketonemia)

Ketosis is a common disease of adult cattle. It typically occurs in dairy cows in early lactation and is most consistently characterized by partial anorexia and depression. Rarely, it occurs in cattle in late gestation, at which time it resembles pregnancy toxemia of ewes (*see* p 1021). In addition to inappetence, signs of nervous dysfunction, including pica, abnormal licking, incoordination and abnormal gait, bellowing, and aggression, are occasionally seen. The condition is worldwide in distribution but is most common where dairy cows are bred and managed for high production.

Etiology and Pathogenesis: The pathogenesis of bovine ketosis is incompletely understood, but it requires the combination of intense adipose mobilization and a high glucose demand. Both of these conditions are present in early lactation, at which time negative energy balance leads to adipose mobilization, and milk synthesis creates a high glucose demand. Adipose mobilization is accompanied by high blood serum concentrations of nonesterified fatty acids (NEFAs). During periods of intense gluconeogenesis, a large portion of serum NEFAs is directed to ketone body synthesis in the liver. Thus, the clinicopathologic characterization of ketosis includes high serum concentrations of NEFAs and ketone bodies and low concentrations of glucose. In contrast to many other species, cattle with hyperketonemia do not have concurrent acidemia. The serum ketone bodies are acetone, acetoacetate, and β-hydroxybutyrate (BHB).

There is speculation that the pathogenesis of ketosis cases occurring in the immediate postpartum period is slightly different than that of cases occurring closer to the time of peak milk production. Ketosis in the immediate postpartum period is sometimes described as **type II ketosis**. Such cases of ketosis in very early lactation are usually associated with fatty liver (*see* p 1018). Both fatty liver and ketosis are probably part of a spectrum of conditions associated with intense fat mobilization in cattle. Ketosis cases occurring closer to peak milk production, which usually occurs at 4–6 wk postpartum, may be more closely associated with underfed cattle experiencing a metabolic shortage of gluconeogenic precursors than with excessive fat mobilization. Ketosis at this time is sometimes described as **type I ketosis**.

The exact pathogenesis of the clinical signs is not known. They do not appear to be associated directly with serum concentrations of either glucose or ketone bodies. There is speculation they may be due to metabolites of the ketone bodies.

Epidemiology: All dairy cows in early lactation (first 6 wk) are at risk of ketosis. The overall prevalence in cattle in the first 60 days of lactation is estimated at 7%–14%, but prevalence in individual herds varies substantially and may exceed 14%. The peak prevalence of ketosis occurs in the first 2 wk of lactation. Lactational incidence rates vary dramatically between herds and may approach 100%. Ketosis is seen in all parities (although it appears to be less common in primiparous animals) and does not appear to have a genetic predisposition, other than being associated with dairy breeds. Cows with excessive adipose stores (body condition score ≥3.75 out of 5) at calving are at a greater risk of ketosis than those with lower body condition scores. Lactating cows with subclinical ketosis (*see* p 1027) are also at a greater risk of developing clinical ketosis and displaced abomasum than cows with lower serum BHB concentrations.

Clinical Findings: In cows maintained in confinement stalls, reduced feed intake is usually the first sign of ketosis. If rations are offered in components, cows with ketosis often refuse grain before forage. In group-fed herds, reduced milk production, lethargy, and an "empty" appearing abdomen are usually the signs of ketosis noticed first. On physical examination, cows are afebrile and may be slightly dehydrated. Rumen motility is variable, being hyperactive in some cases and hypoactive in others. In many cases, there are no other physical abnormalities. CNS disturbances are noted in a minority of cases. These include abnormal licking and chewing, with cows sometimes chewing incessantly on pipes and other objects in their surroundings. Incoordination and gait abnormalities occasionally are seen, as are aggression and bellowing. These signs occur in a clear minority of cases, but because the disease is so common, finding animals with these signs is not unusual.

Diagnosis: The clinical diagnosis of ketosis is based on presence of risk factors (early lactation), clinical signs, and ketone bodies in urine or milk. When a diagnosis of ketosis is made, a thorough physical examination should be performed, because ketosis frequently occurs concurrently with other peripartum diseases. Especially common concurrent diseases include displaced abomasum, retained fetal membranes, and metritis. Rabies and other CNS diseases are important differential diagnoses in cases exhibiting neurologic signs.

Cow-side tests for the presence of ketone bodies in urine or milk are critical for diagnosis. Most commercially available test kits are based on the presence of acetoacetate or acetone in milk or urine. Dipstick tests are convenient, but those designed to detect acetoacetate or acetone in urine are not suitable for milk testing. All of these tests are read by observation for a particular color change. Care should be taken to allow the appropriate time for color development as specified by the test manufacturer. Handheld instruments designed to monitor ketone bodies in the blood of human diabetic patients are available. These instruments quantitatively measure the concentration of BHB in blood, urine, or milk and may be used for the clinical diagnosis of ketosis.

In a given animal, urine ketone body concentrations are always higher than milk ketone body concentrations. Trace to mildly positive results for the presence of ketone bodies in urine do not signify clinical ketosis. Without clinical signs, such as partial anorexia, these results indicate subclinical ketosis. Milk tests for acetone and acetoacetate are more specific than urine tests. Positive milk tests for acetoacetate and/or acetone usually indicate clinical ketosis. BHB concentrations in milk may be measured by a dipstick method that is available in some countries, or by the electronic device mentioned above. The BHB concentration in milk is always higher than the acetoacetate or acetone concentration, making the tests based on BHB more sensitive than those based on acetoacetate or acetone.

Treatment: Treatment of ketosis is aimed at reestablishing normoglycemia and reducing serum ketone body concentrations. Bolus IV administration of 500 mL of 50% dextrose solution is a common therapy. This solution is very hyperosmotic and, if administered perivascularly, results in severe tissue swelling and irritation, so care should be taken to ensure that it is given IV. Bolus glucose therapy generally results in rapid recovery, especially in cases occurring near peak lactation (type I ketosis). However, the effect frequently is transient, and relapses are common. Administration of glucocorticoids, including dexamethasone or isoflupredone acetate at 5–20 mg/dose, IM, may result in a more sustained response, relative to glucose alone. Glucose and glucocorticoid therapy may be repeated daily as necessary. Propylene glycol administered orally (250–400 g/dose [8–14 oz]) once per day acts as a glucose precursor and is effective as ketosis therapy. Indeed, propylene glycol appears to be the most well documented of the various therapies for ketosis. Overdosing propylene glycol leads to CNS depression.

Ketosis cases occurring within the first 1–2 wk after calving (type II ketosis) frequently are more refractory to therapy than cases occurring nearer to peak lactation (type I). In these cases, a long-acting insulin preparation given IM at 150–200 IU/day may be beneficial. Insulin suppresses both adipose mobilization and ketogenesis but should be given in combination with glucose or a glucocorticoid to prevent hypoglycemia. Use of insulin in this manner is an extra-label, unapproved use. Other therapies that may be of benefit in refractory ketosis cases are continuous IV glucose infusion and tube feeding. (*See also* p 1018.)

Prevention and Control: Prevention of ketosis is via nutritional management. Body condition should be managed in late lactation, when cows frequently become too fat. Modifying diets of late lactation cows to increase the energy supply from digestible fiber and reduce the energy supply from starch may aid in partitioning dietary energy toward milk and away from body fattening. The dry period is generally too late to reduce body condition score. Reducing body condition in the dry period, particularly in the late dry period, may even be counterproductive, resulting in excessive adipose mobilization prepartum. A critical area in ketosis prevention is maintaining and promoting feed intake. Cows tend to reduce feed consumption in the last 3 wk of gestation. Nutritional management should be aimed at minimizing this reduction. Controversy exists regarding the optimal dietary characteristics during this period. It is likely that optimal energy and fiber concentrations in rations for cows in the last 3 wk of gestation vary from farm to farm. Feed intake should be monitored and rations adjusted to meet but not greatly exceed energy requirements throughout the entire dry period. For Holstein cows of typical adult body size, the average daily energy requirement throughout the dry period is between 12 and 15 Mcal expressed as net energy for lactation (NE_L). After calving, diets should promote rapid and sustained increases in feed and energy consumption. Early lactation rations should be relatively high in nonfiber carbohydrate concentration but contain enough fiber to maintain rumen health and feed intake. Neutral-detergent fiber concentrations should usually be in the range of 28%–30%, with nonfiber carbohydrate concentrations in the range of 38%–41%. Dietary particle size will influence the optimal proportions of carbohydrate fractions. Some feed additives, including niacin, calcium propionate, sodium propionate, propylene glycol, and rumen-protected choline, may help prevent and manage ketosis. To be effective, these supplements should be fed in the last 2–3 wk of gestation, as well as during the period of ketosis susceptibility.

In some countries, monensin sodium is approved for use in preventing subclinical ketosis and its associated diseases. Where approved, it is recommended at the rate of 200–300 mg/head/day.

SUBCLINICAL KETOSIS

Subclinical ketosis is defined as high serum ketone body concentrations without observed clinical signs. Subclinically affected cows are at increased risk of clinical ketosis and displaced abomasum and are also less fertile than those with normal serum ketone body concentrations. Furthermore, they appear to have reduced milk production. Determination of serum β-hydroxybutyrate (BHB) concentrations is considered the best way to detect and monitor subclinical ketosis, because the cow-side tests mentioned above are insufficiently sensitive and specific in detecting subclinical increases in serum BHB concentrations. Serum concentrations may be determined spectrophotometrically by traditional clinical laboratory means. The BHB concentrations in blood or serum samples are reasonably stable; thus, rigorous sample handling precautions are not necessary to transport the specimens to the laboratory. The test is sensitive to hemolysis, however, so hemolysis should be avoided during sample collection, and serum should be separated from the clot before shipment to the laboratory.

In addition to laboratory determination by spectrophotometry, handheld devices manufactured to monitor blood ketone body concentrations in human diabetic patients have been evaluated for use in monitoring subclinical ketosis in cows. These instruments use whole blood rather than serum for BHB determination, making them particularly practical for on-farm use. The whole blood BHB concentration is very close to the serum concentration, so the interpretation of results obtained from either the handheld device or laboratory analysis is similar.

Diagnosis of subclinical ketosis requires definition of a concentration above which cows are considered to be subclinically ketotic. Concentrations between 1,000 μM (10.4 mg/dL) and 1,400 μM (14.6 mg/dL) are used. Recommended strategies for herd-level testing are to test at least 12 animals in the first 60 days of lactation. If >10% are subclinically ketotic, it should be considered evidence of a herd-level problem and prompt a review of nutritional management. Some farms use the handheld BHB meters to test all cows in early lactation. Cows diagnosed with subclinical ketosis are treated with propylene glycol. Such an approach is labor intensive but has been demonstrated to reduce further disease occurrence in subclinically ketotic animals and to improve milk production in treated animals. Such an approach should not replace sound nutritional management procedures.

MALIGNANT HYPERTHERMIA

(Porcine stress syndrome)

Malignant hyperthermia (MH) is a rare, life-threatening, inherited disorder that can lead to metabolic disease of skeletal muscles in susceptible animals after exposure to triggering agents such as halogenated inhalation anesthetics, depolarizing neuromuscular blocking drugs, stress, and/or exercise. A mutation in the ryanodine receptors (RYR1 locus) on the sarcoplasmic reticulum that surrounds myofibrils of skeletal muscles alters the function of calcium release channels, which results in massive release of calcium into the cytoplasm of the myofibrils. As a result, generalized, extensive skeletal muscle contraction occurs, leading rapidly to a potentially fatal hypermetabolic state known as an MH episode. More than 300 RYR1 variants have been identified, and 31 of those mutations have been confirmed to cause MH according to the molecular genetic guidelines of the European Malignant Hyperthermia Group. Different mutation loci within the RYR1 receptors have been shown to be responsible for MH syndrome in different species.

Etiology and Clinical Findings: MH is considered to be a clinical syndrome rather than a single disease, because research indicates that multiple environmental and genetic factors cause a complex of pathophysiologic events. Contrary to general belief, a full-fledged MH episode, with a sudden and rapidly progressive course of symptoms, does not occur frequently. In most cases, MH is a subtle disorder. Pigs and people seem to be most susceptible, but MH has also been reported in dogs, cats, and horses. In people and dogs, both parents must carry the mutant chromosome for the autosomal recessive gene to result in clinical expression in offspring. In pigs, the mutant autosomal gene is dominant, so that a single copy of the mutant chromosome, carried by either parent, can result in clinical expression in the offspring, ie, 50% of offspring are susceptible to MH.

Interestingly, most MH-susceptible animals, including people, do not suffer from signs of muscle disease in everyday life. In people, the incidence of MH episodes during anesthesia is between 1:5,000 and 1:50,000 per 100,000 anesthetic events. The MH episode may develop at first exposure to an anesthetic triggering agent, but in some cases, as many as three exposures must occur before a full-fledged MH crisis develops. In domestic animals, it is unclear whether multiple exposures to the triggering agent are required before developing a full-fledged episode. This is because the clinical signs of MH can be so subtle that the episode goes unrecognized.

MH can occur at any time during anesthesia or in the early postoperative period. The clinical signs of MH are often a sudden and dramatic rise in body temperature and end-tidal CO_2 ($ETCO_2$), followed by muscle fasciculation, muscle rigidity, tachypnea, tachycardia, arrhythmias, myoglobinuria, metabolic acidosis, renal failure, and often death. The prognosis is usually poor once clinical signs are recognized. Triggering agents of MH include stress (eg, excitement, transportation, and preanesthetic handling), exercise, halogenated inhalation anesthetics (eg, halothane, isoflurane, sevoflurane, and desflurane), and depolarizing neuromuscular blocking drugs (eg, succinylcholine). Of the halogenated inhalation anesthetics, halothane is claimed to be the most potent triggering agent, and it is no longer used in western countries. The use of succinylcholine, another potent triggering agent, has been gradually restricted by international anesthesia societies.

In **pigs**, MH is also referred to as porcine stress syndrome. Breed susceptibility varies, with Pietrain, Portland China, and Landrace pigs very susceptible to MH, and Large White, Yorkshire, and Hampshire pigs much less so. In the past, halothane was the most frequently reported trigger of MH in pigs. Isoflurane has been reported to trigger MH in pigs of susceptible breeds, but only one instance of isoflurane-induced MH has been reported in a potbellied pig. Sevoflurane-induced MH also has been reported in purebred Poland China pigs. Episodes of MH induced by desflurane have been reported in Large White, Pietrain, and Pietran-mixed pigs. There have been no reports of isoflurane- or sevoflurane-induced MH in cattle.

In **dogs**, MH syndrome has been reported in Pointers, Greyhounds, Labrador Retrievers, Saint Bernards, Springer Spaniels, Bichon Frises, Golden Retrievers, and Border Collies. There are distinct differences in the clinical signs of MH seen in dogs and those in pigs and people. The first obvious indication of an imminent MH episode in dogs is the rapid and dramatic increase in CO_2 production, as evidenced by a sudden increase in $ETCO_2$ concentration. Body temperature may increase during the episode, but this occurs much later than the increased $ETCO_2$. In a study in which a colony of Doberman-German Shepherd-Collie dogs were challenged with halothane/succinylcholine, the dogs that developed MH syndrome all had a mutation on the calcium-release channels in the RYR1 receptors. However, this mutation was identified on a different loci (T1640) than that responsible for MH syndrome in pigs (R614C) and in people (CFA01). Another mutation, RYR1V547A, has also been shown to be involved in MH syndrome in dogs. The incidence rate of MH syndrome associated with anesthesia in dogs is reported to be 2.1% in Canada, 0.43% in the USA, and 0.23% in England, with a mortality rate of 0.11% in both Canada and the USA.

MH syndrome in **horses** is difficult to recognize, because it can easily be confused with other myopathies commonly associated with anesthesia in horses. Unlike in pigs, dogs, and people, signs of MH syndrome in horses tend to be slow to develop and are often observed only after ≥3 hr of anesthesia. In addition to the clinical signs of anesthetic-related MH seen in other species, intraoperative cardiac arrhythmia (eg, premature ventricular contraction), postanesthetic myositis, and increased serum potassium and CK have also been seen in MH-affected horses. Clinical signs similar to those of MH syndrome such as hypercarbia, increased body temperature, and hyperkalemia, are also seen in horses with hyperkalemic periodic paralysis (*see* p 1047), a genetic mutation of sodium channels. Thus, a definitive diagnosis should be confirmed by in vitro contracture test (IVCT) or DNA analysis. Prognosis of horses suffering an MH episode during or after anesthesia is usually poor because of the lack of response to symptomatic treatments and difficulty in management of complications such as myositis, fractures, and/or seizures.

Diagnosis: Currently, the gold standard for diagnosis of MH is IVCT, which is based on muscle fiber contracture in response to triggering agents such as halothane or caffeine. However, IVCT requires a surgical procedure (ie, muscle biopsy), is expensive and available only at specialized testing centers, and may produce equivocal as well as false-positive and false-negative results. DNA analysis is an alternative to the IVCT; it requires only a small blood sample to be sent to an accredited diagnostic laboratory to screen for RYR1 mutation. An animal is diagnosed as MH susceptible if 1 of the 31 known causative mutations is detected. However, the diagnostic classification of many RYR1 mutations remains difficult because their pathophysiologic impact with regard to initiating an MH episode is not yet clear. Therefore, an IVCT is required to exclude MH susceptibility in case of an unclassified RYR1 mutation or if RYR1 mutation is absent. Other minimally invasive diagnostic tests for identification of MH susceptibility are in development

Treatment and Prevention: Because of few effective drugs available to treat MH, stress before anesthesia should be minimized, and using anesthetics that are known triggering agents should be avoided to prevent an MH episode in susceptible animals. Total IV anesthesia and/or regional/local anesthetic techniques can be safely used as alternative procedures to allow surgery on MH-susceptible animals. Drugs that can be safely administered to MH-susceptible animals include phenothiazine derivatives (eg, acepromazine), butyrophenone derivatives (eg, droperidol, azaperone), benzodiazepine derivatives (eg, diazepam, midazolam, zolazepam), α_2-agonists (eg, xylazine, detomidine, dexmedetomidine, romifidine), dissociative anesthetics (eg, ketamine, tiletamine-zolazepam), propofol, etomidate, opioids (eg, morphine, hydromorphone, fentanyl, butorphanol, buprenorphine), N_2O, nondepolarizing neuromuscular blocking drugs (eg, atracurium, vecuronium, rocuronium), and local anesthetics (eg, lidocaine, mepivacaine, bupivacaine). MH-susceptible animals should be kept calm and stress minimized by administering effective preanesthetic medication before induction and maintenance of anesthesia. Azaperone at 0.5–2 mg/kg, IM, provided 100% protection against MH in susceptible Pietrain pigs.

Treatment of MH is most effective when signs of MH (eg, muscle rigidity, sudden rise in body temperature and $ETCO_2$) are recognized early and treated aggressively. Treatment is largely symptomatic and includes immediate discontinuation of inhalation anesthetic and use of ice packs and alcohol baths. Controlled ventilation using a machine flushed free of anesthetic agent should also be instituted as soon as possible to remove excessive CO_2 and maintain normal blood pH and acid-base status. Dantrolene (a specific ryanodine receptor antagonist) has proved effective for treatment (1–3 mg/kg, IV) and prophylaxis (5 mg/kg, PO, up to 10 mg/kg) of MH. Animals with cardiac arrhythmias, such as tachycardia or severe premature ventricular contractions, can be treated with lidocaine (1–2 mg/kg, IV), if needed. Calcium chloride and calcium gluconate are not recommended. Hyperkalemia should be treated with controlled ventilation, and 50% dextrose (0.5 mL/kg, IV) and/or insulin (0.25–0.5 U/kg, IV) can be administered to promote movement of extracellular potassium into cells. Sodium bicarbonate (1–2 mEq/kg, IV) can be administered to maintain normal blood pH in the presence of metabolic acidosis. Balanced electrolyte solutions, 5% dextrose in water, and normal saline are acceptable for supportive fluid therapy; Ringer's lactate with added calcium should not be used. Dantrolene should be administered to affected animals. Testing for disseminated intravascular coagulation, which often results when body temperature exceeds 41°C (105.8°F), is prudent, as well as observation of the urine for myoglobinuric renal failure due to severe muscle damage. Affected animals should be closely monitored for signs of MH for 48–72 hr, because 25% may experience recrudescence.

TRANSPORT TETANY IN RUMINANTS

(Railroad disease, Railroad sickness, Staggers)

Transport tetany occurs after the stress of prolonged transport, typically in cows and ewes in late pregnancy, although it is also seen in lambs transported to feedlots and in cattle and sheep transported to slaughter. Crowded, hot, poorly ventilated transport vehicles (railroad cars or trailers) with minimal or no access to feed or water appear to predispose animals to the condition; however, prolonged travel by foot is also a risk factor. The disease is characterized by recumbency, GI stasis, and coma, and is generally fatal.

Although cows in late gestation are most commonly affected, the disease is also seen in cows that have recently calved, as well as in bulls, steers, and dry cows. Risk factors include heavy feeding before shipment, deprivation of feed and water for >24 hr during transit, and unrestricted access to water and exercise immediately after arrival. Exposure to hot environmental conditions is also associated with an increased incidence. Although the specific cause of tetany is unknown, the condition may be a form of acute hypocalcemia precipitated by late pregnancy and early lactation, or by fasting before or during transit. Physical stress is undoubtedly related. Hypomagnesemia may be a precipitating factor in cattle and a contributing factor in sheep.

Clinical signs in cattle may occur while in transit or as long as 48 hr after arrival. Early clinical signs include restlessness and excitement, trismus, and grinding of teeth. A staggering gait may be seen, and later, if recumbent, cattle often demonstrate paddling of the hindlegs. Rumen hypomotility and GI stasis are seen, and animals become completely anorectic. Tachycardia and rapid, labored respiration may develop. Abortion may be a complication. Cattle that do not recover gradually become more obtunded to the point of coma and die within 3–4 days. Moderate hypocalcemia and hypophosphatemia may be seen in cattle. Some sheep are hypocalcemic and hypomagnesemic, but others show no measurable biochemical abnormalities. No specific lesions are found at necropsy other than lesions associated with prolonged recumbency, most commonly ischemic muscle necrosis. In lambs, early signs include restlessness, staggering, and partial hindlimb paralysis followed by lateral recumbency. Death can occur rapidly or after 2–3 days of recumbency. In lambs, mild hypocalcemia may be noted. Recovery rates are fair even with treatment. The relationship of clinical signs with transport or forced, prolonged exercise is diagnostic.

Some animals respond to treatment with combinations of parenteral calcium, magnesium, and glucose. IV injections of calcium borogluconate (25% solution at 400–800 mL/cow or 100 mL/ewe) or calcium borogluconate with magnesium sulfate (5% solution, same volumes) can be administered slowly. A dose of 50 mL/day can be given SC to affected lambs in feedlots. Repeated injections may be warranted, but failure to respond is common (50%) and most likely due to concurrent muscle necrosis. Additional treatment considerations include IV administration of large volumes of polyionic fluids such as lactated Ringer's solution. Animals should be offered good quality feeds (eg, alfalfa hay), fresh water, and soft bedding with good footing underneath. Sedation may be necessary if animals are hyperexcitable or convulsing.

If prolonged transport times of cows or ewes in advanced pregnancy is unavoidable, animals should be fed a restricted diet several days before shipment, then provided adequate feed, water, and rest periods during transport. Administration of ataractic agents (unless transport is to slaughter) such as promazine hydrochloride before loading is recommended, especially for nervous animals. Upon unloading at the destination, animals should be allowed limited access to water for the first 24 hr and minimal exercise for 2–3 days.

MUSCULOSKELETAL SYSTEM

LARGE ANIMALS

SMALL ANIMALS

MUSCULOSKELETAL SYSTEM INTRODUCTION

The musculoskeletal system consists of bones, cartilage, muscles, ligaments, and tendons. Primary functions of the musculoskeletal system include support of the body, provision of motion, and protection of vital organs. The skeletal system serves as the main storage system for calcium and phosphorus and contains critical components of the hematopoietic system. Many other body systems, including the nervous, vascular, and integumentary systems, are interrelated, and disorders of one of these systems may also affect the musculoskeletal system and complicate diagnosis.

Diseases of the musculoskeletal system most often involve motion deficits, functional disorders, and lameness. The degree of impairment depends on the specific problem and its severity. Skeletal and articular disorders are by far the most common and have the greatest economic impact. In horses and dogs, musculoskeletal injuries are a major source of debilitating pain, economic loss, and loss of athleticism. Degenerative joint disease is much more common and has a greater economic importance than acute traumatic injuries or respiratory diseases in performance horses. Several studies estimate that problems involving the fetlock and carpal joints account for 25%–28% of horses lost from training. In addition, tendon injury is a common debilitating injury in performance horses. The healing response is prolonged, and the resultant repair tissue is usually of inferior mechanical strength. Consequently, the prognosis for return to previous levels of performance is poor. In dogs, cranial cruciate ligament injury with resulting osteoarthritis is the most common musculoskeletal injury resulting in lameness. Although perhaps less common, primary muscular diseases, neurologic deficits, toxins, endocrine aberrations, metabolic disorders, infectious diseases, blood and vascular disorders, nutritional imbalances or deficits, and occasionally congenital defects are diagnosed as well.

DISORDERS OF MUSCLE

The structural and functional unit of skeletal muscle is the motor unit. It consists of a ventral motor neuron with its cell body in the central horn of the spinal cord and its peripheral axon, the neuromuscular junction, and the muscle fibers innervated by the neuron. Each of these components must be functionally intact for the muscle to contract properly. The ventral motor neuron is the final common pathway conducting neural impulses from the CNS to the muscle.

The transmission of a nerve impulse at the neuromuscular junction involves massive release of acetylcholine from small synaptic vessels, where it is stored. The acetylcholine fills the synaptic cleft between the nerve terminal and the muscle fiber membrane, where most of it is destroyed by cholinesterase within a fraction of a second. This short period of activity is sufficient to excite the muscle fiber membrane, which results in a significant increase in membrane permeability to sodium ions and allows rapid influx of sodium into the muscle fiber. The sodium ion increases the endplate potential, which elicits electrical currents that spread to the interior of the fibers, where they cause a release of calcium ions from the sarcoplasmic reticulum. The calcium ions initiate, in turn, the chemical events of the contractile process. When this occurs in all the muscle fibers innervated by each motor neuron (possibly thousands), muscle contraction results.

Normal muscle, comprising many motor units, is dynamic, and its function and structure can be influenced by many diseases. Complete paralysis, paresis, or ataxia may be caused by primary muscular dysfunctions of infectious, toxic, or congenital origin. However, in most instances the primary disorder can be attributed to the nervous system (eg, tetanus, rhinopneumonitis, canine distemper, protozoal myelitis), with the muscular system merely representing the effector organ. Disorders that affect the neuromuscular junction (eg, myasthenia gravis, hypocalcemia, hypermagnesemia) can result in muscle fatigue, weakness, and paralysis. The neuromuscular junction can also be affected by muscle-relaxing drugs (eg, curare, succinylcholine, M99), certain antibiotics, and toxins (eg, botulism, tetanus, venoms).

Disorders primarily of the muscle membrane and, to some extent, of the actual muscle fibers are called myopathies. Muscle membrane disorders may be hereditary (eg, myotonia congenita in goats) or acquired (eg, vitamin E and selenium deficiencies, hypothyroidism, and hypokalemia). Myopathies involving the actual muscle fiber components include muscular dystrophy, polymyositis, eosinophilic myositis, white muscle disease, and exertional rhabdomyolysis. Various laboratory tests, eg, histopathologic examination, determination of serum enzyme levels, electromyographic studies, thermography, and determinations of conduction velocity, are very useful in confirmation of a specific diagnosis.

DISORDERS OF TENDONS

Tendons act as bridging and attachment structures for the muscles; some bridge long gaps between the muscle bellies and target bone and, therefore, are prone to injury themselves, especially because they are often loaded to the extreme and are only minimally capable of elastic elongation. A prime example is the superficial flexor tendon of horses, which is frequently injured by partial tearing that leads to tendinitis. Another acquired injury of tendons involves traumatic disruptions. Because of the relatively poor blood supply of both tendons and ligaments, healing is always prolonged with inelastic scar tissue, and the injured tendon never returns to its original strength. Therefore, management of tendon and ligament injuries requires patience with conservative longterm rehabilitation. Reinjury is common.

DISORDERS OF BONE

Bone diseases are generally congenital or hereditary, nutritional, or traumatic. Congenital disorders include in utero malformations and atavisms, such as polydactyly or persistent ulnae or fibulae in foals; examples of genetic defects are atlanto-occipital malformations in Arabian horses or certain cases of spinal ataxia (*see* p 1228), canine hip dysplasia, and abnormal bone formation such as that caused by parathyroid hypoplasia.

Bone defects due to nutrition are caused primarily by imbalances or deficiencies in minerals, particularly the trace minerals such as copper, zinc, and magnesium. *Calcium and phosphorus concentrations* must also be present in the correct ratio. Osteomalacia represents the classic example of imbalanced or deficient calcium and phosphorus intake. Other nutritional disorders are caused by excessive protein intake of growing animals. Either deficiency or excess intake of certain vitamins, particularly vitamins A and D, may influence growth and development of bone. Aseptic physitis or special osteochondrotic conditions of the physes may be caused by zinc toxicity or copper deficiency.

Traumatic causes of bone disorders represent the vast majority of cases and include fractures, fissures, periosteal reactions as a result of trauma, sequestrum formation, and insertion desmopathies or tendinopathies, respectively. Lack of weight bearing, lameness, reduced motion, instability, pain, heat, or swelling usually accompany these disorders.

DISORDERS OF JOINTS

Articulations are divided into synarthrodial joints and diarthrodial joints. Synarthrodial joints are osseous components united by fibrous tissue or cartilage. Synarthrodial joints are practically immovable and are rarely associated with joint disease other than fractures. Diarthrodial joints are mobile; the opposing bone ends are covered by articular hyaline cartilage and are separated by a joint cavity filled with synovial fluid. Articular cartilage serves to distribute weight-bearing forces and to minimize friction between adjacent skeletal components during movement. Normal synovial fluid and articular cartilage express a glycoprotein to provide boundary lubrication to the articular cartilage and synovial membrane during weight bearing. The synovial fluid also nourishes the articular cartilage.

Diarthrodial joints are most frequently involved in pathologic changes. These changes can involve the joint capsule, synovial membrane, hyaline articular cartilage, and subchondral bone. Damage to intra-articular ligaments and the menisci in the stifle joint can affect the stability of the joint and propagate damage to the joint. Joint disorders may be caused by trauma, chronic inflammation, developmental factors, or infections. Severe trauma frequently results in luxation, subluxation, fracture, or instability of a joint. Direct penetration of the joint capsule may also lead to septic arthritis, which is characterized by an increase in synovial WBCs resulting in an increased concentration of proteolytic enzymes within the synovial fluid. The severe inflammatory response within the joint can quickly lead to breakdown of the articular hyaline cartilage. Bacterial and fungal infections involving synovial structures are typically recognized based on their extreme heat, swelling, pain localized to the joint, and lameness that is often severe. All cases of synovial sepsis require immediate and aggressive treatment to preserve the joint.

Developmental defects include osteochondritis dissecans, equine ataxia, angular limb deformities, and lumbar disc syndrome in certain breeds of dogs. Extension of physitis into the adjacent joint and damage due to continuous abnormal weight bearing in animals with angular limb deformities are other inciting causes of joint disease.

Chronic inflammation of joints and surrounding structures is most common in articulations associated with locomotion. Joint homeostasis involves the simultaneous synthesis and degradation of extracellular matrix components of the cartilage. The responses of the synovial membrane and articular cartilage are critical to accommodate the mechanical and chemical demands placed on the joint. In pathologic conditions, the biosynthetic activity of the cells does not compensate for the loss of matrix components through mechanical and enzymatic degradation. This results in a net loss of cartilage and compromised joint function.

Osteoarthritis is a degenerative, progressive disease of diarthrodial joints. It has a multifactorial etiology; aging, trauma, mechanical forces, conformation, hormonal, and genetic factors contribute to varying degrees. It is a major cause of musculoskeletal pain, morbidity, and decreased performance in all species. Although pathologic changes occur in multiple joint tissues, loss of articular cartilage is the hallmark of the disease.

Cartilage damage is recognized clinically when sufficient joint damage occurs to cause synovitis or lameness. As damage accumulates, cartilage fibrillation or complete eburnation can occur at areas of high stress. Histologically there is loss of proteoglycan staining, decreased cell viability, and advancement of the tidemark of calcified cartilage. The loss of proteoglycans is accompanied by an increase in cartilage matrix water content and a reduction in stiffness. The biomechanically compromised cartilage is more susceptible to further damage.

Corticosteroids and NSAIDs have been widely used for symptomatic treatment of osteoarthritis. The benefit of these drugs is minimized in extensive cartilage loss in which chondrocyte replacement is an issue, and their inappropriate use may exacerbate the progression of degenerative change. Several medications have specific chondroprotective actions to treat articular cartilage damage. Structure-modifying osteoarthritis drugs (eg, glycosaminoglycans, pentosan polysulfate, hyaluronic acids) slow down the progression of osteoarthritis by mitigating the rate of cartilage degradation and enhancing matrix synthesis. Intra-articular hyaluronic acid administration reduces synovial inflammatory effects and may also reestablish boundary lubrication within the joint cavity. The autogenous substance interleukin receptor antagonist protein (IRAP) has been used effectively to control joint inflammation in some horses.

DIAGNOSIS AND TREATMENT OF MUSCULOSKELETAL DISORDERS

In all cases of musculoskeletal pain and lameness, diagnostic procedures to determine the nature, extent, and exact location of the injury must be performed. Evaluation of the source of pain and lameness always starts with a thorough history, inspection, and physical examination to look for sources of heat, swelling, and pain on manual palpation. Hoof testers should be applied to determine whether pain is present within the hoof capsule. Next, the gait and locomotion of the animal are evaluated. In a weight-bearing lameness, the lame leg always bears less weight and often has a shorter duration of bearing weight. In swinging leg lameness, the lame leg abducts or adducts to avoid flexion of a painful joint. These findings can be measured objectively using a force plate or a gait analysis system. In horses, flexion tests of joints followed immediately by lameness evaluation at a trot may help localize pain. After determining which limb is lame, diagnostic analgesia (intra-articular or perineural) can be used to localize the painful gait to a specific anatomic structure or a region of the affected limb. After localization, diagnostic imaging techniques can be performed to evaluate the soft-tissue structures and bones. These diagnostic procedures include radiography, ultrasonography, MRI, CT, nuclear imaging, and thermography. When joint sepsis is suspected, synovial fluid analysis of affected joints is necessary for diagnosis. After these procedures, a diagnosis can be made, treatment instituted, and a prognosis given based on the diagnosis, extent of disease, and expected response to therapy.

Therapeutic options for diseases of the musculoskeletal system include rest, restricted or modified activity, immobilization of diseased or injured structures in splints and casts, NSAIDs, corticosteroid administration, physical therapy, acupuncture, extracorporeal shock wave therapy, and surgical repair. Therapeutic options for management of musculoskeletal disorders have greatly expanded during the past few years with the use of regenerative medicine, in which growth factors and mesenchymal cell therapy have been used to augment healing. A return to a useful life for many animals is possible when diagnosis and subsequent treatment is done early in the disease process.

CONGENITAL AND INHERITED ANOMALIES OF THE MUSCULOSKELETAL SYSTEM

Congenital and inherited anomalies can result in the birth of diseased or deformed neonates. Congenital disorders can be due to viral infections of the fetus or to ingestion of toxic plants by the dam at certain stages of gestation. The musculoskeletal system can also be affected by certain congenital neurologic disorders.

MULTIPLE SPECIES

Contracted Flexor Tendons

Contracted flexor tendons are probably the most prevalent abnormality of the musculoskeletal system of newborn foals and calves. An autosomal recessive gene causes this condition. In utero positioning may also affect the degree of disability.

At birth, the pastern and fetlocks of the forelegs and sometimes the carpal joints are flexed to varying degrees due to shortening of the deep and superficial digital flexors and associated muscles. A cleft palate may accompany this condition in some breeds. Slightly affected animals bear weight on the soles of the feet and walk on their toes. More severely affected animals walk on the dorsal surface of the pastern and fetlock joint. If not treated, the dorsal surfaces of these joints become damaged, and suppurative arthritis develops. Rupture of the common digital extensor can occur as a sequela. This condition should be differentiated from arthrogryposis.

Mildly affected animals recover without treatment. In moderate cases, oxytetracycline may be administered to relax the flexor muscles, and a splint can be applied to force the animal to bear weight on its toes. The pressure from the splint must not compromise the circulation, or the foot may undergo ischemic necrosis. Frequent manual extension of the joints, attempting to stretch the ligaments, tendons, and muscles, helps treat these intermediate cases. Severe cases require tenotomy of one or both flexor tendons. A bandage cast may sometimes be indicated. Extreme cases may not respond to any treatment.

Dyschondroplasia

Dyschondroplasia of genetic origin is seen in most breeds of cattle. The forms range from the so-called Dexter "bulldog" lethal,

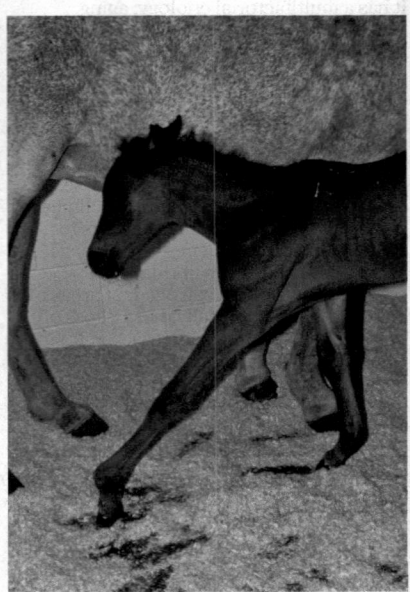

Ruptured common digital flexor tendon as a sequela of contracted flexor tendons in a foal. *Courtesy of Dr. Reid Hanson.*

in which the calf is invariably stillborn, to mildly affected animals.

The **brachycephalic dwarfs** common in Hereford cattle in the 1950s largely have been eliminated through genetic selection. Short faces, bulging foreheads, prognathism, cleft palate, large abdomens, and short legs are characteristic. They are approximately half normal size. The **dolichocephalic dwarf**, most commonly seen in Angus cattle, is of the same general body conformation as the brachycephalic dwarf, except that it has a long head and does not have either a bulging forehead or prognathism. The short-faced calves are frequently referred to as "snorter" dwarfs because of their labored and audible breathing. Both types are of low viability and susceptible to bloat. Their carcasses are undesirable, and they are rarely kept except for research purposes.

Dyschondroplasia of the appendicular and axial skeletons also is seen in dogs. The former is reported in Poodles and Scottish Terriers, the latter in Alaskan Malamutes, Basset Hounds, Dachshunds, Poodles, and Scottish Terriers. In some breeds (Bassets, Dachshunds, Pekingese), the appendicular dyschondroplastic characteristics are an important feature of breed type. In Malamutes, the condition is accompanied by anemia.

Dystrophy-like Myopathies

Numerous examples of progressive myopathies have been described in animals; many are heritable, and many resemble various types of muscular dystrophy in people. Affected muscles have a variety of degenerative and atrophic changes. In Meuse-Rhine-Yssel cattle of Holland, a progressive fatal myopathy of the diaphragm and intercostal muscles has been described. Another dystrophy in cattle is weaver syndrome in Brown Swiss. Hyperplasia, commonly called double muscling (*see* p 1045), is a congenital myopathy found in some European breeds of cattle. Progressive myopathies have been reported in Merino sheep in Australia (an inherited autosomal recessive), in Pietrain pigs (Pietrain creeper syndrome), and in dogs, cats, chickens, turkeys, and mink. Inherited muscular dystrophy of mice and hamsters has been studied extensively; the hamsters have severe myocardial lesions and serve as a model for studies of cardiomyopathy.

Several types of muscular dystrophy are seen in dogs. An X-linked Duchenne-like muscular dystrophy is reported in Golden Retrievers in the USA and in Irish Terriers in Europe. Affected dogs, generally males, develop progressive muscular weakness, dysphagia, stiffness of gait, and muscular atrophy. Microscopically, the distinctive change is lack of dystrophia, a protein concentrated in the sarcolemma and essential for normal membrane function. Some dogs die with accompanying cardiomyopathy. A similar X-linked dystrophy with a lack of dystrophia is described in cats. A second type of dystrophy involves Labrador Retrievers in North America, Europe, and Australia. Clinical signs, which include stiffness, exercise intolerance, and muscular atrophy, develop by 6 mo of age. Autosomal recessive inheritance is implicated. A further dystrophy was described in dysphagic Bouviers in Europe.

Glycogen Storage Disease

(Glycogenosis)

Glycogen storage disease (GSD) is the result of defects in the processing of glycogen synthesis or breakdown within muscles, liver, and other cell types. GSD can be genetic or acquired. Genetic GSD is caused by any inborn error of metabolism (genetically defective enzymes) involved in these processes. In livestock, acquired GSD is caused by intoxication with the alkaloid castanospermine. Progressive muscular weakness and inability to rise properly may be seen in animals with GSDs. Five of the 11 types of GSDs characterized in people have been identified in animals (types I, II, III, VII, and VIII). Affected species include cattle, sheep, dogs, cats, horses, Japanese quail, rats, and mice. Type II glycogenosis in Shorthorn and Brahman cattle has been well documented and is inherited as an autosomal recessive disorder. Affected cattle develop muscular weakness and die at 9–16 mo of age, often with accompanying cardiomegaly and congestive heart failure. Morphologic and biochemical study reveals extensive intralysosomal and cytoplasmic glycogen deposits. Corriedale sheep and Lapland dogs also develop type II glycogenosis.

Myophosphorylase deficiency (type V glycogenosis) is an autosomal recessive disorder in Charolais cattle. Affected cattle show exercise intolerance and may have increased serum activities of skeletal muscle–origin enzymes.

Muscular Steatosis

Muscular steatosis is a condition in which muscle fibers have been replaced by fatty deposits and is seen occasionally in cattle, sheep, and pigs at slaughter. Sometimes the occurrence of muscular steatosis is indicated before slaughter by an abnormal gait, but usually the condition is not found until a carcass is butchered. The condition may be difficult to establish, and it is often only the restriction of muscular steatosis to a single muscle group in an otherwise poorly marbled carcass that makes it conspicuous. In pigs, there is evidence that the onset of muscular steatosis is accompanied by lipid accumulation in muscle fibers. No clinical disease results, and the cause is unknown. The gross lesions are symmetric, pale areas in affected muscles, especially of the back, neck, and upper limbs. Microscopically, many muscle fibers are replaced by fat cells.

Myopathy Associated with Congenital Articular Rigidity

(Arthrogryposis)

This syndrome, one of the more common congenital defects of calves, is characterized by rigid fixation of the limbs in abnormal postures; it often produces dystocia. The muscle weakness and imbalance of muscle power around the joints elicits a physiologic compensatory collagenic response, which replaces atrophied muscle fibers with connective tissue and thickens the joint capsule sufficiently to result in prenatal fixation of limb segments at the joint. Affected animals may have other anomalies, including hydrocephalus, palatoschisis, and spinal dysraphism. The condition may be lethal, but some mildly affected animals recover completely. The muscle lesions may be primary in some types of the disease, but the neural lesions generally are primary, and the muscular alterations represent denervation atrophy. Congenital articular rigidity is seen in cattle, sheep, horses, and pigs. Numerous etiologic factors have been recognized. In cattle, these include viral (Akabane virus [*see* p 620], bluetongue virus [*see* p 738]) and plant (*Lupinus* sp, *see* p 3018) teratogens, and a heritable recessive trait in Charolais (*see* ARTHROGRYPOSIS, p 1045). In sheep, plant (locoweed) and viral (Akabane, Wesselsbron [*see* p 775] teratogens, Rift Valley fever [*see* p 768]), parbendazole exposure, and inherited autosomal recessive primary myopathies of Merino and Welsh Mountain lambs may cause congenital articular rigidity. In pigs, the condition may be inherited as an autosomal recessive, or result from deficiency of vitamin A or manganese or from exposure of pregnant sows to plant toxins (eg, tobacco, thornapple, hemlock, and black cherry).

Osteochondrosis

Osteochondrosis is a disturbance in endochondral ossification that is sometimes classified as dyschondroplasia. The immature articular cartilage may separate from the underlying epiphyseal bone, which sometimes dissects completely free and floats loose in the synovial cavity, resulting in accompanying synovitis or the retention of pyramidal cores of physeal cartilage projecting into the metaphysis. Often, these two lesions are seen simultaneously in the same bone. The disease develops during maximal growth when the biomechanical stresses are greatest in the immature skeleton (4–8 mo in dogs, 80–120 lb [36–54 kg] in pigs). It is most common in large and giant breeds of dogs (*see* p 1195) and in rapidly growing pigs (*see* p 1161), horses (*see* p 1148), turkeys, and chickens (*see* p 2932).

Osteogenesis Imperfecta

Osteogenesis imperfecta is a generalized, inherited bone defect in cattle, dogs, and cats, characterized by extreme fragility of bones and joint laxity attributable to any of a large number of possible mutations of type I collagen. The mechanical properties of the "soft" part of the collagen/mineral composite in the bone appear to be altered. The long bones are slender and have thin cortices. Calluses and recent fractures may be present. The sclera of the eyes may be bluish. The inheritance is most likely polygenic.

Osteopetrosis

Osteopetrosis is a metabolic bone disease characterized by a systemic increase in skeletal mass. It is a rare disease that appears to be inherited as a simple autosomal recessive trait in Angus, Simmental, Dutch Holstein-Freisian and Hereford cattle. It is also seen in dogs and foals. It is characterized by premature stillbirth 10 days to 1 mo before term, brachygnathia inferior, impacted molar teeth, and easily fractured long bones. Bone marrow cavities are absent and replaced by primary spongiosa. The fetal-like abnormal intramedullary bone consists of chondro-osseous tissue. Foramina of the skull and long bones are hypoplastic or aplastic. The cranium is thickened and compresses the brain. Extensive mineralization is present in vessel walls and neurons of the brain. Diagnosis is confirmed by a longitudinal bisection of long bones revealing the diaphyses filled with a plug of bone instead of marrow.

Syndactyly and Polydactyly

Syndactyly, or mule foot, is the partial or complete fusion of the digits of one or more feet. Reported in numerous cattle breeds, it is most prevalent in Holsteins and is inherited as a simple autosomal recessive condition. The forefeet are affected most often, but one or all four feet may be affected. Animals affected with syndactyly walk slowly, usually have a high-stepping gait, and may be more prone to hyperthermia.

Polydactyly is a genetic defect of cattle, sheep, pigs, and occasionally horses. In its most common form, the second digit is developed but the medial dewclaw is missing. The toes may be fused to give rise to polysyndactyly. Rarely one or all four limbs have the condition. Polydactyly in cattle appears to be polygenic, with a dominant gene at one locus and a homozygous recessive at another.

CATTLE

Arthrogryposis

Arthrogryposis is ankylosis of the limbs, usually combined with a cleft palate and other growth deformities. It is seen in all breeds of cattle, particularly Charolais. At birth, affected calves exhibit joints fixed in abnormal positions and frequently have scoliosis and kyphosis. They are usually unable to stand or nurse. Muscle changes, notably atrophy, have also been seen. In the spinal cord, necrosis of neurons and lesions of the white matter may be seen. Arthrogryposis has more than one etiology and pathologic entity. The arthrogryposis syndrome in Charolais is caused by an autosomal recessive gene with complete penetrance in the homozygous state. Teratogens identified as causing arthrogryposis include plants such as lupines (anagyrine as the toxic agent) that are ingested by pregnant cows between day 40 and 70 of gestation. Prenatal viral infections with the Akabane (*see* p 620) or bluetongue (*see* p 738) virus can also cause arthrogryposis.

Brown Atrophy

(Xanthosis, Lipofuscinosis)

In dairy cattle with brown atrophy, the skeletal muscles and myocardium are yellow-brown to bronze. The masseter muscles and the diaphragm are affected most frequently. No clinical disease results. Certain breeds (eg, Ayrshire) are more predisposed than others. Microscopically, brown lipofuscin pigment granules accumulate under the sarcolemma or centrally in the muscle fibers. The inheritance pattern of one affected and three normal offspring suggests that this condition may result from inheritance of a simple recessive gene.

Double Muscling

Double muscling is an overdevelopment of the musculature of the shoulder, back, rump, and hindquarters, separated by deep creases, particularly between the semitendinosus and biceps femoris, and between the longissimus dorsi muscles of either side. Necks of double-muscled cattle are shorter and thicker, and their heads appear smaller. Associated disorders include hypoplastic reproductive tracts, delayed reproductive age of maturity, and lengthened gestation and increased birth weights combined with dystocia. The condition is seen in various beef breeds, including Charolais, Santa Gertrudis, South Devon, Angus, Belgian Blue, Belgian White, and Piedmontese. Double muscling is caused by a pair of incompletely recessive genes that result in the inhibition of myostatin activity in various degrees of the condition. Succinic dehydrogenase activity is significantly decreased in affected calves.

Limber Leg

Limber leg is a hereditary condition of Jersey cattle, apparently controlled by a simple lethal autosomal recessive gene. Some affected calves are born dead. Living calves appear normal at birth but are unable to stand because of incompletely formed muscles, ligaments, tendons, and joints. The shoulder and hip joints can be rotated in any direction without apparent discomfort. Diagnosis is based on signs, necropsy findings, and identification of carrier animals.

Perosomus Elumbis

Perosomus elumbis is an occasionally found congenital anomaly of unknown etiology that is characterized by partial or complete agenesis of the lumbar, sacral, and coccygeal area and accompanied by posterior bimelic arthrogryposis characterized by ankylosis of joints with associated malformations of the musculature. Affected calves cannot use their hindlegs and must be euthanized. The defect is suspected to be inherited. A reduced number of vertebrae has been reported rarely but also has been claimed to be a genetic defect. The condition has also been reported in sheep and pigs.

Spine Defects

There are several defects of the spinal column that include short spine lethal, atlanto-occipital fusion, kyphosis (dorsal arching of the back), lordosis (ventral), scoliosis (lateral), and torticollis (twisted). These defects may occur alone, in combination with, or associated with defects of other body systems, particularly of the CNS.

HORSES

Angular Limb Deformities

In these congenital or acquired skeletal defects, the distal portion of a limb deviates laterally or medially early in neonatal life. In utero malposition, hypothyroidism, trauma, poor conformation, excessive joint laxity, and defective endochondral ossification of the carpal or tarsal and long bones have been implicated. One to four limbs may be affected, depending on the severity of the condition.

The carpus is affected most frequently, but the tarsus and fetlocks are occasionally involved. The deviation is obvious but varies in severity. A lateral deviation (valgus) of up to 6° of the distal portion of a limb may be regarded as normal. Most foals are asymptomatic, but lameness and soft-tissue swelling can accompany severe deviations. Outward rotation of the fetlocks invariably accompanies carpal valgus. Foals with defective ossification of the carpal cuboidal bones or excessive joint laxity are frequently lame as the legs become progressively deviated. Affected limbs must be palpated carefully to detect ligament laxity and specific areas that may be painful.

Diagnosis should include a precise determination of the site and cause for the deviation. The distal radial metaphysis, physis, epiphysis, or cuboidal bones may be the site of deviation. Radiography helps detect physeal flaring, epiphyseal wedging, and deformation of carpal bones. Mildly affected foals frequently improve spontaneously.

Treatment depends on the severity of the condition and tissues affected. Excessive joint laxity, with or without cuboidal carpal bone involvement, requires tube casts or splints. The fetlock and phalangeal region should not be included in the casts, which should protect the weak joint from trauma but allow restricted exercise to maintain tendon and ligament tone. Such limb support may be required for as long as 6 wk.

Physeal and epiphyseal growth disturbances are also amenable to surgical correction through hemicircumferential transection and periosteal elevation of the distal radius on the concave side of the defect or through transphyseal bridging of the physis on the convex side. These surgeries must be performed before the physeal growth plates close (as early as 2–4 mo of age for fetlocks), and success depends on continued growth and development of the bones. Sequential examinations and radiographs are necessary to follow spontaneous improvement or to establish a need for surgery.

Without treatment, the prognosis for severe carpal valgus is poor. The conformational anomaly leads to early degenerative joint disease. Likewise, deformity of the cuboidal carpal bones contributes to a poor prognosis. However, with early detection, careful evaluation, and proper surgical treatment, most foals respond favorably.

Digit Malformation

Digital malformations include supernumerary digits (polydactyly), hypoplasia of phalanges, such as the navicular bone, and bipartite and tripartite navicular bone in which there is incomplete ossification of the navicular bone.

Dwarfism

Dwarfism is the lack of appropriate growth, resulting in a smaller horse. A dwarf horse can be proportionate or disproportionate. Proportionate dwarfs are a result of a deficiency in growth hormone, whereas disproportionate dwarfs are a result of abnormal thyroid hormone levels. The latter results in a foal with musculoskeletal immaturity, characterized by delayed cuboidal bone development, a large head, silky hair coat, floppy ears, and mandibular brachygnathia. Determination and interpretation of either growth hormone assays or thyroid hormone function is not entirely developed or understood in horses, hence the importance of clinical diagnosis. Efforts toward characterizing thyroid function and growth hormone levels should be undertaken to prevent overdiagnosis of this condition. A nitrate toxicity theory has been confirmed in certain foals born with "congenital hypothyroid syndrome."

Glycogen Branching Enzyme Deficiency

Glycogen branching enzyme (GBE) deficiency may be a common cause of neonatal mortality in Quarter horses and related breeds that is obscured by the variety of clinical signs that resemble other equine neonatal diseases. Affected foals lack the enzyme necessary to store glycogen in its branched form and therefore cannot store sugar molecules. The disease is fatal; heart muscle, brain, and skeletal muscles are unable to function. Clinical signs of GBE deficiency may include transient flexural limb deformities, stillbirth, seizures, respiratory or cardiac failure, and persistent recumbency. Leukopenia, high serum CK, AST, and γ-glutamyl transferase are present in most affected foals. Gross postmortem lesions are inconclusive. Muscle, heart, or liver samples contain abnormal periodic acid-Schiff–positive globular or crystalline intracellular inclusions in amounts proportional to the foal's age at death. Accumulation of an unbranched polysaccharide in tissues is suggested by a shift in the iodine absorption spectra of polysaccharide isolated from the liver and muscle of affected foals. Skeletal muscle total polysaccharide concentrations are reduced, but liver and cardiac muscle glycogen concentrations are normal. Several glycolytic enzyme activities are normal, whereas GBE activity is virtually absent in cardiac and skeletal muscle, as well as in liver and peripheral blood cells. GBE activities in peripheral blood cells of dams of affected foals and several of their half-siblings or full siblings are ~50% of controls. GBE protein in liver is markedly reduced to absent in affected foals. Pedigree analysis supports an autosomal recessive mode of inheritance.

Hernias

Hernias are defects in the muscle wall that permit intestines/organs to move into an abnormal location. An umbilical hernia is the incomplete closure of the abdominal wall at the umbilicus. Larger umbilical hernias should be surgically repaired to prevent incarceration of bowel. A congenital diaphragmatic hernia is an opening in the thoracic diaphragm, permitting the displacement of abdominal organs into the thorax. These hernias usually go undetected until the horse is presented for GI signs (colic) rather than respiratory issues. Inguinal hernias are commonly seen in certain breeds, particularly Standardbred and draft horses. They are most common in male foals, and a large scrotal sac is seen. Affected horses rarely present with signs of colic. The hernia should be reduced on a daily basis, and most cases will resolve in 4–6 mo. In cases presented with signs of colic or when there is edema in the inguinal/ventral area (ruptured hernia), surgical repair is advised.

Hyperkalemic Periodic Paralysis

Hyperkalemic periodic paralysis (HYPP) is marked by sudden attacks of paralysis which, in severe cases, may lead to collapse and sudden death. It is an inherited missense mutation in the gene encoding the alpha chain of the adult skeletal muscle sodium channel, resulting in increased sodium permeability across the skeletal muscle cell membrane. Quarter horse, Paint horse, and Appaloosa progeny tracing back to the Quarter horse sire "Impressive" can be affected with this disease and must be eliminated from any reproductive program. Most affected horses are heterozygotes. A sequela of HYPP in horses that undergo general anesthesia is malignant hyperthermia syndrome (*see* p 1027).

Spine Defects

Skeletal malformations include scoliosis (lateral deviation of the back), synostosis (fusion of vertebrae), lordosis (ventral dorsal deviation of the back), kyphosis (dorsal deviation of the back), torticollis (twisted neck), and wry nose (twisted nose). Although all of these conditions are uncommon in foals, congenital scoliosis is encountered most frequently. On clinical examination, it is often difficult to assess the severity. A better appreciation of the condition can be obtained by radiographic examination. In mild cases, improvement is spontaneous and may be complete. Even in the more severe cases, there is rarely any obvious abnormality in gait or maneuverability. However, these foals frequently are not raised because they appear unlikely to be able to withstand being ridden or worked.

Another occasional congenital deformity is that of synostosis (fusion of vertebrae), which may be associated with secondary scoliosis. Radiography is necessary for confirmation.

Congenital lordosis (swayback) is associated with hypoplasia of the intervertebral articular processes. In adult horses, degrees of acquired lordosis and kyphosis (roachback) are occasionally seen, which contribute to back weakness. Diagnosis is based on the clinical appearance and can be confirmed by radiography, which reveals an undue curvature of the vertebral column, usually in the cranial thoracic region (T5–10) in lordosis and in the cranial lumbar region (L1–3) in kyphosis.

Other, less common skeletal malformations include incomplete closures of the bony spinal canal (cervical meningomyelocele, spina bifida) and hydrocephalus (abnormal accumulation of fluid in the cranial vault with resultant enlargement of the head).

Tying-up Syndrome

(Equine rhabdomyolysis syndrome, Exertional rhabdomyolysis, Myoglobinuria)

See also p 1178. Tying-up syndrome in Thoroughbreds is an inherited abnormality in the way calcium is regulated by membrane systems in the skeletal muscle. The narrow genetic origin of Thoroughbreds and the common lineage of the pedigrees of horses with tying-up would support the possibility of an inherited trait. The disease might lie dormant unless specific factors trigger the calcium regulatory system to malfunction. Initiating events include stress, excitement, lameness, high-grain diets, and exercise at submaximal speeds.

A different form of tying-up is **polysaccharide storage myopathy** (PSSM). It is characterized by the accumulation of glycogen polysaccharides in skeletal muscle. The recent identification of a genetic mutation for PSSM revealed that there are actually no less than two forms of this disease. A form of PSSM called type 1 PSSM is caused by a mutation in the glycogen synthase gene. Type 1 PSSM occurs in many Quarter horses and related breeds, draft breeds, some Warmblood breeds, and several other breeds. It has not been identified in Thoroughbreds to date. This mutation causes the muscle to continually make glycogen. Consequently, when beginning exercise, horses have trouble switching over to burn glycogen for energy rather than storing glycogen in their muscles. Affected horses develop stiffness, muscle cramping, and soreness with light exercise probably due to a deficit of energy generation in their muscles. Some horses with this disorder also have an increased sensitivity to insulin, further increasing storage of glycogen in the muscle. PSSM type 1 horses are often calm, sedate horses that tie-up after a lay-up, especially when fed grain. They tend to be found in disciplines such as halter and pleasure horse performance and do not usually perform well at speed.

Type 2 PSSM has a slightly different microscopic appearance, and the genetic cause is yet unknown. It occurs in Quarter horse–related breeds, Warmbloods, and likely other light horse breeds, possibly including Thoroughbreds. Whereas type 1 PSSM can be diagnosed by a DNA-based blood or hair root test, type 2 PSSM requires examination of a muscle biopsy. Treatment of both forms of PSSM involves supplying horses with an alternative source of energy such as fat rather than sugar. Eliminating grain and sweet feed completely and feeding fats such as rice bran or vegetable oils stabilizes blood sugar and provides fat for energy metabolism. It is essential that horses with PSSM be turned out as much as possible and exercised often, even if only for 10 min/day. Horses with mild to moderate clinical signs might be able to return to full athletic performance with careful dietary and management changes, which include regular daily exercise without extended periods of inactivity. Breeding horses with PSSM has at least a 50% chance of passing the trait on to offspring.

SHEEP

Spider Lamb Syndrome

Hereditary chondrodysplasia, or spider lamb syndrome, is an inherited, semilethal, musculoskeletal disease affecting lambs primarily of Suffolk or Hampshire breeds. Because the syndrome is a recessive genetic disorder, a lamb is afflicted only if both parents pass on the mutation. Thus, it is critical to identify carriers, which are structurally normal animals with only one copy of the mutation. The location of the locus causing spider lamb syndrome is along the distal end of ovine chromosome 6. This mutation causes an inactivation of normal fibroblast growth factor receptor 3, which produces skeletal overgrowth in animals homozygous for the gene. Lambs have pronounced medial deviation of the carpus and hock and are unable to stand without distress. Pathologic changes in the skull reveal a rounding of the dorsal silhouette, producing a "Roman nose" appearance and a narrowed elongation of the occipital condyles. The thoracic and lumbar vertebrae are moderately kyphotic, which causes a dorsal rounding of the backline. The sternebrae are dorsally deviated, leading to a flattening of the sternum. The forelimbs have a medial deviation of the carpal joints with a bowed radius and ulna and irregular thickening of the growth plate cartilage. The hindlimbs have medially deviated hocks and bowed tibiae, which also have thickened, irregular growth plates. Muscle atrophy is also predominant. The regulation of liver insulin-like growth factor (IGF) and IGF-binding proteins may be involved in the physical manifestations of this disorder. It is suggested that the condition is inherited in a simple autosomal recessive pattern.

PIGS

Splayleg

(Spraddleleg, Myofibrillar hypoplasia)

In splayleg, a condition of neonatal pigs, the hindlegs are spread apart or extended forward because of weakness of the adductor muscles relative to the abductors. The condition is seen at or soon after birth and can present in a number of forms. In the "stars" form, both sets of limbs are splayed out sideways, such that the pig cannot stand and can move about only by crawling or shuffling. The most common form of the condition is hindleg splays; the back legs splay out sideways and forward, causing the pig great difficulty in standing on its hind end. Many will "dog sit" and shuffle around on their backsides. This can lead to considerable skin trauma and secondary infection. Front leg splays also occur. The hindlimbs work normally, but the front legs splay out sideways such that the pig moves around with its chin on the ground. Such pigs have great difficulty nursing, and mortality levels are high. The incidence of splayleg is greater in the Landrace than in other breeds.

Histologically, there is a continuous gradation in myofibrillar content between normal and severely affected muscles. Myofibrils in affected fibers are scanty and small in cross section. No other morphologic or histochemical abnormalities have been detected. The cause of the condition remains obscure. Newborn piglets of hybrid stock tested for defects of neuromuscular transmission by stimulation electromyography reveal that congenital myofibrillar hypoplasia is not primarily a myasthenia-like syndrome, but that either excitation-contraction coupling or the contractile mechanism itself is primarily affected.

Selection for increased litter size indirectly increases the genetic potential for sows to create a uterine environment more likely to produce litters with splayleg pigs and should be treated as a trait of the sow, rather than of the individual pig. Affected pigs are susceptible to overlaying, starvation, and chilling because of poor mobility. Mortality may reach 50%. Genetic influence has been demonstrated. There are significant differences in the incidence among litters of different sires and breeds. It is seen more frequently in males than females and in pigs of lower birth weight. The syndrome also may be produced if glucocorticoids are administered during pregnancy, and it appears possible that stress-sensitivity of the heavily muscled parent(s) may be a contributing factor. However, any cause of stretching of the adductor muscles increases the incidence. Stretching can result from slippery or sloping floors, struggling while legs are caught in cracks in the floor, or as the result of damage to nerve pathways from intrauterine viral infections. Mycotoxins have been suggested to play a role in some cases. The general nutrition of the sow (choline, methionine, and vitamin E levels) may influence the incidence, but benefits from feeding supplements to sows is questionable.

The clinical signs are distinctive. In utero infections with hemagglutinating encephalitis virus, enteroviruses, other viruses, and postpartum bacterial meningeal infection and trauma should be considered. The affected muscles are generally hypoplastic, and the small muscle fibers contain few myofibrils, as would be found in muscles of normal fetuses nearing parturition. Frequently affected muscles include the semitendinosus, longissimus dorsi, and triceps.

Dry, nonslippery floors should be provided, with no cracks in which the legs can become trapped, especially for the first 2 days. Pigs should be protected from injury by the sow, and adequate suckling should be ensured. In affected piglets, the hindlegs should be secured together above the hocks with a loose "figure 8" of adhesive tape for 2–4 days. Appropriately treated pigs usually recover within a week, although few recover if the front legs are also affected. Glucocorticoids should not be administered late in gestation. Highly susceptible blood lines should be eliminated.

SMALL ANIMALS

Apodia

Few reports of apodia have appeared in the literature. It is likely that this condition occurs more frequently than is documented, but affected animals probably either die, are euthanized by breeders without being brought to a veterinarian, or are just not reported. Congenital absence of the forearm or hand is a relatively common abnormality in people. Most defects are transverse (amelia) and unilateral. Lower limb deformities are less common and also usually unilateral. No familial tendencies have been seen, and intrauterine amputation by amniotic bands is thought to be a common cause of amelia. Longitudinal limb deficiency, or hemimelia, probably results from defective development of the embryonic limb bud.

Few cases of hemimelia in dogs and cats have been reported. Radial agenesis appears to be the most common of these defects. Affected animals have medially directed angular deformities of the affected limbs. There may be complete or partial agenesis of either one or both radii with a compensatory increase in the diameter of the ulna. Tibial agenesis is less common. The fibulae are markedly enlarged in affected animals.

Ectrodactyly Syndrome

Maldevelopment of the central rays of the limbs may produce longitudinal splitting of the extremities. Split hand or foot may be sporadic, but autosomal dominant and recessive forms of this condition, sometimes termed the "lobster claw" defect, have been described. The defect also occurs as part of several syndromes. Splitting is most common between the first and second metacarpals, although all variations have been seen. Other abnormalities associated with this defect include digit contractures, digit aplasia, and metacarpal hypoplasia and fusion. No breed or sex predilection has been noted. Studies of this defect in cats indicate that it is inherited as an autosomal dominant with variable expressivity.

Polydactyly

In dogs and cats, preaxial polydactyly is by far the more common form (an additional digit or digits on the medial side of the paw). In cats, it is inherited as an autosomal dominant trait with variable expressivity. A similar inheritance pattern appears to apply to the occurrence of multiple dewclaws in dogs, as is seen in Great Pyrenees. Lateral polydactylism occurs less frequently. There is no apparent clinical significance to these conditions, other than an increased propensity for traumatic injury of the partial supernumerary digits.

Syndactyly

Syndactyly involves bony and/or soft tissue union of two or more digits, with varying degrees of involvement. Few cases of syndactyly in dogs and cats have been reported. Because few clinical problems are associated with the malformation, this syndrome is probably more common than reported.

DYSTROPHIES ASSOCIATED WITH CALCIUM, PHOSPHORUS, AND VITAMIN D

The principal causes of osteodystrophies are deficiencies or imbalances of dietary calcium, phosphorus, and vitamin D, as well as dysregulation of parathyroid hormone (PTH) activity. Their interrelationships are complex and not easily defined.

The primary source of calcium and phosphorus is the diet. These elements are absorbed in amounts depending on the source of the minerals, intestinal pH, and dietary levels of vitamin D, calcium, phosphorus, iron, and fat. If vitamin D or its activity is decreased, calcium and phosphorus absorption are reduced. Vitamin D is obtained either through the diet or by production when the skin is exposed to sunlight (ultraviolet radiation). Before vitamin D can be used, it must be processed into its metabolically active form in two consecutive hydroxylation steps by the liver and kidney. Vitamin D_3 (cholecalciferol) acts primarily on the GI tract to increase absorption but also affects the bone, thereby increasing availability of elemental calcium. Through a negative feedback loop, it also contributes to the regulation of PTH secretion.

PTH secretion occurs in response to a low circulating calcium ion concentration and depends on the availability of magnesium. The target organs of PTH are the kidneys, bones, and intestines. In the kidneys, PTH promotes renal tubular absorption of calcium while enhancing the renal excretion of phosphorus, as well as the activity of 1α-hydroxylase, the enzyme responsible for activation of vitamin D_3 in the kidney. In the intestine, PTH promotes absorption of calcium. PTH also facilitates mobilization of calcium and phosphorus from bone by allowing utilization of calcium from the osteoid matrix. In ruminants, PTH increases the salivary excretion of phosphorus in exchange for bicarbonate.

Specific bony lesions are associated with abnormalities in absolute or relative amounts of vitamin D, calcium, phosphorus, and PTH. Often, in addition to the deficiency or excess in one element, this also causes a secondary pathology due to feedback mechanisms, altered ratios, or concomitant metabolic deficiencies. Specific disease syndromes can be classified as nutritional, metabolic, or genetic in nature. Classic examples of nutritional osteodystrophies are rickets, osteomalacia, enzootic calcinosis, or hypervitaminosis D. Fibrous osteodystrophy and hyperparathyroidism are common metabolic osteodystrophies. Genetic osteodystrophies can be caused by defects in phosphate transporters or genetic abnormalities in the hormonal regulation of phosphorus homeostasis. Examples of genetic defects associated with osteodystrophies include X-linked hypophosphatemia and hereditary hypophosphatemic rickets.

NUTRITIONAL OSTEODYSTROPHIES

RICKETS

Rickets is a disease of the bony growth plate and thus only affects young, growing animals. The most common causes are dietary insufficiencies of phosphorus or vitamin D. Calcium deficiencies can also cause rickets, and while this rarely occurs naturally, poorly balanced diets deficient in calcium have been said to cause the disease. As in most diets causing osteodystrophies, the abnormal calcium:phosphorus ratio is most likely the cause.

Clinical Findings and Lesions: The characteristic lesions of rickets are failure of both vascular invasion and mineralization in the area of provisional calcification of the physis. This pathology is most obvious in the metaphyses of the long bones. There may be a wide variety of clinical signs, including bone pain, stiff gait, swelling in the area of the metaphyses, difficulty in rising, bowed limbs, and pathologic fractures. On radiographic examination, the width of the physes is increased, the nonmineralized physeal area is distorted, and the bone may show decreased radiopacity. In advanced cases, angular limb deformity can be seen due to asynchronous bone growth.

Animals fed all-meat diets are commonly affected. Kittens fed beef heart exclusively develop locomotor disturbances within 4 wk, even though the high content of digestible protein (>50% on a weight basis) and fat promotes rapid growth, the animals appear well nourished, and their coat maintains a good luster. The predominant clinical signs are reluctance to move, posterior lameness, and ataxia. The kittens often stand with characteristic deviation of the paws. The skeletal disease becomes progressively more severe after 5–14 wk. The kittens become quiet and reluctant to play; they assume a sitting position or sternal recumbency with the hindlimbs abducted. Normal activities may result in the sudden onset of severe lameness due to incomplete or folding fractures of one or more bones. Lameness is the initial functional disturbance in growing dogs and may vary from a slight limp to inability to walk. The bones are painful on palpation, and folding fractures of long bones and vertebrae are common.

Swine kept in confined housing are susceptible to rickets because of their rapid growth rate combined with lack of exposure to sunlight. Furthermore, diets for market swine are formulated to maximize growth of lean muscle mass with little consideration of requirements for bone formation.

Diets with excessive amounts of calcium (three times normal concentrations) have caused rickets-like signs in growing Great Danes. Several other bone pathologies such as retained cartilaginous cores, osteochondrosis, and stunted growth were seen in these dogs as well.

Diagnosis: Typical microscopic lesions associated with rickets are impaired endochondral ossification, which are most prominent in fast-growing bones. Growth plates are widened and irregular, and joints appear enlarged. Trabecula of the spongiosa are thinner, predisposing to infarctions and hemorrhage. Radiographic examination of large bones and joints is the most reliable in vivo diagnostic tool for rickets. The radiopacity of rachitic bones is characteristically less than that of normal bone. Growth plates appear widened and irregular.

Plasma alkaline phosphatase activity is commonly increased. Concentrations of serum phosphorus and vitamin D may be altered depending on the primary cause of rickets. In cases associated with phosphorus or vitamin D deficiencies, concentrations of these compounds in serum are subnormal. Hypocalcemia is seen in advanced stages.

Treatment: Correction of the diet is the primary treatment for rickets. The prognosis is good in the absence of pathologic fractures or irreversible damage to the physes. If the animals are housed, exposure to sunlight (ultraviolet radiation) will also increase production of vitamin D_3 precursors.

Many homemade diets for dogs are deficient in minerals and have altered calcium:phosphorus ratios. Therefore, a high-quality commercial food, or one designed by a credentialed veterinary nutritionist, is recommended.

OSTEOMALACIA

(Adult rickets)

Osteomalacia has a pathogenesis similar to that of rickets but is seen in mature bones and associated with disruption of normal bone remodeling. Because bones mature at different rates, both rickets and osteomalacia can be seen in the same animal. Osteomalacia is characterized by an accumulation of excessive unmineralized osteoid on trabecular surfaces.

Clinical Findings: Animals with osteomalacia are unthrifty and may exhibit pica. Nonspecific shifting lamenesses are common. Fractures can be seen, especially in the ribs, pelvis, and long bones. Spinal deformation such as lordosis or kyphosis may be seen.

In horses, nutritional osteodystrophy is known as **bran disease**, **miller's disease**, and "**big head**." The diet of pampered horses is often too high in grains and low in forage; such a diet is high in phosphorus and low in calcium. Many of the obscure lamenesses of horses have been attributed to nutritional osteodystrophy. The pathologic changes are similar to those in other species, with the provisos that the bones of the head are particularly affected in severe cases and that gross or microscopic fractures of subchondral bone (with consequent degeneration of articular cartilage and tearing of ligaments from periosteal attachments) are dominant clinical signs. Unilateral facial deformity due to secondary (nutritional) hypoparathyroidism has been reported in a 1-yr-old filly.

Nutritional osteodystrophy can occur in cattle grazing on arid, infertile soils deficient in phosphorus if they are not given adequate mineral supplementation. Affected animals are unthrifty and have a rough hair coat. Weight loss, shifting limb lameness, limb deformities, and spontaneous fractures are the most common clinical findings. Pica may predispose affected animals to esophageal obstruction, reticuloperitonitis, botulism, or other intoxications.

Diagnosis: To establish a firm diagnosis of osteomalacia, the diet should be evaluated for calcium, phosphorus, and vitamin D content. There is radiographic evidence of generalized skeletal demineralization, loss of lamina dura dentes, subperiosteal cortical bone resorption, bowing deformities, and multiple folding fractures of long bones due to intense localized osteoclast proliferation. Levels of hydroxyproline, an amino acid released into blood during bone mineralization, can be determined to assess the extent of ongoing bone mobilization. If dietary calcium and phosphorus content cannot readily be determined (eg, in grazing animals), soil or fecal samples can be analyzed as crude proxies for dietary intake of these minerals.

Laboratory values used to assess renal function should be within normal limits in animals with nutritional osteodystrophy.

Treatment: Animals with osteomalacia should be confined for several weeks after initiation of the supplemental diet. Response to therapy is rapid; within 1 wk the animals become more active, and their attitude improves. Jumping or climbing must be prevented, because the skeleton is still susceptible to fractures. Restrictions can be lessened after 3 wk, but confinement with limited movement is indicated until the skeleton returns to normal (response to treatment should be monitored radiographically). Complete recovery can be achieved within months in animals with no or only minor limb and joint deformities.

ENZOOTIC CALCINOSIS

(Enteque seco, Enteque ossificans, Espichamento, Espichacao, Manchester wasting disease, Naalehu disease, Weidekrankheit)

Enzootic calcinosis is a disease complex of ruminants and horses caused by plant poisoning or mineral imbalances and characterized by extensive calcification of soft tissues. The prevalence of the disease in cattle varies widely (10%–50%) in areas of Argentina, Brazil, Papua-New Guinea, Jamaica, Hawaii, and Bavaria. It is said to cause up to 60% mortality and affect 17% of the sheep in southern Brazil and Mattewara (India), respectively. Incidence elsewhere (Australia, Israel, South Africa, and southern USA) is less well documented, and in many areas enzootic calcinosis is rare or nonexistent.

Etiology and Pathogenesis: Known causes of enzootic calcinosis fall into two categories: plant poisonings and mineral imbalances in the soil, the first probably being the more important. *Cestrum diurnum* (wild jasmine, day-blooming jessamine, king-of-the-day), *Trisetum flavescens* (golden oats or yellow oat grass), *Nierembergia veitchii*, *Solanum esuriale*, *S torvum*, and *S malacoxylon* contain 1,25-dihydroxycholecalciferol (calcitriol) glycoside or a substance that mimics its calcinogenic action. Studies indicate that *S malacoxylon* has the required enzyme systems for synthesis of calcitriol from vitamin D_3.

The imbalance of minerals in certain soils, as well as at higher altitude (up to 1,500 m above sea level), have been thought to be the main etiologic factors; higher altitude is considered to favor the growth of plants like golden oats at the expense of other plants less suited for this location.

Osteodystrophy of bulls after prolonged intake of excessive calcium is a similar condition; calcification of the cardiovascular system associated with aging and such cachectic diseases as tuberculosis is not identical. Excessive vitamin D_3 and normal or excessive calcium intake induces aortic calcification and atherosclerosis in ruminants.

Normally, the conversion of 25-hydroxycholecalciferol (calcifediol) to calcitriol in the kidneys is controlled by a feedback mechanism. The calcitriol-like factor in the leaves of plants bypasses this mechanism, and more calcium is absorbed than can be accommodated physiologically. Hypercalcemia promotes calcitonin production, calcinosis, and osteoporosis.

Changes in plasma calcium, phosphorus, and magnesium are different in different species. Horses develop hyperphosphatemia; plasma calcium remains normal but rises with excess doses of calcitriol. In cattle and small ruminants, high serum inorganic phosphorus with increased or normal serum calcium concentrations have been reported in animals with enzootic calcinosis.

Clinical Findings: Enzootic calcinosis is progressive and chronic, extending for weeks or months. The earliest signs are stiffness and shifting limb lameness, most pronounced when the animal rises after prolonged rest. Forelimbs are particularly affected, and some animals even walk or graze on their knees. The distal joints become abnormally straight. When affected animals are forced to walk, their gait is awkward, stiff, and slow, and their steps are short. After walking only short distances, breathing becomes shallow and diaphragmatic, the nostrils are flared, and the head and neck are extended. Tachycardia is a common finding, and heart murmurs may be audible on auscultation. Jugular venous pulse is prominent in some cases.

As the disease progresses, the animal loses weight and becomes weak, listless, reluctant to stand, or even recumbent. The coat becomes shaggy, dull, and faded, particularly in cattle. There is wasting of muscles, a prominent skeleton, tucked up abdomen, kyphosis, and raised tailhead. Appetite is usually unimpaired but sometimes becomes depraved. Calcification of vessels is sometimes palpable on rectal examination.

Osteodystrophy is seen in calcinosis due to *T flavescens* and *C diurnum* toxicities in Bavarian cattle and Florida horses, respectively. Severely affected horses stand with forelimbs somewhat abducted and luxated caudally at the shoulder joints. The flexor tendons, particularly the suspensory ligaments, are painful. Fetlock joints are overextended to varying degrees.

Lesions: Degeneration and calcification of soft tissues are seen, with emaciation and varying amounts of excess fluid in the thoracic and abdominal cavities and pericardial sac. The cardiovascular system is the first to be involved, followed by lung, kidney, and tendons. The heart and aorta show the most pronounced abnormalities. The left side of the heart is more affected than the right. Calcification of the bicuspid valves results in valve insufficiency and systolic heart murmurs. White, elevated plaques of irregular size and shape are seen on the luminal surface; in advanced cases, these are seen throughout the length of the aorta and its main branches. Mineral deposits are found on the pleura, on the surface and edges of the diaphragmatic and apical lobes of lungs, in the renal artery and pelvis of the kidney, and on the ligaments and tendons (particularly of the forelimbs). Capsular thickening and irregular erosions of articular surface of cartilage and joints are seen, especially of the carpus and hock.

The basic histologic evidence is necrosis and calcification of connective tissue, followed by cellular proliferation in the affected area.

Diagnosis: Diagnosis of enzootic calcinosis is usually based on the history, combined with clinical signs such as emaciation, lameness, and listlessness, as well as cardiac and respiratory abnormalities, but may be difficult at early stages. Abnormal serum calcium, phosphorus, and magnesium concentrations and increased activity of alkaline phosphatase in combination with the presence of plants with calcinogenic action in the feed or on pasture are further clues.

Imaging techniques such as radiography and ultrasonography can be used to visualize soft-tissue calcification.

Treatment and Control: No practical treatment reversing soft-tissue calcification is currently available. Removal of the causal factor(s) is essential, but when the disease is associated with the mineral content of the soil, control may be difficult. Change of pasture, forage, and environment may effect clinical improvement. Careful pasture management to limit the density of calcinogenic plants can effectively reduce the disease prevalence. Feeding oat grass hay cut after blooming rather than having animals graze on oat grass pasture may reduce the problem, because calcinogenicity of the plant decreases with maturity and with drying. Experimentally, daily administration of 15 g of aluminum hydroxide, PO, prevented the development of calcinosis in sheep fed *T flavescens*.

VITAMIN D_3 TOXICITY

Iatrogenically induced calcinosis, in the form of vitamin D_3 toxicity, is a condition occasionally reported in cattle that is very similar to enzootic calcinosis. Parenteral administration of vitamin D_3 10–14 days before the predicted calving date is considered an effective strategy to prevent periparturient hypocalcemia (milk fever) in dairy cows. Because of the narrow margin between therapeutic and toxic doses, vitamin D_3 toxicity can occur either after a single overdose or after repeated therapeutic doses injected at short intervals. Commonly, toxicity is due to the repeated injection of therapeutic doses in cows that did not calve within 2 wk of the initial treatment and thus are considered at increased risk of developing periparturient hypocalcemia.

Clinical Findings: Animals with vitamin D_3 intoxication become anorectic, lose weight, and develop acetonemia within 2–3 wk after the overdose. Tachycardia, shallow breathing, and lameness, followed by weakness, recumbency, and even death can be seen in animals with vitamin D_3 toxicosis.

Lesions: Lesions are consistent with soft-tissue calcification described under enzootic calcinosis (*see* p 1053).

Diagnosis: Diagnosis of vitamin D_3 toxicity is usually based on a history of repeated vitamin D_3 injections in combination with the clinical signs mentioned above.

Treatment and Control: No practical treatment for vitamin D_3 toxicity is currently available. Education of producers concerning the risks and toxic dose of parenterally administered vitamin D_3 will help avoid accidental overdoses.

METABOLIC OSTEODYSTROPHIES

FIBROUS OSTEODYSTROPHY

(Rubber jaw syndrome)

Primary Hyperparathyroidism

In primary hyperparathyroidism (*see* p 564), there is excess production of parathyroid hormone (PTH) by an autonomous functional lesion in the parathyroid gland. The normal control mechanisms for PTH secretion by the concentration of blood calcium are lost, and the parathyroid produces excess PTH despite increased levels of blood calcium. This disease is encountered infrequently in older dogs, and it does not appear to be a sequela of renal secondary hyperparathyroidism (*see* p 1056).

PTH acts on cells of the renal tubules initially to promote the excretion of phosphorus and retention of calcium. A prolonged increased secretion of PTH results in accelerated osteocytic and osteoclastic bone resorption. Mineral is removed from the skeleton and replaced by immature fibrous connective tissue. Fibrous osteodystrophy is generalized throughout the skeleton but is accentuated in local areas such as the cancellous bone of the skull. The increased PTH levels also inhibit the renal tubular resorption of phosphorus.

The lesion in the parathyroid gland in dogs is usually an adenoma, occasionally a carcinoma, composed of active chief cells. Usually, adenomas are single, light brown-red, and located in the cervical region near the thyroid gland.

Clinical Findings: In primary hyperparathyroidism, lameness follows severe osteoclastic bone resorption, and fractures of long bones occur after minor physical trauma. Compression fractures of weakened vertebral bodies may exert pressure on the spinal cord and nerves, resulting in motor and sensory dysfunction.

Facial hyperostosis with partial obliteration of the nasal cavity (by poorly mineralized woven bone and highly vascular fibrous connective tissue) and loss or loosening of teeth has been seen in dogs. This may result in an inability to close the mouth properly and development of gingival ulcers. The maxillae and rami of the mandibles often are coarsely thickened by the excess woven bone. Bones of the skull are markedly thinned by the increased resorption and have a characteristic "moth-eaten" appearance radiographically. In advanced cases, the mandible can be twisted gently due to loss of osteoid and severe fibrous osteodystrophy—hence the name "rubber jaw" syndrome.

Lesions: Histologic demonstration of a rim of normal tissue and a partial to complete fibrous capsule in an enlarged parathyroid suggests an adenoma rather than focal hyperplasia. Chief-cell carcinomas tend to be larger than adenomas and fixed to the underlying tissues due to local infiltration of neoplastic cells.

Diagnosis: Although other laboratory findings may be variable when diagnosing primary hyperparathyroidism, hypercalcemia is consistent and results from accelerated release of calcium from bone. The blood calcium in healthy dogs is ~10 ± 1 mg/dL, depending on age and diet (and assay method). Serum calcium values consistently >12 mg/dL indicate hypercalcemia. Dogs with primary hyperparathyroidism usually have a serum calcium of ≥12–20 mg/dL. The blood phosphorus is low or in the low-normal range (≤4 mg/dL). The urinary excretion of phosphorus, and often of calcium, is increased and may result in nephrocalcinosis and urolithiasis. Accelerated bone matrix metabolism is reflected by increased urinary excretion of hydroxyproline. Serum alkaline phosphatase activity may be increased in animals with overt bone disease. Demonstration of increased levels of PTH by a species-specific assay in an adult to aged dog with hypercalcemia, hypophosphatemia, and evidence of generalized bone disease provides conclusive evidence of primary hyperparathyroidism. PTH can be measured by sensitive radioimmunoassays or immunoradiometric assays.

The intact PTH assay or dual-site assays can be performed using either serum (preferred) or plasma that has been separated and frozen (–70°C [–94°F] in either glass or plastic tubes) as soon as possible after collection. Using this method, circulating levels of PTH in most animals are near 20 pg/mL (dogs, 20 ± 5 pg/mL; cats, 17 ± 2 pg/mL), with levels in nonhuman primates being slightly lower (normal values also vary among laboratories). PTH assays that use antibody generated against the carboxy terminal end of the human molecule usually give less consistent results in animals other than people.

Differential diagnoses include other causes of hypercalcemia, such as vitamin D intoxication (overdosage), enzootic calcinosis (*see* p 1052), malignant neoplasms with osseous metastasis, and humoral hypercalcemia of malignancy (*see* p 563). The hypercalcemia of hypervitaminosis D may be as high as that in primary hyperparathyroidism but is accompanied by varying degrees of hyperphosphatemia and normal serum alkaline phosphatase activity. Skeletal disease usually is absent, because the increased concentrations of blood calcium and phosphorus are derived principally from augmented intestinal absorption rather than from bone resorption.

Malignant neoplasms with osseous metastases may cause moderate hypercalcemia and hypercalciuria, but the alkaline phosphatase activity and serum phosphorus level usually are normal or only slightly increased. These changes are believed to be due to the release of calcium and phosphorus into the blood from areas of bone destruction at rates greater than can be cleared by the kidneys and intestine. Bone involvement is more sharply demarcated and localized to the area of metastasis. Osteolysis associated with tumor metastases results not only from a physical disruption of bone by proliferating neoplastic cells but also from local production of humoral substances that stimulate bone resorption, such as prostaglandins and interleukin-1.

Primary parathyroid hyperplasia has been described in German Shepherd pups. The condition was associated with hypercalcemia, hypophosphatemia, increased immunoreactive PTH, and increased fractional clearance of inorganic phosphorus in the urine. Clinical signs include stunted growth, weakness, polyuria, polydipsia, and a diffuse reduction in bone density. IV infusion of calcium fails to suppress the autonomous secretion of PTH by the diffuse hyperplasia of chief cells in all parathyroids. Lesions include nodular hyperplasia of thyroid C cells and widespread mineralization of the lungs, kidneys, and gastric mucosa. The disease is inherited as an autosomal recessive.

Hypercalcemia also may be associated with multifocal osteolytic lesions associated with septic emboli, complete immobilization, osteosarcoma, hypoadrenocorticism (Addison-like disease), hypocalcitoninism due to a destructive thyroid lesion, chronic renal disease, hemoconcentration, or hyperproteinemia. Hypercalcemia is detected occasionally in dehydrated animals but usually is mild. It is attributed to fluid volume contraction that results in hyperproteinemia and increased concentrations of ionized and nonionized calcium; it resolves rapidly after fluid therapy.

Treatment: The objective in treating primary hyperparathyroidism is to eliminate the source of excessive PTH production. An attempt should be made to identify all four parathyroid glands before excising any tissue. Single or multiple adenomas should be removed in toto. If all identifiable parathyroids in the cervical region appear to be of normal or smaller size, and the diagnosis is reasonably certain, surgical exploration of the thorax near the base of the heart may be necessary to localize the parathyroid neoplasm.

Removal of the functional parathyroid lesion results in a rapid decrease in circulating PTH levels, because the half-life of PTH in plasma is <15 min. Because plasma calcium levels in animals with overt bone disease may decrease rapidly and be subnormal within 12–24 hr after surgery, they should be monitored frequently. Postoperative hypocalcemia (≤6 mg/dL) can result from the following: 1) depressed secretory activity of chief cells due to suppression by the chronic hypercalcemia or injury to the remaining parathyroid tissue during surgery, 2) abruptly decreased bone resorption due to decreased PTH levels, and 3) accelerated mineralization of osteoid matrix formed by the hyperplastic osteoblasts, which was previously prevented by the increased PTH levels (known as "hungry-bone syndrome"). Infusions of calcium gluconate to maintain the serum calcium between 7.5 and 9 mg/dL, plus feeding high-calcium diets and supplemental vitamin D therapy, corrects this serious postoperative complication. If hypercalcemia persists for ≥1 wk after surgery, or recurs after initial improvement, a second adenoma or metastases from a carcinoma should be suspected.

Renal Secondary Hyperparathyroidism

Renal secondary hyperparathyroidism is a complication of chronic renal failure characterized by increased endogenous levels of parathyroid hormone (PTH). It is more common than primary hyperparathyroidism. In contrast to primary hyperparathyroidism, renal secondary hyperparathyroidism tends not to be autonomous. It is seen frequently in dogs, occasionally in cats, and rarely in other species.

With progressive renal disease, serum hyperphosphatemia develops as the glomerular filtration rate decreases. Hyperphosphatemia leads to lower serum concentration of ionized calcium. Renal synthesis of calcitriol is also reduced. Calcitriol normally acts on the intestine and kidneys to maintain normal calcium levels. Decreased ionized calcium and calcitriol concentrations cause an increase in serum PTH concentrations. As glomerular filtration rate decreases with advancing renal disease, PTH concentrations progressively increase, leading to the clinical manifestations of renal secondary hyperparathyroidism.

Clinical Findings: The predominant signs of renal insufficiency (eg, vomiting, dehydration, polydipsia, polyuria, and depression) are usually present. Skeletal lesions range from minor changes with early (or mild) renal disease to severe fibrous osteodystrophy of advanced renal failure. The volume of affected bones usually is normal (isostatic), particularly in older dogs because of the slow onset of renal failure and lower metabolic activity of bones. Hyperostotic bone lesions, such as facial swelling, may be seen in younger dogs in which deposition of unmineralized osteoid by hyperplastic osteoblasts and production of fibrous connective tissue exceed the rate of bone resorption.

Skeletal involvement is generalized but not uniform. Lesions become apparent earlier and reach a more advanced stage in certain areas, such as cancellous bones of the skull. Resorption of alveolar bone occurs early and results in loose teeth, which may be dislodged easily and interfere with mastication. As a result of accelerated resorption of cancellous bone of the maxilla and mandible, bones become softened and pliable ("rubber jaw" syndrome), and the jaws fail to close properly. This often results in drooling and protrusion of the tongue. Severely demineralized mandibles are predisposed to fractures and displacement of teeth from alveoli. Long bones are less dramatically affected. Lameness, stiff gait, and fractures after minor trauma may result from increased bone resorption.

Lesions: All parathyroid glands are enlarged, initially due to hypertrophy of chief cells and subsequently by compensatory hyperplasia. Although the parathyroids are not autonomous, the concentration of PTH in the peripheral blood often exceeds that of primary hyperparathyroidism. Changes such as osteoclastosis, marrow fibrosis, and a higher concentration of woven osteoid may be seen histologically. Severe hypercalcemia, hyperphosphatemia, and high concentrations of PTH seen in advanced disease may cause osteosclerosis.

Diagnosis: Renal secondary hyperparathyroidism is diagnosed by laboratory abnormalities consistent with renal insufficiency accompanied by an increase in serum PTH. Radioimmunoassay of PTH that must be species specific is commercially available for most companion animal species and horses. Assays that measure fragments of the PTH molecule should not be used, because the concentration of biologically inactive metabolites of PTH increases with renal failure.

Treatment: Treatment options for renal secondary hyperparathyroidism include dietary modification, administration of calcitriol (the bioactive metabolite of vitamin D_3) in combination with oral supplementation of phosphate binders, and management of the underlying renal disease. Prescription diets with restricted dietary phosphorus are available. Oral calcitriol (1.5–3.5 ng/kg/day) has reversed hyperparathyroidism of chronic renal failure, but calcitriol therapy is contraindicated with hyperphosphatemia or hypercalcemia. (Special compounding of calcitriol is needed, because the dosages currently available commercially are much larger than those needed clinically.) Dietary phosphorus binders are used to decrease the amount of phosphorus available for absorption in the intestines and should be administered with meals. This therapy is especially important during calcitriol supplementation, because calcitriol increases the absorption of phosphorus and calcium.

Prognosis: If untreated, secondary hyperparathyroidism results in irreversible hypertrophy of the parathyroid glands, a condition also known as tertiary hyperparathyroidism. In this stage, hyperparathyroidism becomes unresponsive to treatment and requires surgical extirpation of the hypertrophic parathyroid glands.

HYPOPARATHYROIDISM

In hypoparathyroidism (*see* p 570), either subnormal amounts of parathyroid hormone (PTH) are secreted, or the hormone secreted is unable to interact normally with target cells. It has been recognized primarily in dogs, particularly in smaller breeds such as Miniature Schnauzers, but other breeds may be affected.

Various pathogenic mechanisms can result in inadequate secretion of PTH. Parathyroid glands may be damaged or inadvertently removed during thyroid surgery. After damage to the glands or their vascular supply, adequate functional parenchyma often regenerates, and clinical signs subsequently disappear.

Idiopathic hypoparathyroidism in adult dogs usually is the result of diffuse lymphocytic parathyroiditis that causes extensive degeneration of chief cells and replacement by fibrous connective tissue. Other possible causes of hypoparathyroidism include destruction of parathyroids by primary or metastatic neoplasms in the anterior cervical area, and atrophy of parathyroids associated with chronic hypercalcemia. The presence of numerous distemper virus particles in chief cells of the parathyroid gland may contribute to the low blood calcium in certain dogs with this disease. Agenesis of the parathyroids is a rare cause of congenital hypoparathyroidism in pups. Certain cases of idiopathic hypoparathyroidism in animals (including people) with histologically normal parathyroids may be due to lack of the specific enzyme in chief cells that converts the pro-PTH molecule to the biologically active PTH secreted by the gland. In other cases, an immune-mediated mechanism may be involved, because a similar destruction of secretory parenchyma and lymphocytic infiltration has been produced experimentally in dogs by repeated injections of parathyroid tissue emulsions.

Pseudohypoparathyroidism is a variant seen in people, but it is uncertain whether it is seen in other animals. Target cells in kidney and bone are unable to respond to normal or increased amounts of PTH, and severe hypocalcemia develops even though the parathyroid glands are hyperplastic.

Clinical Findings and Lesions: The functional disturbances and clinical manifestations of hypoparathyroidism primarily are the result of increased neuromuscular excitability and tetany. Bone resorption is decreased because of the lack of PTH, and blood calcium levels diminish progressively (4–6 mg/dL). Affected dogs are restless, nervous, and ataxic, with weakness and intermittent tremors of individual muscle groups that progress to generalized tetany and convulsions. Blood phosphorus levels are increased substantially, owing to increased renal tubular reabsorption. Calcification of microvasculature, intracerebral calcification, decreased mental function, cataracts, osteopenia, and ligamentous ossification have been associated with chronic hypoparathyroidism.

In the early stages of immune-mediated lymphocytic parathyroiditis in dogs, there is infiltration of the gland with lymphocytes and plasma cells and nodular regenerative hyperplasia of remaining chief cells. Later, the parathyroid gland is replaced by lymphocytes, fibroblasts, and capillaries, with only an occasional viable chief cell.

Diagnosis: Diagnosis of hypoparathyroidism is based on clinical signs of increased neuromuscular excitability, severe hypocalcemia, and often moderate hyperphosphatemia in a nonparturient animal, as well as on the response to therapy. Some of the signs (eg, tetany) and laboratory data (eg, hypocalcemia) are similar to those of puerperal hypocalcemia (*see* p 992). However, puerperal hypocalcemia usually is accompanied by hypophosphatemia and a low-normal or subnormal blood glucose concentration as a result of the associated intense muscular activity.

Treatment: The neuromuscular tetany should be treated initially by restoring blood calcium levels to near normal by IV administration of calcium gluconate. One recommended therapeutic regimen is 10 mL of 10% calcium gluconate in 250 mL of 0.9% saline administered at 2.5 mL/kg/hr for 8–12 hr. Care must be taken not to administer the calcium too rapidly because of its cardiotoxic properties. Longterm maintenance of blood calcium levels in the absence of normal PTH secretion should be attempted by feeding diets high in calcium and low in phosphorus and that are supplemented with calcium (gluconate or lactate) and vitamin D_3.

Large doses of vitamin D_3 (≥25,000–50,000 U/day, depending on the weight of the dog) may be required initially to increase the blood calcium level in hypoparathyroid animals, because the lack of PTH diminishes the rate of formation of the biologically active vitamin D metabolite in the kidney. To prevent hypercalcemia and extensive soft-tissue mineralization, the dosage of vitamin D should be carefully adjusted after frequent determination of the serum calcium level. After adjusting the dosage of vitamin D, a 4- to 5-day interval should precede the next blood calcium determination. Once the blood calcium level has returned to normal, substantially lower dosages of vitamin D are indicated for longterm maintenance; in some dogs, only dietary calcium supplementation is required for longterm stabilization.

SARCOCYSTOSIS

In sarcocystosis, the endothelium and muscles and other soft tissues are invaded by Apicomplexan protozoans of the genus *Sarcocystis*. As the name implies, *Sarcocystis* spp (from Greek *sarkos*: muscle and *kystis*: cysts) form cysts in muscles of various intermediate hosts—people, horses, cattle, sheep, goats, pigs, birds, rodents, camelids, wildlife, and reptiles. The cysts vary in size from a few micrometers to centimeters, depending on the host and species. Most *Sarcocystis* spp infections are distributed worldwide.

Etiology, Transmission, and Pathogenesis: *Sarcocystis* spp normally develop in two-host cycles consisting of an intermediate host (prey) and the final host (predator). Species-specific prey-predator life cycles have been demonstrated for cattle-dog (*S cruzi*), cattle-cat (*S hirsuta*), cattle-human (*S hominis*), sheep-dog (*S capracanis, S hircicanis*), sheep-cat (*S gigantea, S medusiformis*), goat-dog (*S capracanis, S hircicanis*), goat-cat (*S moulei*), pig-dog (*S meischeriana*), pig-human (*S suihominis*), pig-cat (*S porcifelis*), horse-dog (*S fayeri*), llama-dog (*S aucheniae*), pigeon-hawk (*S calchasi*), and others. *S sinensis* has been detected affecting muscles of buffalo and cattle, but its final host remains unknown. Some wildlife may serve as intermediate hosts (such as raccoons, rodents, birds, etc) or final hosts (coyotes, opossums, snakes, etc) for some species of *Sarcocystis*.

About 1–2 wk after ingesting muscle tissue that contains *Sarcocystis* cysts (sarcocysts), the final host begins to shed infective sporocysts in the feces; shedding continues for several months. After ingestion of sporocysts by a suitable intermediate host, sporozoites are liberated and initiate development of schizonts in vascular endothelia of mesenteric arterioles and mesenteric lymph nodes. Merozoites are liberated from the mature schizonts and produce a second generation of endothelial schizonts in capillaries from several organs. Merozoites from this second generation subsequently invade the muscle fibers and develop into the typical sarcocysts. Initially, sarcocysts contain only a few metrocytes—round, noninfective parasites that give rise to the banana-shaped infective bradyzoites found in mature cysts beginning 2–3 mo after infection. Sarcocysts of some species are easily visible with the unaided eye (*S aucheniae, S hirsuta, S gigantea*). The presence of such sarcocysts as well as those of zoonotic species can cause condemnation of the carcass during meat inspection. Sarcocysts of other species remain microscopic, even though tremendous numbers of cysts may be present in the muscles. The identification of different species could be achieved by molecular studies and cyst wall morphology (mainly ultrastructure).

S cruzi produce microscopic cysts, principally in myocardium, and can affect 100% of some cattle populations. *S hirsuta* has been primarily responsible for cattle condemnation for visible sarcocysts. *S meischeriana* is the most important species affecting pigs and may affect meat quality. Macroscopic cysts of *S aucheniae* are an important cause of condemnation of llama meat. Sarcocysts are easily recovered from esophagus, diaphragm, and heart muscle.

In general, *Sarcocystis* spp infections are considered of low pathogenicity except induced infection with *S cruzi* sporocysts from canine feces, which may cause acute disease in calves; eosinophilic myositis in cattle; and abortions, stillbirths, and deaths in pregnant cows. Two cases of necrotic encephalitis in heifers have been reported. Similar pathogenicity has been demonstrated for *S tenella* in lambs and ewes and for *S miescheriana* in pigs. An outbreak of myositis affecting 20 ewes with flaccid paralysis was a result of heavy *Sarcocystis* infection. Immune status of the host and the dose of sporocysts may be the most important factors for the development of clinical disease. Pathologic changes in myocardium and skeletal muscles were more pronounced in cows with lymphatic leukemia. "Immunization" using small doses of sporocysts appears to prevent development or reduce severity of clinical disease in sheep when challenged with large doses later (premunitive immunity). In dogs, a longer prepatent period and shortened patent period resulted after repeated infection. Pigs can also have persistent acquired immunity after immunization infections.

People may also serve as intermediate hosts and suffer myositis and vasculitis, but this tissue phase is rare, and the source of such human infection has never been determined. Human intestinal illness as final host, with clinical signs of nausea, abdominal pain, loss of appetite, vomiting, and diarrhea that lasted as long as 48 hr, has followed ingestion of sarcocysts of *S suihominis* in uncooked pork and *S hominis* in uncooked beef. Differentiation between cysts of *S sinensis* and *S hominis* in beef is extremely important to avoid unjustified rejections.

Clinical Findings: *Sarcocystis* spp infections are quite prevalent in farm animals; however, there have been few outbreaks of clinical disease. Most animals are asymptomatic, and the parasite is discovered only at slaughter. In cattle severely affected by *S cruzi*, the signs include fever, anorexia, cachexia, decreased milk yield, diarrhea, muscle spasms, anemia, loss of tail hair, hyperexcitability, weakness, prostration, and death. Cows infected in the last trimester of pregnancy may abort. After recovery from acute illness, calves failed to grow well and eventually died in a cachectic state. Anemia, hepatitis, and myocarditis were the primary lesions in acute ovine sarcocystosis after experimental challenge with *S tenella* sporocysts. Cases of encephalomyelitis in sheep were associated with a *Sarcocystis* sp infection. After recovery from acute illness, some sheep may lose their wool. *S tenella* may also induce abortion in sheep. At necropsy, acutely affected animals have hemorrhage of the serous membranes of the viscera and myocardium. *Sarcocystis* spp infections are probably most important in growing ruminants and swine, in which they can result in subclinical anemia and reduced weight gain.

Equine protozoal myeloencephalitis (EPM, *see* p 1309) is caused principally by *S neurona* in American horses. Only asexual stages of this parasite have been found in horses, and they may be located in neurons and leukocytes of the brain and spinal cord. Opossums (*Didelphis virginiana* and *D albiventris*) are its definitive hosts. Clinical signs in horses include gait abnormalities such as ataxia, knuckling, and crossing over. Muscle atrophy of the hindlimb, which is usually unilateral, is frequent. The lesions are typically focal, and brain-stem involvement is common. Depression, weakness, head tilt, and dysphagia are other possible signs. EPM can mimic many neurologic diseases. Horses may also develop a myopathy. Multifocal myositis has been reported and is possibly due to another *Sarcocystis* species with horses as the intermediate host, *S fayeri*. PCR is an important diagnostic method. *S calchasi* can produce pigeon protozoal encephalitis with severe brain lesions and muscle cysts at the same time.

Control: Livestock become infected by sporocysts from the feces of carnivores. Because most adult cattle, sheep, and many pigs harbor cysts in their muscles, dogs and other carnivores should not be allowed to eat raw meat, offal, or dead animals. Supplies of grain and feed should be kept covered; dogs and cats should not be allowed in buildings used to store feed or house animals. Amprolium (100 mg/kg/day for 30 days), fed prophylactically, reduced illness in cattle inoculated with *S cruzi*. Prophylactic administration of amprolium or salinomycin also protected experimentally infected sheep. Therapeutic treatment of the chronic stage (tissue cysts) has been ineffective. Vaccines are not available. Experimental work demonstrated that infected pork and beef could be made safe for consumption by cooking at 70°C (158°F) for 15 min or by freezing at –4°C (24.8°F) for 2 days or –20°C (-4°F) for 1 day.

Pyrimethamine and sulfadiazine (1 mg/kg/day and 20 mg/kg/day, respectively, for 120 days or longer) is the traditional therapy to treat horses with EPM. Diclazuril and toltrazuril (5 mg/kg) are potentially useful prophylactic agents against *S neurona*.

ARTHROPATHIES IN LARGE ANIMALS

See also LAMENESS IN CATTLE, p 1066; HORSES, p 1096; SHEEP, p 1166; GOATS, p 1092; and PIGS, p 1151.

ARTHRITIS

Arthritis is a nonspecific term denoting inflammation of a joint. All joint diseases of large animals have an inflammatory component to varying degrees. Arthritic entities of importance include traumatic arthritis, osteochondritis dissecans, subchondral cystic lesions, septic (or infective) arthritis, and osteoarthritis (also called degenerative joint disease).

Traumatic Arthritis

Traumatic arthritis includes traumatic synovitis and capsulitis, intra-articular chip fractures, ligamentous tears (sprains) involving periarticular and intra-articular ligaments, meniscal tears, and osteoarthritis. Traumatic arthritis is seen in all breeds of horses worldwide.

Clinical Findings and Diagnosis: Traumatic synovitis and capsulitis is inflammation of the synovial membrane and fibrous joint capsule associated with trauma. Typically, the horse is an athlete and presents with synovial effusion in the acute stage, along with general thickening and fibrosis in the more chronic stage. Lameness varies from a mild gait change to severe lameness. Traumatic synovitis and capsulitis is differentiated from other traumatic entities by use of radiography to exclude osteochondral fractures or disease. Tearing of ligaments or menisci (in femorotibial joints) can often be excluded only by diagnostic arthroscopy. Osteochondral fractures are diagnosed with radiographs. Osteoarthritis is the progressive loss of articular cartilage and can be the consequence of any or all of these traumatic entities (*see also* p 1063). Osteoarthritis is diagnosed with radiographs when the changes are sufficiently severe to demonstrate loss of joint space (associated with articular cartilage loss), subchondral sclerosis, and osteophyte or enthesophyte formation. Lesser degrees of osteoarthritis can be defined only with diagnostic arthroscopy. Clinical signs of osteochondral fractures are similar to those of synovitis and capsulitis, as well as those of osteoarthritis; differential diagnosis of these entities is based on radiographs and, in some cases, arthroscopy.

Arthritis generally results in pain and altered function of the joint. If the process is active or acute, there is usually synovial effusion, and the surrounding tissues are swollen and warm. In more severe cases, manipulation of the joint causes pain. In more subtle cases, flexion tests are required to elicit lameness. As the disease process becomes chronic, the range of motion is reduced with fibrous thickening of the joint capsule. Radiographic evaluation is necessary for positive confirmation of a number of disease entities. Arthroscopy is used to accurately assess the amount of damage to the articular cartilage and to establish a prognosis.

Treatment: Treatment of acute traumatic synovitis and capsulitis includes rest and physical therapy regimens such as cold water treatment, ice, passive flexion, and swimming. NSAIDs (usually phenylbutazone) are used routinely. In more severe cases, the joint is lavaged to remove inflammatory products produced by the synovial membrane, as well as articular cartilage debris that exacerbates the synovitis. Joint drainage alone, without lavage or injection of medication, provides only short-term relief.

Various intra-articular medications have been used. Corticosteroids are the most potent anti-inflammatory agents and are effective in acute traumatic arthritis. However, there are differences in the adverse effects between various corticosteroids and various dosages. Betamethasone products and triamcinolone acetonide are effective with no deleterious adverse effects. Methylprednisolone acetate is more potent and longer acting than the other two drugs but has significant adverse effects that cause degenerative changes in the articular cartilage. Intra-articular sodium hyaluronate has been used effectively for mild to moderate synovitis and has a chondroprotective effect, but it is less effective in severe synovitis or when intra-articular fractures are present. Use of an IV formulation of hyaluronic acid (systemic dose 40 mg) in clinical cases appears to be effective, and this is supported by research data in a controlled model of arthritis in horses. Polysulfated glycosaminoglycans (PSGAGs) are also used frequently for traumatic arthritis entities. PSGAG is effective for synovitis and can help prevent ongoing degeneration of articular cartilage. Although effectiveness of PSGAG when used intra-articularly (250 mg) has scientific support, effectiveness when used IM (500 mg) is less certain. The use of pentosan polysulfate (PPS) at 3 mg/kg, IM, has been shown to be effective as a disease-modifying drug with experimental equine osteoarthritis and has been extensively used in clinical cases outside the USA. Biologic therapies such as autologous conditioned serum are also becoming more commonly used.

Horses with osteochondral chip fragmentation (most commonly seen in the carpus and fetlock joints) are treated with arthroscopic surgery to minimize the ongoing development of osteoarthritis. Fragments are removed, and defective bone and cartilage debrided. Rest periods of 2–4 mo follow, and physical therapy regimens are instituted in the convalescent period. The success rate in returning horses to previous performance level is high when secondary osteoarthritic changes are minimal at the time of surgery. Osteochondral chip fragments that are amenable to arthroscopic surgery and have successful results include those associated with the distal radius or carpal bones; dorsoproximal first phalanx; proximal palmar/plantar first phalanx; apical, abaxial, and basilar fragments of the proximal sesamoid bones; fragmentation of the distal patella in the femoropatellar joint; chip fragments of the tibiotarsal joint; and fragments of the extensor process of the distal phalanx (coffin joint).

Osteochondritis Dissecans

For a complete discussion of equine osteochondrosis, *see* p 1148.

In osteochondritis dissecans (OCD), a focal area of the immature articular cartilage is retained, and the matrix in the basal area of this region becomes chondromalacic and acellular. The immature articular cartilage separates from the underlying trabecular bone. The chondral fracture extends horizontally and vertically until a flap is formed. Synovial fluid gains entrance to the underlying medullary space, and subchondral cysts may form (usually only in larger animals). The flap of immature articular cartilage may stay separated and loose, break away completely ("joint mice"), or reattach by endochondral ossification to the underlying bone, especially in pigs, and result in a wrinkled articular surface. The latter occurs only if the joint is rested or protected, which permits reestablishment of the circulation necessary for endochondral ossification. If the flap is torn free by joint motion, it may be ground into smaller pieces during locomotion and disappear, whereas the larger plaques may become attached to the synovial membrane, become vascularized, and ossify. The resultant articular defect, in time, fills with fibrocartilage.

Etiology: The exact cause of OCD is unknown but is assumed to be multifactorial. Factors include genetic predisposition, fast growth, high caloric intake, low copper and high zinc levels, and endocrine factors.

Clinical Findings: The most common sites of OCD, which usually is seen in young animals, are the femoropatellar joint, tibiotarsal (tarsocrural) joint, fetlock (metacarpophalangeal and metatarsophalangeal) joints, and the shoulder.

Animals with OCD of the shoulder usually present when <1 yr old with severe forelimb lameness and possibly some muscular atrophy. Animals with OCD in the other joints usually present with synovial effusion and varying degrees of lameness. Diagnosis is confirmed with radiographs.

Diagnosis: The history, age, breed, sex, and clinical signs provide useful information; however, radiographs are required to substantiate a diagnosis of OCD.

Treatment: Treatment of OCD depends on the location and degree of involvement. Femoropatellar joint lesions are associated with the lateral trochlear ridge of the femur, medial trochlear ridge of the femur, or distal patella. They are amenable to arthroscopic surgery, which is recommended in all cases except early lesions characterized by flattening (without fragmentation) <2 cm long on the lateral trochlear ridge. In the tarsocrural joint, OCD lesions are seen in decreasing frequency on the intermediate (sagittal) ridge of the tibia, lateral trochlear ridge of the talus, medial malleolus of the tibia, and medial trochlear ridge of the talus. All lesions are amenable to arthroscopic surgery, and the prognosis is usually good. Surgery is recommended when synovial effusion is present. Lesions without fragmentation in the metacarpophalangeal or metatarsophalangeal joints can be treated conservatively, and most affected animals recover well. If a fragment is present, arthroscopic surgery is recommended. In the shoulder, surgery is usually recommended, although milder cases have been managed conservatively with success. The prognosis with arthroscopic surgery is generally less favorable in the shoulder than in other joints.

Subchondral Cystic Lesions

Subchondral cystic lesions are seen in the femorotibial joint and in the fetlock, pastern, elbow, shoulder, and distal phalanx. The diagnosis is usually made on the basis of localization of lameness with intra-articular analgesia (synovial effusion is variable) and confirmed with radiographs.

Subchondral cystic lesions are most frequent in the femorotibial joint, followed by the fetlock joint. Surgery (arthroscopic) is currently recommended in the femorotibial joint whenever a complete cystic lesion is present. Smaller, dome-shaped or flattened lesions are usually treated conservatively in the initial period. Athletic soundness is achieved in 65%–70% of these horses. Intralesional injection of corticosteroids under arthroscopic visualization, in preference to debridement as done previously, achieves superior results. In cases with collapsed edges to the cystic lesion at arthroscopic surgery, or in cases unresponsive to therapy, arthroscopic debridement with augmentation with fibrin, growth factors, and mesenchymal stem cells have been used. Surgery is usually recommended for subchondral cystic lesions of the distal metacarpus in the fetlock but not as consistently as in the femorotibial joint. Single lesions associated with the pastern and elbow joint are treated conservatively and have a fair prognosis. If possible, surgery is recommended for cystic lesions of the distal phalanx (results with conservative treatment are very poor).

Septic Arthritis

(Infective arthritis)

Etiology and Epidemiology: Septic or infective arthritis results from sequestration of bacterial infection in a joint. Infection of a joint develops in three main ways: 1) hematogenous infection, which is common in foals, calves, and lambs (commonly referred to as navel ill); 2) traumatic injury with local introduction of infection; or 3) iatrogenic infection associated with joint injection or surgery (usually in horses). Navel ill is only one example of a hematogenous route of infection, which can also be gained from GI or pulmonary sources.

Clinical Findings and Diagnosis: Septic arthritis is usually characterized by severe lameness and distention of the joint with cloudy, turbid synovial fluid that contains >30,000 WBC/mm^3 and a total protein level of >4 g/dL.

In foals, hematogenous osteomyelitis often accompanies septic arthritis. Septic arthritis in foals has been classified into type S (septic joint only), type P (involving osteomyelitis of the adjacent growth plate as well), or type E (involving osteomyelitis of the epiphyseal and subchondral bone). Various organisms may be involved.

In young lambs, *Actinobacillus seminis* causes polyarthritis, as do *Chlamydia psittaci* and *Erysipelothrix insidiosa*. The latter can follow docking, castration, or navel infection. Viruses and mycoplasma may also be etiologic agents in food-producing animals.

In mature goats, caprine arthritis and encephalitis virus (*see* p 747) is an important cause of infective arthritis. In young goats, *C psittaci* and *Mycoplasma mycoides* are frequent causes.

Bacterial (including *Mycoplasma*) arthritides are seen in young pigs. In newborn pigs, septic arthritis usually is due to intrauterine or navel infection with *Escherichia coli*, *Corynebacterium*, *Streptococcus*, or *Staphylococcus* spp. Control is best directed toward reducing the possibility of infection from the environment. Older pigs sometimes develop arthritis as a sequela of infection with *Haemophilus*, *Erysipelothrix*, or *Mycoplasma* spp. Although diagnosis in the early stages is not difficult, the more chronic stages can be confused with articular lesions produced by dietary hypervitaminosis A.

Traumatic injury to joints with contamination and progression to infection is common in horses, and various species of bacteria are involved. Infection associated with intra-articular injection or surgery occurs in horses and is usually associated with *Staphylococcus aureus* or *S epidermidis*.

Treatment: Septic arthritis requires prompt treatment to avoid irreparable damage. Systemic broad-spectrum antibiotics are indicated; the initial choice is based on the most likely pathogen but is subject to change based on culture and sensitivity tests. Systemic antibiotic treatment is often combined with intra-articular antibiotics (to achieve more effective sterilization of the joint) and other local therapy, including joint lavage (initially) and arthroscopic debridement and drainage. Adjunctive treatment with NSAIDs (eg, phenylbutazone) is also done. The effectiveness of treatment is monitored carefully with clinical signs and repeat synovial fluid analyses.

Osteoarthritis

(Degenerative joint disease)

Etiology and Epidemiology: Osteoarthritis is a progressive degradation of articular cartilage and represents the end stage of most of the other diseases discussed above if treatment is ineffective or the initial problem is too severe. For this reason, prompt diagnosis and correct management of traumatic synovitis and capsulitis, intra-articular fractures or traumatic cartilage damage, osteochondritis dissecans, subchondral cystic lesions, and septic arthritis are critical.

Clinical Findings and Diagnosis: Lameness can be localized with analgesia to the affected joint. There are varying degrees of synovial effusion, joint capsule fibrosis, and restricted motion (decreased flexion). Radiographic signs of osteoarthritis include decreased joint space, osteophytosis, enthesitis, and subchondral sclerosis. In less severe cases, articular degradation requires definition with arthroscopy.

Treatment: Treatment of osteoarthritis is most commonly palliative and includes the use of NSAIDs, polysulfated intra-articular glycosaminoglycans, intra-articular corticosteroids, IV hyaluronic acid, and IM pentosan polysulfate. The use of intra-articular autologous conditioned serum has also been validated. Physical therapy regimens may prove useful. Arthroscopy is commonly performed to diagnose the extent of articular cartilage loss, as well as to treat primary conditions such as articular cartilage separation, meniscal tears, and ligamentous injury. In advanced cases of osteoarthritis, surgical fusion (arthrodesis) may be performed on selected joints.

Surgical fusion of the proximal interphalangeal joint (pastern) or distal tarsal joints can effect athletic soundness. Fetlock arthrodesis is also done in valuable animals and makes them comfortable and capable of breeding. Treatment is usually unsuccessful in chronic cases in bulls and cows, but restricted exercise and careful feeding and nursing prolong the life of and can be worthwhile for valuable breeding animals.

BURSITIS

Bursitis is an inflammatory reaction within a bursa that can range from mild inflammation to sepsis. It is more common and important in horses. It can be classified as true or acquired. True bursitis is inflammation in a congenital or natural bursa (deeper than the deep fascia), eg, trochanteric bursitis and supraspinous bursitis (fistulous withers, *see* below). Acquired bursitis is development of a subcutaneous bursa where one was not previously present or inflammation of that bursa, eg, capped elbow over the olecranon process, shoe boil over the point of the elbow, and capped hock over the tuber calcaneus.

Bursitis may manifest as an acute or chronic inflammation. Examples of acute bursitis include bicipital bursitis and trochanteric bursitis in the early stages. It is generally characterized by swelling, local heat, and pain. Chronic bursitis usually develops in association with repeated trauma, fibrosis, and other chronic changes (eg, capped elbow, capped hock, and carpal hygroma). Excess bursal fluid accumulates, and the wall of the bursa is thickened by fibrous tissue. Fibrous bands or a septum may form within the bursal cavity, and generalized subcutaneous thickening usually develops. These bursal enlargements develop as cold, painless swellings and, unless greatly enlarged, do not severely interfere with function. Septic bursitis is more serious and is associated with pain and lameness. Infection of a bursa may be hematogenous or follow direct penetration.

The pain in acute bursitis may be relieved by application of cold packs, aspiration of the contents, and intrabursal medication. Repeated injections may result in infection. Treatment of chronic bursitis is surgical (and is done arthroscopically (bursoscopy). In infected bursitis, systemic antibiotics as well as local drainage are required.

Capped Elbow and Hock

Capped elbow and hock are inflammatory swellings of the subcutaneous bursae (acquired bursitis) located over the olecranon process and tuber calcaneus, respectively, of horses. Frequent causes include trauma from lying on poorly bedded hard floors, kicks, falls, riding the tailgate of trailers, iron shoes projecting beyond the heels, and prolonged recumbency.

Clinical Findings and Diagnosis: Circumscribed edematous swelling develops over and around the affected bursa. Lameness is rare in either case. The affected bursa may be fluctuating and soft at first but, in a short time, a firm fibrous capsule forms, especially if there is a recurrence of an old injury. Initial bursal swellings may be hardly noticeable or quite sizable. Chronic cases may progress to abscessation.

Treatment: Acute early cases may respond well to applications of cold water, followed in a few days by aseptic aspiration and injection of a corticosteroid. The bursa may also be reduced in size by application of a counterirritant or by ultrasonic or radiation therapy. Older encapsulated bursae are more refractory. Surgical treatment (usually curettage and drainage) is recommended for advanced chronic cases or for those that become infected. A shoe-boil roll should be used to prevent recurrence of a capped elbow if the condition has been caused by the heel or the shoe. With capped hock, behavioral modification so the horse does not kick the stall offers the only hope of permanently resolving the problem.

Fistulous Withers and Poll Evil

Fistulous withers and poll evil are rare, inflammatory conditions of horses that differ essentially only in their location in the respective supraspinous or supra-atlantal bursae. This discussion is of fistulous withers but, except for anatomic details, also applies to poll evil. In the early stage of the disease, a fistula is not present. When the bursal sac ruptures or when it is opened for surgical drainage, and secondary infection with pyogenic bacteria occurs, it usually assumes a true fistulous character.

Etiology: The condition may be traumatic or infectious in origin. Agglutination titers support an infectious etiology. *Brucella abortus* can sometimes be isolated from the fluid aspirated from the unopened bursa.

Clinical Findings: The inflammation leads to considerable thickening of the bursa wall. The bursal sacs are distended and may rupture when the sac has little covering support. In more chronic, advanced cases, the ligament and the dorsal vertebral spines are affected, and occasionally these structures necrose.

In the early stage, the supraspinous bursa distends with a clear, straw-colored, viscid exudate. The swelling may be dorsal, unilateral, or bilateral, depending on the arrangement of the bursal sacs between the tissue layers. It is an exudative process from the beginning, but no true suppuration or secondary infection occurs until the bursa ruptures or is opened.

Treatment and Prevention: The earlier treatment is instituted, the better the prognosis. The most successful treatment is complete dissection and removal of the infected bursa. The expense of the protracted treatment required in chronic cases often exceeds the value of the animal. *Brucella* vaccines have not proved helpful. Sodium iodide therapy is of limited value.

CHLAMYDIAL POLYARTHRITIS-SEROSITIS

(Transmissible serositis)

Chlamydial polyarthritis-serositis is an infectious disease that affects sheep, calves, goats, and pigs. Chlamydial polyarthritis of sheep was first described in Wisconsin and has since been recognized in the western USA, Australia, and New Zealand. The disease was identified in calves from the USA, Australia, and Austria, and in pigs from Austria, Bulgaria, and the USA.

Etiology and Epidemiology: Strains of the causal agent, *Chlamydia psittaci*, isolated from affected joints of sheep and calves, are identical, but strain-specific antigens in their cell walls distinguish them from those that cause abortions in sheep and cattle (*see* p 1332).

The GI tract is of prime importance in the pathogenesis of chlamydial polyarthritis (*see* p 598). The disease has been reproduced experimentally by oral inoculation. Because chlamydiae can be recovered from the feces of clinically healthy calves and lambs, it is most likely the GI tract wherein the host and parasite stay frequently in balance. If there is a shift in favor of the chlamydiae, then a systemic infection and chlamydemia ensues; the ultimate site of replication is the synovial membrane. The GI tract also has been infected after experimental intra-articular inoculations. Chlamydiae are excreted in the feces and urine and transmitted via ingestion or, in some cases, inhalation.

Clinical Findings: Chlamydial polyarthritis is seen in lambs on range, on farms, and in feedlots. Morbidity may be 5%–75%. Rectal temperatures are 102°–107°F (39°–41.5°C). Varying degrees of stiffness, lameness, anorexia, and a concurrent conjunctivitis (*see* p 506) may be seen. Affected sheep are depressed, reluctant to move, and often hesitate to stand and bear weight on one or more limbs, but they may "warm out" of stiffness and lameness after forced exercise. Incidence of the disease in sheep on range is highest between late summer and early winter.

The disease affects cattle of all ages, but calves 4–30 days old are affected more severely. Calves may have fever, are moderately alert, and usually nurse if carried to the dam and supported while sucking. They invariably also have diarrhea, which can be severe. Affected calves assume a hunched position while standing; their joints usually are swollen, and palpation causes pain. Navel involvement and nervous signs are not seen.

Chlamydial polyarthritis has been recognized in older pigs as well as in young piglets. The affected piglets become febrile and anorectic and may develop nasal catarrh, difficulties in breathing, and conjunctivitis. This condition has not been clearly differentiated from other infections that lead to polyserositis and arthritis in pigs.

Lesions: The most striking tissue changes are in the joints. In lambs, enlargement of the joints is not often noticed, but in chronic advanced cases, the stifle, hock, and elbow may be slightly enlarged. In calves, periarticular subcutaneous edema along tendon sheaths and fluid-filled, fluctuating synovial sacs contribute to enlargement of the joints. Most affected joints of lambs or calves contain excessive, grayish yellow, turbid synovial fluid. Fibrin flakes and plaques in the recesses of the affected joints may adhere firmly to the synovial membranes. Joint capsules are thickened. Articular cartilage is smooth, and erosions or evidence of marginal compensatory changes are not present. Tendon sheaths of severely affected lambs and calves may be distended and contain creamy, grayish yellow exudate. Surrounding muscles are hyperemic and edematous, with petechiae in their associated fascial planes.

Diagnosis: The history and careful examination of the pathologic changes in the joints and other organs can be of diagnostic value. Cytologic examination of synovial fluids or tissues may reveal chlamydial elementary bodies or cytoplasmic inclusions. Isolation and identification of the causative agent from affected joints confirms the diagnosis. Bacteriologic cultures of affected joints are usually negative, but *Escherichia coli* or streptococci occasionally may be isolated. If the joints of young calves are arthritic, and if navel lesions are absent, chlamydial polyarthritis should be considered.

Clinical and pathologic features distinguish chlamydial polyarthritis from most other conditions that cause stiffness and lameness in lambs. Lambs with mineral deficiency or osteomalacia usually are not febrile. The abnormal osteogenesis in these two conditions and the distinct lesions of white muscle disease are virtually pathognomonic. In arthritis caused by *Erysipelothrix rhusiopathiae*, there are deposits on and pitting of articular surfaces, periarticular fibrosis, and osteophyte formation. Laminitis due to bluetongue virus infection (*see* p 738) can be differentiated clinically and etiologically. Detailed microbiologic investigations are required to differentiate chlamydial arthritis from mycoplasmal arthritis.

Treatment and Prevention: If begun early, therapy with long-acting penicillin, tetracyclines, or tylosin appears to be beneficial. More advanced lesions do not respond satisfactorily. Feeding chlortetracycline at 150–200 mg/day to affected lambs in feedlots reduces the incidence of chlamydial polyarthritis. No approved vaccines are available.

TENOSYNOVITIS

Tenosynovitis, an inflammation of the synovial membrane and usually the fibrous layer of the tendon sheath, is characterized by distention of the tendon sheath due to synovial effusion. It has a number of possible causes and clinical manifestations. The various types of tenosynovitis include idiopathic, acute, chronic, and septic (infectious). Idiopathic synovitis refers to synovial distention of tendon sheaths in young animals, in which the cause is uncertain. Acute and chronic tenosynovitis are due to trauma. Septic tenosynovitis may be associated with penetrating wounds, local extension of infection, or a hematogenous infection.

Clinical Findings and Diagnosis: There are varying degrees of synovial distention of the tendon sheath and lameness, depending on the severity. Horses are markedly lame in septic tenosynovitis. Chronic tenosynovitis is common in horses in the tarsal sheath of the hock (thoroughpin) and in the digital sheath (tendinous windpuffs). These two entities must be differentiated from synovial effusion of the tarsocrural and fetlock joints, respectively.

Treatment: In idiopathic cases, no treatment is initially recommended. Acute cases with clinical signs may be treated symptomatically with cold packs, NSAIDs, and rest. Tenoscopic surgery is often used to treat specific conditions within the tendon sheath that give rise to tenosynovitis symptoms. Application of counterirritants and bandaging has been used in more chronic cases. Septic tenosynovitis requires systemic antibiotics and drainage. If adhesions develop between the tendon sheath and the tendon, persistent effusion and lameness is the rule.

LAMENESS IN CATTLE

DIAGNOSTIC PROCEDURES

The lesions that cause lameness in dairy cows result in intense pain and are a major animal welfare issue. Lameness also causes stress, which debilitates and reduces productivity. The financial impact of lameness includes losses from decreased production, cost of treatment, prolonged calving interval, and possibly nursing labor. Loss of milk of 1.7–3 L/day for up to 1 mo before and 1 mo after treatment (because of pain) plus milk discarded because of antibiotic therapy must also be considered. Lame cows are more reluctant to use automatic milking systems and show visible signs of stress when forced to do so.

At least 10% of cows in a herd are culled for reasons related to lameness. Rearing replacement heifers is expensive, and replacement animals are not initially as productive as mature cows. Cows in poor condition have a greater predisposition to lameness. Cows that are lame before breeding have a reduced ability to conceive, and cystic ovaries are much more common in lame cows. Lame cows are less aggressive in their struggle for feed and are more likely to die early or be culled.

Considerable funds are being invested in bovine lameness research; within the next decade, national databases detailing bovine lameness are expected to become increasingly available as a management tool. Although the lameness data are being collected primarily by hoof trimmers, veterinarians should be familiar with this information to continue to play a leading role in management of bovine lameness.

PHYSICAL EXAMINATION OF A LAME COW

Visual Appearance of the Standing Animal: Abrasions or swellings on the limbs suggest a prior traumatic event. Decubital lesions (to the knee or more often the hock) might indicate prolonged periods of recumbency or difficulty when rising. Cubicle design should be reviewed. Muscular atrophy, particularly noticeable in the gluteal region, can be associated with a painful condition such as arthritis. Cows experiencing extreme pain can lose body condition rapidly.

Stance or posture can change as the bearing surface of the claw wears or there is a painful lesion in the foot. In a normal stance, the point of the hock (tuber calcanei) lies directly beneath the pin bone (ischial tuber) when viewed either from the side or from behind. Approximately 60% of the body weight is borne by the forelimbs. A lame animal adjusts its posture to relieve pain.

The following principles illustrate specific examples of changes in stance or posture related to lameness: 1) A painful abscess in a lateral hind claw causes the cow to abduct that limb. 2) Pain in the heel of the hind foot forces the cow to hold its foot to the rear, a posture known as "camping back" or retraction. 3) After a cow has spent much time walking on concrete, the lateral hind claw may become overburdened (excessive buildup of solear horn). This forces the hock to turn inward, a posture referred to as "cow hocked." 4) Pain in the toe, which occurs in laminitis, causes the cow to hold its hind feet further forward than normal, a posture referred to as "camping forward" or protraction. This posture can be confused with a conformational defect referred to as "sickle hock," in which the angle of the hock is <160°. 5) When the angle of the hock is <180°, the posture is referred to as "post leg," an undesirable conformational characteristic associated with arthritis. 6) When the hind feet are held closer together than normal (adducted), pain in the medial claw is indicated. The cow is said to be "standing narrow." This posture is often confused with a trait of conformation called "bow leg." Standing narrow can be a sign of laminitic-related lesions in the medial claw.

These principles of abnormal posture can be used to deduce the region of the foot in which the seat of lameness is located. Use of hoof testers may be one way to confirm the observation. For example, if there is pain in the toe, the retraction phase of the stride (when the foot passes behind the phase of vertical weight-bearing) is reduced considerably. In contrast, if there is pain in the heel, the protraction phase of the stride is reduced, or the foot is not carried as far forward as normal. Usually, the gait of one limb can be compared with that of the contralateral limb when viewed from the side. However, lameness simultaneously present in contralateral limbs tends to appear less severe than is actually the case. It is not unusual in cases of subacute laminitis for all limbs to be affected more or less equally. In these cases, no specific gait change is seen, but the cows tend to place their feet carefully with each step, ie, they "plod" or have a stilted gait.

Examination of the Claw: In cows exposed to concrete surfaces for a prolonged period, the sole of the lateral claw is likely to be worn flat and become much wider than that of the medial claw. Such soles are highly subject to trauma.

To facilitate examination of a completely flat claw, the surface of the sole should be washed and examined carefully for black marks by exploring with a hoof knife. If the sole is heavily caked with mud or manure (eg, cows at pasture or confined in corrals or straw yards), it is quicker and easier to cut off a layer of superficial horn together with the caked material to expose fresh horn beneath. Particular attention should be paid to the abaxial white line area. Removal of large amounts of sole horn is contraindicated in the diagnostic phase of an examination. The interdigital space should be evaluated by separating the claws and examining carefully for evidence of a foreign body, fibroma, footrot, interdigital dermatitis, or digital dermatitis.

LOCOMOTION SCORING

Locomotion scoring is a useful tool as part of a routine herd health evaluation or in a detailed herd lameness investigation.

Most farmers will detect between only 25% and 40% of truly lame cows; this underestimation of lameness prevalence means that the economic consequences of lame cows are less obvious to farmers than those caused by mastitis (loss of milk) and fertility problems. Cows in the early stages of sole ulcer, white line disease, and toe necrosis syndrome show only slight signs of lameness; if these lesions can be identified in their early stages, they can be treated and preventive measures instituted.

Locomotion scoring identifies slightly lame cows as well as those more obviously lame. Therefore, use of locomotion scoring can demonstrate the real extent of the problem.

Herd assessments should be done when the cows are walking on level, unobstructed walkways that give the observer a clear view. Locomotion scoring is frequently performed when the cows are leaving the milking parlor. In addition, milkers should note any cow standing in the milking parlor with an arched back, because it is highly probable that such cows are lame. Any cow lying down for an abnormally long time (>70–80 min/bout) should also be noted for special attention.

Locomotion scoring is a 5-point system based on both gait and posture: 1) Normal: The cow is not lame; the back is flat. 2) Mildly lame: The back is slightly arched when walking. 3) Moderately lame: The back is arched when both standing and walking. The cow walks with short strides in one or more legs. 4) Lame: The lame cow can still bear some weight on the affected foot. 5) Severely lame: The back is arched; the cow refuses to bear weight on the affected foot and remains recumbent. (Some observers use a 4-point scoring system, referring to normal as zero.) The repeatability of locomotion scoring is acceptably high among experienced observers.

As the locomotion score increases, milk yield decreases; however, the composition of the milk (fat, protein) remains unaffected.

COMPUTERIZED RECORDING OF DIGITAL LESIONS

Recording foot lesions by hoof trimmers is one of the most valuable advances in hoof health care and can be used to demonstrate the seriousness of the problem. In many cases, the data indicate the risk factors to be investigated. Any defect in the animal's environment that leads to some stress or foot abnormality is considered a risk factor. When a risk factor has been identified, control measures can be instituted before the problem becomes difficult to control. Lameness in cattle is a clinical sign of pain with many possible causes that require investigation. Methods to record lesions and rating severity are not yet standardized, but computer programs are available. In many countries, as many as one-third of hoof trimmers can provide this service and accurately identify and describe the severity of foot lesions.

In one survey, 86% of lesions recorded were found in the lateral claw of hindlimbs and 14% in the forelimbs; 73% of forelimb lesions were observed in the medial claw.

The National Database in Denmark also contains information about milk yield, reproductive status, health, etc. The prevalence of lesions must be interpreted carefully, because not every cow with a lesion will show signs of lameness. However, an abnormally high incidence of lesions may forecast lameness to come. The findings would indicate the urgency with which preventive measures should be implemented. The incidence of lesions varies considerably between countries and between regions of the same country. Lesion incidence also changes with different management system practices (eg, tie stall and free stall) as well as with variations during seasons of the year.

The annual herd incidence of lameness can be extremely high; in unique cases as many as 60% of the cows are affected at least once. However, even a 10%–15% incidence represents a significant economic loss.

DISTAL DIGITAL ANESTHESIA FOR DIAGNOSTIC AND SURGICAL PROCEDURES

For distal digital analgesia (used for surgical or diagnostic procedures), the dorsal site is located on the dorsal axis proximal to the interdigital space close to the metacarpal or metatarsal phalangeal joint. The needle should be placed with care (because the proper digital artery can be found at the dorsal site), and 10 mL of 2% lidocaine injected. If the needle is inserted deep into the interdigital space, the nerves of the flexor surface can be reached. This obviates the necessity of a flexor site block for simple procedures. The distribution of the nerve supply to the axial face of the digits of the forelimb is not constant, which makes this technique unreliable for digital analgesia of the forelimb.

The preferred flexor site is a little lower than the dorsal site because it is difficult to pass a needle through the partially cartilaginous palmar/plantar ligament. The medial and lateral sites are located at the level of the dewclaws, and the needle is inserted dorsally (horizontal in the standing animal) from a point 2.5 cm slightly proximal to the dewclaws. For the flexor site and the medial and lateral sites, ~5–8 mL of 2% lidocaine is injected. For surgery of the digit (eg, amputation), the dorsal, palmar/plantar, and medial or lateral sites are used, depending on the claw. For interdigital surgery (eg, removal of corns), both the dorsal and palmar/plantar sites are used. Differential diagnosis can be aided by selective anesthesia of the nerves of the digit.

There are four sites used for regional nerve blocks in the front and hind feet. The site selected should be perfused with 10 mL of 2% lidocaine using an 18–20 gauge needle.

Intravenous regional analgesia is frequently used for lengthy surgical procedures such as arthrodesis. Sedation and restraint is advised. A tourniquet is applied just below the hock or knee, the hair is clipped, and the skin sterilized from a site over a vein. Lidocaine (10–30 mL) without epinephrine is injected to produce analgesia within ~10 min. The tourniquet should never be kept in place for >60 min. When surgery is complete, the tourniquet should be loosened gradually to prevent a flood of anesthetic suddenly entering the general circulation. Concurrent injection of antibiotic may be helpful.

RADIOGRAPHY

Radiography of the Digital Region: Radiography can help identify the site of lameness and provide information about the stage to which the pathology has progressed. This helps to determine the most advantageous treatment. When pathologic changes are seen in the region of the distal interphalangeal joint, tissue damage is often rapid and severe.

Before a radiograph is taken, the interdigital space and both claws should be cleansed thoroughly, and both claws lightly trimmed. If this is not done, false images or shadows may mask abnormalities present in the claws. The digits can be viewed radiographically using four angles or projections.

In the dorsopalmar/plantar projection, the image produced shows all of the major bones and joints without overlap. This view allows diagnosis of many diseases of the bovine foot.

In the oblique projection, the plate is positioned beneath the claw, and the head of the machine is placed dorsad to the digits and rotated backward at a 45° angle. Because cattle have two digits that overlap one another when viewed radiographically from the side, an abnormality may be unclear or obscured. The oblique view allows the digit to be viewed from such an angle that one claw appears to be behind the other, which gives a much clearer picture than can be obtained when the digits are superimposed. Because each digit is projected differently on an oblique view, it is best to compare two radiographs of oblique views taken at comparable but opposite angles.

The lateromedial or mediolateral projection is generally of much less value than the oblique view. However, because positioning is relatively easy, this view is useful to evaluate fractures, fracture repairs, and luxations.

In the axial projection, a lateromedial or mediolateral view of a single claw is accomplished by placing a nonscreen film (eg, a paper "cassette") between the digits. This view produces a good image of the affected distal phalanx and, if interdigital soft-tissue swelling is not too great, the distal interphalangeal joint.

Radiographic Analysis and Interpretation: A number of factors should be considered in radiographic analysis and interpretation. Age differences can be seen radiographically as differences in skeletal development. In calves, physes are present in the distal metacarpus and metatarsus and at the proximal ends of the proximal and middle phalanges. In a very young calf, the distal phalanges may be incompletely ossified so that the bones appear small, and their distal ends are rounded and indistinct. The subchondral bone may appear indistinct and finely irregular; this should not be mistaken for the subchondral bone lysis seen in septic arthropathy.

Diseases stimulating periosteal new bone in cattle (such as corkscrew claw and postrecovery septic arthritis) can cause marked changes in bone contour and increased bone opacity.

Slight bony changes at articular margins and musculotendinous attachments are commonly seen on radiographs of older cattle. Roughening of the distal surface of the distal digit is a normal sign of aging. Changes that occur during the normal aging process should not be confused with active bony changes.

Reactive new bone (osteophyte, enthesiophyte, or exostosis) that has been present for some time has a distinct border and a rough outline, and the opacity is normally even. Active new bone has an indistinct border and a rough outline, and the opacity is uneven.

Diffuse loss of bone opacity occurs in subacute laminitis, nutritional bone disease, and after limb immobilization. Focal or localized loss of bone opacity occurs in bone infection (osteomyelitis) or inflammation (osteitis), early fracture healing, and with defects in endochondral ossification (osteochondrosis).

Increase in joint width is caused by the presence of increased fluid in the joint. However, this is less evident if the animal is bearing weight at the time the radiograph is taken. To confirm that the joint is in fact wider than normal, it may be compared with the contralateral joint.

Indistinctness and loss of opacity of the subchondral bone are often associated with joint infections. Loss of opacity is often irregular. For this reason, a single radiograph is unlikely to detect this pathology; therefore, several radiographs taken from different angles are usually advised. Comparison between suspect and known normal joints is recommended. Subchondral bone may be indistinct in a young animal.

Radiography is important to evaluate the progress of a fracture repair. A radiograph taken immediately after a fracture has been realigned is the basis for future evaluations, and subsequent radiographs are essential if nonunion or bone infection is suspected.

Loss of bone opacity is difficult to recognize with certainty in metabolic and nutritional diseases. Because all of the bones in the body may be equally affected, it is not helpful to compare one bone with another. In an adult animal, cancellous regions in the bone ends may become coarser or "granular" in appearance as smaller bone trabeculae are resorbed. In the diaphysis of a normal bone in both immature and adult animals, the cortex is thickest at midshaft and becomes thinner toward both ends. If the cortex at midshaft approaches the thinness of the proximal and distal diaphyses, generalized osteopenia must be suspected.

Soft-tissue swelling can be demonstrated on radiographs only in the early stages of a septic disease. The characteristics of a soft-tissue swelling may indicate the location of a lesion and the tissues involved, muscle or tendon disease, cellulitis or edema, or dark gas shadows (eg, a sinus or a cap of an abscess).

ARTHROCENTESIS AND ARTHROSCOPY

Arthroscopy enables visualization of the interior surfaces of a joint for diagnostic or surgical purposes. Arthrocentesis is a procedure by which synovial fluid may be removed from a joint for examination. Local anesthetic can be introduced to ascertain whether painful lesions are present in the joint. Intra-articular therapy permits medication to be deposited into the joint. Because this procedure may be painful, a nerve block at a higher level is recommended.

For the distal interphalangeal joint, the needle is inserted lateral to the common or long extensor tendon, which inserts into the extensor process of the distal phalanx. The entry point is just proximal to the coronary band. For the pastern joint (proximal interphalangeal joint), the needle is inserted lateral to the extensor tendon. For the fetlock joint (metacarpophalangeal or metatarsophalangeal joint), the needle is directed downward close to the bone and between it and the interosseous (suspensory) ligament. The joint can also be entered from the dorsal surface in a similar manner to the distal joints; however, the flexor pouch is more capacious than the dorsal one. For the digital synovial sheath (sheath of the deep flexor tendon), the needle is directed downward behind the interosseous ligament.

For the stifle joint, it is advisable to use two sites because in some animals the lateral femorotibial compartment may not communicate with the rest of the joint. The first site is close behind the lateral patellar ligament (lateral femorotibial compartment), and the needle should be directed caudally. The needle is inserted in the second site between the medial and middle patellar ligaments and directed slightly down and toward the large medial lip of the trochlea (femoropatellar and medial femorotibial compartments).

RISK FACTORS INVOLVED IN HERD LAMENESS

Lameness is a clinical sign of different diseases or disorders. For each condition, the range of causal risk factors and their severity varies; therefore, each condition has its own epidemiologic study. The importance of each factor differs depending on the system of management, be it total confinement, less restrictive systems, or totally pastoral. Management factors can usually be controlled, whereas factors such as ambient temperature, humidity, and rainfall must be taken into consideration but cannot be controlled entirely.

The diseases and disorders that affect the feet of dairy cows fall into two broad categories: those caused by infectious agents and those attributable to management.

The following variables can be controlled: nutrition/water, walking surfaces, resting and stress (cow comfort, social confrontation, stocking density), cleanliness/hygiene (prevalence of infectious agents/moisture/irritants), human care (hoof trimming, footbathing, lesion recording, farmer education), and genetic considerations.

If lameness has become a significant problem on a farm, it is invariably too late for a quick resolution. The first step is to immediately obtain the services of a competent hoof trimmer who preferably uses a chute side computerized lesion recording system (*see* p 1068).

Objective methods to assess risk factors have been developed; progress is needed to develop more objective methods to assess human care, farmer awareness, facility hygiene, and the stressors to which cows are subjected.

Heritability: Correlations between genetics and lameness are being investigated in several European countries. It is thought that different lesions may have different degrees of heritable susceptibility. There is even some proof that the benefits of hoof trimming have a heritable component.

In Sweden a "Bull Index" has been created so that farmers may select sires whose progeny have a low predisposition for lameness.

Nutrition: Subacute ruminal acidosis (SARA) is a common problem in high-producing dairy herds. Volatile fatty acids (VFAs) produced by microorganisms in the rumen are absorbed by rumen papillae. The papillae shrink during the dry period and need to be developed by lead feeding. If the surface of the papillae is inadequate, the pH of the rumen contents drops.

Successfully managing SARA depends on the quantity and digestibility of the carbohydrate fed. The more rapidly carbohydrate is digested, the more rapidly rumen acidosis will develop. Finely ground or moist grains are more digestible than dry, cracked grain. Corn silage is frequently used in dairy production. Sometimes the energy content of the silage is completely underestimated, with disastrous results. Slug feeding once a day is contraindicated, and the more frequently concentrates are fed the better. Sudden changes in the diet or formulation of the diet are extremely dangerous. Component-fed cows should be given up to 7.5% of their body wt in concentrates around calving. After calving, it is safest if rations are not increased by more than 0.25 kg/day for multiparous cows and by 0.20 kg/day for primiparous cows to a maximum of 14–16 kg (30–36 lb).

The quality and quantity of fiber fed could be more important than the carbohydrate component of the diet. Fiber can, depending on its physical characteristics, stimulate rumination. If the carbohydrate:fiber ratio is >50% carbohydrate, the animal is increasingly at risk of ruminal acidosis. If the percentage of acid detergent fiber for the complete ration is <20%, risk of ruminal acidosis also increases. If the particle length of silage is cut too short (25% cut <5 cm long), the contribution of effective fiber is reduced.

If a nutritional problem is suspected, a "walk around" should be done. Feed storage facilities should be evaluated for clues. For example, different batches of feed may be of different textures or colors. Changing from one silage storage unit to another can indicate a possible sudden change in diet characteristics. Sometimes feed is purchased off-farm even from several different suppliers.

The manure should not contain fiber particles <1 cm of undigested grain. This can be checked by placing 2 cups of manure in a fine mesh kitchen sieve and washing the material through with water from a hose. Feces should not contain mucin/fibrin casts, be foamy, or contain gas bubbles. The feces in the same feeding group should not vary from firm to diarrhea. Rumenocentesis can be performed as a last resort.

There should be a drinking station for every 15 cows. The water supply should be clean and free of static electricity. A high level of iron in drinking water can affect palatability.

Walking Surfaces: Walking surfaces are another important contributing cause of lameness. The Nordic countries have pioneered the use of rubber matting. One UK study showed that cows enter and exit the milking parlor more rapidly on rubber matting than on concrete. In addition, sole horn wears less on rubber than on concrete. Of course, rubber is fully effective only if kept free of slurry. Installing rubber matting is expensive but a reasonable recommendation. The best flooring system from the perspective of lameness is slats with rubber caps, but this is reasonable only for new installations or major upgrades.

Resting, Stress, Cow Comfort, Social Confrontation, Stocking Density: These risk factors together with other physical stressors have been referred to as ecopathologic factors or an Animal Suitability Index. These terms refer to an assessment tool for housing conditions based on seven spheres of influence: walking, feeding, socializing, resting and comfort, behavior, hygiene, and care. Ecopathology, therefore, is evaluation of space allowance, cubicle dimensions, stall base, bedding, stall and pen measurements, type of flooring, slipperiness, stocking density, cleanliness, hoof trimming and footbathing, feed bunk space, water supply, walking surface conditions, and mobility locomotion score.

Under normal conditions, a healthy cow rests 10–11 hr/day. Resting periods usually last just longer than 1 hr, during which time the cows ruminate and thus digest their feed. Lameness, depending on its severity, tends to increase both the lying time and the number of lying bouts.

Anything that inhibits a cow from lying down is of particular concern. This can be assessed rapidly by use of the Cow Comfort Index (CCI), which should be calculated 1 hr before milking. The number of cows lying in a stall should be divided by the number of cows standing or in any way touching the stall. It is assumed that cows standing and touching the stall are showing a desire to rest; thus, the higher the CCI, the more probable there is a problem. If the incidence of noninfectious lameness is also high, then cow comfort is a risk factor to be dealt with. Cows not involved in calculating the CCI are those drinking, eating, or just walking. Unwillingness to lie down because of remembered discomfort is another reason for prolonged standing. However, inability to exercise reduces the amount of oxygen and nutrition delivered to the claw.

Stall size is important but varies depending on the frame size of the cows in a herd. The partitions must be of space-sharing design. If the overall slope of the stalls is adequate, the cows will lie with their hindlimbs all running in the same direction.

Cows prefer sand stalls above all other surfaces. The sand keeps cows cool and provides good footing to rise. Mattresses filled with rubber crumbs are acceptable; concrete covered with straw or sawdust and hard rubber mats are less desirable.

When a cow rises, she is forced to lunge forward; anything that makes that difficult should be corrected. Neck rails (never cables) should be 37–43 in. above the stall. A brisket board is important, and flexible *structures* are available to reduce the risk of hematomas of the brisket. Loose house stalls built facing a wall are a poor configuration. Cows should not be forced to lie or stand with their hindlimbs in the alley.

Stress is a factor that can and has been measured in cows. Stress may play a role in causing lameness, and lameness itself is a cause of stress. Stress may also be an etiologic factor in both reproductive failure and in some types of mastitis infections. Social confrontation may be a surprising cause of stress. The matriarch cows dominate the pecking order. Presumably, a submissive animal is somewhat stressed when confronted by a dominant animal in a narrow alley. Prolonged standing, waiting in line to drink, or spending >3 hr in the holding yard each day are commonly overlooked factors. Overstocking increases the occasions on which cows of significantly different dominance will face one another. This is particularly noticeable when heifers are first admitted to the milking herd. This may also be the first time heifers ever encounter concrete. Heifers should always be given 1 mo to adapt to concrete before the added stress of facing dominant cows. Alleys should never be <12 ft wide, feed alleys 13 feet wide, and loafing alleys 14 feet. There must be more cubicle stalls and feeding standings than there are cows. All too commonly, a building built to hold 50 cows is modified to take 100–150 cows, with resulting catastrophic overstocking.

Cleanliness and Hygiene: When the prevalence of digital dermatitis is unacceptably high, contamination should be reduced, especially if the hind ends of the cows are caked in muck. Possibly the most commonly used slurry removal system is the scraper fixed to the front of a tractor. Although this system is acceptable, it is commonly not done often enough. Automatic scrapers are costly to install and subject to mechanical breakdowns. The overall effectiveness of flushing systems remains questionable.

The presence of any slurry during a clinician visit should evoke comment.

Farmer Education: Priority must be given to improving farmers' knowledge and increasing their willingness to implement recommendations, including routine examination (by the farmer) of the herd for lame cows. However, in the UK and France, lack of time and labor are reported as the most important barriers to detecting and treating lameness.

Special efforts should be made to help farmers understand the gravity and complexity of an increasing herd lameness problem. Information pamphlets, regional seminars, and hands-on on-farm demonstrations with a hoof trimmer and nutritionist involved can all be useful.

PREVENTIVE PROCEDURES

FOOTBATHS

Dry cows (and infected heifers) should be included in the footbathing routine.

Permanent, concrete footbaths may measure 3 m (10 ft) long and 0.2–0.6 m (8–24 in.) wide. The sides of the bath should not slope inward and should be 15–25 cm (6–9 in.) deep. Cows prefer to use footbaths that have a bottom close to floor level; therefore, a built-up block "rounded lip" could be considered in the design. The medicated solution should be a minimum of 8–10 cm (3–4 in.) deep. Drainage from the bath should be provided to ensure the foot can be properly cleansed. To avoid blockage, the drain hole should be 10–20 cm in diameter and located at the lowest point of the bath.

Footbaths should be located in relation to the exit from the milking parlor in a frost-free environment with, ideally, an area suitable to drain chemicals from the feet to avoid contaminating the bedding. At all costs, deviation from the normal free flow of cow progression should be avoided.

Prewashing the feet before entering the footbath has been increasing in popularity. Ideally, the wash bath should be located before the cows enter the milking parlor. This allows time for washing fluid to drain before cows enter the chemical bath. The dimensions should be similar to those of the medication bath.

Use of a footbath is not a substitute for either good hygiene or claw trimming. However, if digital dermatitis is endemic on a farm, regular use of a footbath is mandatory.

Plastic, fiberglass, or metal portable footbaths should be avoided. A hoof mat, consisting of a sheet of foam plastic encased in a perforated plastic cover, is also available. The foam is soaked in medication that squirts up between the claws when the cow walks on the mat. There are no recent reports on the effectiveness of this device.

Fully automated power spray washers are claimed to be extremely economical in the use of water, and they require no operator. They deliver soapy water, and some users believe this device alone reduces the incidence of foot disease.

Chemical Agents for Footbaths:

Formalin 4% is the least expensive footbath solution for the control of interdigital phlegmon (footrot). Some cows will refuse to enter a formalin footbath if the solution is stronger than 4%. Formalin has been found of value to control digital dermatitis. The solution should be changed after the passage of ~200 cows, more frequently if the bath is heavily contaminated with manure. Formalin has good bacteriostatic activity and some potential to harden the epidermis. However, it is ineffective at temperatures <13°C.

Formalin generates strong fumes that irritate the lungs of milkers and can taint milk. It should never be used in baths located near the milking parlor.

The stronger the formalin solution used, the more effective it is, but the danger of a chemical burn on the cow's skin is also greater. If the hair on the foot appears to be standing on end or the skin is pink, bathing should be suspended. Normally, cows can tolerate twice daily baths for 3 days using a 3% solution. The treatment should be repeated every 3 wk. Higher concentrations should only be used for the most resistant conditions.

Formalin is regarded as a hazardous waste, and land disposal restrictions should be checked and followed. Formalin must never be released into sewer systems, because sewer treatment plants may have problems and contaminated drinking water could be released. However, formalin is said to break down in 7 days in sludge or slurry; even then, it is wise to wait until it is diluted to one part formalin in three parts sludge before spreading it on arable land. Preferably, the land selected should not have a high water table. Unused formaldehyde concentrate should be returned to the vendor.

Footbathing with a 5% solution of **copper or zinc sulfate** controls interdigital dermatitis and is of some value in controlling footrot (interdigital phlegmon). There are two grades of copper sulfate, and the pentahydrate grade should be used. The solution must be prepared 5 hours before use. Prewashing of the cow's feet is advised, and the solution should be changed after the passage of ~200 cows.

Copper has a strong affinity to be bound by soil, the organic matter in manure, and soil minerals. Hence, much of the copper found in soil is unavailable for plant uptake. Once the copper reaches a high level in the soil, the process cannot be reversed. Therefore, plants stunted by high levels of copper have a lower nutritional value to cattle. Copper sulfate footbath solutions may be tagged to slurry at the highest practical dilution and spread widely on the land.

The sulfates are quite rapidly deactivated by combining with the proteins in manure.

The use of **antibiotics** in footbaths has been a popular past strategy for the treatment, control, and prevention of digital dermatitis. Few reports on the use of antibiotics in footbaths appear in the current literature. Antibiotics are expensive and deteriorate in contaminated solutions. The type of antibiotic used in footbaths should be changed at intervals of ~6 mo to avoid development of resistant strains of the causal organisms. However, treatment may be given for 2–3 days and repeated once after 7 days. Formalin footbaths may be used alternately if more aggressive treatment is necessary. Antibiotics used in footbaths do not result in detectable levels of drug in the bloodstream or milk. Antibiotic sprays or powders are still used for topical treatments.

A new generation of chemical agents has been developed for use in footbaths, but claims of effectiveness have not yet been adequately substantiated in controlled trials. Foams are also available but the cost of associated equipment is considerable. Foams keep the chemical agent in contact with lesions better than liquid products.

FUNCTIONAL CLAW TRIMMING

The role of the professional claw trimmer has changed significantly during the past decade. The introduction of chute-side computerized data collection is providing valuable data; however, it also requires additional training in lesion identification. Close collaboration between trimmer and veterinarian is beneficial for both as well as for the dairy industry overall.

Over time, the claws of cows wear, changing the shape of the sole, which in turn makes the foot unstable. The two claws become unbalanced both longitudinally and laterally. As changes develop in the lateral claw, it becomes "overloaded," the heel horn may become thicker (overburdened), and posture is compromised. Therefore, the objective of trimming is to reduce excessive weight bearing on load-bearing claws.

Under normal circumstances, horn growth keeps pace with wear. The growth/wear rate at the heel is greater than at the toe. Horn that is dry tends to be extremely resistant to wear and may grow longer than normal. Thus, the claws of cattle maintained in straw yards tend to become overgrown. Conversely, the claws of cattle maintained in extremely wet conditions are softer than normal and more prone to wear and damage. If the cows are housed on concrete surfaces, the lateral hind claw tends to wear less than the medial.

If claws are routinely correctly trimmed, longevity of the herd may be extended. Trimming can be expected to decrease milk yield by up to 2 lb/day for 2 days but should be restored or even increase in a similar period. Decrease in milk yield is partly due to disruption in the cow's feeding routine and handling. To some extent, variations in milk yield reflect on the skill of the trimmer. Trimming should be avoided in any location close to the milking parlor, and individuals handling the cows should never attempt trimming. Unskilled claw trimming will negatively affect the claw health of a herd and should be avoided. All claws should be evaluated before trimming. On average, the front (dorsal surface) wall of a hind claw measures ~7.5 cm long from apex to hair line. When the dorsal wall increases in length, the dorsal surface of the claw tends to become concave (buckles like the instep of a human shoe). This causes greater weight-bearing to be transferred to the posterior aspect of the claw, increasing pressure on the flexor process of the distal phalanx, the point beneath which sole ulcers develop. The longer the toe, the greater the stress on the flexor system. When the claws are short and the dorsal wall is >7.5 cm, there is considerable risk that the thickness of the sole at the apex will be less than the desirable 7 mm. Thinning of the apex of the sole of short-clawed animals should be avoided.

Foot trimming of every cow in a high-production, intensively managed herd is recommended every 5 mo. Recording and reporting (to the veterinarian) the types of lesions observed will prompt early treatment and timely introduction of preventive measures.

PREVALENT LAMENESS DISORDERS IN INTENSIVELY MANAGED HERDS

Although there are many important lesions, most lameness protocols are based on data from digital dermatitis, sole ulcer, white line disease, toe necrosis/apical syndrome, and sole hemorrhage. Early identification of lesions permits early treatment, which significantly reduces the recovery period.

The incidence of lameness in pastured dairy cattle in New Zealand is extremely low; the risk factors associated with housing do not exist in that country. Pasture management is also common in Chile.

DIGITAL DERMATITIS

(Hairy warts)

Digital dermatitis is the most common disease of the feet of mature dairy cattle and is endemic in intensively managed dairy operations worldwide. It tends to mask or overshadow other more painful lesions present concurrently. Incidence is low in pastoral settings such as in New Zealand and Chile. The presence of the disease in beef cattle appears to be minimal.

Clinical Findings: Two main types of lesions are seen. The erosive/reactive form is seen more commonly in Europe, whereas the proliferative or wart-like form is more prevalent in North America. Both forms cause varying degrees of discomfort and may give rise to severe lameness. Both forms can be seen in the same animal. The two forms likely represent different stages of the same disease process.

Explosive outbreaks can occur when affected cows are introduced to previously unaffected herds.

Treponema-like organisms can be observed in microscopic samples isolated from most lesions. However, the number of strains of *Treponema* affecting cattle can be as high as 80, some of which may be oral or rectal. It would be wise not to incriminate just one strain as the cause because of the numerous manifestations of digital dermatitis. Digital dermatitis is likely to be polytreponemal (eg, *T phagedenis*, *T vincentii*, and *T denticola*).

Digital dermatitis is much more prevalent if hygiene is poor and the feet are exposed frequently to slurry. It is widely believed that a number of predisposing bacteria are involved. It has been postulated that the once ubiquitous *Dichelobacter nodosus* may be an important synergizing agent; *Campylobacter* spp and *Prevotella* spp may also be involved in the etiology.

Skin maceration and the presence of a semi-anaerobic environment are important predisposing factors. Many treponemes are found in the deeper layers of the epidermis, some of which are believed to reach these layers of the epidermis via hair follicles.

A relatively weak immune response has been detected in naive cattle.

Lesions: Lesions are most common in the region of the flexor commissure of the interdigital space. Less typically, lesions have been seen on the dorsal surface of the foot as well as around the dewclaws. One or both hind feet are most commonly involved, although forefeet can be affected. Lesions vary considerably in size and appearance both within a herd and in different parts of the world.

The following system has been developed to classify the stages of this disease: M0 = normal skin; M1 = early, small circumscribed red to gray epithelial defects of <2 cm in diameter preceding the acute stage, appearing between acute episodes or within the margins of a chronic M4 lesion; M2 = acute, active ulcerative ("strawberry-like") or granulomatous (red-gray) lesions >2 cm in diameter and sometimes surrounded by white halo-like tissues, which may be slightly papillomatous; M3 = the healing stage occurring within 1–2 days after topical therapy, with the lesion covered with firm, scab-like material; M4 = the chronic stage in which the epithelium is thickened and/or proliferative (filamentous or scab-like) and several centimeters in diameter.

Treatment: Acute lesions are initially treated topically. The lesion should be scrubbed clean with a stiff brush and soapy water, rinsed, and dried. An antibiotic powder such as oxytetracycline is applied and protected by a gauze pad or a small feminine hygiene pad held in place by a waterproof bandage or a reinforced nylon device (booties) that can be affixed with hook-and-loop-tape closures. Multiple treatments are usually necessary. Oxytetracycline treatment has not resulted in detectable residual levels of the antibiotic in blood or milk. Extremely high parenteral antibiotic dosages have been reported to help resolve severe lesions.

Once a lesion has started to heal, topical dressings may be sprayed on with a pressurized backpack spray unit. Soluble oxytetracycline or lincomycin-spectinomycin (66 g and 132 g/L of water, respectively) produces the best results. Contamination of the lesion must be avoided at this stage. Although apparent resolution can be achieved, recurrence seems almost inevitable, and farmers should be so advised.

Control: There are no effective vaccines. The following methods are used in control: 1) Automatic power washing of the feet with soapy water before entering the milking parlor. 2) Passage through a medicated footbath after passing through the milking parlor with a 30-min drainage period. 3) Diligence in ensuring the environment is regularly freed from slurry and liquid contamination. 4) If digital dermatitis is not present, replacement animals should not be introduced and the herd should not be exposed to vectors such as unsterilized instruments or visitors' dirty boots.

PODODERMATITIS CIRCUMSCRIPTA

(Sole ulcer)

Sole ulcer is generally regarded as the most important, prevalent, and costly of the noninfectious lesions. All too frequently, it is the cause of culling. Sole ulcers commonly affect one or both lateral hind claws, predominantly in heavy, high-yielding dairy cattle kept under confined conditions. A sole ulcer is a circumscribed lesion located in the region of the sole/bulb junction, usually nearer the axial than abaxial margin. Damage to the dermis is associated with a circumscribed zone of localized hemorrhage and necrosis. The incidence is variable, but in some herds up to 40% of mature cows can be affected.

Recently, *Treponema*-like organisms have been identified in these lesions.

Etiology and Pathogenesis: Sinking of the claw due to activation of matrix metalloproteinase, which is a feature of subclinical laminitis, is the major predisposing factor. As the space between the flexor process of the pedal bone narrows, the corium is crushed, causing ischemic necrosis and compromising horn production. This results in a hole forming in the sole. As the damaged corium undergoes repair, granulation tissues erupt through the hole in the sole. Because this condition is strongly associated with subclinical laminitis, some softening of the sole horn will occur. This increases the rate of horn wear. The sole horn also softens under very unhygienic conditions when horn is exposed to the fluid component in slurry.

Iatrogenic forms of the lesion are produced when inexperienced claw trimmers remove too much horn from beneath the heel (and/or the posterior region of the abaxial wall), resulting in abnormal pressure on the dermis. Excessive wear of the softened sole horn flattens and thins the sole.

Heel erosion is another potential contributing cause of a sole ulcer. Normally, weight is borne by the anticoncussive qualities of the bulb of the heel, but if heel erosion occurs, weight-bearing may be transferred forward to the region beneath the flexor process. Sometimes, a displaced pad of horn slips over to the vulnerable area, causing abnormal pressure over the flexor process of the distal phalanx.

Clinical Findings: The progress and severity of lameness are variable and often masked in bilateral cases, depending on the size of the lesion and extent of the secondary infection. Because the lateral hind digit is usually involved, the limb is often held slightly abducted with weight-bearing on the unaffected medial digit. In tie stalls, the hind toes may be rested on the edge of a curb in an attempt to relieve pressure on the heel-sole junction. On flat surfaces, an affected cow stands with the hindlimbs camped back. Some cows may shake the affected foot frequently, whereas those with bilateral lesions may continually shift weight from limb to limb and frequently lie down.

The earliest stages of this lesion may be discovered during routine claw trimming. As sole horn is removed from over the typical site, a hemorrhagic lesion may be exposed. The clinical lesion varies from a soft, slightly discolored area that may be painful under pressure to a distinct bright red knob of granulation tissue. This is often the stage at which lameness becomes severe enough to be noticed. Once the corium is exposed, infection can invade the deeper structures of the claw and spread proximally to involve the navicular bursa,

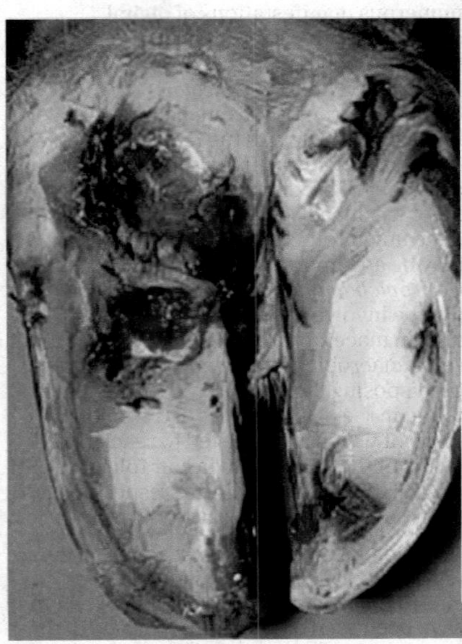

Sole ulcer over flexor process of distal phalanx. The heel has been lost due to heel erosion. *Courtesy of Dr. Paul Greenough.*

resulting in necrosis of the flexor tendon and ligaments of the navicular bone. A retroarticular abscess may develop, which may be further complicated by infection of the distal interphalangeal joint (*see* p 1088). Rupture of the flexor tendon leads to dorsal rotation (upward) of the toe ("cocked toe"). In complicated cases, infection may progress up the deep flexor tendon sheath.

Treatment: Treatment must be aimed at removing pressure from the affected area. Skillful therapeutic claw trimming is highly effective. This procedure lowers the entire bearing surface of the lateral claw, which transfers loading to the sound medial claw. Applying a "lift" has become the accepted treatment for this condition. The simplest form of lift is a wooden or rubber block glued or nailed to the unaffected medial claw, thereby removing all weight-bearing from the ulcer region. Recently, various models of easier-to-apply plastic slippers have been developed. Care must be taken when applying either a block or a slipper to avoid the sharp, hard, rear edge of the device from causing pressure under the sole. Blocks should be removed after ~1 mo to avoid causing damage to the sole.

Protruding granulation tissue need not be excised and must not be treated with any caustic agent, because this can retard healing. Bandages should not be applied, because this results in continued weight-bearing at the ulcer site. Furthermore, covering the lesion causes it to remain moist and promotes maceration and bacterial infection.

Many ulcers never fully resolve, and affected cows may have chronic, low-grade lameness and need corrective foot trimming 3–4 times/yr for their productive lives.

Prevention and Control: Because the development of sole ulcers is intimately related to subclinical laminitis, the latter should be investigated and appropriate control measures instituted (*see* p 1083).

WHITE LINE DISEASE

White line disease is almost as prevalent as sole ulcer and can be just as difficult to treat satisfactorily. Together with sole ulcers, white line disease commonly affects one or both lateral hind claws, predominantly in heavy, high-yielding dairy cattle kept under confined conditions. White line disease is characterized by hemorrhage into or separation (avulsion) of the abaxial wall, most commonly at the heel-sole junction. The corium becomes infected through this lesion.

White line disease is often referred to as also being present in the apical region. Technically, this is true, but this type of lesion will be described as a component of the toe necrosis syndrome (*see* below).

Clinical Findings: The affected cow may adduct its hindlimb(s). The abaxial wall may seem a little longer than normal, and occasionally there may be slight swelling and erythema of the coronary band above the heels.

The lateral claw of the hind foot (often both) is usually involved. If bilateral, the disease may remain unnoticed until lameness is more pronounced in one limb than the other. Because the outer hind claw is affected, the limb is swung away from the body during each stride. The cow may stand with the medial claw bearing weight. White line separation without complications is frequently seen at claw trimming. The degree of pain and lameness depends on the rate of development and extent of the subsolar abscess. Routine examination of the sole must include the complete exploration of the abaxial white line region. Black marks must be explored with the tip of a hoof knife as potential sites for track formation. Discharge of pus from the skin/horn junction above the abaxial wall is always reason to suspect a white line lesion. In these cases, the white line must always be examined very carefully.

Etiology and Pathogenesis: The lamellar/laminar arrangement is longest behind the wall on the dorsal side of the hoof. This arrangement gets shorter toward the heel and more or less disappears at the abaxial groove. That is not to say that the collagenous fibers cease to exist in the other regions of the dermis; it can be postulated that adhesion between wall and corium could be less intense. At the same time, beneath the bulbar region is the structure known as the digital cushion. During locomotion, the digital cushion is compressed and expands toward the abaxial wall. Thus, this region is not only structurally weaker than more dorsal areas but is also subjected to a different set of pressure and mechanical stresses. The white line is composed of very soft horn, which fills the spaces between the lamella at the most distal extremity of the wall. It is postulated that stretching of collagen fibers, combined with sinking of the pedal bone, accounts for the hemorrhage into the white line so frequently seen.

Solid foreign bodies may lodge in the softened, widened white zone. They may push through to the corium beneath and introduce infection; however, the presence of a foreign body is not essential for the lesion to develop.

There are three possible sequelae of localized infection: 1) a localized abscess may develop; 2) infection may be forced proximally to form a track that may discharge at the coronary band; and 3) the infected track may, as it forces its way proximally, infect other structures, depending on the site of the initial infection. An anterior track can infect the distal interphalangeal joint directly. Tracks forming closer to the heel are likely to cause infection of the bursa of the deep flexor tendon. Invariably, the bursa ruptures into the retroarticular space, and an abscess develops in this location. Infection of the distal interphalangeal joint and the tendon sheath of the deep flexor tendon may follow. Necrosis and avulsion of the insertion of the deep flexor tendon into the distal phalanx are frequent complications. These cases are easily detected as the apex of the pedal bone unrestricted by the flexor tendon tips up.

Swelling of the heel bulb represents the most advanced form of white line disease; it is frequently misdiagnosed as footrot (often presented as a case of footrot resistant to treatment). Footrot causes the whole foot to swell evenly to the fetlock; in contrast, a retroarticular abscess leads to enlargement of only one heel bulb.

Treatment: During a claw examination, any black mark in the white line must be cut out until healthy horn is exposed. For a local abscess, removal of an elliptical segment of the wall adjacent to the lesion aids free drainage by providing a self-cleansing abaxial opening. Cream-colored pus may indicate a corporeal response to tissues tearing as collagen fibers stretch and the pedal bone sinks. In contrast, if the pus is black, it is likely that infection has penetrated from the outside.

Abscessation at the coronary band is usually indicative that white line disease is present. The same applies to a retroarticular abscess. Cases of nonhealing white line disease have been reported.

TOE NECROSIS SYNDROME

The term toe necrosis syndrome covers three different etiologies for a condition having a similar appearance. The three different etiopathologies are not completely understood. However, *Treponema*-like organisms have been isolated from all of these lesions.

Etiology and Pathogenesis: Lesion 1–As subclinical laminitis progresses, in some cases the distal phalanx will rotate. Movement of the apex of the pedal bone will cause tearing of tissues, with resultant hemorrhage. In extreme instances, the tip of the bone will prolapse through the apex of the sole. Many cows with a rotated digit also have a ridge (the reaction ridge) running around the wall. The ridge is similar in location to a hardship groove and is displaced distally in a similar manner. Osteomyelitis of the distal phalanx can be seen in complicated cases.

Lesion 2–Many cases have been reported anecdotally in which the anterior half of the sole has been worn down almost paper thin. Hemorrhage from bruising is seen through the thin horn at the apex. Breakdown of the horn and formation of an abscess have been reported. One probable cause is a painful lesion in the heel, which forces the cow to throw most of its weight onto the anterior part of the sole.

Lesion 3–The incidence of apical necrosis can be quite high in young feedlot cattle, many of which become recumbent and die of pneumonia. The condition is sporadically reported in mature cows.

The main blood supply to the digit is the very large axial digital artery, which is vulnerable to pressure from the sharp proximal edge of the axial wall. This artery connects with the terminal arch that penetrates across the bone. Necropsy reveals that necrosis occurs distal to this artery, and radiographs tend to suggest the same thing. The terminal artery marks the margin at which pathologic fractures of the distal digit can be seen.

Necrosis of the apex of the pedal bone is extremely common in yearling beef calves after transportation over long distances. In either case, it is suspected that standing for long periods is the cause. Current laws in North America require that cattle be unloaded and watered every 40–52 hr. It is thought that long periods of standing without exercise allow the blood to pool in the feet and damage the tissues. During locomotion, the coronary cushion with the aid of venous valvules functions as a pump to return blood to the general circulation.

Treatment and Control: Treatment is cost effective only in animals with no obvious complication. The cavity should be cleansed, dried, and packed with an antibiotic powder. If no changes occur after a few days, the lesion may be covered with methyl methacrylate. If the bottom of the lesion is black, a probe should be inserted; if necrotic tissue can be detected, 1–2 cm of the apex of the toe should be removed under regional anesthesia with hoof cutters. The condition of the pedal bone should be visible. If necrosis of the bone is confirmed, a further 1–2 cm of toe should be removed. If the wound bleeds profusely, it is likely that necrosis is not extensive. When hemorrhage is minimal, it is probable that necrosis of the bone is extensive or a physiologic fracture is present. There are several reports of the toe (not the claw) having been amputated with satisfactory recovery. Systemic antibiotics and application of a lift to the sound claw is advised. If the wound is obviously contaminated, the lesion should be packed with a hygroscopic mixture (50% magnesium sulfate and 50% glycerin) and bandaged for a maximum of 24 hr, after which the lesion should be thoroughly dried, dressed with antibiotic powder, and closed with methyl methacrylate.

SOLE HEMORRHAGE

Sole hemorrhage is by far the most common noninfectious lesion in lame cows. It is regarded as a typical sign of laminitis but is frequently overshadowed by bruising of the sole. Blood stains in the sole of the hoof are the most commonly seen abnormality of the sole. When subclinical laminitis was first described, sole hemorrhage was considered to be an invariable clinical sign. It was thought that the arteriovenous shunts in the solear papillae were compromised, allowing blood to perfuse down the tubules, giving a brush-like appearance. Since then, solear hemorrhages have increased in prevalence. This may be due to cows being forced to stand on concrete for longer periods than previously. Bruising/trauma is more likely to occur if the horn is softened by moisture, or if the quality of the horn is reduced because of some nutritional error or because the thickness of the sole is reduced too much during hoof trimming. Interpreting the true cause of solear hemorrhages can be important.

THIN SOLE

As the term "thin sole" implies, the anterior region of the sole has worn very thin due to excessive weight bearing on that region. An innovative method to treat "thin sole" begins by drilling a 10-mm hole through the center of a wooden block. The claw to be treated is thoroughly dried. Next, a fast-setting adhesive is applied along the border of the axial and abaxial wall. The objective is to create a ridge on the wall that does not involve either the white line or sole. This layer is allowed to dry and harden before a second application of fast-acting adhesive is made. The block is set in place and held by a self-adhesive bandage until the fixative has fully set. Sufficient soft setting material is then injected through the hole in the block to entirely fill the space and exert very gentle pressure on the dermis.

HEEL EROSION

(Slurry heel)

Heel horn erosion is seen as a change in the appearance of the surface of the bulb of the heel. Because heel horn erosion alone does not always cause lameness, the true incidence is unknown. However, subjective observations suggest that once cows have been exposed to copious slurry, the incidence of heel erosion rapidly approaches 100%. In some cows, heel horn erosion advances to a point at which complications develop and lameness may be apparent.

Etiology and Pathogenesis: The etiology is unknown. Heel horn erosion is perhaps more commonly seen in herds in which subclinical laminitis has been diagnosed and in herds affected by digital dermatitis. It is also more commonly seen during the winter, particularly when the claws are exposed to an unhygienic, moist environment (eg, intensively managed dairy units).

Clinical Findings: The first lesions seen are small circular erosions <0.5 cm in diameter. As the condition advances, these lesions merge, and ridges form parallel to the hair line on the axial surface of the bulb. Invariably, the color of the roughened area is black. At this stage, the cow is not lame.

In the secondary phase, the appearance of the heel varies. In some cases, there is a buildup of horn beneath the heel. Simultaneously, there may be a loss of horn under the axial part of the bulbs. The excessive accumulation of horn is often more pronounced in the lateral claw and causes the hock to turn in (cow-hocked stance). This stance resolves after therapeutic claw trimming. Generally, the condition is progressive unless corrected. The disturbance interferes with shock absorption, and the animal throws more and more weight forward. A common concurrent lesion is a sole ulcer. In other cases, erosion completely denudes the heel of

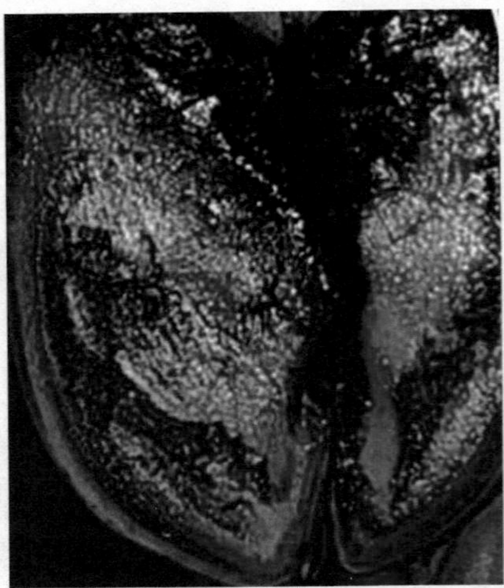

Heel erosion with a wide claw and black necrotic horn. Part of the sole over-reaching the interdigital space. *Courtesy of Dr. Paul Greenough.*

horn—a process that also interferes with shock absorption and can be associated with a sole ulcer. *Treponema*-like organisms have been observed in microscopic samples of heel horn.

Heel horn erosion must not be confused with separation of the heel, which is the result of the escape of pus from an abscess close to the heel.

Treatment and Control: Both heels should be reduced to the same height by paring away excess horn. Careful attention must be paid to maintaining the bearing function of the abaxial wall and sloping the sole toward the axial border.

Attention to hygiene and reduction of slurry are essential. The claws of dairy cows should be trimmed twice each year. A weekly footbath (where permitted, 3%–5% formalin), starting no later than October in the northern hemisphere, should be provided.

OTHER DISORDERS OF THE INTERDIGITAL SPACE

INTERDIGITAL DERMATITIS

(Stable footrot, Slurry heel, Scald)

Since the widespread appearance of digital dermatitis, interdigital dermatitis is rarely reported. This may imply that the causal organism of interdigital dermatitis may be implicated in the etiology of digital dermatitis.

Etiology and Pathogenesis: Interdigital dermatitis is caused by a mixed bacterial infection, but *Dichelobacter nodosus* has been considered to be the most active component. *D nodosus* is an anaerobe and exceptionally proteolytic. The source of the infection is the cow itself, and the infection spreads from infected to noninfected cows through the environment. *D nodosus* cannot survive for >4 days on the ground but can persist in filth caked onto the claws, creating an anaerobic environment. The bacteria first invade the epidermis of the skin between the claws but do not penetrate to the dermal layers. As the condition progresses, the border between the skin and soft heel horn at the posterior commisure disintegrates, producing lesions similar to ulcers or erosions. At this stage, the lesions cause discomfort. In tied systems, the hindlimbs are affected more often than the forelimbs. In loose housing systems, the distribution between fore- and hindlimbs is about equal. Animals on slatted floors are affected less often than animals on solid floors.

Clinical Findings: The early stages of the condition appear as an exudative dermatitis. The exudate oozes to the commissures of the interdigital space and forms a crust or scab, which may be observed occasionally on the dorsal surface of the digits. As the condition progresses, the animal shows discomfort by "paddling," or constantly moving from one foot to the other. If the heels of the hind feet are especially painful, the limbs are held further back than normal. True lameness does not develop until a complicating lesion is present. After a prolonged period, during which the animal has avoided bearing weight on the heel, the horn beneath the heel increases in thickness and some aberrations of gait result. In dairy cows, interdigital hyperplasia (corns, fibroma) may be caused by the chronic irritation of the interdigital space. Often, the fibroma develops on one side of the interdigital space.

Foot-and-mouth disease can be confused with interdigital dermatitis if the interdigital space is not always examined carefully.

Treatment: Systemic therapy, including the use of antibiotics, is not cost effective. In severe cases, the lesions should be cleaned and dried, after which a topical bacteriostatic agent is applied, eg, a 50% mixture of sulfamethazine powder and anhydrous copper sulfate. Alternatively, an animal can be confined in a footbath for 1 hr, bid for 3 days.

Control: Good management and housing systems that keep claws dry and clean are most important. Regular foot trimming helps avoid complications. Footbathing, beginning in late fall and before clinical cases can be identified during high-risk periods, is essential in herds known to be infected. Weekly footbathing may be sufficient in the late fall, but the frequency may have to be increased in late winter.

INTERDIGITAL PHLEGMON

(Footrot, Foul in the foot)

Footrot is a subacute or acute necrotic infection that originates in the interdigital skin, leading to cellulitis in the digital region. Footrot has a worldwide distribution and is usually sporadic. It may be endemic in intensive beef units or in cattle at pasture. The incidence varies according to weather, season of year, grazing periods, and housing system. Footrot is presented less commonly today than decades ago, partly because more cases are treated by farmers and partly because dairy cows spend much less time at pasture. However, on average, footrot accounts for up to 15% of foot diseases.

The appearance of footrot in loose housing systems has been reported.

Etiology and Pathogenesis: Injury to the interdigital skin provides a portal of entry for infection. Maceration of the skin by water, feces, and urine may predispose to injuries.

Fusobacterium necrophorum is considered the major cause of footrot. It can be isolated from feces, in which it may survive as a saprophyte, which may explain why control is difficult. It can also survive in moist soil.

F necrophorum is a gram-negative, nonspore-forming, nonflagellated, nonmotile, pleomorphic anaerobic bacteria. It has a lipopolysaccharide endotoxin capable of necrotizing activity. There are three subspecies and a number of genotypes, each of which targets different tissues. When PCR assays become more widely available, the genotypes will be more readily identifiable.

Other organisms, such as *Dichelobacter nodosus*, *Staphylococcus aureus*, *Escherichia coli*, *Trueperella pyogenes*, and possibly *Bacteroides melaninogenicus* can also be involved.

Clinical Findings: Research suggests that the incubation period of footrot can be a week. The fore- or, more commonly, the hindlimbs can be affected, but more than one foot is rarely involved at the same time in mature cows. However, footrot can occasionally develop in several feet in calves. The first sign is swelling and erythema of the soft tissues of the interdigital space and the adjacent coronary band. The inflammation extends to the pastern and fetlock. Typically, the claws are markedly separated, and the inflammatory edema is uniformly distributed between the two digits. The onset of the disease is rapid, and the extreme pain leads to increasing lameness. In severe cases, the animal is reluctant to bear weight on the affected foot. Fever and anorexia are seen. The skin of the interdigital space first appears discolored; later, it fragments with exudate production. As necrosis of the skin progresses, sloughing of tissue is likely to follow. A characteristic foul odor is produced.

If the disease proceeds unchecked, weight loss is severe and milk yield is significantly reduced. Milk production may not recover during the current lactation. Open lesions can be infected with secondary invaders. If the necrotic lesion is located in the anterior region of the interdigital space, the distal interphalangeal joint can become infected.

Hematogenous infection of the tissues of the interdigital space may account for peracute cases of footrot, which are referred to as either "blind" or "super foul." This form of footrot is characterized by the initial absence of a skin lesion, extreme pain, and the tendency to progress despite aggressive therapy.

Treatment: Most treated animals recover in a few days. Good results are obtained with penicillin G, IM, for 3 days. Treatment should be administered as soon as signs are observed. However, the label dosage may be inadequate to effect a rapid resolution, and increased dosages may be needed, requiring increased withdrawal times. Treatment of "super foul" must be particularly aggressive. Early cases respond well to single doses of long-acting oxytetracycline.

Sodium sulfadimidine solution IV or trimethoprim/sulfadoxine, IV or IM, bid for 3 days, can also be used. A single oral administration of a long-acting bolus containing baquiloprim/sulfadimidine may be suitable to treat beef cattle.

High concentration of an agent in the target tissues can be achieved by a regional IV injection (*see* p 1068). Positive results have been obtained with penicillin or oxytetracycline.

Local treatment is essential for some longstanding cases and in all instances in which the anterior region of the interdigital space has been compromised. The lesion must be thoroughly cleansed, but it is inadvisable to curette or otherwise remove necrotic tissue surgically. The dorsal pouch of the distal phalangeal joint is very superficial at this point. A nonirritant bacteriostatic agent (such as nitrofurazone or a sulfa preparation) should be applied as a topical dressing. The application of gauze, cotton batting, or bandages is contraindicated. However, the lesion can be protected and immobilized by binding the digits together with a bandage. The entire digital region can be protected from contamination if it is enclosed in a plastic bag fixed in place with an adhesive bandage. However, prolonged protection is not advocated, because the enclosed lesion tends to macerate further. Bandages, if used, should be replaced daily.

Prevention and Control: Animals actively shedding infectious organisms should be isolated until signs of lameness have disappeared. If this is not possible, a waterproof dressing or protective boot should be applied; however, animals wearing protective boots should be monitored carefully to avoid additional damage. Boots should be disinfected between use.

Because busy traffic areas are invariably heavily contaminated, steps should be taken to ensure that areas around drinking troughs, gateways, and tracks are adequately drained. Animals at pasture might be moved to a clean, dry area, or possibly housed during periods of heavy rainfall. Contaminated concrete must be frequently cleaned and scraped free of manure.

Preventive use of a footbath with an antiseptic and astringent solution (eg, copper or zinc sulfate [7%–10% in water]) has given beneficial results. Formaldehyde solution (3%–5% in water) can also be used. Ethylenediamine dihydroiodide has been used as a feed supplement for prevention, but the results are extremely uncertain. Vaccines against *F necrophorum* have failed because of the weak immune response to the bacterium. High levels of zinc fed as a supplement have a beneficial effect by improving epidermal resistance to bacterial invaders.

INTERDIGITAL HYPERPLASIA

(Corns)

Etiology and Pathogenesis: In heavy beef breeds, the condition is thought to result from stretching of the insertions of the distal interphalangeal ligament. The claws splay, and the interdigital skin is stretched. When not involved in weight bearing, the skin folds outward and subcutaneous scar tissue develops. In these cases, a mass tends to develop in the axis of the interdigital space. The mass may become so large that it touches the ground and may become necrotic. There may be a heritable disposition in some breeds such as Herefords.

Corns are reported frequently in dairy cows when their feet are continually exposed to slurry, chronic irritation, or have interdigital dermatitis. Organization of areas of irritated skin on one side or other of the dorsal commisure accounts for development of corns in dairy cows.

Interdigital hyperplasia affects forelimbs. Lameness results more often than not. As the lesion becomes larger, its surface may become excoriated, sore, and infected.

Treatment: In simple cases, treatment may be unnecessary. For surgical removal, the animal should be sedated, and dorsal and flexor regional nerve blocks administered (*see* p 1068). Surgery can be performed with the animal standing or in lateral recumbency. After preparation of the surgical site, a tourniquet is applied and the claws separated manually or with retractors. The mass is removed, leaving as much of the interdigital skin as possible. If any fat protrudes when the claws are pressed together, it should be removed. Care must be taken to avoid cutting deep structures such as the distal interphalangeal ligament. After surgery, the wound should be dressed with an antibiotic powder and the claws bandaged closely together. Some field reports suggest considerable success with wiring the toe together. Movement of the wound or separation of the claws must be avoided until ~10 days after surgery. Cryosurgery is also an option.

DISORDERS OF THE HORN CAPSULE AND CORIUM

The genetic relationships between what are now considered to be lamanitic-related claw disorders have been found to be moderate to high.

LAMINITIS

Equine and bovine laminitis are distinctly different. Although acute laminitis occurs in both species and can be caused by grain overload, other etiologies can affect the equine laminae. A major difference between the two species is anatomic, in that the lamellar/laminar surface of the equine hoof is considerably more extensive than that of the cow.

For **chronic laminitis**, *see* p 1086.

Subclinical laminitis is almost certainly an incorrect descriptor for the disorder(s) observed. The condition has been referred to as claw horn disruption, but use of this term is misleading.

Subclinical laminitis is of considerable economic importance to the dairy industry, because it predisposes mature animals to sole ulcer, white line disease, or the toe necrosis syndrome. It has been seen in most developed countries and is of greatest concern in high-production, intensively managed herds.

Clinical Findings: There are no definitive clinical signs of subclinical laminitis. However, in any group of cows presented with the same set of insults, a few cows may show slight signs of the subacute form of the disorder. Some cows with subacute laminitis may walk in a deliberate, careful manner with the legs carried beneath the animal when walking. When standing, such animals tend to draw all four feet under the body. Erythema and edema (puffy foot) of the skin above the coronary band and around the dewclaws in freshly calved cows may indicate a transitory laminitis-like insult and that the cows are being introduced to concentrate too rapidly. Hoof testers may evoke some response.

Sole hemorrhages are an invariable clinical sign of clinical laminitis, but such hemorrhages due to trauma are more common; therefore, this sign must be interpreted carefully (*see* p 1079).

Etiology: The etiology of subclinical laminitis in cattle is not understood. The classic hypothesis suggests that high levels of carbohydrate in the diet (*see* p 225) invoke an increase of *Streptococcus bovis* and *Lactobacillus* spp, which induce a state of acidosis in the rumen. This causes gram-negative organisms to die and release vasoactive endotoxins. Rumenitis is frequently associated with ruminal acidosis. High levels of histamine in the blood have been found in the early stages of the disorder. It is probable that subacute ruminal acidosis is one key factor in development of laminitis, because managing subacute ruminal acidosis (SARA) helps control the incidence of subclinical laminitis.

Contemporary thinking is that as production levels increase, cows become more sensitive to risk factors. A risk factor in this case is any physical insult causing stress. This probably leads to the release of bioactive messengers into the bloodstream. One important risk factor is trauma; many clinicians are convinced that hard flooring is equal in importance to nutritional problems. Care must be taken when dry cows and heifers are introduced to concrete after being accustomed to soft flooring.

Pathogenesis: Although the release of biologic messengers into the bloodstream is known, identification of the agents that play a part in laminitis is ongoing. Epidermal growth factor (EGF) receptors are present in the basement membrane of the corium of the claw. EGF is liberated in large quantities from the GI tract when it is damaged (eg, rumenitis) and could be involved in the pathogenesis of laminitis. In addition to its mitogenic effect, EGF can inhibit the differentiation of keratinocytes in vitro. Inhibited differentiation of keratinocytes of the hoof matrix is a dominant morphologic feature in the early stages of laminitis. This supports the hypothesis that laminitic histopathologic changes result from an inadequate regulation of gelatinase activity, resulting in selective degradation of basement membrane components due to failure of the basement membrane–epidermis attachment.

More recent investigations have studied the role of matrix metalloproteinase (MMP) activity in the pathophysiology of laminitis. It is not known which endotoxins are involved in releasing MMPs. It is known that MMPs play some part in allowing collagen fiber supporting the distal phalanx to stretch. During the peripartum period, hormones such as relaxin are generated. Correct management of nutrition around calving is critical. In early calving heifers, it is possible growth hormones could have a complicating role.

Whatever the biologic messengers, they appear to affect two different types of tissues: the papillary or solear dermis and the collagen fibers of the laminae. This results in two distinctly different pathologies. The first is disruption of normal keratogenesis, and the second, abnormal MMP activity, results in sinkage and/or rotation of the digit.

The pathophysiologic process associated with compromised horn production starts when vasoactive toxins or other biologic agents reach the corium. Arteriovenous shunts may be paralyzed, pressure inside the claw rises, and the walls of the vessels are damaged. Blood or blood fluids escape and soak into the claw horn, staining it either pink or yellow. Hemorrhagic staining of the horn tubules of the sole give a "brush mark" appearance. Mural thrombi form, reducing blood flow and causing oxygen deprivation and an insufficient nutrient supply to the keratin-producing cells. Thrombus formation is a characteristic feature of laminitis. The resulting horn is soft and prone to damage, infection, and scar formation.

The second pathophysiologic process involves MMP release and stretching of the collagen fibers of the suspensory apparatus of the digit. Collagen fibers originate in horny corrugations (lamellae) on the inner surface of the hoof wall and insert into those areas of the distal phalanx that have no periosteum. Thus, the pedal bone is "suspended" from the wall of the hoof. The lamellae are arranged to increase the surface area from which the fibers originate. The vascular tissue and germinal layer, the laminae, are interleafed between the lamellae. In areas of the wall and sole where there are no lamellae, the tissues of the dermis are referred to as corium. Whether laminitis is truly an inflammatory process could be questionable.

As the collagen fibers stretch, the pedal bone is displaced. Occasionally, the pedal bone will rotate and the apex of the bone will prolapse through the apex of the sole. Perhaps more frequently, the whole bone will "sink," causing the space between the flexor process and the sole of the claw to narrow and increasing the possibility of a sole ulcer developing.

Frequently, young animals appear to recover from laminitis. This may be because new blood vessels develop to form collateral circulation and take over the function of those that have been damaged. Nevertheless, each time an animal has a bout of laminitis, more scar tissue is formed and the animal is less able to recover from the next insult.

Treatment and Control: Treatment for subclinical laminitis is impractical, because diagnosis in an individual animal is not possible at the time of the causative insult(s).

Controlling subclinical laminitis (*see* p 1083) in a high-production, intensively managed dairy herd requires a systematic epidemiologic study.

DOUBLE SOLE

In double sole, one sole is present while a new sole grows beneath, ie, there is complete shut-down of horn production for an undetermined short period of time.

Etiology and Pathogenesis: A new sole grows beneath an existing one when fluid forms between the dermis and epidermis. This fluid can result from bruising of the sole under conditions such as prolonged walking on rough roads. The fluid may be pus from a subsolar abscess. Double sole has been seen in cattle suddenly changed from a mainly forage diet to one rich in concentrates. Double sole can be confused with underrunning of the heel, which is a frequent sequela of white line disease. Double sole has also been seen after feeding moldy hay.

Treatment and Control: Treatment is simple unless mismanaged. The abaxial wall must remain completely intact and only a portion of the sole covering the bulb cut away. The sole beneath is extremely soft and vulnerable to damage; therefore, the animal should be confined to a well-strawed stall until the new horn has hardened, after which more of the sole may be removed.

Sudden changes in the quality of the forage should be avoided.

FOREIGN BODY IN SOLE

A stone or fragment of glass or metal penetrating almost through the sole will cause pain due to pressure on the corium and, if not removed, will lead to infective coriitis.

If the foreign body penetrates through to the corium, infection is introduced to the dermal level, and an abscess develops. The rapidity of onset and severity of the lameness depends to some extent on the location of the sole penetration. In the apical and subapical region, the lesion is located between the distal phalanx and the nonresilient sole. As the abscess develops, interungular pressure increases rapidly. Thus, the onset of lameness is rapid, and pain is severe. Acute lameness may cause the animal to stand with the foot off the ground or with the toe lightly touching. A differential diagnosis is fracture of the distal phalanx.

In the sub-bulbar region, the corium is located between the digital cushion (a flexible structure) and the soft, resilient horn of the bulb. The onset of lameness is relatively slow, and the pain is significant but not severe. The pus in the abscess tends to spread over a wide area through the fascial plane and to cause separation of the skin-horn junction at the heel. A moist discharge from this area may be the first indication of the lesion. This is referred to as "underrunning of the heel," a condition that can be confused with double sole (*see* above).

Treatment: The foreign body should be removed and the track cored out to the corium with a fine-pointed hoof knife. Creating a large hole is inappropriate. Pus is often released under considerable pressure. Antibiotic should be squeezed into the cavity, which closes rapidly. The opening should not be plugged but covered with elastic waterproof material to prevent blockage with mud or manure.

Treatment consists of removing the foreign body if still present. The detached horn should not be stripped off in its entirety. Part of the detached horn may be removed, but the abaxial wall must be left intact to bear weight and spare the exposed, newly forming sole. Bandaging may not be required, but the animal should be housed in a well-strawed area for a few days.

VERTICAL FISSURES

(Sandcrack)

Sandcracks are vertical fissures or cracks in the wall of the claw. They account for ~0.2% of lesions of the claws of dairy cows. In western Canada, the average incidence in mature beef cows is ~20%. In individual herds, the incidence can be as high as 60%. No breed differences have been recorded. The lesion is extremely unsightly, which can be a considerable drawback for beef cattle producers who wish to sell their animals.

Clinical Findings: Vertical fissures occur almost exclusively in the lateral fore claw. In dairy cows, fissures are usually small and confined to the proximity of the coronary band. In beef cattle, they are more extensive, mostly starting at the coronary band and/or running part or all of the way to the bearing surface. In herds with the highest incidence of this disorder, lesions are also observed to start from a horizontal groove in the middle of the claw.

Etiology: The etiology remains uncertain. The incidence is highest in mature, heavy cows. Bending or buckling of the claw around one or several horizontal grooves probably creates mechanical stresses that cause rupture of the claw wall.

In beef cattle in the prairies, it is theorized that the most probable cause is a rapid change from a winter diet low in protein and high in fiber to one high in protein and low in fiber.

Treatment: Most sandcracks are not painful and require no treatment. However, if the origin of the lameness can be traced to a claw in which a sandcrack is present, routine treatment of the crack is appropriate.

A crack at the coronary band can split open, allowing infectious organisms to enter. The protrusion of granulation tissue through such a lesion can be quite troublesome. The dorsal pouch of the distal interphalangeal joint is extremely superficial at this point. The joint is very vulnerable, and lesions at this location should never be ignored. Superficial horn should be pared away and an astringent dressing applied (50% mixture of a sulfa powder and anhydrous copper sulfate). Pressure should be applied using cotton batten held tightly in place by a narrow, adhesive elastic bandage encircling the entire coronary band.

The fissures often have ragged edges that may be twisted and gape open. Sometimes, the edges move and pick up a foreign body. Cosmetic treatment may be requested in the case of show animals. The axial wall at the tip of the claw should be cut back so that the weight is borne only by the abaxial portion of the wall. The ragged edges of the fissure should be trimmed, ideally with the cutting disk of a grinding tool. In selected cases, a fissure can be immobilized with an application of methyl methacrylate after the two edges of the fissure have been laced together with steel wire.

HORIZONTAL FISSURES

Horizontal fissures result from disruption of horn production at the dermis beneath the coronary band, leading to a defect in the integrity of the wall. These fissures run parallel to the coronary band. The defect varies in severity from a shallow groove (hardship groove) to a complete fracture (fissure) of the wall. A comparable anomaly is seen as a band of horn differing in appearance from the remainder of the claw. One form of the band is seen in animals stressed after weaning (weaning groove) or during a period of nutritional deprivation. The fissure moves distally as the claw grows, and the distal portion becomes progressively more mobile (thimble) until it fractures, leaving a "broken toe." A series of grooves can destabilize the vertical strength of the dorsal wall, causing it to bend (buckled toe).

Etiology: Fissures are believed to be caused by a wide variety of stressors, including a difficult calving, an acute febrile disease, or a sudden, relatively short-term but significant change in nutrition. A ridge may indicate an event such as compensatory growth.

Clinical Findings: The horizontal groove or fissure is an important indicator of metabolic disturbance. The date on which the causal insult occurred can be calculated by measuring the distance from the hair line to the fissure and dividing that number by the growth rate of the claw. In mature dairy cows, the rate of growth of the wall measured along the dorsal flexure of the claw is ~0.5 cm/mo. Growth rates are more rapid in young animals, in animals on intensive feed, and during the summer months.

Treatment: No treatment is possible except when very deep fissures form a thimble, which is extremely painful. In these cases, the loose horn should be removed with pincers; regional anesthesia may be needed.

CORKSCREW CLAW

A corkscrew claw is twisted throughout its length in a configuration that displaces the abaxial wall by up to 360°. One or both lateral hind claws may be affected in cows >4 yr old. Although corkscrew claws are rarely seen in bulls, many believe there is a heritable component.

Pathogenesis: Bone molding is seen in the distal phalanx, but it is not known whether this is a matter of cause or effect. Periarticular exostoses develop around the distal interphalangeal joint, possibly resulting from strain of the distal abaxial collateral ligament. Pressure from the exostosis on the dermis of the wall probably accounts for the excessive growth of the abaxial wall.

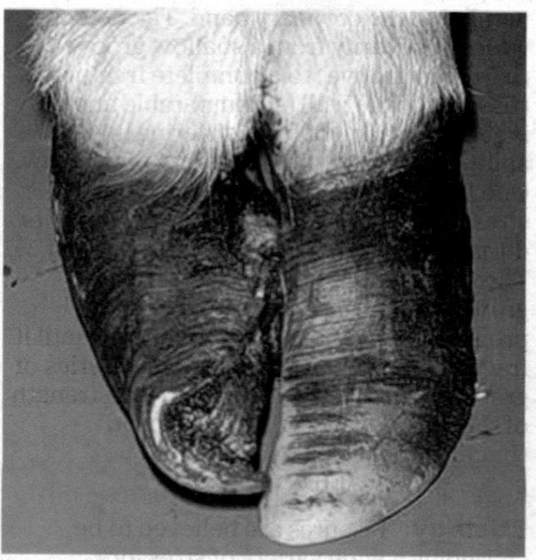

Corkscrew claw. *Courtesy of Dr. Paul Greenough.*

Treatment: Correctly trimming a corkscrew claw requires much skill. The horn formation is extremely hard and difficult to cut. The abnormally narrow shape of the distal phalanx makes it difficult to pare the claw without causing bleeding at the toe. The strategy is to shorten the claw as much as possible without causing bleeding. Next, the horn wall that is displaced beneath the claw is cut away. Then, so far as is possible, the horn is shaped to approximate normal. Trimming helps the animal get around for a while but does not "cure" the condition. Affected animals should ultimately be culled.

SLIPPER FOOT

A slipper foot is named for its alleged likeness to a Persian slipper. The claw is flat and curled upward to form a square end. The horn is heavily ridged and has lost its shine, and the coronary band is rougher and darker than normal. Although there is no objective evidence to support the theory, the slipper foot is probably synonymous with chronic laminitis and may be a sequela of either acute or subclinical laminitis. Treatment is always disappointing. The claw can be shaped to approximate normal, but invariably it collapses and serious sequelae follow. Animals with slipper foot should be culled as soon as economically appropriate.

DISORDERS OF THE BONES AND JOINTS

ANKYLOSING SPONDYLOSIS

In ankylosing spondylosis, exostoses develop on the ligament of the ventral aspect of the lumbar vertebrae, primarily in older bulls. Fracture of the exostosis and associated vertebrae causes pressure on the spinal cord, which results in severe ataxia or paralysis. There is no treatment.

DEGENERATIVE ARTHROPATHY

This nonspecific condition affecting mainly the hip and stifle is characterized by degeneration of articular cartilage and eburnation of subchondral bone, joint effusion, and fibrosis with calcification of the joint capsule.

Etiology: Many causes and predisposing factors influence the development of degenerative joint lesions. There is almost certainly an inherited predisposition to the condition. Certain conformations, eg, straight hocks in beef bulls, are also incriminated. Joint instability after trauma is a common cause. Nutritional factors involved in some cases, such as rations high in phosphorus and low in calcium, influence the strength of subchondral bone. Copper deficiency or fluoride poisoning also may act similarly. Forced traction of a calf in breech presentation can impede the blood supply to the hip joint, and arthritis may result. The role of infection is unclear. Infectious arthritis in calves usually produces severe changes in the hock, but degenerative arthropathy rarely involves this joint.

Bulls fed high-grain diets for show may become lame when as young as 6–12 mo, but most cases are first noticed at 1–2 yr.

Clinical Findings: Onset is gradual (later in bulls), and both hip joints are usually affected; stifle involvement is rare. Lameness to the point of incapacitation, with crepitation of degenerate joints, may develop in a few months; however, correlation between pathologic changes and clinical signs is poor. The earliest changes occur in the acetabulum and on the dorsomedial surface of the femoral head.

In the stifle, the medial condyle of the femur shows the earliest changes. Because degenerative arthropathy may result from any of several initiating factors, a specific diagnosis may be difficult.

Radiographic, cytologic, and microbiologic evaluation of the synovial fluid are useful diagnostic aids. Arthroscopy of articular surfaces and ligaments may help attain a definitive diagnosis and prognosis.

Treatment: Changes in the joints are usually irreversible by the time of diagnosis. Palliative treatment of valuable breeding animals should be undertaken with the knowledge that the condition or predisposing factors may be inherited. The diet should be carefully analyzed and, if necessary, corrected. This is especially important in fast-growing animals, in which adequate exercise is indicated and overfinishing should be avoided.

COXOFEMORAL LUXATION

Luxation of the coxofemoral joint is usually upward. It is seen in cows riding each other. The affected limb appears shorter than the contralateral limb. The hock is turned inward and, when trying to walk, the animal appears to be dragging one foot behind the other.

Treatment: Resolution is possible, provided that the head of the femur or the rim of the acetabulum has not been fractured. The animal should be deeply sedated to the level of recumbency. A rope should be looped around the groin of the affected limb, which should be uppermost. The free ends of the rope should be tied around a tree or some other fixed object, and traction should be applied to forcibly extend the limb. Downward pressure should then be applied to the hock, which should be strongly rotated outward (upward) until the head of the femur slips back into the acetabulum. Traction should be applied at several angles until the head of the femur clicks back into the acetabulum. If the head of the femur or the rim of the acetabulum is fractured, there will be considerable crepitation, and the head of the great trocanter will displace as soon as traction is stopped.

PATELLAR LUXATION

Intermittent fixation of the patella on the upper part of the femoral trochlea results in a characteristic jerky action of one or both hindlimbs. The limb remains in caudal extension for a longer period than normal and may even be dragged for a few steps before clicking forward to a normal posture. In young animals, the condition may resolve spontaneously. For luxations that do not resolve, medial patellar desmotomy should be performed.

FETLOCK DISLOCATION

Fetlock dislocation is seen in young cattle when they cross cattle guards (grillwork laid over a pit as a gate substitute). Tranquilization or light anesthesia facilitates replacement of dislocated structures. A padded, fiberglass cast maintained in place for 3 wk usually promotes a satisfactory recovery.

HIP DYSPLASIA

Hip dysplasia, a bilateral malformation of the hip joint, is often associated with secondary osteoarthritis. It may be present at birth. However, abnormal gait may develop in rapidly growing animals. Usually, it is possible to rock the hindquarter to produce a click as the head of the femur pops in or out. Radiography may confirm the diagnosis in young animals. There is no treatment.

FRACTURES

Bone fractures occur in cattle of all ages, but they are most common in those <1 yr old. Corrective procedures may be justified economically in this age group, provided that joints are not involved. External fixation techniques or Thomas splints have been used successfully. In selected cases, percutaneous transfixation or internal fixation may be attempted.

Fractures of major long bones in adult cattle usually are not treated. The tuber coxae may fracture when cattle are hurried through narrow doorways. In these cases, spicules of bone may penetrate the skin, or unsightly distortions of the flank can result. Fractures of the proximal and intermediate phalanges may be considered for treatment in tractable, young adult cattle.

Fracture of the distal phalanx is relatively common in adult cattle. Onset of lameness is rapid, and the pain is usually severe. If the medial digit is involved, the animal may seek relief from the pain by crossing its legs. Natural recovery is prolonged, and because most such fractures extend into the distal interphalangeal joint, a debilitating arthritis may develop at the fracture site. If treatment is undertaken, the sound digit should be elevated on a wooden block and the affected digit immobilized in a flexed position to the block using methyl methacrylate adhesive.

SEPTIC ARTHRITIS OF THE DISTAL INTERPHALANGEAL JOINT

Most frequently, one of the causal lesions is present and the transition from the initial lesion to the joint infection is readily apparent. However, when a swollen foot is treated before the cause has been established, a joint infection may have been ongoing for weeks before the true nature of the condition is diagnosed. If aggressive treatment of a footrot case does not lead toward resolution within 3 days, septic arthritis should be suspected. Increased pain, together with swelling of the anterior region of the coronary band in cases of sandcrack and white line disease, is suggestive of joint infection. Using regional analgesia and strict aseptic technique, an aspirate of the joint can be collected and examined for infection. A radiograph may indicate an abnormal separation of the joint surfaces.

Etiology: Infection enters the distal interphalangeal joint via three possible main sites: 1) the dorsal commissure of the interdigital space, via penetrating trauma or complicated footrot (interdigital phlegmon); 2) sandcracks; or 3) white line disease or retroarticular abscess.

Treatment: Digital amputation is indicated in animals that have a limited life expectancy, eg, old or poor-producing animals. The procedure is simple, quick, can be performed in standing animals under regional analgesia, and in most cases, produces rapid relief. Amputation is performed through the skin with an embryotomy wire placed as close to the skin-horn junction as possible. Hemorrhage is arrested by means of a tight bandage.

Alternatively, in the case of valuable animals, arthrodesis to fuse the distal and middle phalanges may be attempted. General anesthesia is recommended. A 1-cm canal is drilled through the abaxial wall into the joint, and a second canal is drilled from the causal lesion into the joint. The joint cavity is enlarged by curettage, and a drainage tube drawn through. Continuous irrigation with sterile saline should be performed for 2–3 days. A wooden block is then applied to the sound claw and the affected digit immobilized by fixing it to the block with methyl methacrylate. Immobilization is further facilitated by encasing the digital region in a cast. The cast is removed after 4 wk.

SEROUS TARSITIS

(Bog spavin, Puffy hock)

Serous tarsitis is characterized by three soft, fluctuating swellings between the ligaments of the femorotarsal joint. In some instances, this condition is heritable. It does not cause pain or lameness. In later life, there may be a predisposition to arthritis. Serous tarsitis is diagnosed by depressing the swelling of the joint capsule at one location and palpating the fluctuation that is seen at another. There is no successful treatment.

NEUROLOGIC DISORDERS ASSOCIATED WITH LAMENESS OR GAIT ABNORMALITIES

SUPRASCAPULAR PARALYSIS

This rare condition results from paralysis of the supraspinatus and infraspinatus muscles caused by damage to the sixth and seventh cervical nerves. Acute trauma to the prescapular area (eg, struggling into a head gate) produces a nonspecific ataxia immediately after the injury. Several days after the injury, the muscles may show signs of wasting, indicating the possibility of permanent damage.

Chronic injury to the nerves causes marked wasting of the muscles within weeks. A specific gait aberration develops. The stride is shorter than normal; when weight is borne on the limb, it tends to swivel. In some cases, the cause may be nerve compression in or around the vertebrae (eg, an abscess or fracture), which may be identified on radiographs.

If the trauma is complicated, primary treatment must be directed toward resolving the immediate problem. However, if the clinical presentation suggests that the injury is localized to the nerve, immediate treatment with steroids or other anti-inflammatory agents is appropriate.

RADIAL PARALYSIS

Distal radial paralysis results in an inability to extend the carpus and digit. Proximal radial paralysis prevents the animal from extending the elbow, carpus, and fetlock to bear weight.

Etiology: The proximal radial nerve may be injured by stretching close to the brachial plexus, in which case the triceps muscles as well as the extensors of the carpus and digits may be compromised. The damage is frequently associated with casting an animal with ropes or with any situation in which the forelimb is accidentally restrained and the animal struggles violently to free itself. Either distal or proximal radial paralysis can result from prolonged recumbency in very heavy animals.

The distal radial nerve is vulnerable to injury in the musculospiral groove of the humerus, either from fractures or deep, soft-tissue trauma. A lesion of the nerve proximal to the sulcus for the brachial muscle causes proximal radial paralysis.

Clinical Findings and Diagnosis: In proximal radial paralysis, the elbow drops, the carpus and fetlock are in partial flexion, and the limb is usually dragged. In distal radial paralysis, because the triceps muscles remain functional, dropping of the elbow is minimal. However, paresis affecting carpal and fetlock position is present.

Treatment: Rapid improvement can be expected in most cases. Animals should be confined in a generously bedded stall. Anti-inflammatory drugs may be helpful, particularly in the early hours after the initial trauma. If skin sensation in the forelimb has been completely lost, the prognosis is guarded. When the condition persists for ≥2 wk, damage is likely permanent and the prognosis is grave.

ISCHIATIC PARALYSIS

(Sciatic paralysis)

Damage to the ischiatic and obturator nerves after intrapelvic parturient trauma may cause recumbency after calving. It may be a component of the downer cow syndrome. The tibial and peroneal nerves are branches of the ischiatic nerve that can be damaged at extrapelvic sites.

OBTURATOR PARALYSIS

Passage of a calf through the pelvis exerts pressure on the obturator nerve. The close association of the obturator nerve with the origin of the ischiatic nerve can complicate interpretation of clinical signs.

Clinical Findings: Because the adductors are innervated by the obturator nerve, an animal adopts a base-wide stance or, in recumbency, a sitting position with both hindlimbs extended forward. There is considerable risk that the adductor muscles will be damaged and that permanent recumbency will result. In addition to the base-wide stance, knuckling of the fetlock may be present. This indicates injury of the ischiatic nerve. Both conditions may contribute to downer cow syndrome (*see* p 1188).

Treatment: If obturator paralysis is recognized early enough, vigorous measures should be adopted to prevent complications involving the adductor muscles. The animal should be immediately transferred to a site where there is good footing (eg, a base of tenacious manure over which clean straw has been spread) to prevent slippage during attempts to rise. The hindlimbs can be tied together with a soft nylon strap fixed below the hocks. The limbs are restrained from "spreading" >3 ft (1 m) apart.

FEMORAL PARALYSIS

In femoral paralysis, paralysis of the quadriceps muscles, which extend the stifle, and partial paralysis of the psoas major muscle, which flexes the hip, are seen.

Clinical Findings and Diagnosis: Femoral nerve paralysis is seen in large, newborn calves (eg, Charolais, Simmental) after the use of mechanical force during an assisted birth. Reduced quadriceps tonicity reduces tension on the patella, with the result that a lateral patellar luxation may develop. Atrophy of the quadriceps soon becomes obvious and, although the patella can be replaced easily, the animal has extreme difficulty walking. The condition may affect one or both limbs. Prognosis is related to the severity of the clinical signs.

Treatment: Despite a fair or good prognosis, the animal may be unable to suckle unaided. The animal should be maintained in a well-bedded area, and colostrum given as soon as possible after birth. A radiographic study should be done to exclude fractures. The administration of anti-inflammatory drugs may be useful.

PERONEAL PARALYSIS

Peroneal paralysis results in paralysis of the muscles that flex the hock and extend the digits.

Clinical Findings: The peroneal nerve is the cranial division of the ischiatic nerve. It passes superficially over the lateral femoral condyle and the head of the fibula, which makes it vulnerable to external trauma or pressure from recumbency. An affected animal stands with the digit knuckled over onto the dorsal surface of the pastern and fetlock. The hock may appear to be overextended. In mild cases, the fetlock tends to knuckle over intermittently during ambulation; however, this may also occur if the animal is experiencing pain in the heels.

In severe cases, the dorsal surface of the hoof may be dragged along the ground, and sensation to the dorsum of the fetlock is often decreased. Testing of reflexes may demonstrate that hock flexion is absent, but stifle and hip flexion are normal. This would not be the case if the ischiatic nerve was involved.

Treatment: Most cases resolve naturally. However, if the condition is associated with long periods of recumbency, care must be taken to avoid exacerbation of the initial injury.

TIBIAL PARALYSIS

In tibial paralysis, there is paralysis of the extensors of the hock and flexors of the digits.

Etiology: The tibial nerve is the caudal branch of the ischiatic nerve, which, in its proximal course, is well protected by the gluteal muscles. Distally, it progresses beneath the tendon of the gastrocnemius muscle and can be damaged when the tendon is traumatized.

Clinical Findings: The hock joint is overflexed (dropped hock syndrome) and the fetlock is partially flexed. The gastrocnemius appears to be longer than normal and gives the impression that it or its tendon could be ruptured. The fetlock tends to be buckled, but the animal can walk and bear weight, although its attempts to do so are awkward. Compared with that seen in peroneal nerve injury, the gait disturbance is mild, but the postural disturbance could be permanent.

Treatment: The use of anti-inflammatory drugs may be of value in the early stages. However, the primary efforts should be directed toward ensuring that the animal does not injure itself further, by maintaining it on surfaces with good footing.

SPASTIC SYNDROME

Episodic, involuntary muscle contractions or spasms involving the hindlimbs are associated with postural and locomotor disturbances as well as spasticity. The condition may progress to posterior paresis or hindlimb paralysis. It is seen most frequently in Holstein and Guernsey cattle 3–7 yr old. Spastic syndrome is regarded as a genetic disease, possibly due to an autosomal dominant gene with incomplete penetrance. The pathology and pathophysiology remain obscure.

Clinical Findings: Clinical signs may vary in severity, duration, and frequency. Usually, some stimulus provokes the onset of clinical signs, such as the effort associated with rising or any factor that induces a significant emotional reaction. Pain, particularly in the feet or joints, may precipitate an attack. During an attack, the animal may be unable to move forward, stands trembling, and characteristically extends its hindlimbs backward. Between episodes, the animal can ambulate normally.

Treatment: Spastic syndrome is progressive, and because of the possibility of genetic transmission, animals (particularly bulls used for artificial insemination) are best eliminated as soon as a positive diagnosis is made. Palliative treatment for animals in the peak of production may be helpful. Mephenesin (30–40 mg/kg, PO, for 2–3 days) may be given during an episode. Phenylbutazone may also have beneficial effects.

SPASTIC PARESIS

(Elso heel)

Spastic paresis is a progressive unilateral or bilateral hyperextension of the hindlimb(s). It is seen sporadically in most breeds of cattle. Post-legged cattle are most frequently affected. Attempts to move are believed to simultaneously trigger contractions of both extensors and flexors of the limb. Spastic paresis is currently considered to be inherited via a recessive gene(s) with incomplete penetrance.

Clinical Findings: The disease may be seen within the first 6 mo of life. As the animal ages, the gastrocnemius muscles gradually contract. The hock and stifle become increasingly extended. Over a period of months, the hindlimbs become so stiff that the animal walks with short, pendulum-like steps. If only one limb is affected, the animal stands with the affected limb camped back and the sound limb held toward the midline to maintain balance. If both hindlimbs are affected, the animal may attempt to bear more weight on the forelimbs by holding them well back and simultaneously arching its back.

The quadriceps muscle has been implicated in the pathology of this disorder and can be distinguished from the form of the disorder affecting the gastrocnemius through use of a femoral nerve block.

Treatment: There is no successful medical treatment. Because spastic paresis is heritable, affected animals (especially breeding bulls) should be eliminated from the herd. Palliative surgical treatment may be attempted, although ethical issues should be considered when breeding stock is involved. The procedures, usually performed on calves, include complete tenotomy of the gastrocnemius tendon, which results in a dropped hock; complete tibial neurectomy, which results in sufficient relief to permit a steer to be finished for slaughter; and partial tenectomy of the two insertions of the gastrocnemius muscle and the calcanean tendon sheath, which overcomes the problem of the dropped hock.

SOFT-TISSUE DISORDERS CAUSING LAMENESS

CARPAL HYGROMA

Carpal hygroma is a localized swelling of tissues, including the precarpal bursa, dorsal to the carpal joint. It results from intermittent mild trauma to the precarpal area caused by lack of bedding or a poorly designed manger. *Brucella abortus* may be isolated from the false bursa of some cases in countries where this organism has not been controlled. The lesion is a firm swelling, possibly fluctuating and up to several inches in diameter, located over the dorsal aspect of the carpus. The hygroma is a lesion that is very difficult to resolve. The first step is to ascertain radiographically whether there is more than one cavity. Each cavity should be drained and infiltrated with a long-acting corticosteroid preparation. Surgical removal is messy, with little guarantee of a successful outcome. Introducing irritant materials into the cavity has had uncertain results. If the animal is milking and eating well, hygromas should be left untreated.

RUPTURE OF THE GASTROCNEMIUS MUSCLE

Rupture of the gastrocnemius muscle or tendon is relatively rare. It is most likely to be associated with deficiencies of calcium, phosphorus, and vitamin D. Prolonged recumbency, with resulting myositis and struggling to rise, occasionally precipitates rupture of these muscles. Occasionally, the condition has been associated with pyelonephritis, which presumably causes a myositis, weakening the muscle enough to permit rupture. Injections of irritating medicaments into the gastrocnemius muscle may cause necrosis and rupture.

The hock remains flexed. When the muscle is completely ruptured, the standing animal rests the hock and distal portion of the limb on the ground or walking surface, which is diagnostic, although rupture of the Achilles tendon may produce an identical gait.

Successful treatment is extremely unlikely in heavy adult animals. A leg cast or splint that maintains the hock in extension, supplying adequate vitamins and minerals, and proper nursing may be successful, but a long recovery period is required.

RUPTURE OF THE PERONEUS TERTIUS MUSCLE

The peroneus tertius muscle can be forcibly avulsed from its insertion by accidents associated with mounting or, more frequently, by the inexperienced use of ropes to restrain a hindlimb.

The hock is abnormally extended, while the stifle remains flexed. The animal cannot advance the limb normally, the calcanean tendon is flaccid, and the hooves may be dragged. The site of avulsion may be painful to the touch. A specific diagnostic feature is that the limb can be pulled backward without any resistance from the animal.

The condition may improve slowly if the animal is confined in a stall (loose) for several months.

TARSAL CELLULITIS

(Concrete hock)

Tarsal cellulitis is characterized by a firm, subcutaneous swelling on the lateral aspect of the hock that has little effect on joint mobility. It can include the formation of a false bursa. The condition is caused by severe abrasion of the skin and subcutaneous tissue overlying bony prominences. The skin may be excoriated by contact with concrete and particularly sharp curbs. Superficial abscesses must be drained extremely cautiously, because there is considerable danger of entering the joint. Padding and bandages should always be applied. Poultices rapidly reduce acute swelling.

LAMENESS IN GOATS

Abnormality of gait is a sign common to many diseases and conditions. A complete history is important for diagnosis and should include incidence and duration in the herd, nutrition, feed changes, method of rearing, and recent introductions to the herd. (*See also* HEALTH-MANAGEMENT INTERACTION: GOATS, p 2147.)

Some causes of lameness may be associated with systemic disease. Therefore, a thorough physical examination should always be performed, followed by a detailed examination of all four limbs, with a specific assessment of gait and mobility in an attempt to localize locomotor problems. In goats, as in other species, locomotor difficulties usually involve the musculoskeletal system directly, but conditions of the nervous system can mimic musculoskeletal disease and should be considered during the clinical examination.

The hoof of the affected leg(s) should be examined, and excess horn material removed to leave a level, weight-bearing surface. If the feet have not been trimmed recently, or the goats have been on soft ground or bedding, excess horn commonly overgrows from the walls, toes, and heels, and folds over the sole. With severe neglect, "sled-runner" or "Turkish slipper"–type hooves with elongated toes may cause the goat to walk on its heels. The following should be noted during foot trimming: any portion of the horn that is abnormally *thickened*, any underrunning of the heel or sole, any abnormal wear of one claw, or any abnormal or necrotic smell.

After trimming, the feet should be scrubbed clean and inspected for puncture wounds, foreign bodies such as stones or clover burrs caught in the interdigital space, or pus from a discharging abscess. Inspection should include the coronary band or coronet.

The rest of the leg should be palpated carefully, including the bones, tendons, and muscles. Any muscle atrophy or restriction of movement should be noted, and contralateral limb structures should be compared for signs of asymmetry. The joints also should be checked for heat, swelling, or pain.

If the clinical examination suggests joint involvement, it may be necessary to aseptically sample fluid from an affected joint for visual examination, cytology, Gram stain, and culture and sensitivity tests. Joint fluid containing pus alone, or with Gram-stained bacteria, indicates joint-ill; fibrin and pus combined suggest *Mycoplasma* spp; clear or cloudy joint fluid with many mononuclear cells suggests caprine arthritis-encephalitis virus (CAE, *see* p 747).

A blood or serum sample may also be useful to establish the underlying cause of lameness. In joint-ill, the WBC count is high due to neutrophilia. Blood calcium, phosphorus, and vitamin D levels may help diagnose epiphysitis or rickets, although blood levels often return to normal before the affected goat is examined. If CAE is suspected, the presence of antibody can be checked; however, false negatives may be seen during severe stress, and positive tests may be coincidental to another cause of lameness if seroprevalence of the CAE virus is high in the herd of origin.

Radiography may be helpful. In epiphysitis, the growth plates should be checked; there is also lateral deviation of the radii and occasionally thinness of the bone. In CAE virus infection, the initial swelling of the soft tissue surrounding the affected joint may be followed by calcium deposits in the swollen periarticular tissue, joint capsule, ligaments, tendons, and tendon sheaths. Later changes may include mild periarticular osteophyte production, "joint mice," and rough extensions of the periarticular bone proximally and distally.

Some of the more important conditions that cause lameness in goats are discussed below, listed in alphabetical order. The differential diagnosis in any case of lameness is influenced by geographic location, herd history, management practices, and other relevant factors.

CAPRINE ARTHRITIS AND ENCEPHALITIS

Caprine arthritis and encephalitis (CAE) virus infection has emerged during the past 35 yr as a major cause of disease, primarily in European breeds of dairy goats under intensive management. All breeds of goats are susceptible to this retrovirus, and prevalence of infection is related to exposure to virus. Two distinct forms of locomotor problems are seen. A neurologic form of the disease is seen in young goats, usually 2–4 mo old but as old as 1 yr. It is characterized by a progressive paresis with incoordination leading to paralysis, usually involving the hindlimbs and later the forelimbs. In older, adult goats, the virus infection manifests as a chronic, progressive arthritis involving one or more joints and usually involving the carpal joints. The initial sign is usually swelling of the affected joint(s), followed by progressive degeneration of articular and periarticular tissues with calcification, leading to decreased range of motion, ankylosis, and overt loss of mobility.

For a more detailed discussion, *see* p 747.

CONTRACTED TENDONS IN KIDS

Contracted tendons in newborn kids are seen sporadically in goats of all breeds throughout the world, usually with unexplained causation. However, there are two specific, inherited conditions of goats that result in contracted tendons of newborns.

A usually bilateral, congenital condition that is a genetic defect is seen in Angoras in Australasia. It is due to a recessive autosomal allele that must reach a certain level before affected animals appear; the time between purchase of a carrier buck and appearance of affected kids may be 5–6 generations. Either the fore- or hindlimbs are affected. In rare cases, only one forelimb is twisted. In severe cases, the kid is either unable to stand or walks on its fetlocks. In less severe cases, the kid may move relatively easily with fetlocks that are permanently partly flexed. In mild cases, the limbs may gradually be splinted straighter and straighter until the kid is able to bear weight on its feet.

Anglo-Nubians in the USA, Canada, Australia, and New Zealand can have a rare genetic condition called β-mannosidosis. At birth, affected kids have varying degrees of fixed flexion of the forelimbs and fixed extension of the hindlimbs. They can see, bleat, and suckle if held up to the teat. Their withdrawal reflexes are normal or depressed, and there is intention tremor, especially of the head. There may be nystagmus, deafness, and facial abnormalities. At necropsy, cutting the tendons allows free movement of the limbs. Histologic examination reveals typical lesions of lysosomal storage disease characterized by cellular vacuolation. Affected kids have no plasma levels of β-mannosidase, and both parents have levels half the normal range.

COPPER DEFICIENCY

Copper deficiency may cause locomotor difficulties in goats in two distinct ways. Abnormal bone growth with increased bone fragility can predispose to fractures of long bones. Independently, a neurologic condition known as enzootic ataxia or swayback develops, in which copper deficiency of kids in utero or after birth results in permanent myelin degeneration in the spinal cord, leading to progressive incoordination and paralysis with failure of mobility. Clinically, this appears similar to the neurologic form of caprine arthritis-encephalitis virus (*see* p 747) infection in young kids. Copper status of the ration needs to be evaluated, and copper supplementation provided as necessary.

EPIPHYSITIS

(Bent leg, Windswept)

Epiphysitis may result from imbalance in the calcium:phosphorus ratio. It is seen in young, rapidly growing kids (more often in males than in females) and in young does in late pregnancy or in the early stages of their first lactation. These does are young (eg, 12 mo), extremely heavy milkers, or carrying twins or triplets. Epiphysitis is sometimes compounded by rickets (*see* p 1051).

Clinical Findings and Diagnosis: Epiphysitis starts with lateral or medial bowing of one or both radii. Later changes may consist of lateral deviation of the digits on the fore- or hindfeet; lameness and reluctance to walk; an arched back; and soft swelling and pain in the carpal, metacarpophalangeal, tarsal, and metatarsophalangeal joints. Diagnosis of epiphysitis can be confirmed with radiography.

Conditions that have been implicated in its cause include an excess of dietary calcium with a calcium:phosphorus ratio of >1.4:1 (generally >1.8:1), excess protein intake, excess dietary iron, indoor housing of kids, or lack of vitamin D caused by prolonged overcast weather and low vitamin D levels in the feed. Carotene has an antivitamin D effect. Vitamin D has poor stability in prepared feed, especially when mixed with minerals. Alfalfa is high in calcium (1.4% calcium to 0.2% phosphorus) and protein. Owners frequently feed kids milk for prolonged periods because of a lack of commercial outlets for milk.

Treatment and Control: Once the probable cause(s) is identified, the diet should be corrected and the appropriate supplement given—usually injectable vitamin D and/or phosphorus or oral balanced calcium/phosphorus supplements.

Predisposing factors also must be corrected. The diet of growing kids should be changed to slow growth rate. The mating of young does <7 mo of age should be discouraged, and buck kids should be separated from doe kids by 3 mo of age to avoid unplanned matings. The diet for young does in milk with limb deformities should be corrected to allow for normal bone growth. Proper nutritional management stops limb deformities from worsening, and such deformities self-correct over time in most does.

FOOTROT AND FOOT SCALD

Footrot and foot scald are serious problems of sheep and can also have a major adverse impact on goats under certain management conditions (*see* p 2147).

JOINT-ILL

Several joints of kids can be involved in joint-ill, a nonspecific bacterial infection. Bacteria that have been incriminated are mainly gram-positive and include staphylococci, streptococci, *Corynebacterium* spp, *Actinomyces* spp, and *Erysipelothrix rhusiopathiae*, as well as gram-negative coliforms.

Environmental bacteria gain entry to the neonate's circulation, usually via the umbilical cord. Other methods of entry include contamination of breaks in the skin or via the GI or respiratory tract. Predisposing factors include lack of routine dipping of the umbilical cord; poor sanitation in the kidding pens; or does kidding in overcrowded, dirty conditions. *E rhusiopathiae* are soil-living bacteria that may persist on farms or in pens used by sheep or pigs. *Mycoplasma* infection is also a differential diagnosis (*see* p 1095).

Clinical Findings: With joint-ill, more than one joint is hot, swollen, and painful. Often, the affected limb(s) cannot bear weight, and kids with more than one leg affected may be unable to stand. The more commonly affected joints include the carpus, shoulder, hock, and stifle. Generally, there is a fever but no reduction in appetite. Sometimes the navel area is inflamed, but often there is no visible abnormality. An abscess may form on the navel long after the kid has recovered. The WBC count may be increased with a left shift.

If the condition becomes chronic, the limbs are stiff, some joints may be ankylosed, and overall growth is poor. At this stage the temperature is normal.

Treatment: To be successful, treatment must be given early and, when possible, antibiotic selection should be based on culture and sensitivity testing. Frequent injections of high doses of parenteral antibiotics given for ~1 wk may effect a cure if combined with careful nursing. Joint lavage with saline and antibiotic solutions may enhance therapeutic outcome in select cases. Complications should be prevented by providing soft bedding, frequently turning any kid unable to stand, and massaging the affected joints. If ankylosis starts to develop, the kid should be supported in a sling for short periods as frequently as possible.

In large, commercial herds, treating severely affected kids may not be economically justified, and humane euthanasia should be considered. Many that do recover remain unthrifty for the rest of their lives.

Control: Hygiene at parturition is essential. A deep bed of clean sawdust, wood shavings, or straw should be provided; it is often better to allow the doe to kid on fresh pasture if the weather is warm.

The umbilical cords of newborn kids should be dipped several times in strong, 7% tincture of iodine. Cords should be dipped each time the kid is handled in the first 24–48 hr. Owners should clean their footwear before entering kidding pens. Kids must receive adequate colostrum at birth.

LAMINITIS

(Founder)

Laminitis in goats is seen worldwide, but the incidence is lower than that in dairy cattle and horses. Predisposing causes include overeating or sudden access to concentrates, high-grain and low-roughage diets, or high-protein diets. Laminitis can also develop as a complication of acute infections such as mastitis, metritis, or pneumonia, especially after kidding.

When laminitis is severe, the affected goat is lame and reluctant to move; there is a fever, and all four feet are hot to the touch. Touching the coronary band elicits a severe pain reaction. In less severe cases, only the forefeet are affected. Laminitis can become chronic if the initial phase is not diagnosed or treated successfully. The onset is insidious, but eventually the goat is seen walking on its knees, with "sled-runner" deformities of its hooves.

In acute laminitis, the predisposing condition, if identifiable, must be corrected promptly. The laminitis is treated with analgesics such as daily parenteral flunixin meglumine, and hosing or soaking the affected feet is also useful. Although antihistamines are frequently used, their effectiveness in treatment of laminitis in goats remains unproved. Similarly, the use of corticosteroids is controversial because they may contribute to laminitis in horses, and they should not be used in pregnant does because of the risk of abortion. Chronic laminitis with deformed hooves is treated by routine, vigorous foot trimming.

MYCOPLASMOSIS

See also CONTAGIOUS AGALACTIA, p 1352, and CONTAGIOUS CAPRINE PLEUROPNEUMONIA, p 1474. Kids infected with *Mycoplasma mycoides mycoides* (large colony variant) or other *Mycoplasma* spp may show severe lameness with multiple hot swollen joints, weight loss, pyrexia, and poor coats. Some have diarrhea, and some have increased lung sounds and respiratory rates. Affected kids are generally 2–4 wk old. Morbidity and mortality rates of 90% and 30%, respectively, have been reported. Adult does with *Mycoplasma* infection may have mastitis and polyarthritis. Treatment is with tetracycline, tylosin, or tiamulin, but prognosis for complete recovery is guarded.

TRAUMA

Goats, in general, are agile creatures, but if frightened they may attempt impossible jumps, with resultant fractures or other injuries. Yards designed for goats that are infrequently handled should have a visual as well as physical barrier. Chain-link fences are often associated with limb fractures when used for goat enclosures. Fortunately, most fractures of the lower limbs heal rapidly with normal casting. Shearing of Angoras is a source of potential problems when the shearer's comb cuts into or through the Achilles tendon. Orthopedic procedures suitable for large dogs can be used. If goats are attacked by dogs or wild canines and survive, they often have multiple traumatic injuries that can include fractures.

Some IM injections can cause problems. For example, mixed clostridial vaccines can cause severe soft-tissue swelling and lameness for ≥48 hr. Irritant drugs can damage nearby nerves and cause lameness, particularly when thin or young goats are injected in the thigh muscles and the sciatic nerve is affected. In some cases of severe mastitis, especially gangrenous, there is a hindlimb lameness on the affected side as the doe changes her gait because of swelling and pain in the udder.

WHITE MUSCLE DISEASE

See also NUTRITIONAL MYODEGENERATION, p 1172. Most kids affected by white muscle disease have been in good condition and are 2–3 mo old (range, 1 wk to 4 mo). Commonly, sudden death is associated with cardiac muscle damage. Other kids are depressed, reluctant to move, and appear stiff, with a "sawhorse" stance, or become recumbent. Muscles, especially of the hindlimbs, are firm and painful to the touch. Treatment is with selenium and vitamin E injection in acute cases.

LAMENESS IN HORSES

Lameness is defined as an abnormal stance or gait caused by either a structural or a functional disorder of the locomotor system. The horse is either unwilling or unable to stand or move normally. Lameness is the most common cause of loss of use in horses. It can be caused by trauma, congenital or acquired disorders, infection, metabolic disorders, or nervous and circulatory system disease.

Lameness is not a disease per se but a clinical sign. It is a manifestation of pain, mechanical restrictions causing alteration of stance or gait, or neuromuscular disease. Pain is the most common cause of lameness in all horses. Mechanical lameness is best typified by complete upward fixation of the patella with its characteristic gait abnormality but can also be the result of fibrotic myopathy of the semitendinosus muscle or of restrictions caused by annular ligaments, adhesions, or severe fibrosis.

It is critical to correctly determine the cause of the lameness, because treatment varies greatly depending on the cause. For example, the mechanical lameness of complete upward fixation of the patella will not respond to analgesics, whereas lameness caused by pain often responds to systemic or local analgesics and anti-inflammatory drugs. Some causes of lameness produce very characteristic and classically described gaits. In fibrotic myopathy, a mechanical lameness, the affected limb is pulled back and down quickly before the end of the protraction phase, giving the impression that the foot "slaps down" on the ground. The signs are most obvious at the walk. In stringhalt, a neuromuscular disorder, the affected limb is hyperflexed during the cranial or swing phase, while the stepwise caudal jerking movement before foot contact does not occur. Unfortunately, many causes of lameness do not produce a characteristic gait abnormality, making diagnosis a challenge.

Pain-related lameness can be classified as weight bearing (supporting leg) or nonweight bearing (swinging leg) lameness. Although lameness is most often observed as a weight-bearing deficit, it may be composed of both. A supporting leg lameness is seen when the horse reduces the amount of time or reduces the amount of force applied to the weight-bearing limb. The most consistent and easily recognized clinical signs of lameness are the head nod associated with forelimb lameness and the sacral rise, also called a pelvic rise or hip hike, associated with hindlimb lameness. Hindlimb lameness should be assessed from the side as well as from behind, because this provides an opportunity to assess arc of foot flight, duration of protraction and retraction phases, length of weight-bearing phase, and the presence or absence of a sacral rise. Forelimb lameness should be observed from the front and side. Hindlimb and forelimb lameness in many horses will be accentuated when the horse is worked in a circle with the affected limb on the inside.

Factors that predispose horses to lameness include physical immaturity, which may occur in premature or dysmature foals, and training older foals before maturity. Other factors include preexisting developmental orthopedic disease (eg, osteochondrosis, flexural limb and angular limb deformities); poor conformation; improper hoof balance or shoeing; failure to adequately condition performance horses; monotonous repetitive stresses on bones, tendons, ligaments, and joints in performance horses; hard, slippery, or rocky surfaces upon which horses work; and extremely athletic activities. Inciting factors in lameness include direct or indirect trauma, fatigue resulting in incoordination of muscles (which often occurs in racehorses at the end of races), inflammation, infection, and failure to recognize early disease before it creates significant pain.

Lameness in one part of a limb often results in secondary soreness in another area of the same limb and may result in lameness of the contralateral forelimb or hindlimb from overuse due to compensation. The entire horse should be evaluated for secondary lameness even when the cause of the primary problem is obvious. Secondary lamenesses are very common in performance horses but may occur in all types of horses. A dramatic example of a secondary lameness occurs when biomechanical laminitis develops in the normal contralateral limb of a horse with limited weight bearing from a severe orthopedic problem causing shifting of weight from the injured limb to the normal limb.

THE LAMENESS EXAMINATION

A systematic investigation of a lame horse may be time consuming when the cause is not obvious. The examination benefits from standardized facilities such as a level, firm, nonslip surface to walk and trot the horse and a soft support area to lunge and ride the horse. The examiner must be knowledgeable in equine anatomy, normal conformation and gaits, regional anesthesia, and imaging techniques and be able to recognize forelimb and hindlimb lameness.

The examination begins with a comprehensive medical history; type, age, and training regimen may give important clues to the lameness, as will the time since onset of lameness, interim management, and any suggestions that the lameness may improve with either rest or exercise. The interval since the last shoeing should also be noted. Response to anti-inflammatory or analgesic medications may provide useful information. Results of hematologic and biochemical analyses may shed light on other problems that influence overall performance.

Although valuable, modern diagnostic imaging techniques are no substitute for detailed visual inspection and thorough manual palpation of the limbs in weightbearing and nonweightbearing positions. Conformation should be evaluated and the horse visually checked for symmetry, swellings, muscle loss, abnormal stance, and obvious injuries. The trunk and limbs should be palpated for heat, pain, swellings, and joint effusion. The high degree of variation between horses should be remembered, and comparison with the contralateral limb should always be done, although the latter may not necessarily be a useful control. The reaction of the horse to palpation and the range of flexion and extension of all joints should be noted. The feet should be thoroughly examined, including compression of the walls and sole with hoof testers. Wear patterns of shoes and feet should be noted. A number of abnormalities such as broken toe/pastern axis; mismatched hoof angles; under-run, contracted, and sheared heels; and disproportionate hoof size are seen more frequently in lame than in sound horses. Shoes should be left on during the initial stages of the examination, because removing them might make the horse footsore and preclude further examination with the horse being trotted or ridden. Shoes should be removed for complete and thorough examination of the foot when the lameness has been localized to the foot and any exercise needed for diagnosis has been completed.

The back and neck should be thoroughly examined with the horse restrained and standing square on a level surface. Flexibility and extensibility of the back can be checked by alternately pinching the midline in the midthoracic and sacrococcygeal regions, whereas lateral flexion can be checked by turning the horse short around its own axis.

Examination during exercise is often required to localize the lameness to a specific limb or site and to evaluate the response to diagnostic regional anesthesia. If lameness is major and acute and a fracture is suspected, exercise should not be undertaken or a catastrophic breakdown may result. Similarly, diagnostic regional anesthesia should not be performed when a fracture is suspected. It is important to determine whether the horse may have been given analgesic medication before the lameness examination.

Recognition of lameness is a key skill to successful diagnosis. The most consistent sign of a unilateral forelimb lameness is the head nod. The head and neck of the horse rise when the lame forelimb strikes the ground and is weightbearing, and fall when the sound limb strikes the ground. The sacral (pelvic) rise is the most consistent and easily observed sign of hindlimb lameness. The entire pelvis and sacrum rise when the lame limb strikes the ground and is weight bearing, and fall when the sound limb strikes the ground. Both head nod and sacral rise serve to reduce concussion on the lame limb. A computerized, handheld gait analysis system that objectively measures the head nod and sacral rise is available to detect lameness and is being used by some veterinarians.

The horse should initially be examined by walking and jogging in hand with a loose line to the halter so that the movement of the horse is not restricted. A firm, nonslippery surface (eg, hardpack fine gravel) is ideal to trot on a straight line and to lunge on a firm surface. It also provides an opportunity to listen to the footfall and consider this information along with the visual appraisal. However, feet of different sizes and shapes and different shoes make slightly different impact sounds, often rendering these sounds of little diagnostic value. Frequently, lameness is more pronounced when the horse is worked in a circle. Circling can be done on a lunge line, free exercise in a large round pen, in hand, or under saddle. Lungeing on asphalt or concrete predisposes the horse to slipping and injury but may be done in selected cases to accentuate a very subtle hoof or lower limb lameness. Both forelimb and hindlimb lameness may become worse when the horse is circled; most of the time, the lameness is accentuated when the affected limb is on the inside of the circle.

Flexion tests are useful diagnostic tools. The range of movement and response to passive flexion, along with any suggestion of increased lameness or onset of lameness after flexion, should be observed. The distal phalanges in both forelimbs and hindlimbs should be flexed independently of the carpus and hock to obtain maximal information. Bending pressure should be firm but not excessive, which can create false-positive responses. All tests should be done on both sound and lame limbs for comparison. Consistency should always be applied, and individual experience used. A single positive flexion test without associated lameness may not be of significance.

To establish consistency, the entire examination should involve the same handler, the same bitting when the horse is under saddle, and the same surfaces under foot. The horse should be controlled so that it is trotting at a useful, repeatable pace to evaluate the lameness. Very slight sedation of nervous or fractious horses with 3 mg romifidine or 100 mg xylazine may result in a horse with a more relaxed outline and allow a better assessment without seemingly influencing the degree of lameness. Slowing down the pace at the trot often illustrates a subtle lameness better, because the horse loses its momentum and struggles with suspension in the affected limb(s).

A ridden assessment of the horse may be necessary, particularly with a subtle lameness that can only be observed under saddle. A multiple-limb lameness without an obvious single-limb lameness may also be detected. The clinical signs may be minor (eg, the horse refusing certain movements or activities, slight head tilts, or tail swishing). However, a good rider can, often inadvertently, hide a problem by his or her inherent expertise and ability to "correct" difficulties.

Occasionally, a horse appears to be sound when lunged and ridden, but the rider feels that the performance is impaired. In such cases, it may be worth working the horse on concomitant analgesic or anti-inflammatory medication at therapeutic levels for an adequate period (eg, phenylbutazone 2–3 g/day, PO, for 7–14 days) to assess whether improvement occurs. Some clinical signs purported to be caused by lameness are training problems. If improvement on medication occurs, the medication should be withdrawn and diagnostic anesthesia used beginning in an arbitrary limb, most often a forelimb. In this way, multiple-limb lamenesses (as many as four), often mimicking the clinical picture associated with back pain, can be evaluated and treated.

Diagnostic regional anesthesia (*see* p 1101) should be used to determine the area of pain in all lame horses in which the lameness can be localized to a specific limb but not to a specific site on the limb. A consistently observable lameness must be present for the clinician to evaluate response to anesthesia.

Because lameness may be caused by neuromuscular disorders, a complete neurologic examination should be part of the lameness examination whenever an obvious painful or mechanical cause has not been found. The examination should include evaluation of cranial nerve and upper and lower motor neuron function.

Observing the horse execute movements such as turning short, backing, "hopping" on one forelimb (with the other forelimb held up), negotiating a curb, turning in tight circles, and walking uphill and downhill should be done. These tests help determine whether reduced proprioception, weakness, or spasticity may be the cause of the gait abnormality.

IMAGING TECHNIQUES

Imaging techniques provide important pathologic and physiologic information necessary to treat specific conditions. Imaging can be divided into anatomic and physiologic methods. Anatomic imaging methods include radiology, ultrasonography, CT, and MRI. Physiologic imaging methods include scintigraphy and thermography. When diagnostic analgesia has failed to eliminate the lameness, the lameness is too subtle for localization by diagnostic analgesia, or the horse is not amenable to handling or injection, physiologic imaging techniques may help narrow the problem to a specific region. Anatomic imaging methods can then be used to evaluate those areas. Imaging may also help prevent injury. This requires early detection of the physiologic changes associated with injury. Although frequent use of an anatomic imaging method can detect change in one region, physiologic imaging allows assessment of the entire horse on a routine basis.

Anatomic Imaging Techniques

Radiologic techniques are the methods most commonly used to evaluate lameness in horses. Plain film radiography used to be the standard, but it has been replaced by computed radiography in equine practice. Computed radiography can be divided into indirect and direct. Indirect uses a special plate instead of film. The plate stores energy that is then read by a computer to produce the image. Direct digital radiography also uses a special plate, but the radiation is converted to a digital signal and sent directly to a computer. Direct digital radiography produces images faster, but both share the advantages of fewer retakes, a lower radiation requirement, and post processing techniques that eliminate contrast problems. Radiography requires multiple projections to evaluate any area. It allows assessment of bony tissues and reflects both acute and chronic changes. Occasionally, radiographic techniques that provide more information are needed. Contrast radiography provides information about articular cartilage and surfaces and is of particular value in determining whether subchondral cysts communicate with the joint and in delineating subcutaneous tracts. More recently, these techniques have been used to delineate changes in the navicular bursa and have produced 60% more information than plain radiography. Pathologic diagnoses are usually made by radiography in conjunction with clinical examination.

The goal of radiology, regardless of system used, is to examine the region sufficiently to fully evaluate the anatomic structure. Diagnostic films require preparation, positioning, and production. Preparation involves readying the object to be radiographed. In most cases, this requires the object to be clean and all foreign materials removed (eg, any iodine-based products on the limb will cause artifacts on the radiograph). For radiographs of the hoof, the shoe may need to be removed and the sulci packed, in addition to cleaning.

Positioning is critical; the object must be evaluated from a sufficient number of angles to ensure adequate evaluation. Minimally, this means two radiographs 90° apart. Many of the limbs require more views for adequate evaluation. Examination of those projections may necessitate further views to better assess any areas of interest. For instance, the equine foot, fetlock, and carpus require five projections, whereas the pastern and hock require four. The upper limbs of the horse require fewer projections. This is not because these are less complex areas; rather, the size of the horse makes it difficult to get more projections. Two views can usually be made of the elbow and the stifle. For the shoulder joint, usually only one view is possible. For the hip, anesthesia is usually required. However, digital radiography has made it possible to take standing hip projections on young horses and those with smaller muscle mass.

Production of good radiographs requires the correct exposure of the film. Proper kVp and mA settings, as well as proper focal film distance, are critical. Unfortunately, these factors vary and depend on the particular x-ray machine and the film or electronic system used. For ambulatory equine practitioners, another factor that must be considered is the electricity output in the barn where the images are taken—older barns may not have sufficient electrical output for the x-ray generator to make the desired exposure. New computed radiography systems that are battery operated can avoid these types of electrical problems.

Ultrasonographic examination can be used to assess any soft tissues. Like radiography, the area to be examined should be evaluated in two planes 90° apart. Selection of a probe should take into account the depth, contour, and location of the tissue to be examined. The deeper the tissue to be evaluated, the lower the wavelength of the probe used. The higher the wavelength, the greater the detail that can be achieved. For examination of superficial and deep flexor tendons or the suspensory ligament, a 7.5–10 MHz linear probe is best. Examination of complex anatomic areas such as the foot or pelvic region requires a convex linear probe. Examination of the pelvic region internally requires a rectal linear probe.

Ultrasonography is most useful in the evaluation of tendons and ligaments but can also be used to evaluate muscle and cartilage. In all cases, tissue fiber alignment and echogenicity are the factors used to determine anatomic disruption. Generally speaking, loss of fiber alignment and decreased echogenicity are signs of acute injury; increased echogenicity is generally thought to indicate chronic conditions. However, if any questions arise during the examination, the opposite limb or area can be examined to compare changes. For the novice ultrasonographer, it is a good idea to compare the right and left sides before making an ultrasonographic diagnosis.

Assessment of anatomic changes serves as the basis for any pathologic diagnosis, as well as being important in determining prognosis. For these purposes, radiography and ultrasonography are complementary. Radiography provides information regarding bony tissues, whereas ultrasonography provides information about the soft tissues that connect bone or provide support.

MRI and CT are high-detail anatomic imaging tools. Their use is becoming more common in equine lameness evaluations. MRI in particular has become quite popular. Two types of MRI are available: low-field and high-field magnets. High-field scanners produce a stronger signal and higher resolution pictures in a shorter time than low-field scanners. However, some low-field scanners can be used to examine the standing, sedated horse, whereas high-field scanners require the horse to be anesthetized. The standing units can only be used to evaluate from the carpus and hock distally. Because of the slower image acquisition with the low-field scanners, motion can be a problem. MRI provides sliced images of the anatomic region of interest. The slices are usually in three different planes: axial (transverse), sagittal (longitudinal), and dorsal. MRI of orthopedic disease is performed in several acquisition sequences. Each sequence displays different anatomic, physiologic, and pathologic information. The most common sequences are the proton density and the T1-weighted and T2-weighted images. Proton density provides the most anatomic detail. T1-weighted images highlight the structural characteristics of bone and soft tissues, whereas T2-weighted images emphasize the fluid characteristics of tissues and are sensitive for detecting synovial effusions, cysts, and edema. Special sequences can further clarify or highlight a lesion. For instance, fat-suppressed sequences are used to evaluate edema in high-fat signal areas such as the bone marrow.

CT is a technology that uses very small x-ray beams from many different angles around the body (called a slice) that are reconstructed by computer to produce an image. Because the images are in slices, there is less interference from surrounding anatomy. Therefore, the CT scanner provides the clearest images possible of the limbs, joints, nasal passages, skull, sinus cavities, and neck. These images improve the clinician's ability to accurately define and identify the extent of abnormalities of these regions.

Physiologic Imaging Techniques

These techniques provide images that reflect physiologic processes. Unlike anatomic imaging, which reflects structure, physiologic imaging techniques assess metabolism or circulation. Thermography and scintigraphy allow examination of the entire horse. When combined with a thorough clinical examination, these methods help identify injuries that may otherwise go undetected.

Thermography is the pictorial representation of the surface temperature of an object. It is a noninvasive technique that measures emitted heat in the form of infrared radiation and helps detect inflammatory changes that may contribute to lameness. Relative blood flow dictates the thermal pattern; normal thermal patterns can be predicted based on vascularity and surface contour. Skin overlying muscle is also subject to temperature increase during muscle activity. Circulation is invariably altered in injured or diseased tissues. Thermographically, the "hot spot" associated with the localized inflammation generally is seen in the skin directly overlying the injury. However, diseased tissues may have a reduced blood supply due to swelling, vessel thrombosis, or tissue infarction. With such lesions, the area of decreased heat is usually surrounded by increased thermal emissions, probably due to shunting of blood. The American Academy of Thermology has published guidelines for the use of infrared thermography in veterinary medicine. The purpose of the guidelines is to provide criteria for the production of reliable and repeatable thermal images.

During scintigraphy, polyphosphonate radiopharmaceuticals are given IV. Their distribution is then measured by a gamma camera, which measures the radiation emitted from the radiopharmaceutical after it is distributed through the body. The polyphosphonates bind rapidly to exposed hydroxyapatite crystal, generally in areas where bone is actively remodelling. Because inflammation causes an increase in blood flow, capillary permeability, and extracellular fluid volume, inflamed tissues accumulate high levels of radiopharmaceutical during the soft-tissue phase of scintigraphy, allowing evaluation of soft-tissue injuries. During the bone phase, the radiopharmaceutical accumulates in areas of increased remodelling or vascularity. Because injured bone is remodelled more rapidly, scintigraphy helps detect lesions in bone and ligaments, particularly to identify enthesopathy (damage to the insertions of tendons and ligaments on bone).

ARTHROSCOPY

(Tenoscopy, Bursoscopy)

Arthroscopy is the accepted way to perform joint surgery in horses and is a valuable tool in the diagnosis of joint disease. Arthroscopic surgery can be used to remove bone and cartilage fragments, debride damaged ligaments and menisci, assist the repair of articular fractures with internal fixation, debride or inject subchondral bone cysts, repair cartilage, and debride and flush contaminated or septic synovial cavities. Arthroscopy is a valuable method to evaluate intrasynovial structures and is particularly useful to evaluate soft-tissue structures such as ligaments, cartilage, menisci, and synovial membranes. It should be used in concert with other diagnostic methods, including high-quality radiographs, ultrasonography, and CT and MRI when available. Diagnostic arthroscopy is the most sensitive and specific tool for intra-articular evaluation in horses. Athroscopes of 2.5–5 mm diameter can be placed in all joints of the equine limbs; however, not all areas of every joint can be examined. The arthroscope has also been used to examine, diagnose, and perform surgery on structures within the digital, carpal, and tarsal tendon sheaths (tenoscopy) and in the navicular, calcaneal, and bicipital bursas (bursoscopy).

Advantages of arthroscopy compared with standard surgical procedures include the use of small stab incisions for placement of the arthroscope and instruments, the ability to view numerous areas of the joint, easy operations on more than one joint during the same surgical procedure, less trauma to periarticular soft tissues, less pain, reduced convalescent times, and reduced complications.

Diagnostic and surgical arthroscopy is technically demanding, and extensive experience is necessary to become proficient. Good knowledge of joint anatomy and good hand-eye coordination and spatial awareness are essential characteristics of successful surgeons.

Most arthroscopic procedures are performed with the horse under general anesthesia. Many surgeons prefer dorsal recumbency to allow surgical access to all sides of the joint, to allow surgery on multiple joints and limbs, and to control hemorrhage. Routine aseptic surgical preparation and draping is necessary. Basic equipment required for arthroscopy includes an arthroscope and insertion sleeve, light source and cable, fluid pump for joint distention, egress cannula, and an assortment of hand instruments for intra-articular procedures. A video camera and video screen are highly recommended to decrease the risk of contamination, to improve visualization and depth perception, and to allow capture of images and videos. Triangulation techniques are used to optimize manipulation of intra-articular instruments.

Arthroscopy, bursoscopy, and tenoscopy are often used to evaluate and treat contaminated synovial cavities. The techniques facilitate wound debridement, removal of fibrin and foreign debris, and copious flushing of the cavities without inducing more trauma from a major incision. The normal intrasynovial environment can recover quickly. Bursoscopy of the navicular bursa has greatly reduced the need for the streetnail procedure to treat punctures of the navicular bursa and has reduced the morbidity of calcaneal infections after injury to the hock. Tenoscopy has improved the recovery rate of septic tenosynovitis in horses.

REGIONAL ANESTHESIA

Regional anesthesia is a valuable diagnostic aid used to localize lameness when, after a thorough clinical examination, the site of pain remains uncertain. Localizing pain allows other diagnostic procedures, such as anesthesia of a joint, radiography, ultrasonography, CT, scintigraphy, or MRI to be used more effectively and economically to identify the cause of lameness. Additionally, use of regional anesthesia allows some surgical procedures to be performed without the need for general anesthesia, and it can be used to provide temporary, humane relief of pain.

Lidocaine HCl (2%) and mepivacaine HCl (2%) are the local anesthetic agents most commonly used to induce regional anesthesia during the lameness examination. Mepivacaine HCl is preferred by most clinicians, because it causes less tissue reaction than lidocaine HCl. Bupivacaine HCl is used to induce regional anesthesia for humane relief of pain, because it provides anesthesia that lasts 4–6 hr.

The choice of anesthetic agent may depend on its duration of action. The anesthetic effect of mepivacaine HCl, which lasts 90–120 min, makes this agent valuable for examining a horse with lameness in multiple limbs or if multiple sites of pain on a limb are suspected. Lidocaine HCl, which has an anesthetic effect of only 30–45 min, might be the preferred local anesthetic agent when different techniques of diagnostic analgesia are likely to be used during the lameness examination.

Most nerves below the carpus or hock are anesthetized using a 25-gauge, 5/8-in. (1.59-cm) needle. A 1½-in. (3.8-cm), larger-gauge needle (eg, 22- or 20-gauge) is used to anesthetize nerves located more proximally on the limb. If a relatively large-gauge needle is to be used, SC deposition of a small amount of local anesthetic solution, using a 25-gauge needle, may avoid resentment by the horse when the larger-gauge needle is inserted.

To avoid broken or bent needles during perineural administration of local anesthetic solution, the needle should always be inserted detached from the syringe. Spinal needles are flexible and more likely to bend than break and, thus, safer to use if there is a possibility the horse may move the limb. Using a flexible needle is especially important when the difference in range of movement between skin and deeper tissues is large, in case the horse moves during injection. Luer-lock syringes should not be used because they are difficult to attach to the needle after it is inserted, and this type of syringe cannot be detached quickly from the needle to prevent the needle from being pulled out, bent, or broken if the horse moves during the procedure. The needle should be directed distally during insertion when anesthetizing nerves in the distal portion of the limb. Directing the needle proximally may result in proximal migration of anesthetic solution and unintended anesthesia of more proximal branches of the nerve, thus confusing the results of the examination.

When the goal of regional anesthesia is to identify a site of pain below the carpus or hock, only the smallest effective volume of anesthetic solution should be administered to avoid inadvertent anesthesia of adjacent nerves. When the nerve can be palpated subcutaneously, a very small volume of local analgesic solution can be used because the solution can be placed more accurately into the fascia surrounding the nerve.

Before regional anesthesia is performed, the horse should be consistently and sufficiently lame so that any improvement in gait can be detected. Lungeing or riding the horse may exacerbate a subtle lameness. The lameness of some horses improves or resolves during exercise; for these horses, a false-positive response to regional anesthesia may result if the horse has not been sufficiently exercised before it is examined. If a horse is subtly lame, using a wireless, inertial sensor–based system designed to evaluate lameness allows objective interpretation of results of diagnostic analgesia.

Relief of pain and resolution of lameness after local anesthetic solution is

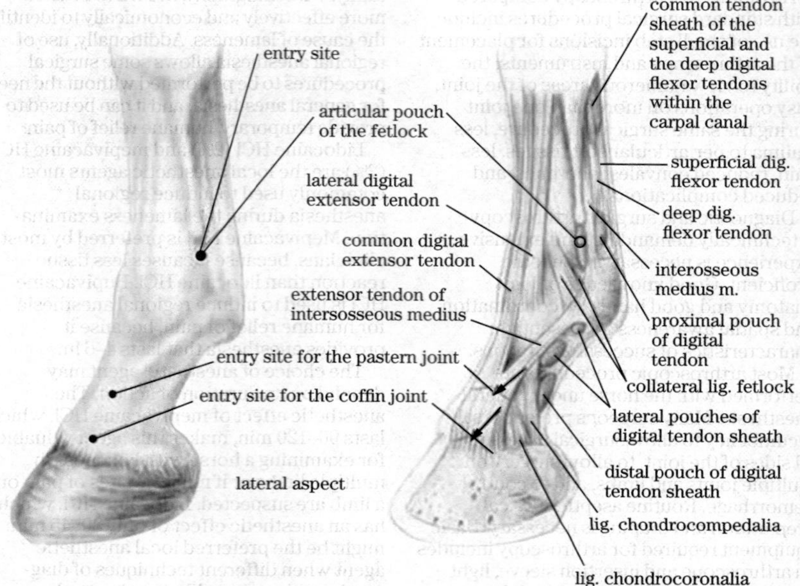

Arthroscopy and arthrocentesis joint entry sites in the digit, lateral aspect, horse. *Illustration by Dr. Gheorghe Constantinescu.*

administered into the fascia surrounding a nerve in the distal portion of the limb usually occurs within 5 min, but anesthesia of larger nerves in the proximal portion of the limb may take 20–40 min. Results of a regional nerve block can be misinterpreted if the horse's gait is assessed before the onset of pain relief. When assessing the effects of anesthesia of nerves in the distal portion of the limb, the clinician should keep in mind that anesthetic solution might migrate up the nerve to anesthetize more proximal structures, thus confusing the results of the examination. To avoid this complication, the gait should be evaluated within 15 min after administering a regional nerve bock in the distal portion of the limb. When a regional nerve block is administered in the proximal portion of the limb, the horse may develop a gait abnormality or stumble because of altered proprioception. When nerves above the hock or carpus are anesthetized, it may be prudent to assess the horse's gait on a soft surface or after bandaging the distal portion of the limb so that abrasion to skin over the dorsum of the fetlock is avoided if the horse stumbles.

If the gait is unchanged after regional anesthesia, the effectiveness of the nerve block should be determined by checking for skin sensation within the dermatome expected to be desensitized. Skin sensation is assessed by pressing the tip of a ballpoint pen, key, or similar instrument over the skin covering the region intended to be desensitized. For a fractious horse, skin sensation is more safely checked with the limb held or from a distance using a blunt instrument taped to a 3-ft pole. A well-behaved, stoic horse may not react to stimulation of skin even though regional anesthesia was ineffective. For such a horse, reaction to cutaneous stimulation should be assessed before regional anesthesia is performed, or reaction to cutaneous stimulation of the same dermatome on the contralateral limb should be assessed.

When performing regional anesthesia, especially in the distal portion of the limb, local anesthetic solution can be administered inadvertently into a blood vessel, joint, tendon sheath, or bursa. Aspiration before injection may indicate that the needle has been placed within a blood vessel. Administering the anesthetic solution as the needle is withdrawn decreases the likelihood of depositing the solution in an unintended structure and results in deposition of the solution in more than one tissue plane, which increases the likelihood of the solution contacting the nerve.

Opinions vary concerning the amount of skin preparation necessary before administering regional anesthesia. For short-haired horses, the site of injection is often prepared by wiping the site with cotton pledgets or gauze sponges soaked in 70% isopropyl alcohol until a pledget or sponge appears clean. If the site of injection is particularly dirty, it should be scrubbed with antiseptic soap. The consequences of a nonsterile, SC injection are usually minimal, but inadvertent, nonsterile injection of a tendon sheath or joint could result in septic synovitis.

Regional anesthesia of the distal portion of the limb can be accomplished in most horses using minimal restraint, but for fractious horses or for horses previously subjected to regional anesthesia, using a lip twitch or lip chain is prudent. The twitch works best when applied immediately before placing the needle. If this does not provide sufficient restraint, xylazine (0.2 mg/kg) or detomidine (10 mcg/kg) can be given IV. Acepromazine has no analgesic effect and, therefore, is less likely to ameliorate lameness than is a sedative, such as xylazine or detomidine, which provides some analgesia. In fact, some clinicians claim that acepromazine accentuates subtle lameness, possibly by making the horse less aware of its environment and, therefore, more aware of pain in the lame limb. The degree to which sedation or tranquilization interferes with assessment of gait depends on the severity of lameness and the skill of the clinician performing the examination.

Restraining the horse in stocks to administer regional anesthesia of the distal portion of the limb increases the likelihood of injury to the clinician. Regional anesthesia of the distal portion of the limb usually requires multiple injections, which is most safely accomplished with the limb held. When a nerve block is performed with the horse's limb on the ground, the contralateral limb can be lifted off the ground to enhance the safety of the procedure for the clinician.

When anesthetizing the foot of a forelimb, most clinicians prefer to hold the limb while facing in the opposite direction as the horse; however, some clinicians prefer to anesthetize the foot while facing the same direction as the horse. When facing the same direction as the horse, the foot can be held between the clinician's knees to free both hands for the procedure, but the clinician is at risk of injury if the horse swings its limb caudally. When the clinician faces the opposite direction as the horse, the procedure is performed using one hand because the other hand must hold the limb.

Nerve blocks performed distal to the fetlock of the pelvic limb are most safely performed with the pelvic limb stretched caudally and held on the thigh of the clinician performing the block.

Complications of regional nerve blocks are rare but include a broken needle shaft, SC infection, and infection of a synovial structure adjacent to the nerve anesthetized. Local anesthetic solution is detectable systemically, which could create a problem for a horse participating in a competition if the horse's serum is examined for the presence of drugs.

Regional Anesthesia of the Forelimb

Because perineural analgesia should start distally and progress proximally, the **palmar digital nerve (PDN) block** is the most commonly performed regional nerve block of the forelimb. The PDN block is performed with the limb held. The needle is inserted directly over the palpable neurovascular bundle ~1 cm proximal to the cartilage of the foot. The needle is directed distally, and 1.5 mL of local anesthetic solution is deposited near the junction of the nerve and the cartilage of the foot. The PDN block is sometimes called a "heel block," but this terminology is erroneous because the block anesthetizes the entire foot, including the distal interphalangeal (coffin) joint. For a few horses, the PDN block may also cause at least partial anesthesia of the proximal interphalangeal (pastern) joint, especially if a large volume of local anesthetic solution (eg, >3 mL) is injected.

If the horse's gait does not improve after a PDN block, some clinicians next administer a **semi-ring block at the pastern** to anesthetize the dorsal branches of the digital nerve that supply the foot. Because the dorsal branches of the digital nerve contribute little to sensation within the foot, a semi-ring block at the pastern is unlikely to improve the gait if a PDN block failed to improve it.

Most clinicians proceed to a **basisesamoid nerve block** if the horse's lameness is not reduced with a PDN block. With this regional nerve block, the palmar nerves are anesthetized at the level of the base of the proximal sesamoid bones, before the nerve branches into the dorsal and palmar digital nerves. When performing an abaxial sesamoid nerve block, 2.5–3 mL of local anesthetic solution is deposited at the base of the proximal sesamoid bones over the neurovascular bundle, which is easily palpated at this location. More proximal deposition of local anesthetic solution may anesthetize a portion of the fetlock joint. Positive response to a basisesamoid nerve block, performed after a PDN block has failed to ameliorate lameness, localizes the site of pain causing lameness to the pastern.

The low **palmar nerve block**, or **low 4-point block**, is performed after a negative response to the abaxial sesamoid nerve block. This nerve block is usually performed with the horse bearing weight on the limb, but it can also be performed with the limb held. The medial and lateral palmar nerves are anesthetized, using a 25-gauge, 5/8-in. needle, by depositing 2 mL of local anesthetic solution over each palmar nerve where it lies subcutaneously at the dorsal border of the deep digital flexor tendon. The palmar nerves should be blocked at the level of the metacarpus to avoid the possibility of misdirecting a needle into the digital flexor sheath, which often extends proximally to the level of the end of the splint bones. When the palmar nerves are blocked at the level of the middle of the metacarpus, the communicating branch that connects them, the ramus communicans, should also be blocked with 1 mL of local anesthetic solution. Blocking one palmar nerve proximal to the ramus communicans and the other distal to it allows sensory impulses to propagate through the ramus from the side blocked proximal to the ramus and then proximally through the palmar nerve blocked distal to the ramus. Though easily palpated on the forelimb, the ramus communicans is often nonexistent or impossible to palpate on the pelvic limb. To complete the 4-point block, 1–2 mL of local anesthetic solution is deposited SC at the distal end of each splint bone, where the palmar metacarpal nerve lies next to the periosteum of the third metacarpal bone. A positive response to a low 4-point block, performed after a negative response to an abaxial sesamoid nerve block, localizes the site of pain causing lameness to the fetlock.

The **high palmar nerve block**, or **high 4-point block**, can be performed when the low 4-point block fails to improve lameness. With the limb bearing weight, the medial and lateral palmar and palmar metacarpal nerves are anesthetized slightly distal to the level of the carpometacarpal joint. To anesthetize a palmar nerve, a 25-gauge, 5/8-in. needle is inserted through fascia to where the nerve lies near the dorsal border of the deep digital flexor tendon, and 3–5 mL of anesthetic solution is deposited over the nerve.

Anesthetizing the medial and lateral palmar nerves alone desensitizes the flexor tendons and inferior check ligament. With the limb held or bearing weight, the palmar metacarpal nerves are anesthetized slightly

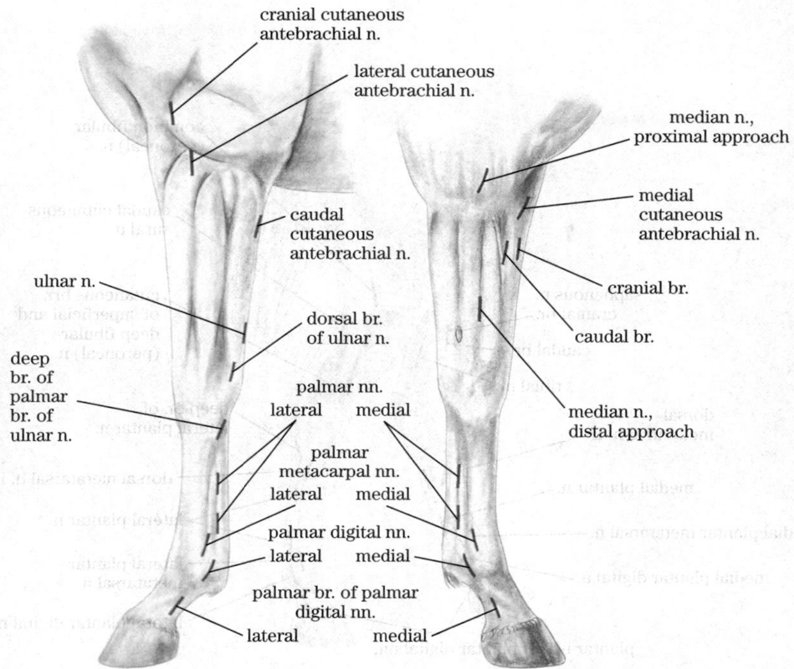

Landmarks for nerve block of the forelimb, horse. *Illustration by Dr. Gheorghe Constantinescu.*

distal to the level of the carpometacarpal joint by inserting a 20- to 22-gauge, 1 ½-in. needle into the angle formed by the junction of the third metacarpal bone and the second or fourth metacarpal bone. Anesthetizing the medial and lateral palmar metacarpal nerves alone desensitizes the splint bones and their interosseous ligaments and the proximal aspect of the suspensory ligament.

An easier alternative to the high palmar nerve block, when the site of pain causing lameness is suspected to be in the proximal portion of suspensory ligament, is the **lateral palmar nerve block**, which is performed, with the limb bearing weight, by inserting a 25-gauge, 5/8-in. needle over the lateral palmar nerve where it courses over the medial aspect of the accessory carpal bone. The needle is inserted in a medial to lateral direction at the distal third of a palpable groove, and 2 mL of local anesthetic solution is deposited. Because the medial and lateral palmar metacarpal nerves arise from the deep branch of the lateral palmar nerve distal to this site, the structures they innervate, such as the proximal aspect of the suspensory ligament, are desensitized.

If the site of pain causing lameness cannot be localized by performing the previously discussed nerve blocks, most clinicians perform joint blocks of the carpus, elbow, or shoulder. The order in which these synovial structures are desensitized is not important. The median and ulnar nerves are sometimes anesthetized simultaneously as part of a lameness evaluation to exclude pain below the elbow as the cause of lameness, but more commonly, they are anesthetized along with the medial cutaneous antebracheal nerve to allow surgery of the limb without the need for general anesthesia.

Regional Anesthesia of the Pelvic Limb

Techniques to administer regional anesthesia of the distal portion of the pelvic limb are

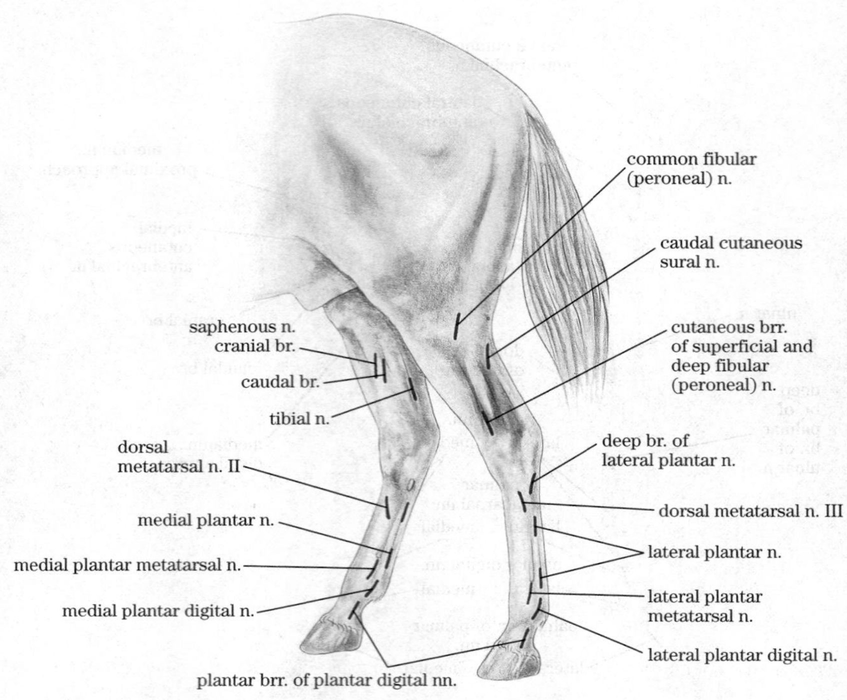

Landmarks for nerve block of the horse pelvic limb. *Illustration by Dr. Gheorghe Constantinescu.*

slightly different than the techniques to administer regional anesthesia of the forelimb, because branches of the deep peroneal (fibular) nerve of the pelvic limb supply additional innervation to this region. These branches, the medial and lateral dorsal metatarsal nerves, course adjacent to the extensor tendon and innervate the dorsal aspect of the laminar corium. After depositing local anesthetic solution for a low 4-point nerve block at the level of the distal aspect of the splint bones, the needle is redirected dorsolaterally or dorsomedially, parallel to the bearing surface of the foot, and an additional 2 mL of local anesthetic solution is deposited SC to anesthetize the medial or lateral dorsal metatarsal nerves. Most lamenesses of the pelvic limb, however, can be evaluated accurately without anesthetizing the dorsal metatarsal nerves.

The **high plantar nerve block** is administered, using techniques similar to those used to administer the high palmar nerve block, ~1 cm distal to the tarsometatarsal joint. When the proximal aspect of the suspensory ligament is suspected to be the site of pain causing lameness, 3–4 mL of local anesthetic solution can be deposited through a 20- to 23-gauge, 1-in. needle, axial to the lateral splint bone and ~1 cm distal to the tarsometatarsal joint, between the tendon of the deep digital flexor muscle and the suspensory ligament. The solution diffuses to anesthetize the deep branch of the lateral plantar nerve, which branches into the medial and lateral plantar metatarsal nerves that supply the proximal aspect of the suspensory ligament.

Depending on results of flexion tests or causes of lameness typical for the particular athletic function of the horse, the clinician may proceed to joint blocks or to more proximal regional nerve blocks. The peroneal and tibial nerves can be blocked simultaneously to exclude pain in the hock or regions distal to the hock as a cause of lameness, or the blocks can be performed separately to gain added insight as to the possible site of pain. If lameness is ameliorated after a tibial nerve block, but not after a low 4- or 6- point block, the suspensory ligament is a likely source of pain. If lameness is ameliorated after a peroneal (fibular) nerve block, but not after a low 4- or 6- point block, one or more of the tarsal joints are the likely source of pain.

The **tibial nerve** is blocked ~10 cm above the point of the hock on the medial aspect of the limb, where it lies in fascia on caudal surface of the deep flexor muscle, cranial to the Achilles tendon. Twenty mL of mepivacaine HCl is deposited through a 20-gauge, 1½- in. (3.8-cm) needle at this site, in at least several planes in the fascia surrounding the nerve. The deep peroneal nerve can be blocked on the lateral aspect of the limb ~4 in. above the point of the hock in the groove formed by the lateral and long digital extensor muscles. A 20-gauge, 1½-in. needle is directed slightly caudally until it contacts the caudal edge of the tibia, and 20 mL of mepivacaine HCl is deposited.

DISORDERS OF THE FOOT

OSSEOUS CYST-LIKE LESIONS IN THE DISTAL PHALANX

Osseous cyst-like lesions in the distal phalanx can result in a lameness that varies from mild to severe and may be unresponsive to anti-inflammatory medication. There is no apparent breed or sex predisposition. The cysts are commonly first diagnosed in young horses (1–3 yr old) but may be diagnosed in older horses. It is unknown whether the cysts have a developmental or traumatic origin. They are most commonly located in the subchondral bone either in the extensor process or along the joint surface close to the midline; the cysts may communicate with the distal interphalangeal joint. The lameness may be exacerbated with distal limb flexion, and it usually responds to intra-articular anesthesia of the distal interphalangeal joint if the cysts communicate with the joint. The lameness may respond to palmar digital nerve anesthesia but more commonly requires a more proximal nerve block (eg, abaxial sesamoid) for resolution of the lameness. Diagnosis is confirmed by radiography and/or CT. Differential diagnoses include keratoma, navicular disease, and primary degenerative joint disease of the distal interphalangeal joint. Surgical treatment includes arthroscopic debridement; extracapsular (through the hoof wall) approaches to the cysts have been used in less accessible lesions. Secondary fracture of the extensor process has been reported to occur due to a cyst in that region. Some horses return to performance status, whereas others are used for alternative purposes such as breeding.

BRUISED SOLE AND CORNS

Bruising on the solar surface of the foot usually is caused by direct injury from stones, irregular ground, or a poorly fitting shoe. Horses with flat feet or either thin or dropped soles are predisposed to bruising, usually at the toe or around the periphery of the sole. Bruising in the caudal sole at the buttress (the angle between the wall and the bar) is termed a corn. Bruising commonly occurs with no abnormalities present on the keratinized sole, although solar changes may be present ranging from some red staining of the inner solar epidermis (due to minor hemorrhage) to the palpable presence of serum either under the solar epidermis or seeping through it. If untreated, the affected area can become infected (ie, a subsolar abscess). Persistent, nonresponsive bruised sole dorsal to the apex of the frog suggests possible distal displacement of the distal phalanx secondary to laminitis.

A "corn" is most common in the forefeet on the inner buttress and can be caused by 1) the heel of a shoe improperly placed (heel of branch bent excessively toward frog); 2) a shoe left on too long, causing pressure on the buttress; or 3) shoes fitted too closely at the quarters or too small for the foot. Corns are described as dry (only mild bruising), moist (serous exudate present), or suppurative (infected or abscessed). Bruising may be associated with lameness, depending on the severity. When the foot is raised and the solar surface freed of dirt and loose horn, a discoloration, either red or reddish yellow, may be noted. Pressure on the affected area with hoof testers usually causes varying degrees of discomfort, again depending on the severity of the lesion.

Treatment of sole bruising is intended to remove pressure and protect the bruised area. In horses predisposed to corns, proper shoeing with branches that fit well on the hoof wall at the quarters and heels (and extend to the caudal aspect of the buttress) will decrease the incidence of lesions. In horses predisposed to bruising due to dropped soles, application of a wide-webbed shoe beveled on the solar surface (made concave relative to the solar surface) to avoid solar pressure will help protect the sole. Additionally, a pad can be placed on the foot to protect the sole. In horses with painful corns, the affected heel can be unweighted by trimming the wall and insensitive sole to minimize contact with the shoe until healed; a bar shoe can also help disperse pressure away from the trimmed area.

If the bruise/corn is suppurating, ventral solar drainage, usually established with a hoof knife, is usually adequate to allow healing. If the affected subsolar area is large, the abscess can usually be addressed by establishing small areas of drainage (~1 cm in diameter) at opposite sides of the affected area (established by probing), followed by lavage with saturated Epsom salt solution via either a 14-gauge catheter or teat cannula attached to a 60-mL syringe, repeated daily or every other day until healed. This is usually more effective than foot baths or application of poultices. The sole should be covered until the solar surface is covered by tough epithelium (horn). Parenteral antibacterial therapy is of questionable value unless cellulitis is present proximal to the coronary band.

CANKER

Canker is a chronic hypertrophy and apparent suppuration of the horn-producing tissues of the foot, involving the frog and the sole. The cause is unknown. Although frequently described as a disease seen in animals kept in moist or unsanitary environments, it is also encountered in well-cared-for animals. The disease can be observed in both front- and hindfeet. It most commonly starts in the caudal frog, where the affected area consists of an inflamed granulation tissue with proliferative epithelium, often appearing as fronds. The affected tissue is commonly covered by caseous exudate, which may be foul smelling. The surface of the lesion is irregular, with a characteristic, cauliflower-like vegetative growth. The disease process may extend to the sole and even to the wall, showing no tendency to heal.

Treatment requires sharp debridement down to normal tissue, attempting to maintain any normal epithelium. All loose horn and affected tissue should be removed. After debridement, an antiseptic or antibiotic dressing should be applied daily; good results have been reported using a solution of 10% benzoyl peroxide dissolved in acetone. Metronidazole is commonly applied topically with the benzoyl peroxide/acetone treatment. A clean, dry wound environment must be maintained to allow healing, which may take weeks or months. Close attention is required over the healing period; if any questionable areas appear, they must be aggressively addressed.

FRACTURE OF NAVICULAR BONE

Navicular bone fractures are usually a result of trauma or excessive concussion to the foot, but the cause is not always known. It is much less common than distal phalanx fracture and is more commonly seen in the forelimb. Although pain is variable, hoof testers usually induce a painful response over the frog. Lameness is severe with acute fractures, but it may be less in a chronic fracture in which a fibrous union has presumably failed. The lameness usually is markedly improved by palmar digital nerve block (which blocks both the navicular region and the coffin joint). Radiography confirms the diagnosis, in which a sagittal fracture is usually found medial or lateral to the midline; care must be taken to pack the sulci of the frog to avoid artifacts that appear as navicular bone fractures.

Conservative treatment is prolonged rest with corrective shoeing to apply a dramatically raised heel (up to 12°); however, a bony union at the fracture site is seldom satisfactory, and the prognosis is guarded to poor. Surgical repair by lag screw has been described to have a better prognosis.

FRACTURE OF DISTAL PHALANX

(Fracture of third phalanx, os pedis, or coffin bone)

Fracture of the distal phalanx is a fairly common injury that occurs most commonly at high speed (ie, during a race) or less commonly from kicking a firm object (eg, a stall wall). The fracture is caused by concussion and produces a sudden onset of lameness. The lameness is severe if the fracture is intra-articular but may be less severe if only a wing (or solar margin of the distal phalanx) is fractured with no articular component. Distal phalangeal fractures occur more frequently in the forelimb but are also common in the hindlimb. Intra-articular fractures may be easily isolated to the foot; lameness is commonly associated with joint effusion. Nonarticular fractures may require compression of the foot with hoof testers and possibly unilateral palmar digital nerve anesthesia for localization. Lameness is exacerbated by turning the horse or making it pivot on the affected leg. If the fracture does not extend into the joint, the lameness may improve considerably after 48 hr of stall rest.

The clinical signs may be suggestive, but the diagnosis is confirmed by palmar digital nerve block and radiographic imaging. Radiographic confirmation may be difficult immediately after the injury, because the fracture is only a hairline at this stage. Often, more than two views are required before the fracture line is evident. Repeating the radiography several days or weeks later (to allow bone resorption) and using oblique views may be necessary to confirm the presence and exact site of the fracture. Additionally, if the suspected fracture is in a wing of the distal phalanx, unilateral palmar digital nerve anesthesia may be performed to localize the lameness to that side. Determining whether the fracture extends into the distal phalangeal joint is important. Scintigraphy and MRI are other imaging options if a definitive diagnosis is not possible by radiographs.

Conservative treatment of 6–9 mo rest is usually all that is required for fractures not involving the joint. Fractures often heal with a fibrous union, so that, even though the horse returns to soundness, radiographic evidence of the fracture remains. A straight bar shoe with a clip well back on each quarter can be applied to limit expansion and contraction of the heels. In young horses (<3 yr old), fractures into the joint may heal satisfactorily, provided a 12-mo rest period is given. Older horses (>3 yr old) have a much less favorable prognosis, and insertion of a cortical bone screw using interfragmentary compression across the fracture site is indicated; however, infection is a frequent complication, because an extracapsular approach is required. Many fractures heal in the presence of infection, but the screw must be removed at a second surgery to restore the horse to complete working soundness. Unilateral palmar digital neurectomy of racehorses with nonarticular wing fractures has been used to allow return to competition without the delay for complete healing.

KERATOMA

(Keraphyllocele)

A keratoma is a benign mass made up of keratin that is situated between the hoof wall and distal phalanx. The cause is unknown. Although keratomas originate at the level of the coronary band, the condition may be difficult to detect until the growth is well advanced and located in the wall far distal to the coronary band. There is commonly bulging of either the coronary band or the hoof wall over the keratoma, depending on its position within the foot. Pressure from the keratoma causes well-demarcated bone resorption of the distal phalanx (usually appears that a "bite" has been taken out of the solar margin in most cases), which can usually be visualized best via the 65° dorsopalmar radiographic view of the distal phalanx. Surgical removal of the mass is indicated. Once localized, it is best to resect the mass through an approach through the hoof wall versus from a solar approach.

LAMINITIS

(Founder)

Equine laminitis is a crippling disease in which there is a failure of attachment of the epidermal laminae connected to the hoof wall from the dermal laminae attached to the distal phalanx. Because the laminae are responsible for suspending the distal phalanx within the hoof wall, laminar failure in combination with the downward forces of the weight of the horse and distracting forces such as the tension from the deep digital flexor tendon commonly results in a catastrophic displacement of the distal phalanx, resulting in severe lameness. Laminitis affects all breeds of horses.

Etiology and Pathogenesis: Three main disease states are thought to be associated with laminitis: 1) diseases associated with sepsis or endotoxemia, 2) endocrinopathic laminitis encompassing both equine metabolic syndrome (including pasture-associated laminitis, *see* p 1006 and pituitary adenoma), and 3) supporting limb laminitis. The pathogenesis of laminitis remains controversial and most likely varies widely between these three primary causes. A fourth, less common cause is ingestion of shavings (sometimes inadvertently used for bedding) from black walnut heartwood; the pathophysiology of this type of laminitis appears similar to that of sepsis-related laminitis. The diseases causing systemic sepsis in sepsis-related laminitis are diseases commonly associated with gram-negative bacterial (or polymicrobial) sepsis and include ingestion of excess carbohydrate (grain overload), acute postparturient metritis (retained fetal membranes), colic (anterior enteritis, large colon volvulus), and enterocolitis. Laminitis secondary to equine metabolic syndrome most commonly occurs in overweight horses and ponies and is commonly exacerbated when grazing lush pastures. It is possible that laminitis occurring from an acute intake of lush pasture may be a combination of sepsis-related laminitis (similar to grain overload) and metabolic syndrome. Supporting limb laminitis can occur any time the horse places excessive weight on one limb for an extended period because of inability to use the other limb (eg, post-operative orthopedic procedures, radial nerve paralysis, or a septic joint or tendon sheath).

The basic cause of laminar failure in laminitis is a failure of attachment of the laminar basal epithelial cells (LBECs) of the epidermal laminae to the underlying dermal laminae. Although this failure was thought to be primarily due to breakdown of the matrix molecules in the basement membrane and dermis (to which the LBECs attach) by matrix metalloproteases, studies have questioned the importance of matrix metalloproteases. It appears that the LBECs may primarily be losing attachment to the underlying dermal laminae due to dysregulation of the hemidesmosomes (the adhesion complexes on the basal side of the LBECs that attach the cells to the underlying matrix molecules of the basement membrane) and possibly the associated cytoskeleton. Inflammatory mediators and enzymes (eg, proinflammatory cytokines, cyclooxygenase-2) are markedly increased in the laminae in the early stages of sepsis-related laminitis and may injure the LBECs or cause cellular dysregulation, leading to loss of attachment. Hypoxia and ischemia due to aberrant vascular flow is also likely to play a role in LBEC dysfunction in sepsis-related laminitis but appears to occur later in the disease process.

The pathophysiology behind laminitis associated with equine metabolic syndrome is not as well researched as sepsis-related laminitis, but work indicates that inflammatory signaling does not play a major role and that dysregulation of the LBECs is likely to result from insulin-related signaling, possibly through growth factor receptors such as IGF-1 receptor. The pathogenesis of supporting limb laminitis is only now being intensively investigated. These studies indicate that the central pathophysiologic factor in supporting limb laminitis is decreased laminar blood flow due to a lack of movement of the supporting limb because of pain in the opposite limb.

After loss of integrity of the laminar attachments, the distal phalanx can undergo three types of displacement depending on the forces placed on the foot and the pattern of laminar injury. Symmetrical distal displacement of the entire phalanx (usually termed "sinking") occurs when there is circumferential loss of laminar attachments, most commonly seen in severe cases of sepsis but also seen in equine metabolic syndrome. Palmar rotation of the distal margin of the distal phalanx (usually termed "rotation") is the most common displacement seen, and most likely occurs due to a combination of loss of the dorsal laminar attachments (while maintaining some laminar integrity in the quarters and heels) and tension on the deep digital flexor tendon. Rarely, uniaxial/unilateral distal displacement of the distal phalanx occurs, most commonly to the medial side in the forelimb; this displacement can only be visualized on an anterior-posterior radiograph of the foot. In laminitis related to sepsis and equine metabolic syndrome, the forelimbs are most commonly affected, although the hindlimbs can also be affected in severe cases. In supporting limb laminitis, either a front or rear foot is affected depending on which opposite limb has the weight-bearing problem.

Clinical Findings: Classically, laminitis is considered acute, subacute, or chronic. Acute laminitis is classically defined as the initial few days of clinical signs of laminitis (usually <3 days) in a horse in which the distal phalanx has not undergone displacement. Subacute laminitis is commonly used to define laminitis in which clinical signs have continued >3 days, but the horse still has no distal phalangeal displacement. Chronic laminitis is classically defined as the case in which distal phalanx displacement has occurred regardless of the duration of the disease. Early in laminitis, the horse is depressed and anorectic and stands reluctantly. Resistance to any exercise is marked, and the normal stance is altered in attempts to relieve the weight borne by the affected feet. If only the forelimbs are affected, the horse will stand with the forelimbs placed far forward (to decrease the weight on the front digits); the hindlimbs also are placed more forward to support more of the weight of the horse. If forced to walk, the horse shows a slow, crouching, short-striding gait. If all four limbs are affected, the animal will appear "camped out," with the forelimbs placed more forward than usual and the hindlimbs placed more caudally than usual. Each foot, once lifted, is set down as quickly as possible.

In the acute stage of laminitis, the entire hoof wall may be warm. An exaggerated and bounding pulse can be palpated and may be visible in the digital arteries. Pain can cause muscular trembling, and a fairly uniform tenderness can be detected when pressure is applied to the sole (most commonly in the toe region). The pulse rate (60–120/min) and respiratory rate (80–100/min) are commonly increased, primarily because of pain. Lameness is usually moderate to severe at this time. In exceptionally severe cases, for which the prognosis is unfavorable, a blood-stained exudate may seep from the coronary bands. These clinical signs do not always occur in endocrinopathic laminitis because of the insidious nature of the disease process, which can occur over months or years; the first clinical sign in many of these horses is toe bruising due to solar compression by the slowly displacing distal phalanx. Radiographic evidence of displacement of the distal phalanx can be present as early as the third day after the onset of disease in horses with sepsis/endotoxemia. However, an MRI study has shown that, in the acute case, the horse may have normal-appearing distal phalanx on radiographs, despite destruction of the entire dorsal laminar attachment that is visible on MRI.

Subacute cases may exhibit any or all of the above clinical signs but to a lesser degree. Often, there is only a mild change in stance, with reluctance to walk and some increased sensitivity to concussion on the soles of the affected feet. There may be no demonstrable heat in the coronary band or increase in digital pulse. The acute and subacute forms of laminitis tend to recur at varying intervals and may develop into the chronic form.

During and immediately after displacement of the distal phalanx (classically termed chronic laminitis once displacement occurs, regardless of the temporal aspect of the disease course), the horse is usually extremely lame and may spend a great deal of time recumbent. In severe cases, the foot may prolapse through the sole cranial to the frog, or the coronary band may separate; both occurrences gravely affect the prognosis. Longterm cases of chronic laminitis are characterized by changes in the shape of the hoof and usually follow one or more attacks of the acute form. Especially with cases of rotation of the distal phalanx, bands of irregular horn growth (laminitic rings) may be seen in the hoof, close at the toe and diverging at the heel (due to minimal hoof growth from the dorsal coronary band). The hoof itself becomes narrow and elongated, with "dishing" of the dorsal surface of the hoof wall with a steep angle to the hoof wall proximally and a much more horizontally oriented wall distally.

As the displacement of the distal phalanx progresses in longterm cases, the sole becomes flattened or somewhat convex in outline on the ground surface immediately cranial to the apex of the frog. The gait is similar to that already described, and when standing, the body weight is continually shifted from one foot to the other. Radiography commonly reveals rotation and some bony resorption of the dorsal solar margin of the distal phalanx in longer term cases.

Diagnosis: In acute laminitis, diagnosis is usually straightforward and is based on the history (eg, grain overload) and posture of the horse, increased temperature of the hooves, a hard pulse in the digital arteries, and reluctance to move. Abaxial sesamoid nerve blocks of the forelimb digits in the very lame horse allow assessment of possible involvement of the hindfeet (by walking the animal a few steps) and enable full assessment of the soles of both feet (for solar prolapse, etc). These nerve blocks also make it possible to obtain good quality lateral and anterior-posterior radiographs of the foot without severe duress to the horse. Lidocaine should be used for the nerve block, because it will last only a short time (ie, not long enough for the animal to move excessively and further damage the laminae); applying a temporary pad to the foot not being radiographed (to protect that foot) is also recommended. Gross observation and distinct measurements of the hoof wall and sole thicknesses from the radiographs allow determination of whether distal displacement, rotation, both distal displacement and rotation, or unilateral sinking has occurred. Depending on the radiographic diagnosis of the type of phalangeal displacement present, there is usually time while the nerve block is still effective to apply a temporary type of pad or shoe.

Treatment: Acute laminitis constitutes a medical emergency, because phalangeal displacement can occur rapidly. Despite prompt therapy, the prognosis is guarded until recovery is complete and it is evident that the hoof architecture is not altered. Most animals should be administered NSAIDs, with flunixin meglumine being the drug of choice if the horse is still systemically ill (ie, enterocolitis). Phenylbutazone is usually used in the early chronic stage when the horse is lame but does not have signs of systemic disease such as sepsis/endotoxemia. Close attention to the potential toxicities of NSAID therapy, particularly with phenylbutazone, is required. Because phenylbutazone accumulates in the tissue (unlike flunixin or most other NSAIDs), it is best to skip a day every 5–7 days to "clear the system" (flunixin can be administered that day). NSAIDs should be used according to label instructions and, if used in combination, the dosage of each drug should be reduced accordingly. Another option for treatment of chronic laminitis in horses at risk of renal or GI complications is the COX-2-selective NSAID firocoxib. Other options for analgesia include detomidine, butorphanol, morphine, or a constant-rate infusion of a "cocktail" of sedatives and analgesics.

For treatment of possible ongoing ischemia, acepromazine is the only drug found to effectively increase digital blood flow in some studies; however, this has been questioned again by a study using laminar microdialysis catheters in which urea clearance (an indicator of blood flow) was not changed in horses administered acepromazine. In a horse at risk of or in the early stages of sepsis-related laminitis, digital hypothermia (cooling of the foot by placing it directly in ice water) has been popularized again by several experimental studies consistently demonstrating efficacy in protection of the structural integrity of the lamellar tissue; in one clinical study of enterocolitis cases in two hospitals, risk of developing laminitis was decreased 10-fold in septic/endotoxemic horses in which continuous digital hypothermia was performed.

During the first 2–3 wk, it is important to remove standard shoes, because shoes place the majority of stress on the hoof wall and therefore the laminae. The feet should be padded with a soft, resilient substance such as a 1- to 2-in. thick piece of closed-cell foam cut to the diameter of the foot. Pads to provide sole support can also be made from different putties available to farriers. Decreasing padding (or beveling the pad) in the region dorsal to the apex of the frog decreases the stress on the dorsal laminae. Styrofoam insulation (2 in. thick) can be used in small equids but usually provides minimal support in larger animals. Other temporary shoes (eg, Redden Ultimate and wooden or EVA clog) that can be applied without severe concussion can provide different physical properties depending on the type of displacement (and veterinarian/farrier preference) in the first few weeks.

Shoeing laminitic horses with metal shoes is usually not a good option until ~3–4 wk after the onset of laminitis, when the laminar structure may be stabilizing. The type of shoeing depends on the type of displacement. In a horse with distal phalangeal rotation, an attempt is made to begin realigning the palmar surface of the distal phalanx to the sole, while not allowing excessive forces on the laminae. The breakover of the shoe is moved as far caudally as possible, and some of the caudal hoof (from the frog apex caudally) is removed to allow realignment to the sole. This may have to be performed in combination with raising of the heel (with wedge pads, etc), which still allows alignment of the distal phalanx to the solar surface while avoiding excessive changes in relation to the ground surface, thus preventing excessive tension on the deep digital flexor tendon and therefore the dorsal laminae. It may be appropriate to place some type of resilient putty on the solar surface to provide support to the distal phalanx in horses in which some degree of laminar instability is still suspected. Multiple types of shoes can be used, including heart bar shoes, egg bar shoes, and natural balance shoes. Steward clogs are an important option for treating horses with distal displacement of the distal phalanx; these allow the horse to maximize comfort because of being beveled in multiple directions (and therefore minimizing laminar stress). Some farriers/clinicians also use clogs in cases of rotation of the distal phalanx.

Surgical options include deep digital flexor tenotomy, to neutralize the pull of the deep digital flexor tendon, and dorsal hoof wall resections. Deep digital flexor tenotomy is most commonly performed in cases of chronic rotation that do not respond to the above shoeing techniques; it should always be accompanied by aggressive derotation via rasping of the caudal foot. The farrier and veterinarian must address subluxation of the coffin joint subsequent to deep digital flexor tenotomy in most cases (usually by applying adequate heel wedging to neutralize the subluxation). Hoof wall resections are performed much less frequently than in the past. Generally, only a partial hoof wall resection is performed (usually on the distal hoof wall) because of the severe digital instability caused by removing the entire dorsal wall in an extensive hoof wall resection.

NAVICULAR DISEASE

(Palmar foot pain, Podotrochlosis, Podotrochlitis)

Navicular disease is one of the most common causes of chronic forelimb lameness in the athletic horse but is essentially unknown in ponies and donkeys. Navicular disease is a chronic degenerative condition of the navicular bone that involves 1) focal loss of the medullary architecture (with subsequent synovial invagination), 2) medullary sclerosis combined with damage to the fibrocartilage on the flexor surface of the bone, 3) traumatic fibrillation of the deep digital flexor tendon from contact with the damaged flexor surface of the bone with adhesion formation between the tendon and bone, and 4) enthesiophyte formation on the proximal and distal borders of the bone.

Etiology: The pathophysiology of navicular disease is unknown. The syndrome is likely due to a complex pathogenesis rather than a specific disease entity, although the greatest consensus appears to support a biomechanical component (causing increased bone medullary pressure) and possibly a vascular component. There appears to be a hereditary predisposition, indicated by the sharp decrease in incidence of the disease in Dutch Warmbloods after certification of stallions with severe navicular changes for breeding was disallowed. It is considered to be a disease of the more mature riding horse, commonly not appearing until 8–10 yr of age.

Navicular disease is overrepresented in some breeds (eg, Warmblood horses, Quarter horses, and Thoroughbreds) and rare in others (eg, Arabians, Friesians). It is usually a progressively deteriorating condition after onset. Conformation of the distal limb is likely to play a large role in the disease process and degree of lameness. Excessive pressure on the navicular bone occurs with a "broken back" hoof-pastern axis, usually accompanied by an underrun heel and excessively long toe. This conformation, leading to excessive concussion between the flexor tendon and the navicular bone, may also cause navicular bursitis, with direct damage to the fibrocartilage of the flexor surface and the collagenous surface of the flexor tendon itself.

Clinical Findings and Diagnosis: The disease is usually insidious in onset. An intermittent lameness is manifest early in the course of the disease. Because disease is bilateral, there may be no obvious head nod to the lameness when the horse is trotted in a straight line, with only a shortened stride present. Lameness is usually exacerbated by lungeing the horse in a circle in both directions, with the inside foot usually exhibiting the greatest lameness. In early stages of the disease, the lameness may not be visible even at a lunge until a nerve block is performed on one of the two digits (ie, the two lame feet cancel each other out). A flexion test of the distal forelimb may produce a transient exacerbation of lameness.

Clinical diagnosis is mainly based on presentation of the horse (age, breed commonly at risk) and, importantly, on the lameness examination, including a characteristic response to palmar digital nerve anesthesia. These horses are rarely positive to hoof testers (11% positive in one study). The lameness can be eliminated by palmar digital nerve block, except in some horses with extensive secondary moderate to severe damage to the deep digital flexor tendon (pain can radiate proximal to the palmer digital nerve block with this pathology). However, because this nerve block anesthetizes the entire sole and coffin joint in addition to the heel, response to the block itself is not diagnostic. A transfer of lameness to the other forelimb, which also is eliminated by a palmar digital nerve block, is necessary for a tentative diagnosis of navicular disease. Anesthesia of the navicular bursa is much more specific but is not as commonly performed during a lameness examination because of the pain involved in performing the injection (needle passes through the deep digital flexor tendon) and the complexity of the injection (usually done under radiographic guidance). Radiographic changes are variable and do not always correlate with the severity of lameness. Thus, they may not be as important in the diagnosis as the lameness examination (although they can be). Radiographs may demonstrate a range of degenerative changes involving the navicular bone: marginal enthesiophytes, enlarged synovial fossae (so-called vascular channels) of variable size and cysts due to loss of medullary trabecular bone, general sclerosis of the medullary cavity, and flexor surface changes (observed on "skyline" radiographic view), including erosions and loss of a defined cortex.

Treatment: Because the condition is both chronic and degenerative, it can be managed in some horses but not cured. The most common effective treatments include NSAID administration and corrective shoeing. Phenylbutazone is the most commonly used NSAID, but it must be used with caution because of adverse effects (renal and GI injury). If used daily, it may be best to take the horse off the drug one day a week to allow the body to clear some of the accumulated drug; the horse can be given flunixin for that day. Another option in horses at increased risk of NSAID complications is the COX-2-selective NSAID firocoxib, which is fairly effective for orthopedic and articular pain. With severe lameness, rest is indicated.

Foot care should include trimming and shoeing that restores normal phalangeal alignment and balance; response to corrective shoeing commonly takes ~2 wk. The principal object of shoeing is to decrease the pressure on the navicular bone. The shoeing technique that most effectively decreases pressure on the navicular area is raising the heel (usually performed with wedge pads or a wedged shoe). Rolling the toe of the shoe further relieves the pressure on the navicular bone. The egg bar shoe does not decrease navicular pressure in sound horses on a hard surface but has been reported to effectively decrease forces on the navicular bone in some horses with navicular disease or collapsed heels. Additionally, egg bar shoes are likely to more effectively decrease forces on the navicular area on soft surfaces (that horses are normally worked on); they are purported to work somewhat like a snowshoe by not allowing the heel to sink as deeply into a soft surface as a foot with a standard shoe would. Natural balance shoes are ineffective at decreasing navicular pressure.

Injection of the coffin joint with corticosteroids will markedly improve soundness in ~1/3 of horses (for an average of 2 mo), whereas injection of corticosteroid into the navicular bursa is reported to resolve the lameness for an average of 4 mo in 80% of horses that do not respond to standard treatments (phenylbutazone, shoeing, and coffin joint injection). Increased incidence of rupture of the deep digital flexor tendon has been reported with multiple intrabursal injections. Isoxsuprine hydrochloride is ineffective as a vasodilator when administered orally and has little therapeutic value.

Palmar digital neurectomy may provide pain relief and prolong the usefulness of the horse, but no neurectomy should be considered curative. Digital neurectomy has a high incidence of severe complications such as painful neuroma formation and rupture of the deep digital flexor tendon. Catastrophic injury to the distal limb in horses brought back to a high level of athletics after neurectomy has resulted in death of the rider. Other surgical procedures for navicular disease are unproved.

Although the prognosis is guarded to poor, a carefully designed therapeutic regimen, including corrective shoeing, NSAID therapy, and navicular bursa injections (and/or possibly coffin joint injections), can prolong the usefulness of most horses and the competitive status of many. Over months or years, most affected horses reach a point of nonresponsiveness to treatment.

PEDAL OSTEITIS

Pedal osteitis is a radiographic finding of demineralization of the solar margin of the distal phalanx, commonly associated with widening of vascular channels near the solar margin, which is best observed on a 65° proximal-distal dorsopalmar radiographic view. Although the term is usually used to describe changes in the dorsal distal (toe) solar margin, it can be used to describe bone resorption of any aspect of the solar margin of the distal phalanx. The bony resorption usually occurs due to chronic or repeated pressure and/or inflammation of the affected region. The resorption can be focal due to a focal lesion such as a keratoma, or it can be more diffuse in states such as chronic toe bruising, in which the entire distal margin of the toe may appear "moth-eaten" due to extensive bone resorption at the solar margin. Resorption in the toe region commonly occurs in chronic laminitis cases in which displacement of the distal phalanx results in inadequate sole depth between the ground surface and solar margin of the distal phalanx, resulting in chronic trauma and inflammation of that region of the phalanx and surrounding soft tissue (ie, sole bruising or chronic subsolar sepsis). Because the bone resorption is usually permanent, the radiographic finding does not indicate current pathology and may be due to a pathologic state that occurred years ago. Therefore, it is essential that a thorough examination be performed, including application of hoof testers to the entire solar margin of the foot and a lameness examination with nerve blocks if lameness exists. (The entire solar surface, including the toe, will be anesthetized with a palmar digital nerve block.)

Navicular disease is an important differential diagnosis to pedal osteitis–associated toe bruising, because toe bruising is also commonly bilateral and both conditions respond to a palmar digital nerve block. Radiography is helpful in diagnosis and in differentiation from navicular disease. Pedal osteitis associated with chronic subsolar abscess is usually aseptic, with the sepsis isolated to the soft tissue. Radiographic signs of sequestration or severe focal lucency in the same region as the subsolar sepsis may indicate septic pedal osteitis, but lucency can also be an artifact caused by subsolar gas once an abscess is drained (an unopened abscess usually has a tissue density). Curettage of the affected distal phalanx should be avoided unless it is documented to be septic.

Local treatment (ie, curettage of the affected area) is necessary only if there is an active septic process associated with the radiographic changes of pedal osteitis. General treatment of nonseptic cases should be directed at the primary disease that caused the resorption (eg, corrective shoeing for chronic laminitis cases with distal phalanx displacement that predisposes to solar margin bruising).

PUNCTURE WOUNDS OF THE FOOT

(Subsolar abscess, Septic navicular bursitis)

Puncture wounds are common in horses and are the most common cause of subsolar sepsis. Most puncture wounds result only in sepsis of the subsolar soft tissue (ie, subsolar abscess) but can be catastrophic when the puncture is in the frog and travels deep enough to enter synovial structures such as the navicular bursa, the distal interphalangeal joint, or possibly the deep digital flexor tendon sheath.

Puncture of the sole by a foreign body is associated with introduction of pathogenic microorganisms that lead to subsolar abscess formation. Lameness is usually severe; the degree of lameness may be similar to that of a fracture. The horse may stand pointing the affected foot. There is commonly a prominent digital pulse in the affected limb. If allowed to progress, the abscess may travel proximally to rupture at the coronary band; there will usually be edematous swelling proximal to the coronary band before rupture. Diagnosis is made by confirming the site of pain by pulling the shoe, using hoof testers, and picking or paring the suspect area to locate the foreign body or its dark tract. If a foreign body is found in the frog, it may be best to obtain a lateral radiograph of the foot to assess the structures penetrated before removing the offending object. If a tract is found in the frog, it should be probed and a radiograph taken with the probe in place. Because puncture wounds in or near the frog commonly enter a synovial structure, they constitute a serious problem requiring rapid, aggressive diagnosis and therapy. If a synovial structure is entered, the horse should be placed on broad-spectrum antibiotics and transported to a facility capable of advanced surgical and medical techniques; the affected synovial structure should be lavaged with sterile polyionic solution as soon as possible (within hours).

If a puncture wound is noted in the solar area, ensuring adequate drainage from the site helps prevent abscess formation. If there is a suspected abscess but no tract is found, the foot can be poulticed in an attempt to promote organization of the abscess for localization. If a tract is found that leads to a subsolar abscess, adequate drainage should be established with a hoof knife; the drainage hole should be kept as small as possible (~0.5–1 cm diameter) to avoid a prolapse of sensitive corium. Some farriers and veterinarians prefer to drain the abscess through the hoof wall (instead of the sole) if possible. Once the abscess has been entered, it should be probed to determine its extent; a palmar digital nerve block will usually be necessary before probing and lavage of the area. If the abscess underruns a large area of the foot, another small ingress/egress hole can be made at the farthest extent of the abscess from the original entry point, and lavage can be performed by placing a 14-gauge catheter or teat cannula into the affected subsolar space and flushing with saturated Epsom salt solution (made by adding Epsom salts to boiling water or saline until some salt crystals sit on the bottom of the container and will not go into solution). If a chronic subsolar abscess has developed, this treatment may have to be repeated daily to every other day for several treatments. The foot should be protected until there is full healing/epithelialization of the solar region entered; healing appears to be much more rapid and is easier to treat if the abscess is entered through the wall instead of the sole. All horses with puncture wounds should be immunized against tetanus. Local and systemic antibiotic therapy are not necessary for a sole abscess but should be considered with swelling above the coronary band (indicating septic cellulitis) and must be used aggressively if sepsis of a synovial structure is present.

PYRAMIDAL DISEASE

(Extensor process fracture, Buttress foot)

Fragmentation of the extensor process of the distal phalanx is thought to occur due to trauma, osteochondrosis, or presence of separate centers of ossification. Forelimbs are more commonly affected than hindlimbs. The fracture fragments are usually intra-articular but are commonly nondisplaced; they may be adhered to the extensor tendon. The fragments may be incidental findings, but they may also cause lameness. The close association of the extensor process with the distal interphalangeal joint can result in secondary arthritis if the fragments are not removed. Fractures can be removed either via arthroscopy or arthrotomy; arthroscopic removal of small fragments carries a good prognosis. With large, untreated fractures, an enlargement of the toe region just above the coronary band is usually present, which results in the "buttress foot" or pyramidal appearance to the foot. Systemic anti-inflammatory medication may be beneficial.

QUITTOR

(Coronary sinus)

Quittor is a chronic, septic condition of one of the collateral cartilages of the distal phalanx characterized by necrosis of the cartilage and one or more sinus tracts extending from the diseased cartilage through the skin in the coronary band region. It is seldom encountered today but was common in working draft horses in the past. Quittor usually follows injury to the limb on the medial or lateral aspect of the lower pastern (immediately proximal to the coronary band, over the proximal extent of the cartilage), by means of which infection is introduced into the traumatized collateral cartilage. This leads to localized sepsis or abscessation of the cartilage. The cartilage may also become infected through a quarter crack (*see* below). The first sign is an inflammatory swelling over the region of the collateral cartilage, which is followed by sinus formation and intermittent drainage. During the acute stage, lameness occurs.

Surgery to remove the diseased tissue is required, but care must be taken not to enter the distal interphalangeal joint. Local or parenteral antibiotic therapy (or both) without surgery is likely to fail. In the absence of any therapy, poor drainage, cartilage necrosis, and recurrent abscessation lead to chronic lameness and extension to deep structures. The prognosis is unfavorable if the disease progresses to involve the distal interphalangeal joint.

QUARTER CRACK

(Sandcrack)

Cracks in the hoof wall are thought to occur primarily because of excessive forces placed on the hoof wall and the germinal tissue of the coronary band. It is proposed that shoeing does not allow the hoof wall to expand normally with weight bearing and that quarter cracks commonly form at the placement of the caudal nail, because the hoof wall will deform caudal to the nail but not cranial to it. This would place abnormal forces on the laminar tissue and the germinal tissue of the coronary band at that point, resulting in a defect in horn growth that appears as a crack. The same excessive force on a quarter can occur with a shoe in which the branch is too short (either due to placement of a shoe that is too small or to an inappropriate interval between resetting the shoe), resulting in excessive pressure and wall stress at the point where the shoe ends on the quarter. Toe cracks are also thought to occur in shod horses due to the fact that the toe expands abnormally between the cranial-most medial and lateral nails, leading to disruption of tubule formation at the coronary band.

A crack in the horn emanating distally from the coronary band is the most obvious sign. Lameness may be present, depending on the degree of wall instability or the presence of submural sepsis. If infection is established, there may be a purulent discharge and signs of inflammation and lameness.

Therapy first involves proper trimming of the foot to remove abnormal forces on the coronary band and wall. Once the farrier and veterinarian are satisfied that the foot is responding to the corrective trimming and shoeing (including the application of a bar shoe), the crack should be debrided (usually with a rotary tool), and any moisture or sepsis treated with appropriate antiseptic and/or astringent agents (eg, 2% iodine) until the crack is dry. Multiple wires are then applied across the crack to stabilize it. The wires can be placed either around sheet metal screws placed in the hoof wall on either side of the crack or through small holes drilled through the horn of the hoof wall on each side and exiting through the crack. The crack can be filled with either a resilient acrylic or putty, but it is critical that there be no moisture or sepsis present. Fenestrated tubing can be placed between the deepest aspect of the crack and the acrylic to allow for drainage. The hoof is then bandaged until new horn formation is evident.

SCRATCHES

(Greasy heel, Dermatitis verrucosa)

Scratches is a chronic, seborrheic dermatitis characterized by hypertrophy and exudation on the caudal surface of the pastern and fetlock. It often is associated with poor stable hygiene, but no specific cause is known. Heavy horses (eg, draft horses) are particularly susceptible, and the hindlimbs are affected more commonly. Standardbreds can be affected in the spring when tracks are wet.

Scratches may go unnoticed if hidden by the "feather" at the back of the pastern. The skin is itchy, sensitive, and swollen during the acute stages; later, it becomes thickened and most of the hair is lost. Only the shorter hairs remain, and these stand erect. The surface of the skin is soft, and the grayish exudate commonly has a fetid odor. The condition can become chronic, with vegetative granulomas. Lameness may or may not be present; it can be severe and associated with generalized cellulitis of the limb. As the condition progresses, there is thickening and hardening of the skin of the affected regions, with rapid hypertrophy of subcutaneous fibrous tissue.

Persistent and aggressive treatment is usually successful. This consists of removing the hair, regular washing and cleansing with warm water and soap to remove all soft exudate, drying, and applying an astringent dressing. If granulomas appear, they can be cauterized. Cellulitis requires systemic antibiotic therapy and tetanus prophylaxis.

WHITE LINE DISEASE

(Hollow wall, Seedy toe, Onychomycosis)

In white line disease, the hoof wall separates from the underlying laminae (stratum internum) at the level of the stratum medium (tubular horn). The separation likely starts as a result of abnormal wall stress due to poor foot conformation or trimming (eg, long toe, underrun heels) and can start at the toes, quarters, or heel. Opportunistic bacteria and fungi may be present in the fissures in the hoof wall. The outer surface of the wall may appear sound, but on dressing the foot from the solar surface, there is commonly a separation of the hoof wall from the underlying laminae. Tapping on the outside of the wall at the toe elicits a hollow sound over the affected portion. Lameness may be present in severe cases, in which loss of support of the distal phalanx results in displacement similar to that seen in laminitis.

The diagnostic evaluation includes a thorough physical examination and lateral and dorsopalmar radiographs to assess the extent of separation of the hoof wall and any displacement of the distal phalanx. For treatment, corrective trimming is critical to remove abnormal stresses on the hoof wall, followed by removal of the entire extent of the separated hoof wall to the point that firm, healthy adhesion of the hoof wall to the underlying stratum internum can be seen. This hoof wall debridement is performed with a combination of hoof nippers, hoof knives, and possibly a rotary tool. With proper debridement, there may be no need for antiseptic or astringent treatment. However, topical treatment with tincture of iodine is commonly performed daily for at least a week. Additionally, commercial equine foot formulations that produce chlorine dioxide can also be used. Corrective shoeing is critical to provide adequate support to the remaining foot, while removing stress from the affected regions; a heart bar or egg bar shoe in combination with a resilient putty in the caudal two-thirds of the sole (to provide distal phalanx support) may be necessary if displacement of the distal phalanx is a concern.

SHEARED HEELS

In sheared heels, there is severe acquired imbalance of the foot with asymmetry of the heels. When viewing the caudal aspect of the foot, one heel is higher than the other side; the higher side commonly has a more vertical hoof wall. When viewed from the side, the coronary band does not gradually angle toward the ground surface in a cranial-to-caudal direction (the normal appearance) on the higher side. Some horses with sheared heels are lame. Hoof cracks, deep fissuring between the bulbs of the heel, and thrush frequently accompany the problem. Sheared heels are most likely caused by abnormal forces being placed on one side of the foot and are seen frequently in horses with abnormal limb or foot conformation on the affected foot or feet.

Corrective trimming and shoeing, in an attempt to restore proper heel alignment and foot balance, are required and entail floating the heel on the higher heel. A full bar shoe to increase ground surface area while protecting the affected quarter and heel is used. Several shoe resettings may be required before improvement is evident. The prognosis is good in uncomplicated cases if the corrective measures are consistently applied until new hoof growth occurs.

SIDEBONE

(Ossification of the collateral cartilages)

Sidebone is ossification of the collateral cartilages of the distal phalanx; it occurs most often in the lateral cartilage. It is most common in the forefeet of heavy horses working on hard surfaces. Repeated concussion to the quarters of the feet is purported to be the cause. Some cases arise from direct trauma. Sidebone is usually an incidental radiographic finding and rarely causes lameness. If sidebone is a cause of lameness, the lameness should entirely subside with a unilateral palmar digital nerve block on the affected side.

When lameness is present, corrective shoeing to promote expansion of the quarters and to protect the foot from concussion may be of value. Grooving the hoof wall on the affected side has been reported to help reduce lameness. If sidebone is documented as a cause of lameness, unilateral palmar digital neurectomy may be indicated if the horse does not respond to corrective shoeing and trimming.

THRUSH

Thrush is a degeneration of the frog with secondary anaerobic bacterial infection that begins in the central and collateral sulci. The central sulcus is more commonly involved if the horse has sheared heels; the lateral sulci are primarily involved in most cases of thrush (without sheared heels). The affected sulci are moist and contain a black, thick discharge with a characteristic foul odor; the borders of the frog are commonly necrotic. These signs alone are sufficient to make the diagnosis. Although many describe the primary etiology as a moist environment with poor hygiene, it is more likely caused by poor foot conformation or trimming and lack of exercise (thought to help "clean out" the sulci when the weight of the horse pushes down on the frog and surrounding structures) than from lack of hygiene in the stall. However, a moist environment should be avoided in animals with thrush.

Treatment should begin by providing dry, clean flooring and thorough debridement of the frog and sulci. Additionally, the foot needs to be balanced, and affected horses placed on a regular exercise schedule in a dry area. An astringent solution (eg, copper sulfate solution) may be applied with daily hoof cleaning. Commercial equine foot formulations that produce chlorine dioxide can also be used. If granulation tissue or sensitive tissue is exposed, astringent solutions should be avoided; a paste made of metronidazole tablets can be applied instead to the affected areas in combination with foot bandaging. The prognosis is usually favorable with appropriate changes in shoeing and exercise.

DISORDERS OF THE PASTERN AND FETLOCK

FRACTURES OF THE FIRST AND SECOND PHALANX

Fractures of the first/proximal phalanx (P1) may occur in any type of horse used for performance. They may be small osteochondral "chip" fractures along the dorsal margin of the proximal joint surface, sagittal (complete or incomplete), or comminuted. Another category involves fragments of the palmar or plantar proximal aspect of P1, which may be associated with osteochondrosis.

"Chip" fractures of the dorsoproximal aspect of P1 typically involve the medial aspect of the joint and occur in horses that exercise at speed. These fractures are normally traumatic in origin and result from hyperextension of the fetlock joint. Acute lameness and increased effusion in the fetlock joint along with sensitivity to firm flexion of the fetlock are clinical signs that a fracture may be present and radiographic examination indicated. In nonracing breeds, a chip fracture may be present on radiographs, but its clinical significance should be determined with diagnostic analgesia before being implicated as a source of lameness.

The cause of proximopalmar and proximoplantar osteochondral fractures is questionable; one thought is that they are from osteochondrosis, the other is that they are fractures. Axial fractures are classified as type I fractures and are generally articular. Type II fractures are located abaxially and typically have minimal articular cartilage present. Type I fractures are generally associated with lameness at speed with clinical signs similar to those of dorsoproximal P1 fractures. These fractures are more common in the hindlimb, and intra-articular diagnostic analgesia is often needed to implicate these fractures as a cause of lameness.

Diagnosis is confirmed by radiography. A number of oblique radiographic views may be necessary to ensure visibility of the fractures. For palmar or plantar osteochondral fractures, oblique radiographic views with the beam raised ~20° from horizontal may be more helpful for identification. The diagnosis of sagittal or comminuted fractures of P1 is typically straightforward, with marked lameness and swelling. Incomplete, short sagittal fractures can be more difficult to diagnose and may require special radiographic views off of dorsopalmar/plantar and/or nuclear scintigraphy in the initial stages, because the fracture line may be difficult to detect radiographically.

Osteochondral "chip" fractures can be removed arthroscopically with an excellent prognosis if no other abnormalities within the joint exist. Routine, nondisplaced sagittal P1 fractures can be repaired by internal fixation using screws placed in lag fashion via stab incisions. More complex P1 fractures typically require open reduction and repair via lag screws to allow accurate realignment of the articular surface of the fetlock to limit postoperative arthritis. Careful attention should be paid to the fracture configuration to ensure that all components are incorporated in the repair. In some circumstances, CT may aid an

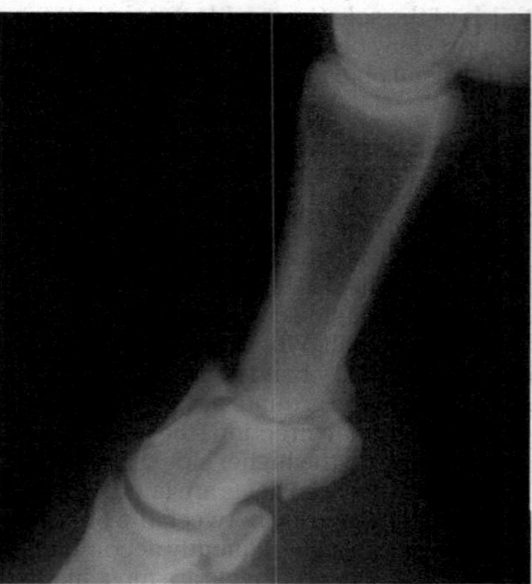

Comminuted fracture of the second phalanx in a horse. *Courtesy of Dr. Matthew T. Brokken.*

accurate diagnosis and reconstruction of the fracture. Conservative treatment of severely comminuted fractures involves immobilization with a plaster or fiberglass cast for up to 12 wk, with or without the use of transfixation pins through the third metacarpal/tarsal bone. Complications of P1 fracture repair include implant failure, poor alignment at the fracture site leading to secondary arthritis, and contralateral limb laminitis.

Fractures of the second/middle phalanx (P2) are most common in Quarter horses and typically affect the hindlimbs. Whereas osteochondral "chip" fractures are common off of proximal P1, osteochondral fractures are relatively uncommon off of P2. The most common fractures of P2 are either palmar/plantar eminence fractures of proximal P2 or comminuted fractures. Treatment of most P2 fractures is either with internal fixation with a combination of plate(s) and screws and/or a transfixation pin cast. Residual lameness typically is present and depends on the degree of osteoarthritis that develops in the distal interphalangeal joint and, to a lesser extent, the proximal interphalangeal joint (if not arthrodesed in the fracture repair). Prognosis depends on how comfortable the horse will be after fracture stabilization to limit the risk of contralateral limb laminitis.

FRACTURES OF THE PROXIMAL SESAMOID BONES

Fractures of the proximal sesamoid bones are classified according to their location in the bone. The most common sesamoid fractures in Standardbreds and Thoroughbreds are apical. They are caused by overextension and often are associated with suspensory ligament damage. The lateral proximal sesamoid in the hindlimb of Standardbreds may be fractured as a result of torque forces induced by shoeing with a trailer-type shoe. Other fractures include mid-body, basilar, abaxial, axial, or comminuted, and they may involve one or both sesamoids. Most, apart from some abaxial and base fractures, are articular. Clinical signs include heat, pain, and acute lameness, which is exacerbated by flexion of the fetlock. There is often hemarthrosis and synovial effusion of the metacarpal/tarsophalangeal joint. Diagnosis is confirmed radiographically. Of Thoroughbred racehorses ≥2 yr old, 82% of horses with apical sesamoid fractures removed arthroscopically ran at the same or at an improved level. Horses with apical fractures of the forelimb medial proximal sesamoid are less likely to race after fragment removal. The presence of suspensory desmitis (*see* p 1122) in the affected limb also decreases the prognosis after surgery. Horses with apical sesamoid fractures in the forelimbs are less likely to race than those with fractures in the hindlimbs (55% vs 86%). Size and shape of apical sesamoid fractures does not appear to affect racing performance. Mid-body fractures typically require reduction using lag screw(s) fixation with a prognosis of 75% (44% in another study) to return to racing. The prognosis for basilar fractures involving a portion of the sesamoid is fair compared with that for fracture of most of the base or in horses with associated articular disease (poor prognosis). Complete disruption of the suspensory apparatus, including fractures of both sesamoid bones, is a catastrophic injury that may be accompanied by vascular compromise; however, some horses can be salvaged for breeding by surgical arthrodesis of the fetlock joint.

OSTEOARTHRITIS OF THE PROXIMAL INTERPHALANGEAL JOINT

Osteoarthritis of the proximal interphalangeal joint (high ringbone) is a common cause of lameness in many types of horses used for a variety of disciplines. The osteoarthritic process can start as a single traumatic episode or as a result of "wear and tear," or overuse. Other causes of osteoarthritis of this joint are infection and developmental orthopedic disease. The proximal interphalangeal joint is a lower motion joint that is somewhat unforgiving to high loads placed upon it. Osteoarthritis is characterized by cartilage loss and periarticular new bone formation. In the chronic, progressive osteoarthritic pastern, lameness is typically subtle at first and becomes more noticeable as the disease progresses. Radiographic findings may include periarticular new bone formation, subchondral lysis and/or sclerosis, and loss of joint space (typically the medial aspect of the joint). In the early stages of disease, diagnostic analgesia is typically required to localize the lameness. In addition, a positive response may be seen on lower limb flexion. Oral or intra-articular anti-inflammatory medication may relieve the signs of lameness temporarily. The use of intra-articular ethanol injection into the proximal interphalangeal joint has been described. If surgical fusion is not an option, multiple injections were successful in some horses for facilitated ankyloses. Surgical arthrodesis of the pastern joint is frequently required to successfully restore performance. Typically, this involves a combination of plate(s) and screw(s). In a retrospective study of 53 horses that had a proximal interphalangeal joint arthrodesis using a combination plate-screw technique (81% forelimb, 95% hindlimb), 87% of horses with follow-up were used as intended. Deterioration of articular cartilage within the metacarpal/tarsophalangeal joint is a common injury in racehorses and can lead to development of periarticular osteophytes, enthesophytes, and joint space collapse. In young, training horses, periosteal bone can form on the dorsal aspect of the distal metacarpus and the proximal aspect of the proximal phalanx, often involving the joint capsule (osselets). Osteoarthritis is often secondary to a primary abnormality such as a chip fracture or osteochondrosis (*see* p 1140). Treatment typically has two goals: reducing pain and minimizing further joint deterioration. The judicious use of anti-inflammatories (eg, NSAIDs, corticosteroids) can provide pain relief. Newer biologic therapies (platelet-rich plasma, stem-cell therapy, interleukin-1 receptor antagonist protein) may help slow down or arrest the progression of osteoarthritis. In severe, advanced cases, arthrodesis of the joint is necessary to provide pain relief.

PALMAR/PLANTAR METACARPAL/ METATARSAL NONADAPTIVE BONE REMODELING

This condition affects the subchondral bone of the palmar/plantar aspects of the distal metacarpal/metatarsal condyles and is a common cause of performance-limiting lameness in Standardbred and Thoroughbred racehorses. It is thought to be a stress remodeling response to high-level activity in young racehorses and is associated with lameness referable to the fetlock region. Typically, the lameness improves with a block of the palmar/plantar metacarpal/ metatarsal nerves proximal to the fetlock. Intra-articular analgesia of the fetlock joint can have varying results and is less reliable to improve lameness. Radiographic signs may be minimal, and the changes are identified earliest using nuclear scintigraphy, CT, or MRI. Treatment consists of controlled exercise.

SESAMOIDITIS

The sesamoid bones are maintained in position by the branches of the suspensory ligament proximally and by a number of sesamoidean ligaments distally. Because of the great stress placed on the fetlock during fast exercise, the abaxial portion of the proximal sesamoid bones is susceptible to stress-related injury. Sesamoiditis is a clinically distinctive condition; however, it is poorly characterized pathologically.

The clinical signs are similar to, but less severe than, those resulting from sesamoid fracture. Depending on the extent of the damage, there are varying degrees of lameness and swelling. Pain and heat are evident on palpation and flexion of the fetlock joint. Radiographic evidence of sesamoiditis involves periarticular osteophytes, entheseophytes, focal osteolysis, and enlarged vascular channels (or linear defects in the abaxial margin of the proximal sesamoid bones). Grading scales for sesamoiditis exist and particularly note the vascular channels on radiographs. Severity of sesamoiditis on radiographs has been linked to a decrease in racing performance in one study. In another study, when radiographic signs of significant sesamoiditis were present, horses had a 5 times greater risk of developing clinical signs of suspensory ligament branch injury with onset of training.

The recommended treatment is enforced rest and symptomatic treatment to combat inflammation and soreness. The insertion of the suspensory ligaments should also be carefully evaluated by ultrasonography for concurrent lesions.

CHRONIC PROLIFERATIVE SYNOVITIS

(Villonodular synovitis)

Proliferative synovitis is the enlargement of the fibrocartilaginous pad on the dorsoproximal aspect of the joint capsule attachment of the fetlock joint. The cause of this inflammation is thought to be from repetitive trauma from exercise. Typically, this condition is found most frequently in racing Thoroughbreds, but it may also develop in Standardbreds and nonracing breeds. Clinical signs include fetlock joint effusion, firm swelling over the dorsoproximal aspect of the fetlock joint, lameness, and decreased range of motion and a positive response to firm flexion of the fetlock.

Diagnosis can be suspected by palpation. Radiography can be used to identify associated osteolysis at the proximal aspect of the dorsal mid-sagittal ridge of the distal third metacarpal bone on the lateromedial projection. The radiolucency is a result of the damage to the cortical bone from the overlying fibrous mass. Ultrasound examination can also be performed, and the synovial pad is considered abnormal if it is >4 mm thick, has rounded distal margins, or if hyperechoic regions are found within the pad. Treatment is surgical excision via arthroscopy.

DIGITAL SHEATH TENOSYNOVITIS

Tenosynovitis of the digital flexor tendon sheath is common in all types of working horses. Chronic digital sheath tenosynovitis may be bilaterally symmetric in the hindlimbs in horses with minimal clinical significance ("windpuffs"). The digital sheath encompasses the superficial and deep digital flexor tendons and extends from the distal one-third of the metacarpus/metatarsus distally to just proximal to the navicular bursa. Asymmetric tendon sheath effusion typically indicates a problem. Lameness degree is variable, depending on the structure(s) involved, and may increase with exercise. Horses are typically sore on firm flexion of the distal limb. Although some cases of tenosynovitis are primary and respond to conservative therapy with or without treatment of the sheath with corticosteroids and/or hyaluronic acid, others are secondary to lesions of structures contained within the sheath. Ultrasonographic examination of the entire digital flexor tendon sheath, including the intersesamoidean ligament and distal sesamoidean ligaments, is recommended and typically leads to a diagnosis. However, marginal tears of the deep digital flexor tendon (typically dorsolateral in the pastern) and tears of the manica flexoria can be difficult to diagnose via ultrasound but are confirmed through tenoscopic examination of the sheath. Verification of site of lameness should be confirmed via intrathecal injection of analgesia.

Palmar/plantar annular ligament constriction can be primary due to desmitis of the ligament or secondary to longstanding tenosynovitis or enlargement of the flexor tendons contained within the fetlock canal. Clinical signs are similar to those of other causes of tenosynovitis and include pain on palpation, swelling, and lameness, especially after forced flexion of the distal limb. Careful ultrasonographic examination is recommended to assess accompanying pathology. Treatment can be either conservative (ie, steroids) or surgical (palmar/plantar annular ligament desmotomy). Surgery is best performed tenoscopically, which allows visualization of the remainder of the sheath for primary pathology and assessment of the degree of constriction.

Other common causes of tendon or ligament pathology distal to the fetlock include desmitis of the distal sesamoidean ligaments (oblique and straight), deep digital flexor tendon, superficial digital flexor tendon, and the distal digital annular ligament. Any of these conditions can result in tenosynovitis of the digital sheath and can typically be diagnosed using ultrasonography or MRI.

DISORDERS OF THE METACARPUS

TENDINITIS

(Bowed tendon)

Inflammation of a tendon can be acute or chronic, with varying degrees of tendon fibril disruption. Tendinitis is most common in horses used at fast work, particularly racehorses. The problem is seen in the digital flexor tendons and is more common in the forelimb than in the hindlimb. In racehorses, the superficial digital flexor is involved most frequently. The primary lesion is a central rupture of tendon fibers with associated hemorrhage and edema.

Etiology: Tendinitis usually appears after fast exercise and is associated with overextension and poor conditioning, fatigue, poor racetrack conditions, and persistent training when inflammatory problems in the tendon already exist. Improper shoeing may also predispose to tendinitis. Poor conformation and poor training also have been implicated.

Clinical Findings and Diagnosis: During the acute stage, the horse is severely lame and the involved structures are hot, painful, and swollen. In chronic cases, there is fibrosis with thickening and adhesions in the peritendinous area. The horse with chronic tendinitis may go sound while walking or trotting, but lameness may recur under hard work. Ultrasonography delineates the cross-sectional and longitudinal extent of the tendinitis.

Treatment: Tendinitis is best treated in the early, acute stage. The horse should be stall-rested, and the swelling and inflammation treated aggressively with cold packs and systemic anti-inflammatory agents. Some degree of support or immobilization should be used, depending on the amount of damage to the tendon. Intratendinous corticosteroid injections are contraindicated. When a distinct hypoechoic or anechoic core lesion is present on ultrasound examination, tendon splitting has been recommended (the rationale is to decrease intratendinous pressure due to serum or hemorrhage). Cases also have been treated with shock wave therapy, intralesional injection of fat-derived stromal cells or cultured bone marrow–derived mesenchymal stem cells, or platelet-rich plasma products. The levels of evidence for these modalities are variable. The horse should be rehabilitated using a regimen of increasing exercise. Superior check ligament desmotomy has been used as an adjunctive treatment to minimize recurrence of the problem before the horse is returned to training.

Other treatments for chronic tendinitis have included superficial point firing (of questionable benefit) and percutaneous tendon splitting. Annular ligament desmotomy is also used when tendinitis occurs within the confines of the digital tendon sheath.

The prognosis for a flat-racing Thoroughbred racehorse to return to racing after a bowed tendon is guarded, regardless of treatment. However, increasing success is seen with eventers, show jumpers and show hunters, and dressage horses, respectively.

SUSPENSORY DESMITIS

Injuries of the suspensory ligament (interosseous muscle) are common in forelimbs and hindlimbs of horses. Lesions are typically classified as affecting the proximal, body, or branches of the suspensory ligament.

Proximal Suspensory Desmitis: The term proximal suspensory desmitis (PSD) is restricted to lesions confined to the proximal one-third of the metacarpus. PSD can occur unilaterally or bilaterally and is a common injury in all types of athletic horses. Injury to the proximal suspensory ligament and/or its attachment to the proximal palmar aspect of the third metacarpal bone typically results in sudden onset lameness that seems to improve within a few days. Lameness varies from mild to moderate and is typically not severe unless there is substantial involvement of the ligament and its attachment (avulsion of the palmar cortex). If the horse has bilateral PSD, there may be less overt lameness but more loss of action of the horse. Lameness is typically more noticeable on soft ground and with the affected leg on the outside of the circle. Response to distal limb and/or carpal flexion tests is variable. Pressure applied to the proximal palmar metacarpal region may elicit pain; however, this response/reaction *should* be compared with that of the other limb to determine significance.

Diagnosis of PSD usually requires localization with diagnostic analgesia, because typically horses do not have clinical signs (eg, heat, pain, swelling) that allow lameness to be localized to this region. There are multiple techniques to desensitize the proximal aspect of the palmar metacarpus. However, there is confusion interpreting the results of subcarpal analgesia because of the lack of specificity of local analgesic techniques. After lameness has been localized, radiographs as well as ultrasonographic examination of the region should be performed. Ultrasound of the proximal suspensory should be critically compared with that of the other limb, remembering that bilateral lesions do exist. Nuclear scintigraphy can help detect osseous injury at the proximal suspensory attachment, but negative scintigraphic images do not exclude the presence of PSD. MRI is also extremely useful to detect subtle changes in the proximal suspensory ligament that may not be visible or conclusive with ultrasonography. In addition, MRI allows accurate examination of the osseous structures adjacent to the suspensory ligament (metacarpal bones and distal carpal bones).

In contrast to hindlimb PSD, most horses with acute forelimb PSD respond well to rest and a controlled exercise program for 3–6 mo (~90% return to function). Premature return to work typically results in recurrence/persistence of lameness. Horses with chronic PSD may require a longer rehabilitation program or adjunct therapy (NSAIDs, shockwave, regenerative therapies) to return to consistent work.

Desmitis of the Body of the Suspensory Ligament: This is principally an injury of racehorses. Injuries usually affect the forelimbs of Thoroughbreds and the forelimbs and hindlimbs in Standardbreds. Soreness on palpation of the forelimb suspensory ligament is quite common in horses with lameness associated with a more distal limb problem; however, structural abnormality of the ligaments is only rarely identifiable ultrasonographically. Clinical signs vary and involve enlargement of the ligament, local heat, swelling, and pain. Diagnosis is usually based on clinical signs and can be confirmed ultrasonographically. Treatment is aimed at reducing inflammation by systemic NSAIDs, hydrotherapy, and controlled exercise. Shockwave therapy, platelet-rich plasma, and stem-cell therapy have also been used for suspensory body lesions.

Desmitis of the Branches of the Suspensory Ligament: This relatively common injury is seen in all types of horses in forelimbs and hindlimbs. Usually only a single branch in a single limb is affected, although both branches may be affected, especially in hindlimbs. Foot imbalance is often recognized in affected horses, and this may be a predisposing factor.

Clinical signs depend on the degree of damage and the chronicity of the lesion(s) and include localized heat and swelling. Swelling is often due to local edema of the affected branch. Effusion can be present in the adjacent palmar/plantar fetlock joint and/or the digital flexor tendon sheath. Pain is usually elicited either by direct pressure applied to the injured branch or by flexion of the fetlock. Lameness is variable and may be absent.

Diagnosis is based on clinical signs and ultrasonographic examination. Radiographic examination should also be performed to evaluate the attachment of the suspensory branch on the proximal sesamoid bones. Low 4-point diagnostic analgesia as well as intra-articular analgesia of the fetlock joint (varying degrees based on the location of the branch injury) improves lameness. Ultrasonography can detect a range of abnormalities, including enlargement, alteration of shape, and alterations in echodensity.

Management depends on the severity of the signs and on the breed and use of the horse. Shockwave therapy, local anti-inflammatories, ligament splitting, and regenerative therapy have all been used with varying results. Strict attention to foot balance is also critical in management of these lesions. Clinical signs may take ≥6 mo to improve, and the condition may recur. Prognosis for reinjury or persistence of lameness is worse in horses that are hyperextended in their fetlocks at rest or in horses with marked periligamentous fibrosis around the branch on ultrasound.

INFERIOR CHECK DESMITIS

The accessory ligament of the deep digital flexor tendon (inferior check ligament [ICL]) is a strong fibrous band that is the direct continuation of the common palmar ligament of the carpus. Desmitis of the ICL may be seen alone or develop secondarily to injury to the superficial digital flexor tendon. In horses with severe ICL damage, the deep flexor tendon may also be affected. Injury to the ICL appears to be more common in adult or aged horses, affirming that degenerative aging changes may predispose the ligament to injury. Injury is relatively uncommon in racehorses and is common in ponies and Warmbloods (show jumpers and dressage). Injury of the ICL is usually unilateral. Diagnosis is typically from clinical examination, with swelling in the proximal one-third of the metacarpus dorsal to the superficial digital flexor tendon. Ultrasonographic examination is typically confirmatory, with areas of enlargement, fiber pattern disruption, and loss of the normal border of the ligament. Injury to the ICL is usually treated with rest and controlled exercise, along with possible shockwave and/or intralesional injection of platelet-rich plasma or stem cells. Desmotomy of the ICL has also been performed in horses that have not responded to conservative therapy.

BUCKED SHINS

"Bucked shins" are part of the disease complex known as dorsal metacarpal disease. Bucked shins is a painful, acute periostitis on the dorsal surface of the third metacarpal bone. It is seen most often in the forelimbs of young Thoroughbreds (2-yr-olds) in training and racing, and less commonly in Standardbreds and Quarter horses. This injury can occur bilaterally and usually occurs sequentially, with the left leg being affected first because horses are trained and raced in North America in a counterclockwise direction. Bucked shins may be the result of high-strain cyclic fatigue caused by excessive compression on a bone that has not remodeled enough to tolerate the stress placed on it. Stressed bone forms a new layer of bone at the point of stress. This new bone is weaker and, in the process of rapid bone formation, the periosteum becomes elevated and inflamed.

Diagnosis is typically by clinical examination and history (soreness over the dorsal aspect of the cannon bone, soreness after high-speed work or the first race, or soreness the day after). Radiography is beneficial to determine the amount of periosteal reaction and if actual stress fracture(s) are present in the dorsal cortex. Treatment typically consists of altering the training schedule to short bursts of speed work 2–3 times a week. Rest from training is also important until the soreness and inflammation resolve. The acute inflammation may be relieved by anti-inflammatory analgesics and application of cold packs. Screw fixation with or without osteostixis is the method of choice to treat radiographically demonstrated stress fractures.

EXOSTOSES OF THE SECOND AND FOURTH METACARPAL BONES

(Splints)

Splints primarily involve the interosseous ligament between the large (third) and small (second) metacarpal (less frequently the metatarsal) bones. The reaction is a periostitis with production of new bone (exostoses) along the involved splint bone. Possible contributory factors include trauma from concussion or injury, strain from excess training (especially in the immature horse), faulty conformation, imbalanced or overnutrition, or improper shoeing.

Splints most commonly involve the second metacarpal bone. Lameness is seen only when splints are forming and is seen most frequently in young horses. Lameness is more pronounced after the horse has been worked. In the early stages, there is no visible enlargement, but deep palpation may reveal local, painful, subperiosteal swelling. In the later stages, a calcified growth appears. After ossification, lameness disappears, except in rare cases in which the growth encroaches on the suspensory ligament or carpometacarpal articulation. Radiography is necessary to differentiate splints from fractured splint bones.

Complete rest and anti-inflammatory therapy is indicated. Intralesional corticosteroids may reduce inflammation and prevent excessive bone growth. Their use should be accompanied by counterpressure bandaging. If the exostoses impinge against the suspensory ligament, surgical removal may be necessary.

FRACTURES OF THE SMALL METACARPAL (SPLINT) BONES

Fractures of the second and fourth metacarpal (splint) bones are not uncommon. The cause may be from direct trauma, such as interference by the contralateral leg or a kick, but often accompany or follow suspensory desmitis and the resulting fibrous tissue buildup and encapsulation of the distal, free end of the bone. The usual site of these fractures is through the distal end, ~2 in. (5 cm) from the tip. Immediately after the fracture occurs, acute inflammation is present, usually involving the suspensory ligament. Lameness is typically noted (may be severe initially), which may recede after several days rest and recur only after work.

Diagnosis is confirmed by radiography. Ultrasound examination of the suspensory ligament may also be beneficial to determine a more accurate prognosis as well as guide a rehabilitation program. Surgical removal of the fractured tip and callus is the treatment of choice. Fractures involving the proximal one-third of the bone may require surgical stabilization of the bone to prevent carpal instability, particularly if the fracture involves the second metacarpal bone. Prognosis is based on severity of the

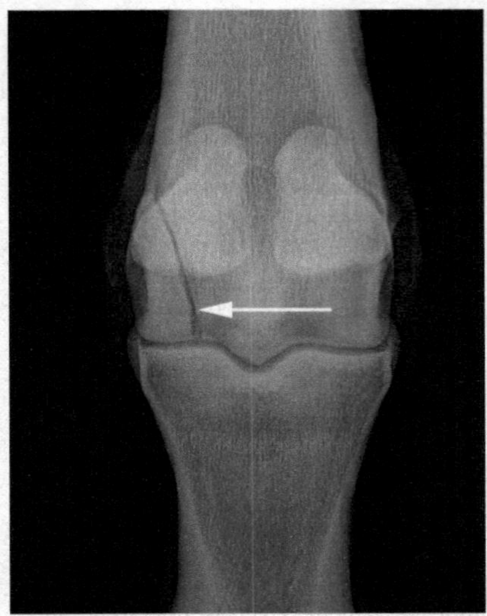

Lateral condylar fracture of the distal third metacarpal bone (arrow) in a horse. *Courtesy of Dr. Matthew T. Brokken.*

associated suspensory desmitis, which has a greater bearing on future performance than the splint fracture itself.

FRACTURE OF THE THIRD METACARPAL (CANNON) BONE

The most common site of major fracture of the third metacarpal bone is in the distal articulation (condylar fractures). Vertical fractures in the sagittal plane of the distal cannon bone (condylar fractures) occur predominately in young racehorses. Most condylar fractures are in the lateral condyle. In Thoroughbreds, condylar fractures of the third metacarpus are at least twice as common as third metatarsal fractures, but in Standardbreds, the ratio of metacarpal to metatarsal fractures is nearly equal. Nearly all lateral condylar fractures originate from the mid to midaxial portion of the lateral condyle and traverse toward the lateral cortex. In contrast to medial condylar fractures, lateral condylar fractures rarely spiral into the diaphysis of the cannon bone. Medial condylar fractures nearly always extend toward the axial aspect of the cannon bone. Clinical signs are straightforward, with acute lameness after exercise (or race) with marked effusion in the fetlock joint. Radiographic examination should include a full series of the fetlock as well as a flexed dorsopalmar view. For medial fractures, complete examination of the entire cannon bone should be performed.

Lateral condylar fractures can be treated conservatively by casting, but the treatment of choice is compression of the fracture, with screws placed in lag fashion to minimize or avoid osteoarthritis. For medial condylar fractures, in addition to lag screw fixation distally, a plate is placed up the remaining metacarpus.

The most common major long bone fracture in horses is fracture of the diaphyseal cannon bone. Typically, these fractures result from trauma incurred while the horse is pastured with other horses. Open reduction and internal fixation is the preferred treatment choice, because the lack of soft-tissue coverage over an unstable fracture typically causes these types of fractures to become open when simply cast or with a coaptation splint.

DISORDERS OF THE CARPUS

The carpus involves three articulations: the radiocarpal (antebrachiocarpal), intercarpal (middle carpal), and carpometacarpal joints. Problems are localized to the carpal area based on lameness, swelling, synovial effusion and pain on palpation, and responses to flexion and diagnostic analgesia. Visualization and palpation are important to determine the site of swelling in the carpus (eg, synovial fluid in the joint or tendon sheath or swelling in the subcutaneous space). Light palpation with fingers with the horse standing and with the leg raised is beneficial in determining the specific area of fluid accumulation. Knowledge of the normal anatomic boundaries of the structures is important.

Diagnostic analgesia of the carpal joints is usually done intra-articularly. The antebrachiocarpal and middle carpal joints can be injected easily. The carpometacarpal joint communicates with the middle carpal joint; therefore, local analgesia in the middle carpal joint provides analgesia of the carpometacarpal joint. There is considerable distal palmar outpouching of the carpometacarpal joint; with time, analgesia will diffuse into the area of the proximal suspensory ligament, thus leading to confusing results.

Radiography of the carpus is critical for specific diagnoses and should include flexed lateral as well as skyline views of the distal row of carpal bones (as well as proximal row/distal radius in some horses).

FRACTURE OF THE CARPAL BONES

Osteochondral fractures (carpal chip fractures) of the carpal bones are a common

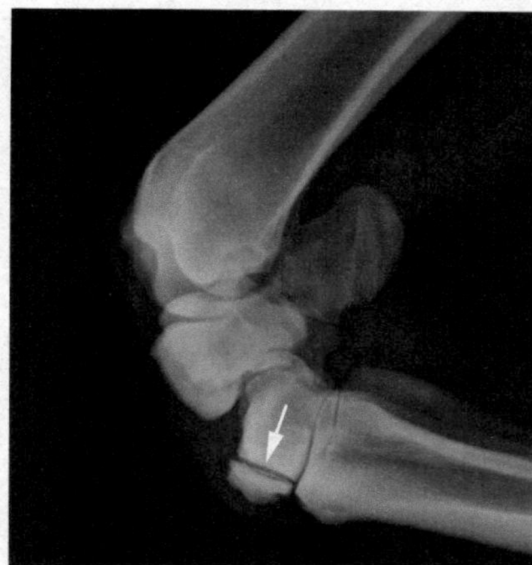

Flexed lateral radiograph of a horse with a slab fracture of the third carpal bone (arrow).
Courtesy of Dr. Matthew T. Brokken.

cause of lameness in racehorses. The primary etiologic factor is trauma, usually associated with fast exercise. Chips typically occur on the dorsal aspect of the joint. In the middle carpal joint, the most frequent sites are the distal radial carpal bone, proximal third carpal bone, and the distal intermediate carpal bone. In the radiocarpal joint, the most common locations are the proximal intermediate carpal bone, distal lateral radius, proximal radial carpal bone, and the distal medial radius. Diagnosis is based on clinical signs of synovitis and capsulitis and radiographic demonstration of osteochondral chip fragment(s). Arthroscopic surgery is the treatment of choice. The overall prognosis is highly dependent on the degree of articular cartilage damage within the joint identified on arthroscopy.

Carpal Slab Fractures

Slab fractures extend from one articular surface to another articular surface. In the carpus, slab fractures occur in both frontal and sagittal planes. The most common fracture is a frontal slab fracture of the radial facet of the third carpal bone, followed by fractures of the intermediate facet and both facets of this bone. The treatment of choice is lag screw fixation for fractures >10 mm or removal of the fracture fragments if they are thin or not amenable to lag screw fixation.

Accessory Carpal Bone Fractures

These are less common than other fractures in the carpus. Lameness is typically acute and severe, and there may be synovial effusion in the carpal sheath and, less commonly, the radiocarpal joint. Radiographs confirm the diagnosis. These fractures are typically treated conservatively; however, if the fracture is articular and fragmented, surgical removal of the fragments has been performed. Fibrous union may enable a horse to return to athletic activity.

SUBCHONDRAL BONE DISEASE OF THE THIRD CARPAL BONE

Degeneration and necrosis of the subchondral bone is common in racehorses and may precede slab fractures of the third carpal bone. The condition was initially identified in the proximal articular surface of the third carpal bone and is considered to be a consequence of cyclic trauma. Clinical signs include lameness, reduced performance, and effusion of the middle carpal joint. Horses typically improve with intra-articular analgesia of the middle carpal joint. A skyline view radiograph is critical for diagnosis and typically shows lysis and sclerosis in the third carpal bone (typically radial facet). Arthroscopic examination is the treatment of choice, with removal of the abnormal cartilage and subchondral bone.

TEARING OF THE MEDIAL PALMAR INTERCARPAL LIGAMENT

This injury, first described in 1990, most commonly involves the medial palmar intercarpal ligament but may involve the lateral palmar intercarpal ligament. A typical presentation is synovitis and capsulitis unresponsive to therapy or the presence of carpal chip fragments with an untoward amount of lameness. Diagnosis is made arthroscopically, and treatment is arthroscopic debridement of the torn fibers. Prognosis depends on the degree of tearing, as well as lack or presence of concurrent subchondral bone damage.

OSTEOARTHRITIS OF THE CARPUS

Radiocarpal and/or middle carpal osteoarthritis typically appears with chronic thickening of the joint capsule and usually associated decreased range of motion. *Radiographic changes* develop slowly, and usually the degree of articular cartilage compromise is severe. Cases that can possibly lead to osteoarthritis should be treated aggressively and correctly. Treatment

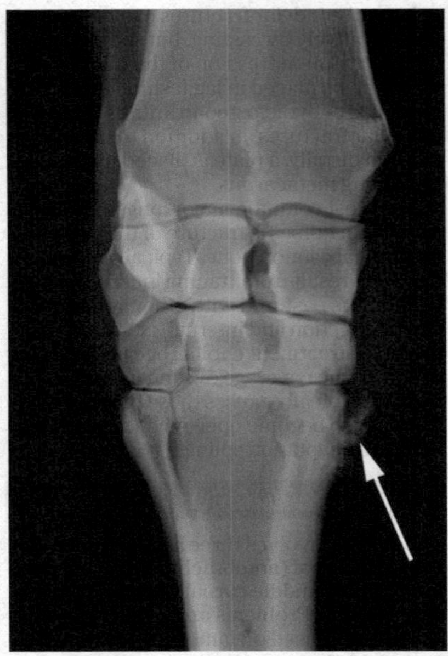

Marked new bone proliferation (arrow) in a horse with osteoarthritis of the carpometacarpal joint. *Courtesy of Dr. Matthew T. Brokken.*

of severe osteoarthritis is largely palliative. Osteoarthritis of the carpometacarpal joint has been described mainly in Arabian and Quarter horses. This condition typically affects the medial aspect of the joint and is characterized by lameness (minimal at first), firm swelling over the medial aspect of the distal carpus, and response to intra-articular analgesia of the middle carpal joint. Radiographs typically show periarticular new bone proliferation (sometimes marked) over the proximal second and/or third metacarpal bone, lysis and/or sclerosis of the bones surrounding the medial carpometacarpal joint, and possible loss of the medial joint space. Treatment consists of conservative therapy (systemic and/or intra-articular anti-inflammatories) and possible facilitated arthrodesis with use of passage of drill bits across the joint. (*See also* OSTEOARTHRITIS, p 1063.)

DISTAL RADIAL EXOSTOSIS AND OSTEOCHONDROMA OF THE DISTAL RADIUS

Exostosis of the caudal aspect of the distal radial physis can cause tenosynovitis of the carpal sheath and damage to the deep digital flexor tendon. Exostosis is differentiated from an osteochondroma based on its location and histologic appearance. Osteochondromas are present on the caudal aspect of the distal radius metaphysis normally 2–4 cm proximal to the distal radial physis. Osteochondromas also have hyaline cartilage remnants present on histologic examination (exostosis do not have hyaline cartilage). Irrespective of origin, these two conditions can cause lameness (swinging leg) and carpal sheath tenosynovitis.

Diagnosis is generally made by radiography, but ultrasonic examination may be helpful to define the presence of soft-tissue injury. The condition can be treated successfully via tenoscopy of the carpal sheath with removal of the protruding mass and identification and debridement of any concomitant damage to the deep flexor tendon. The prognosis is good and depends on the degree of soft-tissue damage.

CARPAL HYGROMA

A carpal hygroma is a subcutaneous swelling over the cranial/dorsal aspect of the carpus. Typically, a history of trauma to the carpus is noted. The swelling is typically aseptic, but risk of infection can develop after drainage or injection. Typically, a hygroma is a cosmetic blemish, and lameness is not usually present. The diagnosis is made by palpation and visualization. Injection of contrast material into the hygroma and subsequent radiographic examination outlines the extent of the hygroma. Communication between joint and hygroma is confirmed or excluded through fluid injection into the carpal joints. Hygromas can be treated in the early stage with drainage, steroid injections, and bandaging. When infection is present, surgical resection of the infected tissue is recommended.

RUPTURE OF THE COMMON DIGITAL EXTENSOR TENDON

This condition occurs in foals and may be present when the foal is born or develop in the first weeks of life. It can be primary or secondary to carpal or fetlock flexural deformities (*see* p 1150). Affected foals have a characteristic soft/fluid swelling over the dorsolateral aspect of the carpus and distal radius. Ultrasound examination is confirmatory. Management involves stall rest and preventing secondary tendon contracture with the use of bandaging with or without PVC splints to prevent knuckling, if appropriate. Prognosis is excellent in foals without concurrent flexural deformities or cuboidal bone abnormalities.

DISORDERS OF THE SHOULDER

Shoulder lameness in horses is less common than many owners expect. Although cases are often described as having a typical gait (reduced protraction/cranial phase, wearing of the toe, a swinging lameness), they are still difficult to diagnose simply from analysis of the animal's walk or trot. However, almost all cases have atrophy of the proximal limb muscles (especially supraspinatus, infraspinatus, the cranial shoulder muscles, and muscles of the cranial antebrachium) beyond that which would normally be expected for lameness caused by distal limb disease. This is associated not with shoulder pathology per se, but is a general feature of proximal limb lameness. Intra-articular anesthesia, medication, and centesis can be accomplished by passing a 90-mm spinal needle between the cranial and caudal parts of the lateral tuberosity of the humerus, angling caudodistally, from above; an ultrasound-guided technique is also described. Radiography is limited to the mediolateral projection, with the limb extended, and in some cases oblique projections (usually caudolateral-craniomedial or proximocranial-proximodistal). Ultrasonography is essential for full assessment of the shoulder region, particularly the soft tissues.

DEVELOPMENTAL DISEASES

Developmental orthopedic disease manifests in the scapulohumeral (shoulder) joint principally as subchondral cyst-like lesions (bone cysts) affecting the glenoid of the scapula or as osteochondritis dissecans of the humeral head. Also, a condition almost exclusive to miniature ponies, caused by dysplasia of the joint and attributable to hypoplasia of the joint surfaces, results in instability and secondary arthritis.

Subchondral Cyst-like Lesions: Bone cysts may develop in the glenoid, or socket, of the shoulder joint. They may or may not communicate with the shoulder joint and respond variably to intra-articular anesthesia. Although part of the developmental orthopedic disease complex, signs may not be apparent until the animal is mature. In common with other manifestations of this syndrome, lameness may not become a feature until the animal begins work (typically breaking in or early ridden exercise). Occasionally, bone cysts may be a cause of lameness in an older horse, having remained quiescent for most of the animal's life; the reason for these later onset cases is not clear.

Diagnosis is made by localization with intra-articular anesthesia, by exclusion of lower limb disease, or occasionally by gamma scintigraphy. Radiographs should document the lesion, although some cysts are too small to be seen.

Treatment in young horses consists of rest in the hope the cyst will remodel to become nonpainful; however, this happens only rarely. Intra-articular medication can provide relief from lameness but usually only transiently. Some disease-modifying preparations show promise (eg, autologous conditioned serum), and some clinicians favor the use of systemic glycosaminoglycans. Surgical debridement is difficult in most cases, because the cyst location and articular cartilage damage that causes secondary osteoathritis may limit its effectiveness; however, it can be very successful. Injection of corticosteroids directly into the cyst via an extra-articular approach could be appropriate, but the lack of 3-dimensional imaging of this region in horses makes the approach hard to plan.

Osteochondritis Dissecans: Derangement of cartilage and bone development on the humeral head can result in weakness within the articular cartilage that may lead to erosion or formation of a free flap of cartilage. Typically, the caudal part of the head is affected, or at least it is the part most evident on radiographs. In other joints, osteochondritis dissecans often can be treated successfully with arthroscopic debridement. Unfortunately, access to the shoulder joint is severely restricted, and in most cases the full extent of the lesion cannot be seen or treated. Clinical resolution in all but the mildest cases in young horses is rare. Rest and various medications have been tried, with little documented success.

Scapulohumeral Dysplasia: Seemingly unique to the miniature breeds, this condition arises from a mismatch between the size of the glenoid and humeral head. This causes instability of the joint and secondary arthritis. Although undoubtedly a developmental problem, probably with a significant degree of heritability, many cases do not present until the animal is an adult, and the history is often of sudden onset lameness. On physical examination, proximal limb muscle atrophy is often profound and lameness considerable. These factors, along with the breed *disposition and the often*-present sign of resentment of proximal limb manipulation, make localization straightforward. Radiographs reveal the presence of osteoarthritis and variable subluxation of the scapulohumeral articulation. Oblique views may demonstrate deep erosion of the humeral head in severe cases. The generalized destruction of the joint produces a "hot spot" on a bone scan, if performed. There is no simple treatment. Most cases present at such an advanced stage that even palliative care is impossible; euthanasia on humane grounds should be considered in such situations. Surgical arthrodesis has been described but is rarely performed.

FRACTURES

Serious trauma can result in fracture to any part of the shoulder region. However, the main sites affected are the supraglenoid tuberosity of the scapula (which serves as the origin of the biceps brachii muscle), the mid to distal scapula, and the proximal humeral metaphysis.

Supraglenoid tuberosity fractures, if complete, invariably displace in a craniodistal direction, because of the pull of the biceps. Large fractures can be surgically repaired. However, this is not easy, because the fragments are often difficult to reduce and the implants are both difficult to place and prone to failure during recovery from anesthesia or during convalescence. Smaller fragments can be removed, but the involvement of the biceps tendon of origin has to be resected. Very large fragments can involve the joint surface. Cases usually present with severe lameness and a history of trauma (eg, a fall during jumping or collision with a fixed object). On manipulation, there is often a sense of disarticulation between the lower limb and shoulder as the biceps is disrupted. Crepitus may be felt. In most cases, because the inciting cause is significant trauma, other signs such as soft-tissue abrasions or swelling will pinpoint the shoulder as the site of pain. Radiographs will reveal the fracture, and ultrasonography can be very useful to assess the biceps tendon. Management varies and depends on intended use, age, size of fragment, size of horse, etc. The prognosis for restoration of normal function is guarded. The size of the fragment, degree of displacement, presence/absence of articular involvement, degree of biceps disruption, and intended use of the horse are probably the most important prognostic factors.

Mid to distal scapula fractures occur through trauma or, in racehorses, as stress fractures associated with cumulative cyclical fatigue. Trauma can result in complete or (presumably because of the flexibility of the bone, especially in foals) incomplete fractures. Radiographs rarely help, because of the difficulty in obtaining diagnostic images of the area. Ultrasonography can accurately assess the integrity of the bone surface and is the technique of choice. Scintigraphy can also detect the injuries. Comminuted fractures can occur, and the prognosis worsens with increased complexity of the fracture. Simple, nondisplaced, or minimally displaced fractures usually heal well with rest alone.

Ultrasonography can be used to monitor healing. Stress fractures are almost always incomplete and heal very well, carrying an excellent prognosis for return to training. Very rarely, scapula fractures manifest as severe, unstable, comminuted injuries necessitating euthanasia on humane grounds. The clinical appearance is key to making a decision in these circumstances; although painful, scapula fractures with a good prognosis cause no observable limb instability.

Deltoid tuberosity fractures are seen infrequently. They are usually the result of trauma, often a kick from another horse, and may involve a wound and variable amounts of infection within the injury. Lesion-oriented oblique radiographs and ultrasonography define these injuries, and affected horses usually recover fully with rest alone, although surgical debridement of infected bone may be required in rare cases.

Stress fractures affect the proximal humerus also, almost exclusively in the caudal metaphyseal region. They are an uncommon but important cause of lameness in racehorses (the craniodistal metaphysis of the humerus is also affected, *see* p 1051). The typical history is one of sudden onset, often moderate to marked lameness closely associated with recent exercise, in an animal usually but not always in faster work. Lameness is usually transient, and the horse generally becomes sound within a short time (days to a week). If exercise resumes, lameness recurs. Localization is difficult; many are detected after the lower limb has been eliminated as the source of pain, or with scintigraphy. Radiographs can identify periosteal and endosteal new bone at the site of injury. Recovery is usually uncomplicated and complete with a few weeks' rest. Prolonged confinement may be counterproductive, and light exercise (walking only) may be introduced surprisingly quickly once the initial painful period has subsided. The injury remains evident on radiographs long after the bone is strong enough to withstand exercise, but a gradual smoothing and resolution of the callus will be seen as remodelling proceeds. Undetected humeral stress fractures can result in failure of the bone during exercise and complete breakdown, necessitating euthanasia.

BICIPITAL BURSITIS

The biceps brachii tendon runs over the cranioproximal humerus, protected by a synovial bursa. Inflammation of this structure can cause lameness and is usually secondary to a more serious inciting cause. Trauma to the proximal humerus, cystic lesions in the underlying bone, and injury to the tendon itself will cause secondary bursitis; it is important to recognize the primary lesion and treat appropriately. Occasionally, idiopathic primary bursitis arises and responds very well to medication of the bursa with corticosteroids. Bacterial contamination and, rarely, fungal infections can cause bicipital bursitis. In most cases, a wound in the vicinity of the bursa alerts the clinician to this possibility but, very rarely, closed sepsis can occur. Treatment for septic bursitis follows the same pattern as for other synovial structures. Radiography and ultrasonography complement each other in the diagnosis and management of primary and secondary bursitis. Repeat examinations may be necessary if a primary lesion cannot be detected, because it may become obvious with time. Scintigraphy is useful in cases in which the primary lesion remains elusive, because small areas of bone damage or cavitation can go undetected radiographically.

INFECTION

Sepsis of the shoulder joint occurs most commonly as a result of penetrating injury. Diagnosis and treatment proceed as for other joints. In foals (and rarely, weanlings or yearlings) infection can spread hematogenously and become established in the growth plates or ends of the bones (physeal or epiphyseal infection). These infections, provided they are not associated with contamination of the synovial structures, can be treated with high levels of antimicrobials systemically before resorting to surgical intervention. Methods to provide high quantities of antimicrobials at the site of infection exist (eg, intraosseus perfusion).

SUPRASCAPULAR NEUROPATHY

(Sweeney)

This syndrome describes the physical appearance of the horse's shoulder. It is not a diagnosis in itself, because there are a number of potential causes. The most common cause is injury to the suprascapular nerve.

All cases have atrophy of the supraspinatus and infraspinatus muscles that cover the scapula. This results in the scapular spine becoming prominent; in severe cases, the muscles virtually disappear. The atrophy is unusual in that it is often profound and very localized, which are hallmarks of an injury to a single lower motor nerve. The nerve involved is the suprascapular. Although the site of damage is rarely documented clinically, most cases involve trauma to the cranial shoulder at the point where the nerve is exposed to potential compression as it courses over the cranial aspect of the scapula. The severity of damage determines the degree of atrophy and the chances of recovery. If nerve function is severely compromised, the shoulder joint becomes unstable (it is a synarthrosis with no true collateral ligaments, relying on the surrounding muscles to support it) and the joint "pops out" sideways as the horse bears weight. This subluxation does not appear overtly painful to the horse, but if the joint cannot be stabilized, it may have significant implications for the longterm health of the joint and the horse's athletic career.

Therapy is aimed at maintaining muscle health during the period of nerve recovery and maximizing neurogenesis. Horses should be restricted to stable rest or a very small paddock. Complete immobilization may negatively impact the nerve and muscles, but activity probably hastens joint degeneration. A surgical procedure to remove part of the scapula over which the nerve courses has been described, aiming to provide optimal conditions for nerve recovery. This should be considered, but its usefulness is open to debate. Muscle stimulation, under the guidance of a trained physiotherapist, will help to limit muscle fibrosis and may encourage nerve regeneration. The vast majority of cases seem to be a result of neuropraxia or axonotmesis (based on clinical observations and rates of recovery), and function is recovered with time. However, this process can take many months, and frequently some loss of muscle bulk will remain. The prognosis seems most affected by duration of injury before diagnosis, degree of atrophy at diagnosis, and willingness of the owner to perform time-consuming physical treatments for many months.

Other causes of sweeney include disuse atrophy (which does not appear focal and is rarely severe), brachial plexus injury (which usually disrupts a number of nerves; atrophy is not focal but observable in a number of muscle groups), and caudal cervical disease resulting in spinal nerve radiculopathy (in which a number of motor nerves are also affected so that other muscles atrophy). Careful assessment of the muscles involved and radiography of the neck and shoulder will aid differentiation. Scintigraphy is useful for rapid screening of the proximal limb and cervical and thoracic vertebra for damage that may have an adverse effect on prognosis.

OSTEOARTHRITIS OF THE SHOULDER

Degenerative joint disease affecting the shoulder joint poses the same problems here as it does elsewhere. If no primary cause is identified that is amenable to correction and if radiographic signs (periarticular osteophytes, etc) are established, it is safe to assume that cartilage destruction is well underway. Signs can be ameliorated, but not cured, with use of anti-inflammatory, analgesic, and disease-modifying therapies.

DISORDERS OF THE ELBOW

Elbow lameness is rare but should always be considered if the source of pain cannot be isolated to the distal limb. Synoviocentesis is achieved via lateral approaches either close to the collateral ligament or into the caudal pouch. Radiography is limited to mediolateral (limb extended) and craniocaudal projections (weightbearing). Ultrasonography allows inspection of the lateral joint margins and collateral ligament as well as the medial collateral ligament (limb flexed and abducted). Lameness originating from the elbow is not generally considered to produce characteristic gait changes, but disuse muscle atrophy may be more evident than expected with lower limb lesions. Occasionally, loss of definition or discomfort may be appreciable during careful palpation.

DEVELOPMENTAL ORTHOPEDIC DISEASE

Cyst-like lesions occur in the proximal radius (usually medial) and less commonly the distal humerus. They are most commonly seen in young animals, similar to cysts in other locations, and the usual treatment regimens of rest, intra-articular medication, and controlled exercise are used. As with the shoulder, access arthroscopically is limited. Extra-articular approaches to the proximal radius have been tried but have the same limitations as the shoulder, although in practice, when orthogonal radiographic projections can be obtained, there is more chance of building a three-dimensional impression of their size and location. Treatment options are limited.

Other types of developmental orthopedic disease in the elbow joint, seen commonly in other species, are rare or unrecognized in horses.

FRACTURES

Significant trauma can result in breakage of any type, but the most commonly encountered fracture of the equine elbow affects the olecranon of the ulna. Stress fractures affect the craniodistal metaphysis of the humerus in racehorses.

Olecranon fractures in mature horses occur as a result of external trauma and may be incomplete (rare), complete but non- or minimally displaced, or complete and significantly displaced. A number of fractures are also open, as a result of the trauma that caused them. In cases of incomplete or nondisplaced fractures, conservative therapy can be rewarding, although some will displace during convalescence. Most authorities recommend cross-tying the horse to prevent it from getting up and down during the first 6–8 wk of box stall rest. The use of splints and Robert Jones bandages is more controversial—a "pendulum effect" can result from increased weight on the lower limb, possibly doing more harm than good. Many olecranon fractures displace under the influence of the triceps muscle and require internal fixation to repair. The use of a tension band plate is most common, with reported success rates for return to athletic function of ~75%.

Fractures of the ulna in foals are less liable to displace and may therefore be treated more commonly with rest alone. If such fractures are displaced, tension band plates can be applied, but their use must be monitored carefully because they will interfere with growth of the limb (the proximal radial physis fuses at 11–24 mo of age) and must be removed as soon as satisfactory healing has been achieved. An unusual but potentially difficult injury to diagnose and treat occurs when the proximal ulnar epiphysis is avulsed due to Salter Harris type 1 or 2 injury of the physis, which fuses at 24–36 mo of age. In some cases, the epiphysis is retracted so far proximally that it does not appear on the standard mediolateral radiograph and can be missed. Less dramatic injuries of this type can be managed conservatively, but significant displacement requires surgical intervention.

Treatment and prognosis may be influenced by whether the fracture enters the elbow joint or not. To determine this, careful assessment of high-quality radiographs is needed.

Stress fractures at the craniodistal metaphysis of the humerus, just above the elbow, occur in racehorses. The history is often similar to that for fractures of the proximal humerus and other stress fractures. Mediolateral radiographs will often detect periosteal and endosteal reaction at the predilection site. This can also be documented ultrasonographically. Scintigraphy is a sensitive method to detect fractures that cannot be seen on radiographs. Management is tailored to the comfort of the horse and severity of the initial injury but proceeds as for other injuries of this type with a careful return to exercise, balancing structural integrity with biomechanical requirements for healing.

OSTEOARTHRITIS

Degenerative joint disease of the elbow joint, in the absence of an inciting primary lesion, is managed as described for the shoulder and other joints (*see* p 1051). Some horses present with lameness localized to the elbow joint by diagnostic anesthesia with little or inconclusive abnormalities evident with imaging. It has been reasonably proposed that these horses may be suffering from subchondral bone damage.

COLLATERAL LIGAMENT INJURY

Most commonly detected laterally, probably for biomechanical and imaging reasons, these injuries can be detected with ultrasonography. Medial collateral ligaments are more difficult to image but can be assessed. Radiographs may document new bone (enthesiophytes) associated with injury. A number are found by scintigraphy, associated with a "hot spot" even in the absence of radiographic changes. Prognosis depends on the severity of the injury. At this time, no proven therapies exist to augment ligament healing. A number of treatments have been tried, including intra-articular medication, periligamentous injection of biologics (eg, platelet-rich plasma), systemic disease-modifying drugs, and extracorporeal shockwave therapy.

DISORDERS OF THE METATARSUS

BUCKED SHINS/DORSAL CORTICAL FRACTURES OF THE THIRD METATARSAL BONE

Modelling and stress remodelling of the dorsal cortex of the third metatarsal bone occur in young racehorses but, unlike in the third metacarpal bone, it is rarely associated with clinical signs of lameness. Dorsal cortical fractures of the third metatarsal bone are rare but may occur in Thoroughbred or Standardbred racehorses.

EXOSTOSES OF THE METATARSAL BONES

Exostoses of the metatarsal bones (splints) are common and may or may not be associated with lameness. Splint exostoses may be caused by direct trauma or instability between metatarsal bones. Large exostoses on the proximal lateral aspect of the second or fourth metatarsal bones are common and usually asymptomatic. Axially located splint exostoses on the proximal end of the second or fourth exostoses may impinge on the proximal end of the suspensory ligament or on the lateral and medial plantar metatarsal nerves and be associated with lameness.

Lameness is usually mild and can be alleviated by infiltration of local anesthetic solution around the exostosis or by perineural analgesia of the lateral and medial plantar metatarsal and lateral and medial plantar nerves.

Management of horses with symptomatic splint exostoses includes local cold therapy (cold hosing, icing, etc), bandaging, and administration of NSAIDs. Infiltration of corticosteroids around the exostosis may be beneficial in some cases. Surgical excision of persistently painful exostoses by periostectomy, ostectomy of exostosis without removing the parent splint bone, adhesiolysis, and fasciotomy can be performed successfully if exostoses involve the axial aspect and encroach on or are adhered to the suspensory ligament.

DIAPHYSEAL FRACTURE OF THE THIRD METATARSAL BONE

Diaphyseal fractures of the third metatarsal bone usually result from direct trauma (eg, kicks) or may result from propagation of medial condylar fractures. Prognosis depends on age and size of horse, configuration of fracture, integrity of the vascular supply, involvement of the metatarsophalangeal or tarsometatarsal joint, and degree of contamination. Prognosis for adult horses with open, comminuted fractures of the third metatarsal bone is poor, but in those with closed, mildly comminuted or oblique fractures, internal fixation may be possible (although often limited by financial constraints). Prognosis in foals with simple or mildly comminuted fractures of the mid diaphyseal third metatarsal bone after internal fixation with two plates is fair.

INCOMPLETE LONGITUDINAL FRACTURES OF THE PLANTAR ASPECT OF THE THIRD METATARSAL BONE

Stress reaction and incomplete longitudinal fractures of the plantar aspect of the third metatarsal bone may occur due to stress-related bone injury at the origin of the suspensory ligament. These are usually associated with increased uptake of radionuclide on bone scintigraphy and are clearly demonstrable on MRI.

FOCAL BONE REACTION AND AVULSION FRACTURES OF THE THIRD METATARSAL BONE

Focal bone reaction and avulsion fractures of the third metatarsal bone at the site of the proximal attachment of the suspensory ligament are not uncommon. They may be solitary injuries or, more frequently, are associated with proximal suspensory ligament desmitis. These injuries are frequently found in sports horses. Severity of lameness is variable, and localizing signs are usually not evident. Diagnostic analgesia is necessary to localize the pain. Some fractures may be evident radiologically, whereas in other horses scintigraphy or MRI is necessary to confirm the diagnosis. Conservative treatment with rest and a controlled ascending exercise program is usually recommended. However, recurrence of lameness is common, particularly in horses with concurrent proximal suspensory desmitis; in these horses, neurectomy of the deep branch of the lateral plantar nerve may be the only chance to resume sustained athletic performance.

FRACTURES OF THE SECOND AND FOURTH METATARSAL BONES

Fractures of the second and particularly the fourth metatarsal bones are common and usually arise from direct trauma (eg, kick from another horse). Simple, comminuted, and displaced fractures occur and are often associated with overlying wounds. Diagnosis is confirmed by radiography.

Most second and fourth metatarsal bone fractures will heal with conservative treatment despite comminution and infectious osteitis with appropriate antimicrobial therapy, wound care bandaging, and rest. Rest of 4–6 mo may be necessary in horses with open or infected fractures. Segmental ostectomy may be indicated in horses with chronic discharging wounds and sequestrum development. Complete removal of severely comminuted fourth metatarsal bones has been reported as successful, although persistent lameness may result. Internal fixation of the fractures of the proximal end of the second metatarsal bone may be indicated in some cases with marked displacement and instability of the fracture fragments. Open fractures of the proximal end of the second and fourth metatarsal bones may result in sepsis of the tarsometatarsal joints, which requires aggressive antimicrobial therapy and appropriate treatment.

Simple fractures of the distal end of the second and fourth metatarsal bones, just above the "button of the splint bone," are usually associated with desmitis of the branches of the suspensory ligament.

ENOSTOSIS-LIKE LESIONS OF THE THIRD METATARSAL BONE

Enostosis-like lesions of the third metatarsal bone appear as intense focal areas of increased uptake of radionuclide on scintigraphic examination after injection of ^{99m}Tc–labelled methylene diphosphonate. Radiologically, they appear as round or irregularly shaped areas of increased radiopacity within the medullary cavity. They are usually asymptomatic and rarely cause lameness. Lameness, if present, usually improves with rest and administration of NSAIDs.

DISORDERS OF THE TARSUS

FAILURE OF OSSIFICATION OF THE DISTAL TARSAL BONES

Incomplete ossification of the central and third tarsal bones is most common in premature or twin foals and is characterized by a "sickle-hock" appearance. It may occur unilaterally or bilaterally. Radiologically, the partially ossified cuboidal bones appear smaller and more rounded than normal. Early recognition and treatment are important to prevent crushing of the bones and resultant progressive osteoarthritis. Cylinder tube casts can be used with good results to protect the immature bones until they have ossified.

OSTEOARTHRITIS OF THE DISTAL TARSAL JOINTS

Degenerative joint disease or osteoarthritis of the tarsometatarsal, distal intertarsal (and less commonly the proximal intertarsal joint), colloquially known as "bone spavin," is a common cause of lameness or poor performance in horses from all disciplines. Lameness may be unilateral or bilateral, and pathology may develop in one joint only, or two or even three concurrently. Distal hock joint pain may be a sequela of incomplete ossification of the central and third tarsal bones; certain conformational abnormalities (sickle hock, cow hocked, or excessively straight hock conformation) are also believed to be predisposing. It has been proposed that degenerative joint disease of the distal tarsal joints may be caused by excessive compression and rotation of these joints as the horse jumps or stops. In Icelandic horses, bone spavin is thought to be heritable.

In most horses, few clinical signs are evident on physical examination, although in horses with more chronic distal hock pathology, the soft tissues over the medial aspect of the distal hock joints may be appreciably thickened. Lameness varies from subtle loss of performance without overt lameness to moderate or severe lameness. A characteristic gait related to lameness from the distal hock joints has been described as adduction of the hindlimb with an abrupt abduction occurring just before the limb contacting the ground; this has been referred to as a "stabbing" gait, which, although frequently evident, is not pathognomonic. Horses can exhibit this gait with lameness originating from other causes, and distal hock pain may also present with a different gait. Lameness may be exacerbated when the horse is on a circle, with some horses showing more lameness with the affected limb on the inside and some with the limb on the outside. A proximal limb flexion test will exacerbate lameness in some, but not all, horses with distal hock joint pain.

Diagnostic analgesia should be used to localize the source of pain. Most, but not all, horses with degenerative joint disease of the distal tarsal joints will improve after intra-articular analgesia of the distal tarsal joints. A negative response to intra-articular analgesia of the distal tarsal joints does not preclude distal hock joint pain. Perineural analgesia of the superficial and deep fibular and tibial nerves can be useful to confirm hock pain.

Radiography is useful to confirm the diagnosis. Radiologic changes may be evident in only one or two projections; therefore, a minimum of four standard orthogonal radiographic projections of the hock should be taken. Radiographic changes include narrowing or loss of joint space, sclerosis of the subchondral bone, lysis of the subchondral bone, periarticular osteophyte formation, and periosteal new bone formation. The severity of lameness and degree of radiologic change are poorly correlated. In those horses in which distal hock joint pain is suspected but there is little radiologic change, scintigraphy of the tarsus may reveal an increased focal uptake of radionuclide in the distal tarsal bones.

The aim of treatment is to provide pain relief so that the horse may remain in work. It has been suggested that by maintaining the horse in work, the distal hock joints will eventually ankylose and the horse will become pain free. However, progressive radiologic ankylosis is rarely observed and has not occurred in lame horses without intervention.

Conservative treatment involves systemic NSAIDs, intra-articular medication with corticosteroids, with or without hyaluronan, remedial trimming and farriery, and adaptation of the work program. Systemic treatment with polysulfated glycosaminoglycan (PSGAG), hyaluronan, or oral nutraceuticals may be used as adjunctive therapy.

Tiludronate, a bisphosphonate compound that inhibits osteoclastic activity, has been advocated for use in horses with distal hock pain. There are few controlled studies with this medication and, in a small double-blind clinical study, only one of eight horses improved with administration of tiludronate for distal tarsal inflammation or arthritis.

Extracorporeal shockwave treatment (ESWT) has also been used in treatment of distal tarsitis. Both focused and radial portable units are available. In one retrospective study of 74 horses with osteoarthritis of the distal tarsal joints treated with ESWT, 80% of the horses showed improvement in lameness but only 18% of horses became sound.

Intra-articular injection of sodium monoiodoacetate (MIA) has been used for chemical arthrodesis of the distal intertarsal and tarsometatarsal joints. MIA inhibits chondrocyte glycolysis and causes chondrocyte death. Contrast arthrography is necessary to ensure accurate needle placement and that no communication with proximal joints is present before injection of MIA. After injection, pain control is important, because severe pain is often present for 4–18 hr. Several studies have shown that 75%–85% of horses have been free of lameness with radiographic evidence of joint fusion at ~6 mo after treatment. However, when horses were followed for several years after treatment, the success rate decreased and a significant number of horses developed arthritis of the proximal intertarsal and tarsocrural joints. Other complications, including persistent swelling, septic arthritis, skin sloughing, and increased lameness, have been reported. Therefore, this technique is difficult to recommend because of the initial severe pain and significant possible complications. Intra-articular injection of ethyl alcohol to achieve arthrodesis has also been reported, although more longterm follow-up studies are required to evaluate its usefulness and safety.

In horses that do not respond to conservative treatment, a number of surgical techniques have been reported. These include cunean tenectomy, subchondral forage, neurectomy, and several different techniques of surgical arthrodesis.

Cunean tenectomy may result in a temporary improvement in lameness but is unlikely to restore soundness. It is believed to reduce the pressure over the medial aspect of the distal tarsus and cunean bursa and to reduce the rotational and shear stress over these joints during contraction of the tibialis cranialis muscle.

The most common surgical technique used in treatment of distal tarsal osteoarthritis is facilitation of fusion of the affected joints. Drilling across the distal intertarsal and tarsometatarsal joints is the most frequently used procedure to promote distal tarsal arthrodesis. Initial techniques described a more aggressive procedure, with 60% of the articular cartilage removed. Significant postoperative pain was associated with this procedure, and a more conservative approach using three drill tracts is currently recommended. Return to full athletic performance usually takes 10–12 mo. Retrospective studies evaluating this technique report ~60% of horses successfully return to their previous level of performance.

Both neodymium:yttrium aluminium garnet (Nd:YAG) and 980-nm diode laser have also been used to facilitate arthrodesis of the distal tarsal joints. Several studies have shown that horses treated with laser-facilitated arthrodesis are more comfortable after the procedure than when surgical drilling or MIA is used. It has been theorized that the superheating that occurs with the laser may cause thermal damage to nerve endings and diminish postoperative pain. Intra-articular drilling with diode-laser treatment has also been recommended, because the drilling should stimulate more bone production and fusion, whereas the laser reduces the postoperative pain.

Surgical stabilization in addition to intra-articular drilling of the distal tarsal joints has been proposed to have a superior clinical result versus intra-articular drilling alone. Lag screws or a screw and plate combination have been used. One study reported a success rate of 89% of horses returning to soundness versus 60% with drilling alone; however, only a small number of cases were reported.

Neurectomy of the deep fibular nerve and a partial neurectomy of the tibial nerves may be performed to relieve pain associated with the distal hock joints, with ~60% of horses undergoing surgery returning to full athletic function.

OSTEOARTHRITIS OF THE TALOCALCANEAL JOINT

Osteoarthritis of the talocalcaneal joint is rare. There are frequently no localizing signs. Lameness is usually partially improved by intra-articular analgesia of the tarsocrural joint and alleviated by perineural analgesia of the fibular and tibial nerves. Diagnosis is confirmed by radiography, with radiologic changes of subchondral sclerosis, lysis, and joint narrowing evident within the talocalcaneal joint. The prognosis for return to athletic soundness with conservative management is poor. Surgical arthrodesis has resulted in improvement in lameness but not complete resolution of signs.

OSTEOARTHRITIS OF THE TARSOCRURAL JOINT

Osteoarthritis of the tarsocrural joint may be seen as a primary disease or develop secondary to trauma, osteochondrosis, or osteoarthritis of the distal hock joints. It is usually associated with joint effusion. Lameness may vary from mild to severe and is usually improved by intra-articular analgesia of the tarsocrural joint. In horses with primary osteoarthritis of the tarsocrural joint, often no radiologic abnormalities are evident, and diagnosis is based on arthroscopic examination. Response to intra-articular medication with corticosteroids and hyaluronan is often disappointing, and prognosis for return to athletic soundness is guarded to poor.

SYNOVITIS/CAPSULITIS OF THE TARSOCRURAL JOINT

(Bog spavin)

Acute or chronic synovitis of the tarsocrural joint resulting in distention of the joint capsule may occur due to osteochondrosis, degenerative joint disease, trauma, poor joint conformation, hemoarthrosis, or infection, or it may be idiopathic. Lameness may or may not be present, depending on the etiology. Diagnosis is based on clinical signs and a positive response to intra-articular analgesia of the tarsocrural joint if lameness is present. Radiographs should be taken to exclude OCD and other radiologically evident pathology, and ultrasonography should be done to assess the periarticular soft-tissue structures. Synoviocentesis of the tarsocrural joint should be performed if sepsis or hemoarthrosis is suspected. Idiopathic synovitis may be diagnosed in the absence of lameness or radiologic change.

Idiopathic synovitis rarely interferes with use of the horse but may be considered an unacceptable cosmetic blemish. Idiopathic synovitis may be managed by draining the synovial fluid and medicating the joint with intra-articular corticosteroids. Pressure bandages should be applied afterward to provide joint compression, and the horse stall rested for 2 wk. However, in approximately half of horses, effusion will recur and a persistent cosmetic blemish remains. Intra-articular injection of atropine (8 mg) may sometimes help.

OSTEOCHONDROSIS OF THE TARSOCRURAL JOINT

Osteochondrosis dessicans (OCD) of the tarsocrural joint is common in many breeds of horses, especially Warmbloods and Standardbreds. OCD of the tarsocrural joint may or may not be associated with lameness and is associated with variable amounts of joint effusion. Diagnosis is confirmed by intra-articular analgesia of the tarsocrural joint if lameness is present and by demonstrating radiologic changes. Few of the common OCD lesions in the hock will heal spontaneously after 5 mo of age, so arthroscopic surgical removal is usually advised. Prognosis for full return to athletic function after surgery is good. If left untreated, fragments may come loose, resulting in cartilage damage and acute signs of effusion and lameness.

OCD lesions in the tarsocrural joint are most commonly seen on the distal intermediate ridge of the tibia. Lesions at this site do not cause lameness unless significant effusion occurs or fragments become loose. Dislodged fragments may become lodged in the dorsal part of the proximal intertarsal joint. Arthroscopic removal of the fragments is usually associated with a good outcome.

OCD lesions of the distal end of the lateral trochlear ridge are most commonly seen in heavy horses and Standardbreds. Lesions can be large and, if loose, cause acute onset of severe lameness and effusion. Large or loose lesions should be removed arthroscopically, and even large lesions can be removed with a good prognosis. Prognosis is determined by the proximal and axial extent of the lesion.

Medial malleolar OCD lesions usually cause more lameness and effusion than the more common OCD lesions on the distal intermediate ridge of the tibia. They are usually seen on the axial aspect of the medial malleolus and may be overlooked on dorsoplantar radiographs. Early arthroscopic removal of fragments is recommended to prevent erosive lesions from developing on the medial trochlea of the talus. Arthroscopic surgery usually has a good prognosis for return to athletic function.

Lateral malleolar fragments are usually traumatic and are only rarely (1%) OCD lesions.

OSTEITIS OF THE CALCANEUS

Osteitis of the end of the tuber calcanei may be seen after traumatic injury and subsequent infection. This most often occurs after a kick from another horse or when the horse kicks a fixed object, such as a wall. Osteitis causes moderate to severe lameness, cellulitis, and tarsal tenosynovitis. Concurrent sepsis of the calcaneal bursae, tarsocrural joint, or tarsal sheath may occur. Diagnosis is confirmed by radiography; however, radiologic signs of focal osteolysis may take days or weeks to develop and, therefore, sequential radiographs are recommended. Treatment involves debridement of any bony lesions, endoscopic lavage of infected synovial cavities, and wound debridement combined with appropriate local and systemic antimicrobial therapy.

FRACTURES OF THE DISTAL TARSAL BONES

Fractures of the central and third tarsal bones occur most commonly in Standardbred or Thoroughbred racehorses. Fractures usually cause acute-onset severe hindlimb lameness. Lameness is exacerbated by hock flexion. Acute fractures may be associated with heat, swelling, and pain on palpation over the distal tarsal bones; there may be tarsocrural joint effusion. Diagnosis is made by radiography, but fractures may not be visible until 7–14 days after injury when fracture line bone resorption has occurred. CT or bone scintigraphy can be useful for diagnosis if fracture is suspected but not evident radiologically. Variable fracture configurations can occur. Horses can be treated surgically with lag screw fixation or conservatively, depending on configuration of fracture. Prognosis depends on fracture configuration.

FRACTURE OF THE TALUS

Sagittal fractures of the talus are rare and have been most commonly reported in racehorses. Lameness is usually moderate to severe and associated with tarsocrural joint distention. Fractures in racehorses usually arise in the proximal aspect of the sagittal groove of the talus and are often incomplete. Fractures after trauma are usually comminuted. Prognosis depends on fracture configuration.

FRACTURE OF THE FIBULAR TARSAL BONE (CALCANEUS)

Fractures of the fibular tarsal bone are uncommon and usually the result of trauma. Small chip fractures may be successfully removed. Complete body and physeal fractures are difficult to repair, although they have been repaired with bone plates and tension band wiring. Horses with open, comminuted fractures have a grave prognosis and warrant humane euthanasia.

FRACTURE OF THE LATERAL MALLEOLUS OF THE TIBIA

Lateral malleolar fractures are usually traumatic. Small, well-rounded fragments are occasionally seen; they are considered likely to be a form of OCD and are usually asymptomatic. Small or minimally displaced fractures may be managed conservatively. Surgical removal of fragments may result in a quicker recovery. Some fragments may be removed arthroscopically, although some require an open approach through the lateral collateral ligament of the tarsocrural joint. Larger fragments may be successfully repaired by lag screw fixation.

TARSAL JOINT LUXATION

Complete luxation or subluxation of the tarsocrural, talocalcaneal-centroquartal, and tarsometatarsal joint may occur with or without concurrent tarsal bone fracture as the result of severe trauma. Horses may be salvaged for breeding or retirement to pasture by reducing the luxation under general anesthesia and applying a full limb cast for 6–8 wk followed by a further 4–8 wk of immobilization in a heavily padded bandage. Restricted range of motion of the hock and progressive osteoarthritis means these horses are unlikely to return to athletic use.

DESMITIS OF THE COLLATERAL LIGAMENTS OF THE TARSUS

Collateral ligament injury is usually the result of trauma or a fall. Lameness varies from mild to severe, depending on the severity of injury. Flexion of the hock is usually resented and will exacerbate lameness. Effusion of the tarsocrural joint and periarticular swelling are evident. Lameness may be improved by intra-articular analgesia of the tarsocrural joint. Diagnosis is confirmed with ultrasonography. Increased uptake of radionuclide at the proximal and distal attachments of the damaged ligament may be evident on scintigraphy, and enthesiopathy may be apparent radiologically in horses with chronic injury. Conservative treatment is recommended, with physical and chemical anti-inflammatory treatments in the acute stages and then a period of stall rest (4–6 mo) followed by a controlled ascending exercise program. Prognosis depends on the severity of injury.

RUPTURE OF THE FIBULARIS (PERONEUS) TERTIUS

The fibularis (peroneus) tertius is a tendinous structure that originates from the extensor fossa of the femur and runs over the craniolateral aspect of the tibia to insert on the dorsoproximal aspect of the third metatarsal bone, the calcaneus, and the third and fourth tarsal bones. It is part of the reciprocal apparatus of the hindlimb, which means there is concurrent flexion and extension of the hock and stifle. Rupture of the fibularis tertius may occur as a result of hyperextension of the limb and usually occurs in the middle of the crus, or laceration may occur on the dorsal aspect of the tarsus. Avulsion of the origin on the fibularis tertius is rare in mature horses but may occur in young animals.

Clinical signs are pathognomonic, because rupture of the fibularis tertius means horses are able to extend the hock while the stifle is flexed. Horses are able to bear weight on the affected limb. At walk, the gastrocnemius and superficial digital flexor muscles appear rather flaccid, and there is a characteristic dimple on the caudodistal aspect of the soft tissues of the crus. At trot, an obvious lameness is usually evident, with delayed protraction of the limb due to overextension of the hock.

Diagnosis is usually based on clinical signs and can be confirmed with ultrasonography.

Conservative treatment with 3–4 mo of stall rest followed by slow and careful reintroduction to exercise usually results in complete resolution of signs and return to athletic soundness.

STRINGHALT

Stringhalt is a gait abnormality characterized by exaggerated upward flexion of the hindlimb that occurs at every stride at walk. The gait abnormality usually lessens at trot and is not evident at canter. It may occur unilaterally or bilaterally. All degrees of hyperflexion are seen, from mild, spasmodic lifting and grounding of the foot, to extreme cases in which the foot is drawn sharply up until it touches the belly and is then struck violently on the ground. In severe cases, there is atrophy of the lateral thigh muscles. In Australian stringhalt and lathyrism, the condition may be progressive and the gait abnormality may become so severe that euthanasia is warranted. Mild stringhalt may be intermittent. The signs are most obvious when the horse is sharply turned or backed. In some cases, the condition is seen only on the first few steps after moving the horse. The signs are often less intense or even absent during warmer weather. Although it is regarded as unsoundness, stringhalt may not materially hinder the horse's ability to work, except in severe cases when the constant concussion gives rise to secondary complications. However, the condition may make the horse unsuitable for some equestrian disciplines (eg, dressage).

The etiology is unknown, but lesions of a peripheral neuropathy have been identified in the sciatic, peroneal, and tibial nerves. Severe forms of the condition have been attributed to lathyrism (sweet pea poisoning) in the USA and possibly to flat weed intoxication in Australia.

Diagnosis is based on clinical signs but can be confirmed by electromyography. If the diagnosis is in doubt, the horse should be observed as it is backed out of the stall after hard work for 1–2 days. False stringhalt sometimes appears as a result of some temporary irritation to the lower pastern area or even a painful lesion in the foot.

When intoxication is suspected, removal to another paddock may be all that is required. Many of these cases apparently recover spontaneously. In chronic cases, tenectomy of the lateral extensor of the digit, including removal of a portion of the muscle, has given best results. Improvement may not be evident until 2–3 wk after surgery, and not all cases respond. This is not surprising, because the condition is a distal axonopathy. Other methods of treatment include large doses of thiamine and phenytoin.

CURB

Curb is a term used to describe a number of soft-tissue injuries that cause swelling on the distal plantar aspect of the tarsus. Traditionally, the term "curb" is used to describe enlargement of the (long) plantar ligament on the plantar aspect of the calcaneus, but curb-like swelling may also be caused by peritendinous-periligamentous inflammation, superficial or deep digital flexor tendinitis, or a combination of injuries. Curb is primarily an injury of racehorses, particularly Standardbreds, and conformational abnormalities may be predisposing. Lameness varies from absent to severe, depending on the structure involved and the extent of the injury. Diagnosis of the exact nature of the injury is confirmed by ultrasonography. In most cases, treatment involves local anti-inflammatory therapy and NSAIDs in the acute phase and then rest and a controlled exercise program thereafter.

DISORDERS OF THE TARSAL SHEATH

(Thoroughpin)

The tarsal sheath is the synovial sheath of the lateral digital flexor tendon at the level of the hock. Tenosynovitis of the tarsal sheath (colloquially called thoroughpin) is common and can be caused by a wide range of lesions.

Idiopathic thoroughpin results in mild to moderate effusion of the tarsal sheath and is most commonly seen in young horses. Effusion may arise from acute inflammation in nearby tissues or edema in the distal limb (sympathetic effusion). It is not usually associated with lameness and tends to resolve spontaneously, although it may be recurrent or persistent.

Thoroughpin may occur as a result of direct trauma (eg, kick or hitting a fence), leading to acute inflammation and hemorrhage in the tarsal sheath. This may occur with or without concurrent damage to the lateral digital flexor tendon. Intrathecal hemorrhage results in pain and inflammation. Chronic inflammation may lead to synovial hypertrophy, fibrosis, and intrathecal adhesions between the lateral digital flexor tendon and parietal lining of the sheath. Primary sprain injuries of the lateral digital flexor tendon may also occur. Infectious tenosynovitis after a penetrating injury and resulting in synovial sepsis may also occur.

Treatment of thoroughpin depends on the underlying cause. Treatment of acute tenosynovitis, in the absence of tendinous or bony pathology, involves rest, systemic or local anti-inflammatory drugs, and cold therapy. Intrathecal medication with hyaluronan and/or corticosteroids may be useful in more severe cases. Intrathecal corticosteroids are contraindicated if there is tendon pathology. Horses with tenosynovitis associated with bony fragments, intrathecal ossicles, tearing or fraying of the lateral digital flexor tendon, or adhesions are candidates for tenoscopic surgery. Horses with infectious tenosynovitis require lavage of the tarsal sheath (best performed tenoscopically), plus appropriate systemic and local antimicrobial therapy.

FALSE THOROUGHPIN

False thoroughpin is a term used to describe a number of swellings that may develop in the distal region of the crus or tarsus and cranial to the gastrocnemius tendon. These may be seen unilaterally or bilaterally and are more common on the lateral aspect of the limb. These discrete swellings do not extend distal to the hock and cannot be balloted from lateral to medial. The swellings vary in size and may be acute or insidious in onset and may or may not be associated with lameness.

The causes of false thoroughpin vary and are not well understood. False thoroughpins are usually solitary, fluid-filled sacs; they may be multiloculated with a wall of variable thickness and may have fibrous bands traversing them. They may develop secondary to local hemorrhage or due to herniation of the tarsal sheath, gastrocnemius, or calcaneal bursae.

Ultrasonography is useful to assess the extent and nature of these swellings. Positive-contrast radiography can be used to determine whether the swellings are discrete or communicate with other structures.

In many horses, the lesions are not associated with lameness, so no treatment is required and the horses may stay in work. In some animals, low-grade lameness may occur. Intrathecal medication with corticosteroids may improve lameness in some horses, although swelling and lameness will often recur; in these cases, surgical excision may be curative.

LUXATION OF THE SUPERFICIAL DIGITAL FLEXOR TENDON FROM THE TUBER CALCANEI

Luxation or subluxation of the superficial digital flexor tendon from the point of the hock may occur after disruption to the retinaculum that attaches the tendon to the calcaneus. Luxation or subluxation more commonly occurs laterally but may occur medially. Rarely, the superficial digital flexor tendon may split sagitally, and part of the tendon luxates medially and part laterally.

Lameness is usually acute and severe in onset and associated with marked swelling over the point of the hock. Horses may become panic-stricken in the acute stages if the tendon is moving on and off the os calcis, and they may kick out frequently with the affected limb. In some horses, the tendon will resume its normal position when the horse is standing but luxate or subluxate as the horse moves; in other horses, the tendon remains permanently displaced. Diagnosis is based on careful observation and palpation and can be confirmed by ultrasonography.

In the acute stages, sedation and analgesia are important. If the tendon remains permanently displaced laterally (or medially), treatment involves prolonged stall rest (4–6 mo), possibly with the limb immobilized in a heavily padded full limb bandage or cast. Lameness usually improves, but the horse may be left with a mechanical lameness causing a jerky hindlimb action that may limit its use as a dressage horse, although horses may be able to jump or race. Horses with a persistently medially displaced tendon usually have a greater degree of mechanical lameness and a poorer prognosis for return to athletic function.

In horses in which the tendon is unstable and subluxates on and off the tuber calcanei, endoscopy of the calcaneal bursa reveals disruption of both the medial retinacular/calcaneal insertion of the superficial digital flexor tendon and its associated fibrocartilage, with disruption of the medial wall of the bursa creating or establishing communication with an acquired subcutaneous bursa. Treatment is by radical resection of the disrupted fibrocartilage and division of remaining attachments of the fibrocartilage or retinacular insertions with the unstable main body of the superficial digital flexor tendon, thereby creating a stable lateral subluxation. Although repair or reconstruction techniques have been reported, results have been unreliable. Permanent stable subluxation eliminates anxiety and usually results in a "sound" functional horse.

GASTROCNEMIUS TENDINITIS

Tendinitis of the gastrocnemius tendon is a rare cause of hindlimb lameness in a horse. Injury usually occurs distally, although rarely at the musculotendinous junction. Lameness may be sudden or gradual in onset, and the severity of lameness varies depending on the severity of injury. Distention of the calcaneal (or intertendinous) and gastrocnemius bursa is common. Lameness is usually exacerbated by a proximal limb flexion test.

Lameness is usually improved by perineural analgesia of the tibial nerve, and diagnosis is confirmed with ultrasonography.

Conservative treatment with stall rest and controlled exercise for 6–12 mo is usually indicated. Horses with mild to moderate lesions have a reasonable prognosis for return to athletic work, but the prognosis for horses with more severe lesions is guarded.

CALCANEAL BURSITIS

The calcaneal (intertendinous bursa) lies between the tendons of the gastrocnemius and superficial digital flexor muscles proximal to the hock and extends on the plantar aspect of the calcaneus to the level of the distal tarsus. In most horses, there is a communication between the calcaneal and gastrocnemius bursa and, in approximately a third of horses, with the subcutaneous bursa.

Inflammation and distention of the bursa may or may not be associated with lameness. It may be idiopathic, secondary to trauma or intrathecal hemorrhage, or occur in association with gastrocnemius tendinitis. Septic bursitis may occur secondary to infectious osteitis of the calcaneus or after a penetrating injury.

Horses with septic bursitis need to be treated aggressively with surgical debridement and lavage and appropriate antimicrobial therapy. Horses with aseptic bursitis may be treated with rest, drainage, and intrathecal medication with corticosteroids; results are variable.

CAPPED HOCK

Capped hock is due to distention of the subcutaneous bursa or development of an acquired bursa over the tuber calcanei. This usually results from repetitive trauma (eg, kicking or leaning on stable walls) and is not usually associated with lameness. Occasionally, a subcutaneous abscess may arise as the result of a penetrating injury and lead to painful swelling and lameness. Treatment of an abscess requires surgical excision and appropriate antimicrobial treatment.

DISORDERS OF THE STIFLE

OSTEOCHONDROSIS

Osteochondrosis (*see* p 1148) is a common cause of stifle lameness in young horses. Lesions in the stifle most commonly occur on the lateral trochlear ridge of the femur but may also occur on the medial trochlear ridge, in the intertrochlear groove, or on the patella. Lesions are often bilateral and probably develop in the first 6 mo of life. In severe cases, joint effusion and lameness may be evident in foals or yearlings. In less severe cases, clinical signs may not become evident until the horse starts athletic work. In mild cases, clinical signs may be absent. The severity of lameness varies from absent to severe and is often acute in onset. Effusion of the femoropatellar joint is common. Diagnosis may be confirmed by demonstration of radiographic or ultrasonographic changes or by arthroscopy.

Mild lesions in foals have been shown to heal with conservative treatment. More severe lesions in foals may require arthroscopic debridement, but care should be taken not to remove too much of the subchondral bone. In horses with larger defects or fragmentation, arthroscopic surgery is the treatment of choice to remove osteochondral fragments and poorly attached or loose cartilage and to debride abnormal subchondral bone.

In adult horses, the prognosis after surgery for return to athletic soundness is fair to good but depends on the severity of the lesions and the size of the defect in the subchondral bone.

SUBCHONDRAL CYSTIC LESIONS

Subchondral cystic lesions most commonly occur in the stifle in the medial femoral condyle. Osseous cyst-like lesions may also occur in the proximal tibia. The pathogenesis of these cysts is poorly understood, but they may develop after trauma to the articular surface or as a result of osteochondrosis. Lesions often present in young horses but can be seen at any age. The severity of lameness varies from mild to severe and may be acute in onset. Lameness may be intermittent, particularly in older horses. In some horses there is mild effusion of the medial femorotibial joint, but in many horses no localizing signs are evident. Intra-articular anesthesia of the femorotibial joints may produce partial improvement.

Diagnosis is usually confirmed by radiography. Medial femoral subchondral cystic lesions are most evident on caudocranial projections and may appear as a variably sized round or oval radiolucent defect in the subchondral bone. Some lesions are surrounded by an obvious sclerotic rim. In some horses, only a very small defect is evident radiographically in the medial femoral condyle; this may be a precursor to subchondral cystic lesions. Defects in the surface of the medial femoral condyle may be evident ultrasonographically in some horses. Subchondral cystic lesions in the proximal tibia are usually smaller and most evident on lateral, lateral oblique, or caudocranial radiographic projections.

Nonarticular osseous cyst-like lesions or small lesions may respond to conservative treatment, including rest, systemic NSAIDs, and intra-articular corticosteroids. If horses do not respond to conservative treatment, surgery is indicated. Some surgeons advise injection of corticosteroids into the lining of the cyst under arthroscopic or ultrasonographic guidance to decrease the shedding of inflammatory enzymes and mediators into the joint; others advise arthroscopic debridement of the cyst to remove the contents and lining.

The prognosis for return to athletic function in horses with subchondral cyst-like lesions of the medial femoral condyle after injection of the lining of the cyst under arthroscopic guidance has been reported to be fair, with 64% returning to athletic use in one study irrespective of the age of the horse. The prognosis for return to athletic function after debridement of the cyst seems to vary with the horse's age. The prognosis for athletic soundness in horses

<3 yr old was better (~64%) than in horses >3 yr old (35%) at the time of surgery in one large, multicenter retrospective study.

MENISCUS AND MENISCAL LIGAMENT INJURIES

Injuries to the menisci and the meniscal ligaments are a common cause of stifle lameness in adult horses. Lesions range from mild fibrillation of the meniscal ligaments and surface of the menisci, causing low-grade, chronic lameness, to severe tears of the meniscal ligament and menisci, causing acute and severe lameness. The medial meniscus is more commonly affected.

Effusion of the femorotibial joints is a common, associated clinical sign. In most horses, lameness is significantly improved by intra-articular anesthesia of the femorotibial joints. Subtle radiographic changes may be evident with enthesiophytes or lytic areas at the site of attachment of the meniscal ligament or dystrophic mineralization within the meniscus. Osteoarthritic changes may be evident in horses with chronic or severe injuries. Ultrasonographic examination may be useful to demonstrate meniscal injury.

Arthroscopic examination is indicated in horses that do not respond to conservative treatment (ie, rest and anti-inflammatory medication followed by controlled rehabilitation). Arthroscopy allows assessment of the extent and severity of injury, although only the cranial and caudal poles of the menisci are visible arthroscopically. Arthroscopy also allows torn or fibrillated fibers of the meniscal ligaments to be debrided and flaps of meniscus or fibrillated meniscal tissue to be removed.

The prognosis for return to athletic function depends on the severity of injury. Overall, ~50% of horses with meniscal and meniscal ligament injury return to athletic use. However, in horses with severe tears that extend beneath the femoral condyle and horses with concurrent osteoarthritis, the prognosis is considerably poorer.

CRANIAL AND CAUDAL CRUCIATE LIGAMENT INJURIES

Complete rupture of a cruciate ligament is usually a catastrophic injury resulting in severe lameness and joint instability. Strains and partial rupture of the cranial and caudal cruciate ligaments may result in variable lameness, depending on the severity of injury. Effusions of the femoropatellar or femorotibial joints are sometimes present. Lameness is usually improved by intra-articular anesthesia of the femorotibial joints. In some horses, radiographic changes may be evident at the sites of attachment of the ligament with enthesiophyte formation or focal areas of radiolucency. Ultrasonography of the cruciate ligaments is difficult but may demonstrate some lesions. However, in many horses, diagnosis is confirmed only by arthroscopic examination.

Conservative treatment involving rest, systemic NSAIDs, and intra-articular corticosteroids is indicated in horses with acute injuries. If horses do not respond to conservative treatment, arthroscopic surgery is recommended to debride loose and torn ligament fibers.

The prognosis for return to athletic function depends on the severity of injury. Horses with complete rupture have a grave prognosis. Horses with moderate to severe injuries have a poor prognosis for return to athletic function, whereas horses with mild injuries have a fair prognosis.

COLLATERAL LIGAMENT INJURIES

Rupture or sprain of the medial or lateral collateral ligaments of the stifle is usually the result of an acute traumatic episode in which the distal limb is forced medially or laterally, thereby stressing the ligaments. Rupture or sprain is more common in the medial collateral ligament than in the lateral collateral ligament. Concurrent injury of the menisci or cruciate ligaments is common, particularly in severe injuries. Lameness depends on the severity of the injury but is usually quite severe initially. Localized edema and joint effusion is seen, particularly in the acute stages. Flexion tests of the stifle usually exacerbate lameness. Clinical signs usually improve within a few days unless there is significant joint instability. Intra-articular anesthesia of the ipsiaxial femorotibial joint will not always alleviate lameness. If the ligament rupture is complete, stressed caudocranial radiographs of the stifle may demonstrate joint widening on the affected side. Enthesiophyte formation at the origin or insertion of the ligament may be evident radiographically in chronic cases. Diagnosis is usually confirmed by ultrasonographic examination.

Horses with mild sprains may be treated conservatively with stable rest and anti-inflammatory medication for 6–8 wk, followed by a controlled, ascending exercise rehabilitation program for a further 6–8 wk. Horses with mild sprains and no joint instability have a fair prognosis for return to athletic use. The prognosis for horses with severe injury is poor.

INTERMITTENT UPWARD FIXATION OF THE PATELLA AND DELAYED PATELLA RELEASE

Intermittent upward fixation of the patella occurs when the medial patellar ligament remains hooked over the medial trochlear ridge of the femur and locks the reciprocal apparatus with the limb in extension. A horse with upward fixation of the patella stands with the hindlimb fixed in extension with the fetlock flexed. The leg will usually release with a sudden snap or jerking movement.

Some horses demonstrate a milder form of this condition. In these horses, there is delayed release of the patella during limb protraction, most commonly evident as the horse moves off or in downward transitions. This appears as a jerky movement of the patella. Horses with recurrent upward fixation or delayed release of the patella may develop chronic, low-grade lameness due to stifle soreness and may be reluctant to work on soft, deep surfaces or up or down hills.

Upward fixation or delayed release of the patella is most commonly seen in young horses and ponies, particularly if they are in poor body condition and poorly muscled. Straight hindlimb conformation may predispose to this condition. It may also be seen in older horses that have had trauma to the stifle region, particularly if the horses are stabled or have been inactive.

Diagnosis is based on recognition of typical clinical signs. In some horses, upward fixation of the patella may be induced by pushing the horse backward or manually pushing the patella proximally. Radiographs of the stifle should be taken in horses with femoropatellar joint effusion and lameness to establish concurrent or secondary pathology.

To release an upward fixated patella, the horse should be pushed backward while simultaneously pushing the patella medially and distally. Alternatively, pulling the limb forward with a rope around the pastern may unlock the patella. If upward fixation of the patella is intermittent and not causing lameness, a conditioning program should be instituted. This involves daily lungeing or riding of the horse, appropriate to its age and type, as well as ensuring an adequate plane of nutrition, good dentistry, and anthelmintic administration. Stable rest is contraindicated, and the horse should be turned out to pasture as much as possible. Remedial foot trimming to ensure the foot is well balanced and shoeing with a bevel-edged shoe with or without a lateral heel wedge may be beneficial. A significant proportion of horses will improve with maturity and conservative treatment, although signs may recur if the horse undergoes prolonged stall rest.

Medial patellar ligament desmotomy is indicated in horses that do not respond to conservative treatment or in horses with lameness caused by upward fixation of the patella. Medial patellar ligament desmotomy is most often performed in the sedated horse under local anesthesia, although some surgeons prefer general anesthesia. After surgery, the horse should be restricted to stable or small stall rest for 2 mo to reduce the risk of complications. Fragmentation of the apex of the patella is the most common complication after surgery (*see* below); if it results in lameness, it may be treated arthroscopically with good results. Other complications include lameness, local swelling, or even patella fracture. The prognosis after medial patellar ligament desmotomy is generally considered to be good, with recurrence of the condition rare. Medial patella ligament splitting, which involves making numerous small incisions in the ligament, has also been used successfully to manage these horses.

FRAGMENTATION OF THE PATELLA

Fragmentation of the apex of the patella usually occurs secondary to medial patellar desmotomy for management of upward fixation of the patella. Lesions are believed to develop due to patellar instability as a result of the surgery. The severity of lameness varies from mild stiffness to moderate lameness. A proximal limb flexion test usually exacerbates lameness, and femoropatellar joint effusion is usually present. Lameness is localized by diagnostic anesthesia of the femoropatellar joint, and diagnosis is confirmed by radiography. Arthroscopic debridement of the apex of the patella with removal of the osteochondral fragments is the treatment of choice. Prognosis is reasonable but depends on the severity of the condition.

PATELLAR LUXATION

Lateral luxation of the patella is a rare, inherited condition in foals caused by a recessive gene. Luxation of the patella in adult horses is unusual and likely to be traumatic in origin. Lateral luxation is more common than medial luxation and may be more likely in horses or foals with hypoplasia of the lateral trochlear ridge of the femur. The condition may be unilateral or bilateral and varies in severity from intermittent luxation that readily reduces to persistent luxation that cannot be reduced.

Severely affected foals are unable to extend the stifle and so adopt a characteristic crouching position. If the condition is less severe, foals or horses may be reluctant to flex the stifle and thus demonstrate a stiff hindlimb gait. Diagnosis can be confirmed by radiography.

Although a number of surgical treatments have been reported, the prognosis in adult horses and in horses with concurrent osteoarthritis is poor. The prognosis for athletic function in foals may be slightly better.

PATELLAR LIGAMENT INJURIES

Patellar ligament injuries are rare but may be seen in jumping horses. The middle patellar ligament is the most commonly affected. Lameness is variable but may be severe in acute cases. Clinical signs are often subtle; femoropatellar joint effusion, periligamentous thickening, and edema are inconsistent findings. In many horses, lameness is unchanged by intra-articular anesthesia of the femoropatellar joint; therefore, diagnosis is confirmed by ultrasonography. Treatment is prolonged rest (up to 6 mo). Lameness is often slow to resolve and may recur.

GONITIS AND OSTEOARTHRITIS

Mild to moderate inflammation of the femorotibial and femoropatellar joints of unknown origin is common. Severity of lameness varies. Synovitis and capsulitis may result from athletic sprain of the joints. Mild trauma to the articular cartilage, menisci, or any of the ligaments of the stifle may produce mild to moderate synovitis. Mild synovitis usually responds to rest and intra-articular and systemic anti-inflammatory drugs. If joint inflammation and lameness persist, further diagnostic investigation and arthroscopic examination are advisable to assess concurrent or causative injuries and to prevent ongoing degenerative joint disease and development of osteoarthritis.

Osteoarthritis of the femorotibial or femoropatellar joints may follow any of the causes of stifle lameness described and usually results in persistent lameness of varying severity. Diagnosis is confirmed with intra-articular anesthesia and radiography. Radiographic changes include periarticular remodeling with osteophyte formation and remodeling of the joint margins (particularly the medial tibial plateau), changes in the subchondral bone, narrowing of the joint space, and dystrophic mineralization of the soft tissues. The prognosis for athletic soundness in horses with osteoarthritis of the stifle is poor, and treatment is usually palliative. Newer techniques for arthroscopy and regenerative therapy may offer some hope for severely affected joints.

CHONDROMALACIA OF THE FEMORAL CONDYLES

Chondromalacia of the femoral condyles is being increasingly recognized in sports horses. Horses typically present with poor performance or low grade, often bilateral, hindlimb lameness with pain referable to the stifle. Lameness or loss of performance usually becomes evident in younger horses as their work intensity increases. Frequently, there are no localizing signs, although mild effusion of the medial femorotibial and/or femoropatellar joints may be evident. Typically there are no radiologic or ultrasonographic signs evident. Arthroscopic examination of the femorotibial joints reveals abnormally soft, irregular, cracked, pitted, and poorly attached articular cartilage over all or part of the femoral condyles. Generally, the prognosis for sustained return to athletic soundness is guarded. More studies are required to determine the best form of surgical intervention in management of these horses.

FRACTURES

Fractures of the Patella

Fractures of the patella usually result from direct trauma, most commonly when a horse is kicked by another horse or hits a fixed obstacle while jumping. Prognosis depends on fracture conformation. Sagittal fractures of the medial pole of the patella are most common. These fractures are usually intra-articular and involve the attachment of the parapatellar fibrocartilage of the medial patellar ligament. Complete horizontal fractures are rare but considered serious injuries because of fragment distraction due to the massive pull of the extensor muscles. Complete sagittal fractures may be more amenable to internal fixation, because there is less distractive force.

Fracture of the patella usually results in marked lameness initially, with swelling and edema over the patella and effusion of the femoropatellar joint. In less severe or nonarticular fractures, lameness may improve within a few days. Diagnosis is confirmed by radiography. Standard radiographic projections of the stifle, together with a cranioproximal-craniodistal oblique projection of the patella, are used to determine fracture configuration.

Management options depend on fracture configuration. Horses with small, nondisplaced, nonarticular fractures may be treated conservatively with stable rest for 6–8 wk and have a good prognosis for return to athletic function. Articular fractures of the medial pole of the patella can be removed arthroscopically or via an arthrotomy and are also considered to have a good prognosis. Larger, mid-body sagittal or horizontal fractures require repair by internal fixation. These injuries carry a risk of catastrophic breakdown during anesthetic recovery but can have a favorable outcome.

Fractures of the Tibial Tuberosity

Fractures of the tibial tuberosity are not uncommon. There is little soft tissue covering this area, and fractures usually result from direct trauma. Fracture configuration may range from small fragments off the cranial proximal part of the tuberosity to large fractures of the whole of the tuberosity extending into the femorotibial joints. Fracture of the tibial tuberosity usually results in marked lameness initially with localized swelling and edema. Lameness will often improve within a few days. Diagnosis is confirmed by radiography.

Small and nondisplaced fractures may heal with conservative treatment. Stable rest for 6–8 wk is advised. During the first 2–3 wk, the horse should be prevented from lying down by tying or the use of slings to prevent fragment displacement. Larger intra-articular fractures should be repaired by internal fixation. Fractures generally have a good prognosis for return to athletic function if appropriately managed.

Fractures of the Femoral Condyles and Femoral Trochlear Ridges

Fracture of the femoral condyles is usually the result of direct trauma. Large, intra-articular, displaced fractures in adult horses are catastrophic and have a grave prognosis. However, traumatic fragmentation of the femoral condyles or trochlear ridges can also occur. Such injuries usually result in acute onset, moderate to severe lameness with joint effusion. Diagnosis is confirmed by radiography. Treatment involves surgical removal of the fracture fragments to prevent development of osteoarthritis. This is usually achieved arthroscopically but may require arthrotomy. The prognosis is usually considered to be good after surgery, so long as there is no significant concurrent soft-tissue damage.

DISORDERS OF THE HIP

Disorders of the coxofemoral joint are relatively rare causes of lameness in horses. Most cases are traumatic in origin, secondary to falls or being cast (within a stall) in recumbency, although septic arthropathies and developmental disorders of the joint have been occasionally reported. Regardless of the etiology of the primary disease, secondary osteoarthritis of the coxofemoral joint is a common sequela, which will frequently result in permanent lameness.

Lameness is the predominant presenting clinical sign of any coxofemoral disease. Although the lameness can be subtle, more frequently a moderate to severe lameness (non-weight-bearing) is seen at presentation. In severe cases, the horse will often stand with the limb partially flexed. With any degree of chronicity, atrophy of the muscles of the hindquarters, such as the gluteals and quadriceps, is often moderate to marked. In cases of coxofemoral subluxation, the leg will be held in a semi-flexed position with an obvious outward rotation of the stifle and toe and an inward rotation of the point of the hock. In complete coxofemoral luxations, the same rotational abnormality in limb position is observed, and additionally the leg will appear shorter, which is best identified by the point of the hock being displaced proximal to that of the contralateral limb. Most horses with coxofemoral pathology show some pain on proximal limb flexion or abduction. Rectal examination is generally unrewarding, although in some cases of acute fracture, a hematoma or alteration in the bony architecture is palpable per rectum. Intra-articular local anesthesia of the coxofemoral joint is frequently used to identify the joint as the cause of lameness, particularly in cases of chronic lameness. Although this technique can be technically challenging, ultrasonography can help guide needle placement.

Definitive diagnosis of coxofemoral pathology usually requires some form of diagnostic imaging. Bone scanning (nuclear scintigraphy) is commonly used to identify the coxofemoral joint as the site of pathology. This technique is highly sensitive for identification of the involvement of the joint but has a low specificity for identification of the pathology within the joint. Percutaneous ultrasonography can provide considerable information on the coxofemoral joint, although its use at this site is technically challenging. Radiography can be very rewarding, especially in smaller horses and ponies, although optimal views require general anesthesia. Because of the risk of using general anesthesia in horses with serious limb injuries, such imaging is only rarely performed. A number of techniques are available to radiograph the coxofemoral joint in the standing horse, using either a ventrodorsal or lateral oblique views. Arthroscopy of the coxofemoral joint is possible, although it is technically challenging in most adult horses and ponies; acceptable joint visualization can be obtained by most operators in foals.

LUXATION OF THE COXOFEMORAL JOINT

Luxation of the coxofemoral joint is relatively rare in horses because of the strong ligamentous support provided to the joint by the round ligament and the accessory femoral ligament, as well as the fibrocartilaginous lip that surrounds the acetabulum. In horses, this injury is usually secondary to trauma. Luxations are much more common in small ponies, such as Shetland ponies, in which luxation of the coxofemoral joint has been frequently described secondary to upward fixation of the patella. Fracture of the dorsal acetabular rim may accompany the dislocation. Luxations are usually accompanied by a characteristic alteration in limb appearance. Luxations of the coxofemoral joint are best managed by closed reduction under general anesthesia, although this is likely to be successful only if the reduction is performed soon after the injury. It can be difficult to maintain the reduction in place through recovery from general anesthesia, and although the use of surgical techniques or Ehmer slings has been advocated, no single technique has been shown to be successful. The prognosis for return to athletic function after coxofemoral luxation is very guarded. In small ponies, closed reduction has allowed animals to become comfortable pasture animals.

PELVIC FRACTURE

Pelvic fractures are relatively common in horses and ponies and can occur as a consequence of trauma or stress from athletic training. Fractures involving the acetabulum almost always occur as a consequence of trauma and usually present as a severe lameness, which is frequently non-weight-bearing at the time of injury. Crepitus may be difficult to appreciate, even during passive flexion of the limb or rectal examination. Radiography can be diagnostic, but the difficulties of obtaining such images means that diagnosis is usually achieved by a combination of nuclear scintigraphy and ultrasonography. In particular, ultrasound diagnosis of pelvic fractures has advanced considerably and is now considered the first-line method to assess pelvic fractures. Fractures of the acetabulum, in contrast to other types of pelvic fractures, carry a poor prognosis for return to athletic function, because such fractures are frequently displaced and invariably lead to osteoarthritis. The only treatment is usually prolonged (6–9 mo) rest followed by symptomatic therapy for any resultant osteoarthritis.

OSTEOARTHRITIS AND OTHER COXOFEMORAL JOINT DISEASES

Osteoarthritis (OA) of the coxofemoral joint is usually secondary to major trauma such as luxation or fracture of the joint. Occasionally, idiopathic OA is diagnosed as a cause of chronic lameness. Cases of osteochondrosis or bone cyst formation within the coxofemoral joint have been reported, which can lead to secondary OA. Septic arthritis of the coxofemoral joint is seen occasionally in foals as a consequence of hematogenous spread or idiopathically in adult animals.

In cases of established OA, treatment is usually symptomatic, using NSAIDs, intra-articular corticosteroids, or other symptomatic treatments. In cases of septic arthritis, treatment should consist of surgical debridement and lavage in conjunction with local and systemic antimicrobial therapy. In cases of OA, full recovery is unusual. Successful treatment of septic arthritis is possible in foals but unlikely in adult horses unless diagnosed quickly and treated aggressively.

DISORDERS OF THE BACK AND PELVIS

Back problems are a major cause of poor performance and gait abnormalities in sport and race horses. Although it is often possible with the history and clinical (physical and dynamic) examination to suspect functional abnormalities of the vertebral column, definitive diagnosis of the cause of the pain is a challenge. There is undoubtedly a complex relationship between subtle (usually bilateral) hindlimb lameness, back pain, and poor performance. It can be challenging practically to differentiate and definitively determine the relative importance of differing orthopedic pathologies in such cases.

Once back pain is suspected or established in a horse, identification of the cause requires imaging procedures. This discipline has seen major advances, particularly relating to integrating radiographic, ultrasonographic, and nuclear scintigraphic findings. In addition, there is greater understanding of the relationships between identification of specific imaging findings and the possibly of such findings leading to pain.

SPINAL PROCESSES AND ASSOCIATED LIGAMENTS

Kissing Spines

The most common location of kissing spines is the vertebral segment between T10 and T18, although these lesions are also identified between L1 and L6. Abnormal findings can be seen in the dorsal part of the spinous processes where their identification is easy; they include kissing and overriding lesions. Different grades can be identified (grade 1: narrowing of the interspinal space; grade 2: densification of the margins; grade 3: bone lysis adjacent to the margins; grade 4: severe remodeling). Abnormal findings can also be seen in the ventral part of the spinous processes and may involve the interspinal ligaments or be associated with osteoarthrosis of the articular processes. Their severity can be established using the same grading system; their clinical incidence seems higher.

The incidence of kissing spines seems to vary according to the discipline/use of the horse and biomechanical effects of specific gaits and exercises on the back. In general, these lesions are commonly found in racing Thoroughbreds and seem to be tolerated in many of them. They are quite rare in Standardbreds, but when present, their likelihood of causing pain seems higher. Intermediate frequency and signs are seen in sport horses. Kissing spines can be found in performance race and sport horses without back pain and even with normal thoracolumbar active and passive mobilization. Thus, in each case, the clinical significance of these lesions must be carefully assessed. Diagnosis can be aided by injection of local anesthetic into the affected interspinous spaces. Medical management includes local injections of steroids and/or shockwave therapy, as well as rehabilitation using tolerated exercises after progressive warm-up at a slow canter. Surgical treatment has been advocated for this condition, with surgical resection of the affected spinous processes being most commonly performed and being described as efficacious in managing this condition. A number of differing techniques have been described for this surgical management.

Fractures

Multiple fractures of the spinous processes of T4–T10 are sometimes seen in horses that have reared and fallen over backward. The summits and centers of ossification are fractured and displaced laterally. After the initial pain and local reaction have subsided, recovery is often satisfactory, with usually no permanent effect on performance, although a persistent deformation of the withers may require some adaptation of the saddle.

Desmopathies

(Supraspinal ligament injuries)

Acute or subacute desmopathies can be identified ultrasonographically, because they demonstrate dorsoventral or transverse thickening of the ligament, altered echogenicity, and obvious alteration of the linear longitudinal pattern. They can be seen both in the median plane or asymmetrically. In old or chronic injuries, the ligament often remains thicker, with a reduced echogenicity and an irregular architectural pattern. Hyperechogenic images with or without acoustic shadows are compatible with mineralization or calcification of the supraspinous ligament. Alteration of the bone surface of the top of the spinous processes indicates insertional desmopathy (enthesopathy) of the supraspinous ligament. The significance of findings can be difficult to definitively prove, because ultrasonographic abnormalities can be seen in healthy as well as injured horses.

ARTICULAR PROCESS–SYNOVIAL INTERVERTEBRAL ARTICULATION COMPLEXES

The articular process-synovial intervertebral articulation complex is located dorsally to the vertebral canal. It is composed of the caudal articular process of one vertebra, the synovial joint (with articular cartilage, synovial fluid and membrane, and articular capsule) located at the base of the interspinal space, and the cranial articular process of the following vertebra. It is also known as the dorsal articular facet joint. Osteoarthritis of this joint has been described radiographically, with a number of different types described, with sclerosis, periarticular new bone, and narrowing of joint space frequently being identified. Commonly two to five joints are affected, usually in the caudal thoracic and cranial lumbar region. In some cases, there will be abnormal nuclear scintigraphic uptake of the region, which can aid with diagnosis. Further ultrasonographic abnormalities can be identified, particularly relating to periarticular osteophytes and proliferation. Treatment and management include periarticular ultrasonographic-guided injections of steroids, use of NSAIDs, and rehabilitation using exercise protocols after progressive warm-up at a slow canter.

VERTEBRAL BODIES AND DISCS

The most common lesion of vertebral bodies and discs is ventral, ventrolateral, or lateral bony proliferation (often called vertebral spondylosis); it is mainly found in the mid-thoracic area (mostly between T11 and T13) but can also be seen in the lumbar area. They can be found on asymptomatic horses but can also be responsible for acute pain or chronic back stiffness. Spondylosis is a rare cause of back pain; in one survey, only 3.4% of 670 horses with back pain demonstrated this abnormality. Congenital abnormalities with vertebral body deformation (triangular or trapezoidal shape) are rare and usually found in the thoracic vertebrae. Vertebral body osteomyelitis, leading to neurologic signs, can be seen in the thoracolumbar spine in foals. Vertebral body fractures occur in horses that have had severe trauma or falls, particularly in racehorses in jumping races. Complete or partial paraplegia results from damage to the spinal cord. The prognosis is usually grave.

MUSCLE STRAIN AND SORENESS

See also MYOPATHIES IN HORSES, p 1176.

Damage to the muscles is probably the most common cause of back soreness in horses. This most commonly involves the longissimus dorsi muscle, which acts to extend and laterally flex the vertebral column. All or part of the longissimus muscles usually are strained during ridden exercise, and clinical signs are associated with altered performance and acute or chronic back pain. The principal sites of damage are the caudal withers and cranial lumbar regions (just in front of and behind the saddle area). Most of these injuries respond to rest and physiotherapy, although several weeks may be needed for full recovery. Abnormalities of the thoracolumbar musculature are also frequently seen in exertional rhabdomyolysis (tying-up syndrome, *see* p 1178).

LUMBOSACRAL JUNCTION ABNORMALITIES

Abnormal findings of the lumbosacral junction causing back pain are often detected with ultrasonography and include 1) congenital abnormalities such as lumbosacral ankylosis (sacralization of L6) or intervertebral ankylosis between L5 and L6; 2) disc degenerative lesions, especially affecting the lumbosacral disc (lesions include fissuration or cavitation of the disc, dystrophic mineralization, and ventral herniation); 3) intervertebral malalignment (spondylolisthesis) of the lumbosacral joint or the joint between L5 and L6; and 4) intertransverse lumbosacral osteoarthrosis (periarticular osteophytes or remodeling at the joint margins).

SACROILIAC JOINT ABNORMALITIES

Acute and severe strain of the sacroiliac ligaments is associated with a history of injury and severe pain in the pelvic or sacroiliac region, often with marked hindlimb lameness. Subacute or chronic sacroiliac strain and osteoarthrosis of the sacroiliac joint cause typical back soreness. There is often a history of poor performance, with an intermittent, often shifting, hindlimb lameness. This may be associated with some restriction in hindlimb action and dragging of the toes of the hindlimb(s).

A diagnosis of sacroiliac pain and lesions can be made in clinical practice with a combination of physical examination and exclusion of other causes of lameness. A demonstration of improvement in gait after local anesthetic infiltration of the sacroiliac joint region is occasionally performed to confirm diagnosis. Ultrasonographic assessment of the ventral aspect of the sacroiliac can be performed using a rectal probe. Abnormal ultrasonographic findings seen at the ventral aspect of the sacroiliac joint in clinical cases include bone modeling of the sacrum and/or ileum, narrowing of the joint space, remodeling or periarticular osteophytes of the caudal border of the articular surface of the sacrum and caudal articular margin of the ileum, periarticular bone fragmentation, and ventral sacroiliac ligament desmopathy and enthesopathy.

Treatment and management of sacroiliac disease is usually supportive and nonspecific. Therapies include periarticular injections of steroids and rehabilitation using progressive warm-up at a slow canter and exercises that develop the gluteal muscles.

DEVELOPMENTAL ORTHOPEDIC DISEASE

Developmental orthopedic diseases of horses constitute an important group of conditions that includes osteochondrosis, physeal dysplasia, acquired angular limb deformities, flexural deformities, and cuboidal bone malformations.

OSTEOCHONDROSIS

(Osteochondritis dissecans, Dyschondroplasia)

Osteochondrosis is one of the most important and prevalent developmental orthopedic diseases of horses. Although its specific etiology is not known, it is considered to arise from a focal disturbance in endochondral ossification, with subsequent trauma or physiologic loading resulting in lesion formation. The term osteochondrosis is currently used to describe the clinical manifestation of the disorder; however, the term dyschondroplasia is preferred when referring to early lesions.

Osteochondrosis has a multifactorial etiology that includes rapid growth, high carbohydrate diet, mineral imbalance, and biomechanics (ie, trauma to cartilage). Genetics has been implicated, with some breeds predisposed (eg, Standardbred and Swedish Warmblood). The condition mainly affects articular growth cartilage, but the metaphysis may also be involved. If the physeal metaphyseal cartilage is affected, bone contours and longitudinal growth are disturbed (*see* p 1149). Dyschondroplasia at articular surfaces may progress to formation of cartilage flaps or osteochondral fragments (osteochondrosis). At some sites, subchondral cysts may develop (*see* p 1062). Axial skeletal involvement includes vertebral articular facets, which may be associated with stenosis of the vertebral canal and, therefore, ataxia and proprioceptive deficits (ie, wobbler syndrome), but the relationship between these conditions is not clear.

Clinical Findings: The clinical signs of equine osteochondrosis are difficult to characterize specifically because of the wide range of lesions and sites involved. In young horses, many cases have no detectable clinical signs and are identified only on presale radiographs. Furthermore, lesions of dyschondroplasia may not progress to osteochondrosis, and radiographically observed osteochondrosis lesions may resolve over time without producing clinical signs. In severe cases, other signs of developmental orthopedic disease also may be apparent.

The most common presenting sign of osteochondrosis is a nonpainful distention of an affected joint (eg, gonitis, bog spavin). The exceptions to this are joints in which swelling is difficult to detect (eg, shoulder joint, medial femorotibial joint), in which case lameness is more often the first sign observed. Clinical signs may be divided broadly into two categories: those seen in foals <6 mo old and those seen in older animals. Often the first sign noted in foals is a tendency to spend more time lying down. This is accompanied frequently by joint swelling, stiffness, and difficulty keeping up with other animals in the paddock. An accompanying sign may be the development of upright conformation of the limbs. Fetlock osteochondrosis is particularly seen in younger foals (<6 mo old).

Lameness is usually absent or mild except for those sites mentioned above for which the earlier sign of joint swelling is difficult to detect. For example, lesions in the shoulder frequently result in moderate to severe lameness, muscle atrophy, and pain on joint flexion. In the stifle, some horses with subchondral bone cysts in the medial femoral condyle present with lameness severe enough that a fracture may be suspected, and swelling may only be detected on careful examination. More severe signs are also observed when osteochondral fragments come loose within the joint. This is often seen in yearlings or older horses that present with stiffness, flexion responses, and varying degrees of lameness. These signs are usually associated with the onset of training.

Diagnosis: Clinical diagnosis can often be made on the basis of signalment and signs.

More definitive diagnosis requires use of some specific clinical aids. Radiographic examination has been the traditional way to confirm diagnosis; however, early lesions involving cartilage without significant subchondral bone damage may not be visualized. In the distal limb, oblique views may be helpful; in the hock, because the most common site of a lesion is the distal intermediate ridge of the tibia, the best view is a plantarolateral/dorsomedial oblique. Ultrasonographic examination of the swollen joints can help delineate articular damage and synovial inflammation and determine whether osteochondral fragments are intra- or extra-articular. The most accurate way to confirm diagnosis is by arthroscopy, and most of the predilection sites are accessible.

Scintigraphy has limitations in growing horses because of normal high activity in physes and sites of active endochondral ossification. It is a useful technique to detect subchondral cysts and secondary degenerative changes in older horses. MRI is ideal for diagnosis of both early and late lesions but is usually not necessary. Also, sites that are most diagnostically challenging are generally in the proximal limb, where access is difficult. Clinical pathology and the evaluation of synovial fluid is rarely helpful but can be used to eliminate inflammatory causes of swollen joints.

Treatment and Management: Management of osteochondrosis depends on the site and severity of signs. Mild cases recover spontaneously, and a conservative approach may be appropriate. In young animals (<12 mo old), this involves restricted exercise for some weeks combined with reduced feed intake to slow the growth rate. Particular care should be taken to ensure appropriate mineral supplementation (eg, in cases of suspected copper deficiency). It is controversial whether correcting the diet, once signs have developed, will actually assist resolution, but it may help limit or prevent further cases on stud farms. Intra-articular medication with hyaluronic acid may be beneficial, but injection of long-acting corticosteroids is not recommended in young, growing horses.

Cases considered for surgery are treated arthroscopically. This technique has been successful in most affected sites, particularly the hock, stifle, and fetlock. Damaged cartilage, osteochondral fragments, and compromised subchondral bone are removed and the joint flushed extensively with sterile fluid. Prognosis after removal of discrete osteochondral fragments is good. In cases with more extensive osteochondral damage, prognosis depends on the extent of the joint surface that must be removed. Prognosis is poor for cases with instability resulting from joint surface loss or in which secondary osteoarthritis (degenerative joint disease) is advanced. This is often the case with shoulder osteochondrosis because of the difficulty in detecting early signs. Cases involving subchondral cysts have a guarded prognosis, because these cysts are often in important weightbearing areas of the joint, and restoration of the joint surface is rarely possible.

PHYSITIS

(Epiphysitis, Physeal dysplasia, Dysplasia of the growth plate)

Physitis involves swelling around the growth plates of certain long bones in young horses. Suggested causes include malnutrition, conformational defects, excessive exercise, obesity, and toxicosis. The condition is seen frequently in well-grown, fast-growing, heavy-topped foals during the summer when the ground is dry and hard, and on stud farms where the calcium:phosphorus ratio in the diet is imbalanced. This suggests that it is a result of overload of the physeal area due to excessive loading or weakened bone and/or cartilage, or a combination of these factors.

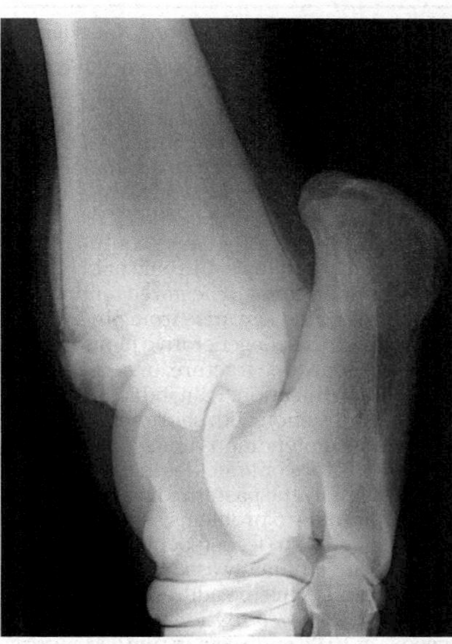

Physitis in the distal tibia of a horse. *Courtesy of Dr. Chris Whitton.*

Physitis most commonly involves the distal extremities of the radius, tibia, third metacarpal or metatarsal bone, and the proximal aspect of the first phalanx. It is characterized by flaring at the level of the growth plate, giving a typical "boxy" appearance to the affected joints. Radiographs aid clinical assessment.

Treatment consists of reducing food intake to reduce body weight or at least growth rate; confining exercise to a yard or a large, well-ventilated loose box with a soft surface (eg, peat moss, deep straw, shavings, or sand); ensuring that the feet are carefully and frequently trimmed; and correcting the diet if necessary. The calcium:phosphorus ratio should be adjusted to 1.6:1, and protein content limited to <10% of dry matter. In general terms, bran should not be fed, and dicalcium phosphate or bone flour (10–30 g daily) should be added to the diet. Vitamin D supplements (PO or parenteral) are indicated, but the dosage must be monitored closely to avoid hypervitaminosis D.

As a preventive measure, older foals or yearlings that are fat or heavy-topped should be watched carefully for clinical signs, especially when the ground is hard and dry. When these conditions prevail, feed rations and exercise should be restricted.

FLEXURAL DEFORMITIES

(Contracted tendons, Club foot, Knuckling)

Flexor tendon disorders are associated with postural and foot changes, lameness, and debility. They may be congenital and therefore identified in newborn foals or acquired at an older age. Uterine malposition, teratogenic insults (arthrogryposis), and genetic defects have been either implicated or proved to cause contracted limbs in newborn foals. Chronic pain is the most common cause of acquired tendon contracture. Pain can arise from physitis, osteochondrosis, degenerative joint disease, pedal bone fracture, or soft-tissue wounds and infection. Pain induces reflex muscle contraction with shortening of the flexor musculotendinous units. The horse walks on its toes or knuckles in the fetlocks or occasionally the pastern joint. Nutritional errors referable to problems associated with bone growth (ie, osteochondrosis and physitis) are intimately associated with the syndrome and must be addressed as part of treatment. (*See also* CONTRACTED FLEXOR TENDONS, p 1042, and ANGULAR LIMB DEFORMITIES, p 1046.)

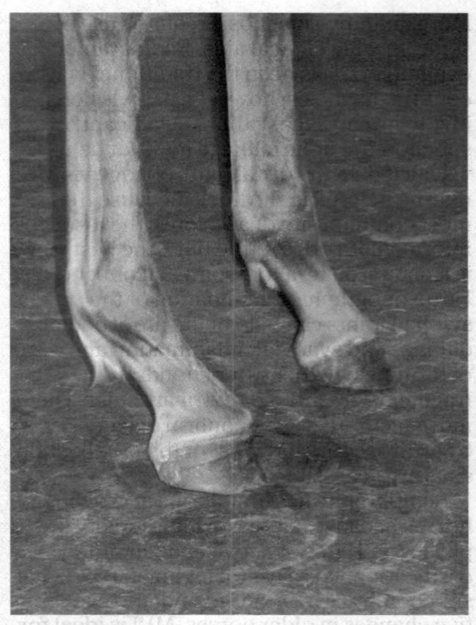

Acquired flexural deformity of the distal interphalangeal joint in a foal. *Courtesy of Dr. Chris Whitton.*

Clinical Findings: Signs vary widely in newborn foals. Some cannot stand, some attempt to walk on the dorsum of their fetlocks, and others can stand but knuckle in the fetlocks or carpi. One foal may improve spontaneously, yet another, seemingly healthy at birth, may become progressively worse. In older foals, onset tends to be rapid; such animals may walk around on their toes with their heels off the ground. A slower onset is characterized by an upright hoof with an elongated heel and concave toe. Physitis frequently is evident in these horses. Involvement of both forelimbs is common, with a tendency to be worse in one leg. Toe abscesses are a frequent complication of the hoof and locomotion changes, and they add to the pain and deformity.

Older horses (1–2 yr old) commonly knuckle in the metacarpophalangeal joints. Yearlings usually are more severely affected and more difficult to treat than younger animals. It is important to attempt to identify any underlying bone or joint disease, but this is often difficult and may have resolved.

Treatment: Mild cases in newborn foals often require no treatment. More severe cases require supportive therapy, and it is essential to correct failure of passive transfer of immunity if the foal has not been able to nurse adequately. Use of splints necessitates careful fitting and management, because rubbing sores are common and can be severe. Casts are generally safer if used only for short periods (5–7 days). High-dose oxytetracycline therapy is commonly used (40–60 mg/kg).

Early acquired cases in older foals and weanlings can be managed conservatively with nutritional correction, proper hoof trimming, and analgesia; however, once the deformity is present for >1 wk, this is rarely successful. Surgical treatment can be simple or complex, depending on the degree of involvement. Desmotomy of the accessory ligament of the deep digital flexor tendon (inferior check desmotomy) is the most successful and commonly used procedure for flexural deformity of the distal limb and does not interfere with future performance. Superior check ligament desmotomy may be included for horses with fetlock deformities. For carpal deformities, sectioning of the tendons of insertion onto the ulnaris lateralis and flexor carpi ulnaris is performed. In hindlimbs, tenotomy of the medial head of the deep digital flexor is performed, because the inferior check ligament is often vestigial. In severe cases, tenotomy of the deep digital flexor tendon can be used as a salvage procedure. Nutritional correction, proper foot trimming, and analgesia are integral to recovery when surgery is performed. The prognosis is fair to good for horses diagnosed early and managed properly.

LAMENESS IN PIGS

Lameness has been an issue in swine production for many years and continues to be a problem worldwide. Although lameness can be caused by congenital or developmental abnormalities, most lameness in production animals is caused by pain associated with infections, trauma-related injuries, or underlying metabolic diseases. As such, it has become an area of focus for swine farm audits of animal well-being. It is also an economic issue, because an increasing prevalence or incidence of lameness in a herd is likely to affect viability, growth, or reproduction of pigs. Pig flow may be affected if farrowing targets are not met because of high rates of breeding stock removal or if growth of grower/finisher pigs is slowed by high lameness incidence. As with diseases of other body systems, lameness problems in a swine herd require a comprehensive approach if a diagnosis (or diagnoses) is to be reached so that preventive or curative measures can be instituted.

Signalment: The types and causes of lameness can vary widely by age of the pig and, to a lesser extent, by gender and breed. Traumatic injury can obviously cause lameness in pigs at any age, but some types of lameness arising from infectious or physiologic causes can have a more limited age range or set of circumstances under which lameness develops. It should also be remembered that some infectious agents can affect and cause lameness in multiple species, so understanding the signalment of not only the group of pigs under evaluation, but also other pigs or species recently in contact or proximity with the affected group, is part of the comprehensive approach required for lameness investigations.

In addition to the signalment of the individual pigs in a population, the signalment of the composite group (ie, demographics) is also an important consideration. Examples of group signalment are the proportion of gilts in farrowing groups because gilts are more likely to pass pathogenic bacteria to their progeny, or the herd immune status with respect to a particular pathogen based on, for example, time since the most recent vaccination against erysipelas. Even the relative body condition of sows going into a cold season can predispose populations to increased or decreased susceptibility to herd health problems.

History: History taking must be thorough and should include information on age of onset, typical clinical signs, and progression of the lameness. Morbidity and mortality associated with any lameness and the number of groups, pens, rooms, or buildings with affected pigs are all relevant. Morbidity information should include treatments and the responses observed. Culling rates can also provide information on morbidity, although recorded reasons for culling sows are notoriously inaccurate. Condemnations at slaughter can be another way to secure objective data on morbidity, when condemnations for limb abnormalities or fractures have a direct bearing on lameness and for polyserositis or downer pigs, which have an indirect bearing on lameness.

Mortality data can be evaluated as an absolute rate or, more usefully, as incidence by stage or week of production. For sows, body condition score at the time of death or euthanasia can help reveal underlying lameness conditions because recorded reasons for cause of death are also prone to inaccuracy, and lame sows tend to lose body condition before death or euthanasia.

The investigation of a lameness problem on a farm also requires an understanding of the operation of the farm itself. The logistics underlying the establishment of the group of pigs under investigation should be explored: the source(s), transport, and placement of the pigs. The history of replacement breeding stock accessions is relevant, especially if new herds of origin or different genetic lines were introduced.

Health program and practices should be considered. It is important to determine whether vaccination or medication protocols were changed. If possible, it is equally important to determine whether protocols were followed correctly. Audits of product consumption or antibody testing for vaccine titers, if available, can be used as verification methods.

Investigating nutrition programs as a possible contributor to lameness problems can become extensive. However, the fundamental questions can be reduced to determining what rations were formulated, mixed, and delivered to the pigs. Problems are relatively rare but possible during each stage of the process. At the formulation stage, lameness problems can result, for example, when book values of phosphorus are different than actual amounts present in the product used, or vitamin D or phytase activities are not at expected levels because of storage, processing, or other issues, which can affect calcium and phosphorus metabolism. At the mixing stage, mills can have time constraints that do not allow adequate mixing of feed batches, so the feed composition can be uneven. At the point of delivery, feed density differences in sow gestation feed can result in over- or underfeeding when volumetric feeders are not adjusted to keep pace with weight and nutrient density changes in the ration.

Experiences with a series of lameness problems collectively referred to as metabolic bone disease—variably concerning problems in calcium, phosphorus, and/or vitamin D metabolism—have put more focus on the need to test feed constituents more thoroughly before inclusion in the diets, to test mixed feed for adherence to the formulation, and to monitor pigs more closely for serum vitamin D levels and bone densities so problems can be detected earlier.

Farm staff have a large role in caring for pigs on farms and, therefore, are a key source of information and possible solutions to lameness problems. Personnel working with the pigs must also be evaluated as possible contributors to lameness problems. Pig handling and movement are obvious potential causes of lameness, so understanding the level of staffing and extent of staff training are important parts of the case history. Observing the interaction between the pigs and the farm staff can help reveal the nature of interactions likely to occur routinely on the farm.

Understanding the farm hygiene practices is important to determine risks of injury and disease from slippery surfaces or contamination from transport vehicles. If bedding is used, determining the sources and management of the bedding is also significant to characterize disease risks.

Finally, the history of diagnostic results for the farm and the area are critically important to have a starting point for further investigation of lameness problems. If possible, the disease history among neighboring farms can help understand disease risks. At a minimum, a review of all the pertinent diagnostic testing results for the specific herd is required.

Clinical Evaluation: Diagnosis of lameness can be complex. At least three body systems (musculoskeletal, nervous, and integumentary) may be affected independently or in combination. Because of the different organ systems potentially involved, a consistent and thorough approach to evaluate all components of lameness is essential. When examining a herd with a locomotor problem, the focus should not be solely on a group of affected pigs. Younger pigs should be evaluated to identify potential underlying causes or predispositions to the problem under investigation. Other groups of pigs of similar ages and older pigs housed in other pens or buildings should also be evaluated to determine whether they have similar or different problems. The conditions potentially causing the problem should not be assumed to be restricted to those most often associated with one particular age group.

When evaluating a population of pigs, it is useful to first consider an inverted pyramid approach of the entire room, followed by pens of pigs and finally individual pig evaluations. The entire room evaluation is intended to provide a general sense of the overall health, activity, and behavior of the group. Pen-by-pen evaluations provide an opportunity to make counts or estimates of the prevalence and severity of the lameness. The individual pig assessments are intended to focus on the specific cause(s) of the lameness.

The pen evaluation is intended to identify the lame pigs. Pigs should be made to move around (in pens or into alleyways), to stand, and if housing allows, to walk, watching for behavior typical of lame pigs. The pen ahead and pen behind the last pigs to stand up and first pigs to lie down should be observed. Pigs that take advantage of the diversion caused by the evaluation to access feed or water should be noted. Abnormal gait and posture, body condition (thin pigs are more likely to be lame), and physical evidence of trauma, infection, or malformation (swelling, vesicles, etc) should be watched for in individual pigs.

If an individual pig warrants a more extensive physical examination, some degree of restraint may be required. If less restraint is sufficient, the pig can remain free in a pen or stall, or a sorting panel can be used to prevent the pig from moving away. If more restraint is needed, small pigs can be lifted or manually held for examination. Larger pigs can be snared or cast using ropes. The advantage of this type of restraint is that it immobilizes the pig. Disadvantages are that the pig is placed in an unnatural posture, excess muscle tone is normally stimulated, and help from additional people is usually required.

Anesthesia is another possible means of greater restraint. The advantage is that muscles are relaxed, allowing manipulation of skeletal structures such as potential fractures. Additionally, muscle mass can be assessed, joint taps or other diagnostic procedures can be performed, and more extensive evaluations such as radiography or other scanning are possible if warranted. Disadvantages are the management of controlled substances used as anesthetics, required withdrawal times, and the challenge of managing recovery from anesthesia with other pigs present or in facilities that may not be set up for such procedures.

Some farms may have lift chutes to immobilize boars, sows, and gilts for foot trimming or other procedures. These chutes allow good restraint with full access to the feet and lower limbs, with none of the disadvantages of chemical restraint. However, availability of lift chutes on sow farms is limited.

A general physical examination of an individual pig for lameness requires a thorough, systematic, and consistent process by individual clinicians. One such approach is to proceed from the bottom up and front to back of the pig, ie, the feet are evaluated first, followed by the limbs and torso in a front-to-back progression.

The feet can be examined most easily when the pig is lying laterally recumbent or lifted (manually for small pigs or using a mechanical chute for sows). Standardized guides exist to score foot lesions by type. Prevalence and severity of foot lesions in a sow herd can be estimated by scoring the feet using statistical sampling. Using a good flashlight enhances scoring foot lesions. Feet may need to be cleaned for pigs housed on non-slatted floors. Exploring lesions by trimming with a hoof knife, clipper, or grinder requires adequate restraint and safety protocols. Foot lesions have been well defined but do not always correlate with lameness on an individual pig basis, because the pain associated with foot lesions depends on exposure or infection of the sensitive tissues underlying the claw, heel, and sole of the toes.

Limb and joint palpation and manipulation should also be conducting using a consistent approach. The amount and type of restraint again depends on age of the pig. Cardinal signs of inflammation, ie, heat, swelling, pain, and redness, should be noted. Strength, range of motion, crepitus, and weight-bearing distribution should be evaluated. Joints embedded in muscle mass (eg, hip, stifle, shoulder) require deep palpation, which may not be possible on large, heavily muscled pigs. Fracture of the head of the femur (epiphysiolysis capitis femoris), a common cause of downer sows, is difficult to diagnose antemortem. Because it is buried under a large muscle mass, even infectious arthritis in the stifle, a site commonly affected by *Mycoplasma hyosynoviae*, can be missed on individual pigs on cursory examination.

The torso can be evaluated and palpated for muscle mass, tone, and symmetry. Ribs should be examined for evidence of fractures or knobby thickening (rachitic rosary), and the spine examined for kyphosis.

A neurologic examination is indicated in cases when neurologic disease is suspected and should be performed in a similar fashion to that for dogs, cows, and horses (*see* p 1213).

Postmortem examination of lame pigs is often required to reach a definitive diagnosis for a herd lameness problem. Field necropsy of baby, nursery, and grower pigs is relatively easy to accomplish. However, for larger finisher pigs, gilts, sows, and boars, the process is laborious because of the size of the animal and the need to examine numerous joints and bones, often including the spine if appropriate to the clinical presentation. At a minimum, developing expertise in opening joints on dead pigs that may not be ideal candidates for diagnostic sampling can help direct diagnostic efforts when more suitable pigs are available. Examination of greater numbers of pigs improves the odds of accurately characterizing the cause(s) of lameness.

Although on-farm necropsies are feasible, it may be better to submit entire or even live pigs to a full-service diagnostic laboratory. In particular, submitting live pigs to a laboratory allows greater odds of successfully culturing live bacteria, which are needed for antimicrobial susceptibility determination or production of autogenous vaccines. Additionally, diagnostic laboratories have the facilities and personnel to perform more complete and careful dissections of joints, the spine, and brain. This is particularly true of sow lameness problems. For example, an extensive dissection of the pelvis is required to reveal an apophysiolysis of ischial tuberosity in young sows with characteristic dog-sitting posture after farrowing. Likewise, vertebral abscessation can be a common cause of downer sows, and the vertebral column must be split sagittally to make a definitive diagnosis of this condition.

If pigs are to be submitted to a diagnostic laboratory, appropriate pigs must be selected and delivered, accompanied by an accurate history and a list of differential diagnoses. Adequate numbers of representative, acutely lame, untreated pigs are essential.

If tissues are to be submitted for a lameness evaluation, the diagnostic laboratory should be contacted to determine what tests will be done and what tissues will be needed. In general, tissues from three euthanized pigs with characteristic clinical signs, acutely affected, and untreated (if available) are a reasonable starting point. Alternatively, three freshly dead pigs can be examined and sampled. Samples should be packaged and identified individually for each pig. Whole blood in EDTA and serum should be collected antemortem if possible. For small pigs, postmortem samples can include intact joints with the skin wiped clean and cooled for transport. For larger pigs, two joint swabs of synovial membranes of affected joints should be collected, along with chilled and formalin-fixed synovial membrane samples. Affected bones can also be submitted chilled.

The bone of choice (based on the recommendation of the laboratory) for bone density determination should be submitted if warranted. Protocols to evaluate bone density using front feet have been developed and may be available in some laboratories.

For suspected neurologic cases, one half of the brain should be submitted chilled and the other half fixed in buffered 10% formalin. Additionally, vertebral sections from the cervicothoracic and lumbosacral region should be submitted chilled, with 5-cm segments of spinal cord also submitted fixed in formalin. If muscle disease is suspected, a sample of diaphragm and muscle from affected areas should be submitted fixed in formalin.

As part of the postmortem examination, a rib should be removed and manually snapped (like a twig) to gain an appreciation of the bone mineral density. Depending on the age of the pig, the rib should snap sharply. With practice, clinicians can develop skill in evaluating bone mineralization in this manner.

Evaluation of affected or cull pigs at a slaughter plant is not usually productive, because processing lines run too fast to evaluate all the elements of the musculoskeletal system, and all joints cannot be thoroughly examined. However, specific conditions can be evaluated even at line speed. For example, rachitic lesions may be apparent on ribs on hanging carcasses. Condemned carcass or euthanized slow or down pigs can sometimes be made available for examination. Some abattoirs are willing to cooperate on specific projects to retrieve lower limbs for investigative purposes if asked.

Environment and Management: Housing and the manner in which pigs and their environment are managed are central to potential lameness problems, especially the interface between the pig and the floor. Flooring type is a major determinant, and all types have forms of lameness associated with them. Dirt and pasture lots can range from too dry to too wet, leading to vertical hoof wall cracks or foot infections, respectively. Bedding can serve as a source of bacteria that cause infectious arthritis, such as *Erysipelothrix rhusiopathiae* in straw bedding. Solid, partial slat, and fully slatted floors also have relative advantages and disadvantages in terms of associated lameness conditions.

In addition to type of flooring, the adjustment and state of repair can have considerable influence on lameness. Holes, gaps, and sharp edges on concrete floors can traumatize the feet and lower legs. Abrasiveness of the flooring surface may be too little, which makes floors slippery and leads to injuries, or too much, which can wear down the claws and promote heel overgrowth.

Cleanliness and moisture are additional factors to evaluate. Buildup of manure in bedded areas can lead to foot infections, whereas excess moisture from misting cooling systems running out of adjustment can lead to softening of the claws, hoof wall cracks, and excess wear.

Interactions among the pigs are also important factors to evaluate. The sourcing and mixing of discrete pig populations can influence whether infectious diseases are maintained as endemic within the population or can become epidemic outbreaks as pigs become susceptible over time with the loss of maternal immunity and have commingling exposure. Stocking density and space for animals to exhibit social behaviors can influence how much aggressive social behavior occurs within groups of pigs. Distance and conditions pigs are required to traverse to access feed and water can affect wear on the feet and trauma to joints.

Group size and stability also have an impact on development of lameness. Sows housed in individual stalls are restricted in terms of movement but tend to develop fewer lameness problems than confined group-housed sows. Pigs kept in very large group sizes have fewer aggressive interactions than pigs housed in small groups. Sorting growing pigs to allow for more variation in size within pens can reduce the time required for social structures to become established at weaning or regrouping times.

Nutrition: Skeletal development may be affected by relatively short-term nutritional deficiencies, especially considering expectations for rapid growth and muscle development in modern hybrid pigs. Problems early in the production cycle may be reflected as abnormal bone growth in nursery or growing pigs, whereas recurrent deficiencies or those seen later in the finishing phase may result in weak bones in slaughter pigs or replacement breeding stock.

During the growing phase, the goal of the nutritional program should be to ensure the development of a strong skeleton so that incidence of spontaneous bone fractures in the finishing barn or during the slaughter process is low, thus preventing large numbers of culls or partial and complete condemnations of carcasses. Fractures of the femur, humerus, ribs, or vertebrae may be induced by strong muscle contractions during the slaughter process; however, if the problem is seen frequently, it may be a reflection of the overall integrity of the skeleton and warrant further evaluation of the minerals and vitamins in the ration. Clinical signs of hypocalcemia can develop before slaughter and can include lameness, including spiral fracture of the femur, leg weakness and posterior paresis, recumbency and paddling, and even sudden death.

In breeding animals especially, foot lesions can cause lameness. Research has demonstrated the need to balance diets carefully for macro and trace minerals, as well as key vitamins such as vitamin D and biotin. Excessive water hardness or high concentrations of iron or heavy metals in water can antagonize trace mineral absorption, leading to foot lesion development.

Viruses: Some acute infectious causes of lameness in pigs can affect pigs of multiple ages. In particular, vesicular diseases caused by several viruses can cause lameness in breeding and growing swine: foot-and-mouth disease, Seneca Valley virus, swine vesicular disease, vesicular stomatitis, and vesicular exanthema all fit this clinical picture. Prevalence and clinical severity among these viruses is variable, but because of the concern over foot-and-mouth, any episode of vesicular disease in pigs is cause for a full diagnostic investigation involving regulatory personnel.

Therapeutic Considerations: Therapies to treat or prevent lameness should, of course, be tailored to the presumed or confirmed underlying cause of lameness but can also be symptomatic to reduce pain and improve function. However, the regulatory landscape for use of products to treat or prevent lameness in pigs is changing. This is true not only for federal regulations regarding use of antimicrobials and analgesics but also for the patchwork of commercial marketing programs that are typically more restrictive on product use through contractual agreements. Thus, any product type, dose, form, and use should be carefully considered in light of pertinent regulations for the jurisdictions in which the pigs are being raised and marketed.

Production practices and conditions are also changing. In certain parts of the world, pig farming is becoming more intensive, whereas others are becoming more extensive. These changes can alter the epidemiology of diseases, posing both a challenge and an opportunity to intervene more effectively to reduce lameness.

Diagnostic regimens are becoming more sensitive, increasing the likelihood of detecting and characterizing disease-causing agents. Distinguishing between presence and significance of a disease-causing agent becomes more difficult, but a more precise understanding of exposure and transmission of agents should help develop more effective control strategies.

Pigs with acute diseases that may result in death typically require parenteral therapy with a drug of choice (using approved products first) based on tentative diagnosis and the clinician's experience until results of a necropsy and antimicrobial sensitivity profiles are available. Virtually all the parenteral products available to treat infections that cause lameness are given IM, with the site of choice behind the ear for all age categories. It may be feasible to provide medication in the water or feed after the initial parenteral treatment. Infectious agents sensitive to a drug in vitro may not be sensitive in vivo, so clinical experience on the farm is essential.

In addition to antimicrobials to treat infectious arthritides, the use of anti-inflammatory agents to relieve pain can be useful and beneficial to the pig. Flunixin meglumine is approved for use in pigs for symptomatic treatment of fever in outbreaks of swine respiratory disease, but anti-inflammatory and analgesic qualities can help relieve pain in a swollen joint or bruised muscle (extra-label). Dexamethasone has been recommended in pigs with streptococcosis and is labeled for glucocorticoid therapy in pigs. Another glucocorticoid, isoflupredone acetate, is specifically approved for musculoskeletal pain that causes lameness in pigs. In a controlled study in Europe, the COX-2 inhibitor meloxicam proved useful to alleviate painful, noninfectious lameness in pigs. This product is approved for use in swine in Canada but not in the USA. All these products are administered by IM injection, so treatment of large numbers of pigs is time consuming and potentially costly. Acetylsalicylic acid and sodium salicylate are allowed for analgesia in swine if manufactured under cGMP and may be a useful adjunct therapy as a water treatment. Additionally, meloxicam and ibuprofen can be compounded from FDA-approved human products. An important consideration with use of any pharmaceuticals in pigs near time of slaughter is observance of withdrawal times recommended by the manufacturer.

Whenever feasible, introduction of a vaccination protocol to protect populations of pigs against a particular infectious agent is desirable. If a suitable vaccine is not commercially available, an autogenous product can be created for some pathogens for use in an individual herd and, provided it is cost-effective, can be used to prevent regular outbreaks of disease. Regular monitoring for causal organisms, serotype, etc, is essential for effective use of either antibacterial agents or vaccines.

Removing lame pigs from competitive group housing environments to hospital pens improves the chances of recovery. Research is inconclusive as to the optimal flooring and husbandry conditions for recovery pens.

PIGS IN FARROWING HOUSES

Neonatal Polyarthritis (Joint-ill): Neonatal septic polyarthritis, which causes death in up to 1.5% of affected pigs, is caused by various facultative and specific pathogens that cause localized infections that precede septicemia. Healthy, suckling pigs typically "paddle" with their legs, abrading the skin of the carpi or coronary bands; an infection often becomes established under scabs that develop. Poor hygiene at tail docking, ear notching, or castration, and careless clipping of needle teeth can also result in localized infections. If an infected wound leads to bacteremia, organisms can cross the synovial membrane, and polyarthritis is likely. Microorganisms can also gain entry to the circulatory system via the tonsils or oropharynx or as a result of an ascending omphalophlebitis. Pigs with exudative epidermitis (*see* p 860) are also prone to polyarthritis, but this may be a reflection of the same skin damage discussed above.

Affected pigs are lethargic and may fail to suckle. Joints are swollen, painful, and warm, and lameness affecting one or more limbs is severe. With time, the soft, fluctuant swellings become firm. At necropsy, the umbilicus should be examined to see whether it is hard and swollen. Typically, cream or green pus is found in and around swollen joints (particularly the elbows, carpi, stifles, and hocks), in the umbilical stalk, and sometimes over the meninges or in the fissure between the cerebrum and cerebellum. Organisms isolated from baby pigs included streptococci (including *Streptococcus suis*), staphylococci, *Actinobacillus suis*, *Trueperella pyogenes*, *Escherichia coli*, and occasionally, *Pasteurella multocida*, *Erysipelothrix rhusiopathiae*, or *Haemophilus* spp. If untreated, affected pigs become runts that fail to thrive in the nursery.

Treatment must be based on bacterial culture and antimicrobial sensitivity profiles and applicable regulations on product use. Antimicrobial therapy should be initiated early in the course of the disease if it is to be effective, and treating all pigs in the group at risk may be prudent, especially if *S suis* is implicated. Penicillins have been the drugs of choice, depending on the causal agent and sensitivity. However, a broader range of drugs is available, including lincomycin, trimethoprim/sulfonamide, and tylosin, provided causal organisms are sensitive. The range of suitable drugs is increased further if streptococcosis caused by *S suis* develops (*see* p 731).

Regardless of the cause of a local infection, if there is an ongoing problem with septic polyarthritis, it is important to observe the practices used in farrowing rooms and to look for opportunities for improvement. An "all-in/all-out" flow of pigs is important, and scrupulous hygiene in farrowing crates helps to reduce environmental contamination and incidence of neonatal polyarthritis. Prevention may be difficult because most types of floors, including those bedded with straw, can cause skin abrasions. Plastic-covered woven wire provides a smooth, relatively soft, self-cleaning floor and may help; plain woven wire is similar if it is smooth. If replacement of flooring is not economically viable, sections of clean, soft carpeting may help reduce skin abrasions.

Separate instruments should be used for teeth and tail clipping, and they should be cleaned and disinfected between pigs, preferably using a dry paper towel. Soaking instruments in contaminated disinfectant solution between pigs or litters promotes contamination and infection. If teeth are not clipped or if there are sharp remnants of clipped teeth, pigs that suckle aggressively can lacerate the faces of other pigs, resulting in pyoderma. Castration equipment must be kept sterile and sharp. If tail stumps are infected, antiseptic solution may be used as a spray to improve hygiene.

Litters from gilts are more prone to neonatal polyarthritis. Colostral protection against this syndrome and other infectious diseases of baby pigs increases as a sow ages. Because pigs in large litters have to compete more to suckle and are, therefore, more prone to lesions on their faces and forelimbs, cross-fostering within 24 hr of birth to balance litter sizes may help. Piglets nursing sows with hypogalactia or agalactia spend more time nursing, leading to more forelimb lesions.

Diseases of the Foot: Neonatal foot lesions fall into two main categories: either the sole or heel is damaged by the floor, or the hoof wall is traumatized by the sow standing on a pig's foot or by entrapment in the flooring.

Bruises or lacerations develop on either the sole or heel. The lesions are associated with worn and rough floor surfaces and with floors that have solid as well as perforated surfaces. Rough flooring can also cause bruising in soft tissue below the hoof wall. If spaces between slats are large, digits can be entrapped, and lameness results from bruising or infection at the coronary band. Pigs on expanded metal floors can incur heel and wall injuries leading to loss of accessory digits. Second and third digits may be damaged as the pigs thrust with their feet during suckling and catch their toes against sharp metal edges. Sharp spicules on woven wire cause lacerations and predispose to infectious laminitis and polyarthritis.

Prevention is based on selecting floors that minimally injure feet or skin. Because of similarities with infectious polyarthritis, the approach to treatment and prevention is similar (*see* above). Improved hygiene within the environment may help reduce septic laminitis and allow injuries to heal.

Muscular Disorders: Splayleg or spraddleleg (*see* p 1049) is precipitated by weakness and immaturity of skeletal muscles at birth because myotubular development is impaired. Forelimbs, hindlimbs, or all four limbs may be affected so that the piglet either walks with difficulty or cannot stand. The disorder appears sporadically in litters, and only a few pigs in a litter are typically affected. There is a hereditary component in European Landrace and, to a lesser extent, in Large

White pigs. Male, premature, and small pigs, and pigs from older sows seem more susceptible. Deficiencies of choline, methionine, and thiamine in the sow's diet may precipitate the syndrome, and zearalanone toxicity via the sow's milk has been implicated, but there is controversy as to the exact cause. To varying degrees, affected pigs are unable to move around and die either because the sow crushes them or they become hypoglycemic because they cannot feed. Alternatively, skin and foot abrasions develop, predisposing to arthritis, polyarthritis, or pododermatitis and osteomyelitis of the digits.

Timely management practices are essential to ensure that pigs can feed and avoid hypoglycemia and hypothermia. If only the hindlimbs are affected, they can be hobbled so that the pig can lever itself up using forelimbs and hop around to nurse. Various hobbles, including a figure-8 tape or bandage, have been successful. Some recommend taping the pelvic limbs so they are directed cranially on the belly. By using the limbs or pushing against a bellyband, the pig potentially develops and strengthens muscles, which can enable to pig to walk after a few days. Hobbles must be removed within a few days of pigs walking, to avoid ischemic necrosis of skin and other tissues as the pigs grow.

Pigs with splayleg may require assistance to suckle colostrum and milk for the first few days of life. Some advocate the use of "hot boxes" to nurture these and other ailing pigs, relying on milk replacers as the main source of food once the pig has had colostrum. Because slippery floors exacerbate the condition, temporary use of sanitized mats may help. Any nutritional deficiency or mycotoxin contamination of food should be addressed.

Iron toxicosis in piglets (*see* p 3077) after injection with iron preparations soon after birth may be associated with muscle fiber fragility, especially if there is a selenium deficiency in the sow and, therefore, the piglet. Inadequate hygiene or technique when baby pigs are injected with an iron preparation can lead to bruising and septic myositis. This problem can be resolved by adequate training of farrowing room staff.

Neurologic Disorders: Meningoencephalocoele and cerebellar hypoplasia interfere with locomotion in affected pigs, as can infections with *Listeria monocytogenes* and *Streptococcus suis*. Thus, *S suis* can cause locomotion problems as a result of meningitis and neurologic signs, or a suppurative arthritis can be the primary complaint. Congenital tremors cause pigs to shake when awake and remain still when sleeping. Either heredity or viral infections may cause the problem. In the USA and other parts of the world, porcine circovirus has been implicated in congenital tremors. The tremors usually are most severe during the first week of life and make it difficult for pigs to nurse. Affected pigs must be assisted with nursing until the tremors subside.

Hereditary and Congenital Disorders: Mycotoxins in the sow's feed can cause arthrogryposis, which leads to deformity of limb bones, but the primary effect may be on neuromuscular function. Pigs affected by hereditary hyperostosis have thickened thoracic limbs and a domed forehead and generally do not survive. Polydactyly and syndactyly are occasional abnormalities that may affect locomotion of the baby pig; syndactylous or mule-footed pigs have been propagated and sold by some producers with no obvious disabilities for the pigs. When causal agents contaminate the feed, sources of these products should be found and avoided; if hereditary disease is suspected, the source(s) of replacement stock must be investigated.

PIGS IN NURSERIES

By the time pigs are weaned, diseases that affected the locomotor system during the nursing phase most likely will have resolved spontaneously, responded to aggressive therapy, or resulted in death. Because pigs that survive episodes of polyarthritis generally remain lame, have one or more swollen "knotty" joints, and are in poor condition, they should be culled.

In a swine producer survey in the USA, CNS and meningitis problems were considered the second most frequent cause of death in weaned pigs, representing 13%–19% of losses. In this survey, *Streptococcus suis* meningitis, Glässer's disease, and edema disease, respectively, were perceived to cause illness or death in one or more pigs in 50%, 17%, and 9% of surveyed herds.

Infectious Arthritis or Polyarthritis: Causes of polyarthritis in this group of pigs usually include *Mycoplasma hyorhinis*, *Haemophilus parasuis*, *S suis*, or *Erysipelothrix rhusiopathiae*, and less commonly *Streptococcus dysgalactiae* subsp *equisimilis*, *Actinobacillus equuli* subsp *equuli*, and other bacteria prone to achieve bacteremia. The birth canal and upper respiratory tract of the sow are often the sources of the organisms for the baby pig, which becomes infected in the farrowing room. *M hyorhinis* and *H parasuis* circulation in the sow herd can be predictive of infection levels in growing pigs. Alternatively, older pigs act as carriers and are a source of infection for their peers. Pigs affected by *E rhusiopathiae* also shed organisms in their feces and urine. Essentially, all are systemic diseases with a septicemic phase, and each may manifest as different clinical syndromes or as a mix of clinical signs.

As with many infectious diseases, management or environmental factors that stress the pig or depress the immune response can precipitate systemic disease or an infectious arthritis. Moving and mixing pigs (particularly if all-in, all-out management is not used); overcrowding; cold, damp, poorly ventilated, or cold, drafty environments; and changing rations are all major stresses that can lead to development of infectious arthritides or neurologic diseases that affect movement. It is also likely that active viral infections associated with porcine reproductive and respiratory syndrome virus (*see* p 729) or circovirus may predispose groups of nursery pigs to bacterial polyarthritis.

Initially, shifting-leg lameness occurs, and joints can be warm, swollen, and painful. If pigs are febrile, they may have no interest in standing and become inappetent. Chronic forms of polyarthritis with polyserositis result in unthrifty, runt pigs and, in the case of chronic erysipelas (*see* p 1160), runt pigs may be lame with hard, swollen joints.

The clinical signs seen in infections caused by *M hyorhinis* and *H parasuis* (Glässer's disease, *see* p 720) are similar, because both cause painful polyarthritis and polyserositis. The conditions cannot be differentiated grossly at necropsy. Infection with *M hyorhinis* usually results in lameness with moderate morbidity and low mortality, but *H parasuis* can cause infection in 50%–75% of pigs and mortality of up to 10%. Outbreaks of Glässer's disease have been particularly severe in SPF and other naive herds. *H parasuis* may also play a part as a primary or concomitant agent in swine respiratory disease complex and cause disease in association with porcine reproductive and respiratory syndrome virus or influenza virus. Fever is associated with mycoplasmosis but can be highest in Glässer's disease (>107°F [41.7°C]) as pigs become anorexic and lame; sometimes *H parasuis* causes neurologic signs.

At necropsy, polyarthritis and polyserositis are seen with both mycoplasma infection and Glässer's disease, and pneumonia may have developed. The initial, exudative response is usually serous or serofibrinous with a mycoplasmal infection; however, it is fibrinous or fibrinopurulent with Glässer's disease. Hence, *M hyorhinis* causes a mild synovitis with villous hypertrophy and hyperplasia; an excess of clear, yellow, or brown synovia; and a serofibrinous pericarditis, pleuritis, and peritonitis. Otitis media has also been reported. With *H parasuis*, a fibrinopurulent synovitis with periarticular edema, polyserositis with pseudomembranes, and sometimes fibrinopurulent meningitis are seen. The articular surfaces are usually unaffected in either condition.

Diagnosis is based on clinical signs, necropsy findings, and detection of the organism. PCR tests are available to detect *M hyorhinis* and *H parasuis*. This is important, because bacterial culture of both bacteria can be challenging if any treatment has been instituted or if the pig has been dead more than a few hours. Treatment for either disease must be aggressive and start soon after the onset of clinical signs if it is to be effective. The effectiveness of treating *M hyorhinis* infections with tylosin, tetracycline, or lincomycin has been variable. Organisms may be susceptible in vitro and resistant in vivo. Treatment of Glässer's disease is discussed in the relevant chapter (*see* p 720). With chronicity, success in treating either disease is unlikely.

Appropriate changes in management to reduce stress, strict all-in/all-out housing, and control of viral infections should all minimize the impact of Glässer's disease. Herds that maintain an SPF status may be free of both *M hyorhinis* and *H parasuis*, but in herds with documented outbreaks of Glässer's disease, morbidity and mortality were high and productivity was decreased. Some 15 serovars of *H parasuis* have been identified, with much strain variation. Vaccination with commercial or autogenous *H parasuis* bacterin may alleviate clinical disease in SPF herds. It is important to vaccinate SPF pigs that are to be shipped to conventional herds with vaccine effective against the serovars present in the recipient herd. There is cross-protection among some serovars. Vaccination of sows against *H parasuis* reduces the prevalence of the problem in nursery pigs through passive immunity.

Streptococcosis: The streptococcal disease of main concern to the pig industry is caused by *S suis* (*see* p 731). Although this organism can cause arthritis, CNS signs and pneumonia are the most common clinical presentations.

Erysipelas: Although acute erysipelas can be seen in nursery pigs, it may be more typical of growing/finishing pigs (*see* p 1160). If the acute form of the disease affects nursery pigs and is not treated appropriately, the subsequent progression of the disease to the chronic form is seen in the grower/finisher pigs. Adequate vaccination protocols are essential to controlling erysipelas. (*See also* SWINE ERYSIPELAS, p 626.)

Vertebral Deformities: Kyphosis or lordosis and cuneiform deformities of vertebrae have been seen in weaned pigs. The condition has been reproduced experimentally using gestation and nursery diets deficient in calcium, phosphorus, and vitamin D. "Humpy back" pigs are seen sporadically in some herds; the spine is curved in the vertical plane such that the lumbar vertebrae are higher than the thoracic vertebrae, and there is a "kink" between the two segments. Rickets is usually not seen clinically until the grower phase, but lesions must be initiated earlier, giving time for typical pathologic changes to develop by ~10 wk of age.

PIGS IN GROWER/FINISHER AREAS

Lameness in pigs is of increasing interest in North American swine production. *Mycoplasma hyosynoviae* in particular has received more attention due, in part, to more intensive diagnostic efforts. Metabolic bone disease has also been an area of focus as problems have arisen after more complex formulations for gestation and grow-finish diets.

Arthritis: Arthritis caused by *Mycoplasma hyosynoviae* and *Erysipelothrix rhusiopathiae* emerge as important causes of lameness in pigs that have been moved to the grower/finisher areas. Again, mixing and moving groups of pigs; overcrowding; cold, drafty environments; or changes in management and feed may precipitate outbreaks of lameness.

In the case of *M hyosynoviae*, the upper respiratory tract of sows and older pigs in peer groups is the likely source. As colostral immunity wanes at 4–8 wk of age, pigs become susceptible to infection. Generally, morbidity is low to moderate, but up to 50% of pigs may be affected; mortality is very low. An acute lameness, lasting up to 10 days, develops in groups of grower/finisher pigs or selected replacement stock. Arthritis may be exacerbated by trauma or stress, and pigs exhibit pain in major joints (eg, elbows, stifles, and hocks) that may develop soft, fluctuant swellings. On necropsy, lesions are restricted to the joints, especially the stifles, and include an excess of clear, yellow synovial fluid that may have fibrin flakes, and yellow synovium with obvious villous hypertrophy. Articular surfaces and periarticular tissues usually are unaffected. *M hyosynoviae* has been isolated at slaughter or necropsy in pigs with degenerative joint disease that is part of the osteochondrosis syndrome, but it is a secondary rather than a causal agent.

Diagnosis is based on the age of onset of clinical disease and clinical signs, including lameness in one or more legs that may be accompanied by fluctuating swelling and puffiness around joints. Typically, pigs are afebrile and there is no evidence of pneumonia, pleuritis, and peritonitis. If a definitive diagnosis is to be made based on detection of the organism, samples of synovium and synovial fluid should be collected from untreated pigs within 3–4 days of the onset of clinical signs. However, *M hyosynoviae* can be cultured from healthy joints and is not always recovered from affected joints.

Lack of a response to penicillin in acute cases has been used to differentiate this disease from erysipelas. Unlike polyarthritis caused by *M hyorhinis*, response to treatment with tylosin and lincomycin is generally good if administered promptly, and tiamulin or tetracycline may be effective where allowed. Mycoplasmal arthritis may exacerbate clinical signs associated with degenerative joint disease and osteoarthrosis and vice versa.

Erysipelas: *Erysipelothrix rhusiopathiae*, the cause of erysipelas, is acquired from healthy carrier pigs or the environment, in which the organism can survive for short periods. Erysipelas can be peracute, acute, or chronic. In the peracute form, pigs die without clinical signs. In the acute form, pigs become febrile and may be lethargic and anorectic and unwilling to rise because of painful joints and cyanosis of the extremities; the latter is associated with vasculitis in peripheral vessels. After 2–3 days, the classic "diamond" skin lesions (focal urticaria) develop over the body surface. In some outbreaks, lameness is seen without the skin lesions. In the chronic form, arthritis progresses such that the stifles and hocks become swollen and feel firm on palpation; skin necrosis can result in extensive sloughing of portions of the integument. In chronic cases, discospondylosis also may develop if intervertebral joints are affected. As the arthritis progresses and joints fuse, pain in the lumbar vertebrae may reduce boar libido. Cyanosis in the extremities in chronic cases may be related to heart valve failure. A presumptive diagnosis of acute disease is based on the clinical signs, of which the "diamond" skin lesions are most consistently useful. All three forms of the disease may be seen in the same herd if the problem has not been investigated and treatment has been delayed.

If the chronic form of erysipelas is investigated as a lameness problem and pigs are necropsied, early changes in the disease process will have subsided (eg, hemorrhages in lymph nodes, kidneys, and muscles). An excess of synovial fluid accumulates during the acute phase, but in chronically affected joints, there is villous hypertrophy and hyperplasia, hyperemia, and periarticular fibrosis. If pannus has formed, the articular surface becomes disrupted. Raised, focal skin lesions progress to sloughed areas and, in extreme cases, the ears and tail may have sloughed. Vegetative, valvular endocarditis is another finding.

Isolation of the causal organism is important for a definitive diagnosis and is most successful if acutely affected, untreated pigs are necropsied and joint fluid is cultured. PCR testing of chronic lesions (eg, endocarditis) can be used to detect the bacteria in chronic cases. A bacterial culture with an antibiotic sensitivity profile is useful during treatment of the herd. Sometimes, a rapid response of the acute condition to penicillin is a diagnostic aid. Provided the *E rhusiopathiae* is sensitive to penicillin, this may still be an economic choice for treatments. However, tylosin and lincomycin are also labeled for treatment of erysipelas, and tetracycline may be successful if the organism is susceptible.

Vaccination with either modified-live or killed organisms effectively controls erysipelas in a herd, and outbreaks may be related to noncompliance with vaccination protocols rather than to changes in the virulence of the causal organism or the nature of the disease. Therefore, any investigation of the problem should begin with a detailed vaccination history to ensure that sows are regularly vaccinated. Even with sow vaccination, infection is seen in grower/finisher pigs in some herds. On these farms, growers must be vaccinated in addition to the sows. In the face of an outbreak, concurrent use of killed vaccine and antibiotic is likely to be the most effective control measure (*see* p 626).

Osteomyelitis: Osteomyelitis can be seen in pigs of any age. If the integument is damaged, sepsis develops and a suppurative lesion extends to the periosteum and bone. Alternatively, organisms can invade bone from the synovium of infected joints. Poor processing or injection techniques can initiate abscesses that can extend into adjacent bone. Disruption of the integrity of the hoof wall initiates cellulitis and osteomyelitis of a phalangeal bone. Ear and flank biting wounds are other foci of infection. Tail biting can result in local infections that ascend the spinal canal and lead to epidural abscesses that can invade and affect vertebral bodies. Lesions and clinical signs may develop slowly.

Depending on the site of infection, the pig may become ataxic and, ultimately, paralyzed in the pelvic limbs. If bones or joints of a limb are affected, the condition is usually chronic and the pig becomes three-legged lame. Young pigs cease to grow.

At necropsy, cream or green caseous pus is seen at the site of the lesion. If *Trueperella pyogenes* is involved, there are abundant pockets of green, semiliquid pus. Other organisms isolated from these abscesses may include streptococci, staphylococci, and enterobacteria. Treatment is not usually feasible, and pigs should be culled for humane reasons. However, when applicable, hygiene can be improved, and problems such as tail biting controlled or prevented.

Osteochondrosis and Osteoarthrosis: Lameness associated with these problems may become clinically relevant by the time the pigs are 4–6 mo old, but the major ramifications are in gilts, sows, and boars (*see* p 1158). Because there is a hereditary component, the importance of these problems increases if affected replacement breeding stock is brought into a herd that was previously free of either condition.

Rickets: Although now uncommon, rickets (*see* p 1051) is occasionally seen, usually associated with a feed formulation or mixing error. Rickets affects rapidly growing, young pigs with a clinical onset at ~10 wk of age. Morbidity is high, and affected pigs become crippled, anorectic, and unthrifty. Limbs are stunted and bowed, joints are swollen, and the head may seem disproportionately large. Long bones of the limbs can spontaneously fracture so that the pig becomes severely lame and unwilling to move. Ribs may fracture. Some pigs develop posterior paresis and sit on the ground if vertebral bodies fracture and damage the spinal cord.

Absolute deficiencies of calcium, phosphorus, or vitamin D, or an imbalance of the calcium:phosphorus ratio causes cessation of mineralization at the metaphysis and thickening of the growth plate and epiphyseal growth cartilage.

On necropsy, bones should be dissected to determine whether there are any fractures or healing fractures, particularly in the ribs, humeruses, and femurs. The costochondral junctions of most ribs are enlarged to form a rachitic rosary, and ribs may bend with moderate manual force. Bone remodeling is inadequate and, radiographically, long bones and ribs are poorly mineralized. Failure of calcification and endochondral ossification results in thickened, irregular growth plates and epiphyseal growth cartilages in which hemorrhages may be seen grossly if slab sections of the ends of long bones are cut on a band saw. In chronic cases, bones can be cut with a knife. A sudden increase in carcass condemnations or partial condemnations because of fractured limb bones, ribs, or vertebrae at slaughter should trigger investigation of rations and their ability to meet the nutritional needs of growing pigs, particularly with some of the fast-growing, lean contemporary hybrids. Ration analysis is useful, but current batches of feed may have been mixed correctly or with different lots of ingredients, thus making it difficult to relate cause and effect. Keeping frozen samples of each batch of feed for retrospective analysis is a good practice.

Although rations can be corrected and vitamin D given parenterally, there is no effective treatment, and attempts to rear large numbers of affected pigs have been economically disastrous. Culling affected pigs may thus be the most cost-effective alternative.

Foot Disorders: On occasion, grower/finisher pigs have overgrown claws or bruises and cracks in the wall or sole of the hoof. The floor type and condition is perhaps the single greatest factor in determining whether lesions develop or resolve. Floors with wide slots enable digits to fall between the slats, causing damage. Floors kept too wet can soften the hoof wall, making them more prone to trauma. If the floor is too smooth, the balance between growth and wear of the horn is lost; if it is too rough, the hoof wall, coronary band, or skin above the *hoof* is damaged so that infectious agents can penetrate the foot or adjacent joints, resulting in abscess formation.

An absolute or intermittent deficiency of biotin results in weak, flaky keratin that makes hoof walls susceptible to cracking; flaky skin accompanies hoof lesion and there is generally poor reproductive performance in the herd. As gilts are prepared for breeding, supplementing biotin may be helpful. Recommended inclusion rates of biotin are 250–400 mcg/kg complete feed. Trace mineral deficiencies or imbalances can also contribute to compromised hoof wall and heel epidermis formation.

Selenium toxicosis can cause coronary band swelling and necrosis in addition to more generalized signs such as anorexia or even paralysis (*see* p 3085). Selenium and ergot toxicity can result in hoof sloughing in pigs.

Nutritional Myopathy (White Muscle Disease): In contemporary systems with adequate ration preparation and storage, nutritional myopathy should not be problematic (*see* p 1174). Although unexpected deaths are typical of selenium and/or vitamin E deficiency, sometimes pigs are found recumbent and unable to rise and walk. At necropsy, a variety of pathologic changes may be seen, including pale muscle masses, epicardial hemorrhages (mulberry heart disease), and a pale, scarred liver with an uneven surface (hepatosis dietetica).

Prevention includes supplementation with selenite so that the total ration concentration is 0.3 ppm selenium. If the condition is diagnosed in a batch of pigs, injectable selenium/vitamin E can be given as a stopgap measure until supplemented feed is part of the nutrition program.

BREEDING GILTS, SOWS, AND BOARS

After reproductive failure, lameness is typically the most important reason for removal of breeding stock from the herd. Lameness in breeding swine can result in the following: 1) higher rate of breeding stock replacement with attendant increased risk of disease introduction; 2) an inability to maintain a breeding schedule due to an unreliable pool of breeding pigs and, ultimately, an impact on pig flow in the grower/finisher area; 3) increased cost of maintaining additional breeding stock; 4) poorer reproductive performance due to regular replacement of lame sows with gilts; 5) poorer growth and feed efficiency in progeny pigs due to a higher proportion of pigs produced by first-parity sows; 6) reduced pigs born alive because of higher stillborn rates in lame sows and reduced subsequent litter size due to poor lactation feed intake; 7) increased preweaning mortality due to clumsy, lame sows that tread or lie on baby pigs; 8) reduced weaning weights of pigs due to reduced feed intake of sows in lactation; 9) reduced salvage value of cull sows due to increased lactation weight loss and sow mortality; and 10) reduced fertility in sound boars that are overworked while others are lame or being replaced. In sum, the impact of breeding herd lameness on the biologic and economic performance of a farm can be substantial.

Many diseases that affect grower/finisher pigs (*see* p 1160) can also affect young gilts and boars selected as breeding stock. Arthritis caused by *Mycoplasma hyosynoviae* or acute or chronic erysipelas can cause an incapacitating lameness. Polyarthritis and polyserositis caused by *M hyorhinis* are seen occasionally in these older pigs. Susceptible, stressed adult pigs can succumb to *M hyorhinis* with a higher fever and a more severe lameness than is seen in nursery pigs. Likewise, *Haemophilus parasuis* can develop as an acute epidemic disease in gilts sourced from herds free of the bacteria after entering a herd endemically infected. High morbidity and even mortality that is quite refractory to treatment can result.

If rickets or skeletal weakness was a problem in the growing phase, pigs that could have been affected should not be retained as breeding stock. Ambulation should be assessed as a component of breeding stock selection. Pigs with conformational abnormalities of their limbs or restricted or abnormal ambulation should be culled. Feet should be evaluated for uniformity among and angulation of the digits and for integrity of the wall, sole, and heel. If any problems are identified, including abnormal traits such as overgrowth of the major or secondary digits in a particular line of pigs, these pigs also should be culled.

Rickets, Osteomalacia, and Osteoporosis: These syndromes can affect older age groups of pigs, with various clinical outcomes. Most pigs, including breeding stock, are slaughtered before their skeleton has fully matured; some growth plates are functional up to 3.5 yr of age and, therefore, are susceptible to rachitic or other changes.

Osteomalacia is characterized by an excess of unmineralized or poorly mineralized osteoid that forms as bone remodeling occurs (or does not occur). Hence, osteomalacia is the component of rickets (*see* p 1161) that affects the growth plate and is described in younger pigs. In contrast, osteoporosis develops when established bone loses mineral and mass by a process of osteolysis, a different pathogenesis from that of either rickets or osteomalacia.

Gilts that have normal skeletal development and are selected as breeding stock must continue to have their nutritional needs met, both for their own growing skeleton and, once pregnant, that of the growing fetuses. This may precipitate as osteomalacia if amounts of calcium, phosphorus, or vitamin D are inadequate or, in the case of the minerals, inappropriately balanced. The problem is further compounded once the sow farrows, due to secretion of calcium in the milk. A first-parity sow may soon draw on her skeletal reserves and become osteoporotic. Because sows can become pregnant within 7 days of weaning, there is little time for recovery of skeletal mass between one breeding cycle and the next, so the skeleton becomes progressively weaker. Limited exercise may also exacerbate calcium mobilization and bone loss. Consequently, in sows late in gestation, during lactation, or soon after weaning, bones that have become weak are susceptible to fractures. It is not surprising that considerable numbers of first- and second-litter sows are culled because of fractures and lameness.

Factors that may lead to bone fractures include entrapment of a limb in or under the bars of a farrowing crate, activity as sows are moved from their farrowing crates, and fighting as new groups of weaned sows reestablish a social order in the breeding or gestation area in group housing conditions. Sows mounted by other sows that are in estrus are also prone to injury. The most frequent sites of fractures are femurs, humeruses, lumbar vertebrae, and occasionally ribs. Whatever the factors that precipitate the fractures, affected sows are in pain and are either severely lame and unwilling to move or paraplegic.

Diagnosis is based on a history of acute lameness or paraplegia in pregnant, lactating, or recently weaned gilts or sows. Sometimes, crepitus can be detected in affected limbs. A neurologic examination can help locate spinal lesions if a sow is paralyzed in the pelvic limbs. Affected sows should be culled or euthanized after an early diagnosis. Prevention through adequate nutrition and exercise for gilts and sows curtails the problem.

Osteomyelitis and Spinal Abscesses: In addition to the causes discussed under grower/finisher pigs, osteomyelitis may also develop secondary to a vertebral fracture or an epiphyseal separation. It is reasonable to assume that occasional "showering" with organisms from superficial wounds, abscesses, or the respiratory or GI tracts can be a source of infection. *Trueperella pyogenes* seems to be a frequent cause of the suppuration and abscessation. Osteomyelitis of the ulnar epiphysis in young boars and sows has been reported.

Vertebral osteomyelitis and epidural abscesses can cause a variety of signs, including nonspecific lameness, hypermetria, ataxia, or bilateral flaccid paralysis of the pelvic limbs. Except for the temporal nature of the infectious process, clinically it is difficult to differentiate a destructive or space-occupying abscess from a fracture. Regardless of underlying cause, recovery is unlikely, and the pigs should be culled.

Osteochondrosis and Leg Weakness Syndrome (Degenerative Joint Disease, Dyschondroplasia):

Degenerative joint disease (DJD) and leg weakness syndrome are generic terms for a clinical syndrome that is a major cause of lameness and culling for lameness in swine breeding stock. Although the conditions are more often investigated in purebred stock, they can cause major losses in commercial pig herds. Given the increased scale of production in many herds and the shift toward pigs that grow faster, are more muscular, and finish heavier, DJD and leg weakness are critical issues.

Osteochondrosis is a specific developmental condition that represents the major cause of DJD. Osteochondrosis is a defect in the development of cartilage of the growth plates or articular cartilage in growing pigs. The pathogenesis of osteochondrosis is increasingly but still incompletely understood. In osteochondrosis, growth plates are more prone to fracture because of areas of retained hypertrophic cartilage that focally thicken and weaken the cartilage. Lesions develop when articular cartilage on the interior aspect of the joint surface becomes necrotic, ostensibly due to loss of vascular supplies. The necrotic cartilage interferes with the advancing ossification front, and the resulting irregular ossification underlying the weight-bearing cartilage surfaces is prone to clefting (displaced cartilage "chips," or osteochondrosis dissecans), exposing the endochondral bone and causing pain and lameness. The developmental lesions have a very high prevalence in young pigs but mostly resolve with age and further development.

Osteochondrosis is apparently seen in all the major breeds of purebred and commercial hybrid pigs. Dyschondroplasia results in deformed long bones, particularly the ulna. Pigs that have valgus deformity or permanently flexed carpi tend to be unsuitable for sale as breeding stock and may be lame. In addition, epiphyseolysis and epiphyseal separation may be precipitated by weakening of underlying growth plates and cause an incapacitating lameness.

Although lesions that precede or develop into DJD or result in limb deformities begin to develop in younger pigs, clinical problems are not usually seen until pigs are >4–8 mo old. Frequently, the fastest growing, most muscular, and heaviest pigs are affected. Given time, some pigs (if not culled) recover from episodes of lameness, but deformities remain. Clinical signs vary with the site and extent of lesions and can range from stiffness and a shortened stride or a stride affected by an angular limb deformity to a three-legged lameness or an inability to stand. Most commonly, these animals have a weight-bearing, shifting lameness because of bilateral lesions that affect multiple joints in the same pig. Pigs that "walk" on flexed carpi usually have severe DJD in the elbows, and pigs that tuck their pelvic limbs under their abdomen in a stance that resembles a "circus elephant balancing on a ball" often have DJD that affects stifles, tibial tarsal bones, or joints on intervertebral processes.

If epiphyseal separation of the femoral head has occurred, the pig has difficulty standing and initially will not use the affected limb. A pig that has unilateral separation of the ischiatic tuberosity also has difficulty standing and a tendency to slip; if both tuberosities are affected, the pig has a hopping gait for a few steps after being lifted and then collapses. The severity of clinical signs in any of these conditions varies, and joints with less extensive lesions appear to be protected by the gait if they are more painful than other degenerating joints. Severe joint lesions also have been seen in pigs that did not appear to be lame.

In pigs that have limb deformities (eg, dyschondroplasia affecting the distal ulnar growth plate), thickened, irregular growth plates are seen on radiographs or at necropsy. In degenerating joints, there is an excess of yellow synovia, and synovial villi may have proliferated. There are various irregularities of the articular surface, including folds in the cartilage, clefts into the cartilage, flaps of cartilage, and in severe cases, craters and exposed subchondral bone. In chronic cases, osteophytes develop, detached fragments of cartilage become embedded in the synovium and start to ossify, and craters fill with fibrocartilage. If vertebral joints are affected, vertebrae eventually fuse. Growth plates that are most severely affected by dyschondroplasia are those of the distal part of the ulna and the ribs, whereas joints most often affected by DJD include the elbow, stifle, and hock, or the intervertebral synovial joints.

Many potential causes of DJD or osteochondrosis have been investigated. There is evidence of a genetic component, because within breeds, specific boars have been identified to have progeny with a higher incidence of osteochondrosis. Breeds and lines of pigs that are heavy and well muscled, particularly in the hams, are commonly affected; therefore, crossbreeding for hybrid vigor (ie, to create faster growing, muscular hybrids) does not solve the problem. The fastest growing pigs in a group seem to have a greater propensity for lesions to develop in either growth plates or joints, but once slower-growing pigs reach the body weight of their faster-growing peers, lesions are comparable. Growth hormone may affect chondrocyte metabolism and thereby influence the onset of articular lesions.

Research into manipulating the energy, protein, and mineral concentrations of the ration in an attempt to influence the development of lesions has been inconclusive, even contradictory. None of the imbalances or deficiencies of nutrients that typically are associated with lesions of cartilage or bone (calcium, phosphorus, and vitamins A, C, and D) seemed to exacerbate osteochondrosis. Deficient or excess zinc and manganese may be causal factors in osteochondrosis, but there is a paucity of evidence from research.

The stress of mixing pigs appears to have little impact on the frequency of osteochondrosis, but trauma from handling or housing conditions have been found to affect clinical osteochondrosis. The culling rate due to lameness for sows kept on solid floors is less than that for those kept on slats, but the benefits of placing pigs with DJD on dirt lots or pasture is equivocal. Although such pigs usually become clinically sound within 6 wk, they are potential carriers of the syndromes.

Because osteochondrosis and DJD interfere with production efficiency, the prognosis for affected pigs is poor. At best, the following practices are recommended: selecting against replacement pigs that are lame or have poor conformation, providing adequate rations for the growth of a strong skeleton, housing gilts in pens with ≥12 sq ft (1.1 sq m) per animal, and promoting exercise on nonslip floors. In problem herds, providing a "hardening off" period for gilts is encouraged. This includes purchasing gilts at <75 kg live weight, restricting their feed intake to slow their growth rate, providing ≥1.1 sq m per animal in pens with solid or only partially slatted floors, waiting to breed gilts until they are 8–10 mo old, and housing gilts in pens until they farrow. If replacements are purchased, suitable breeding stock must be found and inferior pigs rejected at the time of arrival at the farm.

Foot Disorders: Foot lesions can be quite prevalent and severe among sows and boars and have been shown to cause lameness and reduce productivity and longevity of breeding stock. Specific lesions particularly associated with lameness include white line lesions, heel-sole cracks, and heel overgrowth with erosions, but any of the lesions can be significant in individual cases.

As with finishing pigs, floor type and condition are important with respect to lesion development. Housing type and management are also important risk factors for various types of foot lesions. Nutrition, including water quality, can affect the growth rate and quality of the horn wall and heel epithelium.

Bacterial infections of the foot can develop in any age pig but cause serious losses in breeding pigs. Bacterial infections are often a sequelae of foot lesions that allow penetration of bacteria into underlying sensitive foot structures. Foot infections are seen in both confinement and semiconfinement systems, with morbidity of 20%–68%. Often a single limb is affected, and the lameness progresses to the point that the pig is three-legged lame.

Lesions usually develop gradually, and the foot becomes swollen. Lesions vary in severity and can include heel erosions, separation along the white line, toe erosions, sole erosions, vertical hoof wall cracks, deep necrotic ulcers, sinuses at the coronary band, and chronic fibrosis. A mix of organisms has been isolated from the lesions or identified in smears from lesions and tissue sections. These included *Trueperella pyogenes*, *Fusobacterium necrophorum*, *Borrelia suilla*, and a mixture of gram-negative and gram-positive cocci and rods.

A diagnosis is made from the clinical signs and a thorough evaluation of the feet. Ideally, the whole foot should be examined in a recumbent or suitably restrained pig. If there is a herd problem, all sows in crates or pens should be examined. Whenever possible, feet of pigs from affected herds should be evaluated at the slaughterhouse. Superficial examination of some less extensive lesions may lead to inappropriate cause-effect conclusions. Therefore, to ensure that lesions are severe enough to be the cause of the lameness, some pigs can be culled for diagnosis of the problem and their feet sectioned or claws removed after immersing the foot in 140°F water for 60 min to determine whether the soft tissues and bones within the foot are infected.

Treatment of apparent foot infections with penicillin has been commonly practiced (200,000 U into the lesion or 600,000 U, IM), but effectiveness has not been proved and success decreases with chronicity of the lesion. Prevention is a more productive longterm strategy, and it involves improving the nature and cleanliness of the flooring, reducing moisture, resurfacing rough, abrasive areas, and ensuring nutritional adequacy for hoof health. As replacement gilts mature, biotin and trace mineral supplementation enhances the quality and strength of the hoof, and use in breeding sows is recommended.

Trauma: Trauma associated with overexertion can cause detachment of muscle tendons and a proliferative osteitis on the medial humeral epicondyle and the greater trochanter of the femur in sows. Mixing gilts or sows before or after breeding or at weaning commonly results in pigs becoming injured as they reestablish a social order. This can lead directly to fractures of long bones or skin abrasions that may cause secondary bacterial infections.

Traumatic injuries can also result from movement of groups to and from farrowing facilities, especially movements of gilts into farrowing. Gilts typically are more anxious and flighty than older sows. Carrying a heavy, gravid uterus over potentially slippery flooring over some distance poses a high enough risk of injury without adding other stressors. Movement should be calm and deliberate, with small groups of gilts and sows moved at a time to reduce potential injuries.

Sows housed in stalls with concrete slats may tear their dewclaws when they attempt to stand. Treatment with appropriate antibiotics, protection of the wound with a dressing, and isolation in a hospital pen that has clean, deep bedding should enable a lesion to heal. Prevention by trimming elongated dewclaws is a prudent and simple management practice.

LAMENESS IN SHEEP

Lameness in sheep may be caused by a number of systemic diseases, some of which include navel/joint ill (*Escherichia coli* and *Erysipelothrix*), tetanus, white muscle disease, frostbite, chlamydial polyarthritis, rickets, enzootic ataxia (copper deficiency), mastitis, orchitis, nutritional osteodystrophies, selenium toxicosis, laminitis, dermatophilosis, bluetongue, ulcerative dermatosis, and in some countries, foot-and-mouth disease. Weakness, ataxia, and neurologic problems may be misinterpreted as lameness in diseases such as scrapie, listeriosis, and visna. Additional information on differential diagnosis, treatment, and prevention can be found under the specific topics (*see* p 1039 and p 1209).

Lamenesses are often due to injuries. Broken legs are common in young lambs, which are frequently injured inadvertently by adults. Usually, these can be easily splinted and will heal within 3 wk. However, leaving the limb splinted and unobserved for too long may also lead to iatrogenic lameness. The general principles of treatment and prevention of these are the same as in other species.

Lameness can be caused by a group of infections specific to the feet. The most well known of these is contagious footrot, a mixed infection with *Fusobacterium necrophorum* and the obligate pathogen *Dichelobacter nodosus*. The skin between the claws is the primary site of invasion; it is predisposed to infection by breaks in the epidermis from injury or maceration from prolonged exposure to moisture. *F necrophorum* and *Trueperella pyogenes* induce a transient condition called ovine interdigital dermatitis or foot scald, which may lead to more serious problems.

INTERDIGITAL DERMATITIS

(Foot scald)

This necrotizing condition of the interdigital skin usually precedes or accompanies footrot. In Australia, it is considered to be caused by less virulent strains of *Dichelobacter nodosus* and is termed benign footrot (*see* below). Wet weather, damp pastures, and mud are predisposing factors. In milder cases, the interdigital skin is red, hairless, swollen, and moist. In severely affected cases, the integrity of the interdigital skin is compromised, exposing subcutaneous tissues. Suppuration and swelling of the deeper interdigital tissues may develop. Lameness can affect as many as 90% of sheep, and all four feet may be affected. The characteristic smell associated with virulent *D nodosus* infections is not present if *D nodosus* is not present. Healing is rapid when conditions dry out, but the disease may recur when conditions again become wet.

Because scald usually precedes a footrot outbreak, it is prudent to treat the condition as if it were footrot. Other diseases to consider in the differential diagnosis include dermatophilosis (strawberry footrot, *see* p 858), which affects the hairy skin of the coronet and pastern. Viral diseases such as ulcerative dermatitis, contagious ecthyma, and foot-and-mouth disease may be excluded by flock history, clinical signs, electron microscopy, and serology. Currently, the treatment of choice consists of external application of 10% w/v zinc sulfate disinfectants via a footbath or aerosol.

CONTAGIOUS FOOTROT

When there is concurrent invasion by *Dichelobacter nodosus* of foot scald, contagious footrot results. The Australians separate footrot into two categories, benign or virulent, depending on the strain of *D nodosus* present. In the USA, however, benign and virulent footrot are considered to be the same (due to the difficulty of differentiating the two) and are treated accordingly.

Benign Footrot

The infection is confined largely to the interdigital skin, with only minimal underrunning of the adjacent horn. Clinically, benign footrot appears similar to ovine interdigital dermatitis, but *D nodosus* is involved—a situation that is hard to assess because culture of *D nodosus* is difficult and rarely done. The odor, however, is characteristic. Lameness is common but less severe than in virulent footrot. The etiology and pathogenesis are the same, but the strains of *D nodosus* are less virulent and lack the hoof-invasive properties of the strains that cause virulent footrot. *D nodosus* may also be isolated from cattle, but strains affecting cattle usually cause only the benign form of footrot in sheep. The economic effect of benign footrot is much less than that of virulent footrot. Running the sheep through foot baths containing 10% w/v zinc sulfate once every 14 days during the wet season is usually adequate for control. Since the advent of long-acting antibiotics such as tetracycline, their use has been adopted with good results.

Virulent Footrot

Virulent footrot is a specific, chronic, necrotizing disease of the epidermis of the interdigital skin and hoof matrix that begins as an interdigital dermatitis and extends to involve large areas of the hoof matrix. Because the sensitive lamina and its network of capillaries are destroyed by the infection, the hoof wall (corium) loses its blood supply and anchorage to the underlying tissue and becomes detached. Footrot is extremely contagious and, under suitable conditions and susceptible genetics, morbidity may approach 100%. The infection is also rarely found in goats, deer, and cattle. The potential for genetic selection for increased resistance to footrot has been established.

Etiology: *Fusobacterium necrophorum*, a gram-negative anaerobic bacteria, is a normal resident of manure-contaminated environments. Under favorable environmental conditions, it colonizes the moist, macerated interdigital skin and provides ideal conditions for invasion by *D nodosus* at the skin/hoof interface. By action of proteases, *D nodosus*, also a gram-negative anaerobe and obligate pathogen, liquefies the cells of the stratum granulosum and stratum spinosum, causing the separation of the hoof wall from the basal epithelium. It works its way down the interdigital horn to the heel, then to the sole, and finally to the lateral side of the hoof. *D nodosus* has been found to survive <3 wk outside the host, but it can remain sequestered in cavities, cracks, or deformities of the affected foot for the life of the sheep. There are at least 20 different strains of *D nodosus*, with varying pathogenicity. Transmission occurs most rapidly when conditions are warm and moist; however, cold, moist conditions are also conducive to transmission.

Clinical Findings: The most obvious sign is lameness, but the foot is seldom carried or packed. In chronically infected sheep, the hoof becomes gnarled and distorted. When more than one foot is infected, some sheep become recumbent or walk on their knees. Brisket and knees tend to become hairless and ulcerated. Affected sheep do not compete well for food, lose body condition, and produce less wool. Rams with infected hindfeet may be unwilling to breed, and ewes with hindfeet lesions may be unable to bear the weight of a ram at service.

In early cases, examination of the feet generally reveals nothing more than interdigital dermatitis. In slightly more advanced cases, in which the infection has begun to extend into the hoof matrix, there is slight detachment of the hoof wall at the interface of the interdigital skin and hoof. As the disease progresses, the separation of the horn spreads further under the heel and sole. Running one's thumb between the wall and the underlying tissue in the interdigital space often detaches the wall from the heel and sole, revealing a white, slightly moist (but not purulent), odorous substance. Finally, the outer wall is affected. The horny hoof may eventually be attached only at the toe and the coronet on the lateral side of the foot. The odor of the necrotic tissue is characteristic and helps to diagnose the disease. Myiasis is a common sequela during fly season; it may extend to the area of the sheep where the infected feet come into contact with the body when the sheep is recumbent. The clinical disease persists until the environment dries or the sheep are treated. After apparent healing, *D nodosus* remains hidden in small pockets within the foot, where it is detectable only by extensive trimming, and becomes active again when moist conditions recur. These sheep are carriers and generally remain infected for life. Immunity to footrot after infection does not seem to occur, because relapses are the norm.

Diagnosis: In flocks with virulent footrot, underrunning and separation of the hard horn of the hoof of one or more feet, complete with the characteristic odor, is diagnostic. If the problem is discovered early when interdigital dermatitis is the only sign, it should be assumed that the condition is an early stage of contagious footrot, and treatment should be initiated immediately.

Treatment: Treatment efforts may be directed toward temporary control of the disease or total eradication. At certain times, eg, during a wet season, temporary control may be the only realistic goal.

Traditionally, treatment consisted of foot bathing using antibacterial solutions after careful hoof trimming to remove all dead horn and expose infected tissue and bacteria to air. However, foot soaking for 30–60 min has been shown to be more effective even when trimming is not done. In fact, Australian research has shown that trimming may do more damage than good. The most effective solution is 10% w/v zinc sulfate with 0.2% v/v of laundry detergent containing nonionic surfactants such as sodium lauryl sulfate. Aerosol sprays have been used in lieu of foot bathing and include zinc sulfate, tincture of iodine, tetracycline, copper sulfate, formalin, chlorine bleach, and other disinfectants. However, sprays are not as effective as foot bathing or soaking in zinc sulfate.

The advent of long-acting antibiotics used in combination with topical foot treatments has improved recovery and reduced carrier animals. Parenteral treatment using a long-acting oxytetracycline at 13.6 mg/lb gives a duration of effect in cattle of 7–8 days and probably a similar duration of effect in sheep. However, sheep must be placed in a "clean" area (ie, one in which no sheep have been kept for at least 3 wk) or in a completely dry lot after they are run through a foot bath and given the antibiotic. Sheep will become reinfected as soon as the antibiotic is cleared if returned to a contaminated environment. The feet of treated sheep should be examined once a week to identify those not responding to treatment. Sheep that do not respond should be isolated and preferably culled. *D nodosus* is extremely difficult to eradicate from animals that have relapsed numerous times. Furthermore, subclinical or relapsing cases take valuable time to handle, identify, and isolate, and they remain a source of infection for other animals.

Prevention and Control: Animals from unknown premises or auction houses should not be purchased. Any sheep to be added to the flock should be quarantined for several weeks to prevent the spread of footrot and other chronic diseases. During the quarantine period, the animal's feet should be lightly trimmed and examined closely for pockets and other malformations that suggest a previous *D nodosus* infection. Vehicles (eg, trucks, trailers) or facilities in which unknown or infected sheep have been held should be thoroughly cleaned and disinfected before placing uninfected sheep in them. If it is not possible to thoroughly disinfect transport vehicles, zinc sulfate can be liberally scattered over the floor to reduce viable bacteria.

Because the incubation period of footrot is ~14 days, foot bathing at 10-day intervals will control spread of the organism in affected flocks during periods of the year when the sheep are in wet conditions. Footrot has been controlled by placing foot baths with 10% w/v zinc sulfate solution around water troughs, forcing sheep to walk through them and stand in order to drink. Lame sheep should be separated for treatment and not returned to the flock until all evidence of footrot is gone.

D nodosus vaccines accelerate healing in affected sheep and aid in protecting unaffected sheep. They are recommended as an additional tool to control or eradicate the disease. However, their effectiveness depends on the strain(s) causing the infection and those present in the vaccine. No vaccine contains all the various strains of *D nodosus*, and use of vaccination without other means of control will most likely select for strains not contained in the vaccine. Alum-precipitated vaccines require two doses 4–6 wk apart to establish effective immunity, which persists for 2–3 mo. Lesions heal within 4–6 wk if immunity is established. Oil-emulsion vaccines induce immunity within 3 wk of the initial dose and may persist for 3–4 mo. In endemic areas, revaccination is recommended at intervals of 3–6 mo. Reaction to the vaccine is common, resulting in large granulomas and occasional abscesses. Vaccines for *F necrophorum* have not generally shown much benefit in either treatment or prevention. Lately, the vaccine appears to be unavailable in the USA.

Addition of zinc to trace mineral salt, reportedly effective in reducing hoof rot in cattle, has not been shown to be particularly helpful for sheep footrot. However, zinc is important for immunity and skin/hoof health. Providing it in a well-balanced trace mineral mix may be helpful in locations deficient in zinc.

Eradication: A successful eradication program requires planning, commitment, and an investment of time and money. Eradication can be achieved only by eliminating all cases of *D nodosus* infection in a flock and preventing its reintroduction. This may be done by replacing affected stock with footrot-free sheep or by rigorously treating all new infections and culling affected sheep that do not respond readily to treatment. Eradication is easiest when the environment is dry; at other times, treatments should be directed more toward control of transmission. Affected sheep have to be identified by close examination of all four feet; no other diagnostic tests are available (although some exciting European research using PCR and interdigital swab samples is showing great promise as a diagnostic tool). Subclinical cases constitute a major problem. They will relapse as soon as they are placed in wet conditions and the infection spreads rapidly. Other ruminants (goats, deer, cattle) are potential sources of *D nodosus*. If they are in contact with the sheep, they should be considered in the eradication program.

To begin, the feet of all sheep should be trimmed and carefully examined. The flock should then be divided into affected and unaffected groups. Sheep with no visible lesions are foot bathed, isolated, and placed on "clean," dry ground. (This group may have some degree of genetic resistance, and identifying them in some way is recommended. Retaining offspring from this group could further help control the disease.) This group should receive an injection of long-acting tetracycline at 13.6 mg/lb, and any lame sheep should be removed immediately. The group of sheep with footrot lesions are culled or, after careful hoof trimming, the feet are soaked for at least 30 min, and the animals are treated with antibiotic and kept separated from the lesion-free group. This second group should undergo foot soaking once a week for a total of three times and/or be medicated with long-acting oxytetracycline at the time of soaking. At the end of this period, their feet should again be examined and trimmed. Any sheep with an active case of footrot should be culled. This group must be monitored closely during the next wet period to detect any carriers, which are usually the first animals to show lameness. When no relapses have occurred for 1 mo or longer, this group may be placed with the clean flock. However, placing a single active or subclinical case in the clean flock can negate all of the previous hard work.

Australia has implemented an effective eradication program involving many flocks. The program has three phases. The **control phase** is used during periods of active spread or to reduce the number infected. During this phase, vaccination, foot bathing, and parenteral antibiotics can all be used. The **eradication phase** must take place during the dry season and cannot begin until several weeks after the use of all medications has been stopped and 10–12 wk after vaccination. Foot bathing and vaccination tend to mask the presence of infection. During this phase, all four feet of every sheep are inspected every 3–4 wk. Infected sheep can be treated with parenteral antibiotics at the first inspection only. After this, infected sheep are culled at each inspection. This continues until there are two completely negative, consecutive flock examinations. In the **surveillance phase**, all lame sheep in the flock are examined immediately. If footrot is present, the flock goes back to phase 1 or 2 again.

FOOT ABSCESS

(Infective bulbar necrosis, Heel abscess, Bumblefoot)

Bumblefoot is a necrotizing or purulent infection involving the distal interphalangeal soft tissues and sometimes the joint. The incidence is usually sporadic, but as much as 25% of the flock may be affected.

The two organisms most consistently recovered from bumblefoot are *Fusobacterium necrophorum* and *Trueperella pyogenes*. Foot abscesses may develop as a complication of ovine interdigital dermatitis by extension of the necrotic process into the subcutis and then into the distal interphalangeal joint. They also commonly develop after penetration of the interdigital skin by sharp objects (eg, crusted snow, frozen or stiff stubble of alfalfa and grain), bruising of the foot and injury of the skin when slipping on frozen rocks, or even careless paring of the hoof. This joint is vulnerable to infection on the interdigital aspect where the joint capsule protrudes above the coronary border as the dorsal and volar pouches. At these sites, the joint capsule is protected only by the interdigital skin and a minimal amount of subcutaneous tissue.

Foot abscesses often develop when the soil and pastures are wet or frozen. The disease causes an acute lameness that is usually restricted to one foot, which the sheep will not place on the ground. It may be possible to express necrotic material through an opening in the interdigital skin caused by the bacterial invasion, but more commonly the swollen sinuses break open and drain at one or more points above the coronet. If this does not occur, the swelling will have to be lanced. In some instances, movement of the affected digit is exaggerated, indicating that the ligaments about the distal interphalangeal joint have ruptured. Displacement of the digit during locomotion and permanent deformity are likely in those cases.

Acute lameness with the sheep packing a foot, swelling of one digit, and discharging sinuses distinguish foot abscess from footrot.

Early treatment with parenteral long-acting antibiotics is sometimes effective and may prevent joint infection. The therapy aims to maintain the integrity of the joint ligaments by draining the abscess and applying an antibacterial preparation and a self-adhesive bandage. This reduces stress on the ligaments, keeps the lesion out of the mud, and counters the bacterial infection. Although the prognosis for complete recovery is poor, in most cases the foot heals sufficiently to allow adequate locomotion. Once the infection becomes established in the joint, conservative treatment is not effective. However, a toe can be surgically removed (if the other digit is healthy) with relatively good success.

Control depends on early treatment and moving the sheep to avoid conditions that lead to ovine interdigital dermatitis or other causes of abscess. Although *F necrophorum* vaccines are available, they have not proved to be very effective.

IMPACTED OR INFECTED OIL GLAND

Sheep have a sebaceous (oil) gland in the skin of the interdigital space. A thick, oily, translucent secretion is stored in a small pouch lying between the phalanges and is discharged to the skin surface through a duct in the skin. Occasionally, the gland and its contents are mistaken for an abscess. However, the duct can become occluded, causing distention of the oil pouch. It rarely causes lameness. The oil sac also may become infected, resulting in a local cellulitis or abscess that may be confused with bumblefoot. Expression of the contents by manual pressure relieves impaction. Infected glands can then be treated with local or systemic antibiotics or both, depending on the extent and severity of the infectious process. Unlike bumblefoot, this condition generally responds readily to treatment.

INTERDIGITAL FIBROMA

An interdigital fibroma is a mass of fibrous tissue between the toes that may resemble a papilloma. If not removed, it enlarges, spreading the toes. Tendrils grow upward between the first phalanges, causing severe lameness. If the fibroma is detected early, surgical removal (cryosurgery and electrocautery) may be successful; however, by the time it causes lameness, the tendrils cannot be totally removed from between the phalanges, and the fibroma tends to recur.

SEPTIC LAMINITIS

(Lamellar suppuration, Toe abscess)

Septic laminitis is an acute bacterial infection of the laminar matrix of the hoof that is usually restricted to the toe and abaxial wall. The disease is sporadic and the cause variable, but cases due to *Fusobacterium necrophorum* and *Trueperella pyogenes* usually are more severe and extensive than those involving streptococci or other organisms. The organisms probably enter through fissures between the wall and sole and through vertical and horizontal fractures of wall horn. Sometimes, infection is enhanced by impaction with sand, mud, or feces; by overgrowth of the hoof; or by separation of the wall after laminitis.

Forefeet are affected more commonly. Lameness is severe, and the affected digit may be hot and tender. There may be a draining sinus above the lesion at the coronet, or the abscess may be found above the sole on the bottom of the foot. Applying pressure to various sections of the sole with the thumbs will elicit pain and help locate the pocket of infection. Affected sheep usually recover rapidly after paring of the horn to provide dependent drainage.

MYOPATHIES IN RUMINANTS AND PIGS

INFECTIOUS MYOPATHIES

Clostridial Myonecrosis

(Blackleg, Malignant edema, False blackleg, Gas gangrene, Gangrene)

Clostridial infection of skeletal muscle is a noncontagious cause of acute myonecrosis. *Clostridium chauvoei*, *C septicum*, *C sordellii*, occasionally *C novyi* type B, *C perfringens* type A, *C carnis*, or mixed infections involving several agents are common (*see* p 601). *Clostridia* or their spores are ubiquitous in the environment, feces, intestinal tract, and other internal organs of a variety of species. Clostridial myonecrosis may develop after introduction of spores via an IM injection or penetrating wound or through sporulation of organisms already present in muscle when suitable anaerobic conditions are created with muscle trauma. Any skeletal muscle group in the body can be involved, but most infections affect the limb or trunk muscles. Occasionally, muscles such as those around the vulva, tongue, and diaphragm can be involved, or the udder in a cow may be the primary site of sepsis. The release of powerful exotoxins by multiplying clostridia is responsible for the local tissue damage, systemic toxemia, and widespread organ dysfunction. The toxins of *C sordelli* are the most potent of all the clostridial species, and myonecrosis caused by this organism is fatal.

Infections are characterized by a rapid clinical course, fever (104°–106°F [40°–41°C]), lameness, systemic toxemia, tremors, ataxia, and dyspnea, often followed in 12–24 hr by recumbency, coma, and death. Mortality may approach 100%. Initially, the skin over the area may be swollen, hot, and discolored; however, as the disease progresses, the skin over the area may become cool and insensitive with progressive sloughing. Crepitus may be detectable, indicating subcutaneous gas production. If a wound is present, malodorous, serosanguineous discharge may be seen. Hematology and serum biochemical analyses usually reflect hemoconcentration and a stress/toxic leukogram with increased activities of serum CK and serum AST that often do not reflect the toxicity of clostridial myonecrosis. A definitive diagnosis is made from direct smear examination, fluorescent antibody testing, or anaerobic bacterial culture of aspirates of affected tissues. Differential diagnoses include other fulminant disease processes in which there is rapid debilitation or death of the animal.

Clostridial myonecrosis generally has characteristic pathologic lesions that are absent in most other conditions, making diagnosis relatively straightforward. Swelling and autolysis are rapid in animals that have died from clostridial myonecrosis, and the carcass usually has a foul odor similar to that of rancid butter. This odor is a characteristic of most cases of clostridial myonecrosis. *C chauvoei* infection is characterized by engorgement of the subcutis and adjacent tissues with bloodstained fluids and gas bubbles. Cut tissue from the affected area reveals moist, dark-colored muscle in the periphery of the lesion, with lighter-colored, drier muscle with gas bubbles between the separate bundles of muscle toward the center. Lesions are similar in sheep and cattle, except that there is usually less gas and the muscles are not as dry in affected sheep. Myonecrosis resulting from *C sordelli* is most often associated with lesions of the neck or brisket area of cattle; death is frequently so rapid that subcutaneous gas accumulation is rare. In addition to local myonecrosis, animals often have massive subendocardial hemorrhages in the left ventricle of the heart and hemorrhage in the trachea, bronchi, and thymus. Extensive perirenal edema and hemorrhagic renal calyces and severe congestion of the lungs are common findings.

Antibiotic therapy and aggressive surgical debridement may be attempted in the individual animal; however, most cases are usually fatal. Penicillin at a dosage of 44,000 U/kg, IV, every 2–4 hr is given until the animal is stable (1–5 days). Use of specific antitoxins is recommended when possible. Supportive fluid therapy and use of analgesics and anti-inflammatory agents for control of pain and swelling are recommended. Short-acting corticosteroids may be used for initial therapy of systemic and toxic shock, but continued use is contraindicated in the face of overwhelming sepsis.

Vaccination beginning at 4–6 mo in cattle with bacterins containing antigens against two or more clostridial species, including *C chauvoei*, *C septicum*, *C novyi*, *C sordelli*, and *C perfringens* is recommended. For all clostridial species except *C chauvoei*, two doses of vaccine are necessary to establish good protection. Booster vaccinations should be administered every 6–8 mo if protection is to be maintained.

Sarcocystosis

Cysts of *Sarcocystis* are common in the heart, esophageal, and skeletal muscle of cattle, sheep, goats, and other species but rarely cause disease. Heavy infestations of sarcocystis may cause fever, mild anemia, chronic myositis, and muscle wasting. *S cruzi*, *S hirsuta*, and *S hominis* are known to infect cattle, whereas *S ovicanis* and *S capracanis* infect sheep and goats. The most common mechanism for natural infection in cattle is by ingestion of feeds contaminated with infected carnivore feces. (For complete discussion of sarcocystosis, *see* p 1058.)

NUTRITIONAL MYOPATHIES

Nutritional Myodegeneration

(White muscle disease, Stiff lamb disease, Nutritional muscular dystrophy)

Nutritional myodegeneration (NMD) is an acute, degenerative disease of cardiac and skeletal muscle caused by a dietary deficiency of selenium or vitamin E in young, rapidly growing calves, lambs, and kids. Dams usually consumed selenium-deficient diets during gestation. Selenium deficiency appears to be more important than vitamin E in preventing NMD. NMD occurs worldwide in areas where the soil (and therefore the derived grains and forage) is deficient in selenium, and storage conditions do not preserve vitamin E in forages. Soil in the northeastern and eastern seaboards and northwestern regions of the USA are particularly deficient in selenium. Vitamin E deficiency occurs most commonly when animals are fed poor-quality hay, straw, or root crops.

Selenium is an essential component of five antioxidant selenoproteins, and vitamin E acts as an antioxidant within lipid bilayers. Muscle degeneration is the result of oxidant damage to cell membranes and proteins, leading to a loss of cellular integrity. Young, rapidly growing animals usually are affected, although the disease has also been reported in yearling and adult cattle. When cardiac muscle is primarily affected, animals may be found in respiratory distress, have cardiac arrhythmias, or be found dead. In such cases, the clinical course is frequently short, with death occurring commonly in <24 hr despite medical therapy. When skeletal muscle is primarily affected, signs of muscle weakness, stiffness, and difficulty rising are seen. Most affected animals are able to remain standing only for short periods, and locomotor muscles may be firm and painful on palpation. If the respiratory muscles are affected, the animal may show respiratory distress and evidence of increased abdominal effort when breathing. The muscles of the tongue may be involved, resulting in dysphagia. Animals with skeletal NMD often respond favorably to treatment and rest. Improvement is evident after a few days; within 3–5 days, animals can often stand and walk.

Differential diagnoses include infectious diseases resulting in septicemia, pneumonia, and toxemia; cardiac anomalies; cardiotoxic agents such as those found in plants (oleander, senna, yew, white snakeroot, and gossypol toxicity from cottonseed); and the ionophore antibiotics. Other diseases causing stiffness of gait, weakness, and recumbency with no change in mental status include spinal cord compression, cerebellar disease, suppurative and nonsuppurative meningitis/myelitis, polyarthritis, neurotoxins such as organophosphates, tetanus, pelvic fractures, parasitic myositis, clostridial myositis, and traumatic injuries.

Supportive evidence of NMD includes increased levels of CK, AST, and LDH. Definitive diagnosis is based on demonstration of low whole blood selenium (normal range >0.1 ppm) or liver content (normal cattle 0.9–1.75 mcg/g of dry matter, sheep 0.9–3.5 mcg/g dry matter). The critical concentration of vitamin E (α-tocopherol) in plasma is 1.1–2 ppm in large animals. Vitamin E deteriorates rapidly in plasma samples. Therefore, plasma samples for α-tocopherol analysis should be put on ice immediately, protected from light by wrapping in foil, and stored at –21°F (–70°C) if analysis is to be delayed.

Bilaterally symmetric myodegeneration is a consistent finding in NMD. Skeletal muscle degeneration is characterized by pale discoloration and a dry appearance of affected muscle, white streaks in muscle bundles, calcification, and intramuscular edema. The white streaks seen in cardiac and skeletal muscle bundles represent bands of coagulation necrosis or, in chronic cases, fibrosis and calcification. In calves, the left ventricle and septum are most frequently involved, but both ventricles are usually involved in lambs. Histologically, affected muscle fibers may be hypercontracted and fragmented, with some mineralization of muscle fibers and others undergoing macrophage infiltration.

The cardiac form of NMD is often incompatible with life, whereas the skeletal form may respond to injectable selenium products. The label dosage for selenium is 0.055–0.067 mg/kg (2.5–3 mg/45 kg), IM or SC. Dosage of these injectable products should not be greatly increased above that on the label to prevent an inadvertent selenium toxicosis. When using vitamin E/selenium combinations, the amount of vitamin E is insufficient for supplementation; it is present only as a preservative for the solution. Injectable vitamin E products that contain 300 and 500 IU vitamin E per mL as D-α-tocopherol are available. Oral supplementation is the general approach to provide additional dietary levels of vitamin E. Recommended levels of supplementation for calves range from 15 to 60 mg of DL-α-tocopherol acetate per kg of dry feed. Antibiotics may be indicated to combat secondary pneumonia. Provision of adequate energy intake and attention to the fluid and electrolyte balance are critical if recovery is to be successful.

Under current federal regulations in the USA, selenium can be incorporated into the total ration of ruminants and other species to a level of 0.3 ppm. In salt/mineral mixtures formulated for free-choice feeding, selenium can be incorporated at 90 ppm for sheep and 120 ppm for cattle. In certain areas or in herds, levels as high as 200 ppm selenium in salt/mineral mixtures may be necessary to maintain adequate selenium levels. Federal regulations limit the intake of supplemental selenium to 0.7 mg/head/day in sheep and 3 mg/head/day in cattle. The use in ruminants of rumenoreticular boluses, which release a precise amount of selenium daily, is common in many countries; however, under current FDA guidelines such products are not available in the USA. These slow-release boluses can replace supplementation by salt mixtures or by injections and are extremely valuable in extensive grazing systems. Alternatively, individual animals can be supplemented by periodic (30- to 60-day intervals) injections of selenium/vitamin E preparations to help maintain body concentrations and assist in transplacental transfer of selenium.

Regardless of the method of supplementation, periodic blood (or tissue) sampling of animals at risk is recommended to ensure desired levels of selenium. Feeding animals properly prepared and stored hay and grain or allowing access to high-quality, green forage should ensure adequate vitamin E intake.

Hypokalemic Myopathy

Hypokalemic myopathy in dairy cattle occurs when serum potassium concentrations are <2.5 mmol/L, producing severe signs of muscle weakness. Anorexia and enhanced potassium excretion due to the administration of one or more doses of isoflupredone acetate to ketotic cows are common causes of hypokalemia. Isoflupredone acetate has both glucocorticoid and mineralocorticoid activity, resulting in a decrease in mean plasma potassium concentration by 25% 2 days after a single injection (20 mg) and 46% in cows 3 days after two injections.

Clinical signs of hypokalemic myopathy include severe weakness, recumbency, abnormal position of the head and neck, rumen hypomotility or atony, abnormal feces, anorexia, and tachycardia. Cardiac dysrhythmia is also common. Diagnosis is based on clinical signs combined with serum potassium of <2.5 mmol/L. Other common clinical chemistry abnormalities include ketosis, metabolic alkalosis, and increased serum CK and AST activities. Muscle biopsies reveal a vacuolar myopathy.

Restoration of whole-body potassium balance can be difficult, and serum potassium concentrations do not necessarily reflect muscle potassium concentrations. Recommended supplementation includes potassium chloride given IV (16 g/100 kg) and PO (26 g/100 kg) for approximately 5 days. Treatment should also be directed at resolving the primary cause of ketosis and anorexia as well as providing supportive care. Survival has been reported to be 22%–79%.

Nutritional Myopathy of Pigs

(Hepatosis dietetica, Mulberry heart disease)

There are several specific diseases of pigs in which muscle degeneration may be extensive (eg, mulberry heart disease) and others in which the degeneration is frequently less conspicuous (eg, hepatosis dietetica). Yellow fat disease (*see* p 1200) may be seen with accompanying myopathy.

Etiology: Mulberry heart disease and hepatosis dietetica are associated with diets low in selenium or vitamin E. Administration of iron dextran to piglets having low vitamin E status may precipitate a severe myopathy (*see* p 3077) with lesions identical to those of selenium or vitamin E deficiency. Other factors that may increase the selenium requirement include diets with low concentrations of protein (especially sulfur-containing amino acids), diets with an excess of selenium antagonistic compounds, and possibly genetic influences on selenium metabolism. Vitamin E may be less available in diets with high concentrations of polyunsaturated fatty acids, vitamin A, or mycotoxins.

Clinical Findings: These conditions have certain characteristics in common. Losses tend to occur sporadically, and rapidly growing pigs 2–16 wk old are affected. Death almost invariably occurs suddenly and is often precipitated by exercise.

Lesions: In mulberry heart disease, the characteristic lesions are a pericardial sac grossly distended with straw-colored fluid that contains fibrin strands, and extensive hemorrhage throughout the epicardium and myocardium. Microscopically, the heart shows both vascular and myocyte lesions; in addition to interstitial hemorrhage, there is usually extensive myocardial necrosis together with fibrin thrombi in capillaries. If pigs survive for a few days, nervous signs may be seen as a result of focal encephalomalacia.

In hepatosis dietetica, there is often subcutaneous edema and varying amounts of transudate in serous cavities. Fibrin strands adhere to the liver, which has a characteristic mottled appearance caused by irregular foci of parenchymal necrosis and hemorrhage. Acute lesions may appear as scattered, red, swollen lobules and edema of the gallbladder wall. Focal lesions of myocardial necrosis and, less frequently, skeletal myonecrosis may be apparent.

Many pigs that die with selenium or vitamin E deficiency have esophagogastric ulceration or preulcerative changes.

Diagnosis: The history and gross necropsy findings may be distinctive, but histology to demonstrate specific cardiac and skeletal muscle lesions may be necessary. Differential diagnoses for mulberry heart disease include acute septicemic diseases (eg, salmonellosis, erysipelas, and streptococcosis), pericarditis, polyserositis, and edema disease. For hepatosis dietetica, pitch poisoning and gossypol toxicosis should also be considered, as should porcine stress syndrome for pigs with prominent skeletal muscle lesions. Cases of selenium or vitamin E deficiency in pigs can be identified, as in other species, by decreased levels of selenium, vitamin E, and glutathione peroxidase in the serum and tissues and by increased levels of CK and AST in the serum.

Prevention and Treatment: Rations may be supplemented with selenium or vitamin E, or both (as for ruminants). Affected pigs and their herdmates may be given injections of selenium/vitamin E to increase tissue levels rapidly. Injection of sows in late gestation increases tissue levels in newborn piglets.

TOXIC MYOPATHIES

Plant Toxins

Plant toxins affect both cardiac and skeletal muscle. Clinical signs are not specific for the toxin and include anorexia, cardiac failure with tachycardia, dyspnea, diarrhea, stiffness, muscular weakness, recumbency, and myoglobinuria. Myonecrosis may occur when gossypol is fed. Monogastrics, including young calves, should not ingest feed containing >200 ppm gossypol, whereas mature ruminants may tolerate 20 g of gossypol/head/day. *Senna obtusifolia* (sicklepod) is prevalent in the southeastern USA, and ingestion of its seeds by swine or ruminants may cause a degenerative skeletal and/or cardiomyopathy. Trematone is a toxic component of white snakeroot (*Eupatorium rugosum*), which grows in shaded areas of the eastern and central USA, as well as rayless goldenrod (*Isocoma wrightii*), which is common in the Southwest on open pastures. Ingestion of these plants in quantities of ~2% of body weight can cause a fatal cardiomyopathy and severe skeletal muscle degeneration. Trematone remains active in hay and in the stalks of the dead plants on pasture.

Ionophores

Ionophores added to feeds in excess of recommended levels can cause cardiac and skeletal muscle necrosis. Experimental studies have indicated that LD_{50} values for monensin are 12, 17, 26, and 21–36, for sheep, pigs, goats, and cattle, respectively. Feed concentrations of 100 g/ton and 400 g/ton have been fatal to sheep and cattle, respectively. Newborn calves dosed with 100 mg lasalocid tid for cryptosporidiosis experience muscle necrosis. Other ionophores include naracin, salinomycin, and laidlomycin. At necropsy, pale areas of myocardial necrosis and pulmonary congestion are usually prominent in cattle. Pigs and sheep tend to have mainly skeletal muscle lesions that appear quite similar grossly and histologically to those of nutritional myodegeneration. Diagnosis requires history of exposure with development of characteristic clinical and pathologic alterations.

TRAUMATIC MYOPATHIES

Muscle Crush Syndrome of Cattle

Muscle damage commonly accompanies bovine secondary recumbency (*see* p 1188). Tearing of adductor or semitendinosus/membranosus muscles may arise as animals weakened by hypocalcemia attempt to rise. Additionally, the weight of a recumbent animal on dependent muscle groups creates significant increases in intramuscular pressure, resulting in decreased perfusion and ischemia of muscle and nerve. Muscle trauma leads to edema and inflammation, both of which may exacerbate local tissue degenerative changes. Mild increases in serum CK can be expected in recumbent cows, but increases >5000 U/L usually indicate traumatic muscle damage. Treatment requires correcting the underlying cause of recumbency, fluid therapy if renal damage is evident, NSAIDs, good nursing care, adequate footing and bedding, and lifting or rolling the animal several times a day. Aquatherapy using float tanks for cattle also appears to help relieve pressure on muscle groups.

GENETIC MYOPATHIES

Caprine Myotonia

Myotonia congenita in goats is due to an autosomal dominant mutation that has incomplete penetrance in the skeletal muscle chloride channel. Goats with this mutation have been selected for as a breed and are commonly referred to as "fainting goats." Clinical signs ranging from stiffness after rest to marked general rigidity after visual, tactile, or auditory stimulation usually develop by 6 wk of age. These signs remain throughout the animal's life but are not progressive. A diagnosis of myotonia is made by identifying the characteristic "dive bomber" discharges in electromyography and/or by genetic testing.

Congenital Muscular Dystonia in Belgian Blue Cattle

Congenital muscular dystonia in Belgian Blue calves is caused by an autosomal recessive mutation in the gene encoding the neuronal glycine transporter. Affected calves exhibit signs of lateral recumbency, low head carriage, and transient muscle spasms after tactile or auditory stimulation.

Phosphorylase Deficiency in Charolais Cattle

A mutation in the myophosphorylase gene in Charolais cattle produces signs of exercise intolerance and muscle necrosis very similar to nutritional myodegeneration. The disease has been recognized in many countries, including the USA and New

Zealand. Animals become exercise intolerant, may collapse when forced to exercise, and develop muscle necrosis characterized by increased serum CK and prolonged recumbency. Supportive care during episodes has allowed many young animals to survive and, unknowingly to the owner, enter the breeding herd.

Porcine Malignant Hyperthermia

Malignant hyperthermia in swine (*see* p 1027) is due to an autosomal recessive genetic mutation in the skeletal muscle ryanodine receptor 1 gene (*RYR1*) that causes abnormal meat quality in swine. Pietrain, Poland China, and certain strains of Landrace pigs are affected. During transportation or anesthesia, pigs develop increased body temperature, extreme rigidity of the skeletal muscles, and lactic acidosis. At slaughter, affected muscles become pale, soft, and exudative, which diminishes meat quality. A genetic test is available to diagnose affected and carrier animals.

Porcine RN(–) Glycogen Storage Disease

The RN(–) (rendement Napole) phenotype is common in Hampshire pigs. It is due to an autosomal dominant mutation in the protein kinase AMP-activated gamma 3 subunit gene (PRKAG3), which encodes the gamma 3 isoform of AMP-activated protein kinase (AMPK). Clinically, pigs appear healthy; however, the 70% increase in glycogen content in skeletal muscle causes poor meat quality at slaughter.

Pseudomyotonia in Cattle

Bovine congenital pseudomyotonia is an impairment of muscle relaxation induced by exercise that prevents animals from performing rapid movements. Different mutations in the ATP2A1 gene that encodes the Ca^{2+}-ATPase in skeletal muscle sarcoplasmic reticulum have been identified in the Chianina, Belgian Blue, and Romagnola breeds.

MYOPATHIES IN HORSES

Muscle disorders in horses present with a variety of clinical signs ranging from muscle stiffness and pain to muscle atrophy, weakness, exercise intolerance, and muscle fasciculations. The most common clinical presentation is muscle pain, stiffness, and reluctance to move due to rhabdomyolysis. Rhabdomyolysis, defined as disruption of striated skeletal muscle, can broadly be grouped into causes associated with exercise (exertional rhabdomyolysis) and causes unrelated to exercise.

Differential diagnoses for reluctance to move, acute recumbency, and discolored urine include lameness, colic, laminitis, fracture, pleuropneumonia, tetanus, aorto-iliac thrombosis, neurologic diseases resulting in recumbency or reluctance to move, intravascular hemolysis, and bilirubinuria. Causes of non-exercise-associated rhabdomyolysis include infectious (eg, *Clostridium* sp, influenza, *Streptococcus equi*, *Sarcocystis*) and immune-mediated myopathies, nutritional

TABLE 1 DIFFERENTIAL DIAGNOSES OF EQUINE MYOPATHIES

NON-EXERCISE-ASSOCIATED RHABDOMYOLYSIS
Inflammatory myopathies
Clostridial myositis
Influenza myositis
Sarcocystis myositis
Immune-mediated myopathy
Nutritional myopathy
Vitamin E and selenium deficiency

TABLE 1 DIFFERENTIAL DIAGNOSES OF EQUINE MYOPATHIES *(continued)*

- Toxic myopathies
  - Ionophore toxicity
  - *Senna occidentalis*
  - Pasture myopathies
    - Rayless goldenrod/white snakeroot
    - Hypoglycin A in box elder and European sycamore trees
- Traumatic myopathies
  - Compressive anesthetic myopathy
  - Trauma
- Genetic myopathies
  - Glycogen branching enzyme deficiency in Quarter horses
  - Polysaccharide storage myopathy types 1 and 2
  - Malignant hyperthermia in Quarter horses

EXERTIONAL RHABDOMYOLYSIS

- Focal muscle strain
- Sporadic tying-up (overexertion)
- Chronic tying-up
  - Dietary imbalances, vitamins, minerals, electrolytes
  - Polysaccharide storage myopathy types 1 and 2
  - Malignant hyperthermia
  - Recurrent exertional rhabdomyolysis
  - Idiopathic chronic exertional rhabdomyolysis

EXERTIONAL MYOPATHY WITH NORMAL CK

- Mitochondrial myopathy
- Polysaccharide storage myopathy type 2

MUSCLE ATROPHY

- Myogenic atrophy
  - Severe rhabdomyolysis
  - Disuse
  - Cushing disease
  - Immune-mediated myositis (rapid atrophy)
  - Vitamin E–deficient myopathy
  - Homozygous polysaccharide storage myopathy type 1
  - Polysaccharide storage myopathy type 2
- Neurogenic atrophy
  - Equine protozoal myelitis
  - Local nerve trauma
  - Equine motor neuron disease
  - Idiopathic peripheral neuropathy
  - Toxic peripheral neuropathies

MUSCLE FASCICULATIONS

- Pain, fear
- Weakness (botulism, chronic debilitation)
- Electrolyte abnormalities
- Equine motor neuron disease
- Hyperkalemic periodic paralysis
- Hypokalemia
- *Otobius megnini* (ear tick) infestation
- Myotonic dystrophy
- Stiff horse syndrome
- Shivers

myodegeneration (vitamin E or selenium deficiency), traumatic or compressive myopathy, idiopathic pasture myopathy, and toxic muscle damage from the ingestion of ionophores (eg, monensin, lasalocid, rumensin). Plants, including white snake root and vitamin D–stimulating species, should also be considered (*see* TABLE 1). Genetic causes of nonexertional rhabdomyolysis include glycogen branching enzyme deficiency (foals), malignant hyperthermia (Quarter horses), and polysaccharide storage myopathy.

EXERTIONAL MYOPATHIES

Exertional myopathy in horses is a syndrome of muscle fatigue, pain, or cramping associated with exercise. Less common exertional myopathies that cause exercise intolerance without muscle necrosis include mitochondrial myopathies and forms of polysaccharide storage myopathy in Warmblood horses. Most commonly, exertional myopathies produce necrosis of striated skeletal muscle and are termed exertional rhabdomyolysis. Although exertional rhabdomyolysis was previously considered a single disease described as azoturia, tying-up, or cording up, it is now known to comprise several different myopathies, which, despite similarities in clinical presentation, differ significantly in etiopathology.

Clinical signs usually are seen shortly after onset of exercise. Excessive sweating, tachypnea, tachycardia, muscle fasciculations, reluctance or refusal to move, and firm, painful lumbar and gluteal musculature are common signs. Episodes range from subclinical to severe muscle necrosis with recumbency and myoglobinuric renal failure. The severity varies extensively between individuals and to some degree within the same individual. A diagnosis of exertional rhabdomyolysis is based on demonstration of abnormal increases in serum CK, lactate dehydrogenase, and AST.

Exertional rhabdomyolysis can be either sporadic, with single or very infrequent episodes of exercise-induced muscle necrosis, or chronic, with repeated episodes of rhabdomyolysis and increased serum CK or AST with mild exertion.

Sporadic Exertional Rhabdomyolysis

All breeds of horses are susceptible to sporadic exertional rhabdomyolysis. The most common cause is exercise that exceeds the horse's state of training. The incidence of muscle stiffness also has been found to increase during an outbreak of respiratory disease. Dietary deficiencies of sodium, vitamin E, selenium, or a calcium:phosphorus imbalance may also be contributory factors.

A diagnosis of sporadic exertional rhabdomyolysis is made on the basis of a horse with no previous history, or a brief history, of exertional rhabdomyolysis, signs of muscle cramping and stiffness after exercise, and moderate to marked increases in serum CK and AST. Immediately on detection of signs of exertional rhabdomyolysis, exercise should stop and the horse should be moved to a well-bedded stall with access to fresh water. The objectives of treatment are to relieve anxiety and muscle pain and to correct fluid and acid-base deficits. Tranquilizers or opioids may be given. NSAIDs can be given to a well-hydrated horse. Most horses are relatively pain free within 18–24 hr.

Severe rhabdomyolysis can lead to renal compromise due to ischemia and the combined nephrotoxic effects of myoglobinuria, dehydration, and NSAID therapy. The first priority in horses with hemoconcentration or myoglobinuria is to reestablish fluid balance and induce diuresis. In severely affected animals, regular monitoring of BUN and/or serum creatinine is advised to assess the extent of renal damage. Diuretics are contraindicated in the absence of IV fluid therapy and are indicated if the horse is in oliguric renal failure.

Horses should be stall rested on a hay diet with a dietary vitamin and mineral ration balancer supplement for a few days. For horses with sporadic forms of exertional rhabdomyolysis, rest with regular access to a paddock should continue until serum muscle enzyme concentrations are normal. Because the inciting cause is usually temporary, most horses respond to rest, a gradual increase in training, and dietary adjustment. Endurance horses should be encouraged to drink electrolyte-supplemented water during an endurance ride and monitored particularly closely during hot, humid conditions.

Chronic Exertional Rhabdomyolysis

Some horses have recurrent episodes of rhabdomyolysis, even with light exercise. Four forms of chronic tying-up have been identified using muscle biopsies or genetic testing: type 1 polysaccharide storage myopathy (PSSM), type 2 PSSM, malignant hyperthermia, and recurrent exertional rhabdomyolysis.

Type 1 polysaccharide storage myopathy is seen frequently in Quarter horse–related breeds (especially halter and Western pleasure horses), Morgans, and draft horses but is also present in at least 20 other horse breeds. It is caused by a dominantly inherited mutation in the glycogen synthase 1 (*GYS1*) gene. A diagnosis can be made by genetic testing of blood or hair samples. Quarter horse–related breeds and other crossbred or light breeds of horses with type 1 PSSM often develop episodes of rhabdomyolysis at a young age with little exercise. Rest for a few days before exercise is a common triggering factor. Episodes are characterized by a tucked-up abdomen, a camped-out stance, muscle fasciculations, sweating, gait asymmetry, hindlimb stiffness, and reluctance to move. Some horses paw or roll, resembling colic. Serum CK and AST are increased during an episode (usually >1,000 U/L) and, unlike in other forms of rhabdomyolysis, subclinical episodes characterized by persistently abnormal CK levels are common. Clinical signs in draft horses may include loss of muscle mass, progressive weakness, and recumbency. CK and AST may be normal in draft horses with this syndrome. When draft horses develop rhabdomyolysis, CK and AST may be markedly increased, and horses can become myoglobinuric, weak, and reluctant to rise.

Type 2 polysaccharide storage myopathy occurs in light breeds such as Arabians, Morgans, Thoroughbreds, a variety of Warmblood breeds and some Quarter horses. A diagnosis is made by identifying an abnormal pattern of glycogen storage in muscle biopsies in a horse with a negative *GYS1* genetic test. In Quarter horses <1 yr old, it may cause difficulty rising from a recumbent position and increased serum CK activity. Chronic episodes of muscle stiffness, soreness, and muscle atrophy with normal to modest increases in serum CK are common in horses with type 2 PSSM. The most common presentation of this disorder in Warmbloods is a gait abnormality, exercise intolerance, and loss of muscle mass when out of work that is not necessarily accompanied by a concomitant rise in serum CK.

Malignant hyperthermia is caused by an autosomal dominant mutation in the skeletal muscle ryanodine receptor gene (*RYR1*). The mutation is responsible for both anesthesia-related and non-anesthesia-related causes of rhabdomyolysis in Quarter horses. A diagnosis can be made by genetic testing of blood or hair roots. Signs related to inhalation anesthesia include tachycardia, tachypnea, hyperthermia, muscle rigidity accompanied by a severe lactic acidosis, increased serum CK, and electrolyte derangements. Exertional rhabdomyolysis in Quarter horses with malignant hyperthermia can result in sudden death. Signs are preceded by excessive sweating, tachycardia, tachypnea, hyperthermia, and muscle rigidity. Some Quarter horses have both malignant hyperthermia and PSSM, which results in more severe signs of exertional rhabdomyolysis than those seen in horses with PSSM alone.

Recurrent exertional rhabdomyolysis is seen frequently in Thoroughbreds, Standardbreds, and Arabian horses. It is likely due to abnormal regulation of intracellular calcium in skeletal muscles. It appears there is intermittent disruption of muscle contraction, particularly when horses susceptible to the condition are fit and have a nervous temperament. In Thoroughbreds, it is likely inherited as an autosomal dominant trait.

Diagnostic tests to determine the cause of chronic tying-up include a CBC, serum chemistry panel, serum vitamin E and selenium concentrations, urinalysis to determine electrolyte balance, dietary analysis, exercise testing, muscle biopsy, and genetic testing. An exercise challenge test is useful to detect subclinical cases; serum CK is measured before and 4 hr after light exercise. In addition, quantifying the extent of exertional rhabdomyolysis during mild exercise is helpful in deciding how rapidly to reinstate training.

A diagnosis of type 1 PSSM is based on identification of the *GYS1* mutation and/or the presence of muscle fibers with subsarcolemmal vacuoles, dark periodic acid-Schiff (PAS) staining for glycogen, and most notably, amylase-resistant abnormal complex polysaccharide accumulation. A diagnosis of type 2 PSSM is based on the absence of the *GYS1* mutation and the presence of muscle fibers with aggregates of amylase-sensitive PAS-positive staining glycogen and occasionally small amounts of amylase-resistant PAS-positive material. A diagnosis of recurrent exertional rhabdomyolysis is based on history, clinical signs, increases in serum CK and AST, and muscle biopsy.

Horses with type 1 PSSM have constitutively active glycogen synthase that is further stimulated by increased blood insulin concentrations, resulting in high muscle glycogen concentrations. When fed a starch meal, these horses take up a higher proportion of the absorbed glucose in their muscles than healthy horses. Horses with type 2 PSSM also have abnormal glycogen storage, but the cause of this myopathy is unknown. Thus, the ideal diet for PSSM is based on feeding forage at a rate of 1.5%–2% body wt, providing >15% of digestible energy as fat and limiting starch to <10% of daily digestible energy by limiting grain or replacing it with a fat supplement. Caloric needs should be assessed first to prevent horses becoming obese on a high-fat diet. Improvement in signs of exertional rhabdomyolysis for horses with PSSM requires both dietary changes and gradual increases in the amount of daily exercise and turn-out.

Horses with malignant hyperthermia may benefit from premedication with dantrolene (4 mg/kg, PO) 60–90 min before exercise, particularly under hot conditions.

Management of recurrent exertional rhabdomyolysis is aimed at decreasing the triggering factors for excitement and pharmacologic alteration of intracellular calcium flux with contraction. Management changes that may decrease excitement include minimizing stall confinement by using turn-out or a hot walker, exercising and feeding horses with recurrent exertional rhabdomyolysis before other horses, providing compatible equine company, and the judicious use of low-dose tranquilizers during training. A high-fat, low-starch diet is beneficial, possibly by decreasing excitement. In contrast to horses with PSSM, those with recurrent exertional rhabdomyolysis often require higher caloric intakes (>24 Mcal/day). At these high caloric intakes, specialized feeds designed for exertional rhabdomyolysis are necessary, because additional vegetable oil or rice bran cannot supply enough calories for equine athletes in intense training. Hay should be fed at 1.5%–2% body wt, and high-fat, low-starch concentrates should be selected that provide ≤20% of daily digestible energy as nonstructural carbohydrate and 20%–25% of digestible energy as fat.

Dantrolene (4 mg/kg, PO) given 1 hr before exercise may decrease the release of calcium from the calcium release channel. Phenytoin (1.4–2.7 mg/kg, PO, bid) has also been advocated as a treatment for horses with recurrent exertional rhabdomyolysis. Therapeutic levels vary, so oral dosages are adjusted by monitoring serum levels to achieve 8–12 mcg/mL. However, longterm treatment with dantrolene or phenytoin is expensive.

INFECTIOUS MYOPATHIES

Virus-associated Myositis

Necrosis of skeletal and cardiac muscle may occur in association with viral diseases such as equine influenza and equine infectious anemia. In most situations, viral-induced muscle damage represents a component of systemic multiple organ system involvement. Equine influenza 2 has been found to cause severe rhabdomyolysis, and equine herpesvirus 1 has been reported to induce primary muscle stiffness and clinical signs resembling exertional rhabdomyolysis.

Sarcocystis Myositis

Cysts of the sporozoan parasite *Sarcocystis* are present in 90% of esophageal muscles from horses >8 yr of age and in 6% of gluteal muscle biopsies from healthy horses. Occasionally, heavy infestations occur through contamination of feed with canine feces, resulting in signs of fever, anorexia, stiffness, weight loss, muscle fasciculations, atrophy, and weakness. Diagnosis of sarcocystosis requires history, clinical signs, laboratory evaluation, and the demonstration of an inflammatory reaction to immature cysts in muscle biopsies. Treatment includes NSAIDs and drugs such as trimethoprim sulfa and pyrimethamine or ponazuril. (*See also* SARCOCYSTOSIS, p 1058.)

Anaplasma-associated Rhabdomyolysis

Horses that acquire *Anaplasma phagocytophilum* from tick infestations can rarely develop clinical signs of severe muscle stiffness in addition to fever, malaise, and limb edema. Hematologic findings include anemia, thrombocytopenia, neutropenia, morula visible in granulocytes, and marked increases in serum CK and AST levels. A diagnosis is confirmed by PCR testing of blood for *A phagocytophilum*. A direct toxic effect of *A phagocytophilum* on muscle cells is postulated. Treatment should include IV oxytetracycline and supportive care.

Streptococcus equi Rhabdomyolysis

Severe rhabdomyolysis can occur in horses with *Streptococcus equi equi* submandibular lymphadenopathy and/or guttural pouch empyema. A stiff gait is the initial clinical sign, which progresses rapidly to severely painful, firm, swollen epaxial and gluteal muscles. Many horses become recumbent with unrelenting pain that may warrant euthanasia. It is not clear whether myonecrosis is a direct toxic effect of *S equi* on muscle cells or is due to profound nonspecific T-cell stimulation by streptococcal superantigens and the release of high levels of inflammatory cytokines. A diagnosis is based on hematologic abnormalities typical of *S equi* infection, marked increases in CK (>100,000 U/L), and PCR or bacterial culture. Titers to the M protein of *S equi* are low in affected horses, unless they have recently been vaccinated for strangles. At postmortem, large, pale areas of necrotic muscle are evident in hindlimb and lumbar muscles. The histopathologic lesions are characterized by severe acute myonecrosis with a degree of macrophage infiltration. Sublumbar muscles often show the most severe and chronic necrosis, as indicated by greater macrophage infiltration of myofibers. The prognosis becomes guarded if animals become recumbent.

Appropriate therapy includes IV penicillin combined with an antimicrobial that inhibits protein synthesis, such as rifampin. Flushing infected guttural pouches and draining abscessed lymph nodes will diminish the bacterial load. NSAIDs and possibly high doses of short-acting corticosteroids may diminish the inflammatory response. Control of unrelenting pain is a major challenge in horses with severe rhabdomyolysis. Constant-rate infusion of lidocaine, detomidine, or ketamine may provide better anxiety and pain relief than periodic injections of tranquilizers. Horses should be placed in a deeply bedded stall and moved from side to side every 4 hr if they are unable to rise. Some horses may benefit from a sling if they will bear weight on their hindlimbs when assisted to stand.

Clostridial Myositis

A variety of clostridial bacteria can sporulate at the site of an injection or deep wound, causing focal muscle swelling and systemic toxemia in horses. *Clostridium septicum*, *C chauvoei*, *C sporogenes*, and mixed infections are associated with a high fatality rate, whereas *C perfringens* type A has a mortality rate of 20% with early and aggressive treatment. Clostridial spores may lie dormant in skeletal muscle, or spore deposition directly into the tissue may occur in association with penetration. If suitable necrotic conditions exist, the spores convert to the vegetative form, releasing powerful exotoxins. Within 48 hr, horses show depression, fever, toxemia, tachypnea, and swelling and variable crepitus at the injection site. Tremors, ataxia, dyspnea, recumbency, coma, and death may occur in the next 12–24 hr. Myocardial damage occurs in some horses. Hematology and serum biochemical analyses usually reflect a generalized state of debilitation and toxemia (eg, hemoconcentration and a stress/toxic leukogram may be present). Serum CK and AST are usually moderately increased; however, they often do not reflect the toxicity of clostridial myonecrosis.

Ultrasonographic evaluation of swollen areas may reveal fluid and characteristic hyperechoic gas accumulation. Aspirates of affected tissues examined via direct smears or fluorescent antibody staining should show characteristic rod-shaped bacteria. Anaerobic bacterial culture of freshly acquired samples may also be of value. Cut tissue from the affected area may reveal abundant serosanguineous fluid with an odor of rancid butter. At postmortem, swelling, crepitus, and autolysis are rapid, and bloodstained fluid is often seen discharging from body orifices.

Wound fenestration and aggressive surgical debridement over the entire affected area is required for successful treatment. Additional treatment includes high doses of IV potassium penicillin every 2–4 hr until the horse is stable (1 to 5 days), combined with or followed by oral metronidazole along with supportive fluid therapy and anti-inflammatory agents. Extensive skin sloughing over the affected area is common in surviving horses.

Muscle Abscesses

Staphylococcus aureus, *Streptococcus equi*, and *Corynebacterium pseudotuberculosis* are common causes of skeletal muscle abscessation, which develops after penetrating injuries or by hematogenous or local spread of infection. Initially there is an ill-defined cellulitis, which may heal or progress to a well-defined abscess. An abscess may heal, expand, or fistulate, usually to the skin surface with potential for a chronic granuloma with intermittent discharge. Prognosis is usually good for superficial abscesses. Deep abscesses are more difficult to manage successfully. The effect of an abscess on the horse's gait depends on its location and can vary from mild stiffness to severe lameness. Ultrasonography and culture of aspirated fluid are the best means of diagnosis in superficial sites. Abscesses lying deep within muscles can be difficult to diagnose. There may be an increased fibrinogen and nucleated WBCs. The synergistic hemolysin inhibition test, which detects antibodies to

C pseudotuberculosis, can be helpful for detection of internal abscesses. Treatment consists of poulticing, lancing, flushing, and draining. Occasionally, surgical removal may be required for complete excision. If antimicrobial therapy is used, it should be continued for several weeks.

IMMUNE-MEDIATED MYOPATHIES

Infarctive Hemorrhagic Purpura

Purpura hemorrhagica is often associated with mild increases in serum CK activity; however, horses vaccinated for, or exposed to, *Streptococcus equi* within the last month rarely may develop extremely high serum CK activity, variable edema, acute colic, firm swellings within muscle and under the skin, and unilateral lameness. Clinical signs are due to painful infarctions of skeletal muscle, subcutaneous tissue, focal areas of the GI tract, and lungs resulting from a severe immune-mediated vasculopathy. Hematologic abnormalities include leukocytosis, hyperfibrinogenemia, hypoalbuminemia, and marked increases in serum CK and AST. A diagnosis is often established based on clinical signs, a leukocytoclastic vasculitis in skin and affected tissues, and a very high *S equi* M protein titer.

Successful treatment requires early detection, penicillin for 14 days, and prolonged high doses of dexamethasone (0.12–0.2 mg/kg) for at least 10 days, followed by tapering doses of prednisolone at an initial dosage of 2 mg/kg. Without aggressive steroid treatment, the condition progresses to intestinal infarction and death.

Immune-mediated Polymyositis

Immune-mediated polymyositis is characterized by rapidly developing atrophy of the epaxial and gluteal muscles. It is seen in Quarter horses, although other breeds may be affected. The condition shows a bimodal age distribution, affecting horses <8 yr or >16 yr of age. In approximately one-third of affected horses, a triggering factor appears to have been exposure to *S equi* or a respiratory disease. Rapid onset of atrophy of the back and croup muscles is accompanied by stiffness and malaise. Atrophy may progress to involve 50% of the horses' muscle mass within a week and may lead to generalized weakness. Focal symmetric atrophy of cervical muscles has been reported in a pony with immune-mediated polymyositis. Hematologic abnormalities are usually restricted to mild to moderate increases in serum CK and AST. However, in some chronic cases serum muscle enzyme activities are normal. Muscle biopsy of epaxial and gluteal muscles shows lymphocytic vasculitis, anguloid atrophy, myofiber infiltration with lymphocytes, fiber necrosis with macrophage infiltration, and regeneration in acute stages. Biopsies of semitendinosus or semimembranosus muscles may show some evidence of atrophy and vasculitis, but significant inflammatory infiltrates may be absent. The extent of the inflammatory infiltrates in epaxial muscles is such that a diagnosis can often be established from several formalin fixed-core needle biopsy samples. The reason why specific muscle groups are affected is unclear.

Treatment involves antibiotic therapy for horses with concurrent signs of infection and administration of dexamethasone (0.05 mg/kg for 3 days), followed by prednisolone (1 mg/kg for 7–10 days) tapered by 100 mg/wk throughout 1 mo. Serum CK often normalizes after 7–10 days of treatment. Generally, muscle mass gradually recovers throughout 2–3 mo even without corticosteroid treatment. Recurrence of atrophy in susceptible horses is common and may require reintroduction of corticosteroid therapy.

MUSCLE CRAMPING

Muscle cramping is a painful condition that arises from hyperactivity of motor units caused by repetitive firing of the peripheral and/or central nervous system. The origin of the cramp in most cases is believed to be the intramuscular portion of the motor nerve terminals. Most muscle cramps are also accompanied by fasciculations in the same muscle and normal serum CK activity. Muscle cramps can be induced by forceful contraction of a shortened muscle, by changes in the electrolyte composition of extracellular fluid, and by ear tick infestations. In contrast, muscle contractures, like those seen in exertional rhabdomyolysis, are painful muscle spasms that represent a state of muscle contracture unaccompanied by depolarization of the muscle membrane. Muscle contractures are invariably accompanied by markedly increased serum CK activity.

Electrolyte Disturbances

Muscle cramping in endurance horses is most frequent in hot, humid weather. Horses may lose fluids at a rate of up to

15 L/hr in the form of sweat and develop remarkable deficits in sodium, potassium, chloride magnesium, and calcium. Clinical signs of electrolyte derangements include muscle stiffness and periodic spasms of muscle groups. In addition, exhausted horses are often dull, depressed, and clinically dehydrated with increased heart and respiratory rates and persistently increased body temperature. Synchronous diaphragmatic flutter may be seen in association with cramping. Affected horses do not generally develop myoglobinuria or have marked increases in serum CK and AST levels.

Mild muscle cramping is self-limiting, and the signs abate with rest or light exercise. However, exhausted horses with metabolic derangements require immediate treatment, including plasma volume expansion with oral or IV isotonic polyionic fluids and cooling (using water and fans). Because most horses with this condition are alkalotic, administration of solutions containing sodium bicarbonate is contraindicated. Daily direct addition of 2 oz of sodium chloride and 1 oz of potassium chloride to the feed is recommended for horses with recurrent cramping, in addition to electrolyte supplementation before and after endurance rides.

Hypocalcemia

Hypocalcemia is a relatively rare disorder in horses that has also been referred to as lactation tetany, transport tetany, idiopathic hypocalcemia, and eclampsia. Clinical signs, diagnosis, and treatment are discussed elsewhere (*see* p 987). In addition to hypocalcemia, a metabolic alkalosis, hypomagnesemia/hypermagnesemia, and hyperphosphatemia/hypophosphatemia may be present and need correction before a return to normal function is seen. Relapses do occur.

Synchronous Diaphragmatic Flutter

("Thumps")

Synchronous diaphragmatic flutter is due to firing of the phrenic nerve in synchrony with atrial depolarization, causing the diaphragm to contract with each heartbeat. This occasionally produces an audible thumping sound. Inciting causes include endurance exercise, hypocalcemia, hypoparathyroidism, digestive disturbances, and repeated administration of calcium-containing fluids to performance horses. Synchronous diaphragmatic flutter may be a singular occurrence or a chronic recurring problem. The most consistently reported metabolic derangement is low serum ionized calcium concentrations usually associated with hypochloremic metabolic alkalosis. Metabolic alkalosis may alter the ratio of free to bound calcium (increasing calcium binding to protein and decreasing ionized calcium), which possibly induces diaphragmatic flutter.

Most horses undergo rapid remission of signs when given calcium solutions IV. Although hypomagnesemia is often present with synchronous diaphragmatic flutter, horses do not respond to magnesium supplementation unless calcium is administered concurrently. Response to therapy is also reflected by improved mental status, return of appetite, and gut motility. For horses with chronic diaphragmatic flutter, providing chloride, potassium, sodium, calcium, and magnesium during prolonged exercise may help reduce fluid losses and the metabolic alkalosis. Alternative approaches involve reducing dietary calcium for a few days before competition in horses prone to diaphragmatic flutter. This reduction in dietary calcium may stimulate the endocrine homeostatic mechanisms and increase osteoclastic activity. Limiting alfalfa hay, which has a relatively high calcium concentration, may be indicated in chronically affected horses.

Ear Tick–associated Muscle Cramping

Otobius megnini infestations in the ear canal can produce remarkably painful intermittent muscle cramps not associated with exercise that last from minutes to a few hours and often resemble colic. Horses may fall over when stimulated. Between muscle cramps, horses appear to be normal. Percussion of triceps, pectoral, or semitendinosus muscles results in a typical myotonic cramp. Horses have increased serum CK, ranging from 4,000 to 170,000 IU/L. Numerous ear ticks can be identified in the external ear canal of affected horses. *O megnini* is found in the southwestern USA. Without treatment, the spasms continue; however, local treatment of the ear ticks using pyrethrins and piperonyl butoxide results in recovery within 12–36 hr. Acepromazine may be helpful to relieve painful cramping.

Shivers

"Shivers" is a spastic condition of the hind- and occasionally forelimbs of horses that is usually only evident when horses are backing or having their feet picked up. It is most common in adult draft horse breeds, Warmbloods, Warmblood crosses, and Thoroughbreds >16.3 hands tall. The condition is characterized by periodic, involuntary spasms of the muscles in the pelvic region, pelvic limbs, and tail that are exacerbated by backing or picking up the hindlimbs. The affected limb is elevated, abducted, and may actually shake and shiver; the tail head is usually elevated concurrently and trembles. When more severely affected animals are backed up, the hindlimb is suddenly raised, semiflexed, and abducted with the hoof held in the air for several seconds or minutes. The tail is elevated simultaneously and trembles. After a variable period of time the spasms subside, the limb is extended, and the foot is brought slowly to the ground. Some horses will refuse to pick up their hindlimbs and are very difficult to shoe. Suggested causes include genetic, traumatic, infectious, and neurologic diseases, although the exact etiology is unknown. The condition in draft horses is usually progressive and eventually debilitating; in Warmbloods and Thoroughbreds, it usually has less impact on performance and progresses more slowly. There are no known treatments, but avoiding stall rest and keeping horses fit appears helpful.

MYOTONIC DISORDERS

Myotonic muscle disorders share the feature of delayed relaxation of muscle after mechanical stimulation or voluntary contraction due to abnormal muscle membrane conduction. Horses have three known forms of myotonia: myotonia congenita, myotonia dystrophica, and hyperkalemic periodic paralysis (HyPP).

Myotonia Congenita and Dystrophica

The initial signs of myotonia in foals are well-developed musculature and mild pelvic limb stiffness. Bilateral bulging (dimpling) of the thigh and rump muscles is often obvious and gives the impression that the animal is very well developed. Percussion of affected muscles exacerbates the muscle dimpling below a large area of tight contraction that can persist for a minute or more with subsequent slow relaxation. *Myotonia congenita* usually does not show progression of clinical signs beyond 6–12 mo of age, and muscle stiffness may improve with exercise. The cause has not been identified.

Foals with myotonia dystrophica show a progression of signs in the first 1–2 yr of life to include areas of muscle atrophy fibrosis and stiffness that worsens with exercise. Retinal dysplasia, lenticular opacities, and gonadal hypoplasia have been seen in Quarter horse, Appaloosa, and Italian-bred foals with myotonic dystrophy.

A tentative diagnosis of myotonia can be made on the basis of age and clinical signs of stiff gait, muscle bulging, and prolonged contractions after muscle stimulation. Definitive diagnosis of myotonia requires electromyographic examination. Affected muscle manifests pathognomonic, crescendo-decrescendo, high-frequency repetitive bursts with a characteristic "dive bomber" sound. Myotonia dystrophica shows dystrophic changes in muscle biopsies not present in myotonia congenita. Dystrophic changes include ringed fibers, numerous centrally displaced myonuclei, sarcoplasmic masses, and an increase in endomysial and perimysial connective tissue. Fiber type grouping and atrophy of both type I and type II muscle fibers may be present.

Horses with myotonia congenita or dystrophica are rarely serviceable, and euthanasia is usually warranted in dystrophic foals because of the severity of stiffness and atrophy that develop over time. Conclusive evidence regarding the genetic basis of this disorder in horses is still not available.

Hyperkalemic Periodic Paralysis

HyPP is an autosomal dominant trait affecting Quarter horses, American Paint horses, Appaloosas, and Quarter horse crossbreeds worldwide. The point mutation in the voltage-dependent skeletal muscle sodium channel alpha subunit occurs in ~4% of Quarter horses, but this percentage is much higher in halter and pleasure horse performance types.

Clinical signs range from asymptomatic to intermittent muscle fasciculations and weakness and are first identified in foals to horses 3 yr of age. Homozygous horses are often more severely affected and may be identified at a younger age than heterozygotes. A brief period of myotonia is often seen initially, with some horses showing facial myotonia and prolapse of the third eyelid. Muscle fasciculations beginning on the flanks, neck, and shoulders may become more generalized. Although most horses remain standing during mild attacks, weakness with swaying, staggering, dog-sitting, or recumbency may be seen, with severe attacks lasting 15–60 min or longer.

Heart and respiratory rates may be increased, but horses remain relatively bright and alert. Respiratory distress occurs in some horses as a result of upper respiratory muscle paralysis. Once episodes subside, horses regain their feet and appear normal with absent or minimal gait abnormalities. Young horses that are homozygous for the HyPP trait may have respiratory stridor and periodic obstruction of the upper respiratory tract that can be fatal.

Common factors that trigger episodes include sudden dietary changes or ingestion of diets high in potassium (>1.1%), such as those containing alfalfa hay, molasses, electrolyte supplements, and kelp-based supplements. Fasting, anesthesia or heavy sedation, trailer rides, and stress may also precipitate clinical signs. The onset of signs, however, is often unpredictable. Exercise per se does not appear to stimulate clinical signs; serum CK shows no or minimal increases during episodic fasciculations and weakness.

Descent from the stallion Impressive in a horse with episodic muscle tremors is strongly suggestive of HyPP. Hyperkalemia (6–9 mEq/L), hemoconcentration, and hyponatremia are seen during clinical episodes, but a definitive diagnosis requires DNA testing of mane or tail hair. Electromyographic examination of affected horses between attacks reveals abnormal fibrillation potentials and complex repetitive discharges, with occasional myotonic potentials and trains of doublets between episodes. Differential diagnoses for hyperkalemia include delay before serum centrifugation, hemolysis, chronic renal failure, and severe rhabdomyolysis.

Many horses recover spontaneously from HyPP episodes. Owners may abort early mild episodes using low-grade exercise or feeding grain or corn syrup to stimulate insulin-mediated movement of potassium across cell membranes. In severe cases, administration of calcium gluconate (0.2–0.4 mL/kg of a 23% solution diluted in 1 L of 5% dextrose) or IV dextrose (6 mL/kg of a 5% solution), alone or combined with sodium bicarbonate (1–2 mEq/kg), often provides immediate improvement. With severe respiratory obstruction, a tracheostomy may be necessary. Acute death is common, especially in homozygous animals.

Prevention requires decreasing dietary potassium to 0.6%–1.1% total potassium concentration and increasing renal losses of potassium. High-potassium feeds such as alfalfa hay, first cutting hay, brome hay, sugar molasses, and beet molasses should be avoided. Optimally, later cuts of timothy or Bermuda grass hay; grains such as oats, corn, wheat, and barley; and beet pulp should be fed in small meals several times a day. Regular exercise and/or frequent access to a large paddock or yard are also beneficial. Pasture is ideal for horses with HyPP, because the high water content of pasture grass makes it unlikely that horses will consume large amounts of potassium in a short period of time. Complete feeds for horses with HyPP are commercially available. For horses with recurrent episodes even with dietary alterations, acetazolamide (2–4 mg/kg, PO, bid-tid) or hydrochlorothiazide (0.5–1 mg/kg, PO, bid) may be helpful. Breed registries and other associations have restrictions on the use of these drugs during competitions. Some horses have both HyPP and polysaccharide storage myopathy (PSSM) (*see* p 1178), which may result in an episode of rhabdomyolysis during a hyperkalemic paralytic event with subsequent increased serum CK activity and prolonged recumbency.

NUTRITIONAL MYOPATHIES

Nutritional Myodegeneration

Young, rapidly growing foals born to dams that consumed selenium-deficient diets during gestation can develop nutritional myodegeneration (NMD; *see* p 1172). Selenium deficiency has also been implicated in masseter muscle myopathy and occasionally nonexertional rhabdomyolysis in adult horses. Selenium and vitamin E appear to be synergistic in preventing NMD. Clinical signs in foals include dyspnea; a rapid, irregular heartbeat; and sudden death in those with myocardial involvement. Dysphagia, muscle stiffness, trembling, firm muscles, difficulty rising, and myoglobinuria may also be seen. Aspiration pneumonia is a frequent complication. Diagnosis is based on finding moderate to markedly increased serum CK and AST, combined with low whole blood selenium concentrations (<0.07 ppm) or vitamin E (<2 ppm). Hyperkalemia, hyperphosphatemia, hyponatremia, hypochloremia, and hypocalcemia can occur with severe rhabdomyolysis when the normal distinction between extracellular and intracellular compartments is destroyed by massive tissue necrosis. Selenium-dependent glutathione peroxidase formed in RBCs during erythropoiesis also provides an index of body selenium status. Treatment includes IM injection of selenium (0.055–0.067 mg/kg) and either injectable or oral vitamin E (0.5–1.5 IU/kg). Supportive therapy includes administering antibiotics to combat secondary pneumonia, feeding via nasogastric tube, providing adequate energy intake, and maintaining fluid and electrolyte balance.

PLANTS CAUSING MYOPATHIES

Horses ingesting 0.5%–2% body wt of trematone-containing plants are likely to die from skeletal muscle and cardiac muscle necrosis. Horses present with marked depression, weakness, low head posture, and increased cardiac and respiratory rates. Serum AST and CK are often markedly increased, and serum electrolyte abnormalities such as hypocalcemia, hyponatremia, hypochloremia, hyperkalemia, and hyperphosphatemia may be present. Treatment is generally supportive. Trematone (*see* p 1175) has been identified in white snakeroot (*Eupatorium rugosum*) and rayless goldenrod (*Isocoma wrightii*). Trematone remains active in the hay and in the stalks of the dead plants on pasture, so both the fresh and dried forms of the plants should be kept from horses.

Muscle necrosis may also occur in horses ingesting *Senna occidentalis* seeds prevalent in the southeastern USA. Horses develop incoordination, recumbency, and death. Gross skeletal muscle lesions are not present, but histopathologic lesions include segmental myonecrosis.

One of 70 horses poisoned with blister beetles (*see* p 3157) developed muscle necrosis.

Atypical Myoglobinuria

(Pasture myopathy)

Atypical myoglobinuria occurs sporadically in horses kept on pasture, usually with no supplemental feeding. It has been recognized most commonly in the UK and Europe, but a similar syndrome has been seen in North America. It occurs most often in autumn but can occur in early spring; it often follows very windy or rainy weather and a cool spring. Ingestion of seeds of *Acer* species trees such as the box elder (*Acer negundo*) in North America and European sycamore maple (*Acer pseudoplatanus*) are implicated in the pathophysiology of this myopathy. These seeds contain the toxic nonproteogenic amino acid hypoglycin A, the toxic metabolite of which irreversibly binds to multiple acyl CoA dehydrogenases, enzymes essential for metabolism of short- and medium-chain fatty acids and branched-chain amino acids.

The clinical signs are sudden in onset and rapidly progressive, frequently resulting in death. Several horses in a group may be affected, although some may have no signs. Affected horses are reluctant to move, have muscle weakness and fasciculations, and may become recumbent. Choke may be present, and gut sounds may be reduced, with reduction in feces production, although appetite may be unaffected. Heart rates may be markedly increased, and pulmonary edema may be present. The horses do not show signs of pain, despite evidence of widespread myopathy at necropsy. Metabolic and respiratory acidosis, increased cardiac troponin 1, substantial increases in serum CK and AST, and myoglobinuria also are common.

Necropsy reveals widespread myodegeneration in postural and respiratory skeletal muscles and the myocardium. A definitive diagnosis can be made by identifying a pattern of accumulation of short- and medium-chain serum acylcarnitines and specific urine organic acids and glycine conjugates typical of a deficiency in multiple acyl CoA dehydrogenases. Special stains for lipid reveal excessive lipid storage in the heart, diaphragm, and other oxidative postural muscles. Supportive therapy, including antioxidants (eg, vitamin C, vitamin E, riboflavin), and IV fluids containing dextrose are recommended. Fewer than 75% of horses survive.

TOXIC MYOPATHIES

Ionophores

Ionophores are commonly added to ruminant feeds for their growth promotion and coccidiostat properties. Horses, however, are 10 times more sensitive to the toxic effects of ionophores in feed than cattle. When equine feeds are inadvertently contaminated with ionophores or horses eat cattle feed, some animals may die acutely with colic-like signs, myoglobinuria, hypokalemia, cardiac arrhythmia, and tachypnea. Cardiomyopathy is the most common chronic sequela.

TRAUMATIC AND ANESTHETIC MYOPATHIES

Postanesthetic Myopathy

After anesthesia, horses may develop severe muscle pain and weakness in one or more muscle groups. Hypoperfusion of compressed muscle groups with resultant high intracompartmental pressure is the most important causative factor for focal muscle involvement. The dependent triceps muscle is most commonly affected after anesthesia in lateral recumbency, whereas the longissimus dorsi and gluteal muscles are usually affected in horses that have been in dorsal recumbency. Generalized myopathies may develop in horses that were hypotensive during anesthesia. The longer the duration of anesthesia, the higher the risk.

Signs are evident when horses try to stand or may be delayed for up to 2 hr. A dropped elbow stance typical of radial nerve paralysis characterizes triceps myopathy. Gluteal myopathy results in unwillingness to bear weight on the hindlimbs. Horses may appear distressed, with profuse sweating, tachycardia, and tachypnea. The degree of distress depends on the severity of muscle damage. Affected muscles may feel very hard and show localized swelling. Serum CK may be normal immediately after the horse stands but rise substantially and peak ~4 hr after anesthesia. Pain relief is provided by sedation with detomidine, combined with opiate analgesics and NSAIDs. Constant-rate infusions of detomidine or butorphanol may be beneficial for pain control in severe cases. Fluid therapy helps maintain renal perfusion and urine output and ensures adequate muscle perfusion. The prognosis for unilateral myopathy is usually good, although with severe damage there may be residual muscle fibrosis, which may compromise function. The prognosis for generalized myopathy is more guarded.

Prevention requires minimizing the time under general anesthesia, carefully positioning the horse on the operating table, and maintaining arterial blood pressure >60 mmHg using fluid therapy and inotropic agents such as dobutamine (1–5 mcg/kg/min).

Malignant Hyperthermia

The ryanodine receptor gene (*RYR1*) mutation in Quarter horses (*see* p 1178) can cause fatal reactions under general anesthesia that are characterized by marked hyperthermia, acidosis, electrolyte derangements, and muscle necrosis. Unfortunately, once a fulminant episode is underway it is difficult to prevent cardiac arrest. Diagnosis is by clinical signs and genetic testing. Pretreatment with oral dantrolene (4 mg/kg) 30–60 min before anesthesia is the only potential means to prevent an episode.

Fibrotic Myopathy

Fibrotic myopathy describes a classic gait abnormality that develops when horses injure their semitendinosus and semimembranosus muscles at the point of a tendinous insertion during exercise that requires abrupt turns and sliding stops. Trauma (eg, catching a foot in a fence), IM injections, and a congenital form are other potential causes of fibrotic myopathy. Affected muscles in acute cases are warm and painful on deep palpation. Chronically, hardened areas within the muscle may represent fibrosis and ossification. The associated gait abnormality is usually most apparent at the walk and is characterized by an abrupt cessation of the anterior phase of the stride of the affected limb, causing the leg to jerk suddenly to the ground rather than continue its forward motion. The stride has a short anterior phase with a characteristic hoof-slapping gait. The gait reflects a mechanical hindlimb lameness that restricts normal function. Pain is usually not a feature of chronic fibrotic myopathy. Serum CK and AST are usually only mildly increased. In addition to palpation, diagnosis can be confirmed by ultrasonography, thermography, or scintigraphy. Light microscopic evaluation of muscle biopsies is frequently normal in acute cases. Chronically, fibrous replacement of muscle fibers is apparent. Acute cases may benefit from rest and cold therapy followed by deep heating ultrasound and controlled stretching. Chronic cases may require surgical excision or transection of the fibrotic part of the muscle or tenotomy of the tibial insertion of the semimembranosus tendon.

HEREDITARY AND CONGENITAL MYOPATHIES

Mitochondrial Myopathy

A deficiency of Complex 1, the first step in the mitochondrial respiratory chain, was identified in a young Arabian filly with clinical signs similar to those of exertional rhabdomyolisis. However, this horse showed no changes in serum CK level after exercise. A marked lactic acidosis developed even with light exercise, and maximum oxygen consumption was drastically reduced, resulting in marked exercise intolerance. Histopathologic evaluation of muscle biopsies showed an abnormal increase in mitochondrial density, and biochemical analyses revealed a Complex 1 deficiency. The horse has shown slowly progressive signs of muscle atrophy but has otherwise remained healthy at rest.

Glycogen Branching Enzyme Deficiency

Glycogen branching enzyme deficiency (GBED) is a glycogen storage disorder causing abortion, seizures, and muscle weakness in Quarter horse–related breeds caused by an autosomal recessive mutation in the glycogen branching enzyme (*GBE1*) gene. The mutation is carried by 9% of Quarter horses and Paint horses, and at least 3% of abortions are attributed to GBED in Quarter horses. Most foals diagnosed with GBED present at 1 day of age with hypothermia, weakness, and flexural deformities of all limbs. Ventilatory failure may also be a presenting sign in addition to recurrent hypoglycemia and collapse. All foals have died either from euthanasia because of muscle weakness or suddenly because of apparent cardiac arrhythmia. Persistent leukopenia, intermittent hypoglycemia, and high serum CK (1,000–15,000 U/L), AST, and γ-glutamyl-transferase activities are features of affected foals. Gross lesions are not evident, and routine H&E stains of tissues may be normal or show basophilic inclusions in skeletal muscle and cardiac tissues. Frozen sections of muscle, heart, and liver show a notable lack of normal PAS staining for glycogen as well as abnormal PAS-positive globular or crystalline intracellular inclusions. Branching enzyme activity is minimal in skeletal and cardiac muscle as well as liver. A diagnosis is best obtained by confirming the presence of the genetic mutation in tissue samples or by identifying typical PAS-positive inclusions in muscle or cardiac samples. There is no successful treatment.

BOVINE SECONDARY RECUMBENCY

(Downer cow syndrome)

Recumbency in cattle is caused by numerous metabolic, traumatic, infectious, degenerative, and toxic disorders. If treatment of the underlying cause of recumbency is not successful and cattle are unable to rise for >24 hr after initial recumbency, they may develop a secondary recumbency from pressure damage to muscles and nerves, often termed "downer cow syndrome." An alert downer cow does not show signs of systemic illness or depression, is able to eat and drink, and remains in sternal recumbency for no apparent reason. A nonalert downer cow appears systemically sick and depressed. Downer cow syndrome also describes the pathology of pressure-induced muscle and nerve injuries after prolonged recumbency. The most important pathophysiologic event that develops during prolonged recumbency is a pressure-induced ischemic necrosis of the thigh muscles that frequently affects both hindlegs.

Nonambulatory disabled livestock are those that cannot rise from a recumbent position or that cannot walk. This includes, but is not limited to, those with broken appendages, severed tendons or ligaments, nerve paralysis, a fractured vertebral column, or metabolic conditions. Downer cows have been categorized according to potential diseases of the CNS into nonambulatory cows with progressive or nonprogressive neurologic findings.

Etiology and Pathogenesis: In most cases, downer cow syndrome is a complication of periparturient hypocalcemia (milk fever, *see* p 988) in cows that do not fully respond to calcium therapy. Calving paralysis after dystocia may also result in recumbency due to traumatic injury to tissues and nerves inside the pelvic cavity. Regardless of the initial cause of recumbency, all cattle develop pressure-induced damage to muscles and nerves of the pelvic limbs, especially when lying on a hard surface. The hindlimb muscles of the leg the animal is lying on are compressed between the bones and the skin by the physical pressure from the weight of the recumbent cow.

With prolonged recumbency (eg, if treatment of hypocalcemia is delayed), the lymphatic and venous drainage to muscle is decreased because of sustained pressure with no decrease in arterial blood flow. The net result of pressure-induced changes in blood flow is an increase in interstitial fluid volume and pressure within the muscle, because the fascia around each muscle cannot expand sufficiently to accommodate the increase in interstitial volume. In severe and prolonged cases of recumbency, the increase in intramuscular pressure is visible as a firm swelling of the muscle. The resulting compression of muscles, nerves, and blood vessels within an enclosed compartment induces ischemic pressure damage of muscle and nerves, also named compartment syndrome. The severity of pressure damage to the muscles depends on regional anatomic factors (bones), duration of compression, and the surface on which the animal is kept.

Pressure myopathy in downer cows is often complicated by damage to and functional loss of the sciatic nerve and its peroneal branch. The sciatic nerve may be damaged by direct compression against the caudal femur, secondary swelling of the surrounding muscles, or both. The degree of damage to the sciatic nerve is thought to be a critical factor for recovery of downer cows. Damage to the peroneal branch of the sciatic nerve results from direct pressure on the nerve as it crosses over the lateral condyle of the femur.

Experimental sternal recumbency in halothane-anesthetized cattle for 6–12 hr, with the right hindlimb positioned under the body, resulted in a swollen and rigid limb and permanent (terminal) recumbency in 50% of the cases. Cattle able to stand after anesthesia showed hyperflexion of the fetlock, indicating peroneal nerve paralysis, and myoglobinuria with dark brown urine. Necropsy of terminal downer cases revealed extensive necrosis of the caudal thigh muscles and inflammation of the sciatic nerve caudal to the proximal end of the femur.

Additional complications of prolonged recumbency include acute mastitis, decubital ulcers, and traumatic injuries to the limbs (eg, laceration and rupture of muscle fibers in the thigh) from struggling and efforts to rise.

Clinical Findings: Periparturient cows may be found in lateral recumbency, which may indicate an unresolved metabolic problem such as hypocalcemia or hypomagnesemia. Inquiries into the severity and duration of parturition may suggest that the recumbency is at least partially due to exhaustion. In involuntary sternal recumbency, some cows may have a dull, listless appearance. This may indicate hypocalcemia in periparturient mature cows. The second most likely cause of depression is toxemia, the cause of which is most commonly found in the genital tract or mammary gland. Other cows found in involuntary sternal recumbency may be bright and alert in appearance—the most typical demeanor of the true problem downer cow. If the animal is young or not pregnant, the cause is likely to be either physical damage or a rare condition, either of which requires careful, detailed examination.

The environment of the animal can have a bearing on the cause. If the footing is slippery, physical damage to the musculoskeletal system should be suspected. This is much less likely among cows in open space with a dirt or well-bedded surface.

The positioning of the hindlimbs may indicate the cause of the recumbency. Limbs splayed out behind the animal may indicate obturator nerve paresis or paralysis, hip dislocation, or fracture of the femur or tibia. Fracture should be suspected whenever the upper limb is extended sideways in such a manner that a crease is formed in the skin.

Physical Examination: A thorough physical examination should be performed when the cow is first presented. The rectal temperature should be within the normal range. If it is lower than normal, some level of shock might be present. Recession of the eyes into the orbit or persistence of a skin fold for >2 sec indicates dehydration. Pallor of the mucous membranes suggests toxemia, in which case a weak pulse and tachycardia may be present. The respiration of a recumbent cow may be labored by virtue of the pressure of the abdominal contents on the diaphragm.

Vaginal exploration is mandatory in every peripartum, recumbent cow and may lead to discovery of a decomposing fetus. Damage to and infection of the wall of the vagina is common. Metritis and an associated toxemia can contribute to postpartum recumbency.

Rectal exploration is essential for differential diagnosis. The degree of uterine involution should be appropriate for the number of days postpartum. Ballottement of fluid in the organ or lack of tonicity should be noted. Unexpected anomalies may be palpated. Adhesions, lumps of necrotic fat, and enlargement or turgidity of the cervix or vaginal wall are all sequelae of a difficult birth. Hip dislocations and fractures of the pelvis may be palpated per rectum, particularly if an assistant vigorously manipulates the upper limb of a cow in lateral recumbency. Movement of the head of the femur in the obturator foramen may also be detected in cattle with caudoventral hip dislocation. Craniodorsal dislocation of the hip, the most common direction for hip dislocation, or fracture of the femoral neck or proximal femur should be suspected if the affected limb appears shorter than the contralateral limb. Pelvic fractures can be associated with sciatic nerve paralysis, whereas hip dislocation may be associated with some degree of obturator nerve paralysis. If either condition is suspected, the sensory state of the limbs should be evaluated by judicious and humane application of an electric prod to the distal limb. Involuntary sternal recumbency may be associated with lymphosarcoma of the spinal canal, vertebral abscesses, or bizarre traumatic injuries.

Mammary gland examination should always be performed on recumbent cows. A toxic infection of the udder with an organism such as *Escherichia coli* can be a primary cause of recumbency. However, such an infection may be precipitated by the recumbency, especially if the udder is engorged and remains unmilked.

Blood samples are not usually taken when treating routine cases of hypocalcemia. However, hypocalcemia, hypophosphatemia, and hypokalemia should be assumed to be present in all recumbent cattle, and determination of the biochemical status of cattle unresponsive to calcium therapy frequently helps guide treatment and prognosis. Hypokalemia and hypophosphatemia are commonly quoted causes of creeper cows (cows able to crawl but unable to stand). Alert downer cows may have normal serum concentrations of calcium, potassium, magnesium, and phosphorus. Downer cows have increased serum CK, AST, and LDH; cows that do not recover have higher serum AST and CK activities than cows that do recover. Increased serum CK activity is a specific indicator of muscle damage; however, CK activity peaks shortly after the start of muscle damage and declines noticeably within 4 hr. For this reason, increased serum AST activity is the best prognostic indicator in recumbent cattle, with higher AST activities indicating a poorer prognosis. In cattle with severe muscle damage, the urine may contain myoglobin as well as higher than normal concentrations of protein. The age and mean serum concentrations of phosphorus, magnesium, sodium, bilirubin, glucose, and urea are not significantly different between recovering and nonrecovering cows.

Lesions: Ischemic necrosis and rupture of muscles of the thigh region are common necropsy findings in downer cows. Hemorrhage and rupture of adductor muscles may be seen if the animal "spread-eagled" itself while struggling to rise on a slippery surface such as wet or icy concrete. Traumatic and inflammatory injuries to sciatic and peroneal nerves are also found in downer cows. Damage to intrapelvic nerves, such as the sciatic and obturator nerves, account for most cases. Decubital injuries to the lateral aspect of the stifle can be associated with damage to the peroneal nerve.

Treatment: Downer cows are often hypocalcemic. If an apparently hypocalcemic cow does not respond to calcium therapy, potassium, phosphorus, and magnesium should be given as additional treatments pending results of laboratory tests. Monitoring blood mineral status is an important part of downer cow management.

In most cases, recovery depends on the quality of recumbency management and nursing care. Lateral recumbency must be corrected immediately to avoid regurgitation and inspiration of stomach contents. The animal should be rolled into sternal recumbency. However, if this posture is to be maintained, the limb on which the animal has been lying should be drawn from under the body. In other words, if the animal was presented in lateral recumbency on its left side, it should be rolled into sternal recumbency on its right side. Support (eg, straw bale) placed under the shoulder may be required for some animals to maintain sternal recumbency.

Attempting to stabilize a recumbent cow on a concrete surface is highly undesirable but sometimes unavoidable. Bedding the area around and under the cow with wet, sticky manure to a depth of >6 in. is a common practice. At least 10 in. of dry straw should be distributed over the wet mass. If the cow struggles and scrapes the wet manure, exposing concrete, more manure must be added. The manure pack provides good footing but also may soil the skin with urine and manure. Dermatitis can result, and cow comfort is reduced. More seriously, the risk of mastitis resulting from the contaminated environment is very high. A bed of sand >10 in. deep provides a more effective method to house a recumbent cow. A sand bed usually drains well, and good hygiene can be maintained if voided manure is removed several times a day.

Some recumbent cattle appear to lose interest in trying to stand; these cattle may benefit from use of a specially designed flotation tank that has a volume of ~2,500–3,000 L. Cattle are loaded into the flotation tank by being dragged on a mat into the empty tank. Doors are then put in place, and the tank is filled with lukewarm water. Cold or hot water should be avoided, because it can induce hypothermia or hyperthermia. Cattle should be encouraged to stand once the water reaches the level of the scapulohumeral joint. When the cow stands, the musculoskeletal and nervous systems should be thoroughly examined to identify underlying disease processes. Cattle that can support their own weight should be permitted to stand for 6–8 hr; however, the water in the tank should be removed as soon as cattle exhibit trembling. Cattle that remain standing should be encouraged to walk slowly from the tank on a nonslip surface. Cattle able to walk out of the tank after the first flotation treatment are 4.8 times more likely to survive than those that do not walk out of the tank. Cattle that stand on all four limbs during the first flotation treatment are 2.9 times more likely to survive than those that had an asymmetric stance or were unable to stand. Reported success rates in returning recumbent cattle to normal ambulation range from 37%–46%.

Hobbling may be considered in cows suspected to have obturator or sciatic nerve damage to prevent overabduction that can lead to muscular damage. Ropes should never be used for this purpose. A soft nylon strap may be wrapped twice around the middle of each metatarsus, allowing a distance of at least 3 ft between the legs.

Assisting Cows to Rise: On every day of the recumbency, an attempt should be made to bring the cow to its feet. Several simple but effective techniques can be tried. In one method, the clinician stands with feet pressed under the cow at a point below the scapulohumeral joint. A sharp blow is delivered by driving the knees into the muscle mass below and caudal to the scapula. This method must not be used on the thoracic wall unprotected by the muscle mass to avoid fracturing the ribs. If the animal struggles to rise, an assistant should grasp the root of the tail with both hands and lift. Lifting on any other part of the tail may cause damage. Recently calved cows can be motivated to rise if they hear their own calf bawling with hunger. The calf is best restrained close to the cow but out of her sight. Some workers use electric goads and various anecdotal or traditional methods of inflicting pain to stimulate a cow to rise; these measures have a low success rate in inexperienced hands and are not recommended.

The value of hip clamps is controversial. Their proper use requires experience, skill, and a delicate touch. Continual use causes trauma and pain that is counterproductive. The forelimbs support 60% of a cow's weight and, therefore, the use of a canvas sling under the sternum is almost mandatory for consistent success. A chest band is required to prevent the sling from slipping backward. If the sling is suspended from the tine at one end of a fork lift, and the hip clamps from a tine at the other end, minimal trauma results. If a fork lift is not available, a T-bar suspended by a pulley from an overhead beam (or a tripod for animals at pasture) will serve. The jaws of the clamps must be well protected with synthetic foam or rubber secured in place with a wrap of duct tape.

Hip clamps should not be applied too tightly and should lift the cow slowly to allow time for the circulation of the limbs to become reestablished. The device is lifted until the hindfeet just touch the ground. Often, the cow will hang with the limbs slightly flexed. This should not be confused with unilateral flexion, which indicates peroneal paralysis. Next, one assistant on each side of the cow presses a shoulder into the paralumbar fossa while facing the hindlimb. The device is slowly lowered as the assistants attempt to force each hindlimb into a weightbearing posture and to reduce the flexion by manipulating the stifle and hock. As soon as any weight is supported by the two limbs, the device should be lowered 1–2 in. This process may have to be repeated several times.

Even if the cow does not stand, the lifted position provides an opportunity to manipulate the limbs, auscultate for crepitation, and perform vaginal and rectal examinations.

Moving Recumbent Cows: The chances of resolution are considerably enhanced by moving the cow to a location with an earthen floor. In warm, relatively dry weather, the best location for a recumbent cow is grassy pasture, although this means that a method to lift the cow must be readily available. Otherwise, the location selected should have a roof and some protection from the elements. These conditions often exist in a hay barn or implement shed, which may have the added benefit of allowing installation of a pulley system to lift the cow.

Moving the cow requires rolling her into lateral recumbency. The cow can then be slid over dry straw for a short distance by pulling on a rope attached to a lower forelimb and a halter rope. Transportation over longer distances can be accomplished using a suitably prepared farm gate hauled by tractor. The longest dimension of the farm gate is closely applied to the back of the cow still in lateral recumbency. A tarpaulin is placed on the gate to protect the cow from contact with the ground. Dry straw is spread on the tarpaulin, and the cow is rolled over onto the makeshift stretcher. The halter should be tied to the gate to minimize struggling, and a sack placed over the eyes to minimize alarm while the cow is being moved. The tail is best tied to the hock of the upper limb. Once moved, the cow should be restored to sternal recumbency. A few cows, particularly if <12 hr postpartum, will rise immediately after being moved to a location with good footing.

Recumbent cattle should be examined daily to determine any change in ability to rise or bear weight. The chance of improvement is very low if the cow does not show any improvement within 5 days of moving to a location with good footing and correction of any serum electrolyte abnormalities.

Supportive Care of Recumbent Cows: It is vital that recumbent cows be provided with clean water at all times. A shallow rubber feed bowl prevents spillage. If the cow does not drink, she must be given fluid therapy either by drench or parenterally. Every effort must be made to roll the cow from one side onto the other at least three times a day, with more frequent movement being desired. If this is not done, the weight of the cow results in continued ischemia of the muscles of the hindlimb and exacerbation of compartment syndrome.

Protection from the elements is essential. Rain and wind can reduce body temperature considerably and worsen shock if present. A windbreak of straw bales is vital. Straw bedding should be provided to help insulate the cow from the ground. A recumbent cow does not require a warm environment; however, in a cold environment, an inactive animal can gradually succumb to hypothermia.

The downer cows most difficult to treat are those that do not try to eat. A cow that salivates on its feed will not eat it later. Rather than being offered large amounts of feed, the cow should be tempted with sweet hay. This should be cleared away every 30 min if not accepted. Placing bitter-tasting weeds such as ivy or dandelion in the mouth may provoke salivation and an interest in eating. Lettuce and cabbage leaves are accepted by some cows. In extreme cases, the cow can be drenched with rumen contents.

Prevention: Effective strategies to prevent milk fever are important to decrease downer cow syndrome. All dairy cows should be monitored closely around calving for early signs of parturient paresis (*see* p 988). Prophylactic administration of calcium to all cows, beginning with cows entering their second or later lactation, is beneficial in herds with a high incidence of milk fever, especially in smaller farms that cannot implement feeding acidogenic salt diets.

The critical issue seems to be the length of time (several hours) from when clinical signs of milk fever begin until treatment. Every cow that has been successfully treated for hypocalcemia should, if necessary, be moved to a location with a good footing and remain there for 48 hr. Straw over sand provides good insulation and good footing.

Animal Welfare Considerations: Although a cow may rise after being recumbent for >14 days, this does not imply that a cow should be unmonitored for this period. So long as the cow looks bright, occasionally struggles to rise, and continues to eat and drink, recovery is a possibility. However, if the cow becomes listless, shows no interest in feed, or has decubital lesions or starts to lose condition, euthanasia on humane grounds must be considered irrespective of how long she has been recumbent. A cow that has decubital lesions, a poor appetite, or shows signs of wasting is unsuitable for salvage slaughter. Attempting to send animals in this condition to the slaughterhouse is considered an act of cruelty in many countries.

"Dragging" recumbent cows is illegal in some countries. Both veterinarians and producers must be aware of the legal interpretation of the word "dragging." Access to some locations may be so restricted that rolling the animal onto an improvised sled may be impossible. At all times, even when using a sled, great care must be taken to avoid injury to dependent parts of the animal such as the udder, ears, and tail.

LAMENESS IN SMALL ANIMALS

Signs of musculoskeletal disorders include weakness, lameness, limb swelling, and joint dysfunction. Motor or sensory neurologic impairment may develop secondary to neuromuscular lesions. Abnormalities of the musculoskeletal system may also affect other organs of the endocrine, urinary, digestive, hemolymphatic, and cardiopulmonary systems. Evaluation of musculoskeletal disease is aimed at localizing and defining the lesion(s). Diagnosis requires accurate review of the signalment, history, and physical status of the animal. A lameness examination is critical to determine a diagnosis. Useful ancillary tests include radiography, ultrasonography, arthrocentesis, arthroscopy, arthrography, electromyography, and tissue biopsy and histopathology. For subtle lesions, advanced imaging techniques, including bone scans, CT, and MRI, are being used with greater frequency in specialty clinics and university hospitals.

THE LAMENESS EXAMINATION

The lameness examination is a key feature to identify musculoskeletal lesions. Evaluation is performed with the animal at rest, rising, and during locomotion on flat or inclined surfaces. Single- or multiple-limb lameness is noted, with the severity related to the type of activity. With a forelimb lameness, the head is elevated during weight bearing on the unsound limb. The stride is also shortened on the affected side. For hindlimb lameness, the head is dropped during weight bearing on the affected limb. Limbs should be assessed from a distal to proximal manner, and bones, joints, and soft tissue should be palpated. Abnormalities to note include swelling, pain, instability, crepitation, reduced range of motion, and muscle atrophy. In evaluation of a subtle or obscure lameness, serial examinations before and after exercise may be necessary. For fractious animals, sedation may be required; palpation, radiography, and arthrocentesis can often be performed while an animal is sedated with IV butorphanol and acepromazine; propofol; medetomidine (alone or combined with butorphanol or hydromorphone); or a combination of ketamine, diazepam, and acepromazine.

Imaging Techniques: Helpful imaging procedures to diagnose lameness include survey and contrast radiography, ultrasonography, nuclear scintigraphy, CT, and MRI. Animals undergoing these evaluations should be heavily sedated or anesthetized. Survey radiography of affected limbs or the spine requires multiple, orthogonal views. Subtle lesions are often identified after comparison with the contralateral normal limb. The most frequent contrast studies used to evaluate lame animals are arthrograms for joint diseases and myelography for spinal canal disorders. Ultrasonography is useful to evaluate musculotendinous injuries such as bicipital tenosynovitis, Achilles tendon rupture, and muscle contracture. Nuclear scintigraphy, CT, and MRI studies are usually available at private or academic referral centers. Nuclear scintigraphy involves IV injection of a radioactive compound that localizes and highlights periosseous soft tissue and bone lesions. CT imaging permits high contrast and resolution of osseous structures, whereas MRI is helpful to delineate soft tissue and joint injuries. Both can also be used to assess the spinal column, although MRI is a better standard to evaluate nervous tissues.

Arthroscopy: Arthroscopy is a minimally invasive tool used for diagnosis and therapy of lame animals. Advantages of the technique include improved visualization and diagnosis of joint pathology, ability to treat injuries by removal of damaged cartilage or ligament, and reduced surgical dissection. Disadvantages are costs of equipment and development of expertise in its use. Common conditions that can be diagnosed or treated by arthroscopy include osteochondrosis, bicipital tenosynovitis, joint fractures, and cranial cruciate ligament and medial meniscal injuries.

PAIN MANAGEMENT

Control of pain in lame or operative animals involves broad classes of compounds such as NSAIDs and opioids (*see also* PAIN ASSESSMENT AND MANAGEMENT, p 2104). Analgesic agents can be administered via oral, parenteral (including constant-rate infusions), epidural, local, or transdermal routes. Nonpharmacologic pain management strategies include acupuncture therapy, massage, physical therapy, and diet.

Commonly used NSAIDs include deracoxib (4 mg/kg/day, PO), firocoxib (5 mg/kg/day, PO), meloxicam (dogs: 0.1 mg/kg/day, IV, SC, PO; cats: 0.1 mg/kg/day, IV, SC, PO, for 1–3 days), carprofen (2.2 mg/kg, PO, bid), ketoprofen (1 mg/kg/day, PO, IV, SC, IM), etodolac (12.5 mg/kg/day, PO), tepoxalin (10 mg/kg/day, PO), and aspirin (dogs: 22 mg/kg, PO, bid; cats: 10 mg/kg, PO, every 48 hr). The use of NSAIDs is contraindicated in animals with hepatic or renal insufficiency, gastroenteritis, or coagulopathy, and in animals receiving concurrent corticosteroid therapy.

Opioid analgesics bind to μ, κ, and δ receptors in the CNS to provide pain relief. Commonly used opioids include morphine (0.1 mg/kg, IV, IM, SC, every 3–4 hr), oxymorphone (0.05 mg/kg, IV, IM, SC, every 3–4 hr), hydromorphone (0.1 mg/kg, IV, IM, SC, every 2–4 hr), butorphanol (0.1 mg/kg, IV, IM, SC, every 2–4 hr in dogs and cats), and buprenorphine (0.01 mg/kg, IV, IM, SC, tid in dogs and cats, also transmucosal in cats). Opioid narcotics can be given with sedatives such as acepromazine (0.5 mg/kg, IV, IM, SC, every 4–6 hr) for enhanced efficacy of analgesia and sedation. Oxymorphone, hydromorphone, and butorphanol are more potent than morphine. Buprenorphine has the longest duration of action. Another opioid, fentanyl, is most frequently administered via transdermal patches applied for 3 days on shaved areas. Oral opioids used for pain relief include tramadol (5 mg/kg, tid), butorphanol (1 mg/kg, tid), hydromorphone (0.5 mg/kg, tid), codeine (1 mg/kg, tid), and oxycodone (0.3 mg/kg, tid).

Local administration of analgesics involves joint injections with morphine (1 mg diluted in 5 mL of saline), bupivicaine (1 mL/20 kg body wt), or lidocaine (1 mL/20 kg body wt) before joint surgery as a preemptive block of intracapsular pain receptors. Epidural morphine (0.1 mg/kg) in the lumbosacral space is also a useful adjunct for postoperative pain relief in the hindlimbs and for reduced anesthetic requirements. Corticosteroids are considered weak analgesic adjuncts, because they indirectly reduce pain by their primary action as local anti-inflammatory agents at the site of injury. Drugs used include prednisone or prednisolone (1–2 mg/kg/day, PO) or dexamethasone (1–2 mg/kg/day, IV). Their use is contraindicated during concurrent NSAID treatment.

Gabapentin (10 mg/kg, PO, bid) is a calcium channel blocker used to inhibit neurons stimulated by pain; it is useful for treatment of animals with chronic or neuropathic pain. Dexmedetomidine (5 mcg/kg/day, IM) and medetomidine (10 mcg/kg/day, IM) are newer analgesic-sedative, α_2-receptor blocking agents useful to facilitate examinations or diagnostic evaluations.

Joint fluid modifiers (glucosamine, chondroiton sulfate, hyaluronan, pentosan polysulfate, omega-3 fatty acids) have received extensive attention in treating degenerative joint disease and alleviating discomfort. While contraindications and adverse effects are few, scientifically proven efficacy of these compounds is limited and most reports are regarded as anecdotal evidence. Stem cell therapy to alleviate pain and discomfort of diseased joints is also a newer modality for which scientific validity is pending.

ARTHROPATHIES AND RELATED DISORDERS IN SMALL ANIMALS

Many arthropathies are developmental, including aseptic necrosis of the femoral head, patellar luxation, osteochondrosis, elbow dysplasia, and hip dysplasia. Other arthropathies are degenerative, infectious or septic, immune-mediated, neoplastic, or traumatic.

ASEPTIC NECROSIS OF THE FEMORAL HEAD

(Legg-Calvé-Perthes disease)

This deterioration of the femoral head seen in young miniature and small breeds of dogs is associated with ischemia and avascular necrosis of the bone. The exact cause is unknown, although there may be a hereditary component in Manchester Terriers. Infarction of the bone leads to collapse of the femoral head and neck, followed by revascularization, resorption, and remodeling. The lesion is often bilateral.

Clinical signs include hindlimb lameness, atrophy of the thigh muscles, and pain during manipulation of the hip joint. Radiography reveals irregular bone density of the femoral head and neck, collapse, and fragmentation of the bone. Chronic cases have evidence of degenerative joint disease.

Treatment involves surgical excision of the affected femoral head and neck and early postoperative physical therapy to stimulate limb usage. Prognosis for recovery is excellent.

PATELLAR LUXATION

This hereditary disorder in dogs and cats is characterized by ectopic development of the patella medial or lateral to the trochlear groove of the femur. Patellar luxation can be associated with multiple deformities of the hindlimb, involving the hip joint, femur, and tibia. Medial patellar luxations can be involved with a reduced coxofemoral angle (coxa vara), lateral bowing of the femur, internal rotation of the tibia, shallow trochlear groove, and hypoplasia of the medial femoral condyle; lateral luxations cause the reverse changes.

Clinical signs are variable and based on the severity of luxation. Animals of any age may be affected. In general, cats and small and miniature breeds of dogs have a medial luxation, and large dogs have a lateral luxation. Affected animals are lame or ambulate with a skipping gait. Palpation of the stifle joint reveals displacement of the patella. In Grade I, clinical signs are mild and infrequent, and the patella can be manually luxated but easily returns to the trochlear groove. In Grade II, the patella luxates during flexion of the joint and is repositioned during extension, causing animals to have a resolvable skipping lameness. In Grade III, the dislocated patella is more frequently out of, instead of in, the trochlear groove, and lameness is consistent. Bone deformities are evident in these animals. In Grade IV, lameness and limb deformations are most severe. Radiography of affected animals reveals various degrees of limb changes based on the grade of the luxation.

The type of surgery is based on the severity of the luxation and can include both orthopedic and soft-tissue procedures. Useful procedures involve fascial releasing incisions (on the side of the luxation), joint capsule and retinaculum imbrications (on the side opposite the luxation), deepening of the trochlear groove, tibial crest transposition, and fabella to tibial tuberosity derotation sutures. Severe deformations may require femoral or tibial osteotomies, stifle joint arthrodesis, or limb amputation.

Prognosis for recovery is good in mild or moderately affected animals. Concurrent cranial cruciate ligament and medial meniscal injuries should be identified and treated. Cats are less severely affected than dogs and have an excellent prognosis.

OSTEOCHONDROSIS

Osteochondrosis is a developmental disorder of medium and large rapidly growing dogs that is characterized by abnormal endochondral ossification of epiphyseal cartilage in the shoulder, elbow, stifle, and hock joints. Although the exact cause is unknown, excessive nutrition, rapid growth, trauma, and a hereditary component are suspected to be contributing factors. As a result of abnormal maturation and vascularity, basal cartilage cells thicken and weaken, thus leading to cartilage cracks, fissures, and flap formation (osteochondritis dissecans) after minor trauma or normal pressure to the joint. Abnormal cartilage congruency and joint debris lead to a synovitis and subsequent arthritis and continued cartilage breakdown. Cartilage flaps can break loose and attach to the joint capsule or migrate and deleteriously affect joint motion.

Clinical signs are lameness, joint effusion, and reduced range of motion in affected joints or limbs. Locations of the lesions include the head of the humerus (shoulder joint), the medial aspect of the humeral condyle (elbow joint), the femoral condyles (stifle joint), and the trochlear ridges of the talus (hock joint). Additionally, fragmented medial coronoid process and ununited anconeal process in the elbow joint may be related conditions. Radiography is useful in identifying joint lesions; changes may include flattening of joint surfaces, subchondral bone lucency or sclerosis, osteophytosis, joint effusion, and "joint mice." Arthrography can be used to delineate cartilage flaps, and arthroscopy can also be performed to identify and treat cartilage or joint lesions. CT imaging also helps identify subchondral bone changes.

Treatment involves surgical excision of cartilage flaps or free-floating fragments and curettage of subchondral bone to stimulate fibrocartilage formation. Animals with degenerative joint disease may benefit from NSAIDs, eg, aspirin (10 mg/kg, PO, bid), carprofen (2.2 mg/kg, PO, bid), deracoxib (4 mg/kg/day, PO), firocoxib (5 mg/kg/day, PO), meloxicam (0.1 mg/kg/day, PO), tepoxalin (10 mg/kg/day, PO), or etodolac (12.5 mg/kg/day, PO). Joint fluid modifiers such as polysulfated glycosaminoglycan (4.4 mg/kg, IM, twice a week for 4 wk) may also help prevent cartilage degeneration. Prognosis for recovery is excellent for the shoulders, good for the stifle joint, and fair for the elbow and tarsal joints. Concomitant signs of degenerative joint disease, other joint conditions, or instability (hock joint) deleteriously affect recovery.

ELBOW DYSPLASIA

(Ununited anconeal process, Fragmented medial coronoid process, Osteochondrosis of the humeral condyle)

Elbow dysplasia is a generalized incongruency of the elbow joint in young, large, rapidly growing dogs that is related to abnormal bone growth, joint stresses, or cartilage development. One or more of the following lesions may be present in the joint: an ununited anconeal process of the ulna, fragmentation of the medial coronoid process of the ulna, and osteochondrosis of the medial aspect of the humeral condyle. Radiographic grading of dysplastic elbow joints is performed by the Orthopedic Foundation for Animals in the USA and in Scandinavian and European kennel clubs.

Ununited Anconeal Process: This results when there is separation of the ossification center of the anconeal process from the proximal ulnar metaphysis. Fusion should be completed by 5–6 mo of age. The fracture is postulated to result from a biomechanical imbalance of force and movement in the rapidly growing elbow. Initially, the anconeal process is connected to the ulna by a bridge of fibrous tissue, which fragments to form a pseudoarthrosis, and the elbow becomes unstable. This joint laxity continues to damage the articular cartilage, and secondary osteoarthritis results. A hereditary basis has been implicated but not proved.

Lameness develops insidiously between 4 and 8 mo of age; however, some bilateral cases may not be diagnosed until dogs are >1 yr old. Affected elbows may deviate laterally, and the range of motion is restricted. Advanced cases have osteoarthritis, joint effusion, and crepitus. Clinical signs are suggestive, and the diagnosis is confirmed by radiography. A lateral radiograph of the elbow in the flexed position allows visualization of the ununited process. Both elbows should be examined because the condition can be bilateral.

Fragmentation of the Medial Coronoid Process: In this condition of the medial compartment of the canine elbow, the coronoid process fails to unite, either partially or totally, with the ulnar diaphysis and, thus, does not become a part of the articular surface of the trochlear notch. Joint laxity, irritation, and finally osteoarthritis result. This condition and osteochondrosis of the medial humeral condyle are considered to be the most common causes of osteoarthritis of the canine elbow. Bone fragments can be seen by radiography, arthroscopy, or CT.

Osteochondrosis of the Medial Humeral Condyle: This results from a disturbed endochondral fusion of the epiphysis of the medial epicondyle with the distal end of the humerus. The exact cause is unknown, but because the carpal and digital flexors originate from the ventral aspect of this structure, it may represent an epiphyseal avulsion. It results in pain on flexion of the elbow or deep digital palpation and is accompanied by soft-tissue swelling. Radiographically, radiodense structures have been seen caudal and distal to the area of the medial epicondyle.

Treatment: Early surgical treatment is recommended before degenerative joint disease develops. For fragmentation of the medial coronoid process, a medial arthrotomy or arthroscopy is performed and the fragmented process removed. For ununited anconeal process, either a lateral arthrotomy is performed and the ununited process removed, or a midshaft ulnar osteotomy is performed to relieve asynchronous growth and result in union of the process. Reattachment of the process by screw fixation is also an option. For osteochondrosis, the subchondral bone lesion is curetted to stimulate fibrocartilage formation. Prognosis after surgery is good if degenerative joint disease has not developed in the joint. Aspirin or NSAIDs (eg, carprofen, deracoxib, firocoxib, etodolac, meloxicam, tepoxalin) can be used to reduce pain and inflammation. Joint-fluid modifiers (glycosaminoglycans, hyaluronic aid) may be useful.

HIP DYSPLASIA

Hip dysplasia is a multifactorial abnormal development of the coxofemoral joint in dogs that is characterized by joint laxity and subsequent degenerative joint disease. It is most common in large breeds. Excessive growth, exercise, nutrition, and hereditary factors affect the occurrence of hip dysplasia. The pathophysiologic basis for hip dysplasia is a disparity between hip joint muscle mass and rapid bone development. As a result, coxofemoral joint laxity or instability develops and subsequently leads to degenerative joint changes, eg, acetabular bone sclerosis, osteophytosis, thickened femoral neck, joint capsule fibrosis, and subluxation or luxation of the femoral head.

Clinical signs are variable and do not always correlate with radiographic abnormalities. Lameness may be mild, moderate, or severe and is pronounced after exercise. A "bunny-hopping" gait is sometimes evident. Joint laxity (Ortolani sign), reduced range of motion, and crepitation and pain during full extension and flexion may be present. Radiography is useful in delineating the degree of arthritis and planning of medical and surgical treatments. Standard ventrodorsal views of sedated or anesthetized animals can be graded by the Orthopedic Foundation for Animals, or stress radiographs performed and joint laxity measured (Penn Hip). A dorsal acetabular rim view is used by some surgeons to evaluate the acetabulum before reconstructive surgery. Modified ventrodorsal and dorsoventral projections have also been proposed in an effort to mimic the normal standing posture of dogs. Recent reviews of American and international radiographic screening programs have failed to identify a "gold standard." An evaluation shift toward genome screening may yield more promising results in the future.

Treatments are both medical and surgical. Mild cases or nonsurgical candidates (because of health or owner constraints) may benefit from weight reduction, restriction of exercise on hard surfaces, controlled physical therapy to strengthen and maintain muscle tone, anti-inflammatory drugs (eg, aspirin, corticosteroids, NSAIDs), and possibly joint fluid modifiers. Surgical treatments include pectineal myotenectomy to reduce pain, triple pelvic osteotomy to prevent subluxation, pubic fusion to prevent subluxation, joint capsule denervation to reduce pain, dorsal acetabulum reinforcement to reduce subluxation, femoral head and neck resection to reduce arthritis, and total hip replacement for optimal restoration of joint and limb functions. Additionally, femoral corrective osteotomies can be performed to reduce femoral head subluxation, although degenerative arthritis may persist.

Prognosis is highly variable and depends on the overall health and environment of the animal. In general, if surgery is indicated and performed correctly, it is beneficial. Animals on which surgery is not performed may require a change in lifestyle to live comfortably.

DEGENERATIVE ARTHRITIS

(Degenerative joint disease, Osteoarthritis)

Progressive deterioration of articular cartilage in diarthrodial joints is characterized by hyaline cartilage thinning, joint effusion, and periarticular osteophyte formation. Joint degeneration can be caused by trauma, infection, immune-mediated diseases, or developmental malformations. The inciting cause initiates chondrocyte necrosis, release of degradative enzymes, synovitis, and continued cartilage destruction and inflammation. Abnormal cartilage congruency and joint capsule anatomy can further lead to alteration in normal joint biomechanical function. Pain and lameness develop secondary to joint dysfunction or muscle atrophy and to limb disuse. Although more common in dogs, joint degeneration may also be seen in cats.

Clinical signs of degenerative joint disease include lameness, joint swelling, muscle atrophy, pericapsular fibrosis, and crepitation. Radiographic changes in the joint include joint effusion, periarticular soft-tissue swelling, osteophytosis, subchondral bone sclerosis, and possibly narrowed joint space. Arthrocentesis may be unremarkable or yield minor changes in color, turbidity, or cell counts of synovial fluid.

Treatments can be medical or surgical. Nonsurgical therapies include weight reduction, controlled exercise on soft surfaces, and therapeutic application of warm compresses to affected joints. NSAIDs (eg, aspirin, etodolac, carprofen, deracoxib, meloxicam, firocoxib, tepoxalin) reduce pain and inflammation. Caution is advised with longterm NSAID usage in dogs. The most frequently cited adverse effects include GI problems such as inappetence, vomiting, and hemorrhagic gastroenteritis. A carprofen-associated hepatopathy in Labrador Retrievers has also been reported. Corticosteroids also suppress prostaglandin synthesis and subsequent inflammation, but short-term use is advised to prevent iatrogenic hyperadrenocorticism, cartilage degeneration, and intestinal perforation. Joint-fluid modifiers such as glycosaminoglycans or sodium hyaluronate may prevent cartilage degradation. Surgical options include joint fusion (arthrodesis), most frequently performed on the carpus and tarsus; joint replacement, such as total hip replacement; joint excision, such as femoral head and neck osteotomy; and amputation. Prognosis is variable and depends on the location and severity of the arthropathy.

SEPTIC ARTHRITIS

Infectious arthritis is most frequently associated with bacterial agents such as staphylococci, streptococci, and coliforms. Causes include hematogenous spread or penetrating trauma, including surgery.

Other agents producing a septic arthritis include rickettsia (Rocky Mountain spotted fever, ehrlichiosis) and spirochetes (borreliosis).

Clinical signs of septic arthritis include lameness, swelling, pain of affected joint(s), and systemic signs of fever, malaise, anorexia, and stiffness. Radiography may reveal joint effusion in early cases and degenerative joint disease in chronic conditions. Arthrocentesis reveals increased levels of WBCs, especially neutrophils. The synovial fluid may be grossly purulent. Bacterial culture and antimicrobial sensitivity testing may confirm the diagnosis. Serologic testing is used for nonbacterial agents. Treatment is with appropriate IV and oral antibiotics, joint lavage, and surgical debridement in severe cases.

IMMUNE-MEDIATED ARTHRITIS

Inflammatory polyarthritis secondary to deposition of immune complexes can produce erosive (destruction of articular cartilage and subchondral bone) or nonerosive (periarticular inflammation) forms of joint diseases. Rheumatoid arthritis, Greyhound polyarthritis, and feline progressive polyarthritis are examples of erosive arthritides. Systemic lupus erythematosus (SLE) is the most common form of nonerosive arthritis.

Clinical signs are lameness, multiple joint pain, joint swelling, fever, malaise, and anorexia. Clinical signs commonly wax and wane.

Diagnosis is aided by radiography, biopsy, arthrocentesis, and serologic testing. Radiography reveals periarticular swelling, effusion, and joint collapse plus subchondral bone destruction in erosive conditions. Arthrocentesis reveals synovial fluid with reduced viscosity and increased inflammatory cell counts. Biopsy of synovial tissue reveals mild to severe inflammation and cellular infiltrates. Serologic testing is performed for rheumatoid factor and antinuclear antibodies.

Treatment involves anti-inflammatory medications (eg, corticosteroids) and chemotherapeutic agents (eg, cyclophosphamide, azathioprine, or methotrexate). Prognosis is guarded because of relapses and inability to determine the inciting cause of the autoimmune reactions.

NEOPLASTIC ARTHRITIS

Synovial cell sarcoma is the most common malignant tumor involving the joints. The tumor arises from primitive mesenchymal cells outside the synovial membrane. Clinical signs include lameness and joint swelling. Radiography reveals soft-tissue swelling and a periosteal reaction. Pulmonary metastasis is detected in ~25% of animals at initial examination. Biopsy reveals evidence of a soft-tissue tumor. Limb amputation is the treatment of choice, although palliative radiation may be considered for cases with a low tumor burden not involving bone.

POLYARTHRITIS

Polyarthritis involves inflammation of multiple joints and is classified as infectious (septic arthritis, *see* p 1197) or noninfectious (erosive or nonerosive [immune-mediated]). Nonerosive can be idiopathic or breed (Akita) associated, while erosive is characteristic of feline progressive arthritis and rheumatoid arthritis. Clinical signs of a polyarthritis include fever, lameness, swollen joints, lethargy, and inappetence. Diagnosis is by radiography (joint effusion, possible erosive bone destruction) and abnormal (increased cell counts) joint fluid analyses. Treatments involve longterm glucocorticoid therapy or other immunosuppressive medications such as azathioprine or cyclophosphamide. Prognosis in most cases is guarded or poor, with relapses common.

JOINT TRAUMA

Cranial Cruciate Ligament Rupture

Rupture of the cranial cruciate ligament is most frequently due to excessive trauma and a possibly weakened ligament secondary to degeneration, immune-mediated diseases, or conformational defects (straight-legged dogs). Plasmacytic-lymphocytic synovitis is sometimes diagnosed concurrently with ligament injury, but it remains unclear whether it is a cause or effect of the joint instability. Stable (nonsurgical) joints with an early or mild condition can be treated with steroids or an NSAID. Most injuries involve a midsubstance tear (mature dog), although bone avulsion (immature dog) at the origin of the ligament is possible. Instability of the stifle joint after rupture of the cranial cruciate ligament can lead to medial meniscal injury, joint effusion, osteophytosis, and joint capsule fibrosis.

Clinical signs involve lameness, pain, medial joint swelling, effusion, crepitation, excessive cranial laxity of the proximal tibia relative to the distal femur (drawer sign, or positive compression test), and increased internal tibial rotation. Partial cranial crucial ligament tears are characterized by a reduced cranial laxity, usually more pronounced in flexion. Medial meniscal injury may be identified by a clicking sound during locomotion or flexion and extension. A tibial compression test (flexion of the hock and cranial displacement of the tibial tuberosity) can also be used to demonstrate laxity of the cranial cruciate ligament. Radiography reveals joint effusion and signs of degenerative joint disease in chronic injuries. Arthrocentesis may reveal mild cellular increases and hemarthrosis. Arthroscopy can confirm the diagnosis but requires specialized equipment.

Treatments include medical and surgical therapies. Weight reduction, controlled physical therapy, and NSAIDs alleviate pain and discomfort from inflammation and degenerative joint disease. Surgical stabilization of the stifle joint is recommended for active dogs. Extracapsular techniques include fascial suturing, fabella to tibial tuberosity imbrication sutures, cranial transposition of the fibular head, leveling of the tibial plateau, tibial tuberosity advancement, and synthetic grafts. Intracapsular techniques include fascia lata or patellar tendon grafts sutured over the top of the lateral femoral condyle. Medial meniscal injury requires removal of damaged avascular tissue. Postoperative physical therapy is critical for clinical recovery. Prognosis after surgery is good.

Joint Fractures

Traumatic fractures frequently involve the shoulder, elbow, carpal, hip, stifle, and tarsal joints. In immature animals, the weakness of the physis compared with adjacent bones, ligaments, and joint capsule predisposes this area to injury. A Salter-Harris classification scheme (I-V) is often used to describe the location of the fracture relative to the physis and joint. Specific common sites of injury include the greater tubercle and condyle of the humerus, distal ulnar physis, and the head and condyles of the femur. The humeral condyle is also frequently injured in mature Spaniel breeds and characterized by Y or T fracture configurations. This may be related to incomplete ossification and vascularity of the bone.

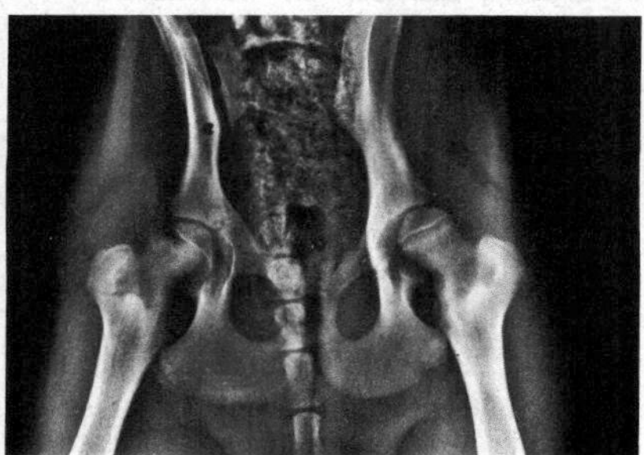

Capital physeal fracture. *Courtesy of Dr. Ronald Green.*

Clinical signs of joint fractures include lameness, pain, and joint swelling. Chronic injuries may be characterized by angular limb deformities if the injury affected an open growth plate. Radiography and CT are useful in delineating the fracture.

The goal of joint fracture treatment is stable anatomic reconstruction to maintain joint congruency and joint and limb functions. Internal fixation with pins, wires, or screws is performed to achieve stable fixation. Prognosis for recovery is good if proper surgical technique has been used and joint trauma has not been excessive.

Palmar Carpal Breakdown

This hyperextension injury secondary to falls or jumps produces excessive force on the carpus, which leads to collapse of the proximal, middle, and/or distal joints secondary to tearing of the palmar carpal ligaments and fibrocartilage. Clinical signs include lameness, carpal swelling, and a characteristic plantigrade stance. External splints or casts may be attempted in mild cases, although surgical treatment is usually required to restore limb function. Surgery involves fusion (arthrodesis) of the affected joints using a bone plate and screws, pins and wires, or external skeletal fixation. A cancellous bone graft is used to enhance bone union, and postoperative support is necessary. Prognosis for recovery is good.

Hip Luxation

Traumatic dislocation of the hip is most frequently a craniodorsal displacement of the femoral head relative to the acetabulum. Clinical signs include lameness, pain during manipulation of the hip joint, and a shortened limb due to dorsal displacement of the femur. Radiography is useful in confirming the luxation and delineating the presence of other fractures in the femoral head or acetabulum. Treatment involves either closed manipulation and postoperative slings to maintain the reduction or open surgical stabilization using sutures or toggle pins. Femoral head and neck resection or total hip replacement can be performed after failed reductions. Prognosis for recovery is usually excellent.

MYOPATHIES IN SMALL ANIMALS

Myopathies can be congenital, hereditary, idiopathic, inflammatory, metabolic, neoplastic, traumatic, or due to nutritional imbalances.

YELLOW FAT DISEASE

(Nutritional steatitis, Nutritional panniculitis)

Yellow fat disease is characterized by a marked inflammation of adipose tissue and deposition of "ceroid" pigment in fat cells. It may be seen alone in cats or with accompanying myopathy in rats, mink, foals, and pigs.

It is believed that an overabundance of unsaturated fatty acids in the ration, together with a deficiency of vitamin E or other antioxidants, results in lipid peroxidation and deposition of "ceroid" pigment in the adipose tissue. Most naturally occurring and experimentally induced cases have been in animals that have had fish or fish by-products as all or part of the diet. The specific cause is believed to be related jointly to the high unsaturation of the fish oil fatty acids and their lack of protection with vitamin E or other antioxidants.

Affected cats are frequently obese, usually young, and of either sex. They lose agility, are unwilling to move, and resent palpation of the back or abdomen. In advanced disease, even a light touch causes pain. Fever is a constant finding, and anorexia may be present.

In mink, kits may be affected with steatitis shortly after weaning and, if untreated, losses may continue until pelting time. Signs appear suddenly; the kits may refuse a night feeding and be dead by morning. Affected mink may refuse their feed and show a peculiar, unsteady hop, followed by complete impairment of locomotion and coma. At pelting, survivors show yellow fat deposits and hemoglobinuria.

The typical laboratory finding is an increased WBC count, with neutrophilia and sometimes eosinophilia. Biopsy of the subcutaneous fat shows it to be yellowish brown and firm. Histologic examination reveals severe inflammatory changes and associated ceroid pigment.

The offending excessive fat source must be removed from the diet. Administration of vitamin E, in the form of α-tocopherol, at least 30 mg daily for cats, or 15 mg daily for mink, is necessary. Antibiotics are of doubtful value, despite the fever and leukocytosis. Parenteral use of fluids is not advisable unless dehydration exists. Because of associated pain, affected animals should be handled as little as possible.

LABRADOR RETRIEVER MYOPATHY

(Centronuclear myopathy)

This inherited (autosomal recessive) condition is characterized by a type 2 muscle fiber deficiency and is now called centronuclear myopathy. Clinical signs are seen at <5 mo of age and include skeletal muscle atrophy, stunted growth, ataxia, and weakness. Signs are progressive until the animal reaches maturity, when they stabilize. Animals may have a normal life span. Diagnosis is by creatinuria, muscle biopsy, and electromyography. Histology reveals increased connective tissue around muscle fibers and staining deficiency of type II fibers. Myotonic discharges are seen with electromyography. There is no effective treatment, although warm housing and L-carnitine supplementation may make affected dogs more comfortable. This condition has different clinical features than exercised-induced collapse in Labrador Retrievers.

GREAT DANE MYOPATHY

Inherited myopathy of Great Danes is a noninflammatory condition of young Great Danes. Affected dogs have been identified in England, Australia, and Canada. An autosomal recessive mode of inheritance is suspected. Clinical signs include exercise-induced tremors, weakness, and muscle wasting. CK activity is usually increased, fibrillation potentials are detected in skeletal muscles, and histopathology reveals a central core myopathy. Treatment is supportive, at best.

FIBROTIC MYOPATHY

Fibrotic myopathy is a chronic, progressive, idiopathic, degenerative disorder affecting the semitendinosus, gracilis, quadriceps, infraspinatus, and supraspinatus muscles, primarily in dogs. The cause is unknown. Affected muscles are characterized by contracture and fibrosis. Normal tissues are replaced by dense collagenous connective tissue. Clinical signs include a nonpainful, mechanical lameness. Neurologic function is normal. Surgical release of affected tissues via tenotomy, myotenotomy, Z-plasty, or complete resection produces inconsistent results. Prognosis is guarded because of recurrence.

MYOSITIS OSSIFICANS

Myositis ossificans is an idiopathic non-neoplastic form of heterotopic ossification of fibrous connective tissue and muscle that frequently affects tissues near the hip joint in Doberman Pinschers. It may be related to a bleeding disorder (von Willebrand disease) in these dogs. Surgical resection of the mineralized mass is usually rewarding.

POLYMYOSITIS

Polymyositis is a systemic, noninfectious, possibly immune-mediated, inflammatory muscle disorder in adult dogs. It may be acute or chronic and progressive. Clinical signs include depression, lethargy, weakness, weight loss, lameness, myalgia, and muscle atrophy. CK may be increased, and electromyography reveals abnormal spontaneous muscle activity. Muscle biopsy reveals myonecrosis, lymphocytic-plasmacytic perimuscular infiltration, phagocytosis, and fiber regeneration. Polymyositis may be associated with megaesophagus and immune-mediated disorders (myasthenia gravis, lupus erythematosus, polyarthritis). Oral corticosteroids (1–2 mg/kg, bid for 3–4 wk) are the treatment of choice; other immunosuppressive agents such as azathioprine or cyclophosphamide can also be used. Prognosis is favorable, although relapses are not uncommon.

MASTICATORY MYOSITIS

(Eosinophilic myositis)

Masticatory myositis is an immune-mediated, inflammatory condition that affects the muscles of mastication. The exact cause is unknown. Specific autoantibodies directed against type II muscle fibers have been detected in affected animals. In acute cases, muscles are swollen, and there is difficulty in opening the jaw. In chronic cases, there is anorexia, weight loss, difficulty in opening the jaw, and muscle atrophy. Diagnostic hematologic values include eosinophilia and increased levels of globulin and muscle enzymes. Electromyography reveals abnormal spontaneous electrical activity in affected muscles. A biopsy sample of the temporalis muscle is usually taken; histologic changes include lymphocytic-plasmacytic cellular infiltrates, muscle atrophy, and fibrosis. Although spontaneous regression can occur, prednisone treatment, on a decreasing dosage schedule (2 mg/kg/day for 2 wk, then 1 mg/kg/day for 2 wk, then 0.5 mg/kg/day for 1 mo) is usually effective. Relapses are common, and long-term (6–8 mo) medication may be required.

FELINE HYPOKALEMIC POLYMYOPATHY

Feline hypokalemic polymyopathy is a generalized metabolic muscle weakness disorder in cats secondary to hypokalemia associated with excessive urinary depletion or inadequate dietary intake. Extracellular hypokalemia causes muscle cell membrane hyperpolarization and secondary excessive permeability to sodium. This leads to hypopolarization of the muscle cell and subsequent weakness.

Clinical signs include generalized weakness, ventroflexion of the neck, abnormal gait, anorexia, and muscle pain. The neurologic examination is normal. Serum chemistries reveal hypokalemia (<3.5 mEq/L) and increased creatinine and CK. The urine has a low specific gravity, and potassium excretion is increased. Treatment is by potassium supplementation, given PO (5–8 mEq/day) or IV in cats with profound hypokalemia. Prognosis is excellent with early diagnosis and treatment.

MALIGNANT HYPERTHERMIA

Malignant hyperthermia (*see* p 1027) is a hypermetabolic disorder of skeletal muscle characterized by catabolism and contracture, usually secondary to inhalant anesthetic agents and stress. It is seen most frequently in heavily muscled dogs. Abnormal calcium regulation, glycogenolysis, and contractile protein activity result in production of heat, CO_2, and lactic acid.

Clinical signs include tachycardia, tachypnea, pyrexia, muscle rigidity, and cardiopulmonary failure. Signs develop 5–30 min after exposure to the anesthetic agent. Treatment consists of immediate cessation of anesthesia and hyperventilation with oxygen. IV fluid therapy, corticosteroids, and ice packs are also used. Dantrolene, a muscle relaxant, may be given at 2–5 mg/kg, IV. Prognosis is poor in severe cases. Urinary output, serum potassium levels, and cardiac function should be monitored.

EXERTIONAL MYOPATHY

(Rhabdomyolysis, Tying-up, Monday morning disease)

This acute exertional myopathy of racing Greyhounds and working dogs is characterized by muscle ischemia secondary to exercise or excitement. Avascularity and lactic acidosis cause muscular lysis, myoglobin release, and a nephropathy.

Clinical signs include muscle pain and swelling 24–72 hr after racing. Severe cases are characterized by stiffness, hyperpnea, collapse, myoglobinemia, and acute renal failure. Urinalysis reveals myoglobinuria; serum potassium, phosphorus, and muscle enzymes are increased. Treatment includes supportive care such as IV fluids, bicarbonate, body cooling, rest, and muscle relaxants (eg, diazepam). Prognosis depends on severity. (*See also* EXERTIONAL MYOPATHIES IN HORSES, p 1178.)

MUSCULAR TRAUMA

Infraspinatus Contracture: Infraspinatus contracture is a uni- or bilateral fibrotic myopathy of the infraspinatus muscle that is usually secondary to trauma in hunting or working dogs. Clinical signs include an acute lameness, pain, and swelling in the shoulder region. The lameness subsides, but a gait abnormality develops 2–4 wk after injury as muscle fibrosis and contracture progress. Clinical signs include a characteristic adduction of the elbow, abduction of the foreleg, and external rotation of the carpus and paw. The limb is circumducted with each stride of the leg. Palpation of the shoulders reveals outward rotation of the humerus as the elbow is flexed. Treatment consists of resection of the fibrous musculotendinous portion of the muscle, including tenotomy of the tendon of insertion. Limb and joint functions are immediately improved, and prognosis for full recovery is excellent.

Tenosynovitis of the Biceps Brachii Tendon: This inflammation of the biceps brachii tendon of origin and associated synovial sheath can be uni- or bilateral. It usually affects mature, large dogs. The mechanism of injury can be direct, indirect, overuse, or migration of osteochondral fragments ("joint mice") from humeral osteochondrosis lesions.

Clinical signs include a progressive or chronic, intermittent lameness that worsens after exercise and improves with rest. The range of motion of the shoulder joint is reduced, and atrophy of the shoulder muscles may be apparent. Acute pain can be elicited by applying digital pressure to the biceps tendon during flexion and extension of the shoulder joint.

Diagnosis can be confirmed by ultrasonography or arthroscopy of the damaged tendon. Radiography can reveal dystrophic calcification of the tendon, osteophytes in the intertubercular groove, or mineralized fragments within the tendon sheath. Contrast arthrography may demonstrate filling defects and irregularities of the synovial sheath. Arthrocentesis may be inconclusive. Diagnosis can also be made by exploration of the tendon and associated sheath.

Acute, mild cases can be treated with rest and oral NSAID and opioids. Acute, severe cases can be treated with intralesional injections of methylprednisolone acetate (20–40 mg) and rest. Chronic cases refractory to multiple corticosteroid injections or cases involving identifiable tendon defects or tears, or "joint mice," are treated by tenodesis (resection and attachment of the tendon to the proximal humerus) and osteochondral fragment removal. Arthroscopic-guided tendon resection has also been described. Prognosis for recovery is good.

Quadriceps Contracture (Quadriceps Tie-down, Stiff Stifle Disease): This serious fibrosis and contracture of the quadriceps muscles develops secondary to distal femoral fractures, inadequate surgical repair, and excessive dissection in young dogs. Adhesions develop between the bone, periosteal tissue, and quadriceps muscles, which lead to limb extension, disuse, osteoporosis, degenerative joint disease, and bone and joint deformations. Clinical signs include hyperextension and cranial displacement of the affected limb. Surgery is usually required to resect fibrous tissues and increase motion of the stifle joint. Bone and soft-tissue reconstructions along with postoperative flexion bandages and physical therapy are required to recover limb function. Prognosis is guarded. Prevention of the condition by accurate, biologic stable repairs of bone fractures is preferred.

Achilles Tendon Disruption (Dropped Hock): This acute, traumatic injury to the common calcaneal tendon (gastrocnemius, superficial digital flexor, biceps femoris, semitendinosus, and gracilis muscle tendons) is seen primarily in mature working and athletic dogs. The common tendon can be ruptured or avulsed from the tuber calcanei of the talus. Ruptures may be partial or complete, and the gastrocnemius tendon component is most frequently affected. Clinical signs include a severe nonweight-bearing lameness, tarsal hyperflexion, and a plantigrade stance. Palpation reveals swelling, pain, and torn or fibrotic tendon ends. Radiography may reveal avulsed bone fragments. Treatment is by surgical repair of torn ends and reattachment of tendinous tissue to the tuber calcanei. External splints or fixators should be used to protect the repair for 4 wk. Prognosis is variable and based on chronicity of the injury, success of the surgery, and expected performance of the dog.

Iliopsoas Muscle Trauma: Trauma to the iliopsoas muscle or tendon of insertion can cause an acute or chronic lameness in active dogs. Physical examination reveals focal pain at the proximal medial aspect of the thigh (attachment of tendon to the lesser trochanter), especially during simultaneous hip joint extension and internal rotation. Ultrasonography reveals disruption of muscle fibers, and radiography may reveal dystrophic calcifications at the region of tendon insertion. Treatment with rest and NSAIDs is helpful.

MUSCLE TUMORS

Primary skeletal muscle tumors can be benign (rhabdomyoma) or malignant (rhabdomyosarcoma). Secondary tumors involved with metastatic spread include lymphosarcoma, hemangiosarcoma, and adenocarcinomas. Local tumors (fibrosarcoma, osteosarcoma, mast cell tumors) can invade adjacent muscle. Lipomas can also invade intermuscular tissue spaces.

Clinical signs include localized swelling and lameness. Diagnosis is confirmed by biopsy and histologic evaluation of the samples. Treatment is by surgical excision or limb amputation; chemotherapy and radiation may be used depending on the tumor type.

OSTEOPATHIES IN SMALL ANIMALS

Osteopathies can be developmental, infectious (osteomyelitis), idiopathic (eg, hypertrophic osteopathy), nutritional, neoplastic, or traumatic.

DEVELOPMENTAL OSTEOPATHIES

Angular Deformity of the Forelimb

(Radial and ulnar dysplasia)

Abnormal development of the radius and ulna can occur secondary to distal (radial, ulnar) or proximal (radial) physeal injury or hereditary breed characteristics (Bulldogs, Pugs, Boston Terriers, Basset Hounds, Dachshunds). Asynchronous growth of the two bones leads to shortened limbs, cranial bowing of the bones, elbow joint subluxation, and valgus or varus deformities in the carpus.

Clinical signs include lameness and reduced painful motion in the elbow or carpal joints. Radiography reveals the bone deformations and closed physes.

Treatment is based on correcting angulation and length of the limb and reestablishing joint congruity. Surgical procedures include corrective osteotomy and stabilization with internal or external implants and tension-releasing osteotomies. Prognosis is good for animals without severe limb deformations.

Craniomandibular Osteopathy

Craniomandibular osteopathy is a non-neoplastic, proliferative bone disorder of growing dogs that affects the mandible and tympanic bullae of Terrier breeds. The cause is unknown, but a genetic basis is suspected. The bone lesion is characterized by cyclical resorption of normal bone and replacement by immature bone along endosteal and periosteal surfaces.

Clinical signs vary in severity and include oral discomfort, weight loss, fever, and painful palpable enlargement of the mandible. Radiography reveals bilateral bone proliferation in the mandibles and tympanic bullae.

Therapy is symptomatic and consists of NSAIDs, opioids, or corticosteroids to reduce inflammation and discomfort, along with a soft-food diet. Prognosis is good with mild bone proliferation and animal maturation.

Hypertrophic Osteodystrophy

(Metaphyseal osteopathy)

Hypertrophic osteodystrophy is a developmental disorder of the metaphyses in long bones of young, growing dogs, usually of a large or giant breed. The exact etiology is unknown. The pathophysiology is based on metaphyseal vascular impairment, leading to a failure in ossification and to trabecular necrosis and inflammation.

Clinical signs include bilateral metaphyseal pain and swelling in the distal radius and ulna, fever, anorexia, and depression. Clinical signs may be periodic. Angular limb deformities may develop in severely affected dogs. Radiography reveals metaphyseal bone lucencies and circumferential periosteal bone formation.

Therapy is symptomatic and aimed at relieving pain (eg, NSAIDs, opioids), reducing dietary supplementation, and providing supportive fluid care. Treatment with corticosteroids (prednisone 0.5 mg/lb, PO, bid for 5 days, then tapered as needed) may be superior to treatment with NSAIDs in Weimaraners.

Multiple Cartilaginous Exostoses

(Osteochondromatosis)

Multiple cartilaginous exostoses is a proliferative disease of young dogs and cats characterized by multiple ossified protuberances arising from metaphyseal cortical surfaces of the long bones, vertebrae, and ribs. The exact etiology is unknown, but hereditary (in dogs) and viral (in cats) causes are suspected. Animals may be asymptomatic, and diagnosis is confirmed by palpation and radiography. Surgical excision of the masses is recommended if clinical signs such as lameness or pain develop.

Panosteitis

Panosteitis is a spontaneous, self-limiting disease of young, rapidly growing large and giant dogs that primarily affects the diaphyses and metaphyses of long bone. The exact etiology is unknown, although genetics (in German Shepherds), stress, infection, and metabolic or autoimmune causes have been suspected. The pathophysiology of the disease is characterized by intramedullary fat necrosis, excessive osteoid production, and vascular congestion. Endosteal and periosteal bone reactions occur.

Clinical signs are acute and cyclical and involve single or multiple bone(s) in dogs 6–16 mo old. Animals are lame, febrile, inappetent, and have palpable long bone pain. Radiography reveals increased multifocal intramedullary densities and irregular endosteal surfaces along long bones. Therapy is aimed at relieving pain and discomfort; oral NSAIDs and opioids can be used during periods of illness. Excessive dietary supplementation in young, growing dogs should be avoided.

Retained Ulnar Cartilage Cores

Retained ulnar cartilage cores is a developmental disorder of the distal ulnar physis in young, large, and giant dogs characterized by abnormal endochondral ossification. As a result, progressive physeal calcification ceases, and forelimb bone growth is restrained. The exact etiology is unknown, although dietary causes are suspected.

Clinical signs include lameness and angular limb deformities. Radiography reveals a radiolucent cartilage core in the center of the distal ulnar physis. Treatments include cessation of dietary supplements and osteotomy or ostectomies of the bone to reduce limb deformation. Prognosis is based on severity of the condition.

Scottish Fold Osteodystrophy

This heritable condition of Scottish Fold cats is characterized by skeletal deformations of the vertebrae, metacarpal and metatarsal bones, and phalanges secondary to abnormal endochondral ossification. Affected cats are lame, and affected bones are deformed and swollen. Treatment is by removal of exostoses. Prognosis is guarded.

OSTEOMYELITIS

Inflammation and infection of the medullary cavity, cortex, and periosteum of bone are most frequently associated with bacteria such as *Staphylococcus* spp, *Streptococcus* spp, *Escherichia coli*, *Proteus* spp,

Pasteurella spp, *Pseudomonas* spp, and *Brucella canis*. Anaerobic bacteria are less frequently isolated and may be part of a polymicrobial infection. Fungal diseases are based on geographic distributions and include *Coccidioides immitis* (southwestern USA), *Blastomyces dermatitidis* (southeastern USA), *Histoplasma capsulatum* (central USA), *Cryptococcus neoformans*, and *Aspergillus* spp (worldwide). Factors contributing to infection include ischemia, trauma, focal inflammation, bone necrosis, and hematogenous spread.

Clinical signs may be acute or chronic. Animals may have lameness, pain, abscessation at the wound site, fever, anorexia, and depression. Radiography can reveal bone lysis, sequestration, irregular periosteal reaction, loosening of implants, and fistulous tracts. Deep fine-needle aspiration, cytology, and blood cultures may also reveal evidence of infection.

Treatment includes both medical and surgical therapies. Long-term oral or injectable antibiotics such as clavulanic acid/amoxicillin (15 mg/kg, bid), cefazolin (30 mg/kg, bid), clindamycin (11 mg/kg, bid), enrofloxacin (15 mg/kg, bid), amikacin (15 mg/kg, bid), or oxacillin (22 mg/kg, tid) are used. Additionally, wound debridement, lavage, and removal of loose implants are recommended. Open or closed wound drainage and delayed autogenous, cancellous bone grafting can also be performed. In chronic, refractory cases, limb amputation may be warranted. Prognosis is variable and based on the severity and chronicity of the infection. Appropriate antimicrobial therapy based on bacterial culture and antibiotic sensitivity testing is mandatory for successful results.

HYPERTROPHIC OSTEOPATHY

Hypertrophic osteopathy is a diffuse periosteal proliferative condition of long bones in dogs secondary to neoplastic or infectious masses in the thoracic or abdominal cavity. The exact pathogenic mechanism is unknown, but periosteal vascularity is reduced.

Clinical signs include lameness, long-bone pain, and signs secondary to body cavity masses. Radiography reveals the primary masses and peripheral bone reactions.

Treatment includes thoracic or abdominal surgery to remove masses and unilateral vagotomy to block the neurovascular reflex associated with bone changes.

NUTRITIONAL OSTEOPATHIES

See also DYSTROPHIES ASSOCIATED WITH CALCIUM, PHOSPHORUS, AND VITAMIN D, p 1050.
Reduced bone mass, bone deformities, exostoses, pathologic fractures, and loose teeth (rubber jaw) are skeletal manifestations of nutritional derangements that affect parathyroid hormone function and calcium and vitamin metabolism. Specific causes such as secondary nutritional or renal hyperparathyroidism, hypovitaminosis D, and hypervitaminosis A can produce lameness. Diagnosis is by serum chemistry analyses, radiography, and identification of underlying nutritional deficiencies. Treatment is aimed at reversing the specific etiology. Surgery is rarely indicated.

BONE TUMORS

Skeletal tumors can be benign or malignant and primary or secondary to metastases or adjacent soft-tissue structures. The most common primary bone tumor is osteosarcoma that affects the distal radius, proximal humerus, distal femur, or proximal tibia.

Clinical signs include lameness, bone swelling, and an acute, nontraumatic pathologic fracture of the bone. Radiography reveals osteolysis, proliferation, and soft-tissue swelling; thoracic radiographs should be performed to delineate metastatic masses. Bone biopsy using a Michelle bone trephine or Jamshidi biopsy needle is imperative in confirming the diagnosis. Less frequently identified tumors include chondrosarcoma, fibrosarcoma, and hemangiosarcoma. Treatment includes limb amputation and chemotherapy with carboplatin, cisplatin, or doxorubicin. Palliative care to reduce pain and discomfort can be provided with oral NSAIDs, opioids, transdermal patches, or radiation therapy. Prognosis is guarded. Untreated animals rarely live more than several months. Amputation and chemotherapy may double the survival times. Median survival times after amputation are 5 mo in dogs and 4 yr in cats. Advanced procedures such as limb sparing and excision of metastases can also (infrequently) be performed.

BONE TRAUMA

Bone fractures are frequently caused by vehicular accidents, firearms, fights, or falls. Fractures can be open or closed and involve single or multiple bones. Characteristics of the fracture—such as simple, comminuted, oblique, transverse, or spiral—are based on disruptive trauma forces (bending, compression, tension, and rotation).

Clinical signs invariably include lameness, pain, and swelling. Radiography is useful in delineating the fracture pattern. Treatments are based on the type of fracture, age and health of the animal, technical expertise of the surgeon, and owner finances.

Young, healthy dogs with incomplete fractures can be treated with external splints or casts. Other injuries are treated with external (fixators) or internal devices, such as bone plates, screws, orthopedic wires, interlocking nails, and pins. Frequently, cancellous bone grafts are used to augment fracture healing in ill or aged patients. Antibiotics are given for open fractures or prolonged repairs. Perioperative analgesics (eg, epidural morphine, narcotic skin patches, systemic narcotics [including constant-rate infusion], oral NSAIDs) are used to alleviate discomfort. Physical therapy or rehabilitation is critical to restore limb function and overall well-being.

Prognosis for recovery is usually good, depending on the nature of the injury and success of repairs; successful wound therapy and monitoring of cardiopulmonary and urologic functions are essential. Followup care includes radiographic and clinical assessments of fracture healing. Internal implants may not need to be removed unless complications such as stress protection, infection, or soft-tissue irritation develop.

NERVOUS SYSTEM

NEF

PARASITIC DISEASES

NERVOUS SYSTEM INTRODUCTION

The nervous system is composed of billions of neurons with long, interconnecting processes that form complex integrated electrochemical circuits. It is through these neuronal circuits that animals experience sensations and respond appropriately.

Neuronal processes that transmit electrical alterations to the neuron cell body are called **dendrites**. Dendrites have receptor sites that receive stimulation or inhibition from outside sources. If electrical stimulation of the cell body reaches a critical threshold, an electrical discharge called an **action potential** develops. The action potential spontaneously travels away from the cell body along an outgoing process called an **axon**. When the action potential reaches the terminal branches of the axon, chemicals called **neurotransmitters** are released. Neurotransmitters either stimulate or inhibit receptor sites on other neurons, muscles, or glands. Although neurons may have a variety of shapes, each one has dendrites, a cell body, and an axon and releases neurotransmitters.

Basic Sensory and Motor Functions

The peripheral nervous system (PNS) is formed by neurons of the cranial and spinal nerves. The central nervous system (CNS) is formed by neurons of the spinal cord, brain stem, cerebellum, and cerebrum.

Groups of neuronal cell bodies in the PNS are called ganglia, whereas those in the CNS are called nuclei. Nuclei form the CNS gray matter. Groups of axons in the CNS form the white matter and are arranged into tracts. The tracts are usually named after their site of origin and termination (eg, the spinocerebellar tract begins in the spinal cord and ends in the cerebellum).

PNS sensory or afferent neurons carry information such as nociception, proprioception, touch, temperature, taste, hearing, equilibrium, vision, and olfaction to the spinal cord or brain stem. CNS sensory neurons carry information to the cerebellum, brain stem, and cerebrum for further interpretation. Important spinal cord and brain-stem sensory tracts include several spinocerebellar, spinothalamic, and spinoreticular tract systems. The spinoreticular tracts begin in the spinal cord and terminate in the reticular formation of the medulla. The dorsal fasciculi gracilis and cuneatus of the spinal cord and the medial and lateral lemniscus of the brain stem are also important sensory tracts. In animals, these sensory tracts may carry fibers from many sensory modalities such as proprioception, nociception (pain), and touch. An alteration in sensation may be due to either CNS or PNS disease.

Reactions to sensory inputs are initiated by efferent or motor neurons in the cerebrum and brain stem called **upper motor neurons** (UMNs). The UMN axons descend to brain-stem and spinal cord segments in tracts named after their site of origination and termination.

The UMNs of the reticulospinal tracts (from midbrain, pons, and medulla oblongata reticular formation) and the rubrospinal tract (from midbrain) are important for voluntary movements of skeletal muscles in domestic animals. The rubrospinal tract mainly functions to facilitate flexors of the limbs, whereas the pontine and medullary reticulospinal tracts have either a facilitative (pontine) or inhibitory (medullary) effect on the extensors. The corticospinal tracts (cell bodies in the cerebral cortex) are most important for voluntary movement in primates. Domestic animals with severe cerebrocortical disease may suffer only transient loss of voluntary movements, because their corticospinal tract has limited influence.

The pontine reticulospinal (from the pons) and vestibulospinal (from vestibular nuclei of the medulla oblongata) tracts facilitate extensor skeletal muscle activity used to support the body. Knowledge of location and function of sensory and motor brain-stem and spinal tracts is essential to localize nervous system lesions and determine their severity. Mild spinal cord compression affects the superficial spinal cord tracts (fasciculus gracilus, cuneatus, spinocerebellar, and vestibulospinal tracts), so initial signs include ataxia and extensor weakness. Important voluntary motor tracts are located in the lateral portions of the spinal cord deep to the spinocerebellar tracts, and paresis or paralysis develops with moderate spinal cord compression. Because many tracts are involved, loss of nociception from the periosteum of the toes and tail (deep pain) occurs when spinal cord lesions are bilateral and severe. This loss of nociception is also an indicator of severe cord injury because those fibers that transmit deep pain are typically nonmyelinated, slow-transmitting C type fibers, which are very resistant to pressure.

Motor neurons with cell bodies in the brain stem, and spinal cord gray matter and axons that travel in the PNS cranial and spinal nerves, respectively, are referred to as **lower motor neurons** (LMNs). Injury to either the UMNs or LMNs results in paresis or paralysis. Brain-stem and spinal cord reflexes are the phylogenetically oldest responses of the nervous system. When the eyelid is touched, it closes; when the toe is pinched, the limb withdraws even before conscious perception intervenes. Only a sensory neuron in the PNS, a connector (internuncial) neuron in the CNS, and an LMN are necessary for a reflex to be present. In a monosynaptic reflex (eg, patellar reflex), only a sensory neuron and LMN are present. During the neurologic examination (*see* p 1213), testing brain-stem and spinal reflexes is helpful to localize CNS and PNS lesions to specific areas. If a reflex is depressed or absent, a lesion must involve the sensory nerve, internuncial neuron, LMN, or muscle at that particular site.

The autonomic nervous system is divided into sympathetic and parasympathetic portions and controls activity in smooth and cardiac muscles and glands. Visceral afferent (sensory) neurons travel in cranial and spinal nerves and sensory spinal cord tracts to the thalamic and hypothalamic regions of the brain stem. UMNs in the hypothalamus descend to LMN cell bodies of the brain-stem nuclei and sacral segments for parasympathetic control and to the intermediolateral gray matter of the spinal cord for sympathetic control.

LMNs of the sympathetic nervous system exit through thoracolumbar spinal nerves (T1 to L4) to affect smooth muscles associated with the pupils, eyelids, orbits, hair follicles, blood vessels, and thoracic and abdominal viscera. **Horner syndrome** (ptosis, miosis, and enophthalmos) is a common finding associated with loss of sympathetic innervation to the eye.

LMNs of the parasympathetic nervous system exit via cranial nerve (CN) III to innervate smooth muscle of the pupils and eyelids, CN VII to the lacrimal and salivary glands, CN IX to salivary glands, and CN X to cardiac muscles and glands and to smooth muscles of all the thoracic and abdominal viscera to the level of the transverse colon. LMNs of the parasympathetic nervous system also exit through the sacral segments to all the viscera in the caudal abdomen, including the bladder and colon. Sacral lesions commonly result in loss of the urinary bladder (detruser) reflex.

Divisions and Effects of Lesions

See also THE NEUROLOGIC EVALUATION, p 1213.
The PNS consists of 26 or more pairs of spinal nerves that correspond to each spinal cord segment and 12 pairs of cranial nerves that correspond to specific brain and brain-stem segments.

The PNS spinal nerves form the brachial plexus to the thoracic limb; the lumbosacral plexus to the pelvic limb; and the cauda equina to the bladder, anus, and tail. Brachial or lumbosacral plexus lesions cause paresis or paralysis of a thoracic or pelvic limb, respectively, with reduced or absent spinal reflexes and reduced or absent sensation of the limb. (*See also* LIMB PARALYSIS, p 1259.) Cauda equina lesions result in an atonic bladder; a dilated, unresponsive anus; and a flaccid, paralyzed tail.

Lesions of all spinal nerves (eg, acute polyradiculoneuritis) result in paresis or paralysis of all four limbs (quadriparesis or quadriplegia, respectively) with depressed or absent spinal reflexes and altered sensation of the limbs. Lesions restricted to PNS cranial nerves result in deficits associated with dysfunction of that particular nerve and no signs of dysfunction in the limbs or other parts of the nervous system.

The spinal cord of dogs and cats is divided into 8 cervical, 13 thoracic, 7 lumbar, 3 sacral, and 5 or more caudal segments. Horses and cows have 6 lumbar and 5 sacral segments, and pigs have 6–7 lumbar and 4 sacral segments. Spinal cord lesions from L4 to S2 cause pelvic limb ataxia, conscious proprioceptive deficits, and paresis or paralysis with depressed or absent spinal reflexes and muscle tone (LMN signs). Sensation may also be depressed or absent below the lesion. Lesions from T3 to L3 cause pelvic limb ataxia, conscious proprioceptive deficits, and paresis and paralysis with normal or exaggerated spinal reflexes (UMN signs). Pelvic limb sensation caudal to the lesion may also be depressed or absent. With spinal cord lesions extending from C6 to T2, thoracic limb spinal reflexes may be depressed or absent, and severe lesions may cause quadriplegia. The spinal reflexes remain intact in the pelvic limbs, but sensation may be affected.

Spinal cord lesions from C1 to C5 cause hemiparesis or hemiplegia (paresis or paralysis of the limbs on one side), or quadriparesis. Spinal reflexes in all four limbs are often preserved. Severe lesions may cause respiratory distress or arrest due to involvement of the UMNs to respiratory muscles in the C5 area.

The brain stem is divided from caudal to rostral into four segments: the medulla oblongata (myelencephalon), the pons (metencephalon), the midbrain (mesencephalon), and the thalamus and hypothalamus (diencephalon).

Similar to lesions of the cervical spinal cord, lesions of the medulla oblongata cause conscious proprioceptive deficits and weakness on the same side (ipsilateral) or both sides with normal or hyperactive limb reflexes. However, involvement of CN nuclei IX, X, XI, or XII localizes the lesion to the caudal medulla oblongata. Involvement of CN nuclei VI, VII, or VIII localizes the lesion to the rostral medulla oblongata. It is rare to have a lesion of the medulla oblongata that does not affect one or more of the cranial nerves as well as sensory and motor tracts.

Pontine lesions cause ipsilateral conscious proprioceptive deficits, hemiparesis or quadriparesis with normal or hyperactive limb reflexes, mental depression from involvement of the ascending reticular activating system (ARAS), and CN V and IV deficits.

The cerebellum is part of the metencephalon and is attached to the dorsal surface of the pons and medulla by rostral, middle, and caudal cerebellar peduncles. The cerebellum coordinates all muscle activity and establishes muscle tone. The flocculonodular lobe of the cerebellum has equilibrium functions and is considered part of the vestibular system. Unilateral lesions of the cerebellum cause ipsilateral dysmetria (hypermetria or hypometria) and a contralateral (paradoxical) head tilt. Bilateral lesions of the cerebellum cause generalized incoordination of the head and limbs, head tremors (intention tremors), and generalized dysequilibrium.

Midbrain (mesencephalon) lesions cause contralateral conscious proprioceptive deficits and hemiparesis. CN III nucleus involvement is present on the ipsilateral side and localizes the lesion to the midbrain. In large, midbrain lesions, the ARAS is affected, and the animal will be stuporous or comatose. If the sympathetic UMNs and parasympathetic LMNs are both affected in the midbrain, the pupils will be midrange size and unresponsive to light.

Diencephalic lesions can be difficult to differentiate from cerebral cortical lesions, because many tracts going to and from the cerebrum pass through the diencephalon by way of the internal capsule. The thalamus, hypothalamus, and subthalamus of the diencephalon have many important structures that alter feeding, drinking, breeding, sleeping, and other behaviors, as well as regulate body temperature. The pituitary gland, which controls many hormonal functions of the body, is connected to the hypothalamus. The ARAS projects through the subthalamus area, in which lesions also produce stupor or coma.

The telencephalon, also called the cerebral cortex, is divided into the neocortex, paleocortex, and archicortex. The paleocortex and archicortex include the olfactory and limbic regions, which provide smell and emotional reactions to all stimuli. The neocortex is divided into the frontal, parietal, occipital, and temporal lobes. The frontal cortex functions include intelligence and fine motor skills (corticospinal tract). Lesions in this area cause dementia, lack of recognition of the owner, difficulty in training, compulsive pacing, circling toward the side of the lesion (adversion syndrome), and motor seizures with contralateral involuntary muscle twitching. Contralateral hopping and placing deficits are also found with frontal lobe lesions. Ascending and descending tracts to and from the frontal lobe form the internal capsule through the region of the basal nuclei and diencephalon. Lesions of the internal capsule can produce the same signs as frontal lobe lesions. The parietal lobe (somesthetic cortex) is for interpretation of general perception, nociception, temperature, and pressure; lesions result in proprioceptive deficits on the contralateral side of the body.

Occipital lobe and optic radiation lesions result in blindness with pupils that respond normally to light. Unilateral occipital lobe and optic radiation lesions result in some degree of visual loss in the contralateral eye, depending on the percentage of crossover of the optic nerve fibers in the optic chiasm of the species (65% in cats; 75% in dogs; 80%–90% in cattle, horses, pigs, and sheep). The pupils still respond normally to light. Blindness with pupils that do not respond to light is associated with lesions of the retina, optic nerve, optic chiasm, or rostral optic tract.

Difficulty in localizing sound is hard to evaluate clinically. It may occur with temporal lobe lesions, as may psychomotor seizures characterized by hysterical running. "Fly-biting" or "star gazing" hallucinations are suspected to occur with lesions in the temporal-occipital region. Aggression occurs when the pyriform area (paleocortex) of the temporal lobe and the underlying amygdaloid nucleus are affected. Aggression can also occur with hypothalamic lesions.

Lesions of the olfactory region may alter feeding or breeding behavior. Slow-growing lesions of the cerebrum and diencephalon often result in few clinical signs because of the adaptability of functions in these areas in animals.

Mechanisms of Disease

Disease processes affecting the nervous system may be congenital or familial, infectious or inflammatory, toxic, metabolic, nutritional, traumatic, vascular, degenerative, neoplastic, or idiopathic.

Congenital disorders may be obvious at birth or shortly after (eg, an enlarged head from hydrocephalus or an uncoordinated gait from an underdeveloped cerebellum). Some familial disorders (eg, lysosomal storage diseases) cause a progressive degeneration of neurons in the first year of life, whereas others (eg, inherited epilepsy) may not manifest for 2–3 yr. (*See also* CONGENITAL AND INHERITED ANOMALIES OF THE NERVOUS SYSTEM, p 1222.)

Infections of the nervous system are due to specific viruses, fungi, protozoa, bacteria, rickettsia, prions, and algae. Noninfectious inflammations such as steroid-responsive meningoencephalomyelitis and meningoencephalomyelitis of unknown etiology (MUE), formerly called granulomatous meningoencephalomyelitis, Pug dog encephalitis, and other CNS inflammatory diseases, may be immune-mediated. Until there is a histologic diagnosis, the term MUE is used.

Toxicity of the nervous system is most frequently caused by organophosphates (*see* p 3064), pyrethrins (*see* p 3063), carbamates (*see* p 3059), bromethalin (*see* p 3167), metaldehyde (*see* p 3070), ethylene glycol (*see* p 3046), metronidazole (*see* p 2696), theobromines (*see* p 2966), sedatives, and anticonvulsants (eg, phenobarbital, bromide). Botulinum, tetanus, and tick toxins, as well as coral and certain other snake venom intoxications, cause neurologic signs.

Metabolic alterations of nervous system function most commonly result from hypoglycemia, hypoxia or anoxia, hepatic dysfunction, hypocalcemia, hypomagnesemia, hypernatremia, hypokalemia, and uremia. Hypothyroidism, hyperthyroidism, hypoadrenocorticism, and hyperadrenocorticism are endocrine disorders that can cause neurologic dysfunction.

Thiamine deficiency results in ataxia, stupor, and coma or seizures in dogs, cats, and cattle. Deficiency of vitamin B_6 may cause seizures.

Trauma to the PNS and CNS causes focal and multifocal neurologic signs from physical damage, hemorrhage, edema, and progressive formation of oxygen-containing free radicals and nervous system destruction that is usually complete in 24–48 hr but lasts as long as 4 days because of the slow influx of inflammatory cells.

Vascular lesions of animals are usually due to septicemia and bacterial embolization of the CNS. Fibrocartilaginous embolization of the spinal cord is common in dogs. Arteriovenous malformations occur occasionally and cause spontaneous hemorrhages. Cerebrovascular disease from arteriosclerosis is rare in domestic animals but has been associated with hypothyroidism caused by hyperlipidemia. Cerebrovascular disease from hypertension is rare but may be seen as multiple cerebral microbleeds with MRI.

Familial degeneration of neurons occurs in lysosomal storage disorders. Degeneration of intervertebral discs that subsequently herniate into the vertebral canal often produces paresis and paralysis in dogs.

Neoplasms of the CNS and PNS are most common in dogs and cats. Astrocytes, oligodendrocytes, and microglia can all become neoplastic and form astrocytomas, oligodendrogliomas, and gliomas. Ependymal cells and the choroid plexus, which line the internal cavities of the CNS and produce CSF, also can become neoplastic and form ependymomas and choroid plexus papillomas. Meningeal cells of the dura, arachnoid, and pial membranes form meningiomas, which are common in dogs and cats. Neurofibrosarcomas are common tumors of the nerve sheaths of peripheral nerves in dogs. Lymphosarcoma is a common metastatic tumor of the PNS and CNS in dogs, cats, and cattle. Hemangiosarcoma is the most common metastatic tumor of the CNS in dogs. (*See also* NEOPLASIA OF THE NERVOUS SYSTEM, p 1267.)

The idiopathic mechanism of disease is reserved for described syndromes with characteristic clinical signs, predictable outcomes, and no known necropsy findings.

THE NEUROLOGIC EVALUATION

An accurate history and thorough physical and neurologic examinations are necessary to evaluate a problem involving the nervous system. An understanding of functional neuroanatomy, neurophysiologic concepts, and mechanisms of disease is a prerequisite for accurate interpretation of clinical findings. Based on the initial clinical assessment, 1) the anatomic location(s) of disease can be determined, and 2) the problem may be defined as diffuse, multifocal, or focal; symmetric or asymmetric; painful or nonpainful; progressive, regressive, waxing and waning, or static; and mild, moderate, or severe. The potential mechanisms of disease must also be considered to determine differential diagnoses. Further diagnostic tests include clinicopathologic tests (on serum, blood, urine, feces, and CSF), diagnostic imaging (including plain and contrast radiography, CT, and MRI), and electrodiagnostic testing.

HISTORY

Neurologic diseases tend to have a species, age, breed, and occasionally a sex predilection. The primary complaints for neurologic problems often include behavioral changes, seizures, tremors, cranial nerve deficits, ataxia, and paresis or paralysis of one or more limbs. Information about the onset, course, and duration of the primary complaint can be used to determine the most probable disease mechanisms. Congenital and familial disorders are most common in purebred animals at birth or within the first few years of life. Inflammatory, infectious, metabolic, toxic, and nutritional disorders can be seen in any species, breed, or age; tend to have an acute or subacute onset; and are usually progressive. Vascular and traumatic disorders have an acute onset and rarely progress after 24 hr. Most degenerative and neoplastic disorders tend to be seen in older animals (except for familial neuronal degeneration) and have a chronic onset and progressive course. Many idiopathic disorders begin acutely and improve throughout a short time. Information about similar familial problems, concurrent or recent systemic disease, vaccination status, other affected animals, diet, possible exposure to toxins or trauma, and past neoplastic disorders may be useful to further support certain mechanisms of disease.

PHYSICAL AND NEUROLOGIC EXAMINATIONS

Evidence of disease in other body systems may be associated with inflammatory, metabolic, toxic, or metastatic neoplastic disorders of the nervous system. Infections of the CNS may not have any signs other than neurologic. External signs of trauma or toxic exposure may support these mechanisms of disease.

The neurologic examination consists of evaluation of the following: 1) the head, 2) the gait, 3) the neck and thoracic limbs, and 4) the trunk, pelvic limbs, anus, and tail. Initially, an attempt should be made to relate all deficits to one focal anatomic lesion.

If abnormalities are found on evaluation of the head, then an initial attempt should be made to explain all limb abnormalities by a lesion above the foramen magnum. If no abnormalities are found on evaluation of the head, but thoracic limb abnormalities are present, then an attempt should be made to explain the abnormalities by a cervical lesion (C1 to T2). Paralysis or paresis of all four limbs with loss of all spinal reflexes (with or without cranial nerve deficits) is often associated with diffuse peripheral nerve or neuromuscular junction disease (*see* p 1238).

Knowledge of specific diseases within a certain mechanism for a given species, age, breed, and sex of animal enables an accurate list of differential diagnoses and a diagnostic plan to be formulated after the history and physical and neurologic examinations are completed. Toxic, metabolic, and nutritional mechanisms rarely produce asymmetric neurologic deficits. The other mechanisms of disease may result in symmetric or asymmetric deficits.

Evaluation of the Head

Mentation, head posture and coordination, and cranial nerve functions are observed during evaluation of the head. Abnormal findings are due to lesions above the level of the foramen magnum in the cerebrum, the brain stem (diencephalon, midbrain, pons, or medulla oblongata), or the cerebellum. Dementia, compulsive pacing, or other behavioral abnormalities and seizures are frequently due to lesions in the cerebrum or diencephalon. Stupor, obtundation, semicoma, or coma may be due to lesions of the cerebrum, diencephalon, or midbrain. A head turn or compulsive circling without a head tilt is also associated with a cerebral or diencephalic lesion on the side toward which the animal turns. A head tilt is due to vestibular system disease (CN VIII, rostral medulla oblongata, or cerebellum). Abnormal head coordination, bobbing, and tremors result from cerebellar dysfunction.

The **cranial nerves** consist of 12 pairs located in specific brain-stem segments; they are simple to test, and test results can help localize disease to that segment. Abnormal findings are produced by lesions of the peripheral cranial nerve or cranial nerve nuclei. If a brain-stem lesion is present, abnormalities are seen in the gait, thoracic or pelvic limbs, and at times mental status. If only a peripheral cranial nerve is affected, there are no changes in gait, the thoracic or pelvic limbs, or mentation. Cranial nerve lesions of one side produce ipsilateral deficits except for lesions of the trochlear nerve (CN IV), which crosses in the midbrain.

I. Olfactory: The olfactory nerves transmit smell.

Tests: The animal's ability to find food or the reaction to chemicals (eg, cloves, benzene, or xylene) should be observed. Substances that irritate the nasal mucosa and the trigeminal nerve endings (eg, alcohol or phenol) should not be used.

Signs of Dysfunction: Inability to find food or respond to nonirritating chemicals is found with disease of the cribriform plate, olfactory bulbs, and olfactory region.

II. Optic: The optic nerves are necessary for vision and also carry the afferent fibers of the pupillary light reflex to the midbrain.

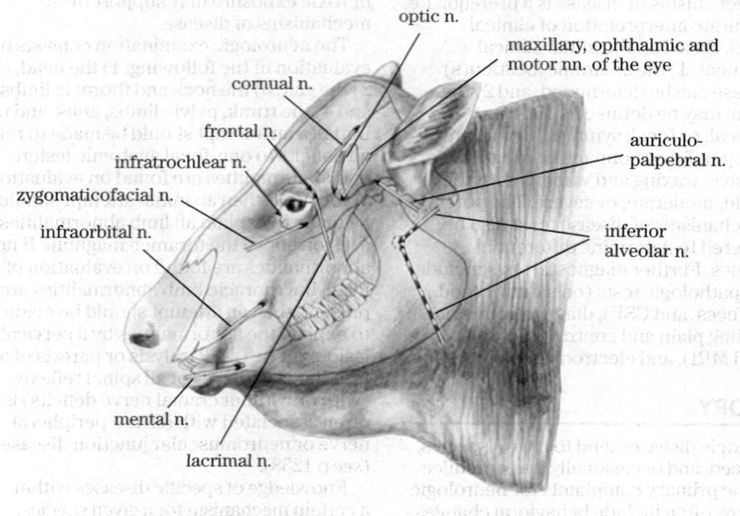

Cranial nerves accessible for nerve block in a bovine head. *Illustration by Dr. Gheorghe Constantinescu.*

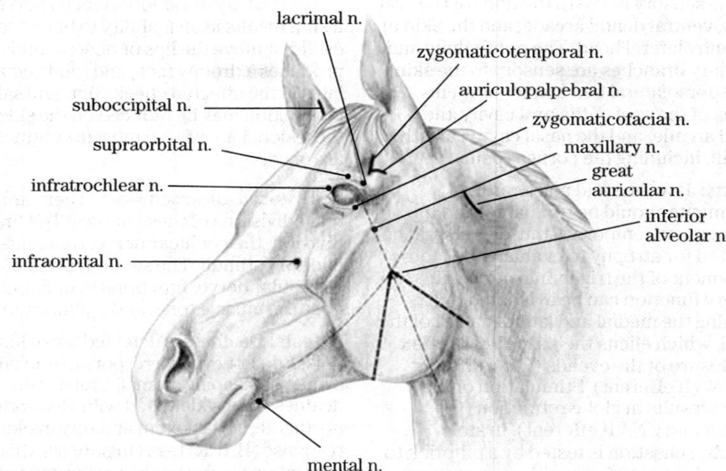

Cranial nerves accessible for nerve block in an equine head. *Illustration by Dr. Gheorghe Constantinescu.*

Visual Tests: Cotton balls can be dropped and the animal observed watching them fall to the floor. The menace response is tested by making a threatening gesture toward each eye, causing the animal to blink. The animal sees the menacing motion (CN II) and blinks the eye (CN VII). In foals and calves this reflex will be evident by 7–10 days of age, whereas in puppies and kittens it may not be present until 10–12 wk. Excessive air currents or touching the eyelashes should be avoided, because this will test response to touch (CN V) rather than vision. Obstacle testing may be necessary when visual acuity is in doubt. It is useful to blindfold one eye at a time to detect blindness of either eye.

Pupillary Light Reflex: A bright focal light is directed into each pupil toward the temporal retina, and the pupil is observed for immediate constriction. The opposite pupil should constrict consensually (a consensual or indirect response) (CN II afferent and CN III efferent).

Ophthalmoscopic Examination: This detects local eye diseases. Chorioretinitis or papilledema may be associated with central or peripheral nervous system diseases. Papilledema is often seen with increased intracranial pressure.

Signs of Dysfunction: Unilateral optic nerve dysfunction results in a decrease or loss of vision and decreased pupillary light reflexes on the affected side. Consensual pupillary constriction of the affected eye should still occur when the other eye is stimulated with light. Unilateral lesions of the optic tract, lateral geniculate nucleus, optic radiation, thalamus, or occipital cortex usually produce a contralateral visual deficit with normal pupillary light reflexes (see above).

III. Oculomotor: These nerves carry efferent parasympathetic fibers from the pupillary light reflex center of the midbrain to the fibers of the ciliary ganglion, which innervate the constrictor muscle of the pupils. They are also efferent to the levator palpebrae muscles; the dorsal, medial, and ventral rectus muscles; and the ventral oblique muscles of the eye.

Tests: The pupillary light reflex test should be performed as described for the optic nerves, and constriction of the pupils to light should be observed. The presence or absence of ptosis of the upper eyelid as well as ventrolateral strabismus should be noted.

IV. Trochlear: These are the motor nerves to the dorsal oblique muscles of the eye.

Test: The eyeballs should be observed for a vertical misalignment (easiest to see in species with a horizontal- or vertical-shaped pupil).

Signs of Dysfunction: Trochlear nerve or midbrain lesions may result in the dorsal aspect of the globe rotating laterally.

V. Trigeminal: These nerves have three branches. The mandibular branch is the motor nerve to the muscles of mastication and the sensory nerve to the floor of the oral cavity, ventral dental arcade, and the skin of the ventrolateral head. The ophthalmic and maxillary branches are sensory to the skin of the dorsolateral head; mucous membranes of the roof of the oral cavity, the dorsal arcade, and the nasal cavity; and the eyeball, including the cornea (pain).

Tests: Jaw tone and masticatory movements should be evaluated, and the masseter and temporalis muscles should be palpated for atrophy to evaluate the motor component of the trigeminal nerve. The sensory function can be evaluated by touching the medial and lateral canthi of the eyelid, which elicits the **palpebral reflex** and closure of the eyelids (CN V afferent and CN VII efferent). Stimulation of the cornea results in globe retraction (CN V afferent and CN VII efferent). In stoic animals, sensation is tested by a pinprick to the nasal mucosa (an avoidance response, turning the head away, will be seen).

Signs of Dysfunction: Lesions of the trigeminal nerves or pons produce temporal and masseter muscle atrophy and/or loss of sensation to the face, cornea, and nasal mucosa. A bilateral lesion of the trigeminal motor nerves produces a dropped jaw.

VI. Abducent: These are the motor nerves to the lateral rectus and retractor bulbi muscles of the eye.

Tests: The eyeballs should be observed for medial strabismus. The corneal reflex should be elicited with the eyelids held open, with the eyeball observed for retraction and the third eyelid observed for prolapse.

Signs of Dysfunction: Lesions of the abducent nerves or rostral medulla oblongata result in medial strabismus and lack of globe retraction.

VII. Facial: These are the motor nerves to the muscles of facial expression (ear, eyelids, nose, and mouth). The sensory part of CN VII is for taste on the rostral third of the tongue. The parasympathetic portion of CN VII innervates the tear glands.

Tests: The menace and palpebral reflexes should be elicited to test orbicularis oculi muscle function. The nose should be examined for deviation (with unilateral lesions). The lip should be pinched to see whether it retracts. The ear should be tickled to see whether it moves. Atropine or another bitter substance may be placed on the distal tongue to test taste. A Schirmer tear test should be performed to evaluate parasympathetic innervation of tear glands.

Signs of Dysfunction: A facial nerve lesion results in an inability to blink the eyelid or move the lips or nose; acutely it produces a droopy face, and food accumulates in the affected cheek. Tear and saliva production may be reduced on the side of the lesion. Later, facial muscle contractures are observed.

VIII. Vestibulocochlear: There are two main divisions of these nerves. The first division, the cochlear nerve, transmits auditory stimuli. The second division, the vestibular nerve, functions to maintain posture, muscle tone, and equilibrium.

Tests: Deafness is detected when loud noises do not evoke a response from an awake or sleeping animal. Unilateral deafness is best detected with electrodiagnostics, ie, a brain-stem auditory evoked response (BAER) test. (In puppies, this evaluation should not be performed before 6 wk of age, because results may be erroneous.) Head tilt, dysequilibrium, and a tendency to circle, fall, or roll to one side develop with unilateral or asymmetric vestibular lesions. The animal should be examined for the presence of spontaneous nystagmus with the head held in a normal position and in a deviated position (positional nystagmus), as well as for abnormal eye position (ventral strabismus) on the affected side when the nose is elevated. Normal vestibular nystagmus (physiologic nystagmus) is seen as a few beats to the left as the head is turned to the left, and to the right as the head is turned to the right.

Signs of Dysfunction: Unilateral lesions of the vestibulocochlear nerves produce dysequilibrium with a head tilt toward the side of the lesion. A spontaneous positional, horizontal, or rotary nystagmus is often present. A positional nystagmus (one in which the character of the nystagmus changes with changes in the animal's position) or a vertical nystagmus are almost always seen with central vestibular disease. A bilateral vestibular lesion results in dysequilibrium on both sides, wide side-to-side excursions of the head (often with no head tilt), loss of normal vestibular nystagmus, and possible deafness. Occasionally, a cerebellar or cerebellar peduncle lesion will result in a head tilt away from the lesion (paradoxical head tilt), but conscious proprioceptive deficits and hemiparesis will be ipsilateral with hypermetria of limbs on the ipsilateral side.

IX. Glossopharyngeal and X. Vagus: The glossopharyngeal and vagus nerves provide sensory and motor control of the pharynx and larynx, and the vagus nerves provide sensory and motor control of the viscera.

Tests: The hyoid bones should be pinched to elicit a gag reflex. The animal should be observed for normal phonation and respiratory sounds.

Signs of Dysfunction: Lesions of the glossopharyngeal and vagus nerves or caudal medulla oblongata result in dysphagia, megaesophagus, or laryngeal paresis or paralysis. A change in phonation also occurs with vagus nerve and nucleus lesions.

XI. Spinal Accessory: These nerves innervate the trapezius, sternocephalic, and brachycephalic muscles.

Tests: The muscles should be palpated.

Signs of Dysfunction: Lesions of the cranial cervical spinal cord or caudal medulla oblongata may result in muscle atrophy. This may be accompanied by weakness when the examiner turns the head away from the side of the lesion.

XII. Hypoglossal: These are the motor nerves to the tongue and geniohyoid muscles.

Tests: The tongue should be observed for muscular control during licking and lapping of water. The tongue curls under to lap water in dogs and cats. In large animals, the tongue may be grasped and pulled side to side to assess its strength.

Signs of Dysfunction: Lesions of the hypoglossal nerves or caudal medulla oblongata may result in deviation or atrophy of the tongue. As with the facial nerve, this deviation of the tongue is at first away from the affected side, then with muscle contracture is toward the affected side.

Evaluation of the Gait

The gait is observed while the animal walks, trots, gallops, turns, sidesteps, and backs up. In large animals, ambulation up and down a grade, on and off a curb, and while blindfolded may accentuate subtle gait deficits. Evaluation of gait is especially important in ambulatory large animals because postural reactions are difficult to obtain because of size and because spinal reflexes usually are not tested unless the animals are recumbent. In small animals, subtle deficits may be detected by postural reaction testing of the limbs (*see* below) and by hemistanding and hemiwalking (standing or walking on one side). Animals with chronic lesions in the cerebral cortex and diencephalon usually have a relatively normal gait but may circle compulsively. Animals with lesions of the midbrain, pons, and medulla oblongata have paresis or paralysis of the limbs, with deficits often more severe on the side of the lesion. Cerebellar lesions produce ataxia and dysmetria. Vestibular dysfunction causes ipsilateral falling, rolling, or circling. If no abnormalities are found on evaluation of the head, but the gait is abnormal, a lesion most likely is located in the spinal cord, peripheral nerves, or muscles.

Evaluation of the Neck and Thoracic Limbs

The neck is examined for pain and, in large animals, atrophy and desensitization to pinprick, which indicate a lesion of the cervical spinal cord. Wheelbarrowing, tonic neck and eye, conscious proprioceptive positioning, placing, hopping, and righting are postural reactions that detect subtle lesions.

Wheelbarrow: The pelvic limbs of small animals are lifted slightly off the ground while keeping body posture as normal as possible, and the animal is evaluated while walking on the thoracic limbs. This test is used to detect subtle deficits of the thoracic limbs. Normal animals should not stumble or knuckle over on the toes as they walk.

Tonic Neck and Eye: With the dog or cat standing, the nose is elevated and the eyes observed to see whether they coordinately adjust to the center of the palpebral fissures. In vestibular dysfunction, the eyeball on the affected side rotates downward (positional strabismus or eye drop). Simultaneously, the thoracic limbs should extend with no tendency to knuckle or collapse, and the pelvic limbs should flex.

Conscious Proprioceptive Positioning: Each foot is displaced by turning it onto its dorsum or by abducting or adducting the limb widely. The animal should immediately replace the leg to a normal position. Lesions of the nervous system often affect conscious proprioception first.

Placing: Small animals may be carried toward a table top; on seeing the table, a normal animal anticipates placing its forepaws on the surface. If blindfolded, the animal should place the forepaws on the table only when the limbs contact the edge of the table. A loss of placing response may be present in subtle dysfunction even when the gait is normal.

Hopping: In small animals, three legs can be held off the ground with normal posture maintained, and the animal forced to move or hop (by being pushed laterally and forward) on the fourth limb. For large dogs and other large animals, one pelvic or thoracic limb opposite the side to be tested is held off the ground. When the animal is pushed toward the side to be tested, it should hop on the limb. Animals will not hop when pushed in a medial direction. Motor and proprioceptive loss, cerebellar incoordination, and cerebrocortical deficiency may be detected.

Righting: The animal is observed to see whether it can right itself from lateral recumbency. A small animal suspended upside down by the hips attempts to hold its head up when the trunk is rotated from side to side and extends its forelimbs to support weight when lowered to the ground. With vestibular dysfunction, the animal twists toward the side of the lesion or curls its head under (bilateral vestibular lesions).

Spinal Reflexes: The spinal reflexes are tested with the animal in lateral recumbency and the limbs relaxed. When the toes or skin of the distal thoracic limb are pinched, that limb should withdraw and the opposite limb usually does not move. This is the **flexor or withdrawal reflex**; it is present if spinal cord segments C6 to T2 and nerves of the brachial plexus are intact. Intramedullary spinal cord lesions at C6 to T2 usually depress or abolish the reflex, but mild extramedullary lesions may produce no change. With lesions cranial to C6, a simultaneous extension of the opposite limb (the **crossed extensor reflex**) may occur when the tested limb flexes. The crossed extensor is a normal reflex; however, an exaggerated response is interpreted as an upper motor neuron (UMN) sign indicating loss of inhibition from the UMN. The **Babinski reflex** is elicited by stroking the palmar surface of the paw in either a carpus to toe or toe to carpus direction. A positive (abnormal) response would be dorsiflexion of the toes, which is interpreted as a UMN sign.

Other tendons (biceps and triceps) and muscles (extensor carpi radialis) may be tapped with a percussion hammer and the response evaluated to test C6 to C7, the musculocutaneous nerve (biceps), and C7 to T2, the radial nerve (triceps, extensor carpi). These reflexes can be difficult to obtain in normal animals, so a reduced response should be interpreted with caution. All reflexes may be normal or exaggerated with lesions above C6.

Muscle Atrophy: Focal muscle atrophy of the limbs or neck localizes the lesion to the cell body in the spinal cord, ventral spinal nerve root, or peripheral axon of the nerve that innervates that muscle.

Sensation: Conscious perception of superficial (skin) or deep (osseous) pain is tested by applying forceps to the skin or bone, respectively, and observing a behavioral response. Such a response indicates that the peripheral sensory nerve and spinal cord, as well as the pathways through the brain stem to the cortex, are intact.

If the evaluation of the head is abnormal, an initial attempt should be made to explain any thoracic limb abnormalities by a lesion above the foramen magnum. If the thoracic limb abnormalities cannot be explained by a lesion in the head, then a multifocal or diffuse disease process (such as an inflammatory, toxic, metabolic, nutritional, traumatic, or metastatic neoplastic disorder) must be present.

If there are no abnormalities on evaluation of the head, and the thoracic limbs are abnormal, then a lesion of the cervical spinal cord or brachial plexus is present. In lesions of the cervical spinal cord, the gait of the thoracic and pelvic limbs is abnormal, and pelvic limb spinal reflexes are normal or exaggerated.

If no abnormalities are found on evaluation of the head and thoracic limbs, then a lesion must be below the T2 spinal cord segment.

Evaluation of the Trunk, Pelvic Limbs, Anus, and Tail

The trunk of the animal is observed for abnormal posture or deviation of the vertebral column, pain, desensitization or hyperesthesia to light pinpricking, and focal muscle atrophy.

Cutaneous Trunci and Panniculus Reflex: Pinpricks applied to the skin of the thorax and abdomen result in contraction of the cutaneous trunci muscle. This reflex arc includes the afferent cutaneous branches of the lumbar and thoracic spinal nerves, a spinal cord tract that ascends to T2, and the LMNs in the lateral thoracic nerve to cutaneous trunci muscles. The reflex is used to localize spinal cord lesions between the site of stimulation and T2.

Postural Reactions: Wheelbarrowing, proprioceptive positioning, placing, and hopping are evaluated on the pelvic limbs in a manner similar to that used for the thoracic limbs. As with the thoracic limbs, these tests require complete integrity of the brain, spinal cord, and peripheral nerves; thus, they are useful to localize lesions and to detect subtle deficits that support the presence of a neurologic lesion.

Spinal Reflexes: The pelvic limb spinal reflexes are more reliable to localize thoracolumbar lesions than are the thoracic limb reflexes. Spinal reflexes are normal or exaggerated with lesions above the reflex arc (UMN) and are depressed or absent with lesions at the level of the reflex (LMN). Percussion of the patellar tendon should cause the stifle to extend if L4 to L6 spinal cord segments and the femoral nerve are intact. Percussion of the gastrocnemius and cranial tibial muscles causes the hock to extend or flex, respectively, and tests the tibial and peroneal nerves, lumbosacral plexus, and L6 to S2 spinal cord segments. A crossed extensor reflex may be associated with lesions above L6 (UMN sign). When the anus is pinched or pricked with a pin, the sphincter tightens and the tail pulls down if S1 to S3 (anus) and caudal (Cd) tail segments and nerves are intact. An atonic (areflexic) bladder, anus, and tail are seen with lesions affecting S1 to Cd5 or the cauda equina. As an incidental finding, the femoral (patellar tendon) reflex may be absent in some geriatric dogs.

Muscle Atrophy: Focal muscle atrophy of the trunk or pelvic limb localizes a lesion to the nerve that innervates that muscle.

Sensation: In moderate to severe spinal cord lesions, superficial sensation may be absent from the cranial aspect of the lesion caudally. In severe spinal cord lesions, deep pain is absent from the periosteum of all toes and the tail.

Schiff-Sherrington Phenomenon: In some animals with acute, severe lesions of the spinal cord between T2 and L3, the pelvic limb paralysis is accompanied by an extensor rigidity of the thoracic limbs when the animal is in lateral recumbency. This occurs because of an interruption of an ascending spinal cord tract from the lumbar intumescence, which inhibits extensors of the forelimb. Although a severe lesion produces this syndrome, the prognosis is probably not hopeless if deep pain sensation can be elicited from the pelvic limbs.

CLINICAL PATHOLOGY

Abnormalities of serum glucose, liver enzymes, BUN, bile acids, ammonia, electrolytes, or blood gases can occur with metabolic dysfunctions. Serum cholinesterase is decreased in acute organophosphate toxicity, and serum lead determinations are increased in lead toxicity. Serum thyroid and cortisol determinations and stimulation tests are useful to detect endocrinopathies. Serum titers or PCRs for viral, fungal, protozoal, and rickettsial organisms can be evaluated. Serum muscle enzymes, especially CK, may be increased in myopathies. Serum acetylcholine receptor antibodies can be detected in dogs and cats with myasthenia gravis, and type II M muscle antibody titers are used to confirm masticatory muscle myositis. Muscle and nerve biopsies are essential for diagnosis and characterization of many neuromuscular disorders. In some cases, brain biopsy is necessary to confirm and characterize an inflammatory or neoplastic process so that proper antimicrobial therapy, chemotherapy, or radiation therapy can be administered.

CEREBROSPINAL FLUID ANALYSIS

The analysis of CSF may further aid in determining the mechanism of a CNS disorder (especially inflammation). The technique of collection is simple and safe with practice. Analysis of CSF requires minimal special equipment. Cell counts and identification should be performed within 30 min after collection, because cells begin to degenerate after that time. Several techniques are available to concentrate or stabilize cells so that a differential cell count can be obtained at a later time.

CSF is collected from the cerebellomedullary cistern or the subarachnoid space in the lumbar region. An increase in protein is often associated with encephalitis, meningitis, neoplasia, or spinal cord compression. Cellular content increases most frequently with inflammation of the CNS. Neutrophils are indicative of bacterial infections, subarachnoid hemorrhage (RBCs are also present), brain abscess or a steroid-responsive suppurative meningoencephalitis, or in some cases, necrosis within a tumor. Increased numbers of lymphocytes, monocytes, and neutrophils are most common in steroid-responsive nonsuppurative meningoencephalitis, meningoencephalitis of unknown etiology (MUE), fungal infections, toxoplasmosis, and neosporosis. Cultures of CSF may demonstrate the causative agent in bacterial and fungal infections. Paired serum and CSF immunoassays for canine distemper virus, cryptococcosis, toxoplasmosis, neosporosis, Rocky Mountain spotted fever, ehrlichiosis, and borreliosis can assist in diagnosis of these infections.

IMAGING

Plain radiographs of the skull and vertebral column are useful to detect fractures, subluxation, infection, or neoplasia of osseous structures. In most infections or neoplastic processes of the brain and spinal cord, plain radiographs are normal. Myelography is used to detect compressive or expansive spinal cord lesions, including herniated or protruded intervertebral discs and spinal cord tumors. CT and MRI scans are useful to evaluate lesions of the brain and spinal cord in small animals. CT scans are helpful to detect changes in bone, acute hemorrhage, and CNS neoplasia. MRI scans are the best to demonstrate soft-tissue changes, eg, neoplasia, abscesses, inflammation, and hemorrhage. MRI is the gold standard for evaluation of lumbosacral disease in small animals. Magnetic resonance angiography can be used to evaluate vascular changes in the CNS.

ELECTRODIAGNOSIS

An electroencephalogram (EEG) is a recording of the electrical activity of the surface of the cerebral cortex, which is influenced by subcortical structures. The EEG is consistently abnormal in hydrocephalus, meningoencephalitis, head trauma, and cerebral neoplasia. An EEG may determine whether seizure discharges are focal or diffuse. The EEG is often normal in idiopathic epilepsy, unless seizures are not well controlled and interictal spikes are present.

An electromyogram (EMG) is a recording of the electrical activity of muscles and is used to evaluate the health of the motor unit. The motor unit consists of the LMN, the nerve root, the peripheral nerve, the neuromuscular junction, and skeletal muscle. The peripheral nerve can be stimulated, and motor and sensory nerve conduction velocities calculated and compared to known normal values to help define the neuropathy as an axonopathy or myelinopathy. Repetitive nerve stimulation may lead to a reduction of the evoked potential in myasthenia gravis. Abnormalities of late waves (F and H) may be associated with disorders of the nerve roots.

The brain-stem auditory evoked response (BAER) is a recording of electrical activity in the auditory pathway from the inner ear receptors through the brain stem to the cerebral cortex. The animal may or may not be awake for this test. No response or a diminished response is seen in auditory nerve disorders associated with hearing loss. Brain-stem disorders may also alter the BAER; it may be abnormal in the Chiari malformation of Cavalier King Charles Spaniels and may also be used as an indicator in determining brain death.

Spinal cord evoked potentials can be used to evaluate spinal cord integrity. These are elicited by stimulating a peripheral nerve and recording the potential as it ascends the spinal cord.

PRINCIPLES OF THERAPY

See also SYSTEMIC PHARMACOTHERAPEUTICS OF THE NERVOUS SYSTEM, p 2590.

Seizure Control: Status epilepticus (continuous or cluster seizures) in dogs and cats may be interrupted by diazepam, given at 0.5 mg/kg (not to exceed 10 mg at one time), IV. Sodium pentobarbital to effect, not to exceed 3–15 mg/kg, IV, may also be used, followed by phenobarbital at 2–4 mg/kg, IV, every 6 hr. A better alternative is to give propofol as a constant rate infusion at 0.1–0.6 mg/kg/min, followed by a loading dose of phenobarbital (if the animal is not already on phenobarbital) of 2–4 mg/kg, IV, every 6 hr for a total of four doses. Diazepam given at 0.5–1 mg/kg/hr as a constant-rate infusion may be used to control persistent status epilepticus. If the animal has a preexisting hepatic condition that precludes the use of phenobarbital, then levetiracitam 40–60 mg/kg may be given IV, SC,or rectally, resulting in a therapeutic blood level that will persist for 9 hr. Oral anticonvulsants should be resumed as soon as possible if currently being given.

Recommended maintenance anticonvulsant therapy in dogs and cats is phenobarbital at 2–4 mg/kg, PO, bid, as needed to control seizures or to maintain serum levels at 15–40 mcg/mL. Dogs can be treated with potassium bromide (KBr), 22–44 mg/kg given with food until the serum level is 1,500–3,000 mcg/mL. Because KBr has a long half-life, if started at maintanance levels, the steady state therapeutic level will not be reached until 3 mo after initiation of therapy. Phenobarbital may become clinically effective in 72 hr, whereas KBr may take several weeks. The longterm efficacy of phenobarbital and KBr is about the same. However, KBr bypasses the liver, so it is preferred in animals with liver disease. Animals taking phenobarbital often have increased liver enzymes and cholesterol levels but decreased thyroid levels; these should be expected and often do not require treatment. KBr has also been linked with megaesophagus and pancreatitis in dogs. A source of KBr is commercially available, or it may be prepared by a compounding pharmacist by mixing KBr crystals in water to give a concentration of 250 mg/mL or by packing the crystals in gelatin capsules. KBr serum levels are affected by the salt content of the diet, so the diet should be consistent; the higher the dietary salt content, the faster the bromide is excreted via the kidneys. KBr has proved more efficacious than phenobarbital in dogs with cluster seizures and for seizures that are difficult to control. Phenobarbital and KBr may be given in combination. Diazepam is not an effective longterm oral anticonvulsant in dogs because of its short half-life; however, a compounding pharmacist can prepare rectal suppositories containing diazepam 0.5–2 mg/kg for home use in dogs with cluster seizures, or the injectable form can be given rectally at 1 mg/kg to prevent trips to emergency clinics. The tertiary anticonvulsants, levetiracitam and zonisamide, are gaining greater favor. Zonisamide especially has shown good efficacy in controlling seizures in those animals with a poor response to phenobarbital and KBr.

KBr may cause asthma in cats, so its use in cats is no longer recommended. Diazepam at 0.5–1 mg/kg, PO, bid, may be used in cats with uncontrolled seizures because of its longer half-life in cats; however, in one report diazepam was associated with fatal hepatic necrosis in cats and thus warrants close monitoring throughout the first few weeks of therapy. Phenobarbital is the anticonvulsant of choice in cats; if seizures are not well controlled, then levetiracitam is added. Acupuncture may be useful to control seizures in all species.

Acute Spinal Cord Injury: Acute spinal cord injury from trauma, intervertebral disc herniation, or fibrocartilaginous embolization resulting in paraplegia must be treated aggressively in dogs to ensure the best chance for recovery. If the dog is seen within the first 8 hr after injury, methylprednisolone sodium succinate or prednisolone sodium succinate is given at 30 mg/kg, IV, followed by 15 mg/kg in 2 and 6 hr, or a constant IV infusion to give a total dose of 60 mg/kg. Steroid use is not advised if it has been longer than 8 hr since the trauma occurred, because there may be more deleterious effects than beneficial ones. Dexamethasone is not used. Oral famotidine at 0.5–1 mg/kg, once or twice daily; cimetidine at 5–10 mg/kg, bid; or misoprostol at 3 mcg/kg, bid, can be used to protect the GI tract. Polyethylene glycol (PEG) 30% solution may be given IV at 2.2 mL/kg, then repeated in 24 hr. PEG is a newer treatment that appears promising. If the injury occurred more than 72 hr before treatment, the benefit of PEG is questionable. For maximal benefit, decompressive spinal surgery should be performed as soon as possible, usually within 24 hr, when indicated.

Anti-inflammatory Drugs: For control of CNS inflammation in dogs and cats unassociated with a virus or other agent, prednisone at 2 mg/kg/day may be given PO. Oral famotidine at 0.5–1 mg/kg, once or twice daily; cimetidine at 5–10 mg/kg, bid; or misoprostol at 3 mcg/kg, bid, is given to prevent GI irritation. If GI ulcers develop and melena is detected, sucralfate (500 mg for cats and dogs <20 kg; 1 g for dogs >20 kg), PO, tid-qid, is given 2 hr apart from other drugs. NSAIDs should never be given in conjunction with steroids, because GI ulceration is common. The dosages of all steroids given should be slowly tapered; abrupt withdrawal should be avoided. Prednisone can be used as longterm maintenance therapy on alternate days to avoid complete suppression of adrenal function. Other chemotherapeutics used for inflammatory CNS disease such as MUE are cytarabine (50 mg/m^2, SC, bid for 2 days, then repeated at 3–4 wk intervals), mycophenolate (10 mg/kg, PO, bid), and cyclosporine (5 mg/kg, PO, bid).

Antiedema Drugs: After cranial surgery and in animals with brain tumors or head injuries that cause a declining neurologic status, 20% mannitol, 0.5–1 g/kg, may be given slowly IV. Mannitol is not given in spinal cord injuries. Use of methylprednisolone sodium succinate as described above for acute spinal cord injury is no longer recommended for head injuries in people, and its use in the veterinary field is declining. For palliative treatment of brain tumors, oral prednisone may be used.

Muscle Relaxants: Diazepam at 0.5 mg/kg or methocarbamol at 40 mg/kg, PO, tid-qid, relieves muscle spasms from intervertebral disc protrusion and other sources of nerve root irritation.

Antimicrobial Therapy: Refer to discussions of specific infections for antimicrobial therapy recommendations.

Nursing Care: Animals with paraplegia and quadriplegia need intensive nursing care. The animal should be maintained on padding and turned every 4–6 hr to avoid decubital ulcers. The bladder must be expressed or catheterized every 6–8 hr.

In paraplegic animals, diazepam may be given to facilitate relaxation of the urinary sphincter, making manual expression of the bladder easier. Urine must be monitored for evidence of cystitis. The skin must be kept clean and free of urine and feces to prevent dermatitis. Quadriplegic animals may need to be hand fed nutritious food and given plenty of water. Manual extension and flexion of joints and muscle massage will help delay contractures and muscle atrophy in paralyzed limbs.

CONGENITAL AND INHERITED ANOMALIES OF THE NERVOUS SYSTEM

Congenital defects of the CNS are, by definition, present at birth. Some congenital defects may be inherited, others may be caused by environmental factors (eg, toxic plants, nutritional deficiencies, viral infections); for many, the cause is unknown. In those animals born with a well-developed nervous system (foals, calves, lambs, pigs), the clinical signs of a congenital neurologic disorder may be recognizable at birth. Kittens and puppies are born with a less well-developed nervous system, and in those species, neurologic signs may not be apparent until they begin to walk. In some inherited neurologic diseases, clinical signs of the disorder are not seen until the animal is an adult (eg, caudal fossa malformation syndrome/syringomyelia, neuronal ceroid lipofuscinosis), even though the defect has obviously been present since birth.

Congenital lesions can be categorized according to the primary region of the CNS affected. **Forebrain disorders** (cerebrum and thalamus) primarily result in clinical signs such as visual disturbances, changes in mental status or behavior, abnormal movements or postures, and seizures. **Cerebellar disorders** usually result in an intention tremor, widebased stance, and incoordination (dysmetria) of the head, trunk, and limbs. **Brain stem disorders** may result in cranial nerve dysfunction, postural disturbances, or vestibular dysfunction. In some cases, brain stem disorders may also result in weakness and proprioceptive gait disturbances, with more severely affected animals exhibiting impaired consciousness. **Spinal cord disorders** do not affect cerebral function or coordination of head movement but may produce weakness, motor dysfunction, or proprioceptive deficits of the limbs, including either dysmetria or reduced proprioceptive placing in more than one limb. (*See also* DISEASES OF THE SPINAL COLUMN AND CORD, p 1245.) **Neuromuscular disorders** include diseases of the peripheral nerves, neuromuscular junction, or muscles. Disorders of these systems can result in signs of weakness and ataxia similar to those seen in spinal cord disease. In addition, they often cause disturbance of reflex function, pain sensation, or marked muscle atrophy. In some cases, these deficits are markedly episodic. **Multifocal disorders** result in combinations of signs from more than one of these categories of neurologic deficits.

CEREBRAL DISORDERS

Large Animals

Anencephaly means that the brain is largely absent at birth. It is a rare disorder but is seen sporadically in calves; the cause is unknown. Because the pituitary gland may also be absent, prolonged gestation (*see* p 1377) of affected calves can occur. Signs include profound lethargy, head pressing, and blindness with normal pupillary reflexes. Cerebral aplasia in calves is usually associated with complete absence of both cerebral hemispheres, and CSF may leak out of a small opening on the midline between the frontal bones.

Exencephaly means that the brain is exposed through a large defect in the skull (cranium bifida). The brain (encephalocele), meninges (meningocele), or both (meningoencephalocele) may protrude through this opening. Encephalocele and meningocele are seen in many species and are known to be inherited in pigs. Defects may be closed or open in terms of communication with the environment through skin defects. Too little information exists to reliably predict outcome and resolution of any deficits. Good surgical outcomes have been achieved in rare case reports of closed meningoencephaloceles; however, safety and quality-of-life issues must be considered, as with any ataxic, seizuring, or mentally inappropriate large animal. When the defects openly communicate externally, CNS infection should be presumed unless proved otherwise.

In **hydranencephaly**, there is a marked loss of cerebral cortical tissue (primarily the neocortex) within a cranial vault of normal conformation. The resultant cavity communicates with the ventricular system, has an incomplete ependymal cell lining, and is filled with CSF. Clinical signs may include lethargy, propulsive circling, head pressing, and blindness. Hydranencephaly develops as a result of the destruction of developing neural tissues and is sometimes accompanied by cerebellar hypoplasia and arthrogryposis. Hydranencephaly is seen sporadically or as an epidemic in calves, lambs, and less commonly in piglets. Known causes include infection in utero with a number of viruses, including Akabane virus (*see* p 620) in ruminants in Australia, Japan, and Israel; bluetongue virus (*see* p 738) in sheep and cattle in North America; Rift Valley fever virus (*see* p 768) and the virus of Wesselsbron disease (*see* p 775) in sheep and cattle in Africa; the Cache Valley virus in sheep in the USA; and the Chuzan virus in calves in Japan. Rarely, bovine viral diarrhea (*see* p 1436) and border disease virus (*see* p 622) produce hydranencephaly in lambs and calves. Hydranencephaly and porencephaly (cystic cavities in the cerebrum) are seen sometimes in lambs with in utero copper deficiency (swayback). It also is seen in a syndrome of prolonged gestation in sheep in Scotland (cause unknown).

Hydrocephalus, an increase in volume of the CSF, can appear similar to hydranencephaly, but in hydrocephalus the ventricles retain a complete ependymal lining. Clinical signs can vary from mild to severe and include seizures, lethargy, or other forebrain abnormalities. There may be extensive expansion of the lateral ventricles in the frontal lobes. Hydrocephalus is seen sporadically in all large animals, although it is relatively common in calves, in which inheritance and vitamin A deficiency have been implicated.

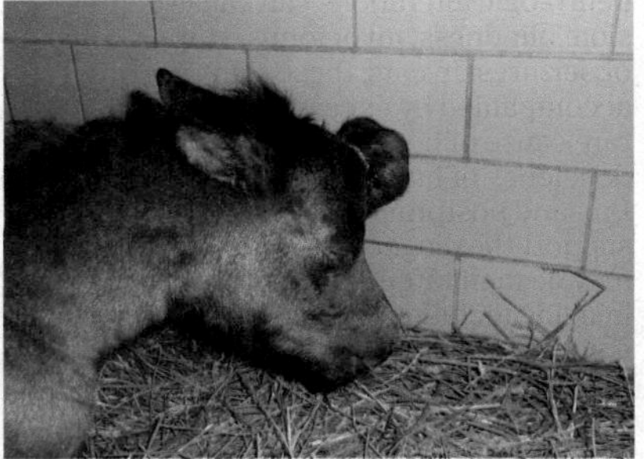

Protrusion of tissue on the forehead of a foal with meningoencephalocele. *Courtesy of Dr. Rebecca Packer and Dr. Paige Jackson, Purdue University.*

Cyclopia is characterized by a single orbital fossa. One cause in lambs is ingestion by the gestating dam of plant alkaloids from *Veratrum californicum*. This malformation also is seen in pigs.

Idiopathic or familial epilepsy has been described in many species. Benign epilepsy is seen in young foals, particularly Arabians, up to 12 mo of age. The foal may present for seizures, head injuries, or postictal blindness. Foals usually recover spontaneously within a few months, but anticonvulsant therapy (phenobarbital, 100–500 mg, PO, bid, for a 50-kg foal) is probably advisable for 1–3 mo, followed by withdrawal over 2 wk. Epilepsy beginning by 1 yr of age has been recorded in Brown Swiss and Swedish Red cattle. Seizures are also seen in young Aberdeen Angus calves; if these calves survive, they show cerebellar signs but become clinically normal by 2 yr of age.

Metabolic disorders and lysosomal storage disorders often cause signs of forebrain dysfunction, along with other neurologic deficits, and are discussed further under multifocal disorders (*see* p 1234). Cerebral signs seem to be most prominent in citrullinemia.

Citrullinemia is a fatal hereditary metabolic defect of Holstein-Friesian calves (mainly in Australia and New Zealand) associated with cerebral cortical edema. It is due to increased citrulline in plasma, caused by deficiency of the urea cycle enzyme argininosuccinate synthetase. Affected calves appear healthy at birth but die of acute neurologic disease in 1–4 days. Signs are sudden in onset and consist of depression, aimless wandering, blindness, seizures, opisthotonos, and recumbency.

Narcolepsy, a disorder of sleep-wake control (typically characterized by excessive sleepiness or sudden paroxysmal attacks of flaccid paralysis with conservation of consciousness), has been reported in several equine breeds, particularly Shetland ponies. The animal is otherwise healthy. During narcoleptic episodes, rapid eye movements occur, and at the same time, the animal may also show cataplexy or sudden loss of muscle tone with collapse.

Small Animals

The same structural anomalies of the brain as described for large animals (*see* p 1222) are also found in small animals.

Hydranencephaly has been described mainly in kittens after in utero exposure to feline panleukopenia virus/parvovirus (*see* p 796). Brain stem malformations and cerebellar hypoplasia may be seen concomitantly.

Hydrocephalus is most common in dogs, particularly in toy and brachycephalic breeds. It can be classified as communicating (nonobstructive), in which CSF can flow freely into the subarachnoid space, or noncommunicating (obstructive). Known causes of noncommunicating hydrocephalus include atresia of the mesencephalic aqueduct, perinatal encephalitis, or adhesions caused by intraventricular hemorrhage at birth. Clinical signs of hydrocephalus usually indicate cerebral dysfunction and often progress, although some animals may remain asymptomatic. The fontanelles are often patent, and affected animals may have ventrolateral strabismus. Blindness due to polymicrogyria (excessive number of smaller gyri) and asymmetric dilatations of the lateral ventricles have been described in Standard Poodles. Hydrocephalus has been observed in Saint Bernard puppies in association with aphakia (absence of the lens) and multiple ocular defects. Imaging by ultrasonography (through the fontanelle), CT, or MRI can provide the diagnosis, and CSF analysis should identify encephalitis. Treatment relies on omeprazole to reduce CSF production or, if necessary, corticosteroids, or surgery to shunt CSF into the peritoneum.

Lissencephaly, an absence or reduction of cerebral gyri, is a rare disorder seen in Lhasa Apsos. It is also seen in association with cerebellar hypoplasia in Irish Setters, Wirehaired Fox Terriers, and Samoyeds and in Korat cats with microencephaly. Clinical signs consist of mild behavioral abnormalities and seizures.

Pug encephalitis is an ultimately fatal disease that may have a familial basis. Affected Pugs show behavioral changes, seizures, and CSF pleocytosis. A similar nonsuppurative, necrotizing encephalitis has been reported in several other toy breed dogs, including Yorkshire Terriers, Chihuahuas, and Maltese Terriers.

Neonatal encephalopathy is an inherited genetic disorder that has been described in Standard Poodles. Poodles appear stunted and weak from birth and begin seizuring at 4–5 wk of age. The disease is fatal. A genetic test is available for diagnosis of this disease in Standard Poodles.

Polymicrogyria is an inherited disease identified in Standard Poodles that results in focal areas of the brain having smaller and more gyri than normal, resulting in disruption of function. The most common clinical signs are visual disturbances, but ataxia, behavioral problems, and hydrocephalus can also be seen. Clinical signs are attributable to the portion of the brain affected by the abnormal gyri.

Idiopathic epilepsy may be inherited in certain breeds, including Beagles, Keeshonden, Irish Setters, Belgian Tervurens, Siberian Huskies, Springer Spaniels, Labrador Retrievers, Golden Retrievers, and German Shepherds. A specific type of seizure known as temporal lobe epilepsy appears to be familial in Cavalier King Charles Spaniels and is characterized by behavioral manifestations such as "fly biting." The diagnosis of idiopathic epilepsy depends on eliminating other causes of seizures, particularly structural brain abnormalities (such as hydrocephalus or juvenile tumors), encephalitis, or metabolic causes (such as hepatic encephalopathy).

Hepatic encephalopathy is usually caused by a congenital portosystemic shunt. The shunt may be a single large vessel, or there may be microscopic shunting of blood within the liver. Breeds often affected include Miniature Schnauzers, Yorkshire Terriers, Cairn Terriers, Australian Cattle Dogs, Old English Sheepdogs, and Maltese Terriers. The clinical signs are usually noticed before 6 mo of age and primarily reflect cerebral dysfunction, including staring into space, inappropriate vocalizing, aggression, and agitation. Advanced neurologic alterations can cause depression, blindness, myoclonus, stupor, coma, or seizures. In cats, these signs are often accompanied by excessive salivation. A rare cause of hepatic encephalopathy is a deficiency of hepatic urea cycle enzymes. Pre- and postprandial bile acid tests may support the diagnosis. Definitive diagnosis may be facilitated by use of radiographic imaging techniques, such as positive contrast portography, CT, transcolonic portal scintigraphy, or diagnostic gray-scale ultrasonography. Blood tests such as the ammonia tolerance test (*see* p 436) should be used with caution in cases of suspected hepatic encephalopathy because of risk of causing an encephalopathic crisis. Resting ammonia levels can be performed; however, ammonia levels have been poorly correlated with both the diagnosis and presence of clinical signs.

Lysosomal storage disorders that commonly cause cerebral signs include ceroid lipofuscinosis and fucosidosis, although there are many other forms of lysosomal storage disorders as well as other inborn errors of metabolism (*see* p 1234). Genetic and enzymatic testing is available for some of these disorders. When specific tests are not available, organic acid screens may support the general diagnosis of metabolic error.

Puppy hypoglycemia is an idiopathic syndrome in toy breeds of dogs that is seen in the first 6 mo of life. It seems to relate to a relative immaturity of the liver, which affects glycogenolysis and can usually be managed by providing frequent meals of a commercial puppy diet. The problem usually resolves as the puppy matures.

Narcolepsy or cataplexy is inherited in Doberman Pinschers, Labrador Retrievers, and Dachshunds and has been described in additional canine breeds. It is rare in cats. Attacks are often stimulated by excitement. It must be differentiated from various types of syncope. Physostigmine (0.025–0.1 mg/kg, IV) potentiates the frequency and severity of cataleptic attacks. Imipramine (0.5–1 mg/kg, PO, tid) can be used to control the severity of the cataplexy.

CEREBELLAR DISORDERS

Large Animals

Arnold–Chiari malformation is a complex malformation of the caudal brain stem and cerebellum and typically consists of herniation of cerebellar tissue through the foramen magnum into the cervical spinal canal. It may be associated with spina bifida, hydrocephalus, or meningomyelocele. It is rare in domestic animals, and the cause is unknown. (A more common variation of this disease is recognized in dogs and appears to be inherited, but this has not yet been proved.) In calves, it may be seen with bilateral elongation and extension of the occipital lobes.

Cerebellar hypoplasia has been described in many species. In utero viral infection (bovine viral diarrhea [*see* p 1436], bluetongue virus [*see* p 738], and swine fever virus [*see* p 713]) during midgestation is the most common cause. Cerebellar lesions may also be seen with bovine fetuses infected with Akabane or Wesselsbron viruses. Clinical or subclinical hydranencephaly and arthrogryposis may accompany the cerebellar disease. The pathologic features include destruction or loss of one or more layers of the cerebellar cortex, particularly the granule and Purkinje cell layers. Prophylactic vaccination of the dam before breeding can prevent the problem. A hereditary cerebellar hypoplasia/dysplasia is seen in Hereford, Shorthorn, Ayrshire, and Angus calves. Cerebellar hypoplasia is present at birth and is nonprogressive, in distinction to the abiotrophies.

Cerebellar abiotrophies have been reported in many species. In abiotrophies, the cerebellar development proceeds normally, and the animal remains unaffected for a period of months or even years before cerebellar neurons begin to die off prematurely. This is in contrast to the cerebellar hypoplasias, in which developing cerebellar germinal cells and neurons are destroyed in utero. In Aberdeen-Angus calves, clinical signs of abiotrophy start early and are accompanied initially by seizures. In Arabian foals and Swedish Gottland ponies, the onset of signs is from birth to 9 mo; in Yorkshire and Large White piglets, 1–3 mo; in Holstein calves, 3–8 mo; and in Merino sheep, 3–6 yr. Most abiotrophies are probably inherited (eg, recessive inheritance for affected Hereford cattle and Welsh Mountain and Corriedale sheep), but toxic causes should also be considered. The latter include locoweed, methylmercury, and exposure to organophosphates in utero (*see* p 3064). Use of trichlorfon during pregnancy can cause a congenital tremor in piglets due to both cerebellar hypoplasia and hypomyelination.

Hypomyelinogenesis congenita, in which myelination is delayed throughout the CNS, can resemble cerebellar disease due to the severe head and body tremor that usually develops. In contrast to pure cerebellar disease, a persistent fine tremor at rest is usually present as well as a marked intention tremor. Newborn lambs, piglets, and occasionally calves are affected. The condition can be associated with in utero infection by viruses such as the virus of Border disease (*see* p 622) or swine fever virus (*see* p 713) or exposure to trichlorfon (*see* p 3067). Affected lambs are often called "hairy shakers." The condition is inherited in Saddleback and Landrace pigs and in Jersey and Shorthorn cattle. Signs are usually nonprogressive or may resolve completely if myelination has only been delayed.

Swayback or enzootic ataxia is largely due to copper deficiency, although there may be a familial predisposition. Hypomyelinogenesis can occur in utero and cause obtundation, blindness/deafness, falling or lying prostrate, and head tremor in lambs. The condition can be prevented by treating affected ewes in pregnancy. Kids, piglets, and perhaps calves may also be affected.

Small Animals

Cerebellar hypoplasia is seen in kittens after in utero infection with feline panleukopenia virus (*see* p 796). The condition is nonprogressive, and affected cats may make suitable pets. Diagnosis can be obtained antemortem using MRI. Concomitant hydrocephalus or hydranencephaly may also be seen. Cerebellar hypoplasia has also been reported in Chow Chows and is seen in association with lissencephaly in Irish Setters and Wirehaired Fox Terriers.

A selective hypoplasia of the cerebellar vermis is also seen in dogs, and when combined with hydrocephalus and cyst-like dilatation of the fourth ventricle, the condition has been termed the Dandy-Walker syndrome, which may have a familial basis. The cerebellar vermis may be partially or completely absent. Clinical signs are typical of a cerebellar disorder and include tremors, ataxia, and hypermetria. Occasionally signs of head tilt and circling may also be present. Toy Fox Terrier dogs are predisposed to the Dandy-Walker form.

Cerebellar abiotrophies have been described in a number of breeds of dogs. In Samoyeds and Beagles, the signs are apparent at the onset of ambulation; in Australian Kelpies, Rough-coated Collies, and Kerry Blue Terriers, the clinical signs are seen in puppies from 4–16 wk of age; in Brittany Spaniels, Old English Sheepdogs, and Gordon Setters, the signs appear in young or mature adults. Clinical signs include progressive cerebellar ataxia, intention tremor, hypermetria, and possible loss of menace response due to cerebellar involvement. Postural reactions remain normal as with any pure cerebellar disease; however, affected animals may be incoordinated when placing paws. Clinical signs can be differentiated from cerebellar hypoplasia, above, by the onset. Hypoplasia is present since birth (apparent at time of ambulation) and nonprogressive, whereas animals with abiotrophies are born normal and progress after onset.

Bandera syndrome is seen in Coton de Tulear dogs and manifests as a cerebellar ataxia from the time of birth. The cerebellum is anatomically normal. A DNA test is available for this disease in the Coton de Tulear.

Congenital hypomyelination is seen as a familial/inherited disorder in Springer Spaniels, Chow Chows, Weimaraners, and Bernese Mountain Dogs, usually with signs developing around 2–8 wk of age. In the latter three breeds, it is often termed dysmyelination because the clinical signs of whole body tremor usually resolve spontaneously with time. The disorder is rare in cats. The diagnosis can be confirmed using MRI. (*See also* DEMYELINATING DISORDERS, p 1236.)

Caudal occipital malformation syndrome and subsequent **syringomyelia** has been commonly reported in Cavalier King Charles Spaniels and less commonly in other small breed dogs. The malformation is comparable to the Chiari type I malformation described in people and includes a congenital malformation of the occipital bone, resulting in a crowded caudal fossa and cerebellar herniation at the foramen magnum. The subsequent disruption of CSF flow results in formation of syringomyelia. A large proportion of asymptomatic Cavalier King Charles Spaniels have the caudal fossa malformation. Although the malformation is present at birth, clinical signs often do not appear until later in life. Clinical signs vary but commonly include paresthesias (eg, face rubbing, phantom scratching of the back of the head), ataxia, and weakness from syringomyelia. Medical management is often not curative but can be attempted with gabapentin (10 mg/kg, PO, tid) for paresthesias, omeprazole (0.7 mg/kg/day, PO) for reduction of CSF production, and analgesics for pain management. Surgical decompression via caudal occipital craniectomy is preferred as definitive treatment; however, recurrence rates of 25%–47% have been reported.

BRAIN STEM DISORDERS

Small Animals

Congenital vestibular disease has been reported in German Shepherds, English Cocker Spaniels, Doberman Pinschers, and Siamese and Burmese cats. Signs are bilateral and may be accompanied by deafness. This is likely a peripheral syndrome affecting the vestibular apparatus, and labyrinthitis has been identified histologically in some pups. The disorder appears inherited. There is no treatment. Deafness is permanent, although the clinical signs of vestibular dysfunction may improve as the animal learns to compensate.

Canine multiple system degeneration has been identified in Kerry Blue Terriers and Chinese Crested dogs. Clinical signs reflect both cerebellar and brain stem dysfunction, including ataxia, dysmetria, and festination. The disorder is inherited as an autosomal recessive mutation. There is no treatment.

SPINAL CORD DISORDERS

See also DISEASES OF THE SPINAL COLUMN AND CORD, p 1245.

Large Animals

Spinal muscular atrophy is an inherited disorder of Brown Swiss calves. The first clinical sign of spinal muscular atrophy is weakness of the pelvic limbs at 2–6 wk of age; calves (most are female) have difficulty getting up and then become recumbent. The characteristic sign is severe muscle atrophy, especially of the pelvic limbs. Histopathologic examination reveals degeneration and loss of motor neurons in the ventral horns of the spinal cord. Neurogenic atrophy of muscles is a consistent lesion. A similar disorder is seen in red Danish calves of American Brown Swiss lines. It is possible that spinal muscular atrophy and bovine progressive degenerative myeloencephalopathy (BPDME) are in some way related because they can be seen in the same blood lines, but the onset of BDPME occurs after 5 mo of age, and it causes ataxia and dysmetria rather than weakness and muscle atrophy. A motor neuron disease with neurofilament accumulation is seen in horned Hereford cattle in Canada with signs appearing soon after birth that are characterized by general tremors, incoordination, difficulty standing, and hyperesthesia to tactile stimulation. A suspected hereditary lower motor neuron disease with accumulation of neurofilaments also is seen in Yorkshire pigs around 5 wk of age, characterized by pelvic limb paresis progressing to recumbency. There is degeneration and loss of motor neurons throughout the spinal cord and brain stem. A similar condition is seen in young Hampshire pigs.

Bovine progressive degenerative myeloencephalopathy (BPDME, weaver syndrome) is a neurodegenerative disorder of Brown Swiss cattle that is seen in the USA, Canada, and Europe. Four basic criteria are required to establish a clinical diagnosis: 1) onset of bilateral pelvic limb ataxia and dysmetria at 5–8 mo of age; 2) deficient proprioceptive responses, ataxia in all four limbs, and progressive paraparesis; 3) normal spinal reflexes and cranial nerve function and absence of dramatic muscle atrophy; and 4) a familial relationship. The disease was initially described as "weaver" because of the peculiar weaving gait. The histopathologic changes are primarily in the sensory nervous system, in contrast to those of spinal muscular atrophy (*see* above). Spinal dysmyelination causes congenital lateral recumbency and opisthotonos, but spinal reflexes and alertness are normal.

Simmental encephalomyelopathy, which is seen in association with behavioral change (eg, aggression or dullness), has an onset in Simmental and Simmental-cross calves at 5–12 mo of age. The gait abnormality progresses from pelvic limb ataxia to recumbency with opisthotonos, and death occurs within 6 mo. It has been reported in the USA, UK, Australia, and New Zealand. Characteristic lesions consist of symmetric necrosis in the caudate nuclei and in other areas of the brain and spinal cord. Similar multifocal lesions are seen in 1- to 4-mo-old Limousin and Limousin-cross calves (with additional signs of blindness) in Australia and England and in Angus calves in Australia and the USA.

Progressive myelopathy of Murray Grey cattle in Australia is inherited (autosomal recessive), and calves usually show spastic paraparesis and ataxia at birth. Neuronal degeneration is widespread in the brain and spinal cord; primary demyelination also develops in the cord.

Progressive ataxia of Charolais cattle has been reported in the UK and North America. It causes clinical signs that are first noticed between 6 and 36 mo of age and progress throughout 1–2 yr from slight ataxia involving all four limbs to recumbency. Female cattle typically manifest a rhythmic pulsatile pattern of urination. Histologic lesions consist of eosinophilic plaques and myelin breakdown in the white matter of the cerebellum and spinal cord.

Neuraxonal dystrophy (NAD) appears to be inherited in sheep and causes an unsteady, stiff, and swaying gait that progresses to paraparesis and finally tetraparesis. Suffolk and New Zealand Coopworth sheep are affected as lambs 1–6 mo old; Romney sheep are affected at 6–18 mo of age. Merinos develop a very similar disease at 1–4 yr of age. NAD has also been seen in 4- to 7-mo-old Merino lambs. Axonal swellings (spheroids) are typically found in gray matter of brain stem and spinal cord, although in the older Merino sheep, axonal spheroids mainly develop in large white matter tracts of the CNS. NAD of Morgan horses affecting the lateral (accessory) cuneate nucleus usually develops at 6–12 mo of age and causes spastic paraparesis and pelvic limb ataxia. It is presumed to be inherited. NAD affecting several brain-stem nuclei and causing mild pelvic limb ataxia has also been reported in 4-mo-old Hafflinger horses in Germany.

Equine degenerative encephalomyelopathy has been mainly associated with vitamin E deficiency, but it may have a familial basis in Appaloosa horses and other breeds, based on occurrence of clusters of cases. Degeneration of the spinocerebellar tracts results in a slowly progressive, symmetric ataxia and paresis of all four limbs that starts as early as 7 mo of age. (*See also* DEGENERATIVE DISEASES OF THE SPINAL COLUMN AND CORD, p 1245.)

Progressive paresis in Angora goats has been reported in Australia and may have a heritable basis. Clinical signs of spastic paresis and ataxia appear from birth to 4 mo of age and progress to recumbency within a few weeks. Widespread (multisystem) neuronal degeneration is seen at necropsy.

Generalized glycogenosis in Shorthorn (type II) and Brahman (type IIb) cattle and in Corriedale sheep (resembling type II) is a lysosomal storage disease that causes ill thrift, respiratory signs, paraparesis, ataxia, and muscle weakness at 3–9 mo of age.

Cervical stenotic myelopathy (wobbler syndrome) is a compressive cervical spinal cord syndrome caused by vertebral canal stenosis, articular process osteophyte proliferation, and vertebral body tipping that occurs in young, rapidly growing horses. Thoroughbreds, Tennessee Walking Horses, and Warmbloods appear to be predisposed, with males being more commonly affected than females. Overnutrition is an important contributory factor, and the clinical signs often can be reversed in horses <9 mo old by reducing caloric intake and restricting exercise. Clinical signs typically become apparent from <6 mo up to 4 yr of age and include cervical myelopathy, with the pelvic limbs usually affected more severely. Imaging (eg, survey radiography, myelography, CT, MRI) can be used to identify stenotic or proliferative lesions, causing spinal cord compression in the midcervical spine. Treatment usually requires surgical decompression of the spinal cord and, in some cases, vertebral stabilization. Interbody fusion with titanium baskets ("Seattle Slew" implants) has shown more success; however, the prognosis remains guarded. In one study, 77% of horses showed neurologic improvement, with 46% regaining athletic function. Early treatment appears to be associated with improved surgical outcome.

Occipitoatlantoaxial malformation is an inherited disorder (autosomal recessive) in Arabian foals and may also be seen in Miniature horse foals, Holstein calves, and lambs. Clinical signs are progressive ataxia, tetraparesis, and an extended neck posture. Affected foals are usually tetraparetic at birth, although neurologic deficits may not develop for several years. Diagnosis is by radiography. Laminectomy has been reported to be successful in some cases.

Spina bifida is seen in most species and usually results in dysfunction of the tail and anus, incontinence, and sometimes pelvic limb weakness (*see* p 1230).

Small Animals

Spinal muscular atrophy is an inherited lower motor neuron (LMN) disorder in Brittany Spaniels that can have an early (by 1 mo), intermediate (by 4–6 mo), or delayed (>1 yr old) onset. Rottweilers can also develop an early form of spinal muscular atrophy that is referred to as a motor neuron disease. Swedish Lapland puppies are affected at 5–7 wk of age, Stockard paralysis (seen in Great Danes crossed with Bloodhounds or Saint Bernards) has an onset at 11–14 wk, and English Pointers are affected when ~5 mo old. LMN disease also is seen in puppies of other breeds, including Doberman Pinschers and Briquet Griffon Vendéens; a focal form involving the thoracic limb(s) is seen in German Shepherds. Paraparesis or tetraparesis with neurogenic muscle atrophy are the main clinical features. The severe, generalized LMN disease in spinal muscular atrophy closely resembles the signs of a peripheral neuropathy. Loss of motor neurons in the spinal cord is the most striking feature on necropsy. There is no treatment.

Demyelination of Miniature Poodles is presumed to be an inherited disorder involving primarily the spinal cord. This rare condition causes paraparesis at 2–4 mo of age that rapidly progresses to tetraplegia. There is no treatment.

Ataxia of Parson Russell and Smooth-haired Fox Terriers can be confusing, because several forms of disease exist. In general, the diseases affecting these breeds are a spinocerebellar ataxia. The predominant clinical signs are cerebellar (cerebellar ataxia, intention tremor, hypermetria), but histopathologically at necropsy, spinal cord demyelination can be seen. Clinical signs begin to appear at ~2–6 mo of age. In one form of the disease, seizures and myokymia (in which the muscles appear to show verminous movement) can occur. The disease is progressive, although in some cases signs may stabilize but not regress, and some affected animals are able to live a relatively normal life, despite the abnormal movements.

Afghan Hound myelopathy is an inherited disorder that causes both demyelination and necrosis of the spinal cord. Paraparesis develops some time during the first year of life and progresses to paraplegia within 1 wk. The thoracic limbs become involved over the next 1–2 wk. A similar condition is seen in young Kooiker dogs (Dutch Decoy dogs) of either sex, with signs beginning at 3–12 mo of age. Prognosis is poor in both breeds.

Neuraxonal dystrophy is described in both cats and dogs but primarily in Rottweiler dogs (autosomal recessive inheritance). In Rottweilers, onset is between 3–24 mo of age, and the disorder progresses slowly over several years. Signs include cerebellar dysfunction and dysmetria in all four limbs, but with preservation of paw position sense, which should distinguish it from leukoencephalomyelopathy (*see* below) and from advanced motor neuron disease in the same breed. Collie dogs in Australia and New Zealand develop similar clinical signs at 2–4 mo of age. There is also early onset in Papillons and Chihuahuas and in cats (autosomal recessive in domestic tricolored cats). Axonal spheroids, often in specific regions of the brain and spinal cord, are the characteristic pathologic finding of these conditions.

Leukoencephalomyelopathy of Rottweilers has a later onset than neuraxonal dystrophy (*see* above), usually at ~2–3 yr of age. It is possible that the disorders have a similar basis, because animals occasionally may show histopathologic features of both conditions. In leukoencephalomyelopathy, there is no head tremor, and paw position sense is delayed. Bilaterally symmetric areas of spinal cord demyelination are the predominant findings on necropsy.

Calcium phosphate deposition in Great Danes causes mineralization of soft tissues and bone deformity, with dorsal displacement of C7. The resultant compressive myelopathy is seen in puppies 1–2 mo old. This condition is distinct from caudal cervical spondylomyelopathy (*see* below).

Degenerative myelopathy is a painless, slowly progressive myelopathy that occurs commonly in dogs. Clinical signs are typically consistent with a thoracolumbar spinal cord localization with pelvic limb paresis and ataxia, although progression may eventually involve the thoracic limbs. Histopathologic changes include a noninflammatory axonopathy and myelinopathy. German Shepherds, Pembroke Welsh Corgis, Boxers, Rhodesian Ridgebacks, and Chesapeake Bay Retrievers are predisposed. There is no treatment. Physical therapy slows the progression of clinical signs. A mutation has been identified that is associated with increased risk of developing degenerative myelopathy, and a genetic test is available to identify those dogs at higher risk of developing the disease.

Progressive axonopathy of Boxer dogs is an autosomal recessive disorder that causes patellar hyporeflexia, severe dysmetria, loss of paw position sense, and spastic paresis at 1–7 mo of age. Axonal spheroids are widespread in both the central and peripheral nervous system on necropsy. Although this condition causes loss of the patellar reflex, in general, the signs are more suggestive of spinal cord disease than of a peripheral neuropathy. There is no treatment, but affected dogs can live relatively comfortably for a considerable time.

Breed-associated aseptic meningitis (steroid-responsive meningitis-arteritis) has been reported in Beagles, Bernese Mountain Dogs, Boxers, German Short-haired Pointers, and sporadically in other breeds. The main signs are neck pain, pyrexia, and dramatic pleocytosis in the CSF in young dogs. Prognosis is guarded to favorable, especially in dogs with acute disease that are treated promptly using immunosuppressive doses of corticosteroids.

Congenital vertebral malformations include hemivertebrae (shortened or misshapen vertebrae), block (fused) vertebrae, and butterfly vertebrae (having a sagittal cleft). Hemivertebrae are most common in screw-tailed dog breeds and are inherited in German Shorthaired Pointers. Decompressive surgery can be very successful but sometimes needs to be combined with spinal stabilization. **Multiple cartilaginous exostosis** is a benign proliferation of cartilage or bone that can affect the ribs, long bones, or vertebrae and may have a familial basis. **Transitional vertebrae** are often clinically associated with lumbosacral stenosis. Myelography or specialized imaging techniques (eg, CT, MRI) are usually required to confirm spinal cord compression in these congenital conditions. Treatment consists of surgical removal.

Caudal cervical spondylomyelopathy (wobbler syndrome) may have a heritable basis in Borzois (5–8 yr) and Basset Hounds (<8 mo) and probably also Doberman Pinschers (≥2 yr) and Great Danes (<2 yr). Neurologic deficits range from mild ataxia of the pelvic limbs to tetraplegia. Affected dogs often keep their neck flexed ventrally, and there may be caudal cervical pain. Spinal radiographs may show malalignment or remodeling of the vertebrae, narrowing of one or more disk spaces, or spondylosis deformans. CT/myelography or MRI usually reveals a marked stenosis at the cranial orifice of the midcervical or caudal cervical vertebrae. Several surgical techniques can provide stabilization of the vertebrae or decompression of the spinal cord.

Atlantoaxial subluxation is most commonly seen as a congenital disorder in young toy or miniature breeds of dogs and occasionally as a congenital disorder in several large breeds, including Rottweilers and Doberman Pinschers. Signs usually develop within the first few years of life and consist of an acute or slowly progressive onset of neck pain or gait dysfunction, ranging from ataxia to tetraplegia. Radiographic confirmation of diagnosis should be followed by stabilization using ventral fixation. The prognosis is guarded.

Arachnoid diverticuli (arachnoid cysts, arachnoid pseudocysts, meningeal cysts, leptomeningeal cysts, subarachnoid cysts) cause accumulations of CSF and a focal myelopathy in young dogs. The cause is unknown, but some cysts may have a congenital origin. Signs consist of progressive ataxia and weakness. Diagnosis is made by myelography and/or MRI.

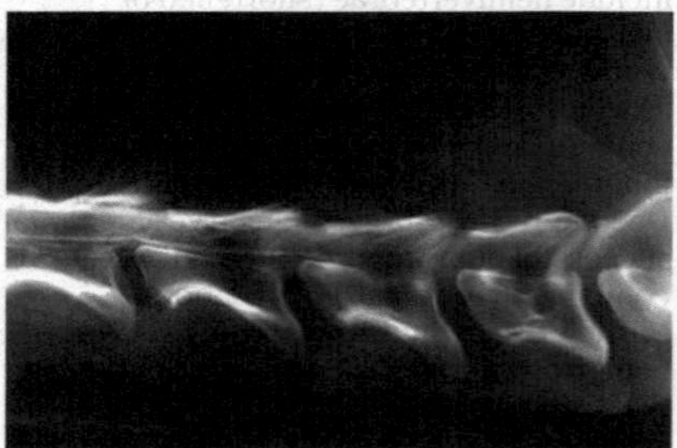

Cervical spondylomyelopathy (wobbler syndrome) in a 6-yr-old Doberman Pinscher. *Courtesy of Dr. Ronald Green.*

Prognosis may be favorable after surgical excision, although recurrence is possible.

Spinal dysraphism or myelodysplasia includes anomalies of the skin, vertebrae, and spinal cord that are secondary to faulty closure of the neural tube. Spinal dysraphism is inherited in Weimaraners. Neurologic deficits are evident by 4–6 wk of age and include paraparesis and a symmetric "bunny-hopping" gait in the pelvic limbs. There is a bilateral flexor reflex; pinching one paw elicits flexion of both pelvic limbs. There may be scoliosis or abnormal hair streams on the dorsal aspect of the neck. Diagnosis is based on clinical signs and imaging techniques such as myelography or MRI. There is no treatment, but neurologic deficits usually do not progress. Similar malformations have been seen in other breeds of dogs and in calves, foals, and lambs.

Syringomyelia is the development of one or more fluid-filled cavities within the spinal cord. **Hydromyelia** is accumulation of fluid within an enlarged central canal of the spinal cord. It is often difficult to differentiate between syringomyelia and hydromyelia, so the term **syringohydromyelia** is often used. Syringohydromyelia causes progressive ataxia and paresis; scoliosis and spinal pain is possible. Causes include trauma, neoplasia, inflammatory conditions, and developmental malformations. The most common cause in dogs is caudal occipital malformation syndrome (*see* p 1226).

Spina bifida occulta is a failure of the neural arch to fuse; if the spinal cord is also involved, it is called **spina bifida manifesta**. The most likely clinical signs of spina bifida are LMN signs in the pelvic limbs and urinary or fecal incontinence. The prognosis for animals with substantial neurologic deficits is poor. Spina bifida can also accompany the **sacrocaudal dysgenesis** that is inherited as an autosomal dominant trait in Manx cats.

Pilonidal sinus (dermoid sinus, dermoid cyst) is another consequence of faulty neural tubulation that appears to be inherited (autosomal recessive) in Rhodesian Ridgeback dogs. The sinus is lined by skin and may communicate with the subarachnoid space, causing possible meningitis or myelitis. Treatment consists of antibiotics and surgical excision of the sinus.

Epidermoid cysts are rare lesions that arise from entrapment of epithelial cells during closure of the neural tube. Myelography or MRI will reveal an intramedullary lesion in a young dog with progressive neurologic deficits.

NEUROMUSCULAR DISORDERS

See also DISEASES OF THE PERIPHERAL NERVES AND NEUROMUSCULAR JUNCTION, p 1238.

Large Animals

Spastic paresis is seen in many breeds of cattle and has been referred to as "contraction of the Achilles tendon," "straight hock," and "Elso heel." (*See also* LAMENESS IN CATTLE, p 1066.) It can be divided into two syndromes, one that affects calves and one that affects adults. In calves, the condition appears to be familial and can be seen in many breeds, with signs beginning between 1 wk and 1 yr of age. It is characterized by extension of the stifle and tarsus and by spastic contracture of the muscles of one or both pelvic limbs. Spasticity primarily affects the gastrocnemius and superficial flexor muscles; in some cases, other muscles of the pelvic limb are involved. The leg is usually held in extension behind the calf and does not touch the ground during walking. The disease is progressive but usually responds to neurectomy of the tibial nerve. The cause is unknown. No lesions are seen in peripheral nerves, and the condition is thought to involve excessive activity of the neuromuscular spindle reflex arc. Adult cattle are affected at 3–7 yr of age. Extensor muscles of the back and pelvic limbs are affected, causing lumbar lordosis and caudal extension of the limbs. This condition is also thought to be familial and is usually progressive. Mephenesin (30–40 mg/kg, PO, for 2–3 days) may produce variable control of signs. Quadriceps muscle hypoplasia as a cause of congenital lameness has been described in Holstein calves. Reduced numbers of spinal cord motor neurons suggest that there is failure to innervate the muscle on the affected side.

Hyperkalemic periodic paralysis (*see* p 1047) is seen in Quarter horses 2–3 yr old and is due to an inherited mutation of the sodium channel. It causes episodes of muscle tremor and sometimes recumbency, both of which may be precipitated by exercise. Hyperkalemia is usually present during an attack, and electromyography can also be helpful for diagnosis. Acetazolamide (0.5–2.2 mg/kg, PO, bid) or hydrochlorothiazide (0.5 mg/kg, PO, bid) may lessen the frequency and severity of attacks.

Myotonia congenita is an inherited/familial disorder in goats and Shropshire lambs and is occasionally seen in horses. It causes muscle rigidity; marked dimpling on percussion of the muscle belly; and a stiff, stilted gait. Electromyography is a useful aid to diagnosis. This disease results from a mutation in a chloride channel.

Muscular dystrophy is an inherited disease in Merino sheep. It results in a slowly progressive stiffness that affects the limbs and neck from 3–4 wk of age onward. Clinically affected sheep have high resting and postexercise concentrations of serum CK and lactate dehydrogenase.

Porcine stress syndrome or malignant hyperthermia (*see* p 1027) is a hypermetabolic and hypercontractile syndrome that, when triggered by anesthesia or stress, produces a sustained increase of intracellular calcium levels within skeletal muscle fibers. This in turn causes muscle stiffness, hyperventilation, hyperthermia, and pale exudative pork. It results from a mutation in a calcium-channel gene that is inherited as an autosomal dominant trait, usually in Landrace pigs.

Small Animals

Hypertrophic neuropathy of Tibetan Mastiffs is an autosomal recessive disease that has been recognized in the USA, Switzerland, and Australia. It causes paraparesis by 8 wk and may progress to tetraparesis. Hyporeflexia is marked, but sensory function is preserved. Demyelination and remyelination are seen on nerve biopsy. Prognosis is guarded. Some puppies regain the ability to walk but remain weak. There is no treatment.

Alaskan Malamute polyneuropathy affects Alaskan Malamutes 10–18 mo old. Clinical signs include exercise intolerance, paraparesis progressing to tetraparesis, muscle atrophy, hyporeflexia, and, in some cases, laryngeal paralysis. Electromyography shows diffuse fibrillation potentials and positive sharp waves. On nerve biopsy, there is axonal necrosis with demyelination. There is no effective treatment, although clinical signs stabilize in some dogs. In most affected dogs, however, progressive disability leads to euthanasia.

Congenital laryngeal paralysis is seen in Bouvier des Flandres (autosomal dominant) and Siberian Huskies, Rottweilers, and Bull Terriers <1 yr old. It results in exercise intolerance and inspiratory dyspnea. Diagnosis is confirmed by visualization on laryngoscopy. Congenital laryngeal paralysis with diffuse peripheral neuropathy is seen in several breeds, including Dalmatians, Rottweilers, and Pyrenean Mountain Dogs (Great Pyrenees). Prognosis is guarded to poor.

Primary hyperoxaluria (l-glyceric aciduria) is a rare, inherited (autosomal recessive) neurofilament disorder of domestic shorthaired cats that results in renal disease and also produces weakness due to a peripheral neuropathy. Signs develop at 5–9 mo of age. A plantigrade stance is the most prominent sign, and spinal reflexes are sometimes reduced. Urine contains increased oxalate and l-glycerate levels. There is no treatment.

Neuropathy of hereditary hyperchylomicronemia (hyperlipidemia) is a suspected autosomal recessive disorder that causes a generalized peripheral neuropathy in cats. Clinical signs do not develop until at least 8 mo of age. The hyperlipidemia results in deposition of lipid granules within nerves, and there is evidence that the clinical signs can be controlled by a low-fat diet. Blood samples from affected cats have the appearance of "cream of tomato soup."

Sensory neuropathy of longhaired Dachshunds (probably autosomal recessive) causes pelvic limb ataxia at 8–12 wk of age. Urinary and GI function may also be disturbed. Paw position sense, spinal reflexes, and pain sensation are depressed, and self-mutilation can occur. There is a loss of myelinated fibers in sensory nerves and in selected areas of the spinal cord. There is no treatment, but affected dogs may have a relatively normal quality of life, provided self-mutilation does not occur.

Sensory neuropathy of Border Collies manifests as ataxia, lack of proprioception, and abnormal sensory testing. Onset is usually at 5–7 mo of age and progresses relentlessly. Euthanasia is the common endpoint. The genetics of this disease are not yet known.

Sensory neuropathy in Pointers is seen in English Pointers (autosomal recessive) in the USA and Shorthaired Pointers in Europe. Self-mutilation of the digits is the main clinical sign, and disease onset is before 6 mo of age. Pain perception is absent in the pelvic limbs and depressed in the thoracic limbs. There is neuronal loss in dorsal root ganglia. Prognosis is poor. There is no treatment.

Inherited polyneuropathy of Leonberger dogs is a distal neuropathy, with an age of onset of 1–9 yr in this breed. Clinical signs include weakness, exercise intolerance, change in bark, and dyspnea. *Pedigree analysis* suggests an X-linked inheritance.

Musladin-Lueke syndrome is a connective tissue disorder affecting muscles, bone, heart, and skin. Clinical signs most prominently reflect muscle fibrosis and contractures. The resulting posture is that of the animal walking on its "tip-toes." This is an inherited recessive disorder, reported in Beagles, for which the genetic mutation has been identified. The abnormal posture is present shortly after birth. Other clinical signs include thickened cartilage of the ear and wide-set eyes. Seizures may occur concurrently. It is not yet known whether the seizures are related to the primary disorder or are a concurrent disorder. There is no treatment. The human counterpart to this disease is progressive and frequently fatal; however, the disease appears to stabilize in dogs.

Congenital myasthenia gravis (autosomal recessive) has been described in Parson Russell Terrier, Smooth-haired Fox Terrier, and Springer Spaniel puppies. It is due to either a deficiency or dysfunction of the acetylcholine receptor, and there is none of the circulating antireceptor antibody seen in the more common acquired form of the disease. Clinical signs usually start at 5–10 wk of age. The characteristic finding is an exercise-induced weakness, often associated with megaesophagus. The prognosis is more guarded than in acquired myasthenia gravis. The congenital disease has also been described in cats. A presynaptic form is seen in 12- to 16-wk-old Gammel Dansk Hønsehund dogs (autosomal recessive). Treatment consists of anticholinesterase drugs.

Scotty cramp (autosomal recessive) causes episodes of muscular hypertonicity in Scottish Terrier puppies. These episodes are exacerbated by excitement, exercise, stress, and poor health and are characterized by a hypermetric gait and arching of the spine, which can cause the dog to somersault when it runs. The disorder seems to be related to faulty serotonin metabolism. Diazepam and promazines help to relieve signs.

Congenital myoclonus of Labrador Retrievers (familial reflex myoclonus) causes muscle spasms/hypertonicity from an early age. Puppies may be unable to walk or even maintain a sternal position due to extensor rigidity. The prognosis is very poor.

Hypokalemic myopathy of Burmese cats (autosomal recessive) causes periodic paralysis or weakness with ventral flexion of the neck. Cats are affected at 3–4 mo of age. Serum CK is markedly increased. Dietary supplementation of oral potassium usually produces a favorable response (eg, potassium gluconate solution at 2–4 mEq or mmol/cat/day, PO, until serum potassium levels are stable).

Myotonia congenita is seen in Chow Chows, Staffordshire Terriers, Great Danes, and Miniature Schnauzers (autosomal recessive) and causes signs similar to those seen in myotonic goats. There is often a degree of muscle hypertrophy, and marked stiffness is seen when dogs first rise. Dimpling is seen on percussion of several muscles, including the tongue. Diagnosis can usually be confirmed by electromyography (characteristic "dive bomber" sound); muscle biopsy changes are mild and nonspecific. Prognosis is guarded, although membrane-stabilizing drugs (procainamide, mexiletine) result in significant improvement.

X-linked muscular dystrophies have been described in Irish Terriers, Golden Retrievers, Miniature Schnauzers, Rottweilers, Samoyeds, German Shorthaired Pointers, Groenendaeler Belgian Shepherds, Brittany Spaniels, Rat Terriers, Labrador Retrievers, Japanese Spitz dogs, and also in cats. All are due to mutations in the dystrophin gene. Males show muscle stiffness, dysphagia, and weakness at an early age, along with a plantigrade stance and muscle atrophy as the animal gets older. Initial muscle hypertrophy may be marked, particularly in cats. Diagnosis is facilitated by the initial massive increases in serum levels of CK and by demonstration of hyalinized and mineralized muscle fibers on biopsy. Prognosis is guarded to poor. Currently, there is no treatment. A novel congenital muscular dystrophy has been reported in cats associated with deficiency of merosin (laminin α_2), in which degenerative changes occur in both muscles and peripheral nerves.

Labrador Retriever myopathy (autosomal recessive) causes a stiff gait and marked muscle atrophy in puppies of both sexes. Signs worsen with cold, stress, or exercise, and affected dogs may be unable to keep their heads elevated in a normal position from as early as 3 mo of age. Tendon reflexes are usually absent. Signs stabilize by 6–8 mo of age, and the prognosis is favorable, so affected dogs can make good pets. There is preferential atrophy of type II muscle fibers.

Dermatomyositis of Collies and Shetland Sheepdogs (inherited as a dominant trait with variable expressivity) causes atrophy and weakness of the masticatory and distal limb muscles from a few months of age, sometimes associated with trismus and megaesophagus. These signs are combined with a dermatitis over the face and extremities. The clinical signs may wax and wane and, in general, do not become severely debilitating. Polymyositis and dermatitis are evident on histopathologic examination. This disorder has also been seen in Beauceron Shepherds, Pembroke Welsh Corgis, Australian Cattle Dogs, Lakeland Terriers, Chow Chows, German Shepherds, and Kuvasz dogs.

Glycogen storage diseases can cause muscle weakness and exercise intolerance in young dogs and cats. Examples include glycogenosis types II (Lapland dogs), III (German Shepherds and Akitas), IV (autosomal recessive in Norwegian Forest cats), and VII (English Springer Spaniels).

Mitochondrial myopathy has been described in Clumber and Sussex Spaniels and in Old English Sheepdogs. Mitochondrial myopathies result in exercise intolerance and collapse, and blood lactate and pyruvate levels are often increased after exercise. Ragged red fibers, indicating increased numbers of mitochondria, may be seen on muscle biopsy. Inherited disorders of carnitine metabolism are another cause of mitochondrial myopathy; they may cause accumulation of lipid vacuoles within muscle fibers.

Nemaline rod myopathy (probable autosomal recessive) in cats causes weakness and later a hypermetric gait at 6–18 mo of age. Patellar reflexes are depressed, and muscle atrophy develops progressively. Large numbers of nemaline rods are found in skeletal muscle fibers. The prognosis is poor. A similar disorder is seen sporadically in young dogs.

Central core myopathy has been described as a cause of weakness, muscle atrophy, and exercise intolerance/collapse in young Great Danes in the UK. Signs begin at approximately 6 mo of age. Prognosis is poor.

Congenital megaesophagus is inherited in Wirehaired Fox Terriers and Miniature Schnauzers and possibly also in German Shepherds, Great Danes, Irish Setters, Newfoundlands, Chinese Shar-Pei, Greyhounds, and Siamese cats. Clinical signs include regurgitation and aspiration pneumonia. Prognosis is guarded.

Devon Rex cat hereditary myopathy (autosomal recessive) is seen in kittens around 4–7 wk old and is characterized by exercise intolerance and passive ventroflexion of the head and neck, which is especially noticeable during locomotion, urination, or defecation. Some cats assume a "dog-begging" position. Megaesophagus is present. Prognosis is guarded.

MULTIFOCAL DISORDERS

Large Animals

Hereditary neuraxial edema with inherited congenital myoclonus (probable autosomal recessive) was first reported in neonatal Polled Herefords and is the result of decreased and/or defective glycine receptors, which provide inhibitory neurotransmission. The calves are alert but unable to rise; they are incoordinated and have coarse, tonic muscular contractions. Sudden stimuli cause vigorous extension of the legs and neck.

Shaker calf syndrome is a neurodegenerative disorder that is seen in Hereford calves. Affected animals show a marked tremor within hours of birth, difficulty in rising, a stiff gait, and loss of voice; signs progress to spastic paraplegia. There is excessive accumulation of neurofilaments within neurons of the central, peripheral, and autonomic nervous systems.

Vitamin A deficiency of sows can cause incoordination, head tilt, pelvic limb paralysis, paddling, and ocular lesions in piglets. Similar signs are seen in congenitally affected calves born from deficient dams.

Generalized Metabolic and Lysosomal Storage Disorders: **Maple syrup urine disease** is a genetic amino aciduria (consistent with a branched-chain ketoacid decarboxylase deficiency) in Hereford calves. Affected calves are dull, become recumbent in 2–4 days, and terminally have opisthotonos. The histologic lesions are severe and consist of generalized status spongiosus in the CNS.

GM$_1$ gangliosidosis is seen in inbred Friesian calves. Clinical signs become evident during the first week of life and include depression, swaying of the hindquarters, reluctance to move, and stiffness. Death occurs in 6–8 mo.

GM$_2$ gangliosidosis causes hypermetria and weakness in Yorkshire piglets within the first 3 mo of life. Death occurs in 4–6 mo.

α-Mannosidosis (autosomal recessive) is seen in Angus, Murray Grey, and Galloway breeds. It produces ataxia, head tremor, aggression, and failure to thrive. There may also be abortions and neonatal death. Most affected calves die within the first year, sometimes shortly after birth. Affected (homozygous) calves have an absolute deficiency of α-mannosidase, and heterozygotes are partially deficient. Mannosidosis can be controlled by identifying and eliminating heterozygotes on the basis of biochemical testing.

β-Mannosidosis causes recumbency and cerebellar signs in newborn Nubian goats and Salers calves.

Ceroid lipofuscinosis is seen in sheep, cattle, and goats. Young Nubian goats show cerebellar signs. Rambouillet sheep show blindness and decreased mentation from 8 mo of age. South Hampshire lambs 9–12 mo old show blindness, depression, head and thoracic limb tremor, and facial twitching and die by 30 mo of age. Devon cattle become blind and weak by 14 mo and die by 4 yr of age. The genetic mutation has been identified in some of these species (Devon cattle, South Hampshire sheep).

Globoid cell leukodystrophy has been reported in polled Dorset sheep 4–18 mo old. Exaggerated tendon reflexes, ascending paralysis, and cerebellar signs may be seen.

Small Animals

Multisystemic chromatolytic neuronal degeneration in Cairn Terriers causes paraparesis in young puppies that progresses rapidly to produce cerebellar involvement with bouts of cataplectic collapse. Degeneration of neurons is widespread in the brain, spinal cord, and sensory ganglia.

Multisystemic neuronal degeneration has also been reported in red-haired Cocker Spaniels and causes abnormal behavior and cerebellar signs. Neuronal changes are found in various brain-stem nuclei. A similar condition is seen in Miniature Poodles (3–4 wk) with signs characterized by rolling from side to side, inability to stand or right into sternal position, periodic opisthotonos, intention tremors, and lack of a menace response associated with neuronal degeneration in the cerebral cortex and cerebellum.

Hydrocephalus in Bull Mastiffs is an inherited disorder that is also associated with abnormal myelin. It results in blindness, abnormal behavior, and cerebellar signs. Bilaterally symmetric spongiform lesions are found in the deep cerebellar nuclei.

Dalmatian leukodystrophy is a rare inherited condition that causes visual deficits with progressive ataxia and tetraparesis at 3–6 mo of age. There is dilatation of ventricles, cavitation of cerebral white matter, and widespread loss of myelin.

Fibrinoid leukodystrophy has been described in two 8-mo-old Labrador Retrievers, a 9-mo-old male Scottish Terrier, a 6-mo-old female Miniature Poodle, and a 13-wk-old Bernese Mountain Dog. It results in progressive ataxia and tetraparesis with personality changes starting at 6 mo of age. Rosenthal fibers are found around blood vessels of the CNS, and the cause seems to be a disorder of astrocyte function. Prognosis is poor.

Spongiform degenerative conditions have been described in young dogs and cats (breeds include Labrador Retriever, Shetland Sheepdog, Samoyed, Silky Terrier, Bull Mastiff, Saluki, Cocker Spaniel, Malinois-Shepherd crosses, Rottweiler, and Egyptian Mau and Burmese kittens) and are often associated with signs of ataxia/hypermetria, head tremors, intermittent contractures, postural abnormalities, and behavioral changes. The underlying pathology relates to spongy degeneration of either white or gray matter. The pathogenesis of these disorders remains uncertain, although a genetic mutation has been identified for a family of Australian Cattle Dogs and Shetland Sheepdogs. Prognosis is poor.

Hereditary quadriplegia and amblyopia in Irish Setters produces signs of head tremor, visual impairment, nystagmus, inability to stand, and seizures beginning at birth.

Lysosomal Storage Disorders:

This clinically rare group of conditions results from deficiency of an enzyme that is essential for the metabolism of a protein, carbohydrate, or lipid substrate, or results from buildup of a byproduct that can be toxic to cells. Clinical signs usually appear early in life, although occasionally the onset is delayed. Specific diseases have been associated with a particular breed, but in theory, any breed could develop any one of these disorders, and many have been described in more than one breed. Considerable phenotypic variation should be expected beyond the classic signs described below. Prognosis is poor for all of these disorders, although gene replacement therapies are being actively investigated. Diagnostic testing is limited except for those diseases in which the enzyme or mutation has been identified or the pattern or organic acids has been recognized. Testing often includes urine metabolic screening, lysosomal enzyme screening, histopathology for specific characteristics in tissue biopsy, or DNA testing for known mutations. Genetics laboratories should be checked for testing availability.

Sphingolipidoses: **Globoid cell leukodystrophy (Krabbe disease)** is seen mainly in Cairn and West Highland White Terriers. Several other breeds of dogs, as well as cats, may be affected. Clinical signs are variable and multifocal, and either an ascending paralysis is seen by itself or combined with a cerebellar disturbance. Death occurs 2–3 mo after the onset of signs. Total protein content of CSF may be increased. Large globoid cells are distributed throughout the white matter of the spinal cord and brain.

GM_1 gangliosidosis is seen primarily in cats, particularly Oriental breeds, and in Beagles, Portuguese Water Dogs, English Springer Spaniels, Alaskan Huskies, and Shibas. Signs of cerebellar dysfunction predominate, and corneal clouding may develop.

GM_2 gangliosidosis or familial amaurotic idiocy (Derry disease) has been seen in German Shorthaired Pointers, Japanese Pointers, mixed-breed cats, and Korat cats. Clinical signs seen at 6 mo of age include behavioral change and visual disturbances. Progressive ataxia and dementia develop later. Clinical signs of ataxia, hypermetria, head tremor, and corneal opacity develop in kittens at ~3 mo of age.

Niemann-Pick disease affects cats and causes cerebellar dysfunction with an associated abdominal enlargement due to hepatosplenomegaly. The neurologic deficits tend to vary with the six subtypes of this disease, ranging from severe cerebellar-like signs (types A and C) to neuropathic signs (type A variant).

Glucocerebrosidosis (Gaucher disease) is a rare disorder of Australian Silky Terriers that produces mainly cerebellar signs at 4–6 mo of age.

Glycoproteinoses: **Fucosidosis of English Springer Spaniels** has been reported in Australia, New Zealand, the UK, and North America. It is characterized by clinical signs of ataxia, personality change, dysphonia, dysphagia, hearing/visual deficits, and seizures. Signs tend to progressively develop from 6 to >24 mo of age. A high proportion of peripheral lymphocytes may show cytoplasmic vacuolation. A DNA-based blood test is available for diagnosis. Prognosis is poor, and there is no effective treatment.

α-Mannosidosis has been seen mainly in cats and may cause retinal and skeletal abnormalities as well as neurologic deficits. Cerebellar signs are the most consistent feature of the otherwise somewhat variable neurologic deficits.

Mucopolysaccharidoses (Types I, II, III, VI, VII): **Mucopolysaccharidosis** is primarily a disorder of cats, although some subtypes affect dogs. This disorder is associated with a flattening of the face, corneal clouding, and multiple bone dysplasias. Plott hounds can also be affected. Several types of this disease are reported; type VI is often associated with progressive paraparesis secondary to focal bony protrusions into the vertebral canal. The skeletal changes are nonprogressive after 9 mo of age, and decompressive surgery may improve the neurologic deficits.

Glycogen Storage Disorders: Glycogenosis (types II, III, IV, VII) and mucolipidosis II are not as well described. English Springer Spaniels, Lapland dogs, German Shepherds, Akitas, and Norweigan Forest cats are among those described. Clinical signs generally include neuromuscular weakness, exercise intolerance, muscle tremors, or dysphagia.

Mucolipidosis II affects domestic shorthaired cats and generally causes skeletal malformations.

Other Storage Disorders: Ceroid lipofuscinosis is characterized by reduced vision, personality change, ataxia, and seizures. Clinical signs typically appear when animals are 12–24 mo old, although some can be older. The condition is an autosomal recessive trait in English Setters, Tibetan Terriers, and Border Collies. It has been reported in many additional breeds of dogs, as well as in Siamese cats. The genetic mutation has been identified in some breeds of dogs. The phenotype and age of onset are variable, and signs tend to slowly evolve throughout several years.

La Fora disease occurs most commonly in miniature Wirehaired Dachshunds but also can affect other breeds, such as Bassett Hounds, Beagles, Poodles, and mixed-breed dogs. It is most well known and genetically understood in the miniature Wirehaired Dachshund, and a genetic test is available for diagnosis in this breed. Clinical signs can include late-in-life onset myoclonic seizures that can in some cases be triggered by visual or auditory stimuli. Other clinical examination findings are not commonly reported.

MISCELLANEOUS CONGENITAL DISORDERS

Large Animals

Pendular nystagmus is seen in various breeds of dairy cattle but appears to have little clinical significance.

Congenital deafness has been reported in horses.

Small Animals

Pendular nystagmus is seen in various breed of Asian cats but appears to have little clinical significance. Compared with pathologic forms of nystagmus, in pendular nystagmus there is no fast or slow phase, and the nystagmus arcs are similar to the pendulum movement of a clock.

Congenital deafness is primarily associated with Dalmatians but has also been recorded in a number of breeds, including Australian Blue Heelers and Shepherds, English Setters, Boston Terriers, and Old English Sheepdogs. It is linked to blue eye color in white cats. The brain stem auditory evoked response (BAER) is a useful diagnostic test primarily used to identify carriers in a litter of affected animals. (*See also* DEAFNESS, p 518.)

DEMYELINATING DISORDERS

Hypomyelination and dysmyelination are disorders of myelin development characterized by axons with thin myelin sheaths, or by axons that are nonmyelinated or have abnormal myelin. There are two possible pathologic classifications: 1) thinly myelinated axons with predominantly normal myelin and occasional *nonmyelinated* axons, or 2) thinly myelinated axons with predominantly abnormal myelin and mainly nonmyelinated axons. These categories have been called hypomyelinating and dysmyelinating disease, respectively, and are characteristic of the congenital myelin disorders seen in young animals. These pathologic changes should not be confused with demyelination, in which there is a breakdown and loss of previously normal myelin. In general, these types of demyelinating diseases do not present clinically as congenital problems.

Etiology and Epidemiology: Demyelinating disorders have been reported worldwide in people, mice, pigs (British saddleback, Landrace), cattle (Hereford, Holstein-Friesian, Jersey, Murray grey, Shorthorn), hamsters, rats, sheep, Siamese kittens, and a number of dog breeds, including Chow Chow, Springer Spaniel, Dalmatian, Samoyed, Golden Retriever, Lurcher, Bernese Mountain Dog, Weimaraner, Australian Silky Terrier, and mixed breeds. This problem has also been documented in a litter of Vizslas and Catahoula Cur dogs.

In utero infection and heredity are the general causes of hypomyelination. The viruses of classical swine fever, border disease, and bovine viral diarrhea have been incriminated, but mechanisms responsible for the hypomyelination have not been defined; these three pestiviruses are closely related members of the family Togaviridae and are transmitted both vertically and horizontally. The inflammatory neuraxial disorders in domestic animals in which demyelination is found are canine distemper, visna, and caprine arthritis encephalitis syndrome. In none, though, does CNS demyelination occur as the predominant central feature of the disorder as it does in human multiple sclerosis. Most toxins that affect myelin cause demyelination. One in particular, trichlorfon, is an organophosphate (*see* p 3064) with a unique toxicity that causes Type A-V porcine congenital tremor syndrome. Pregnant sows treated with trichlorfon during mid and late gestation (days 45–77) produce litters in which up to 90% of the piglets develop a marked tremor syndrome secondary to cerebellar hypoplasia and hypomyelinogenesis. The mortality rate is high.

Other disorders resulting in hypomyelination are hereditary. Almost all of these disorders result in CNS hypomyelination, except in Golden Retrievers, in which hypomyelination of the peripheral nervous system (PNS) has been reported. In CNS hypomyelination, the basic defect involves interference with the functional maturation of oligodendrocytes. The exact mechanisms for the defect are not known, but a point mutation on a critical gene has been found in Springer Spaniels. In PNS hypomyelination, the defect involves Schwann cells.

The genetic basis for the inherited hypomyelination syndromes is not fully defined, but in most instances, males are affected more often and more severely than females. This supports a sex-linked recessive trait or mode of inheritance.

Clinical Findings: Clinical signs from hypomyelination of the CNS can be seen as early as 10–12 days of age and certainly by the time of weaning. Signs include, most notably, a gross whole body tremor that involves the limbs, trunk, head, and eyes. The tremor lessens or disappears when the animal is resting or sleeping but reappears on arousal and increases with excitement. The tremors are very noticeable when the animal is eating and are a severe form of intention tremor. In addition, some animals may have difficulty standing and ambulating and may have weakness in the limbs. Secondary to this, postural test reactions may be deficient. Affected animals appear to have vision and other cranial nerve function, but occasionally a pendular nystagmus or a jerk nystagmus is seen when the globes are voluntarily moved. These neurologic deficits may be so severe in some animals that euthanasia is warranted. In some breeds of dogs, such as Chow Chows and Catahoulas, the signs usually dissipate over the first year of life, and the dogs are normal by 12–18 mo of age. In some dogs, the signs may disappear as early as 12–16 wk of age.

In Golden Retrievers with PNS hypomyelination, the clinical signs include ataxia, paresis, muscle atrophy, and hyporeflexia to areflexia. There is no evidence of CNS hypomyelination in this breed, and tremors are not present.

Lesions: In CNS hypomyelination, gross pathology reveals pallor of the white matter of the brain and spinal cord and possibly a gelatinous appearance. In PNS hypomyelination, the gross changes are minimal and there is no evidence of CNS involvement. In CNS hypomyelination, the microscopic changes include lack of myelin (which is usually severe but not absolute), fewer oligodendrocytes, astrocytes outnumbering oligodendrocytes, oligodendrocytes that differ in appearance from those in healthy animals, and abnormal types of glial cells. In PNS hypomyelination, the microscopic changes consist of paucity of myelinated fibers, fibers with inappropriately thin myelin sheaths relative to the caliber of their enclosed axons, occasional fibers with poorly compacted myelin, Schwann cells with larger than normal cytoplasmic volume, and increased numbers of Schwann cell nuclei.

Diagnosis: The diagnosis of CNS hypomyelination is made primarily from the spectrum of neurologic deficits and signs and the early age of onset. Unfortunately, histopathology is the only definitive method to confirm a diagnosis. In cases with a heritable basis, pedigree evaluation may be helpful. In cases with a viral cause, confirmation may involve immunofluorescent antibody-staining techniques or virus isolation from nervous tissue (or both). In cases of PNS hypomyelination, biopsy of peripheral nerves is beneficial.

Differential diagnoses include disorders that could cause tremors in young animals. The possibilities are numerous, but some of the more common include glycogen storage disease, lysosomal storage disease, cerebellar hypoplasia, encephalitis, hypocalcemia, hypoglycemia, hyperammonemia, toxins (eg, metaldehyde, organophosphates, chlorinated hydrocarbons, fluoroacetate, strychnine, hexachlorophene, bromethalin), and mycotoxins (eg, penitrem-A).

Treatment, Control, and Prevention: There is no specific treatment for hypomyelination. The only means of control and prevention is selective breeding (for heritable syndromes) and immunization (for viral-induced syndromes). If given time to develop normal or further myelin, some animals with congenital hypomyelination syndromes become normal by the age of 12 wk to 18 mo.

DISEASES OF THE PERIPHERAL NERVES AND NEUROMUSCULAR JUNCTION

Diseases of the peripheral nerve and neuromuscular junction include degenerative diseases, inflammatory diseases, metabolic disorders, neoplasia, nutritional disorders, toxic disorders, trauma, and vascular diseases. For a discussion of congenital disorders, *see* p 1222.

DEGENERATIVE DISORDERS

Acquired Laryngeal Paralysis: Laryngeal paralysis (*see* p 1420) is common in middle-aged and older dogs. Large breeds, such as Labrador Retrievers, Golden Retrievers, and Saint Bernards, are predisposed, but small-breed dogs and cats can be affected. In most cases, no underlying cause is identified and the laryngeal paralysis is a component of a generalized polyneuropathy, canine chronic axonal degeneration. A few cases are due to trauma or neoplasia affecting the neck or mediastinum. Hypothyroidism (*see* p 553) is also a potential cause. Clinical signs consist of voice change, laryngeal stridor, and a dry cough. In severe cases, exercise intolerance and episodes of respiratory—especially inspiratory—distress and cyanosis occur. Some affected animals have signs of a more generalized polyneuropathy, such as weakness and proprioceptive deficits.

Diagnosis is based on laryngoscopy with the animal lightly anesthetized. There is a unilateral or bilateral lack of abduction of the arytenoid cartilages and vocal folds during inspiration. Management consists of identifying and treating any underlying disorder. Treatment of idiopathic laryngeal paralysis consists of surgery, such as laryngeal tie back. Surgery does not restore normal laryngeal function but is usually successful in diminishing severe inspiratory dyspnea. A potential complication of surgery is aspiration of food or liquid.

Canine Chronic Axonal Degeneration: Canine chronic axonal degeneration, sometimes called geriatric-onset laryngeal paralysis polyneuropathy, affects middle-aged and older dogs and is characterized by axonal degeneration of peripheral nerves. The cause is unknown. Affected dogs have a wide-based, shuffling gait with ataxia, tetraparesis, and generalized muscle atrophy with decreased spinal reflexes. Laryngeal paralysis is often an early feature. Facial paralysis and dysphagia are also possible. Diagnosis is based on clinical features, electrodiagnostic evaluation showing denervation and slowed motor conduction velocity, and nerve and muscle biopsy showing loss of large-caliber nerve fibers with axonal degeneration and neurogenic muscle atrophy, respectively. It is important to exclude treatable metabolic causes such as hypothyroidism. The neurologic deficits progress slowly over months. There is no specific treatment.

Equine Laryngeal Paralysis: *See* p 1458.

Dancing Doberman Disease: Dancing Doberman disease is a neuromuscular disease that affects Doberman Pinschers of either sex, 6 mo to 7 yr old, and is likely inherited in an autosomal recessive pattern. Initially, affected dogs intermittently flex the hip and stifle of one pelvic limb while standing. Within several months, most dogs alternately flex and extend both pelvic limbs in a dance-like fashion. They often prefer to sit rather than stand. The condition slowly progresses to mild paraparesis, decreased proprioception, and atrophy of the gastrocnemius muscles. The thoracic limbs are not affected. Pathologic changes have been reported in pelvic limb muscles as well as peripheral nerves, and whether this is a primary muscle or nerve disease remains to be clarified. There is no treatment, and signs do not resolve. However, the disease usually does not result in severe disability and does not appear to be painful.

Distal Denervating Disease: Distal denervating disease is a common polyneuropathy of dogs in the UK; it has not been reported elsewhere. The cause is unknown. Any age and breed of dog may be affected. The onset of signs varies from a few days to several weeks. There is progressive tetraparesis, hyporeflexia, and atrophy of proximal skeletal muscles. Sensory deficits are not apparent. Electrodiagnostic evaluation typically shows denervation of limb muscles, relatively normal nerve conduction velocity, and markedly reduced amplitude of M waves. Peripheral nerve biopsies are usually normal, but examination of intramuscular nerves may be diagnostic; distal intramuscular axons degenerate with collateral axonal sprouting. Treatment is supportive, and the prognosis is excellent, with recovery in 4–6 wk. Relapse has not been reported.

Distal Polyneuropathy of Rottweilers: Distal polyneuropathy of Rottweilers is characterized by paraparesis that slowly progresses to tetraparesis, hyporeflexia, and muscle atrophy. The clinical course can be progressive or can wax and wane. Male and female Rottweilers 1–4 yr old have been affected. The cause is unknown. Electrodiagnostic testing shows denervation in distal muscles of the limbs and decreased motor nerve conduction velocity. Nerve biopsy changes consist of axonal necrosis and demyelination, often with infiltrates of macrophages, most severe in distal nerve fibers. Prognosis is poor, although some dogs may temporarily improve with corticosteroid treatment.

Idiopathic Facial Paralysis: Idiopathic facial paralysis is a common disorder that results in unilateral or bilateral paresis or paralysis of the facial muscles in dogs and cats. Cocker Spaniels, Pembroke Welsh Corgis, Boxers, English Setters, and domestic longhaired cats are at increased risk. There is acute onset of unilateral or bilateral inability to blink, drooping ear, drooping upper lip, and drooling from the corner of the mouth. Facial sensation (mediated via the trigeminal nerve) remains intact. Diagnosis is based on clinical features and exclusion of other causes of facial paralysis, including ear disease, trauma, and brain-stem lesions. Pathologic findings consist of degeneration of myelinated axons in the facial nerve. There is no inflammation. The cause is unknown, and there is no specific treatment. Artificial tears often help prevent corneal damage. Partial improvement may occur in a few weeks, but persistent dysfunction is common.

Stringhalt: (*See also* p 1137.) Stringhalt in horses is characterized by brisk, involuntary flexion of one or both pelvic limbs during the protraction phase of the gait. Severity ranges from a mild jerk in the limb to flexion so severe that the affected horse can hardly walk. There may be atrophy of the muscles in the distal aspect of the affected limb(s). Stringhalt is seen in two forms. Ordinary or classic stringhalt is seen sporadically throughout the world, usually as a unilateral problem in individual horses. The cause is unknown. Some cases resolve spontaneously, whereas long digital extensor tenectomy is effective in others.

Australian stringhalt is seen in outbreaks that affect multiple horses in a region and often affects both pelvic limbs. Horses in Australia, New Zealand, and the USA have been affected, usually in late summer or autumn. Australian stringhalt is associated with ingestion of Australian dandelion, European dandelion, and mallow, perhaps due to mycotoxins affecting these plants. Pathologically, the distal aspect of axons in the peroneal and tibial nerves degenerates. Horses with Australian stringhalt usually recover spontaneously when removed from offending pastures.

INFLAMMATORY DISORDERS

Acquired Myasthenia Gravis: Acquired myasthenia gravis is characterized by failure of neuromuscular conduction due to reduction in the number of acetylcholine receptors at the neuromuscular junction. It is caused by the development of circulating antibodies directed against the acetylcholine receptors at the neuromuscular junction. It is fairly common in mature dogs, especially German Shepherds, Golden Retrievers, and Labrador Retrievers, but is uncommon in cats. Three clinical forms exist in animals. The generalized form, which affects 57% of dogs with acquired myasthenia, is characterized by exercise-induced stiffness, tremors, and weakness that resolve with rest. However, weakness is not always associated with exercise. Megaesophagus is common in the generalized form. Focal myasthenia (43% of affected dogs) presents as facial, pharyngeal, or esophageal weakness without generalized weakness. Least common is fulminant myasthenia, which presents as acute, flaccid paralysis and megaesophagus, which rapidly progresses to respiratory paralysis and is usually fatal.

Generalized weakness often resolves quickly after IV administration of edrophonium chloride (0.1–0.2 mg/kg), which is often used as a diagnostic test. Definitive diagnosis is based on the detection of antibodies in serum. Treatment consists of anticholinesterase drugs, eg, pyridostigmine (1–3 mg/kg, PO, bid-tid) or neostigmine (0.04 mg/kg, SC, qid). Immunosuppressive dosages of prednisone and other immunomodulating drugs are recommended in animals that do not respond to anticholinesterase therapy. Megaesophagus is managed with upright feeding and in some cases gastrotomy tube placement for feeding and hydration. Aspiration pneumonia is a frequent complication of megaesophagus and leads to death or euthanasia in ~50% of affected dogs. The prognosis is generally good for animals without pneumonia, and ~85% of dogs will undergo spontaneous remission, evident by a decrease in antibody titer, usually within 6 mo.

Acute Idiopathic Polyradiculoneuritis: Acute idiopathic polyradiculoneuritis primarily affects the ventral nerve roots and peripheral nerves. It is common in dogs and rare in cats. Clinical signs often develop 7–14 days after a raccoon bite or scratch (Coonhound paralysis); however, other affected animals have not been exposed to raccoons. A similar syndrome can develop in dogs and cats within 1–2 wk of vaccination. An immune-mediated reaction to raccoon saliva or other antigen is suspected. Initially, there is a short-strided gait in the pelvic limbs that progresses within 1–2 days to flaccid tetraparesis or tetraplegia and, in some cases, to facial and laryngeal weakness. Occasionally, the thoracic limbs are initially affected. Death from respiratory paralysis can occur in severe cases. Spinal cord reflexes are weak to absent, and severe muscle atrophy is evident within 10–14 days. Pain perception is intact, and some dogs may appear hyperesthetic, showing signs of discomfort on palpation of the trunk or limbs. Mentation and appetite are not affected. Urination, defecation, and tail movement usually remain normal.

Analysis of CSF collected from the lumbar subarachnoid space shows increased protein with a normal cell count. Electromyography shows denervation, and nerve conduction studies show marked dispersion and prolonged latency of F-waves, indicative of slowed conduction in the ventral roots. There is no effective treatment other than nursing care, and corticosteroids are not helpful. Most affected animals begin to improve spontaneously within 3 wk, with complete recovery by 2–6 mo. Animals with severe signs and marked muscle atrophy may recover incompletely. Relapses can occur, especially in hunting dogs that frequently encounter raccoons. Histopathologically, there is inflammation, demyelination, and varying degrees of axonal degeneration in the ventral nerve roots and peripheral nerves.

Chronic Relapsing Idiopathic Polyradiculoneuritis: Chronic relapsing idiopathic polyradiculoneuritis is a rare disease associated with inflammation of the nerves and nerve roots. It affects mature dogs and cats. Exercise intolerance, ataxia, and weakness develop slowly throughout several months. Some animals have spontaneous temporary remissions. Spinal cord reflexes are decreased, and cranial nerves may be affected. In severe cases, decreased sensation is evident. Diagnosis is based on nerve biopsy. There is nonsuppurative inflammation; axonal degeneration; and demyelination of nerves, nerve roots, and, in some cases, dorsal root ganglia. The cause is unknown, although immune-mediated mechanisms are suspected. Corticosteroids help in some cases, but the disease tends to slowly wax and wane, gradually becoming more severe throughout months to years.

Chronic Inflammatory Demyelinating Polyneuropathy: Chronic inflammatory demyelinating polyneuropahy is a fairly common disorder in adult dogs and cats. The cause is unknown. Onset of tetraparesis with hyporeflexia is insidious and sometimes accompanied by cranial nerve dysfunction. Electromyography is usually normal, but nerve conduction velocities are slowed with temporal dispersion. Nerve biopsy shows multifocal paranodal demyelination. Clinical signs usually improve with administration of corticosteroids (eg, prednisone 1–2 mg/kg/day), although signs may relapse when therapy is stopped.

Polyneuritis Equi: Neuritis of the cauda equina (polyneuritis equi) is characterized by inflammation of the sacrocaudal nerves and occasionally other nerves. It is seen in adult horses of all breeds in Europe and North America. The cause is unknown, although an immunologic reaction incited by a viral infection is possible. Affected horses have circulating antibodies against P2 myelin protein. The most consistent clinical signs reflect involvement of the sacrocaudal nerves and include urinary and fecal incontinence, tail paralysis, perineal paresthesia or analgesia, atrophy of the gluteal muscles, mild pelvic limb ataxia, and in male horses, penile paralysis. Affected horses may rub the tail. The thoracic limbs and cranial nerves may also be affected. Diagnosis can usually be based on clinical findings. CSF may be xanthochromic with increased protein content and mononuclear pleocytosis. Sacral fracture should be excluded by rectal examination and radiography. There is no treatment, and the prognosis for recovery is poor. Histopathologically, there is granulomatous inflammation primarily affecting the extradural portions of the sacrocaudal nerves.

Protozoal Polyradiculoneuritis: Protozoal polyradiculoneuritis occurs in dogs, especially puppies, and is caused by infection with *Toxoplasma gondii* (*see* p 685) or *Neospora caninum* (*see* p 663). Transplacental infection is most common, and multiple puppies in a litter can be affected. Affected puppies are normal at birth but by 3–8 wk develop paraparesis and a "bunny-hopping" gait with weak or absent spinal refexes. Over a period of several weeks, the pelvic limbs develop severe extensor rigidity and muscle atrophy. Without treatment, the disease can progress to the thoracic limbs, eventually leading to dysphagia and fatal respiratory paralysis. Serum CK concentration is often increased. Analysis of CSF usually shows increased protein and leukocytes (neutrophils, mononuclear cells, and eosinophils). Serum or CSF antibodies or identification of the organism on muscle biopsy are helpful in diagnosis. Early treatment with clindamycin (15–20 mg/kg, IM, PO, bid) or trimethoprim/sulfadiazine (15 mg/kg, bid) and pyrimethamine (1 mg/kg/day) for 4–6 wk may be effective. The prognosis is poor in dogs with pelvic limb rigidity.

Sensory Ganglioneuritis: Sensory ganglioneuritis affects dogs of any breed, although Siberian Huskies are at increased risk. At 1–6 yr of age, there is ataxia of all limbs with no paresis, dysphagia, regurgitation, and difficulty prehending food. Hyperesthesia and self-mutilation occur in some cases. There is decreased proprioceptive positioning, weak to absent patellar reflexes, and decreased to absent pain perception in the limbs and face. Diagnosis is based on clinical signs, electrodiagnostic testing that demonstrates slowed sensory nerve conduction, and biopsy of a mixed or sensory nerve that shows loss of myelinated axons and endoneural fibrosis. The cause is unknown, but loss of neurons in dorsal root ganglia with infiltration of lymphocytes and macrophages is seen at necropsy. There is no effective treatment; the disease typically progresses and leads to euthanasia.

Trigeminal Neuritis: Idiopathic trigeminal neuropathy is common in dogs and uncommon in cats. It is characterized by acute onset of flaccid jaw paralysis. Affected animals cannot close the mouth and have difficulty eating and drinking. Horner syndrome, facial paresis, and decreased facial sensation are also possible. The cause is unknown. Histopathologically, there is bilateral nonsuppurative inflammation and demyelination in the motor branches of the trigeminal nerve. Affected animals usually recover spontaneously within 3–4 wk. Fluid and nutritional support may be necessary.

METABOLIC DISORDERS

Diabetic Neuropathy: This uncommon complication of diabetes mellitus (*see* p 579) is seen in cats and rarely dogs. Signs include weakness, ataxia, and muscle atrophy. Affected cats often have unilateral or bilateral tibial nerve dysfunction, evident as a plantigrade stance. There are several proposed pathophysiologic mechanisms, but prolonged hyperglycemia seems to be the important underlying factor. Pathologic findings in nerves consist of demyelination with remyelination, axonal degeneration, or both. Diagnosis is based on clinical findings, laboratory evidence of diabetes mellitus, and nerve biopsy. The prognosis is guarded, but partial or complete recovery can occur with insulin therapy.

Hypothyroid Neuropathy: This neuropathy is a potential complication of hypothyroidism in dogs (*see* p 553). Mature dogs, especially large-breed dogs, are predisposed. Several syndromes have been reported, including tetraparesis with proprioceptive deficits and hyporeflexia, vestibular dysfunction, megaesophagus, and laryngeal paralysis. In some cases, classic signs of hypothyroidism (eg, obesity and dermatopathy) are absent, and neurologic dysfunction is the only sign of illness. Pathologic findings in peripheral nerves consist of demyelination or remyelination and axonal degeneration. The pathophysiology is poorly understood and, in some affected dogs with motor deficits, a myopathy may also be present. Diagnosis is based on clinical features, laboratory assessment of thyroid function, and response to thyroid supplementation. In some, but not all, cases, signs resolve within several months of starting thyroid replacement therapy.

NEOPLASIA

Nerve Sheath Tumors: Nerve sheath tumors include schwannomas, neurilemmomas, and neurofibromas. They are seen in most domestic animals but are most common in dogs and cattle. In dogs, tumors often arise in the nerves of the brachial plexus, initially causing unilateral thoracic limb lameness and pain that may be confused with musculoskeletal disease. Pain may be elicited on palpation of the axilla or abduction of the limb; large tumors can be palpated. Muscle atrophy and monoparesis eventually develop. The spinal cord may become compressed by the invasive tumor, causing neurologic deficits in other limbs. The trigeminal nerve is the most frequently affected cranial nerve. This results in unilateral atrophy of the temporalis and masseter muscles and facial dysesthesia or anesthesia. Eventually, brain-stem compression can develop.

Early surgical excision may be curative, although recurrence at the proximal stump of the resected nerve(s) is common. In cattle, nerve sheath tumors are often recognized incidentally in old animals at slaughter. Often, multiple nerves, especially autonomic nerves and cranial nerve VIII, are affected. Peripheral nerves may also be affected by other tumors, including lymphoma and leukemia. (*See also* NEOPLASIA OF THE NERVOUS SYSTEM, p 1267, and PERIPHERAL NERVE SHEATH TUMORS, p 126.)

Paraneoplastic Neuropathy: (*See also* p 1280.) Paraneoplastic neuropathy is associated with neoplasia unrelated to tumor infiltration of nerves. It is most common in dogs with insulinoma but has been associated with a variety of tumors, including bronchogenic carcinoma, multiple myeloma, sarcoma, and adenocarcinoma. The pathogenesis is not well understood but may be related to an immune response directed against the tumor that cross-reacts with nerve components. Clinically, there is paraparesis or tetraparesis that progresses over several weeks with decreased spinal reflexes and muscle atrophy. Diagnosis is based on identifying the underlying tumor, clinical and electrodiagnostic findings of neuropathy, and in some cases, nerve biopsy. Signs may improve with successful treatment of the underlying tumor.

NUTRITIONAL DISORDERS

Pantothenic Acid Deficiency: Pantothenic acid deficiency may develop in animals (particularly pigs) on rations of corn. Clinical signs include pelvic limb ataxia and a "goose-stepping" gait in which the stifles remain extended and the hips flex to lift the limbs off the ground. Pathologic findings consist of degeneration of myelinated fibers in peripheral nerves and chromatolysis and loss of sensory neurons in spinal ganglia.

Riboflavin Deficiency in Chickens: Riboflavin deficiency (curled toe paralysis, *see* p 2941) can develop if feed is not formulated properly. Affected chicks show poor growth, diarrhea, and weakness. There is inability to extend the hocks and progressive inward curling of the toes, so that chicks rest and walk on their hocks. Mortality is high by the third week. At necropsy the peripheral nerves, especially the sciatic nerves, are swollen. Histopathologically, there is hypertrophy of Schwann cells, demyelination, and minimal axonal degeneration. Chickens often recover with riboflavin supplementation unless the curled-toe deformity is longstanding.

TOXIC DISORDERS

Botulism: Botulism is intoxication with a neurotoxin produced by *Clostridium botulinum*. It is seen in horses, cattle, sheep, and birds worldwide. It is uncommon in dogs and pigs. (For a complete discussion, *see* p 605 and p 2889.)

Ionophore Toxicity: (*See also* IONOPHORES, p 1175.) Ionophore toxicity has been seen in cattle, sheep, pigs, dogs, cats, and poultry; horses are particularly susceptible. Lasalocid-contaminated food has caused flaccid tetraparesis with hyporeflexia in dogs. In 1995, cat food contaminated with sialinomycin caused an outbreak of polyneuropathy in ~850 cats in the Netherlands and Switzerland. Affected cats had acute onset of tetraparesis, hyporeflexia, dysphagia, respiratory weakness, and eventual muscle atrophy. Histopathologic findings consisted of degeneration of distal sensory and motor axons. Affected animals usually recover with supportive care and removal of the offending food.

Organophosphate Poisoning: Poisoning involving organophosphates (*see* p 3064) can cause three syndromes. The **acute form** is due to irreversible inhibition of acetylcholinesterase, resulting in increased acetylcholine activation of the nicotinic and muscarinic receptors in the parasympathetic nervous system, nicotinic receptors at the neuromuscular junction, nicotinic receptors of the sympathetic nervous system, and cholinergic pathways within the CNS. Clinical signs of acute toxicity include muscarinic signs (eg, vomiting, diarrhea, salivation, bronchoconstriction, increased bronchial secretions), nicotinic signs (eg, muscle tremor and twitching), and CNS signs (eg, behavioral change, seizures).

The **intermediate form** is primarily manifest as generalized muscle weakness due to accumulation of acetylcholine at the nicotinic neuromuscular junction, causing a depolarizing block. Cats are especially prone to this form of toxicity, most commonly due to chlorpyrifos. Affected cats often do not have obvious signs of acute toxicity, instead developing tetraparesis and ventroflexion of the neck several days after exposure. Mydriasis is common. Diagnosis is based on a history of exposure and the presence of typical clinical signs. Decreased cholinesterase activity in whole blood is supportive. Treatment of acute or subacute toxicity should include administration of atropine (0.2 mg/kg, IM) if dyspnea due to bronchial secretions and bronchoconstriction is present. Atropine will not relieve the nicotinic signs of tremors and weakness, which should be treated with pralidoxime chloride (20 mg/kg, IM or SC, bid). Diphenhydramine (4 mg/kg, IM or PO, bid) may help alleviate muscle weakness. Treatment for several weeks may be necessary.

The **delayed form** of toxicity is associated with degeneration of distal axons in the peripheral and central nervous systems. It is unrelated to inhibition of acetylcholinesterase and is seen only with certain organophosphates. Signs develop several weeks after exposure and are characterized by weakness and ataxia of the pelvic limbs. In horses, laryngeal paralysis has also been reported. There is no specific treatment.

Tick Paralysis: Rapidly progressive paralysis may be caused by several species of ticks (*see* p 1314). Some female ticks produce a salivary toxin that interferes with acetylcholine release at the neuromuscular junction. In North America, *Dermacentor variabilis* and *D andersoni* may affect dogs, sheep, and cattle. In Australia, *Ixodes holocyclus* causes an especially severe form of tick paralysis in dogs, cats, cattle, sheep, pigs, llamas, horses, and occasionally people. In Africa, the major tick associated with paralysis is *I rubicundus*, with cattle, sheep, goats, and rarely dogs affected. A wide variety of ticks affect animals in Europe and Asia.

Clinical signs consist of paraparesis that progresses within 24–72 hr to flaccid tetraplegia, with weak to absent spinal cord reflexes. Sensory perception and consciousness remain normal. Dysphagia, facial paralysis, masticatory muscle weakness, and respiratory paralysis may develop in severe cases. Treatment consists of removal of the tick and application of a topical acaricide to kill any hidden ticks. For all except *I holocyclus* paralysis, prognosis is good, and recovery occurs within 1–2 days. Tick antiserum is available for treatment of *I holocyclus* paralysis, but prognosis is guarded because death from respiratory paralysis may occur despite treatment.

TRAUMA

The immediate effect of injury of a peripheral nerve is a variable degree of dysfunction, depending on the severity of the injury. The mildest form of injury is neuropraxia, which temporarily disrupts function with minimal morphologic alterations in the nerve. Axonotmesis is disruption of axons without disruption of the surrounding connective tissue of the nerve. The most severe form of injury is neurotmesis, which is complete severance of the nerve. With both axonotmesis and neurotmesis, there is subsequent degeneration of the axons distal to the injury site and in a portion of the nerve proximal to the injury site.

Diagnosis of peripheral nerve injuries is based on the history and clinical assessment of the motor and sensory function of the affected nerve(s). Electromyography often helps identify denervated muscles 5–10 days after injury. Nerve conduction studies may also be useful in diagnosis.

Prognosis is guarded. With neuropraxia, complete recovery usually occurs within 3 wk. For function to return after axons are disrupted (axonotmesis, neurotmesis), the nerve must regenerate from the point of injury all the way to the innervated muscle. The growth rate of regenerating axons in the distal stump is 1–3 mm/day. Recovery is unlikely if the severed axons are substantially separated or if scar tissue interferes with axonal growth. Although various anti-inflammatory drugs have been recommended for traumatic nerve injuries, there is little evidence of benefit. Surgery to appose the nerve stumps should be performed promptly in cases in which the nerve has been sharply transected. In instances of blunt trauma, surgical exploration and excision of scar tissue may help. Surgery is often successful in horses with fibrous compression of the suprascapular nerve. Longterm management consists of physical therapy to minimize muscle atrophy and decreased mobility of joints. Bandages or splints may be necessary to help protect the affected limb.

Brachial Plexus Avulsion: Traumatic injury to the C6 to T2 nerve roots that innervate the thoracic limb can lead to brachial plexus avulsion in dogs, cats, and birds. With severe extension or abduction of the limb, the nerve roots stretch or tear from their attachment to the spinal cord. Clinical signs vary with the extent of root involvement. Complete avulsion results in flaccid paralysis of the limb, anesthesia distal to the elbow, ipsilateral Horner syndrome, and ipsilateral loss of the cutaneous trunci (panniculus) reflex. The injured animal bears little or no weight on the limb and drags the dorsal surface of the paw on the ground. Sensation to the ventral surface of the paw is spared if only the cranial nerve roots are affected. Avulsion of the caudal nerve roots causes loss of sensation on the caudal surface of the limb with variable loss on the cranial surface.

There is no treatment, and with complete avulsion, the prognosis is poor. Amputation of the limb may be necessary because of damage from dragging or self-mutilation. Recovery is possible in mild cases in which the roots are contused rather than avulsed.

Peripheral Nerve Injuries: These injuries are some of the most common neuropathies in animals. The **sciatic nerve** or its branches may be injured by pelvic fractures, during or after retrograde placement of intramedullary pins in the femur, or by injections of irritating substances in or near the nerve. Damage to the proximal aspect of the sciatic nerve causes monoparesis with inability to flex the stifle. The hock and digits cannot flex or extend, and weight is supported on the dorsal surface of the foot with the hock excessively flexed. There may be loss of sensation below the stifle except for the medial aspect, which is innervated by a branch of the femoral nerve.

Injury to the **tibial nerve** results in inability to extend the hock or flex the digits as well as reduced sensation over the plantar surface of the foot.

Injury to the **peroneal nerve** results in inability to flex the hock or extend the digits as well as decreased sensation over the craniodorsal surface of the foot, hock, and stifle.

The **femoral nerve** may be injured in calves and foals during dystocia if excessive traction stretches or otherwise damages it. This results in an inability to bear weight on the limb because of an inability to extend the stifle. The patellar reflex is weak or absent. Sensation is lost along the medial surface of the limb (saphenous nerve).

The **suprascapular nerve** is most commonly injured in large animals secondary to trauma of the shoulder region. This results in atrophy of the supraspinatus and infraspinatus muscles and instability of the shoulder joint (sweeney, *see* p 1129). In horses, the nerve may be entrapped by connective tissue that develops in the region of the supraspinous fossa.

Calving Paralysis: Calving paralysis is seen in heifers with oversized fetuses. It has previously been attributed to bilateral compression of the obturator nerve, but damage to the sixth lumbar nerve root, which contributes to the obturator and sciatic nerve, probably accounts for most of the paralysis. Ischemic necrosis of muscles secondary to compression, and ruptures of muscles during attempts to rise, also contribute to the paraparesis. Additionally, metabolic derangements, such as hypocalcemia, may complicate the syndrome. (*See also* BOVINE SECONDARY RECUMBENCY, p 1188.)

Facial Nerve Trauma: Facial nerve trauma is most common in large animals that become recumbent with subsequent compression of the side of the face. It can be caused by pressure from a halter in horses during general anesthesia. There is ipsilateral lip paralysis, deviation of the muzzle to the contralateral side, and weak to absent palpebral reflex. A drooping ear can result from injuries to the proximal aspect of the nerve.

VASCULAR DISEASES

Ischemic Neuromyopathy: Ischemic neuromyopathy is most common in cats with arterial thromboembolism secondary to myocardial disease. It also is seen in dogs with a variety of underlying disorders, including hyperadrenocorticism, hypothyroidism, renal disease, cancer, and heart disease. Occlusion occurs most commonly at the distal aortic trifurcation, resulting in ischemia of muscles and nerves in the pelvic limbs. There is acute, painful paraparesis and an inability to flex or extend the hock. The flexor reflex and, in some cases, the patellar reflex are lost. Sensation distal to the hock is decreased. The gastrocnemius and cranial tibial muscles are often firm and painful. The nails may be cyanotic, and the femoral pulses are weak or absent.

Diagnosis can usually be made based on clinical features. Serum CK is often increased. Doppler ultrasonography helps evaluate blood flow in the distal aorta and femoral arteries. Pathologic changes are present distal to the level of the middle to lower thigh and are characterized as focal muscle necrosis and degeneration of the central portions of the sciatic nerve and its branches. Management consists of analgesics, nursing care, and treatment of any underlying disease (eg, cardiomyopathy). Thrombolytic therapy with streptokinase or tissue plasminogen activator does not improve survival. Anticoagulants, such as unfractionated heparin or low-molecular-weight heparin, are used to reduce continued thrombus formation. Neurologic deficits may improve within 2–3 wk, but 6 mo may be required for complete recovery. Permanent deficits are possible. Approximately 60% of affected cats die or are euthanized during the initial episode. In the cats that survive, the longterm prognosis is guarded (median 12 mo) because of the underlying heart disease and high risk of recurrence of thromboembolism.

DISEASES OF THE SPINAL COLUMN AND CORD

Diseases of the spinal column and cord include congenital disorders, degenerative diseases, inflammatory and infectious diseases, neoplasia, nutritional diseases, trauma, toxic disorders, and vascular diseases. Many of these diseases are discussed in full in other chapters and are only briefly described here. For a discussion of congenital disorders related to the spinal column and cord, *see* p 1222.

DEGENERATIVE DISEASES

Cervical Spondylomyelopathy: Cervical spondylomyelopathy, also called cervical vertebral malformation-malarticulation and wobbler syndrome, is compression of the spinal cord caused by abnormal development of the cervical vertebrae. Genetic factors and possibly nutrition may be involved.

In dogs, there are two forms of the disease, disc-associated wobbler syndrome (DAWS) and bony-associated cervical spondylomyelopathy. DAWS affects middle-aged (mean 7 yr), large-breed dogs, especially Doberman Pinschers. There is ventral compression of the spinal cord due to protrusion of one or more caudal cervical discs, in some cases complicated by congenital stenosis of the vertebral canal or hypertrophy of the ligamentum flavum. Bony-associated compression affects young (several months to 4 yr), giant-breed dogs, including Great Danes, Mastiffs, and Rottweilers. Spinal cord compression is due to bony proliferation of the articular processes and pedicles, usually of the C4 to C7 vertebrae.

Clinical signs can be acute or slowly progressive. Mild cases are characterized by subtle ataxia of all limbs, often evident as a long, protracted stride in the pelvic limbs, with short-strided gait in the thoracic limbs. In severe cases, there is paresis or paralysis of all limbs. Neck pain is variable. Differential diagnoses include congenital anomalies, trauma, meningomyelitis, discospondylitis, and neoplasia. Survey radiographs cannot confirm a diagnosis of cervical spondylomyelopathy but are useful in excluding discospondylitis and bony neoplasia. Definitive diagnosis requires myelography, CT, or MRI.

Nonsurgical treatment is indicated for dogs with mild signs and consists of exercise restriction and prednisone (0.5 mg/kg/day). Signs improve in ~50% of dogs and remained unchanged in ~25% of dogs with nonsurgical treatment. Surgery is indicated in animals with substantial neurologic deficits and in those that do not respond adequately to nonsurgical treatment. The specific technique is based on the changes evident on imaging and include ventral slot with partial discectomy, dorsal laminectomy, or distraction and fusion of affected vertebrae. Overall, ~80% of dogs do well with surgery.

In horses, cervical spondylomyelopathy is the most common noninfectious disease of the spinal cord and occurs in many breeds. Most horses present at <3 yr of age, although they can be affected at any age. The mid-cervical region is most commonly affected, and there is spinal ataxia and tetraparesis. Diagnosis is based on imaging and excluding other causes. Plain radiographs may show abnormal articular facets and stenosis of the vertebral canal. Myelography is necessary for definitive diagnosis and surgical planning. Nonsurgical treatment involves NSAIDs and dimethyl sulfoxide to reduce inflammation. In yearlings, diet modification can help. Surgery most commonly involves ventral fusion of the affected vertebrae. Approximately 80% of affected horses improve with surgery. Owner/rider safety is a major concern in horses with ataxia.

Degenerative Lumbosacral Stenosis: Narrowing of the lumbosacral vertebral canal or intervertebral foramina results in compression of the cauda equina or nerve roots. It is most common in large breeds of dogs, especially German Shepherds, and is rare in cats. It results from degeneration and protrusion of the L7–S1 disc, hypertrophy of the ligamentum flavum, or rarely subluxation of the lumbosacral joint. The cause is unknown, although German Shepherds with congenital transitional vertebrae are at increased risk. Clinical signs typically begin at 3–7 yr of age and may include difficulty using the pelvic limbs, pelvic limb lameness, tail weakness, and incontinence. Pain on palpation or extension of the lumbosacral joint is the most consistent finding. There may be proprioceptive deficits, muscle atrophy, or a weak flexor reflex in the pelvic limbs. Plain radiographs may show degenerative changes, but definitive diagnosis requires MRI, CT, or epidurography. Dogs in which mild pain is the only sign may improve with 4–6 wk of rest. Epidural *injection of methylprednisolone acetate* (1 mg/kg on each of day 1, day 14, and day 42) is effective in ~80% of dogs with pain and minimal neurologic deficits. Surgery is indicated when pain is refractory to medical therapy or there are neurologic deficits. The most common technique is dorsal laminectomy with partial discectomy, but foramenotomy or stabilization is indicated in certain cases. Approximately 70%–95% of dogs improve with surgery, although preexisting urinary incontinence may not resolve.

Degenerative Myelopathy of Dogs: Degenerative myelopathy of dogs, also called chronic degenerative radiculomyelopathy, is a slowly progressive, noninflammatory degeneration of the axons and myelin primarily affecting the white matter of the spinal cord. It is most common in German Shepherds, Pembroke Welsh Corgis, Boxers, Rhodesian Ridgebacks, and Chesapeake Bay Retrievers, but is occasionally recognized in many other breeds. The cause is a mutation in the superoxide dismutase1 (SOD1) gene, inherited in an autosomal recessive pattern with incomplete penetrance. It is similar to familial amyotrophic lateral sclerosis in human patients. Pathologically, there is noninflammatory degeneration of axons in the white matter of the spinal cord, which is most severe in the thoracic region.

Affected dogs are usually >8 yr old and develop an insidious onset of nonpainful ataxia and weakness of the pelvic limbs. Spinal reflexes are usually normal or exaggerated, but in advanced cases there is flaccid tetraparesis and hyporeflexia reflecting lower motor neuron involvement. Early cases may be confused with orthopedic disorders; however, proprioceptive deficits are an early feature of degenerative myelopathy and are not seen in orthopedic disease.

Myelography or MRI and CSF analysis are essential to exclude compressive and inflammatory diseases. A DNA test based on the SOD1 gene is available on the Orthopedic Foundation for Animals Web site. Dogs that are homozygous for the mutation are at risk of the disease and will pass one copy of the mutant allele to their offspring. Heterozygotes are at low risk of the disease but have a 50% chance of passing one copy of the mutant allele to each offspring. Homozygous normals are at low risk of the disease and will not pass the mutation to offspring.

There is no specific treatment and no evidence that glucocorticoids, other drugs, or supplements alter the course of the disease. Most dogs are euthanized because of disability within 1–3 yr of diagnosis.

Equine Degenerative Myeloencephalopathy: Equine degenerative myeloencephalopathy is a progressive neurologic disorder of horses and zebras characterized by diffuse degeneration of axons, myelin, and neurons in the spinal cord and, to a lesser degree, the brain stem. It has been reported in many equine breeds in North America, Australia, and England. The cause is incompletely understood, but a vitamin E deficiency and genetic factors are suspected. Clinical signs usually become apparent during the first year of life and consist of ataxia and weakness in all four limbs, although the hindlimbs may be more severely affected. Clinical signs may stabilize or slowly progress. There is no definitive diagnostic test. Clinical diagnosis is based on clinical features and excluding other causes. Myelography and CSF analysis are normal. Supplementation of pregnant mares and newborn foals with vitamin E is preventive in predisposed families, and affected horses may improve with vitamin E supplementation.

Intervertebral Disc Disease: Degeneration and subsequent herniation of the intervertebral disc results in compression of the spinal cord, spinal nerve, and/or nerve root. It is a common cause of spinal cord disease in dogs, with a lifetime prevalence of ~3.5%. Clinical signs due to disc disease are rare in cats and horses. Chondrodystrophoid breeds of dogs (eg, Dachshund, Beagle, Shih Tzu, Lhasa Apso, and Pekingese) are most commonly affected, with Miniature Dachshunds having a lifetime prevalence of ~20%. In these breeds, there is chondroid degeneration of the discs within the first few months of life. Disc extrusion can occur as early as 1–2 yr of age, and clinical signs are often acute and severe. In contrast, fibroid disk degeneration typically occurs in large breeds of dogs >5 yr old and causes slowly progressive clinical signs.

The most common sites of disc herniation are the cervical and thoracolumbar regions. The predominant sign of cervical disc herniation is neck pain, manifested as cervical rigidity and muscle spasms. There may be thoracic limb lameness or neurologic deficits, ranging from mild tetraparesis to tetraplegia. In thoracolumbar disc herniation, there may be back pain, evident as kyphosis and reluctance to move. Neurologic deficits are usually more severe than those seen in cervical disc disease and range from pelvic limb ataxia to paraplegia and incontinence. In paraplegic animals, the most important prognostic finding is whether there is deep pain perception caudal to the lesion. This is assessed by pinching the toe or tail and observing whether there is a behavioral response, such as a bark or turn of the head. It is important to pinch the bone to stimulate deep pain receptors, not just the skin, which tests only superficial pain. Reflex flexion of the limb must not be mistaken for a behavioral response.

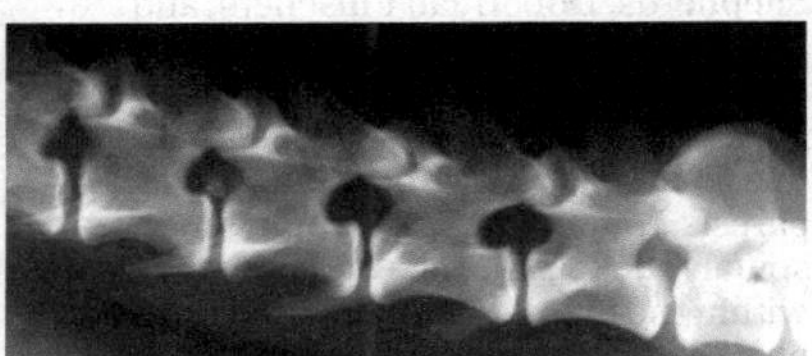

Intervertebral disc extrusion, L3-L4, in a dog.
Courtesy of Dr. William Thomas.

Definitive diagnosis of disc extrusion is based on imaging studies. Spinal radiographs may show narrowing of the affected disc space, intervertebral foramen or articular facets, or radiodense calcified disc material within the vertebral canal. However, radiographs are not sensitive or specific enough for definitive diagnosis, which requires myelography, MRI, or CT. Dogs with pain and minimal to moderate neurologic deficits often recover with 2–3 wk of cage rest. A short course of prednisone (0.5 mg/kg/day for 3 days) is often helpful in relieving pain. The use of anti-inflammatory or analgesic medication without concurrent cage rest is contraindicated, because an increase in the dog's activity may lead to further disc extrusion and worsening of spinal cord compression. Clinical signs recur after conservative therapy in 30%–40% of cases.

In animals with severe neurologic deficits, prompt surgery offers the best chance of recovery (*see* TABLE 1). Other indications for surgery are failure of conservative therapy and recurrent episodes. Hemilaminectomy with removal of the extruded disc material is the most common procedure. Prophylactic fenestration of commonly affected disc spaces (eg, T11 through L4) decreases recurrence in small-breed dogs. Progressive myelomalacia develops in 5%–10% of dogs with paraplegia and loss of deep pain perception. In this syndrome, affected dogs develop flaccid tetraplegia, the level of anesthesia ascends cranially, and respiratory paralysis develops.

Diffuse Idiopathic Skeletal Hyperostosis: Also known as Forestier disease in human patients, diffuse idiopathic skeletal hyperostosis (DISH) is

TABLE 1 RECOVERY RATES AFTER SURGERY FOR INTERVERTEBRAL DISC DISEASE IN DOGS

Patient Type	Recovery Rate
Nonambulatory small-breed dog with thoracolumbar extrusion and intact deep pain	85%–95%
Small-breed dog with thoracolumbar extrusion and loss of deep pain <24 hr	50%
Small-breed dog with thoracolumbar extrusion and loss of deep pain >24 hr	<50%
Nonambulatory large-breed dog with chronic thoracolumbar protrusion	25%–50%
Ambulatory dog with cervical disc disease	95%
Nonambulatory dog with cervical disc disease	65%–95%

characterized by ossification of entheses, the sites where a ligament, tendon, or joint capsule inserts into bone. Radiographic criteria for diagnosis are flowing ossification along the ventrolateral aspect of at least four contiguous vertebrae with relative preservation of disc width and absence of facet joint ankylosis. Approximately 4% of dogs >1 yr old are affected, and the prevelance increases with age. As with spondylosis deformans, Boxers are at increased risk, with a prevelance of ~40%. The thoracic and lumbar regions are most commonly affected. It is unclear how often DISH causes clinical signs, and in many cases the radiographic findings are incidental. However, spinal pain and stiffness is possible and, in those cases, treatment is analgesics as needed.

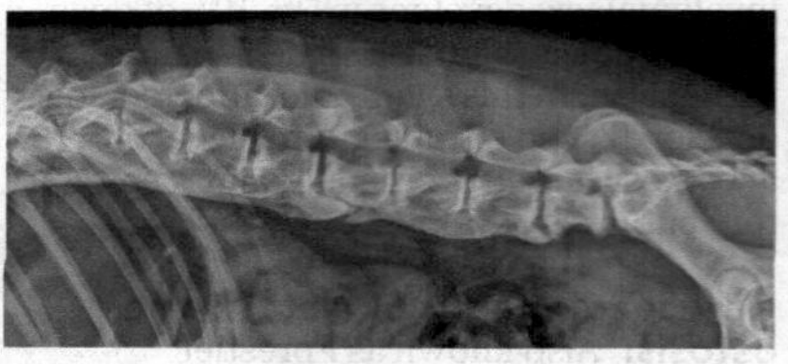
Diffuse idiopathic skeletal hyperostosis (DISH) in a dog. *Courtesy of Dr. William Thomas.*

Equine Motor Neuron Disease:

Equine motor neuron disease is a progressive, noninflammatory degeneration of motor neurons in the spinal cord and brain stem of horses. It is most common in the northeastern USA but has been reported in several areas of North and South America, Europe, and Japan. The cause is uncertain, but vitamin E deficiency is a strong risk factor. Adult horses of any age and breed can be affected, although Quarter horses are affected most commonly. Affected horses typically do not have access to pasture grass and are fed poor-quality grass hay.

Clinical signs consist of generalized symmetric weakness, trembling, and muscle atrophy. Affected horses often stand with their head held low and their feet camped under their body, frequently shifting their weight from one limb to another. Ataxia is not a feature of this disease, in contrast to most spinal cord diseases. Many affected horses have retinal abnormalities, including a distinct reticulated pigment pattern and areas of hyperreflectivity. Electromyography and biopsy of the spinal accessory nerve or the sacrodorsalis caudalis muscle are useful in diagnosis.

There is no specific treatment, but some horses improve partially after 2–3 mo of illness. Horses that lack access to green forage high in vitamin E for prolonged periods should be supplemented with vitamin E.

Degeneration of Motor Neurons:

Degeneration of motor neurons is an inherited or sporadic disease seen in Brittany Spaniels, Pointers, German Shepherds, Doberman Pinschers, and Rottweilers; cats; Hereford, Brown Swiss, and red Danish cattle; Yorkshire pigs; and goats. Also called spinal muscular atrophy, this disease is characterized by progressive paresis, tremor, muscle atrophy, and weak spinal reflexes. The age of onset is typically within the first 1–2 yr of life. Electromyography and muscle biopsy help document muscle denervation, but definitive diagnosis is based on loss of motor neurons in the

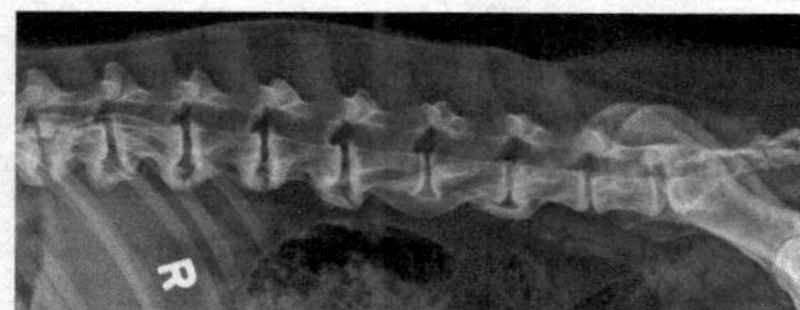

Spondylosis deformans in a dog. *Courtesy of Dr. William Thomas.*

ventral horn of the spinal cord and brain-stem nuclei on necropsy.

Metabolic Storage Disorders: Rare, usually inherited, metabolic disorders can affect the CNS, including the spinal cord. (*See also* CONGENITAL AND INHERITED ANOMALIES OF THE NERVOUS SYSTEM, p 1222.)

Spondylosis Deformans: Spondylosis deformans is a noninflammatory condition characterized by formation of bony projections (enthesophytes) at the location where the annulus fibrosus is attached to the cortical surface of adjacent vertebrae. These bony growths vary from small spurs located several millimeters from the junction between the disc and vertebra to bony bridges that span the disc space, leaving at least part of the ventral surface of the vertebra unaffected. The enthesophytes typically expand laterally and ventrally but not dorsally and therefore rarely affect the spinal cord. The cause is breakdown of the outer fibers of the annulus fibrosis and stretching of the longitudinal ligament. The increased stress at the vertebral attachment of the longitudinal ligament incites bony production.

Spondylosis deformans is seen in dogs, cats, and bulls, and the incidence increases with age. It is uncommon in dogs <2 yr old; by 9 yr of age, 25%–70% of all dogs are affected. It is especially common in Boxers, and a genetic predisposition has been identified in this breed. It is typically an incidental radiographic finding, and there is no correlation between the presence of spondylosis and clinical signs. Rare cases cause spinal hyperesthesia, which should be treated with analgesics.

INFLAMMATORY AND INFECTIOUS DISEASES

Infectious and inflammatory diseases of the spinal column and spinal cord include bacterial, rickettsial, viral, fungal, protozoal, and parasitic infections and idiopathic inflammatory disease. Many of these diseases can also affect the brain (*see* p 1262). Some of the more common infectious and inflammatory diseases in which involvement of the spinal column or cord is a prominent feature are discussed below.

Bacterial Diseases

Discospondylitis is inflammation of the intervertebral disc and adjacent vertebral bodies. **Vertebral osteomyelitis** is inflammation of the vertebra without concurrent disc infection. Both diseases are usually caused by hematogenous spread of bacterial or fungal infection. Immunosuppression may play a role in some infections. Discospondylitis is most common in dogs, especially larger breeds. Osteomyelitis of the lumbar vertebrae can develop in dogs secondary to migration of plant awns. In cats, it is rare and usually due to direct spread of infection from an adjacent wound. Discospondylitis and vertebral osteomyelitis have also been reported in horses, ruminants, and pigs, especially neonates. Infection may be seen at any disc space, and multiple lesions may be seen.

In canine discospondylitis, the most commonly isolated organisms are *Staphylococcus* spp. Other organisms include *Brucella canis*, *Streptococcus* spp, *Escherichia coli*, *Proteus* spp, *Corynebacterium diphtheroides*, *Nocardia* spp, and *Aspergillus* spp. Spinal pain is the most consistent clinical finding. Systemic signs, such as fever, depression, and weight loss, are less common. Neurologic deficits may develop due to spinal cord compression caused by proliferative tissue or, rarely, spread of infection to the spinal cord or pathologic fracture.

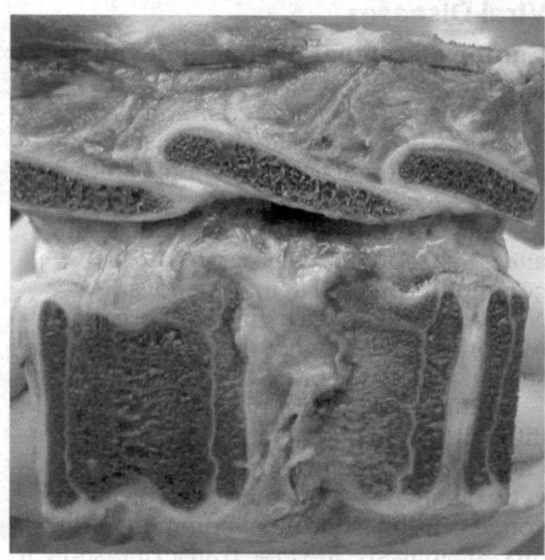

Spinal vertebral body abscess (cross-section). *Courtesy of Dr. Sameeh M. Abutarbush.*

Early radiographic findings consist of destruction of the adjacent vertebral end plates and collapse of the disc space. More advanced lesions also have variable degrees of osteophyte formation. Blood and urine cultures often identify the causative organism. Affected dogs should be tested for brucellosis (*see* p 1402).

Although clinical signs usually resolve within 5 days of treatment with an appropriate antibiotic, treatment should be continued for at least 8 wk. Amoxicillin/clavulanic acid for presumed *Staphylococcus* spp infection is a good choice if cultures are negative.

Rickettsial Diseases

Neurologic abnormalities, including signs of spinal cord dysfunction, are sometimes seen in dogs with rickettsial infection. Dogs with **Rocky Mountain spotted fever** (*Rickettsia rickettsii*, *see* p 806) often have thrombocytopenia, leukocytosis, and a neutrophilic pleocytosis and mildly increased protein on CSF analysis. Diagnosis is based on a 4-fold increase in serum antibody concentration. Dogs with **ehrlichiosis** (*Ehrlichia canis*, *see* p 803) often have thrombocytopenia, anemia, leukopenia, hyperglobulinemia, and mononuclear pleocytosis and marked increase in protein on CSF analysis. A single serum antibody titer is usually sufficient for diagnosis of *E canis*. Treatment of rickettsial myelitis consists of doxycycline or chloramphenicol for 14–21 days. Prognosis is good with early treatment, although neurologic deficits occasionally progress despite treatment.

Viral Diseases

Canine distemper encephalomyelitis (*see* p 777), caused by a paramyxovirus, remains one of the most common CNS disorders in dogs worldwide. Onset of neurologic deficits may be acute or slowly progressive, reflecting the location of the lesion(s) within the CNS. The brain stem and spinal cord are the regions most commonly affected in mature dogs. Neurologic signs are usually not preceded by, nor coincident with, the systemic illness seen in young dogs.

Definitive antemortem diagnosis is difficult. There may be active or inactive chorioretinitis on fundoscopy. A lymphocytic pleocytosis with increased protein concentration is the most common finding on CSF analysis. Reverse transcriptase-PCR on urine or CSF is useful in diagnosis. There is no specific treatment, and the prognosis is poor for severely affected dogs. Vaccination is usually successful in preventing the systemic form of distemper, but previously vaccinated dogs can be affected by the neurologic form.

Caprine arthritis and encephalitis (*see* p 747) is caused by a lentivirus that can also cause pneumonitis and arthritis. CNS disease is most common in goats 2–4 mo old, although older animals may also be affected. There is an acute onset of slightly asymmetric spastic paraparesis that may progress to tetraplegia with exaggerated reflexes. A mononuclear pleocytosis and increased protein in the CSF are present in ~50% of the cases. Serologic testing is helpful in detecting infection, but false-negatives can be seen. Histologically, there is severe nonsuppurative inflammation with demyelination or necrosis, most prominent in the white matter of the spinal cord. There is no treatment, and recovery is unlikely.

A related lentivirus is a rare cause of chronic encephalomyelitis in sheep (**maedi**, *see* p 1475). Affected sheep are usually >2 yr old and suffer an insidious onset of progressive ataxia, paraparesis, or tetraparesis.

Equine infectious anemia (*see* p 699) occasionally produces encephalomyelitis in horses. Neurologic deficits are usually referable to spinal cord disease and include ataxia and weakness in the hindlimbs. The protein concentration of and the number of lymphocytes in the CSF are often increased. Diagnosis is by positive agar gel immunodiffusion testing. There is no treatment, and affected horses are usually euthanized to prevent spread of the disease.

Equine herpesvirus 1 (EHV-1) encephalomyelopathy is a neurologic disorder that affects horses worldwide. The EHV-1 virus infects vascular endothelial cells, particularly those within the CNS, and causes an immune-mediated vasculitis with secondary infarction and hemorrhage throughout the brain and spinal cord. The EHV-1 virus has also been associated with meningoencephalitis in alpacas and llamas. In horses, neurologic signs may be seen as the primary disease or follow rhinopneumonitis or abortion. Any age animal may be affected.

Neurologic deficits have an abrupt onset, vary from mild hindlimb ataxia to paraplegia, and usually do not progress after 24 hr. Urine dribbling, fecal retention, and sensory deficits in the perineum and tail are common. The CSF is often xanthochromic with increased protein content and normal numbers of cells. Diagnosis is based on clinical findings and an increase in antibody concentration in paired serum samples, isolation of virus from nasal or pharyngeal secretions, or PCR testing. There is no specific treatment, but anti-inflammatory agents such as dimethyl sulfoxide, dexamethasone, and NSAIDs may help. Supportive care is important to prevent complications such as urine retention, cystitis, and decubitus. Mildly affected horses often recover with supportive care. Even recumbent horses can eventually recover with meticulous nursing care. Vaccination does not protect from the neurologic form of this disease. (*See also* EQUINE HERPESVIRUS INFECTION, p 1444.)

Feline infectious peritonitis (*see* p 780) is a disease of domestic cats caused by an immune-mediated response to a coronavirus. CNS involvement is common. There are pyogranulomatous lesions involving the neural parenchyma, choroid plexuses, ependyma, and leptomeninges. Clinical signs of spinal cord involvement include spinal hyperesthesia and paraparesis or tetraparesis. Hyperglobulinemia and involvement of other organs, especially the eyes, are common. Serum antibody tests currently available are insensitive and nonspecific. A mixed (neutrophilic and mononuclear) pleocytosis with increased protein concentration is the most common finding on CSF analysis. There is no effective treatment, and prognosis is poor.

Feline leukemia virus–associated myelopathy is seen in some cats infected with the feline leukemia virus (FeLV, *see* p 790) for ≥2 yr. Ataxia and weakness of the pelvic limbs progresses to paraplegia within 1 yr. Other signs include diffuse spinal pain and abnormal behavior. Diagnosis is based on clinical features, FeLV serology, and exclusion of other causes, such as spinal lymphoma and myelitis due to toxoplasmosis or fungal infection. There is no treatment; affected cats are eventually euthanized because of disability. Pathologic findings consist of white matter degeneration, swollen axons, and dilation of myelin sheaths in the spinal cord and brain stem. FeLV antigen is present in the nervous system, indicating that the lesions are due to viral infection.

Teschovirus encephalomyelitis (*see* p 1307), also called Teschen disease, Talfan disease, and porcine polioencephalomyelitis, is caused by a neurotropic teschovirus previously classified as an enterovirus. There is a peracute or subacute onset of hindlimb ataxia and paresis with hyporeflexia, depression, seizures, and death. Older pigs may survive, but mortality is high in young pigs.

Porcine hemagglutinating encephalomyelitis virus is a coronavirus that causes both vomiting and wasting disease (*see* p 728) and an encephalomyelitis. It is most common in piglets <3 wk old, and there is some overlap of these syndromes. The CNS disease starts with several days of vomiting, which is followed by hyperesthesia, muscle tremors, ataxia, paresis, opisthotonos, coma, and death. Histopathologically, there is diffuse nonsuppurative encephalomyelitis, primarily involving gray matter. Diagnosis is based on necropsy or an increase in antibody titer in paired sera. There is no treatment.

Rabies (*see* p 1302) is caused by a neurotropic rhabdovirus that reaches the CNS via peripheral nerves. It produces multifocal, nonsuppurative polioencephalomyelitis in all domestic mammals. Signs of spinal cord involvement include ataxia and progressive paralysis, usually with absent reflexes. Affected animals typically, but not invariably, die with progressive neurologic signs within 2–7 days of illness.

Fungal Diseases

Cryptococcus neoformans is the most common fungus to involve the CNS in animals. Infection is most common in dogs and cats and occurs occasionally in horses. Other fungal organisms may invade the CNS, including *Blastomyces dermatitidis*, *Histoplasma capsulatum*, *Coccidioides immitis*, *Aspergillus* spp, and phaeohyphomycoses. Affected animals often have involvement of other organs, such as the lungs, eyes, skin, or bones. Signs of spinal cord involvement include paresis or paralysis and spinal hyperesthesia. Diagnosis is based on serology, culture, or identifying the organism in CSF or extraneural tissue. Fluconazole is often effective for cryptococcosis and coccidioidomycosis. Itraconazole or amphotericin B is recommended for histoplasmosis and blastomycosis, but the prognosis is guarded to poor. (*See also* FUNGAL INFECTIONS, p 632.)

Protozoal Diseases

Equine protozoal myeloencephalitis (*see* p 1309) is a common disease of horses that produces a nonsuppurative, often necrotizing, meningoencephalomyelitis. Horses are likely an aberrant host for the causative organism, usually *Sarcocystis neurona*, but less commonly, other protozoa cause the disease. Neurologic signs are extremely variable and often asymmetric, reflecting involvement anywhere in the CNS. Ataxia and paresis are common. Other potential signs include obscure lameness, focal muscle atrophy, and cranial nerve dysfunction. Approximately 75% of affected horses improve with treatment, but permanent neurologic deficits are possible and relapse is not rare.

Neosporosis (*see* p 663) is caused by *Neospora caninum*, a protozoan that can cause a nonsuppurative encephalomyelitis, most commonly in dogs. Infection in young puppies typically causes ascending paralysis with rigid contraction of the muscles of one or both pelvic limbs. Other organs, including muscle, liver, and lungs, can be affected. Diagnosis is based on detection of antibodies to the organism by immunohistochemistry or PCR. Early treatment with clindamycin or sulfadiazine and pyrimethamine may be effective, but the prognosis is poor.

Toxoplasmosis (*see* p 685) is caused by *Toxoplasma gondii* and can occasionally cause a nonsuppurative encephalomyelitis in puppies, kittens, and piglets. Diagnosis is based on identifying the organism in tissue or a 4-fold increase in IgG antibody in paired sera. In cats, a high concentration of IgM antibody in serum or CSF supports the diagnosis. Clindamycin or sulfadiazine and pyrimethamine are recommended for treatment.

Parasitic Diseases

Verminous myelitis is inflammation of the spinal cord caused by parasite migration. Organisms include *Parelaphostrongylus tenuis* in sheep, goats, and llamas; *Hypoderma bovis* in cattle; *Strongylus vulgaris*, *Halicephalobus deletrix*, and *Setaria* spp in horses; *Stephanurus dentatus* in pigs; *Cuterebra* spp in cats; and *Baylisascaris procyonis* in dogs. Signs of spinal cord involvement are usually acute, often asymmetric, and may be progressive. Antemortem diagnosis is difficult. Increased eosinophils in the CSF is suggestive, but CSF findings are variable. Treatment with fenbendazole, thiabendazole, or ivermectin is recommended, but the prognosis is guarded. (*See also* CNS DISEASES CAUSED BY HELMINTHS AND ARTHROPODS, p 1310.)

Idiopathic Inflammatory Diseases

Feline nonsuppurative meningoencephalomyelitis (feline polioencephalomyelitis, staggering disease) is a slowly progressive, inflammatory disease of the CNS in domestic cats. It has been reported in North America, Europe, and Australia. The cause is unknown, but an infectious agent, probably a virus, is strongly suspected. The disease causes neuronal degeneration, axonal loss, and demyelination with mononuclear inflammation, most severe in the thoracic segments of the spinal cord. The clinical course is marked by progressive paraparesis of 1–2 mo duration, often with focal hyperesthesia, head tremor, and behavioral changes. Antemortem diagnosis is difficult. There is no treatment, and prognosis is poor.

Granulomatous meningoencephalomyelitis (GME) is an inflammatory disease of the CNS in dogs worldwide. The cause is unknown, although an infectious agent, most likely a virus, is suspected. In the disseminated form, previously called inflammatory reticulosis, there are perivascular accumulations of mononuclear cells and neutrophils. In the focal form, previously called neoplastic reticulosis, there are granulomatous lesions containing primarily reticulohistiocytic cells. Adult dogs of any breed can be affected, but female, small-breed dogs, especially Poodles, may be predisposed.

Clinical signs are variable and may indicate focal or multifocal brain or spinal cord dysfunction. Cervical pain and tetraparesis are the most common signs of spinal cord involvement. Signs are often acute, but the focal form of GME can cause neurologic deficits that slowly progress over the course of several months. The CSF usually has increased protein and pleocytosis, with either mononuclear cells or neutrophils predominating. MRI and CT often show a single or multiple enhancing masses. Tentative diagnosis is based on clinical findings, imaging, CSF analysis, and exclusion of other possible diseases. Dogs often improve with immunosuppressive doses of corticosteroids and other immunomodulating drugs such as cytarabine, cyclosporine, and procarbazine, but relapse is possible, and many dogs eventually become refractory to treatment.

NEOPLASIA

See also NEOPLASIA OF THE NERVOUS SYSTEM, p 1267.

In **dogs**, neoplasms commonly affecting the spinal cord include osteosarcoma, fibrosarcoma, meningioma, nerve sheath tumor, and metastatic neoplasia. A tumor resembling nephroblastoma is seen in young dogs (5–36 mo of age), with German Shepherds affected most commonly. This tumor is consistently located within the

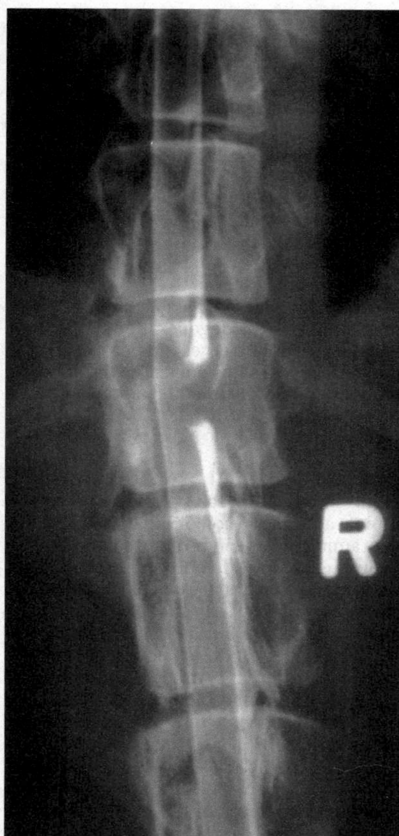

Spinal meningioma, T13, in a dog. Note widening of the contrast column on the right ("golf-tee sign") indicating a mass within the subarachnoid space (myelogram). *Courtesy of Dr. William Thomas.*

dura mater between T10 and L2, causing progressive paraparesis. Diagnosis of spinal neoplasia is based on radiography, myelography, CT or MRI, and surgical biopsy. Surgical excision is possible in some cases, but in general, prognosis is poor.

In **cats**, lymphoma is the most common neoplasia to affect the spinal cord. Adult cats of any age can be affected. There is an acute or slowly progressive onset of signs referable to a focal, often painful, lesion of the spinal cord. Approximately 85% of affected cats have positive test results for feline leukemia virus (*see* p 790), and many have leukemic bone marrow. Myelography, CT, or MRI shows extradural compression. Treatment consists of combination chemotherapy, such as prednisone, vincristine, and cyclophosphamide. Remission is possible in many cases, but longterm prognosis is poor.

In **cattle**, lymphosarcoma may develop in the epidural space at any level, causing spinal cord compression. Often, there is an acute onset of paraparesis or recumbency. Usually, there is other evidence of bovine leukosis (*see* p 743). Definitive diagnosis is based on histopathologic examination.

Neoplasia is a rare cause of spinal cord disease in horses, pigs, sheep, and goats.

NUTRITIONAL DISORDERS

Copper Deficiency: Deficiency of copper causes CNS disease in sheep, goats, and pigs. **Swayback** is the congenital form in lambs and is characterized by degeneration and necrosis of the cerebrum. The acquired form, **enzootic ataxia**, affects lambs, kids, and pigs. Affected animals appear normal at birth but develop progressive paraparesis with hyporeflexia and muscle atrophy within the first few months of life. Other signs include diarrhea and unthriftiness and, in lambs, abnormal fleece. Histologically, there is chromatolysis and loss of neurons and degeneration of axons, primarily in the spinal cord and caudal aspect of the brain stem. Animals may improve with copper supplementation, but permanent neurologic deficits are likely in severely affected animals.

Hypervitaminosis A: Cats fed excess vitamin A, usually from diets consisting largely of liver, develop extensive exostoses, most prominent in the cervical and thoracic spine. Clinical signs include neck pain and rigidity and forelimb lameness. Vertebral lesions are evident on radiographs. Reduction of dietary vitamin A prevents further exostosis but does not significantly reduce the lesions already present.

Thiamine Deficiency: Thiamine deficiency is most common in cats but has also been reported in dogs. Causes include inadequately formulated commercial diets, vegetarian diets, food preserved with sulfur dioxide (which destroys thiamine), and raw fish diets (which contain thiaminase). Affected cats typically exhibit brain dysfunction characterized by vestibular signs, head tremor, ataxia, depression, severe ventroflexion of the head, seizures, and death. Clinical signs in dogs include anorexia, depression, paraparesis, seizures, coma, and death. Pathologic findings are polioencephalomalacia, most prominent in the midbrain. Diagnosis is based on clinical signs, dietary history, and response to thiamine administration (thiamine hydrochloride, 10–20 mg/day, IM, in cats; 25–50 mg/day, IM, in dogs).

TRAUMA

Acute spinal cord injuries are commonly associated with spinal fracture or luxation. Common causes in dogs and cats are automobile accidents, bite wounds, and gunshot wounds. Falls are common causes in horses. Cattle are susceptible to injuries from breeding. Pathologic fractures are common in cattle, sheep, and pigs with malnutrition or vertebral osteomyelitis. Damage to the spinal cord is caused not only by the primary mechanical injury but also as a result of secondary pathologic changes, including edema, hemorrhage, demyelination, and necrosis. These secondary changes are due to biochemical factors, including the release of free radicals, leukotrienes, and prostaglandins that cause further injury to nervous tissue and compromise blood flow to the spinal cord.

Signs of spinal trauma are typically acute and may progress in instances of unstable fractures or luxations. Severe thoracolumbar spinal cord injury may cause paraplegia with increased extensor tone in the thoracic limbs (**Schiff-Sherrington phenomenon**). Radiographs usually demonstrate vertebral fractures and luxations. However, in dogs with trauma, radiographs, compared with CT, reveal only ~75% of spinal fractures, so advanced imaging is indicated in animals with suspected spinal trauma and normal radiographs. Treatment with methylprednisolone may be helpful for animals with severe neurologic deficits if instituted within the first few hours of injury. One protocol is 30 mg/kg, IV, followed 2 hr later by 15 mg/kg, IV, followed 6 hr later by 15 mg/kg, IV, every 6 hr for a total of 24 hr of treatment. Dexamethasone is less effective and is associated with an increased risk of GI ulceration and pancreatitis. NSAIDs have minimal benefit in acute spinal cord injury and increase the risk of complications, especially if used in conjunction with corticosteroids. DMSO (0.5–1 g/kg/day of a 10%–20% solution, given slowly IV for 3 days) is recommended in horses with acute spinal cord injury. Animals with mild neurologic deficits often recover with 4–6 wk of cage or stall rest and analgesics. Surgical reduction and stabilization is indicated for unstable vertebral injuries causing severe neurologic dysfunction. The prognosis is guarded for recumbent horses and cattle. In animals that have lost deep pain perception caudal to the lesion, the prognosis for return of neurologic function is poor.

TOXIC DISORDERS

Arsenic Poisoning: Poisoning can be seen in swine due to an overdose of organoarsenicals, which are often used as feed additives to promote growth and to control swine dysentery. With 3-nitro-4-hydroxyphenylarsonic acid ("3-nitro") poisoning, there is degeneration of the spinal cord, optic nerve, and peripheral nerves. Clinical signs consist of tremors and paraparesis. Mildly affected animals can recover after withdrawal of the offending feed. (*See also* ARSENIC POISONING, p 3071.)

Delayed Organophosphate Intoxication: Intoxication can be seen after oral or topical administration of organophosphate-containing insecticides or anthelmintics, including haloxon. In addition to the acute signs, delayed paralysis can develop 1–4 wk after exposure. Suffolk sheep have an inherited predisposition to this neurotoxicity, because they have low levels of plasma arylesterase activity. Affected animals have progressive, symmetric paraparesis and occasionally become tetraplegic. Diagnosis is based on clinical signs and history of exposure. On histopathologic examination, there is Wallerian degeneration, most prominent in the spinal cord and brain stem. The prognosis for severely affected animals is poor. (*See also* ORGANOPHOSPHATES (TOXICITY), p 3064.)

Sorghum Poisoning: *Sorghum* spp, such as Sorghum, Sudan, and Johnson grass, can cause degeneration of the spinal cord in horses and occasionally in cattle and sheep. The pathogenesis may be related to the high content of hydrocyanide in these grasses. There is ataxia and weakness of the pelvic limbs and incontinence. Urine retention often leads to cystitis and hematuria. Diagnosis is based on clinical features and a history of exposure. Signs may improve with removal of the offending feed, although persistent deficits are possible. (*See also* SORGHUM POISONING, p 3155.)

Tetanus: Tetanus (*see* p 611) is caused by toxins produced by the vegetative form of *Clostridium tetani*. Susceptibility varies markedly among species; dogs and cats are fairly resistant compared with horses. Clinical signs usually develop within

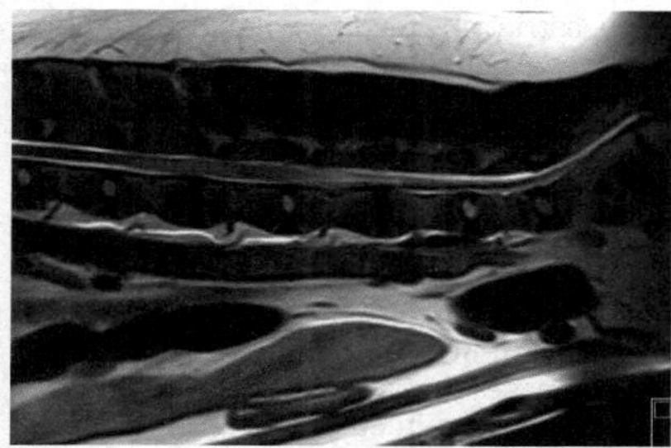

Fibrocartilagenous embolism in a dog, MRI. Note T2 hyperintensity (bright) within the spinal cord dorsal to the L3-4 disc space.
Courtesy of Dr. William Thomas.

5–10 days of infection. These include localized or generalized muscle stiffness and extensor rigidity, dysphagia, protrusion of the third eyelid, and contracted masticatory (lockjaw) and facial (risus sardonicus) muscles. In severe cases, the animal may be recumbent with opisthotonos and reflex muscle spasms. Diagnosis is based on characteristic clinical features. Treatment consists of wound care, antibiotics to kill any remaining organisms, and tetanus antitoxin. In mild cases, prognosis is good with early treatment. In severe cases, death may occur due to respiratory paralysis.

VASCULAR DISEASES

Fibrocartilagenous Embolism: Infarction of the spinal cord can be caused by occlusion of spinal cord arteries or veins (or both) with fragments of fibrocartilage, believed to arise from the intervertebral discs. It is seen primarily in adult dogs, especially large and giant breeds. Miniature Schnauzers and Shetland Sheepdogs also may be predisposed. It is rare in cats, horses, and pigs. Affected dogs have an abrupt onset of gait dysfunction, often occurring during activities such as running or jumping. Deficits are referable to a focal, often asymmetric, lesion in the spinal cord and rarely progress past 12 hr. Spinal pain is typically absent.

Diagnosis is based on clinical findings and MRI, which shows focal T2 hyperintensity within the spinal cord with no compressive lesion. In the acute stage, the CSF may have a mild increase in neutrophils and protein concentration. Mildly affected dogs often improve substantially within 1–2 wk. Prognosis is poor if deep pain perception is absent or if there is no improvement within several weeks.

Postanesthetic Hemorrhagic Myelopathy in Horses: Postanesthetic hemorraghic myelopathy is a rare complication seen in horses positioned in dorsal recumbency under general anesthesia. The cause may be related to impaired venous drainage of the spinal cord due to compression of the caudal vena cava or azygous vein because of the weight of abdominal viscera. There is paraplegia immediately after recovery from anesthesia. Pathologic findings consist of hemorrhagic necrosis of the thoracolumbar spinal cord segments. The prognosis is poor. Positioning the horse slightly tilted off the perpendicular and maintaining adequate blood pressure may help prevent this complication.

DYSAUTONOMIA

FELINE DYSAUTONOMIA

Feline dysautonomia is characterized by widespread dysfunction of the autonomic nervous system. All breeds and age groups are susceptible, although the disease appears to be more common in younger cats. Feline dysautonomia was first reported in 1982 and initially became widespread in the UK (under the name Key-Gaskell syndrome). The incidence has declined considerably, but a few cases were recorded in Europe in the 1990s; sporadic cases have been seen in Dubai, New Zealand, and Venezuela; and a few cases have been reported in the USA, in eastern Kansas and western Missouri. The etiology is unknown. Dysautonomias in horses, dogs, rabbits, and hares share striking similarities to the condition in cats.

Clinical Findings: Affected cats initially are anorectic and often have upper respiratory signs or transient diarrhea. The onset of more definite signs varies from peracute to chronic. Failure of the autonomic system of the GI and urinary tracts can cause esophageal distention and/or dysfunction, gastric and bowel distention and hypomotility, and urinary bladder distention. Other common signs include dilated, nonresponsive pupils, ptosis, and third eyelid protrusion; a dry rhinarium; and reduced lacrimal secretion. In addition, dry oral mucous membranes, prolapse of the nictitating membrane, bradycardia, and urinary or fecal incontinence may be seen. These signs reflect both sympathetic and parasympathetic dysfunction, and there is a wide range in the severity of presenting signs. A dilated anus is sometimes noted, but the underlying somatic lesion is undetermined. Clinical pathology findings are nonspecific.

Lesions: Necropsy may show megaesophagus, diphtheritic mucous membranes, an atonic bladder, and retention of fecal material. During the first few weeks after onset, chromatolysis and neuronal degeneration of pre- and postganglionic sympathetic and parasympathetic neurons is typical. A very specific distribution of chromatolytic autonomic and somatic lower motor neurons is found in the brain stem and spinal cord. The central lesions are identical to those found in the equivalent disease in horses, dogs, rabbits, and hares. Chronic cases can be difficult to confirm because surviving neurons appear normal, and diagnosis depends on an assessment of their numbers relative to surrounding stromal cells.

Diagnosis: Definitive diagnosis depends on histopathologic examination of autonomic ganglia. Clinical confirmation may be aided by contrast radiography (including fluoroscopy) of the esophagus and by reduced lacrimal secretion (<5 mm/min when measured by the Schirmer tear test). Pilocarpine (0.1%) applied to the cornea causes profound miosis within 10–15 min due to denervation hypersensitivity but has no effect on a healthy cat. Dilute (0.5%) phenylephrine reverses the ptosis and protruding third eyelid. Although feline leukemia virus (FeLV, *see* p 790) infection can cause both anisocoria and urinary incontinence, cats with dysautonomia usually show other clinical signs and are FeLV-negative.

Treatment and Prognosis: The main aim of therapy is first to rehydrate the cat and then to maintain adequate fluid balance. Total parenteral nutrition is useful initially but later can be replaced by gastrostomy or nasogastric tube feeding when regurgitation resolves. Maintaining an upright posture after oral intake is important, because the main complication of this condition is inhalation pneumonia. Thrice daily evacuation of the bladder, provision of warmth, use of artificial tears and steam inhalation, and assistance with grooming are all important nursing considerations. Liquid paraffin PO is helpful for constipation but increases the risk of aspiration. Other parasympathomimetics, such as bethanechol (1–2.5 mg, PO, bid-tid), may be of use; however, their effect is crude, and overdosage requires treatment with atropine. Metoclopramide (0.1 mg/kg, IV, or 0.3 mg/kg, SC, tid) may improve gastric emptying.

A small proportion of cats have recovered, and others are able to cope with residual autonomic deficits. Such improvements often require up to 1 yr. In general, the prognosis is poor for severely affected cats.

CANINE DYSAUTONOMIA

Canine dysautonomia is a degenerative polyneuropathy characterized by neuronal degeneration within the autonomic, somatic, central, peripheral, and/or enteric nervous system causing multisystemic effects similar, if not identical, to the dysautonomia in horses, cats, rabbits, and hares. Canine dysautonomia was first described in England in 1983, and there have been no new cases reported in the past decade. Although individual cases have been reported in Scotland, Norway, Belgium, Germany, and Greece, canine dysautonomia is less commonly reported in Europe than in the USA, with higher numbers primarily in the Midwest. In the USA, risk factors were reported to include a rural habitat and spending >50% of the time free outdoors.

Clinical Findings: The most consistent history and physical examination findings are acute-onset vomiting, diarrhea, mild obtundation, inappetence, reduced or absent anal tone, absence of pupillary light responses and lacrimal secretion, mydriasis, and protrusion of the nictitating membrane. Secondary effects of autonomic dysfunction, such as aspiration pneumonia and lethargy, may develop. Weight loss is often dramatic.

Laboratory findings are nonspecific. Pharmacologic testing of the pupils is probably the best single test for confirming the diagnosis. Dilute pilocarpine (0.05% ophthalmic solution) results in rapid pupillary constriction in dogs with dysautonomia because of supersensitivity of the denervated muscle to cholinergic drugs. The prognosis is grave.

LEPORINE DYSAUTONOMIA

Leporine dysautonomia occurs in rabbits and wild hares, and fatal cases have been reported in the UK. Gross lesions are similar to those of equine dysautonomia, including gastric distention, colonic impaction, and weight loss. Histopathologic changes in the central and peripheral nervous systems are almost identical to those found in horses, cats, and dogs.

EQUINE DYSAUTONOMIA

(Grass sickness)

A fatal dysautonomia of unknown etiology, equine grass sickness causes marked reduction of GI motility due to widespread degeneration within the autonomic nervous system. It is seen throughout northern Europe, and a few cases have been diagnosed in the USA in the same geographic area (Midwest) that has a high prevalence of canine dysautonomia.

Grass sickness is seen at any age after weaning and at any time of year, but incidence is highest in spring and in horses 2–7 yr old. Although associated with recently acquired horses kept solely at grass, the condition has very rarely been seen in housed stock. All equidae appear susceptible. Acute, subacute, and chronic forms are recognized, categorized by whether death occurs within 24 hr, 7 days, and 1 wk, respectively. However, chronic cases can survive for weeks or months, and a few cases have recovered. The exact etiology is unknown, but the causal agent is thought to be associated with grazing. A *Clostridium botulinum* toxin may be involved.

Clinical Findings: Horses are afebrile and show tachycardia, ileus, and colic. Patchy sweating and fine muscular fasciculations are often seen over the shoulders and flanks, and penile prolapse may develop. Horses adopt a "tucked up" stance, similar to that seen in equine motor neuron disease (*see* p 1248). In contrast to feline dysautonomia, pupillary light reflexes and tear production are normal. Ptosis, with "droopy" eyelashes, tends to be prominent because of smooth muscle paresis. Rhinitis sicca (dry nose) commonly develops in chronic cases and is considered to indicate a poor prognosis. Affected horses often have dysphagia and esophageal dysfunction, which cause drooling, difficulty passing a stomach tube, nasal reflux of gastric contents, and pooling of barium contrast in the thoracic esophagus. On rectal palpation, the mucosa is dry and tacky, and feces are scant and hard. Distended loops of small intestine and an impacted large colon are seen in the more acute cases. Secondary ileal dilation/impaction and displacement of the large colon can be confusing features. Cachexia can be profound in chronic cases.

Lesions: In acute cases, the stomach and small intestine are markedly distended with fluid (which can result in gastric rupture), and the large intestine is impacted. In chronic cases, the GI tract is usually empty. All forms may show linear ulceration of the esophagus and hard, tarry fecal balls. Neuronal degeneration of pre- and postganglionic sympathetic and parasympathetic neurons is characteristic. A specific distribution of chromatolytic autonomic and somatic lower motor neurons is found in the brain stem and spinal cord.

Diagnosis: No reliable in vivo diagnostic test is available, but dysphagia, tachycardia despite few signs of pain, decreased GI tract motility, a tucked-up stance (chronic cases), and ptosis are useful features. Administration of dilute (0.5%) phenylephrine to one eye should, within 20 min, result in marked decrease in ptosis (most easily seen as a decrease in the angle of the eyelashes to the head when viewed from the front). Biopsies of ileal and rectal tissue (1-cm long, formalin-fixed biopsies preferred) can confirm the diagnosis when examined by a pathologist experienced with grass sickness lesions. Postmortem confirmation of diagnosis depends on histopathologic examination of autonomic ganglia. The cranial cervical ganglia are the most accessible ganglia on postmortem examination and can be found in a fold of mucosal tissue in the caudal wall of the medial compartment of the guttural pouch.

Treatment: A proportion of mildly affected (chronic) cases can survive with dedicated nursing care; a wide variety of feeds should be offered to encourage feed intake. Acute and subacute cases have not survived and should be euthanized on humane grounds. Stabling at-risk stock for part of the day has been recommended.

FACIAL PARALYSIS

Asymmetry of facial expression is common with unilateral lesions of the facial nucleus or nerve in most species. Bilateral facial paralysis may be more difficult to recognize, but affected animals drool and have a dull facial expression. Complete facial paralysis is an inability to move the eyelids, ears, lips, or nostrils. Facial paresis is reduced movement of the muscles of facial expression and indicates milder nucleus or nerve involvement. The nucleus of the facial nerve is located in the rostral medulla oblongata of the brain stem. The facial nerve, cranial nerve VII, exits the brain stem near the vestibulocochlear nerve, passes through the petrous temporal bone, and then exits the skull through the stylomastoid foramen and splits into auricular, palpebral, and buccal branches.

Clinical Findings and Lesions: Clinical signs of facial paralysis vary with the location, severity, and chronicity of the lesion. If a unilateral lesion is located in the facial nucleus or proximal portion of the facial nerve, paresis or paralysis of the eyelids, ears, lips, and nostrils on that side are seen. A lesion of the auriculopalpebral branch of the facial nerve, near the zygomatic arch, results in paresis or paralysis of the eyelids and ear only. A lesion of the palpebral branch of the facial nerve, crossing the zygomatic arch, results in paresis or paralysis of the eyelids only. A lesion of the buccal branch of the facial nerve, as it courses along the surface of the masseter muscles, results in paresis or paralysis of the lips and nostrils only.

In small animals with facial paralysis, the palpebral fissure may be slightly larger on the affected side; in horses and food animals, the palpebral fissure is slightly smaller because of a loss of tone in the frontalis muscles above the eyelid. When the medial or lateral canthus of the eyelids or cornea are touched, the eyelids do not close, but the eyeball will retract into the orbit (if the trigeminal and abducent nerves are functioning properly). The third eyelid will passively elevate as the globe retracts. If both eyes are tested simultaneously, movement on each side can be compared. When the animal is unable to blink the eye, corneal irritation may result in excessive tear production. In acute denervation, the ear carriage is often lower on the side of the lesion in all species, but in chronic denervation with muscle fibrosis and contracture, the ear carriage may be higher. The fibrosis of the auricular muscles can be palpated, and the ear becomes adhered in the abnormal position. In acute lesions, the lips on the paralyzed side may hang loosely, exposing mucosa. When the animal eats or drinks, food and fluids may fall from the lips. The animal may drool excessively, and food may collect between the lips and teeth. In chronic lesions, fibrosis of the lip muscles can be palpated, and the lip on the affected side is higher than on the normal side. In acute, unilateral lesions, the nose deviates away from the side of the lesion, owing to a loss in muscle tone on the affected side. In horses, the affected nostril is unable to dilate on inspiration. In chronic lesions, muscle fibrosis and contracture cause the nose to deviate toward the lesion, and the muscles feel firm and inflexible. Because the facial nerve provides sensory innervation to the distal tongue, a bitter substance such as atropine will not be recognized when placed on the distal tongue.

Often, the parasympathetic portion of the facial nerve is also affected, and tear and saliva production on the side of the lesion is reduced or absent. Reduced or absent tear production, with eyelid paresis or paralysis, can result in corneal exposure with resultant ulceration. In cases of facial nerve paralysis, a Schirmer tear test can be used to determine whether administration of artificial tears is needed. Reduced saliva production can result in dry mucous membranes, and food may collect in the buccal folds. Dryness on the side of the lesion can be detected by simultaneously palpating the mucous membranes on both sides and comparing the degree of moisture.

Other concomitant neurologic deficits can further localize the facial nerve lesion. If the animal has ataxia, hemiparesis, quadriparesis, or conscious proprioceptive deficits associated with facial nerve paralysis, a brain-stem lesion is probable. If the animal has facial paralysis with a head tilt, nystagmus, or other evidence of vestibular deficits, but no hemiparesis, quadriparesis, or conscious proprioceptive deficits, then a lesion of the facial nerve exists as it exits the brain stem or passes through the petrous temporal bone. If a small animal has facial paralysis with ptosis, miosis, and enophthalmos (Horner syndrome), a lesion of the middle ear is likely.

Diagnosis and Treatment: Trauma is a common cause of facial paralysis in all species. In horses, halter injuries and prolonged lateral recumbency may injure the buccal branches of the facial nerve on the side of the jaw and cause unilateral or bilateral paresis or paralysis of the lips and nostrils. Cattle that struggle in stanchions may injure the palpebral branch of the facial nerve as it crosses the zygomatic arch, causing unilateral or bilateral paresis or paralysis of the eyelid(s). Small animals may incur peripheral facial nerve injuries from rough handling, automobile accidents, or surgery such as bulla osteotomy and total ear ablation. Electromyography, including electrical stimulation of the facial nerve, can be used to determine the location and severity of the injury; however, changes will not be evident until 5–7 days after injury.

Therapy for injury may include massage and heat of denervated muscles for 15 min, 2–3 times/day, to maintain their integrity while awaiting any nerve regeneration. Laser therapy, also known as cold laser, low level light therapy, or photobiomodulation, can help nerve regeneration. The facial nerve can regenerate ~1–4 mm/day, so serial neurologic examinations can also help determine the prognosis. If there has been no improvement after 6 mo, the chance of recovery is poor. Horses with collapsing nostrils may require corrective surgery. Species that need the lips for drinking and prehending food must be given deep water containers and wet bulky mashes.

Otitis media is another common cause of facial paralysis in all species, especially in dogs with chronic dermatitis. Otitis externa and a ruptured or diseased tympanic membrane are often seen on otoscopic examination under general anesthesia. Despite an intact tympanum, 16% of animals with acute otitis externa may have otitis media, and as many as 89% of animals with chronic otitis externa may have otitis media (*See also* OTITIS EXTERNA, p 527, and OTITIS MEDIA AND INTERNA, p 531). Skull radiographs, CT, and MRI may be necessary to confirm otitis media. The prognosis can be good if the diagnosis is made early and the animal is treated for 4–6 wk with the appropriate antibiotic, determined by culture and sensitivity on a sample obtained via myringotomy. Corticosteroids should be avoided because they may encourage osteomyelitis. The facial nerve paralysis can be permanent, and longterm administration of artificial tears may be necessary.

Guttural pouch infections (*see* p 1463) can produce facial paralysis in horses. Lesions of the facial nerve nucleus can result in facial nerve paralysis in equine protozoal myeloencephalitis (EPM, *see* p 1309). CSF analysis and titers for EPM are essential for diagnosis and institution of appropriate therapy.

Idiopathic facial nerve paralysis is common in dogs and is diagnosed by excluding other diseases. Otitis media must be excluded with examination and radiographs. Because hypothyroidism (*see* p 553) can cause facial nerve paralysis, levels of thyroxine (T_4) and thyroid-stimulating hormone should be determined in all dogs with facial paralysis. Thyroid replacement therapy may not always resolve facial paralysis in hypothyroid dogs. If there is no infection, thyroid function is normal, and there has been no known trauma, the diagnosis of idiopathic facial paralysis is made. There is no therapy. Artificial tear administration may be necessary. Facial paralysis can be unilateral or bilateral and can resolve spontaneously or be permanent. It can occur on one side, resolve, and then occur on the other side at a later time. Permanent paralysis may be disfiguring but does not affect the quality of life in dogs.

Primary neoplasia of the facial nerve is rare, but dogs and cats can develop a neoplastic process that affects middle ear structures, including the facial nerve. Squamous cell carcinoma and polyps of the middle ear are most common in cats. Otoscopy of the external ear canal under anesthesia with biopsy and histologic examination of abnormal tissue can assist with the diagnosis. CT and MRI of the osseous bulla are necessary to determine the extent of the lesion before surgery. Early radical excision of the tumor and radiation, if indicated, may afford a good longterm prognosis depending on tumor type.

LIMB PARALYSIS

Paralysis of one limb is referred to as monoplegia and is most often associated with diseases of the peripheral spinal nerves. Paralysis of the thoracic limb is usually associated with a lesion of the C6 to T2 nerve roots, the brachial plexus, or musculocutaneous, radial, median, or ulnar nerves. Paralysis of the pelvic limb is usually associated with a lesion of the L4 to S2 nerve roots, the lumbosacral plexus, or femoral, sciatic, peroneal (fibular), or tibial nerves.

Clinical Findings and Lesions: Evaluation of the posture and gait, spinal reflexes, superficial and deep nociception, and muscle mass of the affected limb can localize the lesion to the nerve roots or plexus or to a specific nerve branch. Determining the exact location of the lesion is important for an accurate prognosis because the closer a nerve injury is to the muscle to be reinnervated, the better the prognosis for recovery. In general, nerve root or plexus lesions have a poorer prognosis than do peripheral nerve lesions.

Muscle atrophy from denervation develops within a few days and is faster to develop and more severe than disuse atrophy. With disease of the suprascapular nerve, the supraspinatus and infraspinatus muscles are atrophied; generally, little gait deficit is noted in small animals. However, in horses, the shoulder drops ventrally and rotates laterally, and the hoof may scuff or drag the ground slightly. If the musculocutaneous nerve is affected, the animal is unable to flex the elbow, and the biceps muscle is atrophied. With radial nerve disease, the elbow is dropped, the digits are knuckled onto their dorsal surface, and the limb is unable to bear weight. The thoracic limb flexor reflex (withdrawal reflex) is depressed or absent with lesions of the radial nerve (sensory portion), axillary nerve (shoulder flexion), musculocutaneous nerve (elbow flexion), or median and ulnar (carpal and digit flexion) nerves. The triceps and extensor carpi muscles may also atrophy in radial nerve disease. Superficial and deep digital flexor muscles atrophy with lesions of the median and ulnar nerves. There is little gait abnormality with ulnar nerve injury.

Superficial sensation is tested by observing a behavioral response (such as looking, wincing, crying, or biting) when the skin is pinched with hemostatic forceps or pricked with a needle. Regions of skin sensation associated with specific nerves are less distinct in equine and food animal species than in small animals. A loss of sensation on the rostral skin surface of the thoracic limb from the elbows to the paws indicates radial nerve disease. The skin of the caudal aspect of the limb, from the *elbow to the pads,* is desensitized in median and ulnar nerve disease, and the skin of the lateral aspect of the antebrachium and paw is desensitized with damage to the ulnar nerve.

Deep pain is tested by applying hemostatic forceps to the bones of the digits or hoof testers to the hoof and observing a behavioral response. The presence of deep pain from the fifth digit in small animals indicates integrity of the ulnar nerve. The presence of deep pain from the other digits of the thoracic limb indicates integrity of the radial and median nerves.

The eye on the side of the thoracic limb paralysis will show Horner syndrome (ptosis, miosis, and enophthalmos) when the lesion involves the T1 to T2 nerve roots as they exit the spinal cord. Horner syndrome is manifest in horses by ocular changes and ipsilateral sweating of the face and neck and in cattle by ocular changes and a unilateral loss of moisture on the muzzle.

Inability to extend the stifle to support weight in the pelvic limb is seen with L4 to L5 nerve root or femoral nerve disease; the patellar reflex is reduced or absent, the quadriceps muscle is atrophied, and sensation of the skin is reduced or absent on the medial surface of the limb. Inability to actively flex the stifle, hock, and digits or to extend the hock and digits is seen with lesions of the sciatic nerve, L6 to S2 nerve roots. The animal will support some weight if the femoral nerve is spared but will stand knuckled on the dorsum of the paw or hoof with the hock excessively flexed. If only the peroneal branch of the sciatic nerve is affected, the hock will be overextended and the digits knuckled. If only the tibial branch of the sciatic nerve is affected, the hock will be overflexed and the digits overextended. The prognosis for tibial or peroneal nerve lesions may be better than that for sciatic lesions, so differentiation is important.

The pelvic limb flexor reflex is diminished or absent with sciatic nerve lesions. The gastrocnemius reflex is diminished or absent with lesions of the sciatic or tibial nerve. The cranial tibial muscle reflex is diminished or absent with lesions of the sciatic or peroneal nerve. The distribution of denervation muscle atrophy can indicate whether the sciatic or only one of its branches is involved. Atrophy of gluteal, semimembranosus, semitendinosus, and all muscles below the stifle indicates a lesion of the L6 to S2 nerve roots as they exit the spinal cord. If the gluteal muscles are normal but the others are atrophied, then a lesion of the sciatic nerve is located at the sciatic notch or the proximal two-thirds of the femur. Atrophy of the cranial tibial or gastrocnemius muscles alone indicates a lesion of the peroneal or tibial nerve, respectively. If superficial sensation is reduced or absent on the cranial and caudal aspects of the limb and in the perineal region on the same side, then a lesion of the L6 to S2 nerve roots is likely. With peroneal nerve lesions, superficial sensation on the cranial surface of the hock and tibia and on the dorsal aspect of the foot is reduced or absent. With tibial nerve lesions, superficial sensation of the caudal surface of the hock and tibia and plantar surface of the paw is reduced or absent. Sciatic nerve lesions cause a loss of superficial sensation in the cranial, caudal, dorsal, and plantar regions. A loss of deep pain may be associated with sciatic nerve lesions. Preservation of sensation on the medial aspect of the pelvic limb is attributable to preservation of the saphenous nerve.

Electromyography can be used 7–10 days after a nerve insult to detect denervation in muscles and to outline the distribution of the nerve lesion. Denervation of limb and paravertebral muscles indicates nerve root lesions. Denervation of a specific muscle group indicates a lesion in its respective nerve. Electrical stimulation of the nerve can be used to determine nerve integrity. If some nerve integrity is present, the prognosis is better if motor nerve conduction velocity is normal than if it is slowed.

Diagnosis and Treatment: Trauma is the most common cause of acute monoplegia. Traumatic loss of nerve function may be due to neurapraxia, axonotmesis, axonostenosis, or neurotmesis. **Neurapraxia** is a temporary nerve conduction dysfunction that can last several weeks, but recovery is complete. **Axonotmesis** is rupture of some axons within the nerve but with an intact nerve sheath. Most closed nerve injuries from stretch or compression are a combination of neurapraxia and axonotmesis. Ruptured axons regenerate 1–4 mm/day, but functional recovery depends on the integrity and diameter of the nerve sheath and on the distance between injury and reinnervation sites. Nerves injured >180 mm from their respective muscles may be unable to make anatomic contact. If anatomic contact is made, the nerve sheath contracture, which develops over time, may not leave enough room to develop sufficient myelin to conduct an effective electrical impulse. **Axonostenosis,** or narrowed nerve sheaths with reduced nerve function, may be a sequela of nerve injuries. **Neurotmesis** is total nerve rupture, and surgical reattachment is required for regeneration. If no nerve function is found on the initial neurologic examination, neurapraxia, axonotmesis, and neurotmesis can be difficult to differentiate. Electrical stimulation of a nerve with neurapraxia is usually normal, and the prognosis is good, regardless of the findings of the initial neurologic examination. If the affected nerve does not respond to electrical stimulation distal to the site of the lesion ≥3 days after injury, the prognosis for recovery is guarded. Serial neurologic examinations throughout a 6-mo period are necessary if electromyographic evaluation is not performed.

Injury to the **brachial plexus** or the C6 to T2 nerve roots is common in most species due to direct shoulder trauma or abnormal shoulder abduction (eg, in small animals hit by automobiles). Horses and cattle cast on hard surfaces for foot or other surgeries may develop a brachial plexus injury. If Horner syndrome is present on the same side as a thoracic limb that has lost sensation and is areflexic and paralyzed, a brachial plexus avulsion is likely, and the prognosis for recovery grave. With brachial plexus avulsion, the nerve roots are torn from the spinal cord and cannot be repaired. If there is also no response to radial nerve stimulation, recovery is hopeless. If the limb drags on the ground, it can be held up with a neck sling or amputated in small animals to avoid laceration of the dorsal surface of the paw. Three-legged dogs and cats generally have a good quality of life. If no Horner syndrome is present with thoracic limb paralysis, the prognosis for recovery may be better.

Lumbosacral plexus injuries are less common than brachial plexus injuries but can be associated with automobile accidents or extreme limb abduction. Fractures of long bones can injure peripheral nerves locally. Surgical intervention for pelvic and hip disease and injection injuries are common causes of sciatic nerve injuries. Sustained pressure on the lateral aspect of the stifle can cause peroneal nerve injury. Heat application, massage, and stretching of tendons should be performed for 15 min 2–3 times/day to keep muscles, tendons, and joints healthy while the nerve is regenerating. A light bandage may prevent damage to the foot from dragging, but reduction of circulation should be avoided. No specific therapy is currently available to assist nerve regeneration, but recent studies with laser therapy, also known as cold laser, low level light therapy, or photobiomodulation, has shown some promise in assisting nerve regrowth. In traumatic injuries with accompanying swelling, small animals may be given NSAIDs or a short course of anti-inflammatory oral prednisone at 0.5 mg/kg/day for 5–7 days. This will help reduce edema, which can compromise circulation to the nerve. NSAIDs and corticosteroids should not be used concurrently. NSAIDs can be given to horses to reduce edema. If voluntary movement, nociception, and spinal reflexes improve within 1–2 mo, the prognosis is good. Limb mutilation can be transient in recovering nerve injuries and may be prevented by temporary use of an elizabethan collar. If nerve injury is suspected to be permanent and the animal is mutilating the limb, amputation is recommended in small animals. Enough time should be allowed to pass for possible regeneration of the nerve, typically 3–6 mo, before amputation.

Neoplasia of nerve roots and peripheral nerves can cause a chronic, progressive, often painful paresis of a thoracic or pelvic limb. (*See also* NEOPLASIA OF THE PERIPHERAL NERVES AND NEUROMUSCULAR JUNCTION, p 1242, and NEOPLASIA OF THE NERVOUS SYSTEM, p 1267.) Nerve sheath tumors are common in dogs. Lymphosarcoma of the brachial or lumbosacral plexus is seen in dogs, cattle, and cats. If the nerve roots within the spinal canal are affected, an extramedullary mass may be visualized with a myelogram, CT, or MRI in dogs and cats. Surgical exploration and removal or biopsy are essential to determine diagnosis or prognosis. The longterm prognosis for nerve sheath tumors is poor, even after attempted surgical removal and limb amputation. Nerve sheath tumors often affect multiple nerve roots, and the tumor is difficult to completely remove. If appropriate chemotherapy is instituted for lymphosarcoma, the length and quality of life may be improved. Chemotherapy is not very helpful to treat nerve sheath tumors, but radiation therapy may have some benefit.

Horses with equine protozoal myeloencephalitis (EPM, *see* p 1309) may develop monoparesis and focal muscle atrophy. CSF analysis and CSF and serum EPM titers should be evaluated so appropriate therapy can be administered.

MENINGITIS, ENCEPHALITIS, AND ENCEPHALOMYELITIS

Inflammation of the meninges (meningitis) and inflammation of the brain (encephalitis) are seen in animals and often manifest concurrently (meningoencephalitis). Many of the inflammatory diseases of the CNS of animals are diffuse, involving both the brain and spinal cord (encephalomyelitis and meningoencephalomyelitis). Because many inflammatory processes are disseminated throughout the CNS at the time of clinical observation, differentiation between meningeal-only inflammation vs extension of disease into the neuropil is often difficult to make antemortem. Thus, from a clinical standpoint, any one of these conditions may be the case in an animal with an inflammatory condition of the CNS.

In animals with meningoencephalitis or meningoencephalomyelitis, the clinical signs of meningitis often precede those of encephalitis and may remain the predominant feature of the illness. This is especially apparent in meningitis involving neonates. Causes of meningitis, encephalitis, and meningoencephalitis include bacteria, viruses, fungi, protozoa, rickettsia, parasite migrations, chemical agents, and idiopathic or immune-mediated diseases. In ruminants, generally bacterial infections are more common than other causes of meningitis or encephalitis. In species other than ruminants, especially adult animals, viruses, protozoa, rickettsia, and fungi are as or more frequent causes of meningitis or encephalitis than are bacteria. The appearance of many etiologic agents such as arboviruses, certain rickettsia, and bacteria) are seasonal. Age is an important consideration for bacterial meningitis associated with neonatal sepsis. Even within species (eg, production animals), there can be a difference in risk factors. For instance, sporadic bovine encephalomyelitis (*see* p 1308), caused by *Chlamydia pecorum*, and thromboembolic meningoencephalitis (*see* p 754), caused by *Histophilus somni*, usually occur in feeder beef cattle (6 mo to 2 yr old) and not replacement dairy calves unless managed on feedlots. Vaccine history is also an essential factor in consideration of differential diagnoses in animals with clinical signs of inflammation of the CNS, especially those caused by viruses.

Etiology and Pathogenesis: The incidence of meningitis, encephalitis, and encephalomyelitis is fairly low compared with that of infections of other organs. However, with the recent global expansion of the flaviviruses and tickborne *Anaplasma phagocytophilum* and other vectorborne diseases, the incidence and risk of infectious brain and spinal cord infections of animals has likely increased.

Bacterial Infections: When bacterial infections occur, they are more likely to be sporadic than epidemic. The risk of hematogenously disseminated CNS infections is likely to be low in adult animals because of the blood-brain barrier. Many infections of the nervous system are the result of some injury to its protective barriers. In all species, direct extension of bacterial or mycotic infections into the CNS can develop from sinusitis, otitis media or interna, vertebral osteomyelitis, or discospondylitis. In calves with *Mycoplasma bovis* otitis, meningitis can occur. Infections can also be secondary to migrating grass awns or other foreign bodies, deep bite wounds, or traumatic injuries adjacent to the head or spine; this is common in hunting dogs. Iatrogenic infections are possible from diagnostic and surgical procedures.

Brain abscesses also can arise from direct infections or by septic embolism of cerebral vessels. Pituitary abscesses in ruminants are thought to originate from bacterial invasion of the rete mirabile (intracranial carotid mirabile) surrounding the pituitary gland. In chronic brain abscesses, an adjacent or occasionally diffuse fibrinous leptomeningitis may develop. *Streptococcus equi equi* is one of the most common causes of brain abscessation in horses, and *Rhodococcus equi* abscesses have been described in foals, both of which are secondary to primary infection of lymph or other tissues.

Spontaneous bacterial meningitis or meningoencephalitis develops in dogs rarely, occurs more commonly in food animals, and is most common in septic neonatal animals. Various aerobic bacteria (*Pasteurella multocida*, *Staphylococcus* spp, *Escherichia coli*, *Streptococcus* spp, *Actinomyces* spp, and *Nocardia* spp) and anaerobic bacteria (*Bacteroides* spp, *Peptostreptococcus anaerobius*, *Fusobacterium* spp, *Eubacterium* spp, and *Propionibacterium* spp) have been isolated from animal infections. Bacterial endocarditis with associated septicemia is important in the etiopathogenesis of CNS infection in adult dogs. In Lyme endemic areas, neurologic infection in dogs with *Borrelia burgdorferi* has been implicated. Other non-neonatal hematogenously derived infections are well-recognized disease entities, such as thromboembolic meningoencephalitis of cattle (*Histophilus somni*, *see* p 754), Glässer's disease of pigs (*Haemophilus parasuis*, *see* p 720), and *Haemophilus agni* septicemia in feeder lambs.

Streptococcus suis causes suppurative meningitis of pigs in addition to other syndromes such as pleuritis, epicarditis, and arthritis. (*See also* STREPTOCOCCAL INFECTIONS IN PIGS, p 731.) Several species of *Mycoplasma* cause nonseptic encephalitis in their natural hosts such as goats (*M mycoides*), poultry (*M gallisepticum*), cats (*M felis*), dogs (*M edwardii*), and rodents (*M pulmonis*). Outbreaks of *C pecorum* occur in yearling cattle and cause spontaneous encephalomyelitis with polyserositis and peritonitis. Bacterial meningoencephalitis often affects neonatal animals as a sequela of gram-negative septicemia. Members of the Enterobacteriaceae (*E coli*, *Salmonella* spp, and *Klebsiella pneumoniae*) are the most commonly isolated pathogens, as well as streptococci (commonly *Enterococcus* spp). *Actinobacillus equuli* infection is an important cause of meningoencephalitis in foals. Failure of passive transfer of immunoglobulins is the single most important factor predisposing neonates to omphalophlebitis or enteritis, with subsequent hematogenous spread of the infection to the CNS. *Elizabethkingia* (formerly *Chryseobacterium*) *meningosepticum* is a bacterium that can cause meningitis in newborn and immunocompromised people and animals.

Listeriosis (*see* p 2839), which is caused by *Listeria monocytogenes* and is a common infection in cattle, sheep, and goats and less common in horses, is an example of a multifocal brain stem meningoencephalitis that ascends to the CNS via transaxonal migration in cranial nerves. *Mannheimia haemolytica* and *Pasteurella multocida*, although usually resulting in fibrinous pneumonia and hemorrhagic septicemia in ruminants, occasionally produce a localized fibrinopurulent leptomeningitis. Meningoencephalitis due to *M haemolytica* has also been reported in horses, donkeys, and mules. *Actinomyces*, *Klebsiella*, and *Streptococcus* spp are sporadic causes of meningitis in adult horses.

Viral Infections: Viruses commonly cause nonsuppurative meningitis, encephalitis, and encephalomyelitis. Several viruses are specifically neurotropic or exhibit predilection for the CNS, causing a fulminate or fatal encephalitis, the most notorious being rabies virus infection (*see* p 1302). Although rabies viruses primarily spread to the CNS transaxonally, several other common DNA (adenoviruses, herpesviruses, parvoviruses) and RNA (bunyavirus, lentiviruses, morbilliviruses, alphaviruses, flaviviruses) viruses are likely spread via the bloodstream but exhibit high neuropathogenesis once within the CNS. Both hematogenous and transaxonal routes of spread are thought to occur in flavivirus infections. Recently, minute viruses (Parvoviridae) have been implicated in dogs and nonhuman primates, respectively. Reoviruses cause encephalitis in mice and nonhuman primates. Colorado tick virus, a Coltivirus, has been implicated in infections in domestic species. Most animals have viral species-specific infections that exhibit predilection for the CNS. Rarely, a postvaccination encephalomyelitis in dogs is associated with immunizations against canine distemper virus, rabies virus, and canine coronavirus-parvovirus vaccines. Herpesviruses cause encephalomyelitis syndromes in each of their respective hosts.

Infections Caused by Parasites: Many parasitic agents can cause meningoencephalitis in both large and small animals. Neuropathogenic protozoa include *Toxoplasma gondii*, *Neospora caninum*, and *Encephalitozoon cuniculi* in dogs and cats. *E cuniculi* can cause encephalomyelitis in rabbits. *Sarcocystis neurona* and *N hughesii* are important causes in horses, with *Trypanosoma* spp important in equids outside of the USA. A wide variety of protozoa can infect and cause severe CNS disease in adult cattle, including *Babesia bovis*, *Theileria parva* (theileriosis), and *Trypanosoma* spp, whereas *N caninum* and *T gondii* can cause congenital encephalitis in calves. Free-living amoebae, *Naegleria fowleria*, *Acanthamoeba* spp, and *Balamuthia mandrillaris* are associated with amoebic meningoencephalitis in dogs.

Aseptic suppurative or eosinophilic meningoencephalitis associated with aberrant migration of parasites throughout the CNS can develop in a number of animal hosts. In dogs and cats, CNS infections have been reported with *Dirofilaria immitis*, *Toxocara canis*, *Ancylostoma caninum*, *Cuterebra* spp larva, and *Taenia* spp. A wide variety of nematodes have been reported to cause severe meningoencephalitis in horses, including *Setaria* spp, *Habronema* spp, *Strongylus* spp, *Halicephalobus gingivalis*, and *Angiostrongylus cantonensis* (the rat lungworm). In cattle, migrating *Setaria* and *Hypoderma* larva are commonly implicated. Recently, *A cantonensis* has been identified as a cause of eosinophilic meningoencephalitis in nonhuman primates. *Parelaphostrongylus tenuis* is especially important in goats and llamas.

Fungal Infections: Pathogenic fungi, including *Coccidioides immitis*, *Blastomyces dermatitidis*, and *Histoplasma capsulatum*, can cause meningoencephalitis. Opportunistic invasion with *Cryptococcus neoformans* and *Aspergillus* spp has also been described in several mammalian species. Rarely, other fungi, such as *Candida* spp, *Cladosporium trichoides*, *Paecilomyces variotii*, *Geotrichum candidum*, and dematiaceous fungi (*Bipolaris* sp and *Alternaria* spp) cause meningoencephalitis. Unicellular plants, *Prototheca wickerhamii* and *P zopfii*, can also produce an eosinophilic meningoencephalomyelitis in dogs, cattle, and horses.

Idiopathic/Immune Mediated: Several idiopathic meningoencephalitides are recognized in dogs. Granulomatous meningoencephalomyelitis (*see* p 1252) is a relatively common CNS disease of dogs that most often affects young to middle-aged, small-breed females. A pyogranulomatous meningoencephalomyelitis has been seen in mature Pointer dogs. This acute, rapidly progressive disorder is characterized by extensive mononuclear cells and neutrophils infiltrating the leptomeninges and parenchyma, especially in the cervical spinal cord and brain stem. A necrotizing meningoencephalitis of unknown etiology has been reported in young, adult Pug dogs, as well as in Yorkshire Terriers and Maltese dogs. A steroid-responsive suppurative meningitis affecting mainly young (<2 yr), large-breed dogs and a severe necrotizing vasculitis and meningitis syndrome has been documented in Beagles, Bernese Mountain Dogs, and German Shorthaired Pointers, and both have been identified as possible immunologic disorders with a hereditary predisposition. (*See also* CONGENITAL AND INHERITED ANOMALIES OF THE NERVOUS SYSTEM, p 1222.) An eosinophilic meningoencephalitis that has been described in adult dogs (Golden Retrievers, Rottweilers, and South African Boerboels) and cats is also believed to have an immunologic basis.

Clinical Findings: In the early stages of inflammatory diseases of the CNS, nonlocalizing clinical signs are frequent. In dogs, for example, meningitis can easily be mistaken for intervertebral disc extrusion, polyarthritis, pleuritis, pancreatitis, or pyelonephritis. In horses, initial clinical signs can appear as lameness, myositis, vertebral instability, or even colic. In foals, extreme hyperexcitability and irritability can be an early indication of sepsis in the

CNS. Cattle can demonstrate anorexia, depression, and bizarre behavior.

The usual signs of meningitis are fever, hyperesthesia, neck rigidity, and painful paraspinal muscle spasms. Dogs and occasionally horses display this syndrome acutely and sometimes chronically without clinical signs of brain or spinal cord involvement. However, in diffuse meningoencephalitis due to any agent, depression, blindness, progressive paresis, cerebellar or vestibular ataxia, opisthotonos, cranial nerve deficits, seizures, dementia, agitation, and depressed consciousness (including coma) can develop, depending on the rapidity of onset, pathology, and location of the lesions. Visual deficits, neck pain, seizures, behavioral disturbances, ataxia, weakness, cranial nerve deficits, and depression may be seen in either focal or disseminated CNS disease.

In neonatal infections, omphalophlebitis, polyarthritis, and ophthalmitis with hypopyon can accompany the CNS inflammation. Because of its unusual pathogenesis, listeriosis often causes asymmetric vestibular dysfunction, with head tilt and circling, in addition to other cranial nerve deficits such as facial and pharyngeal paralysis. In histophilosis of cattle, the nervous signs tend to be peracute, with sudden collapse and profound depression of consciousness (stupor or coma); fever and limb stiffness may be the only signs detectable in the prodromal stages. In sporadic bovine encephalomyelitis, calves demonstrate incoordination that can progress to recumbency and opisthotonos.

Lesions: Gross lesions are extremely variable depending on cause and location and whether the disease is diffuse or multifocal. Pathologic changes characteristic of meningitis include diffuse infiltration of leukocytes into the leptomeninges. This can be mild if flaviviral, or florid if granulomatous (thickened) or alphaviral (hemorrhagic). Frequently, the entire subarachnoid space of the brain and spinal cord is inflamed. Vasculitis of meningeal vessels and CNS arterioles may also be apparent. In meningoencephalitis, the inflammation extends into the CNS parenchyma, resulting in leukocyte infiltration with large areas of perivascular cuffing. Necrosis and malacia of the CNS may be seen, with infiltrations of macrophages, neutrophils, and plasma cells. Grossly, this is seen as local areas of discoloration. Listeriosis uniquely causes microabscesses deep within the CNS parenchyma, which consist of accumulations of neutrophils and microglial cell reaction with central liquefactive necrosis.

Diagnosis: Often, there are no related changes in a CBC or serum biochemical profile to indicate CNS infection. The analysis of CSF is the most reliable and accurate means to identify an encephalitis, meningitis, or meningoencephalitis. CSF should be collected whenever history, species, or breed predisposition suggests meningitis or encephalitis, or whenever clinical signs indicate a disseminated or multifocal CNS disorder. Without CSF analysis, an animal exhibiting back or neck pain with an increase in rectal temperature may be misdiagnosed.

Adult large animals and dogs with bacterial meningitis and encephalitis or with steroid-responsive suppurative meningitis typically have a marked neutrophilic pleocytosis in the CSF, with cell counts in the hundreds to thousands. The protein content of the CSF is usually also significantly increased (>100 mg/dL), with an increase in the globulin component of CSF.

Rickettsial infections most often cause a mild to moderate mononuclear pleocytosis, although Rocky Mountain spotted fever can cause neutrophilic inflammation secondary to vasculitis.

In foals with meningitis, the CSF has an increased protein content, and even slight increases in WBCs in the CSF are significant (>10 WBC/μL). Any neutrophils observed on cytology in CSF from a foal warrant treatment with antimicrobials that can obtain high therapeutic levels in the CNS.

Viral infections and listeriosis typically produce a mild to moderate mononuclear pleocytosis in CSF, with an associated increase in protein levels. However, the CSF is normal in rabies virus infections. Herpesvirus infections cause markedly increased proteins and xanthochromia (yellow to reddish discoloration) without dramatic increase in cell count. Feline infectious peritonitis (FIP) in cats and Eastern equine encephalitis in horses are exceptions and can cause markedly high neutrophil counts. In FIP, a markedly high protein concentration (>200 mg/dL) can also be seen.

Parasitic and fungal meningoencephalitides cause eosinophilic or occasionally a highly degenerate neutrophilic pleocytosis. Granulomatous inflammations usually induce moderate to high cell numbers and increased protein in the CSF. The cell population is predominantly mononuclear or a mixed population of neutrophils and mononuclear cells. Distinguishing a granulomatous infection due to a fungal or protozoal organism from granulomatous meningoencephalitis is often difficult. The necrotizing encephalitides typically cause a mild increase in CSF mononuclear cells and protein concentration.

Occasionally, bacteria are seen on cytologic examination of the CSF and identified with Gram stain. Successful culture of bacteria from CSF is more likely in large animals than in dogs. In some cases, serial blood cultures are more successful, especially in foals. Fungi and occasionally protozoa have been identified in CSF, but serology is usually necessary to confirm mycotic and protozoal infections in vivo. Many of these diseases are fatal, and final identification is made at postmortem with in situ identification of the organism.

For premortem etiologic identification, agent-specific testing is recommended; however, most agents, once in the CNS, are not detectable by direct testing through culture or nucleic acid–based testing of body fluids. Serologic testing is available for most viral encephalitides and, in particular, for arboviruses the most reliable test examines IgM in a single sample. Paired serum is required for IgG-based tests, especially those confounded by vaccination. Although CSF analysis is rewarding in terms of clinical pathology, detection of a pathogen within the CSF can also be unreliable depending on the location and pathogen load within the CNS. Culture of the CSF will often yield growth of the organism in bacterial meningitis; however, the detection rate is often <40% for many viruses. Detection of antibody within the CNS can be nonspecific if there is leakage through the blood-brain barrier. IgM detection is likely a more reliable indication of intrathecal antibody production. Most confirmatory testing is performed postmortem if the animal dies.

Treatment: Other than for animals with the probable immune-mediated, steroid-responsive inflammatory CNS diseases and for animals with meningoencephalitis caused by rickettsia and certain bacteria, the prognosis is guarded. The case fatality rate in calves with bacterial meningitis has been reported to be 100%; however, the case fatality rate in foals is much lower.

Appropriate use of antibiotics, according to culture or serology results, is basic to successful therapy. Relapses are common, and prolonged therapy is often necessary. Correction of failure of passive transfer is critical in neonatal large animals. Broad-spectrum antibacterials that can penetrate the blood-brain barrier should be selected, and bactericidal drugs are preferred over bacteriostatic agents. Recommended drugs include ampicillin, metronidazole, tetracyclines, potentiated sulfonamides, fluoroquinolones, and third-generation cephalosporins; higher than normal dosages may be necessary to achieve and maintain adequate concentrations in the CNS. In farm animals, selection of drugs must be based not only on drug efficacy but also on whether the available drug is appropriate for use in a food animal.

For viral infections, the case-fatality rate varies. The most lethal viral infections are rabies (100%) in all mammals, Eastern equine encephalomyelitis in horses (85%–100%), and distemper virus in dogs (50%). Availability of antivirals is limited, and cost can be prohibitive. The most commonly treated viral infection of the CNS is likely that of the neurotropic form of equine herpesvirus 1; however, the prognosis is guarded in recumbent horses.

Mycotic infections of the CNS have been treated successfully in people, but results in veterinary medicine are less rewarding. Treatment with itraconazole or fluconazole may be of benefit, but longterm therapy is required and relapses are frequent. Protozoal infections (eg, toxoplasmosis, neosporosis, sarcocystosis) may respond to a potentiated sulfonamide (trimethoprim, pyrimethamine and sulfonamides). These are commonly used in combination with clindamycin in small animals. However, relapse may occur because of the inability to clear encysted organisms from the CNS. Antiprotozoal medications have been approved for use in horses, such as the triazine analogues, including diclazuril and ponazuril. In balantidiasis, a disease in working donkeys, secnidozole has been shown to decrease fecal cyst counts, which should theoretically decrease the risk of development of CNS disease.

Glucocorticoids are usually contraindicated in animals with meningitis or meningoencephalitis with an infectious etiology; however, a high-dose, short-term course of dexamethasone or methylprednisolone may control life-threatening complications such as acute cerebral edema and impending brain herniation. Immunosuppressive doses of corticosteroids are required for successful therapy of the idiopathic CNS inflammations seen in dogs.

Radiation therapy and immunomodulatory drugs have been used to treat granulomatous meningoencephalitis.

Supportive care should be specific for the needs of the individual animal and may include analgesics, anticonvulsants, fluids, nutritional supplementation, and physical therapy.

MOTION SICKNESS

Motion sickness is characterized by signs referable to stimulation of the autonomic nervous system, including excessive salivation and vomiting. Affected animals may also yawn, whine, or show signs of uneasiness and apprehension; severely affected animals may also develop diarrhea. Motion sickness is seen during travel by land, sea, or air, and signs usually disappear when vehicular motion ceases. The principal causative mechanism involves stimulation of the vestibular apparatus in the inner ear, which has connections to the emetic center in the brain stem. The chemoreceptor trigger zone (CRTZ) and H_1-histaminergic receptors are involved in this pathway in dogs but apparently are less important in cats. Recent evidence has revealed that the neurokinin 1 substance P receptors (NK1) in the emetic center play a major role in motion sickness in both dogs and cats and are more important than the receptors in the CRTZ. Fear of the vehicle may also become a contributory factor in dogs and cats that develop a conditioned response to the event; signs may be seen even in a stationary vehicle. In this situtation, behavioral modification may be needed to eliminate this fear, or the use of drugs that provide a sedative effect may be needed.

In some cases, motion sickness can be overcome by conditioning the animal to travel. In others, ataractic and antinausea drugs can be used with good results. Antihistamines (such as diphenhydramine hydrochloride, dimenhydrinate, meclizine, and promethazine hydrochloride) prevent motion sickness, provide sedation, and inhibit drooling. The centrally acting phenothiazine derivatives (such as chlorpromazine, prochlorperazine, and acepromazine maleate) have antiemetic as well as sedative effects. Cats have no histamine receptors in the CRTZ; therefore, antihistamines are ineffective in treating motion sickness in this species. Motion sickness in cats probably is best treated with an α-adrenergic antagonist (eg, chlorpromazine) instead of a pure H_1-histaminergic antagonist.

Maropitant, an NK1 receptor antagonist, is effective in treating motion sickness in dogs. NK1 receptors are located in the emetic center of the brain stem, which is the source most responsible for the vomiting and nausea of motion sickness. Blocking these receptors is more effective than inhibiting the CRTZ. Therefore, maropitant is probably the drug of choice to treat motion sickness in dogs. Another benefit is that treatment is given once daily. The drug is approved and available in tablet and injectable forms for use in dogs, while only the injectable form is approved for use in cats. Cats should be 16 wk old and dogs 8 wk old before using maropitant.

Phenobarbital and diazepam can be used to produce a general sedative effect if anxiety is a problem. Oral administration of one of these drugs several hours before departure should reduce or eliminate the signs of motion sickness. (*See also* DRUGS TO CONTROL OR STIMULATE VOMITING (MONOGASTRIC), p 2547.)

NEOPLASIA OF THE NERVOUS SYSTEM

Neoplasia of the nervous system has been reported in all domestic animal species. Nervous system tumors have been detected in 1%–3% of necropsies in dogs. In cats, nervous system tumors are less common and are mainly meningiomas and lymphomas. Primary nervous system tumors originate from neuroectodermal, ectodermal, and/or mesodermal cells normally present in (or associated with) the brain, spinal cord, or peripheral nerves. Secondary tumors affecting the nervous system may originate from surrounding structures such as bone and muscle or from hematogenous metastasis of a primary tumor in another organ. Tumor emboli can lodge and grow anywhere in the brain, meninges, choroid plexus, or spinal cord. Dissemination or metastasis of CNS tumors is rare but may occur via the CSF pathways, especially if the tumors are located close to the subarachnoid space or ventricular cavities (eg, choroid plexus papilloma, ependymoma, medulloblastoma, neuroblastoma, pinealoblastoma), or via a hematogenous route such as the dural sinus, with later development of remote metastasis, most often in the lung. Tumors may also spread by direct extension to surrounding tissues, especially bone. The osseous tentorium may be used as a reference point to localize different areas of the brain within the cranial vault. Thus, tumors in the cerebral hemispheres are often referred to as supratentorial or anterior fossa tumors, while those in the brain stem or cerebellum are called infratentorial or posterior fossa tumors.

Classification: Classification of nervous system tumors in animals follows the criteria used for tumors in people and is based primarily on the characteristics of the constituent cell type, its pathologic behavior, topographic pattern, and secondary changes seen within and around the tumor (see TABLE 2).

Immunocytochemical studies and imaging techniques may aid classification. Primary tumors typically grow slowly,

TABLE 2 TUMORS OF THE NERVOUS SYSTEM IN DOGS AND CATS

Tumor Origin	Predilection Sites	Species	Incidence
	PRIMARY TUMORS		
Nerve cells			
Ganglioneuroma (gangliocytoma) Ganglioneuroblastoma Neuroblastoma Primitive neuroectodermal tumors	Variable, eg, cerebellum, cranial nerve roots, eye, cervical ganglion	Dogs	Rare
Neuroepithelium			
Ependymoma	Third and lateral ventricles	Dogs, cats	Uncommon
Nephroblastoma	Meninges, thoracolumbar spinal cord	Dogs (German Shepherd)	Uncommon
Choroid plexus papilloma	Fourth ventricle	Dogs	Common
Neuroglia			
Astrocytoma (fibrillary, protoplasmic, gemistocytic, anaplastic)	Piriform area, convexity of cerebral hemispheres, thalamus, hypothalamus	Dogs (brachycephalic), cats	Common
Oligodendroglioma	Cerebral hemispheres	Dogs (brachycephalic)	Common
Glioblastoma	As for astrocytoma	Dogs (brachycephalic)	Uncommon
Spongioblastoma	Variable, eg, ependymal surfaces, cerebellum, optic nerve and tracts	Dogs (brachycephalic)	Rare
Medulloblastoma	Cerebellum	Dogs, cats	Uncommon
Gliomas (unclassified)	Periventricular areas, especially in cerebral hemispheres	Dogs	Common
Peripheral nerves and nerve sheaths			
Nerve sheath tumors (schwannoma, neurofibrosarcoma, neurofibroma, neurinoma)	Peripheral nerves	Dogs, cats	Common

(continued)

TABLE 2 TUMORS OF THE NERVOUS SYSTEM IN DOGS AND CATS *(continued)*

Tumor Origin	Predilection Sites	Species	Incidence
Meninges, vessels, and other mesenchymal structures			
Meningiomas (fibrous, transitional, psammomatous, angiomatous, papillary, granular cell, myxoid, anaplastic)	Convexities of cerebral hemispheres and floor of the vault	Dogs (dolicocephalic), cats	Common
Angioblastoma	Variable	Dogs, cats	Rare
Sarcoma	Variable	Dogs, cats	Common
Histiocytic sarcoma (focal granulomatous meningoencephalomyelitis reticulosis)	Cerebral hemispheres and brain stem	Dogs, cats	Rare (in dogs)
Pineal gland, pituitary gland, and craniopharyngeal duct			
Pinealoma	Pineal body	Dogs	Rare
Pituitary adenoma	Pituitary gland	Dogs (brachycephalic), cats	Common
Craniopharyngioma	Hypophyseal-infundibular areas	Dogs	Rare
Heterotopic tissues (malformation tumors)			
Epidermoid, dermoid, teratoma, teratoid, intra-arachnoid cyst	Variable (fourth ventricle and cerebellopontine angle for epidermoid, quadrigeminal cistern for intra-arachnoid cyst)	Dogs	Rare
Germ cell tumors	Base of brain above sella turcica	Dogs	Rare
Hamartoma	Variable (eg, hypothalamus)	Dogs	Rare
SECONDARY TUMORS			
Metastatic tumors			
Mammary gland adenocarcinoma, pulmonary carcinoma, prostatic carcinoma, chemodectoma, malignant melanoma, lymphosarcoma, salivary gland adenocarcinoma, hemangiosarcoma, etc	Variable	Dogs, cats	Relatively common
Primary tumors from surrounding tissues			
Osteosarcoma, lipoma, osteochondroma, chondrosarcoma, fibrosarcoma, nasal adenocarcinoma, hemangiosarcoma, multiple myeloma, calcifying aponeurotic fibromatosis, epidermoid cyst, etc	Variable	Dogs, cats	Relatively common

whereas secondary, highly malignant, metastatic tumors and bone tumors generally progress more rapidly. Many animal tumors have characteristics analogous to corresponding human neoplasms; however, 15%–20% of neuroectodermal tumors (especially gliomas) remain unclassified. Many of these are related topographically to the ventricular system and/or subependymal cell nests. As many as 26% of neuroectodermal brain tumors are undifferentiated, as shown by immunocytochemical staining. Although brain tumors are occasionally reported in animals <1 yr old, most are found in mature and aged animals. No sex predilection for nervous system tumors has been identified.

Incidence: The reported incidence of nervous system neoplasia in animals varies. However, such tumors are reported more often in dogs than in other domestic animals. In one survey, 2.83% of 6,175 dogs examined at necropsy had intracranial neoplasia. In another report, incidence of intracranial neoplasia was 14.5/100,000 dogs at risk and 3.5/100,000 cats at risk. A retrospective study of young dogs (<6 mo old) indicated that the three most common sites for neoplasia (in decreasing order) were the hematopoietic system, brain, and skin. Brachycephalic breeds are at increased risk of some neuroectodermal tumors.

Brain Tumors: In dogs and cats, the brain is a more common site of primary tumors of the nervous system than the spinal cord or peripheral nerves. Meningiomas, gliomas (eg, astrocytomas, oligodendrogliomas), undifferentiated sarcomas, pituitary tumors, and ventricular tumors (eg, choroid plexus papillomas, ependymomas) are commonly reported primary brain tumors in dogs. Previously reported cases of neoplastic reticulosis, gliomatosis, microgliomatosis, malignant histiocytosis, or the malignant form of granulomatous meningoencephalomyelitis are now classified as histiocytic sarcomas or lymphomas. Other primary brain tumors (eg, malformation tumors), tumors of nerve cells (eg, neuroblastoma, ganglioneuroblastoma, and ganglioneuroma), pinealomas, craniopharyngiomas (a suprasellar ectodermal tumor that may destroy the pituitary gland), spongioblastomas (*embryonal glioma*), and medulloblastomas are rare. Adult dogs of several brachycephalic breeds—Boxers, English Bulldogs, and Boston Terriers—are often cited as having the highest incidence of brain tumors among domestic animals; glial tumors, including unclassified gliomas, are the most numerous tumors in these breeds. One study of 97 dogs indicated that Golden Retrievers also have a high incidence of brain tumors (especially meningiomas).

Secondary tumors extending into the cranial vault from the nasal sinuses are relatively common in dogs. In some cases, usually those involving caudal nasal tumors, the only clinical signs are neurologic abnormalities such as behavioral changes, circling, paresis, seizures, or visual deficits. Respiratory signs such as epistaxis, nasal discharge, sneezing, dyspnea, stertor, or mouth breathing may develop after neurologic signs or may be absent. Nasal tumor types include adenocarcinoma, anaplastic chondrosarcoma, epidermoid carcinoma, esthesioneuroblastoma, neurofibrosarcoma, neuroendocrine carcinoma, and squamous cell carcinoma. Unlike nasal cavity tumors, tumors that originate in middle or inner ear structures rarely extend into the brain (*see* TABLE 2). Metastatic brain tumors are also commonly recognized in dogs, with hemangiosarcoma being the most common metastatic tumor type. In cats, metastases most frequently originate from mammary carcinomas and lymphosarcomas.

Astrocytomas are probably the most common neuroectodermal brain tumor in dogs. They are usually found in adult dogs, but they have been reported in dogs <6 mo old. They are common in brachycephalic breeds but can be seen in any breed. Astrocytomas consist of relatively large, protoplasmic-rich cells or smaller cells with many processes. The cells tend to be arranged around blood vessels. There are several variants (eg, anaplastic, fibrillary, gemistocytic, protoplasmic, and pilocytic), most of which stain positively for glial fibrillary acidic protein (GFAP), the chemical subunit of the intracytoplasmic intermediate filaments of astrocytes. Regressive changes found histologically include necrosis, mucinoid degeneration, cyst formation, vascular proliferation (often in the form of glomeruloid nests), and multinucleated giant cells. Hemorrhage is rare. Malignant astrocytomas display nuclear polymorphism, mitotic figures, and small cells with dense, hyperchromatic nuclei. In one study using CT, astrocytomas and oligodendrogliomas appeared similar to one another, because both tumors had ring-like, irregular enhancement and poorly defined margins. Differentiating oligodendrogliomas from malignant astrocytomas with MRI has been difficult. In some instances, however, MRI is considered superior to CT in defining diffuse leptomeningeal and low-grade cerebral astrocytomas. Astrocytomas are uncommon in cats; in one report of four cats, the tumors invaded the third and lateral ventricles.

Choroid plexus papillomas are common tumors in dogs, with reported frequency similar to that of glioblastomas (~12% of neuroglial tumors). Developmentally, the choroid plexus epithelium differentiates from the primitive medullary epithelium and is related to the ependymal cells. These tumors are reddish, papillary growths that may bleed. Histologically, they are well defined, grow by expansion, and have a granular papillary appearance. Tumor papillae consist of vascular stroma lined by one layer of cuboidal or cylindrical epithelium. Immunocytochemical studies reveal that these tumors express epithelial but not glial differentiation, based on absence of staining with GFAP. Keratin may be expressed from some of these tumors. In both benign and malignant variants of choroid plexus papillomas, dissemination to other areas of the brain or spinal cord via the CSF pathways may occur after exfoliation. Obstructive hydrocephalus may occur. Meningeal carcinomatosis may follow spread of the tumor in the subarachnoid space. Choroid plexus tumors are seen as well-defined, hyperdense masses with marked, uniform contrast enhancement on CT scans. Marked enhancement, potentially including hemorrhage and mineralization, is also seen with MRI. Choroid plexus papillomas have no apparent predilection for brachycephalic breeds and are rare in cats.

Ependymomas originate from the epithelium lining the ventricles and central canal of the spinal cord. They are rare but have been reported most frequently in brachycephalic breeds. The gray to reddish, soft, lobular masses tend to invade the ventricular system and meninges, which may result in obstructive hydrocephalus. Mestastases within the CSF system may be seen. Ependymomas of the fourth ventricle may encircle the brain stem. Both epithelial and fibrillary varieties have been described. Histologically, cells are isomorphic, with pale or transparent cytoplasm and round, chromatin-rich nuclei. Nucleus-free zones around blood vessels are characteristic. Some ependymomas appear hemorrhagic, with mucinoid degenerative changes and cyst formation. Malignant or anaplastic ependymomas have moderate degrees of pleomorphism and necrosis and may merge into glioblastoma multiforme. In one study, only one of nine ependymomas was positive for GFAP. In a CT study of brain tumors, ependymomas had no definitive distinguishing features.

Gangliocytomas are rare intracranial tumors reported in adult dogs of several breeds. Histologic findings include mature, neuronal-like cells with multiple processes, a central nucleus, and a nucleolus. Neuroblast-like immature cells may also be seen, and occasionally, newly formed myelin sheaths. They seem to be seen most often in the cerebellum. Pure gangliocytomas have no glial elements and do not express GFAP. Mineralization and extensive necrosis accompanied by edema and capillary proliferation may also develop.

Suprasellar **germ cell tumors** are located dorsal to the sella turcica at the base of the brain. They are often intimately associated with the pituitary gland, which may be trapped within or replaced by the germ cell tumor. They are thought to result from extensive migration of germ cells during embryogenesis. Neurologic signs may be acute in onset and may include lethargy; depression; bradycardia; dilated, nonresponsive pupils; ptosis; visual deficits; and blindness. Germ cell tumors may be large—extending from the olfactory peduncles to the pons and pyriform lobes—and may envelop other cranial nerves (eg, nerves III–VII). Histologically, the tumors usually contain a mixture of primitive germ cells, cords resembling hepatocytes, and acini and tubules of tall columnar epithelial cells. They may stain positively for fetoprotein. Affected animals are usually 3–5 yr old; Doberman Pinschers may be at higher risk than other breeds. Some germ cell tumors have been misdiagnosed as pituitary tumors or craniopharyngiomas.

Glioblastoma multiforme, considered to be equated with the more malignant forms of astrocytomas, has been reported with varying frequency in dogs. In one study, the incidence was 12% of 215 neuroglial tumors. Most are large and found in the cerebrum. The tumor cells consist of medium-sized, round or fusiform cells with isomorphic nuclei. Some glioblastomas display considerable pleomorphism, with small and large mononucleated and multinucleated cells. They are locally invasive and destructive, well vascularized, and often contain necrotic zones. Glioblastomas sometimes express GFAP and are most common in brachycephalic breeds.

Hamartomas are formed by disorderly overgrowth of tissues normally present at a site. They are focal malformations resembling neoplasms and have been reported only rarely in dogs, usually as a subclinical finding.

Hematogenous metastatic brain tumors commonly originate from extracranial sites. In dogs, they often develop from carcinomas of the mammary glands, thyroid, bronchopulmonary epithelium, kidneys, chemoreceptor cells, nasal mucosa, squamous epithelium of the skin, prostate, pancreas, adrenal cortex, and salivary glands. Brain metastasis from a transmissible venereal tumor has been reported in a 5-yr-old male mixed breed dog. Common sarcoma metastases in dogs include fibrosarcomas, hemangiosarcomas, lymphosarcomas, and melanoblastomas. Brain metastases may accompany intramedullary spinal cord metastasis in dogs with lymphosarcomas or hemangiosarcomas. In cats, metastases stem most often from mammary carcinomas or lymphosarcomas. Most CNS lymphomas, especially in dogs, are one part of a multicentric disease, with extensive infiltration of the choroid plexus and leptomeninges a common finding. Neoplastic angioendotheliomatosis in dogs is thought to be an angiotropic lymphoma, possibly of the B-cell line. Extraneural tumor cells sometimes localize in the meninges (eg, meningeal carcinomatosis), often in association with intestinal carcinoma or mammary adenocarcinoma.

Histiocytic sarcomas (previously named malignant histiocytosis or primary/neoplastic reticulosis) are rarely reported in dogs. Proliferation and/or infiltration of neoplastic histiocytes in the basiarachnoidal and ventricular areas (bilateral) is a characteristic feature. These cells may also infiltrate the spinal dura mater, arachnoidal space, leptomeninges, and spinal nerve roots. Histologically, the cells may have characteristic histiocytic morphology but exhibit moderate pleomorphism and numerous mitotic figures.

Intracranial intra-arachnoid cysts have been reported in dogs. These rare malformation tumors seem to develop most often in the quadrigeminal cistern. Of the six dogs in one report, three were <1 yr old, four were males, and five of the six weighed <11 kg. One dog had additional developmental anomalies (abnormal corpus callosum and block vertebrae). On CT scans and MRI, the cysts were extra-axial, had sharply defined margins, contained fluid isodense to CSF, and did not show contrast enhancement.

Malformation tumors, including epidermoid and dermoid cysts and teratomas, originate from heterotopic tissue and are rare tumors in dogs. They typically lie close to embryonal lines of closure. Epidermoid and dermoid cysts result from inclusion of epithelial components of embryonal tissue at the time of closure of the neural tube. They reportedly have a predilection for young dogs (eg, 3–24 mo old), although cysts have been found in older dogs. They usually involve the cerebellopontine angle, fourth ventricle, or both. Cysts within the fourth ventricle may secondarily compress the medulla oblongata and cerebellum. Some epidermoid cysts are incidental findings at necropsy.

Histologically, epidermoid cysts may have a multilocular structure; most are lined by stratified squamous epithelium and contain keratinaceous debris, desquamated epithelial cells, and occasional inflammatory cells. In contrast, dermoid cysts contain adnexal structures such as hair follicles, sebaceous glands, and sweat glands. Cysts may measure as much as 2.5 cm in diameter. Because of the tumor's location, dogs may show signs of a pontomedullary syndrome (eg, trigeminal, facial, cerebellar, and/or vestibular dysfunction). Teratomas are well-differentiated germ cell tumors (*see* above) arising from several embryonic germ cell layers.

Medulloblastomas are highly malignant, uncommon neuroectodermal canine tumors that almost always develop in the cerebellum. The tumors tend to bulge into the fourth ventricle, often replacing part of the cerebellar vermis and compressing the midbrain rostrally and the brain stem ventrally. They may infiltrate the meninges, metastasize within the CSF pathways, and cause obstructive hydrocephalus. Histologically, these tumors include sheets of densely packed cells with pale cytoplasm and oval or carrot-shaped nuclei with coarse, granular chromatin. Mitotic figures are common. Regressive changes include pyknosis and karyorrhexis. Although most cases are seen in young dogs, a cerebellar medulloblastoma with multiple differentiation has been described in a 4-yr-old Border Collie.

Meningioangiomatosis is a rare, benign malformation of CNS blood vessels, characterized by proliferation of the vessels and spindle-shaped, perivascular meningothelial cells in the cerebral cortex and brain stem of juvenile and adult dogs. The meningothelial cells stain positively for vimentin, which, along with the presence of mucopolysaccharides and collagen among proliferating cells, suggests a mesenchymal and fibroblastic origin.

Meningiomas are extra-axial tumors. They arise from elements of the dura within the cranial and spinal spaces and are the most commonly reported brain tumors in cats. They are also one of the most common intracranial tumors in dogs, with a reported incidence of 30%–39%. In most studies, meningiomas are seen in dogs >7 yr old and in cats >9 yr old, although they have been seen in young cats (<3 yr old) with mucopolysaccharidosis type I and in dogs <6 mo old. They are often found in dolichocephalic breeds, especially Golden Retrievers. Canine and feline meningiomas have estrogen, progesterone, and androgen receptors. These usually benign tumors tend to grow slowly under the dura mater, although direct brain invasion has been reported.

Pathologic findings include globular, irregular, lobulated, nodular, ovoid, or plaque-like masses ranging in diameter from a few millimeters to several centimeters. Meningiomas are typically discrete and often are firm, rubbery, and encapsulated. They may contain granular calcifications known as psammoma bodies. In addition, there may be focal or massive calcification of the tumor. A substantial proportion of basal and plaque-like meningiomas involve the floor of the cranial cavity, especially when located near the optic chiasm or suprasellar area. They also commonly are found over the convexities of the cerebral hemispheres, less often in the cerebellopontomedullary region, and infrequently in the retrobulbar space (arising from the optic nerve sheath). In cats, common locations include the tela choroidea of the third ventricle and the supratentorial meninges. Cats also have a higher incidence (17%) of multiple meningiomas. Hyperostosis, a thickening of bone adjacent to the meningioma, may develop, especially in cats.

Meningiomas rarely metastasize outside the brain, but may extend into paranasal regions and lungs or be seen as primary extracranial masses as a result of embryonic displacement of arachnoid cells or meningocytes. Those in extracranial locations differ from intracranial meningiomas primarily in their more aggressive behavior and anaplastic/malignant nature. Meningiomas may be distinguishable from tumors within the brain parenchyma on contrast CT scans by their appearance as broad-based, peripherally located masses. Cystic and edematous meningiomas have been detected using CT scans and MRI. When a dural tail (a linear enhancement of thickened dura mater adjacent to an extra-axial mass) is detected by MRI, a meningioma is the most likely cause.

The histologic classification of canine meningiomas includes angioblastic, fibroblastic, meningothelial or syncytial, psammomatous, and transitional. Papillary and microcystic forms may also be seen. The tumors usually consist of large meningothelial cells or fusiform cells arranged in whorls, nests, islands, or stream-like patterns. Cell boundaries are typically ill defined, and the nuclei contain little chromatin. Canine meningiomas commonly have vimentin intermediate filaments. Regressive changes may include cavernous vascular formations, hemorrhage, hyalinization of connective tissue, and deposits of fat, lipopigments, or cholesterol. Many have evidence of focal necrosis with suppuration. This is the likely cause of the reported predominance of polymorphonuclear cells in CSF in many dogs with meningioma.

A grading system in human patients has recently been adapted for dogs and may predict tumor behavior. Grade I tumors are considered benign, grade II tumors are considered atypical, and grade III tumors are considered malignant.

Most feline epitheliomas are meningotheliomatous or psammomatous, often with cholesterol deposits.

In **meningeal sarcomatosis**, sarcomas cause diffuse thickening of the meninges; extensive hemorrhages are common. These rare tumors tend to infiltrate nervous tissue and run along blood vessels. Cell types include lymphoid, plasmacytoid, mature plasma cells, immunoblastic cells, and multinucleate giant cells.

Oligodendrogliomas are common tumors in dogs, particularly in brachycephalic breeds. In one report, they comprised 28% of neuroectodermal tumors. These tumors consist of chromatin-rich, densely packed, round cells with perinuclear halos. Most grow by infiltration and destroy invaded tissue. Capillaries tend to proliferate within these tumors, producing glomerulus-like structures. Regressive changes are similar to those seen in astrocytomas (*see* p 1270). Necrosis and extensive calcification are uncommon. These tumors do not stain with GFAP; in one study, 3 of 11 oligodendrogliomas reacted with myelin-associated glycoprotein, while none reacted with myelin basic protein. Many canine oligodendrogliomas are mixed tumors with areas of astrocytic and, in some cases, ependymal differentiation. The MRI features are similar to those seen with high-grade (malignant) astrocytomas. Oligodendrogliomas are rare in cats.

Pituitary tumors are common in dogs, with an apparent predilection for brachycephalic breeds. They are infrequent in cats. Tumors may be functional or nonfunctional. Either type may cause hypopituitarism by mechanical or functional impairment of remaining pituitary tissue, although this effect is uncommon. Nonfunctional canine pituitary tumors are common and are usually chromophobe adenomas, although adenocarcinomas have also been reported. Functional pituitary tumors associated with the adenohypophysis are typically characterized by pituitary-dependent hyperadrenocorticism (PDH). (*See also* HYPERADRENOCORTICISM, p 543.) Of the cases of pituitary Cushing disease, ≥80% are reportedly associated with a pituitary tumor.

In dogs, these tumors may stem from the pars distalis (80%) or the pars intermedia (20%), because both regions contain cells that can produce adrenocorticotropic hormone. The tumors are generally chromophobic microadenomas (<1 cm in diameter) that do not produce neurologic signs. MRI studies suggest that as many as 60% of dogs with PDH and no neurologic signs have pituitary tumors 4–12 mm in diameter. As many as 50% of dogs with PDH and large chromophobic macroadenomas (>1 cm in diameter on MRI) may not show clinical signs related to an intracranial mass. In one study, seven of eight dogs with pituitary neoplasia that had been treated for PDH for varying periods of time (between 1 and 2 yr) developed neurologic signs, including abnormal behavior (eg, head pressing, lethargy, hiding, wandering, pacing, tight circling, and trembling), seizures, and positional nystagmus. Most pituitary tumors, especially those derived from the pars distalis, tend to grow dorsocaudally because the diaphragma sella is incomplete. Chromophobic canine tumors from the pars intermedia are smaller and less destructive. Dorsal extension of pituitary tumors may lead to compression and obliteration of the infundibulum, ventral portion of the third ventricle, hypothalamus, and thalamus and may eventually impinge on the internal capsule and optic tract. Hypothalamic or median eminence involvement may cause central diabetes insipidus (especially in middle-aged and older dogs with neurologic signs), manifesting as polyuria, polydipsia, and isosthenuria or hyposthenuria. Alteration in water balance results from interference with the synthesis of antidiuretic hormone (ADH) in the supraoptic nucleus or release of ADH into capillaries of the pars nervosa. Although pituitary tumors generally do not lead to visual impairment, acute blindness and dilated, nonresponsive pupils have been noted in seven dogs and one cat with pituitary masses that compressed the optic chiasm.

Approximately 80% of cats diagnosed with Cushing disease have PDH; tumor types include pituitary microadenomas, macroadenomas, and adenocarcinomas. Pituitary acidophil adenomas, especially the large variety, have been associated with acromegaly and nervous system signs (eg, circling, seizures) in cats, accompanied by insulin-resistant diabetes mellitus and high serum growth hormone concentrations.

Histologically, pituitary tumors include polygonal, round, and cylindrical cells arranged in close contact with blood vessels or formed into islands of cells divided by connective tissue. The cell pattern may be uniform, resembling normal pituitary tissue. Many pituitary tumors contain both chromophobic and chromophilic cells. Regressive changes include cyst formation, necrosis, and hemorrhage. MRI with contrast enhancement is extremely helpful to visualize microtumors (3–10 mm in diameter) and macrotumors (≥24 mm) in dogs with PDH, regardless of neurologic signs. MRI and CT scans of pituitary tumors reveal minimal peritumoral edema, uniform contrast enhancement, and well-defined margins; however, tumors <3 mm in diameter may not be visible. Adrenal and pituitary tumors may coexist in dogs with hyperadrenocorticism, complicating test results and making diagnosis and treatment more difficult.

Primary skeletal tumors do not typically cause neurologic signs. Multilobular osteochondroma originates in the flat bones of the skull, usually in older, medium- or large-breed dogs and appears as a firm, fixed mass. It may erode the cranium and compress, rather than infiltrate, underlying brain tissues. Radiographically, the tumor contains nodular or stippled areas of mineralization, resulting in a characteristic "popcorn ball" appearance. Microscopically, the tumor contains multiple lobules of osseous and chondroid tissue. Local recurrence is common in high-grade tumors (78%) and occurs in 30% and 47% of low- and intermediate-grade tumors, respectively. Metastasis frequently occurs (as many as 58%) but usually late in the disease course (>1 yr) and also depends on grade, with rates of 75% in high-grade tumors and 60% in intermediate-grade tumors, as opposed to 30% in low-grade tumors. Vertebral osteochondroma is the spinal cord counterpart.

Vascular malformations are considered developmental lesions rather than true neoplasms and are uncommon in both dogs and cats. They may be located in the cingulate gyrus, pyriform-hippocampal area of the temporal lobe, basal ganglia, cerebellum, occipital lobe, or septum pellucidum and fornix and comprise variable combinations of arteries, veins, and capillaries. The vessels tend to be dilated, sinusoidal in shape, and accompanied by hemorrhages.

Spinal Cord Tumors: Spinal cord tumors are relatively common in cats and dogs. They are generally classified according to their relationship with the spinal cord and meninges as extradural, intradural-extramedullary, or intramedullary. Depending on tumor location, any of the four spinal cord syndromes may be anticipated (eg, cervical, cervicothoracic, thoracolumbar, or lumbosacral syndromes). Regardless of type, the mean age of most dogs with spinal tumors is ~6 yr, and tumors appear to be more common in medium and large breeds. Cats with lymphosarcoma tend to be younger (mean age of ~3.5 yr), possibly because of the infectious etiology (ie, feline leukemia virus) of most cases. However, age alone does not preclude a diagnosis of spinal tumor. The clinical course for the various tumor types and locations is not clearly defined. In one study, the rate of progression was fastest with intramedullary tumors (1.7 wk), followed by extradural tumors (3.4 wk) and intradural-extramedullary tumors (5.7 wk).

Extradural tumors are found outside the dura mater and cause spinal cord compression. They are the most common spinal tumors in both cats and dogs. The most frequent types of canine spinal cord tumors are primary, malignant bone tumors (chondrosarcoma, fibrosarcoma, hemangiosarcoma, hemangioendothelioma, multiple myeloma, osteochondromas or multiple cartilaginous exostoses, and osteosarcoma) and tumors metastatic to bone and soft tissue. Reports of secondary vertebral tumors in dogs include anaplastic tumors, aortic body tumors, bronchogenic carcinoma, chemodectoma, fibrosarcoma, ganglioneuroma, hemangiosarcoma, lymphosarcoma, malignant melanoma, mammary carcinoma, osteosarcoma, pancreatic adenocarcinoma, perianal gland carcinoma, prostatic carcinoma, rhabdomyosarcoma, Sertoli cell carcinoma, squamous cell carcinoma, transitional cell carcinoma, thyroid carcinoma, and tonsillar carcinoma. An extradural ganglioneuroma and its undifferentiated counterpart, ganglioneuroblastoma, have also been reported in dogs.

Primary vertebral tumors are rare in cats, with osteosarcoma being the most frequently reported. Metastatic, extradural spinal cord tumors are unusual in dogs, but extradural lymphosarcoma is the most common spinal tumor in cats. In most cases, these tumors are secondary to lymphosarcoma elsewhere in the body, although primary spinal cord lymphosarcomas have been reported sporadically in dogs. In one study in cats, extraneural involvement was not found in ~50% of the cases, and the tumors were solitary in 22 of 23 cats. A predilection for the thoracic and lumbar vertebral canal was seen, but the tumors may develop in any spinal region. Three of the tumors affected the brachial plexus cervical roots (*see* p 1276). Spinal lymphomas in cats may extend over multiple vertebral bodies and involve more than one level of the spinal cord. Leptomeningeal spinal cord involvement is not common in cats. A tumor termed myxoma-myxosarcoma has been described in four dogs. These malignant tumors resembled soft-tissue myxomas, with polygonally shaped cells with gray, vacuolated cytoplasm that stained positive for S-100 protein antibody. The masses were extradural in three cases and intradural-extramedullary in the other.

Intradural-extramedullary tumors are found in the subarachnoid space and are estimated to account for ~35% of all spinal cord tumors. They are most commonly meningiomas or nerve sheath tumors (eg, neurofibromas, neurilemmomas, and schwannomas) that grow into the vertebral canal and compress the spinal cord. Approximately 14% of CNS meningiomas in dogs (but only 4% in cats) reportedly involve the spinal cord. Tumors may be seen in the cervical, lumbar, or thoracic cord regions. In a report of spinal cord tumors in 29 dogs, nerve sheath tumors were the second most common type after vertebral tumors. In another review of canine spinal tumors, 39 of 60 nerve sheath tumors involved the spinal cord. Nerve sheath tumors often affect the brachial plexus (*see* below).

A primary intradural-extramedullary tumor with a predilection for T10–L2 spinal cord segments in young dogs, particularly retrievers and German Shepherds, has been variously diagnosed as ependymoma, medulloepithelioma, nephroblastoma, or neuroepithelioma. The origin of this tumor is uncertain, and immunocytochemical studies have not supported a neuroectodermal origin. Monoclonal antibody studies suggest it may be a nephroblastoma. Most cases are seen in dogs 5–36 mo old, with males and females affected equally. Clinical signs include a thoracolumbar syndrome. CSF is usually normal, although the protein level was increased in one dog. The extramedullary masses are a tan to grayish white color and 1–3 cm long. They are generally found dorsal and lateral to the spinal cord, may entrap the spinal roots, and may be accompanied by areas of hemorrhage and severe spinal cord compression. Histologic findings include solid sheets of ovoid to fusiform cells interspersed with areas of acinar and tubular differentiation, rudimentary glomeruli, and focal squamous metaplasia.

Intramedullary tumors are the least common of the three categories of spinal cord tumors, with a reported frequency of 15%–24%. Primary glial tumors (eg, astrocytoma, choroid plexus papilloma, ependymoma, oligodendroglioma, and undifferentiated sarcoma) are the most commonly diagnosed. Intramedullary spinal cord metastasis is an uncommon complication of systemic malignancy in dogs, and neurologic signs may be the first indication of systemic malignancy. The mean age of affected dogs is ~6 yr, any part of the spinal cord may be involved, and there may be accompanying brain metastasis.

Malformation tumors rarely affect the spinal cord. In one report, a 2-yr-old, female Rottweiler presenting with a thoracolumbar syndrome had an intramedullary epidermoid cyst. The gray to off-white cyst was ~2 cm long, 1 cm in diameter, and extended from T13 to L2 spinal cord segments. The empty lumen was lined by simple stratified squamous epithelium or, in a few regions, by desquamating keratinized epithelium containing keratohyaline granules. The spinal cord was severely compressed. These cysts may arise from growth of primordial epithelial cells entrapped during closure of the neural tube.

Peripheral Nerve Tumors: Tumors of cranial and spinal nerves and nerve roots are common in dogs, cattle, and horses but are rarely seen in cats. In one report, peripheral nerve tumors accounted for ~27% of canine nervous system tumors. Differing opinions on the cell of origin have led to confusion over the terminology used to describe these tumors. While schwannoma, neurilemmoma, and neurofibroma are common, interchangeable designations, the term malignant peripheral nerve sheath tumors (MPNST) is recommended because many of these tumors are malignant (based on cytologic criteria), and determining the cell of origin is usually impossible. Mid to caudal cervical and/or rostral thoracic nerve roots, especially ventral roots, are the most common sites for MPNST. These tumors frequently involve nerves of the brachial plexus, often appearing as bulbous or fusiform thickenings of one or more nerves. They can spread to other nerves once they advance to the common brachial plexus bundle. The tumors typically result in slow, progressive, unilateral thoracic limb lameness and muscle atrophy, often involving the infraspinatus and supraspinatus muscles. Affected animals may display a unilateral Horner syndrome, pain on leg movement, axillary pain on palpation (an axillary mass may be palpable), and may lick or chew at the foot or carpus of the affected limb. Intradural-extramedullary spinal cord compression is most common with tumors located at the spinal nerve roots, although more peripherally located tumors occasionally may invade the vertebral canal. The trigeminal is the cranial nerve most often affected by MPNST, producing signs of unilateral trigeminal nerve dysfunction (eg, unilateral atrophy of the masseter and temporalis muscles). Brain-stem compression and local vertebral erosion have been reported.

Peripheral nerves may also be affected by other tumor types (eg, giant cell sarcoma with cervical involvement, a malignant tumor of the apocrine sweat glands, and sarcoma extending into the brachial plexus have been described in dogs). Peripheral tumors of neuronal origin, such as ganglioneuromas and their more undifferentiated counterpart, ganglioneuroblastomas, are extremely rare but have caused extradural spinal cord compression in dogs. Sympathetic ganglia are thought to be the source of ganglioneuromas. Lymphosarcomas may involve cranial and spinal nerves and nerve roots in cats and dogs and may extend intracranially. Myelomonocytic neoplasia of the trigeminal nerve and ganglia, leading to a dropped mandible and symmetric atrophy of masticatory muscles, has been reported in dogs. Tumors of the ear canal (eg, ceruminous adenocarcinoma, fibrosarcoma, and squamous cell carcinoma), as well as osteosarcoma of the skull, may affect the facial nerve or one of its branches. Neurofibromas rarely involve the vestibulocochlear nerve. Cranial nerves may be compressed by meningiomas located on the floor of the cranial vault. The vagosympathetic trunk may be compressed by aortic body tumors.

See also DISEASES OF THE PERIPHERAL NERVES AND NEUROMUSCULAR JUNCTION, p 1238.

Clinical Findings: Some of the clinical signs and syndromes associated with various CNS tumors have already been mentioned. Cerebral, hypothalamic/diencephalic, midbrain, cerebellar, pontomedullary, and vestibular syndromes associated with focal discrete intracranial masses might be expected, depending on tumor location. Accurate anatomic localization is possible in many cases, especially in the early stages of tumor growth. However, correlation of clinicopathologic signs with tumor location may be impossible because tumor location may be masked by secondary changes (eg, brain herniation, cerebral edema, hemorrhage, obstructive hydrocephalus, tissue necrosis, and tumor spread within the brain) that independently cause clinical signs. Partial brain herniation may result from increased intracranial pressure and/or shifts in the brain caused by the tumor. Care must be taken to maintain optimal oxygenation and avoid intracranial hypertension during diagnostic tests that involve anesthesia and CSF sampling because of the increased risk of herniation.

Several types of herniation have been described. **Cingulate gyrus herniation** under the falx cerebri toward the unaffected hemisphere leads to compression of the opposite cingulate gyrus. **Occipital or temporal lobe herniation** (primarily the parahippocampal gyrus) under the tentorium cerebelli (caudal transtentorial herniation) often causes dorsoventral and lateral compression of the midbrain at the rostral colliculi and partial occlusion of the mesencephalic aqueduct. Caudal displacement of the diencephalon and midbrain may also occur. Clinical signs include initial pupillary constriction, often followed by mydriasis, tetraplegia, and coma. **Rostral cerebellar vermis herniation** under the tentorium cerebelli (rostral transtentorial herniation) may lead to flattening of the rostral cerebellum, marked compression and rostral displacement of the brain stem, and compression of the temporal cortex. Despite the gross pathology, clinical deficits may be absent. **Cerebellar herniation** (especially the caudal lobe of the cerebellar vermis) through the foramen magnum compresses the underlying medulla oblongata and may cause malacia and hemorrhage. Apnea, hypoxia-induced coma, and tetraplegia may be seen. Concurrent foramen magnum and caudal transtentorial herniation may cause dysfunction in both the midbrain and medulla oblongata. Herniation combined with attenuation of the ventricular system, especially at the level of the mesencephalic aqueduct, can create obstructive hydrocephalus. The increased intracranial pressure may lead to ischemic necrosis of the herniated tissue.

Initially, seizures and behavioral changes may be the only abnormalities associated with tumors involving the rostral cerebrum (eg, olfactory and frontal lobes). Lesions of the frontal and prefrontal lobes may result in no clinical signs. Acute blindness may be the initial clinical sign in animals with tumors in the region of the optic chiasm (eg, pituitary tumors, paranasal sinus carcinoma, polycentric lymphosarcoma, and suprasellar germ cell tumors). Papilledema (often bilateral) is thought to result from a generalized increase in intracranial pressure. A variety of causes (eg, multiple, small metastatic masses from extracranial tumors, especially with malignant melanoma and hemangiosarcoma) may lead to multifocal clinical signs associated with CNS tumors. Other tumors, such as carcinomas (pulmonary or mammary), tend to produce fewer, larger metastases. The cerebrum, hippocampus, and cerebellar cortex are common sites for hematogenous metastases. Extraneural tumor cells sometimes localize in the meninges (eg, meningeal carcinomatosis associated with mammary adenocarcinoma or intestinal carcinoma). Multifocal syndromes may also result from primary CNS tumors in multiple sites, extension of an original tumor to another site, or metastasis via the CSF.

Choroid plexus papillomas and ependymomas tend to obstruct cerebrospinal pathways because of their ventricular orientation, especially when they arise in the fourth ventricle. Neurologic signs associated with ventricular tumors result from the tumor location and the degree of ventricular dilation caused by obstructive hydrocephalus. Clinical signs often are insidious with either of these tumors; the clinical course generally is protracted, ranging from months to years. Extraneural immunoproliferative diseases in dogs and cats (eg, multiple myeloma and macroglobulinemia-associated lymphocytic leukemia) may also result in a range of intermittent cranial neurologic signs, including disorientation, ataxia, intention tremor of the head, visual impairment, circling, and staggering or falling. Intravascular erythrocyte aggregation impairs blood flow in the affected areas and probably leads to the transient signs.

Pituitary tumors are associated with various endocrine signs, including acromegaly, abnormal hair coat, gonadal atrophy, polydipsia, polyuria, and obesity. (*See also*

THE PITUITARY GLAND, p 542). Behavioral changes, circling, paresis, seizures, or visual deficits may result from extension of primary nasal cavity tumors into the cranial vault. Respiratory signs, such as dyspnea, epistaxis, nasal discharge, sneezing, stertor, or mouth breathing, may follow neurologic signs or may not occur at all.

Diagnosis: A variety of diagnostic imaging aids, including plain-film radiography, contrast radiography (eg, myelography), and specialized radiographic techniques such as radionuclide imaging (scintigraphy), CT scans, and MRI are used to diagnose nervous system tumors. These techniques provide information (eg, axial origin, location, shape, pattern of growth, and edema) that can be important when determining prognosis, therapy, and outcome. Bone neoplasia may be observed with plain-film radiography. Intracranial tumors are better evaluated with MRI. Some indices of malignancy (eg, edema, extension of growth across the midline, poor margin definition, and tissue invasion) have been defined using MRI, and many tumor types can be presumptively diagnosed based on location, appearance, and contrast-enhancement patterns. Caution must be exercised, however, because presumptive diagnoses made after imaging are found to be incorrect in ~30% of patients after a histopathologic diagnosis is obtained.

Signs of extradural, intradural-extramedullary, and intramedullary tumors vary on myelography. Extradural lesions are located outside the dura mater, resulting in attenuation of the dural tube and spinal cord. Deflection of the contrast column away from the vertebral canal, resulting in a widened epidural space, confirms an extradural lesion. Intramedullary-extramedullary lesions develop in the subarachnoid space, where they act as wedges, displacing the dura mater toward the bony vertebral canal and the spinal cord toward the contralateral vertebral canal. Contrast material abuts the cranial and caudal margins of the tumor, resulting in a characteristic cup or golf tee appearance. In contrast, intramedullary tumors displace the spinal cord material from within, enlarging the circumference of the spinal cord and attenuating the contrast material in the subarachnoid space surrounding the tumor.

Results from one study suggest that CT is better than survey radiographs to visualize bony changes associated with extradural lesions but that myelography is better than CT to classify spinal cord lesions. In another canine study, MRI was used to determine tumor location in all dogs and bone infiltration in all but one. Localization of tumors in the intradural-extramedullary space was not always possible, however. Myelographic interpretation of intramedullary spinal cord metastasis may be difficult; intramedullary tumors must be differentiated from hemorrhage and spinal cord edema. Classically, myelograms of intramedullary masses reveal widening of the spinal cord shadow and tapering and attenuation of contrast in both lateral and ventrodorsal views.

Electrodiagnostic techniques (eg, electromyography, nerve conduction velocity determination), in conjunction with myelography and imaging techniques, can facilitate diagnosis of peripheral nerve tumors. Myelograms reportedly often are negative in animals with cervical MPNST.

Analysis of CSF may reveal moderate increases in total protein content, total white cell count, and CSF pressure. There is a low frequency of tumor cells in CSF from animals with brain or spinal cord neoplasia, but malignant cells have been reported in dogs and cats with intracranial and spinal cord (extradural and intramedullary) lymphosarcomas.

Prognosis and Treatment: The prognosis for animals with nervous system tumors is generally guarded to poor but depends on the extent of tissue damage, tumor location, surgical accessibility, and rate of tumor growth. Recent improvements in treatment have centered mainly on surgical resection, radiation therapy, and chemotherapy, based on more accurate tumor localization and identification using imaging techniques, such as CT scans and MRI. Better identification and characterization of tumors from tissue biopsies obtained via stereotactically guided biopsy devices may lead to additional improvement. Although success rates for different tumor types and locations are not currently known, cerebral tumors (including meningiomas and ependymomas) without brain-stem signs appear to have the best prognosis, especially in cats. Radiation therapy may be the most successful treatment for a range of intracranial tumors and, if surgery is performed, postoperative radiation therapy may prolong survival times. Radiation therapy is beneficial for treatment of inoperable tumors and may be better than surgery for dogs with infiltrative masses. A retrospective study of 86 dogs with brain tumors showed that dogs treated with ^{60}Co radiation, with or without other combinations of therapy, lived significantly longer than dogs that underwent surgery (some with ^{125}I implants) or dogs that received symptomatic treatment. Dogs with a solitary site of involvement had a better prognosis. Longterm control of primary brain tumors using cytotoxic chemotherapy alone is poor; symptomatic treatment (eg, use of anticonvulsants and/or anti-inflammatory doses of corticosteroids) is palliative at best, with survival time generally measured in weeks. Corticosteroids may relieve signs by reducing edema near the tumor and by causing temporary regression of lymphoid and reticulohistiocytic tumors.

The treatment of choice for meningioma in cats is surgery, because these tumors are usually removable in toto, with postoperative survival times preaching a median of ~2 yr. Recurrence is possible, with reports of up to 20% and with a median disease-free interval of 9 mo; however, second surgical resections are also feasible. In dogs, the ability to completely resect meningiomas is more limited, because tissue invasion is more frequent. The use of surgical aspirator devices and intraoperative ultrasound or endoscopic imaging may improve the surgeon's ability to perform complete removal. Recent reports of dogs with tumors removed by a surgical aspirator and/or endoscopic-assisted removal yielded median survival times of >3–5 yr. In earlier reports, surgical resection alone resulted in median survival times of ~200 days. Postoperative radiation therapy appears beneficial in some studies, with median survival times increasing by ~1 yr over surgery alone. Radiation therapy as a sole treatment, either in standard fractionated courses (usually throughout 3–4 wk) or in stereotactic radiosurgery (SRS) approaches (usually one to four treatments), has also been attempted. Success rates are difficult to determine, because confirmation of tumor type is rarely performed, and only preliminary reports for SRS have been published. Addition of cytotoxic drugs (most commonly hydroxyurea or CCNU) postoperatively or at recurrence may lengthen survival time.

Astrocytic tumors/gliomas are usually not treated surgically because of location but may be treated with radiation therapy, with reported survival times of 6–11 mo. Additionally, newer drugs, such as temozoloamide, which has shown some promise in people, may have some use in the treatment of these tumors in dogs.

Metastatic brain lesions are usually treated palliatively, with a combination of medical therapy, radiation, and/or chemotherapy. More invasive treatments, such as surgery, should be reserved for animals in which the primary tumor is well controlled and no other systemic metastases can be documented.

Most extradural spinal tumors are primary bone tumors, and removal often causes decreased spinal stability, pathologic fractures, or spinal subluxation. In a study of canine malignant extradural tumors, postsurgical survival times were short. A report of 20 vertebral tumors (primary or metastatic fibrosarcomas or osteosarcomas) in dogs treated with combinations of surgery, radiation, and chemotherapy supports a guarded prognosis for dogs with vertebral neoplasia. Median survival time was 135 days, with a range of 15–600 days. Survival time after surgical resection of spinal lymphoma and myxosarcoma in dogs was 560–1,080 days in another report, although some dogs received postsurgical radiotherapy and chemotherapy. Methods recommended to treat spinal lymphosarcoma in cats include focal radiotherapy, surgical cytoreduction, and systemic chemotherapy, including L-asparaginase, cyclophosphamide, vincristine, and prednisone. Longterm results are poor, partly associated with a positive feline leukemia virus status in these patients.

Animals with MPNST have a generally poor prognosis, because only a small percentage of these tumors can be completely resected, and their recurrence rate is high. Metastasis, often to the lungs, is another complication. Early diagnosis of MPNST may lead to better results. Mean survival of 180 days after surgical resection was reported in one study. Many intradural-extramedullary tumors (eg, lipomas and meningiomas) can be successfully removed, with long postsurgical survival. However, intradural-extramedullary tumors that 1) involve spinal cord segments of an intumescence, 2) are ventrally located, or 3) invade adjacent neural parenchyma have a poor prognosis.

Surgical resection is rarely possible for intramedullary masses. However, there are successful reports of removal of a thoracolumbar intramedullary ependymoma and a tumor resembling a nephroblastoma (by exploratory laminectomy, followed by durotomy and myelotomy). Prognosis for dogs with intramedullary spinal cord metastasis is poor because of the frequent presence of disseminated disease, although corticosteroid therapy may lead to temporary improvement.

Peripheral nerve and nerve root tumors can be successfully resected but may necessitate removal of the affected nerve and nerve root. If atrophy of all muscle groups is extreme—as may develop with tumors involving multiple nerves of the brachial plexus—or if more than one root is involved, complete amputation of the limb may be required. Recurrence is common after resection of peripheral tumors, with average time to recurrence of 5 mo in one report. Long-term survival times (18–42 mo) have been reported. Even untreated, dogs with trigeminal nerve tumors can have prolonged survival times (as much as 21 mo in seven dogs). In 45 cats, median survival time was 21.5 mo, with a 20% local recurrence rate.

PARANEOPLASTIC DISORDERS OF THE NERVOUS SYSTEM

Paraneoplastic syndromes are nonmetastatic complications of cancer with effects distant from the primary tumor. They are unrelated to neurologic complications secondary to metabolic or nutritional disorders, infection, cerebrovascular incidents, or adverse effects of treatments. They can affect all parts of the nervous system, including the brain, cranial nerves, spinal cord, dorsal root ganglia, peripheral nerves, and the neuromuscular junction. Some are thought to be immunologically mediated through cross-reactivity by immune cells against antigens expressed by tumors and neural tissues (molecular mimicry), whereas others are related to the production of circulating hormones, peptides, or other substances that exert systemic effects.

Paraneoplastic syndromes affecting the CNS are rarely recognized in animals, but lack of awareness may lead to a low detection rate. Sporadic case reports suggest that brain and spinal cord effects can result from various tumor types. An 8-yr-old, male German Shepherd with a history of acute pelvic limb paralysis, progressive loss of motor function, conscious proprioceptive deficits, loss of superficial and deep pain sensation over the trunk and pelvic limbs, and Schiff-Sherrington-like hyperextension in the thoracic limbs was diagnosed with hepatocellular carcinoma with metastasis to the lungs, liver, spleen, and lymph nodes at necropsy. Severe necrotizing myelopathy was present throughout the gray and white matter of the thoracic spinal cord, including spongy degeneration, gliosis, demyelination, axonal *swelling and degeneration, and neuronal* necrosis. In a second case, a range of neurologic deficits in a 17-mo-old, male Poodle was attributed to hyperviscosity syndrome secondary to macroglobulinemia-associated lymphocytic leukemia. A 3-yr-old Doberman Pinscher developed diencephalic syndrome, associated with a diencephalic tumor (an astrocytoma) that produced growth hormone, resulting in extreme emaciation despite adequate or increased nutritional intake.

Paraneoplastic myasthenia gravis (MG) has been strongly associated with the presence of thymic disease. MG can manifest as systemic weakness, or more focally, especially as megaesophagus. In one review of canine thymoma, 47% of the dogs had MG, 33% had concurrent nonthymic cancer (including pheochromocytoma, mammary adenocarcinoma, or pulmonary adenocarcinoma), and 20% had concurrent signs of polymyositis. Dogs with thymoma-associated MG often have antibodies to nicotinic acetylcholine receptors, which can be used to diagnose and/or monitor treatment response. These dogs may produce autoantibodies to several other neuromuscular antigens, including ryanodine (a skeletal muscle calcium-release channel receptor) and the muscle protein titin. Other tumors that have rarely been reported to cause MG include osteosarcoma, lymphoma, and bile duct carcinoma. MG can improve with immunosuppression or treatment of the underlying tumor but may also be persistent or occur after removal of a thymoma.

An association between myositis (eg, dermatomyositis and polymyositis) and malignant neoplasia in people has been well established. Dogs with malignant tumors such as bronchogenic carcinoma, myeloid leukemia, or tonsillar carcinoma may also have muscular necrosis and low-grade myositis, but the frequency of this potentially paraneoplastic association is unknown. Two dogs with multicentric lymphoma were found to have polymyositis, but the presence of lymphocyte infiltration within the muscle makes differentiating between primary and paraneoplastic disease difficult.

Peripheral neuropathy is commonly associated with neoplasia in people, and is likely so in animals, as well, although less recognized clinically. A large survey on dogs with various malignancies revealed multiple histopathologic changes in the nerve fibers, including paranodal-segmental demyelination, remyelination, axonal degeneration, and myelin globules. Associated tumor types included insulinoma, multiple myeloma, lymphoma, bronchogenic carcinoma, mammary adenocarcinoma, malignant melanoma, thyroid adenocarcinoma, leiomyosarcomas, hemangiosarcomas, undifferentiated sarcomas, and mast cell tumor.

Clinical signs may include reduced or absent spinal or cranial reflexes, flaccid weakness, reduced muscle tone, paralysis of limb or head muscles, and, after 1–2 wk, neurogenic muscle atrophy. Dysphonia may also be present.

Dogs and cats with clinical signs of nervous system disease (or with myositis or necrotizing myopathy confirmed by histopathology) that do not respond to therapy or that relapse should be carefully screened for malignancy, because paraneoplastic syndromes may be the first clinical sign related to tumor presence. Blood tests or imaging may be indicated. Such vigilance may detect tumors at a more treatable stage.

POLIOENCEPHALOMALACIA

(Cerebrocortical necrosis)

Polioencephalomalacia (PEM) is an important neurologic disease of ruminants that is seen worldwide. Cattle, sheep, goats, deer, and camelids are affected. PEM is a pathologic diagnosis and a common end point of several conditions. Historically, PEM has been associated with altered thiamine status, but more recently an association with high sulfur intake has been seen. Other toxic or metabolic diseases (eg, acute lead poisoning, sodium toxicosis/ water deprivation) can result in PEM as well.

Etiology, Pathogenesis, and Epidemiology: Polioencephalomalacia is seen sporadically in individual animals or as a herd outbreak. Younger animals are more frequently affected than adults. Pastured animals can develop PEM, but animals on high-concentrate diets are at higher risk, as are cattle exposed to high levels of sulfur, whether in water, feed (rations with byproducts of corn or beets processing), or a combination. The patterns of PEM occurrence depend on the etiologic factors involved.

PEM has been associated with two types of dietary risks: altered thiamine status and high sulfur intake. Thiamine inadequacy in animals with PEM has been suggested by several types of observations, including decreased concentrations of thiamine in tissues or blood and deficiency-induced alterations of thiamine-dependent biochemical processes (decreased blood transketolase activity, increased thiamine pyrophosphate effect on transketolase, and increased serum lactate). Unfortunately, many of these biochemical features of altered thiamine status are inconsistently observed in cases of PEM, and decreased thiamine status has been observed in diseases other than PEM.

Preruminant animals depend on dietary thiamine. In adult ruminants, thiamine is produced by rumen microbes. Thiamine inadequacy can be caused by decreased production by rumen microbes or factors that interfere with the action of thiamine, eg, plant thiaminases or thiamine analogues. Thiaminases can be produced by gut bacteria or ingested as preformed plant products. They can either destroy thiamine or form antimetabolites that interfere with thiamine function. Thiaminase I, produced by *Bacillus thiaminolyticus* and *Clostridium sporogenes*, and thiaminase II, produced by *B aneurinolyticus*, catalyze the cleavage of thiamine. The latter microorganism proliferates under conditions of high grain intake.

A neurologic disorder in Australia has been associated with the Nardoo fern (*Marsilea drummondii*), which may contain high levels of a thiaminase I enzyme. Other ferns, such as bracken (*Pteridium aquilinum*) and rock fern (*Cheilanthes sieberi*), contain a similar thiaminase I. Although PEM has been produced experimentally by feeding high doses of extracts of such plants, field cases are uncommon, because these plants are unpalatable (*see* p 3089).

Overall, there is not a linear relation among the presence of ruminal and fecal thiaminase, decreased concentrations of tissue and blood thiamine, and development of disease.

A beneficial response to thiamine therapy by PEM-affected animals is sometimes considered evidence of thiamine inadequacy. This thiamine-responsiveness is often seen if treatment is initiated early in the course of the disease. However, the assumption that this response indicates that deficiency of thiamine is the true etiology should be viewed with caution. Large doses of thiamine, beyond maintenance needs, may have nonspecific, beneficial effects in the energy-impaired brain.

PEM associated with high sulfur intake is recognized with increasing frequency. The basis of sulfur-related PEM appears to be the production of excessive ruminal sulfide due to the ruminal microbial reduction of ingested sulfur. Hydrogen sulfide (H_2S) gas, which has the odor of rotten eggs, accumulates in the rumen gas cap. Concentrations can be demonstrated with commercially available H_2S detection tubes via percutaneous gas sampling. Although nonreduced forms of sulfur, such as sulfate and elemental sulfur, are relatively nontoxic, H_2S and its various ionic forms are highly toxic substances that interfere with cellular energy metabolism. The CNS, by virtue of its dependence on a high and uninterrupted level of energy production, is likely to be significantly affected by energy deprivation. When cattle undergo a transition to high sulfur intake, ruminal sulfide concentrations peak 1–4 wk after the change. This pattern is probably due to alterations in ruminal microflora. The occurrence of PEM peaks during the time period when ruminal sulfide concentrations are the highest. Animals with sulfur-associated PEM do not have altered thiamine status.

A variety of sulfur sources can result in excessive sulfur intake, including water, feed ingredients, and forage. Many geographic areas have surface and deep waters high in sulfate. When evaporation occurs, water sulfate concentrations increase. Water consumption by cattle is temperature dependent and increases greatly at high temperatures, leading to increased sulfur intake due to concurrent increases in water consumption and sulfate concentrations in water. Alfalfa, by virtue of its high protein and sulfur-containing amino acid content, can serve as a significant source of sulfur. Although grasses tend to be low in sulfur, some circumstances can result in high sulfate concentrations. Certain weeds, including Canada thistle (*Cirsium arvense*), kochia (*Kochia scoparia*), and lambsquarter (*Chenopodium* spp), can accumulate sulfate in high concentration. Cruciferous plants normally synthesize sulfur-rich products and serve as important sources of excess sulfur. These include turnips, rape, mustard, and oil seed meals. Byproducts of corn, sugar cane, and sugar beet processing commonly have a high sulfur content, apparently due to the addition of sulfur-containing acidifying agents. PEM has been associated with the use of these types of byproducts as feed ingredients. Corn-based ethanol production has resulted in increased availability of corn byproducts that may vary widely in sulfur content. Wet distillers grains plus solubles have been shown to have sulfur content ranging from 0.44%–1.74% sulfur as dry matter. A high molasses-urea diet has been associated with a form of PEM that lacks altered thiamine status.

Clinical Findings: PEM may be acute or subacute. Animals with the acute form often manifest blindness followed by recumbency, tonic-clonic seizures, and coma. Those with a longer duration of acute signs have poorer responses to therapy and higher mortality. Animals with the subacute form initially separate from the group, stop eating, and display twitches of the ears and face. The head is held in an elevated position. There is cortical blindness with absent menace response but normal bilateral pupillary light reflex. Dorsomedial strabismus may develop. Animals may show ataxia and sometimes a hypermetric gait. As the disease progresses, there is cortical blindness with a diminished menace response and unaltered palpebral and pupillary responses. Dorsomedial strabismus may develop. Head pressing, opisthotonos, and grinding of the teeth may also be seen.

The subacute form of PEM is frequently followed by recovery with only minor neurologic impairment. However, in a few cases, the subacute form may progress to a more severe form with recumbency and seizures. Animals that survive the acute form or advanced subacute form often manifest significant neurologic impairment that necessitates culling.

Lesions: Gross lesions are inconsistent and frequently subtle, especially early in the disease. Acutely affected animals may have brain swelling with gyral flattening and coning of the cerebellum due to herniation into the foramen magnum. Slight yellowish discoloration of the affected cortical tissue may be present. The brains of acutely affected animals may also have autofluorescent bands of necrotic cerebral cortex evident on meningeal and cut surfaces of the brain when viewed with ultraviolet illumination. As the pathologic process progresses, the affected cerebrocortical tissue has macroscopically evident cavitation, sometimes sufficient to result in apposition of the pia meninges to the white matter.

The initial histologic lesions are necrosis of cerebrocortical neurons. The neurons are shrunken and have homogeneous, eosinophilic cytoplasm. Nuclei are pyknotic, faded, or absent. Cortical spongiosis is sometimes present in the early phases of the acute form. Vessel cells undergo hypertrophy and hyperplasia. At later stages, the affected cortical tissue undergoes cavitation as macrophages infiltrate and necrotic tissue is removed. A pattern seen in brains of cattle with early, severe, acute sulfur-related PEM features multifocal vascular necrosis, hemorrhage, and parenchymal necrosis in deep gray matter, including the striatum, thalamus, and midbrain.

Diagnosis: The pattern of clinical signs should arouse suspicion of PEM. At necropsy, macroscopically evident cerebrocortical autofluorescent areas under ultraviolet illumination provide a presumptive diagnosis of PEM. Characteristic histologic lesions are confirmatory.

Differential diagnoses for cattle include acute lead poisoning, water deprivation/sodium toxicosis, *Histophilus* meningoencephalitis, rabies, coccidiosis with nervous involvement, and vitamin A deficiency. Differential diagnoses for sheep include pregnancy toxemia, type D clostridial enterotoxemia (focal symmetric encephalomalacia), and listeriosis.

Confirmation of etiology or pathogenesis requires laboratory testing of samples from affected animals or their environment. Assessment of thiamine status is difficult, and results should be interpreted with caution. Few laboratories are capable of routinely measuring thiamine content of blood and tissues, transketolase activity, or the thiamine pyrophosphate effect on transketolase. Demonstration of clinical improvement after thiamine therapy is not adequate evidence for a specific diagnosis.

The possibility of sulfur-associated PEM can be assessed by measuring the sulfur content of the water and dietary ingredients and then estimating the total sulfur intake on a dry-matter basis. The maximal tolerated concentration of sulfur for cattle and sheep depends on the type of diet. For diets >85% concentrate, the maximal tolerable level of total sulfur is 0.3% dry matter. For diets ≥45% forage, the maximal tolerable level of total sulfur is 0.5% dry matter. Because multiple factors are involved in determining the actual risk of developing PEM, these should not be considered as absolute maximal concentrations. Many cattle adapt adequately to sulfur intake levels greater than the maximal tolerable level, although negative effects on performance may occur.

Treatment and Prevention: The treatment of choice for PEM regardless of cause is thiamine administration at a dosage of 10 mg/kg, tid-qid, for cattle or small ruminants. The first dose is administered slowly IV; otherwise, the animal may collapse. Subsequent doses are administered IM for 3–5 days. Therapy must be started early in the disease course for benefits to be achieved. If brain lesions are particularly severe or treatment is delayed, full clinical recovery may not be possible. Beneficial effects are usually seen within 24 hr and sometimes sooner; however, if there is no initial improvement, treatment should be continued for ≥3 days. Reduction of cerebral edema can be attempted with administration of dexamethasone at a dosage of 1–2 mg/kg, IM or SC. Symptomatic therapy for convulsions may be necessary.

Dietary supplementation of thiamine at 3–10 mg/kg feed has been recommended for prevention, but the efficacy of this approach has not been carefully evaluated. During a PEM outbreak, sufficient roughage should be provided. When the problem could be associated with high sulfur intake, all possible sources of sulfur, including water, should be analyzed and the total sulfur concentration of the consumed dry matter estimated. Dietary ingredients or water with high sulfur concentration should be avoided; if this is not possible, then more gradual introduction to the new conditions can improve the chances of successful adaptation.

BOVINE SPONGIFORM ENCEPHALOPATHY

Bovine spongiform encephalopathy (BSE) is a progressive, fatal, infectious, neurologic disease of cattle that resembles scrapie of sheep and goats (*see* p 1288). It was first diagnosed in the UK in 1986. Approximately 200,000 cases of BSE have been diagnosed in cattle, with 97% reported from the UK. In 1992, at the peak of the UK outbreak, 37,280 cases were reported in a single year. Lower incidences were found in cattle native to most European countries and to Israel, Japan, USA, Canada, and Brazil. The economic consequences of the BSE epidemic are important. Countries with BSE cases experienced a dramatic drop of consumer confidence in beef products and trade restrictions of cattle commodities. Since effective control measures have been implemented, BSE incidence has decreased to single cases in 2013.

Etiology: In the 1990s, there was intensive debate on the nature of the BSE pathogen. To date, the most widely accepted hypothesis is that a proteinaceous infectious particle (prion) causes the disease. Prions are misfolded conformational isoforms of host-encoded proteins that induce protein misfolding, protein aggregation, and disease upon transmission to other organisms. This hypothesis is supported by the agent's apparent resistance to heat, freezing, ultraviolet light, and chemical disinfectant procedures effective against bacteria and viruses. Prions are also responsible for scrapie of sheep and goats (*see* p 1288); chronic wasting disease of cervidae (*see* p 1286); transmissible mink encephalopathy (*see* p 1874); and kuru, Creutzfeldt-Jakob disease, fatal familial insomnia, and similar disorders of people. All these conditions are also termed prion diseases, and the related protein is the prion protein (PrP^d, in which d stands for "disease associated"). Based on the anticipated mechanisms that trigger initial PrP^d misfolding, prion diseases are classified as infectious, sporadic, or genetic. The classic type of BSE is caused by infectious prions; however, in the past decade, rare, so-called atypical BSE cases have been described. There is epidemiologic and experimental evidence that classic and atypical BSE differ in their etiology.

Transmission, Epidemiology, and Pathogenesis: Classic BSE develops as a result of foodborne exposure to prions via contaminated animal-source proteins (meat and bone meal [MBM]) in cattle rations. Horizontal transmission is not a significant source of new BSE infections. Calves born to infected cows are at greater risk of acquiring BSE than calves born to noninfected cows; however, this mode of transmission is of minor importance relative to infections acquired through contaminated feed sources. BSE is not transmitted horizontally by contact or aerosols. There is no sex or breed predisposition. In the UK, clinical disease was more common in dairy cows, probably because they were more likely to be fed animal-source protein supplements. Most cases are diagnosed in cattle 3–6 yr old. The incubation period after exposure is ~2–8 yr, and animals as young as 22 mo have been diagnosed with BSE. The details of pathogenesis are unknown, but studies indicate that after oral exposure the agent replicates in the Peyer's patches of the ileum followed by migration, via peripheral nerves, to the CNS. Atypical BSE cases have been described from countries with no apparent classic BSE epidemic. Moreover, animals affected with atypical BSE are relatively old, and the incidence rates do not follow the trends observed for classic BSE. Together, these findings led to the hypothesis that atypical BSE results from spontaneous prion protein misfolding and is not related to ingestion of prion-contaminated feed. However, the mechanisms that induce the spontaneous prion formation remain obscure. It has been postulated that atypical BSE was at the origin of the BSE epidemic in the UK.

BSE has been transmitted experimentally to many animal species by intracerebral inoculation. During the epidemic of BSE in the UK and continental Europe, a few cases were seen in several species of captive-bred wild ungulates and in domestic companion cats as well as in big cats in zoologic gardens. BSE has also been confirmed in two goats, one from France and another from Scotland, but there is no evidence that BSE infected the small ruminant population on a broader scale.

Clinical Findings: Initial clinical signs are subtle and behavioral in nature. The spectrum increases and progresses over weeks to months, with most animals reaching a terminal state by 3 mo after clinical onset. Commonly observed clinical signs include hyperesthesia, nervousness, difficulty negotiating obstacles, reluctance to be milked, aggression toward either farm personnel or other animals, low head carriage, hypermetria, ataxia, and tremors. Weight loss and decreased milk production are common. Yet, in a large portion of affected animals, clinical signs may be nonspecific, and involvement of the nervous system is not obvious in every case.

Diagnosis: Clinical examinations do not provide a definitive diagnosis. In case of a clinical suspicion of BSE, the animal should be euthanized and the brain subjected to neuropathologic examination. In most countries, BSE is a notifiable disease, and a suspect case must be reported to the veterinary authorities. The OIE has nominated OIE Reference Laboratories to assist national authorities of OIE member states in the diagnosis of BSE. Confirmatory diagnostic methods include PrP^d immunohistochemistry and Western immunoblot in brain tissue. The identification of characteristic vacuolar changes by histopathology in specific target structures of the CNS alone is no longer the method of choice for BSE confirmation. In most countries with a BSE case history, active surveillance programs have been established. Approximately a dozen commercial BSE screening tests are available for active disease surveillance: ELISA, Western immunoblot, and immunochromatographic test formats. All these tests are based on the immunologic detection of PrP^d in medulla oblongata samples.

Differential diagnoses include nervous ketosis, hypomagnesemia, polioencephalomalacia, lead poisoning, ingestion of plant or fungal tremoragens, rabies, listeriosis, and other viral and bacterial neuroinfectious diseases. In contrast to these differential diagnoses, BSE typically has a slow onset of clinical signs, with an extended and progressive clinical course. Veterinarians considering BSE as a likely differential diagnosis should contact national veterinary authorities and ensure that definitive postmortem diagnostic tests are performed.

Treatment and Control: There is no effective treatment or vaccine for BSE. Euthanasia is advisable as soon as there is some certainty of the clinical diagnosis, because animals become unmanageable, and their welfare is at risk.

The most effective control measure is prohibition of the feeding of MBM to cattle. MBM supplements for cattle have been banned in many countries as a consequence of the BSE epidemic. Because of the risk of cross-contamination in feed mills, control has been effected in the UK and other European countries by similar statutory prohibitions of the use of MBM in all farm animal diets.

With the drastic decline of classic BSE cases over the past years, there is an ongoing discussion on possible alleviations of the complete MBM ban from feed of animals other then cattle, ie, of pigs and poultry. In this regard, it is important to remember that any reemergence of BSE will remain unrecognized for years because of the extraordinarily long incubation period of the disease. Moreover, with atypical BSE persisting in the cattle population, there is a constant risk of reintroduction of BSE in the population. This highlights the need to maintain a high level of disease awareness as well as effective surveillance and control measures.

Zoonotic Risk: A novel variant of Creutzfeldt-Jakob disease (vCJD) in the human population in Great Britain, initially seen in 1996, has been associated with the emergence of the BSE agent. Cases of vCJD have also been seen outside the UK. A proportion of the affected individuals had been living in the UK, but cases have been seen in Italy and France among people who had not visited the UK. The single person diagnosed with vCJD in the USA was a recent immigrant from the UK, and it is presumed that this person was exposed and infected while residing in the UK. Infection of people is thought to result from eating infected bovine tissues. As a result, many countries have introduced the statutory removal of high-risk bovine tissues from the human food chain and/or banned human consumption of cattle >24 mo old. No cases of vCJD have been seen in laboratory workers, but appropriate safety precautions for handling the BSE agent and conducting necropsies of cattle suspected of being infected are recommended. Safety precautions should primarily be aimed at avoiding accidental exposures.

CHRONIC WASTING DISEASE

Chronic wasting disease (CWD) is a contagious disease of captive and free-ranging deer, elk, and moose that causes progressive, fatal neurodegenerative disease in adult animals. It is a member of the transmissible spongiform encephalopathy (TSE) family of diseases, or prion diseases, that includes bovine spongiform encephalopathy; scrapie of sheep and goats; transmissible mink encephalopathy; and kuru, Creutzfeldt-Jakob disease (CJD), and variant CJD of people. CWD was first identified as a clinical syndrome in the late 1960s among captive mule deer in Colorado; a decade later, it was recognized to be a spongiform encephalopathy with characteristics similar to those of scrapie (*see* p 1288). It is found in free-ranging populations of mule deer, white-tailed deer, and elk (wapiti) in 18 states (USA) and 2 Canadian provinces. Recently, the first cases of CWD in free-ranging moose were diagnosed in Colorado and in Alberta, Canada. CWD has also been found in farmed elk and white-tailed deer in a number of western states and Canadian provinces and a few midwestern states. CWD has been identified outside of North America only once; a few elk imported into Korea from Canada had CWD. Many states and provinces have developed regulations for control and management of CWD in farmed populations, and federal regulations are in place in Canada and the USA. It is a reportable disease in most jurisdictions.

Etiology: CWD is caused by prions. These unconventional pathogens consist solely of protein, namely the misfolded isoform PrP^{Sc} of the normal host-encoded cellular prion protein (PrP^{c}), which is a cell surface glycoprotein with highest expression levels in the CNS. On direct binding of PrP^{c} to PrP^{Sc}, PrP^{c} adopts the disease-associated conformation. In contrast to PrP^{c}, PrP^{Sc} is partially resistant to protease digestion and accumulates within neurons, which eventually leads to neuronal death.

CWD is known to naturally affect mule deer, white-tailed deer, elk, and moose. Transmission after oral inoculation of other *cervid species, eg,* reindeer, has been reported. Experimentally, CWD can be transmitted by intracerebral inoculation to cattle, sheep, goats, domestic ferrets, mink, mice, hamsters, and squirrel monkeys. Transmission efficiency to cattle varies depending on the cervid species from which the CWD-infected brain homogenate used for infection is derived. A large study to investigate susceptibility of cattle by the more natural route of oral or contact exposure began in 1997, and there has been evidence of CWD in the experimentally exposed cattle. Differences in species susceptibility to CWD probably relate to sequence differences among normal host PrP proteins.

Transmission, Epidemiology, and Pathogenesis: CWD is transmitted horizontally. Because prions are highly resistant to environmental and chemical inactivation, they may accumulate in the environment and thus be available to infect susceptible cervids. Consequently, close confinement of farm-raised cervids will likely potentiate the spread of CWD. Likewise, winter feeding of deer and elk will concentrate cervid populations and likely potentiate horizontal transmission. Foraging on feeding grounds contaminated by urine or feces of infected animals or contact with either infected animals or decomposing carcasses of animals with CWD results in transmission of disease to other susceptible cervids. Vertical transmission has also been reported. The agent probably enters a susceptible host via ingestion and is taken up by lymphoid tissues associated with the GI tract. The agent can be detected in lymphoid, nervous tissues, muscle tissue, antler velvet, blood, saliva, urine, and feces. Prions can be detected in the blood and saliva of infected animals as soon as 3 mo after infection. In urine and feces, detection of prions is also possible already at a preclinical stage of the disease. The agent most likely arrives in the brain by retrograde movement up the vagus nerve to the dorsal motor nucleus of the vagus at the obex region of the medulla oblongata. Spongiform lesions in the brain develop first in the vagal nucleus at about the time of onset of clinical disease. This occurs naturally with an incubation period of ~1.5–3 yr; however, incubation periods in all species known to be affected by CWD are influenced by certain PrP polymorphisms. Prevalence in captive herds of deer and elk may reach nearly 100% in heavily contaminated facilities; prevalence in free-ranging cervids is extremely variable, from <1% to 40%, in some hunting areas in Wyoming.

The movement of CWD in populations of free-ranging deer and elk follows natural migration routes, often along waterways and natural corridors. In the past, movement of CWD in farmed deer and elk in commerce was through human-facilitated transportation of animals incubating CWD. Now that programs and regulations are in place in most jurisdictions, movement of CWD in live animals should be curtailed. Surveillance, however, should continue, and submission of samples from hunter-harvested animals may be mandatory in areas with a high prevalence of CWD.

Clinical Findings: Animals with clinical CWD are >16 mo old and show a spectrum of signs. The earliest and most difficult to appreciate are subtle changes in behavior and weight loss. These changes are often detectable only by animal caretakers familiar with the individual animal. As the disease progresses, behavioral changes may include alterations in how the animal interacts with herdmates and caretakers, loss of wariness, somnolence, persistent walking, polydipsia and polyuria, and hyperexcitability when handled. Affected animals may show variable locomotor signs, including ataxia (especially posterior ataxia) and head tremors. Late in the disease, animals may have a low head carriage, drooped ears, and fixed staring gaze; they may hypersalivate and grind their teeth. Death after routine chemical immobilization has been noted. Aspiration pneumonia may be the only presenting clinical sign and is often the cause of death. CWD should be suspected in any adult cervid with aspiration pneumonia. Weight loss is progressive throughout the course of disease, even when adequate feed is present, but it is important to recognize that CWD may be present in cervids that are not emaciated. Death of CWD-affected animals may be precipitated by cold weather or other acute stressors. Affected cervids are more susceptible to hunting, predation, vehicle collisions, and other forms of death by misadventure. Carcasses and offal should be disposed of in a manner that limits the exposure of farm-raised and free-ranging cervids to any potentially infectious material.

Lesions: Lesions are seen in the gray matter of the CNS. Lesions are bilaterally symmetrical and anatomically constant among animals. Spongiform appearance is obvious; vacuolization occurs in neuronal perikarya and neuronal processes. Along with neuronal degeneration, astrocytic hyperplasia and hypertrophy may appear. H&E staining of brains of affected animals reveals amyloid plaques that appear as pale, fibrillar, eosinophilic areas of neuropil and are sometimes surrounded by vacuoles (florid plaques). Detection of PrP^{Sc} in brain sections by immunohistochemistry (IHC) provides a very good way to visualize CWD pathology while maintaining the structural context. A drawback of IHC is that it is not useful in diagnosis of subclinical CWD because spongiform encephalopathy develops about the same time clinical features do. PrP^{Sc} is detected by IHC or immunoblot in a variety of tissues in cervids showing clinical symptoms. Although PrP^{Sc} can be found in regions of the brain not exhibiting spongiform change, typically there is correlation between PrP^{Sc} deposition and spongiform appearance.

Diagnosis: Diagnosis based on clinical signs is not reliable, because they are unspecific and mild at the beginning of disease. Therefore, it depends on detecting disease-associated PrP^{Sc} in CNS or lymphoid tissues. In mule deer and white-tailed deer, the CWD PrP accumulates in the retropharyngeal lymph node before arriving in the brain; thus, it is considered to be the most important tissue to collect for testing. Both brain and lymph node samples should be collected from elk. The correct portion of the brain (ie, the obex, at the caudal end of the fourth ventricle below the cerebellum) must be collected for a meaningful test. The laboratory should be consulted to determine whether the samples must be fixed in 10% buffered formalin, chilled or frozen, or if portions of the samples should be sent both fixed and frozen. Samples should be, and in many jurisdictions are required to be, submitted to certified laboratories to be tested for evidence of CWD. It is good practice either to send the carcass to the diagnostic laboratory or to collect a wide variety of samples, so that if diseases other than CWD are present they will be identified. At a minimum, samples for CWD testing should include brain and retropharyngeal lymph nodes. Many laboratories accept whole heads from cervids for testing. Surveillance programs for free-ranging cervids vary depending on the jurisdiction and are usually conducted by the local wildlife management agency, which should be consulted if CWD is suspected in a free-ranging deer or elk. Surveillance depends mainly on submission of heads from hunter-harvested animals. In some areas, active surveillance is done by taking biopsies from tonsils, retropharyngeal lymph nodes, and recto-anal mucosa-associated lymphoid tissue (RAMALT). Diagnostic tests include detection of PrP^{Sc} by IHC, ELISA, or Western blot in brain and/or lymphoid tissues. In the USA, these tests are run only at USDA-certified laboratories. ELISA is used as a screening test, and IHC, which is considered the preferred test, is used to confirm positive ELISA.

Nevertheless, more sensitive in vivo diagnostic tests are desirable. Using in vitro conversion such as protein misfolding cyclic amplification (PMCA) or real-time quaking-induced conversion assay (RT-QUiC), CWD prions are detectable already at a preclinical stage in specimen that can be obtained antemortem by noninvasive methods, such as blood, urine, feces, or saliva. However, these newly developed assays are not yet certified.

Differential diagnoses for animals suspected of CWD include brain abscesses, traumatic injuries, meningitis, encephalitis, peritonitis, pneumonia, arthritis, starvation and nutritional deficiencies, dental attrition, and anesthetic deaths.

Treatment and Control: There are no treatments available for any TSE. Control in farmed cervids is by depopulation with indemnity and development of a National CWD Herd Certification Program in the USA. This is designed to be a voluntary federal-state-industry cooperative program administered by the USDA Animal and Plant Health Inspection Service. This plan typically requires 5 yr of monitoring to achieve the highest status. The bases for CWD control programs in the farmed cervid industry are individual animal identification, CWD testing in all animals in the herd that die over a certain age, and limiting new herd additions to animals from herds of comparable or higher CWD status.

Control of CWD in free-ranging populations is extremely difficult and varies depending on the location. All jurisdictions have banned movement of live cervids from endemic areas for translocations, and many have regulations on movement of parts of hunted deer and elk. In areas where CWD occurs, attempts at control have included population reduction, test and removal, and intensified surveillance.

Only a few disinfectants and methods of disposal inactivate prions. Fresh household bleach at 50% concentration for 30–60 min or sodium hydroxide (1 M) for 60 min will inactivate the agent and is inexpensive and readily available but may be corrosive to some surfaces and instruments. Additional disinfectants are being considered for general use but are not yet approved. Incineration in a medical incinerator, alkaline digestion in specially designed equipment, and disposal in certified municipal landfills are used for disposal of tissues and carcasses of animals with CWD.

Zoonotic Risk: Although CWD has been present in hunted populations of deer and elk for >30 yr, no case of human CWD has been identified. The risk to people appears to be minimal. The CWD agent has been detected in the muscle tissue of infected cervids. Public health authorities and wildlife management agencies suggest the following precautions for hunters and people handling cervids in areas where CWD is found to further reduce risk of human exposure: do not harvest deer or elk that appear to be sick or abnormal; wear rubber, plastic, or latex gloves when dressing the carcass; avoid contact with brain, spinal cord, and lymphoid tissues; debone the meat when processing; disinfect knives, saws, and tables with 50% bleach; and have the animal tested for CWD. All public health authorities recommend that animals positive for any TSE not be consumed by people or other animals.

SCRAPIE

Classic scrapie, a natural disease of sheep and goats, is seen worldwide except in Australia and New Zealand. It is one of the transmissible spongiform encephalopathies (TSE), related to bovine spongiform encephalopathy and chronic wasting disease of deer and elk, all of which are thought to result from the accumulation of an abnormal form of a cellular protein in the brain. Natural transmission of scrapie to other species has not been shown. In the USA, scrapie primarily affects black-faced sheep breeds (eg, Suffolk, Hampshire, and their crosses), accounting for ~96% of cases. In other countries, the disease is commonly seen in other breeds, including those with white faces.

Etiology, Transmission, and Pathogenesis: An abnormal protein designated as PrP^{Sc}, found in all TSE, appears to convert a normal cellular protein called prion protein (PrP^{C}) to its abnormal form (PrP^{Sc}) in susceptible animals. In sheep, the susceptibility is controlled genetically; however, genetic susceptibility has not been established in goats. As it accumulates within a cell, PrP^{Sc} is deposited as an amyloid plaque in lymphoreticular and nervous tissue, where its accumulation is hypothesized to cause the nervous signs associated with the disease. Although some researchers still do not believe that PrP^{Sc} itself is the disease agent, its presence is a reliable diagnostic test for prion disease.

When PrP^{C} is induced to change to PrP^{Sc}, the conformation of the protein's structure is reconfigured. Although the chemical composition of the molecule is the same, its chemical properties change. The normal protein is soluble in denaturing detergents and is digested by cellular proteases such as proteinase K. However, PrP^{Sc} (as well as the infectivity) is not destroyed by detergents and is resistant to breakdown by rendering processes presently used, heat sterilization temperatures, ultraviolet light, ionizing radiation, and most disinfecting agents. It is only partially inactivated by protease K.

The genetics of scrapie in sheep is located on chromosome 13, and three codons (136, 154, and 171) seem to control most of the susceptibility to scrapie. Codon 136 codes for either valine (V), alanine (A), or threonine (T); 154 codes for arginine (R) or histidine (H); and codon 171 codes for glutamine (Q), lysine (K), H, or R. Resistance to scrapie is correlated with 136A, 154H, and 171R. These small changes in the amino acid components of PrP^{C} apparently enable it to resist reconfiguration. Scrapie is usually related to polymorphisms at codon 171. Among sheep in the USA, 91% of brain samples testing positive for scrapie originated from sheep with the 136/154/171 AARRQQ genotype. However, sheep with codon 136V are at the highest risk of developing scrapie, even when they also carry one R at codon 171. Recently, it was shown that these cases are actually affected by another strain of the agent that at one time was referred to as the V-dependent strain. It was first described in Cheviots by Irish researchers and has been reported in Europe and the USA. The 171RR genotype is considered to be resistant to classic scrapie. Scrapie is also rare in sheep with the 136/171 AAQR genotype. However, at least 83 atypical cases of scrapie from more than 110,000 tested samples have been recorded by The Veterinary Laboratories Agency of Great Britain. These discordant cases, most classified as Nor 98 (first found in Norway in 1998) usually involve only a single sheep in a flock with no obvious contacts between affected flocks. Nor 98 has been seen in sheep with genotypes considered to be resistant, and many of them have one or two of the amino acid leucine (L) at codon 131. This has led to the belief that such cases represent a spontaneous prion disease, analogous to sporadic Creutzfeldt-Jakob disease in people, and that the prion is not transmitted by direct contact. It has been reported in almost every European country, the Falklands, Canada, and New Zealand, even though classic scrapie has not been reported from New Zealand. Eight such cases have been reported in the USA since 2003; the World Health Organization has classified this as a separate disease and declared that it should not affect trade.

The classic disease is naturally transmitted during lambing from infected dams via ingestion of infected placenta or allantoic fluids by flock mates and newborn lambs. Infected males are not believed to transmit the disease, although there is one report of PrP^{Sc} detected in semen of several 131/171 VVQQ and AVQQ V-dependent scrapie affected–rams. This occurred after apparent transmission of scrapie to some of their offspring from 131/171 VVQQ scrapie eyelid and rectal mucosa–negative ewes. However, because of the rarity of 136/171 VVQQ genotype in the USA at this time, it is unlikely that this should be of concern.

The embryo or fetus is not exposed to scrapie while in utero in a scrapie-infected dam, because there is physical separation from PrP^{Sc}-containing allantoic fluid and chorioallantois by the amnion, which remains free of PrP^{Sc} even when the other placental tissues are infected. Lambs delivered via cesarean section from infected dams, kept separate from the allantoic fluid, and isolated from infected sheep remain disease free. Despite the wide distribution of normal prion protein in reproductive, placental, and fetal fluids, PrP^{Sc} has been detected only in the caruncular portion of the endometrium and cotyledonary chorioallantois (the fetal-maternal interface) of pregnant scrapie-infected ewes—but only if both the dam and fetus are of a susceptible genotype. Although tissues of the maternal side of the placenta carry a susceptible prion protein, it requires susceptible prion-containing cells from the fetal side of the placenta for conversion to PrP^{Sc}. However, there can be partial or incomplete anastomosis between fetal blood supply to the cotyledons among fetuses of different genotypes on the same side of the uterine horn, which in rare cases can result in PrP^{Sc} accumulation in cotyledons with resistant genotypes.

Previous contamination of premises is believed to be another source of scrapie infection. Anecdotal accounts abound of flock depopulation and premises decontamination that are followed by recurrence of disease in repopulated infection-free but susceptible sheep.

Clinical Findings: Classic scrapie, which results from ingestion of PrP^{Sc} by a genotypically susceptible sheep, is a longterm, progressive, and debilitating neurologic illness believed to always be fatal. Clinical signs may be noticed 18 mo to 5 yr after exposure and include progressive weight loss with no concurrent loss in appetite, progressive ataxia, fine head tremors (most apparent in the ears), and cutaneous hypersensitivity. Pruritus develops in ~70% of cases. Sheep may assume a vacant, fixed stare or, less often, become suddenly aggressive. Signs of hypersensitivity are often elicited by rubbing or scratching the sheep's back, which induces the sheep to throw its head back, make chewing motions and lick at the air, or compulsively nibble at the limbs below the carpus.

Ataxia is first detected when sheep are running. The hindlimbs appear to be uncoordinated with the forelimbs, and affected animals adopt a bunny-hopping gait. Sheep often have a high-stepping gait in the forelimbs, resembling a prancing horse. As signs worsen, the hindquarters sway while standing.

Clinical signs last from 1 to >3 mo; sheep generally become recumbent because of weakness and incoordination. If helped up, an affected sheep may be able to remain standing for hours but cannot rise unassisted if it falls or lies down. Death follows 1–2 wk after a sheep can no longer right itself. Blindness, resembling that seen with polioencephalomalacia, occasionally develops. The clinical signs of scrapie can vary, depending on the sheep's genotype and the strain of scrapie. The V-dependent strain has a substantially more rapid clinical course of 3–30 days and death in 2–3 days after recumbency. In these cases, weight loss and signs of pruritus are often not seen. This strain, found in the University of Idaho research flock, made up of local flocks found to have scrapie, mainly infects 131/171 VVQQ and 131/171 AVQR sheep. It is probably present whenever scrapie and the 136AV and VV genetics are found together. Most veterinarians or producers would not recognize sheep with the V-dependent gene as having scrapie.

Diagnosis: A complete necropsy should be performed on any sheep dying mysteriously, including submission of the brain for immunohistochemical (IHC) testing for scrapie. Differential diagnoses include caseous lymphadenitis, abomasal emptying disease, Johne disease, ovine progressive pneumonia (visna), dentition problems, and meningitis.

Currently, all diagnostic tests for TSE require infected tissue and the use of antibody reactions. Because animals generally do not produce antibodies against self, antibodies are mostly monoclonal in origin or are made in rodents bred to have no prion protein. IHC and ELISA are used for routine testing. In the EU, ELISA tests are used for slaughter surveillance, but they are not licensed for scrapie testing in the USA. However, several test kits are used for diagnosis of chronic wasting in wild elk and deer. The IHC test is used as a confirmatory test and is considered to be the gold standard worldwide.

Detection of PrP^{Sc} in reticuloendothelial organs (spleen, lymph nodes) before appearance of clinical signs or PrP^{Sc} in the brain is possible. Detection of PrP^{Sc} has been reported in 76% of tonsils examined and 57% of lymphoid tissue specimens collected from the third eyelid of infected sheep. A small percentage of sheep in which the brain contains PrP^{Sc} do not have detectable PrP^{Sc} in the lymph nodes, which may be influenced by genotype or scrapie strain. The atypical strains are not often found in lymphoid tissues.

The palatine tonsil has been used for biopsy and diagnosis; biopsy of the lymph follicles of the third eyelid is simpler and is validated in the USA as a diagnostic test. It yields a high percentage of unreadable samples due to lack of follicles in the sample in as many as 40%–60% of adult sheep. Biopsy of the lymphoid ring in the rectal mucosa has also been validated and yields positive diagnoses in ~55%–65% of positive sheep. Use of the mandibular lymph nodes has not been validated; however, biopsy of that site may be useful diagnostically, because examination of several tissues improves the chances of a positive diagnosis. It has not been established in the course of the disease when the agent will consistently appear in these tissues, but it may be as early as 14 mo after exposure. The interval likely depends on the age of the sheep at exposure and genotype or strain of scrapie.

The pathologic changes associated with scrapie are confined to the CNS and include vacuolation, neuronal loss, astrocytosis, and accumulation of amyloid plaques. However, because histologic changes are often lacking, diagnosis is made on the basis of IHC staining of the obex, other parts of the brain, and/or lymphoid tissue for PrP^{Sc}.

Control: For disinfection, instruments should be soaked in 2.5N NaOH or a disinfectant shown to be effective against abnormal prions. Incineration or digestion by sodium hydroxide are considered appropriate to adequately inactivate infected carcasses.

Individual and premises identification are required for all breeding sheep leaving their original premises as part of the USA mandatory Scrapie Eradication Program. A scrapie slaughter surveillance program initiated by the USDA/APHIS has been underway since 2003 in which brains and lymphoid tissue of aged black-face and black-face crosses and sheep sold for slaughter with signs of scrapie (ataxia, poor body condition scores, alopecia from rubbing) are tested for scrapie by IHC. Sheep found to be positive are traced back to the herd of origin, which is quarantined, and all animals are tested. All positive sheep and those with the 171QQ genotype are euthanized. Animals sold from the flock are also traced and tested. Since the program was initiated, the prevalence of scrapie has decreased 90%, from ~0.5% to ~0.015% as of the end of 2013. The goal is to have the USA declared free of scrapie by 2017.

Voluntary efforts to control and eliminate the disease have been undertaken by producers in the USA by selecting sheep with at least one 171R codon and culling sheep with susceptible genotypes; the expectation is that the remaining sheep will be resistant to scrapie infection. However, some concern has been expressed that reliance on genetics for elimination of the disease may inadvertently select for the atypical strain of scrapie that infects the 171RR genotype. So far there are no data to support that concern.

Rules prohibiting ruminant-to-ruminant protein feeding have been in place in many countries for >10 yr.

EQUINE ARBOVIRAL ENCEPHALOMYELITIS

(Equine viral encephalitis)

Equine encephalitides can be clinically similar, usually cause diffuse encephalomyelitis (*see* p 1262) and meningoencephalomyelitis, and are characterized by signs of CNS dysfunction and moderate to high mortality. Arboviruses are the most common cause of equine encephalitis, but rabies virus, *Sarcocystis neurona* (see p 1309), *Neospora hughesii* (*see* p 663), equine herpesviruses, and several bacteria and nematodes may also cause encephalitis. Arboviruses are transmitted by mosquitoes or other hematophagous insects, infect a variety of vertebrate hosts (including people), and may cause serious disease. Most pathogenic arboviruses use a mosquito to bird or rodent cycle. Tickborne encephalitides are also a differential cause in the eastern hemisphere. Arboviral diseases are ever emerging, and there are arboviruses pathogenic to horses on virtually every continent.

Etiology and Epidemiology of Arboviral Encephalitides:

Alphaviruses: North America is home to some of the most pathogenic encephalitic viruses because of the enduring endemic status of alphaviruses of the family Togaviridae. Endemic species in North, Central, or South America include Eastern equine encephalitis virus (EEEV), Western equine encephalitis virus (WEEV), Highlands J virus, Venezuelan equine encephalitis virus (VEEV), Everglades virus, and Una virus (see TABLE 3). Other alphaviruses associated with equine encephalitis are Semliki Forest virus in Africa and Ross River virus in Australia and the South

TABLE 3 ARBOVIRUSES THAT CAN CAUSE OR ARE LINKED TO EQUINE ENCEPHALOMYELITIS

Virus Species or Variant	Geographic Location	Most Important Reservoir
ALPHAVIRUSES		
North American Eastern equine encephalitis virus	Eastern North America, primarily east of Mississippi river	Birds
Madariaga virus	South America, Caribbean	Rodents
Western equine encephalitis virus	Western South America	Birds, rabbits, and snakes
Highlands J virus		Birds
Venezuelan equine encephalitis virus	Central and South America, Caribbean	Cotton rat and other rodents
Everglades virus	South Florida (USA)	Rodents
Ross River virus	Australia, Papua New Guinea	Marsupial and placental mammals
Semliki Forest virus	East and West Africa	Unknown
Una virus	South America	Birds
FLAVIVIRUSES		
Japanese encephalitis	Asia, India, Russia, Western Pacific	Birds, swine
Murray Valley	Australia, Papua New Guinea	Birds, marsupials, and foxes
Kunjin virus	Australia	Birds (herons and ibis)
St. Louis encephalitis	North, Central, and South America	Birds
Usutu	Europe, Africa	Birds
West Nile	Africa, Middle East, Europe, North, Central, and South America, Australia	Passerine birds
Louping ill	Iberian Peninsula, UK	Sheep, grouse
Powassan	North America, Russia	Lagomorphs, rodents, mice, skunks
Tickborne encephalitis	Asia, Europe, Finland, Russia	Small rodents

Pacific. EEEV has two distinct antigenic variants that are separated longitudinally. The North American variant is the most pathogenic and is found in eastern Canada; all states within the USA east of the Mississippi River and in Arkansas, Minnesota, South Dakota, and Texas; and in the Caribbean Islands. The South American variant is less pathogenic and confined to central and South America and is now called Madariaga virus (MADV).

EEE and WEE viruses are separated in North America primarily latitudinally; however, WEEV is relatively heterogeneous, with several subtypes consisting of WEE, Highlands J virus, Sindbis, Aura, Ft. Morgan, and Y 62–33. Several variants have been found in horses (see TABLE 3). WEE is found in western Canada, states in the USA west of the Mississippi, and in Mexico and South America. WEE previously isolated in the south and eastern USA has been shown to belong to the Highlands J virus serogroup. VEE has six antigenically related subtypes: subtype I, Everglades, Mucambo, Pixuna, Cabassou, and AG80–663. Subtype I serovars AB and C primarily cause epizootics; subtype I and serovar IE caused a large outbreak in Mexico in 1993. Epizootic strains are not generally found in the USA, although there was an epizootic of VEE in 1971. Sylvatic subtype II (Everglades) has been isolated from people and mosquitoes in Florida; subtype III has been isolated in the Rocky Mountains and northern plains states.

The general life cycle of alphaviruses involves transmission between birds and/or rodents and mosquitoes. In North America, theoretically, EEEV is perpetuated in a sylvatic cycle between avian hosts (passerine birds) and mosquitoes, with primary transmission in this cycle via *Culiseta melanura*. Birds do not develop disease but develop sufficient viremia for transmission to mosquitoes unless the bird belongs to an introduced species that in North America includes European starlings, house sparrows, pheasants, and emus. Field work in Alabama indicates that the northern cardinal is the primary target for *C melanura* feeding; however, other mosquitoes (*C erraticus*) are capable of feeding on a wider variety of birds, including robins, chickadees, owls, and mockingbirds. Mammalian reservoirs may also be important during years of high EEEV transmission. Experimental infection of cotton rats, a marshland rat found throughout the Americas, resulted in viremia just being capable of transmitting EEEV, with juvenile rats developing higher titers and 100% mortality to infection.

Horses and people are clinically affected but do not develop viremia sufficiently high enough to transmit virus to mosquitoes and so are considered "dead-end" hosts. However, young animals are more susceptible to EEEV, and it is not known how important non-neural tissues are for harboring high viral infection. Presumed extraneural sites of infection include cardiac tissue and bone marrow. During epizootics, alpacas, llamas, cattle, swine, cats, and dogs can develop disease. Snakes have been identified as a possible reservoir.

Freshwater hardwood swamps are the most associated enzootic niche for EEEV. In the southern USA, which has the highest number of reported annual cases, reemergence within mammalian hosts is associated with "tree farms" that often function as inland freshwater swamps. Nonetheless, EEEV disease occurs frequently in naive horses in southeastern habitats not associated with sylvatic field ecology, so a full understanding of the epizootic cycle still remains to be elucidated. Intense focal activity has been reported in Michigan, Wisconsin, Ohio, Massachusetts, and New Hampshire. In 2005, Massachusetts experienced a human case affected rate more than five times that of the preceding 10 yr; affected people resided within ½ mile of a cranberry bog or swamp associated with forest habitat.

In Central and South America, the principal vectors of MADV belong to *Culex* (*Melanoconion*) spp. These vectors feed on birds, rodents, marsupials, and reptiles, with rodent reservoirs possibly featuring more importantly in this life cycle. Before the year 2000, comparatively few epizootics of disease caused by MADV in horses were recorded in South America, with minimal disease reported in people. Furthermore, there are notable differences in virulence between EEEV strains in South America vs in North America. In 2008 and 2009, larger outbreaks occurred in Central and South America. In northeastern Brazil, 229 horses were affected, with a case fatality rate of 73% and disease severity similar to that of EEEV in North America.

WEE is transmitted primarily by *C tarsalis*, which is found just west of the Mississippi river and throughout the West. This mosquito breeds in sunlit marshes and in pools of irrigation water in pastures. WEE can also be transmitted by the tick *Dermacentor andersoni*. Epizootics of WEE are associated with increased rainfall in early spring followed by warmer than normal temperatures.

Sylvatic VEE viruses are found throughout North, Central, and South America in jungle or swampy areas, Two cycles occur with VEEV, the enzootic cycle and the epizootic cycle. The mosquitoes that serve as the primary vectors for the bird- or rodent-mosquito life cycle are members of the subgenus *Melanoconion* (*C cedecci*). Epizootics are associated with a mutation to a subtype I (AB, C, and possibly E), a change in mammalian pathogenesis, and a change to several bridge vectors. The enzootic cycle centers around sylvatic rodents such as spiny and cotton rats, which have high natural infection rates and can develop viremia high enough to transmit VEEV to mosquitoes. Opossums, bats, and shore birds likely contribute to dispersal of the enzootic virus so that constant cycling occurs. When epizootics occur with mutation of the virus and this change in mosquito vectors, equine infection becomes a predominant feature in the maintenance of epizootic VEE. All mammalian hosts are capable of developing a high-titer viremia of ~106 plaque-forming units/mL for up to 5 days, but the horse is likely to be the most important mammalian host in terms of vector capacity.

Flaviviruses: In general, viruses belonging to the Flaviviridae and Bunyaviridae families are less pathogenic than the Togaviridae; however, viral encephalomyelitis caused by any of these pathogens is a potentially catastrophic illness for any vertebrate host. There are 53 species of flavivirus, and many are clinical pathogens for horses, including Japanese encephalitis, West Nile virus (WNV) encephalitis, Kunjin virus (KUN), and Murray Valley encephalitis virus. Overall, the diseases caused by the Japanese encephalitis serogroup are similar (*see* TABLE 3). All of these viruses are transmitted by a mosquito vector, with *Culex* spp usually the most efficient transmitter. KUN is actually a strain of WNV and is found in Australia, some southeast Asia countries, and New Guinea. Disease in horses caused by Murray Valley fever is geographically restricted to the South Pacific and is sporadic in occurrence.

WNV has the widest geographic distribution of all of the flaviviruses. Prior to 1999, WNV was recognized in Africa, the Middle East, Asia, and occasionally in European countries. In 1999, WNV infection was first recognized in North America. Since then, the virus has spread throughout the USA and parts of Canada and Mexico. WNV isolated from the outbreak in New York in 1999 appears to be closely related to an isolate recovered from geese in Israel in 1998.

Since 2010, continued worldwide spread and reemergence of many flaviviruses, especially WNV, has occurred. As of 2014, WNV is recognized as having seven lineages, with lineage 1 (sublineage 1a, 1b, and 1c) and lineage 2 affecting people and horses. Lineage 1a activity in the USA and Europe dominated much of the end of the 1990s until the mid-2000s, causing neuroinvasive infections in people and horses in Africa, Europe, Australia, Asia, North and Central America, and the Middle East. In 2012, a very large epizootic occurred in the USA, with 5,674 human and 690 equine cases reported. New emergences have occurred *in Greece and Serbia, and the first lineage 1a* case in India was detected in 2012. Lineage 1b viruses are primarily represented by KUN, with Australia undergoing the largest epizootic of arboviral disease in 2011, involving 900 horses. Although multiple pathogens were detected, including KUN, Murray Valley encephalitis virus, and Ross River virus, there was emergence of a new strain of KUN. The 1c viruses are fairly nonpathogenic and found in India. (This sublineage may soon be designated as lineage 5.) Lineage 2 strains, long considered African based and inducing mild disease in horses, is also expanding globally with increased neuroinvasive activity. Neuroinvasive disease due to lineage 2 has emerged across Europe in Hungary, Austria, Italy, and Greece, which had at least four epizootic cycles with cases of neuroinvasive disease identified in horses.

Both wetland and terrestrial birds may be involved in the natural cycle of WNV, with migratory birds thought to introduce the virus into a geographic region. However, a wide range of infected birds (~326) have high, sustained viremia and little or no clinical disease (passerines). Fatal infections among corvids (eg, crows, blue jays, and magpies) have been the hallmark of WNV infection in the USA. Ticks have been demonstrated to be infected with WNV, but their role in natural transmission is unknown. Experimentally, transmission has been documented between cohabitating birds and from oral exposure to WNV in drinking water in birds. Oral transmission has been demonstrated experimentally in several types of raptors.

In people, other important routes of infection include blood transfusions, organ donation, breast milk, and across the placenta. Sporadic infections and illness have also occurred in several other mammalian species, including dogs, cats, camelids, sheep, and squirrels. Oral transmission has been demonstrated experimentally in cats. Farmed alligators have demonstrated disease and mortality due to WNV, and there has also been a report of WNV-induced disease in crocodiles. Alligators are susceptible to oral infection. In addition to birds, only alligators have consistently demonstrated high enough viremia (10^4–10^5 plaque-forming units) to amplify virus, serve as reservoir hosts, and transmit virus back to mosquitoes.

Most equine-associated flaviviruses are maintained in an enzootic transmission cycle between wild birds and mosquitoes, although tickborne encephalitis found in Eurasia can cause disease in horses. Many species of mosquitoes can transmit the equine virulent viruses, although *Culex* spp are principal vectors to maintain enzootic activity. *C pipiens* complex and *C tarsalis* are thought to play the largest role in natural transmission in North America. In the eastern and Midwestern regions of the USA, *C pipiens* is one of the major vectors, whereas in the western regions of the USA, *C tarsalis* is thought to be one of the most efficient vectors.

Bunyaviruses: Cache Valley virus (transmitted by mosquitoes and *Culicoides* sp among rabbits), Main Drain virus (transmitted by *Culicoides varipennis* among hares and rodents in the western USA), and snowshoe hare virus (transmitted by *Culiseta* and *Aedes* mosquitoes among rabbits in southern Canada and northern USA) have all been identified, although infrequently, as the cause of encephalitis in horses.

Clinical Findings of Viral Encephalomyelitis in Equids: The initial clinical signs are similar for the arboviruses; progression of clinical signs and severity of disease are the differentiating features. Initially, horses are quiet and depressed, with clinical neurologic signs generally occurring 9–11 days after infection. Compared with WEE and WNV disease, clinical signs of EEEV (and VEEV) encephalomyelitis more frequently include altered mentation, impaired vision, aimless wandering, head pressing, circling, inability to swallow, irregular ataxic gait, paresis and paralysis, seizures, and death. Spinal signs are often symmetric with ataxia in all limbs, rapidly progressing to quadriparesis, along with intensification of forebrain signs. Many horses progress to recumbence within 12–18 hr of onset of neurologic abnormalities. Most deaths occur within 2–3 days after the onset of signs.

The clinical signs and course of disease are highly variable in WNV disease and other flavivirus encephalomyelitis. Presenting complaints most often include neurologic abnormalities; other common initial complaints include colic, lameness, anorexia, and fever. Initial systemic signs include a mild fever, feed refusal, and depression. Neurologic signs are highly variable, but spinal cord disease and moderate mental aberrations are most consistent. Spinal cord disease manifests as asymmetric, multifocal or diffuse ataxia and paresis. Severe manifestations of WNV may occur independently in the fore- or hindlimbs, unilaterally, or in a single limb. In all clinical studies published to date, for WNV, >90% of affected horses developed some type of spinal cord signs, whereas 40%–60% developed behavioral changes characterized by periods of hyperesthesia, ranging from mild apprehension to overt hyperexcitability, with fractious reactions to aural, visual, and tactile stimuli. Fine and coarse tremors of the face and neck muscles are common, described in 60%–90% of horses. Some horses have periods of cataplexy or narcolepsy that may render them temporarily or permanently recumbent.

Cranial nerve deficits can be seen in all arbovirus infections of horses; these include most cranial nerves with cell bodies located in the mid- and hindbrains. Weakness and/or paralysis of the face and tongue are most frequent. Horses with facial and tongue paresis can be dysphagic, and overt signs of quidding or even esophageal choke can develop. Many horses with severe mental depression and facial paresis will keep their heads low, resulting in severe facial edema. Occasionally, head tilt may be seen. Infrequently in WNV disease, urinary dysfunction ranging from mild straining to stranguria has been reported, making differentiation from equine herpesvirus 1 (EHV-1) more challenging.

During the neurologic phase, horses frequently thrash and injure themselves. Sepsis from trauma in recumbent horses also occurs. Prolonged recumbency leads to pulmonary infections, especially in foals, in which a long duration of slinging and treatment may be pursued more frequently than in large, recumbent animals. Dysphagia leads to decreased water and food intake, with renal damage due to concurrent use of anti-inflammatory drugs. Skin and muscle necrosis are common in recumbent horses. Life-threatening trauma can also occur, including a ruptured diaphragm and fractures.

Lesions: All necropsies on horses suspected of viral encephalitis should be performed with all participants wearing personal protective gear (ie, waterproof gown, boots, gloves, N-95 or N-99 mask, face shield, and hair covering). Gross lesions are most common with EEEV and severe VEEV disease and are characterized by widespread and prominent congestion of the meninges. In other infections, gross lesions are rarer and are limited to small multifocal areas of discoloration and hemorrhage throughout the brain and spinal cord. The brain should be examined microscopically for the presence of meningoencephalitis. In EEEV infection, a severe gliosis with necrosis of the neuropil is seen in the cerebrum and extending through the corona radiata through the hindbrain and cervical spinal cord.

Although mononuclear cells are present, neutrophils are widespread and diffusely distributed. The gliosis is less nodular than in WNV, and when there are accumulations of cells, there is extensive necrosis and often frank microscopic hemorrhage within and around lesions. In milder cases and in WNV infections, microscopically there is a non-necrotizing lymphohistiocytic poliomeningoencephalitis. Slight to severe inflammation, characterized by perivascular cuffing of lymphocytes and monocytes, is usually present. In more severe cases, there can be extravasation of fluid and red blood cells from vessels. Often the distribution of lesions is multifocal, with more severe lesions present in grey matter. In the neuropil, dying neurons often are surrounded by microglial cells. The most severe gliosis and perivascular cuffing is often in the midbrain (thalamus, hypothalamus) and hindbrain (pons and medulla), extending into the cerebellum. Lesions can be multifocal in the spinal cord and can be more severe in the lumbar cord.

Diagnosis: No consistent changes in clinical pathology have been found in equine viral encephalitis. With EEEV and WNV in horses, peripheral lymphopenia is common. Horses are frequently azotemic, likely from decreased food and water intake.

In general, no pathognomonic signs distinguish flavivirus infection in horses from other CNS diseases, and a full diagnostic evaluation should be performed. Confirmation of flavivirus infection with encephalitis in horses begins with assessment of 1) whether the horse meets the case definition based on clinical signs; (2) whether the horse resides in an area in which flavivirus has been confirmed in the current calendar year in mosquitoes, birds, people, or horses; and (3) lack of appropriate vaccination.

In terms of antemortem diagnostic testing, analysis of CSF can be a valuable adjunct to presumptive clinical assessment. CSF analyzed from horses with acute EEEV infection typically shows a neutrophilic pleocytosis with markedly increased total solids. Horses infected with EEEV that are partially immune may have predominantly mononuclear cells, but nondegenerate neutrophils are still present. Although WNV-infected horses can have normal CSF, *if the CSF is abnormal*, there is a mononuclear pleocytosis with moderately to markedly increased total solids. In a few horses with acute infections, virus may be isolated from the CSF. By the time neurologic signs are seen, viremia has ended and detection of virus in the plasma of clinically affected horses is of no value.

Serology is the key to antemortem diagnosis of recent alphavirus and flavivirus infection in horses showing clinical signs. IgM antibody rises sharply and is increased in 85%–90% of horses with clinical arboviral encephalitis. Thus, the IgM capture ELISA is the test of choice to detect recent exposure to these viruses. Neutralizing antibody titers (primarily IgG) develop slowly during this time and stay increased for several months. Although neutralizing antibody tests will differentiate between subtypes of these viruses, and are thus considered the gold standard for confirmatory serology, paired serum samples are essential to detect recent exposure and to differentiate antibody response due to field infection from vaccine responses for any of these viruses. Because virus-neutralizing antibodies appear at the end of viremia and may precede appearance of neurologic signs, paired samples may not show a 4-fold increase in horses while demonstrating neurologic signs. In horses that succumb without premortem and postmortem testing, paired samples from febrile herdmates may be necessary to confirm presence of arbovirus activity within a locale. Maternal antibodies may interfere with neutralizing responses in young foals. This response is confounded by recent vaccination. The most common neutralizing antibody test formats are the classic plaque reduction neutralization test (PRNT) and a microwell format test. Practical application of the microwell vs the PRNT indicates that the endpoint titer in the microwell test can be several logs higher than in the PRNT, so results cannot be compared between samples.

Several postmortem diagnostic assays are available and, although specific, they vary in sensitivity, depending on the virus. The midbrain and brain stem have the highest concentrations of encephalitic viruses, including rabies virus. Immunohistochemistry and PCR testing for EEEV and EHV-1 are relatively straightforward compared with that for WNV. Diagnostic testing continues to confirm the unreliability of detection of virus, even by PCR, because of the low viral load in WNV infection. Often, only a single neuron in one or two sections may yield positive virus staining in the horse by immunohistochemistry. When tested by PCR, the limited viral load dictates accurate testing of appropriate tissues consisting of several locations, including thalamus, hypothalamus, rostral colliculus, pons, medulla, and anatomically identified spinal cord. Viral isolation is still important for molecular epidemiology.

Infectious and noninfectious causes of brain and spinal cord diseases should be considered as differential diagnoses. Infectious causes include alphaviruses, rabies, equine protozoal myeloencephalitis (*see* p 1309), and EHV-1; less likely causes are botulism and verminous meningoencephalomyelitis (eg, *Halicephalobus gingivalis*, *Setaria* spp, *Strongylus vulgaris*). Noninfectious causes include hypocalcemia, tremorigenic toxicities, hepatoencephalopathy, and leukoencephalomalacia.

Treatment: Treatment of viral encephalitis is supportive, because there are no specific antiviral therapies. Management is focused on controlling pain and inflammation, preventing injuries associated with ataxia or recumbency, and providing supportive care. Intervention does not appear to significantly affect the outcome of most fulminate EEEV infections. For WNV, flunixin meglumine (1.1 mg/kg, IV, bid) early in the course of the disease decreases the severity of muscle tremors and fasciculations within a few hours of administration.

Recumbent horses that are mentally alert frequently thrash, causing self-inflicted wounds and posing a risk to personnel. Responses to tranquilizers and anticonvulsant medications are variable, depending on the virus and severity of disease. A sling and hoist may be used to assist horses that are recumbent and have difficulty rising; however, recumbent horses with EEEV generally are too comatose to sling. Dysphagic horses require fluid and nutritional support.

Until equine protozoal myeloencephalitis is excluded, prophylactic antiprotozoal medications may be instituted. Other supportive measures (eg, oral and parental fluids and nutrition for dehydrated and dysphagic horses) are also important. Broad-spectrum antibiotics should be given for treatment of wounds, cellulitis, and pneumonia. Horses with intermittent or focal neuropathies have a better prognosis than those with complete flaccid paralysis or that appear comatose. Efficacy of specific antiviral agents for treatment of naturally occurring WNV or EEEV infection is unknown, even in people. Recent work with passive immunotherapy indicates possible benefit after the onset of clinical signs in WNV models.

Prognosis: Mortality of horses showing clinical signs from EEEV is 50%–90%, from WEEV 20%–50%, from VEEV 50%–75%, and from flavivirus infections 35%-45%. Horses with clinical neurologic signs from alphavirus infection that recover have a high incidence of residual neurologic deficits, whereas many horses that recover from WNV disease have been reported to have no residual neurologic deficits. In EEEV infection, death is frequently spontaneous. With WNV disease, horses are euthanized for humane reasons, but spontaneous death does occur. In EEEV, most surviving horses exhibit longterm neurologic signs. In WNV disease, overt clinical signs in horses that recover can last from 1 day to several weeks; improvement usually occurs within 7 days of onset of clinical signs. Although 80%–90% of owners report that the horse returns to normal function 1–6 mo after disease, at least 10% of owners report longterm deficits that limit athletic potential and resale value. Deficits include residual weakness or ataxia in one or more limbs, fatigue with exercise, focal or generalized muscle atrophy, and changes in personality and behavioral aberrations.

Prevention: Vaccination against alphaviruses and flaviviruses as core annual vaccines are considered the standard of care for all horses in the USA as endorsed by the American Association of Equine Practitioners. Formalin-inactivated whole viral vaccines for EEEV, WEEV, and VEEV are commercially available in bi- and trivalent forms, usually formulated with tetanus toxoid; several now include WNV. Nonvaccinated adult horses require the label priming two injections. For adult horses in temperate climates, an annual vaccine within 1 mo before the start of the arbovirus season is recommended. However, for horses that travel between northern and southern areas affected by the virus, injections should be given two or even three times yearly in active arbovirus seasons. Mares should be vaccinated 1 mo before foaling to induce colostral antibody. If a pregnant mare is naive, the full priming series starting 2 mo before foaling is recommended. However, some mares do not produce colostral antibody if vaccinated for the first time during gestation.

In foals that have received adequate colostrum from vaccinated dams, vaccination should begin at 5–6 mo of age; foals should receive two additional vaccinations at 30 and 90 days after the first one. It is unclear whether maternal antibody interferes with vaccine responses in foals; however, epidemiologic evidence strongly indicates that horses between 4 mo and 4 yr old are highly susceptible to EEEV. If there is early spring (March) activity in the southeastern USA, horses may require three injections throughout the year, especially in horses <5 yr old and in horses that have recently arrived in the southeastern USA. In foals born to nonvaccinated or minimally vaccinated mares, maternal immunity may wane, and vaccination should be performed at 4, 5, and 6 mo of age. In Florida, where the highest numbers of EEEV cases occur, horses of all ages should be vaccinated in January and again in April before the peak of the season. A third vaccination should be administered late in the summer if the season is particularly active. The frequency of vaccination may be minimized to once or twice per year in climates that have short mosquito seasons and in which limited activity has historically been reported.

Currently, several whole inactivated virion vaccines, one recombinant inactivated vaccine, and a canarypox-vectored vaccine are licensed for prevention of WNV viremia in most of the Americas, including the USA and Canada, and Europe. An inactivated virus vaccine is readily available against Japanese encephalitis virus. There is experimental evidence that the canarypox WNV lineage 1 vaccine provides cross-protection against WNV lineage 2 infection. WNV challenge studies indicate that ~10% of properly immunized horses do not produce neutralizing antibodies to WNV and that 2.3%–3% of equine WNV cases seen in the field are in fully vaccinated horses. The duration of immunity from vaccination with the killed, adjuvanted WNV vaccine is unknown.

Protection of horses from arboviruses must also include efforts to minimize exposure to infected mosquitoes. Mosquito mitigation includes applying an insect repellent that contains permethrin on the horses at least daily during vector season, especially at times of day when mosquitoes may be most active. Environmental management is also essential and includes keeping the barn area, paddocks, and pastures cleared of weeds and organic material, such as feces, that might harbor adult mosquitoes. Cleaning water tanks and buckets at least weekly will reduce mosquito breeding areas. Removal of other containers such as flower pots and used tires that may hold stagnant water is essential for reducing the number of mosquitoes in the area.

Options for control of arbovirus infection in other animals emphasize reduction of exposure. Few arbovirus infections have been documented in dogs and cats; however, exposure to EEEV and WNV is detected in both species during arbovirus seasons. In active years, young dogs have been reported to be susceptible to EEEV infection.

Keeping dogs and cats indoors or in a screened area, especially during the time when mosquitoes are most active, reduces exposure. Disposal of dead birds or other small prey that might be eaten may reduce oral exposure.

Clinical cases of both of these diseases have also been recorded in other domestic and exotic animals during active seasons. Emus are exceptionally susceptible to EEEV. These animals are used for the commercial food industry, and infection results in high viremia and high amounts of virus shedding rectally, orally, and in regurgitated material. Vaccination will prevent viremia, shedding, and disease. Camelids are susceptible to WNV, and numerous reports of disease and pathology were recorded as the virus spread across North America. The killed, adjuvanted vaccine marketed for use in horses has been used in camelids without any reports of major adverse effects, and animals have demonstrated production of neutralizing antibody.

Zoonotic Risk: The reporting of these diseases (or suspicion of such) on an international and national basis is a basic duty of all veterinarians to ensure the health and safety of horses and people. As such, a thorough diagnostic investigation to confirm these infections is imperative, irrespective of state resources available for subsidized testing.

People may be infected by most of the arboviruses that commonly cause viral encephalitis in horses. Clinical signs in people vary from mild flu-like symptoms to death. Children, the elderly, and those who are immunosuppressed are the most susceptible. People with neurologic disease due to arboviruses usually have permanent neurologic impairment after recovery. Human disease is reported infrequently and generally follows equine infections by ~2 wk. Veterinarians should be aware of the possibility of human infection and use repellents and other procedures to protect themselves from hematophagous insects when working in sylvatic virus habitats or handling viremic horses. In addition, waterproof clothing (gown, boots, gloves), respirator (N-95 or N-99 mask), face shield, and hair covering are recommended during all necropsies performed on horses suspected of having encephalomyelitis.

LOUPING ILL

(Ovine encephalomyelitis)

Louping ill is an acute, tick-transmitted viral disease of the CNS that primarily affects sheep, but cattle, goats, horses, dogs, pigs, South American camelids, red grouse, and people also can be affected; people can be infected by tick bites or exposure to tissues or instruments contaminated with virus. The disease is seen throughout the rough hill grazings of the British Isles wherever the vector tick, *Ixodes ricinus*, is prevalent. Diseases of sheep indistinguishable from louping ill and caused by similar viruses have been reported in Norway, Spain, Turkey, and Bulgaria, which suggests that the condition may not be restricted to the British Isles.

Etiology and Transmission: The virus belongs to the Flaviviridae family and is part of an antigenically closely related complex of viruses known as the tickborne encephalitides, which are primarily associated with disease in people and distributed throughout the northern temperate regions. Infection is transmitted transstadially by the tick vector; transovarial transmission of louping ill virus does not appear to occur. In sheep flocks, mortality ranges from 60% in newly introduced stock to 5%–10% in sheep acclimatized to the pasture. On farms where the disease is endemic, losses are mainly confined to animals <2 yr old; adults tend to be immune as a result of previous infection, and lambs are protected in their first season by colostral antibody. However, when the disease appears for the first time, or after a lapse of several years, all ages of sheep are susceptible. Mortality is variable in other species but tends to be high in red grouse. All species of vertebrates that come in contact with questing ticks may become parasitized and infected with louping ill virus, but only sheep and grouse develop titers of viremia sufficient to pass the infection to the vector tick. Infection also can be spread through contact with contaminated instruments or tissues. Infected lactating goats can excrete high titers of virus in their milk, which may cause fatal infection of their kids and be a potential human health hazard.

Pathogenesis, Clinical Findings, and Lesions: The course of infection in all species is similar, and varies only in the intensity of viremia and frequency with which clinical signs develop. After inoculation by an infected tick, virus initially replicates in lymphoid tissues, which gives rise to viremia that lasts 1–5 days. Only animals that develop high titers can transfer the virus to ticks. During viremia, a febrile reaction may be present, but overt clinical signs are generally absent until the virus enters the CNS and begins replication, even though the immune response has eliminated the virus from the extraneuronal tissues. The extent of neuronal damage consequent to viral replication determines the severity of signs, from none (subclinical) through varying degrees of neurologic dysfunction to sudden death. Histologic lesions may be present whether or not signs develop. Signs include fine muscular tremors, nervous nibbling, ataxia (particularly of the hindlimbs), weakness, and collapse; death may occur 1–3 days after onset of signs. Peracute deaths may also occur. In some recovered animals, residual paresis or torticollis may persist. All recovered animals are solidly immune for life.

The severity of clinical disease in animals recently infected with *Anaplasma phagocytophilum* (the cause of tickborne fever [*see* p 772]) is markedly increased, presumably because of the immunosuppressive effect of this organism. The accompanying pathology may be complex and associated with secondary bacterial and mycotic infection, accounting for the high mortality experienced when naive flocks are introduced to tick-infested pasture.

No specific gross lesions are present, although secondary pneumonia may develop. Histologic examination of the CNS usually shows a nonsuppurative polioencephalomyelitis with lesions predominantly in the brain stem.

Diagnosis: The disease normally is seen only in animals that have had access to tick-infested pasture; however, the variable clinical picture necessitates differentiation from other conditions that cause locomotor or neurologic dysfunction. Confirmation is by histologic examination of the brain, virus detection in CNS tissue, and serology. As much of the brain and brain stem as possible should be fixed in formaldehyde solution (10% in saline), and sections examined for the characteristic lesions, which can be useful in reaching a presumptive diagnosis. Diagnosis is confirmed by immunohistochemistry using an appropriate monoclonal antibody. For routine diagnosis, virus isolation is now seldom undertaken and has been replaced by reverse transcriptase PCR. This requires a piece of brain stem to be collected into virus transport medium and dispatched to a suitable diagnostic laboratory. Measurement of serum neutralizing and hemagglutination inhibition antibodies also can help reach a diagnosis and for surveys. The presence of IgM antibody in cattle and sheep serum, detected by the hemagglutination inhibition test, provides good evidence that the animal was infected within the preceding 10 days.

Treatment and Control: No specific treatment is available, but nursing, hand-feeding, and sedation may be helpful. An inactivated, tissue culture–propagated vaccine is available and has successfully protected sheep, cattle, and goats. A single injection induces an antibody response that provides protection for <2 yr. Colostrum from the vaccinated ewe prevents infection of lambs in their first months. Generally, all animals to be retained for breeding are vaccinated at 6–12 mo of age. Use of insecticidal dips to protect against exposure to ticks generally is inadequate, although pour-on preparations reduce exposure, and their systematic use may effectively reduce the abundance of ticks and prevalence of virus infection.

Zoonotic Risk: Louping ill virus infection of people can cause severe encephalomyelitis. Symptoms are biphasic; the initial, flu-like symptoms are replaced 4–5 days later with signs of encephalitis. People become infected through the bite of infected ticks or through contact with infected carcasses, sharp instruments, or aerosol. Only a few cases of natural transmission have been reported, most occurring in laboratory workers. Those engaged in the diagnosis or research of this virus should be vaccinated with a human vaccine against tickborne encephalitis virus. Because goats can excrete high titers of virus in their milk, goats kept for milk production in endemic areas must be vaccinated.

PSEUDORABIES

(Aujeszky disease, Mad itch)

Pseudorabies is an acute, frequently fatal disease with a worldwide distribution that affects swine primarily and other domestic and wild animals incidentally. The pseudorabies virus has emerged as a significant pathogen in the USA since the 1960s, probably because of the increase in confinement swine housing or perhaps because of the emergence of more virulent strains. Clinical signs in nonporcine animals are similar to those of rabies, hence the name "mad itch" (pigs do not display this sign). Pseudorabies is a reportable disease and has been successfully eradicated from the vast majority of the USA.

Etiology: Pseudorabies virus is a DNA herpesvirus. The pig is the only reservoir host, but the virus can infect cattle, sheep, cats, dogs, and goats as well as wildlife, including raccoons, opossums, skunks, and rodents. Experimental studies in nonhuman primates indicate that rhesus monkeys and marmosets are susceptible but chimpanzees are not. Reports of human infection are limited and are based on seroconversion rather than virus isolation. Infections in horses are rare. Only one serotype of pseudorabies virus is recognized, but strain differences have been identified using monoclonal antibody preparations, restriction endonuclease assays, and heat and trypsin inactivation markers.

Epidemiology: The virus can be transmitted via nose-to-nose or fecal-oral contact. Indirect transmission commonly occurs via inhalation of aerosolized virus. Infectious virus can persist for up to 7 hr in air with a relative humidity of ≥55%. Data from England indicate that virus may travel via aerosols for up to 2 km in certain weather conditions. Other studies have demonstrated that the virus can survive for up to 7 hr in nonchlorinated well water; for 2 days in anaerobic lagoon effluent and in green grass, soil, feces, and shelled corn; for 3 days in nasal washings on plastic and pelleted hog feed; and for 4 days in straw bedding. The virus is enveloped and, therefore, inactivated by drying, sunlight, and high temperatures (≥37°C [98.6°F]). Dead-end hosts, such as dogs, cats, or wildlife, can transmit the virus between farms, but these animals survive only 2–3 days after becoming infected. The potential role of insects as vectors is being investigated. Birds do not seem to play a role in transmission.

Clinical Findings and Pathogenesis: The clinical signs in pigs depend on the age of the affected animal. Young swine are highly susceptible, and losses may reach 100% in piglets <7 days old. In general, signs of CNS disease (eg, tremors and paddling) are seen. If weaned pigs are infected, respiratory disease is the primary clinical problem, especially if complicated by secondary bacterial pathogens. Pseudorabies virus has been reported to inhibit the function of alveolar macrophages, thereby reducing the ability of these cells to process and destroy bacteria. A generalized febrile response (41°–42°C [105.8°–107.6°F]), anorexia, and weight loss are seen in infected pigs of all ages. Mortality can be very low (1%–2%) in grower and finisher pigs but may reach 50% in nursery pigs. Sneezing and dyspnea are frequently seen, and CNS involvement is reported occasionally. Clinical signs in nonporcine species, such as cats, dogs, cattle, and small ruminants, include sudden death, intense local pruritus, CNS signs (circling, maniacal behavior, paralysis), fever, and respiratory distress.

After natural infection, the primary site of viral replication is nasal, pharyngeal, or tonsillar epithelium. The virus spreads via the lymphatics to regional lymph nodes, where replication continues. Virus also spreads via nervous tissue to the brain, where it replicates, preferentially in neurons of the pons and medulla. In addition, virus has been isolated from alveolar macrophages, bronchial epithelium, spleen, lymph nodes, trophoblasts, embryos, and luteal cells.

Viral excretion begins ~2–5 days after infection, and virus can be recovered from nasal secretions, tonsillar epithelium, vaginal and preputial secretions, milk, or urine for >2 wk. A latent state, in which virus is harbored in the trigeminal ganglia, may exist. In swine with latent infections, shedding may resume after periods of stress such as farrowing, crowding, or transport. Experimentally, corticosteroid injections (dexamethasone, 2 mg/kg, IM) for 5 consecutive days have induced recrudescence.

Lesions: Gross lesions of pseudorabies virus infection are often undetectable. Serous rhinitis, necrotic tonsillitis, or hemorrhagic pulmonary lymph nodes may be seen. Pulmonary edema, as well as pneumonic lesions of secondary bacterial pathogens, may be present. Necrotic foci (2–3 mm in diameter) may be scattered throughout the liver. Such lesions are typically found in young (<7 days old) piglets.

Microscopically, nonsuppurative meningoencephalitis is a characteristic lesion that can be present in gray and white matter. Mononuclear perivascular cuffing and neuronal necrosis may also be present. The meninges are thickened as a result of mononuclear cell infiltration. Necrotic tonsillitis with the presence of intranuclear inclusion bodies, as well as necrotic bronchitis, bronchiolitis, and alveolitis, are commonly seen. Focal areas of necrosis are often found in the liver, spleen, lymph nodes, and adrenal glands of macerated fetuses.

Diagnosis: In addition to the gross and microscopic lesions, other diagnostic aids include virus isolation, fluorescent antibody testing, and serologic testing. Brain, spleen, and lung are the organs of choice for virus isolation. Nasal swabs can be used for isolation of virus from acutely infected animals. The nasal specimens must be stored and transported in cold, sterile saline with antibiotics to suppress bacterial growth. The fluorescent antibody test can be performed using tonsil or brain.

Many serologic tests are now available, including serum neutralization, ELISA, and latex agglutination. Serum neutralization, which is the standard test, requires 48 hr to complete. An ELISA has been developed as a screening assay for large volumes of sera; however, specificity may be poor. False-positive results are typically reassessed using the serum neutralization test. The latex agglutination test, although highly sensitive and rapid, may also have poor specificity. After infection, antibodies can be detected within 6–7 days using the latex agglutination test, within 7–8 days using the ELISA, and within 8–10 days using the serum neutralization test.

A differential ELISA has been used to differentiate antibodies produced as a result of vaccination from those produced as a result of natural infection. The vaccines used in swine are based on the deletion of certain genes (gI, gIII, or gX) from the vaccine virus. Swine vaccinated with a gene-deleted vaccine do not mount an antibody response to the protein coded for by the deleted gene. In contrast, infection with field virus results in antibodies against these proteins.

Colostral antibodies to pseudorabies virus may be present until pigs are 4 mo old (similar to porcine parvovirus). Therefore, paired samples or serologic profiles may be necessary in grower and finisher pigs to assess decreasing levels of maternal antibody and to ensure that pigs are vaccinated at the appropriate time.

Treatment and Control: Although there is no specific treatment for acute infection with pseudorabies virus, vaccination can alleviate clinical signs in pigs of certain ages. Typically, mass vaccination of all pigs on the farm with a modified-live virus vaccine is recommended. Intranasal vaccination of sows and neonatal piglets 1–7 days old, followed by IM vaccination of all other swine on the premises, helps reduce viral shedding and improve survival. The modified-live virus replicates at the site of injection and in regional lymph nodes. Vaccine virus is shed in such low levels that mucous transmission to other animals is minimal. In gene-deleted vaccines, the thymidine kinase gene has also been deleted; thus, the virus cannot infect and replicate in neurons. It is recommended that breeding herds be vaccinated quarterly and that finisher pigs be vaccinated after levels of maternal antibody decrease. Regular vaccination results in excellent control of the disease. Concurrent antibiotic therapy via feed and IM injection is recommended to control secondary bacterial pathogens.

Numerous programs have been developed for eradication of pseudorabies virus. As of 2014, all 50 states in the USA are considered free of the disease in commercial pigs; however, the virus appears to be endemic in feral pig populations and has been identified on game ranches. Effective strategies for eradication of pseudorabies include whole-herd depopulation, a test and removal strategy, and offspring segregation. Although effective, whole-herd depopulation is costly and time consuming. Usually, problems other than pseudorabies virus (eg, genetic improvement) need to be resolved before whole-herd depopulation can be cost effective.

The test and removal strategy consists of blood testing all breeding swine, culling all positive animals, and repeating this procedure until the population tests negative. Naturally infected animals can be culled when such a strategy is used in conjunction with a differential vaccination program. A test and removal strategy can be effective, but it is laborious, and latently infected animals that do not exhibit an antibody response on serologic testing may potentially resume shedding the virus at a later time.

In an offspring segregation program, young piglets (18–21 days old) are removed from vaccinated sows and raised to adulthood at another site. If enough gilts and boars are raised in this manner, the original breeding herd may be depopulated and subsequently repopulated with seronegative replacements. This method also allows seedstock producers to sell animals, even though the breeding herd is infected. In this case, however, all offspring must be individually tested using the serum neutralization test and have negative results before being sold.

RABIES

Rabies is an acute, progressive viral encephalomyelitis that principally affects carnivores and bats, although any mammal can be affected. The disease is fatal once clinical signs appear. Rabies is found throughout the world, but a few countries claim to be free of the disease because of either successful elimination programs or their island status and enforcement of rigorous quarantine regulations. Globally, the dog is the most important reservoir, particularly in developing countries. Integrated veterinary management of local animal populations, by mass vaccination of dogs and community promotion of responsible pet ownership, is the most cost-effective, humane, long-term solution toward eliminating regional canine rabies in a One Health context.

Etiology and Epidemiology: Rabies is caused by lyssaviruses in the Rhabdovirus family. Lyssaviruses are usually confined to one major reservoir species in a given geographic area, although spillover to other species is common. Identification of different virus variants by laboratory procedures such as monoclonal antibody analysis or genetic sequencing has greatly enhanced understanding of rabies epidemiology. Generally, each virus variant is responsible for virus transmission between members of the same species in a given geographic area. To date, >15 different lyssaviruses have been described. Globally, rabies virus is the most important member of the genus.

From an epidemiologic perspective, the name of the mammalian species acting as the reservoir and vector is used as an adjective to describe involvement in the infection process. For example, rabies maintained by dog-to-dog transmission is termed canine rabies, whereas rabies in a dog as a result of infection with a variant from a different reservoir mammal, eg, skunk (or raccoon or fox), would be referred to as skunk (or raccoon or fox, etc) rabies in a dog.

In North America, distinct virus variants are responsible for rabies perpetuation in red and Arctic foxes in Canada and Alaska, raccoons along the eastern seaboard from Maine to Florida, and gray foxes in the southwest, including Arizona, Colorado, and Texas. Two different variants are responsible for rabies in striped skunks, one in the south central states and the other in the north central states, which often extends into the Canadian prairies. Another skunk rabies virus variant is found in California. By comparison, the epidemiology of rabies in bats is complex. In general, each variant found in bats may be characterized with a predominant bat species. Spillover from bats to terrestrial animals is seen infrequently. Most human cases of rabies in the USA in the past decade have been caused by bat rabies virus variants (especially viruses associated with *Lasionycteris noctivagans*, the silver-haired bat, and *Perimyotis subflavus*, the tricolored bat).

Rabies emergence may be affected by changes in virus-host dynamics or human translocation of infected species. For many years, skunks were the most commonly reported rabid animal in the USA, but since 1990, rabid raccoons have been the most numerous. Canine rabies became established in dogs and coyotes (*Canis latrans*) in southern Texas but was eliminated by the end of the 20th century. Canine rabies exists in Mexico, with the potential to spread throughout the USA if reintroduced. Skunk, raccoon, and fox rabies are each found in fairly distinct geographic regions of North America, although some overlap occurs. Bat rabies is distributed throughout the Americas. The vampire bat is an important reservoir in Latin America and is the source of multiple outbreaks in cattle, as well as in people, particularly in parts of Amazonia.

In western Europe, red fox rabies predominated before its elimination by oral vaccination. In parts of eastern Europe, rabies in raccoon dogs is of increasing concern. Bat rabies, maintained by several different lyssaviruses in insectivorous Chiroptera, appears to be widely distributed throughout Europe.

Other wildlife play an important role in the transmission of rabies in certain areas, including different species of mongooses in the Caribbean, southern Africa, and parts of Asia; jackals in parts of Africa; wolves in parts of northern Europe; marmosets in Brazil; and ferret badgers in China.

All rabies reservoirs are also vectors of the virus, but not all vectors are reservoirs. For example, cats can effectively transmit the virus, but no cat-to-cat transmission of rabies perpetuates in lieu of a predominant reservoir (such as infected dogs), and no unique feline rabies virus variant has been documented. However, cats are the most commonly reported rabid domestic animal in the USA. Virus is present in the saliva of rabid cats, and people have developed rabies after being bitten by rabid cats. Reported cases in domestic cats have outnumbered those in dogs in the USA every year since 1990.

Transmission and Pathogenesis: Lyssaviruses are highly neurotropic. Transmission almost always occurs via introduction of virus-laden saliva into tissues, usually by the bite of a rabid animal. Although much less likely, virus from saliva, salivary glands, or brain can cause infection by entering the body through fresh wounds or intact mucous membranes. Usually, saliva is infectious at the time clinical signs occur, but domestic dogs, cats, and ferrets may shed virus for several days before onset of clinical signs. Viral shedding in skunks has been reported for up to 8 days before onset of signs. Rabies virus has not been isolated from skunk musk (spray).

The incubation period is both prolonged and variable. Typically, the virus remains at the inoculation site for a considerable time. The unusual length of the incubation period helps to explain the effective action of local infiltration of rabies immune globulin during human postexposure prophylaxis, even days after exposure. Most rabies cases in dogs develop within 21–80 days after exposure, but the incubation period may be shorter or considerably longer. One recorded case of rabies in a person in the USA had an incubation period estimated reliably of >8 yr.

The virus travels via the peripheral nerves to the spinal cord and ascends to the brain. After reaching the brain, the virus travels via peripheral nerves to the salivary glands. If an animal is capable of transmitting rabies via its saliva, virus will be detectable in the brain. Virus is shed intermittently in the saliva.

Hematogenous spread does not occur. Under most circumstances, there is no danger of aerosol transmission of rabies virus. However, aerosol transmission has occurred under very specialized conditions in which the air contained a high concentration of suspended particles or droplets carrying viral particles. Such conditions have been responsible for laboratory transmission under less than ideal containment situations. There has been a suggestion of rare natural aerosol transmission in a cave inhabited by millions of bats. Oral and nasal secretions containing virus were probably aerosolized from tens of thousands of rabid bats. Aerosol infection may occur via direct attachment of the virus to olfactory nerve endings.

Near the end of the clinical phase, after replication in the CNS, virus may be found in nearly every innervated organ. Rabies has been transmitted by transplantation of tissues and organs from infected people.

Clinical Findings: Clinical signs of rabies are rarely definitive. Rabid animals of all species usually exhibit typical signs of CNS disturbance, with minor variations among species. The most reliable signs, regardless of species, are acute behavioral changes and unexplained progressive paralysis. Behavioral changes may include sudden anorexia, signs of apprehension or nervousness, irritability, and hyperexcitability (including priapism). The animal may seek solitude. Ataxia, altered phonation, and changes in temperament are apparent. Uncharacteristic aggressiveness may develop—a normally docile animal may suddenly become vicious. Commonly, rabid wild animals may lose their fear of people, and normally nocturnal species may be seen wandering about during the daytime.

The clinical course may be divided into three general phases—prodromal, acute excitative, and paralytic/endstage. However, this division is of limited practical value because of the variability of signs and the irregular lengths of the phases. During the prodromal period, which lasts ~1–3 days, animals show only vague nonspecific signs, which intensify rapidly. The disease progresses rapidly after the onset of paralysis, and death is virtually certain a few days thereafter. Some animals die rapidly without marked clinical signs.

The term "furious rabies" refers to animals in which aggression (the acute neural excitative phase) is pronounced. "Dumb or paralytic rabies" refers to animals in which the behavioral changes are minimal, and the disease is manifest principally by paralysis.

Furious Form: This is the classic "mad-dog syndrome," although it may be seen in all species. There is rarely evidence of paralysis during this stage. The animal becomes irritable and, with the slightest provocation, may viciously and aggressively use its teeth, claws, horns, or hooves. The posture and expression is one of alertness and anxiety, with pupils dilated. Noise may invite attack. Such animals lose caution and fear of people and other animals. Carnivores with this form of rabies frequently roam extensively, attacking other animals, including people, and any moving object. They commonly swallow foreign objects, eg, feces, straw, sticks, and stones. Rabid dogs may chew the wire and frame of their cages, breaking their teeth, and will follow a hand moved in front of the cage, attempting to bite. Young pups can seek human companionship and are overly playful, but bite even when petted, usually becoming vicious in a few hours. Rabid skunks may seek out and attack litters of puppies or kittens. Rabid domestic cats and bobcats can attack suddenly, biting and scratching viciously. As the disease progresses, muscular incoordination and seizures are common. Death results from progressive paralysis.

Paralytic Form: This is manifest by ataxia and paralysis of the throat and masseter muscles, often with profuse salivation and the inability to swallow. Dropping of the lower jaw is common in dogs. Owners frequently examine the mouth of dogs and livestock searching for a foreign body or administer medication with their bare hands, thereby exposing themselves to rabies. These animals may not be vicious and rarely attempt to bite. The paralysis progresses rapidly to all parts of the body, and coma and death follow in a few hours.

Species Variations: Cattle with furious rabies can be dangerous, attacking and pursuing people and other animals. Lactation ceases abruptly in dairy cattle. The usual placid expression is replaced by one of alertness. The eyes and ears follow sounds and movement. A common clinical sign is a characteristic abnormal bellowing, which may continue intermittently until shortly before death.

Horses and mules frequently show evidence of distress and extreme agitation. These signs, especially when accompanied by rolling, may be interpreted as evidence of colic. As in other species, horses may bite or strike viciously and, because of their size and strength, become unmanageable in a few hours. People have been killed outright by such animals. These animals frequently have self-inflicted wounds.

Rabid foxes and coyotes often invade yards or even houses, attacking dogs and people. One abnormal behavior that can occur is demonstrated by an animal that attacks a porcupine; finding a fox, or another animal, with porcupine quills can, in many cases, support a diagnosis of rabies.

Rabid raccoons, foxes, and skunks typically show no fear of people and are ataxic, frequently aggressive, and active during the day, despite their often crepuscular nature. In urban areas, they may attack domestic pets.

In general, rabies should be suspected in terrestrial wildlife acting abnormally. The same is true of bats that can be seen flying in the daytime, resting on the ground, paralyzed and unable to fly, attacking people or other animals, or fighting.

Rodents and lagomorphs rarely constitute a risk of exposure to rabies virus. However, each incident should be evaluated individually. Reports of laboratory-confirmed rabies in woodchucks are not uncommon in association with the raccoon rabies epizootic in the eastern USA.

Diagnosis: Clinical diagnosis is difficult, especially in areas where rabies is uncommon, and should not be relied on when making public health decisions. In the early stages, rabies can easily be confused with other diseases or with normal aggressive tendencies. Therefore, when rabies is suspected and definitive diagnosis is required, laboratory confirmation is indicated. Suspect animals should be euthanized, and the head removed for laboratory shipment.

Rabies diagnosis should be done by a qualified laboratory, designated by the local or state health department in accordance with established standardized national protocols for rabies testing. Immunofluorescence microscopy on fresh brain tissue, which allows direct visual observation of a specific antigen-antibody reaction, is the current test of choice. When properly used, it can establish a highly specific diagnosis within a few hours. Brain tissues examined must include medulla oblongata and cerebellum (and should be preserved by refrigeration with wet ice or cold packs). Virus isolation by the mouse inoculation test or tissue culture techniques using mouse neuroblastoma cells may be used for confirmation of indeterminate fluorescent antibody results, but it is no longer in common use in the USA.

Prevention and Control: Comprehensive guidelines for control in dogs have been prepared internationally by the World Health Organization and in the USA by the National Association of State Public Health Veterinarians (NASPHV). They include the following: 1) notification of suspected cases, and euthanasia of dogs with clinical signs and dogs bitten by a suspected rabid animal; 2) reduction of contact rates between susceptible dogs by leash laws, dog movement control, and quarantine; 3) mass immunization of dogs by campaigns and by continuing vaccination of young dogs; 4) stray dog control and euthanasia of unvaccinated dogs with low levels of dependency on, or restriction by, people; and 5) dog registration.

The Compendium of Animal Rabies Control, compiled and updated regularly by the NASPHV, summarizes the most current recommendations for the USA and lists all USDA-licensed animal rabies vaccines marketed in the USA. Many effective vaccines, such as modified-live virus, recombinant, and inactivated types, are available for use throughout the world; in the USA, no modified-live rabies virus vaccines are currently marketed (for any species). Recommended vaccination frequency is every 3 yr, after an initial series of two vaccines 1 yr apart. Several vaccines are also available for use in cats, and a few for use in ferrets, horses, cattle, and sheep. Because of the increasing importance of rabies in cats, vaccination of cats is critical. No parenteral vaccine is approved for use in wildlife. Protective immunity from the commercially available vaccines for domestic species has not been definitively demonstrated in wildlife species.

Until recently, the control of rabies in wildlife populations relied on population reduction of wildlife in an attempt to reduce the contact rate between susceptible animals; however, this proved difficult and often not publicly acceptable, ecologically sound, economically warranted, or programmatically effective. In Europe and Canada, use of oral vaccines distributed in baits to control fox rabies has been widespread and effective. The disease in foxes has been eliminated from most of western Europe and curtailed significantly in Ontario. Use of a vaccinia-rabies glycoprotein recombinant virus vaccine in the USA has successfully eliminated coyote rabies in southern Texas and has limited the western expansion of raccoon rabies from the eastern USA. The license limits use of the vaccine to state or federal rabies programs; it is not available to private veterinarians or for individual animal use. Together with other vaccines, it is also being used to assist in the control of dog rabies in developing countries.

Management of Suspected Rabies Cases—Exposure of Pets: Where terrestrial wildlife or bat rabies is known to occur, any animal bitten or otherwise exposed by a wild, carnivorous mammal (or a bat) not available for testing should be regarded as having been exposed to rabies. The NASPHV recommends that any unvaccinated dog, cat, or ferret exposed to rabies be euthanized immediately. If the owner is unwilling to do this, the animal should be placed in strict isolation (ie, no human or animal contact) for 6 mo and vaccinated against rabies 1 mo before release. If an exposed domestic animal is currently vaccinated, it should be revaccinated immediately and closely observed for 45 days.

Zoonotic Risk: Rabies has the highest case fatality of any infectious disease. When a person is exposed to an animal suspected of having rabies, the risk of rabies virus transmission should be evaluated carefully. Risk assessment should include consideration of the species of animal involved, the prevalence of rabies in the area, whether exposure sufficient to transmit rabies virus occurred, and the current status of the animal and its availability for diagnostic testing. Wild carnivores and bats present a considerable risk where the disease is found, regardless of whether abnormal behavior has been observed. Insectivorous bats, though small, can inflict wounds with their teeth and should never be caught or handled with bare hands. Bat bites may be ignored or go unnoticed, so direct contact with bats could be considered a risk of virus exposure. Any wild carnivore or bat suspected of exposing a person to rabies should be considered rabid unless proved otherwise by laboratory diagnosis; ideally, this includes bats in direct contact with people, such as those found in rooms with sleeping or otherwise unaware persons. Wildlife, including wolf hybrids, should never be kept as pets; if one of those animals exposes a person or domestic animal, the wild animal should be managed like free-ranging wildlife.

Any healthy domestic dog, cat, or ferret, whether vaccinated against rabies or not, that exposes (bites or deposits saliva in a fresh wound or on a mucous membrane) a person should be confined for 10 days; if the animal develops any signs of rabies during that period, it should be euthanized and its brain promptly submitted for rabies diagnosis. If the dog, cat, or ferret responsible for the exposure is stray or unwanted, it may be euthanized as soon as possible and submitted for rabies diagnosis. Since the advent of testing by immunofluorescence microscopy, there is no value in holding such animals to "let the disease progress" as an aid to diagnosis.

Internationally, the World Health Organization recommends several types of cell-culture vaccines for human groups at risk. In the USA, guidelines for human rabies prevention follow recommendations prepared by the Advisory Council on Immunization Practices. Preexposure immunization is strongly recommended for people in high-risk groups, such as veterinary staff, animal control officers, rabies and diagnostic laboratory workers, and, under certain circumstances, some travelers working in countries in which canine rabies is enzootic. Preexposure vaccine is administered on days 0, 7, and 21 or 28. However, preexposure prophylaxis alone cannot be relied on in the event of subsequent rabies virus exposure and must be supplemented by a limited postexposure regimen (two doses of vaccine, IM, on days 0 and 3). For healthy, unvaccinated patients bitten by a rabid animal, postexposure prophylaxis consists of wound care, local infiltration of rabies immune globulin, and vaccine administration on days 0, 3, 7, and 14. When provided in a timely and appropriate manner, modern postexposure prophylaxis virtually assures human survival.

TESCHOVIRUS ENCEPHALOMYELITIS

(Porcine polioencephalomyelitis, Teschen disease, Talfan disease)

Teschovirus encephalomyelitis (formerly known as porcine enteroviral encephalomyelitis) is analogous to human poliomyelitis. Severe disease is now rare; it is seen in eastern Europe and Madagascar but was last reported in western Europe from Austria in 1980. In other countries, sporadic mild disease is reported, or the disease is unrecognized.

Etiology, Epidemiology, and Pathogenesis: Until 1999, viruses causing this disease were classified within the genus *Enterovirus* (family *Picornaviridae*). However, analyses of their complete genome sequences revealed them to be very different from the enteroviruses, and they were reclassified in a new genus, *Teschovirus*, as the species *Porcine teschovirus* (the name was derived from Teschen disease). In 2015, the species was renamed to *Teschovirus A* to remove reference to the host species; however, the virus common name remains porcine teschovirus (PTV). Originally, 11 porcine enterovirus (PEV) serotypes were defined by virus neutralization. Of these, PEV 1–7 and 11–13 have been renamed PTV 1–10. Additional serotypes (PTV 11–13) have also recently been described, and it is likely more serotypes will be discovered in the future. PEV-8 has been reclassified as a member of a new picornavirus genus, *Sapelovirus*. PEV types 9 and 10, which have not been associated with neurologic disease, are distinct from the teschoviruses and remain in the *Enterovirus* genus. PTVs are ubiquitous in swine populations throughout the world. Many strains are nonpathogenic, but most neurotropic strains belong to one of the first three serotypes; serotype 1 includes not only the highly virulent but also many of the less virulent neurotropic strains. Although antigenic subtypes are recognized, they do not distinguish between more or less virulent strains of virus. PTV can survive in the environment for months.

Transmission is by direct or indirect contact with infected pigs. The virulent serotype 1 strain of classical Teschen disease results in high morbidity and mortality in all ages of pigs but apparently has remained confined to certain geographic areas. Mild, sporadic disease is seen elsewhere. Conventional herds are usually endemically infected, and exclusion of teschoviruses from SPF herds is difficult to maintain. Infection is mainly inapparent, and pigs usually become infected at weaning with the decline of passive maternal immunity and mixing of groups. Sporadic clinical cases of nervous disease are seen mainly around this time, although disease is more common in unweaned piglets after introduction of a serotype to which the herd has not been exposed.

Ingested virus replicates in the GI tract and associated lymphoid tissue. There is no destruction of gut epithelium, but virus is shed from multiplication sites into the feces for several weeks. In some pigs, especially those infected with virulent strains, viremia ensues and results in spread of infection to the CNS.

Clinical Findings: In acute virulent infection, clinical signs appear 1–4 wk after exposure in pigs of all ages. Ataxia is often seen first, followed by fever, lassitude, and anorexia. Seizures, nystagmus, opisthotonos, and coma may occur. Paralysis, initially evident as paraplegia but progressing to quadriplegia, is frequent in severe cases. Death is common within 3–4 days of onset of signs.

In mild disease, signs are essentially ataxia and paresis, the latter more rarely progressing to paralysis. Only young pigs (unweaned or weaned) are susceptible, and recovery is frequent.

Lesions: There are no gross lesions. Microscopic changes are most prominent in the gray matter of the brain stem, cerebellum, and spinal cord. The nonsuppurative encephalitis is characterized by neuronal necrosis, neuronophagia, glial foci, and perivascular lymphocytic cuffing. Meningitis is often present over the cerebellum.

Diagnosis: The clinical signs (especially those of locomotor disturbance), epidemiology, and absence of specific gross necropsy findings offer a presumptive diagnosis. The nature and distribution of histologic lesions provide supportive evidence. Acute and convalescent serum samples, taken ≥2 wk apart, may demonstrate a rise in neutralizing or complement-fixing antibodies. Virus isolation from the CNS is required to confirm the diagnosis. Differentiation of severe and milder forms of the disease can be based only on serologic, clinical, and epidemiologic evidence.

Differential diagnoses include the many other viral encephalitides of pigs, particularly classical swine fever, African swine fever, pseudorabies, rabies, and the encephalopathies of edema disease and water deprivation/salt intoxication. The prominent locomotor signs in teschovirus encephalomyelitis also can be confused with several toxic and nutritional neuropathies.

The different serotypes are identified either by virus neutralization, complement fixation, or ELISA using specific antisera. Genome sequence data is available for all the PTV serotypes, and molecular diagnosis by reverse transcriptase-PCR (RT-PCR) and real-time RT-PCR has been described.

Treatment and Control: There is no treatment. Live attenuated vaccine is used for control in areas experiencing severe endemic disease. In the past, eradication measures in central Europe involved ring vaccination and slaughter and also restrictions on importation of pigs and pork products. In many countries, suspected disease must be reported to regulatory authorities. In herds with endemic mild clinical disease, introduction of new breeding stock ≥1 mo before breeding should enhance passive immunity in offspring.

SPORADIC BOVINE ENCEPHALOMYELITIS

(Chlamydial encephalomyelitis, Buss disease, Transmissible serositis)

Sporadic bovine encephalomyelitis (SBE) is reported in various parts of the world. The disease affects cattle and buffalo, resulting in neurologic signs and polyserositis.

Etiology and Epidemiology: SBE is caused by *Chlamydia pecorum* biotype 2. Genetically identical *C pecorum* isolates have been identified from clinical cases in geographically different areas. The *C pecorum* isolates from clinical cases are distinct from those found in the GI tract of asymptomatic animals. Based on these findings, subclinical intestinal infections in cattle and other animals may not be the source of infection in SBE. The disease is most often seen in calves <6 mo old and less commonly in older cattle. Sporadic cases and outbreaks can occur within individual herds. Morbidity rates are most commonly <25%, but can reach 50%. The mortality rate can approach 30% and is highest in calves. Many sick animals die if not treated at an early stage.

Clinical Findings: The incubation period in experimentally infected calves is 6–30 days. The first sign in natural and experimental cases is fever (104°–107°F [40°–41.7°C]). Appetite remains good for the first 2–3 days despite the fever. Afterward, depression, excess salivation, diarrhea, anorexia, and weight loss occur. Nasal discharge and respiratory disease signs due to pleuritis may be seen. Early neurologic signs include stiffness and knuckling at the fetlocks. Calves become uncoordinated and stagger, circle, or fall over objects. Head pressing and blindness are not seen. In the terminal stage, calves are frequently recumbent and may develop opisthotonos. The course of the disease is usually 10–14 days.

Lesions: Lesions are not limited to the brain; vascular damage can be seen in several organs. Serofibrinous peritonitis, pleuritis, and pericarditis are common and are especially pronounced in more chronic cases. Microscopic lesions in the brain consist of perivascular cuffs and inflammatory foci in the parenchyma composed primarily of mononuclear cells.

Diagnosis: A tentative diagnosis can be based on clinical signs and particularly on the presence of serofibrinous peritonitis in the absence of other causes of peritonitis such as intestinal volvulus, intussusception, traumatic perforation of the reticulum, perforated abomasal ulcer, or displaced organs. Differential diagnoses also include rabies, infectious bovine rhinotracheitis with encephalitis, listeriosis, thromboembolic encephalomyelitis, polioencephalomalacia, pseudorabies, paramyxovirus encephalomyelitis, and malignant catarrhal fever. SBE can be diagnosed by PCR detection of *C pecorum* DNA in brain tissue, pleural fluid, pericardial fluid, or peritoneal fluid of affected animals. Diagnosis can also be confirmed by culture in either developing chicken embryos or cell cultures, by histologic changes in brain sections, or by evaluation of tissue impression smears after Giemsa or immunofluorescent staining.

Treatment: The antibiotics of choice are tetracyclines, oxytetracyclines, and tylosin. For treatment to be effective, it must be given as early as possible in high doses (eg, oxytetracyclines at 10–20 mg/kg/day) and for ≥1 wk. If treatment is effective, the fever should drop significantly within 24 hr. No vaccines are available.

EQUINE PROTOZOAL MYELOENCEPHALITIS

Equine protozoal myeloencephalitis (EPM) is a common neurologic disease of horses in the Americas; it has been reported in most of the contiguous 48 states of the USA, southern Canada, Mexico, and several countries in Central and South America. In other countries, EPM is seen sporadically in horses that previously have spent time in the Americas.

Etiology and Epidemiology: Most cases of EPM are caused by an Apicomplexan protozoan, *Sarcocystis neurona*. Horses are infected by ingestion of *S neurona* sporocysts in contaminated feed or water. The organism undergoes early asexual multiplication (schizogony) in extraneural tissues before parasitizing the CNS. Because infectious sarcocysts are only rarely formed, the horse is considered an aberrant, dead-end host for *S neurona*. Like other *Sarcocystis* spp, *S neurona* has an obligate predator-prey life cycle. The definitive (predator) host for *S neurona* in the USA is the opossum (*Didelphis virginiana*). Opossums are infected by eating sarcocyst-containing muscle tissue from an infected intermediate (prey) host and, after a brief prepatent period (probably 2–4 wk), infectious sporocysts are passed in the feces. Nine-banded armadillos, striped skunks, raccoons, sea otters, Pacific harbor seals, and domestic cats have all been implicated as intermediate hosts; however, the importance in nature of each of these species is unknown. Sporadic cases of EPM are associated with *Neospora hughesi*, an organism closely related to *S neurona*. The natural host(s) of this organism have not yet been identified.

Clinical Findings: Because the protozoa may infect any part of the CNS, almost any neurologic sign is possible. The disease usually begins insidiously but may present acutely and be severe at onset. Signs of spinal cord involvement are more common than signs of brain disease. Horses with EPM involving the spinal cord have asymmetric or symmetric weakness and ataxia of one to all limbs, sometimes with obvious muscle atrophy. When the sacrocaudal spinal cord is involved, there are signs of cauda equina syndrome. EPM lesions in the spinal cord also may result in demarcated areas of spontaneous sweating or loss of reflexes and cutaneous sensation. The most common signs of brain disease in horses with EPM are depression, head tilt, and facial paralysis. Any cranial nerve nucleus may be involved, and there may be seizures, visual deficits including abnormal menace responses, or behavioral abnormalities. Without treatment, EPM may progress to cause recumbency and death. Progression to recumbency occurs over hours to years and may occur steadily or in a stop-start fashion.

Lesions: There is focal discoloration, hemorrhage, and/or malacia of CNS tissue. Histologically, protozoa may be found in association with a mixed inflammatory cellular response and neuronal destruction. Schizonts, in various stages of maturation, or free merozoites commonly are seen in the cytoplasm of neurons or mononuclear phagocytes. Also parasitized are intravascular and tissue neutrophils and eosinophils and, more rarely, capillary endothelial cells and myelinated axons. Merozoites may be found extracellularly, especially in areas of necrosis. In at least 75% of clinical cases, protozoa are not seen on H&E-stained sections.

Diagnosis: Postmortem diagnosis is confirmed by demonstration of protozoa in CNS lesions on the basis of distinctive morphology or by immunohistochemical staining. Testing for *S neurona*–specific antibody is the basis for presumptive antemortem diagnosis of EPM. Serologic tests for specific antibodies against whole *S neurona* (eg, indirect fluorescent antibody test) or *S neurona* surface antigens (snSAGs) provide evidence of current or recent exposure to the organism; thus, low or negative serum titers tend to exclude the diagnosis of EPM. Conversely, positive or high serum *S neurona* titers have limited diagnostic utility in that such titers do not clearly distinguish horses with subclinical extraneural infections from those with EPM. In horses with neurologic signs, serum:CSF antibody titer ratios of <1:100 or *C*-ratios >1 are indicative of production of *S neurona* antibody in the CNS and are highly supportive of the diagnosis of EPM. In a few horses with EPM, CSF analysis reveals abnormalities such as mononuclear pleocytosis and increased protein concentration.

Depending on the clinical signs, differential diagnoses may include cervical vertebral stenotic myelopathy, trauma, aberrant parasite migration, equine degenerative myeloencephalopathy, equine herpesvirus 1 myeloencephalopathy, equine motor neuron disease, cauda equina neuritis, arboviral (Eastern or Western equine, West Nile) encephalomyelitis, rabies, bacterial meningitis, hepatoencephalopathy, and leukoencephalomalacia.

Treatment: The FDA-approved treatments for EPM are ponazuril (5 mg/kg/day, PO, for 28 days), diclazuril (1 mg/kg/day, PO, for 28 days), and a combination of sulfadiazine and pyrimethamine (20 mg/kg and 1 mg/kg, respectively, for at least 90 days). The bioavailabilities of ponazuril and diclazuril are improved by concurrent PO administration of corn oil or DMSO. A loading dose of ponazuril (15 mg/kg, PO) may be given on the first day of treatment to rapidly attain therapeutic blood levels. The sulfadiazine/pyrimethamine product must be given at least 1 hr before or after hay is fed. Anemia may develop after prolonged treatment with sulfadiazine/pyrimethamine and is best prevented by providing folate-rich green forage such as alfalfa hay or green pasture. Approximately 60% of horses improve with each type of treatment, but <25% recover completely. Relapses occur commonly up to 2 yr after discontinuation of antiprotozoal therapy. Because immunosuppression/immunodeficiency may be a risk factor for EPM, immunomodulators (eg, mycobacterial cell-wall derivative, levamisole, killed parapox ovis, or transfer factor) are sometimes given as ancillary therapy.

Prevention and Control: No proven preventive is available. A conditionally approved vaccine was marketed, but the license lapsed in 2008 and it is no longer offered. There is interest in using antiprotozoal drugs for prevention; however, evidence-based protocols are not yet available. The source of infective sporocysts is opossum feces, so it is prudent to prevent access of opossums to horse-feeding areas. Horse and pet feed should not be left out; open feed bags and garbage should be kept in closed galvanized metal containers, bird feeders should be eliminated, and fallen fruit should be removed. Opossums can be trapped and relocated. Because putative intermediate hosts cannot be directly infective for horses, it is unlikely that control of these populations will be useful in EPM prevention.

CNS DISEASES CAUSED BY HELMINTHS AND ARTHROPODS

A number of metazoan parasites (helminths and arthropods) are associated with pathology in the CNS and may be categorized as described below.

Immature (Larval) Stages of Parasites of Carnivorous Animals: These developmental stages may induce behavioral changes in the intermediate host that are likely to enhance transmission to the definitive host by means of predation. For example, *Taenia multiceps multiceps* is acquired by the canine definitive host when the dog ingests the infective larval stages of the tapeworm *Coenurus cerebralis* in the brain and spinal cord of the ovine intermediate host. In sheep, *C cerebralis* causes ataxia, which allows the dog (a carnivore) to more easily prey upon the infected sheep.

Immature Stages of Parasites Exhibiting a Neurotropic Affinity: These developmental stages require conditions provided by the host's CNS for their growth and development. For example, *Hypoderma bovis* in cattle can migrate through the spinal cord and adjacent tissues to reach its predilection site, the dorsum of the back.

Erratic or Aberrant Parasites: These parasites are normally found in non-neurologic, predilection sites within the definitive host but, on occasion, may wander erratically into some portion of the CNS. For example, larvae of *Cuterebra* spp are normally found in subcutaneous sites in dogs or cats but may also aberrantly wander into the CNS and localize on the cerebrum or cerebellum.

Incidental Parasites: These parasites are found in a different host than that in which they normally are found. For example, *Parelaphostrongylus tenuis* normally is found in neurologic sites within the definitive host, white-tailed deer, in which the parasite is nonpathogenic. However, in an incidental host, such as moose, elk, or llama, the parasite migrates through portions of the CNS and produces an often fatal neurologic disease.

Facultative Parasites: These parasites are normally free-living within the animal's environment but, on occasion, can develop into a parasitic existence. For example, *Halicephalobus deletrix*, a saprophytic soil nematode that is found free-living in nature, has been reported to produce pathology in the CNS of horses.

Successful chemotherapeutic treatment for cerebrospinal nematodiasis has been reported with diethylcarbamazine at 100 mg/kg (45 mg/lb). Ivermectin and organophosphates kill larval bots and at least some nematodes, but killing parasites in situ within the CNS may provoke additional tissue damage.

Before implementing therapy for a pathogenic helminth or arthropod, other possible causes of neuropathology should be carefully considered. In particular, rabies (*see* p 1302) should always be included in the differential diagnoses. The animal's age, vaccination status, exposure status, and history are factors that should be considered when rendering a diagnosis.

CESTODES

Coenurosis: *Taenia multiceps multiceps* is an intestinal parasite of canids (especially dogs, foxes, and jackals) and occasionally people. Its intermediate hosts include sheep, goats, deer, antelope, chamois, rabbits, hares, horses, and less commonly cattle, which acquire this tapeworm's eggs while grazing. After ingestion, some oncospheres hatch and reach the brain, developing by endogenous budding into a metacestode (larval) stage known as *Coenurus cerebralis*. Initial invasion and development of the oncospheres may be responsible for acute suppurative meningoencephalitis. The fully developed coenurus may be 5–6 cm in diameter and cause increased intracranial pressure, which results in ataxia, hypermetria, blindness, head deviation, stumbling, and paralysis. This clinical condition is colloquially known as gid, sturdy, or staggers. In sheep, palpation of the skull caudal to the horn buds may reveal refraction; surgery to remove the cyst, including its wall, has a reasonable chance of success and is justified in valuable animals. Dogs associated with sheep and other livestock should not be fed the brain or spinal cord from infected animals and should be dewormed regularly.

Cysticercosis: *Taenia solium* is a tapeworm found in the small intestine of people. Its metacestode (larval) stage, a cysticercus, is a large fluid-filled cavity or vesicle or bladder found in the musculature of pigs. This larval stage was once regarded as a separate parasite, and it still retains the scientific name *Cysticercus cellulosae*. In people, this larval stage usually develops in subcutaneous sites and musculature but may be found in nervous tissues, eg, the brain and ocular tissues. Infection in people stems from ingestion of tapeworm eggs in contaminated foods or from dirty hands. In the brain, the parasite usually develops in the ventricles. Infection causes pain, paralysis, epileptiform seizures, locomotor disturbances, and possibly death. The larval cysticerci commonly localize on the meninges and in the neuropil. Treatment of human cysticercosis is by surgical removal of the lesion; however, the prognosis is poor.

Echinococcosis: *Echinococcus granulosus* is a tapeworm found in the small intestine of the canid definitive host. Its eggs are ingested by the intermediate hosts, wild and domestic herbivores, eg, sheep, cattle, and moose. People can also serve as intermediate hosts. After hatching in the intestine of the intermediate host, the oncospheres invade the circulatory system and lodge in various organs (the liver and lungs), where they develop into large, thick-walled, unilocular hydatid cysts that bud protoscolices endogenously. Hydatids have been rarely reported in the CNS of domestic animals and are rare in people, in which they produce symptoms similar to those of a brain tumor.

Foxes are the definitive host for a related species, *Echinococcus multilocularis*. Microtine rodents (such as voles) are the intermediate hosts. This parasite has been rarely found in the brain of people, in which the invasive, thin-walled multilocular hydatid cysts produce innumerable exogenous daughter cysts that bud protoscolices. Surgical intervention is more successful in removing unilocular hydatid cysts of *E granulosus*.

TREMATODES

Paragonimiasis: *Paragonimus westermani* and *P kellicotti*, the lung flukes, have been reported to migrate aberrantly and produce cysts in the brain and spinal cord of pigs, dogs, cats, rats, and people. Flukes in these extrapulmonic sites in dead-end hosts do not produce patent infections.

Schistosomiasis: Schistosomes, or blood flukes, normally deposit their eggs in the small vessels of the gut and urinary bladder, from which they pass into the external environment via the feces or urine. Some eggs, however, may get into the general circulation and reach the CNS, where they become encapsulated. This condition has been noted in people and domestic animals.

Troglotremiasis: *Troglotrema acutum* inhabits the frontal and ethmoidal sinuses of foxes and mustelids in Europe. Flukes live in pairs in cysts in these sinuses. These parasites cause decalcification and atrophy of the bony walls of the sinuses and eventually result in perforation into the cranial cavity. Microorganisms enter the cranial vault, leading to fatal, purulent meningitis. No treatment is available.

NEMATODES

Ascarids

The larvae of some ascarid roundworms, including *Toxocara* spp of dogs and cats and *Baylisascaris* spp of mustelids, can cause CNS disease.

Nervous disorders, frequently associated with ascarid infection in young dogs, may be due to focal lesions in the CNS caused by the death of aberrant arrested larvae of *T canis*. *Toxocara* larvae may also invade the eye and cause ocular larva migrans in people.

Baylisascaris procyonis is the ascarid found in the small intestine of raccoons. It causes larva migrans in both wild and domestic animals in North America and is usually associated with the production of clinical CNS disease. More than 90 species of wild and domesticated animals have been identified as being capable of serving as paratenic (transport) hosts harboring *B procyonis* larvae. Some species, including opossums, skunks, cats, pigs, sheep, and goats, appear to be marginally susceptible or resistant to the neurologic migration. The parasite has been associated with the production of cerebrospinal nematodiasis in people, particularly children; it also has been implicated as a cause of ocular larva migrans.

Filarids

Dirofilaria immitis is often referred to as the canine heartworm but can also infect cats and ferrets. As adults, these parasites usually infect the right ventricle and the pulmonary artery and its fine branches. *D immitis* has been recovered from a variety of aberrant sites, including the CNS of its definitive hosts and the anterior chamber of the eye. (*See also* HEARTWORM DISEASE, p 127.)

Elaeophora schneideri, a filarid of the carotid arteries and its branches, is common in mule deer, primarily in western North America. Microfilariae accumulate in the skin of the head and face; intermediate hosts are tabanid horseflies. Larvae develop in arteries of the leptomeninges before migrating to the carotids. Infection is usually asymptomatic in normal definitive hosts. In wapiti, moose, white-tailed deer, sheep, and goats, worms in the arteries cause degeneration and loss of the endothelium and accumulation of plasma proteins and platelets on and within the intima. Thrombosis, infiltration of the intima, and fibroblastic proliferation may eventually result in occlusion and ischemic necrosis in associated tissues. Necrotic lesions associated with occlusion of leptomeningeal arteries are commonly found in the brain. Neurologic signs include blindness, head deviation, circling, ataxia, and paralysis (*See also* ELAEOPHOROSIS, p 904).

Setaria digitata is found in Asia and is a common parasite of the peritoneal cavity. Microfilariae are found in the blood; mosquitoes are intermediate hosts. Details of development in the normal host are unknown. In cattle, clinical signs do not appear to develop. In horses, goats, and sheep, the developing worms invade the CNS and cause motor weakness, ataxia, lameness, drooping eyelids or ears, and lumbar paralysis. Lesions include focal malacia and degeneration of axis cylinders and myelin sheath in all regions of the CNS.

Setaria cervi has been reported on the leptomeninges of deer in Europe and in the former USSR, often in association with *Elaphostrongylus cervi*. *Setaria* spp have also been found in the CNS of horses. The significance of these findings is unclear.

Filarids may also parasitize avian species. *Splendidofilaria quiscula* is found in the cerebral hemispheres of grackles (*Quiscalus quiscua*) and other birds in North America. *Paronchocerca helicina* is found in the cranial leptomeninges of the snake bird (*Anhinga anhinga*) in the USA.

Metastrongyles

Angiostrongylus cantonensis is a common parasite of the pulmonary arteries of rats in southeast Asia and the south Pacific. Terrestrial, aquatic, and amphibious snails and slugs are intermediate hosts. Paratenic hosts are freshwater prawns, land crabs, coconut crabs, and planarians. Larvae invade the cerebrum and develop in the neural parenchyma for ~2 wk, then enter the subarachnoid space and migrate, ~1 mo after infection, to the pulmonary arteries via the venous system. Neurologic signs are rare in rats with light to moderate infections, but circling, cannibalism, and paraplegia may develop in heavy infections. In endemic areas, people frequently acquire infections by consuming raw or undercooked intermediate or paratenic hosts. In people, this parasite may produce a fatal eosinophilic meningoencephalitis. In Australia, *A cantonensis* has produced an ascending paralysis in puppies. It may be an incidental parasite in dogs.

Gurlita paralysans is found in the spinal veins of cats and has reportedly produced a high incidence of paralysis. It may be an incidental parasite in cats.

Elaphostrongylus cervi is a common parasite of the skeletal musculature of *Rangifer* and *Cervus* spp (reindeer and elk) in the holarctic region, especially Eurasia. It is transmitted through terrestrial snails and slugs and apparently develops for a time in the CNS before migrating to the muscles. Infection is associated with lumbar weakness, paresis, and paralysis in cervids in Sweden and in the former USSR.

Parelaphostrongylus tenuis is found in the subdural space and venous sinuses of the cranium of white-tailed deer in eastern North America. Eggs reach the lungs in the venous blood and develop into larvae, which pass up the bronchial tree and out with the feces. Infective larvae, acquired from terrestrial snails and slugs as the deer feeds, invade the spinal cord and develop for several weeks in the dorsal horns of the gray matter; then, they invade and mature in the subdural space. The infection is usually asymptomatic in white-tailed deer. However, *P tenuis* causes pathology in the CNS of various cervids (moose, caribou, wapiti) and antelope, llamas, sheep, and goats. In these hosts, the parasite produces considerable trauma in the CNS. In addition, eggs deposited in the neural tissue provoke marked inflammatory reactions. Clinical signs consist of lumbar weakness, ataxia, lameness, stiffness, circling, abnormal positions of the head, and paralysis. Signs vary in onset and character in individual animals. Temporary remissions are typical.

Skrjabingylus nasicola and *S chitwoodorum* are found in the frontal sinuses of mustelids, especially mink, weasels, and skunks. Larvae acquired from terrestrial snails and slugs develop for a time in the gut wall, then migrate to the spinal cord. They move on to the leptomeninges to the brain and along the olfactory tracts to the cribriform plate, which they penetrate to reach the frontal sinuses. Their presence on the leptomeninges elicits hemorrhage and leptomeningitis. In heavy infections, some subadult worms may invade the brain and cause neurologic signs, including paralysis.

Rhabditorids

Halicephalobus deletrix is a free-living soil rhabditiform associated with soil and decaying vegetation in the host's environment. This nematode has been reported in the CNS of horses and people. It may reach the CNS through wounds contaminated by soil that contain these nematodes or through abscesses in the oral and nasal cavities. The nematode multiplies in the CNS and is highly destructive of neural tissues. Pathogenicity in the CNS can be attributed to trauma caused by activities of the parasites; the role of excretory and secretory products is unknown. Also, the parasites may transport pathogenic microorganisms to the CNS. Clinical signs are related to the location of and lesions produced by the parasite. Signs resemble viral encephalitis and include motor weakness, ataxia, head deviation, circling, depression, blindness, drooping of the ear or eyelid, loss of the herding instinct, and paralysis. Lesions consist of vasculitis, hemorrhagic necrosis, and malacia.

Miscellaneous Nematodes

Migrating larvae of strongyles (perhaps *Strongylus vulgaris*) have been reported in the CNS of horses. Larvae of *Stephanurus dentatus* rarely invade the CNS of pigs. Larvae of *Trichinella spiralis* were found in the brain in a fatal case of trichinosis in a person. Larvae of *Strongyloides stercoralis* may invade the brain of experimentally infected animals. *Gnathostoma spinigerum* has been found rarely in the CNS of people. *Eustrongylides ignotus* implanted subcutaneously in rats and chickens migrated to the CNS and caused death of the host.

ARTHROPODS

Myiasis is the development of larval dipteran flies (bots and warbles) within the tissues or organs of people and other domestic or wild animals. Myiasis that involves the CNS is rather uncommon except for the larval stages of *Hypoderma bovis*, the cattle heel fly. Its larvae normally burrow between the periosteum and dura mater of the bovine spinal cord during migration to the subcutaneous tissues of the back. Neurologic signs, varying from a transient, stiff, unsteady gait to paralysis, may be seen in cattle given systemic insecticides when the larvae are present in the spinal canal. (*See also* CATTLE GRUBS, p 876.)

The larvae of *Oestrus ovis*, the nasal bot fly of sheep (*see* p 1473), are normally found in the nostrils and paranasal sinuses. They rarely penetrate the ethmoid bone and reach the forebrain. However, it is possible that other factors facilitate entry of larvae into the brain. The bones of the skull may erode. If the brain is injured, clinical signs, such as a high-stepping gait and incoordination, may mimic infection with *Coenurus cerebralis*. This condition is often referred to as false gid. Surgical intervention may be useful but can prove difficult if the larvae are difficult to reach.

Larval *Cuterebra* spp, normally found in subcutaneous sites in dogs or cats, have been known to wander into the CNS and localize in the cerebrum or cerebellum (*see* p 879). Intracranial migrations by larvae of dipteran flies have been reported in people (*Dermatobia hominis*), cattle (*Hypoderma bovis*), and horses (*Hypoderma* spp).

Bots and warbles may move rapidly after death of the host and migrate into tissues far from the site of origin.

Treatment of intracranial myiasis is currently experimental. Surgical and medical therapies to alleviate intracranial myiases have been considered. The efficacy of systemic organophosphates against migrating larvae of *Hypoderma* suggest that organophosphates may effectively eliminate certain dipteran larvae from the nervous system. Parenteral corticosteroids are also recommended to prevent additional inflammatory damage and intracranial pressure throughout the treatment period. Ivermectin (300 mcg/kg on alternate days) used in conjunction with corticosteroids should be considered experimental therapy for intracranial cuterebrosis in cats; it is not approved by the FDA for this use.

TICK PARALYSIS

Tick paralysis (toxicity) is an acute, progressive, symmetrical, ascending motor paralysis caused by salivary neurotoxin(s) produced by certain species of ticks. With some species, other signs of systemic "single organ" toxicity (eg, cardiac, airway, bladder, lung, esophagus, etc) may be seen separate to or within the classic paretic-*paralysis presentation*. People (usually children) and a wide variety of other mammals, birds, and reptiles may be affected. Human cases of tick paralysis caused by the genera *Ixodes*, *Dermacentor*, and *Amblyomma* have been reported from Australia, North America, Europe, and South Africa; these three plus *Rhipicephalus*, *Haemaphysalis*, *Otobius*, and *Argas* have been associated with paralysis to varying degrees in animals.

This toxicity is unique, because it is a pulsed toxin flow associated with repeat tick feeding over a set period of time. Animals are generally affected by paralysis, but there are also very odd presentations of associated toxicity. Deterioration can be unpredictable and rapid in some cases, and some animals may have prolonged and unexplainable recovery. Very severe cases require intensive care, including artificial ventilation, to maximize recovery rates, and generally, only tick removal and use of tick antitoxin serum (TAS) and antibiotics have a major effect on overall mortality.

Etiology, Epidemiology, and Pathogenesis: The potential to induce paralysis has been demonstrated, described, or suspected in 64 species of ticks belonging to 7 ixodid and 8 argasid genera. On the eastern coast of Australia, the paralysis tick *I holocyclus* (and to a lesser extent *I cornuatus* and *I hirstii*, in which morphologic classification has been shown to be unreliable) causes the most severe form of tick paralysis, with a mortality of as much as 10% in dogs (usually 4%–5%), irrespective of therapy.

In North America, *D andersoni* (the Rocky Mountain wood tick) and *D variabilis* (the American dog tick) are the most common causes. Sheep, cattle, and people may be affected, as well as dogs. *D albipictus*, *I scapularis*, *Amblyomma americanum*, *A maculatum*, *R sanguineus*, and *O megnini* may cause paralysis. In fowl, *Argas radiatus* and *A persicus* have caused paralysis. In Africa, *I rubicundus* (Karoo tick paralysis) and *R punctatus* in South Africa, *R evertsi evertsi* and *Argas walkerae* in sub-Saharan Africa, and *R evertsi mimeticus* in Namibia can cause the disease. Cats appear to be resistant to the disease caused by these ticks but are affected by *I holocyclus*. Toxicity is usually less severe (than in dogs), does not include chest complications, and has a better prognosis.

I holocyclus in Australia causes a much more severe disease than that seen in North America and elsewhere. Dogs and cats are affected, as well as sheep, goats, calves, foals, horses, pigs, flying foxes, poultry, birds (ostrich), reptiles (snakes and lizards), and people. Both local (less common) and systemic paresis and paralysis are seen. The natural hosts (bandicoots) are rarely affected, presumably acquiring immunity at an early age. However, without exposure to toxin, they too become susceptible.

Host factors influencing epidemiology include species, sensitivity to toxin, age, acquired immunity, field behavior, concurrent work demands, reaction to environmental factors, skin reactivity, and population density. Antitoxin immunity, starting at least 2 wk after primary tick exposure and lasting a few weeks, can be boosted by further infestations, but chronic tick exposure eventually is associated with a decline in immunity, possibly due to toxin-neutralizing effects by the host. Tick factors include age, toxin absorption and circulation dynamics, paralysis-inducing capability, other toxic effects, sexual activity, rate and volume of secretions, and the frequency of the sucking phase.

The maximal prevalence of tick paralysis is associated with seasonal activity of female ticks, mainly in spring and early summer, but in some areas ticks are active throughout the year. Environmental factors such as temperature and humidity also play a major role in tick morbidity and mortality (ie, ticks are easily killed by both hot/dry and wet conditions). Modern rapid transport of ticks attached to people, animals, or plant material can give rise to isolated cases of tick paralysis, far removed from the particular geographic area (or country) where the ticks are naturally found. The diagnosis may be delayed when such infested animals travel to areas where such paralysis associated with reduced levels of acetylcholine is not typically seen.

Toxicity does not relate directly to tick size, number, or duration of attachment. The clinical signs produced in various hosts depend on several variables, including toxin secretion rate, local site responsiveness, host immunity and susceptibility, and specific organ susceptibility.

Systemic toxicity follows injection of toxin(s) into the host, especially during periods of rapid engorgement, although large numbers of larval or nymphal ticks may also cause the same paralysis of the neuromuscular junction. The toxin is presumed to travel from the attachment site via the lymph to the systemic circulation and thus to all areas of the body, where it has a direct effect on cellular potassium channels and thus on intracellular calcium levels. However, primary hypoventilation is the main cause of death in most severe cases, in which alveolar disease may also be present.

Clinical Findings: In tick paralysis other than that caused by *I holocyclus*, clinical signs are generally seen ~5–9 days after tick attachment and progress over the next 24–72 hr. When *I holocyclus* is involved, clinical signs usually appear in 3–5 days (rarely longer, eg, up to 18 days, possibly with virginal ticks) after attachment and usually progress rapidly throughout the next 24–48 hr. Time periods can vary with *I holocyclus* because of tick factors, environmental humidity, temperature (microclimate), and host factors. Both "shorter onset to severe" signs and delayed "quiet" attachments with minimal signs may be seen. Removal of *I holocyclus* ticks does not immediately halt progression of disease. In severe cases, death from respiratory muscle failure and other respiratory complications can occur within 1–2 days of the onset of signs.

Early signs may include change or loss of voice (due to laryngeal paresis); hindlimb incoordination (presumed to be due to weakness and not central CNS ataxia); change in breathing rhythm, rate, depth, and effort; gagging, grunting, or coughing; regurgitation or vomiting; and pupillary dilation. Dogs with a grunt are believed to have increased airway resistance.

Hindlimb paralysis begins as slight to pronounced incoordination and weakness, which is best observed with the animal turning or walking away from the observer (or when climbing stairs or jumping up). As paralysis progresses, the animal becomes unable to move its hindlimbs and forelimbs, to stand, to sit, to right, and finally to lift its head.

A four-stage classification system based on systemic limb activity may enable clinical predictability. In stage 1, the dog's voice is changed (usually noticed retrospectively), and the dog is weakened but can still walk and stand. In stage 2, the dog cannot walk but can stand. In stage 3, the dog cannot stand but can right. In stage 4, the dog cannot right. Stages 3 and 4 (~30% of cases) indicate a poor prognosis. However, some dogs show few signs because of low levels of toxin or high levels of protective skin or systemic immunology, and some show signs in only one organ (eg, esophageal paralysis). Sensation is usually preserved, but it is increasingly harder to detect the clinical responses to stimuli due to lower motor neuron paralysis. (Visual analog scale scoring is also performed for the neuromuscular junction, overall toxicity, and dyspnea, with highly predictive results).

Breathing abnormalities include choke, upper respiratory tract obstruction, bronchoconstriction (especially seen early in cats), progressive fatigue of respiratory muscles, and aspiration of esophageal and/or gastric contents (due to loss of pharyngeal and laryngeal function), leading to aspiration pneumonia. Aspiration can be significant, and the lung severely affected before any obvious signs. It is possible to have a silent (no crackles), severely pneumonic lung if there is poor airflow into the affected lobe. Some dogs have profound dyspnea, no crackles, and extensive pulmonary radiographic opacity (due to aspiration pneumonia); such cases are usually terminal. Dogs with upper respiratory tract obstruction have a marked expiratory stridor (not the classic inspiratory stridor of primary laryngeal paralysis of large breeds), often with the head and forelegs extended to maximize air flow and exchange. If there is chest disease as well, the animal is usually very dyspneic. A thrill can be felt at or just below the larynx in association with the obstructed expiratory effort and stridor. The upper respiratory tract lesion can be easily missed, especially if the dog is paralyzed. Often the respiratory rate is high and forced. In cats, the doll test can be used to assess upper respiratory tract function. If finger/thumb compression of the chest induces a stridor, then this supports paresis or paralysis, irrespective of other respiratory tract defects. It is essential that any upper respiratory tract obstruction be diagnosed, because the associated workload, anxiety, and resultant fatigue can quickly become terminal.

Paralysis of esophageal muscles develops in most dogs (but not cats), with or without obvious esophageal dilation. Saliva and ingested food or fluid pool in the esophagus and may be regurgitated into the pharynx and mouth. Loss of pharyngeal function makes it difficult for the animal to clear material from the upper respiratory tract, which may then lead to aspiration pneumonia.

Vomiting (with evidence of bile) may occur in *I holocyclus* paralysis; a central action of toxin on the vomiting center has been suggested. Most cases of vomiting reported by owners are probably regurgitation, although drug-induced vomiting can be a complication. Dogs will gag and retch in an attempt to clear secretions and move their head and jaw in an odd way, associated with a characteristic groan, to further attempt clearance of materials.

Body temperature may be normal in the early stages; however, due to the toxin's effect on arteriovenous anastomoses (shunts), normal thermoregulation is lost. This can cause hyper- and hypothermia as animals are affected by local environmental factors. Shivering is also lost in severe cases. Profound hypo- and hyperthermia can occur suddenly and can be easily misdiagnosed; hypothermia clinically resembles tick paralysis in several ways. When body temperature is restored, the level of tick paralysis in some cases can be mild.

Rarely in dogs, acute congestive heart failure can present with extensive pulmonary edema due to diastolic myocardial dysfunction (the myocardium is unable to correctly relax, reducing efficient chamber filling and therefore systolic cardiac output). Venous return may also be reduced, and systemic venous pressure is increased.

Some dogs have a prolonged QT interval on ECG, which can result in a lethal ventricular arrhythmia. The frequency of these unexplained deaths, which follow complete gross clinical recovery, is not known, but most veterinarians who treat many cases report such events.

Cats with moderate to severe toxicity can be anxious. It is essential not to interfere with these animals until they have settled in their cage. If procedures are forced on them, these animals can die from obstructive dyspnea and the (presumed) associated hypoxemia, acidosis, and hypercapnea. Animals can deteriorate if compromised by excessive hospital stress (eg, nursing attention, noise, smell).

Cats may present with an "asthma-like" airway constriction, usually when they are mildly paretic; expiratory wheeze on auscultation, forced abdominal expiratory effort, and very easily induced exercise intolerance are classic signs at this time. These cats often have a positive doll test and will, after a few steps, sit on their hindquarters with the chest in a more upright vertical position than normal, often with an increased respiratory focus or effort. Feline "asthma" can be easily misdiagnosed at this stage if a tick is not found or suspected.

Diagnosis: The presence of a tick in conjunction with the sudden appearance of limb weakness and/or respiratory impairment is diagnostic. The offending tick may no longer be attached, but a "skin crater" (a hole 1–2 mm deep and 1–3 mm wide, surrounded by a variably raised and inflamed area) confirms the diagnosis. Sometimes neither tick nor crater can be found (ticks attached deep in the ear, between toes, or in the mouth or anus may be missed). However, with the appropriate clinical signs, in a known tick area without another obvious cause of lower motor neuron or neuromuscular disease, TAS treatment is still indicated. Recovery after treatment subjectively confirms the provisional diagnosis.

Specific laboratory diagnostic techniques are not available, but procedures that may be generally helpful include a PCV, serum protein, and radiography to assess presence and degree of pulmonary edema, megaesophagus, and pneumonia due to aspiration. Specific signs (eg, congestive heart failure, urethral obstruction) require routine evaluation and treatment of that body area or system.

Botulism, polyradiculoneuritis, acute peripheral neuropathies, snakebite, hypokalemia, and toadfish and ciguatera toxicity are some differential diagnoses. In regions where ticks are endemic, tick paralysis is usually high on the list of differential diagnoses for any flaccid, clinically ascending motor paralysis. It should also be considered in the differential diagnosis of megaesophagus, unexplained vomiting, acute left congestive heart failure (dogs), or "asthma" (cats). The tick season is usually well known for various areas (eg, a local creek) within the environment of a particular practice, and often most tick paralysis cases come from a few, well-defined, highly endemic areas.

Blood and serum values are unchanged in the early stages. Increased PCV (with normal serum protein) indicates a fluid shift into the lungs and a more guarded prognosis. Other changes may include increased levels of blood glucose, cholesterol, phosphate, and CK, and a decrease in blood potassium levels, but none of these changes are specific for tick paralysis or indicate severity or prognosis.

Echocardiography reveals both diastolic and secondary systolic myocardial dysfunction associated with reduced ventricular filling, possibly due to both peripheral venous pooling and poor diastolic myocardial relaxation. Nonstressful radiography gives the best available prognostic support, and pulse oximetry the best continuous assessment of oxygenation. Capnography helps assess the functional level of ventilation. Arterial blood gas analysis (although invasive) gives the best overall assessment of cardiopulmonary function. However, the stress of any such testing should be considered; positioning for chest radiographs (eg, dorsoventral to lateral) can tip animals into a terminal hypoventilatory decline associated with acute respiratory or cardiac arrest.

Treatment: In most infestations (except *I holocyclus*), removal of all ticks usually results in improvement within 24 hr and complete recovery within 72 hr. If ticks are not removed, death may occur from respiratory paralysis in 1–5 days. Removal of *I holocyclus* ticks does not immediately halt progression of disease. Clinical signs can deteriorate for ~24 hr and longer, but most dogs start to improve in 6–12 hr after TAS therapy. In any infestation, removal of all ticks is absolutely necessary. The entire integument should be searched, diligently and repeatedly, especially on long-haired animals or those with thick coats. Most ticks (80%) are located around the head or neck, but they can be found anywhere on the body. Plucking the tick(s) yields the best result (in dogs) and does not induce anaphylaxis.

Therapy for tick toxicity must address primary tick toxemia and paralysis, secondary issues (eg, esophageal reflux, aspiration pneumonia), and potential tertiary factors (eg, chronic weakness, esophageal stricture).

TAS is an immune serum against the toxin (similar to tetanus antitoxin) and is the product of choice. It should be given as early in the disease as possible; subsequent "top up" doses are not effective, because they are too late. For dogs, a minimal dosage of 0.5–1 mL/kg, should be given slowly IV throughout at least 20 min to avoid any shock reaction. Rapid IV use can induce clinical reactions in >80% of dogs. Anaphylaxis can occur unpredictably (as with all products), necessitating the use of high-dose, soluble cortisol and rapid fluid loading, etc. Based on retrospective case studies, cats are believed to be somewhat more susceptible than dogs, presumably with a second dose, a few weeks (not days) after the first dose.

Animals with multiple ticks or in the early stages of paralysis should receive a higher dose, because these cases have the most unbound toxin to neutralize. However, there are no data for the exact dosage rates required, and batch and brand levels of protective immunoglobulin may vary. Severely affected dogs may have less remaining unbound circulating toxin for TAS to neutralize. However, debate persists about the required (possibly less) dose of TAS. It has been suggested that a standard dose should be given, based on the amount needed to neutralize the pulsed toxin flow from one tick rather than on a weight basis; a minimal dose of 10–20 mL is recommended for dogs (and 5–10 mL for cats). However, until the level of remaining unbound toxin in the affected animal and the level of specific protective immunoglobulin can be better assessed, a set dose rate cannot be established (the level of disease is reflective of the level of bound toxin, which is not affected by TAS).

TAS given IP is the best alternative in cats for which the IV route is an issue (eg, respiratory distress, restraint dangers, dyspnea). However, its clinically effective half-life is believed to be short (days not weeks), and it will have no effect if the toxin is already tissue bound and the animal is severely ill or about to become so (with toxin in the perivascular space).

Minimization of stress and anxiety is essential. Acepromazine (0.03 mg/kg) may be given SC before any other medication or handling that may upset the animal. However, high doses should be avoided, especially if the animal is depressed, hypotensive, or hypothermic. (Overdosage may induce hypotension and hypothermia.) Opiates are an alternative (eg, methadone, 0.3–0.5 mg/kg, SC, IM). Oxygen therapy (nonstressful, usually nasal) is implemented (as indicated), but progressive disease requires more intensive therapy.

General anesthesia is indicated in animals that are severely fatigued and dyspneic, to allow for better administration of oxygen, esophageal drainage, and upper respiratory tract suction. Pentobarbitone can be used as a constant-rate infusion or given periodically IV to induce light anesthesia, with repeat doses as needed. Another potential benefit of pentobarbitone may be control of long QT syndrome. The chief benefits of some form of anesthesia (eg, profofol) are to reduce dyspnea, enable muscle rest, and help overcome primary muscle fatigue and general exhaustion. Periods of 6–8 hr of light anesthesia are best, with reassessment of clinical status after each period.

Mechanical or manual ventilation may be required but should be carefully assessed because recovery can be delayed, especially in brachycephalic animals. Longer-term ventilation cases can have a 70% recovery rate. It is essential to assess pulmonary (expired CO_2 levels) and alveolar (pulse oximetry) ventilatory capacity and to be aware of profound respiratory muscle fatigue. Alveolar disease (edema and/or pneumonia) has a poor prognosis in such cases.

Atropine (repeated every 6 hr, lowest dose) can be used if GI and respiratory secretions are excessive, but its effect on tear secretion (and the host's potential for eyelid paralysis, reduced blink reflex, and corneal drying) and cardiac rate and rhythm changes should be considered.

Antiemetic therapy should be used in animals that are vomiting, which is usually a poor prognostic sign. If the animal is regurgitating, the esophagus should be aspirated along with the upper respiratory tract. Correct drainage positioning then becomes a vital factor in helping to avoid aspiration. Care is needed with gastroesophageal reflux cases regarding their chronicity and tissue damage.

Broad-spectrum bactericidal antibiotics are indicated (especially in severe cases) to help avoid development of aspiration pneumonia, but they must be given as soon as possible. Dogs with upper respiratory tract obstruction require either tracheotomy or anesthesia and intubation to overcome the potentially lethal effects of such obstruction.

Diuretics (eg, furosemide) with maximally appropriate oxygen treatment are indicated to treat congestive heart failure. Verapamil (0.1 mg/kg, IV bolus) has been used to help relieve the basic toxic myocardial effect of a failure to relax. The toxin does unbind, so if the animal can be kept free of terminal pulmonary edema (or arrhythmia), the cardiac failure will reverse over a few days, provided routine support is given. Esmolol has been used to treat affected animals that have a long QT interval and the potential for a lethal, unpredictable ventricular arrhythmia.

Fluid therapy should be used with great care, because pulmonary edema can be induced easily. Staying below maintenance levels and ensuring the animal is assessed for edema, both before and during IV fluid therapy, should be routine. Dehydration can occur in tick paralysis but not usually in routine cases until the second day of hospitalization, when increased PCV and protein values may be evident. In small patients, SC or IP fluids can be given if lung status is a concern. Exceptional cases may require extensive rehydration (eg, paralyzed in the sun with high humidity and temperature for a day before presentation), but the extent of the underlying organ dysfunction should be assessed before intensive fluids are given.

The asthma-like disease in cats is hard to reverse, because routine bronchodilators do not seem to be effective.

Muscle fatigue can be reduced (with recovery of some muscle strength) by short periods (6–8 hr) of anesthesia. The animals remain hypercapneic but, with endotracheal intubation and O_2 therapy, can establish reasonable hemoglobin saturation levels (>95%), provided there is no significant alveolar disease.

Intoxicated animals lose their ability to regulate body temperature. Animals that have fallen below 32°C (90°F) for a long period may be hard to resuscitate. Various heating mechanisms are used (hot water bottles, blankets, hot air flow blankets), but peripheral heat absorption cannot occur if arteriovenous anastomoses (shunts) are shut due to the effect of the toxin and the host's vasoconstrictive reaction to hypothermia. Warmth applied at the lower limbs (especially the hindlimbs) will be of maximal benefit; direct application to the groin area may also potentially be useful. Some animals may need warmed fluids, IV or rectally, to reverse a very cold presentation (eg, ≤32°C). Sudden hyperthermia (>42°C) can be seen in hospitalized dogs. They usually show exaggerated head and possibly foreleg movements and signs of anxiousness. With cooling (eg, wet towels, direct fan flow, high rate of air changes), these signs abate.

Because the animal's condition is expected to deteriorate after ticks are removed and TAS is given, hospitalization with minimally invasive monitoring and good nursing care is necessary. The animal should be kept in a quiet, dark, comfortable area of the hospital where it can be easily seen. It should be placed on the sternum to maximize lung function. Lateral recumbency, left side down with the shoulder (not the pharynx or neck) as the highest point, is the best position for drainage. If possible, slight "head down" is also advised. Animals should never be rotated unless it can be done frequently (every 1–2 hr), day and night.

Because the animal cannot void, catheterization is necessary, with the bladder expressed at least twice daily to avoid infection. As with other localized tick toxicity effects, this may persist beyond the period when the animal has generally recovered. Eye protectants should be used to prevent corneal ulceration or dryness (lid closure, artificial tears, contacts). Suction of the pharynx, larynx, and proximal esophagus minimizes upper respiratory tract distress caused by saliva pooling and regurgitation. An esophageal tube may be slowly inserted to remove any pooled material; in some cases, this is voluminous and the tube may possibly prevent choke (seen mostly in brachycephalic breeds with laryngeal blockage by foreign material). Fluid and oxygen therapy should be monitored to avoid overhydration or under-supply, respectively. Nutritional support should be performed carefully to ensure that GI and respiratory function can cope with any offered food and water.

Repeated tick searches should be performed during hospitalization, especially if the animal deteriorates unexpectedly or is slow to recover. Long or matted hair should be clipped, especially about the head and neck. Application of an acaricide may kill any ticks missed in searching. However, the stress of searching, clipping, or bathing can be detrimental in severely affected or nervous animals, in which sedation is recommended.

Prognosis: Appropriate and timely treatment (TAS and antibiotics, especially in severe cases) saves ~95% of affected animals, but ~5% of animals are likely to die despite all treatment efforts, especially those with aspiration, or advanced respiratory paralysis and dyspnea. Most animals (>80%) have only one tick and a large attachment crater. Prolonged recovery and weight loss can be seen with various complications, and death can also occur due to choke, respiratory muscle fatigue, cardiac arrhythmias, congestive heart failure, and cardiopulmonary arrest. Older animals are at greater risk, as are very young pups. Proportionally more severe cases are seen at the start of the season, and a second (close to the first) infestation will be more severe. Dyspnea, crackles, and wheezes are poor prognostic signs, as are high neuromuscular junction scores (3 and 4) or high visual analog scale scores (≥75%) for toxicity or respiratory distress.

Before discharge, the drop test can be used in cats to assess neuromuscular function and three-dimensional gravitational control. Cats should be able to correct a fall from 10–20 cm above the top of the table. Still-affected cats will not correct in time and land more heavily, with the chin hitting the padded table top. Recovered cats land lightly with good head control. Jumping up to and down from the cage can also be used to assess muscle strength in cats. In dogs, jumping down from a cage can induce stridor, indicating unresolved respiratory paresis with forced expiratory air flow, because the unsupported abdominal momentum affects the diaphragm and lung air flow, producing a high-volume expiration. Lifting a dog (with the holder's arms wrapped outside the fore- and hindlegs) with unresolved tick paralysis often produces stridor, indicating abnormal laryngeal function. Animals should be able to eat, drink, and walk normally without any stridor before discharge.

Owners should be advised to continue searching recovered animals for ticks; use appropriate preventive methods to avoid reattachment of ticks; and avoid high temperatures, stress, or strenuous exercise for at least the first month. Smaller, more frequent meals may also be indicated if there was esophageal dysfunction. This rest period especially applies to working farm dogs, in which early overexercise may lead to permanent muscle damage.

Prevention and Control: Owners should not rely solely on chemical control to prevent tick infestation, because no product is totally effective, and a single attached tick can cause the disease. They should be advised about when and where their pets will be at risk; encouraged to thoroughly search the coat daily; keep the coat as short as possible (to aid searching); and understand the efficacy, appropriateness, safety, and limitations of available preventive products (sprays, topical spot-ons, tablets, and collars). Combination therapy (eg, spray and collar) may give better results by using two modes of action, but there are no published data to support this concept.

Attempts to produce an effective vaccine against the *I holocyclus* toxin have so far been unsuccessful, as have been attempts at "in-field" tick control. Specific RNA studies show that ticks vary geographically, and such genetic differences may explain why clinical signs of tick paralysis and visual analog scale toxicity scores can vary between different areas at the same time of the year in the same season.

REPRODUCTIVE SYSTEM

SMALL ANIMALS

REPRODUCTIVE SYSTEM INTRODUCTION

The reproductive system provides the mechanism for the recombination of genetic material that allows for change and adaptation. Manipulation of this system in breeding management programs allows the rapid and dramatic alteration of the conformation and productivity of domestic animals. Theriogenology is the veterinary clinical specialty that deals with reproduction. The reproductive system is incredibly complex in both its anatomy and physiology, and all aspects must be considered when resolving reproductive problems. The differences in the reproductive system between the sexes and among species are extensive. Both sexes have primary sex organs and primary regulatory centers. Gonads and function-adapted, tubular genital organs constitute primary sex organs in both sexes. The pituitary gland and the hypothalamus are the primary regulatory centers; thus, the regulatory function is, in part, neuroendocrine in nature. In pregnant females, the fetoplacental unit has a significant role in maintaining and terminating pregnancy.

For the temporal and physiologic features of the reproductive cycles of selected species, *see* TABLES 1–3.

THE GONADS AND TUBULAR GENITAL TRACT

Both sexes have a pair of gonads (ovaries or testes). However, in birds the right ovary does not develop; only the left ovary and oviduct are present in adult females. The main functions of the gonads are

TABLE 1 APPROXIMATE GESTATION PERIODS

Domestic Animals	Days	Wild Animals	Days
Cat	65	Bear (Black)	210
Cattle[a]		Bison	280
Angus	281	Camel	365-400
Ayrshire	279	Chimpanzee	236
Brahman	292	Coyote	63
Brown Swiss	290	Deer (Mule and White-tailed)	200
Charolais	289	Elephant	660
Guernsey	283	Elk, Wapiti	255
Hereford	285	Giraffe	425
Holstein	279	Gorilla	270
Jersey	279	Hare	36
Limousin	289	Hippopotamus	240
Shorthorn	282	Leopard	95
Simmental	289	Lion	108
Dog	62–64[b]	Marmoset	150
Donkey	365	Monkey (Macaque)	180
Goat	150	Moose	235
Horse[c]	335–342	Muskox	255
Llama, Alpaca[c]	335–365	Opossum	12
Pig	114	Panther	90
Sheep	150	Porcupine	210
Fur Animals	**Days**	Pronghorn	250
Chinchilla	111	Raccoon	63
Ferret	42	Reindeer	225
Fox	52	Rhinoceros (African)	480
Mink		Seal	330
European	41	Shrew	20
American	40–75	Skunk	63
Muskrat	29	Squirrel (Gray)	40
Nutria, Coypu	130	Tapir	390
Otter	270–300[d]	Tiger	103
Rabbit	31	Walrus	450
Wolf	63	Whale (Sperm)	450
		Woodchuck	31

See also SELECTED PHYSIOLOGIC DATA OF LABORATORY ANIMALS, p 1842.

[a] Individuals may range ±7–10 days from these averages.

[b] Gestation period is 58–72 days from breeding at unknown stage of estrus; from day of ovulation (which can be determined by progesterone or LH monitoring), gestation period is 62–64 days.

[c] Individuals may range 20 days from these averages.

[d] 180+ days due to delayed implantation

TABLE 2 APPROXIMATE INCUBATION PERIODS

Domestic Birds	Days	Caged and Game Birds	Days
Chicken	21	Budgerigar	18
Duck	28	Finch	14
Muscovy duck	35	Parrot	26
Goose	28	Pheasant	24
Guinea fowl	28	Pigeon	18
Turkey	28	Quail	16
		Swan	35

gametogenesis and steroidogenesis. Both functions are regulated primarily by gonadotropins released by the anterior pituitary gland under the influence of the hypothalamus. Hypothalamic control of the pituitary is mediated by a peptide, gonadotropin-releasing hormone (GnRH); the secretion and release of GnRH are governed by CNS stimuli and, through a feedback mechanism, by hormones produced by other endocrine organs such as the gonads, pituitary, thyroid, and adrenal glands. (*See also* ENDOCRINE SYSTEM, p 538, et seq.)

The Ovaries: The size and location of the ovaries vary with the species. The ovaries can be directly examined by ultrasonography or by palpation per rectum only in larger animals (eg, cows, mares, and camelids). Once puberty is reached (*see* TABLE 3), the size and form of the ovaries are altered by cyclic functional structures, namely the corpus luteum (CL) and ovarian follicles. Follicle-stimulating hormone (FSH) is responsible for development of ovarian follicles and synthesis of estrogens. Once a certain estrogen level is attained, luteinizing hormone (LH) is released from the anterior pituitary gland in spontaneously ovulating species. This LH release triggers ovulation, which is followed by development of a new CL. The increase of luteal cells parallels an increase in progesterone output. In nonpregnant polyestrous and seasonally polyestrous females, the functional and morphologic life of the CL is terminated by endogenous prostaglandin (PG) $F_2\alpha$ from the uterus. As the CL regresses, a new ovulatory follicle(s) develops, which completes the estrous cycle. The hormonal changes during the estrous cycle can be monitored by laboratory assay of hormones in blood, milk, or feces. Estrual cycling is continuous after puberty unless interrupted by pregnancy and, in some species, by season or lactation during the immediate postpartum period. Cycling may also be blocked by pathologic conditions of the ovaries (eg, nutritional atrophy or ovarian cysts) as well as by uterine disease (eg, pyometra), which may result in persistent luteal function. Estrogens and progesterone act locally, affecting target organs such as the tubular genital tract, and distally, regulating gonadotropin release by a feedback mechanism on both the hypothalamus and anterior pituitary. In addition, they play a prominent role in sexual behaviors, lactation, and the development of secondary sex characteristics.

The Testes: The testes function in both spermatogenesis and secretion of steroid hormones. Spermatogenesis is stimulated by FSH and augmented by androgens, primarily testosterone. Interstitial cells of the testes, under the influence of LH, produce testosterone. Testosterone and its metabolites are required for development and function of accessory glands, copulatory organs, male sex characteristics, and behavior. For optimal spermatogenesis, mammalian testes must descend into the scrotal cavity; however, steroidogenesis occurs in testes that remain within the abdomen, and the libido of cryptorchid males is usually not impaired. Photoperiod affects both sperm cell formation and steroidogenesis in males of species that have a seasonal reproductive pattern. Semen quality, libido, and mating ability are reduced during the seasonally anestrous period of females. Function of the testes can be assessed by evaluation of representative semen samples and hormone assays. Examination and measurement of the testes help predict potential sperm output and may reveal pathologic conditions.

TABLE 3 FEATURES OF THE REPRODUCTIVE CYCLE

Species	Age at Puberty	Cycle Type	Cycle Length	Duration of Estrus
Cattle	10–12 mo, usually first bred ~14-15 mo	Polyestrous all year	21 days (18–24)	18 hr (6–24)
Sheep	6–9 mo	Seasonally polyestrous, early fall to winter	17 days (14–20)	24–36 hr
Goat	5–7 mo	Seasonally polyestrous, early fall to late winter	21 days	24–48 hr
Pig	6–7 mo	Polyestrous all year	21 days (19–23)	40–60 hr
Horse	10–24 mo	Seasonally polyestrous, early spring through summer	~21 days (19–23)	5–7 days
Alpaca	12–18 mo	Polyestrous all year in North America	Not applicable	Up to 36 days
Dog	6–24 mo; earlier in smaller breeds, later in larger breeds	Monestrous all year	6–7 mo	9 days (3–21)
Cat	4–12 mo	Seasonally polyestrous, spring through early fall	14–21 days	6–7 days

The Female Tubular Genital Tract: Except for the vestibule, which develops from the urogenital sinus, the female genital tract is derived from the embryonic paramesonephric ducts. Each of the segments is adapted to fulfill its function. The oviduct acquires the egg(s) and moves the resulting zygote(s) into the uterus, while its secretion provides a proper environment for survival of gametes, fertilization, and the first few critical days of embryonic life. Interference with motility or secretion leads to infertility. Species variation of the bicornual, Y-shaped uterus involves the size of the body and length of horns, which are adapted to accommodate species-specific number and form of fetuses and placentas. The cervix provides a protective barrier that is relatively effective against ascending infections. Morphologic and functional integrity of the uterus and cervix are required to establish and maintain pregnancy and for parturition. Infections contracted at mating or during parturition and the puerperium are common causes of female infertility. Applicability of diagnostic methods for detection of uterine and cervical abnormalities depends on species, size of the animal, and anatomy of the cervix. Clinical diagnosis is by transrectal and abdominal palpation, vaginoscopy, hysteroscopy, radiography, and ultrasonography. In small animals, laparotomy or laparoscopy may be necessary to assist with diagnosis. Laboratory diagnostic aids include microbiologic and cytologic examination of exudate or secretion, histologic examination of biopsies, endometrial cytology, and hormone assays.

The posterior tract, consisting of the vagina, vestibule, and vulva, serves as the copulatory organ and as the last segment of the birth canal. It also provides a pathway for ascending infections, particularly when effectiveness of the vestibulovaginal sphincter or the vulvar labia is lost or reduced because of trauma, relaxation, or defective conformation of the perineal region. Puerperal infections commonly involve the entire tubular tract. In addition,

TABLE 3 FEATURES OF THE REPRODUCTIVE CYCLE *(continued)*

Best Time to Breed	First Estrus After Parturition	Comments
Insemination from midestrus until 6 hr after end of estrus	20–60 days	Ovulation 10–12 hr after end of estrus.
18–20 hr after onset of estrus	Next fall	Ovulation near end of estrus.
Daily during estrus	Next fall	Many intersexes born in hornless strains.
Daily during estrus	4–10 days after weaning	Ovulation usually ~40 hr after beginning of estrus.
Last few days of estrus, just before ovulation; should be bred at 2-day intervals	4–14 (9) days	Ovulation usually 1–2 days before end of estrus. Double ovulation occurs in ~20% of estrous periods, but twins rarely progress to term.
When a large, viable follicle is present	Fertile within 15–20 days	Alpacas are induced ovulators.
Second day after ovulation	4–5 mo	Proestrous bleeding 7–10 days. Ovulation usually 1–3 days after onset of estrus. Ova shed before first polar body has been extruded (primary oocyte).
Daily from day 2 of estrus	4–6 wk	Induced ovulation 24–48 hr after breeding. Pseudopregnancy lasts 40 days. Infertile matings delay onset of next cycle ~45 days.

vestibulovaginal infection perpetuated by urovagina and pneumovagina may sustain chronic infection of the uterus. However, the vestibule and vagina can be inflamed even when the uterus is normal or pregnant. Conversely, in closed-cervix pyometra in cows and bitches, the vagina and vestibule may essentially be normal.

The Male Tubular Genital Tract: In males, the tubular tract provides a pathway for sperm cells and seminal fluid. It begins in the testes as the rete testes and efferent ductules, which exit the testes and merge to become the head, body, and tail of the epididymis; it then continues as the ductus deferens. In mammals, the ductus deferens ascends into the abdominal cavity via the inguinal ring and passes over the dorsal aspect of the bladder to enter the pelvic urethra. The testes in birds are permanently retained in the abdominal cavity. The pelvic and penile urethras are shared as an outlet for semen and urine. Along this pathway, certain segments of the tract have evolved morphologically and functionally to perform additional specific functions. The epididymides are involved in sperm cell maturation and storage and in selective absorption of abnormal spermatozoa. Ampullae and accessory sex glands (ie, seminal vesicles, prostate, bulbourethral glands) contribute to the formation of seminal plasma. The size, form, and function of the accessory sex glands vary among species. The seminal vesicles and the bulbourethral glands are absent in dogs. In bulls, the epididymides and seminal vesicles are common sites of infection. Epididymitis is also common in rams. Prostatic infections, hypertrophy, and malignancy are found primarily in dogs. Pathologic conditions of the epididymides can be diagnosed by scrotal palpation or ultrasonography in most animals. Other diseases or functional disturbances may require evaluation of one or several semen samples. Common semen collection techniques used in veterinary medicine include artificial vagina, electroejaculation, and post-mating recovery from an estrual female. The preferred technique varies with the species and operator preference. The pelvic accessory sex organs can be assessed by transrectal palpation and ultrasonography in large animals and by digital palpation or transabdominal ultrasonography in small animals.

INFERTILITY

Interaction of the CNS, hypothalamus, pituitary gland, gonads, and their target organs results in finely coordinated sequences of physiologic events that lead to estrus and ovulation in females and to ejaculation of fertile semen by males. For optimal results, ovulation and deposition of semen into the female genital tract must be closely synchronized. Failure of any single functional event in either sex leads to infertility or sterility.

The ultimate manifestation of infertility is failure to produce offspring. In polytocous species, a subnormal number of offspring also constitutes infertility. In females, infertility may be due to failure to cycle, aberrations of the estrous cycle, failure to conceive, or prenatal and perinatal death of the conceptus. Major infertility problems in males are caused by disturbances of the production, transport, or storage of spermatozoa; aberration of libido; and partial or complete inability to mate.

Most (if not all) major infertility problems have a complex etiology, and several factors, singly or in combination, can cause reproductive failure. Pathogenesis may be equally complex.

Diagnostic Approach: Because the female bears the offspring, she reflects either success or failure of reproduction. However, the first diagnostic step (regardless of the complaint) is to establish the etiologic role of the female and the male. Additionally, each point of human involvement in the reproductive process, such as observation for estrus, preservation of semen, and insemination methodology, is a potential source of error. Such human errors can be detected or excluded by assessment of performance, with the main emphasis on techniques and procedures and their adequacy and quality.

Diagnostic methods have been developed to test the anatomic and functional soundness of both sexes. These include the signalment, a complete history, and clinical examination, supported by diagnostic aids such as endoscopy, ultrasonography, and laboratory tests (eg, hormone assays, microbiology, cytology, serology, cytogenetic examination, genetic testing, and semen evaluation). The choice of diagnostic methods is determined by the species as well as by the size and temperament of the animal. Decisions with regard to type and extent of laboratory tests are based on history and information gained during the course of clinical examination. In each case of reproductive failure, the diagnostic plan should provide evidence to establish the role of the female, the male, and the breeding management program.

Reproductive problems are seldom accompanied by alarming signs of disease. Furthermore, there is a time interval between when a failure occurs and when it becomes apparent. Examples are intervals between unsuccessful service and return to estrus or failure to give birth. This lag period may allow recovery, yielding negative results on examination. Interpretation of results also must account for species differences and, in species with a seasonal reproductive pattern, the fact that infertility may be physiologic during certain parts of the year.

PRINCIPLES OF THERAPY

See also SYSTEMIC PHARMACOTHERAPEUTICS OF THE REPRODUCTIVE SYSTEM, p 2606, and MANAGEMENT OF REPRODUCTION for the various species, p 2171, et seq.

The increasing demands for production efficiency, along with changes in management systems, have caused a shift in therapeutic strategies in several domestic species. Especially for food and fiber animals, the therapeutic approach of choice often is a combination of pharmacologic agents and correction of management problems targeting the entire herd, with a decreased emphasis on individual animals. This trend is also reflected in the prioritization of disease prevention and implementation of biosecurity programs. The increased use of hormonal pharmacologic agents for reproductive management on a whole-herd basis represents another aspect of this change. Other therapeutic trends in food animals are the result of consumer concerns regarding antimicrobial and hormone residues in tissues and milk, as well as the increasing interest in organic or natural foods.

In small animals, therapeutic strategy has undergone a different but equally dramatic transformation. The individual animal remains the focus of therapeutic efforts, but diagnostic techniques and treatments have become increasingly sophisticated, often reflecting or even presaging advances in human medicine.

More effective therapy for reproductive diseases comes with the risk of propagating a hereditary predisposition for lowered fertility. However, the heritability of most reproductive traits is rather low, so selection programs aimed at improving fertility require a longterm commitment to be successful.

Pharmacologic Control of Reproduction: Exogenous hormone therapy can be used to regulate or control reproduction. This control may take the form of suppression or induction and synchronization of reproductive activity. The same hormone may be used for both purposes. For example, progestogens are used to suppress estrus in the mare, bitch, and queen but are also used in the mare, cow, and sow to induce and synchronize estrus for managed mating programs. Steroid hormones with estrogenic, androgenic, and progestational effects are used in a wide variety of applications.

The gonadotropins and GnRH are used to alter gonadal function. Examples include superovulation of cattle with FSH, induction of ovulation in mares with human chorionic gonadotropin (hCG), and stimulation of testosterone production with GnRH for diagnosis of cryptorchidism in dogs and stallions.

$PGF_2\alpha$ is used primarily to terminate luteal function. Clinical applications include induction or synchronization of estrus in polyestrous species; treatment of pyometra in dogs, cats, and cattle; and induction of abortion in luteal-dependent species such as goats, alpacas, dogs, and cats.

Depending on the species, glucocorticoids, prostaglandin, and oxytocin, alone or in combination, can be used to induce or manage labor. They should be used with caution at the appropriate time and dosage and accompanied by careful observation for any problems that may develop with the dam or fetus.

Assisted Reproductive Technologies: Many of the assisted reproductive technologies commonly used today had their origin in veterinary species as either research or commercial programs. Artificial insemination is commonly used to breed cattle, dogs, sheep, goats, pigs, and horses. Other technologies in use include embryo transfer (*see* p 2239) and in vitro fertilization in cattle and horses. Somatic cell nuclear transfer (cloning, *see* p 2075) is more rarely performed but has been reported for a variety of animal species.

Antimicrobial Treatment: Antimicrobial agents, most commonly antibiotics, are used for treatment of infections of the male and female reproductive tracts in all species (*see also* ANTIBACTERIAL AGENTS, p 2652, et seq). Drug selection should be based, whenever possible, on microbiologic culture and sensitivity tests. The dosage, route of administration, and interval between treatments vary among species. In food animals, proper withholding times must be observed for meat and milk after antibiotic use.

Surgical Treatment: Surgical repair is indicated for acquired conformational damage to the genital system of both sexes. Examples include episioplasty, vestibulovaginal or cervical cerclage, and cesarean section in females and repair of preputial injuries in males. Surgical sterilization is also routinely done, either by gonadectomy in both sexes of most species or by ovariohysterectomy in female cats and dogs.

CONGENITAL AND INHERITED ANOMALIES OF THE REPRODUCTIVE SYSTEM

INTERSEX CONDITIONS

Sex determination of the gonads is important for development of the sex phenotype (internal and external genitalia, secondary characteristics) and sexual behavior. A sex chromosome genotype of XY leads to the development of testes due to the sex-determining region of the Y chromosome (*SRY*) gene. The *SRY* gene induces downstream factors such as *SRY*-box containing gene 9 (*SOX9*), anti-Müllerian hormone, and glial cell line–derived neurotrophic factor in Sertoli cells.

Intersex conditions have been described in several domestic animal species. True hermaphrodites are rare and have both ovarian and testicular tissue and exhibit anomalies of the external genitalia. The chromosomal makeup is variable and may be a chimera, mosaic, or unknown. Pseudohermaphroditism, often referred to as sex reversal syndrome, is more common. Animals have one or the other type of gonad and external genitalia of the opposite sex. Animals may be XY *SRY* negative or XX *SRY* negative. In horses, the most common type is 64XY *SRY* negative. Some cases of sex reversal are believed to be due to a recessive autosomal gene mutation.

The most common intersex condition, the male pseudohermaphrodite, has testicular tissue in the abdominal cavity or beneath the skin in the scrotal region, and external genital organs that resemble those of females. Miniature Schnauzers, Basset Hounds, and rarely, Persian cats may present with pseudohermaphroditism when affected by persistent paramesonephric (Müllerian) duct syndrome. Undescended testes are attached to the uterine horns, and the vasa deferentia are located in the wall of the uterus. There are bilateral oviducts, a complete uterus with a cervix, and a cranial portion of the vagina. Bilateral scrotal testes or unilateral or bilateral cryptorchidism may be present. Affected animals can present clinically with pyometra, urinary tract infection, prostate infection, or Sertoli cell tumor. The diagnosis is confirmed by presence of a 78, XY chromosome constitution, bilateral testes, and the presence of all paramesonephric (Müllerian) duct derivatives. Androgen-dependent masculinization is that of a normal male. Treatment is limited to castration and hysterectomy. The defect is inherited as an autosomal recessive trait in Miniature Schnauzers, and both females and males can be carriers. Homozygous affected dogs with a descended testis are generally fertile and capable of transmitting the trait to all offspring.

Polled intersex syndrome is well described in goats. Polled homozygotic males have decreased fertility due to segmental aplasia of the epididymides. They are often XX *SRY* negative.

Freemartinism: Freemartinism syndrome is well known in cattle but has also been described in sheep, goats, and camelids. It causes sterility in females born co-twin to males; ~92% of all heifers born co-twin to bull calves are sterile. Single-born freemartin females have been reported and are believed to result from the in utero death of a male co-twin. These animals exhibit varying degrees of female-to-male sex reversal of the internal and external genitalia. The tubular genital organs in affected animals range from cordlike bands to near-normal uterine horns. Freemartins have a short vagina that ends blindly without communication with the uterus. The cervix is absent. The ovaries usually fail to develop and remain small. Vascular anastomosis of the chorionic placentas of the two fetuses results in transfer of anti-Müllerian hormone from the male to the female fetus, which inhibits development of the female tract.

Normal and freemartin cattle can be differentiated based on length of the vagina and on the presence or absence of a cervix. In calves 1–4 wk old, the normal vaginal length is 13–15 cm, whereas in a freemartin vaginal length is 5–6 cm. Vaginal length is easily measured by gently inserting a well-lubricated probe with a blunt end into the vagina. Cytogenetic examination can demonstrate XX and XY chromosome patterns in freemartins. The interchange of cells that occurs in the placental circulation between the fetuses can also be demonstrated by detecting two different blood types in a single animal.

Other Chromosomal Abnormalities: Chromosomal abnormalities (XXY) have been described in males with azoospermia due to hypoplasia of the testes, epididymis, and vas deferens. Tortoise-shell or calico male cats possess two X chromosomes (XX/XXY, XY/XXY, or other chimeric or mosaic combination) and are sterile.

MALE GENITAL ABNORMALITIES

Abnormalities of the Testis and Epididymis: **Cryptorchidism** is a failure of one or both testicles to descend into the scrotum. It is seen in all domestic animals; it is common in stallions and boars and is the most common disorder of sexual development in dogs (13%). Cryptorchidism is caused by a combination of genetic, epigenetic, and environmental factors. Bilateral cryptorchidism results in sterility. Unilateral cryptorchidism is more common, and the male is usually fertile because of sperm production from the normally descended testicle. The undescended testicle may be located anywhere from just caudal of the kidney to within the inguinal canal and can be identified by transrectal or transabdominal ultrasonography. Abdominal testicles produce male hormones, and cryptorchid animals have normal secondary sex characteristics and mating behavior. Cryptorchidectomy is recommended for all companion animals because of the suspected inherited nature of the condition and predisposition to testicular neoplasia (seminomas, interstitial cell tumors).

Testicular hypoplasia has been described in several domestic species and is associated with chromosomal abnormalities in some cases. It is common in some family lines in camelids.

Anorchism is the complete absence of development of one or both testes. Unilateral anarchism has been described in horses and camelids. In camelids, the kidney ipsilateral to the missing testis is also missing.

Partial or complete segmental aplasia of the structures originating from the mesonephric duct (epididymis, ductus deferens, ampullae and seminal vesicles) has been described in bulls. Bilateral epididymal hypoplasia has been described in azoospermic stallions and camelids. In camelids, segmental aplasia of the epididymis is often associated with epididymal and rete testis cysts.

Abnormalities of the Penis and Prepuce: **Persistent penile frenulum** is not uncommon. Affected bulls are unable to protrude the penis from the sheath and, in most cases, cannot achieve intromission. Attachment can be minimal (eg, 0.5 cm), or the preputial mucosa can be attached the full length of the ventral raphe of the free part of the penis. Genetic association is suspected in some breeds. Surgical correction should not be performed in bulls intended for seedstock breeding. Many male foals may appear to have a persistent frenulum at birth, but the condition resolves within a few days. If the condition persists, correction should not be attempted until the foal is at least 1 mo old.

Preputial prolapse occurs due to a lack of or a weak preputial retractor muscle in polled breeds. The condition is exacerbated when these breeds are crossed with Brahman cattle.

Congenital short penis has been described in bulls and may be associated with short retractor penis muscles, which prevent full erection. Bulls may breed satisfactorily in the first season, but copulation becomes impossible as their body size increases.

Short retractor penis muscle may occur congenitally or after injury to the penis or prepuce. Affected bulls have normal libido, but during attempted service the penis is only partially protruded from the sheath and the ejaculatory thrust does not occur. Failure of erection in bulls may be a congenital condition but is generally a sequela of trauma and/or hematoma of the penis.

Congenital vascular shunts have been described in bulls with partial erection or erection failure.

Hypospadias is an abnormal opening of the urethra due to failure or incomplete closure of the embryonic urethral groove.

FEMALE GENITAL ABNORMALITIES

Ovarian Abnormalities: The most common congenital abnormality of the ovary is ovarian dysgenesis or ovarian hypoplasia. Ovarian dysgenesis has been described in several domestic animal species and has been associated with various chromosomal abnormalities (monosomy X or Turner syndrome, trisomy XXX, or Klinefelter syndrome XXY). The ovaries are very small and lack follicular activity.

Segmental Aplasia of the Paramesonephric Ducts: The paramesonephric ducts are paired embryonic ducts that develop into the anterior vagina, cervix, uterus, and uterine tube. Segmental aplasia of the paramesonephric ducts results in anomalies of those organs. The aplasia (obstruction) may be located in a segment of the uterine tube, uterine horn, cervix, or vagina. Ovarian development is normal. Accumulation of secretions proximal to the obstruction occurs secondarily (hydrosalpinx, hydrometra, mucometra, colpometra).

Segmental aplasia of the uterus may involve one horn (resulting in a condition called uterus unicornis), both horns, or only part of one horn (which may result in cystic dilatation of the uterine horn anterior to the area of dilatation). Uterus unicornis has been described in several domestic animal species. The condition seems to be relatively common in camelids. These females can become pregnant and carry the pregnancy to term. Cervical aplasia has been described in a few cases but is not as common.

True persistence of the hymen or imperforation of the hymen is the most commonly reported paramesonephric duct anomaly in domestic animals. Fluid accumulates in the vagina and uterus, resulting in protrusion of the hymen at the vulva when the animal is lying down or straining. Hymenal defects are most common in white Shorthorn cattle (white heifer disease).

Cervical Abnormalities: Double external os of the cervix is due to a failure of the paramesonephric ducts to fuse. It may present as a band of tissue caudal to, or in, the external os of the cervix. In other cases, there is a true double external os opening into a single caudal part of the cervical canal. Affected cows usually conceive normally. Rarely, a true double cervix, with a complete septum between the two cervical canals, each opening into its respective uterine horn (uterus didelphys), occurs.

Vaginal and Vulvar Abnormalities:

Vaginal stricture or vestibulovaginal hypoplasia has been described in mares, dogs, and camelids.

Gartner's ducts, located beneath the mucosa of the floor of the vagina, may develop multiple cysts, which are generally of no clinical significance.

Vulvar atresia or hypoplasia (atresia vulvi) has been described primarily in camelids. In extreme cases, the labia are completely fused. The condition is believed to be due to an autosomal recessive gene.

Rectovaginal constriction is a connective tissue disorder of Jersey cattle characterized by stenosis of the anus and/or vestibulovaginal sphincter. Bilateral stenosis of the milk veins has also been described and results in udder edema and ischemic necrosis. It is a simple autosomal recessive defect. Anal stenosis renders transrectal palpation difficult. Affected females experience severe dystocia. The prevalence of the disease has been substantially reduced because of identification of carrier bulls.

ABORTION IN LARGE ANIMALS

Abortion is the termination of pregnancy after organogenesis is complete but before the expelled fetus can survive. If pregnancy ends before organogenesis, it is called early embryonic death. A dead, full-term fetus is a stillbirth (its lungs are not inflated). Many etiologies of abortion also cause stillbirths, mummification, and weak or deformed neonates.

The etiologic diagnosis of abortion in livestock is a difficult and often frustrating task. The diagnostic success rate is relatively low and variable: 30%–40% for bovine, 60%–65% for ovine, 35%–40% for porcine, and from <10% to 90% in equine abortion cases submitted to diagnostic laboratories. The diagnostic success rate in camelids is very low except in outbreaks. Numerous factors complicate diagnosis. Often, abortion follows initial infection by weeks or months, so the causative agent is no longer apparent when abortion occurs. Expulsion may follow fetal death by hours or days, with lesions obscured by autolysis. Fetal membranes and the aborted fetus are usually contaminated by environmental agents before examination. Many sporadic abortions are likely the result of noninfectious (ie, toxic or genetic) causes, about which much less is known than infectious causes; many diagnostic laboratories are not equipped or staffed to deal with these causes of abortion.

Another problem in determining the cause of abortions is improper or inadequate specimen selection and handling. The best specimen is the complete fetoplacental unit in fresh condition, along with maternal serum. The placenta and fetus should be cleaned with water or saline, packed in clean plastic bags, chilled (but not frozen), and rapidly transported to the diagnostic laboratory. In most cases, autolysis proceeds at a much slower rate in fetuses than in carcasses of animals born alive. If chilled as soon as possible, most fetuses will be suitable for examination, even if they do not reach the laboratory for 1–2 days. Fetal pigs, sheep, and goats are usually small enough to transport or ship whole with the placenta. If there are multiple fetuses, three to five should be submitted with their placentas. It is best to submit calves and foals whole, but in many cases it is more convenient to perform a necropsy and collect samples for submission.

The specimens routinely used for testing vary somewhat between diagnostic laboratories, but a basic set of samples that will allow thorough examination includes stomach or abomasal contents; heart blood or fluid from a body cavity; unfixed lung, liver, kidney, and spleen (some laboratories also request tissues such as thyroid glands, thymus, heart, brain, abomasum, and stomach); placenta (if available); and dam's serum. These should be submitted in sterile containers to allow for microbiologic cultures. Because they are always contaminated, placentas should not be mixed with other tissues.

Representative samples of the following should also be submitted in 10% buffered formalin for histopathologic examination: lung, liver, heart, kidney, spleen, brain, skeletal muscle, thyroid, adrenal glands, intestines, and placenta (*see* p 1584). In a large majority of cases, gross lesions other than signs of autolysis (increased pleural and peritoneal fluid and blood-tinged subcutaneous edema) are not present. However, if lesions are found, fresh and formalin-fixed samples of affected tissues should be included.

Most agents, especially bacteria and fungi, infect the placenta and thus gain entry into the amniotic fluid, which is swallowed by the fetus. Stomach contents can be obtained aseptically, making it the best specimen for detection of fungi and most bacteria. Isolation from the stomach contents is much easier than from the placenta, which is always heavily contaminated. Lungs, liver, spleen, and kidneys are also good for culture. Several agents (eg, fungi, *Chlamydia*, *Coxiella*) primarily affect the placenta; failure to include placenta decreases the probability they will be identified. Fetuses sometimes produce antibodies to certain agents (eg, bovine viral diarrhea virus, *Neospora* spp, *Leptospira* spp), and fetal serum or fluid from a body cavity can be tested for antibodies. The presence of precolostral antibodies is evidence of in utero exposure.

A single antibody titer in the dam rarely provides evidence of abortion caused by a particular agent unless background herd titer levels are known. High maternal titers may as likely be the reason an animal did not abort due to that agent, but absence of a titer can be used to exclude an agent. Antibody titers to agents with control programs (eg, *Brucella abortus*, pseudorabies virus) are always significant, even if the abortion was caused by something else. Demonstration of a 4-fold increase in antibody titer is required to prove active infection by a specific agent. Often, abortion occurs weeks or months after initial infection of the dam, and her titer is stable or declining at the time of abortion. Paired serum samples obtained 2 wk apart from 10% of the herd or a minimum of 10 animals often demonstrate seroconversion and provide evidence of active infection in the herd.

ABORTION IN CATTLE

See also MANAGEMENT OF REPRODUCTION: CATTLE, p 2171.

Given the low diagnostic success rate, the high cost of laboratory work, and the low profit margin in both the beef and dairy industries, veterinarians should not attempt to make an etiologic diagnosis in every abortion. Instead, veterinarians should become concerned if fetal loss is >3%–5% per year or per month.

Noninfectious Causes

The actual incidence of abortions in cows due to genetic factors is unknown. Some genetically caused abortions may not have phenotypically recognizable lesions. Most lethal genes cause early abortion or early embryonic death.

Vitamins A and E, selenium, and iron have been implicated in bovine abortions, but documentation based on experiments is available only for vitamin A.

Heat stress causes fetal hypotension, hypoxia, and acidosis. High maternal temperature due to pyrexia may be more important than environmentally induced heat stress.

Although severe trauma may rarely result in abortion (the bovine fetus is well protected by the amniotic fluid), farmers undoubtedly blame too many abortions on the cow "getting bumped."

A number of toxins can cause abortion in cows. Ponderosa pine needles can cause abortion if ingested in the last trimester; the cows may become moribund after delivery and hemorrhage excessively. The main abortifacient compounds in Ponderosa pine needles are isocupressic acid and labdane resin. Locoweed (*Oxytropis* or *Astragalus* sp) contains an indolizidine alkaloid that can affect the corpus luteum, chorioallantois, and neurons, resulting in abortion or deformities. Broomweed (*Guttierrezia microcephala*) ingestion can also cause abortion, as can coumarins from rat poison, many grasses, or moldy sweet clover. Sodium iodide, IV, has been contraindicated in pregnant cows, but no abortions or adverse effects occurred in pregnant cows treated with a single high dose in some studies. Mycotoxins, especially those with estrogenic activity, have been implicated in bovine abortions. Nitrates or nitrites have also been incriminated, but experimental evidence is controversial.

Infectious Causes

Neosporosis: *Neospora caninum* is found worldwide and is the most common cause of abortion in dairy and beef cattle in many parts of the USA. Dogs and coyotes are definitive hosts for *N caninum* and can be the source of infection. Abortion can occur any time after 3 mo of gestation but is most common between 4 and 6 mo of gestation. *Neospora* can be associated with sporadic abortions or abortion storms, and repeat abortions in cows have been reported. Most infections result in an asymptomatic congenitally infected calf. Some infected calves are born with paralysis or proprioceptive deficits. Cows are not clinically ill, and placental retention is not common. The fetus is usually autolyzed or, in a few cases, mummified and rarely has gross lesions. Microscopically, nonsuppurative inflammation is common in the brain, heart, and skeletal muscles. Organisms can be identified in these tissues and the kidneys by immunohistochemical staining and PCR. Many late gestation fetuses have precolostral antibodies. They remain infected for years and possibly for life. Vertical transmission is common. During pregnancy, *Neospora* organisms can become activated and infect the fetus. This is thought to be the most common source of infection. There is no treatment. Strict hygiene to prevent fecal contamination of feed by dogs or coyotes may aid in prevention. A commercial vaccine is available. (*See also* p 663.)

Bovine Viral Diarrhea (BVD): In several surveys, BVD was the most commonly diagnosed virus in bovine abortion cases. The pathology of BVD in the developing fetus is complex. Infection before insemination or during the first 40 days of pregnancy results in infertility or embryonic death. Infection between 40 and 125 days of pregnancy results in birth of persistently infected calves if the fetus survives. Fetal infection during the period of organogenesis (100–150 days) may result in congenital malformations of the CNS (cerebellar hypoplasia, hydrancephaly, hydrocephalus, microencephaly, and spinal cord hypoplasia). Congenital ocular defects have also been seen (cataracts, optic neuritis, retinal degeneration, microphthalmia). After 125 days of gestation, BVD may cause abortion, or the fetal immune response may clear the virus. Diagnosis is by identification of BVD virus by isolation, immunologic staining, PCR, or detection of precolostral antibodies in aborted calves. The virus is present in a wide variety of tissues, but the spleen is the tissue of choice. Rising antibody titers to BVD in aborting animals or herdmates is diagnostic of recent infection. BVD virus is immunosuppressive and is found in many fetuses infected by other agents (eg, bacteria, *N caninum*). Outbreaks of abortions by organisms that normally cause sporadic abortion should raise suspicion of possible concurrent BVD virus infection. Prevention should focus on removal of persistently infected cattle and herd vaccination. (*See also* p 267.)

Infectious Bovine Rhinotracheitis (IBR, Bovine Herpesvirus 1): Infectious bovine rhinotracheitis (IBR) is a major cause of viral abortion in the world, with abortion rates of 5%–60% in nonvaccinated herds. The virus is widespread, causes latent infections, and can recrudesce; therefore, any cow with a positive IBR titer is a possible carrier. The virus is carried to the placenta in WBCs; over the next 2 wk to 4 mo, it causes a placentitis, then infects the fetus and kills it in 24 hr. Abortion can occur any time but usually is from 4 mo to term. Autolysis is consistently present. Occasionally, there are small foci of necrosis in the liver, but in a large majority of cases there are no gross lesions in the placenta or fetus. Microscopically, small foci of necrosis with minimal inflammation are consistently present in the liver. Necrotizing vasculitis is common in the placenta. Diagnosis can be made by immunologic staining of the kidney, lung, liver, placenta, and adrenal glands. IBR virus can be isolated from ~50% of infected fetuses (most successfully from the placenta). In most cases, maternal titers have peaked by the time of abortion. In abortion storms, rising titers can often be demonstrated in herdmates. Control is by herd vaccination; intranasal, modified-live virus, and killed vaccines are available. (*See also* p 1434.)

Leptospirosis: The pathogenic leptospires were formerly classified as serovars of *Leptospira interrogans*, but they have been reclassified into 7 species with >200 recognized serovars. *Leptospira* serovars Grippotyphosa, Pomona, Canicola, and Icterohaemorrhagiae usually cause abortions in the last trimester, 2–6 wk after maternal infection. Serovar Hardjo is host adapted to cattle and can establish lifelong infections in the kidneys and reproductive tracts. In addition to third trimester abortions, serovar Hardjo reduces conception rates in carrier cows and cows bred to carrier bulls.

Although dams may show clinical signs of leptospirosis, most abortions are in otherwise healthy cattle. Abortion rates vary from 5%–40% or more. The leptospires cause a diffuse placentitis with avascular, light tan cotyledons and edematous, yellowish intercotyledonary areas. The fetus usually dies 1–2 days before expulsion and therefore is autolyzed. Occasionally, calves are born alive but weak. Fetuses infected with serovar Pomona may show icterus. There are no specific lesions, but placenta and fetus should be submitted to the laboratory for fluorescent antibody staining or PCR testing for *Leptospira*.

Although maternal titers are probably waning by the time of abortion, an initial titer of >1:800 may be suspicious. Approximately one-third of cows aborting because of serovar Hardjo have titers of <1:100 at the time of abortion. Cows infected with serovar Hardjo can shed the organism in urine throughout life. For other serovars, the dam's urine can be cultured or examined for leptospires within 2 wk of abortion.

For control, sources of infection (such as feed or water contaminated by dogs, rats, or wildlife) should be identified and eliminated. Vaccination with a five-way bacterin every 6 mo provides good protection against serovars Grippotyphosa, Pomona, Canicola, and Icterohaemorrhagiae but does not protect against infection and renal shedding by serovar Hardjo. New monovalent serovar Hardjo vaccines that prevent infection, but do not cure existing infections, are available.

The following treatments have been found to eliminate the renal carrier state: a single injection of oxytetracycline (20 mg/kg, IM), a single injection of tilmicosin (10 mg/kg, SC), ceftiofur (5 mg/kg/day, IM, for 5 days or 20 mg/kg/day, IM, for 3 days), or amoxicillin (15 mg/kg, IM, two injections 48 hr apart).

Leptospirosis is zoonotic, and urine and milk of dams may be infective for up to 3 mo, except for Hardjo, in which case cows can be infective for life if not treated. (*See also* p 646.)

Brucellosis: Brucellosis (Bang's disease) is a threat in most countries where cattle are raised. In the USA, active control programs, including test, slaughter, and heifer vaccination, have greatly decreased its incidence. Brucellosis causes abortions in the second half of gestation (usually ~7 mo), and ~80% of unvaccinated cows in later gestation will abort if exposed to *Brucella abortus*. The organisms enter via mucous membranes and invade the udder, lymph nodes, and uterus, causing a placentitis, which may be acute or chronic. Abortion or stillbirth occurs 2 wk to 5 mo after initial infection. Affected cotyledons may be normal to necrotic, and red or yellow. The intercotyledonary area is focally thickened with a wet, leathery appearance. The fetus may be normal or autolytic with bronchopneumonia. Diagnosis can be made by maternal serology combined with fluorescent antibody staining of placenta and fetus or isolation of *B abortus* from placenta, fetus (abomasal contents and lung), or uterine discharge. Prevention is by calfhood vaccination of heifers.

Brucellosis is a serious zoonosis and a reportable disease, and the appropriate authorities should be contacted. (*See also* p 1348.)

Mycotic Abortion: Fungal placentitis due to *Aspergillus* sp (septated fungi, 60%–80% of cases), or to *Mucor* sp, *Absidia*, *Rhizopus* sp, and a few other nonseptated fungi, is an important cause of bovine sporadic abortion. Abortions occur from 4 mo to term and are most common in winter. It is believed the fungi gain entry through the oral or respiratory tracts and travel hematogenously to the placenta. Placentitis is severe and necrotizing. Cotyledons are enlarged and necrotic with turned-in margins. The intercotyledonary area is thickened and leathery. Adventitious placentation is common. The fetus seldom is autolyzed, although it may be dehydrated; ~30% have gray ringworm-like skin lesions principally involving the head and shoulders. The diagnosis is based on the presence of fungal hyphae associated with necrotizing placentitis, dermatitis, or pneumonia. Fungi can also be isolated from the stomach contents, placenta, and skin lesions. Isolation must be correlated with microscopic and gross lesions to exclude contamination after abortion.

For control, moldy feed should be avoided. (*See also* p 3005.)

***Trueperella pyogenes*:** *Trueperella (Arcanobacterium) pyogenes* causes sporadic abortion at any stage of pregnancy. Rarely, the incidence in a herd may reach epizootic levels. The bacterium is present in the nasopharynx of many healthy cows and in abscesses. It is not normally present, even as a contaminant, in fetuses or fetal membranes, and isolation is almost always significant. It gains entry to the bloodstream and causes an endometritis and placentitis, which is diffuse with a reddish brown to brown color. The fetus is usually autolyzed, with fibrinous pericarditis, pleuritis, or peritonitis possible.

Bronchopneumonia may be evident on histopathology, but *T pyogenes* is best cultured from placenta or abomasal contents. Abortion is usually sporadic, and no effective bacterin is available.

Trichomoniasis: *Tritrichomonas foetus* infection causes a venereal disease that usually results in infertility but occasionally causes abortion in the first half of gestation. Placentitis is relatively mild, with hemorrhagic cotyledons and thickened intercotyledonary areas covered with flocculent exudate. The placenta is often retained, and there may be pyometra. The fetus has no specific lesions, although *T foetus* can be found in abomasal contents, placental fluids, and uterine discharges. Infected cows typically clear the organism within 20 wk, but bulls, especially those infected after 3 yr of age, can become lifelong carriers. There is no legal, effective treatment for individual animals. Herd treatment is based on identifying and segregating pregnant females from "at-risk" females for ≥5 mo and by identifying and culling all infected bulls. Prevention is by artificial insemination or natural insemination using noninfected bulls. A killed, whole-cell vaccine is available for use in cows. (*See also* p 1384.)

Campylobacteriosis: *Campylobacter fetus venerealis* causes venereal disease that usually results in infertility or early embryonic death but occasionally causes abortion between 4 and 8 mo of gestation. *C fetus fetus* and *C jejuni* are transmitted by ingestion and subsequent hematogenous spread to the placenta. Both cause sporadic abortions, usually in the last half of gestation. The fetus can be fresh with partially expanded lungs or severely autolyzed. Mild fibrinous pleuritis and peritonitis may be noted, as well as bronchopneumonia. Placentitis is mild with hemorrhagic cotyledons and an edematous intercotyledonary area. *Campylobacter* spp can be identified by darkfield examination of abomasal contents or culture of placenta or abomasal contents. Isolation and identification of the species involved is important if vaccination is to be instituted. Venereal campylobacteriosis can be controlled by artificial insemination and vaccination. *Campylobacter* spp are zoonotic, and *C jejuni* is an important cause of enteritis in people. (*See also* p 1347.)

Listeriosis: *Listeria monocytogenes* can cause placentitis and fetal septicemia. Abortions are usually sporadic but may affect 10%–20% of a herd. Abortion is at any stage of gestation, and the dam may have fever and anorexia before the abortion; retained placenta is common. The fetus is retained for 2–3 days after death, so autolysis may be extensive. Fibrinous polyserositis and white necrotic foci in the liver and/or cotyledons are common. Diagnosis is by culture of *Listeria* from fetus or placenta. There is no available bacterin. Listeriosis is a reportable disease in many areas and is a serious zoonosis, with spread possible through improperly pasteurized milk. (*See also* p 656.)

Chlamydiosis: *Chlamydia abortus*, the cause of enzootic abortion of ewes, causes sporadic abortion in cattle. Most abortions occur near the end of the last trimester, but they can occur earlier. Placental lesions consist of thickening and yellow-brown exudate adhered to the cotyledons and intercotyledonary areas. Histologically, placentitis is consistently present, and pneumonia and hepatitis can be found in some cases. *C abortus* can be identified by examination of stained smears of the placenta or by ELISA, fluorescent antibody staining, PCR, or isolation in embryonated chicken eggs or cell culture. Organisms can often be identified in the lungs and liver but not as consistently as in the placenta. There are no vaccines for cattle, although they are produced for sheep (*see* p 1338). The bacterium is zoonotic, occasionally producing life-threatening disease and abortion in pregnant women.

Ureaplasma diversum **Infection:** *Ureaplasma diversum* is a common inhabitant of the vagina and prepuce of cattle that also causes abortions. Abortions are usually single, but severe outbreaks occur on occasion. The infection may also result in stillbirths and birth of weak calves. Most fetuses are aborted in the third trimester and are well preserved. The cows are not sick, but retained placentas are common. Placentitis and a necrotic amniotic membrane are common features. The intercotyledonary areas are usually thickened and sometimes contain areas of fibrin deposition and hemorrhage. There are no gross lesions in the fetus. Microscopically, there is nonsuppurative placentitis and pneumonia characterized by accumulations of lymphocytes around bronchi and by diffuse alveolitis. Diagnosis is by isolation of *U diversum* from the placenta, lungs, and/or abomasal contents.

Epizootic Bovine Abortion (Foothill Abortion): Epizootic bovine abortion is localized to the foothill region surrounding the Sacramento/San Joaquin Valley and the Eastern Sierra Nevada range of California, Oregon, and Nevada. Epizootic bovine abortion usually causes a protracted abortion storm affecting primarily heifers or cows recently introduced to the geographic region; however, abortion can occur 3–5 mo after leaving the endemic area. Abortion is usually in the last trimester, and rates may be as high as 60%. The animals abort without illness, and the fetus is seldom autolyzed. Although the etiologic agent has not been definitively determined, it is transmitted by the argasid tick *Ornithodoros coriaceus* and is believed to be an unnamed bacterium in the Myxobacteria family (order Myxococcales). The aborted fetus may have hepatomegaly, splenomegaly, and generalized lymphomegaly. Microscopically, there is marked lymphoid hyperplasia in the spleen and lymph nodes and granulomatous inflammation in most organs. Fetal IgG is increased. Cows seldom abort in subsequent pregnancies, and heifers are often exposed to endemic areas before breeding age in an effort to prevent abortions.

Bluetongue: Bluetongue is caused by an Orbivirus with 24 serotypes and is transmitted by biting midges of the genus *Culicoides*. Historically, bluetongue occurred from approximately latitude 35°S to 40°N, except in the western USA, where it occurs to 45°N. After introduction of an attenuated, live virus serotype 10 vaccine in the 1950s, abortion, mummification, stillbirth, and the birth of live offspring with CNS malformations occurred in cattle and sheep. Since then, multiple bluetongue serotypes have been identified as causes of similar reproductive losses in cattle and sheep. Attenuation of bluetongue virus can increase its ability to cross the placenta. There is evidence that before 2007, reproductive losses were caused by attenuated bluetongue vaccine viruses, either by vaccination of pregnant animals or by spread of vaccine virus in nature by *Culicoides* spp.

In 2006, serotype 8 bluetongue virus appeared, spread, and became endemic across northwestern Europe (north of 50°N), where bluetongue was previously unknown. Beginning in 2007, abortions and birth of "dummy" calves with brain malformations occurred in bluetongue-infected herds; affected calves were documented to have been infected in utero. Since then, many such cases have been reported. Diagnosis is by identification of precolostral antibodies to bluetongue or identification of the virus by PCR. Brain, spleen, and whole blood are the preferred samples from fetuses and neonates for PCR. Control of bluetongue is by vaccination and management procedures to reduce exposure to biting midges. Modified-live and inactivated vaccines are available, but their availability and use varies between countries. (*See also* p 738.)

Other Causes of Abortion: Akabane virus (where present) causes abortion and fetal anomalies. Parainfluenza-3 virus causes abortion in experimentally inoculated seronegative cattle, but is seldom, if ever, diagnosed in field cases of abortion. Occasionally, *Salmonella* spp cause abortion storms. The cows are usually sick, and the fetuses and placentas are autolyzed and emphysematous. Salmonellae can be isolated from the abomasal contents and fetal tissues and from uterine fluids and the dams' feces. *Mycoplasma* spp, *Histophilus somni*, and a wide variety of other bacteria can also cause sporadic abortions in cattle. Schmallenberg virus, discovered in Europe in 2011, belongs to the Simbu serogroup and has been associated with infertility, abortion, and fetal malformation in several ruminant species.

ABORTION IN SHEEP

See also MANAGEMENT OF REPRODUCTION: SHEEP, p 2212.

Abortion in ewes, as in cows, is not always easily diagnosed. Although many of the toxins that cause abortion in cows also cause problems in ewes, others such as *Veratrum californicum* and kale seem unique to the ewe. Subterranean clover (*Trifolium subterraneum*) is a common cause of early embryonic death and abortion in sheep. The major infectious agents causing abortions in sheep are *Campylobacter* sp, *Chlamydia* sp, *Toxoplasma* sp, *Listeria* sp, *Brucella* sp, *Salmonella* sp, border disease virus, and Cache Valley virus.

***Campylobacter* spp Infection (Vibriosis):** Infection with *Campylobacter fetus fetus*, *C jejuni jejuni*, and *C lari* results in abortions in late pregnancy or stillbirths. The route of infection is oral. Ewes may develop metritis after expelling the fetus. Placentitis occurs with hemorrhagic necrotic cotyledons and edematous or leathery intercotyledonary areas. The fetus is usually autolyzed, with 40% having orange-yellow necrotic foci (1–2 cm diameter) in the liver. Fetuses may have accumulated serosanguineous fluid in the thoracic and peritoneal cavities. Diagnosis relies on finding *Campylobacter* organisms in darkfield or fluorescent antibody preparations or by isolation from fetal abomasal contents, liver, and lungs, or from placental smears or in uterine discharge. Identification of the species involved is important, because in some areas *C jejuni* is as common as *C fetus*, and some vaccines do not include *C jejuni*. Strict hygiene is necessary to stop an outbreak. Use of tetracyclines may help prevent exposed ewes from aborting. However, many isolates may be resistant to tetracycline. The disease tends to be cyclical, with epizootics occurring every 4–5 yr; therefore, vaccination programs, which help prevent outbreaks, should be consistently practiced. *C jejuni* is zoonotic and is a common cause of enteritis in people.

Enzootic Abortion of Ewes (EAE): *Chlamydia abortus* is the cause of EAE, which is characterized by late-term abortions, stillbirths, and weak lambs. *C pecorum* is the cause of chlamydial arthritis and conjunctivitis of sheep. EAE occurs worldwide, except for in Australia and New Zealand, and is most important in intensively managed sheep. Abortions occur during the last 2–3 wk of gestation regardless of when infection occurs, and the fetuses are fresh with minimal autolysis. Gross lesions in the fetus are rare and may include ascites, lymphadenopathy, and liver congestion. There is placentitis with necrotic, reddish brown cotyledons and thickened brown intercotyledonary areas covered by exudate. Chlamydial elementary bodies can be found by examination of Gimenez- or Giemsa-stained smears of the placenta or vaginal discharge, but the organisms cannot be differentiated from *Coxiella burnetii*, which occasionally causes abortion in sheep.

Definitive diagnosis is by identification of *C abortus* by ELISA, fluorescent antibody staining, PCR, or isolation. Ewes seldom abort more than once, but they remain persistently infected and shed *C abortus* from their reproductive tract for 2–3 days before and after ovulation. Rams can be infected and transmit the organism venereally. Control consists of isolating all affected ewes and lambs and treating in-contact ewes with long-acting oxytetracycline or oral tetracycline. *C abortus* bacterins are available and reduce abortions. In parts of Europe, a modified-live vaccine is available for use.

C abortus is zoonotic, but human cases are rare. All have involved pregnant women, who developed life-threatening illness. Only in a few cases in which the fetus was delivered by cesarean section did the infant survive. Pregnant women should not work with pregnant sheep, especially if abortions are occurring.

Border Disease: Border disease occurs worldwide and is an important cause of embryonic and fetal deaths, weak lambs, and congenital abnormalities. It is caused by a pestivirus closely related to bovine viral diarrhea (BVD) virus and classical swine fever (hog cholera) virus. Infection of susceptible animals occurs after introduction of persistently infected animals. Venereal transmission from shedding rams is possible. Abortion can occur at any stage of gestation. There are no clinical signs in the dam, except for a mild fever and leukopenia in a few cases. Live infected fetuses usually are undersized, and they often have congenital tremors and an abnormally hairy coat (hairy shaker lambs). Diagnosis is by identification of border disease virus in the placenta or fetal tissues (kidneys, lungs, spleen, thyroid glands, abomasum) by fluorescent antibody staining, virus isolation, or demonstration of precolostral antibodies. No vaccines are available. Inactivated BVD virus vaccines are sometimes used in sheep, but their effectiveness is unproved. (*See also* p 622.)

Cache Valley Virus: Cache Valley virus is a mosquito-transmitted cause of infertility, abortions, stillbirths, and multiple congenital abnormalities in sheep. The virus is endemic in most parts of the USA, Canada, and Mexico. Often, there are epizootics affecting sheep over a wide geographic area that can include several states. The most noticeable effects are stillborn lambs and the birth of live lambs with congenital abnormalities affecting the CNS and musculoskeletal system. Hydranencephaly, hydrocephalus, cerebral and cerebellar hypoplasia, arthrogryposis, scoliosis, torticollis, and hypoplasia of skeletal muscles are common. Infection before 32 days of pregnancy results in early embryonic death. Infection between 32 and 37 days of pregnancy results in musculoskeletal and CNS lesions. Infection between 37 and 48 days results in primarily musculoskeletal lesions. At the time of abortion or birth, the virus is usually no longer viable, and diagnosis is by demonstration of antibodies in precolostral serum or body fluids. Vaccines are not available.

Toxoplasmosis: *Toxoplasma gondii* is a major cause of abortion in small ruminants throughout the world. Ingestion of sporulated coccidian oocytes early in gestation results in resorption or mummification; if ewes contract the disease late in gestation, abortions or perinatal deaths occur. Ewes do not usually appear sick. In an outbreak, there is usually a wide range in gestational age of aborted fetuses. In most cases there are no gross lesions, but in a few cases there are distinct, small, white foci,

1–3 mm in diameter, in some cotyledons. The fetal brain often has focal areas of nonsuppurative inflammation on histology. Fetal serology (indirect hemagglutination inhibition, latex agglutination, or fluorescent antibody) may also be used. Once infected, ewes are immune, so running unbred ewes with aborting ones may allow them to develop immunity. Transplacental transmission is possible. Preventing contamination of feed by cat feces may help reduce exposure. Toxoplasmosis is a zoonosis. (*See also* p 685.)

Listeriosis: Abortion caused by *Listeria monocytogenes* in ewes usually occurs in late gestation. Aborting ewes show variable clinical signs, including fever, depression, and anorexia, and some may succumb to septicemia. There is some necrosis of cotyledons and the intercotyledonary areas, and the fetus is usually autolyzed. Mummification is possible. The fetal liver (and possibly lung) may have necrotic foci, 0.5–1 mm in diameter. Diagnosis is by culture. (*See also* p 656.)

Brucellosis: The major importance of *Brucella ovis* is as a cause of contagious epididymitis in rams. On a flock basis, brucellosis results in infertility, but it also causes late-term abortions, stillbirths, and birth of weak lambs. *B melitensis* is rare in the USA but causes abortion in areas where it is found. *B abortus* occasionally causes abortion in sheep. *Brucella* abortions occur late in gestation, resulting in placentitis with edema and necrosis of the cotyledons and thickened, leathery intercotyledonary areas. Many fetuses aborted due to *B ovis* are alive at the beginning of parturition, although fetuses can be mummified or autolyzed. Most fetuses aborted due to *B melitensis* or *B abortus* are autolytic. Culture of the placenta, abomasal contents, and the dam's vaginal discharge are diagnostic. A vaccine for *B melitensis* is available in some countries. *B melitensis* and *B abortus* are zoonotic. (*See also* p 1348.)

Salmonellosis: *Salmonella* Abortusovis, *S* Dublin, *S* Typhimurium, and *S* Arizona have caused abortions in sheep. *S* Abortusovis is endemic in England and Europe but has not been reported in the USA. The other serotypes occur worldwide. Most ewes are sick and febrile before aborting. There are no specific placental lesions, and the fetus is autolyzed. Diagnosis is by culture of placenta, fetus, or uterine discharge. *Salmonella* spp are zoonotic. (*See also* p 195.)

Bluetongue: Bluetongue virus infection is a cause of abortion, fetal mummification, stillbirth, and congenital brain malformation in lambs. The clinical syndrome, serotypes involved, and diagnosis are the same as for cattle (*see* p 1337). Most, if not all, reproductive failure is caused by attenuated vaccine viruses rather than field viruses. Serotype 8 bluetongue virus has been documented as a cause of abortions and congenital brain malformations in cattle in northwestern Europe, and this is widely regarded as the first confirmed outbreak of transplacental transmission of wild-type bluetongue virus in ruminants. Published studies from Europe have not found evidence that serotype 8 is a significant cause of fetal infection in sheep. However, there are a few anecdotal reports of abortions and congenital anomalies in sheep attributed to serotype 8, and experimentally the virus has been demonstrated to be capable of crossing the ovine placenta. The virus should be considered a potential problem in sheep until more is known.

Control of bluetongue is by management procedures to reduce exposure to biting midges and vaccination. Inactivated and modified-live vaccines are available and widely used, but the availability of each varies between countries. Modified-live vaccines are predominantly used in regions with a long history of bluetongue, such as the USA and Africa, but their use is controversial. If used, the vaccine should not be given to pregnant ewes. Also, the vaccine should not be given when *Culicoides* spp are active, because they can and do transmit the vaccine virus to unvaccinated animals, including pregnant females. Bluetongue virus has a segmented genome, and reassortment viruses are readily produced in animals simultaneously infected or vaccinated with more than one serotype. (*See also* p 738.)

Other Causes of Abortion: Akabane virus (where present) causes abortion and congenital anomalies in sheep and is a differential diagnosis for Cache Valley virus infection. *Coxiella burnetii* causes occasional abortion storms in sheep, with the clinical syndrome and fetal pathology the same as for goats (*see* below). *Neospora caninum* has been reported to cause occasional abortions in sheep, with the lesions resembling those of *Toxoplasma gondii*. Fungal placentitis also occurs but is not as common in sheep as in cattle or horses. Other organisms associated with sheep abortion include Schmallenberg virus, Rift Valley fever, Nairobi sheep disease virus, Wesselsbron disease virus, *Francisella tularensis*, and *Leptospira* sp.

ABORTION IN GOATS

See also MANAGEMENT OF REPRODUCTION: GOATS, p 2182.

Noninfectious causes of abortion in goats include plant toxins, such as broomweed or locoweed poisoning; dietary deficiencies of copper, selenium, vitamin A, or magnesium; and certain drugs such as estrogen, glucocorticoids, phenothiazine, carbon tetrachloride, or levamisole (in late gestation).

Major infectious causes of abortion in goats are chlamydiosis, toxoplasmosis, leptospirosis, brucellosis, *Coxiella burnetii*, and listeriosis. *Campylobacter* causes abortions but is not nearly as important in does as in ewes.

Chlamydiosis (Enzootic Abortion): *Chlamydia abortus* (the agent of enzootic abortion of ewes) is the most common cause of abortion in goats in the USA. In naive herds, up to 60% of pregnant does can abort or give birth to stillborn or weak kids. Abortions can occur at any stage of pregnancy, but most are in the last month. Reproductive failure is usually the only sign of *C abortus* infection, but occasionally there is concurrent respiratory disease, polyarthritis, conjunctivitis, and retained placentas in the flock. Aborted lambs are usually fresh with no gross pathology. Placentitis is usually present and consists of reddish brown exudate covering cotyledons and intercotyledonary areas. Microscopically, necrotizing vasculitis and neutrophilic inflammation are present in the placenta. Chlamydial organisms can be visualized in appropriately stained placental smears, but they cannot be differentiated from *Coxiella burnetii*. Fluorescent antibody or immunohistochemical staining, ELISA, PCR, or culture can be used to definitively identify *C abortus*. The placenta is the specimen of choice, but sometimes the diagnosis can be made by testing liver, lung, and spleen.

During an outbreak, aborting does should be isolated, and tetracyclines given orally or parentally. There is no chlamydial vaccine for goats, but the vaccine for sheep is relatively effective. Like sheep, goats that abort are immune. Sheep that abort due to *C abortus* remain infected for years, if not life, and shed the organism during ovulation; whether this occurs in goats is not known. *C abortus* is zoonotic, occasionally causing serious disease in pregnant women.

Toxoplasmosis: Toxoplasmosis is a common cause of abortion in goats in the USA, and toxoplasmal abortion in goats is similar to the syndrome in ewes. (*See also* p 685.)

Leptospirosis: The most common serovars of *Leptospira interrogans* involved in caprine abortion are Grippotyphosa and Pomona. Although sheep are relatively resistant to leptospirosis, goats are susceptible, with abortions occurring at the time of leptospiremia. Some does have anemia, icterus, and hemoglobinemia; others are afebrile and are not icteric. Diagnosis is by serology or identification of *Leptospira* spp in the dam's urine, the placenta, or fetal kidney. (*See also* p 646.)

Brucellosis: *Brucella melitensis* is the principal organism involved in abortions in animals with brucellosis; *B abortus* is occasionally involved. Abortion may be accompanied by mastitis and lameness and is most common in the fourth month. The placenta is grossly normal, but does may develop chronic uterine lesions. Infection in adults is lifelong, with organisms shed in the milk (*B melitensis* is zoonotic but rare in the USA). In the USA, control is by test and slaughter. Tube agglutination and card tests can be used as screening tests. (*See also* p 1348.)

***Coxiella burnetii* Infection:** *Coxiella burnetii* is increasingly recognized as an important cause of caprine abortion. Occasional outbreaks also occur in sheep. Late-term abortions, stillbirths, and weak lambs are the common presentations. Up to 50% of the flock may be involved. The placenta is covered by gray-brown exudate and the intercotyledonary areas are thickened. Microscopically, there is a necrotizing vasculitis in the placenta, and many chorionic epithelial cells are distended by small, coccobacillary organisms <1 μm in diameter. Infection involves only the placenta; without it, the diagnosis usually cannot be made. Diagnosis is by identification of *C burnetii* by immunologic staining methods, PCR, or by isolation. *Coxiella* is zoonotic, causing Q fever in people. (*See also* p 623.)

Listeriosis: *Listeria monocytogenes* is a common pathogen in goats and causes sporadic abortions. There are no specific fetal lesions, and the fetus is often autolyzed. Does usually show no signs before abortion but may develop severe metritis after abortion. Diagnosis is by isolation from the placenta, abomasal contents, or uterine discharge. In the rare case of a herd outbreak, preventive treatment with tetracycline is recommended. (*See also* p 656.)

Caprine Herpesvirus 1 (CpHV 1): CpHV 1 is closely related to infectious bovine rhinotracheitis virus of cattle and causes sporadic outbreaks of late-term abortions often unassociated with other clinical signs. The virus also causes vulvovaginitis, balanoposthitis, and respiratory disease in adult goats and enteric and systemic diseases in neonatal goats. Fetuses can be fresh or autolyzed and do not contain diagnostic gross lesions. Presumptive diagnosis is by microscopic identification of necrosis with the presence of intranuclear inclusion bodies in the liver, lungs, and other organs. Definitive diagnosis is by identification of CpHV 1 by isolation, PCR, or immunologic staining methods. Not all fetuses contain lesions or virus, so multiple fetuses should be submitted. Infected goats can become latently infected and can shed the virus during times of stress. Vaccines are not commercially available in the USA.

ABORTION IN PIGS

See also MANAGEMENT OF REPRODUCTION: PIGS, p 2201.

Many agents that cause reproductive failure in sows produce a broad spectrum of sequelae, including abortions and weak neonates, as well as stillbirth, mummification, embryonic death, and infertility. Mummification is seen more frequently in swine than in many other species because of the large litter size. If only a few fetuses die, abortion rarely occurs; instead, mummies are delivered at term, along with live piglets or stillbirths.

Noninfectious Causes

High ambient temperature (>32°C [>89.6°F]) is associated with increased returns to estrus, increased embryonic mortality, decreased farrowing rates, and small litters. The effect is greatest if heat stress occurs at the time of breeding or implantation. Increased embryonic mortality and increased irregular return to estrus are seen in pigs bred during the summer. High ambient temperature may play a role, but there is evidence that seasonal low progesterone levels are a major factor.

The estrogenic mycotoxins zearalenone and zearalenol interfere with conception and implantation, causing infertility, embryonic death, and reduced litter size, but rarely, if ever, abortion. Another class of mycotoxins, the fumonisins, causes acute pulmonary edema in swine; sows that recover from the acute disease often abort 2–3 days later.

Other toxic causes of abortions or stillborn pigs include cresol sprays (used for mange and louse control), dicumarol, and nitrates. Nutritional causes of reproductive failure are not well defined. Vitamin A deficiency can cause congenital anomalies and possibly abortions. Riboflavin deficiency can cause early premature births (14–16 days), and calcium, iron, manganese, and iodine deficiencies have been associated with stillbirths and weak pigs.

Carbon monoxide toxicity due to faulty propane heaters has been associated with increased numbers of stillbirths and autolyzed full-term fetuses. Fetal tissues are cherry red; the sows do not appear affected.

Infectious Causes

The major infectious causes of reproductive failure in pigs include porcine reproductive and respiratory syndrome virus, porcine parvovirus, pseudorabies virus, Japanese B encephalitis virus, classical swine fever virus, *Leptospira* spp, and *Brucella suis*.

Porcine Reproductive and Respiratory Syndrome (PRRS): PRRS is caused by an arterivirus. It is of major importance in the USA and throughout most of the world. Most PRRS strains do not cross the placenta until after 90 days of gestation. Consequently, most abortions are near the end of gestation. Affected litters contain fresh and autolyzed dead pigs, weak infected pigs, and healthy, uninfected pigs that often develop respiratory disease within a few days of birth. The sows are often anorectic and feverish a few days before aborting. Concurrent respiratory disease and increased numbers of bacterial infections in the herd are common. Hemorrhage in the umbilical cord, when present, is the only gross lesion associated with PRRS abortions. Not all fetuses are infected, so multiple fetuses should be sampled. Viral antigen is most consistently present in the fetal thymus and in fluid collected from the fetal thoracic cavity. PCR testing of pooled thoracic fluid from three to five fetuses is the most reliable means of diagnosis. Herd management is important in control and prevention. Inactivated and modified-live virus vaccines are available. (*See also* p 729.)

Porcine Parvovirus: Porcine parvovirus is ubiquitous in pigs in the USA and most of the world. Almost all females are naturally infected before their second pregnancy, and immunity is lifelong. Consequently, it is a disease of first-parity pigs. Gilts that are immunologically naive or have high passive antibody titers have the highest risk of reproductive disorders caused by the virus. Infection before day 30 of pregnancy results in early embryonic loss. Fetal infection between 30 and 70 days of gestation can result in death of the fetus and sometimes mummification. Not all fetuses are infected at the same time, and death at different stages of pregnancy is typical. Some fetuses survive and are born alive but persistently infected. Most fetuses infected after 70 days of gestation mount an immune response, clear the virus, and are healthy at birth. Litters with dead fetuses of varying sizes, including mummified fetuses, along with stillborn and healthy pigs born to first-parity gilts, are the hallmark of porcine parvovirus. Diagnosis is by fluorescent antibody testing, virus isolation using lung from mummified fetuses, or demonstration of precolostral antibody in stillborn pigs. Boars shed virus by varying routes, including semen, for a couple of weeks after acute infection and can introduce the virus into a herd. Effective inactivated vaccines are available.

Pseudorabies (Aujeszky Disease, Porcine Herpesvirus 1 Infection): Pseudorabies is a cause of CNS and respiratory diseases. Infection results in latency, and seropositive animals are considered infected. Infection early in pregnancy can result in embryonic death and resorption of the fetuses. Infection later in pregnancy can result in abortion and birth of stillborn and weak pigs. Mummification can occur but is uncommon. There are no gross lesions in most aborted pigs, but a few have pinpoint white foci of necrosis in the liver and tonsils. Diagnosis is by virus isolation, PCR, or fluorescent antibody staining. Effective gene-deleted vaccines that allow serologic differentiation of vaccinated and naturally infected pigs were developed for the eradication program in the USA, but after eradication from commercial pigs was completed in 2003, vaccination was discontinued. Feral pigs in multiple states harbor the virus, and since 2003 there have been sporadic outbreaks of pseudorabies in herds that have contact with feral pigs. These outbreaks are currently controlled by herd depopulation. (*See also* p 1300.)

Japanese B Encephalitis Virus Infection: Japanese B encephalitis is an arthropod-borne disease that causes reproductive failure in pigs and encephalitis in people. The disease is reported primarily in southeast Asia, Indian subcontinent, Indonesia, and Australasian regions. Infected litters can contain dead pigs of various sizes (including mummies), stillborn pigs, weak pigs, and pigs with CNS signs. Hydrocephalus and subcutaneous edema are the most common gross lesions. Diagnosis is confirmed by viral isolation and immunohistochemistry. Viral nucleic acid can be detected in tissue and blood samples using RT-PCR or nested RT-PCR. Pigs are the primary amplifying host for the virus and are vaccinated not only to prevent reproductive failure but also to prevent human infection.

Classical Swine Fever (Hog Cholera): Classical swine fever is caused by a pestivirus eradicated from the USA but still a serious problem throughout much of the world. With highly virulent strains that cause serious maternal illness, abortion is common. With strains of moderate or low virulence, birth of mummified and stillborn pigs, weak pigs, and persistently infected pigs are more common. Fluorescent antibody staining, virus isolation, and PCR are used for diagnosis. Both killed and modified-live vaccines are available, but their use in the USA is prohibited. (*See also* p 713.)

Porcine Circovirus Infection: Porcine circovirus type 2 (PCV2) is found worldwide, is ubiquitous in pigs, and is associated with several conditions, including sporadic outbreaks of late-term abortions and term litters with increased numbers of dead piglets. The dead piglets vary from small, mummified fetuses to stillbirths. Nonmummified fetuses typically have a large amount of serosanguineous fluid in their body cavities. Microscopically, there is myocardial necrosis and/or fibrosis, and PCV2 is present in the heart and other tissues. The incidence of PCV2 reproductive failure is very low; when it occurs the problem soon disappears, perhaps because most pigs are naturally exposed and immune before being bred. Diagnosis is based on presence of PCV2 DNA or antigen in precolostral serum samples from live born piglets. Immunohistochemistry and in situ hybridization are considered the gold standard to detect the agent. Vaccines are available for grower and finisher pigs, but their efficacy in preventing reproductive failure is unknown.

Leptospirosis: *Leptospira interrogans* (especially serovar Pomona) is a major cause of reproductive failure in swine (infertility, abortion, stillbirths, and the birth of weak piglets). Although acute leptospirosis occurs in adult swine, most cases are asymptomatic. Pigs infected with serovars Pomona and Bratislava can become chronic renal carriers. Abortion occurs 1–4 wk after infection, so the abortuses are autolyzed. Mummification, maceration, stillbirths, and weak pigs are also seen. Diagnosis is based on demonstration of leptospires in fetal tissues or stomach contents. However, severely autolyzed fetuses may result in poor fluorescent antibody and immunohistochemistry results. PCR testing has better sensitivity and specificity. Vaccination with a multivalent bacterin every 6 mo helps prevent the disease. Streptomycin was formerly used to eliminate the carrier state and to treat pregnant sows during an outbreak, but it is no longer available for use in food animals. Experimentally, high levels of injectable oxytetracycline, tylosin, and erythromycin and high levels of tetracyclines in the feed have eliminated the carrier state. However, field results indicate that *Leptospira* infection cannot be reliably eliminated with antibiotics. Leptospirosis is zoonotic. (*See also* p 646.)

Brucellosis: *Brucella suis* infection in commercial swine has become rare in the USA as a result of state and federal control programs. However, it is present in feral pigs in multiple states; these represent a source of infection for commercial pigs and people. The route of infection is oral in most cases, but venereal transmission is not uncommon. Infected sows can abort at any stage of gestation, and abortions are not always accompanied by illness. Abortion is probably due to endometritis and fetal infection. There are few fetal or placental lesions, although some fetuses may be autolyzed. Diagnosis is by serology and isolation from the placenta and fetal tissues. No treatment has been uniformly effective. Control is based on test and slaughter. Brucellosis is one of the few venereal diseases recognized in swine. *B suis* causes a serious zoonotic disease. (*See also* p 1348.)

Other Infectious Causes of Abortion: Pigs with foot-and-mouth disease (*see* p 629), African swine fever (*see* p 711), and swine influenza (*see* p 1470) often abort, but they and their herdmates also have clinical signs of those diseases. Enteroviruses and encephalomyocarditis virus have been reported to cause fetal losses in pigs, but they are not considered economically important. Blue eye paramyxovirus is an important cause of abortion, stillbirths, and mummified fetuses in parts of Mexico. Bacteria that cause sporadic abortions include *Staphylococcus aureus*, *Streptococcus* spp, *Erysipelothrix rhusiopathiae*, *Salmonella* spp, *Pasteurella multocida*, *Trueperella (Arcanobacterium) pyogenes*, *Listeria monocytogenes*, and *Escherichia coli*.

ABORTION IN HORSES

See also MANAGEMENT OF REPRODUCTION: HORSES, p 2187.

Noninfectious Causes

The most common noninfectious cause of abortion in horses is **twinning**. Most abortions related to twinning occur at 8–9 mo of gestation and may be preceded by premature lactation. Placental insufficiency ultimately causes abortion of twins. **Umbilical cord abnormalities**, such as torsion due to abnormal length (>100 cm), are commonly diagnosed as a noninfectious cause of abortion, particularly in Thoroughbreds. Diagnosis of abortion due to cord torsion requires evidence of localized swelling or hemorrhage, because torsions occur in some normal births. Signs of fetal circulatory disturbances, such as subcutaneous edema, a swollen, soft liver, and microscopic mineralization of placental vessels, are also signs of umbilical cord obstruction. Various congenital fetal abnormalities have been reported in cases of noninfectious abortions.

Mare Reproductive Loss Syndrome: In spring of 2001, horse farms in Kentucky and neighboring states experienced an explosive outbreak of early abortions and late-term abortions, stillbirths, and weak foals that died within a few days. Simultaneously there was a large increase in fibrinous pericarditis and unilateral uveitis in horses of all ages and both sexes. Together these conditions became known as mare reproductive loss syndrome (MRLS). Analysis of records showed that MRLS had occurred in the area in earlier years. MRLS has since been diagnosed in other states, including New York and Florida. An abortion storm with similar clinical signs and risk factors was recently reported from Australia.

Most early abortions occur at 40–80 days of gestation, with some losses occurring as late as 140 days. A few affected mares have colic, fever, and/or purulent vulvar discharge, but most remain clinically normal. Typically, the first sign is abortion or finding a fetus dead in utero by ultrasound. Most fetuses are expelled within 2 days to 2 wk of dying and are autolytic. Neutrophilic placentitis and metritis are usually present. Most mares rebred during the same breeding season do not become pregnant, but conception is usually normal during the next breeding season. Late-term losses generally occur at 10 mo of gestation to term, and the mare usually does not display signs of impending parturition. Pathologic features of MRLS include the presence of amnionitis and funisitis, with only the amniotic portion of the umbilical cord affected. The placenta and umbilical cord are thickened, edematous, and discolored light brown to yellow. Neutrophilic inflammation of the umbilical cord and placenta are usually present, with the neutrophilic funisitis being characteristic of the syndrome. A variety of bacteria can be isolated from the fetuses, regardless of when they abort, but are not considered causative. Pasture exposure to eastern tent caterpillars (*Malacosoma americanum*) is an important risk factor, and both early and late-term abortions have been reproduced by oral administration of whole caterpillars or their exoskeletons but not their digestive tract. The mechanism causing abortion has not been confirmed. It has been proposed that an unidentified toxin associated with the exoskeleton of these caterpillars is involved, and that bacterial infections are secondary. Alternatively, caterpillar hairs (setae) may penetrate the oral or intestinal mucosa and carry bacteria, resulting in bacteremia with localization in the uterus and other organs. (The horses in the Australian outbreak were exposed to processionary caterpillars [*Ochragaster lunifer*]).

Prevention consists of pasture management to control the numbers of eastern tent caterpillars and other procedures to prevent exposure of pregnant mares to eastern tent caterpillars.

Fescue Grass Toxicosis: Ingestion of fescue infected by the endophyte *Neotyphodium coenophialum* causes prolonged gestation, agalactia, edema and premature separation of the placenta, and perinatal death. Abortion may occur in the last 2 mo of pregnancy due to severe edema and premature placental separation. The placenta is thickened and edematous and does not rupture normally at the cervical star. The chorioallantois precedes the foal through the birth canal instead of remaining attached to the uterus (red bag), resulting in anoxia and death of the fetus. The source of the infected fescue can be pasture, hay, or bedding. (*See also* p 3016.)

Infectious Causes

Infectious causes of abortion include viral diseases (such as equine rhinopneumonitis and equine viral arteritis) as well as bacterial and fungal infections.

Equine Rhinopneumonitis (Equine Herpesvirus 1 Infection): Equine rhinopneumonitis, specifically equine herpesvirus 1 (EHV-1) infection, is the most important viral cause of abortion in horses, although EHV-4 has also been isolated from some cases. The principal mode of transmission of the virus from horse to horse is by direct contact through nasal secretions, reproductive tract discharge, placenta, or the aborted fetus. Short-distance airborne spread of infection is possible. Abortion is usually after 7 mo of gestation and is not preceded by maternal illness. The placenta may be edematous or normal. Gross fetal lesions include subcutaneous edema, jaundice, increased volume of thoracic fluid, and an enlarged liver with yellow-white lesions ~1 mm in diameter. Histologically, these lesions represent areas of necrosis containing intranuclear inclusions. Inclusion bodies are also found in necrotic lymphoid tissues. There is often a necrotizing bronchiolitis. Diagnosis is by fluorescent antibody, PCR, or virus isolation from fetal tissues. Prevention is based on vaccinating at 5, 7, and 9 mo of gestation as well as preventing exposure of pregnant mares to horses attending shows or other equine events. Abortion may occur despite regular vaccination. (*See also* p 1444.)

Equine Viral Arteritis (EVA): Abortion may follow clinical cases of EVA by 6–29 days. Abortion rates can approach 60% in a naive population as the result of direct impairment of placental function and severe fetal infection. Arteritis may be found in the fetal myocardium or placenta, but usually there are no fetal lesions. Stallions can be persistently infected, and EVA can spread venereally (via natural cover or insemination with shipped cooled or frozen semen) or by aerosol. Diagnosis is by a history of EVA shortly before abortion, virus isolation or PCR of placenta and/or fetal tissues, or by seroconversion of the dam. Prevention of EVA is by management to minimize viral transmission in breeding populations and to prevent development of carrier stallions. In the USA, a licensed modified-live virus vaccine is available for use in nonpregnant mares. Antibody titers resulting from vaccination and natural infection cannot be differentiated, and the serologic status of horses can affect their import status. Therefore, the serologic status of breeding horses should be determined before vaccination, and all subsequent vaccinations should be recorded. (*See also* p 701.)

Bacterial Abortion: Bacterial placentitis is by far the most commonly diagnosed cause of abortion in many horse breeding areas. Placentitis is a significant cause of equine late-term abortion, premature delivery, and neonatal death. Except for *Leptospira* spp and nocardioform infections, most cases of bacterial placentitis are ascending. Ascending placentitis is characterized by premature udder development, increased uteroplacental thickness at the level of the cervical star, and mucopurulent vaginal discharge. If placentitis is untreated, placental function is compromised and placental separation ensues, resulting in fetal death and expulsion. In chronic placentitis, the fetus may show intrauterine growth retardation. *Streptococcus equi* subsp *zooepidemicus*, *Escherichia coli*, *Pseudomonas aeruginosa*, *Enterobacter* spp, and *Klebsiella pneumoniae* are the most frequent isolates from the vaginal discharge, uterus, placenta, and fetal stomach contents. Other bacteria have also been reported to cause ascending placentitis in mares, including *Streptococcus equisimilis*, *Enterobacter agglomerans*, α-hemolytic streptococci, *Staphylococcus aureus*, and *Actinobacillus* spp. Examination of the placenta shows an edematous and thickened chorioallantois with fibrinonecrotic exudate at the level of the cervical star.

Leptospira spp placentitis is characterized by diffuse lesions secondary to hematogenous spread. Leptospiral placentitis as a cause of abortion seems to be on the rise in Kentucky, Northern Ireland, England, and South America. Several serovars of *Leptospira interrogans* have been isolated from aborted equine fetuses (eg, Pomona, Grippotyphosa, Bratislava, Pomona type kennewicki, and Hardjo type hardjo-prajitno). In North America, the most common isolate is serovar Pomona type kennewicki, which is carried by several wildlife species, including the striped skunk, raccoon, whitetail deer, and opossum. Most leptospiral abortions occur between 6 and 9 mo of gestation. The placenta is thick, heavy, edematous, hemorrhagic, and occasionally covered with a brown mucoid material on the chorionic surface. Funisitis has also been described in leptospiral abortion. The fetus may have mild to moderate icterus and liver enlargement, and fetal histopathologic lesions may include various degrees of nephritis and hepatitis. Diagnosis is by fluorescent antibody staining of placenta or fetal kidney, liver, or lung and by fetal serology. (*See also* p 652.)

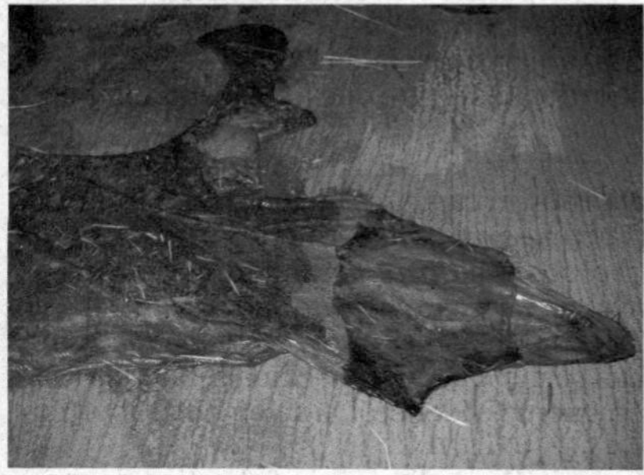

Ascending placentitis in a mare. Note the congested and thick cervical star area.
Courtesy of Dr. Ahmed Tibary.

Nocardioform placentitis is a distinct type of equine placentitis first described in the USA in the late 1980s. Nocardioform placentitis may result in abortion, stillbirth, or birth of weak foals at term. Some mares may exhibit premature mammary gland development and lactation before abortion. Infection of the placenta is generally thought to be a sequela of hematogenous spread of microorganisms from a primary port of entry. The lesion is an extensive and severe exudative, mucopurulent, and necrotizing placentitis, frequently located at the base of the uterine horns or at the junction between the body and horns of the placenta. The affected area is thickened, and its chorionic surface is covered with brown, necrotic, mucopurulent exudate and dotted with white or yellow granular structures. Underneath this mucoid material, the chorionic surface is reddish white, mottled, and roughened. Villous necrosis and adenomatous hyperplasia of the allantoic epithelium, and hyperplasia with or without squamous metaplasia of the chorionic epithelium are frequently seen. Various groups of gram-positive, filamentous, branching bacteria have been implicated as etiologic agents in mares with nocardioform placentitis, including *Nocardia* spp, *Rhodococcus rubropertinctus*, *Amycolatopsis* spp, and *Crossiella equi*. The fetus is often severely underdeveloped as a result of placental insufficiency and does not show any remarkable gross or histologic lesions.

Potomac horse fever (*see* p 283), caused by *Ehrlichia risticii*, may be followed by abortion in mid- to late gestation. There is placentitis, and the placenta is often retained. *E risticii* has been isolated from fetal lymphoid tissues after abortion. Histologically, there is fetal colitis. Identification of this colitis provides a presumptive diagnosis. There is a vaccine for Potomac horse fever, but its efficacy in preventing abortion is not known.

Equine Mycotic Placentitis: Mycotic placentitis in horses is also due to an ascending infection that causes placentitis with a thickened chorioallantois with variable exudate. Causative agents include *Aspergillus* spp, *Mucor* spp, *Candida* spp, *Histoplasma capsulatum*, *Coccidoides* spp, and *Cryptococcus neoformans*. Fetuses aborted in late gestation may be fresh, with evidence of growth retardation. A pale, enlarged liver or dermatitis may be found. Hyphae are found in the placenta, liver, lungs, or stomach contents.

ABORTION IN CAMELIDS

Pregnancy loss is a common complaint in camelid practice. The general approach to diagnosis is similar to that in other species. However, camelids have several unique features of placentation and pregnancy. In nearly all pregnancies, the fetal horn is the left uterine horn, and the placenta is epitheliochorial, microcotyledonary diffuse (such as in the horse), but the allantochorion adheres to the amniotic sac.

Noninfectious Causes

Noninfectious causes of abortion include fetal or placental abnormalities (twinning, umbilical cord torsion, severe deformities, chromosomal abnormalities and placental insufficiency, uterine torsion), luteal insufficiency (hypoluteidism), environmental stressors (severe disease process; long, stressful trip; heat stress), or iatrogenic causes (administration of prostaglandin $F_2\alpha$, corticosteroids, 8-way vaccines). Recurrent loss due to luteal insufficiency has been associated with obesity and possibly hypothyroidism. Presence of large avillous areas suggest placental insufficiency. Twin conceptions are not rare, and most are reduced to singleton or lost by day 45. Abortion of twins is generally seen between 5 and 9 mo of pregnancy.

On a herd basis, severe losses may be seen with nutritional deficiencies (selenium, vitamin A, iodine), or toxicosis (copper, iodine). Lactating and very young maiden females may have an increased incidence of embryo and fetal losses.

Infectious Causes

Viruses: Viral causes of abortion are dominated by bovine viral diarrhea virus (BVDV). However, abortions due to equine herpesvirus 1, equine arteritis virus, and bluetongue virus have been reported. The most common BVDV serotype that affects alpacas and llamas is noncytopathic BVDV-1b. Abortion may occur at any stage of gestation, or a weak, persistently infected (PI) cria may be born prematurely. The birth of a PI animal can have significant effects on a herd of animals. Diagnosis of BVDV infection is based on virus isolation from fetal blood, fetal tissues (lymph nodes), and placenta. Immunohistochemistry may be performed on formalin-fixed tissues. PCR on whole blood samples is commonly used to screen newborn crias.

Bacteria: The most commonly diagnosed infectious causes of pregnancy losses are chlamydiosis and brucellosis (in some parts of the world). *Chlamydia* spp have been identified as a cause of abortion and birth of weak crias in llamas. *C abortus* has been associated with infertility and ovarian hydrobursitis in camels.

Brucellosis (*Brucella abortus* and *B melitensis*) is a common cause of abortion in camelids in some areas of the world.

Other reported bacterial causes of abortion in camelids include leptospirosis (*Leptospira interrogans* serogroups Icterohaemorrhagiae and Ballum), listeriosis (*Listeria monocytogenes*), and campylobacteriosis (*Campylobacter fetus fetus*). Coxiellosis (*Coxiella burnetii*) abortion is suspected to occur but has not been diagnosed definitively.

Nonspecific bacterial infections (*Escherichia coli*, *Streptococcus equi zooepidemicus*) are often isolated from cases of abortion that were due to placentitis.

Protozoa: Reported protozoal causes of abortion in camelids include toxoplasmosis (*Toxoplasma gondii*), neosporosis (*Neospora caninum*), and sarcocystosis (*Sarcocystis aucheniae* and *S cruzi*). Trichomoniasis (*Tritrichomonas foetus*) has been isolated from camels, but there is no strong evidence it is involved in abortion.

Fungi: Sporadic cases of abortion due to *Encephalitozoon cuniculi* and *Aspergillus* spp have been reported.

BOVINE GENITAL CAMPYLOBACTERIOSIS

Bovine genital campylobacteriosis is a venereal disease of cattle characterized primarily by early embryonic death, infertility, a protracted calving season, and occasionally abortion. Distribution is probably worldwide.

Etiology and Epidemiology: The cause is the motile, gram-negative, curved or spiral, polar flagellated, microaerophilic bacteria *Campylobacter fetus venerealis* or *C fetus fetus*. For many years, it was thought that *C fetus fetus* was generally an intestinal organism, only occasionally caused abortion in cattle, and was not a cause of infertility. However, *C fetus fetus* can also be a significant cause of the classic infertility syndrome usually attributed to *C fetus venerealis*. There are several strains of *C fetus fetus*, and the only way to determine whether a strain is a cause of infertility is to test that possibility in a group of heifers. *Campylobacter* spp are very labile and are destroyed quickly by heating, drying, and exposure to the atmosphere. Unless cultured quickly after collection from the animal and grown under microaerophilic or anaerobic conditions, *Campylobacter* spp will not grow.

C fetus is transmitted venereally and also by contaminated instruments, bedding, or by artificial insemination using contaminated semen. Individual bulls vary in their susceptibility to infection; some become permanent carriers, while others appear to be resistant to infection. The primary factor associated with this variability seems to be the age-related depth of the preputial and penile epithelial crypts. In young bulls (<3–4 yr old), in which the crypts have not yet developed, infection tends to be transient, with transmission apparently relying on sexual contact with a noninfected cow within a matter of minutes to days after the initial breeding of an infected cow. Spontaneous clearance in these younger bulls does not seem to be related to any immune response, so reinfection can readily occur. In bulls >3–4 yr old, the deeper crypts may provide the proper microaerophilic environment required for chronic infections to establish.

In cows, the duration of the carrier state is also variable; some clear the infection rapidly, whereas others can carry *C fetus* for ≥2 yr. IgA antibodies are shed in cervical mucus in significant amounts in ~50% of cows for several months after infection and are useful diagnostically. Although most of the genital tract may be free of infection when a cow eventually conceives, the vagina may remain chronically infected through pregnancy.

Clinical Findings: Cows are systemically normal, but there is a variable degree of mucopurulent endometritis that causes early embryonic death, prolonged luteal phases, irregular estrous cycles, repeat breeding, and, as a result, protracted calving periods, assuming the breeding season is long enough to allow for complete clearance and a successful rebreeding. Observed abortions are not common. In herds not managed intensively, disease may be noticed only when pregnancy examinations reveal low or marginally low pregnancy rates but, more importantly, great variations in gestation lengths, especially when the disease has recently been introduced to the herd. In subsequent years, infertility is usually confined to replacement heifers and a few susceptible cows. Bulls are asymptomatic and produce normal semen.

Diagnosis: Campylobacteriosis and trichomoniasis (*see* p 1384) are similar syndromes, and investigations should be directed at both diseases. Systemic antibody responses are not helpful, because they are often due to nonpathogenic *Campylobacter* spp. A vaginal mucus agglutination test (VMAT) is useful, but because of variability in individual responses, at least 10% of the herd or at least 10 cows should be sampled. An ELISA test has been developed for use on vaginal mucus and is said to be more sensitive and able to detect a wider range of antibody responses than the VMAT. Vaginal culture immediately after abortion or infection can be used for diagnosis, but the number of organisms may be low; in addition, because *C fetus* is labile and requires special techniques for isolation, success is limited.

An accurate diagnostic method is to test-breed heifers and then examine them for infection, but this is seldom practical. More often, the preputial cavity and fornix are either scraped and aspirated with an infusion pipette or infused with buffered sterile saline, and the prepuce is massaged vigorously in the area of the fornix. The aspirate or sheath washing is then examined using a fluorescent antibody test and culture. *C fetus* will survive for only 6–8 hr after collection, but inoculation into Clark's or similar media will allow survival for >48 hr. For maximum accuracy, bulls should be sampled twice, ~1 wk apart.

Caution should be exercised when *Campylobacter* spp are isolated from the placenta because of the possibility of contamination by nonpathogenic fecal *Campylobacter* spp. Conversely, failure to successfully isolate *C fetus* from an infected aborted fetus or placenta often results from overgrowth of the colonies by contaminating organisms or the lethal effects of atmospheric oxygen.

Treatment and Control: Vaccination should start as soon as genital campylobacteriosis is diagnosed. Infected cows and cows at risk should be vaccinated. Vaccination of infected cows hastens the elimination of *C fetus* and, although cows may remain carriers, fertility is greatly improved. In routine use, the vaccine should be given once, ~4 wk before breeding starts; because antibody responses are short-lived, cows should be revaccinated halfway through the breeding season. Bulls are vaccinated for the same reason as cows (ie, for treatment as well as for prophylaxis) but are given twice the dose used for cows, 3 wk apart. The infection can also be eliminated in bulls by 1–2 treatments with streptomycin at 20 mg/kg, SC, together with 5 g of streptomycin in an oil-based suspension applied to the penis for 3 consecutive days.

For practical reasons, cows are not usually treated for genital campylobacteriosis. When practical, artificial insemination is an excellent way to prevent or control genital campylobacteriosis. Because *C fetus* has been isolated from cows for >6 mo after the end of pregnancy, it has been suggested that artificial insemination should continue until all the cows in a herd have been through at least two pregnancies.

BRUCELLOSIS IN LARGE ANIMALS

Brucellosis is caused by bacteria of the genus *Brucella* and is characterized by abortion, retained placenta, and to a lesser extent, orchitis and infection of the accessory sex glands in males. The disease is prevalent in most countries of the world. It primarily affects cattle, buffalo, bison, pigs, sheep, goats, dogs (*see* p 1402), elk, and occasionally horses. The disease in people, sometimes referred to as undulant fever, is a serious public health problem, especially when caused by *B melitensis*.

BRUCELLOSIS IN CATTLE

(Contagious abortion, Bang's disease)

Etiology and Epidemiology: The disease in cattle, water buffalo, and bison is caused almost exclusively by *Brucella abortus*; however, *B suis* occasionally is isolated from seropositive cows but does not appear to cause clinical signs and is not contagious from cow to cow. In some countries, the disease in cattle is caused by *B melitensis*. The syndrome is similar to that caused by *B abortus*. *B melitensis* is not present in the USA.

Infection spreads rapidly and causes many abortions in unvaccinated cattle. In a herd in which disease is endemic, an infected cow typically aborts only once after exposure; subsequent gestations and lactations appear normal. After exposure, cattle become bacteremic for a short period and develop agglutinins and other antibodies; some cattle resist infection, and a small percentage of infected cows spontaneously recover. A positive serum agglutination test usually precedes an abortion or a normal parturition but may be delayed in ~15% of cows. The incubation period may be variable and is inversely related to stage of gestation at time of exposure. Organisms are shed in milk and uterine discharges, and the cow may become temporarily infertile. Bacteria may be found in the uterus during pregnancy, uterine involution, and infrequently, for a prolonged time in the nongravid uterus. Shedding from the vagina largely disappears with the cessation of fluids after parturition. Some infected cows that previously aborted shed brucellae from the uterus at subsequent normal parturitions. Organisms are shed in milk for a variable length of time—in most cattle for life. *B abortus* can frequently be isolated from secretions of nonlactating udders.

Natural transmission occurs by ingestion of organisms, which are present in large numbers in aborted fetuses, fetal membranes, and uterine discharges. Cattle may ingest contaminated feed and water or may lick contaminated genitals of other animals. Venereal transmission by infected bulls to susceptible cows appears to be rare. Transmission may occur by artificial insemination when *Brucella*-contaminated semen is deposited in the uterus but, reportedly, not when deposited in the midcervix. Brucellae may enter the body through mucous membranes, conjunctivae, wounds, or intact skin in both people and animals.

Brucellae have been recovered from fetuses and from manure that has remained in a cool environment for >2 mo. Exposure to direct sunlight kills the organisms within a few hours.

Clinical Findings: Abortion is the most obvious manifestation. Infections may also cause stillborn or weak calves, retained placentas, and reduced milk yield. Usually, general health is not impaired in uncomplicated abortions.

Seminal vesicles, ampullae, testicles, and epididymides may be infected in bulls; therefore, organisms are present in the semen. Agglutinins may be demonstrated in seminal plasma from infected bulls. Testicular abscesses may occur. Longstanding infections may result in arthritic joints in some cattle.

Diagnosis: Diagnosis is based on bacteriology or serology. *B abortus* can be recovered from the placenta but more conveniently in pure culture from the stomach and lungs of an aborted fetus. Most cows cease shedding organisms from the genital tract when uterine involution is complete. Foci of infection remain in some parts of the reticuloendothelial system, especially supramammary lymph nodes, and in the udder. Udder secretions are the preferred specimens for culture from a live cow.

Serum agglutination tests have been the standard diagnostic method. Agglutination tests may also detect antibodies in milk, whey, and semen. An ELISA has been developed to detect antibodies in milk and serum. When the standard plate or tube serum agglutination test is used, complete agglutination at dilutions of 1:100 or more in serum samples of nonvaccinated animals, and of 1:200 of animals vaccinated at 4–12 mo of age, are considered positive, and the animals are classified as reactors. Other tests that may be used are complement fixation, rivanol precipitation, and acidified antigen procedures.

Screening Tests: In official eradication programs on an area basis, the *Brucella* milk ring test (BRT) has effectively located infected dairy herds, but there are many false-positive tests. The brucellosis status of dairy herds in any area can be monitored by implementing the BRT at 3- to 4-mo intervals. Milk samples from individual herds are collected at the farm or milk processing plant. Cows in herds with a positive BRT are individually blood tested, and seropositive cows are slaughtered to determine herd status.

Nondairy and dairy herds in an area may also be screened for brucellosis by testing serum samples collected from cattle destined for slaughter or replacements through intermediate and terminal markets, or at abattoirs. Reactors are traced to the herd of origin, and the herd is tested. The cost of identifying reactors by this method is minimal compared with that of testing cattle in all herds. Screening tests, including the brucellosis card (or rose bengal) test and plate test, may be used in markets and laboratories to identify presumptively infected animals, thus reducing the number of more expensive and laborious diagnostic tests.

Brucellosis-free areas can be achieved and maintained, effectively and economically, by using the BRT on dairy herds and through market cattle testing. Adult cattle are sampled at the time of slaughter.

Supplemental tests using sensitive screening methods may be used in cattle in which the brucellosis status is unclear. Use of a battery of these tests improves the probability of detecting infected cattle that have remained in some herds as possible reservoirs of infection. Supplemental tests are also used to clarify the results of plate or card tests, especially in serum samples from vaccinated cattle. These tests, which include complement fixation and rivanol precipitation, are designed to detect primarily the antibodies specifically associated with *Brucella* infection. Another supplemental diagnostic procedure is to test milk samples from individual udder quarters by serial dilution BRT, which can be used to detect chronic infection in udders of cows that may have equivocal serum test reactions.

Control: Efforts are directed at detection and prevention, because no practical treatment is available. Eventual eradication depends on testing and eliminating reactors. The disease has been eradicated from many individual herds and areas by this method. Herds must be tested at regular intervals until two or three successive tests are negative.

Noninfected herds must be protected. The greatest danger is from replacement animals. Additions should be vaccinated calves or nonpregnant heifers. If pregnant or fresh cows are added, they should originate from brucellosis-free areas or herds and be seronegative. Replacements should be isolated for ~30 days and retested before being added to the herd.

Vaccination of calves with *B abortus* Strain 19 or RB51 increases resistance to infection. Resistance may not be complete, and some vaccinated calves may become infected, depending on severity of exposure. A small percentage of vaccinated calves develop antibodies to Strain 19 that may persist for years and can confuse diagnostic test results. To minimize this problem, calves in the USA are mostly vaccinated with a vaccine of Strain RB51. It is a rough attenuated strain and does not cause production of antibodies, which are detected by most serologic tests.

Whole-herd adult cattle vaccination using Strain 19 or RB51 has been practiced in certain high-incidence areas and selected herds in the USA with much success.

Vaccination as the sole means of disease control has been effective. Reduction in the number of reactors in a herd is directly related to the percentage of vaccinated animals. However, when proceeding from a control to an eradication program, a test and slaughter program becomes necessary. *B abortus* has been eradicated from cattle herds in the USA, and all states are considered free of brucellosis.

Brucellosis is endemic in some nondomesticated bison and elk herds in the USA. Transmission of *B abortus* to domestic cattle herds is rare but has occurred in several cattle herds commingling with infected elk in the greater Yellowstone Park area.

BRUCELLOSIS IN GOATS

The signs of brucellosis in goats are similar to those in cattle. The disease is prevalent in most countries where goats are a significant part of the animal industry, and milk is a common source of human brucellosis in many countries. The causal agent is *Brucella melitensis*. Infection occurs primarily through ingestion of the organisms. The disease causes abortion at approximately the fourth month of pregnancy. Arthritis and orchitis may occur. Diagnosis is made by bacteriologic examination of milk or an aborted fetus or by serum agglutination tests. The disease can be eliminated by slaughter of the herd. In most countries where *B melitensis* is endemic, vaccination with the Rev. 1 strain is common. Rev. 1 is an attenuated strain of *B melitensis* and is administered by SC or intraconjunctival routes. *B melitensis* is highly pathogenic for people.

BRUCELLOSIS IN HORSES

Horses can be infected with *Brucella abortus* or *B suis*. Suppurative bursitis, most commonly recognized as fistulous withers or poll evil (*see* p 1064), is the most common condition associated with brucellosis in horses. Occasionally, abortion has been reported. It is unlikely that infected horses are a source of the disease for other horses, other animal species, or people. Brucellosis in horses is very rare in the USA because of elimination of the disease in cattle.

BRUCELLOSIS IN PIGS

Clinical manifestations of brucellosis in pigs vary but are similar to those seen in cattle and goats. Although the disease is often self-limiting, it remains in some herds for years. Brucellosis caused by *Brucella suis* rarely occurs in domestic animals other than pigs. Epidemics of brucellosis in people have been reported among packing-house workers, and the usual source is infected pigs. The prevalence in the USA is sometimes high among feral pigs. The incidence of swine brucellosis among domesticated animals in the USA is very low. Currently there are no known infected domestic swine herds.

Etiology and Transmission: *B suis* is usually spread mainly by ingestion of infected tissues or fluids. Infected boars may transmit the disease during service; the organism can be recovered from semen.

Pigs raised for breeding purposes are sources of infection. Suckling pigs may become infected from sows but most reach weanling age without becoming infected.

Clinical Findings: After exposure to *B suis*, pigs develop a bacteremia that may persist for as long as 90 days. During and after the bacteremia, localization may occur in various tissues. Signs depend considerably on the site(s) of localization. Common manifestations are abortion, temporary or permanent sterility, orchitis, lameness, posterior paralysis, spondylitis, and occasionally metritis and abscess formation.

The incidence of abortion may be 0–80%. Abortions may also occur early in gestation and be undetected. Usually, sows or gilts that abort early in gestation return to estrus soon afterward and are rebred.

Sterility in sows, gilts, and boars is common and may be the only manifestation. Before attempting treatment for other diseases, it is logical to test for brucellosis in herds in which sterility is a problem. Sterility in sows is more frequently temporary but may be permanent. In boars, orchitis, usually unilateral, may occur, and fertility appears to be reduced.

Diagnosis: The principal means of diagnosis in pigs is the brucellosis card (rose bengal) test; however, other serum agglutination tests or complement fixation tests have been used. It is generally accepted that the tests have limitations in detecting brucellosis in individual pigs. Thus, entire herds or units of herds, rather than individual pigs, must be tested in any control program. Low agglutinin titers are seen in almost any size herd, regardless of infection status, and a few infected pigs may have no detectable titer. The card test is usually more accurate than conventional agglutination tests. Supplemental tests designed for cattle may also be used for pigs.

Prevention and Control: Caution should be practiced in the purchase of individual pigs that exhibit a low agglutinin titer unless the status of the entire herd of origin is known. Pigs should be isolated on return from fairs or shows before reentering the herd. Replacements should be purchased from herds known to be free of brucellosis, or they should be tested and isolated for 3 mo and retested before being added to the herd.

There is no vaccine for brucellosis in swine, and no practical recommendations can be made for treatment. Control is based on test and segregation as well as slaughter of infected breeding stock. Brucellosis remains a problem in feral swine and is a potential source of infection for domesticated herds and people.

BRUCELLOSIS IN SHEEP

Brucella melitensis infection in certain breeds of sheep causes clinical disease similar to that in goats (*see* above). However, *B ovis* produces a disease unique to sheep, in which epididymitis and orchitis impair fertility—the principal economic effect. Occasionally, placentitis and abortion are seen, and there may be perinatal mortality. The disease was first described in New Zealand and Australia and has since been reported from many sheep-raising areas of the world. *B ovis* infection among sheep in the USA is rare.

There is no evidence that the disease is present in any other animal species. Rare natural and experimental infections in farmed red deer stags have been reported in New Zealand.

Rams as young as 8 wk have been infected experimentally by various nonvenereal routes. The disease can be transmitted among rams by direct contact. Active infection in ewes is unusual but has developed after mating with naturally infected rams. Contaminated pastures do not appear to be important in spread of the disease. Infection frequently persists in rams, and a high percentage shed *B ovis* intermittently for several years.

Primary manifestations are lesions of the epididymis, tunica, and testis in rams; placentitis and abortion in ewes; and occasionally perinatal death in lambs. Lesions may develop rapidly. In rams, the first detectable abnormality may be a marked deterioration in semen quality associated with the presence of inflammatory cells and organisms. An acute systemic phase is rarely seen in naturally occurring infections. After regression of the acute phase—which may be so mild as to go unobserved—lesions may be palpated in the epididymis and scrotal tunics. Epididymal enlargement may be unilateral or bilateral. The tail of the epididymis is involved more frequently than the head or body, and the most prominent lesion is spermatoceles of variable size containing partially inspissated spermatic fluid. The tunics frequently become thickened and fibrous, and extensive adhesions develop between them. The testes may show fibrous atrophy; these lesions are usually permanent. In a few cases, palpable lesions are transient, while in others, organisms may be present in semen over long periods without clinically detectable lesions.

Because not all infected rams show palpable abnormalities of scrotal tissues (and not all cases of epididymitis are due to brucellosis), the remaining rams must be examined further. Rams shedding organisms, but having no lesions, must be identified by culture of semen. Repeated examinations may be necessary to identify intermittent shedders. Microscopic examination of stained semen smears may also be helpful; fluorescent antibody examination is a highly specific diagnostic aid. Serologic tests used for eradication of disease and certification of animals include indirect ELISA, complement fixation, hemagglutination inhibition, indirect agglutination, and gel diffusion.

Incidence and spread of the disease may be reduced by regular examination of rams before the breeding season and culling of those with obvious genital abnormalities. Because susceptibility in rams increases markedly with age, it is advantageous to keep a young ram flock and isolate noninfected rams from older, possibly infected rams.

Immunization of weaner rams with attenuated (Rev. 1) *B melitensis* has been recommended in some countries. Because infection in ewes apparently originates almost exclusively from service by infected rams, lamb losses through infection of ewes may be controlled economically by restricting vaccination to rams. There is no recommended vaccination in the USA.

Chlortetracycline and streptomycin used concurrently have effected bacteriologic cures. However, treatment is not economic except in especially valuable rams, and even if infection is eliminated, fertility may remain impaired.

CONTAGIOUS AGALACTIA

First recognized in Italy more than 200 years ago, contagious agalactia is primarily a disease of dairy sheep and goats and is characterized by an interstitial mastitis leading to a loss of milk production, arthritis, and infectious keratoconjunctivitis. It is more often seen on farms practicing traditional husbandry. Contagious agalactia is principally caused by the wall-less bacterium *Mycoplasma agalactiae*, but in recent years, *M mycoides capri* (*Mmc*; formerly known as LC), and, to a lesser extent, *M capricolum capricolum* (*Mcc*) and *M putrefaciens* have also been isolated from goats with mastitis, arthritis, and occasionally, respiratory disease. The clinical signs of these infections are sufficiently similar to those of contagious agalactia for the OIE to include them as causes of this listed disease.

Etiology and Epidemiology: Mycoplasmas that cause contagious agalactia can persist for >1 yr after clinical recovery of infected animals, which are the main reservoir of the organism. The introduction of such carriers into a susceptible flock can initially cause high morbidity and mortality. Once established in a herd, young ruminants become infected while suckling. Adults are contaminated via the milkers' hands, milking machines, or possibly by bedding. Other routes of transmission may include aerosols of infective exudates over short distances and ingestion of contaminated water.

Sheep and goats are equally susceptible to *M agalactiae*, but goats are additionally susceptible to *Mcc*, *Mmc*, and *M putrefaciens*. However these mycoplasmas may be found in both animal species in regions where they graze together. In general, clinical disease is more pronounced in goats. Antibodies to *Mcc* and *Mmc* have been detected in South American camelids, but no mycoplasmas have yet been isolated. Because alpacas, llamas, and vicunas develop polyarthritis, pneumonia, and pleuritis, it is likely that mycoplasmas may eventually be found. *Mmc* has also been isolated from cattle, although its role in disease in this species is not clear.

Contagious agalactia has been reported in many countries surrounding the Mediterranean, in particular Portugal, Spain, Greece, Italy, France, Turkey, Israel, and North Africa, as well as in many parts of the Middle East, most notably Iran, India, Mongolia, and parts of South America. Sporadic cases have been reported in the USA.

Clinical Findings and Lesions: The incubation period ranges from 1 wk to 2 mo and can be followed by either an acute disease with fever, neurologic signs, and occasionally death or, more commonly, a subacute or chronic disease characterized by mastitis, arthritis, and infectious keratoconjunctivitis. The infection begins as an interstitial mastitis giving rise to a hot, swollen, and painful udder, followed by a sudden drop in the quantity and quality of milk production. The milk may appear discolored and granular, separating into watery and solid phases, or take on a thick, yellow consistency with milk clots obstructing the teat duct. After several days, the affected udder shrinks because of damage to secretory tissue. Abscesses within the udder and enlargement of the retromammary lymph nodes may also be seen. Generally the clinical condition improves after a few weeks, with partial restoration of udder function, but the quality of milk remains abnormal. In some cases, atrophy and fibrosis lead to permanent loss of milk production.

The acute syndrome may lead to abortion and weak lambs as a result of ingestion of infected milk or starvation brought about by reduced milk production. Arthritis can be seen in adults and the young who find it difficult to keep up with the flock; affected animals may be seen limping or sitting on their carpal joints because of the discomfort. In these animals, the joints are hot, swollen, and painful. Conjunctivitis presents as a discharge of clear exudates from the eyes, followed by corneal opacity, keratitis, purulent exudation, and occasionally ulceration and panophthalmitis. Severe cases may result in irreversible blindness. Necropsy often reveals generalized peritonitis among animals that die during the acute stage. The infected udder is grossly atrophic in either one or both halves. Microscopically, the chronic inflammatory reaction in the stroma shows increased fibrosis and a reduced number of glandular acini. Infected joint capsules are edematous, and the synovium may contain clumps of fibrin. Articular surfaces may be eroded and occasionally ankylosed. In early stages of keratitis, the cornea is edematous and infiltrated with leukocytes; later, abundant purulent exudate infiltrates both the cornea and the ciliary body.

M putrefaciens is common in milking goat herds in western France. It can be isolated from the milk of animals with or without clinical signs, and milk production is usually severely affected. The milk of affected animals has a characteristic smell of putrefaction.

Diagnosis: When a flock is severely affected, clinical diagnosis is easy; the three major signs—mastitis, arthritis, and keratoconjunctivitis—are generally present, although rarely in the same animal. However, an acute form, in which there is septicemia without specific local signs, can confound the diagnosis.

Laboratory diagnosis is the only means of confirmation. Preferred samples from living animals include milk and udder secretions, joint fluid from arthritic cases, eye swabs from cases of ocular disease, and serum for antibody detection. The ear canal is a rich source of pathogenic mycoplasmas. Isolation of mycoplasmas from the blood during the brief mycoplasmaemia stage of the disease is rarely successful. Samples from dead animals should include udder and associated lymph nodes, joint fluid, lung tissue (at the interface between diseased and healthy tissue), and pleural or pericardial fluid. Samples should be kept moist and cool and sent promptly to a diagnostic laboratory. PCR tests, which can be performed directly on clinical samples, including milk, can be used to confirm the diagnosis.

Identification of the organism is usually achieved by the growth inhibition or immunofluorescence tests using hyperimmune rabbit antiserum and, increasingly, by PCR tests that can be performed directly on clinical samples, including milk, within hours. PCR, together with denaturing gradient gel electrophoresis, which can detect all causative mycoplasmas in a single reaction, has been described.

Detection of antibodies in serum by ELISA provides rapid diagnosis of disease but may not be very sensitive in chronically affected herds and flocks. Indirect ELISA, some commercially available, have been used routinely in control programs to screen herds for *M agalactiae* but less so for *Mmc* and *Mcc*. Immuno (Western) blotting can be used to confirm suspect ELISA results and can distinguish field infection from vaccine antibody. In areas believed to be free of contagious agalactia, it is usually necessary to isolate and identify the causative organism to confirm infection. Serologic tests are not widely available for *M putrefaciens*.

A number of other mycoplasmas such as *M arginini*, *M bovigenitalium*, and *M bovis* have occasionally been isolated from mastitic milk and joint fluids, but their role in disease is not known. *M conjunctivae* is a common cause of keratoconjunctivitis but does not affect the udder or joints. Other bacteria causing mastitis include staphylococci, streptococci, *Escherichia coli*, and *Klebsiella*; caprine arthritic encephalomyelitis virus and *Erysipelothrix rhusiopathiae* should also be considered in cases of arthritis.

Treatment, Control, and Prevention: Regular laboratory monitoring of flocks/herds and replacement animals may help to prevent spread or introduction of disease and can be done on serum and/or milk (including bulk tank milk) by serology, culture, or PCR. Culling or isolation of infected animals is generally advised, because udder damage is considered permanent. When this is not possible, hygienic measures, such as improved milking hygiene and pasteurizing milk before feeding to the young, should be implemented.

Antibiotics that inhibit cell wall synthesis (eg, penicillins) are not effective against contagious agalactia. In vitro tests have shown that strains of *M agalactiae* are still sensitive to fluoroquinolones and macrolides. These can bring about clinical improvement, particularly if given early in the disease, but there is always the danger of promoting carrier animals. Resistance to tetracyclines has been reported for some strains of *M agalactiae*. The use of erythromycin and tylosin can destroy milk-producing tissue in small ruminants. In many disease-free countries and regions, a confirmed infected herd is always slaughtered.

In countries bordering the Mediterranean, both attenuated and inactivated vaccines have been used with mixed success. Some have provided protection from clinical disease and have been useful in endemic areas; however, they do not prevent transmission of the mycoplasmas. Generally, the duration of immunity, particularly to the formalinized, inactivated vaccines that are used in Europe, is short. Vaccines containing two or three of the causative agents are now available, but published data on their effectiveness is scarce.

Zoonotic Risk: There is no evidence that contagious agalactia is transmitted to people.

CYSTIC OVARY DISEASE

Among domestic animals, cystic ovary disease (COD) is most common in cattle, particularly the dairy breeds, but it occurs sporadically in dogs (*see* p 1395), cats, pigs, and perhaps mares.

Cystic Ovary Disease and the Corpus Luteum: Three ovarian structures in cattle may include the term "cyst": follicular cysts, luteal cysts, and cystic corpus luteum (CL). However, in contrast to the other two, the structure sometimes described as a cystic CL (a CL with a cavity or "lacunae") actually arises after normal ovulation. CL with a lacunae are a normal stage or variation of CL development and are found in normally cycling and pregnant cows without concurrent abnormal reproductive performance. The lacunae can be compared with the homogeneous, liver-like consistency of the base of a typical CL.

The CL may have an ovulation crown or papilla at its apex; however, 10%–20% of functional, *normal* CL fail to develop this feature.

The two pathologic forms of bovine cystic ovary disease, follicular cysts and luteal cysts, are etiologically and pathophysiologically related but differ clinically. Both are characterized by the presence of a fluid-filled structure >25 mm diameter, persisting for >7 days and associated with abnormal reproductive performance.

FOLLICULAR CYSTIC OVARY DISEASE

(Cystic follicles, "Bulling")

Follicular cystic ovary disease may be defined on a number of levels. Essentially, all signs relate to the disruption of the normal endocrine events of the estrous cycle, through the failure of ovulatory events. Key features include the presence of a thin-walled, fluid-filled structure >25 mm diameter and present for >7 days in the absence of a CL on ultrasonographic imaging of the ovary. Along with occasional behavioral signs of nymphomania, such as short inter-estrus intervals and excessive heat behavior, are endocrine changes, including a suboptimal luteinizing hormone (LH) surge and persistently increased estradiol levels.

Etiology and Pathogenesis: A hereditary predisposition has been implicated in dairy cattle. Cystic ovary disease or syndrome (COD) is commonly considered to be associated with negative energy balance and stress factors in dairy cows that are high milk producers. Genetic predisposition to partition glucose to the udder to prioritize lactose synthesis and milk production is characterized by insulin resistance in Holstein cattle. IGF-1 is a cytokine associated with metabolic influences on reproduction and hence COD. Incidence increases with age. Most cases occur within 3–8 wk of parturition at the first attempted postpartum ovulation, coinciding with peak daily milk production and rapidly decreasing body condition. The reported herd incidence is 5%–25% per lactation, or higher in some problem herds.

During normal proestrus, regression of the CL coincides with development of a selected follicle, while the growth of any additional follicles is inhibited. In animals developing COD, ovulation fails to occur and the dominant follicle continues to enlarge. An important component of the etiology is the failure of positive feedback of follicular estrogen on the hypothalamus via estrogen receptor α to release sufficient GnRH during estrus to trigger an LH surge. The end result is a failure of ovulation at the time of estrus. Moreover, other follicles may grow and form multiple cysts either bilaterally or unilaterally.

Grossly, follicular cysts resemble enlarged follicles, generally defined as varying in size from 25 mm to 50–60 mm in diameter. The size and form of an affected ovary depends on the number and size of cysts present. The cystic ovary is capable, at least initially, of steroidogenesis, and its products vary from estrogens to progesterone to androgens. The actions of the various hormones produced or the absence of the stabilizing action of high progesterone from the normal CL during ~75% of the estrous cycle (or both) are responsible for the changes seen in the genital tract, body conformation, and general behavior.

Clinical Findings: Behavioral aberrations range from frequent, intermittent estrus with exaggerated monosexual drive to bull-like behavior, including mounting, pawing the ground, and bellowing. This behavior may be accompanied by masculinization of the head and neck. Relaxation of the vulva, perineum, and the large pelvic ligaments, which causes the tail head to be elevated, can occur in chronic cases. Some affected cows show these signs, but others may be sexually quiescent; anestrous or subestrous cows are a common presentation.

The affected ovaries generally are enlarged and rounded, but their size varies, depending on the number and size of cysts. Their surface is smooth, elevated, and blister-like. Cysts frequently are multiple and may approach 4–6 cm in diameter. Under the influence of hormones produced by the cystic ovary or the lack of hormones (especially progesterone) normally present during estrous cycles, the uterus undergoes palpable changes, which in turn vary with the duration of the cystic condition. Thus, during the first week, the uterine wall is thickened and edematous as an extension of the preceding estrus. Toward the end of the first week, the uterine wall develops a sponge-like consistency. In chronic cases, atony and atrophy of the uterine wall are common. Occasionally, the uterine horns become markedly shortened. Some degree of mucoid to mucopurulent vaginal discharge is common. Hydrometra, a fluid-filled, extremely thin-walled uterus, is seen occasionally.

Diagnosis: Palpation of the uterus may help differentiate a follicular cyst from a dominant preovulatory follicle; the estrous cow has a coiled, extremely turgid uterus and a follicle. As noted earlier, cystic cows fail to ovulate a preovulatory follicle after undergoing CL regression and, on examination of the reproductive tract, they present with a large follicle, absence of a CL, and absence of a turgid uterus. Ultrasound technology per rectum can be used to differentiate cysts from corpora lutea and may help diagnose cyst type (ie, follicular cyst wall diameter has been described as <3 mm vs luteal cyst wall diameter >3 mm). Larger, multiple cysts are easily identified by rectal palpation. History, conformation, and uterine changes, when present, provide supplemental diagnostic evidence.

Treatment: COD may be frustratingly unresponsive to therapy. Some cysts respond readily to an LH-type hormonal treatment. In the past, human chorionic gonadotropin (hCG) was commonly used. It is most effective at 10,000 USP units IM, although success with lower doses given IM or IV has also been reported.

Hormone therapy with GnRH may be effective at 100 mcg and less antigenic than hCG. To hasten the onset of the first estrus after treatment, prostaglandin (PG) $F_2\alpha$ products can be given 7 days after hCG or

GnRH. Ovulation synchronization protocols combine GnRH and $PGF_2\alpha$ to control follicular dynamics, luteolysis, and ovulation. They allow for fixed timed artificial insemination (TAI) of cattle without the need for estrus detection and have been successfully used to treat cows with cystic ovaries. This protocol consists of giving GnRH, then prostaglandin 7 days later, then a second administration of GnRH 48 hr later, and finally TAI 0–24 hr later. Breeding on the first estrus may reduce recurrence by establishing pregnancy as soon as possible. However, COD recurrence is a risk.

Manual rupture is used, but the potential danger of traumatizing the ovary and causing hemorrhage with subsequent local adhesions should not be overlooked.

Prognosis: After therapy with an LH-type hormone, a normal, fertile estrus can be expected in 15–30 days. With GnRH therapy, 25% of cases required a second treatment, and 5% required a third. One-third of the cases treated for the third time did not respond. Spontaneous recovery is possible and is most common in cases arising during the first 50 days after calving. Likewise, successful treatment encourages perpetuation of the disease in the herd if the offspring are used for breeding. Although COD in cattle clearly has a genetic component, it is unlikely that a single farm using artificial insemination can significantly influence the incidence. In Sweden, progress has been made in reducing the condition through culling and selection procedures for bulls used in artificial insemination, but affected cows are often still treated.

LUTEAL CYSTIC OVARY DISEASE

Luteal cystic ovary disease is characterized by enlarged ovaries with one or more cysts, the walls of which are thicker than those of follicular cysts because of a lining of luteal tissue. Incidence ratios of follicular versus luteal cysts vary greatly because of diagnostic tendencies of individual veterinarians. Classically, luteal COD is defined as the presence of a fluid-filled ovarian structure >25 mm diameter persisting >7 days in the absence of a CL and with a wall diameter >3 mm, usually associated with abnormal reproductive signs. Normal lacunae formation in CL may be incorrectly classified as luteal COD.

Etiology and Pathogenesis: The basic causes of true luteal cysts are believed to be the same as for follicular cysts. The release of luteinizing hormone (LH) may be somewhat greater than that occurring when follicular cysts develop, and sufficient to initiate luteinization of follicles but inadequate to cause ovulation. Luteal cysts may be an extension of follicular cysts such that the nonovulatory follicle is partially luteinized spontaneously or in response to hormonal therapy.

Clinical Findings: Luteal cysts are accompanied by normal conformation and anestrous behavior. Rectal palpation reveals a quiescent uterus characteristic of the luteal phase of the estrous cycle. Luteal cysts are recognized as smooth, fluctuant domes protruding above the surface of the ovary. Usually, they are single structures.

Luteal cysts are differentiated from follicular cysts on the basis of palpable characteristics of both the structure and the uterus and, to some extent, on the cow's behavior. Progesterone assay and ultrasonography can help differentiate between follicular and luteal cysts, although with either method a final diagnostic decision remains somewhat subjective. On attempts to manually rupture the cystic structure, follicular cysts burst or rupture under minimal pressure whereas luteal cysts cannot be ruptured with reasonable force. Both types of cysts respond to LH or GnRH therapy, but $PGF_2\alpha$ will lyse some luteal cysts and generally all diestrual CL structures.

Treatment and Control: The treatment of choice is luteolytic doses of $PGF_2\alpha$ if a correct diagnosis can be ascertained. A normal estrus is expected in 3–5 days. The major limitation of this treatment is the difficulty in accurately estimating the amount of luteal tissue present. If the structure being diagnosed as a luteal cyst is really a developing CL (as discussed above, sometimes called a cystic CL), it may not respond because dairy cows do not become highly responsive to the luteolytic action of $PGF_2\alpha$ until day 6 after estrus. Ultrasound examination is increasingly common and facilitates diagnosis of ovarian structures. Luteal cysts also respond to human chorionic gonadotropin and GnRH therapy that is effective in the treatment of follicular cysts, but the next estrus could occur 5–21 days after treatment. Manual rupture of luteal cysts is not recommended because of the risk of trauma and hemorrhage. Because of poor estrus detection practices on many dairy farms, the treatment of choice for both follicular and luteal cysts is intravaginal progesterone/prostaglandin (a fixed timed artificial insemination protocol) (*see* p 1355). Application of this protocol in affected cows promotes timely breeding after treatment.

CYSTIC OVARY DISEASE AS A HERD PROBLEM

Individual herds may experience exceptionally high rates (~50%) of cystic ovary disease (COD) over a period of months. Determining the cause of these multifactorial episodes is not easy, but the following questions should be addressed: 1) Is the diagnosis accurate, ie, are the structures being identified as cysts really cysts? This can be established via second opinion diagnoses, determination of milk or plasma progesterone levels, ultrasound examination of the ovaries in suspected cases, observing ovarian changes and time of estrous activity after treatment with prostaglandin products, and/or improving diagnostic skills by continuing education. 2) Has the palpation examination schedule for the herd changed? Initiating routine postpartum examinations for all cows and increasing frequency of herd visits can result in an increased apparent incidence. 3) Has the herd incidence of periparturient complications and stress increased? Cows having problems around calving (such as twins, milk fever, dystocia, retained placenta, ketosis, etc) are much more likely to develop cysts. Attempts to reduce these complications are indicated. 4) Have herd genetics been considered? It is well accepted that ovarian cysts are more common in certain lines. 5) Has the nutritional program of the herd been evaluated? Nutritional problems are frequently implicated as a risk factor for COD. Proper nutritional management of dairy herds is always warranted. Monitoring the effects of the nutritional program via a body condition scoring program should be done as part of the effort to reduce ovarian cysts in problem herds. 6) Has management of cows around estrus changed? Social and environmental changes may cause stresses associated with COD.

CYSTIC OVARY DISEASE IN MARES

When diagnosing the reproductive status of mares, it must be remembered that follicles during estrus are normally 4–6 cm in diameter. Ovulation failure can also be seen in mares having irregular estrous cycles during the spring or fall transition phases of the reproductive cycle, but this state is not treated in the same way as the cystic ovary disease condition of cattle. The granulosa cell tumor condition in mares causes marked enlargement of one ovary but differs from cystic ovary disease of cattle.

EQUINE COITAL EXANTHEMA

(Genital horsepox, Equine venereal balanitis in stallions)

Etiology and Epidemiology: Equine coital exanthema is a benign venereal disease of horses that probably occurs worldwide. It affects both sexes and is caused by equine herpesvirus type 3 (EHV-3). This virus has a single antigenic type but also has small and large plaque variants in tissue culture, indicating that variation may occur in the severity of field outbreaks. Although the primary route of transmission is venereal, outbreaks have been documented in which transmission occurred via contaminated supplies and instruments or by the use of a single glove for rectal examination of many mares. It is probably for this reason that EHV-3 has also been isolated from horses that have not been bred.

Equine coital exanthema is probably transmitted only in the acute phase of the disease; after the lesions have healed, horses do not appear to shed the virus. However, the existence of a carrier state is unclear: the scars that persist after healing may identify potential carriers, but such asymptomatic carriers have not been identified. Immunity is short-lived, but evidence from stallions shows that recurrence is not likely within a single breeding season.

Clinical Findings: Clinical signs in mares develop 4–8 days after sexual contact or veterinary examination and are manifest by the appearance of multiple, circular, red nodules up to 2 mm in diameter on the vulvar and vaginal mucosa, the clitoral sinus, and perineal skin. These lesions develop into vesicles and then pustules and eventually rupture, leaving shallow, painful, ulcerated areas that may coalesce into larger lesions. Edema can develop in the perineum and may extend to between the thighs. Occasionally, ulcers will be found on the teats, lips, and nasal mucosa. Secondary bacterial infection of the ulcers by *Streptococcus* spp is common, causing the ulcers to enlarge and exude a mucopurulent discharge. In such cases, the horse may become febrile. Unless secondary bacterial infection occurs, skin healing is complete within 3 wk, but clitoral and vaginal ulcers heal more slowly. Skin lesions persist for long periods as unpigmented scars. However, pregnancy rates are not reduced.

Lesions in stallions are similar to those in mares and are found on both the penis and prepuce. As a result, intromission is painful, and the stallion may be reluctant to copulate. If copulation does occur during the ulcerative stage, the ulcers may hemorrhage into the ejaculate, reducing sperm viability.

Diagnosis: A tentative diagnosis is based on clinical signs and confirmed by identifying (using electron microscopy) the virus in cells from the margin of ulcers. Typical intranuclear herpesvirus inclusion bodies can also be seen in cytologic or histologic preparations. Acute and convalescent samples for serum neutralization or complement fixation tests can also be diagnostic, but these tests must be interpreted carefully because both EHV-1 and EHV-4 have also been isolated from genital lesions.

Treatment and Prevention: Sexual rest is essential to allow ulcers to heal and prevent spread of the disease. The use of antibiotic ointments to prevent secondary infections is also advisable. Affected horses should be isolated until all lesions have healed, and disposable equipment should be used for examinations. During the acute phase of the disease, mares should be bred only by artificial insemination. No vaccine is available. All horses should be examined carefully before they are allowed to breed, keeping in mind that the incubation period is up to 10 days.

MASTITIS IN LARGE ANIMALS

Mastitis, or inflammation of the mammary gland, is predominantly due to the effects of infection by bacterial pathogens, although mycotic or algal microbes play a role in some cases. Pathologic changes to milk-secreting epithelial cells from the inflammatory process often bring about a decrease in functional capacity. Depending on the pathogen, functional losses may continue into further lactations, which may reduce productivity and potential weight gain for suckling offspring. Although most infections result in relatively mild clinical or subclinical local inflammation, more severe cases can lead to agalactia or even profound systemic involvement, resulting in death. Mastitis has been reported in almost all domestic mammals and has a worldwide geographic distribution. Climatic conditions, seasonal variation, bedding, housing density of livestock populations, and husbandry practices may affect the incidence and etiology. However, it is of greatest frequency and economic importance in species that primarily function as producers of milk for dairy products, particularly dairy cattle. (*See also* UDDER DISEASES, p 1385.)

MASTITIS IN CATTLE

Almost any microbe that can opportunistically invade tissue and cause infection can cause mastitis. However, most infections are caused by various species of streptococci, staphylococci, and gram-negative rods, especially lactose-fermenting organisms of enteric origin, commonly termed coliforms. From an epidemiologic standpoint, the primary sources of infection for most pathogens may be regarded as contagious or environmental.

Except for *Mycoplasma* spp, which may spread from cow to cow through aerosol transmission and invade the udder subsequent to bacteremia, contagious pathogens are spread during milking by milkers' hands or the liners of the milking unit. Species that use this mode of transmission include *Staphylococcus aureus*, *Streptococcus agalactiae*, and *Corynebacterium bovis*. Most other species are opportunistic invaders from the cow's environment, although some other streptococci and staphylococci may also have a contagious component. Additionally, contagious transmission infrequently occurs for pathogens typically associated with environmental reservoirs, eg, through the development of host-adapted virulence factors (*Escherichia coli*) or by shedding of overwhelming numbers of bacteria from infected udders (*Trueperella* [formerly *Arcanobacterium*] *pyogenes*).

The bedding used to house cattle is the primary source of environmental pathogens, but contaminated teat dips, intramammary infusions, water used for udder preparation before milking, water ponds or mud holes, skin lesions, teat trauma, and flies have all been incriminated as sources of infection.

Intramammary infections are often described as subclinical or clinical mastitis. **Subclinical mastitis** is the presence of an infection without apparent signs of local inflammation or systemic involvement. Although transient episodes of abnormal milk or udder inflammation may appear, these infections are for the most part asymptomatic and, if the infection persists for at least 2 mo, are termed chronic. Once established, many of these infections persist for entire lactations or the life of the cow. Detection is best done by examination of milk for somatic cell counts (SCCs) (predominantly neutrophils) using either the California Mastitis Test or automated methods provided by dairy herd improvement organizations. SCCs are positively correlated with the presence of infection. Inflammatory changes and decreases in milk quality may start with SCCs as low as 100,000 cells/mL. Although variable (especially if determined on a single analysis), an SCC of ≥280,000 cells/mL in a cow indicates a >85% chance of being infected. Likewise, the higher the SCC in a herd bulk tank, the higher the prevalence of infection in the herd. Herd SCCs <200,000 cells/mL are considered desirable, and lower counts can be attained. Causative agents must be identified by bacterial culture of milk.

Clinical mastitis is an inflammatory response to infection causing visibly abnormal milk (eg, color, fibrin clots). As the extent of the inflammation increases, changes in the udder (swelling, heat, pain, redness) may also be apparent. Clinical cases that include only local signs are referred to as mild or moderate. If the inflammatory response includes systemic involvement (fever, anorexia, shock), the case is termed severe. If the onset is very rapid, as often occurs with severe clinical cases, it is termed an acute case of severe mastitis. More severely affected cows tend to have more serous secretions in the affected quarter.

Although any number of quarters can be infected simultaneously in subclinical mastitis, typically only one quarter at a time will display clinical mastitis. However, it is not uncommon for clinical episodes caused by *Mycoplasma* to affect multiple quarters. Gangrenous mastitis can also occur, particularly when subclinical, chronic infections of *S aureus* become severe at times of immunosuppression (eg, at parturition). As with subclinical mastitis, culture of milk samples collected from affected quarters is the only reliable method to determine the etiology of clinical cases.

Subclinical Mastitis

Epidemiology: All dairy herds have cows with subclinical mastitis; however, the prevalence of infected cows varies from 5%–75%, and quarters from 2%–40%. Many different pathogens can establish a chronic infection in which clinical signs of mastitis will manifest only occasionally. The primary focus of most subclinical mastitis programs is to reduce the prevalence of the contagious pathogens *S agalactiae* and *S aureus*, as well as other gram-positive cocci, most notably *Streptococcus dysgalactiae* (which may also be contagious or an environmental pathogen), *Streptococcus uberis*, enterococci, and numerous other coagulase-negative staphylococci, including *Staphylococcus hyicus*, *Staphylococcus epidermidis*, *Staphylococcus xylosus*, and *Staphylococcus intermedius*. Herds have been identified that have considerable subclinical mastitis caused by gram-negative rods such as *Klebsiella* sp, *Serratia marcescens*, *Pseudomonas aeruginosa*, and other atypical pathogens such as mycotic and algal microbes.

For contagious pathogens, adult lactating cattle are most at risk of infection, either while lactating or during the dry period. The primary reservoir of infection is the mammary gland; transmission occurs at milking with either milkers' hands or milking equipment acting as fomites. Primiparous heifers have been reported to be infected with staphylococci and streptococci before calving, although the prevalence varies greatly among herds and geographic regions. Teat-end dermatitis caused by the horn fly, *Haematobia irritans,* which can harbor *S aureus*, has been associated with increased risk of infection in heifers, especially in warmer climates.

For the contagious pathogens and coagulase-negative staphylococci, there is little or no seasonal variation in incidence of infection.

Treatment: Therapy is given on the premise that treatment costs will be outweighed by production gains after elimination of infection. In the case of contagious pathogens, elimination may also result in a decrease of the reservoir of infection for previously noninfected cows. No significant economic losses will occur as a result of delaying therapy until bacterial culture can be completed. However, many subclinical cases selected as potential therapy candidates have chronic infections; particularly in the case of *S aureus*, prediction of therapeutic outcome by in vitro testing is unreliable. Drug distribution after intramammary administration may not be adequate because of extensive fibrosis and microabscess formation in the gland; it is critical to assess the cow's immune status from a perspective of duration of infection, number of quarters infected, and other variables.

Prevalence of *S agalactiae* infection can be rapidly reduced by treating an entire herd—or more economically, all the infected cows in a herd—with antibacterials. All four quarters of infected cows should be treated to ensure elimination of the pathogen and to prevent possible cross-infection of a noninfected quarter. Cure rates can often be 75%–90%. Labeled use of commercial intramammary products that contain amoxicillin, penicillin, and erythromycin are as efficacious as procaine penicillin G infusions derived from multiple-dose vials. Consequently, use of drugs originating from multiple-dose vials (labeled for systemic therapy) should *not* be used for intramammary therapy, because commercial intramammary preparations have superior quality control standards for sterility and better reliability to predict withholding periods for milk and meat after treatment. It is critical to apply strict aseptic techniques (use of alcohol swabs for teat-end preparation) whenever any intramammary infusion product is administered.

Herds undergoing extensive therapy for *S agalactiae* must be monitored by SCCs and bacteriology to further identify and treat cows not identified or cured during the initial therapy. Usually, 30-day monitoring intervals are successful. A small percentage of cows will not respond to therapy and are best segregated or culled. In addition, failure to use postmilking teat dipping and total dry cow treatment to prevent new infections during the treatment period will ultimately result in reinfection of the herd. Parenteral therapy is not likely to offer any benefit over intramammary therapy.

Most other streptococci also display in vitro susceptibility to numerous antibacterials, especially β-lactam drugs. Despite this apparent susceptibility, many streptococcal infections are not as easily cured as those caused by *S agalactiae*. Generally, subclinical infections caused by *S uberis* and *S dysgalactiae* should be preferentially treated at the end of lactation with intramammary infusions of commercial dry cow products. Cure rates at this time may exceed 75%.

S aureus intramammary infections often result in deep-seated abscesses. Therapy is difficult, because resistance to antibacterials (particularly β-lactams) is more common than with streptococcal infections, and *S aureus* may survive intracellularly after phagocytosis when antibacterial concentrations are reduced. Intramammary infusions may cure only 35%–40% of infections; however, this number will be substantially lower for chronic infections.

The success rate of therapy for chronic subclinical intramammary infections caused by *S aureus* may be increased by using both parenteral and intramammary therapy. However, systemic therapy involves extra-label drug use, and milk and meat withholding periods must be determined judiciously. Therapy should be administered for periods long enough (7–10 days) to allow effective killing of the pathogen. It is most economical and least likely to result in residues in milk if this therapy is applied to dry cows. Depending on susceptibility testing, lipophilic antibacterial drugs that distribute well into mammary tissue, such as oxytetracycline (11 mg/kg/day) are the best candidates for systemic administration, although several studies have found oxytetracycline (administered for 4 days or less) to be ineffective. Cure rates may not be much better than those attained from spontaneous cure, and cure must be defined critically. Affected quarters should be monitored bacteriologically for ≥30 days to encompass the refractory period when bacteria may not be isolated.

Occasionally, premature agalactia will occur in chronically infected quarters, particularly quarters infected with resistant pathogens. Culling may be a practical option for these cows. Alternatively, it is common to dry off the infected quarter and continue to milk the cow. This may have some benefit for genetically superior animals within a herd or for cows that are to be maintained until calving. Anecdotally, the overall milk production from such cows may remain the same. The goal is to eliminate the infection by causing fibrosis of the affected quarter, thus reducing the risk of further pathogenic change or systemic effects on the cow, as well as reducing risk of infection for other cows.

Dry Cows: The dry period of the lactation cycle is a critical time for the udder health of dairy cows. The mammary gland undergoes marked biochemical, cellular, and immunologic changes. Involution of the mammary parenchyma begins 1–2 days after the end of lactation and continues for 10–14 days. During this time, the gland is particularly vulnerable to new intramammary infections. However, the involuted mammary gland offers the most hostile immune environment for bacterial pathogens. Consequently, the dry period is an ideal time to attain synergy between antibacterial therapy and immune function, without incurring the extensive costs typical of lactating cow therapy. Intramammary administration of antibacterials at the end of lactation has been a standard of dairy mastitis management for 30 yr and continues to help reduce the prevalence of mastitis in most dairy herds.

Numerous commercial products are available and include penicillin, cloxacillin, cephapirin, ceftiofur, or novobiocin. One tube per quarter is sufficient and should be administered immediately after the last milking of lactation. Therapy should not be repeated by intramammary infusion; if there is a need to extend therapy, systemic administration should be used as an adjunct to the intramammary infusion. In addition to eliminating existing subclinical infections, one of the most critical roles of dry cow therapy is to prevent new infections. However, most commercial dry cow products have little or no activity against gram-negative pathogens, and their administration at the start of the dry period will not be effective against new infections that begin during the periparturient period. The antimicrobial therapy can be supplemented by subsequent infusion of internal teat sealants that serve as a barrier to help reduce new infections.

Heifers: Many infections in calving heifers are caused by staphylococcal species other than *S aureus*, which have a high rate of spontaneous cure. However, under some herd conditions, a substantial portion of heifers are infected at calving; some of these infections are caused by pathogens such as *S aureus*. Potential sources include milk (fed to calves) and body sites such as tonsils and skin. There is also a geographic risk factor: fly bite dermatitis of the teat end, which compromises this important physical barrier to infection, may play a role in the pathogenesis.

Intramammary infusions of β-lactam antibacterial drugs 7–14 days before expected calving dates have been reported to reduce the rate of intramammary infections at calving. However, longterm benefits on SCCs, milk production, and incidence of clinical mastitis during lactation were found to be highly herd variable and not consistent. Strict teat-end antisepsis should be followed before infusion to prevent contamination; thus, labor to handle animals for treatment can be extensive. This is not a recommended management program for many dairies. However, if herd records indicate that an undesirable proportion of first-lactation animals are infected at calving, particularly with staphylococci, this regimen may be considered.

Prevention: New infections caused by *S agalactiae* and *S aureus* can be prevented by focusing management efforts on milking technique and hygiene. Clean and dry bedding, clean and dry udders at the time of milking, and lack of teat-end lesions all have a positive effect on control. The single most important management practice to prevent transmission of new infections is the use of an effective germicide as a postmilking teat dip. These products should be applied as a dip (rather than a spray) immediately after milking. Other practices that augment teat dipping include use of individual towels for drying teats, gloves for milkers' hands, use of a premilking germicide (spray or dip), attachment of units at the proper time after teat stimulation (60–120 sec), cleaning milking units after an infected cow has been milked, or segregation of infected cows into a separate milk group. This last option may be unrealistic for cattle in free housing that are normally segregated for nutritional or reproductive reasons. Routine milking equipment evaluations should be conducted to ensure that the teat-end vacuum is operating at a proper level and remains stable during milking. Proper pulsator function should be maintained, and liners and rubber air hoses should be replaced as needed.

Proper milking hygiene also reduces the new infection rate of noncontagious pathogens. More importantly for environmental pathogens, cows should be provided dry, clean housing. Emphasis should be placed on bedding and any other practices that reduce the exposure of the teat end to bacteria. Inorganic bedding supports less bacterial growth than cellulose-based material; thus, sand is preferred over sawdust, straw, recycled paper, or manure. In particular, higher incidence of infections caused by *Klebsiella* has been associated with sawdust bedding. Similarly, a higher incidence of infections caused by environmental streptococci has been associated with straw bedding. However, the concentrations of bacteria can vary greatly depending on moisture and presence of organic matter (such as in sand after recycling). Thus, identification of reservoirs of infection should not be based solely on the choice of bedding material. Regular cleaning or changing of bedding, reducing heat stress, removing udder hair, preventing teat trauma, reducing udder edema in periparturient cows by nutritional management of potassium and sodium intake, and preventing frostbite and fly exposure all have a positive impact on environmental mastitis control.

Clinical Mastitis

When the balance between host defenses and invading pathogens causes a marked inflammatory response, clinical signs become apparent. Infections from any pathogen can be clinical or subclinical, depending on the duration of infection, host immune status, and pathogen virulence. Control of clinical mastitis usually focuses on prevention and elimination of pathogens that arise from an environmental reservoir. Thus, the epidemiology and prevention of clinical mastitis is similar to previously discussed concepts regarding control of subclinical mastitis.

Epidemiology: Except for outbreaks of *Mycoplasma*, clinical mastitis in most dairy herds is caused by environmental pathogens. In addition, many clinical mastitis cases are transient, especially those that are initial episodes for a cow and quarter. Thus, from an epidemiologic perspective, assessment of clinical mastitis is based on incidence and not prevalence.

The standard methods to monitor subclinical mastitis, ie, routine somatic cell counts (SCCs) and culture of cows with increased SCCs, are poor predictors of herd clinical mastitis episodes. Cows with high SCCs caused by chronic infections may occasionally display clinical mastitis, although it is usually mild. However, cows with low SCCs are also prone to develop clinical mastitis. Herds with low SCCs may actually have a higher incidence of clinical cases caused by environmental organisms (as high as 30–50 cases/100 cows/yr) than herds with higher SCCs. Similarly, routine culture of milk samples from a cow with a low SCC is a poor indicator of the probability of developing clinical mastitis, especially if the culture yielded no organisms.

Thus, the incidence of clinical cases, and data from each case that may determine risk factors (eg, season, age, stage of lactation, and previous episodes), should be recorded as part of a mastitis control program. Milk samples should be collected from affected quarters and, when feasible, antibacterial susceptibility testing performed. For well-managed herds in which mastitis caused by contagious pathogens has been controlled, a goal for the incidence of clinical mastitis should be 1–2 cases/100 cows milking/mo. Severe mastitis cases should be in the range of 1–2 cases/100 cows milking/yr.

Typically, 3%–40% of milk samples collected from clinical mastitis cases yield no organisms on culture. However, of the samples that do yield organisms, 90%–95% of the isolated bacteria include a wide variety of streptococci, staphylococci, or coliforms. If this is not the case, especially if a single pathogen such as a noncoliform gram-negative rod or a mycotic or algal (*Prototheca* sp) predominates, a point source of infection should be considered.

Severe Clinical Mastitis: Coliforms (lactose-fermenting gram-negative rods of the family Enterobacteriaceae) are the most common cause of this form of mastitis. After infection, coliform numbers in milk increase rapidly, often attaining peak bacterial concentrations within a few hours. A subsequent decline (rapid in most cases but may take several days in truly severe mastitis) in bacterial concentration follows neutrophil migration into the gland. Most coliform infections are cleared from the gland with few or mild clinical signs. However, if bacterial concentrations are increased enough to elicit an acute inflammatory response, systemic involvement is a frequent consequence.

Mastitis caused by coliforms results in a higher incidence of cow death or agalactia-related culling (30%–40%) than mastitis caused by other pathogens (2%). Prognosis for cases of *Klebsiella* infection should be particularly guarded, because these cows are twice as likely to be culled or die than those infected by other coliforms. Thus, primary therapy for severe clinical mastitis should be directed against coliform organisms, although secondary consideration must be given for other causative agents. Supportive care, including fluids, is indicated, and in the case of coliform mastitis, may be the most beneficial component of the therapeutic regimen. Antibacterial therapy is ideally based on identification of the causative pathogen; however, this is not attainable for some hours after initial case recognition. In addition, most antibacterial therapeutic regimens currently used for severe clinical mastitis in the USA are not approved by the FDA.

Many inflammatory and systemic changes seen in severe coliform mastitis result from the effects of release of lipopolysaccharide (LPS) endotoxin from the bacteria and subsequent activation of cytokine and arachidonic acid–derived mediators of inflammation and the acute phase response. By the time therapy is initiated, maximal release of LPS has likely occurred. Thus, the primary therapeutic concern is the treatment of endotoxin-induced shock with fluids, electrolytes, and anti-inflammatory drugs. The IV route is preferred as the initial method of fluid administration. If isotonic saline is administered, 30–40 L are necessary throughout a 4-hr period, which can be difficult under farm conditions. A practical alternative is 2 L of 7% NaCl (hypersaline) administered IV. This induces rapid fluid uptake from the body compartment into the circulation. Cows should then be offered free-choice water to drink, and if at least 10 gal. is not consumed, 5–7 gal. should be pumped into the rumen. Many cows with endotoxic shock are marginally hypocalcemic; thus, 500 mL of calcium borogluconate should be administered SC (to avoid potential complications of IV administration). Alternatively, rapid absorption calcium gels, designed for periparturient hypocalcemia, can be given. If the cow remains in shock, continued fluid therapy should be administered PO or IV as isotonic, not hypertonic, fluids.

If administered early in the course of disease, glucocorticoids may be helpful in cases of mastitis caused by endotoxin-producing coliforms. Administration of dexamethasone (30 mg, IM) to dairy cows immediately after introduction of *E coli* into the mammary gland has been reported to reduce mammary gland swelling and inhibition of rumen motility. Isoflupredone (10–20 mg, IM) has also been shown to reduce local mammary swelling. Cattle are sensitive to glucocorticoid-induced immune suppression; however, it is unlikely that one-time administration of a glucocorticoid will adversely affect cows with endotoxin-induced severe clinical mastitis. Temporary suppression of inflammation as manifested by reduced neutrophil migration may well be beneficial. Care should be exercised in administering these drugs to pregnant animals; however, severe clinical mastitis in and of itself may cause pregnancy loss in cattle.

There is little published research on the use of glucocorticoids for mastitis caused by gram-positive bacteria. It is reasonable to expect that gram-positive infections would be less likely to benefit from the anti-inflammatory activities of glucocorticoids and may even be adversely affected. Intramammary glucocorticoid administration to reduce local inflammation, without affecting the migration of neutrophils into the gland, is an attractive therapeutic option. Although products that combine antibacterial and glucocorticoid drugs for intramammary administration exist in Europe, it is not clear whether clinical benefit is gained when compared with antibacterial therapy alone. As a general guideline, glucocorticoid treatment should be reserved for severe cases of gram-negative mastitis, with a single dose administered early in the disease course.

NSAIDs are widely used in treatment of acute mastitis. Flunixin meglumine, flurbiprofen, carprofen, ibuprofen, and ketoprofen have been studied as treatments for experimental coliform mastitis or endotoxin-induced mastitis. Systemic use of these drugs is preferred over orally administered aspirin, which is not likely to attain effective concentrations in tissue or lead to beneficial results. Dipyrone use in food animals is specifically prohibited by the FDA. Phenylbutazone is prohibited in dairy cattle >20 mo old; the tolerance level for phenylbutazone is zero, and detection of any concentration is an illegal residue. Thus, these two drugs should not be used for anti-inflammatory therapy for mastitis in cattle.

Treatment with ketoprofen improved recovery of cows with acute clinical mastitis in a blinded, placebo-controlled study. Ketoprofen is available as a veterinary product for use in horses, has a high therapeutic index, has favorable pharmacokinetics for use in lactating dairy cattle, and is approved for use in cattle in France; however, it is not labeled for food animal use in the USA. The Food Animal Residue Avoidance Databank (FARAD) recommends withdrawal intervals of 7 days for slaughter and 24 hr for milk, with IV or IM administration, for dosages up to 3.3 mg/kg/day, for up to 3 days.

Flunixin meglumine is labeled for beef and dairy cattle. It is the only NSAID labeled for use in cattle in the USA and is therefore the most logical choice for treating clinical mastitis. In field studies, increased survival and improved milk production have not been demonstrated after treatment of clinical acute mastitis with flunixin meglumine at a dosage of 1.1 mg/kg. However, in studies of experimental mastitis, flunixin meglumine reduced the severity of clinical signs such as fever, depression, heart and respiratory rates, and udder pain. The FDA-approved withdrawal intervals are 4 days for slaughter and 36 hr for milk when used as labeled by IV administration. Because of extensive and unpredictable withdrawal periods, this drug should *not* be administered by IM injection. As with the glucocorticoids, NSAIDs may provide symptomatic relief and promote well-being. Administration early in the course of infection is likely to increase clinical benefit.

Antibacterial therapy may be of secondary importance relative to immediate supportive treatment of endotoxic shock, but it remains an integral part of a therapeutic regimen. Occasionally, coliform infections do result in chronic mastitis. Research suggests that bacteremia may occur in >40% of severe coliform cases. In addition, numerous other pathogens, including gram-positive cocci, cause severe clinical mastitis, which can be difficult to distinguish from cases caused by coliforms at initial presentation.

Selection of an appropriate antibacterial for severe coliform mastitis depends primarily on the susceptibility of the organism to the selected drug and the ability to maintain effective concentrations at the primary pharmacologic target (which, in the case of coliform mastitis, is the plasma compartment of the cow).

In one study, IM gentamicin was not more effective in preventing agalactia or death resulting from severe coliform mastitis, or in improving other clinical outcomes, than IM erythromycin or no systemic antibacterials. Cows experimentally challenged with *E coli* and treated with 500 mg of intramammary gentamicin bid did not have lower peak bacterial concentrations in milk, duration of infection, convalescent SCCs or serum albumin concentrations in milk, or rectal temperatures than untreated challenged cows. In addition, gentamicin readily diffused through the milk-blood barrier, resulting in drug residues in the kidney that could extend beyond 18 mo. Because of zero tolerance for aminoglycoside residues at slaughter, the use of this class of drugs in dairy cattle is *not* recommended.

Oxytetracycline (11 mg/kg/day, IV) improved outcome of cows with clinical coliform mastitis (not necessarily severe) as compared with cows that did not receive systemic antibacterials. Ceftiofur sodium (2.2 mg/kg/day, IM) decreased the mortality and cull rates of cows with severe coliform mastitis. This drug distributes poorly to the mammary gland, supporting the emphasis on treating the cow rather than the mammary gland because of the risk of septicemia.

Intramammary infusion of commercial products that have good activity against gram-positive organisms should be administered to any cow with severe clinical mastitis. This treatment is not likely to affect the outcome of a case caused by coliforms but may provide some benefit for cases caused by gram-positive cocci. The need for antibacterial therapy in cows with grossly abnormal milk, but with improved appetite, attitude, and milk production, should be evaluated critically. Unnecessary extension of therapy in these instances results in increased discarded milk expense for the dairy producer and risk of antibacterials in marketed milk.

Mild Clinical Mastitis: No microorganisms are isolated from 30%–40% of bacteriologic cultures of milk samples collected from cows with clinical mastitis. Many mild mastitis cases that fail to yield bacteria on culture are coliform intramammary infections that resolve before treatment is necessary. In addition, numerous mild clinical mastitis cases are temporary setbacks in the balance between pathogen and host defenses that occurs in more chronic intramammary infections. A "no antibiotic" approach to mild clinical mastitis cases avoids costs of discarded milk and residue risks inherent in antibacterial therapy.

A comparison of cure rate in treated versus untreated cows in a study of three California dairies found bacteriologic cure assessed at 4 and 20 days after treatment with amoxicillin, cephapirin, or oxytocin (no antibacterial) did not differ for mild clinical mastitis cases caused by streptococci and coliforms. However, the rates of both relapses and recurring cases were higher in untreated cows, especially among streptococcal cases. In a Colorado dairy study, a no-antibiotic approach also increased the rate of relapses, with an increase in the incidence of clinical mastitis, prevalence of intramammary infections, and herd SCCs associated with streptococcal infections. If bacterial culture of affected quarters yields no organisms or coliforms, therapy is not likely to be beneficial, whereas if gram-positive cocci are isolated, therapy is recommended.

Common sense and individual herd history should determine the course of therapy for mild clinical mastitis cases in dairy herds. Use of approved commercial intramammary infusions is likely to be the best option. Assessment of success should be based on bacteriologic cure but will be more practically based on return to normal milk. However, the frequency of relapsed cases should be monitored as the best means to determine cures, because many cases will be deemed to have been successfully treated initially but relapse later in lactation. If mastitis recurs regularly in affected quarters in the absence of systemic signs, repeated treatment of what now has become chronic intramammary infection is not warranted. Additionally, augmentation with parenteral therapy for these cases has not been demonstrated to be effective and will not likely overcome the expense of discarded milk, other related treatment costs, and the increased risk of residues in milk and meat. Previous history of clinical cases ("repeat offenders"), long duration of infection (as exhibited by high individual SCCs or extended periods of increased SCCs), and infections caused by nonresponsive pathogens are the greatest risk factors for poor therapeutic outcome. Practitioners should develop a protocol with dairy clients to reduce unnecessary treatment of poor risk cases as listed above and not rely on continued unsuccessful therapy or seeking a "better drug."

If standard regimens achieve less than desired results, it would be better to extend initial therapy for a prolonged period rather than to change to other antibacterial drugs or increase the amount of each dose. Studies have demonstrated improved cure rates for gram-positive cocci, especially coagulase-negative staphylococci and streptococci, when infected quarters were treated with intramammary infusions for up to 8 days as compared with 2 or 5 days. Care should be especially exercised in teat asepsis for extended therapy because of the increased risk of nosocomial infections.

Unusual Pathogens: *Pseudomonas aeruginosa* may cause outbreaks of clinical mastitis. Generally, a persistent infection occurs, which may be characterized by intermittent acute or subacute exacerbations. The organism is found in soil-water environments common to dairy farms. Herd infections have been reported after extensive exposure to contaminated wash water, teat cup liners, or intramammary treatments administered by milkers. Failure to use aseptic techniques for udder therapy or use of contaminated milking equipment may lead to establishment of *P aeruginosa* infections within the mammary glands. Severe peracute mastitis with toxemia and high mortality may follow immediately in some cows, whereas subclinical infections may occur in others. The organism has persisted in a gland for as long as five lactations, but spontaneous recovery may occur. Other than supportive care for severe episodes, therapy is of little value. Culling is recommended for cows.

Trueperella (formerly *Arcanobacterium*) *pyogenes* is common in suppurative processes of cattle and pigs and produces a characteristic mastitis in heifers and dry cows. It is occasionally seen in mastitis of lactating udders after teat injury, and it may be a secondary invader. The inflammation is typified by the formation of profuse, foul-smelling, purulent exudate. Mastitis due to *T pyogenes* is common among dry cows and heifers that are pastured during the summer months on fields and that have access to ponds or wet areas. The vector for animal-to-animal spread is the fly *Hydrotaea irritans*. Control of infections is by limiting the ability to stand udder-deep in water and by controlling flies. Preventive treatment of heifers and dry cows in susceptible areas with long-acting penicillin preparations has effectively reduced infections. Therapy is rarely successful, and the infected quarter is usually lost to production. Infected cows may be systemically ill, and cows with abscesses usually should be slaughtered. (*See also* ACTINOMYCOSIS, p 590.)

Mycoplasma spp can cause a severe form of mastitis that may spread rapidly through a herd with serious consequences. *M bovis* is the most common cause. Other significant species include *M californicum*, *M canadense*, and *M bovigenitalium*.

Onset is rapid, and the source of infection is believed to be endogenous after outbreaks of respiratory disease in heifers or cows. The disease is often seen in herds undergoing expansion in which animals from outside sources have been added. Typically, introduced animals will be asymptomatic carriers and then shed the organism via respiratory or intramammary transmission. Some or all quarters become involved. Loss of production is often dramatic, and the secretion is soon replaced by a serous or purulent exudate. Initially, a characteristic, fine granular or flaky sediment may be seen in the material removed from infected glands. Despite the severe local effects on udder tissue, cows usually do not manifest signs of systemic involvement. The infection may persist through the dry period. Identification of infected cows can be difficult because of the frequent propensity of these cows to become asymptomatic carriers and intermittently shed the organism in milk.

Because there is no satisfactory treatment, affected cows should be segregated during active outbreaks. Routine screening of the bulk tank and milk strings may help identify the presence of infected cows. However, culture of the mammary secretion of cows with clinical mastitis, or recently calved cows, is the most reliable surveillance method. If cows continue to display clinical mastitis or systemic signs, they should be culled. Sanitary measures should be strictly enforced, especially at milking and in hospital/treatment areas. Milk from *Mycoplasma*-infected cows should not be fed to calves, because this may result in respiratory and inner ear infections. Milk replacer or pasteurized milk, rather than discarded milk, should be fed to calves in herds with *Mycoplasma*.

Nocardia asteroides causes a destructive mastitis characterized by acute onset, high temperature, anorexia, rapid wasting, and marked swelling of the udder. Response in the udder is typical of a granulomatous inflammation and leads to extensive fibrosis and formation of palpable nodules. Herd histories suggest that infection of the udder may be associated with failure to ensure asepsis in intramammary treatment of the common forms of mastitis. Slaughter is recommended for infected cows.

Serratia mastitis may arise from contamination of milk hoses, teat dips, water supply, or other equipment used in the milking process. The organism is resistant to disinfectants. Cows with this form of mastitis that continue to display clinical signs should be culled.

Mastitis due to various mycotic organisms (yeasts) has appeared in dairy herds, especially after the use of penicillin in association with prolonged repetitive use of antibiotic infusions in individual cows. Yeasts grow well in the presence of penicillin and some other antibiotics; they may be introduced during udder infusions of antibiotics, multiply, and cause mastitis. Yet, heifers that have never received intramammary infusions may develop yeast mastitis. Signs may be severe, with a fever followed either by spontaneous recovery in ~2 wk or, more rarely, by a chronic destructive mastitis. Other yeast infections cause minimal inflammation and are self-limiting. If mastitis due to yeast is suspected, antibiotic therapy should be stopped immediately. Yeast or other mastitis infections can be reduced if the tip of the plastic infusion tube is only partially (rather than completely) inserted through the teat canal during intramammary therapy.

A chronic, indurative mastitis similar to that caused by the tubercle bacillus has been reported to be caused by acid-fast *Mycobacterium* spp derived from the soil, such as *M fortuitum*, *M smegmatis*, *M vaccae*, and *M phlei* when such organisms are introduced into the gland along with antibiotics (especially penicillin) in oil or ointment vehicles. The oil apparently enhances the invasiveness of these organisms, and such therapy is contraindicated. These organisms otherwise tend to be saprophytic and to disappear from infected quarters, at least by the next lactation. In the meantime, mastitis is usually moderate. Distinct outbreaks do occur and several have been reported, especially with *M fortuitum* and *M smegmatis*.

Prototheca sp are nonpigmented unicellular algae commonly found in wet environments such as streams, stagnant ponds, and marine waters, particularly in humid habitats with organic matter in the soil. In dairy farm environments, they are especially abundant in muddy or wet outdoor runs or lots, resting areas, paths where animals are driven, and pastures contaminated with slurry. Protothecal mastitis in dairy cattle is often chronic and asymptomatic with increased SCCs, although sporadic severe infections occur. Although some infections may spontaneously resolve, longterm carriage with intermittent shedding is common. After initially causing clinical mastitis, infections may be undetectable by culture of milk for several months, only to recur during the subsequent lactation, particularly soon after calving. Therapeutic interventions are unrewarding. Thus, dairy producers have limited ability to predict the progression or affect the outcome of protothecal mastitis and are constrained to management options similar to those used to manage chronic mastitis caused by other pathogens. Therefore, the primary management focus is prevention rather than mitigation of infections. To reduce pathogen exposure to other noninfected cows in the herd, chronic mastitic cows are often culled. The primary causative agent of protothecal mastitis in cattle has been identified as *P zopfii*. Other reports have challenged the absolute exclusivity of *P zopfii* as the etiologic agent of protothecal mastitis, but on a practical basis cows identified as having mastitis caused by *Prototheca* sp are managed in similar fashion, regardless of species or genotype.

Prevention: Bacterins made using core-antigen technology based on J5 mutant *E coli* can help reduce the severity of clinical mastitis caused by coliforms. Vaccination programs using these bacterins should minimally include multiple administration during the dry period to reduce the incidence of clinical coliform mastitis frequently associated with early lactation. Protocols for extended numbers of immunizations of these bacterins may be warranted in herds with high rates of severe mastitis beyond 60 days in milk, because protection often wanes 50–60 days after the last immunization.

MASTITIS IN GOATS

The organisms infecting the udder of goats are similar to those in cows. Coagulase-negative staphylococci are generally the most prevalent and can cause persistent infections that result in increased cell counts and low-grade mastitis with some recurring clinical episodes. The level of infection and incidence of mastitis due to *Staphylococcus aureus* tends to be low (<5%) but can result in persistent infections that do not generally respond to therapy. Streptococcal intramammary infections can occur in both subclinical and clinical cases but are usually much less frequent than in cattle. *Streptococcus agalactiae* is not a common pathogen of mastitis in does.

Mycoplasma infections, primarily *M mycoides* (large colony type) and *M putrefaciens*, sometimes cause serious outbreaks of mastitis in goats (*see* p 1352). The latter also causes septicemia, polyarthritis, pneumonia, and encephalitis, together with serious disease and mortality in suckling kids. *M capricolum* has also been reported to cause severe mastitis in goats and infection in kids. Does usually recover in ~4 wk.

As with cows, gram-negative organisms cause intermittent infections that may be severe but are usually self-limiting. *Trueperella* (formerly *Arcanobacterium*) *pyogenes* sometimes produces multiple, nodular abscesses.

Does can also exhibit signs of mastitis from caprine arthritis and encephalitis (*see* p 747) and ovine progressive pneumonia (*see* p 1475) secondary to systemic infection. Agalactia is common, as is a hardening of the udder from fibrosis.

Programs for diagnosis, control, and treatment of bacterial mastitis in goats are similar to those in cows. However, monitoring subclinical mastitis with somatic cell counts (SCCs) in does is difficult because of poor discrimination between infected and noninfected animals, especially in the later stages of lactation. This is partially because a higher proportion of cells are epithelial in origin in goat milk than in cow milk. As lactation progresses, shedding of epithelial cells into milk increases; thus, SCCs >1,000,000 cells/mL are common in uninfected does in late lactation. Proper milking procedures and good environmental sanitation are needed to reduce the prevalence and spread of infection. Chronically infected goats should be culled, as should goats with *M mycoides* infections and those that do not recover from *M putrefaciens* or *M capricolum* infections.

MASTITIS IN EWES

Mastitis can be an important disease in sheep, with an incidence >2%. In addition to deaths from severe infections, the disease can be a cause of lamb mortality from starvation or of depressed weaning weights of lambs. Peracute, gangrenous (usually due to *Staphylococcus aureus*), acute, subacute, and probably subclinical types occur. The organisms most commonly involved are *S aureus*, coagulase-negative staphylococci, streptococci, *Escherichia coli*, *Mannheimia haemolytica*, and *Trueperella* (formerly *Arcanobacterium*) *pyogenes*.

The principles of diagnosis and treatment used in bovine mastitis can be applied to ewes. Little is known about the control of ovine mastitis, but careful inspection of the mammary glands of ewes before mating to detect and eliminate those with chronic mastitis should be beneficial.

MASTITIS IN MARES

Acute mastitis occurs occasionally in lactating mares, most commonly in the drying-off period, in one or both glands. *Streptococcus zooepidemicus* is the most frequent pathogen, but *S equi*, *S equisimilis*, *S agalactiae*, and *S viridans* are also found. A variety of gram-negative bacteria has also been reported. Marked, painful swelling of the affected gland and adjacent tissues develops, and the secretion is often seroflocculent. Fever and depression may be present. The mare may walk stiffly or stand with hindlegs apart due to the discomfort.

Treatment is similar to that in cows, but when intramammary infusions are used, they should be inserted separately into both orifices of the teat. Systemic therapy has been suggested to include trimethoprim-sulfonamide (based on 5 mg/kg of trimethoprim, PO, bid) or a combination of penicillin (20,000 IU/kg, IM, bid) and gentamicin sulfate (2 mg/kg, IV, tid). Therapy should be continued on the basis of culture and antibacterial sensitivity testing. Without prompt treatment, abscessation or induration of the gland can occur. Little is known about the frequency and persistence of subclinical intramammary infections in mares.

MASTITIS IN SOWS

Mastitis can be important in swine-raising units. Peracute mastitis can affect sows and gilts and is most commonly associated with coliform (*Escherichia coli*, *Enterobacter aerogenes*, and *Klebsiella*) infections. It is most common at or just after parturition, and affected sows have a moderate to severe toxemia. The sow's temperature may increase to 107°F (42°C) or may be subnormal. The affected glands are swollen, purple, and have a watery secretion. Sow mortality is high, and the piglets will die unless fostered or fed artificially. Milk production of recovered sows may be impaired in the next lactation. The treatment of peracute coliform mastitis in sows is similar to that in cows. Ampicillin, dihydrostreptomycin, or oxytetracycline administered systemically have been used. Treatment of lactating sows requires consideration of withholding periods, because affected sows are often culled after weaning.

Subacute mastitis may occur in older sows and lead to induration of one or more glands, impairing the sow's ability to nurse a large litter. This form of mastitis is more likely to be associated with infection by streptococci or staphylococci. Granulomatous lesions in the mammae of sows have been associated with *Actinobacillus lignieresii*, *Actinomyces bovis*, and *Staphylococcus aureus* infections. *Fusobacterium necrophorum* and *Trueperella* (formerly *Arcanobacterium*) *pyogenes* also have been incriminated in sow mastitis. A thorough examination and culture of the mammary glands of the sow are important to diagnose any of the above peracute and subacute types of mastitis. (*See also* POSTPARTUM DYSGALACTIA SYNDROME, p 1373.)

The control of mastitis in sows has not been extensively investigated, but isolating sows in adequately disinfected pens before, during, and for an adequate period after farrowing should help prevent the severe losses associated with coliform mastitis.

METRITIS IN LARGE ANIMALS

ACUTE PUERPERAL METRITIS

In all species, acute puerperal metritis occurs within the first 10–14 days postpartum. It results from contamination of the reproductive tract at parturition and often, *but not invariably, follows* complicated parturition. Important causative organisms in cattle include *Escherichia coli* and *Trueperella (Arcanobacterium) pyogenes*, but culture-independent studies have demonstrated the dominant role of gram-negative anaerobic bacteria such as *Prevotella melaninogenica* and *Fusobacterium necrophorum*. The condition is usually acute in onset. Affected cows, mares, ewes, does, or sows are depressed, febrile, and inappetent. A fetid, watery uterine discharge is characteristic of the condition in cows but may not be conspicuous in other species. Milk production is diminished, and nursing young may show signs of food deprivation.

Acute puerperal metritis responds well to systemic antimicrobial therapy combined, if necessary, with NSAIDs and other supportive measures such as fluid therapy. Cephalosporin antibiotics or penicillin are considered most appropriate for systemic treatment of cows with metritis because they are active against most common pathogens, reach therapeutic levels in endometrial tissues, and may help prevent some of the potential sequelae of metritis and endometritis, such as endocarditis or renal disease. Oxytetracycline requires administration at high levels (11 mg/kg, bid) to maintain uterine tissue concentrations of 5 mcg/g, which is below the minimal inhibitory concentration (MIC) for many strains of pathogenic *T pyogenes*. Drainage of the uterine content may be advantageous but should be attempted only after initiation of antimicrobial therapy; it should be done very carefully because the inflamed uterus may be friable, and manipulation of the uterus may result in bacteremia.

METRITIS AND ENDOMETRITIS

Cows: Several specific diseases are associated with metritis or endometritis. These include brucellosis (*see* p 1348), leptospirosis (*see* p 646), campylobacteriosis (*see* p 1347), and trichomoniasis (*see* p 1384). More often, endometritis is the result of nonspecific infections.

The normal uterus is a sterile environment, in contrast to the vagina, which hosts numerous microorganisms. Opportunistic pathogens from the normal vaginal flora or from the environment may invade the uterus from time to time. A healthy uterus is able to rid itself of these transient infections very efficiently; however, in the immediate postpartum period, the uterus of cows is usually contaminated with a variety of organisms. Within days or weeks postpartum, the sterile uterine environment is reestablished in most animals. In those in which infection persists, chronic or subacute endometritis develops and has a detrimental effect on fertility. The prevalence of subclinical endometrial inflammation in dairy cows seems to exceed the prevalence of uterine infection. The pathogenesis of this form of endometritis is not yet understood, but it is becoming increasingly clear that postpartum uterine diseases, particularly in high-producing dairy cows, are mediated by impaired immune response, probably related to negative energy balance.

In cows, the causative organisms are most often *Trueperella pyogenes*, alone or in association with *Fusobacterium necrophorum* or other gram-negative anaerobic organisms. Signs of infection vary from obvious and persistent purulent exudate from the uterus to inapparent infection. Changes in uterine consistency may occur, but transrectal palpation alone is an insensitive means of diagnosis. The presence of purulent exudate in the vagina does not necessarily confirm endometritis; the source of the exudate may be the cervix or, occasionally, the vagina itself. Manual vaginal examination or use of a device to recover vaginal content may also allow evaluation of vaginal exudates for diagnosis of clinical endometritis. Diagnosis of subclinical (cytologic) endometritis requires use of endometrial cytology, ultrasonography, or endometrial biopsy, because other signs are often absent. Cows with endometritis do not exhibit any systemic signs of illness, and appetite and milk production are usually unimpaired.

For decades, endometritis in cows has been treated with intrauterine infusion. Although infusion of antimicrobials may rid the uterus of bacteria, there is little evidence that it eliminates the endometrial inflammation or restores fertility. Many preparations routinely administered into the bovine uterus are detrimental to uterine tissue. Increased concern about milk and carcass residues, along with poor or uncertain results, should discourage intrauterine therapy as a routine approach to management of bovine endometritis. Intrauterine infusion of cephapirin in a form specially formulated for intrauterine use, and available in many countries (but not the USA), has enhanced fertility in dairy cows with endometritis. Systemic use of antimicrobials for treatment of clinical or subclinical endometritis has not been evaluated.

Cows are more resistant to uterine infection during estrus, and as cows undergo more estrous cycles after parturition, the prevalence of endometritis diminishes. This has led to increased use of prostaglandin $F_2\alpha$ or its analogues, at usual luteolytic doses, for the management of endometritis, although there is little evidence that such use reduces the incidence or effect of endometritis.

Mares: Although profound endometritis accompanies contagious equine metritis (*see* p 1371) in mares, most breeding problems are related to endometritis caused by nonspecific infections. In mares, the most common etiologic agent of endometritis is *Streptococcus zooepidemicus*, but several other organisms may be involved, including *Escherichia coli*, *Pseudomonas* *aeruginosa*, and *Klebsiella pneumoniae*. Yeasts and fungi are incriminated in some cases, particularly in mares with reduced resistance, or as a sequela of exuberant antimicrobial therapy.

Visible exudate is rarely a feature of endometritis in mares. (Contagious equine metritis is a notable exception.) Endometrial inflammation is best confirmed by examination of endometrial cytology or biopsy samples. Additional support of the diagnosis is provided by ultrasonographic demonstration of intraluminal free fluid, especially during diestrus, or by isolation of potentially pathogenic bacteria from appropriately guarded swabs of the endometrium. Because most causative organisms are common commensals, isolation of bacteria alone is not sufficient evidence for diagnosis. Nevertheless, evidence suggests that fertility of mares is impaired if either endometrial cytology or culture is positive.

Intrauterine therapy is still commonly used in mares. Many antimicrobial drugs have been used, and effective doses determined mainly empirically. Some examples include penicillin (5 million U; effective mainly against *S zooepidemicus*), ticarcillin (6 g; broad spectrum), ampicillin (3 g of soluble preparation), gentamicin (2 g, buffered with bicarbonate; effective especially against gram-negative agents), and kanamycin (2 g; effective against gram-negative bacteria). For fungal or yeast infections, 100 mg of amphotericin B or 500 mg of clotrimazole have been effective. Treatment should be continued for several consecutive days, preferably during estrus. Most of the above treatments constitute extra-label drug use in the USA.

Some mares appear particularly susceptible to postbreeding endometritis. These mares accumulate fluid in the uterine lumen after mating or insemination. This is related to persistent endometrial inflammation. In contrast, normal mares have a vigorous, but transient, inflammatory response to mating, and the uterus rapidly regains its sterile, noninflamed status. Postbreeding endometritis may be treated by uterine lavage or by use of oxytocic drugs to rid the uterus of fluid.

Sows: A form of endometritis characterized by profuse vaginal discharge at the onset of estrus has been described in Europe and other regions. The causative agent is usually *Staphylococcus hyicus* or *E coli*, and the disease seems to be transmitted at mating or artificial insemination; signs are seen 15–25 days later during the subsequent proestrus or estrus. Infection may be of long duration, with signs recurring at each estrus. Some sows recover spontaneously, but there does not seem to be any effective treatment for those that do not. At necropsy, copious quantities of purulent exudate may be found in the uterus, making this condition more akin to pyometra (*see* below).

Other Species: Endometritis has been seen in sheep, goats, and camelids. In commercial sheep and goat flocks, diagnosis is seldom made antemortem, and treatment is generally impractical. In animals with a persistent uterine discharge, remnants of a macerated fetus should be considered as a nidus of chronic infection. Endometritis in camelids is usually treated empirically based on treatments for cattle and horses.

PYOMETRA

Pyometra is characterized by accumulation of purulent or mucopurulent exudate in the uterus. In cows, it is invariably accompanied by persistence of an active corpus luteum and interruption of the estrous cycle. In affected mares, the cervix is often fibrotic, inelastic, affected with transluminal adhesions, or otherwise impaired. Mares may continue to cycle normally, or the cycle may be interrupted. Discharge from the genital tract may be absent or intermittent and corresponding to periods of estrus. In general, affected animals do not exhibit any systemic signs of illness, but affected mares may be in poor condition. In both cows and mares, pyometra must be distinguished carefully from pregnancy before treatment is undertaken.

The treatment of choice in cows is administration of prostaglandin $F_2\alpha$ or its analogues at normal luteolytic doses. Expulsion of exudate and bacteriologic clearance of the uterus follows in ~80% of treated cases. Although first-service conception rate after treatment may be low, most cows may be expected to conceive within three or four inseminations. The treatment may need to be repeated in ~20% of cows. No intrauterine treatment is recommended in conjunction with the prostaglandin.

In the face of cervical changes, drainage of the affected equine uterus may be virtually impossible. Lavage of the uterus using large volumes of fluid is recommended; however, the condition frequently recurs, and permanent cure in these cases requires hysterectomy or wedge resection of the cervix to allow continual uterine drainage, a salvage procedure that allows continued use of the mare but renders her infertile.

Pyometra is seen in small ruminants, swine, and other species; diagnosis is rendered more difficult by animal size and management practices. If pyometra is diagnosed, evacuation of the uterus is recommended.

CONTAGIOUS EQUINE METRITIS

Contagious equine metritis (CEM) is an acute, highly contagious venereal disease of horses (and experimentally of donkeys) characterized by a profuse, mucopurulent vaginal discharge and early return to estrus in most affected mares. Infected stallions and chronically infected mares show no clinical signs. The disease is seen primarily in Europe, but technical challenges in propagation of the causative organism prevent accurate determination of the precise distribution of the disease.

Etiology and Transmission: CEM is caused by the gram-negative, microaerophilic coccobacillus *Taylorella equigenitalis*, also known as the contagious equine metritis organism (CEMO). Important strain differences exist; some strains are resistant to streptomycin (a fact that helps isolate this fastidious, slow-growing organism from contaminants), whereas others are sensitive to streptomycin. It is best cultured on chocolate Eugon agar at 37°C in an atmosphere of 5%–10% CO_2 in air. *T equigenitalis* is asaccharolytic but is positive for catalase, cytochrome oxidase, and phosphatase and unreactive to other conventional biochemical tests.

CEM is transmitted primarily at mating, but infected fomites (instruments and equipment) also play a role. Undetected infected mares and stallions are the source of new outbreaks. Infected stallions show no signs and harbor the organism in the smegma of the prepuce and the surface of the penis, especially in the urethral fossa. The transmission rate is exceptionally high; virtually every mare mated by an infected stallion becomes infected.

Clinical Findings: In mares, a copious, mucopurulent vaginal discharge is seen 10–14 days after infected matings. Mares may return to estrus after a shortened estrous cycle. Although the discharge subsides after a few days, mares may remain infected for several months. Chronically infected mares show no signs. Most mares do not conceive at the time of infected mating. If they do, they may infect the foal at or shortly after birth. Foals so infected may become carriers of CEMO when they reach sexual maturity.

Lesions: Lesions consist of edema and hyperemia of the endometrium, the endocervix, and the vaginal mucosa. The microscopic lesions include invasion of the affected tissues by neutrophils during the acute stage, and by lymphocytes, macrophages, and plasma cells later in the course of the infection.

Diagnosis: Diagnosis depends on isolation of the causative organism. Although other bacterial infections of the genital tract of mares may produce a conspicuous vaginal discharge, this is uncommon, and no other venereal pathogen of the equine reproductive tract is as contagious. In mares, swabs for culture should be taken from the endometrium (preferably during estrus) and from the clitoral fossa and sinuses. Swabs from suspected stallions should be taken from the urethral fossa, the urethra, the preputial cavity, the shaft of the penis, and, if possible, the preejaculatory fluid or ejaculate. Stallions should be sampled at least three times before being declared free of CEMO. Test-mating suspect stallions to susceptible mares that are then screened bacteriologically constitutes a satisfactory way to determine CEM status. All swabs should be placed in a transport medium (preferably Amies with charcoal), kept on ice or at 4°C, and delivered to a qualified laboratory within 24 hr (or frozen if transport will take longer). A variety of serologic tests has been developed, but none is yet capable of reliably detecting the carrier status.

Treatment and Control: Stallions can be treated by thoroughly cleaning the extended penis with chlorhexidine surgical scrub and then applying nitrofurazone ointment. This should be repeated daily for 5 days, and the stallion retested at least 10 days after treatment. Most mares rid themselves of uterine infection after a few weeks. Those that become chronically infected harbor the CEMO in the clitoral fossa or sinuses. They can be treated by thoroughly cleaning the clitoral area with chlorhexidine surgical scrub and then applying nitrofurazone ointment (as for the stallion). In some mares, surgical excision of the clitoral sinuses may be required to rid them of infection.

Control of CEM depends on identification of infected carrier animals and on their treatment or elimination from breeding programs. Strict import regulations exist in many countries to avoid the introduction of CEM, and current prevalence of the disease appears to be low.

POSTHITIS AND VULVITIS IN SHEEP AND GOATS

Two common and distinct forms of posthitis and vulvitis are recognized in small ruminants. The first, referred to as enzootic posthitis and vulvitis, is associated with high-protein diets, infection with *Corynebacterium renale* or other urease-producing organisms, locally high concentrations of ammonia, and severe posthitis. The second is referred to as necrotic or ulcerative balanoposthitis and vulvitis. Its cause is unclear, but *Mycoplasma mycoides mycoides* is implicated, as are other *Mycoplasma* spp organisms of the *Histophilus/Haemophilus* group, and potentially viruses, such as caprine herpesvirus 1.

ENZOOTIC POSTHITIS AND VULVITIS

(Sheath rot, Pizzle rot, Enzootic balanoposthitis)

Etiology and Epidemiology: This moderately contagious disease is caused by *C renale*, a gram-positive, diphtheroid bacterium capable of hydrolyzing urea. When protein intake is high, urinary urea concentration increases. Hydrolysis of urea by *C renale* results in local production of large quantities of ammonia, which is believed to irritate the penis, lamina interna of the prepuce, and skin surrounding the preputial orifice. The condition is more common in male castrates, probably because of the hypoplastic nature of the penis, exacerbated in some cases by failure of penile-preputial separation that leads to pooling of urine in the prepuce. If preputial hair is cut too short or becomes caked with mud or organic matter, drainage of urine away from the preputial orifice (normally facilitated by this hair) is impaired, and ulcerative lesions may develop.

The incidence of ulcerative posthitis is highest in Merino and Angora wethers, which is attributed to the long hair or wool surrounding the prepuce in these animals, allowing urine to soak the area, which in turn is conducive to bacterial growth and activity. It is also seen in show rams or rams that have been fit for sale; in this case, the condition is more associated with dietary protein levels. The condition can be transmitted experimentally by infective material from a preputial or vulvar ulcer. Ulcerative posthitis or vulvitis has a seasonal occurrence that varies with local animal husbandry methods. Peak incidence corresponds to the time when animals graze lush green pasture (eg, spring and early summer in New Zealand or autumn and winter in southern Brazil) or are fed or have access to high-protein feedstuffs.

Clinical Findings: In mild cases, signs are limited to swelling of the prepuce. In severe cases, swelling and inflammation interfere with urination and result in straining, which needs to be differentiated from urolithiasis (*see* p 1502). Histologic characteristics are acanthosis, parakeratosis, and hyperkeratosis, followed by leukocyte invasion and ulceration. Ulcers and scabs may be found around the preputial orifice, on the lamina interna of the prepuce, and on the shaft of the penis. Urine and exudate may accumulate in the prepuce. The condition may cause severe discomfort. If the preputial orifice or urethra is occluded, affected animals may die. Ulcerative vulvitis begins with signs of vulvar inflammation, including swelling and redness, and progresses to development of a yellow exudate with ulceration and scab formation around the vulva, vestibule, and caudal vagina. The glans clitoridis may be swollen, red, and ulcerated.

Lesions of ulcerative posthitis or vulvitis should be distinguished from those of granular posthitis or vulvitis (associated with *Mycoplasma* spp or *Ureaplasma* spp, *see* p 1391), herpesviral balanoposthitis or vulvovaginitis, ulcerative dermatosis (*see* p 872 [sheep only]), or contagious ecthyma (orf, *see* p 866 [goats only]). Removal of the scabs of ulcerative posthitis or vulvitis characteristically results in little or no hemorrhage.

Treatment and Control: If possible, affected animals should be isolated from the rest of the herd and not fed a high-protein diet. Lesions should be examined to ensure they do not interfere with urethral patency. Clipping and cleaning hair around the prepuce may be beneficial. *C renale* is usually sensitive to penicillins and cephalosporins, which may be beneficial if practical. Ulcerative posthitis is controlled principally by limiting dietary protein to a level consistent with requirements. If untreated, scarring may be so severe that the penis cannot be extended.

ULCERATIVE BALANOPOSTHITIS AND VULVITIS

(Pizzle disease, Knobrot, Peestersiekte)

Ulcerative balanoposthitis and vulvitis is characterized by ulceration and inflammation of the glans penis and the prepuce, as well as the vulva of affected ewes. The first signs observed may be swelling and bleeding of the prepuce or vulva. On examination, ulcers are seen; these bleed readily when manipulated. In ewes, the ventral aspect of the tail (where it contacts the vulva) may be similarly affected. The condition may spread within a breeding flock to involve a considerable proportion of the animals. The pregnancy rate in affected flocks is depressed.

The cause of ulcerative balanoposthitis and vulvitis is not clear. *Mycoplasma mycoides mycoides* has been isolated from affected sheep. *Trueperella (Arcanobacterium) pyogenes* is frequently present. In some cases *Histophilus ovis* has been isolated. Viruses, such as ovine herpesvirus 2 or, in the case of goats, caprine herpesvirus 1, may be involved.

Affected rams should be removed from the flock and isolated. If practical, affected ewes should also be maintained separately. Rams should be treated with antimicrobials; ewes also respond well to antimicrobial treatment. Irrigation of the prepuce may help prevent preputial adhesions. Tulathromycin has been used successfully. Recovered animals appear to have normal fertility.

POSTPARTUM DYSGALACTIA SYNDROME AND MASTITIS IN SOWS

Numerous etiologies or pathophysiologies can be involved in this syndrome, which is reflected by the use of several different names—mastitis-metritis-agalactia (MMA) complex, agalactia syndrome, dysgalactia syndrome, mammary edema, periparturient hypogalactia syndrome, agalactia toxemia, and puerperal mastitis. However, these names are not synonymous and have often been misused. The syndrome can currently be classified according to the number of mammary glands affected, ie, uniglandular or multiglandular mastitis (including postpartum dysgalactia syndrome [PPDS], MMA complex). (*See also* MASTITIS IN LARGE ANIMALS, p 1358.)

Acute or chronic mastitis of only one or two mammary glands (acute or chronic uniglandular mastitis) in sows is present in nearly all herds. If the entire udder is acutely affected, it can be a primary or a secondary mastitis (acute multiglandular mastitis) as well as mammary edema ("hard udder syndrome"), which is common in primiparous sows.

Due to bacterial effects, acute multiglandular mastitis is usually accompanied by systemic signs and agalactia, whereas hard udder syndrome is not. Both conditions occur within the first 3 days after farrowing and rapidly lead to piglet starvation. Although the problem can be sporadic and limited to a few sows, sometimes it can occur in a greater number of sows and become nearly epidemic.

Differentiating acute multiglandular mastitis and hard udder syndrome can be difficult. For this reason, it is often reported by producers as "acute mastitis."

PPDS is characterized by transitory hypogalactia. It can lead to acute multiglandular mastitis and should be considered as the general cause of lactation failure in the sow. MMA complex is a misnomer and is only part of the more general PPDS. Although the mammary glands are swollen and frequently warmer than normal, grossly detectable primary mastitis is uncommon. Likewise, metritis (more commonly endometritis) is only an occasional finding in some herds. Finally, only rarely is there complete agalactia; most sows continue to produce milk but at a greatly reduced rate (hypogalactia or more correctly dysgalactia). The primary clinical signs of the sow's inability to produce a sufficient amount of milk to meet the needs of the piglets are growth retardation and increased mortality in piglets.

Mammary glands of sows are anatomically different from those of cows. In sows, there are no well-identified gland cisterns (gland sinus) in the mammary glands. There are usually two complete gland systems and two teat orifices per teat. When three orifices are present, one sinus ends blindly at the base of the teat and does not have glandular tissue. There is no muscular sphincter around the teat orifice. Therefore, intramammary treatment by way of the teat opening is impossible. Mammogenesis occurs almost exclusively during the last half of gestation and during the first days of lactation. New glandular tissues are produced during each gestation. For this reason, feeding and nutrition are of major importance during mammogenesis and the end of gestation, and are less important at midgestation.

Opinions differ as to whether the position of the caudal mammary glands should be considered as a risk factor for mastitis development. Most recent findings seem to reject an increased incidence in caudal glands compared with cranial ones.

Infection of a mammary gland during one lactation has no consequences for the next. However, chronic lesions of the teat canal may be present for multiple lactations.

ACUTE MULTIGLANDULAR MASTITIS

This syndrome is seen in all types of herds, including those with excellent hygiene and adequate disinfection practices. It occurs mainly during the first 3 days after farrowing and has major consequences for the piglets. Acute multiglandular mastitis can also follow a specific systemic disease of the sow (eg, septicemia, pseudorabies [*see* p 1300], porcine reproductive and respiratory syndrome [*see* p 729]).

Etiology and Pathogenesis: The etiology is multifactorial. Infections of the mammary gland are more often secondary, and many microorganisms have been identified, including *Escherichia coli*, *Klebsiella* spp, *Enterobacter* spp, *Citrobacter* spp, *Staphylococcus* spp (eg, *S epidermidis*), and *Pseudomonas aeruginosa*. All these microorganisms are common in the environment of sows.

Although many sows in a herd may be severely affected, this type of mastitis is not contagious. After farrowing, the mammary gland is infected by environmental opportunist bacteria. Very few bacteria (often <100 organisms) are enough to colonize the mammary gland.

Major herd risk factors are the sow (PPDS, *see* below), the piglets (uncommon primary form), or the environment (eg, some beddings such as wood shavings can be contaminated by *Klebsiella pneumoniae*).

Some genetic lines of females are more resistant to coliform mastitis than others. The heritability of this characteristic is believed to be ~10%. Selection among the gilts to minimize or eliminate mastitis-prone sows can provide longterm improvement of the herd.

Clinical Findings: Systemic signs such as anorexia, constipation, fever, and depression are common. Local signs include acute induration of the mammary glands as well as severe edema and skin congestion of the mammary region. However, many sows (especially primiparous sows) develop mammary edema without any signs of acute mastitis. Circumstantial evidence suggests that this is usually associated with increasing milk production (often the milk drips during and right after farrowing) to such an extent that piglets are unable to consume all the available milk.

Once acute multiglandular mastitis is established, the secretion (with oxytocin) of milk is no longer possible. Affected sows deny piglets access to the teats by lying on their mammary glands. General signs result from bacterial multiplication and resorption of toxins. Common consequences for the litter include an economically significant increase in preweaning mortality caused by weak piglets, neonatal diarrhea, starvation, hypoglycemia-induced weakness, an increased incidence of crushing by the sow, and increased susceptibility to other diseases due to inadequate maternal immunoglobulin transfer and other problems (eg, runt pigs).

Diagnosis: Early diagnosis is not always easy. Most problem litters are thought to be due to early lactation problems. The primary differential diagnoses are peripartum mammary edema, which is often seen in primiparous sows without any systemic signs, and PPDS, which is less spectacular but affects a greater number of sows. A thorough physical examination, including careful palpation of the mammary glands, should be performed. However, it is necessary to be cautious in the interpretation—hard mammary glands without systemic signs do not always indicate acute mastitis. Although frequently seen, peripartum mammary edema is poorly documented. Sows often appear to be in discomfort and lay down, as do sows with mastitis. However, peripartum mammary edema can certainly lead to an acute multiglandular mastitis. In contrast to the situation in cows, interpretation of cellular modifications in the milk is very difficult in sows.

Treatment and Control: Systemic antibiotic therapy should be started as soon as possible (*see* p 1376). Longterm control of a herd problem also requires identification and correction of risk factors. General antibiotic therapy as well as corticosteroids are useful to reduce the intensity of the inflammatory reaction. Meloxicam has also been shown to improve recovery of the sows. Management techniques to improve hygiene should be implemented as soon as possible. Cross-fostering is often the only effective way to save a litter.

ACUTE UNIGLANDULAR MASTITIS

In lactating or weaned sows, inflammation of a single mammary gland is common. Such uniglandular inflammations are more often noticed in old sows.

Etiology and Pathogenesis: The microorganisms involved are the same as those in acute multiglandular mastitis (*see* above). Sometimes only one or two mammary glands are affected; the cause should be identified. Traumatic lesions or inaccessibility of teats to piglets are common. Piglets suckling inguinal mammary glands of old sows are often unable to reach the teat during the phase of milk ejection. Usually, piglets have selected a specific gland by 24 hr after birth. A piglet suckling a teat affected by acute uniglandular mastitis will show growth retardation, while littermates remain healthy. Milk secretion may be restricted by acquired problems of mammary conformation (as in old sows), traumatic lesions, and other teat abnormalities. Teat lesions may have developed during the previous lactation, the previous weaning-to-estrus interval, or the previous gestation.

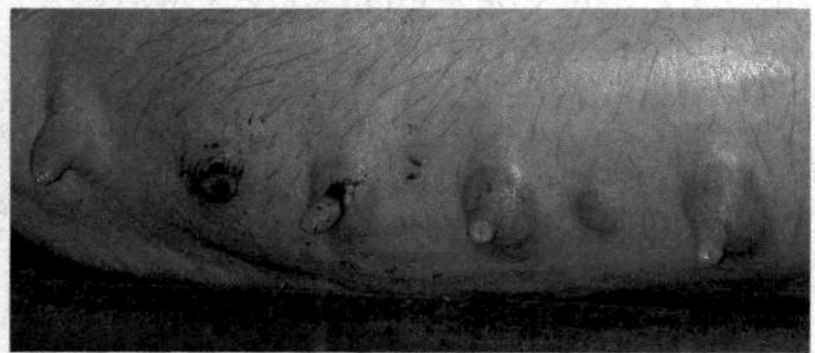

Teat damage as a result of trauma in a sow. *Courtesy of Dr. Glen Almond.*

Diagnosis: The integrity of the mammary gland should be checked before each farrowing. Except for cases associated with inaccessible teats, risk factors involved in the development of blind teats should be identified. Traumatic teat lesions can be the consequence of injuries induced by piglets or other sows, or by slipping on slatted floors, etc. Unfortunately, these primary lesions often go unnoticed until several weeks or months have passed. Size homogeneity within a litter should also be monitored. Any discrepancy or growth retardation in a piglet compared with its littermate could be indicative of mastitis in a mammary gland.

Treatment and Control: The affected gland is lost for the current lactation and sometimes for the next lactation. During subsequent lactations, the number of nursing piglets should be limited, or the sow should be culled.

CHRONIC OR DRY-SOW MASTITIS

Postweaning or dry-sow mastitis is a common type of mastitis that affects one or a few glands. The prevalence among newly weaned sows is 10%–20%. Chronic mastitis is characterized by the formation of abscesses and granulomas in the mammary tissue, which are often seen at weaning or shortly after. A primary pathogen has not been identified. Bacteria commonly enter the mammary glands through teat wounds caused by the piglets' sharp teeth during suckling, fights among aggressive weaned sows grouped in the same pen, or trauma associated with the particular anatomy of inguinal mammary glands of old sows.

POSTPARTUM DYSGALACTIA SYNDROME

Postpartum dysgalactia syndrome (PPDS) is a primary cause of neonatal problems (eg, diarrhea, crushing, runting, inanition, poor growth) but is challenging to characterize because of its multiple manifestations and the difficulty in making an etiologic diagnosis. In a given herd, PPDS affects ~15%–20% of the sows; a higher percentage is uncommon. It is more common in young sows in their first or second parity.

Etiology and Pathogenesis: There are numerous multifactorial etiologies, which complicate the diagnosis and clinical evaluation. Classically perceived as a part of the mastitis-metritis-agalactia (MMA) complex, PPDS should instead be considered a broader pathology. Thus, the MMA complex is essentially a subtype of PPDS, probably the most severe clinically but also the least common.

Evidence suggests that lipopolysaccharide (LPS) endotoxins, a portion of the cell wall of all gram-negative bacteria, play a central role. Bacterial endotoxins can be absorbed from the uterus (eg, endometritis or metritis), mammary glands (eg, acute multiglandular mastitis), or gut (eg, constipation as a consequence of feeding finely ground feed to sows can result in bacterial overgrowth and subsequent absorption of endotoxins from the intestines) and lead to endotoxemia. Identifying the source of the bacterial endotoxins is important to determine the best preventive approach for the particular herd.

The secretion of colostrum is determined by a complex hormonal balance (homeorhesis). LPS endotoxins exert their effects even before farrowing and act with the intervention of the innate immune system (macrophage activation). These changes adversely affect production and secretion of colostrum and milk. In addition, the colostrum is as important for its energy content as it is for its immunoglobulin content. Any decrease in the amount of ingested colostrum will result in consequences for the piglets such as diarrhea, inanition, and poor growth.

Other causes of general hypogalactia that should be considered include acute multiglandular mastitis, udder and teat abnormalities, hypocalcemia (uncommon in sows), and acute (agalactia) or chronic (hypogalactia) ergotism (uncommon in practice). Indeed, ergot derivatives suppress prolactin release.

Risk factors are those associated with stress of the sow and with conditions that lead to bacterial multiplication and subsequent endotoxemia. Such factors are numerous and are linked with different entities (eg, cystitis, metritis, vaginitis, constipation, mastitis).

Genetics can also be a risk factor for PPDS; most recent studies identified susceptibility genes on chromosome 17. Selection among genetic lines should include this parameter.

Clinical Findings: PPDS is seen almost exclusively *within the first* 3 days after farrowing. Associated signs are numerous and vary from herd to herd, as well as within herds. PPDS is commonly associated with fat sow syndrome, prolonged farrowings, large litter sizes, and a high postpartum fever. Management practices reported in herds with a high incidence of PPDS include too much manual intervention during parturition or too many parenteral injections to sows (antibiotics, oxytocin, prostaglandins) or piglets (mainly antibiotics). Moving pregnant sows to the farrowing facilities ≤4 days before the expected farrowing, and feeding sows ad lib during lactation also should be considered risk factors. Piglet losses are due to emaciation or diarrhea (or both), as a consequence of poor nutrition during the first few days postpartum.

Diagnosis: Diagnosis is difficult and based on clinical signs. Clinical examination is best performed while piglets are nursing; milk ejection in affected sows is either absent or of brief duration, which causes the piglets to actively nurse for an extended time. During the initial stages, piglets repeatedly attempt to nurse at frequent intervals and do not settle after nursing. As a result of vigorous nursing efforts, the teats may be traumatized. As the energy reserves of the piglets are depleted, their attempts to nurse decrease, and they often migrate to the warmest portions of the farrowing crate. Crushing by the sow is common. Therefore, litter behavior should be watched closely for a prolonged time when trying to diagnose PPDS.

Mammary tenderness, swelling, and teat damage are consistent with a diagnosis of lactational insufficiency. The mammary glands vary from grossly normal to swollen, firm, and warm to the touch, sometimes with blotched purple skin. Pure bacterial cultures may be isolated from milk samples. Rectal temperature of the sow varies from normal to markedly increased (>40.5°C [104.9°F]). The concept that postpartum rectal temperatures >39.5°C (103.1°F) predict early lactation problems must be questioned. Physiologic hyperthermia observed in lactating sows should not be confused with fever. Reduced appetite or anorexia, constipation, and depression may also be seen. Abnormal and copious vaginal discharges may be seen in some sows (eg, cervicitis, endometritis). Cystitis, metritis, vaginitis, constipation, or mastitis in the sow and diarrhea in neonatal piglets should be considered as a general syndrome (requiring an overall diagnosis) rather than as individual problems.

Treatment and Control: Systemic or local therapeutic intervention (antibiotics, NSAIDs) can sometimes be helpful but only on a short-term basis. Flunixin meglumine may help to counteract the effects of endotoxins. Antimicrobial treatment is usually prescribed before susceptibility can be tested. A broad-spectrum antibiotic is therefore recommended. However, if antibiotics are used longterm, a dependence on them for puerperal fevers, acute mastitis, vaginitis, endometritis, or neonatal diarrhea can develop rapidly and lead to multiresistant bacterial infections. Oxytocin or prostaglandins (or both) can be useful in cases of prolonged farrowing or postpartum endometritis. By far the most effective method is to cross-foster the piglets from affected to healthy sows, as long as the health status of the litters are equivalent. Oxytocin (5–10 U/sow) is occasionally effective in reestablishing lactation if used 4 or 5 times at 2- to 3-hr intervals. In herds in which PPDS is a significant problem, incidence may be reduced by inducing parturition with prostaglandin $F_2\alpha$; this results in rapid induction of labor and dilatation of the teats for a shorter period of time. However, the amelioration is not constant among herds and depends on farm circumstances.

As many risk factors as possible should be identified and corrected or minimized. Systematic manual interventions during farrowing or uterine washings should be limited to only those that are necessary. There is no clear evidence that vaccines have a beneficial effect. Good sanitation tends to decrease the incidence of mastitis in the sow and diarrhea in the piglets, but PPDS is also common in herds in overall good health and with a high level of hygiene.

For chronic mastitis, use of partially slatted farrowing pens and cleaning with disinfectants between batches of sows in the farrowing and breeding areas may be helpful. Cutting or grinding the piglets' teeth after farrowing is not considered a good way to control chronic mastitis. Indeed, it can lead to a high prevalence of mastitis, possibly caused by changes in the oral flora of the piglets or the failure of piglets to suckle as a result of sore mouths from careless cutting of teeth.

PROLONGED GESTATION IN CATTLE AND SHEEP

Parturition is induced by the fetus in both cattle and sheep. It is initiated by rising cortisol levels in the fetus that provoke a cascade of endocrine activity in the dam. Fetal cortisol increases as a result of increased adrenocorticotropic hormone (ACTH) production by the maturing fetal pituitary caused by fetal stressors such as hypoxia and hypercapnia. Gestation length is unique to each fetus, but approximate gestation lengths can be ascribed to each species (*see* TABLE 1, p 1324).

In cattle, gestation length is influenced by factors such as the breed of the cow and bull, calf gender, single vs multiple birth, the parity of the cow, and the fetal genotype. Environmental factors, including nutrition, ambient temperature, and the season of the year, have a smaller influence. The breed of cattle has the greatest influence on gestation length. In European cattle of the *Bos taurus* species, considerable breed variation is recognized (eg, 279 days mean gestation in Holstein-Friesian to 287 days in Charolais). In breeds of the *Bos indicus* species, a slightly longer gestation length is often seen (eg, Zebu cattle have a mean gestation length of 296 days). Within breeds, individual bulls may sire calves with longer gestation length than normal, leading to a higher incidence of dystocia. In sheep, the normal gestation length is 144–150 days.

In many cases, prolonged gestation is incorrectly diagnosed because of human error. The service dates of dairy cattle are normally known. Hence the date of anticipated parturition is calculated and recorded once pregnancy is confirmed. In beef cattle, in which cows often run with a bull, exact calving dates are not known, but individual pregnant cows are expected to calve within a recognized calving season. Individual animals that have not calved at the anticipated time are checked to confirm they are still pregnant and that their pregnancy appears to be normal.

In sheep, the exact lambing date is seldom known unless ewes were served in hand or by artificial insemination. In most flocks the ewes run with rams and, when served, receive a raddle crayon mark on their rumps to indicate that service has occurred. Crayon color is changed at 14- to 17-day intervals, and after later pregnancy confirmation, a lambing date within a 14- to 17-day period is calculated. Individual ewes that fail to lamb are culled or further evaluated for pregnancy.

Miscalculation of the prospective calving or lambing date, failure to record a subsequent service, faulty pregnancy diagnosis, and incorrect identification of animals may lead to a diagnosis of prolonged gestation in an animal that has a normal pregnancy. True prolonged gestation is relatively uncommon; the common denominator is a defective hypothalamic-pituitary-adrenal axis. Suspected cases should be investigated and examined with care. In some cases, the fetus is dead or severely deformed and is of little economic value. The life of the dam may be at risk if prolonged gestation is allowed to continue, and termination of the abnormal pregnancy is recommended.

Diagnosis: When a number of cases of prolonged gestation are seen in a herd or flock, a full investigation should be conducted in an attempt to identify the cause and possibly a preventive program. A genetic abnormality may be determined by a study of pedigrees or by finding an abnormal karyotype in affected fetuses. Possible exposure to toxic plants and viral infection should be investigated. Tests for evidence of pathogenic viruses or serologic evidence of exposure to them may lead to clear evidence of virus involvement. In some cases, the cause of prolonged gestation remains unknown. Evidence of pituitary hypoplasia or compromise may be found, but the underlying cause remains elusive.

Treatment: In a case of suspected prolonged gestation, the dam's breeding records, if available, should be checked to ensure that parturition truly is overdue. Treatment of a case in which gestation is not genuinely prolonged may result in the delivery of a premature fetus that is unlikely to survive. Once the true length of gestation is established, a full clinical examination of the dam should be conducted.

In cattle, rectal examination of the uterus and its contents is an important diagnostic aid. Fetal parts may be palpable, and in some cases it is possible to detect an *abnormal cranium*. An ultrasonographic scan may confirm the presence of fetal abnormalities, including a thin-walled, fluid-filled cranium. The weight of an overdue fetus may cause it to pass under the rumen while still within the uterus, so that it cannot be palpated per rectum.

In some animals, prolonged gestation is accompanied by development of excessive amounts of fetal fluid. The origin of excessive fetal fluid can be assessed by analysis of sodium and chloride levels in an aspirated sample. Amniotic fluid contains sodium at ~120 mmol/L and chloride at ~90 mmol/L. Allantoic fluid contains sodium at 50 mmol/L and chloride at 20 mmol/L. The correlation between hydrops amnion and hydrops allantois and prolonged gestation is tenuous, however. Most fetal giants suffer from oligoamnios.

In true prolonged gestation, the fetus is unlikely to be of any economic value. Treatment should be aimed at fetal delivery with minimal damage to the dam. In cases of fetal giantism, the dam may be distressed by the weight of the fetus and its associated fluids. Painful edema in front of the udder may indicate rupture or impending rupture of the prepubic tendon. A canvas sling support can be placed around the abdomen to prevent further damage until the pregnancy is terminated. General health of the dam should be assessed and economic considerations discussed with the owner before treatment is attempted. Milk production may be compromised.

Successful induction of parturition requires an intact fetal hypothalamic-pituitary-adrenal axis. Pregnancy is maintained in cases of prolonged gestation chiefly by continued production of progesterone by the corpus luteum. Spontaneous induction of birth in cases of prolonged gestation fails as a result of insufficient production of fetal cortisol and the failure of luteolysis to occur. Birth in both cows and sheep can be successfully induced by administering both prostaglandin $F_2\alpha$ (or its synthetic analogue cloprostenol) and the corticosteroid dexamethasone by IM injection. Luteolysis is induced by the prostaglandin, and the maternal hormone cascade that precedes parturition is initiated by the corticosteroid. In cows, 500 mcg cloprostenol and 20 mg dexamethasone are given; in sheep 125 mcg cloprostenol and 16 mg dexamethasone are recommended. A single dose of these two drugs is normally effective. Parturition should begin in 24–72 hr.

Induced parturition should be monitored carefully. Assistance may be required if there is evidence of uterine inertia or damage to the abdominal wall, either of which might make expulsive efforts ineffective. Fetal malposition requiring obstetric assistance may occur once birth begins. If the fetus is very large, dystocia due to fetal-pelvic disproportion may occur, and assisted delivery by careful traction may be attempted. If this is not possible, cesarean section may be required. If the dam is seriously ill but considered well enough to withstand surgery, an elective cesarean without an attempt at vaginal delivery may be considered. Fetal dysmaturity can be a problem, especially in very valuable cloned offspring, and intensive care facilities may be needed.

After fetal delivery, uterine involution may be encouraged by administration of oxytocin. Retention of fetal membranes is managed in the usual way (*see* p 1381). Fluid therapy, antibiotics, and treatment with NSAIDs such as flunixin meglumine may aid recovery and provide analgesia.

PROLONGED GESTATION ASSOCIATED WITH FETAL DEATH

Fetal death may be followed by abortion, fetal maceration, or fetal mummification. In cases of abortion and fetal maceration, the hormonal support of pregnancy is lost. The animal normally shows signs that pregnancy has terminated. An aborted fetus may be found, the dam may show an abnormal vaginal discharge, and she may return to estrus. Fetal bones may be trapped in the uterus and compromise future breeding.

In cases of fetal mummification, fetal death is often not immediately apparent. In such cases, the corpus luteum persists in the ovary, and there is no vaginal discharge and no signs of estrus. The abnormal pregnancy in such animals continues indefinitely. Affected animals are normally identified when owners notice that external signs of late pregnancy, including abdominal enlargement, are less obvious than in other members of a group. Clinical examination reveals that the fetus is dead, although the dam is pregnant. Rectal examination reveals an irregularly shaped, contracted uterus with a fetal mass but no fetal fluid within it. There is no fremitus in the uterine artery. Ultrasonographic examination of accessible parts of the uterus per rectum confirms the diagnosis. The abnormal pregnancy can be terminated by a single IM injection of prostaglandin $F_2\alpha$. The fetus is expelled from the uterus and can be manually removed from the vagina 48 hr later.

In sheep, fetal mummification can be diagnosed by abdominal palpation supported by a transabdominal ultrasonographic scan. Affected animals are normally culled on economic grounds. Treatment can be attempted (*see* above).

PROLONGED GESTATION ASSOCIATED WITH FETAL DEFORMITY

Prolonged gestation associated with fetal deformity cases usually occur as the result of some compromise of the hypothalamic-pituitary-adrenal axis of the fetus, which is no longer able to initiate parturition. The affected fetus may either die and be aborted or live on indefinitely in the uterus. Genetic, infectious, toxic, and unknown causes have been associated with this problem.

Genetic Abnormalities: Prolonged gestation associated with fetal adrenal malfunction is a genetically determined prolonged gestation caused by an autosomal recessive gene of the fetus in Holstein-Friesian cows. The fetal adrenal glands fail to produce corticosteroids at term, in response to fetal ACTH. As a result, the fetus continues to grow until it outgrows its blood supply. Induction with dexamethasone does not induce normal labor and parturition because of insufficient preparation of the birth canal. A cesarean section will save the dam, but the fetus invariably dies due to adrenal insufficiency.

Four further genetic abnormalities associated with prolonged gestation in various breeds of cattle involve fetal pituitary abnormalities. In one condition, severe fetal oversize (fetal giantism) is present. In the second, the calf has severe craniofacial defects and is much smaller than normal. In the third condition, multiple skeletal abnormalities are present. In a fourth condition, genetic abnormalities may occur as a result of cloning.

Prolonged gestation and fetal giantism has been reported in Holstein-Friesian, Ayrshire, and Swedish breeds of cattle. Gestation is prolonged by 21–150 days. Pronounced abdominal enlargement is seen in some cases. There is no attempted parturition unless the fetus dies first after having outgrown its blood supply. Cervical relaxation is poor, and dystocia invariably results. The calf weighs 48–80 kg at birth and shows signs of postmaturity. The coat and hooves are longer than normal, and prominent loose teeth are present in the gums. Breathing is difficult as a result of failure of surfactant release, and the calf may die from hypoglycemia. At necropsy, hypoplasia of the anterior pituitary and adrenal glands is seen.

Prolonged gestation with craniofacial defects in the fetus has been reported in

Holstein-Friesian, Ayrshire, Guernsey, and Jersey breeds of cattle and is thought to be caused by a recessive gene. Affected fetuses cease to grow at 7 mo gestation. There is no spontaneous parturition in affected cattle because of the nonfunctional or absent pituitary gland in the fetus. Calves are usually dead when delivered. Some may show evidence of severe abnormalities of the cranium and face.

Prolonged gestation associated with multiple skeletal abnormalities has been reported in Hereford cattle. Affected calves show evidence of pituitary aplasia or hypoplasia. Arthrogryposis, torticollis, kyphosis, and scoliosis are present, and some calves have cleft palates.

Prolonged gestation associated with cloning has been reported in both fetal calves and lambs produced by somatic cell nuclear cloning. Early placental abnormalities have been detected in a high proportion of such animals, and placentomegaly may be seen in later pregnancy. The abnormality may result in fetal death or, if the fetus survives, in the large offspring syndrome. Spontaneous birth may not occur, and prolonged gestation results. Fetal lung and maternal mammary development is retarded and can compromise fetal survival.

Infectious Causes: Although bovine viral diarrhea virus (*see* p 267) can cause abortion in cattle, it can also produce congenital defects in the fetus. These include cerebellar hypoplasia, anencephaly, and hydrocephaly. Affected calves may be born with severe defects of the CNS, but prolonged gestation occasionally occurs if pituitary function is compromised. The related pestivirus border disease virus (*see* p 622) can produce severe brain and coat abnormalities in fetal lambs. Pituitary compromise in such lambs can lead to prolonged gestation.

Akabane virus (*see* p 620), found in Africa, Australia, the Middle East, and the Far East, can be transmitted by insects to both pregnant cattle and sheep. Bovine fetuses exposed to the virus at 76–104 days gestation may develop hydranencephaly (fluid-filled cavitation of the brain). Exposure to the virus at 105–174 days of pregnancy may cause both hydranencephaly and arthrogryposis. Affected fetuses may have severe brain damage. The cerebral cortex may be absent and the cranial cavity filled with fluid. Cerebellar hypoplasia may be present, and the brain stem is smaller than normal. Compromise of pituitary function in the affected fetus can lead to prolonged gestation.

Bluetongue virus (*see* p 738), found in Africa, Australia, North and South America, and Europe, is also transmitted by insects; infection can occasionally cause prolonged gestation. The fetuses of cows exposed to the virus at 60–120 days of pregnancy developed hydranencephaly, whereas fetuses exposed later in pregnancy developed less severe CNS defects.

Gestation lengths >200 days have been recorded in ewes vaccinated during pregnancy with Rift Valley fever attenuated viral vaccine. Affected lambs developed severe brain defects and skeletal abnormalities. Some ewes developed hydrops amnion by the fourth month of gestation. Ewes in which pregnancy was not terminated developed ketosis.

Toxic Causes: Several plant toxins cause fetal deformity and prolonged gestation when eaten accidentally or fed experimentally. When fed to sheep in early pregnancy, *Veratrum californicum* (skunk cabbage) produces fetal deformities, giantism, and prolonged gestation. Cranial defects and brain and eye abnormalities were seen in fetuses of ewes fed this plant at 14 days of gestation; pregnancy length in some cases was >230 days. The plant contains the amine cyclopamine, which is believed to be responsible for the fetal abnormalities. This plant also contains a number of toxic alkaloids that cause GI disturbance, dyspnea, and convulsions in sheep. *Veratrum album* has similarly caused prolonged gestation and fetal abnormalities in Holstein-Friesian cows in Japan.

An unidentified toxin in the plant *Salsola tuberculatiformis* (cauliflower saltwort) is thought to cause prolonged gestation in sheep. Pregnancy was extended >220 days, and affected lambs showed atrophy of the pituitary, adrenal, and thyroid glands. Fetuses appear to be most susceptible to the toxin in the first and third trimesters of pregnancy. Amniotic fluid continues to increase in volume in cases of prolonged gestation associated with this plant. Physical abnormalities such as cleft palate prevent normal swallowing of amniotic fluid in affected fetuses. Excessive fetal weight and the weight of accumulated fetal fluids may lead to rupture of the prepubic tendon in ewes.

PSEUDOPREGNANCY IN GOATS

Pseudopregnancy is one of the major causes of anestrus in dairy goats during the breeding season. Older, parous does are most often affected. It is characterized by the persistence of a corpus luteum in the absence of a (viable) conceptus in the uterus.

Etiology and Pathogenesis: Failure of luteal regression, either in nonmated cycling animals or in mated does affected by embryonic or fetal mortality, is the key factor in the pathogenesis of the disorder. Pseudopregnancy can also spontaneously develop in unmated animals, even during the nonbreeding season. A genetic predisposition has been postulated, but in a recent study from the UK the incidence of pseudopregnancy in the offspring of affected dams was not significantly different from that in daughters of unaffected does.

Clinical Findings: Hydrometra (accumulation of fluid in the uterus) is the primary clinical feature of pseudopregnancy. It develops during prolonged and continuous exposure to progesterone from the corpus luteum. When not diagnosed, pseudopregnancy can persist for up to several months, and the amount of fluid can reach a volume of several liters. In such cases the distended abdomen will give the false impression that the animal is pregnant; this can also be accompanied by udder enlargement.

Diagnosis: Pseudopregnancy can be diagnosed by ultrasonography. The fluid is recognized as anechoic, black spots of variable size, separated by thin, double layers of tissue that represent sections through the apposing walls of the distended, curved uterine horns. When an abundant amount of fluid is present, these tissue layers can be seen undulating when the examiner shakes the abdominal wall of the doe. During an early ultrasonographic pregnancy diagnosis (20–30 days after mating or insemination), it can be difficult to discriminate between a normal pregnancy and a hydrometra because the embryo or placentomes can be difficult to locate at that stage, and excess fluid may be mistaken for allantoic fluid.

Treatment and Prognosis: Treatment with a luteolytic dose of prostaglandin $F_{2}\alpha$ (or one of its synthetic analogues) induces luteal regression and discharge of the uterine fluid within 1–2 days. If treated during the breeding season, the doe will come into estrus within 2–3 days and can be mated or inseminated again. Sometimes a second injection is necessary to accomplish a complete emptying of the uterus. Pseudopregnancy also may end spontaneously when progesterone production by the (aging) corpus luteum stops. As a result, relaxation of the cervix and stimulation of uterine contractility occur, followed by discharge of the uterine fluid. This latter process has also been described as "cloudburst." The fertility of does appears to be normal after effective treatment with prostaglandins, so culling of affected goats is generally not indicated.

RETAINED FETAL MEMBRANES IN LARGE ANIMALS

(Retained placenta)

COWS

Retention of fetal membranes, or retained placenta, usually is defined as failure to expel fetal membranes within 24 hr after parturition. Normally, expulsion occurs within 3–8 hr after calf delivery. The incidence in healthy dairy cows is 5%–15%, whereas the incidence in beef cows is lower. The incidence is increased by abortion (particularly with brucellosis or mycotic abortion), dystocia, twin birth, stillbirth, hypocalcemia, high environmental temperature, advancing age of the cow, premature birth or induction of parturition, placentitis, and nutritional disturbances.

Cows with retained fetal membranes are at increased risk of metritis, displaced abomasum, and mastitis.

Retention of fetal membranes is mediated by impaired migration of neutrophils to the placental interface in the periparturient period. The impaired neutrophil function extends into the postpartum period and probably mediates the recognized complications of retained fetal membranes. Cows with retained fetal membranes have increased cortisol and decreased estradiol concentrations in late pregnancy. They may also have an altered prostaglandin (PG) E_2:PGF_2 ratio. Uterine contractility is increased in affected cows. (Placental detachment, rather than uterine motility, is responsible for retention of fetal membranes.)

Diagnosis is usually straightforward as degenerating, discolored, ultimately fetid membranes are seen hanging from the vulva >24 hr after parturition. Occasionally, the retained membranes may remain within the uterus and not be readily apparent, in which case their presence may be signalled by a foul-smelling discharge. In most cases, there are no signs of systemic illness. When systemic signs are seen, they are related to toxemia. Uncomplicated retention of fetal membranes is unsightly and inconvenient for animal handlers and milkers but generally not directly harmful to the cow. However, cows with retained fetal membranes are at increased risk of developing metritis, ketosis, mastitis, and even abortion in a subsequent pregnancy. Cows that have once had retained fetal membranes are at increased risk of recurrence at a subsequent parturition.

Manual removal of the retained membranes is not recommended and is potentially harmful. Trimming of excess tissue that is objectionable to animal handlers and contributes to gross contamination of the genital tract is permissible. Untreated cows expel the membranes in 2–11 days. Routine use of intrauterine antimicrobials has not been found to be beneficial and may be detrimental. Although advocated at various times, oxytocin, estradiol, $PGF_2\alpha$, and oral calcium preparations have not been shown to hasten expulsion of retained membranes or to prevent complications. When systemic signs of illness are present, systemic treatment with antimicrobials is indicated. In herds in which incidence of retained fetal membranes is unacceptably high, predisposing causes should be sought and eliminated. Supplementation with vitamin E and selenium for herds in which these nutrients are deficient has been found to be beneficial.

MARES

Equine fetal membranes are normally expelled within 3 hr after parturition, but expulsion may be delayed for 8–12 hr or even longer without signs of illness. The cause of retention of fetal membranes often is not known, but the condition is associated with infection, abortion, short or prolonged gestation, uterine atony, and dystocia. Mares that have retained their fetal membranes appear to be at increased risk of recurrence of the condition, and Friesian mares are particularly predisposed. Retention of just a portion of the fetal membranes entirely within the uterus (usually at the tip of the previously nongravid uterine horn) is less conspicuous but equally likely to result in complications. For this reason, the chorionic surface of the expelled membranes should be examined carefully to ensure they have been completely expelled.

Retention of fetal membranes may mediate development of metritis or even peritonitis. Laminitis is a potential sequela. For these reasons, it is common practice to administer oxytocin (5 U, IM, every 2–3 hr) beginning 3–4 hr after parturition if the membranes have not yet been expelled. Calcium supplementation may be beneficial. Manual removal of retained membranes carries the risk of uterine damage or prolapse and is not recommended beyond gentle tugging to displace already loosened membranes. In cases of prolonged retention of fetal membranes, antimicrobials should be administered prophylactically, along with other therapeutic strategies aimed at preventing laminitis (*see* p 1109). Mares that have recovered from retention of fetal membranes do not generally have lower fertility.

DOES, EWES, AND SOWS

In does and ewes, the incidence of retained fetal membranes increases with larger litter sizes and with assisted parturition. Systemic treatment to guard against infection and gentle traction on exposed membranes may be used. In sows, retained placentae are contained within the uterus and are not visible at the vulva. In this species, entire fetuses may be retained. Usually, the fetus or membranes decompose in situ. This may be accompanied by signs of systemic illness and a purulent vaginal discharge. Although serious or fatal sequelae occasionally occur, the prognosis for recovery and future fertility is surprisingly good. Antimicrobial treatment is indicated in animals with systemic signs of illness.

SEMINAL VESICULITIS IN BULLS

The seminal vesicles are paired accessory sex glands located on the floor of the pelvis, lateral to the ampullae, and dorsal to the neck of the urinary bladder. The vesicles secrete a clear fluid that adds volume, nutrients, and buffers to semen. The term "seminal" vesicle is a misnomer, because the vesicles are not a reservoir for spermatozoa.

Seminal vesiculitis is an inflammation and often an infection of one or both vesicular glands. The purulent material associated with vesiculitis is a contaminant of semen and is a cause for semen to be discarded from bulls collected at an artificial insemination center. Bulls found to have vesiculitis during a breeding soundness examination are considered unsatisfactory breeders. Bulls refractory to treatment efforts should be culled.

Epidemiology: Vesiculitis has been reported in bulls wherever breeding cattle are raised. The reported incidence of vesiculitis in the general population of bulls is 1%–10%. However, incidences of 20% and even 49% have been reported for bulls housed in groups. Bulls of all ages can be affected, but vesiculitis is most frequently seen in yearling bulls presented for a breeding soundness examination or collected for the first time. Because many yearling bulls affected with vesiculitis are culled, it is seen less frequently in adult bulls.

Etiology and Pathogenesis: Vesiculitis is typically considered to be caused by bacterial infection. The most commonly identified bacteria are *Trueperella pyogenes*, *Pseudomonas aeruginosa*, streptococci, staphylococci, *Proteus* spp, and *Escherichia coli*. Other microbial agents implicated include *Mycoplasma bovigenitalium*, *Chlamydia* spp, and viruses.

Postulated pathogenic mechanisms include infectious agents ascending the urethra to the vesicle, descending through the ductus deferens from the testicles or epididymides, or metastasis from another tissue or organ hematogenously. The ascending route of infection is considered unlikely unless the bull has accompanying penile trauma or urethritis. The descending route would be considered if the vesiculitis is ipsilateral to an infectious epididymitis or orchitis. Vesiculitis subsequent to systemic infection, umbilical infection, infectious arthritis, or pneumonia is considered more plausible.

Congenital malformation of the excretory ducts of the vesicles where they open into the urethra at the colliculus seminalis has been reported. A malformation of the excretory duct orifice permits reflux of spermatozoa or urine from the pelvic urethra into the vesicle. If the tubular lining of the vesicle degenerates subsequent to irritation from abnormal material in the ducts, significant local inflammation can result. This noninfectious etiology may account for the poor therapeutic response in some cases.

Clinical Findings: There are usually no external signs of disease. It has been suggested that a bull with a severe acute case or vesicle abscessation may stand with its back arched, have pain on defecation or rectal examination, and show hesitation when mounting. However, such clinical signs are very uncommon.

Diagnosis: Vesiculitis is usually first suspected after collection of a semen sample grossly contaminated with purulent material. If the bull has vesiculitis, the rectal examination typically reveals an enlarged, sometimes irregular, and often fibrotic vesicle. Vesiculitis may be unilateral or bilateral. If vesiculitis is unilateral, there is usually asymmetry in the size of the glands. Infrequently, a vesicle will be abscessed; in such cases, the affected vesicle is markedly larger than the other and may be fluctuant on palpation.

Purulent contamination of semen is not pathognomonic for vesiculitis. A bull with epididymitis, orchitis, or posthitis may also have semen contaminated with purulent exudate. The entire genital tract must be examined to determine a possible cause for the abnormal semen. The prepuce may need to be douched with water or saline before collection of semen to exclude posthitis as a transient cause of pus in semen. Semen may be cultured but, unless collected aseptically after catheterization of the urethra, culture is usually unrewarding because of microbial contamination from the prepuce.

Treatment and Prognosis: Because vesiculitis may have a bacterial etiology, broad-spectrum antibiotics administered at labeled therapeutic dosages are usually administered to affected bulls. There are no published controlled studies that indicate preference of a specific antibiotic for treatment. Prolonged-release antibiotics are preferable because the bull, which can become unruly, does not have to be handled daily. Because vesiculitis is an inflammation as much as an infection, NSAIDs reduce the excretion of purulent material. Transient alleviation of purulent contamination may be achieved during the treatment interval in some bulls, but the prognosis for a longterm cure is guarded to poor. This is particularly true for chronic cases. Spontaneous remission has been seen when vesiculitis was diagnosed in bulls <1 yr old. Semen contaminated with purulent material is not suitable for artificial insemination and should be discarded. Surgical removal of affected vesicles has been done but is a difficult procedure. The prognosis after surgery is fair in yearling bulls; surgery has not been successful in adult bulls with chronic vesiculitis.

TRICHOMONIASIS

Trichomoniasis is a venereal disease of cattle characterized primarily by early fetal death and infertility, resulting in extended calving intervals. Distribution is probably worldwide.

Etiology and Epidemiology: The causative protozoan, *Tritrichomonas foetus*, is pyriform and ordinarily 10–15 × 5–10 μm, but there is considerable pleomorphism. It may become spherical when cultured in artificial media. At its anterior end, there are three flagella approximately the same length as the body of the parasite. An undulating membrane extends the length of the body and is bordered by a marginal filament that continues beyond the membrane as a posterior flagellum. Although *T foetus* can survive the process used for freezing semen, it is killed by drying or high temperatures.

T foetus is found in the genital tracts of cattle. When cows are bred naturally by an infected bull, 30%–90% become infected, suggesting that strain differences exist. Variation in breed susceptibility to trichomoniasis may also exist. Bulls of all ages can remain infected indefinitely, but this is less likely in younger males. By contrast, most cows are free of infection within 3 mo after breeding. However, immunity is not longlasting and reinfection does occur. Transmission can also occur when the semen from infected bulls is used for artificial insemination.

Clinical Findings: The most common sign is infertility caused by embryonic death. This results in repeat breeding, and attending stock persons often note cows in heat when they should be pregnant. This, along with poor pregnancy test results (eg, too many "nonpregnant normal" and late-bred cows) is usually the presenting complaint. In addition to a reduced number of cows estimated to calve during the regular calving season, an increased number of cows with a "nonpregnant abnormal" reproductive tract diagnosis is seen. These include cows with pyometra, endometritis, or a mummified fetus.

Fetal death and abortions can also occur but are not as common as losses earlier in gestation. *T foetus* has been found in vaginal cultures taken as late as 8 mo of gestation and, apparently, live calves can be born to infected dams. Pyometra occasionally develops after breeding.

Diagnosis: History and clinical signs are useful but are essentially the same as those of bovine genital campylobacteriosis (*see* p 1347). Confirmation depends on isolation of *T foetus*, which may be difficult to differentiate from other trichomonads resident in the digestive tract. Diagnostic efforts are directed at bulls, because they are the most likely carriers. Suction is applied to a pipette while it is used to vigorously scrape the epithelium in the preputial fornix. Alternatively, douching with saline or lactated Ringer's solution (without preservatives) can be used. Aspirates or douches, concentrated by centrifugation, are examined using darkfield contrast microscopy. This material is also transferred immediately to the surface of a liquid culture medium such as Diamond medium. Better success culturing the organism has been reported when using commercially available media-filled pouches. In addition, incubating the media beyond the standard 48 hr may also enhance the accuracy of the diagnosis. Sampling every 48 hr for 10 days from the bottom of the tube and examining at 100–400× may reveal the rolling jerky movements of *T foetus*. Studies have examined the possibility of using PCR assays to identify *T foetus* directly from the preputial samples without an intervening culture. These tests are being used by some laboratories to reduce the time required for a definitive diagnosis of trichomoniasis. Some diagnostic laboratories are suggesting that the scraping be placed in phosphate buffered saline before transport to the diagnostic laboratory. A sample prepared in this way can be effectively examined for both trichomoniasis and campylobacteriosis by using a specific PCR application.

Studies suggest that 90%–95% of infected bulls will be positive on culture, and that three successive cultures at weekly intervals will detect ~99.5% of infected bulls. A vaginal discharge (after treatment of pyometra) or vaginal mucus (obtained toward the end of a luteal phase) may also be of diagnostic value.

The number of times the bull battery should be sampled and cultured to ensure the bulls are negative depends on the prevalence of fetal wastage in the cow herd. With more open and late cows, the frequency of testing should increase to improve the probability that bulls are negative for the protozoan.

Treatment and Control: Various imidazoles have been used to treat bulls, but none is both safe and effective. Ipronidazole is probably most effective but, due to its low pH, frequently causes sterile abscesses at injection sites. In addition, bulls are probably susceptible to reinfection after successful treatment. Resistance to ipronidazole may also be a concern. The biggest problem, however, is that the success of treatment is measured by repeated sampling, which may mean the individual bull can never be definitively called negative. Therefore, an unqualified recommendation for the bull's use cannot be given.

Control consists of eliminating the infection from the bull battery by culling all bulls and replacing them with virgin bulls or by testing and culling positive bulls. Repeated testing in older bulls may be unsatisfactory, and it may be prudent to cull them all. Reinfection is prevented by exposing only the uninfected (clean) bulls to uninfected (clean) cows. Clean cows are assumed to be those with calves at foot (even though some infected cows may produce a live calf) and virgin heifers. In situations in which several herds are commingled on the same range, caution must be exercised to ensure that cows and heifers are not exposed to potentially infected bulls at the home ranch before they are turned out on the common grazing pasture.

T foetus can be safely eliminated from semen with dimetridazole.

Vaccines developed some time ago for use in cows and evaluated in the field were not highly effective, especially in the absence of other control measures. However, the efficacy of whole-cell *T foetus* vaccines has recently been critically reviewed. Although there is some evidence to suggest that timely vaccination will improve reproductive performance in heifers, there is a distinct lack of evidence that vaccination will reduce "bull-associated outcomes."

UDDER DISEASES

See also MASTITIS IN LARGE ANIMALS, p 1358, and PSEUDOCOWPOX, p 868.

DISEASES OF BOVINE TEATS AND SKIN

Bovine Ulcerative Mammillitis (Bovine Herpesvirus II and IV): Bovine herpesvirus II and IV (BHV-II, BHV-IV) can cause an acute, ulcerative condition of teat and udder skin of dairy cows that is often referred to as bovine ulcerative mammillitis. BHV-II can occur sporadically or in outbreaks that often have a seasonal association with cold weather and may result in reduced milk production and increased susceptibility to bacterial mastitis.

Clinical signs range from relatively mild, small plaques of edema to severe ulceration. Early signs may vary, but the lesions often begin as one or more thickened, edematous plaques of varying size on the skin of one or more teats. Vesicles develop and may rapidly rupture, leaving a raw, ulcerated area that becomes covered with a dark-colored scab. The scabs tend to crack and bleed, especially if milking is attempted. The lesions are of variable size and can include much of the teat wall and orifice. Teats are generally painful, and affected cows often resist milking, leading to development of mastitis. The greatest incidence is often seen in first-lactation cows, but previously unexposed cows of any age are susceptible. Severe lesions may take several weeks to heal.

Diagnosis is based on clinical signs and confirmed by histopathology or by virus isolation from early lesions. Treatment is directed toward supportive care, because there is no effective therapy for this virus. The use of iodophore-containing teat dips with added emollients may help to inactivate the virus. It is important to isolate affected cows and to use separate milking equipment. Affected animals should be segregated to prevent spread among all animals. The use of separate milking equipment; clean, single-use towels to dry udders; and clean gloves for milking personnel help to prevent spread of the agent to susceptible animals.

Pseudocowpox: Pseudocowpox is a condition of teat skin caused by a poxvirus that results in a characteristic horseshoe-shaped lesion or scab (*see* p 868).

Bovine Warts (Bovine Papillomavirus): Several strains of bovine papillomavirus (BPV1, BPV5, BPV6, BPV9) cause the development of papillomas or fibropapillomas on teats. In some herds, pale, smooth, raised lesions develop frequently on teat skin and may persist indefinitely without causing problems. In other instances, filamentous or frond-like lesions develop at the teat orifice and interfere with milking. Bovine warts are spread by direct or indirect contact, and bovine papillomavirus DNA has been identified in blood, milk, urine, and other biologic fluids obtained from infected animals. Diagnosis is usually made presumptively based on examination of the lesion and exclusion of other causes. In many instances, treatment of warts is *not* necessary, but frond-like lesions that interfere with milking may require excision. The use of autogenous vaccines and virucidal teat dips may be recommended in herd outbreaks.

Teat-end Hyperkeratosis: The development of raised smooth or rough rings at the teat ends of lactating cows is a common occurrence and is associated with the keratin dynamics of the streak canal. Teat ends affected with hyperkeratosis may progress from smooth, doughnut-shaped lesions that do not affect milking to severely hyperkeratotic rings with radial cracks. When teats are severely affected, the ability to properly sanitize teat ends before milking may be compromised. Diagnosis is usually made by clinical examination of affected teats. The degree of hyperkeratosis is often characterized by scoring teat ends using the following scale: 1) no ring, 2) smooth ring, 3) rough ring, and 4) very rough, cracked ring.

The cause of hyperkeratosis is multifactorial; thus, prevention is directed toward a number of potential risk factors. Hyperkeratosis is often associated with cold weather, probably because of changes in peripheral circulation. Risk factors for development of hyperkeratosis include incorrect use of teat sanitizers, exposure of wet teats to cold weather, improper milking machine settings leading to overmilking, inadequate massage phase during milking, and inadequate milk letdown. After underlying risk factors are addressed, affected teats generally recover over several weeks or over a dry period.

Dermatitis: Dermatitis of the udder has a number of causes, including chemical irritants, sunburn, and bacterial infection. The udder can be exposed to chemical irritants from bedding additives (eg, some types of limestone) or chemicals used during milking. The irritation usually resolves after removal of the offending substance, but gentle udder washes and use of emollient products can accelerate healing. Udder impetigo (udder acne) is a bacterial dermatitis characterized by development of small pustules on the skin of the udder and teats. Staphylococci usually can be isolated from the pustules. Treatment of udder impetigo consists of clipping hair from the affected area and washing the skin thoroughly each day until the condition resolves.

Frostbite: Teat skin can chap and crack when wet teats are exposed to cold winds or frozen bedding areas. Exposure of wet skin to subfreezing temperatures may result in frostbite. Skin affected by frostbite becomes swollen and discolored and ultimately develops a leathery texture. In severe cases, the teat skin may slough. Frostbite is best prevented by ensuring that teat skin is dry before allowing cows access to housing areas or pastures during periods of temperatures <0°F. Care should be taken to ensure that all bedding areas that contact teat and udder skin are thoroughly dry. Teat disinfectant products (eg, powder teat dips and other cold weather formulations) specifically designed for extremely cold weather are relatively successful at preventing frostbite after dipping. When liquid dips are used during periods of extremely low ambient temperatures, the teats should be dried before the cows exit the milking facility.

Udder Sores (Necrotic Dermatitis): Moist, foul-smelling, necrotic lesions may develop in areas of tightly adjacent skin of some animals (such as the udder cleft). In heifers, the lateral aspect of the udder and medial aspect of the thigh are often involved. In this area, the udder is pressed tightly against the leg, resulting in chafing, dermatitis, and necrosis. Udder edema is a risk factor for development of this condition and must be treated concurrently. The necrotic skin should be cleaned daily with an antiseptic solution and thoroughly dried. Mild astringents should be applied. A similar condition, which may be associated with infestation by *Sarcoptes* mites, has been seen at the anterior portion of the udder between the two forequarters. Older cows have been reported to be at greater risk than heifers. The swollen, necrotic area may be treated topically with an approved miticide; however, appropriate milk withholding periods must be observed.

PHYSIOLOGIC DISORDERS

Udder Edema: Udder edema is common in high-producing dairy cattle (especially heifers) before and after parturition. Predisposing causes include age at first calving (older heifers are at greater risk), gestation length, genetics, nutritional management, obesity, and lack of exercise during the precalving period. Prepartum diets that contain excessive salt increase the severity of udder edema. Physiologic edema is not usually painful and occurs when pitting edema develops symmetrically in the udder before parturition. Udder edema is a risk factor for development of clinical mastitis and occasionally can become a chronic condition that persists throughout lactation. Treatment should be initiated if swelling threatens the udder support apparatus or if edema interferes with the ability to milk the cow. Edema can be treated by milking cows before parturition. Positive effects of premilking in heifers have been reported, but the practice may predispose older cows to parturient paresis (*see* p 988). Massage, repeated as often as possible, and hot compresses stimulate circulation and promote edema reduction. Diuretics have proved highly beneficial in reducing udder edema, and corticosteroids may be helpful. Products that combine diuretics and corticosteroids are available for treatment of udder edema.

Precocious Mammary Development: Initiation of milk secretion in heifers before calving is occasionally noted. Precocious mammary development in a single gland sometimes results from suckling by herdmates. Symmetric mammary development has been occasionally associated with ovarian neoplasia or exposure to feedstuffs containing estrogen or contaminated by mycotoxins. Removal of contaminated feedstuffs generally results in resolution of the problem.

Failure of Milk Ejection (Milk Let-down): In rare instances, newly calved heifers may have problems with milk ejection. Fear of handling or unfamiliarity with the milking facility or milking procedures is the usual cause. Care should be taken to ensure that animals are handled calmly and gently and that the milking routine provides for adequate stimulation (>20 sec) before attaching the milking unit. Administration of oxytocin (20 IU, IM) may be necessary in some instances, but doses should be gradually reduced to avoid dependence on administration of exogenous oxytocin.

Agalactia: Agalactia is seen occasionally in heifers and can be a primary endocrine problem or a localized problem of the mammary gland. It is occasionally caused by a severe systemic disease or by mastitis caused by *Mycoplasma bovis*. Agalactia has also been associated with cows grazing or eating endophyte-infested fescue.

"Blind" or Nonfunctional Quarters: Nonfunctional quarters are usually the result of a severe mastitis infection, which may occur in dry or lactating cows or in heifers due to suckling by other heifers or calves. Some of these quarters may occasionally return to production in future lactations. Rarely, blind or nonfunctional quarters may be congenital.

Congenital Disorders: Congenital aberrations include many structural defects, but the most significant disorder is

supernumerary teats. These may be located on the udder behind the posterior teats, between the front and hind teats, or attached to either the front or hind teats. Removal of supernumerary teats from dairy heifers is desirable to improve appearance of the udder, to eliminate the possibility of mastitis in the gland above the extra teats, and to facilitate milking. Most are easily removed surgically when the heifer is from 1 wk to 1 yr old (best done at 3–8 mo of age). Supernumerary teats may be surgically removed from preparturient heifers before lactation begins. The incision should be sutured or stapled after excision of the teat.

TRAUMATIC AND STRUCTURAL DISORDERS

Trauma and Laceration: Superficial wounds to the udder and teats may be cleaned with suitable antiseptic solutions and treated as open wounds with frequent application of antiseptic powders or sprays. If the teats are involved, adhesive tape may hasten healing. Wounds involving the teat orifice should be dressed with antiseptic creams and bandaged after milking. Affected quarters are at very high risk of infection, and prophylactic treatment with intramammary antibiotics is recommended to prevent development of mastitis.

Lacerations of the large milk vein should be considered an emergency because of the potential for severe hemorrhage; prompt compression and ligation of these lacerations is recommended.

Deeper wounds of the udder and teats should be promptly (within 6 hr) cleansed and sutured or stapled under local anesthesia with appropriate sedation and restraint. When the wound involves the teat cistern, it may be necessary to insert a self-retaining teat cannula with removable cap into the teat for the first 24 hr to prevent milk seeping through the wound (which would delay or prevent healing) and to aid in milking. The affected quarter should be infused with antibiotic preparations.

Teat Obstructions: Acquired teat obstructions are usually the result of proliferation of granulation tissue after the occurrence of an observed or unobserved teat injury. Teat obstructions are usually recognized when they interfere with milk flow. They can range from diffuse, tightly *adherent lesions* to highly mobile discrete lesions that float throughout the gland cistern. Some "floaters" are caused by formation of small masses from butterfat, minerals, and tissue in mammary ducts during the dry period. These can be recognized by intermittent disruptions in milk flow. They may be removed by forced pressure downward on the teat cistern or by use of specialized instruments inserted through the teat canal. Membranous obstructions in the area of the annular fold at the base of the gland cistern are sometimes seen in heifers. Treatment of these obstructions is generally unsuccessful.

Complete teat obstruction may result when adhesions fill the teat cistern after severe trauma. Treatment is similar to that for stenosis (*see* below), but the prognosis usually is more guarded. In instances of severe injury, milking of the quarter should be permanently discontinued.

Teat stenosis is characterized by a marked narrowing of the teat orifice or streak canal, which makes milking difficult. It usually results from a contusion or wound that produces swelling or formation of a blood clot or scab or from mastitis infections (especially in prelactating heifers). Teat obstructions can be diagnosed initially by careful palpation of the affected gland. Complex teat obstructions or obstructions in valuable animals may require diagnostic imaging such as ultrasonography, contrast radiography, or theloscopy (endoscopy).

Treatment varies depending on severity. Conservative treatment includes the use of teat cannulas and external pressure to remove obstructions, whereas serious cases may require prompt referral to specialists for thelotomy or theloscopy (endoscopic surgery). All injuries to, or surgical procedures on, the teat should be handled carefully to prevent infection. Prophylactic antibiotic infusions of the quarter are indicated when the teat or teat orifice is involved. Permanent fistulas into the teat or gland cisterns are best repaired during the dry period.

Breakdown of Udder Support Apparatus: Rupture of the suspensory ligaments of the udder (usually the medial suspensory ligament) occurs gradually in some older cows and leads to a dropping of the udder floor, resulting in lateral deviation of the teats. Occasionally, acute rupture can occur at or just after parturition. Animals with this condition are at high risk of developing mastitis. There is no successful treatment; supportive trusses generally are not satisfactory. The condition is suspected to have a genetic basis, and these animals are often removed from the milking herd.

Hematomas: Trauma (often related to inadequate housing) can result in contusions and hematomas of the udder. Hematomas usually appear as soft-tissue swellings located anterior to the foreudder or caudodorsal to the rear udder. They may be difficult to differentiate from abscesses. Severe hematomas can result in anemia if not treated. In most instances, hematomas resolve after conservative treatment consisting of pressure wraps and rest. Hematomas should not be incised or drained unless they become infected. Milking should be performed cautiously during the convalescent period. Hematomas that continue to enlarge should be considered an emergency because of the possibility of excessive blood loss and shock.

Abscesses: Subcutaneous abscesses of the udder (not involving the milk-producing tissue) can develop between the skin and the supporting connective tissue of the udder. Diagnosis is by needle aspiration. Abscesses usually develop secondary to wounds, chronic mastitis, infected hematomas, or severe contusions. They should be incised and drained when chronic and near the surface of the udder. The wound should be flushed daily with an antiseptic solution or water under pressure until healing is complete.

Bloody Milk: The occurrence of pink- or red-tinged milk is common after calving and can be attributed to rupture of tiny mammary blood vessels. Udder swelling from edema or trauma is a potential underlying cause. Bloody milk is not fit for consumption. In most cases, it resolves without treatment in 4–14 days, provided the gland is milked out regularly. The occurrence of frank blood in a single quarter is likely the result of severe, acute mastitis (*see* p 1358) or trauma, and milking should be discontinued until hemorrhage is controlled. Intramammary antibiotics should be administered if mastitis is suspected.

Teat Sphincter Inadequacy ("Leakers" or Incontinentia Lactis): High levels of intramammary pressure in high-producing dairy cows may result in milk dripping from teats. Risk factors for milk leakage include high peak milk flow rates, short teats, and inverted teat ends. Shorter intervals or more frequent milking may be recommended when a large proportion of the herd is affected. Occasionally, cows are observed to leak milk continuously. These cows usually have sustained a severe teat injury or have an abnormal streak canal. In general, little can be done to correct this condition, and most of these cows will develop mastitis; it is recommended that persistent leakers be designated for removal from the herd.

UTERINE PROLAPSE AND EVERSION

Prolapse of the uterus may occur in any species; however, it is most common in dairy and beef cows and ewes and less frequent in sows. It is rare in mares, bitches, queens, and rabbits. Invagination of the tip of the uterus, excessive traction to relieve dystocia or retained fetal membranes, uterine atony, hypocalcemia, and lack of exercise have all been incriminated as contributory causes.

Prolapse of the uterus invariably occurs immediately after or within several hours of parturition, when the cervix is open and the uterus lacks tone. Prolapse of the post-gravid uterine horn usually is complete in cows, and the mass of uterus usually hangs below the hocks. The invagination of the contralateral horn, which is prevented from exteriorization by the strong intercornual ligament, can be located by careful examination of the surface of the prolapsed organ. In sows, one horn may become everted while unborn piglets in the other prevent further prolapse. In small animals, complete prolapse of both uterine horns is usual. A contributory cause in sheep may be grazing estrogenic pastures.

In cows, treatment involves removing the placenta (if still attached), thoroughly cleaning the endometrial surface, and repairing any lacerations. Rubbing the surface of the uterus with glycerol helps reduce edema and provides lubrication. The uterus is then returned to its normal position. An epidural anesthetic should be administered first. If the cow is standing, the cleansed uterus should be elevated to the level of the vulva on a tray or hammock supported by assistants, and then replaced by applying steady pressure beginning at the cervical portion (or at the level of the invagination of the nonprolapsed uterine horn) and gradually working toward the apex. Once the uterus is replaced, a hand should be inserted to the tip of both uterine horns to be sure there is no remaining invagination that could incite abdominal straining and another prolapse. Installation of warm, sterile saline solution is useful to ensure complete replacement of the tip of the uterine horn without trauma. If recumbent, the cow should be positioned with the hindquarters elevated by placing her in sternal recumbency with the hindlegs extended backward. When elevating the hindquarters of the cow, care should be taken to lift the prolapsed uterus with the hindquarters to prevent stretching and laceration of the uterine artery.

Replacement of the prolapsed uterus in mares is done in a similar way, usually with the mare sedated but standing, taking care not to perforate the uterus.

In sows and small animals, the uterus may be repositioned by simultaneously manipulating it from outside with one hand and through an abdominal incision with the other. Resection of the uterus is indicated in longstanding cases in which tissue necrosis has occurred. Once the uterus is in its normal position, oxytocin (up to 5 IU, IV, or up to 20 IU depending on species, IM) is administered to increase uterine tone. Administration IV of calcium-containing solutions is indicated in most cases, also as a means of increasing uterine tone. Caslick sutures or other forms of vulvar closure are not useful, because the uterine prolapse begins at the apex of the uterine horn. Prevention of recurrence depends on complete and correct replacement of the uterus and restoration of uterine tone.

The prognosis depends on the amount of injury and contamination of the uterus. The prognosis is favorable when a clean, minimally traumatized uterus is promptly replaced. There is no tendency for the condition to recur at subsequent parturitions.

Complications tend to develop when laceration, necrosis, and infection occur, or when treatment is delayed. Shock, hemorrhage, and thromboembolism are potential sequelae of a prolonged prolapse. In some instances, the bladder and intestines may prolapse into the everted uterus. These require careful replacement before the uterus is replaced. The bladder may be drained with a catheter or needle passed through the uterine wall. Elevation of the hindquarters and pressure on the uterus aid in replacement of bladder and intestines. It may be necessary to incise the uterus carefully (in a longitudinal direction) to replace these organs. In cows, amputation of a severely traumatized or necrotic uterus may be the only way to save the animal. Supportive treatment and antibiotic therapy are indicated.

VAGINAL AND CERVICAL PROLAPSE

Eversion and prolapse of the vagina, with or without prolapse of the cervix, occurs most commonly in cattle and sheep. A form of vaginal prolapse, different in pathogenesis, also occurs in dogs (*see* p 1399). In cattle and sheep, the condition is usually seen in mature females in the last trimester of pregnancy. Predisposing factors include increased intra-abdominal pressure associated with increased size of the pregnant uterus, intra-abdominal fat, or rumen distention superimposed upon relaxation and softening of the pelvic girdle and associated soft-tissue structures in the pelvic canal and perineum mediated by increased circulating concentrations of estrogens and relaxin during late pregnancy. Intra-abdominal pressure is increased in recumbent animals. Added to this, sheep tend to face uphill when lying down, so gravity contributes to vaginal eversion and prolapse. Docking the tails of lambs may damage structures that support the pelvic girdle (eg, coccygeus muscle) and predispose to vaginal prolapse if the tail is docked too short. The tail should be removed at the level of the ventral skin fold, leaving two or three coccygeal vertebrae intact.

The prolapse begins as an intussusception-like folding of the vaginal floor just cranial to the vestibulovaginal junction. Discomfort caused by this eversion, coupled with irritation and swelling of the exposed mucosa, results in straining and more extensive prolapse. Eventually the entire vagina may be prolapsed, with the cervix conspicuous at the most caudal part of the prolapsus. The bladder or loops of intestine may be contained within the prolapsed vagina. As the bladder moves into the prolapsed vagina, the urethra may be occluded. The bladder then fills and enlarges, which hinders replacement of the prolapsed vagina unless the bladder is first drained. The bladder may even rupture with potentially fatal consequences. Vaginal prolapse may be graded as I (intermittent prolapse, especially when recumbent), II (continuous prolapse), III (continuous prolapse of vagina, bladder, and cervix), or IV (grade II or III with tissue damage by trauma, infection, or necrosis).

Although most common in mature animals in late pregnancy, vaginal prolapse can occur in young, nonpregnant ewes and heifers, especially in fat animals. Predisposing factors include grazing estrogenic plants (especially *Trifolium subterraneum*) or exogenous administration of estrogenic compounds (usually in the form of growth-promotant implants). Cervicovaginal prolapse is more common in stabled than in pastured animals, suggesting that lack of exercise may be a contributing factor. Vaginal prolapse may also be a problem in cows subjected to repeated superovulation for embryo recovery due to repeated exposure to supraphysiologic concentrations of estrogens. A genetic component in the pathogenesis of cervicovaginal prolapse is likely, because a breed predisposition exists in both cattle (Brahman, Brahman crossbreds, Hereford) and sheep (Kerry Hill, Romney Marsh). In pigs, vaginal prolapse is often associated with estrogenic activity of mycotoxins.

For replacement of the prolapsed vagina, an epidural anesthetic is first administered. The organ is washed and rinsed, and the bladder emptied if necessary. Usually, this can be achieved by elevating the prolapsus to allow straightening of the urethra; occasionally, needle puncture through the vaginal wall may be necessary. The vagina is well lubricated (glycerol provides lubrication and reduces congestion and edema by osmotic action) and replaced and then held in position until it feels warm again.

Retention is achieved by insertion of a Buhner suture—a deeply buried, circumferential suture placed around the vestibulum to provide support at the point at which the initial eversion of the vaginal wall occurs. The Buhner suture has largely superseded earlier attempts to prevent prolapse by various patterns of sutures in the vulvar lips (which do not prevent the initial eversion of the vagina into the vestibulum) or by methods that relied on placement of a retention device within the vagina (which tend to cause discomfort and further straining). Buhner sutures should generally be removed before parturition to prevent extensive laceration. Modification of the Buhner suture to include an exposed, horizontal mattress–like suture has the advantage of remaining in place even when vestibulovaginal tissues have little holding power, and a traditional Buhner suture may be prone to tear through the dorsal or lateral vestibular wall. The Buhner suture and its modifications attempt to replicate the support normally provided by the constrictor vestibuli muscles that are lacking in cases of prolapse. Permanent fixation of the vagina can be achieved by the Johnson button technique, whereby sutures are placed from the vagina, through the sacrospinotuberal ligament and gluteal muscles, and then anchored in the vagina and on the skin with large, flat discs. This can also be accomplished by anchoring the cervix to the prepubic tendon or iliopsoas muscle. Although the cervical os may be edematous and inflamed, cervicovaginal prolapse seldom interrupts pregnancy and does not specifically predispose to dystocia or postpartum uterine prolapse, which has a different etiology.

Vaginal prolapse in sheep may occur simultaneously in many ewes as a herd problem, making surgery impractical. In these cases, use of a commercially available vaginal retention device (a bearing retainer) may be useful. Sheep may lamb without mishap with these devices in place. Permanent fixation techniques (cervicopexy or vaginopexy) have been described in which the cervix or vaginal wall is anchored to other pelvic structures. They may be useful in individual cases of chronic or recurrent prolapse, but most cases are resolved by a well-placed Buhner suture.

VULVITIS AND VAGINITIS IN LARGE ANIMALS

Contusion and hematoma of the vagina are noted infrequently after parturition in all species but particularly in mares and sows. Occasionally, vaginal hematomas in sows may rupture and cause serious (or fatal) hemorrhage that can be controlled by ligation of the labial branch of the internal pudendal artery. Necrotic vaginitis, vestibulitis, and vulvitis may follow dystocia in all species. Onset of signs, consisting of arched back, elevated tail, anorexia, dysuria, straining, vulvar and perivulvar swelling, and possibly a fetid, serous discharge, begins within 1–4 days of parturition and may persist for 2–4 wk. In most cases, only gentle and conservative treatment is needed. Prophylactic antibiotic treatment is wise, because clostridial or other organisms may proliferate in the damaged tissue and cause tetanus (*see* p 611), blackleg (*see* p 602), or other forms of clostridial myositis. Possible consequences of necrotic vaginitis include permanent stricture of the vagina, transvaginal adhesions, or perivaginal abscessation.

Vestibular lymphocytic follicles, also called granular venereal disease, granular vulvitis, or granular vulvovaginitis, are seen in cows and are characterized by vestibular hyperemia and hyperplasia of the lymphoid nodules of the vestibular mucosa. These lesions do not constitute a specific disease but reflect irritation of the vestibular mucosa. They can be reproduced experimentally by topical application of *Ureaplasma ureolyticum* or *Mycoplasma* spp in goats and cattle.

Infectious pustular vulvovaginitis of cows is caused by bovine herpesvirus 1 (*see* p 1434) and is transmitted by natural service, nasogenital contact, or mechanically by insects such as flies. It is characterized by vaginal lesions. Affected cows show signs of vaginal discomfort (raised tail, frequent urination) and have numerous, round, white, raised lesions of the vestibular mucosa. Within a short time, these lesions progress to pustules and erosions or ulcers. Mucopurulent discharge may be prominent, even in pregnant animals in which pregnancy is uninterrupted. The histologic lesion consists of necrosis of vestibular and vaginal epithelium, with intranuclear inclusion bodies typical of herpesvirus infection. The virus may be secreted in the semen of infected bulls (which have similar lesions of the penis and prepuce). Intrauterine inoculation of the virus produces necrotizing endometritis and cervicitis.

A severe disease characterized by vaginitis in cows and epididymitis in bulls occurs sporadically in eastern and southern Africa, where it is referred to as epivag. The disease is spread by natural mating. In the early stages of infection, cows have intense *vaginitis characterized by* reddened mucosae without ulcers, erosions, or vesicular lesions. A thick, creamy, white to yellow discharge develops. The infection spreads to the uterus and uterine tubes, and salpingitis and fimbrial adhesions frequently result in permanent infertility. Although epivag has been transmitted experimentally by transferring exudate, the cause is unknown.

Necrotic vulvitis has been observed as a severe granulomatous and necrotic lesion centered on the ventral commissure of the vulva of cows, sometimes occurring in outbreak form. It is associated with several pathogens, possibly acting synergistically and, in particular, *Porphyromonas levii*.

Catarrhal bovine vaginitis has been reported from many countries. Although enteroviruses have been associated with this condition, the cause remains unknown. In areas of the world where bovine tuberculosis (*see* p 687) is still endemic, vaginal lesions may be either a primary lesion after service by a bull with genital infection or evidence of uterine disease or of cervicitis.

One cause of vulvitis in sheep is ulcerative dermatosis (*see* p 872), characterized by crusted ulcers of the vulvar skin, penis, prepuce, and facial skin. Posthitis and vulvitis are also caused by the interaction of a high-protein diet and infection with urease-producing organisms, usually *Corynebacterium renale*. *Demodex* mites have been seen in the vulvar skin of sheep; they usually are not associated with lesions but may produce granulomas.

Equine coital exanthema (*see* p 1357) is caused by equine herpesvirus 3. It is an acute disease without systemic signs. Red papules appear in the vaginal and vestibular mucosae 2–10 days after infection, which occurs as a result of mating with an infected stallion. Lesions extend to the perivulvar skin. The lesions progress rapidly to pustules, then ulcerate, and finally heal, leaving depigmented scars. Stallions show similar lesions on the penis and prepuce. The disease causes discomfort and may prevent mating but does not specifically inhibit fertility.

Dourine (*see* p 38) is a venereal disease of horses. Early signs are characterized by edematous swelling of the vulva and secondary vulvovaginitis of the swollen, irritable tissue.

Coital injuries of cows and mares may be attributable to the relatively large size of the penis in these species compared with the vagina. Injuries of the vulva and vagina may be caused by horned cattle. Vaginal injuries in a variety of species have also been inflicted maliciously.

REPRODUCTIVE DISEASES OF THE FEMALE SMALL ANIMAL

See also MANAGEMENT OF REPRODUCTION: SMALL ANIMALS, p 2219.

Most "infertile" dogs are healthy and fertile. Breeding practices should be reviewed before engaging in diagnostic testing for the less common causes of canine infertility. A basic understanding of the reproductive cycle of the bitch is essential to diagnose "infertility" problems related to breeding at the incorrect time, artificial insemination, etc. Most bitches cycle twice a year, with an interestrous interval of at least 4 mo. Bitches with <4 mo between two cycles usually do not get pregnant. Some large breeds (eg, Great Danes) may cycle every 9–12 mo with normal fertility.

The bitch is a spontaneous ovulator, ie, ovulation occurs without any breeding stimulus. The bitch starts cycling with the influence of hormones released from the hypothalamus and pituitary glands. Gonadotropin-releasing hormone (GnRH), released from the hypothalamus, stimulates the release of follicle-stimulating hormone (FSH) and luteinizing hormone (LH). FSH has a primary responsibility for growth of follicles on the ovaries, whereas LH causes ovulation of the follicles.

The **estrous cycle in the bitch** is unique and different from that of other domestic animals. It starts with proestrus, which most breeders refer to as the start of the "season," when spotting or bleeding from the vagina is noticed. During proestrus, the bitch is attractive to males but does not allow breeding. Estrogen produced by ovarian follicles causes changes in the epithelial cells of the vaginal mucosa, which can be examined by vaginal cytology (*see* p 1607). Estrus or time of receptivity follows proestrus, when the bitch accepts the male for breeding. The duration of proestrus and estrus is traditionally considered to be 9 days each, on average, but each phase can range from 2 or 3 to 21 days. During proestrus, the vulvar lips of the bitch are turgid or firm and become soft and "wrinkly" as the bitch nears the time of receptivity. In most bitches, the bloody discharge of proestrus also changes to a straw color as estrus nears, but some may bleed all the way through estrus.

The production of **progesterone** is also unique during the estrous cycle of the bitch. The early rise of progesterone during estrus is from the luteinized follicles of the ovaries and can be used in breeding management. The bitch ovulates ~2–3 days after the LH peak. After ovulation, the follicles are replaced by corpora lutea (CLs), which produce progesterone. The production of progesterone continues throughout diestrus, the phase of the estrous cycle after estrus, regardless of whether the bitch is pregnant. The duration of diestrus is the same as that of pregnancy, ~62–63 days from the LH peak. Unlike in other domestic species, in the bitch there is no production of prostaglandin $F_2\alpha$ from the endometrium to cause luteolysis (CL regression). During diestrus, many bitches go through pseudopregnancy in which they may gain weight and have an enlarged abdomen; other overt signs may be seen, including mammary gland enlargement, as well as prewhelping behavior such as nesting or "adopting" toys and shoes. The pseudopregnancy (or diestrus) is considered a normal occurrence and may not need any treatment.

Ovulation: The ova released during ovulation in the bitch are at the primary oocyte stage, ie, the first polar body has not come out of the ovum and sperm are unable to penetrate the ovum. It takes ~3 days for the ovum to become a secondary oocyte, which can be penetrated by sperm. Sperm can survive as long as 10 days in the bitch's reproductive tract. This can become a diagnostic challenge when a bitch's owner requests a cesarean section 62 days after breeding, because theoretically the gestation period may be only 52 days. A fairly reliable predictor of whelping is hypothermia or a decrease in rectal temperature of 2°–3°F, caused by a progesterone decrease 12–36 hr before. Vaginal cytology can also be used to predict whelping by determination of day 1 of diestrus.

Reproductive Anatomy: Successful vaginal swabbing technique requires knowledge of the unique reproductive anatomy of the bitch. The vagina of the bitch is very long, ~20 cm (9 in.) in a medium-sized bitch. The cervix is located in the abdominal cavity, whereas it is located in the pelvic inlet in other domestic animals (eg, cow, mare). Therefore, the cervix in the bitch cannot be visualized by an endoscope or speculum; a flexible endoscope with a light source is required. This is important to deposit semen transcervical in the uterus for artificial insemination (AI). The size of the uterus and ovaries vary considerably with the breed.

Vaginal Cytology: A clean, cotton tip swab is commonly used to swab the vagina to obtain a cytology sample. An endoscope cone or vaginal speculum can be used to guide the swab. A right-handed person can hold the bitch's vulva with a gloved left hand, opening the vulvar lips with the thumb and middle finger, while using the index finger behind the vulva to support it. The swab is moistened with warm tap water and inserted almost vertically into the vagina, avoiding the clitoral area, up and over the brim of the pelvis. It may be helpful to forward the swab, especially in small size bitches and bitches without serosanguineous discharge. If the swab feels "stuck" in the vaginal folds, it may be pulled back slightly and redirected before proceeding. Once the swab is inserted to a depth of at least 6–10 cm (2–4 in.), it is rolled a few times in one direction (if rotated back and forth, the cotton may unroll and drop in the vagina) and withdrawn. Inserting the swab as deep as possible to reach the cranial part of the vagina (versus the caudal part) minimizes collection of extraneous debris. Getting in a habit of reaching the cranial vagina is also helpful to take samples for vaginal culture and for AI. The swab is rolled on a clean microscope slide, air-dried, and stained; two slides are recommended. Stains that can be used include Wright-Giemsa, Romanowsky, methylene blue, eosin-nigrosin, Gram stain, etc. The slides with smears are dipped 5–7 times in each jar, rinsed with tap water, air-dried, and examined under the microscope. Viewing under 200× magnification first is helpful to get an overall impression of the types and distribution of cells before examining more closely under 400× magnification.

Vaginal Cytology Interpretation: Various theriogenologists, clinical pathologists, and other practitioners have interpreted vaginal cytology of the bitch a little differently. One method is described here. The vaginal mucosa is responsive primarily to estrogens, and so vaginal cytology is useful only during the estrogenic phase of the cycle. **Parabasal cells** are small, round *cells with large* and distinct nuclei. The total area of the cytoplasm part of the cell is smaller than the nucleus. These cells (along with RBCs) are present during proestrus. **Superficial intermediate** cells are larger than the parabasal cells, with small nuclei and irregular/folded borders. Large numbers of these cells are seen during late proestrus to early estrus. **Superficial cells**, also called cornified or anucleated, are the largest of the epithelial cells present during estrus. Under a simple microscope, the nuclei of these cells appear faded or absent. The cells also appear "light in weight," multi-layered, and with folded borders. The appearance of 80%–90% of these cells in the smear is used to indicate that breeding can start. A series of vaginal cytology samples is needed to observe the progressive change in epithelial cells; only one smear is unreliable. Epithelial cells may remain the same for many days in some bitches, whereas they may change within 24 hr in others. In addition, many bitches reach 80%–90% cornification during estrus, but in others cornification never goes above 70%. In these bitches, waiting for 80%–90% cornification will result in loss of breeding during that cycle. Another breeding management tool is the progesterone assay, discussed below. The appearance of neutrophils on the vaginal cytology sample indicates the first day of diestrus, and whelping will occur 57–58 days later. Daily vaginal cytology samples are recommended because in some bitches, the cells change from cornified to superficial intermediate and neutrophils appear within 24 hours.

Progesterone Assay: Progesterone is secreted not only from the CLs but also from the early luteinized follicles of the ovaries. The early rise in progesterone can be used to determine ovulation in the bitch, which occurs ~3 days after the LH peak. The LH peak is very short. LH kits are available, and LH should be checked every day during the expected ovulation time. Progesterone assays are commonly used for canine breeding management. These ELISA-based qualitative test kits are based on a color change that corresponds to a range of progesterone values. Many clinicians prefer to send the blood samples to an endocrinology laboratory for progesterone determination by radioimmunoassay. Progesterone is the same hormone in all species, including people; therefore, blood samples can be analyzed for progesterone in veterinary or human diagnostic laboratories.

The progesterone assay is an excellent tool to determine ovulation time for appropriate breeding. This becomes critical when using chilled transported or frozen-thawed semen for AI. As in vaginal cytology, progesterone concentration is monitored starting a few days after the start of proestrus, projecting ahead using progesterone concentrations of 2–10 ng/mL, with 2–2.9 ng/mL indicative of ovulation in approximately 2 days, 3–3.9 ng/mL in 1 day, and 4–10 ng/mL indicative of ovulation day.

DYSTOCIA

Dystocia refers to abnormal or difficult birth. Causes include maternal factors (uterine inertia, inadequate size of birth canal) and/or fetal factors (oversized fetus, abnormal orientation as the fetus enters the birth canal). The condition occurs more commonly in certain breeds. In one survey (253 whelpings, 1,671 pups born), a high frequency of dystocia (32% of the individual bitches and 27.7% of all the whelpings) in Boxers was reported, mainly due to uterine inertia but also to fetal malpresentations.

Dystocia should be considered in any of the following situations: 1) animals with a history of previous dystocia or reproductive tract obstruction, 2) parturition that does not occur within 24 hr after a drop in rectal temperature to <100°F (37.7°C), 3) strong abdominal contractions lasting for 1–2 hr without passage of a puppy or kitten, 4) active labor lasting for 1–2 hr without delivery of subsequent puppies or kittens, 5) a resting period during active labor >4–6 hr, 6) a bitch or queen in obvious pain (eg, crying, licking, or biting the vulva), or 7) abnormal vulvar discharge (eg, frank blood, dark green discharge before any neonates are born [indicates placental separation]).

To determine the appropriate therapy, the cause of dystocia (obstructive vs nonobstructive) must be determined and the condition of the animal assessed. A thorough history regarding breeding dates, previous parturitions, pelvic trauma, etc, is desirable. The animal should be examined for signs of systemic illness that, if present, may necessitate immediate cesarean section. The normal vaginal discharge at parturition is a dark green color; abnormal color or character warrants immediate attention. A sterile digital vaginal examination should be performed to evaluate patency of the birth canal and the position and presentation of the fetus(es). Radiography or ultrasonography can determine the presence and number of fetuses, as well as their size, position, and viability.

Medical management may be considered when the condition of the dam and fetuses is stable, when there is proper fetal position and presentation, and when there is no obstruction. Oxytocin (3–20 U in bitches, 2–5 U in queens) given IM up to 3 times at 30-min intervals, with or without 10% calcium gluconate (3–5 mL, IV slowly) may promote uterine contractions. If no response follows, a cesarean section should be performed.

Surgery is indicated for obstructive dystocia, dystocia accompanied by shock or systemic illness, primary uterine inertia, prolonged active labor, or if medical management has failed.

FALSE PREGNANCY

(Pseudopregnancy, Pseudocyesis)

False pregnancy is common in bitches and uncommon in queens. It occurs at the end of diestrus and is characterized by hyperplasia of the mammary glands, lactation, and behavioral changes. Some bitches behave as if parturition has occurred, "mothering" by nesting inanimate objects and refusing to eat. The possibility of a true pregnancy should be eliminated by the history, abdominal palpation, and abdominal radiographs and ultrasonography.

The falling progesterone and increasing prolactin concentrations associated with late diestrus are believed to be responsible for the clinical signs. No treatment is recommended, because the condition resolves spontaneously in 1–3 wk. In bitches with discomfort secondary to mammary gland enlargement, alternating cold and warm compresses on the engorged mammae or wrapping the abdomen with an elastic bandage may give relief. Owners should be advised not to milk out the mammary glands, because doing so will only stimulate lactogenesis.

Tranquilizers (eg, diazepam, PO, up to 4 days) may be considered for bitches with significant behavioral changes. Estrogens should not be used because of the potential for bone marrow suppression. Megestrol acetate, a progestin (2.5 mg/kg/day, PO, for 8 days), is the only drug currently approved for treatment of false pregnancy in bitches in the USA. Prolonged or repeated use of megestrol acetate may cause pyometra. Androgens (eg, mibolerone, 16 mcg/kg/day, PO, for 5 days) may decrease clinical signs of false pregnancy in bitches. Mibolerone is not approved for treatment of false pregnancy in bitches in the USA. If owners are distressed by repeated bouts of pseudopregnancy, the bitch should either be bred or undergo ovariohysterectomy.

FOLLICULAR CYSTS

These fluid-filled structures develop within the ovary and result in prolonged secretion of estrogen, continued signs of proestrus or estrus, and attractiveness to males. Ovulation may not occur during this abnormal estrous cycle. Follicular cysts should be suspected in any bitch showing clinical manifestations of estrus for >21 days, or when proestrus plus estrus have lasted for >40 days. Estrous cycles due to follicular cysts in queens may be difficult to differentiate from normal, frequent cycles.

The primary differential diagnosis is functional ovarian granulosa cell tumor. Assessment of vaginal cytology with presence of cornified cells indicates increased serum estrogens.

The treatment of choice is ovariohysterectomy. If the animal is to be bred, induction of luteinization of the cystic follicles may be accomplished by using GnRH (25 mcg, IM) or human chorionic gonadotropin (220 IU/kg, IV, or 1,000 IU, half IV, half IM).

MAMMARY HYPERTROPHY IN CATS

(Fibroadenoma complex, Mammary fibroadenomatosis, Glandular mammary hypertrophy)

This benign condition is characterized by rapid abnormal growth of one or more mammary glands. There are two basic types of hyperplasia of the feline mammary gland—lobular hyperplasia and fibroepithelial hyperplasia. Lobular hyperplasia is seen as palpable masses in one or more mammary glands in intact cats 1–14 yr old. Fibroepithelial hyperplasia occurs in young, cycling, or pregnant cats; in old, intact females and males; and in neutered males after treatment with progestins.

Feline mammary hypertrophy is considered to be a hormone-dependent dysplastic change in the mammary gland. Hyperplasia occurs within 1–2 wk after estrus or 2–6 wk after progestin treatment. The tremendously enlarged glands may appear erythematous, and some of the skin may be necrotic. Edema of the skin and both hindlegs is common, and the condition can easily be confused with acute mastitis.

Ovariohysterectomy or mastectomy is curative, although spontaneous remissions occur. Ovariohysterectomy is followed by regression of the glands and prevents recurrence.

MASTITIS

Mastitis is inflammation of the mammary gland(s) associated with bacterial infection. It occurs in postpartum bitches and less commonly in postpartum queens. Rarely, mastitis is seen in lactating pseudopregnant bitches. Risk factors for developing mastitis include poor sanitary conditions, trauma inflicted by offspring, and systemic infection. Mastitis may be acute or chronic.

Mastitis may be localized (eg, involving a single gland sinus), diffuse in a single gland, or diffuse within multiple glands. The animal may be asymptomatic or critically compromised. Milk from mastitic glands may appear normal grossly or may be abnormal in color or consistency. In acute mastitis, the affected glands are hot and painful. If acute mastitis progresses to septic mastitis, signs of systemic illness such as fever, depression, anorexia, and lethargy may be seen, and the dam may neglect the neonates. In chronic or subclinical mastitis, the main complaint may be failure of offspring to thrive.

Diagnosis is usually evident from the history and physical examination. Microscopic examination of milk may reveal inflammatory cells. Milk from each gland should be evaluated in any postpartum bitch or queen with signs of systemic illness. Before beginning therapy, a milk sample should be collected (or obtained by fine-needle aspiration) for bacterial culture and sensitivity. Culture of milk or fluid expressed from the affected glands yields moderate to heavy growth of *Escherichia coli* or staphylococci.

Broad-spectrum, bactericidal antibiotics should be chosen based on sensitivity tests and with the understanding they will be passed in the milk to the young. Antibiotics such as tetracycline, chloramphenicol, or aminoglycosides should be avoided during lactation unless the neonates are weaned. Cephalexin (5–15 mg/kg, PO, tid) and amoxicillin/clavulanate (14 mg/kg, PO, bid-tid) are recommended as initial therapeutic agents pending culture results. Hot-packing the affected gland encourages drainage and seems to relieve discomfort. Fluid therapy is indicated in animals with septic mastitis that are dehydrated or in shock. An abscessed mammary gland should be lanced, drained, flushed, and treated as an open wound.

Nonseptic mastitis is seen most commonly at weaning. The affected glands are warm, swollen, and painful to the touch, but the animal is alert and healthy. Warm compresses should be applied to the affected glands 4–6 times daily, and the young should be encouraged to nurse from these glands. When galactostasis occurs at weaning, lactation can be diminished by reducing food and water intake of the dam.

The mammary glands should not be stimulated during this time. Appropriate food and water must be provided for the young.

METRITIS

Metritis is postpartem infection of the uterus. Predisposing causes include prolonged delivery, dystocia, and retained fetuses or placentas. *Escherichia coli* is the most common bacterium isolated from the infected uterus; streptococci, staphylococci, *Proteus* sp, and others are isolated less frequently.

The primary clinical sign is purulent vulvar discharge. Bitches or queens with metritis are usually depressed, with signs of fever, lethargy, and inappetence, and may neglect their offspring. Pups may become restless and cry incessantly. Metritis should be considered in any postpartum animal with signs of systemic illness or an abnormal vaginal discharge. A large, flaccid uterus may be palpable. Radiographs should be taken to determine whether fetuses or placentas are retained. The hemogram may show leukocytosis with a left shift.

Treatment includes stabilization with IV fluids, supportive care, and antibiotic therapy based on culture and sensitivity testing of the vulvar discharge. Prostaglandin $F_2\alpha$ (0.1–0.25 mg/kg, SC, for 2–3 days) or oxytocin (5–20 U in bitches, 2–5 U in queens, IM) may help evacuate the uterine contents. Ovariohysterectomy is recommended after initial stabilization if the animal is extremely ill or if future reproduction is unimportant. Otherwise, it should be considered an elective procedure to be performed when lactation has ceased.

OVARIAN REMNANT SYNDROME

Ovarian remnant syndrome refers to clinical signs indicating the presence of functional ovarian tissue in a previously ovariohysterectomized bitch or queen. It is not a pathologic condition but a complication of ovariohysterectomy. It occurs when a retained piece of ovarian tissue revascularizes and becomes functional. The most common presentation is recurrent estrus (eg, vulvar swelling, flagging, standing to be mounted) after ovariohysterectomy.

Differential diagnoses include vaginitis, uterine stump pyometra, and exogenous estrogen therapy. Presumptive diagnosis of ovarian remnant syndrome requires demonstration of a cornified vaginal epithelium in a spayed female. A commercially available luteinizing hormone test can be used to distinguish ovariectomized and sexually intact bitches.

Exploratory laparotomy to find and remove the ovarian remnant is the treatment of choice.

PYOMETRA

Pyometra is a hormonally mediated diestrual disorder characterized by cystic endometrial hyperplasia with secondary bacterial infection. Pyometra is reported primarily in older bitches (>5 yr old), 4–6 wk after estrus.

Etiology: Factors associated with occurrence of pyometra include administration of longlasting progestational compounds to delay or suppress estrus, administration of estrogens to mismated bitches, and postinsemination or postcopulation infections. Progesterone promotes endometrial growth and glandular secretion while decreasing myometrial activity. Cystic endometrial hyperplasia and accumulation of uterine secretions ultimately develop and provide an excellent environment for bacterial growth. Progesterone may also inhibit the WBC response to bacterial infection. Bacteria from the normal vaginal flora or subclinical urinary tract infections are the most likely sources of uterine contamination. *Escherichia coli* is the most common bacterium isolated in cases of pyometra, although *Staphylococcus*, *Streptococcus*, *Pseudomonas*, *Proteus* spp, and other bacteria also have been recovered.

Because queens require copulatory stimulation to ovulate and produce progesterone from corpora lutea, pyometra is less common in queens than in bitches. Administration of medroxyprogesterone and other progestational compounds has been associated with development of pyometra in bitches and queens. Pyometra can develop in uterine tissue left after ovariohysterectomy (stump pyometra). It can also occur secondary to postpartum metritis.

By itself, estrogen does not contribute to the development of cystic endometrial hyperplasia or pyometra. However, it does increase the stimulatory effects of progesterone on the uterus. Administration of exogenous estrogens to prevent pregnancy (ie, "mismate shots") during diestrus greatly increases the risk of developing pyometra and should be discouraged.

Clinical Findings: Clinical signs are seen during diestrus (usually 4–8 wk after estrus) or after administration of exogenous progestins. The signs are variable and include lethargy, anorexia, polyuria, polydipsia, and vomiting. When the cervix is open, a purulent vulvar discharge, often containing blood, is present. When the cervix is closed, there is no discharge and the large uterus may cause abdominal distention. Signs can progress rapidly to shock and death.

Physical examination reveals lethargy, dehydration, uterine enlargement, and if the cervix is patent, a sanguineous to mucopurulent vaginal discharge. Only 20% of affected animals have a fever. Shock may be present.

The leukogram of animals with pyometra is variable and may be normal; however, leukocytosis characterized by a neutrophilia with a left shift is usual. Leukopenia may be found in animals with sepsis. A mild, normocytic, normochromic, nonregenerative anemia (PCV of 28%–35%) may also develop. Hyperproteinemia due to hyperglobulinemia may be found. Results of urinalysis are variable. With *E coli* uterine infection, isosthenuria due to endotoxin-induced impairment of renal tubular function or to insensitivity to antidiuretic hormone (or both) may develop. A glomerulonephropathy caused by immune-complex deposition may result in proteinuria. These renal lesions are potentially reversible once the pyometra is resolved.

Diagnosis: Pyometra should be suspected in any ill, diestrual bitch or queen, especially if polydipsia, polyuria, or vomiting is present. The diagnosis can be established from the history, physical examination, abdominal radiography, and ultrasonography. Vaginal cytology often helps determine the nature of the vulvar discharge. A CBC, biochemical profile, and urinalysis help

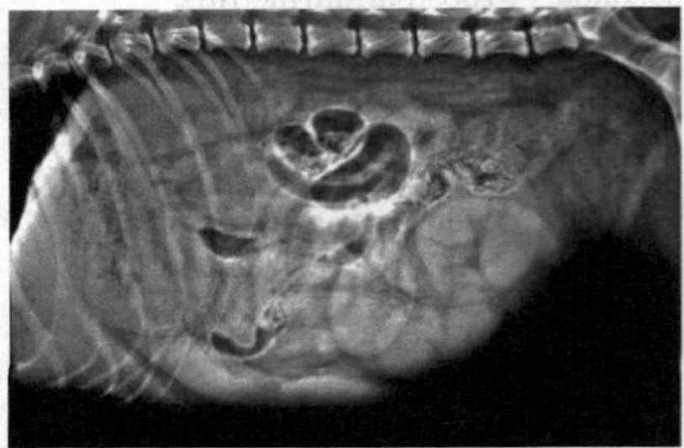
Pyometra in a 10-yr-old Norwegian Elkhound, lateral projection. *Courtesy of Dr. Ronald Green.*

exclude other causes of polydipsia, polyuria, and vomiting; they also evaluate renal function, acid-base status, and septicemia. The uterine exudate should be cultured and sensitivity tests performed. Differential diagnoses include pregnancy and other causes of vulvar discharge, polyuria and polydipsia, and vomiting.

Treatment and Prognosis: Ovariohysterectomy is the treatment of choice for pyometra. Medical management could be considered if preserving the reproductive potential of the bitch or queen is desired. Fluids (IV) and broad-spectrum, bactericidal antibiotics should be administered. Fluid, electrolyte, and acid-base imbalances should be corrected as quickly as possible, before ovariohysterectomy is performed. The bacterial infection is responsible for the illness and will not resolve until the uterine exudate is removed. Oral antibiotics (based on the results of the culture and sensitivity) should be continued for 7–10 days after surgery.

Medical therapy with prostaglandin $F_2\alpha$ ($PGF_2\alpha$) can be used for animals to be bred in the future, although prostaglandins are not approved in the USA for use in cats or dogs. $PGF_2\alpha$ causes luteolysis, contraction of the myometrium, relaxation of the cervix, and expulsion of the uterine exudate. They should probably not be used in animals >8 yr old or in those not intended for breeding. The delay before clinical improvement and the many adverse effects of $PGF_2\alpha$ preclude its use in a severely ill animal. $PGF_2\alpha$ also should be used with caution in bitches or queens with a closed-cervix pyometra because of increased risk of uterine rupture. Pregnancy must be excluded, because prostaglandins can induce abortion.

Naturally occurring $PGF_2\alpha$ (0.25 mg/kg/day, SC, for 5 days) is commonly used. Synthetic analogues (eg, cloprostenol, fluprostenol, and prostalene) are much more potent than natural $PGF_2\alpha$ and have been used to treat pyometra in dogs. Broad-spectrum, bactericidal antibiotics, chosen on the basis of culture and sensitivity tests, should be given for ≥2 wk.

The adverse effects of $PGF_2\alpha$ include restlessness, anxiety, panting, hypersalivation, pacing, tachycardia, vomiting, urination, and defecation. In cats, vocalization and intense grooming behavior also may be seen. These reactions disappear within 2 hr of the injection. The LD_{50} of $PGF_2\alpha$ in dogs is 5.13 mg/kg. Severe ataxia, respiratory distress, and muscle tremors may be seen in queens given 5 mg/kg. If adverse effects are severe, IV fluids at rates appropriate for treatment of shock are indicated. Uterine evacuation after an injection is variable.

Other antiprogestins (eg, aglepristone) are available in some European countries. Clinicians using aglepristone report virtually no adverse effects as compared with prostaglandins. Aglepristone is also used to treat bitches with closed-cervix pyometra. In one study, a dosage of 10 mg/kg given on days 1, 2, and 8 in 15 bitches with closed pyometra led to opening of the cervix after 26±13 hr in all treated animals.

Animals should be reexamined 2 wk after completion of medical therapy. If a sanguineous or mucopurulent vulvar discharge or uterine enlargement is still present, $PGF_2\alpha$ therapy, using the same protocol, may be repeated; however, the prognosis for recovery is much worse. After medical therapy, the prognosis for initial resolution of the pyometra is good if the cervix is open but guarded to poor if closed. Of those animals that respond, as many as 90% of bitches and 70% of queens with open-cervix pyometra may be fertile. Recurrence is likely; 70% of bitches treated medically for pyometra had recurrence within 2 yr. Therefore, the animal should be bred on the next and each subsequent cycle until the desired number of puppies or kittens has been produced, and then spayed. Prostaglandins should not be dispensed for owner administration because of the narrow safety index and the potential to trigger asthmatic events and pregnancy loss in people.

SUBINVOLUTION OF PLACENTAL SITES

Subinvolution of placental sites (SIPS) is abnormal repair of the endometrial placental sites. This disorder is most common in young bitches (<3 yr old) after whelping a first litter. Bitches with SIPS are normal except for hemorrhagic uterine discharge passing from the vulva for several weeks postpartum. Diagnosis is by exclusion; differentials include metritis, vaginitis, and cystitis. Treatment is supportive. Ovariohysterectomy is recommended for bitches that become anemic enough to require transfusion and for bitches not intended for future breeding.

VAGINAL HYPERPLASIA

(Vaginal prolapse)

In vaginal hyperplasia, a proliferation of the vaginal mucosa, usually originating from the floor of the vagina anterior to the urethral orifice, occurs during proestrus and estrus as a result of estrogenic stimulation. Occasionally, the prolapse continues throughout pregnancy or recurs at parturition. The most common sign is a mass protruding from the vulva. Initially, the surface is smooth and glistening, but with prolonged exposure it becomes dry and fissures develop. A slight vaginal discharge may be present. Although the hyperplastic tissue originates near the urethral orifice, dysuria is uncommon. Vaginal hyperplasia interferes with copulation. Reluctance to breed or failure of intromission may be the only clinical sign if the hyperplastic tissue is contained within the vaginal vault. Vaginal hyperplasia resolves spontaneously as soon as estrogen declines.

The diagnosis is made by the history (stage of the estrous cycle) and examination of the vagina. Estrogenic stimulation could be confirmed by cornification of the vaginal epithelial cells, the presence of the characteristic serosanguineous estrous discharge, and the presence of estrous behavior. The differential diagnosis is vaginal neoplasia, which can be excluded by biopsy of the protruding tissue.

If the hyperplastic tissue is not causing problems, therapy is not indicated. However, if it protrudes from the vulva, it should be kept clean and moist and an antibiotic ointment applied. An Elizabethan collar may be necessary to prevent self-trauma. These animals may be bred by artificial insemination. The hyperplasia regresses as soon as the follicular phase of the estrous cycle has passed. Submucosal resection may be necessary if the mass is extremely large or if mucosal damage is extensive. Recurrence is common even after surgical resection. Vaginal hyperplasia resolves within days of removal of estrogen. Rarely, the hyperplasia recurs at parturition, presumably associated with a burst of estrogen. Ovariohysterectomy, the treatment of choice, permanently corrects this condition by removing the gonadal source of estrogen, thus preventing recurrence.

VAGINITIS

Inflammation of the vagina may occur in prepubertal or mature (intact or spayed) bitches. It is rare in queens. Vaginitis usually is due to bacterial infection, which may be secondary to conformational abnormalities such as vestibulovaginal strictures. Viral infection (eg, herpes), vaginal foreign bodies, neoplasia, hyperplasia of the vagina, androgenic steroids (eg, mibolerone), or intersex conditions also may cause vaginitis.

The most common clinical sign is a vulvar discharge. Licking of the vulva, attraction of males, and frequent micturition also may be seen. Signs of systemic illness are not present, and the hemogram and biochemical profile are normal. The absence of these abnormalities helps differentiate vaginitis from open-cervix pyometra, the most important differential diagnosis. The diagnostic evaluation should include a digital examination of the vagina, vaginoscopy, cytology, and if necessary, culture of the exudate, as well as abdominal radiographs or ultrasonography to evaluate the uterus. An anterior vaginal culture may be obtained using a guarded sterile culture swab. The vagina contains normal bacterial flora; therefore, culture results must be interpreted cautiously. A heavy growth, especially of one organism, is probably more significant than a light growth of several organisms.

Predisposing factors such as foreign material or anatomic abnormalities should be corrected. Bacterial infection may respond to local treatment (ie, vaginal douches). Systemic, broad-spectrum, bactericidal antibiotics may be needed for persistent infections. Prepubertal animals often do not require treatment, because the vaginitis nearly always resolves with the first estrus. Therefore, it may be wise to delay elective ovariohysterectomy in affected animals until after their first estrous cycle.

REPRODUCTIVE DISEASES OF THE MALE SMALL ANIMAL

See also MANAGEMENT OF REPRODUCTION: SMALL ANIMALS, p 2219, and PROSTATIC DISEASES, p 1405.

ORCHITIS AND EPIDIDYMITIS

Acute inflammation of the testis or epididymis can be caused by trauma, infection (fungal, bacterial, or viral), or testicular torsion. Infection can be hematogenous or urologic in origin. Clinical signs are pain and swelling of the testes, epididymides, and/or scrotum. There may be wounds or other lesions in the scrotal skin. Orchitis and epididymitis are rare in cats unless due to trauma.

The scrotal contents should be carefully palpated to identify which structures are involved, including the epididymis and testis, but patient discomfort and edema can make palpation difficult. Ultrasonography (with sedation or analgesia as needed) is helpful to further evaluate the affected structures and to confirm the presence of testicular torsion and focal (eg, mass, abscess) lesions in the testis or epididymis. It can also identify less common causes of scrotal enlargement such as scrotal hernia or hematoma.

Diagnostic tests should always include evaluation for *Brucella canis* infection. (*See also* BRUCELLOSIS IN DOGS, p 1402.) Cytologic examination of semen with bacterial and mycoplasmal culture are also helpful, but semen collection from animals that are ill or in pain may be difficult. Testicular or epididymal specimens for cytology and culture may be obtained by fine-needle aspiration. Testicular biopsy for histopathology and bacterial culture may be performed, if needed, after less invasive diagnostic tests have been completed. Because of the greater risk of granuloma formation, epididymal aspiration and biopsy are rarely done. If future reproduction is not of importance, specimens can easily be obtained during castration.

Treatment is difficult unless the underlying cause can be identified. The prognosis for maintaining fertility is guarded despite aggressive therapy because of the potential for irreversible damage to the germinal epithelium, tubular degeneration, development of immune-mediated orchitis, or obstruction of the duct system. These sequelae may take months to occur. Application of cool water packs may decrease testicular damage caused by local swelling and hyperthermia; care must be taken not to damage the scrotal skin. In the case of unilateral involvement, the unaffected testis/epididymis must be protected from damage by heat, pressure, and direct extension of the disease process. Hemicastration may be prudent. If bacterial cultures are positive, appropriate systemic antibiotics should be administered for 3–4 wk. There is no completely successful treatment for *B canis* infection. All antifungal agents interfere with spermatogenesis, either directly or indirectly. The potential for involvement of the prostate by direct extension dictates the use of antibiotics with good prostatic penetration once inflammation has subsided (fluoroquinolones). Culture and sensitivities should refine therapy.

Histopathology may suggest an immune-mediated process (eg, lymphocytic-plasmacytic infiltration); treatment with immunosuppressive drugs has been attempted without success. Chronic *B canis* infection also causes lymphocytic-plasmacytic inflammation. Furthermore, as a result of inhibitory effects on the hypothalamic-pituitary-gonadal axis, glucocorticoids can cause testicular atrophy and infertility. The ischemic damage caused by testicular torsion becomes irreversible within hours. When maintaining fertility is not important, castration is the treatment of choice for orchitis and epididymitis due to any cause. Lesions of the scrotal skin are treated the same as other skin lesions, keeping in mind that resection of scrotal skin can promote thermal damage to the testes.

Chronic orchiepididymitis may develop as a sequela of the acute syndrome, or there may be no previous history of testicular inflammation. Possible causes include those of acute orchiepididymitis, immune-mediated orchitis and epididymitis, neoplasia, and spermatocele or granuloma formation. Most animals are asymptomatic except for infertility. Physical examination often reveals testicular atrophy. Tumors may be palpable. Palpation of the epididymis may reveal induration or enlargement, which may erroneously be interpreted as dramatic relative to the atrophic testis. Epididymal atrophy is uncommon. Ultrasonography can help identify the lesions.

Other noninflammatory causes of testicular atrophy include previous exposure to excessive pressure, heat, cold, and cytotoxic agents. Hormonal causes (eg, glucocorticoids, estrogen from contralateral Sertoli cell tumor, iatrogenic exposure to human transdermal hormone replacement therapy) are also possible.

The prognosis for return of normal fertility in cases of chronic orchitis/epididymitis is grave. If warranted by the dog's value as a stud, the diagnostic and therapeutic plan is as described above for the acute condition.

BALANOPOSTHITIS

Inflammation of the penile or preputial mucosa is common in dogs. The normal preputial secretions usually do not result in overt clinical signs. Mild balanoposthitis, resulting in a slight mucopurulent preputial discharge, is present in many sexually mature dogs, resolves spontaneously, and is of little clinical significance. Diagnostic tests and treatment are not necessary, except as needed for reasonable hygiene. Trauma, lacerations, neoplasia, foreign bodies, urinary tract infection, urolithiasis, or phimosis may result in development of more severe balanoposthitis. A mucopurulent preputial discharge is the most common clinical sign. Excessive licking of the prepuce may also be noted. Swelling of the prepuce and pain are rarely present except in cases of trauma, snake bite, or foreign bodies. If signs of systemic illness are present, the possibility of a more serious concomitant disorder should be considered. Balanoposthitis is rare in cats.

The penis and prepuce should be thoroughly examined, to the level of the fornix, for underlying predisposing factors. The use of saline infusion through a rigid endoscope facilitates this examination, but an otoscope can be used if necessary. Sedation or general anesthesia may be needed. Preputial cytology may be helpful. Bacterial cultures of the preputial cavity, although sometimes difficult to interpret because of the presence of normal preputial flora, may help identify unusual organisms and determine antibiotic sensitivities for refractory cases. Foreign bodies can be submucosal and difficult to see, so tiny tracts should be explored.

Treatment includes correcting any predisposing factors, clipping long hair away from the preputial orifice, and thoroughly flushing the preputial cavity with a mild antiseptic (eg, dilute povidone-iodine or chlorhexidine) or sterile saline solution. If bacterial infection is suspected, an antibiotic ointment may be infused into the preputial cavity for 7–10 days. Recurrence of mild balanoposthitis is common irrespective of therapy. Castration may diminish genital secretions but will not abolish them.

PARAPHIMOSIS

The inability to completely retract the penis into the preputial cavity usually occurs after erection. It is seen most often after semen collection or coitus. The skin at the preputial orifice becomes inverted, trapping the extruded penis and impairing venous drainage. Other causes of paraphimosis include a small preputial opening, priapism, foreign objects around the penis, a constricting band of hair at the preputial orifice, or trauma. Paraphimosis is easily differentiated from priapism (persistent erection without sexual stimulation), congenitally shortened prepuce, congenital deformity of the os penis, or penile neoplasia or hematoma on the basis of physical examination and palpation.

Paraphimosis warrants veterinary intervention if not resolved quickly. The exposed penis quickly becomes edematous, because its venous drainage is compromised. With continued exposure, the mucosa becomes dry and painful. Self-trauma exacerbates the condition. If recognized early, before severe edema and pain develop, paraphimosis is easily treated. Treatment begins with gentle cleansing and liberal lubrication of the exposed penis. The penis is then replaced inside the prepuce by first sliding the prepuce in a posterior direction, extruding the penis further. This everts the skin at the preputial orifice; usually the prepuce then slides easily over the penis. The edema resolves promptly once circulation is restored. Hypertonic solutions can be useful in difficult cases. If the everted prepuce does not slide over the edematous, exposed penis, a cold compress may be applied with gentle digital pressure to act as a pressure bandage. A temporary purse string suture can be placed to keep the penis inside the prepuce.

With paraphimosis due to other causes, or of longer duration, sedation or general anesthesia can be required. It may be necessary to incise the preputial skin to thoroughly examine the preputial cavity, remove restricting material, and relieve venous obstruction. The penis is then replaced in the preputial cavity, and the incision is closed. If the urethra has been damaged, temporary placement of a closed-system indwelling urinary catheter may be needed to prevent stricture formation.

PRIAPISM

Priapism is a persistent erection without sexual stimulation and is diagnosed by physical examination. Partial paraphimosis can also result. Priapism can be caused by myelopathy, drugs, vascular abnormalities, penile masses, or trauma, or it can be idiopathic. It can be ischemic and a medical emergency. If nonischemic and no primary cause is identified, therapy with gabapentin, ephedrine, or terbutaline can be attempted. Castration is not helpful, because priapism is not testosterone mediated.

If necrosis or gangrene is severe, amputation of the penis and prepuce and urethrostomy might be necessary.

PHIMOSIS

An abnormally small preputial orifice, resulting in inability to extrude the penis, can be congenital, or acquired as a result of neoplasia, edema, or fibrosis after trauma, inflammation, or infection. Clinical signs are variable. Usually, the problem is unnoticed until the dog attempts to mate and is unable to copulate. Urine can pool in the prepuce and cause posthitis. Diagnosis is established by physical examination of the prepuce and penis. Treatment depends on severity of the stenosis and intended use of the dog. If the dog is not used for breeding, therapy probably is not needed, although castration should be considered to prevent arousal. Surgical enlargement of the preputial orifice is indicated if the animal is to be used for breeding, if the phimosis contributes to balanoposthitis, or in the unlikely event that phimosis interferes with normal micturition.

BRUCELLOSIS IN DOGS

Although dogs occasionally become infected with *Brucella abortus*, *B suis*, or *B melitensis*, these sporadic occurrences typically are closely associated with exposure to infected domestic livestock (*see* p 1348).

B canis is a cause of abortion at 45–55 days of gestation in kenneled dogs. Dogs are the only definitive host of this organism. Infection has caused a reduction of 75% in the number of pups weaned in some breeding kennels. The disease disseminates rapidly among closely confined dogs, especially at time of breeding or when abortions occur. Transmission occurs via ingestion of contaminated materials or venereal routes. Urine transmission has been reported but seems to be unusual. Both sexes appear to be equally susceptible.

Primary signs are abortion during the last trimester of pregnancy without premonitory signs, stillbirths, and conception failures. Prolonged vaginal discharge usually follows abortion. Abortions may occur during subsequent pregnancies. Infected dogs may develop generalized lymphadenitis and frequently epididymitis, periorchitis, and prostatitis. Spondylitis and uveitis are occasional complications. Bacteremia is frequent and persists for ~18 mo after exposure. Fever is not characteristic.

Diagnosis is based on isolation and identification of the causative agent or by serology. The organisms can usually be readily isolated from vaginal exudate, aborted pups, blood, milk, or semen of infected dogs. The most widely used serologic test is an agglutination test by a tube or slide method. Nonspecific agglutination reactions occur in some dogs. To eliminate nonspecific antibody reactions, the serum is treated with 2-mercaptoethanol and retested. An agar gel immunodiffusion test performed in some laboratories is quite specific. Other tests, such as immunofluorescence and ELISA, have been used sometimes.

Attempts at immunization have not been successful. Control is based on elimination or isolation of infected dogs identified by positive cultural or serologic tests at monthly intervals. Incidence of infection is much lower in kennels where dogs are caged individually. Longterm therapy, eg, with a combination regimen of streptomycin or gentamicin and tetracycline, has been successful in many cases. Neutering of infected dogs is sometimes an alternative to euthanasia.

Prevention of canine brucellosis is done by testing before entry and breeding. The disease is reportable in some states. *B canis* is zoonotic, although cases of human infection are rare and less severe than those caused by the smooth species of the genus. The true incidence is unknown. Diagnostic tests used for smooth species do not cross-react with those for rough species; this may result in a missed diagnosis. In addition, signs of *B canis* infections may resemble those of other diseases. Appropriate measures to prevent exposure should be taken.

MAMMARY TUMORS

The frequency of mammary neoplasia in different species varies tremendously. The dog is by far the most frequently affected domestic species, with a prevalence ~3 times that in women; ~50% of all tumors in the bitch are mammary tumors. Mammary tumors are rare in cows, mares, goats, ewes, and sows. There are differences in both biologic behavior and histology of mammary tumors in dogs and cats. Approximately 45% of mammary tumors are malignant in dogs, whereas ~90% are malignant in cats, and dogs have a much higher number of complex and mixed tumors than do cats.

Etiology: The cause of mammary tumors is unknown in any species except mice, in which an oncornavirus is causative in certain inbred strains. Hormones play an important role in the hyperplasia and neoplasia of mammary tissue, but the exact mechanism is unknown. Estrogen or progesterone receptors (or both) have been reported on mammary tumor cells in animals; these may influence the pathogenesis of hormone-induced mammary neoplasia as well as the response to hormone therapy.

Genetic and nutritional effects on mammary neoplasia have been identified in mice and some people but are still not as well understood in dogs or cats. In people, BRCA1 and BRCA2 are the most important genes significantly associated with mammary tumors. In dogs, one single nucleotide polymorphism (SNP) in exon 9 of BRCA1 and one SNP in exon 24 of BRCA2 were found to be significantly associated with canine mammary tumors. It has been demonstrated that the consumption of red meat, obesity at 1 yr of age, and obesity a year prior to diagnosis are associated with an increased risk of mammary gland tumors in intact or ovariohysterectomized dogs. Obesity is thought to mediate breast cancer risk in postmenopausal women by increasing circulating free estrogen levels as well as through increased local estrogen production by aromatases. It is possible that obesity increases risk of mammary tumors through similar mechanisms in dogs.

From a practical view, all mammary tumors should be regarded as potentially malignant regardless of the size or number of glands involved. Spread of mammary carcinomas in both dogs and cats is primarily to regional lymph nodes and lungs. In dogs, 5%–10% of mammary carcinomas may produce skeletal metastases, primarily in the axial skeleton, but also in long bones.

Canine Mammary Tumors: Mammary tumors in dogs are most frequent in intact bitches; they are extremely rare in male dogs. Ovariectomy before the first estrus reduces the risk of mammary neoplasia to 0.5% of the risk in intact bitches; ovariectomy after one estrus reduces the risk to 8% of that in intact bitches. Bitches neutered after maturity have generally been considered to have the same risk as intact bitches. However, questions remain regarding the impact of ovariohysterectomy at the time of tumor excision. Questions also remain about the timing of such surgery relative to survival. In one study, dogs spayed <2 yr before tumor excision lived 45% longer than either intact dogs or those spayed >2 yr before tumor excision.

The two posterior mammary glands are involved more often than the three anterior glands. Grossly, tumors appear as single or multiple nodules (1–25 cm) in one or more glands. The cut surface is usually lobulated, gray-tan, and firm, often with fluid-filled cysts. Mixed mammary tumors may contain grossly recognizable bone or cartilage on the cut surface.

More than 50% of canine mammary tumors are benign mixed tumors; a smaller percentage of malignant mixed tumors are seen. In the latter, epithelial or mesenchymal components, either singly or in combination, may produce metastases. Histologically, canine mammary gland tumors have been classified by the World Health Organization as carcinomas (with six types and additional subtypes), sarcomas (four types), carcinosarcomas (mixed mammary tumors), or benign adenomas. This classification scheme is based on the extent of the tumor, involvement of lymph nodes, and presence of metastatic lesions (TNM system); it includes unclassified tumors and apparently benign dysplasias. In addition to tumor size and the status and timing of neutering, special stains (including those for the KIT receptor and AgNOR) may have prognostic value.

Feline Mammary Tumors: Mammary tumors in cats are most common in older (average 11 yr) intact females. Cats spayed before 6 mo or 12 mo of age have a 91% or an 86% reduction, respectively, in the risk of mammary carcinoma development than intact cats. Parity does not affect feline mammary carcinoma development. Unlike in dogs, in cats the two anterior or thoracic glands are more frequently involved than the posterior glands.

Histologically, most feline mammary tumors are adenocarcinomas, with tubular or papillary types more common than solid or mucoid types. Mixed mammary tumors and sarcomas are less commonly diagnosed than carcinomas. Benign tumors of the feline mammary gland are relatively infrequent and account for only ~10% of these tumors. The TNM clinical staging system is used for mammary tumors in cats as well as in dogs.

A distinct entity called feline mammary hypertrophy has been noted in cats (*see* p 1396). It affects primarily young, actively cycling, or pregnant cats. It also has been seen in neutered cats, including older males given exogenous progestational drugs (megestrol acetate). The disorder is marked clinically by the rapid growth of one or more mammary glands.

Diagnosis: A mammary tumor is usually suspected on detection of a mass during physical examination. The length of time the mass has been present is usually unknown, but the rate of growth may be helpful in determining prognosis. Palpation of the regional lymph nodes can help determine the extent of spread. Thoracic radiographs, preferably three views (a ventral-dorsal and two laterals), should be taken to detect pulmonary metastases. Fine-needle aspirates may differentiate between inflammatory and neoplastic lesions but may lead to erroneous conclusions and delay of surgery. The diagnosis is determined by histopathology and is important in defining treatment and prognosis.

Treatment and Prognosis: Mammary tumors are treated surgically, although there is no consensus as to the best procedure. Removal of the tumor alone (lumpectomy), simple mastectomy (removal of the affected gland only), modified radical mastectomy (removal of the affected gland and those that share lymphatic drainage and associated lymph nodes), and radical mastectomy (removal of the entire mammary chain and associated lymph nodes) all have their proponents. In dogs, the more involved procedures have not prolonged survival compared with the others, and the advantages of the simpler procedures are obvious. In cats, radical mastectomy has increased the disease-free interval but not survival time.

In theory, the use of anticancer drugs to combat micrometastatic disease (adjuvant chemotherapy) is a reasonable consideration. However, chemotherapy has not been shown to be an effective treatment for mammary tumors in dogs. Part of the difficulty of evaluating the response to adjuvant chemotherapy relates to the fact that only about half of the canine mammary tumors diagnosed as malignant on histopathologic examination actually behave that way. A combination of doxorubicin and cyclophosphamide has been used with limited efficacy in cats. Neither radiation therapy nor antiestrogenic compounds have been effective.

Use of the NSAID piroxicam (0.3 mg/kg/day, PO) as a single agent has been beneficial in treating inflammatory mammary carcinoma, a subtype of mammary tumor in dogs that has been very difficult to manage by surgical or medical means. This is in step with current interest in metronomic low-dose therapy in other malignancies for an antitumor and anti-angiogenic effect.

The prognosis is based on multiple factors. In dogs, most mammary tumors that are going to cause death do so within 1 yr. Sarcomas are associated with shorter survival times than carcinomas. Other factors, including size of tumor, lymph node involvement, and nuclear differentiation, also affect the prognosis. In cats, tumor size is important; cats with tumors >3 cm in diameter have a median survival time of 6 mo, but cats with tumors <2 cm in diameter have a median survival time of >4 yr.

PROSTATIC DISEASES

Disease of the prostate gland is relatively common in intact dogs but less common in other domestic animal species. Benign prostatic hyperplasia is by far the most common disease of the prostate in intact male dogs. Bacterial prostatitis (acute or chronic), prostatic abscesses, prostatic and paraprostatic cysts, and prostatic adenocarcinoma are seen much less frequently and can be seen in castrated males. Depending on the disorder, clinical signs may include tenesmus during defecation, intermittent hematuria, recurrent urinary tract infections, and caudal abdominal discomfort. However, many intact males with benign prostatic hyperplasia (with or without chronic prostatitis) are asymptomatic or present with signs of hemospermia and/or infertility only. Additional nonspecific signs, such as fever, malaise, anorexia, severe stiffness, and caudal abdominal pain, can be seen with acute bacterial infections, abscesses, and neoplasia. Prostatic adenocarcinoma with bony involvement of the pelvis and lumbar vertebrae may cause hindlimb gait abnormalities. Less commonly, prostatic diseases may cause urinary incontinence. Prostatic adenocarcinoma may cause complete urethral obstruction.

Physical examination of the prostate gland should include abdominal and rectal palpation. An enlarged prostate typically is located further cranial than usual and can be found in the caudal abdomen rather than within the pelvic canal. Simultaneous abdominal and rectal palpation allows not only for the cranial aspects of the prostate to be palpated but also for better palpation per rectum because the prostate can be pushed into or near the pelvic canal, which is especially important in large-breed dogs and in males with very enlarged prostates. Size, shape, symmetry, consistency, mobility, and the presence or absence of pain can be assessed by palpation. The normal dorsal sulcus (depression) aids in assessment of shape and symmetry.

Abdominal radiographs may help define the size, shape, and position of the prostate gland. The sublumbar lymph nodes, lumbar vertebrae, and bony pelvis should be evaluated radiographically for evidence of periosteal new bone and bony metastases. A positive-contrast retrograde urethrogram can be done when an abnormal prostate or paraprostatic cyst is difficult to differentiate from the bladder. However, transabdominal ultrasonography is the best imaging modality for evaluation of the prostate, because it allows for evaluation of the prostatic parenchyma and adjacent soft-tissue structures. Increased echogenicity is associated with benign prostatic hyperplasia, chronic bacterial prostatitis, and prostatic neoplasia, whereas areas of mineralization may be secondary to chronic bacterial prostatitis or prostatic neoplasia. Mass lesions within the prostatic urethra and discontinuity of the prostatic urethral wall are both highly suggestive of prostatic neoplasia.

If the dog will not ejaculate, material for cytologic and microbiologic examination can be obtained by prostatic massage. Using aseptic technique, the bladder is catheterized, and all urine removed. The bladder is flushed with saline, and this sample is saved. The catheter is then withdrawn so that the end is caudal to the prostate. The prostate is subsequently massaged per rectum for about 1 minute to release prostatic fluid into the urethra, where it can be collected with the catheter. While occluding the urethral opening, saline is slowly injected. The catheter is then advanced into the bladder as aspiration is performed and another sample is collected. Results of cytologic and microbiologic examination from both prostatic wash specimens should be compared. Prostatic massage may produce septicemia in dogs with acute bacterial prostatitis or a prostatic abscess. Neoplastic cells are often not recovered in specimens obtained by ejaculation or prostatic massage.

Fine-needle aspiration of the prostate gland can be performed transrectally or percutaneously, with or without ultrasonographic guidance. While generally safe and simple, this is not without some risk of penetration of surrounding structures. Biopsy is the most definitive, but also the most invasive, diagnostic procedure to differentiate prostatic diseases. To obtain diagnostic samples, prostatic biopsy should be performed via celiotomy or by a skilled ultrasonographer.

BENIGN PROSTATIC HYPERPLASIA

Benign prostatic hyperplasia (BPH) is the most common prostatic disorder and is found in most intact male dogs >6 yr old as a result of androgenic stimulation or altered androgen:estrogen ratio. It is not known why some males are affected and others are not. In some dogs, hyperplasia may begin as early as 2.5 yr of age and, after 4 yr of age, cystic hyperplasia tends to develop. Clinical signs may be absent, or tenesmus, persistent or intermittent hematuria, or hemorrhagic preputial discharge may occur. The diagnosis is suggested by physical and historical findings and by a nonpainful, symmetrically enlarged prostate. Radiology can confirm prostatomegaly. Ultrasonography should show diffuse, relatively symmetric involvement with multiple, diffuse, cystic structures. Cytologic examination of massage or ejaculate specimens reveals hemorrhage with mild inflammation without evidence of sepsis or neoplasia. Definitive diagnosis is only possible by biopsy. Castration is the treatment of choice; prostatic involution is usually evident within a few weeks and is often complete in several months.

For males intended for use in breeding, medical therapy with finasteride is effective. Finasteride blocks the action of 5 α-reductase, an enzyme that converts testosterone to dihydrotestosterone. Dihydrotestosterone is the biologically active hormone to promote prostatic hyperplasia in both people and dogs. Giving finasteride at 1 mg/kg/day, PO, for 16–21 wk, to laboratory Beagles resulted in a 50%–70% reduction in prostatic hypertrophy with no negative effect on semen quality. Lower dosages of finasteride (0.1 mg/kg/day, PO, for 16 wk) reduced hypertrophied prostate volume by 43%, resolved clinical signs, reduced dihydrotestosterone concentration by 58%, maintained normal testosterone levels, and had no deleterious effect on semen quality, fertility, or libido in a group of nine dogs with prostatic hypertrophy. However, prostatic hypertrophy returns if finasteride administration is discontinued. The low dosage (0.1–0.5 mg/kg) of finasteride correlates to convenient dosing of one 5-mg capsule/day for dogs weighing 10–50 kg.

PROSTATITIS

Inflammation of the canine prostate gland usually is suppurative, and acute prostatitis may result in abscesses. Chronic prostatitis occurs secondary to benign prostatic hyperplasia (*see* p 1406). Various organisms, including *Escherichia coli*, *Staphylococcus*, *Streptococcus*, and *Mycoplasma* spp, have been incriminated. Infection may be hematogenous (acute prostatitis) or ascend from the urethra (chronic prostatitis). Because prostatic fluid normally refluxes into the bladder, a secondary urinary tract infection often accompanies prostatic infection. Acute prostatitis and chronic prostatitis vary based on progression and severity of clinical signs.

Acute prostatitis is associated with malaise, pain, and fever. Dehydration, septicemia, and shock may occur in severe cases. Neutrophilia with a left shift, monocytosis, and/or toxic WBCs may be seen. Ultrasonography shows hypoechoic areas consistent with small pockets of fluid. Ideally, prostatic material is obtained by prostatic massage for cytologic examination and for culture and sensitivity testing. Massage of an acutely infected prostate may release organisms into the blood and cause septicemia. Urinalysis shows hematuria, pyuria, and bacteriuria. The urine should be submitted for culture and sensitivity testing. Often, the urine and prostatic material yield the same organisms.

IV fluid therapy is indicated when acute prostatitis is associated with dehydration or shock. Because the prostate-blood barrier is disrupted in acute prostatitis, antibiotics should be selected on the basis of sensitivity testing and given for 3–4 wk. Enrofloxacin at a dosage of 5 mg/kg, bid, orally is a good empiric treatment choice while awaiting results of microbiologic testing. After the infection is controlled, castration should be considered. In some instances, multiple microabscesses within an infected prostate gland may coalesce into a solitary abscess. Large prostatic abscesses are best treated by surgical drainage and intracapsular omentalization. Urine or prostatic fluid (or both) should be cultured again 2—4 wk after antibiotic therapy to be certain that infection has resolved.

Chronic bacterial prostatitis may cause no clinical signs except recurrent urinary tract infection. Physical abnormalities may be limited to the urinary tract. Rarely, prostatic size and shape may be normal. Microbiologic examination of the third (prostatic) fraction of the ejaculate is more accurate for assessment of chronic bacterial prostatitis than examination of prostatic massage specimens. Dogs with chronic bacterial prostatitis are usually willing to ejaculate. Prostatic fluid and urine should be submitted for cytologic and microbiologic examination.

Chronic bacterial prostatitis will not resolve without also treating for benign prostatic hyperplasia. In fact, most cases of chronic bacterial prostatitis will resolve with only treatment for benign prostatic hyperplasia, whether surgical (castration) or medical (finasteride). Antibiotic therapy alone is unrewarding. Many antibiotics do not diffuse easily into the prostatic parenchyma because of the presence of the blood-prostate barrier. The mild inflammation associated with chronic prostatitis may not impair the blood-prostate barrier, so antibiotics that are non-ionized at neutral pH with high fat solubility (eg, erythromycin, clindamycin, trimethoprim-sulfamethoxazole, or enrofloxacin) are most effective. If antibiotic therapy is implemented, it should be continued for ≥4 wk.

PROSTATIC AND PARAPROSTATIC CYSTS

Large cysts are occasionally found within or adjacent to (paraprostatic) the prostate gland. Paraprostatic cysts result from embryologic remnants of the female reproductive tract found in males that become fluid-filled. The signs are similar to those seen with other types of prostatic enlargement and usually become apparent only when the cyst reaches a size sufficient to cause pressure on adjacent organs. Large cysts may result in abdominal distention and must be differentiated from the bladder and from prostatic abscesses.

Medical treatment is ineffective. Castration alone is unlikely to be of benefit but may be indicated after the cyst has been removed. Total excision of the prostatic cyst is the treatment of choice. If complete excision of the cyst is not possible, the remaining portion of the cyst may be filled with a leaf of omentum secured with sutures. This "omentalization" of the cyst will provide internal drainage and lead to resolution. Surgical excision is preferable to marsupialization, because chronic management of the marsupialization fistula is often problematic.

NEOPLASMS

The most common neoplasm of the prostate is carcinoma arising from ductal or urothelial tissue. Transitional cell carcinoma arising from the prostatic urethra occasionally invades the prostate. Not only does castration not protect against future development of prostatic neoplasia in dogs, but incidence of prostatic neoplasia is higher in castrated dogs.

The clinical signs of prostatic neoplasia may be similar to those of other prostatic diseases. Pain and fever may be present. If the neoplasm infiltrates the urethra, dysuria or urethral obstruction is likely. On rectal palpation, the prostate may be normal in size but feel asymmetrical and nodular. It may also be firmly adhered to the pelvic floor or adjacent structures. Ultrasonographic examination may show an irregularly shaped prostate gland with hyperechoic, heterogenous foci. Gross metastases are present at the time of diagnosis in >80% of dogs with prostatic carcinoma. The most common sites of metastases are the regional lymph nodes, lumbar vertebrae, and bony pelvis. Spread to distant sites (such as the lungs) is uncommon until late in the course of disease. Urethral obstruction caused by prostatic disease in dogs is highly suggestive of neoplasia, as is prostatomegaly in a previously castrated dog. Diagnosis is made by biopsy. Prostatic tumor markers used for human prostatic cancer, such as prostate-specific antigen or prostatic acid phosphatase, are not present in canine prostate glands.

There is no effective curative treatment for prostatic carcinoma in dogs. Because of the high incidence of metastases at the time of diagnosis, and the high incidence of urinary incontinence after prostatectomy in dogs, total prostatectomy is not recommended as a treatment. Radiation therapy for prostatic cancer often results in incontinence due to radiation-induced fibrosis of the urinary bladder. Alternative means of ablating prostatic tissue such as transrectal high-intensity focused ultrasound, transurethral intraprostatic absolute ethanol injections, transurethral laser vaporization, or transurethral electrocoagulation have been successful in experimental studies but have not been performed on dogs with prostatic carcinoma. A relatively simple treatment offered some efficacy for dogs with prostatic carcinoma in one study involving 32 dogs. Treatment with the cyclooxygenase inhibitors piroxicam (0.3 mg/kg/day, PO) or carprofen (2.2 mg/kg, PO, bid) significantly prolonged the median survival time of dogs with prostatic carcinoma compared with dogs receiving no treatment (6.9 vs 0.7 mo).

PROSTATIC CALCULI

When prostatic calculi occur (rarely), there is usually some other prostatic disease as well. Rarely, radiopaque prostatic calculi are incidental findings on abdominal radiographs.

CANINE TRANSMISSIBLE VENEREAL TUMOR

Canine transmissible venereal tumors (TVTs) are cauliflower-like, pedunculated, nodular, papillary, or multilobulated in appearance. They range in size from a small nodule (5 mm) to a large mass (>10 cm) that is firm, though friable. The surface is often ulcerated and inflamed and bleeds easily. TVTs may be solitary or multiple and are almost always located on the genitalia. The tumor is transplanted from site to site and from dog to dog by direct contact with the mass. They may be transplanted to adjacent skin and oral, nasal, or conjunctival mucosae. The tumor may arise deep within the preputial, vaginal, or nasal cavity and be difficult to see during cursory examination. This may lead to misdiagnosis if bleeding is incorrectly assumed to be hematuria or epistaxis from other causes. Initially, TVTs grow rapidly, and more rapidly in neonatal and immunosuppressed dogs. Metastasis is uncommon (5%) and can occur without a primary genital tumor present. When metastasis occurs, it is usually to the regional lymph nodes, but kidney, spleen, eye, brain, pituitary, skin and subcutis, mesenteric lymph nodes, and peritoneum may also be sites.

Because of their homogenous populations of large, round cells with distinctive centrally located nucleoli, TVTs are usually easily diagnosed by cytologic examination of fine-needle aspirates or impression smears or by histopathologic evaluation of biopsies. TVTs may be difficult to distinguish from other round cell tumors, particularly lymphosarcomas, when they occur in extragenital locations. Although TVT has a worldwide distribution, prevalence varies from relatively high in some geographic regions (eg, tropical and subtropical urban environments) to rare in others.

Although spontaneous regression can occur, TVTs are usually progressive and treated accordingly. Complete surgical excision, radiation therapy, and chemotherapy are effective treatments; however, chemotherapy is considered the treatment of choice. Vincristine sulfate (0.5–0.7 mg/m^2, IV, once weekly for 3–6 wk) is reported to be effective. The rate of tumor regression is negatively correlated with tumor size, older age, and season. Usually, total remission can be expected by the sixth treatment. Adriamycin (30 mg/m^2 for dogs weighing >10 kg; 1 mg/kg for dogs weighing ≤10 kg; IV, once every 3 wk) and radiation therapy have been effective for those animals that do not respond to vincristine.

The prognosis for total remission with chemotherapy or radiation therapy is good, unless there is metastatic involvement of organs other than skin. Complete surgical excision often cannot be achieved because of the anatomic location of many of these tumors. Recurrence is likely in such cases unless adjunct radiation or chemotherapy is used.

RESPIRATORY SYSTEM

RESPIRATORY SYSTEM INTRODUCTION

The respiratory system performs several functions. Most importantly, it delivers oxygen to the cardiovascular system for distribution to the body and it removes carbon dioxide. Gas transfer occurs in the alveoli of the lungs, where the air-blood barrier is a thin, permeable membrane. Failure or major dysfunction of gas transfer due to disease processes that compromise this membrane or its air or blood supply have serious effects. In addition to gas exchange, the respiratory system performs numerous other functions, including maintaining acid-base balance, acting as a blood reservoir, filtering and probably destroying emboli, metabolizing some bioactive substances (eg, serotonin, prostaglandins, corticosteroids, and leukotrienes), and activating some substances (eg, angiotensin). The respiratory system also protects its own delicate airways by warming and humidifying inhaled air and by filtering out particulate material. The upper airways also provide for the sense of smell (olfaction) and play a role in temperature regulation in panting animals.

Large, airborne particles are usually deposited on the mucous lining of the nasal passages, larynx, trachea, and bronchi, after which they are carried by the mucociliary "blanket" to the pharynx to be swallowed or expectorated. Small particles may be deposited as deep as the alveoli, where they are phagocytized by macrophages. Defense against invasion by microorganisms and other foreign particles is provided by anatomic structures and by both nonspecific and immunologic mechanisms (both cellular and humoral). These are the factors that determine species and individual susceptibility to disease and that may be manipulated by using various management techniques, vaccines, antimicrobials, and other agents such as interferons and lymphokines. Other mechanical factors include the tortuosity of nasal passages; presence of hairs, cilia, and mucus; the cough reflex; and bronchoconstriction. Cellular defenses include macrophages, which phagocytize invaders and present them (or at least their important antigens) to lymphocytes for stimulation of an immune response, and neutrophils, which often die in their fight against invaders and must be removed along with their potentially damaging enzymes. Secretory defenses include interferon for antiviral defense, complement for lysis of invaders, surfactant lining the alveoli to prevent their collapse and to facilitate macrophage function, fibronectin to modulate bacterial attachment, antibodies, and mucus.

The respiratory system must perform many functions, preferably while expending minimal energy. The required effort is increased by processes that oppose expansion of the lung (eg, fibrosis or hydro-, chylo-, pneumo-, or hemothorax), impede the flow of air (eg, obstructive nasal disease, bronchiolitis, bronchoconstriction, laryngeal paralysis, or pulmonary edema), or thicken the air-blood interface (eg, interstitial pneumonia due to viruses or toxins, pulmonary edema).

The anatomy of the respiratory tract differs markedly among species in the following features: 1) shape of both the upper and lower respiratory tract; 2) extent, shape, and pattern of the turbinate bones; 3) branching patterns of bronchi; 4) anatomy of terminal bronchioles, including collateral ventilation; 5) lobation and lobulation; 6) thickness of pleura; 7) completeness of the mediastinum; 8) relationship of pulmonary arteries to bronchial arteries and bronchioles; 9) presence of vascular shunts; 10) distribution of mast cells; and 11) blood supply to the pleura. Each variation in anatomic structure implies variation in function, which can influence the pathogenesis of respiratory disease in a particular species. The three main groups of species that have similar subgross anatomy of the lung are 1) cattle, sheep, and pigs; 2) dogs, cats, monkeys, rats, rabbits, and guinea pigs; and 3) horses and people.

Marked physiologic variations also exist between different species. For example, cattle are prone to retrograde drainage from the pharynx, are predisposed to pulmonary hypertension and reduced ventilation in a cold environment, have relatively small lungs with low tidal volume and functional residual capacity, and are more sensitive to changes in environmental temperatures than are most other species. These anatomic and physiologic differences largely determine why some pathogens affect only some species (eg, *Mannheimia haemolytica* affects cattle but not pigs) and why pneumonia is very important in some species (cattle, pigs) but less so in others (dogs, cats).

Hypoxia (lowered oxygenation, often termed anoxia) causes clinical signs of respiratory disease. It can result from the following: 1) reduced oxygen-carrying capacity of the blood (anemic anoxia, as in carbon monoxide or nitrite poisoning, or true anemia due to various causes); 2) reduced blood flow (stagnant anoxia, as in congestive heart failure or shock); 3) insufficient alveolar ventilation, mismatching between ventilation and perfusion, shunt or diffusion impairment (hypoxic anoxia, as in pneumonia, pulmonary edema, chronic congestion, pneumothorax, or paralysis of respiratory muscles); or 4) inability of tissues to use available oxygen (eg, histotoxic anoxia, as in cyanide poisoning).

Compensatory mechanisms for hypoxia include increased depth and rate of breathing, which is mediated by chemoreceptors located in the carotid and aortic bodies; contraction of the spleen, which forces more RBCs into the circulation; and increased cardiac stroke volume and heart rate. If cerebral hypoxia develops, respiratory function may be reduced even further due to depression of neuronal activity. Erythropoiesis is also stimulated with chronic hypoxia, although the degree of polycythemia is species dependent. In addition, myocardial, renal, and hepatic functions may be reduced, as may motility and secretions of the intestine. If compensatory mechanisms are inadequate, a vicious cycle may begin in which all body tissues function less efficiently.

CLINICAL SIGNS OF RESPIRATORY MALFUNCTION

Nasal discharge may be serous, catarrhal, purulent, or hemorrhagic, depending on the degree of mucosal or turbinate damage. It indicates increased production of normal secretions, sometimes supplemented by neutrophils (purulent) or blood (hemorrhage). It probably also indicates decreased "grooming" of the nostrils with the tongue when animals are ill. **Epistaxis** (bleeding from the nose) is often caused by vascular rupture, such as in mycotic infection of the guttural pouch or exercise-induced pulmonary hemorrhage in horses, or by intranasal fungal infection or neoplasia, systemic coagulopathy, vasculitis, thrombocytopenia (immune-mediated or a result of rickettsial infection), hyperviscosity syndrome, hypertension, or nasal trauma. **Hemoptysis** (the coughing up of blood) occurs after rupture of pulmonary aneurysms in the lungs of cattle with chronic lung abscesses. Bleeding may also result from polyps, neoplasms, granulomas, trauma, thrombocytopenia, and bracken fern or sweet clover toxicity.

Hyperpnea (an increase in rate and depth of breathing) becomes **dyspnea** when the breathing appears to be labored and causing distress. Hyperpnea, however, is not always a sign of disease (eg, labored breathing after vigorous exercise in an otherwise healthy animal). Infectious respiratory diseases that cause toxemia may further compromise the host, eg, bovine pneumonia due to *M haemolytica*. Dyspnea can be caused by disease of the respiratory tract itself (eg, airway obstruction, pneumonia, bronchitis, or alveolitis) or by other problems (eg, heart failure, acid-base imbalances, thoracic effusions, abnormal oxygen-carrying capacity of the blood, or disorders of neuromuscular function). Labored inhalation seen with obstructive diseases above the thoracic inlet (eg, laryngeal paralysis, cervical tracheal collapse) or with pleural effusions is termed inspiratory dyspnea; labored expiration seen with obstructive diseases below the thoracic inlet (eg, diffuse bronchitis, principal bronchial collapse, or pulmonary edema) is termed expiratory dyspnea. Fixed airway obstructions (eg, tracheal neoplasia, foreign body, or stenosis) or a combination of upper and lower obstructive airway diseases (eg, pleural effusion with congestive heart failure) result in both inspiratory and expiratory dyspnea. Other responses include coughing, clear exudates, and shallow breathing with grunting, often associated with the pain of pleuritis.

CAUSES OF RESPIRATORY MALFUNCTION

Congenital anomalies of the respiratory tract are rare but do occur. Examples include cysts in the sinuses and turbinates, tracheal hypoplasia, nasopharyngeal turbinates, and accessory lungs. A common cause of upper respiratory tract malfunction is **rhinitis** (which results in exudation of neutrophils, macrophages, and fluids), or erosion and ulceration (or both) of the nasal mucosa. It may be caused by viral, bacterial, fungal, or parasitic agents, as well as by hypersensitivity reactions, such as localized allergies and anaphylaxis (*see* p 811). Atrophy of the turbinates (eg, in atrophic rhinitis of pigs) removes a major filtration function and exposes the lungs to much heavier loads of dust and microorganisms. The nasal cavity may be obstructed by tumors, granulomas, abscesses, or foreign bodies. Sinusitis can be a complication of upper respiratory infections, tooth root infection, or dehorning.

Laryngitis, **tracheitis**, and **bronchitis** result in coughing and possibly inspiratory or expiratory dyspnea. Coughing may be nonproductive if the irritation is caused by mucosal erosion, or productive if caused by copious exudate in the major airways. Severe pulmonary edema and emphysema cause extreme respiratory insufficiency.

The most common respiratory disease is **pneumonia**, which is defined as inflammation of the lungs. There are many systems to classify the various types of pneumonia. One useful method is to classify according to the distribution of lesions in the lungs. **Focal pneumonia** has one or more discrete foci in a random pattern, eg, abscessation due to emboli from other sites, tuberculosis, or actinomycosis. **Lobular pneumonia** accentuates the anatomic pattern of lobules, as in bronchopneumonia caused by *Pasteurella multocida*. **Lobar pneumonia** covers large areas of lobes and is often severe (eg, fibrinous pneumonic pasteurellosis of cattle). **Diffuse** or **interstitial pneumonia** often involves the entire lung, as in maedi of sheep or in hypersensitivity reactions. The appearance or cause of a particular pneumonia can be described further, eg, gangrenous, parasitic (verminous), aspiration, etc.

Infection may develop as a result of one or a combination of factors: 1) defense mechanisms are overwhelmed, 2) the infectious agent is highly virulent, 3) the size of the inoculum is large, and/or 4) the animal's defense mechanisms are compromised. The initial problem in many pneumonias is thought to be a sudden change in the normal nasal bacterial flora, which results in a sudden dramatic increase in one or more species of bacteria. Bacterial proliferation is usually caused by a breakdown of the host defenses as a result of stress (eg, transportation, concurrent illness) or cellular insult (eg, viral infection, toxicity). These bacteria are breathed into the lung in large numbers and may overwhelm the normal defense mechanisms, localize, multiply, and initiate inflammation. In addition, stress is often a precursor of viral respiratory infections, particularly in groups of animals that have recently been congregated and stressed by travel, handling, and mixing. Some respiratory viral infections can cause temporary dysfunction of phagocytic mechanisms of the alveolar macrophages. This usually occurs several days after viral exposure. Inhaled bacteria proliferate and pneumonia ensues, often with an overwhelming infection and massive exudation into the alveoli.

Pneumonia also can be caused by direct infection with viruses, bacteria, and fungi, as well as by toxins arriving hematogenously, by inhalation, or by aspiration of food or gastric contents.

Through natural processes, possibly aided by appropriate therapy, the exudate may be removed from the lungs, and the mucosal lesions of the air passages may heal. However, serious sequelae can persist. **Bronchiectasis** is a chronic lesion of the bronchi and parenchyma characterized by irreversible cylindrical or saccular dilatation, secondary infection, and atelectasis. Ulceration of bronchioles caused by viral agents may lead to organized plugs of connective tissue in small bronchioles, a lesion called **bronchiolitis obliterans**, which may cause permanent obstruction, atelectasis, and severe respiratory insufficiency. Constriction of bronchi and bronchioles in chronic allergic bronchitis and bronchiolitis results in similar clinical signs. However, administration of bronchodilators results in rapid relief of airway obstruction in cases of allergic bronchitis (eg, heaves in horses). Some chronic pneumonias (eg, maedi in sheep) are characterized by firm diffuse lesions due to hyperplasia of lymphoid follicles, hyperplasia of smooth muscle around bronchioles, diffuse fibrosis, and diffuse lymphocytic infiltration. Aspiration pneumonia often leads to gangrene, with severe toxemia accompanying the acute inflammatory reaction.

Most infectious pneumonias develop in the anteroventral portions of the lungs. However, infectious agents, as well as neoplasms, can invade the lungs via the blood, which may extensively impair pulmonary function, as can pulmonary edema from chronic heart failure. Pleuritis, empyema, hydrothorax, chylothorax, atelectasis, diaphragmatic hernia, or pneumothorax can also seriously impair respiratory function. Pulmonary thrombosis leads to acute, often fulminant, respiratory failure as a result of a lack of pulmonary arterial blood flow to ventilated regions of the lung. Infarction of the lung can reduce respiratory function but is rare because of the dual blood supply of the organ. Toxic injury, such as in 3-methylindole toxicity in cattle, causes edema, emphysema, and necrosis of alveolar epithelium, followed by compensatory hyperplasia of these cells; the effects on gas exchange result in severe hypoxia and dyspnea.

Although pneumonia is most important, several other thoracic conditions can cause respiratory dysfunction. **Pulmonary edema**, the abnormal accumulation of fluid in the interstitial tissue, airways, or alveoli of the lungs, may occur in conjunction with circulatory disorders, particularly left ventricular failure or increased capillary permeability, occasionally in anaphylactic and allergic reactions, and in some infectious diseases. Head trauma can cause pulmonary edema in dogs. Dyspnea and open-mouth breathing may occur. Animals stand in preference to lying down, lie only in sternal recumbency, or may assume a sitting position. Auscultation of the chest may reveal wheezing and fluid sounds.

Pleuritis (pleurisy) may be caused by any pathogen that gains entrance to the pleural cavity, but it is often an extension of pneumonia. Rapid shallow breathing, fever, and thoracic pain are suggestive of pleuritis. Auscultation of the chest may reveal friction sounds.

Empyema (purulent exudate in the pleural cavity) is caused by pyogenic bacteria or fungi reaching the thoracic cavity via the blood or by extension of a pneumonia, traumatic reticulitis, or penetrating wound of the chest. Cough, fever, pain, and dyspnea may be present.

Hemothorax (the accumulation of blood in the pleural cavity) is usually caused by trauma to the thorax, systemic coagulopathy, or thoracic neoplasia. **Hydrothorax** (the accumulation of transudate in the pleural cavity) is usually due to interference with venous blood flow or lymph drainage. **Chylothorax** (the accumulation of chyle in the pleural cavity) is relatively rare and is seen most often in cats. It may be caused by rupture of the thoracic duct but often is idiopathic. The signs of all three conditions include respiratory embarrassment (eg, rapid shallow breathing with inspiratory dyspnea) and weakness.

Pneumothorax (air in the pleural cavity, *see* p 1664) may be of traumatic or spontaneous origin. Air can enter the pleural cavity through penetrating wounds of the thoracic wall or by extension from pulmonary emphysema or ruptured bullae. The lung collapses if a large volume of air enters the pleural cavity. Bilateral pneumothorax may develop if the mediastinum is weak or incomplete. Inspiratory dyspnea or rapid, shallow breathing is evident.

DIAGNOSTIC TECHNIQUES

Clinical history and physical examination should help to determine the possible cause and site of respiratory disease. Lateral cervical and thoracic radiographs may be helpful when obstructive upper airway disease or fixed airway obstruction is suspected (eg, tracheal foreign body, masses, foreign bodies, or stenosis). Thoracic radiographs are essential in any animal exhibiting lower respiratory signs (eg, cough, rapid shallow breathing, dyspnea), but diagnostic value may be limited in animals that have a large thorax (eg, adult horses or cattle). Arterial blood gas analysis or pulse oximetry may help assess the need for oxygen therapy in an animal with severe dyspnea.

When obstructive upper airway disease is suspected, the diagnostic procedure of choice is endoscopy of the respiratory tract, preferably without sedation. Laryngeal function should be assessed, and the presence of obstructive lesions within the nasopharynx, oropharynx, larynx, trachea, or principal bronchi should be identified.

With diffuse or lobar lung disease, diagnostic procedures include transtracheal wash, bronchoscopy with bronchoalveolar lavage or endobronchial biopsy, and transthoracic fine-needle aspirates of lung or lung biopsy. When bacterial pneumonia is suspected, bacterial culture of transtracheal wash is recommended. Cytologic evaluation of transtracheal or bronchoalveolar lavage fluid may aid in the diagnosis of fungal, parasitic, or allergic lung diseases. Transthoracic fine-needle aspirates of lung often are useful in the diagnosis of fungal pneumonia but have lower yields in the definitive diagnosis of solitary pulmonary lesions. Solitary pulmonary masses often require transthoracic lung biopsy or surgical excision for definitive diagnosis. Transthoracic ultrasonography is a sensitive diagnostic tool for pleural disease (eg, pleural effusion, pneumothorax) and for parenchymal lung disease when lesions are adjacent to the pleural surface.

In dogs or cats with pleural effusions, thoracocentesis should be performed for cytologic and potentially microbiologic evaluation of fluid. In cats, pleural effusions often occur with cardiac disease, so an echocardiography should be performed. In animals suspected to have a chylous effusion, serum and fluid triglyceride levels should be determined. Chylous effusions are associated with fluid triglyceride levels greater than that in serum.

Acute nasal discharge, sneezing, or both, may suggest the presence of infection (viral or bacterial) or a nasal foreign body. Chronic nasal discharge warrants further investigation via radiography (nose, guttural pouches in horses), nasal CT, rhinoscopy, nasopharyngoscopy, or nasal biopsy. Rhinoscopy may be of limited value if copious thick discharge or hemorrhage is present. Bacterial cultures of nasal tissue may be of value if bacterial rhinitis is suspected; however, in some species (eg, dogs and cats) primary bacterial rhinitis is rare and typically occurs secondary to other nasal conditions. Cytologic evaluation of nasal tissue may help diagnose nasal fungal infections. Serologic testing for fungal respiratory infections may be considered, but these findings should correlate with the animal's clinical signs and documentation of the presence of fungal organisms because false-positive and false-negative tests can occur.

CONTROL OF RESPIRATORY DISEASE

Sudden dietary changes, weaning, cold, drafts, dampness, dust, high levels of ammonia, poor ventilation in general, and the mixing of widely divergent age groups all play a role in respiratory disease in groups of animals. Stress and mixing of animals from several sources should be avoided or minimized. Establishing individual animal identification, making accurate clinical and postmortem diagnoses, and maintaining a record system of diagnosis and treatment are important to minimize or control outbreaks of pneumonia. Transportation over long distances is another stress factor that plays a major role in the pathogenesis of respiratory infections in large animals.

Immunization can help control respiratory infection. However, control may be compromised by improper timing, use of ineffective or inappropriate vaccines, or overwhelmingly negative management practices. In most cases, severe insults to the natural defenses cannot be reversed later by therapeutic agents and biologicals.

The mucosal surfaces of the respiratory tract contain lymphoid follicles that exchange cells with other parts of the body. However, most of the lymphocytes in the respiratory lining produce only IgA, whereas the cells in the lymph nodes of the respiratory tract produce IgM and IgG. Depending on the agent involved, various cell- and antibody-mediated immune responses occur in the respiratory tract and include opsonization, agglutination, immobilization, neutralization of toxins and viruses, blockage of adherence to cells, lysis, and chemotaxis. The type of immune response varies because of age, species, and the means to respond to specific virulence mechanisms of the pathogens involved.

Species vary in the type of immune response available at different sites in the respiratory tract. Large antigen droplets may immunize the upper tract with IgA, but small replicating particles may be necessary to immunize the lower tract. To develop adequate antibody levels to protect the lungs, repeated doses of antigen plus adjuvant, or a replicating antigen, are often necessary. These results are seldom achieved under field conditions (eg, many field trials using respiratory vaccines in cattle have not demonstrated statistically significant efficacy).

Environmental management is an essential part of therapy in allergic respiratory diseases. For example, clinical signs in horses with heaves (recurrent airway obstruction, *see* p 1455) or cattle with hypersensitivity pneumonitis (*see* p 1441) may be effectively controlled by preventing exposure to molds present in hay.

PRINCIPLES OF THERAPY

See also SYSTEMIC PHARMACOTHERAPEUTICS OF THE RESPIRATORY SYSTEM, p 2608.

Respiratory disease is often characterized by abnormal production of secretions and exudates and by a reduced ability to remove them. The primary goal of therapy is to reduce the volume and viscosity of the secretions and to facilitate their removal. This can be accomplished by controlling infection and inflammation, modifying the secretions, and when possible, improving postural drainage and mechanically removing the material. Therapeutic methods include altering the inspired air and administering expectorants, antitussives, bronchodilators, antimicrobials, diuretics, and other drugs. However, expectorants have shown little or no beneficial effects in clinical trials.

Hydration should be maintained. Inhalation of humidified air may facilitate removal of airway secretions. Expectorants are sometimes used with the intention of liquefying these secretions. However, they should be used in conjunction with ancillary respiratory therapy such as improved postural drainage, mild exercise, and thoracic percussion, which (in addition to coughing) encourages expectoration and removal of secretions. Mechanical removal of tenacious and viscid secretions by aspiration may be necessary in severe airway obstruction.

Antitussive agents are indicated to relieve the discomfort associated with nonproductive coughing but are contraindicated when secretion of airway mucus is excessive. Products that contain atropine also are contraindicated, at least in theory, because atropine increases the viscosity of airway secretions.

Increased airway resistance caused by bronchial smooth muscle contraction can be alleviated with bronchodilators, which may be indicated in animals with asthma-like conditions and chronic respiratory disease. Methylxanthines, such as theophylline and aminophylline, are effective bronchodilators in species other than cattle (and possibly dogs); however, the therapeutic index is relatively narrow and they are less efficacious than β_2-agonists. Isoproterenol, clenbuterol, and epinephrine are also generally effective, and sodium cromoglycate may be used in horses with inflammatory airway disease. Corticosteroids are highly effective in allergic conditions, but systemic use may result in adverse effects. Aerosolized corticosteroids are efficacious and associated with few to no adverse effects; however, they require an aerosol delivery device (eg, face mask) for proper administration. Antihistamines can be used to alleviate the bronchoconstriction caused by histamine release; however, they are of limited value in large animals. Bronchospasm also can be reduced significantly by removing irritating factors, using mild sedatives, or reducing periods of excitement.

In bacterial infection, antimicrobial therapy should be instituted. The goal is to select either the most effective agent against a specific organism or the least toxic agent of several alternatives. Culture and sensitivity testing of airway secretions provide a worthwhile, although not infallible, guide to determining the appropriate antibiotic. Knowledge of tissue penetration and pharmacokinetic characteristics of the antimicrobial agents is important as well. The following agents have proved effective in the listed species: cattle—oxytetracycline, cephalosporins, fluoroquinolones, macrolides, florfenicol, penicillins, and sulfonamides; sheep and goats—oxytetracycline, cephalosporins, macrolides, penicillins, and sulfonamides; pigs—lincomycin, spectinomycin, penicillins, and sulfonamides; dogs and cats—cephalosporins, chloramphenicol, amoxicillin-clavulanate, aminoglycosides, trimethoprim-sulfamethoxazole, fluoroquinolones, macrolides, and tetracyclines; horses—penicillins, aminoglycosides, cephalosporins, fluoroquinolones, sulfonamides, and tetracyclines (the latter with caution due to an occasional adverse effect of severe diarrhea). Aminoglycosides are useful but can be nephrotoxic. Trimethoprim, usually in combination with a sulfonamide, is useful for respiratory therapy in most species but is not licensed for food-producing animals in the USA. Drugs such as enrofloxacin (approved for small animals and cattle but not for horses in the USA) and ceftiofur are effective for pneumonia.

Broad-spectrum antibiotics should be used if specific bacteria cannot be identified, and once begun, a full course of therapy should be completed. Multiple antimicrobial agents should be used only with full knowledge of the potential drug interactions. Because of residues in food-producing animals, veterinarians must use these products according to label instructions and provide sound advice to producers. Extra-label use of antimicrobials is permitted in some situations and is regulated by the Animal Medicinal Drug Use Clarification Act of 1994.

The hypoxemia caused by most lung disorders usually can be corrected by administering oxygen. However, continuous administration of high concentrations increases the tendency for regional resorption atelectasis, thus worsening the hypoxemia, and can cause pneumonitis on its own. Hypoxemia is often accompanied by variable degrees of hypercapnia and acidemia. Endotracheal intubation and mechanical ventilation may be necessary in animals with acute respiratory failure or in animals that are comatose or apneic. Arterial blood gas and pH determinations, when practicable, are extremely valuable to monitor treatment.

Diuretics are indicated in pulmonary edema. The osmotic diuretics have a minimal action on diuresis, carbonic anhydrase inhibitors (eg, acetazolamide) have a moderate effect, and loop diuretics (eg, furosemide) have a profound effect.

ASPIRATION PNEUMONIA

(Foreign-body pneumonia, Inhalation pneumonia, Gangrenous pneumonia)

Aspiration pneumonia is a pulmonary infection characterized by inflammation and necrosis due to inhalation of foreign material. The severity of the inflammatory response depends on the material aspirated, the type of bacteria aspirated, and the distribution of aspirated material in the lungs.

Etiology: Inappropriate administration of therapeutic agents is a common cause of aspiration pneumonia in large animals and less common in dogs and cats. Liquids given by drench or dose syringe should not be delivered faster than the animal can swallow. Drenching is particularly dangerous when the animal's tongue is drawn out, when the head is held high, or when the animal is coughing or bellowing.

In sheep, poor dipping technique with repeated immersion of the animal's head may cause aspiration of fluid. Calves and lambs may inhale inflammatory debris if affected with diphtheritic stomatitis/laryngitis. The muscles of deglutition may be affected in lambs with nutritional myopathy. Pigs fed fine particulate food in dry environments may inhale feed granules. Aspiration pneumonia in cattle after treatment for milk fever is usually fatal. Cervids affected with chronic wasting disease may develop aspiration pneumonia due to CNS dysfunction. In dogs and less frequently in cats, aspiration pneumonia is generally associated with inhalation of oral ingesta, regurgitated material, or vomitus. Common risk factors for dogs and cats include pharyngeal abnormalities (cricopharyngeal motor dysfunction), esophageal diseases (megaesophagus, gastroesophageal reflux disease, esophageal obstruction), weakened clinical condition, and anesthesia or heavy sedation. Bacteria in aspirated material may initiate acute infection or secondary infection later in disease.

Clinical Findings: A history suggesting recent foreign body aspiration within the past 1–2 days is of greatest value for a diagnosis of aspiration pneumonia. Affected animals separate from the rest of the group and present with pyrexia 104°–105°F (40°–40.5°C), a painful expression, arched back, inappetance, depression, toxic mucous membranes, and an increased respiratory rate (>40–60 breaths/min) with a shallow abdominal component. This is often associated with a purulent nasal discharge that sometimes is tinged reddish brown or green. Milk yield is greatly reduced to zero in lactating animals. Thoracic auscultation reveals reduced lung sounds over affected consolidated lung, with increased breath sounds over normal lung. In cows that aspirate ruminal contents as a consequence of becoming cast with hypocalcemia, toxemia is usually fatal within 1–2 days.

Superficial consolidated lung and overlying lesions of fibrous pleurisy can readily be identified on ultrasound examination using either linear or sector probes connected to 5-MHz machines; pleuritic friction rubs are not audible on auscultation. In dogs and cats, clinical signs may be peracute, acute, or chronic. Cough, dyspnea, tachypnea, or exercise intolerance are seen most frequently. Thoracic radiographs generally show a bronchoalveolar pattern in gravity-dependent ventral lung lobes (right cranial and middle and left cranial lobes); however, radiographic changes may not be seen until 24 hr after acute aspiration.

Lesions: Aspiration pneumonia is usually in the anteroventral parts of the lung; it may be unilateral in animals in which lateral recumbency was the cause of aspiration, or bilateral and centered on airways. In early stages, the lungs are markedly congested with areas of interlobular edema. Bronchi are hyperemic and full of froth. The pneumonic areas tend to be cone-shaped, with the base toward the pleura. Suppuration and necrosis follow. The foci become soft or liquefied, reddish brown, and foul smelling. There usually is an acute fibrinous pleuritis, often with pleural exudate. Animals that survive develop chronic abscesses and fibrous adhesions between the visceral and parietal pleura.

Prevention and Treatment: Broad-spectrum antibiotics should be used in animals known to have inhaled a foreign substance without waiting for signs of pneumonia to appear; however, this rarely occurs in farm animals presented with severe clinical signs. A transtracheal wash can help identify the causative agent for which an antibiotic sensitivity can be obtained. Care and supportive treatment include NSAIDs such as flunixin meglumine. In small animals, oxygen therapy can be useful. Saline nebulization and coupage may assist with generating a productive cough to facilitate clearance of the aspirated material. Despite all treatments, prognosis is poor, and efforts must be directed at prevention.

DIAPHRAGMATIC HERNIA

A break in the continuity of the diaphragm allows protrusion of abdominal viscera into the thorax.

Etiology: In small animals, automobile-related trauma is a common cause of diaphragmatic hernia, although congenital defects of the diaphragm may also result in herniation (eg, peritoneopericardial hernia). In horses, diaphragmatic hernia may occur, less commonly, congenitally or after trauma, dystocia, or recent strenuous activity. Diaphragmatic hernias are extremely rare in cattle.

Clinical Findings: The signs vary, depending on the duration and species affected. Dogs and cats are characteristically dyspneic in the acute case. The degree of dyspnea may vary from subclinical to incompatible with life, depending on the amount of herniated viscera. If the stomach is herniated, it may bloat and the animal may deteriorate rapidly. In chronic cases, systemic signs such as weight loss may be more prominent than respiratory signs. Physical examination findings may include the absence of lung sounds and/or the presence of GI sounds on auscultation of the thorax. Congenital peritoneopericardial hernia is most frequently an incidental finding, although findings may be related to the respiratory or GI systems or due to compromised venous return to the heart.

Horses most frequently present with acute, severe colic secondary to displaced intestines, or with respiratory signs and dyspnea. In cattle and water buffalo, diaphragmatic hernias may be associated with traumatic reticulitis and herniation of the reticulum.

Diagnosis: Careful physical examination, including auscultation and percussion, usually suggests the presence of thoracic disease. The definitive diagnosis is most frequently made from radiographs. Loss of diaphragmatic contour, abdominal viscera in the thorax, and displacement of viscera from the abdomen may be apparent. Radiographic contrast studies may be necessary to make the diagnosis. Barium may be given by mouth (GI series), or water-soluble contrast may be injected intraperitoneally (celiogram). Radiographs may be difficult to obtain in horses and cows; ultrasonography is useful. Samples from abdominocentesis and thoracocentesis, electrocardiographs, and blood work may be obtained, and surgical exploration of the abdominal cavity may be necessary for definitive diagnosis in these species.

Treatment: Surgical repair of the hernia is the preferred treatment. Other areas of trauma may be present. Optimally, the animal should be stabilized before surgery. If the diaphragmatic tear is chronic, it is necessary to be especially careful with anesthesia, because reexpansion pulmonary edema is likely fatal.

LARYNGEAL DISORDERS

See also LARYNGEAL HEMIPLEGIA, p 1458.

Laryngitis, an inflammation of the mucosa or cartilages of the larynx, may result from upper respiratory tract infection or by direct irritation from inhalation of dust, smoke, or irritating gas; foreign bodies; or the trauma of intubation, excess vocalization, or injury from roping or restraint devices (in livestock). Laryngitis may accompany infectious tracheobronchitis and distemper in dogs; infectious rhinotracheitis and calicivirus infection in cats; infectious rhinotracheitis and calf diphtheria in cattle; strangles, herpesvirus 1 infection, viral arteritis, and infectious bronchitis in horses; *Fusobacterium necrophorum* or *Trueperella pyogenes* infections in sheep; and influenza in pigs.

Edema of the mucosa and submucosa is often an integral part of laryngitis and, if severe, the rima glottidis may be obstructed. Edema may also result from allergy, inhalation of irritants, or surgery in the area. Intubation for anesthesia, especially when attempted with inadequate induction or poor technique, is likely to provoke laryngeal edema. Brachycephalic and obese dogs, and dogs with laryngeal paralysis (*see* p 1420) develop laryngeal edema and laryngitis through severe panting or respiratory effort during excitement or hyperthermia. In cattle, laryngeal edema has been seen in blackleg, urticaria, serum sickness, and anaphylaxis. In pigs, it may develop as a part of edema disease. In horses, cattle, and sheep, laryngeal edema may lead to arytenoid chondropathy.

Laryngeal chondropathy is a suppurative condition of the cartilage matrix that principally affects the arytenoid cartilages; it is believed to result from microbial infection, often as a sequela of inhalation of irritants or trauma to the area. In herbivores, trauma can occur when administering medications by bolus or drench or by ingestion of rough foodstuffs; in dogs, trauma can occur from sticks or foreign bodies. Laryngeal chondropathy is characterized by necrosis and ulceration of the laryngeal mucosa, over or just caudal to the vocal cords, and abscessation within the arytenoid cartilage. Initially, there is often acute laryngeal inflammation. Later, there is progressive enlargement of the cartilages that commonly results in a fixed upper airway obstruction with stertorous breathing and reduced exercise tolerance. Laryngeal chondropathy is seen in horses, sheep, and cattle, most often young males. There is a distinct breed predisposition in Texel sheep and Belgian Blue cattle. Laryngeal contact ulcers are common in young feedlot cattle and often result in necrotic laryngitis and chondropathy.

Clinical Findings: A cough is the principal sign of laryngitis when edema is slight and the deeper tissues of the larynx are not involved. It is harsh, dry, and short at first, but becomes soft and moist later and may be very painful. It can be induced by pressure on the larynx, exposure to cold or dusty air, swallowing coarse food or cold water, or attempts to administer medicines. Vocal changes may be evident, especially in small animals. Stridor may result from swelling and reduced motion of the arytenoid cartilages in laryngeal chondropathy. Halitosis and difficult, noisy breathing may be evident, and the animal may stand with its head lowered and mouth open. Swallowing is difficult and painful. Systemic signs are usually attributable to the primary disease, as in infectious bovine rhinotracheitis, in which temperatures of 105°F (40.5°C) may occur. Secondary systemic signs due to inappetance and dehydration rapidly become apparent. Death due to asphyxiation may occur, especially if the animal is exerted.

Edema of the larynx may develop within hours. It is characterized by increased inspiratory effort and stridor arising from the larynx. Respiratory rate may slow as the effort of breathing becomes exaggerated. Visible mucous membranes are cyanotic, the pulse rate is increased, and body temperature rises. Horses may sweat profusely. Dogs with obstructions of the conducting airways may show extreme disturbance of thermoregulation in hot weather; marked hyperthermia is not uncommon. Untreated animals with marked obstruction eventually collapse and often have signs of pulmonary edema.

Diagnosis: A tentative diagnosis is based on the clinical signs, auscultation of the laryngeal region, and exacerbation of stridor by palpation of the larynx. Definitive diagnosis requires laryngoscopy. In conscious horses and cattle, this can be achieved with a flexible endoscope passed per nasum; in dogs and cats, anesthesia or analgesia usually is required. The history and signs usually permit rapid identification of the primary disease and the associated laryngeal involvement. Bilateral laryngeal paralysis, laryngeal abscess, pharyngeal trauma and cellulitis, and retropharyngeal abscesses or masses can cause similar signs.

Treatment: In laryngeal obstruction, a tracheotomy tube should be placed immediately; if a tracheotomy is not possible, airway patency may be established by passage of a pliable tube through the glottis. Corticosteroids should be administered to reduce the obstructive effect of the inflammatory swellings. Concurrent administration of systemic antibiotics is also necessary. In cases in which corticosteroids cannot be used, NSAIDs can be given. Administration of diuretic drugs, eg, furosemide, may be indicated to resolve laryngeal edema and, if present, pulmonary edema. Identification and treatment of the primary disease is essential. Palliative procedures to speed recovery and give comfort include inhalation of humidified air; confinement in a warm, clean environment; feeding of soft or liquid foods; and avoidance of dust. The cough may be suppressed with antitussive preparations, and bacterial infections controlled with antibiotics or sulfonamides. Control of pain with judicious use of an analgesic, especially in cats, allows the animal to eat, and thus speeds recovery. Subtotal arytenoidectomy is an effective remedy for laryngeal chondropathy of horses, although a return to full athletic capacity in competitive horses is uncertain. Tracheolaryngostomies and permanent tracheostomies have been used successfully to salvage cattle and sheep with laryngeal chondropathy but carry significant anesthetic risk. A medical alternative for ruminants is prolonged antibiotic therapy, 14–21 days of parenteral lincomycin (5–10 mg/kg), plus initial, short-acting corticosteroids.

LARYNGEAL PARALYSIS

Laryngeal paralysis is common in dogs and rare in cats. Signs include a dry cough, voice changes, noisy breathing that progresses to marked difficulty in breathing with stress and exertion, stridor, and collapse. Regurgitation and vomiting may occur. Progression of clinical signs is slow, usually taking months to years before respiratory distress is evident. It is a common acquired problem in middle-aged to older, large and giant breeds of dogs, eg, Labrador Retrievers, Irish Setters, and Great Danes. It is seen less often as a hereditary, congenital disease in Bouvier des Flandres, Leonbergers, Siberian Huskies, Bulldogs, and racing sled dogs.

Diagnosis is based on clinical signs; laryngoscopy under light anesthesia is needed for confirmation. Laryngeal movements are absent or paradoxical with respiration. Electromyography shows positive sharp waves, denervation potentials, and sometimes myotonia. Radiographs are not diagnostic. Denervation atrophy is seen on histologic sections of laryngeal muscles.

Differential diagnoses include myositis, recurrent laryngeal or vagal nerve tumor, inflammation, myasthenia gravis, severe hypothyroidism, trauma, and more widespread generalized neurologic degeneration. Therapy is directed at relieving signs of airway obstruction. Tranquilization and corticosteroids are effective temporarily in mild cases. Severe obstruction may require tracheotomy. Definitive therapy is surgical and directed at enlarging the glottic opening. Currently recommended techniques include arytenoid cartilage lateralization, ventriculocordectomy and partial arytenoidectomy, castellated laryngofissure, or permanent tracheostomy. Studies have demonstrated that bilateral ventriculocordectomy through a ventral median laryngotomy has had good longterm treatment success for surgical treatment of idiopathic laryngeal paralysis in dogs, and unilateral aryte-noid lateralization appeared to be a suitable method to treat laryngeal paralysis in cats.

LUNGWORM INFECTION

(Verminous bronchitis, Verminous pneumonia)

An infection of the lower respiratory tract, usually resulting in bronchitis or pneumonia, can be caused by any of several parasitic nematodes, including *Dictyocaulus viviparus* in cattle, llamas, and alpacas; *D filaria* in goats, sheep, llamas, and alpacas; *D eckerti* in deer; *D arnfieldi* in donkeys and horses; *Protostrongylus rufescens* and *Muellerius capillaris* in sheep and goats; *Metastrongylus apri*, *M pudendotectus*, and *M salmi* in pigs; *Oslerus osleri*, *Crenosoma vulpis*, and *Eucoleus aerophilus* in dogs; and *Aelurostrongylus abstrusus* and *E aerophilus* in cats. Other lungworm infections occur but are less common.

Species of *Dictyocaulus* belong to the superfamily Trichostrongyloidea and have direct life cycles. *E aerophilus* belongs to the Trichuroidea and is thought to have a direct life cycle. The others belong to the Metastrongyloidea and, except for *O osleri*, have indirect life cycles.

Some nematodes that inhabit the right ventricle and pulmonary circulation, eg, *Angiostrongylus vasorum* and *Dirofilaria immitis*, both found in dogs in certain areas of the world, may be associated with pulmonary disease. Clinical signs relating to a cardiac or a pulmonary syndrome or to a combination of both may occur.

Epidemiology: Diseases caused by the ruminant *Dictyocaulus* spp are of most economic importance. The cattle lungworm *D viviparus* is common in northwest Europe and is the cause of severe outbreaks of "husk" or "hoose" in young (and more recently, older) grazing cattle. The lungworm of goats and sheep, *D filaria*, is comparatively less pathogenic but does cause losses, especially in Mediterranean countries, although it is also recognized as a pathogen in Australia, Europe, and North America. *D filaria* and *D viviparus* are less pathogenic in alpacas and llamas, although severe infections can cause coughing, dyspnea, depression, and loss of condition. *D arnfieldi* can cause severe coughing in horses and, because patency is unusual in horses (but not in donkeys), differential diagnosis with disease due to other respiratory diseases can be difficult. *M capillaris* is prevalent worldwide and, although usually nonpathogenic in sheep, can cause severe signs in goats. Other lungworm infections cause sporadic infections in various animal species in many countries.

Dictyocaulus spp: Adult females in the bronchi lay larvated eggs that hatch either in the bronchi (*D viviparus*, *D filaria*) or in host feces (*D arnfieldi*) after being coughed up and swallowed. The infective third-stage larvae can develop on pasture within 5–7 days in warm, moist conditions, but typically in summer in temperate northern climates will require 2–3 wk. Once larvae are infective, transmission depends on their dispersal away from the fecal pats.

Dispersal mechanisms are, primarily, mechanical and include rain or, in the case of *D viviparus* and possibly *D arnfieldi*, by the sporangia of the fungus *Pilobolus*. A proportion of infective larvae survive on pasture throughout the winter until the following year but, in very cold conditions, most become nonviable. The principal source of new infections each year is from infected carrier animals, with overwintered larvae providing a secondary but not unimportant contribution in some countries. In the case of *D arnfieldi*, donkeys are the prime source of pasture contamination for horses. Clinical disease in ruminants usually develops on first exposure to sufficient infective larvae; the severity of disease and stimulation of an immune response is related to the number of larvae ingested. In cattle and sheep, this usually occurs during their first season at pasture; however, an increase in the number of older cattle affected has been reported and is attributed to the efficiency of some prophylactic anthelmintic regimens, which eliminates infection and prevents development of a protective immune response. Because transmission of infection to horses requires infected donkeys (patent infections rarely occur in adult horses but may occur in foals and yearlings), first infections can occur at any age in that species. Once infected, adult ruminants generally become immune to further disease, but a proportion maintain subclinical infections during which they act as a source of further pasture contamination. Occasionally, when previously infected adults or groups that have not been exposed to reinfection for >1 yr, and in which immunity may have waned, are exposed to an overwhelming level of infection, clinical disease may recur. In areas of Europe in which cattle are housed during winter and first grazing season calves turned out in late April or May, the first infections can be seen between mid June and late July, but most severe infections generally occur in previously unexposed calves after development of the second generation of infective larvae on pasture between August and early October.

Other Species: *Metastrongylus* spp in pigs require an earthworm intermediate host; thus, infection is confined to pigs with access to pasture and may become more common in previously uncommon areas as a result of organic farming methods. *M capillaris* and *P rufescens* in sheep and goats require slugs or snails as intermediate hosts, which must be eaten for infection to occur. *C vulpis* is acquired by dogs through ingestion of an infected terrestrial snail or slug intermediate host. *A abstrusus* is normally acquired by cats after ingestion of a paratenic host such as a bird or rodent that has previously eaten the infected slug or snail intermediate host. Adults of *O osleri* live in nodules in the trachea of dogs, and larvated eggs laid by adults hatch there. Larvae migrate up the bronchial tree and may pass in the feces; however, these are not active, are often dead or degenerating, and are not an important route of transmission. Infection in domestic dogs is mainly through saliva as the dam cleans her pups. *E aerophilus* in dogs likely has a direct cycle, with larvated eggs being ingested with food or water.

Pathogenesis: The pathogenic effect of lungworms depends on their location within the respiratory tract, the number of infective larvae ingested, and the animal's immune state. During the prepatent phase of *D viviparus* infection, the main lesion is blockage of bronchioles by an infiltrate of eosinophils in response to the developing larvae; this results in obstruction of the airways and collapse of alveoli distal to the block. Clinical signs are moderate unless large numbers of larvae are ingested, in which case the animal may die in the prepatent phase with severe interstitial emphysema and pulmonary edema.

In the patent phase, the adults in the segmental and lobar bronchi cause a bronchitis, with eosinophils, plasma cells, and lymphocytes in the bronchial wall; a cellular exudate, frothy mucus, and adult nematodes are found in the lumen. The bronchial irritation causes marked coughing, and the entire reaction leads to increased airway resistance. A major component of the patent stage is development of a chronic, nonsuppurative, eosinophilic, granulomatous pneumonia in response to eggs and first-stage larvae aspirated into alveoli and bronchioles. This is usually in the caudal lobes of the lungs and is severe when widespread; in combination with the bronchitis, death may result. Interstitial emphysema, pulmonary edema, and secondary bacterial infection are complications that increase the likelihood of death. Survivors may suffer considerable weight loss.

If the animal survives until the end of patency (2–3 mo for *D viviparus*), most or even all of the adult worms are expelled, and the cellular exudate resolves over the ensuing 4 wk. Most animals recover unless secondary infection develops in the damaged lungs during the postpatent phase. In a few animals, clinical signs are exacerbated in the postpatent phase due to development of a diffuse, proliferative alveolitis characterized by hyperplasia of the type II alveolar epithelial cells. The cause is unknown, but it is seen much less often in cattle treated with anthelmintics with a persistent action against *D viviparus* such as the macrocyclic lactones ivermectin, doramectin, eprinomectin, and moxidectin.

D filaria is similar to *D viviparus*, but interstitial emphysema is not a common complication. Bronchial lesions predominate in *D arnfieldi* infections; when an alveolar reaction occurs, as in donkeys or foals, there are lobular areas of overinflation due to intermittent obstruction of small bronchi.

The pathogenic effect of the other lungworms has a similar basis, but frequently such severe clinical signs are not produced, perhaps because of a more restricted localization in the lungs and less severe infections. The patent phase and the associated lesions last >4 mo for some lungworms (*M apri* and *A abstrusus*) but can be >2 yr (*M capillaris*). The lesions in pigs with metastrongylosis are a combination of localized bronchitis and bronchiolitis with overinflation of related alveoli, usually at the tips and midway along the diaphragmatic lobes. Associated with the mass of nematodes in the lumen is hypertrophy and hyperplasia of bronchiolar and alveolar duct smooth muscle with marked mucous cell hyperplasia. Near the end of the patent period (as adult worms are killed), gray-green lymphoid nodules (2–4 mm) are formed; fragments of dead worms may be seen microscopically in these nodules composed of lymphocytes and plasma cells surrounding a central zone of eosinophils.

In *M capillaris* and *P rufescens* infections, chronic, eosinophilic, granulomatous pneumonia seems to predominate; the reaction is in the bronchioles and alveoli that contain the parasites, their eggs, or larvae. They are surrounded by macrophages, giant cells, eosinophils, and other immunoinflammatory cells, which produce gray or beige plaques (1–2 cm) subpleurally in the dorsal border of the caudal lung lobes. Small (1–2 mm), greenish, nodular lesions may also develop. The effect of these lesions in sheep is minor, perhaps because of the predominantly subpleural location. This infection represents the lower end of the pathogenic spectrum for lungworms.

In cats, *A abstrusus* produces nodular areas of granulomatous pneumonia in the caudal lobes that, if sufficiently generalized, can be clinically significant and occasionally fatal; a notable feature is the hypertrophy and hyperplasia of the smooth muscle in the media of pulmonary arteries and arterioles. The nodules of *O osleri*, found in the mucous membrane of the trachea and large bronchi, can produce extreme airway irritation and persistent coughing. *C vulpis* infections result in chronic bronchitis and bronchiolitis, which leads to chronic coughing. *E aerophilus* infections in dogs are usually well tolerated but may cause chronic tracheitis and bronchitis.

In adult animals not previously exposed to infection, the lesions and pathogenesis are the same as in young animals. However, in adults with some degree of immunity, reexposure to the parasite (eg, husk in adult cattle) can result in different lesions. Despite the immune response, many larvae reach the lungs before they are killed in the terminal bronchioles and alveoli. Larvae not killed in the terminal bronchioles may reach the bronchi and cause a bronchitis characterized by marked eosinophilic infiltration of the bronchial walls and greenish yellow exudate in the lumen comprising eosinophils, other inflammatory cells, and parasitic debris. The reaction associated with this process can lead to severe clinical signs if the nodules are numerous and the eosinophilic bronchitis extensive; this is responsible for the reinfection phenomenon.

Clinical Findings: Signs of lungworm infection range from moderate coughing with slightly increased respiratory rates to severe persistent coughing and respiratory distress and even failure. Reduced weight gains, reduced milk yields, and weight loss accompany many infections in cattle, sheep, and goats. Patent subclinical infections can occur in all species.

The most consistent signs in cattle are tachypnea and coughing. Initially, rapid, shallow breathing is accompanied by a cough that is exacerbated by exercise. Respiratory difficulty may ensue, and heavily infected animals stand with their heads stretched forward and mouths open and drool. The animals become anorectic and rapidly lose condition. Lung sounds are particularly prominent at the bronchial bifurcation. In adult dairy cattle, milk yield drops severely, and abnormal lung sounds are heard over the caudal lobes. The reinfection phenomenon in adult dairy cattle is usually seen in the fall; although less severe than in initial infections, the signs are widespread coughing and tachypnea and a marked drop in milk yield.

The signs in llamas, alpacas, sheep, and goats infected with *D filaria* are similar to those in cattle. Pulmonary signs usually are not associated with *M capillaris* or *P rufescens* in sheep, but the former can affect goats similarly to *D filaria*. *D arnfieldi* is associated with coughing, tachypnea, and unthriftiness in older horses but with few if any signs in foals or donkeys.

The main clinical sign of metastrongylosis in pigs is a persistent cough that may become paroxysmal.

Coughing and dyspnea occur with *A abstrusus* infections in cats and *O osleri* or *C vulpis* infections in dogs. Fatalities are relatively uncommon with these lungworms, although they do occur in kittens.

Diagnosis: Diagnosis is based on clinical signs, epidemiology, presence of first-stage larvae in feces, and necropsy of animals in the same herd or flock. Bronchoscopy and radiography may be helpful. Larvae are not found in the feces of animals in the prepatent or postpatent phases and usually not in the reinfection phenomenon (*D viviparus*). ELISA tests are available in some countries. The test is mainly of use in detecting cattle that have not been exposed, rather than as a differential diagnostic tool in acute respiratory disease. In the early stages of an outbreak, larvae may be few in number. First-stage larvae or larvated eggs can be recovered using most fecal flotation techniques with the appropriate salt solutions; however, larvae will crenate if allowed to sit for a long time on the slide before examination, making identification difficult. Bronchial lavage can reveal *D arnfieldi* infections in horses. A convenient method to recover larvae is a modification of the Baermann technique, in which large fecal samples (25–30 g) are wrapped in tissue paper or cheese cloth and suspended or placed in water contained in a beaker. The water at the bottom of the beaker is examined for larvae after 4 hr; in heavy infections, larvae may be present within 30 min.

In domestic pets, detection of first-stage larvae in the feces, either on flotation or with the Baermann technique, *is still the diagnostic technique of choice*. However, in dogs, cats, and horses, because of the relative infrequency of infection in many areas, lungworms may be considered only after failure of antibiotic therapy to ameliorate the condition. Adults of *Dictyocaulus* spp and *M apri* are readily visible in the bronchi during the patent phases of infection. However, examination of smears from bronchial mucus or histologic sections from lesions may be necessary to confirm the diagnosis during other stages of lungworm infection (and also for other lungworms).

Bronchoscopy can be used to detect nodules of *O osleri* or to collect tracheal washings (dogs and horses) to examine for eggs, larvae, and eosinophils.

Necropsy should include examination of the trachea, particularly at the bifurcation, for *O osleri* and the lesions they induce.

Treatment: Several drugs are useful to treat lungworms (*see* TABLE 1). The benzimidazoles (fenbendazole, oxfendazole, and albendazole) and macrocyclic lactones (ivermectin, doramectin, eprinomectin, and moxidectin) are frequently used in cattle and are effective against all stages of *D viviparus*. These drugs are also effective against lungworms in sheep, horses, and pigs. Levamisole is used in cattle, sheep, and goats, but treatment may need to be repeated 2 wk later because it is less effective against larvae during the early stages. Topical formulations containing moxidectin, selamectin, or emodepside and oral fenbendazole have been used successfully in cats for *A abstrusus*. *O osleri* in dogs is a problem, but there is evidence that fenbendazole and ivermectin are effective if treatment is prolonged (fenbendazole). Injectible doramectin along with removal of as many nodules as possible is the current treatment of choice. *E aerophilus* in dogs and cats is similarly difficult to treat, but success has been reported with ivermectin, fenbendazole, or selamectin.

Animals at pasture should be moved off infected pasture, and supportive therapy may be needed for complications that can arise in all species.

Control: Lungworm infections in herds or flocks are controlled primarily by vaccination or anthelmintics. Oral vaccines are available in Europe for *D viviparus* (northeastern areas) and *D filaria* (southeast). Two doses of irradiated infective larvae are given 4 wk apart, with the second dose given at least 2 wk before the start of grazing or exposure to probable infection. Used properly, they prevent clinical disease,

TABLE 1 RECOMMENDED TREATMENTS FOR LUNGWORMS

Parasite	Host	Treatment[a]
Dictyocaulus viviparus	Cattle	Ivermectin, doramectin, moxidectin, eprinomectin, fenbendazole, albendazole, levamisole
D filaria	Sheep, goat	Ivermectin, doramectin, moxidectin, eprinomectin, fenbendazole, albendazole, levamisole
D arnfieldi	Horse, donkey	Ivermectin, moxidectin
Metastrongylus spp	Pig	Ivermectin, doramectin, moxidectin, fenbendazole, levamisole
Aelurostrongylus abstrusus	Cat	Fenbendazole, emodepside, moxidectin, selamectin
Oslerus osleri	Dog	Fenbendazole, ivermectin, doramectin
Eucoleus aerophilus	Dog, cat	Fenbendazole (dog), selamectin (cat)[b]
Crenosoma vulpis	Dog	Febantel, fenbendazole, milbemycin oxime, moxidectin

[a] In severe cases, NSAIDs may also be helpful.

[b] Anecdotal evidence for efficacy but no published evidence or label recommendations.

but some vaccinated animals may become mildly infected to the extent that larvae are excreted and perpetuate further infection.

Anthelmintic prophylaxis has become feasible with the advent of anthelmintics with prolonged activity (eg, ivermectin, doramectin, moxidectin, eprinomectin). With persistent anthelmintics, two or three treatments during the grazing season, the timing of which depends on local grazing practice and epidemiology, are effective and may, by disrupting developing infections, stimulate immunity to the parasite. The use of multiple treatments may delay immunity to *D viviparus* until the animal is adult, when infection (albeit usually less severe) can occur. However, these methods have become popular in that GI parasites are controlled simultaneously.

Other more sporadic infections can be controlled more easily by management, eg, avoidance of grazing horses with donkeys, indoor husbandry of pigs, and by not mixing sheep and goats on the same grazing.

MYCOTIC PNEUMONIA

Fungal infection of the lung may result in an acute to chronic active, pyogranulomatous pneumonia.

Etiology: *Cryptococcus neoformans*, *Histoplasma capsulatum*, *Coccidioides immitis*, *Blastomyces dermatiditis*, *Pneumocystis jiroveci*, *Aspergillus* spp, *Candida* spp, and other less common fungi have been identified as causative agents of mycotic pneumonia in immunocompromised hosts (*see also* FUNGAL INFECTIONS, p 632). Infection is typically caused by inhalation of spores, which can lead to hemolymphatic dissemination. Pulmonary tissues and secretions are an excellent environment for these organisms. Aspergillosis is most commonly associated with sinonasal infection in dogs or sino-orbital infection in cats, with systemic infection being quite rare and seen only in immunocompromised individuals. Cryptococcosis most commonly affects the nasal cavity in cats, with CNS infection less commonly encountered in dogs and cats. The source of most fungal infections is believed to be soil-related rather than horizontal transmission.

Clinical Findings: Mycotic pneumonia is more commonly seen in small animals than in large. The most common course of disease is chronic. A short, productive cough is often present. A thick, mucoid to mucopurulent nasal discharge may be present. As the disease progresses, dyspnea, emaciation, and generalized weakness become increasingly evident. Respiration may become abdominal, with crackles on auscultation. Generalized lymphadenopathy is common in dogs. Multiple cutaneous and subcutaneous nodules with draining tracts may be seen with blastomycosis in dogs. Blastomycosis is often associated with emaciation and diarrhea in dogs, with skin lesions common in cats. Coccidiomycosis is often associated with severe bone pain due to osteomyelitis in dogs, with skin lesions common in cats. Uveitis or granulomatous chorioretinitis may accompany dimorphic fungal infections. (*See also* FUNGAL INFECTIONS, p 632.)

Lesions: Multifocal to coalescing lesions of granulomatous to pyogranulomatous inflammation are present in the lungs or other affected organs. Abscess formation and cavitation may be seen in conjunction with yellow or gray areas of necrosis. Causative organisms are present within macrophages or areas of intense inflammation.

Diagnosis: Thoracic radiographs often disclose a diffuse pattern with tracheobronchial lymphadenopathy in dogs or large focal pulmonary granulomas in cats. If bone pain is present, skeletal radiography shows osteolysis with periosteal proliferation and soft-tissue swelling at infected sites. Abdominal radiography may reveal granulomas or lymphadenopathy. The clinical diagnosis can be confirmed with impression smears of cutaneous draining tracts, fine-needle aspirate of the lung, lymph node aspirates, or CSF tap (cryptococcosis). Special stains can be used to highlight the organisms.

Treatment: Treatment of mycotic pneumonia is often lengthy. Drugs of choice include itraconazole, fluconazole (cryptococcosis), lipid-complexed amphotericin B, and terbinafine (aspergillosis). Newer generation azole antifungals such as voriconazole or posaconazole are more effective for resistant infections or systemic aspergillosis.

PHARYNGITIS

Pharyngitis is an inflammatory condition of the walls of the oro- or nasopharynx. Pharyngitis may develop secondary to viral or bacterial infections of the upper respiratory tract, eg, strangles in horses and distemper in dogs.

In most species, a common pharynx is present at times other than deglutition. The unique caudal pharyngeal-laryngeal anatomy of horses shows complete separation of the pharynx into two components, the nasopharynx and the oropharynx. (*See also* PHARYNGEAL LYMPHOID HYPERPLASIA, p 1459.)

Clinical Findings: Animals affected with pharyngitis have a normal desire to eat and drink but may have difficulty swallowing and appear dysphagic. Animals with secondary peripharyngeal cellulitis and abscessation may be acutely dyspneic secondary to pharyngeal obstruction. For example, foals affected with suppurative pharyngitis secondary to abscessation of the retropharyngeal lymph nodes can become acutely dyspneic and require an emergency tracheotomy.

Diagnosis: The diagnosis of pharyngitis can be made with a complete physical examination, radiography of the skull, endoscopic evaluation of the pharynx, and microbial cultures of draining abscesses or nasopharyngeal swabs for viral isolation. In small animals, oral pain and resistance to having the mouth opened may indicate retropharyngeal abscessation and the presence of a penetrating foreign body or oral or tonsillar neoplasia. Abnormal pharyngeal tissue should be biopsied and submitted for histopathology to exclude pharyngeal neoplasia. In small animals, oral examination and/or endoscopic examination is the best diagnostic tool for pharyngitis. In large animals, the diagnosis of pharyngitis is easily made by endoscopic examination of the upper respiratory tract.

Treatment: Bacterial pharyngitis should be treated with systemic antimicrobials based on microbial culture and sensitivity testing. Abscesses should be drained and lavaged when appropriate. Viral-induced pharyngitis should be managed with antimicrobials to prevent secondary bacterial infections. Animals affected with either bacterial or viral pharyngitis should be treated with NSAIDs. Pharyngitis secondary to foreign bodies should be resolved with removal of the offending object and effective surgical drainage accompanied by excision of necrotic tissue.

Racehorses affected by pharyngeal lymphoid hyperplasia can be treated with topical and systemic anti-inflammatory agents such as flunixin meglumine, phenylbutazone, or dexamethasone. A commonly used topical anti-inflammatory treatment includes prednisolone, DMSO, glycerin, and nitrofurazone. Large pharyngeal masses can also be treated with contact diode laser photoablation. Some veterinarians have also found hyperimmunization helpful in managing pharyngeal lymphoid hyperplasia.

Calicivirus infections in cats may cause mild, moderate, or severe ulceration of the oropharyngeal mucosa. Although specific antiviral therapies are not available, affected cats should be treated with systemic antimicrobials to prevent secondary bacterial infection. Animals that cannot maintain their own hydration because of severe mucosal ulceration may require nutritional and electrolyte supplementation either intravenously or by extraoral alimentation.

PHARYNGEAL TRAUMA

Pharyngeal trauma in ruminants is not uncommon secondary to iatrogenic causes, such as incorrect passage of balling guns or attempts to pass probangs per os. Affected cattle develop severe swelling of the head and proximal neck secondary to diffuse cellulitis caused by penetration of the pharyngeal mucosa. Feed frequently becomes impacted in these areas and can lead to acute dyspnea. Management of pharyngeal trauma in ruminants should include the placement of a temporary rumen fistula to provide extraoral alimentation while the pharyngeal defect heals. Treatment should also include systemic antimicrobials and anti-inflammatory agents. Some affected animals may also require surgical drainage of accumulated feed and abscessation secondary to the foreign material.

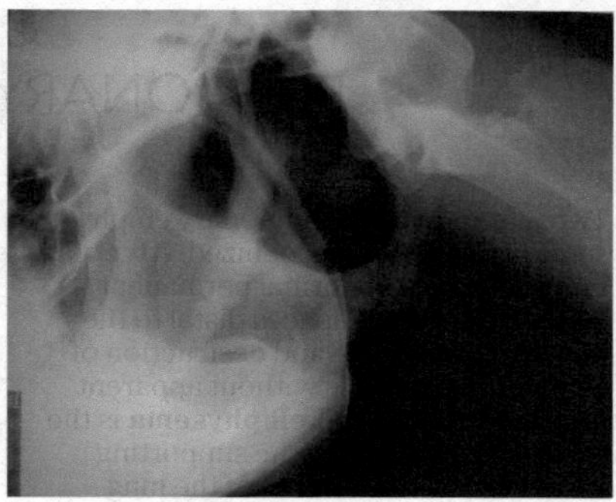

Stylohyoid fracture in a horse. *Courtesy of Dr. Sameeh M. Abutarbush.*

In small animals, oropharyngeal foreign bodies are quite common in dogs but less so in cats. However, cats are prone to ingestion of linear foreign bodies, which may become entangled with the tongue and can be identified with a careful oral examination under sedation or general anesthesia. Penetrating foreign bodies include pins, needles, and pieces of stick or bone fragments. Small animals suspected to have oropharyngeal foreign bodies should be evaluated with an oral examination while sedated or anesthetized and with radiographs or ultrasound to identify all foreign material present. Once identified, pharyngeal foreign bodies may be removed directly via the oral cavity or approached externally.

PULMONARY EMPHYSEMA

Two major forms of pulmonary emphysema are generally recognized. **Alveolar emphysema** is abnormal permanent enlargement of air spaces distal to the terminal bronchiole and destruction of alveolar septal walls without apparent fibrosis. **Interstitial emphysema** is the presence of air within the supporting connective tissue stroma of the lung (interlobular, subpleural, mediastinal, subcutaneous).

Epidemiology and Pathogenesis:

Emphysema affects ~10% of people with chronic obstructive pulmonary disease; the main risk factors are tobacco smoke exposure and α_1-antitrypsin deficiency. In animals, it typically occurs secondary to a primary obstructive pulmonary disease process. While the pathogenesis of pulmonary emphysema is not fully understood, at least three mechanisms have been suggested: 1) an imbalance between protease secreted by neutrophils and macrophages, and antiprotease activity results in destruction of alveolar walls and interstitial matrix; 2) inappropriate maintenance of lung structure and repair follows injury; and 3) the condition develops secondary to obstruction of airways on expiration due to chronic bronchitis/bronchiolitis or congenital abnormality of the airway wall. This creates a "check valve" lesion, in which air is able to enter alveoli on inspiration or through collateral ventilation but is unable to leave freely and causes air trapping.

Recurrent airway obstruction, or "heaves" in horses (*see* p 1455), is associated with chronic bronchitis and bronchiolitis, resulting in alveolar hyperinflation by air trapping. The condition is partially reversible with bronchodilators; however, a small subset of horses develop alveolar emphysema presumably from chronic overdistention of alveolar walls and protease/antiprotease imbalance associated with pulmonary inflammation. Congenital lobar emphysema of dogs (as seen in the Pekingese breed) occurs secondary to aplasia or hypoplasia of bronchiolar cartilage that collapses during expiration, leading to air trapping. Because of well-developed interlobular septa and lack of collateral ventilation, cattle are particularly susceptible to interstitial emphysema. Pulmonary diseases associated with airway obstruction and dyspnea, such as bovine respiratory syncytial virus infection, acute respiratory disease syndromes, such as acute pulmonary edema and emphysema (*see* p 1439), and moldy sweet potato toxicity (*see* p 1442) are commonly associated with interstitial emphysema. Severe interstitial emphysema can cause large gas bullae in all parts of the lung and subcutaneous emphysema as air dissects along fascial planes from the lungs through the mediastinum and thoracic inlet to the subcutis of the back.

Clinical Findings and Diagnosis:

Clinical signs depend on the primary disease process. Often, affected animals present with labored breathing, and auscultation reveals abnormal breath sounds such as wheezes and crackles due to airway disease. The area of thoracic auscultation is typically enlarged due to lung hyperinflation. At necropsy, the lungs do not collapse and stay overinflated. Histology is the only method to differentiate lung overinflation secondary to pulmonary emphysema from air trapping due to airway obstruction from chronic bronchiolitis or bronchitis. Air bubbles (bullae) of various sizes may be seen in the subpleural space and interstitium, as well as around the kidneys and pericardial sac in cattle with emphysema. Pulmonary emphysema affects a small percentage of horses with recurrent airway obstruction (~12%). Lesions may develop as subpleural bullae or emphysema localized to a lobe or diffused lesions.

Minor degrees of emphysema may precede death if there was a prolonged struggle or exaggerated respiration. These agonal changes should be differentiated from antemortem lesions.

Treatment: Emphysema is an irreversible lung lesion; however, therapy directed toward the primary disease process may result in significant improvement of clinical signs, especially by targeting airway obstruction with administration of bronchodilator and anti-inflammatory drugs.

RESPIRATORY DISEASES OF CATTLE

Respiratory disease is among the most economically important diseases of cattle in production on a worldwide basis.

ALLERGIC RHINITIS AND ENZOOTIC NASAL GRANULOMA

Allergic rhinitis is an uncommon disease of cattle that, when chronic, may lead to granuloma formation. The etiology is an allergic reaction to pollen or fungal spores. Signs are seasonal and occur under warm, moist conditions; they include rhinorrhea, sneezing, and a sudden onset of dyspnea. In the chronic stage, multiple granulomas may form on the mucosal surface of the nasal cavity. Cytologic examination of nasal discharges may reveal eosinophils. Treatment should focus on removing the allergen or removing the animal from the allergen. Treatment with corticosteroids to block the hypersensitivity reaction is a consideration.

SINUSITIS

Etiology: Sinusitis in cattle typically involves the frontal or maxillary sinus. Frontal sinusitis is usually associated with dehorning, and maxillary sinusitis with infected teeth. Numerous bacteria have been isolated from sinusitis infections in cattle.

Clinical Findings: Frontal sinusitis may occur immediately after dehorning while the site is still open or months later after the dehorning site has healed. The condition is most often unilateral. Signs may include anorexia, pyrexia, unilateral or bilateral nasal discharge, changes in air flow through the nasal passages, and foul breath. Head carriage may be abnormal. In longstanding cases of frontal sinusitis, there may be distortion of the frontal bone, exophthalmos, and neurologic signs.

Diagnosis: Diagnosis can usually be made on the basis of clinical signs. Percussion may reveal a dull sound over the affected sinus. Radiographs may reveal fluid in the sinus, the presence of dental disease, or bone lysis. Cytology of aspirated material from the affected sinus may reveal purulent material.

Treatment: Sinusitis is treated by draining the affected sinus. Trephine sites should be selected carefully, using appropriate anatomic landmarks. If an infected tooth is the cause of maxillary sinusitis, the tooth can be repelled through a sinusotomy site created with a trephine. Once drainage has been established, the sinus can be lavaged daily with antiseptic solutions. Treatment with parenteral antibiotics is indicated if systemic signs are present. NSAIDs can be given for pain relief, if needed. The prognosis is guarded.

Control: The best control method is to dehorn calves at a young age using a closed dehorning technique. If this is not possible, close attention should be paid to disinfection of surgical instruments between animals, dust control, and fly control.

NECROTIC LARYNGITIS

(Calf diphtheria, Laryngeal necrobacillosis)

Fusobacterium necrophorum, a gram-negative, nonsporeforming anaerobe, is a normal inhabitant of the alimentary, respiratory, and genital tract of animals. The organism is an opportunistic pathogen that causes several necrotic conditions in animals (ie, necrobacillosis), including necrotic laryngitis.

Necrotic laryngitis is an acute or chronic *F necrophorum* infection of the laryngeal mucosa and cartilage of young cattle, characterized by fever, cough, inspiratory dyspnea, and stridor. It occurs primarily in feedlot cattle 3–18 mo of age; however, cases have been documented in calves as young as 5 wk and in cattle as old as 24 mo. Cases are seen worldwide and year round but appear to be more prevalent in fall and winter.

Etiology: Predisposing factors are not fully understood. *F necrophorum*, commonly isolated from laryngeal lesions of affected cattle, is unable to penetrate intact mucous membranes. Laryngeal contact ulcers, a common finding in slaughtered cattle, are thought to provide a portal of entry for *F necrophorum*.

Transmission, Epidemiology, and Pathogenesis: Necrotic laryngitis is most common where cattle are closely confined under unsanitary conditions or in feedlots. The prevalence in feedlot calves is estimated to be 1%–2%. Most cases are sporadic and occur year round, but disease peaks in fall and winter. Mixed upper respiratory tract infections (caused by infectious bovine rhinotracheitis virus and parainfluenza-3 virus; *Mycoplasma* spp; and bacteria, including *Pasteurella* and *Haemophilus*), and the coughing and swallowing associated with these infections, may predispose feedlot cattle to develop laryngeal contact ulcers. These ulcers on the vocal processes and medial angles of arytenoid cartilages are thought to provide a portal of entry for *F necrophorum*.

F necrophorum causes inflammation, necrosis, and edema in the laryngeal mucosa, resulting in variable narrowing of the rima glottidis and inspiratory dyspnea and stridor. If infection extends into the laryngeal cartilage, laryngeal chondritis develops, which may lead to a chronically deformed larynx. Pharyngeal invasion by the organism causes discomfort characterized by painful swallowing motions. Systemic signs of illness have been attributed to the exotoxin produced by *F necrophorum*.

Clinical Findings: Initially, a moist, painful cough is noticed. Severe inspiratory dyspnea, characterized by open-mouth breathing with the head and neck extended, and loud inspiratory stridor are common findings. Ptyalism; frequent, painful swallowing motions; bilateral, purulent nasal discharge; and a fetid odor to the breath may also be present. Systemic signs may include fever (106°F [41.1°C]), anorexia, depression, and hyperemia of the mucous membranes. Untreated calves die in 2–7 days from toxemia and upper airway obstruction. Longterm sequelae include aspiration pneumonia and permanent distortion of the larynx, resulting in a chronic harsh cough and inspiratory dyspnea.

Lesions: Lesions are typically located over the vocal processes and medial angles of arytenoid cartilages. Acute lesions are characterized by edema and hyperemia surrounding a necrotic ulcer in the laryngeal mucosa; lesions may spread along the vocal folds and processes to involve the cricoarytenoideus dorsalis muscle. In chronic cases, lesions consist of necrotic cartilage associated with a draining tract surrounded by granulation tissue.

Diagnosis: Clinical signs are usually sufficient to establish a diagnosis. However, because numerous other conditions can cause signs of upper airway obstruction, the larynx should be visually inspected to confirm a diagnosis. This can be accomplished by means of an orally inserted speculum, laryngoscopy, endoscopy, or radiography, but care must be exercised to avoid further respiratory embarrassment. A tracheostomy should be performed before laryngoscopic or endoscopic examination in cattle with severe inspiratory dyspnea. Differential diagnoses include pharyngeal trauma; severe viral laryngitis (eg, infectious bovine rhinotracheitis); actinobacillosis; and laryngeal edema, abscesses, trauma, paralysis, or tumors.

Treatment and Control: Oxytetracycline (11 mg/kg, IV or SC, bid, or 20 mg/kg of long-acting tetracycline, SC, every 72 hr) or procaine penicillin (22,000 U/kg, IM, bid) are the antimicrobials of choice. NSAIDs (aspirin, 100 mg/kg, PO, bid; flunixin, 1.1–2.2 mg/kg, IV, once daily or divided bid; or ketoprofen, 3 mg/kg/day, IM or IV, for up to 3 days) are used to decrease the fever and laryngeal inflammation and edema. A single dose of dexamethasone (0.2–0.5 mg/kg, IV or IM) may be used to decrease laryngeal edema in animals with severe respiratory distress. A tracheostomy is indicated in cattle with severe inspiratory dyspnea. Good nursing care should be provided. Intravenous fluids may be required in dehydrated animals. The prognosis is good for early cases treated aggressively; chronic cases require surgery under general anesthesia to remove necrotic or granulation tissue and to drain laryngeal abscesses. A 60% success rate has been reported for surgical intervention in advanced cases.

There are no specific control measures for necrotic laryngitis; however, the proposed pathogenesis suggests that control measures for common respiratory pathogens may be beneficial.

TRACHEAL EDEMA SYNDROME OF FEEDER CATTLE

Tracheal edema syndrome is characterized by extensive edema of the mucosa and submucosa in the dorsal membrane of the lower trachea. The etiology is unknown. Proposed causes include respiratory viruses and bacteria, trauma to the trachea from feed bunks, passive congestion and edema from excessive fat accumulation in the thoracic inlet, hypersensitivity reactions, and mycotoxins.

The condition occurs in heavy feeder cattle in the later two-thirds of the feeding period throughout North America but may be most severe in the summer in southern plains (USA) feedlots. Onset is sudden and appears to be associated with an increase in respirations stimulated by hot weather or exercise. The initial signs are a loud inspiratory noise (stridor) and the onset of dyspnea. Forced movement causes the respiratory distress to worsen. The cattle become cyanotic and typically collapse and die of asphyxiation in <24 hr. The disease is usually very sporadic, with small numbers of animals in the population affected.

In the acute form, necropsy lesions include edematous and/or hemorrhagic thickening of the submucosa and mucosa of the dorsal trachea extending from the midcervical area to the thoracic inlet. There is extensive hemorrhage in the trachea but no lung lesions. In the chronic form, lesions consist of hyperemia of the caudal third of the trachea with mucopurulent exudate in the trachea. In fatal cases, the lesion becomes completely obstructive.

Movement and handling of affected cattle should be limited. Antibiotics and corticosteroids are recommended for the acute form, although the efficacy of treatment is not reported. Tracheostomy may be required in severe cases. Providing shade and cooling with fans or water sprays is recommended. Animals that recover are prone to relapse and should be sent to slaughter.

BOVINE RESPIRATORY DISEASE COMPLEX

Bovine respiratory disease (BRD) has a multifactorial etiology and develops as a result of complex interactions between environmental factors, host factors, and pathogens. Environmental factors (eg, weaning, transport, commingling, crowding, inclement weather, dust, and inadequate ventilation) serve as stressors that adversely affect the immune and nonimmune defense mechanisms of the host. In addition, certain environmental factors (eg, crowding and inadequate ventilation) can enhance the transmission of infectious agents among animals. Many infectious agents have been associated with BRD. An initial pathogen (eg, a virus) may alter the animal's defense mechanisms, allowing colonization of the lower respiratory tract by bacteria.

ENZOOTIC PNEUMONIA OF CALVES AND SHIPPING FEVER PNEUMONIA

Enzootic pneumonia and shipping fever pneumonia share many similarities in their respective etiologies and pathogeneses and in general measures for control and prevention.

Enzootic Pneumonia of Calves

(Dairy calf pneumonia, Summer pneumonia of beef calves)

Enzootic pneumonia of calves refers to infectious respiratory disease in calves. The term "viral pneumonia of calves" is sometimes used but is not preferred based on the current understanding of etiology and pathogenesis. Enzootic pneumonia is primarily a problem in calves <6 mo old with peak occurrence from 2–10 wk, but it may be seen in calves up to 1 yr of age. It is more common in dairy than in beef calves and is a common problem in veal calves. It is also more common in housed dairy calves than in those raised outside in hutches. Peak incidence of disease may coincide with decline of passively acquired immunity. Morbidity rates may approach 100%; case fatality rates vary but can reach 20%.

Etiology: The etiology is similar to that for BRD complex in general (*see* p 1431). The pathogenesis involves environmental and management stressors and possibly an initial respiratory viral infection followed by a secondary bacterial infection of the lower respiratory tract. Stress results from environmental and management factors, including inadequate ventilation, mixing by adding calves to an established group, crowding, and nutritional factors such as poor-quality milk replacers. Partial or complete failure of passive transfer of maternal antibodies is an important host factor related to development of disease. Any of several viruses may be involved, and a variety of bacteria may be isolated from affected calves. Mycoplasmal and bacterial agents, including *Pasteurella multocida*, *Mannheimia haemolytica*, and *Mycoplasma bovis*, represent the most frequently isolated pathogenic organisms. The individual viral and bacterial etiologies, clinical signs, lesions, and treatment are discussed under VIRAL RESPIRATORY TRACT INFECTIONS, below, and BACTERIAL PNEUMONIA, p 1436.

Control and Prevention: When calves of varying ages are placed in communal pens, control of enzootic pneumonia is difficult. The severity of the pneumonia may be decreased by improved husbandry, proper housing, adequate ventilation, and good nursing care. Prevention begins with vaccinating the cows against specific respiratory viruses and bacteria 3–4 wk prepartum to improve the quality of colostral antibodies. Calves should receive good-quality colostrum at 8%–10% of body wt in the first 6 hr after birth. Newborn dairy calves should be housed individually in hutches or stalls and fed whole milk or a high-quality milk replacer with a fiber content of <0.25% until 8–12 wk old. The use of calf hutches in dairy herds is the preferred standard for calf housing and has been shown to significantly improve calf respiratory health. However, delivering milk to a large number of hutches in cold weather presents a significant challenge. Single calf housing in naturally ventilated calf barns is the next best alternative. Calves should be vaccinated against respiratory viruses 3–4 wk before the first grouping, although in some situations, the presence of passive immunity may interfere with an active immune response. Calves should be of similar age when assembled into groups, and a group should be limited to ≤10. As calves mature, groups can become larger as the size of the herd, facilities, and available labor dictate. An "all in/all out" management style should be practiced when establishing and terminating a group. Newborn beef calves and their dams should be moved from concentrated calving areas as soon as the calf is nursing well and strong enough to travel. The use of screening systems such as the Calf Respiratory Scoring Chart (University of Wisconsin) may serve as an objective tool to evaluate calves for treatment.

Shipping Fever Pneumonia

Shipping fever pneumonia, or undifferentiated fever, is a respiratory disease of cattle of multifactorial etiology with *Mannheimia haemolytica* and, less commonly, *Pasteurella multocida* or *Histophilus somni* (*see* p 754) being the important bacterials agents involved. Shipping fever pneumonia is associated with the assembly into feedlots of large groups of calves from diverse geographic, nutritional, and genetic backgrounds. Morbidity in feeder calves often peaks within 7–10 days after assembly in a feedlot. Morbidity can approach 35%–50%, and case fatality is 5%–10%; however, the level of morbidity and mortality strongly depends on the array of risk factors present in the cattle being fed.

Etiology: The pathogenesis of shipping fever pneumonia involves stress factors, with or without viral infection, interacting to suppress host defense mechanisms, which allows the proliferation of commensal bacteria in the upper respiratory tract. Subsequently, these bacteria colonize the lower respiratory tract and cause a bronchopneumonia with a cranioventral distribution in the lung. Multiple stress factors are believed to contribute to suppression of host defense mechanisms. Weaning is a significant stressor, and the incidence of this disease is highest in recently weaned calves. Transportation over long distances serves as a stressor; it may be associated with exhaustion, starvation, dehydration, chilling and overheating depending on weather conditions, and exposure to vehicle exhaust fumes. Additional stressors include passage through auction markets; commingling, processing, and surgical procedures on arrival at the feedlot; dusty environmental conditions; and nutritional stress associated with a change to high-energy rations in the feedlot. The individual viral and bacterial etiologies, clinical signs, lesions, and treatment are discussed under VIRAL RESPIRATORY TRACT INFECTIONS, below, and BACTERIAL PNEUMONIA, p 1436.

Control and Prevention: Prevention of shipping fever pneumonia should focus on reducing the stressors that contribute to development of the disease. Cattle should be assembled rapidly into groups, and new animals should not be introduced to established groups. Mixing of cattle from different sources should be avoided if possible; however, in the North American beef industry, this risk factor is almost unavoidable for large intensive feedlots. Transport time should be minimized, and rest periods, with access to feed and water, should be provided during prolonged transport. Calves should ideally be weaned 2–3 wk before shipment, and surgical procedures should be performed in advance of transport; however, the availability of these "preconditioned" calves is quite limited. Cattle should be processed within 48 hr after arrival at the feedlot. Adaptation to high-energy rations should be gradual, because acidosis, indigestion, and anorexia may inhibit the immune response. Vitamin and mineral deficiencies should be corrected. Dust control measures should be used.

Metaphylaxis with long-acting antibiotics such as oxytetracycline, tilmicosin, florfenicol, gamithromycin, tildipirosin, or tulathromycin has been widely adopted as a control measure given "on arrival" to cattle at high risk of developing shipping fever pneumonia. Metaphylaxis on arrival has been shown to significantly reduce morbidity and improve rate of gain and, in some cases, reduce mortality. Mass medication in feed or water is of limited value because sick animals do not eat or drink enough to achieve inhibitory blood levels of the antibiotic, and many of these oral antibiotics are poorly absorbed in ruminants.

On arrival, processing usually involves administration of modified-live vaccines for viral antigens and for bacterial components of shipping fever pneumonia. Because most cases of pneumonia occur during the first 2 wk after arrival, these on-arrival vaccines may not have adequate time to stimulate immunity. When possible, vaccinations for the viral and bacterial components of shipping fever pneumonia should be given 2–3 wk before transport or earlier and can be repeated on entry to the feedlot.

VIRAL RESPIRATORY TRACT INFECTIONS

Parainfluenza-3 Virus

Etiology: Parainfluenza-3 virus (PI-3) is an RNA virus classified in the Paramyxovirus family. Infections caused by PI-3 are common in cattle. Although PI-3 is capable of causing disease, it is usually associated with mild to subclinical infections. The most important role of PI-3 is to serve as an initiator that can lead to development of secondary bacterial pneumonia.

Clinical Findings and Lesions: Clinical signs include pyrexia, cough, serous nasal and lacrimal discharge, increased respiratory rate, and increased breath sounds. The severity of signs worsens with the onset of bacterial pneumonia. Fatalities from uncomplicated PI-3 pneumonia are rare. Lesions include cranioventral lung consolidation, bronchiolitis, and alveolitis with marked congestion and hemorrhage. Inclusion bodies may be identified. Most fatal cases have a concurrent bacterial bronchopneumonia.

Diagnosis: Diagnostic procedures for PI-3 are similar to those for BOVINE RESPIRATORY SYNCYTIAL VIRUS, *see* below.

Treatment and Prevention: Treatment focuses on the antimicrobial therapy directed toward bacterial pneumonia (*see* p 1436). NSAIDs are also a therapeutic consideration.

PI-3 vaccines are available and are almost always combined with bovine herpesvirus 1 (infectious bovine rhinotracheitis). Modified-live and inactivated vaccines are available for IM administration. Vaccines containing temperature-sensitive mutants for intranasal administration are also available.

Bovine Respiratory Syncytial Virus

Etiology: Bovine respiratory syncytial virus (BRSV) is an RNA virus classified as a pneumovirus in the Paramyxovirus family. This virus was named for its characteristic cytopathic effect—the formation of syncytial cells. In additional to cattle, sheep and goats can also be infected by respiratory syncytial viruses. Human respiratory syncytial virus (HRSV) is an important respiratory pathogen in infants and young children. Antigenic subtypes are known to exist for HRSV, and preliminary evidence suggests there may be antigenic subtypes of BRSV. BRSV is distributed worldwide, and the virus is indigenous in the cattle population.

BRSV infections associated with respiratory disease occur predominantly in young beef and dairy cattle. BRSV can be considered as a primary BRD pathogen and is also a component of the bovine respiratory disease complex. Passively derived immunity does not appear to prevent BRSV infections but reduces the severity of disease. Initial exposures to the virus are associated with severe respiratory disease; subsequent exposures result in mild to subclinical disease. BRSV is an important virus in the bovine respiratory disease complex because of its frequency of occurrence, predilection for the lower respiratory tract, and ability to predispose the respiratory tract to secondary bacterial infection. In outbreaks, morbidity tends to be high, and the case fatality rate can be 0–20%.

Clinical Findings and Lesions: Fever (104°–108°F [40°–42°C]), depression, decreased feed intake, increased respiratory rate, cough, and nasal and lacrimal discharge are common. Dyspnea, possibly with open-mouthed breathing, may become pronounced in the later stages of the disease. Subcutaneous emphysema may occur. Secondary bacterial pneumonia is a frequent occurrence. A biphasic disease pattern has been described but is not consistent.

Gross lesions include a diffuse interstitial pneumonia with subpleural and interstitial emphysema along with interstitial edema. These lesions are similar to and must be differentiated from other causes of interstitial pneumonia (*see also* p 1439). Bronchopneumonia of bacterial origin is usually present. Histologic examination reveals syncytial cells in bronchiolar epithelium and lung parenchyma, intracytoplasmic inclusion bodies, proliferation and/or degeneration of bronchiolar epithelium, alveolar epithelialization, edema, and hyaline membrane formation.

Diagnosis: A diagnosis of BRSV requires laboratory confirmation. BRSV is a difficult virus to detect, although chances of isolation may improve when sampling animals in the incubation or acute phases of infection. Although virus isolation is difficult, PCR is a useful and rapid method commonly used to detect the antigen. Other procedures that have proved useful in detection of BRSV antigen are fluorescent antibody and immunoperoxidase staining.

Paired serum samples can be used to establish a diagnosis. However, the antibody titer of animals with well-developed clinical disease may be higher in the acute sample than in the sample taken 2–3 wk later, because the antibody response often develops rapidly, and clinical signs follow virus infection by up to 7–10 days. Single serum samples with high antibody titers from a number of animals in a respiratory outbreak may help diagnosis if coupled with clinical signs. Calves that become infected with BRSV in the presence of passively derived antibody may not seroconvert.

Treatment and Prevention: Treatment focuses on antimicrobial therapy to control secondary bacterial pneumonia (*see* p 1436). There is no specific treatment for the viral interstitial pneumonia. Supportive therapy and correction of dehydration may be necessary. There are anecdotal reports of treatment with antihistamines and/or corticosteroids being of benefit. Most animals will recover in several days without treatment.

General control and prevention are discussed under ENZOOTIC PNEUMONIA OF CALVES AND SHIPPING FEVER PNEUMONIA, p 1431. Inactivated and modified-live vaccines are available and may serve to reduce losses associated with BRSV; however, there is a paucity of field trials to evaluate the efficacy of these vaccines.

Bovine Herpesvirus 1

(Infectious bovine rhinotracheitis virus, Infectious pustular vulvovaginitis, and associated diseases)

Etiology and Epidemiology: Bovine herpesvirus 1 (BHV-1) is associated with several diseases in cattle: infectious bovine rhinotracheitis (IBR), infectious pustular vulvovaginitis (IPV), balanoposthitis, conjunctivitis, abortion, encephalomyelitis, and mastitis. Only a single serotype of BHV-1 is recognized; however, three subtypes of BHV-1 have been described on the basis of endonuclease cleavage patterns of viral DNA: BHV-1.1 (respiratory subtype), BHV-1.2 (genital subtype), and BHV-1.3 (encephalitic subtype). BHV-1.3 has been reclassified as a distinct herpesvirus designated BHV-5.

BHV-1 infections are widespread in the cattle population. In feedlot cattle, the respiratory form is most common. The viral infection alone is not life-threatening but predisposes to secondary bacterial pneumonia, which may result in death. In breeding cattle, abortion or genital infections are more common. Genital infections can occur in bulls (infectious pustular balanoposthitis) and cows (IPV) within 1–3 days of mating or close contact with an infected animal. Transmission can occur in the absence of visible lesions and through artificial insemination with semen from subclinically infected bulls. Cattle with latent BHV-1 infections generally show no clinical signs when the virus is reactivated, but they serve as a source of infection for other susceptible animals.

Clinical Findings: The incubation period for the respiratory and genital forms is 2–6 days. In the respiratory form, clinical signs range from mild to severe, depending on the presence of secondary bacterial pneumonia. Clinical signs include high fever, anorexia, coughing, excessive salivation, nasal discharge that progresses from serous to mucopurulent, conjunctivitis with lacrimal discharge, inflamed nares (hence the common name "red nose"), and dyspnea if the larynx becomes occluded with purulent material. Nasal lesions consist of numerous clusters of grayish necrotic foci on the mucous membrane of the septal mucosa, just visible inside the external nares. They may later be accompanied by pseudodiphtheritic yellowish plaques. Conjunctivitis with corneal opacity may occur as the only manifestation of BHV-1 infection. In the absence of bacterial pneumonia, recovery generally occurs 4–5 days after the onset of signs.

Abortions may occur concurrently with respiratory disease but may be seen up to 100 days after infection. They can occur regardless of the severity of disease in the dam. Abortions generally occur during the second half of pregnancy, but early embryonic death is possible.

In genital infections, the first signs are frequent urination, elevation of the tailhead, and a mild vaginal discharge. The vulva is swollen, and small papules, then erosions and ulcers, are present on the mucosal surface. If secondary bacterial infections do not occur, animals recover in 10–14 days. With bacterial infection, there may be inflammation of the uterus and transient infertility, with purulent vaginal discharge for several weeks. In bulls, similar lesions occur on the penis and prepuce. (*See also* p 1391.)

BHV-1 infection can be severe in young calves and cause a generalized disease. Pyrexia, ocular and nasal discharges, respiratory distress, diarrhea, incoordination, and eventually convulsions and death may occur in a short period after generalized viral infection.

Lesions: In uncomplicated IBR infections, most lesions are restricted to the upper respiratory tract and trachea. Petechial to ecchymotic hemorrhages may be found in the mucous membranes of the nasal cavity and the paranasal sinuses. Focal areas of necrosis develop in the nose, pharynx, larynx, and trachea. The lesions may coalesce to form plaques.

The sinuses are often filled with a serous or serofibrinous exudate. As the disease progresses, the pharynx becomes covered with a serofibrinous exudate, and blood-tinged fluid may be found in the trachea. The pharyngeal and pulmonary lymph nodes may be acutely swollen and hemorrhagic. The tracheitis may extend into the bronchi and bronchioles; when this occurs, epithelium is sloughed in the airways. The viral lesions are often masked by secondary bacterial infections. In young animals with generalized BHV-1 infection, erosions and ulcers overlaid with debris may be found in the nose, esophagus, and forestomachs. In addition, white foci may be found in the liver, kidney, spleen, and lymph nodes. Aborted fetuses may have pale, focal, necrotic lesions in all tissues, which are especially visible in the liver.

Diagnosis: Uncomplicated BHV-1 infections can be diagnosed based on the characteristic signs and lesions. However, because the severity of disease can vary, it is best to differentiate BHV-1 from other viral infections by viral isolation. Samples should be taken early in the disease, and a diagnosis should be possible in 2–3 days. A rise in serum antibody titer also can be used to confirm a diagnosis. It is not possible to detect a rising antibody titer in abortions, because infection generally occurs a considerable length of time before the abortion, and titers are already maximal. BHV-1 abortion can be diagnosed by identifying characteristic lesions and demonstrating the virus in fetal tissues by PCR, virus isolation, immunoperoxidase, or fluorescent antibody staining. Gross and microscopic lesions detected shortly after death may help to establish a diagnosis. PCR methods can be used to identify antigen in a variety of tissues or exudates.

Treatment and Control: Antimicrobial therapy is indicated to prevent or treat secondary bacterial pneumonia. General recommendations for control are discussed under SHIPPING FEVER PNEUMONIA, p 1432. Immunization with modified-live or inactivated virus vaccines generally provides adequate protection against clinical disease. Both IM and intranasal modified-live vaccines are available, but the IM types may cause abortion in pregnant cattle. The intranasal vaccines can be used in pregnant cattle. The IM vaccines are easier to use and often are the vaccines of choice in feedlots. Breeding and replacement heifers and bulls should be immunized when 6–8 mo old, before breeding, and yearly thereafter. Some recommend that young bulls not be vaccinated, because they may be discriminated against when sold for breeding if they have antibody titers. Feeder calves should be immunized 2–3 wk before entry into the feedlot. A number of western European countries have eradicated or are attempting to eradicate BHV-1 from their domestic cattle populations. Eradication of the virus is possible by a combination of serologic surveillance, culling of reactors, biosecurity, and vaccination. To aid in eradication, deletion mutant vaccines have been developed that permit discrimination between antibody produced in response to the vaccine and antibody produced in response to natural exposure.

Bovine Viral Diarrhea Virus

Bovine viral diarrhea virus (BVDV) is an RNA virus classified as a Pestivirus in the family Flaviviridae (*see* p 267). The role of BVDV in BRD as a primary pathogen has been controversial but appears to be that of a virus capable of inducing immunosuppression, which allows for development of secondary bacterial pneumonia. Seroconversion to BVDV after arriving in the feedlot has been reported to be the occurrence of respiratory disease in feedlot calves. Calves that arrive at the feedlot with high titers to BVDV have also been shown to be less likely to develop respiratory disease, and BVDV has been reported to be the virus most frequently associated with multiple viral infections of the respiratory tract of calves. Some studies have shown that the presence of a calf persistently infected with BVDV in a feedlot pen increases the risk of respiratory disease within that pen.

Treatment for acute BVDV infection is supportive and includes antimicrobials to prevent or treat bacterial pneumonia. General principles of control are discussed under ENZOOTIC PNEUMONIA OF CALVES AND SHIPPING FEVER PNEUMONIA, p 1431. Inactivated and modified-live vaccines are available for IM administration. Recently, vaccines containing both the type I and type II genotypes have become available. Vaccination of cows before breeding with modified-live vaccines is an important strategy to prevent the occurrence of persistently infected calves. Testing for persistently infected calves and removing them from the pen has been used as a strategy to reduce the risk of disease within feedlots in high-risk groups.

Other Bovine Respiratory Viruses

Several other viruses may potentially be involved in BRD. Bovine herpesvirus 4 has been implicated in several diseases, including BRD. Bovine adenovirus has been associated with a wide spectrum of diseases, with bovine adenovirus type 3 being the serotype most often associated with BRD. Two serotypes of bovine rhinovirus have been recognized to cause respiratory tract infections in cattle. Other viruses reported to be associated with BRD include bovine reovirus, enterovirus, and coronavirus. Evidence is growing that bovine coronavirus may have a more important role in BRD than previously recognized. Bovine coronavirus may play a role in some outbreaks of calf pneumonia on pasture in beef cow-calf operations.

These viruses have a role similar to that of the other viruses previously discussed; ie, in combination with other stressors, they can serve as initiators of bacterial pneumonia. Vaccines are not available for prevention of these viral respiratory diseases.

BACTERIAL PNEUMONIA

Mannheimia haemolytica–associated Bovine Respiratory Disease

Etiology: *Mannheimia haemolytica* serotype 1 is the bacterium most frequently isolated from the lungs of cattle with BRD. Although less frequently cultured, *Pasteurella multocida* is also an important cause of bacterial pneumonia. *Histophilus somni* is being increasingly recognized as an important pathogen in BRD; these bacteria are normal inhabitants of the nasopharynx of cattle (*see* p 754). When pulmonary abscessation occurs, generally in association with chronic pneumonia, *Trueperella pyogenes* is frequently isolated.

Under normal conditions, *M haemolytica* remains confined to the upper respiratory tract, in particular the tonsillar crypts, and is difficult to culture from healthy cattle. After stress or viral infection, the replication rate of *M haemolytica* in the upper respiratory tract increases rapidly, as does the likelihood of culturing the bacterium. The increased bacterial growth rate in the upper respiratory tract, followed by inhalation and colonization of the lungs, may occur because of suppression of the host's defense mechanism related to environmental stressors or viral infections. It is during this log phase of growth of the organism in the lungs that virulence factors are elaborated by *M haemolytica*, such as an exotoxin that has been referred to as leukotoxin. The interaction between the virulence factors of the bacteria and host defenses results in tissue damage with characteristic necrosis, thrombosis, and exudation, and in the development of pneumonia. The pathogenesis of pneumonia caused by *P multocida* is poorly understood. This organism may opportunistically colonize lungs with chronically damaged respiratory defenses, such as occurs with enzootic calf pneumonia or existing lung lesions of feedlot cattle, and cause a purulent bronchopneumonia. *H somni* may invade the lung and cause pneumonia after damage to the respiratory defenses. This organism is capable of systemic spread from the lung to the brain, myocardium, synovium, and pleural and pericardial surfaces; often, death can occur later in the feeding period (40–60 days after arrival) from involvement of these additional organ systems.

Clinical Findings: Clinical signs of bacterial pneumonia are often preceded by signs of viral infection of the respiratory tract. With the onset of bacterial pneumonia, clinical signs increase in severity and are characterized by depression and toxemia. A combination of clinical signs of depression and fever (104°–106°F [40°–41°C]), without any signs attributable to other body systems, are the classic components of a case definition for early cases of BRD. Serous to mucopurulent nasal discharge; moist cough; and a rapid, shallow respiratory rate may be noted. Auscultation of the cranioventral lung field reveals increased bronchial sounds, crackles, and wheezes. In severe cases, pleurisy may develop, characterized by an irregular breathing pattern and grunting on expiration. The animal will become unthrifty in appearance if the pneumonia becomes chronic, which is usually associated with formation of pulmonary abscesses.

Lesions: *M haemolytica* causes a severe, acute, hemorrhagic fibrinonecrotic pneumonia. The pneumonia has a bronchopneumonic pattern. Grossly, there are extensive reddish black to grayish brown cranioventral regions of consolidation with gelatinous thickening of interlobular septa and fibrinous pleuritis. There are extensive thromboses, foci of lung necrosis, and limited evidence of bronchitis and bronchiolitis.

P multocida is associated with a less fulminating fibrinous to fibrinopurulent bronchopneumonia. In contrast to *M haemolytica*, *P multocida* is associated with only small amounts of fibrin exudation, some thromboses, limited lung necrosis, and suppurative bronchitis and bronchiolitis.

H somni infection of the lungs results in purulent bronchopneumonia that may be followed by septicemia and infection of multiple organs. *H somni* is associated with extensive fibrinous pleuritis in feedlot calves.

Pulmonary abscessation can occur as the pneumonia becomes chronic. Abscesses develop in ~3 wk but do not become encapsulated until 4 wk. *T pyogenes* is frequently cultured from these abscesses.

Diagnosis: Generally, neither serologic testing nor direct bacterial detection are performed, and diagnosis relies on gross necropsy findings and bacterial culture. Because the bacteria involved are normal inhabitants of the upper respiratory tract, the specificity of culture can be increased by collecting antemortem specimens from the lower respiratory tract by tracheal swab, transtracheal wash, or bronchoalveolar lavage. Lung specimens can be collected for culture at necropsy. If possible, specimens for culture should be collected from animals that have not been treated with antibiotics to permit determination of antimicrobial sensitivity patterns. A multiplex PCR has been used to identify a number of bacterial agents implicated with bovine respiratory disease, including *M hemolytica*.

Treatment: Early recognition by trained personnel skilled at detecting the early clinical signs of disease followed by treatment with antibiotics is essential for successful therapy. Treatment protocols should be established so the producer has a standardized approach to identifying and treating cases. Long-acting antimicrobials such as tulathromycin, tilmicosin, florfenicol, and enrofloxacin have label claims to treat BRD and are commonly used as first- or second-line treatment options in feedlot calves. These long-acting antimicrobials allow the feedlot producer to avoid commingling sick animals in a hospital pen, and treated animals can return directly to the home pen. NSAIDs have been shown to be a beneficial ancillary therapy in controlling fever in cases of BRD, but data are lacking in terms of effect on relapse and mortality outcomes. If selection for treatment is late and pulmonary abscessation has occurred, it is difficult to achieve resolution with antimicrobials, and use of a convalescent pen or culling of the animal should be considered.

Control: General principles of control are discussed under ENZOOTIC PNEUMONIA OF CALVES AND SHIPPING FEVER PNEUMONIA, p 1431. The value of *M haemolytica* and *P multocida* bacterins is questionable, and some reports indicate they may even exacerbate the disease. Newer vaccines, which include live culture and subunit vaccines (leukotoxin), show much more promise for disease prevention and may reduce morbidity in high-risk feedlot calves given one dose of vaccine on arrival by as much as 25%; however, trials have not been consistent in all risk categories of feedlot cattle. Ideally, vaccination should be done 3 wk before transport to the feedlot and can be repeated on arrival. In dairy calves, vaccination of the dam may be of benefit by providing passive immunity to the calf. *H somni* bacterins are available, and there is some evidence they are effective in control of BRD in feedlot calves even when only one dose is given on arrival.

Mycoplasmal Pneumonia

Mycoplasma bovis is an emerging cause of respiratory disease and arthritis in feedlot cattle and in young dairy and veal calves. Experimental infections usually result in inapparent to mild signs of respiratory disease, but virulent strains have been identified that cause severe lung disease in calves. However, this does not preclude a synergistic role for mycoplasmas in conjunction with viruses and bacteria in BRD. Mycoplasmas can be isolated from the respiratory tract of nonpneumonic calves, but the frequency of isolation is greater in those with respiratory tract disease. *M bovis* has been associated with otitis media in young calves and a syndrome involving chronic pneumonia and polyarthritis in feedlot cattle. These cattle invariably have a pneumonic lesion, and 40%–60% may also develop a polyarthritis and tenosynovitis that causes severe chronic lameness. The condition results in a chronic disease that does not respond to antimicrobial therapy. A significant proportion of these animals are euthanized because of the chronic nature of the disease. Lesions include chronic bronchopneumonia with caseous and coagulative necrosis. In severe cases, >80% of the lung tissue may be involved. Culture of these organisms requires special media and conditions; growth of the organisms may take up to a week. PCR tests are now available that can detect the mycoplasma within hours, thus greatly speeding up diagnosis. Immunohistochemical tests can also be done on fixed tissue that link the mycoplasma antigen directly with the lung lesion. Vaccines are commercially available for *M bovis*, but their efficacy has not been demonstrated conclusively.

Chlamydial Pneumonia

Chlamydial agents have been implicated in a number of diseases of cattle, including pneumonia. Clinical signs and lesions of bronchopneumonia have been produced by experimental infections. A synergism between *Chlamydia* and *Mannheimia haemolytica* has been demonstrated experimentally. Because this pathogen is infrequently tested for, its overall importance remains undetermined. The organism can be tested for by staining sections of lung lesions with Gimenez stain or by fluorescent antibody. Isolation requires inoculation of yolk sacs of embryonating chicks. Chlamydial agents are sensitive to tetracyclines. (*See also* p 598.)

CONTAGIOUS BOVINE PLEUROPNEUMONIA

Contagious bovine plueuropneumonia is highly contagious and generally accompanied by pleurisy. It is present in Africa, with minor outbreaks occurring in the Middle East. The USA has been free of the disease since 1892, the UK since 1898, and Australia since 1973. The last outbreak of CBPP in Europe was seen in Portugal in 1999. Little is known about the disease in Asia, but China claims that its last outbreak was in 1995.

Etiology: The causal organism is *Mycoplasma mycoides mycoides* small colony type. (*See also* p 1474.) Susceptible cattle become infected by inhaling droplets disseminated by coughing in affected cattle. Small ruminants and wildlife are not important in the epidemiology. Sheep and goats can be naturally infected but have no associated pathology. The organism can also be found in saliva, urine, fetal membranes, and uterine discharges. Transplacental infection of the fetus can occur. Viability of the organism in the environment is poor. The incubation period varies, but most cases occur 3–8 wk after exposure. In some localities, susceptible herds may show up to 70% morbidity, but much lower infection rates (~10%) associated with clinical signs are more common. Mortality is likely to be ~50% in herds experiencing the disease for the first time. Of recovered animals, 25% may become carriers with chronic lung lesions in the form of sequestra of variable size. Because carriers may not be detectable clinically or serologically, they constitute a serious problem in control programs. Breed susceptibility, management systems, and general health of the animal are important factors that influence the infection.

Clinical Findings: In acute cases, signs include fever up to 107°F (41.5°C);

anorexia; and painful, difficult breathing. In hot climates, the animal often stands by itself in the shade, its head lowered and extended, its back slightly arched, and its elbows turned out. Percussion of the chest is painful; respiration is rapid, shallow, and abdominal. If the animal is forced to move quickly, the breathing becomes more distressed and a soft, moist cough may result. The disease progresses rapidly, animals lose condition, and breathing becomes very labored, with a grunt at expiration. The animal becomes recumbent and dies after 1–3 wk. Chronically affected cattle usually exhibit signs of varying intensity for 3–4 wk, after which the lesions gradually resolve and the animals appear to recover. Subclinical cases occur and may be important as carriers. Infected calves may present primarily with polyarthritis that is seen as swelling of joints and lameness.

Lesions: The thoracic cavity may contain up to 10 L of clear yellow or turbid fluid mixed with fibrin flakes, and the organs in the thorax are often covered by thick deposits of fibrin. The disease is largely unilateral, with more than 80%–90% of cases affecting only one lung. The affected portion is enlarged and solid. On section of the lung, the typical marbled appearance of pleuropneumonia is evident because of the widened interlobular septa and subpleural tissue that encloses gray, yellow, or red consolidated lung lobules. Microscopically, this is a severe, acute, fibrinous pneumonia with fibrinous pleurisy, thrombosis of pulmonary blood vessels, and areas of necrosis of lung tissue; the interstitial tissue is markedly thickened by edema fluid containing much fibrin. In chronic cases, the lesion has a necrotic center sequestered in a thick, fibrous capsule, and there may be fibrous pleural adhesions. Organisms may survive only within the inner capsule of these sequestra, and these animals may become carriers.

Diagnosis: Diagnosis is based on clinical signs and the characteristic gross pathologic lesions of the lungs. Complement fixation, latex agglutination, or competitive ELISA tests can be used to aid definitive diagnosis. Confirmation is often by isolation of the mycoplasma followed by growth inhibition or immunofluorescence test using hyperimmune rabbit sera against the mycoplasma, or increasingly by PCR. Confirmation of serologic reactions can be made by immunoblotting test. As soon as an outbreak is suspected, slaughter and necropsy of presumptively infected cattle is advisable.

Control: The disease is reportable by law in many countries from which it has been eradicated by slaughter of all infected and exposed animals. In countries where cattle movement can readily be restricted, the disease can be eradicated by quarantine, blood testing, and slaughter. Where cattle cannot be confined, the spread of infection can be limited by immunization with attenuated vaccine (eg, T1/44 strain). However, the vaccine is effective only if herd coverage within a country is high. Tracing the source of infected cattle detected at abattoirs, blood testing, and imposition of strict rules for cattle movement also can aid in control of the disease in such areas.

Treatment is recommended only in endemic areas because the organisms may not be eliminated, and carriers may develop. Tylosin (10 mg/kg, IM, bid, for six injections) and danofloxacin 2.5% (2.5 mg/kg/day for 3 consecutive days) have been reported to be effective.

INTERSTITIAL PNEUMONIA

This classification represents a group of respiratory diseases characterized by an acute onset of severe respiratory distress and a combination of lung lesions that include pulmonary edema and congestion, interstitial emphysema, alveolar epithelialization, and hyaline membrane formation.

Lungworm infection in cattle (*see* p 1421) can also result in an atypical interstitial pneumonia .

ACUTE BOVINE PULMONARY EMPHYSEMA AND EDEMA

(Fog fever, Bovine atypical interstitial pneumonia)

Acute bovine pulmonary emphysema and edema (ABPEE) is one of the more common causes of acute respiratory distress in cattle, particularly adult beef cattle, and is characterized by sudden onset, minimal coughing, and a course that ends fatally or improves dramatically within a few days. It is a disease involving groups of cattle; morbidity may be >50%, although usually only a small minority develops severe respiratory distress. Typically, ABPEE occurs in the fall, 5–10 days after change to a better, often lush, pasture. A similar condition has been reported when cattle are fed on a wide variety of grasses, alfalfa, rape, kale, and turnip tops.

Etiology: Metabolites of the naturally occurring amino acid L-tryptophan probably are responsible for many outbreaks. In the rumen, L-tryptophan is degraded to indoleacetic acid, which can be converted to 3-methylindole by some ruminal microorganisms. 3-Methylindole is absorbed into the bloodstream and is the source of the pneumotoxicity after metabolism by the mixed function oxidase system, which is very active in the lungs. Apparently, the level of L-tryptophan in crops is most likely to be high in lush, rapidly growing pastures, particularly (but not exclusively) in the fall.

Clinical Findings: ABPEE is most common in adult beef cows but may occur in either sex and in dairy or beef cattle under similar management conditions. Nursing calves are unaffected. Outbreaks usually develop within 5–10 days of a change to better grazing and rarely occur in animals that have been on a field >3 wk.

Mild cases may go unnoticed. Cattle are subdued but still alert; there is tachypnea and hyperpnea, but auscultation is usually unrewarding. Such cattle usually recover spontaneously within days. Severely affected cattle show extensive respiratory distress with mouth breathing, extension of the tongue, and drooling. A loud expiratory grunt is common, but coughing is unusual. In the early stages, auscultation reveals surprisingly soft respiratory sounds. Mild exercise increases dyspnea and may precipitate death. If death does not occur, the animals improve dramatically and resume eating by the third day. At this stage, auscultation reveals harsh respiratory sounds and, in some animals, dorsal (emphysematous) crackles. Some cattle have subcutaneous emphysema extending along the back from the withers. Full clinical recovery may require 3 wk.

Lesions: In affected cattle that have died or been slaughtered in extremis, the lungs are heavy and do not collapse normally. They are widely affected, with various degrees of firmness; there is extensive edema and emphysema, often with the formation of large, air-filled bullae in interlobular and subpleural regions. Submucosal hemorrhages are often present on the larynx and in the trachea and larger bronchi. Histologically, the lesion is characterized by congestion, alveolar edema, hyaline membrane formation, and areas of early alveolar epithelial hyperplasia of type II pneumocytes; occasionally, areas of bronchiolar necrosis may be found. The emphysema is often dramatic and is limited to interstitial fascia, where it is accompanied by edema.

In animals slaughtered after 3 days of illness, the lungs are still heavy and do not collapse normally. They are pinkish gray and of increased firmness; edema and emphysema are inconspicuous or absent. Histologically, widespread alveolar epithelial hyperplasia characteristic of a diffuse, acute, proliferative alveolitis is seen.

Diagnosis: Diagnosis is based on history, signs, and lesions. Because the syndrome is not specific with regard to cause, evidence must be obtained from history of management factors such as change in pasture.

Treatment: Severely affected animals have so little pulmonary reserve that any driving or handling must be done with caution to prevent immediate death. Removal of cattle from the offending pastures may not prevent the development of new cases for the next 4–7 days. No treatment has been identified that will reverse the fully developed lesions of ABPEE.

Control: One approach to control is dietary management, including the following options: 1) avoiding pastures likely to induce ABPEE, 2) feeding hay before turn out on pasture and limiting exposure time on suspect pastures, 3) limiting grazing time and gradually increasing exposure to the pasture over time, 4) using pastures before they become lush, 5) delaying use of lush pastures until after a hard frost, 6) initially grazing pastures with less susceptible stock (cattle <15 mo old or sheep), or 7) using strip grazing.

A medical approach to control involves feeding monensin or lasalocid, which inhibit the bacteria that convert L-tryptophan to 3-methylindole. Treatment with monensin can be started 1 day before introduction to pasture, whereas lasalocid requires a 6-day pretreatment period. These drugs are of no benefit after onset of clinical signs.

ANAPHYLAXIS

Anaphylaxis or Type I hypersensitivity reactions in cattle can result in an atypical interstitial pneumonia. The lung is a major target organ in cattle for Type I hypersensitivity. Clinical signs are those of acute respiratory distress. Cattle that die of anaphylaxis may have lesions consistent with those described for atypical interstitial pneumonia. Treatment is administration of epinephrine; supportive treatment includes anti-inflammatory therapy with corticosteroids or NSAIDs. If pharyngeal or laryngeal edema is present, a tracheostomy may be indicated.

HYPERSENSITIVITY PNEUMONITIS

(Extrinsic allergic alveolitis, Farmer's lung disease)

Hypersensitivity pneumonitis is a condition that appears to be similar to farmer's lung disease in people and occurs in both acute and chronic forms in adult cattle. The human and bovine forms of the disease may coexist on problem farms because of common exposure to dust from moldy hay.

Etiology: The disease occurs when sensitized individuals inhale antigens from thermophilic actinomycetes, commonly the spores of *Micropolyspora faeni*. The actinomycetes proliferate in vast numbers in hay, grain, or other vegetable material that has overheated to ~150°F (65°C) after damp storage (30%–40% moisture content). Dust that contains large numbers of spores is released when this moldy hay is shaken. The small size (1 µm) of the spores allows them to reach the smallest airways and alveoli to provoke a reaction that has been termed a "hypersensitivity pneumonitis"; this is considered to be predominantly a Type III hypersensitivity reaction, although a Type IV hypersensitivity component is suspected (*see* IMMUNOLOGIC DISEASES, p 817 et seq).

Affected herds are found in areas where rainfall is usually significant during the haymaking season, suggesting that a clinical problem may arise only after repeated sensitization and challenge from the spores. Clinical disease tends to arise during the latter half of the winter feeding period and usually only when moldy hay is fed indoors. Under such circumstances, serum antibodies (usually detected by immunodiffusion) to *M faeni* are widespread among adult cattle by the end of each winter feeding period, and many apparently healthy cattle are seropositive. By contrast, few adult cattle are seropositive on other farms on which "good" hay or grass silage is fed.

Clinical Findings: Cattle may succumb to the acute form of the disease over a period of weeks. Usually, only severe acute cases are noticed. There is respiratory distress, anorexia, and agalactia in animals ≥5 yr old; coughing and pyrexia also occur, and adventitious sounds are occasionally heard on auscultation. Death is rare.

The chronic disease usually has a higher morbidity; in most instances, the signs are weight loss, poor production, and persistent coughing. Affected cattle are fairly bright and eat reasonably well, but tachypnea, hyperpnea, and coughing are widespread. Auscultation may reveal cranioventral crackles and sometimes, in more severe cases, scattered rhonchi. Exercise intolerance may be seen, and congestive cardiac failure can develop if pulmonary fibrosis is widespread.

Lesions: The macroscopic lesions are often unremarkable; usually, there is mild peripheral lobular overinflation with diffusely scattered, small, gray, subpleural spots. Although transient pulmonary edema may be a feature of severe acute cases, the histologic lesions consistently found are interalveolar cellular infiltration, epithelioid granulomata, and bronchiolitis obliterans. In some chronic cases, small foci of alveolar epithelial hyperplasia and metaplasia with interstitial fibrosis are found. These areas may extend to include most, if not all, of the lung substance to produce cases clinically indistinguishable from diffuse fibrosing alveolitis (*see* below). Circumstantial evidence suggests that some cases of diffuse fibrosing alveolitis are the end stage of hypersensitivity pneumonitis.

Treatment and Control: Because it is often impossible to completely shield cattle from further challenge, most recover only partially after dexamethasone treatment (1 mg/5–10 kg body wt). However, improvement is usually marked when cattle are turned out in the spring. Prevention is difficult in areas where hay is likely to be wet during the curing process and it is not possible to alter the feeding regimen.

DIFFUSE FIBROSING ALVEOLITIS

Diffuse fibrosing alveolitis is a chronic, progressive respiratory disease of undetermined cause and possibly of multiple etiologies. A proportion of affected cattle are seropositive for precipitating antibodies to *Micropolyspora faeni*, and this condition may represent the end stage of hypersensitivity pneumonitis. Other than the respiratory signs, the animals appear alert and maintain a good appetite until the onset of heart failure in the terminal stages. Signs include coughing, increased respiratory rate, dyspnea, and weight loss. Necropsy findings include right ventricular hypertrophy, interalveolar fibrosis, obliteration of the alveolar spaces, alveolar hyperplasia, bronchitis, and bronchiolitis. There is no treatment.

ACUTE RESPIRATORY DISTRESS SYNDROME OF FEEDLOT CATTLE

An acute respiratory distress syndrome has been described in feedlot cattle with clinical signs and pathologic findings of an atypical interstitial pneumonia. The syndrome occurs sporadically, and the etiology remains undefined. Feedlot heifers seem to be at higher risk of developing the disease than feedlot steers. Bovine respiratory syncytial virus, abnormal production of 3-methylindole in the rumen, dusty conditions, and preexisting lesions of chronic cranioventral bacterial pneumonia have been suggested as causes or contributing factors. Clinical signs include respiratory distress characterized by tachypnea and dyspnea, and affected cattle may be found dead if clinical signs are unobserved. Lesions are those of atypical interstitial pneumonia with prominent emphysema and edema in the lungs. Treatment protocols have not been defined; thus, treatment is symptomatic and supportive. In many cases, emergency slaughter is the most economical option. Management strategies suggested include vaccinating for bovine respiratory syncytial virus, controlling dust in the feedlot, and avoiding abrupt dietary changes.

4-IPOMEANOL TOXICITY (MOLDY SWEET POTATO) AND *PERILLA* KETONE TOXICITY (PURPLE MINT TOXICITY)

Clinicopathologic syndromes indistinguishable from acute bovine pulmonary emphysema and edema (ABPEE, *see* p 1439) occur after ingestion of either moldy sweet potatoes infested with *Fusarium solani*, or the wild mint *Perilla frutescens*. Moldy sweet potato toxicity is caused by the ingestion of a furanoterpenoid toxin produced by sweet potatoes (*Ipomoea batatus*) in response to infestation with the fungus *F solani*; the end result is production of the pneumotoxin 4-ipomeanol. *Perilla* ketone toxicity is caused by ingestion of the leaves and seeds of the plant *P frutescens* (purple mint), which contains a pneumotoxin and is found in the southeastern USA. The pathogeneses of both these conditions are similar to that of ABPEE, as is approach to treatment.

TOXIC GASES

Nitrogen dioxide is a major component of silo gas; in people, the disease associated with exposure to NO_2 is termed silo filler's disease. Exposure of cattle results in respiratory distress and necropsy findings of atypical interstitial pneumonia. Treatment is empirical and includes diuretics, corticosteroids, and antibiotics to prevent pneumonia.

Zinc oxide is produced during oxyacetylene cutting or arc welding of galvanized pipes. These activities in closed facilities in which cattle are housed may result in toxicity characterized by respiratory distress. Lesions are similar to those described for atypical interstitial pneumonia. Treatment is as described for nitrogen dioxide toxicity.

VENA CAVAL THROMBOSIS AND METASTATIC PNEUMONIA

Etiology: Vena caval thrombosis and metastatic pneumonia is associated with multifocal abscesses in the lung as the result of septic embolism of the pulmonary arterial vascular system arising from septic thrombi in the caudal vena cava. The most common cause of vena caval thrombosis is ruminal acidosis leading to rumenitis and subsequent liver abscessation, which may result in a thrombus in the caudal vena cava if the vessel wall is infiltrated by the abscess. Bacteria most frequently involved include *Fusobacterium necrophorum*, *Trueperella pyogenes*, staphylococci, streptococci, and *Escherichia coli*.

Clinical Findings: The condition usually occurs in adult dairy cattle or in feedlot cattle on high-carbohydrate diets. Presenting signs can be acute, manifested by respiratory distress, or chronic, manifested by weight loss and chronic coughing. A common presentation is tachypnea, tachycardia, hemic murmurs, coughing, pale mucous membranes, increased lung sounds, hemoptysis, and epistaxis. Pyrexia and melena may also be present. The case fatality rate is essentially 100%.

Lesions: A thrombus is found in the vena cava, and hepatic abscesses may be noted. A suppurative pneumonia is present with pulmonary abscesses, aneurysms, and blood clots from ruptured aneurysms found throughout the entire lung parenchyma. The generalized distribution of these lesions caused by hematogenous spread is characteristic of this condition.

Treatment and Control: Because of the poor prognosis, treatment is not indicated. If attempted, treatment includes antibiotics and supportive therapy. Control efforts should focus on reducing the incidence of ruminal acidosis, which can result in rumenitis and subsequent formation of liver abscesses.

RESPIRATORY DISEASES OF HORSES

Viral respiratory infections are common in horses; the most notable are equine herpesvirus infection, equine influenza, and equine viral arteritis. The clinical manifestations are similar and include pyrexia, serous nasal discharge, submandibular lymphadenopathy, anorexia, and cough. In addition to respiratory disease, equine herpesvirus type 1 (EHV-1) can cause abortion and neurologic disease, and equine herpesvirus type 5 (EHV-5) is a newly recognized cause of multinodular pulmonary fibrosis. Equine viral arteritis produces respiratory disease, vasculitis, and abortion. Equine herpesvirus type 2 (EHV-2), equine rhinitis virus, and reovirus are ubiquitous viral respiratory pathogens, and infection results in minimal clinical disease. Adenovirus pneumonia is most often seen in association with severe combined immunodeficiency in Arabian foals. Hendra virus (*see* p 1448) is a zoonotic disease of horses identified in Australia; it is rapidly fatal in horses, and close contact is necessary for disease transmission.

Secondary bacterial respiratory infections are primarily initiated by viral disease, because viral respiratory infections impair and/or destroy respiratory defense mechanisms (ie, influenza destroys the mucociliary apparatus, EHV destroys bronchial-associated lymphoid tissue). The most common organisms associated with pneumonia in horses are opportunistic bacteria originating from the resident microflora of the upper respiratory tract. Clinical evidence of a secondary bacterial infection includes mucopurulent nasal discharge, depression, persistent fever, abnormal lung sounds, hyperfibrinogenemia, and leukocytosis. Secondary bacterial disease may result in mucosal bacterial infections (rhinitis and tracheitis) or may produce more serious invasive disease such as pneumonia and pleuropneumonia. *Streptococcus equi zooepidemicus* is the most common opportunistic pathogen of the equine lung, although *Actinobacillus equuli*, *Bordetella bronchiseptica*, *Escherichia coli*, *Pasteurella* spp, and *Pseudomonas aeruginosa* are frequently isolated. *S equi equi*, the causative agent of strangles (*see* p 1453), is a primary bacterial pathogen of the upper respiratory tract and is capable of mucosal invasion without predisposing factors. *Rhodococcus equi* is a primary pathogen of the lower respiratory tract of foals and produces pulmonary consolidation and abscessation. *R equi* pneumonia has been reported in adult horses with a compromised immune system.

Noninfectious respiratory disease is a common, performance-limiting condition that affects adult horses of various ages. **Inflammatory airway disease** is characterized by excessive tracheal mucus, airway hyperreactivity, and poor exercise performance in young horses. The etiology is unclear, but viral respiratory infection (EHV-2), allergy, and environmental factors may play a role in the pathophysiology. **Reactive airway disease (heaves)** is triggered by exposure to organic dusts in older horses with a genetic predisposition to allergic airway disease. Small airways are obstructed by bronchoconstriction and excessive mucus production. The severity of clinical signs ranges from exercise intolerance to dyspnea at rest.

The respiratory system is one of the most accessible body systems to test diagnostically. Endoscopic examination allows direct visualization of the upper respiratory tract, guttural pouches, trachea, and mainstem bronchi. Indications for endoscopic examination include upper airway noise, inspiratory difficulty, poor exercise performance, and unilateral or bilateral nasal discharge. Radiographs of the skull are indicated to investigate facial deformity, abnormalities of the sinus (sinusitis, dental abnormalities, and sinus cyst), guttural pouch (empyema, tympany), and soft-tissue structures (epiglottis, soft palate). The most important techniques for evaluation of lower respiratory tract secretions are transtracheal wash and bronchoalveolar lavage. Transtracheal wash is indicated to obtain secretions for bacterial and fungal culture of the lower respiratory tract. Bronchoalveolar lavage is indicated for cytologic evaluation of the lower respiratory tract in animals with diffuse, noninfectious pulmonary disease. Nasal swab culture is inappropriate for investigation of pulmonary infectious disease but is indicated for horses with suspected strangles infection.

Thoracic radiography and ultrasonography are valuable for assessing lower respiratory tract disease. Thoracic radiography is used to identify abnormalities of the pulmonary parenchyma, mediastinum, and diaphragm. Pulmonary consolidation (pneumonia), peribronchial disease, pulmonary abscessation, interstitial disease, and mediastinal masses (neoplasia, abscess, granuloma) are most easily identified via thoracic radiography. Thoracic ultrasonography is the most appropriate technique to evaluate fluid in the pleural space, peripheral pulmonary consolidation, and peripheral pulmonary abscessation. Ultrasonographic examination can identify the volume, location, and character of pleural fluid or air within the pleural space (pneumothorax). Additionally, it can identify fibrin tags, gas echoes (anaerobic infection), masses, and loculated fluid pockets, and it allows the clinician to determine the most appropriate site for centesis and to formulate a prognosis.

Pleurocentesis is performed in animals with accumulation of fluid in the pleural space and should be conducted with ultrasonographic guidance. Lung biopsy and fine-needle aspiration are invasive procedures and performed only after other diagnostic procedures have been exhausted. Pulmonary neoplasia, pulmonary fibrosis, and interstitial diseases may require lung biopsy to obtain a definitive diagnosis.

Vaccination does not always prevent respiratory infections in horses, but duration and severity is usually lessened in horses that have been vaccinated regularly, depending on factors such as the disease and specific vaccine. Vaccines are commercially available for equine influenza, viral rhinopneumonitis, equine viral arteritis, and strangles. The cost and hazards of each vaccination must be weighed against the probability of exposure and potential disease. Vaccination recommendations and schedules vary according to use of the horse and its potential for exposure to contagious animals. The American Association of Equine Practitioners (AAEP) Infectious Disease Committee has developed guidelines for all core and risk-based equine vaccinations; recommendations are posted on the AAEP Web site.

Regardless of the type of respiratory disease, environmental factors and supportive care are important to aid recovery. A dust and ammonia-free stable environment prevents further damage to the mucociliary apparatus. Highly palatable feeds are indicated to prevent weight loss and debilitation during the treatment and recovery period. Adequate hydration will decrease the viscosity of respiratory secretions, facilitating their removal from the lower respiratory tract. A comfortable, dry, temperature-appropriate environment will allow the horse to rest and minimize the role of the respiratory tract in thermoregulation.

EQUINE HERPESVIRUS INFECTION

(Equine viral rhinopneumonitis, Equine abortion virus)

Etiology and Epidemiology: Equine herpesvirus 1 (EHV-1) and equine herpesvirus 4 (EHV-4) comprise two antigenically distinct groups of viruses previously referred to as subtypes 1 and 2 of EHV-1. Both viruses are ubiquitous in horse populations worldwide and produce an acute febrile respiratory disease upon primary infection, characterized by rhinopharyngitis and tracheobronchitis. Outbreaks of respiratory disease occur annually among foals in areas with concentrated horse populations. Most of these outbreaks in weanlings are caused by strains of EHV-4. The age, seasonal, and geographic distributions vary and are determined by immune status and horse population. In individual horses, the outcome of exposure is determined by viral strain, immune status, pregnancy status, and possibly age. Infection of pregnant mares with EHV-4 rarely results in abortion.

Mares may abort several weeks to months after clinical or subclinical infection with EHV-1. The neurologic form of EHV-1 has demonstrated increasing morbidity and mortality in the documented outbreaks since 2000 and appears to be evolving in virulence and behavior. Therefore, the USDA has designated neuropathic EHV-1 as a potentially emerging disease. The natural reservoir of both EHV-1 and EHV-4 is the horse. Latent infections and carrier states are seen with both virus types. Transmission occurs by direct or indirect contact with infectious nasal secretions, aborted fetuses, placentas, or placental fluids.

Clinical Findings: The incubation period of EHV is 2–10 days. Susceptible horses develop fever of 102°–107°F (38.9°–41.7°C), neutropenia and lymphopenia, serous nasal discharge, malaise, pharyngitis, cough, inappetence, and/or submandibular or retropharyngeal lymphadenopathy. Horses infected with EHV-1 strains often develop a biphasic fever, with cell-associated viremia coinciding with the second temperature peak. Secondary bacterial infections are common and manifest with mucopurulent nasal exudate and pulmonary disease. The infection is mild or inapparent in horses immunologically sensitized to the virus.

Mares that abort after EHV-1 infection seldom display premonitory signs. Abortions occur 2–12 wk after infection, usually between months 7 and 11 of gestation. Aborted fetuses are fresh or minimally autolyzed, and the placenta is expelled shortly after abortion. There is no evidence of damage to the mare's reproductive tract, and subsequent conception is unimpaired. Mares exposed late in gestation may not abort but give birth to live foals with fulminating viral pneumonitis. Such foals are susceptible to secondary bacterial infections and usually die within hours or days.

Outbreaks with specific strains of EHV-1 infection result in neurologic disease (*see* p 1245). Clinical signs vary from mild incoordination and posterior paresis to severe posterior paralysis with recumbency, loss of bladder and tail function, and loss of skin sensation in the perineal and inguinal areas. In exceptional cases, the paralysis may progress to quadriplegia and death. Prognosis depends on severity of signs and the period of recumbency.

Lesions: The pathogenetic mechanisms of EHV-1 and EHV-4 differ significantly. EHV-4 infection is restricted to respiratory tract epithelium and associated lymph nodes; EHV-1 strains develop cell-associated viremia and have a predilection for vascular endothelium, especially the nasal mucosa, lungs, placenta, adrenal, thyroid, and CNS. The neuropathic strain of EHV-1 produces a viremic load 10- to 100-fold higher than that of non-neuropathic strains.

Gross lesions of viral rhinopneumonitis are hyperemia and ulceration of the respiratory epithelium, and multiple, tiny, plum-colored foci in the lungs. Histologically, there is evidence of inflammation, necrosis, and intranuclear inclusions in the respiratory epithelium and germinal centers of the associated lymph nodes. Lung lesions are characterized by neutrophilic infiltration of the terminal bronchioles, peribronchiolar and perivascular mononuclear cell infiltration, and serofibrinous exudate in the alveoli.

Typical lesions in EHV-1 abortion include interlobular lung edema and pleural fluid; multifocal areas of hepatic necrosis; petechiation of the myocardium, adrenal gland, and spleen; and thymic necrosis. Intranuclear inclusions are found in lung, liver, adrenal, and lymphoreticular tissues.

Horses with EHV-1–associated neurologic disease may have no gross lesions or only minimal evidence of hemorrhage in the meninges, brain, and spinal cord parenchyma. Histologically, lesions are discrete and comprise vasculitis with endothelial cell damage and perivascular cuffing, thrombus formation and hemorrhage, and in advanced cases, areas of malacia. Lesions may occur at any level of the brain or spinal cord.

Diagnosis: Equine viral rhinopneumonitis is difficult to clinically differentiate from equine influenza (*see* p 1447), equine viral arteritis (*see* p 701), or other equine respiratory infections solely on the basis of clinical signs. Definitive diagnosis is determined by PCR or virus isolation from samples obtained via nasopharyngeal swab and citrated blood sample (buffy coat) early in the course of the infection.

In cases of suspected EHV-1 abortion, definitive diagnosis is based on PCR, virus isolation, and characteristic gross and microscopic lesions in the aborted fetus. Lung, liver, adrenal, and lymphoreticular tissues are productive sources of virus. Serologic testing of mares after abortion has little diagnostic value. Diagnosis of neuropathic EHV-1 is determined by real-time PCR on samples obtained from nasal secretions, CSF, or neural tissue to detect the neuropathic strain of EHV-1. A presumptive diagnosis can be based on clinical signs and CSF analysis (xanthochromia, albuminocytologic dissociation). Necropsy reveals characteristic perivascular cuffing and hemorrhage in the CNS.

Treatment: There is no specific treatment for EHV infection. Rest and nursing care are indicated to minimize secondary bacterial complications. Antipyretics are recommended for horses with a fever >104°F (40°C). Antibiotic therapy is instituted upon suspicion of secondary bacterial infection evidenced by purulent nasal discharge or pulmonary disease. Most foals infected prenatally with EHV-1 die shortly after birth despite intensive nursing and antimicrobial medication. If horses with neuropathic EHV-1 remain ambulatory or are recumbent for only 2–3 days, the prognosis is usually favorable. Valacyclovir (30 mg/kg, PO, bid) has shown promise in the treatment of affected horses and in prophylaxis during EHV-1 outbreaks. Intensive nursing care is necessary to avoid pulmonary congestion, pneumonia, ruptured bladder, or bowel atony. Recovery may be complete, but a small percentage of cases have neurologic sequelae.

Control: Immunity after natural infection with either EHV-1 or EHV-4 involves a combination of humoral and cellular immunity. Whereas little cross-protection occurs between virus types after primary infection of immunologically naive foals, significant cross-protection develops in horses after repeated infections with a particular virus type. Most adult horses are latently infected with EHV-1 and EHV-4. The infection remains dormant for most of the horse's life, although stress or immunosuppression may result in recrudescence of disease and shedding of infectious virus. Immunity to reinfection of the respiratory tract may persist for as long as 3 mo, but multiple infections result in a level of immunity that prevents clinical signs of respiratory disease. Diminished resistance in pregnant mares allows cell-associated viremia, which may result in transplacental infection of the fetus.

For prevention and control of EHV-4– and EHV-1–related diseases, management practices that reduce viral spread are recommended. New horses (or those returning from other premises) should be isolated for 21 days before commingling with resident horses, especially pregnant mares. Management-related, stress-inducing circumstances should be avoided to prevent recrudescence of latent virus. Pregnant mares should be maintained in a group away from the weanlings, yearlings, and horses out of training. In an outbreak of respiratory disease or abortion, affected horses should be isolated and appropriate measures taken for disinfection of contaminated premises. No horse should leave the premises for 3 wk after recovery of the last clinical case.

Vaccination (EHV-4 and EHV-1) should begin when foals are 4–6 mo old. A second dose is given 4–6 wk later, and a third dose at 10–12 mo of age. Booster vaccinations may be indicated as often as every 6 mo through maturity (5 yr of age). Vaccination programs against herpesviruses should include all horses that travel to high-risk destinations (racetrack, show grounds) and all other horses on the premises. A high-antigen load, inactivated EHV-1 vaccine is recommended to prevent EHV-1 abortion. Vaccine should be administered during months 3, 5, 7, and 9 of pregnancy. Mares are often vaccinated with inactivated EHV-1/EHV-4 at an interval 4–6 wk before foaling. A modified-live EHV-1 vaccine is available to help prevent respiratory disease caused by EHV-1.

Infection by other Herpesviruses: Equine herpesvirus 2 (EHV-2) is ubiquitous in respiratory mucosa, conjunctiva, and WBCs of normal horses of all ages. The pathogenic significance remains obscure. It has been suggested that EHV-2 is the cause of herpetic keratoconjunctivitis and inflammatory airway disease in young horses. Equine herpesvirus 3 (EHV-3) is the cause of equine coital exanthema (*see* p 1357), a benign, progenital exanthematous disease.

Equine gamma herpesvirus 5 (EHV-5) has emerged as the pathogen associated with equine multinodular pulmonary fibrosis (EMPF). The role of EHV-5 in EMPF is unclear (precipitating, causative, incidental). Clinical signs include weight loss, cough, fever (variable), and respiratory difficulty. EMPF is seen primarily in middle-aged horses, although it has been reported in young horses. Physical examination findings include tachycardia, tachypnea, increased respiratory effort (inspiratory), and poor body condition. Wheezes and crackles are often ausculted without a rebreathing procedure. In early cases, EMPF may be mistaken as heaves. In addition to EMPF, EHV-5 has been associated with lymphoproliferative disease and lymphoma. One unusual case report describes a 21-yr-old horse with profound pancytopenia and pulmonary fibrosis; EHV-5 was isolated from the bone marrow of this horse.

Diagnostic testing includes routine blood work, thoracic radiographs, and virus-specific PCR testing on pulmonary secretions (bronchoalveolar lavage) or percutaneous lung biopsy sample. CBC reveals neutrophilic leukocytosis with or without hyperfibrinogenemia and anemia. Findings on thoracic radiographics range from a moderate interstitial pattern to a severe reticulonodular pattern. Differential diagnoses of radiographic images include fungal pneumonia and metastatic neoplasia. Fungal pneumonia typically occurs after primary GI disease with neutropenia, and metastatic neoplasia is rare. The most common antemortem diagnostic test is virus-specific PCR of bronchoalveolar lavage fluid. Percutaneous, ultrasound-guided lung biopsy can be performed to confirm the diagnosis and establish a prognosis. The procedure is not without risk in dyspneic horses. Histopathology reveals multifocal granulomas, type II pneumocyte hyperplasia, and intraluminal cellular accumulation. Advanced pulmonary fibrosis indicates a poor prognosis for survival.

The prognosis for survival is ~50%. Horses with granulomatous inflammation have been successfully treated with antiviral therapy. Valacyclovir (30 mg/kg, PO, tid) and/or acyclovir (10 mg/kg, IV, in 1 L of isotonic crystalloid fluid as a constant-rate infusion over 1 hr, bid × 2 days) appear promising, although sensitivity of the virus to these medications has not been documented. Doxycycline (5-10 mg/kg, PO, once to twice daily) is administered to combat secondary bacterial infection and for its anti-inflammatory properties. Administration of corticosteroids is controversial, although they are commonly used. Corticosteroids (0.08-0.1 mg/kg, IV, every 24–48 hr) may improve disease outcome through reduction of pulmonary cytokines and inflammatory mediators, but they may also cause immunosuppression, which may enhance viral replication and disease severity.

EQUINE INFLUENZA

Etiology and Epidemiology: Equine influenza is highly contagious and spreads rapidly among naive horses. Horses 1–5 yr old are the most susceptible to infection. Orthomyxovirus A/equine-2 was first recognized in 1963 as a cause of widespread epidemics and has subsequently become endemic in many countries, except for New Zealand and Iceland. China, Japan, and Australia experienced devastating epidemics of equine influenza affecting tens of thousands of horses in 2007. Equine influenza had not been reported in China since 1993, in Japan since 1972, and had never been reported in Australia.

Endemicity is maintained by sporadic clinical cases and by inapparent infection in susceptible horses introduced into the population by birth, through waning immunity, or after movement from other areas or countries. A carrier state is not recognized for equine influenza. The clinical outcome after viral exposure largely depends on immune status; clinical disease varies from a mild, inapparent infection to severe disease in susceptible animals. Influenza is rarely fatal except in donkeys, zebras, and debilitated horses. Transmission occurs by inhalation of respiratory secretions. Epidemics arise when one or more acutely infected horses are introduced into a susceptible group. The epidemiologic outcome depends on the antigenic characteristics of the circulating virus and the immune status of a given population of horses at time of exposure. Frequent natural exposure or regular vaccination may contribute to the degree of antigenic drift seen with specific strains of A/equine-2 virus in some parts of the world.

Clinical Findings and Lesions: The incubation period of influenza is ~1–3 days. Clinical signs begin abruptly and include high fever (up to 106°F [41.1°C]), serous nasal discharge, submandibular lymphadenopathy, and coughing that is dry, harsh, and nonproductive. Depression, anorexia, and weakness are frequently seen. Clinical signs usually last <3 days in uncomplicated cases. Influenza virus replicates within respiratory epithelial cells, resulting in destruction of tracheal and bronchial epithelium and cilia. Cough develops early in the course of infection and may persist for several weeks. Nasal discharge, although scant and serous initially, may become mucopurulent due to secondary bacterial infection. Mildly affected horses recover uneventfully in 2–3 wk; severely affected horses may convalesce as long as 6 mo. Recovery may be hastened by complete restriction of strenuous physical activity. Respiratory tract epithelium takes ~21 days to regenerate; during this time, horses are susceptible to development of secondary bacterial complications such as pneumonia, pleuropneumonia, and chronic bronchitis. Complications are minimized by restricting exercise, controlling dust, providing superior ventilation, and practicing good stable hygiene. Primary complications of vasculitis, myositis, and myocarditis are seen infrequently.

Diagnosis: The presence of a rapidly spreading respiratory infection in a group of horses characterized by rapid onset, high fever, depression, and cough is presumptive evidence of equine influenza. Definitive diagnosis can be determined by virus isolation, influenza A antigen detection (patient-side kit), or paired serum samples (hemagglutination inhibition). Nasopharyngeal swabs are obtained for virus isolation and antigen detection. These samples should be obtained soon after the onset of illness. Virus isolation in chick embryos is highly specific but less sensitive for detection of influenza because of bacterial contamination of the sample. Antigen detection is performed using a human influenza A kit, which provides immediate results that are not affected by bacterial contamination.

Treatment and Prevention: Horses that do not develop complications require rest and supportive care. Horses should be rested 1 wk for every day of fever, with a minimum of 3 wk rest (to allow regeneration of the mucociliary apparatus). NSAIDs are recommended for horses with a fever >104°F (40°C). Antibiotics are indicated when fever persists beyond 3–4 days or when purulent nasal discharge or pneumonia is present.

Prevention of influenza requires hygienic management practices and vaccination. Exposure can be reduced by isolation of newly introduced horses for 2 wk. Numerous vaccines are commercially available for prevention of equine influenza. An intranasal modified-live influenza vaccine, designed to induce mucosal (local) antibody protection, has demonstrated protection against natural challenge. This vaccine is temperature sensitive and is not capable of replicating beyond the nasal passages (ie, inactivated by core body temperature). Most commercially available influenza vaccines are inactivated, adjuvanted vaccines recommended primarily for IM administration. A recombinant canarypox-vectored influenza vaccine has also been shown to be effective against influenza challenge. Because the duration of protection provided by current vaccines is limited, booster injections for at-risk adult horses should be administered every 6 mo. Sedentary horses can be vaccinated annually. Foals should be vaccinated with a single modified-live intranasal vaccine or a series of three inactivated vaccines beginning at 6 mo, with booster vaccination in 3–6 wk and again between 10 and 12 mo of age. Broodmares should be vaccinated 4–6 wk before foaling.

EQUINE VIRAL ARTERITIS

Equine viral arteritis (EVA) is caused by an RNA togavirus and produces clinical signs of respiratory disease, vasculitis, and abortion. Horses with EVA infection present with fever, anorexia, and depression. The clinical signs of respiratory infection due to EVA are serous nasal discharge, cough, conjunctivitis, lacrimation, and palpebral, scrotal, and periorbital edema. Clinical signs of disease persist for 2–9 days. Treatment consists of supportive care (support bandages) and NSAIDs for fever and inflammation. Antimicrobial therapy is usually unnecessary. A carrier state occurs in most stallions after natural infection and is primarily responsible for persistence of the virus in the horse population through infectious seminal fluids. Vaccination (modified-live virus) is targeted toward prevention of venereal spread of EVA in breeding animals as opposed to prevention of respiratory disease (*see* p 701).

HENDRA VIRUS INFECTION

(Equine morbillivirus)

Hendra virus (HeV) is the prototype species of a new genus *Henipavirus* within the subfamily Paramyxovirinae and was first identified in Australia in 1994. The viral agent is endemic in specific species of fruit bats (also called flying foxes), and close contact with these bats is suspected to have facilitated transfer of the HeV to horses. Horses are infected by oronasal routes and excrete HeV in urine, saliva, and respiratory secretions.

There have been multiple, sporadic incidents of human and equine disease in Australia occurring in 1994, 1995, 1999, 2004, 2008, and 2009. The case fatality rate in horses and people is high, with reports of 81 horses and 4 people succumbing to Hendra virus infection, including an equine veterinarian investigating an outbreak.

Very close contact is required to transmit the virus among horses and from horses to people, and the virus is not considered highly contagious. Equine veterinarians are considered at occupational risk of contracting HeV. Infected horses develop severe and often fatal respiratory disease, characterized by dyspnea, vascular endothelial damage, and pulmonary edema. Depression, anorexia, fever, respiratory difficulty, ataxia, tachycardia, and frothy, nasal discharge are common clinical signs. (*See also* p 707.) A commercial HeV vaccine for use in horses is available under a Minor Use Permit for release to veterinarians who have completed an online training program. Horses must have a microchip to be vaccinated, and the information must be entered into the HeV Vaccine National Online Registry. The vaccine consists of soluble forms of G glycoprotein of HeV; it does not contain modified or inactivated virus.

PLEUROPNEUMONIA

(Pleuritis, Pleurisy)

Pleuropneumonia is defined as infection of the lungs and pleural space. In most instances, pleural infection develops secondary to bacterial pneumonia or penetrating thoracic wounds. Spontaneous pleuritis (without accompanying pneumonia) is uncommon in horses. In the USA, ~70% of horses with pleural effusion have pleuropneumonia. The primary differential diagnoses for pleural effusion are neoplastic effusions, heart failure, and hydatidosis.

Etiology and Pathogenesis: Viral respiratory infection, long-distance transportation, general anesthesia, and strenuous exercise are common predisposing factors that impair pulmonary defense mechanisms, allowing secondary bacterial invasion. Head restraint results in bacterial contamination and multiplication within the lower respiratory tract within 12–24 hr and may be the single most important predisposing factor for development of pneumonia associated with long-distance transport. Race and sport horses are particularly at risk. Most horses with pleuropneumonia are athletic horses <5 yr old. Exercise-induced pulmonary hemorrhage may contribute to development of respiratory infection by providing a favorable environment for bacterial replication. Acute pulmonary infarction can be the inciting event for equine pleuropneumonia.

Polymicrobial and mixed anaerobic-aerobic infections are common in horses with pleuropneumonia, with more than one organism isolated from transtracheal aspirates. The most common aerobic organisms are *Streptococcus equi zooepidemicus*, *Escherichia coli*, *Actinobacillus* spp, *Klebsiella* spp, *Enterobacter* spp, *Staphylococcus aureus*, and *Pasteurella* spp. Anaerobic bacteria are isolated from 40%–70% of horses with pleuropneumonia; *Bacteroides* spp, *Clostridium* spp, *Peptostreptococcus* spp, and *Fusobacterium* spp are the most common. The etiology of pleural infection in horses is usually bacterial, although *Mycoplasma felis* and nocardial agents have been isolated from pleural effusions.

Clinical Findings and Lesions: Horses with pleuropneumonia present with fever, depression, lethargy, and inappetence. Clinical signs specific to pleuropneumonia include pleural pain (pleurodynia) evident as short strides, guarding, and flinching on percussion of the chest; shallow respiration; and endotoxemia. Horses with pleural pain have an anxious facial expression; stand with their elbows abducted; and are reluctant to move, cough, or lie down. Gait may be stiff or stilted, and some horses grunt in response to thoracic pressure, auscultation, or percussion. Nasal discharge is a variable sign. Putrid breath or fetid nasal discharge indicates anaerobic bacterial infection and necrotic pulmonary tissue. The respiratory pattern is characterized by rapid, shallow respiration due to pleural pain and restricted pulmonary expansion from pleural effusion. A plaque of sternal edema is seen in horses with a large volume of pleural effusion. Horses with toxemia have injected mucous membranes, delayed capillary refill time (>2 sec), and tachycardia. Auscultation reveals a lack of breath sounds in the ventral lung fields and abnormal lung sounds (often crackles) in dorsal lung fields. Cardiac sounds may be muffled or absent or may radiate over a wider area. Although uncommon, pleural friction rubs are most prominent at end-inspiration and early expiration and are detected after thoracic drainage.

Diagnosis: In horses with peracute pleuropneumonia, laboratory findings reflect bacterial sepsis or toxemia and include abnormalities such as leukopenia, neutropenia, left shift, hemoconcentration, and azotemia. Horses with more stable disease have leukocytosis, mature neutrophilia, hyperfibrinogenemia, hyperglobulinemia (chronic antigenic stimulation), hypoalbuminemia (loss in pleural space), and anemia of chronic disease.

Thoracic ultrasonography is ideal for investigation of pleural effusion and is indicated in horses with regions of poor to absent breath sounds, thoracic pain, and/or dull thoracic percussion. Transudative pleural fluid (neoplastic effusion) appears anechoic, whereas more cellular exudate appears echogenic. Gas echoes represent small air bubbles within pleural fluid, which may indicate an anaerobic pleural infection, a bronchopleural fistula, or iatrogenic introduction of air. Pulmonary atelectasis, consolidation, and abscessation can be identified if the lesions are located in peripheral lung fields. Ultrasonographic evidence of a large area of pulmonary consolidation, in conjunction with serosanguineous suppurative pleural effusion, is consistent with pulmonary infarction and necrotizing pneumonia. Adhesions of the visceral to parietal pleura can be visualized using thoracic ultrasonography, and these regions should be avoided during thoracocentesis.

Ultrasonography should be performed before pleurocentesis to determine the best site for maximal drainage and to avoid cardiac or diaphragmatic puncture. Thoracocentesis is performed for diagnostic and therapeutic purposes in horses with pleuropneumonia. Pleural fluid should be drained relatively slowly to avoid hypotension. The hemithorax that appears to contain the most fluid is drained first. Bilateral thoracocentesis is usually necessary. The chest tube may be removed immediately after drainage of the thoracic cavity or may be secured in place to allow continual drainage. Thoracic radiography is indicated after pleurocentesis to evaluate pulmonary parenchymal lesions, mediastinal structures, and the presence/severity of pneumothorax.

Gross examination of pleural fluid includes evaluation of color, odor, volume, and turbidity. Malodorous pleural fluid is associated with necrotic tissue and anaerobic infection and indicates a guarded prognosis. Cytologic evaluation of septic pleural fluid reveals purulent exudate (>90% neutrophils) with increased cellularity (25,000–200,000 cells/μL) and increased total protein (>3 g/dL). Intracellular and extracellular bacteria may be seen, and Gram stain examination is used to direct initial antimicrobial therapy. Bacterial culture and sensitivity should also be performed on transtracheal aspirate samples, which yield positive bacterial cultures more frequently than pleural fluid samples.

Treatment: Management of horses with pleuropneumonia includes daily ultrasound examination to monitor fluid production, evaluate effective drainage, identify isolated fluid pockets, and assess peripheral pulmonary disease. The volume and character of pleural fluid will determine whether single, intermittent, or continual drainage is indicated. Continual drainage is preferable in cases with fibrinous, cellular, malodorous, and/or large volume of effusion. A one-way (Heimlich) valve allows constant drainage of pleural fluid with minimal risk of development of pneumothorax. An indwelling chest tube should remain in place as long as drainage is productive. Medical therapy includes broad-spectrum antibiotics, NSAIDs, analgesics, and supportive care. Broad-spectrum antimicrobial therapy targeting common aerobic and anaerobic bacteria (eg, penicillin, gentamicin, metronidazole) should be instituted pending results of culture and sensitivity. Intrathoracic fibrinolytic therapy has been reported to reduce fibrin deposition and pleural fluid accumulation. In some horses, the pleural infection does not resolve despite weeks to months of antimicrobial therapy and drainage via indwelling chest tubes. Thoracostomy allows manual removal of organized fibrinous material and necrotic lung; however, this technique should be limited to horses with chronic, stable, unilateral disease with resolving infection in the contralateral hemithorax.

Complications associated with pleuropneumonia include thrombophlebitis, laminitis, bronchopleural fistula, pulmonary abscess, and cranial thoracic mass.

The prognosis for horses with pleuropneumonia has greatly improved throughout the past 20 yr because of early recognition, advancements in diagnostic testing, and aggressive therapy. The survival rate is reported to be as high as 90% by some investigators, with a 60% chance of return to athletic performance. The duration of hospitalization is not indicative of outcome; however, a delay in initiation of appropriate therapy by >48 hr promotes development of anaerobic infection and, ultimately, poor response to treatment. Placement of an indwelling chest tube does not limit the prognosis for return to athletic function.

Horses with hemorrhagic necrotizing pneumonia respond poorly to conventional therapy and have a low survival rate.

RHODOCOCCUS EQUI PNEUMONIA

Rhodococcus equi is the most serious cause of pneumonia in foals 1–4 mo old. It is not the most common cause of pneumonia in this age group; however, it has significant economic consequences because of mortality, prolonged treatment, surveillance programs for early detection, and relatively expensive prophylactic strategies. Clinical disease is rare in horses >8 mo old. Compelling epidemiologic data indicate pulmonary infection probably originates within the first week of life. (*See also* p 679.)

Etiology and Pathogenesis: *R equi* is a gram-positive, facultative intracellular pathogen that is nearly ubiquitous in soil. Inhalation of dust particles laden with virulent *R equi* is the major route of pneumonic infection. Development of clinical disease is related to immunocompetency of individual foals; foals that produce little to no detectable γ interferon (IFN-γ) are at risk of developing pneumonia. Manure from pneumonic foals is a major source of virulent bacteria contaminating the environment. Foals with pulmonary infections swallow sputum laden with *R equi*, which readily replicates in their intestinal tract. The pathogenicity of *R equi* is linked to its ability to survive intracellularly, which hinges on failure of phagosome-lysosomal fusion in infected macrophages and failure of functional respiratory burst upon phagocytosis of *R equi*.

Clinical Findings and Lesions: *R equi* infection is slowly progressive, with acute to subacute clinical manifestations. Clinical signs of disease are difficult to detect until pulmonary infection reaches a critical mass, resulting in decompensation of the foal. Pulmonary lesions are relatively consistent and include subacute to chronic suppurative bronchopneumonia, pulmonary abscessation, and suppurative lymphadenitis. At the onset of clinical signs, most foals are lethargic, febrile, and tachypneic. Diarrhea is seen in one-third of foals with *R equi* pneumonia and may be caused by colonic microabscessation. Cough is a variable clinical sign; purulent nasal discharge is less common. Thoracic auscultation reveals crackles and wheezes with asymmetric/regional distribution. Pulmonary regions with marked consolidation lack breath sounds and exhibit dull resonance on thoracic percussion. In foals with subclinical infections, small to moderate-sized abscesses (<10 cm) may resolve spontaneously.

Immune-mediated polysynovitis (eg, stifle and hock effusion) is often seen in affected foals at presentation. Intestinal and mesenteric abscesses are the most common extrapulmonary sites of infection. Foals with abdominal involvement often present with fever, depression, anorexia, weight loss, colic, and diarrhea. Intestinal lesions are characterized by multifocal, ulcerative enterocolitis and typhlitis involving Peyer's patches with granulomatous or suppurative inflammation of the mesenteric and/or colonic lymph nodes. The prognosis for foals with abdominal forms of *R equi* is less favorable than for those with pulmonary disease. Septic physitis and osteomyelitis are less common extrapulmonary sites of infection. Vertebral osteomyelitis may result in pathologic vertebral fracture and spinal cord compression and is a devastating manifestation of *R equi* osteomyelitis. Panophthalmitis, guttural pouch empyema, sinusitis, pericarditis, nephritis, nonseptic uveitis, and hepatic and renal abscessation with *R equi* have been reported.

Diagnosis: Routine laboratory evaluation of CBC and serum chemistry reveals nonspecific abnormalities consistent with infection and inflammation. Neutrophilic leukocytosis and hyperfibrinogenemia are common, and the severity of these findings relates to prognosis. Thoracic radiographic evaluation may reveal a pattern of perihilar alveolization, consolidation, and abscessation. The presence of nodular lung lesions and mediastinal lymphadenopathy in foals 1–4 mo old is highly suggestive of *R equi*. Bacterial culture of transtracheal wash samples is required for definitive diagnosis. Cytologic evaluation of transtracheal wash samples reveals intracellular coccobacilli, indicating that appropriate antimicrobial therapy should be started pending culture results.

Treatment and Prognosis: The combination of erythromycin (25 mg/kg, PO, qid; esters or salts) and rifampin (5–10 mg/kg, PO, bid) has historically been the treatment of choice for *R equi* infection in foals. These antimicrobials may be bacteriostatic, but their activity is synergistic, and the combination has markedly improved survival of foals with *R equi* pneumonia. Rifampin is lipid soluble (able to penetrate abscess material) and is concentrated in phagocytic cells. Erythromycin is concentrated in granulocytes and alveolar macrophages; however, its antimicrobial activity is somewhat inhibited by intracellular pH. Adverse reactions are relatively common in foals treated with the erythromycin-rifampin combination. Diarrhea, idiosyncratic hyperthermia, tachypnea, anorexia, bruxism, and salivation can occur with erythromycin administration, and antimicrobial resistance of *R equi* to erythromycin-rifampin has been reported.

Clarithromycin is the macrolide of choice for foals with severe disease, given the most favorable minimum inhibitory concentration against *R equi* isolates obtained from pneumonic foals (90% of isolates are inhibited at 0.12, 0.25, and 1 mcg/mL for clarithromycin, erythromycin, and azithromycin, respectively). In foals with *R equi* pneumonia, the combination of clarithromycin (7.5 mg/kg, PO, bid) and rifampin is superior to erythromycin-rifampin and azithromycin-rifampin. Foals treated with clarithromycin-rifampin have improved survival rates and fewer febrile days than foals treated with erythromycin-rifampin and azithromycin-rifampin. Reported adverse events of clarithromycin-rifampin include diarrhea in treated foals. The duration of antimicrobial therapy typically is 3–8 wk.

Supportive therapy includes provision of a clean, comfortable environment and highly palatable, dust-free feeds. Judicial IV fluid therapy and saline nebulization facilitates expectoration of pulmonary exudates. NSAIDs should be administered as needed to maintain rectal temperature <103.5°F (39.7°C). Nasal insufflation with oxygen is necessary in foals with severe respiratory compromise. Bronchodilator therapy may or may not improve arterial oxygenation. Prophylactic antiulcer medication is indicated in foals stressed by respiratory difficulty, pain, frequent handling, hospitalization, and transportation.

The survival rate of *R equi* pneumonia is ~70%–90% with appropriate therapy. The case fatality rate without therapy (or with inappropriate antimicrobial therapy) is ~80%. Parameters for discontinuation of medical therapy include clinical signs, serum fibrinogen concentration, and radiographic resolution of pulmonary consolidation and abscessation. Life-threatening, antibiotic-induced enterocolitis, due to *Clostridium difficile*, has been seen in the dams of nursing foals treated with all macrolide preparations.

Prevention: There are several strategies to decrease the incidence of *R equi* pneumonia on endemic farms: early detection of clinical cases, enhanced passive immunity for neonatal foals, and enhanced nonspecific immunity for neonatal foals. Foals should be maintained in well-ventilated, dust-free areas, avoiding dirt paddocks and overcrowding. Pneumonic foals should be isolated and their manure composted. Herd surveillance programs for early detection of pneumonic foals on endemic farms include twice weekly physical examination and auscultation and monthly CBC and fibrinogen concentration. Foals with a WBC count >14,000 cells/μL should be further evaluated via ultrasonographic examination for *R equi*. Administration of hyperimmune plasma might reduce the incidence and severity of *R equi* within the herd, but it is not completely effective in preventing disease. Hyperimmune plasma (1 L) is administered IV within the first week of life, followed by a second liter at ~25 days of age. Foals with low IFN-γ production in the first month of life appear more susceptible to development of clinical disease. Administration of a nonspecific immunostimulant may enhance IFN-γ production and protect this susceptible population. Mass treatment of foals with subclinical infection has resulted in marcolide- and rifampin-resistant strains and should be avoided.

ACUTE BRONCHOINTERSTITIAL PNEUMONIA IN FOALS

Acute bronchointerstitial pneumonia is a sporadic, rapidly progressive disease of foals characterized by acute respiratory distress and high mortality.

Etiology, Epidemiology, and Pathogenesis: The etiology of acute bronchointerstitial pneumonia in foals is not clear. It may result from different insults rather than a single factor, initiate a cascade of events, and result in a final common response of severe pulmonary damage and acute respiratory distress. Warm weather (>85°F [29.4°C]) is a common epidemiologic factor. Many foals have a history of antimicrobial therapy when clinical signs developed. No virus is consistently isolated, and no bacterial agent has been consistently identified. Enteric gram-negative organisms, *Rhodococcus equi*, *Pseudomonas aeruginosa*, and *Pneumocystis jiroveci* have been cultured from the lungs of affected foals.

Clinical Findings and Lesions: The age of affected foals ranges from 1 wk to 8 mo. Acute bronchointerstitial pneumonia has an acute or peracute onset and is accompanied by high fever. The disease is rapidly progressive and may result in sudden death due to fulminant respiratory failure. Foals are unable or reluctant to move and are usually cyanotic. Severe respiratory distress is the most striking clinical sign. Clinicopathologic evaluation of foals with acute respiratory distress should include arterial blood gas, CBC, serum chemistry analysis, and thoracic radiographs. Hypoxemia, hypercapnea, and respiratory acidosis are consistent findings. These arterial blood gas findings quantify the severity of respiratory impairment and are used to monitor response to therapy. The hypoxemia of bronchointerstitial pneumonia is relatively resistant to supplemental oxygen therapy. Bronchointerstitial pneumonia is similar to bacterial pneumonia in that hyperfibrinogenemia and neutrophilic leukocytosis are seen in most foals.

Diagnosis: Physical examination and clinicopathologic findings may appear similar to those of foals with severe *R equi* pneumonia (*see* p 1451), and thoracic radiographic examination may be the most valuable diagnostic test to differentiate *R equi* pneumonia from bronchointerstitial pneumonia. Interstitial pneumonia appears as diffuse to caudodorsally distributed interstitial and bronchointerstitial pulmonary opacities. With advanced disease, the radiographic pattern progresses to include patches of a coalescing alveolar nodular pattern with air bronchograms. Transtracheal aspiration may be prohibitively dangerous to perform on a dyspneic foal but should be done when the foal becomes more stable to obtain samples for bacterial culture/sensitivity, cytologic evaluation, and virus isolation. Cytologic evaluation of tracheal aspirates reveals acute neutrophilic inflammation with or without evidence of sepsis. Bacterial organisms are often recovered from transtracheal aspiration samples or necropsy of foals with bronchointerstitial pneumonia; however, no single organism is consistently recovered.

Necropsy examination reveals diffusely enlarged lungs that fail to deflate upon opening of the thoracic cavity with rib impressions on the visceral pleural surface. The cut surface of lung is mottled, with dark red lung interspersed with more normal-appearing lung tissue and edematous separation of lobules. The most prominent histopathologic findings are severe, diffuse, necrotizing bronchiolitis, alveolar septal necrosis, and neutrophilic alveolitis. Surviving foals develop a proliferative epithelial and interstitial response, including bronchiolar and alveolar epithelial hyperplasia, type II cell hyperplasia, and hyaline membrane formation.

Treatment: Because the cause of bronchointerstitial pneumonia is unknown, therapy is symptomatic. Treatment includes anti-inflammatory therapy, broad-spectrum antibiotics, thermoregulatory control, bronchodilation, supplemental oxygen, and supportive care. Anti-inflammatory therapy with corticosteroids (eg, dexamethasone 0.1 mg/kg/day, IV) appears to improve survival. An alcohol bath, an air-conditioned stall, and/or a fan are used in conjunction with NSAIDs to maintain rectal temperature <103.5°F (39.7°C). The suitability of an antibiotic regimen appears to have little bearing on the outcome of bronchointerstitial pneumonia. Nonetheless, broad-spectrum antibiotic therapy should be instituted to treat existing or impending secondary bacterial infections. Additional supportive therapy includes provision of a clean, comfortable environment; highly palatable, dust-free feeds; and ulcer prophylaxis.

Prognosis: Although mortality is high, affected foals that receive aggressive medical care have a reasonably favorable prognosis for survival (70%). The longterm pulmonary consequences after recovery from bronchointerstitial pneumonia are variable, ranging from undetectable to persistent exercise intolerance.

STRANGLES

(Distemper)

Strangles is an infectious, contagious disease of Equidae characterized by abscessation of the lymphoid tissue of the upper respiratory tract. The causative organism, *Streptococcus equi equi*, is highly host-adapted and produces clinical disease only in horses, donkeys, and mules. It is a gram-positive, capsulated β-hemolytic Lancefield group C coccus, which is an obligate parasite and a primary pathogen.

Etiology and Pathogenesis: *S equi equi* is highly contagious and produces high morbidity and low mortality in susceptible populations. Transmission occurs via fomites and direct contact with infectious exudates. Carrier animals are important for

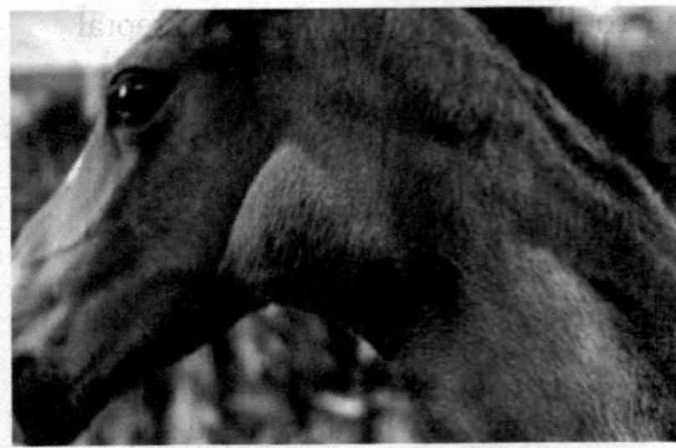

Strangles. *Courtesy of Dr. Thomas Lane.*

maintenance of the bacteria between epizootics and initiation of outbreaks on premises previously free of disease. Survival of the organism in the environment depends on temperature and humidity; it is susceptible to desiccation, extreme heat, and exposure to sunlight and must be protected within mucoid secretions to survive. Under ideal environmental circumstances, the organism can survive ~4 wk outside the host. Under field conditions, most organisms do not survive 96 hr.

Clinical Findings: The incubation period of strangles is 3–14 days, and the first sign of infection is fever (103°–106°F [39.4°–41.1°C]). Within 24–48 hr of the initial fever spike, the horse will exhibit signs typical of strangles, including mucoid to mucopurulent nasal discharge, depression, and submandibular lymphadenopathy. Horses with retropharyngeal lymph node involvement have difficulty swallowing, inspiratory respiratory noise (compression of the dorsal pharyngeal wall), and extended head and neck. Older animals with residual immunity may develop an atypical or catarrhal form of the disease with mucoid nasal discharge, cough, and mild fever. Metastatic strangles ("bastard strangles") is characterized by abscessation in other lymph nodes of the body, particularly the lymph nodes in the abdomen and, less frequently, the thorax. *S equi* is the most common cause of brain abscess in horses, albeit rare.

Diagnosis: Diagnosis is confirmed by bacterial culture of exudate from abscesses or nasal swab samples. CBC reveals neutrophilic leukocytosis and hyperfibrinogenemia. Serum biochemical analysis is typically unremarkable. Complicated cases may require endoscopic examination of the upper respiratory tract (including the guttural pouches), ultrasonographic examination of the retropharyngeal area, or radiographic examination of the skull to identify the location and extent of retropharyngeal abscesses.

Treatment: The environment for clinically ill horses should be warm, dry, and dust-free. Warm compresses are applied to sites of lymphadenopathy to facilitate maturation of abscesses. Facilitated drainage of mature abscesses will speed recovery. Ruptured abscesses should be flushed with dilute (3%–5%) povidone-iodine solution for several days until discharge ceases. NSAIDs can be administered judiciously to reduce pain and fever and to improve appetite in horses with fulminant clinical disease. Tracheotomy may be required in horses with retropharyngeal abscessation and pharyngeal compression.

Antimicrobial therapy is controversial. Initiation of antibiotic therapy after abscess formation may provide temporary clinical improvement in fever and depression, but it ultimately prolongs the course of disease by delaying maturation of abscesses. Antibiotic therapy is indicated in cases with dyspnea, dysphagia, prolonged high fever, and severe lethargy/anorexia. Administration of penicillin during the early stage of infection (≤24 hr of onset of fever) will usually arrest abscess formation. The disadvantage of early antimicrobial treatment is failure to mount a protective immune response, rendering horses susceptible to infection after cessation of therapy. If antimicrobial therapy is indicated, procaine penicillin (22,000 IU/kg, IM, bid) is the antibiotic of choice. Untreated guttural pouch infections can result in persistent guttural pouch empyema with or without chondroid formation.

Prevention: Postexposure immunity is prolonged after natural disease in most horses, and protection is associated with local (nasal mucosa) production of antibody against the antiphagocytic M protein. The clinical attack rate of strangles is reduced by 50% in horses vaccinated with IM products that do not induce mucosal immunity. Local (mucosal) production of antibody requires mucosal antigen stimulation. An intranasal vaccine containing a live attenuated strain of *S equi equi* was designed to elicit a mucosal immunologic response. This attenuated strain is not temperature sensitive (inactivated by core body temperature) like the intranasal influenza vaccine. Reported complications include *S equi equi* abscesses at subsequent IM injection sites (live bacteria on hands of administrator), submandibular lymphadenopathy, serous nasal discharge, and purpura hemorrhagica (*see* p 828).

Control: Clinically affected horses should be physically separated from the herd and cared for by separate caretakers wearing protective clothing. The rectal temperature of all horses exposed to strangles should be obtained twice daily, and horses developing fever should be isolated (and potentially treated with penicillin). Contaminated equipment should be cleaned with detergent and disinfected using chlorhexidine gluconate or glutaraldehyde. Flies can transmit infection mechanically; therefore, efforts should be made to control the fly population during an outbreak. Farriers, trainers, and veterinarians should wear protective clothing or change clothes before traveling to the next equine facility. Additions to the herd should be carefully scrutinized for evidence of disease or shedding (nasopharyngeal culture) and quarantined for 14–21 days. Two negative nasal swab cultures should be obtained during the quarantine period.

Most horses continue to shed *S equi* for ~1 mo after recovery. Three negative nasopharyngeal swabs, at intervals of 4–7 days, should be obtained before release from quarantine, and the minimal isolation period should be 1 mo. Prolonged bacterial shedding (as long as 18 mo) has been identified in a small number of horses. Guttural pouch empyema is the source of infection in most prolonged carrier states. Bacterial culture of nasopharyngeal swab and/or guttural pouch lavage is used to identify persistent carriers.

RECURRENT AIRWAY OBSTRUCTION

(Heaves, Chronic obstructive pulmonary disease)

Recurrent airway obstruction (RAO) is a common, performance-limiting, allergic respiratory disease of horses characterized by chronic cough, nasal discharge, and respiratory difficulty. Episodes of airway obstruction are seen when susceptible horses are exposed to common allergens. Most horses exhibit clinical signs when stabled, bedded on straw, and fed hay, whereas elimination of these inciting factors results in remission or attenuation of clinical signs. The pathophysiology involves small-airway inflammation (neutrophilic), mucus production, and bronchoconstriction in response to allergen exposure.

Etiology: The average age at onset is 9 yr. Approximately 12% of mature horses have some degree of allergen-induced lower airway inflammation. There is no breed or gender predilection; however, there does appear to be a heritable component to susceptibility.

Clinical Findings: Horses present with flared nostrils, tachypnea, cough, and a heave line. The typical breathing pattern is characterized by a prolonged, labored expiratory phase of respiration. Cough may be productive and often occurs during feeding or exercise. The abdominal muscles respond by assisting with expiration, and hypertrophy of these muscles produces the classic heave line. Characteristic auscultatory findings include a prolonged expiratory phase of respiration, wheezes, tracheal rattle, and overexpanded lung fields. Wheezes are generated by airflow through narrowed airways and are most pronounced during expiration. Crackles may be present and are associated with excessive mucus production. Mild to moderately affected horses may present with minimal clinical signs at rest, but coughing and exercise intolerance are noted during performance. Horses with RAO are not typically febrile unless secondary bacterial pneumonia has developed.

Horses from the southeastern USA may demonstrate clinical signs on late-summer pasture, which likely reflects sensitivity to molds or grass pollens. This is referred to as **summer pasture–associated obstructive**

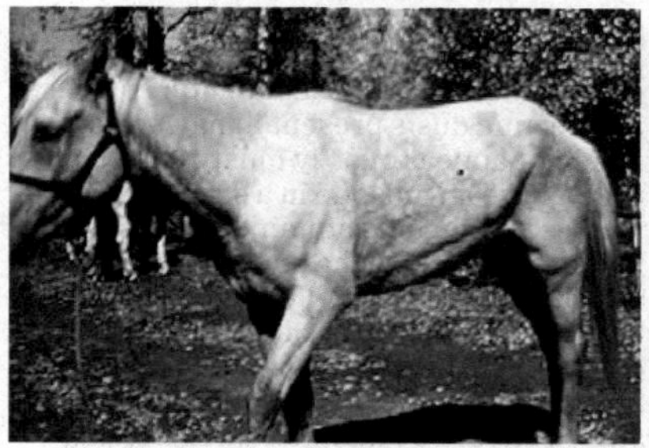

Chronic obstructive pulmonary disease with "heave line" along the costal arch. *Courtesy of Dr. Thomas Lane.*

pulmonary disease. The management is similar to that of a horse with heaves, with the addition of pasture avoidance.

Diagnosis: The diagnosis of RAO is determined in most horses on the basis of history and characteristic physical examination findings. Hematology and serum chemistry results are unremarkable. Radiographic findings in horses with RAO are peribronchial infiltration and overexpanded pulmonary fields (flattening of the diaphragm). Thoracic radiographs are of little benefit in confirming the diagnosis of RAO and may not be necessary in horses with characteristic clinical signs, unless there is no response to standard treatment after 14 days of therapy. However, they may help identify the most important differential diagnoses, including interstitial pneumonia, pulmonary fibrosis, or bacterial pneumonia.

Bronchoalveolar lavage is rarely required for diagnosis of fulminant RAO and is not innocuous in horses that are dyspneic at rest. It is indicated in horses with mild to moderate disease with poor performance and coughing during exercise. Neutrophilic inflammation (20%–90% of total cell count) confirms the presence of lower airway inflammation and differentiates horses with eosinophilic pneumonitis, fungal pneumonia, or lungworm infestation from horses with heaves. Curschmann spirals may be seen on cytologic evaluation and represent inspissated mucus/cellular casts from obstructed small airways.

Treatment: The single most important treatment is environmental management to reduce allergen exposure. Medication will alleviate clinical signs of disease; however, respiratory disease will return after medication is discontinued if the horse remains in the allergen-challenged environment. The most common culprits are organic dusts present in hay, which need not appear overtly musty to precipitate an episode in a sensitive horse. Horses should be maintained at pasture, with fresh grass as the source of roughage, supplemented with pelleted feed. Round bale hay is particularly allergenic and a common cause of treatment failure for horses on pasture. Horses that remain stalled should be maintained in a clean, controlled environment. Complete commercial feeds eliminate the need for roughage. Hay cubes and hay silage are acceptable, low-allergen alternative sources of roughage and may be preferred by horses over the complete feeds. Soaking hay with water before feeding may control clinical signs in mildly affected horses but is unacceptable for highly sensitive horses. Horses maintained in a stall should not be housed in the same building as an indoor arena, hay should not be stored overhead, and straw bedding should be avoided. Horses with summer pasture–associated obstructive pulmonary disease should be maintained in a dust-free, stable environment.

Medical treatment consists of a combination of bronchodilating agents (to provide relief of airway obstruction) and corticosteroid preparations (to reduce pulmonary inflammation). Bronchodilator therapy (β agonists and parasympatholytic agents) will provide immediate relief of airway obstruction until clinical signs of disease are controlled by corticosteroids. Severely affected horses are ideally controlled with aerosolized bronchodilators (eg, albuterol, ipratropium) and systemic corticosteroids (eg, dexamethasone 0.1 mg/kg/day, IV). Horses with mild to moderate airway inflammation can be treated with aerosolized corticosteroids and aerosolized or systemic (clenbuterol) bronchodilators. It is inappropriate to treat RAO with bronchodilators as the sole therapy. NSAIDs, antihistamines, and leukotriene-receptor antagonists have not demonstrated therapeutic benefit.

INFLAMMATORY AIRWAY DISEASE

(Lower respiratory tract inflammation, Small airway inflammatory disease)

Inflammatory airway disease (IAD) describes a heterogeneous group of inflammatory conditions of the lower respiratory tract that appear to be primarily noninfectious. IAD occurs in 22%–50% of athletic horses and is a common cause of impaired performance and interruption of training.

Etiology and Pathophysiology: Proposed etiologies of IAD include allergic airway disease, recurrent pulmonary stress, deep inhalation of dust, atmospheric pollutants, and/or persistent respiratory viral infections, most notably EHV-2. IAD often develops after an overt viral respiratory infection and may result from inability of the immune system to fully eliminate viruses or bacteria from small airways. *Streptococcus pneumoniae* has been isolated from horses with IAD; however, its role in the pathophysiology is unclear, because this population of horses is largely unresponsive (or transiently responsive) to antibiotic therapy.

Clinical Findings: The most common clinical signs are chronic cough and mucoid to mucopurulent nasal discharge. Fever and auscultable pulmonary abnormalities are rarely seen. Horses with IAD demonstrate poor exercise tolerance at maximal speed. Endoscopic examination reveals mucopurulent exudate in the pharynx, trachea, and bronchi.

Diagnosis: Diagnosis of IAD is based on poor race performance and clinical signs. Bronchoalveolar lavage is performed to characterize the type of pulmonary inflammation. Cytologic evaluation of bronchoalveolar fluid will reveal one of the following inflammatory profiles: 1) mixed inflammation with high total nucleated cells, mild neutrophilia (15% of total cells), lymphocytosis, and monocytosis; 2) increased metachromatic cells (mast cells >2% of total cells); or 3) eosinophilic inflammation (5%–40% of total cells). The mixed inflammatory profile likely results from environmental irritation or the consequences of a previous infectious disease.

Treatment: The type of inflammation in bronchoalveolar fluid will dictate the therapeutic plan. Regardless of the cytologic profile, all horses with IAD should receive aerosolized bronchodilator therapy before exercise to avert exercise- or irritant-induced bronchoconstriction. In horses with a mixed inflammatory cytologic profile, administration of low-dose interferon-α is recommended for immunomodulation and antiviral activity. Interferon-α reduces tracheal exudate and improves cytologic profiles in horses with mixed inflammatory IAD. Eosinophilic bronchoalveolar fluid likely represents a Type I hypersensitivity reaction. In addition to tracheal exudates, peripheral eosinophilia, miliary pulmonary opacities, and eosinophilic pulmonary granulomas may be seen in affected horses. If such fluid is identified, parasitic pulmonary disease should be considered in addition to hypersensitivity pneumonitis. Systemic corticosteroid therapy is recommended to reduce pulmonary inflammation in horses with eosinophilic IAD. Mast cell inflammation likely represents a local pulmonary hypersensitivity response and may represent an early form of recurrent airway obstruction (*see* p 1455). In IAD-affected horses with increased mast cells in bronchoalveolar fluid, aerosol administration of an inhaled corticosteroid preparation (beclomethasone or fluticasone) improves clinical signs of respiratory disease.

EXERCISE-INDUCED PULMONARY HEMORRHAGE

(Epistaxis, "Bleeder")

Exercise-induced pulmonary hemorrhage (EIPH) is seen in most racehorses and in many other horses used in equine sports (eg, polo, barrel racing, 3-day events) that require strenuous exercise for short periods of time. Epistaxis is seen in a small proportion (~5%) of horses with EIPH. Blood in the tracheobronchial tree is identified in 45%–75% of racehorses via endoscopic examination, and hemorrhage is detected by cytologic examination of bronchoalveolar lavage in >90% of racehorses.

Etiology: The proposed pathophysiologic mechanism for pulmonary hemorrhage includes high pulmonary vascular pressures during maximal exercise, with resultant thickening of pulmonary vein walls and decreased luminal diameter and increased intravascular pressure at the level of the pulmonary capillaries.

Diagnosis: Endoscopic observation of blood in the airways 30–90 min after exercise provides definitive evidence of EIPH. Other sources of hemorrhage in the upper airway, particularly guttural pouch mycosis (*see* p 1463) and ethmoid hematoma (*see* p 1462), must be excluded during endoscopic examination. If EIPH is suspected and the horse cannot be examined after exercise, cytologic examination of bronchoalveolar lavage fluid for semiquantitative assessment of hemosiderophages is diagnostic. Stains that highlight iron-containing pigments (Prussian blue) facilitate recognition of these cells. Thoracic radiography demonstrates alveolar or mixed alveolar-interstitial opacities in the caudodorsal lung fields; however, radiographic examination of the thorax has little impact on the diagnosis or management of EIPH.

Treatment and Control: Furosemide reduces the incidence and severity of

EIPH in Thoroughbred racehorses. Horses with and without EIPH demonstrate equal improvements in race performance after administration of furosemide, indicating that the drug may enhance performance via mechanisms unrelated to EIPH. Application of nasal dilator bands reduces RBC counts in bronchoalveolar fluid from affected horses running on a treadmill by 33%. Alternative treatments, including procoagulant agents (eg, vitamin K, conjugated estrogens, aminocaproic acid), antihypertensive drugs, rheologic agents (pentoxyphylline), bronchodilators, prolonged rest, dietary supplements (hepseridin-citrus bioflavinoids), and anti-inflammatory drugs, have not demonstrated therapeutic benefit.

LARYNGEAL HEMIPLEGIA

(Roaring, Left laryngeal hemiplegia)

Left recurrent laryngeal hemiplegia is characterized by paresis or paralysis of the left arytenoid cartilage and vocal fold. It manifests clinically as exercise intolerance and inspiratory respiratory noise ("roaring") during exercise. Right-sided hemiplegia and bilateral (paraplegia) arytenoid dysfunction are uncommon.

Etiology and Pathogenesis: Progressive loss of the large myelinated fibers in the distal portion of the recurrent laryngeal nerves results in neurogenic atrophy of the intrinsic laryngeal musculature, the most crucial of which is the cricoarytenoideus dorsalis muscle. Axonal dystrophy of the left recurrent nerve occurs more commonly than the right, perhaps due to its extended length around the base of the heart. Left laryngeal hemiplegia is likely heritable. Less common causes include direct trauma to the recurrent laryngeal nerve, accidental perivascular injection of irritating substances, and plant (eg, *Cicer arietinum* [chick peas] and *Lathyrus* spp) and chemical intoxications. Lead toxicity should be suspected in horses with bilateral laryngeal paralysis. The peroneal nerve (similar length to the left recurrent laryngeal) may be affected with toxic insults, and axonal dystrophy of the peroneal nerve may manifest as stringhalt (*see* p 1137). Although all breeds are affected, prevalence is higher in males and long-necked/larger breeds. The prevalence in young Thoroughbreds presented for sale is estimated to be ~3%–5%.

Loss of neuromuscular control of the abductor muscle results in collapse of the arytenoid cartilage and vocal fold, which reduces the glottal cross-sectional area. The resistance to airflow necessitates greater respiratory effort. Because of the pliable nature of the glottis, the exaggerated subatmospheric pressure in the airway results in further collapse of the arytenoid cartilage and exacerbation of the impedance to airflow. Upon inspiration during strenuous exercise, the affected side is drawn across the midline (by negative pressure in the airway) until it abuts the abducted normal arytenoid, effectively occluding the airway (dynamic collapse). The characteristic inspiratory whistle results from resonance within the open ventricle on the affected side. The harsher stridor, or roar, is produced by vortex shedding from the edges of the arytenoid cartilage and vocal fold.

Clinical Findings and Diagnosis: The principal clinical signs are inspiratory noise during exercise and exercise intolerance. Affected horses are asymptomatic at rest but may have an unusual whinny. Diagnosis is confirmed by endoscopic observation of reduced or absent mobility of the arytenoid cartilage and vocal fold. With laryngeal hemiplegia, the arytenoid cartilage and vocal fold are located in a median position within the laryngeal lumen and are immobile. Asynchronous movements of the laryngeal cartilages occur commonly, with variable clinical relevance. Horses with laryngeal asynchrony, exercise intolerance, and respiratory noise during exercise should have their laryngeal function evaluated endoscopically during treadmill exercise to confirm laryngeal dysfunction.

Differential diagnoses include other pharyngeal conditions that produce upper

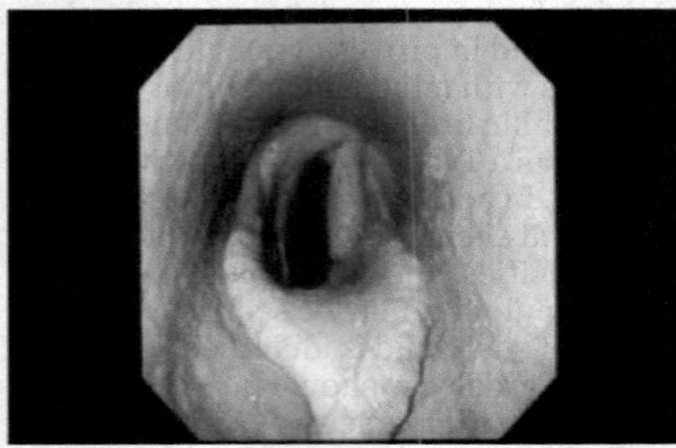

Endoscopic image demonstrating grade IV paralysis of the left arytenoid from a horse with left laryngeal hemiplegia at rest. *Courtesy of Dr. Bonnie R. Rush.*

airway obstruction and exercise intolerance. Most of these conditions are easily differentiated from laryngeal hemiplegia during endoscopic examination. Although arytenoid chondritis may be confused with laryngeal hemiplegia, misdiagnosis can be avoided by observation of the shape and size of the arytenoid cartilages. In arytenoid chondritis, the arytenoids thicken transversely and lose their characteristic "bean" shape. Abduction and adduction are usually limited. The axial (medial) surface of the arytenoid cartilage may be distorted with granulation tissue protruding through the mucosa, and a contact (kissing) lesion may be present on the contralateral arytenoid cartilage. Arytenoid chondritis should always be considered if motility of the right arytenoid is reduced. Radiographic examination of the pharynx may reveal mineralization within the arytenoid cartilages in cases of chondritis.

Treatment: Prosthetic laryngoplasty can stabilize the affected side of the larynx during inspiration and prevent dynamic collapse of the airway during exercise. Laryngeal ventriculectomy performed via laryngotomy, or ventriculocordectomy performed via transendoscopic laser, improves airflow and reduces the "roaring" sound during exercise. Prosthetic laryngoplasty is commonly done in racing horses and is the only technique that satisfactorily reduces the impedance to inspiratory flow. Postoperative complications include chronic cough, chronic aspiration of feed, implant failure, and implant infection. Athletic performance will improve after surgery; however, horses are more likely to experience inflammatory airway disease and exercise-induced pulmonary hemorrhage, have fewer race starts, and are unlikely to develop their predicted performance potential.

PHARYNGEAL LYMPHOID HYPERPLASIA

(Pharyngitis)

Pharyngeal lymphoid hyperplasia is a common condition of the dorsal pharyngeal wall seen in young horses (1–3 yr old). Horses do not have discrete masses of lymphoid tonsillar tissue; rather, they have many small foci or follicles of lymphoid tissue spread diffusely over the roof and lateral walls of the pharynx. In mature horses, these follicles blend with mucosal

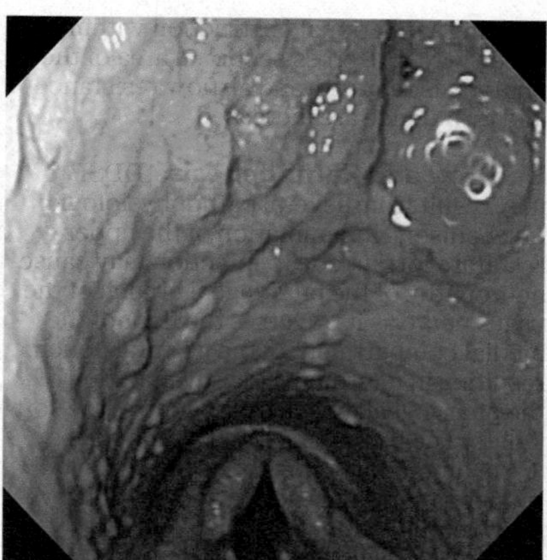

Endoscopic photograph of grade 3.5/4 pharyngeal lymphoid hyperplasia. *Courtesy of Dr. Jan Hawkins.*

tissue and are unnoticeable. In young, maturing horses, lymphoid follicles appear as prominent, raised nodules on the surface of the pharyngeal roof and extend down the lateral walls of the pharynx and cranially into the nasopharynx. Although PLH was once believed to be an important cause of poor performance in racehorses, its clinical significance is now questionable. Virtually all young horses develop hyperplasia of pharyngeal lymphoid follicles; in most cases, this represents a normal immunologic event.

Occasionally, follicles may enlarge and coalesce with surrounding follicles. In these situations, follicles may appear hyperemic or inflamed and may exude mucoid or mucopurulent material. These cases likely represent a mild or subclinical viral infection and may be associated with impaired performance. Signs of pharyngeal pain include reduced appetite and frequent swallowing. Treatment is not necessary in the vast majority of cases; however, rest and NSAID administration are warranted in horses demonstrating pharyngeal pain.

DORSAL DISPLACEMENT OF THE SOFT PALATE

Dorsal displacement of the soft palate (DDSP) is a performance-limiting condition of the upper respiratory tract and is a relatively common cause of upper respiratory noise during exercise. During DDSP, the caudal free margin of the soft palate moves dorsal to the epiglottis, creating a functional obstruction within the airway. The cross-sectional area of the pharynx is reduced, and airflow resistance and turbulence are increased.

Etiology and Pathogenesis: DDSP may result from several pathophysiologic mechanisms. Inflammation of the upper respiratory tract due to infection may cause neuropathy of the pharyngeal branch of the vagus nerve as it traverses the floor of the medial compartment of the guttural pouch, resulting in neuromuscular dysfunction of the pharyngeal muscles that control the soft palate. The retropharyngeal lymph nodes are in direct contact with the pharyngeal branch of the vagus nerve, and retropharyngeal lymphadenopathy may result in compression and irritation. Clinical signs can be induced by local anesthesia of this nerve. Congenital hypoplasia of the epiglottis may contribute to DDSP due to insufficient epiglottal tissue to maintain the position of the caudal border of the soft palate ventral to the epiglottis. Horses that have undergone laryngoplasty for left laryngeal hemiplegia are more likely to develop DDSP.

Clinical Findings: DDSP creates a characteristic gurgling respiratory noise, primarily during expiration, due to vibration of the soft palate. Horses may make no noise at the onset of exercise but displace their palate during high-speed exercise, causing them to "choke down." Head position (flexed) may contribute to displacement.

Treatment: The most effective treatment for DDSP in young horses (2-yr-olds) and horses with evidence of upper respiratory tract infection is rest and anti-inflammatory therapy. Caudal retraction of the tongue elevates the soft palate and pushes the larynx caudally, both of which may predispose to DDSP. Placing a tongue tie during exercise reduces caudal retraction of the tongue. Sternothyrohyoideus myectomy performed in horses prone to DDSP to alter the anatomy of the upper respiratory tract is successful in ~50% of horses. Soft palate resection (staphylectomy) is frequently performed in horses with DDSP and also has a success rate of ~50%; however, the mechanism of improvement after surgery is unclear. Success has been attributed to reduction in the mass of soft palate obstructing the airway, easier replacement of the shorter soft palate to the subepiglottic position, and firming of the caudal edge of the soft palate to keep it ventral to the epiglottis. Palatal sclerotherapy via endoscopic-guided sodium tetradecylally sulfate injection has demonstrated success in a small number of horses, resolving respiratory noise in 7 of 8 horses and improving performance in 6 of 8 horses. A laryngeal tie-forward procedure can be performed to alter the position of the larynx with respect to the caudal edge of the soft palate.

EPIGLOTTIC ENTRAPMENT

Epiglottic entrapment is a less common cause of respiratory noise and exercise intolerance. In this condition, the aryepiglottic fold completely envelops the apex and lateral margins of the epiglottis. The general shape of the epiglottis is visible, and the position (dorsal to the soft palate) is appropriate. However, the distinct serrated margins of the epiglottis and the dorsal epiglottic vascular pattern are obscured by a fold of aryepiglottic mucosa. Clinical signs of epiglottic entrapment include inspiratory and expiratory respiratory noise during exercise and poor exercise performance. Less common signs include cough, nasal discharge, and headshaking. In mature nonracehorses, cough is the most consistent presenting complaint. Diagnosis is determined by endoscopic examination. Surgical correction of epiglottic entrapment is axial division of the aryepiglottic fold to free the epiglottis. Axial transection of the aryepiglottic fold may be performed by transendoscopic contact Nd:YAG laser, transnasal or transoral transection via curved bistoury, or direct excision through a laryngotomy or pharyngotomy. Surgical transection is generally curative, with a relapse rate of 5%. Some affected horses can race successfully with the condition.

SUBEPIGLOTTIC CYST

Subepiglottic cysts are an uncommon cause of respiratory noise in young horses. They are likely present from birth but remain undetected until the horse begins exercise training. These cysts are suspected to arise from remnants of the thyroglossal duct. Clinical signs include respiratory noise and exercise intolerance. Large cysts may produce coughing, dysphagia, and aspiration in foals. Diagnosis is determined by endoscopic examination of the upper respiratory tract. The cyst appears as a smooth-walled, fluctuant mass that contains thick, yellow, mucoid material. Occasionally, the mass is not visible in the nasopharynx, and oral examination under general anesthesia may be required to identify it. Histologically, subepiglottic cysts are lined with a combination of stratified squamous and pseudostratified columnar epithelium. Treatment involves complete removal of the secretory lining of the cyst. Rupture of the cyst results in immediate decompression, but recurrence is common. The most common approach is ventral laryngotomy, although transendoscopic Nd:YAG laser surgery has been used for complete excision.

FOURTH BRANCHIAL ARCH DEFECT

(Rostral displacement of the palatopharyngeal arch)

The extrinsic structures of the larynx, such as the wing of the thyroid cartilage, cricothyroid muscle, and upper esophageal sphincter, develop from the fourth branchial arches. Aplasia or hypoplasia of one or more of these structures may occur unilaterally or bilaterally. Right-sided defects are more common than bilateral or left-sided defects. The severity of clinical manifestation ranges broadly and is based on the degree of the defect. The most common clinical sign is respiratory noise, although mild dysphagia, eructation, and cough have been reported. Palpation of the larynx reveals absence of one or both wings of the thyroid cartilage, resulting in failure of the cricothyroid articulation and a palpable space between the cricoid and thyroid cartilages. Radiographic evidence of a fourth branchial arch defect includes dilation of the cricopharynx with a continuous column of air from the pharynx to the cervical esophagus. Rostral displacement of the palatopharyngeal arch may or may not be detected during endoscopic examination. Endoscopic examination during treadmill exercise may reveal dynamic collapse of the vocal folds. Affected horses are unlikely to become effective athletes. Partial arytenoidectomy may improve airway dynamics sufficiently for pleasure riding.

DISEASES OF THE NASAL PASSAGES

Nasal Septum

Diseases of the nasal septum are rare. Most nasal septal disorders are congenital abnormalities that remain undetected until the horse is exercised. Traumatic injury to the bridge of the nose as a juvenile can produce nasal septal deviation and thickening. Other less common diseases of the nasal septum include amyloidosis, fungal infection, and squamous cell carcinoma.

Thickening or deviation of the nasal septum causes low-pitched stertorous breathing during exercise. Facial deformity may be seen. Septal abnormalities may be detected by palpation, visual inspection, and endoscopic examination. Dimensions of the nasal cavity are difficult to appreciate via endoscopic examination; however, abnormalities of the mucosa are easily identified. Precise dorsoventral radiographs of the skull provide definitive evidence of septal deformity, deviation, and thickening. Histologic examination of any nodules or discrete lesions on the septum will identify tumors, amyloidosis, or fungal infections.

Surgical resection of the nasal septum is the only treatment option in most cases. The entire diseased portion of the septum can be excised using obstetrical wire by transecting the septum on the dorsal, ventral, and caudal border. Hemorrhage is substantial during this procedure (4–8 L), and the nasal passages are packed with sterile gauze soaked in saline or in 1:100,000 epinephrine solution to minimize blood loss. Before the horse recovers from anesthesia, a tracheotomy is performed.

Postoperative care includes parenteral antibiotics and NSAIDs. The packing and tracheotomy tube should be removed 48–72 hr after surgery. All incisions heal by second intention within 3 wk. Horses should be rested for ~2 mo before returning to normal activity. After surgery, most horses make a respiratory noise during work, although less than before surgery, and exercise tolerance is improved. Shortening of the upper jaw, incisor malalignment, or nostril collapse can develop if the procedure is performed in immature horses. Ideally, the surgery should be delayed until maturity.

Nasal Polyps

Nasal polyps are pedunculated growths that arise from the mucosa of the nasal cavity, nasal septum, or tooth alveolus. Polyps are usually unilateral and single but can be bilateral and multiple. They form in response to chronic inflammation by hypertrophy of the mucous membrane or exuberant proliferation of fibrous connective tissue. There is no age, breed, or gender predilection.

Clinical signs are poor airflow through the affected nasal passage; inspiratory dyspnea; unilateral, malodorous, mucopurulent nasal discharge; and low-volume epistaxis. The mass may extend rostrally until it protrudes beyond the nostrils. Polyps are detected via endoscopic and radiographic examination, and histopathologic evaluation of biopsy samples provide a definitive diagnosis. Surgical excision is performed via an incision in the false nostril, a trephine opening, or a bone flap.

Choanal Atresia

Choanal atresia is caused by persistence of the bucconasal membrane that separates the primitive buccal or oral cavity from the nasal pits during embryonic development. Bilateral and unilateral cases have been described in horses. Clinical signs are evident immediately after birth in foals with bilateral disease, because dyspnea is severe and air cannot be detected passing through the nostrils. An endoscope or stomach tube passed through the ventral meatus will be obstructed at the level of the medial canthus of the eye.

Bilateral complete choanal atresia is a life-threatening condition, and a tracheotomy must be performed immediately after birth. It may be possible to perforate a thin membrane by electrocoagulation or laser or by excision through bilateral flaps centered along the midline. Indwelling tube stents should be inserted through both choanae and left in place for 6 wk.

DISEASES OF THE PARANASAL SINUSES

The maxillary sinus is the largest paranasal sinus and is divided by a thin septum into caudal and rostral parts. The frontal sinus has a large communication with the dorsal conchal sinus at its rostral end, thereby forming the conchofrontal sinus. The conchae or turbinates are delicate scrolls of bone that are attached laterally in the nasal passage and contain the conchal sinuses. The caudal and rostral maxillary sinuses have separate openings into the middle nasal meatus, and the caudal maxillary sinus communicates with the frontal sinus through the large frontomaxillary opening. Diseases that originate in one sinus cavity may extend to and involve others.

Most diseases of the paranasal sinuses cause mucopurulent or bloody nasal discharge. Drainage is unilateral, in contrast to disease of the lungs, pharynx, and guttural pouches, because the source of *discharge is rostral to the* caudal border of the nasal septum. Unilateral facial swelling, epiphora, dull percussion of the sinuses, and inspiratory noise are common manifestations of disorders of the sinuses.

On endoscopy, purulent material, a mass, or blood can be seen in the nasal passage originating from the nasomaxillary opening. Lateral and dorsoventral radiographs of the skull may reveal fluid lines, sinus cysts, solid masses, or lytic/proliferative changes associated with dental disease and neoplasia. Oblique projections in a dorsal to ventral direction may be required to improve views of the tooth roots. CT is useful, particularly for ventral conchal sinus disease. Centesis of the maxillary or frontal sinuses is performed to obtain fluid for bacterial culture, sensitivity testing, and cytologic examination. With sedation and local anesthesia, the sinuses can be examined in the standing horse by insertion of an arthroscope (4 mm). A second portal could be used to insert an instrument into the sinus to obtain specimens, debride tissue, and lavage the sinus cavity.

Sinusitis

Primary sinusitis occurs subsequent to an upper respiratory tract infection that has involved the paranasal sinuses. It usually involves all sinus cavities but can be confined to the ventral conchal sinus. This cavity is difficult to detect radiographically and access surgically. Secondary sinusitis can result from tooth root infection, fracture, or sinus cyst. The first molar, fourth premolar, and third premolar (in decreasing frequency) are the most likely to develop tooth root abscesses. Clinical signs of secondary sinusitis closely resemble those of primary sinusitis, including unilateral mucopurulent nasal discharge and facial deformity. Tooth root abscesses typically produce a fetid nasal discharge. Treatment of primary sinusitis involves lavage of the sinus cavity and systemic antimicrobial therapy based on culture and sensitivity results. Secondary sinusitis requires removal of affected cheek teeth or cystic material via sinusotomy.

Ethmoid Hematoma

Progressive ethmoid hematoma is a locally destructive mass of nasal passages and paranasal sinuses of uncertain etiology. The mass resembles a tumor in appearance and development but is not neoplastic. Large hematomas usually arise from the ethmoid labyrinth, and smaller masses arise from the floor of the sinuses. Masses originating in the sinus extend into the nasal passage. An expanding hematoma can cause pressure necrosis of surrounding bone but rarely causes facial distortion; it is primarily seen in horses

>6 yr old. Low-grade, spontaneous, intermittent, unilateral epistaxis is the most common clinical sign. Horses with extensive masses may have reduced airflow through the affected nasal passage and fetid breath. In longstanding cases, the mass may protrude from the nares. In most instances, the lesion can be seen extending into the nasal passages on endoscopic examination, and the extent of the mass can be determined radiographically. Conservative management includes intralesional injection of the mass with 4% formaldehyde. Formalin is injected into the mass using a guarded endoscopic needle. The mass typically regresses rapidly, but recurrence is common. Neurologic signs have been reported after intralesional formalin injection, associated with communication of the hematoma into the calvarium. Surgical excision is achieved via frontonasal bone flap.

Sinus Cysts

Sinus cysts are single or loculated fluid-filled cavities with an epithelial lining. They develop in the maxillary sinuses and ventral conchae and can extend into the frontal sinus. A congenital form has been described. Sinus cysts are typically found in horses <1 yr old but can also be seen in those >9 yr old. The primary clinical signs are facial deformity, nasal discharge, and partial airway obstruction. Radiographs are more likely to identify a sinus cyst than endoscopic examination. Multiloculated densities and fluid lines in the sinuses are observed radiographically; occasionally, dental distortion, flattening of tooth roots, soft-tissue mineralization, and deviation of the nasal septum are seen. Treatment involves radical surgical removal of the cyst and associated conchal lining. Prognosis for complete recovery is good, and the recurrence is low. Some horses may have a permanent, mild mucoid discharge after surgery.

GUTTURAL POUCH DISEASE

Empyema

Guttural pouch empyema is defined as the accumulation of purulent, septic exudate in the guttural pouch. The infection usually develops subsequent to a bacterial (primarily *Streptococcus* spp) infection of the upper respiratory tract. Clinical signs include intermittent purulent nasal discharge, painful swelling in the parotid area, and in severe cases, stiff head carriage and stertorous breathing. Fever, depression, and anorexia may or may not be seen. Diagnosis is determined by endoscopic examination of the guttural pouch. Radiographs of the pharynx demonstrate a fluid line in the guttural pouch and may allow identification of an associated retropharyngeal mass.

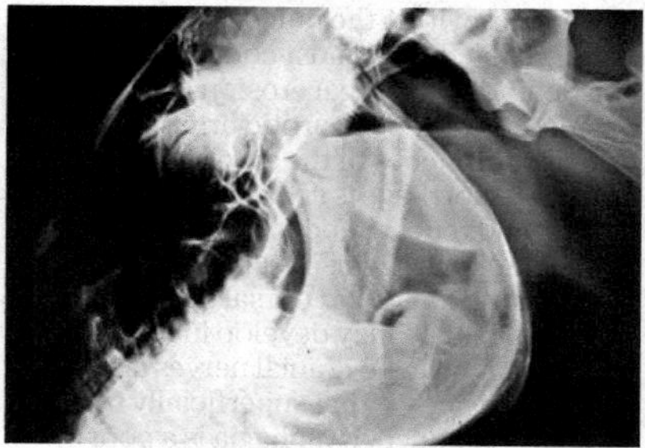

Empyema of guttural pouch, horse, radiograph. *Courtesy of Dr. Ronald Green.*

Systemic antimicrobial therapy alone rarely resolves the infection; guttural pouch lavage is necessary. Penicillin gel (prepared using sodium penicillin) can be administered directly into the guttural pouch and may enhance bacterial clearance. Retropharyngeal abscesses can be resolved by rupturing the abscess into the guttural pouch using an endoscopic blade. If endoscopic rupture into the guttural pouch is unsuccessful, surgical drainage is necessary for retropharyngeal abscessation. Guttural pouch empyema may compress the dorsal pharynx and produce upper airway obstruction. Tracheotomy may be necessary to provide a temporary alternative airway in these cases. If guttural pouch empyema is not treated, chondroid material may form in the guttural pouch and serve as a source of chronic infectious exudate. A small number of chondroids can be removed endoscopically, but accumulations of exudate, chondroid material, or unresolved retropharyngeal abscesses require surgical drainage.

Guttural Pouch Mycosis

Mycotic plaques in the guttural pouch are typically located on the caudodorsal aspect of the medial guttural pouch, over the internal carotid artery. In some instances, fungal plaques may be multiple or diffuse. The most common fungal organism associated with guttural pouch mycosis is *Aspergillus* spp (*see* p 633). Clinical signs arise from damage to the cranial nerves and the arteries within the mucosal lining of the guttural pouch. The most common sign is epistaxis, due to fungal erosion of the wall of either the internal carotid artery (most cases) or branches of the external carotid artery. Hemorrhage is spontaneous and severe, and repeated bouts may precede a fatal hemorrhagic episode. Dysphagia, Horner syndrome, and dorsal displacement of the soft palate may develop in response to fungal damage to cranial nerves and the sympathetic nerve that superficially traverse the guttural pouch. Dysphagia is a poor prognostic indicator and is highly correlated with nonsurvival. Diagnosis is determined by endoscopic examination of the guttural pouch. Treatment consists of topical and systemic antifungal therapy, based on sensitivity testing. Topical antifungal therapy is administered directly on the lesion via infusion through the biopsy channel of an endoscope. A fatal hemorrhagic event can be prevented by occluding the affected arteries along their course through the guttural pouch by means of a balloon-tipped catheter or a coil embolus. It is necessary to occlude the arteries proximal and distal to the lesion to prevent retrograde bleeding from the circle of Willis.

Guttural Pouch Tympany

Guttural pouch tympany is seen in horses ranging from birth to 1 yr of age and is more common in fillies than in colts. A genetic basis of disease has been identified in Arabian and German warmblood breeds. In some cases, the condition is acquired due to inflammation of the upper respiratory tract. The affected guttural pouch is distended with air and forms a characteristic nonpainful swelling in the parotid region. Breathing may become stertorous in severely affected animals. Tympany may result from inflammation or malformation of the pharyngeal orifice of the eustachian tube, which then acts as a one-way valve by allowing air to enter the pouch but preventing its return into the pharynx. Diagnosis is based on clinical signs and radiographic examination of the skull. Severely affected animals may develop a secondary empyema. Tympany is usually unilateral, but bilateral cases have been reported. Medical management with NSAIDs and antimicrobial therapy resolves most cases due to upper respiratory tract inflammation. Surgical intervention is warranted in horses with malformation of the guttural pouch opening and involves fenestration of the membrane that separates the affected guttural pouch from the normal one. This provides a route for air in the abnormal guttural pouch to pass to the normal side and be expelled into the pharynx. The postoperative prognosis is good.

Rupture of the Longus Capitis Muscle

Traumatic rupture of the longus capitis is the second most common cause (after mycosis) of severe hemorrhage from the guttural pouch. The longus capitis muscle is one of the ventral straight muscles of the head. It inserts on the basisphenoid bone at the base of the skull. The point of rupture occurs at the insertion of the muscle dorsal to the guttural pouch. Rupture results from traumatic poll injury (rearing over backward) and produces profuse hemorrhage. Hemorrhage into the retropharyngeal space can cause asphyxia and death. On endoscopic examination, swelling and hemorrhage can be seen in the most rostral and medial aspects of the guttural pouch by retroflexion of the endoscope. On lateral radiographic examination, an avulsion fracture of the basisphenoid bone may be seen overlying the guttural pouch region. Significant neurologic deficits are often seen with this fracture. Treatment involves stall rest for 4–6 wk; broad-spectrum antibiotics are given for 5–7 days for any infection at the site of muscle rupture. Prognosis for full recovery is good, but persistent neurologic signs or recurrent hemorrhage worsens the prognosis.

RESPIRATORY DISEASES OF PIGS

Respiratory diseases of pigs can be classified into two broad categories based on the extent and duration of overt disease: those that affect large numbers of pigs and may be serious but of limited duration, and those that persist in a large number of pigs for indefinite periods. Diseases in the first category can be costly, but the losses are limited rather than ongoing. They include swine influenza (*see* p 1470), classical swine fever (*see* p 713), the pneumonic forms of pseudorabies (*see* p 1300), porcine circovirus-associated disease (*see* p 723), and porcine reproductive and respiratory syndrome (*see* p 729). The causal viruses may persist in a herd, but outbreaks of overt disease tend to be self-limiting.

The most important syndromes in the second category are mycoplasmal pneumonia and pleuropneumonia (*see* p 1467). Atrophic rhinitis, once considered to be a significant cause of respiratory disease in swine, has declined substantially as a result of eradication programs. Salmonellosis and *Haemophilus parasuis* infections may be significant problems in some herds. Moderate levels of atrophic rhinitis caused by *Bordetella bronchiseptica* alone may not be too significant but, when coupled with toxigenic strains of *Pasteurella*, are an important cause of economic loss due to decreased rate of growth and reduced feed conversion in young pigs. Enzootic pneumonia, when caused by mycoplasma alone, is of little consequence; however, when it is combined with secondary infection, eg, *Pasteurella multocida*, the resulting condition may be severe. *Actinobacillus pleuropneumoniae* may be associated with considerable losses in some herds. Migrating worm larvae or the infections listed in the first category often lead to severe problems when they occur with the infections in the second category.

The severity and economic importance of diseases in the second category also are related to population density and to the type and size of herd. They may be of little importance in weanling pig operations but become of major importance in high-density feeder-pig units. Although mortality usually is low, economic damage results from an adverse and uneven effect on growth rate, decreased feed efficiency, and additional costs of drugs, particularly medicated feed. However, when stress can be avoided by proper management, such diseases may result in only minimal losses.

Finally, it must be stressed that respiratory disease problems in pigs are frequently the result of multiple agents (co-infection) and rarely due to the effects of a single pathogen.

It is possible to set up herds free of diseases in the second category by techniques such as SPF repopulation or segregated early weaning, or by buying pigs from a pneumonia-free herd. The latter method is the least expensive, but because the etiology of diseases in the second category is complex, all the pigs should be purchased from one source. This is also true when purchasing weaned pigs for feeder-pig units.

It is difficult to keep herds free of respiratory diseases. Aerosols have been suspected as sources of pathogen entry onto naive farms. Organisms such as *Mycoplasma hyopneumoniae* have been postulated to be transmitted over distances of as far as 2 miles, depending on climate, terrain, and density of pigs in the locality; however, this assumption is based on speculation and use of mathematical models rather than on experimental data.

Closed herds, ie, buying in no live animals (using artificial insemination or embryo transfer to bring in new genetic material), help establish immunity to present organisms and avoid introduction of new infections, strains, or serotypes. Multiple site production or an "all-in/all-out" policy, in which the entire barn or air space is emptied before refilling, can very effectively minimize the potential effect of chronic pneumonia.

Respiratory disease is endemic in many herds. The main control factors are stress management, stocking density, ventilation, temperature control, and freedom from mixing and moving. Multiple site production or "all-in/all-out" and closed-herd management practices greatly decrease the need for preventive and therapeutic medication.

ATROPHIC RHINITIS

Atrophic rhinitis is characterized by sneezing, followed by atrophy of the turbinate bones, which may be accompanied by distortion of the nasal septum and shortening or twisting of the upper jaw. Its significance has declined substantially, and it is no longer considered a major health risk to swine herds.

Etiology: The etiology is complex and involves at least two organisms. Various infections (eg, inclusion body rhinitis and pseudorabies) and noninfectious agents (eg, dust or high ammonia levels) cause sneezing and tear-staining, usually without leading to atrophic rhinitis. *Bordetella bronchiseptica* has long been implicated as a major cause. This bacterium is not host-specific, although strains that cause atrophic rhinitis are generally isolated only from pigs. Dogs, cats, rodents, and other species may harbor *B bronchiseptica* for long periods, but their role in the spread of atrophic rhinitis in pigs is uncertain.

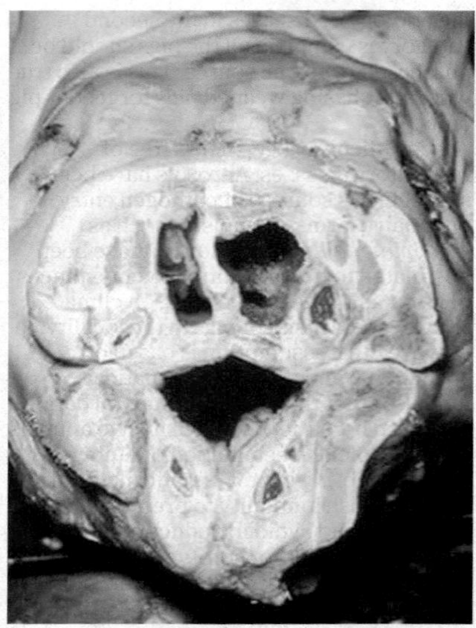

Atrophic rhinitis in a pig. The nasal turbinate bones have been completely destroyed after natural infection with type D toxigenic *Pasteurella multocida*. Courtesy of the Department of Pathology, University of Guelph.

Toxigenic strains of *Pasteurella multocida* (type D), often acting with *B bronchiseptica*, cause permanent turbinate atrophy and nasal distortion. Both organisms can cause clinical atrophic rhinitis.

The disease has been divided into two forms: **nonprogressive** atrophic rhinitis, due to *B bronchiseptica*, is mild and transient and probably does not greatly affect the animal's growth and performance; **progressive** atrophic rhinitis, due to toxigenic *P multocida*, is severe, permanent, and usually accompanied by poor growth.

Outbreaks of disease usually follow either the introduction of infected pigs or mixing of pigs from different sources. Piglets may be affected at any age, especially with *P multocida*, which also may infect mature animals. Crowding, inadequate ventilation, mixing and moving, and other concurrent diseases are important contributory factors in intensification of the disease.

Clinical Findings: Acute signs, which usually appear at 3–8 wk of age, include sneezing, coughing, and inflammation of the lacrimal duct. In more severe cases, nasal hemorrhage may occur. The lacrimal ducts may become occluded, and tear stains then appear below the medial canthi of the eyes. Some severely affected pigs may develop lateral deviation or shortening of the upper jaw, whereas others may suffer some degree of turbinate atrophy with no apparent outward distortion. The degree of distortion can be judged from the relationship of the upper and lower incisors if breed variations are considered. In addition to the above clinical signs, outbreaks frequently impair growth rate and feed conversion.

The severity of atrophic rhinitis in a herd depends largely on the presence of toxigenic strains of *P multocida*, the level of management, and the immune status of the herd. The latter is related to both vaccination status and the parity distribution of the sow herd, because younger sows tend to shed more organisms and produce less lactogenic immunity for their nursing piglets than do older multiparous sows.

Lesions: The degree of atrophy and distortion is best assessed by examining a transverse section at the level of the second premolar tooth (the first cheek tooth, up to 7–9 mo of age); some recommend additional parallel sections. In the active stages of inflammation, the mucosa has a blanched appearance, and purulent material may be present on the surface. In later stages, the nasal cavities may be clear, but there may be variable degrees of softening, atrophy, or grooving of the turbinates; deviation of the nasal septum; and asymmetric distortion of the surrounding bone structure.

Diagnosis: The signs and lesions are commonly the basis for diagnosis; however, the presence of toxigenic strains of *P multocida* should be confirmed. Routine monitoring is done in some breeding herds by measuring the degree of turbinate atrophy and giving the herd an atrophy score. Atrophic rhinitis must be differentiated from necrotic rhinitis (*see* p 1468).

Control: It is rarely possible to keep herds entirely free from mild outbreaks of sneezing, and a low level of aberrant turbinates and nasal bones at necropsy is common, even in herds that show no clinical signs of rhinitis. When atrophic rhinitis rises to an unacceptable level in a herd, control measures are usually strategic: chemoprophylaxis, vaccination, temporary closure of the herd to introduction of new pigs, and improved management (eg, better ventilation and hygiene, less dusty feed). Chemoprophylaxis usually includes administration of antibacterial drugs to all sows, particularly before farrowing, as well as programs of repeated medications for newborn piglets and sometimes for newly weaned pigs. Medication of weaner and grower rations, and sometimes sow rations, is often helpful. Drugs commonly used are ceftiofur, sulfonamides, tylosin, and tetracyclines.

Bacterins against toxigenic *P multocida* and *B bronchiseptica* have been developed. Both toxoid vaccines and bacterin-toxoid mixtures are available against *P multocida*; although both give satisfactory results in most herds, infection can be best prevented with bacterin-toxoid mixtures. Typically, sows are vaccinated 4 and 2 wk before farrowing, and the young pigs at 1 and 4 wk of age. However, vaccination schedules recommended by the manufacturer should be followed. A high level of colostral immunity is acquired by piglets nursing vaccinated sows. An intranasal vaccine using modified-live strains of *B bronchiseptica* is also available for young pigs.

MYCOPLASMAL PNEUMONIA

(Enzootic pneumonia)

Mycoplasmal pneumonia is a chronic, clinically mild, infectious pneumonia of pigs, characterized by its ability to become endemic in a herd and to produce a persistent dry cough, retarded growth rate, sporadic "flare-ups" of overt respiratory distress, and a high incidence of lung lesions in slaughter pigs. It occurs worldwide.

Clinical outbreaks of mycoplasmal pneumonia may impair growth rate and feed conversion. This effect is enhanced when large numbers of pigs are closely confined in poorly ventilated buildings under poor husbandry conditions. The effects of the disease are uneven and unpredictable and place limits on the efficiency and flexibility of large production units. However, in swine units with good disease control measures, mycoplasmal pneumonia may remain largely subclinical and is of little economic importance.

Etiology and Epidemiology: The terms "viral pneumonia" and "enzootic pneumonia" are frequently used to describe a characteristic disease syndrome now known to be caused primarily by *Mycoplasma hyopneumoniae.* The pleomorphic organism is fastidious, smaller than most bacteria, and difficult to see clearly under ordinary light microscopes. It can be cultured in specially prepared media, but isolation from field cases is difficult. It is rapidly inactivated in the environment and by disinfectants, but it may survive longer in cold weather. It appears to be host-specific.

Mycoplasmal pneumonia is also frequently complicated by other mycoplasmas, bacteria, and viruses, which affect the severity of the disease. Certain strains of *M hyorhinis*, and perhaps some viruses, may themselves act as primary agents to produce a syndrome resembling the pneumonia caused by *M hyopneumoniae.*

In most countries that use modern pig-farming methods, the lungs of 30%–80% of the pigs slaughtered show pneumonic lesions of the type associated with mycoplasmal infection. Pigs of all ages are susceptible, but within a herd, pigs become infected in the first few weeks of life either by their dam or by other young pigs after mixing. Transmission to lactating piglets can occur from sows of all parities but is most prevalent in first-parity (gilt) litters. In addition, with the adaptation of segregated (multisite) production, the onset of the disease has been delayed and may be most evident in the finishing stage at ~18–20 wk of age. The incidence of lung lesions is highest in pigs 3–5 mo old. Immunity develops slowly, followed by regression of the lung lesions. Older growing and mature pigs may recover completely.

Clinical Findings: In herds in which the disease is endemic, morbidity is high, but clinical signs may be minimal and mortality is low. Coughing is the most common sign and is most obvious when pigs are roused. Individual pigs or groups sporadically develop severe pneumonia. A common predisposing factor is a change of weather, but other stresses (eg, transient viral infections, parasitic migration, and mixing pigs) may also cause outbreaks. The disease is usually more severe when it first enters a naive herd.

Lesions: Affected lungs are gray or purple, most commonly in the apical and cardiac lobes. Old lesions become clearly demarcated. The associated lymph nodes may be enlarged. Histologically, inflammatory cells are present in the bronchioles; there is perivascular and peribronchiolar cuffing and extensive lymphoid hyperplasia.

Diagnosis: Clinical, pathologic, and epidemiologic findings are usually adequate for diagnosis. *M hyopneumoniae* can be demonstrated in impression smears of the cut surface of affected lung, identified by fluorescent antibody technique, and sometimes isolated and identified in culture. Serologic tests, principally the complement fixation test, and ELISA are occasionally used on a herd basis, but results may be difficult to interpret. A PCR test to detect *M hyopneumoniae* in nasal and bronchial swabs has been developed and appears to be very sensitive and specific.

Control: When the disease first enters a herd, mass treatment with antibiotics (eg, tylosin, lincomycin, tiamulin, or a tetracycline) helps to control the severity of signs. When disease increases in endemic herds, treatment of individual pigs with antibiotics usually results in remission, presumably by controlling secondary bacteria.

Inactivated mycoplasmal cultures have been developed as bacterins and consist of whole-cell preparations as well as new subunit bacterins. These induce excellent protection against development of gross lesions and significantly reduce clinical signs (coughing) in growing pigs. Data indicate that prefarrowing vaccination of sows with *M hyopneumoniae* vaccines significantly reduces colonization of suckling piglets.

The economic effects of the disease can be reduced, and sometimes eliminated, by improvements in housing and husbandry, particularly ventilation and overcrowding, along with medication and vaccination. "All-in/all-out" management of pigs from birth to market is extremely effective at reducing negative effects of disease; following this practice improves growth performance and reduces lung lesions.

In large intensive units, starting with foundation stock free of mycoplasmal pneumonia and adopting strict precautions against direct and indirect contact with pigs from other herds is advisable. Unfortunately, many herds set up in this way do not remain free of mycoplasmas for very long, particularly in areas with a high density of pigs. Field observations suggest that infection can be windborne for at least a mile between large herds in cold, wet weather.

In the USA and parts of Europe, most herds free of mycoplasmal pneumonia were established by the pig repopulation technique. More recently, some have been established by segregated early weaning. The biggest problems with these herd programs are the breakdown rate and the difficulty of monitoring herds that claim to be free of mycoplasmal pneumonia. Hypotheses for these outbreaks suggest that the organism may never have been successfully eliminated in certain herds, but rather coexisted within the population at an undetectable level for extended periods. Use of nasal swab PCR technology has demonstrated presence of the organism in pigs free of clinical signs, lesions, and antibodies. Analysis of tracheal sections from these pigs by electron microscopy has indicated presence of the organism on the cilia.

NECROTIC RHINITIS

(Bullnose)

Necrotic rhinitis is an uncommon, sporadic disease of young pigs characterized by suppuration and necrosis of the snout, arising from wounds of the oral or nasal mucosa. Confusion exists in the literature because of the use of the misnomer "bullnose" to also describe atrophic rhinitis (*see* p 1465).

Etiology: *Fusobacterium necrophorum* is commonly isolated from the lesion and undoubtedly contributes to the disease, but other types of organisms are frequently present. They gain entry through damage to the roof of the mouth, often as a result of clipping the needle teeth too short or using blunt clippers.

Clinical Findings and Lesions: Signs include swelling and deformity of the face, occasionally hemorrhage, snuffling, sneezing, foul-smelling nasal discharge, sometimes involvement of the eyes with lacrimation and purulent discharge, loss of appetite, and emaciation. Generally, only one or two pigs in a herd are affected.

The facial swelling usually is hard, but incision reveals a mass of pinkish gray, foul-smelling necrotic tissue, or greenish gray tissue debris, depending on the age of the lesion. The nasal and facial bones become involved, and facial deformity may be marked.

Diagnosis: Necrotic rhinitis is readily differentiated from atrophic rhinitis by the bulging type of facial distortion seen in the former. The character of the exudate and its location within the tissue of the snout or face are also distinctive of necrotic rhinitis.

Prevention and Treatment: Prevention is directed toward avoiding injuries to the mouth and snout, improving pig processing techniques, and improving sanitation. When the disease occurs repeatedly, needle teeth should be clipped carefully.

If the condition is advanced, treatment may not be advisable. Early surgical intervention and packing the cavity with sulfonamide or tincture of iodine may be useful. In young pigs, sulfamethazine given PO is of value.

PASTEURELLOSIS

Pasteurellosis is most commonly seen in pigs as a complication of mycoplasmal pneumonia (*see* p 1438), although swine influenza, Aujeszky disease, *Bordetella bronchiseptica*, or *Haemophilus parahaemolyticus* may also cause changes in the lungs that lead to disease caused by *Pasteurella* spp. The causative organism usually is *P multocida*. A normal inhabitant of the porcine upper respiratory tract, it produces an exudative bronchopneumonia, sometimes with pericarditis and pleuritis. Primary, sporadic, fibrinous pneumonia due to pasteurellae, with no epidemiologic connection with mycoplasmal or other pneumonia, may also be seen in pigs. In both primary and secondary forms, chronic thoracic lesions and polyarthritis tend to develop. Diagnosis is based on necropsy findings and recovery of pasteurellae from the lesions. Nontoxigenic strains of capsular type A are the predominant isolates from cases of pneumonia. Toxigenic strains of *P multocida*, in the presence of *B bronchiseptica*, are now associated with atrophic rhinitis (*see* p 1465).

Septicemic pasteurellosis and meningitis occasionally occur in piglets. *Mannheimia haemolytica* has been recovered from aborted fetuses, and septicemia may also occur in adult pigs. There are no distinctive lesions, and the pathogenesis is obscure. Porcine strains of *M haemolytica* are often untypeable and do not belong to the common ovine and bovine serotypes. However, some outbreaks in the UK have been associated with close contact with sheep.

Control of the secondary, pneumonic form of the disease is generally based on prevention or control of mycoplasmal pneumonia. Early and vigorous therapy with antibiotics, or in combination with sulfonamides, is indicated to prevent chronic sequelae of all forms of the disease. An increasing resistance to some antibiotics has been noted among the pasteurellae.

PLEUROPNEUMONIA

Pleuropneumonia is a severe and contagious respiratory disease, primarily of young pigs (≤6 mo old), although in an initial outbreak, adults also may be affected. It has a sudden onset, short course, and high morbidity and mortality. It occurs worldwide and appears to be increasing in incidence, although some reports suggest that severity is declining in countries where it has been long established.

Etiology: The causal organism is *Actinobacillus pleuropneumoniae*. To date, 15 serotypes have been identified; they vary widely in virulence and significance across countries. Historically, serotypes 1, 5, and 7 have been prevalent in the USA. Transmission is mainly by nose-to-nose contact, and many recovered pigs are carriers. Clinical signs develop within 4–12 hr in experimental infections. Aerosol transmission is limited.

Clinical Findings: Onset is sudden, and in herds that have not been infected previously, spread is rapid. Some pigs may be found dead without having shown clinical signs. Respiratory distress is severe; there are "thumps," and sometimes open-mouth breathing with a blood-stained, frothy nasal and oral discharge. Fever up to 107°F (41.5°C), anorexia, and reluctance to move are typical signs.

Although primarily a disease of growing pigs, *A pleuropneumoniae* infection may be fatal in adults or cause sows to abort. The course of the disease varies from peracute to chronic. Morbidity may reach 50%, and in untreated cases, mortality is high. Survivors generally show reduced growth rates and persistent cough.

Once established in a herd, the disease may be evident only as a cause of reduced growth rate and pleurisy at the abattoir, although acute disease exacerbations may occur. However, severe lesions may not always be accompanied by equally severe clinical signs. Deaths in transit and carcass condemnation may result. Concurrent infection with mycoplasma, pasteurellae, porcine reproductive and respiratory syndrome, or swine influenza virus is common.

Lesions: The pneumonia is usually bilateral. The characteristic lesion is a severe fibrinonecrotic and hemorrhagic pneumonia with accompanying fibrinous pleuritis. Fibrinous pleuritis and pericarditis may be severe. In acute cases, the lungs are dark and swollen and ooze bloody fluid from the cut surface; hemorrhagic, even necrotic, bullae of various sizes may be present. The trachea may contain blood-stained froth. In chronic cases, the lesions are more organized and localized. Extrathoracic lesions are uncommon.

Diagnosis: An explosive disease onset is suggestive and, when combined with clinical signs and gross lesions, often justifies a tentative diagnosis. Concurrent infections, eg, with pasteurellae, may complicate diagnosis. In herds that have been exposed and have developed at least a degree of immunity, the pattern may be less distinctive. Many serologic tests, including complement fixation and ELISA, have been used to confirm a herd diagnosis or detect carriers, but results are not always straightforward. A definitive diagnosis depends on isolation and identification of *A pleuropneumoniae*, a gram-negative coccobacillus that requires V factor (NAD) supplementation for growth. A *Staphylococcus aureus* nurse colony can provide the necessary factor. PCR testing is also available and provides better sensitivity than direct culture.

Treatment and Control: Rapidity of onset and persistence in infected herds make treatment difficult. Ceftiofur, tilmicosin, tetracyclines, synthetic penicillins, tylosin, and sulfonamides have been used. The first treatment should be parenteral, followed by medication given in water or feed, which also may protect contact pigs.

Because survivors frequently remain carriers, control is difficult, although good results are being claimed for some vaccines. Segregated early weaning, "all-in/all-out" management, reduced stocking rates when possible, and improved ventilation are recommended. In herds free of the disease, replacements should be purchased from herds free of *A pleuropneumoniae*; if the disease proves difficult to control, herd depopulation and repopulation should be considered. Serologic testing effectively detects previously infected herds but may not identify carrier animals.

SWINE INFLUENZA

(Hog flu, Pig flu)

Swine influenza is an acute, highly contagious, respiratory disease that results from infection with type A influenza virus. Field isolates of variable virulence exist, and clinical manifestation may be determined by secondary organisms. Pigs are the principal hosts of classic swine influenza virus. (Human infections have been reported, but porcine strains of influenza A do not appear to easily spread in the human population. However, deaths have occurred in immunocompromised people.) In 2009, a pandemic strain of H1N1 influenza A virus spread globally; it infected people, swine, and poultry, as well as a small number of dogs, cats, and other animals. The disease in swine occurs commonly in the midwestern USA (and occasionally in other states), Mexico, Canada, South America, Europe (including the UK, Sweden, and Italy), Kenya, Mainland China, Japan, Taiwan,PRC and other parts of eastern Asia.

Etiology: Swine influenza virus (SIV) is an orthomyxovirus of the influenza A group with hemagglutinating antigen H1 and neuraminidase antigen N1 (ie, H1N1). Recently, new subtypes of SIV have been reported (H3N2, H1N2, and H2N3). Influenza B and C viruses have been isolated from pigs but have not caused the classic disease. The classic type A infection with isolates of mild virulence may favor replication of pseudorabies virus (*see* p 1300), *Haemophilus parasuis* (Glässer's disease, *see* p 720), *Actinobacillus pleuropneumoniae* (*see* above), and *Mycoplasma hyopneumoniae* (*see* p 1467), any of which may complicate outbreaks. The mixing of carrier and nonimmune pigs is an important predisposing factor. The virus is unlikely to survive outside living cells for >2 wk except in cold conditions. It is readily inactivated by disinfectants.

Transmission and Epidemiology: In North America, outbreaks are most common in fall or winter, often at the onset of particularly cold weather. In warmer areas of the world, infection may occur at any time. Usually, an outbreak is preceded by one or two individual cases and then spreads rapidly within a herd, mainly by aerosolization and pig-to-pig contact. The virus survives in carrier pigs for up to 3 mo and can be recovered from clinically healthy animals between outbreaks. In antibody-positive herds, outbreaks of infection recur as immunity wanes. Up to 40% of herds may contain antibody-positive pigs. Carrier pigs are usually responsible for the introduction of SIV into previously uninfected herds and countries.

Pathogenesis: The spectrum of infection ranges from subclinical to acute. In the classic acute form, the virus multiplies in bronchial epithelium within 16 hr of infection and causes focal necrosis of the bronchial epithelium, focal atelectasis, and gross hyperemia of the lungs. Bronchial exudates and widespread atelectasis, grossly appearing as plum-colored lesions affecting individual lobules of apical and intermediate lobes, are seen after 24 hr. The lesions continue to develop until 72 hr after infection, after which the virus becomes more difficult to demonstrate. Losses in reproduction associated with primary outbreaks appear to be secondary, because virus has been recovered only rarely from the fetus.

Clinical Findings: A classic acute outbreak is characterized by sudden onset and rapid spread through the entire herd, often within 1–3 days. The main signs are depression, fever (to 108°F [42°C]), anorexia, coughing, dyspnea, weakness, prostration, and a mucous discharge from the eyes and nose. Mortality is generally 1%–4%. The overt course of the disease is usually 3–7 days in uncomplicated infections, with clinical recovery of the herd almost as sudden as the onset. However, virus may continue to cycle among pigs when clinical signs are suppressed by immune responses. Some pigs may become chronically affected. In herds that are in good condition, the principal economic loss is from stunting and delay in reaching market weight. Some increase in piglet mortality has been reported, and effects on herd fertility, including abortions in late pregnancy, may follow outbreaks in nonimmune herds.

Lesions: In uncomplicated infections, lesions usually are confined to the thoracic cavity. The pneumonic areas are clearly demarcated, collapsed, and purplish red. They may be distributed throughout the lungs but tend to be more extensive and confluent ventrally. Nonpneumonic areas are pale and emphysematous. The airways contain a copious mucopurulent exudate, and the bronchial and mediastinal lymph nodes are edematous but rarely congested. There may be severe pulmonary edema, especially of interlobular septae, or a serous or serofibrinous pleuritis. Histologically, the lesions, when fully developed, are primarily those of an exudative bronchiolitis with some interstitial pneumonia.

Diagnosis: A presumptive diagnosis can be made on clinical and pathologic findings, but confirmation depends on detection of viral RNA via PCR, molecular sequencing, or demonstration of virus-specific antibody. Virus can be isolated from nasal secretions in the febrile phase or from affected lung tissue in the early acute stage. A retrospective diagnosis can be made by demonstrating a rise in virus-specific antibodies in acute and convalescent serum samples using the hemagglutination inhibition test. Both H3 and H1 subtype antigens should be included. This test is also used for herd surveys. To diagnose uncomplicated influenza infection, conditions such as pasteurellosis, pseudorabies, porcine reproductive and respiratory syndrome, and chlamydial and *Haemophilus* infections must be excluded.

Treatment and Control: There is no effective treatment, although antimicrobials may reduce secondary bacterial infections. Expectorants may help relieve signs in severely affected herds. Vaccination and strict import controls are the only specific preventive measures. Good management practices and freedom from stress, particularly due to crowding and dust, help reduce losses. Commercially available killed vaccines that contain both H1N2 and H3N2 subtypes appear to induce a strong protective immune response.

RESPIRATORY DISEASES OF SHEEP AND GOATS

Upper Respiratory Tract: Diseases of the upper respiratory tract of sheep and goats include sinusitis caused by the larvae of *Oestrus ovis*, nasal foreign bodies, and nasal tumors. Clinical signs associated with sinusitis may include some or all of the following: unilateral or bilateral, serous to mucopurulent nasal discharge; decreased or lack of airflow through one or both nostrils; coughing; sneezing; and mild to severe respiratory distress. The types of nasal neoplasms reported include adenopapillomas (nasal polyps), adenomas, adenocarcinomas, lymphosarcomas (goats), and squamous cell carcinomas (sheep).

Enzootic nasal tumor is caused by an exogenous retrovirus referred to as enzootic nasal tumor virus (ENTV). It can be transmitted experimentally by tumor homogenates, which would explain the widespread occurrence of this condition within some flocks. This type of tumor generally affects mature animals (2–4 yr old), although it has been reported in animals as young as 4 mo old. The lesion may be unilateral or bilateral, resulting in either unilateral or bilateral serous, mucoid, or mucopurulent nasal discharge. Advanced unilateral tumors may cause deviation of the nasal septum, resulting in bilateral nasal discharge. Affected animals show progressive signs of dyspnea (inspiratory), including open-mouth breathing, decreased airflow as measured at the nares, dullness on percussion over the turbinates, sneezing, and head-shaking. Stridor may also be caused by compression of the larynx by enlarged retropharyngeal lymph nodes associated with abscessation of the head. Laryngeal chondritis also results in inspiratory dyspnea of varying severity. With advancing tumor growth, exophthalmos and facial deformity may occur. Metastatic spread is uncommon. Outcome depends on the tumor type, condition of the animal, and extent of the lesion, but in most commercial situations the animal is culled for animal welfare and commercial reasons. Surgical removal of a noninvasive tumor is rarely undertaken.

The most common problems associated with the pharynx are trauma and abscessation. Pharyngeal trauma usually results from overly aggressive use of equipment used to administer boluses. Injuries may result in the formation of discrete abscesses or extensive and diffuse cellulitis, both of which can interfere with swallowing and possibly lead to respiratory difficulty or distress. Bacteria commonly isolated after an incident of pharyngeal trauma include *Trueperella*, *Pasteurella multocida*, *Mannheimia haemolytica*, and *Fusobacterium*.

Laryngeal chondritis is an obstructive upper respiratory tract disease characterized by severe dyspnea most commonly encountered in meat-breed rams 18–24 mo old. Acute onset of severe respiratory distress with marked inspiratory effort and stertor is caused by edema of the arytenoid cartilages of the larynx, resulting in narrowing of the lumen. Affected sheep stand with the neck extended, head held lowered with flared nostrils, and mouth open; they are reluctant to move because of dyspnea. Delayed identification and/or inadequate duration of antibiotic therapy may result in abscess formation within the arytenoid cartilages.

Lower Respiratory Tract: The most common problem associated with the lower respiratory tract is pneumonia. Pneumonias can be caused by viruses, bacteria, or parasites. They can be acute, chronic, or progressive.

Viruses associated with acute pneumonia include parainfluenza type 3 (PI-3), adenovirus, and respiratory syncytial virus. These viral pneumonias most often affect lambs and kids.

PI-3 is an enveloped RNA virus (family Paramyxoviridae) that induces a mild interstitial pneumonia. Clinical signs may include coughing, serous nasal and/or ocular discharge, fever (104°–106°F [40°–41°C]), and an increased respiratory rate. The single PI-3 serotype for sheep that has been identified is distinct from the bovine PI-3 serotype. Infection with this virus can be confirmed by its isolation from nasal swabs from affected animals, or by comparison of acute and convalescent serum antibody levels. Treatment is usually not warranted in mildly affected animals. In severely affected animals in which secondary pathogens are suspected, antimicrobial therapy is recommended using drugs with efficacy against the most likely organisms, such as *P multocida*, *M haemolytica*, and *Mycoplasma* sp. There are no PI-3 vaccines specifically designed for use in small ruminants.

Chronic, progressive viral pneumonia is most common in adults and includes progressive interstitial retroviral pneumonia (in sheep, ovine progressive pneumonia or maedi [*see* p 1475]; in goats, pneumonia induced by arthritis encephalitis virus [*see* p 747]) and ovine pulmonary adenocarcinoma (*see* p 1477), also known as jaagsiekte or the contagious lung tumor of sheep and, infrequently, of goats.

Chronic, progressive, proliferative changes in the lungs are usually associated with the lentiviruses (family Retroviridae), or so-called slow-virus infections. In both progressive pneumonia and pulmonary adenocarcinoma, the entire lung can change in a gradual process of abnormal cellular proliferation. In affected sheep, the loss of functional lung tissue results in progressive dyspnea, anorexia, and weight loss.

M haemolytica, *P multocida*, *Mycoplasma* spp, *Chlamydia pneumoniae*, and *Salmonella* spp are associated with either primary or secondary bronchopneumonia in sheep and goats. Both *P multocida* and *M haemolytica* can be cultured from the upper respiratory tract of normal sheep and goats. Not all factors predisposing to acute respiratory diseases are known, but acute viral infections in a susceptible population can alter the protective mechanisms in the respiratory tract so that certain bacteria may invade lung tissue, multiply, and cause serious disease. An initial infection with PI-3 virus may predispose an animal to infection with pathogenic *M haemolytica*. Also, *Mycoplasma ovipneumoniae* alone can cause a mild bronchopneumonia; however, it is often isolated along with *M haemolytica* from sheep and goats with severe pneumonia, suggesting that the *Mycoplasma* may predispose the lung to invasion by this organism. Additionally, introduction of new animals, high-density stocking, poor ventilation, and a sudden change to a high plane of nutrition can act as stress factors that predispose to development of pneumonia.

Caseous lymphadenitis (*see* p 63) caused by *Corynebacterium pseudotuberculosis* may result in abscessation of the lungs and mediastinal lymph nodes. This can result in a progressive debilitation in sheep and goats with or without obvious clinical signs of respiratory disease.

Parasitic or verminous pneumonias of sheep and goats are most commonly caused by infection with *Dictyocaulus filaria*, *Muellerius capillaris*, or *Protostrongylus rufescens*. (*See also* p 1421.) In contrast to the acute viral and bacterial pneumonias, which result in a bronchopneumonia affecting the anterior ventral portion of the lungs, verminous pneumonia affects the margins of the diaphragmatic lung lobes. *Dictyocaulus* has a direct life cycle, whereas *Protostrongylus* and *Muellerius* have indirect life cycles and rely on a variety of snails and slugs to serve as intermediate hosts. Adult forms of *Dictyocaulus* and *Protostrongylus* live in bronchi but rarely cause clinical signs. Adult *Muellerius* live in alveoli and lung parenchymal tissue and are considered the least pathogenic of the three lungworms. *Muellerius* appears to cause more problems for goats than for sheep.

Diagnosis of lungworm infection requires Baermann examination of fecal material (*See also* p 1619). Treatment for lungworm infection is rarely indicated; however, it is likely that sheep with such infections will also carry other nematodes that will cause parasitic gastroenteritis and limit production.

SHEEP NOSE BOT

The sheep nose bot fly, *Oestrus ovis*, is a cosmopolitan parasite that, in its larval stages, inhabits the nasal passages and sinuses of sheep and goats. Its geographic distribution is worldwide.

The adult fly is grayish brown and ~12 mm long. The female deposits larvae in and about the nostrils of sheep without alighting. These small, clear-white larvae (initially <2 mm long) migrate into the nasal cavity; many spend at least some time in the paranasal sinuses. The larval period, which is usually shortest in young animals, lasts 1–10 mo. When mature, the larvae leave the nasal passages, drop to the ground, burrow down a few inches, and pupate. The pupal period lasts 3–9 wk, depending on the environmental conditions, after which the fly emerges from the pupal case and pushes its way to the surface. Mating soon occurs, and the female begins to deposit larvae.

Clinical Findings: Once the larvae begin to move about in the nasal passages, a profuse discharge occurs, at first clear and mucoid, but later mucopurulent and frequently tinged with fine streaks of blood emanating from minute hemorrhages produced by the hooks and spines of the larvae. Paroxysms of sneezing accompany migrations of the larger larvae. Larvae present in the sinuses are sometimes unable to escape; they die and may gradually become calcified or lead to a septic sinusitis. However, the principal effects are annoyance, with a resulting reduction in grazing time, and loss of condition. Usually only 4–15 larvae are found, although many more may be present.

To avoid the fly's attempts at larval deposition, a sheep may run from place to place, keeping its nose close to the ground, sneeze and stamp its feet, or shake its head. Commonly, especially during the warmer hours of the day when the flies are most active, small groups of sheep gather and face the center of a circle, heads down and close together.

Treatment: Ivermectin at 200 mcg/kg, PO or SC, is highly effective against all stages of the larvae.

CONTAGIOUS CAPRINE PLEUROPNEUMONIA

Contagious caprine pleuropneumonia is a highly fatal disease that occurs in goats in the Middle East, Africa, and Asia. It was seen for the first time on European soil in Thrace, Turkey, in 2002, but does not appear to have spread to neighboring countries, Greece and Bulgaria. Outbreaks have recently been reported in sheep and captive wildlife, including gazelles and small ruminants.

Etiology: *Mycoplasma capricolum capripneumoniae* (*Mycoplasma* biotype F38) is the causative agent. It appears to be transmitted by infective aerosol. Morbidity can be 100%, and mortality 60%–100%. The disease is introduced into a new region by healthy carriers. Gathering or housing animals together facilitates spread of the disease.

Pneumonia and pleuropneumonia can be caused by other mycoplasmas, including *M mycoides capri*. Taxonomic change means this subspecies also includes *M mycoides mycoides* large colony type. Morbidity and mortality rates are generally lower with *M mycoides capri*, and joint and udder infections may also be seen.

Clinical Findings: Weakness, anorexia, cough, hyperpnea, and nasal discharge accompanied by fever (104.5°–106°F [40.5°–41.5°C]) are often found. Exercise intolerance progresses to respiratory distress, with open-mouth breathing and frothy salivation. A septicemic form of the disease without specific respiratory tract involvement has been described.

Lesions: Typically, there is an excess of straw-colored pleural exudate and acute fibrinous pneumonia. Consolidation is sometimes confined to one lung. The distention of interlobular septa by serofibrinous fluid, commonly seen in infections caused by *M mycoides capri*, is rarely seen in contagious caprine pleuropneumonia. In antibiotic-treated or recovered animals, the predominant lesion is a sequestrum similar to that seen in contagious bovine pleuropneumonia.

Diagnosis: The clinical signs, epidemiology, and necropsy findings are used to establish a diagnosis. The causative organism should be isolated and identified, but isolation may be difficult, and special media is required for culture. PCR, which can be performed directly on the pleural fluid or affected lung, has greatly facilitated the diagnosis of contagious caprine pleuropneumonia. Serologic tests are complement fixation, passive hemagglutination, and ELISA; the latex agglutination test can be done in the field directly on whole blood as well as on serum samples in the laboratory. Serologic cross-reactions may occur with other members of the *Mycoplasma mycoides* cluster.

Control: Quarantine of affected flocks is desirable. Vaccines are available in some countries, and good to excellent protection has been reported. Treatment with tylosin at 10 mg/kg/day, IM, for 3 days, has been effective, as has oxytetracycline (15 mg/kg).

PASTEURELLA AND *MANNHEIMIA* PNEUMONIAS

Bronchopneumonia caused by *Pasteurella multocida* or *Mannheimia haemolytica* has a cranioventral lung distribution and affects sheep and goats of all ages worldwide. It can be particularly devastating in young animals around weaning. It is a common cause of morbidity and mortality in lambs and kids, especially in those that have not received adequate colostrum or in which passive colostral immunity is waning. The disease appears to occur most often in animals that have undergone recent stress such as transportation, weaning, change of diet, or commingling with animals from unrelated farms. *Bibersteinia trehalosi* (formerly *Pasteurella trehalosi*) causes septicemia in lambs 4–9 mo old (systemic pasteurellosis). (*See also* PASTEURELLOSIS OF SHEEP AND GOATS, p 765.)

Etiology: *P multocida* and *M haemolytica* are commensals of the upper respiratory tract that can cause pneumonia either alone or in conjunction with other organisms. Primary infections with respiratory pathogens such as parainfluenza type 3, adenovirus, respiratory syncytial virus, *Bordetella parapertussis*, or in particular *Mycoplasma ovipneumoniae* appear to predispose to secondary infection with *Pasteurella* and *Mannheimia*.

Pathogenesis: Stress appears to be an important factor that allows *Pasteurella*, *Mannheimia*, *Mycoplasma ovipneumoniae*, other bacteria, and viruses to multiply and impair the normal physical defense mechanisms, facilitating invasion of lung tissue and development of pneumonia. In calves, alveolar macrophage function is impaired after viral pneumonia. This results in decreased clearance of inhaled bacterial pathogens, allowing them to become established. Pathogen-host interactions result in tissue damage, especially because of massive influx of neutrophils. As these neutrophils are lysed, enzymes are released that cause more lung tissue damage. This mechanism may be similar to that of *Pasteurella* and *Mannheimia* pneumonias in sheep and goats.

Clinical Findings: Acute respiratory disease caused by *M haemolytica* is uncommon in adult sheep, unless there is a predisposing problem such as ovine pulmonary adenocarcinoma or other viral infection. Clinical signs include acute onset depression, lethargy, and inappetance and are consistent with profound endotoxemia. Sudden death may occur without clinical signs having been observed. Affected sheep are typically separated from the remainder of the flock and are easily caught and restrained. On approach, they may show an increased respiratory rate with an abdominal component.

Affected sheep are typically febrile (>40.5°C [104.9°F]). The mucous membranes are congested, and there may be evidence of dehydration with sunken eyes and extended skin tent duration. Auscultation often does not reveal significant changes other than an increased respiratory rate. Rumen contractions are reduced or absent. There may be evidence of diarrhea. Frothy fluid may be noted around the mouth during the terminal stages.

Lesions: There are subcutaneous ecchymotic hemorrhages over the throat and ribs. The lungs are heavy, swollen, and purple-red in peracute cases, and the airways contain blood-stained froth. Cases of longer duration show anteroventral consolidation and fibrinous pleurisy.

Diagnosis: At necropsy, testing whether lung tissue sinks (pneumonia) or floats (normal) remains a useful screening test. In acute cases, cultures obtained from tracheal swabs or washes or from lung tissue or associated lymph nodes are diagnostic. Histopathologic examination is useful, especially if other types of pneumonia (eg, retrovirus interstitial pneumonia in adult sheep and goats) are also suspected. In chronic cases, bacterial cultures may be less rewarding; *Pasteurella* or *Mannheimia* may have been the initial problem, but results of cultures taken later may reveal *Trueperella pyogenes*, a common causative agent of lung abscesses.

Treatment and Control: Whenever possible, treatment should be based on bacterial culture and sensitivity, especially in herd or flock outbreaks, when valuable animals are involved, or in acute or chronic cases when initial therapeutic attempts have failed. Commonly recommended antibiotics include oxytetracycline (10 mg/kg/day of non-long-acting product, or 20 mg/kg once of the long-acting product), florfenicol (20 mg/kg, every 48 hr), and tylosin (10–20 mg/kg, once to twice daily). Therapy should continue for at least 24–48 hr after body temperature has returned to normal. Duration of treatment usually is 4–5 days. Tilmicosin and other macrolide antibiotics can also be used but are considerably more expensive than oxytetracycline. Acute cases may also benefit from the use of NSAIDs (eg, flunixin meglumine or ketoprofen) in conjunction with antibiotic therapy for control of endotoxemia and inflammation.

Inadequate ventilation, crowding, commingling of animals from various farms (feedlot or sale barn situations), poor nutrition, failure of passive transfer of antibodies, transportation, and other stresses have all been associated with pneumonia outbreaks. Control and prevention lies with correction of the predisposing factors whenever practical.

Prevention of pasteurellosis is best attempted using vaccines incorporating iron-regulated proteins; because these proteins are antigenically similar, they confer cross-protection against other serotypes. Breeding ewes require a primary course of two injections 4–6 wk apart followed by an annual booster 4–6 wk before lambing. However, this vaccination regimen provides only passive immunity to the lambs for up to 5 wk. Lambs can be protected by two doses of vaccine administered from 10 days of age, because colostral antibody does not interfere with development of active immunity.

PROGRESSIVE PNEUMONIA

(Maedi, Zwoegersiekte, La bouhite, Graaff-Reinet disease)

Ovine progressive pneumonia and maedi-visna are chronic diseases of sheep caused by lentiviruses (family Retroviridae) that are structurally and antigenically similar. Progressive pneumonia virus and maedi (meaning "dyspnea") virus induce chronic progressive pneumonias that present with similar clinical signs. Visna (meaning "wasting") is the term used in many parts of the world to refer to the neurologic form of the disease in sheep, resulting initially in unilateral pelvic paresis, progressing to paralysis. A closely related lentivirus-induced disease in goats, caprine arthritis and encephalitis (CAE, *see* p 747), affects the nervous system and joints. Reported seroprevalence for lentiviral infection in sheep varies widely, ranging from 49% in the western USA to 9% in the north Atlantic region. This variation has been reported in other countries as well and may result from varied climatic conditions (arid vs more lush climates) and management (range conditions vs close confinement).

Etiology and Pathogenesis: The causal lentivirus, which persists in lymphocytes, monocytes, and macrophages of infected sheep in the presence of a humoral and cell-mediated immune response, can be detected by several serologic tests. Seropositive sheep and goats must be considered infected and capable of transmitting the virus. Transmission occurs most commonly via the oral route, usually by ingestion of colostrum or milk that contains virus, or by inhalation of infected aerosol droplets. Intrauterine infection is thought to occur infrequently. All breeds of sheep and goats appear susceptible; however, some resistance to lentivirus infection may exist within breeds. Management practices can influence morbidity rates.

Clinical Findings: Signs rarely occur in sheep <2 yr old and are most common in sheep >4 yr old. The disease progresses slowly, with wasting and increasing respiratory distress as the main signs. Coughing, bronchial exudate, depression, and fever are seldom evident unless secondary bacterial infection occurs. A noninflammatory, indurative mastitis may occur. The encephalitic form of visna causes head tilt and circling, whereas the spinal form causes unilateral pelvic limb proprioceptive deficits progressing to paresis and eventually to complete paralysis.

Lesions: Macroscopic lesions of progressive pneumonia are confined to the lungs and associated lymph nodes. The lungs do not collapse when the thorax (with obvious rib indentations) is opened and are abnormally firm and heavy (~2 kg; 2–4 times normal weight). Early lung changes may be difficult to detect, but later in the disease, lungs are mottled by gray and brown areas of consolidation. The mediastinal and tracheobronchial lymph nodes are greatly enlarged and edematous. Interstitial pneumonia, perivascular and peribronchial lymphoid hyperplasia, and hypertrophy of smooth muscle are seen throughout the entire lung. CNS lesions, when they occur, are those of meningoleukoencephalitis with secondary demyelination. All lesions are progressive and result from the cellular immune response of the host, and not directly from viral damage.

Diagnosis: Differential diagnoses of progressive pneumonia include pulmonary adenocarcinoma, pleural abscesses, and pulmonary caseous lymphadenitis. Ultrasonographic examination is very useful to differentiate these various types of pneumonias in the live animal. Listeriosis, scrapie, cerebrospinal nematodiasis, and space-occupying lesions should be considered when the neurologic form (visna) of the disease is seen.

In the live animal, agar gel immunodiffusion and ELISA tests are used. The competitive inhibition ELISA is reported to be highly sensitive and specific; it has been reported to produce false-negative results in animals very recently infected. Serologic testing is considered a useful tool to detect infected sheep, especially if the disease has been confirmed in the flock by histopathologic examination or virus isolation. PCR and virus isolation are sensitive and specific techniques to detect virus. However, both are more expensive and time consuming than serologic testing.

Control: Currently, there is no practical, effective treatment, and no vaccines are available. Therefore, the only means for control and prevention is serologic testing and removal of positive animals. Because of the long incubation period and time to seroconversion, retesting animals once a year, or even twice a year, is recommended. In addition to the test and cull approach, consideration should be given to raising neonates in isolation from their dams, especially if the dam is seropositive. Lambs should be fed colostrum from seronegative sheep, or heat-treated sheep colostrum, and raised on milk replacer, milk from seronegative ewes, or heat-treated sheep milk.

OVINE PULMONARY ADENOCARCINOMA

(Jaagsiekte, Sheep pulmonary adenomatosis)

Ovine pulmonary adenocarcinoma (OPA) is a contagious, viral, neoplastic disease of the lungs of sheep and more rarely of goats. It has been reported from Europe, Asia, Africa, and South and North America.

Etiology: OPA is an infectious neoplastic lung disease resulting from infection with a beta retrovirus called Jaagsiekte sheep retrovirus (JSRV). The virus replicates predominantly in the tumor cells, is released into the airways, and is found in respiratory secretions. Transmission of JSRV occurs predominantly through the aerosol route by inhalation of infected respiratory secretions, although the virus may also be transmitted via colostrum and milk.

Clinical Findings: The period of incubation after natural infection extends over months, so clinical signs generally become evident when sheep are 2–4 yr old. However, disease may be seen in lambs 8–12 mo old that are progeny of infected dams. The tumors produce clinical signs when they become sufficiently large or numerous enough to interfere with respiration. Affected sheep lose weight and show increasing respiratory distress and panting. Crackles are audible over a much larger area than the distribution of OPA lesions determined ultrasonographically. Coughing is not prominent, and infected animals are afebrile unless secondary infection develops. During the advanced stages of clinical disease, the tumor mass may occupy up to 60% of lung parenchyma. Clinical disease ends in death after many months but sometimes within 1–2 days due to secondary pasteurellosis.

Lesions: Tumors are confined to the lungs and, rarely, the associated lymph nodes. They vary from small nodules to extensive solid areas that involve the ventral parts of one or more lobes and are firm, gray, flat, and sharply demarcated. Copious amounts of white, frothy fluid are present in the air passages. Histologic changes are caused by uncontrolled proliferation of columnar-shaped type II pneumonocytes and similar cells in the bronchioles (Clara cells).

Diagnosis: Chronic weight loss, dyspnea, crackles, and copious amounts of serous nasal discharge from accumulated lung fluid in an adult sheep that is afebrile are highly suggestive clinical signs of OPA.

During the advanced stages of clinical disease, several mL of a clear, frothy fluid may flow freely from both nostrils when the sheep's head is lowered during feeding; this quantity may exceed 50 mL if the hindquarters are raised when the head is simultaneously lowered (colloquially referred to as the "wheelbarrow test"). This test causes affected sheep considerable distress and must be discontinued as soon as some clear fluid appears at the nostrils; euthanasia is warranted immediately once this positive result is obtained. Not all cases of OPA produce this fluid in detectable amounts even in the advanced stages of disease. Therefore, a negative wheelbarrow test should not be considered conclusive, although a positive wheelbarrow test is pathognomonic for OPA.

There is presently no commercial confirmatory serologic test for OPA. The PCR test has been used in research on OPA for several years. However, whereas the test is highly sensitive in laboratory assays, it fails to detect JSRV in most infected sheep other than overt clinical cases. This is because there are few infected cells in the blood during the early stages of disease progression. Bronchoalveolar lavage has been used on sedated sheep to collect cells from the airways, followed by DNA extraction and PCR testing. Although this method appears to offer better sensitivity than the blood test, the sample collection method does not lend itself to routine on-farm large-scale testing.

Ultrasonography can be used to differentiate chronic lung pathologies and support a diagnosis of OPA, including superficial lung lesions as small as 1–2 cm in diameter. The first indication of changes in the superficial lung parenchyma caused by OPA is the abrupt loss of the bright linear echo formed by normal aerated lung tissue (visceral or pulmonary pleura) to be replaced by a hypoechoic area in the ventral margins of the lung lobes at the fifth or sixth intercostal spaces.

Control: No specific treatment or vaccine is available. Affected sheep must be culled as soon as clinical suspicions are confirmed by ultrasonographic examination of the chest. Antibiotic therapy may temporarily improve the clinical appearance of those sheep with significant secondary bacterial infection. Good biosecurity is essential to minimize the risks of introducing OPA to unaffected farms with purchased sheep. At this time, the best that can be recommended once a diagnosis is confirmed is removal of all animals showing signs suggestive of pulmonary adenomatosis. However, subclinically infected sheep serve as a reservoir for the virus. Maintaining sheep in single-age groups is the most important management factor to reduce clinical disease.

RESPIRATORY DISEASES OF SMALL ANIMALS

Respiratory diseases are common in dogs and cats. Although clinical signs such as coughing and dyspnea are commonly referable to primary problems of the respiratory tract, they may also occur secondary to disorders of other organ systems (eg, congestive heart failure).

Both young and aged animals are at increased risk of developing respiratory disease. At birth, the respiratory and immune systems are incompletely developed; this facilitates the introduction and spread of pathogens within the lungs, and alveolar flooding may occur. In aged animals, chronic degenerative changes that disrupt normal mucociliary clearance and immunologic anergy may render the lungs more vulnerable to airborne pathogens and toxic particulates.

A varying flora of indigenous commensal organisms (including *Pasteurella multocida*, *Bordetella bronchiseptica*, streptococci, staphylococci, pseudomonads, and coliform bacteria) normally reside in the canine and feline nasal passages, nasopharynx, and upper trachea, and at least intermittently in the lungs, without causing clinical signs. Opportunistic infections by these bacteria may occur when respiratory defense mechanisms are compromised by infection with a primary pathogen (eg, distemper, parainfluenza virus, or canine type 2 adenovirus in dogs, and rhinotracheitis virus or calicivirus in cats), other insults (eg, inhalation of smoke or noxious gases), or diseases such as congestive heart failure and pulmonary neoplasia. Secondary bacterial infections complicate the management of viral respiratory infections of both dogs and cats. Pathogens may continue to reside in the respiratory tract of convalescent animals. When stressed, these animals may relapse; they can also act as a source of infection for others. Poor management practices (eg, overcrowding) are often associated with poor hygienic and environmental conditions, and the resultant stress increases both the incidence and severity of infections. Conditions that favor the spread of infections often occur in catteries, kennels, pet shops, boarding facilities, and humane shelters.

Congenital abnormalities, such as stenotic nares, elongation of the soft palate, nasopharyngeal turbinates, and tracheal stenosis, can cause respiratory dysfunction. Neoplastic masses, degenerative changes of the airways, and tracheal collapse can result in dyspnea and other clinical manifestations of respiratory disease.

Tracheal collapse is most common in toy and miniature breeds of dogs and rare in cats. The cause is unknown. Affected animals have a nonproductive, honking, chronic cough and inspiratory or expiratory dyspnea. Frequently they are obese and may have concurrent cardiovascular or other pulmonary disease (especially chronic bronchitis). Weight loss (if obese) is critical in management. Other measures include exercise restriction, reduction of excitement and stress, and medical therapy, eg, antitussives, antibiotics, bronchodilators, and corticosteroids.

ALLERGIC PNEUMONITIS

Allergic pneumonitis is an acute or chronic hypersensitivity reaction of the lungs and small airways.

Etiology: An underlying cause is rarely determined in pulmonary hypersensitivity reactions in dogs and cats. Type I or immediate hypersensitivity is probably the most common mechanism, although Type III and IV mechanisms may also be involved (*see* IMMUNOLOGIC DISEASES, p 817 et seq). The cellular infiltrate is typically eosinophilic; however, mixed inflammatory infiltrates consisting of mononuclear cells, eosinophils, and neutrophils, or predominantly lymphocytic infiltrates can be seen.

Eosinophilic bronchopneumopathy (formerly pulmonary infiltration with eosinophilia [PIE], *see* p 825) is a group of diseases associated with both pulmonary-associated and peripheral eosinophilia. Not all types of allergic pneumonitis, however, are associated with eosinophilic bronchopneumopathy. Causes of eosinophilic bronchopneumopathy include migrating parasites, reaction to microfilariae of heartworms, lungworms, chronic bacterial or fungal infections (eg, histoplasmosis, aspergillosis), viruses, external antigens, and unknown precipitating factors. Canine heartworm (*see* p 127) pneumonitis occurs when dogs become sensitized to microfilariae. A similar reaction may be seen in cats with heartworms. Migrating intestinal parasites and primary lung parasites may induce either subclinical or mild signs of allergic pneumonitis.

Pulmonary nodular eosinophilic granulomatous syndrome is a rare, severe eosinophilic bronchopneumopathy–like syndrome that occurs in dogs and is most often associated with heartworm infection or possibly an uncontrollable progressive form of eosinophilic bronchopneumopathy. In this condition, a severe granulomatous hypersensitivity reaction to microfilariae (or other antigen) results in mixed alveolar and interstitial pulmonary infiltrates plus variably sized, multiple pulmonary nodules scattered throughout the lung fields. Associated pathology may include eosinophilic granulomatous lymphadenitis, tracheitis, tonsillitis, splenitis, enteritis, gastritis, and pericholangitis. Pulmonary hypersensitivity also may be caused by drugs and reactions to inhaled allergens; however, this is poorly documented in small animals.

Clinical Findings: Chronic cough is the most common sign. It may be mild or severe, productive or nonproductive, and progressive or nonprogressive. Weight loss, tachypnea, dyspnea, wheezing, exercise intolerance, and occasionally hemoptysis may be seen. Severely affected animals may exhibit moderate to severe dyspnea and cyanosis at rest. Auscultation varies from unremarkable to increased breath sounds, crackles, or wheezes. Fever is usually absent. The degree of dyspnea and coughing is related to the severity of inflammation within the airways and alveoli.

Diagnosis: This is based largely on history and on radiographic and clinicopathologic findings. Thoracic radiographs frequently show irregular patchy alveolar infiltrates and increased bronchial and interstitial markings. Radiographic evidence of heartworm disease or parasitic pulmonary disease may suggest an underlying cause. Typical hematologic changes are mild leukocytosis, variable peripheral eosinophilia (4%–50%), and occasionally basophilia. Fecal analysis and an occult heartworm test are indicated when lung parasitism or heartworm disease is suspected. Bronchoalveolar lavage for cytologic analysis, culture, and detection of larval forms is often helpful. In allergic pneumonitis, bronchoalveolar lavage cytology generally reveals a predominance of eosinophils. Bacterial cultures of aseptically collected lavage specimens are commonly negative.

Treatment: When an underlying cause can be found, elimination of the offending agent and a short-term course of glucocorticoids resolves the problem. Prednisolone beginning at 1–2 mg/kg, PO, tapered over 10–14 days is often sufficient. When eosinophilic bronchopneumopathy is secondary to heartworm disease or pulmonary parasites, treatment with prednisolone before or during treatment for the parasite controls the pulmonary signs. When an underlying cause cannot be determined, prolonged therapy with prednisolone for 3–12 wk is often required. When severe bronchoconstriction is suspected, bronchodilators or β_2-agonists may be helpful. Severely dyspneic animals may require short-term oxygen therapy.

CANINE INFLUENZA (FLU)

Etiology, Epidemiology, and Transmission: Two strains of the canine influenza virus (CIV) have been identified, H3N8 and H3N2. The H3N8 strain was first identified in the USA in 2004, and the H3N2 strain was identified only in Asia until 2015, when an outbreak occurred in the USA. Outbreaks are most common when dogs are in close contact, eg, kennels, shelters, dog parks.

CIV is spread via respiratory secretions, contaminated objects (eg, water bowls), and people moving between infected and uninfected dogs. The incubation period is usually 2-4 days from exposure to onset of clinical signs, when dogs are most contagious; ~20% of infected dogs remain asymptomatic but can still shed virus.

Clinical Findings and Diagnosis: Most exposed dogs (80%) develop mild infection, with a cough that persists 1-3 wk and may be similar to the cough of canine infectious tracheobronchitis (*see* p 1491). Other possible clinical signs include ocular and nasal discharge, sneezing, fever, lethargy, and anorexia. Some dogs become severely ill, with high fever (104°-106°F), pneumonia, and secondary bacterial infection. The mortality rate is <10%.

There is no rapid test for specific diagnosis. Nasal or pharyngeal swabs from dogs ill for <3 days can be submitted for PCR testing. After 4 days of illness, PCR testing may result in false-negatives, because the time of maximal virus shedding has passed. Serum antibodies to CIV may be detected as early as 7 days after onset of clinical signs. The best method for confirmation of infection is serologic testing with acute and convalescent serum samples.

Treatment, Prevention, and Control: Treatment is largely supportive; most dogs recover in 2-3 wk. Additional treatment (eg, antimicrobials, NSAIDs) is warranted to combat secondary bacterial infection, pneumonia, and other complications.

H3N8 canine influenza vaccines are available, but whether they protect against the H3N2 strain is unknown. Two vaccines for H3N2 canine influenza are available under conditional license from the USDA.

Routine infection control practices and good hygiene within facilities are key to preventing spread. CIV can persist in the environment for 1-2 days but is readily killed by common disinfectants. There is no evidence of transmission of CIV from dogs to people.

CANINE NASAL MITES

The canine nasal mite, also known as *Pneumonyssoides caninum* or *Pneumonyssus caninum*, has been reported worldwide, including the USA, Canada, Japan, Australia, South Africa, Italy, France, Spain, Norway, Sweden, Finland, Denmark, and Iran.

Etiology and Epidemiology: The canine nasal mite has most commonly been reported in dogs and has also been reported in a silver fox. There does not seem to be a breed, age, or sex predilection, although one report suggested that dogs >3 yr old were affected more often and that large-breed dogs had a higher incidence than small-breed dogs.

The mites live in the nasal passages and paranasal sinuses. The complete life cycle of *P caninum* is not known or understood. Transmission is thought to be via direct and indirect contact between dogs. There is no evidence to suggest that *P caninum* presents a zoonotic risk.

Clinical Findings: The most common clinical signs associated with nasal mite infestation include epistaxis, sneezing, reverse sneezing, impaired scenting ability, facial pruritus, nasal discharge, head shaking, and stridor. Other reported clinical signs include coughing, restlessness, and collapse. These signs are not specific for nasal mite infection and may indicate many types of upper respiratory disease.

Diagnosis: Differential diagnoses based on the clinical signs include many upper respiratory diseases such as rhinitis (idiopathic, secondary bacterial, parasitic, or fungal), oronasal neoplasia, dental disease (oronasal fistula), nasal foreign body, or nasopharyngeal disease (foreign body or mass lesions). To exclude concurrent systemic disease, a CBC, serum chemistry profile, and urinalysis should be performed. If epistaxis is present, a one-stage prothrombin time, partial thromboplastin time, and buccal mucosal bleeding time should be considered in addition to a platelet count.

Imaging of the nasal chambers via nasal/dental radiographs should be considered. Alternative imaging modalities such as CT provide excellent images of the nasal cavity and paranasal sinuses. More invasive diagnostic procedures such as rhinoscopy, retroflex nasopharyngoscopy, nasal flushing, and nasal biopsy must be delayed until after imaging, because iatrogenic changes may be hard to distinguish from primary disease.

Rhinoscopy and nasal flushing are the most useful diagnostic tools. Flexible rhinoscopes allow observation of the nasal choanae. This area is best visualized by putting a u-bend in the rhinoscope (retroflexed view) and advancing it into the oral cavity until it can be hooked under the soft palate. Gentle traction is applied, and the endoscopist can view the nasal choanae or the caudal nasal passages as they enter the nasopharynx. Flooding the nasal chambers with anesthetic gas or oxygen to encourage the mites to migrate toward the nasopharynx and the endoscope has been described.

Nasal flushing may also help identify *P caninum*. This is generally performed with the dog under general anesthesia with a cuffed endotracheal tube in place. The oropharynx is packed with gauze, and saline is flushed through the external nares with a Foley catheter or a tight-fitting syringe to collect fluid from the oropharynx. Retrograde flushing can be done by placing a modified catheter behind the soft palate, occluding the nasal pharynx, and flushing with saline. This allows fluid to be collected via the external nares. In both cases, the fluid should be evaluated using an illuminated magnifying lens to look for mites.

The definitive diagnosis of nasal acariasis can be made via endoscopy or nasal flushing if the mites are identified. This does not, however, determine whether the disease is primary or secondary.

Treatment: No drugs are currently approved for the treatment of *P caninum*; however, ivermectin (200–400 mcg/kg, SC or PO), milbemycin oxime (1 mg/kg, PO, three times at 10-day intervals), and selamectin (topical) have been suggested. The optimal treatment regimen has yet to be determined. Treatment has been reported to be effective in >85% of cases, and the prognosis is excellent. However, treatment may not completely eliminate clinical signs, particularly if infection is suspected rather than demonstrated. In these cases, it is probable that the signs are the result of a concurrent upper airway disease. Treatment is based on definitive diagnosis, but empirical therapy has also been performed based on a high index of suspicion.

FELINE RESPIRATORY DISEASE COMPLEX

Feline respiratory disease complex includes those illnesses typified by rhinosinusitis, conjunctivitis, lacrimation, salivation, and oral ulcerations. The principal diseases, feline viral rhinotracheitis (FVR; feline herpesvirus type 1), feline calicivirus (FCV), *Chlamydia felis*, *Mycoplasma felis*, or combinations of these infections, affect exotic as well as domestic species. Feline pneumonitis (*Chlamydia psittaci*) and mycoplasmal infections appear to be of lesser importance. Feline infectious peritonitis (*see* p 780) typically causes a more generalized condition but may cause signs of mild upper respiratory tract infection.

FVR and caliciviruses are host-specific and pose no known human risk. Human conjunctivitis caused by the feline chlamydial agent has been reported.

Etiology: Most acute feline upper respiratory infections are caused by FVR virus, although FCV may be more prevalent in some populations. Dual infections with these viruses may occur. Other organisms such as *C felis*, *Mycoplasma* spp, and reoviruses are believed to account for most of the remaining infections or further complicate FVR or FCV infection. Concurrent *Bartonella henselae* also may further complicate infection.

Natural transmission of these agents occurs via aerosol droplets and fomites, which can be carried to a susceptible cat by a handler. Convalescent cats may harbor virus for many months. Calicivirus is shed continually, while infectious FVR virus is released intermittently. Stress may precipitate a secondary course of illness. The incubation period is 2–6 days for FVR and FCV, and 5–10 days for pneumonitis.

Clinical Findings: The onset of FVR is marked by fever, frequent sneezing, conjunctivitis, rhinitis, and often salivation. Excitement or movement may induce sneezing. The fever may reach 105°F (40.5°C) but subsides and tends to fluctuate from normal to 103°F (39°C). Initially, a serous nasal and ocular discharge occurs; it soon becomes mucopurulent and copious, at which time depression and anorexia are evident. Severely debilitated cats may develop ulcerative stomatitis, and ulcerative keratitis develops in some. Signs may persist for 5–10 days in milder cases and as long as 6 wk in severe cases. Generally, the mortality is low and prognosis good except for young kittens and aged cats. The illness often is prolonged, and weight loss may be marked. FVR often is complicated by secondary bacterial infections; abortions and generalized infections also have been associated with disease.

There are many serologically related strains of feline caliciviruses. They appear to have a predilection for the epithelium of the oral cavity and the deep tissues of the lungs. Some caliciviruses are nonpathogenic. Some induce little more than salivation and ulceration of the tongue, hard palate, or nostrils; others produce pulmonary edema and interstitial pneumonia. Clinically, it is often impossible to differentiate FVR from FCV infection. Two strains may produce a transient "limping syndrome" without signs of oral ulceration or pneumonia. These strains produce a transient fever, alternating leg lameness, and pain on palpation of affected joints. Signs occur most often in 8- to 12-wk-old kittens and usually resolve without treatment. The syndrome may occur in kittens vaccinated against FCV; no vaccine protects against both of the strains that produce the "limping syndrome."

Calicivirus has also been found in cats with lymphocytic-plasmacytic gingivitis and stomatitis (*see* p 217). The superficial lesions heal rapidly, and appetite returns 2–3 days after onset. The clinical course usually is 7–10 days. An acute febrile response, inappetence, and depression are common signs. Serous rhinitis and conjunctivitis also can occur.

C felis infections characteristically produce conjunctivitis (*see* p 506); infected cats sneeze occasionally. Fever may develop as the disease progresses beyond serous lacrimal discharge to mucopurulent conjunctivitis, lymphoid infiltration, and epithelial hyperplasia. Convalescent cats may undergo relapses.

Mycoplasma spp may infect the eyes and upper respiratory passages, characteristically producing severe edema of the conjunctiva and a less severe rhinitis.

The occurrence of severe viral upper respiratory disease is rare in adult, properly vaccinated cats. These cats should be tested for other upper respiratory diseases and, less commonly, concurrent immunodeficiency diseases, including feline leukemia virus and feline immunodeficiency virus.

Lesions: Lesions generally are confined to the respiratory tract, conjunctivae, and oral cavity. In FVR, the conjunctivae and nasal mucous membranes are reddened, swollen, and covered with a serous to purulent exudate. In severe cases, focal necrosis of these membranes may be seen. The larynx and trachea may be mildly inflamed. The lungs may be congested, with small areas of consolidation; however, pulmonary changes are rarely remarkable in FVR except possibly in stressed, young kittens. The characteristic histologic lesion of FVR is the acidophilic intranuclear inclusion body. During the early stage of illness, inclusions may be present in sites of epithelial necrosis on the tongue, nasal membranes, tonsils, epiglottis, trachea, and nictitating membranes. Inclusion bodies are transitory. Inclusions are not seen in calicivirus infections.

The characteristic lesion caused by FCV is ulceration of the oral mucosa. Lesions on the tongue or hard palate initially may appear as vesicles, which subsequently rupture. Ulcerations are occasionally found on the epithelium covering the median nasal septum. The more virulent caliciviruses destroy epithelial cells of the bronchioles and alveoli, which causes acute pulmonary edema that progresses through seropurulent bronchiolar hyperplasia and interstitial pneumonia.

Early in the clinical course of feline pneumonitis, the causative organism may be identified in Giemsa-stained conjunctival smears or scrapings. The elementary bodies are intracytoplasmic. Mycoplasmas occur as extracellular coccoid bodies often seen on the surface of conjunctival epithelial cells.

Diagnosis: The presumptive diagnosis is based on such typical signs as sneezing, conjunctivitis, rhinitis, lacrimation, salivation, oral ulcers, and dyspnea. FVR tends to affect the conjunctivae and nasal passages, caliciviruses the oral mucosa and lower respiratory tract. Chlamydial infections result in chronic, low-grade conjunctivitis. These characteristics may be obscured in mixed infections. Cytologic examination of Giemsa-stained conjunctival scrapings is of value for the identification of chlamydiae and mycoplasmas. A definitive diagnosis is based on isolation and identification of the agent. The oropharyngeal mucosa, external nares, and conjunctival sacs are the preferred sampling sites. However, diagnosis of FVR may be difficult, because virus is shed intermittently and because seroprevalence and virus isolation rates are similar in ill and clinically normal cats. Samples of ocular, nasal, or caudal pharyngeal secretions for PCR may help establish a diagnosis and causative agent.

Treatment: Treatment is largely symptomatic and supportive, but broad-spectrum antibiotics are useful against secondary bacterial invaders (eg, amoxicillin with clavulanic acid, cephalosporins, trimethoprim-sulfa, fluoroquinolones, tetracyclines, chloramphenicol) as well as directly against *C felis* and *M felis*. Tetracyclines and fluoroquinolones are the most effective against *C felis* and *M felis*. Nasal and ocular discharges should be removed frequently for the comfort of the cat. Nebulization or saline nose drops may aid in the removal of tenacious secretions. Nose drops containing a vasoconstrictor (eg, two drops of ephedrine sulfate [0.25% solution] in each nostril, bid) and antibiotics may help reduce the amount of nasal exudate. Prolonged use of nasal decongestants, however, may result in rebound nasal congestion and worsening of clinical signs. A bland ophthalmic ointment containing antibiotics (tetracyclines in *C felis* infections) is indicated 5–6 times daily to prevent corneal irritation produced by dried exudate. If corneal ulcers develop in FVR infections (herpetic keratitis), ophthalmic preparations containing idoxuridine or acyclovir are indicated in addition to other antibiotic ophthalmic preparations. Lysine

(250 mg, PO, bid-tid) interferes with herpetic viral replication and may reduce the severity of FVR infection. If dyspnea is severe, the cat can be placed in an oxygen tent. Fluids may be indicated to correct dehydration, and force-feeding may be necessary. Esophagostomy and gavage may be appropriate for alimentation in severely debilitated cats. Antihistamines (eg, chlorpheniramine maleate, PO, bid [8 mg for adults, 4 mg for kittens]) may be beneficial early in the course of the disease.

Prevention: Two types of modified-live virus FVR-FCV vaccines are available. The first type is intended for parenteral administration; cats >9 wk old should be vaccinated twice, with a 3-wk interval. Kittens should be vaccinated at intervals of 3–4 wk until they are ≥12 wk old. In adult cats, revaccination with a single dose every 1–3 yr is indicated.

The second type of vaccine is administered to healthy cats by instillation into the conjunctival cul de sacs and nasal passages. Owners should be advised that cats inoculated oronasally may sneeze frequently for 4–7 days after vaccination. Kittens vaccinated when <12 wk old should be revaccinated when reaching this age. Annual revaccination with a single dose is recommended.

Modified-live virus FVR-FCV vaccines intended for parenteral administration are available in combination with either chemically inactivated or modified-live virus feline panleukopenia vaccines. A parenterally administered vaccine composed entirely of inactivated viruses also is available.

Vaccines containing either chick-embryo- or cell-line-origin *C felis* are administered parenterally. A single dose is recommended for cats >12 wk old; younger kittens should be revaccinated when they reach 16 wk. All should be revaccinated annually. These vaccines are indicated in catteries or on premises where *C felis* infection has been confirmed. The chlamydial vaccines are available in combination with FVR-FCV and panleukopenia vaccines. Systematic vaccination and control of environmental factors (such as exposure to sick cats, overcrowding, and stress) provide good protection against upper respiratory disease.

LUNG FLUKES

Paragonimus kellicotti and *P westermani* usually are found in cysts, primarily in the lungs of dogs, cats, and several other domestic and wild animals. They also have been found rarely in other viscera or the brain. Infection is most common in China, southeast Asia, and North America. *P westermani* is a parasite of people and other animals in China and other countries in the Far East.

The adult flukes are fleshy, reddish brown, oval, and ~14 × 7 mm. The eggs are golden brown, oval, distinctly operculated, and ~100 × 60 μm. The eggs pass through the cyst wall, are coughed up, swallowed, and passed in the feces. The life cycle includes several snails as the first intermediate host, and crayfish or crabs as the second. Dogs and cats become infected by eating raw crayfish or crabs that contain the encysted cercariae. After penetrating the intestinal wall and wandering in the peritoneal cavity, the young flukes pass through the diaphragm to the lungs, where they become established.

Infected animals may have a chronic, deep, intermittent cough and eventually become weak and lethargic, although many infections pass unnoticed. Finding the characteristic eggs in feces or sputum is diagnostic. The location in the lungs is ascertained by radiography. Aberrant infections can be identified serologically.

Fenbendazole (50 mg/kg/day, PO, for 10–14 days) or less preferably albendazole (25 mg/kg, PO, bid for 14 days) reduce the number of eggs deposited and eventually kill the parasites. Praziquantel (25 mg/kg, PO, tid for 3 days) may also eliminate lung flukes in dogs.

LUNG NEMATODES

See also LUNGWORM INFECTION, p 1421.

Aelurostrongylus abstrusus

Aelurostrongylus abstrusus, the most common lungworm of cats, is found in many parts of the world, including the USA, Europe, and Australia. They are small parasites (males 7 mm, females 10 mm), deeply embedded in the lung tissues. The eggs are forced into alveolar ducts and adjacent alveoli, where they form small nodules and hatch. Once the larvae escape, they are coughed up, swallowed, and passed in the feces. The larvae seen in the feces of infected animals are tightly coiled, have an undulating tail with a spine, and are <400 μm long. The life cycle includes snails or slugs as first intermediate hosts, and frogs, lizards, birds, or rodents as transport hosts of encysted larvae. When one of these transport hosts is eaten, the larvae migrate from the stomach to the lungs via the peritoneal and thoracic cavities. They reach the lungs within 24 hr and are seen in the feces in ~1 mo.

Although prevalence can be high, clinical and diagnostic signs are often lacking. Chronic wasting, cough, dyspnea, and pulmonary wheezes may be seen. The lungs usually have solidified, gray, raised nodules 1–10 mm in diameter; generalized alveolar disease has been seen in chronic cases. Treatment is difficult and not often necessary, but fenbendazole (50 mg/kg/day, PO, for 10–14 days) or ivermectin (400 mcg/kg, SC, twice at a 3-wk interval) may be effective.

Capillaria aerophila

Although usually parasites of the frontal sinuses, trachea, bronchi, and rarely nasal cavities of foxes, *C aerophila* are found in dogs and other carnivores. They are 25–35 mm long. The females produce eggs with bipolar plugs that resemble those of whipworms; however, their shells are colorless to greenish and pitted. The eggs are laid in the lungs, coughed up and swallowed, and passed in the feces. The eggs can be identified from either tracheal washes and bronchoalveolar lavage or fecal flotation. The life cycle is direct; dogs become infected through consumption of feed or water contaminated with larvated eggs. After hatching in the intestine, the larvae reach the lungs and bronchi via the circulatory system. They mature ~40 days after infection.

Clinical signs include coughing, sneezing, and nasal discharge. Treatment may be attempted using fenbendazole (50 mg/kg/day, PO, for 10–14 days) or ivermectin (200 mcg/kg, SC, twice at a 3-wk interval).

Filarids

Oslerus osleri are tracheal worms of dogs, usually found in thin-walled nodules around the bronchial bifurcation. They have been found in the USA, South Africa, New Zealand, India, Great Britain, France, and Australia. The males are ~5 mm long, and the females 10–15 mm. The life cycle is direct, and an infected bitch can transfer larvae in her saliva to her pups while licking and cleaning them. On ingestion, the larvae pass to the blood and are carried to the lungs and bronchi.

A persistent, dry cough is the most common clinical sign. Coughing may later become severe, with respiratory distress. *Finding larvae in the feces is diagnostic,* but because these larvae are lethargic and few in number, bronchoscopy is a better method. Surgical excision of the nodules combined with administration of fenbendazole, levamisole, or thiabendazole has effectively treated infected dogs. Chemotherapy alone can be successful but does not always result in a complete cure.

Filaroides hirthi is similar to *O osleri* but is found in the lung parenchyma. The females are oviparous. Adults are found in nests in the lung parenchyma, where a focal granulomatous reaction occurs. Diagnosis of low-grade infection can be difficult. Zinc sulfate flotation is usually more successful than using a Baermann apparatus. Treatment with fenbendazole (50 mg/kg/day, PO, for 10–14 days) or less preferably albendazole (25 mg/kg, PO, bid for 5 days and repeated in 2 wk) has reportedly been effective. Ivermectin (200 mcg/kg, SC, twice at a 3-wk interval) may also be effective.

NEOPLASIA

Tumors of the Nose and Paranasal Sinuses

Tumors of the nose and paranasal sinuses account for 1%–2% of all canine or feline tumors. The incidence in dogs is twice that in cats; incidence is also higher in males of both species than in females. The mean age at time of diagnosis is 9.5–10 yr for dogs and 12 yr for cats. In dogs, nasal tumors are nearly all malignant, and slightly >60% are carcinomas, of which adenocarcinoma is the most common. In dogs, the ethmoturbinates tend to be the site of predilection. Dolichocephalic and mesocephalic breeds appear to be at higher risk than brachycephalic breeds. In cats, ≥90% of nasal tumors are malignant, the most common being lymphoma and the second most common being carcinomas. Tumors of the nose and paranasal sinuses typically are very invasive locally and metastasize infrequently; metastasis is more likely in carcinomas and usually occurs late in the disease. Common sites of metastasis are regional lymph nodes, lungs, and brain. Invasion of the paranasal sinuses tends to be greater in dogs than in cats. In general, survival of untreated animals is 3–5 mo after diagnosis.

Chronic nasal discharge is the most common clinical finding; it may be mucoid, mucopurulent, or serosanguineous. Initially, discharge is unilateral but often becomes bilateral. Periodic sneezing, epistaxis, and respiratory stertor may occur. Facial and oral deformities result from destruction of bony or soft-tissue sinonasal structures. Retrobulbar extension of these tumors results in exophthalmos and exposure keratitis. Secondary epiphora may occur if the nasolacrimal duct is blocked. Late in the disease, CNS signs (eg, disorientation, blindness, seizures, stupor, and coma) may develop if the tumor extends into the cranial vault.

Diagnosis is based on history and clinical findings and elimination of other causes of nasal discharge, sneezing, or facial deformation. Nasal radiographs or CT typically show increased density of the nasal cavity and frontal sinuses as well as evidence of bone destruction. CT is vastly superior to plain radiography in diagnosis of chronic nasal diseases. Definitive diagnosis is based on biopsy of tumor tissue, either with blind biopsy based on CT lesion localization or on rhinoscopic visualization with direct biopsy. Nasal hydropulsion using a high-pressure saline infusion into the nose often yields diagnostic samples and, if large volumes of tumor tissue break free, nasal obstruction will be relieved immediately.

Treatment largely depends on tumor type and extent of disease. The treatment of choice for canine nasal adenocarcinoma is radiation therapy. Aggressive surgical excision, chemotherapy, radiation therapy, or combinations for other tumor types afford a more favorable prognosis when diagnosis is made early.

Tumors of the Larynx and Trachea

Tumors of the larynx and trachea are rare in dogs and cats. Tumors of the larynx most frequently reported in dogs are oncocytoma, squamous cell carcinoma, mast cell tumor, melanoma, and osteosarcoma; in cats, they are squamous cell carcinoma, lymphosarcoma, and adenocarcinoma. Benign inflammatory polyps of the larynx also are seen in dogs and cats. Tumors of the trachea are particularly rare. Osteochondral dysplasia of the trachea (osteochondroma) is a benign tumor of the trachea primarily seen in dogs <1 yr old. Other benign mesenchymal tumors, carcinomas, and sarcomas are occasionally seen.

The most common signs of tumors of the larynx include inspiratory dyspnea, stridor, voice change (hoarse bark or loss of voice), coughing, and exertional dyspnea. Findings typically associated with tumors of the trachea are coughing, dyspnea, stridor, and rarely hemoptysis. Laryngeal and tracheal tumors may be associated with signs of fixed upper airway obstruction (inspiratory and expiratory dyspnea). The degree of dyspnea often relates to the degree of luminal obstruction.

Diagnosis is made from the history and clinical findings and by eliminating other causes of upper airway obstruction or coughing. The tumor mass may be seen radiographically or on laryngoscopy or tracheoscopy. Definitive diagnosis is made on biopsy.

Surgical excision and resection is the treatment of choice. Radiation therapy may be palliative for radiosensitive tumors such as squamous cell carcinoma, mast cell tumor, and lymphoma. Surgical resection of tracheal osteochondral dysplasia in dogs is curative.

Primary Lung Tumors

Primary lung tumors are rare in dogs and cats; however, the reported incidence of lung carcinomas has increased at least 100% during the last 20 yr. This is attributed to an increased average life span, better detection and awareness, or possibly increased exposure to environmental carcinogens. Most primary lung tumors are diagnosed at a mean age of 10–12 yr in dogs and 12 yr in cats. There is no consistent breed or sex predilection in either species. Primary lung tumors usually originate from the terminal bronchioles and alveoli; they occasionally develop as a second coincidental tumor, which may make differentiation between primary and metastatic disease difficult.

Of the primary lung tumors in dogs and cats, ≥80% are malignant. Adenocarcinoma and alveolar carcinoma are the most common types. Primary lung sarcomas and adenomas are rare in both species. Metastatic spread of primary lung tumors is generally to other areas of the lungs, tracheobronchial lymph nodes, bone, and brain. Intrapulmonary spread via the airways occurs in ~50% of dogs with adenocarcinoma. Metastatic spread to the pleurae, pericardium, heart, and diaphragm may occur; miscellaneous extrathoracic sites include liver, spleen, and kidney. Dogs with papillary (bronchoalveolar) adenocarcinoma have a better prognosis than those with other lung tumors; however, histologic grade and detection of clinical signs are the most important determinants of prognosis and survival. Both recurrence and metastasis tend to occur earlier and with greater frequency in dogs with moderately or poorly differentiated tumors.

Clinical Findings: Primary lung tumors have variable manifestations, which depend on the location of tumor, rapidity of tumor growth, presence of previous or concurrent pulmonary disease, and awareness of the owner. Common signs include cough, inappetence, weight loss, reduced exercise tolerance, lethargy, tachypnea, dyspnea, wheezing, vomiting or regurgitation, pyrexia, and lameness. The most common clinical findings in dogs are cough, dyspnea, lethargy, and weight loss, although 25% of dogs with primary lung tumors have no clinical signs related to the tumor. Coughing is uncommon in cats; nonspecific signs, such as inappetence, weight loss, and tachypnea and dyspnea, are more common. In either species, tachypnea or dyspnea indicates massive tumor burden or pleural effusion. Pleural effusion is particularly common in cats with primary lung tumors. Lameness may be due to hypertrophic osteopathy (unusual in cats) or to metastasis to bone or skeletal muscle. Thoracic auscultation may be normal, reflect increased breath sounds compatible with pulmonary airway disease, or be muffled because of pulmonary consolidation or pleural effusion.

Diagnosis: One-third or more of primary lung tumors are recognized incidentally during radiography for other problems, or at necropsy. Thoracic radiographs are essential for a tentative diagnosis in those animals exhibiting compatible clinical signs. Primary lung tumors in dogs may occur as single or multiple circumscribed mass lesions, as a diffuse lung pattern, or as a lobar consolidation. In cats, single circumscribed mass lesions are less common, whereas a diffuse lung pattern or lobar consolidation is more frequent. Pleural fluid accumulation is common in cats and less frequent in dogs. In either species, chest wall involvement and hilar lymphadenopathy may be seen. Tentative diagnosis can be made by excluding other causes of pulmonary disease with similar radiographic lung patterns. Definitive diagnosis requires biopsy.

Treatment: Surgical resection of tumor via lobectomy of diseased lung lobes is the treatment of choice. Inoperable lesions or metastatic disease may be controlled with chemotherapy. Overall median survival time for dogs having surgical treatment for primary lung tumor is 120 days. Mean survival time for operable primary lung tumors without node involvement in dogs is 12 mo; if the lymph nodes are involved or multiple tumors are found at the time of diagnosis, survival time is only 2 mo. Recurrence or metastasis of tumor is a common cause of death.

Metastatic Tumors of the Lungs

A localized tumor may extend to the lungs by dissemination through hematogenous or lymphatic routes or by direct extension of tumor cells. Certain primary tumors, such as mammary adenocarcinoma, osteosarcoma, hemangiosarcoma, and oral melanoma, most commonly metastasize to the lungs. The lungs may be the only site of metastasis, or there may be concurrent metastasis in other organs; in the former, the diagnostic approach is to identify an occult primary tumor or to carefully review the medical history for disclosure of previous tumor removal. Because pulmonary metastasis occurs late in the clinical course of a malignant tumor, prognosis is poor.

The signs of metastatic pulmonary disease are similar to those of primary lung tumors except that coughing is less common. Severity of signs depends on the anatomic location of the tumor and whether the lesions are solitary or multiple.

Establishing a diagnosis is similar to that for primary lung tumors. Because of the limitations of routine radiography, small lesions (≤3 mm in diameter), which are present in ≥40% of cases with pulmonary metastasis, may not be seen. Thoracic CT can identify lesions not seen radiographically.

Radiography of the chest should precede removal of tumors with a known high incidence of metastatic spread to the lungs. The major goal of cancer therapy is prevention of metastasis rather than cancer eradication. Slow-growing or solitary metastatic lesions are best treated by surgical excision. Chemotherapy or radiation therapy may be useful with certain tumor types not amenable to surgical resection. Overall, the prognosis for animals with pulmonary metastasis is poor.

PNEUMONIA

Pneumonia is an acute or chronic inflammation of the lungs and bronchi characterized by disturbance in respiration and hypoxemia and complicated by the systemic effects of associated toxins. The usual cause is primary viral infection of the lower respiratory tract.

Canine distemper virus, adenovirus types 1 and 2, parainfluenza virus, and feline calicivirus cause lesions in the distal airways and predispose to secondary bacterial invasion of the lungs. Parasitic invasion of the bronchi, as by *Filaroides*, *Aeluros-*

trongylus, or *Paragonimus* spp may result in pneumonia. Protozoan involvement, eg, by *Toxoplasma gondii* (*see* p 685) or *Pneumocystis jiroveci*, is rarely seen. Tuberculous pneumonia, although uncommon, is seen more often in dogs than in cats. The incidence of mycotic granulomatous pneumonias is also higher in dogs than in cats. Cryptococcal pneumonia has been described in cats. Injury to the bronchial mucosa and inhalation or aspiration of irritants may cause pneumonia directly and predispose to secondary bacterial invasion. Aspiration pneumonia (*see* p 1417) may result from persistent vomiting, abnormal esophageal motility, or improperly administered medications (eg, oil or barium) or food (forced feeding); it may also follow suckling in a neonate with a cleft palate.

Clinical Findings: The initial signs are usually those of the primary disease. Lethargy and anorexia are common. A deep cough is noted. Progressive dyspnea, "blowing" of the lips, and cyanosis may be evident, especially on exercise. Body temperature is increased moderately, and there may be leukocytosis. Auscultation usually reveals consolidation, which may be patchy but more commonly is diffuse. In the later stages of pneumonia, the increased lung density and peribronchial consolidation caused by the inflammatory process can be visualized radiographically. Complications such as pleuritis, mediastinitis, or invasion by opportunistic organisms may occur.

Diagnosis: Analysis of bronchoalveolar lavage fluid is valuable for the diagnosis of bacterial infections. Cytologic examination can demonstrate the animal's immune response and indicate the intracellular or extracellular location of bacteria. Bacterial culture and sensitivity testing is required and may include anaerobe and mycoplasma culture, especially in refractory cases. A viral etiology generally results in an initial body temperature of 104°–106°F (40°–41°C). Leukopenia, often expected, may not be seen in many viral respiratory infections (eg, canine infectious tracheobronchitis, feline calicivirus pneumonia, feline infectious peritonitis pneumonia). A history of recent anesthesia or severe vomiting indicates the possibility of aspiration pneumonia. Acutely affected animals may die within 24–48 hr of onset. Mycotic pneumonias are usually chronic in nature. Miliary nodules seen at necropsy may suggest protozoal pneumonia.

Treatment: The animal should be placed in a warm, dry environment. Anemia, if present, should be corrected. If cyanosis is severe, oxygen therapy may be used, administered by means of an oxygen cage, with a concentration of 30%–50%. Empirical antimicrobial chemotherapy should be initiated and changed if needed based on results of culture of bronchoalveolar lavage fluid. Supportive therapy should be instituted as needed and may include oxygen supplementation, pulmonary physiotherapy (nebulization and coupage), and bronchodilators. If no response is seen after 48–72 hr of therapy, the treatment plan should be reassessed. Antimicrobial chemotherapy should be continued 1 wk after clinical and radiographic signs resolve.

Animals should be reexamined frequently. Chest radiographs should be repeated at regular intervals to monitor recurrence or note a primary underlying disease process and to detect complications such as lung consolidation, atelectasis, or abscessation.

PULMONARY THROMBOEMBOLISM

See also THROMBOSIS, EMBOLISM, AND ANEURYSM, p 141.

Pulmonary thromboembolism (PTE) is an obstruction of one or more pulmonary vessels by a blood clot. The actual incidence of PTE is uncertain, although in critically ill animals or in those with certain disease states (eg, immune-mediated hemolytic anemia, corticosteroid administration, bacterial infections, protein-losing enteropathy or nephropathy, neoplasia, trauma, feline infectious peritonitis, diabetes mellitus, hyperadrenocorticism, hypothyroidism, disseminated intravascular coagulation, dirofilariasis) the incidence is considerable, and PTE is underdiagnosed. Mortality rates of PTE in animals are uncertain but probably significant. Survival depends on early diagnosis and early appropriate therapy.

Thromboemboli in the venous circulation become trapped in the pulmonary vasculature and, if occlusion is substantial, pulmonary and hemodynamic sequelae result. Animals with preexisting cardiac or respiratory compromise may be affected earlier or more severely. The acute pulmonary consequences of PTE include ventilation-perfusion mismatch, hypoxemia, hyperventilation, and bronchoconstriction. Hemodynamic consequences of PTE are related to the magnitude of the obstruction and presence of coexisting cardiopulmonary disease. Myocardial ischemia, arrhythmias, or right ventricular failure may result. Decreased cardiac output may ensue with severe obstruction to pulmonary arterial blood flow as a result of decreased venous cardiac return.

In dogs, PTE is associated with protein-losing nephropathy, heartworm disease, endocarditis, cardiomyopathy, necrotizing pancreatitis, hypercortisolism, immune-mediated hemolytic anemia, sepsis, diabetes mellitus, neoplasia, atherosclerosis, trauma, and major surgical procedures. Cardiomyopathy and neoplasia are most commonly associated with PTE in cats.

Clinical Findings: Clinical signs are nonspecific and most often subclinical or may be mild to profound, reflecting the severity of cardiorespiratory compromise. Dyspnea, tachypnea, and depression are commonly seen. Coughing, cyanosis, hemoptysis, collapse, shock, and sudden death can occur.

Diagnosis: Diagnosis is often difficult because PTE can resemble many other conditions, including pneumonia, pulmonary edema or hemorrhage, neoplasia, or pleural effusion. Routine diagnostic tests such as thoracic radiography or arterial blood gas analysis are nonspecific and rarely confirm diagnosis. Arterial blood gas analysis will identify hypoxemia present in 80% of dogs, although response to oxygen is variable. Thoracic radiographs can be normal in 9%–27% of dogs and in 9% of cats with PTE. Abnormal radiographic findings with PTE include alveolar or interstitial pulmonary infiltrates or regional hypovascular lung areas. However, thoracic radiographs that underestimate the degree of clinical respiratory compromise should raise suspicion of PTE. Blood gas analysis may reveal hypoxemia and hypocapnia, indicating inefficient gas exchange, but the presence of normal blood gas values does not exclude PTE. Echocardiography can aid in assessment, demonstrating changes suggestive of PTE and pulmonary hypertension (dilation of the right ventricle, pulmonary artery, inferior vena cava; right ventricular hypokinesis; tricuspid regurgitation; abnormal septal wall motion). A normal echocardiogram does not exclude diagnosis of PTE. Spiral CT angiography or selective pulmonary angiography remain gold standards for diagnosis of PTE in people, but these advanced imaging studies are available at few veterinary institutions.

Treatment: Therapy should begin as soon as possible and include support of respiratory and cardiovascular systems, prevention of thrombus development and recurrence, and possibly thrombolysis. Oxygen supplementation and bronchodilators are indicated when dyspnea is evident or when arterial oxygen saturation is <92%. Although anticoagulants such as warfarin or unfractionated or low-molecular-weight heparin do not lyse existing thrombi, their use is indicated to inhibit thrombus propagation and prevent recurrent venous thrombosis. Antiplatelet drugs such as aspirin or clopidogrel can be given together with, but not in lieu of, anticoagulant therapy. Sildenafil may benefit animals with documented pulmonary hypertension. Thrombolytic therapy can rapidly cause clot lysis and improve cardiovascular function and hemodynamic stability, thereby reducing mortality in animals with massive PTE and shock. Veterinary experience with thrombolytic agents such as streptokinase and tissue plasminogen activator is limited.

RHINITIS AND SINUSITIS

Inflammation of the mucous membranes of the nose and sinuses may be acute or chronic.

Etiology: Viral infection is the most common cause of acute rhinitis or sinusitis in dogs and cats. Feline viral rhinotracheitis (FVR), feline calicivirus (FCV), canine distemper, canine adenovirus types 1 and 2, and canine parainfluenza are most frequently incriminated. Chronic states exist for FVR and FCV, with intermittent shedding associated with stress. Bacterial rhinitis or sinusitis frequently is a secondary complication. Primary bacterial rhinitis is extremely rare in dogs. It may result from infection with *Bordetella bronchiseptica* in dogs. Bacterial rhinitis appears to be a common complicating factor in cats with chronic rhinosinusitis, although exposure to environmental aeroallergens may also play a role. Allergic rhinitis or sinusitis is a poorly defined atopy that may occur seasonally, possibly in association with pollen production, or perennially, probably in association with house dusts and molds. Smoke aspiration, inhalation of irritant gases and dusts, or foreign bodies lodged in the nasal passages also may cause acute rhinitis.

Chronic rhinitis is commonly complicated by secondary bacterial colonization or infection because the primary nasal disease results in increased mucus production and altered mucociliary clearance of debris within the nose. Underlying causes of chronic rhinitis include idiopathic chronic inflammatory disease (lymphoplasmacytic rhinitis), trauma, parasites (*Cuterebra*), foreign bodies, neoplasia, or mycotic infection. In cats, chronic rhinosinusitis is a frequent sequela of acute viral infections of the nasal and sinus mucosa that result in hyperplastic glandular and epithelial changes. Rhinitis or sinusitis may result when an apical tooth root abscess extends into the maxillary recess. Mycotic rhinosinusitis may be caused by *Cryptococcus neoformans*, *Aspergillus* spp, and *Penicillium* spp. Cats are more often affected with *Cryptococcus* spp than dogs, whereas aspergillosis is frequent in dogs but rare in cats.

Clinical Findings: Acute rhinitis is characterized by nasal discharge, sneezing, pawing at the face, respiratory stertor, open-mouth breathing, and/or inspiratory dyspnea. Lacrimation and conjunctivitis often accompany inflammation of the upper respiratory passages. Affected tissues are often hyperemic and edematous. The nasal discharge is serous but becomes mucoid as a result of secondary bacterial infection. If inflammatory cells infiltrate the mucosa, the discharge may become mucopurulent. Sneezing, in an attempt to clear the upper airways of discharge or exudate, is seen most frequently in acute rhinitis and tends to be intermittent in chronic rhinitis. Aspiration reflex ("reverse sneeze"), a short paroxysmal episode of inspiratory effort in an attempt to clear the nasopharynx of obstructing material, may also be seen.

Respiratory stertor, open-mouth breathing, and inspiratory dyspnea occur when the nasal passages are narrowed from inflamed mucosa, glandular elements, and secretions. An acute unilateral nasal discharge, possibly accompanied by pawing at the face, suggests a foreign body. Neoplastic or mycotic disease is suggested by a chronic nasal discharge that was initially unilateral but becomes bilateral or that changes in character from mucopurulent to serosanguineous or hemorrhagic. Approximately 35% of cats with nasal cryptococcosis have facial deformity (dorsal lump) of the rostral aspect of the nose. Head shyness or facial pain is more commonly associated with fungal rhinitis in dogs.

Diagnosis: Diagnosis is based on history, physical examination, radiographic findings (especially CT), rhinoscopy, nasal biopsy, deep nasal tissue culture, and elimination of other causes of nasal discharge and sneezing. Advanced imaging studies and biopsy may identify a specific etiologic diagnosis for nasal discharge (eg, fungal rhinitis, neoplasia, foreign body) in as few as 36% of cats and 63% of dogs with chronic nasal disease.

Serum titer for cryptococcal antigen is a very specific and sensitive test for nasal cryptococcosis. Serologic evaluation for aspergillosis is more problematic in that negative test results do not exclude infection. Nasal tissue culture for *Aspergillus* may also result in false-positive results; as many as 30% of normal dogs and 40% of dogs with nasal neoplasia have positive culture results. The combination of seropositivity for and culture identification of *Aspergillus* is highly suggestive of infection, although negative test results do not exclude nasal aspergillosis. Direct sampling of visualized suspected fungal plaques may potentially yield *Aspergillus* hyphae in all cases.

Treatment: In mild or acute cases, supportive treatment may be effective. Severe cases of rhinosinusitis in kittens or adult cats may require parenteral fluids to prevent dehydration, and nutritional support via a nasogastric tube to maintain weight. Chronic secondary bacterial rhinosinusitis may be treated with antimicrobial chemotherapy for 3–6 wk. Intermittent use of vasoconstrictive nasal decongestants usually provides only temporary relief of congestion.

Mycotic rhinosinusitis requires antifungal therapy based on identification of a fungal etiologic agent. Fluconazole (50–100 mg/day, PO) or itraconazole (50–100 mg/day, PO) may be effective for treatment of nasal cryptococcosis in cats. Oral antifungal agents have variable efficacy in treatment of dogs with nasal aspergillosis, although voriconazole (4 mg/kg, PO, bid) alone or in combination with terbinafine (15 mg/kg, PO, bid for 1 mo) may be effective. Topical intranasal infusions of enilconazole or clotrimazole or combined clotrimazole solution and cream depot therapy instilled via the frontal sinuses have success rates as high as 50% for the first treatment and 90% with two treatments, although reinfection or relapse may occur.

Animals that do not respond to medical therapy may require surgery consisting of sinusotomy or rhinotomy, lavage, and biopsy to reestablish definitive diagnosis. Radiation therapy is the most viable treatment for intranasal neoplasia.

TONSILLITIS

Etiology: Tonsillitis is common in dogs but rare in cats. In dogs, it seldom occurs as a primary disease, but when present it is most frequently seen in small breeds. It usually is secondary to nasal, oral, or pharyngeal disorders (eg, cleft palate); chronic vomiting or regurgitation (eg, from megaesophagus); or chronic coughing (eg, with bronchitis). Chronic tonsillitis may be seen in brachycephalic dogs in association with pharyngitis accompanying soft palate elongation and redundant pharyngeal mucosa. Chronic tonsillitis in young dogs is thought to represent maturation of pharyngeal defense mechanisms.

Escherichia coli, *Staphylococcus aureus*, and hemolytic streptococci are the pathogenic bacteria most often cultured from diseased tonsils. Plant fibers or other foreign bodies that lodge in the tonsillar fossa may produce a localized unilateral inflammation or a peritonsillar abscess. Other physical and chemical agents may cause irritation of the oropharynx and one or both tonsils. Tonsillitis may also accompany neoplastic tonsillar masses because of physical trauma or secondary bacterial infection.

Clinical Findings and Diagnosis: Tonsillitis is not always accompanied by obvious clinical signs. Fever and malaise are uncommon unless consequent to systemic infection. Gagging, followed by retching or a short, soft cough, may result in expulsion of small amounts of mucus. Inappetence, listlessness, salivation, and dysphagia are seen in severe tonsillitis.

Tonsillar enlargement may range from protrusion just out of the crypts to a mass of sufficient size to cause dysphagia or inspiratory stridor. A septic, suppurative exudate may surround the tonsil, which may be reddened with small necrotic foci or plaques. Tonsillitis usually is a sign of generalized or regional inflammatory disease; therefore, primary tonsillitis should be diagnosed only after underlying diseases have been excluded. Squamous cell carcinoma, malignant melanoma, and lymphosarcoma are common in canine tonsils and should be distinguished from tonsillitis. Tonsillar lymphosarcoma generally results in bilateral symmetric enlargement, whereas nonlymphoid neoplasia is usually unilateral.

Treatment: Prompt systemic administration of antibiotics is indicated for bacterial tonsillitis. Penicillins are often effective, but in refractory cases, culture and sensitivity testing may be needed. Mild analgesics are appropriate for severe pharyngeal irritation, and a soft, palatable diet is recommended for a few days until the dysphagia resolves. Parenteral administration of fluids is required for those animals unable to take food by mouth.

Tonsillectomy is rarely required for chronic primary tonsillitis but provides permanent relief. Other indications for tonsillectomy include tonsillar neoplasia and tonsillar enlargement that interferes with airflow (eg, in brachycephalic breeds).

TRACHEOBRONCHITIS

Tracheobronchitis is an acute or chronic inflammation of the trachea and bronchial airways; it may be primary or secondary depending on the etiologic agent. Bronchitis may extend from the bronchioles to the lung parenchyma.

Etiology: Canine infectious tracheobronchitis (kennel cough, *see* p 1491) is often secondary to viral infection of the respiratory system. Other causes of tracheobronchitis in dogs include parasites, eg, *Aelurostrongylus abstrusus* (also in cats), *Capillaria aerophila*, *Crenosoma vulpis*, and *Oslerus osleri*.

Tracheitis may be secondary either to diseases of the oropharynx or to chronic coughing related to heart disease or noncardiac pulmonary disease. Other causes include smoke aspiration and exposure to noxious chemical fumes. Exacerbation of a chronic bronchitis affecting middle-aged and older dogs may follow sudden changes in the weather or other environmental stresses. Feline bronchial asthma (allergic bronchitis) is a syndrome in cats with similarities to asthma in people. Young cats and Siamese and Himalayan breeds are most affected. Feline asthma is associated with airway hyperresponsiveness, airflow obstruction, airway remodeling, and eosinophilic airway inflammation. Asthma in cats is induced by an aberrant immune response with upregulation of cytokines, leading to IgE production. Foreign bodies in the airway and developmental abnormalities such as laryngeal deformities may predispose to bronchitis. Chronic bronchitis most often affects small breeds of dogs, although it is also seen in large breeds. It is characterized by persistent cough for at least 2 mo in the absence of specific pulmonary disease. Bronchiectasis may occur as the end stage of chronic bronchitis in dogs. Recognition of tracheobronchitis as an often secondary disease syndrome underlies the importance of diagnosis and control of an associated primary disease.

Clinical Findings: Spasms of coughing are the outstanding sign. These are most severe after rest or a change of environment or at the beginning of exercise. On auscultation, respiratory sounds may be essentially normal. In advanced cases, inspiratory crackles and expiratory wheezes are heard. Body temperature may be slightly increased. The acute stage of bronchitis passes in 2–3 days; the cough, however, may persist for 2–3 wk. Severe bronchitis and pneumonia are difficult to differentiate; the former often extends into the lung parenchyma and results in pneumonia. Feline bronchial asthma may result in cyanosis and dyspnea and may be accompanied by eosinophilia.

Lesions: During the acute and subacute inflammatory stages, the air passages are filled with frothy, serous, or mucopurulent exudate. In chronic bronchitis, they contain excessive viscid mucus. The epithelial linings are roughened and opaque, a result of diffuse fibrosis, edema, and mononuclear cell infiltration. There is hypertrophy and hyperplasia of the tracheobronchial mucous glands and goblet cells. The act of coughing is an attempt to remove the accumulations of mucus and exudate from the respiratory passages.

Diagnosis: The diagnosis is made from the history and clinical signs and by elimination of other causes of coughing. In chronic bronchitis, chest radiographs may show an increase in linear and peribronchial markings. Bronchoscopy reveals inflamed epithelium and often mucopurulent mucus in the bronchi. In addition, the procedure allows collection of biopsy and swab samples for in vitro assay. Bronchial washing is an additional diagnostic aid that may demonstrate causative agents or significant cellular responses (eg, eosinophils).

Treatment: In mild or acute cases, supportive therapy may be effective, but treatment of concurrent disease is also indicated. Rest, warmth, and proper hygiene are important. Broad-spectrum antimicrobial chemotherapy is indicated for treatment of cough when infection is documented. Corticosteroids are the mainstay of therapy to reduce airway inflammation in dogs with chronic bronchitis. Persistent, nonproductive coughing is best controlled by antitussives that contain codeine. If conservative medical management is unsuccessful, laboratory tests and radiographs of the thorax and cervical trachea should be evaluated to eliminate other differential diagnoses. Bronchoalveolar lavage or transtracheal wash for cytology and culture sensitivity may be indicated to identify an etiologic agent and to determine appropriate antimicrobial chemotherapy. Pulmonary physiotherapy consisting of sodium chloride nebulization and gentle coupage may loosen secretions and stimulate expectoration. A bathroom environment with steam from a hot shower may be substituted for nebulization.

Oral (prednisolone, dexamethasone) or inhaled (fluticasone, budesonide) corticosteroids are indicated for treatment of feline asthma. Bronchodilators (albuterol, terbutaline) may be considered for adjunctive therapy in combination with glucocorticoids but not as sole therapy for feline asthma. Feline aerosol chambers and inhaler therapy are available for aerosol drug delivery in cats with feline asthma. Cyprohepatidine, an antiserotonergic drug, has been suggested; however, studies have failed to show significant reduction in eosinophilic airway inflammation. Experimental studies suggest that cyclosporine A therapy may hold promise to inhibit development of eosinophilic airway inflammation and airway remodeling through inhibition of T-cell activation and cytokine synthesis. Avoidance of environmental aeroallergens (eg, cigarette smoke, perfumes, pollens, molds, dust) must be considered in management of these cats.

Infectious Tracheobronchitis of Dogs

(Kennel cough)

Infectious tracheobronchitis results from inflammation of the upper airways. It is a mild, self-limiting disease but may progress to fatal bronchopneumonia in puppies or to chronic bronchitis in debilitated adult or aged dogs. The illness spreads rapidly among susceptible dogs housed in close confinement (eg, veterinary hospitals or kennels).

Etiology: Canine parainfluenza virus, canine adenovirus 2 (CAV-2), or canine distemper virus can be the primary or sole pathogen involved. Canine reoviruses (types 1, 2, and 3), canine herpesvirus, and canine adenovirus 1 (CAV-1) are of questionable significance in this syndrome. *Bordetella bronchiseptica* may act as a primary pathogen, especially in dogs <6 mo old; however, it and other bacteria (usually gram-negative organisms such as *Pseudomonas* sp, *Escherichia coli*, and *Klebsiella pneumoniae*) may cause secondary infections after viral injury to the respiratory tract. Concurrent infections with several of these agents are common. The role of *Mycoplasma* sp has not been clearly established. Stress and extremes of ventilation, temperature, and humidity apparently increase susceptibility to, and severity of, the disease.

Clinical Findings: The prominent clinical sign is paroxysms of harsh, dry coughing, which may be followed by retching and gagging. The cough is easily induced by gentle palpation of the larynx or trachea. Affected dogs demonstrate few if any additional clinical signs except for partial anorexia. Body temperature and WBC counts usually remain normal. Development of more severe signs, including fever, purulent nasal discharge, depression, anorexia, and a productive cough, especially in puppies, indicates a complicating systemic infection such as distemper or bronchopneumonia. Stress, particularly due to adverse environmental conditions and improper nutrition, may contribute to a relapse during convalescence.

Diagnosis: Tracheobronchitis should be suspected whenever the characteristic cough suddenly develops 5–10 days after exposure to other susceptible or affected dogs. Severity usually diminishes during the first 5 days, but the disease persists for 10–20 days. Tracheal trauma secondary to intubation may produce a similar but generally less severe syndrome. Thoracic radiographs are essential to determine the severity of disease and to exclude other causes of cough.

Treatment: Preferably, affected dogs should not be hospitalized because the disease is usually highly contagious (and also self-limiting). Appropriate management practices, including good nutrition, hygiene, and nursing care, as well as correction of predisposing environmental factors, hasten recovery. Cough suppressants containing codeine derivatives, such as hydrocodone (0.25 mg/kg, PO, bid-qid) or butorphanol (0.05–0.1 mg/kg, PO or SC, bid-qid), should be used only as needed to control persistent nonproductive coughing. Antibiotics are usually not needed except in severe chronic cases; cephalosporins, quinolones, chloramphenicol, and tetracycline are preferable because they reach effective concentrations in the tracheobronchial mucosa. When needed, the antibiotic should be selected by culture and sensitivity tests of specimens collected by transtracheal aspiration or bronchoscopy. Antibiotics given PO or IM may not significantly reduce the numbers of *B bronchiseptica* in the distal trachea or major bronchi. Thus, in severely affected dogs that are not responsive to parenteral antibiotics, kanamycin sulfate (250 mg) or gentamicin sulfate (50 mg) diluted in 3 mL of saline may be administered by aerosolization bid for 3 days. Aerosolization treatment should be preceded by administration of bronchodilators. Endotracheal injection of antibiotics (eg, gentamicin) is a possible alternative to aerosolization. Corticosteroids may help alleviate clinical signs but should be used concurrently with an antibacterial agent; they are contraindicated in severely ill, coughing dogs.

Prevention: Dogs should be immunized with modified-live virus vaccines against distemper, parainfluenza, and CAV-2, which also provides protection against CAV-1. Commercial products frequently combine these agents and may include modified-live parvovirus and leptospiral antigens. An initial vaccination should be given at 6–8 wk and repeated twice at 3- to 4-wk intervals until the dog is 14–16 wk old. Revaccination should be performed annually. When the risk of *B bronchiseptica* infection is significant, a live, avirulent, intranasal vaccine or parenteral products containing subunit bacterial extracts should be used. A combination of an avirulent *B bronchiseptica* and a modified-live parainfluenza vaccine is available for intranasal use. One inoculation is administered to puppies >3 wk old.

URINARY SYSTEM

URINARY SYSTEM INTRODUCTION

Primary functions of the urinary system include: 1) excretion of waste products of metabolism; 2) maintenance of a constant extracellular environment through conservation and excretion of water and electrolytes; 3) production of the hormone erythropoietin, which regulates hematopoiesis, 4) production of the enzyme renin, which regulates blood pressure and sodium reabsorption; and 5) metabolism of vitamin D to its active form (1,25-dihydroxycholecalciferol).

Many abnormalities of the urinary system can be diagnosed from the signalment, history and physical examination findings, serum chemistry profile, urinalysis, and aerobic bacterial urine culture. The history should include information regarding changes in water consumption, frequency of urination, volume of urine produced, appearance of urine, and behavior of the animal. It is also important to obtain information about historical and current drug administration, appetite, diet, changes in body weight, and previous illnesses or injuries.

The physical examination should include palpation of the bladder and examination of external genitalia. In dogs, rectal examination should be performed to evaluate the urethra in both sexes and the prostate in male dogs. Rectal examination in cats may not be feasible because of their small size; however, the kidneys are generally easier to palpate in cats than in dogs. A full neurologic examination should be performed on all animals with micturition disorders. Additional diagnostic tests, such as CBC, blood gas analysis for acid-base status, blood pressure, urine protein:creatinine ratio, iohexol clearance test, survey abdominal radiography, abdominal ultrasonography, contrast studies of the upper and lower urinary tract, cystoscopic examination of the urinary bladder, and renal biopsy may also provide valuable information.

Urinalysis: One of the most important diagnostic tests for evaluation of urinary tract disorders is a urinalysis. (*See also* p 1615.) Urine may be collected by one of four methods: spontaneous micturition, manual compression of the urinary bladder, catheterization, and cystocentesis. Each method has advantages and disadvantages (*see* TABLE 1). A urinalysis should include method of collection, urine specific gravity, color, turbidity, pH, glucose, ketones, bilirubin ictotest, occult blood, protein, and leukocytes (urine dipstick leukocyte tests are unreliable in cats). Urine specific gravity should be obtained using a refractometer. Microscopic examination of urine sediment should include RBCs, WBCs, epithelial cells, renal casts, bacteria, yeast, parasitic ova, fat, sperm, and crystals. Delay in analyzing urine samples can result in artifacts (eg, changes in urine pH, formation of crystals, etc), so it is important to note the time when the sample was collected and the time when it was analyzed. If a sample will not be analyzed immediately, it should be refrigerated.

Protein in urine should be evaluated in light of the specific gravity. Protein in a concentrated urine sample may not be significant, whereas the same amount in a dilute sample may be significant. Urine dipsticks provide a semiquantitative assessment of protein and can be influenced by urine pH. Therefore, they should be used only as a screening test for protein, not as a definitive diagnosis of proteinuria. A urine protein:creatinine ratio from a single urine sample or from a 24-hr urine sample is required to quantitate the amount of protein in urine. In dogs, the following International Renal Interest Society (IRIS) guidelines should be used for interpretation of urine protein:creatinine ratios. In dogs, <0.2 = nonproteinuric, 0.2–0.5 = borderline proteinuric, and >0.5 = proteinuric; in cats, <0.2 = nonproteinuric, 0.2–0.4 = borderline proteinuric, and >0.4 = proteinuric. Urine

TABLE 1 ADVANTAGES AND DISADVANTAGES OF URINE COLLECTION METHODS

Method of Collection	Advantages	Disadvantages
Spontaneous micturition	No risk (eg, trauma, bacterial infection) to animal. Avoids iatrogenic hematuria.	May contain debris (eg, bacteria, exudate) from lower urinary and genital tract. If bacterial growth appears on urine culture, must differentiate between urethral contamination and urinary tract infection. Quantitative urine culture required.
Manual compression of urinary bladder	Provides method to obtain urine sample when voluntary micturition has not occurred.	May induce trauma to urinary tract, resulting in hematuria. May be stressful for animal, especially if bladder is painful. If bacterial growth appears on urine culture, must differentiate between urethral contamination and urinary tract infection. Quantitative urine culture required.
Catheterization	Provides method to obtain urine sample when other methods of collection have failed.	Potential for trauma to urinary tract, especially urethra. More invasive than other methods; sedation may be required. Risk of introducing bladder infection. If bacterial growth appears on urine culture, must differentiate between urethral contamination and urinary tract infection. Quantitative urine culture required. Least desirable method of urine collection.
Cystocentesis	Preferred method of collection for urine culture. Avoids contamination of sample from lower urinary tract.	Potential risk of trauma if performed incorrectly or animal moves during procedure. Potential for iatrogenic hematuria. More invasive than spontaneous micturition. Potential for bacterial contamination of sample if needle penetrates colon during procedure.

protein:creatinine ratios must be interpreted in the context of other information from the urinalysis. Inflammation and hematuria can falsely increase urine protein:creatinine ratios, although hematuria generally has minimal effects.

Bacterial Culture of Urine: A urinalysis is unreliable to exclude a urinary tract infection (UTI). Not all UTIs are associated with an inflammatory response. In addition, >10,000 bacterial rods/mL and >100,000 bacterial cocci/mL of urine are required to consistently find bacteria in a urine sample using light microscopy. Approximately 25%–30% of all dogs with UTI have urine bacterial counts below these figures at the time of specimen collection, so urine culture is important to exclude a UTI.

Urine samples for bacterial culture may be obtained by the same methods used to obtain samples for urinalysis; however, the preferred method is cystocentesis. Urine obtained by cystocentesis should be sterile. If urine samples are collected by methods other than cystocentesis, a quantitative urine culture should be requested. If the sample is collected by spontaneous micturition or manual compression, significant numbers of bacteria are present if ≥100,000 colony forming units (CFU)/mL of urine in dogs or ≥10,000 CFU/mL of urine in cats are detected. Samples with >10,000–90,000 CFU/mL in dogs and >1,000–10,000 CFU/mL in cats are suspicious for a UTI. If the sample is collected by catheterization, ≥10,000 CFU/mL in dogs and ≥1,000 CFU/mL in cats is significant, whereas samples containing 1,000–10,000 CFU/mL in dogs and 100–1,000 CFU/mL in cats are suspicious for a UTI.

Serum Chemistry Profile: Evaluation of serum chemistries, including BUN, creatinine, calcium, phosphorus, bicarbonate, and serum electrolytes, is useful in many urinary tract disorders and can provide a crude indication of glomerular filtration rate (GFR). Although increases in BUN and creatinine are supportive of renal dysfunction, these tests are influenced by nonrenal factors as well. For example, dehydration can cause increases in BUN and serum creatinine not associated with renal failure. BUN can also be influenced by diet and GI bleeding and is considered inferior to creatinine to evaluate GFR. Serum creatinine levels can be falsely decreased in animals with severe muscle wasting and falsely increased in animals with severe muscle damage. Although BUN and serum creatinine increase as GFR decreases, this relationship is not linear. Large changes in GFR early in renal disease cause only small increases in BUN and serum creatinine, whereas small changes in GFR in advanced renal disease may be associated with large changes in BUN and serum creatinine.

Additional Diagnostic Tests: More sensitive methods to detect renal dysfunction include plasma clearance tests (eg, inulin clearance), radionuclide techniques, endogenous creatinine clearance, and exogenous creatinine clearance. However, these tests are impractical to perform routinely in clinical practice. The iohexol clearance test is a recently developed alternative to detect renal dysfunction. It entails recording an accurate body weight, administering a precise amount of iohexol IV, and accurately timing the collection of blood samples as directed after administration. This test does not require timed collection of urine samples or special equipment. Plasma clearance of exogenous creatinine has also recently been validated for use in dogs.

Depending on the cause of the urinary tract disorder, radiographic procedures, sonographic examination, and cystoscopic examination of the bladder may provide additional valuable information. The kidneys have a limited range of responses to disease; therefore, renal biopsies are rarely useful when evaluating renal dysfunction. An exception to this is in animals with significant proteinuria.

Blood gas analysis or serum bicarbonate levels provide useful information on acid-base status, especially in animals with renal dysfunction. Metabolic acidosis is a common problem in chronic renal failure and can result in protein catabolism.

PRINCIPLES OF THERAPY

Diseases of the urinary system can result from a variety of pathologic processes, and appropriate therapy (as discussed in the following chapters) depends on the location, severity, and cause of the problem. *See also* SYSTEMIC PHARMACOTHERAPEUTICS OF THE URINARY SYSTEM, p 2617. If the condition is not life threatening, appropriate diagnostic samples should be collected before initiating therapy. It is important to remember that some diagnostic tests and treatments have the potential to cause significant harm. If the specific cause cannot be determined, nonspecific and supportive therapy (eg, monitoring fluids, treating acidosis) should be instituted.

CONGENITAL AND INHERITED ANOMALIES OF THE URINARY SYSTEM

Congenital and inherited anomalies of the urinary system comprise a group of anatomic defects that, although uncommon, may have subclinical to serious functional consequences.

RENAL ANOMALIES

Renal Dysplasia and Hypoplasia: These defects are most common in dogs and have been reported in many breeds, including Alaskan Malamutes, Bedlington Terriers, Chow Chows, Cocker Spaniels, Doberman Pinschers, Keeshonden, Lhasa Apsos, Miniature Schnauzers, Norwegian Elkhounds, Samoyeds, Shih Tzus, Soft-coated Wheaten Terriers, and Standard Poodles. Renal dysplasia is rare in cats, lambs, and horses. In pigs, renal dysplasia may be idiopathic or associated with nutritional avitaminosis A.

Renal dysplasia may be unilateral or bilateral. Animals affected bilaterally generally die in the early neonatal period, whereas animals affected unilaterally typically develop hypertrophy of the contralateral kidney. The kidneys are usually small, firm, and pale; they may have a uniformly diminished renal cortex. Histologic examination reveals immature glomeruli, primitive tubules, and secondary inflammatory lesions, especially interstitial fibrous connective tissue.

Polydipsia and polyuria usually precede signs of uremia. Dwarfing may be noticed if the onset of renal failure occurs within the first few months of life. Urinalysis, hemogram, and blood chemistry changes are the same as in other chronic, progressive renal diseases. Uremia is usually identified between 6 mo and 2 yr of age. The diagnosis is suspected based on the breed and age of disease onset and is confirmed by renal biopsy. Treatment is aimed at managing the associated chronic renal failure.

Renal Agenesis: Renal agenesis, the complete absence of one or both kidneys, is always accompanied by ureteral aplasia and may be associated with aplastic reproductive tissues on the same side. The condition is typically an incidental finding so long as the other kidney functions normally; frequently, the contralateral kidney undergoes compensatory hypertrophy. Renal agenesis is believed to have familial predisposition in Beagles, Shetland Sheepdogs, and Doberman Pinschers. Unilateral renal agenesis is the most common congenital kidney condition in pigs; it is less common in sheep, cattle, and goats. Bilateral agenesis results in early perinatal death.

Polycystic Kidneys: Multiple cysts form within the renal parenchyma, and such kidneys are usually grossly enlarged on palpation. This condition may be associated with hepatic biliary cysts in both dogs and cats. Polycystic kidneys may cause no clinical signs or lead to progressive renal failure. This condition is familial in Beagles, Bull Terriers, Cairn Terriers, and West Highland White Terriers. Polycystic kidneys are an autosomal dominant inherited trait in Persian cats and domestic long-haired cats. Polycystic kidneys are also hereditary in pigs and may alternatively be associated with avitaminosis A. Polycystic kidneys are rare in cattle and horses and very rare in sheep. Diagnosis is based on physical and radiographic findings, ultrasonic examination, or exploratory laparotomy. Pyelonephritis may be seen concurrently and precipitate renal insufficiency.

Simple Renal Cysts: These solitary, unilocular cysts generally do not communicate with the renal collecting system; the rest of the kidney is normal. The origin of these cysts is uncertain. They are usually an incidental finding in all domestic species.

Perirenal Pseudocysts: Perirenal pseudocysts are accumulations of fluid that develop external to the renal parenchyma. They have been identified in cats. Their origin is unknown. The accumulated fluid may be located between the renal parenchyma and the renal capsule or between the renal capsule and a thin-walled fibrous sac attached to the capsule. They are termed pseudocysts rather than cysts because they are not lined by epithelium. Because only a limited number have been examined histologically, it is unknown whether all perirenal fluid-filled structures are pseudocysts. The fluid contained within these structures is not urine or lymph but is described as a transudate. Clinical signs are characterized by progressive abdominal enlargement. Abdominal palpation reveals a large, firm, nonpainful mass located in the area of the kidneys. Renal function tests and urinalysis are typically normal; however, a mild azotemia may occur. Diagnosis is made by excretory urography or ultrasonography. Treatment involves exploratory surgery to confirm the diagnosis, drainage of the pseudocyst fluid, and resection of as much of the pseudocyst wall as possible. The prognosis appears to be good; however, only a limited number of cases have been evaluated.

Miscellaneous Renal Anomalies: Double or multiple renal arteries are seen in ~5% of dogs. Other congenital defects include renal malpositioning, renal fusion, and nephroblastoma. Nephroblastoma is an embryonal tumor and is rare in domestic animals except pigs. It may cause no problems but may be very large and cause abdominal distention.

URETERAL ANOMALIES

Ectopic Ureter: This defect is most commonly reported in 3- to 6-mo-old dogs, with female dogs affected 8 times more frequently than male dogs. In dogs, ectopic ureter has a reported incidence of 0.016%–0.045%. In horses, ectopic ureter is the most common congenital anomaly affecting the urinary tract; as in dogs, it is significantly more common in fillies than in colts. Ectopic ureters are infrequently identified as a clinical problem in cattle, sheep, or pigs. Other anomalies frequently associated with ectopic ureter include hydroureter, hydronephrosis, renal hypoplasia, bladder hypoplasia, and urethral sphincter incompetence. Continual dripping of urine is the classic sign, although animals with unilateral ectopic ureter may void normally; the inability to void normally suggests bilateral ectopic ureters. A low-grade vaginitis or vulvitis may also be present due to urine scalding. Involved ureters may open into the urethra, the uterus, or the vagina. Unilateral ectopic ureter is seen with equal frequency on right and left sides, and involvement is bilateral in ~25% of cases. Ectopic ureters generally result from disruption of development of the mesonephric and metanephric duct systems. A genetic component is suspected on the basis of identifying high-risk breeds (West Highland White Terriers, Fox Terriers, and Miniature and Toy Poodles) and a familial occurrence in Siberian Huskies and Labrador Retrievers. Diagnosis is confirmed by IV urography that traces the course of the ureter.

Successful surgical treatments usually involve transplantation of affected ureters into the bladder, or ureteronephrectomy. A recent review of surgically repaired ectopic ureters in female dogs indicated that factors including left- or right-sided ectopic ureter, unilateral or bilateral ectopic ureter, presence of hydroureter, or presence of urinary tract infections were not significant to influencing postoperative incontinence. Another study showed that female dogs with ectopic ureters treated by cystoscopic-guided laser ablation had a 47% postoperative success rate based on their maintaining urinary continence. Additional medical management further improved the urinary continence rate to 77%. Indications for ureteronephrectomy may include severe ipsilateral renal disease such as hypoplasia, *hydronephrosis, or* pyelonephritis in the presence of a normally functioning contralateral kidney. Important postoperative complications are persistent incontinence, hydronephrosis, and dysuria. Incontinence occurs most often in cases of bilateral ectopic ureters and may be due to abnormal development of the bladder neck and urethra. An adrenergic agent such as phenylpropanolamine (0.5–1.5 mg/kg, PO, bid-tid) may help minimize the incontinence.

Miscellaneous Ureteral Anomalies: Less frequently recognized ureteral anomalies include aplasia, duplication, and ureterocele. Ureteroceles are characterized by dilation of the submucosal ureter segment within the bladder. Diagnosis is by excretory urography. Appropriate therapy is ureteronephrectomy if the lesion is unilateral with secondary hydronephrosis and hydroureter. If the proximal ureter and kidney are normal, excision or incision of the ureterocele, in addition to ligation of any ectopic distal channel, has been successful.

BLADDER ANOMALIES

Urachal Remnants: Congenital anomalies resulting from incomplete urachal closure include patent urachus, urachal diverticulum, umbilical urachal sinus, and intra-abdominal urachal cyst. These conditions may be seen in any domestic species but are most frequently a clinical problem in cats, dogs, and horses. Clinical signs and appropriate therapy depend on the type of anomaly. Patent urachus is typically associated with continuous urinary incontinence, urine scalding of the ventral abdomen, and development of bacterial urinary tract infections. Urachal diverticula also predispose to urinary tract infection by serving as a nidus for bacteria. Definitive diagnosis of both disorders is by positive contrast cystography. Treatment consists of surgical resection and 2–4 wk of appropriate antibiotic therapy when indicated. Surgical resection is the standard treatment for umbilical urachal sinuses and intra-abdominal urachal cysts.

Miscellaneous Bladder Anomalies: Bladder duplication, dysplasia, hypoplasia, agenesis, and exstrophy (congenital eversion) have been reported and are often associated with other urinary tract defects. Diagnosis is by physical examination, observation of micturition, and contrast radiography. Clinical signs and therapy depend on the type of anomaly.

URETHRAL ANOMALIES

Congenital or hereditary urethral anomalies are uncommon in all domestic species; they include urethral agenesis, imperforate urethra, hypospadias, epispadias in combination with bladder exstrophy, urethral duplication, urethral diverticula, urethrorectal fistula, and urethral stenosis.

Hypospadias: This developmental defect results from failure of the urethral grooves to fuse during phallus elongation. The urethral opening is ventral and caudal to the tip of the penis and is classified on the basis of anatomic localization as glandular, penile, scrotal, perineal, or anal. The penis or scrotum may be underdeveloped as well. This uncommon anomaly is most frequently seen in male dogs; the highest prevalence is seen in Boston Terriers, suggesting a genetic basis. The condition is also rarely seen in bulls. Clinical signs depend on the site of the urethral meatus and include urine scalding and complications of increased susceptibility to urinary tract infection. Although surgical correction also depends on the site of the urethral meatus, a modification of the prescrotal urethrostomy is generally useful.

Urethrorectal and Rectovaginal Fistulas: These congenital anomalies predominantly affect dogs, cats, and horses. The anomalies are more common in males than females; males are more likely to develop urethrorectal fistulas, whereas in females the rectovaginal fistulas predominate. In dogs, English Bulldogs seem to have a breed predisposition, possibly as a congenital defect due to abnormal separation of the embryonal cloaca into the urethra and rectum. Clinical signs include hematuria and dysuria secondary to urinary tract infection. Simultaneous passage of urine from the anus and urethra during micturition may be noted. Appropriate therapy consists of surgical correction and concurrent management of urinary tract infection.

INFECTIOUS DISEASES OF THE URINARY SYSTEM IN LARGE ANIMALS

BOVINE CYSTITIS AND PYELONEPHRITIS

(Contagious bovine pyelonephritis)

Bovine cystitis is an inflammation of the urinary bladder of cattle that may ascend the ureters to cause infection of the kidneys (pyelonephritis). A similar condition is seen in sheep. The condition is sporadic and worldwide in distribution. Cystitis and pyelonephritis are most often seen after parturition (in one study, the average days to onset after parturition was 83), with multiparous cows being at highest risk. In locations where the disease has been studied, the prevalence is low (<1%–2%). Cystitis and pyelonephritis are rare in male cattle.

Etiology and Pathogenesis: Formerly, the most common causative agents were the *Corynebacterium renale* group of bacteria, including *C renale*, *C cystitidis*, and *C pilosum*, as well as *Escherichia coli*; however, *E coli* and *Trueperella* (formerly *Arcanobacterium* or *Corynebacterium*) *pyogenes* are now the bacteria most frequently isolated from cows with pyelonephritis. Other opportunistic and environmental bacteria may be involved, including staphylococci and streptococci.

The most common causative bacteria are ubiquitous in the environment and are common inhabitants of the vagina and prepuce. Pyelonephritis develops from an ascending infection from the bladder. Cystitis may be present without involving the ureters or ascending to the kidney until some event occurs that compromises the defense mechanism of the ureteral mucosa. The organisms attack or colonize the mucosal lining of the bladder and ureters usually after some traumatic insult (such as parturition or abnormal deformity of the vaginal tract). The stresses of parturition, peak lactation, and a high-protein diet (which increases the pH of the urine and is therefore conducive to colonization of the urinary tract by *Corynebacterium* spp) are all contributing factors. Routine catheterization of the bladder with nonsterile catheters may facilitate transmission of *Corynebacterium* spp from cow to cow. The decrease in the frequency of urinary catheterization has been associated with a decreased prevalence of *Corynebacterium* spp as a cause of pyelonephritis.

Clinical Findings and Lesions: The first sign observed may be the passage of blood-stained urine in an otherwise healthy cow. As the infection proceeds up the ureters, causing inflammation and subsequent involvement of the kidney, the animal exhibits discomfort manifest by frequent attempts to urinate, anorexia, a slight fever, loss of production, colic with restlessness, tail switching, polyuria, hematuria, or pyuria. In chronic cases, the animal may show colic, diarrhea, polyuria, polydipsia, stranguria, and anemia. As the disease progresses, the bladder becomes thickened and inflamed. The ureters become thickened and dilated with a purulent exudate. The involved kidneys develop multiple small abscesses on the surface that may extend into the cortex and medulla.

Diagnosis: Diagnosis is based on clinical signs; hematuria; a history of recent parturition; palpation of the left kidney for enlargement, loss of lobulation, and pain; ultrasonographic inspection of the kidneys, ureters, and bladder; endoscopic inspection of the bladder for detection of cystitis; microscopic examination of the urine for WBCs and bacteria; dipstick screening for proteinuria and hematuria; and quantitative urine culture to identify the organism. The right kidney cannot be palpated per rectum, except for the caudal pole in Jersey cows and heifers. In early acute cases of pyelonephritis, enlarged ureters and involvement of the kidney may not be detectable on palpation per rectum. Typically, only one kidney is affected.

Treatment: Early diagnosis and prompt, sustained treatment are needed for a successful recovery. A catheterized urine sample should be taken for culture and antimicrobial susceptibility testing. The treatment of choice for pyelonephritis due to *Corynebacterium* spp is penicillin (22,000 IU/kg, IM, bid) or trimethoprim-sulfadoxine (16 mg combined/kg, IM, bid) for ≥3 wk. The dosage, frequency, and length of administration for both of these drugs is extra-label, and adequate precautions must be taken to prevent antibiotic residues from entering the human food supply. *E coli* infections require a broad-spectrum antimicrobial. Ceftiofur (1.1–2.2 mg/kg/day, IM or SC) or gentamicin (2.2 mg/kg, IM, bid) for ≥3 wk have been used successfully in some cases. Because of the extremely long tissue-depletion time, the aminoglycosides may not be indicated in food-producing animals. Manipulation of urine pH may theoretically be of value because *E coli* grow best in acidic urine (pH <7), whereas *Corynebacterium* spp grow best in alkaline urine (pH >7). Nonazotemic animals with pyelonephritis confined to one kidney may benefit from unilateral nephrectomy.

Even though the organisms are ubiquitous in the environment, affected animals should be isolated from the herd to restrict buildup of organisms. Because of suspicion that bulls may act as mechanical vectors of *Corynebacterium* spp, artificial insemination in herds with multiple animals affected may be considered.

PORCINE CYSTITIS–PYELONEPHRITIS COMPLEX

Porcine cystitis-pyelonephritis complex, a leading cause of mortality in sows, has been reported throughout the world. Increased incidence appears to be correlated with changes in management, particularly the adoption of confinement housing for gestating sows. Distinguishing features of endemic cystitis and pyelonephritis within a herd include lack of a temporal relationship between the vulvar discharge and the estrous cycle, minimal effect on herd fertility, low morbidity, high mortality, and an increased frequency in advanced-parity (6+) sows.

Etiology and Pathogenesis: A wide variety of bacteria has been isolated from cases of porcine cystitis and pyelonephritis, including *Escherichia coli*, *Arcanobacterium pyogenes*, and *Streptococcus* and *Staphylococcus* spp. These endogenous and opportunistic organisms typically inhabit the lower urinary tract and are often referred to as being responsible for nonspecific urinary tract infections. *Actinobaculum suis*, a specific urinary pathogen, is an important cause of ascending infection in swine. Formerly classified in the genera *Eubacterium* and *Actinomyces*, *A suis* is a gram-positive, rod-shaped bacterium that grows well under anaerobic conditions and is a commensal organism of the porcine urogenital tract. *A suis* is fimbriated, and the short, wide urethra of the sow enhances accessibility to the bladder.

Once within the bladder lumen, the alkalinity of the environment increases due to the cleavage of urea into ammonia via the urease enzyme. The increased pH enhances bacterial proliferation and inflames the mucosal surface. The alkaline environment also inhibits the growth of competitive microflora and promotes precipitation of urinary salts and crystals, particularly struvite. Such precipitates not only further increase inflammatory changes in the bladder mucosa but also provide a nidus for bacterial growth and protection from antibiotics and host defense mechanisms.

Although the primary means of accessibility to the kidneys is not yet completely understood, it is hypothesized that damage to the ureteric valves secondary to bacterial products (possibly originating from *E coli*) may predispose affected animals to pyelonephritis.

Epidemiology: Problems frequently encountered in confinement facilities that hasten the development of porcine cystitis are the reduced availability of water, increased fecal contamination of the perineal area, excessive weight gain, and leg injuries, all of which result in a reduced frequency of urination and enhanced bacterial survival in the urogenital tract. The problem may not be as prevalent in outdoor, loose housed sows; however, data are lacking. *A suis* has been isolated from the preputial cavity of boars at slaughter, the vaginal tract of neonatal piglets sampled immediately after parturition, and the vaginal tract of sows sampled throughout all stages of production. It may also be isolated from voided urine, contaminated parturition sleeves of farrowing attendants, pen floors of farrowing and nursery rooms, and the boots of stockpersons working in the breeding area. The organism is ubiquitous, and the vaginal tract can become colonized anytime during the life of the pig.

Clinical Findings: Clinical signs vary according to the severity and phase of the disease. In acute and severe cases, affected pigs may be found dead, probably from acute renal failure. Symptomatic animals are usually afebrile and may show anorexia, hematuria, and pyuria. The urine is typically reddish brown with a strong odor of ammonia. Urinary pH may increase from normal values of 5.5–7.5 up to 8–9. Animals that survive the initial infection frequently experience weight loss and reduced productivity secondary to end-stage renal disease, resulting in premature removal from the breeding herd. Inflammatory reaction on the mucosal surface of the bladder may be catarrhal, hemorrhagic, purulent, or necrotic, and the bladder wall may be thickened. Struvites can also be found in the lumen. The ureters, often filled with exudate, may increase to as much as 2.5 cm in diameter. Unilateral or bilateral pyelonephritis or pyelitis is the primary lesion in the kidneys. The pelvic region of the kidney, frequently distended with blood, pus, and foul-smelling urine, often shows irregular ulceration and necrosis of the papillae. In longstanding cases of pyelonephritis, fibrosis ultimately replaces inflammation.

Diagnosis: Cystitis and pyelonephritis in live animals can best be presumptively diagnosed when frequent micturition of bloodstained and cloudy urine can be observed. Examination of the urine sediments may reveal the presence of inflammatory cells, RBCs, granular renal casts, bacteria, and crystals. Because of the striking gross lesions, confirmation of the diagnosis is usually not difficult. To properly isolate the causative organism, care must be taken during sample collection to minimize exposure to oxygen. In the field, the bladder should remain unopened, and the neck of the bladder should be sealed with umbilical tape. Similar care should be taken with renal tissue. Lesions of pyelonephritis can be demonstrated by examination of one kidney; the other should remain unopened with the ureter sealed as previously described. Cultures should be grown on colistin nalidixic acid agar at 37°C (98.6°F) under anaerobic conditions for 5–7 days. If the culture is to be done at a distant location, swabs can be placed into Kary Blair anaerobic transport media for shipment. A PCR test for *A suis* has been described and appeared to have better sensitivity than direct culture. Data indicate detection of 1–2 CFU/mL of urine, and the pathogen can be successfully detected in samples of sow urine and boar preputial cavity.

Treatment and Prevention: Treatment of urinary tract infections may be successful if the correct antibiotic is administered early in the disease course. Penicillin and ampicillin are often the drugs of choice because of their effectiveness in alkaline conditions and their propensity for excretion through the urinary tract. Dosages of 2.2 mg/kg are typically administered IM for 3 days. Water-soluble ampicillin can be administered at 2.3 mg/kg for 5 days, although bioavailability is questionable and cost may become an issue. Acidification of the urine through oral administration of feed-grade citric acid has been reported. Results showed a reduced incidence of clinical urinary tract disease, as well as highly significant (P <.0001) differences in urinary pH and bacterial concentration/mL of urine in medicated versus nonmedicated groups. A level of 70 mg of citric acid was administered daily for 14 days with no palatability problems.

Maintaining excellent hygiene during breeding and parturition, as well as throughout the gestation period, is critical to prevent urinary tract disease. Facilities must be properly designed to reduce the spread of pathogens within the breeding herd and to allow for efficient removal of feces from the environment. Free-choice water should be available at all times, because restricting water availability through use of intermittent delivery systems or poor husbandry results in an increase in abnormal urine parameters in gestating sows, including decreased urine output, increased specific gravity (>1.026), and increased creatinine concentration. Finally, because a higher degree of urinary tract disease can be seen in older sows, proper culling procedures are important to ensure that an optimal parity distribution is maintained within breeding herds.

SWINE KIDNEY WORM INFECTION

Etiology: *Stephanurus dentatus* are stout-bodied worms (2–4.5 cm long) found encysted in pairs along the ureters in the perirenal fat and in the kidney. The kidney worm is found worldwide, particularly in tropical and subtropical areas. It is primarily a parasite of swine raised outdoors in the southeastern and south central USA. The eggs hatch shortly after being passed in the urine and reach the infective stage in 3–5 days. The larvae are susceptible to temperature extremes, desiccation, and sunlight. Infection is by skin penetration or ingestion of the infective larvae (earthworms may serve as paratenic hosts). The larvae enter the liver, where they migrate extensively for 3–9 mo. Larvae then penetrate the capsule and migrate through the peritoneal cavity to the perirenal area, where they find their way into the ureters, kidney, and perirenal fat. Occasionally, some larvae errantly migrate to other tissues and organs or to developing fetuses. Infections usually become patent in 9–16 mo but may be found as early as 6 mo.

Clinical Findings and Diagnosis: When present in large numbers, kidney worms may adversely affect growth. The principal economic loss results from condemnation of organs and tissues affected by migrating larvae. The most severe lesions are usually in the liver, which shows cirrhosis, scar formation, extensive thrombosis of the portal vessels, and a variable amount of necrosis. Kidney and lung damage are also possible.

When worms are in the kidney or in cysts that open into the ureter, eggs may be recovered in the urine. Prepatent infections are difficult to diagnose, and a definitive diagnosis depends on demonstration of the worms or lesions at necropsy.

Control: Good control practices are indicated in areas where the worm is found. Because of the long prepatent period, control may be achieved with a "gilts only" breeding program, which prevents patent infection from developing. Older boars are replaced with young boars from clean herds, and only gilts are bred and then sold after weaning. Eradication is possible within 2 yr. More commonly, anthelmintics and sanitation (rearing on concrete or in confinement) are used to control kidney worm.

Ivermectin (in-feed for 7 days at 1.8 g/ton), fenbendazole (in-feed for 3–12 days at 9 mg/kg/day), or levamisole (in-feed at 0.36 g/ton) are effective against *Stephanurus* sp. Doramectin (single injection at 300 mcg/kg) is also approved for use against this worm.

NONINFECTIOUS DISEASES OF THE URINARY SYSTEM IN LARGE ANIMALS

UROLITHIASIS

For a more general introduction to urolithiasis, *see* p 1525.

Urolithiasis in Ruminants

Uroliths in cattle, sheep, and goats are common. Although uroliths can be found anywhere within the urinary tract, urethroliths are responsible for most clinical problems. Obstruction induced by urethroliths causes urine retention and leads to bladder distention, abdominal pain, and eventual urethral perforation or bladder rupture, with death from uremia or septicemia. It is an important disease of feeder animals but is also seen in mature breeding animals. Urolithiasis is seen most often during winter in steers and wethers on full feed, or on range during severe weather conditions with limited water intake, especially when the water has a high mineral content. Obstructive uroliths are common in male goats, regardless of feed, season, or other risk factors. Urolithiasis has no specific geographic distribution, and the different urolith types reflect the mineral distribution of the feed. Uroliths occur in either sex, but obstructive urolithiasis develops primarily in males because of anatomic differences.

Etiology and Pathogenesis: Ruminant urolithiasis is considered primarily a nutritional disease. The prevalence of urolithiasis in the USA is highest in calves, lambs, and kids castrated at an early age and fed high-grain diets with roughly a 1:1 calcium:phosphorus ratio or a diet high in magnesium. Ruminants fed high-grain diets with a low calcium:phosphorus ratio are at increased risk of developing struvite uroliths, whereas ruminants grazing on silica-rich soil are predisposed to form silica uroliths. Diets high in calcium (eg, subterranean clover) may result in calcium carbonate uroliths, while plants such as halogeton or tops from the common sugar beet may be a factor in calcium oxalate formation. The mineral composition of water, in concert with dietary mineral imbalances, probably contributes more to initiating urolith formation than does the lack of water itself. A definitive diagnosis of urolithiasis in a single animal suggests that all males in the population are at risk of the disease. Struvite calculi have the apperance of sand, whereas calcium carbonate calculi and calcium oxalate are distinct, round stones.

The distal aspect of the sigmoid flexure of cattle and the sigmoid flexure and urethral process of sheep and goats are the most common sites for uroliths to lodge. Irritation at the site of lodging causes inflammation and swelling that contributes to urethral occlusion. Castration of young males also predisposes to urolith-induced urethral obstruction by removing hormonal influences necessary for mature development of the penis and urethra.

Clinical Findings: Clinical signs may be associated with partial or complete urethral occlusion. Animals with partial obstruction dribble blood-tinged urine after prolonged, painful (stranguria) attempts at urination; before complete occlusion occurs, urine may dry on the preputial hairs and leave detectable mineral deposits. Animals with complete urethral obstruction exhibit tenesmus, tail twitching, weight shifting, and signs consistent with colic. Inappetence, bloat, depression, and rectal prolapse also may be seen. Affected steers may elevate the tail and show urethral pulsations just ventral to the rectum. Goats may vocalize.

Common sequelae of complete urethral obstruction include urethral perforation, hydronephrosis, or urinary bladder rupture. Bladder rupture often results in death from uremia. The disease course may be 5–7 days. Although urethral perforation may also cause uremia and death, it is not uncommon for the ventral abdominal skin to necrose and slough, allowing a pseudo-urethra to develop.

Diagnosis: Diagnosis based on the history, clinical signs, and physical examination is usually straightforward. Hypersensitivity in the region of the sigmoid flexure may be evident. Palpation may identify abnormal pulsations of the urethra and tissue swelling associated with the obstruction. Rectal palpation may reveal an enlarged, distended bladder, or the bladder may be nonpalpable, consistent with bladder rupture. Examination of the urethral process in sheep and goats may reveal the occluding urolith. In small ruminants, the distended bladder can be felt by abdominal palpation and visualized on ultrasound examination. Calcium carbonate and calcium oxalate calculi can be seen on radiographs of the urethra in small ruminants; struvite calculi are not seen on radiographs. If early clinical signs of obstructive uropathy are missed, the animal may show only inappetence, depression, subcutaneous swelling along the penis, or uroperitoneum; abdominal distention due to uroperitoneum must be differentiated from ruminal tympany, peritonitis, peritoneal tumors, uterine hydrops, and GI tract obstructions. Ballottement allows detection of the fluid, and when viewing the animal from behind, the abdomen appears symmetrically enlarged and pear-shaped. Ultrasound examination of the abdomen reveals a large amount of hypoechoic fluid.

Confirmation of ruptured bladder is obtained by examining fluid collected by abdominocentesis and finding that the amount of creatinine in peritoneal fluid is two times or more that in plasma. Subcutaneous swellings along the prepuce and ventral abdomen due to a perforated urethra must be differentiated from traumatic injury, subcutaneous abscesses, and umbilical or ventral hernias. In breeding animals, preputial lacerations with prolapse and sheath infection, and hematoma of the penis must also be differentiated. In animals with clinical signs of acute colic, other causes of abdominal pain must be eliminated; these diseases include indigestion, stasis or obstruction of the GI tract, primary enteritis, abomasal ulcers, and coccidiosis.

Treatment and Control: Treatment of obstructive urolithiasis generally involves establishing a patent urethra and correcting fluid and electrolyte imbalances. In many instances, surgical management of the obstruction is all that is necessary; however, severely uremic and depressed animals require rehydration and correction of acid-base and electrolyte abnormalities, especially hyperkalemia or hyperammonemia. If a rupture of the urinary tract has occurred, hyponatremia, hypochloremia, hyperphosphatemia, and metabolic alkalosis with variable potassium concentrations are found. Treatment with IV normal saline is indicated. The volume of fluid administered should be calculated to correct clinical dehydration. Once the animal is rehydrated and any rupture repaired, fluid therapy may be continued to encourage diuresis.

Animals with an intact urethra and bladder that have early clinical signs of obstructive urethral disease may benefit from conservative therapy using antispasmodics and tranquilizers. This is believed to relax the retractor penis muscles with straightening of the sigmoid flexure. However, conservative therapy is only rarely beneficial in small ruminants and is warranted only in cases of acute or partial obstruction without evidence of urethral or bladder damage; it should not be used in complicated or advanced cases. Uroliths trapped within the urethral process of sheep and goats may be removed by gentle manipulation or by amputation of the urethral process. Proper restraint, tranquilization, and a regional anesthetic are necessary. The techniques vary, but the typical procedure requires exteriorization of the penis. Although amputation may be effective, relief is typically temporary (<2 days) in most animals, because obstruction recurs due to the presence of multiple uroliths.

Perineal urethrostomy has also been recommended as an effective surgical technique in castrated males. Short-term complications associated with perineal urethrostomy may include postoperative hemorrhage, surgical wound dehiscence, and subcutaneous urine accumulation. Urethral stricture is a common longterm complication. Transection of penile attachments to the pelvis may decrease risk of postoperative stricture. In addition, perineal urethrostomy is associated with loss of breeding ability in intact males. In more complicated cases, such as those with urethral perforation, amputation of the penis proximal to the sigmoid flexure or near the perineal area may be necessary as a salvage procedure. Animals that develop urethral perforation also require drainage of accumulated subcutaneous urine; this is accomplished by lancing the skin overlying the area of accumulated urine. Topical antiseptics and fly repellents may be applied to these ventral lacerations, and parenteral antibiotics are recommended to prevent infection.

Cystotomy followed by dietary management is believed to be a more effective longterm solution to urolithiasis in sheep and goats than is perineal urethrostomy. Cystotomy allows removal of multiple urocystoliths, permits bidirectional urethral flushing, and poses less risk of urethral stricture. Tube cystotomy is generally considered the treatment of choice, allowing time for the calculi to be expelled spontaneously. An intact urethral process, absence of abdominal fluid, and serum potassium concentration <5.2 mEq/L have all been associated with improved survival after tube cystotomy in small ruminants.

If the bladder is ruptured, the ability to urinate must be restored and uremia corrected. In animals with substantial uroperitoneum, the peritoneal cavity should be slowly drained using a teat tube or trocar. Urine removal may also reduce the severity of peritonitis and make the animal more comfortable. Fluid, electrolyte, and acid-base homeostasis normally returns within 24 hr after restoration of a patent urinary system. Persistent uremia indicates the possibility of hydronephrosis or ascending pyelonephritis or both. A urethrostomy should be performed to provide unobstructed passage of urine. Attempts to surgically repair the ruptured bladder have been largely unsuccessful because of the chronic distention before the rupture. The bladder may heal spontaneously after urethrostomy and removal of abdominal fluid; however, these animals are best salvaged within 3–4 mo to avoid further complications. Despite treatment, some animals cannot pass urine effectively, and the uroperitoneum recurs. These animals may be treated by performing tube cystotomy followed by appropriate antibiotic and fluid therapy.

Several measures to prevent the formation of urethral calculi have been recommended. Most important for struvite calculi prevention are to increase urinary chloride excretion, decrease urine pH, and provide a calcium:phosphorus ratio of 2:1 in the complete ration. Intensive concentrate feeding, such as in many finishing programs, frequently leads to urolith formation and urethral obstruction. Thus, any feeding program that incorporates concentrate feeding must include appropriate calcium supplementation. Adjunct measures to minimize the formation of urethral calculi include adding sodium chloride up to 4% of the total ration. This promotes increased sodium and chloride concentration in the urine, water intake, and urine dilution, which increases the mineral solubility. Ammonium chloride can be used as a urinary acidifying agent (7–10 g/head/day for a 30-kg lamb or kid; 50–80 g/head/day for a 240-kg steer). Complete rations with dietary cation-anion difference (DCAD) are also used to prevent struvite calculi; these rations are high in chloride. Urine acidification antagonizes magnesium-ammonium-phosphate crystal formation and has been shown empirically to be a useful preventive measure. Lower calcium diets should be used if calcium carbonate or calcium oxalate is a concern.

In operations with a significant problem of urolith formation, evaluation of the ration is the most important measure that can be taken to reduce the incidence. Commercial anionic dietary supplements are available for small ruminants.

Urolithiasis in Horses

Urolithiasis is a less common condition in horses than in small ruminants or steers. The disease can affect immature horses but is seen most frequently in adults. There is no breed predilection. Urolithiasis is seen more frequently in males than in females, which has been attributed to anatomic differences between the male and female urethra.

Equine uroliths have a diameter of 0.5–21 cm, weigh as much as 6.5 kg, and are found most often within the bladder. Most equine uroliths are composed of calcium carbonate, in various hydrated forms, with either calcium phosphate or struvite uroliths occasionally noted. Calcium carbonate uroliths have two separate clinical forms. The first form is a concretion of salts and mucoproteins that varies in consistency from friable to firm. These uroliths are usually yellow and oval or irregularly shaped; they frequently have a rough or spiculated surface and are generally soft enough to be fragmented during surgery. The second calcium carbonate form is a firm concretion that is hard and resistant to fragmentation and is typically smooth and white. There appears to be no difference in chemical composition between these forms.

Etiology: The mechanism of urolith formation in horses is unknown, although the alkaline pH and high mineral content of normal equine urine may favor crystal formation and precipitation. Normal equine urine also contains large amounts of mucoproteins, which may serve as a cementing substance to adhere crystals. Consumption of feed and water high in mineral content may increase urinary solute concentrations and thereby promote crystallization and precipitation. Multiple nephroliths may develop in horses with renal papillary necrosis (associated with NSAID administration while dehydrated) and mineralization of the papillae.

Clinical Findings: Clinical signs depend on the urolith location. Most uroliths are located in the bladder and cause dysuria, pollakiuria, and hematuria. Hematuria is most evident after exercise and toward the end of a voided urine stream. Affected horses frequently stretch out to urinate and may maintain this posture for variable periods before and after micturition. Additional signs may include scalding of the perineum in females or of the medial aspect of the hindlimbs in males. Geldings and stallions may protrude the penis flaccidly for prolonged periods while intermittently dribbling urine. Affected horses may occasionally exhibit recurrent bouts of colic or an altered hindlimb gait. Urethral obstruction may also develop as the result of a trapped urolith and is typically accompanied by restlessness, sweating, varying degrees of colic, and frequent attempts to urinate. The bladder is distended on rectal examination. In most fatal cases, a single large urolith, occasionally accompanied by smaller ones, is found in the bladder; less frequently, the urolith may be found lodged at the bladder neck or the ischial arch. Nephroliths are occasionally found via ultrasonography in horses with cystic calculi; owners of such horses should be informed that obstruction may recur.

Bilateral nephroliths are not uncommon in adult horses that have been used for performance. Intermittent chronic obstruction of ureters will eventually cause renal failure, resulting in weight loss and anorexia.

Diagnosis: Tentative diagnosis of urolithiasis is usually based on the history and clinical signs and confirmed most easily by rectal palpation of a firm, ovoid, intravesicular mass at or near the neck of the bladder. In most cases, urolith palpation is not difficult, because clinical signs are rarely evident until the stone is several centimeters in diameter. Transrectal ultrasonography with a 7.5 MHz linear probe allows visualization of the stone. If ultrasound examination cannot be performed, the distended bladder should be catheterized to facilitate palpation and eliminate the possibility of urethroliths, urethral stricture, or smegma impaction of the urethral sinus. Urinalysis frequently reveals RBCs, neutrophils, calcium carbonate crystals, and proteinuria. Cystoscopy, ultrasonography, and radiology are not essential for detection of urocystoliths in horses but may provide additional diagnostic or prognostic information. Ultrasonography is necessary to identify nephroliths. Ureteroliths and cystic calculi can usually be palpated during rectal examination.

Treatment: Several surgical procedures have been described for urocystolith removal. Surgical options include midline or paramedian laparotomy and cystotomy, pararectal cystotomy, subischial urethrostomy, urethral sphincterotomy, and laser or shock wave lithotripsy. Selection of a procedure is dictated by the size, location, and number of uroliths; the sex and physiologic status of the horse; and the availability of surgical facilities. Bladder rupture, although uncommon in adult horses, may occur due to urethral obstruction or recumbency or after foaling in mares.

UROPERITONEUM IN FOALS

Uroperitoneum is defined as urine leakage into the peritoneal space. In foals, this most commonly results from tearing of the bladder during parturition, prolonged recumbency while being treated for a neonatal illness, or rupture of the urachus secondary to umbilical abscessation. Ureteral or urethral tears are rare. Some studies indicate a higher incidence of bladder rupture in males than in females, possibly because the narrower pelvis and the longer, narrower urethra of colts is a predisposing factor. Urachal rupture occurs both in males and females. Traumatic bladder rupture is thought to be caused by uterine contractions on a full bladder as the foal passes through the birth canal. Although most ruptured bladders at birth are thought to be traumatic, the presence of *smooth* edges and absence of hemorrhage around the tear in some foals might suggest a congenital origin (developmental defect of the bladder wall). Most bladder tears are located on the dorsum of the bladder. In the case of a ruptured urachus, infection in the umbilical stump can weaken the urachal wall and result in leakage of urine into the abdomen or subcutaneously near the umbilicus. Prematurity, neonatal encephalopathy, cystitis, ascending infection, abdominal trauma, failure of passive transfer, and sepsis may predispose the foal to bladder rupture.

Clinical Findings: Foals generally appear normal at birth but progressively become lethargic, tachycardic, and tachypneic throughout 24–48 hr. Signs may not appear for a longer period in foals with a ruptured urachus. As the condition progresses, the abdomen becomes noticeably distended, and ballottement may produce a fluid wave. Most foals attempt to urinate often, with small amounts of urine being produced. This stranguria is often misinterpreted as straining to defecate. Other foals may be anuric or urinate normally.

Diagnosis: Ultrasonographic abdominal examination and blood and peritoneal fluid analysis can be helpful in diagnosis. Foals usually have a neutrophilic leukocytosis. Serum hyperkalemia combined with hyponatremia and hypochloremia are seen because of the high concentration of potassium and low levels of sodium and chloride in the urine, which rapidly equilibrate across the peritoneum. An ECG may show broad QRS complexes and very tall T waves due to hyperkalemia. The increased serum potassium predisposes the foal to bradycardia and cardiac arrhythmias (AV block, atrial standstill, and cardiac arrest) if not corrected. Serum BUN and creatinine values can be normal but usually are increased. Blood gas analysis may also be normal or reveal a metabolic acidosis. Abdominal fluid is pale yellow and copious and can easily be detected on ultrasonographic evaluation. The creatinine level in the peritoneal fluid is at least double that in the serum. This test is the most accurate in diagnosing the problem. If laboratory testing is not available, 10 mL of methylene blue can be injected into the bladder via a urinary catheter. If the bladder is patent to the peritoneal space, dye should be seen in the peritoneal fluid within 15 min.

The clinical signs of progressive depression and stranguria can confuse the diagnosis. Differential diagnoses include septicemia (*see* p 2089), hypoxic ischemic encephalopathy/neonatal encephalopathy (*see* p 2094), persistent meconium impaction (*see* p 2096), or colic (*see* p 248) for other reasons.

In the case of a urachal rupture, abdominal ultrasonography may be helpful to establish an etiologic diagnosis. Ultrasonography of the umbilical remnants may suggest the presence of infection or abscessation. A large amount of fluid in the abdomen is also seen. Rarely, neonatal foals may become azotemic because of rupture of one or both ureters. Accumulation of urine in the retroperitoneal area can be seen via ultrasound.

Treatment: Surgery is necessary to correct the defect and, in uncomplicated cases, is very successful. The foal should be stabilized before surgery. Potassium >6 mEq/L should be lowered preoperatively by either 500 mL of normal saline, sodium bicarbonate plus 10% dextrose throughout 30–40 min, or sodium bicarbonate administration alone. All of these treatments help drive potassium into cells. If the potassium is >8 mEq/L or the above treatments are unsuccessful, administration of insulin at 0.1 mg/kg, IV, in dextrose and saline and/or peritoneal fluid drainage can be considered.

The bladder should be repaired using absorbable sutures. Because surgical staples have migrated into the bladder and become the nidus for stone formation at a later date, they should not be used. If the umbilical structures are enlarged (indicating infection), they should be removed at the time of surgery and cultured. After surgical correction of the bladder, an indwelling urinary catheter may be placed for 48 hr to decrease bladder distention and leakage of urine at the repair site; however, this is rarely done on a first repair.

If a bladder rupture is recognized early in an otherwise healthy foal and the foal is stabilized appropriately before surgery, the prognosis for recovery is good to excellent, with success rates as high as 95%. In septic or premature foals, in which complications such as peritonitis, incisional complications, adhesions, and anesthetic death are encountered more frequently, the prognosis is fair. All recumbent foals should be considered at high risk of bladder rupture and may require prophylactic indwelling catheterization.

RENAL TUBULAR ACIDOSIS IN HORSES

Etiology: Type 1 renal tubular acidosis (RTA) is a sporadic disorder in horses. The RTA may be preceded by drug therapy for another condition or renal injury, or there may be no predisposing cause. RTA may be transient or recurring. Genetic predisposition is unproved but possible in some cases.

Clinical Findings and Diagnosis: Signs include acute onset of depresson, anorexia, muscle trembling, and tachycardia and/or arrhythmia. There are many differential diagnoses for these clinical signs, so serum chemistry testing and urinalysis are necessary. There is a severe metabolic acidosis, marked hyperchloremia, and hypokalemia with equine RTA. The urine pH is neutral to alkaline.

Treatment: Administration of sodium bicarbonate IV and PO is generally successful in correcting the metabolic acidosis. Potassium supplementation may be critical if the serum potassium concentration is <2.5 mEq/L or if the horse is trembling or has cardiac arrhythmias. Treatment throughout a few days may result in complete resolution in some horses, but others may require continued supplementation with sodium bicarbonate administered PO.

URETHRAL DEFECTS CAUSING HEMATURIA IN ADULT MALE HORSES

Etiology: The cause of the urethral defects is not proved, but they are believed to occur because of high pressure in the corpus spongiosum at the end of urination in geldings or during ejaculation in stallions.

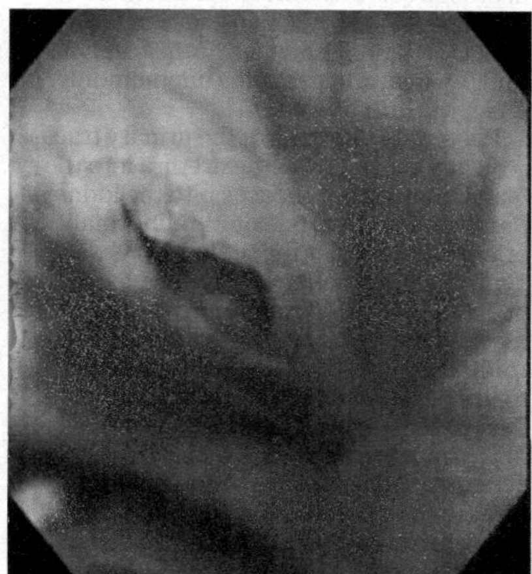

Endoscopic examination of the urethra of an adult Quarter horse gelding that had hematuria at the end of urination. The defect in the urethra is dorsal and at the level of the ischial arch. *Courtesy of Dr. Thomas J. Divers.*

This high pressure may cause a "blow-out" tear in the urethral mucosa.

Clinical Findings and Diagnosis: The clinical signs are limited to hematuria at the end of urination, associated with contractions of the bulbourethral muscle in geldings or with hemospermia and decreased fertility in stallions. All breeds may be affected, although the disorder seems more common in Quarter horses.

Diagnosis is based on clinical signs and urethral endoscopic findings. The urethral defect is seen in most cases on the dorsal convex surface of the urethra at the level of the ischial arch.

Treatment: Some cases may heal spontaneously, but most continue with intermittent hemorrhage; anemia is rare. Breeding rest is recommended for stallions. Subischial urethrostomy or subischial incision into the spongiosum penis reduces vascular pressure in the corpus spongiosum during urination, allowing the defect to heal. A buccal mucosal graft was used to repair the defect in a stallion.

INFECTIOUS DISEASES OF THE URINARY SYSTEM IN SMALL ANIMALS

Most infectious diseases of the urinary system in small animals are aerobic bacterial infections. Common organisms include *Escherichia coli*, *Staphylococcus*, *Enterococcus*, and *Streptococcus*. Less common organisms causing infection include *Klebsiella*, *Proteus*, and *Pseudomonas*. *Pasteurella* is more common in cats than dogs. *Mycoplasma* is an uncommon cause of urinary tract infection and is usually found as a coinfection with bacteria. Leptospirosis is a worldwide zoonotic disease caused by filamentous bacteria that infect the kidney and many other organs. Fungi, yeast, and parasites uncommonly infect the urinary system.

Bacterial infections of the urinary tract typically ascend from the urethra into the bladder and in some cases into the kidneys. Predisposing factors include abnormalities of urine flow (eg, urine retention), decreased urothelial defense mechanisms, decreased systemic immune defense mechanisms, or inadequate urine concentration. Female dogs are more susceptible to urinary tract infections than male dogs, except for bacterial prostatitis in older, uncastrated male dogs. Dogs with concurrent diseases (eg, chronic kidney disease or hyperadrenocorticism) are at greater risk. Cats are relatively resistant to bacterial cystitis compared with dogs. Less than 2% of cats 1–10 yr old with lower urinary tract signs have a positive culture for bacterial infection. Adults cats with clinical signs of lower urinary tract pain and inflammation typically have a noninfectious cause, such as idiopathic cystitis, interstitial cystitis, or urinary bladder stones. Geriatric cats, immunosuppressed cats, or those with systemic diseases (eg, chronic kidney disease, hyperthyroidism) are more prone to bacterial urinary tract infections. Urinary tract pathogens, except for *Leptospira interrogans*, are not considered zoonotic. However, the potential for multidrug-resistant bacteria to localize in the urinary system is a concern for both animal and human health. Subtherapeutic treatment regimens and inappropriate antibiotic selection are contributing factors. Animals that receive chronic antibiotic treatment or are immunocompromised may (rarely) become infected with *Candida* spp. Systemic fungal infections (eg, blastomycosis, aspergillosis, protothecosis) can involve the urinary system; the kidneys and prostate are the most likely sites.

BACTERIAL CYSTITIS

Bacterial cystitis is infection and inflammation of the urinary bladder. Clinical signs are pollakiuria, hematuria, dysuria, and urinating in inappropriate places. Hematuria may be more noticeable at the end of the urine stream. An animal may exhibit pain on palpation of the caudal abdomen, and the bladder may feel thickened or irregular. Bacterial cystitis is occasionally diagnosed in an asymptomatic animal when a routine urinalysis is performed. Chronic glucocorticoid administration, hyperadrenocorticism, chronic kidney disease, and diabetes mellitus may be associated with asymptomatic urinary tract infections. Occasionally, animals with no concurrent disease will have bacteria in the urine without evidence of a true infection (ie, bladder mucosal invasion and inflammation); this condition is termed asymptomatic bacteriuria.

Urinalysis often shows increased protein and hemoglobin on the urine dipstick analysis. The WBC part of the dipstick (ie, nitrate) is inaccurate in dogs and cats and should not be used. The urine pH may be alkaline (7.5–9) if the bacteria are urease positive (eg, *Staphylococcus* or *Proteus*). However, an alkaline urine pH by itself is not abnormal, because diet and other factors can affect urine pH. Urine sediment should be examined microscopically. Increased numbers of WBCs, RBCs, and/or bacteria are consistent with cystitis. Bacteria can be confused with stain precipitate; filtering the stain or evaluating the sediment without staining is advised. Lack of visible bacteria in the sediment does not exclude urinary tract infection.

If clinical signs and/or urinalysis are suggestive of infection, a urine culture and antimicrobial susceptibility test should be performed. Cystocentesis is the preferred method for sample collection, followed by sterile urethral catheterization or a midstream free catch into a sterile collection cup. A quantitative culture is necessary to interpret the result, unless the sample was collected by cystocentesis. Ideally, the culture should be set up within 2 hr of collection. If the laboratory is off-site, the sample should be refrigerated and processed by the laboratory within 24 hr. If the specimen cannot be refrigerated, commercial collection kits that contain preservatives can be used to maintain a stable bacterial population at room temperature for 24 hr. Laboratories that can provide both quantitative culturing and a minimum inhibitory concentration–based method for antimicrobial susceptibility testing are preferred.

Antibiotic regimens for infections involving soft tissues, such as bacterial cystitis with prostatic involvement, should be similar to pyelonephritis (*see* below). Simple bacterial cystitis is treated for 2 wk with a broad-spectrum antibiotic that achieves a high concentration in the urine. Appropriate initial choices include amoxicillin (10–20 mg/kg, PO, bid-tid), cefadroxil (22–30 mg/kg, PO, bid), cefpodoxime (5–10 mg/kg/day, FDA approved for dogs only), ormetoprim-sulfadimethoxine (27 mg/kg, PO, day one, then 13.5 mg/kg/day, PO), or cefovecin (8 mg/kg, SC, day one, which may be repeated once 7 days later). A repeat urine culture 3–7 days after oral therapy or on day 21 if cefovecin is used is recommended. If positive, another antibiotic based on the new susceptibility test results is given for a longer treatment period (eg, 3–4 wk). Very resistant or recurrent infections should be treated for 4–6 wk. Every course of treatment should be followed by a urine culture, even if the signs have resolved. In animals that have a history of chronic or recurrent infections, a urine culture should be done 3–7 days and 3 mo after successful therapy. If both of these cultures are negative, then a urine culture should be repeated at 6 and 12 mo after therapy. Because resistance to antibiotics can develop during therapy, antimicrobial susceptibility testing should be performed on every positive urine culture.

Animals with recurrent bacterial cystitis should be evaluated for an underlying cause. A recurrent infection caused by the same bacterial organism is termed a relapse and is essentially a treatment failure. This is typically caused by inappropriate antibiotic therapy (ie, wrong drug, dosage, or treatment duration) and often occurs because of an unrecognized complicating factor (eg, deep-seated bladder wall infection, bladder polyps, renal or prostatic involvement, concurrent disease). A recurrent infection in which different organisms are causative is termed a reinfection and is usually caused by host defense problems such as disorders of micturition (eg, urethral incompetence), anatomic abnormalities (eg, hooded vulva, patent urachus, ectopic ureters, uroliths), and/or concurrent disease (eg, chronic kidney disease, hyperadrenocorticism, chronic glucocorticoid administration). Abdominal radiographs are frequently diagnostic for uroliths but negative survey films should be followed by ultrasonography, cystoscopy, and/or double-contrast cystourethrography to exclude radiolucent urocystoliths, anatomic defects, polyps, and neoplasia. The history may reveal chronic glucocorticoid use. A serum biochemical profile, CBC, and complete urinalysis are important to exclude predisposing systemic diseases, such as chronic kidney disease, hyperadrenocorticism, and diabetes mellitus. Other diagnostic considerations include feline immunodeficiency virus, feline leukemia virus, and hyperthyroidism in cats or hyperadrenocorticism in dogs.

In cases that respond to therapy but continue to have frequent bouts of cystitis without an identifiable cause, low-dose prophylactic antibiotics can be used to prevent ascending bacteria from establishing an infection according to the following protocol: 1) a therapeutic course of an antibiotic for the current infection is completed, 2) no antibiotics are given for 3 days, to allow collection of urine for a culture after treatment, and 3) the prophylactic protocol is immediately started. Prophylaxis consists of using a broad-spectrum antibiotic (eg, amoxicillin, cefadroxil) at one-third of the total daily dose, given at bedtime, indefinitely. Every 6–8 wk, the antibiotic should be stopped for 3–7 days to obtain a sample for repeat urinalysis and culture. Every new infection should be treated with a therapeutic course of an antibiotic based on culture and susceptibility results. The treatment antibiotic will likely be different than the prophylactic antibiotic. Oral cranberry extract and D-mannose may be useful adjuncts. The most valuable therapeutic antibiotics (eg, fluoroquinolones, second- or third-generation cephalosporins) should be reserved for resistant infections. If the recurrent infection is resistant to the prophylactic antibiotic, this antibiotic can still be used for future prophylaxis after the infection is eradicated. Encouraging frequent voiding during the daytime is helpful to prevent recurrent infections. The major disadvantage of using a prophylactic antibiotic protocol is development of multidrug-resistant bacteria.

PYELONEPHRITIS

Kidney infection (pyelonephritis) is usually due to ascending bacteria, although hematogenous spread is possible. The organisms and predisposing causes are similar to those of bacterial cystitis. Renoliths and ureteroliths, which impede the normal flow of urine out of the renal pelvis, may be contributory. Animals at risk of pyelonephritis are the very young, the very old, the immunosuppressed, or those with inadequate urine-concentrating ability. In many instances, an underlying cause is not identified. Virulence factors associated with specific bacterial strains play a role in allowing colonization of the urothelium, especially with pyelonephritis caused by *Escherichia coli*. The fact that pyelonephritis is usually ascending and bilateral suggests that these virulence factors are more important than previously recognized.

Animals with acute pyelonephritis may exhibit kidney or flank pain, fever, malaise, and sometimes vomiting, polyuria, and polydipsia. Urinalysis shows proteinuria, pyuria, bacteriuria, and/or hematuria. WBC casts may be present in fresh urine sediment. The urine culture is usually positive; the CBC may show leukocytosis with a left shift. The biochemical profile may be normal or show azotemia (prerenal or renal) and/or hyperglobulinemia. The animal may be in kidney failure. Chronic pyelonephritis is more difficult to recognize, because clinical signs may be subtle or absent. Polyuria and polydipsia are frequent. In many cases, the disease goes unrecognized until kidney failure occurs. Although abnormalities in the urinalysis are present, they are often less dramatic than with acute kidney infection. A single urine culture can be negative if bacterial numbers are low. Other useful diagnostic tests include abdominal ultrasonography and IV pyelography. Both studies may show dilation of one or both renal pelvises secondary to inflammation and partial obstruction. Asymmetric renal size and architectural changes with renal pelvic dilatation is highly suggestive of chronic pyelonephritis. In some cases, nephropyelocentesis via ultrasonographic guidance is useful to obtain a sample of urine from the dilated renal pelvis for analysis and culture.

Pyelonephritis should be treated aggressively with broad-spectrum antibiotics, based on urine culture and antimicrobial susceptibility testing, for 4–8 wk. The infection may respond to the same antibiotics recommended for cystitis, but more frequent administration (eg, amoxicillin tid rather than bid) and/or higher dosages are indicated. A fluoroquinolone or a combination of a fluoroquinolone with a β-lactam antibiotic is often effective. Dosages should be the same as for other soft-tissue infections. Animals that are febrile, anorectic, dehydrated, or azotemic should be hospitalized to provide IV antibiotics and fluid therapy. Fluid therapy may prevent acute pyelonephritis from progressing to azotemic acute kidney injury and will improve renal perfusion and uremic signs in animals already experiencing uremia. Animals with acute pyelonephritis may recover normal renal function, depending on the amount of damage that occurred before treatment. In cases of chronic pyelonephritis with a severely hydronephrotic, nonfunctional kidney, a nephrectomy may be the treatment of choice once the animal has been stabilized. This will remove the source of infection and hopefully save the opposite kidney. IV pyelography and/or renal scintigraphy are useful to assess the relative function of each kidney. If both kidneys are severely affected, medical management alone is the only alternative. Recovery to chronic, stable renal failure is possible in many cases.

The urine should be cultured during the first 5–7 days of therapy to assess antibiotic efficacy. A urinalysis and culture should be repeated 3–7 days after therapy, and then monthly for 3 consecutive months. If all of these cultures are negative, the interval between urine cultures may be gradually lengthened. Animals with pyelonephritis are at high risk of persistence or recurrence of infection and for secondary infections at other sites (eg, bacterial endocarditis and discospondylitis).

INTERSTITIAL NEPHRITIS, GLOMERULONEPHRITIS, AND VASCULITIS

Acute interstitial nephritis in dogs is caused most often by *Leptospira interrogans* (*see* p 650). Cats rarely develop leptospirosis, and clinical signs are less severe than in dogs. Other infectious causes of nephritis in dogs include *Leishmania donovani* and *Borrelia burgdorferi*. These systemic vectorborne diseases are endemic in specific geographic areas. Glomerulonephritis is the predominant renal pathology, so these are considered immune complex diseases rather than true urinary tract infections. Toxoplasmosis can cause pyogranulomas in the kidneys or elsewhere in the urinary system. Systemic infectious diseases that cause vasculitis in cats or dogs (eg, feline infectious peritonitis, Rocky Mountain spotted fever) may also cause kidney disease.

CAPILLARIA PLICA INFECTION

Capillaria plica may infect the urinary bladder, and occasionally the ureters and renal pelvises, of dogs and cats. Distribution is worldwide, and wild animals appear to be the primary hosts. A similar but less common organism, *C felis cati*, is also found in cats. Dogs and cats become infected by eating earthworms that contain the first-stage larvae. Mature *Capillaria* are threadlike, yellowish, and 13–60 mm long. The eggs are colorless, operculated, have a slightly pitted shell, and are 63–68 × 24–27 μm in size. Most dogs and cats are asymptomatic. Some animals show signs of pollakiuria, urinary incontinence, and urinating in abnormal places. The eggs are shed in the urine and may be found in the urine sediment. Microscopic hematuria and increased numbers of epithelial cells may also be present. Reported treatments include levamisole, fenbendazole, albendazole, and ivermectin. The treatment of choice is unknown, but a single dose of ivermectin at 0.2 mg/kg, SC, is likely to be effective. It is not FDA approved for this use and is contraindicated in Collie breeds. The parasite may be self-limiting in the absence of reinfection.

GIANT KIDNEY WORM INFECTION IN MINK AND DOGS

Mink are the most common definitive host for *Dioctophyma renale*, the largest known nematode, which has a worldwide distribution. Many other species, including dogs and people, can become infected. The definitive host contracts the parasite by ingesting encysted larvae in raw fish (eg, pike, bullhead) or frogs or by ingesting an infected annelid worm. The larvae penetrate the bowel wall and migrate first to the liver and later to the kidneys. In dogs, the parasite often fails to reach the kidneys and may be found free in the abdominal cavity. Kidney worms grow larger in dogs than in mink, reaching up to 103 cm.

Female worms are larger than male worms, and both are blood red. Both male and female worms must be present in the same kidney to complete the life cycle. Barrel-shaped, yellow-brown eggs with a thick, pitted shell measuring 71–84 × 45–52 μm are shed into the urine.

In the kidneys, the worm(s) cause obstruction, hydronephrosis, and destruction of the renal parenchyma. The right kidney is most commonly affected. Kidney failure can result if both kidneys are parasitized. Chronic peritonitis, adhesions, and liver disease are also possible. Clinical signs are hematuria, pollakiuria, weight loss, and renal or abdominal pain. Urinalysis may reveal proteinuria, hematuria, and pyuria. Ultrasonography or IV pyelography shows the enlarged hydronephrotic kidney(s). The diagnosis is made by finding the eggs in the urine sediment if both sexes of the nematode are present in the kidney and the ureter is patent. Alternatively, exploratory laparotomy may reveal the diagnosis. Worms may be found in the peritoneal cavity, between the lobes of the liver, or within the affected kidney(s) via nephrotomy.

Unilateral nephrectomy is the treatment of choice if the opposite kidney is unaffected. Preventing ingestion of raw fish or other aquatic organisms is recommended in areas where the parasite is known to infect wild animals.

NONINFECTIOUS DISEASES OF THE URINARY SYSTEM IN SMALL ANIMALS

RENAL DYSFUNCTION

Failure of the filtration function of the kidneys leads to the development of azotemia (an excess of nitrogenous compounds in the blood), which may be classified as prerenal, renal, postrenal, or of mixed origin. Prerenal azotemia develops whenever mean systemic arterial blood pressure declines to values <60 mmHg and/or when dehydration causes plasma protein concentration to increase. Conditions that may lead to development of prerenal azotemia include dehydration, congestive heart failure, and shock. Prerenal azotemia generally resolves with appropriate treatment, because kidney structure has not been altered, which allows normal function to resume once renal perfusion has been restored. Renal azotemia refers to a reduction in glomerular filtration rate (GFR) of ~75% during acute or chronic primary renal (or intrarenal) diseases. Postrenal azotemia develops when the integrity of the urinary tract is disrupted (eg, bladder rupture) or urine outflow is obstructed (eg, urethral or bilateral ureteral obstruction). Once adequate urine flow is restored, postrenal azotemia will resolve.

Chronic Kidney Disease

Chronic kidney disease (CKD) involves a loss of functional renal tissue due to a prolonged (≥2 mo), usually progressive, process. Dramatic changes in renal structure may be seen, although structural and functional changes in the kidney are only loosely correlated. CKD often smolders for many months or years before it becomes clinically apparent, and it is invariably irreversible and frequently progressive. Although congenital disease results in a transient increase in prevalence in animals <3 yr old, the prevalence increases with advancing age from 5–6 yr. In geriatric populations at referral institutions, CKD affects as many as 10% of dogs and 35% of cats. The prevalence in the general small animal population is likely to be lower, perhaps 1%–3%. Several breeds of dogs and cats are associated with heritable CKD (*see* p 1496). There is no apparent breed or sex predisposition for nonheritable CKD in dogs or cats.

CKD is generally classified into various stages (*see* TABLE 2) based on laboratory tests and clinical signs. In Stage 1, a process is damaging the kidneys but azotemia and clinical signs have not developed. Unfortunately, renal disease is uncommonly detected at this stage. In Stage 2, the disease has progressed, GFR has fallen to <25% of normal, and azotemia is present, but clinical signs are not yet seen. However, this stage may be associated with impaired urine-concentrating ability and increased urine volume. Stage 3 occurs when GFR has declined further, azotemia is present, and clinical signs are often seen. Stage 4 reflects further progression and severe azotemia, with clinical signs present. This staging system applies to CKD only.

Substaging Based on Blood Pressure: Systemic hypertension is present in ~20% of dogs and cats with CKD and is associated with target organ damage in the kidneys,

TABLE 2 CLASSIFICATION OF STAGES OF KIDNEY DISEASE

Stage[a]	1	2	3	4
	Nonazotemic Kidney Disease	Mild Renal Azotemia	Moderate Renal Azotemia	Severe Renal Azotemia
Creatinine (mg/dL)				
Dogs	<1.4	1.4–2.0	2.1–5.0	>5.0
Cats	<1.6	1.6–2.8	2.9–5.0	>5.0

[a] Stages are as recommended by the International Renal Interest Society.

TABLE 3 SUBSTAGES OF CHRONIC KIDNEY DISEASE BASED ON ARTERIAL BLOOD PRESSURE (AP) MEASUREMENTS AND RISK OF TARGET ORGAN DAMAGE

Substage[a]	AP0	AP1	AP2	AP3
	No or minimal risk	Low risk	Moderate risk	High risk
Blood pressure (mmHg)				
Systolic	<150	150–159	160–179	>180
Diastolic	<95	95–99	100–119	>120

[a] Substages are as recommended by the International Renal Interest Society. Other modifiers that may be added to the AP substage: C = evidence of end organ damage or complications present; T = patient presently being treated.

eyes, CNS, and cardiovascular system. It is recommended that animals with CKD be substaged on the basis of blood pressure measurements (*see* TABLE 3).

In general, animals in substage AP3 and those in substage AP2 with preexisting target organ damage (eg, retinal injury or CKD) should be considered candidates for antihypertensive therapy.

Substaging Based on Proteinuria: The routine dipstick evaluation of urine for protein is not particularly specific, because many of the positive reactions (⅓ in dogs and ⅔ in cats) are false-positives. Although it is a useful screening test, a positive result should be followed with a more specific test, such as the sulfosalicylic acid test, the urine protein:creatinine ratio, or albumin-specific assays.

Species-specific antibodies for albumin have led to development of highly specific and sensitive assays for the detection and measurement of urine albumin concentrations. Microalbuminuria is defined as a urine protein content that leads to a negative reaction for the routine urine dipstick and a positive reaction with a species-specific antibody test. Animals with microalbuminuria frequently exhibit or subsequently develop kidney disease, systemic inflammatory or metabolic disease, neoplasia, or infectious diseases.

Proteinuria is an important finding and is associated with a poor prognosis in aged animals and in those with CKD. Changes in the magnitude of proteinuria represent a good marker for the efficacy of antihypertensive therapy. Animals with CKD should also be substaged on the basis of proteinuria (*see* TABLE 4), using the protein:creatinine ratio.

Etiology: Attempting to identify the primary process causing the kidney disease, especially in Stages 1 and 2, is important to form a prognosis and treatment plan. Known causes of CKD include diseases of the macrovascular compartment (eg, systemic hypertension, coagulopathies, chronic hypoperfusion), microvascular compartment (eg, systemic and glomerular hypertension, glomerulonephritis, developmental disorders, congenital collagen defects, amyloidosis), interstitial compartment (eg, pyelonephritis, neoplasia,

TABLE 4 SUBSTAGES OF CHRONIC KIDNEY DISEASE BASED ON PROTEINURIA

Substage[a]	N	BP	P
	Nonproteinuric	Borderline	Proteinuric
Dogs	<0.2[b]	0.2–0.5	>0.5
Cats	<0.2	0.2–0.4	>0.4

[a] Substages are as recommended by the International Renal Interest Society.

[b] Urine protein:creatinine ratio

obstructive uropathy, allergic and immune-mediated nephritis), and tubular compartment (eg, tubular reabsorptive defects, chronic low-grade nephrotoxicity, obstructive uropathy). Many causes of chronic, generalized renal disease are associated with progressive interstitial fibrosis. The severity of interstitial fibrosis is positively correlated with the magnitude of decline of GFR and negatively correlated with the prognosis. The glomerular, tubulointerstitial, and vascular lesions found in animals with generalized CKD are often similar, regardless of the initiating cause, particularly in Stage 4. At this point, renal histology may show only marked interstitial fibrosis, which may be called chronic interstitial nephritis or tubulointerstitial fibrosis. This term describes the morphologic appearance of kidneys with end-stage chronic disease of any cause. Because acute kidney injury may progress to a chronic condition, any cause of acute kidney injury is also a possible cause of CKD.

Clinical Findings: Generally, no clinical signs are seen as a direct result of disease until ≥75% of nephron function has been impaired (Stages 3 and 4). Exceptions are chronic kidney diseases that develop as part of a systemic disease with clinical signs referable to involvement of other body tissues (eg, systemic lupus erythematosus, systemic hypertension), chronic kidney diseases accompanied by nephrotic syndrome, or those associated with marked renal inflammation and capsular swelling leading to flank pain and occasionally to vomiting. Usually, the earliest clinical signs commonly attributable to renal dysfunction are polydipsia and polyuria, which are not seen until the function of approximately two-thirds of the nephrons has been impaired (late Stage 2 or early Stage 3). Further destruction of renal tissue leads to azotemia without new clinical signs in Stage 2, and finally to the clinically apparent uremic syndrome in Stage 4. Initially, uremia is associated with occasional vomiting and lethargy. As the disease progresses within Stages 3 and 4 throughout months (dogs) to years (cats), anorexia, weight loss, dehydration, oral ulceration, vomiting, and diarrhea become fully manifest. Loose teeth, deformable maxilla and mandible, or pathologic fractures may be seen with renal *secondary osteodystrophy* (*see* p 1056), but these are uncommon and generally seen only in young dogs with end-stage congenital renal disease. Physical examination and imaging studies of animals in Stages 3 and 4 usually reveal small, irregular kidneys, although normal to large kidneys can be seen in animals with neoplasms, hydronephrosis, or glomerulonephritis. Mucous membranes are pale in late Stage 3 and Stage 4, due to the presence of a nonregenerative, normocytic, normochromic anemia.

Diagnosis: In Stages 1 and 2, diagnosis is often missed or made incidentally during imaging studies or urinalyses conducted for other purposes. In Stages 3 and 4, the BUN, serum creatinine, and inorganic phosphorus concentrations are increased. Potassium depletion, due to renal potassium wasting combined with inadequate intake and the kaliuretic effects of acidosis, is frequently seen in cats and occasionally in dogs. Hyperkalemia associated with oliguria and anuria may be noted in terminal Stage 4 or whenever marked prerenal azotemia is concurrent with CKD. Systemic hypertension and associated complications develop in ~20% of affected cats and dogs and can occur at any stage. Osteoporosis may be seen radiographically, although this late finding is generally not helpful for diagnosis.

The urine specific gravity may range from 1.001–1.060 in dogs and 1.005–1.080 in cats, depending on body needs for water homeostasis; the normal range overlaps the abnormal or inappropriate range. In animals with dehydration and normal renal function, urine specific gravity should be >1.030 in dogs and >1.035 in cats. The inability to produce concentrated urine when challenged by dehydration is an early sign of CKD; however, dogs with primary glomerular disease, and some cats, may become azotemic while retaining the ability to concentrate urine to a specific gravity >1.035. Even so, concentrated urine is rarely seen when the serum creatinine is >4 mg/dL in an animal with azotemia of renal origin.

The polydipsia and polyuria of CKD must be differentiated from diseases that cause primary polydipsia (eg, psychogenic polydipsia, hyperthyroidism) or interfere directly with the urine-concentrating mechanism. This includes conditions that lead to retention of solute in tubular fluid (eg, diuretic administration, diabetes mellitus), central diabetes insipidus, and nephrogenic diabetes insipidus (eg, hyperadrenocorticism, hypercalcemia, pyometra, diseases causing septicemia). Adrenal insufficiency leads to a urine-concentrating defect and may thus be confused with Stage 2 and 3 renal disease, because prerenal azotemia may be caused by the vomiting, diarrhea, and polydipsia associated with hypoadrenocorticism. Hyperkalemia, hyponatremia, and/or reduced plasma Na^+ to K^+ ratio helps establish a tentative diagnosis of adrenal insufficiency, which must be confirmed by hormonal assay(s). Also, animals with hypoadrenocorticism improve rapidly in response to proper therapy.

Combinations of survey radiography, abdominal ultrasonography, serial clinical pathology tests, including urinalyses and urine cultures, and blood pressure measurements should be performed to evaluate the severity of disease, establish a prognosis, monitor the response to therapy, and identify complicating factors. Specific renal function tests and renal biopsy may be helpful to identify the exact cause in Stages 1–3, but the presence of advanced pathologic changes in Stage 4 is nonspecific and often precludes identification of an underlying cause by histologic studies. This condition in late Stage 4 is often described as end-stage renal failure clinically and as chronic, generalized nephritis pathologically. CKD should be distinguished from the more readily reversible acute disease. Frequently, differentiation may be accomplished with an appropriate history, physical examination, and laboratory findings, although a renal biopsy may be required. However, therapy for CKD caused by a range of morphologic lesions is similar, so renal biopsies may not be warranted unless marked proteinuria is present or a treatable cause is suspected.

Treatment: With appropriate therapy, animals can survive for long periods with only a small fraction of functional renal tissue, perhaps 5%–8% in dogs and cats. Recommended treatment varies with the stage of the disease. In **Stages 1 and 2**, animals usually have minimal clinical abnormalities. Efforts to identify and treat the primary cause of the disease should be thorough. The identification and supportive treatment of developing complications (eg, systemic hypertension, potassium homeostasis disorders, metabolic acidosis, bacterial urinary tract infection) should be aggressively pursued. The systemic hypertension seen in ~20% of animals with CKD may be seen at any stage and is not effectively controlled by feeding a low-salt diet. The usual antihypertensive medications for blood pressure substages AP2 and AP3 (*see* TABLE 3) are a calcium-channel blocker such as amlodipine besylate (0.25–0.5 mg/kg/day, PO) or an angiotensin-converting enzyme (ACE) inhibitor such as enalapril or benazepril (0.5 mg/kg, once daily in cats and bid in dogs) or an angiotensin-receptor blocker (ARB) such as telmisartan (1 mg/kg, once daily in cats and bid in dogs). If an ACE inhibitor is used in conjunction with a renal diet, potassium should be carefully monitored. Hyperkalemia may develop, particularly in Stage 4, and dietary change or dosage adjustment should be considered if serum potassium exceeds 6.5 mEq/L. While ACE inhibitors (or ARBs) and calcium-channel blockers may be administered together, a calcium-channel blocker is usually recommended as initial therapy in cats and an ACE inhibitor (or ARB) in dogs. In addition to providing a continuous supply of fresh drinking water and encouraging (and documenting) adequate dietary intake, body condition scoring should be used routinely to assess adequacy of intake. Animals in this stage should be fed standard, commercially available maintenance diets, unless they are markedly proteinuric (*see* below). All affected animals should be reevaluated every 6–12 mo, or sooner if problems develop.

In **Stages 2 and 3**, the principles for management of complications are the same, except that the animal should be evaluated every 3–6 mo. These evaluations should include hematology, serum biochemistries, and urinalysis. Because dogs and cats with CKD are prone to development of bacterial urinary tract infections, urine culture should be performed annually and any time urinalysis suggests infection. The progressive nature of this disease produces a vicious cycle of progressive renal destruction. Measures that may slow this progression include dietary phosphorus restriction, dietary fish oil supplementation, antihypertensive agents (for hypertensive dogs and cats), and administration of ACE inhibitors or ARBs (proteinuria substage P; *see* TABLE 4). Dietary restriction of phosphate and acid load is essential in this stage, and specialized diets for management of kidney disease should be fed. Potassium citrate or sodium bicarbonate, given PO, may be indicated if the animal is severely acidotic (plasma bicarbonate <15 mEq/L) or remains acidotic 2–3 wk after diet change. If dietary restriction of phosphorus is unsuccessful in maintaining a normal level of serum phosphorus within 2–3 mo, phosphate-binding gels containing calcium acetate, calcium carbonate, calcium carbonate plus chitosan, lanthanum carbonate, or aluminum hydroxide should be administered with meals to achieve the desired effect. There is also a clear rationale for the inclusion of dietary n-3 polyunsaturated fatty acids in these stages.

In **late Stage 3 and Stage 4**, all of the principles of managing the preceding stages apply, except that the animal should be evaluated every 1–3 mo. Dietary restriction of protein may relieve some of the signs of uremia. High-quality protein (eg, egg protein) should be fed at a level of 2–2.8 g/kg/day for dogs and 2.8–3.8 g/kg/day for cats. Commercial diets formulated for cats and dogs with CKD generally meet this recommendation. Administration of a proton pump inhibitor such as omeprazole (0.5–1 mg/kg/day, PO) or an H_2-receptor antagonist such as famotidine (5 mg/kg, PO, tid-qid) decreases gastric acidity and vomiting. Anabolic steroids, such as oxymethalone or nandrolone, have been administered to stimulate RBC production in anemic animals, but this is not effective.

Recombinant erythropoietin and other erythropoiesis-stimulating agents (eg, darbopoietin, continuous erythropoietin receptor activator) may stimulate RBC production, but antierythropoietin antibodies develop in ~50% of animals treated with the human recombinant erythropoietin, epoetin alfa, and may result in refractory anemia. Darbopoietin may be less likely to produce this effect and may be preferred. Until species-specific products become generally available, erythropoietin administration is now recommended only for animals with clinically apparent signs of anemia (eg, weakness, marked lethargy not attributable to other factors), which generally occurs at a hematocrit <20%.

Fluid therapy with polyionic solutions, given IV or SC in the hospital or SC by owners at home, is often beneficial in animals with intermittent signs of uremia. Oral vitamin D administration may reduce uremic signs and prolong survival, particularly in dogs. However, vitamin D administration requires prior resolution of hyperphosphatemia (goal is serum phosphorus <6 mg/dL), and it may induce hypercalcemia. Probiotic medications and certain dietary fibers may enhance gut catabolism of nitrogenous compounds and uremic toxins. Feeding tubes may help manage chronic anorexia. Euthanasia or renal replacement therapy (renal transplantation and/or dialysis) should be carefully considered if therapy does not improve renal function and alleviate signs of uremia.

Acute Kidney Injury

Because not all animals with acute kidney injury (AKI) will be identifed or exhibit azotemia, AKI has replaced the older term, acute renal failure. Animals with AKI are most often presented to the veterinarian when a sudden, major insult damages the kidneys. The principal causes are toxins (eg, ethylene glycol, aminoglycoside antibiotics, hypercalcemia, hemoglobinuria, melamine-cyanuric acid, grapes or raisins, NSAIDs), ischemia (eg, embolic showers from disseminated intravascular coagulation or severe prolonged hypoperfusion), and infection (eg, leptospirosis, borreliosis).

Clinical Findings: Mild AKI often goes unrecognized; severe initial or repeated bouts may lead to CKD. Most often, AKI is recognized in advanced stages and is characterized clinically by anorexia, depression, dehydration, oral ulceration, vomiting and/or diarrhea, or oliguria. Physical examination findings often reveal dehydration but otherwise are usually not remarkable, although pain is occasionally elicited on palpation of the kidneys, which may be normal in size to slightly enlarged.

Diagnosis: A history of hypotension, shock, or recent exposure to known nephrotoxins in an animal with sudden-onset uremia is the typical clinical picture of an animal with acute kidney disease. The presence of poorly concentrated urine (specific gravity 1.007–1.030) despite dehydration and/or azotemia suggests renal dysfunction. Differentiating between chronic and acute kidney disease (and establishing a specific cause in acute kidney disease) is important, because the prognosis and specific therapy may differ. Animals with AKI usually have a compatible history and other urinalysis abnormalities; marked cylindruria is a frequent and definitive finding. Other urinalysis findings may include the presence of a large number of renal epithelial cells and leukocytes in the urine sediment, glucosuria, crystalluria, enzymuria, and/or myoglobinuria/hemoglobinuria. Animals with AKI generally have increased serum urea nitrogen, creatinine, and inorganic phosphorus concentrations and metabolic acidosis. Oliguria or anuria after rehydration, which is often associated with hyperkalemia, is a poor prognostic sign; in contrast, polyuric animals have a better prognosis, although they may become hypokalemic. The kidneys are typically normal in size and shape and an anemia is often, but not always, absent—findings that may help differentiate acute from chronic kidney disease.

After injury, the kidney has considerable potential for functional regeneration through the process of compensatory hypertrophy and adaptive hyperfunction. In animals with CKD, it is likely that most of this regenerative process has occurred before the initial diagnosis. In contrast, animals with AKI have considerably more potential for improvement of renal function, if they can be sustained through a uremic episode. The duration of the uremic episode may be substantial with some nephrotoxins (eg, 1–3 wk with aminoglycoside antibiotics and 4–8 wk with ethylene glycol). A renal biopsy may be of value in assessment of the severity, extent, cause, and potential reversibility of the disease.

As a disease process, AKI is a spectrum, and the International Renal Interest Society recommends that patients with AKI be categorized primarily on the basis of serum creatinine. Animals with Grade I AKI have nonazotemic AKI (serum creatinine ≤1.6 mg/dL). Animals with Grades II–V AKI exhibit varying degrees of azotemia, with serum creatinine levels of 1.7–2.5 mg/dL in Grade II, 2.6–5 mg/dL in Grade III, 5.1–10 mg/dL in Grade IV, and >10 mg/dL in Grade V.

Treatment: Severe AKI that necessitates medical intervention is a serious condition, with a survival rate of ~50%. If the cause is known, specific therapy should be instituted, eg, 4-methylpyrazole or ethanol for ethylene glycol toxicity in dogs (*see* p 3046). Fluid therapy is indicated for all dehydrated and inappetant animals. A polyionic fluid such as lactated Ringer's solution is satisfactory unless hyperkalemia is present, in which case normal saline is recommended. Sodium bicarbonate may be cautiously added to the fluids to correct acidosis.

In oliguric or anuric animals, therapy to promote increased urine volume is often recommended if the animal is well hydrated and urine production is <0.5 mL/kg/hr. This approach has been questioned because urine flow may increase without corresponding increases in renal blood flow and GFR. Administration of excess fluid to an animal in the maintenance phase of oliguric renal failure may result in life-threatening pulmonary and cerebral edema. Nonetheless, efforts to increase renal blood flow and GFR may enhance urine production and do have a role in the management of these animals. For this therapy, urine production must be quantitatively monitored closely via an indwelling urethral catheter. Monitoring central venous pressure is advised to prevent overhydration. A sequential approach generally includes an initial slight overhydration by administration of a test dosage of polyionic solution IV at 50 mL/kg. If this fails to yield adequate urine flow within 3 hr, further measures include osmotic diuresis (10% or 20% mannitol or dextrose, 0.5–1 g/kg, IV, as a slow bolus throughout 15– 30 min, alternated with infusion of lactated Ringer's solution, 30 mL/kg, IV, throughout 30 min). Subsequent measures generally include furosemide (2 mg/kg, IV, which can be doubled and then tripled at 2-hr intervals if urine production does not increase above the target of 0.5 mL/kg/hr). However, furosemide may worsen the severity of AKI caused by aminoglycosides. Finally, renal vasodilators (dopamine diluted in 5% dextrose, IV, to provide 1–5 mcg/kg/min) plus furosemide (2 mg/kg, IV) may be tried for 2 hr. Dopamine may lead to ventricular arrhythmias, and high doses of dopamine may cause renal vasoconstriction. Dopamine produces minimal renal vasodilation in cats and calcium channel blockade (eg, amlodipine besylate, 0.25–0.5 mg/kg, or diltiazem, 1–3 mg/kg) may be preferred. If attempts to restore urine flow fail, aggressive measures should be discontinued to avoid overhydration. Daily fluid therapy based on maintenance and rehydration needs is continued until renal function and clinical condition improve. Feeding tube placement greatly facilitates patient management at this stage and should be implemented for any animal with marked renal azotemia (serum creatinine >10 mg/dL after rehydration).

A second therapeutic option, rather than the aggressive measures discussed above, is to proceed directly to fluid therapy with polyionic solutions while waiting for renal regeneration. Again, feeding tube placement for parenteral nutrition should be implemented in anorectic animals with marked azotemia. Peritoneal dialysis or hemodialysis may be necessary if none of the above measures restores urine production.

GLOMERULAR DISEASE

Glomerular disease is a well-recognized cause of chronic kidney disease (CKD) in dogs, may produce acute kidney injury in dogs, and is also occasionally seen in cats with CKD. These animals should be staged and substaged as recommended above (*see* TABLE 2, TABLE 3, and TABLE 4). Animals with primary glomerular disease as a cause of CKD may have somewhat different clinical and laboratory abnormalities than those with primary tubulointerstitial disease. Although uncommon, urine specific gravity may be inappropriately high for the degree of renal dysfunction, a condition referred to as glomerulotubular imbalance. Damage to the glomerular basement membrane results in albuminuria, which may lead to hypoalbuminemia. Animals may then exhibit signs related to hypoalbuminemia (eg, peripheral edema, hypercoagulability with thrombosis, hypercholesterolemia) instead of or in addition to uremia.

Secondary glomerulopathies, observed as sequelae of systemic or glomerular hypertension in animals with Stage 3 or 4 CKD, are common. Although the overall prevalence of a primary glomerulopathy as an inciting cause is not known, it is apparently more common in dogs than cats.

Immune-mediated glomerulonephropathy is characterized by deposition or in situ formation of immune complexes in the glomerular capillary wall, which then incite inflammatory changes (*see* p 828). In one study of dogs, the mean age of presentation for glomerulonephritis was 4–8 yr; 55% were males, and there was no breed predilection. Immune-mediated glomerulonephritis has been associated with neoplasia, rickettsial diseases, systemic lupus erythematosus (SLE), heartworm disease, pyometra, chronic septicemia, and adenovirus infection, but it is usually idiopathic. Although multifactorial in origin, the glomerular disease associated with hyperadrenocorticism and diabetes mellitus in dogs is rarely attributable to immune complex formation.

In one study of cats with glomerulonephritis, the mean age at presentation was 3–4 yr; 75% were males, and there was no breed predisposition. Primary glomerular disease in cats is most frequently associated with chronic infection by feline leukemia virus (FeLV), feline immunodeficiency virus (FIV), or feline infectious peritonitis (FIP) virus but has also been reported in association with neoplasia and systemic inflammatory diseases. The relatively young age and predilection for males reflects the high prevalence of FeLV infection as a cause in reported feline cases.

Familial glomerulopathies as a primary cause of CKD have been reported in several breeds of dogs, including Bernese Mountain Dogs, English Cocker Spaniels, English Springer Spaniels, Doberman Pinschers, Greyhounds, Lhasa Apsos, Poodles, Rottweilers, Samoyeds, Shih Tzus, and Soft-coated Wheaten Terriers. These are not immune complex diseases, although some are characterized by proteinuria and associated clinical abnormalities that *resemble those caused* by immune-mediated glomerulonephropathy. Several of these breeds of dogs have genetic defects in collagen structure and function (types III or IV), analogous to hereditary nephropathies in people such as Alport syndrome (hereditary nephritis).

Most cases of amyloidosis (*see* p 592) in dogs and cats, including familial amyloidosis in Chinese Shar-Pei and Abyssinian cats, are reactive, or secondary, amyloidosis. In this form of the disease, amyloid A protein is deposited in various tissues after serum levels increase as a result of chronic inflammation. When the kidneys are affected, amyloid deposition in the nonfamilial forms in dogs usually occurs in the glomerulus. However, in Shar-Pei, at least 25% of Abyssinian cats, and in many domestic cats with the nonfamilial form of this disease, amyloid is found primarily in the medullary interstitium, where it interferes with the renal concentrating mechanism and is more likely to produce nonproteinuric CKD than protein-losing glomerular amyloid deposition. In contrast, glomerular amyloidosis usually leads to marked proteinuria. The nonfamilial form of amyloidosis usually affects middle-aged to older dogs and cats. Beagles, Collies, and Walker Hounds are reported to be at increased risk. Animals with the familial form of the disease are usually diagnosed at a younger age.

Clinical Findings: Glomerulopathy often leads to proteinuria (primarily albuminuria) and can produce hypoproteinemia, ascites, dyspnea (due to pleural effusion or pulmonary edema), and/or peripheral edema, which may be referred to as the nephrotic syndrome. Protein wasting can produce preferential loss of lean body mass that may be apparent on careful physical examination. Severe or chronic glomerular disease is a cause of CKD; most dogs and many cats with glomerular disease eventually develop Stage III or IV disease. Systemic hypertension may be more prevalent in proteinuric CKD and may be seen at any stage.

Proteinuria may result in loss of antithrombin III through the glomerular basement membrane, leading to a hypercoagulable state in dogs. Proteinuria also contributes to mild thrombocytosis and platelet hypersensitivity, which contribute to coagulation abnormalities in affected dogs, generally when plasma albumin levels are ≤1 g/dL. Severe dyspnea secondary to pulmonary thromboembolism or other sequelae of thrombotic disease may be seen in dogs with glomerulonephritis or amyloidosis. It is unclear whether a hypercoagulable state also exists in proteinuric cats, because clinical signs from hypercoagulability have not been reported in cats.

Diagnosis: The BUN, creatinine, and phosphorus concentrations are usually increased, although the degree varies with the stage of CKD at the time of diagnosis. Animals should be staged and substaged on the basis of measurements of blood pressure (*see* TABLE 3), proteinuria (*see* TABLE 4), and serum creatinine (*see* TABLE 2). Marked proteinuria with edema may be seen in the presence or absence of azotemia. Physical findings are usually nonspecific except that ascites, pleural effusion, and/or peripheral, pitting, nonpainful, subcutaneous edema are evident in some animals (75% of cats and 15% of dogs). Although uncommon, urine specific gravity may be inappropriately high for the degree of renal dysfunction. A urine protein:creatinine ratio >2 suggests a glomerular origin. If the sediment examination eliminates inflammatory urinary tract disease and hemorrhage as the source of proteinuria, then the degree of increase may help distinguish tubular proteinuria (typical ratio value of 0.5–2), glomerulonephritis (typical ratio value of 0.5–15), and glomerular amyloidosis (typical ratio value of 0.5–40). However, substantial overlap exists in these ranges, and a variety of glomerulopathies such as focal segmental glomerulosclerosis in dogs have yet to be well characterized. Further, the ratio tends to be low in the initial stages of a glomerulopathy, increases in severity as the disease progresses, and then decreases terminally as GFR falls to very low levels in late Stage 4 disease.

Renal biopsy is required to determine the type of glomerular disease. Membranous glomerulonephritis is reported most frequently in cats; there is a roughly equal distribution of histologic findings in dogs, with glomerular amyloidosis; focal segmental glomerulosclerosis; and membranous, proliferative, and membranoproliferative glomerulonephritis all represented. The degree of proteinuria does not always correlate with the severity of the histologic lesions or the degree of azotemia. Systemic hypertension develops in an unusually large proportion of animals with protein-losing glomerulonephritis; therefore, blood pressure should be determined in all animals with evidence of glomerular disease.

A careful search should be made for an inciting disease process. Abdominal and thoracic radiographs, ultrasonography, and specialized serologic tests can exclude various inflammatory, infectious, and neoplastic diseases. In dogs with glomerulonephritis, this includes tests for SLE (eg, antinuclear antibody titer and LE prep) and appropriate antigen or antibody screening tests for other infectious agents and heartworm disease; in cats, tests for infection with FeLV, FIV, FIP, SLE, and heartworm disease should be included.

Treatment: There are six basic principles for treatment of glomerulonephropathies: 1) If a cause of immune complex disease can be identified, it should be treated. 2) Manifestations of the nephrotic syndrome, if present, should initially be managed by therapies designed to reduce proteinuria. This includes a renal diet low in protein and salt and subsequently, if needed, judicious use of diuretics. 3) Antithrombotics (eg, aspirin) should be considered for hypoalbuminemic (plasma albumin <1 g/dL) dogs but not cats, as well as for dogs with low serum levels of antithrombin III (<30% of normal). In dogs with marked proteinuria and serum albumin <2 g/dL, low-dose aspirin therapy (2.5–5 mg/kg/day, PO) is appropriate, unless melena is present or gastric ulceration is suspected. However, aspirin is bound to plasma proteins and is eliminated via the kidneys, so the lower end of the dosage range should be used in hypoalbuminemic dogs. 4) Because proteinuria may promote interstitial fibrosis, treatment to limit glomerular loss of protein is warranted and may include dietary protein restriction, n-3 polyunsaturated fatty acid supplementation, and administration of an angiotensin-receptor blocker (eg, telmisartan 1 mg/kg/day, PO) or angiotensin-converting enzyme inhibitor (eg, benazepril or enalapril, 0.5 mg/kg, PO, once daily in cats and bid in dogs). 5) Efforts to reduce the magnitude and consequences of glomerular immune complex deposition should be considered, especially in animals with biopsy-confirmed glomerular inflammation and no known primary antigenic stimulus. Immunosuppressive drugs (eg, mycophenolate, azathioprine, cyclophosphamide, cyclosporine) can be used in dogs with glomerulonephritis, although results are variable. For amyloidosis, dimethylsulfoxide and colchicine have been tried, without consistent results. These anti-inflammatory drugs should be administered only on a trial basis with owner consent. Corticosteroids seem to be beneficial only in mild glomerulopathy; they may worsen proteinuria in other glomerulopathies and should be avoided in animals with amyloidosis, because they are reported to enhance amyloid deposition. 6) Manifestations of CKD should be monitored and managed in accordance with the stage of disease (*see* p 1512).

Prognosis: Although one study found that mean survival time of dogs with glomerulonephritis was 87 days, the prognosis with early diagnosis and appropriate therapy is much better. In a recent study of dogs with glomerulonephritis, those receiving a placebo medication survived beyond the entire 6-mo duration of the study. The prognosis for animals with amyloidosis is guarded but variable, with reported mean survival times ranging from 49 days to 20 mo.

RENAL TUBULAR DEFECTS

Renal Acidosis

The form of metabolic acidosis that occurs in acute kidney injury and Stages 2–4 of chronic kidney disease, referred to as uremic acidosis, is due to reduced urine-acidifying ability of diseased kidneys. In uremic acidosis, although the ability of individual tubular cells to reabsorb bicarbonate and/or secrete hydrogen ions may be normal, there is generally far less total cell mass present. Acid accumulates if the animal is under metabolic or dietary acid pressure, which is common in carnivores. This is particularly problematic in cats, which are often fed acidifying maintenance diets.

Rare renal tubular defects in dogs and cats may result in hyperchloremic metabolic acidosis, referred to as **renal tubular acidosis**. Two types of renal tubular acidosis have been described in dogs and one in cats. In Type I (distal), the ability of the distal tubule to secrete hydrogen ions against a concentration gradient is defective; in Type II (proximal), the ability to reabsorb bicarbonate in the proximal tubule is reduced. Type I has been reported in both species; Type II has also been described in dogs in conjunction with other proximal tubular defects in acquired (gentamicin nephrotoxicosis and an idiopathic form) and heritable (Fanconi syndrome, *see* p 1520) forms.

Type I renal tubular acidosis has been associated with demineralization of the skeleton (due to buffering of excess hydrogen ions) and nephrolithiasis (due to hypercalciuria from bone resorption) in dogs. Diagnosis is based on the presence of hyperchloremic metabolic acidosis with a urinary pH that is inappropriately high for the degree of systemic acidosis in the absence of bacterial urease modification of urine. Failure to produce acid urine in the face of metabolic acidosis or after oral ammonium chloride loading is diagnostic; however, this challenge test is contraindicated in animals that are already severely acidotic. Type II renal tubular acidosis is diagnosed by demonstrating increased urinary fractional excretion of bicarbonate when plasma bicarbonate levels are normal or decreased; this test is not practicable in the clinical setting and diagnosis is presumptively based on history, signalment, and clinical pathology findings.

Therapy consists of oral administration of an alkalinizing agent sufficient to maintain normal blood pH (1 mEq bicarbonate equivalent/kg/day for Type I and 1–6 mEq bicarbonate equivalent/kg/day for Type II, PO). Therapy is more problematic in dogs with Type II renal tubular acidosis, because supplemental bicarbonate is readily lost in the urine.

Fanconi Syndrome

Fanconi syndrome is a generalized proximal tubular reabsorptive defect resulting in excessive loss of many solutes in the urine. It has been reported as an acquired condition in dogs (chicken jerky treat ingestion, gentamicin nephrotoxicosis, and an idiopathic form) and in a heritable form in a variety of breeds (most notably Basenjis), in which it develops gradually in adults of both sexes. There is excessive urinary loss of glucose, sodium, potassium, phosphorus, uric acid, bicarbonate, albumin, and amino acids. Blood glucose concentrations are normal. Serum electrolytes are normal early in the disease, but hypophosphatemia, hypokalemia, and metabolic acidosis are seen in the later stages.

Clinical signs include polydipsia, polyuria, and weight loss. Signs of uremia may be present if the animal is in Stage III or IV chronic kidney disease. Diagnosis is based on documentation of increased urinary fractional excretion of glucose, sodium, potassium, phosphorus, and bicarbonate in the presence of normal plasma concentrations. Hypoalbuminuria is likely to be present, because the proximal tubule normally reabsorbs the small amount of albumin that traverses the glomerular filtration barrier. Differential diagnoses include simple renal glucosuria and chronic kidney disease from other causes. The microscopic renal changes in the heritable form are not remarkable in the early stages but progress to nonspecific findings characteristic of chronic kidney disease. A genetic marker has been developed. A treatment regimen to reverse the tubular defect has not been described. The histologic appearance of the acquired forms of Fanconi syndrome vary, depending on the cause.

Oral supplementation of sodium chloride (5–10 mg/kg/day, PO), potassium (potassium citrate 10–30 mg/kg/day, PO), and alkali (sodium bicarbonate 10–30 mg/kg/day, PO) is indicated if the corresponding serum concentration is low. Dogs with acute or chronic kidney disease should be treated symptomatically as appropriate. The heritable disease is slowly progressive despite therapy and usually results in death from uremia.

Renal Glucosuria

This is usually a congenital defect in proximal tubular handling of glucose that results in glucosuria despite normal blood glucose concentration. Affected animals may be asymptomatic, have polydipsia and polyuria, or have recurrent or severe urinary tract infections due to bacterial colonization in the presence of glucose. Diagnosis is made by demonstrating persistent glucosuria despite a normal blood glucose concentration and by identifying no other renal reabsorptive abnormalities. This disease is so uncommonly recognized that little is known about its biologic behavior. The general consensus is that it is not progressive and does not require treatment, except that some animals with heritable Fanconi syndrome may initially exhibit glucosuria as the only clinically apparent renal reabsorptive defect.

OBSTRUCTIVE UROPATHY

Even though the kidneys would otherwise be able to function normally, obstruction of urine flow at any point below the level of the kidneys leads to accumulation of metabolic wastes and postrenal azotemia/uremia. Obstruction of the urethra by uroliths in dogs and by matrix-crystalline plugs in young male cats and obstruction of a ureter by a urolith in geriatric cats are the three most common causes, although uroliths, tumors, or blood clots may obstruct the ureters (or urethra) in either species.

Hydronephrosis is characterized by dilatation of the renal pelvis as the result of partial or complete obstruction of outflow of urine from one or both kidneys. When the obstruction is acute, complete, and bilateral, morphologic changes in the kidneys are less extensive, because the period of survival is short. In unilateral or partial obstruction, the animal often survives long enough for severe pressure atrophy of the renal parenchyma and cystic enlargement of the affected kidney to develop. Hydroureter commonly develops when the obstruction is located lower in the tract. Increased hydrostatic pressure results in atrophy of functional renal parenchyma. The pseudodiverticula of the renal pelvis disappear first; later, even the cortex may atrophy. The affected kidneys eventually become grossly enlarged, functionless sacs, filled with urine or serous fluid that may harbor bacteria.

Clinical Findings: Animals with urethral obstruction frequently exhibit pollakiuria, stranguria, and hematuria; abdominal pain may be marked. Signs of uremia develop rapidly and include vomiting, dehydration, hypothermia, and severe depression. The bladder is distended and painful on palpation, and a urethral catheter cannot be readily passed. Bradycardia or cardiac arrhythmias due to hyperkalemia may be present, particularly if plasma potassium is >7 mEq/L. Because compensatory hypertrophy of the nonaffected kidney results in a nonazotemic state, unilateral ureteral obstruction commonly is undiagnosed, unless the animal has accompanying renal disease or the enlarged, hydronephrotic kidney is palpated during physical examination and/or seen on radiologic or ultrasonographic imaging studies.

Diagnosis: The history, clinical signs, and physical examination usually provide a straightforward diagnosis of urethral obstruction. Ureteral obstruction should be suspected in any acutely uremic cat, including those with a history of chronic kidney disease. Excretory urography or abdominal ultrasonography are necessary to establish a diagnosis in animals with bilateral or unilateral ureteral obstruction. Serum potassium levels should be determined immediately in animals with cardiac arrhythmias. An ECG can provide presumptive evidence of hyperkalemia (bradycardia; tall, peaked T waves; increased PR interval; widened QRS complex; atrial standstill) if laboratory results are delayed.

Treatment: The urethral obstruction should be relieved (*see* p 1525). Fluids given IV improve renal function and correct electrolyte and acid-base abnormalities. Normal saline is preferred but not required in hyperkalemic animals. Unless the animal is markedly hyperkalemic (serum potassium >7 mEq/L), has cardiac arrhythmias, or is known to have preexisting kidney disease, it is often best to avoid overcorrection by allowing plasma potassium and acid-base balance to return toward normal via restoration of renal excretory function for 12 hr before administering therapy specifically intended to correct these abnormalities. In animals with severe hyperkalemia and cardiac arrhythmias, bicarbonate (0.5 mEq/kg, given slowly IV over 5 min) or regular insulin and dextrose infusions can be given to drive potassium intracellularly. Because of a postobstructive diuresis that lasts for 1–5 days, hypokalemia and/or dehydration are often seen within 24–48 hr after correction of urethral obstruction. Plasma electrolytes, body weight, urine output, hematocrit, and plasma total solids should be monitored daily, with the type and quantity of fluid administered adjusted appropriately.

Surgery is often necessary to correct complete ureteral obstruction. When possible, the obstruction should be removed to reestablish urine flow. In some cases, ureteroliths will pass through the ureters, eliminating the need for surgery. This may require partial ureteral resection and reimplantation, particularly in cats, which have very small and friable ureters. In some cases, unilateral nephrectomy may be required, but a kidney should not be removed without clear evidence that the contralateral kidney is capable of sustaining life. Preferred evidence includes the estimation of GFR in the contralateral kidney but could alternatively be based on the following criteria: normal renal size, shape, and consistency on ultrasonography; presence of normal vascular and excretory phases on excretory urography; normal renal ultrasonographic examination; and normal renal biopsy.

NEOPLASIA

Neoplasms of the Kidney

Neoplasms of the kidney are uncommon and represent ~0.5%–1.7% of all neoplasms in dogs. Benign neoplasms are uncommon, usually incidental findings at necropsy, and generally of little clinical significance. Adenomas, lipomas, fibromas, and papillomas have been reported.

Primary malignant renal neoplasms (except nephroblastomas) are most common in middle-aged to older animals. No breed predilection has been found, except for heritable predilection for the development of bilateral, multifocal cystoadenocarcinomas in German Shepherds, generally between 5–11 yr of age. The most common primary malignant renal neoplasm is carcinoma, which originates from the renal tubular epithelium. Usually, it is unilateral, located at one pole of the kidney, and well demarcated. Size varies from microscopic to several times that of the normal kidney, and color may be yellow, white, or gray. Renal carcinomas metastasize early to various organs; the opposite kidney, lungs, liver, and adrenals are involved most commonly.

Nephroblastomas (embryonal nephroma, Wilms' tumor) arise from vestigial embryonic tissue. They are seen in young animals and, in dogs, are most commonly diagnosed at <1 yr of age. There is no breed predilection. Males are affected twice as commonly as females. Nephroblastomas are usually unilateral but are occasionally bilateral. They can grow to immense size; it is not uncommon to have virtually the entire abdomen occupied by tumor. Metastasis may occur to regional lymph nodes, liver, and lungs.

Transitional cell carcinomas arise from transitional epithelium of the renal pelvis, ureter, bladder, or urethra (*see* p 1523). Other primary malignant renal neoplasms are uncommon and include hemangiosarcomas, fibrosarcomas, leiomyosarcomas, and squamous cell carcinomas.

The kidneys are a common site of metastatic or multicentric neoplasms. Metastatic lesions may be unilateral or bilateral. Lymphosarcoma is the most common multicentric tumor involving the kidneys. As many as 50% of dogs and cats with lymphosarcoma have renal lesions and, in some cases, only the kidneys or kidneys and brain are affected. Renal involvement is usually multifocal or diffuse, interstitial, and bilateral, and results in large, irregular kidneys. Lymphosarcoma in cats frequently is associated with infection by feline leukemia virus.

Clinical Findings: Signs are nonspecific and may include weight loss, anorexia, depression, and fever. Bilateral neoplasms may uncommonly destroy sufficient renal tissue to cause chronic kidney disease and associated signs of uremia. Astute owners may notice "lumps" in their animal's abdomen or abdominal enlargement. Persistent hematuria, usually microscopic, may occur. Rarely, renal tumors may produce excessive erythropoietin, which results in erythrocythemia (*see* p 43).

Diagnosis: History and clinical signs may indicate a mass in the area of the kidneys or renomegaly, which can be confirmed by ultrasonography or radiography, although an excretory urogram or renal arteriogram may be required. Radiographs of the thorax may reveal metastatic disease. Neoplastic cells occasionally can be found in the urine sediment. A tissue sample suitable for a diagnosis may be obtained via catheterization. Cystoscopic biopsy can be an effective method to obtain a diagnostic sample in dogs with transitional cell carcinoma of the bladder and urethra, especially females. Percutaneous needle aspiration and cytologic examination may be sufficient for the diagnosis of lymphosarcoma in cats and dogs, particularly when there is diffuse involvement or with ultrasonographic guidance when multifocal disease occurs. Histologic examination of tissue obtained by cystoscopy, needle biopsy, or surgical wedge biopsy is often necessary to determine the type of tumor.

Treatment: Ultrasound-guided endoscopic diode laser ablation holds promise as a palliative treatment for dogs with transitional cell carcinoma of the urinary tract. Otherwise, treatment of all renal neoplasms except lymphosarcoma involves surgical removal; unilateral nephrectomy is usually required. Lymphosarcoma is best managed by combination chemotherapy (*see* p 40). Chemotherapy is generally ineffective against renal tumors other than lymphosarcoma.

Neoplasms of the Lower Urinary Tract

Neoplasms of the ureters, bladder, and urethra are uncommon in dogs and rare in cats. The low incidence in cats may be due to a difference in tryptophan metabolism that results in low urinary concentrations of carcinogenic tryptophan metabolites. The mean age of affected dogs and cats is 9 yr.

In the lower urinary tract, primary neoplasms are more likely to be malignant than benign. Papillomas, leiomyomas, fibromas, neurofibromas, hemangiomas, rhabdomyomas, and myxomas are found infrequently.

Among primary malignant neoplasms of the lower urinary tract, transitional cell carcinomas are diagnosed most frequently in both species. Squamous cell carcinomas, adenocarcinomas, fibrosarcomas, leiomyosarcomas, rhabdomyosarcomas, hemangiosarcomas, and osteosarcomas also are found. Transitional cell carcinomas may be solitary or multiple papillary-like projections from the mucosa or may develop as a diffuse infiltration of the ureter, bladder, prostate, and/or urethra. Cystic transitional cell tumors are more common in certain breeds of dogs, particularly Scottish Terriers, have been associated with prior therapy with cyclophosphamide, and may be linked to exposure to herbicides and older-generation insecticides. Transitional cell tumors are highly invasive and metastasize frequently, most commonly to the regional lymph nodes and lungs. Ureteral and bladder neoplasms can cause chronic obstruction to urine flow with secondary hydronephrosis. Urethral tumors are more likely to cause acute obstructive uropathy. Intractable secondary bacterial urinary tract infections are commonly associated with neoplasms of the bladder and urethra.

Clinical Findings: Hematuria, dysuria, stranguria, and pollakiuria are the most common signs. Animals with ureteral obstruction and unilateral hydronephrosis may show signs of abdominal pain and have a palpable, enlarged kidney. Signs of uremia may be apparent in animals with bilateral ureteral obstruction and hydronephrosis or with urethral obstruction. The bladder wall may be thickened, and a cord-like urethra or urethral mass(es) may be palpable rectally.

Diagnosis: History and clinical signs are highly suggestive of lower urinary tract disease in animals with tumors of the bladder or urethra. Urinalysis frequently reveals hematuria, and there may be evidence of secondary infection. Chronic, uncomplicated urinary tract infections must be differentiated from those associated with neoplasms. Neoplastic cells may be found in the sediment, particularly with transitional cell carcinomas. For bladder tumors in dogs, the veterinary bladder tumor antigen test may be helpful, although false-positives do occur. A cystourethrogram, retrograde urethrogram, or ultrasonography is generally necessary to determine the location and

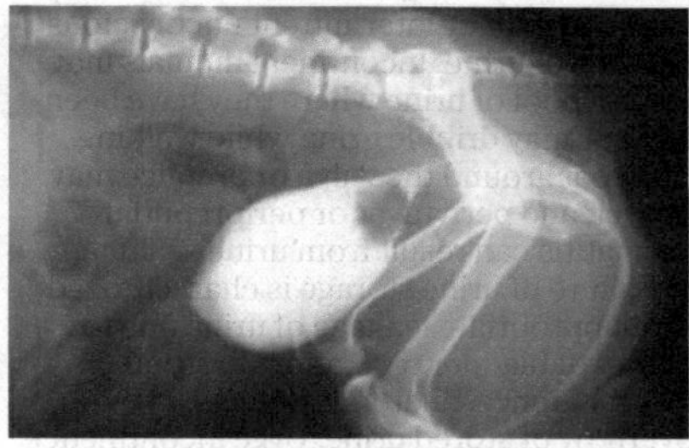

Transitional cell carcinoma in trigone area of canine bladder, contrast radiograph. *Courtesy of Ontario Veterinary College.*

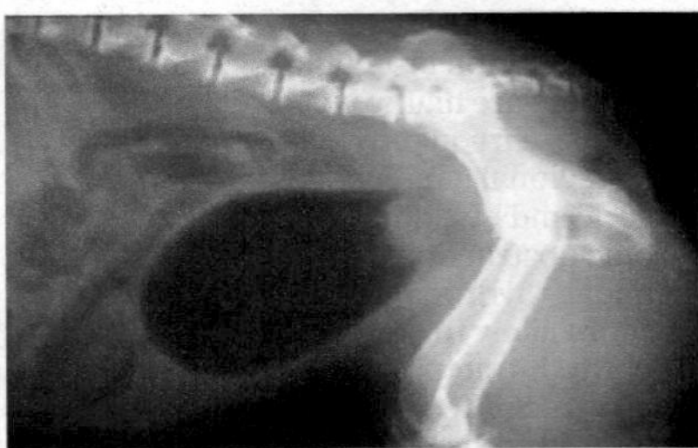

Transitional cell carcinoma in trigone area of canine bladder, pneumocystogram. *Courtesy of Ontario Veterinary College.*

extent of the tumor. Biopsy of the tumor is required for definitive diagnosis.

Treatment: Excision of the tumor, if possible, is the most beneficial therapy. Transitional cell carcinomas are frequently located at the trigone of the bladder or in the urethra and may necessitate radical reconstructive surgery of the lower urinary tract. Prognosis is poor for these animals, even with surgery, because recurrence and metastasis occur rapidly. Radiation therapy and/or chemotherapy with piroxicam, cisplatin, doxorubicin, vinblastine, chlorambucil, or mitoxantrone will generally prolong the life of affected animals. Dogs with transitional cell carcinoma, including those being treated for the tumor, are predisposed to development of bacterial urinary tract infections, and routine urine cultures are indicated.

DISORDERS OF MICTURITION

Disorders of micturition result from a dysfunction in the storage or voiding of urine and may be neurogenic or non-neurogenic in origin. Urinary incontinence is the failure of voluntary control of micturition, with constant or intermittent unconscious passage of urine. Incontinent animals may leave a pool of urine where they have been lying or may dribble urine while walking. The coat around the vulva or prepuce may be wet, and perivulvar or peripreputial dermatitis can result from urine scalding.

Failure of urine storage is characterized by inappropriate leakage of urine due to failure of bladder relaxation, urethral incompetence, anatomic defects, or overflow of stored urine. Urge incontinence is seen with detrusor irritability, usually associated with cystitis. The most common non-neurogenic incontinence is attributed to deficiency of sex hormones in neutered animals, particularly female dogs, and is referred to as hormonal-responsive urethral incompetence. Idiopathic urethral sphincter incompetence also is seen. Urinary incontinence associated with anatomic defects may be detected in animals at an early age. For example, an animal with a unilateral congenital ectopic ureter may void normally but "dribble" urine intermittently, whereas animals with bilateral ectopic ureters are less likely to void normally. Paradoxical urinary incontinence may develop when there is a partial obstruction of the urethra leading to bladder distention and overflow incontinence.

Failure of normal voiding is characterized by frequent attempts to urinate with stranguria and passage of only small amounts of urine. Inability to urinate can be due to mechanical obstruction of the urethra by calculi, neoplasms, or strictures; detrusor atony from overdistention of the bladder; or neurologic disease. Animals with abnormalities of the voiding phase may develop overflow incontinence due to dribbling of urine associated with bladder overdistention.

Neurologic causes of micturition disorders can be categorized as upper (UMN) or lower motor neuron (LMN) lesions. Lesions in the sacral spinal cord, pelvic nerve, and detrusor atony lead to LMN signs, which are often characterized by a distended, easily expressed bladder. Dysautonomia in cats is a multisystemic disease characterized by widespread disruption of autonomic system functions, including urinary incontinence of LMN origin. Damage to the thoracolumbar spinal cord or disease of the cerebrum, cerebellum, or brain stem can lead to UMN signs, characterized by a distended bladder that is difficult to express. Another neurologic cause of inability to urinate is functional obstruction (detrusor-sphincter reflex dyssynergia), which occurs when there is incoordination of the normal micturition reflex; this is believed to result from overdischarge of sympathetic nerve impulses to the urethral sphincter, resulting in a failure of urethral relaxation during detrusor contraction. Animals with neurogenic incontinence may leak urine (LMN) and/or develop overflow incontinence due to dribbling of urine associated with bladder overdistension (any neurogenic cause).

Diagnosis: Clinical signs are usually suggestive of a micturition disorder. The history should include age of onset, whether the animal is intact or neutered, age at neutering, current medication, and history of previous urinary tract disorders. A thorough physical and neurologic examination is indicated, and the act of voiding should be observed, including estimation of initial and final bladder volume.

Animals with LMN lesions or an atonic bladder have a large, distended bladder that can be expressed with minimal pressure. Animals with mechanical or functional obstruction or with spinal lesions causing UMN signs also have a large distended bladder, but urine cannot be readily expressed. Caution must be exercised when attempting to express urine from these animals to avoid rupturing the bladder. Plain or contrast radiography, cystoscopy, or ultrasonography are necessary to determine the type and location of mechanical obstruction.

Animals with functional obstruction (reflex dyssynergia) generally exhibit pollakiuria with interrupted urine stream, distended urinary bladder, no identifiable structural cause of obstruction, and overflow incontinence; the neurologic examination is generally abnormal. A catheter can easily be passed into the bladder in animals with functional obstruction but will not pass in animals with mechanical obstruction.

Treatment: Accurate diagnosis or localization of the lesion is essential for appropriate pharmacologic management. Animals with hormonal incontinence can be treated with the appropriate sex hormone (eg, diethylstilbestrol in females and testosterone in males). The dosage should be adjusted to the minimum required to maintain continence. Diethylstilbestrol may be difficult to obtain. Alternatively, an α-adrenergic agonist drug (eg, phenylpropanolamine, 2–4 mg/kg/day in divided doses) can be given to animals with urethral incompetence alone or in combination with an estrogenic compound. Although ephedrine is another α-agonist shown to be effective in the treatment of urinary incontinence in female dogs, its use is more often associated with adverse effects of anxiety and excitability. Pseudoephedrine is apparently not effective for this purpose. Urge incontinence (detrusor instability) is treated with anticholinergic drugs such as oxybutin chloride (0.5 mg/kg/day, PO) or propantheline (dogs <20 kg, 7.5 mg/day; dogs >20 kg, 15 mg/day; cats, 7.5 mg every 72 hr). Cholinergic drugs such as bethanechol are used in animals with detrusor atony. Functional obstruction is treated with sympatholytic drugs (eg, phenoxybenzamine, 2.5–10 mg, 1–3 times/day); cholinergic drugs may also be necessary.

Complete mechanical obstruction of the urethra is a medical emergency and should be relieved by catheterization and retropulsion of the obstructing material into the bladder or by surgery. Animals with detrusor atony from overdistention but without neurologic lesions benefit from decompression of the bladder by placement of an indwelling urinary catheter for 3–7 days. This may be done continuously or intermittently. Those with neurogenic atony, which usually does not respond to medical management, may require manual expression of the bladder or catheterization several times daily.

UROLITHIASIS

Some mineral solutes precipitate to form crystals in urine; these crystals may aggregate and grow to macroscopic size, at which time they are known as **uroliths** (calculi or stones). Uroliths generally contain an organic matrix that is believed to vary minimally among uroliths and that constitutes ~2%–10% of the stone's chemical composition. The remaining 90%–98% of the urolith is composed of minerals that vary depending on the type of urolith. **Urolithiasis** is a general term referring to stones located anywhere within the urinary tract. Uroliths can develop in the kidney, ureter, bladder, or urethra and are referred to as nephroliths, ureteroliths, urocystoliths, and urethroliths, respectively.

Uroliths in all animal species are composed of ~10 different minerals. Identification of the minerals in uroliths by qualitative analysis is unreliable. The type of minerals in uroliths can be readily identified by optical crystallography, infrared spectroscopy, and/or x-ray diffraction. Minerals found in uroliths have a chemical name and often a mineral or crystal name (*see* TABLE 5). Variation in urine characteristics over time can result in more than one crystal type within a single urolith. In such instances, the urolith core corresponds to conditions that were present when the urolith initially formed, and the outer layers correspond to more recent conditions.

Mechanisms involved in stone formation are incompletely understood in dogs and cats. However, three main contributing factors are 1) matrix—the inorganic protein core may facilitate initial urolith formation, 2) crystallization inhibitors—organic and inorganic crystallization inhibitors may be

TABLE 5 UROLITH NAMES

Mineral Name	Chemical Formula	Chemical Name
Struvite	$MgNH_4PO_4 \bullet 6H_20$	Magnesium ammonium phosphate hexahydrate
Whewellite	$CaC_2O_4 \bullet H_20$	Calcium oxalate monohydrate
Weddellite	$CaC_2O_4 \bullet 2H_20$	Calcium oxalate dihydrate
Hydroxyapatite	$Ca_{10}(PO_4)_6(OH)_2$	Calcium phosphate (hydroxyl form)
Urate	$C_5H_4N_4O_3$	Urate
Ammonium urate	$NH_4 \bullet C_5H_4N_4O_3$	Ammonium urate
Sodium urate	$Na \bullet C_5H_4N_4O_3 \times H_2O$	Sodium urate monohydrate
Cystine	$(SCH_2CHNH_2COOH)_2$	Cystine
Silica	SiO_2	Silica
Xanthine	$C_5H_4N_4O_2$	Xanthine

lacking or dysfunctional in animals with uroliths, and 3) precipitation crystallization factors—a complex relationship among urine solutes and other chemical factors in the urine can lead to conditions favoring crystallization. Regardless of the underlying mechanism(s), uroliths are not produced unless sufficiently high urine concentrations of urolith-forming constituents exist and transit time of crystals within the urinary tract is prolonged. For selected stones (eg, struvite, cystine, urate), other favorable conditions (eg, proper pH) for crystallization must also exist. These criteria can be affected by urinary tract infection, diet, intestinal absorption, urine volume, frequency of urination, therapeutic agents, and genetics.

Clinical signs associated with urolithiasis are seldom caused by microscopic crystals. However, formation of macroscopic uroliths in the lower urinary tract that interfere with the flow of urine and/or irritate the mucosal surface often results in dysuria, hematuria, and stranguria. Nephroliths often are asymptomatic unless pyelonephritis exists concurrently or they pass into the ureter. Ureteral obstruction may produce signs of vomiting, lethargy, and/or flank and renal pain, particularly if there is acute total obstruction with distention of the renal capsule. The only clinical sign associated with unilateral urethroliths may be pain, which can be difficult to detect in dogs and cats. If these initial signs of ureteral obstruction do not lead to a diagnosis, unilateral ureteral obstruction may result in hydronephrosis with loss of function of the ipsilateral kidney. Ureteroliths may also precipitate a uremic crisis in cats with previously compensated chronic renal failure. Because clinical signs of renal dysfunction are generally not apparent until two-thirds or more of total functional renal parenchyma is lost, clinical signs may not be seen except in the following situations: 1) both ureters are obstructed, 2) there is contralateral chronic kidney disease, or 3) a renal infection develops. Unilateral ureteroliths may be identified serendipitously during abdominal imaging studies or surgery.

Abdominal palpation can help detect urocystoliths; the bladder wall may be thickened, and a grating sensation may be felt when the bladder is palpated. Although palpation may reveal a single large urolith or multiple uroliths by their crepitation, it cannot dependably identify all animals with uroliths; urethral calculi may be detected by rectal palpation or located by passing a catheter. Because multiple uroliths may be present throughout the urinary tract, a complete radiographic examination of the tract is indicated; radiodense calculi >3 mm in diameter are usually visible on radiographs. Urate, and occasionally cystine, uroliths may be radiolucent, requiring contrast radiography or ultrasonography to confirm their presence. Urinalysis, including identification of crystals on microscopic examination of fresh, warm urine and bacterial culture and sensitivity testing, is a critical part of the evaluation and may help determine the type of urolith present. Ultrasonography and cystoscopy may also be useful.

Urethral Obstruction: Urethral obstruction is common in male dogs and cats. It may occur suddenly or may develop throughout days or weeks. Initially, the animal may frequently attempt to urinate and produce only a fine stream, a few drops, or nothing. Animals may also exhibit extreme pain manifested by crying out when attempting to urinate. Complete obstruction causes uremia within 36–48 hr, which leads to depression, anorexia, vomiting, diarrhea, dehydration, coma, and death within ~72 hr. Urethral obstruction is an emergency condition, and treatment should begin immediately.

If the bladder is intact, it is distended, hard, and painful; care should be used when palpating the bladder to avoid iatrogenic rupture. If the bladder has ruptured, it cannot be palpated and urine can sometimes, but not always, be obtained from the abdominal cavity by paracentesis. Animals with spontaneous bladder rupture may appear temporarily improved because the pain associated with bladder distention has been relieved; however, peritonitis and absorption of uremic toxins and potassium occur rapidly and lead to depression, abdominal distention, cardiac arrhythmias, and death.

Hyperkalemia and metabolic acidosis are life-threatening complications of urethral obstruction. An ECG (to record cardiac rhythm and rate) and a serum potassium are indicated. Initial emergency care involves immediate relief of obstruction by catheterization and fluid therapy with normal saline. Occasionally, an obstruction at the external urethral orifice can be dislodged by gentle massage. Sometimes, when a portion of the urethra is dilated with fluid under pressure and then suddenly released, urethral calculi can be flushed out. The urolith nearly always can be flushed back into the bladder by using the largest catheter that can be easily passed to the calculus, occluding the distal end of the urethral lumen around the catheter, and infusing a sterile mixture of equal parts of isotonic saline solution and an aqueous lubricant. If the urethrolith cannot be flushed back into the bladder, a urethrotomy should be performed to remove the obstructing stone(s). Depending on the clinical circumstances, the urethrotomy site may be sutured or a permanent urethrostomy created. Calculi flushed back into the bladder should be removed by cystotomy to prevent recurrence, although in some cases they can be dissolved. The stone should be sent for quantitative analysis, with the animal managed medically to prevent stone recurrence based on the results.

Canine Urolithiasis

The most common canine uroliths are magnesium ammonium phosphate, calcium oxalate, or urate; less common uroliths include cystine, silica, calcium phosphate, and xanthine. While general management includes surgical removal and medical management, the appropriate treatment protocol depends on the location of the urolith and its chemical composition, as well as on patient-specific factors. Nephrolithiasis is generally not associated with an increase in the rate of progression of kidney injury; thus, it is recommended that animals with nephrolithiasis be managed without surgery in most cases.

Struvite Stones: The most common urinary stones in dogs are composed of struvite. The mineral composition is mostly struvite ($MgNH_4PO_4 \cdot 6H_2O$), but frequently, small amounts of carbonate-apatite and ammonium urate are present. In most cases, struvite uroliths form in association with urinary tract infections with urease-producing *Staphylococcus* or *Proteus* spp. Although they are frequent in cats, sterile struvite uroliths rarely form in dogs. They have been detected in a family of English Cocker Spaniels, suggesting a genetic predisposition.

Medical management involves dissolution and prevention of stone formation. In both instances, the aim of treatment is to reduce the concentrations of NH_4^+, Mg^{2+}, and PO_4^{-3} in urine. For dissolution, urine should be extremely undersaturated for struvite; for prevention, the degree of struvite saturation should be sufficiently low to make crystallization unlikely. The choice between surgery, lithotripsy, and medical treatment may not be easy. Owner compliance, the animal's acceptance of the diet, availability of lithotripsy, practice philosophy, and knowledge of the indications and contraindications are necessary to make a decision. If stone dissolution is prolonged or fails, it may be more costly than surgical treatment. Surgical removal of uroliths is often incomplete, with small, hidden uroliths often inadvertently left in the urinary tract serving as a nidus for recurrence.

Before beginning stone dissolution by medical therapy, a physical examination, CBC, serum chemistry profile, urinalysis, urine culture and sensitivity, abdominal radiographs to document stone size, and blood pressure measurement (if possible) should be performed. Contraindications to stone dissolution include heart failure, edema, ascites, pleural effusion, hypertension, hepatic failure, renal failure, and hypoalbuminemia. However, chronic kidney disease is not always a contraindication for dissolution of struvite nephroliths.

Dissolution Protocol: While the use of urinary acidification to reduce urine pH to <6 and other individualized dietary maneuvers may prove effective, a few commercially available diets that are generally nutritionally balanced promote struvite stone dissolution. Dogs fed these rations generally have reduced intake of protein, phosphate, and magnesium and a high intake of sodium. This results in osmotic diuresis, reduced daily urea output, and enhanced urine volume. The low urinary urea concentration is one of the most important features of such diets and also reduces ammonia production by the action of urease-producing bacteria. No other food, including treats, should be fed, and adequate fresh water should be available at all times.

Urease-producing urinary tract infections must be treated. The choice of antibacterial should be based on sensitivity testing when possible. Most *Staphylococcus* and *Proteus* infections are sensitive to levels of amoxicillin or ampicillin achieved in the urine of healthy dogs. A urease inhibitor can be given but is not usually necessary. Concurrent treatment with a urease inhibitor such as acetohydroxamic acid enhances the rate of struvite stone dissolution, particularly when antibiotic resistance precludes effective antibacterial sterilization of the urine. A reasonably safe dose of acetohydroxamic acid appears to be 12.5 mg/kg, PO, bid. A reversible, mild hemolytic anemia has been seen in dogs given higher dosages.

After ~4 wk of treatment, a physical examination, serum chemistry profile, urinalysis, and abdominal radiographs or ultrasonography should be repeated. The stone dissolution protocol should be discontinued if severe adverse effects develop, although a mild degree of hypoalbuminemia is to be expected and can be tolerated. With good compliance, the following results can be anticipated: urine pH <6.5, urine specific gravity <1.025, serum urea <10 mg/dL. The radiographic stone size should be compared with the size on previous radiographs. Routine testing should be repeated every 4 wk until 4 wk after the stone is no longer visible radiographically; this generally takes 8–12 wk but may take as long as 20 wk. Stones that fail to reduce in size after 8 wk of treatment are probably not composed of struvite and should be treated another way, although failure could also result from poor treatment compliance. Renal stones tend to dissolve more slowly than bladder stones.

The recurrence rate after surgical treatment of struvite uroliths has been reported to be ~20%–25%, with most recurrences within 1 yr. When surgery is performed to remove multiple small struvite calculi, removing all stone material is often difficult. In such cases, a 4-wk dissolution protocol starting at the time of suture removal aids in preventing recurrence due to residual crystalline material. Once the urinary tract is free of stones, prevention strategies are much more likely to be successful.

Prevention Protocol: The key to prevention of recurrence in animals with a struvite stone associated with infection is to achieve and maintain sterile urine. Routine testing of urine pH by the owner is important. If fresh urine is alkaline, a urinalysis and culture should be done, with the dog treated appropriately if an infection is present.

Once stone dissolution is completed, a prevention program can be considered. The aim is to prevent urinary tract infections with urease-producing microbes. The concentration of major struvite solutes in urine should also be reduced. A commercially available diet may be fed to lower urinary phosphate and magnesium and to maintain an acidic urine. Urease-producing infections should be eliminated, after which owners should regularly check the pH of the first voided urine in the morning after an overnight fast; in most dogs on a normal diet, the urine will be acidic. Checking urine pH weekly is sufficient.

Calcium Oxalate Stones: Calcium oxalate uroliths have been increasing in frequency in dogs. Although they may develop in any breed, Miniature Schnauzers, Lhasa Apsos, Yorkshire Terriers, Bichon Frises, Shih Tzus, and Miniature Poodles may be predisposed. Most affected dogs are 2–10 yr old. Hypercalciuria leading to calcium oxalate stone formation can result from increased renal clearance of calcium due to excessive intestinal absorption of calcium (absorptive hypercalciuria), impaired renal conservation of calcium (renal leak hypercalciuria), or excessive skeletal mobilization of calcium (resorptive hypercalciuria).

Absorptive hypercalciuria is characterized by increased urine calcium excretion, normal serum calcium concentration, and normal or low serum parathormone concentration. Because absorptive hypercalciuria depends on dietary calcium, the amount of calcium excreted in the urine during fasting is normal or significantly reduced when compared with nonfasting levels. Renal leak hypercalciuria has been recognized in dogs less frequently than absorptive hypercalciuria. In dogs, renal leak hypercalciuria is characterized by normal serum calcium concentration, increased urine calcium excretion, and increased serum parathormone concentration. During fasting, these dogs do not show a decline in urinary calcium loss. The underlying cause of renal leak hypercalciuria in dogs is not known. Resorptive hypercalciuria is characterized by excessive filtration and excretion of calcium in urine as a result of hypercalcemia. Hypercalcemic disorders have been associated only infrequently with calcium oxalate uroliths in dogs.

Routine laboratory determinations should include serum calcium, phosphate, total CO_2, and chloride to eliminate the possibility of hyperparathyroidism and renal tubular acidosis. Dissolution of calcium oxalate stones by medical means has not currently been established. Treatment requires surgical removal or lithotripsy followed by preventive strategies.

Prevention Protocol: Recurrence is a major problem with calcium oxalate uroliths. An "ideal" diet is considered to be low oxalate, low protein, and low sodium and would maintain urine pH at 6.5–7.5 and urine specific gravity <1.020. A few commercially available canned foods achieve these goals and may minimize the risk of recurrence. Potassium citrate may be added as needed to assure the urine pH is within the desired range; water may be used to provide appropriate reduction in urine concentration. If these urine conditions are achieved and calcium oxalate crystals are still seen in warm, fresh urine, then vitamin B_6 and/or thiazide diuretics can be considered (although of unproven efficacy). Effectiveness of therapy should be reevaluated at 1- to 4-mo intervals by urinalysis. Chlorothiazide diuretics may also be of value.

Urate Stones: Ammonium urate stones are most common in Dalmatians and in dogs with congenital portosystemic vascular shunts. The formation of ammonium urate calculi depends on the urine concentrations of urate and ammonium and on other poorly understood factors. Dalmatians do not convert most of their metabolic urate to allantoin and thus excrete the bulk of nucleic acid metabolites as relatively insoluble urate. The biologic mechanism responsible for decreased hepatic conversion of urate to allantoin lies not in reduced uricase activity but in reduced hepatic transport of urate; the rate of urate hepatic transport is approximately three times faster in breeds other than Dalmatians. The net result is that only 30%–40% of urate is converted to allantoin in Dalmatians compared with ~90% in other breeds.

Dalmatians fed a diet high in animal protein excrete a net acid load in the urine, and urinary ammonium output is subsequently increased. The combined high concentration of ammonium and urate in urine increases the risk of formation of ammonium urate stones. The excretion of acidic metabolites of an animal protein diet is believed to be important in this process, because urinary ammonium excretion is enhanced and ammonium urate is insoluble. Urate output has been reported to be the same in Dalmatians that form stones and in those that do not, although in some studies the methods used to determine urine uric acid concentrations were unreliable. In dogs with a portosystemic vascular anastomosis, increased urinary ammonium output may partially be due to the increased filtered load of ammonia, because plasma levels of ammonia tend to be increased.

Dissolution Protocol: Urine alkalinization minimizes renal ammonia production; the goal is to achieve a urine pH >7. If required, urine alkalinization can be achieved by administering $NaHCO_3$, 1 g (¼ tsp)/5 kg, PO, tid, with food. Potassium citrate, administered to effect (25–50 mg/kg/day) is an alternative, more palatable alkalinizing agent.

Urinary urate output should be reduced. This can be accomplished by feeding a low-purine, low-protein commercial diet. In addition, the xanthine oxidase inhibitor allopurinol (15 mg/kg, PO, bid) may be administered to ensure the nucleic acid metabolite load is excreted as a combination of xanthine, hypoxanthine, uric acid, and allantoin, rather than almost entirely as urate. However, the effectiveness of allopurinol in reducing urinary urate output is variable, and urinary urate levels should be measured (although this may be difficult). Allopurinol must be used cautiously in dogs with hepatic disease or primary renal failure, because it is metabolized to its active form in the liver and is excreted via the kidneys. It is important that diets high in purines not be fed to dogs receiving allopurinol because xanthine uroliths may result.

Urine volume should be increased to reduce the concentration of all dissolved solutes in urine. This can be achieved by feeding canned diets restricted in protein. By reducing formation of urea, renal medullary urea concentration declines, interfering with the countercurrent system of urine concentration. Adding salt, 1 g (¼ tsp)/5 kg, daily to the diet, or mixing water with the food are additional methods. Salt should not be given to animals with hypertension but otherwise poses little risk in normotensive dogs without chronic kidney disease, proteinuria, or hypoalbuminemia.

Prevention Protocol: Prevention strategies aim to reduce the concentration of ammonium and urate in urine to levels unlikely to induce flocculation.

A low-protein, low-purine diet should be fed to reduce urinary urate output. Alkalinization should be used as needed to ensure alkalinuria. Treatment with allopurinol (10 mg/kg/day, PO) can be considered. Ideally, allopurinol is not needed as a supplement to dietary management; however, if urate crystals persist, a low-maintenance dose of allopurinol is appropriate.

These dissolution and prevention strategies were developed for use in Dalmatians in which hepatic conversion of urate to allantoin is reduced but the liver is otherwise normal. They may not be safe for use in dogs with portosystemic vascular shunts. Such dogs tend to develop hypoalbuminemia, edema, and ascites when fed a low-protein diet. The safety of allopurinol in these dogs has not been established. In addition, alkalinization can predispose to hepatic encephalopathy because of increased GI absorption of dietary protein metabolites.

Cystine Stones: Stones composed almost entirely of cystine form in dogs that have a renal tubular amino acid reabsorption defect known as cystinuria. Healthy dogs demonstrate 97% fractional reabsorption of cystine, whereas affected dogs excrete a much greater proportion of the filtered cystine load and may even exhibit net cystine secretion. Cystine is a relatively insoluble amino acid; therefore, in high concentration it may precipitate and form stones. Despite excessive urinary loss of cystine in cystinuric dogs, plasma cystine levels remain the same as in healthy dogs; in fact, the only morbidity or mortality associated with the inherited defect of cystine reabsorption is urolith formation. Identification of cystine crystals by urinalysis indicates the dog is at risk of forming cystine uroliths. For poorly understood reasons, not all cystinuric dogs develop uroliths. However, the absence of uroliths does not preclude their future development, and preventive measures are indicated.

Cystinuria is thought to be inherited as a sex-linked trait. However, in Newfoundlands it is transmitted as a simple autosomal recessive trait. The defect has also been reported in Dachshunds, Basset Hounds, English Bulldogs, Chihuahuas, Yorkshire Terriers, Irish Terriers, and mixed-breed dogs. Cystinuria has been recognized almost exclusively in male dogs, except in Newfoundlands. A urine cystine concentration of >75 mg/g creatinine in nonfasted dogs is predictive of susceptibility to cystine urolithiasis.

Cystine solubility depends on urine pH, with solubility increasing rapidly when urinary pH is >7.5. Dogs fed meat-based diets tend to excrete acidic urine, which leads to urine cystine supersaturation.

Cystinuria is a lifelong defect of tubular reabsorption and cannot be cured. Cystine stones tend to recur within 1 yr without management to prevent recurrence, and they often recur despite attempts at prevention.

Dissolution and Prevention Protocols: Urinary cystine output should be reduced. Protein-restricted alkalinizing diets have been associated with reducing the size of cystine urocystoliths. Urinary cystine concentration can also be reduced by administering N-(2-mercaptoproprionyl)-glycine (2-MPG, tiopronin) or penicillamine. 2-MPG should be given at 15–20 mg/kg, PO, bid, for dissolution, and at 10–15 mg/kg, PO, bid, for prevention. Penicillamine (15 mg/kg, PO, bid) can be substituted for 2-MPG; unfortunately, ~40% of dogs treated with penicillamine exhibit anorexia and vomiting. The vomiting may be partially resolved by giving the medication with meals; however, a severe reduction in dosage or complete withdrawal is often necessary.

The urine should be alkalinized to a pH >7.5. Sodium bicarbonate added to the diet at 1 g (¼ tsp)/5 kg, tid, readily accomplishes this, but because sodium supplementation may enhance cystinuria, potassium citrate (20–75 mg/kg, PO, bid) is preferred.

Urine volume can be increased by mixing water with the food. Salt should not be added to the diet, because increased sodium excretion may cause increased cystine excretion. If urine volume is adequate and the urine pH is maintained above 7.5, most cystinuric dogs will pass urine that is only slightly supersaturated or undersaturated for cystine. Under such conditions, only relatively small doses of 2-MPG or penicillamine may be necessary to achieve 24-hr undersaturation.

Silica Stones: Early reports indicated a predominance of silica stones in German Shepherds, but many breeds have now been implicated. Urethral obstruction in males is the most common presenting problem, but signs similar to those associated with other types of uroliths also may be noted. The mean age at occurrence is ~6 yr. The stones are usually multiple and develop in the bladder and urethra. Silica uroliths are radiopaque. They frequently, but not always, have a characteristic "jackstone" appearance. Identification requires spectrographic analysis and cannot be made with kits for qualitative stone analysis.

The role of diet in spontaneously occurring silica urolithiasis has not been determined, although plants are often an abundant source of silica. If the diet of an affected dog is known to be high in silica, or if silica urolithiasis has been recurrent, a dietary change should be recommended. Only general management principles can be suggested for silicate urolithiasis. Additional salt and/or water should be added to the diet to induce diuresis and to lower the urine solute concentration. When present, urinary tract infections should be eliminated. Diets high in plant proteins should be avoided.

Feline Lower Urinary Tract Disease

(Feline urologic syndrome)

Hematuria, pollakiuria, and stranguria are the characteristic clinical signs of feline lower urinary tract disease (FLUTD) in cats. Although the specific underlying cause of this common syndrome is often not identified, associated conditions include urinary tract infection, neoplasia, trauma, urethral plugs, urolithiasis, and sterile cystitis (feline interstitial cystitis).

Feline Urolithiasis: Feline urolithiasis is a common disease seen with equal frequency in both sexes. Until recently, it was thought that most uroliths in cats were small and resembled sand or were gelatinous plugs that differed from typical uroliths in that they contained a greater amount of organic matrix, giving them a toothpaste-like consistency. Matrix-crystalline plugs are most commonly found within the urethra near the urethral orifice and are primarily responsible for urethral obstruction. Recently, prevalence of urolithiasis with grossly observable stones composed primarily of calcium oxalate has increased in cats. The most common feline uroliths are calcium oxalate, magnesium ammonium phosphate, and urate.

Urolithiasis is usually suspected based on clinical signs of hematuria, dysuria, or urethral obstruction. Urinalysis, urine culture, radiography, and ultrasonography may be required to differentiate uroliths from urinary tract infection or neoplasia. Radiography, cystoscopy, or ultrasonography are critically important to detect uroliths, because only ~10% of feline urocystoliths can be detected by abdominal palpation. Uroliths with a diameter >3 mm are usually radiodense; however, because smaller uroliths are common, double-contrast radiography may be required for detection. Radiographic evidence of uroliths is seen in ~20% of cats with hematuria or dysuria.

The usual clinical approach to grossly observable urocystoliths is surgical removal or lithotripsy where available, followed by dietary therapy instituted as a preventive measure. For sterile struvite uroliths, medical dissolution is the preferred treatment. Nephrolithiasis is not associated with an increase in the rate of progression of feline kidney injury, and cats with nephrolithiasis are generally managed without surgery.

Calcium Oxalate Stones: Calcium oxalate uroliths are the most common feline uroliths and the most common nephrolith, although their underlying cause is unknown. Common management schemes that involve feeding urine-acidifying diets with reduced magnesium have reduced the incidence of feline struvite urolithiasis. Magnesium has been reported to be an inhibitor of calcium oxalate formation in rats and people; thus, the reduced magnesium concentration in feline urine may partially explain the increase in calcium oxalate stones in cats.

Medical protocols that promote calcium oxalate dissolution are not known; therefore, surgery and lithotripsy are the primary means for removal (small bladder stones may be eliminated by voiding urohydropulsion). However, some calcium oxalate uroliths, especially those in the kidneys, may not cause clinical signs for months to years. Because of the unavoidable destruction of nephrons during nephrotomy, this procedure is not recommended unless it can be established that the stones are a cause of clinically significant disease. Recurrence remains problematic. A variety of diets has been formulated to restrict the formation of calcium oxalate uroliths and should be considered appropriate for maintenance in cats with nephroliths and after the removal of urocystoliths. Diets that reduce the likelihood of formation of both struvite and calcium oxalate stones are commercially available. Eliminating any associated urinary tract infections, avoiding mineral and vitamin C and D supplementation, and encouraging water consumption are critical.

Struvite Stones: Three distinct types of struvite uroliths are recognized in cats: amorphous urethral plugs with a large quantity of matrix, sterile struvite uroliths (which form perhaps as a result of certain dietary ingredients), and struvite uroliths that form as a sequela of urinary tract infection with urease-producing bacteria. Struvite uroliths induced by infection are less common than sterile struvite uroliths. An additional type of struvite urolith in cats consists of a sterile struvite nidus that predisposes to urinary tract infection with urease-producing bacteria and subsequent formation of infected struvite laminations around the sterile nidus.

Treatment of sterile struvite urolithiasis focuses on reducing the urine pH to ≤6 and on reducing the urine magnesium concentration by feeding magnesium-restricted diets. Reducing urine pH and magnesium concentration is best accomplished by feeding a commercially available prescription diet formulated for this purpose. Some diets are formulated to reduce the formation of both struvite and calcium oxalate stones. Generally, neither sodium chloride nor urine acidifiers should be given concurrently with these diets, because they are already supplemented with sodium chloride and formulated to produce aciduria. In addition, these diets should not be fed to cats that are acidemic, have azotemia of any cause, or have cardiac dysfunction or hypertension. Urolith size should be monitored every 4 wk by radiographs or ultrasonography, and crystalluria by urinalysis. Struvite crystals should not form if therapy has been effective in producing urine that is undersaturated with magnesium, ammonium, and phosphate. Because small uroliths may not be detected radiographically, the calculolytic diet should be continued for ≥4 wk after radiographic documentation of urolith dissolution. If treatment does not induce complete dissolution of uroliths, it is likely that either the wrong mineral component was identified, the nucleus of the urolith is composed of a different mineral than the outer portion of the urolith, or the owner is not complying with therapeutic recommendations.

Other Feline Stones: Ammonium urate, uric acid, calcium phosphate, and cystine uroliths are less common in cats, but ammonium urate and uric acid account for ~6% of feline uroliths. Although a renal tubular reabsorptive defect and portovascular anomalies have been incriminated as causes in a few cases, the cause of most urate uroliths in cats has not been established. Nonetheless, formation of highly acidic and concentrated urine associated with consumption of diets high in purine precursors (especially liver) appears to be a risk factor.

Medical protocols that consistently promote dissolution of ammonium urate uroliths in cats have not been developed, and surgery remains the most common method of removal. For small stones, voiding urohydropulsion may be effective. Prevention should include feeding a diet low in purine precursors and promoting formation of less acidic urine that is not highly concentrated. Although allopurinol may reduce the formation of urate in cats, studies of the efficacy and potential toxicity of allopurinol in cats are required before meaningful guidelines can be established.

Sterile Cystitis (Feline Interstitial Cystitis): Feline interstitial cystitis is generally taken to be synonymous with sterile cystitis of unknown cause. The underlying cause of this disorder is unknown, although anxiety and altered neurohormonal factors have been implicated.

Diagnosis is by exclusion of other causes of lower urinary tract disease in cats, such as obstruction by urethral plugs, bacterial urinary tract infection, neoplasia or other mass lesions, and urolithiasis. Diagnostic tests to exclude these conditions may include radiographs, ultrasonography, urinalysis, urine culture, and cystoscopy.

Because the cause of feline interstitial cystitis is unknown, the goal of treatment is to reduce the severity and frequency of episodes of cystitis. Therapeutic considerations include reduction of stress through environmental changes, dietary adjustments (eg, use of canned preparations), pheromones applied topically in the environment, and analgesics (eg, butorphanol, 0.2–0.4 mg/kg, PO, bid-tid). Other medications (eg, amitriptyline, 5–12.5 mg/cat, PO, once or twice daily; clomipramine, 0.5 mg/kg/day, PO; fluoxetine, 1 mg/kg/day, PO) have yielded mixed results.

BEHAVIOR

BEHAVIORAL MEDICINE INTRODUCTION

An animal's "behavior" is the product of its genetic composition, the environment in which the animal functions, and the animal's experience (particularly in the pre- and postnatal environment through the primary socialization period). This section focuses primarily on the diagnosis and treatment of abnormal behavior of domestic animals. For each species, normal social behavior is outlined, followed by a description of common behavioral disorders.

The minimum behavioral welfare requirements for the housing and enrichment of farm, zoo, and laboratory animals, known as the five freedoms, are equally important for family pets. These include freedom from hunger and thirst; discomfort; pain, injury, or disease; fear and distress;

and freedom to express normal species behaviors. When these needs are not fully addressed, welfare is compromised and both health and behavior problems arise.

In companion animals, behavior problems weaken the pet–owner bond, resulting in a decreased owner commitment to pet care. They are a primary reason for pet relinquishment and euthanasia. Yet studies show that many owners do not report behavior changes to their veterinarian, and most veterinarians neglect to inquire about them. Thus, screening for any behavioral changes or emerging behavior problems should be done at each veterinary visit to ensure that the behavioral health, physical health, and welfare of the pet are being effectively and humanely managed.

INTEGRATING BEHAVIORAL SERVICES INTO VETERINARY PRACTICE

Each veterinary visit should include screening questions to determine whether there are any behavior concerns or any change in behavior from previous visits. In addition to enabling the veterinarian to assess the health and welfare of the pet, this initiates a dialogue with clients about behavior and lets them know that behavior is central to good veterinary care. Recording responses to behavior questions at each visit allows a baseline to be established for future comparison.

A basic behavior screening questionnaire is a simple way to collect information. Questionnaires should be standardized so no topic is left uncovered and so data can be compared from visit to visit. When used continually from the pet's first visit, these tools allow for early detection and intervention. Addressing behavioral concerns early provides the best chance to manage the problem and prevent a minor issue from becoming more serious and deeply entrenched. If behavioral signs (eg, barking, growling, lunging, housesoiling) are identified during the visit, the veterinarian will need to determine whether there are underlying medical issues, whether the behaviors are normal and in context or abnormal and out of context, and whether they are manageable for the household, either to begin offering behavior guidance or, when indicated, to refer the client for *further counseling*.

Behavioral services should be offered using an integrated team approach. Staff can help with behavioral screening (questionnaires) and provide pet selection advice and preventive guidance for new pet owners. Veterinarians or staff with sufficient skills and training can offer client education about how to prevent and manage undesirable behaviors and classes to help pet owners socialize and train their pets. A good set of resource materials and links to Web sites that provide appropriate and sound behavioral guidance can supplement the advice provided.

Veterinary behavioral technicians can oversee the preventive counseling and training services offered by a veterinary hospital. They can also play an integral role during behavioral consultations by taking the history, demonstrating behavior modification techniques and products, and conducting case followup and ongoing support. Information sources for veterinarians, technicians, and staff interested in veterinary behavior are listed in TABLE 1.

Veterinarians also have a vested interest in how clients train their pets. Trainers should have a sound background on species-typical behaviors, as well as how behaviors can be shaped and modified through the principles of learning that apply to all species. The Association of Pet Dog Trainers, the American Humane Association, and the American Veterinary Society of Animal Behavior have published guidelines for appropriate and humane training and behavior modification. Certified trainers can be found at www.ccpdt.org and www.karenpryoracademy.com, and advocates of force-free dog training at www.petprofessionalguild.com. However, even with a certified trainer, veterinarians should observe and talk with the trainer to ensure that the methodologies used are humane, effective, and appropriate for the individual owners and pets. Having an active discussion about training with each dog owner can help the owner to understand the principles of learning and how to differentiate those trainers who use undesirable techniques from those who use humane, reward-based techniques.

GLOSSARY OF BEHAVIORAL TERMS

Abnormal Behavior: These activities show dysfunction in action and behavior. Alternatively, the terms behavior problem, behavior pathology, mental health disorder, or emotional disorders might be used. By comparison, many behavioral complaints are normal behaviors that are undesirable to owners (eg, garbage raiding, jumping up, predation, herding, guarding).

TABLE 1 BEHAVIOR RESOURCES FOR VETERINARIANS AND TECHNICIANS

Organization	Web Site
BEHAVIOR ASSOCIATIONS	
American Veterinary Society of Animal Behavior	www.avsabonline.org
Companion Animal Behaviour Therapy Study Group	www.bvba.org.uk
European Society of Veterinary Clinical Ethology	www.esvce.org
Society of Veterinary Behavioral Technicians	www.svbt.org
Australian Veterinary Behaviour Interest Group	www.ava.com.au/avbig
BEHAVIOR CERTIFICATION GROUPS	
American College of Veterinary Behaviorists	www.dacvb.org
European College of Animal Welfare and Behavioural Medicine	www.ecawbm.org
Australian and New Zealand College of Veterinary Scientists	www.anzcvs.org.au
Academy of Veterinary Behavioral Technicians	www.avbt.net

Abnormal Repetitive Behaviors: Abnormal repetitive behaviors are a heterogenous group of behaviors that include both stereotypies and compulsive/impulsive behaviors (*see* below). Although these two categories of behavior have similarities in clinical presentation and perhaps neurophysiology, they are not synonymous. In addition, underlying medical conditions might cause or contribute to these signs. Thus, until a definitive diagnosis is made, the term abnormal repetitive behavior is a descriptive term for any of the behaviors that are maladaptive, repetitive or fixed, and pathologically abnormal. Although categories overlap, clinical signs have been described as oral/ingestive (eg, pica, polyphagia, licking, gulping), neurologic/hallucinatory (eg, fly snapping, light chasing), locomotory (eg, spinning, pouncing), and self-directed (eg, acral lick dermatitis, psychogenic alopecia).

Aggression: Aggression can be defined in a narrow sense (attack) or in a broader sense as agonistic behavior. In the latter case, aggression can be appropriate or inappropriate, in context or out of context, inter- or intraspecific, or a challenge or contest that results in deference or in combat and resolution.

Anxiety: Anxiety is the apprehensive anticipation of future danger or misfortune, which may be accompanied by both behavioral and somatic signs (vigilance and scanning, autonomic hyperactivity, increased motor activity and tension).

Compulsive or Obsessive-Compulsive Disorders: Compulsive behaviors are abnormal and repetitive, may be variable in form, and are often fixated on a goal. They may be exaggerated, sustained, intense, and difficult to interrupt or have an element of dyscontrol in either the initiation or continuation of the behavior or the inhibition or switching between behaviors. They are generally derived from normal behaviors such as grooming, predation, ingestion, or locomotion. Compulsive disorders might initially arise in situations of frustration or conflict but become compulsive when they persist or arise outside the original context. There appears to be a genetic predisposition to the development of certain compulsive behaviors (eg, wool sucking in Oriental breeds of cats, tail chasing in German Shepherds, flank sucking in Dobermans). There is likely an alteration in serotonergic activity for most compulsive disorders in dogs and cats. However, there can be a wide range of presentations, and multiple neurotransmitters have been implicated (eg, dopamine, opiates). This may indicate an altered course of disease over time or that the diagnosis encompasses more than one disorder. Drugs that inhibit serotonin reuptake are generally most effective to enhance serotonin transmission and inhibit dopamine activity. Brain areas of interest include the prefrontal cortex and amygdalae.

Conflict: Conflict arises when a pet has competing motivations or is motivated to perform more than one opposing behavior. This might occur when a dog is motivated to greet but is fearful of approach, perhaps because of previous unpleasant experiences (eg, yelling, hitting, pinning). The resultant behavior might be either a displacement behavior (*see* below) or aggression (when fear is an overriding factor).

Displacement Behavior: This type of activity is generally a normal behavior that is performed out of context, or is "displaced," because the animal is unable—physically or behaviorally—to execute another activity or otherwise occupy itself. This is less specific than redirected behavior (*see* below), in which the intended behavior is directed toward another target. When displacement activity occurs, the behavior may be out of context with the situation (eg, circling, air snapping, or even urination). Displacement behaviors may arise from conflict or frustration or be a vacuum activity.

Dominance: Dominance is a concept frequently misapplied. The ethological concept of dominance refers to competitive control over a resource in a limited circumstance and to the ability of a higher-ranking animal to displace a lower-ranking one from that resource. Rank is usually defined by an ability to control the resource or by access and ability to restrict matings; however, extra-pair copulation is almost always more common when assessed by DNA analysis than it was believed to be on the basis of behavioral observations.

Dominance is not interchangeable with hierarchical rank. Ranks, particularly those that are linear and in which a "dominant" animal is identified, are largely artifacts of experimental or manipulated situations. A "dominant" animal is *not* the one engaged in the most fighting and combat. Most high-ranking animals seldom have to contest their right of access to a resource. Instead, high-ranking animals are usually better identified by the character and frequency of deferential behaviors exhibited by others in their social group and by their ability to respond appropriately to a variety of social and environmental circumstances. Thus, confident and assertive postures and signaling of one individual in a pair might be described as dominant if the response of the second individual is deferent or subordinate. However, dominant/subordinate does not describe the relationship between the pair, unless the response is consistent across resources and interactions. While this terminology applies to communication and signaling between members of a species (eg, dog-dog), it does not "translate" to communication between species (eg, dog-human).

Fear: Fear is a feeling of apprehension associated with the presence or proximity of an object, individual, or social situation. Fear is part of normal behavior and can be an adaptive response. The determination of whether the fear or fearful response is abnormal or inappropriate must be determined by context. For example, fire is a useful tool, but avoidance of fire is an adaptive response. If a pet is fearful of stimuli that are innocuous, such as walking on certain types of surfaces or going outdoors, such fear would be irrational and, if it were constant or recurrent, probably maladaptive. Fears usually occur as graded responses, with the intensity of the response proportional to the proximity of the stimulus. A sudden, all-or-nothing, profound, abnormal response that results in extremely fearful behaviors is usually called a phobia.

Frustration: This state arises when an animal is motivated to engage in a sequence of behaviors that it is unable to complete because of physical or psychological obstacles in the environment. When pets are frustrated—such as a cat that cannot gain access to an outdoor cat that it sees through the window, or a dog that cannot get to a stimulus on the other side of a door or fence—the resultant behavior can be a redirected behavior (eg, attack of another family pet or owner), a displacement behavior (eg, stereotypic pacing), or signs associated with anxiety (eg, whining or howling). Another example of goal frustration is the dog or cat that chases a laser light toy but is unable to finish the sequence or achieve any goal. This frustration may lead to obsessive chasing of other lights and shadows.

Phobia: Most fearful reactions are learned and might be unlearned with gradual exposure, although a lack of sufficient previous exposure, consequences of previous exposure, and genetic factors all play a role in how quickly or completely the unlearning might be achieved. Phobias involve sudden, all-or-nothing, profound, abnormal responses that result in extremely fearful behaviors (catatonia, panic). Phobias may develop over time—some animals develop increasingly more intense fears with repeated exposure (eg, storm phobias). However, once established, they are associated with immediate and intense anxiety when the stimulus is presented. Once a phobic event has been experienced, any event associated with it or the memory of it is often sufficient to generate the response (eg, wind, rain, or darkening sky and storm phobias). Although fears may diminish with repeated exposure and no untoward consequences, phobias can remain at or exceed their former high level for years even without reexposure. The genesis for such events in dogs is usually either extremely frightening or traumatic, or the dog itself has profound internal problems with fear (eg, genetic predisposition) so that responses to unfamiliar stimuli are excessive. Owner responses might inadvertently aggravate the problem, either by further encouraging the behavior or by adding to the fearful emotional state if the outcome for the pet is unpleasant (eg, owner anger or punishment). Phobic situations are either avoided at all costs or, if unavoidable, are endured with intense anxiety or distress.

Redirected Behavior: Redirected behavior activities are directed away from the principal target and toward another, less appropriate target. When the animal is in a state of emotional arousal and is unable to reach the appropriate target, the behavior can be redirected to an alternative target if the animal is interrupted.

Stereotypic Behaviors: A stereotypy is a perseverant repetition of behaviors that are unvaried in sequence and have no obvious purpose or function. They usually derive from contextually normal maintenance behaviors (eg, grooming, eating, walking). The behaviors have been reported commonly in farm, zoo, and laboratory animal species and arise in situations of conflict or frustration related to confinement or husbandry practices. They may arise when the environment is barren or stress evoking, when the animal lacks the opportunity to display a full range of species-typical behaviors, with maternal deprivation, and as a result of neurologic disorders. It is thought that some stereotypic behaviors, at least in their early stages, may provide a mechanism for the pet to cope. For example, non-nutritive suckling in calves may assist digestive processes. Stereotypys might be associated with basal ganglia dysfunction and can be induced by dopaminergic stimulation of the striatum.

Vacuum Activity: When an animal is highly motivated to perform an instinctive behavior but there is no available outlet, a vacuum activity may be exhibited (flank sucking, licking, etc). These activities have no apparent useful purpose.

DIAGNOSIS OF BEHAVIORAL PROBLEMS

Veterinarians must have an understanding of the behavior and development of the species, the principles of learning, and the signs of fear and anxiety to differentiate normal behavior from abnormal behavior. When presented with an animal with undesirable behavior, the first step is to exclude any medical problems that might be causing or contributing to the behavioral signs. In addition, while it is common to consider the effects of disease on behavior, stress can cause alterations in behavioral, physiologic, and immune responses, which can have variable effects on health and behavior with increasing chronicity. Stress leads to alterations in the hypothalamic-pituitary axis and in levels of dopamine, serotonin, norepinephrine, and prolactin. In animals, stress can cause or contribute to feline interstitial cystitis; dermatologic, respiratory, and GI disorders; and behavior problems such as compulsive disorders, exaggerated fear responses, and psychogenic polydipsia and polyphagia.

Diagnosis of any behavioral problem requires the identification of all behavioral and medical signs, history taking, a physical and neurologic examination, and any diagnostic tests indicated to exclude underlying medical conditions that might cause or contribute to the signs (*see* TABLE 2).

If there is no underlying medical cause for the behavioral signs, then a comprehensive behavioral history is required to determine the diagnosis, prognosis, and treatment options. The history should include: 1) sex, breed, and age of animal (breed predispositions); 2) age at onset of condition or complaint; 3) duration of condition or complaint; 4) description of undesirable behavior; 5) frequency (hourly, daily, weekly, monthly); 6) duration of bouts; 7) any changes in pattern, frequency, intensity, and duration of bouts; 8) corrective measures tried and the response, if any; 9) any activities that stop the behavior (eg, animal collapses); 10) 24-hr schedule of animal and

TABLE 2 MEDICAL CAUSES OF BEHAVIORAL SIGNS

Medical Condition	Behavioral Signs
Illness or disease	Altered personality, lethargy, depression, withdrawal, anorexia, reduction in grooming, altered social relationships, altered response to stimuli
	NEUROLOGIC
Central (affecting forebrain, limbic/temporal, and hypothalamic), rapid-eye movement sleep disorders	Altered awareness and response to stimuli, loss of learned behaviors, housesoiling, disorientation, confusion, altered activity levels, temporal disorientation, vocalization, change in temperament (fear, anxiety, aggression), altered appetite, altered sleep cycles, interrupted sleep (aggression/waking/activity)
Peripheral (neuropathy)	Self-mutilation, irritability, aggression, circling, hyperesthesia
Focal seizures/temporal lobe seizures	Repetitive behaviors, self-trauma, chomping, staring, altered temperament (eg, intermittent states of fear or aggression), tremors, shaking, interrupted sleep
Sensory dysfunction	Altered response to stimuli, confusion, disorientation, altered sleep cycles, irritability, aggression, vocalization, housesoiling
	METABOLIC / ENDOCRINE
Feline hyperthyroidism	Irritability, aggression, urine marking, increased activity, night waking
Canine hypothyroidism	Lethargy, decreased response to stimuli, irritability, aggression
Hyperadrenocorticism	Panting, night waking, housesoiling, irritability, polyphagia, anxiety
Diabetes/hyperglycemia	Housesoiling, night waking
Functional ovarian and testicular tumors	Androgen-induced behaviors: males—aggression, roaming, marking, sexual attraction, mounting; females—nesting or possessive aggression of objects
Hepatic or renal encephalopathy	Signs associated with affected organ, anxiety, irritability, aggression, altered sleep, housesoiling, mental dullness, decreased activity, restlessness, increased sleep, confusion
Anemia or electrolyte imbalances	Pica
Pain	Altered response to stimuli, decreased activity, restlessness/inability to settle, vocalization, housesoiling, aggression, irritability, self-trauma, waking at night
Gastrointestinal	Licking, polyphagia, pica, coprophagia, housesoiling (fecal), wind sucking, tongue rolling, unsettled sleep, restlessness
Urogenital	Housesoiling (urine), polydipsia, waking at night
Dermatologic	Psychogenic alopecia (cats), acral lick dermatitis (dogs), nail biting, hyperesthesia, other self-trauma

owner, as well as any day-to-day variability; 11) environment and housing; 12) animal's familial history; and 13) anything else the owner thinks is relevant. In farm animals, questions should be framed within the context of the problem so that housing, management, group or herd behavior, production, and perhaps reproduction are addressed.

For each behavior problem, the "ABC" should be considered, ie, the antecedent, or what precedes the behavior; the behavior, or the description of the problem; and the consequences, or what happens immediately after the behavior. With maturity and learning, the animal's response to a stimulus may be modified; thus, the initial events may be just as important to evaluate as the more recent events.

History might be collected in part by having the owner complete a history questionnaire before the visit, especially with respect to data about the home and housing, family, daily schedule, training, husbandry, and background. However, further interactive questioning and discussion with those responsible for the animal's care, housing, and training are required to further evaluate the progress and development of the problem from the initial event to the present time. Having the owners bring video clips of the behaviors can further help provide insight as to the diagnosis, prognosis, and how the problem might be managed or improved.

Additional information about the pet's personality, relationship with the owner, response to stimuli, and owner's response might be gained during the visit by observation of the pet and how it interacts with the owners. Although provoking the pet is generally contraindicated because any further repetition of the problem is ill advised for the pet and might lead to further learning, a controlled interactive assessment might include how the animal responds to other animals and people, sounds, a child-like doll, or handling, including physical examination, petting, or the application of products such as a head halter, muzzle, or body harness. The pet's response to commands can be assessed during the visit, as well as the types of treats or toys most likely to positively affect the pet.

PROGNOSIS OF BEHAVIORAL PROBLEMS

Client understanding and compliance are critical if animals with behavioral disorders are to improve. Because the strategy to modify undesirable behavior requires that the owner be prepared and capable of identifying each situation and substituting a more desirable response, the initial approach should be to avoid or prevent the provocative situation. The predictability of the problem, the ability of the owners to implement initial preventive strategies, the expectations as to what might be achieved, the pet's temperament, how the pet's behavior will need to be modified over time, and the practicality of implementing the program considering the environment, family, and pet should all be reviewed and must be both acceptable and practical for the owners. In addition, special consideration will need to be given in cases of aggression to evaluate risk and ensure safety. (For guidelines on risk factor assessment, *see* www.esvce.org.)

TREATMENT OF BEHAVIORAL PROBLEMS

In production animals, treatment focuses on group management, environmental or housing modifications, and in some cases removing individual animals out of or to other groups. Specifics are covered in the relevant species discussions.

In companion animals, the treatment of behavior problems varies with diagnosis and prognosis. In general, the program begins with prevention and avoidance of problems, while the owner develops effective strategies to modify the pet's behavior so that it might gradually be reintroduced to the problem situations while achieving a desirable outcome. Initially, prevention is necessary to avoid further compromising the pet's welfare and to ensure safety in cases of aggression. Repetition of the behavior further aggravates the problem if the pet successfully accomplishes its intended goal (eg, escape or retreat from the stimulus), while each exposure in which the outcome is unpleasant can condition further anxiety. Improvement is generally a slow and gradual process; therefore, owners must have realistic expectations of what might be achieved. Modifications to the environment may be required, so that the pet can be kept away from the stimuli (or the sights or sounds of the stimuli) that incite the problem or from the areas in which the problem occurs. Modifying the pet's behavior is accomplished by applying the principles of learning and behavior modification, primarily achieving and rewarding desirable outcomes along with use of products that improve safety, reduce anxiety, or help to achieve the desired response more effectively (eg, muzzles, head halters, no-pull harnesses, etc). Drugs and natural products may also be indicated for some pets and some problems.

Behavior Modification Principles

The most commonly used behavioral techniques include habituation, extinction, desensitization, counterconditioning, response substitution, and shaping. Flooding is often talked about but seldom used because it is likely to make most animals worse. While punishment is frequently used with varying degrees of success, few people correctly use this technique, and there are both humane and safety issues with the use of positive punishment. For punishment to be successful, the aversive stimulus (eg, startling with a loud noise, spraying compressed air) must occur sufficiently close to the onset of the behavior that the probability of the behavior occurring in the future is lessened. Often, punishment is more about the owner's anger than about changing the behavior. In addition, some dog owners have been ill advised by training advice that advocates confrontation, with the intent of asserting leadership (dominance). In fact, numerous studies have demonstrated that punishment-based training and confrontational techniques are more likely to lead to fear, avoidance, and increased aggression.

Most of the humane, passive, or positive techniques involved in behavior modification are not hard to learn and together with preventive strategies are very successful. In fact, dogs trained with rewards have fewer behavior problems, less fear, and less avoidance than dogs trained with punishment. The following is a short review of the basic principles involved in the techniques and their associated strategies.

Classical Conditioning: The pairing of an unconditioned stimulus with a neutral stimulus results in a conditioned stimulus and a conditioned response. Classical conditioning can occur in both positive and negative ways. Examples of a positive conditioned emotional response are the pairing of a clicker with favored treats (for clicker training) or a doorbell signaling visitors (for pets enthused about meeting new people).

Problems arise when a fearful conditioned emotional response is established *toward a previously neutral stimulus* (visual, odor, auditory, animate, inanimate) by repeated pairing with a fear-producing stimulus. Once this occurs, the stimulus itself will elicit the fear response, eg, a doorbell paired with the arrival of unfamiliar people (for pets fearful of visitors), or a doorbell paired with verbal or physical discipline applied by the owner for barking or jumping up (pinning, leash corrections). Similarly when a pet lunges or barks when meeting new people on the street or at the front door, the use of positive punishment to inhibit the behavior (such as choke collars, prong collars, shock, pinning) may condition a new response in which unfamiliar people become a fear-evoking conditioned stimulus. A visit to the veterinary clinic that may begin as a neutral situation may quickly become fear evoking if it is associated with unpleasant outcomes or is further enhanced by owner anxiety. In addition, all of the stimuli associated with the event (sights, sounds, smells) also become conditioned stimuli for fear. In much the same way, rain, wind, darkening skies, and lightning can quickly become conditioned fear-evoking stimuli for pets fearful of thunder.

Counterconditioning and Desensitization: Counterconditioning involves the consistent and repeated pairing of a stimulus that evokes an unpleasant response with something that is emotionally positive until a positive association is made. To be successful, counterconditioning should be coupled with desensitization in which the stimulus is minimized or reduced to a level that does not evoke the fear response (eg, by reducing volume, increasing distance, changing the environment, or modifying the stimulus to something less threatening). Once a positive association is made, rewards can be paired with stimuli of gradually increasing intensity.

Desensitization and counterconditioning are extremely time consuming. The exercises must be constantly repeated, so that the response is altered to a positive one. All stimuli that evoke fear (sights, sounds, odors, tactile) must be considered. Clients often want both quicker fixes and less work. However, moving too quickly provokes anxiety and sabotages any behavior modification program.

Operant Conditioning: Operant conditioning is a method based on making an association between a behavior and consequences of that behavior. The results either increase or decrease the likelihood of future responses. There are four types of behavior-consequence relations: positive and negative punishment and positive and negative reinforcement. Reinforcement increases the likelihood a behavior will be repeated, and punishment leads to a reduction in behavior. Negative refers to the removal of a stimulus, and positive refers to the application of a stimulus.

Positive reinforcement training occurs if behavior is increased by something applied (generally something pleasant or appealing); **negative reinforcement** occurs if behavior is increased by something removed (generally something unpleasant). In positive reinforcement training, a reward should be given immediately and consistently until the behavior is reliably repeated. If the behavior is to be trained on command or cue, a word or hand signal should then be added before the behavior-reward sequence. Once learned, behavior can be reinforced on a variable schedule, so that the period of time or number of responses before the reward is given is varied. Rewards are used for positive reinforcement, but a reward is not synonymous with positive reinforcement. A reward is anything desirable to the pet, from an activity such as petting, walking, or play, to an item such as a toy, food, chew, or treat. However, unless there is a clear relationship between the behavior and the reward (timing, consistency, contiguity), then the reward does not achieve the goal of positively reinforcing behavior.

Negative reinforcement must not be confused with punishment, because punishment decreases behaviors and reinforcement increases behaviors. One example of negative reinforcement is avoidance or escape behavior. For example, if an animal anticipates an unpleasant outcome (eg, meeting another dog, veterinary visit), then the aversive outcome will not occur if the animal retreats. Similarly, if the owner puts pressure on a head halter until the desired behavior is achieved (eg, sit, back up), the release of tension is negative reinforcement. One potential consequence of negative reinforcement is that if a pet's threats or aggression lead to removal of a stimulus (eg, dog, delivery person, owner), the behavior is reinforced by the retreat of the stimulus.

Positive punishment occurs when a behavior decreases when something is applied (generally something unpleasant), and **negative punishment** occurs when a behavior is decreased when something is removed (generally something pleasant or appealing). In positive punishment, if behavior does not decrease after the first few applications, then the punishment is not being appropriately timed or the behavior is too strongly motivated to be deterred by punishment. Positive punishment applied by a person (owner, trainer) is intended to cause the pet to become fearful of repeating the behavior. However, a potential consequence is that the pet becomes fearful or defensive to the punisher or to an approaching hand. Relationships with people should always remain positive! Also, if an unpleasant consequence occurs only when the owner is present, the behavior may continue in the owner's absence. Another problem with positive punishment is that punishment paired with exposure to a stimulus (barking at cars, meeting other dogs on walks) can result in a conditioned fear of the stimulus (*see* above).

Punishment cannot be used to achieve desirable behaviors, only to stop what is undesirable. If the goal is to make the pet fearful of repeating a behavior (eg, garbage raiding, taking things from counters, chewing plants) or to keep the pet away from an area (room, couch, bed), then environmental punishment or pet-activated punishment (eg, motion detector alarms or sprays, upside-down carpet runners, aversive tastes, double-sided tape, or bark-activated sprays) or remote punishment (eg, spraying water while out of sight, remote-activated alarm or spray) might be most appropriate. However, before focusing on how to stop what is undesirable, the owner should first focus on providing a desirable alternative (eg, where to sleep, where to climb, what to chew).

Negative punishment is the reduction of a behavior by the removal of something pleasant. For example, if the pet is receiving affection or play when an undesirable behavior begins (eg, play biting, mouthing, mounting), the immediate removal of the play or affection will "negatively" punish the pet. However, unless the pet can determine what behavior leads to the removal of play, the behavior may actually intensify because of frustration at not receiving its reward.

Second-order Reinforcers: Signals that can be used at a distance to convey that the reward is coming are second-order reinforcers. Commonly used second-order reinforcers are words (eg, "Good dog!"), clickers, or whistles. By repeatedly and continuously pairing these with a primary reward such as a toy or treat, second-order reinforcers can elicit the same response that the reward would, as long as the pairing is repeatedly maintained. Clicker training requires frequent practice and excellent timing, but once achieved the animal can be reinforced each time the desired behavior is observed. Clicker training is an excellent way to immediately "mark" desirable responses, gradually shape new or more desirable behaviors (eg, longer, more relaxed), or associate a positive emotional response with the stimulus. (A useful resource is www.clickertraining.com.)

Premack Principle: When a more desirable behavior is made contingent on a less desirable behavior, the less desirable behavior is more likely to be repeated. Thus, the more desirable behavior serves as the reinforcer. For example, if a pet wants to go out or cross the street for its walk, the owner can train a sit-stay before each of these behaviors. A horse or dog that wants to walk ahead can be taught that walking on a slack rein or leash will result in this behavior.

Overlearning: Overlearning is the repeated evocation and expression of an already learned response. It is a phenomenon frequently used in training for specific events but may be underused in preventing fearful responses in dogs. Overlearning accomplishes three things: it delays forgetting, it increases the resistance to extinction, and it increases the probability that the response will become a "knee-jerk" one, or response of first choice, when the circumstances are similar.

Shaping: Shaping works through gradual approximations and allows the animal to be rewarded initially for any behavior that resembles the desired behavior. For instance, when teaching a puppy to sit, providing a food reward for a slight squat will increase the probability that squatting will be repeated. This squatting behavior is then rewarded only when it more closely resembles a sit, and finally, when it becomes a true sit. Shaping can also be used to reward an increase in duration of or progressively more relaxed behaviors.

Extinction: The ending of a behavior once all reinforcement is removed is termed extinction. For example, if people pet a dog that jumps up on them for attention, the behavior continues; if they stop, the dog will eventually extinguish its response because the reward is no longer there. However, any form of intermittent reinforcement—even occasional petting of the dog in response to its jumping—will prolong the performance of the response. Valuable rewards, a long history of performance, and intermittent reinforcement all increase resistance to extinction. Owners also must be prepared for the intensity of the behavior to initially increase before it is extinguished. Giving in will make extinction even more difficult as the animal learns that higher intensity behaviors achieve the desired outcome.

Habituation: Habituation is a gradual lessening of a response to a stimulus. Usually this occurs with repeated presentation of a stimulus whereby the animal learns that it does not signal anything important. For example, horses placed in a pasture bordering a road may at first run away when traffic passes but eventually learn to ignore it. Stimuli associated with potentially adverse consequences are more difficult to extinguish with habituation than other stimuli. In prey species, responses to sounds associated with predators would be difficult to habituate, because they have been selected for and generally are adaptive. If the fear response is too intense, instead of habituation the animal may become increasingly more fearful of the stimulus. This is termed **sensitization**.

If an extended interval has occurred since the time an animal last experienced a stimulus to which it had habituated, the animal may again react when reexposed to the stimulus. This is termed **spontaneous recovery**.

Flooding: This is used to treat fears of harmless stimuli by forcing the animal to stay in the presence of the stimuli until the fear is extinguished. This procedure is seldom effective and has welfare implications in dogs, because it initially enhances fear and cannot be stopped until all physiologic and emotional signs of fear are gone. If done improperly, flooding may therefore increase problem behaviors. In practice, a controlled level of flooding is quite often used as a component of behavior modification, in which the stimulus is presented at a level that is low enough to cause mild fear and the pet is not removed until it habituates. This can then be combined with reinforcement, ie, the pet is positively reinforced or the stimulus removed (negative reinforcement) when the fear response subsides or abates.

Response Substitution: This involves the replacement of an undesirable response with a desirable one. For example, high-value rewards can be used to train desirable target behaviors that are alternatives to the undesirable behavior. However, if the behavior is part of the pet's natural repertoire (eg, greeting, barking), it can be particularly difficult to train alternative behaviors. Specific examples of response substitution include training a dog to sit or lie down as an alternative to jumping up, mounting, or play biting; or to sit, walk on loose leash, or back up for dogs forging ahead or running out the door. Training should begin in a variety of environments where success can be most readily achieved. The desired endpoint for the new response is for the animal to be quiet and calm. Therefore, the owner must learn to read the look in the eyes, body posture, facial expressions, and breathing to be able to gradually shape the desired behavior. Training could then move to environments with increasing distractions and locations where the problem is most likely to arise. Alternatively, the pet might be enticed to engage in a behavior that is incompatible with the undesirable behavior, eg, teaching the dog to fetch a toy when visitors arrive instead of jumping up.

To replace the undesirable behavior with one that is desirable, response substitution can be coupled with desensitization by beginning training with stimuli of low enough intensity while training the target behaviors (eg, relaxation) with high-value rewards. However, for pets that are fearful or anxious, the focus should be on desensitization and counterconditioning to change the pet's emotional state rather than the behavioral response.

PRINCIPLES OF PHARMACOLOGIC AND NATURAL TREATMENT

Psychotropic drugs and natural products can be used to reestablish a more stable emotional state and improve trainability in animals that are anxious, fearful, or overly reactive. Drugs might also be effective in the treatment of behavior that is abnormal, pathologic, or lacking impulse control. In addition, drugs may be indicated to improve compromised welfare. However, whereas drugs can improve the animal's emotional state and facilitate new learning, only with concurrent behavior modification can new neuronal pathways be established, new behaviors learned, and fearful responses to stimuli changed to positive ones.

Evidence-based decision making is a way to provide the best information and treatment options. Treatment should be selected using the evidence combined with the clinician's expertise regarding the animal, client, and problem. Very few drugs have been adequately tested in rigorous, randomized, controlled trials for use in veterinary behavioral therapy. In fact, most drugs used in veterinary behavioral therapy are human drugs, very few of which have had pharmacokinetics established for animal species. This can lead to inaccurate assumptions with respect to dosage, duration of effect, contraindications, and adverse effects. In addition, there is a wide range of published dosages based on the application, individual variability, and desired outcome. Therefore, practitioners should remain current with the most recent veterinary behavior literature with respect to indications, recommended dosages, evidence of efficacy, potential adverse effects, and contraindications before dispensing any of these medications. (For dosing guidelines, *see* TABLE 3). Depending on the drug and patient, compounding may be required to achieve an appropriate dosage and formulation for administration; however, reformulation may alter a drug's pharmacokinetics, safety, efficacy, and stability. Recent studies on the use of transdermal preparations of behavioral drugs such as fluoxetine, amitripyline, and buspirone have found little to no absorption of transdermal preparations versus oral dosing.

A variety of natural products have been used to treat anxiety; however, only a few have demonstrated any evidence to support efficacy. Products that have published studies indicating potential therapeutic effects to calm and reduce underlying fear and anxiety include the canine appeasing pheromone (Adaptil®), the feline cheek gland pheromones (Feliway® and Felifriend®), a feline pheromone that might aid in scratching post training (Feliscratch®), L-theanine (Anxitane®), α-casozepine (Zylkene®), a diet supplemented with α-casozepine and L-tryptophan (Royal Canin Calm™ Feline and Canine), a product combining *Magnolia officinalis* and *Phellodendron amurense* (Harmonease®), a *Souroubea* sp supplement (Sin Susto™), as well as perhaps melatonin, and lavender aromatherapy.

A physical examination and blood and urine tests should be part of a minimum database before dispensing drugs to ensure there are no underlying medical problems that may be causing or contributing to the behavioral signs, or that might have an impact on drug selection and use. For tricyclic antidepressants and selective serotonin reuptake inhibitors, 4 wk may be required to achieve optimal therapeutic effect.

TABLE 3 DRUG DOSAGES FOR BEHAVIORAL THERAPY IN DOGS AND CATS

Drug	Dog Dosage	Cat Dosage
TRANQUILIZER		
Acepromazine	0.5–2 mg/kg, prn[a] to tid	0.5–2 mg/kg, prn
BENZODIAZEPINES		
Alprazolam	0.01–0.1 mg/kg, prn to qid	0.125–0.25 mg/cat, prn to tid
Clonazepam	0.1–1 mg/kg, bid-tid	0.05–0.2 mg/kg, one to three times/day
Clorazepate	0.5–2 mg/kg, prn to tid	0.2–1 mg/kg, one to two times/day
Diazepam	0.5–2 mg/kg, prn (eg, every 4–6 hr)	0.2–1 mg/kg, prn to tid[b]
Lorazepam	0.025–0.2 mg/kg/day to prn	0.025–0.08 mg/kg, one to two times/day
Oxazepam	0.2–1 mg/kg, one to two times/day	0.2–0.5 mg/kg, one to two times/day
TRICYCLIC ANTIDEPRESSANTS		
Amitriptyline	1–4 mg/kg, bid	0.5–2 mg/kg/day
Clomipramine	1–3 mg/kg, bid[c]	0.25–1 mg/kg/day[c]
Doxepin	3–5 mg/kg, bid-tid	0.5–1 mg/kg, one to two times/day
Imipramine	1–4 mg/kg, one to two times/day	0.5–1 mg/kg, one to two times/day
SELECTIVE SEROTONIN REUPTAKE INHIBITORS		
Fluoxetine	1–3 mg/kg/day[c]	0.5–1.5 mg/kg/day
Fluvoxamine	1–2 mg/kg, one to two times/day	0.25–0.5 mg/kg/day
Paroxetine	0.5–2 mg/kg/day	0.25–1 mg/kg/day
Sertraline	1–3 mg/kg/day or divided bid	0.5–1.5 mg/kg/day
β-BLOCKER		
Propranolol	0.2–3 mg/kg, prn to bid	0.2–1 mg/kg, tid
α_2-AGONIST		
Clonidine	0.01–0.05 mg/kg, prn to bid	
AZAPIRONE		
Buspirone	0.5–2 mg/kg, one to three times/day	0.5–1 mg/kg, one to three times/day

(continued)

TABLE 3 DRUG DOSAGES FOR BEHAVIORAL THERAPY IN DOGS AND CATS *(continued)*

Drug	Dog Dosage	Cat Dosage
SEROTONIN ANTAGONIST REUPTAKE INHIBITOR		
Trazodone	3–8 mg/kg, prn to tid	
ANTICONVULSANTS		
Carbamazepine	4–8 mg/kg, bid-tid	2–6 mg/kg, one to two times/day
Gabapentin	5–30 mg/kg, bid-tid	3–10 mg/kg, bid-tid
Levetiracetam	20 mg/kg, tid	10–20 mg/kg, tid
Phenobarbital[d]	2–5 mg/kg, bid (to 10 mg/kg, prn for sedation)	1–3 mg/kg, bid
Potassium bromide[d]	10–40 mg/kg/day, or divided bid	Not recommended
GLIAL MODULATOR		
Propentofylline[e]	2.5–5 mg/kg, bid	
MONOAMINE OXIDASE INHIBITOR		
Selegiline[c,e]	0.5–1 mg/kg/day (in morning)	0.5–1 mg/kg/day (in morning)

[a] prn = as needed

[b] Rare reports of hepatic necrosis with diazepam in cats and potentially with other benzodiazepines

[c] Licensed and labeled for veterinary behavior use in some countries

[d] Titrate upward if inadequate clinical improvement and serum levels not adequate

[e] Licensed and labeled for cognitive dysfunction in some countries

NORMAL SOCIAL BEHAVIOR AND BEHAVIORAL PROBLEMS OF DOMESTIC ANIMALS

HORSES

SOCIAL BEHAVIOR

Horses are social animals that under feral conditions (or on pasture) live in bands (harems) that consist of several mares, their offspring up to 2–3 yr of age, and at least 1 and as many as 6 adult males. The core of the group is the mares, which stay together even if the stallion leaves or dies. The group size ranges from 2 to 21 horses; multiple-male bands are larger than single-male bands. Groups are not limited to a specific geographic area and will travel in search of resources. Colts and fillies leave the group usually before 2 yr of age (when they become sexually mature), stay alone for a few months, and then join a different group or establish a new one. Some colts may form a “bachelor band” with up to 16 males, and later join other groups in which the stallion has died or been chased away.

Hierarchy in horses appears to be linear (with occasional triangular relationships) and not necessarily based on age, weight, height, gender, or time in the group. These are important factors when considering problems in stabled horses, and attentive management is required before introducing horses to each other. Offspring of high-ranking mares appear to be high-ranking later in life, which might indicate both genetic and experience components. Hierarchical rank in females is determined by observing group behavior (eg, seeking out resources such as water holes). Females make the decision about whether to leave or to stay within a band based on factors such as assessment of food resources or number of stallions in the group. High-ranking females can successfully interfere with the nursing of foals by lower-ranking females. Mares have preferred associates, are preferentially groomed, and will groom certain individuals. As in many other species, hierarchy in horses is based on deference by lower-ranking animals, not fighting.

The highest-ranking stallion in a band does most of the breeding, because it is the first to secure access to a receptive female and the first to displace a female from another band. In the absence of conception, horses cycle every 21 days during the spring and summer. There are three phases of sexual behavior in horses: courtship, mating, and postmating behavior. During courtship the stallion will approach the mare, prance, sniff her, nuzzle her, and groom her. The mare may squeal, kick, or move away to show the stallion she is not ready, or she may stand still, deviate her tail, and urinate, leading the stallion to mount her. Pasture breeding can achieve 100% success rates, versus 50%–60% for "in hand" or controlled breeding. This is probably because of familiarity between the horses, higher fertility of the mare, and less aggression between horses.

Ovulation usually occurs 36 hr before estrous behavior ends. Gestation lasts 315–365 days, with an average of 340 days. Factors that affect gestation length include nutrition, time of year (shorter time for late summer breeding), and gender (slightly longer for colts). Mares usually deliver at night, even when provided with artificial light. Bonding between mare and foal occurs in the first 24 hr. Most nursing behavior is initiated by the foal and terminated by the mare, especially in the first month.

During the first month of life, foals show maximal dependence on their dams and have minimal contact with other horses. They spend most of the time resting near the dam. The socialization period is 2–3 mo of age; the foal starts playing with other foals and explores its environment. It is important to provide gentle handling during the first 42 days of life. At this time, snapping (teeth clapping) peaks. This is a behavior shown by foals toward adult horses, presumably to reduce aggression. It may also be a displacement nursing behavior, such as air nursing. Snapping is not the same behavior as smacking, which is an aggressive behavior or threat. Allogrooming also peaks at this time.

From 4 mo of age, the foal starts developing independent relationships and spends more time in adult maintenance behaviors such as grazing and resting while standing. There are sex differences in play; colts mount more and fight more than fillies, who focus on grooming and running. Colts groom only fillies, while fillies groom both sexes.

BEHAVIORAL PROBLEMS

Many behavioral problems are associated with confinement. Under free-ranging circumstances, horses wander and spend >60% of their day foraging. The remainder of their time is spent resting (standing or lying down), grooming, or engaging in another activity. This same pattern is seen under barn conditions; even with free choice of grain, horses will eat many small meals a day. Horses are highly social animals that require contact with others for normal daily maintenance and well-being. Isolating horses can lead to development of problems. The main goal of managing behavior problems in horses is to identify the deviation from normal equine behavior and correct it.

Aggression

Aggression is a common problem in horses and includes chasing, neck wrestling, kicks and bites, and other threats. Signs of aggression include ears flattened backward, retracted lips, rapid tail movements, snaking, pawing, head bowing, fecal pile display, snoring, squealing, levade (rearing with deeply flexed hindquarters), and threats to kick. Submissive horses respond by avoiding, lowering the neck and head, clamping the tail, and turning away from the aggressor.

Aggression to People: This behavior is seen mostly in stalls in which the horse feels confined in a small space that is also easily defended. The varieties of aggression toward people include fear, pain induced, sexual (hormonal), learned, and dominance related. Some horses, especially young ones, play with each other while showing signs of aggression such as kicking and biting. Although benign to other horses, this can be dangerous to people.

The first step in managing equine aggression is identifying the cause, and if possible, removing it. Training and positive reinforcement to establish control over the horse are also used, along with desensitization and counterconditioning. Dominance-related aggression in horses is different from canine status-related aggression (also known as dominance aggression) in that it is not context-dependent. Environmental management is important as well; good management should include sufficient resources such as space, food, and water. Some horses are considered to have pathologic dominance aggression; they will attack other horses and people that are near them. These horses should be separated completely from other people or horses and have a poor prognosis.

Aggression Toward Other Horses: Aggression toward other horses is mostly associated with sexual competition, fear, dominance, or territory (protecting the group and resources). As with aggression toward people, some horses may be pathologically aggressive toward other horses. The first step is separation of aggressive horses from other horses, and keeping subordinate away from dominant horses. Separation is achieved by solid walls or two fences to avoid kicks through the fence. Horses should have sufficient resources, and desensitization and counterconditioning is the best treatment approach. In cases of sexually related aggression, castration and progestins (eg, medroxyprogesterone 70–80 mg/300 kg/day) can help. Adverse effects of such treatment should be weighed carefully, and the horse should be monitored closely. Adding tryptophan to the daily ration or administering selective serotonin reuptake inhibitors (SSRIs) may be helpful in some cases. Punishment should be avoided.

Maternal Aggression: Aggression by mares toward people is normal during the first few days after parturition. This behavior is hormonally driven and usually wanes with time. Mares should be familiarized with their caretakers before delivery and have minimal contact with other people after delivery. No treatment is required in most cases.

Aggression While Breeding: Stallions that are aggressive when used for breeding are often overused or used out of season. Stallions can develop preferences for mating and may not be compatible with the chosen mare; changing the mare may help. If stallions were stabled with mares when they were colts, they may have some social inhibition for mating, and forced mating can result in aggression. The goal of treatment is to treat the main cause of aggression; changing the mare (because of preferences) or artificial breeding can also be attempted. Physical restraint (eg, hobbles) and desensitization can help as well. Clicker training has been used successfully to desensitize stallions with this problem.

Stereotypic Behaviors

Compulsive behaviors in horses can be divided into movement-related behaviors and oral behaviors. They can be called stereotypic because they are repetitive, occupy a large part of the daily activity, and serve no function. Confinement and poor management practices are the primary contributing factors. In addition, bedding, feed, and social contact influence stereotypic behaviors. Horses that have more social contacts, are fed more roughage and more than one type, are fed two or more times daily, and are bedded on straw are less prone to these behaviors. Cribbing and wood chewing are examples of oral behaviors, whereas weaving, stall walking, and pawing are examples of locomotor stereotypies. Horses with one stereotypic behavior are likely to exhibit another. In Thoroughbreds, these behaviors are commonly seen in mares and 2-yr-old foals.

Cribbing (Aerophagia, Windsucking): When cribbing, the horse usually grasps an object in the stall (such as the water bucket) with its incisors, flexes its neck, and sucks air into the pharynx. Some horses will aspirate or swallow the air. In some cases, horses will suck air without grasping any object. Feeding highly palatable food (eg, grains, molasses) is associated with cribbing. Lack of exercise is also associated with cribbing; endurance horses are less likely to do it than race or dressage horses. Thoroughbreds are more prone to cribbing than other horses. The rate of cribbing is higher in confined horses; however, even if the horse is turned to pasture once the behavior is established, it will persist. It is possible that GI discomfort can lead to cribbing. One of the major complications of cribbing is damage to the incisors. Other problems include gastroduodenal ulcers and epiploic foramen entrapment. In most cases, cribbing is a benign behavior that does not affect the horse's welfare and does not require treatment. Close to 10% of foals 20 wk of age will start cribbing when weaned and placed in stalls. Those kept on pasture will not start. It has been speculated that horses can learn cribbing by watching other horses; however, no clear evidence exists.

Cribbing can be diagnosed by finding U-shaped pieces missing from fences and horizontal surfaces in the stall, and worn incisors and enlarged neck muscles in horses that crib. In some cases, the caretaker may directly observe the behavior. Management should include more roughage, exercise, and social contact. Turning confined horses to pasture may help, and providing toys and stimulation is also advocated. Placing a strap around the horse's neck behind the poll will apply pressure each time the horse tries to flex its neck. This essentially punishes the horse for cribbing, with the punishment associated with the behavior and not the caretaker. Alternatively, an open-end muzzle can be applied. This will allow the horse to eat and drink but prevent it from grasping objects to crib on. Some horses find a way to crib with the muzzle (eg, grasping a linear object, such as a stick), and most horses seem to tolerate the strap better than the muzzle. Keeping stalls free of horizontal surfaces and objects that the horse can grasp can help minimize cribbing. A variety of surgeries have been suggested to manage cribbing; however, the varying success rates and negative impact on animal welfare are significant disadvantages.

Wood Chewing (Lignophagia): Like a horse that cribs, a wood-chewing horse will grasp pieces of wood with its incisors, but unlike in cribbing, it will swallow the pieces. The definitive cause of wood chewing is lack of roughage in the diet. Confinement, high-concentrate diets, and lack of exercise and stimulation increase incidence of wood chewing. Horses on pasture normally spend 8–12 hr/day grazing, while confined horses *spend <3–4 hr/day feeding*. Wood chewing increases in cold, wet weather. Providing more roughage, exercise, stimulation, toys, or social contact can reduce incidence of this behavior. Eliminating exposed wood and covering fence edges with wires and taste repellents can also help minimize wood chewing.

Geophagia (Pica): Most horses will ingest sand or dirt. Soil that is ingested is richer in iron and copper than other soils, and this may attract the horse. Ingestion of stones can become a serious problem, because it can lead to intestinal obstructions. Management should include increasing roughage and exercise and providing salt blocks and toys.

Polydipsia: Polydipsia in horses is similar to behavior seen in dogs (*see* p 1568). The most common presenting complaint is a wet stall due to frequent urination. It is important to exclude medical causes (eg, diabetes insipidus).

Stall Walking and Weaving: These behaviors are seen in confined horses, serve no purpose, are hard to interrupt, and are usually slower than other types of movement. Horses that stall walk usually walk in circles in the stall, and when released to a larger space (eg, pasture or barn) continue to circle in a small area. Tying the horse to prevent walking will only transform the behavior into weaving, ie, lifting the legs and shifting weight and head position from side to side in the same spot. Possible causes of stall walking include lack of exercise and social contact and claustrophobia. Stress and anxiety appear to aggravate the problem. Treatment should focus on increasing exercise and stimulation, providing social contact, and turning the horse to pasture. Providing thick bedding and feeding more than twice daily can help as well. In extreme cases, SSRIs might be necessary to control the problem. Providing a large mirror in the stall in front of the horse can help decrease weaving.

Stall Kicking: Horses may kick the walls of the stall because of boredom, aggression, or frustration. The horse may kick in anticipation when food is being prepared but is out of reach. When the horse is then fed, the behavior is reinforced. The horse may also be frustrated when it cannot achieve its goals (eg, exercise, mating, or social contact). It is possible that this behavior is a form of self-mutilation. Many horses that kick and make holes in the walls of the stall also eat wood from these holes. Treatment should be directed toward eliminating the underlying cause. Treatment for aggressive kicking is discussed earlier (*see* p 1546), and for most other causes the treatment is similar to that for stall walking (*see* above). Owners should never reinforce kicking by providing food when the horse kicks. Providing more social contact, exercise, and stimulation can also help.

Pawing: Similar to kicking but less dangerous, pawing or digging may be a result of frustration and anticipation. This could also be a displacement behavior. Changing the floors to concrete may stop pawing; however, it will not change the motivation to do so, and some horses (especially stallions) may rear up instead of pawing. Treatment is similar to that for kicking (*see* above).

Head Shaking: A head-shaking horse shakes or jerks its head uncontrollably, without any apparent stimulus. Some horses will also snort, rub their head on objects, and display an anxious expression. Most commonly, horses shake up and down. There are five grades to this problem: 1) intermittent signs, mainly facial twitching; 2) moderate signs with noticeable shaking such that can interfere with riding; 3) advanced stage, and difficult to control; 4) uncontrollable and unrideable horse; and 5) dangerous behavior with bizarre patterns. In most cases, the horse looks as if it has nasal mites or is being attacked by biting flies. Many medical conditions can cause head shaking (eg, seizures, respiratory tract diseases and parasites, ear and eye disease, GI disorders, pain, trauma, nasal foreign bodies), and these must be excluded. Behavioral causes of head shaking include an improper bit, an incompetent rider, fear and anxiety, dressage leading to extreme cervical flexion, and compulsive disorders. Geldings seem to be affected more frequently than stallions or mares. Management should include treating any underlying medical problem, desensitization and counterconditioning, and potentially use of SSRIs.

Self-mutilation: Some horses hurt themselves by biting or kicking the abdomen with their hindlegs. Some of these horses also vocalize. Underlying causes include displacement behavior, self-reinforced behavior, and redirected behavior. Skin diseases and pain can also lead to self-mutilation and must be excluded. This problem seems more common in young males (<2 yr old) and may possibly be triggered by environmental stressors. Management should include sufficient stimulation and exercise and increased social contact.

Fear and Phobia

Like dogs, horses can have fears and phobias. The two main presentations are noise and location or environment phobias. Horses have an innate fear of new things (neophobia) that explains some behavior issues such as trailer-related problems (*see* below). The management is similar to that in dogs and cats (*see* p 1565).

Trailer-related Problems: There are two main presentations of trailer-related problems: loading into the trailer and travelling. Horses may be afraid to load into a trailer because of innate factors (eg, neophobia, a dark interior, instability of the trailer, noise) and/or learned factors (eg, previous accident, motion sickness, previous punishment while loading). A horse may load into a trailer readily but misbehave while inside. This could be because the horse finds it difficult to keep its balance while the trailer is moving, anticipates a stressful event such as a race after the trailer ride, or has motion sickness. In a small number of cases, horses are reluctant to leave the trailer. Heart rate and salivary cortisol levels have been shown to increase during and after trailering.

The best approach to managing trailering problems is slow desensitization and counterconditioning using food and treats. This may take a long time and may not be suitable for an acute problem. Desensitization should be done long before the expected trailer ride. Punishment should be avoided, because it may aggravate the situation and be dangerous for both the horse and the caretaker. Some horses prefer to see their environment and may load better in a rear-facing trailer. Horses are herd animals and learn from each other; having a horse with a trailer-related problem view another horse loading can facilitate learning. Foals should be loaded with their mothers at an early age. Sedatives such as xylazine can be used in acute situations; however, the horse may not learn to load or ride better while drugged and may be less able to balance itself for the ride and any performance after the ride.

Sexual Behavioral Problems

Silent Heat: Behavioral anestrus is a common problem in young mares, especially during the first cycle. The ovaries are normal on palpation, and ovulation occurs normally. However, the mare will not accept the stallion. Causes include environmental stressors and mating preference. Presenting several stallions may help, and if the mare is still nursing a foal, weaning may help.

Nymphomania: Medical conditions that can cause excessive sexual behavior in mares include granulosa cell tumor and persistent ovarian follicles. These conditions should be differentiated because a persistent follicle may resolve without treatment (although it may require treatment with gonadotropins or luteinizing hormone or increasing daylight to ≥16 hr), whereas granulosa cell tumors require surgical resection. Excessive estrous behavior is manifested as squatting and urinating frequently, receptiveness to males, and exposing the clitoris ("winking"). Some granulosa cell tumors produce testosterone, leading to stallion-like behavior (eg, aggression, mounting, flehmen, and urine marking). Management should be directed toward the underlying problem.

Psychic Estrus: Mares with psychic estrus show estrous behavior without any of the physiologic correlates of heat. Treatment is as for nymphomania (*see* above).

Poor Libido: Overused stallions, submissive stallions presented to aggressive mares, and stallions with previous negative experiences may be unwilling to mate. Masturbation is a normal behavior in horses; colts will start mounting within the first few weeks of their lives. Ejaculation is rare, and fertility rates are unaffected. Some owners use various devices to stop masturbation; these essentially punish the horse for masturbating and cause pain. They can cause fear while trying to breed and predispose the stallion to poor libido. Management should be directed toward eliminating the underlying problems. The stallion should be presented with teaser mares, should be well rested and fed, and have increased social contact with mares on pasture. Using an artificial vagina to desensitize the stallion can help, and treatment with anxiolytics such as diazepam may address underlying anxiety. Other cases may require semen collection and artificial insemination.

Stallion-like Behavior in Geldings: Approximately 50% of geldings show some stallion-like behavior, including courting and mounting females, flehmen, fighting, and attacking foals. The brain of the male horse is masculinized before birth; therefore, some of these behaviors do not require androgens to be expressed. Some geldings may achieve erection and intromission while mounting the mare. In advanced cases, the horse should be checked for pituitary adenoma. Normally, the testosterone level should be <0.2 ng/mL. Treatment includes separation, progestins, and SSRIs.

Eating Disorders

Coprophagia: Eating feces is mainly seen in foals during the first 8 wk of life. Foals usually consume fresh feces of their mothers, and it is believed that maternal pheromones play a role in this behavior. Deoxycholic acid is found in feces and may help protect against infantile enteritis and aid in deposition of myelin. The behavior may also provide vitamin B and introduce normal intestinal flora. In adults, the behavior is mainly associated with a low-roughage diet.

Obesity: Decreased exercise and overfeeding a palatable and highly concentrated diet can lead to obesity. On pasture, horses spend 8–12 hr grazing while moving from place to place; confined horses spend <3–4 hr. Increasing exercise, social contact, and roughage can help maintain appropriate body weight.

Anorexia: Horses are herd animals, and any changes in social relationships or the environment can increase stress and lead to anorexia. Appropriate weaning of foals is also important to prevent anorexia. Submissive horses may not eat near aggressive horses if they have previously been attacked. Management should be directed toward the underlying problem. Increasing social contact and separating affected animals from aggressive horses can help.

Foal Rejection

There are three types of foal rejection: 1) avoidance, seen mainly in primiparous mares that appear fearful of the foal—the mare will not attack the foal but will not allow suckling; 2) intolerance of suckling, which is seen in primiparous mares or mares with a painful udder; and 3) aggression toward the foal, in which mares exhibit stallion-like behavior and may kick and bite the foal. There may be a genetic factor for this type of aggression in Arabians and Morgans. Some mares paw at the foal to stimulate them to stand, and this should be differentiated from aggression.

The most important aspect of treatment is to protect the foal. In extreme cases, the foal should be supplied with colostrum within the first 12 hr and then bottle fed or cross-nursed to another mare. Restraining a primiparous mare and letting the foal suckle may teach the mare that nursing is pleasurable and encourage her to let the foal nurse without restraint. Avoiding any disturbances while the mare is nursing the foal is paramount for successful nursing. Any evidence of mastitis or retained placenta should be addressed. For an aggressive mare, appropriate restraints such as a barrier or tying should be considered. Feeding the mare treats while the foal nurses can help desensitize her. In some cases, stimulating maternal behavior by separating the mare from the foal or faking a threat to the foal (eg, other horses, dogs) can help. Medications such as acepromazine, xylazine, diazepam, and progestins may help; however, these drugs can enter the milk and affect the foal.

CATTLE

SOCIAL BEHAVIOR

Range cattle live in groups of cows and calves; males are often separated until breeding season. Dominance in cattle is based on age, sex, weight, presence of horns, and territoriality. Breed also seems to play a role—heavier dairy cattle are dominant to lighter breeds, while lighter beef cattle are dominant to heavier breeds. When a heavier and older cow is introduced into a group, it is usually subordinate to existing members of the group. In large herds, triangular relationships between cows exist. In dairy cattle, hierarchies change constantly as cows are added or removed from the herd. Once a hierarchy is established, overt aggression is reduced.

Very little is known about vocal communication of cattle; most commonly noted are the moo, call, hoot, and roar. A distressed cow or calf will call or hoot, an aggressive bull may roar, and a hungry calf will give a high-intensity "menh."

Under natural conditions, cows cycle throughout the year, with peak activity between May and July and low activity between December and February (northern hemisphere). The heat cycle is usually 18–24 hr and generally begins in the evening. Common estrous behaviors include reduced food intake, increased movement, flehmen, standing behind another cow and resting the chin on its back, and increased licking and sniffing. Aggression and mounting also increase during the cycle. Heat detection is an important practice, especially in dairy cattle, in which artificial insemination is common. There are many methods to augment the detection of heat, including placement of dyes on cows' backs that will stain the estrous cow's ventral torso and pedometers that record increased movement. On some farms, a teaser bull is still in use. Bulls on pasture will graze alongside proestrous cows; the bull will stand head to head with the cow or may rest his head on her back. As estrus progresses he will try to mount, licking her vulva and showing flehmen.

Parturition normally occurs at night on pasture, and the calf normally starts suckling in <3 hr. The newborn calf spends most of its time near the dam until it is ~4–6 mo old, when it forms unstable groups with other calves. Cows maintain bonds with their calves even when the next calf is born. On pasture, heifers are weaned when ~8 mo old and bull calves when ~11 mo old. Social status increases with age, and social relationships are not stable until at least 1 yr of age.

BEHAVIORAL PROBLEMS

Most behavioral problems in cattle involve breeding or aggression and are related to poor management practices, confinement, and lack of enrichment.

Breeding-related Problems

Silent Heat: Silent heat occurs most often in heifers during the first cycle. Physical signs of heat (eg, vaginal discharge, vulvar relaxation, and behavioral signs) are absent. Estrus detection methods (*see* above) can help identify cows in heat. In recent years, the use of freemartins and dogs for detection of estrus has gained popularity.

Nymphomania: Increased sexual behavior occurs mainly in high-producing dairy cows that are 4–6 yr old and have had 1–3 calves. These cows usually mount other cows excessively, act like bulls, and have a significant decrease in milk production. In most cases nymphomania is associated with follicular cysts, and treatment with luteinizing hormone or chorionic gonadotropin is useful.

Masturbation: Masturbation in bulls normally does not affect fertility. The bull will have a partial erection, arch its back, and perform pelvic thrusts. Because this does not lead to increased aggression or reduced fertility, no treatment is needed. Increases in exercise and stimulation can reduce the frequency.

Poor Libido: Many diseases of bulls can lead to poor libido; therefore, the first step in managing impotence is excluding and treating possible diseases. Bulls with poor libido may refuse to mount, avoid estrous cows, and be unable to develop an erection. Behavioral causes for impotence include inexperience in young bulls that attempt breeding an aggressive cow, bulls that are used too frequently for semen collection, and the stress of a new environment. Using a new teaser bull or, preferably, a teaser cow in estrus can stimulate these bulls to breed. Allowing the bull to watch other bulls mounting may increase arousal. Food rewards (eg, molasses) may help as well. In many cases impotent bulls should be eliminated from breeding programs, or alternative ways of semen collection such as electroejaculation should be used.

Buller Steer: Buller steers are steers mounted by others. This problem is seen in ~3% of feedlot steers and seems related to both hormonal and crowding factors. Steers are usually implanted with anabolic steroids, most commonly stilbesterol or estrogen, which can lead them to mount others. However, the level of these hormones in the buller is usually lower. In large, overcrowded groups of steers, the number of bullers is higher. This problem may also be related to dominance; the more dominant and aggressive steers mount others. Erection and intromission rarely occur. Both the buller and the mounting steer may fail to gain adequate weight because of psychological stress and increased activity. Removing the buller is the most common solution. Adding hiding places, placing overhead electric wires, providing sufficient food and water to avoid conflict, and painting odiferous material on the back of the buller also can help reduce incidence of this behavior.

Aggression

Aggression in cattle is usually a result of fear, learning, and hormonal state. Aggression between cows is worse than that between bulls. Horned cattle will bunt (push or strike with the horns) and strike an opponent on the side. Polled cows will use their head as a battering ram. Two cows can fight for a long period with resting periods in between. Each cow will rest while pushing its muzzle between the udder and hindquarter of the other cow to immobilize it. Aggression toward people usually includes bunting, kicking, and crushing. Aggressive and dangerous animals should be culled.

Aggression in Bulls: Bulls are notorious for their unpredictable aggression. Some bulls may mount others, and these may respond with aggression. Such fights can end with serious injuries and even death, especially if the bulls are horned. Dairy bulls are commonly more aggressive (and also larger and heavier) than beef bulls. The bull may paw and dig in the ground, and horned bulls may kneel on the front legs and dig using their horns. Because hand-reared bulls are more aggressive toward other bulls, it is thought that inadequate socialization may contribute to this behavior. Aggressive bulls should be separated from others and perhaps culled if dangerous to people.

Kicking: Kicking is mainly a problem in beef cattle and is seen most commonly in heifers. Beef cattle are not selectively bred for gentleness and are handled minimally. These animals can be dangerous when placed in pens or cages for examination and may cause severe injuries. Such animals should be handled carefully and potentially sedated. Food rewards can be offered for calm behaviors.

Nursing-related Behaviors

Intersuckling: Non-nutritional suckling is a common problem in calves; the suckling calf will suck on other calves or the cow on any available appendage or skin tag. This can lead to skin irritation and even umbilical hernias (if the suckling calf suckles on the umbilical sheath of another calf). Poor nutrition may influence development of this behavior (increasing roughage can minimize the problem). Penning or isolating suckling calves does not solve the problem; the calf will continue to suckle on buckets or engage in self-suckling. The problem is more common in calves weaned after 6 days of age. Non-nutritional suckling occurs mostly after feeding; providing dry teats next to the feeding area can help reduce incidence of this behavior. Other ways to minimize this behavior include placing a serrated nose ring in the suckling calf, applying repellent materials to suckled areas, and fitting a muzzle. These may prevent suckling but do not reduce the motivation to do so, and calf welfare should be considered.

Cross-fostering: In some cases, it is necessary to cross-foster a calf. Dairy cows are more likely to refuse a new or unfamiliar calf than beef cows. Bonding between the cow and calf is based on fetal fluid and visual cues; therefore, covering the new calf with drapes soaked with amniotic fluid or the skin of the cow's own dead calf or blindfolding the cow can help. Encouraging the cow with food rewards can also help.

Miscellaneous Behavior Problems

Reluctance to Enter the Milking Parlor: Reluctance to enter the milking parlor is a problem related mainly to management. When dairy cows accustomed to milking with simultaneous feeding in a stanchion barn are moved to free stalls and are not fed when milked, they may refuse to enter the parlor. Previous negative experience (eg, mastitis, aberrant electric shock, punishment from the handler) can also play a role. In addition, changing the side from which the cow is normally milked can increase anxiety and even aggression. Providing more grain feeding, a calm environment, and possibly a preferred cow "mate" can help minimize the problem. Similar problems can arise with the introduction of electric squeeze gates.

Food Throwing: The underlying cause of food throwing is not well understood. The affected animal grabs food with its mouth and throws it on its back. One possible explanation is maintenance behavior that is meant to reduce biting flies in the presence of docked tails. The diet mixture may also play a role; the problem is seen more commonly in cattle fed a total mixed ration.

Tongue Rolling: Tongue rolling occurs mainly in veal cattle and is most likely a stereotypic behavior resulting from confinement. The affected calf flicks its tongue outside and rolls it back inside the mouth, followed by swallowing saliva. One study showed that veal calves that displayed tongue rolling had no abomasal ulcers, while those that did not show this behavior had ulcers. This may indicate that the behavior reduces stress. However, calves that showed tongue rolling as well as those that did not had abomasal erosions. Increasing stimulation (eg, adding sucking teats) may reduce incidence of this behavior.

SWINE

SOCIAL BEHAVIOR

Pigs are social animals that under free-ranging conditions live in groups of approximately eight individuals. The groups typically consist of three sows and their offspring. Boars are solitary. A hierarchy is formed at social maturity. Sows in the same group cycle at the same time and participate equally in group maternal behavior; one sow will remain with the piglets while the others forage. Communal nesting is also found under free-ranging conditions. In confined pigs, a hierarchy is formed as early as 1 wk of age. Piglets will fight newly introduced piglets in the pen. Piglets also form a teat rank by the end of the first week of life; the dominant piglet suckles on the first pair of teats and gains weight faster. Once the teat order is formed, the hierarchy remains stable as long as the same piglets remain in the same group. Normally, the heavier pig is more dominant. It appears that both genetics and experience play a role; dominant sows give birth to dominant piglets. Once a hierarchy is formed, fighting is mostly replaced with threats. Weaning takes place within the first 3–4 mo of the piglet's life, but in mass production environments, it can take place as early as 3–4 wk of age.

Sows normally have two estrous cycles per year and farrow twice. Pheromones and the sight of a boar are major factors in inducing cycles in gilts. In postfarrowing sows, weaning helps induce estrus; boars can be used to detect females in heat. The boar is usually highly vocal (courting song) and exhibits flehmen when an estrous female is present. Boars will nuzzle the head, shoulders, flank, and anogenital area of sows during courtship. Normally, boars urinate several times and produce thick saliva rich in pheromones. Boars raised without the presence of other pigs show low sexual performance.

Communication in pigs is mainly vocal; there are ~20 different recognized sounds. The grunt is one of the most common sounds, given in response to familiar sounds or while looking for food (rooting). A short grunt is given when the pig is excited, whereas a long grunt is a contact call and normally associated with pleasurable stimuli. When pigs are aroused they may squeal, and they may scream when hurt. Dominant pigs bark at subordinate pigs as a threat. Visual signals in pigs are not well developed. The tail position indicates the well-being of the pig. A tightly curled tail is an indication of a healthy pig, and a twitching tail indicates skin irritation. In mass production environments, tails are normally clipped to avoid tail biting (*see* below). Olfactory signals are highly developed in pigs. There are sex differences; sows can detect lower concentrations of smell and pheromones than boars. When introducing a new pig into an existing group, the resident pigs investigate the newcomer by nosing it. Pigs can form social ranks when they are blindfolded, which indicates the importance of olfactory and vocal communication.

Socialization in piglets starts at ~5 wk of age with conspecifics and at 14 wk of age with other species. Pigs 14–17 wk old are most sensitive, and any negative or unpleasant experience during this period can delay sexual maturity, leading to late first farrowing. In free-ranging conditions, grouping promotes foraging, nursing, and protection against predators. Pigs under free-range conditions will also choose one place to defecate. In commercial production, the most noticeable group behavior is in newborn piglets, which huddle when cold.

BEHAVIORAL PROBLEMS

Many behavioral problems in swine are related to confinement or stress. The treatment is usually directed toward managing social groups, establishing normal conditions when possible, and maintaining welfare.

Aggression

Aggression Toward Other Pigs: Piglets show aggression to other piglets within the first week of life while forming a teat order. Later, introducing new pigs into a group may lead to aggression as the pigs establish social ranks. Pigs may spend 1–2 min nosing each other, vocalizing, and then biting until one of the pigs retreats. It may take several days to establish a hierarchy in older pigs. Once the hierarchy is established, fights are rare and ranks are preserved mostly by threats from the dominant pig and submissive gestures from subordinates (eg, twisting the head away). During estrous cycles, sows may show severe aggression toward newly added sows. Submissive sows show the least estrous behavior, have small litters, and lose weight (most likely due to low nourishment). Most aggression in pigs seems to be related to resources such as food. Crowding and limited amounts of food increase aggression. During breeding, boars may fight and become very vocal; boars will strut shoulder to shoulder, champ their jaws (producing pheromone-rich saliva), then finally face each other and attack. Serious injuries may result, especially among boars that still have their tusks. Breed likely plays a role; Large Whites are more aggressive than Hampshires, which are more aggressive than Durocs. Body fat percentage may also be a factor; breeds with lower body fat are more aggressive when handled.

Management includes slow introduction of new pigs into existing groups, provision of shelters where subordinate pigs can hide, provision of sufficient resources and toys, and application of boar pheromones. Most producers keep lights dim in the pen to reduce aggression. Using tranquilizers such as azaperone (2.2 mg/kg) or amperozide (1 mg/kg) can help reduce aggression but may not be economical. Lithium (an antipsychotic) has been used successfully.

Tail Biting: Tail biting is seen mostly in confined pigs. Overcrowding and boredom seem to be the main causes. Free-ranging pigs spend 5–10 hr daily looking for food and rooting, whereas pigs kept in pens consume meals in a short time. Slatted floors without bedding, low-salt diets, and low-iron soil seem to predispose pigs to tail biting. Once the problem starts, blood from the injured tail seems to arouse the other pigs and can even lead to death of the victim but rarely advances to pure cannibalism. Most losses are due to secondary infections that result in culling. Management includes removing the biting pigs (if there are only a few of them) and providing stimulation such as straw bedding to root, toys, and corn on the cob to chew. Most commercial producers dock piglets' tails; however, this does not reduce the motivation for tail biting, and pigs may bite the stump or ears instead.

Cannibalism: Mostly seen in primiparous gilts, cannibalism accounts for 4% of piglet deaths and is estimated to affect ~18% of litters. It is most common immediately after parturition when the sow is stressed. Usually, the sow will bark to warn piglets walking by her head and then later attack them, biting them to death. Farrowing crates have been used successfully to reduce the incidence of cannibalism. Azaperone (2.2 mg/kg) has been used for treatment as well.

Crushing Piglets: Heavy sows may lie on their piglets, killing them. This normally occurs when there are weak, underdeveloped, or sick piglets that cannot move fast enough to avoid the sow. However, it is also a breeding and management problem—sows are naturally intensely protective mothers that will prevent the handler from attending to the piglets; selective breeding for less-protective sows has resulted in sows less devoted maternally. Management includes providing appropriate farrowing crates with slopes and bars on the sides that allow the piglets to move away from the sow and prevent the sow from rolling over on the piglets. In addition, heat lamps provide the piglets with an alternative heat source and motivation to rest away from the sow.

Breeding-related Problems

Reproductive problems are usually associated with management of boars and sows and estrus synchronization. These problems are fairly unusual in pigs because of rigid genetic control of sexual behaviors. Mating preferences are an important factor in breeding management of pigs.

Poor Libido: Poor libido in boars can be caused by nutritional problems (deficiencies or overfeeding) and behavioral causes such as stress or fear. Exposing a boar to an aggressive female can result in low sex drive. Socialization, visual social contact with affiliative sows for a few days (in pens across from each other, not next to each other), and appropriate nutrition are the keys to successful management.

Failure to Reproduce: This is seen mainly in confined gilts, and stress seems to play an important role. Regrouping or overcrowding increases stress levels as well. These two factors (confinement and crowding) lead to chronic stress, delayed puberty, and failure to reproduce. In contrast, acute and mild stress such as transport and gentle handling accelerate estrous cycles.

Refusal to Nurse: Normally, the sow lies in lateral recumbency and grunts to attract the piglets to nurse. Mastitis is the most common reason sows refuse to nurse piglets. A physical examination is necessary to exclude this and other medical conditions. The sow lies sternally, preventing the piglets from accessing the teats. Mastitis is typically seen during late phases of lactation when the farrowing crates are removed. Sows with postpartum dysgalactia syndrome and mastitis (*see* p 1373) are usually too weak to move and prevent the piglets from nursing. However, these sows usually do not eat, and their piglets do not gain weight. Piglets of such sows should be transitioned to milk replacers and solid food. This can be encouraged by mixing sow's milk with the food or sweetening the food.

Stereotypic Behaviors

Stereotypic behaviors are not common in pigs and mostly relate to management, boredom, and nutrition. The most common stereotypic behaviors include rubbing nasal secretions on the floor or another pig, bar biting by confined sows, and polydipsia. Environmental enrichment in early stages is usually successful. Feeding smaller quantities more frequently and providing toys, bedding to root, corn on the cob, and clean tires can be enriching and mentally stimulating for pigs.

SHEEP

SOCIAL BEHAVIOR

Sheep are a prey species, and their only defense is to flee. Sheep display an intensely gregarious social instinct that allows them to bond closely to other sheep and preferentially to related flock members. Flock mentality movements protect individuals from predators. Flocks include multiple females, offspring, and one or more males. Ewes tend to stay in their maternal groups for life, whereas rams may form transient, unstable, and easily disbanded bachelor herds. If most rams in a group die because of fights or diseases, those remaining join another group. Under standard grazing situations, sheep graze together in casual affiliations; social hierarchies are not as apparent as they are for cattle.

Flock dynamics are apparent in groups of four or more as evidenced by willingness to follow a leader or flee in unison. When escape is prevented, even a ewe may charge or threaten by hoof stomping. Separation from the flock can cause stress and panic. Isolation from other sheep can cause severe stress and should be avoided. Mirrors can be used in the absence of other sheep.

Males in rut will physically challenge one another for social rank and breeding privileges. Social rank depends on the presence and size of horns, body mass, and height at the withers and hocks. Age may also play a role, because the mortality of lambs from yearling ewes is extremely high. Higher-ranking males concentrate on courting females when in rut and do not graze to the extent lower-ranking rams do. Groups of 40–50 ewes/adult ram and 25–30 ewes/juvenile ram are common management choices. Mortality in rams is five times that in ewes. Generally, subordinates and lower-ranking rams are excluded from breeding, unless lower-ranking animals outnumber the higher-ranking male and serve to distract or otherwise occupy him (this need not be cooperative). While the higher-ranking male usually has larger horns, the role of the demographic environment (ie, the number of lower-ranking males in the group) prevents an extreme selection response for these secondary sex characteristics.

In large groups of sheep or in sheep on large pastures, more subordinates are likely to mate. In tightly confined, relatively small groups, the role the social order plays in mating is critical, and owners should understand that lower-ranking rams may not mate under such conditions.

Sheep are seasonally polyestrous and reach puberty at 7–12 mo. Mating behavior includes nudging, kicking, or pawing with the front legs, low stretching, and pushing. These same behaviors and head-to-head banging with horn clashing occur in conflicts between males.

Artificial weaning occurs at 10 wk of age, but these lambs recognize and will return to the ewes after a 2-mo separation. Sheep are naturally weaned at 6 mo of age, usually when their mother again comes into heat. Ewe lambs continue to follow the dam, but ram lambs do not.

Sheep are likely to be more intelligent than generally regarded. They respond readily to food calls, may problem solve, learn their names, carry packs, and can even be clicker trained. Sheep may be grazed on open, unfenced areas and may heft (remain in home field) to a limited area as a learned behavior by lambs from their ewes. Sheep possess specialized neural mechanisms in the right temporal and frontal lobes of the brain and may recognize familiar human or ovine faces for as long as 2 yr.

BEHAVIORAL PROBLEMS

Homosexuality: Homosexuality is a normal behavior in sheep and is seen in up to 30% of all rams. Incidence of homosexuality is decreased in rams raised in heterosexual groups and in rams that have experience with ewes, but it still persists. It is unclear to what extent such behaviors are facilitated by a sex ratio that has been skewed for mating purposes.

Lamb Stealing: Ewes can steal the lambs of others before their own parturition and then reject their own lamb when it is born. Lambs seek out soft, warm, hairless areas (regardless of where they are), which can help with raising orphaned lambs but render *stealing easier.* Individual pens or partial barriers can usually prevent theft. Ewes will sequester the lambs at first, and providing them a shelter where this can be done will help. The smell of the wool is important to the ewe for individual lamb recognition, as is the shape and color of the lamb's head. Ewes are more likely to accept lambs that have familiar head coloration.

Lamb Rejection: Lamb rejection can be associated with the social hierarchy or due to behavioral, physiologic, or environmental stresses (eg, rain) at delivery. The smell of the wool is important to the ewe, and lambs that smell unfamiliar are more likely to be rejected. Experimental results show that lambs whose heads have been altered are at risk of rejection. Alteration of the tail does not have the same effect. If the rejection is noted sufficiently early, using a stanchion to confine the ewe with the lamb can address the problem. Tranquilization may be needed.

Cross-fostering: Cross-fostering can be a successful solution for abandoned, rejected, or orphaned lambs. Cross-fostering is best addressed by fooling the ewe, using cervical stimulation (using balloons that stimulate oxytocin release and maternal behavior). Covering the lamb to be fostered with a t-shirt that the ewe's own lamb has worn can provide an appropriate olfactory cue, as can the skin of the ewe's own dead lamb.

Stereotypic Behaviors: In sheep, stereotypic behaviors include wool-sucking, intersucking, and self-sucking (tails or udder).

GOATS

SOCIAL BEHAVIOR

Social behavior in goats is similar to that in sheep, and horns also play a major factor in caprine social rankings. Goats also hide early in life but, unlike cows, spend more time away from the nannies for the first 6 wk than for the next 6 wk. The nanny initiates early approaches, and the kid initiates the later ones. Sexual behavior of goats differs slightly from that of sheep. Billy goats throw their head up in the air and ventroflex their neck when they ejaculate. They also frequently urinate on their front legs, which they then rub on the doe as part of the courtship ritual. The scent of female urine is important and is transported into the vomeronasal organ during flehmen.

BEHAVIORAL PROBLEMS

Behavioral problems are not commonly reported in goats, perhaps because adult males are expected to charge people if their turf is traversed. Behavioral problems may actually be more rare (as opposed to less frequently reported) in this group, because their maintenance conditions more closely mimic those in a free-ranging situation. Domestication may have had less of an impact on the social patterns of goats than is true for other species.

Self-suckling: Goats that abort late in pregnancy or those that have a second pregnancy subsequent to nursing can self-suckle. The latter situation may be illuminating, because the behavior did not occur when the nanny was nursing. Treatment involves behavioral and environmental enrichment, social companionship that is stable before pregnancy, and possibly some antianxiety medications.

Stereotypic Behaviors: Stereotypic behaviors in goats are similar to those in sheep (*see* above). Goats separated from a group may develop competitive "rearing" or elevation.

CHICKENS

SOCIAL BEHAVIOR

Free-ranging chickens are social animals. In these groups, hens and chicks are the core, while roosters live independently. Social maturity occurs at ~1 yr of age, although most chickens are sent to slaughter before this age. Free-ranging chickens show more aggressive behaviors than battery chickens do. Rank is based on multiple factors (eg, size, age, color, and social environment). A new or foreign chicken is lower in rank than a chicken on home ground. Both nesting and food intake are genetically controlled behaviors, and chickens are selected for high food intake. Hens will form nests if supplied with nesting material. An adult chicken that has never used a nesting box will use one if provided.

BEHAVIORAL PROBLEMS

Aggression and feather pecking or plucking are the two most common behavioral problems in chickens. They may be related and possibly have similar underlying components, including stress, overcrowding, and competition over resources such as food. Both conditions can be managed by addressing the underlying problem and in some cases by removing the instigator. Providing enrichment and changing the social structure by removing or adding individuals may help as well. In rare cases, aggression can advance to cannibalism (*see* p 2873). Broilers and free-ranging chickens are more likely to show these problems because egg-laying chickens in mass production are usually confined to small groups.

Aggression can manifest as pecking at the head and face or as pecking at and pulling feathers. Chickens have sharp and strong beaks that may lead to severe injuries. Reducing daylight in battery conditions, adding tryptophan to the food, and beak trimming can minimize aggression. Beak trimming is a symptomatic treatment, however, and may raise welfare concerns.

Grooming and feather care are part of normal hygiene in chickens and can also be social activities. Dust baths can help reduce the incidence of feather picking.

DOGS

SOCIAL BEHAVIOR

The dog's social structure has been referred to as a pack hierarchy, but this does not accurately or entirely describe the relationship of dogs with other dogs or with people.

Scientific studies into the behavior of wild wolves have established that the wolf pack is actually a family unit, with the adult parents guiding the activities of the group. The dog likely originated from the grey wolf 12,000–14,000 yr ago, although the origins of domestication may extend back 30,000 yr. Communication and relationships are established through a language of visual signals (body postures, facial expressions, tail and ear carriage, and piloerection), vocalization, scents, and pheromones. However, domestication and selective breeding have led to extensive variation not only from wolf to dog but also between breeds and individuals in morphology, breed traits, temperament, behavior problems, variation in behavioral neoteny, and social signaling. In fact, Huskies retain most of the social signaling repertoire of wolves, German Shepherds less than ⅔, and Cavalier King Charles Spaniels the least. Thus, it may be difficult for dogs (and people) to read and interpret the signals of other dogs, especially those of different breeds. Early and frequent socialization with a wide variety of dogs is therefore an important component of intraspecific communication.

The term dominance (*see* p 1536) does not describe the relationship between two individuals; it is a relative term established by the value of the resource to each individual and the cumulative effects of learning.

Hierarchy in dogs is neither static nor linear, because the motivation to obtain and retain a specific resource, together with previous learning, defines the relationship between two individuals for each encounter. Stability is maintained by deference and not by agonistic behaviors. Only in those relationships in which one individual consistently defers to another across resources and interactions might a linear hierarchical relationship between the individuals be described. Although this terminology applies to the intraspecific communication and signaling between members of a species (eg, dog-dog), it does not "translate" to communication between species (eg, dogs-people).

Relationships with people are not established by dominant/submissive social signaling; they are a result of genetics, early handling, and socialization and shaped by learning and consequences. In fact, dogs have acquired an ability and readiness to respond to human behavior not found in wolves, even if the wolf pup is hand raised and socialized. In turn, dog owners must learn to read canine visual signaling and vocalization to understand when dogs want to engage and when they do not, as well as to train and reward relaxation and to safely and effectively modify fearful and aggressive behaviors.

Canine Development

The first important period of development is the neonatal period, which extends into the third week of life. Puppies are born with closed eyes and limited motor ability. Puppies are altricial; therefore, in the first few weeks, maternal care is critical. Grooming by the mother arouses the puppy to eat, stimulates elimination, and helps to keep the puppies in the nest. Good maternal care results in an increased ability to handle stress and increased maturation of the nervous system. Similarly, mild stress in the form of gentle human handling during the first 2 wk of life can improve cardiovascular performance and resistance to disease. Handled puppies also mature faster, perform better in problem-solving tasks, and are better able to withstand stress as adults. In contrast, moderate to severe prenatal and neonatal stress as well as maternal separation can have a sensitizing effect on the hypothalamic-pituitary-adrenal axis. Feeding the bitch a diet enhanced with docosahexaenoic acid during the neonatal and prenatal periods has been shown to improve the puppy's brain and retinal development and trainability.

Between the neonatal and socialization period is a transition period, during which the eyes open and puppies begin to develop motor skills. At this time, interactions with littermates are important for development of social skills.

The next period of development (socialization or sensitive period) extends from 3–4 wk to ~12 wk of age. During this period, the puppy is most sociable and will most readily habituate to dogs, people, other animals, and the environment (sights, sounds, odor, touch, taste). Between 3 and 8 wk of age, puppies start exploring their environment and continue to refine social skills with their littermates and other dogs. Weaning is normally completed at 7 wk of age, and at ~8 wk of age puppies start developing a preference for elimination locations.

As the socialization period winds down, puppies make attachments less easily. Therefore, a lack of adequate socialization and enrichment during the sensitive period can contribute to excessive responses to stimuli, including fear and aggression. Spending the first 7–8 wk with the mother and littermates plays an important role in the development of social skills with other dogs. However, if exposure to people, other pets, and new environments does not begin before the end of the socialization period, the dog may become socially maladjusted and unable to cope and communicate. Proper development of social skills can be accomplished in part by adopting puppies into the new home at ~8 wk of age and enrolling in puppy socialization classes before 12 wk of age, so that the puppy can be exposed to a range of dogs, people, and other stimuli (eg, novel surfaces, noises, odors, moving objects, uniforms, and handling) in a controlled, instructional, and positive environment. Similarly, visits to the veterinarian or groomer, car rides, visitors to the home, and the use of sound desensitization recordings provide additional opportunities for exposure. Dog appeasing pheromone and the presence of another dog may also ease adoption into a new home. If there are any signs of fear, every effort should be made to overcome the fear by finding the limits (threshold) the dog will tolerate and using food and treats or toys to try to ensure a positive outcome. Continued exposure to a wide variety of stimuli with positive outcomes should be continued to adulthood.

The third (juvenile) period extends from ~3 mo to 1 yr of age. Domestic dogs reach sexual maturity at 6–9 mo (later in some giant breeds) and social maturity at 12–36 mo of age. Social relationships are established to minimize conflicts within the group. Although heredity and previous socialization play important roles in the behavior of an individual, positive exposure to a wide range of animate and inanimate stimuli during this period should minimize development of fear and anxiety.

Domestic dogs are nonseasonal breeders and have on average two heat cycles/yr (range one to four). If the female does not get pregnant, she will go through hormonal changes as if she were pregnant, known as false pregnancy or pseudocyesis, which can be associated with overt physiologic and behavioral changes, including lactation, nesting, and protective aggression of objects such as toys.

Counseling to Prevent Undesirable Behaviors

Veterinarians and staff should work with breeders, trainers, pet stores, and shelters to ensure that the newly adopted dog gets off to the right start. For puppies, this includes advice on socialization, normal canine behaviors (eg, jumping up, play biting, elimination) and how they can be managed, a household environment that provides appealing but safe outlets for all of the dog's behavioral needs (eg, chewing, social play, object play, rest), guidance on canine communication, and learning principles of reinforcement-based training. The goal should be to reinforce desirable behaviors and to ignore or prevent undesirable behaviors. Clicker training can be particularly useful to immediately mark and reward desirable behavior and gradually shape behaviors that more closely approximate the final outcome (duration, relaxation).

Oral behaviors are a common problem, because puppies have a behavioral need for exploration and play. Therefore, providing constructive social activities that do not include mouthing or biting of people, such as tug games, retrieving, walking and running, chasing, hide and seek, playing with other dogs, and training for rewards, gives the dog something positive on which to focus. A head halter is also an option for better control of the head and muzzle. Another way to manage oral stimulation and exploration is to provide chew toys, food-stuffed toys, and food-dispensing toys. When the puppy cannot be effectively supervised, the household should be set up to ensure success (and avoid failure). Preventing undesirable behaviors while providing the dog with options acceptable to the owners and the dog gives the dog control to make choices, reduces uncertainty and anxiety, and prevents undesirable behaviors. Of particular value to establish a safe haven is a crate, exercise pen, or room to provide security and safety for the dog when it cannot be supervised or wants to be alone. A daily routine can be established that provides stability and predictability for the dog, beginning with meeting the dog's social and physical needs, followed by sessions of inattention during which the dog is given the opportunity to nap and rest or to engage in exploratory play with its food and chew toys. By confining the dog to a crate, pen, or room during these "inattention" times, the dog learns to spend time on its own; this also may prevent damage to property, housesoiling, and even separation anxiety. Undesirable behavior might alternatively be prevented through environmental management (eg, child gate, shutting doors, tie downs, deterrent devices). Neutering males may also help to prevent testosterone-influenced behaviors such as urine marking, mounting, and roaming.

BEHAVIORAL PROBLEMS

When behavior of dogs is undesirable, there are three levels of consideration: 1) Behaviors within the normal range for the species, age, and breed. In these cases, the owners need guidance on how to effectively manage the behaviors. 2) Behaviors more difficult or challenging, because they might fall within or just beyond the range of what is considered normal but are particularly intense or difficult to manage. Examples include mouthing, urine marking, mounting, barking, chasing, predation, or overactivity. Also in this category might be what could be normal for the breed but unsuitable for the family and home (ie, mismatch). These cases require behavior assessment and counseling to ensure the owners have a realistic understanding of what might be achieved and to implement treatment strategies, including environmental management and behavior modification, to achieve an acceptable level of improvement for both the owners and the pet. 3) Behaviors that are abnormal or pathologic, as a result of emotional disorders or mental health issues. These may have developed as a result of genetic factors, stressful perinatal environment (prenatal, neonatal), insufficient early socialization, medical conditions affecting brain health and development, or particularly traumatic environmental events. For these pets, the prognosis may be guarded, and owner expectations altered to achieve an acceptable outcome. Treatment generally requires both environmental management and behavioral modification, often in combination with medication (natural products, diet, drugs) to improve underlying pathology and facilitate learning.

The process to diagnose behavior problems and their treatment with behavior modification and drugs has been previously described (*see* p 1539). If the problem is determined to be a normal but undesirable behavior, the owners will need counseling on how to effectively provide for the pet's needs and how to reinforce what is desirable while preventing what is undesirable. For most canine behavior management problems, counseling from veterinary staff or trainers and quality resources are required, as well as hands-on guidance from a trainer. Trainers should be selected based on their credentials and screened to ensure they use reinforcement-based training techniques. Positive punishment–based techniques should not be used in training, because at best they serve only to suppress undesirable behavior and can lead to fear, avoidance, and even aggression. Management issues include inappropriate play (eg, nipping or mouthing of people); unruly behavior (eg, pulling, lunging, jumping up, mounting, overactivity); and some forms of barking, destructive behaviors, and housesoiling.

If the problem is determined to be an emotional disorder or abnormal behavior, resolution will require a combination of behavior modification techniques, modifications to the environment to prevent further problems, and medications to help reestablish a more normal mental state and facilitate new learning (*see* p 1539).

Fears and Phobias

Fear is a normal response to an actual or perceived threatening stimulus or situation. Anxiety is a response to fear and agitation, or apprehension when the animal anticipates a threat or fearful situation. Phobia is an exaggerated fear response (*see* p 1536). The fear response may include panting and salivation, tucked tail, lowered ears, gazing away, low body posture, piloerection, vocalization, or displacement behaviors such as yawning or lip licking. While avoidance and escape is one strategy, some dogs use aggression to remove the fear-evoking stimulus and are reinforced by success (negative reinforcement).

Some of the more common presentations include the following: 1) fear of other dogs, especially those that are unfamiliar, appear threatening to the dog, or with which the dog has had an unpleasant experience; 2) fear of unfamiliar people, especially those who are novel or look, act, or smell different than those the dog is accustomed to (eg, young children); 3) fear of inanimate stimuli such as loud or unfamiliar noises (eg, construction work, trucks, gunshot), visual stimuli (eg, umbrellas, hats, uniforms), environments (eg, backyard, park, boarding kennel), surfaces (eg, grass, tile or wood floors, steps), or a combination of stimuli (eg, vacuum cleaners, car rides); and 4) fear of specific situations such as veterinary clinics or grooming parlors. Some dogs have a more generalized anxiety, in which the fearful reaction is displayed in a wide range of situations to which a "normal" pet would be unlikely to react. Although there can be a genetic component to fear and anxiety, prenatal and neonatal stressors, including maternal separation, lack of socialization (ie, unfamiliarity), or a previous unpleasant outcome during encounters with the stimulus (or similar stimuli), can also be causative factors.

Phobic responses in dogs are generally associated with loud noises (eg, thunder, fireworks, gunshots) and the stimuli associated with these events, including rain, lightning, and perhaps even static or pressure changes associated with a thunderstorm. Some fears (eg, veterinary clinics, going outdoors, entering certain rooms, or walking on certain types of flooring) may become so intense that they meet the definition of a phobia.

Separation Anxiety: It is estimated that ~14% of dogs have separation anxiety, or an inability of the pet to find comfort when separated from family members. The problem may be primary (eg, hyperattachment, dysfunctional attachment) as the puppy ages and matures; in fact, the chances of the problem developing can be reduced by having puppies regularly spend time during the day on their own (preferably in a safe haven). In other cases, the anxiety about being left alone is secondary to an event such as a change in the household or dog's daily routine, or associated with an underlying state of anxiety along with other behavioral issues such as noise phobias and separation anxiety. Anxiety may lead to destructive behavior (particularly at exits or toward owner possessions), distress vocalization, housesoiling, salivation, pacing, restlessness, inability to settle, anorexia, and repetitive or compulsive behaviors. The behaviors are exhibited when the dog is left alone and generally arise within the first 15–30 min after departure. A video recording can be an invaluable diagnostic aid to visualize the behavior and determine whether there are other concurrent signs of anxiety (autonomic stimulation, increased motor activity, and increased vigilance and scanning). The diagnosis requires that other common causes of the signs be excluded (eg, incomplete housetraining, exploratory play and scavenging, external stimuli leading to arousal and anxiety, noise aversion, or confinement anxiety). Many pets with separation anxiety begin to exhibit signs as the owner prepares to depart (eg, putting on shoes, getting keys, going to the door). When the owner is home, the dog may crave constant contact or proximity to the owner. When the owner returns, the welcoming responses are commonly exaggerated and the dog is hard to calm down.

Abnormal Repetitive Behaviors

Abnormal repetitive behaviors may actually comprise a number of conditions with different pathogeneses, including compulsive disorders, stereotypies, neurologic disorders, and other forms of behavioral pathology. Therefore, until a diagnosis is made, the term abnormal repetitive behavior may better describe the clinical presentation.

Compulsive disorders may be repetitive, stereotypic, locomotory, grooming, ingestive, or hallucinogenic behaviors that occur out of context to the time and situation in which they take place, and occur in a frequency or duration that is excessive. There may be lack of control over onset or termination. Although it can be debated whether animals can obsess, they do perceive and experience concern; therefore, the term obsessive-compulsive has also been used to describe this disorder. The diagnosis should start with a description and observation of the behavior, including video recordings if necessary. Because there is likely a genetic component for many compulsive disorders, the signalment and age of onset is also important. For example, German Shepherds and Bull Terriers are known to spin or tail chase, while a genetic locus for flank sucking has been identified in Doberman Pinschers. The problem may first arise as a displacement behavior when the dog is frustrated, conflicted, or highly aroused. Lack of predictability in the daily routine, alterations in the environment, unpredictable consequences, lack of sufficient outlets for normal behaviors, and chronic or recurrent anxiety might be initiating factors. At this point, if the owners can teach appropriate acceptable alternative responses (eg, sitting before greeting or play as an alternative to spinning) and provide constructive alternatives (eg, feeding from toys), the problem might be resolved. However, as the frequency or intensity increases, the behavior may become compulsive. The diagnosis is considered to be a compulsive disorder when the behavior interferes with normal function or when it becomes independent of (or emancipated from) the inciting stimulus. There is likely altered serotonin transmission.

Stereotypies are defined as repetitive behaviors that are unvaried in sequence and have no obvious purpose or function. They may arise when the environment lacks sufficient outlets for the dog to engage in normal behaviors, or when caused by maternal deprivation or as a result of a neurologic disorder. It is possible that stereotypic behaviors, at least in their early stages, may provide a coping mechanism for the pet. Stereotypies might be induced by dopaminergic stimulation.

Although most dogs respond to drugs that inhibit serotonin reuptake including the SSRIs and clomipramine, alterations in other neurotransmitters may play a role, eg, dopamine, endorphins, *N*-methyl-D-aspartic acid (NMDA). Because medical problems might be the cause of the signs, these should first be excluded. In cases in which the physical examination, history, and diagnostic testing do not clearly identify the cause, a therapeutic response trial might be indicated (eg, anticonvulsants to exclude focal seizures as a cause of fly snapping or light chasing; clomipramine or fluoxetine to exclude compulsive disorders). *See also* TABLE 4.

Aggression

Aggression is the most common problem in referral practices across North America, approximating 70% of the caseload. It is also a major human concern, because at least 5 million people are referred to the hospital each year in the USA alone for treatment of dog bites. Most forms of aggression, except for predation, are

TABLE 4 CLINICAL PRESENTATION AND MEDICAL DIFFERENTIALS FOR COMPULSIVE DISORDERS

Compulsive Disorder Signs	Medical Differentials	Diagnostic Tests / Therapeutic Trials
Ingestive: pica, licking, sucking, swallowing (glugging)	GI, food intolerance	Endoscopy, food trial, steroid trial, GI protectants
Polyphagia, polyuria, polydipsia	Urogenital/renal, hepatic, endocrine	Blood and urine testing, hormonal assays, modified water deprivation test
Dermatologic/self-trauma: nail biting, flank sucking, acral lick dermatitis, pyschogenic alopecia, tail mutilation	Atopic dermatitis, bacterial or parasitic hypersensitivity, adverse food reaction, parasite, infection, neuropathy, pain	Dermatologic tests (eg, skin scraping, trichogram, fungal culture, biopsy), therapeutic response trial
Neurologic: spinning, star gazing, pouncing, fly snapping, light or shadow chasing	Focal seizure, neuropathy	Neurologic tests (eg, MRI), therapeutic seizure therapy trial (eg, levetiracetam, potassium bromide, phenobarbital)

distance-increasing behavior (ie, the dog is attempting to actively increase the distance between itself and the stimulus). There are many types of aggressive behaviors with different motivations; however, fear, anxiety, conflict (uncertainty), genetics, and learned responses generally play a role in most cases; however, in some cases the behavior may be abnormal or pathologic. The effects of early development (prenatal, postnatal), socialization, and previous experience all play a role in development of aggression.

Aggression refers to threatening behavior or harmful attacks and can range from subtle changes in body posture, facial expressions, and vocalization to biting. Dogs that are easily aroused are at high risk of aggression, because their decision-making is affected by their physiologic state (ie, flight or fight). For treatment to be effective, the pet's anxiety and arousal must first be managed by avoiding situations or staying below the threshold at which aggression might arise. Some or all of a combination of reward-based training, behavior products that can help to better manage the pet, and medications to help achieve a behavioral state most conducive to new learning is required to successfully modify the behavior to achieve desirable outcomes *and countercondition the* pet to the stimuli that incite aggression.

Before treating aggression, the practitioner must assess the potential risk of injury. All stimuli that might incite aggression should be accurately identified to ensure initial safety. Predictability is a critical issue in prognosis, both to prevent further incidents and to develop a stimulus gradient for treatment. The signalment, environment, history, and target of the aggression also provide invaluable information as to whether the problem might be safely and effectively managed. The type of aggression is an additional factor; some can be managed and improved, whereas others require prevention. Finally, the clinician must assess the ability of the owner to effectively and safely prevent the problem. Aggression that is unpredictable, arises during relatively benign interactions, involves targets that cannot realistically avoid exposure to the aggressive dog (eg, young children, other household pets), or is performed by a large dog or in an uninhibited manner worsens the prognosis. Any medical condition that might cause or contribute to aggression must be identified, because they are important factors in diagnosis, prognosis, and treatment. (*See* www.esvce.org for risk assessment guidelines.)

Fear-related Aggression: Fear is the underlying cause of most forms of canine aggression. It is triggered by a stimulus that is threatening to the dog. When the aggression is a direct response to a challenge or confrontation, it might be referred to as defensive aggression. Fearful dogs may try to avoid the stimulus but become aggressive if they cannot escape (eg, leashed, confined, cornered, or physically grasped), are motivated to maintain their place (eg, on property, between the owner and stimulus, near food or toy), or if they learn that aggression is successful at removing the threat. Inadequate socialization, learning, genetics (temperament), reinforcement of aggressive behavior (eg, retreat of the stimulus), and associating a negative outcome with the stimulus (eg, punishment) can all lead to the development of fear-related aggression. The diagnosis is based on identifying signs of fear as well as the history beginning with the first event, because dogs can exhibit fear at the initial exposure but with time may display a more offensive form of aggression (without threats) when they learn it can be successful. (For treatment of fear-related and other types of aggression, *see* p 1565.)

Possessive Aggression (Resource Guarding): Possessive aggression is most likely to arise when a person or an animal approaches the dog while it is in possession of something it wants to retain. Pets in the process of ingesting or chewing an object might be more likely to display aggression, but the behavior can also be seen in dogs near an object. Aggression is most commonly displayed when in possession of highly motivating food, treats, chew toys, stolen items, or even sleeping places. While genetics and early experience play a role in development, the relative value of the object to the pet and the threat of losing the object to another dog or person determine whether the pet is likely to be possessive. Items that are novel or scarce may be more desirable. Fear and defensive behavior also play a role if the owners threaten, punish, or confront the pet when it takes an object or has it in its mouth. The dog may also learn that it can successfully retain the object with aggression.

The problem might be prevented by tossing the puppy high-value treats whenever the owner approaches or passes by the food bowl, and by offering a high-value treat or toy whenever the puppy voluntarily gives up another toy or chew. Food bowls, toys, and chews should not be removed by confrontation, because this can contribute to an increase in anxiety and aggression when approached. In adult dogs, the problem should be managed by preventing access to these items or confining the dog when it is given items over which it might be possessive and by training the dog to give and drop on cue (beginning with items of low value for high-value rewards). If safety is an issue (ie, the dog may hurt itself by chewing on the item), it may be possible to trade the object for one of higher value. Providing more toys and multiple small meals (eg, in feeding toys) may reduce the value and novelty of the resource.

Play Aggression: Aggressive play is a normal puppy behavior, which may persist into adulthood as a result of genetics, neotinization, and learning. When puppies play aggressively with other puppies, they may nip and bite but will generally resolve the conflicts among themselves. However, if the problem becomes excessive, owner intervention may be required to redirect the dog's activities into other forms of play (eg, feeding toys) or to interrupt the behavior with commands or a leash and head halter. If play with people escalates to biting, the interaction can be immediately stopped (negative punishment) and resumed when oral play ceases (positive reinforcement). Alternatively, a leash and head halter or verbal distraction ("off") can be used to interrupt play biting. In all interactions, the puppy should be taught to sit before given anything of value (eg, food, toys, affection). In addition, the puppy should be engaged in regular alternative acceptable forms of play, including fetch, tug games, and manipulation and chew toys. Punishment should not be used to stop play, because it can lead to fear of the owner, defensive aggression, or conflict-induced aggression, or serve as inadvertent reinforcement for some puppies.

Redirected Aggression: Aggression is directed toward a third party when the dog is prevented or unable to exhibit aggression to its primary target. This type of aggression is most commonly described when the dog bites the owner as he or she grasps or restrains the dog when trying to prevent or break up a dog fight. Similarly, dogs that might be aggressive toward a veterinarian might bite the person restraining the dog. Redirected aggression arises as a result of the frustration or interruption of other forms of aggression or arousal.

Irritable/Conflict/Impulse Control Aggression: Aggression directed toward family members is often mislabeled as dominance or status-related aggression. However, aggression toward family members generally arises from fearful or defensive behaviors, resource guarding, redirected behavior, or situations of conflict (competing emotional states and unpredictable consequences). In some dogs, the problem may be traced back to the owner's attempts to inhibit excessive play aggression (*see* above).

When a dog successfully uses aggression to achieve a goal (retaining a resource) or remove a threat, the pet learns that aggression is successful (negative reinforcement). If the owner continues to threaten, confront, challenge, or punish the pet, some dogs may inhibit their responses, but a large proportion become more aggressively defensive. When dogs are resting or sleeping, chewing on a favored object, or no longer desirous of human affection, they may respond with either deferent displays or threats. However, if the owner continues to approach, tries to remove the resource, or attempts to pet the dog despite its signaling, aggression may escalate and future signaling may be lost. The owner-pet relationship can quickly deteriorate as the dog becomes more wary and defensive while the owner becomes more fearful and/or confrontational.

Genetic factors and early experience likely also play a role; many of these dogs are easily aroused, excessively fearful, or may have emotional disorders or behavioral pathology (*see* below). Other cases are primarily a result of learning. Aggression when grabbing the collar or during bathing, nail trimming, or ear cleaning is a defensive response. Interrupting a pet that is aroused may lead to redirected aggression. Therefore, when a dog is presented for aggression toward family members, it can be difficult to determine the dog's underlying motivation because each incident has added to prior learning, fear conditioning, and underlying conflict. Dominance might refer to the relationship between two individuals of the same species within a social group, as described by actions, interactions, and intraspecific communication/signaling. These relationships are not established by aggression of the dominant individual but rather by the deferent signaling of others. Relationships between species, particularly dogs and people, are established through early socialization, the personality of the individual, and what it learns from its observations and interactions with family members. Physical techniques intended to assert dominance (eg, pinning, rolling over) and verbal discipline (yelling "no") are therefore ill advised and can result in fear, anxiety, and further aggression.

Dogs with impulse control aggression may respond with aggression to relatively benign interactions with family members. In some lines of English Cocker Spaniels and English Springer Spaniels, this aggression is associated with alterations in serotonin in blood samples or CSF.

When aggression is excessive, unpredictable, and disproportionate to the level of threat, safety is a serious concern and the prognosis generally guarded. However, when behavior is abnormal or pathologic, substantial improvement might be achieved with a combination of drugs (eg, SSRIs) and behavior modification.

Aggression Toward Other Dogs: Dogs in the same group or household usually avoid conflict without aggression. Communication is based on dominant and submissive signals, with the deference of one of the two individuals to avoid escalation of the encounter. Dominance is a relative concept— the dog that displays deferent signaling may vary between resources and situations. Aggression between individuals living in the same household is generally an abnormal behavior caused by fear and anxiety, redirected aggression, impulse dyscontrol, or poor intraspecific communication skills as a result of genetics or lack of early socialization and compounded by experience and learning. Redirected aggression and competition over a valued resource may also lead to aggression between dogs in the home.

Owners may play a role by inadvertently supporting or encouraging a dog during an encounter in which it would normally defer. Age or illness may also play a role, if the way in which one dog signals or responds to the other is altered. Male-to-male aggression may have underlying hormonal factors that can be improved by neutering; however, learning may play a role in maintaining aggression.

If any situations arise in which the dogs are unable to resolve conflicts without aggression or injury, behavioral guidance should be sought. Aggression toward unfamiliar dogs and those that are not members of the family group are likely fearful, possessive, protective, or territorial.

Territorial/Protective Aggression: Aggression may be displayed when the dog is approached in its territory. Territory can be stationary (eg, yard, home) or mobile (eg, car). What defines the behavior as territorial is that the dog does not display fear to similar stimuli when outside its territory. Fear, anxiety, defensive, and possessive behaviors may all be components, because the pet is most likely to display the behavior toward unfamiliar stimuli, and the motivation to escape or avoid (flight) is decreased or absent when the pet is on its own property. Learning (negative reinforcement when the stimulus retreats) and fear conditioning (unpleasant outcomes such as yelling, discipline, and confinement) can also play a role.

Predatory Aggression: This is one of the most dangerous types of aggression, because there is usually no warning. The attack is intended to kill prey, and the bite is uninhibited. The sequence of events may include stalking, chasing, biting, and killing. Young children and babies may be at risk because their size and behaviors mimic those of prey. Although extensive socialization to a species might reduce predation toward that species, the behavior may be enhanced when predatory individuals are together in a group. Predation is a normal and dangerous canine behavior; thus, any dog that exhibits the behavior must be prevented from opportunities to repeat it.

Pain-induced and Medical Causes of Aggression: Any disease that causes pain or increases irritability (eg, dental disease, arthritis, trauma, allergies) can lead to aggression. The dog may become aggressive when it is handled or anticipates handling. Organ dysfunction (eg, renal, hepatic), CNS disease, and endocrinopathies (eg, hyperadrenocorticism, functional testicular and ovarian tumors, and thyroid dysfunction) might also contribute to irritability and aggression. (*See also* TABLE 2.) While hypothyroidism is more likely associated with lethargy, dermatologic signs, and heat seeking in the early stages, it has been suggested that dogs might display an increase in aggression, particularly toward family members. Treatment should likely be reserved for cases in which diagnostic tests are also consistent with hypothyroidism, because excessive supplementation could lead to a hyperthyroid state (with associated medical and behavioral consequences). Treating the medical problem may resolve the aggression, but the behavior, once learned, may persist.

Maternal Aggression: Maternal aggression may be seen in intact females with a litter of puppies or in females with pseudocyesis. It can be directed toward people or other animals. Signs of aggression arise when the bitch's puppies or toys that mimic puppies are protected, and the aggression should resolve when the hormonal state returns to normal and/or the puppies are weaned. The term maternal aggression has also been used to describe the aggression or cannibalism directed toward the puppies by the bitch. Although the problem may have a genetic component, it is reported to occur more frequently after a first litter. Ovariohysterectomy can prevent further incidents.

Treatment of Fears, Phobias, Anxiety, and Aggression

Before implementing specific therapy to manage, improve, or resolve a behavior problem, some common elements that apply to most cases should be considered. The initial discussion should focus on 1) an understanding of normal behavior as it relates to the problem, 2) learning to read canine body language and facial expressions, 3) ensuring that all of the dog's needs are adequately being met, 4) reviewing the principles of learning and reinforcement-based training (predictable consequences), and 5) managing both the environment and the dog to prevent further incidents. The cause, diagnosis, and motivation behind the behavior should be reviewed. Finally, the owner should be given a prognosis with realistic expectations for both short- and longterm outcomes.

In most cases, treatment focuses on changing the dog's emotional response with the stimulus (counterconditioning) and/or replacing the undesirable response with one that is desirable using reinforcement-based techniques (response substitution). However, dogs that are highly aroused respond with autonomic fight-or-flight responses and tend to make reflexive responses. Therefore, arousal must be reduced before treatment can proceed. This can be achieved by training the dog to settle on cue, by minimizing the intensity of the stimulus during exposure (desensitization), or by using management devices such as head halters that can change the dog's focus and help it to settle, and with drugs or natural products that reduce anxiety and behavioral pathology. Early intervention with medication may be necessary to achieve success and can be in the best interest of the fearful, anxious, or phobic dog.

There are common elements to the treatment of fear, anxiety, phobias, and most types of aggression. The first step in the treatment program is to identify each situation stimulus or interaction in which the problem might arise, so that a preventive program can first be implemented. Prevention ensures safety (eg, in aggression cases), prevents further damage to the household or injury to the dog, avoids further anxiety-evoking situations for the dog, and ensures no further aggravation of the problem through fear conditioning (ie, unpleasant outcomes) and learning (ie, negative reinforcement if the stimulus retreats).

Prevention can be most effectively achieved by identifying and avoiding any situation in which the dog might be exposed to the stimulus. A leash and head harness, leash and body harness, or verbal commands (when effective) can also prevent access to the stimulus. If avoidance cannot be ensured and aggression is a possibility, then a basket muzzle might be the best alternative.

A common starting point to begin to reduce anxiety, improve communication and training, teach self-control, and allow the dog to control its consequences/outcomes is to establish a program of structured interactions in which the dog is not given anything it values (or wants) until it sits (or lies down). If the owners' response is consistent and predictable by ensuring the dog sits (or lies down) every time a treat (food or toy) is given, the leash is attached, the dog goes in and out of the door or car, or the dog wants affection, the dog will soon learn that the sit or down action is required to get the reward, at which point gradually longer and more relaxed responses can be taught. This is sometimes termed structured interactions, predictable consequences, learn to earn, or "saying please."

Because the ultimate goal is to successfully expose the dog to controlled levels of the stimuli while achieving calm and positive outcomes, it is necessary to determine what behaviors need to be trained to achieve desirable outcomes during exposure training. For example, if problems arise indoors, the dog may first need to learn a focused sit, a relaxed down, and a mat command (or other location such as room or crate). A drop or give command and a come or recall may also need to be trained. When problems arise outdoors, sit and focus or down and settle may also be useful, but loose leash walking, backing up, or turning and walking away may be the best options for stimulus exposure. These behaviors should be learned *reliably* and *consistently* in a variety of environments with a minimum of distractions before the owners proceed to a graduated stimulus exposure (*see* p 1540 and p 1542).

By identifying a range (gradient) of the dog's most favored rewards, the most desirable can be used for training and shaping new behaviors that approximate the final goal; less-motivating rewards can then be used to ensure immediacy and timing of previously learned commands. In addition, a way to minimize and control the intensity of the stimulus will also need to be designed (eg, volume, distance, location). Exposure exercises can then be implemented by setting up situations in which high-value rewards are used to reinforce the desired behavior and condition a positive response during exposure to low-intensity stimuli and gradually proceeding through more intense stimuli. Setbacks can be avoided by determining the level of stimulus intensity at which a calm and positive outcome can be achieved and reinforced, and with the use of management devices such as a head halter (sit, reorient head, turn and walk away) or front control body harness (turn away from the situation) to ensure safety and success. Drugs and natural therapeutics might be used concurrently in dogs with excessively intense or abnormal behaviors to enable the successful implementation of behavior modification.

For noise phobias, controlled exposure can best be achieved through recordings that can be gradually increased after each successful session of desensitization and counterconditioning. Concurrent behavioral management to reduce stimuli (with sound proofing, ear covers, eye covers, crate covers, or white noise) and develop a safe haven to help the dog settle might also help the dog to cope. For separation anxiety, once a regular routine of play, exercise, and training is established, any additional reinforcement should focus on shaping gradually longer inattention sessions when the dog rests or occupies itself with favored chew and food- or treat-filled toys, ideally in a comfortable safe haven (bed, crate, or room) where the owners can house the dog while gradually increasing their time away. Any attention- or affection-soliciting behavior should be ignored, unless the dog is sitting or lying down calmly (sit for all interactions) or resting on its bed or mat. Visual and auditory cues that signal departure should be avoided if possible; alternatively, they can be decoupled from departure by exposing the dog while remaining home, and associating with play and treats (counterconditioning). In addition to preventive and environmental management strategies and behavior modification, drugs or natural therapeutics can be used to reduce underlying fear, anxiety, arousal, reactivity, or impulse dyscontrol to help facilitate learning; to improve underlying behavioral pathology; and in many cases to improve the behavioral well-being of the dog.

For impulsivity, generalized anxiety disorders, excessive stimulus anxiety, and phobias, selective serotonin reuptake inhibitors (SSRIs) and tricyclic antidepressants (TCAs) are commonly used. Because fluoxetine has been evaluated in and licensed for dogs, it is generally the first choice of the SSRIs, although fluvoxamine, sertraline, paroxetine, and citalopram might be alternatives when fluoxetine is insufficiently effective or adverse effects such as anorexia are an issue. SSRIs are also used to treat compulsive disorders. Among the TCAs, clomipramine is licensed for use in dogs and is an alternative to fluoxetine for the treatment of anxiety disorders and phobias. Because clomipramine is the most selective of the TCAs to inhibit serotonin reuptake, it could be used for compulsive disorders, as an alternative to SSRIs. Other TCAs might be selected for their more potent antihistaminic effects (eg, doxepin, amitriptyline), whereas imipramine has been used as an aid in improving sphincter control with behavioral incontinence. Although the full effect might not be achieved for 3–4 wk, some effect might be noted in the first week. For some compulsive disorders, especially those in which there is a self-traumatic component, gabapentin or carbamazepine might be used concurrently, whereas in those cases in which focal seizures might be causing the behavioral signs, levetiracetam, phenobarbital, or potassium bromide might be used in a therapeutic response trial.

When an anxiety-evoking event can be predicted (eg, thunderstorms, fireworks, owner departure, visit to the veterinarian, car ride, exposure to dogs or strangers on a walk, visitors coming to the home), a benzodiazepine can be given with the antidepressant ~1 hr before the event. Because benzodiazepines have variable effects and relatively short half-lives, their efficacy, dose, and duration should be determined in advance of their therapeutic use. Clonidine, trazodone, or propranolol are other options that might be used adjunctively with SSRIs ~1 hr before an expected fear-evoking event (eg, thunder, fireworks, owner departure). In some refractory anxiety cases, trazodone, clonidine, a benzodiazepine such as clonazepam, or perhaps gabapentin might be used concurrently with an SSRI.

Buspirone, a nonsedating anxiolytic, is another option for ongoing use. Caution should be exercised when using anxiolytics, because some may disinhibit fearful dogs, which could lead to increased confidence and aggression.

Selegiline, which is licensed in North America for treatment of cognitive dysfunction syndrome in dogs, is also licensed for treatment of emotional disorders or chronic anxiety in Europe.

Natural products might be used alone or adjunctively with drugs or other natural products to help calm or reduce anxiety, although evidence of efficacy is more limited. A number of studies support the use of pheromone therapy. Adaptil™ simulates the intermammary-appeasing pheromones produced by the lactating bitch and is available as a spray, diffuser, or collar. Pheromones have been used for anxiety associated with car rides, veterinary visits, separation anxiety, storm and fireworks aversions, and to reduce the stress of adoption and aid socialization. A calming or anxiety-modulating effect has been reported for alpha-casozepine (Zylkene®, a milk protein hydrolysate), Harmonease® (containing *Magnolia officinalis* and *Phellodendron amurense*), L-theanine (Anxitane®) and Sin-Susto™ (a *Souroubea* plant blend), and aromatherapy (with lavender). In addition, studies with L-tryptophan in combination with a low-protein diet have demonstrated a possible reduction in some forms of aggression. A commercial diet also has been developed that combines L-tryptophan and alpha-casozepine (Royal Canin Calm®) that might aid in reducing stress and anxiety.

Hyperactivity

Although hyperactivity or attention deficit disorder has been poorly documented in dogs, there have been published case studies of dogs with excessive motor activity and an altered ability to acquire new tasks (learn), sometimes accompanied by stereotypic behaviors. It may be particularly difficult to train such dogs to behaviorally settle. There may also be signs of sympathetic activity even at rest (eg, increased heart and respiratory rate, vasodilation). Affected dogs may respond to treatment with methylphenidate. If no improvement with an initial dose of 0.25–0.5 mg/kg, bid, the dosage can be gradually increased every few days to a maximum of ~2 mg/kg until a measurable therapeutic response is seen (reduced motor activity, heart rate, respiratory rate, repetitive activities), provided no adverse effects develop. Differential diagnoses include impulse control disorders that might respond to SSRI therapy, and normal behaviors in dogs with behavioral needs that are not being adequately met. In fact, it can be quite challenging to meet these needs in some breeds and individuals, depending on the home and family.

Destructive Behaviors

Many of the destructive behaviors, including chewing, stealing, garbage raiding, and digging, are normal exploratory behaviors that arise when the dog is unsupervised and not otherwise engaged in more desirable activities. A regular daily routine with sufficient reward training, exercise, and social enrichment can help to ensure that these behaviors do not arise when the owners are home, although varying degrees of supervision may be required. When the owners cannot supervise the dog, it should be provided with adequate outlets for exploratory play in the form of chews, food-stuffed toys, or manipulation toys, or in the case of outdoor dogs, perhaps even a designated area for digging. These dogs may also need to be confined away from the areas in which problems might arise or housed in crates, pens, or runs to prevent access to potential targets of destruction. Some dogs engage in destructive behaviors because of anxiety (eg, separation anxiety, confinement, noise phobias). Together with the history, videotaping or camera monitoring is generally the best way to diagnose behavior problems that occur when the owner is absent, as well as assess response to treatment.

Eating Disorders

Behavioral problems related to ingestion include those in which food intake is excessive (polyphagia), inadequate (hyporexia), or too fast (gorging); water intake is excessive (polydipsia); and nonfood items (pica) or feces (coprophagia) are eaten. Medical causes should be excluded first. Some dogs that scavenge do so as a normal component of food acquisition and are reinforced by success. Coprophagia may occasionally have a medical cause, but normal maternal behavior includes consumption of feces and *urine of young puppies. In addition,* as part of exploratory behavior, many dogs are attracted to and may ingest feces, compost, and prey (dead or live). Similarly, although some dogs with pica and polyphagia have compulsive disorders, many dogs, especially puppies, begin to chew and ingest nonfood items as part of investigative and exploratory behavior.

Dogs with hyporexia may have an anxiety disorder, and some may develop specific taste preferences and aversions that reduce what they will eat.

Many feeding problems can be improved through a work-for-food program in which dogs are given food as reinforcers for training, with the balance placed inside toys that require chewing or manipulation to release the food. This encourages exploration, makes feeding an enjoyable, time-consuming, and mentally challenging activity, and can limit the quantity consumed and prevent gorging. As with most behavior problems, correcting feeding problems needs to be accompanied by management strategies to prevent access to potential targets at any time the dog cannot be supervised or actively engaged in other chew and play behaviors.

Elimination Behavioral Problems

Housesoiling: Dogs may soil in inappropriate locations because of inadequate or insufficient training, as a marking behavior, or as a result of fear or anxiety. However, pain, sensory decline, cerebrocortical disease including cognitive dysfunction, or any medical condition that leads to increased volume, more frequent elimination, pain on elimination, or lack of control, must first be excluded as potential causes or contributing factors.

A detailed behavioral history is necessary to determine whether the dog has ever been housetrained. If not, a housetraining regimen should be reviewed in which the focus is solely on reinforcement of elimination in desirable locations rather than punishment of elimination in inappropriate locations. This requires the owner to accompany the dog to its elimination area (eg, outdoors), reinforce elimination, supervise the dog indoors to prevent or interrupt any attempts at elimination (perhaps with the aid of a leash to ensure continuous supervision), and return the dog to its elimination site at appropriate intervals or if there are signs that the dog is ready to eliminate (eg, sniffing, heading to the door, sneaking away). When the owner is not able to supervise, a combination of scheduling (ensuring that the dog eliminates before departure and having someone return to take the dog to its elimination area before it must eliminate) and confinement training/prevention are required.

Dogs can either be confined away from areas where they might eliminate or kept in an area where they will not eliminate, such as a pen, room, or crate, where the dog eats, plays, or sleeps. Alternatively, the dog can be provided with an indoor elimination area (eg, paper, indoor puppy potty) within its confinement area where it can relieve itself when the owner is gone. Puppies obtained from pet stores or any location where they have been extensively caged may be more difficult to housetrain, because they have never had to inhibit elimination and may have learned to play with or eat feces.

Marking Behavior: Although marking is most often seen in intact males as a form of social and olfactory communication, it is also seen in females (especially when in heat) and in neutered males and females, often as an overmarking of other odors (eg, where other pets have urinated, or on items such as blankets with the residual odor of other dogs, people, or cats). Some dogs will mark when they visit unfamiliar households, especially when another dog's odor is present. There is often a typical posture of a raised or partially raised leg when the surface to be marked is vertical. Fecal marking is uncommon.

Although marking is likely a component of normal communication, it is unacceptable when it occurs indoors. Neutering intact males will reduce the behavior, and good supervision can prevent or inhibit most marking. As with housesoiling, dogs should be confined away from areas that might be marked when owners are not able to supervise. Marking that is related to anxiety may be reduced by identifying and treating the cause, perhaps with the aid of drugs or natural products that reduce anxiety.

Excitement, Submission, and Conflict-related Elimination: Dogs may eliminate when they are overly excited, such as when greeting people. Some dogs will urinate when showing submissive postures (eg, crouching to the ground or turning over to expose the belly) or when highly aroused. Because loss of urine control may be associated with a concurrent desire to both greet and show deferential behavior, many cases may be due to conflicting behavioral motivations. Treatment should focus on avoiding the stimuli (reaching, approach, eye contact) that incite the behavior and avoiding any punishment during greeting, which would add to fear and conflict behaviors. Acceptable alternative behaviors that are incompatible with excitable greeting or deferent postures can be taught, such as a relaxed sit, or any game or "trick" the pet may have learned such as fetch or giving a paw. Phenylpropanolamine might increase sphincter control, whereas imipramine may improve control and reduce anxiety.

Other Elimination Disorders: Dogs with separation anxiety or other fears and phobias (eg, thunderstorm phobia, firework phobia) may soil during these times.

Aging and Cognitive Dysfunction

The aging process is associated with progressive and irreversible changes in body systems that can affect behavior (*see* TABLE 2). In older dogs, these might include hepatic or renal failure, endocrine disorders (eg, Cushing disease), pain, sensory decline, or any disease affecting the CNS (eg, tumors) or circulation (eg, anemia, hypertension). To diagnose the cause of behavioral signs in a geriatric dog, a detailed history, physical examination, neurologic evaluation, and diagnostic tests are required to exclude potential medical causes of the presenting signs. Many owners do not report these signs, perhaps because the owners think they are insignificant or assume little can be done. Yet in one study, 30% of dogs 11–12 yr old and nearly 70% of dogs 15–16 yr old had signs consistent with cognitive dysfunction syndrome (CDS). A more recent Internet survey estimated CDS in 14.2% of dogs >10 yr old, with prevalence increasing with age, but >85% of these had not been diagnosed. It is therefore essential that owners be informed of the importance of reporting signs when they arise and for veterinarians to take a proactive approach in asking owners about behavior at each visit. Early detection provides the best opportunity to improve signs and slow the decline of cognitive function.

Aging dogs may exhibit a decline in cognitive function (memory, learning, perception, awareness) that manifests as one or more of a group of clinical signs. These are sometimes referred to by the acronym DISHA and include disorientation, interactions, sleep-wake cycles, housesoiling, and activity changes (which may be decreased or increased and repetitive). In addition, anxiety, agitation, and altered responses to stimuli are frequently reported. The first and most prominent sign of brain aging is a decline in learning or memory, which is generally impractical for pet owners to assess. However, neuropsychologic testing of older dogs has documented memory decline beginning at 6–8 yr of age and learning deficits by 9 yr of age. CDS in dogs is analogous to the early stages of Alzheimer disease in people, both in clinical signs and brain pathology. As with people, some dogs show minimal to no clinical impairment with age, whereas others develop varying degrees of deficits.

Treatment should first focus on environmental enrichment (both physical and mental stimulation), which has been shown to slow cognitive decline and improve the signs of CDS. Selegiline is a monoamine oxidase B inhibitor that may improve the signs of CDS by enhancing dopamine and other catecholamines in the cortex and hippocampus and by decreasing free radical load. Propentofylline, which is licensed in Europe and Australia for the treatment of dullness, lethargy, and depressed demeanor in old dogs, may increase blood flow and inhibit platelet aggregation and thrombus formation.

A number of natural products, including diets and supplements, have also been shown to have beneficial effects in improving the signs and potentially slowing cognitive decline. Two such diets are Canine b/d®, which is supplemented with fatty acids, antioxidants, and DL-alpha-lipoic acid and L-carnitine to enhance mitochondrial function, and a specialized Purina One® diet that uses botanic oils containing medium-chain triglycerides to provide ketone bodies as an alternative source of energy for aging neurons.

Other natural supplements that have demonstrated efficacy in improving cognitive function include Senilife®, which contains a combination of phosphatidylserine, *Ginkgo biloba*, resveratrol, and vitamins E and B_6; Activait®, which contains phosphatidylserine in combination with α-lipoic acid, carnitine, fatty acids, glutathione, and other antioxidants; *S*-adenosyl methionine (Novifit®); and apoaequorin (Neutricks®), a calcium-buffering protein found in jellyfish.

CATS

SOCIAL BEHAVIOR

Cats are social animals that, in feral conditions, live in groups consisting mainly of queens and their litters. The density of the group depends partly on food resources. Because cats have been exposed to less selective breeding than dogs, there is far less breed diversity and a much narrower range of differences in both physical and behavioral traits. Most cats are solitary hunters that prey on rodents and other small animals, which is likely why their coexistence with people is so successful. Kittens usually learn to prefer to hunt prey that their mother hunted. Kittens may also develop limited food preferences based on texture and taste if not given a variety of foods when young.

In free-range conditions, multiple generations of related females can live together, which also allows for communal rearing of kittens. Kittens may stay with the social group until 12–18 mo old. Sexual maturity is reached by ~6 mo of age. Queens are induced ovulators and generally cycle seasonally (most often from winter to summer) about every 3 wk if not bred. Weaning occurs at 5–8 wk of age. Although some kittens may suckle much later, this is more likely to be social than nutritional. Early weaning of kittens leads to earlier onset of play and predation.

The socialization period of cats is much shorter than that of dogs and may begin to wane by 7–9 wk of age. During this narrow window, exposure to cats, other animals, people, and a variety of stimuli in the environment is important for prevention of fear. Kittens handled extensively by people at 2–7 wk of age may be friendlier, more outgoing, and have fewer problems with aggression. Hand-reared kittens may lack feline social skills and may be hyperactive in object and social play; however, if a kitten is reared with other cats in the home and provided with play sessions with wand-type toys, these problems may be prevented. Genetics, especially those of the father, also play a strong role in personality. Cats may be behaviorally categorized as active, playful and aggressive, calm and sociable, or timid and shy.

Social play, including biting, chasing, and play fighting, begins around 4 wk of age, peaks at 6–9 wk, and declines at 12–14 wk. Social play may be directed at people, especially if there are no other cats with which to play. Object play begins around 6–8 wk and peaks at ~18 wk of age. Object play simulates the predatory sequence and includes stalking, chasing, pawing, pouncing, and biting and can be directed at objects or social partners.

Cats may develop preferences for particular elimination substrates. Many cats dig before and after elimination (which may be a visual mark or to bury urine and feces). Cats are strongly influenced by scents and may respond by marking with urine (spraying) or feces, scratching as both a visual and scent mark, or rubbing sebaceous glands of the cheeks or body in the environment or on other cats. Urine marking, roaming, and fighting with other cats may be androgen influenced, in which case these problems may be prevented or resolved by neutering.

BEHAVIORAL PROBLEMS

As with dogs, undesirable behavior might be 1) normal behavior but undesirable for the owners (eg, climbing, scratching, and excessive nocturnal activity); 2) behaviors that fall within the range of normal but are at or near the limits, excessive in intensity or frequency, and particularly challenging or disturbing for the home environment (eg, play biting, petting-induced aggression, overexuberant play, play/predation, vocalization, asocial, litter box avoidance); or 3) behaviors that are abnormal, pathologic, or incompatible with living in the home (eg, intercat aggression, fear and avoidance, urine marking). In most cases of normal but undesirable behaviors, the owners require guidance and resource material on meeting the behavioral needs of cats and understanding learning principles to reinforce what is desirable while preventing what is undesirable. When behaviors are at or near the limits of normal, a more in-depth behavior assessment is needed to discuss realistic goals for what might be achieved, how the environment might be managed, and how the behavior might be modified. In some households, it may be impractical to make the changes necessary to achieve an endpoint that meets the owner's needs. In cases when the behavior is abnormal or incompatible with the home environment, a behavior consultation is required to diagnose, determine the prognosis, implement behavior and environmental modifications, and dispense drugs or supplements when indicated to achieve a sufficient level of improvement for the owner and the cat. The most common behaviors seen by veterinary behaviorists are elimination (undesirable toileting and marking) and aggression. Because aggressive encounters in cats may be overt or subtle and passive, their frequency may be seriously underestimated.

For both prevention and treatment, it is important to first ensure that the behavioral needs of the cat are adequately met. This is a particularly important consideration for cats housed exclusively or primarily indoors. Although individual variability in expression can be extensive, a cat's primary behavioral needs include eating (hunting), drinking, elimination, security, play and exploration, climbing, perching, and scratching. Specifically, hunting and feeding needs might be better addressed by giving food in small portions throughout the day and placing food or treats inside toys that require some manipulation to release the food (batting, chasing, rolling, pawing). To add an element of hunting, the cat can be given opportunities to chase, pounce on, and bite toys the owner dangles or pulls in front of the cat.

Play appears to be motivated by two mechanisms: an initial interest if the toy possesses appropriate characteristics (texture, small size) and rapid habituation. Owners should find a number of toys that interest the cat and play with several different toys until the cat's interest wanes. Cats may also be offered small toys for batting and chasing; boxes or containers to explore; appealing outlets to climb, perch, and scratch; and perhaps an occasional catnip toy (to which 50%–75% of cats respond).

Teaching the basics of reinforcement-based training allows owners to focus on rewarding desirable behaviors (eg, where to eliminate, climb, scratch, or perch). Clicker training (*see* p 1540) can be particularly useful to immediately time (mark) desirable behaviors and gradually shape outcomes that more closely approximate the final goal. Punishment should be avoided, because it can cause fear and anxiety toward the owners or fear of handling and petting and, at best, will stop the undesirable behavior only when the owner is present. Provided all of the cat's needs are adequately met, the best approach to stop repetition of the undesirable behavior can be to prevent access to areas where problems might arise. Another alternative is to teach the cat to avoid the area by making it unpleasant with taste (eg, cayenne pepper), odor (eg, citrus), substrate (eg, upside-down carpet runner, double-sided sticky tape), or perhaps a motion-activated device (eg, alarm, air spray).

Diagnosis and Treatment

Assuming all possible medical causes have been excluded, a thorough history is necessary to diagnose, determine the prognosis, and develop an appropriate treatment program. In cats, especially those with elimination and marking problems, it is particularly important to assess the environment either by visiting the home or having the owners diagram the home so that it can be determined how the environment affects the problem and how it might be modified to improve the situation.

Response substitution (training an alternative desirable behavior) can be a useful approach if the cat is reward trained with food or favored toys to respond to one or more simple commands (eg, come, sit). A leash and harness can be used as an aid in training as well as a way to prevent undesirable behaviors and ensure safety. For fearful behavior, access to the stimuli should be prevented, at least in the short term. For example, if cats are fearful or aggressive with other cats or visitors, confinement away from the stimulus is an essential first step to ensure safety as well as to prevent further aggravation of the problem. This generally involves housing the cat in its own room with litter, toys, bedding, and food. When the cat is calm and comfortable, it might then be possible to gradually reintroduce the cat using favored toys, treats, or food for counterconditioning.

Drugs for fearful behaviors that could be used on an ongoing basis include fluoxetine, paroxetine, or clomipramine; buspirone or other tricyclic antidepressants (TCAs) or selective serotonin reuptake inhibitors (SSRIs) might be an alternative. A benzodiazepine such as alprazolam might be used on an as-needed basis for situational anxiety such as car rides. Because of the range of individual variability in behavioral effects and adverse effects, trials with different benzodiazepines should be done in advance to determine which drug and dose achieves the desired effect and for how long. Caution is necessary, particularly with the use of diazepam, for any indication of anorexia or depression, because rare cases of acute and potentially fatal hepatic dysfunction have been reported. In some situations, a benzodiazepine such as clonazepam might be considered on an ongoing basis for a more immediate anxiety reduction and to enhance appetite for counterconditioning. Natural products including the F3 cheek gland pheromone (Feliway® [available as diffuser or spray]), L-theanine (Anxitane®), alpha-casozepine (Zylkene®), and a diet containing both alpha-casozepine and L-tryptophan (Royal Canin Calm Feline™) might also be used alone or adjunctively with drugs or other natural products to help calm, reduce anxiety, or reduce the stress associated with environmental change. The F4 cheek gland pheromone (Felifriend®), associated with social marking (bunting) of cats, is also available as a topical gel in some countries to reduce fear of people or other cats. With intercat aggression, buspirone or a benzodiazepine might increase the confidence of the victim cat during reintroductions. However, anxiolytic drugs could disinhibit and increase aggression.

Housesoiling

With housesoiling, the first step is always to exclude medical problems, because any condition that affects urine volume, frequency, control, or ability to access the litter box can contribute to soiling. Evaluating the behavioral history is then the primary process to make the diagnosis, determine the prognosis, and develop a treatment plan. Important aspects of the history include whether the elimination is urine or feces, whether urine deposits are vertical (spraying) or horizontal (soiling), duration and frequency of the problem, signalment and temperament of the soiling cat, when and where the cat eliminates, litter box details (number, placement, cleaning, substrate, size), the cat's daily routine, and its home environment.

Urine Marking (Spraying): Spraying is emission of a stream of urine onto vertical surfaces, usually accompanied by elevation and quivering of the tail and in some cases treading of the feet. Marking on horizontal surfaces (eg, owner's clothing, bedding, or countertops) is less common. Spraying is much more commonly seen in male cats, and neutering will reduce or eliminate it in most cats, although ~10% of neutered males continue to mark. Marking may be due to anxiety, such as might arise with introduction of a new cat; a change in schedule, environment, or family (eg, renovations, new furnishings, new baby, marriage or divorce); or unfamiliar visual, auditory, or olfactory stimuli.

Treatment can include a combination of prevention, environmental modification, behavior modification, and medication. Providing more litter boxes and more litter box locations, cleaning the soiled areas with bacterial or enzymatic cleaners, and cleaning the litter box more frequently may reduce or eliminate marking in some cats. Punishment is contraindicated, because it increases fear and anxiety in an already anxious animal. Unless the stimuli inciting marking or the underlying factors contributing to the marking can be effectively resolved, most cats are likely to require drug therapy with either fluoxetine or clomipramine (buspirone or other SSRIs or TCAs might be an alternative). Feliway® feline pheromones in the form of a spray on marked locations or a diffuser in the environment might also effectively reduce marking alone or in combination with drugs.

Inappropriate Elimination: Soiling on horizontal surfaces with urine, feces, or both, can be a problem in males and females. Cats that consistently return to the same location or substrate may have a location or substrate preference. Cats that do not use their litter for urine, feces, or both may be avoiding the litter itself, the litter box, or its location. A common cause of avoidance is any medical problem that might cause painful elimination, increased frequency, lack of control, or difficulty accessing the litter box. If medical problems have been excluded or treated and the problem persists, the focus should then be on the behavioral history. Avoidance might arise because of aspects of the substrate (texture, depth, scent, cleanliness), box (size, shape, hood), or location that reduce appeal; unpleasant experiences at or near the box (eg, insufficient cleaning, noises, pain due to medical problems); or difficulty in gaining access to the box. Although anxiety may not be an inciting factor for inappropriate elimination, cats may avoid the litter or box if fearful (ie, personality) or when there is conflict between cats in the home (whether active or passive). Although substrate, litter box, and location preferences may arise secondary to avoidance, some cats may actually have a preference for a particular odor, texture, or location.

Treatment should focus on providing a litter, box, and site that is most appealing to the cat; reducing or preventing the use of the soiled location; and resolving the underlying factors contributing to the soiling. Appeal might be improved by identifying and resolving potential deterrents (eg, undesirable location, fear-evoking stimuli such as furnace noise, or limited access such as a shared washroom), adding additional boxes or additional sites, finding a more appealing location for the litter, improving access to the litter (eg, larger box, ease of entry, ease of exit), and finding out which litter (eg, sand, clumping, clay, soft towel, scented) and box type (eg, size, shape, height, covered, self-cleaning) is preferred by offering the cat choices to decide. Access to the soiled location might be prevented by blocking access to the area, or the appeal reduced by using odor counteractants in the soiled area, making the area unpleasant (eg, double-sided sticky tape, upside-down [nubs-up] carpet runner), or changing the function of the area (play, scratching, feeding, sleeping).

Aggression

Aggression Toward People: Aggression toward owners may be fear induced or related to play or predation. Cats that bite during petting may have a low tolerance for physical contact, and some cats bite to keep people from approaching or handling them when they are resting, sleeping, or eating (which may be a learned, fear, or social issue). Aggression may be particularly intense if the cat is approached when it is aroused. When the arousal is due to a stimulus to which the cat cannot gain access (eg, another cat outside, loud noise), the cat may redirect its aggression to any person who approaches.

Some cats display abnormal and out-of-context social responses, including aggression, when approached or handled. This may have a genetic component that is compounded by insufficient socialization, lack of adequate maternal care, inadequate early handling, and fear-evoking or traumatic early experiences. However, at the time of presentation, most aggression also has a learned component, because any unpleasant response on the part of the owner (eg, fear, punishment) will cause increased fear, whereas retreat of the owner negatively reinforces the behavior. Aggression toward strangers most often has a fear component.

Aggression Toward Other Cats: Cats may display aggression toward other cats due to play, predatory behavior, redirected behavior, fear, and perhaps as a status-related behavior in which cats use aggression to retain control of sleeping areas, common areas, or possessions. Ultimately, the relationship that develops between any pair of cats will be affected by learning, because fearful responses by either cat can increase aggression, as will retreat of one of the cats (negative reinforcement). Aggression toward unfamiliar cats is most often a fear response but may have a territorial component.

Treatment: The first step is to ensure that further injuries are prevented. Avoidance (physical, visual, and preferably olfactory separation of cats that are fighting) is paramount, and early intervention is best. Although some cats will need to be separated at all times until they are calm enough to be reintroduced, if there are particular times or situations when conflicts arise, it might be necessary to separate the cats only at these times. Only after the cats are calm (which can take days to months) can desensitization and counterconditioning with favored rewards begin (ie, play with toys, treats). Desensitization and counterconditioning might first begin with odors by grooming each cat with a brush or towel used on the other, and by feeding each cat separately in a common area on opposite sides of a partition (glass, screen, or solid door) and then in a common area at sufficient distance that the cats can be calm and take food or play with toys. Training one or both cats to wear a leash and harness can help to ensure safety and distance during reintroductions, while a bell on the aggressor can help the victim be aware of its whereabouts. Providing more three-dimensional space, including climbs and perches, and ensuring sufficient resources at sufficient distance to facilitate avoidance can further decrease conflict. Reward training limited to a few selected verbal cues (eg, come, sit, go to your room) can further aid in managing the cats during introductions or in diffusing potentially aggressive situations. Punishment should be avoided, because it increases fear and anxiety in cats. Drugs might also be indicated (*see* p 1565).

Feline Compulsive Disorders

Abnormal repetitive behaviors in cats are derived from normal behaviors such as stalking, chasing, grooming, etc. These may be exacerbated by stress or anxiety such as alterations in relationships with people or other cats, or may be inadvertently aggravated by the owners either reinforcing or punishing the behavior (increasing conflict and anxiety). If these behaviors occur out of context or in a frequency or duration in excess of that needed to accomplish the task, a diagnosis of compulsive disorder should be considered. Medical problems must be excluded, because they can be responsible for many of the same signs. For example, self-mutilation, excessive grooming, and/or self-directed aggression can be due to any condition that might cause neuropathic pain or pruritus such as adverse food reactions, atopic dermatitis, and parasitic hypersensitivity.

Cats that suck, lick, chew, or even ingest non-nutritive substances—including natural materials such as wool or cotton, synthetic fabrics, plastic, rubber, paper, cardboard, and string—may have a compulsive disorder if the problem becomes sufficiently frequent or intense; however, disease processes, in particular those that might affect the GI tract, should first be excluded. Oriental breeds develop pica, particularly sucking of woolen objects, more frequently than other cats. Hallucinatory and locomotory compulsive disorders are less common than in dogs; however, painful conditions and any disease process affecting the neurologic system first need to be excluded.

Cats often improve with modifications to the environment that provide more control and predictability and increased enrichment, combined with medications that augment the amount of brain serotonin such as fluoxetine and clomipramine.

Hyperesthesia

Hyperesthesia may not be a specific disorder but rather a sign of underlying medical or behavioral problems. Most commonly, the skin along the lumbosacral area may twitch or ripple. There may be excessive self-grooming, hissing or biting at the back or flank, and intensive tail wagging. Some cats cry, dash away, and even defecate. These episodes arise when the cat is highly aroused and may be incited by physical contact or external stimuli. A compulsive disorder is a consideration when the intensity, frequency, and duration of these problems is sufficiently severe. However, medical causes such as neuropathic pain, dermatologic conditions, myopathies, and focal seizures can also present with similar signs. Therefore, a therapeutic response trial for neuropathic pain, seizures, pruritus, or compulsive disorders might be part of the diagnostic process.

Fear

Fear may arise in cats as a result of genetic factors, lack of sufficient early socialization and exposure, or fear-evoking experiences. The fear may be of unfamiliar people, unfamiliar cats, dogs, noises, or places and situations such as car rides, veterinary visits, and unfamiliar environments. Some cats may also be fearful of familiar people and cats. This may be evidenced as threatening displays and overt aggression (*see* above) or avoidance, withdrawal and hiding, and possibly spraying.

Treatment should begin with identification and avoidance of any situation, stimulus, approach, or handling that might lead to fear. When the cat is sufficiently calm, gradual improvement might be achieved with desensitization and counterconditioning. Drugs might also be indicated (*see* p 1573).

Aging and Cognitive Dysfunction

Aging and younger cats have similar behavior problems; however, the likelihood of a pathophysiologic underlying condition is higher in older cats. Many diseases, including those affecting the CNS, metabolic and endocrine systems (eg, renal disorders, hyperthyroidism), sensory decline, and pain (eg, arthritis), may present with behavioral signs. Once medical problems have been excluded or treated, behavioral therapy may be required. Behavior problems in senior pets may be more difficult to resolve because of a decline in cognitive function, medical problems that cannot be entirely resolved, and drug contraindications or adverse effects.

Cognitive dysfunction syndrome (CDS) is less commonly reported in cats than in dogs. Yet in one study, ~35% of cats >11 yr old displayed at least one sign of CDS, and 50% of cats >15 yr old showed two or more signs. Brain changes are similar to those seen in CDS in dogs (*see* p 1569). Environmental enrichment and mental stimulation is paramount to prevent and treat CDS. Medications, diets, and supplements might also improve the signs of CDS or slow its progression. Although no drugs or diets are licensed for feline CDS, selegiline and propentofylline have been used off-label. Both S-adenosyl methione (Novifit®) and a commercial diet containing antioxidants, arginine, B vitamins, and fish oil have demonstrated improvement in learning and memory in geriatric cats. Cognitive supplements containing antioxidants, vitamins, and phosphatidylserine (Senilfe®, Activait®) have also been developed for cats.

THE HUMAN-ANIMAL BOND

Companion animals are commonly considered to be family members, and the human-animal bond has become a household term. More than half of all households in the USA have at least one dog or cat, and most pet owners have more than one pet. Cats outnumber dogs as companion animals, and many veterinary practices serve only cats. Yet, a 2008 study of the care pets receive reported that dogs were seen by a veterinarian more than twice as often as cats, even in households with both species.

Households with children are the most likely to have pets. Most couples also have pets, including retired couples, who have recently shown a growth rate in pet ownership. Currently, fewer than half of single persons have a pet. In dealing with owners, using approaches that incorporate the entire family is an important feature of a successful veterinary practice.

With the growing awareness of the human-animal bond, the roles of pets as service and therapy animals are expanding into new areas and fill many of the same support functions that people do. Service dogs assist people with various disabilities, including mobility, visual, or hearing impairments. The dogs may also detect and alert people to impending seizures or abnormal blood glucose levels.

The human-animal bond has also increased focus on ensuring that animals receive adequate consideration and care. Albert Schweitzer's concept of "reverence for life" has become a standard for decision-making concerning animals. Acknowledgment of the human-animal bond has become a cornerstone of veterinary practice, and evidence suggests that practitioners who pay close attention to the various aspects of the human-animal bond will thrive both financially and in terms of finding their work enjoyable and rewarding.

VETERINARY FAMILY PRACTICE

The evolution of the role of pets in human affairs has opened new opportunities for veterinarians, especially those in family practice. Owners become deeply attached to and care about the health and well-being of their companion animals. Their expectations for veterinary care are becoming similar to the care ideally provided in human medicine, particularly as high-tech medicine expands within veterinary specialties. In addition, the current increased importance of animals changes the nature of veterinary practice to include the entire family, and a sophisticated level of family support is expected by many clients. The style and emphasis of companion animal practices have shifted, as reflected in the term "veterinary family practice."

Practices that include the entire family build lifelong relationships with families and their animals. Clients look forward to consistently seeing the same veterinarian. A new animal brought into the family is the occasion to discuss the animal's life cycle with the family and provide an overview that can optimize the likelihood of a positive human-animal relationship with few behavioral problems. Veterinarians no longer just treat the animal; emotional needs of the family are addressed along with the medical needs of the pet.

Many families with companion animals have young children, particularly families that have both a dog and a cat. Animals are acknowledged to play a central and formative role in children's lives. In some studies, pet-owning preadolescents scored higher on measures of self-esteem and autonomy. Practitioners may consider incorporating children into their communications with the family and making it easy for families with children to be comfortable during veterinary visits (eg, providing a play area in the waiting room or planning for children to be present in or visibly near the examination room). Hospitals providing extended care for animals with complex diagnostic procedures and treatment plans that require hospitalization sometimes find entire families coming in to offer support to the animal, perhaps spending hours with the pet; these hospitals may want to plan accommodation for such families.

Providing areas for relaxation, softer light in public areas, and comfortable seating in exam rooms without barriers from the medical staff are some features that improve client satisfaction. Impeccable cleanliness also matters. Veterinary practices that exhibit these values demonstrate the understanding that medical interventions carry emotional consequences and that medical competence and providing emotional support go hand-in-hand.

Studies have shown that communication has a key role in the owner-pet and client-veterinarian bond, because it affects the care pets receive. Effective communication significantly affects the loyalty of the pet owner to the veterinarian. Pet owners are more concerned with the health and well-being outcomes for the animal, whereas veterinarians often emphasize time and services in their communications. Clients value the genuine love and interest veterinarians show for the animals. The veterinarian's empathetic concern expressed through effective communication builds relationships with clients and enhances client satisfaction. Focus groups have revealed that clients expect veterinarians to educate them, explaining important information clearly and in various formats. Clients want to be provided options and offered a respectful partnership with the veterinarian in the health care of their pet. They expect interactive, two-way communication that includes listening and asking relevant questions. Clear recommendations and effective communication of their rationale also lead to better adherence to medical and treatment plans.

A strong owner-animal bond is associated with greater attention to veterinary care. Owners feel strongly about the quality of life of their pets, as revealed in studies involving surgery or medical problems of pets. Owners want effective pain management for the animal before, during, and after surgery, including spaying or neutering, even though they may not wish to administer such medication at home. People feel that a good quality of life for their pets includes mobility, play or mental stimulation, health, and companionship. Owners of dogs with heart disease expressed extreme concern regarding their inability to subjectively assess whether their pet is suffering. Teaching owners to assess and improve the animal's quality of life is an important aspect of veterinary care and client education. Veterinarians and owners can use a quality of life scale (eg, the HHHHHMM Scale to monitor the pet's hurt, hunger, hydration, hygiene, happiness, mobility, and more good days than bad) as an aid in assessment. A strong majority of owners indicate they would trade their pet's longevity for quality of life. Among variables of quality of life, the pet's ability to interact with the owners was the most important.

Good communication skills also build strong client-veterinarian bonds, and successful veterinarians pay close attention to their nontechnical competencies, including interpersonal relationship-building skills. Such skills enable veterinarians and staff members to facilitate clients' understanding of medical situations and preventive medicine throughout the animal's life, from encouraging clients to attend puppy socialization classes to preparing clients to provide palliative care or deal with end-of-life issues. Follow-up communication can also improve client adherence, which is generally lower than believed by veterinarians. Curricula for veterinary students increasingly include opportunities to develop communication skills, allowing students to practice engaging clients, asking open-ended questions, offering reflective listening and empathy, educating clients, meeting clients' and patients' needs, and emphasizing support and partnership.

Despite optimal communication skills, research has unfortunately shown that veterinarians inevitably encounter owners who are inattentive, neglectful, over-involved, or completely cost-driven, as well as pets that are uncontrolled, dangerous, or dirty, adding to medical and emotional problems. Almost all veterinarians feel they were not prepared by their education and training to deal with such nonmedical issues. Making plans in advance and developing specific protocols for interventions can prepare the veterinary staff with strategies for these situations.

HUMAN HEALTH BENEFITS OF PET OWNERSHIP

Animal companionship both relaxes and entertains people. Pets can provide both social support and status. In coming to know their clients, veterinarians can assess the importance of the pet to a family and the extent to which the family members benefit from the potential psychosocial effects of living with an animal. The pet's contribution may be magnified for vulnerable people, such as older adults who are facing increasing disabilities and losses of close companions and family. During stressful periods in people's lives, many studies have reported that pets offer meaningful comfort that is protective against depression and loneliness. Older women score more favorably on measures of mental health, and college-aged women report less loneliness if living with a companion animal rather than alone.

Similar comforting effects of animal companions, whether cats or dogs, in warding off depression were reported for patients with Alzheimer disease. The same is true for men with AIDS who had a companion animal and were cared for at home and whose social lives were shrinking. Older people experiencing typical life stresses are less affected (as measured by number of medical visits) when they have a companion dog, suggesting that a dog can be a stress buffer that softens effects of adverse events on the person. Of course, pets require caregiving, and the reciprocal caregiving exchanged with the animal can also allow the person to nurture and feel needed, while also feeling nurtured. The animal's constancy bolsters courage during setbacks, because the animal's affection is unaffected by factors such as the person's physical capabilities or mood.

Companion animals facilitate social interactions with other people and an overall positive social involvement. The socializing effects of dogs have been documented in public settings and also among people with a variety of disabilities. A companion animal provides a person who has few friends with an ally in making new human acquaintances, while also creating a richer family environment with enhanced companionship. Even one person with an animal lives in a family unit and is greeted or recognized on arrival home.

The motivating role of animals is a further antidote to depression. Many people are inspired to walk their dogs, volunteer to take animals into nursing homes for visits, or just actively nurture an animal, whereas without the animal they may be less involved and engaged in living or even depressed. Walking a dog and being outdoors where other social contact arises are two healthful effects of living with a canine companion. Research projects and community programs in many parts of the USA and elsewhere are seeking to raise the popularity of dog walking as an approach toward improving human health and lessening human disease, including diabetes and cardiovascular problems.

The daily comfort, socialization, and relaxing motivation offered by an animal also are associated with cardiovascular benefits. Blood pressure decreases transiently when a person relaxes with, talks to, or just watches an animal. When human patients with increased blood pressure were given medication and randomly assigned pets, those patients with pets performed better on stressful tasks, indicating a lower response to stress in this group; however, blood pressure scores did not differ in those with pets and those without. Several studies show longterm health correlates with animal companionship, although the animals were not randomly assigned to the people but rather were chosen by them or their families.

Cardiovascular measures were better among pet owners than nonowners in a large Australian study. Two studies reported that pet ownership was related to decreased mortality. Survival for 1 yr after heart attack was found to be more likely among people with companion dogs, along the lines of human social support.

ANIMAL-ASSISTED INTERVENTIONS: THERAPY, ACTIVITIES, AND EDUCATION

The field called animal-assisted therapy originated when the public began to take animals into nursing homes and other facilities to share them with residents. Unless medically supervised, these programs are termed "animal-assisted activities," whereas those directed as part of medical treatment are termed "animal-assisted therapy." An emerging area is animal-assisted education, in which animals are provided to help improve classroom behavior or learning of children. Procedures to screen animals and provide training for the people involved are offered and have been standardized by Pet Partners (formerly the Delta Society). However, programs that train and certify "therapy animals" (mainly dogs) are not legislatively required as part of a certification process; likewise, there is no conventional educational process for individuals seeking to work in this area. Therapy dogs have no special rights of public access and are not granted special privileges in housing or transportation.

An accreditation process has been developed for instructional programs serving health professionals through the International Association for Animal-Assisted Therapy. The University of Denver offers social work students an emphasis in animal-assisted therapy. Some individuals within human health professions, such as clinical psychology, social work, occupational therapy, physical therapy, and/or nursing, have incorporated animal-assisted activities and therapy with therapy dogs into their professional practice.

A much larger number of people continue to volunteer to bring their animals into facilities, often with some screening process and training organized by local groups. Such groups often benefit from veterinary assistance and leadership in developing appropriate screening methods for selection and preparation of both animals and people participating in these programs.

SERVICE OR ASSISTANCE DOGS AND OTHER WORKING DOGS

If periodic exposure to an animal via animal-assisted activities, therapy, or education is healthful for someone with special needs, more frequent or continual exposure may offer even greater benefits. Service or assistance dogs are trained to perform specific tasks in partnership with people who have disabilities. In addition to guide dogs for people with visual disabilities, hearing dogs for people with hearing disabilities, and service dogs for people using wheelchairs, dogs can assist people with many other disabilities, such as detecting an impending seizure, detecting high or low blood glucose levels in a person with diabetes, or helping to stabilize a child with autism. A growing role of service dogs is as psychiatric service dogs, assisting persons with mental illness such as post-traumatic stress disorders, schizophrenia, bipolar disorder, agoraphobia (fear of open spaces), or anxiety. Other working dogs assist in law enforcement, agricultural or bomb sniffing, search and rescue, or war tasks. Service and assistance dogs have legally protected special access to use public transportation through the Department of Transportation and for housing through the Department of Housing and Urban Development. Some working dogs are kenneled in a facility when not working, although many police dogs live with the families of their handlers. Dogs range from being purpose-bred with extensive training, to being shelter-sourced with minimal formalized training. Significant investments of money and time are required for the specialized training and development of working partnerships with these dogs. As they forge working partnerships with their dogs, the handlers inevitably become emotionally bonded. Formally trained assistance or service dogs can have several trainers or handlers in their early lives, but after being placed, typically spend the rest of their lives with a single handler, providing assistance to the handler while also offering relief and comfort to other family members.

Also based on "equal accommodation" for people with disabilities, "emotional support animals" (ESAs) are another category of animals assured legally protected special access to transportation and housing if they provide a nexus of support for someone with a disability; however, they lack the broader aspects of public access provided to service dogs. Handlers of ESAs (and psychiatric service dogs) may be asked by landlords or transportation personnel to provide documentation from their medical professionals that they have a disability alleviated by the ESA. ESAs require no special training; they naturally offer special support. ESAs are not limited to dogs but can be of various species so long as they are helping the person who has the disability.

With limited oversight of service dogs and ESAs in the USA, permissive enforcement of requirements, and an expanding array of service dogs and ESAs, dogs of many different breeds and body sizes are providing meaningful support to people with a variety of disabilities. Smaller dogs are easier to manage for people who are frail or live in small apartments, and they may be sufficient for a person's needs, eg, in their capacity to retrieve dropped items. Informed veterinarians can offer wise counsel in these matters to people with disabilities regarding the needed training, medical care, and breed selection. This service is valuable, because the growing demand for service dogs has resulted in some cases of poorly trained dogs at high prices being presented for sale as purported service dogs.

Working dogs are extremely precious and valuable to their handlers. When a medical crisis arises with such a dog, the veterinarian is often the closest professional at hand and may need to provide support to the handler as well as the animal. Treatments that adversely affect performance, especially for an extended period, disrupt functioning of both the dog and the person. If the individual has a disability, special accommodation may be required for communication and veterinary instructions. Treatments not involving an emergency should be planned well in advance, with consideration of the handler's needs and schedule. Attentive listening and respect, although essential for all clients, assumes particular importance in these relationships.

Although no legal or regulatory process certifies assistance dogs, Assistance Dogs International is one organization engaged in developing international standards. Curricula for professionals interested in continuing education in this area are being offered by the Bergin University of Canine Studies in Santa Rosa, California (formerly the Assistance Dog Institute), leading to a Master of Science in Canine Life Sciences.

ANIMAL WELFARE

Reducing or preventing the incidence of animal pain or distress and promoting animal well-being (and even pleasure) are overall goals of animal welfare. These goals pertain to animals on farms or in laboratories as well as companion animals. Aversive handling, even if infrequent, can have stressful consequences. Veterinarians are often the first contacts when someone seeks help for animals being badly treated or receiving inadequate care.

Intentional, deliberate abuse of animals is an extreme marker of a likely pattern of abuse elsewhere within a family. Veterinarians who report suspected animal abuse sometimes can avert similar abuse of other vulnerable family members, especially children or older adults. Two studies reported that >90% of veterinarians would report cases of suspected animal abuse to authorities. Most agreed that animal abuse in families would tend to be linked with abuse or mistreatment of children or older adults.

Although occasionally seen by veterinarians, outright abuse appears less common than the neglect, poor husbandry, or lack of essential medical care of animals, some of which may be inadvertent. A serious problem occurs with animal hoarders who may be mentally ill. The person, perhaps without awareness, acquires more animals than they can possibly care for properly. Some communities routinely combine efforts of animal control and mental health agencies when dealing with such cases.

A major, widespread societal problem of animal welfare is the abandoning and killing of companion animals. Relinquishment of animals that would be adoptable has decreased, yet the problem remains widespread. Many studies have shown that behavioral problems of animals and owners' lack of knowledge of how to adequately care for an animal increase the likelihood of relinquishment. Veterinary teams can provide leadership and education about more realistic expectations of companion animals and can encourage earlier intervention if problems arise.

Despite the growing population of dogs and cats, the number of veterinary visits has been decreasing, raising concerns about whether pets are getting adequate veterinary care. Cats receive less veterinary care then dogs; a 2011 study found that 40% of cats had not been to a veterinarian within the past year, compared with 15% of dogs. Most of these cat owners said their pet "hated" going to the veterinarian. A cat's resistance to veterinary visits can be addressed by facilitating transport in carriers; making the visit, examination, and treatment more comfortable for the cat and owner; or considering mobile veterinary services.

Some emotionally charged issues and social conflicts pertaining to animals reflect contrasting perspectives on animal welfare. How best to deal with feral cats and their kittens can be a contentious question when weighed against the impact on songbirds and other wildlife. Another emerging concern is the possible adverse medical effect of early neutering for some breeds of dogs, such as a potentially increased incidence of hip dysplasia or certain cancers. Although early neutering curtails unwanted reproduction, other options also could be offered to owners to manage reproduction. As contentious topics regarding animal welfare arise in communities, veterinary professionals are those more prepared to offer reasoned and informed leadership to address problems.

EUTHANASIA, PET LOSS, AND GRIEF FOR OWNERS AND VETERINARIANS

When a beloved animal companion dies or is ill, people are likely to feel stress, sorrow, and grief. This may include the animal's family and neighbors in the community, as well as the veterinary team that provided care. The significance of pets dying and the consequent emotional impact on owners is clearly profiled within the veterinary profession, and educational materials and support groups, hotlines, and counseling are available. The relatively short life span of dogs and cats means that owners face losing several animals during a lifetime.

An extra burden comes in assuming responsibility for the moment of death by euthanasia. The desire or perceived duty to relieve pain and suffering may need to be weighed against the feeling of some owners about the wrongness of killing or a religious argument for reverence for life. The difficulty of this decision overlays the loss with feelings of guilt and the thought that there must have been some other step that could have been taken. Even with family support, these feelings may not be assuaged. Among married couples in one study, approximately half of the wives and more than a quarter of husbands reported they were quite or extremely disturbed by the death of the family pet.

As an alternative to euthanasia, it is important to offer instruction in palliative care for owners prepared to provide it. Procedures developed in hospice care can assure high-quality, end-of-life care with pain relief for animals, and help the family as well. The technical aspects of treatment no longer override the compassionate care, as a specific approach is often offered to deal with the family's and pet's distress.

Owners are also concerned about the care of their pet's remains. Veterinarians offer the available choices, with information about the final disposition of the pet's remains. After a cremation, some owners are concerned to know that the ashes they receive are, in fact, those of their own pet. Veterinarians' communication with clients concerning questions around euthanasia and the care of pet remains is especially important, as is providing support during the mourning process.

Compassionate veterinarians include themselves in the circle of remembrance of their clients' animals and respect the families' regard for the animal throughout the relationship. Many grieving owners need a year of recovery to pass through the holidays and family traditions before somewhat accepting a loss, and veterinarians may consider sending a remembrance card to the family after a year.

SELF-CARE FOR VETERINARIANS

Notwithstanding the anguish that pet owners experience, the process of animals dying, especially the act of performing euthanasia, poses an emotionally wearing duty for veterinarians as well. A recent USA survey found that a veterinarian typically euthanizes more than seven animals per month, sharply contrasting with a study of veterinarians in Japan, where the median number of euthanasias in the previous year was one, and 20% of Japanese veterinarians had not euthanized any pets that year. In one study, euthanizing animals resulted in perpetration-induced traumatic stress for 11% of the study sample of veterinarians, veterinary nurses/technicians, and research and animal shelter staff. Lower levels of stress were reported among those who were more satisfied with their social support and had worked longer with animals. Most veterinarians in another study reported having been clinically depressed. In one study, almost all veterinarians felt they were untrained in explaining euthanasia to clients. Almost half regretted a specific occasion of euthanasia, and most private practitioners reported feeling guilty after performing euthanasia. After euthanizing their own pets, a majority of veterinarians felt depressed, and 30% felt guilty. These figures were higher among female veterinarians, suggesting that its impact may have risen with the gender shift of the profession.

A major concern with regard to the mental welfare of veterinarians is the suicide rate, which is higher than that of the general population. The suicide rate of veterinarians in the UK is four times that of the general population; although precise figures are not available, similar problems are arising in the USA. Risk factors mentioned in the UK include the initial entry into a helping profession, routine involvement with euthanasia and knowing the means to perform it, and the contagion of emotional stress. This work became the lynchpin for VetLife: Looking After the Veterinary Profession (www.vetlife.org.uk/), a Web site to support the well-being of veterinarians and to address personal and professional issues.

Increasingly, veterinary students and practitioners realize the value of ongoing monitoring of their own self-care and make use of instruments such as a Self-Care Assessment Worksheet. This brief inventory offers support to keep one's life in balance with a detailed inventory of physical, psychological, emotional, spiritual, and professional self-care.

CLINICAL PATHOLOGY AND PROCEDURES

CP

COLLECTION AND SUBMISSION OF LABORATORY SAMPLES

Each veterinary diagnostic laboratory offers a unique set of diagnostic tests that is subject to frequent changes as better tests become available. The increasing availability of tests based on newer molecular biology techniques is an excellent example of this trend. The protocols for sample collection and submission are therefore also subject to change. The practitioner and diagnostic laboratory staff *must* maintain good communication to complete their diagnostic efforts efficiently and provide optimal service to the client. Practitioners must be specific and clear in their test requests. The laboratory staff can provide guidance when there are questions regarding sample collection and handling, as well as offering assistance in interpretation of test results. Most diagnostic laboratories publish user guidelines with preferred protocols for sample collection and submission, but the following broad recommendations are fairly standard.

Regardless of the type of submission, a detailed case history should be included with the samples to assist laboratory personnel in determining a diagnosis. The information should include owner, species, breed, sex, age, animal identification, clinical signs, gross appearance (including size and location) of the lesion(s), previous treatment (if any), time of recurrence from any previous treatment, and morbidity/mortality in the group. If a zoonotic disease is suspected, this should also be clearly indicated on the submission form to alert laboratory personnel. The submission form should be placed in a waterproof bag to protect it from any fluids that might be present in the packaged materials. Waterproof markers should be used when labeling specimen bags and containers. When packaging samples, the use of breakable containers should be avoided, but properly padded glass tubes are commonly shipped. The basic principles of good shipping practices include the use of sturdy containers, clearly labeled to contain biologic diagnostic specimens; ideally, this should be a styrofoam container within a cardboard box. Any coolant packs should be sealed within plastic bags and accompanied by adsorbent material within the container. If dry ice is used, this should be noted on the cardboard box label, and the stryofoam lid should *not* be sealed with tape. A "triple barrier" approach can be applied to most diagnostic specimens. One barrier is the outer cardboard box; another is the inner styrofoam container or perhaps sealable plastic bags (with adsorbent material). Note that if air shipment of samples is anticipated, then International Air Transport Association (IATA) requirements include specialized bags capable of withstanding 95 kilopascals of pressure. The third barrier is around the sample itself. Liquid samples should not be shipped in plastic bags; a sealable tube or jar should be used. The top of these fluid-filled containers should be sealed with tape. The tube/jar is then placed in a sealable plastic bag with some adsorbent material in case of leakage. Fresh tissue samples are similarly placed within a second bag (third barrier) containing some adsorbent material. Use of appropriate padding material within the box will protect sample integrity while preventing coolant packs from crushing samples. Regulations regarding shipping of biologic samples vary according to country but in the USA are mainly in the purview of the Department of Transportation, Hazardous Materials Regulations. Also, IATA restricts the volume of formalin that can be shipped in any single shipping container to <1 L in total and <30 mL per jar.

Histology: Tissues for microscopic examination collected either via biopsy or during necropsy can be critical to obtaining a diagnosis. Use of this relatively rapid and inexpensive diagnostic technique can often result in substantial savings in time, money, and animal life. The increasing number of immunohistochemical (IHC) tests that can be applied to formalin-fixed tissue has further reinforced the utility of this diagnostic technique.

Autolyzed tissues are generally useless for histopathologic examination; prompt necropsy examination and organ sampling are critical. Tissue should *not* be frozen before fixation. Other than CNS tissues (*see* below), samples collected for histology should never be >1 cm thick (preferably 5–7 mm) and must be placed immediately into ≥10 times their volume of phosphate-buffered 10% formalin to ensure adequate fixation. Tissues collected for histologic examination should be representative of any lesions present and, in the case of cutaneous punch biopsies and biopsies obtained via endoscopic collection, should be centered directly on the grossly visible lesions. Wedge biopsies or tissue samples collected at necropsy should include some of the apparently normal surrounding tissue; the interface between normal and abnormal may provide key information. Excisional biopsies of small tumors (<1.5 cm) may be cut in half. Larger tumors may be sliced like bread so that formalin can penetrate to the face of each slice. Alternatively, several representative samples (7 mm wide, including the interface of normal and abnormal) may be collected. The tissues should remain in fixative for ≥24 hr; after this initial fixation, the samples may be placed in a smaller volume of fresh formalin for shipment if necessary. Prolonged fixation can adversely affect IHC testing, so samples should be shipped promptly if IHC tests are anticipated. Histologic samples should be shipped in unbreakable containers and packed in a manner that prevents spillage during shipment. *Fixed tissues should be protected from freezing.*

Specific tissues collected at necropsy require additional attention. Because the GI mucosa decomposes rapidly, short sections of gut collected at necropsy must be opened lengthwise to allow adequate fixation. If spinal cord is to be submitted, the dura mater should be carefully incised lengthwise to permit more rapid penetration to the cord. Fixing the brain poses a special dilemma, especially if a neuroanatomic location of the lesion(s) within the organ could not be determined antemortem. Ideally, a whole, intact fixed brain is required for complete histopathologic analysis. Immersion of the brain for many days in a very large volume of formalin is required to adequately fix such a specimen, so brains are commonly transported in an only partially fixed state. If the specimen can be shipped by overnight delivery, it may be acceptable to send a chilled, carefully packaged, unfixed brain, which can then be processed at the diagnostic laboratory. Often, the brain is halved longitudinally and one-half sent unfixed (fresh), properly refrigerated, for microbiologic tests, while the other half partially fixes in transit. This method can prove unsatisfactory if a solitary unilateral lesion is involved. Slicing the brain into widths suitable for rapid fixation introduces considerable fixation artifact and should be avoided if possible; fixing the intact/halved brain in a large volume of formalin for >24 hr is preferred.

Microbiology: Any specific agents that are of interest in the diagnostic investigation should be mentioned on the submission form; some agents have requirements (eg, anaerobic culture, special media) that would not be used in most laboratories unless the pathogen was cited as a differential diagnosis. Laboratory techniques and capabilities for microbiologic examination vary; available tests include bacteriologic culture, fungal culture, virus isolation, in-situ hybridization, a variety of PCR methods, fluorescent antibody tests, latex agglutination tests, Western blotting, ELISA, and many others. Most tests, including the newer molecular biology techniques, rely on either the growth/visualization of intact viable organisms or the detection of the nucleic acids and proteins of these pathogens. Therefore, unfixed specimens (tissue, fluid, etc) should be collected aseptically and shipped promptly to avoid degradation. If PCR testing is to be performed, it is particularly important to avoid cross-contamination between multiple animals in a submission; this applies to tissues, fluids, and even dissection instruments. Furthermore, swabs destined for PCR analysis should not be placed in agar or charcoal-based transport media. Calcium alginate swabs should be avoided. Instead, cotton or dacron swabs should be shipped in a tube with a few drops of sterile saline or viral transport media.

Some test protocols may permit pooling of organ specimens from an individual, but for the vast majority, it is preferable that each tissue be collected into separate sterile, clearly labeled bags or tubes for shipping. Gut samples must never be pooled in a container with other tissue samples. Tissues and fluids for most microbiologic assays may be frozen before shipment, but generally freezing is undesirable if samples can be chilled and delivered directly to the laboratory within 24 hr. Exceptions to this rule include analysis for certain toxins, such as those of *Clostridium perfringens* and *C botulinum*, in which degradation of the toxin must be prevented by prompt freezing after collection. Adequate refrigerant should be provided so that samples remain chilled (or frozen) until they reach the laboratory.

Toxicology: If a known toxin is suspected, a specific analysis should always be requested—laboratories cannot just "check for poisoning." A complete description of clinical and epidemiologic findings may help differentiate poisoning from infectious diseases that can simulate poisoning. For a list of appropriate samples for many of the more common toxicities, *see* TABLE 1. The most critical samples to be collected are generally stomach contents, liver, kidney, whole blood, plasma/serum, and urine, but exceptions exist, such as cerebral tissue for cholinesterase analysis. For some investigations, the diagnosis requires analysis of feed or water. If there is doubt about sample submission procedures, the laboratory should be contacted.

TABLE 1 GUIDELINES FOR SUBMITTING SAMPLES FOR TOXICOLOGIC EXAMINATION

Suspected Poison or Analysis	Specimen Required	Comments
Ammonia	Whole blood or serum Urine Rumen contents	Frozen Frozen Frozen (or may add 1–2 drops saturated $HgCl_3$)
Anticoagulants (warfarin and related compounds)	Whole blood Liver Feed Stomach contents	Heparin or EDTA Refrigerated
Arsenic	Liver Kidney Urine Ingesta Feed	
Chlorates	Stomach contents Urine Feed	Frozen, in airtight container
Chlorinated hydrocarbons	Cerebrum Ingesta Body fat Liver Kidney	Use only glass containers Avoid contamination Refrigerated or frozen
Cholinesterase	Serum Cerebrum	Frozen
Copper (and Ni, Fe, Co, Cr, and Tl)	Kidney Liver Serum Feed Whole blood Feces	
Cyanide	Forage Whole blood Liver	Rush to laboratory or ship promptly, frozen in airtight container
Dicoumarol	Forage Liver	
Ethylene glycol	Serum Urine Kidneys	Fresh plus fixed in formalin

(continued)

TABLE 1 GUIDELINES FOR SUBMITTING SAMPLES FOR TOXICOLOGIC EXAMINATION *(continued)*

Suspected Poison or Analysis	Specimen Required	Comments
Fluorides	Bone Water Forage Urine	Best to send affected bone(s)
Herbicides (many)	Treated weeds Urine Ingesta Liver or kidney	
Ionophores	Feed Rumen contents Heart Skeletal muscle	 Fixed in formalin Fixed in formalin
Lead (also Hg, Mo, Ni, and Tl)	Kidney Whole blood Liver Urine	 Heparinized blood preferred
Mercury and molybdenum	Kidney Whole blood Liver Feed	*See* LEAD, above
Mycotoxins	Grain, forages Liver, kidney	Consult with laboratory personnel on specific tests
Nitrate	Forage Water Body fluids (eg, aqueous humor)	Refrigerated
Organophosphates (and carbamates)	Feed Ingesta Urine	Also send urine, blood, and stomach contents from clinically normal animals
Oxalates	Fresh forage Kidney	Do not macerate; freeze Fixed in formalin
Phenols	Gastric or rumen contents	In airtight container
Polychlorinated (and polybrominated) biphenyls	Fat Cerebrum Feed	
Rumen pH	Ingesta	Frozen
Selenium	Whole blood Feed Liver Hair clippings	Heparinized
Sodium (NaCl)	Brain Serum CSF Feed	Other half fixed in formalin
Sodium fluoroacetate (1080)	Stomach contents Liver	Frozen

(continued)

TABLE 1 GUIDELINES FOR SUBMITTING SAMPLES FOR TOXICOLOGIC EXAMINATION *(continued)*

Suspected Poison or Analysis	Specimen Required	Comments
Strychnine (and some other convulsants such as bromethalin)	Liver Kidney Stomach contents	
Sulfates	Water Brain	 Fixed in formalin
TDS (total dissolved solids)	Water	
Triaryl-PO_4	Ingesta Feed	
Urea	Feed	*See* AMMONIA, above
Vitamin A (also D and E)	Liver Serum	 Frozen
Vitamin D_3 (rodenticides)	Kidney	
Zinc	Liver Kidney Serum	 Use "trace minerals" tubes
Zinc phosphide	Liver Gastric contents	Frozen

Tissues or fluids for chemical analysis should be as fresh as possible and kept refrigerated. For some analyses, freezing is critical to prevent degradation of volatile chemicals, and in rare instances a chemical preservative is required.

If legal action is a possibility, all containers for shipment should be either sealed so that tampering can be detected or hand-carried to the laboratory and a receipt obtained. The chain of custody must be accurately documented.

If feed or water is suspected as the source of poisoning, samples of these and any descriptive feed tag should accompany the tissue samples. If at all possible, a representative composite sample of the feed should be submitted from the suspect lot or shipment. In some instances, if an adequate amount of involved feed is available, some of it may be fed to experimental animals in an effort to reproduce the signs and lesions seen in the field cases.

Hematology: Routine studies require anticoagulated whole blood and several blood smears. Blood smears should be prepared immediately after the sample has been collected to minimize cell deterioration. Anticoagulated blood should be kept refrigerated; blood smears should not. EDTA is the anticoagulant of choice for a CBC because it best preserves the cellular components of the blood and prevents platelet aggregation. Blood for coagulation testing should be collected into a blue top tube, which contains sodium citrate. After mixing, the sample should be centrifuged for 5 min, and then plasma should be removed and transferred to a clean tube without anticoagulant. The plasma should be kept frozen until the time of analysis. Whole blood should not be frozen because this causes cell lysis and gross hemolysis, which interfere with testing.

Clinical Chemistry: Most clinical chemistry tests require serum, but an occasional test may require plasma. Anticoagulants present in plasma may interfere with tests; therefore, serum should always be submitted unless plasma is specifically requested. Because lipemia can interfere with a number of chemistry tests, dogs and cats should be fasted for 12 hr before samples are collected.

For serum samples, the blood should be drawn into a red top tube or a separator tube. The sample should be held at room temperature for 20–30 min to allow complete clot formation and retraction. Incomplete clot formation may cause the serum to gel due to latent fibrin formation. The clot should be separated from the glass by gently running an applicator stick around the tube walls ("rimming"). The sample should then be centrifuged at high speed (~1,000 g; 2,200 rpm) for 10 min. Rough handling of the sample or incomplete separation of erythrocytes from serum may promote hemolysis, which can interfere with certain tests.

If the sample has been collected into a serum separator tube, centrifugation will cause a layer of silicon gel to lodge between the packed cells and the serum. The gel layer should be inspected to ensure the integrity of the barrier, and re-centrifugation is recommended if there is a visible crack in this layer. If a red top tube has been used, the serum should be removed and transferred to a clean tube. Serum should be refrigerated or frozen until analyzed.

Many commercial laboratories provide sample containers and mailers.

Serology: Serology generally requires serum, but plasma is often satisfactory. Samples should be collected as described for clinical chemistry tests and should always be free of hemolysis. In some instances, paired samples may be required for an adequate diagnosis. The acute sample should be collected early in the course of the disease and frozen. The convalescent sample should be collected 10–14 days later, and both samples should be forwarded to the laboratory at the same time.

Cytology: Air-dried smears are usually acceptable. Rapid air drying of smears minimizes cell distortion, thereby enhancing diagnostic quality. However, depending on the method of staining used, some laboratories prefer alcohol-fixed smears. Samples can be obtained by fine-needle aspiration or by scraping. Imprints (touch preparations) of external lesions can also be used, although these tend to have a greater degree of contamination. Aspirated material should always be smeared before air drying. Smears of fluid can be prepared using a traditional blood smearing technique. Highly cellular fluids may be smeared directly; fluids of low cellularity should be centrifuged to concentrate the cells. Thick material or viscous fluid is more readily smeared using a squash technique in which a second glass slide is placed over the aspirated material and then slid rapidly and smoothly down the length of the lower slide.

Blood or cytologic smears should never be mailed to the laboratory in the same package with formalin-fixed tissues because formalin vapors will produce artifacts in the specimen. Many laboratories now offer immunocytochemical testing, and proper handling of cytologic submissions is required for reliable results. Usually air-dried, unfixed smears will suffice, but in some instances shipping of samples in tubes containing a transport media is recommended.

Fluid Analysis: Analysis of various effusions and fluids usually includes determination of protein content, total cell count, and cytologic examination. Other tests may be performed depending on the source or appearance (eg, chylous fluid) of the effusion. A sample of effusion/fluid should be collected into an EDTA (purple top) tube for routine analysis. A second sample should be collected into a serum (red top) tube if any biochemical analyses (eg, triglyceride, cholesterol, lipase for chylous effusions) are to be performed or if a bacterial culture is desired (eg, joint fluid). These samples should be shipped chilled but not frozen. Smears for cytologic examination (*see* above) should be prepared from a drop of the fluid immediately after the sample has been collected to minimize cell deterioration and other in vitro artifacts. Samples of CSF should be collected into small EDTA tubes and *shipped immediately with high priority*; the cytologic value of CSF samples degrades rapidly and the low cellularity makes examination of direct smears unrewarding. If sufficient CSF is available, then a red top tube sample may be useful for serology or culture attempts.

Genetic Analysis: Tests based on the detection of specific genetic features range from karyotype analysis to the identification of specific genes. The laboratory offering the test should be contacted to determine the specifics of sample collection and handling; required samples range from hair to skin or blood. Many blood-based analyses require collection into yellow-topped acid-citrate-dextrose tubes and overnight shipment of the chilled tubes to the laboratory. Tissue samples for genetic analysis should be unfixed and shipped immediately after collection. As with most molecular techniques, aseptic collection and the prevention of cross-contamination between samples is critical for reliable test results.

DIAGNOSTIC PROCEDURES FOR THE PRIVATE PRACTICE LABORATORY

Numerous laboratory tests can be done in a private practice laboratory. Use of a commercial laboratory versus in-house testing should be evaluated to determine whether in-house testing is practical and economical. Because the availability of diagnostic laboratories and their reporting intervals may be problematic (eg, nights and holidays), performing some diagnostic screening tests in-house is often desirable. However, because the people performing these tests often have minimal technical training, quality control procedures must be rigorous. The time and care that must be devoted to quality control issues may preclude in-house testing in many practices. Errors may occur not only in testing procedures but also in sample collection and handling and in recording results.

Tests can be done using either manual or automated methods. Manual methods tend to be time consuming and are more subject to human error. Automated and semiautomated systems are available but are more expensive. Factors to be considered include instrument and reagent costs (including materials for calibration and quality control), availability of personnel training, technical support, and instrument maintenance and service. Although service contracts can cost up to 10% of the purchase price of an instrument, they are often cost-effective because of the expense of instrument repair.

CLINICAL BIOCHEMISTRY

Clinical biochemistry refers to the analysis of the blood plasma (or serum) for a wide variety of substances—substrates, enzymes, hormones, etc—and their use in diagnosis and monitoring of disease. Analysis of other body fluids (eg, urine, ascitic fluids, CSF) is also included. One test is very seldom specific to one clinical condition, and basic checklists of factors affecting the most commonly requested analytes are given below. Thus, rather than six tests that merely confirm or deny six possibilities, a *well-chosen group of six tests can provide* information pointing to a wide variety of different conditions by a process of pattern recognition. Biochemistry tests should be accompanied by full hematology, because evaluation of both together is essential for optimal recognition of many of the most characteristic disease patterns (*see* p 1610).

Before samples are collected, a list of differential diagnoses should already be established based on the history and clinical examination. Then, additional appropriate tests can be added to the basic panel below.

Making a diagnosis entails establishing a list of differential diagnoses based on the history and clinical examination. Based on this list, tests can be selected to include or exclude as many of the differentials as possible. Yet more tests may be necessary until only one of the original list remains to determine the diagnosis. If all differentials are excluded, then the list must be reevaluated. It is not good practice to order tests without a sensible differential list unless the animal presents without definitive clinical signs.

Basic Test Panel: Most veterinary laboratories offer a basic panel of tests, which represents a minimal investigation applicable to most general situations. For small animals, a typical panel includes total protein, albumin, globulin (calculated as the difference between the first two analytes), urea, creatinine, ALT, and alkaline phosphatase (ALP). In addition, a yellow color seen in the plasma should be considered an indication to measure bilirubin. This panel may be modified as appropriate for other species, eg, glutamate dehydrogenase (GDH) and/or γ glutamyl transferase (γGT) are more appropriate "liver enzymes" for horses and farm animals, or it may be more appropriate to concentrate primarily on muscle enzymes (CK and AST) in athletic animals.

Total protein level increases due to dehydration, chronic inflammation, and paraproteinemia. It decreases due to overhydration, severe congestive heart failure (with edema), protein-losing nephropathy, protein-losing enteropathy, hemorrhage, burns, dietary protein deficiency, malabsorption, and some viral conditions (especially in horses).

Albumin level increases due to dehydration. It decreases due to the same factors as total protein, plus liver failure.

Urea level increases due to excess dietary protein, poor quality dietary protein, carbohydrate deficiency, catabolic states, dehydration, congestive heart failure, renal failure, blocked urethra, and ruptured bladder. It decreases due to low dietary protein, gross sepsis, anabolic hormonal effects, liver failure, portosystemic shunts (congenital or acquired), and inborn errors of urea cycle metabolism. Urea measurement is used especially to indicate renal disease and to a lesser extent liver dysfunction.

Creatinine level increases due to renal dysfunction, blocked urethra, and ruptured bladder. It decreases due to sample deterioration. Animals with a high muscle mass have high-normal creatinine concentrations, whereas animals with a low muscle mass have low-normal creatinine concentrations. Creatinine measurement is used especially for renal disease.

ALT is present in the cytoplasm and mitochondria of liver cells and, therefore, increases due to hepatocellular damage. It has a half life of 2–4 hr and rises higher than AST but recovers quicker. There are minor increases with muscle damage and hyperthyroidism.

ALP level increases due to increased bone deposition, liver damage, hyperthyroidism, biliary tract disease, intestinal damage, hyperadrenocorticism, corticosteroid administration, barbiturate administration, and generalized tissue damage (including neoplasia). The most common causes for an increase is raised levels of circulating steroids and biliary disease. The half-life is 72 hr in dogs but only 6 hr in cats. Levels in the cat are generally much lower than in the dog, and *any* increase in cats is considered significant. In dogs, ALP levels in the thousands of units are usually associated with increased steroid levels. ALP and ALT levels rarely rise above 1,000 units, even in severe liver disease.

GDH level increases in hepatocellular damage, particularly hepatic necrosis, in horses and ruminants.

γGT increases in longer-term liver damage; it is particularly useful in horses and ruminants.

CK, the classic "muscle enzyme," increases markedly in rhabdomyolysis and aortic thromboembolism. Slight level increases are reported in hypothyroidism. Only a very small amount of muscle damage such as bruising or IM injections can result in high serum CK levels. In dogs and cats, unless investigating specific muscle disease, increased levels are generally of no clinical significance.

AST level increases in both muscle and liver damage but is of less value than ALT. The half-life is 5 hr in dogs and 77 min in cats. It is also reported to increase in hypothyroidism.

Most of the above parameters are associated with liver function/dysfunction and are frequently overinterpreted. In small animals, increases in ALT and ALP levels can reach four times normal and still be associated only with fatty change, a nonspecific finding and not, in most cases, a primary liver problem. Some laboratories also frequently receive liver biopsies from dogs that have significant increases in liver enzymes and bile acids >80 but that have normal histologic morphology. The reason for this is unknown.

In general, plasma enzyme levels decrease due to sample deterioration. Uncommonly, atrophy or fibrosis of an organ may result in unusually low plasma activities of the relevant enzymes.

Additional Tests: Further tests may be added to the basic panel, according to the principal presenting signs, to create panels for polydipsic animals, collapsing animals, etc. These panels are structured so that the patterns of abnormalities typical of all the likely differential diagnoses applicable to the situation can be discerned. For example, a polydipsia panel may add calcium, glucose, and cholesterol. Calcium allows recognition of hyperparathyroidism and other causes of hypercalcemia (which causes polydipsia and renal insufficiency), glucose may indicate diabetes mellitus and contributes to the pattern characteristic of hyperadrenocorticism, and cholesterol also adds to the appreciation of the "Cushing pattern." Renal failure is covered by the tests already included in the basic panel. In contrast, in a panel for a "collapsing animal," calcium and glucose may be added to screen for hypocalcemia or hypoglycemia. Sodium and potassium are included to screen for hypoadrenocorticism or hypokalemia. Analytes that might be considered for incorporation in such expanded profiles are described below.

Sodium level increases due to Conn syndrome (hyperaldosteronism), restricted water intake, vomiting, and most causes of dehydration. It decreases due to hypoadrenocorticism, loss of any high-sodium fluid such as some forms of renal disease, and insufficient sodium provision during IV fluid therapy.

Potassium level increases due to hypoadrenocorticism and severe renal failure (especially terminal cases). It decreases due to Conn syndrome, chronic renal dysfunction, vomiting, diarrhea, and insufficient potassium provision during IV fluid therapy. Congenital hypokalemia occurs in Burmese cats.

Chloride level increases in acidosis, and in parallel with increases in sodium concentration. It decreases in alkalosis, vomiting (especially after eating), and in association with hyponatremia.

Total CO_2 (bicarbonate) level increases in metabolic alkalosis and decreases in metabolic acidosis. It is less useful to assess respiratory acid/base disturbances.

Calcium level increases due to dehydration (which is also associated with increased albumin), primary hyperparathyroidism (neoplasia of parathyroid gland), primary pseudohyperparathyroidism (neoplasms producing parathormone-related peptide [PRP], usually perianal adenocarcinoma or some form of lymphosarcoma), bone invasion of malignant neoplasms, thyrotoxicosis (uncommon), and overtreatment of parturient paresis. It decreases due to hypoalbuminemia, parturient paresis, oxalate poisoning, chronic renal failure (secondary renal hyperparathyroidism), acute pancreatitis (occasionally), surgical interference with parathyroid glands, and idiopathic (autoimmune) hypoparathyroidism.

Phosphate level increases due to renal failure (secondary renal hyperparathyroidism). Decreases are seen in some downer cows and as part of the stress pattern in horses and small animals.

Magnesium level increases are rarely seen, including during acute renal failure. It decreases in ruminants due to dietary deficiency, either acute (grass staggers) or chronic, and diarrhea (uncommon).

Glucose level increases due to high-carbohydrate meals, sprint exercise, stress or excitement (including handling and sampling stress), glucocorticoid therapy, hyperadrenocorticism, overinfusion with glucose/dextrose-containing IV fluids, and diabetes mellitus. It decreases due to insulin overdose, insulinoma, islet cell hyperplasia (uncommon), acetonemia/pregnancy toxemia, acute febrile illness, and idiopathically (in certain dog breeds).

β-Hydroxybutyrate level increases in diabetes mellitus. It is a major component of ketoacidosis and as such is also increased in acetonemia/pregnancy toxemia and extreme starvation. It can be measured in both blood and urine.

Bilirubin level increases due to fasting (benign effect in horses and squirrel monkeys, may be caused by hepatic lipidosis in cats), hemolytic disease (usually mild increase), liver dysfunction, and biliary obstruction (intra- or extrahepatic). Theoretically, hemolysis is characterized by an increase in unconjugated (indirect) bilirubin, whereas hepatic and post-hepatic disorders are characterized by an increase in conjugated (direct) bilirubin; however, in practice this differentiation is unsatisfactory. Better appreciation of the source of the jaundice is gained from bile acid measurements.

Bile acid levels increase when hepatic anion transport is impaired, usually during liver dysfunction (bile acids are more sensitive than bilirubin to hepatic impairment) and in the presence of a portosystemic shunt (congenital or acquired). The latter condition is characterized by a marked increase in bile acid concentration after feeding, from a fasting concentration that may be normal. It also increases in bile duct obstruction; very little increase is seen in feline infectious peritonitis or mild cases of hepatic lipidosis. Very high levels can sometimes be seen without structural histologic changes. The reason for this is not known.

Cholesterol level increases due to fatty meals, hepatic or biliary disease, protein-losing nephropathy (and other protein-losing syndromes to some extent), diabetes mellitus, hyperadrenocorticism, and hypothyroidism. It decreases in some cases of severe liver dysfunction and occasionally in hyperthyroidism.

Lactate dehydrogenase is a ubiquitous enzyme with a number of isoenzymes; electrophoretic separation of isoenzymes is necessary to locate the source of increased activity. It is therefore of very limited value in general clinical practice.

Sorbitol dehydrogenase level increases in acute hepatocellular damage in horses but is a very labile analyte.

α-Amylase level increases in acute pancreatitis but in dogs is also increased in chronic renal dysfunction. It is therefore of limited use in the diagnosis of pancreatitis. Pancreatic lipase immunoreactivity is now the test of choice for diagnosis of pancreatitis in dogs and cats. Amylase is not a useful indicator of pancreatitis in cats.

Lipase level increases in acute pancreatitis in dogs (longer half-life than amylase) and also occasionally in chronic renal dysfunction. Lipase (routine assay) is not a useful indicator of pancreatitis in cats.

Immunoreactive trypsin (trypsin-like immunoreactivity) level decreases in exocrine pancreatic insufficiency in dogs. It will also increase (irregularly) in pancreatitis.

Tests for Pancreatic Disease:

Pancreatitis: **Serum amylase and lipase activities** have been used for several decades to diagnose pancreatitis in both people and dogs. Unfortunately, neither of these tests is both sensitive and specific for pancreatitis in dogs. In one study, significant serum amylase and lipase activities remained after total pancreatectomy, indicating there are sources of serum amylase and lipase activity other than the exocrine pancreas. Also, clinical data suggest a specificity for pancreatitis of only ~50% for both of these markers. Many nonpancreatic diseases, such as renal, hepatic, intestinal, and neoplastic diseases, can lead to increases in serum amylase and lipase activities. Steroid administration can also increase serum lipase activity and cause variable responses in serum amylase activity. Thus, in dogs, measurement of serum amylase and lipase activities are of limited usefulness for diagnosis of pancreatitis. Serum amylase and/or lipase activities that are 3–5 times the upper limit of the reference range, in animals with clinical signs consistent with pancreatitis, are suggestive of such a diagnosis. However, it is important to note that ~50% of dogs that fulfill these criteria do not have pancreatitis. In cats, serum amylase and lipase activities are of no clinical value for diagnosis of pancreatitis. Although cats with experimental pancreatitis can show an increase in serum lipase activity and a decrease in serum amylase activity, these changes are not consistent in cats with spontaneous pancreatitis. In one study of 12 cats with severe forms of pancreatitis, not a single cat had serum lipase or amylase activity above the upper limit of the reference range.

Serum trypsin-like immunoreactivity (TLI) concentration measures mainly trypsinogen, the only form of trypsin circulating in the vascular space of healthy individuals. However, trypsin, if present in the serum, is also detected by these assays. Serum TLI concentrations can be measured by species-specific assays that have been developed and validated for both dogs and cats. In healthy animals, serum TLI is low, but during pancreatitis an increased amount of trypsinogen leaks into the vascular space, which can lead to an increase in serum TLI concentration. Trypsin that has been prematurely activated may also contribute to this increase. However, both trypsinogen and trypsin are quickly cleared by the kidneys. In addition, any prematurely activated trypsin is quickly removed by proteinase inhibitors, such as α_1-proteinase inhibitor and α_2-macroglobulin. In turn, α_2-macroglobulin-trypsin complexes are removed by the reticuloendothelial system. Thus, the serum half-life for TLI is short, and a significant degree of active inflammation is required to increase serum TLI concentration. Because of the limited sensitivity of serum cTLI and fTLI concentrations for canine and feline pancreatitis, respectively, and because only a limited number of laboratories measure these assays routinely, serum TLI concentration is of limited usefulness for diagnosis of pancreatitis in dogs and cats.

Pancreatic lipase immunoreactivity (PLI) concentration measures the concentration of classical pancreatic lipase in the serum. This is in contrast to serum lipase activity, which measures the enzymatic activity of all triglyceridases present in the serum, regardless of their cellular origin. Assays to measure PLI in canine (cPLI) and feline (fPLI) serum have been developed and validated and are commercially available. Serum PLI is highly specific for exocrine pancreatic function. Also, serum PLI is far more sensitive for diagnosis of pancreatitis than any other diagnostic test currently available.

A patient-side semiquantitative assay for diagnosis of canine pancreatitis is also available. A test spot that is lighter in color than the reference spot suggests that pancreatitis can be excluded. A test spot darker in color than the reference spot raises the suspicion of pancreatitis and should prompt the clinician to measure a serum cPLI concentration in the laboratory.

Other tests for diagnosis of pancreatitis in dogs and cats have been evaluated, including plasma trypsinogen activation peptide (TAP) concentration, urine TAP concentration, urine TAP:creatinine ratio, serum α_1-proteinase inhibitor trypsin complex concentration, and serum α_2-macroglobulin concentration. However, none has been shown to be of clinical usefulness.

Exocrine Pancreatic Insufficiency: In the past, several fecal tests have been used to diagnose exocrine pancreatic insufficiency (EPI). Microscopic fecal examination for fat and/or undigested starch or muscle fibers are at best useful to suggest maldigestion. However, in light of wide availability of tests to diagnose EPI, microscopic fecal examination is no longer justified. Fecal proteolytic activity had been used to diagnose EPI in small animals for several decades. Most of these methods, particularly the radiographic film clearance test, are unreliable. One method, which uses pre-made tablets to pour a gelatin agar, is considered most reliable. However, false-positive as well as false-negative results have been reported. The clinical use of fecal proteolytic activity is limited to species for which more specific assays to estimate pancreatic function are not available and in areas where the more accurate and sophisticated tests are not available.

Serum TLI concentration is the diagnostic test of choice for EPI in both dogs and cats. Assays for TLI measure trypsinogen circulating in the vascular space. In healthy animals, only a small amount of trypsinogen is present in serum. However, in dogs and cats with EPI, the number of pancreatic acinar cells is severely decreased. Serum TLI concentration decreases significantly and may even be undetectable. The reference range for TLI in dogs is 5.7–45.2 mcg/L with a cut-off value of ≤2.5 mcg/L considered diagnostic for EPI. Similarly, the reference range for TLI in cats is 12–82 mcg/L, with a cut-off value of ≤8 mcg/L considered diagnostic. Rarely, animals with serum TLI concentrations below the cut-off value for EPI do not have clinical signs of EPI. This is probably because of the functional redundancy of the GI tract. At the same time, many dogs and cats with chronic diarrhea and weight loss have mild decreases in serum TLI concentration. Most of these animals have chronic small-intestinal disease and should be investigated accordingly. However, a small number of these dogs and cats may have EPI. If there is no evidence of small-intestinal disease in such patients, a trial therapy with pancreatic enzymes and reevaluation of serum TLI concentration after 1 mo is indicated.

PLI is also highly specific for exocrine pancreatic function and could be used to diagnose EPI. However, initial studies showed there is a small degree of overlap in serum PLI concentrations between healthy dogs and dogs with EPI, making the measurement of PLI slightly inferior to that of TLI for accurate diagnosis. In view of these findings, PLI assays for both dogs and cats have been optimized toward higher concentrations, and the current assays are no longer suitable for diagnosis of EPI in dogs or cats.

A **fecal canine elastase concentration** assay has been developed and validated but is inferior to the widely used TLI measurement.

Handling of Samples: Most biochemistry tests can be performed on either serum or heparinized plasma. A few (eg, insulin) require serum, whereas potassium is best measured on heparin plasma separated immediately after collection. Glucose measurement requires fluoride/oxalate plasma. Suitable collection tubes with and without anticoagulant are available commercially. Plastic tubes are satisfactory for blood in anticoagulant, but clotted blood must be collected either into glass tubes or plastic tubes specially coated to prevent the clot from adhering to the vessel walls.

Samples for biochemical analysis should be separated as soon as possible after collection to minimize artifacts caused by hemolysis and leakage of intracellular fluid components (eg, potassium) out of the cells. Samples in anticoagulant may be centrifuged immediately, but clotted samples need at least 30 min to allow the clot to form. Fluoride/oxalate samples hemolyze very readily because the cells can no longer respire, so timely separation is especially important. Proprietary gels or plastic beads assist with separation, and these may be incorporated into the collection tube or added before centrifugation.

Larger bucket-type centrifuges will accept almost any type or size of tube, but the rotors require careful balancing. They should be spun at 3,000 rpm for 10 min. Dual-purpose, high-speed microhematocrit centrifuges are favored for in-practice use, because they separate samples more quickly and the same machine can be used to measure PCV. However, they can handle only a limited range of small-volume tubes.

Some "gel-tube" products may provide a permanent separation of serum or plasma; otherwise, this must be separated into a fresh tube. The new tube must be adequately labeled. Samples may then be sent to a professional laboratory or analyzed in the practice.

Point-of-Care Tests: A number of biochemical analytes may be estimated in the practice without the need for large analytical instruments.

Total protein level is measured by refractometry, using the same instrument as is used to measure urine specific gravity, provided the instrument has a total protein scale. It is also valid for protein measurement of ascitic and pleural fluids. The readout may be in g/dL, in which case multiplying the result by 10 will yield the SI unit of g/L.

Urea level may be estimated by chromatographic reaction strips, which correlate well with standard laboratory methods. A rapid whole-blood color comparison strip is also available, but these read only up to ~20 mmol/L and are thus of limited use. A dedicated reflectance meter for urea estimation is not available.

Glucose meters for use on whole blood are widely available for home use by human diabetic patients. These yield acceptably accurate results on animal blood, although an unexpected hypoglycemia should be confirmed by a professional laboratory. Fresh whole blood may be used, but fluoride blood or plasma is the preferred sample if analysis is not immediate.

Ketone levels may be estimated on either urine (preferred sample) or plasma/serum. This can be achieved by using the ketone patch of a urine dipstick, giving a qualitative result. However, there are a number of point-of-care instruments for measurement of blood glucose and ketone levels, including specifically β-hydroxybutyrate.

Triglyceride levels may be visualized in a plasma or serum sample as lipemia. If the milkiness rises to the top of the tube on storage, chylomicrons are present. Otherwise, the milkiness is caused by triglycerides. This is a qualitative judgment but is nevertheless useful, especially in equine patients.

Bilirubin level may also be appreciated by eye in most species. Equine and bovine plasma is normally yellow, which makes determination problematic, but in other species, any yellow color is abnormal and indicates an increased bilirubin level. Visual assessment of the depth and shade of color may provide additional information.

Other point-of-care tests include **C-reactive protein** as a marker for inflammation and **cardiac troponin** as a marker for cardiac muscle damage.

For emergency in-clinic use, the most important analytes beyond these simple basics are sodium and potassium. A dedicated ion-specific electrode meter is the best way to measure these. Instruments are available that can analyze whole blood, although great care must be taken to avoid artifacts due to unappreciated hemolysis. Critical care meters are also available that can estimate a variety of analytes, including glucose, urea, and electrolytes; however, these have not been extensively validated on nonhuman blood, and results should be interpreted with caution.

The Practice Laboratory: Extending in-practice analysis beyond these emergency basics requires a dedicated instrument capable of measuring multiple analytes. Two types are available—those based on transmission/absorbance photometry (wet chemistry) and those based on reflectance photometry (dry-reagent chemistry). Transmission/absorbance photometry is the reference method on which all reference values and interpretive guidelines are based. Reflectance photometry methods do not always compare well with the reference method and are best confined to simpler tests such as glucose and urea. For wider applications, such as enzyme analysis, wet chemistry instruments are preferred.

In-clinic analysis is inevitably more expensive than the same investigations done by a professional laboratory, and the range of analytes available is more restricted. Additionally, the level of accuracy or reliability is likely to be lower. Therefore, it is still best practice to regard in-practice analysis as an interim emergency investigation, with the results to be confirmed as appropriate by a professional laboratory. Detailed case laboratory evaluation of nonemergency patients is best referred to a professional laboratory from the outset, for reasons of cost, accuracy, range of analytes available, and the assistance of the clinical pathologist in interpretation of the results.

If in-clinic analysis is to be relied on for general case laboratory evaluation, meticulous attention must be paid to quality assurance. Samples of known composition must be run at least daily for each analyte, in both normal and pathologic ranges; unless these are within the tolerance limits, no patient samples should be tested. Participation in an external quality assessment program is also strongly recommended. Employing a trained technician will address some of these issues but has implications for availability of results during off hours and holidays. The veterinarian in charge of the laboratory is responsible for all the results issued and incurs a legal liability to prove accuracy and reliability. If these cannot be guaranteed to the same standard as a referral laboratory, then results should not be relied on without external confirmation.

CLINICAL MICROBIOLOGY

In-house microbiology can be a valuable asset to practitioners, providing quick results with minimal investment. Expensive equipment and materials are not usually necessary for recovery of common aerobic or facultatively anaerobic bacterial pathogens, such as *Staphylococcus* spp, *Streptococcus* spp, and coliforms. Although microbiologic media is not difficult to prepare, it may be more convenient to purchase from a scientific supply house. Most bacteria will grow readily on standard media (blood agar and MacConkey agar plates) when incubated aerobically. Basic equipment should include an incubator, refrigerator, Bunsen burner or portable gas torch, and microscope with low, high, and oil immersion objective lenses. Materials should consist of inoculating loops, prepared microbiologic media, microscope slides, Gram-stain reagents, 3% hydrogen peroxide, oxidase reagent, microbial identification systems, and a current veterinary microbiology textbook.

Specimen Selection and Collection: Although it is not always easy to obtain optimal specimens when working with animals, certain practices can ensure the best possible specimen under the circumstances. Application of the following principles should result in acceptable specimens that produce high-quality microbiology results: 1) Specimens must be obtained aseptically from a site that is representative of the disease process. 2) Swabs are the most common specimen collected, but they are generally not the specimens of choice, because they may become contaminated with commensals during the collection process and they provide a small sample volume. Swabs are most useful to obtain specimens from skin pustules, ears, conjunctiva, deep within draining tracts or wounds, soft-tissue infections, or the reproductive tract. 3) A sufficient quantity of material should be collected to permit adequate examination. 4) Specimens must be collected at the proper time in the disease process and before initiation of antimicrobial therapy to maximize pathogen recovery. 5) If specimens are not immediately cultured after collection, they should be refrigerated.

Specimen Processing: Microbiologic testing should include both direct and microscopic examination and culture of the specimen. Gram-stained smears should be examined using oil immersion to determine the correct reaction. Generally, both solid (agar) and liquid (broth) media should be inoculated. Solid media permit colony isolation, rough bacterial quantitation, and selection or differentiation of normal flora from potential pathogens, whereas broth media allow for recovery of small numbers of organisms.

Clinical specimens should be inoculated onto both general purpose and selective media to maximize bacterial recovery. Plates containing trypticase/tryptic soy agar with 5% sheep blood are the most widely used types of general purpose media. Selective and/or differential media include MacConkey agar (gram-negative bacteria), mannitol salt agar (staphylococci), and phenylethyl alcohol agar (gram-positive bacteria). Microbiologic media should be stored in the refrigerator but allowed to warm to room temperature before inoculation.

Transfer of specimens to plated media depends on the type of specimen. Liquid specimens are inoculated by use of a sterile syringe or pipette. Swabs are generally plated directly by rolling the swab over an area ~2 cm in diameter. Feces are inoculated by dipping a swab into the specimen. Surgical biopsy specimens may be touched directly to the agar surface.

Bacterial identification methods depend on obtaining isolated colonies. The most common technique to achieve isolation is to streak plates using a wire loop. After the specimen has been inoculated onto a plate, a wire loop is flamed, cooled, and passed at a 90° angle several times through the initial area of inoculation. The plate is rotated 90°, the loop is flamed and cooled, and the process is repeated three more times. This results in four quadrants on the plate, which enable quantitation of the relative numbers of bacteria present in a given sample after colonies appear.

After inoculation, plates and tubes should be labeled and placed in an incubator set at 35°–37°C. Plates are incubated with their lids down to prevent condensed water from dropping down from the lid onto the agar surface, which can result in confluent bacterial growth.

Bacterial Identification: The first step in culture evaluation is the visual examination of plated media. Most bacteria produce visible colonies in 24 hr, although some require 48–72 hr. Inspection includes examination of colonial morphology, noting both the types and numbers of colonies and any hemolytic reactions on blood-based agar. Further classification is based on the presence or absence of growth on differential or selective media.

After the evaluation of plated media, examination of Gram stains made from each different colony type is performed. Those reactions, combined with colonial morphology, may allow for the presumptive identification of organisms. If more than one colony type is present, subcultures of each are made. A single colony is streaked to a plate of nonselective medium. This will ensure a pure culture of the unknown organism, which is required for biochemical characterization and identification.

Several microbial identification systems are commercially available. Systems may be manual or automated. Each usually contains a complete package for identification of a particular group of organisms. There are specific systems for staphylococci, streptococci, corynebacteria, nonfermenting gram-negative rods, and *Enterobacteriaceae*. All are useful to conduct a wide variety of biochemical tests simultaneously. Most manual systems consist of plates or strips made up of a series of wells or cups that contain test substrates. A pure culture of the unknown organism in suspension is added to the test wells. The strips are incubated aerobically at 37°C for 24–48 hr. The wells are viewed for colorimetric changes, and a biocode is generated from scoring the test results. This numeric code is compared with those in the system database to obtain an identity for the test organism. Most systems are adequate for identification of common, rapidly growing aerobic to facultatively anaerobic veterinary pathogens.

Antimicrobial Susceptibility Testing:

Antimicrobial susceptibility testing is indicated when the susceptibility of a pathogen cannot be reliably predicted based on the clinician's experience or the identity of the pathogen, or if the antimicrobial agent of choice would not be acceptable for therapeutic use. There are two common procedures to determine the antimicrobial susceptibility of bacteria that are able to grow aerobically within 24 hr, and both have been accepted by the Clinical and Laboratory Standards Institute (CLSI). The first procedure is qualitative and is based on the agar disk diffusion method of Bauer and Kirby. The second procedure is quantitative and involves dilutions of antimicrobial agents, which are tested either in liquid or solid agar media. The latter is referred to as the minimal inhibitory concentration test.

The agar disk diffusion method is more widely used to test the common, rapidly growing aerobic to facultatively anaerobic pathogenic bacteria and lends itself better to in-house testing. The Bauer-Kirby method is based on the diffusion of an antimicrobial agent impregnated within a paper disk through an agar medium. Briefly, a suspension of actively growing test organism is standardized to a turbidity equivalent to 0.5 on the McFarland scale. Within 15 min of standardization, a sterile swab is dipped into the bacterial suspension and a dry Müeller-Hinton agar plate is inoculated by streaking the swab over the entire surface three times. To ensure an even distribution of the inoculum, the plate is rotated ~60° each time. Antimicrobial disks are placed on the plate and gently pressed down to ensure their close contact with the agar surface. Inverted plates are placed in an incubator at 35°C. Plates are examined after 18 hr of incubation. Zones of complete inhibition are measured in millimeters. The zone sizes around each drug are compared with those published by the CLSI in document VET01-S2: *Performance Standards for Antimicrobial Disk and Dilution Susceptibility Tests for Bacteria Isolated from Animals* to make an interpretation of susceptible, intermediate, or resistant for each agent tested.

Reliable antimicrobial susceptibility testing results can only be obtained by following standardized procedures set forth in CLSI document VET01-A4: *Performance Standards for Antimicrobial Disk and Dilution Susceptibility Tests for Bacteria Isolated from Animals, Second Informational Supplement*. Any procedural deviation may lead to erroneous results. It is imperative to properly store antimicrobial susceptibility test disks and test media and to ensure quality control for each test. Any clinic that does not regularly perform testing on a weekly basis may wish to use a veterinary diagnostic laboratory for this procedure instead.

CYTOLOGY

Cytology is a useful clinical tool for investigation of disease processes, and the techniques and their interpretation have developed into an entire discipline. This discussion is a brief guide to enable practitioners to prepare samples and undertake basic interpretation; it refers mostly to small animals, but the basic principles apply to all species.

Cytology should be considered a guide. Characteristics of the cells may not be sufficient in many instances to yield a definitive diagnosis or indicate the probable behavior of the lesion. These may require examination of the overall architecture of the tissue, for which cytology is not appropriate. If complex, expensive, or life-threatening therapy is being considered, then the diagnosis should if possible be confirmed by histology.

Techniques

Full cytologic interpretation requires a good quality sample. A substantial minority of samples collected by practitioners are unsuitable for full interpretation. The technique appears to be simple, but consistently obtaining good-quality samples requires practice. If samples are sent to a laboratory for interpretation, sending more than one is recommended. In addition, staining and examining one of the preparations in-house helps to monitor the quality of the samples taken and make a provisional diagnosis. This requires a good staining technique and a good quality microscope with a range of objectives, including oil immersion.

Staining: The stains and techniques used for cytology preparations in a practice setting are the same as those used for hematology preparations. The traditional stains for cytology preparations are modified Wright stain (Wright-Giemsa) and May-Grunwald Giemsa. Over the past few years, good-quality rapid Romanowsky stains have been developed for cytology and hematology and are often used by veterinary diagnostic laboratories. Many different brands of rapid stain have been developed, so trying a number of products to see which stain is best suited to a practice is recommended. Poor preparations are not always the fault of the collection technique; the stain may be the problem. Stains deteriorate with use and require regular renewal. Many slides can be adjusted by returning a finished stained slide to the stain for deeper color reaction, or if overstained, can have some color removed by placing the slide in alcohol. Formalin-fixed cytology preparations must be stained with either H&E or Papanicolaou stain. If samples are sent to a laboratory for interpretation, the submission form should indicate whether formalin has been added.

Fine-needle Aspiration: The aim of fine-needle aspiration is to obtain a high cell harvest with minimal artifactual damage or blood contamination. The basic sampling kit consists of 21- and 25-gauge needles and 3-, 5-, and 10-mL syringes. Precise technique and choice of equipment depends on physical characteristics of the lesion and whether blood contamination is a problem.

The *basic technique* uses a 25-gauge needle and a 10-mL syringe. The needle is inserted into the lesion and repeatedly redirected to sample a number of areas while applying a small amount of suction on the syringe. Suction is released before withdrawing the needle. If suction is continued on withdrawal, the cell sample is violently sucked into the barrel of the syringe, causing cell rupture. Sample size is often very small and may be present only within the lumen of the needle and not in the syringe. When the sample has been obtained, the syringe is removed, filled with air, reattached, and used to gently express the sample onto a clean, dry, glass slide. Expressing the sample forcefully will rupture cells. Another slide is placed on top of the sample and pulled lengthways to spread the sample to a monolayer. Additional pressure should not be applied, because this also may cause rupture of the cells. Thicker areas are not a concern; the edges will often be thin enough to examine individual, nonoverlapping cells. The sample should be air dried as quickly as possible to reduce the effects of shrinkage; a hair dryer can be used for this purpose, but heating the sample must be avoided.

This technique can be adapted to different situations. If blood contamination is a problem, the size of the syringe and amount of suction can be reduced or the syringe removed altogether. This is particularly a problem with bone marrow aspiration but is common with all cytology samples and is thought to be due to excessive suction on the syringe. If blood contamination is unavoidable, the blood can be centrifuged. However, if the sample is directly smeared, a feathered edge should be examined, because this is where the heavier cells from the tissue tend to congregate. Blood contamination can often be decreased with the use of a very fine needle (25 gauge); this increases the chance of collecting enough cells for interpretation.

An alternative technique uses a needle without a syringe; no difference in the cell harvest between these two techniques has been shown. The needle is inserted without the syringe and repeatedly redirected to sample different depths and directions within the lesion. The cells are detached by the cutting edge of the needle and enter the needle lumen by capillary action. After withdrawal of the needle, a syringe containing air is reattached and used to gently express the sample. This technique is also particularly useful to sample fragile cells, such as lymphoid cells from lymph nodes. A far better cell harvest is obtained from splenic lesions with this technique than by applying suction. In addition, there is greater sensitivity in placement of the needle, which is especially useful for small lesions.

Certain tissues tend to give a very low cell harvest. These are usually composed of mesenchymal cells (connective tissue) that tightly adhere to each other and therefore do not exfoliate easily. For these lesions, a larger bore needle and increased suction may be necessary. However, a needle with a bore >21 gauge tends to provide a tissue core more suitable for histologic interpretation than cytology.

Impression Smears: Impression smears are often used for ulcerated surface lesions. They are of limited value, because they usually sample only the surface inflammatory exudate and rarely include cells from deeper tissues. A better use of this technique is at the time of biopsy to allow an immediate assessment of the lesion before fixation and processing of the tissue sample. The cut surface of the excised sample is blotted a number of times to remove surface blood and serum, and the dried surface is applied to a clean, dry slide with gentle pressure. A number of areas can be prepared on a single slide. The preparations should be quickly air dried and then stained.

Body Fluid Evaluation: Once a body fluid (eg, urine, pleural or peritoneal fluid) is obtained, a cytospin preparation is by far the best method of cell concentration. However, few practices have access to a cytospin, so centrifugation of the preparation and sampling of the centrifuged sediment is the usual method of cell concentration. Once the slide has been prepared, it should be rapidly air dried before staining.

If the fluid is to be sent to a laboratory, adding a few drops of formalin (the concentration is not critical) helps preserve cells and prevent bacterial overgrowth during transit. Severe bacterial overgrowth obscures the cells, and their metabolic products tend to destroy cells in cytology preparations. This is particularly useful for bronchoalveolar lavage samples and urine, which often contain infectious agents and are prone to bacterial contamination at sampling. The laboratory must be advised of the presence of formalin, which excludes the use of Romanowsky stains. Adding EDTA to help preserve cytology samples is often recommended, but the effect is minimal.

Cells in CSF samples degenerate very quickly and are usually present in very low numbers. Cytospin preparations are almost essential for CSF examination; this can usually be achieved only in a reference laboratory. The addition of a few drops of 10% formalin preserves the cells in CSF very well during transit.

Interpretation of Cytology Samples

Cytology interpretation can be guided by an algorithm that also covers the common questions asked by clinicians. From a clinical viewpoint, it is often not necessary to complete all stages of this algorithm. For example, a simple differentiation of inflammation from neoplasia may be sufficient to allow a decision on the next stage of case management. Full cytology interpretation may require the services of a diagnostic laboratory, and a definitive diagnosis often requires histopathology. Some lesions cannot be definitively diagnosed by cytology. If in doubt or if the cytologic interpretation does not correlate with the clinical picture, histology is essential for full interpretation. Whenever the diagnosis is in doubt, biopsy is indicated.

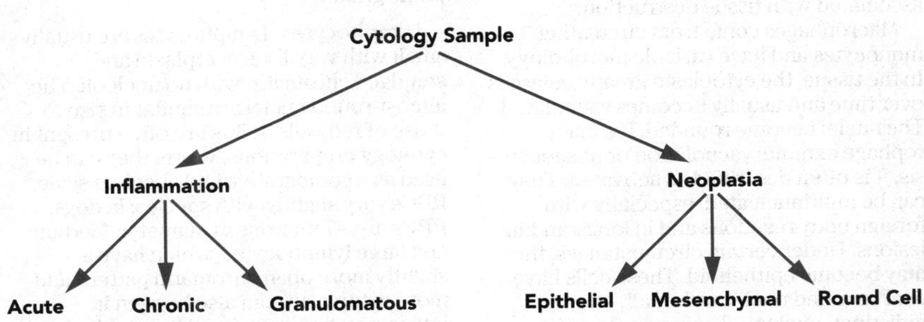

Algorithm to interpret cytology samples.

Inflammation: Recognition of basic inflammatory cells—neutrophils, eosinophils, lymphocytes, macrophages, and plasma cells—is essential for interpretation of cytology samples. Some tumors contain a large number of inflammatory cells, but these are very uncommon, even when there is tumor necrosis. The presence of only inflammatory cells in a sample usually indicates a primary inflammatory lesion. Ulceration produces inflammation on the surface of neoplastic lesions, but even in this case the inflammatory cells typically do not extend deeply into the underlying neoplasm. A small percentage of mast cell tumors, however, are composed almost entirely of inflammation, hemorrhage, and edema with only a small number of mast cells. These can be difficult to identify even by histology.

Neutrophils: These are the first cells to arrive in an area of inflammation, and they continue to be attracted to the site as long as the inflammatory stimulus lasts. Large numbers of neutrophils indicate acute inflammation and often are accompanied by smaller numbers of macrophages. This pattern is most often caused by infection or foreign body reaction, including furunculotic reactions directed against hair and keratin embedded in the soft tissue. If fluids are not examined immediately, bacteria, if present, will begin to proliferate, but phagocytosis of bacteria does not occur after sampling. Therefore, if the bacteria are truly pathogenic, they should be within the cytoplasm of the phagocytic cells. The cells' cytoplasm may contain RBCs, tissue debris, or foreign material.

Macrophages: Macrophages arrive at a site of inflammation within 2–3 hr and are not necessarily an indicator of chronicity, although they often increase with time. They phagocytize bacteria and also larger structures, such as fungi, cellular debris, and foreign material. These cells are often associated with tissue destruction.

Macrophages come from circulating monocytes and have variable morphology. In the tissue, the cytoplasm greatly enlarges over time and usually becomes vacuolated. The nuclei become rounded. If a macrophage exhibits vacuolation or phagocytosis, it is often described as activated. They can be multinucleated, especially with foreign body reactions and in longstanding lesions. Under certain circumstances, they may become epithelioid. These cells have oval or round nuclei and small, often indistinct, nucleoli. Their cytoplasm is expanded but uniformly stained and not vacuolated. They can look epithelial, and great care must be taken when interpreting such cells. However, they do not normally form clusters, which is a key factor in differentiation from epithelial cells.

Macrophages are almost always seen in bronchoalveolar lavage fluid (they come from the alveoli) and body cavity fluids (part of the modification process), joints (a normal component but increased in disease), and cyst contents (a nonspecific reaction).

Eosinophils: Eosinophils have segmented nuclei and eosinophilic cytoplasmic granules. They vary slightly between species and are generally slightly larger than neutrophils. In cytology preparations, it can occasionally be difficult to distinguish poorly stained eosinophils from neutrophils, because the granules can become indistinct and the cytoplasm of degenerating neutrophils become more acidic, giving a more eosinophilic staining reaction. They are often seen in association with mast cells. Eosinophils are associated with allergies and also are prominent in parasitic diseases, superficial cutaneous viral infection in cats, and fungal infections. They are the predominant cell type in specific eosinophilic conditions such as eosinophilic granuloma in cats (rarely in dogs), canine eosinophilic folliculitis and furunculosis, and eosinophilic collagenolytic granuloma in horses. Some cases of canine cutaneous mast cell tumors have a very high proportion of eosinophils and very few mast cells (<5% of cases).

Of the most commonly encountered veterinary species, rabbits and guinea pigs have inflammatory cells equivalent to neutrophils in other species, but have eosinophilic cytoplasmic granules. These are called heterophils. They can be difficult to distinguish from eosinophils. The cellular equivalent to neutrophils in birds and reptiles are also heterophils with eosinophilic granules.

Lymphocytes: Lymphocytes are usually small with very little cytoplasm and smudged chromatin with no nucleoli. The almost-round nuclei are similar in size to those of red cells. RBCs are often present in cytology preparations, where they can be used as a comparative and absolute scale. RBCs vary slightly with species; in dogs, RBCs are ~7 microns in diameter. Medium and large lymphocytes, which have a slightly more open chromatin pattern and more cytoplasm, can also be seen in inflammatory processes. Along with plasma cells, lymphocytes are part of the chronic inflammatory response and tend to arrive in tissue a few days after the acute inflammation has begun. However, they are not specific for a particular stimulus and are mostly small lymphocytes. If mostly medium to large cells are present, lymphoma is a possibility. However, even large lymphoblastic cells can be seen in low numbers in inflammatory processes. Normal and reactive lymphocytes in body fluids often appear larger than the same cells from soft tissue.

Multinucleated Cells: These cells are large and have larger numbers of nuclei with one to three small nucleoli and vacuolated cytoplasm. They develop from macrophages (*see* above) and tend to appear late in the course of inflammation. The cytoplasm should be examined for the presence of fungal organisms and for foreign material. These cells are usually seen in small numbers mixed with other inflammatory cells as part of a granulomatous reaction. Multinucleated cells are much less specific in birds and reptiles, in which they are common in many focal inflammatory lesions, irrespective of cause, and can appear quite early in the inflammatory process.

Fibroblasts: Fibroblasts are not inflammatory cells, but they are frequently seen in association with inflammation. They will proliferate as part of the repair reaction associated with any tissue damage and appear in an inflammatory lesion after ~2 days. Classically, fibroblasts and fibrocytes are elongated cells with pointed tails of cytoplasm. They have round or oval nuclei, indistinct nucleoli, and moderate amounts of uniform, pale blue-staining cytoplasm. The cytoplasmic boundaries are indistinct, giving a "wispy" appearance. When fibroblasts are aspirated from tissue, the cells often become round and lose their spindle shape, but a small number, especially cells in groups, retain their elongated shape. Reactive fibroblasts cannot be definitively distinguished cytologically from low-grade spindle cell tumors. If found in association with inflammatory cells, spindle cells are most often reactive. If found in large clumps with no apparent stimulus, they are more often neoplastic (but neoplasia cannot be excluded). Because fibroblasts and fibrocytes are the principal connective tissue cell, they are tightly adherent to each other, and cell harvest tends to be low.

Neoplasia:

Inflammatory lesions are characterized by cells from different populations. The presence of cells that are predominantly of the same population indicates normal tissue, hyperplasia, or neoplasia. Ideally, the first stage in evaluation of a cytologic sample for neoplasia is to determine the tissue type from which the cells have come. If this is not possible, it is necessary to simply determine the likely behavior of the cells. This can often be done without specifically identifying the cell type. The following checklist includes features that can be examined to determine tissue type and likely behavior of the lesion: 1) cell numbers, 2) cell distribution within the smear, 3) cell shape, 4) nucleus:cytoplasm ratio, 5) pleomorphism (both nuclear and cytoplasmic), 6) number, shape, and size of nucleoli, and 7) cytoplasmic content such as melanin, metachromatic granules, fat, etc. Classification of the cell type and likely behavior may require a tissue biopsy. With few exceptions, histology will be necessary for a definitive diagnosis and is always necessary to assess mitotic index and to grade a tumor.

There are three basic tissue types: epithelial, mesenchymal (supporting or connective tissue), and round cells.

Epithelial Cells: Epithelial cells are round, cuboidal, or polygonal and tend to adhere tightly to each other and exfoliate in clusters or sheets. They have a sharp cytoplasmic outline and exfoliate in moderate numbers. Cells with more than one nucleus are uncommon.

Mesenchymal Cells: Mesenchymal cells are tightly adherent and usually exfoliate in low numbers as single cells or small aggregates. They are classically spindle shaped but usually round up and become

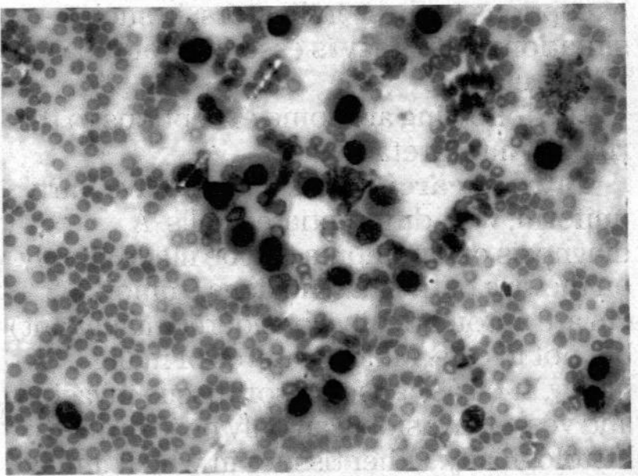

Within the usual blood contamination, there are cells that are well separated and nonadherent; this is typical of round cell tumors. *Courtesy of Abbey Veterinary Services.*

plump when removed from the body, particularly when they are lying singly within the smear. The spindle shape is often more apparent in small aggregates. They tend to appear "wispy" because of indistinct cytoplasmic boundaries. Binucleate cells are not uncommon.

Round Cells: Round cells have little or no adherence in the body. They typically exfoliate in large numbers and lie individually in the smear without clumping. Cells of this category include mast cells, lymphocytes, histiocytes, plasma cells, and cells of transmissible venereal tumors.

Tumor Evaluation: To distinguish benign from malignant tumors, the amount of variation in certain characteristics within the cell population must be assessed. In general, the more malignant the cell, the less differentiated it becomes and the more variation there is in the cell morphology. Benign tumors have cells that are often uniform in size with a uniform nucleus:cytoplasm ratio; they strongly resemble or are identical to the cell of origin. The more malignant the cells become, the more variation is seen in these criteria. Nuclear criteria are the major indicators of malignancy.

Criteria for malignancy include the following: variation in cell size and shape, increased cell exfoliation, increased nuclear size, increased nucleus:cytoplasm ratio, variation in nuclear size and an increase in multinucleated cells, increased mitosis with abnormal mitotic figures, a coarse and often clumped chromatin pattern, altered shape of the nucleus due to close approximation of a nucleus from an adjacent cell (nuclear moulding), and large and often multiple nucleoli of irregular and abnormal shape. There are a number of exceptions to these indicators; in such situations, histology is essential for full interpretation.

The following are some exceptions to the rules of interpretation:

Thyroid carcinomas usually have fairly uniform, well-differentiated cells. A diagnosis of carcinoma can be made simply on the size of the mass in dogs (tumors >3 cm are automatically considered malignant) but not in cats. Major features of malignancy, such as capsular, soft-tissue invasion and vessel invasion, can only be identified histologically. Other tissues in which it may be impossible to differentiate benign from malignant cells include **apocrine gland carcinomas, basal cell tumors, melanomas**, and proliferative lesions of the liver.

Unlike most malignant tumors, **lymphoma** is commonly characterized by a uniform population of cells that are larger than normal lymphoid cells. Therefore, variation in morphology is not necessary for a diagnosis of malignancy with this tissue type. If there is marked variation and small lymphocytes are present, then that is more typical of hyperplasia.

Some normal structures, such as hepatoid glands, have more than one cell type (reserve and terminal cells) and can therefore show variation in morphology, and benign tumors of hepatoid glands can have a similar mixture. Nuclear morphology, however, maintains benign features.

Many **mammary tumors** can show marked variation in cell morphology but histologically would be classified as benign. Indicators of mammary tumor behavior are architectural features, such as local tissue invasion and invasion of vessels. These cannot be assessed using cytology. These exceptions often make cytologic interpretation unreliable, particularly for these types of tissues.

Most **spindle cell tumors** do not metastasize but are locally aggressive and often difficult to remove. The criteria for malignancy are often less important with respect to the behavior of these tumors than for the epithelial tumors.

Common Cytology Results: Some specific features of cytology preparations can provide a more accurate interpretation of the sample. Listed below are some common results and their interpretation.

Mature Fat Cells: Mature fat cells are seen in benign lipomas and mature body fat. It is not possible to differentiate these

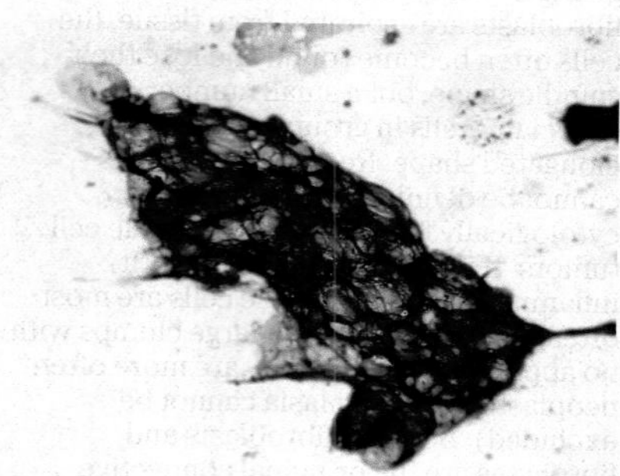

These typical balloon-like fat cells are characteristic of benign lipoma and mature body fat. Both involve the same cells and cannot be distinguished on cytology. *Courtesy of Abbey Veterinary Services.*

cytologically. Fat cells are mesenchymal cells, and because they tend not to exfoliate well, they are usually present in low numbers. If a sample has come from the center of a nodular mass, fat cells are diagnostic for lipoma. These clear-staining, balloon-like cells are often in clusters, folded, and overlapping.

Spindle Cells: It is usually not possible to differentiate reactive spindle cells from those of spindle cell neoplasia. Indicators of neoplasia include absence of a reactive stimulus, such as inflammation or hemorrhage, and a higher cell population with more numerous and larger clumps of cells. Greater variation in cell morphology indicates more aggressive behavior. When removed from their tissue, they often round up and can be mistaken for round cells, but there are usually some distinctly spindle cells in most preparations.

Keratin: Keratin includes nucleated and terminally differentiated non-nucleated squamous epithelial cells. Keratin can be a contaminant from the surface of the skin of the animal or the skin of all handlers of the sample and is a common artifact. It can also be sampled from cutaneous keratin-filled cysts, which are always benign and very common, particularly in dog skin. Large, densely packed clumps of keratin in restricted areas in the center of the slide suggest that keratin is not an artifact but has been sampled from the lesion.

Blood: Blood is a common artifact of fine-needle aspiration but can also come from blood-filled spaces in tissue. These can be non-neoplastic, such as hematomas, aneurysms, or severe bruising, or neoplastic lesions such as hemangiomas and hemangiosarcomas. The presence of spindle cells does not adequately differentiate neoplastic from non-neoplastic causes of hemorrhage (*see* above). Spindle cells produce the neoplastic blood vessels in hemangiosarcomas, but especially in young dogs, they can occasionally produce a very cellular capsule to a soft-tissue hematoma. The capsule contains very active fibroblasts, but they are not neoplastic. Blood that has come directly from the vascular system normally contains significant numbers of platelets. Using a 25-gauge needle can help decrease blood contamination. Blood is almost always seen in aspiration from parenchymatous organs, such as the liver, spleen, kidneys, and bone marrow.

No Cells: Lack of cells is a common problem of fine-needle aspiration. If the technique is practiced properly, absence of cells can indicate mesenchymal cell proliferation (including lipomas), because these structural cells within the body are tightly adherent cells that do not exfoliate well.

Cells with Cytoplasmic Granules: The most important type among cells with cytoplasmic granules is the **mast cell**, given that mast cell tumors are common in dogs. These are medium-sized cells with round nuclei. With Romanowsky stains, the granules are dark blue or purple, small (about the size of bacteria), and usually found in large numbers in the cytoplasm. Less-differentiated mast cells have fewer granules. Cytology cannot be used to grade mast cell tumors; grading always requires histology, because it does not depend on only cell morphology. The cells are fragile, and often there are large numbers of granules in the background that have been released from damaged cells. In dogs, eosinophils are often present and very occasionally can be the dominant cell type; however, they are less common in other species. Mast cell tumors in horses have similar cytology to those in dogs, but in cats the cells in mast cell tumors are often smaller, more uniform, and have less distinct granulation.

Thyroid cells can also have dark granules, usually blue or black. These tyrosine granules are very small, low in number, and can be difficult to see. Larger black granules are associated with **melanomas**. Cytology cannot differentiate benign from malignant melanomas; however, melanomas on haired skin in dogs are usually benign and those on nonhaired areas, such as the lips, feet, and mouth, are usually malignant. Basal cell tumors also often contain cells with melanin, especially in cats. These tumors are usually benign and cytologically can sometimes be difficult to distinguish from melanomas. Melanin can also be seen in **macrophages (melanophages)**, sometimes in large amounts, but it is usually in much larger clumps within the cytoplasm rather than fine granules that are seen in melanocytes. Very fine magenta granules can sometimes be seen in **osteoblastic cells** from osteosarcoma. Golden, granular material accumulates in the cytoplasm of macrophages when there has been hemorrhage into soft tissue (hemosiderophages). **Liver cells** can sometimes contain bile, which stains very dark, and occasionally long, thin strands of dark material can be seen where canaliculi have become filled with bile.

Cells with Cytoplasmic Vacuoles: A large, single vacuole is seen in fat cells. In normal or benign cells, the nuclei are small and often indistinct, and the cells are often folded like a collapsed ball. Smaller cells with larger, more prominent nuclei and some cytoplasm in addition to clear, often small vacuoles are more suggestive of malignancy.

Cells with multiple, small vacuoles with a foamy appearance include macrophages, sebaceous glandular cells, and salivary cells. It can be very difficult to differentiate these; the site and other clinical features can be a deciding factor in interpretation.

Differentiation of Round Cell Tumors: Round cell tumors include mast cells, plasma cells, lymphocytes, histiocytic cells, and transmissible venereal tumor cells. **Mast cells** have distinctive granules within the cytoplasm and are usually easily identified; if they are the dominant cell type, this is diagnostic for a mast cell tumor. In rare cases, mast cells can have few or no granules in the cytoplasm. **Lymphoid cells** classically have a very high nucleus: cytoplasm ratio; few other cells have this feature. Neoplastic, lymphoid cells are medium size to large, with a nucleus at least 1.5 times the size of an erythrocyte. Nucleoli are often multiple, sometimes quite prominent. However, the rare cases of small-cell lymphoma have cells indistinguishable from normal lymphocytes.

Cells of a **histiocytoma** (Langerhans cells) are not especially histiocytic cytologically. They are round cells with a small to moderate amount of pale-staining cytoplasm. They are fairly uniform and have nuclei that are eccentric within the cell. Nucleoli are indistinct. True **histiocytic cells** are slightly more problematic to interpret. These are part of the cell line that includes the antigen-presenting cells, such as macrophages and Langerhans cells, but can range from inflammatory and reactive cells to highly malignant round cell tumors. They tend to be larger than the other round cells with more cytoplasm, sometimes are vacuolated, and can have oval or indented nuclei. Infiltrates of histiocytic cells are often problematic, even with a full-tissue biopsy examination, and always require histologic examination to assess behavior.

Neoplastic plasma cells include cells of **myeloma**. These are usually well differentiated and have most of the characteristics of normal plasma cells. When neoplastic, they are found in large numbers with few other cell types present. Benign nodular proliferations of plasma cells, **plasmacytomas**, show more marked pleomorphism and often differ markedly from normal plasma cells. Many have a slightly histiocytic appearance, and these can be difficult to distinguish cytologically. These cells have a round nucleus and a coarse chromatin pattern, which sometimes becomes clumped around the nuclear membrane. The nucleus is often eccentric with an intensely basophilic cytoplasm and paranuclear pale Golgi zone.

Cells of **transmissible venereal tumors** tend to have a moderate amount of cytoplasm (more than found in lymphoblasts), often with small vacuoles. Nuclear chromatin is coarse, with one or two fairly prominent nucleoli. Mitotic figures are often numerous. Unlike most cytology preparations of neoplastic lesions, they tend to have moderate variation in the nucleus:cytoplasm ratio.

Cytology of Specific Sites:

Lymph Nodes: Normal, hyperplastic, and early neoplastic lymph nodes have a mixed population of cells. Cells are predominantly small lymphocytes with variable numbers of medium and large lymphoid cells and some plasma cells. A uniform population of cells indicates neoplasia. Lymph node aspirates often have a population of cells that are much paler staining and larger, with some cells completely losing their cytoplasm. These cells are in varying stages of degeneration and should be ignored. Size in comparison with RBCs is useful. Normal mature lymphocytes or small neoplastic lymphocytes (rare) have nuclei the same size as RBCs. However, neoplastic lymphoid cells have nuclei at least 1.5 times the diameter of RBCs. Lymphomatous lymph nodes may still contain a significant number of normal lymphoid cells. The proportion of smaller mature lymphocytes must then be compared with the larger immature cells to differentiate hyperplasia from neoplasia. The proportion considered significant varies, but in general, most cytologists consider a diagnosis of lymphoma when immature cells are >50% of the cell population. Some cytologists require a higher percentage of immature cells, particularly if there is only one lymph node enlarged. If there is doubt, a biopsy should be performed. Histopathologic confirmation of diagnosis is essential if therapy for lymphoma is considered and is always needed for full grading.

Submandibular lymph nodes are often difficult to assess. They drain the buccal and nasal areas and are subject to strong antigenic stimuli. They frequently undergo hyperplasia, often histologically atypical, especially in cats. Cats also develop unusual neoplastic conditions affecting this node, such as the T cell–rich B-cell lymphoma and Hodgkin-like lymphoma, both of which have a majority of normal lymph node cells. For these reasons, great care must be taken in the interpretation of lesions involving the submandibular lymph nodes, because false-negative and false-positive results for neoplasia are not uncommon.

Aspirates from suspected enlarged submandibular lymph nodes often yield only large foamy cells, which are salivary cells. This result can be due either to sampling error or to hypertrophy of the salivary gland in cases of sialoadenosis. The cause of sialoadenosis is not understood, but a significant minority of submandibular aspirates contain only these cells.

Body Cavity Fluids: Meaningful analysis of fluids from body cavities requires total protein (measured with a handheld refractometer), total cell count, and a differential of cell types present (*see* TABLE 2). Pure transudates are rare, because they rapidly become modified by leakage of fluid from lymphatics or blood vessels and attraction of mixed inflammatory cells. Transudates attract activated macrophages with varying numbers of nondegenerate neutrophils. The lymphocytes that may also be present are classified as small, but most look slightly larger than circulating lymphocytes and are part of the reactive process of the fluid in the body cavity. In addition, when fluid accumulates in the body cavity, the lining mesothelial cells proliferate and are shed into the fluid. These cells are large, often multinucleated, vary in appearance, and often are seen in groups with large nucleoli. They sometimes form grape-like clusters with a narrow, pale space between the cells. These features are usually considered to be associated with malignancy, but in this case, the cells are simply reactive and not neoplastic. Care must be taken to differentiate these mesothelial cells from neoplastic cells within the body fluid. A small number of these cells typically have a corona around the cytoplasmic envelope (giving a fuzzy outline); this is a distinguishing feature of mesothelial cells.

Mesothelial cells can be present in very large numbers, especially in pericardial fluid. Malignant mesotheliomas are rare in domestic species, but it is not possible to differentiate neoplastic from reactive mesothelial cells on cytologic examination. The degree of polyploidy is not a distinguishing feature.

Mixed inflammatory cells increase in number as a transudate becomes modified and are present in large numbers in an exudate. Mesothelial cells would be expected in this type of sample, and it can therefore be useful to look for a second population when checking for neoplasia. Smoothly demarcated aggregates of atypical cells with no narrow spaces between the cells may indicate a second population of carcinoma cells.

Tracheal or Bronchoalveolar Lavage (BAL): **Respiratory epithelial cells** are seen in BAL from healthy and diseased animals. The epithelial cells may retain their original structure with a ciliated surface and basal nuclei, but they often appear round with indistinct cilia.

Macrophages are usually the dominant inflammatory cell type in BAL from healthy animals. These come from deep in the alveoli and are part of the normal defense mechanisms. They greatly increase with fluid accumulation in the lung (eg, cardiovascular insufficiency) and in inflammatory conditions, where they are accompanied by other inflammatory cells. Debris, foreign material, hemosiderin, RBCs, and microorganisms can sometimes be seen in the cytoplasm of these cells. Macrophages containing hemosiderin in people are called heart failure cells, but their cause is less specific in domestic species. There are increased numbers of macrophages in many subacute and chronic lung disorders.

TABLE 2 CHARACTERISTICS OF TRANSUDATES AND EXUDATE

	Total Protein (g/dL)	Cell Count (cells/mL)
Transudate	<2.5	<1,500
Modified transudate	2.5–7.5	1,000–7,000
Exudate	>3.0	>7,000

In healthy dogs and cats, **neutrophils** contribute <5% of cells in BAL preparations. Neutrophils are nonspecific inflammatory cells in the respiratory system and do not necessarily indicate infection. They can be the most numerous cells in an inflammatory reaction, even in cases of allergy. However, when neutrophils are present, the cytoplasm should always be examined carefully for the presence of any infectious agent. Bacteria can also sometimes be seen in the extracellular parts of the smear, but extracellular bacteria are often contaminants from the pharynx.

Great care must be taken to differentiate **eosinophils** from neutrophils in BAL preparations because the granules are often faint and difficult to identify. Eosinophils can comprise up to 5% of cells in BAL from healthy dogs but may reach 10% in healthy cats. Eosinophils that comprise >10% of cells indicate an allergic respiratory disease, although lungworms and heartworms can also cause this reaction. With lungworm infestation, larvae are sometimes present as large coiled structures.

Nucleated and nonnucleated **squamous cells** are commonly seen in BAL preparations and are often associated with bacteria on the cell surface. This indicates contamination from the pharynx. Bacteria are normal inhabitants of the pharynx, in particular *Simonsiella*, which are very large, ladder-like organisms. Their presence confirms contamination from the pharynx. If bacteria are present along with squamous epithelial cells, it may not be possible to conclude whether the bacteria are from the respiratory tree or the pharynx. Bacteria in the cytoplasm of neutrophils confirms a significant infection.

Synovial Fluid: Full examination of synovial fluid should include protein content, mucin clot formation, viscosity, cell count and differential, and direct cytologic examination. It is usually not feasible to perform all of these tests in a practice setting, but cytologic examination and physical examination can usually give a good estimate of the results of most of these tests. Cytology, therefore, is the most useful single test in synovial fluid examination.

Sampling technique requires the following equipment: a 3-mL syringe, a 21- or 25-gauge needle, clean glass slides, and various collection tubes (plain, EDTA, and heparin). This technique always requires a degree of sedation, and a sterile technique is essential. Each joint has a recommended site for aspiration (beyond the scope of this discussion) and generally requires slight flexion or hyperextension. The needle attached to the syringe is slowly advanced into the joint space and, taking care not to scratch the articular surface, gentle suction is applied. Normal joint fluid is viscous and sticky and of small volume. The volume of fluid, however, depends on the size of the animal, the joint sampled, and the degree of effusion into the joint. When sample size is sufficient, it is essential to release the suction on the syringe before withdrawing the needle.

Sample handling is critical; because many tests can be performed on synovial fluid and cytology is the most important, sometimes the sample volume is so small that no other test is possible. Therefore, a plain smear should always be made and quickly air dried as soon as the sample is obtained. Most tests can be performed on samples without anticoagulant (a plain red-topped tube), or the sample can be left in the sampling syringe. However, blood contamination, hemarthrosis, and inflammatory effusion introduce fibrin into the joint, and the sample may clot. Placing part of the sample into an EDTA tube can prevent this, but EDTA can interfere in the mucin clot test and, for this reason, a heparinized sample may also be necessary.

Results of cytology preparations can indicate the number of cells present, the type of cell and the differential, the presence of tumor cells, and the presence of bacteria. They can also give an indication of viscosity. In fluid of normal or increased viscosity, cells tend to align in rows in the direction of the smearing; this is described as windrowing.

In healthy animals, **cell counts** vary widely (eg, 0–4,400/mL in dogs), but they are usually very low. Counts >500/mL in dogs generally indicate a significant increase. Normal synovial fluid contains ~2 cells/high-powered field (400× magnification). In the vast majority of cases where there is an increased cell content, cell numbers are either low (up to 4 or 5 cells/high-powered field) in degenerative joint disease or very high in septic or autoimmune arthritis. Intermediate equivocal results are extremely uncommon.

Cell types include joint mononuclear cells, which are a mixture of circulating monocytes, tissue macrophages, and synovial lining cells. It is not possible, or even necessary, to differentiate these cells, because they all have a similar morphology and all react to similar stimuli. Cytoplasmic vacuolation of these cells, and especially the presence of phagocytosis of debris or RBCs, indicate activation, a feature not seen in normal joint mononuclear cells. In degenerative joint disease, synovial fluid usually contains only macrophages, occasionally with extremely low numbers of neutrophils.

Hemorrhage is common in synovial preparations but is frequently an artifact. True hemarthrosis provides a synovial fluid sample that is uniformly contaminated with blood at the time of sampling. If the blood contamination occurs at the very end of the sampling procedure with clear fluid initially, this is most likely artifact. In addition, in true hemarthrosis, RBCs may be seen in the cytoplasm of macrophages. Artifactual blood contamination will also introduce WBCs, such as neutrophils, making interpretation of inflammatory cells in the sample difficult, although blood contamination still gives only a low cell number.

Neutrophils are present in large numbers in both septic arthritis and autoimmune joint disease. These two conditions can usually be differentiated by the clinical history. In septic arthritis, bacteria are sometimes found within the cytoplasm of phagocytic cells. The absence of bacteria, either within cytology preparations or by culture, does not exclude bacteria as a cause of arthritis. False-negative results for bacteria are not uncommon.

Lymphocytes are often present in very small numbers in inflammatory processes but are not specific for a particular cause.

Osteoclasts are very occasionally seen when there has been erosion of the articular cartilage with exposure of the underlying bone.

Neoplastic cells in joint fluid are rare, although joints can be the site of both primary and secondary tumors.

Macrophages increase with any damage to a joint, especially in cases of degenerative joint disease. Cytoplasmic vacuolation of these cells, and especially the presence of phagocytosis of debris or RBCs, indicate macrophage activation, a feature not seen in normal joint mononuclear cells. In degenerative joint disease, synovial fluid often contains only macrophages.

Nasal Cavity: The cytology of nasal flush preparations is similar to that seen with BAL preparations. A small number of respiratory epithelial cells are usually flushed out along with exudate. A predominance of eosinophils may indicate inhaled allergens, parasites, or fungi and may occasionally indicate bacteria or neoplasia. The presence of eosinophils in the nasal cavity therefore is less indicative of a specific process than in some other sites, eg, the trachea or bronchi.

Neutrophils are the most common exudative cell but, as with BAL, often indicate secondary infection. In the case of intranasal neoplasia, cells with neoplastic characteristics (*see* p 1601) may be present, but absence of these cells does not exclude neoplasia. Only a minority of neoplastic processes erode the overlying respiratory epithelium and allow exfoliation of neoplastic cells.

Similarly, absence of fungal hyphae within the preparation does not exclude fungal infection. Unless fungal plaques are sampled directly for both cytology and culture, false-negative results are common. Viral inclusions are rarely seen.

Vaginal Cytology: This can be used to identify the various stages of the canine estrous cycle, but results must be interpreted in conjunction with the animal's behavior. A sample of exfoliated cells is obtained from the vaginal vault cranial to the urethral orifice with a cotton-tipped swab or glass rod. Cells are gently rolled onto a glass slide, air dried, and stained. Features to be identified include neutrophils, bacteria, RBCs, and the types of epithelial cells. Epithelial cells (in increasing order of differentiation) are parabasal, small and large intermediate cells, and superficial cells. Parabasal cells are small, with central round nuclei, indistinct nucleoli, a relatively narrow band of cytoplasm, and a nucleus:cytoplasm ratio of ~1:1. Small intermediate cells have a similar nucleus but a much larger amount of cytoplasm. Large intermediate cells have a similar nucleus with very large amounts of cytoplasm and an angular, irregular outline. Superficial cells also have large amounts of cytoplasm, but their nuclei are pyknotic (small and contracted) or absent.

The stages of the estrous cycle change gradually. If a preparation does not conform exactly to a specific part of the cycle, judgment must be made regarding what stages are present. In **proestrus**, all types of epithelial cells are present along with neutrophils, RBCs, and mucus. As proestrus progresses, the epithelial cells increasingly approach terminal differentiation (superficial cells), and neutrophils slowly decrease. Bacteria are often present in large numbers. In **estrus**, >90% of epithelial cells are superficial cells, with no background mucus. There are large numbers of bacteria, but no neutrophils. In **diestrus**, parabasal and intermediate cells are >80% of the total epithelial cells. Variable numbers of neutrophils and bacteria are present but usually fewer than in proestrus. It can be difficult to differentiate some stages of proestrus from diestrus. In **anestrus**, parabasal and intermediate cells predominate. Neutrophils and bacteria are rare. RBCs do not help differentiate the stages of estrus.

Cerebrospinal Fluid: Interpretation of CSF cytology is difficult, because it can be hard to obtain enough well-preserved cells for examination before the sample deteriorates. Cell counts in normal CSF are low (0–5 cells/µL in dogs and 0–8 cells/µL in cats). However, there is a large variation in cell counts between individuals; counts can also vary between cysternal and lumbar taps in the same individual. Because the albumin level of CSF is ~20% of that found in serum, the cells that are present rapidly degenerate. Cell counts should ideally be done and morphology examined within 1 hr of collection.

Because of the low cell numbers, the use of an automated cell counter is usually not appropriate. A hemocytometer can be used for cell counts, and a cytocentrifuge for cytology preparations. A simplified sedimentation technique (description of which is beyond the scope of this discussion) to concentrate cells onto a slide is suitable for practice use. The presence of more than one or two nucleated cells in a plain smear of CSF should be considered potentially significant.

In CSF, an increase in nucleated cells is called **pleocytosis**. There is tremendous variation and overlap in both the degree of pleocytosis and the types of cells present in both infectious and noninfectious conditions in the CNS. Interpretation should be integrated with the other clinical details of the case. If neutrophils and/or macrophages are present, the cytoplasm of the cells should be searched for bacteria and fungi. The absence of organisms or pleocytosis does not exclude infection, and noninfectious conditions in the CNS can also produce a neutrophilic pleocytosis.

Apart from lymphoma, it is rare to find neoplastic cells in CSF. If noninflammatory cells are present in the CSF, they should be interpreted using the basic principles detailed above.

Urine Cytology: Urine can be examined as a wet preparation or as a dried cytology smear. Because of the absence of staining in a wet preparation, these are better limited to examination for crystals and RBCs. Although nucleated cells may be seen, in most cases they cannot be identified and are better examined using a dried cytology smear.

There are at least 10 common forms of urinary crystals. Identification is not discussed here but may be readily accomplished by use of good reference illustrations. (*See also* UROLITHIASIS, p 1525.)

Because cells in urine rapidly degenerate, particularly if bacteria are present, centrifuged preparations of urine samples should be examined rapidly after sampling. If this is not possible, boric acid is often added to urine to prevent degeneration and bacterial overgrowth, although its effect may be very limited. If a delay between sampling and examination is likely, a better preservation method is the addition of a few drops of formalin; however,the traditional Romanowsky stains cannot then be used. H&E stain is a better alternative for formalin-fixed samples.

Normal urine usually has very few nucleated cells. Single urothelial cells are occasionally present. Squamous epithelial cells are also seen in urine and come from the terminal urethra, vagina, vulva, and preputial epithelium. Squamous metaplasia of bladder epithelium after chronic inflammation is very rare.

Neoplastic cells in urine samples are almost always epithelial. They are rounded polygonal cells, often clumped, with marked variation in morphology, especially the nucleus:cytoplasm ratio. Uniform cells are more likely to be normal. Mildly pleomorphic cells can be associated with hyperplasia (eg, some cases of polypoid cystitis).

The inflammatory cells seen in cystitis are almost exclusively neutrophils. Eosinophils are seen in some rare, specific inflammatory conditions, but macrophages are very uncommon even in chronic conditions. By far the most common cause of inflammation is infection, so the cytoplasm of the neutrophils should be examined carefully for bacteria. It is very uncommon to see a significant neutrophil component accompanying neoplasia or calculi.

RBCs are commonly seen with neoplastic and inflammatory diseases of the bladder but are also often seen without an indication of other pathology. This can be a sampling artifact but is also a common finding in cases of interstitial cystitis. In cats, this term is often used synonymously with feline urologic syndrome, but interstitial cystitis also is seen in dogs and people, suggesting other unknown pathogenic factors that can cause this condition. Persistent hematuria without cytologic evidence of neoplasia or inflammation may indicate interstitial cystitis.

See also URINALYSIS, p 1615.

Liver Cytology: Although cytology is a popular method to investigate liver disease, there is disagreement on its usefulness. Blood contamination is found in most samples and may overshadow inflammatory infiltrates by introducing circulating WBCs. Diagnosis of many hepatic diseases relies on architectural features and the distribution of the changes within the liver rather than on the morphology of individual cells. Finally, in some hepatic disorders, hepatocytes proliferate without significant changes in their individual morphology (*see* below). These factors limit the amount of information that can be obtained from cytology of liver tissue.

Sampling methods are similar to those used for other organs. Sampling is usually performed under guidance of ultrasound, but blind sampling can be performed at the tenth intercostal space at the level of the connection of rib to rib cartilage. Bleeding during this procedure is not a significant risk.

In the healthy liver, hepatocytes are plump, polygonal rounded cells with a diameter of 25–30 microns. Nuclei are central and round with a single large, prominent nucleolus. A few cells are binucleated. There is a large amount of blue-staining cytoplasm that usually appears granular.

Changes in the metabolism of liver cells can be seen within the cytoplasm. The presence of numerous small, discrete vacuoles or one large vacuole indicates accumulation of fat. This has several potential causes and is prominent in feline hepatic lipidosis syndrome, starvation, pregnancy, and diabetes mellitus. Enlarged hepatocytes with a pale granular-staining cytoplasm but no discrete vacuoles are characteristic of excess glycogen storage. This is most often caused by increased levels of circulating steroids.

Bile stasis and pigment accumulation (eg, iron) can also be assessed by examination of the cytoplasm. Hepatocytes normally accumulate lipofuscin pigment, noted as small, fairly uniform, dark-staining granules, whereas bile and often hemosiderin tend to appear as slightly larger dark-staining bodies within the cytoplasm. Bile accumulation within the canaliculae (canalicular plugs) can also occasionally be seen. These appear as black ribbons on the surface of hepatocytes.

Cytologic interpretation of inflammation is difficult because of the inevitable blood contamination of samples. Inflammation should be considered significant only if it is present within clusters of hepatocytes. Although the individual inflammatory cells can be recognized, it is not possible to indicate which part of the liver is principally affected. Neutrophils can be seen in diffuse hepatitis and also in more focal cholangitis. Small, mature inflammatory lymphocytes are usually seen in periportal inflammatory conditions, such as lymphocytic pericholangitis in cats and chronic active hepatitis in dogs. Macrophages can also be seen in the chronic inflammatory conditions and also in certain infections. Phagocytic cells should be investigated for the presence of organisms within the cytoplasm, but this is uncommon in liver disease.

Primary proliferative nodular hepatocellular lesions include regenerative hyperplasia, nodular hyperplasia, adenoma (hepatoma), and hepatocellular carcinoma. Biliary proliferations can appear as cysts, adenomas, or carcinomas. Bile duct cells tend to be smaller than hepatocytes with less cytoplasm. They are cuboidal or low columnar cells that occasionally produce tubular structures within cytology samples. The cytoplasm is also more uniformly pale staining and not significantly granular. Nucleoli are smaller and less distinct. Significant cell harvest from cystic bile ducts is uncommon because most of these lesions are simply cystic space rather than cellular. If a significant number of biliary epithelial cells are obtained, neoplasia is most likely. However, malignant bile duct cells are more commonly uniform in size and shape and, therefore, do not always show the morphologic features usually associated with malignancy.

Hepatocellular proliferation is a difficult area of interpretation, because hepatocytes in benign proliferative lesions are very similar to those in well-differentiated carcinomas and indeed often cannot be differentiated even from normal hepatocytes. Only in cases with poorly differentiated pleomorphic cells can an adequate interpretation of malignancy be made. The benign and non-neoplastic proliferations always have the same morphology as normal hepatocytes. Therefore, false-negative results for proliferative lesions within the liver are common. Cytology is thus of limited value for nodular hepatocellular lesions.

Cytology can be a useful technique for diagnosis of round cell tumors in the liver. Even with severe inflammatory lesions, lymphocytes are present in low numbers and are generally small, mature lymphocytes. A large population of medium and large lymphoid cells indicates lymphoma. No other condition will give this result.

The other common round cell tumor that can affect the liver (particularly in cats but also occasionally in dogs) is mast cell tumor. The granules within mast cells are metachromatic, facilitating diagnosis. Aspirates of normal liver may contain a few mast cells, but in neoplasia they are usually present in large numbers. If other cells are obtained from cytology preparations, they should be interpreted using the principles described above.

Kidney Cytology: Normal renal aspirates have almost a pure population of renal tubular cells. These are uniform, medium-sized cells of ~17–20 microns with central nuclei, small indistinct nucleoli, and a moderate amount of pale-staining cytoplasm. In cats, lipid droplets within the cytoplasm are a common, normal feature. The cells can be present either singly or in clusters and can occasionally be seen as tubular structures. They sometimes contain small, dark granules within the cytoplasm.

Renal lymphoma is the most common neoplastic disease of the kidney in cats and dogs. Because the cells are usually widely distributed within the tissue, false-negative results with cytologic examination are uncommon. Diagnosis can be made using the criteria described above. Primary renal tumors are uncommon.

Cystic lesions include renal cysts, most commonly seen in cats but also occasionally in dogs, and hydronephrosis. In both disorders, cell harvest is usually low, with a large amount of fluid. The cellular component of the sample is rarely helpful in identifying further the nature of the cystic structure.

Most inflammatory lesions in the kidney are chronic and produce fibrous connective tissue. Cell harvest from these lesions is usually exceedingly low, and cytology is not typically a useful technique. Pyogenic inflammation can sometimes be diagnosed. Cytology may help diagnose feline infectious peritonitis, although diagnosis using serologic techniques is more common. Because of the usually severe and widespread nature of the inflammation, cell harvest is usually high. The wide mixture of inflammatory cells present in feline infectious peritonitis, with a predominance of neutrophils, along with an appropriate history, are typical of the disorder.

Mammary Cytology: Cytology is useful to differentiate inflammatory from neoplastic nodular lesions within mammary tissue. Mammary tumors are not commonly inflamed. It is less useful to differentiate the neoplastic conditions.

Neoplastic lesions must be interpreted using the criteria listed above (*see* p 1601). The criteria most useful to determine the behavior and prognosis of a mammary tumor are local tissue and vessel invasion, not cell morphology. These are best assessed histologically rather than cytologically. Therefore, cellular morphology is not necessarily a good guide to tumor behavior. In cats, malignant cells are often uniform and do not exhibit the normal malignant features; the size of the malignant tumor is the most useful prognostic indicator.

CLINICAL HEMATOLOGY

Hematology refers to the study of the numbers and morphology of the cellular elements of the blood—the RBCs (erythrocytes), WBCs (leukocytes), and platelets (thrombocytes)—and the use of these results in the diagnosis and monitoring of disease. (*See also* HEMATOPOIETIC SYSTEM INTRODUCTION, p 4.)

Red Blood Cells: Three RBC measurements are routinely done: packed cell volume (PCV), the proportion of whole blood volume occupied by RBCs; hemoglobin (Hgb) concentration of whole lysed blood; and RBC count, the number of RBCs per unit volume of whole blood. Although these are separate estimations, they are in effect three ways to measure the same thing, and it is incorrect to attempt to interpret them as separate variables. Inasmuch as they do vary in relation to each other, they allow calculation of two further meaningful parameters, mean corpuscular volume (MCV) and mean corpuscular hemoglobin concentration (MCHC).

MCV varies widely between mammalian species, from ~15 fL in goats to ~90 fL in people. Avian and reptilian red cells are even larger, up to 300 fL. Nevertheless,

$$\text{MCV (fL)} = \frac{\text{PCV(decimal fraction)} \times 1{,}000}{\text{RBC}(\times 10^{12}/\text{L})}$$

$$\text{MCHC (g/L)} = \frac{\text{whole blood hemoglobin concentration (g/L)}}{\text{PCV(decimal fraction)}}$$

MCHC varies little with species (or erythrocyte size), at ~330 g/L.

Several artifacts can cause significant and potentially misleading alterations to measured RBC parameters: 1) old samples cause RBCs to swell, thus increasing PCV and MCV and decreasing MCHC; 2) lipemia causes a falsely high Hgb reading, and hence a falsely high MCHC; 3) hemolysis causes PCV to decrease while Hgb remains unchanged, again leading to a falsely high MCHC; 4) underfilling of the tube causes RBCs to shrink, causing PCV and MCV to decrease and MCHC to increase; 5) autoagglutination causes a falsely low RBC count, and hence a falsely high MCV.

Visual description of RBC morphology on a Romanowsky stain also provides useful diagnostic information. The most common terms include 1) normocytic—cells are of normal size; 2) macrocytes—abnormally large cells, usually polychromatophilic; 3) microcytes—abnormally small cells, usually caused by a lack of hemoglobin precursors; 4) anisocytosis—variation in size of cells due to macrocytes, microcytes, or both; 5) normochromic—cells are of normal color; 6) polychromasia—variation in color of the cells, which usually describes the appearance of large, juvenile, bluish-staining polychromatophilic macrocytes (these broadly correspond to the "reticulocyte" seen with new methylene blue staining, in which the reticulum represents the remnants of the nucleus); 7) hypochromasia—decrease in staining density of the cells, usually due to a lack of hemoglobin precursors, especially iron; and 8) annulocyte—extreme form of hypochromic cell with only a thin rim of hemoglobin.

PCV is the variable usually used to assess the basic status of the erythron—increased in polycythemia, decreased in anemia—although if a sample is too hemolyzed to allow measurement of PCV, a meaningful Hgb measurement may still be obtained. RBC count as such should not be interpreted clinically.

An abnormally high PCV (polycythemia) may be relative, due to a change in the proportion of circulating RBCs to blood plasma without any change in the size of the erythron, or absolute, due to a real increase in erythron size. Absolute polycythemia may be primary (eg, polycythemia vera or, rarely, erythropoietin-producing tumors) or secondary (a consequence of disease in another organ system). (*See also* POLYCYTHEMIA, p 43.)

Polycythemia vera and erythropoietin-producing tumors should be suspected only when PCV is very high, normally >0.7. The former is characterized by normal, mature RBCs and a normal (or low) erythropoietin concentration, whereas the latter may show a regenerative RBC picture with high erythropoietin concentration. Relative polycythemia may also be associated with very high PCV values, and normal, mature RBCs. Secondary polycythemia generally shows a more modest increase in PCV, often with evidence of regeneration (more so when the cause is pulmonary or cardiac, less so when the cause is hormonal). It is often possible to make the differential diagnosis of polycythemia on clinical grounds.

Abnormally low PCV (anemia) may be caused by loss of blood (hemorrhage), breakdown of RBCs in circulation (hemolysis), or lack of production of RBCs by the bone marrow (hypoplasia or aplasia). Presentation varies according to whether the condition is acute or chronic. Aplastic anemia is always chronic in onset, because anemia occurs gradually as existing cells reach the end of their lifespan. (*See also* ANEMIA, p 7.)

In acute hemorrhagic anemia, external blood loss is easily appreciated clinically, but blood loss into a body cavity may be determined only on paracentesis. Initially, all hematologic parameters may be normal, because it may take 12 hr for fluid shifts to produce a decrease in the PCV. Within a few days, RBCs become regenerative, with juvenile forms appearing in circulation (except in horses, in which circulating evidence of regeneration is not readily appreciable). These consist of polychromatophilic macrocytes and normoblasts (nucleated RBCs). Late normoblasts have a small, nonviable nucleus and a moderate amount of cytoplasm colored similarly to that of the polychromatophilic macrocytes, whereas early normoblasts have a larger, viable nucleus and scanty cytoplasm. These are most easily distinguished from lymphocytes by their more densely staining nucleus.

If substantial amounts of blood have been lost from the body, the RBC picture may become hypochromic. Thus, this type of anemia shows an increase in MCV and a decrease in MCHC. If bleeding is into a body cavity, hypochromasia may not be evident because hemoglobin precursors will be recycled. However, slight jaundice may be seen as the sequestered cells are broken down. Some sequestered cells may also be returned to the circulation intact, if somewhat misshapen.

In acute hemolytic anemia, PCV will decrease immediately, and in the early stages some jaundice will be evident. In the very early stages, even a sample collected with extreme care may be markedly hemolyzed. As with hemorrhagic anemia, the RBCs will become regenerative within a few days, with polychromatophilic macrocytes and nucleated RBCs evident. Because hemoglobin precursors are not lost from the body, true hypochromasia is not seen.

Chronic hemorrhagic anemia may be difficult to appreciate if blood is lost in the feces or urine, or due to bloodsucking ectoparasites. Anemia may be severe, and the RBC picture will be regenerative on presentation. Hypochromasia is usually very marked. In very longstanding conditions, depletion of iron and other hemoglobin precursors can become so marked that most of the cells are microcytic, and MCV may paradoxically decrease. Intermittent intra-abdominal hemorrhage leads to a somewhat different picture, because blood shed into the peritoneal cavity can be returned to the circulation. PCV may therefore recover quickly (until the next episode), and signs of depletion of hemoglobin constituents do not emerge.

In chronic hemolytic anemia, RBCs are regenerative on presentation, except that some cases of autoimmune hemolytic anemia (AIHA) paradoxically show little or no regeneration until treatment has been initiated. Hypochromasia is less marked than in hemorrhagic conditions, and misshapen RBCs (including target cells and folded cells) are more common. The spherocyte, in which the erythrocyte loses its classic biconcave shape, is essentially pathognomonic for AIHA. Jaundice may be absent, because the products of the destruction of the RBCs may be cleared by the reticuloendothelial system and the liver as quickly as they are formed.

Hypoplastic and aplastic anemia may be mild if RBC production is merely depressed secondary to some other disease. Protein, mineral, or vitamin deficiencies may cause hypoplastic anemia, but these are more likely to be secondary to another disease (eg, chronic hemorrhage or malabsorption) than simple dietary deficiency. Other diseases may cause depression of erythropoietin production, eg, renal failure, deficiencies of hormones that usually stimulate erythropoietin production (eg, hypothyroidism, hyperadrenocorticism), and chronic, debilitating conditions (eg, chronic infections, chronic parasitism, and neoplasia). RBC morphology is nonregenerative and may be hypochromic if a deficiency state is involved. Paradoxically, vitamin B_{12} and/or folic acid deficiency produces a macrocytic RBC picture due to early maturation arrest of the erythrocytes. Neoplasia of the bone marrow may cause severe anemia as erythropoietic elements are crowded out, but some regeneration may be seen as the remaining bone marrow attempts to compensate. In this case, other bone marrow cell lines will also be affected.

True aplastic anemia refers to a failure of the entire bone marrow. The shorter-lived granulocytes and platelets decrease first, followed by a progressively severe anemia that is normocytic and normochromic.

White Blood Cells: The WBCs consist of the granulocytes (neutrophils in most mammals, called heterophils in rabbits, reptiles, and birds [and these look like eosinophils in smears]; eosinophils; and basophils) and the agranulocytes (lymphocytes and monocytes). Although each type is traditionally counted by determination of its percentage of the total WBC population, meaningful interpretation requires that the absolute number of each type be calculated by multiplying the total WBC count by the fraction attributable to the individual cell type. Percentages of each cell type alone are not helpful. An increased percentage that is due to an absolute decrease in another cell type is not an increase at all.

Mature **neutrophils** have a lobulated nucleus, but when demand is high, immature cells with an unlobulated band nucleus (no constriction of the nucleus is more than half the width of the nucleus) may be released into circulation. They function as phagocytes and are important in infectious conditions and in inflammation. Increased neutrophil counts (neutrophilia) are caused by inflammation, bacterial infection, acute stress, steroid effects, and neoplasia of the granulocytic cell line (granulocytic leukemia can be difficult to differentiate from a simple neutrophilia without special stains or bone marrow biopsy). Decreased neutrophil counts (neutropenia) are caused by viral infections, toxin exposure (including foodborne toxins), certain drugs (eg, carbimazole and methimazole), autoimmune destruction of neutrophils, bone marrow neoplasia not involving the granulocytes, and bone marrow aplasia.

Eosinophils are characterized by prominent pink-staining granules on a Romanowsky stain. They inactivate histamine and inhibit edema formation. Increased eosinophil counts (eosinophilia) are caused by allergic/hypersensitivity reactions, parasitism, tissue injury, mast cell tumors, estrus, and pregnancy or parturition in the bitch. Some large dog breeds (eg, German and Belgian Shepherds, Rottweilers) normally have a relatively high eosinophil count. Extremely high eosinophil counts (hypereosinophilic syndrome), possibly due to an out-of-control hypersensitivity reaction, and eosinophil leukemia (a form of chronic myeloid leukemia) are also described. Decreased eosinophil count (eosinopenia) is almost always caused by the action of glucocorticoids, either endogenous or therapeutic.

Basophils are rare in most species and are characterized by blue-staining granules on a Romanowsky stain. They are more easily seen in cattle. They are closely related to mast cells and, like them, initiate the inflammatory response by releasing histamine. An increased basophil count (basophilia) accompanies eosinophilia in some species as part of the hypersensitivity reaction.

Monocytes are large cells with blue-gray cytoplasm, which may be vacuolated, and a kidney bean-shaped or lobulated nucleus. Their main function is phagocytosis, and they are essentially identical to tissue macrophages. An increased monocyte count (monocytosis) may occur in any chronic disease, especially chronic inflammation, and may be very marked in neoplasia. Monocytes also increase as part of the steroid response in dogs.

Lymphocytes mainly develop outside the bone marrow in the lymph nodes, spleen, and gut-associated lymphoid tissue. They are the smallest of the WBCs, with a round, evenly staining nucleus and sparse cytoplasm. Larger, reactive lymphocytes can be seen after antigenic stimulation, and care must be taken to differentiate them from neoplastic lymphocytes. Their primary function is immunologic, including both antibody production and cell-mediated immune responses. Some survive only a few days, but many are long-lived. The number in circulation is a balance between populations in the blood, lymph, lymph nodes, and splenic follicles and does not necessarily reflect changes in lymphopoiesis. An increased lymphocyte count (lymphocytosis) may occur for physiologic reasons, especially in cats, but significant increases usually indicate leukemia. Immature or bizarre cells may also be recognized. Decreased lymphocyte counts (lymphopenia) are usually due to an effect of corticosteroids, either endogenous (stress or Cushing disease) or therapeutic, and may also accompany neutropenia in some viral infections, especially the parvoviruses. Lymphopenia may also be a feature of solid-organ lymphosarcomas, when leukemia is absent.

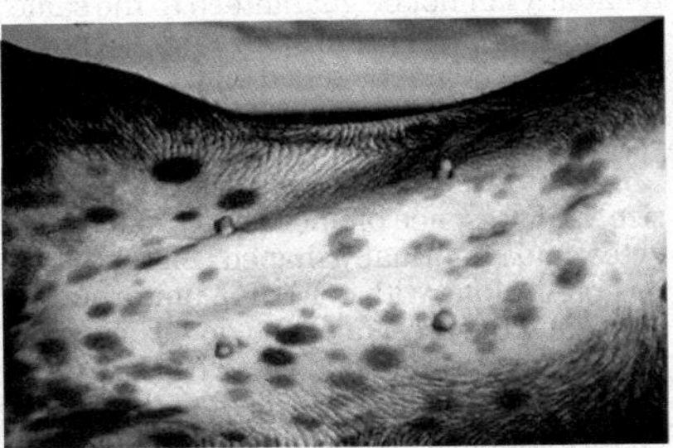

Ecchymotic lesions on the abdomen of a dog. *Courtesy of Ontario Veterinary College.*

Platelets: Mammalian platelets are pale blue granular fragments (much smaller than RBCs) shed from multinucleate megakaryocytes in the bone marrow; avian and reptilian platelets are true cells with nuclei. They maintain the integrity of the endothelium and act as part of the clotting process to repair damaged endothelium, where they ensure mechanical strength of the clot.

Increased platelet counts (thrombocytosis) occur as a reaction to consumption after injury, when large juvenile platelets may also appear; after splenectomy, as splenic stores are liberated to the circulation; after vincristine treatment, which increases platelet shedding from megakaryocytes; and in megakaryocytic leukemia.

Decreased platelet counts (thrombocytopenia) are caused by autoimmune reactions, thrombotic/thrombocytopenic purpura, bone marrow suppression and aplasia, bone marrow neoplasia, and equine infectious anemia. Signs are petechiation and ecchymosis more than frank hemorrhage, and little may be seen until the platelet count is <20 × 10^9/L. Platelet functional abnormalities present similarly, but platelet numbers and morphology are normal.

Blood Sample Preparation and Evaluation: In-house hematologic investigations, with a minimum of specialist equipment, can provide almost as much information as a full laboratory analysis, although some estimations are qualitative rather than quantitative.

Blood for hematology should be collected into tubes containing EDTA anticoagulant and immediately mixed well to avoid clotting. Larger (2.5 mL) tubes yield better results than the smaller (1 mL) pediatric tubes and are less likely to clot. Nevertheless, it is essential to fill the tube exactly to the mark, so smaller tubes may be unavoidable for small patients. WBC morphology deteriorates most quickly, especially in equine blood, so if the sample cannot be analyzed immediately, a thin blood smear should be submitted to the laboratory with the blood sample.

PCV is measured by microhematocrit, which is the reference method. A capillary tube is filled ¾ full with well-mixed blood and sealed at one end; heat-sealing is best if a Bunsen burner is available, otherwise a proprietary clay pad is used. The tube is spun in a high-speed microhematocrit centrifuge for 6 min, and the PCV is read using a microhematocrit reader with a sliding cursor. The appearance of the plasma (eg, normal, icteric, hemolyzed, lipemic) and the thickness of the buffy coat, which gives a very rough guide to total WBC count, should be noted.

Further information is obtained from a blood film. This is made by using one slide, with a corner broken off as a spreader, to pull a small drop of blood across a clean slide into a thin film. A suitable film is thin (one erythrocyte thick) and tapers to a feathered edge before the far end of the slide. The broken corner of the spreader slide ensures two straight edges parallel to the long edges of the slide. Immediately after the film is spread, it is dried quickly by fanning the slide in the air. Air-dried smears can be sent to the laboratory in a slide mailer or stained and examined in the practice. Commercial rapid Romanowsky-type stains merely require the slide to be dipped in three colored solutions in succession. Cell morphology is clear and comparable to more permanent stains such as Leishman or May-Gruenwald-Giemsa, although quality deteriorates after a few days. The slide should be allowed to dry naturally or dried with a hair dryer (not wiped dry), and examined under oil immersion.

Clinically useful information may be easily achieved in-house for all hematologic variables. The main deficiency is the absence of a numerical WBC count, and hence of numerical values for the differential WBC count. This may be acceptable for an interim emergency investigation, and a WBC count using a hemocytometer slide may be attempted. A mirrored slide with an Improved Neubauer ruling may be used, with a cover slip fitted so that Newton rings are visible on both sides. The blood sample is diluted 1:20 with Turck fluid or a similar diluent. An automatic pipette capable of dispensing 0.95 mL and 0.05 mL (50 μL) should be used to ensure an accurate dilution. The sample should be mixed well and allowed to stand for 10 min while the stain is taken up by the cells. The chamber of the hemocytometer is then filled by using a capillary (PCV) tube. The number of cells in each of the four large corner squares of the grid are counted, and the total divided by 20 to calculate the total WBC count $\times 10^{9}$/L.

Several hematologic instruments are available for in-practice use. Those based on centrifugation, in which WBC measurements are made by spreading a stained buffy coat, are not true hematology analyzers, but give approximate counts. Although a numerical estimate of total WBC count is provided, the differential WBC count cannot distinguish between lymphocytes and monocytes, and results do not always correlate well with standard methods. This method is appropriate only as an emergency approximation, and a blood film must always be examined in addition. It is also wise to check the PCV by microhematocrit.

Impedance counters (Coulter principle) are used by diagnostic laboratories and perform well in experienced hands. However, it is difficult to achieve optimal performance without trained technical staff. Instruments not based on the Coulter principle should be avoided for veterinary use, because their results do not necessarily compare well on nonhuman samples. Instruments providing automated differential counts perform poorly on nonhuman blood, and results must never be accepted without also checking a blood film. No hematology laboratory should be without the facility for examining blood films, and a blood film should be examined for every patient sample. Quality assurance issues are the same as those for biochemistry laboratories (*see* p 1590). If accuracy and reliability cannot be guaranteed to the same standard as the referral laboratory, then results should not be relied on without external confirmation.

Red Blood Cells: The size, uniformity of size, and presence of microcytes, macrocytes, and abnormally shaped cells should be noted, along with cell color, uniformity of color, and the presence of hypochromasia, polychromasia, and nucleated RBCs. An overall descriptive assessment of the RBC picture should be made, including the degree of regeneration or hypochromasia, if any.

White Blood Cells: A qualitative estimate of numbers should be made (ie, very low, low, normal, high, very high). This can be remarkably consistent with practice. The proportions of each cell type can be estimated, or preferably, a formal differential count of 100–200 cells performed. Unusual or abnormal WBC forms (eg, band or toxic neutrophils), or pathologic cells (eg, prolymphocytes, lymphoblasts, or mast cells) should be noted.

Platelets: A qualitative estimate of platelet numbers, based on how many can be seen in a typical high-power field (oil immersion) should be made. Several fields should be examined, more if numbers appear low. Results can be ranked as none seen (on entire slide), rare (very few on entire slide), low in number (<5 per high-power field), adequate (5–20 per high-power field), or abundant (>20 per high-power field). Normal platelet numbers in the horse are about half those of other species. In a sample more than a few hours old, platelets may clump into rafts, leaving areas of the slide apparently devoid of platelets. Slides should be scanned for rafts before reporting platelet numbers as low. Enlarged or macroplatelets should also be noted.

URINALYSIS

Urinalysis is an important laboratory test that can be readily performed in veterinary practice and is considered part of a minimum database. It is useful to document various types of urinary tract diseases and may provide information about other systemic diseases, such as liver failure and hemolysis. Urine may be collected by cystocentesis, urethral catheterization, or voiding. Urine should be evaluated within 30 min, but if this is not possible, it may be refrigerated for up to 24 hr or submitted to an outside diagnostic laboratory; however, this may result in crystal precipitation. Refrigeration does not alter urine pH or specific gravity. If cytologic evaluation is required and a delay in preparing the slides is anticipated, then a preservative should be added. A few drops of 10% formalin (exact concentration not necessary) is better than boric acid. However, the usual Romanowsky stains are unsuitable with formalin; if submitting to an outside laboratory, it should be communicated that formalin has been added.

Urine Appearance

Color: Normal urine is typically transparent and yellow or amber on visual inspection. The intensity of color is in part related to the volume of urine collected and concentration of urine produced; therefore, it should be interpreted in context of urine specific gravity. Significant disease may exist when urine color is normal. Abnormal urine color may be caused by presence of endogenous or exogenous pigments, but it does not provide specific information. Interpretation of semiquantitative reagent strips, which are colorimetric tests, requires knowledge of urine color because discolored urine may result in a false-positive result. Equine urine may turn brown after a period of time.

Clarity: Urine is typically clear but may become less transparent with pigmenturia, crystalluria, hematuria, pyuria, lipiduria, or when other compounds such as mucus are present. Depending on the cause, increased turbidity may disappear with centrifugation of the sample.

Odor: Normal urine has a slight odor of ammonia; however, the odor depends on urine concentration. Some species, such as cats and goats, have pungent urine odor because of urine composition. Bacterial infection may result in a strong odor due to pyuria; a strong ammonia odor may occur if the bacteria produce urease.

Urine Chemistries

Urine must be at room temperature for accurate measurement of urine specific gravity and for chemical analysis. These tests are usually done before centrifugation; however, if urine is discolored or turbid, it may be beneficial to perform these tests on supernatant (*see* p 1617).

Specific Gravity: Specific gravity is defined as the ratio of the weight of a volume of liquid to the weight of an equal volume of distilled water; therefore, it depends on the number, size, and weight of particles in the liquid. It is different from osmolality, which depends only on the number of particles in the liquid; measurement of osmolality requires specialized instrumentation.

The urine specific gravity (SG) is determined using a refractometer designed for veterinary samples, which includes a scale calibrated specifically for cat urine. SG for species other than cats should be determined using the scale for dogs. In healthy animals, SG is highly variable, depending on fluid and electrolyte balance of the body. It is normally at least 1.015. Interpretation of SG, therefore, depends on the clinical presentation and serum chemistry findings. (*See also* URINARY SYSTEM INTRODUCTION, p 1494.) An animal that is dehydrated or has other causes of prerenal azotemia will have hypersthenuric urine with an SG >1.025–1.040 (depending on species). Dilute urine in a dehydrated or azotemic animal is abnormal and could be caused by renal failure, hypo- or hyperadrenocorticism, hypercalcemia, diabetes mellitus, hyperthyroidism, and diuretic therapy. In cases of diabetes insipidus, values <1.010 can be expected. Glucosuria increases the SG despite increased urine volume.

Semiquantitative, Colorimetric Reagent Strips: Reagent strips such as Multistix® or Chemstrip ® can be used to perform several semiquantitative chemical evaluations simultaneously. They are used routinely to determine urine pH, protein, glucose, ketones, bilirubin/urobilinogen, and occult blood. Some reagent strips include test pads for leukocyte esterase (for detection of WBCs), nitrite (for detection of bacteria), and SG; these are not valid in animals and should not be used. Reagent strips are adversely affected by moisture and have a limited shelf life. Bottles should be kept tightly capped, and unused strips should be discarded after their expiration date.

Urine pH: Urine pH is typically acidic in dogs and cats and alkaline in horses and ruminants, but varies depending on diet, medications, or presence of disease. Reagent strip colorimetric test pads for pH determination are accurate to within ~0.5 pH units. For example, a reading of 6.5 means the actual pH is likely to be between 6.0 and 7.0. Portable pH meters are more accurate than pH colorimetric test pads. A bacterial urinary tract infection with a urease-producing microbe will result in alkaluria. Urine pH will affect crystalluria because some crystals, such as struvite, form in alkaline urine, whereas other crystals, such as cystine, form in acidic urine.

Protein: The protein test pad uses a color indicator (tetrabromophenol blue), which detects primarily albumin in urine. Results range from 10 mg/dL to 1,000 mg/dL. Proteinuria can occur from prerenal (fever, strenuous exercise, seizures, extreme environmental temperature, and hyperproteinemia), renal (primarily glomerular and occasionally tubular disease), or postrenal (inflammation, hemorrhage, and infection) causes. A positive reaction must be interpreted in light of SG, pH, and urine sediment examination. For example, a trace amount of protein in concentrated urine is less significant than a trace amount of protein in dilute urine. Alkaluria will give a false-positive reaction. Likewise, presence of other proteins, such as Bence-Jones proteins, will give false-negative results. Proteinuria can be measured using sulfosalicylic acid precipitation, which detects albumin and globulins; however, it is not accurate in dogs and cats. If proteinuria is present with an inactive urine sediment, its significance can be verified and quantitated by dividing the urine protein concentration by the urine creatinine concentration (urine protein to urine creatinine ratio [UP:UC]). Interpretation of a UP:UC is as follows: <0.5:1 (dogs) and <0.4:1 (cats) is normal, 0.4 or 0.5–1:1 is questionable, and >1:1 is abnormal. With primary renal azotemia, a UP:UC >0.5:1 in dogs and >0.4:1 in cats is considered abnormal. A semiquantitative microalbuminuria test is available to detect urinary albumin in the range of 1–30 mg/dL. It uses ELISA technology specific for canine or feline albumin. Because of minor species differences in albumin, there are different kits for dogs and cats. The microalbuminuria test detects lower concentrations of albumin than a standard dipstick test pad. Hematuria must be macroscopic to increase the microalbuminuria or UP:UC; however, pyuria increases both.

Glucose: Glucose is detected by a glucose oxidase enzymatic reaction that is specific for glucose. Glucosuria is not present normally because the renal threshold for glucose is >180 mg/dL in most species and >240 mg/dL in cats. With euglycemia, the amount of filtered glucose is less than the renal threshold, and all of the filtered glucose is reabsorbed in the proximal renal tubules. Glucosuria can result from hyperglycemia (due to diabetes mellitus, excessive endogenous or exogenous glucocorticoids, hepatocutaneous syndrome, or stress) or from a proximal renal tubular defect (such as primary renal glucosuria or Fanconi syndrome). If glucosuria is present, blood glucose concentration should be determined. False-negative results can occur with high urinary concentrations of ascorbic acid (vitamin C) or with formaldehyde (a metabolite of the urinary antiseptic, methenamine, which may be used for prevention of bacterial urinary tract infections). False-positive results may occur if the sample is contaminated with hydrogen peroxide, chlorine, or hypochlorite (bleach).

Ketones: Ketones are produced from fatty acid metabolism and include acetoacetic acid, acetone, and β-hydroxybutyrate. The ketone test pad detects acetone and acetoacetic acid, but not β-hydroxybutyrate (which can be measured in blood and urine using a point-of-care instrument or a biochemistry analyzer). The test pad contains nitroprusside that reacts with acetoacetic acid and acetone to cause a purple color change; it is more sensitive to acetoacetic acid than acetone. Ketonuria is associated with primary ketosis (ruminants), ketosis secondary to diabetes mellitus (small animals), consumption of low-carbohydrate diets (especially in cats), and occasionally with prolonged fasting or starvation. A false-positive reaction can occur with presence of reducing substances in urine.

Bilirubin/Urobilinogen: When hemoglobin is degraded, the heme portion is converted to bilirubin, which is conjugated in the liver and excreted in bile. Some conjugated bilirubin is filtered by the glomerulus and excreted in urine. In dogs, but not cats, the kidney can metabolize hemoglobin to bilirubin and secrete it. Male dogs have a higher secretory ability than females. Dipstick reagent pads use diazonium salts to create a color change and are more sensitive to conjugated bilirubin than unconjugated bilirubin. Bilirubinuria occurs when conjugated bilirubin exceeds the renal threshold as with liver disease or hemolysis. In dogs with concentrated urine, a small amount of bilirubin can be normal. Pigmenturia and phenothiazine may result in a false-positive reaction; false-negative reactions may occur with large amounts of urinary ascorbic acid (vitamin C).

Urobilinogen, formed from bilirubin by intestinal microflora, is absorbed into the portal circulation and excreted renally. A small amount of urinary urobilinogen is normal. Increased urinary urobilinogen occurs with hyperbilirubinemia; a negative test may be seen with biliary obstruction. However, the test is not specific enough to be clinically useful.

Occult Blood: The occult blood test pad uses a "pseudoperoxidase" method to detect intact RBCs, hemoglobin, and myoglobin. A positive reaction can be due to hemorrhage (hematuria), intravascular hemolysis (hemoglobinuria), or myoglobinuria. The latter two processes can be distinguished by examination of plasma: plasma will appear pink to red after intravascular hemolysis, whereas myoglobin is rapidly cleared from plasma, resulting in clear plasma. As with other colorimetric test pads, discolored urine may yield false-positive results. A positive result should be interpreted with microscopic examination of urine sediment.

Urine Sediment

Microscopic examination of urine sediment should be part of a routine urinalysis. For centrifugation, 3–5 mL of urine is transferred to a conical centrifuge tube. Urine is centrifuged at 1,000–1,500 rpm for ~3–5 min. The supernatant is decanted, leaving ~0.5 mL of urine and sediment in the tip of the conical tube. The sediment is resuspended by tapping the tip of the conical tube against the table several times. A few drops of the sediment are transferred to a glass slide, and a cover slip is applied. Examination of unstained urine is recommended for routine samples. Microscopic examination is performed at 100× (for crystals, casts, and cells) and 400× (for cells and bacteria) magnifications. Contrast of the sample is enhanced by closing the iris diaphragm and lowering the condenser of the microscope. Stains such as Sedistain® and new methylene blue can be used to aid in cell identification but may dilute the specimen and introduce artifacts such as stain precipitate and crystals. Use of a modified Wright stain increases the sensitivity, specificity, and positive and negative predictive values for detection of bacteria. For some tests, air dried, stained smears are necessary.

Red Blood Cells: In an unstained preparation, RBCs are small and round and have a slight orange tint and a smooth appearance. Normal urine should contain <5 RBCs/field at 400× magnification. Increased RBCs in urine (hematuria) indicates hemorrhage somewhere in the urogenital system; however, sample collection by cystocentesis or catheterization may induce hemorrhage.

White Blood Cells: WBCs are slightly larger than RBCs and have grainy cytoplasm. Normal urine should contain <5 WBCs/field at 400× magnification. Increased WBCs (pyuria) can occur due to inflammation, infection, trauma, or neoplasia. Catheterization or collection of voided urine may introduce a few WBCs from the urogenital tract.

Epithelial Cells: Transitional epithelial cells, a common urine contaminant derived from the bladder and proximal urethra, resemble WBCs but are larger. They have a greater amount of grainy cytoplasm and a round, centrally located nucleus. In a voided urine sample, squamous epithelial cells may be seen. They are large, oval to cuboidal in shape, and may or may not contain a nucleus. Occasionally, neoplastic transitional cells may be seen in an animal with a transitional cell carcinoma. Neoplastic squamous cells may be seen in an animal with a squamous cell carcinoma.

Cylindruria (Casts): Casts are elongated, cylindrical structures formed by mucoprotein congealing within renal tubules and may contain cells. Hyaline casts are pure protein precipitates; they are transparent, have parallel sides and rounded ends, and are composed of mucoprotein. They may occur with fever, exercise, and renal disease. Epithelial cellular casts form from entrapment of sloughed tubular epithelial cells in the mucoprotein; they may be seen with renal tubular disease. Granular casts are thought to represent degenerated epithelial cellular casts. Waxy casts have a granular appearance and are thought to arise from degeneration of longstanding granular casts. They typically have sharp borders with broken ends. Other cellular casts include RBC casts and WBC casts and are always abnormal. RBC casts form because of renal hemorrhage. WBC casts form because of renal inflammation, as with pyelonephritis. Fatty casts are not common but can be seen with disorders of lipid metabolism, such as diabetes mellitus. A few hyaline or granular casts are considered normal. However, presence of cellular casts or other casts in high numbers indicates renal damage, and may be one of the earliest laboratory abnormalities noted with toxic damage to renal epithelial cells (eg, gentamicin, amphotericin B).

Infectious Organisms: The presence of bacteria in urine collected by cystocentesis indicates infection. Small numbers of bacteria from the lower urogenital tract may contaminate voided samples or samples collected by catheterization and do not indicate infection. Bacterial rods are most easily identified in urine sediment. Particles of debris may be mistaken for bacteria. Suspected bacteria can be confirmed by staining urine sediment with Gram stain; however, aerobic culture is best to confirm a bacterial urinary tract infection. Rarely, yeast and fungal hyphae and parasitic ova may be seen in urine sediment. Their presence is not always associated with clinical disease. Parasitic ova observed include those of *Stephanurus dentatus*, *Capillaria plica*, *C felis*, and *Dioctophyma renale*. Additionally, microfilariae of *Dirofilaria immitis* may be seen in urine sediment.

Crystals: Many urine sediments contain crystals. The type of crystal present depends on urine pH, concentration of crystallogenic materials, urine temperature, and length of time between urine collection and examination. Crystalluria is not synonymous with urolithiasis and is not necessarily pathologic. Furthermore, uroliths may form without observed crystalluria. Many urine samples are examined at room temperature, which may alter the number of crystals present, and the result may not represent the situation in vivo.

Struvite crystals are commonly seen in canine and feline urine. Struvite crystalluria in dogs is not a problem unless there is a concurrent bacterial urinary tract infection with a urease-producing microbe. Without an infection, struvite crystals in dogs are not associated with struvite urolith formation. However, some animals (eg, cats) do form struvite uroliths without a bacterial urinary tract infection. In these animals, struvite crystalluria may be pathologic. Struvite crystals appear typically as "coffin-lids" or "prisms"; however, they may be amorphous.

Calcium oxalate crystalluria occurs less commonly in dogs and cats. If persistent, it may indicate an increased risk of calcium oxalate urolith formation, which has been increasing in some countries throughout the past few years. (*See also* UROLITHIASIS, p 1502, and p 1525.) However, calcium oxalate and calcium carbonate crystalluria is common in healthy horses and cattle. Calcium oxalate dihydrate crystals appear as squares with an "X" in the middle, or "envelope-shaped." Calcium oxalate monohydrate crystals are "dumb-bell" shaped. An unusual form of calcium oxalate crystals is typically seen in association with ethylene glycol toxicity (*see* p 3046). These crystals are found in neutral to acidic urine. They are small, flat, and colorless and are shaped like "picket fence posts."

Ammonium acid urate crystals suggest liver disease (eg, portosystemic shunt). These crystals occur in acidic urine and are yellow-brown spheres with irregular, spiny projections; however, they may also be amorphous. Certain species, such as birds and reptiles, and certain breeds of dogs, specifically Dalmatians, can normally have ammonium acid urate crystalluria.

Cystine crystals are six-sided and of variable size. They are seen in acidic urine. Presence of cystine crystals represents a proximal tubular defect in amino acid reabsorption. Cystinuria has been reported in many breeds of dogs and rarely in cats. Dachshunds, Newfoundlands, English Bulldogs, and Scottish Terriers have a high incidence of cystine urolithiasis.

Bilirubin crystals occur with bilirubinuria; however, they may be normal in small numbers in dogs.

Lipids: Fat droplets are commonly present in urine from dogs and cats and may be mistaken for RBCs. They often vary in size and tend to float on a different plane of focus than the remainder of the sediment. They are not considered to be pathologic.

Spermatozoa: Spermatozoa may be seen normally in urine collected from reproductively intact male dogs.

Plant Material: Occasionally, plant material may be seen in urine samples collected by voiding. When present, they indicate contamination of the urine sample and are not pathologic.

Bladder Tumor Antigen Test

The bladder tumor antigen test can be used to screen for transitional cell carcinoma in dogs. The results are not specific for transitional cell carcinoma, and non-neoplastic disease (eg, urinary tract infections, hematuria, etc) can give positive results. A negative test, however, is meaningful in that a transitional cell carcinoma is not likely to be present. This test may be useful for routine screening of dogs at higher risk of developing transitional cell carcinoma (eg, Scottish terriers) that do not have other signs or laboratory findings of lower urinary tract disease. This tests for the presence of basement membrane fragments and is a color reaction using a commercial test kit.

PARASITOLOGY

Internal Parasite (Endoparasite) Diagnosis in Small Animals: Diagnosis of internal parasites in small animals is typically performed by examination of feces for parasite eggs. Fecal samples should be fresh, preferably collected from the animal during the act of defecation or from the rectum using a fecal loop during the physical examination. Specimens should be submitted to a diagnostic laboratory in a sealed container, labeled with proper identification. Specimens should be fixed in 10% formaldehyde solution or sent chilled. Other preservative solutions (eg, sodium acetate formalin, polyvinyl alcohol, available in commercial mailer kits) better preserve protozoa and facilitate special staining (eg, trichrome, iron hematoxylin).

Routine examinations should be done by both direct fecal smear and fecal flotation. Direct smears are prepared by mixing feces (an amount of feces fitting on one-half the tip of a wooden applicator stick) with 1 drop each of saline (for motile organisms) and Lugol's iodine stain (to see internal morphologic structures, eg, those of *Giardia*), and covering with separate coverslips on the same slide. Flotation methods concentrate diagnostic stages and provide a cleaner final preparation, using ~2 g of feces. Sugar (specific gravity [SG] 1.27) and sodium nitrate (SG 1.39) are commonly used flotation media. Zinc sulfate flotation (SG 1.18), repeated on 3 consecutive days, is the method of choice to reveal *Giardia* cysts, which are intermittently shed in feces. Motile nematode larvae may be collected and concentrated by Baermann sedimentation; a convenient method is to place ~2 g of feces on several sheets of cotton gauze in a tea strainer suspended in the wide end of a large, conical funnel fitted with a rubber tube and stopcock. The funnel is filled with warm tap water or saline for 1 hr before sediment examination. Larvae descend within the funnel due to gravity and are collected from the end of the stopcock for microscopic examination. Special procedures, such as formalin-ethyl acetate sedimentation, may be used for parasitic larval stages that do not float well. Sheather's sugar (SG 1.30) can be used to detect small oocysts of *Cryptosporidium* (4–6 μ) or *Toxoplasma* (12 μ) by focusing just under the coverslip. Oocysts "float up" to the under-surface of a coverslip placed on the slide for 10 min before examination.

A direct smear using 1 drop of blood can be used to detect motile microfilariae of *Dirofilaria immitis*, but this should not be the sole means of detection. More accurate examination of blood may be done by a modified Knotts' test: 1 mL blood is added to 9 mL of 2% formalin solution in a 15-mL tube and centrifuged at 1,500 rpm. The supernatant is discarded and a drop of methylene blue stain is mixed with the sediment "button," which is pipetted onto a microscope slide, covered with a coverslip, and examined to differentiate microfilariae of *D immitis* from those of the nonpathogenic *Dipetalonema reconditum*. Commercial filtration and staining procedures are effective alternatives to the modified Knotts' test. Animals on heartworm preventive become amicrofilaremic, and an occult heartworm test using a commercially available ELISA for circulating uterine antigen of adult female *Dirofilaria* is the method of choice for treated dogs. Feline dirofilariasis cannot be reliably diagnosed by microfilaremia or antigenemia tests, because heartworm numbers are typically too low; antibody titers to *D immitis* are used to detect prior exposure and possible current infection in cats.

Internal Parasite (Endoparasite) Diagnosis in Livestock: Fresh fecal samples from livestock should be collected from pasture or, preferably, per rectum using plastic gloves. Samples should be placed in a properly identified, sealed specimen jar. A representative number of herd samples should be collected from a minimum of 10 animals to account for the typical high individual variation in numbers of eggs shed. Samples can be combined after thorough mixing to enable examination of a single herd composite sample.

Quantitative fecal egg counts by the modified Wisconsin centrifugal flotation procedure or similar methods can be used to estimate relative infection burden for nematodes of the "GI parasite complex" (eg, trichostrongylid larvae of cattle), while also detecting coccidia and other parasites such as lungworm larvae and tapeworms. Three grams of feces are placed in a container, suspended in ~15 mL water, strained through a gauze square into a 15-mL tube, and centrifuged (1,500 rpm for 3 min). The supernatant is decanted and the sediment mixed with saturated sugar solution, filling the tube enough to form a positive meniscus before placing a 22 × 22 mm coverslip on the lip of the test tube. The tube is centrifuged again at low speed (1,500 rpm for 5 min). The coverslip, with the surface film containing eggs, is removed and transferred to a microscope slide for counting of trichostrongylid eggs in cattle feces or strongylid eggs in horse feces. The total is divided by 3 to derive eggs/g (EPG). Other parasites are noted, if present, with a general abundance designation of +1 (few), +2 (small number), +3 (large number), or +4 (too numerous to count).

A saturated solution of table salt (SG 1.20) is an inexpensive alternative medium for diagnosis of livestock parasites, although salt may be highly corrosive to metal surfaces. Magnesium sulfate (SG 1.20) is the preferred medium for swine feces. Special slides containing chambers with etched areas of known volume are also used to estimate EPG, especially for small ruminants. Feces in a strained solution (usually saturated salt) are introduced into each chamber with a Pasteur pipette, and the eggs are counted under low-power magnification. A commonly used counting slide is the McMaster slide, which has two chambers, each with a volume of 0.15 mL under the etched area. For example, if 3 g of feces are mixed with 42 mL of concentrate solution, then each egg counted is multiplied by 50 to yield the number of EPG in the fecal sample. Acceptable correlation between the EPG and the relative worm burden is often possible in young animals, although low (<5 EPG) or negative counts are typically found in adult animals. In young cattle, which generally have EPG counts 10 times that of adult animals, EPG counts >50 reflect a moderate infection, and EPG counts >500 indicate a heavy burden and a need for treatment.

Because fluke eggs do not float readily, quantitative fecal sedimentation procedures are usually used. Two grams of feces are mixed with 35 mL soapy solution (2% liquid detergent) and strained through gauze into a 50-mL centrifuge tube. The tube is filled with soapy water and allowed to stand for 3 min, after which ½ of the supernatant is discarded. This is repeated 2–3 times until the supernatant is clean. All but 15 mL is poured off, 2 drops of new methylene blue are added, and the eggs counted with a dissecting microscope in a gridded Petri dish or by examining several coverslipped microscope slides. The eggs of the liver fluke, *Fasciola hepatica*, can be differentiated from those of *Paramphistomum* spp, the rumen fluke, by the golden color, more barreled shape, and slightly larger size of eggs of *F hepatica* versus the gray color, more pointed end, and smaller size of the usually nonpathogenic rumen fluke. Commercial sieve-sediment kits can reduce sample preparation time by 50%. In cattle, *Fasciola* EPG counts >3 suggest economic losses; EPG >10 may be associated with clinical signs.

External Parasite (Ectoparasite) Examination in Small Animals and Livestock: Animals with dermatoses should be evaluated by examining for ectoparasites or evidence of their presence. For example, fleas may not be seen on a cat or dog, but small black flecks of flea excrement (flea frass or flea "dirt") that produce a reddish stain when placed on a moistened paper towel may be noted. Skin must sometimes be scraped to diagnose parasites. A scalpel blade is used for the deep scrapings (until blood oozes) needed to demonstrate parasites that live in burrows (eg, *Sarcoptes*) or hair follicles (*Demodex* spp). The scraped material is placed in a drop of mineral oil on a slide, and the entire area under the coverslip is scanned under low-power magnification. A few drops of 10% potassium hydroxide solution may be added to clear debris and allow better visualization.

SEROLOGIC TEST KITS

In-house serologic test kits continue to improve in reliability, ease of use, and types available. They include tests for infectious disease by measuring either antigens or antibodies. Antibody levels can also be measured to establish the presence of adequate protection to an infectious agent. However, these levels are not an absolute measure of protection. High serum antibody levels do not always confer protection, and low levels do not always indicate susceptibility to infection. The level of cell-mediated immunity is also important. Measurement of hormone levels also use serologic tests. Many of these tests are ELISA that may be microwell or membrane-based, but other types, including immunomigration, immunochromatography, and agglutination tests, are also available. Sample requirements may be plasma, serum, whole blood, feces, or saliva, depending on the test format.

Feline Leukemia Virus (FeLV): Serologic testing for FeLV is important to identify infected cats and prevent transmission of the virus (*see* p 790). Testing is also recommended before vaccination against FeLV, because vaccination of infected cats will not limit development or transmission of disease. Most currently available in-house diagnostic kits are designed to detect soluble FeLV-specific *gag* protein p 27, which is produced in large amounts during viremia. The time between infection and the presence of detectable antigen varies but is likely to be within 28–30 days. Vaccination against FeLV will not yield a positive test result when antigen tests are used, nor will the presence of maternally derived antibodies in kittens. Testing serum, plasma, or whole blood is considered more reliable than testing saliva or tears. Most test kits have positive and negative controls incorporated into the kit, so technical problems with running the test may be detected.

A negative result on a screening test is very reliable; however, false-positive results may occur with the tests of soluble antigen, especially in a population of cats with a low incidence of disease. A true positive result may reflect either transient or persistent viremia, so clinical decisions should not be based on a single test result. Confirmation of positive results, especially in asymptomatic cats, should be pursued by additional testing such as soluble antigen testing using a kit from a different manufacturer or immunofluorescent antigen testing on blood or bone marrow. Cats with discordant results should be retested using both test methods in 60 days and should probably be considered potentially infective until their status is clarified.

Some cats previously thought to have cleared infection have been identified using real-time PCR, which is a very sensitive method to detect cell-associated FeLV proviral DNA or viral RNA. These cats are proviral DNA positive but FeLV antigen negative and are unlikely to shed virus or develop clinical disease. However, proviral FeLV could be transmitted in blood transfusions, so potential feline blood donors should be PCR negative for FeLV.

Feline Immunodeficiency Virus (FIV): Because the concentration of FIV antigen in the blood of infected cats is often very low, in-house diagnostic tests are designed to detect anti-FIV antibodies rather than antigen. Test kits yield a positive or negative result for antibody rather than a titer. Antibodies usually develop within 60 days of infection, but this period is quite variable, and a few infected cats do not develop detectable antibody levels. Once present, antibodies appear to be present for >2 yr, except for those transiently detectable in kittens that have maternally derived antibodies. A kitten <6 mo of age that tests positive should be retested after 6 mo of age for this reason. If the test is still positive, the kitten is most likely infected.

With the currently available ELISA in-house test kits, sensitivity is high. However, these tests cannot distinguish between antibodies produced in response to vaccination with FIV vaccine and those produced by natural infection. An ELISA test that appears to successfully discriminate between antibodies produced in response to vaccination and those produced in natural infections has been developed but is not available for commercial use. A reasonable approach is to use the in-house test as a screening test. A negative result is a fairly reliable indicator that the cat is not infected. Positive results, especially in asymptomatic cats, should be confirmed by another test such as Western blot if available. Kittens born to vaccinated queens are antibody-positive for a variable length of time.

Canine Parvovirus (CPV): Both ELISA and immunomigration test kits are available for detection of CPV antigen in feces. These tests are fairly specific for the virus, but dogs that have been recently vaccinated may transiently shed antigens detected by the test kits. The sensitivity is somewhat lower for several reasons. Fecal shedding occurs for only ~7–10 days, beginning on day 3–5 after exposure, so virus is not always detectable in dogs with clinical signs. Blood in the feces as well as the formation of antigen-antibody complexes, with antibodies from the blood or exudate present in the gut, may be associated with false-negative results. It appears that in-house test kits may have decreased sensitivity to the new CPV2c strain.

Although in-house test kits for diagnosis of CPV are not licensed for use in cats, several studies have shown they can be used to detect feline panleukopenia virus in cat feces. The specificity and sensitivity are not known. Some cats test positive after vaccination, even when inactivated virus vaccines are used.

In-house tests for assay of anti-CPV antibodies have become available to evaluate the need for revaccination and the presence of possibly interfering maternal antibodies. These tests are not intended to diagnose parvovirus infection and do not distinguish between natural exposure and vaccine-induced antibodies. Currently available test kits include ELISA and immunochromatographic tests. They are semiquantitative and use color changes in positive control wells compared with color changes in samples to determine relative antibody levels. The level of anti-CPV antibody protective against infection is not known, but results are interpreted based on protective titers measured by other methods. PCR is widely available for detection of virus in feces.

Canine Distemper Virus (CDV): In-house test kits for determination of antibodies to CDV are available, usually in combination with canine parvovirus antibody testing. These tests are semiquantitative ELISA for anti-canine distemper IgG in serum or plasma. They may be used to evaluate the need for revaccination and to determine the level of maternal antibody present in puppies. They are less useful for diagnosis of infection with CDV. An immunochromatography-based assay for CDV antigen has been developed and has good sensitivity and specificity, especially when conjunctival swabs are the sample used; sensitivity and specificity are somewhat less for blood and nasal swabs. This assay is not currently available as an in-house test kit.

***Borrelia burgdorferi*:** Lyme disease (*see* p 659) is caused by the tickborne spirochete *B burgdorferi*. In general, diagnostic tests for this infection have had several potential problems, including relatively high levels of positive results in clinically healthy animals, persistence of antibodies after apparent resolution of clinical disease, interpretation of antibody titers in vaccinated dogs, and the fact that detectable antibody may not be present until 4–6 wk after exposure. An in-clinic ELISA test kit for detection of anti–*B burgdorferi* antibodies in serum or plasma minimizes some of these problems by using a synthetic peptide (C_6) based on a conserved *B burgdorferi*–specific protein. This protein is important in inducing a humoral immune response by 3–5 wk after natural infection in dogs. Vaccination does not induce a cross-reactive immune response to this antigen, so assays using the C_6 protein are able to distinguish vaccine-induced antibodies from those produced in response to natural infections. C_6-based assays are also more specific than previous tests, because there is no cross-reactivity with other tickborne agents or with autoimmune antibodies.

A currently available in-house test assay for anti–*B burgdorferi* antibodies is a screening test that gives only a positive or negative result and is thus not quantitative. Although licensed for dogs, this test kit also has been validated in cats and horses. Quantitative assays, performed in reference laboratories, can be used to monitor treatment efficacy (ie, detection of decreasing antibody titers), but these results are not always conclusive.

***Ehrlichia canis*:** Canine ehrlichiosis (*see* p 803) is a tickborne disease caused by one of several species of *Ehrlichia*. It can be associated with thrombocytopenia, anemia, and neutropenia as well as other nonspecific clinical signs. Although identification of *Ehrlichia* morulae in leukocytes can be diagnostic for this infection, serologic assay for detection of antibodies is more common and has better sensitivity. In-house tests for ehrlichiosis are either qualitative (giving only a positive or negative result) or semiquantitative tests for antibodies to *E canis*. Those currently available are ELISA to be performed on serum, plasma, or whole blood. The test kits use either recombinant analogues of major outer membrane proteins of *E canis* or whole *E canis* proteins as the antigen. The different *Ehrlichia* species stimulate antibodies that appear to cross-react in these assays, for the most part. Because anti–*E canis* antibodies may be very long-lived and may be present in subclinical infections, detection of these antibodies does not distinguish between exposure and *Ehrlichia*-induced illness and cannot reliably indicate success of response to therapy.

Brucella canis: *B canis* is not a problem in some countries, and tests are not always readily available. However, infection may be subclinical, or it may cause a variety of clinical signs, including abortion, infertility, and discospondylitis (*see* p 1402). Infection most often occurs during mating; thus, testing of breeding animals is important in disease prevention. A rapid slide agglutination test that includes a 2-mercaptoethanol (2-ME) step to reduce false-positive results by eliminating nonspecific IgM reactions is available as an in-house diagnostic kit. This assay detects serum antibody to surface antigens of the bacteria. Reports of sensitivity and specificity of this test vary depending on the confirmatory test used. ELISA and immunochromatographic assays have been developed for qualitative and semiquantitative tests for anti–*B canis* antibodies. Positive results obtained using any of these test kits should be confirmed with PCR or blood culture.

Heartworm Antigen—Dogs: Serologic testing for heartworm antigen in dogs is more sensitive than screening for microfilaremia and, in addition, can detect occult infections. Heartworm antigen is first detectable at ~5 mo after infection and will usually precede microfilaremia by a few weeks; however, this time frame may be shifted later in animals on macrocyclic lactone preventives and those with low numbers of worms. Antigen test formats available include ELISA and immunochromatographic assays. Serum or plasma may be used in all kits, and some may be performed using whole blood. Some test kits can be stored at room temperature, whereas others must be stored refrigerated and brought to room temperature before use. Batch testing and single sample testing are both available. All of the test kits have very high specificity. False-positive results are most often due to technical problems such as inadequate washing or failure to read the results at the optimal time. Manufacturer's instructions should be closely followed with any of the test formats.

Sensitivity varies from one test to another and is affected by worm load, worm gender (a female antigen is detected, thus male-only infections will not be detected), and maturity of female worms. None of these tests has 100% sensitivity. When unexpected false results are obtained on an antigen test, additional testing, using a different format, is recommended.

After adulticide treatment, antigenemia should become undetectable by 6 mo. However, it can take more than a month for some adult heartworms to die, so a positive antigen test at 5–6 mo after treatment does not necessarily indicate treatment failure. The test should be repeated 2–3 mo later.

Heartworm Antibody and Antigen—Cats: Heartworm disease in cats is substantially different from the disease in dogs, and recommendations for serologic testing are consequently different. Cats tend to have a much lower worm burden—often only one or two worms. Cats also have single-sex infections more frequently than do dogs. Circulating microfilaremia is rare in cats, and microfilariae have a shorter life span. These differences are often attributed to a more effective feline immune response to heartworm infection. However, heartworms can cause serious disease in cats.

Heartworm antigen tests are less sensitive for detection of infection in cats than they are in dogs, with a reported sensitivity of 50%–80%. Therefore, a negative antigen test does not exclude heartworm infection. Antibody testing is also available and can be useful as a screening test, but the presence of antibody does not confirm feline heartworm disease. Transient exposure to larvae will stimulate production of antibody; many early infections are cleared spontaneously, and adult heartworms never develop. A combination of testing for both heartworm antigen and anti-heartworm antibody results in much higher sensitivity and specificity than using either test method alone. Combination testing is warranted in cats with clinical signs of heartworm disease when results of a single test are not conclusive.

Test kits for detection of heartworm antigen and anti-heartworm antibody in cats are marketed in several formats. These can use either plasma or serum and are qualitative or semiquantitative.

Canine and Feline Pregnancy Diagnosis—Relaxin: The only known pregnancy-specific hormone in the bitch and queen is relaxin, which is produced by the placenta when a fertilized egg is implanted. Relaxin is first detectable in the plasma around day 20–25 after fertilization. It is not present in pseudopregnant or nonpregnant bitches or queens. Relaxin levels peak by approximately day 40–50 of gestation and drop at parturition, but they may remain detectable for up to 50 days during lactation. In-clinic test kits to measure relaxin include microwell ELISA and immunomigration qualitative tests requiring serum, plasma, or whole blood. The assays appear to have very good specificity, ie, a detectable level of relaxin is not found in nonpregnant animals. False-negative results have been reported in some bitches carrying very small litters or in those with one or more nonviable puppies.

Canine and Feline Luteinizing Hormone—Ovulation Timing and Ovariectomy Status: In the bitch, serum luteinizing hormone (LH) is normally present in very low levels except for a dramatic rise just before ovulation. Ovulation occurs 2 days after this LH surge, and the LH level returns to baseline within 24–40 hr of peaking. Serum progesterone levels begin to rise at the time of the LH surge. A bitch will be fertile between 4–7 days after the LH surge, with the most fertile period on days 5 and 6. In addition, the LH surge determines the gestation period, with parturition occurring between day 64 and 66 after the surge. The LH surge may occur anywhere from 3 days before to 5 days after the onset of estrous behavior, so it cannot be reliably predicted by behavior.

Ovulation timing by measurement of LH requires daily testing, which usually begins when >50% of vaginal epithelial cells are cornified, based on vaginal cytology. There is occasionally a false LH peak not followed by ovulation, but it will also not be followed by an increase in progesterone. For that reason, assays of both LH and progesterone are recommended for most accurate ovulation detection. An increased LH concentration not followed by increased progesterone levels is considered a proestrus fluctuation, and testing for ovulation should continue.

A currently available in-clinic kit to measure LH concentrations in serum is essentially qualitative, with a serum level of <1 ng/mL being read as negative and a level of >1 ng/mL considered positive. The test is an immunochromatographic assay.

Ovariectomized bitches and queens have serum concentrations of LH >1 ng/mL. Because this LH concentration is also seen in intact bitches about to ovulate, a single high LH concentration does not confirm reproductive status, but a low LH concentration indicates a nonovariectomized animal.

Canine Ovulation Timing—Progesterone: Serum progesterone begins to increase after the LH surge with a modest increase on the day before ovulation and a further increase to 4–10 ng/mL on the day of ovulation. Progesterone continues to increase and stays increased throughout pregnancy or diestrus. As the rise in progesterone is more constant compared with LH, daily testing is not necessary. It is recommended that testing begin in late proestrus and continue every 2–3 days until a high range is reached, indicating ovulation.

The test kits for in-clinic progesterone testing are semiquantitative ELISA with preovulatory concentrations designated according to the kit used. Some kits are designed to give two additional progesterone ranges (intermediate and high), whereas others indicate only preovulatory and "ovulatory day or later" levels. In comparison with other test methods, the in-house test kits are less accurate, particularly in the range of roughly 1.5–10 ng/mL, which is the range of interest for earliest detection of ovulation. Accuracy is greater at higher progesterone levels. As mentioned above, measurement of both LH and progesterone is recommended for most accurate breeding management.

Thyroxine: Assay of total serum thyroxine (T_4) may be used as a screening test for canine hypothyroidism or as a diagnostic test for feline hyperthyroidism. (*See also* THE THYROID GLAND, p 552.) In addition, T_4 concentrations are measured when monitoring therapy for hypo- or hyperthyroidism. An in-house ELISA test kit, which uses an additional instrument to read results, provides semiquantitative information about T_4 concentration in canine and feline sera. The assay is run at one of two "dynamic ranges," depending on the predicted range of results. Published studies comparing this assay with other test methods for T_4 vary in their conclusions. It is recommended that T_4

concentrations be periodically measured in stored pooled serum of cats and dogs to monitor whether assay performance is consistent. It is probably still better to use a commercial laboratory for thyroxine measurement.

Almost all (99%) of total T_4 is bound to protein in the blood and therefore not biologically accurate. Free T_4 levels are a more accurate test of thyroid function in cats and dogs.

Foal Immunoglobulin (IgG): Measurement of foal serum IgG concentration within the first 24 hr after birth can be useful in preventing disease related to failure of passive transfer of IgG in colostrum from mare to foal. Use of foal-side testing procedures can facilitate prompt diagnosis and treatment. A foal serum IgG level of >800 mg/dL is generally considered optimal, with <200 mg/dL indicating failure of passive transfer. Concentrations of 200–800 mg/dL are considered evidence of partial transfer.

Although radial immunodiffusion is considered the most accurate test for IgG concentration, it takes much longer (5–24 hr) than many of the other test methods and thus is not as useful as an indicator of the need for therapeutic intervention. More rapid screening tests include the zinc sulfate turbidity test, glutaraldehyde clot test, and ELISA test kits.

The zinc sulfate test estimates IgG in serum based on its precipitation when added to a zinc-containing solution. Turbidity generally becomes visible when IgG levels are 400–500 mg/dL. This test takes ~1 hr and may be performed with zinc sulfate solutions made in the clinic, or reagents for the test may be purchased as a test kit.

The glutaraldehyde clot test requires the addition of 1 volume of serum to 10 volumes of 10% glutaraldehyde and examination of the tubes at timed intervals up to 60 min. The presence of IgG in the serum causes a solid clot to form in the tube. Clot formation in <10 min generally correlates to an IgG concentration of >800 mg/dL, whereas a positive reaction within 60 min is interpreted as an IgG concentration of >400 mg/dL. Both of these test methods use serum, rather than plasma, so time for the blood to clot and separation of serum must be added to the time needed to perform the test.

ELISA test kits for in-house or foal-side testing can use either serum or whole blood as the sample and take ~10 min. Most are semiquantitative, with color changes corresponding to IgG concentrations of <400 mg/dL, 400–800 mg/dL, or >800 mg/dL. One quantitative handheld colorimetric immunoassay is currently available.

Reports of sensitivity and specificity among these methods vary. In general, sensitivity in identifying foals with IgG concentrations <400 mg/dL appears to be acceptable for all methods. Thus, there are few foals with total failure of passive transfer that would not be identified by any of these methods. Specificity is less acceptable for some of the methods, and treatment of some foals that did not need it might be instituted based on the results.

Calf Immunoglobulin: Measurement of IgG concentration in neonatal calf serum is important for the same reasons described for foals. However, IgG levels in calves are different from those in foals, with >1,000 mg/dL considered evidence of adequate passive transfer and <1,000 mg/dL indicating failure of passive transfer. Radial immunodiffusion is the gold standard for accurate measurement of serum IgG in calves (as in foals), but the length of time required to complete this assay makes it less useful than other methods. Other methods include zinc sulfate and sodium sulfite turbidity tests, glutaraldehyde coagulation test, measurement of total serum solids by refractometry, and a lateral flowthrough ELISA test kit.

The sodium sulfite and zinc sulfate turbidity tests are both based on the precipitation of high-molecular-weight proteins in these solutions. Serum is used as the sample, and tests are read after 15–30 min of incubation. Results of these tests vary in sensitivity and specificity depending on the endpoint chosen, and technical difficulties with reagents can decrease test performance. The glutaraldehyde clot test is performed as in foals, with no clot formation at 60 min indicating failure of passive transfer.

Measurement of serum total protein by refractometer is a fairly reliable indicator of adequate passive transfer in healthy, well-hydrated calves. A level of 5.2 g/dL is roughly equivalent to an IgG concentration of 1,000 mg/dL.

A commercially available ELISA test kit uses serum as the sample and takes ~20 min. The assay is qualitative in that it indicates an IgG concentration of >1,000 mg/dL or <1,000 mg/dL. Sensitivity and specificity are reasonably good, and this test is less influenced by factors such as calf dehydration or reagent instability than some other methods. Manufacturer recommendations for storing and using the kits must be followed.

DIAGNOSTIC IMAGING

RADIOGRAPHY

Radiography comprises the majority of diagnostic medical images generated in veterinary practice, but other imaging modalities such as ultrasonography, CT, MRI, and nuclear imaging are also very important and commonly available in specialty practices and academic centers. Imaging provides a large amount of information by noninvasive means. It does not alter the disease process or cause unacceptable discomfort to the animal. Although radiography itself is painless, sedation is often desirable to reduce anxiety and stress associated with the procedure, to promote acquisition of good diagnostic studies with minimal repeats, and to control pain associated with manipulation in animals with painful disorders such as fractures and arthritis.

Equipment: Radiographs are made using a specialized type of vacuum tube that produces x-rays. The tube current, measured in milliamperes (mA), and voltage, measured in kilovolts (kV), determine the strength and number of x-rays produced and are two of the three exposure factors that can be set on most x-ray machines. Kilovoltage potential (kVp) is the highest potential voltage achieved at any given kV setting.

Higher kV settings produce more penetrating beams in which a higher percentage of the x-rays produced penetrate the subject being radiographed. There is also a decrease in the percentage difference in absorption between tissue types. This results in decreased contrast (long-scale contrast) on the final image. High kVp techniques are most useful for studies of body regions with many different tissue densities (eg, thorax). Higher kVp techniques are appropriate for larger and thicker animals with limitations. Increasing kV is not a linear function, and small increases in kVp settings may substantially increase the number of x-rays penetrating the animal. However, for a number of reasons relating to the production and absorption of x-rays, this effect is much less dramatic above 85 kVp.

Increasing the mA setting on the machine increases the number of x-rays produced. The energy spectrum of the x-ray beam is essentially unchanged, as are the relative numbers of x-ray photons penetrating tissues of different densities such as bone, soft tissue, and fat. However, the amount of darkening on the image is related to the total number of photons reaching it. Therefore, increasing mA increases image contrast. Changes in mA settings are relatively linear; increased contrast is desirable when tissue densities are similar (eg, soft-tissue components of the musculoskeletal system). However, increasing mA generally results in more heat loading on x-ray tubes, thus limiting exposure times and reducing tube life.

The third major parameter in making a radiographic exposure is exposure time. Increasing the exposure time increases the number of photons produced and hence the darkness of the image. For exposures in the general diagnostic range, this is a linear function; as is the case with increasing mA, increasing exposure time generally results in greater heat loading of the x-ray tube than increasing kVp, once again potentially shortening tube life.

All three of the above parameters are interdependent, with exposure time and mA so much so that the term milliampere-seconds (mAs) is usually used to indicate the product of these two factors. Increasing the mA and decreasing the exposure time by a proportionate amount results in a radiograph less likely to be degraded by motion. As a rule, it is best to minimize the exposure time but maintain an appropriate mAs and scale of contrast. Increasing kVp increases the number of photons penetrating the subject and so darkens the image. This effect can be used within limits to correct an underexposure. The converse is likewise true.

When correcting a previously unsatisfactory image, underexposure or overexposure should be corrected for by adjusting the mAs when examining areas of high contrast (skeleton) or by adjusting the kVp when examining areas of low contrast (thorax). This will maintain the same relative contrast for that anatomic area while adjusting the film darkness.

Establishing a technique chart to take radiographs makes it easy for the operator to arrive at a technique by simply correcting a standardized protocol for the size of the animal being examined and the anatomic area under consideration. It also ensures that radiographs of the same anatomic region will have a consistent appearance from animal to animal. A technique chart must be made for each machine. However, some generalizations can be made. Exposure factors for the thorax should have mAs values ≤5 unless the animal is very large. Values of 10 for the abdomen and 15–20 for skeletal studies are appropriate. In many modern x-ray machines, the technique chart is built into the machine. The operator need only enter the species, body part, and thickness, and the machine automatically sets the technique. This is convenient and reduces mistakes in technique, but the settings may need to be altered to suit the specific equipment, film-screen (detector) speed, and the viewer's preferences (eg, contrast level).

Automatic exposure control (AEC) is a system in which the operator sets the kVp and mA, and the machine terminates the exposure at the appropriate time. If used properly, this system results in nearly identical image exposures between animals. However, appropriate kV settings are needed, and consistent animal positioning is critical. Identical positioning between animals is required to achieve identical images. Placing the heart or lungs over the AEC sensor results in radically different appearing radiographs. AEC is probably most effective when large numbers of images are being done of the same anatomic area by the same personnel.

X-ray machines are equipped with collimators that allow adjustment of the size of the beam to the size of the area being radiographed. This reduces the amount of scatter radiation generated, improving image contrast and detail. Scatter radiation is also the major source of radiation exposure to operators, so proper collimation is important to reduce this risk.

When a radiograph is made, some of the x-rays are scattered. When the object being radiographed is ≥10 cm thick (15 cm for digital systems), scattering becomes a problem by causing unwanted exposure of the x-ray film. A grid, which is a thin plate made up of alternating thin strips of lead and plastic, can be placed between the animal and the film to reduce the scattered x-rays from exposing the film. The ability of a grid to remove scattered radiation is measured by the grid ratio. The grid ratio is determined by the height of the lead strips divided by the distance between them. A grid with an 8:1 ratio will eliminate more scattered radiation from exposing the film than will a grid with a 6:1 ratio if both have the same number of lead lines per centimeter.

Digital recording is rapidly increasing in usage, but radiographic images have traditionally, and still are, commonly stored on specially optimized film. However, even the best silver halide film is relatively insensitive to x-rays. For that reason, the x-ray film is usually placed between specially designed phosphorescent screens—panels composed of microscopic phosphorescent crystals embedded in a plastic matrix that directs propagation of the phosphorescent light toward the film. These screens are much more sensitive to x-rays than is film. When the x-ray strikes a crystal, it causes the crystal to phosphoresce, and the light exposes the film secondarily. This process of recording the x-ray image is much more efficient than using film alone and markedly reduces radiation exposure to the subject (sometimes by a factor of 100 or more) and the operator. It also reduces the amount of scatter radiation recorded on the image. The screens and film are contained in a lightproof cassette, which is transparent to x-rays.

Screens and film must be matched for spectral emission and sensitivity. Films produced by one company are generally not optimally sensitive to screens made by another, and it is inadvisable to mix screen and film brands. Screen and film combinations come in different speeds. The larger the crystals in a screen are, the more likely it is to interact with an x-ray and the greater the amount of light produced. Unfortunately, larger crystals also produce larger areas of light, which decreases the detail of the film. Likewise, film with larger silver halide grains is more sensitive to the light creating the exposure but also reduces the detail or resolution of the final image. Therefore, fine grain films are matched to fine crystal screens, resulting in very detailed images that take more radiation to produce. The converse is true for large grain film and large crystal screens.

The speed of these combinations is designated by a rating of 100–1,600, with 100 being relatively slow but with very good detail and 1,600 being very fast but with limited detail. Film-screen combinations with speeds of 200–800 are generally used in veterinary medicine; 200-speed systems are used for small body parts and skeletal imaging, whereas 800-speed systems are used for large abdomens in small animals and thoracic radiography in large animals. Choice of the proper speed system for a specific use is based not only on the area being radiographed but also on the capabilities of the machine. Small, portable x-ray machines can be used for larger body parts with fast film-screen combinations, substantially improving the utility of these machines.

Use of radiographic film is rapidly being phased out except for special purposes, with digital image capture likely leading to a cessation of film production for most purposes. As advances in digital detector systems continue, it is likely that images produced on digital detector plates will be indistinguishable in detail and quality from those acquired on film. It is already becoming difficult to find film cassettes and screens for medical radiography sold by primary vendors.

Darkroom: As digital image capture replaces radiographic film, darkrooms will no longer be required. However, because radiographic film is still used by many veterinary practices, a brief description of darkroom procedures is provided.

Once the film is exposed, it must be processed in a darkroom to make the latent image recorded on the film visible and fixed so that the image remains unchanged once the film is brought into the light. Care should be taken to be sure no exterior light enters the darkroom. Even very small amounts of white light will markedly fog a film and decrease its diagnostic quality. Safelights used to illuminate darkrooms include filters that remove the frequencies of the light to which the film is sensitive, so the film will not be exposed. Films vary in their spectral sensitivity; therefore, when replacing a safelight filter, the spectral requirements of the filter must be specified.

Automatic processing systems improve processing quality and consistency and reduce the processing time compared with traditional hand film developing. Relatively few films processed per week can justify the purchase of an automated processing system. In any case, film processing must be done in strict accordance with the specified time and temperature requirements of the film being used. These requirements have been standardized for many years, and automated systems are designed to meet them.

Whether processing is manual or automated, the chemicals must be handled with care. Contamination of the darkroom with chemicals can ruin film, screens, and clothes. Fumes from the chemicals may be harmful, and some people may be more sensitive than others, especially to the fixer solution. Cross contamination of the developer solution with fixer inactivates it and requires replacement of the developer. Improper handling of chemicals results in many artifacts on films as well as potential health hazards to the operators.

Filmless Radiography: Image recording systems do not require the use of film, screens, or processing chemicals. They have several advantages over conventional film radiography: 1) radiographs cannot be lost if adequate data safeguards are used; 2) there is no need for film storage and its attendant space and environmental requirements; 3) the process allows for manipulation and enhancement after the image has been recorded; 4) images can be transmitted electronically to a remote location for immediate interpretation; 5) the images are generally available more quickly, usually within 30 sec; and 6) there is no need for a darkroom.

These systems can be divided into two categories: **computed radiography** (CR), in which a semiconductor plate contained in a cassette is exposed in the usual fashion and then read electronically inside a special reader that detects the magnitude of electrostatic charge on each of the semiconductor elements within the plate; and **direct digital radiography** (DR), in which a cesium iodide scintillator array absorbs the x-rays, producing a light pulse detected by a large array (millions) of amorphous silicone photodiode/transistor elements. In both systems, the electrical output from each of the detector elements is proportional to the number of x-rays that strike the detector element and is mathematically quantifiable, hence the term "digital images." In both systems, the data produced are processed by a computer, which generates the image on a monitor according to a previously determined processing algorithm that is specific to the region being radiographed. Processing algorithms are critical to the development of diagnostic images. In many displaced systems, the algorithm can be altered to provide enhancement of various features of the image. The digital images are then stored electronically and made available to any computer with access to the image archive.

The difference between the two systems lies in the intermediate step of exposing a plate in CR, which is then placed in a reader. These plates must be replaced periodically because of wear created during the reading process. There is also the issue of whether the latent image recorded by the reader is an accurate representation of the true image.

The portability of the cassettes is an important benefit in practice situations in which radiographic images are produced in multiple places. CR systems are also still considerably less expensive than all but the simplest DR systems and generally still have higher resolution capabilities, which may be important for imaging smaller anatomic parts.

DR systems are very complex electronically and subject to the same insults as any complex electronic system. They are particularly sensitive to shock and electronic interference. However, when properly cared for, DR systems are durable and reliable. They do not require handling of the image recording plate, which reduces wear and tear on the system. Their main advantage over CR is image display speed. DR systems have been developed that do not require a cable to communicate between the detector and the computer processing the data into an image. The cable has been replaced by wireless communication on specified electrical magnetic frequencies that are unlikely to be interfered with by other electromagnetic devices such as cell phones and electronic equipment. Although they are still much more expensive than systems incorporating a cable connection between the detector and computer, such systems are particularly suited for use in equine ambulatory practices. Images can also be sent to the storage system in a wireless manner in many areas.

The flexibility and reliability of digital radiography systems, whether wireless or wired, have improved to the point that they are almost universally used in human radiology departments as well as in many veterinary hospitals. As DR systems grow in capability, reliability, ease of use, and resolution, and decrease in cost, it is expected they will eventually replace both CR and traditional film systems. Although currently DR still cannot match the spatial resolution of either standard speed film or CR systems, newer systems are narrowing the gap. This low spatial resolution is offset to a large degree by improved contrast resolution. Because of their inherent high contrast, direct digital systems are also becoming the choice imaging device for very large animals.

The advent of digital imaging has led to the development of special image storage systems and formats. The data stored on computers must be protected from loss and corruption. Loss of data can be guarded against by storing identical sets of data on different computers in different geographic locations and/or by copying the data files to optical storage media that are then kept in a safe location. Protection of the data from corruption is a more thorny issue. Because images stored in a digital format are easily manipulated by various computer programs, it is possible that they could be altered (accidentally or deliberately) to reflect a different situation than the actual one. For this reason, many electronic image formats are not recognized as legal documents and are not acceptable in a court of law. Because of this potential for alteration or abuse, a special medical image format has been developed and agreed on by the American College of Roentgenology, the American College of Veterinary Radiology, and others as the standard format for medical image generation and storage. This is the Digital Imaging and Communication in Medicine (DICOM) III format. The key feature of this format is the presence of a hidden header in the image file that records all manipulations of the image or the header each time the image is saved. The header also contains a large amount of information about the patient and production factors of the image, which must be specified before creation of the image. This makes accidental or malicious manipulation of the image much easier to trace. Another and even more important benefit of the DICOM III format is that it makes images easily transferable to other sites for referral interpretation or patient referral. No digital imaging system should be purchased that does not conform to the DICOM III standard.

A common misconception associated with digital radiography is that it results in decreased radiation requirements to provide a diagnostic image. Although there has been some progress in this direction, most current digital radiography systems require essentially the same amount of radiation to produce a diagnostic image as with film. The computer system will attempt to reconstruct the image with the proper level of contrast and edge enhancement; however, data poor images will often lack detail despite this enhancement.

Animal Restraint: Animals must be adequately restrained and positioned to obtain quality radiographic images. People dressed in appropriate protective apparel may manually restrain animals; however, manual restraint should be kept to a minimum. In some states, manual restraint is not allowed except under explicitly defined circumstances. Sedation or short-acting anesthesia is often necessary and usually desirable if medical circumstances permit it. Chemical restraint lessens the need for and intensity of manual restraint, which leads to fewer poor or unacceptable radiographs and usually shortens the time required to complete the examination. In many instances, animals can be restrained and positioned using sandbags, tape, and foam pads. With some practice, it is often possible to complete the radiographic examination in essentially the same time it could have been performed using manual restraint, with the added benefit that the animal is less likely to injure personnel or itself.

Animal motion may also be minimized by decreasing exposure time and maximizing mA to achieve the required mAs for the body region examined. Other technical adjustments, such as increasing the kVp or shortening the film focus distance, may be made in some cases. However, major changes in film focus distance will likely cause serious degradation of the image. In most instances, it is preferable to chemically immobilize the animal as long as there is not a medical contraindication.

Paradoxically, the development of DR systems that allow images to be viewed within 30 sec of production has led to an increase in the number of radiographic images typically produced. Because the images do not have to be processed in a darkroom or through secondary systems such as in CR, individuals making the images often attempt to improve positioning of the animal multiple times. Particularly in instances when the animal is being manually restrained, there is a proportional increase in radiation exposure to both the animal and the holders. This can be avoided by taking a few extra seconds to properly position the animal for the first image.

Proper positioning is also important to maximize the diagnostic content of the x-ray examination. In many cases, improper positioning or radiographic examination can result in a misdiagnosis or inability to appreciate major lesions. Perhaps the best example of this is in thoracic radiography. Both right and left lateral recumbent radiographs are recommended in dogs and cats. This is done because positioning of the animal on its side results in rapid relocation of fluids to and atelectasis of the downside lung. The result is compression and increased *radiographic opacity* of the dependent lung. Soft-tissue nodules, sometimes of considerable size, can be obscured by this phenomenon. Similarly, lesions affecting the pylorus may be more evident on a left lateral radiographic examination of the abdomen than on a right lateral. Another example of positioning affecting interpretation is frequently encountered when evaluating the coxofemoral joints for hip dysplasia in dogs. If the legs are excessively abducted, the femoral necks will appear thickened, mimicking the production of osteophytes and potentially leading to a misdiagnosis. Radiography of the spine without the aid of anesthesia in an acutely paraparetic or paraplegic animal may result in inability to properly position the animal for optimal visibility of vertebral structures because of the pain such positioning produces.

Radiation Safety: Radiographic examinations must be performed with proper respect for radiation safety procedures. Diagnostic x-ray machines are potent sources of radiation and can, if improperly used, result in injurious exposure to personnel over time. The exposure factors used in modern x-ray systems are substantially lower than those used in the past but can still result in injury. It is never acceptable to hold animals without the use of lead-impregnated aprons and gloves to decrease exposure to the hands and body of personnel from scattered radiation. Leaded gloves should not be used within the primary beam of the x-ray machine. These gloves and aprons reduce exposure from scatter radiation by a factor of ~1,000 but reduce exposure from the primary beam by only a factor of ~10. Thyroid shields are considered mandatory, and eye shields in the form of lead-impregnated plastic "glasses" are also recommended, especially when radiographing large animals, because the exposures used are sometimes quite high and the orientation of the beam is more likely to be horizontal. Upper limb, cervical spine, and skull studies in horses are particularly likely to result in substantial exposure to anyone holding the film/detector or the horse.

Proper collimation of the x-ray beam is an important and integral part of radiation protection. If the x-ray beam extends beyond the animal, then that radiation contributes to increased scatter radiation and personnel exposure. Any image in which the entire field of the detector or film is exposed is probably under-collimated, unless the animal extends to the limits of the detector. In addition, with digital radiography systems, excessive amounts of exposure outside the subject can result in false interpretation of the data by the reconstruction algorithm and substantially degrade image quality. If this occurs, the exposure must be repeated with proper collimation to achieve an acceptable image. In most instances, the x-ray beam should be collimated to ~1 cm outside the subject limits to provide optimal image quality and radiation protection for personnel.

Pregnant women and any personnel <18 yr old should refrain from direct involvement in taking radiographic images whenever possible. If a pregnant woman is directly involved in taking radiographs, she should wear an apron that completely encircles her abdomen.

Although federal and state authorities have set maximal limits for both extremities and whole-body radiation exposure for occupationally exposed personnel, the principal of "as low as reasonably achievable" (ALARA) should always be adhered to. The currently set limits allow occupational whole-body exposure to be roughly the same as that which occurs from environmental sources. However, in many veterinary teaching hospitals with large radiographic case loads, the occupational exposure is held to <10% of the permitted values by use of proper protective equipment and radiographic techniques. There is no reason for veterinarians or technicians in private practice to ever receive exposures approximating the allowed limits unless they are heavily involved in specialized interventional radiography.

Individuals involved in taking radiographic images should be monitored for radiation exposure. This is essential to identify and correct conditions that can result in excessive radiation exposure to personnel. Monitoring of exposure also provides evidence of proper adherence to radiation safety standards if questions arise as to whether an employee's medical condition could be related to radiation exposure. Several companies provide this service for a relatively nominal fee.

Interpretation of Images: Radiographic images are complex two-dimensional representations of three-dimensional subjects that are generated in a format unfamiliar to the average individual. Substantial experience and attention to detail is required to become proficient in interpretation. The start of radiographic interpretation is a properly positioned and exposed study. Studies that are poorly or inconsistently positioned are difficult to interpret, and improper technique further decreases the amount of information obtained from the radiograph.

Although interpretation is aided by experience, conscious use of a systematic approach to evaluation of the image will improve the reading skill of even very experienced individuals and ensure that lesions in areas not of primary interest or near the edge of the image are not missed. However, many studies have shown that experience is the best teacher with regard to evaluation of radiographs. So, although anyone will become more adept at image interpretation with time, those individuals who interpret large numbers of images will be the most proficient. Even proficient individuals can miss lesions that are unfamiliar to them or so-called "lesions of omission." A lesion of omission is one in which a structure or organ generally depicted on the image is missing. A good example of this is the absence of one kidney or the spleen on an abdominal radiograph. Therefore, particular attention to systematic evaluation of the image is very important. It is perhaps best to begin interpretation of the image in an area that is not of primary concern. For instance, when evaluating the thorax of an animal with a heart murmur, the vertebral column and skeleton should be evaluated first because if a substantial lesion is identified for the heart, it is possible that the skeletal structures may not be examined.

It is essentially impossible to evaluate radiographs without a preexisting bias as a result of knowledge of the history, physical examination findings, and previously performed laboratory results. This bias can easily promote under-evaluation of the image by focusing on only the area of interest associated with the bias.

Interpretation of radiographic images depends on a pleural knowledge of anatomy and understanding of disease pathology. Anatomic changes, such as in size, shape, location/position, opacity, and margin sharpness represent the basis of radiographic interpretation. In addition, the degree of change, whether generalized throughout an organ or associated with other abnormalities, must be evaluated. The presence of lesions that do not affect the entirety of an organ, such as focal enlargement of the liver or focal opacification of the lung field, are strongly suggestive of localized disease such as tumors or bacterial infections. Conversely, lesions causing generalized change throughout an organ such as the liver or kidneys are most suggestive of a systemic disease such as viral infections or toxicities. Combinations of lesions in different locations or organs also help narrow down the potential diagnosis. Careful attention to the basic principles of interpretation and use of a careful systematic approach will often provide answers not readily apparent on initial examination.

Once all of the lesions on the study are identified, a rational cause for those lesions can be formulated. The maximum amount of information is derived from the radiographic study when interpretation is done in light of the clinical and clinicopathologic information available. In this way, the most likely cause for the animal's condition can be determined. However, many diseases can cause similar radiographic lesions, and radiographs must be interpreted in light of the entire gestalt of lesions present and not based on any single lesion if multiple abnormalities are present. In many cases, it is appropriate and advisable to seek the opinion of a radiologist for interpretation of radiographic images, particularly as the number of radiographic studies available and potential diagnoses proliferate.

Contrast Procedures: Radiographic exposure of film alone lacks sufficient contrast to evaluate many structures; therefore, contrast procedures are used to increase the native contrast of organs and lesions, to separate them from surrounding tissues. Contrast media are radiopaque compounds that have extremely low toxicity, although there are well-recognized hemodynamic alterations seen after administration of IV contrast agents. These consist of primarily a reflex hypotension followed by a rebound mild hypertension. In extreme cases, the hypotension can lead to vascular collapse and even anaphylaxis. This effect is thought to be primarily associated with the hypertonic nature of ionic contrast agents and is markedly less evident when nonionic agents are used. For this reason, nonionic agents have almost completely replaced the ionic agents as IV contrast material. IV and intra-arterial contrast agents are generally iodine based and increase the opacity of the blood, making vascular structures visible. Iodinated contrast agents are cleared primarily by the kidneys, making the collecting system of the urinary tract visible. Orally administered agents, primarily barium sulfate–based compounds, outline the mucosa and lumen of the GI tract. Intrathecal contrast agents are also iodine based and allow evaluation of the spinal cord and meninges. Many of these contrast procedures have been largely supplanted by modern imaging procedures, but many of them are still the best way to image the structures they are designed to evaluate and should not be forgotten if modern imaging procedures fall short. Many contrast procedures do not require special equipment and can be performed in the average veterinary practice, but interpretation is best performed by someone with extensive experience and training in the interpretation of radiographic images.

ULTRASONOGRAPHY

Ultrasonography is the second most commonly used imaging format in veterinary practice. It uses ultrasonic sound waves in the frequency range of 1.5–15 megahertz (MHz) to create images of body structures based on the pattern of echoes reflected from the tissues and organs being imaged. Several types of image formats can be displayed. The most familiar one (and the one that creates the actual image of anatomy) is B-mode grayscale scanning. The sound beam is produced by a transducer placed in contact with and acoustically coupled by means of a transmission gel to the animal. An ultrashort pulse of sound is directed into the animal, after which the transducer switches to the receive mode. Echoes occur as the sound beam changes velocity while passing from a tissue of one density to one of another density, even when the change occurs at nearly microscopic levels. The greater the change in velocity, the greater the strength of the echo. A small percentage of these echoes are reflected back to the transducer, which then reconverts the energy of the echoes into electrical impulses recorded by the computer in the ultrasound machine. The strength of the echo, the time required for the echo to return after the pulse, and the direction the sound beam that was sent are all recorded. Using information from multiple echoes, the machine creates an image that represents the appearance of the tissues when cut in the same plane on an anatomic specimen. In modern scanning systems, the sound beam is swept through the body many times per second, producing a dynamic, real-time image that changes as the transducer is moved across the body. This real-time image is easier to interpret and allows the examiner to scan continuously until a satisfactory image is obtained. The image may then be frozen and recorded in a digital format, which also allows for recording of short segments of the real-time scan. As for radiography and all other medical imaging systems, the standard, accepted, legal format for digital images is the DICOM III standard.

Ultrasonography cannot be used to scan gas-filled or bony tissues. The sound beam is totally reflected at soft tissue/gas interfaces and absorbed at soft tissue/bone interfaces. Gas and bone also "shadow" any other organs beyond them. Bowel gas can inhibit imaging of adjacent abdominal organs, and the heart must be imaged from locations that do not require the sound beam to pass through the lungs.

Sonographic imaging is also limited in regard to the depth of tissue that can be examined. Most scanners will display tissues to a depth of ~24 cm, but the image is often quite noisy at that depth. This is because most tissue echoes do not return directly to the transducer but are reflected in some other direction. By a depth of 24 cm, the loss of energy from the sound beam results in echoes so weak that the scanner cannot separate the returning echoes from the background electronic noise. In addition, some echoes that are not directly reflected may return to the transducer by reflection from a tissue outside the beam path. Such echoes require longer to return to the transducer and are depicted at a spurious location, adding noise to the image. Low-frequency transducers can scan deeper than high-frequency transducers, but resolution is decreased. There is much less loss of beam intensity in fluid media such as the urinary bladder, so if the beam passes through such a fluid media, the maximum scanning depth may be increased at the expense of temporal resolution.

Although ultrasound can be used to evaluate most soft tissues, the heart and abdominal organs still constitute the majority of examinations performed in small animals. In scanning of the abdomen, the abdominal structures should be systematically evaluated. Each sonographer develops his or her own system of completely evaluating the abdomen. Systematic evaluation ensures that all structures are scanned. In the past, organs such as the adrenal glands and pancreas were seen only if diseased and enlarged, but modern ultrasound machines operated by an experienced sonographer produce images of such quality that the normal adrenal glands, pancreas, and lymph nodes can be imaged.

Ultrasonography also is widely used to evaluate the soft tissues of the musculoskeletal system. In Equidae, ultrasound is used to detect and evaluate the presence of tears in the tendons and ligaments of the legs. Examination of joints and the margins of bones around the joints in both large and small animals is also widely performed and yields information not available from standard radiographic evaluation. Of course, ultrasound cannot be used to evaluate the bones themselves, so the two imaging methods are complementary. In small animals, soft-tissue lesions of the ligaments, tendons, joint capsule, and articular cartilage of the shoulder and stifle joints are readily detectable by an experienced examiner. Most joints and muscles can be evaluated by ultrasonography if the operator is familiar with the normal anatomy and the manner in which pathology of those structures is manifest on the image.

Changes in the size and shape of organs, tissues, and structures are evident in most cases, but evaluation of the echo pattern is based on comparison with that of other organs and tissues the examiner has scanned in other animals. The person evaluating the scan must have a firm idea, developed from experience and comparison with known normals, of the normal echo pattern for each organ scanned with each transducer. The echo pattern will change between transducers because of changes in axial and transaxial resolution as well as transducer design. Comparison of the echogenicity of several tissues must be made, because any organ may have increases or decreases in the echogenicity of its parenchyma. Diseased organs may be either uniformly altered in echogenicity or exhibit focal or multifocal changes. Focal changes are usually easier to detect than uniform changes. Sonographic lesions are sometimes quite characteristic of a given disease process, but more often the changes are nonspecific. Although ultrasonography can be quite sensitive to detection of disease, the changes are not specific for a given disease in most cases unless a characteristic change in anatomic presentation is detected along with changes in echogenicity.

Ultrasound technology has improved the ability of sonographic examinations to detect diseases previously not well characterized by sonographic evaluation. Pancreatitis is a primary example, and in the past 10 years, sonographic evaluation of the pancreas has become a mainstay of assessing animals with suspected pancreatic disease. However, it does not always agree with clinical pathologic evaluation or physical examination. In some cases, the physical examination and pathologic data will suggest pancreatitis, but it is not detected on sonographic examination. This is probably due to the great difficulty of interrogating the entire pancreas using ultrasound. In other cases, chronic pancreatitis may be indicated by the sonographic examination but poorly characterized by clinical pathologic data because of the chronic status of the disease. Cushing disease is also frequently difficult to interpret on the basis of sonographic examination or any other imaging modality because of the problems of benign adenomas that have no clinical significance in the adrenal glands and because in true Cushing disease the adrenal glands are being overdriven by a pituitary adenoma and are not themselves structurally abnormal. Other instances of increased usage of ultrasound are in the evaluation of other soft tissues such as muscle and tendon injuries as well as cartilage injuries in various joints such as the shoulder and stifle.

Ultrasonography can also be used to direct biopsy instruments to acquire tissue for a specific pathologic diagnosis. This obviates the need for an open surgical exploration in many cases. Lesions buried within large organs such as the liver and kidneys that might not be detectable at surgery may be detected and biopsied with ultrasonographic guidance. Presurgical diagnosis permits more thorough and specific planning of surgical procedures and presurgical treatment of lesions. These procedures can frequently be safely performed under heavy sedation and analgesia. Ultrasound-guided biopsy and aspiration of lesions can also be performed in large animals without the need for general anesthesia.

Echocardiography: Echocardiography is ultrasonic evaluation of the heart. In the past, it was done using the M-mode format of displaying ultrasound information. A narrow beam of sound is projected into the heart, and the echo pattern and strength are displayed onto a persistence screen with the x-axis of the display representing time (y-axis is depth), similar to the familiar format of an ECG. The pattern and amplitude of movement of the walls of the chambers of the heart and valves can be evaluated, as well as the size of the respective structures along the path of the sound beam. The M-mode format has very high temporal resolution and thus is especially excluded to evaluation of rapidly moving structures such as heart valve leaflets. Considerable experience is required to obtain and interpret diagnostic studies. The M-mode examination has been coupled with real-time B-mode studies to improve the accuracy of beam placement and add additional information, such as shape of the chamber.

Ultrasonographic images are also used to acquire quantitative information about cardiac function. Measurement of specified parameters may be made on either the M-mode scan or on the two-dimensional B-mode image. Mathematical formulas are then applied to determine values for cardiac output, ventricular contractility, ejection fraction, ventricular wall stiffness, and other cardiac functions.

Doppler ultrasound makes use of the familiar phenomenon that sound emitted from a moving object such as a train has a different apparent frequency to someone standing still relative to the moving object. If the object is moving away from the observer, the frequency of the sound is lower; conversely, if the emitter is moving toward the observer, the frequency of the sound is higher. The same is true of diagnostic ultrasound. Echoes from moving RBCs change the frequency of the sound reflected back to the transducer. The amount by which the frequency is shifted is proportional to the velocity of the RBCs; whether it is a positive or negative frequency shift is used to determine blood flow direction. This is used to identify valvular regurgitation (insufficiency), increased flow velocity (as in stenosis), or abnormal movement of the blood in the heart or vessels elsewhere in the body.

Doppler signals may be displayed in two formats. In the first, spectral Doppler, a sound beam is used to evaluate a specific small volume within the vessel of interest. This display resembles the M-mode display except that the frequency shift, or velocity, is substituted on the y-axis. It also shares high temporal resolution capabilities of the M-mode format. The second way to display Doppler frequency shifts is to select a larger area of the scan and a real time B-mode image, encoding the velocities and direction as a color spectrum. The color (usually red or blue) depicts blood flow direction, and the hue depicts mean flow velocity. This allows evaluation of larger areas, but at the price of lower temporal resolution. For this reason, color-encoded B-mode flow studies are used to guide placement of spectral sample volumes to acquire more accurate and complete information. Thus, Doppler studies complement and improve the accuracy and specificity of echocardiograms. Quantitative evaluation of spectral Doppler studies also allows the examiner to determine values such as pressure gradients across valves and stenotic areas or resistance to flow of blood entering an organ. In some cases, abnormal blood flow patterns can be detected before obvious anatomic lesions are present.

Contrast Ultrasonography: Ultrasound contrast agents increase the reflectivity of blood and any tissue through which blood flows. Enhancement of blood reflectivity is usually accomplished by injection or formation of transient microscopic bubbles in the plasma. The increase in echogenicity is related to the amount of blood flowing through the tissue. The bubbles are quickly absorbed into the plasma and therefore do not constitute an embolism hazard. The ability to evaluate the vascularity of a tissue provides additional information about the type of lesion present. For instance, granulomas generally have poorer blood flow than normal tissue and do not enhance as much as the surrounding tissue, whereas tumors may enhance more and retain the contrast for a longer time than the surrounding tissue. Contrast agents hold great promise for improving both the sensitivity and specificity of ultrasonographic examinations. However, they are extremely expensive, which precludes their use in all but special instances or funded research.

COMPUTED TOMOGRAPHY

In computed tomography (CT), an x-ray tube moves around the body and continuously projects a thin fan of x-rays through the body. Electronic detectors opposite the tube continuously monitor the number of x-rays passing through the body and the angle at which the beam is being projected. The number of x-rays reaching the detector changes as the beam passes through different tissues because of the tube movement. A computer mathematically evaluates the data and determines the most probable density of any point within the volume of tissue scanned. The density is generally measured in terms of Hounsfield units, which divide the entire spectrum of possible densities into 4,000 levels extending from a value of –1,000 to +3,000. Air is considered to have a value of –1,000, water is at 0, and lead or some other heavy metal is at +3,000. Because these units represent the degree to which the x-ray beam is attenuated, the image generated is really an attenuation map, which is what is displayed on the monitor and stored as a digital file by the computer. Together, all of the attenuation points make an image of the cross-section of the portion of the body through which the beam is passed. This tomographic image is usually referred to as a **slice**, and each of the individual attenuation points in the image is referred to as a **voxel** (volume element). The animal is then moved a specified number of millimeters, and the process repeated. By sequentially scanning a body area, the entire volume of interest can be imaged without any superimposition of structures. CT also has much better contrast discrimination than standard radiographs, so structures such as individual parts of the brain or individual muscle bellies are seen as separate and distinct on the CT scan. X-ray contrast media is frequently used to further enhance the contrast between structures and help characterize lesions.

Modern multislice CT scanners can acquire up to 620 cross-sectional images at once; each rotation may be as short as ¼ sec. These systems are capable of continuous rotation (helical or spiral scanning), in which motion of the patient through the scanner occurs in concert with the rotation of the scanner. These systems can perform a complete scan of the abdomen or thorax in a person on a single breath hold (~10 sec) and with appropriate ECG-based control can provide CT images of a beating heart during all portions of the cardiac cycle. The image reconstruction time is short, and the entire study can be completed in less time than was required to acquire a single image 15 years ago. Some veterinary practices now have 8- to 64-slice scanners installed, and the actual scan takes less time than it takes to position the animal on the scanning table. Even with such extraordinarily fast systems, veterinary patients must still be anesthetized and immobilized to perform most studies, but the period of anesthesia is short and the value of the information derived is great. Although studies have been published in which fully awake or minimally sedated animals were imaged, scans performed in this manner lack controlled positioning and reflect movement and are therefore difficult to interpret. This type of study should be reserved for instances in which the animal is severely obtunded by its medical condition or for the rare instances in which sedation would significantly alter the status of the tissues (such as an attempt to evaluate the effect of drug intervention in an asthmatic cat).

As with conventional radiography, the use of nonionic contrast agents can markedly improve the diagnostic accuracy and sensitivity of CT. For vascular studies, the contrast dosage is also substantially less than that used in conventional radiographic angiography. The utility of contrast enhancement on CT imaging is so important that nearly all CT studies of soft-tissue structures such as the brain or abdominal organs are contrast enhanced. Obtaining a contrast-enhanced image after a nonenhanced study allows comparison of the two images to give insights into the hemodynamic and physiologic changes present.

Modern reconstruction algorithms also allow three-dimensional reconstruction of structures with a given density. Bones can be depicted without the overlying soft tissues, and vascular structures that have been contrast enhanced can be depicted without any overlying tissues. Newer scanners can produce images of vessels that rival those obtained by conventional contrast angiography.

In addition to some of the imaging procedures unique to CT, this modality is replacing conventional radiography for evaluation of some structures and diseases traditionally assessed by radiography. CT scans of the skull in any species are far more informative and diagnostic than any conventional radiograph because the complex anatomy of the skull, which results in a pattern of overlying structures on a radiograph, is vastly simplified on a CT scan, making the diagnosis much more specific and accurate and improving treatment results. CT scanning is also rapidly replacing myelography for evaluation of spinal cord disease because of its greater safety and speed as well as being able to directly image the discs and vertebrae. CT scanning is also receiving much attention as a screening procedure to evaluate the lungs and other anatomic areas for evidence of distant metastasis in cancer patients. Metastatic lesions in the lung are far more evident at a smaller size on CT scans than on conventional radiographs. If a CT scan is performed after detection of metastatic lesions on radiographs, the CT scan will almost always find more nodules than are evident on the radiographic images.

CT scans of the feet and legs of horses can detect structural changes in bones and hoof structures that are not readily evident on even detailed radiographic images of the same body part. Unfortunately, no scanners currently can scan the abdomen or thorax in adult horses.

CT is also used to guide the acquisition of biopsy and aspirate of samples from many areas of the body, including the lungs and brain, that cannot be approached using *ultrasound* or other imaging modalities. The same type of approach may be used to perform image-guided therapy of some diseases such as radiofrequency ablation of tumor nodules in the liver. Such image-guided treatment obviates the need for a surgical procedure, reducing the impact of treatment on the patient.

CT scans are used to detect structural changes deep within the body, including tumors, abscesses, vascular abnormalities, occult fractures, and hematomas. Modern, high-speed scanners are also used to evaluate dynamic physiologic processes such as blood flow, changes in respiratory volume, and intestinal dynamics. The radiologist must have a firm knowledge of anatomy and physiology to ascertain the identity of structures in any plane through the body and evaluate changes in its anatomy or physiology. Knowledge of physiology and artifacts are also important in evaluating CT scans. Extensive experience and training are required to become adept in performing CT procedures and deriving the most information from the images. As the utility and availability of scanners has increased, veterinary medicine has seen a great jump in the number and quality of instruments available for use in veterinary patients.

MAGNETIC RESONANCE IMAGING

Magnetic resonance imaging (MRI) is the newest form of imaging in general use today. In this imaging modality, a powerful magnet, up to 60,000 times as strong as the magnetic field of the earth, is used to transiently align the hydrogen atoms in the body with the magnetic field. All atoms with odd atomic numbers are affected, but the effect on hydrogen overshadows the effect on other natural elements within the body. If the hydrogen atoms are then subjected to a radiofrequency (RF) pulse of the proper frequency, the alignment of these atoms is then deflected to one side or reversed. Once the RF pulse is turned off, the hydrogen atoms realign with the magnetic field. The rate at which they do this is restricted by (and characteristic of) the molecule of which they are a part. During this relaxation or realignment phase, the hydrogen atoms emit radio waves that can be detected by highly sensitive equipment. The frequency of these waves depends on the strength of the magnetic field. By using a second set of magnets referred to as the gradients, the magnetic field of the scanner can be arranged in such a way that each small discrete volume (voxel) has a different field strength. Because the RF emitted by the relaxing hydrogen atoms depends on the strength of the magnetic field in which it is located, each of these volumes can be represented by a unique frequency. Then, by evaluating the signal strength and duration for each frequency, the chemical composition of each voxel can be estimated. In practice this is done by representing the signal strengths for each volume on a monitor, much as is done with CT. The signal strength from each volume element is very small, so many repetitions or pulses of the RF field are required to provide a statistically significant determination of the relative signal strength from the volume elements. Thus, each scanning sequence may require several minutes to perform. Sequential examination of slices through the body is done the same way CT examinations are performed. MRI differs from CT in that the data for all the slices in the volume being imaged are acquired simultaneously; however, previously only one set of planes is acquired at a time, but recent developments in scanner technology allow acquisition of volume data sets. Scans are typically acquired in more than one of the three orthogonal planes, with different magnet pulsing sequences to highlight different types of tissue. Also, unlike CT, MRI scans are seldom reformatted to project oblique planes, although three-dimensional rendering may be done either on the scanner's computer or a stand-alone workstation.

MRI does not use ionizing radiation and thus has gained rapid and wide use in pediatric imaging in human medicine. Although this is less of a concern in veterinary medicine, the ability to obtain diagnostic images without the use of ionizing radiation is desirable for veterinary personnel.

MRI scanners are extremely sensitive to the presence of certain metals such as iron and cobalt. The presence of such materials within the patient can markedly degrade the quality of the image, even to the point that it is not possible to develop an image at all. Although surgical stainless steel now in use has minimal ferromagnetic properties, it can still distort the image somewhat. Even the small amount of iron present in identity chips can produce significant artifacts on the images. For this reason, animals to be subjected to MRI scanning should have radiographs of the area of interest before being placed in the MRI scanner. The presence of metallic foreign material in the GI tract or soft tissues can easily result in a nondiagnostic study. An exquisite example of this is the presence of a steel shotgun or BB gun pellets; the presence of even a single such pellet may totally degrade the images. Another potential source of such artifacts could be stainless steel sutures or hemoclips. Depending on their chemical composition, such materials may or may not significantly alter the images.

MRI interpretation requires a firm knowledge of sectional anatomy as well as knowledge of the physics of the imaging system. Because this type of imaging is based on chemical composition of the body rather than density, it provides exquisite detail and contrast of body structures. However, the duration of data acquisition limits its use in areas of substantial movement, such as the chest and upper abdomen, although recent improvement in scanner technology has largely done away with this limitation. MRI does not image cortical bone well and therefore is of limited use in the evaluation of bony lesions, although it is quite applicable to imaging of bone marrow and cartilage. Like CT, MRI was initially used primarily for neuroimaging and is still the mainstay of imaging in that area. Another major area of MRI usage is in evaluation of blood vessels deep within the body, particularly those of the legs, neck, and head. Because of its exquisite sensitivity to the changes in tissue organization and composition as well as density, MRI is also used frequently for joint and muscle imaging, where it has become a valuable tool in assessment of joint integrity because of its unique ability to image cartilage and ligaments. This has led to great interest in developing and promoting MRI imaging of equine extremities if the issue of motion can be overcome.

Contrast enhancement of MRI scans is common when imaging the brain and other soft tissues. It can frequently permit the radiologist to make a relatively specific diagnosis regarding the etiology of the lesions seen on the scan. In other instances, the contrast images are the only ones that reveal the presence of a lesion. The agents used are specifically designed for use in MRI and are different from those used in CT and radiography.

In the past, MRI systems were large and expensive to purchase, install, and maintain, but many smaller, low-field-strength magnets are available, including some specifically designed for use in veterinary medicine. Dedicated equine extremity scanners are available, and although these instruments are relatively expensive, they are within financial reach of many large practices, especially those specializing in imaging and neurology. The use of lower field strengths will reduce the construction requirements of MRI facilities to house these instruments but comes at the price of longer scan times and decreased image resolution.

The length of time required to complete MRI scans and the exquisite sensitivity of MRI to motion dictates that studies be performed under general anesthesia. Because powerful magnets are used, ferromagnetic material may not be brought into the room because of safety considerations. For veterinary patients, injectable anesthesia may be used if special anesthesia machines, oxygen tanks, and monitoring equipment are unavailable. Injectable anesthesia may not be appropriate for all patients, so facilities dedicated to veterinary patients are well advised to have appropriate anesthetic equipment. The cost of such equipment is minor compared with that of developing the MRI facility itself.

Because of their exquisite sensitivity to radiofrequency signals, MRI systems must be shielded from all extraneous signals of this type. This requires installation of specialized shielding material in the walls of the room in which the MRI is located. Further, the larger, more advanced systems with higher field strength typically require liquid helium as a coolant to minimize signal noise from within the machine itself and to maintain a superconductive magnetic field. The construction of an MRI facility must be done under the direction of a qualified architect and engineering firm.

MRI scanners should be operated by technologists specially trained in operation of these instruments. Many factors must be taken into account when preparing an animal for an MRI. This training is not part of either the veterinary curriculum or the veterinary technical curriculum and must be acquired by attending special training sessions or preferably as part of the training program in a school of radiologic technology. Having well-trained technologists to perform these studies will greatly improve the quality of the scans and promote the use of these instruments for a wider variety of imaging applications.

Because of the expense of acquiring and maintaining these instruments (especially those with field strength of 1 Tesla or above), the technical complexity of MRI imaging, and the special training and experience required to interpret the images, MRI scanning systems are generally found only in large private and academic referral specialty practices.

NUCLEAR MEDICINE IMAGING

(Nuclear scintigraphy)

Although it has been around for >50 yr, nuclear scintigraphy is still relatively unused in veterinary medicine. The reason is because it uses radionuclides, which are both expensive and heavily regulated. In addition, the images derived from the studies are physiologic in nature and therefore quite unfamiliar to most veterinarians. This is unfortunate, because nuclear scintigraphy provides information on pathologic and physiologic processes that cannot be obtained by other means.

Nuclear medicine imaging involves dosing the patient with a very small amount of a gamma ray–emitting radioisotope. The location and distribution of the radioisotope within the body is then detected with a gamma camera, a device specifically designed to collimate and detect gamma rays. The isotope may be injected, ingested, or inhaled as appropriate for the study being performed. The radioisotope is usually part of a larger molecule that has a specific affinity for the tissue or organ of interest. For instance, some organic phosphonates have an affinity for bone, and isotopes bound to sulfur colloids will localize in the liver and spleen. Very few radioisotopes have direct affinity for a given tissue; iodine is the notable exception and localizes very strongly in the thyroid. Inhaled gases or aerosols localize in the airways and lungs and may or may not be absorbed into the bloodstream. In veterinary medicine, the most commonly used isotope is metastable technetium 99 (^{99m}Tc), although radioactive iodine, indium, and thallium are also used in specific instances.

The data collected by the gamma camera can be displayed directly on a monitor or projected onto a film or a digital file as a permanent record. Most modern systems send the data to a computer system for analysis, which allows enhancement of count differences and determination of organ margins. The operator can select regions of interest to analyze for isotope content and rate for accumulation over time. When the study uses a radiopharmaceutical that is metabolized or has a limited residence time in an organ, organ function can be determined. These dynamic studies can be used to evaluate the function of organs such as the lungs, kidneys, and heart. Such studies may reveal abnormalities that static forms of anatomic imaging cannot detect. Functional imaging is the great strength of nuclear medicine and allows disease detection earlier and more readily than anatomic imaging systems. Advanced MRI studies can emulate this functional aspect of scintigraphic imaging in some cases, but those systems are much more limited in scope and availability, as well as costing an order of magnitude more.

Single photon emission computed tomography (SPECT) and positron emission tomography (PET) are advanced scintigraphic imaging techniques widely used in human medicine for detection and evaluation of many diseases. In both of these techniques, a CT-like cross-sectional image based on the deposition of radionuclides within the body is generated. Such images have greater sensitivity than planar images and improved specificity as well.

PET imaging in particular has seen tremendous growth in the last decade and is routinely used in the staging and evaluation of many diseases, especially cancer. This technology, which is based on the use of positron-emitting isotopes of lighter elements such as oxygen, nitrogen, carbon, and fluorine, can evaluate the metabolism and localization of these elements with great sensitivity. PET imaging is available at most academic centers, and its use exceeds that of traditional nuclear scintigraphy in some centers. These instruments are extremely sensitive and can often define the presence of or characterize the extent of some disease processes long before they can be evaluated by anatomic imaging systems such as MRI or CT. When these images are combined with CT or MRI images, tremendous sensitivity for the detection of numerous diseases results.

The major issue with using nuclear medicine imaging in veterinary medicine is not the availability of gamma cameras or the technical expertise required to operate them. Cameras are readily available on the used market, and training of technologists to operate them is not prohibitively complex. Rather, it is the regulations surrounding the acquisition and use of radiopharmaceuticals. All use must be strictly documented and, unlike in human medicine, the veterinary patient generally must remain in the hospital after the study is performed to allow the agents to be mostly cleared from the body. A second reason for limited use is the physiologic nature of the lesions, which results in images of poor spatial resolution even though they are exquisitely sensitive to some disease processes. The special training required for interpretation of these images is provided as part of a veterinary radiology residency program available at only a few centers.

DISPOSAL OF CARCASSES AND DISINFECTION OF PREMISES

When animals die or are slaughtered on farms, carcasses and parts that are unfit for use as food should be disposed of properly. Safe and environmentally responsible disposal of animal carcasses, whether an individual death or during significant mortality events, is an essential consideration. Premises should be promptly cleaned in a manner that prevents any infectious or toxic health hazard to domestic or wild animals or people. Information on the safe and lawful disposal of carcasses can be obtained from local environmental protection agencies. When the circumstances under which death has occurred suggest a transmissible disease or toxic hazard, the nearest animal health official should be notified immediately.

As general precautions, persons handling carcasses and disinfectants should wear protective clothing and be properly equipped to complete the tasks of disposition and disinfection. The method of disposal should preclude contamination of soil, air, and water. Hides and other parts of animals that have succumbed to infectious diseases or toxins should be safely disposed of and not retained for use.

There are restrictions on carcass disposal for cattle ≥30 mo old because of specified risk materials (tissues in which prions that cause **bovine spongiform encephalopathy** [BSE] concentrate). Sheep or cattle diagnosed with or suspected of being affected by **scrapie** (*see* p 1288) or BSE (*see* p 1284), respectively, must not be rendered. The preferred means of disposal for these animals is incineration, although they may also be buried (*see* below).

Rendering: Ordinarily, rendering is a safe, rapid, and economical method of disposal of carcasses. Renderers are required to use equipment and methods that prevent health hazards. Local regulations specify requirements for transportation of carcasses to rendering plants. During transportation, biosecurity must be considered to avoid spreading infectious agents into the environment.

Burial: When a site acceptable to the local environmental protection agency is available, burial is usually the preferred method of disposal. In selecting a burial site, it is necessary to consider the adequacy of soil depth and to avoid underground electrical cables, water pipes, gas pipes, septic tanks, and water wells. The prevention of secondary toxicosis or exposure to infectious agents to scavengers or groundwater must be considered (eg, the burial of a carcass infected with blastomycosis could potentially contaminate the soil thereafter). The burial pit or trench should be at least 2.3 m wide and 3 m deep (7 × 9 ft). The pit is a cave-in hazard and must not be entered without proper shoring, and any other appropriate precautions should be taken. At this depth, 1.3 m^2 (15 ft^2) of floor space will accommodate a mature bovine or equine carcass, 5 mature pigs or sheep, 100 mature chickens, or 40 mature turkeys. For each additional meter (3 ft) in depth, the number of animals per 1.3 m^2 of floor space may be doubled. Contaminated litter, soil, manure, feed, milk, or other material should be placed in the pit with the carcasses and covered with at least 2 m (6 ft) of soil. The covering soil should not be compacted. Decomposition and gas formation cause cracking, bubbling, and leaking of fluids from a compacted burial site. The soil should be mounded and neatly graded.

Burning: Burning in an incinerator that is operated in compliance with local laws and ordinances is an excellent means to dispose of one or a few carcasses and is the preferred means for sheep with scrapie and *cattle with BSE.*

Burning carcasses in an open site should be done only when legally permitted. Burning poultry carcasses should be considered only when burial is not feasible. The burn site should be away from public view and on flat, open ground that is clear of buildings, hay or straw stacks, overhead cables, and shallow underground pipes or cables. Locations upwind from houses, farm buildings, roads, or populated areas, and those from which precipitation runoff may contaminate the environment, should be avoided.

Carcasses must be placed on a quantity of combustible supporting materials sufficient to reduce them completely to ashes. The material must also be arranged in a manner to permit an adequate flow of air to the fire. Gasoline or other highly volatile combustible liquids should not be used.

To prepare the fire bed, an area of ground should be staked out to accommodate the number of carcasses to be burned: 8 × 3 ft for each mature cow or horse, 5 mature pigs or sheep, 100 mature chickens, or 40 mature turkeys. The fire bed burns best if at a right angle to the prevailing wind.

Under favorable conditions, burning should be complete in 48 hr. Additional combustible material should be added as needed. When the fire has died out, the ashes should be buried and the area cleaned, graded or plowed, and prepared for seeding.

Other Disposal Methods: Composting, fermentation, and dry extrusion methods have been developed to process certain dead animals and animal waste, destroy pathogenic organisms, reduce volume, and produce feedstuffs. Local environmental protection agencies and state agriculture departments should be consulted concerning the acceptability of these and other possible alternative disposal methods.

Disinfection of Premises: Removal and safe disposal of manure, feed, and debris by burial or burning, followed by thorough scraping and cleaning of all buildings and equipment, must precede the application of chemical disinfectant. Except for steam cleaning, cleaning with aqueous solutions is practical only at temperatures above freezing. A cleaning agent such as trisodium phosphate or sodium carbonate dissolved in hot water will facilitate cleaning. All traces of the cleaning agent must be rinsed away with clear water before disinfectant is applied. Provision must be made to contain and safely dispose of cleaning solutions, rinse water, and disinfectant.

Disinfectants recommended for general use on surfaces free of organic matter are sodium or calcium hypochlorite (1,200 ppm available chlorine), iodine, phenol, and quaternary ammonium compounds. Newer disinfectants use a combination of products (eg, quaternary ammonia and glutaraldehyde) to enhance efficacy. Information on disinfectants for specific animal disease agents can be obtained from state or federal animal health agencies. Disinfectants should bear the approval statement of the Environmental Protection Agency in the USA or of a similar agency in other countries. Label instructions for application must be followed.

EUTHANASIA

Euthanasia is the term used to describe ending the life of an animal in a way that eliminates or minimizes pain and distress. Animal slaughter, depopulation, and humane killing are distinguished from euthanasia, because they are performed for reasons different than sparing an animal from unresolvable painful or distressful conditions. Euthanasia of animals is a common procedure performed by veterinary professionals, and because of the seriousness of the action, it deserves appropriate consideration. Some of the most difficult euthanasia decisions that veterinarians are required to make involve the euthanasia of healthy animals when no other alternative for their care can be identified. A veterinarian must be fully prepared to speak frankly about the animal's condition and be knowledgeable about all possible alternative care resources when interacting with animal owners, caretakers, and control professionals. Recognizing the importance of a "good death" in the humane termination of an animal's life, many countries and professional organizations have developed guidelines and recommendations for animal euthanasia; some are more specific for certain species and environmental settings. Most recommendations emphasize certain factors that personnel performing euthanasia should consider when selecting the best method of euthanasia. These factors include: 1) ability of the method to induce loss of consciousness and death with minimal pain and distress; 2) time required to induce loss of consciousness; 3) reliability; 4) safety of personnel; 5) irreversibility; 6) compatibility with intended animal use and purpose; 7) documented emotional effect on observers or operators; 8) compatibility with subsequent evaluation, examination, or use of tissue; 9) drug availability and human abuse potential; 10) compatibility with species, age, and health status; 11) ability to maintain equipment in proper working order; 12) safety for predators or scavengers should the animal's remains be consumed; 13) legal requirements; and (14) environmental impacts of the method or disposition of the animal's remains.

To be able to understand and help others to understand euthanasia, personnel performing euthanasia should be well informed of established definitions of the more important physiologic and psychological states that may be observed during euthanasia. The American Veterinary Medical Association Panel on Euthanasia accepts the following important definitions: 1) anesthetic-induced unconsciousness is the loss of the righting reflex; 2) pain is a conscious experience; 3) distress is an animal's response to stimuli that interferes with its well-being and comfort. Thus, biological functions (urination, defecation), unintentional movements (limb paddling), and vocalizations after administration of an appropriate euthanasia method, and subsequent recumbency are not necessarily signs of perceived pain or distress. Loss of physiologic function and death should occur in the following order to help prevent fear and distress: 1) rapid loss of consciousness, 2) loss of motor function, 3) arrest of respiratory and cardiac functions, and finally 4) permanent loss of brain function. If loss of motor or respiratory and cardiac function precedes loss of consciousness, as might be the case if paralytic agents are used, animals may become fearful and experience distress. In some species, particularly rabbits and chickens, tonic immobility may be induced by fear, and care must be taken to not confuse this behavioral response with loss of consciousness.

In addition to the selection of the method of euthanasia, the euthanasia administrator should consider the natural behavior of the species. For virtually all species, being placed in a novel environment before euthanasia is stressful. Therefore, a euthanasia approach that can be applied in familiar surroundings may help reduce distress. Gentle restraint, careful handling, and talking during euthanasia often have a calming effect on animals accustomed to human contact. These techniques may also be effective coping strategies with personnel and owners. In some species, sedation may assist in achieving the best conditions. The emotional attachment between animals and their owners or caretakers requires an additional layer of professional respect and care. Discussing euthanasia openly with personnel allows everyone the opportunity to understand that the best interests of the animal, owners, and caretakers have been considered.

Regardless of the method of euthanasia selected, personnel performing euthanasia must confirm death and dispose of the carcass in a legal manner that does not contaminate food sources or the environment. Confirming death may best be accomplished by an adjunctive method (thoracotomy, decapitation) performed after the loss of consciousness. Using an adjunctive method may be especially important when euthanizing ectothermic animals, because their heartbeat and respiration are difficult to assess.

For a list of acceptable methods and agents for euthanasia of different species of animals, *see* TABLE 3. The AVMA Guidelines for Euthanasia 2013 provide additional details, as well as references for specific technical and safety information.

TABLE 3 AGENTS AND METHODS OF EUTHANASIA BY SPECIES

Species	Acceptable Methods[a]	Acceptable Methods with Conditions[b]
Aquatic invertebrates	S 6.3[c]: Immersion in anesthetic solution (magnesium salts, clove oil, eugenol, ethanol)	S 6.3: Adjunctive methods (second step) include 70% alcohol and neutral-buffered 10% formalin, pithing, freezing, boiling
Amphibians	S 7.3: As appropriate by species—injected barbiturates, dissociative agents, and anesthetics as specified, topical buffered tricaine methanesulfonate or benzocaine hydrochloride	S 7.3: As appropriate by species—inhaled anesthetics as specified, CO_2, penetrating captive bolt or firearm, manually applied blunt force trauma to the head, rapid freezing
Avian species (*see also* Poultry, below)	S 5: IV barbiturates	S 5: Inhaled anesthetics, CO_2, CO, N_2, Ar, cervical dislocation (small birds and poultry), decapitation (small birds) S 7.5: Gunshot (free-ranging birds)
Cats	S 1: IV barbiturates, injected anesthetic overdose	S 1: Barbiturates (alternative routes of administration), inhaled anesthetic overdose, embutramide, T-61, CO[c], CO_2[c], gunshot[c]
Cattle	S 3.2: IV barbiturates	S 3.2: Gunshot, penetrating captive bolt
Dogs	S 1: IV barbiturates, injected anesthetic overdose	S 1: Barbiturates (alternative routes of administration), inhaled anesthetic overdose, embutramide, T-61, CO[c], CO_2[c], gunshot[c]

(*continued*)

TABLE 3 AGENTS AND METHODS OF EUTHANASIA BY SPECIES *(continued)*

Species	Acceptable Methods[a]	Acceptable Methods with Conditions[b]
Finfish	S 6.2: Immersion in buffered benzocaine or benzocaine hydrochloride, isoflurane, sevoflurane, metomidate, quinaldine sulfate, buffered tricaine methanesulfonate, 2-phenoxyethanol, injected pentobarbital, rapid chilling (appropriate zebrafish/ research setting)	S 6.2: Eugenol, isoeugenol, clove oil, CO_2-saturated water (aquarium-fish facilities/fisheries), decapitation/ cervical transection/manually applied blunt force trauma followed by pithing, rapid chilling followed by adjunctive method (aquarium-fish facilities), maceration (research setting)
Equids	S 4: IV barbiturates	S 4: Penetrating captive bolt, gunshot
Marine mammals	S 7.4: Injected barbiturates (captive)	S 7.4: Inhaled anesthetics (captive) S 7.6: Gunshot, manually applied blunt force trauma, implosive decerebration (free ranging)
Nonhuman primates	S 2.3, S 7.4: Injected barbiturates or anesthetic overdose	S 2.3, S 7.4: Inhaled anesthetic, CO, CO_2 (as appropriate by species)
Poultry	S 3.4: Injected barbiturates and anesthetic overdose	S 3.4: CO_2, CO, N_2, Ar, cervical dislocation (as anatomically appropriate), decapitation, manual blunt force trauma, electrocution, gunshot, captive bolt
Rabbits	S 2.4: IV barbiturates	S 2.4: Inhaled anesthetic overdose, CO_2, cervical dislocation (as anatomically appropriate), penetrating captive bolt
Reptiles	S 7.3: As appropriate by species—injected barbiturates, dissociative agents, and anesthetics as specified; topical buffered tricaine methanesulfonate or benzocaine hydrochloride	S 7.3: As appropriate by species–inhaled anesthetics as specified, CO_2, penetrating captive bolt or firearm, manually applied blunt force trauma to the head, rapid freezing
Rodents	S 2.2: Injected barbiturates and barbiturate combinations, dissociative agent combinations	S 2.2: Inhaled anesthetics, CO_2, CO, tribromoethanol, ethanol, cervical dislocation, decapitation, focused beam microwave irradiation
Small ruminants	S 3.2: Injected barbiturates	S 3.2: Gunshot, penetrating captive bolt
Swine	S 3.3: Injected barbiturates	S 3.3: CO_2, CO, N_2, Ar, gunshot, electrocution, nonpenetrating captive bolt, manually applied blunt force trauma

Reprinted, with permission, from the AVMA Guidelines on Euthanasia 2013 Edition. *Note:* Initial "S" references with associated numbers in table entries refer to specific areas of more detailed information in the AVMA Guidelines, available at www.avma.org/KB/Policies/Documents/euthanasia.pdf.

[a] Acceptable methods are those that consistently produce a humane death when used as the sole means of euthanasia.

[b] Acceptable methods with conditions are those that may require certain conditions to be met to consistently produce humane death, may have a greater potential for operator error or safety hazards, are not well documented in the scientific literature, or may require a secondary method to ensure death.

[c] Not recommended for routine use.

MEAT INSPECTION

Inspection of meat by qualified individuals to eliminate unwholesome, adulterated, or mislabeled meat or meat products from the food supply protects consumers from the physical, infectious, and toxic hazards that may originate in food animals, the environment, or people. The standard procedures do not cover every possibility concerning the acceptability of carcasses, organs, or other animal parts; personal judgment is also required to ensure that only wholesome, unadulterated product is approved for food. (*See also* CHEMICAL RESIDUES IN FOOD AND FIBER, p 2518.)

Inspection activities are divided into premortem, postmortem, and processing inspection.

PREMORTEM INSPECTION

Premortem inspection is conducted at the abattoir on the day of slaughter to detect and condemn animals that are unfit for slaughter and to note signs or lesions of disease that may not be apparent after slaughter (eg, rabies, listeriosis, or heavy metal poisoning). During inspection, animals should be confined in a lighted enclosure so that they can be clearly observed at rest and in motion. The animals must not be allowed to enter into any area of the facility where slaughtering, dressing, or handling of edible products is performed until they have been inspected and found to be acceptable candidates for human consumption. Gates, chutes, and equipment must be available to segregate abnormal animals for closer examination and proper identification.

Seriously crippled animals, animals commonly termed “downers,” and disabled or moribund animals are not acceptable candidates for slaughter as food. Rectal temperatures should be verified on any animal suspected of being febrile. Body temperature should be <106°F (41°C) for pigs and <105°F (40.5°C) for cattle, sheep, goats, horses, and mules. Animals with signs or lesions that do not warrant immediate condemnation can be identified as “suspects” so that their carcasses and viscera can be inspected separately. Certain animals may be retained to allow recovery from minor diseases or to permit depletion of residues of biologic substances and chemicals. Animals that may have been treated with or exposed to substances that may make the edible tissues unfit for human food should not be slaughtered for such.

Animals that have reacted to a test for anaplasmosis, leptospirosis, or tuberculosis are unacceptable as food. The temperature of bovine tuberculosis reactors should be taken on premortem inspection.

Animals suspected of having a foreign disease or parasite should be held and reported immediately to the nearest federal or state health official.

Animal welfare and humane slaughter concerns are increasingly important to the livestock industry. Slaughtering plants in the USA are routinely observed to ensure full compliance with provisions of the Humane Methods of Slaughter Act of 1978 and related regulations. Humane handling of livestock before slaughter is necessary and includes methods of stimulation, nonabuse by plant workers, provision of food and water, safe pen construction, nonslip floors, and protection from adverse weather conditions.

Most large meat producers require compliance with humane slaughter regulations. Therefore, these animals must be rendered insensible to pain by a single blow, gunshot, or an electrical, chemical, or other method that is rapid and effective before shackling, hoisting, or cutting.

Recognized ritual slaughter methods, such as halal and kosher, are exempted from these requirements.

POSTMORTEM INSPECTION

Animals should be inspected immediately after slaughter and evisceration for possible changes and lesions that indicate unsuitability of the meat for food. Postmortem examination requires observation of all parts of the carcass, dressing procedures, equipment, and facilities to prevent contamination of edible parts. The inspector must ensure that condemned carcasses and parts are disposed of safely. The following are unacceptable for human food: lactating mammary glands, laryngeal muscles, thyroid glands, and lungs. Brains, cheek meat, and head trimmings from animals that were stunned by lead, sponge iron, or frangible bullets, and carcasses suspected of containing antibiotics, sulfonamides, or other residues are also unacceptable. CNS tissue and spinal cords must be discarded to eliminate the threat of bovine spongiform encephalopathy in the food supply.

Routine postmortem inspection should include the following procedures.

Cattle: *Head*: Incise and visually examine the left and right atlantal, mandibular, parotid, and suprapharyngeal lymph nodes. Examine two incised layers of both masseter muscles. Examine and palpate tongue. *Viscera*: Examine abdominal viscera and mesenteric lymph nodes. Examine and palpate ruminoreticular junction. Examine esophagus and spleen. Incise and examine anterior, middle, and posterior mediastinal lymph nodes and right and left bronchial lymph nodes. Examine and palpate costal and ventral surfaces of the lungs. Incise heart from base to apex through interventricular septum, and examine and cut inner and outer surfaces. Incise and examine hepatic lymph nodes. Incise bile duct in both directions and examine contents. Examine and palpate dorsal and ventral surfaces and renal impression of liver. *Carcass*: Examine internal and external surfaces. Palpate internal iliac and superficial inguinal or supramammary lymph nodes. Examine and palpate diaphragm and kidneys.

Calves and Veal: *Head*: Incise and examine suprapharyngeal lymph nodes. *Viscera*: Examine and palpate bronchial and mediastinal lymph nodes, heart, and lungs. Examine spleen. Examine and palpate dorsal and ventral surfaces of the liver, and palpate hepatic lymph nodes. Examine abdominal viscera. *Carcass*: Examine exposed inner and outer surfaces. Palpate the kidneys and internal iliac lymph nodes.

Sheep and Goats: *Head and Carcass*: Examine body cavities and outer surfaces. Palpate back and sides of carcass. Examine head, neck, and, shoulders. Palpate prescapular lymph nodes. Examine and palpate kidneys. Palpate femoral, popliteal, and superficial inguinal or supramammary lymph nodes. Incise lymph nodes when necessary to exclude caseous lymphadenitis. *Viscera*: Examine abdominal viscera, esophagus, mesenteric lymph nodes, omental fat, and spleen. Examine bile duct and gallbladder and their contents. Examine and palpate liver and costal and ventral surfaces of lungs. Palpate bronchial and mediastinal lymph nodes. Examine and palpate heart.

Pigs: *Head*: Examine head and cervical muscles. Incise mandibular lymph nodes. *Viscera*: Examine and palpate mesenteric lymph nodes and spleen. Palpate portal lymph nodes. Examine dorsal and ventral surfaces of the liver. Palpate left and right bronchial and mediastinal lymph nodes. Examine and palpate dorsal and ventral surfaces of the lungs. Examine and palpate heart. *Carcass*: Examine external and internal surfaces and incise any suspected abnormalities. Examine and palpate kidneys.

Poultry: Examine external surfaces for dressing defects, bruises, and disease lesions. Palpate tibias for bone diseases. Examine internal surfaces, kidneys, and lungs in place. Examine viscera and palpate heart, liver, and spleen.

Horses: *Head*: Examine surfaces. Palpate, incise, and examine mandibular, pharyngeal, and parotid lymph nodes; guttural pouches; and tongue. *Viscera*: Examine and palpate lungs and bronchial and mediastinal lymph nodes, and incise any suspected abnormalities. Examine and palpate spleen, liver, and portal lymph nodes. Incise hepatic duct. Examine remaining viscera. *Carcass*: Examine internal and external surfaces. Palpate superficial inguinal or supramammary and internal iliac lymph nodes. Examine and palpate kidneys and diaphragm. Examine and incise the internal abdominal walls for possible parasitic cysts. Examine spinous processes of thoracic vertebrae, supraspinous bursa, and first two cervical vertebrae for fistulous conditions. Examine axillary and subscapular tissues of white and gray horses for melanosis.

GENERAL CONDEMNATIONS

Livestock clearly showing at premortem inspection any irreversible disease or condition that justifies condemnation as unfit for use as food should be humanely destroyed and disposed of (*see* p 1639).

Carcasses contaminated by physical, infectious, or toxic agents should not be approved for use as food. Carcasses with generalized conditions or diseases, including cancers, that have so altered the normal characteristics of the meat as to cause it to be inedible or sufficiently abnormal to be reasonably considered unfit for food should not be approved. Localized conditions that do not affect the wholesomeness of the entire carcass should be removed by trimming so that the remainder of the carcass can be used for food.

Special Considerations for Tuberculosis: The entire carcass should be condemned when there is evidence of tuberculosis. This includes when an active lesion is present; the animal is cachectic; a lesion is present in muscle, intermuscular tissue, bone, joint, abdominal organs other than the GI tract, or in a lymph node associated with these parts; extensive lesions are present in the thoracic or abdominal cavity; lesions are multiple, acute, and actively progressive; and the nature or extent of lesions does not indicate localization.

An organ or part should be condemned when it or its corresponding lymph nodes contain lesions. When lesions in pigs are localized and are found at only one primary site of infection, such as the cervical lymph nodes, the unaffected parts are acceptable for food after condemnation of the affected organ or part. Even though certain carcasses minimally affected with tuberculosis may be considered safe after commercial cooking, this procedure is not recommended for carcasses that are not inspected in facilities inspected by federal or state officials.

DETECTION OF UNWHOLESOME MEAT

Meat for human consumption should be prepared from animals that were healthy and have been exsanguinated. Animals having physical, infectious, or toxic agents that may be hazardous to human health or that are otherwise unwholesome in their tissues should not be used for food. Fitness for food can be determined by a comprehensive evaluation that may include chemical, histologic, microbiologic, organoleptic, and toxicologic examinations.

Meat should be examined under light of adequate intensity. Foreign objects on the surface or visible within the tissue should be collected for further examination. Items such as feathers, fibers, hair, insect larvae, or parasites may provide valuable data on the species, origin, and handling of the meat. Color, odor, and texture should be noted. Meat should be firm, and cut surfaces should be glossy. Gray or green discoloration may indicate bacterial action. Dark red meat may result from postmortem retention of blood in animals that were not exsanguinated. A stable, bright red color may indicate the unwholesome addition of sulfite. Ultraviolet light may be used to visualize rodent urine and fluorescent substances produced by certain spoilage bacteria. Areas of bruising, hemorrhage, or inflammation should be readily recognized. Odors from contaminating chemicals, fish, urine, or other sources are unacceptable. When there is uncertainty about odors, a possible unwholesome odor can be enhanced by boiling or frying the meat.

Histologic examination may be used to evaluate abnormalities caused by physical, infectious, or toxic agents. Similarly, microbiologic examination may be used to evaluate spoilage and determine the presence of infectious organisms capable of causing illness in consumers. Chemical and toxicologic examinations should be done when the presence of adulterative or toxic substances is suspected. It may be necessary to increase random microbial testing of meat products to ensure their freedom from bacterial contamination.

ABATTOIR SANITATION

Abattoir buildings, equipment, personnel, and operating procedures should assure the continued wholesomeness and freedom from adulteration of carcasses and meat. Floors, walls, and ceilings should be constructed of materials and in a manner that allows sanitary operation and thorough cleaning. An ample supply of hot and cold water and cleaning materials should be conveniently available for slaughtering, cleaning, and personal hygiene. Water of at least 180°F (82°C) should be available to sanitize equipment and tools after cleaning. Equipment, knives, and utensils that have contacted diseased carcasses should be cleaned and sterilized before being used again. Waste-water drainage, with proper trapping and sewage disposal, should be adequate to maintain the abattoir in a sanitary condition. Ventilation should be sufficient to assure that edible product areas are free of noxious odors. Access of flies, rodents, and other vermin should be prevented. Lighting should be maintained at an intensity adequate for cleaning and inspection. Equipment should be of such material and so constructed as to be readily and thoroughly cleaned and should be properly maintained. Separate, clean containers for edible and inedible materials should be provided at convenient locations. Racks or tables should be provided for heads. Personnel should wear clean garments and follow all hygiene and sanitation procedures.

PREPURCHASE EXAMINATION OF HORSES

See also THE LAMENESS EXAMINATION, p 1097.

Prepurchase examinations are often requested by a potential buyer of a horse. The objective is to reduce the buyer's risks in relationship to the general health and athletic soundness of the horse for sale. The examination is not meant to guarantee soundness of the horse but is an attempt, on the part of the examining veterinarian, to ascertain any preexisting problem or any potential problem that may affect future soundness (eg, degenerative joint disease).

The examining veterinarian should have experience with the specific breed and discipline, as well as knowledge of the purpose and level of exercise for which the horse is being purchased. Ideally, the examiner should also be aware of any related organizational regulations that may influence the prepurchase examination. All notes generated during the examination should be kept in the buyer's file, and a report should be generated for the buyer. The examination should be conducted in a thorough and organized manner, because prepurchase examinations are a common cause of litigation from dissatisfied buyers. The major problems related to litigation are lack of understanding of the prepurchase examination process and the client's unrealistic expectation of a secure investment.

Pre-examination Issues: At the onset, the roles of all involved parties (eg, buyer, trainer, legal agent) in the purchase of the particular horse should be defined. Trainers may or may not have legal agent status. The trainer does have the potential to be responsible for assessing the buyer's expectations for the horse's athletic future and also whether the horse is suitable for the buyer. If an agent is representing the buyer, the examining veterinarian should encourage all information gathered to be communicated to the buyer, along with the report. Buyers of horses have different levels of experience and practical expectations. The veterinarian should ascertain the particular buyer's expectations and define the limitations of the examination, emphasizing that the examination does not eliminate risks.

The buyer is the owner of the information but needs to maintain a level of confidentiality so that the reputation of the horse is not potentially altered because of inappropriate dissemination of medical information. Through requests by the buyer or the buyer's agent, the seller and/or the seller's veterinarian may agree to provide the horse's medical history to the examining veterinarian. These medical records are returned at the end of the examination. The potential examination and its procedures should be thoroughly reviewed with the buyer and seller verbally and with written explanatory documents. Written release forms for riding the horse, payment, and the seller's permission for any interventional procedures, such as sedation for radiographs, shoe removal, hair clipping, etc, should be obtained before the examination. Partial examinations should not be encouraged. Trial periods are often acceptable and encouraged, especially if the seller can be assured of the horse's safety. One option is to house the horse in a mutually known, professionally managed barn. The seller may request that the horse be insured.

Traditionally, it is recommended that the examining veterinarian have had no contact with the horse or seller in a previous medical or personal role. However, this is often not possible when the horse is being sold within a small community or within the same boarding barn. In such situations, the relationship of the veterinarian to all parties involved should be clearly stated. The opposite situation can occur when the horse is being purchased out of town and the examining veterinarian is not the routine veterinarian for the buyer. The examining veterinarian may want to have the buyer's routine veterinarian review the examination report and any ancillary information, such as radiographs, laboratory tests, etc. Also, if any particular question arises during the examination, an opinion from a board-certified veterinary specialist might be indicated.

If the veterinarian has working knowledge of competition rules related to the discipline in which the horse is being purchased (eg, height requirements), he or she should explain how these rules may apply to the prepurchase examination. The veterinarian should counsel the buyer to learn the specific rules and verify "cards" that belong to the pony or horse. Having the buyer verify any rule requirements may help reduce future problems.

State and international disease testing and other requirements should be reviewed with the buyer and complied with by the examining veterinarian. Drug testing should be offered to the buyer and its limitations discussed. If the horse is purchased at a competition, or the seller is not known to the buyer, drug testing should be strongly recommended. Even when a buyer does not wish to have drug testing, examiners often collect blood at the time of the examination and store the serum or plasma frozen. It would then be available if any questions arose after the purchase.

Prepurchase examinations of performance horses often are conducted under several different conditions of training. The ideal situation is that the horse is currently active in the particular level of competition for which it is being purchased. However, prepurchase examinations can involve some inherent predictability, even though they are not classically meant for prediction of a horse's health. The following are examples of conditions an examiner may face. Any of these or other modifying conditions should be included in the examination notes: 1) A horse is currently in early training for a specific athletic endeavor and the buyer is ultimately looking to have the horse compete at a higher level. 2) A horse is coming off a lay-off period and has been back in work for only a brief period of time. 3) An older horse that has some infirmities and is being purchased as a schoolmaster by a less experienced rider, in which case the physical demands will potentially decrease with the new buyer. 4) A horse is being purchased for a financial investment. 5) A horse is being purchased as a pleasure or trail horse for a moderate or light workload but the horse's attitude is extremely important. In each of these conditions, different approaches are needed, and different questions should be asked and understood by the examiner.

Examinations of pretraining and brood stock present different issues to the examining veterinarian. The examiner must be alert to potential limiting conditions of the suckling, weanling, or yearling that would diminish its ability to perform its potential future work. In examining mares and stallions, experience with reproductive examination procedures is needed. (*See also* BREEDING SOUNDNESS EXAMINATION OF THE MARE, p 2189, and BREEDING SOUNDNESS EXAMINATION OF THE MALE, p 2230.) In all situations, thorough knowledge of the rules of the specific breed and any governmental disease regulations is critical.

History: *The simplest way for the veterinarian to accumulate history before the examination is to have the seller complete and sign a history form. This helps to legally bind the seller in the transaction and gives* information that may or may not have been known to the buyer, his or her agent, or the examining veterinarian. A similar questionnaire can be devised for the buyer as to his or her expectations, potential use, and previous experience with the horse in question. Examples of such forms are readily available on the Internet and may be modified as needed.

Physical Examination: The examination for a performing horse can be divided into four sections. The first part is observing the horse in the stall. The second includes observing the horse on a lead strap at a walk and a trot on a straight line, doing flexion tests, and in a circle with a long line. The third part of the examination involves observation of the horse while it is being ridden. The fourth part includes diagnostic procedures such as radiography and ultrasound.

In the UK, there is a standardized 5-stage vetting procedure: Stage 1, preliminary examination; Stage 2, trotting up in hand; Stage 3, strenuous exercise ridden or longed to evaluate conditioning, heart, breathing, and strains that might be expressed; Stage 4, a period of rest for as long as 30 min to evaluate heart and lung recovery, during which time paperwork such as identification can be completed; and Stage 5, a second trot in hand and foot evaluation.

Phase 1: The key to any successful prepurchase examination is having a systematic, consistent routine. At some point during the first part of the examination, a thorough identification of the horse should be recorded. This can be a written description of its color and age verification with inspection of the teeth. Digital photographs are easily adapted and helpful in prepurchase identification. Notations of markings and any other permanent peculiarities to the horse's body are also beneficial. The most common markings include a star, stripe, blaze, or snip on the face of the horse. Any white markings on the legs should also be described. Other markings that are valuable to record include whorls on the face and neck, brands, and tattoos. The presence of any scars, splints, or joint effusion should be noted. In some cases, brands or tattoos can give information, such as age (eg, American Jockey Club tattoos have an alphabet letter before the number; "A" represents the years 1971 and 1997, "B" 1998). The date, time, and place of the examination should also be recorded. The initial part of the examination ideally should be done in a stall or area out of direct sunlight, dark enough for an ophthalmologic examination. Temperature and pulse recordings, auscultation of the heart and lungs, and oral examinations can be done in the quiet and controlled confines of the stall. It is also worth looking in the stall for wood chewing, the character of the manure and feed, and/or oral medication remaining in the feed bucket.

Phase 2: The second phase of the examination outside the stall can begin with general body and skin condition. The body condition score (1–9) can be assigned a number from thinness (1) to obesity (9). Scores of 4, 5, or 6 are considered normal. Each of the front and hind feet should be thoroughly examined; mismatching, abnormal foot conformations, flares, dishing, type of shoeing, and rings should be noted. Photographs that document body condition scoring and feet can be part of the examination and may simplify a written description. Next, visual observation and palpation of the limbs, hoof examination (including hoof testers), passive and active flexion tests, and watching the horse move on different surfaces on a straight line and in a circle should be done. It is also valuable to perform a basic neurologic examination.

Phase 3: Many examiners feel it is helpful to watch the horse being ridden to exclude any subtle unsoundness. It also gives the examiner some observations and insight into the potential of the rider, if it is the buyer. These observations are worth noting, even though it is the trainer's and buyer's responsibility to determine the suitability of the horse. It is in this portion of the examination that the British Equine Veterinary Association recommends exerting the animal at a level appropriate for its age and fitness. Having the horse hand gallop for 5–10 min so the examiner can evaluate breath sounds and perform cardiac auscultation is recommended. Young or untrained horses can be longed. The horse is then monitored during recovery. Next, the jogging in hand is repeated so that any subtle lameness that might have been accentuated during the exercise stage can be detected. All observations are duly recorded in the report.

Phase 4: The fourth part of the examination should include any diagnostic procedures necessary to determine soundness, including radiographs (particularly of the feet, hocks, and stifles), ultrasonography, and nuclear scans. (*See also* THE LAMENESS EXAMINATION, p 1097.) Radiography is the most common diagnostic procedure performed. A recent retrospective analysis of radiography in equine prepurchase examinations suggests that higher radiographic grades (eg, 2–3) in the navicular bone and distal phalanx are associated with lameness, whereas similar grades in the tarsus were less likely to be associated with lameness.

Report of Findings: A summary report should be prepared and provided to the buyer. There are many published samples of these reports, available in letter or check-off list form. The report should describe any abnormal or undesirable findings and include an opinion as to the functional effect of these findings. Tests that were recommended to but declined by the buyer should be noted in the final report. The American Association of Equine Practitioners publishes guidelines for reproduction, medications, sale issues such as cryptorchidism, dental malocclusions, postsale examination of the upper respiratory tract of horses intended for racing, radiograph custody, and sale disclosure. Specific guidelines to report prepurchase examinations are also included. The British Equine Veterinary Association also publishes guidelines to conduct a prepurchase examination.

PREPURCHASE EXAMINATION OF RUMINANTS AND SWINE

See also BIOSECURITY, p 2068.

The buying and selling of cattle, sheep, goats, cervids, and swine are critical to the continuing vitality of the global livestock industry, and the health of animals to be sold or moved to other premises is extremely important. The purchaser, the seller, state and federal animal health officials, and others engaged in livestock transactions want assurance that the animals are healthy and will not introduce disease into the new herd or area.

Within the USA, every state has specific animal health requirements that must be satisfied to legally move an animal into the state. Because these requirements frequently change in response to a state's efforts to protect their animal populations, it is always recommended that the Office of the State Veterinarian in the destination state be contacted before a move. Animals that arrive in a state without the proper health certification will likely be quarantined until the proper tests and inspections can be accomplished. In some rare instances, the animals may be destroyed because of the risk they pose to the state's animal populations.

The state of destination may require additional statements about the animals in the shipment. These statements, which generally provide additional information about the animals and their origin, are added to the body of the certificate of veterinary inspection (CVI). A permit number may also be required for some species. Collectively, these additional documents provide assurances that the animals meet or exceed the requirements of the state.

Because of continuing progress in eradication programs for brucellosis, tuberculosis, and pseudorabies in the USA, many states have been declared free of these diseases by the USDA. Once a state is designated as "free," other states may waive the requirement for an individual animal test for these diseases and will instead receive the animals based on the state of origin's status. If a herd or flock has been declared free of a disease, including classification as accredited-free, certified-free, or qualified-free, many states will waive an individual animal test for the specific disease.

Electronic CVI, especially when coupled with radiofrequency identification (RFID) devices used as official identification, reduce the time necessary to prepare and distribute the required paperwork. Although RFID devices are not currently required for interstate movement of animals, a recognized form of official identification for each animal is required. If a state has specific identification requirements, they can be determined when contact is made with the state of destination's animal health official.

Countries also have specific health regulations for imported animals. These regulations have been developed to protect their animal populations for many of the same reasons individual states have established specific importation requirements in the USA. Global standards for the movement of animals and animal products are developed by the OIE.

The chief veterinary official (CVO) for each country is responsible for protecting the health of the animal populations in that country, as well as the public health in the case of zoonotic diseases. Animal health requirements for the destination country can be obtained by contacting the CVO of that country or more simply by contacting the office of the USDA Area Veterinarian in Charge (AVIC) located in nearly every state. The AVIC has access to the animal health requirements for all foreign destinations. Most of the CVI prepared for animals being shipped to a foreign country must bear the endorsement of the AVIC before the animals leave the state of origin. Animals that are not accompanied by the proper documentation will be detained or refused at the border or point of debarkation.

It is not unusual for an exhibition, sale, or private treaty agreement to have requirements for animal movement that exceed those of the state or country of destination. To determine these unique requirements, the host of the event or the buyer of the animal should be contacted.

The USDA veterinary accreditation program facilitates the movement of animals by enlisting private veterinary practitioners. This system has reduced the need for state and federal animal health agencies to provide these essential services to livestock producers. The accredited veterinarian is ultimately responsible for the completeness of any document prepared and for certifying that the animals have been inspected and are not showing signs of infectious, contagious, or communicable diseases.

In the examination of any animal before sale, several points should be emphasized: 1) The veterinarian is working for the person paying the fee and reports only to that person. The person responsible for compensating the veterinarian should be informed of the cost before the inspection. 2) The purpose for which the animal is to be used should be clearly established before the examination. 3) The examining veterinarian must be knowledgeable not only in the care and treatment of animals but also aware of the purpose for which they will be used.

Because legal action against the examining veterinarian is a possibility, a veterinarian may choose not to provide a written report for prepurchase examinations. However, a written record of findings should be made, because it may be needed at a future date. The responsibility of the veterinarian is to supply information and identify abnormalities; the prospective purchaser must make the decision whether to purchase. The prospective purchaser may also select a second veterinarian to perform an additional inspection.

The examination is divided into three parts: history, clinical examination, and special examinations or diagnostic procedures.

History: A complete history should be obtained by questioning the seller, examining the seller's records, and observing the remainder of the herd or flock and the management conditions. The animal's breed, sex, age, color, markings, tattoos, ear tags, brands, and other identification aids should be noted. If applicable, registration papers should be checked and the animal's identity definitively established.

For a breeding animal, the records of its sire and dam also should be considered, including their breeding ability, the possibility of heritable defects in the line to which each belongs, and, if dead, the cause of death. Also, breeding records of the animal itself should be reviewed to determine its fertility. Breeding records of the herd of origin of the animal should be examined for evidence of disorders that may affect reproduction. If the animal is an adult female, the breeding dates and stage of pregnancy, if applicable, should be noted.

Records should be examined to determine whether the animal has had any previous diseases, injuries (and their severity), or surgical procedures. Previous vaccinations, their type, and date of administration should be noted. The health of the herd or flock of origin and possible contacts with other animals before the sale should be determined, because animals so exposed could be in the incubation period of disease. It should also be established whether the animal received any drugs or medication that could alter its normal state. If this cannot be established in the history, it may be prudent to perform assays for suspected medication.

Clinical Examination, Special Examinations, and Diagnostic Tests: All areas of the body and their functions should be examined. The clinical examination should establish the current state of the animal's health and condition of each body system.

As previously discussed, some diagnostic tests are performed at the time of sale to satisfy the requirements of the state or country of destination, but additional diagnostic tests and special examinations may be required by the seller, buyer, or others involved in the transaction. It may also be necessary to conduct additional testing as indicated by the findings of the clinical examination. When certain diseases are not present in the seller's geographic area but are endemic in the purchaser's area, vaccination (if available) for those specific diseases is frequently required before movement. The CVI prepared after the examination must accurately reflect the findings of the accredited veterinarian.

If a male is to be purchased for breeding purposes, a complete breeding soundness examination (*see* p 2230) should be conducted.

RADIATION THERAPY

Radiation therapy has seen dramatic increases in demand and sophistication in recent years, which has led to creation of a board specialty in radiation oncology, granted by the American College of Veterinary Radiology. The sophistication and scope of both veterinary imaging and radiation therapy has advanced to the point that only a few radiologists now actively practice in both the fields of imaging and therapy.

Historically, radiation therapy was delivered using orthovoltage x-ray machines or very large activities of 64-cobalt and 137-cesium. Except for a few specialized instances, orthovoltage x-ray machines have fallen from favor because of the intensity of adverse radiation reactions associated with their use and their limited flexibility. Cobalt and cesium are no longer used because as long-lived isotopes they are extremely dangerous and

TABLE 4 SELECTED COMMON NEOPLASMS THAT CAN BE TREATED WITH RADIATION THERAPY

Tumor Type	Radiosensitivity	Comments
Nasal adenocarcinoma	Intermediate	Usually respond well but often recur
Nasal squamous cell carcinoma	Low	Response is often minimal
Nasal chondrosarcoma	Intermediate to high	Some subtypes respond better than others
Nasal osteosarcoma	Low	Response may be better if after surgery
Oral melanoma	Low to intermediate	Poor response usually unless after surgery
Oral squamous cell carcinoma	Low	Especially poor in cats; aggressive treatment required
Osteosarcoma	Low	Metastatic disease in >90%; pain palliation
Chondrosarcoma	Intermediate	Best when small; metastasis a problem
Fibrosarcoma	Low to intermediate	Depends on tissue of origin
Injection-related fibrosarcoma	Low to intermediate	Best if done after first surgery, poor later
Thyroid carcinoma	Intermediate to high	Usually respond very well; ^{131}I possible
Thyroid adenoma	High	Treat with ^{131}I (>95% cure)
Salivary adenocarcinoma	Intermediate	Usually respond well, especially in cats
Brain tumor – meningioma	Intermediate to high	Usually stabilizes mass; good clinical result
Brain tumor – glioma	Low to intermediate	Depends on size, location, and clinical signs
Brain tumor – lymphoma	High	Most effective treatment for CNS lymphoma
Brain tumor – metastasis	Intermediate	Effective but short term due to other disease
Spinal cord mesenchymal tumor	Intermediate	Reasonable response but dose limited by cord
Spinal neurofibrosarcoma	Low to intermediate	Short-term response good but commonly recur
Lymphosarcoma	High	Excellent response but can only treat locally
Cutaneous lymphoma	High	Often curative
Nasal lymphoma	High	Good response, often very durable
Thymoma	Low to high	Low for scirious form, high for lymphocytic

(continued)

TABLE 4 SELECTED COMMON NEOPLASMS THAT CAN BE TREATED WITH RADIATION THERAPY *(continued)*

Tumor Type	Radiosensitivity	Comments
Mediastinal chemodectoma	Low	Large masses, dose limited by heart and lungs
Adrenal neoplasias	Low	Difficult to accurately localize treatment
Transitional cell carcinoma	Intermediate	May respond well initially but recur
Prostatic adenocarcinoma	Low to intermediate	Data available on response is quite variable
Mast cell tumors	Intermediate to high	Very good for low grade, less for high grade
Peripheral nerve sheath tumor	Intermediate to high	Strongly recommended after surgery
Soft-tissue sarcoma	Low to high	Improves control after surgery, not alone
Lick granuloma	Intermediate to high	Treatment of last resort, often works well
Transmissible venereal tumor	High	Very good control even for large tumors
Equine sarcoid	High	Used in refractory tumors, brachytherapy
Equine nasal carcinoma	Intermediate to high	Beam treatment effective, very few sites
Equine ocular squamous cell carcinoma	Intermediate to high	Best treatment when bone involved

heavily regulated in most of the world. Today, it is virtually impossible to purchase these sources because of public safety concerns.

Veterinary radiation therapy practices today almost exclusively use linear accelerators as the source of the ionizing radiation used to treat neoplasia and occasionally specific benign diseases. These machines produce powerful x-rays and electron beams with energies of 4–20 million electron volts. The x-rays are used to treat deep-seated tumors, whereas electron beams are generally used to treat tumors of the skin and subcutis. Linear accelerators are complex machines that require the support of a medical physicist to maintain safe and effective use. This increased support load is offset by the machine's flexibility and speed, which is necessary as treatment techniques become more sophisticated and complex.

Computerized treatment planning systems are now used by veterinary radiation oncologists to improve the localization and distribution of the therapeutic beam within the patient. This reduces the dose to healthy tissues relative to the dose to the neoplastic tissue being treated, increasing cure or control rates and reducing the severity of healthy tissue complications. These programs are best used in conjunction with CT or MRI images, which determine the position and extent of the tumor within the body and its relative position to healthy structures. Many hours of work may be required to generate a treatment plan for a large, complex tumor.

Patients are then treated in precisely the same position as they were in for the CT or MRI. Repeatability of positioning is of paramount importance and can be achieved by using special positioning devices in conjunction with careful landmarking. Proper patient positioning is then confirmed using an imaging system integrated with the linear accelerator. Once proper positioning is confirmed, the treatment can be administered. Great attention to detail is necessary during this part of the treatment, because even small changes in position can have profound effects on the distribution of the radiation dose delivered. This is especially true in CNS tumors, in which the lesion diameter may be only 1 cm.

Except in rare instances, all radiation therapy treatments using external sources of radiation must be delivered with the patient immobilized by general anesthesia. Because the plane of anesthesia required is light and the procedures are typically of a relatively short duration, this repeated anesthesia is well tolerated, and complications are few with proper observation and monitoring. This requirement for anesthesia is rarely if ever a contraindication for implementing a course of radiation therapy.

A typical course of radiation therapy consists of multiple doses of radiation delivered on different days. This is done to allow healthy tissues to heal somewhat between doses. Healthy tissues have a greater ability to repair radiation damage than neoplastic tissues; therefore, use of multiple small doses of radiation, although it has a cumulative effect, favors survival of healthy over neoplastic tissues. Most radiation therapy regimens designed with curative intent use 15–20 individual doses (fractions) of radiation. Each dose of radiation may be delivered using several different fractions of radiation of differing size, shape, and intensity. In cases when the tumor is too advanced to be controlled by radiation, palliative therapy using larger doses and fewer fractions of radiation may be used to retard the tumor's growth or reduce associated pain. Such a palliative approach may also be used when mandated by owner finances.

Whenever possible, removal of a tumor by surgery is preferred. However, in many instances, large neoplasms, or those in critical areas such as the brain, are not amenable to complete or even partial surgical removal. Even when a tumor is grossly removed, microscopic foci of neoplastic cells often extend beyond the limits of the surgical field. This is more common for some tumor types than for others. In all of these instances, radiation therapy, often in combination with chemotherapy, is useful in treating the remaining cancer. Radiation therapy is often the treatment of choice for brain tumors, nasal tumors, and other neoplasms of the head and neck in which even partial *resection* may be extremely disfiguring or carry a high risk of mortality. It may be the only treatment option for cancer of the vertebral column and pelvic canal. Radiotherapy is also used to treat tumors in the mediastinum and soft tissues of the skin and subcutis either before or after surgery. It is seldom used in the treatment of lung neoplasia or in the treatment of neoplastic disease of the abdominal cavity because of the mobility of tumors in these areas. However, treatment of mediastinal tumors and those of the pelvic canal, such as thymoma and prostatic carcinoma, are possible and may well be indicated. As the sophistication of radiotherapy techniques increases, more and more types of neoplasia are being treated at least in part by radiation therapy.

In many instances, radiation therapy, especially when combined with surgery and chemotherapy, may be curative. However, radiation therapy can delay the development of disease or control its expansion in many instances. Radiation oncologists typically talk in terms of control rate rather than cure. Sometimes, the control may be relatively short lived, and recrudescence of the tumor occurs within months after completion of the treatment regimen. In other cases, control may last several years or even until other disease processes supersede the neoplastic disease. Unfortunately, it is seldom possible to predict even within an individual tumor type which patients will experience good control and which ones will not. Continual advances in the evaluation of genetic markers within tumors hold the promise of being able to predict this in the future.

Because of the risk of serious and potentially life-threatening complications associated with this treatment modality, the complexity of the equipment and sophistication of the radiation therapy procedures should only be prescribed by and administered under the supervision of a veterinarian with special training, experience, and certification in the field of veterinary radiation oncology. A veterinary radiation oncologist should also be consulted any time further treatment is contemplated for neoplasia that has been treated by radiation therapy. This is particularly important if surgery within the radiation field is being considered.

Brachytherapy is the implantation of radioactive sources into the tumor to achieve radiation therapy. It is seldom used for treatment of cancers in animals because of the difficulties associated with maintenance of the sources and keeping the sources in place within the tumor. The notable exception to this is the use of radioiodine to treat thyroid adenomas in cats and adenocarcinomas in dogs. Radioisotopes developed for treatment of metastatic osseous neoplasia in people are also useful in the treatment of primary and metastatic bone cancer in dogs and cats. Such "nuclear oncology" treatments are being continually developed for use in human medicine and are directly applicable to veterinary patients as well. In fact, these treatments are typically developed in veterinary patients before being introduced into human medicine.

Implantable radiation sources that are so small (microns or even nanometers) that they are permanently implanted within the body blur the margins between radiation therapy and nuclear medicine. The implantation of such sources comes under the heading **interventional radiology**. Interventional radiology procedures such as catheter placement and CT guidance of source implantation are used to introduce both macroscopic and microscopic scale brachytherapy sources into neoplasms located deep within the body. Targeting of such agents is accomplished either by using sources of sufficient size to be locally retained within the tissue or capillaries of the tumor or by targeting them specifically to tumor cells using monoclonal antibody labeling. These techniques have been around for many years but have not received widespread attention in veterinary medicine because of the cost of both the agents and the equipment required for their implantation. However, in recent years there has been a marked upswing in the interest in such interventional radiology procedures for both treatment and diagnosis, not only of cancer but also of many other conditions. Such techniques may well increase the interest in and availability of brachytherapy procedures. Because of the risk of excessive radiation exposure and contamination of the patient or hospital, these procedures should be performed only by veterinarians with appropriate training, experience, and support in a properly licensed facility.

A full list of appropriately trained and accredited veterinarians as well as a list of radiation therapy facilities can be obtained through the American College of Veterinary Radiology or the American Veterinary Medical Association.

The radiosensitivity of virtually any neoplasm is higher in minimal or microscopic disease. Some neoplasms respond well initially but tend to recur at some time after radiation therapy. The time to recrudescence is highly variable between and within tumor types.

EMERGENCY MEDICINE AND CRITICAL CARE

EMERGENCY MEDICINE INTRODUCTION

Emergency patients present special challenges because their underlying disease processes can cause immediate, life-threatening problems that require rapid and aggressive intervention. In addition, the full extent of the animal's illness, injuries, or toxicity may not be evident for 24–48 hr or more after initial presentation.

Problems can arise from an acute illness, toxicity, or injury; from a chronic illness that has decompensated; or from an unexpected complication of a concurrent illness. The status of all postoperative patients should be considered critical until life-threatening anesthetic or surgical complications are excluded. The golden rule of emergency medicine is to treat the most life-threatening problems first.

Variables that contribute to the overall success of emergency treatment include the severity of the primary illness or injury, the amount of fluid or blood lost, age of the animal, previous health problems, the number and extent of associated conditions, time delay in instituting therapy, the volume and rate of fluid administration, and the choice of fluids (eg, crystalloid, blood components, or synthetic colloids). Therapy must be done at the right time, in the right amount, and in the right order. Therapeutic failures are generally a result of failing to act expeditiously at a crucial moment.

Emergency care often begins with the owner's initial telephone call. Instructing the owner on first aid and transport procedures can be life-saving for the animal. The clinic and staff must be in readiness, especially if more than one animal in critical condition arrives at the same time. The primary survey, or **triage** (*see* below), requires a quick and accurate assessment and decision regarding the stability of the animal. As life-threatening airway, breathing, and circulation problems are identified, immediate treatment is initiated. Once the animal has been stabilized, a more systematic and organized approach to the history and physical examination (secondary survey) and more specific diagnostic and therapeutic procedures aimed at the underlying cause can be done.

FIRST AID AND TRANSPORT

Owners can provide significant medical assistance at the scene of the injury. At the time of the initial telephone call, the owner should be questioned about the level of consciousness, breathing pattern, type of injury or toxicity, and even some aspects of the animal's perfusion (eg, gum color, level of responsiveness, heart rate). The first concern is for the safety of the owner. Placing a light cloth over the head of the animal can lessen external stimuli that may cause fearful and aggressive reactions. Owners can be instructed as to how to muzzle most dogs using a long strip of fabric if there are no facial injuries or respiratory distress. Cats can be placed in dark boxes to minimize stress during transport; the box should have holes large enough so that the cat can be observed. It is vital that the owner adequately restrain the pet before starting any first aid procedures to ensure the safety of the owner and pet.

When moving the animal, motion of the head, neck, and spine should be minimized. A flat, firm board of wood, cardboard, or thick fabric can be used to provide support. Radiographs can also be taken through these materials without having to move the animal when it arrives at the hospital.

Rapid detection of cardiopulmonary arrest (CPA) in an unconscious animal can be difficult for owners. The pet's lack of response to external stimuli or presence of limp body tone are unreliable indicators of CPA. Instructing owners to feel for a pulse or heart rate can delay intervention. Instead, owners can be instructed to watch for chest excursions and to touch the cornea or eyelids to elicit a corneal or palpebral reflex in an unconscious pet, with absence of one or both indicative of CPA.

Mouth-to-nose resuscitation and chest compressions (*see* p 1670) may provide enough respiratory and circulatory support to maintain life during transport. If the animal is cyanotic and collapsed (and was pawing at the face), an upper airway obstruction may be present; the owner should be instructed how to perform a Heimlich maneuver or sudden chest compression to relieve the obstruction and then to manually clear the airway. If the animal is unconscious and not breathing, the owner should be instructed to close the animal's mouth, place their lips over the animal's nostrils, and initially give 3–4 strong breaths. If the animal's breathing does not become spontaneous, the owner should breathe for the animal at a rate of 10 breaths/min. The owners can also be instructed to compress the esophagus behind the mandible on the left side so that most of the air will go down the airway instead of into the stomach. Chest compressions should be initiated at a rate of 100–120/min. A compression: ventilation ratio of 30:2 can be performed. This necessitates another person to drive during transport.

Owners should be asked whether hemorrhage is ongoing or whether bleeding was seen at the site of injury. Pulsating arterial bleeding should be controlled by direct digital pressure and then by a pressure bandage. Any long pieces of fabric or gauze can be used. Often, washcloths and hand towels are adequate when applied with mild pressure. Additional material can be placed over the original bandage if it becomes soaked with blood. If the bleeding from a limb is venous (dark, oozing), the limb can be elevated above the heart. Tourniquets should be used only on appendages (eg, limbs, tail) when compression wraps have failed to control bleeding. The tension on the tourniquet must be relaxed to allow blood flow to the distal limb and then retightened every 5–8 min.

Penetrating foreign objects (eg, sticks, arrows) should be left in place during transport; however, care should be taken to guard against movement of the object to prevent further injury. It is often necessary to stabilize the shaft of the penetrating object just outside the body and, holding it firmly, cut off the shaft, leaving a portion exposed so it can be easily located.

In dogs with fractures below the elbow or stifle with significant displacement—and, therefore, concern for movement causing damage to muscle, nerve, vessels, or bone—support can be provided during transport. Once the pet has been adequately restrained, the owner can make a support splint from a rolled newspaper or magazine, which is secured in place by long pieces of fabric or duct tape.

Animals with altered mentation after trauma should be transported with the head level with the body or elevated 20°. There should not be any jerking or thrashing motions, and manipulations of the neck or occlusion of the jugular veins should be minimized.

If a toxic ingestion is present, the owner should be instructed to bring the animal immediately to a veterinarian. Instructing an owner by phone to administer hydrogen peroxide or other substances carries the risk of further injury such as a vagal response (resulting in collapse and bradycardia), choking on vomitus, aspiration pneumonia, further toxic injury from caustic substances, or mucosal injury from hydrogen peroxide administration. If possible, the container of the likely toxin should be brought in.

READY AREA

A central area of the clinic should be designated as the "ready area," where resuscitation therapeutics and equipment are organized and available for immediate use. Front desk and triage staff should be aware of presenting conditions that require immediate evaluation by a veterinarian. All members of the veterinary team must be familiar with the ready area and location of all necessary emergency equipment and medications. Regular drills should be organized for emergency situations such as CPA with subsequent cardiopulmonary resuscitation efforts to ensure everyone knows his or her role and to improve techniques. An emergency treatment or "crash" cart should contain endotracheal tubes of various sizes, a laryngoscope, syringes of different sizes with 18- or 20-gauge needles attached, and drugs for cardiac resuscitation. Oxygen and a small and large bag-valve-mask apparatus or other ready access to oxygen (such as an anesthetic machine flushed free of anesthetic gas) should be immediately available, so positive-pressure ventilation can be started. Other necessary materials include hair clippers, surgical scrub, tape, intravenous and intraosseous catheters with flushing solutions, intravenous isotonic crystalloids, pressure infusion bags, synthetic colloids, bandage material, and trauma transport materials. Additional beneficial equipment includes a defibrillator, monitoring devices (ECG, SpO_2, $ETCO_2$, and indirect blood pressure), a suction unit with Yankauer and whistle tip suction attachments, and warming devices.

EVALUATION AND INITIAL TREATMENT OF THE EMERGENCY PATIENT

PRIMARY SURVEY (TRIAGE) AND RESUSCITATION

Triage is the art of assigning priority to emergency patients and their problems based on rapid assessment of historical and physical parameters (*see* TABLE 1). *Several historical* or observed problems warrant transfer of the animal to the treatment area regardless of physical findings. These problems include known or suspected trauma, poisonings, profuse vomiting or diarrhea, urethral obstruction, labored breathing, cardiopulmonary arrest, seizures, loss of consciousness, severe alterations in mental state, acute inability to walk, excessive bleeding, prolapsed organs, potential snake bite, heat prostration, open wounds exposing extensive soft tissue or bone, anemia, burns, dystocia, shock, and disease that may rapidly decompensate such as gastric dilatation and volvulus and allergic reactions.

TABLE 1 PARAMETERS TO EVALUATE DURING TRIAGE

Parameter	Evaluation	Significance
Mucous membrane color	Pink	Normal PCV and adequate perfusion
	Pale or white	Anemia or shock
	Cyanotic	Severe hypoxemia
	Yellow	Increased serum bilirubin due to hepatic disease or hemolysis
Capillary refill time	1–2 sec	Normal perfusion and rapidity with which capillaries refill with blood
	>2 sec	Poor perfusion or peripheral vasoconstriction
	<1 sec	Hyperdynamic states; could be associated with fever, heat stroke, distributive shock, or early compensatory stage of hypovolemic shock
Heart rate	70–120 bpm (small dogs) 60–120 bpm (large dogs) 120–200 bpm (cats)	Normal heart rates; indicate that at least one component of cardiac output is normal
	Bradycardia	Decreased cardiac output and subsequent poor perfusion; cats in particular develop bradycardia (<120 bpm) in shock; an irregular, slow heart beat can be associated with imminent cardiac arrest, severe arrhythmias, or metabolic derangements (hyperkalemia, hypocalcemia, etc)
	Tachycardia (dogs >180 bpm, cats >220 bpm)	Compromised diastolic filling; sinus tachycardia often results from hypovolemic shock or pain; tachycardia that is irregular or associated with pulse deficits usually indicates an arrhythmia, and an ECG is indicated
Pulse rate and quality	Strong and synchronous with each heart beat	Normal; both femoral and digital pulses should be palpated
	Irregular	Usually indicative of a cardiac arrhythmia
	Bounding	Hyperdynamic (compensatory) state of shock
	Weak or absent	Decreased cardiac output, peripheral vasoconstriction, decreased pulse pressure, or thromboses
Level of consciousness	Alert and responsive to surroundings	Normal overall neurologic and metabolic state
	Depressed or obtunded (less responsive to visual and tactile stimuli, sleepy appearance but still arousable)	Can be caused by any illness or decreased perfusion; may be mild, moderate, or severe

(*continued*)

TABLE 1 PARAMETERS TO EVALUATE DURING TRIAGE *(continued)*

Parameter	Evaluation	Significance
	Stupor (arousable only with painful stimuli)	Severe neurologic or metabolic derangements
	Comatose (unarousable with any stimuli) or seizures (usually associated with whole body convulsions, salivation, facial tremors, possibly involuntary urination and defecation)	Abnormal cerebral electrical activity from primary neurologic disease or secondary to metabolic derangements seen in diseases such as diabetes, hepatic encephalopathy, hypoglycemia, or toxin exposure; accurate history or prior health problems, current medications, and possible toxin exposure important
Level of pain	Vocalization, changes in behavior (avoidance, aggression), or physical changes (tachycardia, dilated pupils, etc)	Clinical signs can be similar to those seen in compensatory stage of shock; pain delays healing and must be treated.

Airway, breathing, and circulation are evaluated sequentially, followed by examination for sources of hemorrhage, and determination of the level of consciousness and level of pain. The most common reasons for an animal in catastrophic distress include 1) airway—airway obstruction or disruption; 2) breathing—cyanosis from tension pneumothorax, alveolar flooding (edema fluid or blood), severe bronchoconstriction with air trapping or brain-stem pathology affecting ventilation; and 3) circulation—shock (decreased perfusion), cardiopulmonary arrest, extreme bradyarrhythmias or tachyarrhythmias, cardiac tamponade, and acute intravascular volume loss usually due to internal or external hemorrhage.

Airway

Life-threatening airway pathology (catastrophic or severe) includes complete large airway obstruction and partial obstruction of the large and small airways.

Diagnosis: Animals with complete large airway obstruction are unconscious and apneic. Partial large airway obstruction causes noisy breathing (stridor or stertor), heard without the aid of a stethoscope. Cyanosis and anxiety are often present with loud referred airway sounds heard throughout the thorax on auscultation. Compromise of the extrathoracic airway (nasal passages, pharynx, larynx, or cervical trachea) causes inspiratory stridor; compromise of the intrathoracic trachea or bronchi causes expiratory stridor. Stertor is most common with pharyngeal disease. Possible causes of large airway pathology include foreign bodies, edema, laryngeal paralysis or paresis, tracheal collapse, elongated soft palate, aspiration of stomach contents, neoplasia, and pharyngeal hematomas. Animals with severe small airway obstruction have labored breathing with an expiratory push of the diaphragm, cyanosis, and anxiety. Auscultation reveals high-pitched wheezes throughout the lung field. In severe life-threatening situations, the animal is cyanotic, open-mouth breathing, collapsed, and asphyxiating. Common causes include anaphylactic reactions; asthma (cats); and bronchial obstruction from edema, mucus, exudates, or foreign material.

Treatment: Unconscious, apneic animals require immediate tracheal intubation. The clinician should be practiced in orotracheal intubation of animals in dorsal, lateral, and sternal recumbency. If an obstruction is present, it must be immediately relieved (with suction, manual removal, or the Heimlich maneuver) or bypassed via emergency tracheotomy. Once an airway is established, confirmed, and secured, ventilation is initiated with 100% oxygen via a bag-valve-mask. Should auscultation during ventilation detect absent or muffled lung sounds indicative of pleural fluid or air, immediate thoracocentesis is warranted. Heart sounds and pulses are checked and, when absent, cardiopulmonary resuscitation (*see* p 1670) is initiated.

With partial large airway obstruction, flow-by oxygen is delivered through oxygen tubing at a high flow rate aimed at the open, panting mouth until an airway is secured or, if appropriate, a transtracheal or nasotracheal oxygen line is placed. Heavy sedation using a narcotic/tranquilizer (eg, butorphanol 0.2–0.4 mg/kg with or without acepromazine 0.01–0.05 mg/kg) combination may be used to relieve anxiety and struggling, to allow a cursory examination of the pharynx and larynx, and to remove pharyngeal foreign bodies. When tracheal intubation is necessary, general anesthesia should be induced using rapid-acting IV anesthetics such as etomidate (0.5–3 mg/kg), ketamine/diazepam combination (5–20 mg/kg and 0.1–0.4 mg/kg), or propofol (6–8 mg/kg to effect). The ability of the laryngeal cartilages to abduct during inspiration should be assessed during intubation and a full oropharyngeal examination performed when time allows. A tracheotomy is necessary when pharyngeal, laryngeal, or tracheal pathology prevents orotracheal intubation or when prolonged intubation is anticipated. A transtracheal catheter can be used to provide oxygen support during stabilization. When the airway pathology lies within the thoracic cavity, airway patency must be established down to the bifurcation of the trachea. Once the airway is established, it should be secured with a tie and inflation of the cuff mechanism, as well as confirmed with at least two of the following methods: palpation of the tube within trachea in the cervical region, ausculation of the lungs and visualization of chest wall movement when a breath is administered, visualization of the tube entering the airway, placement of an end-tidal CO_2 monitor, or radiographs.

Cyanosis from small airway obstructive disease is treated by providing oxygen by flow-by, hood, or nasal cannula and sedation with a narcotic/tranquilizer combination. Epinephrine is given for its bronchodilatory effects both in anaphylaxis (0.01–0.02 mg/kg, IV) and in life-threatening asthma (0.02 mg/kg, IM). Corticosteroids (prednisone sodium succinate, 15 mg/kg, IV, or dexamethasone, 2–4 mg/kg, IM or IV) are given for allergic bronchitis, asthma, or severe swelling of the larynx or pharyngeal tissues. Other bronchodilators, such as aminophylline or terbutaline, are given IM, or albuterol can be given by nebulization in the case of an animal in crisis.

Breathing

Diagnosis: Compromised breathing in both dogs and cats manifests with an increased respiratory rate and effort, immediately followed by a change in the respiratory pattern. Postural changes (orthopnea) follow; dogs stand with the elbows abducted and the back arched or high on the rear haunches with the head and neck extended, whereas cats may sit crouched on all four limbs with the sternum slightly elevated. Obvious labored, open-mouth breathing, and changes in mucous membrane color (gray and/or blue [cyanosis]) develop last and indicate significant loss of pulmonary function and impending pulmonary arrest.

The location of the pathology—pleural space or parenchymal disease—can be determined at presentation by careful observation of the breathing pattern and auscultation of the thorax. This will direct resuscitative efforts. Taking radiographs or performing stressful diagnostic procedures before the animal has been stabilized can lead to rapid decompensation.

Pleural space disease causes asynchronous breathing. The chest expands on inspiration as the abdomen is pulled inward, then the chest moves inward on expiration as the abdomen expands. In cats, breathing is slower and more deliberate than in dogs. The respiratory pattern is the same whether air, fluid, or abdominal contents are in the pleural space. Thoracic auscultation reveals muffled lung sounds over the affected regions.

Lung parenchymal disease causes quiet, smooth breathing, with the chest and abdominal wall moving in the same direction. Inspiration and expiration are equally labored unless concurrent small airway edema or constriction adds an expiratory push. Cats demonstrate rapid, shallow synchronous breathing, often with movement of the cupula. Thoracic auscultation reveals louder than normal lung sounds in early phases. As disease progresses, harsh lung sounds with moist crackles and rales are heard over the affected lungs. Pulmonary edema may be cardiogenic, often accompanied by a murmur, gallop, or arrhythmia noted on auscultation and mild hypothermia. Other differential diagnoses include CNS disease, pneumonia (viral, parasitic, fungal, or bacterial), aspiration, pulmonary contusions, or hemoglobin abnormalities. Noncardiogenic pulmonary edema may be caused by seizures, electrocution, after an acute airway obstruction (such as after choking or near-drowning) and acute lung injury, or respiratory distress syndrome.

Thoracic radiography should be performed only when the animal is able to tolerate the procedure. Radiographs can help differentiate many of these diseases;

however, imaging should not delay therapy. Some animals may be more tolerant of ultrasonography. The thoracic focused assessment with sonography (TFAST) technique may be used to identify pleural fluid and air, examining both hemithoraces between the fifth and sixth ribs ventrally and between the seventh and ninth ribs dorsally. A pneumothorax may be present when the "slide sign" is absent; this is a linear movement noted between the visceral and parietal pleura and requires practice to identify.

Treatment: Oxygen is administered immediately via flow-by, mask, hood, or oxygen cage techniques. Sedation with a narcotic/tranquilizer combination (butorphanol 0.2–0.4 mg/kg, IV or IM, with or without acepromazine, 0.05 mg/kg, IV or IM) can relieve struggling and anxiety. Longterm continuous supplemental oxygen is best provided by a nasal oxygen catheter. The intranasal oxygen catheter is placed after topical anesthetic has been instilled into the nostril where the tube is to be inserted. Humidified nasal oxygen flow rates of 50–100 mL/kg/min deliver 40%–60% inspired oxygen while allowing the animal to be examined and the underlying disease treated. Nasopharyngeal or nasotracheal catheters or bilateral nasal cannulas may provide higher percentages of inspired oxygen. If cyanosis and decompensation persist or work of breathing is profound, intubation and positive-pressure manual ventilation or mechanical ventilation with 100% oxygen is necessary.

Catastrophic pleural space disease with rapid cardiovascular decompensation, absent lung sounds throughout the thorax, and a barrel-shaped chest suggests tension pneumothorax. A routine thoracocentesis is often inadequate for these animals, so an intercostal incision or placement of a large-bore catheter is necessary: lidocaine is injected for local anesthesia, a small skin incision is made between ribs (at the seventh to eighth intercostal space), and hemostats are used to enter the pleural space, relieving the tension within the thorax. This allows cardiovascular filling and lung reexpansion. The open pneumothorax is then managed by placing a chest tube and surgically closing the intercostal incision.

When breathing is severely compromised *by pleural air or fluid* without tension pneumothorax, the pleural space should be drained by thoracocentesis. The intended site is clipped and aseptically prepared (when time permits). If fluid is expected, the needle is inserted ventrally between the sternum and costochondral junction. When air is to be recovered, the needle is inserted into the dorsal half of the thorax, above the costochondral junction. A local anesthetic is placed into the skin, subcutaneous tissue, and intercostal muscle at the site to be tapped. After the needle is inserted just through the skin, a drop of saline is placed in the hub of the needle. The needle is then gradually inserted straight into the thorax (with the needle perpendicular to the chest wall) until the saline in the needle hub moves. The movement of the saline in the hub indicates that the pleural space has been entered, although this may not always occur. The needle is immediately directed so that it lies against the parietal pleura. This prevents laceration of the lung by the needle as the lung reexpands. As soon as the pleural space is entered, the evacuation apparatus (an IV extension set, 3-way stopcock, and syringe) is attached and aspiration begins. In animals in which the pleural space cannot be emptied (eg, tension pneumothorax, ongoing hemorrhage) or when repeated chest taps are required within minutes to hours, an indwelling chest tube should be placed for continuous closed suction until the problem resolves or futher therapy is performed.

Lung parenchymal disease is primarily treated using oxygen supplementation, sedation to relieve anxiety, and therapy directed at the underlying cause. Cardiogenic edema is usually associated with a gallop, murmur (determined by auscultation), arrhythmia, and/or mild hypothermia and responds well to furosemide administration (1–4 mg/kg, IV, every 1–2 hr) in all but the most severe of cases. Furosemide is more effective when delivered as a constant-rate infusion (1–2 mg/kg/hr). Cardiogenic edema can benefit from venodilation from nitroglycerin ointment (¼ in. for cats and ½ in. for larger dogs) applied topically to a shaved area of the abdomen, inguinal region, or directly to a mucous membrane; severely affected animals with normal blood pressure may benefit from a balanced vasodilator (nitroprusside, 0.5–10 mcg/kg/min), tapered up slowly and monitoring blood pressure continuously to keep the mean arterial pressure >85 mmHg. After initial stabilization, further diagnostic procedures (eg, thoracic radiography and echocardiography) aid in determining the cause and specific therapy. Animals with proteinaceous fluid (such as occurs with noncardiogenic pulmonary edema, respiratory distress syndrome, pneumonia, etc) will not respond to simple diuretic therapy. If oxygen supplementation does not maintain PaO_2 >60 mmHg (pulse oximetry or SpO_2 >90%), or if $PaCO_2$ ≥60 mmHg, or if there is moderate to severe increases in work of breathing despite oxygen therapy, then manual or mechanical positive-pressure ventilation is required.

If respiratory failure is imminent with pulmonary fluid visible in mouth or nares, then intubation, airway suctioning, and manual bag-valve-mask ventilation with 100% oxygen are required. Elevated or postural pulmonary parenchymal evacuation (EPPE) can be performed with two or more people elevating the pet vertically, head down, while guarding the endotracheal tube. The thoracic cavity is manually compressed to assist airway and lung fluid drainage. Manual ventilation with 100% oxygen and suction of the airway should be performed between EPPE efforts.

Circulation

Diagnosis: Animals with circulatory compromise have alterations in their physical perfusion parameters (ie, heart rate, mucous membrane color, capillary refill time [CRT], rectal temperature, pulse quality, and level of consciousness). Careful auscultation of the heart for a murmur, gallop, arrhythmia, or muffled heart sounds and of the lungs for evidence of fluid is important to help identify heart failure as a cause of poor perfusion. Measurement of arterial blood pressure, central venous pressure, central venous PaO_2, and serum lactate provide objective data for reaching resuscitation endpoints and monitoring trends of change after resuscitation.

In the early compensatory stages of hypovolemic shock in dogs, there is a rapid heart rate, pink to red mucous membranes, rapid CRT, and bounding pulses; the animal is most often alert and responsive. Animals with a significant amount of pain or anxiety may appear to be in compensatory shock; pain medications are warranted, and time for the animal to acclimate to the environment is helpful. This stage is rarely identified in cats. Tachycardia is often the first and only sign, so persistent tachycardia must be considered a sign of decreased perfusion and addressed as such. As the pathology progresses, dogs begin to have pale mucous membranes, prolonged CRT, weak pulses, tachycardia, and a decreased level of responsiveness—the classic signs of the middle or early decompensatory stage of shock. Cats have gray mucous membranes, slow CRT, weak or absent pulses, hypothermia, and a normal or low heart rate. As shock approaches the terminal stages, the heart rate slows in both dogs and cats, and animals begin to lose consciousness. Clinical signs in this terminal stage include heart failure, pulmonary edema, severe hypotension, oliguria, and abnormal respiratory patterns. Cardiopulmonary arrest is a common sequela.

Treatment: The therapeutic goal is to deliver oxygen and substrate to the tissues. This requires a heart that effectively pumps blood and adequate hemoglobin, intravascular volume, vascular tone and patency, as well as sufficient oxygen and substrate for cellular metabolism. General guidelines for treatment of hypovolemic and distributive shock are described below, but modifications may be needed for specific animals or disease processes.

Oxygen Supplementation: Oxygen (at least 40%–60% inspired concentration) should be administered by flow-by technique, mask, hood, nasal cannula, endotracheal tube, or transtracheal catheter.

Hemostasis: Control of ongoing hemorrhage is essential for stabilization and often required before restoration of circulation. The animal must be carefully and thoroughly examined for any evidence of external hemorrhage. Direct pressure should be immediately placed over the bleeding skin site, and bleeding arteries clamped. When blood slowly oozes from a skin wound, a compression bandage should be placed. If more aggressive hemostasis is required, a blood pressure (pneumatic) cuff or tourniquet can be temporarily placed until coagulation occurs or surgical intervention is used to stop the bleeding. Tourniquets should not remain in place for >10 min.

Intrathoracic or abdominal hemorrhage may be dfficult to detect and may be exacerbated when blood pressure and circulation are restored. The focused abdominal sonography for trauma (FAST) technique may be used to rapidly identify free abdominal fluid, focusing the probe on the ventral midline caudal to the xiphoid, over the urinary bladder, and on the right and left dependent flank regions. A four-quadrant abdominocentesis can be performed if ultrasound is not immediately available. The TFAST may be used to identify pleural fluid as well.

Ongoing abdominal hemorrhage is initially managed by small volume fluid resuscitation to low-normal endpoints and abdominal counterpressure (*see* p 1667). Ongoing intrathoracic hemorrhage should be managed with thoracocentesis or a thoracostomy tube to evacuate the blood and to allow measurement of the volume lost. Exploration of these body cavities may be required for assessment and definitive hemostasis if a coagulopathy is not present. PCV of thoracic or abdominal fluid the same or higher than that of peripheral blood confirms hemorrhage. Significant volumes of cavitary hemorrhage may be collected in sterile, empty IV bags or blood transfusion bags for autologous blood transfusion, if necessary.

Intravascular Volume Replacement: Intravenous or intraosseous catheters are used, with multiple catheters placed for rapid, large-volume infusion in dogs >30 kg body wt. Isotonic crystalloids can be administered by repeated low-volume boluses (10–15 mL/kg) until desired endpoints of resuscitation are reached (eg, low-normal cardiovascular parameters). However, the interstitium is at risk of fluid overload with crystalloids alone. The concurrent use of colloids and crystalloids can reduce the amount of crystalloid required, rapidly expand the intravascular space with a smaller volume of fluid infused, and reduce the amount of fluid extravasating into the interstitial spaces of vital organs (eg, lung, brain). Isotonic crystalloids are given with hydroxyethylstarches (eg, hetastarch) or stroma-free hemoglobin. Whole blood, stroma-free hemoglobin, or packed red cells are necessary during initial volume resuscitation when hemorrhage has been significant.

Small volume resuscitation to low-normal endpoints (measured perfusion parameters) is used to avoid volume overload or hypertension and is ideal for animals with head injury, pulmonary edema or contusions, abdominal or intrathoracic hemorrhage, heart disease, and all cats in hypovolemic shock. Isotonic crystalloids are given (10–15 mL/kg, IV), followed by hetastarch or stroma-free hemoglobin (dogs 5 mL/kg, IV; cats 1–5 mL/kg, IV, slowly), repeating the colloid infusion, to effect. The least amount of crystalloids and colloids possible are used to obtain and maintain a systolic blood pressure of 90 mmHg, restore a normal heart rate, and improve CRT and pulses. For an in-depth explanation, *see* p 1675.

Pain Control: Analgesia is provided *during initial fluid* resuscitation for optimal cardiovascular response and relief of anxiety. Narcotics are administered systemically, and local anesthetics can be infiltrated into the affected area. (*See also* p 2104.)

Warming: Animals in shock should be warmed during fluid resuscitation until rectal temperatures are >98°F. This is best accomplished by increasing the environmental temperature using warm air blowers or hot water bottles with blankets, warm water blankets, and IV fluid line warmers. Gastric, peritoneal, or urinary lavage may be needed for severe hypothermia. Surface warming is instituted only after initial volume resuscitation has provided enough intravascular volume to offset the peripheral vasodilation. Care must be taken in animals with cardiogenic shock or pericardial disease to avoid excessive peripheral vasodilation, because this may exacerbate a relative hypovolemia (due to decreased cardiac output).

Corticosteroids: Corticosteroids are administered when a deficiency is suspected (ie, Addisonian crisis, critical illness–related corticosteroid insufficiency). High-dose steroid administration has not been proved to reduce mortality in hypovolemic, septic, or cardiogenic shock and has been associated with increased morbidity, so it is not recommended.

Cardiovascular Support: Pharmacologic agents (positive inotropes, systemic vasodilators, and vasopressors) can be used when fluid infusion has adequately replaced intravascular volume (ie, central venous pressure >5–8 cm H_2O) but fails to restore blood pressure and perfusion, or when poor cardiac contractility is thought to contribute to hypotension. A positive inotropic agent can be administered to increase cardiac contractility in diseases such as sepsis and dilated cardiomyopathy (eg, dobutamine, initially at 2–5 mcg/kg/min, and the dosage titrated for optimal cardiac output). Stroma-free hemoglobin (dogs 5 mL/kg; cats 1–3 mL per cat, slowly) can be administered, and repeated as indicated, for its colloid effect as well as its mild vasopressor effect; it is particularly useful in animals with concurrent anemia. The initial resuscitation doses may be followed by a slow constant-rate infusion (dogs 10–15 mL/kg/day; cats 1–3 mL/hr up to 5 mL/kg/day) to maintain perfusion if the initial dose was successful and further support is anticipated. Pressor agents delivered as an IV constant-rate infusion such as dopamine (5–20 mcg/kg/min), norepinephrine (0.05–2 mcg/kg/min) or vasopressin (extra-label, 1–4 mU/kg/min) are other options to support blood pressure; they should be delivered in the smallest dosage needed to maintain arterial systolic pressure >90 mmHg. The blood flow to the kidneys and GI tract, as well as other organs, may have been significantly impaired during shock. Urine output, heart rate, blood pressure, ECG, pulse intensity, and mucous membrane color should be closely monitored, because further vasoconstriction can worsen organ blood flow and function. If organ function declines or if arrhythmias become a problem, the IV drip should be stopped.

Hindlimb and Abdominal Binding: When ongoing abdominal hemorrhage is suspected from trauma, hindlimb and abdominal counterpressure can improve perfusion. This procedure compresses the arteries and arterioles within the bound regions, increasing regional vascular resistance, and produces abdominal tamponade, thereby effectively slowing or arresting hemorrhage and redirecting blood flow from the venous capacitance vessels in the caudal half of the body to the more central (core) circulation. Hindlimb and abdominal counterpressure can be performed by placing a rolled towel or rolled cotton between the legs and along the ventral midline of the abdomen. This prevents the wrap from impairing ventilation or fracturing the spleen or liver. If time permits, a urinary catheter is placed. The hindlimbs and abdomen are then firmly wrapped with padded bandage material or towels, beginning at the toes of the hindlimb and moving cranially toward the xiphoid, taking care not to impede respiration. The bandage should be secured with tape or stretch bandage material wrapped in a spiral pattern starting caudally and moving cranially. Abdominal binding should be avoided in cases of intrathoracic or intracranial hemorrhage. Once perfusion has stabilized, the wrap is removed slowly by sections (releasing one section every 15 min) from the abdomen, starting at the most cranial portion and moving caudally. Any signs of decompensation warrant rapid rebinding of the region last unwrapped.

SECONDARY SURVEY

The secondary survey of emergency patients is the process of obtaining significant and thorough historical information, performing a complete physical examination, and collecting general diagnostic information. These data are used to direct the formulation of a specific diagnostic, therapeutic, and monitoring plan.

The **history** should be recorded in a concise format. The presenting complaint is obtained from the owner, who can provide information such as when the animal was last completely normal. A chronology of the daily progression of abnormalities since the onset of signs can be useful. Background information includes past medical problems, toxicities, medications, drug and food sensitivities, blood transfusions, the date of last vaccinations, and other preventive care. Other organ systems not seemingly involved should also be historically evaluated. Details of the specific disease process are obtained and may help direct diagnostics and care.

A complete **physical examination** should be performed, working from head to tail. Particular attention is given to heart and lung auscultation for abnormalities, and to abdominal, rectal, and joint palpation for pain or enlargements. A complete neurologic and orthopedic examination is often warranted. Acute abdominal pain requires localization of the pain and auscultation of the abdomen for bowel sounds to localize the problem to the reticuloendothelial, reproductive, urinary, or GI systems; the peritoneal space; or the muscle, skin, nerves, or fat around the abdominal wall. Fever of unknown origin directs examination to the peritoneal cavity and to the reproductive, urinary, pulmonary, and cardiovascular systems.

An initial **minimum database** should consist of a PCV, total solids, glucose, and BUN. Other important diagnostics include urinalysis (before fluid administration), venous or arterial blood gas, an electrolyte panel, a CBC, and a serum chemistry panel. When coagulation disorders are suspected or surgery is anticipated, blood smears to estimate platelet number, buccal bleeding time to evaluate platelet function, and a clotting profile such as an activated clotting time or prothrombin time and activated partial thromboplastin time are warranted.

A deficit in any of the first three components of the primary survey (ie, airway, breathing, circulation) will quickly result in anaerobic metabolism due to poor oxygen delivery to the tissues. This can rapidly result in a type A lactic acidosis. Lactate can be accurately, easily, and rapidly measured with several point-of-care analyzers. Normal lactate values in dogs and cats are <2 mmol/L. Lactate levels normalize rapidly with treatment of the underlying condition of poor oxygen delivery to the tissues and is associated with improved survival. Lactate can be used along with other parameters as an endpoint of resuscitation in hypovolemic animals. Initial increases in blood lactate have been reported to be associated with an increase in complications and mortality in certain diseases in small animals.

SPECIFIC DIAGNOSTICS AND THERAPY

TRAUMA

Diagnostic and therapeutic efforts in emergency situations can be directed by the nature of the trauma. Blunt trauma is commonly associated with thoracic and abdominal bleeding, organ rupture, fractures, and neurologic injuries. Penetrating trauma is typically localized to the path of the penetrating object, which is rarely a straight line. Falling from a height causes long bone and facial bone fractures as well as thoracic and abdominal injuries. A dog bitten by a larger dog can have deep-penetrating bite wounds, spinal injuries, major abdominal and thoracic trauma (even without penetrating wounds), and tracheal rupture from the shearing forces sustained during thrashing motions. Resuscitation of the airway, breathing, and circulation; control of hemorrhage; and pain relief are followed by a careful evaluation of the nervous system, chest, abdomen, integument, and musculoskeletal system.

The traumatized animal should be approached as if multiple injuries are present. The neck and spine should be immobilized until a thorough examination for spinal fractures or luxations is made. Thoracic auscultation for cardiac arrhythmias and the presence and quality of lung sounds should be done to identify chest injuries. The abdomen should be palpated for pain, fluid, or hernias. Extremity fractures should be supported by bandages or splinted to prevent further injury. Significant swelling may indicate ongoing hemorrhage. Because many internal injuries may not be apparent for a significant amount of time after the initial trauma occurs (12–48 hr), close monitoring is essential to allow early detection of potentially life-threatening problems. An animal that appears normal and stable on initial examination may have substantial underlying injury, making monitoring of at least physical examination parameters in the hospital (eg, respiratory and heart rates, mucous membrane color, and mentation) appropriate.

Initial diagnostic evaluation should include the minimum database before fluids are administered, if possible. Point-of-care tests should minimally include a PCV, total solids, BUN test strip, and blood glucose. When hemorrhage first occurs, the peripheral blood PCV may be normal or even increased with a normal or decreased relative total protein level; this is a clinical indication of hemorrhagic shock in dogs and occurs because of splenic contraction. This release of RBCs into circulation may occur faster than interstitial to intravascular fluid shifts; therefore, serial PCV and total solid measurements should be monitored after trauma. Both PCV and total solids will decrease as hemorrhage and subsequent crystalloid/colloid resuscitation continues. An extended initial database includes arterial or venous blood gases, electrolyte panel, blood lactate, and prothrombin time/partial thromboplastin time. This baseline information is used to create the initial treatment plan and to provide the baseline for subsequent monitoring. Ionized hypercalcemia has been associated with a poorer prognosis after trauma and may warrant more intensive monitoring. Survey lateral radiographs of the chest and abdomen at presentation can demonstrate the initial changes resulting from thoracic and abdominal trauma. Orthogonal views should be performed as the animal's condition dictates. Ultrasound examination of the abdominal and thoracic cavities may provide additional information about internal injuries and can often be performed while fluid resuscitation is initiated.

Some scoring systems have been developed for trauma, such as the animal trauma triage score; this system assigns a number from 0 (slight or no injury) to 3 (severe injury) in the following categories: perfusion, cardiac, respiratory, eye-muscle-integument, skeletal, and neurologic. In one study assessing >200 dogs evaluated after vehicular trauma, dogs that died or were euthanized had signficantly higher scores (median 6) than those that survived (median 2); higher scores were also associated with higher cost of care.

Thoracic Trauma

Pulmonary contusions, pneumothorax, cardiac arrhythmias, pleural hemorrhage, pericardial hemorrhage, rib fractures, flail chest, and diaphragmatic hernia are some of the potentially life-threatening complications that must be considered in thoracic trauma. Oxygen supplementation and analgesics allow careful physical examination. An ECG, thoracic radiographs, blood gas analysis, and diagnostic or therapeutic centesis help determine the extent and severity of the problems.

Severe pulmonary contusions cause hypoxemia, labored breathing in a pattern consistent with parenchymal disease, and crackles and rales on pulmonary auscultation. If the animal does not improve with supplemental oxygen, pain medications, and fluid therapy, then tracheal intubation and positive-pressure ventilation with 100% oxygen are indicated. The airway should be suctioned to evacuate blood and debris that are obstructing the flow of air.

Labored breathing with asynchronous movement of the chest and abdomen and dull or quiet lung sounds is consistent with pleural air or fluid and warrants immediate thoracocentesis. Thoracocentesis should be performed before taking radiographs in animals with respiratory distress, because animals may struggle and decompensate while radiographs are being taken; assessment with ultrasound may be less stressful but should not delay therapy. When a negative pressure cannot be achieved, repeated thoracocentesis or continuous drainage of the pleural space by chest tube is required. Large quantities of whole blood removed on thoracocentesis or ongoing leakage of air after 72 hr of pleural drainage are indications for surgical exploration of the chest. Large volumes of blood aspirated during a centesis may be collected into an IV bag or blood transfusion bag, because they may be used for autologous blood transfusion.

The thoracic focused assessment with sonography technique (TFAST) can help diagnose pneumothorax, hemothorax, or thoracic wall trauma and provides an alternative to radiographs when performed by a skilled sonographer familiar with ultrasonographic changes associated with these injuries. The chest cavity should be palpated for rib fractures with displaced bone, flail segments, avulsion of ribs, torn intercostal muscles, and herniations. When flail segments impair ventilation, the segment is stabilized by securing it to an external frame or cast, formed to the shape of the chest. Penetrating bite wounds over the chest should be explored under anesthesia for debridement and drain placement; if the wound is penetrating, the thorax may be surgically entered to inspect damage to underlying tissue, repair or debride that tissue as necessary, lavage the thoracic cavity, and place a thoracostomy tube before closure.

As the animal's condition allows, thoracic radiographs (two or three views) should be performed to assess for injury to the lungs. Many of the above-listed injuries may show up on routine radiographs; however, radiographic evidence of pulmonary contusions may not appear until 12–24 hr after the initial injury.

The heart should be ausculted and an ECG evaluated for arrhythmias. Arrhythmias may not be present at the time of injury but develop 12–48 hr after the event as myocardial contusions and hypoxemia affect the cardiac conduction system. Common arrhythmias seen after thoracic trauma include sinus tachycardia, ventricular premature contractions, and ventricular tachycardia. Treatment with lidocaine or other antiarrhythmic medications is warranted if the arrhythmias impair perfusion, if the rate is rapid and sustained (>180 bpm in dogs), if ventricular premature contractions are multiform, or if there are prefibrillatory rhythms (R on T phenomenon, torsades de pointes, ventricular flutter).

Abdominal Trauma

The extent and severity of abdominal injuries are often not initially apparent, unless there is visceral herniation outside the body cavity. The abdominal surface should be examined closely for evidence of bruising, abrasions, lacerations, protrusions, localized swelling, herniations, distention, and pain. Animals with evidence of abdominal pain that are in shock are considered to have intra-abdominal hemorrhage until proved otherwise. Rupture or laceration of the spleen or liver are the most common sources of intra-abdominal hemorrhage. However, all abdominal organs are susceptible to the shearing forces from blunt trauma. Other common sources of abdominal bleeding include avulsed mesenteric vessels, damaged muscle, or avulsion of the kidneys in the retroperitoneal space.

Approximately 40 mL/kg (just less than half of the circulating blood volume) is necessary before free blood in the abdominal cavity will be evident by palpation or visual inspection; this volume is associated with signs of poor perfusion (shock). Smaller volumes of abdominal fluid may be apparent with radiographs, abdominocentesis, or ultrasound of the abdomen. Abdominal distention from hemorrhage may become apparent if aggressive fluid resuscitation increases blood pressure and disrupts one or more blood clots that provided hemostasis. Small volume fluid resuscitation to achieve a low-normal blood pressure endpoint (90 mmHg systolic) is indicated to avoid sudden increases in arterial or venous pressures. When ongoing abdominal hemorrhage is confirmed, hindlimb and abdominal binding (*see* p 1667) is indicated early to reduce the amount of hemorrhage until hemostasis is accomplished.

After injury of any abdominal organ, clinical signs of organ dysfunction or hollow viscus rupture typically develop over a period of hours but may be longer or shorter depending on the nature of the injury. Acute abdominal pain is a key physical finding. Survey abdominal radiographs can demonstrate organ displacement, distention, rotation, or free abdominal gas or fluid. Fluid can be recovered by four-quadrant abdominocentesis. Using the focused assessment with sonography technique (FAST, *see* p 1665), even small amounts of free fluid in the abdomen can be identified and aspirated using ultrasound guidance.

When free fluid is not readily identified, a diagnostic peritoneal lavage can be done. A fenestrated catheter is placed into the peritoneal space, and warm isotonic saline (20 mL/kg) is infused into the abdomen. The fluid is allowed to dwell for several minutes and distribute throughout the abdomen; it is then drained and evaluated.

Clear fluid indicates that the possibility of significant abdominal hemorrhage is minimal. Fluid with a 1% PCV indicates mild abdominal hemorrhage, whereas fluid with a PCV >5% indicates significant abdominal hemorrhage that warrants careful monitoring.

Fluid obtained from the abdomen should be examined cytologically for evidence of WBCs, plant or meat fibers, and free or intracellular bacteria. Biochemical evaluation for creatinine and potassium, bilirubin, amylase, and phosphorus help identify urinary system rupture, gallbladder rupture, pancreatic injury, or ischemic bowel, respectively. Abdominal fluid glucose that is 20 mg/dL or more below peripheral blood glucose is characteristic of a septic peritonitis and warrants exploratory surgery. The abdominocentesis, peritoneal lavage, or FAST scan can be repeated in several hours if fluid from the first assessment did not indicate a significant problem but the clinical signs continue or progress. Retroperitoneal, fascial, or intramuscular (body wall) hemorrhage or hemorrhage into the GI system can be more challenging to identify.

Criteria for emergency exploratory laparotomy include ongoing hemorrhage; inability to stabilize shock; organ rotation, entrapment, or ischemia; diaphragmatic hernia; and evidence of organ rupture or peritonitis. Some simple bladder ruptures may be amenable to medical management and placement of a urinary catheter. Surgery to repair a diaphragmatic hernia should not be delayed, particularly with gastric displacement into the thoracic cavity, respiratory compromise, or ongoing hemorrhage.

Retroperitoneal, severe fascial compartment hemorrhage (associated with pelvic fractures), or hemorrhage into a hollow viscus is suspected in acutely traumatized animals that still have signs of a declining PCV/total solids, nonresponsive hemorrhagic shock, and no significant findings on abdominocentesis, peritoneal lavage, or FAST scan. Radiographs typically show expansion and loss of detail in the retroperitoneal space. An IV pyelogram should be done to help delineate disruption in the renal vascular supply or in the retroperitoneal portion of the ureter before proceeding with exploratory surgery in this situation.

CARDIOPULMONARY RESUSCITATION

The success of cardiopulmonary resuscitation (CPR) efforts depends on many factors, including the underlying cause of the arrest, the timeliness and effectiveness of the intervention, and the preparedness of the team administering CPR. Overall prognosis of recovery from cardiopulmonary arrest (CPA) with CPR efforts is as high as 35%–44%; however, only <10% of animals survive to discharge. Animals with CPA associated with anesthesia have a better prognosis. The American College of Veterinary Emergency and Critical Care developed the first set of guidelines for veterinary CPR; this effort was termed the Reassessment Campaign on Veterinary Resuscitation (RECOVER) and is available at www.acvecc-recover.org. CPR is divided into several sections: prevention and preparedness; basic cardiac life support (BCLS) promoting oxygenation, ventilation, and circulation; advanced cardiac life support (ACLS) using electrocardiographic evaluation of cardiac rhythms, administration of drugs, and defibrillation when necessary; monitoring during CPR; and postresuscitation management, which involves intensive monitoring of common complications after arrest as well as diagnosis and treatment of underlying conditions that led to the cardiopulmonary arrest.

Prevention and Preparedness

In an effort to have the entire veterinary team prepared for CPR on any animal, RECOVER guidelines recommend standardization and regular audit of resuscitation equipment as well as immediate availability of cognitive aids and descriptive CPR algorithms (eg, dose charts, checklists), which are available through the RECOVER website. Cognitive skill training and didactics should be incorporated for all veterinary team members on a regular basis. Assigning a leader and having specific leadership training, including debriefing after any CPR efforts, are recommended as well. Each team member should be familiar with available medical equipment and his or her role during CPR.

Basic Cardiac Life Support

When CPA is recognized, CPR efforts should begin immediately. Early recognition and intervention is essential. Palpation of pulses is not recommended before initiating compressions, because this will delay intervention. Mouth-to-nose resuscitation should be performed until endotracheal intubation and positive-pressure ventilation with 100% oxygen can be accomplished. The compression to ventilation ratio should be 30:2. Once the airway is established, it is imperative to confirm placement with thoracic auscultation, visualization, palpation, and $ETCO_2$ monitoring, as well as to secure the tube with a tie-in. Ventilations should be provided at a rate of 10 breaths/min, with a volume of 10 mL/kg and an inspiratory time of 1 sec. Ideally, these breaths are provided with a portable bag-valve-mask apparatus.

Simultaneous with ventilation, circulation should be promoted in small animals by compressing the chest externally. Compressions should be performed with the animal in lateral recumbency (or dorsal recumbency for barrel-chested animals, such as Bulldogs). Compressions should be performed over the widest part of the thorax using the "thoracic pump" technique. In keel-shaped animals (such as Greyhounds or cats), compressions may be performed directly over the heart (at the fourth and fifth intercostal space) using the "cardiac pump" technique. The compression rate should be 100–120 compressions/min regardless of size. Each compression should be delivered quickly in a cough-like fashion and should compress the chest wall ⅓ to ½ of the width and allow full recoil of the chest. When the cardiac pump technique is used, direct compression of the ventricles of the heart contribute to forward blood flow; in the thoracic pump technique, changes in thoracic pressure are the important mechanism to generate forward blood flow. Simultaneous ventilations and compressions should be done in 2-min cycles; individuals performing the ventilation and compressions should change functions every 2 min to prevent fatigue and less-effective compressions. Interruptions to chest compressions to assess ECG or auscult the heart should be minimal. Interposed abdominal compressions may be added for animals without abdominal disease if adequately trained staff is available. This is performed by placing both hands on the abdomen and compressing quickly, timing the compression to be done between chest compressions.

The goal is to improve venous return to the heart during the diastolic phase of the compression cycle. Monitoring CPR (*see* below) may necessitate a change in CPR technique.

Advanced Cardiac Life Support

In ACLS, an ECG is obtained to characterize arrhythmias, followed by drug administration or defibrillation as indicated. The purpose is to reestablish electrical and mechanical activity of the heart. The major arresting rhythms in veterinary medicine include sinus bradycardia, asystole, pulseless electrical activity (PEA, previously termed electromechanical dissociation), and ventricular fibrillation or flutter. Drugs are selected based on the arrhythmia or known/suspected underlying disease and can be administered by intravenous, intraosseous, or intratracheal routes (*see* TABLE 2). Drugs that can be administered intratracheally include naloxone, atropine, vasopressin, epinephrine, and lidocaine (best remembered by the acronym NAVEL); the dosage for all drugs is usually doubled when administration is intratracheal. Intracardiac administration of drugs is no longer recommended, because arrhythmias, myocardial hemorrhage, and myocardial vessel laceration may occur.

If the animal is known or suspected to be hypovolemic, isotonic balanced crystalloid solutions should be rapidly infused to restore volume and promote perfusion. Synthetic colloids such as hetastarch, hydroxyethyl starch, dextran 70, or stroma-free hemo-

TABLE 2 DRUGS AND DEFIBRILLATION USED IN CARDIOPULMONARY RESUSCITATION

Drug	Dosage[a]	Indications
Epinephrine	Low dose (0.01 mg/kg) every 3–5 min early in CPR; high dose (0.1 mg/kg) after prolonged CPR; 10 times the dose may be required when given intratracheally	Asystole, ventricular fibrillation, PEA[b]
Atropine	0.1 mL/5 lb (0.5 mg/mL solution)	Sinus bradycardia, asystole, or PEA associated with high vagal tone
Sodium bicarbonate	1 mEq/kg (1 mEq/mL solution)	Severe metabolic acidemia associated with prolonged (>10–15 min) cardiopulmonary resuscitation efforts (must be adequately ventilated to be effective), hyperkalemia
Calcium gluconate	1 mL/5–10 kg (2% solution without epinephrine)	Routine use not recommended; treat cases with documented hypocalcemia (or severe hyperkalemia)
Amiodarone	5 mg/kg	Refractory ventricular fibrillation or pulseless ventricular tachycardia
Magnesium sulfate	30 mg/kg	Hypomagnesemia, torsades de pointes
Lidocaine	2–4 mg/kg	Pulseless ventricular tachycardia, ventricular fibrillation resistant to defibrillation
Vasopressin	0.4–0.9 U/kg	Combined with or as a substitute for epinephrine every 3–5 min (asystole, bradycardia, PEA)
Naloxone	0.02–0.04 mg/kg	To reverse opioids
Defibrillation	4–6 joules/kg external (monophasic), 2–4 joules/kg external (biphasic), 0.2–1 joules/kg internal	Single shock, resume CPR efforts immediately after for one cycle (2 min), dose escalation may occur

[a] Dosage should be doubled if given via intratracheal route.

[b] PEA = pulseless electrical activity

globin rapidly expand the intravascular volume with much smaller infusion volumes required. Overzealous fluid administration can result in fulminant pulmonary edema due to poor myocardial contractility and arrhythmias. Fluids should not be administered to euvolemic animals, because the increase in central venous pressure may reduce myocardial and cerebral blood flow. Metabolic alterations such as hyperkalemia, hypocalcemia, and severe acidosis should be treated when evident but not otherwise.

Impedance threshold devices may be considered an adjuvant to therapy and used only on animals weighing >10 kg.

If closed chest BCLS is unsuccessful (as determined by lack of spontaneous respiration or inability to generate detectable forward blood flow) after 5–10 min, open-chest CPR (*see* below) is indicated. Instances when open-chest CPR is indicated during initial BCLS include unwitnessed arrest, recent abdominal or thoracic surgery, suspected pleural or pericardial disease, trauma or pathology of the chest or abdominal wall with blood loss, diaphragmatic hernia, and in larger dogs in which external compressions are unlikely to generate an adequate forward blood flow.

Arrhythmias of Cardiac Arrest

Asystole: Asystole appears as a flat line on the ECG and suggests complete absence of electrical activity. In arrest situations known or suspected to be associated with hyperkalemia, calcium gluconate should be administered. Regular insulin at 0.2 U/kg, followed by glucose at 1–2 g/U of insulin, diluted to 25%, temporarily reduces serum levels of potassium. Epinephrine or vasopressin, with or without atropine can be administered in an attempt to generate impulses. Fine ventricular fibrillation may look like asystole, and for this reason, open-chest heart massage and direct observation of myocardial activity are warranted early with this arrhythmia; if fibrillation is visualized, defibrillation is indicated.

Ventricular Flutter: This rhythm is more chaotic than ventricular tachycardia and is prefibrillatory. Lidocaine is the drug of choice to block the excited focus. If lidocaine is ineffective after two boluses and perfusion is absent, defibrillation may be required.

Ventricular Fibrillation: This rhythm implies that multiple foci within the ventricles are firing rapidly and independently, resulting in no coordinated mechanical activity. There are no ventricular contractions and no cardiac output. The goal is to abruptly stop the electrical activity and allow one strong (hopefully normal) electrical rhythm to take over. Defibrillation is more successful when there are few, strong foci (coarse fibrillation) than when there are multiple, weak foci (fine fibrillation).

Pulseless Electrical Activity (PEA): The ECG tracing can be normal or show an arrhythmia (commonly a bradyarrhythmia of ventricular or supraventricular origin), but the heart has no muscular activity associated with the electrical activity, ie, no contractions and no cardiac output and, subsequently, no pulses. In this arrhythmia, it is vital that thoracic auscultation be performed in tandem with central pulse (femoral arterial) palpation and ECG evaluation. There are no heart sounds or pulse activity. However, severe hypovolemia, pericardial effusion, and significant accumulation of fluid or air in the pleural cavity can prevent detection of normal heart sounds. The ECG associated with these conditions demonstrates tachyarrhythmias, in contrast to the usually normal or slow rate of PEA. Atropine and epinephrine or vasopressin may be given in an attempt to correct this arrhythmia. Defibrillation may be attempted with pulseless ventricular tachycardia.

Sinus Bradycardia: Sinus bradycardia on the ECG has P, QRS, and T waves that appear normal, except they occur at a much slower rate. This arresting rhythm may be caused by many disease processes, such as high vagal tone due to GI, urinary, or thoracic disease, and hyperkalemia due to urinary obstruction or rupture and prolonged CPA with CPR efforts. Treatment of known or suspected hyperkalemia with calcium gluconate, insulin, and dextrose with or without sodium bicarbonate may be necessary. Atropine is indicated in this arrhythmia.

If the CPA is believed to be associated with drug administration, a reversal agent should be administered in addition to treating arrhythmias in ACLS. Benzodiazepines such as diazepam and midazolam are reversed with flumazenil, opioid medications such as fentanyl and morphine-related drugs can be reversed with naloxone or partially reversed with butorphanol, xylazine can be reversed with yohimbine, and dexmedetomidine can be reversed with atipamezole. If inhalant anesthesia was used, it should be discontinued and the anesthetic circuit flushed with fresh oxygen.

Open-Chest Cardiopulmonary Resuscitation

(Emergency thoracotomy)

If possible, a quick clip of the hair along the intended incision site is helpful. Usually, there is no time for a full aseptic preparation of the area. A scalpel blade or Mayo scissors are used to incise the skin and subcutaneous tissues along the cranial border of the fourth or fifth rib from the spine to sternum. A Carmalt forceps or Mayo scissors are used to bluntly dissect through the underlying muscle tissues and push through the pleura. Ventilations should be discontinued momentarily, and the instrument should be guarded with a thumb and forefinger as the pleura is entered to prevent injury to the heart or lungs. After the pleura is entered at the ventral aspect of the incision, Mayo scissors are used to incise the muscles dorsally along the entire length of the intercostal space, along the cranial aspect of the rib. Care should be taken to avoid incising the internal thoracic vessels running parallel and lateral to the sternum. After the chest cavity is opened, manual ventilations should continue, and the pericardiodiaphragmatic ligament elevated and incised with scissors, extending the incision dorsally to just ventral to the phrenic nerve. The heart is then lifted out of the pericardial sac and observed for any coordinated spontaneous contractions. If no cardiac contractions are noted, the heart is grasped with one or both hands and compressed progressively from the apex to the base. The compression is then released to allow the cardiac chambers to refill with blood. If fine or coarse fibrillation of the heart muscle is noted, internal defibrillation should be performed.

The descending aorta can be isolated and temporarily cross-clamped to direct blood flow to the brain. Aortic cross-clamping can be performed with atraumatic vascular clamps or by using a modified Rommell tourniquet, passing a rubber tube, latex tube, or umbilical tape around the aorta with the assistance of curved hemostats and then clamping on the tube to occlude aortic flow. Aortic cross-clamping can be performed for 10 min without serious complications (from lack of blood flow to the spinal cord).

An ECG is evaluated and drugs given as indicated during ACLS procedures. Return of spontaneous circulation allows lavage of the thorax with large quantities of sterile, warm, isotonic saline; placement of a thoracostomy tube; and surgical closure of the thorax. Cardiovascular support (*see* p 1665) is frequently required to maintain circulation while the underlying cause of the arrest is treated.

Monitoring

End-tidal CO_2 ($ETCO_2$) should be measured in intubated patients at risk of having CPR and is a useful monitoring tool during CPR efforts. Using an $ETCO_2$ reading along with visualization, palpation, and auscultation can help confirm endotracheal intubation. $ETCO_2$ may also be an early indicator of return of spontaneous circulation (ROSC) and effectiveness of CPR efforts (when minute ventilation is consistent). An $ETCO_2$ of <10 mmHg indicates esophageal intubation, ineffective CPR technique, incorrect placement of endotracheal tube, or hyperventilation (if adequate perfusion is established). An $ETCO_2$ reading of 12–18 mmHg indicates an ROSC, and a reading of >45 mmHg may indicate hypoventilation or increased CO_2 delivery to the lungs after ROSC occurs.

Routine monitoring of ECG is essential during CPR to allow identification and specific therapy of arrhythmias. Palpation of pulses either to detect CPA or to monitor effectiveness of CPR efforts is not recommended because of the insensitive nature of this test. Use of Doppler monitoring (on eyes or peripheral arteries) to detect CPA or monitor efforts of CPR is also not recommended.

Use of blood samples may help guide therapy in some instances during CPR. Centrally collected samples are ideal; however, most patients do not have a central catheter. Peripheral blood samples do not necessarily reflect the central circulation but may help guide therapy in some instances (such as hyperkalemia). It is not recommended to monitor with arterial gas samples or pulse oximetry; these require pulsatile arterial flow, which is inadequate during CPR.

Close monitoring of an animal after arrest is vital, because significant abnormalities of acid-base and electrolytes (especially hyperkalemia) are common and may require additional treatment. Parameters such as ECG, blood pressure, neurologic status, pulse oximetry, $ETCO_2$, and venous blood gases should be monitored closely. Blood pressure support with dopamine, dobutamine, other pressor agents, or stroma-free hemoglobin, as indicated, may be required to maintain cardiac output. Body temperature, glucose, and lactate may provide additional information.

With anaerobic metabolism that occurs during shock and cardiopulmonary arrest, blood lactate levels (*see* p 1686) rise dramatically (normal levels are <2 mmol/L). With ROSC, lactate levels may rise dramatically and then resolve with appropriate treatment.

Postresuscitation Care

Routine use of large volumes of fluids is not recommended and should be avoided in animals with congestive heart failure. It is important to use resuscitation endpoints during post-CPA care to normalize venous oxygen content, lactate, blood pressure, central venous pressure, PCV, and oxygen saturation. Medications to help reduce cerebral edema, such as mannitol and furosemide, can be administered after CPA and are often recommended to help decrease cerebral edema. Routine mechanical ventilation is not routinely recommended but reasonable in animals that are hypercapneic or hypoxemic. Vasopressors and positive inotropes are reasonable when needed. Animals with open-chest CPR will require control of hemorrhage, pleural lavage, placement of a chest tube, perioperative antibiotics, and closure of the thoracic cavity. A large percentage of animals that sustain a CPA will have another episode of CPA. Treatment of the underlying condition that led to the CPA is essential to help prevent recurrence.

FLUID THERAPY

Cardiac function; intravascular volume; and vascular tone, integrity, and patency are critical to normal circulation. An abnormality in one or more of these components of circulation leads to stimulation of the sympathetic nervous system, which results in compensatory changes to maintain perfusion. The hemodynamic and cellular changes that develop as a result of these abnormalities are called shock. As shock progresses, oxygen and substrate delivery to the tissues becomes insufficient to meet energy requirements for cellular maintenance and repair. If shock progresses and cellular energy demands cannot be met, the ensuing organ failure leads to death. Early recognition of the type and stage of shock is vital to establishing a successful fluid therapy plan; timely intervention with appropriate therapy will prevent or decrease organ injury and/or death.

Shock is typically classified into three categories: hypovolemic, cardiogenic, and distributive. Hypovolemic shock develops when there is a blood volume deficit ≥15%; this may be from hemorrhage or other fluid losses (eg, as occurs with severe vomiting and diarrhea). Cardiogenic shock results when the heart fails as a pump; common causes include pulmonary emboli, cardiac tamponade, valvular insufficiency, cardiomyopathy, and cardiac arrhythmias. Distributive shock is caused by maldistribution of blood flow away from the central circulation as a result of peripheral vasodilation; it can be caused by conditions such as anaphylaxis, corticosteroid deficiency (hypoadrenocorticism and critical illness–related corticosteroid insufficiency), and systemic inflammatory diseases that lead to systemic inflammatory response syndrome (SIRS). The different types of shock may have different hemodynamic profiles during the early and middle stages. Frequently, more than one type of shock is present, with hypovolemia likely to play a role in each form. Rapid and aggressive fluid resuscitation yields the best outcome, with hemostasis used as required. In veterinary patients, many stages and categories of shock will respond to fluid resuscitation alone; medications such as antiarrhythmics and inotropes may be necessary for primary cardiogenic shock, and vasopressor agents may be necessary for distributive shock. The ability to create an effective fluid resuscitation plan depends on an understanding of the different body fluid compartments and the dynamics of fluid movement and distribution between fluid compartments.

BODY FLUID COMPARTMENTS AND FLUID DYNAMICS

There are three major fluid compartments; intravascular, interstitial, and intracellular. Fluid movement from the intravascular to interstitial and intracellular compartments occurs in the capillaries. A capillary "membrane," which consists of the endothelial glycocalyx, endothelial cells, and the subendothelial cell matrix, separates the capillary intravascular space from the interstitial fluid compartment. This capillary "membrane" is freely permeable to water and small-molecular-weight particles such as electrolytes, glucose, acetate, lactate, gluconate, and bicarbonate. Gases such as oxygen and carbon dioxide diffuse freely through this membrane to enter or exit the intravascular compartment.

The interstitial compartment is the space between the capillaries and the cells. Fluids support the matrix and cells within the interstitial space. The intracellular compartment is separated from the interstitial space by a cell membrane. This membrane is freely permeable to water but not to small- or large-molecular-weight particles. Any particle movement between the interstitium and the cell must occur through some transport mechanism (eg, channel, ion pump, carrier mechanism).

Fluids are in a constant state of flux across the capillary endothelial membrane, through the interstitium, and into and out of the cell. The amount of fluid that moves across the capillary "membrane" depends on a number of factors, including capillary colloid oncotic pressure (COP), hydrostatic pressure, and permeability, which is dictated by factors such as the endothelial glycocalyx and pore sizes between the cells. The natural particles in blood that create COP are proteins: primarily albumin but also globulins, fibrinogen, and others. The hydrostatic pressure within the capillary is the pressure forcing outward on the capillary membrane generated by the blood pressure and cardiac output. Fluid moves into the interstitial space when intravascular hydrostatic pressure is increased over COP, when membrane pore size increases, or when intravascular COP becomes lower than interstitial COP.

THE FLUID RESUSCITATION PLAN

In hypovolemic shock, compensatory neuroendocrine responses are initiated to restore blood volume and meet metabolic demands that occur during acutely decreased cardiac output states, increasing ATP demands. When perfusion continues to be compromised despite these mechanisms, cells can no longer generate ATP, compensatory mechanisms become exhausted, and decompensatory shock ensues. An adequate fluid resuscitation plan is necessary to optimize survival.

The fluid resuscitation plan should include the following steps: 1) determine where the fluid deficit lies, 2) select fluid(s) specific for the patient, 3) determine resuscitation endpoints, and 4) determine the resuscitation technique to be used.

Determination of the Fluid Deficit

Loss of fluid volume from the intravascular fluid compartment is manifested by poor perfusion (shock) and inadequate tissue oxygenation. This volume deficit results in a lower vessel wall tension. Decreased wall tension in the aortic arch and carotid arteries results in decreased stimulation of the baroreceptors. This decreased rate of firing, sent via the glossopharyngeal and vagus nerves to the medulla oblongata, results in decreased inhibition (stimulation) of the sympathetic system. Stimulation of the sympathetic nervous system is manifested by clinical changes in heart rate, pulse intensity, blood pressure, capillary refill time, mucous membrane color, level of consciousness, and rectal temperature. These physical perfusion parameters, combined with blood pressure, are used clinically to detect intravascular volume deficits. Most animals with an intravascular deficit (poor perfusion) also have concurrent extravascular (interstitial and intracellular) deficits.

Fluid deficit in the interstitial and intracellular spaces causes clinical signs of dehydration. Physical findings are used to estimate the percentage of dehydration. Semidry oral mucous membranes, normal skin turgor, and eyes maintaining normal moisture indicate 4%–5% dehydration. Dry oral mucous membranes, mild loss of skin turgor, and eyes still moist indicate 6%–7% dehydration. As dehydration becomes more severe, significant quantities of fluid shift from the intravascular space into the interstitium, causing concurrent perfusion deficits with dehydration. Dry mucous membranes, considerable loss of skin turgor, retracted eyes, acute weight loss, and weak rapid pulses (concurrent intravascular deficit) indicate 8%–10% dehydration. Very dry oral mucous membranes, complete loss of skin turgor, severe retraction of the eyes, dull eyes, possible alteration of consciousness, acute weight loss, and thready, weak pulses indicate ≥12% dehydration.

The physical guidelines to estimate dehydration are misleading in two common clinical situations. Chronically emaciated and geriatric animals may have metabolized the fat from around the eyes and the collagen in the skin, resulting in poor skin turgor and sunken eyes despite normal hydration. Animals with rapid fluid loss into a third body fluid space (a space within the body cavity where fluid from the local interstitial and intravascular spaces leak) have rapid fluid shifts from the intravascular compartments into these spaces before clinical evidence of interstitial fluid loss is seen. Both situations require evaluation of mucous membrane and eye moisture, PCV, and total solids before dehydration can be estimated.

Selection of Fluids

Fluids must be administered that will concentrate within the body fluid compartment where the volume deficit lies. Crystalloids are water-based solutions with small-molecular-weight particles, freely permeable to the capillary membrane. Colloids are water-based solutions with a molecular weight too large to freely pass across the capillary membrane. Colloids are thought of as intravascular volume replacement solutions, and crystalloids as interstitial volume replacement solutions.

Crystalloids: The small-molecular-weight particles in crystalloids are primarily electrolytes and buffers (*see* TABLE 3). When the sodium concentration of the solution is equivalent to that of the (red blood) cell, the solution is called isotonic. Intravascular administration of isotonic crystalloids (eg, lactated Ringer's, 0.9% saline) will result in interstitial volume replacement and minimal intracellular fluid accumulation. More than 75% of the isotonic crystalloid administered IV can move into the extravascular space within 1 hr in a healthy animal. This is because of the normal fluid shifts between fluid compartments. Hypotonic fluids (eg, 5% dextrose in water, half-strength saline) will result in intracellular water accumulation and should not be used as resuscitation fluids. Hypertonic solutions (eg, 7% NaCl) contain higher concentrations of sodium and are best used when hydration is normal and concurrently with other fluids.

Crystalloids are considered buffered when they contain molecules (such as acetate, gluconate, and lactate) that are converted to bicarbonate in the liver, equilibrating the pH of the fluid to normal blood pH (7.4). Normal saline (0.9%) is isotonic but not buffered; it is used initially for specific clinical problems, including hyponatremia, hypernatremia, hypercalcemia, hypochloremic metabolic alkalosis, head trauma, and oliguric renal failure.

Crystalloids are considered balanced when they contain electrolytes in addition to Na and Cl (such as K, Mg, Ca), making them similar to plasma. Lactated Ringer's is an example of a balanced solution; normal saline is not balanced.

The particular crystalloid to administer is determined by the measured or estimated sodium and potassium concentrations and by the osmolality of both the animal's serum and the fluid to be administered (*see* TABLE 3). Most clinical problems will benefit from the use of buffered, balanced, isotonic crystalloids (eg, lactated Ringer's) as part of the resuscitation fluid plan.

Sodium Content: When serum sodium measurements are normal, a balanced isotonic electrolyte solution can be used for volume replacement. Serum sodium levels that are moderately to severely decreased (<130 mEq/L) or moderately to severely increased (>170 mEq/L) may contribute to serum osmolality changes and result in neurologic abnormalities. Care must be

TABLE 3 CRYSTALLOIDS

Crystalloid	Tonicity	Na^+	Cl^-	K^+	Ca^{+2}	Osmolality (mOsm/L)	pH
Lactated Ringer's solution	Isotonic	130	109	4	3	273	6.7
Plasmalyte-A®	Isotonic	140	103	5	0	294	7.4
Normosol-R®	Isotonic	140	98	5	0	295	7.4
Normal saline (0.9%)	Isotonic	154	154	0	0	308	5.7
Dextrose (2.5% in 0.45% saline)	Isotonic	77	77	0	0	280	4.5
Dextrose (5%) in water	Hypotonic	0	0	0	0	253	5.0
Hypertonic saline (7.5%)	Hypertonic	1,232	1,232	0	0	2,464	5.2
Normosol-M® with 5% dextrose	Hypertonic	40	40	13	0	363	5.2

Electrolyte units are mEq/L.

taken not to increase or decrease the sodium concentration too quickly, which may result in cerebral edema or dehydration (and can lead to intracranial hemorrhage). In general, sodium concentrations should not be altered by >0.5 mEq/L/hr or 8–12 mEq/L/day. This allows for increased or decreased osmolality of neurons to adjust over time and avoids cerebral edema or dehydration. Crystalloids are also classified as either replacement or maintenance fluids. Replacement fluids are intended to replace fluids lost from the body (such as through hemorrhage, vomiting, diarrhea, etc) and often contain a sodium concentration near that of plasma (such as lactated Ringer's or 0.9% saline); these fluids result in excessive concentrations of sodium if given over prolonged periods of time (>24–72 hr) or for animals with free water loss; however, they are ideal resuscitation fluids for animals with sodium-rich fluid losses. Maintenance fluids contain significantly less sodium (such as half-strength saline or 5% dextrose in water) and are intended for animals that have free water loss or require prolonged fluid administration. Replacement fluids given to an animal with free water deficits or for prolonged periods of time (without access to water) will result in hypernatremia and hyperosmolarity.

Serum sodium alterations with fluid administration (Δ[Na]) can be estimated using the following formula:

$\Delta[Na] = ([Na]_{fluid} - [Na]_{patient}) / (\text{total body water} + 1)$, in which total body water = 0.6 × body wt (kg)

In animals with decreased serum sodium content, volume replacement should be with isotonic saline (0.9%) or other replacement/isotonic fluids. Increased serum sodium values most commonly reflect a loss of solute-free water. The animal should be perfused and hydrated using isotonic saline or other replacement/isotonic fluids. The free water can then be replaced, if necessary, using 2.5% dextrose in half-strength lactated Ringer's, 2.5% dextrose in half-strength saline, 0.45% saline, or 5% dextrose in water when hypernatremia persists. This must be done carefully, and the sodium concentration lowered slowly. Desmopressin may be required if hypernatremia persists after appropriate fluid therapy, especially when the animal has hyposthenuria or head injury.

Potassium Content: When serum potassium estimates are normal, a balanced electrolyte solution can be used. Unless severe, hypokalemia can be difficult to recognize clinically. Few clinical situations warrant potassium supplementation beyond the content of lactated Ringer's or Plasmalyte-A® during initial volume replacement. Once the animal has been stabilized, potassium chloride should be added to the fluids, administered at ≤0.5 mEq/kg/hr. This rate may be increased when severe hypokalemia (<2 mEq/L) is associated with catastrophic clinical signs, (eg, respiratory distress/hypoventilation from paresis of the diaphragm or generalized lower motor paresis or paralysis). The serum potassium level must be closely monitored with more rapid infusions. More commonly, potassium chloride is added to 1 L of balanced isotonic crystalloids

TABLE 4 GUIDELINE FOR POTASSIUM SUPPLEMENTATION IN DOGS AND CATS

Serum Potassium Concentration (mEq/L)	mEq KCl to Add to 1 L of Maintenance Fluids
<2.0	80
2.1–2.5	60
2.6–3.0	40
3.1–3.5	25–30
3.6–5.0	20
>5.0	none

administered as maintenance fluids based on serum potassium concentration (*see* TABLE 4). Serum potassium concentration should be monitored closely during continued therapy. Potassium phosphates may be used if a concurrent phosphorus deficiency is present.

In animals with hyperkalemia, fluids should be selected carefully. When oliguric renal failure is suspected as the cause of the hyperkalemia, potassium-free solutions, such as 0.9% saline, are used for volume replacement. Clinical conditions requiring potassium-free solutions include oliguric renal failure, heat stroke, adrenal insufficiency (Addison disease), and massive muscle breakdown. After volume replacement and fluid diuresis resolve the hyperkalemia, a balanced electrolyte solution should be used. These solutions have a normal pH and promote potassium excretion. Recent evidence suggests that with hyperkalemia secondary to feline urinary obstruction, any isotonic balanced fluid can be used, with minimal concern for increasing serum potassium as long as the underlying obstruction is treated.

Osmolality: Osmolality is defined as the number of solute particles per unit of solvent. Serum osmolality can be calculated using the following formula:

$$\text{Osmolality (mOsm/kg)} = 2([Na^+] + [K^+]) + [\text{glucose}]/18 + [\text{BUN}]/2.8$$

Normal serum osmolality is 290–310 mOsm/L. Fluids that do not contribute significantly to serum osmolality should be used for volume replacement.

Hyperosmolar solutions include hypertonic saline, Normosol-M® with 5% dextrose, or any isotonic fluid that has glucose or hypertonic saline added. Except for hypertonic saline, the hyperosmolar glucose-containing solutions are meant to be maintenance solutions used in animals in which fluids are not shifting rapidly from the vascular compartment to a third body fluid space. They are usually not used as volume replacement solutions.

Hypertonic saline provides a supranormal concentration of sodium and is generally given in a 3%, 7%, or 7.5% IV solution. The effect is to rapidly draw water from the interstitial space into the intravascular space, rapidly expanding the intravascular volume. Hypertonic saline may also decrease cellular swelling and improve myocardial contractility. If the animal has concurrent interstitial fluid deficits (dehydration) or a disease that results in free water loss (eg, hyperthermia, diabetes, etc), administration of hypertonic saline could result in severe hyperosmolality with neurologic complications. Because hypertonic crystalloid solution will leak into the interstitium in <1 hr, combining hypertonic saline with a colloid is recommended to offset the interstitial edema resulting from interstitial extravasation.

Colloids: When colloids are to be administered, it must be decided whether a natural colloid (eg, plasma, albumin, or whole blood) or a synthetic colloid (*see* TABLE 5) is to be used. When the animal requires RBCs, clotting factors, antithrombin III, or albumin, blood products are the colloids of choice.

When the initial goal is to rapidly improve perfusion in an animal with adequate RBCs, a synthetic colloid can achieve the desired volume expansion rapidly. Choices of synthetic colloids include dextran, hydroxyethyl starch (HES), and stroma-free hemoglobin.

Dextrans are polysaccharides composed of linear glucose residues. They are produced by the enzyme dextran sucrase during growth of various strains of *Leuconostoc* bacteria in media containing sucrose. Dextrans are isotonic and can be stored at room temperature. Dextran is broken down completely to CO_2 and H_2O by dextranase present in spleen, liver, lung, kidney, brain, and muscle at a rate approaching 70 mg/kg every 24 hr. In normal dogs, dextran 70 increases plasma volume 1.38 times (138%) the volume infused.

Hemostatic changes in healthy experimental dogs given dextran 70 include an increase in the buccal mucosal bleeding time and partial thromboplastin time and a decrease in von Willebrand factor antigen and factor VIII coagulant activity, without clinical bleeding. Dextran copolymerizes with the fibrin monomer, destabilizing clot formation. Blood glucose levels may be increased during dextran metabolism. Dextran 70 may cause a change in the total solids value that does not reflect actual protein content and may interfere with blood crossmatching. Moderate to life-threatening reactions in dogs have been rare. Dextran 70 is being used much less commonly in favor of other colloids, and dextran 40 is not recommended because it is known to cause renal injury.

Hydroxyethyl starch (HES) is the parent name of a polymeric molecule made from a waxy species of either corn or potatoes and is composed primarily of amylopectin (98%). HES molecules vary in size from ten thousand to several million daltons (average 70–670 thousand daltons). The disappearance of HES molecules from the body depends primarily on their rate of enzymatic degradation by α-amylase and subsequent renal excretion. Other methods of elimination include absorption by tissues (liver, spleen, kidney, and heart), uptake by the reticuloendothelial system, and clearance through bile. Blood α-amylase–mediated hydrolysis (primarily at the C6 position) reduces the molecular weight to <72,000 daltons; these smaller particles are more osmotically active but eliminated at a faster rate through the kidney. Metabolism of HES retained in tissue is probably performed by cytoplasmic lysosomes. An increase in serum amylase is to be expected without alteration in pancreatic function.

Along with molecular weight, the degree of molar substitution, which is the number of glucose units on the starch molecule that have been replaced by hydroxyethyl units, is the major determinant of how long the different types of HES survive in the blood. Molar substitution rates vary from 0.35 to 0.7, and the higher the molar substitution, the longer the half-life in blood. The position of the molar substitution also impacts half-life; this can occur at the C2, C3, and C6 positions. Stereotactically, substitution at the C2 site impedes degradation by amylase, prolonging the half-life of HES; this is often referred to as the C2:C6 ratio. Higher ratios imply impeded breakdown and therefore longer half-lives in blood. When hetastarch (the most common HES) is infused at 25 mL/kg in healthy dogs, the initial increase in plasma volume is 1.37 times (137%) the volume infused; most hetastarches will expand plasma volume 100%–150%. Intravascular persistence is significantly greater than that of dextran 70, with 38% of hetastarch remaining, compared with 19% of dextran, 24 hr after infusion. Administration by constant-rate infusion may provide a constant supply of larger molecular weight particles, perhaps maintaining and augmenting plasma COP and intravascular volume in animals with albumin loss or increased capillary permeability. Most HES molecules may persist in the body for 2–7 days.

TABLE 5 SYNTHETIC COLLOIDS

Colloid	In Solution with	Molecular Weight (daltons)[a]	C2:C6 Ratio	Colloid Oncotic Pressure (mmHg)	Suggested Upper Limit (dose/kg/ day)	Concentration (%)
Dextran 70	0.9% NaCl	70,000 (10,000–80,000)	NA	59	20 mL	6
Hextend™ (670/0.7)	Lactated electrolyte solution	670,000 (20,000–2,500,000)	5:1	25–30	20 mL	6
VetStarch™/ Voluven™ (130/0.4)	0.9% saline	130,000 (110,000–150,000)	9:1	36	50 mL	6
HESPAN® (600/0.4)	0.9% saline	600,000 (450,000–800,000)	5:1	25–30	20 mL	6
Stroma-free hemoglobin (Oxyglobin®)	Modified lactated Ringer's solution	65,000–130,000 (up to 500,000)	NA	20	See text	13

NA = not applicable

[a]Average, followed by range in parentheses.

Hydroxyethyl starches favor retention of intravascular fluid and prevent washout of interstitial proteins. In hypooncotic situations, HES infusion has a great advantage over other colloids because the larger molecules remain intravascular, limiting pulmonary fluid flux. It is nontoxic and nonallergenic in dosages as high as 100 mL/kg in dogs. Many cats have a moderate reaction—nausea and occasional vomiting—with rapid infusion. However, when hetastarch is given slowly (throughout 5–15 min), this adverse effect is minimal. Renal injury, reported to occur from an osmotic nephrosis in people, has been poorly documented in dogs and cats, and allergic reactions are rare.

Hetastarch is associated with minor alterations in laboratory coagulation measurements but not with clinical bleeding unless daily minimal dosages (20–50 mL/kg/day) are exceeded. Molecular weight seems to have the biggest impact on coagulation, with larger molecular weight starches impacting coagulation to a greater degree. The proposed mechanisms of impact on coagulation include "coating" platelets or impeded platelet receptor signalling, dilution of coagulation factors, and interference with von Willebrand factor/factor VIII interaction. Dilutional effects on coagulation, cells, and proteins are produced in response to the volume expansion of the plasma. Animals that receive large volumes of HES solutions may have more oozing if surgery is performed, and diligent hemostasis is warranted.

A variety of HES solutions are currently available, each with its own advantages and disadvantages based on its molecular composition.

Stroma-free hemoglobin (Oxyglobin®) is a polymerized bovine hemoglobin-based solution that increases plasma and total hemoglobin concentration. This solution is indicated for the treatment of anemia and hypovolemia with tissue hypoxia. It has colloidal properties similar to those of hetastarch and exerts mild vasopressor activity, believed to be through scavenging of nitric oxide, a potent constitutive and inducable vasodilator. The dark hue of the solution causes discoloration of the serum (and sometimes the urine) that can interfere with some serum chemistry tests, depending on the type of analyzer and reagents used. Bilirubinuria will be present. Dosages ≤30 mL/kg/day have been approved for dogs, with the rate of infusion <10 mL/kg/hr. When given to an animal with a normal blood volume, administration must be slow and carefully monitored to avoid volume overload resulting from the colloidal and pressor properties of the solution. Oxyglobin has also been used in cats as infusions (4–25 mL/kg/24 hr) and/or rapid infusions (1–5 mL/cat). Anecdotally, the pressor effects in cats seem pronounced, and blood pressure should be monitored. Oxyglobin has been associated with development of pulmonary edema, pleural effusion, and respiratory distress, particularly in cats with underlying heart disease.

Lyophilized canine albumin is available as a 5% lypophilized solution that can be reconstituted. It has been administered to dogs with septic peritonitis and hypoalbuminemia and has been demonstrated to increase oncotic pressure, measured albumin levels, and Doppler-measured blood pressure, with increased albumin levels persisting for as long as 24 hours. Minimal adverse effects have been noted. Replacement volume in mL of albumin 5% solution (50 mg/mL) can be calculated using the following formula:

body wt (kg) × 90 mL/kg × (target albumin level [eg, 2 mg/dL] – patient's current albumin level) × 0.2 g/dL

It may also be administered as a more concentrated solution (16% or 166 mg/mL) for hypotensive patients, at a dosage of 800 mg/kg throughout 6 hr. Human serum albumin is available as well and has been used with success in critically ill veterinary patients; however, when administered to healthy animals, severe adverse effects, including multiple organ failure, have been noted.

Blood products are important in many situations (*see* p 17). Animals that need clotting proteins may require frozen (or fresh frozen) plasma or cryoprecipitate, which contains concentrated amounts of factor VIII and von Willebrand factor; platelet-rich plasma may be necessary for platelet deficiencies. Animals with severe anemia or blood loss may require whole blood or packed red blood cells. Cavitary hemorrhage may allow collection of blood either with centesis or in surgery for autologous blood administration when banked blood is not available.

Fluid Selection: Interstitial and intracellular volume deficits (dehydration) are replaced by the administration of crystalloids. Intravascular volume (perfusion) deficits can also be replaced with crystalloids alone. However, when large quantities of isotonic crystalloids are rapidly administered IV, there is an immediate increase in intravascular hydrostatic pressure, a decrease in intravascular COP, and extravasation of large fluid quantities into the interstitial spaces. By administering colloids in conjunction with crystalloids during fluid resuscitation of perfusion deficits, less total fluid volume is required (crystalloids reduced by 40%–60%), there is less tendency toward fluid overload, and resuscitation times are shorter.

Many conditions can increase capillary permeability and cause systemic inflammation (SIRS), including parvoviral diarrhea, other severe GI disease, pancreatitis, septic shock, massive trauma, heat stroke, cold exposure, burns, snake bite, and systemic neoplasia. Hetastarch or stroma-free hemoglobin are the colloids of choice for intravascular volume resuscitation when there is increased capillary permeability and loss of albumin through the capillary membrane. Using crystalloids alone in animals that require large volumes for resuscitation or that have increased capillary permeability will result in significant interstitial edema.

Many of these animals also have third-space fluid losses, most likely due to significant regional inflammation, that result in massive fluid requirements and make it difficult to predict the volume required to maintain fluid balance.

Determination of Resuscitation Endpoints

There are no "standard" formulas for crystalloid or colloid infusion that will guarantee complete volume resuscitation in a small animal. Variables such as renal function, presence of a third body fluid space, brain injury, lung injury, heart disease or failure, continued losses, or closed cavity hemorrhage require that fluid resuscitation rate and volumes be individualized for the patient. Sufficient volumes of fluid should be administered to reach desired endpoints of resuscitation. This has also been termed early goal-directed therapy. The endpoints typically reflect perfusion status and include heart rate, blood pressure, central venous pressure, mucous membrane color, capillary refill time, and pulse intensity. A resolution of an increased blood lactate to <2 mmol/dL supports adequate tissue oxygenation. More advanced endpoints, which can be used if additional instrumentation is available, include a central venous pressure of 5–8 cm H_2O, central venous oxygen saturation >70%, and a urine output of at least 1–2 mL/kg/hr.

Shock will deplete cellular energy stores, with subsequent cellular and organ dysfunction. Restoring the circulation to "normal," with normal oxygenation and perfusion parameters, may not be enough to allow sufficient ATP production for repair as well as maintenance. When an animal is suspected of having a disease process related to SIRS, such as vasodilation, increased capillary permeability, or depressed cardiac output, resuscitation endpoints are chosen for supranormal resuscitation (*see* TABLE 6). The goal is to deliver oxygen and glucose to the cells in higher than normal concentrations to promote sufficient energy production for both repair and maintenance of the cells.

There are situations, however, when supranormal resuscitation can be detrimental. Increased vessel wall tension can dislodge a life-saving clot in the vasculature of a traumatized animal, exacerbating hemorrhage. Brain and lung edema or hemorrhage can be worsened by aggressive and sudden increases in hydrostatic pressure. Hypotensive resuscitation provides endpoints that are at the lower limit of normal (*see* TABLE 6). The goal is to administer the smallest volume of fluids possible to successfully resuscitate the intravascular compartment while minimizing extravasation of fluids into the interstitium (especially brain or lungs), titrating the amount of preload to minimize excess fluid load to a potentially disabled heart, and reducing the probability of dislodging clots. Small-volume resuscitation techniques should be used to reach hypotensive resuscitation endpoints.

Determination of Appropriate Resuscitation Technique

Large- and small-volume techniques are used to reach endpoints discussed above. These doses of fluids should be administered throughout 10–15 min as a rapid IV infusion, and then the animal should be reassessed for restoration of normal clinical perfusion parameters and objective measurements of perfusion. Continual reassessment and titration of fluid doses will achieve resuscitation from shock in most cases (while the underlying disease is investigated and therapy instituted). Dogs in hypovolemic shock that require supranormal endpoint values can benefit from large-volume resuscitation techniques. Typically, an initial infusion of 20–50 mL/kg of buffered, balanced isotonic crystalloids

TABLE 6 RESUSCITATION ENDPOINTS

Monitored Parameter	Endpoints: "Supranormal" (high-end resuscitation)	Endpoints: "Hypotensive" (low-end resuscitation)
Blood pressure		
Systolic	90–120 mmHg	80–90 mmHg
Mean arterial	80–90 mmHg	60–80 mmHg
Central venous pressure	6–8 cm H_2O	3–5 cm H_2O
Heart rate[a]		
Dog	<140 bpm	<140 bpm
Cat	160–200 bpm	160–200 bpm
Capillary refill time	1–2 sec	1–2 sec
Pulse intensity (femoral)	Strong	Strong
Resuscitation technique		
Dog	Large volume	Small volume
Cat	Small volume	Small volume
Clinical indications	SIRS diseases Cortisol deficiency (hypoadrenocorticism, critical illness-related corticosteroid insufficiency) Anaphylaxis	Heart failure Closed cavity hemorrhage Ongoing hemorrhage Brain disease Lung edema Oliguric renal failure

[a] After appropriate analgesia

is given, followed by 5–15 mL/kg of a hydroxyethyl starch solution. When stroma-free hemoglobin is selected as the colloid, the dosage is 5 mL/kg. Additional colloids can be administered using small-volume intravascular resuscitation techniques if perfusion has not improved to the desired supranormal endpoints after the initial large volume dose of fluids. Colloids should be added immediately in any animal with proteinaceous fluid losses (SIRS disease, GI fluid losses, etc).

Whole blood products can be administered by large-volume resuscitation techniques in catastrophic hemorrhagic situations. However, initial administration of stroma-free hemoglobin will allow for a slower administration of whole blood and less chance for transfusion reaction from rapid whole blood administration.

Small-volume resuscitation techniques are recommended in hypovolemic cats and any dog with closed cavity hemorrhage, head injury, pulmonary contusions or edema, cardiogenic shock, or oliguric renal failure. An initial dosage of balanced isotonic crystalloids (10–15 mL/kg for dogs; 5–10 mL/kg for cats) is given. An HES solution can be administered (5 mL/kg in dogs; 2–5 mL/kg in cats) throughout 1–5 min as well. The perfusion parameters are reassessed, and the initial bolus dose repeated as needed until the resuscitation endpoint is reached. When stroma-free hemoglobin is used as the colloid in dogs, the dosage is 2–5 mL/kg. Stroma-free hemoglobin is not approved for use in cats, but it has been used successfully at a dosage of 1–5 mL/cat (0.25–1 mL/kg) given slowly throughout 5 min.

Hypothermia, especially in cats, can significantly limit the cardiovascular response to endogenous sympathetic stimulus (catecholamines) and to fluid resuscitation. Active external warming with circulating water blankets should be done once fluid resuscitation has been initiated. Additional warming techniques such as warm water bottles, fluid line warmers, and warm air blowers can be used to warm cats. Aggressive volume administration without active warming of hypothermic cats can result in pulmonary edema despite continued hypotension.

ASSESSMENT OF RESUSCITATION EFFORTS

Once the fluid therapy plan is underway, ongoing assessment is critical. If adequate fluids have been administered and reasonable resuscitation endpoints have not been reached, several causes should be considered: inadequate volume administration, ongoing hemorrhage, third body fluid spacing, heart disease or pericardial fluid, severe vasodilation, vasoconstriction, organ ischemia, hypoglycemia, hypokalemia, arrhythmias, severe acidemia or alkalemia, decreased venous return, severe anemia, endocrine disease (hypoadrenocorticism or critical illness related to corticosteroid insufficiency), hypothermia, or brain pathology. These variables should be rapidly assessed and corrected. If a central venous pressure (CVP) line is available, it should be checked to see whether CVP is near the endpoints assigned (TABLE 6). If not, or if no CVP is available, a fluid challenge can be given. This typically consists of a bolus (10–15 mL/kg) of crystalloids and a bolus (5 mL/kg) of hetastarch. If the perfusion parameters improve with this challenge, then the likely cause of the nonresponsive shock is inadequate volume, and colloids are titrated to reach the desired endpoints. Ultrasound, with an experienced ultrasonographer, may be useful to assess cardiac function and/or volume status in select patients.

If fluid volume appears adequate and underlying etiologies have been addressed and treated and the animal is still hypotensive, vasopressors can be used. Oxyglobin® can be given at the dosages listed above if it has not yet been used. If stroma-free hemoglobin fails to increase the blood pressure, then dopamine is administered at 2–15 mg/kg/min as a constant-rate infusion; alternative vasopressors include norepinephrine, vasopressin, and phenylephrine. These medications are weaned once blood pressure has stabilized.

MAINTENANCE FLUID PLAN

Maintaining intravascular fluids after resuscitation from hypovolemic shock and during systemic inflammatory response syndrome disease conditions causing increased capillary permeability can be a challenge. Hydroxyethylstarch solutions or Oxyglobin® can be administered as a constant-rate infusion at 0.5–1 mL/kg/hr in dogs, or 0.25–1 mL/kg/hr in cats. Newer HES solutions may be administered at higher rates (2 mL/kg/hr) without impacting coagulation. The dosage is adjusted to maintain an adequate mean arterial pressure and CVP. The amount of crystalloids administered with colloids must be reduced by 40%–60% of what would be administered if crystalloids were used alone. The maintenance fluid plan should address three ongoing requirements: replacement of lost interstitial volume (rehydration), maintenance fluids (for normal homeostasis), and replacement of ongoing losses. The volume of rehydration fluids required is determined by reassessing hydration parameters after resuscitation, using the following formula: % dehydration × body wt (kg) × total body water (0.6). This volume is commonly administered throughout 4–12 hr with standard isotonic, balanced electrolyte replacement fluids.

Maintenance fluid requirements (40 mL/kg/day for larger animals and 60 mL/kg/day for smaller animals) are added to the rehydration rate. With prolonged parenteral fluid administration, usually throughout a course of days, serum sodium may increase, and maintenance fluids (eg, half-strength saline or 5% dextrose in water) may be needed to replace free water deficits.

Ongoing or increased fluid losses vary substantially and must be estimated and replaced. Ongoing losses can be estimated by measuring urine and fecal output, nasogastric tube suction, or vomitus volume. Insensible losses, which can be increased with fever, or higher metabolic demands can increase the maintenance rate by 15–20 mL/kg/day.

Monitoring Fluid Therapy

All animals receiving fluids should have a physical examination, including assessment of hydration and body weight, with urine production checked at least twice per day, more frequently in the critically ill. Overzealous administration of crystalloids can manifest as increased respiratory rate and effort, crackles or wheezes on auscultation, serous discharge from the nares, chemosis, jugular vein distention or pulsations, shivering, edema, hypertension (>140–150 mmHg systolic), increased CVP (>8–10 cm H_2O), significant increase in body weight (>12%–15%), and rapid and/or dramatic decrease in PCV and total solids. In animals with urinary catheters, urine output can be monitored and compared with fluid administration volumes. Monitoring CVP, pulmonary capillary wedge pressures, and cardiac output variables may be helpful in selected animals, although pulmonary artery catheters are rarely placed. Monitoring electrolytes and PCV/total solids may provide an objective measurement of fluid balance.

When parenteral fluid administration is to be discontinued, the animal should be able to maintain hydration by voluntary drinking and eating or tolerate enteral supplementation (through a feeding tube) or subcutaneous fluid administration. Tapering the volume infused IV throughout 24–48 hr allows the renal medulla to reestablish the osmotic gradient and helps prevent excessive fluid loss through diuresis.

MONITORING THE CRITICALLY ILL ANIMAL

Anticipation, not reaction, is the key to successful management of critically ill animals. Animals must be effectively treated and actively monitored to detect or prevent organ compromise *before* organ failure occurs. This often requires aggressive and repeated fluid resuscitation and support throughout the course of definitive therapy.

Tissue hypoxia and organ compromise or failure can be a direct result of the primary disease or can be secondary to the disease or its therapy. Organs frequently affected include the heart and blood vessels, kidneys, lungs, GI tract, and liver. When the disease process is multisystemic, problems such as malnutrition and coagulopathies must be anticipated. Optimal care requires a thorough and methodical approach to diagnostic procedures, monitoring, specific therapeutics, and supportive care.

THE RULE OF 20

The Rule of 20 is a list of 20 critical parameters that should be evaluated at least daily in all critically ill animals; many of these should be assessed several times per day. Using the Rule of 20 ensures that the clinical status and therapeutic strategy for each animal is comprehensive and meets the animal's ongoing needs. Like any monitoring tool, the Rule of 20 is not a static concept but a dynamic one; the specifics of each parameter will change with advancements in laboratory testing, understanding of disease pathology, and current concepts in critical care. In addition, the systems examined in the Rule of 20 are not singularities; each is impacted by and can impact other parameters, so each parameter should be assessed while considering the patient as a whole. Some more recent applications of the Rule of 20 include monitoring of blood lactate levels, adrenal function, body fluid glucose levels, and ultrasonographic assessment techniques. Diagnostic tools that are currently being investigated and may apply to the Rule of 20 in the future include biomarkers such as cardiac troponins, C-reactive protein, etc.

Fluid Balance: The goal of fluid therapy (*see* p 1675) is to provide adequate perfusion (intravascular volume) and hydration (interstitial volume) without overloading the interstitial space. Peripheral perfusion can be assessed by physical parameters such as heart rate, mucous membrane color, pulse quality, and mentation, as well as by measured parameters such as blood pressure, central venous pressure, urine output, and blood lactate measurements. Hydration can be assessed by physical parameters such as mucous membrane and corneal moistness and skin turgor, and by measured values such as body weight. Animals with systemic inflammatory response syndrome (SIRS) diseases may require more fluid than expected because of peripheral vasodilation and loss of endothelial integrity, making the administration of colloids with crystalloid solutions optimal. When treating fluid deficits, intravascular deficits should be addressed rapidly first; interstitial deficits should be treated using standard calculations to correct dehydration and monitor ongoing losses.

Oncotic Pull/Albumin: Albumin provides the major intravascular oncotic pull in the normal vasculature. In conditions in which there has been massive blood loss or leakage of plasma proteins due to an exudative process, albumin is lost from the intravascular space. This loss of intravascular oncotic pressure combined with increased capillary permeability associated with many SIRS diseases requires treatment using synthetic colloids that have a higher molecular weight than that of albumin. Colloid oncotic pull (COP) can be measured with colloid osmometry but is not commonly available in veterinary practice. Formulas are available to calculate COP based on plasma protein levels, but they are not reliable predictors of measured COP. Normal COP in dogs is ~20 mmHg. In patients with moderate to severe decreases in COP or in total proteins, natural and synthetic colloids should be administered. Examples of natural colloids include plasma, concentrated human or canine albumin, and stroma-free hemoglobin. Examples of synthetic colloids include dextrans and hydroxyethyl starches. Newer understanding of the endothelial cell function and the impact of the endothelial glycocalyx may present novel therapeutic options in the future.

Part of the oncotic activity normally provided by albumin can be provided by synthetic colloids, but only albumin can perform other functions such as drug, cation, and hormone transport, as well as contribute to acid/base balance. Albumin can be lost with a variety of diseases (GI, renal, or SIRS); in addition, it is a negative acute-phase protein, so production of albumin drops during critical illness. Interstitial albumin stores are drawn upon to replace serum albumin, and a low serum albumin reflects a total body deficit of albumin. Albumin levels <2 g/dL have been associated with a poor prognosis; however, it is not known whether restoring albumin levels improves survival. Plasma and albumin transfusions are often administered to supplement the albumin to reach a target of 2 g/dL, but large volumes of plasma are required. Lyophilized canine serum albumin is now available in 100-g vials, making replacement of albumin more cost-effective and with lower total volumes than plasma transfusions. Human albumin products have been used in critically ill dogs but may result in severe organ dysfunction when given to healthy dogs. Interstitial albumin stores must be replenished as well as intravascular levels, so multiple units of plasma or albumin may be necessary to increase serum albumin levels.

Glucose: The goal is to maintain glucose between 80 and 120 mg/dL. Septic animals are at an increased risk of hypoglycemia that can be severe enough to cause hypotension or neurologic dysfunction ranging from weakness to stupor or seizures. Other causes of hypoglycemia include inadequate nutrition, glycogen storage diseases, heat stroke, young age, small size, severe liver disease or portosystemic vascular anomalies, certain neoplasias, hypoadrenocorticism, and iatrogenic insulin administration. Dextrose supplementation is warranted in any animal that is hypoglycemic. Solutions with a dextrose concentration >5% are best administered through a central line. Animals with clinical hypoglycemia despite administration of solutions with high dextrose concentrations should be assessed for insulinoma and may benefit from glucagon infusions. A difference of >20 mg/dL in blood glucose values and abdominal fluid glucose values has high sensitivity and specificity for septic peritonitis in animals who have not recently had surgery.

Insulin treatment of hyperglycemia in diabetic animals is important to offset ketoacidosis or hyperosmolar complications. Constant-rate infusion (CRI) of regular insulin can result in the slow and controlled lowering of blood glucose (to help avoid rapid changes of blood osmolality); close monitoring of blood glucose levels should be performed. Tight control of increased blood glucose has improved neurologic outcome after head trauma in critical human surgical patients but not in human medical patients; in addition, increased incidences of hypoglycemia may occur with tight glucose control. Acutely traumatized animals are prone to insulin resistance because of large amounts of circulating cortisol and epinephrine and may develop hyperglycemia severe enough to require treatment with insulin. The benefit of tight blood glucose control has not been clearly demonstrated in veterinary medicine.

Electrolytes and Acid-Base Balance: Hypokalemia can be a contributing factor in weakness and ileus of critically ill animals. These animals commonly have reduced oral intake and/or increased GI and urinary losses of potassium that require potassium supplementation in the IV fluids. Hyperkalemia can be a life-threatening complication of urinary tract rupture or obstruction, renal failure, reperfusion injury, or massive cellular death. Hyperkalemia commonly results in bradyarrhythmias and can be temporarily treated with calcium gluconate and insulin, concurrently with dextrose and/or sodium bicarbonate. The underlying pathology that led to hyperkalemia must be addressed. Other important electrolytes to monitor include sodium, ionized calcium, phosphorus, magnesium, and chloride; all can be increased or decreased in critically ill animals and may affect other body systems (such as neurologic acid/base balance, serum osmolality, the cardiovascular system, and RBCs). The anion gap (AG) can be calculated when blood electrolytes are measured: AG = [Na] + [K] – [HCO_3] – [Cl]. Normal AG values are between 12 and 24 mEq/L. An increased AG indicates there is some unmeasured anion present in the blood, which may include ketones, lactate, uremic compounds, or toxins (eg, salicylates, ethylene glycol, ethanol, methanol, indomethacin, isoniazid, paraldehyde, propylene glycol). The most common cause of metabolic acidosis is lactic acidosis caused by poor perfusion leading to anaerobic metabolism. Lactate production results in an equimolar production of hydrogen ions and subsequent alterations in blood gas values (metabolic acidosis). Lactate measurements can be easily performed with handheld or benchtop analyzers. Resolution of hyperlactatemia with adequate fluid resuscitation is often associated with improved survival. Treatment involves maximizing blood flow and tissue oxygen delivery. Rarely is the administration of sodium bicarbonate ($NaHCO_3$) warranted for perfusion-related acidosis. Once perfusion and hydration are corrected, the acid-base status is reassessed.

If severe metabolic acidosis (as occurs with ketosis or uremia) persists and HCO_3 remains below ~12 mEq/L after perfusion has been restored, slow administration of fluids with $NaHCO_3$ supplementation is warranted, restoring serum values to >15 mEq/L. The dosage of $NaHCO_3$ is calculated as follows:

mEq $NaHCO_3$ = 0.3 × (target $NaHCO_3$ [eg, 15] – patient $NaHCO_3$) × body weight in kg

Serum bicarbonate levels are carefully monitored to meet patient requirements.

Oxygenation and Ventilation: Pulmonary function can be compromised in critical illness for a variety of reasons (pneumonia, acute respiratory distress syndrome, thromboembolism, congestive heart failure, etc). Early diagnostic tests (eg, imaging, blood work, tracheal washes, urine blastomycosis antigen testing, etc) for targeted therapeutics will help limit extension of pulmonary disease. Aspiration pneumonia is a particular challenge, because it is most commonly a "second hit" disease (secondary to another systemic illness); therapeutics (such as antiemetics, prokinetics, or use of nasogastric tubes) to prevent aspiration pneumonia should be used whenever appropriate. Arterial blood gas measurement is the "gold standard" method to detect hypoxemia or hypercarbia. Pulse oximetry (SpO_2) is a noninvasive way to determine the oxygen saturation of hemoglobin. Supplemental oxygen and/or therapeutic ventilation may be indicated with SpO_2 values <96%. Hypercarbia can be detected using end-tidal CO_2 through an endotracheal tube or nasal catheter and has been shown to correlate with arterial CO_2 levels in animals. Serial monitoring is recommended in the initial management of animals with respiratory compromise to determine the adequacy of oxygen supplementation and the need for mechanical ventilation. If hypoxemia is unresponsive to oxygen supplementation (PaO_2 <60 mmHg or SpO_2 <90%) or hypercarbia is present ($PaCO_2$ >60 mmHg), or if respiratory effort (work of breathing) is substantially increased, manual or mechanical ventilation is necessary. Ventilation should not be delayed until respiratory failure or arrest. Prognosis for animals that require ventilation is variable; those with hypoxemia from congestive heart failure or hypoventilation from metabolic disease (eg, hypokalemia) or cervical spinal disease have a better prognosis than those that require ventilation for hypoxemia due to primary pulmonary disease. Invasive (arterial sampling) and noninvasive ($ETCO_2$/SpO_2) blood gas measurements should be performed during mechanical ventilation to determine need for adjustment of the ventilator settings.

Level of Consciousness/Mentation/Neurologic Status: A decline in an animal's level of consciousness warrants investigation to exclude metabolic causes, such as hypoglycemia, hyperglycemia, hepatic encephalopathy, acidosis, electrolyte or osmotic derangements, or sudden development of hypertension, hypotension, or shock. An increase in intracranial pressure can result from intracranial hemorrhage, fluid overload (cerebral edema), primary brain/meningeal disease, and/or ischemia. The drugs the animal is receiving should be carefully evaluated for adverse effects that can lead to altered mentation or level of consciousness. Cerebral edema may be responsive to medical management with furosemide and concurrent mannitol therapy. Steroids may be indicated in certain inflammatory diseases (eg, meningitis, neoplasia), and antibiotics in infectious disease (eg, toxoplasmosis). Craniotomy may be needed in animals not responsive to medical management. Cerebral perfusion pressure = mean arterial pressure – intracranial pressure. Elevating the head 15° and avoiding procedures that may increase venous pressure and subsequently intracranial pressure is essential. Maintaining normal oxygenation/ventilation, blood pressure, glucose level, and serum osmolality is essential for animals with brain disease. Neurologic status may be evaluated using a scoring system assessed on a regular basis, such as the modified Glasgow Coma Scale; lower scores are associated with a poorer prognosis.

Spinal injury that is severe enough to cause paralysis (particularly with lack of deep pain sensation) and inability to ventilate and ambulate, and that has not responded to medical management (such as anti-inflammatory medications) warrants immediate imaging and surgical intervention. Loss of deep pain is associated with a poor return to function. Serial neurologic examinations should be performed in any animal with neurologic disease.

Blood Pressure: Blood pressure should be monitored via direct or indirect methods. The goal is to maintain organ perfusion by maintaining a minimum mean arterial blood pressure >60 mmHg (systolic >90 mmHg). In hypotensive animals with adequate cardiac function, treatment consists of intravascular volume infusion (*see* p 1675), oxygen administration, and pain control. Hypotension unresponsive to intravascular volume replacement can be due to one or more of the following: hypoglycemia, acidosis, alkalosis, electrolyte disorders (eg, potassium, calcium, magnesium), brain-stem pathology, cardiac arrhythmias, metabolic toxins (eg, hepatic, renal), ongoing fluid loss, relative hypoadrenocorticism (eg, cortisol deficiency), heart or pericardial disease, excessive vasodilation, and excessive vasoconstriction. The need for cardiac support with positive inotropes should be assessed. An experienced ultrasonographer may be able to assess ventricular and/or capacitance vessel size to provide an estimate of preload and contractility. Once intravascular volume (central venous pressure >8 cm H_2O) and cardiac function are assessed as adequate, vasopressor therapy with CRI of dopamine (5–15 mcg/kg/min) or norepinephrine (0.05–2 mcg/kg/min), beginning at the lower end of the dosage range and increasing by increments of 0.2–0.5 mcg, is recommended. Stroma-free hemoglobin can be infused for its pressor effects.

Objective measurements of global perfusion may also include lactate monitoring; animals with a significantly increased lactate concentration may have a poorer prognosis. Studies have demonstrated that serial lactate monitoring as pathology is treated is more useful than a single measurement. Central venous oxygen measurement is another objective measurement of global perfusion; normal values are 70–80 mmHg, whereas lower values may indicate increased oxygen extraction.

Hypertension is a relatively uncommon condition in veterinary medicine, but it can lead to catastrophic problems such as retinal detachment or neurologic derangements from intracranial hemorrhage. Hypertension can exacerbate proteinuria in animals with chronic kidney disease. Moderate to severe hypertension can be treated with oral antihypertensive agents such as angiotensin-converting enzyme inhibitors (eg, benazepril), calcium channel blockers (eg, amlodipine), direct arterial dilators (eg, hydralazine), or systemic injectable antihypertensive agents such as nitroprusside (0.5–10 mcg/kg/min), titrated to effect. Blood pressure must be monitored constantly to assess response to therapy with nitroprusside. Chronic hypertension that is rapidly decreased may result in decreased renal perfusion.

The American College of Veterinary Internal Medicine classifies risk of target-organ damage from hypertension into four categories based on systolic blood pressure: I: <150 mmHg = minimal risk; II: 150–159 mmHg = mild risk; III: 160–179 mmHg = moderate risk; and IV: >180 mmHg = severe risk.

Heart Rate, Rhythm, Contractility, and Myocardial Injury: The electrical and mechanical systems of the heart should be evaluated separately. Specific antiarrhythmic drug therapy should be instituted based on an accurate ECG diagnosis when perfusion is compromised by an arrhythmia and the first-line therapy of oxygen supplementation and analgesics has been unsuccessful in controlling the arrhythmia. Arrhythmias can occur for a variety of reasons, such as SIRS diseases, splenic disease, organ torsion (eg, gastric dilatation-volvulus), and electrolyte abnormalities (eg, hyperkalemia); the underlying condition must be treated/investigated as well. Some ventricular rhythms (such as ventricular premature contractions and accelerated idioventricular arrhythmias) may not necessarily require immediate therapy. Indications for treatment of a ventricular rhythm include tachycardia (rates >160–180 bpm), clinical signs of poor perfusion (low blood pressure, poor pulse quality, etc), multiform arrhythmias, and R-on-T phenomenon. Other tachyarrhythmias may respond to class I, II, III, or IV antiarrhythmics; bradyarrhythmias can be challenging to treat medically and may require pacemaker placement. An echocardiogram can be performed to evaluate cardiac contractility in SIRS diseases and to detect underlying cardiac diseases. If cardiac contractility is decreased, dobutamine at 5–10 mcg/kg/min (dogs) or 2.5–5 mcg/kg/min (cats) should be considered to provide inotropic support if there is evidence of poor cardiac output. Recent studies have demonstrated that dogs with mitral valve disease and dilated cardiomyopathy have a poorer prognosis if their cardiac troponins (cTnI) and/or natriuretic peptide (NT-pro-BNP) is increased. However, these tests are not available in all hospitals and do not necessarily direct therapy, or diagnose or differentiate disease processes.

Temperature: Body temperature is considered part of the initial clinical database and should be measured regularly in every critically ill animal. A variety of diseases can result in increased or decreased body temperature. Temperature is measured most accurately and consistently with a rectal thermometer.

Increased temperatures can be seen with environmental exposure (eg, heat stroke), increased activity (eg, exercise, excitement), and infectious, inflammatory, or neoplastic diseases. Severe increases of temperature (>105.5° [40.8°C]), particularly when prolonged, can lead to severe metabolic disease such as hemorrhagic diathesis, disseminated intravascular coagulation, and SIRS diseases, which may lead to multiorgan dysfunction. Effective means of cooling animals include fluid therapy, using wet towels with fans, and placing alcohol in paw pads. Animals should not be immersed in cold water, because this causes peripheral vasocontriction and decreases core heat dissipation. Fever of unknown origin warrants a systemic evaluation (*see* p 1015).

Hypothermia is most commmonly associated with anesthesia in small animals; however, severe systemic disease (particularly in cats) and environmental exposure may be contributing factors. Mild hypothermia can be a common sequela of severe cardiovascular disease and is a prognostic marker in cats with limb thromboembolism. Temperature is a vital parameter to monitor and treat in cats with clinical signs of shock, and active warming is an essential component of therapy. Therapeutic hypothermia may have some neuro-sparing effects in animals with traumatic brain injury or in postresuscitation (CPR) care; however, further investigation is needed. In animals with induced hypothermia, blood flow to most organs can be significantly decreased, and coagulation may be affected.

Altered body temperature is part of the definition of SIRS-type diseases; other parameters include an increased or decreased heart rate, increased or decreased WBC count, and an increased respiratory rate.

Coagulation: Disseminated intravascular coagulation (DIC) can develop in any animal that has undergone a period of relative vascular stasis as occurs during shock, severe tissue or capillary damage such as that which occurs with trauma, exposure of capillary endothelial cells to circulating inflammatory mediators as occurs during sepsis or SIRS, or moderate to severe alterations in body temperature. In the early stages of DIC, there may be few or no clinical signs. However, as DIC progresses, its effects are obvious and catastrophic. The goal is to detect DIC in the early stages and to slow or prevent its progression.

Early DIC is characterized by a hypercoagulable stage in which serum antithrombin (AT) levels are decreased and the coagulation cascade is activated by any of the precipitating causes. Activation of the coagulation cascade throughout the body rapidly depletes the clotting factors and the blood platelet count as platelets are incorporated into the clots. At this stage, the prothrombin time and partial thromboplastin time may be decreased, but this is a challenging stage to identify and diagnose. However, this rapidly progresses to a hypocoagulable stage as the coagulation factors are consumed. In this late stage, the prothrombin time and partial thromboplastin time (or activated clotting time) are prolonged, and fibrinogen degradation products are increased.

Treatment of DIC focuses on treating the underlying disease and removing the stimulus for continued activation of the coagulation cascade. In the early hypercoagulable stages, treatment focuses on maximizing the function of AT, which is the most abundant natural inhibitor of the serine proteases of the coagulation cascade. When AT levels are adequate, heparin can be administered SC (50–100 U/kg, tid). If AT levels are <60% of normal, then plasma transfusions should also be given to increase the level to ≥80%. In animals with diseases known to predispose to DIC, coagulation parameters and platelet counts should be monitored. Thomboelastography (TEG) provides another means of global assessment of the clotting cascade and may be a useful tool with suspected hypo- or hypercoagulable states; hypercoagulable states are challenging to diagnose, and TEG is one of the few methods that may provide an accurate assessment.

Thrombosis occurs without DIC when there are alterations in Virchow's triad: endothelial injury, blood stasis, and hypercoagulable states. Abnormalities in one or more of these components may be seen with vascular anomalies, atrial enlargement, severe systemic illness (SIRS, immune-mediated hemolytic anemia), trauma, neoplasia, renal disease, hyperadrenocorticism, and as a primary disease in Greyhounds. The most common severe manifestations of hypercoagulability are aortic and pulmonary thromboemboli. Pulmonary thromboemboli should be suspected when significant hypoxemia is present with minimal lung changes on thoracic radiographs. Anticoagulation therapy and oxygen support should be implemented, and oxygenation and ventilation monitored. Arterial thromboembolism can occur in cats with underlying heart disease. Antithrombotics are warranted in these cases; options include aspirin and/or clopidogrel, heparin (low molecular weight or unfractionated), or warfarin. Most of these drugs require close monitoring of clotting times to achieve therapeutic goals. This disease can be painful, and opioid medications are often warranted as well as monitoring for reperfusion injury.

Disease states that result in relative hypocoagulability may include anticoagulant rodenticide ingestion, fulminant liver failure, severe thombocytopenia, snake bites, dilutional hypocoagulability from fluid and colloid administration, and congenital defects in the coagulation cascade such as von Willebrand disease, hemophilia A or B platelet defects (Boxers), or hyperfibrinolysis (Greyhounds). Therapy should be specific to the inciting cause; plasma products are often necessary to correct life-threatening coagulopathies.

Red Blood Cell and Hemoglobin Concentration: Because Hgb carries most of the oxygen in the blood, maintaining adequate Hgb levels is essential to maintaining adequate oxygen delivery. When anemia is associated with clinical signs of tachycardia, increased respiratory rate, altered mentation, severe lethargy/weakness, and hypotension, then packed RBCs, whole blood, or stroma-free hemoglobin should be administered to bring the PCV to >20% or the Hgb level to >7 g/dL. In some cases of hemolytic or chronic anemia, the PCV can be maintained at a lower percentage before transfusion is required if there are no corresponding clinical signs. In animals that require multiple blood sampling (such as diabetic patients) or very small animals, blood sampling should be minimized to prevent iatrogenic blood loss. Optimal hemoglobin levels have not been determined; however, conservative transfusion managment in people (Hgb goal of 7 g/dL or PCV of 20%) has improved survival benefit over more liberal transfusion goals (Hgb of 10 g/dL or PCV of 30%).

Except in the case of acute, life-threatening hemorrhage, before an RBC-containing blood product is administered, a crossmatch should be performed to ensure a safely administered transfusion. Even type-specific or "A-negative" blood may not be antigenically appropriate for some dogs, because many antigens are present on canine RBCs. If multiple transfusions are anticipated, blood typing should be performed as well. Only type-specific blood should be administered to cats. In dogs and cats with acute cavitary (pleural or peritoneal) hemorrhage, blood may be salvaged from the cavity with aspiration (via centesis or exploratory surgery when indicated) and an autologous blood transfusion administered through a blood filter.

Rarely, disease states may result in altered hemoglobin (such as methemoglobinemia) or altered oxygen-carrying capacity (such as carboxyhemoglobinemia), often recognized by altered mucous membrane color (muddy or brick-red, respectively). Despite normal measured hemoglobin concentrations, oxygen is not being delivered to tissues in these animals, and oxygen supplementation is necessary along with treatment of the underlying disease.

An alternative means to increase oxygen-carrying capacity of the blood is a commercial stroma-free hemoglobin-based oxygen carrier (HBOC) such as Oxyglobin®. Monitoring PCV is not an adequate assessment of oxygen delivery after use of HBOCs.

Animals with a PCV >55% (other than sight hounds and at high altitudes) may have microvascular sludging (due to the altered blood rheology) and hypertension (which impairs microvascular delivery of oxygen to the tissues). This occurs most commonly with hemorrhagic gastroenteritis. Treatment with IV fluids, and phlebotomy in cases of absolute polycythemia, are performed to improve microvascular flow and oxygen delivery to the tissues.

Renal Function: In animals that have had a hypotensive episode, are receiving potentially nephrotoxic medications, or have primary renal compromise, renal function should be evaluated daily. Urinalysis performed on a sample collected before fluid administration will help to assess renal function. Normal urine output is 1–2 mL/kg/hr and can be closely monitored with an indwelling urinary catheter. Animals in polyuric renal failure are most often managed medically; however, animals in oliguric (<0.8 mL/kg/hr), anuric (<0.03 mL/kg/hr), or relative oliguric (less than expected) renal failure may require peritoneal or hemodialysis to maintain fluid and electrolyte balance. Serial measurement of serum BUN, creatinine, electrolytes, and phosphorus will detect changes and help guide therapy. Serial urinalyses to detect glucosuria, proteinuria, or renal tubular casts help evaluate acute tubular injury before the damage progresses to overt renal failure and azotemia. If urine output monitoring with a catheter is not possible, then estimating urine output by measuring absorbent pads or litterboxes is neccesary. Body weights should be recorded regularly. Additional necessary diagnostics may include urine culture and susceptibility testing, urine protein to creatinine ratio, or specific testing for renal-specific disease (eg, ethylene glycol, leptospirosis). Animals may also be monitored using a scoring system to provide additional "objective" monitoring: the International Renal Interest Society has a staging system to monitor dogs and cats with chronic renal disease based on serum creatinine, blood pressure, and proteinuria.

Infection Identification/Prevention and Treatment and Immune Status: Strict aseptic technique should be observed when examining or treating animals that are neutropenic or receiving immunosuppressive drugs. These animals should be isolated from other animals and handled by a single person who adheres to appropriate barrier nursing techniques (washes hands, wears gloves and gown before handling the animal, etc). All veterinary staff should be encouraged to wash hands between patients, treat wounds in a clean manner, and administer IV injections only after swabbing an IV port with an alchohol swab. Educating hospital staff on appropriate patient handling techniques may help limit development of nosocomial infections, which develop 48 hr after hospital admission.

Ultimately, antibiotic selection should be based on the results of culture and susceptibility testing, but empiric treatment, based on site of infection and suspected type of bacteria, is necessary pending these results. Empiric therapy may be based on common organisms found at the affected site and/or Gram stain and cytologic examination, which should be performed immediately. Repeat culture and susceptibility testing may be necessary in animals not responding to therapy as expected or if prolonged antibiotic therapy is anticipated.

In animals that have sustained a hypotensive episode or have a GI disease that would allow bacterial translocation, broad-spectrum bacterial coverage should be provided until the results of culture are available or the risk of systemic infection has passed.

An antibiotic protocol should be established for veterinary hospitals to minimize the number of antibiotics administered empirically on a routine basis to reduce the development of resistant organisms in the hospital environment and to improve their susceptibility patterns. Limiting use of specific classes of antibiotics or having rotating schedules may help limit development of microbial resistance. Periodic environmental cultures and facility-based monitoring of culture and susceptibility results for evidence of nosocomial infections and bacterial resistance patterns can help identify and control sources of infection and limit development of resistance. A first-generation cephalosporin (eg, cefazolin, 22 mg/kg, tid) is useful for gram-positive and gram-negative infections; an alternative choice is an aminopencillin with a β-lactamase inhibitor (such as clavulanic acid or sulbactam), which has good gram-negative, gram-positive, and anaerobic coverage at 20–30 mg/kg, tid. If a resistant bacteria is suspected, gentamicin (3–5 mg/kg/day, IV) can be given to more specifically target gram-negative organisms after hydration and perfusion have normalized; a fluoroquinolone (eg, enrofloxacin at

5–10 mg/kg, IV, once or twice daily) is an alternative. The once-daily dosage is less likely to cause toxicity and has the same antibacterial effect as a divided dosage schedule. Metronidazole (7.5–15 mg/kg) given slowly IV over 20 min every 6–8 hr is used for suspected anaerobic infections. If multiple antibiotics are started, the antimicrobial spectrum should be narrowed and antibiotic choice adjusted as soon as the organism's susceptibility pattern is identified. Recurrent infections should be investigated for an underlying pattern of resistance, nidus of infection, or immune-compromising disease.

Newer generations and classes of antibiotics, such as carbapenems (eg, imipenim), third-generation cephalosporins (eg, ceftazidime), and vancomycin should be reserved for use in animals with bacterial infections demonstrated to be resistant to other antibiotics.

WBC counts performed on a semiregular basis (every 48–72 hr) may indicate an appropriate response to infection/inflammation or patient deterioration.

Various molecular or "bio" markers have been investigated in SIRS-type diseases to help understand and stratify disease. High mobility group box 1 protein and C-reactive protein have been associated with poor outcome or diagnosis of SIRS-type disease; however, how that information affects therapy has yet to be determined. Plasma interleukin 1B and IL-6 have been demonstrated to have some prognostic value in cats with sepsis.

GI Motility and Mucosal Integrity: Critically ill animals, even those without a primary GI disease, are prone to gastric atony, ileus, and gastric ulceration. Auscultation for bowel sounds should be performed three times a day. Metoclopramide (1–2 mg/kg/day as a CRI) is useful because of its central antiemetic effects and its ability to increase progressive gastric and intestinal motility. Other motility modifiers to consider include cisapride, ranitidine, and erythromycin. Motility modifiers should be avoided if gastric or intestinal obstruction is suspected or has been confirmed.

Placement of a nasogastric tube to allow removal of accumulated gas and fluid reduces the possibility of aspiration of refluxed gastric contents and allows continuous decompression. The nasogastric tube also can be used to introduce small amounts of a glucose and electrolyte solution or a liquid diet to provide nutrition directly to enterocytes, which helps prevent gastric ulceration and intestinal mucosal compromise with secondary bacterial translocation. Antiemetics are used in animals that continue to vomit frequently despite placement of a nasogastric tube, thus improving patient comfort and reducing the incidence of aspiration, vagal-induced collapse, and bradycardia that can accompany the vomiting reflex. Metoclopramide blocks the dopaminergic receptors in the chemoreceptor trigger zone (CRTZ) and central vomiting center and acts peripherally by promoting gastric emptying. Ondansetron and dolasetron are potent antiemetics that block serotonin receptors and act at the CRTZ and the central vomiting center; they are administered at 0.6–1 mg/kg/day. Maropitant is an NK_1 receptor antagonist that blocks vomiting at the CRTZ, vomiting center, and peripheral receptors, administered at 1 mg/kg/day, SC, or 2 mg/kg/day, PO. Vomiting refractory to all other treatments in an otherwise stable animal with normal blood pressure can be treated with chlorpromazine (dogs: 0.05–1 mg/kg, IV, every 4–8 hr; cats: 0.01–0.025 mg/kg, IV, every 4–8 hr). A combination of antiemetics that have different mechanisms of action is often required to arrest refractory emesis in severe illness; in animals that require multiple antiemetics, an obstructive disease should be excluded.

GI ulceration often accompanies critical diseases such as hypotension, hypergastrinemia associated with liver and kidney disease, drug toxicities, neurologic disease, and respiratory disorders requiring ventilation. Histamine$_2$-receptor antagonists such as ranitidine and famotidine, and proton-pump inhibitors such as omeprazole and pantoprazole should be administered to treat gastric ulcers. However, changing the pH of the stomach can change its microbial flora. Agents such as sucralfate and barium are administered to bind to esophageal and gastric erosions and ulcers. Misoprostol may help prevent NSAID-induced ulceration when toxic levels of NSAIDs are ingested.

Drug Dosages and Metabolism: An active medications list should be kept with each animal's medical record and carefully reviewed daily for potential drug interactions, drug dosages, and possible adverse effects. If renal or hepatic function is compromised, or if protein (albumin) binding capacity is decreased, some drug dosages should be decreased to account for altered metabolism, elimination, or protein binding. The daily review also should ensure that the dosage has been calculated correctly and that it is appropriate for the animal's current weight and body condition score. The sudden onset of any new clinical signs should be investigated in light of the medications and their potential adverse effects.

Nutrition: When nutritional needs are not met, animals rapidly develop a negative energy balance, which can result in GI dysfunction, organ dysfunction, poor wound healing, and even death. Direct enteral nutrition will improve the normal GI barrier, function, and motility. Enteral feeding is always preferred, and most animals tolerate trickle flow feeding techniques. Short-term options include syringe or forced feeding; however, this can lead to food aversion and is not comfortable for most critically ill animals. Easy to place and well-tolerated, short-term feeding tubes that allow trickle feeding include nasogastric, nasoesophageal, and nasojejunal. Nasogastric tubes also allow gastric suctioning to monitor GI function and may limit continued vomiting and risk of aspiration pneumonia; nasojejunal tubes can be challenging to place. Long-term feeding tubes include esophagostomy, pharyngostomy, gastrotomy, or jejunostomy tubes. Each of these tubes are well tolerated by most animals, and all require anesthesia to place; the esophagostomy is a minor surgical procedure, and gastrostomy tubes can be placed with endoscopic assistance.

Feeding by trickle flow is initiated with small volumes of a dilute veterinary liquid diet solution. If an animal has been starved for an extended period of time, nutrition should be increased slowly (by 25%–33% of daily caloric requirements per day) to avoid the hyperglycemia, hypokalemia, hypophosphatemia, and hypomagnesemia seen with refeeding syndrome.

For the first 12–24 hr, the diet should be calculated to provide ¼ to ⅓ of the daily caloric requirement and is diluted 1 part liquid diet to 2 parts water (or electrolyte solution). This volume is delivered by CRI over 12–24 hr or divided into small boluses every 2–4 hr. Before each bolus feeding and every 6 hr during a CRI, the feeding tube should be suctioned to determine whether any residual volume is present that would necessitate decreasing the volume infused or adding prokinetic agents. After suctioning or administering a liquid diet, the tube should be flushed with saline. If this initial feeding is tolerated, the concentration is increased to 2 parts liquid diet mixed with 1 part water during the next 12–24 hr. If this is tolerated, then the undiluted diet can be delivered to provide the full caloric requirements. As the animal recovers, bolus feeding can be introduced by gradually decreasing feeding frequency and increasing volumes.

When nutritional needs cannot be met by enteral feeding, parenteral feeding is used. Partial parenteral nutrition, consisting of amino acid and carbohydrate solutions, can be infused through a peripheral vein, providing part of the animal's caloric requirements in a readily metabolizable form. Total parenteral nutrition (including the lipid component) must be delivered through a central venous catheter, because high osmolarity of the solutions may cause phlebitis and RBC lysis. In animals with prolonged anorexia, vitamin supplementation may also be necessary.

Appetite stimulants, such as the serotonin antagonist cyproheptadine and the serotonin agonist mirtazapine, are commonly used but with varying success. Oral benzodiazepines may cause hepatotoxicity in cats and are not good alternatives; injectable benzodiazepines may be used as a short-term solution for animals with rapidly resolving disease. The use of appetite stimulants provides inconsistent food intake and is not recommended as the primary way to administer nutrition in critically ill animals.

Pain Control: Pain activates the stress hormone systems of the body and contributes to morbidity and mortality. Signs of pain are quite variable in animals; these may include decreased normal behavior (decreased appetite, ambulation, grooming, etc), development of abnormal behaviors (vocalizing, inappropriate urination, altered posture, signs of agitation or aggression, etc), reaction to touch, and altered objective physical parameters (increased heart rate, pale mucous membranes, dilated pupils, etc), which can mimic signs of shock. (*See also* SYSTEMIC PHARMACOTHERAPEUTICS OF THE NERVOUS SYSTEM, p 2590, and PAIN MANAGEMENT, p 2104.) Animals that may not show obvious signs of pain but are known to have a painful condition should receive analgesics as part of their treatment (*see* TABLE 7). Preemptive administration of analgesics is recommended, when possible. Pain should be assessed using a validated pain assessment tool and monitored on a regular basis during the course of hospitalization to ensure adequate analgesia.

Analgesia in critically ill animals can safely be provided by opioids titrated to effect. Opioids provide potent analgesia (given IV, IM, or SC) with minimal cardiovascular adverse effects, and their actions are reversible with antagonists (eg, naloxone). Long-acting opioids are best avoided in unstable animals. Reports of IV morphine causing hypotension due to histamine release do not seem to be clinically significant if the drug is given

TABLE 7 ANALGESICS USED IN EMERGENCY PRACTICE

Drug	Dosage	Comments
Morphine	Dogs: 0.05–0.4 mg/kg, IV, every 1–4 hr; 0.2–1 mg/kg, IM or SC, every 2–6 hr; 0.1 mg/kg diluted with 0.9% saline administered epidurally at 0.23 mL/kg, every 8–24 hr	Incremental IV bolus technique: dogs—increments of 0.1 mg/kg until analgesia appears adequate; cats—increments of 0.02 mg/kg. In dogs, this can be followed by CRI at 0.1 mg/kg/hr that can be increased incrementally if needed. Rapid IV injections may cause histamine release.
	Cats: 0.05–0.2 mg/kg, IM or SC, every 2–6 hr	
Oxymorphone/ hydromorphone	Dogs: 0.02–0.1 mg/kg, IV, every 2–4 hr; 0.05–0.2 mg/kg, IM or SC, every 2–6 hr	Minimal cardiovascular effects; may cause panting or emesis
	Cats: 0.02–0.05 mg/kg, IV, every 2–4 hr; 0.05–0.1 mg/kg, IM or SC, every 2–6 hr	Can be given as a CRI with the dose divided over 4 hr
Fentanyl	Dogs: 2–10 mcg/kg, IV, every 30–60 min; 2–20 mcg/kg/hr, IV as a CRI	With short half-life, fentanyl is best administered as a CRI.
Fentanyl transdermal patch	12.5 mcg/hr for animals <2.5 kg body wt; 25 mcg/hr for animals 2.5–10 kg body wt; 50 mcg/hr for animals 10–20 kg body wt; 75 mcg/hr for animals 20–30 kg body wt; 100 mcg/hr for animals >30 kg body wt	The patches cannot be cut. More than one patch may be used in larger animals. Injectable repository fentanyl solutions may be an alternative if available.
Butorphanol	Dogs: 0.2–0.5 mg/kg, IM, IV, or SC, every 1–3 hr	Has a ceiling effect; short duration of effect (1–2 hr) in most dogs
	Cats: 0.1–0.4 mg/kg, IM, IV, or SC, every 1–6 hr	Can be given as a CRI with the dose divided over 4 hr
Buprenorphine	Dogs: 0.005–0.02 mg/kg, IM or IV, every 1–6 hr	May be more difficult to reverse
	Cats: 0.005–0.01 mg/kg, IM, IV, or sublingual, every 4–8 hr	Sublingual absorption reported to be excellent in cats
Methadone	0.1–0.5 mg/kg IV, IM, or SC every 4–6 hr	Less vomiting than morphine, less panting than hydromorphone

over 5–10 min or as a CRI. Other medications such as hydromorphone, oxymorphone, and fentanyl can be given without this risk. CRI provides constant analgesia and is often more convenient and less painful than intermittent IM or SC injections. In cats, injectable buprenorphine is absorbed systemically after sublingual administration. Neuroleptanalgesia can be provided by combination of an opioid with a sedative (eg, benzodiazepine) or tranquilizer (eg, acepromazine) in animals without contraindications to these medications.

For longterm control of pain, transdermal fentanyl patches or repository fentanyl injections are used but require up to 12 hr to reach therapeutic blood levels; analgesia must be provided by injection until adequate blood levels have been reached.

If pain is not adequately controlled with opioids alone, then ketamine, an NMDA receptor antagonist, can be delivered by CRI with the opioids. Ketamine may have variable effects on the cardiovascular system, making patient selection crucial, and it should not be used as a sole agent for pain relief. Lidocaine, a local anesthetic, can be used as an adjunct for systemic pain relief when delivered as a CRI and combined with ketamine and/or an opioid. Some investigation into using maropitant as an adjunctive analgesic agent is promising, because it decreased anesthetic requirements during noxious stimuli in dogs.

Local pain relief can be provided using local infiltrative or nerve blocks on extremities. Intermittent infusions of bupivicaine administered through thoracotomy tubes or abdominal catheters can provide pleural and peritoneal analgesia. Epidural injections by needle or infusions by catheter can provide pain relief from pelvic, hindlimb, and abdominal injuries or disease.

NSAIDs are rarely used in critically ill animals because of their effects on the GI tract, kidney, and liver; however, they may be appropriate in animals with significant fevers or orthopedic injury that are not systemically ill. α_2-Agonists (such as dexmedetomidine) provide sedation as well, but case selection is critical because of the significant cardiovascular adverse effects. Other oral classes of medication that are well tolerated for mild to moderate pain include tramadol, amantidine, and gabapentin. Adjuvant methods of pain relief may include placing ice packs on regions of swelling, acupuncture, laser therapy, or massage.

Nursing Care: Providing nursing care to critically ill animals requires a skilled, knowledgeable, attentive, and highly trained nursing staff. Recumbent animals should be turned from one side to the other every 4 hr or maintained in variations of sternal recumbency to prevent decubital ulcers and atelectasis. Physical therapy 3–4 times a day is important to maintain range of motion and muscle tone and blood flow; this can be provided through massage, passive range of motion, encouraged activity, etc. Activity may also improve GI motility and provide a time when animals can urinate and defecate outside of their kennel. Catheters should be labeled and marked with the date of placement, and catheter sites should be inspected on a routine basis for signs of infection or displacement. When catheters are removed, the entrance site should be inspected for inflammation/infection. Urine and fecal soiling should be immediately cleaned. Recumbent animals require regular inspection and cleaning to prevent urine scalding of the skin; tail wraps minimize contamination from diarrhea. Nursing care must be tailored to the specific condition(s). A well-trained nursing staff can recognize deterioration or alterations in an animal often before the attending clinician because of the substantial amount of hands-on time with the patients.

Wound Care and Bandage Changes: Bandages, essential to cover wounds, should be changed whenever they become soiled or wet. Distal limb edema can be improved by placing light compression wraps that are changed every day. (*See also* WOUND MANAGEMENT, p 1701.) Open wounds should be bandaged on arrival to prevent further contamination or nosocomial infection until surgical debridement can be done. Areas of skin swelling or bruising should be marked to determine progression or resolution of the pathology.

Tender, Loving Care: Owner visits should be encouraged. Animals should be handled and spoken to kindly to minimize stress and anxiety. Having familiar items such as toys or blankets from home are helpful for some pets. Consolidating several treatments at one time and turning down the lights at night, when the animal's condition permits, allow the animal some time to rest and sleep undisturbed.

OPHTHALMIC EMERGENCIES

Ophthalmic emergencies require rapid diagnosis and appropriate and often aggressive therapy for maintenance of vision.

TRAUMATIC PROPTOSIS

Traumatic proptosis may follow blunt trauma (eg, being hit by a car, fight with another animal). During trauma, the globe is luxated from the orbit, and eyelid spasms prevent its retraction. Secondary orbital hemorrhage and swelling displace the globe further from the orbit. Corneoconjunctival drying and malacia follow. Prognosis depends on pupil size and reflexes, duration of exposure, other globe or orbital damage, breed (brachycephalics are predisposed), and other systemic trauma. Approximately 40%–60% of dogs, but very few cats, recover vision. Treatment begins by providing moisture to lubricate the exposed corneoconjunctiva. General anesthesia followed by a lateral canthotomy and complete temporary tarsorrhaphy with usually two or three interrupted horizontal mattress sutures (placed at one-half thickness of the eyelids) and stents should be followed by systemic antibiotics and corticosteroids as well as topical antibiotics and mydriatics (if miosis is present). Sutures and stents are removed only when a brisk blink reflex returns (usually 7–21 days), or more conservatively, a single suture every 2–3 days until all have been removed. Premature suture removal results in lagophthalmia and persistent and often progressive corneal ulceration. Complications include corneal ulceration, enophthalmia, optic nerve degeneration, keratoconjunctivitis sicca, and medial rectus muscle injury.

TRAUMATIC RETROBULBAR HEMORRHAGE

Orbital and ocular contusion can produce retrobulbar hemorrhage sufficient to damage the orbital vasculature and cause exophthalmos, iridocyclitis, and lagophthalmos. This occurs most often in dogs, horses, and cats. The exophthalmos and resultant lagophthalmos are associated with an impaired blink reflex and acute exposure

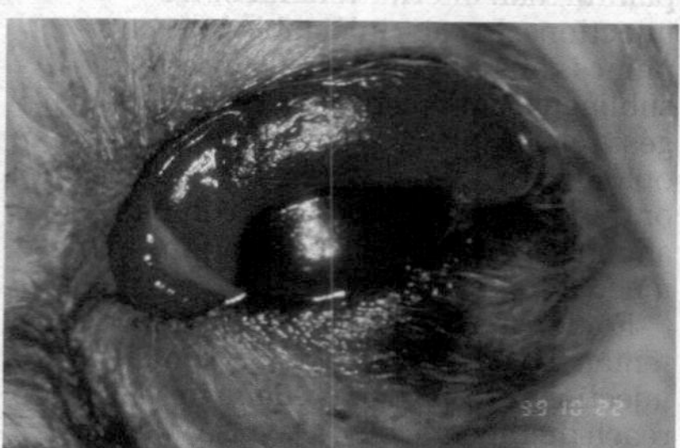

Traumatic retrobulbar hemorrhage, dog; hemorrhage displaces the globe forward but not sufficiently to produce proptosis. *Courtesy of K. Gelatt.*

ulcerative keratitis. Subconjunctival and intraocular hemorrhage may also be present, and the latter can prevent intraocular examination. Corneal and scleral lacerations should be excluded by ophthalmic examination, and B-scan ultrasonography to detect retinal detachment is recommended in eyes with intraocular hemorrhage.

Medical and surgical therapy consists of topical and systemic antibiotics and corticosteroids, mydriatics if pupillary dilation is necessary, and a complete temporary tarsorrhaphy to protect the cornea until a brisk blink reflex returns. Prognosis is guarded, because secondary glaucoma and phthisis bulbus are not infrequent. Intraocular hemorrhage is usually allowed to reabsorb.

EYELID LACERATIONS

Eyelid lacerations should be reapposed as soon as possible. Lacerations involving the lid margin require exact apposition to prevent longterm v-shape defects and an impaired lid function. Small dogs and cats require a single layer of sutures (usually single interrupted 4-0 silk sutures), whereas large and giant breeds require a two-layer closure; the deep layer involves the tarsus and orbiculis oculi muscle (single interrupted 4-0 absorbable sutures) and the superficial layer (skin) apposed with simple interrupted 4-0 silk sutures (remove after 7–10 days). Horses require double-layer closure. When skin sutures are in place, the lid must be protected from self-trauma by either an Elizabethan collar (dogs and cats) or hard eye cup (horses). Because the blink response is often impaired by the swollen lid, a temporary tarsorrhaphy is necessary to protect the cornea. Postoperative therapy often includes topical antibiotics and corticosteroids, as well as systemic antibiotics and NSAIDs.

CORNEAL FOREIGN BODIES

Corneal foreign bodies are seen most frequently in dogs, cats, and horses. They are usually organic material, but sand, metal, and glass foreign bodies are also seen. Presenting signs include variable blepharospasm, tearing, and a variable secondary iridocyclitis (aqueous flare, miosis, iridal swelling, ocular hypotony, and possible hypopyon). Ophthalmic examination reveals a foreign body on the conjunctival surface, in the posterior third eyelid fornix, or on or in the cornea. Foreign bodies that adhere to the ocular surfaces are usually removed under topical anesthesia with either vigorous irrigation or small serrated ophthalmic forceps. If the foreign body has embedded within the deeper corneal layers or has penetrated into the anterior chamber, general anesthesia is required for careful removal from either the anterior corneal surface or the anterior chamber. The corneal wound is apposed with simple interrupted 7-0 to 8-0 absorbable sutures. Postoperative therapy includes topical and systemic broad-spectrum antibiotics, mydriatics, systemic NSAIDs, and if necessary, drugs to reduce intraocular pressure. Prognosis for vision is usually good. Infrequent complications include variable corneal scar formation, septic endophthalmitis, cataract formation, and secondary glaucoma.

PENETRATING INTRAOCULAR INJURIES

Penetrating intraocular injuries with retained foreign bodies are seen most frequently in dogs and cats. They are often associated with lead pellets and bullets that partially or totally traverse the ocular tunics, but splinters or spines (eg, cactus) can also cause a penetrating injury. Pellets or bullets usually cause self-sealing, slightly tan corneal defects; may cause intraocular hemorrhage; and may traverse the lens and posterior segment wall. Perforation of the lens can lead to rapid cataract formation, especially when the anterior lens capsular tear is >2 mm long. Vitreal and retinal hemorrhage and retinal detachments are likely. Ophthalmic ultrasonography and orbital radiology are most helpful to assess pellet location and the integrity of the intraocular and orbital tissues. Anterior lens laceration and rupture is also a common sequela of cat claw injuries in young dogs.

Penetration of the anterior lens capsule (lacerations >2 mm) requires lens removal as soon as possible, because escape of lens material causes gradually intensifying lens-induced uveitis that often progresses to secondary glaucoma and phthisis bulbus. The posterior segment changes usually resolve provided the retina eventually reattaches. Focal retinal degeneration in the area of retinal penetration and detachment is common. Prognosis is guarded and based, in part, on the response to therapy and gradual clearing of the intraocular media.

Therapy is directed at controlling the post-traumatic inflammation and maintaining normal levels of intraocular pressure. Mydriatics and topical and systemic antibiotics and corticosteroids are administered to control the uveitis. Intraocular hemorrhage is allowed to resolve, with anterior chamber hemorrhage usually disappearing in ~1–2 wk and the vitreal hemorrhage resolving in 3–6 mo.

DEEP STROMAL CORNEAL ULCERS, DESCEMETOCELE, AND IRIS PROLAPSE

Most corneal ulcerations readily heal with appropriate antibiotic, antiproteinase (often topical serum), and mydriatic therapy. However, corneal ulcers detected late in the disease process, complicated by other ocular diseases, or given inadequate topical therapy can progress. These require surgical intervention using a conjunctival graft or, more recently, the commercially available porcine small-intestinal submucosa or experimental amniotic membranes. Deep corneal ulcers, descemetocele, and iris prolapse are seen with some frequency in dogs, cats, and horses. These conditions require immediate surgical support of the weakened cornea, because they can threaten or seriously compromise corneal integrity. Brachycephalic breeds and dogs with keratoconjunctivitis sicca are most vulnerable. These corneal defects often develop in the center of the cornea and can markedly impair vision. Important diagnostic aids are the Schirmer tear test to measure aqueous tear production and topical fluorescein to determine the extent of the corneal ulcer. Corneal culture and cytology can assist in choosing topical and systemic antibiotics. Secondary anterior uveitis with aqueous flare, miosis, ocular hypotony, and hypopyon is common.

Corneal ulcer depth must be accurately estimated using magnification, focal illumination using a slit-beam, and topical fluorescein. Central corneal ulcers are more vulnerable, because they require more time for the healing response and vascularization. Adequate ulcer debridement is essential for successful adherence of a conjunctival graft. The corneal ulceration (stromal, descemetocele, or iris prolapse) is covered with the bulbar conjunctival graft (360°, 180°, bridge, or pedicle) that appears most appropriate.

For full-thickness corneal ulcers with iris prolapse, conjunctival grafts are also used, but the postoperative corneal opacity is usually larger and more dense. Postoperative therapy includes topical and systemic broad-spectrum antibiotics, systemic NSAIDs or corticosteroids, and mydriatics. Treatments are gradually tapered and administered for 4–8 wk. Postoperative complications include variable corneal scar and pigmentation, anterior and/or posterior synechiae, secondary cataract formation, and rarely bacterial endophthalmitis.

CORNEAL LACERATIONS

Corneal lacerations are seen most frequently in dogs and horses and infrequently in cats. Bites, self-inflicted trauma, and other accidents can partially or totally penetrate the cornea. Partial-thickness corneal lacerations are usually highly painful and require apposition with simple interrupted absorbable sutures to the healthy cornea. Excision of the lacerated section is not recommended.

For full-thickness corneal lacerations, signs usually include pain, blepharospasm, tearing, a corneal defect, and variable iris prolapse. Marked aqueous flare, hyphema, miosis, and distortion of the pupil are common. Often, the size of the iris prolapse is much larger than the underlying corneal laceration. Prognosis depends on size and position of the corneal laceration, other ocular tissue involvement, gender (horse), age of the animal, duration of the injury, and other systemic injuries. If the entire eye cannot be examined directly, B-scan ultrasonography is used.

The corneal laceration is apposed with simple interrupted 7-0 to 8-0 absorbable sutures. To provide additional protection and support, the sutured laceration may be covered with a third eyelid flap, bulbar conjunctival graft, or partial temporary tarsorrhaphy. Postoperative therapy to control the secondary iridocyclitis consists of topical and systemic antibiotics, systemic NSAIDs, and mydriatics. Postoperative complications include variable and often dense corneal scarring, cataract formation with posterior synechiae, secondary glaucoma, phthisis bulbus, and bacterial endophthalmitis.

GLAUCOMA

Animals are usually presented with high-pressure glaucoma because intraocular pressure (IOP) >40–60 mmHg results in clinical signs of buphthalmia, mydriasis, corneal edema, episcleral venous congestion, and variable ocular pain. The underlying glaucoma may be either open or narrow-closed angle, and either acute or chronic. Dog breeds most often affected with primary glaucoma include the American Cocker Spaniel, Basset Hound, Chow Chow, Akita, Chinese Shar-Pei, Norwegian Elkhound, and Samoyed. In cats, glaucoma is often associated with anterior uveitis, whereas in horses the risk factors are age >10 yr old, anterior uveitis, and breed (Appaloosa). Although globe enlargement (buphthalmia) is detected fairly early in dogs, buphthalmia in horses and cats is often missed until the glaucoma has progressed.

Diagnosis depends on clinical signs and accurate tonometry. The Tono-Pen® and TonoVet® applanation tonometers are the most versatile. Gonioscopy and other diagnostic methods are used to evaluate the anterior chamber angle and the posterior segment, including the optic nerve head.

The goals of therapy are to rapidly lower IOP and to preserve as much vision as possible. Immediate referral to a veterinary ophthalmologist is often helpful. Short-term treatment includes mannitol (1–2 g/kg, IV), topical β-blockers and carbonic anhydrase inhibitors, systemic carbonic anhydrase inhibitors, and either prostaglandin analogues or miotics (pilocarpine or demecarium). The beneficial effects of the topical medications are not usually apparent until IOP is

<30 mmHg. If mannitol treatment does not lower IOP within 2–4 hr, anterior chamber paracentesis under general anesthesia may be attempted. Longterm therapy usually includes topical and systemic ocular hypotensive medications, laser cyclophotocoagulation, cyclocryotherapy, and anterior chamber shunts.

ANTERIOR LENS LUXATION

Anterior lens luxation usually affects middle-aged dogs of the terrier breeds and is seen most frequently in Smooth and Wire Haired Fox Terriers and Jack Russell Terriers. It is associated with zonular defects in the terrier breeds (associated with the ADAMTS17 mutation), whereas in other breeds with inherited cataract formation it is associated with advanced cataract (hypermature) formation. These secondary glaucomas appear as acute corneal edema, increased IOP, blepharospasm, tearing, and ciliary flush. Often, the lens is in front of the pupil and often totally within the anterior chamber. Pupillary blockage with vitreous adherent to the posterior lens capsule and iridocorneal angle closure are common and can markedly increase IOP within the posterior segment. Applanation tonometry from the central cornea may yield erroneous low IOP levels. Direct examination of the posterior segment is not usually possible, and B-scan ultrasonography may be used to evaluate the vitreous and retina.

Treatment consists of lowering IOP to normal levels (usually with mannitol, 1–2 g/kg, IV); transpupillary aqueous humor flow may be reestablished with moderate dilation with 10% phenylephrine. Lens removal, preferably by phacoemulsification or intracapsular extraction, is performed as soon as possible. Postoperative treatment consists of topical and systemic antibiotics and corticosteroids and maintenance of a moderate but moving pupil. IOP is closely monitored and any increases treated with topical β-blockers, topical and systemic carbonic anhydrase inhibitors, and prostaglandin analogues. Longterm postoperative complications include anterior uveitis, secondary glaucoma, and retinal detachment.

ANTERIOR UVEITIS

(Red eye)

Anterior uveitis or iridocyclitis is most common in dogs, cats, and horses but is uncommon in other species. It is often confused with other inflammatory conditions of the cornea and/or conjunctiva. It presents clinically as acute photophobia, pain, blepharospasm, a congested and red conjunctiva, corneal edema, reduced intraocular pressure, miosis, aqueous flare (increased levels of proteins and inflammatory cells in the aqueous humor) to frank hypopyon, and/or hyphema. Chronic anterior uveitis, in addition, may exhibit anterior and posterior synechiae, irregular pupil shape, cataract formation, and secondary glaucoma associated with peripheral anterior synechiae and/or annular posterior synechiae and iris bombé.

Anterior uveitis may be associated with trauma, systematic diseases (especially when bilateral), cataract formation, primary and metastatic neoplasia, and other causes. Prognosis and therapy depends on the cause. Therapy usually includes mydriatics, topical and systemic antibiotics, corticosteroids or NSAIDs, and other drugs to target specific pathogens. Prognosis is usually favorable for acute anterior uveitis but guarded for recurrent or chronic anterior uveitis (eg, uveodermatologic syndrome in dogs, Golden Retriever uveitis, or equine recurrent uveitis) because of the high likelihood of developing secondary cataracts, refractory glaucoma, and phthisis bulbus.

ACUTE VISION LOSS

Acute loss of vision may occur with many ophthalmic and CNS diseases, usually with abrupt onset of blindness, anisocoria, mydriasis, and loss of both direct and indirect pupillary light reflexes. Bilateral loss of vision is more common, but unilateral vision loss can occur particularly when the other eye is blind. For acute vision loss, large amounts of the retina must be involved; lesions of the optic nerve can cause blindness, because the disease process can be quite localized. The rod or cone photoreceptors may be preferentially affected initially and cause either night or day vision loss. Evaluation includes thorough ophthalmic and general physical examinations, because many systemic diseases may cause blindness. Because visual field evaluations cannot be performed in animals, subjective tests for vision are necessary and include the menace test, dazzle reflex, maze test in both light and dark illumination, electroretinography, and visual evoked potentials. *See* TABLES 8 and 9.

TABLE 8 CLINICAL GUIDE FOR ACUTE BLINDNESS IN DOGS

Diagnosis	Clinical Signs	Affected Visual Pathway	Etiology
Sudden acute retinal degeneration syndrome	Acute-onset blindness, dilated pupils, ± PLR[a]	Outer retinal layers	Unknown; Miniature Schnauzer and Dachshund have increased risk; increased alkaline phosphatase, ALT, and cholesterol
Optic neuritis	Acute-onset blindness, both eyes affected, dilated pupils, ± PLR	Optic nerve disc, retrobulbar	Part of systemic disease (eg, canine distemper, mycosis [cryptococcosis, blastomycosis], protothecosis, granulomatous meningoencephalomyelitis), neoplasia, trauma, orbital cellulitis
Retinal detachment	Acute blindness, hemorrhage	Neurosensory retina	Systemic hypertension, multiple intraocular myeloma
Intracranial disease	Normal eyes, acute blindness ± PLR	Optic chiasm	Pituitary masses, ± paranasal masses, meningiomas, lymphosarcoma
Central blindness	Acute blindness, normal PLR	Optic tracts, occipital cortex	Cardiac arrest during anesthesia, seizures, severe head trauma
Slow vision loss	Progressive loss of vision/PLR	Retrobulbar visual tracts	Hydrocephalus, CNS neoplasia, granulomatous meningoencephalomyelitis

[a]Pupillary light-induced reflexes

TABLE 9 CLINICAL GUIDE FOR ACUTE BLINDNESS IN CATS

Diagnosis	Clinical Signs	Affected Visual Pathway	Etiology
Retinal detachment	Acute blindness, hemorrhage	Neurosensory retina	Systemic hypertension, intraocular
Intracranial diseases	Normal eyes, acute blindness ± PLR[a]	Optic chiasm	Pituitary masses, ± paranasal masses, meningiomas, lymphosarcoma
Central blindness	Acute blindness, normal PLR	Optic tracts, occipital cortex	Cardiac arrest during anesthesia, seizures, severe head trauma
Slow vision loss	Progressive loss of vision/PLR	Retrobulbar visual tracts	Hydrocephalus, CNS neoplasia

[a]Pupillary light-induced reflexes

OPTIC NEURITIS

Optic neuritis may be divided into papillitis (an inflamed optic nerve head visible with an ophthalmoscope) and retrobulbar optic neuritis, which includes mydriasis, absence of pupillary reflexes, and blindness without any ophthalmoscopic abnormalities. Flash electroretinography, combined with visual evoked potentials, and fluorescein angiography may be used to confirm optic neuritis. A CBC, blood chemistry profile, neurologic examination, radiology, and vitreous and CSF analyses may be indicated.

Papillitis is common in 1) granulomatous meningoencephalitis in dogs; 2) systemic viral, bacterial, and fungal infections in dogs, cats, horses, and cattle; and 3) trauma. It appears as a swollen optic nerve head with blurred margins, variable hemorrhages, and exudates. Peripapillary retinitis is often present and appears as a translucent to opaque retina adjacent to the optic disk. Therapy is directed at the underlying systemic disease. Systemic corticosteroids may be used for the optic neuritis. A positive response includes return of the pupillary reflexes and normal pupil size in several days, followed by vision a few days later.

SUDDEN ACQUIRED RETINAL DEGENERATION (SARD)

SARD occurs in dogs. Clinical findings include acute loss of vision (often occurring throughout several days), widely dilated and poorly responsive to nonresponsive pupils, and a normal-appearing ocular fundus. Dogs affected most often are middle-aged and sometimes have liver disease and hyperadrenocorticism with clinical signs of weight gain, polyuria, polydipsia, and polyphagia. Electroretinography indicates loss of outer retinal function; complete retinal and optic nerve degeneration becomes apparent ophthalmoscopically throughout several weeks. There is no effective treatment.

RETINAL DETACHMENT

Retinal detachment is being diagnosed more commonly and is an important cause of vision loss (either unilateral or bilateral). It is an important postoperative complication of cataract and lens surgery. Once retinal detachment is detected, immediate medical and/or surgical treatment can reduce the resultant retinal degeneration and facilitate restoration of vision. Contributing factors include breed (eg, Shih Tzu with vitreal syneresis), previous cataract or lens removal, trauma (dogs, horses, and cats), systemic hypertension (cats and dogs), and systemic mycoses (dogs and cats). History, complete ophthalmic and systemic examinations, CBC, blood chemistry profile, and other diagnostic tests are important to determine the underlying cause. Ophthalmoscopy, B-scan ultrasonography, electroretinography, and blood pressure measurement are important diagnostic tests for retinal detachment.

Exudative nonrhegmatogenous retinal detachments may resolve with resolution of the inflammatory or hemorrhagic intra- and subretinal exudates. Some retinal degeneration usually occurs, but vision may return. Retinal detachments secondary to Collie eye anomaly (*see* p 502) may be treated successfully by diode laser photocoagulation of the surrounding normal retina. Repair of rhegmatogenous retinal detachments, characterized by retinal breaks (holes and tears), may be attempted using vitreoretinal techniques that are routine in people, including intraocular gases, silicone oil, scleral buckling, and laser or cryoretinopexy.

WOUND MANAGEMENT

Wound healing is the restoration of the normal anatomic continuity to a disrupted area of tissue. An understanding of the normal process of wound healing is essential to make sound decisions in the management of wounds. Correctly using the principles of wound management helps avoid premature wound closure and its potential complications.

Wounds may be classified as clean, contaminated, or infected. Clean wounds are those created under aseptic conditions, eg, surgical incisions. The number of bacteria present can determine the difference between contaminated and infected wounds. As a guideline, $>10^5$ bacteria per gram of tissue is considered adequate to cause infection. The level of contamination, blood supply, and the cause of the wound all contribute to development of the necessary conditions for infection, and each case must be assessed individually.

GENERAL PRINCIPLES OF WOUND HEALING

Although there are many types of wounds, most undergo similar stages in healing that are mediated by cytokines and other chemotactic factors within the tissue. The duration of each stage varies with the wound type, management, microbiologic, and other physiologic factors. There are three major stages of wound healing after a full-thickness skin wound.

Inflammation is the first stage of wound healing. It can be divided into several phases, resulting in the control of bleeding and the resolution of infection. During the initial phase, vasoconstriction occurs immediately to control hemorrhage, followed within minutes by vasodilation. During the second phase, cells adhere to the vascular endothelium. Within 30 min, leukocytes migrate through the vascular basement membrane into the newly created wound. Initially, neutrophils predominate (as in the peripheral blood); later, the neutrophils die off and monocytes become the predominant cell type in the wound. Debridement is the next phase of wound healing. Although neutrophils phagocytose bacteria, monocytes, rather than neutrophils, are considered essential for wound healing. After migration out of the blood vessels, monocytes are considered macrophages, which then phagocytose necrotic debris. Macrophages also attract mesenchymal cells by an undefined mechanism. Finally, mononuclear cells coalesce to form multinucleated giant cells in chronic inflammation. Lymphocytes may also be present in the wound and contribute to the immunologic response to foreign debris.

Proliferation is the second stage of wound healing. It consists of fibroblast, capillary, and epithelial proliferation phases. During the proliferation stage, mesenchymal cells transform into fibroblasts, which lay fibrin strands to act as a framework for cellular migration. In a healthy wound, fibroblasts begin to appear ~3 days after the initial injury. These fibroblasts initially secrete ground substance and later collagen. The early collagen secretion results in an initial rapid increase in wound strength, which continues to increase more slowly as the collagen fibers reorganize according to the stress on the wound.

Migrating capillaries deliver a blood supply to the wound. The center of the wound is an area of low oxygen tension that attracts capillaries following the oxygen gradient. Because of the need for oxygen, fibroblast activity depends on the rate of capillary development. As capillaries and fibroblasts proliferate, granulation tissue is produced. Because of the extensive capillary invasion, granulation tissue is both very friable and resistant to infection.

Epithelial cell migration begins within hours of the initial wound. Basal epithelial cells flatten and migrate across the open wound. The epithelial cells may slide across the defect in small groups, or "leapfrog" across one another to cover the defect. Migrating epithelial cells secrete mediators, such as transforming growth factors α and β, which enhance wound closure. Although epithelial cells migrate in random directions, migration stops when contact is made with other epithelial cells on all sides (ie, contact inhibition). Epithelial cells migrate across the open wound and can cover a properly closed surgical incision within 48 hr. In an open wound, epithelial cells must have a healthy bed of granulation tissue to cross. Epithelialization is retarded in a desiccated wound.

Remodeling is the final stage of wound healing. During this period, the newly laid collagen fibers and fibroblasts reorganize along lines of tension. Fibers in a nonfunctional orientation are replaced by functional fibers. This process allows wound strength to increase slowly over a long period (as long as 2 yr). Most wounds remain 15%–20% weaker than the original tissue. However, the urinary bladder and bone regain 100% of their original strength after wounding and repair.

INITIAL WOUND MANAGEMENT

The first step in wound management is assessment of the overall stability of the animal. Obvious open wounds can detract attention from more subtle but potentially life-threatening problems. After initial assessment, the animal should be stabilized. First aid for the wound should be performed as soon as safely possible. Active bleeding can be controlled with direct pressure. A pneumatic cuff, instead of a tourniquet, should be used in cases of severe arterial bleeding; the cuff should be inflated until hemorrhage is controlled. Use of a cuff avoids neurovascular complications that can be associated with narrow tourniquets.

Treatment for any local wound should be guided by the fundamentals of debridement, infection or inflammation control, and moisture balance. The wound must be protected from further contamination or trauma by covering it with a sterile, lint-free dressing. The delay between examination and definitive debridement should be minimized to decrease bacterial contamination. If the wound is infected, a sample should be collected for culture and sensitivity testing. Antibiotic therapy should be instituted in all cases of dirty, infected, or puncture wounds. A broad-spectrum bactericidal antibiotic, eg, a first-generation cephalosporin, is generally recommended pending culture results. Analgesia is also indicated for pain relief.

Wound Lavage: Irrigation of the wound washes away both visible and microscopic debris. This reduces the bacterial load in the tissue, which helps decrease wound complications. Assuming the solution is nontoxic, the most important factor in wound lavage is use of large volumes to facilitate removal of debris. The recommended lavage is a moderate pressure system using a 35-mL syringe and a 19-gauge needle that delivers lavage fluid at 8 lb/sq in. The use of antibiotics in the lavage fluid is controversial.

The ideal lavage fluid would be antiseptic and nontoxic to the healing tissues. Although isotonic saline is not antiseptic, it is the least toxic to healing tissue. Surgical scrub agents should not be used because the detergent component is damaging to tissue. Dilute antiseptics can be used safely. Chlorhexidine diacetate 0.05% has sustained residual activity against a broad spectrum of bacteria while causing minimal tissue inflammation. However, gram-negative bacteria may become resistant to chlorhexidine. Stronger solutions of chlorhexidine are toxic to healing tissue. Povidone-iodine 1% is an effective antiseptic, but it has minimal residual activity and may be inactivated by purulent debris. (*See also* ANTISEPTICS AND DISINFECTANTS, p 2738.)

Debridement: After wound preparation and hair removal, debridement can be performed. Skin and local tissue viability should be assessed. Skin that is blue-black, leathery, thin, or white is associated with nonviability. Necrotic tissue should be sharply excised. The debridement may be done in layers or as one complete section of tissue. Tissues that have questionable viability or are associated with essential structures such as neurovascular bundles should be treated conservatively. Staged debridement may be indicated. In addition to sharp dissection, debridement may be performed mechanically (with wet-to-dry dressings), enzymatically, or biologically (maggot therapy).

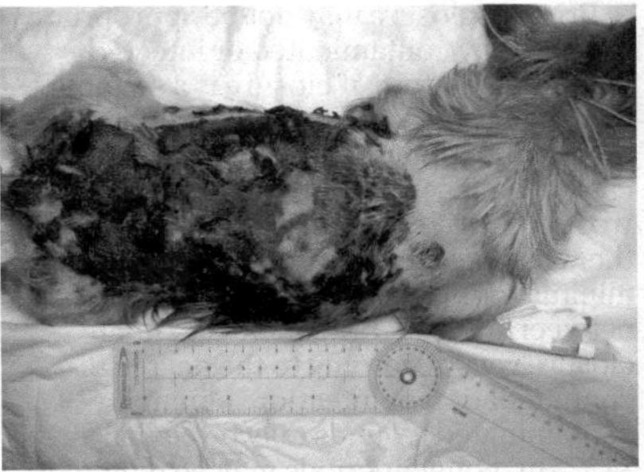

Thermal burn injury in a dog. *Courtesy of Dr. Kevin Winkler.*

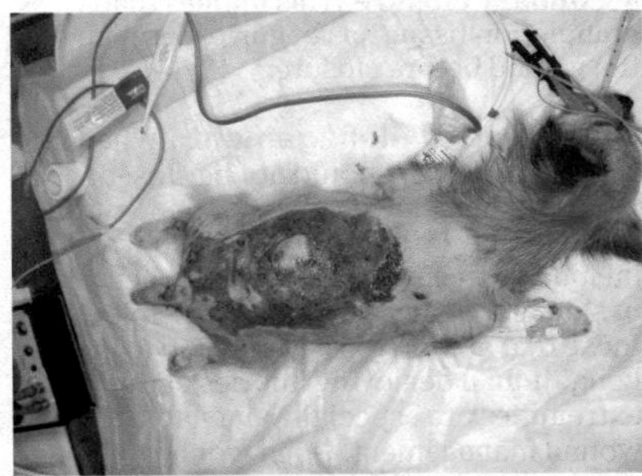

Thermal burn injury after surgical debridement in a dog. *Courtesy of Dr. Kevin Winkler.*

After initial inspection, lavage, and debridement, a decision must be made whether to close the wound or to manage it as an open wound. Considerations include the availability of skin for closure and the level of contamination or infection. If the wound is left open, it should be managed for optimal healing.

Wound Closure: Although **primary closure** is the simplest method of wound management, it should be used only in appropriate situations to avoid wound complications. Wounds may be closed with suture, staples, or cyanoacrylate. Clean wounds that are properly debrided usually heal without complication. With a primary closure, the layers should be individually closed to minimize "dead space" that might contribute to seroma formation. The types of suture and suture patterns used depend on the size and location of the wound and on the size of the animal.

Primary closure may not be appropriate for a grossly contaminated or infected wound. Therefore, if closure is a suitable goal, it may be delayed until the contamination or infection is controlled. The wound can be managed short-term as an open wound until it appears healthy. At that time, the wound can be safely closed with minimal risk of complications. The time between initial debridement and final closure vary according to the degree of contamination or infection. Minimally contaminated wounds may be closed after 24–72 hr. Longer periods may be required for heavily infected wounds.

Wounds that are closed >5 days after the initial wounding are considered to be **secondary closure**. This implies that granulation tissue has begun to form in the wound before closure.

Open Wound Management: When a wound cannot or should not be closed, open wound management (ie, second-intention healing) may be appropriate. Such wounds include those in which there has been a loss of skin that makes closure impossible or those that are too grossly infected to close. Longitudinal degloving injuries of the extremities are especially amenable to open wound management. Open wound management enables progressive debridement procedures and does not require specialized equipment (such as may be needed with skin grafting). However, it increases cost, prolongs time for healing, and may create complications from wound contracture.

Open wound management is based on repeated bandaging and debridement as needed until the wound heals. Traditional therapy calls for wet-to-dry dressings initially. The initial wide meshed gauze dressings help with mechanical debridement at every bandage change. Until a granulation bed forms, the bandage should be changed at least once daily. In the early stages of healing, the bandage may need to be changed as often as twice daily. After granulation tissue develops, the bandage should be changed to a dry, nonstick dressing so the granulation bed is not disrupted. Both the granulation bed and the early epithelium are easily damaged, and disruption of the granulation bed delays wound healing.

With the concept of moist wound healing, bandaging is combined with autolytic debridement to promote wound healing. The use of moist wound dressings keeps white cells healthier, allowing them to aid in the debridement process. A variety of dressings is available. Alginate dressings are commonly used in the exudative wound to stimulate granulation tissue. Hydrogels are used to maintain moisture levels in drier wounds. Foam dressings may be used to absorb excessive exudate or protect granulation beds. These newer dressings are changed only every 2–5 days.

Sugar Dressings: Sugar has been used as an inexpensive wound dressing for more than three centuries to control odor and infection. The use of sugar is based on its high osmolality drawing fluid out of the wound and inhibiting the growth of bacteria. The use of sugar also aids in the debridement of necrotic tissue while preserving viable tissue. Granulated sugar is placed into the wound cavity in a layer 1-cm thick and covered with a thick dressing to absorb fluid drawn from the wound. The sugar dressing should be changed once daily or more frequently whenever “strike-through” is seen on the bandage. During the bandage change, the wound should be liberally lavaged with warm saline or tap water. Sugar dressings may be used until granulation tissue is seen. Once all infection is resolved, the wound may be closed or allowed to epithelialize. Because a large volume of fluid can be removed from the wound, the animal’s hemodynamic and hydration status must be monitored and treated accordingly. Hypovolemia and low colloid osmotic pressure are complications that may be associated with this therapy.

Honey Dressings: Honey has also been used for wound dressings over the centuries. Honey’s beneficial effects are thought to be a result of hydrogen peroxide production from activity of the glucose oxidase enzyme. The low pH of honey also may accelerate healing. Honey used for wound healing must be unpasteurized, and the source of the honey appears to be a factor in its effectiveness. Manuka honey may be the best option for wound care. The contact layer wound dressings should be soaked in honey before application. The bandage should be changed daily or more frequently as needed.

DRAINS

Drains are used to direct fluid out of a wound or body cavity. Passive drainage techniques require gravity or capillary action to draw fluid from the wound or cavity. Penrose drains are soft, flat, commonly used passive drains made from latex. These drains must be placed in gravity-dependent locations to ensure proper function. A firmer drain can be constructed from a red rubber or silicone tube. Active drains require some type of negative pressure to pull fluid from the wound. Red rubber or silicone drains can be used with a closed system, and low-pressure suction maintained with the intermittent use of low-pressure pumps or handheld rechargeable devices. Negative-pressure wound therapy is based on this theory to remove purulent debris and speed closure of an open wound. The use of active, closed-drain systems decreases the likelihood of ascending infection that can be associated with passive drains. Drains should be left in place until the draining fluid decreases in quantity and no longer appears purulent. The fluid can be evaluated by cytologic examination.

BANDAGES

The goals of bandaging include limiting hemorrhage, immobilizing the area, preventing further trauma or contamination of the wound, preventing wound desiccation, absorbing exudate, controlling infection, and aiding in mechanical debridement of the wound. When constructing bandages, several principles must be followed to avoid complications. The bandages should be sufficiently padded, applied evenly and snugly, composed of three layers (primary, secondary, and tertiary), and placed to avoid traumatizing the newly formed granulation tissue or epithelium.

The first or primary layer directly contacts the wound to allow tissue fluid to pass through to the secondary layer. The first layer may be adherent or nonadherent. A nonadherent bandage is usually a fine mesh or foam, nonstick material and is indicated when a healthy granulation bed has developed. This layer prevents tissue desiccation and causes minimal trauma. An adherent bandage uses a wide mesh material that allows tissue and debris to become incorporated into the bandage. This debris is then removed with the bandage change. Adherent bandages are classified as dry to dry, wet to dry, or wet to wet based on the composition of the primary layer. Dry-to-dry bandages consist of dry gauze applied to the wound. The bandages are painful to remove but enable excellent tissue debridement. Wet-to-dry bandages are made with saline-moistened gauze placed directly on the wound. They are also painful to remove but result in less tissue desiccation than dry-to-dry bandages. Wet-to-wet bandages tend to damage the tissue bed by keeping it too moist. Newer bandage materials may be impregnated with various materials, such as silver, to help control infection.

The secondary layer of a bandage absorbs tissue fluid, pads the wound, and supports or immobilizes the limb. This layer is frequently composed of cast padding or roll cotton. The tertiary layer functions to hold the primary and secondary layers in place, provide pressure, and keep the inner layers protected from the environment. This layer is composed of adhesive tape or elastic wraps.

SURGICAL TECHNIQUES

Advancement flaps can be used to move skin and relieve tension. The simplest type of advancement flap involves sliding skin to cover an adjacent defect. These flaps are elevated without regard to their vascular supply. Flap survival depends on the subdermal vascular plexus from the flap base and revascularization from the recipient bed. With subdermal plexus flaps, the vascular supply is affected by the width of the flap base. A high length/width ratio decreases the likelihood of survival, because blood supply will not reach the distal end of the flap. Any flap placed in tension carries a high risk of failure.

The basic advancement flap technique is known as the **single pedicle advancement flap**. Two slightly divergent incisions are made perpendicular to the defect. The tissue is undermined, advanced, and sutured to close the original defect. For larger wounds, two single pedicle flaps are safer than one large flap. Two advancement flaps are combined to form the "H" plasty. There are several other well-described flap techniques, including the bipedicle advancement flap and the "V-Y" advancement flap. In each of these techniques, the coverage depends on stretching the skin over the defect. For this reason, the use of these techniques may be limited by vascular supply or the regional anatomy, such as the area around the eyelids.

Flaps designed to incorporate a direct cutaneous artery are known as **axial pattern flaps** (arterial pedicle grafts). The flaps can be used to cover a large area of tissue and carry along a new blood supply to ensure flap survival. Muscle-based pattern flaps can also be used to reconstruct a body wall defect in addition to covering a loss of skin. The surviving area of axial pattern flaps is 50% greater than a corresponding subdermal plexus flap and therefore allows coverage of a larger area. Because axial pattern flaps are based on arteries, they must have consistent landmarks and do not cover all regions of the body. The best described of the axial pattern flaps is based on the caudal superficial epigastric artery. Based in the caudal aspect of the abdominal wall, this flap can extend cranially to include mammary glands 2 through 5. Other commonly used flaps include the thoracodorsal, omocervical, and deep circumflex iliac artery flaps.

Free skin grafts are used for cases with massive tissue loss such as large burns or degloving injuries. The grafts are best used as a split mesh. This allows drainage and helps prevent seroma formation. Skin grafts will not remain viable if laid over squamous epithelium, denuded bone, cartilage, or tendon. The grafts must have a healthy, vascularized bed. Initially, nutrition for the flap is maintained because capillary action pulls serum into the dilated capillaries of the skin graft, creating graft edema. Anastomosis with recipient bed vessels (inosculation) begins within 48–72 hr of surgery. The edema may worsen immediately after inosculation, because arterial supply is established before venous return. The edema should resolve as normal blood flow returns to the flap by day 4–6 after surgery.

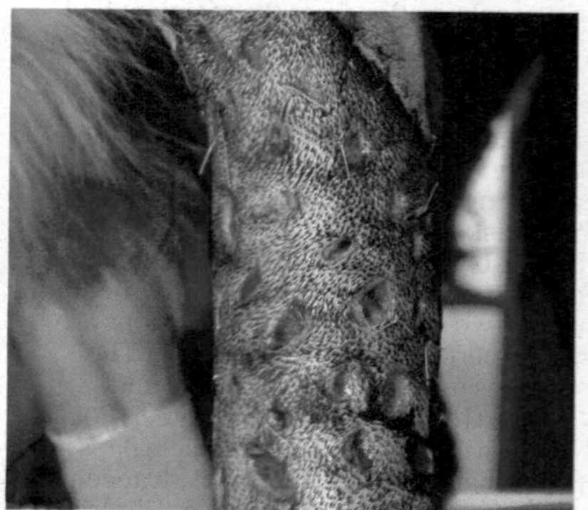

Appearance of a free skin mesh graft 24 hr after surgery. *Courtesy of Dr. Kevin Winkler.*

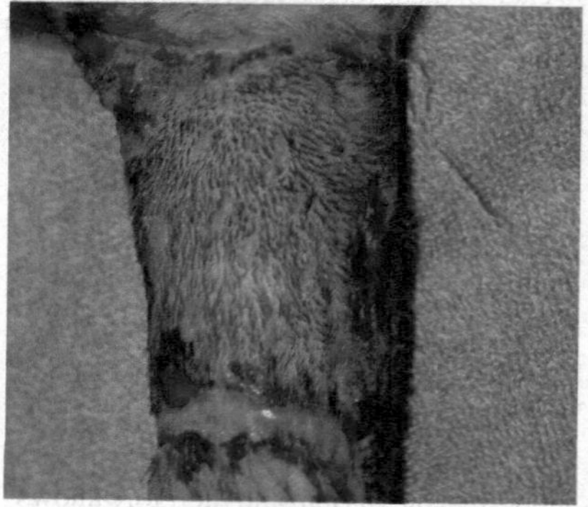

Appearance of a free skin mesh graft 3 wk after surgery. *Courtesy of Dr. Kevin Winkler.*

All skin flaps and grafts require a clean, healthy recipient bed for survival. This is especially important for subdermal plexus flaps and free tissue transfers, because they do not contain a direct cutaneous arterial supply. The recipient bed must be free of debris, infection, and necrotic tissue.

Although flaps may have well-described anatomic markers, determining their viability may not be as easy. The simplest, but least accurate, methods to assess a flap's viability are subjective measures, including the assessment of color, warmth, sensation, and bleeding. Purple color cannot be used as a predictor of viability. Contused, purple skin is often viable. Progression from deep purple to black indicates necrosis. Skin temperature may be affected by the state of vasodilation and is therefore not an accurate method to assess viability. Viable flaps may bleed from a cut surface, as may nonviable flaps that still have some arterial function but poor or no venous return. After a flap is moved, it may develop edema for the first few days until venous vascularization is completed. Newer techniques and medications being developed for wound care include platelet-rich plasma, extracorporeal shock wave therapy, stem cell therapy, microcurrent stimulation, and a variety of growth factors. Their efficacy has not yet been completely demonstrated.

FACTORS THAT INTERFERE WITH WOUND HEALING

Factors that interfere with wound healing may be divided by source into physical, endogenous, and exogenous categories.

Physical factors that affect wound healing include temperature and mechanical forces. Temperature affects the tensile strength of wounds. Ideal conditions allow wound healing to occur at 30°C. Decreasing the temperature to 12°C results in a 20% loss of tensile wound strength. Mechanical forces include pressure and sheer force. Pressure can compromise blood flow in the region, decreasing oxygen levels in the tissue. Sheer forces result in tearing of the vessels. Because adequate oxygen levels are required for appropriate wound healing, anything that interferes with blood flow will slow wound healing. Low levels of oxygen interfere with protein synthesis and fibroblast activity, causing a delay in wound healing. Oxygen levels may also be compromised by other physical factors, including hypovolemia, the presence of devitalized tissue, hematomas, and excessively tight bandages.

Endogenous factors typically reflect the overall condition of the animal. Anemia may interfere with wound healing by creating low tissue oxygen levels. Nutrition has a significant overall effect on the body. Although the ideal nutritional level for wound healing is unknown, hypoproteinemia delays wound healing when the total serum protein content is <2 g/dL. Because wound healing is a function of protein synthesis, malnutrition can alter the healing process. The addition of DL-methionine or cysteine (an important amino acid in wound repair) can reverse delayed wound healing. Uremia can interfere with wound healing by slowing granulation tissue formation and inducing the synthesis of poor quality collagen. Obesity contributes to poor wound healing through decreased blood supply and with poor suture holding in the subcutaneous fat layers.

Exogenous factors include any external chemical that alters wound healing. Cortisone is commonly implicated in wound complications. Corticosteroids markedly inhibit capillary budding, fibroblast proliferation, and rate of epithelialization. Similar to cortisone, vitamin E adversely affects wound healing by slowing collagen production. Vitamin C is required for hydroxylation of proline and lysine. Zinc is required for epithelial and fibroblastic proliferation; however, excessive zinc delays wound healing by inhibiting macrophage function. Other factors that may slow wound healing include radiation, alkylating agents (eg, cyclophosphamide, melphalan), inappropriate concentrations of antiseptics, and NSAIDs. Although most NSAIDs are thought to be safe in wound healing, it has been suggested that agents selective for COX-2 inhibition may slow fracture healing.

MANAGEMENT OF SPECIFIC WOUNDS

Lacerations: Uncomplicated simple lacerations are usually managed by complete closure if they are not grossly contaminated. The wound should be thoroughly lavaged and debrided as necessary before closure. If tension is present on the wound edges, it should be relieved by tension-relieving suture techniques, sliding tissue flaps, or grafts. Deep lacerations may be treated according to the same principles, depending on the extent of the injury. Damage to underlying structures (eg, muscles, tendons, and blood vessels) must be resolved before closure. If a laceration is grossly contaminated with debris, primary closure of the wound may not be indicated. Contaminated wounds may be closed with drains or treated as an open wound.

Bite Wounds: Bite wounds are a major cause of injuries, especially in free-ranging animals. Cat bites tend to be small, penetrating wounds that frequently become infected and must be treated as an abscess with culture, debridement, antibiotics, and drainage. Dog bites have a more varied presentation. Because of the slashing nature of dog bite injuries, the major tissue damage is usually found beneath the surface of the wound. Although only small puncture marks or bruising may be evident on the surface, ribs may be broken or internal organs seriously damaged. The animal should be thoroughly examined and stabilized before definitive wound care is begun. The wound should be surgically extended as far as necessary to allow a thorough examination and determination of its extent before a decision on the repair can be made. After a proper assessment, debridement can be performed. Unless en bloc debridement is performed, complete wound closure is usually not recommended because the sites are considered contaminated. Closure can be accomplished with drains, as a delayed closure, or by second intention depending on the extent of the injury.

Degloving Injuries: Degloving injuries result in loss of skin and a variable amount of deeper tissue. These injuries are a result of a shear force on the skin. Sources include fan belt injuries and loss of tissue during an accident with a motor vehicle. With a physiologic degloving injury, the skin is still present but completely freed from the underlying fascia. If the injury results in a loss of blood supply to the skin, necrosis may develop later. In an anatomic degloving injury, the skin is torn off the body. Degloving injuries frequently require marked and repeated debridement. Differentiating viable and nonviable tissue may be a problem in the early wound debridement process. An attempt should be made to salvage tissue in which viability is questionable. Subsequent debridement can be used to remove any necrotic tissue. With orthopedic injuries that typically accompany degloving injuries, final stabilization may be delayed until local infection is under control.

Gunshot Injuries: In gunshot injuries, most of the damage is not visible. As the projectile penetrates, it drags skin, hair, and dirt through the wound. If the projectile exits the body, the exit wound is larger than the entrance wound. The amount of damage caused by the projectile is a function of its shape, aerodynamic stability, mass, and velocity. High-velocity projectiles tend to produce more damage as a result of impact-induced shock waves that move through the tissue. The shock waves create blunt force trauma that results in tissue and vascular damage.

Gunshot wounds are always considered to be contaminated, and primary closure is generally not recommended. These wounds should be managed as open wounds or by delayed primary closure. After initial assessment and stabilization of the animal, the wound may be explored to evaluate the extent of damage and to determine a plan for repair. If the projectile caused a fracture, the method of repair depends on the location and type of fracture. External fixation, bone plates, and intramedullary nails are common choices for rigid stabilization of the fracture so that the soft tissues may be appropriately managed. Gunshot wounds to the abdomen are an indication for exploratory celiotomy. Gunshot wounds to the thorax may require a thoracotomy if hemorrhage or pneumothorax cannot be conservatively managed.

Pressure Wounds: Pressure wounds or decubital ulcers develop as a result of pressure-induced necrosis. Pressure wounds can be extremely difficult to treat and are best prevented. Preventive measures include changing the position of the animal frequently, maintaining adequate nutrition and cleanliness, and providing a sufficiently padded bed. Factors that predispose to pressure wounds include paraplegia, tetraplegia, improper coaptation, and immobility. Mild ulcers may be managed with debridement and bandaging to prevent further trauma to the affected site. More severe wounds require extensive surgical management. After debridement and development of a granulation bed, an advancement flap or pedicle graft may be required for closure.

EQUINE EMERGENCY MEDICINE

Equine emergencies can be challenging for veterinary practitioners and emotionally charged for owners. There is also the inherent possibility of injury to the owner and veterinarian because of the sheer size of the animal and the "fight or flight" reflexes of an injured horse. Problems can be reduced by educating owners about emergency preparedness and first aid procedures. The most common types of equine emergencies are abdominal pain (colic), trauma, lacerations, and acutely ill foals.

EQUINE EMERGENCY PROCEDURES

Emergency Fluid Therapy

Conditions that may require emergency fluid replacement include injuries with concurrent blood loss, exhaustion, acute rhabdomyolysis, hyperthermia, and circulatory shock secondary to systemic illness. Fluids may be needed for maintenance purposes when oral intake is physically not possible. Replacement fluids are required when excessive losses have been incurred or ongoing fluid losses anticipated.

Design of a fluid therapy regimen requires consideration of the volume required, the type of fluids needed, and the route and rate of administration. The volume to be administered over 24 hr can be calculated using the following formula: volume to administer (L) = maintenance rate (60 mL/kg/day) + estimated fluid deficit (body wt [kg] × estimate of dehydration) + estimate of ongoing losses. Maintenance fluid requirements are ~1 L/hr for adult horses (~450 kg) but are much lower if the animal is not eating. Dehydration can be estimated by using clinical and laboratory parameters (*see* TABLE 10). These numbers should be considered in relation to the horse's age and clinical condition and are only an estimate of the deficit. For example, a nervous horse may have a transiently high heart rate in response to excitement and an increased PCV because of splenic contraction.

TABLE 10 PHYSICAL AND LABORATORY PARAMETERS FOR ESTIMATION OF DEHYDRATION IN THE HORSE

Estimated Dehydration	Heart Rate (bpm)	Capillary Refill Time (sec)	PCV (%)	Total Protein (g/dL)	Plasma Creatinine (mg/dL)	Skin Elasticity (sec)	Sunken Eyes	Mucous Membrane Moisture/Color
6%	40–60	2	40	7	1.5–2	2	+/-	Moist/Pink
8%	61–80	3	45	7.5	2–3	2–3	+/-	Tacky/Pink
10%	81–100	4	50	8	3–4	3–4	+	Dry/Red
12%	>100	>4	>50	>8	>4	>4	++	Dry/Cyanotic

Ongoing losses are difficult to estimate, because losses from the GI tract are hard to measure. The equine GI tract secretes and resorbs the equivalent of the extracellular fluid volume (~30% of body wt) on a daily basis. If small-intestinal ileus or obstruction is present, the amount of gastric reflux obtained can be easily quantitated to gauge losses. If the large intestine is not resorbing water (eg, diarrhea), fluid losses can be significant but difficult to measure. With severe diarrhea, ~50% of the extracellular fluids can be lost daily.

The formula to calculate volume of fluid to administer provides only a crude estimate of needs; volumes administered should be adjusted based on responses to treatment, such as heart rate, pulse quality, capillary refill time, urine production, PCV, serum total protein, creatinine, and lactate. Reassessment is required to adjust the daily fluid requirements for any horse receiving supplemental fluids, and the timing should be dictated by the horse's clinical condition. In horses in severe shock, cardiovascular parameters may need to be monitored continually (eg, every 15 min) until improvement is noted. In horses with severe ongoing fluid losses (eg, diarrhea, anterior enteritis), cardiovascular parameters should be reassessed every 4 hr and laboratory parameters measured as frequently as 4 times a day until the horse stabilizes.

After determination of volume required, the type of fluid to be administered should be selected. Fluid choices include crystalloids (fluids containing substances that freely cross the capillary membrane) and colloids (fluids retained in the vascular space for a certain number of hours because of their larger molecular size). Crystalloids are most commonly used for replacement fluid therapy, whereas colloids are more often reserved for resuscitation purposes. (*See also* FLUID THERAPY, p 1675.)

Two general types of crystalloids are available: balanced electrolyte solutions (BES), which are solutions of electrolytes in concentrations similar to those in plasma, and saline solutions, which contain only sodium chloride. Although considered a crystalloid, dextrose solutions are rarely used alone, and are usually added as a supplement to a BES when indicated by the needs of the individual horse. The decision to choose BES or saline can be based on a serum chemistry profile. Saline is chosen if the sodium concentration is <125 mEq/L, if there is a metabolic alkalosis, or if the potassium is >5.9 mEq/L (eg, acute hyperkalemic periodic paralysis, uroabdomen). In most emergent cases, however, a BES is used.

The addition of colloids to a fluid therapy regimen serves two purposes: it prevents edema formation caused by hypoproteinemia, and it maintains the intravascular fluid volume. Plasma products that contain antibodies to treat or prevent a variety of conditions (including endotoxemia, *Rhodococcus equi* pneumonia, West Nile virus infection, clostridial diseases, and snake envenomation) are also available. Colloid solutions are available in natural or synthetic forms. Natural colloids are plasma, serum products, or albumin. In general, fresh or fresh frozen plasma is selected when an increase in colloid oncotic pressure is needed, and coagulation factors or specific anticoagulants such as antithrombin III are required. Albumin solutions are not commonly administered to horses, because the intravascular half-life of albumin in diseases with compromised vascular permeability is short. They also do not have the added benefits of whole plasma. Synthetic colloids include dextran and hydroxyethyl starch. The synthetic colloid most commonly administered to horses is hydroxyethyl starch (hetastarch). It is used to increase plasma oncotic pressure, and its effect is best evaluated by clinical response (decreased edema) or increased oncotic pressure (measured by colloid osmometry). A refractometer that measures total protein cannot be used to monitor the effect of synthetic colloid administration.

The goal of fluid therapy for treatment of shock is to rapidly expand circulating blood volume to improve tissue perfusion and oxygen delivery. Isotonic crystalloids should be administered at a dosage of up to 60–80 mL/kg in the first hour (equal to the circulating blood volume) for maximal benefit. This fluid rate, the "shock dose," should be given in boluses of 20 mL/kg (approximately 10 L at a time), and the horse should be reassessed between each bolus to determine whether additional boluses are needed. Because of the large volumes of BES required, hypertonic fluids or colloids may be given first to immediately support the circulation until the shock dose of crystalloids can be administered. At a dosage of 2–4 mL/kg, hypertonic saline (7.5%) can rapidly expand the circulating volume by redistributing extravascular fluids into the vascular space. Because of redistribution, hypertonic solutions have a short duration of effect (~45 min) in horses. Colloid solutions can be used for a more sustained effect. Hydroxyethyl starch has been reported to increased oncotic pressure for up to 24–36 hr. However, dosages of colloids >10 mL/kg/day have caused coagulopathies. For resuscitation, a combination of hypertonic saline (4 mL/kg) and hetastarch (4 mL/kg) may have the most beneficial and sustained effects.

The flow rate of fluids through an administration set is directly proportional to the diameter of the line and inversely proportional to the viscosity of the fluid and the length of the infusion set. Polytetrafluoroethylene or polyurethane 14–gauge catheters are routinely used in horses. A rate of 7 L/hr can be achieved when fluids are >2 feet above the jugular vein, and faster rates can be achieved through gravity flow if the fluid bags are raised even higher. For more rapid flow, 10- or 12-gauge catheters with large-bore connection sets can be used, but 10-gauge catheters are more thrombogenic. Other ways to increase fluid administration rates include cannulating both jugular veins or using a pressure bag system or peristaltic pump. Complications of peristaltic pumps are endothelial damage and an increased risk of venous thrombosis.

An alternative route of fluid administration is use of an indwelling nasogastric tube. Case selection is key, and horses that are in shock, are >8% dehydrated, or have positive net gastric reflux are not candidates for oral fluids. Equine electrolyte solutions are preferred, or a homemade mixture can be formulated using 5.27 g sodium chloride, 0.37 g potassium chloride, and 3.78 g bicarbonate per liter of water. The daily fluid rate is divided into boluses and administered using a bilge pump. The horse should be checked for reflux before administration. Volumes <8 L every 2–4 hr are typically well accepted. If a smaller gauge feeding tube is in place, a continuous delivery system from a nonsterile IV set and fluid bags or a carboy can be used, and the rate should be determined in a manner similar to that of an IV infusion rate.

Nasogastric Intubation

Nasogastric intubation is an essential and possibly life-saving procedure performed routinely in cases of equine colic to decompress the stomach and to provide therapy. After the horse is adequately restrained, the nasogastric tube is passed into the ventral meatus, using the thumb to keep the tube directed correctly. If a hard structure is encountered (eg, the ethmoid or nasal turbinates) and the tube is difficult to pass, the tube should be redirected more ventrally. Once the pharynx is reached, a soft resistance is felt when the tube contacts the larynx and/or esophageal opening. The horse's head is flexed at the poll, and the tube can be turned 180° so that the curvature of the tube is directed dorsally toward the esophagus. Swallowing is stimulated with gentle pressure against the esophageal opening or by blowing small puffs of air into the tube, and the tube is then passed into the esophagus by coordinating with the swallow reflex.

Once the tube is in the esophagus, mouth suction on the tube will be met with negative resistance. The tube may also be palpated in the proper position dorsal to the larynx or on the left side of the neck above the jugular vein. If the tube is in the trachea, shaking the trachea will result in a "rattle." If the horse coughs, or if air is noted when suction is applied by mouth, the tube should be withdrawn into the pharynx and the procedure repeated until the tube is correctly positioned. Once the tube is confirmed in the esophagus, intermittently blowing into the tube will help to dilate the esophagus and facilitate insertion into the stomach. The tube is advanced into the stomach until level with the twelfth rib. If difficulty is encountered in passing the tube through the cardia, 60 mL of mepivicaine may be injected into the tube and followed with air or water.

Once the tube is in place, if there is no spontaneous reflux, the stomach should be lavaged. It should not be assumed that any excess fluid in the stomach will drain spontaneously. Medications should never be administered by nasogastric tube without checking first for net reflux. To do so, the tube is filled with ~2 L of water using a pump or funnel with gravity flow to establish a siphon effect, the pump removed, and the end of the tube directed downward to verify the presence of gastric contents. Subtracting the amount of water pumped in from the amount of fluid obtained determines the "net" reflux. Horses should be lavaged with at least 8 L of water to confirm lack of net reflux before any therapy is administered.

Net nasogastric reflux is not normal. Occasionally, a small amount of reflux (<1 L) is obtained if a horse has had an indwelling nasogastric tube. In most horses with colic, >2 L net reflux is abnormal. When reflux is obtained, the amount, character, and timing in relation to the onset of colic should be noted, as well as any clinical response to gastric decompression.

Typically, reflux accompanies small-intestinal ileus, either functional or mechanical. Lesions of the proximal small intestine or pylorus produce large amounts of reflux early in relation to the onset of colic. With lesions of the distal jejunum and ileum, there is initially no reflux, but nasogastric reflux usually becomes productive several hours after the onset of colic. Occasionally, large-colon disorders can be associated with net reflux if the colonic distention exerts pressure on the duodenum as it courses over the base of the cecum. Foul-smelling, fermented, or copious bloody reflux is associated with anterior enteritis and should be treated as a biohazard because of the association of this disease with clostridial and *Salmonella* spp organisms. With mechanical obstruction, including strangulating lesions and ileal impactions, the reflux is usually composed of fresh feed material and intestinal secretions. Reflux originating from the small intestine is alkaline, whereas reflux composed of gastric secretions is acidic. Because gastric outflow obstruction is rare in horses, pH is usually not measured.

Response to gastric decompression should be noted. Horses with functional ileus show signs of relief, and the heart rate may decrease in response to decompression. Horses with a mechanical obstruction usually remain in pain, although some do respond. The rest of the physical examination of horses with reflux should focus on determining whether functional or mechanical ileus is present. The amount of reflux obtained should be noted after each decompression, and the volume of fluids given IV adjusted accordingly. Horses with functional ileus generally need gastric decompression every 2–4 hr. The nasogastric tube should be left in place only as long as required, because it can cause pharyngeal and laryngeal irritation. Esophageal rupture has been described in severe cases.

Abdominocentesis

Abdominocentesis is important in the evaluation of abdominal disease (eg, weight loss, colic, peritoneal effusions, or postoperative complications). Ultrasonography can be used to determine the best location to obtain a fluid sample, which can be collected using an 18-gauge needle, a catheter, or a teat cannula through a stab incision. Most commonly, the sample is obtained just to the right of midline, caudal to the descending pectoral muscle on the dependent abdomen. This will prevent the site of the abdominocentesis from interfering with a surgical incision if an exploratory laparotomy is needed, and it will also help to avoid the spleen. The body wall is much thicker off midline, and the length of the instrument used to sample the fluid should be considered. A needle tap should be avoided with severe small-intestinal distention to reduce the risk of bowel puncture and iatrogenic peritonitis. The fluid is collected using sterile technique and placed in a tube with anticoagulant for analysis and in a culture tube if peritonitis is suspected. It is useful to shake out the EDTA from the tube before sampling, because EDTA will falsely increase the total protein.

Normal values for abdominocentesis include a total protein <2.5 g/dL and WBC counts of <5,000 cells/μL. Repeated abdominocentesis will not significantly alter these values above reference ranges. On cytology, neutrophils comprise most of the cells; the remainder are lymphocytes, macrophages, and peritoneal cells. With intestinal strangulation, protein increases in the first 1–2 hr. After 3–4 hr of strangulation, RBCs are present, and after ≥6 hr, WBCs increase gradually as intestinal necrosis progresses. Degenerate neutrophils will be noted on cytology, and the gross appearance is serosanguinous. Peritoneal lactate is also increased with intestinal ischemia (>4 mmol/L) or is found to increase over time if serial abdominocenteses are performed.

Enterocentesis sometimes occurs, especially in cases of sand colic, and should be differentiated from intestinal rupture. With enterocentesis, cytology reveals plant material, bacteria, and debris but few cells. The horse's clinical condition is not consistent with rupture, although in early rupture (~2–4 hr), clinical signs of endotoxemia (eg, depression, tachycardia, congested mucous membranes, shock) may not be seen. Cytology of abdominal fluid compatible with intestinal rupture shows a large number of toxic and degenerate neutrophils, in addition to bacterial organisms, plant material, and bacteria that have been phagocytized by neutrophils.

Blood contamination that occurs during the procedure should be differentiated from internal hemorrhage or severely devitalized bowel. Blood from skin vessels or an abdominal vessel usually swirls in the sample and spins down when centrifuged, leaving the sample clear. Fresh blood contamination shows platelets, which are not present in blood >12 hr old. If the spleen is accidentally punctured, centrifugation of the sample reveals a PCV the same or higher than the peripheral PCV. In internal hemorrhage, the blood in the sample is hemolyzed, there are no platelets, and erythrophagocytosis may be seen. When centrifuged, the supernatant will remain reddish. Abdominal ultrasound will reveal fluid swirling on the abdomen. If vascular compromise of the bowel occurs, hemolysis of RBCs that leak from damaged capillaries will result in a serosanguineous fluid, with a red supernatant after a spin.

Abdominal surgery increases the total protein and WBCs in the abdominocentesis. With a sterile peritonitis, the WBC count will remain increased for up to 2 wk, and cell counts of 40,000 cells/dL have been reported at 6 days after surgery. Neutrophils will appear nondegenerate on cytology, and there are no bacteria. The total protein peaks at 6 g/dL 6 days after surgery and may remain increased for 1 mo. After an enterotomy, or resection and anastomosis, degenerate neutrophils and occasional bacteria may be seen in the first 12–24 hr but should resolve in time. If septic peritonitis is present, clinical signs will be consistent with bacterial infection (eg, fever, depression, anorexia, ileus, colic, endotoxemia). The WBC and total protein in the abdominocentesis will be markedly increased. On cytology, >90% of cells are neutrophils and will appear degenerate. Free and phagocytized bacteria are seen. A serum–peritoneal glucose difference >50 mg/dL or a peritoneal fluid pH <7.2 with a peritoneal glucose <30 mg/dL is supportive of a diagnosis of peritonitis.

Trocarization

Trocarization is useful to decompress the abdomen when abdominal compartment syndrome is suspected (increased intra-abdominal pressure resulting in severe abdominal distention, dyspnea, and perfusion abnormalities). Trocarization is performed only for distention of the cecum and large intestine, and never to decompress the small intestine or stomach. Thus, it is necessary to identify the segment of intestine involved before the procedure. In adult horses, this is done by transrectal palpation combined with transabdominal ultrasound. Abdominal auscultation may note a "ping" after percussion indicative of a gas-filled organ. In foals or small horses, radiographs and/or ultrasound can be used. The distended segment of large intestine must also be against the body wall so it can be safely reached. The most common site for trocarization is the upper right flank, just cranial to the greater trochanter at the location of the cecal base. Ultrasound is used to confirm a gas-filled structure at the chosen site, to avoid other organs or large blood vessels.

In adult horses, a 14-gauge, 12.5-cm over-the-needle catheter is typically used, whereas in neonates, a 5-cm needle may be adequate. The area is clipped, sterilely prepared, and infiltrated with a local anesthetic. The catheter is inserted aseptically and attached to a long extension set that is placed in a nonsterile cup of water to monitor progress. Gas released will produce bubbles, and the catheter may be repositioned as the bowel decompresses. A successful trocarization may take >30 min to decompress the bowel. When removing the catheter, an antibiotic (usually ~5 mL of gentamicin) is infused as the catheter is withdrawn.

Complications after trocarization include peritonitis, hemorrhage, and a local subcutaneous abscess. The horse should be observed for 48 hr for signs of peritonitis, including abdominal pain and fever. Peritonitis is confirmed with abdominocentesis and treated with systemic broad-spectrum antibiotics until it is resolved. Hemorrhage is typically self-limiting, and local abscesses can be drained percutaneously.

Tracheostomy

Tracheostomy is used as an emergency procedure for conditions resulting in acute upper airway obstruction (eg, arytenoid chondritis, snakebite). The incision site is selected at the junction of the proximal and middle third of the neck, above the "V" formed by the paired sternomandibularis muscles. If possible, the skin should be clipped, aseptically prepared, and infiltrated with a local anesthetic. In acute respiratory distress, this may not be possible, and the procedure is performed without sterile preparation.

The incision (6–8 cm) is made on midline, through the skin and between the paired sternothyrohyoideous muscles. The trachea is exposed, and a transverse incision is made between two tracheal rings, taking care to avoid the tracheal cartilages. The incision will extend to ~30% of the circumference of the trachea. If the horse's head is elevated or extended, the tracheal incision should be made caudal relative to the skin incision, to avoid covering the tracheostomy site when the head is lowered. A J-type silicone tracheostomy tube may be used and secured in place to the mane with gauze. The cuff should not be inflated, unless the horse is to be ventilated, to prevent tracheal necrosis. Alternatively, a self-retaining tube may be preferred because of the tendency of J-tubes to fall out.

The tracheostomy tube should be removed, cleaned, and replaced twice a day or more often if secretions occlude the lumen. Petroleum jelly applied to the surrounding skin will help to reduce skin scalding. Complications are rare (eg, cartilage deformity, intraluminal granulation tissue, mucosal structure) but can be reduced by removing the tube as soon as possible. One method to determine when the tube can be removed is to temporarily occlude the lumen by hand and observe whether the horse can breathe without it. After tube removal, the site is cleaned with saline twice daily and allowed to heal by second intention. The trachea will generally close in 10–14 days and heal completely in 3 wk.

EQUINE TRAUMA AND FIRST AID

Common emergencies involving the musculoskeletal system include fractures, luxations, lacerations, puncture wounds, synovial infections, and exertional rhabdomyolysis. Although many of these conditions cannot be treated in the field, an accurate diagnosis and provision of appropriate emergency treatment are essential for the possibility of a successful outcome.

Fractures and Luxations

A thorough physical examination is warranted but may be complicated by the severity of the injury and other factors (eg, pain, anxiety, exhaustion, dehydration, owner/trainer anxiety). The goals of initial coaptation of fractures are to relieve anxiety, prevent further injury, and allow for safe transportation for additional evaluation and possible treatment. Emergency coaptation of unstable limbs is key and should be performed before radiographic evaluation or transportation to a surgical facility.

Initial Assessment: Fractures or luxations should be suspected if a loud crack is heard, if there is acute, non-weight-bearing lameness, or if the limb has an abnormal angulation or is visibly unstable. The extent of the physical examination should be dictated by the situation, to avoid further injury to the horse or bystanders. If the horse is recumbent, full assessment of the limb should be completed before attempting to stand the horse. If the horse is standing, examination of the limb should be completed before attempting to move the horse. With an unstable fracture, the limb should be stabilized before any other treatment.

Sedation or a twitch can be used to aid restraint for the examination. For sedation, an α_2-agonist such as xylazine or detomidine can be used. Because α_2-agonists often cause the horse to lean forward, which may increase the weight on an injured forelimb or decrease the ability to manipulate the limb, the minimal effective dose is preferred to reduce ataxia. However, up to double the standard dose regimen may be required to achieve effective sedation after maximal exercise or if the horse is excited. Butorphanol may be used for horses not well controlled by α_2-agonists alone. Acepromazine should be reserved for euvolemic horses because of its hypotensive effects. If the horse is recumbent and a serious injury is suspected, general anesthesia can be safely induced using sedation with xylazine followed by induction with ketamine and diazepam or tiletamine-zolazepam. Before sedation or anesthesia, the circulatory system should be briefly assessed by evaluating heart rate, mucous membrane color, capillary refill time, and pulse quality. A heart rate >80 bpm accompanied by a delayed capillary refill time and poor peripheral pulse quality indicate the need for IV fluid support. Laboratory determination of biochemistry profile indices are becoming more commonly available in field situations. If available, parameters of hydration and electrolyte balance are useful to dictate fluid volume and type.

For limb stabilization, it is useful to divide the limbs into four levels, which help define the method of coaptation. Level 1 injuries involve the distal metacarpus/metatarsus and phalanges and include the fetlock joint and extensor and flexor tendon injuries located at the level of the metacarpus and metatarsus. Level 2 injuries involve the mid-metacarpus to distal radius, the carpal joint, and the mid- to proximal metatarsus. Level 3 injuries involve the mid- to proximal radius in the forelimb or the tarsus and tibia in the hindlimb. Level 4 injuries are noted in the forelimb proximal to and including the elbow joint, or in the hindlimb proximal to and including the stifle joint.

The presence of a fracture can be determined by instability, crepitus, abnormal angulation, palpation of bone fragments, or direct visualization of the fractured bone. Luxation should be suspected when there is abnormal lateral-to-medial motion at the level of a joint. Radiographs are indicated to confirm the presence or absence of a fracture or luxation but only after coaptation has been applied. If radiographic equipment is unavailable on site, the horse should be transported to a referral facility for further examination. Hairline or stress fractures can be difficult to demonstrate radiographically, particularly in field conditions. Therefore, in the presence of severe lameness with pain localized to a long bone, external coaptation should be applied before moving the horse, to avoid catastrophic displacement of an incomplete fracture.

Emergency Treatment: Therapeutic aims of the initial management of traumatic injuries are to relieve anxiety, immobilize the fracture or luxation for transportation, prevent further damage, and provide safe transportation. The principles of emergency *coaptation of traumatic* injuries in horses include appropriate wound care before application of external coaptation, provision of adequate padding to prevent skin abrasions, immobilization of the joint below and above the area of injury, prevention of lateromedial and craniocaudal motion, and never ending a splint in the middle of a long bone segment or at the end of a fracture line.

Wounds should be carefully cleaned and debrided. A nonstick gauze bandage can be applied and held in place with conforming gauze. Cotton padding is applied to the entire length of the segment to be immobilized and held in place with gauze, followed by elastic bandage material. The bandage should be snug, to avoid loosening with compression of the cotton material. Splints are then applied and held in place, ideally with fiberglass casting tape. This is particularly useful in stabilizing a luxation. If casting tape is unavailable, heavy tape (duct tape or medical white tape) can be used. The splints must be well padded to avoid the development of sores.

Immobilization of Level 1 Injuries: Level 1 injuries include phalangeal fractures, distal metacarpus and metatarsal fractures, sesamoid fractures, fetlock, pastern or coffin bone luxations, or severance of one or more flexor tendons. Not included are fractures of the coffin bone; they are supported by the hoof capsule and do not require a splint. Although technically level 1 injuries, extensor tendon lacerations require a different mode of splint application and are discussed separately.

Forelimb and hindlimb immobilization differ slightly because of the presence of the reciprocal apparatus in the hindlimb. In forelimb injuries, immobilization is best accomplished by aligning the cannon bone with the phalanges to establish a straight, weight-bearing column. The horse will bear weight, although not fully weight bearing, on its toe. To bandage the limb, an assistant holds the leg by the radius, allowing the limb distal to the carpus to hang in a straight line to facilitate bandaging. A modified Robert-Jones bandage is placed using cotton combine bandage, brown gauze, and elastic bandaging material to form a light bandage that will allow for soft-tissue swelling. Each layer of bandaging material is wrapped separately and in the same direction to prevent shifting of the splint. A splint is applied to the cranial aspect of the limb, extending from toe to carpus using 4–6 layers of overlapping, nonelastic tape (eg, white medical tape, duct tape). The splint should be padded proximally to prevent skin injury. If lateral to medial instability is noted, a lateral splint may be added or casting tape applied over the splint.

In the hindlimb, the reciprocal apparatus prevents extension of the distal limb if the horse is non-weightbearing. Therefore, the limb is best immobilized by applying the splint on the caudal aspect of the limb, from the toe, on the plantar aspect of the hoof, to the point of the hock. Dorsal alignment of the bony column will not be possible and is not necessary for adequate coaptation. Bandaging and splinting techniques are otherwise similar to those used for the forelimb.

A commercially available splint (Kimsey Legsaver®) may be used for some level 1 fractures or tendon injuries; however, it does not provide enough lateral-to-medial stability for joint luxations or severely comminuted fractures. The splint is readily available in a number of sizes, easy to apply, and effective to achieve immediate immobilization. Two configurations are available: one with a slightly forward-angled bar for a flexed position of the forelimb, and one with a backward angle at the level of the fetlock to improve weight bearing. The forward angle is more effective for most fore- and hindlimb injuries, when weight bearing is not advantageous. Nonslip tape should be placed on the foot plate after application to make it less slippery, particularly on cement floors.

Lacerations or rupture of the extensor tendons, unlike flexor tendons, require a different type of splint. When both extensor tendons are completely disrupted, the horse will knuckle over, which can lead to injury of the dorsal aspect of the fetlock and further disrupt any associated wound. In this instance, external coaptation is needed to prevent knuckling over at the fetlock. A splint is applied to the cranial aspect of the fore- or hindlimb with the hoof flat on the ground to prevent joint flexion.

Immobilization of Level 2 Injuries:

Examples of level 2 injuries include mid to proximal cannon bone fractures, carpal bone fractures, distal radial fractures, and wounds of the carpus. The goal of coaptation is to prevent angulation and place the carpus in extension. In level 2 injuries of the forelimb, a moderately thick Robert-Jones bandage is applied up to the elbow, wrapping each layer separately to prevent slipping. The bandage should be ~3 times the diameter of the limb when finished, so that the entire splint lies flat against the bandage over its length. Two splints are applied, at a 90° angle, one lateral and one caudal. The splints should extend from the floor to the elbow, and the hoof should be flat on the floor. In hindlimb injuries, as in the forelimb, the bandage should be 3 times the diameter of the limb and extend from the floor to the stifle. Two splints are needed. One splint will extend from the floor to the stifle laterally. However, because of interference with the reciprocal apparatus and the angulation of the hock, the caudal splint cannot extend to the stifle but should stop at the point of the hock.

Immobilization of Level 3 Injuries:

Level 3 injuries include fractures of the mid to proximal radius, tarsus, or tibia. Because of the nature of the fracture, the flexor muscles of the limb become abductors, resulting in a valgus angulation. The medial aspect of both the radius and tibia does not have a sufficient muscle mass to help prevent penetration of the skin by fractured bone, and open fractures are common. The goal of external coaptation is to prevent abduction of the limb and soft-tissue injury. On the forelimb, the splint is applied similar to that in level 2 injuries; however, the lateral splint must extend from the ground to the withers. The caudal splint is the same, extending up to the elbow. The lateral splint above the bandage should be well padded to improve fit and prevent skin injury. Once the horse is standing on the trailer, the splint can be secured to the chest with nonelastic tape in a figure-8 configuration for further stability, if needed. On the hindlimb, the splint is similar to that for a level 2 injury; however, the caudal splint is not needed, and the lateral splint should extend to the level of the tuber coxae. The splint can be a wide wooden board or a contoured metal splint made of electrical conduit. Adequate padding should be placed wherever the splint contacts skin above the bandage. Placing the hoof in extension can facilitate splint application.

Immobilization of Level 4 Injuries:

Level 4 injuries include fractures of the scapula, humerus, femur, and pelvis. They also include olecranon fractures and radial nerve paralysis because these injuries disrupt the passive stay apparatus in the forelimb. The flexion of the carpus that results can cause injury to the dorsal aspect of the limb and eventually tendon contracture. For forelimb fractures and radial nerve paralysis, a level 2 bandage and a caudal splint from the ground to the elbow is used to fix the carpus in extension. Although the fracture is not directly stabilized by this splint, it will prevent tendon contraction and allows the horse to prop the leg, which reduces anxiety. External coaptation is not indicated for fractures of the hindlimb at this level. The joint above and below the fracture cannot be immobilized, preventing fracture stabilization. Bandaging will only distract the fracture and make it more awkward to move the horse. Hematoma and soft-tissue swelling around the site of injury will provide functional immobilization. If the pelvis is fractured, the need for transportation and further diagnostics should be discussed, because motion during transit may displace fracture fragments, resulting in fatal hemorrhage.

Guidelines for Safe Transportation

Before loading an injured horse, proper functioning of the vehicle should be assessed, the horse stabilized, and the injury immobilized as described. A low ramp facilitates loading and unloading. The trailer ideally should be brought to the horse if possible for loading. Once loaded in the trailer, the horse will lean on the wall and partitions to help balance and to reduce the load on the injured leg. It is never advised to transport a horse loose in a trailer or in a makeshift stall. A sling can be placed under the abdomen to help reduce the weight bearing on the limb. Many trailers have standing stalls at 45° angles (slant load trailers), which help horses balance during transport. If a regular, straight-load trailer is used, the horse should be loaded facing backward for a forelimb injury and forward for a hindlimb injury, to help cushion sudden stops. The head should be loosely tied, in case the horse falls, and a hay net provided to reduce anxiety. Frequent stops should be made to check on the status of the horse and provide drinking water. If significant cardiovascular compromise exists, IV fluids can be administered while in transit.

If the horse is severely injured and needs to remain recumbent, it can be pulled onto the trailer after stabilizing the limb using a large tarp or blankets as a glide. The horse should be kept sedated during transport to avoid further injuries. A head protector, hay bales, or a bandage can be used to protect the head from self-trauma, and the down eye should be padded with a towel or blanket. The halter should be padded or removed to reduce the risk of facial nerve paralysis, with lower limb bandages applied to the remaining limbs to avoid trauma *caused by paddling.* Foals can be transported in recumbency with the help of restraint by a handler either in a trailer with the mare or separated from the mare in the vehicle with a handler.

Wounds and Lacerations

Wounds and lacerations are common in horses. The steps involved in management of these injuries include control of hemorrhage, identification of all involved structures, and evaluation of the need for referral. Referral to a surgical facility is recommended if there are tendon injuries, penetration of a synovial structure, extensive degloving injury, severe blood loss, neurologic signs, or involvement of the thoracic or abdominal cavity. In addition to wound management, tetanus prophylaxis, analgesia, and appropriate antimicrobial therapy are indicated. If severe blood loss has occurred, cardiovascular support should be provided before and/or during transportation.

Assessment: A brief physical examination should be completed before addressing the primary problem. If the wound is located on the limb, the presence and degree of lameness should be noted as indicators of a potentially more serious injury and the need for coaptation. The following characteristics are then evaluated: location, hemorrhage, configuration, penetration of a body cavity or synovial structure, and/or involvement of tendons. Assessment should first include application of a sterile, water-based lubricant, clipping of the hair, sterile preparation of the skin, and lavage of the wound. Wounds over joints, tendon sheaths, or tendons (particularly flexor tendons), puncture wounds, and those that expose or penetrate bone should be explored thoroughly for injury to important underlying structures. Hemorrhage may need to be controlled before further wound assessment is possible. Pressure bandages may be applied, and if the vessel can be located, it should be temporarily clamped or ligated. Certain wound configurations may significantly damage the blood supply to the skin and subcutaneous tissues and result in sloughing (eg, an inverted "V" configuration, crushing injuries with significant bruising). Wounds over the chest or abdomen may penetrate important organs. In the case of thoracic wounds, development of an open or closed pneumothorax can lead to severe respiratory distress. Any horse with chest trauma and dyspnea should have all open wounds sealed with plastic, airtight bandages and evaluated for a pneumothorax.

The potential involvement of a synovial structure should be immediately determined. The horse should be restrained and sedated as needed for the procedure. A site of entry into the joint or tendon sheath remote from the wound is chosen, clipped, and aseptically prepared. Using sterile technique, saline or a balanced electrolyte solution is injected into the synovial compartment. The amount needed to achieve distention and back-pressure can vary from a few milliliters, in the case of the distal tarsal joints, to >100 mL for the femoropatellar joint. All compartments of the joint should be assessed. Synovial structure involvement may be confirmed if leakage of the injected solution is noted from the wound. If communication is not noted, the solution is aspirated from the joint, and the structure is injected with a prophylactic dose of an antibiotic (eg, amikacin). In chronic wounds or injuries caused by a puncture, the communication with the synovial cavity may have sealed. Horses should be reevaluated for increased lameness, heat, or effusion over the next 3–5 days, which could be evidence of an insidious infection. If there is significant edema, swelling, or skin trauma over all points of entry, the synovial structure should not be tapped to avoid the possibility of iatrogenic infection. In these cases, close monitoring or direct probing of the wound with a sterile instrument and radiographic assessment may be diagnostic.

Extensor tendon injury of the distal limbs results in the inability to appropriately place the hoof on the ground, and knuckling over. This suggests involvement of both extensor tendons in the proximal metacarpus or metatarsus, or the common digital extensor tendon more distally. Flexor tendon injuries result in hyperextension of the fetlock (superficial digital flexor), lifting of the toe (deep digital flexor), or complete dropping of the fetlock to the ground (severance or rupture of the suspensory ligament). For this to be seen, the horse must bear weight on the limb at least transiently, but this is not advised. In complete suspensory breakdown, severe stretching of the digital vessels can lead to thrombosis and avascular injury and necrosis of the distal limb. It is important to support the fetlock and not allow weight bearing until the limb is stabilized in a flexed position.

The goals of initial wound care are to decontaminate the wound as much as possible and prevent further contamination during transportation. After clipping and sterile preparation of the intact skin, the injured tissue is lavaged with sterile saline and cleaned by sharp debridement of gross contamination. The wound should be dressed with a sterile, nonstick bandage and a support wrap or padded bandage. Immobilization of the limb (*see* p 1714) will be needed if there is injury to a supporting structure (bone, tendon) or significant instability (luxation).

Pneumothorax: A penetrating chest wound can result in development of a pneumothorax and lead to respiratory distress. If untreated, pneumomediastinum can result, and this or the primary pneumothorax can be fatal. On examination, a restrictive pattern to the respirations is noted. Auscultation of the thorax will reveal a lack of breath sounds in the dorsal lung fields. Because of the incomplete mediastinum in horses, a unilateral chest wound can lead to bilateral pneumothorax. An open pneumothorax is managed by providing a temporary seal over the chest wound. The wound is cleansed and bandaged with a layer of airtight plastic wrap and sealed with elastic adhesive tape. The chest is then evacuated by inserting a 14-gauge catheter, using aseptic technique, in the dorsal aspect of the 12th intercostal space. Aspiration can be facilitated by use of a 3-way stopcock and 60-mL syringe or by negative suction. A closed pneumothorax may require an indwelling chest tube and Heimlich valve until the cause is resolved.

Hemothorax: Hemothorax is a possible complication of a penetrating chest wound and can lead to respiratory distress similar to that seen in pneumothorax. Auscultation of the thorax will reveal a lack of breath sounds in the ventral lung fields, with muffled heart sounds. If dyspnea is noted, the hemothorax should be drained; however, if ventilation is adequate the chest should not be tapped, and the blood will gradually resorb. To evacuate the chest, a 14-gauge catheter or thoracic trocar is placed using aseptic technique in the ventral aspect of the 6th–8th intercostal space. Ultrasound helps guide placement, to prevent accidental penetration of vital structures. Aspiration can be facilitated by use of a 3-way stopcock and 60-mL syringe or provided by passive drainage with a Heimlich valve. Complications of trocarization can include pleuritis due to introduction of bacteria, continued hemorrhage, and hypovolemic shock if the fluid in the third space is removed too quickly. Conservative fluid therapy should be provided for cardiovascular support, and a transfusion may be needed.

Penetrating Abdominal Wounds: Penetration of the abdominal cavity is a serious and potentially fatal injury that can lead to hemorrhage, penetration of an abdominal organ, or development of peritonitis. If a penetrating wound is suspected, it should be sterilely prepared, cleansed with saline and low-pressure lavage, explored for the presence of a foreign body, and debrided. A transabdominal ultrasound may reveal free fluid. Abdominocentesis can be performed to detect fecal contamination, indicating a ruptured viscus, or internal hemorrhage. However, abdominocentesis may not be diagnostic initially, because indicators of peritonitis (eg, increased total protein, WBCs, bacterial organisms) take several hours to develop. The wound should be bandaged, and broad-spectrum systemic antibiotics and pain management initiated. In the presence of a large wound, or if the abdominal musculature is involved, the abdomen can be supported with a compressive support bandage.

Head Injuries

Head injuries can result in severe CNS damage. Injuries can be primary (eg, contusion, laceration, fracture, hemorrhage) or secondary (eg, subsequent edema, reperfusion injury, secondary necrosis). Therapy of head injury is designed to minimize secondary CNS damage.

Causes of head injury in horses include direct trauma from a fall or blows to the head. A common cause of head injury is when the horse falls over backward onto the poll. Injuries associated with this fall include basisphenoid fractures and avulsion of the ventral straight muscles (longus capitus and/or rectus capitus ventralis muscles) from the base of the skull. Basisphenoid fractures can result in acute optic nerve damage and cerebral signs. Temporary or permanent blindness may result. Rupture of the ventral straight muscles may cause severe epistaxis, requiring transfusion, and avulsion fractures at the muscular insertion onto the skull may contribute to additional CNS injury.

The diagnosis is made by radiographs or CT to identify skull fractures, avulsion fractures, or a soft-tissue opacity in the guttural pouch (consistent with a hematoma from rupture of the ventral straight muscles). Endoscopy may show hemorrhage from the guttural pouch originating from the base of the stylohyoid bone or medial wall of the guttural pouch. Hematomas may be noted in the guttural pouch septum where the ventral straight muscles lie. Hemorrhage caused by fractures may also be seen draining from the ethmoid turbinates.

Treatment: Treatment of head injuries is mainly supportive to reduce secondary CNS damage. Horses with head injuries can be severely ataxic and should be handled and moved with extreme caution. If the horse is recumbent, short-term general anesthesia is best to transport the horse to a referral facility for further evaluation. Opioids should be avoided for sedation of horses with head trauma because of the risk of decreased cerebral perfusion pressure. The horse should be given IV fluids to maintain normal blood pressure and reduce the risk of cerebral ischemia. Diuretics are contraindicated. If hypoventilation develops, the horse should be intubated, and ventilation assistance provided to prevent hypercapnea. If the blood-brain barrier has been breached by a fracture, broad-spectrum antibiotics should be started. NSAIDs are administered to minimize inflammation, and seizures should be managed with diazepam (0.5–0.44 mg/kg, IV) or phenobarbital (5–15 mg/kg, given slowly IV). Although controversial for traumatic brain injury in human medicine, corticosteroids may be indicated in the acute phase of injury (eg, dexamethasone, 40–100 mg, IV). DMSO (1 g/kg, IV, in 5 L balanced electrolyte solution every 12 hr) has also been used to minimize secondary edema and decrease intracranial pressure. More effective for treatment and prevention of edema is 20% mannitol (1 mg/kg, IV, every 6–12 hr) or 7.5% hypertonic saline (4–6 mL/kg, IV, every 6–12 hr). Magnesium (0.05 mg/kg, IV, over 30 min) has also been proposed as a therapeutic agent to reduce cerebral ischemia.

Ocular Injuries

Ocular injuries are usually traumatic in origin and include periocular lacerations, corneal lacerations, foreign body penetrating injuries, and direct blows to the eye, causing retinal detachment. (*See also* OPHTHALMIC EMERGENCIES, p 1696.) Evaluation of acute ocular injury includes a thorough evaluation of the structures of the eye (including the eyelids, conjunctiva, cornea, and lens), a fundic examination, and evaluation of cranial nerve function to assess the degree of damage. Vision can be assessed by the menace response and obstacle course testing. Oculomotor, trochlear, and abducens nerve function are assessed by the position of the eye and pupillary light responses. Facial nerve and sympathetic innervation to the eye are assessed by eyelid tone and position of the eyelashes.

Treatment of acute ocular injuries includes minimizing pain and inflammation, preventing infection, and preventing further injuries. If penetration by a foreign body is suspected, rapid surgical intervention is indicated. Eyelid lacerations should be sutured, with assistance of a palpebral nerve block and local infiltration of an anesthetic. Sutures should be placed carefully to prevent corneal abrasion, and skin should be preserved during debridement. Anti-inflammatory medications administered to minimize pain and inflammation include NSAIDs and topical osmotic agents. Pain from pupillary spasm can be minimized by dilating the pupil with atropine and covering the eye to prevent myosis in bright sunlight. Acute injuries can be associated with corneal ulceration and secondary bacterial or fungal invasion. Use of broad-spectrum topical antibiotic and an antifungal medication may prevent secondary infection of a corneal ulcer. Horses that are acutely blind cannot move around their environment well. Further injury should be prevented by protecting the blind eye and by careful handling.

Thermal injuries

Thermal injury to a horse is rare. Most cases involve barn fires, lightning, electricity, caustic chemicals, or friction. Most burns are superficial, easily managed, inexpensive to treat, and heal in a short time.

Classification: Like those in people, burns in horses are classified according to the depth of injury. First-degree burns involve only the most superficial layers of the epidermis. These burns are painful and characterized by erythema, edema, and desquamation of the superficial layers of the skin. The germinal layer of the epidermis is spared, and the burns heal without complication.

Second-degree burns involve the epidermis and can be superficial or deep. Superficial second-degree burns involve the stratum corneum, stratum granulosum, and a few cells of the basal layer. Tactile and pain receptors remain intact. Because the basal layers remain relatively uninjured, superficial second-degree burns heal rapidly with minimal scarring, within 14–17 days. Deep second-degree burns involve all layers of the epidermis, including the basal layers. These burns are characterized by erythema and edema at the epidermal-dermal junction, necrosis of the epidermis, accumulation of WBCs at the base of the burn zone, eschar (slough produced by a thermal burn) formation, and minimal pain. The only germinal cells spared are those within the ducts of sweat glands and hair follicles. Deep second-degree burn wounds may heal spontaneously in 3–4 wk if care is taken to prevent further dermal ischemia that may lead to full-thickness necrosis.

Third-degree burns are characterized by loss of the epidermal and dermal components, including the adnexa. These burns, when fresh, range in color from white to black. There is fluid loss and a marked cellular response at the margins and deeper tissue, eschar formation, lack of pain, shock, wound infection, and possible bacteremia and septicemia. Healing occurs by contraction and epithelialization from the wound margins, or acceptance of an autograft. These burns are frequently complicated by infection.

Fourth-degree burns involve all of the skin and underlying muscle, bone, ligaments, fat, and fascia.

Pathophysiology: After severe burns, there is a dramatic cardiovascular effect termed burn shock, which resembles hypovolemic shock. Local and systemic capillary permeability increases dramatically in response to heat and the release of cytokines, prostaglandins, nitric oxide, vasoactive leukotrienes, serotonin, histamine, and oxygen radicals. Because heat is slow to dissipate from burn wounds, it is often difficult to accurately evaluate the amount of tissue damage in the first 24–72 hr after injury. The extent of the burn depends on the size of the area exposed, while the severity relates to the maximum temperature the tissue attains and the duration of overheating. This explains why skin injury often extends beyond the boundaries of the original burn.

Management: Administration of isotonic fluids, at a rate of 4 mL/kg/% burn, in the first 24 hr (one-half of which is given in the first 8 hr) is recommended, but fluid resuscitation is best titrated to maintain stable and adequate blood pressure. An alternative is to use hypertonic saline solution (4 mL/kg) followed by administration of isotonic fluids. If there has been smoke or heat inhalation injury, crystalloid administration should be limited to the amount that normalizes circulatory volume and blood pressure. Continuing to administer electrolyte solutions at the same rate after burn shock has resolved leads to edema, which counters any improvement in cardiovascular dynamics. During fluid administration, hydration, lung sounds, and cardiovascular status should be monitored carefully by clinical assessment and PCV and total protein measurement.

Flunixin meglumine (0.25–1 mg/kg, IV, 1–2 times daily) is an effective analgesic. Firocoxib (0.1 mg/kg/day, PO) is a COX-2 inhibitor for horses. Although COX-2 inhibitors would seem beneficial in the management of burn patients, firocoxib is approved only to alleviate musculoskeletal pain. Human studies have found a synergistic effect of ketamine and morphine to ameliorate pain of skin burn injuries. Pentoxyfylline (8 mg/kg, IV, bid) is used to improve the flow properties of blood by decreasing its viscosity. Administration of dimethylsulfoxide (DMSO) at 1 g/kg, IV, for the first 24 hr, may decrease inflammation and pulmonary edema. If pulmonary edema is present and is unresponsive to DMSO and furosemide treatment, dexamethasone can be administered once at 0.5 mg/kg, IV.

The cornerstones of therapy for smoke inhalation injury are maintenance of airway patency, adequate oxygenation and ventilation, and stabilization of hemodynamic status. Antibiotics and corticosteroids do not influence survival rates and should not be routinely administered. Systemic antimicrobials are indicated only for proven infections, the incidence of which increases 2–3 days after smoke inhalation. Procaine penicillin IM is effective against oral contaminants colonizing the airway. If signs of respiratory disease worsen, a transtracheal aspirate should be submitted for culture and sensitivity testing, and the antibiotic regimen adapted accordingly. Horses with suspected significant smoke inhalation should be observed closely for several hours and hospitalized if burns are extensive. Successful treatment depends on continual patient reassessment, as well as early and aggressive care.

First-degree burns are generally not life-threatening and thus simply managed. Second-degree burns are associated with vesicles and blisters. These vesicles should be left intact, because blister fluid provides protection from infection and an intact blister is less painful than the denuded exposed surface. An antibacterial dressing such as silver sulfadiazine is applied to the wounds while an eschar is allowed to form. Third-degree burns can be difficult to manage. The horse's systemic condition should be stabilized as rapidly as possible before undertaking wound management. Destruction of the dermis leaves a primary collagenous structure called an eschar. The eschar does not prevent bacterial contamination or evaporation of heat or water. The eschar should be covered with an antibacterial agent twice daily. Wound contraction does not occur while the eschar is intact. The eschar is sloughed by bacterial collagenase activity within 4 wk. The exposed bed can then be grafted or allowed to contract.

Although bacterial colonization of large burns in horses is not preventable, the wound should be cleansed 2–3 times daily, and a topical antibiotic reapplied to reduce the bacterial load to the wound. Occlusive dressings should be avoided because of their ability to produce a closed wound environment, which may both encourage bacterial proliferation and delay healing. Amnion can decrease the pain of the wound and is antibacterial. It is more useful in areas of the body where it can be firmly pressed into the wound, such as the distal limbs. Additionally, circulation to the burned areas is often compromised, making it highly unlikely that parenteral administration of antibiotics can achieve therapeutic levels within the wound.

The most commonly used topical antibacterial for the treatment of burns is silver sulfadiazine in a 1% water miscible cream. It is a broad-spectrum, antibacterial agent able to penetrate the eschar. Silver sulfadiazine is active against gram-negative bacteria, especially *Pseudomonas*, with additional effectiveness against *Staphylococcus aureus*, *Escherichia coli*, *Proteus*, Enterobacteriaceae, and *Candida albicans*. It causes minimal pain on application but must be used twice a day because it is inactivated by tissue secretions.

Many burn patients suffer pruritus such that measures must be taken to prevent self-mutilation of the wound. Reserpine (2.5 mg, PO, for 7–10 days), normally used in horses as a long-acting tranquilizer, can effectively decrease the urge to scratch by successfully breaking the itch-scratch cycle. Weight loss of 10%–15% during the course of illness is indicative of inadequate nutritional intake. Gradually increasing concentrate, adding fat in the form of vegetable oil, and offering free-choice alfalfa hay increase caloric intake.

OTHER COMMON EQUINE EMERGENCIES

Esophageal Obstruction

(Choke)

Intraluminal esophageal obstruction is a common emergency in horses and is caused by impaction of ingested feed material. The most frequent sites of impaction are the proximal esophagus and just cranial to the thoracic inlet. Predisposing factors include bolting of feed, poor dentition, recent sedation, poor feed quality, recent feed changes, and dehydration. *See also* ESOPHAGEAL OBSTRUCTION, p 215.

Diagnosis: Clinical signs of choke include nasal discharge containing saliva and feed material, hypersalivation, coughing, retching, signs of colic, or frequent attempts to swallow. The horse may be observed repeatedly stretching and extending the head and neck. Esophageal obstruction is identified by palpation of a foreign body in the neck, passage of a nasogastric tube, or esophageal endoscopy. In refractory cases, radiography and contrast radiography may be used, particularly if a foreign body, stricture, diverticulum, or esophageal rupture is suspected. Ultrasonography may identify thoracic changes consistent with aspiration of feed.

Treatment: Once the presence of an obstruction has been confirmed, the horse should be muzzled, and feed and water withheld. Acute, simple obstructions may resolve with sedation and consequent relaxation of the esophageal musculature. An α_2-agonist such as xylazine or detomidine provides good muscle relaxation. Oxytocin (0.11 mg/kg, IV) has been demonstrated to provide good esophageal relaxation and has been used to resolve esophageal obstructions. Adverse effects may include mild signs of colic, and this drug should not be given to pregnant mares. The obstruction should resolve within 1 hr after administration of a muscle relaxant. If the horse is dehydrated, IV fluids may also help to resolve the obstruction.

If the obstruction has not resolved within ~1 hour after sedation, or if the choke is chronic (>3 hr duration), the horse should be sedated again to allow the head to drop for lavage of the esophagus. A nasogastric tube is passed, and gentle lavage with water is performed to flush the esophagus. Mineral oil should never be used because of the risk of aspiration pneumonia. An esophageal lavage tube (a nasogastric tube with a cuff) is useful to help resolve the obstruction and reduce feed aspiration. Alternatively, a cuffed endotracheal tube can be passed through the nasal passages and into the esophagus, and a smaller nasogastric tube used for lavage. These procedures can be repeated intermittently and can be aided by general anesthesia. If unsuccessful, an endoscope can be used to identify the obstruction and facilitate manual removal using endoscopic forceps.

After the obstruction has been relieved, endoscopy can be used to assess the esophageal mucosa. Circumferential ulceration can lead to stricture formation with recurrence of obstruction. Horses that have been choked are at risk of recurrence in the 2–4 wk after the initial event, even without visible esophageal damage. Feeding a slurried, pelleted diet or grass can prevent recurrence. When the esophagus has been damaged, narrowing is maximal 30 days after the obstruction. Before attempts are made to resolve a potential stricture, the horse should be managed medically with dietary modification for 60 days to allow for remodeling of the scar tissue. Broad-spectrum antibiotics are administered to prevent or treat aspiration pneumonia, along with anti-inflammatory drugs and tetanus prophylaxis. Sucralfate (20–40 mg/kg, PO, tid-qid) has been advocated to facilitate healing of esophageal ulceration.

Rectal Tears

Rectal tears are serious and possibly life-threatening injuries in horse. Prevention is key, but if a rectal tear occurs, appropriate and timely referral can result in a successful outcome. Rectal tears are classified into four grades based on the number of layers involved. Grade I tears involve the mucosa and submucosa only; grade II involve the muscularis only, with a mucosal-submucosal hernia; grade III involve the mucosa, submucosa, and muscularis, leaving the serosal layer intact; and grade IV involve all layers of the rectum, including the serosa. In the case of grade III tears, further classification is made based on the location of the tear; grade IIIa tears leave the visceral peritoneal intact, and grade IIIb tears are located dorsally in the mesentery. Most tears resulting from rectal palpation are located dorsally and extend into the mesocolon. Retroperitoneal tears are rare but have been reported. Fecal contamination often occurs with grade IV tears, but bacterial translocation and peritonitis is still possible with grade III tears. *See also* RECTAL TEARS, p 190.

Diagnosis: A rectal tear is suspected when there is sudden loss of resistance during palpation and when a copious amount of fresh blood is present on the rectal sleeve. Blood-tinged mucus usually indicates mucosal irritation only. If a tear is suspected, the severity should be immediately assessed and measures taken to initiate treatment or referral.

The horse should be sedated for assessment of the tear, and an epidural performed if there is any straining. N-butylscopolammonium bromide (0.3 mg/kg, IV) may be given to decrease peristalsis. A lidocaine enema may also reduce straining. A speculum should not be used, because it can worsen the tear. Digital palpation (preferably bare handed) is then carefully performed. A thin flap of tissue indicates a tear through only the mucosa. If a large cavity with a thin membrane is noted, a grade III tear is present. If intestine can be palpated, the tear is a grade IV. Visual confirmation can be made carefully using colonoscopy.

Treatment: Grade I and II tears can be medically managed with antibiotics, a laxative diet (mineral oil, mashes of complete pelleted feeds or alfalfa pellets, fresh grass) and analgesics (flunixin meglumine) to facilitate defecation. Select grade III tears can be managed similarly, if necessary because of financial restrictions, but also require daily manual evacuation for up to 3 wk. Peritonitis is a risk, repeat epidurals are required, and the time commitment is substantial. For the best outcome, grade III and IV tears should be referred to a surgical facility. However, it is essential to prevent fecal contamination of the abdomen during transportation; therefore, rectal packing is highly recommended. The horse is sedated and an epidural performed using a combination of xylazine and mepivicaine. A tampon composed of a 7.5-cm stockinette filled with moist, iodine-soaked cotton, coated with surgical lubricant is inserted until it is located at least 10 cm cranial to the tear. The stockinette should be inserted before filling it completely to avoid enlarging the tear. The anus is then temporarily occluded with a purse-string suture or towel clamp. The horse should be given systemic, broad-spectrum antibiotics, NSAIDs, and appropriate tetanus prophylaxis. Prevention of fecal contamination by grade III and IV tears during referral has a direct influence on the success of the outcome.

At the referral facility, the tear is reassessed to identify additional damage sustained during transportation. An abdominocentesis is performed to check for peritonitis. After assessment, several *treatment options* are available. For grade II tears with no fecal contamination that are at risk of forming a diverticulum, primary repair using a rectal approach can be attempted using one-handed sutures. The horse should be monitored carefully for development of a perirectal abscess, which will require surgical drainage. For retroperitoneal tears with fecal contamination, the tear can be packed with iodine-soaked gauze and the cavity cleaned out daily. In mares, the cavity can be drained into the vagina, and the tear closed primarily. A laxative diet and analgesics are provided to decrease the pain of defecation. The most serious complication of retroperitoneal tears is development of an abscess that migrates forward into the abdominal cavity. This is prevented by ensuring appropriate drainage into the rectum or vagina.

For grade III or IV tears in a caudal location, primary repair using sutures through a rectal approach can be attempted. A successful repair of a grade IV tear using a linear stapling device has been reported. This approach requires that the abdomen has minimal to no contamination. Alternatively, these tears can be treated through a ventral midline approach, followed by an antimesenteric incision in the caudal small colon and repair through the lumen. A celiotomy has the advantage of a large-colon enterotomy and lavage, thus reducing the fecal load on the suture line.

Grade III and IV tears can also be treated by insertion of a rectal liner using a ventral midline celiotomy. Rectal liners are made of a plastic ring glued to a rectal sleeve. The liner is introduced rectally by a nonsterile assistant and sutured to the small colon using an external circumferential suture pattern that allows the ring to slough in ~10 days, resulting in a small-colon anastomosis. The liner diverts the normal fecal passage until the tear has healed. In other cases, a loop colostomy can be performed to maintain patency of the distal segment. The colostomy is performed as the first step; after the tear has healed, colonic continuity is reestablished using a second surgical procedure. In all fecal diversion procedures, an attempt is made to close or approximate the tear. Laparoscopic suturing of rectal tears has been described experimentally.

Postcastration Evisceration

Postcastration evisceration is always a risk after open castrations, but the risk is increased in draft horses, in Tennessee Walking horses and Standardbreds (because of their larger inguinal rings), or after castration of an adult stallion. Evisceration typically occurs within 4 hr of castration, but is a risk for up to 6 days after surgery.

Diagnosis: Evisceration of omentum or small intestine is first identified by a structure hanging out of the surgical incision. It is important to instruct the owner to keep the horse quiet and to support the eviscerated structure(s) with a towel to avoid further stretching or damage. Examination quickly reveals what structure is involved, so that treatment can be initiated.

Treatment: For omental evisceration, the horse is restrained, and rectal palpation performed to ensure that only the omentum is involved. Prolapse of the omentum can usually be managed by sedation and emasculating the omentum as far proximal as possible. For more severe cases, the horse is placed under short-term general anesthesia, and the omentum and scrotum cleaned and sterilely prepared. The omentum is emasculated as proximal as possible, and the scrotum packed with gauze and closed. Systemic antibiotics and NSAIDs are administered, and the packing removed in 2 days. Barring complications, antibiotics are discontinued on day 3.

If the small intestine is eviscerated, a short-term general anesthetic is given. The intestine is copiously lavaged and examined for damage. Avulsion of the mesenteric vessels or intestinal compromise require resection. The scrotum should be sutured closed over the eviscerated bowel, and the horse referred to a surgical facility. If the intestine appears healthy, it is replaced in the abdomen, which often requires dilation of the internal inguinal ring. Care should be taken to replace the intestine within the peritoneal cavity through the inguinal canal, and not through a separate, iatrogenic opening. If the herniation cannot be reduced confidently, the scrotum should be packed, sutured closed, and the case referred.

If the herniation can be reduced, the inguinal canal and scrotum are packed with sterile gauze, taking care to prevent introducing gauze into the abdomen, and the scrotum is sutured closed. A short segment of gauze is left exposed. Alternatively, the external inguinal ring and vaginal tunic can be sutured closed primarily instead of packing. Systemic, broad-spectrum antibiotics and NSAIDs are administered, and the horse monitored closely for development of colic or ileus, which may indicate intestinal devitilization. Should that occur, the horse must be referred for abdominal exploratory surgery. If the horse progresses well, the packing can be removed in 48 hr, and antibiotics discontinued 24 hr after removal. It is advised to perform a rectal examination before removing the packing to ensure herniation has not recurred and the intestine has not adhered to the packing material.

NEONATAL INTENSIVE CARE AND EMERGENCIES

Initial Assessment

Early recognition of abnormalities is of utmost importance for successful management of critically ill foals. (*See also* MANAGEMENT OF THE NEONATE, p 2087.) Immediately after birth, the cardiovascular and respiratory systems of the foal must adapt to extra-uterine life. These critical events can be undermined by factors such as inadequate lung development, surfactant deficiency (primary or secondary), viral or bacterial infection, placental abnormalities, in utero hypoxia, and meconium aspiration.

Spontaneous breathing should begin within 1 min of birth, and many foals attempt to breathe as soon as the thorax clears the mare's pelvic canal. During the first hour of life, the respiratory rate can be >60 breaths/min but should decrease to 30–40 breaths/min within a few hours. Auscultation of the thorax shortly after birth reveals a cacophony of sounds as airways are gradually opened and fluid is cleared. End-expiratory crackles are consistently heard in the dependent lung during and after periods of lateral recumbency. It is not unusual for a newborn foal to appear slightly cyanotic during the adaptation period, but this should resolve within a few minutes of birth. Similarly, the heart rate of a healthy newborn foal has a regular rhythm and should be at least 60 bpm after the first minute. Occasionally, arrhythmias (atrial fibrillation, wandering pacemaker, atrial or ventricular premature contractions) may be ausculted but should resolve within 15 min after birth. A continuous holosystolic, or machinery, murmur heard for the first few days after birth over the left side of the heart is consistent with patent ductus arteriosis. Various other systolic murmurs, thought to be flow murmurs, may be heard during the first week of life. Murmurs that persist beyond the first week of age, those that are loud (>2/6), or murmurs that cause exercise intolerance or hypoxemia should be investigated more thoroughly.

Foals are normally nonresponsive to stimulation while in the birth canal. This lack of responsiveness has led to the presumption of fetal death during dystocia. Diagnostics, including palpation of a pulse in the tongue, neck, or limb, or palpation and auscultation of the thorax for a heartbeat should be performed to confirm the foal has died. If the foal's nose is accessible during parturition, nasotracheal intubation will allow measurement of CO_2 tension in the expired gas. A long endotracheal tube (size 7–12 mm outer diameter) with an inflatable cuff should be used. The tube is passed blindly into the ventral meatus using a finger to guide the tube. Proper placement can be determined by palpation of the throat. The cuff is inflated, and manual ventilation is performed with either 100% oxygen or room air. CO_2 tension is measured continuously with a capnograph or a single-use end tidal CO_2 monitor. End-tidal CO_2 varies in foals during parturition, depending on cardiac output and ventilation frequency, but it should be consistently >20 mmHg and is usually closer to 30 mmHg. Once manual ventilation of a living foal is established, it must continue until the foal is delivered.

The righting reflex is present as the foal exits the birth canal, as is the withdrawal reflex. Cranial nerve responses are intact at birth, but the menace response may take as long as 2 wk to fully develop. Absence of a menace reflex should not be considered diagnostic of visual deficits in newborn foals. The suckle reflex should be strong by 10 min of birth. Within 1 hr of birth, healthy foals demonstrate auditory orientation with unilateral pinna control. The normal pupillary angle is ventromedial in the newborn; this angle gradually becomes dorsomedial throughout the first month of life. Foals may attempt to rise within 20 min of birth; most should stand on their own within 1 hr and nurse by 2 hr. Some foals defecate shortly after standing, but many will not attempt to defecate until after successfully suckling, about 3 hr after birth. First urination is more variable, with fillies usually urinating before colts. It is not unusual for colts not to "drop" their penis when urinating for the first few days of life because of the persistence of a normal tissue frenulum within the prepuce. The penis should not be forced from the prepuce; the frenulum will resolve without treatment.

The gait of the newborn foal is hypermetric, with a wide-based stance. Extreme hypermetria of the forelimbs, usually bilateral but occasional unilateral, has been seen in some foals associated with perinatal hypoxia and ischemia, but this gait abnormality usually resolves without specific therapy within a few days. Spinal reflexes tend to be exaggerated in the neonate. Foals also exhibit an exaggerated response to external stimuli (eg, noise, sudden movement, touch) for the first few weeks of life.

Dystocia and Resuscitation

Most newborn foals make the transition to extra-uterine life easily. However, for those with difficulties (eg, dystocia, premature placental separation), it is of utmost importance to recognize and institute appropriate resuscitation procedures. A modified Apgar scoring system has been developed as a guide to initiate resuscitation and estimate the level of fetal compromise (*see* TABLE 11). A brief physical examination should also be performed before starting resuscitation, because of humane issues concerning resuscitation of foals with serious birth deformities (such as severe limb contracture and hydrocephalus, among others).

The initial assessment begins during the presentation of the foal in the birth canal. Although the following applies primarily to the birth of a foal from a high-risk pregnancy, quiet and rapid evaluation can be performed during any attended birth.

TABLE 11 MODIFIED APGAR SCORE FOR EQUINE NEONATES

Clinical Evaluation (first 20 sec of life)	Score: 1	Score: 2	Score: 3
Heart rhythm and rate	Regular, >60 bpm	Irregular, <60 bpm	Absent
Respiration	Regular	Irregular	Absent
Response to external stimulation (nose, ear)	Sneeze, ear flick	Grimace, weak ear flick	Absent
Muscle tone	Active, sternal	Some ability to flex limbs	Limp, lateral

The goal in the normal birth of a healthy foal is to minimally disturb the bonding process between mare and foal. This also applies to a high-risk birth, although some disruption of normal bonding is inevitable.

The strength and rate of any palpable peripheral pulse should be evaluated as the foal presents. The apical pulse should be assessed as soon as the thorax clears the birth canal. Bradycardia (pulse <40 bpm) is expected during forceful uterine contractions, but the pulse rate should rapidly increase once the chest clears the birth canal. Persistent bradycardia is an indication for rapid intervention.

The fetus is normally hypoxemic compared with the newborn foal, and this hypoxia is largely responsible for the maintenance of fetal circulation by generation of pulmonary hypertension. During normal parturition, mild asphyxia occurs and results in fetal responses that lead to a successful transition to extra-uterine life. If more than mild asphyxia occurs, the fetus is stimulated to breathe in utero; this is known as primary asphyxia. If the initial breathing effort resulting from the primary asphyxia is not effective, a second gasping period occurs within several minutes known as secondary asphyxia. If asphyxia does not improve, the foal enters a stage called "secondary apnea," which is irreversible unless resuscitation is initiated. Therefore, the first priority of neonatal resuscitation is establishing an airway and breathing for the foal. Foals that are not spontaneously breathing are assumed to be in secondary apnea.

The airway should be cleared of the fetal membrane as soon as the nose is presented. If meconium staining is present, the airway should be suctioned before delivery of the foal is complete, and before the foal breathes spontaneously to prevent aspiration. Suction should be continued to the level of the trachea if aspiration of the nasopharynx is productive. Suctioning should be brief and gentle; overzealous suctioning worsens hypoxia, which causes secondary bradycardia or cardiac arrest through vagal reflexes. Suctioning should stop once the foal begins to breathe spontaneously.

If the foal does not breathe or move spontaneously to right itself within seconds of birth, tactile stimulation is necessary (eg, drying with a towel). If tactile stimulation does not result in spontaneous breathing, the foal should be intubated immediately and manually ventilated. Mouth-to-nose ventilation can be used if nasotracheal tubes or a bag-valve-mask is not readily available. Hyperventilation with 100% oxygen is suggested to be the best choice to reverse fetal circulation; however, evidence from human medicine suggests there are no apparent disadvantages in using room air instead.

Almost 90% of foals requiring resuscitation respond to ventilation alone and require no additional therapy. Nasotracheal intubation can be started while the foal is in the birth canal if the foal is not delivered rapidly (eg, dystocia). This blind technique may require some practice but can be lifesaving. The nasotracheal tube also provides a convenient site for administration of intratracheal medications, such as epinephrine. Once breathing is spontaneous, humidified oxygen should be provided via nasal insufflation at 8–10 L/min.

Chest compressions should be started if the foal remains bradycardic despite ventilation or if a nonperfusing rhythm is palpated. The foal should be placed on a hard surface in right lateral recumbency with the topline against a wall or other support to keep the foal from sliding. The resuscitator's hands are placed over each other either directly over the heart (the cardiac method) or at the highest point of the chest (the thoracic method). The cardiac method is theorized to push blood forward by directly compressing the heart, whereas the thoracic method pulls blood forward by altering the intrathoracic pressure; both methods are valid in the foal. Compressions are provided at a rate of 80–120 per min, depressing the thorax 40% of its diameter, and allowing the chest to fully recoil. The first round of compressions should last 30–60 sec to allow for assessment of progress and addition of medications; after that, each round of compressions should last 2–3 min, followed by a 10-sec break to allow for assessment of heart rate, pulses, and rhythm. If the foal's heart does not start immediately after compressions cease, the resuscitator should switch out to prevent fatigue, and compressions are continued. Breaths should be provided by an assistant at a rate of 8–10 per min during cardiac compressions, or 2 breaths for every 30 compressions if the resuscitator is alone. If the foal is not resuscitated after 10–15 min of compressions, cerebral hypoxia is likely to have made further resuscitation efforts futile.

Because ~5% of foals are born with fractured ribs, assessment for the presence of rib fractures should be performed before starting chest compressions. Some of these fractures can be identified by palpation. Fractures typically occur between ribs 3 and 8, are usually multiple and consecutive, and are located in a relatively straight line along the part of the rib with the greatest curvature just dorsal to the costochondral junction. Unfortunately, their location over the heart can make chest compressions a potentially fatal exercise. Foals with rib fractures should be placed in lateral recumbency with the fractured ribs down for compressions. After resuscitation, ultrasound can be used to identify rib fractures that have escaped detection by palpation, or new fractures caused by compressions. Ultrasound is the most sensitive diagnostic tool to identify rib fractures.

Drug therapy should be started if a nonperfusing rhythm persists for >30–60 sec in the face of chest compressions. Epinephrine remains the drug of choice at a dosage of 0.01–0.02 mg/kg, IV. If given through the nasotracheal tube, the dosage should be 0.05–0.1 mg/kg. Epinephrine can be repeated every 2–3 min during compressions, coinciding with the 10-sec assessments between rounds of compressions. Vasopressin (0.6 U/kg, every 10–20 min) is gaining attention as a cardiovascular resuscitation drug, but experience in foals is limited. Atropine is not recommended in bradycardic newborn foals, because the bradycardia is usually secondary to hypoxia. Atropine can also increase myocardial oxygen debt if hypoxia is not corrected. Doxapram is not recommended for resuscitation of newborns, because it does not reverse secondary apnea.

Immediately after birth, the foal must adapt to independent thermoregulation. In response to the catecholamine surge associated with birth, uncoupling of oxidative phosphorylation occurs within the mitochondria, releasing energy as heat. This nonshivering thermogenesis is impaired in newborns undergoing hypoxia or asphyxiation, and in those ill at birth. Human infants born to mothers sedated by benzodiazepines are similarly affected, a consideration in the choice of sedative and preanesthetic medications in mares with dystocia or undergoing cesarean section. In addition to nonshivering thermogenesis, thermoregulation in the healthy foal is supported by a high *metabolic rate, a thick* hair coat, fat stores, and the ability to shiver within minutes of birth. Heat losses by convection, radiation, and evaporation are quite high in most areas where foals are delivered, resuscitated, and managed, and care must be taken to ensure that cold stress is minimized in newborn and critically ill foals. The foal should be dried and placed on dry bedding once resuscitation is compete. Supplemental heat in the form of radiant lamps or warm air circulating blankets may be required.

Fluid therapy should be used conservatively in postpartum resuscitation. The neonate is not volume depleted unless excessive hemorrhage has occurred. Some compromised newborns are actually hypervolemic. Because the renal function of the equine neonate is substantially different from that of adult horses, fluid therapy cannot simply be scaled down. If IV fluids are required for resuscitation and blood loss is identified, administration of 20 mL/kg of a polyionic, isotonic, glucose-free fluid over 20 min (~1 L for a 50-kg foal) can be effective. Indications for this shock bolus include poor mentation, poorly palpable peripheral pulses, and development of cold distal extremities compatible with hemorrhagic shock. The foal should be assessed after the initial bolus, and additional boluses (up to three) administered as needed. Glucose-containing fluids can be administered after resuscitation at a rate of 4–8 mg of glucose/kg/min (~120 mL/hr, 10% dextrose in balanced electrolyte solution to the average 50-kg foal), particularly in the obviously compromised foal. This therapy is indicated to maintain blood glucose levels, resolve metabolic acidosis, and support cardiac output, because myocardial oxygen stores have likely been depleted.

Prematurity, Dysmaturity, and Postmaturity

Traditionally, prematurity in horses is defined as a birth at <320 days gestation. However, normal gestation length ranges from 310 days to >370 days in some mares, which makes it difficult to define maturity based solely on gestational age. Premature foals are small, with a fine, silky hair coat, generalized muscle weakness, joint and tendon laxity, incomplete cuboidal bone ossification, a domed forehead, and floppy ears. Foals born post-term, but small, are termed dysmature. These foals may also exhibit the characteristic signs of prematurity. Dysmature foals may have been classified in the past as "small for gestational age" and are thought to have suffered from placental insufficiency. A postmature foal is a post-term foal that has a normal axial skeletal size but is thin to emaciated. The hair coat is generally long, and the teeth may have erupted in utero. Postmature foals are usually healthy foals that have been retained too long in utero, perhaps due to an abnormal signaling of readiness for birth. Postmature foals become more abnormal the longer they are maintained in utero, and they may suffer from placental insufficiency. They are most commonly born to mares ingesting endophyte-infested fescue (*see* p 3017).

Prematurity, dysmaturity, and postmaturity may all be associated with high-risk pregnancy. Iatrogenic causes include early elective induction of labor (based on inaccurate breeding dates) or interpretation of late-term colic or uterine bleeding as ineffective labor. Most often, the cause is idiopathic. Even if undetermined, the cause may continue to affect the foal after birth. All body systems may be affected by prematurity, dysmaturity, and postmaturity, and thorough evaluation is necessary.

Respiratory failure is common in these foals and is related to immaturity of the respiratory tract, poor control of respiratory vessel tone, and weak respiratory muscles, combined with poorly compliant lungs and a greatly compliant chest wall. It is usually not due to a surfactant deficiency. Most foals require oxygen supplementation and positional support for optimal oxygenation and ventilation. Effort must be expended to maintain these “floppy foals” in sternal recumbency. Some may require mechanical ventilation.

These foals also require cardiovascular support but are frequently unresponsive to commonly used pressors and inotropes, including dopamine, dobutamine, epinephrine, and vasopressin. Careful use of these drugs and judicious IV fluid therapy are necessary. Renal function, reflected in low urine output, is often initially poor because of a delay in making the transition from fetal to neonatal glomerular filtration rates. The delay can be due to true failure of transition or secondary to a hypoxic or ischemic insult. Fluid therapy should be used cautiously in these cases; an initial fluid restriction may be required to avoid fluid overload.

Many premature, dysmature, or postmature foals have suffered a hypoxic insult and present with all of the disorders associated with perinatal asphyxia syndrome, inducing neonatal encephalopathy (*see* p 2094). Treatment is similar to that of term foals with these problems. These foals are also predisposed to secondary bacterial infections and must be examined frequently for signs consistent with early sepsis or nosocomial infection.

The GI system of these foals is not usually functionally mature because of a primary lack of maturity or secondary to hypoxia. Dysmotility and varying degrees of necrotizing enterocolitis are common, as are hyperglycemia and hypoglycemia. Hyperglycemia is generally related to stress, increased levels of circulating catecholamines, and a rapid progression to gluconeogenesis, whereas hypoglycemia is associated with diminished glycogen stores, the inability to engage gluconeogenesis, sepsis, and hypoxic damage. Endocrine function may be immature, particularly regarding the hypothalamic-pituitary-adrenal axis, and contributes to metabolic derangements. If possible, enteral feeding should be delayed until metabolic and cardiorespiratory parameters are stable, and parenteral nutrition provided. When enteral feeding is initiated, small volumes should be provided first and slowly increased throughout several days.

Musculoskeletal problems are frequent, particularly in premature foals, and include significant flexor laxity, periarticular ligament laxity, and decreased muscle tone. Premature foals frequently exhibit flexor laxity combined with decreased cuboidal bone ossification that predisposes them to crush injury of the carpal and tarsal bones if weight bearing is not strictly controlled. Physical therapy, in the form of assisted standing and controlled exercise, is indicated in the management of these problems; however, care should be taken to ensure that the foal does not become fatigued and stand in abnormal positions. Splints and casts only increase laxity in the limbs, although light bandages over the fetlock may be necessary to prevent injury if flexor laxity is severe. Glue-on shoes may help improve the weight-bearing axis. If tube casts are used, they should not extend below the fetlock to minimize laxity, and they should be changed regularly to prevent sores. These foals are also predisposed to angular limb deformities and must be closely monitored for development of this problem as they mature. Postmature foals may be affected by flexural contracture deformities, most likely due to decreased intrauterine movement as they increase in size. (*See also* FLEXION DEFORMITIES IN HORSES, p 1150.)

The overall prognosis for premature, dysmature, and postmature foals remains good with intensive care and attention to detail. Many foals survive and become productive athletes. Complications associated with sepsis and musculoskeletal abnormalities are the most significant indicators of poor athletic outcome.

Neonatal Encephalopathy

A wide spectrum of clinical signs is associated with neonatal encephalopathy, ranging from mild depression with loss of suckle reflux to grand mal seizures. Affected foals are typically healthy at birth but show signs of CNS abnormalities within a few hours. However, the timing of onset of clinical signs varies; some foals are obviously abnormal at birth, and some do not show clinical signs until 24 hr of age. Neonatal encephalopathy is commonly associated with adverse peripartum events, including dystocia, placentitis, twinning, and premature placental separation. However, some foals have no known evidence for the cause of the hypoxic event, suggesting that unrecognized in utero hypoxia occurred. (*See also* p 2094.)

Therapy for the various manifestations of hypoxia and ischemia involves control of seizures and cerebral edema; support of cerebral perfusion; correction of metabolic abnormalities; maintenance of normal blood gas values, tissue perfusion, and renal function; treatment of GI dysfunction; prevention, recognition, and early treatment of secondary infections; and general supportive care. Seizures must be controlled, because they increase cerebral oxygen consumption by 5-fold. Diazepam (0.1–0.44 mg/kg, IV) and midazolam (0.04–0.1 mg/kg, IV slow) can be used for emergency therapy, but the foal must be monitored for respiratory depression. For severe or persistent seizures, phenobarbital (2–3 mg/kg, IV, bid-tid) or a constant-rate infusion of midazolam (2–5 mg/hr for a 50-kg foal) may be instituted.

Sepsis

Sepsis in foals can be quite subtle initially, and the onset of clinical signs is variable depending on the pathogen involved and the immune status of the foal. Common pathogens include gram-negative bacteria, although gram-positive infections have been identified. Failure of passive transfer of immunity can contribute to development *of sepsis in foals at risk.* The current recommendation is that foals have an IgG level >800 mg/dL for passive transfer to be considered adequate. Other risk factors for development of sepsis include any adverse event at the time of birth, maternal illness, or any abnormalities in the foal. Although the umbilicus is frequently implicated as a major portal of entry for infectious organisms, the GI tract may be the primary site of entry. Other portals of entry include the respiratory tract and wounds.

Early signs of sepsis include depression, decreased suckle reflex, increased recumbency, fever, hypothermia, weakness, dysphagia, failure to gain weight, increased respiratory rate, tachycardia, bradycardia, injected mucous membranes, decreased capillary refill time, shivering, lameness, aural petechiae, and coronitis. Survival rates of foals treated for sepsis have improved, but infection must be recognized early for the possibility of a good outcome. The pathogen involved can also affect survival. Gram-negative species are more commonly diagnosed, but gram-positive septicemia is being recognized more frequently, and multiple organisms may be involved. It is important to identify the organism early in the course of the disease. Blood cultures should be obtained, as well as samples from synovial fluid, CNS, peritoneal fluid, urine, and tracheal aspirates if localized signs are present. Until antimicrobial sensitivity patterns for the pathogen involved are obtained, broad-spectrum antimicrobial therapy should be started. IV amikacin (25–30 mg/kg/day, IV) and penicillin (22,000–44,000 U/kg, IV, qid) are good first-line choices, but renal function must be monitored closely. Other first-line antimicrobials include high-dose ceftiofur sodium (2–10 mg/kg, IV, tid-qid) or ticarcillin/clavulanic acid (50–100 mg/kg, IV, qid).

Failure of passive transfer should be treated, if present, with hyperimmune plasma. Intranasal oxygen insufflation at 5–10 L/min should be provided even if hypoxemia is not present, to decrease the work of breathing and provide support for the increased oxygen demands associated with sepsis. Mechanical ventilation may be necessary in cases of severe respiratory involvement seen with acute lung injury or acute respiratory distress syndrome. If the foal is hypotensive, pressor agents or inotropes may be administered by constant-rate infusion. Inotrope and pressure therapy is generally restricted to referral centers, where the infusions and the foal's blood pressure can be closely monitored. NSAIDs are used by some practitioners, as are corticosteroids in specific circumstances. Use of these drugs should be judicious, because they may have several negative consequences, including, but not limited to, renal failure and gastric or duodenal ulceration. Antiulcer medications are controversial, because critically ill, recumbent foals typically have an alkaline gastric pH but may be useful once the foal is ambulatory.

Supportive care is important in treatment of septic foals. Foals should be kept warm and dry, and turned at 2-hr intervals if recumbent. Every attempt should be made to keep the foal sternal to improve respiratory function and reduce atelectasis. Feeding septic foals can be a challenge if GI function is abnormal; total parenteral nutrition may be needed. If at all possible, foals should be weighed daily and blood glucose levels monitored frequently. Some foals become persistently hyperglycemic on low glucose infusion rates. These foals may benefit from constant-rate infusions of insulin. Recumbent foals must be examined frequently for decubital ulcers, corneal ulcers, and for heat and swelling associated with the joints and physes. Physical therapy or passive range of motion exercises should be provided.

The prognosis for foals in the early stages of sepsis is fair to good. Once the disease has progressed to septic shock, the prognosis becomes less favorable, although short-term survival rates are similar to those seen in human patients. Long-term survival and athletic outcomes are fair. Racing-breed foals that make it to the track perform similarly to their age-matched siblings.

EXOTIC AND LABORATORY ANIMALS

EXL

AMPHIBIANS

The class Amphibia is composed of three orders: Anura (frogs and toads), the largest with >3,500 species; Caudata (salamanders, newts, and sirens) with ~375 species; and Gymnophiona (caecilians) with ~160 species.

ENVIRONMENT AND *HUSBANDRY*

Captive amphibians require proper environmental conditions to remain healthy. Natural stressors, including temperature change, food availability, and habitat loss, combined with anthropogenic stressors, such as exposure to pesticides, fertilizers, heavy metals, nitrogenous wastes, and acidification, likely increase amphibian susceptibility to disease, contributing to the large population losses documented in recent years. As ectotherms, amphibians thermoregulate by shuttling back and forth between different temperatures in their environment. The range of temperatures necessary for proper metabolism, called the preferred optimal temperature zone

(POTZ), varies among species. Metabolism, including the regulation of immune function and digestion, can be adversely affected if animals are kept at temperatures outside of their POTZ. Infectious diseases and malnutrition are common problems in tropical amphibians kept at suboptimal temperatures.

Amphibians require moisture to prevent desiccation. Aquatic amphibians may be accommodated in aquariums with appropriate areas for swimming. Terrestrial amphibians need a shallow container of water in the enclosure. Moisture may also be provided by incorporating small streams, waterfalls, or ultrasonic humidifiers into enclosures, or by misting frequently with a spray bottle. Because amphibians have a semipermeable skin that readily absorbs potentially harmful substances, the water must be clean and free of toxins such as chlorine, ammonia, nitrite, pesticides, and heavy metals. Chlorine can be removed from tap water by placing the water in a barrel and circulating it through a carbon filter for ≥24 hr before use. Some municipal water supplies may include chloramines. The chloramine bond must be split with specific dechlorinizing agents, after which water can be filtered to remove the chlorine. External canister filters or under-gravel filters help maintain water quality in tank waterfalls, streams, and ponds.

Substrates that can be used include gravel, soil, sphagnum moss, and mulch. Gravel should be either too large to be swallowed or small enough to be easily passed in the feces. Soils with chemical additives such as fungicides must not be used. Substrates such as sphagnum moss, untreated hardwood mulches, and leaf litter can be used, but cedar and pine mulches have toxic oils and should be avoided. Some amphibians cannot tolerate low pH and may develop skin irritation if they come into contact with peat moss and sphagnum moss. Heating soils to 200°F for 30 min is recommended to kill arthropods, such as trombiculid mites, and helminth parasites. Freezing substrates at <32°F also effectively removes many infectious organisms.

Adequate ventilation (1–2 fresh air changes/hr) is needed to prevent disease in amphibians. Live plants are recommended furnishings for terrestrial amphibians as they purify the air, remove organic wastes in the soil, filter light, generate humidity, and provide hiding and perching places. Aquatic plants oxygenate the water, remove nitrogenous waste, provide hiding places, and are often a source of nutrition for larval amphibians. Full-spectrum lighting using bulbs that emit biologically active ultraviolet-B (280–320 nm) is recommended to prevent metabolic bone disease. Bulbs must be changed every 6–8 mo or according to the manufacturer's specification.

Longterm maintenance of most captive amphibians requires live food. Although most adult terrestrial and aquatic amphibians feed on invertebrates, including earthworms, bloodworms, black worms, white worms, tubifex worms, springtails, fruit flies, fly larvae, mealworms, and crickets, some amphibians feed on vertebrates and require live minnows, guppies, goldfish, or neonatal mice or rats. Vitamin and mineral supplements are necessary to prevent nutritional disease. These are commonly administered by "gut loading" insects, using commercially available diets high in calcium or by coating insects with powdered multiple-vitamin preparations that include vitamin D_3 and calcium (also known as "dusting").

Bleach (30 mL/L of water) can be used to disinfect tools and housing materials. A minimum of 30 min of contact time is recommended, after which the tools should be thoroughly rinsed with fresh water and preferably dried before use. Several sets of tools should be kept on hand when working with more than one colony of animals. Humidifiers and spray bottles must be disinfected weekly to remove potentially pathogenic bacteria, including *Pseudomonas* spp and *Aeromonas* spp.

CLINICAL TECHNIQUES

All possible routes of escape from the examination room, such as ventilation ducts and sink drains, should be blocked before handling amphibians. Recommended supplies include a mist bottle containing dechlorinated water, which can be used to keep amphibians moist when handled, dip nets, a small air pump with airline and air stone, a water quality test kit, a small room humidifier, tryptic soy broth blood culture vials, the anesthetic tricaine methanesulfonate, and a microliter syringe. Fine-tipped culture swabs, glass slides, coverslips, scalpel blades of various sizes, an assortment of needles and syringes, sterile red-rubber tubes, and sterile saline should also be readily accessible.

The history should include a description of the animal's diet and appetite; environmental conditions of the animal's habitat, including humidity, temperature, water quality measures, and lighting regimen; social structure and reproductive status; the recent introduction or loss of animals; and the use of medications. Problems noted by owners should be described in detail. A review of food and water quality records is useful to identify important trends. A water sample from the animal's enclosure should be analyzed for ammonia, nitrite, pH, hardness, alkalinity, and copper using a simple test kit readily available from most pet stores. Owners must take and record air and water temperatures at the time of water collection.

Before handling, the animal's body condition, agility, posture, and behavior should be noted. Parasitic or microbial infections, malformation, or nutritional deficiencies may cause asymmetry. Loss of muscle mass commonly occurs as a result of improper nutrition, improper environmental temperatures, or chronic disease (eg, mycobacteriosis, chromomycosis, microsporidiosis). Neurologic impairment may be detected by first watching the animal move about its enclosure and then assessing its response to the introduction of stimuli. Neurologic impairment may also be suspected if an amphibian is unable to maintain equilibrium or exhibits an abnormal swimming pattern. When handled, most normal amphibians attempt to escape, withdrawing limbs that are grasped. Placed upside down, most species will attempt to right themselves. Touching the eyes typically elicits a blink reflex or withdrawal of the globe.

A cool, bright light and magnification are required when performing a physical examination. The mouth can be opened using the edge of an index card, a plastic card, or a rubber spatula. The color of the mucous membranes should be evaluated and any lesions noted (eg, retrobulbar injury, orogastric intussusception). Ulcerations, erythema, hemorrhage, and pigment loss in the skin may indicate poor husbandry, trauma, or infections (microbial or parasitic). Improper substrate or sanitation leading to bacterial and fungal infections can cause lesions on the feet. Touch preparations or skin scrapings of affected areas are easily made and can be stained with Wright-Giemsa and Gram stains for cytologic evaluation. Heart rate can often be determined by watching the skin overlying the xiphoid or using a hand-held 8-MHz transcutaneous Doppler system. Because pulmonic respiration (if present) depends on positive-pressure ventilation from buccal pumping, respiratory rate should be assessed by watching the rapid movements of the intermandibular space. The nares should be free of obstruction from mucus, which may indicate respiratory disease. *Rhabdias* spp, a nematode that has a direct life cycle, is a common cause of respiratory infections in captive amphibians. Eggs or larvae may sometimes be detected in oropharyngeal mucus. Ocular lesions are often detected and may include conjunctival, corneal, iridal, and lenticular changes. Corneal diseases, including nonspecific keratitis and lipid keratosis, are common. Corneal scrapings are easily collected for cytologic examination. Panophthalmitis and uveitis are associated with systemic or localized infection. A sample of aqueous or vitreous humor can be collected with a small-gauge needle for cytology and for bacterial and fungal culture. Coelomic palpation may detect retained egg masses, bladder stones, foreign bodies, or neoplasms. Hydrocoelom and subcutaneous edema (anasarca and ascites) are common and may be caused by lymph heart failure; cardiac failure; renal, GI, or hepatic disease; neoplasia; microbial infection; parasitism; toxicosis; improper environmental conditions; or other unknown factors. Collection of fluid for biochemical analysis, cytologic evaluation, and culture for bacteria and fungi is recommended. Blood collected from the ventral abdominal vein, lingual vein, femoral vein, coccygeal vein, or by cardiac puncture and placed into lithium heparin can be used for hematologic evaluation. A volume equal to 1% of the body weight of a healthy amphibian and 0.5% of the body weight of a sick amphibian may be taken. Normal values have not been established for most species of amphibians. Urine may be collected for analysis from those anurans that urinate when first restrained. Fecal samples uncontaminated by environmental organisms may be collected from species such as dart frogs by feeding the animal just before placing it on a clean, moist paper towel. Direct and float examinations are useful to identify protozoa and metazoa.

Treatments are administered orally, topically, or by injection. Oral administration requires firm restraint and opening the mouth with a piece of waterproof paper or thin piece of plastic (such as a credit card). Guitar picks, which come in a variety of thicknesses, work well. Small amphibians can be dosed accurately using a microliter syringe. Many drugs may be administered topically; the skin of most amphibians will absorb drugs directly. Some drugs, such as enrofloxacin, may be irritating, and alternative routes may be preferable. Treatments may also be delivered topically by placing the amphibian in a medicated bath. Bubble wrap or other nonabrasive material placed strategically over the amphibian may be needed to keep it in contact with the solution. Injections are typically given intracoelomically, into the lymph sacs, or intravenously.

Anesthesia: Anesthesia may be required for further examination or for diagnostic and surgical procedures. Response to anethesthics depends on individual health and species of the animal. Tricaine methanesulfonate, ketamine hydrochloride, propofol, halothane, isoflurane, and sevoflurane may be used. Routes of administration include immersion bath, topically, or parentally. Inhalant anesthetics are typically used topically or via an immersion bath, because they are readily absorbed through the skin. Larger amphibians can be intubated and maintained on anesthetic gas. Parental anesthetics are typically injected IV, IM, intracoelomically, or into the dorsal lymph sac. Injections into the rear limbs are avoided because of the presence of a renal-portal system. Heart rate can be monitored in most amphibians using an ultrasonic Doppler positioned over the heart. A baseline heart rate should be established before initiating anesthesia. Because amphibians can breathe through the skin, observing gular movement is less rewarding. Tricaine methanesulfonate is a fine white crystal that is highly soluble in water. It can be prepared and stored as a 10 g/L stock solution, which is diluted just before use. Administration is by bath, because most amphibians will absorb tricaine through the skin. The dosage used for many large amphibians is 2–3 g/L for induction. For short procedures, the amphibian should be immediately removed and rinsed with fresh water. For longer procedures, the amphibian may be placed into a maintenance solution of 100–200 mg/L after it has been induced. In smaller amphibians, an induction dosage of 100–200 mg/L is safer. Aeration must be provided in the anesthetic solution to avoid hypoxia. Tricaine produces an acidic solution that must be buffered to a pH of ~7 using sodium bicarbonate, sodium hydroxide, or sodium hydrogen phosphate. Isoflurane gas can also be bubbled into an anesthetic bath placed in a sealed container; this will allow both percutaneous and inhalation absorption. Ketamine hydrochloride injected percutaneously or into the dorsal lymph sac at a dosage of 75–125 mg/kg body wt can be used; however, a surgical plane of anesthesia can be difficult to maintain, and recoveries are long. Intracoelomic injections of propofol at a dosage of 35–45 mg/kg body wt will also provide sedation to anesthesia.

INFECTIOUS DISEASES

Bacterial Diseases: "Red-leg" syndrome commonly refers to the hyperemia of the ventral skin that accompanies systemic infection in amphibians. Saprophytic, gram-negative bacteria such as *Aeromonas*, *Pseudomonas*, *Proteus*, and *Citrobacter* spp typically cause red-leg. Viruses, fungi, and other pathogens may cause similar lesions. Ventral hyperemia is a nonspecific sign and may also be seen with toxicosis. Malnourished, newly acquired amphibians that are maintained in poor-quality water or other inappropriate environmental conditions are particularly susceptible. Clinical signs include lethargy; emaciation; ulcerations of the skin, nose, and toes; and characteristic cutaneous pinpoint hemorrhages of the legs and abdomen. Hemorrhages may also be seen in the skeletal muscles, tongue, and nictitating membrane. In acute cases, these signs may be absent. Histologic evidence of systemic infection may include inflammatory or necrotic foci in the liver, spleen, and other coelomic organs. Blood or, if present, coelomic fluid, should be taken for culture before beginning therapy. Individuals can be treated initially with enrofloxacin

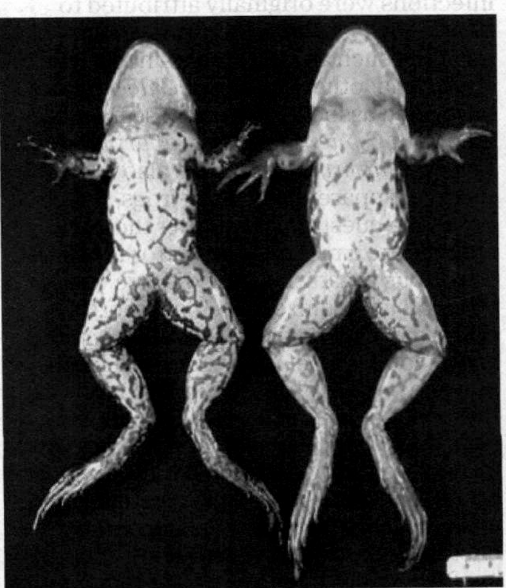

Red-leg syndrome in two leopard frogs. The larger frog is more severely affected. *Courtesy of Research Animal Diagnostic Laboratory, University of Missouri.*

(5–10 mg/kg/day, PO or IM), oxytetracycline (50 mg/kg, PO, bid), or chloramphenicol (50 mg/kg, PO, bid) before receiving culture and sensitivity results. If fungal infection is suspected, a 0.01% itraconazole bath (3.5 L fresh water mixed with 35 mL itraconazole solution; 5 min/day for 8 days) may be effective.

Mycobacteriosis, caused by acid-fast bacilli, including *Mycobacterium fortuitum*, *M marinum*, *M chelonea*, *M abscessus*, *M avium*, *M szulgai*, and *M xenopi*, is found principally in debilitated amphibians. Although often an infection of the integument, ingestion of infectious organisms may also lead to GI disease and systemic infection. Affected amphibians may exhibit gray nodules in the skin, liver, kidneys, spleen, lungs, and other coelomic organs. Infected amphibians may eat well but still lose weight. Acid-fast bacilli may be detected in feces and oropharyngeal mucus. A premortem diagnosis can be made by finding acid-fast bacilli in animals with external lesions. Culture of mycobacteria requires special media such as Lowenstein-Jensen agar (cultured at 23°, 30°, and 37°C) but is frequently unsuccessful. In cases in which staining is inconclusive, confirmation using PCR is recommended. Treatment is not recommended for this potentially zoonotic disease, and euthanasia should be considered.

Chlamydiosis is a serious infection of amphibians. Based on histologic lesions and the presence of inclusion bodies, these infections were originally attributed to *Chlamydia psittaci*. Using molecular methods such as PCR, it has since been shown that other species of *Chlamydia* have been associated with these infections, including *C pneumoniae*, *C abortus*, and *C suis*. *Chlamydia* spp have also been found in apparently healthy frogs, which raises the question of whether these animals are a reservoir or vector for these infectious organisms. The disease was originally recognized in a mass mortality of African clawed frogs (*Xenopus laevis*) fed uncooked beef livers. Infected frogs may die peracutely or exhibit lethargy, dysequilibrium, cutaneous depigmentation, petechiae, and edema. Histologically, intracytoplasmic basophilic inclusion bodies can be identified in sinusoidal lining cells of the liver and spleen. Secondary bacterial infections are frequently present in affected amphibians and must be treated appropriately. Antibiotic treatment, including doxycycline (5–10 mg/kg/day, PO) or oxytetracycline (50 mg/kg/day, PO), may be effective against chlamydial infection.

Fungal Diseases: Many of the fungi that infect amphibians are difficult to distinguish grossly because they produce similar clinical effects, including lethargy and skin ulcerations. Some fungi can be identified via the examination of a wet mount prepared from a skin scraping, whereas others require culture, histology, and special stains. Treatment includes proper hygiene and the use of topical or systemic antifungal agents such as itraconazole. Other antifungal drugs such as fluconazole may also be effective.

Chytridiomycosis is the most serious fungal infection in amphibians and has been implicated in the decline of wild and captive frog, toad, and salamander populations around the world. The causative agent, *Batrachochytrium dendrobatidis* (Bd), is a nonhyphal zoosporic fungus identified in specimens preserved as far back as 1938, yet it was not until the 1990s that the organism was associated with large losses of Australian frogs. Chytrids are typically found in moist environments, where they feed on decomposing organic matter or are parasitic to plants and invertebrates. Amphibians are the only known vertebrate host for chytrid fungi. Postmetamorphic anurans are affected far more than caudates or larval amphibians. Tadpoles are usually subclinical, because Bd infects only tissues that contain keratin. Anuran larvae have keratin only in their mouthparts, which may become depigmented and sometimes damaged. Most caudate larvae do not have keratinized mouthparts. As larvae undergo metamorphosis and their skin becomes keratinized, Bd can spread over the animal, infect the stratum corneum of the epidermis, and cause mortality. The "drink patch," specialized skin located in the ventral pelvic region that absorbs water, and the digits are especially affected. Diagnostic samples are best taken from these regions for this reason. Because pathogenicity of Bd appears to decline above 25°–27°C, it is speculated that some amphibian populations living at higher elevations have disappeared because of the cooler temperatures associated with the winter months and possibly climate change. Although the exact mechanism of infection is unknown, Bd causes skin hyperkeratosis and subsequent sloughing, osmoregulatory disruption, electrolyte disruption, and cardiac arrest. Infection intensity (>10,000 zoospores) appears to be associated with mortality. Some amphibians, including the bullfrog (*Rana catesbeiana*) and the African clawed frog (*Xenopus laevis*) are less susceptible to Bd and may serve as reservoirs for the disease. Mobile zoospores contribute to the loss of whole populations of amphibians. Clinical signs include abnormal posture, anorexia, lethargy, dehydration, hyperemia, excessive shedding of skin, pupillary miosis, and muscle incoordination. These signs may be mild to absent in infected caudates, emphasizing the importance of performing diagnostic tests. Visualizing the spherical, single-celled organisms in skin scrapings stained with Wright-Giemsa or Gram stains using a light microscope is diagnostic, but the organisms are not always readily seen. Real-time PCR performed on swabs of the integument or pieces of skin is diagnostic and provides rapid assessment of presence and quantity of zoospores. This is useful in screening and management of amphibian populations at risk, such as those undergoing transport or quarantine. On histopathology, zoosporangia containing zoospores are associated with hyperkeratosis and underlying dermal infection. Treatment includes the topical administration of itraconazole (0.01% bath for 5 min/day for 10–11 days) and maintaining animals well within their normal thermal range. The use of terbinafine (0.01% bath buffered using bicarbonate to a pH of 7.2–7.4 for 5 min/day for 5 days) may also be effective. If appropriate for the species, raising environmental temperatures for captive populations to >23°C may help halt the infection while medicated baths are used to eliminate Bd. Systemic antifungal drugs appear to be ineffective in treating this infection of the epidermis. Bd is a World Organization for Animal Health (OIE) notifiable disease.

Saprolegniasis refers to disease caused by several genera of opportunistic fungi or "water molds" that infect the gills and/or skin of aquatic and larval amphibians. When in water, newly affected animals appear to have a whitish cotton-like growth on their skin. As the fungal mat ages, it may become greenish due to the presence of algae. Once removed from water, the fungal mat collapses and is difficult to see. Other signs include lethargy, respiratory distress, anorexia, and weight loss. Skin ulcerations may occur as the infection progresses. A diagnosis of saprolegniasis is made by finding hyphae and the thin-walled zoospores in a skin scrape. Treatment with a malachite green dip (67 mg/L for 15 sec, once daily for 2–3 days) or copper sulfate (500 mg/L for 2 min, once daily for 5 days, then once weekly until healed) may be effective. Treatment of eggs with methylene blue may be effective. Secondary bacterial and parasitic infections may be present in animals with dermal ulcers. Poor water quality conditions should be corrected.

Chromomycosis is caused by pigmented or black fungi from several genera (eg, *Cladosporium*, *Fonsecaea*, *Phialophora*, *Ochroconis*, *Rhinocladosporium*, and *Wangiella*). These fungi may be found in organic substrates such as topsoil and decaying plant matter. Disease is either cuteaneous or disseminated systemic; both have been seen in captive and wild populations of amphibians. Signs may include anorexia, weight loss, granulomatous skin lesions or ulcers, coelomic distention, and neurologic disease. Diagnosis is usually made postmortem by finding disseminated granulomas with pigmented fungal cells and hyphae. Culture is frequently unsuccessful; histopathology may be necessary to confirm the diagnosis. Treatment using itraconazole (10 mg/kg/day, PO, for 30 days) may be given, but the prognosis is poor once the infection is disseminated.

Zygomycosis, caused by fungi of the class Zygomycetes (*Mucor* spp, *Basidiobolus* sp, and *Rhizopus* spp), affects both wild and captive populations of anurans. Clinical signs include lethargy and multifocal hyperemic nodules with fungal growth on the ventrum. Disease progresses rapidly and results in mortality within 2 wk. Zygomycetes are found in the environment, especially soils and decaying matter, and are a normal component of the amphibian's GI tract. Successful treatment has not been reported, but advanced antifungal agents may be tried.

Mesomycetozoans are fungus-like microrganisms at the animal-fungal boundary. Those reported in the literature to infect amphibians include *Amphibiothecum* (previously *Dermosporidium*), *Amphibiocystidium*, and *Ichthyophonus*; however, continued molecular characterization of these organisms is ongoing, resulting in nomenclature changes and taxonomic reorganization. *Amphibiothecum* and *Amphibiocystidium* are spore-forming organisms that typically produce a nonlethal infection in anurans. Clinical signs include multifocal nodules and pustules, usually on the ventrum, that resolve in 4–8 wk. Microscopically encysted spores contain large cytoplasmic vacuoles. *Ichthyophonus* is pathogenic to salamanders and frogs living in the eastern half of the USA. Pre- and post-metamorphic life stages are infected. Clinical signs include muscle swelling in the thigh, rump, and tail and may appear nodular, especially in tadpoles. Debilitation may lead to mortality, especially in adults. Diagnosis is based on histopathology or finding characteristic spores through microscopic examination of material from the lesions. There is no treatment other than supportive care.

Parasitic Diseases: Many of the protozoa and metazoa found in and on amphibians are not associated with disease unless the host amphibian is stressed or immunocompromised. Recently caught or transported amphibians are particularly susceptible to parasitism, as are those kept in poor hygienic conditions and outside their POTZ. Parasites with indirect life cycles tend to die out when wild-caught amphibians are brought into captivity if the intermediate or final host is not present. Conversely, infections by parasites with a direct life cycle may be magnified in a closed environment. Excellent hygiene is essential for parasite control and includes the routine removal of sloughed skin, fecal material, uneaten food, and carcasses from animal enclosures.

External parasites may be found by close examination of amphibians using magnification and a bright, cool light. A skin scrape or biopsy may be required to identify parasites causing nodules or epidermal lesions. Internal parasites are often identified through examination of fresh fecal samples. Some small frogs are translucent enough to allow the visualization of nematodes using transillumination. In some cases, metazoan and protozoan parasites are found only at necropsy. Finding flagellates, ciliates, and opalinids in the feces is normal and does not require treatment in healthy amphibians. Although many larval nematodes found in the feces are nonpathogenic, treatment is recommended because pathogenic and nonpathogenic species cannot be readily distinguished.

Most protozoans found in the GI tract, including ciliates, opalinids, and flagellates, are commensals. The ciliate *Tetrahymena*, although normally nonpathogenic, has been associated with mortality of salamanders. Trichodinids may be found in the urinary bladder or on the skin of amphibians and require treatment. Hemoflagellates are occasionally found and generally nonpathogenic but can result in anemia. Greater-than-normal loads of GI flagellates and other protozoa may be found in debilitated amphibians and require treatment aimed at restoring balance and not eliminating the protozoa. External dinoflagellates (eg, *Piscinoodinium*) and flagellates (eg, *Ichthyobodo*) can cause significant mortality, especially in larval amphibians. Fecal samples collected by placing the amphibian on clean, moist paper towels helps to prevent contamination from free-ranging protozoa. Cloacal wash, gill clips, and skin scrapes are also diagnostic. Treatment using metronidazole is often effective for external and GI organisms. Sporozoans such as coccidia (*Eimeria* and *Isospora*) and microsporidians (*Microsporidium*, *Pleistophora*, and *Alloglugea*) may be incidental findings or parasitic. Clinical signs are nonspecific and include poor body condition and wasting. Myxozoa occasionally cause disease in amphibians and result in specific host/disease agent lesions. Treatment efforts are focused on providing supportive care.

Metazoa parasites include myxozoa, helminths, and arthropods. Myxozoa infections in amphibians generally do not cause mortality. Helminths that are pathogenic to amphibians include trematodes (*Ribeirola*, *Clinostomum*) and nematodes (*Rhabdias*, *Strongyloides*, *Pseudocapillaroides*). Arthropods, such as the common fish parasites *Argulus* and *Lernaea*, may infect amphibian aquatic life cycle stages, whereas ticks and mites affect postmetamorphic terrestrial animals. Larval dipterid flies may consume amphibian eggs and embryos and feed on the tissues of adults. Two of the most significant metazoan infections in captive amphibians are caused by *Rhabdias* sp and *Pseudocapillaroides xenopi*.

Rhabdiasis, caused by the lungworm *Rhabdias* sp, commonly causes pulmonary damage and secondary infections in captive amphibians. This nematode has a direct life cycle with free-living phases. Adult worms live in the lungs, where they deposit larvated eggs that are coughed up, swallowed, and then excreted into the environment. Infective L_3 larvae then burrow through the skin of a new host, where they mature and migrate to the lungs. Affected animals may appear anorectic, thin, and generally debilitated. A premortem diagnosis may be made by finding ova or worms in oral and nasal secretions. Infection should be suspected when nematode larva and larvated eggs are found in fresh feces from an animal with clinical signs. When rhabdiasis is suspected, treatment using fenbendazole (100 mg/kg/day, PO, for 2 days then repeated 12–14 days later) or ivermectin (200–400 mcg/kg, PO, once, repeated 12–14 days later) is recommended. After the second of each 2-day fenbendazole treatment or each dose of ivermectin, the animals should be moved into a newly established environment to prevent reinfection from free-living life stages. Some reactions to fenbendazole have been reported, so animals should be monitored closely and treatment discontinued if necessary.

The capillarid nematode *Pseudocapillaroides xenopi* burrows into the skin and is known to affect colonies of the aquatic African clawed frog. Signs include discoloration, roughening, pitting, and ulceration of the skin. As the infection progresses, lethargy, anorexia, and skin sloughing occur. Diagnosis is made by finding small, white nematodes beneath the mucus on the skin; skin scrapings may show larvae and ova. Treatment by adding thiabendazole (0.1 g/L) to the water may be effective. Levamisole and other anthelmintics may also be effective. Frequent water changes with removal of shed skin containing the parasite are required to prevent the amplification and spread of infection to cage mates.

Viral Diseases: Renal adenocarcinomas (Lucké tumors), caused by ranid herpesvirus-1, are relatively common in leopard frogs (*Rana pipiens*) wild-caught in the northeastern and north central USA. Few frogs with tumors are seen in the summer, because viral replication is temperature-dependent. Virus particles and intranuclear inclusion bodies are seen when frogs are in hibernation, at 41°–50°F (5°–10°C). Metastasis of the tumor to liver, lungs, and other organs is common; both the primary and metastatic tumors can become very large. There is no treatment. The neoplasm is a model of herpesvirus-induced cancer.

Ranaviruses, which are DNA-based viruses in the genus *Ranavirus*, family Iridoviridae, have been identified as the cause of mass mortality in wild populations of anurans and caudates across the world. Environmental conditions, reservoir species, persistence in the environment, direct and indirect transmission, stress, and host immunity contribute to the impact of ranaviruses on amphibian populations. Species of *Ranavirus* that infect amphibians include frog virus 3 (FV3) and FV3-like viruses, *Bohle iridovirus*, and *Ambystoma tigrinum* virus. These viruses are highly virulent and may produce 90%–100% mortality in tadpoles and adults. Transmission occurs through exposure to contaminated water or soil, contact with infected individuals, and consumption of infected tissues. Fish and reptiles (especially turtles) are reservoirs for ranaviruses. Clinical signs are nonspecific, develop rapidly in a large number of cohorts, and include abnormal swimming behavior, swelling of the limbs or body, edema, hydrocoelom, erythema, ventral skin hemorrhage (especially in the hind region), and occasionally skin ulcerations. Lesions may appear very similar to those of bacterial dermatosepticemias. The original viral lesions may be overwhelmed by secondary invaders, and many outbreaks of "red-leg" may have had underlying and undiagnosed viral infection. Death typically results from multiple organ failure. Amphibian larvae undergoing metamorphosis or recently metamorphosed juveniles seem to be most susceptible to infection. For this reason, mortality events often occur in the spring/summer. Survivors appear to acquire some immunity to future infections. Diagnosis is made using PCR, primary cell culture, and/or microscopy. Ranaviruses can persist in the aquatic environment without a host for weeks, which contributes to their ability to infect naive amphibian populations and emphasizes the need for biosecurity measures when transporting amphibians or working in environments where the virus exists. Disinfection using bleach (1%) and chlorhexidine (0.75%) are effective. Ranavirus disease is notifiable to the World Organization for Animal Health (OIE).

NONINFECTIOUS DISORDERS

Nutritional Diseases: Metabolic bone disease is frequently seen in amphibians consuming nonsupplemented invertebrates. Except for earthworms, most invertebrates used as food have an inverse calcium:phosphorus ratio. This results in mandibular deformity, long bone fracture, scoliosis, and eventually tetany and bloating. Diagnosis is made radiographically by finding thinning cortices of long bones, mandibular and hyoid bone deformities, pathologic fractures, and in severe cases, GI gas. Treatment includes correcting the diet and administering calcium glubionate 1 mL/kg/day, PO, for 30 days. Full-spectrum lighting with biologically active ultraviolet-B light should be provided. Vitamin D_3 can also be administered in severe cases. Starvation, resulting in weight loss, lethargy, and dehydration, must be treated by providing proper nutrition through assist feeding.

Thiamine deficiency is seen in amphibians fed frozen fish containing thiaminase. Clinical signs include tremors, seizures, and opisthotonos. Initial treatment is the administration of thiamine at 25–100 mg/kg, IM or intracoelomic, followed by thiamine 25 mg/kg body wt, PO, with each meal. Thiamine deficiency can be prevented by

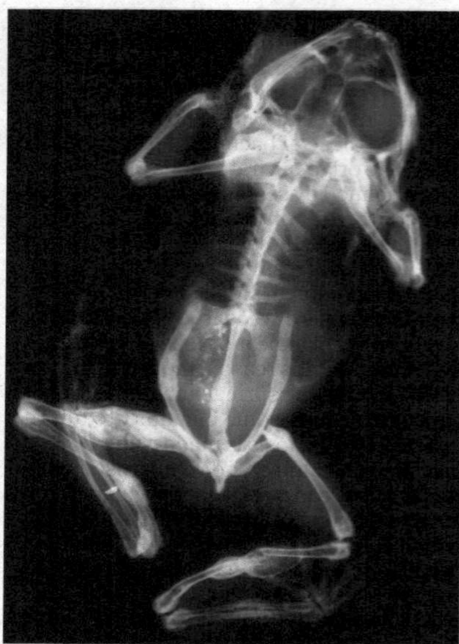

As metabolic bone disease in amphibians advances, pathologic fractures of the long bones are readily seen on radiographs.
Courtesy of the National Aquarium.

routinely supplementing diets with 250 mg thiamine/kg of fish fed.

The carotenoids, including vitamin A, are not synthesized by amphibians and must be provided through diet. Excessive levels of vitamin A have been hypothesized to interfere with vitamin D metabolism and contribute to metabolic bone disease, whereas deficiency has been associated with lethargy, wasting, and inability to use the tongue to catch prey due to the development of squamous metaplasia of the tongue (short tongue syndrome). Treatment includes providing vitamin A supplementation and force feeding a proper diet.

Obesity is a disease. Overfeeding is the primary cause of obesity; many amphibian species will continue to consume prey as long as it is available and without regard for their energy needs. The oversized fat bodies may be palpated within the coelomic cavity; however, in females, ultrasound may be necessary to differentiate enlarged fat bodies from egg masses. Treatment for active species includes enlarging the size of the enclosure to allow increased activity. Maintaining the amphibian at the upper end of its POTZ will accelerate metabolic rate and increase caloric use. Reducing caloric intake also may be used to control weight.

Neoplasia: Spontaneous neoplasia occurs in most organ systems but is rare except when caused by pollutants or an infectious agent, such as the virally induced Lucké renal carcinoma that affects populations of northern leopard frogs (*see above*) or epidermal papillomata in the Japanese firebelly newt. With increasing longevity in captivity and better health care, it is likely that more cases of neoplasia will be identified.

Trauma: Traumatic injuries are common in captive amphibians and include lacerations, bone fractures, internal bleeding, desiccation, and the loss of digits, limbs, or tail. Rapid assessment followed by supportive care is required for a successful outcome. Desiccation is common in amphibians that escape their enclosure or do not receive proper care. For smaller amphibians (<30 g), most fractures can be managed conservatively with cage rest. For larger amphibians, the use of external or internal fixation may be beneficial. Pain management must be considered in traumatic cases. The presence of opioid receptors suggests using opioids may be beneficial (buprenorphine, 0.02 mg/kg, IM, SC, or PO). NSAIDs may also be used (meloxicam, 0.2 mg/kg) and appear to provide pain relief.

EMERGENCY CARE

Initial emergency support includes providing fluid therapy, oxygen, and an environment of proper temperature and humidity. Placing the animal in a shallow bowl of isotonic or slightly hypotonic fluid enables transdermal uptake. Equal parts 2.5% dextrose in 0.45% sodium chloride and lactated Ringer's solution is effective. Coelomic, IV, or interosseus fluids may be given by bolus to larger animals at 5–10 mL/kg. In the absence of known exposure to an organophosphate, seizuring animals should be treated for hypocalcemia (calcium gluconate, 100 mg/kg, IM, IV, SC, or intracoelomic, once or twice daily), organophosphate toxicity (atropine, 0.1 mg/kg, SC or IM as needed), and thiamine deficiency (vitamin B_1 25–100 mg/kg, IM or intracoelomic as needed). If sepsis is suspected, antibiotic administration (eg, enrofloxacin 5–10 mg/kg/day, PO, SC, IM, or intracoelomic) should be initiated. Treatment for traumatic injuries is directed at minimizing blood loss, providing fluid therapy and respiratory support (doxapram 5 mg/kg, IM or IV as needed), and reducing pain (buprenorphine 0.02 mg/kg, IM, SC, or PO, or meloxicam 0.2 mg/kg), followed by corrective therapy.

AMPHIBIANS AS LABORATORY ANIMALS

Amphibians have long been used as laboratory animals. In an effort to enable scientific research while maintaining humane and ethical principles, the 8th edition of *The Care and Use of Laboratory Animals* (National Research Council, National Academies Press, 2011) provides organizations conducting research on animals, including aquatic animals, with information regarding environment, housing, management, and veterinary care. This guide should be consulted when using amphibians in research. (*See also* LABORATORY ANIMALS, p 1836.) Species that are captive born and readily available from commercial suppliers include the African clawed frog (*Xenopus laevis*, *X tropicalis*), the African dwarf frog (*Hymenochirus boettgeri*), the fire-bellied toad (*Bombina orientalis*), the axolotl (*Ambystoma mexicanum*), and the tiger salamander (*A tigrinum*). Wild-caught species collected by researchers or vendors for use in the laboratory include the northern leopard frog (*Rana pipiens*, sometimes called the grass frog), bullfrog (*R catesbeiana*), cane toad (*Bufo marinus*, sometimes called the marine toad), and the mud puppy (*Necturus maculosus*). Other North American ranid frogs are sometimes used. When collecting or importing amphibians, it is important to abide by state laws and obtain all required permits.

Pelleted diets are available for some aquatic species, like African clawed frogs, bullfrogs, and axolotls, making it easier to feed large groups. These foods must be stored in a cool, dry location to maintain freshness. Uneaten food should be removed after all animals appear satiated to avoid fouling the tank. Handling and research protocols should be developed to minimize stress to the animals. Overcrowding must be avoided to maintain sanitation, prevent disease transfer, and reduce social stress.

Most aquatic species used for laboratory studies are kept in large, recirculating systems that have multiple tanks using a common water supply. Water is filtered, sent to individual tanks, and then returned for filtration and disinfection. Proper water quality is maintained using one or more types of filtration. These include a mechanical filter to remove suspended waste material, a biofilter to convert nitrogenous wastes to less toxic compounds, and a chemical filter to remove dissolved organic compounds. The addition of an ultraviolet sterilizer to inactivate microorganisms is highly recommended. Bulbs must be kept clean and changed every 6–8 mo for the ultraviolet sterilizer to remain effective. Ozone, a potent oxidant, may also be used with caution to remove suspended organic material and potential pathogens from the water.

Ammonia toxicosis is common in systems that have not established a good biofilter. Amphibians exposed to inappropriate levels of ammonia typically produce excess mucus, become dull in color, and attempt to escape. Amphibians should be removed from the contaminated water and rinsed thoroughly with dechlorinated and well oxygenated fresh water. A diagnosis can be confirmed if the source water has ammonia at levels >0.5 ppm, although toxicity can be seen at levels >0.1 ppm for some species. Many tropical fish stores sell test kits that check for ammonia.

AQUACULTURE

Aquaculture is the production of marine and freshwater organisms under controlled conditions. Hundreds of different species of aquatic animals are raised in aquaculture and include fish and aquatic invertebrates cultured for food, the aquarium hobby, bait, recreational fisheries, research, private ponds, and stock enhancement of wild populations. Animal aquaculture was valued at $137.7 billion (USD) worldwide in 2012, with China's production valued at $66 billion and the USA's at $1 billion. Within the USA, major commercial commodities include channel catfish, centered around the Mississippi Delta; rainbow trout in the north/northwest, including Hagerman Valley, Idaho; Atlantic salmon in the Pacific northwest and Atlantic northeast; aquarium fish with production centered in Florida; baitfish in Arkansas; and goldfish and koi production scattered throughout the USA. In addition, other public and private entities, including research facilities, public aquaria, and hobbyists, are breeding numerous other species.

PRODUCTION METHODS

Aquaculture production methods vary greatly, but regardless of method, a good understanding of water quality and chemistry, species requirements, and systems design and operation will facilitate good management. Production can be divided into two major categories: land-based and open-water systems. Land-based facilities use tanks and ponds to house and raise fish. Tank systems can be flow-through, in which continuous replenishment of "new" water comes from a well, reservoir, or other central water body; recirculating, with reuse of system water after filtration to remove nitrogenous wastes and dissolved and suspended particulates; or a combination of the two. Indoor, land-based tank systems afford much greater control over water quality, predators, and pests than outdoor facilities, but often house fish at much higher densities.

Design and management of recirculating aquaculture systems (RASs) requires greater technical knowledge than for flow-through systems (*see* Southern Regional Aquaculture Center [SRAC] Fact Sheet 4708 [https://srac.tamu.edu]). Most RASs typically incorporate biologic filtration and mechanical filtration components, although some also include some type of chemical filtration and in-line sterilization. Biologic filters rely on the establishment of two sets of nitrifying bacteria on biofiltration surfaces to transform ammonia, a by-product of protein and nucleic acid metabolism by fish from food, first into nitrite (a toxic intermediate), and then into nitrate, considered a much less toxic compound (although levels of nitrate may be problematic for invertebrates and, at higher levels, fish). More advanced systems include a denitrification component that transforms nitrate into nitrogen gas that is released into the atmosphere. Mechanical filters remove particulates to reduce their negative effects on water quality and fish health, and to improve water clarity, which facilitates observations. Chemical filtration is used to change the concentration of specific ions or compounds in the water (eg, ion-exchange resins such as those used in softeners to remove calcium, or zeolite to bind ammonia). Ultraviolet (UV) sterilization units and ozone are common choices for aquaculturists who wish to include in-line disinfection of system water. UV sterilizers act optimally at a wavelength of 254 nm and disrupt pathogen DNA. Systems with these components typically include a system bypass loop to feed a portion of total system water into these disinfection units. UV sterilizing units must be designed and rated to deliver a specific "zap dose" to target a specific pathogen or pathogen group. Component maintenance, water clarity, wattage, and water flow through the UV sterilizer all contribute to the efficiency of the unit. Although there are exceptions, in general the larger and more complex a pathogen is, the greater the zap dose required to kill it. Ozone units use highly reactive O_3 to break apart microorganisms. However, because ozone can be very harmful to fish, it must be removed from the water before it is returned to the system. Ozone is also a human health hazard, so protocols to safeguard human health should be implemented. *See also* AQUATIC SYSTEMS, p 1766.

Pond systems include earthen and lined ponds typically filled from wells, aquifers, or surface water bodies. Ponds have minimal water exchange and rely on good management of their more "natural" systems to maintain acceptable water quality and control aquatic weeds, algae, and other pond life. Nitrifying bacteria are found on surfaces in the pond. Important key water quality parameters—oxygen, carbon dioxide, and pH—can vary widely throughout the day in a pond because of photosynthesis by phytoplankton (algae) and other plant life. During the day, photosynthesis increases oxygen levels. However, during the evening, when photosynthesis has ceased, oxygen is consumed by all organisms in the pond, including algae and higher plants, resulting in lower levels. At the same time, increased production of carbon dioxide (without consumption through photosynthesis) results in lowering of pH. During the day, these trends are reversed. Any ammonia levels in a pond will have increased toxicity as pH rises throughout the day. Other challenges in pond production include pests and predators, such as snails, otters, birds, amphibians, and reptiles, as well as nontarget fish, all of which can also act as reservoirs or vectors for pathogens or intermediate hosts. *See also* AQUATIC SYSTEMS, p 1766.

Channel catfish, tilapia, hybrid striped bass, shrimp, crawfish, baitfish, and ornamental fish are raised in ponds, tanks, or a combination of the two. Some species, including rainbow trout, require higher oxygen concentrations and are raised in land-based raceways.

Open-water aquaculture includes production in net pens or sea cages placed in oceans, bays, lakes, or reservoirs. Open-water systems rely on good flushing, dilution, and natural processes occurring within the given water body to maintain acceptable culture parameters. In many cases, land-based systems are used for reproduction and early life-stage growout for "open water aquaculture" species. Open-water systems do have a number of challenges. Water quality in the main body of water cannot be controlled. Access (by boat in many cases) and logistics are more complex because of location within a larger body of water. Biofouling (growth of algae, bacteria, other invertebrates) on nets can reduce water exchange and degrade water quality within the net or cage. Pests and predators can be more difficult to control, as can human theft or vandalism. Disease management is also more complex because of increased environmental restrictions in natural water bodies and treatment logistics (eg, modifications such as "tarping" (placing a large polyethylene liner over or under a net to hold water for temporary bath/immersion treatments).

Open-water systems are used for final grow-out stages of clams, oysters, mussels, Atlantic salmon, flounder, pompano, cobia, and other marine species. Production of some freshwater species (eg, tilapia) may also use net pens set in lakes, ponds, or reservoirs for growout.

PRODUCTION MEDICINE AND BIOSECURITY

General veterinary approaches in aquaculture parallel those for other production animals, such as large animals and poultry. When working with fish, disease prevention is always more rewarding than treatment. Once fish are sick, accurately identifying all present problems can be difficult, and treatment must be administered early in the course of an epizootic to be effective.

A comprehensive program of fish health management should be based on the principles of good husbandry and biosecurity. Good husbandry practices, including water quality, systems management, and nutrition, facilitate health and prevent disease. Consequences of poor husbandry are magnified in production aquaculture because of the greater size and density of populations in a production setting than in a hobbyist or aquarium display system. Population health is the focus (although valuable broodstock may warrant individual care), with preventive medicine of critical importance. Populations can vary from several individuals to millions, with many facilities averaging thousands to hundreds of thousands within any given defined population.

Biosecurity underlies critical fish health management practices for disease prevention and management (*see* SRAC Fact Sheets 4707, 4708, and 4712 [https://srac.tamu.edu/index.cfm/viewAllSheets/]). Good biosecurity will minimize the risk of introduction and spread of an infectious disease into and within a facility, as well as minimize the risk that diseased animals or infectious agents will leave the facility and spread to other sites. Major biosecurity goals include good animal management, obtaining and maintaining healthy stocks through good sourcing and husbandry, pathogen management, and people management through education and awareness for staff and visitors. *See also* BIOSECURITY, p 2068.

Animal Management: Eggs and animals should be from a reputable supplier, and animals should be screened for species-specific health parameters and diseases of concern. Previous testing and other relevant historical and husbandry information should be obtained for any lots of fish entering a facility. New fish should undergo quarantine to prevent spread of disease. Water quality, other environmental conditions (such as choice of holding units, density, water flow, lighting, and sound), and nutrition should be optimized for the facility's goals and species.

Pathogen Management: Water source is a major risk factor for disease introduction, with protected water sources (ie, sources that do not have fish or other potential pathogen reservoirs) having low to zero risk of carrying diseases of concern. Examples of protected water sources include those from deep wells or disinfected municipal supplies. Protected water sources are preferable to unprotected sources, such as surface waters from a lake or river. Risks from unprotected sources can be mitigated (eg, through filtration, UV sterilization, chlorination, and/or ozonation) to make them safer.

Efforts to maintain as clean an environment as possible, including minimal accumulation of organic debris, proper disinfection of nets and equipment, and thorough disinfection of fish-holding units between groups of fish, help minimize disease outbreaks by optimizing water quality and reducing pathogen loads and reservoirs (*see* below). Familiarity with common diseases for a given species, as well as potential disease reservoirs and relevant diagnostics and control are important. Some pathogens, such as the bacteria *Aeromonas hydrophila* and the ciliated protist *Trichodina*, are considered ubiquitous and opportunistic, whereas others may result in significant morbidity and mortality (eg, *Streptococcus* spp or *Amyloodinium*), and/or have regulatory consequences (eg, infectious salmon anemia or spring viremia of carp, a foreign animal disease in the USA). Quarantine of new fish at temperatures permissive for significant diseases will facilitate determination of presence of specific pathogens. Isolation of diseased populations, use of equipment dedicated to a specific group, and system and equipment sanitation and disinfection are important methods of pathogen management.

People Management: Important components of a good biosecurity program include owner and staff education, awareness, and commitment to principles of biosecurity. Written protocols and rules for workers and facility visitors help solidify understanding and accountability. Increasingly, facilities are making the effort to develop written biosecurity, health management, and disaster management plans. Interested veterinarians should be familiar with aquaculture systems and be able to evaluate these protocols, as well as staff and visitor adherence to them through general biosecurity audits.

Cleaning and Disinfection: Proper cleaning and disinfection are critical components of a good fish health management program. There are a number of good references for cleaning and disinfection in aquaculture settings (*see* SRAC Fact Sheet 4707: Biosecurity in Aquaculture, Part 1, Tables 1 and 2 [https://srac.tamu.edu], and Guide to Using Drugs, Biologics, and Other Chemicals in Aquaculture, Table 5 [www.fws.gov/fisheries]).

Cleaning and disinfection of tanks and equipment starts with general cleaning and removal of dirt and organic debris. Organic debris, including biofilms, and dirt can shield pathogens from disinfection. Liquid household bleach (3%–6% NaHClO) delivered at 35 mL/gal. of water creates a concentration of 200 mg/L. Granular bleach (HTH, calcium hypochlorite) is more stable than household bleach and is often used on commercial farms. It is available in three different concentrations: 15%, 50%, or 65% available chlorine. The target dose of chlorine for disinfection is 200 mg/L for at least 1 hr. This concentration can be achieved by mixing 1.4 g of the 15% product/L of water, 0.4 g/L of the 50% product, or 0.32 g/L of the 65% product. These products are strong oxidizers, and precautions listed on the label or relevant Material Safety Data Sheet should be followed when handling them. A 1-hr contact time at 200 mg/L will destroy most organisms of concern, including most viruses. Bleach should not be used in closed areas containing live fish, because the volatile compound may get into the solution and kill fish in nearby tanks. Mycobacteria are refractory to bleach disinfection because of their waxy cell wall. Spraying equipment and contact surfaces with alcohol after treatment with bleach should effectively eliminate mycobacteria, although access to some surfaces (eg, PVC pipework) and associated biofilms may be difficult. In these instances, it is understood that major reduction in pathogen numbers is the key goal. Another commonly used aquaculture disinfectant, Virkon® Aquatic (active ingredient 21.4% potassium peroxymonosulfate and 1.5% sodium chloride), is highly effective at 1%–2% concentrations and considered much less toxic to fish (manufacturer directions must be followed). Quaternary ammonium compounds such as Roccal® and benzalkonium chloride are also excellent disinfectants and can be used at concentrations of 500 mg/L for 1 hr, but residual films should be rinsed off completely. Both Virkon Aquatic and quaternary ammonium compounds are more suitable for net dips and net disinfection.

NECROPSY AND DIAGNOSTIC TECHNIQUES

For information on fish physiology, *see* AQUARIUM FISHES, p 1779. General methods for clinical evaluation of aquacultured species are similar to those used in aquarium fish. However, for more structured surveillance and pathogen testing, more uniform and standard methods may be required. OIE-accepted diagnostic methods for reportable diseases are described in *The Manual of Diagnostic Tests for Aquatic Animals* (also known as the OIE *Aquatic Manual* [www.oie.int]). Another good reference with standards for necropsy and diagnostics is The American Fisheries Society Fish Health Section Blue Book (2014 Ed.) *Suggested Procedures for the Detection and Identification of Certain Finfish and Shellfish Pathogens* (www.afs-fhs.org). Depending on the specific goals for testing (disease diagnostics, health certification, surveillance) and on the ultimate recipient of any testing results (eg, another state agency vs another country), one or both provide excellent information on methodology. Most veterinary practitioners will require additional laboratory support for more advanced diagnostics (eg, virology, histopathology, bacteriology). Therefore, it is important that the laboratory is qualified and, for USDA-APHIS relevant documentation, approved by the USDA-APHIS to run specific diagnostic tests for aquaculture species.

THE NATIONAL AQUATIC ANIMAL HEALTH PLAN

The U.S. National Aquatic Animal Health Plan (NAAHP) (www.aphis.usda.gov) was developed to facilitate the legal movement of all aquatic animals, their eggs, and products in interstate and international commerce; protect the health and thereby improve the quality and productivity of farmed and wild aquatic animals; ensure the availability of diagnostic, inspection, and certification services; and minimize the impact of diseases when they occur in farmed or wild aquatic animals. The NAAHP is a federal guidance document intended to help direct federal, state, and tribal efforts in the areas listed above. Work is ongoing to continue to refine and implement relevant and urgent aspects of the NAAHP.

USDA-APHIS is the lead federal agency for commercial aquaculture and the protection of aquatic animal health. See the focus on fish health Web site (www.aphis.usda.gov/focusonfish/) for useful links to access additional information on the USDA-APHIS aquaculture program.

The OIE sets the standards for members of the World Trade Organization with regard to determination of internationally reportable diseases and their management, and monitors these diseases with the cooperation of member nations (*see* the Aquatic Animal Health Code [www.oie.int]).

REPORTABLE DISEASES AND REGULATORY CONCERNS

With increased regulation of ornamental and aquacultured fish in the USA, there are additional needs for professional veterinary services, including USDA health certification (*see* below) for movement of animals. Implementation of the NAAHP should more clearly define the role of veterinary practitioners in the future. USDA-APHIS provides voluntary training to practitioners who wish to work in this area and is developing a special aquatic certificate for accredited veterinarians. Information on federal regulations pertaining to fish medicine is available at www.aphis.usda.gov. State law may be more restrictive than federal law, and there is significant variation in state regulations regarding importation of aquatic animals. The State Veterinarian or State Animal Health Officer is the ultimate resource for information on state animal health regulations.

Currently, USDA-APHIS has adopted the reportable disease list of the OIE (www.oie.int) as reportable in the USA (*see* TABLE 6, p 1786). If a USDA-APHIS reportable disease is suspected, appropriate samples should be collected as per the OIE Aquatic Manual. Practitioners should stay informed of changes in the status of diseases of regulatory concern, because they are liable if they have a case that is not reported. Regulated fish diseases of greatest concern to aquatic animal veterinarians in the USA include koi herpesvirus, spring viremia of carp, and viral hemorrhagic septicemia. Notification of reportable aquatic diseases should be made directly to the State Veterinarian and to the USDA Area Veterinarian in Charge.

Health Certification: A major role of the aquaculture veterinarian is health certification of many animals leaving a facility. Movement of animals may be intrastate, interstate, or international. Specific testing and general health requirements for aquaculture exports vary according to region, state, country, and species. In some instances, only a visual inspection is required, whereas in others statistically determined sample sizes and more standardized diagnostic methods are necessary. Level of required oversight also varies. Some countries require only evaluation and signature by a licensed veterinarian, whereas others require the oversight and acknowledgement of the national competent authority. USDA-APHIS is the competent authority for commercial aquaculture in the USA and provides information on specific import/export requirements by country (www.aphis.usda.gov). For importing countries requiring USDA-APHIS oversight, veterinarians must be licensed to practice in the USA and obtain veterinary accreditation (Category 2 accreditation is required for aquaculture) through USDA-APHIS for evaluation of aquaculture species. USDA-APHIS is also tasked to protect aquaculture in the USA from foreign disease introduction. For facilities within the USA that import fish, USDA-APHIS determines health requirements for incoming shipments, with fish, crustacean, molluscan, and amphibian diseases of concern listed by the OIE currently considered reportable by USDA-APHIS; however, not all of these are program diseases with specific actions required for positive cases.

THERAPEUTIC CONSIDERATIONS

Although improvement of water quality, nutrition, and other general husbandry factors may be enough to improve the health of a population, chemotherapeutics are often required to ameliorate disease outbreaks. Management of fish diseases is challenging because of basic logistics, including the aquatic environment, numbers of fish, and routes of administration, and also because of the pharmacologic and regulatory complexities of chemotherapeutic usage in fish.

One major point of confusion among veterinarians, more critical because of impacts on the aquatic environment, is the difference between a drug and a pesticide. Drugs are regulated by the FDA, whereas pesticides are regulated by the Environmental Protection Agency (EPA). According to the Federal Food Drug and Cosmetic Act definition, the term "drug" can be defined four ways: 1) articles recognized in the official United States Pharmacopoeia, official Homoeopathic Pharmacopoeia of the United States, or official National Formulary, or any supplement to any of them; or 2) articles intended for use in the diagnosis, cure, mitigation, treatment, or prevention of disease in man or other animals; 3) articles (other than food) intended to affect the structure or any function of the body of man or other animals; and 4) articles intended for use as a component of any of the aforementioned articles.

The EPA regulates water and effluents and controls the use of pesticides against "pests." A "pest" is defined by the Federal Insecticide, Fungicide and Rodenticide Act (FIFRA) as "any insect, rodent, nematode, fungus, weed" or "any other form of terrestrial or aquatic plant or animal life or virus, bacteria, or other microorganism (except viruses, bacteria, or other microorganisms on or in living man or other living animals)."

Legally, a drug is a compound that works in or on the fish, whereas a pesticide works in the water. Challenges occur for one of two reasons: 1) certain pathogens, and in particular some parasites, including the fish louse *Argulus* spp and anchorworm *Lernaea* spp, have life stages off the host and in the environment; and 2) certain compounds, such as copper and diquat, are legal pesticides but are also drugs effective against some pathogens.

FDA-approved Drugs, Indexed Drugs, Pesticides, and Regulatory Concerns

FDA-approved therapeutic options for fish are limited but increasing. The FDA Web site (www.fda.gov) is the best resource for basic information on the status of drugs and chemicals, particularly those intended for aquaculture use. In addition, the FDA has listed several compounds as being of "low regulatory concern." These compounds, although not fully approved, are considered innocuous enough for use in food fish. Of these, salt is the most important. A few compounds, including copper sulfate and potassium permanganate, are not FDA approved but are legally available for limited use in food fish as part of a supplementary FDA data collecting process as Investigational New Animal Drugs. For more information, see https://srac.tamu.edu/index.cfm/event/viewAllSheets/, specifically the link for SRAC Fact Sheet 4709 (Investigational New Animal Drug [INAD] Exemptions and the National INAD Program [NIP]). Another category is drugs on the *Index of Legally Marketed Unapproved New Animal Drugs for Minor Species* (the *Index*). Fish are considered by the FDA to be a minor species. The process of placing drugs on the *Index* involves the use of an expert panel and is intended to increase legal access to unapproved drugs intended for non-food-producing minor species (including non-food fish) and non-food early life stages of food-producing minor species (www.fda.gov). Currently, the only two fish drugs on the *Index* are Aquacalm™ (metomidate), a fish sedative/anesthetic, and Ovaprim® (GnRH + domperidone), a spawning aid also used to "spawn out" egg-bound females under some conditions. *See* TABLE 1 for a summary of the approval status and withdrawal times of drugs used in aquaculture in the USA. Practitioners are encouraged to visit the FDA Web site frequently for the most current information.

Finally, a number of compounds that are not FDA approved are used in pet fish practice under controlled conditions. These drugs have no legal status and have no place in food animal practice. A term formerly used by the FDA, "regulatory discretion," has fallen out of favor, but it does provide some explanation of the FDA's current approach to use of unapproved, non-Indexed drugs. The primary concerns are degree and magnitude of impact on human and environmental safety, and regulatory action against any illegal use will be weighed against those two measures (*see* www.fda.gov for additional guidance).

In addition to being aware of FDA concerns, fish practitioners should be familiar with environmental regulations for drugs and pesticides. Federal and state environmental regulations are of greatest importance when treating outdoor ponds.

Considerations include potential for entry of treated water into natural water bodies or the water table and potential effects to nontarget species. Compounds labeled pesticides are regulated in the USA by the EPA and therefore cannot be used under extra-label drug use provisions regulated by the FDA (ie, these compounds cannot be used in a manner beyond their specific label, which would have to include an aquatic use section).

Three FDA-approved antibiotics are currently available for use in aquacultured food fish in the USA. Some of these products can be useful in ornamental fish, especially koi; however, extra-label use of FDA-approved medicated feeds is not permitted under current law. Recognizing the need to deliver some medications in a medicated food for fish, the FDA has indicated that it would not normally consider regulatory action against a veterinarian using medicated fish food in an extra-label manner if the following criteria are met: 1) the extra-label use is for treatment of a minor species as defined by federal law; 2) in an aquatic species, the use of medicated feed in an extra-label manner is limited to products approved for use in other aquatic species; and 3) a valid veterinarian-client-patient relationship is clearly established.

Veterinarians should also be familiar with the Veterinary Feed Directive (VFD). This is of particular interest to practitioners in rural areas, who may be asked to write prescriptions for aquacultured fish. For a veterinarian to issue a VFD order, there must be a valid veterinarian-client-patient relationship, and the veterinarian must have examined the fish and identified a bacterial disease that would be treatable with the VFD drug (eg, florfenicol). Extra-label use of the VFD drug, including use for species or pathogens not indicated on the label, is prohibited by law. However, VFD drugs may be legally accessible through enrollment in the appropriate INAD (*see* above).

A small group of compounds have been designated by the FDA as "high regulatory priority," meaning their use is likely to result in enforcement action. These drugs either have human or environmental safety concerns or are related to compounds considered critical for human health and disease. The most important of these compounds are chloramphenicol, the nitrofurans, fluoroquinolones and quinolones, steroid hormones, and malachite green. These compounds should never be used in food animals for any reason, and their use in nonfood species is discouraged.

Antibiotics

Aquaflor® is an approved medicated feed containing florfenicol for use against specific pathogens in enteric septicemia (*Edwardsiella ictaluri*) in channel catfish, coldwater disease (*Flavobacterium psychrophilum*) in salmonids, furunculosis (*Aeromonas salmonicida*) in freshwater-reared salmonids, streptococcal septicemia in freshwater-reared warmwater finfish, and columnaris disease (*Flavobacterium columnare*) in freshwater-reared finfish. It is marketed as a VFD product. This broad-spectrum antibiotic has excellent efficacy against many gram-negative bacteria and gram-positive streptococci, although as a VFD drug extra-label use is forbidden. However, as discussed, for INAD data collection purposes, use may be permitted in other species and for other indications in certain situations. The withdrawal time is 15 days.

Oxytetracycline dihydrate (Terramycin® 200 for Fish) is an in-feed medication approved 1) to control mortality in freshwater-reared salmonids due to coldwater disease associated with *F psychrophilum*, 2) to control mortality in freshwater-reared rainbow trout due to columnaris disease associated with *F columnare*, and 3) to mark skeletal tissue in Pacific salmon. All approved uses require a 21-day withdrawal period for harvest-size food fish species.

Ormetoprim sulfadimethoxine (Romet-30®) is an in-feed treatment approved by the FDA to control furunculosis (*A salmonicida*) in salmonids, for which a 42-day withdrawal period is required, and to control enteric septicemia of catfish (*E ictaluri*) in channel catfish for which a 3-day withdrawal period is required. Romet-30 can be used extra-label as long as there is a veterinarian-client-patient relationship and veterinary oversight.

Hydrogen peroxide 35% (Perox-aid®) is administered by immersion and is FDA approved for use in finfish to control bacterial gill disease (caused by *F branchiophilum*) in salmonids, external columnaris (caused by *F columnare*) in freshwater-reared coolwater finfish and catfish, and fungal infection (saprolegniasis) of freshwater-reared finfish eggs. These are common external infections in fish that may follow handling or be associated with high organic load or other water quality perturbations for the affected species. Hydrogen peroxide is used as a short-term, continuous-flow bath. Treatments are administered daily or on consecutive alternate days for three

TABLE 1 DRUGS USED IN AQUACULTURE IN THE USA – APPROVAL STATUS AND WITHDRAWAL TIMES

Active Ingredient	Trade Name	Generic Use
Florfenicol	Aquaflor®	Antibiotic
Oxytetracycline dihydrate	Terramycin-200®	Antibiotic
Ormetoprim sulfadimethoxine	Romet-30®	Antibiotic
Hydrogen peroxide (35%)	PEROX-AID®	Antimicrobial (gills and skin only)
Chloramine-T	HALAMID Aqua®	Antimicrobial (gills and skin only)
Diquat	Reward®	Herbicide Antibiotic (gills and skin only)
Formalin	Formalin-F™ Formalin-B Parasite-S®	Parasiticide (gills and skin only)
Copper sulfate ($CuSO_4$)		Parasiticide (gills and skin only)
Potassium permanganate ($KMnO_4$)		Parasiticide (gills and skin only)
Diflubenzuron	Dimilin®	Parasiticide (external crustaceans)
Tricaine methanesulfonate	Tricaine-S®	Anesthetic
Eugenol	Aqui-S20E®	Anesthetic
Metomidate	Aquacalm®	Sedative
Chorionic gonadotropin	Chorulon®	Spawning aid
sGnRHa + domperidone	Ovaprim®	Spawning aid

treatments. An initial bioassay is recommended before treating a large group of fish. Paddlefish are sensitive, and use of hydrogen peroxide is not recommended. Other sensitive species include northern pike, pallid sturgeon, and in some instances, walleye. Hydrogen peroxide can be used extra-label, and experimental use has been attempted in other species and for other indications, including as a parasiticide (*see* UF/IFAS EDIS publication *Use of Hydrogen Peroxide in Finfish Aquaculture* [http://edis.ifas.ufl.edu/fa157]). There is no required withdrawal time after treatment with Perox-aid®.

Other Chemotherapeutic Drugs

Formalin: Formalin is FDA approved for use in finfish and penaeid (saltwater) shrimp. Several brands have received FDA approval for aquaculture use. Methanol may be added to formalin products as a preservative. "Pure" 100% formalin is, technically, water saturated with ~37%–40% formaldehyde gas. Formalin eliminates protistan parasites and monogeneans from the external surface of fish. It also has some efficacy against external fungal infections. It can be used as a prolonged bath at concentrations of 15–25 mg/L. The lower concentration is recommended for pond

TABLE 1 DRUGS USED IN AQUACULTURE IN THE USA – APPROVAL STATUS AND WITHDRAWAL TIMES *(continued)*

Application Method	Approval Status[a]	Withdrawal Time
Medicated feed	FDA approved[a] (Veterinary Feed Directive)	15 days
Medicated feed	FDA approved	21 days
Medicated feed	FDA approved	42 days in salmonids; 3 days in catfish
Immersion	FDA approved	None
Immersion	FDA approved	None
Immersion Immersion	EPA INAD required	5 days in channel catfish, muskellunge, tiger muskellunge, northern pike; 30 days in all others
Immersion	FDA approved	None
Immersion	INAD required	7 days
Immersion	INAD required	7 days
Immersion	EPA[a] (restricted use pesticide)	Not for use in food fish
Immersion	FDA approved	21 days
Immersion	INAD required	72 hours
Immersion	The *Index*	Not for use in food fish
Injection	FDA approved[a] (prescription only)	None (broodstock)
Injection	The *Index*	Not for use in food fish

[a]Approval status is of January 8, 2015. Practitioners should check the FDA Web site (www.fda.gov) frequently for the most current information.

use, because formalin removes dissolved oxygen from the water. Vigorous aeration during formalin treatment is essential. When treating at ≤25 mg/L, a water change is not necessary after chemical administration. At this concentration, formalin has minimal impact on biofiltration; however, if ammonia is tested using Nessler's reagent, a very high reading may be seen for several days. This is an artifact caused by the interaction of the two compounds. Use of the salicylate method to test ammonia is suggested when formalin has been used in a system. Short-term baths with formalin can be provided at concentrations up to 250 mg/L for 30 min, but a bioassay and close observation during treatment is essential because 250 mg/L may be lethal in some fish. At water temperatures >77°F (25°C), the concentration should not exceed ~170 mg/L. If adverse reaction to the chemical becomes apparent, the fish should be immediately placed in clean water. If formalin is allowed to chill to <45°F, a white precipitate, paraformaldehyde, will form. Because paraformaldehyde is highly toxic to fish, formalin should never be used if a precipitate or cloudiness is seen. Formalin is carcinogenic and potentially toxic to workers; material safety data sheets should be on hand in businesses where the chemical is used, and employees should be informed of appropriate safety precautions.

There is no required withdrawal time after treatment with formalin.

Chloramine-T: Chloramine-T (HALAMID Aqua®), a biocide and mild disinfectant, has been approved by the FDA for three indications: 1) to control mortality in freshwater-reared salmonids caused by bacterial gill disease associated with *Flavobacterium* spp, 2) to control mortality in walleye due to external columnaris disease (*F columnare*), and 3) to control mortality in freshwater-reared warmwater finfish due to external columnaris disease (*F columnare*). No withdrawal period is required before harvest.

Hypersalinity and Hyposalinity: Hypersalinity (for freshwater systems) and hyposalinity (for marine systems) are often used in aquaculture and can be effective methods for control of some parasites. Hypersalinity in freshwater typically involves use of sodium chloride, which is considered "low regulatory priority." In some instances, dilution of seawater may be used. Sodium chloride effectively mitigates nitrite toxicity (*see* AQUATIC SYSTEMS, p 1766) to reduce osmoregulatory stress in freshwater fish and to control some protistan and copepod parasite infestations. In some instances, seawater may be used. Salt is not generally practical for use in production ponds because of their large volume, except for control or prevention of nitrite toxicity, but it can be used in ornamental ponds that are not more than several thousand gallons. Salt is commonly used in recirculating aquaculture systems.

Copper Sulfate: Copper sulfate ($CuSO_4$) is currently an INAD not yet approved by the FDA; however, a number of compounds containing $CuSO_4$ have been approved by the EPA as algicides for use in aquatic sites. Technically, the chemical form of the commonly used blue crystal copper sulfate is $CuSO_4 \bullet 5H_2O$ (copper sulfate pentahydrate), but for purposes of brevity, the formula $CuSO_4$ will be used here, and this blue compound referred to as "copper sulfate."

Copper sulfate is currently designated as "of moderate regulatory concern" and is used in food fish practice. $CuSO_4$ has been used for many years as a parasiticide and is particularly useful in large production ponds because of its relatively low cost. Copper is highly toxic to fish, and safe use depends on knowing both the volume of water to be treated and the total alkalinity, as well as potential species sensitivities.

In freshwater systems, the concentration of $CuSO_4$ is considered 100% active, and application should be based on the total alkalinity (TA) of the water. If TA is <50 mg/L, copper sulfate cannot be used safely. If TA is 50–250 mg/L, a safe concentration of $CuSO_4$ can be determined by dividing the TA by 100. For example, if TA = 100 mg/L, a safe concentration of $CuSO_4$ would be 1 mg/L. If TA is >250 mg/L, the concentration of $CuSO_4$ should not exceed 2.5 mg/L. $CuSO_4$ also has algicidal activity. Rapid death of an algal bloom can precipitate catastrophic oxygen depletion. Use of $CuSO_4$ in ponds not equipped with supplemental aeration is risky. Use of $CuSO_4$ is hazardous if a pond has a heavy algal bloom (secchi disk ≤18 in.) or if the water is already deficient in oxygen because of other factors (eg, cloudy weather, heavy stocking density, or high water temperature).

Copper in marine systems, by contrast, is dosed according to level of free copper ion (Cu^{2+}). Therapeutic concentrations are based on maintaining a longterm dosage range of 0.15–0.2 mg/L of free Cu^{2+}. As discussed earlier, "blue" copper sulfate is actually $CuSO_4 \bullet 5H_2O$, so for purposes of marine systems, copper sulfate is considered 25% active ingredient (the molecular weight of free copper is ~25% of the entire compound). Because copper is toxic and because treatment periods for susceptible marine pathogens often last for ≥2–4 wk, copper should be added to a system slowly at 0.05 ppm/day to reach the target range of 0.15–0.2 mg/L over the course of 3–4 days. This allows the fish's body to acclimate and activate detoxifying pathways to reduce toxic effects. Free copper levels should be monitored daily. Copper is highly toxic to many invertebrates, and even with slow acclimation some saltwater species are still fairly sensitive. The following formula can be used to calculate the grams of copper sulfate required to treat a marine tank: volume (in gal.) × 0.0038 × desired concentration × 4 = g of $CuSO_4$.

Chelated copper compounds (copper sulfate or copper ion chelated with another chemical) have also been used in some circumstances, but caution should be used for legal reasons and when dosing for treatment. Copper can be removed from a system with water changes or by filtering water through activated carbon. Food fish must undergo a 7-day withdrawal period after treatment before harvest.

Potassium Permanganate: Potassium permanganate ($KMnO_4$) is an INAD, and $KMnO_4$ is used as an external parasiticide, fungicide, and bactericide. It is a strong oxidizing agent and "burns" organic material off the external surface of fish. Overuse, particularly multiple uses within a short period of time (more than once a week) will kill fish. The concentration of $KMnO_4$ used varies with the permanganate demand of the water. In aquaria or ornamental ponds with very clear water, a concentration of 1–2 mg/L is usually safe and effective. Permanganate demand is greater in water with a high organic load. To determine the permanganate demand, a bioassay can be performed: the water to be treated is placed in small containers, and $KMnO_4$ is added in incremental concentrations of 2 mg/L. The correct concentration for therapeutic use will be the lowest concentration that maintains a pink color for 4–8 hr. If the concentration of $KMnO_4$ required is >6 mg/L, then the organic load is excessive, and sanitation practices should be evaluated. $KMnO_4$ has little impact on biofilters when applied at ≤2 mg/L. Potassium permanganate is more toxic as salinity of the water increases, and use in marine systems is not recommended. Food fish must undergo a 7-day withdrawal period after treatment before harvest.

Diquat: Diquat (Reward®), first registered as a contact herbicide (pesticide), has been used for many years to control columnaris disease (*F columnare*) in fish. Only recently has it come under greater FDA scrutiny and become an INAD for control of *Flavobacterium* species associated with bacterial gill disease and columnaris disease. Withdrawal times for harvestable food fish species are 5 days for channel catfish, muskellunge, tiger muskellunge, and northern pike, and 30 days for all other fish species.

Diflubenzuron: Diflubenzuron (Dimilin®), a chitinase inhibitor used to control crustacean parasites, is a restricted use pesticide that can be applied only by licensed pesticide applicators. Dimilin is labeled for control of anchorworms on ornamental fish and baitfish commercially produced in ponds and tanks. Fish being raised for human consumption should not be exposed to diflubenzuron.

Anesthetics/Sedatives

Tricaine Methanesulfonate (MS-222, TMS): Tricaine methanesulfonate (approved product Tricaine-S®) is a benzocaine derivative and is the only FDA-approved fish anesthetic. TMS is approved for the temporary immobilization of fish, amphibians, and other aquatic, cold-blooded animals. In fish intended for human consumption, TMS can only be used in members of the Ictaluridae, Salmonidae, Esocidae, and Percidae, and water temperature should not exceed 10°C (50°F). Withdrawal period if used in these species is 21 days.

Eugenol: Eugenol (Aqui-S20E®, active ingredient 10% eugenol), one component of several found naturally in clove oil, is an INAD intended for use as an anesthetic/sedative. Although eugenol is not approved, it is currently allowed for use in freshwater fisheries work as a zero-withdrawal fish anesthetic. However, if used in aquaculture, the withdrawal time is 72 hr. A related compound, isoeugenol (Aqui-S®), is not allowed for use in the USA because of carcinogenicity concerns.

Metomidate: Metomidate hydrochloride (Aquacalm®) is a fish sedative on the FDA-CVM *Index of Legally Marketed Unapproved New Animal Drugs for Minor Species* (the *Index*), labeled for the sedation and anesthesia of ornamental finfish. It is not legal for use in food fish species.

Spawning Compounds

Chorionic Gonadotropin: Chorionic gonadotropin (Chorulon®) is FDA approved for use as an aid to improve spawning function in male and female brood finfish. This is the only spawning aid approved by the FDA for use in food fish species. There is no withdrawal time if used according to label instructions on broodfish. Veterinarians may work as part of a team for fish hatcheries and may be asked to help obtain spawning hormones. Chorionic gonadotropin is a prescription drug and is restricted to use by or on the order of a licensed veterinarian.

Gonadotropin-releasing Hormone (sGnRHa) + Domperidone: Salmonid GnRH analogue + domperidone (Ovaprim®) is on the *Index* and labeled for use as a spawning aid in ornamental finfish broodstock. This product cannot be used in food fish species.

INFECTIOUS DISEASES

Some fish pathogens may be more common in or adapted to a given species, genus, or family; however, many are ubiquitous and have broad host ranges. Environmental factors, including type of rearing system and production method, influence pathogen variety and prevalence within a given unit and facility. Many pathogens can infect fish regardless of rearing system and production method, but the following sections describe pathogens that may be more problematic under certain conditions.

Ponds: Most production ponds are outdoor and earthen (dirt or clay lined) and, over time, become high in organic loading as a consequence of feeding, fish growth, waste accumulation, and other related processes. In Florida, smaller ponds facilitate periodic cleaning, whereas much larger catfish ponds in the southeast are logistically much more difficult to clean. Although fish in production ponds are certainly susceptible to a wide spectrum of parasites, high organics favor sessile ciliates, including *Heteropolaria/Epistylis*, *Apiosoma*, and *Ambiphyra*, which attach to fish but feed on bacteria and other nutrients in the water column. Other protist parasites that thrive in rich, organic environments include the trichodinids (eg, *Trichodina*, *Tripartiella*), and *Tetrahymena*. *Uronema*, the marine counterpart to *Tetrahymena*, also thrives in highly organic waters.

Fish cultured in outdoor ponds are much more susceptible to infection by metazoan parasites with indirect life cycles because of the presence of final hosts and intermediate hosts that permit completion of the life cycle. These include digeneans, myxozoa, nematodes, and cestodes. The presence of birds and snails facilitate infestations by digeneans, requiring fish and snails as intermediate hosts and aquatic birds as the final host. *Bolbophorus damnificus* is an important digenean parasite of channel catfish, the final host of which is the American white pelican, and the intermediate hosts are the ram's horn snail and the fish. *Centrocestus formosanus*, another important digenean parasite infecting the gills of numerous fish species, uses a wading bird, such as the green heron or great egret, or the cone snail (*Melanoides tuberculata*) to complete its life cycle.

Oligochaetes, annelid worms, are also much more prevalent in highly organic waters. *Henneguya ictaluri*, a myxozoan parasite and the causative agent of proliferative gill disease in channel catfish, requires the oligochaete *Dero digitata* to complete its life cycle. *Eustrongylides*, a nematode parasite that infects wading birds as adults, has an indirect life cycle that may involve either an oligochaete worm and a fish or just a fish. Juvenile, pond-reared fish can be adversely affected when heavily infected with this organism. Other fish, reptiles, or amphibians may serve as paratenic hosts by feeding on infected fish and carry or transport the parasite.

Bacterial diseases, such as those caused by *Edwardsiella ictaluri* and *Streptococcus* spp, as well as viral diseases may be more difficult to control once they infect a pond population because of logistical challenges with pond disinfection.

Recirculating Aquaculture Systems: Recirculating aquaculture systems (RASs), by contrast, are situated within enclosed facilities with more limited access by potential final or intermediate hosts. Parasites with direct life cycles are more common and dangerous in an RAS, because RASs used in production tend to have greater fish densities and by definition recycle water, which results in closer fish-to-fish contact and greater buildup of parasite numbers within the system. Once a parasite infects a fish within an RAS, it becomes magnified, and disease can spread rapidly. *Ichthyophthirius multifiliis* ("ich"), *Cryptocaryon irritans* ("salt water ich"), and *Amyloodinium* (marine velvet disease) can spread rapidly within an RAS. Similarly, egg-laying monogeneans such as *Dactylogyrus* sp and *Neobenedenia* sp, the capillarid nematodes (which have direct life cycles), and microsporidia also can spread rapidly within an RAS.

Bacterial and viral diseases are also much more problematic in RASs, partly because microbial flora can be much less diverse and skewed than in more natural pond systems. Mycobacteriosis and streptococcosis have caused significant morbidity and mortality in RASs, which can favor their growth, amplification, and formation of reservoirs. Certain environmental conditions promote mycobacterial growth, including warm water temperatures, low dissolved oxygen levels, acidic pH, high soluble zinc, high fulvic acid, and high humic acid. Many of these conditions—especially the low dissolved oxygen, low pH, and an organically rich environment—are present in intensive aquaculture systems. Closed conditions and higher stocking densities enhance the potential for spread and amplification. Biofilms on the tanks, in pipework, and in filtration systems, as well as organics, inaccessible or overlooked mortalities, and detritus, can serve as reservoirs.

Net Pens/Cage Culture: Open ocean net pens, or cage culture systems within large reservoirs or lakes, have their own unique challenges. Under ideal conditions, "open" access through the net or cage structures is intended to make use of the vast surrounding water body and allow for dilution of solid and dissolved wastes. However, this "open" access also facilitates direct or indirect contact with pathogens endemic to the water body. Smaller wild fish or other organisms may directly enter and intermingle with the farmed species, or pathogens themselves may flow directly into the structure through the water or on other vectors. The higher densities found in net pens and cages can then magnify the disease through close contact and facilitate spread.

Salmonid producers, during marine grow-out phases, can have significant losses caused by sea lice and infectious salmon anemia, among others. *Neobenedenia* and other monogeneans are a major problem in warmwater marine systems. Bacterial diseases such as vibriosis are common in net pens, and emerging viral diseases, including those caused by iridoviruses (including megalocytiviruses) and betanodaviruses, are of increasing concern in marine open ocean systems because of potential for transmission from wild populations.

PARASITIC DISEASES

Protists Infecting Gills and Skin: For information on protists infecting the gills and skin of fish, *see* p 1799. Information presented here is relevant to fish reared in intensively cultured systems. As previously mentioned, trichodinids are indicators of poor sanitation and/or overcrowding. These organisms are commonly found in cultured fish, especially in systems with high stocking densities, high organic loads, and minimal (or no) in-line sanitation (eg, UV or ozone). When fish are heavily infested, losses will occur. In these cases, chemical treatment alone may not be adequate for complete control. Addressing management problems that favor infestation should be incorporated into the treatment plan. Decreasing organic material is essential for treatment efficacy, because these organisms can be protected from chemical treatment by "hiding" within organic debris.

Ambiphyra and *Apiosoma* are sessile ciliates found on the skin, gills, and fins of fish. These are common in pond-reared fish and also have a predilection for organically rich environments. They are not generally found on marine fish. In high numbers, these parasites can cause significant epithelial damage, predisposing fish to opportunistic pathogens in the environment and compromising respiration and osmoregulation. Infested fish demonstrate flashing, decreased appetite, loss of condition, and hyperplasia of infested epithelial surfaces. Severe infestation of the gills is particularly damaging. These organisms can be controlled with a single treatment of formalin, copper sulfate, potassium permanganate, or a salt dip. Excessive crowding and poor sanitation are frequently associated with heavy infestations and should be corrected.

For identification of protists affecting external surfaces of cultured fish, *see* p 1799. Control strategies are determined by the species affected and their intended use, the type of system the fish is housed in, cost of treatment, and environmental considerations.

Internal Protistan Parasites: For information on flagellated parasites (diplomonads such as *Spironucleus*, and kinetoplastids such as *Cryptobia iubilans*), *see* INTERNAL PROTISTAN PARASITES, p 1803. These parasites are also common in the GI tract of susceptible aquaculture species. The use of chemical treatment to control these organisms is not feasible in food fish; however, improvements in environmental conditions and husbandry will decrease morbidity and mortality.

Opalinids, larger "cilate-like" parasites commonly found in the GI tract, may be found occasionally in kissing gourami, discus, some catfishes, and other species. Considered commensal by some, these may or may not be associated with disease.

Internal Metazoan Parasites: Myxosporean (Myxozoa) diseases significant in aquaculture include whirling disease and proliferative kidney disease (PKD) of salmonids and proliferative gill disease ("hamburger gill disease") of channel catfish. Whirling disease is caused by *Myxobolus cerebralis*. Fish are infected as fingerlings when the parasite infects cartilage in the vertebral column and skull, resulting in visible skeletal deformities. Affected fingerlings typically show rapid tail-chasing behavior (whirling) when startled. The disease is also sometimes called "blacktail," because the peduncle and tail may darken significantly. Recovered fish remain carriers. Adults do not show behavioral signs, but skeletal deformities associated with infection do not resolve. The disease can be prevented by purchasing uninfected breeding stock and maintaining them in an environment free of the intermediate hosts (tubifex worms). A presumptive diagnosis of whirling disease is made by detection of spores from skulls of infected fish. Diagnosis may be confirmed histologically or serologically. Whirling disease is of regulatory concern in some states.

PKD is one of the most economically important diseases affecting salmonid industries of North America and Europe. Rainbow trout are particularly susceptible. PKD is caused by *Tetracapsuloides bryosalmonae*, a myxosporidian with four distinct polar capsules. It occurs most commonly in the summer when water temperatures are >12°C, and the parasite primarily infects yearling and younger fish. Clinical signs include lethargy, darkening, and fluid accumulation indicated by exophthalmos, ascites, and lateral body swelling. Infected fish are frequently anemic, resulting in gill pallor. Grossly, the posterior kidney appears gray, mottled, and significantly enlarged. Presumptive diagnosis can be based on observation of suspect organisms, 10–20 μm in diameter, in Giemsa-stained wet mounts of kidney tissue. Histologic examination of infected tissue, stained with H&E, and immunohistochemistry are required for confirmation. There is no treatment, but fish that recover from the infection are resistant to subsequent outbreaks. Infected stocks in nonendemic areas should be depopulated, the premises sanitized, and disease-free stock obtained for replacement. Avoidance is the best preventive measure.

Proliferative gill disease ("hamburger gill disease") is a myxosporean infection of channel catfish caused by *Aurantiactinomyxon ictaluri*. The organism has a complex life cycle, with the oligochaete worm *Dero digitata* serving as the intermediate host. Channel catfish may be aberrant hosts for *A ictaluri*, and the disease usually occurs in new ponds or previously infected ponds that have been drained and refilled. Although proliferative gill disease can cause catastrophic mortality approaching 100%, losses may be as low as 1%. Disease occurs at water temperatures of 16°–26°C, and mortality is exacerbated by poor water quality, particularly low dissolved oxygen or high levels of un-ionized ammonia. Gills of affected fish are severely swollen and bloody. A presumptive diagnosis can be made from a wet mount of infected tissue, in which filaments appear swollen, clubbed, and broken. Cartilaginous necrosis is strongly supportive of a diagnosis of proliferative gill disease; however, histology is required for confirmation. Quantitative PCR has also been used diagnostically.

Platyhelminthes (Flatworms): Flatworms (Platyhelminthes: monogenea, digenea, leeches, turbellaria, *see* p 1807) are also of concern in aquaculture.

Monogeneans, including gyrodactylids, dactylogyrids, ancyrocephalids, and capsalids, have all been identified in numerous aquacultured species.

Gyrodactylus salaris is a reportable disease of salmonids but has not been reported in the USA. Any gyrodactylid found on a salmonid species should be identified well enough to determine whether it is *G salaris*. *Neobenedenia* and *Benedenia* are important monogeneans in marine aquaculture.

Although treatments will vary depending on the aquaculture setting and species of parasite and fish host, formalin is approved for use in food fish. Hyposalinity for marine species, including freshwater dips, can help reduce loading on fish, but environmental reservoirs (eg, eggs) will need to be controlled as well. *Neobenedenia* was controlled in one study when salt levels were reduced to ≤15 g/L for 5 days and ≤18 g/L for 7 days. Hydrogen peroxide is not approved for use against monogenean infestations in food fish but can be used extra-label under the supervision of a veterinarian. Doses are experimental (*see Use of Hydrogen Peroxide in Finfish Aquaculture* [http://edis.ifas.ufl.edu/fa157] for some reported doses). Freshwater monogenea can be treated with formalin or saltwater dips to remove a majority of parasites from fish, but environmental stages (eg, eggs) will also require control.

Digeneans have complicated life cycles, with several larval stages that infect one or more hosts. As discussed above, fish raised in outdoor aquaculture systems are more likely to become infested by this group of parasites. With rare exceptions, the first intermediate host is a mollusc, without which the life cycle generally cannot be completed. The final host for many common freshwater aquacultured fish digenean parasites is a wading bird. A diagnosis usually can be established by gross or microscopic examinations that reveal the cercarial, metacercarial, or adult worms in any of the tissues or body cavities of the fish. Fish tend to form pigmented tissue encapsulations that encyst the parasites. Depending on the color of the cysts in the skin, the condition is called black, white, or yellow grub disease. Heavily parasitized fish often are weak, thin, inactive, and feed poorly. In many cases, low level infestations may not result in significant morbidity but will prevent sale of fish for aesthetic reasons. Treatment is not recommended.

Pond-reared, juvenile, tropical fish may develop severe gill disease from metacercarial cysts of the digenean *Centrocestus formosanus* in gill tissue. Although acute death is occasionally seen, infected fish more commonly die during harvest or shipping when they may be exposed to suboptimal dissolved oxygen concentrations. If only a small percentage of gill tissue is infested, then fish may be clinically normal. Treatment of infected fish has not been successful; however, prevention of the disease by elimination of the intermediate host, the freshwater snail *Melanoides tuberculata* (common name, the red-rimmed melania), has been effective.

Bolbophorus confusus is a digenean trematode that causes morbidity and mortality in channel catfish fingerlings in production ponds in Mississippi, Louisiana, and Alabama. The definitive host of *B confusus* is the white pelican, and the first intermediate host is the ram's horn snail (*Heliosoma* spp). Cercariae released from snails encyst in fish tissue, forming metacercariae in any tissue, but most are found in skin and skeletal muscle of the peduncle of juvenile channel catfish. Severe disease (mortality up to 95%) occurs when metacercariae encyst in visceral organs, particularly the posterior kidney and liver. Involvement of these organs can result in a presentation similar to that of enteric septicemia or channel virus disease, characterized by fluid accumulation in the abdomen and exophthalmia. Skin and muscle lesions typically result in raised bumps that are white to reddish in color. The presence of digenea in skeletal muscle can result in condemnation of affected carcasses by processing plants.

Other Vermiform Internal Parasites: **Acanthocephalids** (thorny-headed worms) are common in wild fish as both larval tissue stages and adult intestinal parasites. They are most common in salmonid and marine fish. Arthropods are the first intermediate host. Adult acanthocephala are easily recognized by their protrusible proboscis, armed with many recurrent hooks.

Pentastomids, which may present as either "white grub"–like lesions externally or within the body cavity in numerous organs, have been identified in aquacultured aquarium fish species, including swordtails. Fish are infected with the larval or "nymph" stage, and the final hosts are aquatic reptiles (turtles, snakes, alligators). Under the microscope, pentastome nymphs appear as thick, stout, curved, and "segmented" worms (*see Pentastomid Infections in Fish* [http://edis.ifas.ufl.edu/fa090]). Fish often show no behavioral changes and may have minimal morbidity or mortality, but fish cannot be sold for aesthetic reasons. Treatment is not recommended, but management involves removal of final hosts from the system.

Crustacean Parasites: Crustacean parasites, including *Argulus*, *Lernaea*, and *Lepeophtheirius*, can become significant problems in aquaculture (*see* p 1808). Treatment of these organisms is not feasible for food fish species.

BACTERIAL DISEASES

Common Bacterial Pathogens (*Aeromonas, Vibrio,* and *Edwardsiella*): Common bacterial pathogens (*see* p 1808), *Aeromonas hydrophila*, *A salmonicida*, *Vibrio* spp, *Edwardsiella ictaluri*, *E tarda*, *Streptococcus* spp, and other related gram-positive cocci, can also infect aquaculture species. Organisms that may have previously been identified as *E tarda* have now been recognized as new organisms with biochemical characteristics very similar to those of *E tarda*. Two new groups are also recognized, *E piscicida* and *E piscicida*–like bacteria, which have been associated with disease in channel catfish and freshwater game fish (*see* below). Treatments for food fish species are limited to the species and disease indicated on the label of approved drugs, although approved forms of oxytetracycline and Romet® can be used extra-label under the supervision of a veterinarian. Florfenicol (Aquaflor®) is the only drug approved for use against streptococcal infections in freshwater-reared, warmwater finfish; however, extra-label use of this product is prohibited. Enrollment in an INAD program may allow limited use of florfenicol for indications and species beyond the current label. *See* https://srac.tamu.edu/index.cfm/event/viewAllSheets/, SRAC 4709 (Investigational New Animal Drug [INAD] Exemptions and the National INAD Program [NIP]). Appropriate withdrawal periods before harvest must be followed when used in food fish species (*see* TABLE 1, p 1750). Vaccines are available for a number of bacterial pathogens and species indications. Under supervision by a veterinarian, licensed commercial vaccines can be used off-label (*see Use of Vaccines in Finfish Aquaculture* [http://edis.ifas.ufl.edu/pdffiles/fa/fa15600.pdf]).

Yersiniosis: Yersiniosis (enteric redmouth disease) is a serious acute or chronic bacterial disease of intensively cultured salmonids. The etiologic agent is *Yersinia ruckeri*. Signs are darkening and hemorrhage of the mouth (red mouth), skin, anus, and fins. Chronic signs are associated with inappetence, exophthalmos, swelling, and degenerative changes of internal organs. Mortality rates are variable but are exacerbated by poor water quality and related stressors. Diagnosis is by isolation and identification of pure cultures of the organism obtained from the internal organs of infected fish. Fish that survive remain carriers and may cyclically shed bacteria, particularly when exposed to stressful conditions and water temperatures of 15°–18°C. Depopulation of infected fish and avoidance of introduction of infected fish can be recommended, but preventive vaccination is the usual procedure in endemic areas. Yersiniosis can be treated successfully with antibiotics, which should be selected based on a sensitivity test. Therapy should be continued for at least 14 days.

***Edwardsiella piscicida* and *E piscicida*–like Diseases:** *Edwardsiella ictaluri* causes **enteric septicemia of catfish**, the most important infectious disease in the channel catfish industry. Infection occurs in the spring and fall when water temperatures are 22°–28°C, and mortality may be exacerbated by handling stress, chemical treatment, or poor water quality. The disease occurs in two forms: the enteric (or intestinal) form and the meningeal form. In the enteric form, infected fish may develop skin lesions characterized by massive petechial hemorrhage around the mouth, operculum, and eyes, or they may develop measles-like, red, punctate lesions along the body wall. There is a hemorrhagic enteritis, and the intestine may be hemorrhagic and fluid- or gas-filled. Liver lesions are common and may be evident as multifocal areas of necrosis, abcessation, or hemorrhage. In contrast, in the meningeal form, few external signs may be seen in infected fish. The bacteria enter the CNS through the olfactory system, and affected fish develop severe meningitis. In fingerlings, the inflammation may be severe enough to erode the skull, resulting in the characteristic "hole-in-the-head" lesion. Fish affected with the meningeal form may demonstrate bizarre behavior, including spinning, erratic swimming, and general disorientation. Diagnosis is based on bacterial culture and isolation. Brain culture is indicated whenever *E ictaluri* is suspected. *E ictaluri* will grow on blood agar incubated at 25°C for 48 hr. Antibiotic therapy should be based on results of sensitivity testing. Vaccination is available for channel catfish fingerlings.

There has been a significant change in understanding of fish diseases caused by an organism historically identified as *E tarda*. This organism is the causative agent of **emphasematous putrifactive disease of catfish**. The name is descriptive of the most common lesions, an ulcerative dermatitis associated with a malodorous, gas-producing bacteria. *E tarda* is an enteric bacterium that is ubiquitous in terrestrial and aquatic environments. It has been associated with enteric disease in mammals, including people, as well as birds, reptiles, and fish. Recent molecular work has demonstrated that several different organisms that may have been previously identified as *E tarda* are likely causing many of the disease outbreaks attributed to *E tarda* in fish. These newly recognized taxa, *E piscicida* and *E piscicida*–like organisms, are considered important emerging diseases in the channel catfish industry. They can present not only as an ulcerative dermatitis but also can cause a systemic granulomatous disease with gross and microscopic lesions very similar to those seen in mycobacteriosis (*see* p 1760). Granulomatous disease attributed to *E piscicida* tends to result in hepatic lesions, which are not typical of mycobacteriosis. Histologically, the granulomas contain gram-negative and acid-fast negative rods. Molecular testing is required to confirm a diagnosis of *E piscicida* or *E piscicida*–like infection. The disease will respond to antibiotics, but it is unclear whether fish can clear bacteria sequestered in granulomas. These environmental bacteria thrive in organically rich environments, so sanitation may need to be addressed as part of the management strategy. For aquariums and recirculating systems, UV filtration may help decrease numbers of bacteria in the environment.

Columnaris and Related Diseases: The taxonomic grouping of bacteria causing columnaris disease, coldwater disease, and bacterial gill disease has undergone significant revision in recent years based on genomic studies. The primary causative agent of each of these important diseases has been moved into the genus *Flavobacterium*, although other genera have also been implicated. These gram-negative, rod or filamentous bacteria have a distinctive gliding motion. Skin or gill lesions have slimy or cotton-like surface exudates, which usually cover surface necrosis, ulcerations, and marginal hemorrhages.

Flavobacterium columnare, the most prominent member of this group responsible for **columnaris disease**, is most common in warmwater species of fish. A presumptive diagnosis can be made from visualization of typical organisms on wet mounts of infected skin or gill tissue. Columnaris disease can be confirmed by isolation of the organism on Ordal's or other cytophaga media. Sensitivity tests are difficult to perform, because *F columnare* will not grow on Müller-Hinton media. If the disease is diagnosed early in the course of infection, treatment with potassium permanganate or hydrogen peroxide may be effective. If the disease becomes chronic, it may have become systemic, in which case treatment with florfenicol or oxytetracycline is recommended. Columnaris disease can be prevented by reducing organic loading and avoiding traumatic injuries. A vaccine is currently available in the USA for use in channel catfish and largemouth bass.

A similar organism affecting marine fish was previously grouped with *F columnare* but has been given its own genus and is now named *Tenacibaculum maritimum*. Potassium permanganate may not be a good option in warmwater marine finfish because of its increased toxicity at higher salinities.

Flavobacterium psychrophilum causes **coldwater (peduncle) disease**, or bacterial coldwater disease, in salmonids and other coldwater species. Rarely, warmwater fish exposed to cold temperatures may be affected. Disease is most severe at water temperatures of 4°–10°C, and signs should not be seen at temperatures >18°C. Skin lesions usually begin on the dorsal and posterior surfaces of the fish but may be found on any part of the body. Advanced cases show necrosis and ulceration of the peduncle, and underlying musculature will be exposed. As the disease progresses, the infection becomes systemic, typically involving the spleen, kidney, and liver. Confirmed diagnosis is possible after isolation of *F psychrophilum* using cytophage media (15°–20°C for 3–6 days), or by immunohistochemistry or PCR. Outbreaks can be controlled with oxytetracycline.

Bacterial gill disease, caused by *F branchiophilum*, is most frequently reported in young cultured salmonids or fish cultured under conditions of high organic loading. It has been seen occasionally in aquarium fish. It may be initiated by crowding and poor water quality, particularly high organic loads, high ammonia levels, and silt. Gills appear swollen and mottled, with patchy areas of bacterial growth that can be confirmed by microscopic examination of direct gill smears. Hyperplasia, adhesions, and deformity of the gill lamellae can be seen. In young fish affected with the disease, mortality is high and morbidity sustained. Prevention efforts include improving water quality and avoiding overstocking. A single treatment with potassium permanganate, followed by addition of salt to the system (2–5 ppt) may help control losses, but sanitation is critical for longterm resolution of the problem. Antibiotic therapy may be used as needed to control secondary bacterial problems.

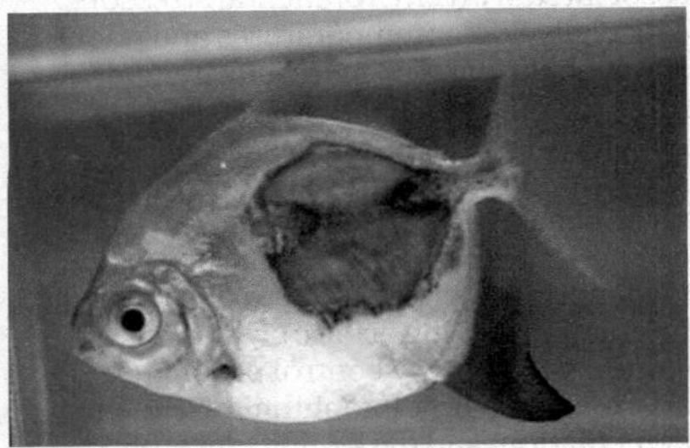

Erosion typical of columnaris disease in a silver dollar. *Courtesy of Dr. Ruth Francis-Floyd.*

Bacterial Kidney Disease: Bacterial kidney disease is economically important in cultured salmonids. The cause is *Renibacterium salmoninarum*, an obligate intracellular bacteria that is one of the relatively few gram-positive organisms that causes disease in fish. Bacterial kidney disease is a chronic disease affecting juveniles (6–12 mo old) and prespawning adults, with clinical signs very similar to those of mycobacteriosis. Clinically, infected fish appear lethargic and darkened and may have coelomic distention, pale gills (anemia), and vent hemorrhages. Typical lesions include grayish, localized, or conglomerate granulomata in the viscera, especially the kidney or body wall; exophthalmos; blindness; cystic cavities in musculature; and emaciation. A presumptive diagnosis can be based on visualization of small, gram-positive rods in kidney imprints. Definitive diagnosis requires isolation and identification of the bacteria by using a selective medium that contains cysteine and incubating at 15°C for 3–6 wk. *R salmoninarum* is transmitted both horizontally and vertically, and fish that survive an epizootic remain carriers. Infected female fish should be injected with erythromycin (11–20 mg/kg, IM) 14–60 days before spawning to prevent vertical transmission. Erythromycin (100 mg/kg for 10–21 days) is effective when administered in feed early in the course of an outbreak; however, it is not FDA approved for this use. Obtaining disease-free stock and preventing contamination by infected wild fish are the best preventive measures.

Mycobacteriosis: Mycobacteriosis (*see also* p 1810) is an important disease in aquaculture because of its typically chronic nature (although acute and subacute presentations can occur) and the lack of effective antibiotics. External or internal masses, nodules, or granulomas are a common presentation in aquaculture species. Important differential diagnoses for a suspect case of mycobacteriosis, based on identification of granulomas in tissue, are *Edwardsiella piscicida* (*see* p 1758) and francisellosis (*see* below). Further, although granulomatous lesions are typical of mycobacteriosis, they are not always seen. In some species, and under some conditions, granulomas may not be present. Instead, caseous ("pus-like") lesions may be seen, or histologically, only a histiocytic inflammatory response (increased macrophages/tissue phagocytes without granuloma formation) may be apparent. Acid-fast stains and/or culture are necessary to exclude mycobacteriosis in cases with chronic morbidity/mortality and chronic inflammation but no granulomas. In addition, processing differences (including the decalcification method, if necessary, and the type of acid-fast stain used) may affect staining characteristics of mycobacteria.

Rickettsia and Rickettsial-like Diseases: Rickettsial disease associated with *Piscirickettsia salmonis* has been described in salmonid species from Chile, Norway, Ireland, and Canada. Rickettsial-like organisms have been reported in tilapia, sea bass, and blue-eyed plecostomus. Rickettsial disease can result in acute mortality, affecting up to 95% of fish with few gross signs. In tilapia, acute mortality may be triggered by sudden drops in temperature. Chronic disease is manifest by nonspecific external lesions, including anorexia, pale gills, and skin lesions. Internally, lesions are more typical, with granulomatous lesions possible throughout the viscera. The most characteristic lesions may be found in liver and kidney tissue and appear as gray to yellow mottled areas with ring-shaped foci. Visceral lesions are grossly similar to those seen in advanced cases of mycobacteriosis, and differentiation is important. Histologically, intracellular organisms may be seen in macrophages and hematopoietic tissue in the liver, spleen, and kidney. Blood or tissue smears stained with Giemsa or acridine orange may reveal the intracellular organisms, often appearing as paired, curved, gram-negative rods in macrophages or hepatocytes. *Rickettsia*-like organisms can be isolated using a variety of cell lines; however, confirmation of a suspect case may also be based on serology.

Transmission of rickettsial-like diseases in fish is not understood. In terrestrial species, a vector is often required; however, *R salmonis* has been demonstrated to survive for 14 days in seawater, suggesting that horizontal transmission in the absence of vectors may be possible in aquatic species. Oxytetracycline is the treatment of choice, although it is unclear whether an advanced case can be completely resolved with antibiotic treatment. *Rickettsia*-like organisms do not appear to be a zoonotic threat, because they do not seem able to survive at mammalian body temperatures.

Francisellosis: Francisellosis, an important emerging bacterial disease caused by *Francisella noatunensis*, has been identified as the primary cause of disease in a variety of aquacultured and wild-caught species, including tilapia, hybrid striped bass, Atlantic cod, Atlantic salmon, various grunt species, ornamental cichlids, fairy wrasses, and blue-green damselfish. In tilapia, francisellosis is often associated with environmental stressors, especially cooler temperatures and poor water quality, and so increasing temperatures (for indoor facilities) may help mitigate the disease. Many signs and necropsy findings are grossly similar to those seen in mycobacteriosis. The disease can be acute, with few clinical signs and high mortality, or subacute to chronic, with fish demonstrating erratic swimming, spiraling, buoyancy control problems, anorexia, lethargy, exophthalmia, anemia, petechiation, and darkening. Severely infected fish may have necrotic or nodular gills with red and white patchiness, and histologically, portions of the gill may also be severely hyperplastic with consolidation of secondary lamellae. On necropsy, the spleen and kidney typically have a granular or nodular (granulomatous) appearance, and most other organs can also be affected. Francisellosis should be another differential diagnosis for granulomatous disease in fish. Identification is supported by history, clinical signs, species affected, and presence of non-acid-fast bacterial organisms that are Giemsa positive and weakly gram negative. Because *Francisella* does not grow on routinely used media (such as blood agar), confirmation requires PCR of affected tissue and/or culture on various special media, all of which include increased levels of cysteine (or cystine) and glucose. Culture and sensitivity should be performed by a microbiologist and laboratory with expertise in this pathogen for identification and to determine sensitivity patterns. Because *Francisella* is intracellular and causes granulomatous disease, chemotherapy may be less effective, unless the disease outbreak is identified very early in its course. Optimization of husbandry, including increasing temperatures when possible, may help reduce morbidity and mortality.

MYCOTIC DISEASES

The "fungi" and "fungi-like organisms" (*see* p 1811) can affect aquacultured species. A number of these pathogens, previously lumped together as "fungi" based on similarity in morphology and saprophytic lifestyle, are unrelated taxonomically. The more common "water molds," including *Saprolegnia* and *Aphanomyces*, are not true fungi but members of the Oomycota (Oomycetes). This distinction is important, because a more precise understanding of the biology of each group should lead to more targeted, effective management and chemotherapy.

Another true pigmented fungus, *Veronaea botryosa*, has been identified and described as the cause of a phaeohyphomycosis in aquacultured white sturgeon and Siberian sturgeon. Affected fish had one or more of the following clinical signs: abnormal orientation, buoyancy control problems, coelomic distention, reddening of the skin, emaciation, and ulceration of the skin or eye. Internal pathology included hemorrhages throughout the coelom, the presence of serosanguineous fluid, and organomegaly with nodules or cysts in multiple organs. Wet mounts of affected tissues often revealed presence of fungal hyphae, and positive confirmation was based on culture characteristics and identification by PCR. The disease appears to be linked to environmental stressors that may include temperature.

In general, systemic fungal infections in aquacultured species do not respond well to treatments. External infections of *Saprolegnia* may require environmental/handling modifications in addition to chemotherapy. For food fish use, specific commercial formalin and hydrogen peroxide products are FDA approved for use against fungus on fish eggs. Use of these products on other life stages is extra-label and requires veterinary oversight.

Mycotoxins: *See also* p 1811. As in other species, mycotoxin contamination of feeds is associated with disease in aquaculture species. Specifically, exposure to aflatoxin-contaminated feed causes serious disease in rainbow trout. Aflatoxin is produced by fungi in the genus *Aspergillus* and is commonly associated with use of oil-seed crops such as corn, cottonseed meal, and peanuts. Toxin production may be associated with improper storage, with high humidity (>14%) and high temperatures (>27°C) being significant risk factors. Affected trout may have a grossly distended abdomen, and necropsy findings reveal a hepatoma or hepatic carcinoma. Liver lesions have been reported after exposure to concentrations as little as 1 mg/kg. Disease has been induced experimentally in tilapia at higher concentrations and/or extended exposure periods. In one study, tilapia fed 10 mg/kg for 8 wk had liver pathology and when fed 100 mg/kg for 8 wk, hepatic necrosis and mortalities were seen. In another study, tilapia fed 0.245 mg/kg over the course of 20 wk demonstrated reduced growth and liver pathology. Presence of the toxin can be confirmed using high-performance liquid chromatography (HPLC) or ELISA. Commercial test kits are also available.

VIRAL DISEASES

The identification and characterization of previously undescribed viral diseases in aquaculture is increasing because of recent technologic advances and increasing expertise in the aquatic veterinary field. Viruses (*see* p 1812) may also affect susceptible species in aquaculture settings. Again, management options are limited but vary depending on the type and pathogenicity of the virus, species susceptibility, reportability, and whether the virus is considered endemic or exotic. In general, no approved or effective treatments exist for viral diseases in aquaculture species. Temperature manipulations are problematic, especially because of concerns over latency and potential recrudescence. Vaccine development for economically important viruses is ongoing, and some vaccines exist for some viruses either in the USA or internationally. Additional viruses of importance to aquaculture are described below.

Herpesviruses (Alloherpesviruses)

Herpesviruses (alloherpesviruses) are also important pathogens in aquaculture (*see also* p 1812). Herpesviruses have been identified in a number of different aquacultured species, including cyprinids and various cichlid species.

Channel Catfish Virus Disease: Channel catfish virus (CCV) disease is an acute, virulent herpesvirus infection of fry and fingerling channel catfish that can cause mortality of >80% at water temperatures ≥25°C in small fish (≤5 cm). As fish age, mortality decreases, and clinical infection in fish >1 yr old is rare. Acute infection often includes a recent history of a stressful event such as handling or transport, low dissolved oxygen, or chemical treatment. Infected fish show signs of ascites, exophthalmos, and hemorrhages in fins. The cell line of choice for virus isolation is channel catfish ovary, followed by serum neutralization to confirm identification. Typical cytopathic effects include cell fusion, syncytia formation, and intranuclear inclusions. There is evidence for vertical transmission of CCV; consequently, survivors of an epizootic should not be used for broodstock. Although CCV can cause severe mortality when an outbreak is in progress, the annual number of cases of CCV in the catfish industry is relatively low.

Novirhabdoviruses

Infectious Hematopoietic Necrosis: Caused by a novirhabdovirus in the family Rhabdoviridae, infectious hematopoietic necrosis is listed as an OIE notifiable disease. It is endemic in salmonid (*Oncorhynchus* spp) populations in the Pacific Northwest and Alaska and has been reported in Atlantic, chum, chinook, sockeye, and kokanee salmon and in cutthroat, steelhead, and rainbow trout. Lake trout and Arctic char, members of the genus *Salvelinus*, appear resistant. The disease has also been reported in parts of Europe and Asia. Most epizootics have been attributed to importation of infected eggs or fry.

Acute disease in fry <2 mo old may result in high mortality (>90%) with few external signs. Disease usually occurs at water temperatures of 10°–12°C, although outbreaks occasionally occur at temperatures >15°C. Typical signs include lethargy with sporadic hyperexcitability, including whirling. Sick fish may be darkened with distended abdomens, exophthalmia, pale gills, and mucoid fecal casts. Important differential diagnoses include infectious pancreatic necrosis and viral hemorrhagic septicemia. Hematopoietic tissue in the kidney and spleen are most severely affected by necrosis.

Risk factors include age (fish <2 mo old are more susceptible), density, and water temperature. Hauling young fish around dams in trucks may be a significant risk factor because of crowding during transit. Although most disease outbreaks have been reported in freshwater, active disease has occurred in Atlantic salmon housed in sea cages. Diagnosis is by viral isolation (from kidney and spleen of young fish and ovarian fluid of broodstock), with confirmation by serum neutralization. Rapid serologic tests are becoming more available. A nonlethal test involving viral isolation from mucus has been reported. The disease is transmitted horizontally through the water, and vertical transmission is suspected. Asymptomatic carrier fish serve as reservoirs of infection. A vaccine is available in the USA for use against this pathogen.

Viral Hemorrhagic Septicemia: Viral hemorrhagic septicemia (VHS) is caused by a novirhabdovirus in the family Rhabdoviridae and is a highly regulated disease in the USA. VHS can be divided into several different strains based on genotype: VHS strain IVa is the predominant strain in USA aquaculture; strain IVb (*see* below) has been identified in wild stocks only in the USA and Canada; and strains I, II, and III are found primarily in Europe and Asia. The disease causes marked necrosis of hematopoietic tissue in the kidney, particularly the anterior kidney, but largely spares excretory tubules in the posterior kidney. Rainbow, brook, and lake trout (genus *Salvelinus*) and Atlantic salmon and brown and golden trout (genus *Salmo*) are susceptible. The virus also causes disease in a variety of freshwater and marine coldwater fish, including pike, turbot, white fish, and sea bass. VHS also is found in free-ranging marine fish in the Pacific northwest, including anadromous salmon (coho and chinook), as well as haddock and cod in the North Sea.

The disease occurs in three forms: acute, chronic, and nervous. Acute mortalities occur in rainbow trout fry <3 g and <30 days old. In these fish, the kidney is swollen and the anterior segment is necrotic and pale. The liver may be pale with hemorrhagic mottling, and systemic hemorrhage may be visible in the eyes, skin, skeletal muscle, and viscera. The most notable lesion is widespread hemorrhage in the liver, adipose tissue, and within skeletal muscle. Moribund fish lie on the bottom of the tank and may exhibit sporadic flashing and corkscrew swimming behavior. As fish age, mortalities drop from 80%–100% to 10%–50%. The chronic form is a persistent infection with low RBC and WBC counts; virus can be isolated from all tissues. Chronically infected fish may exhibit few visible external signs. The nervous form of the disease has been reported primarily in cultured freshwater fish but has also been reported in marine fish.

The optimal temperature for active infection is 9°–12°C; the virus is unable to replicate at temperatures >15°C. The cell line of choice for virus isolation is bluegill fry (BF-2). Viral identification is confirmed by serum neutralization. Newer diagnostic tests include immunofluorescence, ELISA, and PCR. VHS is a highly regulated disease, with disease-free geographic regions defined in Europe. No vaccine is commercially available. Veterinarians working with zoologic collections must ensure that susceptible species received from endemic areas are properly tested and certified disease free.

In 2005, a new strain of VHS, VHS IVb, was identified in the Great Lakes and caused widespread morbidity and mortality of only wild stocks. Affected species included muskellunge, Chinook salmon, brown trout, freshwater drum, black crappie, bluntnose minnow, gizzard shad, largemouth bass, smallmouth bass, blue gill, yellow perch, and channel catfish. Signs of VHS IVb can be nonspecific. Some affected fish have no clinical signs, but exophthalmia, ascites, hemorrhages (in the eyes, skin, gills, fin base), and behavioral changes may be seen.

To date, no aquacultured specimens have been found to be infected with this strain, but veterinarians should be aware of it and avoid introducing stocks or water from infected/unprotected systems.

Iridoviruses

Viral Erythrocytic Necrosis: Viral erythrocytic necrosis has been reported in >20 species of marine and anadromous fish (both cultured and free ranging) and is characterized by erythrocytic degeneration. Affected species include Pacific herring, Atlantic cod, and Pacific salmonids (chum, pink, coho, and Chinook), steelhead trout, and cultured eels in Taiwan. The disease is chronic, and external signs may be subtle or nonexistent. Sick fish are anemic, which may result in pale gills and internal organs. Severity of the disease is related to age and species of fish, with juveniles <1 g most severely affected.

The characteristic lesion is a single eosinophilic cytoplasmic inclusion body in the circulating erythrocytes of anemic fish. The inclusions are best visualized from Giemsa-stained fresh blood smears. To date, the agent has not been successfully isolated. Histologically, increased hematopoietic activity may be evident in the kidney, and round cytoplasmic inclusions (0.8–4 μm) are found in circulating RBCs. Inclusions stain pink or magenta with Giemsa. Other degenerative changes may be evident in RBCs, including cytoplasmic vacuolation and margination of nuclear chromatin. Hemolytic anemia with concurrent hemosiderosis and erythroblastosis has been reported in moribund Pacific herring. Multinucleated giant erythroblasts may occasionally be seen in peripheral blood, and macrophages may phagocytize abnormal erythroblasts. A presumptive diagnosis is based on the presence of typical cytoplasmic inclusions in circulating RBCs of anemic fish. Confirmation requires visualization of hexagonal virus particles in cytoplasm of affected RBCs using transmission electron microscopy. A marine reservoir is suspected but has not been identified. Vertical transmission is suspected because of the high prevalence of infection in fry from infected broodstock.

Epizootic Hematopoietic Necrosis: The ranaviruses are an important group within the family Iridoviridae and, as a group, include viruses that can infect fish, amphibians, and reptiles. One of these causes epizootic hematopoietic necrosis (EHN), which so far has been reported to cause disease only in fish and is listed as a notifiable disease by OIE. First reported in redfin perch in Australia in the spring of 1984, it has since been shown to cause disease, albeit less severe, in rainbow trout. Similar viruses have been reported in sheatfish in Germany and black bullhead catfish in France and Italy.

EHN is endotheliotropic, producing necrotic lesions in the endothelium of blood vessels and some visceral lesions. Behavioral signs include lethargy, darkening, and erratic swimming. Mortality occurs after 4–5 days. The most consistent lesion associated with EHN is focal necrosis of hematopoietic tissue in the anterior kidney and liver. Necrotic hematopoietic cells may be visible within blood vessels. Presumptive diagnosis is based on clinical signs and isolation of the suspect agent in cell culture. Bluegill fry (BF-2) is the cell line of choice. Detection may also be accomplished using ELISA, immunofluorescence, or electron microscopy. Epizootics of EHN in redfin perch are most common in the spring and summer and almost exclusively involve juvenile fish. Survivors seem to be resistant to future infection. There is no evidence of vertical transmission of EHN, and redfin perch carriers have not been detected. An unidentified reservoir and carrier host is suspected. Fomite transmission of EHN has been demonstrated, and birds have also been shown to carry infected material.

Largemouth Bass Virus: This ranavirus was isolated from moribund largemouth bass in South Carolina in 1995. It was previously isolated from largemouth bass in several Florida lakes but had not been directly associated with disease. It has been found in largemouth bass in most southeastern and many midwestern states. The disease is not well understood, because the virus is commonly isolated from tissues of clinically normal fish. In the 1995 fish kill, ~1,000 fish died over a 2- to 3-mo period in an area that encompassed >66,000 hectares. Lesions were nonspecific and are still poorly described. Fat-head minnow (FHM) is the cell line of choice for isolation of virus.

Megalocytiviruses: The megalocytiviruses are another very important and emerging group of viruses within the family Iridoviridae (*see* MEGALOCYTIVIRUSES, p 1814). They have been associated with disease in freshwater angelfish and gourami species, as well as in numerous other aquacultured freshwater and marine food and aquarium fishes, including oscars and other cichlids (family Cichlidae), swordtails, sailfin mollies, and other common live-bearers (family Poeciliidae), and Banggai cardinalfish. Numerous marine and freshwater food and game finfish species are also naturally susceptible to infection by megalocytiviruses, including jacks and pompanos (several species, family Carangidae), mackerels and tuna (several species, family Scombridae), grouper (several species, family Serranidae), cobia (*Rachycentron canadum*), largemouth bass (*Micropterus salmoides*), barramundi (*Lates calcarifer*), redfish (*Sciaenops ocellatus*), hybrid striped bass (*Morone saxatilis* × *M chrysops*), and gray mullet (*Mugil cephalus*).

Clinical signs are nonspecific but include lethargy, anorexia, darkening, abnormal swimming (including spinning) or position in the water, increased respiration, coelomic distention, ulceration, hemorrhages/petechiae, pale gills/anemia, fin erosion, white feces, and moderate to heavy mortalities. Higher temperatures may be associated with some outbreaks.

Diagnosis is based on clinical signs, history, histopathology, and PCR identification (many of these viruses have not been successfully cultured). Histopathology often includes areas of acute, diffuse, severe coagulative necrosis in some tissues, and/or variable amounts of necrosis and mild inflammation. Large, finely granular basophilic to amphophilic intracytoplasmic inclusions are most commonly identified in spleen and kidney, although in severe infections, liver, heart, oral cavity, thymus, bone, gills, skeletal muscle, submucosa of the GI tract, and gonads are also affected.

There is currently no treatment for megalocytiviruses other than depopulation. A vaccine is available internationally but not yet available in the USA.

Other Viruses

Infectious Salmon Anemia: Infectious salmon anemia is reportable to USDA-APHIS and the OIE. The first report was from farmed Atlantic salmon on the west coast of Norway in 1984. Affected fish were lethargic and severely anemic (PCV <5% in moribund fish). The causative agent is an orthomyxovirus. Acute outbreaks result in high mortality. Initial signs include lethargic fish hanging around the edges of the cage. As the disease progresses, moribund fish lie on the bottom.

Diagnosis is based on clinical signs, with emphasis on anemia (PCV <10%), the gross appearance of a dark liver, and hepatic necrosis. Confirmation can be by viral isolation using the SHK-1 cell line. Virus may be visualized in endothelial cells of cardiac blood vessels using transmission electron microscopy. The agent is enveloped, slightly pleomorphic, and ~100 nm in size. Suspected cases can also be verified using an immunofluorescent antibody technique on frozen tissue. Transmission is horizontal, and virus is shed in skin, mucus, feces, and urine. Sea lice (*Lepeophtheirus salmonis*) may be a vector; disease outbreaks seem worse when sea lice are present. There is no evidence of vertical transmission. Sea trout have been proposed as a possible reservoir of infection. Protective immunity has been demonstrated in salmon that survive an outbreak. Vaccines are available internationally but may not confer complete protection. The disease is heavily regulated in Norway and now in the USA, where the USDA should be notified immediately of any suspected cases.

Infectious Pancreatic Necrosis: Infectious pancreatic necrosis is an acute, systemic, contagious disease of salmonid fry and fingerlings caused by a birnavirus. The virus is the archetype of the aquatic birnaviruses, which are further subdivided into two serotypes, A and B, that do not cross-react using serum neutralization. The serotype B group currently consists of only 10 isolates, all European in origin. In contrast, the A serotype contains >200 isolates that have been further subdivided into 9 serotypes, A1–A9. Morbidity and mortality occur only in young animals, usually <3 g; however, virus can be isolated from survivors for the duration of their lives, resulting in a persistent carrier state. Recrudescence of disease in survivors has not been reported. The virus is vertically and horizontally transmitted, widespread, and reported worldwide, except in Iceland and Australia. Rainbow trout are highly susceptible to disease. In the USA, striped bass and their hybrids are recognized as potential carriers. Other species affected include freshwater eels (*Anguilla* spp), yellowtail, turbot, sea bass, and menhaden, as well as aquatic invertebrates including molluscs and crustaceans. Brook trout are believed to be reservoirs of infection in the USA.

Clinical infection is nonspecific. Diseased fish may be anorectic, ataxic, and display a corkscrew swimming pattern. Externally, fish are darkened; exophthalmia and external petechiation may be evident. Internally, petechiae may be visible on viscera; the gut is typically empty and may contain a yellow exudate. Fecal pseudocysts may be evident in the water column. Histologically, focal areas of coagulative necrosis involve acinar and islet cells of the pancreas and hematopoietic cells of the kidney. Intracytoplasmic viral inclusions may be visible in pancreatic acinar cells. Infection should be confirmed with viral isolation followed by serum neutralization. Most fish cell lines are susceptible. The virus can also be identified using fluorescent antibody, complement fixation, and ELISA techniques. There is no treatment for infected fish, but avoidance can be accomplished by purchase of SPF stocks, quarantine, and disinfection of eggs with iodophores (20–50 mg/L). Infectious pancreatic necrosis is not regulated by the USDA, but state regulations exist in various parts of the country.

Salmonid Alphaviruses: Salmonid alphaviruses are the cause of pancreas disease and sleeping disease in Atlantic salmon, rainbow trout, and brown trout. To date, reports have been from Norway and parts of the UK, although farmed fish in other countries in Europe have also been affected. This suite of diseases and the etiologic agent are reportable to USDA-APHIS and the OIE, and this disease is considered a foreign disease to the USA. As the disease names suggest, pathology involves necrosis and loss of exocrine pancreatic tissue, as well as changes in heart and skeletal muscle. Mortality rates vary from minimal to >50% in severe cases. As a sequela, a percentage of surviving fish may become slender and long runts. Survivors may also become carriers; however, vertical transmission is still under debate, and horizontal transmission is considered the main route of infection. A vaccine is available in affected countries.

Viral Nervous Necrosis (Betanodaviruses): The betanodaviruses are an emerging group of viruses infecting >40 different species of primarily marine fish worldwide. Susceptible species include red drum, cobia, barramundi, tuna, groupers, flatfishes, surgeonfishes, lemonpeel angelfish, the orbicularis batfish, and tilapia. The resulting disease is also known as viral nervous necrosis (VNN) and viral encephalopathy and retinopathy. A few freshwater species have also been reported as susceptible. Betanodaviruses can infect tropical, subtropical, or cold-temperate species, with species susceptibilities and optimal temperature ranges varying depending on the strain of the virus. Four different genotypes are currently recognized, and VNN is reportable to USDA-APHIS and the OIE. As a group, betanodaviruses can infect fish at temperatures ranging from approximately 15°–30°C.

Younger life stages (larvae, fry, fingerlings) are more frequently affected, although older, market-size fish may become affected. Losses can range from 15%–100%. Betanodaviruses are somewhat unique in that, as the disease name suggests, their target tissue is the CNS.

Consequently, clinical signs include abnormal swimming or spinning, vertical position in the water, flexing of the body, muscular tremors, and darkening or lightening of the skin. Hyperinflation of the swim bladder is also often seen, with affected fish positively buoyant and found near the surface. Traumatic lesions resulting from abnormal swimming may be secondary sequelae. Betanodaviruses can be spread horizontally and vertically, and live or frozen fish fed to broodstock or grow-out stages may be a potential source of infection. Other sources of infection include wild invertebrates and contaminated water. Egg disinfection may help reduce impact of the disease. A commercial vaccine may be available internationally, but none is currently available in the USA.

Histopathologically, in properly fixed samples of affected CNS tissue (brain, spinal cord, retina of the eye), the presence of severe vacuolation is a hallmark of the disease. Disease and pathogen confirmation is based on clinical signs, species, histopathology, immunofluorescent antibody techniques, and PCR.

AQUATIC SYSTEMS

A fundamental assessment in working with aquatic species is examination and evaluation of the life support system sustaining the animals. This is a critical step in the clinical examination of any aquatic species, not just fish. The emphasis of this chapter is on aquarium and aquaculture systems, but the principles may be applied to life-support designs for all aquatic organisms.

Water quality management is a basic component of successful maintenance of aquatic organisms. Information is presented on normal parameters, as well as on environmental diseases of fish.

TYPES OF AQUATIC SYSTEMS

There are three basic types of aquatic systems, broadly defined as "open," "semi-open," or "closed." An open system has incoming water from some source (eg, surface water, well water, or city water) flowing through the culture facility one time, then discharged. Raceway and cage systems are examples of open systems. Semi-open systems have some capacity to recirculate water, which requires some type of treatment, but fresh water from an external source may be added as needed to supplement the treated water. Closed systems can be natural, such as static outdoor ponds, or can be highly engineered; intensive aquaculture systems depend on extensive filtration of water before recirculation. Aquariums are typically considered closed systems; however, the complexity of design and carrying capacity of individual systems vary greatly.

Basic housing units for fish may be outdoor ponds, raceways, cages, or aquarium systems (which may include recirculating system designs). The selection of a housing unit will be determined by available resources and facilities, as well as the goals of the owner.

Outdoor ponds are typically constructed in clay-based soils, or they may have a type of plastic liner to retain water. In Florida, there are also "water table ponds," which have a certain amount of horizontal flow of ground water into and out of the pond. Production ponds vary greatly in size, but a good design maximizes surface area while minimizing depth (ideally <6 ft). This design decreases the risk of stratification that can result in catastrophic "turnover" events (*see* p 1771). Ideally, an aeration device should be available for all outdoor ponds. In the southeastern USA, most aquaculture production ponds range from 0.1–20 surface acres of water, whereas recreational fishing ponds usually have a smaller surface area but may be quite deep, substantially increasing the risk of stratification and turnover.

Ornamental ponds may vary from a few hundred gallons to many thousands. Larger ponds (>10,000 gal.) are usually easier to manage from a water quality perspective and are more forgiving of an owner who may overstock or overfeed the fish. Most larger ponds have water provided from a well or city water source and are operated as closed systems. Supplemental aeration is also very important for these systems and is often provided by a waterfall, stream, or other aesthetic means of moving water.

Clinicians should not only test dissolved oxygen (DO) when evaluating an ornamental pond but also assess water movement. In poorly maintained systems, filters will become clogged and flow rates can decrease dramatically. Poor flow rates result in poor performance by biofilters and, ultimately, system failure with consequent rises in total ammonia nitrogen concentrations. Poor flow rates are also often associated with low levels of DO and an inability to maintain oxygen concentrations near saturation. If the pond depends on a waterfall as the primary source of aeration, and flow rates decline, the aeration capability is also compromised. Shade may be an important consideration when evaluating an ornamental pond. Lack of shade can result in rapid and extreme heating of water, especially if the pond is shallow. Hot water is not only detrimental in its own right, but it also does not hold oxygen well, increasing the risk of oxygen depletion. Shade trees around a koi pond may contribute to leaf litter and organics in the pond. Preventing predation is another important consideration when designing an ornamental pond. Typically, fish housed in these units are very colorful and may be very attractive to birds (including owls), as well as to mammalian predators such as raccoons or otters. In Florida, reptiles (eg, alligators) may also prey on ornamental fish. Some type of visual barrier to minimize the detection of colorful fish by birds can help, as can pond design features or other structures that limit the ability of wading birds to access the pond. An electric perimeter fence located 12–18 in. off the ground may keep small mammals or crocodilians out of an owner's yard, protecting the fish and other pets.

Other types of systems, more typical of aquaculture production, include cages and raceways. A raceway system is typically a series of long, narrow, and relatively shallow concrete or earthen tanks. Water enters the unit at one end and is discharged at another. Often, these use some source of surface water, such as a flowing river, for growout of the fish. Advantages of raceway systems include capacity for heavier stocking densities than ponds of a corresponding volume. Disadvantages include concerns about bringing pathogens or contaminants onto the farm and discharging nutrient waste, pathogens, or treatment chemicals in the effluent. Cage production is most common in open water, with the salmon industry being a prime example. Typically, large cages are placed in protected bays for the grow-out phase of the operation. Alternatively, new technologies allow cage systems to be completely sunk in deep water, decreasing the risk of damage from wind and wave action. Advantages of cage production include tidal water exchange, which would not require pretreatment to be suitable for the fish. Disadvantages include potential damage to equipment or escape of fish during storms, potential contamination in the event of a chemical spill or harmful algal bloom, and concerns about adverse environmental impacts by the aquaculture operation itself. Global use of cage culture technology is increasingly important as marine food fish are cultured more intensively.

AQUATIC LIFE SUPPORT SYSTEM COMPONENTS

The basic components of a life support system are a vessel that houses the animals, and if water is to be recirculated, the filtration components, and a sump or reservoir (area to collect water before and/or after treatment). Understanding these component parts can help the practitioner appreciate the basic design and how it may impact animal health and disease management. Additional study is required for clinicians who plan to develop greater knowledge and skills for aquatic practice.

There are three basic types of filtration: biologic, mechanical, and chemical. All recirculating systems have biologic and mechanical components, and most also include a chemical component. Some types of filters provide more than one of these functions and may be dual purposed in the design. Practitioners should familiarize themselves with basic filtration and more complex system designs as their experience grows.

Biologic Filtration: Biologic filters remove nitrogenous waste from the system. Fish excrete ammonia directly from the bloodstream via passive diffusion across the gill epithelium. Biologic filters provide substrate and massive surface area for nitrifying bacteria to live. These bacteria are ubiquitous in the environment and grow well when nitrogenous compounds (ammonia and nitrite) are present in the water column. These bacteria require both oxygen and a carbonate source, which must be provided by the water and filter design. Examples of biologic filters are plastic plenums placed in the bottom of home aquaria, fluidized bed filters common in commercially designed systems, and an array of bead and sand filters sold for use in ornamental pond and aquaculture units.

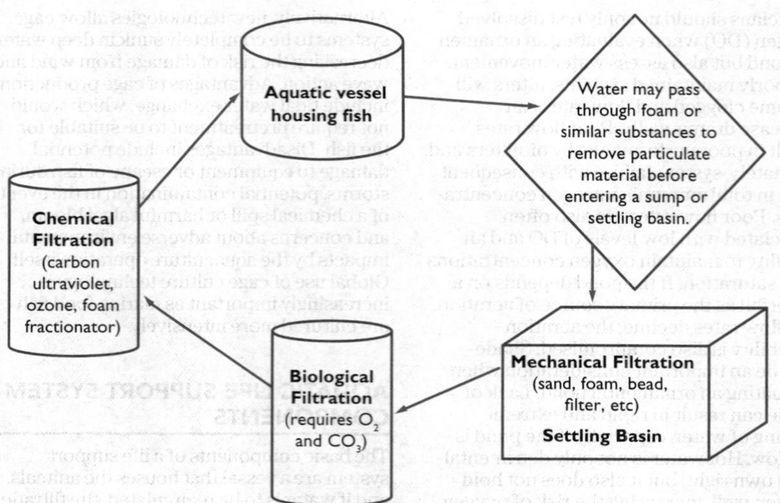

Generic schematic of a basic aquatic life support system. Mechanical filtration should precede biofiltration. Mechanical filters help prevent channeling and anoxia in biofilters by removing large particulate matter. Biofilters must have a lot of surface area for nitrifying bacteria. Chemical filtration, although not required in all designs, polishes and cleans water before it is returned to the vessel housing the fish. *Courtesy of Dr. Ruth Francis-Floyd.*

Mechanical Filtration: Mechanical filters are always placed before biologic filters in the system design. Mechanical filters typically receive water leaving the vessel housing animals and remove large particulate matter before water comes into contact with the biofilter. Large particles can clog a biofilter, resulting in channeling and development of anoxic areas that greatly compromise function of the unit. Mechanical filters can be as simple as floss or foam pads receiving a stream of water, or much more complex. Sand and bead filters are commonly used and have dual functions of mechanical and biologic filtration.

Chemical Filtration: Chemical filters provide a way to treat the water. Activated carbon is very commonly used to remove toxins and colored compounds from aquarium water, which helps maintain clarity. Activated carbon filters may also be placed on inflowing water to remove chlorine and/or chloramine from city water. Activated carbon filters can also be used to remove treatment chemicals from water *before discharge to city sewers*. Other examples of chemical filters include protein skimmers and foam fractionators, which are commonly used in marine systems to remove proteinaceous waste (decreasing the load on the biofilter); ultraviolet light, which removes potentially pathogenic organisms from the water column; and ozone, which clarifies water and kills microbes. Ozone is common in large commercial aquaria and requires a de-gassing area before the treated water comes back into contact with fish. Malfunction of ozone units can be hazardous to people as well as animals housed in aquarium systems.

EQUIPMENT NEEDED FOR SYSTEM AND WATER ANALYSIS

To competently assess a system's design takes some practice, but a basic understanding and analysis can be accomplished by keeping in mind the component parts and their functions. Site visits are essential to understanding how a system has been put together. In addition to assessing the design and functionality of a system, a site visit allows the opportunity to assess maintenance and cleanliness, both critical aspects of animal husbandry. The importance of a DO meter cannot be overstated when assessing an aquatic system. Oxygen concentration should be measured in the area housing the animals, and it should also be used to help identify areas prone to anoxia because of equipment problems, poor maintenance, or design flaws.

Water quality testing equipment is a requirement for aquatic practice. Good quality testing kits are commercially available at reasonable prices. Tests can be run quickly, providing data in a timely manner. Basic requirements include a means to test temperature, DO, carbon dioxide (CO_2), chlorine, chloramine, ammonia, nitrite, nitrate, pH, total alkalinity, total hardness, and salinity. Testing for freshwater and marine systems is similar; however, the ammonia test often sold for freshwater use requires the use of Nessler's reagent, which has two distinct disadvantages: it contains mercury and therefore must be treated as hazardous waste, and it does not work in marine systems. Alternatively, an ammonia test using an ammonium salicylate reagent is recommended. Chlorine test kits (free and total chlorine) are not included in many kits marketed to the aquaculture industry and need to be ordered separately. Also, a copper test kit and a refractometer (to measure salinity) should be on hand for use in marine systems. If a practice has enough cases to warrant the investment, an electronic oxygen meter is strongly recommended. If working in a rural area where well water is commonly used, test kits for iron and hydrogen sulfide should be considered. For true specialty practices, investment in a saturometer for detection of supersaturation is also suggested.

ENVIRONMENTAL HISTORY

As with all aspects of medical analysis, a good history is critical in establishing a diagnosis. Specific questions are important to assess the environmental quality and may play an important role in treatment recommendations. First, a thorough description of animal housing should include the volume, design of the system, and source of water. The number and size of animals stocked, species (fish and non-fish), new additions, use of quarantine, decorations, plants, and previous medications are part of the case history and may also be relevant to assessment of environmental quality and system design. Owners can be asked to bring fish and water samples to the clinic, or the practitioner may wish to visit the site. Site visits allow the system to be more accurately evaluated and the behavior of fish to be readily observed. If a site visit is not possible, the owner can be asked to provide a video and/or photos of the system (including filtration) and the fish, both affected and unaffected. If fish are brought into the clinic for examination, a separate water sample should be provided in a plastic bag or clean, plastic water bottle. If the source water is from a municipal water supply, a second sample should be collected in a glass bottle for chlorine/chloramine testing. Water samples collected by the owner should be capped under the surface of the water without any gas bubbles visible. A minimum of 1 quart of tank water should be requested for regular analysis, and a second smaller sample (<100 mL) in a glass container for chlorine testing. If desired to use for recovery after anesthesia of the animal, a larger volume of tank water may be requested.

ENVIRONMENTAL DISEASES

Because poor water quality is the most common cause of environmentally induced diseases, some way to assess water quality is essential. Inexpensive test kits are easy to use and provide reasonably accurate information. Professional aquaculturists or advanced tropical fish hobbyists should be encouraged to purchase and use their own water-testing equipment. Pet fish owners often rely on pet stores to do the water testing; however, many pet stores have very limited capabilities in this area, use less accurate tests, and may be unable to accurately interpret results.

Veterinarians practicing fish medicine should have a comprehensive understanding of the dynamics and management of water quality, including general guidelines for acceptable water quality parameters (*see* TABLE 2). In addition to temperature, basic parameters of water quality can be grouped into four major categories: dissolved gases, nitrogenous compounds, pH and carbonate compounds, and salinity. The significance of water quality parameters varies with the type of system, species, and stocking density. Low DO and high ammonia are the two water quality parameters most likely to directly kill fish. Water quality interactions are dynamic and complex. Indirect relationships can lead to toxicity from other parameters, such as the effect of rising pH on (increased) ammonia toxicity, or there can be indirect relationships between water quality and certain infectious agents. For example, low or inappropriate temperature can be associated with fungal diseases of fish. A classic example is *Fusarium solani* infection of bonnethead sharks, which has been managed by raising the environmental temperature to >80°F (27°C).

TABLE 2 "NORMAL" REFERENCE RANGES FOR ROUTINE WATER QUALITY ANALYSIS

Parameter	Freshwater	Saltwater
Dissolved oxygen	Saturation[a]	Saturation
Carbon dioxide	<12 mg/L	<12 mg/L
pH	6.5–9.0	7.8–8.3
TAN (total ammonia nitrogen)[b]	0 mg/L	0 mg/L
Toxic un-ionized ammonia (NH_3)[b]	0 mg/L	0 mg/L
Nitrite	0 mg/L	0 mg/L
Nitrate	<20 mg/L	<70 mg/L
Total alkalinity (carbonate fraction)	>100 mg/L $CaCO_3$	>250 mg/L $CaCO_3$
Total hardness (Ca and Mg primarily)	>20 mg/L $CaCO_3$	>250 mg/L $CaCO_3$
If source water is from municipal water supply:		
Total chlorine (free chlorine + chloramines)	0 mg/L	0 mg/L
Free chlorine	0 mg/L	0 mg/L

[a] Dissolved oxygen in ponds will fluctuate on a diurnal basis. Concentrations <5 mg/L are dangerous. Mortality will be species-specific and related to time of exposure but may be observed at ≤4 mg/L. Oxygen saturation at room temperature (25°C [77°F]) and sea level will be 8.27 mg/L in freshwater and 6.75 mg/L in seawater (35 ppt or chlorinity of 20 ppt).

[b] Under most circumstances, freshwater fish can tolerate total ammonia concentrations <1 mg/L, whereas saltwater fish will usually tolerate TAN <0.5 mg/L. Un-ionized ammonia concentrations <0.05 mg/L are not considered harmful.

See TABLE 3 for an overview of common environmental diseases of fish.

Chlorine, Chloramine, and Other Toxicants: Aquatic organisms are sensitive to a wide variety of toxicants, particularly **chlorine** and **chloramine**, which are common additives to city water. Chlorine is also used to disinfect tanks and equipment. Chloramine is a form of chlorine that has been stabilized by amination. When treated for removal of the chlorine molecule, ammonia is released into the system. Both compounds are highly toxic to fish, with adverse effects seen at chlorine concentrations as low as 0.02 mg/L and mortality at 0.04 mg/L. A simple colorimetric test is available to measure chlorine and chloramine in aquatic systems. No chlorine or chloramine should be detected at any time live animals are present. Water samples for chlorine testing should be tested onsite; however, if that is not possible, they may be transported in glass bottles. The chemical can be transient and difficult to detect, so a negative test result may not completely exclude some contamination in the system being evaluated.

To test for chlorine and/or chloramine, kits are available that measure both free and total chlorine. Free chlorine measures hypochlorous acid (HOCl) and the hypochlorite ion (OCl^-), which is the active property in bleach. Total chlorine measures free chlorine plus chlorine that is tied up as chloramine. Water treated with chloramines alone will test negative for free chlorine but have high amounts of total chlorine detectable; therefore, testing for both is important. When chloramines are treated with sodium thiosulfate to eliminate the chlorine, ammonia is released into the system. In such an instance, repeated water changes (each of which requires dechlorination, releasing additional ammonia) can result in high ammonia levels that also may be toxic. A properly conditioned biofilter should be able to metabolize the ammonia as it is released, but a new or damaged bacterial bed will not be able to manage the influx of ammonia from repeated deamination of chloramines. This problem can be overcome by using a dechlorinator specifically designed to deal with chloramines by also binding the ammonia byproduct. Effective use of dechlorination products requires testing water for both free and total chlorine before and after use. Following label instructions on products sold from pet stores usually effectively removes these chemicals; however, in rare instances more chlorine/chloramine than expected may be present in municipal water supplies. Treatment of water supplies will vary, and boluses of chlorine or chloramine may be sent through water lines as part of maintenance protocols in some circumstances. Further, inaccurate calculation of the volume to be treated can also lead to poor performance or failure of dechlorination products.

Chronic exposure to sublethal concentrations of chlorine is a surprisingly frequent problem, even for experienced aquarists. Veterinarians should test water for chlorine (free and total) every time a sample is submitted from a tank that uses a municipal water supply as source water. Clinical indications of sublethal chlorine exposure are nonspecific but may include ragged fins, excess mucus on skin and gills, cloudy corneas, behavioral signs such as lethargy or irritation, and sometimes a history of low chlorine level and chronic mortality.

Other toxicants include hydrogen sulfide and heavy metals. **Hydrogen sulfide** usually is a problem in poorly maintained tanks in which the sediments are not cleaned frequently enough, allowing anoxic areas to develop. Cleaning or other disturbance of these areas can release hydrogen sulfide into the water column, resulting in acute and catastrophic mortality. Another common source of hydrogen sulfide is well water; if this is the case, a distinctive "rotten egg" smell can sometimes be detected. Hydrogen sulfide is volatile and transient, so unless a water sample is collected at the time of the problem, a confirmed diagnosis may not be possible. Acute mortality has been reported at concentrations of 0.5 mg/L, but any detectable hydrogen sulfide should be considered a significant problem.

Heavy metals in water can result in acute, or more often, chronic mortality. If household plumbing includes copper piping, some copper may leach into the water. If released in sufficient volume, this may cause a fish kill. Problems are most likely when water has been allowed to stand in pipes. A copper test of suspect water should confirm the problem. Solutions include running the water before it is placed into the aquarium, or special filtration (eg, activated carbon) to remove metals.

Zinc toxicity has been associated with use of stainless steel vessels to house fish. It has also been reported rarely from public exhibits in which coins were allowed to collect on the substrate or to be ingested by fish.

Dissolved Gases: Of the dissolved gases, oxygen is the most important. In outdoor production ponds, photosynthesis by algae is the primary source of oxygen. A diurnal cycle is established, which coincides with photosynthetic activity. During daylight hours, when photosynthesis occurs, oxygen levels rise and CO_2 levels fall. At night, respiration is the driving force, resulting in a decrease in DO and an increase in CO_2. Most finfish thrive when the DO concentration is >5 mg/L. When DO is <5 mg/L, fish become stressed; depending on species, size, and duration of exposure, a fish kill may result. Cardinal signs of a fish kill caused by hypoxia include sudden, significant mortality, usually noticed early in the morning (when oxygen levels are lowest); often, large fish are affected more than small fish. Fish that are hypoxic often school near the surface of the water and may be seen trying to gulp air, a behavior referred to as "piping." Differential diagnoses for piping includes low DO, high nitrite, and gill disease.

Although low DO is most common early in the morning in outdoor ponds, it can occur at any time. Other common causes of low DO in ponds are cloudy weather, death of an algal bloom, excessive feeding, overstocking, and pond turnover. Unrecognized overstocking can occur in koi ponds if fish spawn successfully and offspring survive and are retained in the system. Pond turnover is a common cause of catastrophic mortality in pond fish. It occurs most frequently in deep ponds (>6 ft) and involves a phenomenon referred to as stratification. Water at the bottom of the pond cools, and a temperature gradient, called a thermocline, develops between warm surface water and cool bottom water. The thermocline acts as a physical barrier between the surface water (epilimnion) and bottom water (hypolimnion). Because photosynthesis, and hence oxygen production, occurs at the surface, the hypolimnion becomes hypoxic and develops a biologic oxygen demand. When the pond is mixed, or "turns over," the oxygen is removed as the biologic oxygen demand of the hypolimnion is satisfied. This sudden removal of oxygen can result in oxygen depletion and a fish kill. The most common cause of pond turnover in the southern USA is a summer thunderstorm, in which energy released from cold rain coupled with wind and wave action is sufficient to mix the pond. Fish kills in Florida have occurred after hurricanes and have been attributed to pond turnover. Pond turnover can also be caused by seining, aeration, or other management

TABLE 3 COMMON ENVIRONMENTAL DISEASES OF FISH

Disease	Problem	Behavioral Signs
Low dissolved oxygen	Hypoxia	Piping at surface; large fish affected more than small ones
Gas bubble disease	Supersaturation (often N_2 gas)	Lethargy, buoyancy problems
Carbon dioxide toxicity	CO_2 >40 mg/L	Lethargy at surface
Ammonia toxicity (new tank syndrome)	Un-ionized ammonia >1 mg/L pH >8	Lethargy, anorexia, spinning, convulsive swimming
Nitrite[a] toxicity	NO_2 >0.1 mg/L[a] Low chloride (freshwater)	Piping at surface
Nitrate[b] toxicity	NO_3–N ≥70 mg/L Low (no) iodine, O_3	Lethargy
Old tank syndrome	Total alkalinity (TA) ~0 mg/L pH <6, high total ammonia nitrogen (TAN)	Lethargy, poor appetite
Lack of minerals	Total hardness <20 mg/L Use of distilled water	Sudden death
Chlorine toxicity	Detectable chlorine	Acute: sudden death Chronic: lethargy, irritation
Hydrogen sulfide toxicity	Detectable H_2S (rotten egg smell)	Acute: sudden death Chronic: lethargy, poor appetite/growth
Copper toxicity	Cu^{2+} >0.2 mg/L Low alkalinity	Sudden death
Zinc toxicity	Coins in exhibit Stainless steel, acidic pH	Lethargy, anorexia
Stray voltage	Electrical short, mechanical problem	Irritation, mortality

[a] There is tremendous species-specific variation to nitrite toxicity. Environmental conditions, especially chloride concentration, can mitigate the effects. Most test kits measure mg/L NO_2–N. To convert to NO_2 (mg/L) concentration, this value must be multiplied by 3.3.

[b] Most test kits measure mg/L NO_3–N. To convert to NO_3 (mg/L) concentration, this value must be multiplied by 4.4.

practices that result in mixing of the epilimnion and hypolimnion. Fish kills caused by pond turnover can be avoided by performing a weekly oxygen profile during periods of greatest risk (usually during hot, summer weather). If stratification is detected, the pond should be aerated or mixed to break down stratified layers before a significant oxygen demand layer can develop. Turnover events resulting in localized areas of low DO are common causes of wild fish kills during the summer in lakes, ponds, and even rivers in the southern USA. Although rare, stratification-related phenomenon can occur in aquariums and other aquatic systems. Under some conditions, flow rate, current patterns (related to tank design), and oxygen demand can cause layering (ie, stratification) and consequent focal areas of anoxia.

When assessing DO and aeration in indoor systems or exhibits in which the primary source of DO is an aeration device, and water is clear, the percent saturation

TABLE 3 COMMON ENVIRONMENTAL DISEASES OF FISH *(continued)*

	Mortality	
Physical Signs	**Acute**	**Chronic**
Flared gills, dark	Catastrophic mortality	Ongoing
Gas bubbles in gill capillaries, fins, and eyes; exophthalmos ("popeye")	Catastrophic mortality	Ongoing
None	Yes	Yes
Darkened	Catastrophic mortality	Ongoing
Gills and blood dark brown color	Yes	Yes
Swelling around throat ("goiter")	No	Yes
None	No	Yes
None	No	Yes
Acute: none Chronic: excess mucus, cloudy eyes, gill inflammation/ necrosis	Catastrophic mortality	Ongoing
None	Catastrophic mortality	Ongoing
None	Catastrophic mortality	Ongoing
None Enlarged abdomen (coins in GI tract)	Not usually	Yes
Broken back	Yes	Yes

should be considered along with the total DO reading. The amount of oxygen that water can hold in saturation varies with water temperature, salinity, and altitude. Of these three factors, water temperature is the most important. As any of these variables increase, the amount of oxygen in solution at saturation decreases. Saturation tables are available to determine percent saturation for a given DO if temperature, salinity, and altitude are known. Many modestly priced oxygen meters now provide data on the concentration of DO (mg/L) as well as the percent saturation. If oxygen saturation is <100%, it may indicate inadequate aeration for the bioload or sanitation problems (development of anoxic, organic-rich areas within the system). In either case, an inability to maintain a system at, or very near, 100% oxygen saturation requires correction. Most fish do well if DO is >5 mg/L; however, the percent saturation should be considered an indicator of the system's health.

Gas bubble disease is caused by supersaturation of water with dissolved gases. Although oxygen and/or CO_2 can contribute to supersaturation, the predominant gas contributing to the problem is usually nitrogen. Gas bubble disease can result in acute catastrophic or chronic mortality. It may occur transiently and can be difficult to confirm. Supersaturation should be considered when unexplained mortality is encountered in an aquarium setting. One common source of supersaturation is the use of well water that contains high concentrations of nitrogen (gas) or CO_2. This problem is easily remedied by aerating the water before it comes into contact with the fish. Common causes of gas bubble disease in public aquaria include the use of cavitating pumps, leaks in plumbing on the intake side (allow for gas to enter and be forced under pressure through the pump), and sometimes excessive turbulence in cold water exhibits. In these cases, the supersaturation is caused by atmospheric nitrogen gas. Gas bubble disease is manifest by exophthalmos and the presence of tiny gas emboli within fins, corneas, or other tissue. The presence of gas emboli within gill capillaries is diagnostic. Treatment of gas bubble disease is vigorous aeration to volatilize excess gas and correction of underlying mechanical problems. Confirming a case of supersaturation can be extremely difficult, especially if mortality was acute and gas emboli cannot be detected in tissue. Sometimes, tiny gas bubbles may be visible on the inside of the glass in an aquarium, suggesting a lot of gas is in the water column. A saturometer will measure all dissolved gases and is the best tool for direct detection of the condition. If DO of the system is known, this equipment can be used to calculate the concentration of nitrogen gas present. Permanent correction of the problem includes identification and correction of the source of the excess gas.

CO_2 can be toxic to fish at concentrations >12 mg/L. The concentration of CO_2 in solution in ground water is typically <10 mg/L. Water from affected systems often is acidic (pH <7). A quick field test for excessive CO_2 involves vigorous aeration of a bucket of suspect water for 1 hr. A significant increase in pH (ie, >1 unit) over the hour is indicative of excess CO_2. Fish exposed to high concentrations of CO_2 may be quite lethargic and even disoriented. Hybrid striped bass exposed to toxic levels of CO_2 (~40 mg/L) at the surface have been observed with their backs out of the water. These fish reacted dramatically to salt added to the affected tank by trying to jump out of the water. When CO_2 is high in the water column, fish are not able to release it from the bloodstream, resulting in hypercarbia and acidemia. The condition is exacerbated by low concentrations of DO. Nephrocalcinosis and visceral granuloma were reported in salmonids exposed to a high level of CO_2 in the water, leading to metabolic acidosis and urinary and tissue precipitation of calcium, around which extensive granulomas developed. Treatment for CO_2 toxicity is increased and vigorous aeration. Stocking density should be assessed and may need to be decreased.

Nitrogenous Compounds: Nitrogenous wastes enter the aquatic system directly from excretion by fish, decomposition of organisms in the water, or degradation of fish food. Fish foods are generally very high in protein, often >38%, and can add significant quantities of nitrogen to a system. Nitrogen is eliminated from fish by passive diffusion of ammonia (NH_3) from gill capillaries. Once NH_3 is released into the water, it enters the nitrogen cycle, a natural process in which bacterial populations change ammonia to nitrite (NO_2) and then to nitrate (NO_3). Nitrate is most commonly removed from aquariums by water changes. In large, commercial systems, discharge of salt water to municipal water supplies is not allowed, and nitrate accumulates. It can be removed by anaerobic filtration, which converts NO_3 to nitrogen gas (N_2), which is volatile and quickly leaves the system. These anaerobic filters are expensive and can be challenging from the design perspective, so they are not common except in very large exhibits. Plants or algae, if present in a system, will use nitrogen products directly. Toxicity of each of these parameters is discussed below.

NH_3 is highly toxic and frequently limits fish production in intensive systems. It is also dynamic, and when it enters the aquatic system, an equilibrium is established between NH_3 and ammonium (NH_4^+). Of the two, NH_3 is far more toxic to fish, and its formation is favored by high pH (>7) and water temperature. When pH exceeds ~8.5, any NH_3 present can be dangerous. In general, a normally functioning aquatic system should contain no measurable NH_3 because as soon as it enters the system, it should be removed by aerobic bacteria in the environment. Ammonia test kits do not typically measure NH_3 directly but instead measure the combination of NH_3 and NH_4^+, referred to as total ammonia nitrogen (TAN). A TAN <1 mg/L is usually not cause for concern unless the pH is >8.5. However, if the amount of NH_3 is increased, an explanation should be sought. The amount of toxic NH_3 present can be calculated using the TAN, pH, and water temperature. When NH_3 levels exceed 0.05 mg/L, damage to gills becomes apparent; levels of 2 mg/L are lethal for many fish. Fish exposed to ammonia may be lethargic and have poor appetites. Acute toxicity may be suggested by neurologic signs such as spinning, disorientation, and convulsions.

Overfeeding or malfunction (death) of a biologic filter are common causes of increased NH_3. If possible, a water change (≥50%) should be done as soon as high NH_3 levels are detected. When changing water to alleviate NH_3 toxicity, it is imperative to consider whether source water contains chloramines, because this can contribute to increased NH_3 concentrations. If TAN is extremely high (ie, >5 mg/L) and pH is acidic (ie, <6), fish should be moved to a clean system (tempered for pH and temperature) to avoid a sudden shift from NH_4^+ to NH_3 as the pH rises during the water change. Feeding should be discontinued or significantly reduced until the problem has been corrected.

Two conditions encountered in pet fish medicine are characterized by high NH_3 concentrations, appropriately called new tank syndrome and old tank syndrome. **New tank syndrome** occurs when NH_3 levels rise during the first 2–3 wk after a new system is set up, because the biofilter has not had time to develop. In this situation, the NH_3 concentration will be increased, but all other parameters should be within normal limits. Beginning aquarists are likely to overstock and overfeed new systems, resulting in significant NH_3 spikes and, subsequently, sick or dying fish. Daily monitoring of TAN coupled with frequent water changes to manage NH_3 will be necessary until the biofilter cycles. Maturation of the biofilter will be indicated by decreasing concentrations of TAN and increasing concentrations of NO_2 (which will decrease as the filter conditioning process is completed). Damage to a biofilter can be caused by use of antibiotics or other chemicals and result in a similar situation. It usually takes ~6 wk for a new biofilter to cycle. When this time frame is extended, there may be complications attributed to poor design, use of chemicals, or lack of adequate oxygen and carbonate (alkalinity) in the filter bed. To prevent new tank syndrome, aquarists use several "tricks" to get biofilters started. These include purchasing commercially available nitrifying bacteria from a reputable source, "feeding" the bacteria with fish food or ammonium chloride before adding fish, or adding fish slowly to the new system.

Old tank syndrome is less frequently recognized. It is characterized by extremely high NH_3 levels (TAN may be >20 mg/L), extremely low pH (usually <6, may be <5 in severe cases), and a complete absence of alkalinity. The condition is caused by complete exhaustion of buffering capacity within a system, usually precipitated by improper management over a period of months. Over time, the biofilter bacteria acidify the water through the nitrification process. As the buffering capacity (alkalinity) is exhausted, organic acids that have accumulated drop the pH, and the acidic environment kills the biofilter, leading to an accumulation of NH_3. When correcting such a situation, it is important to eliminate as much "bad" water as possible and avoid a shift in residual NH_3-H to the toxic un-ionized state (NH_3) as pH rises. A simple water change under such circumstances can result in catastrophic mortality as pH rises above 7 and ammonium shifts to un-ionized (toxic) ammonia. Over-the-counter products that chemically remove or bind NH_3 can help prevent mortality, but the system must be thoroughly cleaned and restarted. It will take several weeks for the system to recover.

The second breakdown product in the nitrogen cycle is nitrite (NO_2), which is also toxic to fish. Most test kits actually measure nitrite-nitrogen rather than nitrite. A conversion factor of 3.3 can be used to calculate the actual nitrite concentration ($3.3 \times$ mg/L NO_2–N = mg/L NO_2). NO_2 can enter the bloodstream passively across the gill epithelium. It complexes with hemoglobin to form methemoglobin, resulting in methemoglobinemia, or **brown blood disease**. As in other species, RBCs containing methemoglobin are unable to transport oxygen, resulting in a physiologic hypoxia regardless of oxygen content in the water. There are species-specific differences in fishes' susceptibility to NO_2 toxicity (eg, centrarchids [bass, bluegill, etc] are refractory). Marine fish were thought to be protected from NO_2 toxicity by salts in their environment; however, red drum have developed brown blood disease in the presence of NO_2. A tentative diagnosis of brown blood disease can be made by observing the characteristic chocolate brown color of the gills, although this change is not detectable until methemoglobin levels are substantial. In severe cases, the color of blood samples will also be abnormally dark. Methemoglobin concentrations in the blood can be determined, although this is not necessary for clinical management. A water quality test can confirm the presence of NO_2. Fish affected with methemoglobinemia typically show signs of hypoxia, often manifest by piping.

The most rapid treatment for NO_2 toxicity is a water change, but this is not feasible in large ponds. Increasing chloride (Cl^-) concentration in the water creates a competitive inhibition at the gill epithelium between Cl and NO_2. Many ornamental ponds and aquaria are maintained with residual chloride levels because of the addition of salt (1–3 ppt) as a relatively permanent treatment. In these cases, nitrite is less likely to be a problem, because chloride levels are increased by the residual salt concentration. In freshwater production ponds for channel catfish, a ratio of 6 parts Cl to 1 part NO_2 has effectively prevented or treated methemoglobinemia caused by nitrite exposure. The absorption of Cl^- across the gill membrane reduces the amount of NO_2^- entering the bloodstream; consequently, the percentage of hemoglobin converted to methemoglobin is decreased, resulting in immediate relief to the fish and a cessation of mortality usually within 24 hr. To determine the amount of salt required to increase chloride levels in large ponds, the concentrations of NO_2 and Cl present must be measured by commercial test kits. The concentration of Cl needed (mg/L) = (6 × NO_2) – Cl present. Once the necessary concentration of Cl^- to be added is known, the volume of water can be calculated in acre-feet or gallons (1 acre foot = 1 surface acre, 1 foot deep or 325,850 gal.), and salt can be added to achieve the desired Cl level (4.5 lb of salt will add Cl at 1 mg/L to 1 acre-foot of water, or 1 lb of salt will add 1 mg/L Cl to 72,411 gal.). In aquariums and garden ponds, a water change and filter maintenance are recommended to correct nitrite problems; however, salt may still be used to halt mortality during a sudden increase in NO_2 exposure for many freshwater fish.

Although considered less toxic than ammonia or nitrite, chronic exposure to nitrate (NO_3–N) has been associated with development of goiter in some species of elasmobranchs. As mentioned earlier for the nitrite test kit, most test kits for nitrate actually measure NO_3–N. To convert to the actual NO_3 concentration, this number must be multiplied by a correction factor of 4.4. Practitioners should read the literature carefully to distinguish reports of NO_3-N versus NO_3 concentrations. Chronic exposure to NO_3-N concentrations of 70 mg/L resulted in histologic evidence of goiter in white spotted bamboo sharks within 29 days of exposure. Chronic exposure to NO_3–N of 35 ± 5.12 mg/L resulted in development of overt goiter and 100% mortality of brown spotted bamboo sharks and 18% mortality of white spotted bamboo sharks in a recirculating system after ozone was added. Goiter is a complex disease, and there seem to be species-specific differences in susceptibility that are not well understood. Contributing factors include inadequate dietary iodine or environmental iodide, ozonation, and nitrate exposure. Goiter is characterized by a ventral midline swelling in the cervical region of elasmobranchs. Diagnosis can be confirmed by measuring T_4. In healthy (no clinical or histologic evidence of goiter), captive, white spotted bamboo sharks housed in a natural seawater system, T_4 was 14.77 ng/mL (range of 9.57–30.50 ng/mL in five animals). Lower levels have been reported in sharks with visual evidence of goiter. If an animal is necropsied, thyroid tissue can be evaluated histologically to confirm the diagnosis. Nitrate is well recognized as a goitrogenic compound and may be present in fairly high concentrations (>70 mg/L NO_3-N) in recirculating aquarium and aquaculture systems. Nitrate blocks the uptake of iodine by the thyroid gland, resulting in an inability to produce thyroid hormone and constant stimulation of the glandular tissue. Fish and elasmobranchs absorb micronutrients, including iodine, from the water column. In an ozonated system, the problem is exacerbated because iodine is converted to iodate (IO_3), which is not biologically available. Dietary supplementation of iodine at 10–30 mg/kg/wk is recommended for elasmobranchs to prevent development of goiter. Environmental iodine should be maintained with concentrations of 0.15 µM (0.01–0.02 mg/L) iodide (I^-). Potassium iodide (Lugol's solution) has been used to increase environmental iodide concentrations in public aquaria. Goiter occurs in teleosts and other aquatic species but is not as easily recognized. The body shape of many elasmobranchs allows for easy recognition of the problem during a visual examination.

pH and Carbonate Compounds: The carbonate cycle is an important concept in water quality management, and its complexity is reflected in the dynamic interactions between CO_2, pH, total alkalinity, and total hardness. In aquatic systems containing algae or plants, CO_2 fluctuates on a diurnal basis, similar but opposite to fluctuations in DO. As CO_2 concentration changes, the pH of the water also changes. As CO_2 concentration decreases during daylight hours, pH rises, peaking in late afternoon. Conversely, as CO_2 concentration increases during the night, pH falls, reaching its lowest level just before daylight. A diurnal pH change from 6.5 to 9 is not unusual in a freshwater fish pond with a healthy algal bloom. Most freshwater fish can tolerate reasonable fluctuations in pH, and the lethal limits for many species are approximately 4 and 10. Marine fish are much less tolerant of pH fluctuations the marine environment is much more stable, with a pH of 8.2–8.3. For marine tanks, a pH in the range of 7.8–8.5 is usually considered normal.

Although fish kills caused by improper pH are rare, hydrated lime ($Ca[OH]_2$) is sometimes added to freshwater ponds by mistake. $Ca(OH)_2$ will rapidly increase the pH to >10, killing all fish present. Correct liming of ponds is mentioned briefly below.

CO_2 released into an aquatic system enters the carbonate cycle: $H_2O + CO_2 \leftrightarrow H_2CO_3 \leftrightarrow H^+ + HCO_3^- \leftrightarrow 2H^+ + CO_3^{2-}$. The process is driven by the presence of carbonate (CO_3^{2-}) in the system, which is measured by testing the total alkalinity (TA). For most fish, water should be of moderate alkalinity, 100–250 mg/L. When TA is <50 mg/L, water is considered low in alkalinity, and buffering ability will not be adequate to prevent major pH fluctuations. Toxicity of copper sulfate, an algicide and effective parasiticide, is closely associated with TA, and the compound cannot be used safely if TA is <50 mg/L. To raise alkalinity, dolomite ($CaCO_3$ and $MgCO_3$) or agricultural limestone ($CaCO_3$) may be added to the system. Dolomite is most convenient for small systems and can be purchased in 50-lb bags and used to effect. Baking soda ($NaHCO_3$) can also be used to increase alkalinity in small systems. To raise alkalinity in outdoor ponds, agricultural limestone is commonly used; the method is similar to "liming" a pasture. Soil samples can be tested to determine how much lime needs to be added, but in general 1–2 tons per surface acre works well. The limestone should be unloaded on the bank of the pond and then usually has to be moved into the water using a shovel and boat. It does not need to be distributed throughout the entire surface area of the pond, but it takes several weeks to get into solution. Consequently, the alkalinity will change slowly, so it should be monitored for several days, or weeks if necessary, after the addition of these compounds. Lack of alkalinity can impair biologic filtration, resulting in accumulation of ammonia in a system. Alkalinity should be ≥100 mg/L in freshwater systems and ≥250 mg/L in saltwater systems.

Total hardness (TH) should not be confused with TA. Both TH and TA are reported as mg/L of $CaCO_3$. The difference is that the test for TA measures the HCO_3^-, OH^-, and CO_3^{2-} fraction, and the test for TH measures the calcium (Ca^{2+}) fraction. The test for TH also measures other divalent cations in the system, including magnesium, manganese, iron, and zinc. TH is important in determining the amount of calcium available to young fish. Calcium chloride, dolomite, or agricultural limestone can be added to water to increase calcium concentration. For channel catfish, TH >20 mg/L is required for normal skeletal growth and development. Fish absorb minerals from the water column; therefore, use of water with very low TH, which can be caused by use of deionized water, can result in poor growth and mortality.

Salinity: The salinity of seawater is determined by a complex array of salts. Seawater is ~3% salt, which is 30 ppt (30 g/L). For marine fish, many of the micronutrients present in seawater are essential, so it is necessary to buy or make "sea salts." In freshwater, salinity may be increased using table or water softener salt (NaCl). Salt is often used in freshwater systems to reduce osmoregulatory stress or to eliminate certain ectoparasites. Salinity can be measured with a clinical refractometer or with a hydrometer purchased from a pet store. It is important not to confuse the chloride (Cl^-) test, which is used in assessment of NO_2:Cl in freshwater systems with high nitrite, with salinity. The chloride test measures ppm chloride; if any salinity at all is present in the water (ie, salt has been added), the test will not work properly because the amount of chloride present is so high. The easiest way to calculate the amount of salt needed to increase salinity is to calculate the total volume in liters (3.8 L = 1 gal.), remembering that 1 g/L = 1 ppt. Most non-pond freshwater systems can be maintained with a residual salinity of 1–3 ppt, whereas most saltwater systems will have a salinity of 30–33 ppt. Some freshwater species (eg, wild-caught Amazonian fish) may not tolerate permanent exposure to the low levels of salt mentioned above.

Temperature: Environmental temperature is extremely important to the health and well-being of fish and other aquatic species. As poikilotherms, fish have a very limited ability to control body temperature, and physiologic systems are designed to work optimally at species-specific temperature ranges. Sudden changes in temperature, of even just a few degrees, can result in compromise of immunity and increased pathogenicity of some infectious agents. Some fish (eg, channel catfish or koi) are very tolerant of a wide range of environmental temperatures; however, this does not imply that drastic temperature fluctuations are acceptable even for these species. Others, such as discus, thrive in only a very narrow temperature window. When evaluating housing and husbandry, practitioners should know the temperature at which animals are being housed and confirm that it is appropriate for the species. Suboptimal environmental temperature is an important component in some fungal infections. Many infectious agents, especially viruses, have specific temperature windows at which they cause clinical disease and mortality. Fish infected but maintained at temperatures above or below these optimal ranges are more likely to survive infection but may become carriers. When handling or transporting fish, moderating temperature change is essential. A general rule is 1°F, or even 1°C, per hour as a maximum change. Some fish may tolerate more or less of a change over time.

ENVIRONMENTAL CONSIDERATIONS FOR SELECTED INFECTIOUS DISEASES

A number of infectious diseases have specific environmental parameters that can substantially enhance the impact of an outbreak or make an outbreak more difficult to control. A few of the more significant examples are mentioned below.

Mycobacteria: *Mycobacterium* spp is an important infectious pathogen of fish and other aquatic organisms. There have been many species of *Mycobacterium* identified in fish; however, all are nontuberculous and most are environmental. Typically, environmental conditions common in aquaculture favor growth of *Mycobacterium*. These conditions include low DO concentrations, accumulation of organic debris and particularly biofilms, as well as acidic pH. Mycobacteria are hydrophobic because of their thick, waxy cell walls and tend to adhere to surfaces and each other. Once infected fish are present in a system, these animals may continually shed the organism in feces and cells released from external lesions. Ultraviolet light (ie, UV filtration) may decrease the number of these bacteria in the water column, which may help decrease transmission; correction of these environmental factors can also enhance control efforts. In aquaculture, infected fish are almost always culled. In display aquaria, however, the decision may be made to maintain infected fish. In these cases, environmental management can be an important part of the protocol developed for the care of affected animals. Maintaining oxygen concentration near saturation and avoiding acidic and organically rich environments in the presence of some type of disinfection on the system (eg, UV or ozone) can greatly enhance the quality of an exhibit populated with mycobacteria-positive fish. In this situation, the exhibit should be clearly labeled as mycobacteria-positive, and employees should be properly trained to minimize risk of disease transmission from the contaminated exhibit to personnel working in the area or to other systems or animals.

Bacterial Gill Disease: Bacterial gill disease is an important disease of cultured salmonids and has been reported in other species, including hybrid striped bass. It is rare in aquarium fish. It is caused by bacteria in the genus *Flavobacterium* and other closely related genera and is manifest by gill pathology (hyperplasia, clubbing of gill filaments) and subsequent mortality. However, bacterial gill disease has an important environmental component, and mechanical damage to gill epithelium, which may be caused by excessive crowding and debris in the water column, is believed to be an important predisposing factor. Cleaning the environment, removing debris, and decreasing stocking density all contribute to a positive treatment outcome. Correcting these underlying problems also prevents recurrence of the condition. Potassium permanganate can be useful in removing organic detritus from an affected freshwater system. However, caution is advised, because this treatment may cause mortality in fish already compromised with significant gill damage.

The Role of Temperature in Infectious Diseases: Many infectious diseases of fish occur in a specific "temperature window," and adjusting temperature may be an important part of successful treatment. For example, *Fusarium solani* is a fungus that has been linked to suboptimal environmental temperatures in bonnethead sharks. Infected sharks must have environmental temperatures raised above 80°F (27°C) to control or prevent the infection. *Saprolegnia*, a common fungus-like oomycete of freshwater and brackish water fish, is also often associated with suboptimal environmental temperature. Raising water temperature a few degrees may significantly improve response to treatment. Clinicians are encouraged to determine optimal environmental temperature when fish are observed with this condition and to make appropriate corrections if needed.

Temperature is also critical in control of most viral diseases of fish. Two important diseases of koi, spring viremia of carp (SVC) and koi herpes virus (KHV), have strong temperature predilections. This should always be kept in mind when working with these popular pets. It should be remembered that KHV is a warm water disease. Infected koi typically develop disease when water temperatures are in the range of 64°–81°F (18°–27°C). Fish with KHV typically exhibit significant gill lesions and signs of hypoxia. In contrast, SVC is a cool water disease, typically occurring at water temperatures of 41°–64°F (5°–18°C). Both of these diseases are reportable at the state and federal levels. Although KHV is considered endemic in the USA, SVC is a foreign animal disease, and the USDA will impose quarantine and forced destruction of fish if an infection is confirmed. Consideration of water temperature is an important first step when confronted with a disease in this species.

Almost all viral diseases of fish have specific temperature ranges at which they cause active disease. Clinicians must familiarize themselves with diseases of concern and the temperatures at which they occur in the species at hand.

Excessive Organic Load: Organic debris can accumulate because of poor husbandry or poor system design. Detection of accumulated detritus can be surprisingly difficult when areas of "dead space" exist in a system, because these areas are often not directly visible. Environmental parameters that suggest this problem include an inability to maintain DO concentrations at or near saturation. Further, total alkalinity and pH may be lower than that in source water. All of these changes suggest a substantial amount of decomposition of organic matter is occurring somewhere in the system. Pet owners or aquarists may need to break the system down to locate and remove the accumulated material.

In these systems, a presenting disease problem may be infestation of external surfaces of the fish with *Trichodina*, a common ciliate. *Trichodina* is often considered a bio-indicator of suboptimal conditions that may include overcrowding, overfeeding, and excessive organic debris (ie, a dirty system). Thoroughly cleaning the system, removing detritus, and correcting design flaws when possible are important to correct these problems. Treating the parasite without correcting system problems will result in continual recurrence and frustration. Other infectious agents that may be observed in the presence of poor sanitation include sessile ciliates such as *Epistylis*, *Heteropolaria*, *Ambiphyra*, and *Apiosoma*. Saprophytic fungi and fungi-like diseases (eg, the oomycete *Saprolegnia*) may also be seen when hygiene is a concern.

Infectious Sequelae of Environmental Disease: Fish that survive a severe environmental insult, such as an acute hypoxic event, are at increased risk of opportunistic bacterial infections. Common infections that may occur 1–2 wk after an insult could include infections with *Aeromonas hydrophila* and *Pseudomonas fluorescens* in freshwater systems, and *Vibrio* spp in marine systems. Given this possibility, it may be prudent to treat valuable fish with a broad-spectrum antibiotic with general efficacy against gram-negative organisms after survival of a significant insult. In many cases, good water and a quiet environment will be sufficient for recovery, but when in doubt, the use of antibiotics may be justified, especially if they can be provided in feed. Once fish start to break with an infection, they often go off-feed, making treatment much more difficult.

AQUARIUM FISHES

Aquatic medicine has emerged as a recognized specialty within the practice of zoologic medicine. Fish medicine, an important component of the aquatic specialty, is evolving, with distinct subspecialties of aquaculture and production medicine (*see* AQUACULTURE, p 1743) as well as pet and exhibit fish medicine that focuses on individual animals. This chapter focuses on pet and exhibit fish medicine.

The business of ornamental fishes, which includes specimens that may be added to zoologic collections, can be broadly divided into freshwater and marine species. Most pet fishes are freshwater, and many are farm raised in the USA, Asia, or elsewhere. Many fish sold through the pet trade are imported to the USA. Except for a small number of species such as some clownfishes (*Amphiprion* spp), dottybacks (*Pseudochromis* spp), gobies (primarily *Elacatinus* spp), blennies (primarily *Meiacanthus* spp), and seahorses (*Hippocampus* spp), most marine fishes are wild caught.

The trade in ornamental fishes is a global industry, and fishes are often moved through several dealers before reaching a wholesale or retail outlet. The source of these fishes is an important consideration when designing quarantine protocols and anticipating the types and severity of disease that may be seen in recently acquired animals. Some fish species, whether marine or freshwater, are particularly prone to parasitic and bacterial infection during the quarantine period (first 30 days), including the first few weeks after arrival in a pet store or home aquarium.

Cyprinids such as koi and fancy goldfish for ornamental ponds are popular pets and typically respond well to veterinary care. Many of the highest quality are imported from Japan (koi) or China (fancy goldfish) and may have significant value (up to several thousand dollars for show-quality koi). Many are large enough for clinical manipulation, are quite hardy, and often have significant emotional value to their owners. These fish are susceptible to several diseases of regulatory concern, most notably spring viremia of carp and koi herpesvirus, which are both reportable diseases.

Clinical management of individual pet fish, exhibit animals, and valuable broodstock has changed dramatically in recent years. Advances include use of nonlethal methods to diagnose disease and more sophisticated treatment options. Radiology and ultrasound are particularly well suited for use in aquatic species, as are CT and MRI. They are especially valuable for evaluation of the gas bladder, investigation of internal masses, and more. Development of blood culture techniques to accurately identify bacterial agents and perform susceptibility tests before starting antibiotic therapy has been useful to decrease the need to euthanize, or surgically biopsy, an animal to achieve an accurate diagnosis. Surgical advances, including use of exploratory laparotomy and gas bladder repairs, have salvaged animals that previously would have been euthanized.

The equipment needed to treat fish in a veterinary practice is modest. In addition to equipment already on hand (eg, microscope, glass slides and cover slips, basic surgical or dissecting tools), water quality parameter testing equipment is needed (*see* AQUATIC SYSTEMS, p 1766).

TABLE 4 COMMON PARASITIC DISEASES OF SELECTED FISH FAMILIES

Parasite	Cyprinidae	Characidae
Ciliates		
"Ich"	√	√
Chilodonella		
Tetrahymena		
"Flagellates"		
Ichthyobodo	√	
Piscinoodinium	√	
Spironucleus		
Cryptobia		
Coccidia	√	
Myxozoans		√
Cestodes	√	
Monogeneans	√	√
Gyrodactylids	√	√
Ancyrocephalids		√
Dactylogyrids	√	
Nematodes		√

Note: A table cell that is not marked does not mean the parasite is not seen in that family.

In addition to these basic tools, a practice should have a few fish tanks for use as hospital systems. These can be 10- or 20-gal. tanks with simple foam filters and aeration pumps. A dechlorinator such as sodium thiosulfate should be on hand if the practice uses water that contains chlorine or chloramine. In addition, tricaine methanesulfonate (MS-222) and baking soda should be available for sedation or anesthesia. Other useful equipment includes a 1-L plastic graduated cylinder for measurement of water volume, a balance to weigh out anesthetic, and a battery-powered aeration pump if an anesthetized fish is to be moved around the clinic for radiology, surgery, or other procedures. For surgery, a 10- to 20-gal. tank works well as a receptacle. An egg crate lighting panel, or a plexiglass or plastic cover with small holes drilled in it, can be placed over the tank to allow water to flow over the fish and back to the tank. The fish can be positioned in a v-shaped foam "bed," and a small, submersible aquarium pump and flexible tubing can be used to circulate anesthetic-treated, aerated water out of the tank and over the gills. Use of equipment that can be sterilized after each patient is advantageous.

Veterinarians who offer fish medicine should be aware of evolving regulatory concerns, including the current USDA accreditation programs. In addition, aquarium fishes are susceptible to several reportable diseases, which include spring viremia of carp (*see* p 1813), koi herpesvirus (*see* p 1812), epizootic ulcerative syndrome (*see* p 1803), and red sea bream iridovirus (*see* p 1814).

FISH FAMILIES

This brief introduction to fish families is intended to provide veterinarians new to fish medicine with information on anatomy and pathogens common to those families. Fishes can be first split into two major groups: the cartilaginous fishes such as sharks and stingrays, and the bony fishes. To further divide them, bony fishes commonly kept as pets or display animals usually belong to one of the two subcohorts of Ostariophysi or Neoteleostei.

For an overview of common parasitic and viral diseases of aquarium fish, *see* TABLES 4 and 5. Susceptibility of specific families of fish to specific pathogens is implied; however, the absence of mention of a

TABLE 4 COMMON PARASITIC DISEASES OF SELECTED FISH FAMILIES *(continued)*

Loricariidae	Cichlidae	Poeciliidae	Osphronemidae
√			
√			
		√	√
	√		
	√		√
	√		
		√	
	√	√	√
√	√	√	√
	√	√	
	√	√	

TABLE 5 COMMON VIRAL DISEASES OF SELECTED FISH FAMILIES

Virus	Cyprinidae	Characidae
Rhabdovirus		
Spring viremia of carp	Koi, goldfish	
Herpesviruses		
Carp pox	Koi	
Koi herpesvirus	Koi	
Herpesviral hematopoietic necrosis	Goldfish	
Iridoviruses		
Megalocytivirus		
Lymphocystivirus		

Note: A table cell that is not marked does not mean the virus is not seen in that family.

specific pathogen does not mean that other families of fish are refractory.

Ostariophysi

Fishes that belong to this subcohort are considered to be basal fishes; this does not mean they are primitive. They have a unique chemical alarm system associated with their skin. If the epithelium is damaged, a material called schreckstoff is released by specialized club cells in the epidermis. It induces a flight response when detected by nearby related fishes. These fish also have cellular bone, which lends itself well to fracture stabilization techniques.

Ostariophysians are physostomous, which means they have a pneumatic duct that connects the anterior lobe of the gas bladder to the dorsum of the esophagus.

Another unique feature of ostariophysians is the presence of a Weberian apparatus, which amplifies sound. This apparatus consists primarily of a small series of auditory bones connected to the gas bladder.

Ostariophysi includes popular aquarium fishes that belong to the families Cyprinidae and Loricaridae and the order Characiformes.

Cyprinidae: The family Cyprinidae contains more fish species than any other family of freshwater fishes, and many are popular as pet fishes. Cyprinids have a widespread distribution, including Asia and North America. Representative cyprinids include goldfish, koi, barbs, danios, most of the freshwater sharks (eg, redtail, rainbow, and bala), and rasboras.

The primary distinguishing anatomic features of this family are the lack of a stomach and a dual-lobed gas bladder. They also often have a diffuse hepatopancreas, and the posterior kidney is usually positioned between the two lobes of the gas bladder. The absence of a stomach means attention must be given to feeding practices, and the bioavailability of some oral drugs may be lower. Cyprinids benefit from several feedings per day. Related to feeding, buoyancy control is a common problem in fancy goldfish such as orandas, ryukins, etc, due to aerophagia. This can be avoided by feeding sinking feeds.

Mycobacterial disease is a frequent problem in zebrafish (danio) research colonies but can also be seen in other cyprinids. Columnaris disease, caused by *Flavobacterium columnare*, is frequently a source of high mortality in koi and zebrafish. *Edwardsiella ictaluri* is also a problem in zebrafish.

Microsporidia (*Pseudoloma*) is a fungal parasite of concern in zebrafish.

Characiformes: The primary representatives of this order are the tetras, such as neon, cardinal, etc. Unlike the cyprinids, characins have a stomach and pyloric caeca. They usually have a single-chambered gas bladder. Although they are similar to the smaller cyprinids externally, most members of Characiformes have a small adipose fin.

Mycobacteriosis and columnaris are common bacterial diseases of characins.

Microsporidia (*Pleistophora*) is a fungal parasite of concern in tetras.

TABLE 5 COMMON VIRAL DISEASES OF SELECTED FISH FAMILIES *(continued)*

Loricariidae	Cichlidae	Poeciliidae	Osphronemidae
	√		
	√	√	√
	√		

Loricariidae: Originating from South America, this family contains the popular armored catfishes, the plecos (short for plecostomus) and the small *Otocinclus* commonly kept in planted tanks. Their scales are modified into plate-like scutes. They usually have a ventrally located mouth. Most are omnivorous, with some being herbivorous. Although some plecos such as the genus *Panaque* are said to be obligate wood-eaters in the hobby literature, some sources indicate this is not true. Accordingly, these fishes have a long intestine. Many of the plecos are able to obtain oxygen through their stomach after swallowing air at the water surface.

Callichthyidae: Another group of popular armored catfishes, including the genus *Corydoras*, belongs to this family. Like the loricariids, the scales of these fishes are modified into armor-like scutes. They have small barbels on either side of the mouth. Axillary glands are located beneath the skin of the shoulder and are the source of the venom that causes punctures by their pectoral fins to be painful. These fishes often scurry to the water surface to ingest air; oxygen is then absorbed via the intestine.

Corydoras spp appear to be very susceptible to infection with *F columnare*.

Neoteleostei

This subcohort of fish families contains the more advanced fishes. Unlike the ostariophysians, the members of this superorder do not have alarm signal cells in their epidermis. In addition, these fishes have acellular bone and lack the Weberian apparatus. Most have a single-chambered gas bladder and are physoclistous, which means the gas bladder does not have a connection to the esophagus except at hatching.

Many popular aquarium fishes belong to families in Neoteleostei, such as Cichlidae, Poeciliidae, and Osphronemidae.

Cichlidae: This large family contains many popular aquarium fishes, including the freshwater angelfish, discus, oscar, and many more. Most cichlid species originate from Central or South America or Africa. These fish are often very colorful, particularly those originating from the African Rift Lakes. Many cichlid species are aggressive and territorial, requiring substantial cover to minimize injury caused by interspecific aggression. Wild-caught Amazonian cichlids (eg, freshwater angelfish and discus) generally prefer soft water and slightly acidic environments, whereas most African Rift Lake species thrive under hard water and slightly basic conditions.

Cichlids have a single-chambered gas bladder, which often is severely reduced in riverine species from Africa.

Cichlids are usually hardy and well adapted to aquariums. Many species are prone to intestinal parasitism from the flagellate *Spironucleus*. African cichlids may be infected with *Cryptobia iubilans*, which causes a granulomatous gastritis, and some affected fish become extremely emaciated. Monogeneans are common findings on the gills of tank-raised discus.

Poeciliidae: This is another popular family of aquarium fishes, which includes guppies, swordtails, platies, and mollies. Some are euryhaline, such as the guppy and the molly, whereas the swordtail and platy are stenohaline to freshwater. These fishes are adapted to feed primarily at the water surface.

Poeciliids are susceptible to the bacterial diseases *F columnare* and epitheliocystis.

Osphronemidae: This family, which includes gourami, paradise fish, and bettas, is well-adapted to life in shallow, slow-moving to stagnant water. This group of fishes has a unique air-breathing apparatus often called a labyrinth organ that consists of plates covered in respiratory epithelium. It is located above the gills in the branchial cavity and is deliberately filled with air when these fishes rise to the air-water interface. The bulk of the oxygen required is obtained via the labyrinth organ, and if these fishes are held so they cannot reach the air-water interface, they will drown.

The endocommensal *Protoopalina* is often seen in the intestine.

These fishes are susceptible to *F columnare*.

For an overview of common parasitic and viral diseases of aquarium fish, *see* TABLES 4 and 5. Susceptibility of specific families of fish to specific pathogens is implied; however, the absence of mention of a specific pathogen does not mean that the other families of fish are refractory.

MANAGEMENT

Many management principles applied to other species are equally relevant for fish, including taking a good history, considering appropriate diagnostic techniques, and being cognizant of therapeutic options, water quality issues, and quarantine and biosecurity procedures.

Physiology

Fish are poikilothermic, and all physiologic processes are greatly influenced by water temperature. In freshwater, the internal tissues of fish are hyperosmotic to the environment, whereas in saltwater they are hypoosmotic. Surface injuries to the skin make osmoregulation more difficult and may be of serious consequence because of the loss of fluid balance and circulatory collapse.

The structure of the fish kidney varies with the species; generally it is divided into an anterior "head" kidney, which is usually located anterior to the gas bladder, and a posterior "caudal" kidney, which is retroperitoneal and ventral to the vertebral column. Hematopoietic, renal, and endocrine tissues are found in the kidney, with hematopoietic tissue located cranially and excretory tissue located caudally. Divalent ions are excreted principally via the kidney, and monovalent ions and nitrogenous excretions via the gills. Accordingly, lesions of the kidney and gills may seriously interfere with respiration, excretion, and fluid balance.

The gas bladder (also known as the swim or air bladder) in bony fish, which originates as an appendage of the foregut, regulates body buoyancy and may also be used for sound production. Physostomous fish have an open connection between the swim bladder and the GI tract, whereas physoclistous fish do not. Although a single chamber in most fish, the gas bladder consists of dual chambers in cyprinids and three chambers in cod and suckers belonging to the genus *Moxostoma*.

A sensory lateral line system along the sides of the body and head receives stimuli from the aquatic environment and mediates adaptive responses through the CNS.

Fish depend on increases in environmental temperature for efficient antibody production during infections (or after vaccinations), when most pathogens are replicating at a more rapid rate. The optimal temperature for antibody production varies with the species of fish (tropical, temperate, or coldwater). Extremes in environmental temperature (above or below that of the natural habitat) inhibit antibody production. Like T lymphocytes in other vertebrates, those in fish are responsible for cell-mediated immunity. Immunity is not as age dependent in fish as it is in other animals; young fish are usually immunocompetent and can be vaccinated successfully. Antibodies are found in the mucus of the fish skin and GI tract.

Although vaccination of fish against specific diseases has been economically important in preventing losses, there is a need for improved methodology. Advances include increased use of autogenous vaccines; several companies will work with veterinarians and their clients to develop custom vaccines for specific situations. A few vaccines (eg, for *Aeromonas salmonicida*) are available or in development for pet fish, particularly koi.

History

As with all species, a good history is critical to establish a diagnosis. Questions of particular interest for fish cases include the number of animals affected, whether one species or multiple, the chronicity of the problem, and a thorough description of animal housing and care, including the volume and design of the system (*see* AQUATIC SYSTEMS, p 1766), number and size of animals stocked, species, new additions, use of quarantine, and previous medications. Owners can be asked to bring fish and water samples into the clinic, or the practitioner may wish to visit the site. Site visits allow the system to be more accurately evaluated and the behavior of fish readily observed. If fish are brought to the clinic, the owner should provide an animal showing the signs of concern. A live animal can be transported in a cooler with a battery-powered aerator. A separate water sample should be provided in a plastic bag and transported on ice. A minimum of 1 quart of tank water should be requested for analysis. If desired for recovery after anesthetizing the animal, a larger volume of tank water may be requested. Recently deceased specimens have diagnostic value and may be submitted to the veterinary clinic, or the owner may be directed to submit these to a laboratory experienced in fish necropsy and diagnostic testing (*see* below). Water samples should be submitted with necropsy specimens.

Necropsy and Diagnostic Techniques

Although the same principles are used in necropsy of fish as in other animals, great emphasis is placed on an accurate and thorough history, premortem signs, fresh necropsy material, and direct microscopic examination of fresh tissue smears and squash preparations. Fish decompose quickly, and many saprophytic microorganisms reproduce rapidly in the decaying tissues, which complicates isolation of pathogens unless samples are collected immediately after death. A general fish necropsy may include blood collection (premortem); biopsy of gill, skin, and fin tissues; bacterial or viral culture of internal organs; and histology. A veterinary clinic or diagnostic facility familiar with fish necropsy protocols and aquatic microbiology should be used. Whenever possible, live fish should be submitted. If the fish has just died, the eyes should be clear and the gills normal in coloration and texture. There should be no "dead fish" smell; however, some moribund fishes may have a strong odor. Freshly dead fish should be placed in a sturdy plastic bag and submitted on ice. A water sample should always be submitted with the fish. An animal that has died and been placed in a freezer has limited diagnostic value, but freshly dead frozen fish may be useful for bacteriology, virology, or toxicology testing.

Fresh tissue samples of gill filaments, skin mucus, and fins should be collected, prepared as a wet mount, and examined under a light microscope at 40×, 100×, and 400×. Fresh water should be used to prepare wet mounts of external tissues from freshwater fish, and saltwater should be used to prepare wet mounts from marine fish. If uncertain, water from the tank or from the submitted water sample should be used. Ensuring that the salinity used to prepare mounts is similar to the salinity present in the environment should allow organisms to remain viable long enough for identification. Distilled water should not be used for tissue samples. Tissue should be examined for morphology and for the presence of parasites, bacteria, or fungal elements. Microscopic examination of internal organs is also recommended if the fish has been euthanized. Unstained sections of stomach and intestine should be examined for presence of parasites, and the lower intestine should be examined for flagellates. Unstained sections of spleen, anterior and posterior kidneys, and liver should be examined for presence of parasites, granulomas, or other anomalies. Wet-mount examination of fish tissues is crucial for diagnosis of most parasites.

Blood can be collected from a number of sites, and hematologic parameters measured. In fish >25–100 g, depending on species, the caudal vessels of the caudal peduncle, the duct of Cuvier (common cardinal vein), and the dorsal and ventral aortas are easily accessible. For smaller specimens that are to be euthanized, blood can be collected in a hematocrit tube immediately after euthanasia by severing the caudal peduncle and exposing the caudal vessels. Use of hematology and serum chemistry is limited, because normal values for many fish species are not readily available; however, the information may still be clinically useful. Lithium heparin is the anticoagulant of choice for most fish species, although EDTA is preferred for ictalurid catfishes, and plasma may be used for biochemistry tests. Serology may be diagnostic in certain cases (eg, heavy metal toxicity). Whole blood (1–2 drops) can be incubated in brain heart infusion broth at room temperature on an electric rotator. If cloudiness indicative of bacterial growth develops, a loop of the blood-broth mix can be used to attempt primary isolation of a systemic bacterial pathogen.

Fish should be euthanized and opened under sterile conditions. A sterile swab of posterior kidney, or other organ of interest, may be shipped to a laboratory in transport media, but primary isolation directly onto an enriched media (eg, tryptic soya agar enriched with 5% sheep blood) is preferable. Although blood agar supplemented with salt is helpful for marine fish, it is not necessary if an enriched blood agar is used. Ordal's or similar cytophaga media should be available for isolation of myxobacteria (slime bacteria, including *Flavobacterium columnare*). Sabouraud agar is an excellent all-purpose media for isolation of fungal agents. Lowenstein-Jensen or Middlebrook media is recommended for isolation of *Mycobacterium* spp. Mueller-Hinton is the media of choice for susceptibility testing of most common bacteria isolated from fish. If abscesses or other obvious anomalies are visible, those sites should also be cultured.

TABLE 6 FISH DISEASES OF REGULATORY CONCERN IN THE USA

Disease	Causative Agent	Susceptible Species
Viral hemorrhagic septicemia (Egtved disease)	*Novirhabdovirus* Family: Rhabdoviridae	Primary: salmonids (*Oncorhynchus* spp), turbo, herring and spat (*Clupea* spp), Japanese flounder Secondary: grayling, whitefish, pike, Atlantic and Pacific cod, haddock, many freshwater, marine, and estuarine species
Infectious hematopoietic necrosis	*Novirhabdovirus* Family: Rhabdoviridae	Primary: cultured salmonids (*Oncorhynchus* spp); lake trout and char (*Salvelinus* spp) are resistant
Spring viremia of carp	*Vesiculovirus* Family: Rhabdoviridae	Primary: carp (including koi, goldfish), sheatfish (European catfish), orfe, tench
Epizootic hematopoietic necrosis	*Ranavirus* Family: Iridoviridae	Primary: redfin perch Secondary: rainbow trout (wild and farmed fish)
Red sea bream iridoviral disease	*Megalocytivirus* Iridoviridae	Red sea bream, many other estuarine species, other marine species

In general, bacterial or fungal cultures taken from fish tissue should be incubated at room temperature (25°C). Some agents of concern will not grow at all at 37°C, the standard temperature for incubation of cultures taken from mammals. Agents of zoonotic concern, such as *Mycobacterium*, can be dual incubated at both 25°C and 37°C. An acid-fast stain should be available for bench-top staining of granulomatous material which, when positive, is strongly suggestive of *Mycobacterium*. If fish are seen spinning or showing other behavioral indications of neurologic disease before death, brain cultures are indicated.

If viral disease is suspected, appropriate tissues may be collected. Specimens should include both fresh tissues placed in reagent ethanol and frozen tissues. Several viral diseases are of regulatory concern to veterinarians practicing fish medicine in the USA (*see* TABLE 6).

TABLE 6 FISH DISEASES OF REGULATORY CONCERN IN THE USA *(continued)*

Clinical Signs and Pathology	Temperature Range	Status in USA
Acute form: nonspecific hemorrhaging (eyes, fins, skin), darkening, exophthalmia, ascites Chronic form: few signs Neurologic form: spinning/flashing Gross: enlarged spleen, ascites, necrotic kidney Histologic: focal necrosis of kidney liver, spleen; hemorrhage in muscle	9°–12°C (48°–54°F) optimal	Present in wild populations, sporadic, limited distribution; endemic in Pacific Northwest and Alaska (wild salmonids, haddock, and cod); emerging disease in Great Lakes region
Rapidly increasing mortality (fish <1 yr), lethargic but sporadic bursts of rapid swimming occur, protruding vent, fecal casts, exophthalmic, pale gills, darkening, abdominal distention/ascitic fluid (possibly bloody)	10°–12°C (50°–54°F) optimal; rare >15°C (59°F)	Present in western USA, sporadic, limited distribution; endemic in Pacific Northwest and Alaska (wild salmonids); also present in parts of Europe and Asia
Nonspecific: darkening, exophthalmic, pale gills, distended abdomen, ascites, hemorrhage (gills, skin, eye), petechiae in organs (including swim bladder), protruding vent with thick mucoid fecal cast Coinfection with *Aeromonas* or other bacteria common	12°–22°C (54°–72°F)	USA is free (last occurred in captive fish in 2004, wild fish in 2007); occurs in eastern Europe, Russia, China, and Middle East
Acute and high mortality of redfin perch; darkening, ataxia, lethargy, hemorrhage around nares; morbidity and mortality of rainbow trout less severe Histologic: necrosis, renal hematopoietic tissues	Redfin perch: >12°C (54°F) Rainbow trout: 11°–17°C (52°–63°F) Experimental: 8°–21°C (46°–70°F)	Has never occurred in USA; endemic in Australia
Severe anemia, lethargic, pale gills, enlarged spleen		Has never occurred in USA; occurs in Japan and Taiwan,PRC

TABLE 6 FISH DISEASES OF REGULATORY CONCERN IN THE USA *(continued)*

Disease	Causative Agent	Susceptible Species
Infection with HPR-deleted or HPR0 Infectious salmon anemia	*Isavirus* Family: Orthomyxoviridae	Atlantic salmon Brown trout, sea trout, rainbow trout
Infection with salmonid alphavirus (pancreas disease or sleeping disease)	*Alphavirus* Family: Togaviridae	Atlantic salmon, rainbow trout, brown trout
Koi herpesvirus	Herpesviridae Cyprinid herpesvirus-3	Common carp and hybrids, including koi and ghost carp
Epizootic ulcerative syndrome (mycotic granulomatosis)	*Aphanomyces invadans*	Atlantic menhaden, striped mullet, many other freshwater and estuarine species; snakeheads, barbs (*Puntias* spp) sensitive; gouramis, goldfish and other ornamentals susceptible; tilapia resistant
Gyrodactylus (*Gyrodactylus salaris* only)	Monogenea *Gyrodactylus salaris* only	Atlantic salmon, rainbow trout, brook trout, North American lake trout, brown trout, grayling arctic char

Tissue sections no larger than 1 cm^3 should be placed in 10% neutral buffered formalin for histopathology. After 24 hr of fixation, they should be removed and placed in reagent alcohol in case molecular diagnostic techniques will be required.

Therapeutic Considerations

Therapy for pet and ornamental fish is often based on environmental management followed by the use of targeted therapy to control specific pathogens. Use of prophylactic medication in the absence of diagnostic testing is strongly discouraged and may contribute to resistant bacterial infection and other complications.

Drug therapy can be provided via several routes of administration, including exposure by bath (adding medication to water), medicated feed, injection, or topical administration. Generally speaking, bath and topical treatments are most useful for external infections, whereas medicated food and injection are most appropriate for internal infections.

Using a bath treatment requires accurate measurement of the volume of water to be treated. Volume of a rectangular tank is calculated by multiplying measurements of the length, width, and depth. Volume of a circular tank is calculated by multiplying 3.14 by the radius squared by the depth. To calculate directly into liters, measurements should be in cm and multiplied by 0.001. If the measurements are made in feet, the result will be in cubic feet; cubic feet can be converted to gallons by multiplying by 7.481. If the container is oddly shaped, volume may be calculated mathematically, but it may be easier to purchase a flow meter to measure the volume required to fill the tank. Alternatively, the volume of inflowing water per minute can be measured by determining how long it takes to fill a 1-L graduated cylinder (or 5-gal. bucket). Using that information, determining how long it takes to fill a tank or ornamental pond can provide a fairly accurate assessment of volume.

Some medicated feeds can be purchased commercially for aquaculture or pet fish. Custom-made medicated feeds can be prepared for use in ornamental fish. Flake, pellet, or gel diets can be used as a base for medicated food for pet fish. Cooking oil spray is an effective binder for use with

TABLE 6 FISH DISEASES OF REGULATORY CONCERN IN THE USA *(continued)*

Clinical Signs and Pathology	Temperature Range	Status in USA
Pale gills, severe anemia (PCV <10%), swollen liver (black/brown color), ascites, petechiae of viscera, mesenteric fat, swim bladder	In vitro: Maximum replication 15°C (59°F) No replication 25°C (77°F)	Present in northeast USA, sporadic, limited distribution; endemic in Maine, New Brunswick, Scotland, and Norway
Necrosis of exocrine pancreas, heart and skeletal muscle changes	12°–15°C (54°–59°F)	Has not occurred in USA; detected in Ireland, UK, France, Germany, Italy, Spain, Switzerland, Poland, and Norway
Severe necrosis gill tissue	22°–25.5°C (72°–78°F) optimal[a]	Present in USA, sporadic, widely distributed
Necrotizing deep ulcers (penetrate body wall), granulomatous tissue response; deep ulcers with red centers, white rims; invasive nonseptate hyphae (culture possible but difficult)	<25°C (77°F) (reduced salinity also contributes in brackish systems)	Present in USA, sporadic, limited distribution
		Has never occurred in USA

[a] Mortalities stop at >30°C (86°F), but survivors remain carriers.

pelleted or flake foods for ornamental fish. The addition of medication to commercially available gel diets is easily done as the gel cools. In general, medication should not be added when the gelatin is hot, because some medications, particularly oxytetracycline, are heat labile.

Injections can be given either IM or intracoelomic (IC). IM injections are given in the epaxial muscles, lateral to the dorsal fin. Injection of some drugs can cause muscle necrosis, so it is important to alternate injection sites and to limit injections to every 3 days unless required more often. To administer IC injections, fish should be placed head downward in dorsal recumbency to move internal organs away from the injection site, which should be anterior to the anus, just off the ventral midline. Topical treatments, usually in ointment form, should be applied directly to the external lesion(s). The fish can be manually restrained, usually without removing the entire animal from the water. The area to which the treatment is applied should be held out of the water for several seconds (<1 min) to allow some absorption before returning the fish to the water. Repeated applications may be necessary.

Sunburn can occur in surface-swimming fish or can be induced (even in bottom-dwelling species) by feeding photodynamic drugs such as phenothiazine, although ultraviolet light penetrates water poorly. Affected fish will have visible lesions along the dorsal surface. Providing shade solves the problem.

FDA-approved Drugs and Regulatory Concerns: FDA-approved therapeutic options in fish are limited; however, there has been significant progress in approvals in the past few years, and this trend is expected to continue. The FDA Web site (www.fda.gov/cvm/aqualibtoc.htm) is the best resource for current information on the status of drugs and chemicals. In many cases, therapeutic management of fish other than catfish or salmonids requires extra-label use of drugs. A new mechanism called indexing is being developed by the FDA to allow for legal use of nonapproved drugs in ornamental fish. The following information is intended for use in pet fish medicine.

TABLE 7 FDA-APPROVED DRUGS FOR AQUACULTURE USE IN THE USA (2014)

Drug	Species	Indications
IMMERSION		
Formalin (Parasite-S®, Formalin-F™, Formacide-B)	All finfish	Control external protozoa (*Chilodonella, Ichthyobodo, Epistylis, Ichthyophthirius, Ambiphyra, Trichodina* spp), *Tetrahymena* spp and monogeneans (*Cleidodiscus, Dactylogyrus, Gyrodactylus* spp)
	All finfish eggs	Control fungi of the family Saprolegniaceae
	Penaeid shrimp	Control protozoan parasites (*Bodo, Epistylis*, and *Zoothamnium* spp)
	Salmon, trout, and esocid eggs	Control fungi of the family saprolegniaceae
Hydrogen peroxide (35% PEROX-AID®)	Freshwater-reared finfish eggs	Control mortality due to saprolegniasis
	Freshwater-reared salmonids	Control mortality due to bacterial gill disease (*Flavobacterium branchiophilum*)
	Freshwater-reared coolwater finfish and channel catfish	Control mortality due to external columnaris disease (*Flavobacterium columnare*)
Oxytetracycline hydrochloride (OxyMarine, Oxytetracycline HCI Soluble Powder-343®, Terramycin-343 Soluble Powder, PENNOX 343, TETROXY Aquatic)	Finfish fry and fingerlings	Mark skeletal tissues, most often otoliths, of finfish fry and fingerlings for identification purposes
Tricaine methanesulfonate (Tricaine-S®)	Fish, amphibians, and other aquatic poikilotherms	Temporary immobilization

TABLE 7 FDA-APPROVED DRUGS FOR AQUACULTURE USE IN THE USA (2014) *(continued)*

Dosage Regimen	Comments
	IMMERSION
Tanks and raceways: salmon and trout: above 50°F: up to 170 µL/L for up to 1 hr; below 50°F: up to 250 µL/L for up to 1 hr. All other finfish: up to 250 µL/L for up to 1 hr Earthen ponds: 15–25 µL/L indefinitely	Drug must not be subjected to temperature <40°F. Do not apply to ponds when water is warmer than 80°F, there is a heavy phytoplankton bloom, or dissolved oxygen is <5 mg/L. Ponds may be re-treated in 5–10 days if needed. Do not treat ponds containing striped bass. Test on a small number from each lot to check for any unusual sensitivity to formalin before proceeding.
All finfish eggs: 1,000–2,000 ppm for 15 min; Acipenseriformes: up to 1,500 ppm for 15 min	Preliminary bioassay should be conducted to determine species sensitivity.
Tanks and raceways: 50–100 µL/L for up to 4 hr daily Earthen ponds: 25 µL/L as single treatment	Drug must not be subjected to temperature <40°F. Do not apply to ponds when water is warmer than 80°F, when there is a heavy phytoplankton bloom, or when dissolved oxygen is <5 mg/L. Ponds may be re-treated in 5–10 days if needed.
1,000–2,000 ppm for 15 min	Preliminary bioassay should be conducted to determine species sensitivity.
Coldwater and coolwater: 500–1,000 mg/L for 15 min in a continuous flow system daily on consecutive or alternate days until hatch Warmwater: 750–1,000 mg/L for 15 min in a continuous flow system daily on consecutive or alternative days until hatch	Initial bioassay on a small number is recommended before treating entire group.
100 mg/L (30 min) or 50–100 mg/L (60 min) daily on alternate days for 3 treatments	Initial bioassay on a small number is recommended before treating entire group.
Fingerling and adults (except northern pike and paddlefish): 50–75 mg/L (60 min) daily on alternate days for 3 treatments Fry (except northern pike, pallid sturgeon, and paddlefish): 50 mg/L (60 min) daily on alternate days for 3 treatments	Use with caution on walleye. Initial bioassay on a small number is recommended before treating entire group.
200–700 mg oxytetracycline hydrochloride (buffered) per liter of water for 2–6 hr	
15–330 mg/L (fish) 1:1,000 to 1:20,000 (other poikilotherms)	Powder is added to water; concentration depends on desired degree of anesthesia, species, size, water temperature and softness, stage of development. Preliminary tests of solution should be made with a few fish; 21-day withdrawal time (fish); laboratory or hatchery use only in other poikilotherms; water temperature >50°F (10°C)

TABLE 7 FDA-APPROVED DRUGS FOR AQUACULTURE USE IN THE USA (2014) *(continued)*

Drug	Species	Indications
INJECTABLE		
Chorionic gonadotropin (Chorulon®)	Male and female brood finfish	Help improve spawning function
MEDICATED ARTICLE/FEED		
Florfenicol (Aquaflor®)	Freshwater-reared finfish	Control of mortality due to enteric septicemia of catfish associated with *Edwardsiella ictaluri*, streptococcal septicemia in freshwater-reared warmwater finfish, columnaris disease in freshwater-reared finfish
Oxytetracycline dihydrate (Terramycin-200® for Fish)	Pacific salmon	Mark skeletal tissue, most often otoliths, of finfish fry and fingerlings for identification purposes
	Freshwater-reared salmonids	Bacterial coldwater disease (*Flavobacterium psychrophilum*)
	Scaled warm freshwater-reared finfish	Control bacterial hemorrhagic septicemia (*Aeromonas liquefaciens*) and pseudomonas disease (*Pseudomonas*)
	Cool freshwater-reared finfish	Control bacterial hemorrhagic septicemia (*Aeromonas liquefaciens*, furunculosis (*Aeromonas salmonicida*), and pseudomonas disease (*Pseudomonas*)
	Lobster	Control gaffkemia (*Aeroccocus viridans*)
	All freshwater-reared finfish	Control of columnaris disease
Sulfadimethoxine-ormetoprim (Romet-30®)	Salmonids	Control furunculosis (*Aeromonas salmonicida*)
	Catfish	Control enteric septicemia (*Edwardsiella ictaluri*)
Sulfamerazine	Rainbow, brook, and brown trout	Control furunculosis (*Aeromonas salmonicida*)

Note: This is an abbreviated summary. For complete labeling, see the package insert. Approval applies only to the specific drug that is the subject of a new animal drug application (NADA); active ingredients from other sources (eg, a bulk drug from a chemical company or similar compounds made by companies other than those specified in the NADA) are not approved new animal drugs. Approval applies only to use of the drug for the indications and manner specified on the label.

TABLE 7 FDA-APPROVED DRUGS FOR AQUACULTURE USE IN THE USA (2014) *(continued)*

Dosage Regimen	Comments
INJECTABLE	
50–510 IU/lb males; 67–1,816 IU/lb females	IM injection up to 3 doses; total dose not to exceed 25,000 IU in fish intended for human consumption; restricted to use by or on the order of a licensed veterinarian
MEDICATED ARTICLE/FEED	
10 mg/kg/day for 10 consecutive days	Veterinary Feed Directive drug; 12-day withdrawal time
250 mg/kg/day for 4 days	Salmon <30 g; in feed as sole ration; 7-day withdrawal time
2.5–3.75 g/100 lb/day for 10 days	In mixed ration; water temperature not <48.2°F; 21-day withdrawal time
2.5–3.75 g/100 lb/day for 10 days	In mixed ration; water temperature not <62°F; 21-day withdrawal time
1 g/lb medicated feed for 5 days	In feed as sole ration; 30-day withdrawal time
50 mg/kg/day for 5 days	In feed; 42-day withdrawal time
50 mg/kg/day for 5 days	In feed; 3-day withdrawal time
10 g/100 lb/day for up to 14 days	In feed; 21-day withdrawal time; not currently available

Antibiotics: Antibiotics can be delivered to pet fish through any of the treatment routes listed; however, medicated food is most common and usually most effective. Common antibiotics used in pet or ornamental fish include oxytetracycline, potentiated sulfa drugs, and enrofloxacin (in koi and exhibit fish). For approved dosages and withdrawal times, *see* TABLE 7. Oxytetracycline (Terramycin® 200) can be fed at a dosage of 55–83 mg/kg/day for 10 days to control many gram-negative bacterial infections, including columnaris disease. Because oxytetracycline has been on the market for many years, there may be significant resistance to it in some bacterial isolates. Romet®-30 (sulfadimethoxine and ormetoprim) also is effective against many gram-negative organisms, with less resistance. Palatability can be a problem when feeding medicated food to sick fish, which may have a poor appetite.

Florfenicol is available as Aquaflor® for use in medicated feed (*see* AQUACULTURE, p 1743).

Erythromycin is not FDA approved for use in fish but is an excellent antibiotic for fish infected with gram-positive bacteria, particularly *Streptococcus*. Erythromycin can be fed at a dosage of 100 mg/kg/day, for 14 days. Palatability may be a concern with erythromycin-medicated feed. Erythromycin has been used in management of bacterial kidney disease of salmonids and streptococcal infections in food and nonfood species. FDA permission is required for use in food animals.

Delivery of antibiotics in a bath treatment is not generally recommended because of unknown or limited efficacy and damaging environmental effects (ie, antibiotics tend to kill the biofilter). Oxytetracycline (100–400 mg/L for 1 hr, daily for 10 days) has some efficacy when delivered in a bath. Oxytetracycline in a bath treatment is chelated by hard water and is therefore ineffective in marine systems. Enrofloxacin has been used as a bath at 2.5–5 mg/L for 5 hr, daily for 7 days. Water changes are recommended after the 5-hr contact time, and the drug may be chelated by hard water. Kanamycin has also been used as a bath treatment at dosages of 50–100 mg/L for 5 hr, repeated every 3 days for three treatments, with water changes recommended after the 5-hr contact time. Nephrotoxicity is a concern in fish treated with aminoglycosides. Many other options are discussed in the literature.

Injection is the most effective way to control the amount of antibiotic delivered to a fish. Enrofloxacin can be delivered IC at a dosage of 5–10 mg/kg, and the higher dosage can be repeated every third day, minimizing handling. Three treatments are generally recommended. When using enrofloxacin, the less concentrated dose (22.7 mg/mL) is recommended, even for use in large fish, because of adverse tissue reactions with the concentrated dose. If injection volume is excessive, more than one injection site can be used. Other injectable antibiotics include amikacin (5 mg/kg, IM, every 3 days for a total of three treatments). As with other aminoglycosides, nephrotoxicity may be a concern. Erythromycin (10 mg/kg/day, IM, for 3 days) can be used to treat gram-positive infections in large fish.

Use of topical ointments containing antibiotics can be practical in pet fish. Some seem to absorb fairly quickly, but if treating a substantial wound, it may be appropriate to cover it with a waterproof compound. Frequent application of antibiotic ointment (eg, twice a day) can work well to treat superficial ulcers in pet fish.

Parasiticides: Several brands of formalin (37% formaldehyde in aqueous solution, not 10% formalin used for fixation of tissues for histology) are FDA approved as parasiticides for use in finfish and penaeid (saltwater) shrimp (*see* TABLE 7). These products are usually used as a prolonged bath at concentrations of 15–25 mg/L. Vigorous aeration during formalin treatment is essential. A concentration of 25 mg/L is equal to 2 drops/gal. or 1 mL/10 gal. (useful for delivering formalin to aquarium fish).

Salt is categorized as of "low regulatory concern" by the FDA and has many uses in fish medicine, including destruction of single-celled protozoans and management of osmoregulation. Salinity is typically measured as parts per thousand (ppt) or g/L (1 ppt = 1 g/L). Seawater is typically 32–37 ppt salt. By increasing or decreasing the amount of salt to which a freshwater or marine fish is exposed, osmoregulatory stress can be minimized and many parasites eliminated. For freshwater fish, a 30 ppt dip for 0.5–10 min, depending on species, is an effective ectoparasiticide and is strongly recommended when moving fish. When fish show signs of distress, commonly manifested by rolling on their side, they should be removed from the bath. The use of salt is a quick and effective way to minimize the introduction of some protistans into a system with new fish. A solution of 5–10 ppt salt is recommended for transportation of freshwater fish; most species will tolerate this concentration for several hours or days. Permanently increasing salinity to 2–3 ppt in a freshwater system can minimize some parasitic protistans. Salt is not generally practical for use in production ponds, except for control or prevention of nitrite toxicity, because of their large volume, but it can be used in ornamental ponds that are not more than several thousand gal. Less information is available on lowering salinity for marine fish; however, freshwater dips adjusted for temperature and pH are often recommended when moving animals. Lowering salinity to 16–18 ppt can be very useful when treating some parasitic diseases, particularly *Cryptocaryon*.

In saltwater systems, copper is sometimes applied in a chelated form, because it stays in concentration longer. Chelated compounds may be difficult to use safely and require careful monitoring. Copper sulfate ($CuSO_4$) can be used to treat marine fishes, but the concentration of active copper (Cu^{2+}) must be closely monitored (test kits are available) and should be maintained at 0.18–0.2 mg/L for up to 3 wk. When using over-the-counter products in marine aquaria, label directions should be followed. Cu^{2+} concentrations should be tested at least once a day.

Copper is extremely toxic to invertebrates and plants, which must be removed before the water is treated. Finally, copper will adversely impact the nitrifying bacteria in biofilters, and a transient increase in ammonia and nitrite should be expected for weeks to months after treatment. Monitoring of ammonia and nitrite until measurable concentrations subside is recommended.

Organophosphates have been used in nonfood fish practice for decades to control monogenea, parasitic crustaceans, and leeches. Organophosphates can be used in freshwater systems, for ornamental fishes only, at concentrations of 0.25 mg/L as an indefinite bath. Most compounds are sold as 37.3% active ingredient liquid. Toxicity and efficacy are affected by pH, with more acidic pH resulting in increased toxicity. For this reason, an increased dosage may be necessary in marine systems (pH 8–8.3), with concentrations up to 1 mg/L used by some facilities. Some veterinarians add atropine (0.1 mg/kg, PO, IM, or IC) to the food of sensitive freshwater fishes and marine exhibit fish before treatment with organophosphates. Because of environmental concerns, organophosphates should not be used in outdoor ponds, unless specific provisions for such use exist in state law and are followed by the veterinarian. After treatment with organophosphates, most facilities hold water for up to 96 hr before allowing any discharge, and divers are usually restricted from entering exhibit tanks for at least 48 hr. Organophosphates may not be used in food fish in the USA.

Diflubenzuron is a chitin synthesis inhibitor effective against anchor worms (*Lernaea*), fish lice (*Argulus*), and other crustacean parasites in aquarium fish only. It is used as a prolonged bath at concentrations of 0.03 mg/L. It has a fairly long half-life (>1 wk), and treated water should be retained for 28 days and then run through a carbon filter before discharge.

Metronidazole is used to control intestinal protozoans and can be delivered in a medicated food or as a bath when fish are anorectic. Although very effective against *Spironucleus* spp, metronidazole does not seem to be effective against gastric infections with *Cryptobia iubilans*. A concentration of ~7 mg/L (~250 mg metronidazole dissolved in 10 gal. of water) can be administered daily for 5 days. A daily water change a few hours after treatment is recommended. Metronidazole can be administered in medicated feed at 50 mg/kg, PO, for 5 days. Metronidazole may not be used in food fish in the USA.

Fenbendazole has been used to control intestinal helminths in fish. A dosage of 25 mg/kg, delivered in food for 3–5 days, has been commonly recommended, but efficacy has not been evaluated in controlled trials. When fenbendazole has been used in a bath treatment, high mortality has occurred. Consequently, this use is not recommended. Levamisole administered in a bath treatment at a concentration of 2 mg/L is also used by some clinicians. These compounds may not be used in food fish in the USA.

Praziquantel is selective for flatworms, so consequently is used to control cestodes and external monogeneans. The most common use of praziquantel is as a prolonged bath in large marine aquaria for control of capsalid monogeneans. It is applied at a concentration of 5 mg/L and may remain active for several weeks. Treated water should be run through an activated carbon filter before discharge. Praziquantel can also be administered PO at a dosage of 35–125 mg/kg for up to 3 days or as a short-term bath treatment at a concentration of 10 mg/L for 3 hr. Efficacy has been demonstrated in yellowtail kingfish fed praziquantel at a dosage of 50 mg/kg/day, for 7 days. Use of praziquantel is not permitted in food fish in the USA.

Chloroquine has been used to control *Amyloodinium* spp in ornamental marine fish. It is applied as a prolonged bath at concentrations of 10 mg/L. Efficacy in recirculating systems seems to be very good; however, there are essentially no data on treatment intervals, effects on biofilters, or other basic husbandry effects. Weekly examination of fish, including biopsy of infected tissue, is recommended to assess treatment efficacy. Some aquarists have used chloroquine (10–15 mg/L for 7 days; follow-up with 10 mg/L may be required) coupled with decreased salinity (16–18 ppt) as a treatment for *Cryptocaryon* in marine fish. Results are mixed, but advantages include decreased labor, because intensive water testing is not required (as is the case for Cu^{2+}). Use of chloroquine is not permitted in food fish in the USA. Treated water should be run through a carbon filter before discharge.

Anesthetics: Tricaine methanesulfonate (MS-222) is the most commonly used anesthetic for fish. An FDA-approved product is available. MS-222 is used to sedate, anesthetize, or euthanize fish. It should always be buffered with baking soda (sodium bicarbonate) at a ratio of 2 parts baking soda to 1 part MS-222. *See also* p 1753.

Eugenol and clove oil (an over-the-counter product, usually 84% eugenol) have become popular with pet fish enthusiasts as anesthetics. These products are not FDA approved for use in fish in the USA, and use in food animals is prohibited. When eugenol at concentrations of 50, 100, and 200 mg/L was compared with MS-222 in red pacu, it resulted in effective immobilization of fish; however, there was concern about analgesia, prolonged recovery, and a narrow margin of safety, especially at higher concentrations. Use of both MS-222 and eugenol resulted in hypoxemia, hypercapnia, respiratory acidosis, and hyperglycemia in red pacu. Aqui-S® is a product approved for sedation of fish in other countries, and it is currently being investigated in the USA as an anesthetic for non-food fish. The active ingredient is isoeugenol, but evidence of carcinogenicity in laboratory animals has caused the use of this product in any food fish to be strictly prohibited. The US Fish and Wildlife Service has an active INAD program assessing the potential use of Aqui-S in non-food fish.

Euthanasia: Veterinarians should follow the AVMA Guidelines for Euthanasia of Animals (*see* p 1641). When using overdoses of MS-222 for euthanasia, the pH should be carefully ascertained before use; the sodium bicarbonate buffering can be variable because of the type of water used to make up the euthanasia solution.

Surgical Considerations

Increasingly, surgery is an option for management of some medical problems in pet or exhibit fish, including neoplastic disease, failure to ovulate (ie, "egg bound" fish), and gas bladder repair for buoyancy problems. Fish skin does not have the subcutaneous tissue that provides flexibility to domesticated animal tissue; therefore, wounds are not usually treated by surgical closure but instead allowed to heal by second intention. The clinical evaluation before surgery is similar to that in other species, although there may be more emphasis on imaging and less on blood work. Radiology and ultrasound work very well in fish, and use of these techniques before an invasive surgical procedure is recommended.

Descriptions in the literature show how a fish may be positioned for a surgical procedure. For smaller animals, such as koi, a foam "bed" is easily constructed and can be covered with something as simple as clear plastic wrap so that the fish does not lose skin, scales, or mucus from direct contact with the foam. The "bed" can be positioned over an aquarium using a plastic tray with holes to allow water drainage. A pump can move water containing an anesthetic solution (usually MS-222) from the aquarium through a small tube or catheter and across the fish's gills. Ideally, dissolved oxygen, ammonia, and pH should be monitored in the anesthetic solution. The fish can be covered with a clear plastic surgical drape (avian drapes work well), followed by fairly minimal preparation of the incision site. Plucking scales along the incision line and carefully cleaning the area with a sterile swab soaked in sterile saline may be all that is required. Very dilute disinfectants such as povidone-iodine or chlorhexidine can be used, but if the fish is clean this is probably not necessary (or recommended) because the normal mucus has significant antibacterial properties.

Absorbable sutures are generally not recommended in fish, because they may persist for significant periods of time (>1 yr in some cases). Monofilament material and a needle with a cutting edge generally work well. The simple interrupted suture pattern works well to close fish skin, but other techniques can be used successfully. Skin sutures should be removed when the incision site has healed, generally at 3–4 wk. Surgical staples have been used successfully in fish. Results using cyanoacrylate tissue adhesive have been mixed because of a significant inflammatory reaction seen in some species. If postoperative antibiotics are used, enrofloxacin delivered via IC injection at a dosage of 5 mg/kg is a good option but can only be given to non-food fish. Butorphanol given at 0.1–0.4 mg/kg, IM, and meloxicam at 0.15 mg/kg, IM, have been used for postoperative pain control in non-food fish. Increasing the salinity in freshwater systems to 1–3 ppt (g/L) is strongly recommended during the recovery and healing periods. Most freshwater fish should be able to tolerate a salinity of 3 ppt (3 g/L) on an almost indefinite basis.

Quarantine and Biosecurity

Quarantine is strongly recommended for pet fish and certainly for animals intended for display in public aquaria. A 30-day period is the minimum time for quarantine, but longer periods may be necessary. Quarantined animals should be handled only when contact with all other animals is finished for the day. Quarantined animals should have their own designated equipment (ie, nets, buckets, siphons, etc) and be kept separate from other animals. Disinfectant should be used on equipment and in footbaths at entry points to the quarantine area.

When receiving fish, a thorough history should be obtained regarding previous treatment or disease outbreaks. Fish should be examined early in the quarantine period; a visual examination may suffice, but for valuable specimens a full clinical examination, including recording the weight of the animal and completing gill, skin, and fin biopsies, is recommended. Moribund fish should be examined, and dead fish necropsied. Prophylactic use of antibiotics may be warranted in some shipments, especially recently imported marine specimens. Treatment with praziquantel for monogeneans is often prudent with marine fish as well. Goldfish commonly have significant monogenean infestations, and treatment with formalin or praziquantel may be appropriate. Koi should be quarantined to prevent introduction of koi herpesvirus (KHV), a serious and reportable disease, to established populations. Koi should be quarantined for a minimum of 30 days at a temperature of 75°F (24°C). Fish that become ill during quarantine should be tested for KHV (*see* p 1812).

Quarantine is not useful for some pathogens, but that does not mean it should not be done. Examples are mycobacteria, which at this time cannot be detected with nonlethal tests, and many viruses, microsporidia, and myxozoans. These diseases are usually detectable using necropsy techniques if quarantined animals that die are thoroughly examined. Quarantine is most useful for detection of external parasites and some internal parasites that can be detected by examination of feces.

Biosecurity for the Home Aquarium: For a modest investment, a hobbyist can set up a quarantine tank using an inexpensive 10-gal. tank, sponge filter, small aeration pump, and heater. Once fishes have cleared quarantine, the tank and equipment should be disinfected and stored dry until needed again. During the quarantine period, separate nets and siphon hoses should be used exclusively for the quarantine tank. Before purchasing new fish, the hobbyist can run the previously disinfected sponge filter in an established tank that is free of disease to inoculate the sponge with nitrifying bacteria. This practice will help avoid the common water quality problems that occur in newly set up aquaria.

Common Water Quality Problems in Hobbyist Aquaria

New tank syndrome (*see* p 1775) usually occurs within the first 6 wk after a new fish hobbyist sets up a tank. Owners may report everything was fine for several weeks, and then the fishes suddenly become lethargic, anorectic, and frequently die. Although parasites may be present in newly purchased fishes, it is critical to perform a complete analysis on a water sample from the affected tank. Often total ammonia nitrogen (TAN) or nitrite, or both, are high enough to result in toxicity. Treatment should include decrease in feeding, water changes, the addition of chloride for nitrite toxicity, and evaluation of adequate biofiltration. It can take up to 8 wk for a biofilter in a tropical fish tank to become established. New tank syndrome can be avoided by several methods. One method, known as fishless cycling, is to completely set up the tank but with no fish addition; ammonia is added to achieve a concentration of at least 1–5 mg/L. This will initiate the "cycling" process, which should be monitored by regular testing for ammonia, nitrite, and nitrate. Once no ammonia or nitrite is present, fish can be added safely. Another method is to slowly add several fish to the tank over several months, although this can result in high ammonia or nitrite levels if not done carefully.

Old tank syndrome (*see* p 1775) can occur when water changes are small and infrequent. In some cases, no water is exchanged, and the practice of "topping off" is done by adding water to the tank to replace what has evaporated. Although this can occur in any tank, it is more frequent in tanks that are inhabited by large, carnivorous fishes. These fishes eat large, high-protein meals, frequently in the form of other fish, and consequently excrete large amounts of TAN. Consequently, the biofilter uses up bicarbonate to transform TAN to nitrite and nitrate, and the bicarbonate depletion decreases total alkalinity. This results in either a gradual or dramatic drop in pH. If the former, the fishes will adapt to the slow change often with no outward sign of distress. If the pH decline is rapid, the result could be death for the resident fishes.

The water quality parameters of total hardness, nitrate, total alkalinity, and pH are often abnormal. Total hardness (TH) and nitrate are usually significantly higher than normal. TH of the tank water should be compared with TH of the water used for water changes. Total alkalinity and pH are usually significantly lower. Often TAN will be high because of inadequate bicarbonate for the nitrogen cycle. If the fish are still alive, the water quality parameters should be returned to normal by performing daily small water changes to avoid pH shock. From that point on, the tank should receive regular, large water changes to prevent a recurrence of the problem.

NUTRITIONAL DISEASES

With so many species of fishes kept in home and public aquaria, providing good nutrition is a challenge. (*See also* p 2307.) A major hurdle is that nutritional requirements are known for only a handful of fish species. Given the vast diversity in fishes, it is dangerous to assume what is good for one type of fish will be good for a similar but unrelated fish. At the basic level, it can at least be determined whether the fish is carnivorous, omnivorous, or herbivorous. However, beyond that, the amount of protein and lipids required is unknown. In general, many fishes have a higher requirement for protein than other vertebrates.

Inadequate nutrition can result in poor growth, deformities, a depressed immune system, hepatic lipidosis, and impaired metabolism. Iodine deficiency can result in thyroid hyperplasia, which has been seen in both elasmobranchs and teleosts. The condition may be caused by an overt nutritional deficiency or may be associated with chronic nitrate exposure and/or the application of ozone (*see* AQUATIC SYSTEMS, p 1766).

Hepatic lipidosis is a common problem seen in captive fishes and can occur for multiple reasons. Examples include starvation, a high percentage of carbohydrates in the diet, a high amount of lipids, and rancidity.

Fish require ascorbic acid, delivered in the feed. Most foodstuffs for fish should be supplemented with a stabilized form of ascorbic acid. Inadequate dietary vitamin C can result in a condition called "broken back disease" by some farmers and hobbyists. Severely affected fish exhibit extreme scoliosis. Less obvious, but detectable on wet mount examination (100×) of gill tissue, is "bent" or deformed cartilage, which may also indicate a history of ascorbic acid deficiency.

Feeding a wide variety of feeds is one way to try to meet the nutritional requirements. Live feeds can be varied with diverse commercially prepared feeds. This practice will also help prevent animals from eating only one type of feed. Fishes that feed at the surface should be fed feeds that float, whereas bottom-dwellers should be fed items that rapidly sink. The feed should be in particles easily ingested by the fish. Flaked feeds may be too large for a small-mouthed fish to easily ingest. Such feeds can be crushed to enable easy ingestion. In contrast, feeding

TABLE 8 PROTISTAN PARASITES OF FISHES

	Parasites	Tissue	Susceptible Species
External ciliates (motile)	*Ichthyophthirius* (FW), *Cryptocaryon* (SW)	Gills, skin, fins	All
	Trichodina (FW, SW), *Chilodonella* (FW), *Brooklynella* (SW)	Gills, skin, fins	All
	Tetrahymena (FW), *Uronema* (SW)	Skin, eye, muscle	All ("guppy killer")
External (sessile)	*Ambiphyra, Apiosoma, Epistylus*	Gills, skin, fins	Primarily pond fish
External flagellates	*Ichthyobodo, Cryptobia* (*see also* Internal flagellates)	Gills, skin, fins	All

flaked feed to a large fish like an oscar or other cichlid will result in a messy tank, because larger fish cannot easily ingest enough flaked feed to meet their requirements.

When feeding a mixed population of fishes, as is typical in hobbyist tanks, several types of feed items may be required to meet the needs of the fishes. Often, popular bottom-dwelling fishes such as loricariids and *Corydoras* catfish are expected to survive on the leftovers from the other fish. This is not an acceptable practice, and these fish should receive targeted feeding.

Another consideration is quantity of feed fed. Ideally, adult fishes should be fed 3% of their body weight daily for maintenance. Fry and fingerlings can be fed up to 5% of their body weight daily. Various types of feeds have dramatically different weights. For example, flaked feeds tend to be much lighter than pelleted feeds. Pelleted feeds come in different sizes and can be floating or sinking.

Most aquarium fishes should be fed at least daily, except for carnivorous fish that ingest large meals. These may be fed once or twice a week.

Careful attention must be paid to storage of feeds. Fish feeds usually have a high protein and oil content, which can deteriorate rapidly. Dry feeds should be kept in a pest-proof container and in an area of low humidity and temperature. High humidity and high temperature result in degradation of the diet, promotion of mold growth and potential mycotoxin production, and rancidity. Many feeds can be frozen, which will prolong their shelf-life. A feed container kept at room temperature should be discarded after 2 mo of opening. Commercial feeds stored in the freezer should be discarded after 6 mo. Commercial frozen feeds such as brine shrimp, bloodworms, mysids, glassworms, etc, should be discarded after 1 yr. If thawed, these feeds should not be refrozen.

PARASITIC DISEASES

All of the major groups of animal parasites are found in fish, and apparently healthy wild fish often carry heavy parasite burdens. Parasites with direct life cycles can be important pathogens of cultured fish; parasites with indirect life cycles frequently use fish as intermediate hosts. Knowledge of specific fish hosts greatly facilitates identification of parasites with marked host and tissue specificity, whereas others are recognized because of their common occurrence and lack of host specificity. Examination of fresh smears that contain living parasites is often diagnostic.

The most common parasites of fish are protistans (*see* TABLE 8). These include species found on external surfaces and species found in specific organs. Most protistans have direct life cycles.

Protistans Infecting Gills and Skin

Ciliates: Ciliated protozoa are among the most common external parasites of fish. Most ciliates have a simple life cycle and

TABLE 8 PROTISTAN PARASITES OF FISHES *(continued)*

Signs	Diagnosis	Treatment
White spot disease; no spots visible if on gills only	Wet mount	FW—formalin, $CuSO_4$; SW—formalin, Cu^{2+}, decreased salinity, chloroquine (efficacy not completely demonstrated)
High respiration rate, piping, excess mucus, flashing, loss of condition	Wet mount	FW—formalin, $CuSO_4$; SW—formalin, Cu^{2+}
Mucus, flashing, intra-ocular lesions, popeye	Wet mount	External as above; improve sanitation Internal: no treatment
Excess mucus, flashing, piping, loss of condition	Wet mount	Formalin, $KMnO_4$, $CuSO_4$ Management—decrease crowding, correct sanitation
Blue slime, flashing, piping, excess mucus, loss of condition	Wet mount	Formalin, $CuSO_4$, $KMnO_4$, salt

TABLE 8 PROTISTAN PARASITES OF FISHES *(continued)*

	Parasites	Tissue	Susceptible Species
External dinoflagellates	*Piscinoodinium* (FW), *Amyloodinium* (SW)	Gills, skin	Tiger barbs, many marine fishes, including clownfish and red drum
Internal flagellates	*Spironucleus*	Intestine	All cichlids, bettas, gouramis, other aquarium fishes
	Cryptobia iubilans	Stomach	African cichlids
	Trypanosoma	Blood	Wild-caught loricariids
Coccidia	Various genera	Intestine	Multiple

Note: FW = freshwater; SW = saltwater

divide by binary fission. Ciliates can be motile, attached, or found within the epithelium. The most well-known organism in the latter group is *Ichthyophthirius multifiliis*, which has a more complex life cycle than the other ciliates.

The infection caused by *I multifiliis* is referred to as "ich" or "white spot disease." *I multifiliis* is an obligate pathogen that cannot survive without the presence of living fish. All fish are susceptible, and a similar appearing parasite, *Cryptocaryon irritans*, is seen in marine species. *I multifiliis* is readily transmitted horizontally via direct exposure to infected fish or via fomites (nets, etc). Fish that survive an outbreak may be refractory in future outbreaks but may also serve as a source of infection to previously unexposed individuals. The parasite invades epithelial tissue of gills, skin, or fins, leaving a small wound and visible white spot or nodule where each parasite encysts. The organism causes substantial damage because of its unique life cycle (*see* below), which allows a rapid intensification of infection. Infected fish are extremely lethargic and covered with visible white dots. Mortality can be rapid and catastrophic. Infections confined to gill tissue may not be recognized by nonprofessionals (because white spots are not grossly visible) but are easily diagnosed using gill biopsy techniques. The organism is identified using a light microscope at magnification of 40× or 100×. It is large (0.5–1 mm), round, covered with cilia, and has a characteristic horseshoe-shaped macronucleus. Its characteristic movement varies from constantly rotating to ameboid-like.

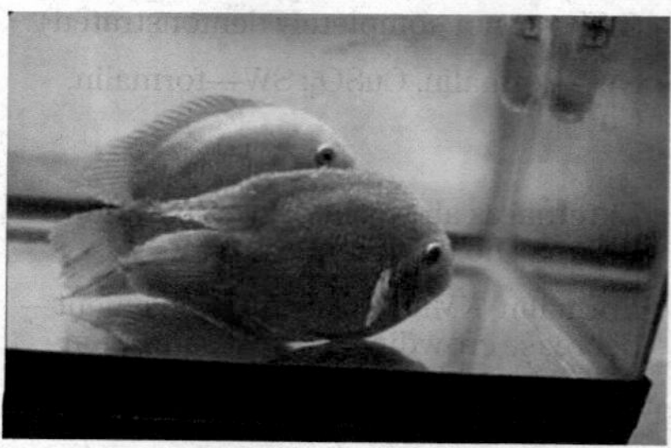

Typical white spots characteristic of "ich" on gold sevrums. *Courtesy of Dr. Ruth Francis-Floyd.*

Ich infections require immediate and thorough medical treatment. Formalin or copper are often drugs of choice. Over-the-counter medications for pet fish often contain formalin and malachite green and are effective but, because of regulatory concerns regarding the use of malachite green, should not be dispensed by the veterinarian. Multiple chemical treatments (with intervals determined by water temperature) are required for successful treatment of *I multifiliis*. At warm temperatures typical of home aquaria (eg, >26°C), infected fish should be treated every 2–3 days. Constant chemical exposure for at least 3 wk is generally recommended to control *Cryptocaryon* in marine systems; lowering salinity to 16–18 ppt is often helpful.

I multifiliis has a direct life cycle but has massive reproductive potential from each adult parasite. Adults leave the fish host and encyst in the environment, releasing hundreds of immature parasites (tomites) that must find a host within a specific time frame (days for warmwater fish, weeks for

TABLE 8 PROTISTAN PARASITES OF FISHES *(continued)*

Signs	Diagnosis	Treatment
Mortality, lethargy, piping; "velvet" (if on skin)	Wet mount	Copper sulfate, chloroquine (nonfood fish only); freshwater dips for marine food fish
Weight loss (anorexia), mortality of fry and juveniles	Wet mount	Metronidazole (nonfood fish only)
Extreme weight loss, anorexia	Wet mount, histology	None; management—correct sanitation, feeding, stocking density, cull affected fish
Anemia, mortality	Wet mount	
Weight loss, mortality	Histology	Sulfamethazine (efficacy questionable)

coldwater fish), determined by water temperature. For this reason, leaving a system fallow is one way to prevent reinfection. While encysted, parasitic life stages are refractory to chemical treatment, but cysts can be removed by thorough cleaning and removal of debris from gravel substrates.

Two important groups of ciliates are motile and move on the surface of skin and gills of fish: *Chilodonella* spp (which has a marine counterpart, *Brooklynella* spp) and the trichodinids, which are found on both freshwater and marine fish. Fish with chilodonelliasis typically lose condition, and copious mucous secretions may be noticed in areas where infestation is most severe. If gills are heavily infested, the fish may show signs of respiratory distress, including rapid breathing and coughing. The gills may be visibly swollen and mucoid. Infected fish may be irritated as evidenced by flashing (scratching) and decreased appetite. *Chilodonella* can be easily identified from fresh biopsies of infected tissues. They are 0.5–0.7 mm, are somewhat heart-shaped with parallel bands of cilia, and move in a characteristic slow spiral. *See* TABLE 8 for treatment.

Several genera of peritrichous ciliates have been grouped together and are collectively referred to as the trichodinids. These include *Trichodina*, *Trichodinella*, *Tripartiella*, and *Vauchomia* spp. Clinical signs associated with trichodinid infestation are similar to those of chilodonelliasis, although secretion of mucus is not usually as noticeable. Trichodinids are easily identified from biopsies of infected gill or skin tissue. They are readily visible using a light microscope at 40×–100×. Trichodinids move along the surface of infested tissue and appear as little saucers or, from a lateral view, as little bubbles. The body of the organism may be cylindrical, hemispherical, or discoid. Trichodinids are characterized by an attaching disc with a corona of denticles on the adoral sucker surface. For treatment of trichodinids, *see* TABLE 8. Infestations of *Trichodina* often indicate poor sanitation and/or overcrowding, so chemical treatment alone may not be adequate for complete control.

Tetrahymena corlissi, another ciliate, may be motile and surface dwelling but is also occasionally found within tissue, including skeletal muscle and ocular fluids. Somewhat similar to *Tetrahymena* are the scuticociliates that affect marine fishes. *Uronema* and *Miamiensis*, like *Tetrahymena*, are teardrop-shaped ciliates that, although primarily found on external tissues, can be very invasive. *Tetrahymena* spp are pear-shaped and 10–20 μm long, with longitudinal rows of cilia and inconspicuous cytostomes. External infestations of *Tetrahymena* spp are not uncommon on moribund fish removed from the bottom of a tank or aquarium and are often associated with an environment rich in organic material. As long as *Tetrahymena* spp are restricted to the external surface of the fish, they are easily eliminated with chemical treatment and sanitation. When they become established internally, they are not treatable and can cause significant mortality. Fish with intraocular infections of *Tetrahymena* spp develop extreme exophthalmos. The parasite is readily identified by examining ocular fluids with a light microscope.

Ambiphyra, *Apiosoma*, and *Epistylis* spp are sessile peritrichs that do not feed on the fish host; instead, they attach to the fish, which is often debilitated, and use their cilia to filter and ingest bacteria and small microorganisms in the water column. When seen in low numbers, they cause little harm; however, in high numbers they can cause irritation. Their presence on a fish usually indicates a rich, organic environment. Often, just performing large water changes will diminish the population. Salt can also be used to help control the numbers. *Ambiphyra* and *Apiosoma* are solitary but can be seen in large groups on a heavily infested fish. *Epistylis*, *Vorticella*, and *Carchesium* are colonial stalked peritrichs.

Flagellates: *Ichthyobodo* spp are some of the most common and smallest (~15 × 5 μm) flagellated protistan parasites of the skin and gills. A kinetoplastid protist, they are flattened, pear-shaped organisms with two flagella of unequal lengths. These parasites can be found on freshwater or marine fish from a broad geographic range. Ichthyobodo move in a jerky, spiral pattern, and free-swimming organisms are fairly easy to identify in direct smear preparations. Once attached, the organism can be difficult to see, but movement typical of a flickering flame may be seen under 400× and is characteristic. Affected skin often has a steel-gray discoloration due to copious mucus production ("blue slime disease"), and gills may appear swollen. Behavioral signs of infestation include lethargy, anorexia, piping, and flashing. *Ichthyobodo* is readily controlled with salt, formalin, copper sulfate, or potassium permanganate baths. Because the parasite has a direct life cycle, a single treatment should be adequate. If reinfestation occurs, sanitation and quarantine practices should be evaluated.

One of the most serious health problems of captive marine fish is the parasitic dinoflagellate *Amyloodinium* spp. Its freshwater counterpart, *Piscinoodinium* spp, is less common but can also result in high mortality. These parasites produce a disease that has been called "velvet," "rust," "gold-dust," and "coral disease" because of the brownish gold color they impart to infected fish. The pathogenic stages of the organism are pigmented, photosynthetic, nonflagellated, nonmotile algae that attach to and invade the skin and gills during their parasitic existence. When mature, these parasites give rise to cysts that contain numerous flagellated, small, free-swimming stages that can initiate new infections. Control of *Amyloodinium* is challenging, and the prognosis is guarded. Copper sulfate is the only therapeutic option for food animals in the USA, and repeated treatments are necessary to break the life cycle. The disease is particularly problematic in clownfish. The treatment of choice in ornamental fish is chloroquine, delivered at 10 mg/L as an indefinite bath.

Oomycota: Although the oomycetes (water molds) share some morphologic traits with the true fungi, they are more closely related to diatoms, opalinids, and

TABLE 9 COMMON METAZOAN PARASITES OF FISHES

	Parasites	Tissue	Susceptible Species
Myxozoans (IH)	*Myxosoma cerebralis* (whirling disease)	Head, cartilage, backbone	Rainbow trout, salmonids
	Ceratomyxa shasta	Posterior intestine	Salmonids (Pacific NW)
	Aurantiactinomyxon ictaluri (PGD, HGD)	Gill	Channel catfish
	Henneguya	Gill	Channel catfish, other
	Sphaerospora auratus (renal dropsy)	Kidney	Goldfish (pond-reared)
	Proliferative kidney disease	Kidney	Rainbow trout, all salmonids
Monogeneans	*Gyrodactylus* (live bearer, except in Loricaridae)	Skin, fins	Goldfish, koi (predisposed)

labyrinthulomycetes. Of the many genera of water molds, *Saprolegnia* and *Aphanomyces* are the most frequently associated with disease in freshwater fishes. These primarily saprophytic organisms are common to freshwater fish around the world. *Saprolegnia* commonly infects fish eggs and traumatized external tissues of live fishes. Gross signs are grayish white, cotton-like growths on the skin, gills, eyes, or fins that may invade deeper tissues of the body. Fishes exposed to water temperatures below their optimal range are especially susceptible to *Saprolegnia* infection. Microscopically, saprolegniasis can be recognized by making direct smears from the infected tissues and observing the large nonseptate filaments. The sexual stages of the organism can be seen only in cultures of the organism and are required for specific identification. Sabaroud's dextrose agar is acceptable for primary isolation of oomycetes, including the genus *Saprolegnia*. Preventive measures include removal of predisposing causes, eg, improper temperature, inadequate sanitation, excessive chemical treatment, or the presence of dead, infected fish and decaying organic material. If the environment is clean, the temperature is appropriate for the species, and skin pathogens have been eliminated, a single treatment with potassium permanganate, formalin, or hydrogen peroxide is often adequate to control external saprolegniasis. There are some effective over-the-counter products sold through the pet trade that contain malachite green. These dilute solutions should be effective in the home aquarium but should not be dispensed by the veterinarian and should never be used on food animals. Use in zoologic collections is also discouraged.

Epizootic ulcerative syndrome (EUS), caused by *Aphanomyces invadans*, is a reportable disease and endemic to much of the USA.

Internal Protistan Parasites

Flagellates: *Spironucleus* spp are common, small (~9 µm), bilaterally symmetric, flagellated (four pairs) diplomonad protists most frequently found in the intestinal tract of finfish. Among ornamental fishes, the cichlids are highly susceptible. However, they are also frequently seen in the intestinal tract of gourami and some catfishes. Pathogenicity of these organisms is variable and correlated with the number present. If there is a loss of condition, or >15 organisms are seen per low-power field on wet mounts of intestinal tissue or contents, then treatment is strongly recommended. The only treatment available for spironucleosis is metronidazole (use only in ornamental species), which should be given orally but can be administered as a bath if fish are anorectic. Chronic infections have been seen in fish maintained in unsanitary or crowded conditions.

Cryptobia and *Trypanosoma* spp are slender, elongated (6–20 µm), actively

TABLE 9 COMMON METAZOAN PARASITES OF FISHES *(continued)*

Signs	Diagnosis	Treatment
Blacktail, skeletal deformity	Histology, isolation of parasite	None; regulatory concern
Weight loss, distended and hemorrhagic vent	Wet mount, histology	None; regulatory concern
Mortality, piping	Wet mount, histology	None
None, severe hypoxia	Wet mount	None
Mortality, severely enlarged and cystic kidney	Histology	None
Lethargy, darkening, fluid accumulation, exophthalmia	Wet mount, histology	None
Excess mucus, flashing, weight loss	Wet mount	Praziquantel in nonfood fishes, formalin

TABLE 9 COMMON METAZOAN PARASITES OF FISHES *(continued)*

	Parasites	Tissue	Susceptible Species
	Family: Ancyrocephalidae Family: Dactylogyridae (egg layers)	Gills	Goldfish, koi, angelfish, discus (predisposed), channel catfish
	Capsalids; *Benedenia*, *Neobenedenia* (egg layer)	Cornea, gills, skin	Marine tropicals, other marine species, marine angelfish (predisposed)
	Polyopisthocotylea	Gill	Striped bass
Trematodes (IH usually mollusc)	Heterophyidae	Gill	Redtail shark, black shark, rainbow shark, angelfish (FW), other pond-reared fish, aquarium fish
	Clinostomum	Skeletal muscle	Largemouth bass, centrarchids, hybrid striped bass
	Bolbophorus confusus	Skeletal muscle, viscera	Channel catfish
	Posthodiplostomum	Viscera, heart, posterior kidney	Largemouth bass, bluegill, centrachids, salmonids, other fish
	Diplostomum	Eye (lens)	Fish are IH (unspecified species)
Cestodes	*Diphyllobothrium latum*	Viscera, musculature	Salmonids, other FW species
	Corallobothrium	Intestine (adult)	Channel catfish
	Proteocephalus ambloplitis	Ovary (larval stage)	Largemouth bass
	Bothriocephalus acheilognathi	Intestine (adult)	Carp, aquarium fish
Acanthocephalids	*Acanthocephalus*	Intestine	Wild-caught salmonids, wild-caught marine fish
Nematodes (fish as DH)	*Capillaria*	Intestine	Angelfish, discus, other aquarium fish
	Camillanus	Posterior intestine	Largemouth bass, other centrarchids
	Philometra	Posterior intestine	Aquarium fish
Nematodes (fish as IH)	*Eustrongylides*	Encysted in coelom	Angelfish, other aquarium species
	Contracaecum	Encysted in viscera	Largemouth bass, centrarchids
Leeches	Leech	Skin	FW game fish, aquarium fish

Note: FW = freshwater; IH = intermediate host; DH = direct host; $KMnO_4$ = potassium permanganate

TABLE 9 COMMON METAZOAN PARASITES OF FISHES *(continued)*

Signs	Diagnosis	Treatment
Piping, coughing, weight loss, skin lesions	Wet mount	Praziquantel in nonfood fishes, formalin
Eye lesions, flashing, weight loss, mortality	Wet mount	Praziquantel in nonfood fishes, formalin
Pale gills, piping, mortality	Wet mount	Praziquantel in nonfood fishes, formalin
Flared gills, hypoxia, piping, do not tolerate shipping and handling	Wet mount	
Yellow grub	Direct visualization, wet mount	
None	Direct visualization, wet mount	
None	Direct visualization, wet mount	None
Cataracts, blindness	Direct visualization, histology	None
Adhesions, sterility (if gonads affected)	Direct visualization, wet mount	Praziquantel in nonfood fishes
None	Direct visualization, wet mount	Praziquantel in nonfood fishes
Sterility	Direct visualization, wet mount	Praziquantel in nonfood fishes
Weight loss, enteritis, mortality	Direct visualization	Praziquantel in nonfood fishes
Enteritis, mortality	Direct visualization	
Weight loss, pot belly	Direct visualization, wet mount	Fenbendazole, levamisole
Visualize worms protruding from anus	Direct visualization	Fenbendazole, levamisole
Visualize worms protruding from anus	Direct visualization	Fenbendazole, levamisole
Weight loss, pot belly	Direct visualization	
Often none	Direct visualization	
Anemia, weight loss	Direct visualization	None

motile, biflagellated kinetoplastid protistans easily detected in fresh blood and tissue smears of both marine and freshwater finfish. Hematozoic forms are generally described as *Trypanosoma* and have a well-developed undulating membrane. Trypanosomes can be transmitted by leeches and have been associated with anemia in blue-eyed plecostomus *Panaque suttoni* and other wild-caught loricariids. *Cryptobia iubilans* has been associated with granulomatous disease in African cichlids and discus. Clinical disease is manifest by severe weight loss and cachexia. Clinically affected fish should be culled. Presumptive diagnosis can be made from microscopic examination of fresh tissue. Typically, granulomas will be found in the stomach, which may be visibly thickened. Acid-fast positive material will not be found in granulomas caused by *Cryptobia*. Motile flagellates may be visible using magnification of 400× or greater.

Sporozoans: Coccidiosis, although common in freshwater or marine finfish, is rarely diagnosed in live fish. Many species of finfish are affected. Species of the genera *Cryptosporidium*, *Eimeria*, and *Goussia* have been frequently reported in both freshwater and marine fishes. The life cycles of many fish coccidia are unknown, and some involve more than one host to complete their development. In addition to intestinal infection, the internal organs may be affected; sporulated *Eimeria*-like oocysts and sexual and asexual stages can be found in direct smears and histologic sections of the internal organs.

A number of *Eimeria* species are found in skates and rays. Of these, *E southwelli* has caused high mortality in cownose rays (*Rhinoptera bonasus*), although it has been reported in other species of rays. Infected cownose rays often present with pale skin and loss of weight despite normal appetite. Fluid obtained by aspiration of the coelomic cavity should be examined for presence of coccidia. Treatment with toltrazuril 10 mg/kg/day, PO, for 5 days may help control but not eliminate infection. This parasite is highly prevalent in wild-caught cownose rays.

Heavy intestinal infection of *Goussia* spp has been associated with high mortality in comet goldfish (*Carassius auratus*). Affected fish are lethargic, frequently lay on their side, and have pale feces. Clumps of cells in the intestine can be visualized on a wet mount, but histopathology is required for diagnosis.

Sulfamethazine, at 22–24 g/100 kg of fish wt/day in the feed for 50 days at 50°F (10°C), is used to treat food fish (21-day withdrawal time) in some countries. An FDA-approved form of this drug is not currently available in the USA. For aquarium fish, 10 ppm sulfamethazine in the aquarium water once a week for 2–3 wk has been reported to be preventive, but safety and efficacy data are sparse.

Metazoan Parasites

Metazoan parasites include the myxozoans, helminths, and crustaceans, and are common in both wild and cultured fish (*see* TABLE 9). Fish frequently serve as intermediate or transport hosts for larval parasites of many animals, including people. Helminths with direct life cycles are most important in dense populations, and heavy parasite burdens are sometimes found. In general, heavy parasite burdens seem to be more common in fish originating from wild sources.

Myxozoans: Although originally thought to be single-celled organisms, myxozoans are multicellular and closely related to Cnidaria. They are common fish parasites and have life cycles that use invertebrates as definitive hosts and fishes for multiplication. Hence, myxozoan infections are often more common in wild fish or fish reared intensively in outdoor fish ponds. The organisms tend to be host- and tissue-specific. Accordingly, expression of the disease is related to the specific pathogen and host and location within the host. For example, coelozoic myxozoans that reside in cavities typically cause little pathology, unlike the histozoic forms that reside in tissues. Myxozoan-infected fish in captive display aquaria are not able to transmit the infection unless the necessary intermediate hosts are present.

Myxozoans are divided into two groups, Myxosporea and Malacosporea, and members of both groups are infective to fishes. Although a few cases of direct life cycle have been reported, myxosporeans usually have an indirect life cycle, with oligochaete or polychaete worms used as a definitive host. In contrast, bryozoans are used as a definitive host by the malacosporeans.

There are two important myxosporean infections of ornamental fish. "Renal dropsy of goldfish" is caused by the myxosporean *Sphaerospora auratus*. The disease is characterized by renal degeneration and ascites and is usually diagnosed by identification of spores in histologic sections of the kidney. Affected fish present with extreme abdominal distention but may have few other clinical signs. Radiographs may reveal a mass in the area of the posterior kidney; definitive diagnosis is made at necropsy and confirmed histologically. No practical treatment is available. *Henneguya*, a myxosporean occasionally found in ornamental fish, causes white nodular lesions that are usually found in gill tissue and may be grossly visible. *Henneguya* is easily identified by the forked-tail appendage of the spore, seen microscopically. If ponds are dried and limed heavily, infection can be eliminated, apparently by reduction of the intermediate hosts. Aquarium infection can be self-limiting in the absence of intermediate hosts. Although an occasional cyst may be considered an incidental finding, severe damage has been associated with diffuse distribution of interlamellar cysts.

Myxosporean diseases significant in aquaculture include whirling disease and proliferative kidney disease of salmonids and proliferative gill disease ("hamburger gill disease") of channel catfish. Whirling disease is caused by *Myxobolus cerebralis*. Fish are infected as fingerlings when the parasite infects cartilage in the vertebral column and skull, resulting in visible skeletal deformities. Affected fingerlings typically show rapid tail-chasing behavior (whirling) when startled. The disease is also sometimes called "blacktail," because the peduncle and tail may darken significantly. Recovered fish remain carriers. Adults do not show behavioral signs, but skeletal deformities associated with infection do not resolve. Whirling disease can be prevented by purchasing uninfected breeding stock and maintaining them in an environment free of the definitive hosts (tubeficid worms). A presumptive diagnosis of whirling disease is made by detection of spores from skulls of infected fish. Diagnosis may be confirmed histologically or serologically. Whirling disease is of regulatory concern in some states.

Monogeneans: Monogeneans have direct life cycles and are common, highly pathogenic, and obligatory parasites most commonly seen on skin and gills. The preferential location of some species is in internal organs such as the esophagus, stomach, posterior kidney, or urinary bladder. Freshwater parasites tend to be ~0.1–0.8 mm long and are best seen microscopically; however, several important species parasitizing marine fish are significantly larger and may be visible grossly. The worms can be identified by their characteristic hold-fast organ, the haptor, which is armed with large and small hooks. Aquarium and cultured fish are subject to a rapid buildup of parasites by continual infection and worm transfer to other fish in the tank or pond. Although many species are host specific, the more common types seen in aquaria are less selective. The two most common monogeneans in freshwater aquaria are gyrodactylids and ancyrocephalids. *Gyrodactylus*, a common parasite of many ornamental fishes, primarily gives birth to live young and is usually found on skin; the ancyrocephalids lay eggs and parasitize the gills. Dactylogyrids are egg-laying gill monogeneans commonly seen in cyprinid fishes, especially goldfish and koi. High numbers of any of these monogeneans can result in catastrophic mortality of infested fishes.

The capsalids are a large group of monogeneans that affect brackish and marine fishes and include the genera *Neobenedenia* and *Benedenia*, which are important monogeneans in marine fishes. They attach and graze on skin and gill and the cornea. The capsalids lay sticky eggs easily transmitted via fomites. Monogenean-infected fish may show behavioral signs of irritation, including flashing and rubbing the sides of their bodies against objects in the aquarium. Fish become pale as colors fade. They breathe rapidly and distend their gill covers, exposing swollen, pale gills. Localized skin lesions appear with scattered hemorrhages and ulcerations. Ulceration of the cornea may become evident if the eyes are involved. Mortality may be high or chronic.

Praziquantel (5 mg/L, prolonged bath) is the treatment of choice for monogenean infection in freshwater and marine ornamental fish. Formalin is the only treatment option for food fish. When using formalin, multiple treatments at weekly intervals are recommended for egg-laying monogeneans, because eggs are resistant to chemical treatment. Organophosphates (0.25 mg/L, prolonged bath) have been used successfully in ornamental fish in the past, but treatment with praziquantel is considered more effective. Organophosphates should be avoided in systems containing elasmobranchs and some characins and cichlids. Many monogeneans on marine fish can be partially removed using freshwater dips for 1–5 min, depending on the tolerance of the species; however, eggs will not be damaged or removed. To prevent the disease, introduction of infected fish should be avoided.

Trematodes: Trematodes belong to the phylum Platyhelminthes, and this class contains two subclasses, Aspidogastrea and Digenea, both of which contain members that infect fishes. Also known as flukes, this group of flatworms has a complex life cycle that includes a variety of host animals, typically beginning with a mollusc. Fishes can be a second intermediate or final host, depending on the requirements of the trematode species. Although adults may be found in the intestine of infected fish, it is more common to see the metacercarial stage in fishes. This stage is usually considered to cause little harm to the host but much depends on the site of encystment. For example, large numbers of metacercariae encysted in gill tissue can be detrimental to normal function.

Nematodes: Nematodes are common in wild fish exposed to the intermediate hosts. Fish may be definitive hosts for adult nematodes, or they may act as transport or intermediate hosts for larval nematode forms (anisakids, eustrongylids, and others) that infect higher vertebrate predators, including people. Encysted or free nematodes can be found in almost any tissue or body cavity of fish. Aquarium and cultured pond fish may be heavily infected if crustacean intermediate hosts are present. *Cyclops* and *Daphnia* spp are common intermediate hosts for *Philometra* sp, a nematode that is pathogenic for guppies and other aquarium fish. These blood-red worms can be seen in the swollen abdominal cavity and protruding from the anus of affected fish (red worm disease). *Capillaria* spp are commonly found in aquarium fish, particularly freshwater angelfish. Heavy infections in juvenile angelfish have been associated with poor growth rates and an inability to withstand shipping and handling. Treatment with fenbendazole (25 mg/kg for 3 days) is recommended, but efficacy has not been firmly established. Levamisole (10 mg/L) administered as a bath treatment for 3 days has also been recommended.

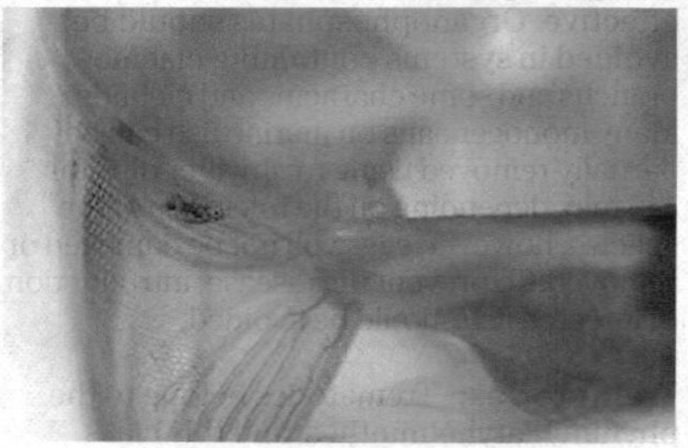

Small, gray speckled fish louse (*Argulus* spp) attached to the tail fin of a fancy goldfish. *Courtesy of Dr. Louise Bauck.*

Ivermectin can be highly toxic to aquarium fish, particularly cichlids, and its use is discouraged.

Leeches: Leeches are parasitic bloodsuckers of fish and also serve as vectors for blood parasites of fish (eg, *Trypanosoma*, *Cryptobia*, and haemogregarines). They can produce a debilitating anemia due to chronic blood loss and disease. Leech infestations are most common in wild fish, but aquarium and pond infestations can occur by introduction of infested fish, plants, etc. Heavily infested fishes have been observed to swim primarily at the water surface, often with their dorsum exposed. Fishes exhibiting this behavior also suffer from ulcerative lesions of the exposed skin. Organophosphates (0.25 mg/L, prolonged bath) are somewhat effective but not approved for use in food fish. Further, environmental regulations may restrict use in outdoor ponds. Multiple treatments may be required to control leeches, because eggs are resilient and juveniles may continue to hatch. Preventive measures include avoiding leeches (ie, effective quarantine). Infestations in recreational fishing ponds are often self-limiting.

Crustaceans: Parasitic crustaceans include copepods and branchiurans. Some copepods, such as the anchor worm, are obligatory parasites of finfish during specific stages of their complicated life cycle. They lose their copepod form, including their appendages, and become rod- or sac-like structures specifically adapted for piercing, holding, feeding, and reproducing. Grossly, they appear as barb-like attachments to the skin or gills, where they feed on blood and tissue fluids. They can cause hemorrhage, anemia, and tissue destruction, as well as provide a portal of entry for other pathogens. Many different species of these parasites can be found on freshwater and marine fish. The anchor worms, *Lernaea* spp, are commonly found in a wide variety of aquarium- and pond-reared fish, including goldfish and other cyprinids. *Ergasilus* spp infest the gills.

The branchiurans, often called lice, have flattened bodies adapted for rapid movement over the skin surface. By means of hooks and suckers, they periodically attach for feeding by inserting the piercing mouth part (stylet) into the skin. Sea lice (*Lepeophtheirus salmonis*) are a significant disease problem of pen-reared salmonids. Consultation with a salmonid health specialist is suggested if these parasites are encountered, because treatment options are limited and environmental concerns are significant. *Argulus* spp are commonly found on aquarium, pond-reared, and wild freshwater fish.

As a chitin synthesis inhibitor, diflubenzuron is the most effective treatment for crustacean parasites. It is applied once at the rate of 0.03 mg/L and has a long half-life. Because of this and the toxicity of diflubenzuron to all crustaceans, treated water must be retained for 28 days before release. Organophosphates are somewhat effective in controlling crustacean parasites, but legal restrictions constrain clinical use (*see* p 3064). Some success has been achieved in treating freshwater fish for parasitic copepods by giving infected fish a 3% (30 ppt = 30 g/L) salt dip (<10 min, remove fish when it rolls) followed by 5 ppt (5 g/L) salt added to the affected tank for 3 wk. The increased salinity kills immature forms as they hatch. Diflubenzuron and organophosphates are not approved for use in food fishes.

BACTERIAL DISEASES

Epidemics of bacterial diseases are common in dense populations of cultured food or aquarium fish. Predisposition to such outbreaks frequently is associated with poor water quality, organic loading of the aquatic environment, handling and transport of fish, marked temperature changes, hypoxia, or other stressful conditions. Most bacterial pathogens of fish are aerobic, gram-negative rods. Diagnosis is by isolation of the organism in pure culture from infected tissues and identification of the bacterial agent. Sensitivity testing before antibiotic use is recommended.

Aeromonas, Pseudomonas, and Vibriosis: A number of bacteria produce a similar syndrome, generically referred to as **hemorrhagic septicemia** and characterized by external reddening and hemorrhage in the peritoneum, body wall, and viscera. Morbidity and mortality are highly variable, depending on predisposing conditions such as low dissolved oxygen, other water quality problems, handling stress, or trauma. Ulcerative lesions are common as disease progresses, and mortality can be significant if stress is not controlled. Antibiotic therapy is recommended if fish are dying. Common bacterial isolates from affected fish include *Aeromonas* and *Pseudomonas* spp, which are more common in freshwater animals, and *Vibrio* spp, more commonly isolated from marine fishes. Control is based on removal of predisposing factors. If antibiotic therapy is warranted, drug selection should be based on sensitivity testing when possible.

Aeromonas salmonicida, a gram-negative, nonmotile rod, is the causative agent of **goldfish ulcer disease** and **furunculosis** in salmonids and is a very important disease of koi and goldfish. The disease also occurs in freshwater and marine species other than the groups mentioned above. In the acute form, hemorrhages are found in the fins, tail, muscles, gills, and internal organs. In more chronic forms, focal areas of swelling, hemorrhage, and tissue necrosis develop in the muscles. These lesions progress to deep crateriform abscesses that discharge from the skin surface. Liquefactive necrosis develops in the spleen and kidney. Diagnosis is made by isolating and identifying a pure culture of the organism from infected tissue. Avoidance through use of good quarantine practices, and vaccination when appropriate, is preferable to treatment. Successful treatment is possible, based on appropriate antibiotic therapy. Blood culture is an effective and nonlethal method for effective identification and sensitivity testing of *A salmonicida* isolates from valuable koi. Commercial vaccines are available for prevention of *A salmonicida* in salmonids and koi, but information on efficacy in koi is limited.

Vibriosis is a potentially serious, common systemic disease of many cultured, aquarium, and wild marine and estuarine fishes; it is less common in freshwater fish. Three genera of the family Vibrionaceae are frequently associated with infection in fishes: *Vibrio*, *Listonella*, and *Photobacterium*. These genera can result in hemorrhages and ulcerations of the skin, fin, and tail; hemorrhagic and degenerative changes of internal organs; and other systemic changes. Diagnosis requires identification of pure isolates from infected tissues. Isolation of *V cholerae* from fish is not uncommon and should not cause alarm as long as the isolate is the non-O type. Preventive measures include minimizing stress and crowding. Coldwater vibriosis (Hitra disease), a serious problem in sea farming of salmonids, is characterized by high mortality, resistance to drug therapy, and stress mediation. The etiologic agent is *Aliivibrio salmonicida*. Because members of this family are ubiquitous in marine environments, avoidance is difficult. Preventive vaccination with formalin-killed *Vibrio* is used in the salmonid industry. Antibiotic therapy should be based on results of sensitivity testing.

Edwardsiella: *Edwardsiella ictaluri* is commonly associated with disease in channel catfish; however, it is also responsible for high mortality in zebrafish, both in research laboratories and aquarium fish. It is an obligate pathogen and can be transmitted by direct contact with infected fish, water, and feces. Clinical signs of disease in infected zebrafish include hemorrhaging in the skin, pale gills, lethargy, and splenomegaly. On histopathology, bacteria frequently can be found in high numbers in spleen, anterior and posterior kidneys, nares, and forebrain. It can be isolated on standard culture media, but it is slow-growing. Coinfections with *Aeromonas* spp are common; *Aeromonas* spp are fast growers and can easily overgrow *E ictaluri*.

Although more commonly reported in aquacultured fish species, **epitheliocystis** is seen in aquarium fishes and is frequently seen in discus (*Symphysodon* spp), oscar (*Astronotus ocellatus*), and occasionally other pet fishes. Epitheliocystis is caused by an obligate intracellular bacteria in the order Chlamydiales. Infection most frequently involves the gills and occasionally the skin. Infections are more common in freshwater-reared fish species. Epitheliocystis should be suspected if colorless spherical structures (infected, hypertrophied cells) that have granular contents are seen on gill biopsy or skin scraping. Histopathologic examination typically reveals basophilic hypertrophied cells. Clinical signs are variable and depend on severity of infection. Heavily infected fish may be lethargic and dyspneic. Oral oxytetracycline has been used to successfully control infections.

Flavobacterium: *Flavobacterium columnare*, the member of this group responsible for **columnaris disease**, is most common in warmwater species of fish. A presumptive diagnosis can be made from visualization of typical organisms on wet mounts of infected skin or gill tissue. There are several strains of this bacterium, which range from low to high virulence. As yet unidentified water quality conditions predispose susceptible fishes to infection with the virulent strain. Mortality can be acute, and by the time the condition is seen it may be difficult to control.

Gram-positive Bacterial Infections: These infections of concern to fish culturists and aquarists may be caused by *Streptococcus* and related genera *Lactococcus*, *Enterococcus*, and *Vagococcus*. Infections are uncommon but can cause significant mortality (>50%) when they do occur. Chronic infections may continue for weeks, with only a few fish dying each day. Species known to be susceptible include salmonids, assorted marine fish (eg, mullet, sea bass), tilapia, sturgeon, and striped bass. Susceptible aquarium species include rainbow sharks, red-tailed black sharks, rosy barbs, danios, and some tetras and cichlids. In general, all fish should be considered susceptible. A characteristic manifestation of *Streptococcus* infection is neurologic disease, often manifest by spinning or spiraling in the water column. Brain and kidney cultures from suspect fish should be incubated on blood agar at 25°C for 24–48 hr. Gram stains of pinpoint bacterial colonies reveal typical chains of gram-positive cocci, which allow a presumptive diagnosis. Confirmation requires definitive identification of the organism. Antibiotic therapy should be based on sensitivity testing. Erythromycin is often the drug of choice, but it is not FDA approved for this use. Sources of infection may be environmental or include live foods, such as tubeficid worms, amphibians, or previously infected fish. Future epizootics can be prevented if the source of infection is identified and eliminated. *Streptococcus iniae* has been isolated from tilapia and aquarium fish and has zoonotic potential. Autogenous vaccines are available for use in aquaculture facilities.

The zoonotic gram-positive bacterium *Erysipelothrix rhusiopathiae* is frequently associated with rostral ulceration in cyprinids such as tiger barbs (*Puntigrus tetrazona*) and rosy barbs (*Pethia conchonius*). It usually responds well to treatment.

Mycobacteria: Mycobacteriosis is a chronic or acute, systemic, granulomatous disease of aquarium fish and cultured food fish, particularly those reared under intensive conditions. Predisposing environmental factors include low dissolved oxygen, low pH, and high organic load, all found in recirculating aquaculture systems. Correct use of ultraviolet light as a way to disinfect system water reduces bacterial counts and can be a useful tool to control infection in exhibit animals. The causative bacteria can be any number of species of *Mycobacterium*, including *M chelonae*, *M marinum*, and *M fortuitum*. Syngnathids (sea horses) are particularly susceptible, but the disease can be seen in any fish. These weakly gram-positive, acid-fast, nonmotile bacteria are difficult to grow but can be isolated using Löwenstein-Jensen or Middlebrook media after incubation at 25°C for 3–4 wk. Signs

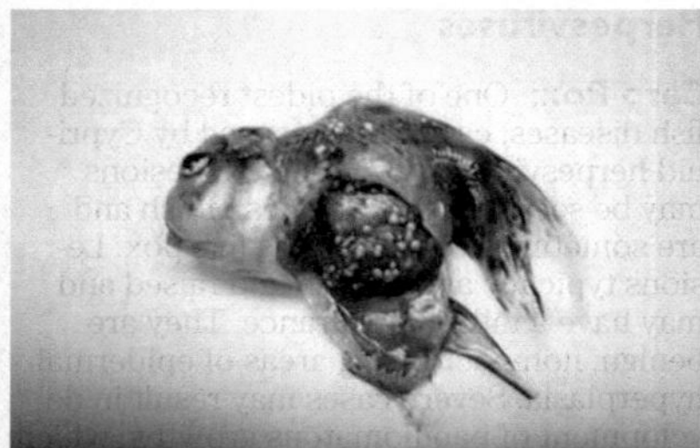

Granulomatous lesions typical of *Mycobacterium* in a fancy goldfish. *Courtesy of Dr. Ruth Francis-Floyd.*

are variable and nonspecific; they can include emaciation, ascites, skin ulceration and hemorrhages, exophthalmos, paleness, and skeletal deformities. On necropsy, gross lesions of viscera consist of grayish white, necrotic foci that sometimes coalesce to form tumor-like masses. Granulomas may not be grossly visible and are often found first on wet mounts, especially of anterior kidney and spleen, or other viscera from infected fish. A presumptive diagnosis is based on visualization of acid-fast rods in granulomatous material from suspect lesions. Definitive diagnosis requires isolating and identifying the bacteria. There are no effective treatments that eliminate mycobacteria in fish. Mycobacteria can cause zoonotic infections, and aquarists should be informed of potential risks if handling or cleaning contaminated fish or exhibits. An infected aquarium should be disinfected before other fish are added. Bleach is not an effective disinfectant against mycobacteria; disinfection with alcohol or phenolic compounds is recommended.

MYCOTIC DISEASES

Aquatic fungi often are considered secondary tissue invaders that follow traumatic injuries, infectious agents, or environmental insults such as poor water quality or low water temperatures. Because many fungi grow on decaying organic matter, they are especially common in the aquatic environment.

For more information on *Saprolegnia* and other members of the Oomycota, which are fungus-like protists, *see* p 1761.

Fusarium solani is emerging as an important cause of disease in captive marine fish, particularly elasmobranchs. This organism is found in aquatic plants and soils in tropical and subtropical regions. Clinical disease has been reported in bonnethead and scalloped hammerhead sharks, as well as several species of marine fish, including angelfish and parrotfish. Disease is associated with low water temperatures (<80°F or 27°C). Bonnethead sharks are particularly susceptible and develop erosions and granulomatous lesions along the head. Resolution of lesions requires warming the affected animals to a more appropriate temperature for the species.

Closely related to true fungi, **microsporidia** are tiny, obligate intracellular, spore-forming parasites with single polar filaments. They are common parasites of finfish and are host- and tissue-specific; they can also infect helminth parasites of fish. The spores are extremely resistant, and microsporidia are considered nontreatable. Microsporidia have a direct life cycle; therefore, horizontal transmission in an aquarium is likely. Some species of microsporidia cause the formation of xenomas; a xenoma results in the hypertrophy of an infected cell and its nucleus and is often surrounded by fibrous connective tissue by the host.

The spores are very hardy and can remain infective in water for many months. Ingestion of the spores is the primary route of infection, but entry through other portals, eg, damaged skin or gills, and transovarial transmission are possible.

Recommendations for management of microsporidian disease include removal of older and moribund animals from a population, ultraviolet sterilization, and strict biosecurity. Depopulation and disinfection are recommended for elimination of microsporidian infections.

Ovipleistophora ovariae infects ovarian tissue of golden shiners (bait fish), resulting in sterility. The organism has no intermediate host and is transmitted horizontally (through ingestion of infective spores) or vertically (through infected ova). Fertility declines as fish age, eventually resulting in sterility. Grossly, infected ovarian tissue appears marbled. Diagnosis is confirmed by examination of a wet mount of suspect tissue, revealing presence of microsporidian spores.

Neon tetra disease is caused by *Pleistophora hyphessobryconis*, which infects the skeletal musculature of a number of species of aquarium fish, including tetras, angelfish, rasboras, barbs, and zebrafish. Infected fish may exhibit abnormal locomotion caused by muscle damage, and muscle tissue may appear marbled or necrotic at necropsy. The spores are readily visualized in wet mounts of infected tissue.

The microsporidia *Pseudoloma neurophilia* infects zebrafish and can be problematic in research facilities and the pet industry. The nervous system and skeletal muscles are the most common sites of infections, but occasionally other organs such as gonads are affected. A common presentation is lordosis, but some fish may present with a grossly distended body with pale epaxial musculature caused by a massive number of parasites. Often, fish may be heavily infected yet show no clinical signs of disease. Xenomas are not formed with this microsporidia. Fish are infected by ingesting spores from an infected fish or during spawning activity, when spores may be released from an infected ovary. It is unknown whether this parasite can be transmitted vertically. An important source of infective spores is tank debris.

A number of microsporidia belonging to the genus *Glugea* are associated with disease in a disparate group of host fishes, including seahorses, flounder, and sticklebacks. Infection with the members of this genus results in xenoma formation.

VIRAL DISEASES

Descriptions of viral diseases of fish are rapidly expanding. Viruses are being reported in new species, and interpretation of the significance of findings is also changing. Several viral diseases of ornamental fish are reportable (*see* TABLE 6, p 1787).

Although viruses of homeothermic animals are cultured at uniform temperatures, fish viruses have wider, but specific, temperature tolerances in fish cell cultures at lower temperatures. Because of this relatively defined temperature range, variation in temperature may enable control, although often it merely induces latency. Because many viral diseases of fish are geographically limited, regulatory agencies and fish farms in disease-free areas consider them exotic diseases and require certification of introduced stocks. Many result in high mortality in young fish and little or no losses in adults, which may become carriers. For these reasons, avoidance of carriers and certification of SPF replacement stocks are frequently required. Specific testing procedures are available. Most vaccines used for control of fish diseases are for bacterial agents; however, use of vaccines to control some viral diseases is being introduced. Drugs are not effective; however, antibiotics and other drugs may be used to control secondary bacterial infections. Management techniques that minimize stress and crowding, biosecurity measures, and temperature manipulation hold the greatest promise for control of piscine viral diseases.

Herpesviruses

Carp Pox: One of the oldest recognized fish diseases, carp pox is caused by Cyprinid herpesvirus-1 (CyHV-1). Pox lesions may be seen on other species of fish and are sometimes referred to as fish pox. Lesions typically are smooth and raised and may have a milky appearance. They are benign, non-necrotizing areas of epidermal hyperplasia. Severe cases may result in development of papillomatous growths, which may be a site of complicating bacterial infection. Generally, lesions are self-limiting and of minimal clinical significance. Carp pox can be a significant problem in koi because their aesthetic quality, and hence market value, is severely compromised. For the serious koi enthusiast, fish affected with carp pox should be culled, preferably during quarantine. Surgical removal of the lesions has not been rewarding.

Koi Herpesvirus: Koi herpesvirus (KHV), caused by Cyprinid herpesvirus-3 (CyHV-3), was first recognized in 1996. It is widespread in the USA and considered endemic. Confirmed cases must be reported to the State Veterinarian and the USDA Area Veterinarian in Charge. Because the disease is endemic, regulating bodies report its occurrence to the OIE, but they do not require specific action, such as depopulation, when the disease is reported.

KHV causes clinical disease in koi and common carp. Goldfish and grass carp are refractory to clinical disease but may serve as carriers. Koi that are exposed, but survive, may also serve as carriers. Clinical disease is seen at water temperatures of 72°–81°F (22°–27°C), with maximal mortality at temperatures of 72°–78°F (22°–25.5°C). Mortality rates can reach 80%–100%. Fish of any age are susceptible, but mortality rates may be higher in younger fish, especially fry. The most obvious lesions are seen on gill tissues, which are severely affected and develop a mottled red and white appearance with obvious hemorrhage in some cases. Affected fish are lethargic, swim at the surface, and may show behavioral signs of respiratory distress. The presence of severe bacterial or parasitic disease may mask the fact that KHV is the primary cause of gill lesions. The disease is transmitted horizontally by exposure to sick or carrier fish and also by exposure to contaminated water, substrate, or equipment.

When KHV is suspected, affected fish can be shipped to a laboratory for confirmation. Freshly dead specimens shipped on ice and received within 24 hr should be adequate.

PCR or virus isolation and identification can be used to confirm the infection in dead animals. Because of the value of koi, there is significant demand for nonlethal testing protocols. Blood, gill tissue from biopsy, feces, or mucus may be used to assess the status of moribund fish. It is important to note these tests can result in false-negatives if performed on clinically normal fish. Indirect tests using blood samples, including ELISA or virus neutralization, are less straightforward. Negative test results could indicate a true negative or, alternatively, that the infection is in its early stages and the fish has not yet developed a measurable antibody response. A negative test result could potentially be obtained from a previously infected fish that has had a decrease in circulating antibody; however, such a fish could still function as a carrier. There is a misconception among some hobbyists that a negative blood test is an adequate screening test to exclude carrier status. Practitioners should communicate this clearly to owners, because it is easily misunderstood.

If KHV infection is confirmed in a population of koi, depopulation is strongly recommended. Surviving fish are carriers and can serve as a source of infection for naive fish. Although mortality decreases or stops as water temperature approaches 86°F (30°C), survivors will retain carrier status and therefore put other populations at risk.

Prevention of KHV is best accomplished with careful quarantine protocols. A minimum quarantine of 30 days at 75°F (24°C) is recommended to minimize the chance of introducing KHV to an established population of koi. If disease develops during the quarantine period, fish should be evaluated with special consideration for excluding KHV. After quarantine, a new fish may be placed in an isolated area with a few fish from the established population and monitored for signs of disease for at least 2 wk as an added precaution. If koi are taken to shows, quarantine protocols should be followed every time they return. Koi enthusiasts should be strongly encouraged to attend English-style shows (versus Japanese-style shows), where competing fish are not placed in a common container.

Herpesviral Hematopoietic Necrosis: This condition of goldfish is caused by Cyprinid herpesvirus-2 (CyHV-2). It is probably widespread throughout the USA, but it is not a reportable disease. Clinically ill goldfish often are anorectic and exhibit pale gills and ascites. At necropsy, the spleen and kidneys (anterior and posterior) are often enlarged. As is typical for herpesviruses, survivors can be carriers and exhibit clinical signs of disease if subjected to stressors. Water temperatures between 10° and 22°C will result in replication of the virus that can be detected with quantitative PCR. There is no treatment.

Herpesvirus of Angelfish: A herpesvirus of angelfish (*Pterophyllum* spp) has been detected by electron microscopy of skin from moribund angelfish. Affected fish produce copious amounts of skin mucus that gives affected fish a grey sheen. Often, these fish have multiple parasitic infestations and bacterial infections, similar to that of KHV in koi. It is suspected that survivors are carriers.

Rhabdoviruses

Viral Hemorrhagic Septicemia (VHS): This reportable disease is caused by a *Novirhabdovirus* and is a member of the family Rhabdoviridae. This disease is listed by OIE as notifiable. Most of the reported hosts are not ornamental fishes, but koi were shown to be susceptible experimentally to genotype IVb. This genotype affects a diverse group of fishes in the Great Lakes region of North America.

Spring Viremia of Carp (SVC): This acute, virulent, usually hemorrhagic disease of cultured carp is caused by a *Vesiculovirus* that, like VHS, is a member of the Rhabdoviridae family. The disease is listed as notifiable by the OIE. Historically, it was reported in Europe and the former USSR; however, several outbreaks have been reported in the USA between 2002–2007, in both wild fish and cultured ornamental koi. SVC is considered a foreign animal disease in the USA and must be reported. It causes disease in common carp, including koi, as well as grass, bighead, silver, and crucian carp. Limited experience suggests that common goldfish may be susceptible.

Clinical signs are nonspecific and may include darkening of the skin, exophthalmia, ascites, pale gills, hemorrhage, and a protruding vent with thick mucoid fecal casts. Pinpoint hemorrhage in the swim bladder is indicative of SVC, if present. Coinfection with *Aeromonas* or other systemic bacteria may obscure the presence of the virus. The bacterial component of the infection can be controlled with antibiotics; however, depopulation of affected or exposed fish is required in the USA. The disease causes death in both adult and young fish. Clinical disease occurs at cool temperatures, 54°–72°F (12°–22°C), an important distinction from KHV. The virus is readily isolated in common fish cell lines and identified by serum neutralization and fluorescent antibody tests.

Iridoviruses

Lymphocystis Disease: This typically chronic, viral infection of wild or captive marine and freshwater fish is caused by an icosahedral DNA virus of the Iridoviridae family. Infection may be manifest by benign, cauliflower-like lesions typically located on fins. The disease affects a wide range of fish and is generally considered to have a global distribution. Within the aquarium trade, painted glass fish and marine tropical fishes such as the anemonefishes (Pomacentridae), marine angels (Pomacanthidae), and butterflyfishes (Chaetodontidae) are susceptible. Presumptive diagnosis is based on the presence of enlarged fibroblasts (up to 1 mm), which are easily visualized with a light microscope. Microscopic examination typically reveals the appearance of grape-like clusters of virus-laden cells. Diagnosis is confirmed histologically. Feulgen-positive cytoplasmic inclusions and a hypertrophied nucleus are pathognomonic. The disease is usually self-limiting but is of aesthetic concern.

Megalocytiviruses: Several other iridoviruses have been described in ornamental fish. Megalocytiviruses consist of two major groupings, red sea bream iridovirus (RSIV) and infectious spleen and kidney necrosis virus (ISKNV). RSIV has been found in >30 other marine fishes so far; many of the affected species include some tropical fishes kept in aquaria. RSIV is a reportable disease. ISKNV includes megalocytiviruses that primarily affect ornamental freshwater fishes. ISKNV is not currently reportable.

A megalocytivirus has been described in freshwater angelfish (*Pterophyllum scalare*), but the agent has not been isolated. It can result in high mortality. An iridovirus has also been isolated in the USA from gourami in the genus *Trichogaster* using a tilapia heart cell line. This virus does not grow on FHM cells or other common cell lines used for isolation of fish viruses. The gourami virus has been associated with systemic disease and mortality of *T trichopterus* and *T leeri* gourami. Efforts to fulfill River's postulates were supportive although not conclusive. Clinical disease with the USA gourami megalocytivirus appears to be more severe at water temperatures ≥30°C, based on very limited information. A megalocytivirus is known from dwarf gourami *Trichogaster* spp, but it is not known whether it is the same virus that affects gourami in the USA.

Other Viruses:

Koi sleepy disease is also known as carp edema virus. Caused by a poxvirus, it was first seen in Japan in 1974 and has since occurred in other countries, including the USA. Affected fishes appear lethargic, lay on their sides, and have thin body condition. Mortality is usually low but can be variable. Gill hyperplasia is a common histopathologic finding. Infected koi can recover, but it is unknown whether they retain a carrier state.

NEOPLASIA

Neoplastic diseases similar to those found in other animals are found in fish. Their incidence frequently is higher in some geographic areas and in certain species. Some tumors are genetically mediated, such as the malignant melanoma of the platy-swordtail cross, and possibly the pseudobranch tumor of cod, thyroid tumors, malignant lymphosarcoma of northern pike, and fibromas or sarcomas of goldfish. Liposarcomas have been reported in captive-bred clownfish, and pigmented tumors of unknown origin have been seen in wild Hawaiian marine butterflyfishes, *Chaetodon miliaris* and *C multicinctus*. Both species are popular in the marine aquarium hobby. Although the reported incidence of tumors in sharks, skates, and rays is low, neoplasia does occur.

Gonadal tumors are important neoplastic disorders of fishes and have been reported in koi and northern pike. Typically, fish present with a swollen abdomen, and, depending on the severity of disease, there may be significant loss of condition. The presence of a mass can be confirmed with ultrasound. Biopsy of tissue may not offer a clear diagnosis. Laparotomy of affected fish often reveals a circumscribed mass of gonadal tissue. Fish that are not excessively debilitated are excellent surgical candidates for removal of the mass.

Viruses, especially retroviruses, have been associated with neoplasia in fishes. Two examples of viral-induced neoplasia have occurred in tropical fishes. Viral particles have been found in fibromas on the lips of freshwater angelfish. Debulking the tumor can allow affected fish to feed normally. Bicolor damselfish neurofibromatosis, a fatal disease, was reported in 1991 in wild *Stegastes partitus* found on the reefs of south Florida; it is believed to be a viral-induced tumor. Although not reported in captive bicolor damselfish, it has the potential to occur.

BACKYARD POULTRY

Raising backyard poultry (*Gallus domesticus*) in urban environments is a growing trend in the USA. In developing countries, backyard poultry represent ~80% of poultry stock, often consisting of indigenous unselected breeds of various ages, with various species mixed in the same flock. This serves to meet household food demands and is an additional source of income. Modern day USA backyard poultry owners often view their birds as companion animals, in contrast to poultry raised for commercial production. A 2010 USDA study in four cities (Los Angeles, Denver, Miami, New York) found that 0.8% of all households owned chickens, and nearly 4% of households without chickens planned to have chickens in the next 5 yr. As backyard poultry ownership becomes increasingly popular, owners must be properly educated about how to keep their flocks healthy; thus, more veterinarians must be capable of providing this education.

All commercial and domestic chickens originate from the red jungle fowl (*Gallus gallus*), which was domesticated in Southeast Asia many centuries ago. Today, hundreds of different chicken breeds are bred for different purposes and are characterized by meat-type, egg-laying type, and dual purpose. Meat-type chickens are characterized by rapid growth rate and good meat yield, versus egg-laying chickens, which are selected for good egg production. Dual purpose chickens, such as Plymouth Rock, New Hampshire, Rhode Island Red, Wyandotte, and Orpington, are reasonably good for both egg and meat production, making them a suitable choice for backyard chickens for most owners. Purchasing chicks and other poultry from a reputable hatchery or breeder is recommended to get off to a good start and prevent future problems. Purchasing from hatcheries or breeders that participate in the National Poultry Improvement Plan (NPIP) is recommended, because these flocks are routinely tested for diseases such as *Salmonella* Pullorum and *S* Gallinarum (*see* p 2865). A list of certified hatcheries and breeders can be found by contacting official state poultry associations. In addition, prospective owners are encouraged to physically visit the breeder flock or hatchery of purchase to ensure only healthy birds are brought into the backyard flock.

Many backyard flock owners have multiple ages and/or species of birds. Mixing birds of different species and from different sources increases the risk of introducing disease, and it is preferable to keep only birds of similar ages and species together ("all in/all out"). If multiple ages and/or species are kept on a property, efforts should be made to minimize contact between groups by keeping them in separate locations. Separating new or returning birds for at least 4–6 wk is necessary to monitor for signs of illness. Practicing good biosecurity (*see* p 2068) is also key for good poultry health.

PHYSICAL EXAMINATION

Before conducting a physical examination, the bird's appearance and behavior should be observed from a distance and within the flock. A healthy bird should be bright, alert, and interacting with the flock, with good appetite and free of abnormal behavior. Chickens and other domestic fowl can be restrained for examination by reaching over the back and holding the wings down. Then, the bird should be picked up and the fingers inserted between the legs while supporting the breast with the other hand. Restraining the bird upside down is not ideal, because it may increase its stress level and also cause regurgitation, as well as result in broken

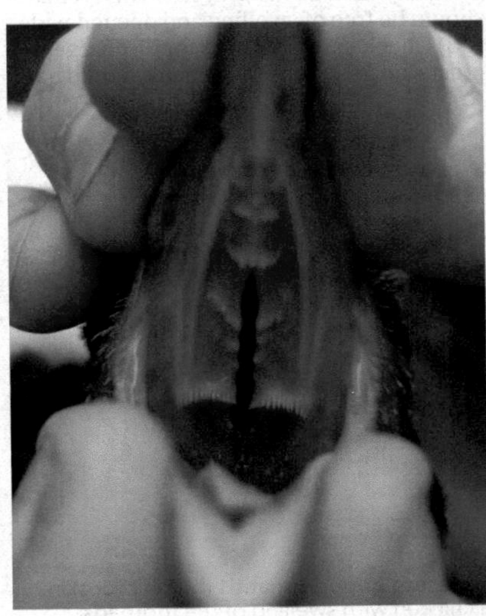

Open mouth of a healthy chicken. *Courtesy of Dr. Patricia Wakenell.*

bones if bones are brittle from low calcium. The bird should be kept as calm as possible to prevent injury to both the bird and the handler. A chicken catcher, which is a wire hook used to grab birds by the legs, can also be used. For larger birds such as turkeys, the handler can fold his or her arms and upper body over the wings and back of the bird, hug firmly, and lift. It is important to remain low to the ground when handling bigger birds; grabbing these birds by their wings or legs can be dangerous and easily cause injury during struggling. For waterfowl such as ducks and geese, it is easiest to use the neck as a catching handle; however, once the bird is caught, it should be picked up by grabbing the wings together behind the back and using the other hand to support the abdomen. Smaller flight birds, such as quail, chukar partridges, and pheasants, can first be restrained by careful use of a net or towel and then holding the wings or legs. Catching birds on the first attempt minimizes stress.

Physical examinations should be performed using a systematic approach.

1) Examine the head and neck. The comb should be bright red, slightly warm, turgid, and free of scabs and lesions. The bird should hold its head high and have good muscle tone.

2) Observe the eyes, and check for any discharge or cloudiness that may indicate illness. The eyes of a healthy adult bird should be clear and bright and have a copper-red iris and a round pupil with well-defined margins. Young chicks generally have a blue-gray iris. The eyelids should be free of swelling and opened wide.

3) Check external nares for discharge, crusts, and scratches. The beak should be smooth and free of cracks, and the tips should come to a point.

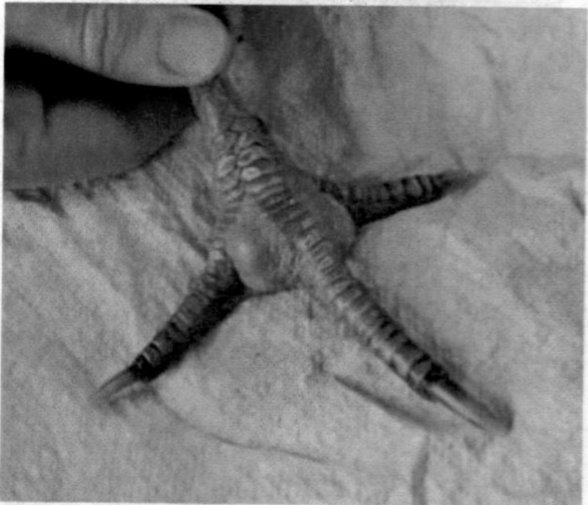

Subacute pododermatitis (bumblefoot) in a chicken with swelling of the footpads.
Courtesy of Dr. Patricia Wakenell.

4) Open the mouth and check for ulcers and mucosal lesions on the tongue and mucosal membranes at the commissures of the beak.

5) Check the color of the earlobes to predict the color of the eggs the hens will produce. Hens that have white earlobes generally produce white eggs, and hens that have red earlobes generally produce brown or other pigmented eggs.

6) Evaluate the feathers to check for feather loss and how they are distributed. Loss of feathers around the back and back of the neck may indicate mating behavior by roosters. Check feathers at the base of the feather shaft to look for parasites such as lice, mites, and nits (lice egg packets). Feathers around the vent should be clear and free of blood or feces. Pasting of the vent with loose feces may indicate enteric disease. Check for scabs and blood around the vent, which are evidence of vent pecking and cannibalism.

7) The two small bones at the sides of the vent are the pubic bones. They should be flexible and have space in between. If hens are in lay, this distance should be the width of three or four fingers. When the hen is not laying, the pubic bones are usually stiff and close together (distance between is one finger width or less).

8) Check the legs and feet. The scales should be smooth and closely adhered to each other. If scales are raised and crusty, there may be a scaly leg mite infestation. Check the footpads for scratches, swellings, or ulcers caused by footpad dermatitis or pododermatitis (bumblefoot).

MANAGEMENT

Environment: Backyard poultry ownership laws and regulations vary by city, county, and neighborhood. Some cities and homeowner's associations have specific rules about chicken ownership, whereas other cities permit chicken ownership with no limitations on the number or type of chickens. It is important to know the regulations and to keep peace with the neighborhood about owning poultry.

It is crucial to fence in backyard poultry to keep them at home and to protect them. Domestic chickens are easy prey for predators such as cats, dogs, skunks, hawks, and foxes. The fencing should extend into the ground at least a foot to prevent predators such as raccoons and foxes from digging under the fencing. Water holes and vegetation should be avoided around the coop, because they encourage waterfowl, insects, rodents, and other vermin to the area, which can harm poultry and spread disease. It is wise to cover the top of the enclosure to protect the birds from predators that fly or climb, as well as to prevent exposure to wild fowl that may transmit disease.

Overcrowding should be avoided; space allocation must consider and allow for growth of the birds. Enough indoor space should be available to prevent overcrowding during inclement weather. The type of bird will help determine the type of housing. Most breeds of chickens are hardy, although meat-type birds are usually sturdier than egg layers. Show breeds often do not have hybrid vigor and require heated or cooled housing. Minimum space requirements should be determined not only by size of bird but also for activity levels. However, in general, laying hens and larger chickens need a minimum of 1.5–2 sq ft of space inside and 8–10 sq ft in outside runs. Ducks and geese need much more space, 3–6 sq ft inside and 15–18 in outside runs.

Floor type is an important consideration in building a coop, and owners need to be cognizant about how to work with various materials. Putting the birds on dirt is cheap and easy, but manure is hard to remove and can become a muddy mess without proper maintenance. When the soil gets wet or contaminated, the dirt must be tilled and new soil added after topdressing the old dirt with lime or bleach to prevent parasite and microbial overgrowth. Wood is another option, but it must be in good condition, because old wood may rot and harbor pathogens, and exposed splinters can result in injuries. In addition, wood should not be treated, because chemicals such as lead can be harmful to birds. Concrete flooring is the best for permanent coops, because it is easy to clean, impervious to vermin, and a good barrier to predators. However, it is the most expensive and takes the most effort to maintain. It is also important to use good, absorbent litter material for bedding in the houses. The litter should be clean, dry, and free of mold. Good litter choices include pine shavings, rice and nut hulls, chopped straw, and ground corncobs. Litter can get very wet around the drinkers, and proper removal of caked litter is necessary. Wet litter encourages growth of pathogens, such as bacteria, fungi, and parasites, as well as leads to problems such as footpad dermatitis. Dry litter creates a dusty environment and may cause tracheal irritation. Ideally, litter should contain 20%–25% moisture; a quick test is to grab a handful of litter and see whether the litter clumps briefly and then crumbles apart. Wet litter and high ammonia levels can lead to serious welfare issues, including ammonia burns of the cornea, footpad dermatitis, breast blisters, and skin burns. The US Environmental Protection Agency (EPA) recommends that people and animals not be exposed to 25 ppm of ammonia for ≥8 hr. Adequate ventilation allows for moisture to be properly removed from the bedding.

Chickens have a body temperature of 105°–109°F (40°–43°C) and start to feel heat stress at environmental temperatures >75°F. In temperature extremes, poultry will modify their behavior to stay in their thermoneutral zone (55°–75°F). The ideal temperature range for poultry is 65°–75°F, with a relative humidity of up to 40%. To encourage good air circulation, windows should be put up on the south or east side of the barn, with a narrow ledge on the windows to prevent birds from roosting and defecating in the area. Using misters and fans will help keep the poultry cool during the hot summer months, and a well-insulated barn will keep birds warm during the winter.

Nutrition: The biggest expense in raising poultry is the cost of feed. However, good feed is a sound investment, because unbalanced diets will reduce performance levels and may result in nutritional diseases. Common issues in backyard flocks are insufficient water quality or amount, prolonged storage and degradation of vitamins and minerals, dilution of balanced and complete nutrition with scratch or supplemental feed, and feeding diets for the wrong life stage. Poultry require 1.5–3.5 parts water for every 1 part of feed consumed (up to 5–6 times for waterfowl) and require more in hot weather. Poultry will not consume feed if the amount of water is inadequate, which can lead to serious health problems. Poultry owners also have to consider the possibility of bacteria (eg, coliforms) and other contaminants in the water, including arsenic, calcium, chlorine, copper, fluorine, iron, lead, magnesium, mercury, nitrates, nitrites, sodium, sulfate, and zinc.

Vitamin and mineral deficiencies seen in poultry are discussed in more detail in the poultry section (*see* p 2936 and p 2930). The most common vitamin deficiency problems in backyard flocks are caused either by not using a vitamin premix in the diet or by using a vitamin premix beyond its shelf-life, resulting in loss of efficacy. Typically, fat-soluble vitamin deficiencies, especially vitamin D_3, will become clinically evident before water-soluble vitamin deficiencies. The most common presentation of birds with vitamin D_3 deficiency is skeletal abnormalities (rickets) that can present in a flock as mortality, loss of condition, and birds that are lame or reluctant to move because of scoliosis, soft and pliable bones, or lack of bone strength. Owners should be advised to purchase quality feed, store it correctly (avoid temperature extremes to prevent vitamins and minerals from denaturing), and use it within the expiration date. Feed should be stored in a dry, cool area to avoid vitamins from breaking down and to prevent mold/fungal growth. Using a black light to check for fluorescence in corn grains is a quick way to screen for harmful mycotoxins. If poultry owners wish to mix their own feed, the most common range of inclusion for a vitamin/mineral premix would be 3–10 pounds of premix per ton of feed. Most feed and premixes are available in large quantities and expire in 3–6 mo (as short as 2 mo in the summer), and poultry owners need to be aware of the dangers of feeding old and improperly stored feed.

Backyard poultry owners need to know how much feed each bird will consume a day to predict when to order the next batch of feed. A day-old chick will eat approximately the amount of feed that can fit on the surface of a US quarter, and an adult laying hen should eat no more than a quarter of pound of feed per day. In contrast, a meat-type bird may consume close to twice as much feed as an adult layer. However, overfeeding or giving feed ad lib can result in musculoskeletal disorders. Using commercial broiler breeds in a backyard setting is strongly discouraged, because these birds need to be on very strict feed restriction to avoid metabolic disease. Birds with access to outdoors will supplement their diet by foraging and eating insects. In addition, many poultry owners choose to supplement their birds' diet with table scraps and scratch grains. Scratch should not be overfed, because it may cause the birds not to eat a balanced diet. Fat scraps should be avoided also, because they promote fatty liver and acute death from liver rupture. Signs of low or inadequate nutrient density include slow growth, slow or lack of egg production, and feather loss. Although foraging behavior may be desired, the birds should still receive most of their diet from a balanced, complete ration.

The type of feed recommended varies with the species, age, and use of the bird. For some species of birds, finding the appropriate feed ingredients can be difficult. In general, gamebird owners who cannot find the appropriate gamebird starter feed can substitute a turkey poult starter feed, which is typically high in protein (25%–28% crude protein). It is critical to not feed layer diets to nonlaying, growing birds, because the inadequate protein levels and high calcium content (3.5%–6%) may result in irreversible renal damage. Thus, one of the most common problems seen in mixed-age flocks is urolithiasis (gout). Causes of gout include infectious bronchitis virus, feeding excessive levels of sodium bicarbonate, mycotoxicosis, and more often, feeding a high-calcium (adult layer) diet to an immature bird. Diets for growing birds (pre-lay) are typically 0.8%–1.2% calcium, whereas laying birds require 3.5%–6% calcium because of the nutritional demand for laying eggs (a typical egg requires ~2 g of calcium). However, it is important for adult layers to have adequate calcium to avoid osteoporosis (cage-layer fatigue) and thin-shelled eggs.

LAYING AND REPRODUCTION

For laying hens, nest boxes just large enough to fit one "seated" hen are desirable. If eggs are to be collected for consumption, efforts need to be made to decrease broodiness in the hens. The term "broody" refers to a hen that stops laying eggs in order to sit on the eggs, even when no eggs are present. As soon as this behavior is noticed, the hen should be moved to a wire cage. Broody hens can have an aggressive temperament, and caution must be taken during handling. Most hens put into cages become less broody in 2–3 days. Without intervention, hens may remain broody for 3–4 wk.

Backyard flocks raised under natural light will stop laying once hours of daylight become shorter and undergo a molt period lasting 3–4 mo or longer. Artificial lighting may be used for layers to lay eggs during the winter months, which will increase the number of eggs laid during that period but not the total number of eggs laid by the hen. Light schedules are usually 13-hr days, or lights on all night. Hens will be stimulated to start laying again as hours of daylight increase, not with continuous lighting. Supplemented lighting increases the risk of cannibalism in birds not individually caged. Chickens will lay eggs for ~1 yr before going into a molt. As long as feather loss is not associated with insect infestation, reddened or abraded skin, poor nutrition, or open wounds, an "unusual molt" can be assumed for lengthy or bizarre-appearing feather loss. If desired, this is also the time hens can be culled from the flock. In general, even the best hens will approach only ~70% of their former production level in their subsequent production period. All hens should molt at least once a year. If the hens do not naturally molt, molt can be induced by decreasing hours of light.

Incubation and Hatching of Eggs: Probably the largest determinant in deciding whether to buy hatched chicks or hatch within the backyard flock is the desired size of the flock. For small flocks, inexpensive, easy-to-operate incubators/hatchers are available at farm stores or through mail order catalogs. When first starting out, as many as 50% of the eggs may not hatch, thus making egg space a concern if a large hatch is needed. Most home incubators have good temperature control but inadequate humidity control. Chicken eggs can withstand changes in humidity during incubation; however, other species such as turkeys are much more sensitive to poor humidity control. With home incubators, temperature should be regulated for at least 2–3 days before the eggs are placed. During incubation, the temperature should be checked twice daily (fluctuations between 98°F and 101°F are fine for chicken eggs; temperature requirements for other species should be researched before incubation) and the water pan kept full. Eggs (except dark shelled) should be candled at least once during incubation, typically after the first mortality peak at 7–10 days of embryonation. Candling consists of shining a light through the egg to determine embryo viability by detecting movement of the embryo and presence of blood vessels. Fertile eggs will candle dark except for the air cell (air sac) with visible blood vessels and a live embryo. Infertiles or "yolker" eggs will candle through with only a slight shadow for the yolk and have no internal structures and no embryonic development. Embryos that died with no positive development can also candle this way. Dead or nonviable embryos may have a blood ring around the embryo, caused by the movement of blood away from the embryo after death.

Dead eggs can be removed before possibly exploding. Eggs need to be turned ~4 times/day until the last few days before hatch (embryonation day 18 for chicken eggs). It helps to know approximate incubation periods of the poultry of interest to gauge when to provide adequate interference for a successful hatch. For example, the incubation period for chickens is 21 days, for Bobwhite quail 23–24 days, for guinea fowl 27–28 days, for ducks 28 days, and for geese 28–33 days. If eggs do not hatch, examination of the dead embryos can yield some clues as to the cause.

Common problems include early deaths (infertile eggs, too long or improper storage of eggs before incubation, extreme temperature fluctuation), late deaths but not pipped (extreme temperature fluctuation, poor humidity), pipped but dried and stuck to the egg shell (generally poor humidity in late incubation, hatching period, weakened embryos from temperature fluctuations), and pipped but drowned in egg fluids or malpositioned embryos (turning malfunction during incubation). Once the chicks are hatched, they should not be moved until dry and fluffed. Occasionally, chicks will hatch that have not completely absorbed their yolk sac and/or intestines. These chicks have a poor chance of survival, and euthanasia is warranted. If possible, all chicken chicks should be vaccinated for Marek's disease (*see* p 2849).

VACCINATION

For the small flock owner, vaccination is generally necessary only if the birds have had disease problems in the past, may possibly be exposed to other birds (eg, at poultry shows, meat swaps, or wild bird access), or if new birds are introduced to the flock (open flock). Birds should not be vaccinated for a disease not present in their local area, because this will only introduce new organisms into the flock. Also, a sick bird's immune system is compromised and unable to withstand the stress of vaccination.

If certain diseases are a problem in a backyard flock, vaccination may be recommended after veterinary consultation. Marek's disease is present in almost every flock, and vaccination of chickens is strongly recommended in all cases; vaccination is key for control and is inexpensive. Backyard poultry owners may purchase chicks from hatcheries and request their chicks be vaccinated at hatch with serotype 3, or they can vaccinate their own chicks if hatched onsite. Because the virus is ubiquitous and spreads through feather dander, vaccinating birds at hatch before they are most susceptible (2–7 mo) is critical to establish early immunity. There are three serotypes of Marek's disease: 1, 2, and 3. Because most backyard chickens are vaccinated only for serotype 3, they may not be fully protected. Vaccination does not prevent infection or shedding of the field virus.

COMMON MANAGEMENT-RELATED DISEASES

Birds are prey animals, so early signs of illness may be subtle and difficult to discern. Some early signs of illness include changes in eating and drinking habits; dull feathers; soiling of the feathers around nares, vent, shoulders, or eyes; swelling around or discharge around the eyes; discharge from the eyes or nares; abnormal feces; favoring or lameness in limbs; or decrease in activity.

Cannibalism: Pecking or cannibalism (*see* p 2873) is one of the most frustrating and common problems to control in floor-reared birds. Certain species such as pheasants and quail are notorious for cannibalism, often leading to individual cages as the only housing option. Certain breeds can be more aggressive than others within specific species. Cannibalism usually does not begin in chicks <2–3 wk old, although in young chicks, it is generally the result of insufficient feed or diarrhea (soiled or pasty vents). In mature birds, methods to control cannibalism include reducing lighting, reducing bird density, increasing the number of feeders, and trimming the beaks. If an individual bird has been pecked severely on the skin and separate housing is not available, spraying or painting the affected area with tree pruning tar (pruning sealer) is a quick remedy. After the sealer has been sprayed or painted on the affected area, the bird should be restrained until the sealant is dry. The tar protects the exposed area from fluid loss, is nontoxic on open wounds, and has the advantage of "identifying" the perpetrators by staining their beaks black. If small numbers of birds are the aggressors, these birds can be given red spectacles that attach to their nares, red contact lenses, or have their beaks retrimmed to reduce trauma in other birds.

Trauma: This is the most common condition of backyard poultry and includes predator injury, entrapment of limbs in cages or other equipment, cannibalism, crushing injuries (stepped on, trapped in doors, etc), and self-mutilation (spurs, beak, nails). Most adult poultry are highly resilient and seem able to recover from severe injuries if the wound has not penetrated into the respiratory or abdominal cavity. Supportive therapy includes providing warmth (via brooder lamp), adequate hydration, and force-feeding warm molasses/sweetened feed. Hydration can be encouraged by offering a half concentration powdered milk instead of water. Superficial wounds can be treated with antibiotic cream and parenteral antibiotics. Most poultry will show evidence of recovery in 2–3 days. If there is no improvement after a few days, the prognosis for full recovery is generally poor.

Fatty Liver: Although all laying birds retain more fat in their livers than non-layers or males, fatty liver (*see* p 2820) is characterized by extreme fat deposition, sudden drop in egg production, and increased mortality. The hens are often obese and have pale combs, and the wattles and combs may be covered with dandruff. The cause is thought to be a combination of fatty feed and decreased exercise. Hens and poultry fed predominantly scratch diet (poultry treats, table scraps) are predisposed. Mortality is due to liver rupture and hemorrhaging, with large blood clots found in the abdomen on necropsy. Treatment is by prevention; most backyard birds have adequate outdoor access for exercise, but the diet must be controlled. Lipotrophic agents and dietary supplements (alfalfa, wheat bran, fish meal, dried brewer's yeast, soybean mill feed, vitamin E, and torula yeast) have been used with inconsistent results.

Cage Layer Fatigue (Osteoporosis): Cage-layer fatigue (*see* p 2897) is common in chickens, Coturnix quail, and Khaki Campbell ducks. Birds are unable to stand and have brittle bones. The ribs are often deviated in a sigmoid shape or fractured at the junction of the sternum and vertebra. Paralyzed birds are alert and responsive unless dehydrated. Possible causes include vitamin D_3, calcium, and phosphorus deficiencies and/or imbalances. Birds may die acutely (often from fractured spinal vertebrae and severed spinal cords) or can rapidly (4–7 days) recover after placement on the floor with easy access to food and water. With backyard poultry, treatment with vitamin D_3 IM or calcium gluconate IV can be helpful. Oyster shells and other large particle calcium sources can be added to the diet ad lib to prevent this condition. The oyster shell must not be ground so small that it passes through the intestinal tract, because it is essential to have slow release of calcium from larger particles being ground in the gizzard. The strain of bird and type of housing also affect incidence. The key is to ensure good nutrition (and good cortical bone formation) just before onset of lay. However, prolonged increase in dietary calcium before production can result in urolithiasis and/or a permanent cessation of parathyroid gland activity.

Cloacal Prolapse or "Vent Blow-Out": The vent will prolapse temporarily during normal delivery of an egg. However, slow retraction due to obesity or in poorly developed hens (those that come into lay too early) will attract cannibalism, trauma, and edema formation, which will often prevent retraction. Typically, these chickens are culled, and prevention is practiced by controlling obesity, stocking density of cages, lighting schedules, precocious onset of lay, and proper beak trimming. For backyard poultry, stopping lay (reduced light, sharp reduction in feed), isolating from other birds, and keeping the vent clean until retraction are sometimes effective in mild cases. If chicks are hatched in the fall, increasing light in the spring can induce them to come into lay when they are physically immature. Controlling light is extremely important in this circumstance.

Egg Binding: Egg binding is common in pullets brought into production too early or in obese hens. It can range from a temporary egg-binding observed in pullets that lay large eggs to complete obstruction of the oviduct. There can be eggs in the abdominal cavity (retropulsed); single or multiple eggs in the oviduct; or shell membranes, shells, and yolk/albumin concretions in the oviduct. The impaction can generally be identified on abdominal palpation, ultrasound, and/or radiographic examination. Commercial hens are culled. Backyard poultry can sometimes be treated by external reduction (smashing) of the egg within the oviduct and natural elimination, or by surgical removal of the entire oviduct (not ovary). Wrapping the bird in a warm towel and massaging the abdomen toward the vent after use of generous amounts of lubrication around the cloaca can sometimes induce propulsion if the binding is caught early enough. The surgical approach is generally midline; care should be taken to minimize damage to the air sacs. After removal of the oviduct, eggs deposited into the abdominal cavity will be absorbed. Most hens will assume male characteristics (crowing, aggression, spurs) after surgery and are called "pollards" (genetically female, phenotypically male).

COMMON INFECTIOUS DISEASES

The following list includes some of the more common conditions encountered in backyard poultry practice.

Parasitism

As in other species, the common parasites in poultry are mites, lice, ticks, worms, and protozoa. Two common mites of poultry are the Northern fowl mite (*Ornithonyssus sylviarum*) and the red mite (*see also* p 2877). The Northern fowl mite is most commonly found around the vent, tail, and breast. These mites are easily observed as small, reddish-brown flecks. Red mites (*Dermanyssus gallinae*) feed only at night, making daytime diagnosis difficult. They can be found in cracks and seams near bedding areas and appear like flea dust or salt and pepper–like deposits. Red mites cause feather loss, irritation, and anemia. Several types of lice live on poultry, and lice or nits can be seen at the base of the feathers. In severe infestations, growth and egg production can be affected. Insecticides are available for treatment. Fowl ticks (*see* p 2876) comprise a group of soft ticks that parasitize many species of poultry and wild birds. Ticks are easily missed, because they spend relatively little time on the bird. Heavy infestations can cause anemia or tick paralysis, and ticks can be vectors for *Borrelia anserina* (spirochetosis). Spraying of buildings with insecticide is the treatment of choice.

Roundworms and tapeworms are the most common internal poultry parasites and are generally the result of soil contamination and poor management. Unless infestations are heavy, clinical disease is usually not evident. A fecal examination should be performed before treatment to assess levels of infestation (and monitor effectiveness of treatment), because most domestic poultry will have some degree of internal parasitism. Piperazine can be used for roundworms, although its effectiveness can be minimal and drug resistance is a problem; off-label fenbendazole or levamisole can be used for tapeworms. These compounds should not be used in laying hens. Proper litter management will reduce parasite loads and reinfection. As in commercial poultry production, control of coccidia is one of the more costly problems in raising backyard poultry. Coccidia are found primarily in the intestinal tract of most poultry but are also found in the kidney in geese. Coccidiosis is generally seen in young birds (1–4 mo old), although it can be seen in any bird >10–14 days old. Signs include diarrhea that is often bloody and frequently leads to loss in production, general malaise, and death. Coccidia thrive in moist, heavily soiled litter, and disease is often a result of too high a density of birds. Prevention is by supplying coccidiostats in the feed, which can be given to birds as early as in their starter diet. Outbreaks can be treated with treatment dose of selected coccidiostats and extra-label sulfa drugs. Sulfa drugs have a long withdrawal period and should not be used in laying hens. Routine yearly fecal examinations are recommended for all backyard flocks. (*See also* COCCIDIOSIS, p 2791).

Viral Diseases

Marek's Disease: Marek's disease (MD) is a common viral disease of chickens, both in commercial production and backyard flocks (*see* p 2849). The primary lesions are tumors of the viscera, muscle, skin, and peripheral nerves. Nerve lesions can be an early indicator of the disease and result in a condition termed "range paralysis." Birds with visceral tumors often have cachexia as the only clinical sign. Tumors of the muscles and skin are frequently palpable. Tumors that affect the eyes (ocular Marek's) could be seen as a grayish color change in the pupils or irregular margins of the pupils, with lack of proper pupillary light reflex. MD cannot be treated but can be prevented by vaccination at hatch. When backyard poultry are acquired or hatched onsite, every attempt should be made to vaccinate for MD. Vaccinations may not be effective if administered to birds >1–2 wk old. Clinical MD generally affects birds 4–14 wk old; however, it is not uncommon in older birds, and death loss is often sporadic rather than explosive. If tumors are found in the viscera of deceased birds, carcasses should be submitted to a diagnostic laboratory for differential diagnosis between MD and avian leukosis (*see* p 2851), another common lymphoid tumor disease. Avian leukosis is seen in birds >14 wk old, and tumors are similar to those found with MD. Avian leukosis has no treatment or vaccination.

Infectious Bronchitis: Infectious bronchitis virus (IBV; *see* p 2909) causes a rapidly spreading respiratory disease in young chicks. Production is reduced and egg shell abnormalities are seen in laying hens. Certain strains of IBV also cause kidney disease. Chicks infected early in life may have permanent damage to the oviduct, so they do not produce eggs or become false layers (*see* p 2897). IBV is highly transmissible, but most birds recover with supportive treatment. Antibiotics can be administered in the water to prevent secondary infection. Vaccines are available; however, backyard chickens are usually not vaccinated unless they come in contact with other chickens.

Newcastle Disease: Newcastle disease virus (NDV; *see* p 2856) affects numerous species of birds and is the reason for quarantine regulations for birds entering the USA. Exotic NDV is highly fatal and is not present in the USA at this time. Past outbreaks have resulted in the slaughter of thousands of birds. Milder forms of NDV are present in the USA and are primarily characterized by respiratory disease and a drop in egg production. Mortality is variable and depends on the strain of the virus. As with infectious bronchitis virus, vaccination is available but is generally given to backyard poultry only if exposed to other birds.

Fowlpox: Fowlpox virus (*see* p 2824) causes crusty and nodular lesions primarily on the unfeathered portions of the bird. Occasionally, poxvirus can cause lesions in the mouth and trachea, causing death due to suffocation (wet form). If the bird recovers, immunity is generally lifelong. Not all pox outbreaks are caused by fowlpox virus but can be caused by related strains such as turkey pox, psittacine pox, quail pox, etc. Strains are usually species specific but can occasionally affect other species (eg, pigeon pox). One strain may not cross-protect with another. Vaccination is available and should be given to flocks on premises with a previous history of pox or with presence of pox in nearby birds. Poxvirus is transmitted through contact of infected lesions with open wounds and by insect bites (mosquitoes), and insect control is key to prevent spread.

Avian Encephalomyelitis: Avian encephalomyelitis (AE; *see* p 2888) is seen in chickens, turkeys, pheasants, and quail. It primarily affects chicks 1–3 wk old. Nearly all commercial flocks are infected, but clinical disease is low because of maternal antibodies. AE can be transmitted vertically in eggs laid between 5 and 13 days after infection and is an enteric infection under natural conditions. The spread is more rapid in floor-raised birds than in cage-raised birds. There is no treatment, and vaccination of breeders (both chicken and turkey) for maternal antibodies to protect the young during early life is critical to prevention. Because many specialty breeders, particularly those that sell stock to an intermediate supplier, do not vaccinate, AE is a fairly common viral disease in backyard poultry. Vaccination should be given after 8 wk of age but by at least 4 wk before production.

Bacterial Infections

Salmonellosis: In general, *Salmonella* Pullorum (*see* p 2865) and *S* Gallinarum (fowl typhoid; *see* p 2866) cause the greatest problem for poultry, whereas *S* Typhimurium, *S* Enteritidis, *S* Heidelberg, and *S* Kentucky are important in terms of public health. *S* Pullorum is egg transmitted, causes a diarrheal disease in young chicks and poults, and results in high mortality. Adult birds are asymptomatic carriers. Diagnosis is based on disease history and isolation of the bacteria. Prevention is achieved by purchasing birds from a breeder flock that is NPIP certified (National Poultry Improvement Plan) clean of *S* Pullorum and typhoid. Treatment is not recommended, because it can cause birds to become carriers. Fowl typhoid is seen in chickens, turkeys, and many other game and wild birds. Fowl typhoid is similar in disease presentation and diagnosis to *S* Pullorum, although mature birds can show clinical signs of fowl typhoid. Clinical signs are infrequently observed in poultry infected with *S* Enteritidis and *S* Typhimurium, although most paratyphoid *Salmonella* infections are asymptomatic in most poultry. Flocks can be monitored by obtaining egg samples and environmental samples to culture the organism.

Colibacillosis: Colibacillosis (*see also* p 2814) is caused by *Escherichia coli* and is usually secondary to other infections such as infectious bronchitis virus and mycoplasmosis. *E coli* is seen in most species and age groups. A wide variety of clinical signs affecting the respiratory, reproductive, and intestinal systems can be seen. Vigorous adherence to biosecurity and sanitation programs can effectively prevent the organism from causing disease. Many antibiotics can be used for treatment, and sensitivity to the antibiotic should be tested. Treatment is usually successful if the disease is in the early stages.

Mycoplasmosis (Chronic Respiratory Disease): Chronic respiratory disease in poultry (primarily chickens and turkeys) is generally caused by *Mycoplasma gallisepticum* infection (*see* p 2841). *M gallisepticum* is a reportable disease in turkeys in select states in the USA. Pathogenicity of *M gallisepticum* is enhanced by infection with other organisms. Clinical signs of respiratory disease develop slowly in a flock, and feed consumption drops. Infection of the sinuses with purulent exudate (swollen face) is common in turkeys. Serology and isolation and identification of the organism can be used for diagnosis. Prevention, as with the salmonellae, rests with establishment of a clean flock by eliminating the infected flock, completely sanitizing the premises, and obtaining clean stock. Vaccination is available on a state-by-state basis. Treatment is expensive, and the disease often recurs after treatment is stopped. Other important mycoplasmas in poultry include *M synoviae* (infectious synovitis) and *M meleagridis* (venereal infection and airsacculitis).

Fungal Diseases

Aspergillosis: Aspergillosis (*see also* p 2901), or brooder pneumonia, is seen in many poultry and other species of birds. Birds <3 wk old are most commonly affected, and infection is obtained from hatchers or brooders contaminated with fungal spores. Morbidity is variable, and mortality can be high in clinically affected birds. Culturing the fungus or demonstrating typical fungal hyphae in fresh preparations from lesions are used for diagnosis. Prevention is accomplished by thoroughly cleaning hatchers, incubators, waterers, feeders, and ventilation fans and by keeping litter clean and dry. Treatment is expensive and may not be effective. Ketaconazole and nystatin have been used.

Favus: Favus, or ringworm, also known as white comb, is a fungal disease caused by *Microsporum gallinae*, which is of minor importance in all fowl, especially chickens and turkeys. Affected birds have small, white, chalky deposits on the comb, which can enlarge and coalesce to form a dull white, moldy layer that could be several millimeters thick. The disease is self-limiting, and the comb heals after several months. Typically, if the disease is limited to the comb, the health of the bird is not affected, but if feathered portions are involved, the bird may become emaciated and die. Favus is a public health concern.

Antibiotic Usage

Antibiotics are readily available in feed stores and online poultry supply sites; however, use of antibiotics must be carefully considered. Each antibiotic is labeled for different species and the use of the poultry, and administering the correct dosage may be difficult. In some instances, antibiotics are useful to treat and control disease. Certain antibiotics such as chloramphenicol, glycopeptides, and fluoroquinolones are prohibited for extra-label use in food animals, including backyard poultry. A veterinarian should be consulted; judicious use of antibiotics may be recommended after appropriate diagnostics. However, vaccination, good biosecurity, good management, proper sanitation practices, and a good plane of nutrition are key to control of disease and are far more effective than antibiotic usage.

FERRETS

The domestic ferret (*Mustela putorius furo*) is in the order Carnivora, family Mustelidae, and has been in captivity for more than 2,000 years. Ferrets are used as research animals, often in studies of the respiratory system and as a model for *Helicobacter* sp infection. They have become popular pets in recent years in the USA. They are also used as hunting animals in Europe, Australia, and New Zealand.

MANAGEMENT

The male ferret (hob) can weigh as much as 2 kg when intact, with an average weight of 1.2 kg when neutered. The female (jill) can weigh as much as 1.2 kg when intact, with an average weight of 0.8 kg when spayed. Sexual maturity is reached at 4–8 mo and occurs in the first spring after birth. The vast majority of ferrets are spayed or neutered before 6 wk of age, primarily because females are induced ovulators and can develop severe hyperestrogenemia if not bred. Ferrets also have less of the musky smell that is characteristic of Mustelids if they are gonadectomized early in life. The anal scent glands are usually removed at the time of the neuter or spay. Most physiologic data for ferrets are similar to those of the domestic cat, except that creatinine should not be >0.9 mg/dL in ferrets. Ferrets require high levels of fat and protein in the diet and should be fed commercial ferret food or high-quality cat or kitten food. Most adult ferrets have a large spleen. This is usually caused by extramedullary hematopoiesis and is nonpathogenic; ultrasonography and aspiration can be used for a definitive diagnosis.

Vaccination: Ferrets are vaccinated annually for rabies and canine distemper. There is one FDA-approved rabies vaccine for ferrets in the USA. It should be given to ferrets >16 wk old and repeated annually. If this vaccine is unavailable, a recombinant vaccine should be substituted. Canine distemper vaccines for ferrets should be of chick embryo or recombinant origin. Vaccines of mink or ferret culture (eg, most multivalent vaccines for dogs) should not be used, because they may cause seroconversion and disease. There is currently one FDA-approved distemper vaccine in the USA for ferrets. Ferrets should be vaccinated at ~8, 10, and 12 wk of age and then yearly. Vaccine reactions occur frequently in ferrets; vaccinated animals should be monitored for 20–30 min after vaccination, and only one vaccine (ie, rabies or distemper) should be given at a time. Ferrets raised commercially are often vaccinated for *Clostridium botulinum* type C at 6–8 wk old.

INFECTIOUS DISEASES

Bacterial Diseases: *Helicobacter mustelae* is found in the stomach and duodenum of all ferrets after weaning. It is an opportunistic pathogen and can induce chronic, persistent gastritis and ulcer formation similar to the disease in people. Gastric lymphoma may occur in chronic cases. Clinical signs include inappetence, vomiting, bruxism, diarrhea, melena, and hypersalivation. Lethargy, weight loss, and dehydration can also occur. These animals may be painful on cranial abdominal palpation because of the ulcers induced or enhanced by the presence of this bacterium. Definitive diagnosis requires examination of tissue from surgical or endoscopic biopsy but is not commonly performed because of the ubiquitous nature of this organism in the ferret GI tract. Silver stains and urease tests should be performed on the biopsy specimens when attempting to determine a definitive diagosis. A molecular assay is available for fecal samples. Treatment is with multidrug regimens, including amoxicillin (20 mg/kg, PO, bid), metronidazole (20 mg/kg, PO, bid), and bismuth subsalicylate (1 mL/kg, PO, bid). Clarithromycin (25 mg/kg/day, PO) and omeprazole (1 mg/kg/day, PO) can be used for refractory cases. Treatment is usually for 21 days. Because of the opportunistic nature of this pathogen, it is important to look for underlying problems such as gastroenteritis, foreign bodies, or stress. Treatment for *Helicobacter* is commonly initiated when gastroenteritis or foreign bodies are diagnosed or when a gastrotomy is peformed.

Lawsonia intracellularis can cause a proliferative bowel disease, especially in younger ferrets. Signs include diarrhea, weight loss, and rectal prolapse. Treatment is with chloramphenicol (25 mg/kg, PO, bid) for 14–21 days.

Salmonellosis in ferrets is rare but associated with feeding raw or undercooked meat or unpasteurized milk. Signs include bloody diarrhea, conjunctivitis, and anemia. *Salmonella* Typhimurium, *S* Newport, and *S* Choleraesuis may be involved. Treatment is with aggressive supportive care and antibiotics. Ferrets are susceptible to *Mycobacterium avium*, *M bovis*, and *Mycobacterium tuberculosis*. Intradermal testing is not reliable. Bacterial cystitis is rare in ferrets and is usually associated with urolithiasis and prostatomegaly. *Escherichia coli*, *Staphylococcus aureus*, and *Proteus* spp are most commonly identified. Bacterial pneumonias in ferrets are caused by *Streptococcus zooepidemicus*, *Mycobacterium* spp, and gram-negative bacteria such as *E coli* and *Klebsiella pneumoniae*. Other bacterial infections are similar to those seen in other carnivores.

Viral Diseases: Ferrets are susceptible to **canine distemper virus**. Transmission is by aerosol or exposure to infected secretions. Clinical signs begin 7–10 days after infection and start as fever and dermatitis on the chin and inguinal area, progressing to anorexia, erythema of mucus membranes, and mucopurulent ocular and nasal discharge. Brown crusts on the face and eyelids and hyperkeratosis of the footpads also occur. Respiratory signs develop and progress rapidly. Diagnosis is by history, clinical signs, and positive immunofluorescent antibody testing or histopathology. Mortality is close to 100% and typically occurs 12–14 days after infection.

The **human influenza virus** causes fever, lethargy, anorexia, nasal discharge, sneezing, and depression in ferrets. Treatment is supportive and includes antibiotics for secondary infections, antihistamines, and amantadine (6 mg/kg, nasally, bid). Recovery is usually within 7–14 days.

Two coronaviruses cause disease in ferrets. The ferret enteric coronavirus causes **epizootic catarrhal enteritis**. This disease is highly transmissible and is often brought into a group of ferrets by an asymptomatic juvenile animal. Clinical signs begin 2–14 days after introduction of the new ferret or exposure through fomites and include anorexia, vomiting, green or mucoid diarrhea, melena, dehydration, lethargy, and weight loss. The disease is most severe in older ferrets, which may take months to fully recover. The virus causes blunting of the intestinal villi and consequent maldigestion and malabsorption. Definitive diagnosis is difficult, although scanning electron microscopy of the feces may identify coronavirus. Increased ALT and alkaline phosphatase may occur secondary to hepatic lipidosis. Treatment is supportive and includes fluids, nutritional support, broad-spectrum antibiotics, and GI protectants. Prevention is by quarantine of new ferrets, thorough cleaning of new bedding and toys, and washing hands and changing clothes after handling other ferrets.

A second related coronavirus called ferret systemic coronavirus causes a systemic pyogranulomatous inflammatory disease resembling the dry form of feline infectious peritonitis. This disease is seen in young ferrets (average age 11 mo) and is progressive throughout several weeks to months. Clinical signs include anorexia, weigh loss, diarrhea, and enlarged intra-abdominal and, less commonly, peripheral lymph nodes. Hypergammaglobulinemia, anemia, and CNS signs can be seen as the disease progresses. This disease was initially called disseminated idiopathic myofasciitis because of the white nodules found in many tissues on necropsy. These nodules are pyogranulomatous inflammation and involve many organs, including peritoneum, adipose tissue, viscera, and blood vessels. A pyogranulomatous pneumonia has also recently been reported. Treatment is supportive with immunosuppressants such as prednisolone and anecdotal reports of use of polyprenyl immunostimulants, which have resulted in some increase in survival time. Average survival time is ~2 mo.

Aleutian disease is a parvovirus originally seen in mink, but at least two distinct ferret strains of the virus have been identified (*see* p 1872). The virus causes immune complex deposition in organs, which results in a variety of nonspecific clinical signs such as progressive weight loss, weakness, ataxia, hepatomegaly, and splenomegaly. A severe hypergammaglobulinemia is the most consistent finding on blood work. A presumptive diagnosis is based on clinical signs and hyperglobulinemia. The two most common tests for the virus antibody are counterimmunoelectrophoresis and immunofluorescent antibody tests. Definitive diagnosis is difficult, because many apparently normal ferrets have positive titers. The organism has been found in the urine, feces, and blood of symptomatic and asymptomatic animals. Treatment with anti-inflammatories and immunosuppresants such as prednisolone and cyclophosphamide can be considered and may have clinical benefit. Treatment of infected mink kits with gamma globulin–containing Aleutian disease virus antibody has decreased mortality rates, but this treatment has not been attempted in ferrets. There is currently no vaccine available for this disease in ferrets.

Fungal Diseases: Ferrets are susceptible to *Microsporum canis* and *Trichophyton mentagrophytes*. Transmission is by direct contact or fomites and is often associated with overcrowding and exposure to cats. Infection is more common in kits and young ferrets and is often seasonal and self-limiting. A pyogranulomatous dermatitis and fungal pododermatitis has been associated with *Microsporum nanum*. Other fungal diseases in ferrets include cryptococcal meningitis and blastomycosis causing granulomatous meningoencephalitis. Fungal pneumonia is uncommon in ferrets but can be caused by *Blastomyces dermatitidis* and *Coccidioides immitis* in endemic areas. Cryptococcosis from *Cryptococcus bacillisporus* and *C neoformans* var *grubii* has been diagnosed in ferrets. Signs include pneumonia, pleuritis, rhinitis, and regional lymph node enlargement.

Parasitic Diseases: Ear mites are the most common ectoparasite in ferrets and are caused by *Otodectes cynotis*. The same ear mite is found in dogs and cats, and it can be passed between species. Diagnosis and treatment are as for dogs and cats (*see* OTITIS EXTERNA, p 527). Fleas are also common in ferrets and can be transmitted between ferrets and other household pets. Diagnosis is by visualization, and treatment is the same as for dogs and cats (*see* FLEAS AND FLEA ALLERGY DERMATITIS, p 880). Many of the long-acting topical treatments, such as fipronil, last longer in ferrets because of the increased sebum in the coat. Mange in ferrets is caused by *Sarcoptes scabiei* and can be seen as a generalized dermatitis or can be limited to the feet, toes, and pads in a pedal form unique to ferrets.

Heartworm disease, caused by *Dirofilaria immitis*, can be found in ferrets, especially if given outdoor access in endemic areas. Disease can be caused by even a single worm. Clinical signs include lethargy, coughing, dyspnea, and ascites. Ferrets are typically infected with a very small number of worms (1–20), making diagnosis difficult. Echocardiography is warranted, because the parasites often obstruct blood flow and cause right-side heart failure. Echocardiography may also be helpful in identification of the worms in the right ventricle, pulmonary arteries, and vena cavae. Peripheral microfilaremia is uncommon in ferrets; therefore, antigen testing is more beneficial. Treatment using longterm antithrombotic drugs and adulticides can be done but may cause problems. Low-dose ivermectin (0.05 mg/kg, SC, monthly until clinical signs and microfilaremia resolve) is the current recommended treatment (*see* HEARTWORM DISEASE, p 127).

Coccidiosis can cause disease in young ferrets including diarrhea, lethargy, and rectal prolapse. Diagnosis and treatment are similar to those in dogs. Rectal prolapse can also occur with coccidiosis and usually resolves after treating the underlying disease. Topical hemorrhoidal creams may be helpful.

NEOPLASIA

Cutaneous mast cell tumors are probably the most common nonendocrine tumor in ferrets. These tumors can appear anywhere on the body but typically affect the trunk and neck. The tumor appears as a raised, irregular, and often scabbed mass. Systemic signs are rare, but the tumors may bleed when scratched. Treatment is by excision. Local treatment with strontium may also be beneficial.

Lymphoma is common in ferrets and can affect many organ systems, including the lymph nodes, spleen, liver, heart, thymus, and kidneys. Disease of the spine and CNS has also been seen. Lymphoma of young ferrets is often rapidly progressive, whereas it is often a chronic disease in adults. Clusters of lymphoma have been seen in related or cohabitating ferrets, and a viral agent is suspected in those cases. Diagnostics should include a CBC, chemistry panel, radiographs, ultrasonography, and aspirates of any suspected tissues. Treatment protocols for ferrets have not been standardized but can include removal of the neoplastic tissue if possible, chemotherapy, and/or radiation therapy. Immunosuppression is a common problem with chemotherapy in ferrets, and frequent CBCs are imperative with any treatment protocol.

Chordomas and chondrosarcomas have been reported in ferrets. Chordomas typically appear as firm masses on the tail. They may become ulcerated from dragging on the ground but otherwise cause few problems. These tumors have also been reported at the cervical region, causing paresis and ataxia. Surgical removal is suggested when possible. Chondrosarcomas can develop anywhere along the spine, ribs, or sternum and tend to cause spinal cord compression and associated clinical signs. Treatment should include removal, if possible.

Splenomegaly is common in adult ferrets and is usually caused by extramedullary hematopoiesis; however, lymphoma and hemangiosarcoma can occur. An irregular or firm spleen should be investigated with ultrasonography and aspiration.

ENDOCRINE DISORDERS

Insulinomas are very common in ferrets >2–3 yr old. These functional tumors of the pancreatic β cells cause increased insulin levels, resulting in hypoglycemia and its associated clinical signs such as weakness, lethargy, posterior paresis, hypersalivation, bruxism, and seizures. Diagnosis is based on demonstration of hypoglycemia and corresponding normal or increased insulin levels. Other blood tests are usually normal. Ultrasonography is only occasionally useful in demonstrating these pancreatic masses. Medical and surgical treatments are possible, but there is no cure, and owners should be made aware of the chronic and progressive nature of this disease. Surgical treatment involves removing discrete tumors via nodulectomies or partial pancreatectomy. Microscopic tumors within the entire pancreas are common; therefore, removal of the entire tumor is unlikely. A period of euglycemia occurs after surgery in some cases, but most cases require continued medical treatment. Major benefits of surgery are decreased severity of signs, ease of management, and moderately increased survival time. Medical management includes use of prednisone (0.5–2 mg/kg, PO, bid) and diazoxide (5–30 mg/kg, PO, bid) to counteract the effects of the tumor; however, this does not affect the tumor directly. Prednisone increases resting blood glucose levels and down-regulates peripheral insulin receptors, whereas diazoxide decreases insulin release from the β cells and competes at peripheral insulin receptors. These drugs can be used independently or synergistically. Typically, prednisone is used first until the dosage approaches 2 mg/kg and then diazoxide is added. Medical treatment is lifelong, and glucose levels should be monitored 5–7 days after changing doses and at least every 3 mo afterward.

Hyperadrenocorticism in ferrets is caused by excessive secretion of the sex hormones progesterone, testosterone (in the form of androstenedione), and estrogen by the zona reticularis of the adrenal gland. It can be seen in ferrets as young as 1.5 yr old. The most common clinical sign is hair loss beginning on the tail and rump and progressing up the flank and head.
In females, a swollen vulva and enlarged mamillae may also be seen, whereas males may develop aggression and stranguria secondary to prostatic enlargement. Bone marrow suppression may be seen in either sex, with severe hyperestrogenemia. A presumptive diagnosis is made after history and physical examination. The enlarged adrenal glands are often palpable cranial to either kidney. CBCs and chemistry panels are typically normal. Radiographs are not useful, because the masses do not calcify as commonly as in other species. Ultrasonography can demonstrate enlargement of the gland(s). Definitive diagnosis requires measurement of the three sex hormones, which can be performed in a panel (at University of Tennessee).

Medical and surgical treatments exist. Surgical removal of the adrenal gland(s) is more likely to be curative than medical management, but there is still a recurrence rate of ~40% after surgery. The left gland is easier to remove, because the right gland is closely associated with the caudal vena cava. If both sides are affected, a subtotal adrenalectomy can be performed. Histology of these glands may reveal hyperplasia, adenoma, or adenocarcinoma. Functionally, all three grades are similar, and metastasis is unlikely. Hypoadrenocorticism may develop if both adrenal glands are completely or partially removed. This may be treated with mineralocorticoid and glucocorticoid supplementation. Medical management of hyperadrenocorticism is aimed at reducing the clinical signs but does not affect the adrenal tumor itself. Leuprolide acetate is the most common drug used. The mechanism is not completely understood but is probably related to down-regulation of peripheral hormone receptors. Leuprolide is a repositol formulation of a GnRH agonist that is formulated in 1-mo (100–400 mcg, IM) and 4-mo (2–4 mg, IM) preparations. Owners should be advised that this is a lifelong treatment to control the clinical signs of the disease. Recently, some clinicians have treated hyperadrenocorticism medically only during breeding months, typically November to March. Deslorelin acetate, a similar GnRH agonist, is also available. This is a longer-acting implant that lasts 10–17 mo. This drug is well tolerated by ferrets. Melatonin can also be used at 1 mg per ferret per day, orally or in an injectable, repositol formulation, which is reported to last 4 mo. This drug counteracts the alopecia and may help with other signs as well, but, like leuprolide, is only symptomatic treatment. Drugs used to control sex hormone levels in people are beginning to be used in ferrets and show promise in controlling clinical signs.

OTHER NONINFECTIOUS DISEASES

Gastric foreign bodies are common in ferrets because of the animal's inquisitive nature. Foreign bodies are usually soft rubber or plastic items but can also be trichobezoars. Clinical signs include anorexia, bruxism, hypersalivation, cranial abdominal pain, diarrhea, and melena. Vomiting is more common with gastritis than with foreign bodies. Diagnosis is with plain or contrast radiography. Treatment involves surgical or endoscopic removal. Gastritis should be treated after removal of the foreign body.

Dilated cardiomyopathy can occur in ferrets, usually those >4 yr old. Clinical signs can be similar to those of insulinoma, so both should be excluded when examining a ferret with lethargy, weakness, ascites, increased respiratory effort, or exercise intolerance. Diagnosis is by radiography and echocardiography. Treatment is based on echocardiographic abnormalities and includes furosemide, digoxin, enalapril, benazepril, and pimobendan. A formulary should be consulted for dosing instructions.

Renal disease in ferrets is similar to that in other species. Renal cysts are common in adult ferrets and usually do not cause a problem unless present in large numbers. Uroliths can develop in ferrets fed diets high in plant proteins and are usually composed of struvite.

HEDGEHOGS

Hedgehogs are in the family Erinaceidae, within the order Insectivora. The central African hedgehog (*Atelerix albiventris*), also known as the white-bellied, four-toed, or African pygmy hedgehog, is native to dry, open habitats in central and eastern Africa. They are nocturnal and very active, jogging for miles in search of invertebrate prey. In the USA, it is illegal to own a hedgehog as a pet in some states and municipalities; in other states, a permit is required. Additionally, a USDA permit is required to breed, transport, sell, or exhibit hedgehogs.

Anatomy, Physiology, and Behavior:

The dorsum is covered in a dense coat of keratin spines; each spine has a basal bulb that firmly attaches it within the follicle, with a narrowed portion at the skin surface. Healthy spines are difficult to pull from the follicle without breakage. The spined skin has a thin and hairless epidermis and a thick, fibrous dermis with much fat and few blood vessels. A wary hedgehog will raise the spines and crouch. If a hedgehog is frightened, contraction of the panniculus muscle pulls the loose spiny skin over the entire body. The panniculus is thickened at the rim to form the orbicularis, a purse-string–like muscle that closes the spined skin over the animal. For selected physiologic data for African pygmy hedgehogs, *see* TABLE 10.

Hedgehogs have brachydont teeth. The first incisor in each quadrant is large and projects forward, and there is a gap between the maxillary first incisors. The stomach is simple, and a vomiting reflex is present. The male has a conspicuous prepuce that opens mid-abdomen. There is no scrotal sac; the testes are located in a para-anal recess surrounded by fat and can be palpated in reproductively active males. The female urogenital opening is a few millimeters cranial to the anus. The uterus is bicornuate with a single cervix and no uterine body. Hedgehogs are polyestrous and breed throughout the year in captivity. Ovulation is believed to be induced, and sterile matings with pseudopregnancy may occur. Hedgehogs are born hairless, with closed eyes and ears; at birth the spines are covered by a membrane that is removed within the first few hours of life.

Hedgehogs are adept at climbing, digging, swimming, and jogging. While they have sensitive olfaction and hearing, their sense of vision is not as well developed. Foraging hedgehogs normally emit a variety of snuffling sounds; agitated hedgehogs make a loud hissing sound that may be punctuated with various puffing and cough-like sounds. With intense distress, a scream may be emitted. With patience, most hedgehogs learn to accept handling.

Hedgehogs demonstrate a unique behavior called self-anointing, or anting. This behavior may be elicited by a variety of substances, particularly those with a strong odor. The hedgehog takes the material into the mouth,

TABLE 10 PHYSIOLOGIC DATA FOR AFRICAN PYGMY HEDGEHOGS

Average body weight	Male: 400–600 g Female: 300–400g
Life span	Average 4–6 yr, may live to 8 yr
Body temperature	95.7°–98.6°F (35.4°–37.0°C)
Adult dental formula	2 (I 3/2:C 1/1:P 3/2:M 3/3) = 36 (variations have been noted)
GI transit time	12–16 hr
Heart rate	180–280 bpm
Respiratory rate	25–50 bpm
Age at sexual maturity	2–3 mo
Reproductive life span	Male: throughout life Female: 2–3 yr
Gestation	34–37 days
Litter size	3–4 (range 1–9)
Birth weight	10–18 g
Eyes open	14–18 days
Deciduous teeth eruption	Begins on day 18; all deciduous teeth erupted by 9 wk
Permanent teeth eruption	Begins at 7–9 wk
Age at weaning	5–6 wk (start eating solids at 3 wk)

mixes it with frothy saliva, and applies the mixture to its spines with the tongue. The purpose of this behavior is unknown.

MANAGEMENT

Housing: Wild hedgehogs are solitary; as pets they are usually maintained in individual cages. Some fanciers successfully house multiple animals together, but this can lead to disproportionate feeding and injuries from fighting. Healthy hedgehogs are very active; 2 × 3 ft are minimal floor dimensions. Hedgehogs are able to climb and can escape through small holes, so the cage must be secure and lidded. Glass tanks and plastic-bottomed cages with wire walls are suitable, provided that the wire spacing is sufficiently close. Widely spaced wires can lead to limb entrapment or death if the hedgehog's head becomes ensnared by its spines. A hiding place is essential. The cage substrate should be soft and absorbent. Recycled newspaper bedding is a good choice; aspen shavings, alfalfa pellets, and hay are other options. Wire, cedar, corncob, and dusty or scented substrates are not recommended, and cloth bedding poses a risk of limb entrapment. The substrate should be 3–4 in. deep to allow for digging.

Ambient temperature should be 72°–90°F (22°–32°C); 75°–85°F (24°–29°C) is optimal. Hedgehogs may go into a torpid state if too cool or too warm; this is believed to be unhealthy for pet hedgehogs. A heating pad placed underneath the enclosure or a ceramic reptile heater may be used. Low humidity (<40%) is preferred. Hedgehogs avoid bright light; however, a day cycle of 10–14 hr of mild light should be provided. Although some owners may attempt to convert their pets to a diurnal schedule, most remain nocturnal.

Some hedgehogs use a litter tray; natural plant litters used for cats make the best litter substrate. Clay, clumping-type litter, or sand may stick to the animal and should not be used. Many hedgehogs defecate in their hide boxes and exercise wheels, so daily spot cleaning is often necessary. Exercise wheels with solid metal or plastic running surfaces are highly recommended. Hedgehog legs can become entrapped in wire wheels. Hedgehogs should be let out daily for exercise. Cardboard tubes, straw, safe climbing structures, swimming tubs, and other toys provide interest. Dirty hedgehogs may be bathed with a mild pet shampoo and use of a soft-bristle vegetable brush.

Diet: The ideal diet is a commercially prepared hedgehog food. If hedgehog food is not used, premium food for less active cats or dog food are alternatives. Food should be rationed to prevent obesity. Depending on the animal's weight and activity, 3–4 tsp (15–20 mL) of the main diet is typically fed daily. Growing animals and reproductively active females may be fed ad lib, and calcium-rich foods are recommended.

In addition to the main diet, ~1–2 tsp (5–10 mL) of varied moist foods and/or invertebrate prey (eg, canned cat or dog food, cooked meat or egg, low-fat cottage cheese, mealworms, earthworms, waxworms, gut-loaded crickets) and ~1 tsp (5 mL) of vegetable/fruit mix (eg, beans, cooked carrots, squash, peas, tomatoes, leafy greens, banana, grape, apple, pear, berries) should also be provided daily. Invertebrate prey and dry food items may be hidden in the bedding to promote foraging. Hedgehogs should not be fed raw meat or eggs, which may harbor *Salmonella*. Milk can cause diarrhea. Vitamin or mineral supplementation is not necessary for hedgehogs fed a commercial diet. Hedgehogs are often slow to accept new foods, and diet changes must be made with care. Fresh water should be available at all times. Most hedgehogs can learn to drink from water bottles.

Breeding and Neonatal Care: Females should be at least 6 mo old before breeding. A weight gain of ≥50 g within 3 wk of breeding suggests pregnancy. At 30 days, abdominal and mammary enlargement may be detected. Infanticide and cannibalism of the young can occur; the female needs strict privacy from other hedgehogs and people starting ~5 days before delivery and continuing 5–14 days after parturition.

In cases of lactation failure or abandonment, fostering of the pups (or "hoglets") to another dam with similarly aged pups is usually successful. If a surrogate dam is unavailable, a canine milk replacer may be fed through a feeding tube or syringe; however, hand-rearing of hedgehogs is associated with high mortality. Weaning generally occurs at 5–6 wk, and the young may be moved to separate cages at 8 wk. Daily handling starting at 3 wk will result in hedgehogs that remain tame.

Restraint and Examination: Because most hedgehogs roll up when restrained, a thorough examination usually requires chemical restraint. Before sedation, the hedgehog should be observed in the examination room. Healthy, untroubled hedgehogs should be active and walk with the ventrum raised off the table, but weak or wary hedgehogs tend to crouch. The nose is normally moist and active. Respiration is normally silent, except when the hedgehog hisses in defense. Normal feces are dark brown and very soft to pellet-like. The skin in the spiny areas may have a mildly dry or flaky appearance, but excessive flaking, quill loss, erythema, and crusting are abnormal.

Once the hedgehog is sedated or anesthetized (eg, with isoflurane at a light plane), the remainder of the examination can be performed. Hydration may be assessed by eyelid turgor. The eyes should be clear, and the pinnal margins should be free of crusting or ragged edges. The teeth should be white and the gingiva a uniform pink. The oral cavity and tongue should be inspected for ulcers, foreign material, and masses. Normal lymph nodes are difficult to palpate, but they may become enlarged in cases of neoplasia or infection. The heart should have a regular rhythm and no murmurs, and a femoral pulse should be palpable. The abdominal contour should be flat but may be distended by obesity, organomegaly, masses, or fluid. The prepuce or vulva should be checked for inflammation, discharge, or adherent debris. Testicles may be palpable in the para-anal area. The toes should be inspected for encircling fibers and overgrown nails.

Clinical Techniques: The jugular vein can be used to collect blood samples; its anatomic location is similar to that in other small mammals. Alternatively, the cranial vena cava may be used, but there is a greater risk of cardiac puncture because of the relatively cranial position of the hedgehog heart. The femoral, lateral saphenous, or cephalic veins may be used for injections or to collect small samples (up to 0.5 mL).

SC injections can be given in the spiny or furred areas; the furred skin is more elastic and vascular but less accessible. The dermis under the spiny skin is poorly vascularized, so drugs or fluid given in this location may not be absorbed for several hours. The junction of furred and spined skin provides an accessible and reliable site. IM injections may be given in the triceps, quadriceps, gluteal, or orbicularis muscles. IV catheters are usually dislodged if the animal curls. An intraosseous catheter may be placed in the tibial crest using a 22- or 25-gauge needle or 1-in. spinal needle; the catheter remains accessible even when the animal is curled.

Radiography may be useful, but the hedgehog's spines can obscure detail. For lateral views, the spines can be pulled away from the chest and abdomen and secured with a large plastic clip. Anesthesia is generally required for proper positioning.

Oral medication may be difficult to administer. Some animals accept liquid medications that have been compounded with fruit flavor. Alternatively, medication may be injected into mealworms or mixed with a favorite food. Applying topical medications is complicated by the presence of spines and self-grooming, and some odors may initiate anting behavior (*see* p 1828).

A cage temperature of 80°–85°F (27°–29°C) is recommended for ill hedgehogs. Voluntary feeding is facilitated by providing the animal's customary diet and by offering live invertebrates. Anorectic animals should be fed a high-calorie canine or feline diet via syringe or tube. For ongoing assisted feeding, a pharyngostomy or esophagostomy tube can be placed.

Hedgehogs are not bacterial fermenters, and there are no particular concerns regarding antibiotic use. For appropriate drugs and dosages in this species, consult the *Exotic Animal Formulary* (2013) or other sources.

Anesthesia and Surgery: A 4- to 6-hr fast is recommended before anesthetic procedures longer than 20 min. Isoflurane is commonly used for induction and maintenance. Hypersalivation may occur, and premedication with atropine is advised. Ketamine, diazepam, midazolam, xylazine, and toletamine/zolazepam have also been used but may prolong recovery. Tracheal intubation may be indicated for longer or oral procedures and is accomplished with a 1.0–1.5 mm endotracheal tube, Teflon IV catheter, or feeding tube.

Spines are removed by clipping or with steady traction. Hedgehogs may self-mutilate traumatic or surgical wounds; prompt primary closure with subcuticular sutures should be used whenever possible. Bandages and dilute chlorhexidine baths are well tolerated. If the cutaneous muscle is damaged, it must be closed in a separate layer. Contraction of the rolling-up musculature can cause wound dehiscence. Elizabethan collars are not practical.

Ovariohysterectomy is similar to the procedure in other mammals, although substantial fat surrounds the ovaries and mesosalpinx. Castration is performed through a para-anal skin incision over each testicle; a closed technique is preferred.

Preventive Medicine: Hedgehogs have a short life span and often hide signs of illness; therefore, examinations (under isoflurane anesthesia) every 6 mo with blood testing are recommended. A 2-yr-old hedgehog should be considered geriatric. There are currently no vaccines labeled for use in hedgehogs. Because hedgehogs are not usually housed in mixed gender groups, castration and ovariohysterectomy are not generally requested or recommended. The incidence of uterine and mammary tumors is a concern; however, the effect of early age ovariohysterectomy on tumor reduction is unknown.

DISEASES

Sick hedgehogs with a variety of illnesses, including acariasis, dental problems, pneumonia, gastric ulceration, neoplasia, and hepatic disease, often present with nonspecific clinical signs such as lethargy, weakness, and anorexia. This frequent presentation serves to emphasize the importance of diagnostic testing, even if anesthesia is required.

Cardiovascular and Hematologic Diseases: Dilated cardiomyopathy (*see* p 115) is a common postmortem finding, with an incidence of 38% in captive African hedgehogs. The etiology is not known; however, genetic and nutritional causes have been suggested. Affected hedgehogs are typically ≥3 yr old, although it may be seen in animals as young as 1 yr of age. Males are slightly overrepresented. Signs include dyspnea, decreased activity, weight loss, an auscultable murmur, ascites, and acute death. Radiographs typically demonstrate varying degrees of cardiac enlargement, pulmonary edema, pleural effusion, hepatic congestion, and abdominal fluid. Common gross necropsy findings associated with cardiovascular disease in hedgehogs include cardiomegaly, hepatomegaly, pulmonary edema and/or congestion, hydrothorax, ascites, and pulmonary or renal infarcts. Normal echocardiographic measurements have been published for the African pygmy hedgehog. These reference intervals, along with subjective evaluation of wall motion and chamber size, can be used to confirm the diagnosis of dilated cardiomyopathy. Hematologic and biochemical testing are useful to screen for concurrent problems and to monitor the effects of therapeutic agents. Therapy with furosemide, enalapril, and digoxin may be helpful. Alternatively, furosemide, pimobendan, and supplementation with oral carnitine have been used. The longterm prognosis for hedgehogs with congestive heart failure is poor.

Saddle thrombus and pulmonary thromboemboli have been seen. Myocardial mineralization and splenic extramedullary hematopoiesis may exist in pet hedgehogs with concurrent diseases; the clinical significance of these lesions is unknown. Congenital erythropoietic porphyria was reported in a 6-mo-old male inbred pet African hedgehog.

Gastrointestinal and Hepatic Diseases: GI obstructions are most often caused by ingestion of rubber, hair, or carpet fibers. Signs include acute anorexia, lethargy, and collapse. Vomiting may be present but often is not. Diagnosis of obstruction is complicated by the fact that gaseous dilation of the GI tract can be a nonspecific finding in ill hedgehogs. A fatal intestinal mesenteric torsion has also been reported. Alimentary inflammation, including esophagitis, gastritis, enteritis, colitis, and gastric ulceration with perforation, has also been seen. Most of these hedgehogs had nonspecific signs such as decreased appetite and weight loss; vomiting and diarrhea were not seen. A case of gastroesophageal intussusception and megaesophagus has been reported in a hedgehog. This animal's clinical signs included dyspnea, vocalization, and salivation; vomiting ensued before death.

Enteritis may be caused by *Salmonella* or other bacteria. Salmonellosis in hedgehogs may be clinically silent or may cause diarrhea, weight loss, decreased appetite, dehydration, lethargy, and death. Diagnosis should be confirmed with fecal culture, using *Salmonella*-enriching medium. Although treatment is indicated in hedgehogs with clinical signs of disease, owners should be advised of the zoonotic potential and the risks of creating antibiotic resistance. Alimentary candidiasis (*Candida albicans*) and cryptosporidiosis are other reported infectious diseases. Although numerous species of nematodes, cestodes, and protozoa have been identified in wild hedgehogs, their significance in pets appears to be minimal.

Diarrhea also can be associated with some commercial diets or inappropriate foods such as milk. GI neoplasia, particularly lymphosarcoma, is relatively common. Other considerations for GI signs include dietary change, toxins, hepatic disease, and malnutrition. Hedgehog digestion does not rely on bacterial fermentation, and there is no evidence of antibiotic sensitivity as is seen in herbivorous mammals. Hematochezia should be clearly differentiated from urinary or vaginal bloody discharge.

Hepatic lipidosis is relatively common and may be a sequela of cardiomyopathy, neoplasia, starvation, obesity, toxicosis, pregnancy, or infectious disease. Signs may include lethargy, inappetence, icterus, diarrhea, and signs of hepatic encephalopathy. Diagnosis is supported by testing for hepatic enzymes, plasma bilirubin, and bile acids. Radiography and ultrasound-guided liver aspirates may also be performed. Treatment for hepatic lipidosis is similar to that in other species. Other important causes of liver failure include primary and metastatic hepatic neoplasia. Hepatic necrosis caused by human herpes simplex virus 1 was reported in a hedgehog that received dexamethasone.

Integumentary Diseases: Acariasis caused by *Caparinia* spp (psoroptic mite) is very common. Infestation with *Notoedres* spp (sarcoptic mite) has also been reported in hedgehogs. Signs include lethargy, decreased appetite, hyperkeratosis, seborrhea, quill loss, loose quills, and white or brownish crusts (mite droppings) at the base of the quills and around the eyes. Hedgehogs may scratch or rub themselves, but many individuals do not have obvious pruritus. Some animals have subclinical infestations. Diagnosis is confirmed by identifying mites and eggs (nits) via skin scraping. Treatment consists of ivermectin or a combination of ivermectin and amitraz. All bedding must be removed, and cage furnishings disinfected or discarded. During treatment, the cage is lined with paper that must be changed daily. All hedgehogs in the home should be treated concurrently.

Pet hedgehogs may be infested with fleas; however, cat and dog fleas generally do not infest African pygmy hedgehogs. This is likely because of the hedgehog's low body temperature. Treatment consists of topical or systemic flea control agents. Shampoo and powder products that are safe for kittens appear to be safe for hedgehogs. Tropical rat mites, *Ornithonyssus bacoti*, may also cause flaky skin and loss of spines; fipronil spray is an effective treatment.

Dermatophytosis is a common clinical disease in African pygmy hedgehogs; however, infection without significant clinical signs is also possible. Dermatophytes (*Trichophyton erinacei*, *T mentagrophytes*, *Microsporum* spp, and *Arthroderma benhamiae*) cause crusting dermatitis, especially around the face and pinnae. Quill loss may also be noted. Although some animals may scratch with the hindlimbs or rub against stationary objects, many individuals do not display signs of pruritus. Some infections are secondary to other dermatopathies, such as acariasis or trauma. Diagnosis is confirmed by culturing spines in dermatophyte test medium. Treatment consists of topical antifungal agents, with systemic griseofulvin or ketoconazole if needed. Lime-sulfur dips may also be used. Other hedgehogs in the home may be subclinically infected, and treatment of all animals is recommended.

Contact dermatitis may result from unsanitary bedding. Cellulitis has been linked to secondary myositis and sepsis; the primary cause in most of these cases was trauma. *Staphylococcus simulans* was reported to cause dermatitis characterized by a broad, well-circumscribed area of hyperkeratosis and alopecia on the back of a hedgehog. Allergic dermatitis has been anecdotally described; restricted antigen diets, antihistamines, and glucocorticoids may be helpful. Pruritus may be observed with development of new spines, as occurs in young hedgehogs. Pemphigus foliaceus has been reported; loss of spines, flaking skin, moist erythema, and epidermal collarettes were seen. Dexamethasone injections were reported to be an effective treatment.

Skin neoplasia is common. Squamous cell carcinoma, lymphosarcoma, and sebaceous gland carcinoma have been described. Papillomas of suspected viral etiology have been reported; recurrence in other sites after excision is common. Cutaneous and subcutaneous nodules may also be caused by abscesses, mycobacteriosis, and *Cuterebra* larvae.

Musculoskeletal Diseases: Myositis secondary to cellulitis has been reported. Osteoarthritis has also been seen. Bone cysts should be considered as a differential for mandibular masses, along with neoplasia and trauma. Fractures can occur when a limb becomes entrapped in a wire cage or exercise wheel. Splinting can be performed for distal limb fractures. Surgical correction may also be performed, but any fixation device must be able to withstand the hedgehog's strong rolling-up mechanism. Lameness may be caused by ingrown toenails, arthritis, nutritional deficiencies, pododermatitis, constriction of a foot or digit by fibrous material, neurologic disease, or neoplasia.

Neoplasia: Neoplasia in hedgehogs is very common in both sexes. A variety of tumor types affecting every body system has been reported. According to one survey, the body systems in which most tumors were found were the integumentary, hemolymphatic, alimentary, and endocrine systems. The most common tumors are mammary gland tumors, lymphosarcoma, and oral squamous cell carcinoma. The median age at time of diagnosis is 3.5 yr, although tumors may be seen in animals as young as 2 yr old. In one survey, >80% of the tumors were malignant. Proliferative uterine tumors or polyps are common and are associated with vaginal bleeding, hematuria, and weight loss. Ovariohysterectomy allows prolonged survival of hedgehogs with uterine tumors. Some sarcomas have been associated with retroviral infection.

Signs depend on the location and severity of disease and may include palpable masses, weight loss, anorexia, lethargy, diarrhea, dyspnea, and ascites. Diagnosis is based on cytology or histopathology. Diagnostic imaging and blood testing may help determine the extent of the disease and establish a prognosis. Treatment generally includes surgical excision and supportive care, although other treatment modalities may be helpful. Not every mass in pet hedgehogs is neoplastic; for example, abscesses, bone cysts, papillomas, and uterine polyps are seen.

Neurologic Diseases: Neurologic signs (particularly ataxia) may be caused by torpor, hepatic encephalopathy, postpartum eclampsia, malnutrition, trauma, intervertebral disc disease, toxins, infarcts, infectious causes (eg, parasitic migration, rabies), otitis media, demyelination, polioencephalomalacia, or neoplasia.

Hedgehogs kept in cold (or sometimes excessively high) temperatures may enter a state of torpor or dormancy. In this state, the hedgehog has a greatly diminished response to stimulation, decreased heart and respiratory rates, and possibly increased susceptibility to infection. Dormancy can last for several weeks, during which the hedgehog may have periods of activity with ataxia.

Hypocalcemia may result from postpartum eclampsia, malnutrition, or for unknown reasons, and usually responds to calcium supplementation.

Intervertebral disc disease has been reported. Both cervical and lumbar lesions have been identified; multiple discs were affected in each of these hedgehogs. Radiographic findings included spondylosis, disc-space narrowing, and disc mineralization. Necropsy findings included degeneration of the nucleus pulposus and annulus fibrosus, dorsal extrusion of disc material, and mineralization of the nucleus pulposus.

One case had evidence of fibrocartilaginous embolism. Temporary improvement with corticosteroids has been described in two cases of intervertebral disc disease.

Vestibular signs may be caused by otitis media/internal or central neurologic disease.

Demyelinating paralysis (wobbly hedgehog syndrome) occurs in as many as 10% of pet hedgehogs. Onset can occur at any age but is more common in animals <2 yr old. An early sign is the inability to close the hood. This progresses to mild, intermittent ataxia. The signs gradually increase in severity and include falling, tremors, exophthalmos, scoliosis, seizures, muscle atrophy, self-mutilation, and severe weight loss. The paralysis usually ascends from hindlimbs to forelimbs and usually leads to complete paralysis within 9–15 mo after the onset of signs. Death occurs within 18–25 mo. Appetite is usually normal until the terminal stages, when most hedgehogs become dysphagic. The diagnosis is confirmed at necropsy. Histopathologic lesions include vacuolization of white matter (cerebrum, cerebellum, brainstem, and spinal cord), axonal swelling, degeneration of spinal cord ventral tracts, and axonal and myelin degeneration in brain white matter. Peripheral nerves may also be involved. Inflammation of the CNS is not associated with wobbly hedgehog syndrome. The etiology is unknown, but a hereditary basis is suspected. Numerous treatments have been attempted without success. Euthanasia is warranted when the quality of life is compromised. A single case of pneumonia virus of mice in an African hedgehog with suspected wobbly hedgehog syndrome, resulting in nonsuppurative encephalitis with vacuolization of the white matter, has been reported.

Nutritional Disorders: Obesity is common. Healthy hedgehogs should be able to roll up completely, without any fat deposits protruding. Treatment includes reducing high-fat foods, rationing the main diet, and increasing exercise. Weight reduction should be gradual to prevent hepatic lipidosis, and owners should monitor their pet's weight. Nutritional excess or deficiency may occur with unbalanced diets; for example, calcium deficiency may result from a diet consisting mainly of invertebrates. Moist diets may predispose hedgehogs to periodontal disease. Other nutritional diseases are uncommon.

Ocular Diseases: Hedgehogs are prone to corneal ulcers and other ocular injuries. Diagnosis and treatment are as for other species, although administration of topical medication can be difficult. Blind hedgehogs navigate their captive environments with minimal detriment to their quality of life.

According to one report, ocular proptosis is relatively common and carries a poor prognosis for viability of the eye. Hedgehogs have a shallow orbit that may predispose them to proptosis, especially if excessive fat accumulation or orbital inflammation is present. Concurrent neurologic disease may result in ocular trauma.

Oral and Dental Diseases: Oral neoplasia, particularly squamous cell carcinoma, is common in hedgehogs. Dental disease, including calculus, gingivitis, and periodontitis, is also common. Periodontal disease is often associated with a bacterial component. The addition of abrasive items to the diet (eg, hard kibble, charcoal, or bone) and antibiotics are recommended for prevention and treatment of periodontal disease, respectively. Dental prophylaxis, periprocedural antibiotics, and tooth extraction may be necessary to treat severe dental disease. If advanced periodontal disease requires extraction of all the teeth, hedgehogs can be maintained on soft food. Tooth fractures and dental abscesses are also seen. *Actinomyces* infection has been reported; anaerobic culture and treatment should be considered for dental abscesses in hedgehogs.

Excessive tooth wear occurs in older hedgehogs, and hedgehogs with this condition should be fed a soft diet. Hedgehog teeth do not grow continuously and should not be trimmed. Hedgehogs are susceptible to wedging of hard items (eg, peanuts) against the palate. Stomatitis may develop in males that bite their mates; treatment is with soft food and antibiotics.

Otic Diseases: Pinnal dermatitis is common; skin crusts, accumulated secretions, and a ragged pinnal margin may be seen. Dermatophytes and acariasis are important causes; other possibilities include nutritional deficiencies, dry skin, seborrhea with hyperkeratosis, and extension of ear canal disease. Ear mites (*Notoedres cati*) are occasionally seen; signs, diagnosis, and treatment are as for cats (*see* p 921). Bacterial or yeast otitis externa is also seen; these infections are often secondary to acariasis or another cause of chronic inflammation. Signs include purulent discharge, odor, and sensitivity of the face and ear. Otic cytology, skin scrapings, cleansing, and topical antimicrobial/anti-inflammatory therapy are used as for other species. Otitis media/interna can also be seen.

Reproductive Diseases: Posthitis may be caused by substrate entrapment in the prepuce. Hemorrhagic vulvar discharge is often caused by uterine neoplasia or endometrial polyps. Pyometra and metritis have been reported. Dystocia also is seen and treated as in other small mammals. Premature births occasionally occur; the prognosis for young without a suckling reflex is poor. Agalactia may be suspected if neonates lose condition within 72 hr after birth. Diagnosis may be confirmed by attempting to express the mammary glands; however, this usually requires anesthesia and may cause the dam to abandon or cannibalize her young. Causes of agalactia include malnutrition, stress, lack of oxytocin, inadequate mammary development in young females, and mastitis. Supportive care for weak neonates includes warming to normal body temperature over 1–3 hr, fluid support, and caloric support once normothermia has been achieved.

Respiratory Diseases: Predisposing factors for upper and lower respiratory tract infection are suboptimal environmental temperature; aromatic, dusty, or unsanitary bedding; concurrent disease causing immunocompromise; and aspiration of material from an oral infection. Signs include nasal discharge, increased respiratory noise, dyspnea, lethargy, inappetence, and sudden death. Radiographs, hematologic testing, and culture of tracheal or lung lobe aspirates are useful in diagnosis. Treatment includes antibiotics, nebulization, supportive care, and correction of underlying problems. Differential diagnoses for dyspnea are pulmonary neoplasia and cardiac disease.

A case of fatal corynebacterial bronchopneumonia has been reported in a pet African hedgehog. *Pasteurella* spp and *Bordetella bronchiseptica* can cause respiratory infections in European hedgehogs and are possibly important in *Atelerix* as well. Lungworms can also cause pneumonia, but this is unlikely in indoor pets. The existence of cytomegalovirus in African hedgehogs has been questioned; in any case, it is highly unlikely in domestically raised pets.

Urinary Diseases: Cystitis and urolithiasis cause changes in urine color, stranguria, pollakiuria, inappetence, and lethargy. Urinalysis with culture and radiographs should be obtained. Renal disease is also common (50% prevalence in a necropsy survey) and in many cases may be secondary to systemic disease. Genetic or dietary factors may contribute to the high prevalence. Nephritis, tubular necrosis, nephrocalcinosis, glomerulosclerosis, renal infarcts, polycystic kidneys, neoplasia, and various glomerulonephropathies have been identified. Signs associated with renal disease tend to be nonspecific, although polyuria and/or polydipsia may be noted. Diagnosis should be based on urinalysis and serum chemistry panels. Treatment consists of correcting the underlying cause, fluid therapy, and supportive care.

Zoonoses: Several strains of *Salmonella* are found in pet hedgehogs, including *S* Tilene, *S* Typhimurium, and *S* Enteritidis. Many cases of transmission to people have been documented, particularly in young children. It should be assumed that all pet hedgehogs can carry and transmit *Salmonella*. Because infected animals may shed intermittently, a negative culture cannot exclude the carrier state. Treatment aimed at eliminating the carrier state is unlikely to be successful and may lead to antibiotic resistance.

Human dermatophytosis from pet hedgehogs is also well documented. African pygmy hedgehogs can be subclinical carriers of *Trichophyton mentagrophytes* var *erinacei*, *Microsporum* spp, and *Arthroderma benhamiae*. In addition, some people are extremely sensitive to contact with African hedgehog spines and develop transient, markedly pruritic urticaria after handling a hedgehog.

Wild African hedgehogs are susceptible to foot-and-mouth disease. To prevent introduction of this disease to the USA, importation of African hedgehogs was banned by the USDA in 1991.

Rabies has not been reported in wild or captive African hedgehogs, but the salivation that occurs during anting is occasionally mistaken as a sign of rabies. A single report of rabies in a wild European hedgehog exists.

Human herpes simplex virus 1 was recovered from the liver of a pet African hedgehog that died acutely after glucocorticoid treatment for intervertebral disc disease. Monkeypox virus DNA was recovered from an African hedgehog housed with many other exotic species at a pet distributor facility in Illinois. *Candida* infection of the footpads and intestine of the African pygmy hedgehog has been reported. Acute intestinal cryptosporidiosis has been reported. A single case of Chagas' disease (*Trypanosoma cruzi*) was reported in a captive African hedgehog housed outdoors in Texas.

African pygmy hedgehogs are considered susceptible to a variety of infectious agents, based on susceptibility observed in other hedgehog species. Possible bacterial zoonoses include *Yersinia pseudotuberculosis*, *Y pestis*, *Mycobacterium marinum*, *M avium intracellulare*, *Coxiella burnetii* (Q fever), and *Leptospira* spp. Possible viral zoonoses include Crimean-Congo hemorrhagic fever, arboviral tickborne encephalitides, and paramyxoviruses of the Morbillivirus group. *Chlamydia psittaci* and *Toxoplasma gondii* have been isolated from wild European hedgehogs.

LABORATORY ANIMALS

REGULATORY REQUIREMENTS

Most American laboratories must adhere to two main sets of animal welfare regulations: the Animal Welfare Act (AWA; created in 1966) and the Public Health Service Policy on Humane Care and Use of Laboratory Animals (PHS Policy; originally enacted in 1985).

The Animal and Plant Health Inspection Service (APHIS) of the USDA oversees enforcement of the AWA, which covers the care of research animals and includes guidelines for the oversight and conduct of studies intended to minimize or prevent pain or distress of laboratory animals. The AWA also regulates zoos, exhibitors, animal dealers, and those who transport animals in commerce. All warm-blooded species are regulated by the AWA, whether alive or dead, except for domestic mice and rats bred for scientific purposes, birds, and farm animals used in agricultural research. Provisions for veterinary care have existed under the AWA since 1970; requirements for exercise for dogs and ensuring the psychological well-being of nonhuman primates were added in 1985. The AWA is enforced through a self-reporting mechanism along with routine, unannounced inspections by APHIS. Failure to meet the requirements of the AWA can result in fines, citations, criminal proceedings, or revoked registration with disqualification to use AWA-regulated species in research.

The PHS Policy is based on a set of research animal care standards, the *Guide for the Care and Use of Laboratory Animals*, first published in 1963. The PHS Policy requires institutions to use this guide as a basis for developing and implementing institutional programs for research involving animals. The PHS Policy has been modified only once, in 2002, while the Guide, now in its 8th edition, was last revised in 2011. The policy applies to all research institutions awarded federal grants and covers all vertebrate animals, not just those that are warm-blooded. Regulatory compliance is based on a system of self-regulation whereby institutions must provide the following to federal officials: a written Animal Welfare Assurance that describes their compliance with the PHS Policy, updates via an annual report, timely reporting of all incidents of noncompliance, and site visits for-cause or other purposes. Failure to adhere to PHS Policy can result in revocation of federal funding for some or all research projects at the institution.

The 8th edition of the *Guide for the Care and Use of Laboratory Animals*, released in 2011, at 220 pages represented a 76% increase in information, guidance, and prescribed action from the content of the 7th edition (1996). It is organized into five chapters that cover the subject areas of 1) key defining concepts, including applicability, a brief review of the ethical principles in the humane care and use of animals in research, and clarifying definitions; 2) articulation of the basics of an animal care and use program, most prominently oversight structure, salient aspects of safety, and requirements for training; 3) the environment, housing, and management of research animals; 4) veterinary care; and 5) animal research facility design and physical plant operation. While there were abundant changes in the Guide from the 7th to 8th edition, most momentous were the unprecedented responsibility delegated to the attending veterinarian (AV) for the welfare of any animal in research at all times during experimentation and in all phases of the animal's life and in establishing the unambiguous and absolute authority of the AV to prescribe treatment and other interventions, including removal of subjects from experimentation. Other significant additions addressed the accordance of cage space allocated to breeding rodents, the genetic management of rodent breeding colonies to ensure authenticity, the care of aquatic species, and an enhanced emphasis on the training of personnel when applicable in proper animal care and methods of use, particularly in aseptic surgery and humane euthanasia technique.

Program Accreditation: The Association for Assessment and Accreditation of Laboratory Animal Care International (AAALAC), a private, nonprofit organization that promotes the humane treatment of animals in science through voluntary accreditation and assessment programs, was incorporated in 1965. More than 890 companies, universities, hospitals, government agencies, and other research institutions in 37 countries have voluntarily earned AAALAC accreditation as of 2013. Institutions that seek AAALAC accreditation are subject to comprehensive peer review of their animal care and use program every 3 years; this accreditation is given credence by the National Institutes of Health as a means of demonstrating compliance with PHS Policy.

Veterinary Care: Under provisions of the AWA, all persons who use animals in research or for exhibition, sell them at the wholesale level, or transport them in commerce must have established programs of veterinary care and animal husbandry. APHIS requires the owner of each licensed and registered facility to define a program of veterinary care (PVC), including the employment of an AV. In cases in which the AV is not a full-time employee, the facility owner must prepare a written PVC and schedule an appropriate frequency of visits by the AV. These visits must be on at least an annual basis. Whatever the employment arrangement, the facility owner must give the AV sufficient authority to ensure adequate veterinary care. The PVC must incorporate appropriate facilities, personnel, equipment, and services to meet this standard; ensure the availability of emergency, weekend, and holiday care for animals; include the requirement for the daily observation of all animals by employees to assess the animals' health and well-being; and define channels for the direct and frequent communication between facility personnel and the AV.

Responsibilities of the AV include using suitable methods to prevent, control, diagnose, and treat diseases and injuries; providing adequate guidance and training of personnel who care for animals regarding handling, immobilization, anesthesia, analgesia, tranquilization, and euthanasia; and ensuring that the pre-procedural and post-procedural care of animals is in accordance with established veterinary medical and nursing procedures. Beyond these general responsibilities, the AV is responsible for reviewing the facility's PVC at least once a year to ensure that the following meet contemporary standards of veterinary care for each species: vaccinations, handling of biologics and drugs, product safety assurance, parasite control, emergency care, euthanasia methodology, nutrition, pest control and product safety, quarantine procedures, exercise (dogs only), environmental and social enrichment (nonhuman primates only), water quality (when marine mammals are involved), and, for wild or exotic animals, capture and restraint methods.

Institutional Animal Care and Use Committee: Since 1985, the AWA and PHS Policy have required that Institutional Animal Care and Use Committees (IACUC) oversee not only the care, but also the use, of animals in research. The responsibilities of the IACUC are delineated in these laws and the associated federal policy and regulations. According to the AWA, the IACUC must consist of at least one veterinarian with training in laboratory animal science and expertise in the species under consideration, at least one practicing research scientist, and at least one person not affiliated with the institution. The PHS Policy requires a minimum of five members, including at least one of each of the following: veterinarian, scientist, nonscientist, and nonaffiliated member.

Each IACUC has three main areas of responsibility: review of research protocols; semiannual evaluations of the institution's animal care and use, which includes inspections of animal housing areas and laboratories where animal procedures are performed; and judiciary activities such as investigating animal welfare concerns and adjudicating disagreements. Review of research protocols by the IACUC involves considering the merits of the animal study in the context of a broad range of complex, scientific, animal welfare, and veterinary topics. The IACUC also has the responsibility to monitor the compliance of ongoing studies and the authority to suspend research not performed in accordance with the conditions or with unforeseen negative consequences. Since 1985, the IACUC has been the primary means of animal welfare oversight within research institutions in the USA.

Emergency Preparedness: History shows that animal research facilities are regularly and often unpredictably subject to the effects of natural events, manmade actions, or failures of technology that imperil animals, experiments, and facilities. While principles of disaster preparedness and response have been integral to the Guide since its 7th edition, in 2013 the USDA instituted requirements for emergency and disaster preparedness and response plans and mandated training programs for appropriate personnel. As such, the Guide and USDA policy in conjunction make it mandatory that each institution craft and train personnel in a comprehensive emergency operations and disaster responsiveness plan.

ANIMALS USED IN RESEARCH

Research institutions registered under the AWA are required to submit an annual report to APHIS that details, among other specifications, a listing of the common names and the numbers of reportable species used. In 2010, there were 1,104 research institutions in the USA registered under the requirements of the AWA. These institutions reported the total use of 1,134,693 regulated animals. The most abundant species used were guinea pigs (213,629), rabbits (210,172), and the combination of several species of hamsters (145,895) of which >90% were estimated to be of the Syrian variety. Other animals used included nonhuman primates (71,317), dogs (64,930), pigs (53,260), domestic cats (21,578), sheep (13,271), and a combination of marine mammals, other farm animals, and other species not identified (341,214). There is no federal reporting requirement for mice, rats, birds, amphibians, or fish, making precise numbers difficult to determine. Research subjects of these species, for the most part, are obtained via a combination of in-house breeding colonies and from commercial vendors, with production and sales data from the latter being proprietary and not disclosed publicly. Wild-caught birds and aquatic species sometimes may be captured for experimental purposes. Since 2000, the estimated total number of mice and rats used for research purposes annually in the USA has ranged fairly consistently from 20 to 30 million. There are millions of zebra fish and thousands of amphibians, likewise, used annually.

The domestic mouse, *Mus musculus* and related subspecies (*see* MICE AND RATS AS LABORATORY ANIMALS, p 2032), is popular as a mammalian research model because of its small size, adaptability, docility, low husbandry costs, fecundity, well-defined health and genetic backgrounds, and relative ease of genetic manipulation. The development of genetic engineering techniques of inserting foreign genes (transgenes) into the mouse genome and the ability to delete genes, leading to what are known as "knockout" mice, profoundly increased the use of mice as research subjects. Since these advances, countless mutant genotypes of mice have been developed, ranging from subtle defects in immune function to full-fledged, inherited diseases virtually homologous with those of higher mammals.

Among other rodents, the domestic Norway rat (*Rattus norvegicus*) is second only to the mouse as a research subject. Rats (*see* p 2032) share many of the attributes of mice that make them attractive for use in research, but because they are larger than mice, they are suited for a greater variety of manipulations. Numerous mutant and inbred strains and outbred stocks of rats are used in a broad array of studies, including topics such as aging, cancer, reproductive physiology, drug effects, behavior, addiction, alcoholism/cirrhosis, arthritis, brain and nerve injury, hypertension, embryology, teratology, endocrine diseases, neurophysiology, infectious disease, stroke, organ transplantation, and surgically induced disease. The genetic engineering of mutant rat types, however, has lagged behind mice and is only beginning to show effect.

Excluding mice and rats, guinea pigs and rabbits are the most common mammals used in research, although their numbers have declined from peaks in the 1980s. Although the guinea pig (*Cavia porcellus*) was among the first animals to be used in medical research, its popularity has diminished relative to that of mice and rats because of its long gestation period (59–72 days), small litter size (2–5), poor vascular access, and difficulties in anesthesia. Guinea pigs are still used in notable ways in immunology, in vaccine and infectious disease research, and as hearing models. Rabbits are used most often in product safety testing; for polyclonal antibody production; and in studies of vision, orthopedics, and cardiology.

In addition to the Syrian hamster (*Mesocricetus auratus*), a few other species of hamsters are used in research, including the Armenian, Siberian (Djungarian), Chinese, European, and Turkish species. Hamsters are readily available, reproduce easily, and are relatively free of spontaneous diseases but susceptible to many induced viral diseases. They are used for studies of obesity, induced carcinogenesis, prostatic disease, toxicity, infectious diseases (including slow viruses), dental caries, chronic bronchitis, and teratogenesis.

Other rodent species used in research include gerbils, deer mice, chinchillas, cotton rats, rice rats, multimammate rats, Egyptian spiny mice, degus, voles, and woodchucks, among others.

While rodent models are unarguably the most common for scientific use, larger animal models provide unique opportunities for biomedical research. Dogs are used in studies of cardiology, endocrinology, orthopedics, prosthetic devices, surgical techniques, pharmacokinetics, and product safety. Since use of dogs began declining in 1984, livestock have been used more frequently. This has been a consequence of regulatory and public pressure related to the use of dogs, but it is also due to attributes of comparative anatomy and physiology that make livestock more conducive to particular investigations. For example, swine are used for cardiovascular research (particularly atherosclerosis), in studies of digestive physiology, as surgical models, and for xenotransplantation. Sheep are used for studies of neonatal development, human vaccine improvement, asthma pathogenesis and treatment, drug delivery, circadian rhythms, and surgical techniques.

Nonhuman primates remain critical in studies of vision, the neurosciences, infectious diseases, vaccines, and product safety testing. In recent years, they have become increasingly valuable as models of immunodeficiency virus infection and the neurodegenerative diseases associated with aging.

Although the absolute number of cats used in research has been in steady decline since 1980, cats are still important models in the neurosciences and in the study of infectious diseases.

The most important aquatic species used in research are the zebra fish and the African clawed frog.

Other species used in scientific research include goats, calves, horses, ferrets, armadillos, opossums, domestic and wild birds, reptiles, amphibians, other species of fish, and invertebrates.

MANAGEMENT

Consistently delivered quality programs of husbandry and veterinary care provide the foundation that enables valid scientific research. For proper management of research animals, the animal care and research staff must be responsible, sensitive to the animals' health and well-being, well trained in the humane care and use of laboratory animals, highly motivated, experienced, and diligent in performing their duties and responsibilities. Standard operating procedures must be established, and training and supervision provided to assure a consistently applied and uniformly high level of animal care. Within research facilities, environmental conditions must be carefully controlled so that, along with conscientiously applied programs of animal care and use, the best possible conditions for conducting research are provided. The *Guide for the Care and Use of Laboratory Animals* is still the primary reference for information on basic principles and standards for laboratory animal management.

Laboratory rodents that are disease- and pathogen-free and that do not possess antibodies indicative of past infection are readily available from commercial vendors. Procuring such animals from high-quality sources, transporting them in filtered shipping containers, and maintaining them in facilities with both physical and procedural barriers to the introduction of infectious agents are effective measures to prevent disease within a colony that may confound or ruin experiments.

Although there are colonies of some species of primates that are free of most agents that cause infectious disease in these species, many primates used are of feral or wild origin. For this reason, appropriate quarantine, isolation, and conditioning programs should be implemented in addition to the program followed in the importers' facilities.

Housing: Cages, pens, or runs should provide adequate space to allow for normal physiologic needs, permit postural adjustments, and meet requirements for species-specific behavior. When possible, compatible groups of social animals should be housed together. Primary enclosures should be constructed of durable materials, easily cleaned and sanitized, and designed for comfort and safety. Static microisolation (filter top) cages and more advanced individually ventilated caging systems have been used widely for rodent housing to impede cage-to-cage transmission of infectious agents. However, infection can be transmitted horizontally or vertically from parents to progeny in breeding colonies; naive mice introduced for cross-breeding and back-crossing can perpetuate infection; and experimental mice potentially can be exposed to pathogens via a contaminated environment, shared watering valves, research devices, or when taken to laboratories. Individual ventilation of cages serves to delay deterioration of the environment within the cage and maintain a more consistent and wholesome microenvironment; it also saves space in the facility and can be engineered to minimize odors, allergens, dust, and heat exhausted into the macroenvironment. A potential drawback of ventilated cages is that hairless genotypes and neonates may be prone to chilling. This risk can be reduced by providing nesting material.

Federal law in the USA requires that laboratory dogs have an opportunity to exercise regularly and have sensory contact with other dogs unless restricted by experimental or behavioral considerations. Housing for nonhuman primates must provide social and environmental enrichment to promote psychological well-being compatible with the experimental and practical constraints of the housing situation. Successful enrichment strategies for nonhuman primates have included pair or group housing; variation in the dietary content and method of presentation; diversification of the internal cage environment with ancillary apparatus (eg, perches, swings, or ladders); provision of devices to enhance visual, auditory, or tactile stimulation; and participation in challenging, nonaversive behavioral laboratory studies. Efforts to extend and adapt environmental enrichment practices to other laboratory animal species warrant consideration and have been implemented in many institutions.

Temperature, relative humidity, ventilation rates, lighting conditions (spectrum, intensity, and photoperiod), gaseous pollutants (eg, ammonia), and noise should be carefully controlled at all times and monitored as appropriate. Unstable environmental conditions can have a profound effect on the comfort, well-being, and metabolism of animals and therefore on the quality of experimental data derived. In general, temperature should be maintained at 68°–79°F (20°–26°C) for most rodents; 61°–72°F (16°–22°C) for rabbits; 59°–64°F (15°–18°C) for ferrets; 64°–84°F (18°–29°C) for primates, dogs, and cats; and 61°–81°F (16°–27°C) for most farm animals and poultry. Within these ranges, optimal systems should maintain temperatures within ±1°F of the set point. Relative humidity should be maintained at 30%–70% for most species and preferably within 10% of the set point. Ventilation rates should be 10–15 fresh air changes/hr. Air should not be recirculated unless it has been treated to remove particulate and gaseous contaminants. Lighting should be distributed evenly and sufficiently intense to promote animal well-being and to allow personnel to observe the animals and to perform all husbandry and sanitation duties safely and effectively. Diurnal or day-night cycles, as determined by species' requirements, should be controlled by automatic timers to maintain *circadian and neuroendocrine* regulation. The microenvironment within certain types of caging may be very different from that of the macroenvironment of the room. Carefully conducted research is needed to more precisely define the optimal environmental and social conditions for each species or group of species at the cage level.

Bedding: Bedding materials should be nonirritating, absorbent, free of chemical contamination and pathogens, and unpalatable. Adequate quantities should be used to dilute and limit contact with excreta, promote air quality and other environmental factors by suppressing microbial growth, and keep animals dry and clean between changes of bedding or caging. The major types of contact bedding used are derived from ground corncobs, hardwood chips, recycled paper, heat-treated softwood shavings, and virgin cellulose. Untreated softwoods are not recommended because they contain volatile oils that may alter hepatic enzyme systems and affect certain kinds of research. Depending on research requirements, bedding may be sterilized by autoclaving or irradiation before use or used as is.

Feeding: Feed should be of adequate quantity, palatable, free of contaminants, nutritionally adequate, easily accessible, and provided using means that meet behavioral needs according to specific species requirements. Feeds specifically manufactured for research animal use are preferred, because they are more likely to be uniformly constituted, free of contaminants, of known shelf life, and mill dated. Feed should be manufactured, transported, stored, and used in ways that minimize its deterioration, contamination, or infestation. Most small animals consume food in relation to their energy requirements as influenced by the environment and dictated by their genotype and are fed ad lib; rabbits, laboratory carnivores, swine, aquatic amphibians, and primates may be restricted to measured quantities of feed each day. As a general rule, laboratory animals minimally consume 4%–6% of their body weight in food daily. In addition to commercially prepared and usually pelleted natural ingredient diets of varying specification (eg, quality control and assurance of ingredients), semisynthetic or completely synthetic diets and all-liquid preparations can be formulated for use in certain kinds of research. Autoclavable or irradiated diets are available for rodents and can be used when sterilization of feed is desired.

Water: Potable, uncontaminated water should be provided in adequate quantities to meet specific species requirements. Quality assurance programs that measure pH, hardness, chemical content, and microbial load are recommended. Highly purified, deionized, acidified, chlorinated, or sterile water may be required under certain experimental or husbandry conditions. Water is usually provided ad lib in manually filled or automated watering devices. Particularly in the housing of rodents, an automated water supply enhances the advantages of ventilated caging systems and reduces operational costs/expenses, increases safety for animal care technicians, saves labor, reduces disruptions of the mice by caretakers, and provides consistently high water quality. The drawback of the use of automated drinking water supply for rodents is the risk of hypothermia, drowning, or dehydration of cage inhabitants as a consequence of failure of the in-cage water delivery valve.

Water quality is the most important environmental variable for aquatic species and a key determinant of health. Inadequate water quality or fluctuations of water temperature are physiologic stressors that impact the intake, digestion, and use of food; alter the immune system; and predispose to opportunistic infection. Water for aquatic vertebrates should be free of nitrite, ammonia, and chlorine, with total coliform counts not exceeding 200/mL. The pH should be 6.5–8.5. Although aquatic amphibians may be maintained in small containers of standing water, water recirculation with biologic filtration and periodic partial replenishment with fresh water, just as with fish, are helpful in suppressing bacterial counts and preventing the build-up of toxic chemicals. The ideal water temperature range for maintaining the aquatic amphibians used most popularly in research, the tetraploid South African clawed frog (*Xenopus laevis*) and the axolotl (*Ambystoma mexicanum*), is 65°–72°F (18°–22°C). For *X tropicalis*, a smaller, more rapidly maturing, diploid species of clawed frog from forested west Africa, water temperature should be 70°–85°F (21°–29°C). (*See also* AMPHIBIANS, p 1734.) Zebrafish and other tropical species used in research are best maintained at a consistent water temperature within the range 80°–90°F (27°–32°C).

Sanitation: A uniformly high level of animal enclosure and facility sanitation is mandatory to ensure that animals are clean and dry, air quality is adequate (without using masking agents), and primary enclosure surfaces and accessories are clean. Housing rooms and ancillary support space should be cleaned and sanitized as often as necessary to keep them free of dirt, debris, and potentially harmful contamination. For rodents in solid-bottom cages, usually 1–3 changes per week will suffice; for rodents, rabbits, and nonhuman primates in suspended cages over excreta pans and for mice in ventilated caging systems, cage changes every other week should be adequate. For larger animals, excreta and soiled bedding should be removed daily, and primary enclosures cleaned and sanitized daily, or at minimum every other week. Water bottles and other watering or feeding devices should be cleaned and sanitized at least weekly. Automated watering devices on cages, racks, or in rooms should be designed and programmed to flush continually or regularly or they should be manually drained, rinsed, and sanitized at regular, frequent intervals. Heating cages and other equipment to 180°F (82.2°C) or using appropriate chemical disinfection (eg, hypochlorite solutions) kills nonspore-forming pathogenic bacteria and viruses. All caging and other equipment should be rinsed thoroughly after treatment with detergents or disinfectants. The effectiveness of the programs of sanitation should be evaluated regularly using appropriate microbiologic, organic material detection systems or other means.

Vermin Control: Professionally directed programs to prevent, identify, and eradicate or control insects or escaped, feral, or wild rodents must be instituted, regularly scheduled, and consistently documented. The use of pesticides should be as a last resort and generally be confined to areas not used for animals or for storage of feed or bedding. If these agents are used in proximity to animals or their food and bedding, researchers should be informed of the use. Relatively inert substances, such as silica aerogel or boric acid powder, are recommended and are useful for control of crawling insects, eg, cockroaches.

COLONY MONITORING

While most commercially reared rodents, some rabbits, and relatively fewer dogs, cats, and primates can be obtained as SPF animals, resident animal colonies must be monitored for naturally occurring disease as a measure of the effectiveness of the prevention and control program. Investigators should be informed regularly as to the health status of their research animals. In addition to monitoring for infectious disease, a quality assurance program should monitor for genetic integrity, especially for inbred mouse strains that are bred and maintained in the research facility, as well as for environmental factors (quality of feed, water, and bedding; efficacy of sanitation programs; air handling and quality; lighting; noise; etc) that can affect colony health.

Colony health monitoring consists of a defined program of regular physical and laboratory evaluations of animals within a unit, as well as a morbidity and mortality reporting system that enables timely identification of potential problems. Thorough investigations of illnesses, deaths, and unusual experimental outcomes in a colony are essential components of such a program. For selected physiologic data of some laboratory animals, *see* TABLE 11.

While certain general principles apply, a health monitoring program must be specifically developed for each species maintained in a facility. For example, generally, all primates are quarantined and isolated on arrival. Physical examinations, tuberculin testing, and baseline hematologic and other clinical pathologic tests should be performed. In addition, serologic evaluation for Macacine herpesvirus type 1 (formerly Cercopithecine herpesvirus type 1, Herpervirus simiae, B virus), simian retroviruses, and other specific agents may be performed, depending on the species of primate. Primates should be released from quarantine only when both the health status and suitability for use are determined. Furthermore, primates should have regular health surveillance screens, each consisting of defined elements. Depending on the nature and value of the colony and research use, screenings may range from quarterly to semiannual or annual in frequency. (*See also* NONHUMAN PRIMATES, p 1876.)

For colony-bred rats and mice, programs for disease monitoring can consist of any or all of the following: vendor surveillance, quarantine and isolation evaluation, ongoing clinical and postmortem evaluation during the course of studies, sentinel animal programs, and evaluation at termination of the study. In addition, all transplantable tumors, cells, or other biologic products destined for animal passage should either be screened for murine and zoonotic pathogens or colony management practices used to appropriately isolate animals receiving these materials. Of particular concern to colony health is the occasional and justifiable need to obtain animals from less well-defined sources, such as an investigator's colony at another institution or other nonapproved source. The presence of infectious agents either in transplantable tumors or noncommercial animal sources can pose a substantial threat to resident colonies and personnel. Colony monitoring of rodents is typically based on serology, bacteriologic, and parasitic evaluations supported by the evaluation of environmental, fecal, and fur samples through the use of molecular biologic techniques such as PCR.

Although the use of filter top caging technology to impede cage-to-cage transmission of infectious agents in rodent colonies has resulted in a dramatic reduction in enzootic disease transmission and protection of naive animals from epizootics, it has created challenges for

TABLE 11 SELECTED PHYSIOLOGIC DATA OF LABORATORY ANIMALS[a]

Species	Gestation Period (days)	Litter Size	Age and Body Weight at Sexual Maturity
Mice	19–21	6–10	6 wk (20–30 g)
Rats	21–23	6–14	2–3 mo (0.2–0.3 kg)
Guinea pigs	59–72	1–4	3–4 mo (0.4–0.5 kg)
Hamsters, golden	15–18	4–10	2 mo (85–110 g)
Gerbils	25	2–9	3 mo (60–100 g)
Rabbits	30–33	4–12	5–6 mo (3–4 kg)
Squirrel monkeys	150	1	3–5 yr (0.6–1.1 kg)
Rhesus monkeys	164	1–2	3–4 yr (5–11 kg)
Chimpanzees	227–235	1	7–10 yr (40–50 kg)
Baboons	164–186	1	4–7 yr (11–30 kg)

[a] *See also* TABLE 3, FEATURES OF THE REPRODUCTIVE CYCLE, p 1326.

[b] Typical of an average adult; varies with body mass index, number of animals per cage, moisture in feed, temperature, etc.

[c] Results obtained under anesthesia.

sentinel programs. Because most diseases of laboratory rodents do not cause clinical signs and there can be high and unpredictable turnover of research rodents, health surveillance programs are traditionally based on the premise that infectious agents can be transmitted to sentinels, which can then be tested for a variety of pathogens. This provides assurance that the research colonies are free of specific pathogens and alerts personnel to the presence of infection. Before the widespread use of filter top caging, dedicated sentinels in open cages were readily exposed to airborne fomite particles and true aerosols from infected animals in the colony.

The same filter tops that protect colony animals from contagion, however, also hinder the exposure of sentinels to these same agents. For many reasons, dedicated sentinels are preferred over the alternative of monitoring colony rodents. State-of-the-art sentinel programs have thus come to rely on the regular exposure of sentinels to soiled bedding as the means of exposure to colony animals. This indirect exposure has been found to be suboptimal for the detection of many bacterial pathogens, agents transmitted by true aerosol, and fur mites. Agents that are shed intermittently, those with a self-limited, single window of shedding, those that require a high dose to be infective, and those that may deteriorate rapidly are difficult to detect by exposure to soiled bedding. The sentinels themselves may add confounding influences if their age or genetic background makes them relatively resistant to infection.

The primary contemporary challenges to the health of research rodents—particularly mice—are the noroviruses, parvoviruses, *Helicobacter* spp, pinworms, and fur mites that infect or infest colonies, perturbing biologic processes and introducing variation into research data. For the most part, these agents, along with mouse hepatitis virus , are thought to have gained entry to research colonies largely via the trading of live mice of unique genotypes between institutions. The situation has been complicated by the inability of quarantine programs to reliably detect these agents. However, there is a body of substantial, compelling, anecdotal evidence that nonsterilized diets may be a source of introduction for some pathogens (eg, mouse parvovirus). Murine norovirus has been shown to be the most widespread virus in domestic mouse colonies. The virus likely existed in research mice for decades, but it was not described until 2003. Mouse parvovirus was definitively discovered 10 years earlier. These viruses may persist for lengthy periods in mice and can contaminate and remain infectious in the environment for months, making them ideally suited to persevere in colonies kept in filter top cage systems.

TABLE 11 SELECTED PHYSIOLOGIC DATA OF LABORATORY ANIMALS[a] *(continued)*

Usual Life Span (yr)	Average Body Temperature (°C)	Heart Rate (bpm)	Water Consumption (per day)[b]
1–3	37	310–840	4–7 mL
2–3	37.5	300–500	30 mL
3–4	38	230–380	150 mL
2–3	37	280–410	30 mL
3–4	39	250–360	4 mL
5–7	39	200–300	300–700 mL
16–20	39	300–380[c]	70–110 mL
15–30	38	120–180[c]	0.2–1 L
20–30 (males) 30–40 (females)	37	60–120[c]	2.2–2.7 L
30–40	39	95–145[c]	1–1.5 L

LLAMAS AND ALPACAS

The four members of the South American camelids (SACs) are the llama, alpaca, guanaco, and vicuña. Although their progenitors originated in North America, these species evolved in the South American Andes, with the wild guanaco and vicuña serving as the foundation stock for the domesticated llama and alpaca, respectively.

Mature, average alpacas weigh 60–80 kg and stand 76–97 cm at the withers. Alpacas are primarily used as fiber-producing animals. The fiber grows rapidly and ideally requires shearing every 12–24 mo. Mature llamas are significantly larger animals, weighing an average of 120–200 kg and standing 102–127 cm at the withers. Llamas were primarily developed as pack animals and can carry loads of 25–40 kg. Both domestic SACs are meat staples for indigenous peoples. Males and females of both species have approximately similar mature weights. Guanacos are similar in size to llamas but weigh somewhat less. Unlike llamas and alpacas, in which coloration patterns vary markedly, guanacos and vicuña have a "wild pattern" characterized by a light brown or tan coat over the neck, back, and outside of the legs, with white on the underbelly and medial surface of the legs. Vicuñas are slightly taller than alpacas, with a longer neck, much shorter fiber, and a characteristic "bib" of long fibers in the chest region. Vicuñas have extremely fine fiber and are managed and protected in much of South America.

All SACs have 74 chromosomes and can interbreed, producing fertile F1 progeny. The most common, naturally occurring cross is a llama-alpaca mating, producing a "huarizo" that is intermediate in size, body characteristics, and fiber quality. Recent attempts to increase fiber quality and quantity have involved alpaca-vicuña crosses resulting in paco-vicuñas. Intact male llamas and alpacas are called studs (machos in Spanish), whereas castrated males are referred to as geldings. Females are called females (hembras in Spanish). The neonates and young up to 6 mo of age are called crias, whereas juveniles are called tuis in the local Quechua language.

Most llamas have characteristic "banana-shaped" ears, a level back, and a high tail set. There are no distinct llama breeds, but several types based on fiber length and crimp have emerged. A "suri-style" llama has recently been introduced into the North American market.

In contrast, there are two morphologically distinct types of alpacas: the Huacaya and Suri. The more common Huacayas have a lofted fiber coat with variable coverage down the legs and around the face. Suri have a flat-lying corded fiber structure ("dreadlocks") with less coverage on the head. Alpacas have shorter "spear-shaped" ears, a lower tail set, slightly more humping to the back, and a sloping rear end that results in a slight sickle hock appearance.

SACs are most closely related to the Old World camelids (Bactrian and Dromedary), having the same number of chromosomes, similar anatomy and physiology, and general patterns of disease susceptibility. Although conventional ruminants are frequently used as reference points for drug dosage extrapolation, disease susceptibility, and management decisions, it is important to remember that SACs and common domestic ruminants are not the same.

MANAGEMENT

Llamas and alpacas are adaptable to a wide climatic range and have been successfully raised in regions with winter temperatures as low as –20°C (–4° F) if reasonable wind shelter is provided. Heat stress is a significant problem if animals have moderate to heavy fiber coats and are subjected to high temperature and humidity. Shearing, leaving remaining fiber at least 2 cm long to prevent sunburns, and providing access to shade and sufficient water usually allow SACs to handle moderately high temperature and humidity. Air conditioning, misters, and damp sand pits are helpful to maintain heavy fiber coats in warm, humid climates. Llamas and alpacas can adapt well to damp climates as long as the temperature does not get too high, and few problems of either footrot or "rain scald" are encountered.

Llamas and alpacas can be housed with other species, including sheep, goats, and horses. Individual llamas (ideally geldings) have been successfully used as guard animals with sheep flocks and goat herds. Llamas and alpacas are herd animals and do poorly if isolated from cohorts or other animals; ill animals should be housed with

TABLE 12 SELECTED DRUGS USED IN LLAMAS AND ALPACAS

Drug	Dosage	Comment
SEDATION/ANESTHESIA		
Xylazine	0.1–0.2 mg/kg, IV	For sedation
	0.3–0.4 mg/kg, IV	For recumbency
Butorphanol	0.1–0.2 mg/kg, IM or IV	For sedation
KXB: ketamine (4 mg/kg), xylazine (0.4 mg/kg), and butorphanol (0.04 mg/kg)	1 mL/22.5 kg, IM (llamas) 1 mL/18 kg, IM (alpacas)	Mix 1,000 mg ketamine with 100 mg xylazine and 10 mg butorphanol; if needed to maintain anesthesia, ½ initial dose can be given IV in the medial saphenous vein
ANTIBIOTICS		
Aqueous procaine penicillin	20–40,000 units/kg, SC	
Long-acting tetracycline	18–20 mg/kg, SC, every 2–3 days	
Ceftiofur	2.2 mg/kg, IM or IV, bid	
Trimethoprim/ sulfamethoxazole	3/15 mg/kg, IV, bid	
Ampicillin sodium	6 mg/kg, IM or IV, bid	
Enrofloxacin	5 mg/kg, IV, bid	
Gentamicin	0.75 mg/kg, IV, tid	
	4–5 mg/kg/day, IV	
Tobramycin	4 mg/kg/day, IV	
Amikacin	12 mg/kg/day, IV	
REPRODUCTIVE		
hCG[a]	5,000 IU	
GnRH	1 mcg/kg	
Cloprostenol	100–150 mcg, IM, repeated in 24 hr	
Dinoprost tromethamine	5 mg, SC, repeated in 24 hr	
ANTHELMINTICS		
Ivermectin	0.2 mg/kg	
Pyrantel pamoate	18 mg/kg	
Fenbendazole	5–10 mg/kg	
Clorsulon	7–14 mg/kg	
Albendazole	10 mg/kg	

TABLE 12 SELECTED DRUGS USED IN LLAMAS AND ALPACAS *(continued)*

Drug	Dosage	Comment
COCCIDIAL		
Ponazuril[b]	20 mg/kg/day for 3 days	Ideally should be followed by sulfadimethoxine, 55 mg/kg, SC on day 1, then 27.5 mg/kg, SC, for 2 additional days
GASTRIC		
Omeprazole	0.4 mg/kg, bid	
MANGE, LOCAL THERAPY		
Mixture of:		Shake before use and apply mixture to local lesions with a paint brush every 5 days for 5 treatments
Mineral oil	2 oz	
DMSO, 10%	2 oz	
Ivermectin, injectable	4 mL	
Gentamicin	1 g	

[a] Human chorionic gonadotropin

[b] For treatment of *Eimeria macusaniensis*

herdmates if appropriate. If sufficient space is available, large groups of males (or females) can be pastured together. In the presence of nonpregnant females, however, intact males and recently castrated geldings will commonly spend much of their time fighting, typically biting at the ears, neck, and scrotum. Llamas and alpacas generally do not destroy fences and can usually be confined behind a 1.5-m or 1.2-m fence, respectively. Barbed wire is not needed for containment, and electric fences have been successfully used.

A somewhat unique behavioral characteristic of SACs is the use of communal dung piles. Animals urinate and defecate on the same pile, with favorite sites being in the depths of barns and other inconvenient locations. Normal feces are pelleted and firm. Unless forage becomes very limited, animals will not graze in areas around or downstream from dung piles. The urethral diameter in both males and females is relatively small, and the process of urination takes much longer than in other species of comparable size.

Handling: Llamas and alpacas are highly trainable, and most animals can be easily taught to come into a barn or corral for food. An arm around the base of the neck and another arm holding the tail or flank region on the opposite side can restrain many animals. Halter-trained SACs can be easily led into a smaller area for examination and treatment. Specially designed llama chutes should be used for reproductive examinations and other potentially uncomfortable procedures. In contrast, alpacas respond better to most procedures if assistants, and not restraint chutes, are used to hold the animals. With both llamas and alpacas, it is particularly important to maintain control of the animal's head. The neck is very muscular and can move with amazing speed. Sedation is not needed for most procedures. A small catch pen crowded with animals will afford adequate control to administer injections and perform body condition scoring.

Feeding and Nutrition: Mature males, and most females during midgestation, will maintain appropriate body condition on 10%–14% crude protein grass hay with total digestible nutrients (TDN) of 50%–55%. Late gestation and heavily lactating females require a slightly higher percentage of crude protein and TDN of 60%–65%. Under basal conditions, most camelids eat 1.8%–2% of body wt/day on a dry-matter basis. Legumes are usually not needed and may contribute to obesity. Palpating the amount of tissue over the lumbar vertebrae and ribs can best assess body condition. Body condition is generally scored from 1 (thin) to 9 (fat), with 5 being ideal.

Seasonal vitamin D deficiency, characterized by diminished growth, angular limb deformities, kyphosis, and a reluctance to move, can be a problem in heavily fibered animals raised in regions with poor sun exposure during winter months. The problem is most severe in rapidly growing, fall-born crias. Serum phosphorus of <3 mg/dL, a calcium:phosphorus ratio of >3:1, and vitamin D concentrations of <15 nmol/L in crias <6 mo old are diagnostic. Normal phosphorus and vitamin D concentrations in this age group are 6.5–9 mg/dL and >50 nmol/L, respectively.

To date, there does not appear to be a nutritional justification for routinely incorporating ionophores into the diet of camelids. However, because pelleted or mixed-grain feeds intended for camelid consumption may be formulated in the same facilities that handle ionophores, camelid feed has been accidentally contaminated. Such an incident resulted in a high incidence of death, and other health compromises to animals exposed during the period of consumption are not fully known. Routine and effective purging of feed milling facilities should allow for production of camelid feed without contamination; however, human error and equipment failure can still compromise any feed product.

Copper toxicity is a much greater concern than copper deficiency in camelids. Although there is a requirement for copper in camelid diets, mistakes in formulation and use of multiple supplements without full knowledge of total copper intake has resulted in toxicity. Most reported cases of toxicity have been due to chronic intake rather than acute deaths.

Anesthesia: There are several options for sedation and anesthesia of camelids (*see* TABLE 12). Generally, alpacas require more drug than llamas to achieve the same results. For short procedures, it is usually not necessary to withhold food and water; however, when deemed necessary, both should be withheld at the same time, reducing the tendency to regurgitate.

Xylazine can be used for sedation without recumbency. Higher dosages will result in recumbency and provide a light plane of anesthesia for 20–30 min. Simultaneous administration of xylazine, ketamine, and butorphanol usually provides 20–30 min of recumbent restraint. Butorphanol can provide sedation of short duration and is especially useful for head, ear, and dental procedures.

Llamas and alpacas tolerate general anesthesia well and usually do not require tranquilization before induction. Induction and maintenance of anesthesia is similar to that in other domestic species; however, tracheal intubation requires some practice.

Clinical Pathology: Hematology and clinical chemistries are similar to those in other species, with a few significant differences. Camelid RBCs are relatively small and elliptical and may produce anomalous results when evaluated using an automated cell counter. Normal PCV is 27%–45%, normal RBC counts are 10.1–17.3 × 10^6/μL, and normal WBC counts are 8,000–21,400/μL.

Basal glucose concentrations in llamas and alpacas are more typical of monogastric species than ruminants. Basal levels are 82–160 mg/dL, but glucose levels >300 mg/dL are common after stressful events. For additional hematologic and serum biochemical reference ranges, *see* TABLES 6 and 7, p 3176.

Drug Use: No drugs are currently approved for use in llamas and alpacas, so all use is extra-label. SACs in North America have the potential to be food animals, making drug withdrawal time a consideration. *See* TABLE 12 for antibiotics that have been used for treatment of sensitive bacteria in SACs.

Although drug use in exotic species is commonly based on approaches used in other species and often has favorable results, adverse outcomes have prevailed with numerous drugs in camelids.

Camelids are prone to lidocaine toxicity, so its use should be minimized. If deemed necessary, lidocaine should be diluted to 0.5% and used sparingly; the total dose should not exceed 4 mg/kg (1 mL of 2% lidocaine/5 kg). Lidocaine toxicity is characterized by lethargy, ataxia, slow and labored breathing, weakness, hypotension, and diminished response to stimuli. Diazepam should be available and administered at 0.1–0.5 mg/kg in case of lidocaine toxicity.

Although dexamethasone is used in other animals to stimulate surfactant activity in fetal lungs, as little as 0.5 mg in pregnant camelids has consistently caused fetal death and complications, including retained placenta and uterine prolapse. Virtually any steroid-containing product that a female camelid comes in contact with, especially during the third trimester, will cause abortion. Even a cria with steroid cream on the muzzle nursing a dam has caused abortion.

Tilmicosin has caused enough deaths in camelids to warrant the recommendation that it should not be used in these species. The cardiovascular system is the target of toxicity, which may be due to calcium channel blockade.

The prolonged-release form of ceftiofur has produced neurologic changes, including blindness. IV administration should be avoided. However, many camelids have been successfully treated SC without problems.

Normally used to reverse xylazine sedation, tolazoline has produced severe signs, including initially anxiety, hyperesthesia, profuse salivation, and tachypnea. Convulsions, hypotension, and GI hypermotility resulting in diarrhea also develop. Doses >2 mg/kg are incriminated, as well as too rapid IV administration. Because death has also resulted after administration of tolazoline, use of yohimbine is likely a better approach.

Dinoprost tromethamine (prostaglandin $F_2\alpha$) use in camelids has often resulted in rapid death, likely due to bronchiolar constriction and pulmonary edema.

Leptospirosis 5-way killed vaccine has caused type 2 hypersensitivity and anaphylaxis in camelids. Similar reactions have been reported occasionally in cattle and swine, so it is likely that sensitivity will increase in camelid herds in which vaccination against leptospirosis is indicated.

Atropine, whether administered locally in the eye or parenterally, has resulted in pupillary dilation observed to persist in camelids for as long as a week. Treated animals must be kept out of direct sunlight until pupillary response is normal.

Camelids have relatively thin skin, and use of topical eprinomectin can result in dermatitis and blisters.

After a llama herd was treated for biting lice with topical permethrin 10%, some animals were observed to be breathing hard and drooling; recovery was uneventful.

Although numerous potential adverse effects from therapeutic use of trimethoprim-sulfamethoxazole have been reported in the literature, it appears that acute death after IV administration is rare. The rate of administration or existing condition being treated may be a predisposing factor in the outcome.

Commonly and immediately after camelids are injected with B-complex vitamins or levamisole, they demonstrate signs of hyperexcitement and itching. In the case of multiple procedures or administration of several injections, those anticipated to sting should be done last.

REPRODUCTION

Reproductive Physiology

Females: Relative to body size, the nonpregnant reproductive tract of SACs is relatively small. Uterine morphology is similar to that of a mare, with relatively short horns and uterine body. The cervix can be felt on rectal palpation and has two or three cartilagenous rings. The urethra opens onto the floor of the vagina. A suburethral diverticulum is present.

Ovarian activity typically begins at 10–12 mo of age. Camelids are induced ovulators. At the onset of puberty, follicular waves occur, with a dominant follicle developing every 12–14 days. Because of the small size of females and the potential for dystocia associated with early breeding, females are usually not bred until they are >18 mo old and weigh 40 kg (alpaca) or 90 kg (llama). When a female is truly receptive, she will usually assume a position of sternal recumbency (cushing) within seconds to a few minutes after introduction of a male and allow the male to breed. While mounting, the male will typically begin a vocalization described as "orgling." The volume of the ejaculate is relatively small (2–5 mL) and is mostly deposited directly into the body of the uterus after cervical dilation. Ejaculation occurs over an extended period of time. An ovulation induction factor in the semen stimulates reflex ovulation ~24–30 hr after mating. A functional corpus luteum (CL) is present 2–3 days after ovulation. The fertilized oocyte is usually found in the uterus by day 7 after mating, with implantation occurring by ~30 days of gestation. The type of placentation is diffuse epitheliochorial, developing in both horns. Although ovulation occurs from either ovary, uniquely, ~95% or more of the pregnancies are carried in the left horn. Live births of twins are extremely uncommon, with most twin pregnancies being resorbed or aborted early in gestation.

A female with a functional CL will aggressively refuse the male's efforts to mount. An indication of pregnancy is the female's rejection of the male if he is reintroduced >15 days after the initial breeding. Progesterone concentrations of >1 ng/mL are typical in females with a functional CL and can be used for confirmation of both ovulation at 6–9 days after mating and of pregnancy at >21 days after mating. Persistent CL are periodically seen and account for most false-positive results when using serum progesterone for pregnancy confirmation. Rectal palpation for pregnancy diagnosis is practical in llamas at >45 days of gestation. It is usually not possible to safely perform rectal palpation in alpacas, unless the palpator has small hands. Pregnancy can positively be diagnosed by transrectal ultrasound from ~28 days of gestation, although it is possible to be suspicious as early as 10–12 days based on presence of fluid and to be reasonably sure by day 21 when a hyperechoic "embryo" is seen. Ultrasonographic transabdominal approach from 45–60 days can be expected to produce positive results.

Normal gestation in camelids is ~342 ± 10 days, with alpacas being somewhat shorter. Most normal births (>70%) occur in the morning. Dystocias due to excessively large crias are rare. There are few reliable indications of pending delivery. Stage I labor typically lasts 1–6 hr and may be accompanied by increased frequency of urination, increased "humming," and separation from the herd. Stage II labor is rapid (typically <30 min), with delivery of a cria weighing 5.5–8 kg (alpaca) or 11–16 kg (llama). Stage III should be complete within 4–6 hr. All stages are usually longer in a first-time delivery. Retained placentas are rare. Uterine involution begins shortly after birth, and most females can conceive within 14–21 days after delivery. Females have four teats and do not exhibit significant mammary enlargement during the prepartum period. Mastitis is rare.

Males: Both testicles should be fully descended at birth. Testes should be at least 2 × 4 cm and 3 × 6 cm in mature alpacas and llamas, respectively. Relative to body size, the testes are smaller than those of many other domestic livestock species and are held close to the body wall. The urethra is relatively small and contains a urethral diverticulum at the level of the ischial arch, making retrograde catheterization difficult to impossible. The unstimulated prepuce points backward, accounting for the rear-directed urination, while the forward-pointing penis is fibrous, with a sigmoid flexure. A cartilaginous process is present at the tip of the penis, and the urethra opens 1–2 cm back from the tip. Urinary calculi are relatively uncommon and have a poor prognosis because of the small urethral diameter (3.5–5 French).

Although androgen production may begin at <8 mo of age, and some sperm can be collected by vaginal retrieval as early as 14 mo of age, normal preputial adhesions prevent full penile extension and copulation until ≥18–24 mo of age. Most males enter breeding programs when 18–24 mo old, and most are fertile by 30 mo of age. Sexual maturity may be later in alpacas than in llamas.

Semen evaluation is difficult in camelids because of the small total volume of semen and the dribble ejaculation. Although males can be trained to mount a phantom or dummy equipped with an artificial vagina, semen collection usually requires heavy sedation or anesthesia and electroejaculation. Semen collection, even from males of known fertility, is inconsistent. The most reliable semen evaluation is afforded by postbreeding retrieval from the vagina of a receptive dam.

Management of Reproductive Problems

Fertility problems are relatively common in llamas and alpacas. Although most problems primarily involve females, problems with males include hypoplastic testes, penile injuries, and heat stress, which is characterized by scrotal edema, decreased activity, and reluctance to breed. After heat stress, fertility can be permanently impaired or reduced for up to 6 wk. Shearing, adequate shade, and sufficient water help prevent the problem. When working with inexperienced males, vaginal intromission should be visually confirmed.

Because of the relatively high incidence of congenital anomalies, anatomic problems must be considered as causes of infertility in nulliparous animals. In multiparous animals, vaginal strictures, uterine infections, and cervical damage are also relatively common. Complete uterine strictures are possible sequelae of dystocia. The diagnostic approach to all these conditions is similar to that used in mares, except that rectal palpation cannot usually be safely done in alpacas unless sedated. If uterine biopsies or cultures are appropriate, they should be performed when the dam has a dominant follicle, which relaxes the cervix.

Rupture of a mature follicle (>7 mm) can reliably be induced with human chorionic gonadotropin or GnRH. Increased progesterone concentration (>1 ng/mL) 7 days after copulation or hormonal treatment is indicative of CL formation. Although persistent CL have been identified, they are relatively rare. Prostaglandin treatment will result in regression of a persistent CL and abortion throughout gestation. Induction of parturition with prostaglandins or glucocorticoids is not recommended. Rapid death of llamas and alpacas has occurred after prostaglandin therapy, especially at high doses and when administered by other than SC route.

HERD HEALTH

Neonatal Care: Crias should be on their feet and attempting to nurse within 2 hr after birth and every 1–2 hr thereafter for the first few days. While weight gain for the first 24 hr postpartum may be minimal, thereafter llamas should gain 250–500 g/day and alpacas 100–250 g/day. Healthy crias should approximately double their birth weight by 1 mo of age.

Routine cria care should include weighing and single dipping the navel in 7% tincture of iodine or 0.5% chlorhexidine three times during the first 24 hr after birth. If appropriate for the area, supplemental selenium could be provided by injection (0.5 mg for alpacas, 1 mg for llamas). At birth is an ideal time to take a blood sample if there is any concern of failure of passive transfer of colostral antibodies. Having a baseline sample to measure PCV and total proteins to compare with a subsequent sample at 24 hr will provide valuable information regarding failure of passive transfer and hydration.

Parasite Control: Parasite control programs vary according to climatic conditions, population density, and parasite load, and should be developed according to local conditions.

No drugs have been approved for use in SACs. However, anthelmintics that are generally recognized as safe and effective include ivermectin, pyrantel pamoate, and fenbendazole. Parasite resistance has developed in all ruminant species, making it necessary to develop a strategic deworming program, particularly in locations where the meningeal worm is present. Liver flukes can be a significant problem. Control with clorsulon or albendazole is usually effective, although repeated clorsulon treatment every 6–8 wk may be necessary.

Vaccinations: Most vaccination protocols for SACs have been empirically derived. Most animals should receive *Clostridium perfringens* type C and D vaccinations and tetanus toxoid. In regions where liver fluke (*Fasciola hepatica*) infections or snake envenomations are a problem, use of polyvalent vaccines against *C novyi*, *C septicum*, *C sordellii*, and *C chauvoei* are warranted. One successful approach has been to give an initial vaccination at 3 mo of age, a booster 30 days later, and annual boosters thereafter. Llamas and alpacas are immunocompetent at birth, so neonatal vaccination can begin in the first week of life, followed by two boosters at 3-wk intervals.

Abortions secondary to *Leptospira* spp infections are regionally a problem and can usually be prevented using an initial vaccination, followed by boosters twice a year. Killed rabies vaccines have been used with unknown efficacy in endemic areas. Any attempt to control other viral diseases (including West Nile virus infection) should only involve use of killed vaccines.

Dental Development and Care: The dental pad of llamas and alpacas is similar to that of a cow. At birth, the first two pairs of lower incisors are normally through the gum line; lack of eruption is one indication of prematurity. The central, middle, and lateral mandibular deciduous incisors are replaced at ~2–2½, 3–3½, and 4–6 yr, respectively, although determining age by the teeth is notoriously inaccurate in these species.

A unique feature of SACs is the development of the upper I3 and upper and lower canine teeth on both sides into "fighting" teeth that may grow to >3 cm long. The teeth can cause serious damage to other males during fights and usually need to be cut flush to the gum with obstetrical wire or a grinder beginning with eruption at 18–24 mo of age and repeated as needed in intact males. If castration is to be performed, eruption of the fighting teeth signals an ideal time to schedule both procedures. Growth of fighting teeth usually stops after castration. Fighting teeth in most females barely penetrate the gumline and seldom, if ever, need to be cut. Tooth extraction to avoid periodic trimming is impractical because of very deep, curved roots.

The incisors are open-rooted in alpacas and continue to grow throughout life. Poor occlusion of the incisors and dental pad necessitate periodic tooth trimming and appears to be more of a problem in alpacas than in llamas. Cheek teeth are rooted, normally sharp, and do not require regular floating. Premolar and molar occlusion should be checked and problems corrected in older animals exhibiting difficulty in chewing or weight loss.

Abscessed lower second premolar and first and second molars are seen as a hard, well-developed swelling on the lateral surface of the mandible over the affected teeth. A draining tract may or may not be present. The area is usually not painful on palpation, and most animals maintain body condition. No bacterial agent has been consistently isolated from the abscesses. Prolonged antibiotic therapy is palliative, although rarely curative. Tooth extraction usually requires making a lateral incision over the affected teeth, splitting the tooth because of the divergent roots and repelling the tooth into the oral cavity. Care should be taken during extraction to avoid mandibular fracture.

Nail Trimming: Some animals rarely need foot care, whereas others require nail trimming every 2–3 mo. Diet, genetics, and environment likely play a role. The nails should be trimmed flush with the bottom of the pad. Occasionally and especially with overgrown toes, "quicking" may occur but generally is inconsequential.

DISEASES

Congenital and Inherited Anomalies

Although few congenital anomalies have conclusively been shown to be genetic in origin, it is assumed that defects inherited in other species are probably inherited in SACs as well. Accordingly, this should be considered in breeding decisions. Facial and cardiac defects are reported to be the most frequent inherited anomalies. A historically narrow gene pool is likely the reason that congenital defects are relatively common in SACs. Affected individuals commonly have more than one defect.

Choanal atresia, a condition caused by failure of the inner nares (choanae) to open during embryologic development, is the most widespread congenital defect. It can be unilateral or bilateral and may result in complete or partial blockage. Accordingly, the primary clinical presentation is a variable degree of respiratory distress in the neonate. Distress becomes more apparent during nursing, and crias commonly gasp as milk is inhaled. Surgical correction is not recommended.

Wry face is characterized by a slight (<5°) to severe (>60°) lateral deviation of the maxilla. The mandible may or may not have a similar deviation. When severe, occlusion of the nares and lack of apposition of the incisors and dental pad usually necessitate euthanasia of the cria. There appears to be a relationship of this defect to choanal atresia, in that they occasionally occur together.

Ocular and **ear** conditions include juvenile cataracts (seen occasionally), blocked nasolacrimal ducts, and an association between blue eyes and deafness in some lines of white animals. Fused (tip or base) and short ("gopher") ears are recognized heritable defects, the latter appearing to be a dominant trait.

Cardiac defects are relatively common, with ventricular septal defects heading the list.

Numerous **musculoskeletal defects** have been identified, including syndactyly and polydactyly. Arthrogryposis, rotated talus, angular limb deformities of the front limbs, and tendon laxity are also seen.

Other congenital anomalies identified in llamas and alpacas include **atresia ani**, **atresia coli**, **umbilical hernias**, and several different types of **tail defects**, including a pronounced lateral deviation of the tail at the base.

Urogenital defects are much more common in SACs than in other species. Significant defects in females include uterus unicornis, hypoplastic ovaries, double cervices, segmental aplasia of the vagina or uterus, and clitoral hypertrophy suggesting intersex conditions. Unilateral absence of a kidney is periodically seen, commonly in association with choanal atresia. Total absence of kidneys has also been seen. Congenital conditions in males include hypospadia, retained testicles, testicular hypoplasia, persistent frenulum, ectopic testicles, and corkscrew penis.

Bacterial Diseases

Brucellosis, tuberculosis, and Johne's disease (paratuberculosis) have been identified in SACs, although the naturally occurring incidence of these infections is low. There are reported cases of both type C and D *Clostridium perfringens*, which has prompted the use of toxoid vaccination as a routine measure in most herds. Although SACs are not apparently highly susceptible to tetanus, most herd vaccinations using the C/D toxoid include tetanus toxoid.

C perfringens type A is a very important pathogen under stressful circumstances, especially in South America, and results in a high death rate in crias <4 wk old. Enterotoxogenic strains of *C perfringens* type A are believed to be particularly lethal. Clinical signs are similar to those of type A infections in other species, with a rapid onset of neurologic changes followed shortly by death.

Anthrax has been diagnosed in SACs, but vaccination should only be done in endemic areas using a killed product.

Respiratory infections in North America caused by bacteria remain relatively rare, but in South America the condition referred to as alpaca fever is caused by *Streptococcus zooepidemicus*. The onset of this condition is often preceded by stressful conditions.

Individual cases and herd problems with abscesses caused by *Corynebacterium pseudotuberculosis* have been reported. Contact with sheep and shearing wounds are likely contributing factors.

Viral Diseases

Most camelids are seropositive for a presumptively nonpathogenic adenovirus that is specific to llamas. Occasionally, an animal will develop a titer to bovine viral diarrhea virus, and a few animals have developed a mild diarrhea, respiratory disease, and even abortion presumably in response to the virus. Exposure during pregnancy also can lead to persistent infection in crias. Equine herpesvirus 1 infections with associated neurologic signs and blindness have been seen in a small number of SACs, particularly when cohabitating with equids. Growing numbers of neurologic cases in SACs have been found to be due to Eastern equine encephalomyelitis virus. Bluetongue virus likely will emerge as a clinical entity in SACs as it evolves with greater distribution and pathogenicity. An outbreak in 2007 of respiratory disease, principally in alpacas, was found to be due to what is referred to as alpaca respiratory coronavirus. Stress conditions often predispose to the onset of clinical presentations that vary from mild upper respiratory tract disease to severe respiratory disease and death.

During the spread of West Nile virus across North America, SACs were found to be susceptible, with most developing a titer consistent with exposure. Some became severely affected and died. Naive and immunosuppressed animals are most likely to be at risk. West Nile virus vaccines approved for horses have been found to produce a good immune response. SACs can also contract foot and mouth disease, although clinical disease is usually relatively mild; the carrier status of infected animals is presumed to be of short duration.

Mycoplasma Infection

A common condition that was formerly referred to as eperythrozoonosis is now known to be caused by *Mycoplasma haemolamae*. A high percentage of the SAC population has been exposed by insect vectors, contaminated needles, or transplacentally. Animals with a healthy immune system develop a state of premunity (infected but immune); they demonstrate the organism in RBCs only when stressed or truly immunosuppressed. PCR diagnostic tests are available. Treatment of clinically affected anemic animals with long-acting tetracyclines does not entirely clear the infection but improves the anemia.

Fungal infections

As with most animals, ubiquitous contact with fungal organisms in SACs will occasionally lead to clinical disease. Notable clinical possibilities include coccidioidomycosis, candidiasis, aspergillosis, cryptococcomycosis, mucormycosis, and mycotoxins. The most significant fungal infection in SACs is coccidioidomycosis; it is an endemic problem in the southwest USA, potentially affecting all resident animals (as well as the human population). An important consideration is that SACs showing chronic respiratory signs even in nonendemic locales may have been exposed during shows or breeding time while in endemic areas.

Gastrointestinal Diseases

The oral cavity and esophagus of SACs are unremarkable. The stomach has three distinct compartments (C-1, 2, and 3) that do not correlate directly with the four chambers of the ruminant stomach. Although not classed as ruminants, they do eructate, regurgitate, and remasticate and would be

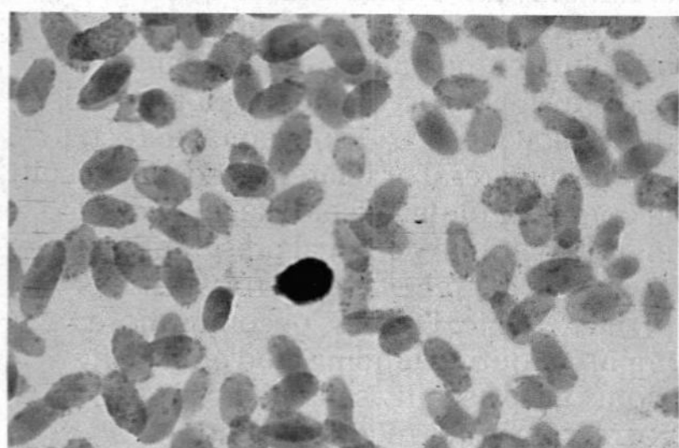

Mycoplasma infection in llama RBCs. *Courtesy of Dr. LaRue Johnson.*

considered as foregut fermenters in C-1 and 2. Only the distal fifth of C-3 is analogous to the acid-secreting monogastric stomach. The spiral colon is generally a flat, single spiral prone to blockage when the centripetal loop turns to become centrifugal.

Megaesophagus: Moderate to severe dilatation of the esophagus is relatively common in llamas and alpacas, especially after instances of choking. Signs include chronic weight loss frequently associated with postprandial regurgitation or "frothing" of food. There is no identified age or sex predilection, and no consistent cause has been established. A suspected case of megaesophagus should be confirmed with barium contrast radiography. No treatments (surgical or changes in feeding practices) have been consistently successful. The longterm prognosis is fair to poor, with some animals maintaining condition for an extended period and others continuing to lose weight.

Stomach Atony: Gastric atony is an occasional problem of unknown cause. Signs include decreased or complete cessation of food consumption, loss of body condition, and depression. Other GI problems, including diarrhea, may be present. Supportive therapy, including fluids, is frequently helpful. Lack of food for 3–5 days also usually causes the death of bacteria and protozoa in C-1 and C-2. Transfaunation (0.5–1 L) of camelid C-1 or strained rumen contents (sheep or cow), administered by gavage, frequently results in a dramatic improvement in appetite and reestablishment of appropriate flora.

Ulcers: Partial and complete thickness erosions of the acid-secreting distal portion of C-3 and most proximal portion of the duodenum occur. Signs may include decreased food consumption, intermittent to severe colic, and depression. Although the cause has not been clearly established, stress appears to be a significant component, with problems often developing 3–5 days after change of environment affecting social structure, serious injuries, and illnesses.

No reliable premortem diagnostic procedures are available; treatment is usually based on history and clinical signs. Theoretically beneficial oral medications have not proved effective. Parenteral administration of omeprazole reduces acid production. Stress reduction, including clinical housing with a cohort animal, parenteral antibiotics, and supportive therapy, are helpful.

Hepatic Disease: The visceral surface of the liver normally has multiple fissures, whereas the parietal surface is smooth and lobation is indistinct. There is no gallbladder. SACs appear to be particularly susceptible to *Fasciola hepatica*, with fecal shedding beginning 10–12 wk after infection. Clinical signs can include ill thrift, diminished growth, and acute death. Icterus is rarely seen. Increased serum bile acids (>25 μmol/L) and enzyme concentrations (normal, alkaline phosphatase 15–121 IU/L and AST 66–235 IU/L) are also diagnostically useful.

Hepatic lipidosis is a relatively common problem in SACs. Clinical signs associated with liver failure in other species are frequently seen, although acute death without prior indication of pending problems also has been reported. The cause is not clearly established, but stress and/or abrupt decrease or change in food consumption appear to play a role. Treatment is symptomatic. Mortality in untreated animals is frequently high.

Small- and Large-intestinal Diseases: Diarrhea is relatively uncommon in llamas and alpacas. Shortly after birth, SAC crias may experience a mild diarrhea due to abundant dam milk production, essentially a substrate purge. The primary recognized infectious causes of diarrhea in neonates include rotavirus, coronavirus, cryptosporidia, and enteropathogenic strains of *Escherichia coli*. Some crias also have a transitory diarrhea 2–3 wk after birth, at about the time they experience new food matter. At this same time, some crias develop colic signs due to blockage in the spiral colon. Diarrhea in older neonates is more likely associated with *Eimeria* spp infection, especially associated with the stress of weaning. Identified causes of diarrhea in older animals include *Yersinia pseudotuberculosis*, *Salmonella* spp, *Giardia* spp, and *Cryptosporidium parvum*. Treatment options are the same as for other species (ie, fluid and electrolyte replacement and appropriate antibacterials).

Diarrhea in adult SACs is relatively rare but often accompanies a change of feed. Serious conditions characterized by diarrhea include eosinophilic enteritis, infection with *Eimeria macusaniensis* or *Mycobacterium paratuberculosis*, or severe nematode parasitism. Compared with that in cattle with Johne's disease, the clinical course in SACs tends to be short and fatal. When diagnosed by fecal examination,

E macusaniensis must be promptly treated, because infection can cause marked debilitation. Although variable, current therapy recommendations include oral ponazuril followed by parenteral sulfadimethoxine.

Lymphosarcoma is the only neoplasia found with significant frequency in SACs. It can occur as either a juvenile lymphoma or a primitive malignant round cell tumor. Clinical signs and course vary depending on organ involvement.

Respiratory Diseases

Auscultation of llamas and alpacas is difficult and frequently unrewarding. Little air movement is heard under normal conditions, and identification of areas of infection, congestion, or consolidation is typically difficult. Lateral radiographs may be required for diagnosis of pneumonia. Bacterial infections of the lung are relatively rare, with *Streptococcus* and *Corynebacterium* spp being the most common isolates.

Chronic obstructive pulmonary disease appears to be increasing in frequency. Animals allowed to live to their expected life span is a factor, but feeding practices can contribute to onset as well as exacerbation of clinical signs—coughing, shortness of breath, and expiratory dyspnea. Therapy includes changing the feeding regimen to reduce dust, molds, and pollen. Bronchodilators and steroids may be helpful but remain unproved.

Skin Diseases

Unique features of normal camelid skin histologically include a marked vascularity and significant presence of eosinophils. Several skin conditions are shared with sheep and goats, including ringworm, contagious ecthyma, dermatophilosis, and occasionally pizzle rot.

Shearing Injury and Sunburn: Complications associated with shearing are common. Lacerations may occur where there are loose folds of skin, eg, near the axilla. These often heal uneventfully with or without suturing. Hot shears may cause burns that lead to thick scabs, usually on the dorsum of the back, that may resemble "wool rot." A history of shearing by a novice often helps confirm the diagnosis. Antibiotic ointment is generally beneficial for these *iatrogenic lesions.*

Sunburn also can occur after shearing, especially in light-skinned animals. If found in the acute stage, protection from further exposure and application of aloe vera lotion have proved useful. Later appearance of sunburned sites varies from mild peeling to ulcers.

Ulcerative Pododermatitis: Llamas and alpacas kept in moist conditions develop "immersion foot," characterized by footpad blistering and sloughing, with variations depending on infection by anaerobic bacteria. Debridement, antiseptics, and foot protection may be required for prolonged periods to facilitate resolution. Treatment with penicillin is always indicated unless unique bacterial isolates are involved. These cases require a relatively long healing period.

Mange, Lice, and Ticks: All four genera of mange mites (ie, *Sarcoptes*, *Psoroptes*, *Chorioptes*, and *Demodex*) have been diagnosed in camelids. Alopecia, hyperkeratosis, and scaling accompanied by pruritus tend to characterize all species. The clinical signs may resemble those of zinc deficiency. Deep skin scrapings or biopsies are ideal to make a definitive diagnosis. Although various options for therapy exist, most mange cases will respond to routine parenteral doses of ivermectin repeated every 10–14 days. Oral therapy does not appear to be as effective. *Chorioptes* infestation may require higher doses repeated every 14–21 days and local therapy. Refractory *Sarcoptes* cases involving the lower legs have benefited from the same topical treatment.

With louse infestation, it is important to determine whether pediculosis is due to biting (*Damalinia breviceps*) or sucking (*Microthoracius cameli*) lice. This can be accomplished with the aid of a hand lens or microscope. Use of transparent tape to retrieve lice for diagnosis from within the depths of wool can be attempted. Sucking lice can be treated with injectable ivermectin as per routine mange therapy. However, biting lice are not affected by parenteral ivermectin. Topical application of synthetic pyrethrin preparations has been effective, but critical doses for these species have not been established. Preventive measures for lice and mange include routine treatment of new herd additions as well as animals visiting and returning for breeding purposes or from shows. Ticks have caused tick paralysis as is seen in other species. In addition, ticks gaining access to ears have caused inner ear afflictions resulting in Horner syndrome as well as encephalitic death.

Copper Deficiency: Copper deficiency is characterized by depigmentation of fiber with a wiry or steely texture. Juveniles grow poorly and are predisposed to infections. Confirmation of deficiency is best based on comparison of liver copper levels with species normals. Therapy requires dietary supplementation. However, excessive supplementation will cause copper toxicity, which has been diagnosed more commonly than deficiency.

Dorsal Nasal Alopecia (Dark Nose Syndrome): The most common clinical sign of dorsal nasal alopecia is usually alopecia over the bridge of the nose. The skin is normal or variably scaly, hyperpigmented, and thickened. Dark-haired animals are predisposed, presumably because insects prefer the warmer surface of a dark background. In some animals, the condition may be secondary to rubbing the nose; in others, it may be a fly bite exacerbation. Systemic or topical steroids produce some transient response, but steroids may cause abortion in camelids. In northern climates, the condition tends to spontaneously improve during winter months. Alopecia of the ears has also been seen, particularly in black alpacas.

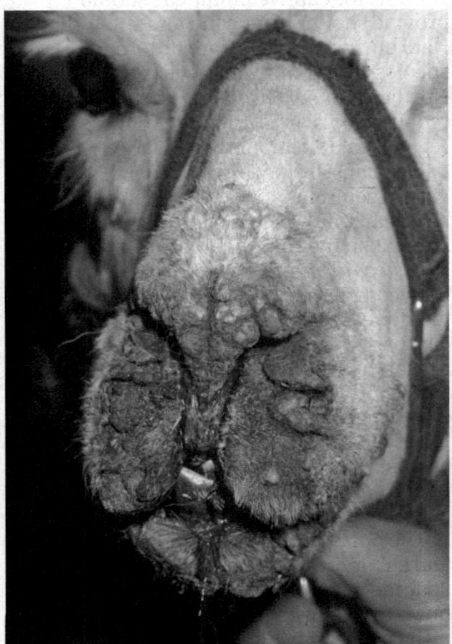

Perinasal munge in a llama. *Courtesy of Dr. LaRue Johnson.*

Idiopathic Hyperkeratosis (Zinc-responsive Dermatosis): Onset of idiopathic hyperkeratosis is possible at any age. The lesions appear as nonpruritic papules with a tightly adherent crust. Papules progress to plaques and then large areas of thickening and crusting. Lesions are most common in the less densely haired areas of the perineum, ventral abdomen, inguinal region, medial thighs, axilla, and medial forearms, but the face may also be involved. The signs may wax and wane. Diagnosis is by skin biopsy. Treatment is 1 g zinc sulfate or 2–4 g zinc methionine per day. Calcium supplementation should be minimized and alfalfa hay discontinued. Affected animals may be zinc responsive but not deficient.

Idiopathic Nasal/Perioral Hyperkeratotic Dermatosis (Munge): Most animals with munge are 6 mo to 2 yr old at onset. Variable degrees of hyperkeratosis (heavy, adherent crusts) in paranasal and perioral regions are seen. Less commonly, the bridge of the nose and periocular and periaural regions are affected. Inflammatory lesions may wax and wane. Differential diagnoses include viral contagious pustular dermatitis, dermatophilosis, dermatophytosis, bacterial dermatitis, and autoimmune/immune-mediated disease. Treatment is directed at resolving secondary bacterial infections (ie, daily 10% povidone iodine scrubs plus application of 7% tincture of iodine). If lesions do not respond to antibiotics, adding topical glucocorticoid preparations or intralesional triamcinolone acetonide (2 mg/mL) may be beneficial. Some animals do not respond to any of the described therapies, including those with juvenile llama deficiency syndrome, which has been shown to affect both llamas and alpacas; in these cases, an evaluation of the immune response is indicated.

MARINE MAMMALS

Marine mammals are a diverse group of species that include cetaceans, pinnipeds, sirenians, sea otters, and polar bears. The cetaceans consist of two major groups with different physiology and anatomy: toothed whales (Odontocetes) and baleen whales (Mysticetes). The pinnipeds consist of three major groups: true seals (Phocidae), eared seals (Otariidae), and walruses (Odobenidae). Sirenians (Sirenidae) are of a single family that includes manatees and dugongs. The sea otter (*Enhydra lutris*) is a marine member of the Mustelidae, and the polar bear (*Ursus maritimus*) is the only member of the Ursidae that is considered marine.

Few pharmaceuticals or vaccines are approved for use in marine mammals. Many recommendations can be made based on personal experience or published reports, but clinicians should be cautious in their application.

MANAGEMENT

The general rule in maintaining marine mammals in captivity is to duplicate their natural environment as closely as possible. Most live in marine habitats, although some species migrate into freshwater; Baikal seals (*Phoca sibirica*) and five species of river dolphins have adapted completely to freshwater habitats. Manatee subspecies vary in the time they spend in freshwater, but the dugong (*Dugong dugong*) is completely marine.

Marine cetaceans should be kept in water with a salinity of 25–35 g/L, preferably using balanced sea salts. Water for captive marine cetaceans should be maintained as close to the pH of mid-ocean waters (8–8.3) as possible. Freshwater cetaceans and seals require water similar to that of their natural habitat. In the USA, the Marine Mammal Protection Act of 1972 specifies that coliform bacterial counts of water for captive marine mammals must be ≤1,000 MPN (most probable number/100 mL).

Marine mammals kept in the extremes of their temperature tolerance range are more susceptible to environmental and infectious disease. In general, cetaceans and pinnipeds are better adapted to cold than to heat, but species-specific tolerances differ. Inappropriately combining different species for display purposes can result in compromises that jeopardize the well-being of some species.

Good air quality, especially in indoor facilities (10–20 air changes/hr) is as important as good water quality. Photoperiods, light spectral and intensity requirements, sound tolerances, and flight distance requirements are not well established for any cetacean. Extremes in any of these factors should be considered detrimental in the absence of specific data.

Environmental requirements of pinnipeds are similar to those of cetaceans except that pinnipeds can "haul out" on land. Although captive pinnipeds can be kept in freshwater, saltwater pools that meet the specifications listed above for cetaceans are preferred. Most pinnipeds obtain their metabolic water requirements in food and do not require access to freshwater if provided fish with a high fat content. However, it is common practice to allow pinnipeds access to potable water.

Pools for captive pinnipeds should provide shelter from wind and some shade. Haul out requirements are different for each species, and some pinnipeds (eg, the Northern fur seal [*Callorhinus ursinus*]) require very specific timing of access to land (eg, only at the pupping season).

Sirenians are warmwater species with water requirements similar to those of cetaceans, although the most common sirenian in the USA, the Florida manatee (*Trichechus manatus latirostris*), migrates between marine and freshwater environments seasonally. Manatees do better in captivity if salinity is changed seasonally to match migration in the wild.

In captivity, the sea otter thrives best in a cold marine water system. Because the fur of the sea otter is its major protection against hypothermia, the water must be kept free of oils and organic material that could mat or damage the coat.

The polar bear naturally lives on arctic and subarctic ice. It has successfully adapted to subtropical climates in captivity but is more susceptible to dermatologic disease in warm climates. Polar bears traditionally have been provided with freshwater in captivity. Proper attention to filtration and water quality is beneficial.

Restraint: Marine mammals must be restrained for thorough examinations. Trained cetaceans and pinnipeds can be taught behaviors to facilitate examination and collection of diagnostic samples. For these animals, the presence of familiar attendants is important.

For complex procedures or untrained animals, the safest approach to restraining a cetacean is to remove it from the water. Captive enclosures should allow water drainage so that cetaceans can be stranded without the use of nets. As the animal begins to lose buoyancy in the draining water, it should be positioned over thick foam pads to minimize struggling and injury. Nets are an alternative for corralling small cetaceans kept in sea pens or encountered in the wild; however, experienced personnel are required to minimize the risk of drowning or injury to the animal or staff. Netted cetaceans are placed on foam or specially designed stretchers or floats that can suspend the animal above water level.

Small cetaceans (dolphins) can often be restrained by the weight of three or four attendants—one person controls the peduncle of the tail fluke and the others apply weight to the animal's body. The pectoral fins should be folded alongside the animal in a natural position to avoid permanent damage. In larger cetaceans (whales), the powerful tail fluke may be secured with mechanical restraints.

Capturing pinnipeds is generally easier on dry ground, although small animals can be captured in the water with end-release hoop nets. Larger animals should not be netted in water but should be coaxed or driven from the water or have the water drained from their pool. On land, hoop nets can be used on larger animals. Cargo nets, baffle boards, and "come-along" poles also can be helpful. Once captured, small seals can be restrained for some procedures by an experienced handler sitting on the seal's back and holding the head. Larger pinnipeds or more complex procedures require an appropriately designed squeeze cage.

Sirenians are relatively docile; problems in restraint are generally due to their bulk and weight, and caution is recommended because they tend to roll. They can be handled in much the same way as cetaceans. Sea otters can be restrained like most other large mustelids. Hoop nets can be used to remove them from pools. Once they are out of the water, restraint bags, squeeze boxes, or other restraint devices for small wild carnivores can be used. Polar bears are large and dangerous, and manual restraint is not advised.

Anesthesia: Physiologic adaptations to diving and marine environments make general anesthesia of cetaceans and pinnipeds difficult. Anesthetic drugs commonly used in other animals often have narrow margins of safety or cause unexpected reactions in marine mammals. Tranquilizers, sedatives, and anesthetics should be administered to marine mammals only by personnel experienced in their use. Specialized anesthetic machines and respirators (apneustic plateau) are required for cetaceans. Sirenians rarely require general anesthesia or tranquilization for treatment. Sea otters can be sedated with diazepam (0.2 mg/kg body wt) or tiletamine-zolazepam (1 mg/kg). A combination of fentanyl (0.22 mg/kg) and diazepam (0.07 mg/kg) has been successful for sample collection in wild sea otters. Narcotic recycling has been seen. Surgical anesthesia can be obtained with higher dosages of fentanyl-diazepam (0.33 mg/kg/0.11 mg/kg); tiletamine-zolazepam (2 mg/kg); or halothane, isoflurane, or sevoflurane, with or without nitrous oxide. Polar bears are routinely immobilized with etorphine, tiletamine-zolazepam with or without medetomidine, ketamine with xylazine, or a variety of other agents used IM. The required dose is highly dependent on the individual animal and environment.

ENVIRONMENTAL DISEASES

Corneal Edema: Corneal opacity is frequent in captive pinnipeds kept in either freshwater or saltwater; it is also seen in captive cetaceans but is rare in wild animals. It can be due to various environmental problems. Transient cases can be caused by simply moving an animal to freshwater from saltwater or vice versa. Lack of shade and excessive bright light have been implicated. Poor water conditions (eg, high bacterial loads or overuse of oxidative disinfectants in the water) also have been associated with the disease. Nutritional deficiencies have been suggested as causes, but response to supplementation with vitamin C or A has not been dramatic. Feeding other oral antioxidants (leutin, grape seed extract) as a preventive measure is being evaluated. The condition is usually self-limiting if the underlying insult to the cornea is removed early enough in the pathogenesis.

Corneal Ulcers: Corneal ulcers are common in captive pinnipeds and cetaceans. They can be the result of direct trauma or the sequelae of unresolved or untreated cases of corneal edema.

Diagnosis is by observation of epithelial defects on corneas stained with fluorescein. Culture of the lesion (bacterial, fungal) before therapy can help direct treatment of nonresponsive cases with associated infections. In trained animals, small lesions can be treated topically. In untrained animals, subconjunctival injections of antibiotics and steroid are required. Oral docycyline is being used in some pinniped cases to stabilize the cornea, and topical cyclosporine or tacrolimus is being used in tractable animals with some success in reducing recurrence. Extensive lesions benefit from protection by suturing the eyelids. Deep ulcers or lacerations in danger of eroding Descemet membrane should be stabilized with a thin methylacrylate patch. As in corneal edema, successful resolution and prevention of recurrence depend on removal of the underlying cause.

Foreign Bodies: Many captive marine mammals develop the habit of swallowing objects dropped into their pools. In cetaceans, the opening to the second compartment of the stomach is small, and foreign objects remain in the first compartment. In pinnipeds, the small pylorus prevents passage of most foreign bodies. Frequently, no clinical signs are evident. On occasion, anorexia, regurgitation, or lethargy may be seen. Diagnosis is often made by having witnessed the animal swallow an object. Smaller animals can be radiographed; in small cetaceans, the esophagus can be palpated to establish the presence of foreign bodies. Animals occasionally regurgitate foreign bodies; however, assisted removal is usually indicated. Removal is usually best performed by gastroscopy, which is also used as a method of diagnostic confirmation. All efforts should be made to prevent ingestion of foreign bodies. Training animals to retrieve for reward as a displacement to swallowing foreign objects is thought to be beneficial.

Gastrointestinal Ulcers: GI ulcers are a significant problem in captive marine mammals and are also found in free-ranging marine mammals. Ulcers of the first compartment of the cetacean stomach are a common necropsy finding and pose less severe clinical problems than do ulcers of the pyloric region or proximal duodenum. Gastric ulcers in pinnipeds frequently progress to perforation, which results in peritonitis and subsequent death. Gastric ulcers also are found in sirenians. Although ulcers in cetaceans perforate less frequently than in pinnipeds, they should be treated as a serious problem. Various causes, including parasitic damage and increased histamine content of spoiled fish, may be involved in the cause of a GI ulcer, but the disease in captive animals should be considered associated with environmental or stress-related conditions. Dramatic environmental changes, including changes of personnel or companion animals, can precipitate serious GI ulceration in cetaceans or pinnipeds.

Clinical signs include lethargy, partial anorexia, abdominal splinting, pallor, and occasionally regurgitation. Animals with bleeding ulcers show anemia and possibly leukocytosis. Diagnosis generally is based on identification of mammalian RBCs in gastric washes; confirmation is by endoscopic visualization of the lesions. Palliative treatment of nonperforating ulcers usually consists of administration of histamine blockers and alumina gel–based antacids with or without simethicone, along with frequent small meals. The underlying cause must be identified and corrected for successful resolution. Management of perforating ulcers with resulting peritonitis includes intensive broad-spectrum antibiotic and fluid therapy. As in people, stress-induced GI ulcers are more likely to develop in marine mammals that have previously had an ulcer.

Trauma: Traumatic lesions (eg, cuts, wounds from gunshots or propeller blades) are common in marine mammals. Propeller injuries are a major problem in manatees, which commonly enter heavily navigated recreational waters in Florida. Traumatic wounds should be cleaned, debrided, and generally allowed to heal as open wounds unless body cavities are breached. Antibiotics should be administered during convalescence to prevent gross infection. Maintenance of good water quality and a high plane of nutrition is beneficial to the healing process. Large wounds frequently heal uneventfully.

Oil Exposure: Exposure of marine mammals to spills of petroleum hydrocarbons is a major concern. Sea otters are particularly susceptible to such exposure because of their natural grooming habits and their lack of an insulating blubber layer. Hepatotoxicity, renal toxicity, GI damage, and loss of homeothermic ability are important effects of exposure to petroleum hydrocarbons; however, the most devastating effects are due to direct pulmonary damage from inhalation of volatile hydrocarbons.

Experimental evidence suggests cetaceans and pinnipeds will avoid petroleum spills if possible (unlike sea otters) and are relatively resistant to toxicities from direct skin contact. Ingestion of large quantities of oil by these species is unlikely, and although baleen fouling occurs in mysticete whales, it usually resolves within 24–36 hr. Pinnipeds and cetaceans are susceptible to severe pulmonary damage due to inhalation of volatile hydrocarbons as are other mammals, including people. Efforts to reduce human exposure to hydrocarbons when dealing with oil-contaminated animals is a top priority. Treatment of exposed animals includes removal of oil from both the skin (using mild detergents, eg, 2% New Dawn) and the GI system (activated carbon gavage), along with physiologic supportive therapy. For sea otters, use of warm wash water and provision of soft freshwater reduces recovery time. It is critical to recognize that capture, transport, and holding stresses appear to lower the threshold of hydrocarbon toxicity in these animals.

NUTRITION AND NUTRITIONAL DISEASES

Generally, captive animals fed a diet that is solely or primarily fish are provided dead fish that have been frozen. The logistics and difficulty in providing this diet can lead to some special nutritional concerns. All fish are not of equal nutritional value; diets consisting of a single species of fish are unlikely to provide balanced nutrition for any animal. Similarly, one diet will not serve all piscivores equally. Only fish suitable for human consumption should be fed. (*See also* NUTRITION: EXOTIC AND ZOO ANIMALS, p 2297.)

Storage and thawing of frozen fish must be monitored carefully. Feed fish should be held at or below −19°F (−28°C) to slow deterioration of their nutritional value through oxidation of amino acids and unsaturated lipids. Dehydration of frozen fish can also be a problem for animals that obtain their water from food. Fatty fish should not be stored >6 mo. Few fish, with the possible exception of capelin, should be stored >1 yr. To retain optimal vitamin content and reduce moisture loss, frozen fish should be thawed in air under refrigeration. Thawing in water leaches away water-soluble vitamins. Thawing at room temperature encourages bacterial growth and spoilage.

The energy requirements of marine mammals vary with age, environmental temperatures, and condition. Young, growing bottlenosed dolphins and smaller pinnipeds generally require 9%–15% of their body wt in high-quality fish per day. Older animals may need only 4%–9% of their body wt for maintenance. Larger species (whales, elephant seals) generally require less food per unit body weight (2%–5% of body wt) as adults.

Sirenians thrive on a diet of hydroponic grass and various lettuces and vegetables, supplemented with high-protein monkey chow, carrots, bananas, and multivitamin-mineral supplements used particularly to balance calcium to phosphorus ratios. It is thought that sirenians ingest considerable animal protein incidentally during grazing in the wild. Intake requirements have been estimated at 7%–9% of body wt daily. Sirenians are generally fed several times a day to accommodate their grazing feeding pattern.

Sea otters are usually fed diets consisting of various invertebrates (echinoderms, molluscs, occasional crustaceans) and fish. Adult animals require ~25%–30% of their body wt in food each day.

Polar bears in the wild have high-lipid diets, particularly in winter when they subsist heavily on seals. They are considered to have an exceptional dietary requirement for vitamin A, and some dermatologic conditions respond to daily supplementation of 20,000–1,000,000 IU in the diet. Polar bears are commonly fed large amounts of fish in captivity.

Neonatal Nutrition: Young, unweaned marine mammals are frequently encountered in strandings and must be fed a diet resembling their dam's milk. In captivity, neonates may be abandoned by their parents and require artificial rearing. The milk of marine mammals has a high lipid content. Most species are carbohydrate intolerant, and neonates fed formulas with carbohydrates develop severe, life-threatening bacterial gastroenteritis. Most neonatal marine mammals also require immense caloric density in replacement milks. Milk replacement formulas based on commercial component-based milk replacers (eg, Zoologic® Milk Matrix) have begun to supplant some of the very complex scratch-made formulas used in the past. When confronted with a marine mammal neonate to raise, contacting one of the major marine mammal rescue centers for advice is recommended.

Phocid and otarid seals can be reared on the same milk replacer–based formulas. Pinniped pups should be fed every 4 hr in their first week of life; gradually, the amount of formula fed should be increased and the feedings dropped to five per day. Harbor seal (*Phoca vitulina*) pups should be tube fed until 2–3 wk old, when they can be weaned to small pieces of fish. Elephant seal pups require tube feeding until they are 4 wk old, when weaning can begin. California sea lion (*Zalophus californianus*) pups can be force fed fish as early as 4 wk of age and be free feeding by 6 wk.

Neonatal walruses (*Odobenus rosmarus*) have been reared on milk replacer–based formulas, as well as on whipping-cream base extended with ground molluscs (clams) rather than fish. They also seem to tolerate carbohydrates reasonably well. Walruses have a much longer nursing period than other pinnipeds.

Neonatal cetaceans have longer nursing periods than pinnipeds. Success at bottle rearing has improved with experience, and individuals from species ranging from common dolphins (*Delphinus delphis*) to gray whales (*Escrichtius robustus*) have been reared successfully. The fat content of cetacean milks varies considerably; bottlenose dolphin (*Tursiops* spp) milk is ~17% fat (half that of most pinniped milks); beluga whale (*Delphinapterus leucas*) milk, 27%; harbour porpoise (*Phocoena phocoena*) milk, 46%; and mysticete blue whale (*Baleanoptera musculus*) milk, 42%. Formulas based on commercial component milk replacers supplemented with ground fish and oils have been fed successfully to bottlenose dolphins and harbour porpoises using a lamb's nipple or stomach tubing.

Neonatal sirenians begin to nibble sea grasses shortly after birth but may continue to nurse up to 18 mo. They can be reared on artificial milks with early weaning. Neonatal sea otters also have been reared successfully from birth on artificial formulas. Neonatal polar bears are extremely altricial and are a challenge because of an apparently immature immune system. Polar bear milk is high in fat (31%) and contains minimal lactose. Polar bears have been successfully reared on formulas with a whipping-cream or oil base.

Thiamine Deficiency: This can be seen in any piscivorous animal. Thiamine in the food is destroyed by the activity of thiaminase enzymes or antithiamine substances in the fish being fed. These active enzymes can also destroy supplemental thiamine placed in fish if the fish sits for long periods before feeding. Clinical signs of thiamine deficiency are primarily of CNS disturbances. Affected animals may show anorexia, regurgitation, or ataxia. The condition can progress to seizures, coma, and death.

Animals with signs of thiamine deficiency respond rapidly to IM injection of thiamine hydrochloride (up to 1 mg/kg body wt), followed by oral supplementation. Control usually involves supplemental thiamine at 25 mg/kg food, preferably administered 2 hr before a main feeding.

Vitamin E Deficiency (Steatitis, White Fat Disease): The antioxidant properties of vitamin E are believed to play an important role in maintaining the integrity of cellular membranes. Oxidative processes during the storage of fish destroy vitamin E and other antioxidants. Steatitis has been induced experimentally in phocid seals, and relationships between vitamin E deficiency and hyponatremia are suspected. Captive piscivores commonly are supplemented PO with vitamin E at a rate of as much as 100 mg/kg of feed, which generally maintains high serum levels of the vitamin. This does not appear necessary if feeder fish are properly stored and thawed.

Hyponatremia (Salt Deficiency, Addison Disease): Hyponatremia in pinnipeds is closely related to adrenal exhaustion and development of Addison disease, which links the syndrome to environmental stressors rather than to a simple primary salt deficiency. It is most common in pinnipeds maintained in freshwater exhibits but can be seen in animals kept in saltwater. It is more common in phocid seals but occurs in otarids and other marine mammals. Signs include periodic weakness, anorexia, lethargy, incoordination, tremor, and convulsions. Serum sodium levels can fall to <140 mEq/L. Severely affected animals may collapse in an Addisonian crisis, which can be fatal.

Emergency therapy consists of sodium chloride infusion and replacement corticosteroids. Longterm management of advanced cases requires mineralocorticoid supplementation in conjunction with oral sodium chloride supplements and periodic monitoring of serum sodium levels. Provision of saltwater pools and supplementation of sodium chloride (3 g/kg food) in the diet of captive pinnipeds maintained in freshwater pools should be considered a poor second choice. Animals on salt supplementation should have continuous access to freshwater.

Histamine Toxicity (Scombroid Poisoning, Mackerel Poisoning): Scombroid fish (mackerel, tuna) and other dark-fleshed fish have a short shelf life, even when frozen at low temperatures. A complex of substances, including histamine formed by bacterial decarboxylation of the large amount of histidine found in the flesh of the fish, is responsible for the signs seen in affected marine mammals. The toxicity can also occur with nonscombroid fishes, including poorly handled herring, anchovies, or pilchard. It is most common in pinnipeds but is seen in other marine mammals. Clinical signs include anorexia; lethargy; a red, inflamed mouth or throat; and conjunctivitis and increased lacrimation. Occasionally, vomiting, diarrhea, pruritus, urticaria, or postures indicative of abdominal pain are seen. Antihistamines, including cimetidine, may provide symptomatic relief, but the condition is generally self-limiting, and the animal begins feeding within 2–3 days. In more severe or acute cases, epinephrine is effective in counteracting the histamine reaction. Cortisone and diphenhydramine hydrochloride can be beneficial in the face of respiratory difficulty. Control consists of avoiding scombroid fish in the diet or paying careful attention to their quality, storage, and handling when used.

BACTERIAL DISEASES

Actinomycetes: Nocardiosis (*see* p 666) is commonly reported in debilitated marine mammals. Several species of *Nocardia* have been described from both captive and free-ranging marine mammals of many species, both pinniped and cetacean. Diagnosis is usually postmortem, and most affected animals present with a systemic form of disease. Infections due to *Actinomyces* or *Arcanobacterium* spp are receiving considerable attention and have also have been diagnosed in many marine mammal species. *Arcanobacterium phocae* has been implicated in pathology in stranded California sea lion, common dolphin, gray seal, harbor seal, northern elephant seal, and sea otter. *Arcanobacterium animalium* has been isolated from harbour porpoise, To date, most cases are diagnosed postmortem, but the infection may be underreported.

Brucellosis: Since the 1990s, previously unknown strains of *Brucella* have been found in free-ranging pinnipeds and cetaceans from many countries. Two species have been classified: *B ceti* (cetaceans) and *B pinnipedialis* (seals). There appears to be host preferences.

Pathologic findings include placentitis, orchitis, abortion, mastitis, pneumonia, subcutaneous lesions, arthritis, meningoencephalitis, and hepatic and splenic necrosis. Transmission may be horizontal and vertical.

The bacteria possess the same surface antigens commonly used for diagnosis in livestock. The prevalences of marine mammal brucellosis are not known, but cases appear to be widespread. The role of environmental factors in the emergence of marine mammal disease is unknown.

There is some evidence of potential for zoonotic infections, and there have been a few cases of human infections from marine mammals in those with contact with tissues. In one case, the cultured organism from the blood of a laboratory worker matched a marine mammal strain she was working with. Three other human cases in which marine mammal–associated *Brucella* strains were isolated had no documented contact with marine mammals but histories of eating raw shellfish or fish and contact with raw fish bait.

Clostridial Myositis: Severe myositis due to infections with *Clostridium* spp has been diagnosed in captive killer whales, pilot whales, bottlenose dolphins, California sea lions, and manatees. All marine mammals are probably susceptible. The disease is characterized by acute swelling, muscle necrosis, and accumulations of gas in affected tissues, accompanied by a severe leukocytosis. Untreated, it can be fatal. Diagnosis is based on detection of gram-positive bacilli in aspirates of the lesions and is confirmed by anaerobic culture and identification of the organism. Treatment includes systemic and local antibiotics, surgical drainage of abscessed areas, and flushing with hydrogen peroxide. Commercially available inactivated clostridial bacterins are used routinely in some facilities, although efficacy in marine mammals has not been studied. Botulism has been reported in captive California sea lions during an endemic outbreak of the disease in waterfowl. Affected animals stopped eating and appeared unable to swallow several days before dying.

Pneumonia: The chief cause of death in captive marine mammals (other than polar bears) is believed to be pneumonia. Most cases of marine mammal pneumonia have significant bacterial involvement, and most organisms cultured from terrestrial species have been identified in marine mammals. Pneumonia often can be considered the result of mismanagement, although even in carefully managed captive animals pneumonia-associated mortality is common. Marine mammals require good air quality, including high rates of air exchange at the water surface in indoor facilities. Tempered air or acclimation to cold temperatures is also important to prevent lung disease, even in polar species. Animals acclimated to cold temperatures are usually quite hardy; however, sudden transition from warm environments to cold air, even with warmer water, can precipitate fulminating pneumonias, particularly in nutritionally or otherwise compromised animals. Clinical signs include lethargy, anorexia, severe halitosis, dyspnea, pyrexia, and marked leukocytosis. The disease can progress rapidly. Diagnosis is usually based on clinical signs and confirmed by response to therapy, although bronchoscopy and fine-needle aspirates are being used more extensively to establish the cause of pneumonic disease in marine mammals. Treatment consists of correction of environmental factors and appropriate intensive antibiotic and supportive therapy.

Erysipelas (Diamond Skin Disease): Erysipelas can be a serious infectious disease of captive cetaceans and pinnipeds and has been recognized in wild harbour porpoises, bottlenose dolphins, and harbor seals. The organism, *Erysipelothrix rhusiopathiae*, which causes erysipelas in pigs and other domestic species, is a common contaminant of fish. A septicemic form of the disease in marine mammals can be peracute or acute; affected animals die suddenly either with no prodromal signs or with sudden depression, inappetence, or fever. A cutaneous form that causes typical rhomboidal skin lesions is a more chronic form of the disease. Animals with this form usually recover with timely antibiotic treatment.

Necropsy of peracute cases generally fails to reveal grossly discernible lesions other than widespread petechiation. Diagnosis is based on culture of the organism from the blood, spleen, or body cavities. Arthritis has been found in animals that have died with the chronic form.

Treatment of the peracute and acute forms has rarely been attempted, because the absence of prodromal signs obscures the diagnosis. Animals with the dermatologic form usually recover with administration of penicillins, tetracyclines, or chloramphenicol and supportive treatment.

Control seems primarily related to provision of high-quality fish that is properly stored and handled. Vaccination is controversial, and vaccine breaks can occur. Vials of killed erysipelas bacterin should be cultured for surviving organisms before use in marine mammals. Modified-live bacterins should be avoided for the initial vaccination. Fatal anaphylaxis can occur on revaccination. For this reason, some vaccination programs have been reduced to one-time administration even though antibody titers fall below the presumed effective level.

If cetaceans are to be revaccinated, sensitivity tests should be performed by injecting a small amount of bacterin submucosally on the lower surface of the tongue. Hypersensitive animals develop swelling and redness at the injection site within 30 min. Because the vaccine is extremely irritating, no more than 3–5 mL should be used at any one site, even in nonsensitive mammals. A long needle (≥2 in. [5 cm]) should be used to assure that the vaccine is deposited in the muscle and not between muscle and blubber, or a sterile abscess can result. Bacterin should be administered in the dorsal musculature anterior and lateral to the dorsal fin. Administration posterior to the dorsal fin can result in a severe tissue reaction, immobilizing the animal for several days. To maintain high antibody titers, a booster after 6 mo and annual revaccination are required.

Leptospirosis: This has been diagnosed in otarid pinnipeds and bears. In seals, the disease is characterized by depression, reluctance to move, polydipsia, and pyrexia. It may also cause abortions and neonatal deaths in California sea lions and Northern fur seals. Lesions include a severe, diffuse, interstitial nephritis, with renal tubules packed with spirochetes. The gallbladder may contain inspissated black bile, but hepatitis may not be apparent grossly. Hyperplasia of Kupffer cells, erythrophagocytosis, and hemosiderosis are seen histologically. Gastroenteritis can be a feature. Antibodies to various *Leptospira* serovars (including *L* Canicola, *L* Icterohaemorrhagiae, *L* Autumnalis, and *L* Pomona) have been identified in many species, including sea otters and manatee. Treatment in pinnipeds is similar to that in dogs (*see* p 650). Control in captive animals requires serologic examination of new animals during quarantine. Captive animals can be vaccinated in endemic areas. Leptospirosis is zoonotic, and appropriate precautions should be taken.

Streptothricosis (Dolphin Pseudopox, Cutaneous Dermatophilosis): Streptothricosis, a subcutaneous bacterial infection with *Dermatophilus congolensis*, has been reported in pinnipeds and polar bears. It must be distinguished from sealpox. Simultaneous infections of streptothricosis and pox have been recorded in sea lions. Cutaneous streptothricosis usually manifests as sharply delineated nodules distributed over the entire body and usually progresses to death. Diagnosis is based on demonstration of the organism in biopsies or culture. Treatment with prolonged high dosages of systemic antibiotics can be successful.

Sporothrix schenckii, the cause of a subcutaneous mycosis, has been reported in Pacific white-sided dolphins (*Laegenorhynchus obliquidens*).

Mycobacteriosis: Marine mammals are susceptible to various mycobacteria. Evidence points to mycobacterial disease being possibly endemic in free-ranging otarids off the coast of Australia. Originally thought to be caused by *Mycobacterium bovis*, subsequent molecular assessment places the isolates from free-ranging southern hemisphere pinnipeds in a unique cluster assigned its own species in the *M tuberculosis* complex. Subantarctic fur seals (*Arctocephalus tropicalis*) are thought to be the common link in the spread of *M pinnipedii* to other pinniped species because they cohabit with the other known affected species, Australian sea lions (*Neophoca cinerea*) and New Zealand fur seals (*Arctocephalus forsteri*). Otherwise, mycobacteriosis has been a disease of captivity. Pinnipeds, cetaceans, and sirenians have developed disease due to *M bovis*, *M smegmatis*, *M chitae*, *M fortuitum*, *M chelonae*, and *M marinum*. Cutaneous and systemic forms are seen. There are strong indications that immunosuppression may be involved in development of infections by the atypical mycobacteria.

Intradermal testing with high concentrations of bovine or avian purified protein derivative tuberculin can be used to screen exposed animals; however, anergy occurs and the usefulness is controversial. In pinnipeds, injections in the webbing of the rear flippers should be read at 48 and 72 hr. ELISA screening has identified antibodies in seals but requires further evaluation before it can be considered a screening test. Diagnosis is made by culture and identification of the organism from lesion biopsies, tracheal washes, or feces. Mycobacteriosis in marine mammals is an emerging disease and is possibly of public health significance. (*See also* TUBERCULOSIS AND OTHER MYCOBACTERIAL INFECTIONS, p 687.)

Mycoplasmosis: *Mycoplasma* spp have been isolated from the teeth, wounds, and respiratory tracts of seals. They have been associated with respiratory disease historically but can be found in healthy animals. They are frequently cultured from animals concurrently infected with respiratory viruses.

Miscellaneous Bacterial Diseases: Marine mammals are probably susceptible to the entire range of pathogenic bacteria. *Pasteurella multocida* has caused several outbreaks of hemorrhagic enteritis with depression and abdominal distress, leading to acute death in dolphins and pinnipeds. It has also been reported to cause pneumonia in pinnipeds. In dolphins, *Mannheimia haemolytica* has been incriminated in hemorrhagic tracheitis that responded to chloramphenicol therapy.

Plesiomonas shigelloides has been responsible for gastroenteritis in harbor seals. *Burkholderia pseudomallei* has caused serious fatal outbreaks of disease in various marine mammals in captivity in the Far East. *Salmonella* spp have caused fatal gastroenteritis in manatees and beluga whales. Staphylococcal septicemia has caused the death of a dolphin with osteomyelitis of the spine (pyogenic spondylitis). Another case of intradiscal osteomyelitis, due to *Staphylococcus aureus*, was treated successfully with a prolonged course of cefazolin sodium and cephalexin. *S aureus* also has been incriminated in a fatal pneumonia in a killer whale. *Vibrio* spp infect slow-healing wounds of cetaceans managed in open sea pens.

MYCOTIC DISEASES

Captive marine mammals seem particularly prone to fungal infections (*see* p 632). Most appear to be secondary to stress, environmental compromise, or other infectious disease. Some systemic mycoses have distinct geographic distributions. Diagnosis is based on clinical signs and confirmed by identification of the organism in biopsy or, preferably, culture. Wet mounts in lactophenol or cotton blue may render an immediate diagnosis with some of the morphologically distinct fungi. Tissue smears cleared in warm 10% potassium hydroxide can be examined to identify characteristic fruiting bodies or hyphae.

Topical medication of pinnipeds for dermatophytosis is feasible. Smaller cetaceans can be kept out of water in a sling for 2–24 hr, if areas of the body not being treated are kept moist. Otherwise, systemic therapy is used.

Aspergillosis: Fatal pulmonary aspergillosis has been diagnosed in several species of cetaceans, including bottlenose dolphins and killer whales, and in several pinnipeds, including Antarctic fur seals (*Arctocephalus gazella*), harbor seals, and California sea lions. In addition to disseminated aspergillosis, case reports of aspergillomas of the inner ear have been reported in free-ranging harbour porpoise, and cutaneous aspergillosis has been seen in gray seals (*Halichoerus grypus*) with concomitant mycobacteriosis. The respiratory form has been a postmortem diagnosis. Cutaneous lesions have responded to topical povidone-iodine with ketoconazole therapy (10 mg/kg/day, PO).

Candidiasis: This common mycotic disease in captive cetaceans occurs secondary to stress, unbalanced water disinfection with chlorines, or indiscriminate antibiotic therapy. Candidiasis is also reported in pinnipeds and has been found in cultures of wild cetacean blow holes and stomachs. In clinical disease in cetaceans, the lesions usually are found around body orifices. At necropsy, esophageal ulcers are often found, particularly in the area of the gastroesophageal junction. In phocid pinnipeds, inflammation at the mucocutaneous junctions, particularly at the commissures of the mouth and around the eyes, anus, and vulva, is the common presentation. Diagnosis is based on identification of the yeast in cultures or biopsy. Candidiasis generally responds well to ketoconazole (6 mg/kg/day, PO) along with correction of any environmental deficits. Supplementation with prednisolone (0.01 mg/kg) may be appropriate to compensate for ketoconazole inhibition of glucocorticoid production. Fluconazole (2 mg/kg, bid) has also been used successfully. One anecdotal report suggests a possible toxic reaction to ketoconazole in a northern elephant seal (*Mirounga angustirostris*). Early detection and treatment is usually successful. Another opportunistic yeast, *Cryptococcus neoformans*, has been diagnosed in fatal advanced pulmonary disease in a bottlenose dolphin. Prolonged treatment with itraconazole (120 days) at routine mammalian doses was ineffective despite serum drug levels above the suggested therapeutic range.

Dermatophytosis: Mycotic dermatitis due to *Trichophyton* spp or *Microsporum canis* generally responds to topical povidone-iodine, oral griseofulvin, or both.

Lobomycosis: This disfiguring cutaneous disease is caused by infection with *Lacazia loboi*. The disease has been reported only in people and in Atlantic bottlenose Sotalia (*Sotalia fluviatilis*) dolphins. Culture of the organism has not been possible. Excisional therapy and systemic antifungal drugs have been used with varying success. Zoonotic transmission is strongly suspected in a case of a European handler of an infected dolphin. Most human cases have no history of marine mammal contact. Differential diagnoses include sporotrichosis, chromomycosis, paracoccidiodomycosis, and other fungal diseases characterized by extensive granuloma formation.

Systemic Mycoses: The systemic mycoses of marine mammals are a zoonotic risk, and precautions should be taken to prevent infection when handling dead and diseased animals. Cystofilobasidiales has caused fatal disease in a California sea lion. Blastomycosis has caused fatal disease in bottlenose dolphins, California sea lions, a Stellar sea lion (*Eumetopias jubatus*), Northern fur seals, and polar bears. Fatal systemic histoplasmosis has been reported in a captive harp seal (*Pagophilus groenlandicus*), a bottlenose dolphin, and a Pacific white-sided dolphin. Coccidioidomycosis has been found in bottlenose dolphins, California sea lions, and sea otters. Blastomycosis has been successfully treated with intensive management, including 70 days of itraconazole (3.5 mg/kg/day, PO) combined with antibiotic and supportive therapy when indicated.

Zygomycetes: Dermatologic conditions caused by various *Fusarium* spp have been reported in pygmy sperm whales (*Kogia breviceps*), Atlantic white-sided dolphins (*Laegenorhynchus acutus*), harbor seals, gray seals, California sea lions, and northern elephant seals. Diagnosis is based on culture or organism identification from biopsy. Cases have responded to ketoconazole (5 mg/kg/day for 10 days), fluconazole (0.5 mg/kg, bid for 21 days), or itraconazole (1 mg/kg/day for 120 days).

Mucor spp and *Entomophthora* spp have caused fatal disease in bottlenose dolphins, harbour porpoises, and harp seals. Other zygomycetes have been diagnosed as a cause of fatal disseminated disease in various species of marine mammals. Localized fusariomycosis has been successfully treated in a captive beluga whale (*Delphinapterus leucas*) using voriconazole after surgical debridement. These infections should be considered diseases of debilitated animals; the underlying cause of the low host resistance to these opportunistic infections must be corrected if therapy is to be successful. Amphotericin B has been the therapy of choice for zygomycete infections, but newer imidazoles warrant consideration and may have clinical efficacy despite laboratory tests of resistance.

PARASITIC DISEASES

Marine mammals are susceptible to all of the major groups of parasites, including various nematodes, trematodes, cestodes, mites, lice, and acanthocephalans. Clinical experience with many of these is limited, whereas others are commonly seen in recently captured specimens.

Acanthocephalans: Cetaceans are the primary host of *Bolbosoma* spp but can be infested with parasites of the genus *Corynosoma*, which have pinnipeds and sea otters as primary hosts. *Bolbosoma* spp have been reported in pinnipeds. *C enhydra* has only been reported from sea otters. Diagnosis is by detection of eggs in feces, but clinical disease and therapy are not well documented. Three species of *Profilicollis* (also found in birds) are reported to cause peritonitis associated with intestinal perforation in sea otters. Mortality usually occurs before the parasite produces ova. Premortem diagnosis is problematic. No successful treatment has been reported.

Acariasis: Nasal and lung mites are found in phocid and otarid seals. Lung mites cause rattling coughs. Nasal mites cause nasal discharge but apparently little discomfort. Diagnosis is made by identifying the mite in nasal secretions or sputum. The life cycles of these mites are not completely known. Infections have been cleared rapidly with two injections of ivermectin at 200 mcg/kg, 2 wk apart. Treatment of infected animals eliminates the problem in captive enclosures without environmental treatment.

Mites have been associated with large, roughened lesions of the laryngeal area of cetaceans, but their overall significance or treatment is unknown.

Demodectic mange has been diagnosed in California sea lions. Nonpruritic, alopecic lesions with hyperkeratosis, scaling, and excoriation develop on the flippers and other body surfaces that contact the substrate. Diagnosis is made by deep skin scrapings and identification of the mite. Secondary bacterial infection that results in pyoderma is seen in chronic cases. Treatment is the same as in dogs (*see* p 920). Predisposing factors in pinnipeds are unknown. The mites are not readily transmitted among contact animals.

Heavy infestations of sucking lice are common in wild pinnipeds and can cause severe anemia. The lice can be seen grossly and are readily transmitted. They are highly sensitive to ivermectin as well as to chlorinated hydrocarbon insecticides. Rotenone powder is also effective. The affected animal must be removed from the water, allowed to dry before being dusted, and kept out of the water for ≥12 hr. Treatments must be repeated in 10–12 days. Animals in captivity can be freed of parasites if no new sources of infestation are introduced.

Lungworm: Lungworms are common in all pinnipeds. Sea lions have *Parafilaroides decorus*, whereas true seals are usually parasitized by *Otostrongylus circumlitus*. The latter parasite is also found in the hearts of some phocids; however, it does not produce a microfilaremia. Both of these parasites use fish as intermediate hosts. There are at least four species of lungworms in various cetacean hosts, including *Halocercus lagenorhynchi*, which has caused prenatal infections in Atlantic bottlenose dolphins.

Lungworm infection can be diagnosed by examination of feces or bronchial mucus. Anorexia, coughing, and sometimes blood-flecked mucus are the first signs of pulmonary parasitism. Treatment of *P decorus* infection consists of mucolytic agents administered intratracheally, antibiotics to treat any concomitant bacterial pneumonia, ivermectin, and concurrent prednisone or dexamethasone. Diagnosis of *O circumlitus* in elephant seals is complicated by mortality occurring after generalized clinical signs of depression, dehydration, and neutrophilia before the parasites become patent and first-stage larvae can be detected in sputum or feces.

Some treatment success has been reported using intratracheal administration of levamisole phosphate (5 mg/kg/day for 5 days); however, combined therapy with ivermectin and fenbendazole given 3 days after initiation of therapy with dexamethasone, antibiotics, and mucolytic agents may be more effective. Cetacean lungworms probably are also susceptible to levamisole and ivermectin; however, the sudden deaths of two beluga whales injected IM with levamisole phosphate suggest this drug administered by that route may be contraindicated. A percentage of pinnipeds also show neurologic reactions to IM injection of levamisole; PO or SC administration has been recommended.

Lungworm infections often remain asymptomatic for long periods, with clinical signs appearing only when an animal becomes debilitated for other reasons. In captivity, lungworm infections are usually self-limiting if larvae are not introduced in fresh fish intermediate hosts. Feeding frozen fish prevents reinfection.

Heartworm: Heartworms of the genus *Acanthocheilonema* are a common necropsy finding in pinnipeds. Phocid seals are affected by *A spirocauda*, and otarids are infected subcutaneously by *A odendhali*. Transmission of *A spirocauda* is thought to be by the seal louse (*Echinophthirius horridus*). Both groups of pinnipeds can be infected with the canine heartworm, *Dirofilaria immitis*, in endemic areas; however, phocid seals are abnormal hosts. Dirofilariasis is diagnosed by identifying microfilariae in the blood. Transmission is thought to be by the same mosquitoes that bite dogs. A graded regimen of levamisole phosphate progressing to a high dosage (40 mg/kg/day for 1 wk) has successfully cleared infection in captive pinnipeds, with the advantage of oral administration. Prevention in endemic areas has been successful with oral administration of ivermectin (canine dosages) monthly or diethylcarbamazine (3.3 mg/kg) weekly in food during the mosquito season (*see also* p 127).

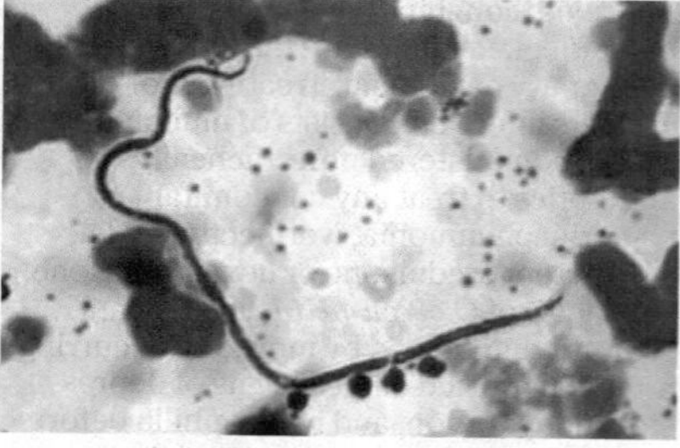

Acanthocheilonema microfilariae. Courtesy of Dr. James McBain.

Other Nematodes: The Anasakidae are pathogenic nematodes found in the stomach of marine mammals. Granulomas form at their attachment sites and can lead to blood loss, ulceration, and ultimately perforation and peritonitis. Raw fish is most often incriminated as the source of infection. Infections with *Contracaecum* spp are common in wild cetaceans and pinnipeds. Polar bears in captivity are prone to heavy ascarid infection. Gastric nematodes can be successfully treated with oral dichlorvos (30 mg/kg), fenbendazole (11 mg/kg), or mebendazole (9 mg/kg) given twice, 10 days apart. Ivermectin may be considered.

Hookworms (*Uncinaria* spp) are found in pinnipeds. Severe infections are known in fur seals. Newborn fur seal pups are infected via colostrum. Disophenol (12.5 mg/kg) or ivermectin (100 mcg/kg) injected SC have been effective against these parasites.

Many species of a large spirurid nematode (*Crassicauda* spp) infect the cranial sinuses, major vessels, kidneys, and mammary gland ducts of cetaceans. Successful treatments are not documented but are potentially possible with systemic parasiticides. The dual intermediate host requirement of these species in captivity usually means these infections are self-limiting.

Cestodiasis: *Diphyllobothrium pacificum* is commonly found in sea lions, and heavy infection is thought to cause intestinal obstruction. Praziquantel (10 mg/kg) is an effective treatment. Other cestodes commonly seen include *D lanceolatum* in phocid seals, *Diplogonoporus tetrapterous* in all pinnipeds, and *Tetrabothrium forsteri* and *Strobilocephalus triangularis* in cetaceans. Cetaceans are also commonly infected with subcutaneous tapeworm cysts throughout the blubber. These usually are the larval forms of tapeworms of sharks. Several species of cestodes are reported in sea otters and polar bears but are not known to have clinical significance.

Trematodiasis: Fluke infections are common in pinnipeds and cetaceans; *Nasitrema* spp are found in the nasal passages and sinuses of cetaceans. Ova of these trematodes have been associated with necrotic foci in the brains of animals showing behavioral aberrations and have been incriminated as a cause of localized pneumonia in cetaceans. Infections are often accompanied by halitosis and brown mucus around the blowhole and occasionally by coughing. Diagnosis is based on demonstration of typical operculated trematode ova in blowhole swabs or feces. Oral praziquantel (10 mg/kg, two treatments 1 wk apart) is usually effective. Reinfection can be prevented by not feeding fresh or live fish.

Zalophotrema hepaticum is an important hepatic trematode of California sea lions; it causes biliary hypertrophy and fibrosis of the liver. Signs are usually seen in adults and include icterus, lethargy, and anorexia. Bilirubinemia and increased serum hepatic enzymes are common. Diagnosis is based on identification of trematode ova in the feces. Treatment with praziquantel (10 mg/kg) or with bithional (20 mg/kg) has been successful.

Various other trematodes infect the stomach, intestines, liver, pancreas, and other abdominal organs of marine mammals. Pancreatic fibrosis due to trematodiasis is a common necropsy finding.

Coccidiosis: Coccidia (*Eimeria phocae*) have been found in harbor seals with a fatal, bloody diarrhea. Clinical disease with this parasite is thought to be rare unless the host is stressed through capture, handling, or husbandry changes. At least two new species of intestinal coccidia have been identified in California sea lions. A coccidian, *Cystoisospora delphini*, has been reported as the cause of enteritis in bottlenose dolphins; however, some consider the parasite to have been a fish coccidia not associated with the disease. *E trichechi* reported from the Amazonian manatee (*Trichechus inunguis*), and *E nodulosa* reported from the Florida manatee, are also not associated with disease. These coccidia are probably susceptible to anticoccidial drugs used against other species, eg, amprolium. (*See also* p 203.)

Sarcocystis: *Sarcocystis neurona* is found in high prevalence in the California population of sea otters. Infection can be asymptomatic or cause severe encephalitis characterized by generalized neurologic signs. No successful treatment of neurologic cases has been reported. *Sarcocystis* spp have been found in the muscles of many cetacean, otarid, and phocid species and are often not associated with any recognized clinical signs. Successful treatment has been reported in an adult California sea lion with myositis using ponazuril (10 mg/kg/day, PO) for 28 days and prednisolone in the first 5 days of therapy.

Toxoplasmosis: *Toxoplasma gondii* is known to infect the California population of sea otters, causing disease that ranges from asymptomatic infection to severe encephalitis. Fatal meningoencephalitis due to *T gondii* has also been reported in a Florida manatee and disseminated disease in Antillean manatees. *Toxoplasma* spp encephalitis is also reported in harbor seals and Northern fur seals. Disseminated toxoplasmosis is reported in California sea lions. *T gondii* is reported from Atlantic bottlenose, Risso's (*Grampus griseus*), striped (*Stenella coeruleoalba*), and spinner dolphins, and serologic evidence of toxoplasmosis is being discovered in an ever-widening array of marine mammal hosts, including polar bears. No successful treatment has been reported. Transplacental transmission has been reported in a Risso's dolphin.

VIRAL DISEASES

Adenovirus: Adenovirus has been isolated from a sei whale (*Balaenoptera borealis*), beluga whale, and bowhead whales (*Balaena mysticetus*). A novel otarine adenovirus 1 has been isolated from California sea lions affected with hepatic disease, and adenovirus particles have been reported in walrus and fur seals. Fatal disease associated with adenovirus infection has been reported in California sea lions, South African fur seals, and South American sea lions. No disease was noted in the cetaceans.

The most prominent histologic lesion in all cases was hepatic necrosis. Massive coagulation necrosis without apparent zonal distribution was seen in some animals. Basophilic intranuclear inclusions in hepatocytes or granular amphophilic intranuclear inclusions in Kupffer cells were seen. No evidence of adenovirus was detected in the lungs. Adenovirus from California sea lions is not known to cause disease in people.

Caliciviruses (San Miguel Sea Lion Virus): Caliciviruses have been isolated from otarid seals, walrus, Atlantic bottlenose dolphins, and opaleye fish

(*Girella nigricans*). The marine caliciviruses appear to be serotypes of vesicular exanthema of swine virus (VESV, *see* p 738). Several species of mysticete cetaceans have antibodies to different serotypes of VESV. By 4 mo of age, most California sea lions have neutralizing antibodies to one or more of the serotypes. Opaleye fish are probably responsible for the endemic status of caliciviruses in marine mammals that inhabit the coastal waters of California. To date, infections have not been diagnosed in marine mammals in the Atlantic Ocean.

The most consistent lesion in marine mammals is skin vesicles. In pinnipeds, the vesicles are most prevalent on the dorsal surfaces of the fore flippers. In dolphins, vesicular lesions have been seen in association with "tattoo" lesions and old scars. Vesicles are 1 mm to 3 cm in diameter. They usually erode and leave shallow, fast-healing ulcers, but occasionally vesicles regress and leave plaque-like lesions. Treatment is supportive only; skin lesions usually resolve without treatment. Infection may cause premature parturition in pinnipeds. Affected pups have interstitial pneumonitis and encephalitis and fail to thrive.

Inoculation of marine caliciviruses into pigs causes vesicular lesions identical to those seen in vesicular exanthema. In people, heavy exposure to marine caliciviruses can result in neutralizing antibodies. Localized lesions in an accidental laboratory exposure as well as isolation of calicivirus from a clinically ill primate indicate that these viruses should be handled carefully.

Herpesvirus: Herpesviruses isolated from pinnipeds include phocid herpesvirus 1 (PhHV-1), an alpha herpesvirus, and four gamma herpesviruses, phocid herpesvirus 2 (PhHV-2), Hawaiian monk seal herpesvirus, Otarid herpesvirus 1, and Northern elephant seal herpesvirus. Herpesviruses have been identified in a wide range of cetaceans, some associated with encephalitis and others with various skin lesions.

Young harbor seals from Atlantic waters infected with PhHV-1 develop nasal discharge, inflammation of the oral mucosa, vomiting, diarrhea, and fever, followed by coughing, pneumonia, anorexia, and lethargy that can result in death in 1–6 days. Morbidity can approach 100% in stressed seals in crowded conditions; mortality is ~50%. The incubation period appears to be 10–14 days. Pacific harbor seals with PhHV-1 tend to develop signs related to adrenal and hepatic dysfunction.

PhHV-2 has been associated with recurring circumscribed areas of alopecia ~0.5 cm in diameter in gray seals. Herpetic lesions in beluga whales are generally circular, as much as 2 cm in diameter, and may appear slightly depressed with a target appearance or be raised and proliferative. The centers of some lesions are necrotic or may contain verrucous growths. Systemic infections have not been documented in the cetaceans.

Diagnosis is often made at necropsy or by clinical signs and observation of characteristic intranuclear inclusion bodies in biopsies of early skin lesions. In seals, interstitial pneumonia caused by herpesvirus must be distinguished from bronchial pneumonia caused by influenza virus.

In systemic herpesvirus infection, therapy is supportive. In a documented epidemic, oral acyclovir did not eliminate the infection but appeared to significantly shorten clinical signs in primary infections. Vaccination with 1 mL of trivalent poliovirus vaccine to control recrudescence of suspected herpesvirus lesions has been used with some success; although it reduced the severity of recrudescence in seals, there is a potential public health risk because live poliovirus may be shed after vaccination. Stress and immunosuppression are associated with recrudescence of latent infections. There is no evidence that the herpesviruses of pinnipeds or cetaceans are zoonotic.

Influenza Virus: Four different influenza A viruses have been isolated from harbor seals and two other subtypes from a stranded pilot whale. H1N1 has been isolated from a northern elephant seal. Serologic evidence of exposure to influenza virus exists for a wide range of marine mammals. Infection is probably common. Only nonspecific clinical signs were reported in the stranded pilot whale, which had difficulty maneuvering, was emaciated, and was sloughing skin. Disease due to influenza virus in seals is better characterized. Even well-fed captive animals become weak, incoordinated, and dyspneic. Swollen necks due to fascial trapping of air escaping through the thoracic inlet is reported. Occasionally, white or bloody nasal discharge is evident. The incubation period during epidemics in harbor seals is ≤3 days. Many factors probably contribute to the explosive nature of the reported epidemics. High population densities and unseasonably warm temperatures contribute to high mortality.

In harbor seals, influenza pneumonia is characterized by necrotizing bronchitis and bronchiolitis and hemorrhagic alveolitis. In the pilot whale, the lungs were hemorrhagic and a hilar node was greatly enlarged. For differential diagnosis, *see* HERPESVIRUS, above.

The virulence of epidemics has precluded attempts at intensive supportive care. People whose eyes were contaminated while doing necropsies, or by being sneezed on by affected seals, have developed keratoconjunctivitis within 2–3 days, and identical virus has been recovered. All affected people have recovered completely within 7 days without developing any antibody titers, which suggests that the reaction is local, as occurs with Newcastle disease virus.

Morbillivirus: Phocid seals are susceptible to canine distemper virus (*see* p 777) and to a closely related but distinct morbillivirus (phocine distemper virus [PDV]). Generally, young seals are affected and show depression, anorexia, crusting conjunctivitis, nasal discharge, and dyspnea. Pneumonia develops, and mortality can be high in previously unexposed animals. Outbreaks in wild harbor seals have been extensive in the North Sea. Seals vaccinated with canine distemper vaccine have been rendered immune to challenge with the virus (suspension of organ material) obtained from dead wild seals.

A delphinoid distemper virus (cetacean morbillivirus [CMV]), closely related to rinderpest (*see* p 771) and peste des petits ruminants (*see* p 766), has been implicated in the deaths of harbour porpoises and common dolphins off the coast of the UK, striped dolphins in the Mediterranean, and bottlenose dolphins in the western Atlantic and Gulf of Mexico. Pilot whale calves, white-beaked dolphins (*Laegenorhynchus albirostris*), harp seals, hooded seals (*Cystophora cristata*), and Mediterranean monk seals (*Monachus monachus*) have been affected by PDV and/or CMV infections. In the wild, harp seals and pilot whales have been incriminated as apparent reservoirs of PDV and CMV, respectively.

Therapy is supportive. Mortality in naive populations is high, often due to secondary infections facilitated by the immunosuppressive impact of active morbillivirus infection. Vaccination with a subunit vaccine is practiced in European rescue centers and appears to be protective, but this approach has not been applied in North America, in large part due to lack of availability of the appropriate vaccine.

Poxvirus: Poxvirus has been identified morphologically in skin lesions of both captive and free-ranging pinnipeds and cetaceans of a wide range of species. Lesions in California sea lions, harbor seals, and gray seals are probably due to parapoxviruses; lesions in South American sea lions (*Otaria byronia*) and Northern fur seals are probably not. An orthopox virus has been isolated from pox-like lesions on a gray seal. Poxvirus has also been associated with skin lesions in Atlantic bottlenose dolphins, Atlantic white-sided dolphins, killer whales, dusky dolphins, long-beaked common dolphins (*Delphinus capensis*), Hector's dolphins (*Cephalorhynchus hectori*), and Burmeister's porpoises (*Phocoena spinipinnis*), among others.

Outbreaks typically occur in postweanling pinnipeds recently introduced into captivity. The incubation period is 3–5 wk. A break in the epithelial surface may be required to start an infection. Lesions can recur. Small, cutaneous, raised nodules (0.5–1 cm in diameter) occur on the head, neck, and flippers of affected pinnipeds. These may increase to 1.5–3 cm in diameter during the first week and may ulcerate or develop satellite lesions during the second week. After the fourth week, lesions begin to regress, although nodules are reported to persist as long as 15–18 wk. Areas of alopecia and scar tissue may remain after resolution.

Cutaneous poxvirus infections in cetaceans can develop on any part of the body, but lesions are most common on the head, pectoral flippers, dorsal fin, and tail fluke. They range from ring or pinhole lesions to black, punctiform, stippled patterns ("tattoo" lesions). Ring or pinhole lesions appear as solitary, 0.5–3 cm, round or elliptical blemishes, which sometimes coalesce. They are usually light gray and may have a dark gray border, although the reverse color pattern is also seen. Lesions may persist for months or years without apparent ill effects.

Major differential diagnoses include cutaneous streptothricosis and calicivirus. Diagnosis is based on the presence of eosinophilic, intracytoplasmic inclusion bodies in lesion biopsies and is confirmed by identification of typical poxvirus particles by electron microscopy.

Poxviruses of marine mammals do not appear to cause systemic infections. Although animals with cutaneous poxvirus lesions have died, other factors were responsible. Therapy to control secondary bacterial infections is indicated only when skin lesions suppurate. The parapoxviruses of pinnipeds can cause isolated lesions on the hands of people not wearing gloves during contact with infected animals.

Miscellaneous Viral Diseases: A ringed seal (*Phoca hispida*) in Norway was diagnosed with rabies, which was confirmed by immunofluorescent examination of the brain. At the time, there was an epidemic of rabies in foxes in the area. Other rhabdoviruses isolated from cetaceans, which are not recognized by antisera to representatives of the *Lyssavirus*, *Ephemerovirus*, or *Vesiculovirus* genera, may be related to rhabdoviruses of fish.

Papillomavirus infections have been reported in a wide range of cetaceans, including narwals (*Monodon monoceros*) and several species of mysticete whale. Lesions are typical of those found in terrestrial species. No therapy is known. Lesions are usually self-limiting.

Hepadnavirus infection with a hepatitis B–like agent has been documented in a Pacific white-sided dolphin with a long history of recurrent illness in captivity. No evidence of zoonotic transmission was identified.

Endogenous gamma retroviruses have been identified in the genome of killer whale, bottlenose dolphin, Atlantic white-sided dolphin, long-finned pilot whale, striped dolphin, short-beaked common dolphin, Risso's dolphin, harbour porpoise, and white-beaked dolphin. The only retrovirus cultured and characterized to date in a marine mammal was a spumavirus isolated from recurring skin lesions in a California sea lion that subsequently died of *Pasteurella* pneumonia complicated with herpesvirus.

Coronavirus infections have been associated with pneumonia epizootics in wild Pacific harbor seals. A coronavirus has also been identified in a beluga whale.

An enterovirus of unknown pathogenicity isolated from a rectal swab of a California gray whale has been reclassified as a calicivirus. Antibodies, unassociated with disease, against human influenza virus (after challenge) and poliomyelitis virus were found in bottlenose dolphins. Enterovirus has been found associated with tongue lesions in bottlenose dolphins.

Severe enteritis and vomiting that rapidly led to death in a captive beluga whale were suggestive of parvovirus enteritis, but no virus was isolated.

NEOPLASTIC DISEASES

Tumors in marine mammals are infrequent, although a wide variety has been reported. They are of little consequence except for malignant lymphoma in harbor seals, in which horizontal transmission can occur in a closed population, and transmissible venereal tumor of California sea lions.

MINK

MANAGEMENT

Mink (*Mustela vison*) are housed individually in raised, wire mesh pens. A nest box with a hole for entry is attached outside or placed within the pen. Wood used for the nest box should not be painted or treated with wood preservatives. Soft, awn-free marsh hay, clean straw, untreated dry wood shavings, or fine wood-wool make suitable nest material. Nest boxes should be cleaned and nest material replaced as required, especially before whelping. Sheds are used throughout the year and should admit natural daylight. There should be plenty of air circulation and shade in the warmer months.

Mink feed may be supplied as a wet gruel placed on top of the wire mesh or as a commercially prepared, dry, pelleted ration placed in feed hoppers. During the weaning and postweaning periods, food is supplied on feeding trays or placed on an adjustable wire nest box cover for small kits that cannot reach the top of the pen. Fresh water should always be available. Watering cups fastened to the outside of the pen with a lip protruding inside are used. Automatic, heated, recirculating watering systems with individual nipples are most commonly used in sheds.

Cold storage facilities are necessary to freeze and store the meat portion of the ration. A day's supply of fish and meat by-products is thawed, commercial cereal and vitamins added, and the combined ration mixed with water to a consistency that will remain on the wire of the pen without dropping through. Ready-mixed feeds may be delivered daily, either ready to feed or in frozen blocks that are thawed as required. Dry pelleted diets are used on some ranches for part or all of the year.

Ranchers usually keep one male for each five female breeders. Mink are seasonal breeders, with reproductive activity controlled by increasing periods of daylight. Artificial lights in the sheds must be used with caution, because they may adversely affect photoperiod and interfere with the normal reproductive cycle. In the northern hemisphere, the breeding season begins in late February or early March and lasts ~4 wk. Mating should occur within 1 hr after the female is placed in the male's pen. If fighting ensues, they should be separated. Ovulation is induced by mating. Females mated before mid-March are usually mated again after 7–8 days, often with an additional mating the following day; thus, individual females may be mated two or three times. Ova from two matings have been known to develop in the same litter. Implantation of the fertilized ova is delayed, so the apparent gestation period is 40–75 days. The implantation period can be altered by using artificial light after breeding.

Mink have one annual litter of 1 to 12 kits (average 5). Most kits are born during the last week in April and the first 2 wk in May. Kits are blind, hairless, and weigh ~10 g when born but grow rapidly throughout the summer to reach a weight of ~1,200 g (females) or 2,600 g (males) by October. Kits are weaned at ~6–8 wk of age and may be separated shortly thereafter and housed in single pens. Adult mink are extremely agile, strong, and vicious. Handling requires the use of special leather gloves or wire catching cages.

Mink kits are vaccinated when at least 6–8 wk old with a 3-way vaccine containing *Pseudomonas* bacterin, botulism, and mink enteritis virus, and again when at least 10 wk old with a modified-live distemper vaccine. Breeders should be revaccinated in December or January before the breeding season.

Pelt collection usually is done in November or December. The most humane way to kill mink is with pure cooled carbon monoxide in cylinders. In the USA, mink farms are certified under the strict criteria for the humane treatment of animals by the Fur Commission USA.

BACTERIAL DISEASES

Botulism: Botulism (*see* p 605) occasionally causes heavy losses in unvaccinated mink that consume feed containing type C toxin. Usually, many mink are found dead within 24 hr of exposure to the toxin, while others show varying degrees of paralysis and dyspnea. Necropsy findings are nonspecific and related to death from respiratory paralysis. Diagnosis is confirmed by inoculation of serum or filtered tissue from affected mink into mice. The immunotype of the botulism toxin is type C in almost all outbreaks.

Toxic feed should be removed and sampled for testing, and stored feed or ingredients tested for the toxin. Recovered mink are not immune to further challenge. Annual vaccination of kits (at 6–8 wk) and breeders with vaccines containing type C botulism toxoid, *Pseudomonas* bacterin, distemper, and mink virus enteritis vaccines is highly recommended.

Hemorrhagic Pneumonia: *Pseudomonas aeruginosa* may result in serious losses. Mink of all ages are affected, particularly during the stress of fall molt. Mink are usually found dead with no prodromal signs. A bloody nasal exudate may be seen at the time of death. Gross lesions include a severe hemorrhagic pneumonia with swelling and consolidation of one or more lung lobes. Treatment involves immediate vaccination of the entire herd. A *Pseudomonas* bacterin is included in the recommended 3-way vaccine (*see* above).

Escherichia coli has become the more common cause of hemorrhagic pneumonia in mink as a result of vaccination against *Pseudomonas*. Gross and clinical signs are indistinguishable from those of *Pseudomonas*. Bacterial culture is the only way to determine which pathogen is present. Exposure to *E coli* most frequently comes from contaminated water, but it may also be feedborne. Underlying viral infections such as influenza, Aleutian disease, and distemper must be excluded. Antibiotic sensitivities are a must to assist with treatment selection, because sensitivity patterns for *E coli* in mink vary greatly.

Urinary Infections and Urolithiasis: Urinary tract infections, commonly called "plum bladders," cause serious losses in females in late spring (during pregnancy and lactation) and in males in late summer and autumn (during the rapid growth and furring period). Several predisposing factors have been suggested, including contamination of food, cages, or nest boxes by pathogenic bacteria; decreased water intake; or increased ash intake.

Mink may die without showing signs, but a large, distended bladder can be palpated grossly, or they may have difficulty in urinating or dribble urine. Occasionally, hematuria may be seen. Necropsy findings include acute hemorrhagic cystitis or pyelonephritis, usually associated with calculi (magnesium ammonium phosphate) in the bladder or kidneys. Various organisms, including staphylococci, coliforms, and *Proteus* sp, have been isolated.

In severe outbreaks, culture and antibiotic sensitivity tests should be done, and medication added to the feed. Good sanitation to reduce environmental contamination and increasing the water supply help prevent the condition. When a continual problem exists (with magnesium ammonium phosphate calculi), feed-grade (75%) phosphoric acid may be added to the feed (0.8 lb/100 lb [8 g/kg] of wet mixed feed), from March to early June and from mid-July to October, to reduce the urine pH. Feed and urine pH should be monitored to keep urine pH at ≤6. Feed pH should not be <5.1.

Mastitis: A variety of bacteria, mainly staphylococci, streptococci, and *Escherichia coli*, are involved in mastitis in mink. Staphylococcal mastitis typically results in abscessation of affected glands or subclinical disease evidenced only by mild diarrhea in the kits. *E coli* causes a peracute, necrotizing mastitis similar to that seen in dairy cattle. Predisposing factors include poor nest box and cage sanitation, rough or sharp edges to the entrance of nestboxes, and high bacterial contamination of feed. Treatment and prevention involve improving management and treating individual animals or the herd with appropriate antibiotics based on sensitivity testing.

Miscellaneous Bacterial Diseases: Various diseases or signs of disease, including septicemia, pneumonia, purulent pleuritis, abortions, abscesses, cellulitis, and enteritis, occur sporadically; occasionally, they may become herd problems. Many bacteria, including *Proteus*, *Klebsiella*, and *Campylobacter* spp, coliforms, streptococci, staphylococci, and salmonellae, have been isolated.

Treatment should be based on antibacterial sensitivity tests. Drugs may be administered parenterally or in the feed or water. Dosage can be estimated on the basis of body wt; female mink weigh ~2–3 lb (0.9–1.4 kg), and males ~5–6 lb (2.3–2.8 kg). Dosages recommended for cats should be used and adjusted for weight. However, some sulfonamides (eg, sulfaquinoxaline and sulfamethazine) and streptomycin should not be used in mink. Trimethoprim/sulfadiazine causes abortions in pregnant female mink.

The source of infection should be determined and eliminated. Enteritis often is caused by contaminated or spoiled feed and dirty nest boxes. Abscesses are often caused by injury from wire or splintered wood in the pens, awns in hay or straw used for bedding, or spicules of bone in the feed. Outbreaks of tularemia, anthrax, brucellosis, tuberculosis, and clostridial infections have been caused by feed contaminated with tissue of animals that have died or are carriers of these infections. Careful selection of feed ingredients and disinfection of equipment and pens are important in prevention and control of many infections. Dead stock should not be used as mink feed.

VIRAL DISEASES

Aleutian Disease (Plasmacytosis): Aleutian disease is a parvovirus infection characterized by poor reproduction, gradual weight loss, oral and GI bleeding, renal failure and uremia, and high mortality. All color phases of mink may be infected, but light color phases genetically derived from the Aleutian color phase are most susceptible. The causative parvovirus is not related to mink viral enteritis (*see* below). Transmission occurs in utero and by direct or indirect contact with infected mink.

After infection, immunoglobulin levels frequently increase markedly. Immunoglobulins are unable to neutralize the virus; immune complexes form and deposit in various tissues, resulting in immune-complex glomerulonephritis and arteritis. Gross pathologic changes include splenomegaly, renal changes (varying from swelling and petechiation to atrophy and pitting), and enlargement of mesenteric lymph nodes. Histologic lesions include plasma cell infiltration in the kidneys, liver, spleen, lymph nodes, and bone marrow; bile duct proliferation; membranous glomerulonephritis; and fibrinoid arteritis. Kits from dams negative for Aleutian disease virus may die from acute interstitial pneumonia.

Aleutian disease is controlled through a test and slaughter program. Positive mink are identified by blood testing for specific antibody by counterimmunoelectrophoresis or lateral flow ELISA. All positive mink should be culled. Mink to be kept for breeding stock should be tested in late fall (before selection of breeding stock and pelting) and in January or February (before breeding). New introductions to the herd should be tested.

Genetic selection of resistant mink using a quantitative ELISA and/or iodine agglutination test is being used to increase survivability and reproduction. These tests identify mink with hypergammaglobulinemia for culling. The quantitative ELISA identifies overall antibody levels to Aleutian virus, allowing mink with lower antibody levels to be selected for breeding.

There is no vaccination or effective treatment. The virus is present in the saliva, urine, feces, and blood of infected mink. Pens should be steam cleaned and dipped in or sprayed with 2% sodium hydroxide. Equipment should be disinfected after handling, vaccinating, or testing mink on infected farms. Raccoons and flies may serve as vectors, and their control is essential.

Distemper: Mink of all ages are susceptible to canine distemper virus (*see* p 777). The incubation period is 9–14 days. The virus may be recovered from infected mink 5 days before clinical signs appear. Recovered mink may continue to shed the virus for several weeks. Transmission may be direct (through contact or aerosol) or indirect.

Clinical signs include nasal and ocular discharge; hyperemia, thickening, and crustiness of the skin on the muzzle, feet, and ventral abdominal wall; neurologic signs (convulsions and "screaming fits"); or a combination of these. Histologic ELISA, immunohistochemistry, or fluorescent antibody examination may reveal intracytoplasmic or intranuclear inclusions or distemper antigen in epithelial cells of the bladder, kidneys, bile ducts, intestine, lungs, trachea, and occasionally brain. Recent outbreaks have required PCR confirmation, because immunohistochemistry testing was negative.

In outbreaks, affected mink should be culled, and the balance of the herd vaccinated as soon as possible. Deaths from neurotropic distemper may occur until 12 wk after vaccination. Kits should be vaccinated prophylactically when 11–12 wk old with a modified-live vaccine. Ordinarily, adults are vaccinated at the same time.

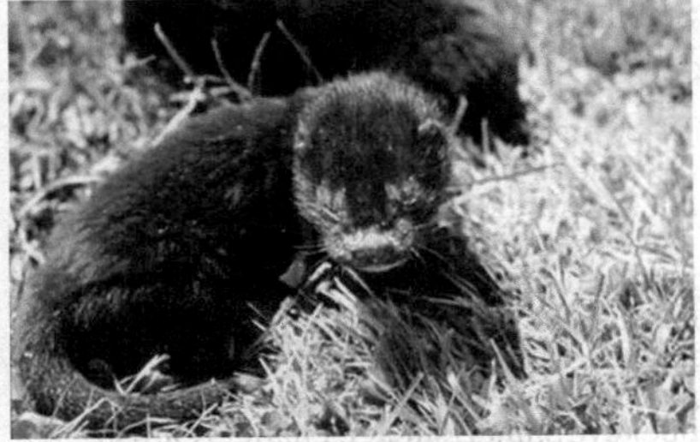

Mink kit showing signs of canine distemper, including heavy nasal and ocular discharge with eyelids that are swollen and sealed shut. *Courtesy of Dr. John Gorham.*

Mink Viral Enteritis: Mink viral enteritis is a highly contagious disease caused by a parvovirus related to, but not identical with, that of feline panleukopenia (*see* p 796). All ages are susceptible, but the disease is most serious in kits. Transmission usually occurs by the fecal/oral route; the incubation period is 4–8 days.

Clinical signs include sudden anorexia; depression; watery, mucoid, blood-tinged diarrhea; dehydration; and death. Characteristic gross lesions include a flaccid, dilated, hyperemic small intestine with liquid fetid contents. Some mink may die suddenly with no gross lesions. Intestinal lesions are characterized by erosion of surface mucosa, blunting and attenuation of villi, and dilation of crypts. Ballooned epithelial cells may contain inclusion bodies similar to those of feline panleukopenia. A fluorescent antibody procedure is used to confirm the diagnosis. Splenic and lymph node lesions include lymphoid depletion and necrosis.

Early in an outbreak, all mink showing signs should be culled or isolated, and all clinically healthy mink should be vaccinated immediately. Affected mink can be treated PO with a mixture of kaolin, pectin, and neomycin. Mink viral enteritis can be prevented by vaccination. All mink should be vaccinated when they reach at least 6–8 wk old with a combination 3-way vaccine containing mink viral enteritis, botulism, and *Pseudomonas*. Annual vaccination is recommended.

Influenza: The first case of influenza was identified in the USA in mink in October 2010. Since then, it has become a frequent cause of disease on mink ranches. Influenza usually presents with coughing and sneezing heard in areas of the ranch. Losses usually increase due to secondary bacterial infections. Influenza has also affected newborn kits, presenting as increased respiration and significant death losses. Exposure to influenza can come from multiple sources. Raw pork, poultry products, and sick employees may all be avenues for virus introduction. Treatment consists of treating secondary infections to mitigate losses. Spread across the ranch usually takes 2–6 wk. After the disease runs its course, >90% of mink have been shown to be antibody positive.

Aujeszky Disease (Pseudorabies): Aujeszky disease occurs occasionally in mink fed pork products contaminated with pseudorabies virus (*see* p 1300). Mortality may be high, and clinical signs are referable to the CNS (tonic and clonic convulsions, excitement alternating with depression, and self-mutilation in some cases). Diagnosis is confirmed by virus isolation or serology. Because contaminated pork is the usual source of infection, all pork products should be cooked before being fed to mink.

Astrovirus (Shaky Mink Syndrome): Astrovirus infection is a self-limiting neurologic disease seen sporadically in mink kits from mid June to mid July. Usually, the condition is limited to one kit per litter, with an incidence of 0.1%–2%. Higher incidence has been reported on a European ranch. Kits have tremors, and histopathology shows meningoencephalitis. Mortality is low and appears to be caused by inability of the mink to eat or drink because of the shaking. Early in the disease, astrovirus can be identified, but later the mink clear the virus and are negative. Lesions and clinical signs do not improve, and euthanasia of affected mink is warranted for welfare concerns.

Epizootic Catarrhal Gastroenteritis: Millions of mink have been affected by an agent (most likely a coronavirus) that causes an acute catarrhal gastroenteritis. The disease usually occurs in adult dark mink. Outbreaks occur most frequently during times of stress, eg, early fall molting, spring mating, and whelping seasons. Clinical signs (mucus in the feces and partial anorexia) rarely last longer than 5–6 days. Death may occur if the affected mink are immunosuppressed by Aleutian disease virus. There are no commercially available vaccines. Treatment is symptomatic and of questionable value. It is important to differentiate this condition from mink viral enteritis.

PRION DISEASE

Transmissible Mink Encephalopathy: This progressive neurologic disease of mink is rare, but mortality may reach 60%–90% of the ranch population. The incubation period is 8–12 mo. Mink usually bite compulsively, are incoordinated and somnolent, scatter feces in the pen, and flip their tails up over their backs (like squirrels). Histologic lesions of the brain are spongiform changes of the gray matter, astrocytosis, and neuronal vacuolation. The demonstration of disease-specific prion protein in nervous tissues aids in the diagnosis. Although the means of transmission is unknown, "downer" cattle are suspected to be the source of the agent. There are no vaccines or treatment.

NUTRITIONAL DISEASES

Steatitis or myositis (yellow fat disease, *see* p 1200) occurs in young, rapidly growing mink as a result of excessive, rancid, unsaturated fatty acids and a deficiency of vitamin E in the diet. Affected mink may be found dead, or they may exhibit slight locomotor disturbances followed by death. Necropsy findings include yellow, edematous internal or subcutaneous fat that contains an acid-fast pigment. It is more common to find myoglobinuria and dark red bladders (resembling plum bladder). Histopathology shows myositis and cardiomyopathy. Hepatic vitamin E levels <15 mcg/g can lead to acute death. Control consists of removal of the source of the rancid fats and polyunsaturated oils and proper storage of feed. Stabilized vitamin E may be administered in the feed (15 mg/mink) for 4 wk, and affected kits should be injected parenterally with 10–20 mg of vitamin E for several days. Feeding a nutritionally sound diet with added vitamin E is preventive.

Chastek paralysis (thiamine deficiency) results from feeding certain raw fish that contain the enzyme thiaminase. These include whitefish, freshwater smelt, carp, goldfish, creek chub, fathead minnow, buckeye shiner, sucker, channel catfish, bullhead, minnow, white bass, sauger pike, burbot, and saltwater herring. Affected mink gradually become anorectic, lose weight, and die after terminal convulsions and paralysis. Fish that contain high levels of thiaminase should be thoroughly cooked at 181°F (83°C) for ≥5 min, or fed raw as a portion of the diet only on alternate days. Mink injected with thiamine hydrochloride, 50 mg, SC, recover rapidly. Adequate thiamine (brewer's yeast) should be included in the ration.

Rickets occurs due to the rapid growth rate of kits when rations are deficient in vitamin D, calcium, or phosphorus. Affected kits usually crawl unsteadily in a frog-like posture, have rubbery bones, and are smaller than normal. The diet should be supplemented as required, and severely affected kits may be treated individually. (*See also* p 1051.)

Nursing disease is a metabolic disease that affects lactating mink ~40 days after whelping. It is characterized by rapid dehydration, serum electrolyte imbalances, renal shutdown, and death. Treatment can be successful if affected females are identified as soon as they begin refusing feed and rehydrated with IP or SC sterile fluids. The disease is multifactorial; although there appears to be a genetic predisposition in certain light color mutations, it is more severe in females with large litters and during hot weather. Often, affected females have concurrent subclinical mastitis. Adequate water, environmental cooling systems, fostering kits from large litters to make litter size more manageable for the female, and early weaning help prevent this condition.

Cotton underfur usually indicates anemia and may be caused by feeding certain fish (Pacific hake, coalfish, whiting) that interfere with iron metabolism in mink, which affects melanin pigment formation. Thoroughly cooking the offending fish at 181°F (83°C) for ≥5 min or feeding it on alternate days prevents the condition.

Biotin deficiency, which can cause gray underfur and loss of guard hair, is seen when high levels of uncooked eggs, particularly turkey eggs, are fed. Avidin, a factor present in eggs, inactivates biotin, a vitamin required for pigmentation and hair growth. Affected mink may be injected with 1 mg biotin twice weekly for 4 wk, and biotin may be added to the ration. Biotin deficiency can be prevented by cooking eggs at 196°F (91°C) for 5 min.

POISONING

Lead poisoning (*see* p 3078) may be seen in mink that have ingested lead-containing paint from wire or other equipment. Affected mink gradually lose weight and die within 1–2 mo with clinical signs consistent with either gastroenteritis or CNS disturbance. Individual mink may be treated with calcium edetate as a chelating agent. All sources of lead should be removed.

Insecticides other than pyrethrum, piperonyl butoxide, and rotenone may be highly toxic to mink. Even these insecticides should not be used on mink <8 wk old, or where such mink can contact them (eg, nest boxes). Other insecticides should be avoided whenever possible. (*See also* p 3058.)

Wood preservatives (chlorinated phenols, cresols) can cause death of kits in the first 3 wk of life and occasionally of older mink. They should not be used where mink can chew on treated wood (pens, nest boxes, or nest litter). Shavings used as nest-box litter should not contain wood preservatives.

Diethylstilbestrol causes reproductive failure and a high incidence of urinary tract infections in mink and should not be included in the ration. Similarly, thyroid and parathyroid glands included in meat trimmings fed to mink may result in reproductive failure if present at high levels.

Chlorinated hydrocarbons and **polychlorinated biphenyls** contained in the ration can cause reproductive failure. Mink appear to be exquisitely sensitive to **polybrominated biphenyls**; 1 ppm in the ration has caused litter size and offspring viability to decrease. (*See also* p 3056.)

Dimethylnitrosamine (DMNA) is hepatotoxic in mink. In the past, addition of sodium nitrate as a preservative to herring meal resulted in formation of DMNA, which causes hepatic degeneration, ascites, and extensive internal hemorrhage.

Sulfaquinoxaline upsets normal blood-clotting mechanisms of mink and causes extensive internal hemorrhage. **Streptomycin** is toxic to mink.

Salt toxicity is seen in young kits starting on solid food. Affected kits become dehydrated and show CNS signs such as tremors or seizures. The most common cause is increased salt levels in feedstuffs. By-product from the cheese, poultry, fish, and processed sandwich meat industries contain higher than expected salt concentrations. Prevention is accomplished by testing feed and ingredients for salt levels and removing ingredients with high salt concentrations and supplemental salt.

MISCELLANEOUS DISEASES

Fur clipping and **tail biting** are common in mink and may be caused by captivity. Fur clipping decreases the value of the pelt, and tail biting frequently results in fatal hemorrhage. There is no effective treatment. All mink demonstrating these behaviors should be culled.

Urinary incontinence (wet belly disease) is a nonfatal condition that usually affects obese males in the late summer and autumn. It is characterized by dribbling of urine and staining of the pelt around the urinary orifice. Because affected areas of the pelt must be discarded, the condition is of economic importance. The cause is unknown, but genetic strain, high dietary fat level, and obesity appear to have the greatest influence on incidence. Affected mink should have an ample water supply.

Starvation and **chilling** cause death in mink fed inadequate fat or provided with too little feed during the winter and early spring. Affected mink are thin and may run until they collapse and die, or they may be found dead in their cages. Such deaths usually occur after the environmental temperature decreases suddenly, especially in the early spring when mink are being brought into breeding condition. Necropsy reveals emaciation and an absence of body fat, in some cases accompanied by hepatic lipidosis and gastric ulceration. This results from improper management and must be differentiated from infectious diseases.

Gray diarrhea in mink clinically resembles chronic pancreatic necrosis in dogs and is characterized by a ravenous appetite and passage of large amounts of gray, fetid feces. Affected mink appear to die of starvation. No pancreatic abnormalities, viruses, bacteria, or parasites have been demonstrated to be causes. Treatment is of questionable value.

Gastric ulcers and **hepatic and renal lipidosis** are common in mink and usually are associated with high levels of dietary fat or with other diseases or stresses that result in several days of inappetence (eg, during late gestation, the period of weaning kits, or the fall period of furring up). Renal lipidosis is commonly seen in mink implanted with melatonin. Treatment involves B vitamins (either feeding or via injection) and increasing the protein quality of the feed.

Hereditary diseases such as hydrocephalus, hairlessness, "screw neck," "bobbed tails," Ehlers-Danlos syndrome, hemivertebrae, and tyrosinemia occur occasionally. Culling the sire, dam, and littermates of affected mink is necessary for control.

Coccidiosis (*see* p 203) occasionally causes losses in young mink. Affected mink have diarrhea, blood-tinged feces, dehydration, and weight loss. Coccidiostats may be used to control outbreaks. Coccidiosis can be prevented through good sanitation and regular manure removal.

Myiasis develops in mink when flies of *Wohlfahrtia* spp lay maggots directly on the skin of kits. The larvae penetrate the skin and produce inflammation and lesions that resemble abscesses. Affected kits become restless, lose condition, and may die. Malathion dust (5%) placed beneath the litter in the nest boxes beginning a few days before the flies appear may help prevent infestation. It should not be used before whelping or until the kits are 1 wk old. Treatment may be repeated once after a 2-wk interval. (*See also* CUTEREBRA INFESTATION IN SMALL ANIMALS, p 879.)

NONHUMAN PRIMATES

This overview presents a working knowledge of the common families of nonhuman primates maintained in captivity. More species than ever are now promulgated and maintained in captivity, and many are kept in private facilities. Prosimians such as *Lemur catta* (ring-tailed lemur) and New World monkeys such as *Cebus albifrons* (white-fronted capuchin) are commonly encountered in practice. The nonhuman primate species most widely used in research are the macaques, *Macaca mulatta* (rhesus monkey), *M fascicularis* (cynomolgus monkey), and *M nemestrina* (pig-tailed monkey); some African species, primarily *Chlorocebus aethiops* (African green monkey, vervet) and *Papio* spp (baboons); and some of South American origin, *Saimiri sciureus* (squirrel monkey) and *Aotus trivirgatus* (owl monkey). *Saguinus* spp (marmosets) and *Callithrix* spp (tamarins, marmosets), also of South American origin, have had more limited use in research but are common in the pet trade.

Increased restrictions on exportation or reduced availability of nonhuman primates from countries of origin have led to decreased importation. Importation of nonhuman primates into the USA is prohibited except for scientific, educational, and exhibition purposes.

Nonhuman primates are natural hosts for a variety of infectious agents, many of which are zoonoses, and are also susceptible to many human infectious diseases, such as measles and tuberculosis. Consequently, newly acquired nonhuman primates should be quarantined for 1–3 mo before research use or introduction into established colonies, to permit adequate evaluation of their health status and to allow adaptation to the laboratory environment. The basic principle of quarantine is to completely isolate each group of animals and not mix animals from different shipments or sources without restarting the quarantine period. Nonhuman primates imported into the USA must undergo a 31-day minimum primary import quarantine in a facility registered with the CDC. Imported animals that die or become severely ill and require euthanasia during this quarantine period must be necropsied and the deaths reported to the CDC, Division of Quarantine. In clinical practice, any new nonhuman primate should be tested for tuberculosis, and a routine fecal examination and trichrome stain should be done. Depending on the species, routine tests such as those for cytomegalovirus, herpes simiae, and herpes simplex (1, 2, etc) also can be run at this time. Many of the nonhuman primates seen in clinical practice are infants and are immunocompromised; they are highly susceptible to common cold and influenza viruses as well as streptococcal infections and should be isolated from people with upper respiratory signs.

For nonhuman primate therapeutics, *see* TABLE 13.

TABLE 13 NONHUMAN PRIMATE THERAPEUTICS[a]

ANTIBIOTICS	
Amoxicillin	11 mg/kg/day, IM or SC; 11 mg/kg, PO, bid; 62.5 mg, PO, bid (lemurs)
Metronidazole	25–50 mg/kg, PO, bid for 10 days (gastroenteritis and inflammatory bowel disease)
Azithromycin	40 mg/kg, PO, once, then 20 mg/kg/day, PO, for 5 days
Cefazolin	25 mg/kg, IM or IV, bid for 10 days
Ceftriaxone	50–100 mg/kg, IM or IV, bid
Doxycycline	2.5 mg/kg, PO, bid for one day, then 2.5 mg/kg/day, PO
Minocycline	2–15 mg/kg/day, PO
Enrofloxacin	5 mg/kg, IM or PO, once to twice daily for 10 days
Erythromycin	30–50 mg/kg, IM or PO, bid-tid
Gentamicin	3–5 mg/kg, IM or IV, bid for 5-7 days
Penicillin G potassium + penicillin G benzathine	20,000–60,000 U/kg, IM, once to twice daily (higher dosage in lemurs)
Trimethoprim-sulfamethoxazole	15–50 mg/kg, PO or IM, bid; sulfamethoxazole at 20 mg/kg, PO, bid (higher dosages for lemurs)
PARASITICIDES	
Fenbendazole	50 mg/kg/day, PO, for 5 days, repeated in 2 wk
Ivermectin	200–300 mcg/kg, SC, IM, or PO, repeated in 14 days
Mebendazole	22 mg/kg/day, PO, for 3 days, repeated in 14 days (for *Giardia* sp)
Metronidazole	30–50 mg/kg, PO, bid for 5–10 days

TABLE 13 NONHUMAN PRIMATE THERAPEUTICS[a] *(continued)*

Praziquantel	5 mg/kg, IM, PO, or SC, once (15–20 mg/kg, PO or IM, for some cestodes; 40 mg/kg, PO or IM, for trematodes)
Thiabendazole	100 mg/kg, PO, once, repeated in 14 days (owl monkeys); 50 mg/kg/day, PO, for 2 days (*Strongyloides*); 75–100 mg/kg/day, PO, for 10 days (*Entamoeba, Balantidium*) in great apes
ANESTHETICS AND ANALGESICS	
Ketamine hydrochloride	10–15 mg/kg, IM, for restraint only; ketamine (15 mg/kg) with diazepam (1 mg/kg), IM, or ketamine (8 mg/kg) with midazolam (0.2–1 mg/kg), IM, for additional muscle relaxation
Ketoprofen	2 mg/kg/day, IV or IM
Inhalant gas (isoflurane, halothane)	1%–2%; maintenance of surgical plane of anesthesia
Flunixin meglumine (analgesic)	0.5–2 mg/kg, IV, IM, or SC, bid
Buprenorphine	0.005–0.01 mg/kg, SC, IM, or IV, bid-qid (great apes) 0.015–0.02 mg/kg, IM, SC, tid-qid (New World primates)
Butorphanol tartrate	0.02 mg/kg, SC, qid (New World primates); 0.02 mg/kg (not to exceed 0.3 mg total), IM (chimpanzees); may cause profound respiratory depression
Dexmedetomidine	40 mcg/kg, IM, for anesthesia in combination with ketamine at 20–30 mcg/kg, IM (lemurs) or at 2–6 mg/kg, IM (macaques and baboons)
Midazolam	0.05–0.1 mg/kg, IV (slow) or IM: 0.1–0.5 mg/kg, IM (with ketamine helps prevent seizures in lemurs); 5 mg/animal, IM (chimpanzees)
Oxymorphone (opioid analgesic)	0.025–0.075 mg/kg, IM or IV, every 4–6 hr (New World primates); 0.15 mg/kg, SC, IM, or IV, every 4–6 hr (Old World primates); 1–1.5 mg/animal, SC or IM, every 4 hr (chimpanzees)
Propofol	2.5–5 mg/kg, IV bolus induction, 0.3–0.4 mg/kg/min constant-rate infusion (baboons and macaques); 7–8 mg/kg, IV bolus (marmosets, larger nonhuman primates); 1–2 mg/kg, IV bolus (chimpanzees), followed by infusion to effect; oxygen support always available
Tiletamine-zolazepam	3–5 mg/kg, IM, for restraint only (great apes), severe ataxia noted during recovery: 1–2.5 mg/kg, IM (New World primates); 1.5–3 mg/kg, IM (macaques)

[a] All are extra-label uses.

BACTERIAL DISEASES

Gastrointestinal Diseases: The bacteria most commonly associated with GI disease in nonhuman primates are *Campylobacter jejuni* and *Shigella* spp. Occasionally, enterotoxigenic *Escherichia coli, Pseudomonas aeruginosa, Yersinia* spp, *Lawsonia intracellularis, Salmonella* spp, *Aerobacter aerogenes*, and *Aerobacter hydrophila* are implicated. Nonhuman primates may be intermittent, asymptomatic carriers of any of these organisms. *Helicobacter* spp have been implicated as a cause of gastritis, anorexia, and vomiting.

GI diseases may be major problems in captive nonhuman primates. Clinical signs include watery or mucoid, blood-tinged feces, rapid dehydration, emaciation, and prostration. Smaller primates will dehydrate and become hypoglycemic very rapidly. In many privately owned nonhuman primates, dietary indiscretion is common, and the owner should be asked about irregular feeding habits. Rectal prolapse is an occasional sequela. Helminths or pathogenic protozoa may be a complicating factor. Fecal assays and trichrome stains should be done, and appropriate anthelmintics administered. Mortality can be extremely high in acute outbreaks unless treatment is instituted promptly to restore and maintain normal fluid and electrolyte balance. The most common lesions at necropsy are hemorrhagic enteritis, enterocolitis, colonic ulcers, or simply colitis.

Severe clinical signs and death are generally due to dehydration, hypokalemia, and metabolic acidosis. Hydration should be restored and maintained with parenteral electrolyte solutions. Although medications may often be easily administered parenterally, potassium, B vitamins, electrolytes, bismuth subsalicylate, and antibacterial agents can be administered PO or by nasogastric tube in most nonhuman primates. Culture and identification of the infecting organisms and assessment of antibiotic sensitivity may be needed for effective therapy. Metronidazole at 25–50 mg/kg, PO, bid, may be instituted until culture results are obtained. Enrofloxacin (5 mg/kg/day) or the combination of trimethoprim (4 mg/kg) and sulfamethoxazole (20 mg/kg), administered as a total daily oral dosage for 10 days, is useful to treat shigellosis. Azithromycin (30–50 mg/kg, IM, bid for 7–14 days) is recommended to treat *Campylobacter*-associated diarrhea.

Pneumonia: Upper respiratory diseases of bacterial origin can cause widespread illness, and bacterial pneumonia is associated with increased mortality, particularly in newly imported or immature nonhuman primates. Causative agents include *Streptococcus pneumoniae*, *Klebsiella pneumoniae*, *Bordetella bronchiseptica*, *Haemophilus influenzae*, and various species of streptococci, staphylococci, and pasteurellae. Both New World and Old World infant primates are highly susceptible to cross-species transfer from people. Many times, caretakers have had a history of an upper respiratory infection, so adequate history on presentation is important. Infants that are handreared frequently present with aspiration pneumonia from bottle feeding, and appropriate cultures and radiographs will be needed.

Pneumonia may accompany or follow other primary diseases (eg, dysentery or respiratory viral infection). Clinical signs may include coughing, sneezing, dyspnea, mucoid or mucopurulent nasal discharge, pyrexia, lethargy, anorexia, and weight loss. The principal lesions seen at necropsy are those of bronchopneumonia or lobar pneumonia. Empiric antibiotic therapy with azithromycin, trimethoprim/sulfamethoxazole, penicillin, or cephalosporin (either of the latter two in combination with an aminoglycoside) generally is indicated. Cultures from pharyngeal swabs or transtracheal lavage are useful to isolate the causative agent and determine the specific antibiotic sensitivity. Intensive nursing and other supportive therapy, such as fluid and oxygen administration, may also aid recovery in select cases.

Tuberculosis: All nonhuman primates are susceptible to tuberculosis, although major differences exist in the prevalence of cases in different species. Most cases of tuberculosis in nonhuman primates have been reported in Old World primate species such as rhesus monkeys. Reports in New World species such as squirrel monkeys are much less frequent. The incidence of tuberculosis is <1% among quarantined Old World primates, but 45% of cases (especially cynomolgus monkeys) may not be diagnosed until after the first 30 days of quarantine. Clinical signs are not a reliable indication of the severity of tuberculosis in monkeys. A monkey that appears healthy may have extensive miliary disease involving thoracic and abdominal organs; signs of debilitation may appear only shortly before death. However, advanced tuberculosis should be suspected in animals that cough; lose appetite or weight; and/or have enlarged or draining lymph nodes, skin wounds that fail to heal, or abdominal masses. A testing program is mandatory; a tuberculin skin test (intradermal tuberculin skin test), using mammalian old tuberculin (MOT) is the only USDA-approved tuberculin test for nonhuman primates and is the primary diagnostic method for routine surveillance. Intradermal injection of 0.1 mL of MOT using a 26-gauge needle in the palpebrae is an approved USDA method; 0.5 mL may be used in marmosets and tamarins. The injection sites are observed at 24, 48, and 72 hr after injection. Grading systems can be found in the Guidelines for the Prevention and Control of Tuberculosis in Nonhuman Primates on the National Institutes of Health Web site. If palpebral swelling is present with a lid droop, this may be interpreted as positive. Tuberculin tests should be done on all nonhuman primates on arrival at the facility and at 2-wk intervals thereafter until at least three consecutive negative tests have been recorded for the entire group. The last test should be administered within 14 days of the release from quarantine and introduction into an established colony.

The time from initial infection to skin-test conversion depends on the route of exposure, the infecting inoculum, and the strain of organism, but usually occurs within 3–4 wk in rhesus monkeys. Late in the disease, anergy can result in a negative skin test. Anergy may also be induced by concurrent viral infection, such as measles, or immunosuppressive disease. Infected nonhuman primates may also develop latent tuberculosis. These animals appear healthy, are not infectious, and are often skin-test negative. Latent tuberculosis may be reactivated in response to environmental stressors or other immune modulation, leading to active disease and potential transmission.

After their release from quarantine, all nonhuman primates should be skin-tested at least semiannually, and quarterly testing is recommended for research animals. Captive animals in private settings and New World primates may be tested annually. Radiographic examination of the chest may aid diagnosis in well-established cases but is unreliable because lesions rarely calcify or cavitate as they do in people. Additional diagnostic tests, such as culture, PCR, and staining of a gastric lavage or transtracheal wash sample, ELISA, and comparative abdominal skin testing with avian and atypical tuberculins, may aid in diagnosis. Biopsies of positive or suspicious abdominal tests may be useful in identifying true delayed-type hypersensitivity reactions. Because of the public health risk, euthanasia is recommended for all positive reactors. Tuberculosis should then be confirmed at necropsy. When a positive case is identified, the entire group of exposed nonhuman primates in a maintenance colony should be quarantined, and skin testing at 2-wk intervals implemented. Privately owned animals should be quarantined away from small children and untrained personnel. For animals in quarantine, the period should be restarted and testing should be continued. All personnel working with any nonhuman primates or in primate facilities should have regular skin tests.

MYCOTIC DISEASES

See also FUNGAL INFECTIONS, p 632.

Microsporum spp and *Trichophyton* spp rarely infect institutional nonhuman primates. In clinical practice with privately owned nonhuman primates, it is more common. Topical treatment of ringworm with undecylenic acid ointment or 1% tolnaftate cream, bid for 2–3 wk, may help, but nonhuman primates often orally remove any topical medications, making treatment ineffective. Administration of griseofulvin at 25 mg/kg/day, PO; ketoconazole at 5–10 mg/kg, PO, bid for 30 days; or fluconazole at 2–3 mg/kg/day, PO, for 30 days is also very effective. *Candida* spp are common saprophytes of the skin, GI tract, and reproductive tract; they act as facultative pathogens in debilitated nonhuman primates. Ulcers or white, raised plaques may be seen on the tongue or mouth; the fungus may also attack fingernails. Oral lesions must be differentiated from those of trauma, monkeypox, or herpesvirus infections. A topical cream containing nystatin is effective in superficial infections. Oral nystatin (200,000 U, qid, continued for 48 hr after clinical recovery) is effective for candidiasis of the GI tract. *Dermatophilus congolensis* infection has been reported in owl monkeys. Papillomatous lesions are seen on the face and extremities. The infection is transmissible to people. Aspergillosis may develop in various nonhuman primate species, and the organism usually is a facultative pathogen in immunocompromised hosts. Treatment with voriconazole or terbinafine is empirical. In endemic regions of the western and southwestern USA, *Coccidioides immitis* has been associated with fungal pneumonia and disseminated mycosis ("valley fever") in monkeys and apes after exposure to airborne spores of this soil fungus.

PARASITIC DISEASES

Newly imported nonhuman primates harbor numerous parasites. Some are commensal; others can be made self-limiting by strict sanitation and good husbandry. However, some can cause serious diseases or debilitation and should be removed by specific treatment. Captive-raised New World primates housed indoors (ie, with their caretakers) are rarely found to have intestinal parasites; however, this may not be the case when they associate with sandboxes and various outdoor enclosures. Fecal examinations should be part of the routine clinical annual examination.

Arthropods: Pulmonary acariasis (*Pneumonyssus* spp) is common in wild-caught Asian and African primates, particularly rhesus monkeys and baboons.

Infection is rare in laboratory-raised or captive, privately raised nonhuman primates. The life cycle of *Pneumonyssus* spp is not well understood. Infestations usually do not produce serious symptomatic disease, although they may cause sneezing and coughing. Lesions include dilation and focal chronic inflammation of terminal bronchioles. The gross lesions may occasionally be confused with tuberculous granulomas. Ivermectin (200 mcg/kg, SC, PO, IM, repeated in 14 days) has been used for treatment in closed breeding colonies.

Mange mites (*Psorergates* spp, *Sarcoptes scabiei*) or sucking lice (*Pedicinus obtusus*) are seen occasionally, particularly in feral animals, and may produce dermatoses. Systemic treatment with ivermectin, 200 mcg/kg, PO, SC, IM, repeated every 3 wk, or topical treatment with pyrethrin, repeated after 3 days if necessary, is recommended. Use of more toxic topical parasiticides should be avoided because of the possibility of ingestion during grooming. Fleas are commonly seen in New World primates that are associated with dogs or cats in the environment. Premise control measures must be instituted, and baths with a pyrethrin-based shampoo will temporarily remove fleas from the animal's haircoat.

Helminths: *Oesophagostomum* may cause characteristic granulomatous nodules in the large bowel associated with development of the worms and with an immune reaction of the host. The nodules may rupture and cause peritonitis. *Strongyloides* and *Trichostrongylus* are invasive—adults may cause enteritis and diarrhea, larvae may cause pulmonary lesions during migration. These helminths, as well as *Trichuris*, can be treated effectively with thiabendazole at 100 mg/kg, administered PO at intervals of 2–4 wk; ivermectin at 200 mcg/kg, SC, repeated in 14 days; or febendazole at 50 mg/kg/day, PO, for 3 days and repeated in 14 days. The effectiveness of anthelmintic treatment is enhanced by aggressive environmental hygiene practices. *Prosthenorchis* is an acanthocephalan, common in Central and South American nonhuman primates, that burrows into the mucosa of the ileocecal junction and sometimes perforates the bowel or causes obstruction when present in large numbers. Cockroaches are intermediate hosts, and their elimination, along with strict sanitation, is essential for control of infection. *Dipetalonema* and *Tetrapetalonema* are filarid worms found in the peritoneal cavity of New World species; large numbers may be present with very limited host reaction. Lungworms such as *Filaroides* are commonly found in many South American monkeys.

Cestodes: *Bertiella studeri* and other enteric cestodes may be found in animals of feral origin and are treated effectively with praziquantel (5 mg/kg, IM, PO, or SC, once). For some cestodes, 15–20 mg/kg, PO or IM, once, will be needed. Somatic larval (cystic) cestodiasis has been reported. Flukes may cause respiratory, GI, and hematologic signs. *Schistosoma* sp is a blood fluke, whereas *Fasciola* sp infect the liver and may cause hepatic disease and abscessation (more common in Old World primates). The intermediate hosts are snails and crustaceans, which are ingested through contaminated water or food. This is of zoonotic concern. Praziquantel at 40 mg/kg, PO or IM, in a single dose has been effective.

Protozoa: Nonhuman primates may serve as hosts of various intestinal amebae. *Entamoeba histolytica* is the principal pathogenic form in nonhuman primates (as in people). It has only rarely been reported as pathogenic in monkeys, mostly in South American spider and woolly monkeys. However, it can be a serious infection in marmosets and has caused serious enteritis in great apes. In a heavy infection, it may cause severe enteritis and diarrhea, and cysts may be demonstrated in the feces in large numbers. The fecal trichrome stain is a useful tool to diagnose these types of infections, which are often overlooked in a direct or flotation fecal examination. *Giardia* inhabit the upper small intestine and may cause watery diarrhea. Treatment with metronidazole (50 mg/kg/day, PO, for 5–10 days) is recommended. *Cryptosporidium parvum* may also cause diarrhea in nonhuman primates, mainly in young animals. Successful treatment in marmosets with paromomycin has been reported. This infection is usually self-limiting in immunocompetent hosts.

Blood parasites, such as *Plasmodium*, *Leishmania*, and *Trypanosoma* spp, are also found. Generally, there is an equilibrium between the parasite and the natural host, with infections rarely causing overt clinical disease. Transmission of simian malarias to people, although rare, has occurred in areas where the appropriate mosquito vectors are present. Some nonhuman primate species (eg, owl monkeys) are excellent models for malarial research.

Naturally occurring toxoplasmosis (*Toxoplasma gondii*) has been reported in Central and South American primates. Clinical signs of infection tend to be nonspecific (lethargy, anorexia, diarrhea). Hepatic focal necrosis and fibrinous pneumonia with edema are common histologic findings. *Toxoplasma* can be demonstrated in blood smears in acute cases. (*See also* p 685.)

VIRAL DISEASES

A number of herpesviruses affect nonhuman primates; many exist as latent or subclinical infections in reservoir hosts but cause severe disease or death when transmitted naturally to other hosts. All macaques are considered to be potential shedders of Cercopithecine herpesvirus type 1 (Herpesvirus simiae, B virus). The infection is generally subclinical or mild (conjunctivitis or oral vesicles) in *Macaca* spp but usually causes a fatal encephalitis and encephalomyelitis in people. Transmission may occur via a bite, scratch, or contamination of a superficial wound or mucous membranes (eg, conjunctiva) with infectious saliva, conjunctival secretion, or genitourinary secretions. Human fatalities due to B virus encephalitis illustrate the importance of using appropriate precautions and personal protective equipment to prevent direct or indirect contact with macaque secretions and body fluids. Captive-born and raised animals should still be screened when first presented in a clinical setting and subsequently every year afterward in a private facility.

Saimiriine herpesvirus type 1 (herpesvirus T) causes mild herpetic lingual ulcers and stomatitis in squirrel monkeys, but fatal epizootics have followed natural transmission to owl monkeys and marmosets. The human herpesvirus, herpes simplex virus type 1, causes a mild infection in people and certain other primates, but owl monkeys, gibbons, capuchins, and tree shrews (*Tupaia glis*) are highly susceptible and may die; signs may include ulcerations of the mucous membrane or skin, conjunctivitis, meningitis, or encephalitis. Human caretakers with oral lesions should be replaced until the infection regresses, and any interaction with the public should be *discouraged*.

Naturally occurring, clinically silent infections of hepatitis A virus (enterically transmitted hepatitis virus) have been seen in chimpanzees (*Pan troglodytes*) and monkeys. Increased AST and ALT values are of diagnostic significance in nonhuman primates. Human infections have been contracted from chimpanzees.

Because some vaccines are not available to protect nonhuman primate colony personnel or the primates against herpes and some viral hepatitis infections, exposure should be prevented. This is best accomplished by carefully training personnel in the handling of nonhuman primates, using personal protective equipment (clothing, face masks, goggles or shields, and gloves), separating primates in species-specific rooms, and paying strict attention to hygienic standards. In private facilities, prescreening the primates by serologic and PCR testing is recommended.

Several other viruses commonly produce clinical disease in newly imported primates. Rubeola infection (measles) acquired via human contact can assume epizootic proportions. The virus causes a nonpruritic, exanthematous rash on the face, chest, and lower portions of the body; it may also cause interstitial giant-cell pneumonia, rhinitis, conjunctivitis, and, particularly in New World monkeys, gastroenteritis. Marmosets are extremely susceptible, and children, especially, should not be encouraged to interact with this species. There is no specific treatment. Vaccination of infant rhesus monkeys and other macaques with human measles vaccine is recommended. Modified-live measles vaccine can cause disease in marmosets and is *not* recommended. Monkeypox and other poxvirus infections may be seen in primate colonies. Monkeypox is a reportable, zoonotic disease characterized by a maculopapular rash and variolous pustules (*see* p 2419). Affected monkeys usually survive; after recovery, they are immune to challenge.

Immunosuppressive disease in nonhuman primates may be caused by a number of retroviruses, including several orthoretroviruses formerly called type C and type D oncornaviruses, and several simian immunodeficiency viruses (SIVs). The SIVs are lentiviruses closely related to human immunodeficiency virus 1 (HIV-1) and HIV-2. Unique isolates have been found in different species of nonhuman primates. SIVs are of low pathogenicity in the natural hosts, African species, and infections are often clinically silent but may cause devastating disease similar to AIDS in macaques after cross-species transmission. SIV has been demonstrated to infect people, although the longterm consequences of infection are unknown. Infection with orthoretroviruses in the genus *Betaretrovirus* (formerly the type D retroviruses SRV, 5 serotypes) may cause an immunodeficiency predisposing to a complex of diseases such as fibromatosis, atypical mycobacteriosis, intestinal cryptosporidiosis, pneumocystic pneumonia, disseminated cytomegalovirus infection, and candidiasis in colonies of macaques. Infection with oncornaviruses in the genus *Deltaretrovirus* (formerly type C retrovirus) results primarily in lymphoproliferative disease, and rarely T-cell lymphoma, in Old World monkeys and apes. There is great host-interspecies variation in clinical signs and susceptibility from virus to virus. Transmission between nonhuman primates is via direct or indirect contact with infected blood and other body fluids or from dam to offspring.

Hemorrhagic viral zoonoses, such as Ebola, Marburg, and mosquitoborne yellow fever, are risks with wild-caught animals. An important differential diagnosis for these zoonoses is simian hemorrhagic fever. This *Arterivirus* infection is subclinical in African monkeys but is highly contagious and fatal for Asian species. Hemorrhagic necrosis of the proximal duodenum is a pathognomonic lesion. Captive populations that ultimately are housed in private facilities are a low risk.

NUTRITIONAL DISEASES

See also NUTRITION: EXOTIC AND ZOO ANIMALS, p 2287.

All laboratory nonhuman primates are susceptible to vitamin C deficiency. Hypovitaminosis C may cause immunosuppression and increase susceptibility to infectious diseases before clinical signs of the deficiency appear. Commercial monkey diets contain vitamin C that is stable for 3 mo after the diet is milled and packaged, if properly stored. Supplemental sources are green leafy vegetables and citrus fruits. Orally administered human pediatric vitamin preparations that contain ascorbic acid are readily accepted. Daily intake of vitamin C at 3–6 mg/kg prevents scurvy. Scurvy should be treated with ascorbic acid at dosages of 25–50 mg/kg/day until clinical signs resolve and dietary consumption of adequate vitamin C is restored. Primates require vitamin D to prevent rickets and osteomalacia. Asian and African primates can use provitamin D_2 (in plant materials); Central and South American primates (New World) cannot and require provitamin D_3. Commercial diets specifically formulated for New World primates should be the main component of the diet of these animals. Fish-liver oils provide an adequate source of D_3, or as little as 1.25 IU/g of diet can be added to the ration. Exposure of monkeys to sunlight facilitates conversion of vitamin D to active forms. Without adequate D_3, New World primates may develop secondary nutritional hyperparathyroidism (*see* p 1054).

MISCELLANEOUS CONDITIONS

Diabetes: Diabetes is frequently seen in clinical practice. The genus *Cebus* is overrepresented. Causes of diabetes vary from obesity (carbohydrate overload), genetic predisposition, and overall poor dietary choices. The animal should be brought to the hospital fasting; laboratory tests should include a CBC, serum chemistries, a urinalysis, levels of insulin and fructosamine, and a glycosylated hemoglobin. The caretaker should be educated on dietary restrictions and the availability of newer commercial diets for these animals. Blood glucose readings can be obtained at home by the caretaker, and both oral and parental medications administered with little effort.

Acute Gastric Dilatation: Life-threatening bloat occurs sporadically in captive nonhuman primates and may be associated with feeding after a prolonged fast or periods of water restriction or accidental overfeeding. Etiologic factors include intragastric fermentation associated with *Clostridium perfringens* and abnormal gastric function. Monkeys become acutely ill, with clinical findings similar to those seen in small animals (*see* p 384). Acute gastric dilatation is often fatal without emergency treatment. The stomach must be evacuated and fluids replaced, in like volume, with electrolyte solution given parenterally. Shock and dehydration usually occur and require prompt treatment. Periodic evacuation of the stomach may be necessary for several days until GI function is normal. Metabolic alkalosis may result from continued loss of hydrochloric acid. Adequate sodium, chloride, and potassium must be provided via parenteral fluid therapy.

Tetanus: Infection with *Clostridium tetani* is a risk with free-ranging and outdoor-housed monkeys, particularly as a consequence of fighting, parturition, frostbite, and other forms of skin trauma. Immunization with tetanus toxoid should be considered for populations at risk. Marmosets are routinely vaccinated with adsorbed human product or equine product at 0.25 mg, IM, every 5 yr. (*See also* TETANUS, p 611.)

Intestinal Adenocarcinoma: The number of aged nonhuman primates maintained in captivity has increased in recent years, primarily due to improvements in husbandry, nutrition, and veterinary care, but also because of an emphasis on animal models for aging research. This increase in the aged nonhuman primate population, particularly macaques, has been associated with an increase in the incidence of intestinal adenocarcinoma, which may exceed 20% in animals >30 yr old in some colonies. Decreased appetite, weight loss, anemia, and a palpable abdominal mass are common clinical findings. Tests for fecal occult blood are often positive. Radiographic examination may show changes associated with partial obstruction. Surgical biopsy is diagnostic for adenocarcinoma. The location of these tumors is most commonly the ileocecocolic junction, rarely in the small intestine. Histologic lesions include a thickened intestinal wall and constriction of the lumen (so-called "napkin ring" lesion), with variable signs of hemorrhage and ulceration. Metastatic lesions are uncommon, and some animals respond favorably to surgical excision.

Trauma: Trauma from cagemate aggression or self-mutilation (biting or hair pulling) may occur occasionally, as may thinning of the hair due to self-induced alopecia. Trauma is also very common in captive nonhuman primates in clinical practice. Animals that live with other species in the domestic environment may be subjected to wounds inflicted by dogs and cats. Massive soft-tissue injury, such as that which occurs from these attacks, may cause increased loads of bacteria into the bloodstream, as well as acute blood loss and shock causing coagulopathy and endothelial disruption. This complicated chain of events causes hypothermia, acidemia, and inflammation and should be treated as a life-threatening emergency. Rapid control of *hemorrhage, correcting* the hypothermia, early blood component administration, and high-volume fluid therapy are indicated to avert continued ischemia and renal shutdown; antibiotics should be given to prevent infection and sepsis. Measures should be taken to enhance the psychologic well-being of nonhuman primates (eg, group housing, exercise pens, shelters, foraging activities, and cage toys), and animals in social groups should also be provided facilities for refuge and escape.

PSYCHOLOGICAL WELL-BEING AND ENVIRONMENTAL ENRICHMENT

Providing for the psychological as well as the physical well-being of nonhuman primates maintained in captivity is a high priority. Psychological well-being is enhanced by appropriate social companionship (ie, compatible conspecifics); opportunities to engage in behavior related to foraging, exploration, and other activities appropriate to the species, age, gender, and physical condition of the animal; and housing that allows typical movement and resting postures. When home cages are of the minimum legal size, enlargements or added exercise areas should be encouraged. Interactions with human caretakers should be generally positive and not a source of undue stress. Well-designed and implemented environmental enrichment programs should meet these basic requirements, with the objective of minimizing traumatic injuries due to aggressive interactions, reducing the incidence of stereotypic and self-injurious behaviors, and ameliorating preexisting abnormal behaviors. Results of attempts to manage self-injurious behavior (eg, self-biting, hair plucking) with drugs such as benzodiazepines or haloperidol have been inconsistent, and longterm management is generally unrewarding. Socialization, which may involve visual and auditory stimuli as well as physical contact, appears to provide substantial benefit to most species of nonhuman primates, and should be provided within the constraints of research protocols and daily management practices. Additional enrichment options include forage boards or other food-related enrichment devices, manipulation mirrors, and a variety of cage toys provided on a rotating schedule to maintain novelty. Animal behavioral assessments as well as periodic review and evaluation of the effectiveness of enrichment program components should be performed by appropriately trained individuals.

PET BIRDS

Advances in avian medicine have changed the emphasis from infectious diseases and emergency medicine to wellness care. Nutrition and behavior are important components of the health of psittacine birds and play a major role in pet bird wellness programs. Mass importation of wild-caught psittacine birds was curtailed in the mid-1980s, and the current pet bird population is comprised primarily of captive-bred parrots. This has resulted in novel medical concerns and unique behavioral challenges. The knowledge base regarding psittacine and other pet bird diets and husbandry continues to increase, as does the importance of providing a psychologically suitable environment for these complex animals. Pet birds are intelligent and social animals adapted for flight. Keeping solitary pet birds in small indoor cages, with limited opportunity for exercise, has both physical and psychological consequences.

Veterinarians have a responsibility not only to diagnose and treat disease but also to educate bird owners on how to provide the best care for and prevent disease in their bird. Preventing disease entails providing a proper diet, an appropriate size cage and perches, proper sanitation, and environmental enrichment (ie, toys, foraging opportunities, social interaction).

A cage provides living space as well as protection and security. It should be large enough to not only house the bird and provide ample room for climbing and playing but also to accommodate toys, foraging opportunities, and multiple perches of different sizes and textures. Owners should purchase the largest cage possible (considering space and cost), while following minimum size recommendations (TABLE 14). Cages must be large enough to accommodate multiple perches and ensure that birds will have adequate room to move around and exercise.

MANAGEMENT

Managing pet birds in the clinical setting can be challenging. The ability to "mask" clinical signs of illness until late in the disease process often results in birds presenting much sicker than owners realize. Because of this, birds are also riskier patients to evaluate. Birds have a much higher metabolism than mammals, and oxygen deprivation can occur during restraint, treatment, or diagnostic sampling. Owners should be informed of the risks of handling and sampling and the need for a step-by-step approach through the physical examination and diagnostic testing. Placing severely debilitated birds in a warm oxygen incubator or cage while obtaining the history and before physical examination may be warranted. In all avian examinations and diagnostic procedures, being prepared with all needed items for examination, sample collection, and treatments before restraining the bird is important. This includes a light source, oral speculum, gram scale, stethoscope, syringe and needle for venipuncture, blood tubes, and fluids for administration. If a bird is extremely stressed, in pain, or not used to handling, sedation before diagnostic testing may be warranted.

TABLE 14 MINIMUM CAGE SIZE AND BAR SPACING RECOMMENDATIONS

Bird	Cage Size (inches [length × width × height])	Bar Spacing (inches)
Budgerigar, cockatiel, lovebird, parrotlet	20 × 20 × 30	0.5
Conure, *Poicephalus* spp, caique, miniature macaw	36 × 24 × 48	0.75
African grey parrot, Amazon parrot, small cockatoo	40 × 30 × 60	0.751
Macaw, large cockatoo	48 × 36 × 66	1.5

History: Having the owners bring a pet bird in its own cage for examination is desirable but often impractical. Alternatively, owners can be asked to bring photos or videos of the cage set-up, as well as recent papers from the cage floor so the droppings can be examined. The history should include the type and size of cage, cage bar size and spacing, type of substrate and how often it is changed, frequency of cleaning food and water bowls, where the cage is located in the home, and temperature and humidity of the cage environment. The diet that is offered, the foods that are actually eaten, and any recent changes in diet or appetite should be noted. A complete history also should include the source of the bird and whether it was hand or parent raised; exposure to other birds or pets, including client-owned birds and birds outside the home; length of ownership and history of previous owners; how much time the bird is outside of its cage and if it is monitored during this time; exposure to outdoors; and time spent in interaction with people or other birds in the household.

The length of time a bird has been in the household is usually inversely proportional to the probability that illness will be caused by a primary infectious disease. Newly acquired birds or those exposed to other birds outside the household via bird shows or pet store visits are most likely to be affected by contagious diseases. Chronic malnutrition and secondary infections are more common in birds without recent exposure to potentially infectious birds. Malnutrition is a major cause of subclinical disease in birds, which often becomes clinical when a secondary infection occurs.

Clinical signs of illness can be difficult to detect in birds. However, astute owners may recognize minor behavioral differences in their bird, such as not vocalizing in the morning or decreased interaction with family members. These changes should be considered potential signs of illness. Owners with less experience or less interaction with their birds are less likely to notice these early signs. Feathers can effectively mask even severe emaciation or abdominal distention. Owners may also notice other signs of illness, such as changes in droppings or vocalizations, or if the bird appears to be sleeping more. Veterinarians who see avian patients should be able to identify common species of pet birds (cockatoos, Amazon parrots, macaws, conures, etc) and be familiar with normal species-specific behaviors. For example, parrots of *Pionus* spp often make rapid sniffing noises when stressed that can be mistaken for respiratory distress.

Physical Examination: The bird should be observed in the cage or carrier before manual restraint. Observation should be done from a nonthreatening distance (several feet away). The bird's stance and breathing pattern should be noted. Is it perching and standing on both legs? Is it alert? Are the eyes open or closed? Are the feathers fluffed or sleek? Is there a wing droop? Is the tail bobbing up and down (a sign of increased respiratory effort)? Is the bird open-mouth breathing? A respiratory rate should be obtained at this time. The normal resting respiratory rate for pet birds varies with size and species, with the rate ranging in smaller birds (<300 g) from 30–60 beats/min and in larger birds (400–1,000 g) from 15–30 beats/min. If the bird is showing signs of respiratory distress, it should be placed in a warm, oxygenated incubator before restraint.

Birds should be restrained in a manner that minimizes stress and does not cause undue fear. If the bird is used to being handled, often a towel can be slowly and gently placed over the bird. If an owner has worked with the bird at home with a towel, the veterinarian may ask the owner to towel the bird and then hand it off for examination or testing. Minimizing restraint time, talking to the bird in a quiet voice, and moving slowly can help with many birds. Baby birds or hand-raised cockatoos often can be examined with minimal to no restraint. Many pet birds will step out of the cage or on to a hand and can be gently toweled. Some nervous birds may benefit from sedation for examination and diagnostic testing. Birds that are not handled routinely (breeding or aviary birds) may have to be gently toweled directly from the cage or carrier.

Restraint of psittacine birds involves immobilizing the head, generally with a thumb on one side of the mandible and the

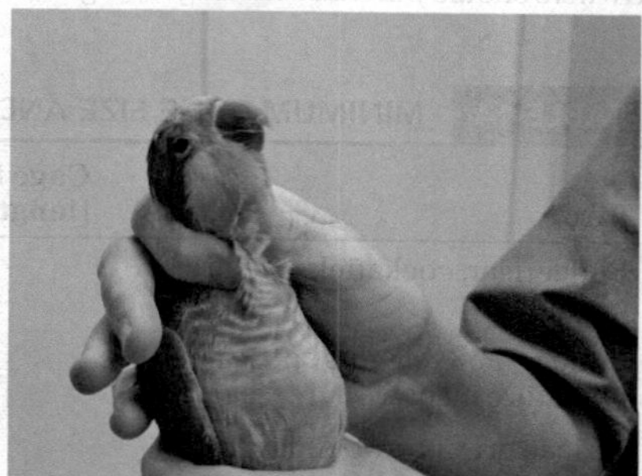

Restrained Quaker parakeet. *Courtesy of the Schubot Exotic Bird Health Center.*

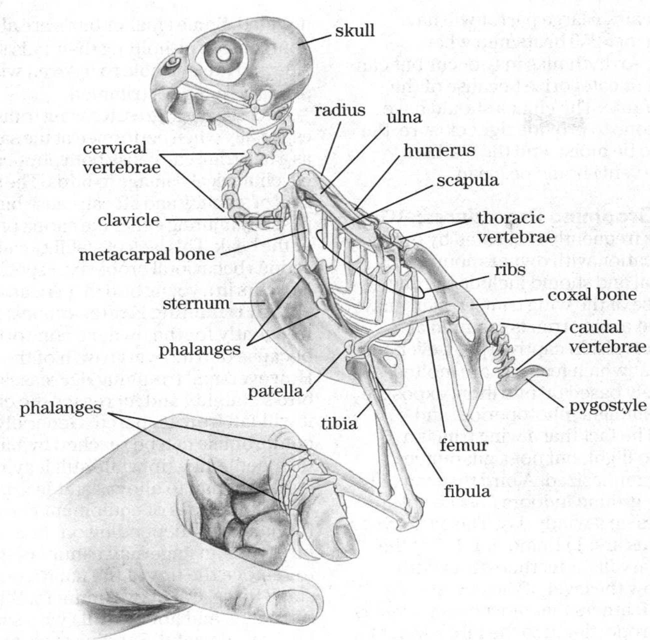

Skeleton of a budgerigar. *Illustration by Dr. Gheorghe Constantinescu.*

index or middle finger on the other. The feet and the distal reminges (primary wing feathers), if not trimmed, are held by the opposite hand in medium to large parrots. This leaves the thorax and abdomen free to expand with respiration. If the primary wing feathers have been trimmed, a towel may be useful to prevent the wings from flapping during restraint. Birds should be observed closely during restraint; all birds can become stressed, and obese birds can overheat, especially when held in a towel. If respirations become increased or labored, or if the bird becomes weak, the bird should be returned to its cage.

As soon as the bird has been restrained, the crop should be palpated to determine whether food or fluids are present. If the crop is full, the holder should monitor for any signs of regurgitation during restraint. Diagnostic procedures may need to be delayed until the crop empties. An accurate weight is critical to monitor health, body condition, and recovery from illness and to determine fluid therapy, nutritional needs, and medication dosages. Ears, eyes, nares, and oral cavity should all be examined and appear clean, with no exudate, masses, or swellings. The choana on the roof of the oral cavity should have intact sharp papilla. Exudate around the nares can indicate respiratory or sinus infection, and debris on the feathers of the head or face can indicate vomiting or regurgitation. The condition of the feathers and skin should be noted, including the symmetry and integrity of the beak and nails. Overgrown beak and nails can indicate poor husbandry, nutrition, or liver disease. The integument of the feet should be intact, without excessive wear, callous, or ulceration. Excessive wear of the plantar surface of the feet can indicate inadequate perching or poor nutrition. Excessive wear or callous unilaterally may indicate a problem with the contralateral foot.

Body condition can be determined by palpating the pectoral muscles. A keel scoring system from 1–5 is often used, with 1 as very thin, 5 as obese, and 3 as an appropriate score for most pet birds. Severely obese birds may deposit fat over the neck, thighs, and abdominal cavity. Wings and legs should extend and flex fully, and grip strength should be symmetrical.

Respiratory rate should be monitored throughout the examination; respirations may increase with hyperthermia, stress, or obesity. Respirations should normalize within 3–4 min after the bird has been released. Heart rate is rapid in restrained birds; typically, a large parrot will have a heart rate of >250 beats/min when restrained. Arrhythmias may occur but can be difficult to categorize because of the rapid heart rate. The cloaca should have sufficient tone to provide tight closure, the skin should be moist, and the feathers around the vent should be clean.

Routine Grooming Procedures: **Wing clipping** is frequently requested by owners. Communication with owners about wing trims is vital and should include the degree and purpose of the wing trim. Owners may assume that a wing trim is required at regular intervals. In captivity, however, the frequency at which feathers are molted varies widely based on nutrition, exposure to natural sunlight, photoperiod, and humidity. The fact that a wing trim is a deterrent to flight, but not a guarantee, should be emphasized. A bird that can only glide to the ground indoors may be able to fly outdoors on a windy day. The basic types of wing trims are: 1) Removing 4–7 of the distal primary flight feathers from both wings, below the level of the coverts. The number of feathers that must be removed is inversely proportional to the bird's weight. 2) Leaving 1–4 distal primary feathers and removing the remainder of the primaries from both wings. This clip has fallen out of favor, but some owners have used it for many years. If it has worked well for their bird, it may be wise to continue its use. 3) Removing a variable number of primary feathers from just one wing. This clip is unnecessarily severe and not recommended. Some smaller birds are able to compensate by holding their tails to the side and are still able to fly even with all primary reminges trimmed.

Excessively aggressive wing trims, especially when performed at the same time as a nail trim, can cause both physical and psychological damage to birds. The sudden lack of stability and lift can cause birds to fall, possibly injuring either the carina of the keel or the beak. This lack of stability can lead to serious behavioral problems, especially when it occurs in a young bird that is learning to fly.

Nail trimming is often requested, frequently for the owner's comfort and not because of true overgrowth of the nails. However, nail trimming decreases the bird's stability and increases the chance it will fall from its perch. Generally, a compromise can be reached by blunting the needle-like tip while still leaving sufficient nail to allow a stable grip.

Various types of equipment can be used for nail trims, depending on the size of the bird. Human fingernail trimmers work well to remove the tips of the nails from very small birds. Cat claw trimmers, White's nail trimmers, and hobby drills with sanding bits are all useful. Sanding tools are also excellent to remove excess keratin that can accumulate on the lateral surfaces of the beak. **Beak trimming** is sometimes necessary because of an overgrown upper or lower beak. Birds with beak deformities often have underlying nutritional deficiencies, disease, or previous trauma. Healthy birds provided adequate environmental abrasive surfaces rarely require beak trims.

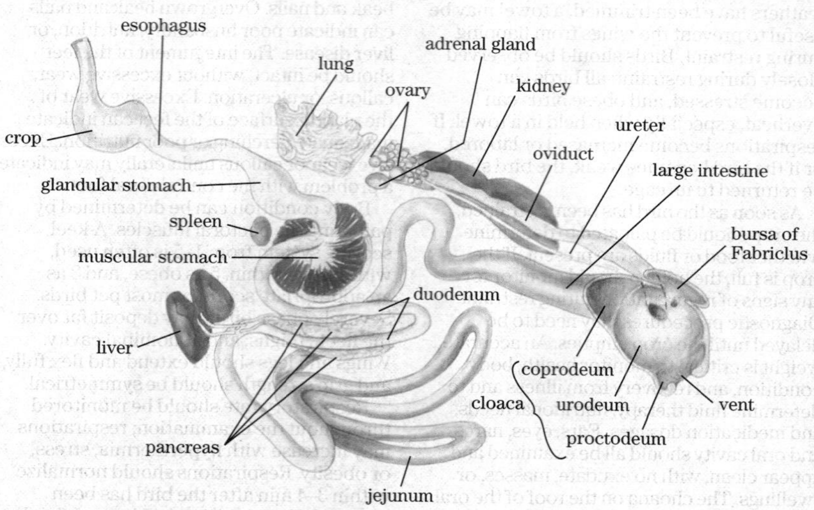

Viscera, budgerigar. *Illustration by Dr. Gheorghe Constantinescu.*

Concrete (cement) perches are available in various sizes and textures. These can work well for medium-sized psittacine birds (~250–700 g) when a suitable size is selected and properly placed in the cage. These perches can eliminate the need for both nail trimming and removal of excess keratin from the beak. The perch should be placed where the bird is forced to stand for brief periods (eg, in front of a food bowl or treat cup). To avoid irritation to the plantar surfaces of the feet, the concrete perch should not be the main perch on which the bird sits to preen or sleep.

In previous decades when parrots were widely imported, open-rolled steel bands were used to identify the location at which they were quarantined. Now most birds are **leg banded** (using closed bands) as chicks for individual identification. Bands present certain hazards to the bird, but removal also entails some risk if the proper equipment is not available. The open (gap present), rolled, steel quarantine bands are extremely strong and require removal by a full-size bolt cutter with sharp edges. The closed aluminum bands placed on young, captive-raised birds must be stabilized to prevent twisting while being cut. These bands require two cuts to remove; a sharp, properly designed instrument for removal decreases the danger of leg trauma. Full-circle plastic bands can be removed in the same manner. **Microchipping** is replacing or augmenting banding as a means of identification. The standard for placement of these chips in psittacine birds is in the left pectoral muscles. Adverse reactions or failures in birds have been infrequent; the intramuscular placement reduces the risk of microchip migration. Although microchipping is relatively safe in large parrots with good breast muscle (>150 g), it is riskier in smaller birds. Microchipping small birds (<150 g) has resulted in bleeding and death.

Clinical Pathology: Hematologic testing and plasma biochemical analysis are especially important in birds, because physical examination tends to be less revealing than in other animals. The quantity of blood that can be drawn depends on the weight and health of the bird. Blood collection should be limited to 1% of body wt. Blood is usually collected from the right jugular vein, which is larger than the left. The basilic (wing) vein can also be used but is prone to hematoma formation. In medium to large psittacine birds, seabirds, and poultry, the medial metatarsal vein can also be used. Coating a syringe with an anticoagulant before collection may be helpful in smaller species in which sample collection may take longer but can cause artifacts in the blood smear, affecting the differential cell count.

The normal PCV varies between psittacine species. For example, cockatiels normally have a higher PCV than many other species, averaging 50%–55%. Cockatoos (*Cacatua* spp), however, often have a PCV in the 40%–45% range.

Anemia can be a result of blood loss or decreased production. Blood loss can occur in cases of trauma or severe organ disease or in idiopathic cases such as conure bleeding syndrome. Response to blood loss anemia may include the presence of immature erythrocytes and anisocytosis along with increased polychromasia. Decreased RBC production can occur with any chronic disease, and the anemia is often nonregenerative. Toxins such as lead or oil ingestion can result in hemolytic anemia.

Polycythemia is rare in birds and is defined as a PCV >70%. It has been reported in birds with chronic respiratory diseases and in macaws with pulmonary hypersensitivity syndrome, a condition that occurs in macaws housed in poorly ventilated areas with birds that produce large amounts of powder down such as cockatoos, cockatiels, and African grey parrots.

Avian RBCs are nucleated, so traditional mammalian methods of WBC determination are not adequate. Various diluents (eg, Eosinophil Unopette®, Natt-Herricks® solution) are available to enable accurate WBC determinations. Estimated WBC counts are less accurate but can be useful when the individual performing the estimate produces blood smears of consistent quality and thickness. Normal total WBC counts vary with species and age (*see* TABLE 15). Adult cockatiels often have total WBC counts of $4{,}000–7{,}000 \times 10^3/\mu L$. Adult macaws are usually at the high end of the normal avian range ($12{,}000–15{,}000 \times 10^3/\mu L$).

For many avian species, reference values for WBC counts are still being determined. A leukocytosis, and the differential or type(s) of WBCs that are increased, can identify underlying disease and give an indication of the most likely causes. The differential count in birds can be affected by bacterial, fungal, and viral diseases, as well as toxins. The types of avian WBCs are the heterophil, eosinophil, monocyte, and basophil.

Heterophils are equivalent to mammalian neutrophils, with much the same function. Avian heterophils contain lysosomal enzymes and are bactericidal and phagocytic. They are the first cells to respond to any infectious or inflammatory disease process. Instead of forming a liquid purulent material, avian heterophils form an inspissated, caseous material. This caseous material is then walled off by macrophages and fibrous tissue to form a granuloma. Heterophilia can occur during infection or from stress. Heteropenia is often associated with an overwhelming infection or viral disease.

Lymphocytes function in antibody and antigen production and cellular and humoral immune reactions. Lymphocytosis may occur in chronic infections (chlamydial, fungal, mycobacterial) or with lymphoid neoplasia. In some species (eg, canaries and Amazon parrots), up to 70% of the WBCs are normally lymphocytes. Lymphopenia is often associated with viral diseases (eg, circovirus or polyomavirus) or sepsis.

Monocytosis is often associated with chronic granulomatous diseases such as chlamydial, fungal, or mycobacterial infection. Eosinophilia has been reported with parasitic diseases and has also been associated with delayed hypersensitivity reactions. Basophilia can occur during inflammatory conditions and chronic infection.

Physiologic differences in birds create variations from accepted mammalian normal values for many **biochemical measurements**. Because of the excretion of uric acid rather than urea as the primary product of protein metabolism, uric acid levels are significantly higher in birds than in mammals, whereas BUN is significantly lower. Uric acid may be increased in severe renal disease or with articular gout (*see* p 1926). Severe dehydration may increase uric acid levels, but levels return to normal with rehydration. No reliable biochemical indicator is currently available to detect early renal impairment.

Serum or plasma glucose is higher in birds than in mammals, with levels of 250–400 g/dL common, depending on species. Levels that indicate diabetes also vary with species and individuals but often are >700–800 g/dL (*see* p 1925).

Hepatic enzymes measured commonly include AST and LDH, which have normal values several times those of mammals (AST, 10–400 U/L; LDH, 75–450 U/L). Measurement of CK is often performed concurrently to differentiate increased values of AST due to muscle necrosis from those due to hepatic damage. LDH is a short-lived enzyme of limited usefulness in detection of hepatic necrosis. ALT levels are very low compared with those in mammals (5–15 U/L); however, increased levels can indicate hepatocellular necrosis. Birds have low bilirubin reductase levels; therefore, total bilirubin is normally also very low, and increases with hepatic disease are not consistent (total bilirubin range 0–0.1 mg/dL). Birds also do not become icteric with hepatic disease as do mammals; they excrete biliverdin through their kidneys, resulting in yellow or lime-green urates. Bile acid measurements are useful indicators of hepatic function, with levels <100 μmol/L considered normal for most avian species (depending on the laboratory). Establishing reference values for different avian species will enhance the usefulness of bile acid assays.

TABLE 15 NORMAL HEMATOLOGIC VALUES IN SELECTED PET BIRD SPECIES

Bird	Sample Size (n)	WBC × 10^3/μL	PCV
African grey parrots (*Psittacus erithacus*)	176	8–11	42–50
Amazon parrots (*Amazona* spp)	155	7.5–12.5	44–49
Budgerigars (*Melopsittacus undulates*)	57	2.5–6.5	42–53
Cockatiels (*Nymphicus hollandicus*)	212	3.0–7.8	45–57
Cockatoos, umbrella (*Cactua alba*)	115	5–13	38–48
Conures (*Aratinga* spp)	62	7.5–11.5	42–49
Eclectus parrots (*Eclectus roratus*)	44	7.0–11.7	41–49
Lovebirds (*Agapornis* spp)	31	4.5–9.0	39–51
Macaws (*Ara* spp)	146	8.5–15.5	41–52
Pionus parrots (*Pionus* spp)	28	7.0–11.5	44–51
Quaker/monk parrots (*Myiopsitta monachus*)	62	5.5–12.5	38–48
Senegal parrots (*Poicephalus senegalus*)	26	6.5–12.0	37–49

Note: Samples were obtained at wellness examination. No other concurrent disease was detected or treated, except for behavioral concerns.

Calcium and phosphorus values are similar to those found in mammals. These levels may increase up to 3-fold in hens in preparation for egg laying (ie, calcium ~30 mg/dL and phosphorus >10 mg/dL), usually with a relatively normal ratio of these minerals. Total solids as measured via refractometer are significantly lower in birds than in mammals, with levels of 3–5.5 g/dL normal for most species. Total solids can also increase in reproductively active hens.

Cholesterol and triglyceride reference ranges are still being evaluated, but reference values are ~180–250 mg/dL for cholesterol and 51–200 mg/dL for triglycerides. Increased levels of both triglycerides and cholesterol have been reported in birds fed a high-fat diet. High levels can also be seen in reproductively active females and may be a risk factor in birds that develop atherosclerosis. Omega-3 fatty acids added to the diet as well as dietary restriction and conversion to a pelleted diet have been shown to reduce hypertriglyceridemia and hypercholesterolemia.

Hematology and Plasma Biochemistry of the Neonate: Neonates have some important differences from mature birds in their hematologic and biochemical parameters. Neonates have a lower PCV (20%–30%). The normal adult range is present beginning at 10–12 wk in most species. Neonates have a lower total protein (1–3 mg/dL) and concomitant lower plasma albumin concentrations than adults. A high WBC count (20,000–40,000 cells/uL) is common in neonates; the normal adult range is present at 9–11 wk of age. Neonates also have lower uric acid values and higher alkaline phosphatase and CK concentrations than adults.

Routine Medical Procedures: Injections can be given by several routes. SC injections are used for fluid administration, some vaccinations, and many routine medications such as antibiotics. Preliminary studies show that the SC route may be as effective as IM injections for most medications, without the associated muscle necrosis. To ensure that the medication or fluid being injected is actually deposited subcutaneously, the skin must be clearly visualized; use of alcohol to wet the skin and feathers is recommended to aid in visualization. Insulin syringes (50 U or 0.5 mL) with 27-gauge needles are invaluable for accurate dosing when small quantities must be administered. SC fluids are often used in birds. To maximize their absorption and minimize discomfort, fluids should be warmed to 102°–106°F. Sites of administration are the lateral flank, the inguinal web, and the back. Maintenance fluids are estimated at 50 mL/kg divided bid-tid. In dehydrated birds, 50% of the total daily maintenance can be administered SC (25 mL/kg) and repeated every 6–8 hr until hydration is reestablished.

IM injections are given into the pectoral muscles in most pet birds; leg muscles are also used in some species, particularly raptors. The muscle fibers of birds are more vascular and tightly packed than those of mammals, making both muscle necrosis and inadvertent IV injection more likely.

IV injections are occasionally indicated in birds. Common medications administered IV are some antibiotics, amphotericin B, chemotherapeutic drugs, contrast media, and fluids.

Indwelling catheters can be placed in the jugular, basilic, or medial metatarsal veins for constant-rate infusions or intermittent fluid administration. Intraosseous (IO) catheters can also be inserted, generally in the proximal tibiotarsal bone or distal ulna. A standard hypodermic needle may be used (usually 25-gauge for initial entry, followed by a second 22-gauge needle sutured in place), or a spinal needle with stylet may be used for large birds. Without a stylet or second needle, a bone plug may obstruct the needle. The IO or IV catheter is intermittently flushed with warm saline whenever fluids are not being infused. Maintaining an IV catheter in an avian patient can be challenging, and IO catheters are often preferable for longterm fluid therapy. However, fluid therapy via IO catheters can be painful to the bird, especially after 1–2 days.

Crop (gavage) feeding may be used to meet caloric needs in anorectic birds. Commercial formulas are available and convenient to use. Adequate hydration and normal body temperature (103°–106°F [39°–41°C]) must be established before initiating crop feeding to prevent desiccation of the crop food and GI stasis. In adult birds, generally 30 mL/kg can be administered tid-qid. Baby birds have a much more distensible crop and will hold ~10% of their body weight per feeding (100 mL/kg). Oral medications may be added to the crop feeding or given directly by mouth. The technique of holding the bird so that the medication is administered into the commissure of the mouth and rolls onto the tongue will minimize stress, loss of medication, and the danger of aspiration. Medicating birds can be quite difficult for owners; wrapping the bird in a towel for administration of medication can be stressful for both the bird and the owner and, in some cases, adversely affect the human-bird bond. Compounding medications to make them more palatable and in a smaller volume can be very helpful in using oral medications. Mixing the flavored medication with favorite foods, juice, or baby food can also help ensure compliance. Medications administered in the water are indicated only in special circumstances such as small flocks of birds or aviary birds not used to handling and would require daily netting and restraint, or in special cases in which an owner cannot handle a bird. Enrofloxacin and doxycycline in drinking water generally provide adequate blood levels for efficacy. However, lack of accurate dosing, stability of the medication, and palatability make this route undesirable in most cases.

Sedation is sometimes desirable for diagnostic or treatment procedures to reduce stress and minimize fear. Midazolam administered at 0.5–1 mg/kg, IM, or 1–2 mg/kg intranasally (IN) is a safe and effective sedation protocol in most pet birds; flumazenil (0.02–0.1 mg/kg, IM or IN) may be given to reverse the effects. If the bird is thought to be in pain or discomfort, butorphanol (0.5–3 mg/kg, IM or IN, depending on species) may be given alone or with midazolam. Amazon parrots often require the higher dosage (2–3 mg/kg) of butorphanol, whereas raptors require the lower dosage (0.5 mg/kg). Isoflurane or sevoflurane anesthesia delivered by face mask can also be used alone or in conjunction with sedation for more prolonged procedures or painful treatments.

Intubation in birds is relatively easy, because the absence of an epiglottis facilitates visibility of the tracheal opening and arytenoids. Fasting before anesthesia should be of minimal duration; fasts of 4–6 hr are typical. Regardless of the duration of the fast, the crop should be palpated for the presence of food or fluid before anesthesia. Delayed crop emptying is common in clinically ill birds. If anesthesia must be administered to a bird with food or water still in the crop, fluid should be removed by a feeding tube if possible, and the head should be elevated for the duration of anesthesia, regardless of whether the bird is intubated. Endotracheal tubes should be uncuffed, because the absence of a tracheal ligament increases the risk of tracheal necrosis if a cuff is overinflated. Even an uncuffed tube can cause tracheal damage or necrosis; therefore, after the bird is intubated, head movement should be minimized. A small animal ventilator can be used for most birds as small as 100 g and can greatly improve ventilation during anesthesia. If a mechanical ventilator is not available, manual intermittent positive-pressure ventilation will increase oxygenation in anesthetized birds. A capnograph, pulse oximeter, and Doppler are also useful for anesthetic monitoring. The normal body temperature of most psittacines is 103°–106°F (39°–41°C). Birds tend to lose body heat rapidly when anesthetized, and maintaining body temperature during prolonged anesthesia or surgery is crucial for recovery. Birds with feather loss are more at risk of hypothermia. Water warming blankets under the bird or Bair Huggers™ can be used effectively to maintain body temperature. An emergency drug sheet and emergency drugs should be readily available whenever a bird is anesthetized.

Environmental management is very important; severely ill birds benefit greatly from increased environmental temperature and humidity (eg, use of commercial incubators with temperature and humidity controls). For at-home emergencies, a warm environment can be created by wrapping clear plastic wrap around three sides of the cage and placing an electric heating pad on the remaining side, being sure the bird cannot reach the pad. Digital thermometers with remote probes can provide accurate monitoring of environmental temperatures. A quiet location, away from the sound of barking dogs and other excessive activity, will decrease stress.

The cage arrangement can be critical for ill birds. If a perch is supplied, the food and water must be elevated so that the bird has ready access without having to climb down from the perch. Often, it is best to remove perches entirely from the cage of an ill bird and place the food and water container on the cage floor so that the bird has easy access and does not expend energy simply trying to maintain a perched position.

PEDIATRIC DISEASES

Birds are classified by their maturity level at hatching. Parrots, doves, and finches are altricial, hatched without feathers, with eyes closed, and helpless. Poultry, ratites, and waterfowl are born precocial, with down feathers, open eyes, and the ability to walk and feed themselves at hatching. Psittacine neonates are completely dependent on the parent birds for warmth and food; they also lack a functional immune system and are more susceptible to disease. Because of these characteristics, proper husbandry and nutrition of the chick and parents is critical for their health and survival.

Today, chicks are either parent raised (most small parrots such as budgerigars and lovebirds) or hand raised (large parrots). There are advantages and disadvantages with both methods. Most aviculturists believe that hand-raised parrots make better pets and that incubator hatching and hand raising reduces the incidence of some infectious diseases. Disadvantages of hand raising can include stunting and an increase in husbandry-related diseases such as crop stasis or aspiration pneumonia. Many avian veterinarians and behaviorists also believe that hand raising may lead to behavioral issues because chicks cannot learn species-specific behaviors from parent birds and become imprinted on people.

The health of a chick depends on many factors, such as the health of the parents, genetics, the incubation process, nutrition (type of food, temperature, and consistency), environment (humidity, warmth, and cleanliness), and exposure to infectious diseases. When an ill neonate is presented, the history of not only the chick, but also of its parents, the aviary, and the nursery are important. Is the chick being hand fed or parent fed? Is the chick incubator hatched? How old is the chick? Is the nursery closed, or are chicks taken in from other facilities? What is the temperature and humidity of the nursery? What is the type of food fed, its consistency, temperature, amount fed, and frequency of feedings? What are the cleaning practices?

General environmental temperature guidelines are for newly hatched psittacine chicks, 92°–94°F; unfeathered chicks, 90°–92°F; pin-feathered chicks, 85°–90°F; and fully-feathered and weaned chicks, 75°–80°F.

A diet of 25%–30% solids should be fed to chicks >2 days old (more dilute formula for newly hatched), with the environmental temperature between 102°–106°F. Most medical issues arise in young birds in the first week of life, at fledging, or at weaning.

Physical examination of the chick can typically be done with minimal restraint, and the chick should be kept warm throughout the examination. The crop should be palpated at the beginning of the examination. Birds with food in their crop should be handled carefully to reduce the risk of regurgitation and/or aspiration. Mentation and body weight (a growth chart should be requested from the breeder if possible) should be noted. Before they fledge, chicks have little musculature over their keel bone; therefore, the muscle and subcutaneous fat over the hips, elbows, and toes should be evaluated. It should be determined whether the ears and eyes are open, or when they opened, if known.

The skin, feather quality, and distribution of the feathers should be examined. Healthy chicks have yellowish pink skin, and feathers first appear on the head, wing, and tail. Abnormal feather growth or delayed or abnormal opening of eyes can be a sign of stunting. Stress bars (lucent areas across the vane of the feathers) indicate a period of stress when that portion of the feather was forming. These are common during weaning, so a few stress bars are not uncommon. A large number of stress bars may indicate an underlying illness or condition.

The oral cavity should be moist with no plaques or lesions, and the choana should be examined for blunting of the choanal papilla, which can indicate hypovitaminosis A or chronic respiratory disease. The crop may be quite full in a neonate. The veterinarian should observe for crop contractions and ask when the chick was last fed and how much was fed, to determine whether the crop is emptying normally. Nestlings have a normally distended abdomen because of an enlarged proventriculus and ventriculus from being fed large amounts of formula. Chicks should be handled carefully to avoid placing excess pressure over their abdomen.

The spine, neck, wings, legs, and feet should be examined for abnormal curvature or weakness and evaluated for normal posture. The vent should be clean of debris.

Aspiration Pneumonia: Aspiration pneumonia is one of the most common causes of respiratory disease in hand-fed psittacine birds. Chicks can aspirate while being fed large quantities of liquid formula, especially when being fed by an inexperienced person. Aspiration often occurs as birds begin to wean.

Clinical signs include increased respiration, respiratory distress, poor feeding response, and depression. Depending on the age and size of the chick, a CBC and radiographs may aid in the diagnosis; however, diagnosis is often based on history and physical examination findings.

Treatment consists of oxygen therapy, nebulization, antibiotics, antifungals, warmth, supplemental fluids, and anti-inflammatory drugs. Prognosis is guarded.

Bacterial Disease: The normal gut microflora in chicks is primarily gram-positive bacteria. The presence of large numbers of gram-negative bacteria or budding yeast indicates infection. Bacterial infections can occur from multiple sources: an unsanitary environment, inappropriate storage of formula, and use of unclean feeding utensils.

Clinical signs can include crop stasis, poor feeding response, regurgitation, depression, and dehydration. Diagnosis is based on clinical signs and results of a fecal or crop Gram stain, CBC (leukocytosis, monocytosis), and culture and sensitivity testing.

Treatment is with antibiotics, based on culture and sensitivity results if available, and supportive care. Neonates on antibiotics often develop secondary yeast infections; therefore, prophylactic treatment with an antifungal drug such as nystatin or fluconazole may be warranted (*see* TABLE 18, p 1901).

Yeast Infection: *Candida albicans* can be present in low numbers in a healthy chick but may proliferate in the presence of antibiotic treatment, malnutrition, stress, or immunosuppression. It is the most common fungal infection in young birds and can result in thickening of the crop mucosa, which may be palpable externally and has been described as "Turkish towel in appearance."

Clinical signs are crop stasis, poor feeding response, and depression. There may be lesions or plaques in the oral cavity. Intestinal or gastric candidiasis can result in malabsorption. Diagnosis is with fecal or crop cytology revealing large numbers of budding yeasts.

Treatment is with antifungal medications. Antifungals should be given to baby birds prophylactically when on antibiotic therapy to prevent yeast overgrowth (*see* p 1899).

Viral Disease: The most common viral diseases in psittacine chicks are polyoma virus, avian bornavirus, proventricular dilatation disease and circovirus, and psittacine beak and feather disease (*see* p 1908).

Foreign Bodies: Foreign bodies can be found in young birds, including ingestion of substrate, toys, or feeding tubes. Diagnosis is based on clinical signs, history, and radiographs or CAT scan results. Treatment may require an ingluviotomy to gain access to the mucosal surface and lumen of the crop, proventriculus, or ventriculus. Removal of a foreign body, such as a feeding tube, is the most common indication for this procedure in pediatric birds. In larger or older birds, a rigid endoscope may be necessary to visualize and extract upper GI foreign bodies. The endoscope may be used either orally or through an ingluviotomy incision, depending on the accessibility of the foreign body.

Crop Stasis: Crop stasis, defined as the inability of the crop to empty in a normal time frame, is a common condition in hand-fed chicks. Crop stasis can occur due to poor husbandry and nutritional practices or primary disease. Environmental temperatures that are too cold or inadequate humidity can lead to crop stasis, as can feeding formula that is too cold or thick. All aspects of the nursery and feeding practices should be evaluated.

Clinical signs include a distended crop, dehydration, poor feeding response, regurgitation, and depression. Diagnosis is based on physical examination findings, palpation of the crop, and cytology and/or culture of the crop contents.

Treatment may include physically emptying the crop, fluid therapy, antibiotics and /or antifungals, and providing smaller, more dilute, and more frequent feedings once the crop is emptying.

Crop Burns: Crop burns result from feeding baby bird formula that is too hot. This can occur when a microwave oven is used to heat the formula (not recommended because of the formation of hot spots within the formula). Mild cases may result in red and inflamed skin in the area of the crop. Second- and third-degree burns will be acutely inflamed and blistered and may lead to tissue necrosis and fistula formation. In subacute cases, birds may be presented with food draining from a fistula through the crop wall and skin. Diagnosis is based on history, clinical signs, and physical examination findings. Treatment includes antibiotics, supplemental fluids, anti-inflammatory drugs, and nutritional support. Surgical repair is often required but should be postponed until the burned area is well demarcated (usually several days); repair involves debriding devitalized tissues, separating the crop wall from overlying skin, and closing the two layers separately. Prognosis is good if the remaining crop wall is sufficient for closure and the esophagus is intact.

Esophageal and Pharyngeal Trauma: Esophageal and pharyngeal trauma occurs from improper hand-feeding technique, either with the syringe tip or a rigid feeding tube. This leads to tissue trauma, cellulitis, and distribution of food into subcutaneous tissues. Birds may present depressed, anorexic, cold, and dehydrated, with poor feeding response. Swelling may be palpable in the neck area. Diagnosis is based on the history of hand feeding and oral or endoscopic examination to identify the puncture site.

Surgically opening the pockets, flushing the wounds, and allowing for drainage is important in treatment, along with antibiotics, analgesics, anti-inflammatory drugs, and supportive care. Prognosis depends on severity of the lesion, amount of food deposited in the tissues, and how quickly the lesion is detected and treated. In severely traumatized cases, prognosis is guarded to poor.

Hepatic Lipidosis: The liver relative to total body weight is typically larger in neonates than in adult birds, so some degree of hepatomegaly is normal in chicks. However, neonates with hepatic lipidosis typically have the following characteristics: 1) they are usually still being hand fed, often with a commercial formula to which the owners have added peanut butter, oil, or some other high-fat food, and 2) they are usually heavy for their age and exhibit severe respiratory distress. These birds must be handled gently and minimally. Cool oxygenation is the best first step. They have virtually no air sac capacity, and the stress of feeding and breathing at the same time may exceed their oxygen reserves. Drastically reducing the quantity of crop food per feeding, adjusting the content of the formula, and adding lactulose to the formula are the general nutritional changes required. Parenteral fluid supplementation will help keep the initially hyperthermic bird hydrated. When possible, blood samples should be submitted to check for concurrent infection or other diseases.

Failure to Thrive: Hereditary, congenital, and husbandry issues may affect the growth of young birds. Stunted chicks are thin, and the head is disproportionately large. Toes, wings, and hips are thin; eye and ear openings may be delayed. The skin may be dry and without adequate subcutaneous fat. Abnormal feather patterns (swirls) may develop on the head of a stunted chick. Stunting can develop early, in the first 30 days, or shortly after purchase from the breeder. Usually stunting is caused by husbandry and nutritional issues, often because of handlers inexperienced at hand feeding. Inappropriate quantities of hand-feeding formula, incorrect temperature, and incorrect consistency of the formula cause reduced feeding response and/or GI stasis. Birds purchased soon after arriving at the pet store are often mistakenly labeled as "weaned." In nature, these birds would be eating partially on their own but still receiving supplementation from their parents. When such a bird is sold to an uninformed owner, it usually takes a few days to a few weeks for the bird's insufficient food intake to create noticeable debilitation and weakness. These birds may also have underlying problems, eg, decreased hepatic function or immunosuppression.

Diagnosis is based on the history and physical examination findings. Treatment is supportive (fluids, nutritional support, and warmth). Antibiotics or antifungal drugs may or may not be needed, based on diagnostic test results. Some of these birds will survive, but many will not.

Splayleg or Rotational Leg Deformity: The term splayleg is a catchall for deformities of the legs in young birds. Often, there are laxities of the ligaments of the stifle and/or angular deformities of the femur, tibiotarsus, and tarsometatarsus. Causes are poorly documented, but risk factors include nutritional deficiencies (consistent with those of metabolic bone disease, *see* p 1917) and insufficient support or substrate in the enclosure.

Various methods of external coaptation have been devised and are most successful when the bird is young. Placing the chick in a deep enclosure with a suspensory device or cloth that allows the leg to be directed vertically or taping the legs together in a "hobble" may be corrective if implemented early. Stifle subluxation can develop because of disruption of the cruciate and /or collateral ligaments. Surgery (osteotomy and external skeletal fixator) may be used for rotational deformities.

Beak Deformities: Mandibular prognathism commonly occurs in several birds from the same clutch and is seen most commonly in cockatoos. If detected early, the hand feeder may be able to correct prognathism by pulling the beak upward and out for several minutes, several times a day. In older chicks, the condition may require a prosthetic that pulls the upper beak out and over the lower beak. This can be cumbersome and painful, and the prosthetic often needs to be reapplied. Trans-sinus pinning is a more recent and more reliable method of correction but carries some risk.

Scissor beak is a lateral deviation of the upper or lower beak. This may be caused by improper incubation temperature or possibly genetic factors in some chicks. If detected early, mild scissor beak can be corrected by manually placing a counter force on the beak for several minutes 2–3 times daily. More severe defects may require placing a beak prosthetic.

Constricted Toe Syndrome: Constricted toe syndrome is fairly common in neonates, often affecting more than one digit. An annular band of fibrous tissue forms at a joint of the digit, impeding circulation. The cause is unknown, although either excessively low or high humidity and septicemia have been proposed. This syndrome is most common in *Eclectus* parrots and macaws, usually in chicks housed in environments with inadequate humidity.

When detected early, debriding the annular band and applying a moist dressing is often effective. In more severe cases, small longitudinal incisions can be made on the medial and lateral surfaces of the affected toe to allow for swelling and to promote circulation. If circulation loss is severe and necrosis is apparent, amputation may be necessary. NSAIDs can be used to reduce inflammation and pain. A bandage will protect the site from contamination and secondary infection. Early detection and intervention is critical in successful treatment.

Toe Malposition: Toe malposition usually involves the lateral or fourth toe, which points forward instead of backward. If discovered early, malposition is easily corrected by taping the toe in a normal position. In young birds, the foot can be bandaged with the toe pointing backward in the normal position for several days. Older chicks may need prolonged bandaging.

Cryptophthalmia (Eyelid Atresia): Cryptophthalmia is most commonly seen in cockatiels and is often observed in clutch mates. The condition is usually bilateral. The eyelids, if present, are generally normal in conformation but greatly reduced in length, leading to small to nonexistent palpebral fissures. If the palpebral fissure is sufficient to allow functional vision, no correction is needed or recommended. Extending the palpebral fissure by conjunctival eversion can be performed with modest success when the palpebral aperture is absent or reduced and functional vision is compromised.

"Lockjaw": *Bordetella avium* is the causative agent of a syndrome that can appear in clutch mates, most commonly in cockatiels. Bacterial invasion from the sinuses progresses to the skeletal muscle of the mandible, resulting in a myositis and "lockjaw." Treatment is antibiotics and supportive care. Manually opening the beak can be difficult, so feeding and medicating the bird can be challenging. Prognosis is guarded to grave.

Choanal Atresia: Choanal atresia is seen most commonly in African grey parrots but has also been documented in other species. With choanal atresia, the communication between the nares, infraorbital sinus, and the choana is incomplete or absent. Clinical signs are increased mucus accumulation and possible infection in the nares and sinuses. Blunted choanal papilla may be detected on oral examination. Diagnosis is by endoscopic examination of the choana.

Atresia can be treated by creating an opening in the choana through the nares with an intramedullary pin. A red rubber feeding tube is then threaded through the nares, out the choana, and back behind the head of the bird and is left in place for 2–3 wk. This procedure is usually performed in stages, beginning with a small tube first and following with a larger tube.

BACTERIAL DISEASES

Bacterial diseases are common in pet birds and should be considered in the differential list of any sick bird. Inappropriate husbandry and nutrition are often contributing factors. Neonates and young birds are especially susceptible. GI and respiratory infections are most common and can lead to systemic disease.

Normal bacterial flora of companion birds include *Lactobacillus*, *Corynebacterium*, nonhemolytic *Streptococcus*, *Micrococcus* spp, and *Staphylococcus epidermidis*.

The most commonly reported pathogens are gram-negative bacteria (*Klebsiella*, *Pseudomonas*, *Aeromonas*, *Enterobacter*, *Proteus*, and *Citrobacter* spp, *Escherichia coli*, and *Serratia marcescens*). *Pasteurella* spp have been reported as possible septicemic agents in birds attacked by pet cats or rats. *Mycobacterium* and *Chlamydia* are common intracellular bacterial pathogens. Infections with *Salmonella* spp are occasionally seen.

The most common gram-positive bacterial pathogens are *Staphylococcus aureus*, *S intermedius*, *Clostridium*, *Enterococcus*, *Streptococcus*, and other *Staphylococcus* spp. Methicillin-resistant *S aureus* (MRSA) is rare but has been documented. *Mycoplasma* spp have been implicated in chronic sinusitis, often found in cockatiels. This organism is difficult to culture, and the true incidence is unknown. Staphylococci and streptococci (especially hemolytic strains) and *Bacillus* spp are thought to be responsible for several dermatologic conditions in psittacine birds. Staphylococci are often isolated from lesions of pododermatitis (bumblefoot) in many avian species.

Clostridial organisms are common secondary invaders of damaged cloacal tissue in birds with cloacal prolapse or papillomatosis. Several specific syndromes of birds can arise from various species of clostridia. A Gram stain or anaerobic culture is necessary to identify these organisms.

Diagnosis is based on clinical signs and results of cytologic examination and culture of tissue or swab samples. A Gram stain is used to identify normal flora, yeast, and spore-forming bacteria. Culture is needed to identify specific organisms and their sensitivity to antibiotics. Samples can be obtained from the respiratory, GI, urinary, and reproductive tracts. Sample sites for culture and cytology include the choanal slit, sinus, cloaca, wounds, conjunctiva, internal organs (via ultrasound-guided fine-needle aspirates, endoscopic examination, or surgery), and blood.

Treatment is based on location of infection and results of culture and sensitivity testing. See TABLE 16 for a partial list of frequently recommended antimicrobials.

Chlamydiosis

(Psittacosis, Ornithosis)

Chlamydia psittaci is an obligate intracellular bacterium that can infect all companion birds but is especially common in cockatiels, budgerigars, and parrots. Current state and federal regulations governing the testing, reporting, treatment, and quarantine for *Chlamydia* should be followed.

TABLE 16 ANTIMICROBIALS USED IN PET BIRDS

Antimicrobial[a]	Dose, Route, and Frequency[b]
Amikacin sulfate	15 mg/kg, IM, bid
Amoxicillin/clavulanate	125 mg/kg, PO, tid
Azithromycin	50 mg/kg/day, PO
Ceftazidime sodium	75 mg/kg, IM, tid
Ciprofloxacin	25 mg/kg, PO, bid
Clindamycin	100 mg/kg, PO, bid for 5 days to treat *Clostridium*
Doxycycline	25 mg/kg, PO, bid for 45 days[c]
Doxycycline injectable, 20 mg/mL	75–100 mg/kg, IM or SC, every 5 days, then weekly for six treatments[c]
Enrofloxacin	15–20 mg/kg, PO or IM, bid
Metronidazole	25 mg/kg, PO, bid for 14 days for *Giardia*, *Clostridium*
Marbofloxacin	2.5 mg/kg/day, PO
Trimethoprim/sulfamethoxazole	50–100 mg/kg, PO, bid

[a] Most are unapproved for use in birds, and caution is indicated.

[b] May vary with etiology and species treated

[c] Duration and dosage for treatment of *Chlamydia*

The incubation period of *C psittaci* is from 3 days to several weeks. The organism is excreted in the feces and in nasal and ocular discharge of infected birds. Although labile in the environment, the organism can remain infectious in organic debris for >1 mo.

Clinical signs range from asymptomatic carriers to severe disease and may include ocular, nasal, or conjunctival irritation and discharge; anorexia; dyspnea; depression; dehydration; polyuria; biliverdinuria; and diarrhea. Clinically ill birds may have a leukocytosis, monocytosis, and increased AST and bile acid concentrations. Radiographs may reveal hepatomegaly, splenomegaly, or airsacculitis.

Diagnosis of *C psittaci* can be challenging, especially in the absence of clinical signs. Few laboratories will culture the organism. Various antibody and antigen tests are available, but these have limitations. Serologic tests available include indirect fluorescent antibody, complement fixation, ELISA, and fluorescent antibody. A positive serologic test result is evidence that a bird has been infected but might not indicate active infection. Exposed but clinically normal birds may produce appreciable antibody titers. Acutely ill birds may not mount an antibody response, also yielding false-negative results. These factors make an antibody test an insufficient screening tool for chlamydiosis in birds when used alone. Because of the intracellular nature of *Chlamydia* and the reduction in numbers of organisms that accompanies antibiotic use, false-negative results of antigen tests are common. With the advent of PCR testing, diagnosis of *Chlamydia* is more readily accomplished, and attempts to culture the organism or identify elementary bodies in tissue specimens are rarely done. Laboratories should be consulted before shipment to identify appropriate samples and shipping methods. Because of the difficulty in diagnosing *Chlamydia*, a single test method may not be adequate, and a PCR assay of a combined conjunctival, choanal, and cloacal swab sample, in conjunction with a serologic test, is recommended.

Doxycycline is commonly used for treatment of *Chlamydia* infection. Because the treatment period required to eliminate the organism is uncertain, treatment for 45 days is recommended. Dietary calcium sources should be reduced if doxycycline *is administered orally*. Clinically ill birds should be treated with oral or injectable doxycycline initially to establish therapeutic drug levels quickly. Formulations of doxycycline in the food or water and chlortetracycline-impregnated seeds or other foods are available or can be manufactured to treat infected flocks. A doxycycline-medicated feed for budgerigars can be created by combining 300 mg of doxycycline hyclate (from capsules) with 1 kg of a mixture of oats, millet, and sunflower oil (1 part cracked steel oats is mixed with 3 parts hulled millet; add 5–6 mL of sunflower oil per kg of the oat/seed mixture). Fresh medicated mix should be made daily and fed as the sole diet for 30 days. Doxycycline may also be added to the water for cockatiels (200–400 mg doxycycline hyclate/L of water), Goffin's cockatoos (400–600 mg/L), and African grey parrots (800 mg/L). A doxycycline syrup, using a monohydrate- or calcium-syrup formulation, can be given at 40–50 mg/kg/day, PO, to cockatiels, Senegal parrots, and blue-fronted and orange-winged Amazon parrots; in African grey parrots, Goffin's cockatoos, blue and gold macaws, and green-winged macaws, the recommended dosage is 25 mg/kg/day, PO. These indirect modes of antibiotic administration depend on ingesting sufficient quantities of antibiotics to maintain effective blood levels, which may not always occur. Only certain formulations of doxycycline can be given IM or SC. Doxycycline injectable has been successful at 75–100 mg/kg every 5–7 days for 6 wk.

Because *C psittaci* is transmissible to people, the zoonotic risk must be considered when designing the diagnostic and therapeutic plan. Current state and federal regulations governing the testing, reporting, treatment, and quarantine for birds infected with *Chlamydia* should be followed. A compendium of control measures is available at www.nasphv.org/documentsCompendia-Psittacosis.html.

Avian Mycobacteriosis

Avian mycobacteriosis infections are usually caused by *Mycobacterium avium* and *M genavense*. *Mycobacterium intracellulare*, *M bovis*, and *M tuberculosis* are less commonly reported. Psittacine birds most commonly infected are brotogeris parakeets and Amazon parrots. Avian mycobacteriosis is a chronic progressive disease affecting the liver and GI tract. Clinical signs include anorexia, weight loss, depression, and diarrhea. Birds with early infections may show few clinical signs.

Diagnosis of mycobacterial infection can be challenging and is most reliably done by acid-fast staining, culture, and/or DNA probe of a biopsy specimen. Biopsy of the liver, intestines, spleen, or a suspected mass is recommended; however, PCR testing of ultrasound-guided fine-needle aspirates of the liver may be diagnostic. Avian mycobacteria are difficult to culture, so a negative culture result does not exclude infection. A fecal acid-fast stain has poor sensitivity but may identify birds shedding large numbers of organisms; PCR testing of a fecal sample is a more sensitive test method. Most birds will have a significant leukocytosis with a monocytosis. Radiographs may reveal hepatomegaly and splenomegaly. Granulomas may occur that may be confused with tumors.

If infected birds are in a multiple bird collection, determining whether other birds are infected can be difficult. Husbandry and sanitation should be assessed. High-risk birds should be isolated and monitored by serial examinations (weights), CBCs, and fecal acid-fast stains or PCR testing.

Treatment involves combination antibiotic therapy for 6–12 mo or longer. Owner compliance is critical and should be discussed at length before beginning treatment. Use of multiple antibiotics (typically three) is recommended, because mycobacterial organisms are prone to developing antibiotic resistance. Antibiotics in differing combinations that have been used successfully are rifabutin (45 mg/kg), clarithromycin (60–85 mg/kg), ethambutol (30 mg/kg), and enrofloxacin (20–30 mg/kg). All combinations are used daily.

Birds with advanced disease and granuloma formation have a poor prognosis. Although human infection has not been associated with exposure to birds, precautions should be taken for zoonotic risk, especially in immunocompromised people.

MYCOTIC DISEASES

Fungal diseases are common in companion birds. Often, they are a secondary infection in an already ill or immunocompromised bird. The most common fungal diseases are respiratory tract infections caused by *Aspergillus* spp and GI tract infections caused by *Candida* spp. *Macrorhabdus* is an unusual fungus that affects the GI tract and occurs most commonly in small pet birds (budgerigars, lovebirds, finches, parrotlets, and cockatiels).

Candidiasis

Candidiasis is a common fungal disease seen in pet birds. The etiologic agent is the opportunistic yeast *Candida albicans*, which commonly affects the GI tract. Although *C albicans* is the most common isolate, others including *C tropicalis*, *C parapsilosis*, *C glabrata*, and *Hansenula* spp may also be found and may be refractory to treatment.

C albicans is not generally considered a primary pathogen. Small numbers of *Candida* are commonly found in the GI tract of birds and may become pathologic when normal digestive flora are disrupted by immunosuppression. (*See also* CANDIDIASIS, p 2791.)

Candidiasis most commonly affects unweaned chicks. Those on broad-spectrum antibiotics are most at risk. Neonatal cockatiels are considered most susceptible. Infection may be endogenous, because of yeast overgrowth, or caused by oral inoculation of large numbers of *Candida*, either by parental feeding or by hand feeding with utensils that are inadequately cleaned.

Clinical signs in adult birds are typically mild and may include mild weight loss, lethargy, and dull plumage. Young birds may have more severe disease, especially if they are immunocompromised. Clinical signs in juvenile birds include anorexia, crop stasis, white plaques in the oral cavity, regurgitation, and weight loss. Localized infections in the oral cavity can lead to difficulty swallowing or halitosis. With severe infections, there may be complete crop and GI stasis. Thickening of the crop may develop (Turkish-towel appearance). Infection of the proventriculus and ventriculus can also occur and may lead to more severe clinical signs such as weight loss, regurgitation, diarrhea, and depression. *See* TABLE 17 for differential diagnoses for regurgitation in birds.

Diagnosis of candidiasis is by identifying *Candida* spp on a Gram, Romanowsky-type, or new methylene blue stain of the feces, crop contents, or regurgitated material. Scrapings or impression smears may also be performed to diagnose suspected yeast infections of the skin. In severe cases, when tissue invasion has occurred, the budding yeast will produce hyphae that can be seen in scrapings obtained from the crop or pharynx, or from the feces.

Often candidiasis is secondary to poor husbandry and an unclean environment. If a reservoir of exogenous *Candida* is present (eg, poor nest box or feeding tube hygiene), then eliminating the source of the *Candida* is critical. In neonates with crop stasis, the crop must be emptied and smaller amounts fed until the crop stasis has resolved. Metoclopramide may help

TABLE 17 DIFFERENTIAL DIAGNOSES FOR REGURGITATION IN PET BIRDS

Problem	Species Commonly Affected	Common Agents (if known)	Typical Signs
Toxicosis	Various	Lead, zinc, pesticides, medications	Vomiting, abnormal droppings, lethargy, possible CNS signs
Oral upper GI irritation	Cockatiels, various	Plants (*Pothos*, *Philodendron*), various medications, other caustic materials	Lethargy, ptyalism, passive regurgitation of water, erythema of tongue and pharynx
Proventricular dilatation syndrome	Macaws, miniature macaws, African grey parrots, cockatoos, others	Avian bornavirus	Weight loss, vomiting, seeds in feces, possible CNS signs
Bacterial GI infections	Various	Gram-negative bacteria	Vomiting, watery droppings, lethargy
Candidiasis	Cockatiels, lovebirds, others	*Candida* spp	Regurgitation, crop distention, oropharyngeal and crop lesions
Trichomoniasis	Budgerigars, cockatiels, doves, others	*Trichomonas* spp	Regurgitation, mouth and crop lesions (white matter), mucus in crop
Ventricular, proventricular, or crop obstruction	Cockatoos, macaws, *Eclectus* parrots, cockatiels, others	Wood shavings, corncob bedding, other bedding, fibers, foreign bodies, ascarids	Vomiting, depression, weight loss
Proventricular adenocarcinoma	Various	Neoplasm	Vomiting, weight loss, lethargy, severe pain, sudden death
Internal papillomatosis	Amazons, macaws	Psittacine herpesvirus 1	Vomiting, straining to defecate, secondary cloacal and choanal infections
Abdominal mass	Budgerigars	Renal or gonadal mass—usually neoplasia	Weight loss, lameness, vomiting
Behavioral	Various	Courtship behavior	Regurgitation on mirror, owner, toy, or cagemate

crop motility and prevent regurgitation. After identifying and resolving any predisposing factors, treatment with nystatin or fluconazole should be initiated. Nystatin (300,000 IU/kg, PO, bid) is commonly used for treatment because of its low cost and low toxicity. Disadvantages are poor taste and large volume required. Because it is fungistatic and not absorbed from the GI tract, it is only effective when in direct contact with infected tissue, so it is often administered tid before feeding. If the yeast is resistant to nystatin or the bird is difficult to medicate, then fluconazole (20 mg/kg, PO, every 48 hr) is available for systemic treatment.

Flock treatment has historically been accomplished with use of chlorhexidine at

10 mL/gal. of drinking water for 1–3 wk. Because chlorhexidine is a disinfectant, its use will also deplete the normal digestive flora. Acidification of the upper GI tract by use of apple cider vinegar has also been reported to resolve *Candida* overgrowth.

See TABLE 18 for some antifungal drugs used in pet birds.

Aspergillosis

Aspergillosis is an opportunistic infection that typically occurs in immunocompromised hosts (malnutrition, especially vitamin A deficiency) or when birds are exposed to large numbers of aerosolized spores. It is not transmitted bird-to-bird. *Aspergillus fumigatus* is the most common species isolated; *A flavus* and *A niger* are also found. *Rhizopus*, *Penicillium*, *Mucor*, and *Scedosporium apiospermum* can cause similar signs and are more difficult to diagnose and treat. Predisposing factors for developing infection include species predilection (African grey parrots, Amazon parrots, cockatiels, and macaws), aspiration of food or medications, immunosuppression (underlying disease), moldy bedding or feed, and use of corticosteroids. Poor hygiene and inadequate ventilation,

TABLE 18 ANTIFUNGALS USED IN PET BIRDS

Antifungal[a]	Dosage	Route, Frequency
Amphotericin B	1 mg/kg intratracheal; 0.25–1 mg/mL sterile water for nebulization	Given intratracheally once daily; nebulized 10–20 min, bid
	1.5 mg/kg	IV, tid
Amphotericin B suspension	100 mg/kg	PO, bid × 30 days
Clotrimazole	2 mg/kg	Given intratracheally, once daily × 5 days
	10 mg/mL (1%)	Nasal flush; nebulized for 30 min bid
Enilconazole	1 mg (0.05 mL/kg of a 1:10 dilution)	Given intratracheally, once daily × 7–14 days
	0.1 mL/kg in 5 mL sterile water	Nebulize for 30 min, 5 days on, 2 days off
Fluconazole	5–15 mg/kg	PO, bid
	20 mg/kg	PO, every 48 hr × 3 treatments
Griseofulvin	10 mg/kg	PO, bid
5-Flucytosine	20–75 mg/kg	PO, bid
F-10[b] (quaternary ammonium disinfectant)	1.5/400 mL distilled water	Nebulization for cutaneous and possibly respiratory fungus
Itraconazole	5–10 mg/kg	PO, once to twice daily (lower dosage, and use cautiously in African grey parrots)
Ketoconazole	10–30 mg/kg	PO, bid
Terbinafine	10–15 mg/kg 1 mg/mL solution	PO, bid Nebulization for 30 min
Nystatin oral suspension (100,000 U/mL)	300,000–600,000 U/kg	PO, bid
Voriconazole	12–18 mg/kg	PO, bid

[a] Most are unapproved for use in birds, and caution is indicated.

[b] Quaternary ammonium and biguanidine compound; nontoxic, ampholytic surfactant

especially in warm, humid climates, can also increase the incidence of disease.

Clinical Findings: Clinical signs depend on the site of infection. Most infections occur in the upper respiratory tract, air sacs, lungs, trachea, and syrinx. Systemic infections occur when the infection spreads to internal organs, including bone, liver, kidneys, or brain. Eye and skin infections can also occur. Anorexia and weight loss are often present. Respiratory signs may include dyspnea, tail bobbing, exercise intolerance, and voice change. Rhinitis caused by *Aspergillus* appears similar to bacterial rhinitis or sinusitis. A Gram stain or modified Wright's stain of lesions or debris often demonstrates fungal hyphae. Infraorbital sinusitis caused by aspergillosis often must be surgically debrided before therapy is effective. Extensive or chronic fungal sinusitis may lead to osseous changes and permanent malformation of the upper respiratory architecture. Extension of infection to the brain can cause CNS signs.

Tracheitis due to aspergillosis can occur in immunocompromised birds. *Aspergillus* granulomas often form in the syrinx of psittacine birds and raptors and are particularly challenging to treat. Changes in vocalization may occur before dyspnea is observed, and often these birds will stretch out their necks while breathing. Lower respiratory disease, including airsacculitis, often involves invasion by *Aspergillus* spp. Granulomas of the air sacs or the coelomic cavity are also common, usually in the caudal thoracic or abdominal air sacs. These lesions may require surgical resection.

Diagnosis: Diagnosis can be challenging but should be pursued because treatment is longterm and costly. Aspergillosis should be considered in any pet bird presenting with signs of upper or lower respiratory disease, wasting disease, or marked leukocytosis/monocytosis. A leukocytosis/monocytosis combined with clinical signs and radiographic findings can provide a strong presumptive diagnosis in suspect cases. Often birds with chronic disease will be anemic. A radiograph may reveal airsacculitis, granulomas, or severe pulmonary disease. A CT scan or MRI is more likely to reveal more subtle or diffuse disease. Serologic testing is of limited use; antibody and antigen titers, including galactomannan antigen testing, often result in false-negative or false-positive results. A false-negative often occurs because of immunosuppression, so consultation with the laboratory regarding interpretation is important. PCR testing to detect specific *Aspergillus* DNA is a much more sensitive method to confirm infection and is more suitable for immunocompromised birds because detection of antibodies is not involved. Plasma protein electrophoresis showing increased β-globulin levels is consistent with aspergillosis. Definitive diagnosis may require direct visualization of lesions either by surgery or endoscopy and confirmation by biopsy, cytology, and/or fungal culture of lesions. Low fungal viability may yield a negative culture despite confirmation by cytologic results.

Treatment: Treatment varies depending on the site of infection. An acute tracheal infection with obstruction by an aspergilloma is an emergency that may require placing an air sac tube. After tube placement, syringeal or tracheal plaques are removed with a rigid endoscope. Amphotericin B can then be instilled intratracheally at 1 mg/kg through the glottis, and treatment with systemic antifungals and nebulization should be started. Amphotericin B is the only fungicidal agent available and can be used in nebulization, as a nasal flush, intratracheally, and in IV administration. For nebulization, a concentration of 0.25–1 mg/mL of sterile water can be used. Nasal and sinus flushes are generally more dilute at 0.05 mg/mL of sterile water. Amphotericin should not be diluted with saline, because this decreases its potency.

Flushing the nares and sinus with unmedicated sterile water or saline before medicating may allow samples to be obtained for cytologic examination and culture. Several flushes of unmedicated warm isotonic saline or sterile water should be done before a final infusion of the medicated mixture. Care must be exercised to maintain the bird's head in a downward position to avoid the potential for aspiration of the infected debris into the lower respiratory tract.

Itraconazole (5–10 mg/kg, PO, once to twice daily) is the most commonly used azole for systemic infection. African grey parrots are more sensitive to adverse effects of itraconazole, especially regurgitation and anorexia, and should be dosed at 5 mg/kg/day, PO. Terbinafine (10–15 mg/kg, PO, bid) can be used in lieu of or in conjunction with itraconazole. Clotrimazole can be used for nebulization in conjunction with systemic therapy (10 mg/mL, nebulized 15–30 min

2–4 times/day). Voriconazole (12–18 mg/kg, PO, bid) is being used for resistant strains of *Aspergillus*.

If fungal granulomas are identified and the lesions are accessible, debulking endosurgically or treating the lesions topically with amphotericin B may improve the outcome. Birds undergoing treatment should be monitored closely for adverse effects of many antifungal drugs, which can include depression, anorexia, and liver dysfunction. Hepatic enzyme, bile acids, and uric acid concentrations should be monitored every 4 wk during treatment. Treatment success may be difficult to determine, but serial CBCs and radiographs may be helpful. Treatment with oral drugs should be continued for 2–4 wk after clinical signs have resolved. Birds with aspergillosis often have underlying disease problems and may be immunocompromised, which may affect treatment and recovery. Thickened and scarred air sacs that develop during and persist after infection can provide an ideal environment for disease recurrence.

Macrorhabdus ornithogaster Infection

(Macrorhabdosis, Megabacteria, Avian gastric yeast)

Macrorhabdus ornithogaster most often affects the proventriculus and ventriculus of smaller companion birds (eg, budgerigars, parrotlets, lovebirds, cockatiels, and finches). Previously described as a bacterium, this organism has a worldwide distribution and varies widely in pathogenicity.

Clinical Findings and Diagnosis: Clinical signs of infection are weight loss, regurgitation, lethargy, passage of undigested food, and diarrhea. These clinical signs may mimic proventricular dilatation disease. Mortality may be high, but birds may recover. In birds that recover, relapses and potential shedding of the organism in the feces are likely. This disease is often seen in conjunction with immunosuppression (eg, polyomavirus and circovirus infection, or associated with poor husbandry). Asymptomatic infection is common.

Diagnosis is made by examining a wet mount of a fresh dropping at 10–50× magnification with the stage condenser mostly closed to increase contrast. The large, rod-shaped organisms are approximately 2–4 μm wide and 60–90 μm long. Many birds are asymptomatic and shed low numbers of organisms, whereas sick birds tend to shed large numbers. Birds may shed the organism intermittently, so a negative fecal examination does not exclude infection. Wet mount, modified Wright's, or Gram stain of a fecal sample often reveal organisms. *M ornithogaster* appears as a large, gram-positive rod, with mottling or stippling throughout its length. Although the size and length may vary, organisms recovered from the droppings are generally several magnitudes larger than the normal digestive bacilli found in birds. Selected veterinary laboratories offer both visual identification and PCR testing. *M ornithogaster* does not grow on conventional fungal media. Radiographs may reveal a dilated proventriculus. Necropsy lesions may include thinning of the isthmus, proventricular dilation and ulceration, thickening of the proventricular wall, mucus production, and softening of the koilin layer of the ventriculus.

Treatment and Control: The goals of treatment are to reduce the number of organisms and improve the general health and immunocompetence of the bird. Amphotericin (100 mg/kg, PO, bid for 30 days) has had the highest treatment success rate, but failures are common, especially with a shorter duration of treatment. Acidification of the proventriculus (apple cider vinegar, vitamin C) has been reported to create an environment less conducive to proliferation of *Macrorhabdus*. Voriconazole has been successful (anecdotal) at 10 mg/kg, PO, bid.

Treatment with sodium benzoate in the drinking water has been anecdotally reported to be successful but still experimental. Sodium benzoate at 1 tsp/L water for 5 wk cleared the infection in nonbreeding budgerigars, but in budgerigars that were rearing chicks in high environmental temperatures >90°F, treatment with ½ tsp/L water resulted in neurologic signs and death of the adult budgerigars because of their increased water intake. The current recommendation for treatment of *Macrorhabdus* with sodium benzoate is ½ tsp (2.5 g) of sodium benzoate powder/L of water (used as only water source and made fresh daily). If the birds are not drinking the medicated water, the dose should be decreased to ¼ tsp (1.25 g)/L of water, and slowly increased back to ½ tsp over the next few days. Feces should be rechecked at 14 days; if *Macrorhabdus* organisms are still present, the dose should be increased over several days to 1 tsp (5 g)/L. Feces should be rechecked at 30 days. The lower dose of ¼ to ½ tsp powder/L of water should be used in birds housed outdoors in summer (temperatures >90°F [32.2°C]) and in birds feeding chicks. Gloves should be worn when handling medication.

Asymptomatic carriers are common. Artificial incubation of eggs and hand feeding nestlings can help establish a pathogen-free flock.

Malassezia spp

Malassezia spp have been reported in birds with feather picking and dermatologic conditions. In suspect cases, biopsy or cytology should be performed. Culture is often unrewarding. The recommended treatment is fluconazole at 5–10 mg/kg, PO, once to twice daily. Topical therapy with either dilute chlorhexidine 0.1% spray or clotrimazole may be used alone or in conjunction with systemic treatment.

Cryptococcus neoformans

Cryptococcosis is worldwide in occurrence and caused by a saprophytic fungus, *Cryptococcus neoformans*. This fungus is uncommon in avian species, but it has been isolated from the fecal droppings of wild birds, particularly pigeons, and from feces of canaries and psittacine birds. *C neoformans* infection has been reported in Columbiformes, a Moluccan cockatoo, a thick-billed parrot, a green-wing macaw, and an African grey parrot. Veterinarians should be aware that not only can birds be carriers of the disease and become ill but also that *C neoformans* is zoonotic. Most human infections with *C neoformans* occur in immunocompromised individuals and are associated with environmental exposure, although cases have been reported in which contact with a pet bird appeared to be the source of infection.

Clinical signs of *Cryptococcus* infection include weakness, lethargy, anorexia, diarrhea, and dyspnea. With CNS involvement, neurologic signs such as blindness and paralysis may occur. Clinical diagnosis can be difficult. A definitive diagnosis requires demonstrating the organism on cytologic or histologic examination or culture. The organism is a round to oval yeast with a mucopolysaccharide capsule. A mucoid gelatinous exudate may be noted within the respiratory tract, coelomic cavity, sinuses, brain, or within the long bones.

Treatment recommendations for birds include amphotericin B, itraconazole, ketoconazole, fluconazole, or voriconazole. Fluconazole or voriconazole are the drugs of choice for CNS or ocular infections.

Rhodotorula mucilaginosis

Rhodotorula mucilaginosis is a yeast occasionally seen in skin infection in raptors (falcons). It causes yellowish brown crusty areas of the skin in the axillary or inguinal areas. Untreated lesions may develop into hyperkeratotic proliferative growths. Diagnosis is based on physical examination findings and results of cytologic or histopathologic examination and culture of infected tissues.

Treatment involves excision of proliferative lesions and topical antifungal therapy. Antibiotics may be necessary to prevent secondary infections, and analgesics or anti-inflammatory drugs may be warranted for pain.

Miscellaneous Mycoses

Dermatophytosis, including *Trichophyton* and *Microsporum* spp is occasionally reported in pet birds. Treatment protocols for dogs and cats are used (*see* p 874). Histoplasmosis and mucormycosis are also occasionally reported in pet birds.

PARASITIC DISEASES

See also POULTRY, p 2780 et seq.
Parasitic disease has become less common in captive parrots throughout the past 20 yr with the restrictions against importation of wild-caught birds; many pet birds now are incubator hatched, hand raised, and have little to no access to the outdoors or to other birds. Commonly reported parasitic diseases include protozoal infections such as giardiasis in cockatiels, sarcocystis in larger parrots, and mites in budgerigars and passerines.

Parasites of the Circulatory System

See also BLOODBORNE ORGANISMS, POULTRY, p 2780.

Protozoa: *Haemoproteus* was previously documented with great frequency in imported *Cacatua* spp. *Leucocytozoon*, *Plasmodium*, and *Atoxoplasma* spp are all seen occasionally in various species, most commonly in raptors, canaries, and Columbiformes, and are currently not of major significance in psittacines. Atoxoplasmosis is still diagnosed in canaries.

Parasites of the Gastrointestinal System

Giardiasis: Giardiasis has been reported in many species of birds but is most commonly seen in cockatiels. Adult birds may be latent carriers. Transmission is presumably direct (ingestion of infective cysts). Affected cockatiels occasionally exhibit feather pulling in the axillary and inner thigh regions, along with vocalization. A true causal relationship between giardiasis and these clinical signs has not been proved. Droppings of affected cockatiels may be voluminous and aerated (a "popcorn" appearance).

There are several ways to diagnose *Giardia* spp infection: the zinc sulfate flotation test of feces to detect cysts, the direct saline smear of fresh feces to detect motile trophozoites, and an ELISA test for *Giardia* spp antigen in feces. Because the presence of cysts is variable, serial tests may be needed. The accuracy of the *Giardia* spp SNAP test designed for people is unknown.

Metronidazole (50 mg/kg/day, for 5–7 days) or carnidazole (20 mg/kg/day, PO, for 1–2 days) is the recommended treatment. In cockatiels, treatment of giardiasis with fenbendazole at dosages extrapolated from dogs has been anecdotally reported to cause death.

Trichomoniasis: Trichomoniasis has been reported in many orders of birds, including Columbiformes, Galliformes, Falconiformes, Psittaciformes, and Passeriformes. *Trichomonas gallinae* (called frounce in birds of prey and canker in Columbiformes) is occasionally seen in pet birds, notably budgerigars. Clinical signs may include anorexia, dysphagia, weight loss, and dyspnea. Whitish yellow, caseous lesions adherent to the mucosa of the oropharynx, crop, and esophagus may be seen in raptors and Columbiformes. Budgerigars generally do not have grossly visible oral lesions but do have increased salivation and regurgitation. Transmission is by direct (parents feeding young) or indirect (ingestion of contaminated food and water) contact; raptors may become infected by ingesting infected pigeons or doves.

Microscopic examination of a warm saline mount of material from the oral cavity may reveal the flagellated organism. Treatment protocols include carnidazole (20 mg/kg, PO, once), ronidazole (6–10 mg/kg/day, PO, for 14 days), or metronidazole (50 mg/kg/day, PO, for 5 days).

Other Protozoal Diseases: Other protozoan parasites such as coccidia are much more common in gallinaceous or Columbiforme birds, although coccidial oocysts are seen occasionally in psittacine and passerine birds.

Cryptosporidiosis has been seen in a variety of avian species but is thought to be a secondary rather than a primary pathogen. Transmission of *Cryptosporidium* spp is through ingestion or inhalation of sporulated oocysts. Because of the small size and low shedding rate of *Cryptosporidium* spp, diagnosis can be difficult, but a Sheather's sugar flotation test is best. An acid-fast stain can also be used to detect the organism. Clinical signs may involve the GI, respiratory, or urinary tract, especially in immunosuppressed birds. Treatment for cryptosporidiosis in birds is not described.

***Plasmodium* spp** infection (malaria) is highly pathogenic in gyrfalcons, canaries, and penguins. *Plasmodium* is spread by mosquitoes. Clinical signs may be none to weakness and death. Treatment for malaria, if needed, is with chloroquine.

Atoxoplasmosis is a highly pathogenic protozoal disease that causes hepatomegaly and splenomegaly in canaries, with coccidia-like oocysts shed in the feces. The host becomes infected by ingesting the oocysts. Infected birds may be asymptomatic or exhibit anorexia, weight loss, diarrhea, and depression. Clinical disease is typically more severe in fledgling birds, whereas adults are often asymptomatic. Diagnosis is made by fecal flotation (best in adults), buffy coat smear with Romanowsky stain, liver impression smear, or PCR testing of feces. Treatment options are toltrazuril (12.5 mg/kg/day, PO, × 14 days) or sulfachlorpyridazine (150–300 mg/L drinking water, 5 days/wk × 2–3 wk).

Other protozoan parasites such as **coccidia** are much more common in gallinaceous or Columbiforme birds, although coccidial oocysts are seen occasionally in psittacine and passerine birds.

Roundworms: Various genera and species of roundworms infect pet birds, and wild birds may transmit nematodes to captive parrots housed outdoors. Transmission is direct by ingestion of embryonated ova. Clinical findings include loss of condition, weakness, emaciation, and death; intestinal obstruction is common in heavy infections. Diagnosis of intestinal nematode infection is by fecal flotation, although shedding of ova may be intermittent. Ivermectin (0.2 mg/kg, PO, SC, or IM, repeated in 10–14 days), pyrantel pamoate (4.5 mg/kg, PO, repeated in 10–14 days), or fenbendazole (20–50 mg/kg, PO, repeated in 14 days) are generally effective. In warm climates where exposure via outdoor aviaries is likely, routine deworming (every 6 mo) with one of these anthelmintics is often practiced.

Cestodes: Cestodes are uncommon in domestically bred birds. The most common pet birds infected with tapeworms are cockatoos, African grey parrots, and finches. Intermediate hosts are most likely insects and arachnids of various types, earthworms, and slugs. Infected birds are asymptomatic or are unthrifty, with or without diarrhea. Diagnosis is based on visualization of eggs on a fecal flotation.

Praziquantel (5–10 mg/kg, PO or IM, once) is the recommended treatment. Recurrence is rare in cases in which the intermediate host is not indigenous to the area where the bird is housed.

Parasites of the Integumentary System

Scaly Face (Leg) Mite: *Knemidocoptes pilae* (also *Cnemidocoptes pilae*) is common in budgerigars and rare in all other psittacine species. In budgerigars, white, porous, proliferative encrustations involving the corners of the mouth, cere, beak, and occasionally the periorbital area, legs, or vent are typical. In passerine birds (particularly canaries and European goldfinches), crusts form on the legs and surfaces of the digits ("tassel foot"). The mites can be recovered from facial scrapings of budgerigars, although the clinical appearance is generally pathognomonic. In passerines affected with *Knemidocoptes*, skin scrapings of the legs often result in hemorrhage and are generally not recommended. Ivermectin (0.2 mg/kg, PO or IM) or moxidectin (0.2 mg/kg, PO or topically) is generally effective. The treatment is repeated in 2 wk.

Feather Mites: Psittacine birds are seldom affected by feather mites. Occasionally, infestation with the red mite (*Dermanyssus gallinae*) may be found in outdoor aviaries, especially in nest boxes. A causative relationship between mites and feather picking is often assumed by owners of feather-picking birds, although this is rarely the case. More commonly, behavioral, husbandry, and/or systemic factors are linked to feather loss (*see* p 1927).

Mite-infested birds may be treated with pyrethrin sprays, 5% carbaryl powder, or ivermectin (0.2 mg/kg, PO or IM) repeated in 2 wk. Nest box treatment includes mixing 5% carbaryl powder into the nest box substrate. Cages should be cleaned thoroughly, and wooden nest boxes should be discarded and replaced.

Parasites of the Respiratory System

Air Sac Mites: *Sternostoma tracheacolum* parasitizes the entire respiratory tract, most frequently of canaries and gouldian finches. The mites are found in the trachea, syrinx, lungs, and air sacs. All stages of the mite are found within the respiratory tissues. The life cycle is poorly understood.

In mild infections, birds are usually asymptomatic; in heavy infections, audible dyspnea (high-pitched noises and clicking), sneezing, tail bobbing, and open-mouthed breathing are noted. Copious amounts of saliva are seen in the oropharynx, and ptyalism may be present. Signs are exacerbated by handling, exercise, and other stresses. Mortality can be high. Transillumination of the trachea in a darkened room occasionally reveals the mite. Response to treatment can help reach a diagnosis.

When the recovery of an individual bird is paramount, treatment should be administered quickly and with minimal handling. Ivermectin (0.2–0.4 mg/kg, PO or IM) repeated in 2 wk or moxidectin (0.2 mg/kg, PO or topically) repeated in 2 wk may be administered.

Sarcocystosis: Sarcocystosis is a major cause of mortality in parrots housed outdoors in the southern USA. In severely affected areas, even indoor birds can be infected via contaminated food. The oocysts of this protozoan parasite are passed from infected opossum feces by insects (eg, flies, cockroaches) or mice and rats into the feed cups or enclosure of the birds. The feces of these transport hosts are then consumed by the birds, and a rapidly fatal disease can develop. Old World species are immunologically naive to this disease, and a high mortality rate is observed in untreated birds such as cockatoos, African grey parrots, and *Eclectus* parrots. Cockatiels are also susceptible, and renal as well as pneumonic lesions are often noted at necropsy in this species. Although not contagious, cases tend to occur in clusters because the infected opossum feces are spread via insects around the aviary grounds. Large die-offs have been documented.

Clinical signs are lethargy, passive regurgitation of water, respiratory distress, weakness, ataxia, and anemia. In Old World parrots (eg, cockatoos, African grey parrots), disease occurs in the early stages of infection as the parasite is undergoing schizogony or merogony (asexual reproduction) in the lung. This causes lung damage, and the birds die acutely with or without signs of respiratory distress. In New World parrots (eg, macaws, conures), the organism encysts in the muscle or CNS, causing weakness, ataxia, or neurologic signs. The disease can manifest as an asymptomatic or clinically apparent muscular disease, cardiac disease, acute pulmonary disease, or encephalitis. Encephalitis (paresis, intention tremors, and head tilt) has been seen in psittacines and raptors.

No specific diagnostic test is available, although results of plasma protein electrophoresis may indicate infection (marked increase in β-globulin concentrations with or without a marked increase in gamma globulin concentrations). An indirect immunofluorescence antibody (IFA) test has been developed that may aid in antemortem diagnosis of the nonperacute form of sarcocystosis in psittacine birds. The sensitivity and specificity of the IFA test ranges from 83%–86%. Results of muscle biopsy may be conclusive for the encysted stages but is not commonly performed. When a muscle biopsy is done, the quadriceps muscle has been reported to be a better biopsy site than the pectoral muscle. Increases in enzyme activities of LDH, AST, and CK have been reported.

Protracted treatment with trimethoprim/sulfa (30 mg/kg, bid) and pyrimethamine (0.5 mg/kg, PO, bid) has had limited success. Response to treatment is generally monitored by serial PCV sampling. Newer drugs used to treat infection by the related protozoa, *Sarcocystis neurona*, that affects horses have not yet been evaluated for treatment in birds.

Gross necropsy findings include increased lung density, hemorrhage, and renal lesions. Clinical signs may also reflect CNS involvement. Histopathologic samples should include lung, kidney, muscle, and CNS tissue if neurologic signs are apparent.

VIRAL DISEASES

Avian Polyomavirus

(Papovavirus, Budgerigar fledgling disease, Psittacine polyomavirus)

Avian polyomavirus (APV) primarily affects young birds. There are two primary forms of the disease based on species affected: budgerigar fledgling disease and a nonbudgerigar polyoma infection. Both are characterized by peracute to acute death of preweaned neonates. Adult birds typically are resistant to infection; they will seroconvert and shed the virus for up to 90 days, then clear the infection. The incubation period is 7–10 days.

The typical presentation of budgerigar fledging disease is a well-fleshed juvenile, just before fledgling age, with acute onset of lethargy, crop stasis, and death within 24–48 hr. Other clinical signs are cutaneous hemorrhage, abdominal distention, and feather abnormalities. Surviving budgerigars >3 wk old often exhibit feather dystrophy (French molt or feather dusters). In other species of psittacines <4 mo old, the infection is also often fatal. Older nonbudgerigar psittacines may have subclinical disease or hemorrhages and coagulopathies. Prevalence of the virus in adult psittacines, including budgerigars, is thought to be high.

Antemortem diagnosis is accomplished with DNA probes of cloacal swab and blood samples and virus-neutralizing antibody tests of blood samples to identify birds with previous viral exposure. Diagnosis in a flock setting is typically based on clinical signs, signalment, and necropsy findings.

Gross necropsy findings in deceased chicks often include pale skeletal musculature and subcutaneous ecchymotic hemorrhages. The kidneys and liver are enlarged and may be pale, congested, and mottled, or have pinpoint, white foci. Petechial or ecchymotic hemorrhages may also be present on viscera, particularly the heart. The heart is sometimes enlarged and may show hydropericardium. Intranuclear inclusion bodies are often seen in the liver, kidneys, heart, spleen, bone marrow, uropygial gland, skin, feather follicles, etc.

Aviary control methods include avoiding the housing of budgerigars or lovebirds on premises where other species are bred, adhering to standard hygiene procedures, preventing access to the nursery by visitors, and not introducing birds into the aviary without 90 days quarantine and testing. Eliminating APV infection from an infected budgerigar aviary is challenging. First, all breeding must be stopped for 6 mo. The presence of infected neonates, fledglings, and adults propagates the disease. During this time, adult birds are moved to a noninfected area while the entire aviary is disinfected. Nest boxes should be disinfected or discarded and replaced. After 6 mo, adult breeding birds can be returned to a clean aviary and breeding resumed.

Pet store prevention should include separating neonates from different sources, purchasing birds from sources where polyomavirus testing and vaccination are performed, and ideally, not purchasing or selling unweaned birds.

Treatment is supportive care. A vaccine is available. For breeding birds, two doses of the vaccine are administered at a 2-wk interval; this should be done off-season. The manufacturer recommends administration of the first dose when the chick is >35 days old, with a booster vaccination in 2–3 wk.

Psittacine Beak and Feather Disease

Psittacine beak and feather disease (PBFD) is caused by a psittacine circovirus. The virus was first recognized in the 1970s in cockatoos with beak and feather lesions. Since then, it has been recognized in most species of parrots and also in Passeriformes and Columbiformes. Infected birds shed virus in their feathers, feather dander, feces, and oral secretions. Transmission occurs by inhalation and/or ingestion of the virus and can occur vertically. The virus is very stable in the environment, so fomites can be a significant source of infection. The name is not as representative of the current typical clinical presentation, which often does not include beak abnormalities and is less likely to have the severe, classic feather abnormalities seen in cockatoos when the disease was first documented. Use of screening PCR tests has greatly decreased the prevalence of the virus in captive bred *Cacatua* spp. However, disease is still seen in African grey parrots, *Eclectus* parrots, lovebirds (*Agapornis*), lorikeets, and other species, but is rare. The natural infection appears to occur primarily in juvenile birds, with few instances of clinical infection seen in birds >3 yr old.

In the classic PBFD infection, the first indication of the presence of disease is a lack of powder down on the beak. The virus causes abnormal formation of growing feathers and immunosuppression. Feathers are pinched or clubbed at their base and may have hemorrhage within the developing shaft. The feathers fall out easily and grow back slowly or not at all. The distribution of affected feathers depends on the age of the bird and the stage of the molt when infected. Pigment loss may occur in colored feathers. The bird may live with these lesions for months to years. As the disease progresses, the immune system is affected, and most birds die of secondary infections. A peracute form of the disease occurs in young birds, which develop enteritis and pneumonia, lose weight, and die. African grey parrots may develop a pancytopenia, because the virus attacks the bone marrow. These birds die suddenly with viral inclusions in the thymus, bursa, and bone marrow.

Diagnosis is based on clinical appearance; results of PCR testing of feces, feather dander, or blood; and biopsy of affected feather follicles showing basophilic intracytoplasmic inclusions. Testing by PCR may detect infection in birds that still appear healthy. These birds may subsequently become ill or may mount an effective response to the virus. Because of the stability of the virus, PCR analysis can also be used for environmental testing. Quarantine and retesting are recommended for PCR-positive, asymptomatic birds. At necropsy, affected birds often have no gross lesions internally, but intranuclear or intracytoplasmic inclusions may be seen histologically in the feathers, bursa, thymus, liver, or other organs.

There is no specific treatment for PBFD, and treatment of infected birds is supportive. The contagious nature of PBFD and its generally terminal outcome in clinically affected birds warrant isolation and eventual euthanasia in most clinical cases. Strict hygiene with attention to dust control, screening protocols including PCR testing of both birds and the environment, and lengthy quarantines are highly recommended in breeding facilities with susceptible species. All new susceptible birds should be tested before introduction to the aviary. In infected breeding colonies, removing all eggs for cleaning and artificial incubation may also be required. Since the development of a PCR-based assay, prevalence of the disease has decreased.

Pacheco's Disease

(Pacheco's herpesvirus)

Psittacine herpesvirus is an alpha herpesvirus that is the causative agent of Pacheco's disease and internal papillomatosis in parrots. Pacheco's disease causes a viral hepatitis seen predominantly in New World species (Amazon parrots, macaws, and conures). Internal papillomatosis occurs in parrots that have survived Pacheco's disease. Papillomatosis is most commonly observed in macaws, Amazon parrots, conures, and hawk-headed parrots. Disease is associated with stress, which can cause clinically healthy carriers to shed virus and initiate infection in susceptible birds, as often occurs during introduction of new birds, relocation, or in those with underlying illness or during breeding. It is spread by direct contact, aerosol, or fecal contamination of food or water, with an incubation period of 3–14 days. The outcome of the infection depends on the genotype of the virus, the species of bird infected, and the bird's overall health. Infected birds become chronic carriers and will remain persistently infected and intermittently shed the virus throughout their lives. Old World species are less likely to be either inapparent carriers or clinically susceptible. Patagonian species and some *Aratinga* spp may be natural hosts in the wild, and some individuals of these species may asymptomatically shed virus when stressed. Other species can also act as carriers.

Terminal signs include acute death in well-fleshed birds and bright yellow urates with scant feces. Other clinical signs are diarrhea, green urates, lethargy, regurgitation, weakness, and depression. Diagnosis in the live bird can be done by DNA probes of combined oral and cloacal swabs or blood samples. Increases in plasma AST activity and marked leukopenia have been reported.

Because of the acute nature of the disease, gross histologic lesions may not be evident. However, most affected birds will have hepatomegaly, splenomegaly, and renomegaly. The liver may be mottled or grossly discolored. Ecchymotic and petechial hemorrhages may be present on the pericardium and within the mesenteric fat. Intranuclear inclusions are seen histologically in the liver, spleen, intestinal epithelium, and pancreas. Primary differential diagnoses for Pacheco's disease include acute salmonellosis, polyomavirus, and psittacine reovirus. Acyclovir (80 mg/kg, tid, or 400 mg/kg in feed) can be used during an outbreak; however, the risk of increased transmission because of handling is great. Autogenous vaccines have been developed during outbreaks and have effectively decreased morbidity and mortality. An inactivated vaccine is available.

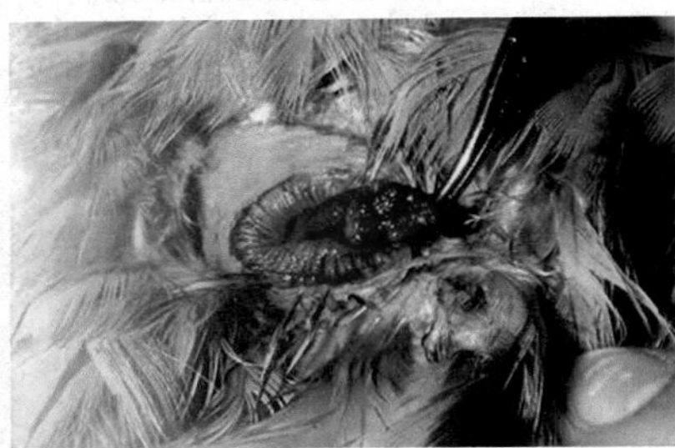

Cloacal papilloma, gross lesion, in a blue-fronted Amazon parrot. A red proliferative mass commonly originates from just inside the rim of the cloacal opening. *Courtesy of Dr. Louise Bauck.*

The lesions of **papillomatosis** are predominantly present in the oral and cloacal mucosa but may also be found internally in the intestinal tract, or less commonly, in the conjunctiva or bursa. Owners usually first notice blood from a papilloma in the droppings, and/or the papilloma prolapses through the cloaca. Lesions may be mild or severe (ulcerated and bleeding) and often wax and wane. Ulcerated lesions may need to be cauterized or surgically removed, although they typically recur. Treatment is supportive, such as analgesics, cautery, and antibiotics to prevent secondary infection. Antiherpesviral drugs are not curative and do not appear to impact the course of disease.

Other Herpesvirus Infections: **Amazon tracheitis** is also caused by a herpesvirus, although the incidence of this infection is low. Other clinically significant herpesviruses include the strain responsible for papillomatous foot lesions in *Cacatua* spp and the depigmentation lesions noted on the feet of macaws.

Avian Bornavirus/Proventricular Dilatation Disease

(Macaw wasting disease)

Proventricular dilatation disease (PDD), also known as macaw wasting disease, neuropathic ganglioneuritis, lymphoplasmacytic ganglioneuritis, psittacine encephalomyelitis, and most recently avian bornavirus (ABV), was first recognized in the late 1970s in macaws imported into the USA and Germany. The disease primarily affects macaws, conures, and African grey parrots, although all parrots are probably susceptible. The causative agent of this disease is avian bornavirus.

The common presentation of affected birds is chronic weight loss (often following an initial increase in appetite), passage of undigested food (most easily recognized when whole seeds are found in the droppings), and regurgitation. A dilated proventriculus may be seen radiographically. Neurologic signs (convulsions, tremors, weakness, ataxia, blindness) may occur in some species, with or without concurrent GI signs. Clinical signs may be slowly progressive or develop acutely. Outbreaks are sporadic, with a low morbidity and a high mortality.

Before the discovery of ABV as the causative agent of PDD, the only antemortem diagnosis was identification of lymphoplasmacytic infiltrates in the tissues of affected birds, most commonly with a crop biopsy. Histopathologic lesions can be present in the brain, spinal cord, peripheral nerves, nerves of the GI tract, heart, adrenal gland, lungs, and kidneys. Transmission is fecal/oral, and positive results of PCR testing of choanal, cloacal, or fecal swabs confirms the presence of ABV. Serologic assays such as ELISA can also confirm exposure. Although the presence of ABV in the droppings indicates shedding, many birds are positive for ABV with no clinical signs of PDD. If or when these birds may develop disease is unknown.

Because shedding of the virus is intermittent, one negative result of fecal or cloacal PCR testing does not exclude disease. Testing at least three times at weekly intervals, with all three tests being negative, is best before declaring a bird negative for ABV. Differential diagnoses are heavy metal toxicosis, foreign body intestinal obstruction, internal papillomatosis, internal neoplasia, and GI infections (including bacterial and fungal proventricular infections).

Clinicopathologic findings vary, but increased plasma CK activity and mild lymphocytosis, monocytosis, or heterophilia may be seen. Proventricular biopsies in affected birds are prone to dehiscence and are not done routinely. Crop biopsy is a less invasive diagnostic tool and may be useful if the collected sample contains sufficient innervation to be diagnostic; however, a negative crop biopsy does not exclude the presence of PDD.

Treatment for PDD includes providing easily digestible foods and may be aided by administration of an NSAID (eg, meloxicam, celecoxib). Isolation of positive birds is important in disease prevention. Testing by PCR (a minimum of three tests) and separating positive birds from negative birds is a recommended control measure, although the number of false-negative tests (due to intermittent shedding) makes this a long and potentially difficult task. ABV is not a long-lived virus in the environment; therefore, good hygiene and ultraviolet light can help to limit spread of disease in a home or aviary setting.

Poxvirus Infections

Poxviruses are large DNA viruses that induce intracytoplasmic, lipophilic *inclusion bodies* (Bollinger bodies) in the epithelial cells of the integument, respiratory tract, and oral cavity. All birds are considered susceptible to poxvirus infection, but many companion and aviary birds are rarely exposed to a susceptible strain. Because of import restrictions, poxvirus in blue-fronted Amazon parrots is no longer commonly seen. In pet bird practice, veterinarians will generally encounter only canary, lovebird, and pigeon poxviruses and fowlpox (*see* p 2824), which have specific host ranges. Poxviruses are environmentally stable, increasing the likelihood that a viable organism will come into contact with a susceptible host. Poxviruses cannot penetrate intact skin, and a break in the skin or mucous membrane must be present for infection to occur.

Poxvirus infection may cause cutaneous, diphtheritic, or systemic infections based on the strain of virus, route of exposure, affected species, and age and health of the bird. The cutaneous form appears as nodular proliferations or wartlike lesions on the unfeathered skin around the eyes, beak, nares, and legs. The diphtheritic form is characterized by lesions on the mucosa, tongue, pharynx, and larynx. The septicemic form is characterized by a ruffled appearance, depression, cyanosis, anorexia, and wartlike tumors of the skin. The cutaneous form is most commonly seen in psittacines and raptors.

Clinical signs depend on the form of disease, location of the lesions (eye, oral, ear), and overall health of the bird and may include lethargy, respiratory distress, partial blindness, difficulty eating, weight loss, emaciation, and skin lesions. Diagnosis of poxvirus infection is typically confirmed through history, physical examination findings, and histologic findings of Bollinger bodies in affected tissues.

Treatment is usually nonspecific and may include supportive care, fluids, parenteral vitamin A, ophthalmic ointments for eye infections, assisted feedings, and antibiotics to prevent or treat secondary infections. Lesions on the skin may need daily cleaning. Transmission is via insect vectors (mosquito bites) or other entry through breaks in the skin. Therefore, mosquito control and indoor housing are vital to prevent outbreaks. Vaccines for canarypox, fowlpox, and pigeonpox are available but are specific for their host species.

Viscerotropic Velogenic Newcastle Disease

(Exotic Newcastle disease)

Viscerotropic velogenic Newcastle disease (VVND, *see* p 2856), caused by a paramyxovirus group 1, affects most avian species and is a significant threat to the poultry industry. Transmission is by respiratory aerosols, fecal contamination of food or water, direct contact with infected birds, and fomites.

Birds may be asymptomatic or die acutely. Clinical signs include depression, anorexia, weight loss, sneezing, nasal discharge, dyspnea, conjunctivitis, bright yellow-green diarrhea, ataxia, head bobbing, and opisthotonos. In prolonged cases, unilateral or bilateral wing and leg paralysis, chorea, torticollis, and dilated pupils also may be seen. Primary differential diagnoses include other paramyxoviruses (non-Newcastle), psittacine proventricular dilatation syndrome, and heavy metal toxicosis. Lesions include hepatomegaly, splenomegaly, petechial or ecchymotic hemorrhages on serosal surfaces of all viscera and air sacs, airsacculitis, and excess straw-colored peritoneal fluid. Diagnosis is traditionally via viral isolation, but agar gel immunodiffusion tests that can be performed on whole blood or serum are available.

Only symptomatic treatment is possible and thus not advised. If suspected, VVND must be reported to appropriate federal and state authorities. Vaccination is prohibited in birds entering the USA, because it does not eliminate the carrier state and hampers viral detection during quarantine.

Other Paramyxovirus Infections:

There are several less pathogenic strains of paramyxovirus. Paramyxovirus groups 2 and 3 are endemic in aviculture. Paramyxovirus group 2 causes mild illness in passerines and a more serious disease in psittacines. Clinical signs in psittacines include tracheitis, pneumonia, and enteritis. Paramyxovirus group 3 is reported most frequently in *Neophema* spp, lovebirds, and gouldian finches and typically causes mild disease. Clinical signs may be absent, and disease results in acute death. In disease of longer duration, respiratory signs, pancreatitis, and torticollis may occur.

Diagnosis is the same as for paramyxovirus group 1. Treatment for paramyxovirus groups 2 and 3 infections is supportive care. The vaccine for paramyxovirus group 1 should not be used in psittacines, because it can cause fatal reactions.

West Nile Virus

West Nile virus (WNV) infection is an arthropodborne virus in the genus *Flavivirus* (family Flaviviridae). WNV was first reported in birds in the USA in August 1999. Many species of birds can be infected, and it has been reported in >320 species of birds. The American crow (*Corvus brachyrunchus*) and other corvids have suffered particularly high morbidity and mortality. Other affected species include canaries, psittacines, and raptors. Although psittacines appear to be somewhat resistant, the disease has been reported in parakeets, cockatoos, conures, rosellas, caiques, lorikeets, and a King parrot. Affected parrots have been adults housed outdoors with documentation of mosquito populations present. Mosquitoes (*Culex* spp) are the principal vectors of disease.

Clinical signs include depression, anorexia, weight loss, head tremors, ataxia, blindness, seizures, and death. Juvenile birds are the most commonly affected. Ophthalmologic findings in raptors are anterior uveitis, exudative chorioretinal lesions, and chorioretinal scarring.

Antemortum diagnosis can be difficult. Initial diagnosis may be based on clinical signs, species, and age; however, many diseases may cause similar clinical signs. Serologic tests (serum neutralization) may indicate antibody response to infection. Paired samples submitted 2 wk apart may reveal a rise in antibody levels and give a more definitive diagnosis. Adult birds may have high circulating antibody levels in endemic areas. Diagnosis is often determined at necropsy. The brain and kidney are the preferred tissues to submit for histopathologic examination.

There is no specific treatment for WNV in birds. Some birds may improve with supportive care (fluids, feeding, antibiotics/antifungals as needed) and time. A vaccination protocol using a recombinant vaccine has been successful in some birds. The recommendation is vaccination of captive birds 2–4 wk before mosquito season, with a booster 3 wk after the initial dose.

During the mosquito season, birds should be housed indoors or in completely covered outdoor facilities. Mosquito netting and mosquito traps should be used, and any standing or stagnant water sources eliminated.

Avian Influenza

Avian influenza is caused by an orthomyxovirus. Because of the zoonotic potential of some strains and the recent discovery of new mutations, this virus may become a more significant pathogen. Both the zoonotic potential and the economic effects on the poultry industry are causes for concern. (*See also* AVIAN INFLUENZA, p 2902.)

GERIATRIC DISEASES

Until recently, geriatric medicine has been a neglected area of avian medicine. Infectious diseases, inadequate diets, and poor husbandry meant that most pet birds did not live long enough to develop geriatric conditions. As the knowledge base of avian medicine, nutrition, and proper husbandry has grown, so has the life span of pet birds increased. Most pet birds have the potential to live 20–80 yr, depending on their size (with smaller birds having a shorter life span and larger birds a longer life span). With pet birds living longer, the incidence of geriatric-onset diseases, including cataracts, neoplasia, arthritis, and cardiovascular disease, has increased.

Cataracts

Cataracts occur in many species of psittacine birds as they age, notably macaws, Amazon parrots, and cockatiels. These species may be prone to cataracts or may be overrepresented in the older pet bird population. If the onset of cataracts is gradual, adaptation to decreased vision usually occurs; if not, clinical signs can be depression, inactivity, and reluctance to come out of or move around in the cage.

The eyes of older birds should be examined annually to detect early changes in lens opacity. Because of the small size of the exposed cornea and pupil in psittacines, and the numerous acquired diseases that can occur, screening by an ophthalmologist is recommended. Cataracts often develop secondary to infection or trauma or may be age related. Uveitis may also be present. Additional ophthalmic conditions that may be encountered in geriatric birds are keratoconjunctivitis sicca, corneal ulcerations, third eyelid abnormalities, hypopyon, anterior uveitis, conjunctival granulomas, infection of the conjunctiva (eg, *Chlamydia*, *Mycoplasma*, poxvirus), Harderian gland adenoma, and lymphoma.

In large psittacine birds, surgical removal of cataracts is successful in many cases. The bird's general health and the degree to which the cataracts affect its quality of life should be evaluated before surgery. Commonly used mydriatics are not useful in birds because of the skeletal (as opposed to smooth) muscle found in the iris. In any bird with decreased vision, minimal alteration of the home environment is critical. Early cataracts, especially if uveitis is present, may be painful. NSAIDs, either ocular drops (flurbiprofen) or systemic (meloxicam, celecoxib), or both, can be used to reduce inflammation and pain.

Arthritis

Septic and traumatic arthritis may occur at any age. Septic arthritis is most common in the digits. Osteoarthritis is also common in geriatric birds and can lead to other issues such as pododermatitis if not caught early and treated. The weight of the bird, its general physical condition, previous injuries, and any concurrent medical conditions can all contribute to the onset and severity of arthritis. Concurrent pododermatitis is often present and may be both a cause and result of decreased activity. Malnutrition, which decreases the integrity of the plantar epithelium, and concurrent obesity are often present in affected birds. The cage environment, especially the variety, diameter, and texture of perches, can be important in providing comfort and stability for arthritic birds while preventing or minimizing pododermatitis. If possible, the nails should be left with sharp points to add strength and stability to the grip. Wings should not be clipped, to help with balance.

Clinical signs vary, depending on the location of the arthritis and the severity of disease. Birds may exhibit lameness or be less active. A flighted bird may not want to fly or may not fly as well. The bird may not be perching normally or may fall off perches. Other signs of arthritis are swollen or warm joints, decreased range of motion, feather picking or mutilation, or excessive vocalization.

Diagnosis is based on clinical signs, physical examination findings, and imaging (radiographs or CT scan). Radiographic lesions include narrowing of the joint space, sclerosis of the subchondral bone, misalignment of the joint, and osteophyte formation. CT scans help determine the severity of the bony changes. Commonly affected joints are the tarsus, stifle, and phalangeal joints. The joints of the thoracic limb appear to be less commonly affected.

A multimodal treatment plan is recommended, incorporating both medical and nonmedical modalities. Medical treatment includes the use of NSAIDs, chondroprotectants, and possibly opioids. The most common NSAID used in avian medicine is meloxicam (0.5–1 mg/kg, PO, once to twice daily), a COX-2 inhibitor. Potential adverse effects of NSAIDs are renal ischemia, so they should be used with caution longterm and at the lowest therapeutic dose possible. Anecdotally, glucosamine (20 mg/kg, PO, bid, or 35 mg/kg, PO, once daily or every other day) or polysulfated glycosaminoglycan (5 mg/kg, IM, once weekly for 4 wk then monthly) has been used successfully. The latter should be used carefully, because some birds have had fatal coagulopathies from the injections.

Opioids may be necessary for acute exacerbations of a chronic arthritic condition or for conditions not responding initially to NSAIDs. Tramadol (15–30 mg/kg, PO, bid-qid) or butorphanol (0.5–3 mg/kg, IM, every 4 hr (depending on species of bird), may be used until the NSAIDs take effect.

Additional management includes husbandry changes, a weight loss and exercise plan, a healthier diet (rich in omega-3 fatty acids), and physical therapy. Encouraging flighted birds (without clipped wings) to fly in a safe environment is the best form of exercise. If a safe environment is not possible, encouraging climbing, walking, or even stepping up multiple times can be exercise for parrots. Foraging for food, by putting multiple foraging boxes on opposite sides of the cage or enclosure, promotes exercise. If the bird is overweight, then weight loss is essential, because studies have shown that obesity is a risk factor for osteoarthritis in many species. This may involve converting the bird slowly to a pelleted diet with added essential fatty acids. Fatty acids may have an anti-inflammatory effect and be renal protective. Flax seed oil (0.1–0.2 mL/kg/day, PO) is recommended as the best source of fatty acid supplementation for birds. Other husbandry changes, such as changes in perch texture or diameter or padding perches, can be helpful in birds with weak or painful legs or feet.

Articular gout is also common in older birds (*see* p 1926). Differentiation between arthritis and articular gout is critical because of the vast differences in progression, quality of life, and prognosis.

Pododermatitis

Pododermatitis, or bumblefoot, is a relatively common condition of older pet birds. It is a general term for any inflammatory or degenerative condition of the avian foot and can range from mild redness to bony changes. Bumblefoot develops most commonly when birds are either housed with inappropriate perching or secondarily to an injury in one leg, which causes the bird to shift its weight to the other (good) leg and creates increased pressure and potential ulceration on the plantar surface of the foot. Birds most at risk are birds with leg fractures; arthritis of a hip, stifle, or tarsal joint; and obese birds or birds on a poor diet (eg, vitamin A deficiency). These are the same conditions that can predispose a bird to arthritis. Bumblefoot is often a sequela of osteoarthritis. Pododermatitis is a progressive disease. A localized hyperemic lesion develops, followed by ulceration and, if untreated, abscess formation and osteomyelitis. Initially, the skin on the metatarsal and digital pads becomes flattened and smooth. The skin may become proliferative and then ulcerate, allowing bacterial access, which leads to inflammation and infection. As the infection progresses, tendon sheaths become affected, and osteomyelitis and septic arthritis develop.

Birds may present with lameness, depression, and anorexia due to the inflammation, pain, and infection. Diagnosis is based on clinical signs, physical examination findings, radiographs, and culture results. Affected birds should be examined thoroughly for predisposing injuries or illness.

Treatment includes correcting inappropriate husbandry (adding padded perches or perches covered with artificial grass) and conversion to a healthier, preferably formulated diet. Weight loss and exercise should be encouraged in obese birds (flying, climbing, or walking). In early cases, this may be all that is necessary.

As the disease progresses, a bandage may be necessary to relieve the pressure on the lesion. The lesions should be kept clean. Strict sanitation of the perches and feet is important to prevent bacterial infections. If a scab is present, it should be softened and removed or surgically debrided. Antibiotic use should be based on results of culture and sensitivity testing. *Staphylococcus* spp is most commonly identified; other reported bacteria include *Escherichia coli* and *Proteus* spp. Effective antibiotics are amoxicillin/clavulanate (125 mg/kg, PO, tid), enrofloxacin (10–15 mg/kg, PO, bid), and marbofloxacin (5 mg/kg/day) for 10–14 days. Pain management is important and includes a combination of NSAIDs and/or opioids, depending on the severity of disease and after any surgical debridement. One regimen is meloxicam (0.5–1 mg/kg, once to twice daily) along with tramadol (15–30 mg/kg, PO, bid-tid), and, in severe cases or after surgery, butorphanol (0.5–3 mg/kg, IM, every 4 hr, depending on species). Local anesthetics may be helpful after surgery.

Renal Disease

Renal disease may be seen at any age, but older birds are more likely to develop renal insufficiency. Causes are multiple and include glomerulonephropathies, renal tubular gout, and chronic bacterial nephritis.

Clinical signs include weight loss, depression, polyuria, polydipsia, and articular gout. Diagnosis is made based on a persistent hyperuricemia before and after fluid therapy. Imaging (radiographs or CT scan) may demonstrate small or large kidneys with or without mineralization. Occasionally, urethroliths may be seen. Renal biopsy is necessary for definitive diagnosis.

Treatment includes supportive care (fluid therapy) and antibiotics as needed based on diagnostics. Colchicine (0.04 mg/kg, PO, bid) and allopurinol (10–30 mg/kg, PO, bid) have successfully treated certain disease processes. After stabilization, conversion to an appropriate diet should be initiated. Essential fatty acids (omega 3) at 0.1–0.22 mL/kg/day, PO, have been used anecdotally to manage renal disease in birds.

Cardiac Disease

As birds live longer and diagnostic techniques improve, cardiac disease is being diagnosed more frequently. It can be difficult to detect and may mimic other problems, such as respiratory disease. Cardiac disease has been associated with atherosclerosis in pet birds, and potential risk factors are a sedentary lifestyle, a high-fat diet, and hypercholesterolemia.

Clinical signs are weakness, depression or lethargy, increased respiratory rate and effort, or tachycardia. With right-side heart disease, hepatomegaly and ascites are common. Disease also may be subclinical, then present acutely, with the bird arresting when diagnostic tests or treatments are attempted. In birds, right-side cardiac disease is more prevalent than left-side.

Consultation with a cardiologist on any avian patient with suspected cardiac disease is advised. Diagnosis of the cardiovascular abnormality and forming a therapeutic plan requires knowledge of avian anatomy and physiology and a cardiologist's diagnostic skills and pharmacologic recommendations. Radiographs and cardiac ultrasound can aid in the diagnosis.

The stress of handling can increase intracardiac blood flow velocity 300% in avian patients; therefore, inhalant anesthesia or sedation is preferred over manual restraint for performance of echocardiograms in all but the most docile birds. The equipment necessary for echocardiology in birds includes an ultrasound unit with Doppler function, 100 frames/sec minimum speed, and microcurved or phased array probes with a minimum 7.5 MHz frequency. Anatomic constraints in birds also limit the echocardiograph windows available. Parameters for chamber sizes, blood flow velocities, functional contractility, and valvular insufficiency have been determined for several species, and studies are ongoing in this area.

Reported therapies include enalapril (0.25–0.5 mg/kg/day, PO), furosemide (0.15–2 mg/kg, PO, SC, or IM, once to twice daily), pimobendan (6 mg/kg, PO, bid), and digoxin (0.01-0.02 mg/kg, PO, bid). Although most avian therapeutic regimens are still extrapolated from those used in mammals, numerous reports indicate that cardiac drug therapy can improve cardiac function, thereby increasing the quality and length of life.

Pulmonary Hypertension: The cardiovascular system of birds differs anatomically and physiologically from that of mammals. The right atrioventricular valve is a single, muscular valve with no chordae tendinae. The physiologic responses that maintain low pulmonary vascular resistance (both vascular distensibility and vasculature recruitment) are absent in birds, resulting in the inability of the pulmonary vasculature to accommodate increased cardiac output by either altering vascular diameter or changing the percentage of vascular channels being used. This may be, at least in part, responsible for the high incidence of pulmonary hypertension syndrome in poultry (*see* p 2871) as well as right-side heart disease in psittacines. Studies on the impact of pulmonary hypertension in broiler hens have demonstrated that the response to pulmonary arterial hypertension in chickens involves an increase in two vasoactive substances: a vasodilator and a vasoconstrictor. The vasoconstrictor predominates over the vasodilator in broiler hens susceptible to pulmonary hypertension. For geriatric psittacine patients with pulmonary hypertension, vasodilator therapy should be explored. Macaw asthma may theoretically cause pulmonary hypertension, both from chronic capillary hypoxia and subsequent polycythemia.

Atherosclerosis: Atherosclerosis is a proliferative lesion of the tunica media and tunica intima of elastic and muscular arteries. Atherosclerotic plaques cause abnormal vascular flow and loss of endothelial integrity. These changes in vessel walls can initiate thrombosis. In birds, lesions are primarily in the aorta and brachiocephalic arteries. Atherosclerosis is common in psittacine birds. It is generally a geriatric condition, except in African grey parrots, in which this disease has been observed in very young birds. Amazon parrots, macaws, and African grey parrots seem to be particularly susceptible.

Predisposing factors appear to include age (most affected birds are 10–15 yr old), sedentary lifestyle, and a high-fat diet. Clinical signs are rarely reported in birds, and the condition is often associated with sudden death. Clinical signs that may be seen are exercise intolerance, dyspnea, episodic weakness, and neurologic signs (eg, seizures, tremors, paresis). At necropsy, grossly thickened arterial walls are seen.

Diagnosis can be difficult. Radiographically, the right aortic arch may be enlarged, with increased density. Lipemia is often present, and marked increases in cholesterol and triglyceride concentrations may be seen. Unfortunately, definitive antemortem tests are lacking.

Medical treatment is anecdotal. A variety of treatments have been advocated to lower cholesterol levels, but none appears to be consistent in its efficacy. Isoxsuprine (10 mg/kg/day, PO) has been used anecdotally with some success. Essential fatty acids (flax seed oil at 0.1–0.2 mL/kg/day, PO) have been advocated and used to reduce cholesterol and inflammation.

Liver Disease

Liver disease can affect birds of any age but is more common in geriatric birds. Hepatic lipidosis is most common, possibly resulting from longterm feeding of an inappropriate (high-fat) diet. Chronic liver disease can result in fibrosis of the liver and decreased liver function and failure.

Clinical signs of liver disease are anorexia, lethargy, overgrown beak and nails with bruising, biliverdinuria, discolored feathers, and, in later stages, ascites. Birds often are overweight or have a history of being obese. Clinical pathology may reveal high liver enzyme levels (AST) and bile acids, a nonregenerative anemia, and high triglyceride and cholesterol concentrations. Imaging (radiographs or CT scan and/or ultrasound) may reveal hepatomegaly or microhepatica. Liver biopsy may be necessary to confirm the diagnosis and determine etiology and prognosis.

Treatment involves supportive care (fluid therapy), antibiotics as needed, and medications to support hepatic function such as silymarin (milk thistle) (100–150 mg/kg, PO, bid) and ursodeoxycholic acid (10–15 mg/kg/day, PO).

NEOPLASTIC DISEASES

Neoplasia occurs with some frequency in pet birds of all ages and includes cancer of the skin, sinuses, oral cavity, GI tract, lungs, air sacs, liver, spleen, kidneys, reproductive tract, bone, vascular and connective tissue, and brain. The incidence of cancer is likely to rise as pet birds age. Often, external tumors can be seen on physical examination and diagnosed by fine-needle aspirate and cytology or biopsy. Internal neoplasia often requires imaging (radiographs, ultrasound, or CT scan), endoscopic examination, or exploratory surgery to determine the type and extent of the neoplasia. Treatment protocols are becoming more successful but are still extrapolated from other species and often have been performed in only one or two birds. More information (clinical studies and research) is needed on diagnostic tests, treatments (including adverse effects), and prognosis of neoplasia in companion birds.

Pseudoneoplastic Skin Conditions

Xanthomas are not neoplasms but locally invasive subcutaneous, yellow, fatty masses in the skin. Xanthomas are rarely found in internal organs. The distal wing, keel, and the sternopubic area are common locations, although xanthomas may be found anywhere. Cockatiels and budgerigars are overrepresented, although xanthomas are seen in most psittacine species. The lesions may be pruritic and may be associated with lipomas or sites of chronic irritation. The cause is unknown; however, dietary improvement, including sufficient vitamin A, has been curative in less advanced cases. Xanthomas tend to be vascular. Therapy includes surgical resection, although in large masses closure may be difficult, and strict attention to hemostasis must be observed. Amputation is recommended for xanthomas on the wing tip.

Lipomas occur most frequently in budgerigars, rose-breasted cockatoos, Amazon parrots, and cockatiels. These benign, soft, yellowish, encapsulated subcutaneous masses are most often located on the keel or in the sternopubic area. If traumatized, they may become inflamed or necrotic. Lipomas can grow rapidly and result in ulceration of the overlying skin. Treatment includes conversion to a low-fat diet, weight loss in obese birds, and surgical excision. Recurrence is common with incomplete removal.

Cutaneous, Subcutaneous, and Other Neoplasms

Fibrosarcomas may be lobular, subcutaneous masses without skin involvement or may be seen as erythemic skin lesions. They may also develop in the oral cavity, bone, or abdominal cavity. Fibrosarcomas tend to be locally invasive and recurrent. Surgical excision followed by radiation and chemotherapy has shown some success.

Liposarcomas are malignant tumors of the lipocytes and have rarely been reported in pet birds. They have been described in cockatiels, budgerigars, a conure, an African grey parrot, and a quaker parakeet. They are similar in appearance to lipomas (yellowish, gray mass) but are firmer, more infiltrative, and vascular. Cytologic examination may not differentiate between a lipoma and liposarcoma, so surgical biopsy is recommended. Therapy includes surgical excision, although recurrence is common with incomplete removal.

Squamous cell carcinoma (SCC) is a malignant tumor comprised of moderately undifferentiated to poorly differentiated squamous cells. SCCs are most common on the skin and beak, in the oral cavity, esophagus, or crop, and on the distal wing and phalanges. These tumors tend to be locally invasive. Cutaneous SCCs often appear as proliferative masses or woundlike ulcers. Tumors often develop at sites of chronic irritation. It has been experimentally demonstrated that inflammation can promote neoplastic proliferation. SCCs of the uropygial gland can occur and result in enlargement of the gland and ulceration. SCCs of the beak result in overgrowth and deformation of the beak. Tumors involving the sinuses or oral cavity typically have poorly defined borders and are associated with necrosis and hemorrhage.

Clinical signs of SSCs of the sinus or oral cavity are dyspnea, dysphagia, anorexia, exophthalmos, and nasal discharge. Clinical signs of birds with SSCs of the crop or esophagus include anorexia, regurgitation, and depression. Cutaneous SCCs tend to be locally aggressive and recur, but there are few reports of metastasis. Tumors are often associated with chronic (secondary) bacterial and fungal infections. Diagnosis is based on imaging (radiographs, CT scan) and fine-needle aspirate and cytology or biopsy of the lesion.

Recommended treatment is surgical excision with or without radiation therapy. Cobalt-60 radiation therapy and intralesional carboplatin and cisplatin have had limited success in treatment of SCCs. Radiation therapy with a strontium-90 probe has had some success in treatment of SCCs of the uropygial gland after surgical excision or debulking.

Musculoskeletal neoplasms reported in psittacines include osteosarcoma, chondroma, chondrosarcoma, hemangioma, and leiomyosarcoma. Wide surgical resection is the suggested treatment.

Internal carcinomas include **ovarian neoplasia** (various cell origins), **renal carcinoma**, **hepatic adenocarcinoma**, and **hepatobiliary adenocarcinoma** (related to papillomas in Amazon parrots).

Clinical signs of coelomic tumors include anorexia, weight loss, depression, and/or dyspnea (from organ enlargement and compression of air sacs). Gastric carcinomas, generally diagnosed at necropsy, are often found at the proventricular-ventricular junction. Death from gastric neoplasia may be caused by hemorrhage, gastric perforation and sepsis, endotoxic shock, or inanition and subsequent wasting. Diagnostic tests include radiographs with or without barium contrast, CT scan, or ultrasound with fine-needle aspirate and cytology or biopsy.

Both carboplatin and cisplatin have been used successfully in various forms of internal carcinoma. Toxicity studies with cisplatin in cockatoos indicate that psittacine tolerance for this drug may be greater than that of mammals. Several cases of ovarian neoplasia have been treated with GnRH agonists (leuprolide or deslorelin implant) with some success.

Pituitary adenomas are most prevalent in budgerigars and cockatiels but have been observed in other psittacine species. Tumors may cause acute neurologic conditions (eg, seizures, opisthotonos, ataxia, blindness, and difficulty flying). Affected birds may also show signs related to the pituitary hormone(s) affected (eg, adrenocorticotropic hormone [ACTH] associated with polydipsia and polyuria). Diagnostic tests are of limited use. Pituitary tumors are typically diagnosed based on species and clinical signs and are confirmed at necropsy.

Thymoma and thyroid adenocarcinomas have been reported in several psittacine species. Primary **pancreatic neoplasias** of variable cell origins have been reported.

Lymphoma/lymphosarcoma is the most common lymphoid neoplasia in psittacine and passerine birds. Multicentric lymphosarcoma is most common, whereas lymphocytic leukemias occur rarely. Lymphoma can involve the spleen, liver, kidneys, GI tract, skin, bone, oviduct, lungs, sinuses, thymus, testes, brain, mesentery, trachea, and pancreas. The liver is most commonly affected, followed by the spleen and kidneys. Numerous reports of exophthalmos in psittacines, particularly young African grey parrots, have been diagnosed as retrobulbar lymphoma. Cutaneous lymphoma often occurs on the head or neck. Lesions are grayish yellow, diffuse or multifocal, and may resemble xanthoma or inflammation. Clinical signs vary based on location of the tumor but may include depression, anorexia, weight loss, coelomic distention, paresis, lameness, blindness, regurgitation, or dyspnea. Canaries often present for having stopped singing.

Diagnosis is based on physical examination findings, imaging (radiographs with or without contrast, ultrasound, or CT scan) and fine-needle aspirate or biopsy of affected organs, masses, or bone marrow. A CBC often reveals leukocytosis or lymphocytosis rather than a leukopenia. Anemia (PCV <35%) is commonly reported. No evidence of retroviral activity has been associated with psittacine lymphoma.

Treatment has included surgical excision with or without chemotherapy. Chemotherapy regimens have included one or more of the following: corticosteroids, orthovoltage x-ray, chlorambucil, doxorubicin, L-asparaginase, cyclophosphamide, α-interferon, and/or vincristine sulfate. Diphenhydramine and dexamethasone have been used to reduce the incidence of allergic reaction or anaphylaxis. Although chemotherapy and radiation therapy have been successful, treatment success overall has been variable.

Primary respiratory neoplasia is uncommon in psittacines, except for a mixed pulmonary tumor reported in cockatiels. Metastatic pulmonary neoplasia may occur.

Chemotherapy and Radiation Therapy Agents

Most reports of chemotherapy in birds have demonstrated both higher tolerance for chemotherapeutic agents than expected and less tumor response than desired. Anecdotal reports indicate that neoplasia in birds is more resistant to radiation than that in mammals. Very few case reports and even fewer research reports are available for chemotherapy or radiation therapy protocols in birds. Because very little is known about chemotherapy and radiation in birds, a current literature search and consultation with a veterinary oncologist are recommended before treatment of a pet bird diagnosed with cancer. In addition to the antineoplastic drugs that have been used in birds discussed below, *see* ANTINEOPLASTIC AGENTS, p 2722.

Vincristine was used in the chemotherapeutic regimen of an African grey parrot with malignant lymphoreticular neoplasia, a Moluccan cockatoo with lymphoma, and a Pekin duck with lymphoma and leukemia.

Cisplatin/carboplatin was evaluated in eight sulfur-crested cockatoos. A dose of 1 mg/kg infused over 1 hr was tolerated well, and plasma levels were in a therapeutic range. Adverse effects were weight loss, regurgitation, and bone marrow suppression. Intratumoral cisplatin and radiation therapy were used to treat fibrosarcoma in a macaw. Intralesional cisplatin was used unsuccessfully in treatment of SCC in a Buffon's macaw. Carboplatin was used successfully to treat a bile duct carcinoma in a yellow-naped Amazon parrot and pancreatic duct adenocarcinoma in a green-winged macaw.

L-Asparaginase was used to treat lymphoma in a Moluccan cockatoo. Adverse effects associated with treatment were weight loss, lethargy, anorexia, and regurgitation. Doxorubicin was used successfully in a blue-fronted Amazon parrot with osteosarcoma. Doxorubicin in combination therapy was unsuccessful in treating lymphoma in a Moluccan cockatoo. Chlorambucil was used successfully in treatment of cutaneous pseudolymphoma in a blue and gold macaw. Cyclophosphamide has been used to treat lymphoma in a Moluccan cockatoo.

Radiation therapy has been used in birds with variable results (*see* p 1651).

NUTRITIONAL DISEASES

Proper nutrition for companion birds historically has been and continues to be a concern for avian veterinarians, aviculturists, and owners. Although avian nutrition has greatly improved in the past decades, nutritional disease is still common in pet birds. The availability of formulated diets and hand-feeding formulas have been pivotal in improving avian nutritional health, but many birds are still fed inadequate diets. The two most common reasons for malnutrition in companion birds are feeding diets that allow the birds to choose what they want to eat (either mixtures of seeds/nut and pellets, or table foods the owner considers healthy) and feeding pure seed or seed-based diets. Feeding a mixture of pellets and seeds is also common, resulting in selective eating and consequently inadequate nutrient consumption.

Many of the illnesses seen in pet birds have their basis in malnutrition. This includes hepatic disease, renal insufficiency, respiratory impairment, musculoskeletal disease, and reproductive problems. For additional information on nutrition in pet birds, *see* p 2288.

Obesity: Obesity is common in companion birds. High-fat diets (seeds, nuts, and many table foods), overabundance of food, and a sedentary lifestyle are all contributing factors. Obesity is typically defined as a bird being 20% over ideal weight, with a body condition or keel score of 4 out of 5 (*see* p 1887). Galahs, macaws, Amazon parrots, and quaker parrots are prone to obesity. Clinical signs may not be evident but include lameness (pododermatitis and/or arthritis) and respiratory issues from excessive abdominal fat.

Obese birds should be converted to a pelleted diet with portion control. Exercise should be encouraged by providing a larger cage with multiple food bowls around the cage to encourage movement. Rope or spiral rope perches will encourage climbing and balance. A flight cage outdoors should be provided for flighted birds, and walking or climbing stairs encouraged for non-flighted birds. Obese birds are more prone to arthritis, fatty liver disease (hepatic lipidosis), atherosclerosis, and cardiac disease.

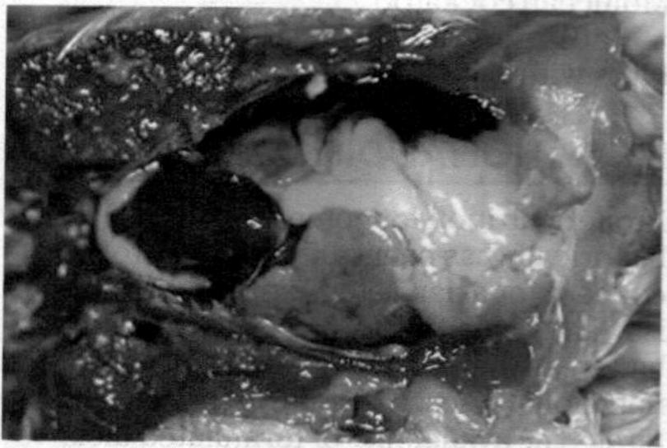

Fatty liver disease (hepatic lipidosis), gross lesions, in a cockatiel. A pale liver is located beneath the heart, nestled in a pad of abdominal body fat. *Courtesy of Dr. Louise Bauck.*

Vitamin A Deficiency: Vitamin A plays an important role in avian health and is crucial for a healthy immune system. Hypovitaminosis A causes squamous metaplasia of epithelium within the oropharynx, choana, sinuses, GI tract, urogenital tact, reproductive tract, and uropygial gland as well as hyperkeratosis of the feet. All-seed diets and even mixed diets of ½ seeds and ½ pellets are deficient in vitamin A.

Clinical signs are nasal discharge, sneezing, periorbital swelling, conjunctivitis, dyspnea, polyuria, polydipsia, poor feather quality, feather picking, and anorexia. Birds may have absent or blunted papilla of the choanal slit. White plaques (hyperkeratosis) may develop in and around the mouth, eyes, and sinuses. In chronic epithelial conditions (eg, pododermatitis, sinusitis, and conjunctivitis) that have been refractory or recurrent, often vitamin A deficiency is the primary cause. Birds with reproductive disease on poor diets should be considered deficient.

Treatment involves treating secondary infections, supplementing with vitamin A, and converting the bird to a good quality pelleted diet. Parenteral vitamin A can be given (100,000 U/kg, IM). Vitamin A precursors, such as spirolina, sprinkled daily over the food are a safe way to supplement diets deficient in vitamin A. The diets of all pet birds should be evaluated for vitamin A content.

Iodine Deficiency: Goiter, or thyroid hyperplasia, occurs in budgerigars on all-seed diets deficient in iodine. This condition is no longer common because of the availability of pelleted and fortified diets. Classic signs are respiratory stridor, wheezing, or clicking due to the pressure of the thyroid on the syrinx. Lugol's iodine (1 drop/250 mL of drinking water) can be used until conversion to a pellet or fortified seed diet is accomplished and clinical signs have subsided.

Calcium, Phosphorus, and Vitamin D_3 Imbalance: Seed-based diets are well known for their calcium:phosphorus imbalance and amino acid deficiencies. Sunflower seeds, which tend to be selected preferentially by many psittacines, are low in calcium, deficient in essential amino acids, and high in fat. Safflower seeds are actually higher in fat content than sunflower seeds, contrary to popular belief, and also contain inadequate amino acids and calcium.

Metabolic Bone Disease (Nutritional Secondary Hyperparathyroidism): Nutritional secondary hyperparathyroidism can occur in young and older pet birds. Because the calcium to phosphorus ratio in most seeds is poor (high phosphorus and low calcium), birds on a seed diet become seriously depleted. The effects of a calcium-deficient diet are often compounded by inadequate exposure to unfiltered sunlight in birds housed indoors, resulting in vitamin D_3 deficiency as well. In young birds, especially African grey parrots, hypocalcemia may present as osteodystrophy, with curvature and deformation of the long bones and vertebrae. African grey parrots are also prone to an acute hypocalcemia syndrome that is associated with both hypocalcemia and hypovitaminosis D_3.

Clinical signs include weakness, ataxia, tremors, depression, seizures, and pathologic fractures. In reproducing birds, eggs are often thin-shelled, egg production and hatchability are decreased, and embryonic death occurs. Calcium deficiency can lead to cessation of egg laying, egg binding, or cloacal prolapse. Diagnosis is based on decreased total and ionized plasma calcium levels and radiographic evidence of decreased bone density or pathologic fractures. Serum 25-hydroxycholecalciferol levels can also be measured and are usually low.

Treatment is supportive care, calcium and vitamin D supplementation, conversion to an appropriate diet, and exposure to ultraviolet light, preferably natural sunlight. If pathologic fractures are present, splinting or bandaging may be necessary, along with cage rest, NSAIDs, or analgesics. Initial treatment should consist of calcium gluconate (100 mg/kg, IM).

Pet birds should have exposure to natural sunlight when possible. Owners should provide an outdoor cage that provides opportunities for climbing and/or flight and access to direct sunlight. Birds should be monitored closely when outdoors, even in a cage, because many predators can injure a pet bird through cage bars.

Vitamin D Toxicosis: Although excessive oral calcium intake is not thought to cause clinical problems in most cases, excessive oral vitamin D_3 can cause harmful calcium accumulation in tissues such as the kidneys. Supplements should be used carefully, especially in susceptible species (eg, macaws).

Iron Storage Disease: Iron storage disease refers to disease that occurs with excessive iron accumulation in the liver. Hemachromatosis is reserved for cases associated with actual pathology. As iron levels within the liver increase, hepatic lysosomes are damaged and release ionic iron, resulting in oxidative damage to membranes and proteins. Iron storage disease is common in mynahs and toucans, and in certain zoo birds such as birds of paradise; it has been occasionally reported in pet psittacine species, particularly lories. Iron storage disease is associated with excessive intake of dietary iron. However, not all birds are affected when fed similar diets, and stress or genetic factors may also play a role. Certain foods rich in vitamin C, such as citrus fruits, increase dietary iron uptake. Current dietary iron recommendations for toucans and mynahs are <50–100 ppm.

Clinical signs are anorexia, weight loss, depression, distended abdomen with ascites, dyspnea, and biliverdinuria. The liver, spleen, and heart are the most commonly affected organs. Circulatory failure, ascites, and hypoalbuminemia are often seen clinically. Diagnosis is by liver biopsy.

Treatment includes periodic phlebotomy, iron chelation, and dietary modification. Recommending low-iron diets routinely for pet mynahs and toucans is prudent (commercial formulas are available). Foods high in vitamin C should be avoided. Supplementation with chelators such as tannins, fiber, and phytates has been suggested.

Additional Nutritional Concerns: In addition to the well-documented nutritional deficiencies in diets designed for psittacines, described above, the following dietary concerns should also be noted: 1) the potential sensitivity of individual birds to dyes and preservatives added to some seed and pelleted foods; 2) the high incidence of hepatic lipidosis, atherosclerosis, and right-side heart failure in sedentary captive birds consuming primarily seed diets; 3) the occurrence of hepatic fibrosis and cirrhosis secondary to aflatoxicosis from improperly stored seed and pet-grade peanuts; 4) the difference between food provided by well-meaning owners for their birds to eat (table foods, formulated pelleted diet, vegetables, etc) and what the birds actually consume (seed); and 6) the low palatability of most vitamin and mineral supplements added to water, which are not only ineffectual but can lead to decreased water consumption and dehydration.

Foods that owners should be advised to avoid feeding their birds at any time are chocolate, caffeinated beverages, alcohol, junk food (salt, sweets), milk products, onions, avocados, and apple seeds.

Wild birds spend many hours a day foraging for food. Captive and pet birds usually consume all of their caloric needs at one food bowl, with very little time or energy expended. To promote a healthier lifestyle for companion birds, foraging opportunities should be provided that increase activity, promote a healthier diet, and stimulate birds intellectually. Owners need to provide a cage large enough for the bird to climb and play in, with rope or other perches that stimulate activity and balance. Multiple small food bowls should be placed throughout the cage to encourage movement. Foraging toys with food bits promote activity as well. An outdoor flight cage that allows natural sunlight and increased activity is ideal.

REPRODUCTIVE DISEASES

Birds are oviparous, meaning they lay and incubate eggs. Chicks may be precocial (hatched with downy feathers and able to eat on their own soon after hatching) or altricial (featherless and completely dependent on being fed by parent birds until weaned). Passerine and psittacine birds are altricial. Sexual maturity occurs from 6 mo of age in smaller birds to 3–5 yr in larger parrots. Most hens have only a left ovary and oviduct and are heterogametic (the female determines the sex of the chick). The male has two testes located internally cranial to the cranial pole of the kidney.

Most wild birds have a specific breeding season. Captive and pet birds breed at any time based on environment (photoperiod), nutritional status, and absence or presence of a mate (bird) or perceived mate (human) and/or nest box. Females store calcium in their bones (hyperostosis), which is later used in egg shell production. Ovulation occurs in response to increasing levels of estrogen and luteinizing hormone. The oviduct is composed of four segments: the infundibulum, where fertilization occurs; the magnum, where albumen is deposited; the isthmus, where the inner and outer shell membrane is added; and the uterus (shell gland), where calcification of the shell occurs. The entire period of egg formation takes ~24 hr. Most pet birds lay 2 to 4 eggs in a clutch, although indeterminate layers such as cockatiels and budgerigars can produce much larger clutches.

Most pet birds are not sexually dimorphic, so determining the sex requires endoscopic examination or DNA sexing. Common reproductive problems in pet birds include behavioral issues, failure to reproduce, excessive egg production, dystocia (egg binding), impacted oviduct, egg yolk peritonitis, cloacal prolapse, and neoplasia.

Behavioral Problems: Behavioral problems that can be related to reproductive issues include feather picking, mutilation, and excessive screaming. These behaviors can also occur for other reasons, so a full evaluation must be done to determine the cause. Behavioral problems are most common in hand-raised parrots overly bonded to their owners. Psittacines are intelligent, social animals. In the wild, most live in flocks, have a set breeding season (based on temperature, photoperiod, humidity), and raise chicks with their mate. In captivity, most pet birds are kept all year at stable temperatures and are provided adequate food, which is often high in fat. This can promote breeding behavior year round.

Many hand-raised parrots are overly bonded to their owner at sexual maturity, resulting in sexual frustration that may lead to over-grooming behaviors and excessive contact calls (screaming) when the owner leaves the room or house. Some of these over-stimulated (excessively handled and petted) birds begin laying eggs or masturbating early, leading to egg binding or cloacal prolapse (*see* p 1922) along with feather destructive behavior or screaming.

Significant behavior modifications may need to be implemented (*see* p 1927) along with conversion to a pelleted diet. In some cases, a GnRH agonist may be necessary to decrease production of reproductive hormones. This should ideally only be done along with implementing necessary behavioral modifications.

Excessive or Chronic Egg Laying: Excessive egg laying is when a bird has repeat clutches, lays more eggs than normal, or produces more eggs than is normal. It is common in small birds, eg, budgerigars, lovebirds, and especially cockatiels. Affected birds typically are on a high-fat and high-calorie diet. Other birds typically are housed either in the same cage or close by, or birds are overly bonded to the owner. They often have an extended photoperiod (>12 hr). In some color mutations, there may be a genetic predisposition.

Clinical signs may not be evident, with only a history of excessive egg laying, or the bird may present nonperching, weak, depressed, and tail bobbing (indicating dyspnea), with decreased defecation or voluminous droppings. Birds often have a wide-based stance, are broody, and may have pathologic fractures from hypocalcemia. Excessive egg laying, if untreated, often leads to more serious reproductive issues such as dystocia, impacted oviduct, egg-yolk peritonitis, or cloacal prolapse.

Diagnosis is based on the history, physical examination findings, high plasma calcium levels, and radiographic findings of hyperostosis and/or evidence of an egg. Reproductively active birds often have high cholesterol, triglyceride, and total protein concentrations.

Treatment involves decreasing day length to 8 hr of daylight, conversion to a pelleted diet, removal of nest boxes and any toys the bird may be overly bonded to, removal of any mate, and discussion with the owner of appropriate handling of their bird. Calcium supplementation and a GnRH agonist may be needed to reduce the production of reproductive hormones. Usually, leuprolide acetate (800 mcg/kg, IM, every 3 wk for three injections, then prn) is administered. If the above changes and medications are unsuccessful, then a salpingohysterectomy may be necessary. This will prevent egg laying but not always ovulation, because it is impossible in birds to remove all ovarian tissue. Prognosis is good with early cases that respond to management, dietary changes, and GnRH agonists.

Egg Binding: Dystocia (egg binding) is a common occurrence in captive hens, most notably in cockatiels, budgerigars, and lovebirds. Usually, these birds are chronic egg layers, and calcium deficiency (resulting in misshapen or soft-shelled eggs) is a factor. Other causes include vitamin A deficiency, oviductal disease or neoplasia, abdominal wall herniation, being a first-time layer, and genetic factors. An inappropriate environment and lack of a nest box can be contributing factors for some birds. Egg binding may also be seen in large psittacines, although excessive egg laying is not as commonly associated with the condition in these birds. Obesity, general nutritional inadequacy, behavioral factors, and husbandry conditions may be involved. Egg-bound birds often present as emergencies. These birds should receive supportive care (ie, rehydration, parenteral calcium, increased humidity, and warmth) before attempting extraction of the egg.

Clinical signs include a bird on the bottom of the cage, depression, closed eyes, bobbing tail, and dyspnea. The abdomen may be distended. An egg is not always palpable. Diagnostic tests may need to wait until the bird is stable; they include a CBC, plasma biochemical profile (including ionized and total calcium), and radiographs. These tests may need to be done stepwise in a critical patient.

Medical treatment includes fluid therapy, parenteral calcium supplementation, analgesics, and/or NSAIDs, and continued maintenance in a warm humid incubator. Oxytocin and the avian equivalent arginine vasotocin both cause uterine contractions and induce oviposition, as can prostaglandins F or E. If the egg is adherent to the uterine wall or unable to be passed (often due to swelling, adhesions, or collection of feces and urates), administration of these drugs could theoretically lead to uterine rupture, but this has rarely been reported.

If medical management fails, then sedation, inhalant anesthesia, and manual extraction may be required. With the bird under anesthesia, the cloaca is lubricated with sterile jelly. Barring adherence of the egg to the uterus, steady digital pressure applied between the end of the sternum and the egg will cause the slow descent of the egg. At this point, the uterus will often evert and reveal the white pinhole where the uterine opening is located. This opening will gradually dilate. Very seldom will any additional pressure or manipulation be required. After the egg is delivered, the uterus typically will normally involute. If oviposition does not occur with digital pressure or because of a soft-shelled egg, ovocentesis is indicated. After aspiration, firmer shells are collapsed and carefully removed or allowed to pass. Postoperative care includes antibiotics, NSAIDs, and a GnRH agonist to reduce further egg laying. After egg extraction, the hen may continue to be depressed, with labored breathing, and often will not appear clinically normal for up to 24 hr. A second egg may be produced by the following day, so repeated palpation is indicated.

Surgical intervention (salpingohysterectomy) is warranted if the egg is severely adhered to the oviduct, multiple eggs are present, or the egg is ectopic. Prognosis for egg binding is fair to good if medical treatment or manual extraction of the egg is effective. Husbandry, nutritional, and behavioral issues as discussed under excessive egg laying (*see* above) need to be addressed.

Impacted Oviduct: An impacted oviduct is often a sequela of dystocia or salpingitis.

The oviduct becomes impacted with excess mucin, albumen, and soft-shelled or malformed eggs. These materials often become adhered to the oviduct wall and become inspissated. Clinical signs are depression, anorexia, distended abdomen, and possibly dyspnea.

Diagnosis is based on a history of chronic egg laying or dystocia. Imaging (radiographs, CT scan, or ultrasound) may reveal an enlarged oviduct. Hyperostosis may be present. The bird may have a leukocytosis and high total protein, cholesterol, and triglyceride concentrations. Treatment is supportive (fluids, analgesics, NSAIDs, and antibiotics). Surgery is recommended but is high risk.

Cystic Ovarian Disease: Birds with cystic ovarian disease often present with a history of previous egg production, but egg laying may not have occurred for several years. Cystic ovarian disease is most commonly seen in budgerigars and canaries.

Clinical signs may include depression, inactivity, abdominal distention, ascites, and often dyspnea. Abdominal palpation often reveals distention with ascitic fluid.

Diagnosis is similar to other reproductive diseases. The fluid is usually a transudate, although it should be examined for evidence of secondary infection or egg-yolk peritonitis. Careful aspiration of fluid from the ventral midline may relieve respiratory distress. Imaging (radiographs or ultrasound) when the bird is stable will often demonstrate hyperostosis of the femurs and other long bones. On the lateral view, the ventriculus will be displaced cranially, and a space-occupying mass will be noted in the renal and gonadal area. Ultrasonography can often detect cystic follicles, in addition to normal follicular development.

Treatment is supportive care, abdominocentesis if ascites is present, antibiotics, and GnRH agonists to reduce reproductive hormone production, stimulate atresia of the follicles, and decrease cyst size and production. Surgery may not be needed if there is no concurrent infection or neoplasia.

Egg Yolk Coelomitis: Egg yolk coelomitis is another common sequela of chronic reproductive disease. It can occur after salpingohysterectomy because of the *inability to completely* remove the ovary and the potential for ovulation to occur into the coelomic cavity. Other causes are ectopic ovulation, salpingitis, neoplasia, cystic hyperplasia, or ruptured oviduct. Egg yolk, along with bacteria (eg, *Escherichia coli*, *Staphylococcus*) in the coelomic cavity results in infection. Egg yolk coelomitis causes a severe inflammatory reaction and can lead to an egg-related pancreatitis or a yolk emboli (which can resemble a stroke). This occurs most commonly in cockatiels.

Clinical signs are similar to other reproductive disorders, but typically abdominal distention and ascites are present. Birds often present severely compromised and require supportive care before diagnostic testing. A leukocytosis and monocytosis may be present. Imaging (radiographs or ultrasound) may reveal an enlarged oviduct or a fluid-filled abdomen. Endoscopic examination may be diagnostic but should be done only by an experienced clinician in a bird with ascites. Abdominocentesis may need to be performed to relieve dyspnea. Other treatments include fluids, antibiotics, analgesics, anti-inflammatories, a warm incubator, and oxygen as needed. Many birds will improve with supportive care and antibiotics, but some may require salpingohysterectomy. Prognosis is fair with medical management and becomes guarded to grave with surgical intervention.

Cloacal Prolapse: Cloacal prolapse can occur in any bird that strains frequently. It is seen in egg-bound hens and in adult cockatoos, typically males. The exact cause is not known, but the following characteristics have been associated with most cases: 1) hand-raised birds, 2) delayed weaning or continued begging for food, 3) close attachment to at least one person, 4) signs of either a child/parent or a mate/mate relationship with the owner, who may not be aware of these signs, and 5) a tendency to hold the feces in the vent for prolonged periods (eg, overnight), rather than defecating in the cage or when the bird has been taught to defecate on command. Cockatoos independent of people do not have this medical problem.

If detected and treated early, surgery combined with behavioral modification may correct the problem and prevent secondary infections and other complications. Treatment includes cleaning exposed tissue, carefully debriding any necrotic or infected tissue, using hyperosmotic fluids to reduce swelling, and gently replacing the tissue. Stay or transcutaneous sutures may be required for several days and are more effective if combined with GnRH agonists and changes in management (eg, reduced handling of pet cockatoos by owners). Owners may be unwilling to alter their behavior, because often their attraction to the bird is because the bird is willing to allow stroking and cuddling. If the bird still perceives its owner as either a parent or mate, it will continue to strain and the problem will likely recur. Behaviors that should be avoided include stroking the bird, especially on the back (ie, petting); feeding the bird warm foods or food by hand or mouth; and cuddling the bird close to the body. If an owner is serious about trying to change their bird's behavioral patterns, consultation with a board-certified veterinary behaviorist who is experienced with psittacines is advisable.

In severe cases, where the vent is flaccid, vent reduction and/or cloacopexy may need to be performed but should only be done with behavior modification. Females may require salpingohysterectomy, because the vent reduction and cloacopexy may not allow passage of an egg.

Reproductive Failure: Most owners do not breed their pet birds, but reproductive failure is an issue for aviculturists who do. When evaluating a pair of birds for reproductive failure, a complete history is important. Is this a bonded pair (do they sit close to each other and allopreen, etc)? How long have they been together? Have they had a successful clutch in the past? What is their diet? Are the cage size, nest box, and perches appropriate for the species of bird? Most pet birds prefer an enclosed nest box and a stable perch for breeding. Is the owner certain of the sex? One of the most common reasons birds do not reproduce is same-sex pairs. Confirming the sex by DNA testing or endoscopic examination (to evaluate health and status of reproductive organs) is important. Common findings during endoscopy include same-sex pairings, immature birds, and reproductive disease. Physical examination, hematologic testing, and biochemical profiles are recommended to determine overall health. Treatment will depend on the examination and diagnostic findings and may include alterations in the environment or medical therapy if indicated.

Medical and Surgical Management: In many cases of reproductive disease, birds with moderate to severe disease require intensive nursing and supportive care. Often, physical examination and diagnostic tests must be postponed until the bird is stabilized in a warm (85°–90°F) oxygen incubator with supportive care. Procedures may need to be done in a stepwise fashion over time to minimize stress. Treatments may include warm parenteral fluid therapy, nutritional support, analgesics, anti-inflammatories, and antimicrobials (based on results of a Gram stain or culture and sensitivity testing). Some birds may require surgery. Reproductive surgery in birds is complicated by the difficulty in removing the ovary. Because of the position of the ovary cranial to the kidney, near the left adrenal gland and major vasculature, removing the entire ovary is not possible. The standard approach to the avian reproductive tract is a left coeliotomy. Endoscopic orchidectomy and salpingohysterectomy have been described but require specialized training.

TABLE 19 DRUGS USED IN AVIAN REPRODUCTIVE DISEASE

Drug	Type/Class	Dosage
Calcium gluconate (10%)	Calcium supplement	50–100 mg/kg, SC, IM
Calcium glubionate	Calcium supplement	25 mg/kg, PO, bid
Leuprolide acetate	GnRH agonist	700–800 mcg/kg, IM, every 2–3 wk
Deslorelin acetate	GnRH agonist	4.7-mg and 9.5-mg implants SC, dorsal back between scapulas every 3–6 mo
Oxytocin	Hormone	5–10 U/kg, IM; may repeat once
Dinoprostone	Prostaglandin E_2	0.02–0.1 mg/kg, topically to uterovaginal sphincter
Dinoprost tromethamine	Prostaglandin F_2	0.02–1 mg/kg, IM, intracloacal once

TOXICOSES

Heavy Metal Toxicosis: **Lead toxicosis** is commonly reported in companion birds as well as in free-ranging avian species, especially waterfowl. In pet birds, toxicosis often occurs from ingestion of metal in the home, such as blinds, costume jewelry, mirror backings, bird toys, hardware cloth, and curtain weights. Ingested lead degrades in the ventriculus and then is slowly released into the GI tract and blood. The lead is stored in soft tissues and bone and is slowly excreted over time. Lead toxicosis affects numerous biochemical processes in birds.

Clinical signs vary depending on the amount of lead ingested and may include anorexia, weight loss, regurgitation, diarrhea, depression, ataxia, weakness, seizures, blindness, polyuria, and polydipsia. *Amazona* spp, *Aratinga* spp, *Eclectus* parrots, and some other species may develop hemoglobinuria.

Diagnosis is based on clinical signs, biochemical analysis, hematologic findings, blood lead levels, and diagnostic imaging. Hematologic testing may reveal a microcytic, hypochromic anemia. Increased concentrations of AST, total protein, uric acid, and CK may be present. Radiographs may reveal metallic densities within the GI tract. However, the absence of metal in the GI tract does not exclude toxicosis. A blood level >50 mcg/dL (0.5 ppm) is considered diagnostic of lead toxicosis. Blood lead levels >20 mcg/dL (0.2 ppm) with clinical signs is considered consistent with lead toxicosis. Lead levels of 3–6 ppm or higher are considered significant in tissue (kidney, liver, brain, or bone).

Treatment includes supportive care (fluids, nutrition, etc) and chelating therapy with calcium edetate disodium (Ca EDTA) (30–35 mg/kg, SC or IM, bid) for 3–5 days until asymptomatic (with fluid therapy), followed by oral treatment with dimercaptosuccinic acid (DMSA) (25–35 mg/kg, PO, bid) or, less commonly, D-penicillamine (30–50 mg/kg, PO, bid). Midazolam or diazepam may be necessary for control of seizures. Bulk diets (with psyllium, peanut butter) may assist in removal of lead from the GI tract. In severe cases, flushing of the GI tract under general anesthesia may be necessary. Sources of lead in the environment must be removed.

Lesions associated with lead toxicosis seen on postmortem examination include demyelination of peripheral nerves, vascular necrosis, renal nephrosis, hemosiderosis in multiple organs, and focal areas of vascular damage in the cerebellum.

Zinc toxicosis is frequently reported in pet birds. Sources of zinc include any galvanized toys, chains, mesh, bells, keys, and pennies (post 1982). Galvanized wire contains mainly zinc, but some may also contain lead.

Clinical signs of zinc toxicosis include anorexia, GI disease, weakness, regurgitation, polydipsia, and polyuria. Diagnosis is based on history and clinical signs and an increased blood zinc level. Radiographs may reveal metallic densities within the GI tract. Blood samples for zinc analysis should be collected in glass or all-plastic syringes and tubes. Rubber stoppers on serum tubes and the grommets on some plastic may artifactually increase the zinc levels in the collected sample. Blood zinc levels >2 ppm are diagnostic for zinc toxicosis.

Treatment of zinc toxicosis is similar to lead toxicosis with supportive care, Ca EDTA, DMSA, and D-penicillamine. The source of zinc should be determined if possible and removed from the environment. Zinc is not stored in the bone like lead, so it chelates faster than lead.

Polytetrafluoroethylene Toxicosis: Polytetrafluoroethylene (PTFE) gas poisoning occurs commonly in pet birds housed in or near kitchens. The gas is released from nonstick cookware such as Teflon® when the pans are overheated, at temperatures reaching 280°C (536°F). Other sources of PTFE include irons, ironing board covers, some self-cleaning ovens, heating elements from some reverse cycle heat pumps, and some heat lamps. *See also* POLYTETRAFLUOROETHYLENE (POISONINGS IN POULTRY), p 2862, and SMOKE INHALATION, p 3022.

Often, the only clinical sign is acute death. Other signs depend on the level of exposure and size of the bird. Small birds often die suddenly with minimal exposure. Larger birds may present with dyspnea, wheezing, ataxia, weakness, in respiratory distress, or seizuring. With a large enough exposure, large birds can die acutely. Diagnosis is based on a history of exposure and sudden death, or a history and clinical signs consistent with exposure.

Treatment is supportive with a warm, oxygenated incubator, fluids, NSAIDs, broad-spectrum antibiotics, and diuretics. Prognosis is guarded. Necropsy often reveals severe hemorrhage and congestion of the lungs.

Tobacco: Passive inhalation of tobacco smoke (second-hand smoke inhalation) or contact with tobacco on hands, fingers, hair, or clothes of smokers can lead to chronic respiratory disease and dermatologic problems on the face and feet of pet birds.

Clinical signs may include coughing, sneezing, nasal and ocular discharge, dyspnea, conjunctivitis, or feather destructive behavior and mutilation. Ingestion of tobacco products has led to hyperexcitability, seizures, and death. Diagnosis is based on history, clinical signs, and response to treatment.

Treatment will depend on severity of clinical signs. For birds that are dyspneic or showing neurologic signs, supportive care and oxygen may be needed. If the bird has ingested tobacco, activated charcoal may be warranted. Treatment involves removing the bird from the exposure and placing it in a smoke-free environment. Owners who smoke should wash their hands before handling their birds.

Other aerosols, including some carpet fresheners, plastics either melted or burned in a microwave oven, perfumes, deodorizers, votive candles, and new heating duct systems may also be irritating or toxic to caged birds.

TRAUMATIC INJURY

Trauma is a common presentation for avian patients. Cat or dog bite wounds or large birds attacking smaller birds all occur frequently. Pet birds allowed to roam or fly freely in the house can become injured flying into walls, windows, or ceiling fans, or falling off shoulders, play gyms, or the top of their cage. Birds can also be injured in their cage. A foot or band may get caught in a toy or in the bars. Other common traumatic injuries include puncture wounds, lacerations, fractures, limb amputations, and crushing injuries.

Stabilization is paramount; birds presenting with trauma are often cold and stressed and have suffered blood loss. The bird should be placed in a warm, oxygenated incubator immediately after presentation and observed from a distance. Is there respiratory distress (tail bobbing) or open-mouth breathing? Is there active bleeding? Is the bird able to perch? Is it using both legs? Is there a wing droop?

After the initial assessment, the clinician must decide whether to maintain the bird in the incubator or oxygen, perform a brief physical examination and begin immediate supportive treatments, or perform a more thorough physical examination with or without diagnostic tests. Before picking up the bird, a detailed plan must be determined, and then all items set up ahead of time for anticipated treatments and diagnostics.

Examination and treatments may need to be done in steps, placing the bird back in the oxygenated incubator to recover if it becomes stressed or weak at any point during handling or treatments. Emergency treatments include warm fluids (SC, IV, or intraosseous), analgesics, anti-inflammatories, and antibiotics. Maintenance fluids are estimated at 50 mL/kg divided bid-tid. In dehydrated birds, 50% of the total daily maintenance can be administered SC (25 mL/kg) and repeated every 6–8 hr until hydration is reestablished. Often, birds are stressed and in pain and may benefit from sedation for diagnostic testing and treatments. In stressed birds, midazolam (0.5–1 mg/kg, IM, or 1–2 mg/kg, intranasally), with or without butorphanol (0.5–1 mg/kg, IM or intranasally) can be used.

Often with trauma cases, diagnostic tests or extensive treatments or surgery should be postponed until the bird is stable, which may take 12–48 hr. All birds with trauma should be treated with the goal of the bird's survival first and treatment of traumatized tissue second. For example, a bird that has been struggling for hours with its leg band caught, with possibly a fractured tibiotarsal bone, is in more danger of dying from stress related to the prolonged struggling than from the fracture.

Diagnostic tests should be based on physical examination findings and may include radiographs to determine whether fractures or luxations are present.

With predator bite wounds, antibiotic therapy consisting of treatment for both anaerobic and aerobic bacteria is crucial to increase the chances of a successful case outcome.

MISCELLANEOUS DISEASES

Diabetes Mellitus: Diabetes mellitus (DM) is an uncommon disease of pet birds and can be challenging to diagnose. Normal glucose levels in birds are significantly higher than those in mammals (200–400 mg/dL). Birds often have a significant hyperglycemia with stress, which can occur when handled or restrained. Glucosuria can occur at 600 mg/dL in birds, so birds with a stress hyperglycemia can also have glucosuria without a diagnosis of DM. Therefore, a persistent hyperglycemia and glucosuria need to be documented for a diagnosis of DM in birds.

Controlling blood glucose levels is a balance between the activity of glucagon and insulin within the pancreas. In mammals, pancreatic disease often leads to DM and is due to a lack of or resistance to insulin, which causes the blood glucose to rise. The cause of hyperglycemia and DM in birds is less clear. Blood glucose levels in some birds (granivorous birds) seem much more responsive to glucagon levels than to insulin levels, whereas other bird species may be more responsive to insulin. It is still debatable and may depend on the species as to whether DM in birds is caused by abnormalities with insulin, glucagon, or both.

Clinical signs of DM in pet birds include polyuria, polydipsia, increased glucose levels in the blood and urine, and weight loss. DM is often seen in conjunction with obesity or pancreatic or reproductive problems and may be transient in such cases. A persistent hyperglycemia and glucosuria need to be documented for a diagnosis of DM. Diagnosis is based on persistent increases in blood glucose (>700–800 mg/dL) and glucosuria, along with clinical signs of disease.

Treatment includes converting the bird to a healthier (pelleted) diet and limiting treats. Response of birds to mammalian insulin is variable, and insulin treatment is generally less effective in birds than in mammals. Regular insulin at 0.1–0.2 U/kg has been used successfully to stabilize birds. Longer-acting insulins (NPH or ultra-Lente) at 0.067–3.3 U/kg, once to twice daily, have been used for longterm control. Bird owners are often reluctant to give injections to their birds, so often oral antidiabetic medications are used. Glipizide (0.5 mg/kg, PO, bid, or 1.25 mg/kg/day, PO) and metformin (100–500 mg/L of drinking water) have been used anecdotally. Water intake, urine output, weight, and glucosuria should be monitored to determine whether the treatment protocol is effective. In some cases, dietary conversion and weight loss can result in resolution of the clinical signs, reducing or eliminating the need for oral medications or insulin.

Gout: Gout is the abnormal deposition of uric acid in the body. Uric acid is the major end product of protein breakdown in birds. It is produced and secreted primarily in the kidneys and liver and eliminated by tubular secretion. Elimination is independent of glomerular filtration rate. Hydration has only a minimal effect on plasma uric acid levels; therefore, hyperuricemia can be an indicator of renal disease in birds. Gout typically occurs secondarily from increased plasma uric acid levels. Articular gout occurs in the joints (most often the metatarsal and phalangeal joints) of birds, and visceral gout occurs on the serosa of various organs and is commonly found on the pericardium, liver, and spleen.

Clinical signs of articular gout are pain, lameness, swelling in the joints, depression, anorexia, and dehydration. Visceral gout is rarely diagnosed antemortem and is typically found at necropsy. Acute death is often the only clinical sign. The serosal surface of various organs and the renal tubules are the locations of uric acid deposition. Diagnosis of articular gout is by identifying gout tophi—whitish yellow, subcutaneous, and intra-articular deposits that demonstrate uric acid crystals on staining. Uric acid levels commonly are increased.

Treatment includes fluid therapy to reduce uric acid levels and analgesics for pain. Articular gout tends to be severely painful. If effective pain control cannot be accomplished, euthanasia should be considered. Surgical removal of these tophi is not practical in most cases, because they are extremely vascular and the risk of fatal hemorrhage is high. Additionally, unless the underlying condition can be identified and corrected or controlled, new tophi will appear very rapidly. Allopurinol (10–30 mg/kg/day, PO) and colchicine (0.04 mg/kg, PO, once to twice daily) may be useful in control of articular gout. The genetic, nutritional, or environmental factors that predispose a bird to gout are not fully understood. However, current treatment of birds with increased uric acid levels include conversion to an appropriate diet (this may be a pelleted diet in some species) or a diet change to whole grains, seeds, fruits, and vegetables for some smaller birds such as cockatiels and budgerigars (for whom a pelleted diet may be a factor in renal disease). Essential fatty acids (omega 3) at 0.1–0.22 mL/kg/day, PO, have been used anecdotally to manage renal disease in birds.

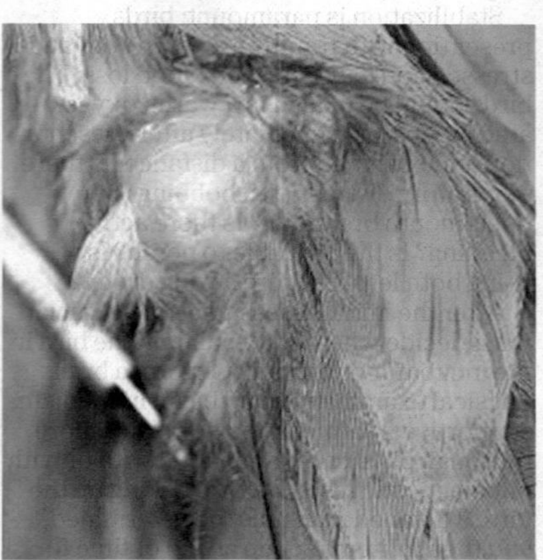

This macaw has a single, large ingrown feather or feather cyst. Canaries are commonly affected with multiple feather cysts. *Courtesy of Dr. Louise Bauck.*

Feather Cysts: Feather cysts are ingrown feathers that result in a granulomatous mass. Recurrence is common unless the extensive dissection of the feather follicle is accomplished. In birds with multiple affected feathers, such as the genetically predisposed Norwich canary, this is not practical.

Feather Destructive Behavior: The phrase "feather plucking" is commonly used to describe behavior that ranges from mildly excessive preening to self-mutilation. Management of this condition is frequently challenging. Feather plucking seldom has a single etiology, and it is prudent to thoroughly explore all possible contributing factors, including underlying medical problems. Good communication concerning feather plucking in birds at the onset will help owners realize that this is a complicated behavior that is difficult to stop. The goal should be to improve the health of the bird and to reduce (or eliminate) the plucking behavior if possible.

Possible medical causes for feather plucking include: 1) Endoparasites (especially giardiasis in cockatiels) and, rarely, tapeworms or roundworms. 2) Ectoparasites (rarely). 3) Hepatic disease, with associated pruritus. 4) Coelomic cavity granuloma or mass. 5) Neoplasia, which typically causes localized plucking of the area associated with an underlying mass. 6) Folliculitis or dermatitis that is primary, or secondary to excessive plucking and/or mutilation. Bacteria, viruses, fungi, or yeasts may be involved. 7) Allergies. Although difficult to confirm, a change in environment or diet when allergens are suspected may lead to a decrease in plucking and a tentative diagnosis by elimination. 8) Endocrine abnormalities, the most likely being hypothyroidism. However, hypothyroidism is overdiagnosed in part because of the lack of established normal values for avian thyroid levels, the low range for baseline T_4 noted in birds, and difficulty in obtaining a reliable thyroid-stimulating hormone (TSH) response test. Nevertheless, some obese birds that demonstrate a lack of weight loss after a rigid diet, accompanied by poor quality feathers and infrequent molts, may be thyroid deficient. The plucking exhibited by these birds is often an attempt to rid themselves of old, damaged feathers. 9) Heavy metal toxicosis, notably zinc. Barbering and feather plucking from zinc ingestion have been hypothesized. Many of these cases lack radiographic evidence of heavy metal and require a blood zinc analysis for diagnosis.

Malnutrition is likely a more common contributing factor to feather plucking than the medical conditions listed above. Basic seed and table food diets often create multiple nutritional deficiencies. These deficiencies cause abnormal skin and feather development resulting in plucking behavior, as well as myriad other medical problems that may occur. The dyes and preservatives added to seeds and most pelleted diets may be a factor for some birds. The relatively low humidity in most households also has a drying effect on the skin. Being deprived of natural sunlight, fresh air, humidity, and the normal light/dark cycle has negative physiologic and psychologic effects on birds.

A diagnostic evaluation for a bird with feather destructive behavior may include a CBC, biochemical profile, viral testing, skin biopsy, radiographs, and/or endoscopic examination. Behavioral feather picking should be determined only after a complete evaluation that excludes as many medical causes as possible.

Treatment is based on the findings of the diagnostic evaluation. A hormonal bird may need an injection of leupolide acetate, a GnRH agonist, to reduce reproductive behavior, along with environmental changes (*see* p 1920).

Although treatment of medical and environmental factors may reduce the severity of feather plucking, a strong behavioral component is often involved. Treatment of some of the above-mentioned problems may lead to initial improvement, followed by a relapse. Psychologic stressors can lead to feather plucking as a displacement behavior. Unfortunately, once the stress has been relieved, the habit may still remain. Feather plucking does not occur in the wild, where birds are occupied with finding food, maintaining their social status in the flock, seeking a mate, avoiding predators, and breeding and raising young. Therefore, often the best-kept birds, which have all their apparent needs met, will pluck feathers for behavioral reasons. Psychologic conditions that may cause feather plucking in birds vary. Overstimulation may cause plucking in a nervous bird. Another bird that plucks from boredom may feel both stimulated and slightly threatened by increased activity in the home and stop plucking to pay attention to the environment and guard itself against potential predators. Birds that reach sexual maturity may begin to pluck as an outlet for their increased energy and agitation. Owners of these birds often report that their birds show more cage territoriality, more aggression toward family members, and potentially, sexual behavior toward a perceived human mate or inanimate objects.

All feather destructive behavioral issues require a multimodal treatment approach that involves proper nutrition, enrichment, providing foraging opportunities and, in some cases, psychotropic medications (*see* TABLE 20). Neither of these categories of drugs tends to produce longterm positive results, and adverse effects may be seen. As is true of most medications administered to pet birds, these drugs are not approved by the FDA.

Psychotropic drugs should not be used alone but only in conjunction with dietary modifications, enrichment, and foraging opportunities. In addition, changes may need to be made in the owner/bird interactions. Dietary modifications include both conversion to a healthier formulated diet and providing foraging opportunities for the bird. Owners can place food in multiple food dishes throughout the cage or hide food inside foraging toys to stimulate normal foraging behavior. Enrichment can be provided in the form of natural branches, toys, wood to chew on, multiple play gyms throughout the house, natural sunlight, and ideally a flight cage to encourage activity. Exercise should be encouraged, either through flight or walking and climbing activities. Rope and boing perches stimulate activity and balance. Teaching birds tricks such as waving, dancing, and recall can provide intellectual stimulation and positive interaction between the owner and bird.

In addition to traditional medical therapies, acupuncture has been reported to be helpful in some cases. Dietary supplementation with omega fatty acids has been reported to be helpful. Whether this is due to the antiprostaglandin effect or a true fatty acid deficiency is not certain.

TABLE 20 PSYCHOTROPIC MEDICATIONS USED FOR FEATHER PLUCKING IN PET BIRDS

Medication[a]	Dosage	Comments
	PSYCHOTROPIC MEDICATIONS	
Amitriptyline	1–2 mg/kg, PO, once to twice daily	Maximal effects may require treatment for several weeks.
Clomipramine	1 mg/kg/day, PO	Effects similar to those of amitriptyline but may be effective in some cases in which amitriptyline is not.
Diazepam	2.5–4 mg/kg, PO, as needed	Limited usefulness; most birds require a dose that causes sedation to inhibit plucking.
Haloperidol	0.15 mg/kg, PO, once to twice daily for larger birds; 0.2 mg/kg, PO, bid for smaller species	Serious adverse effects, including anorexia, hepatic dysfunction, and CNS signs have been reported; most often used in cockatoos.
Fluoxetine	2 mg/kg/day, PO, once to twice daily	Effectiveness reported to vary; maximal effects may require treatment for several weeks.
	HORMONES	
Medroxyprogesterone acetate	—	Decreases sexual behavior; not recommended because of serious adverse effects, including weight gain, polyuria, polydipsia, lethargy, hepatopathy, diabetes mellitus, and death.
GnRH agonist, eg, leuprolide acetate	300–800 mcg/kg, IM	Decreases sexual behavior by negative feedback, reducing production of sex hormones.

[a] All are extra-label usages.

An ideal medical treatment is not likely to be found for feather plucking in captive birds. Environmental manipulation, ensuring quality nutrition, and psychologic adaptations suited to the species and temperament of the bird offer the best hope to reduce this syndrome. Consultation with a board-certified behaviorist familiar with psittacines may be indicated.

Hypersensitivity Pneumonitis:
A respiratory condition similar to chronic obstructive pulmonary disease (COPD) has been reported in macaws (primarily Blue and Gold macaws). These birds often have a history of being housed with birds that produce large amounts of powder down, such as cockatiels and cockatoos in poorly ventilated environments. The birds may also have secondary bacterial or fungal infections.

Clinical signs include increased respirations, exercise intolerance, dyspnea, respiratory distress, and cyanosis of the facial skin.

Diagnosis is based on a history of being housed with feather down–producing birds in poor ventilation with respiratory disease and often polycythemia (>60%–70%). Pulmonary biopsy is diagnostic. Histopathologic lesions are confined to the lower respiratory tract. The most prominent lesion is atrial smooth muscle hypertrophy and some atrial loss due to fusion and epithelial bridging.

Treatment is supportive care and removal of the bird from the offending environment. Improved ventilation and separation from birds that produce powder down is critical. NSAIDs such as meloxicam (0.5–1 mg/kg, PO, once to twice daily) may help reduce inflammation. Albuterol (0.05 mg/kg, PO, bid) has been used anecdotally. Birds should be housed to reduce stress and minimize exertion. Often, birds with confirmed pulmonary hypersensitivity will not have a normal life expectancy.

POTBELLIED PIGS

Potbellied pigs (PBPs) have a short to medium wrinkled snout, small erect ears, large jowls in proportion to the head, short neck, pronounced potbelly, swayed back, and straight tail with a switch at the end. The CON and LEA lines of PBPs at 1 yr of age should not be >18 in. at the withers (ideal height ≤14 in.) or weigh > 95 lb (ideal weight ≤ 50 lb). The life span of PBPs is probably 8–20 yr with ~10–15 yr typical. Very small or obese PBPs may have a shortened life span. For hematologic and serum biochemical reference ranges, *see* TABLES 6 and 7, pp 3176 and 3178.

The term "teacup" pigs has no strict definition, and it is difficult to make an educated guess of mature size without seeing the parents and grandparents, which is rarely possible. Mature size is also heavily influenced by adequate nutrition. In general, when pigs are "selected for smaller size," in addition to nutritional stunting, many other possible problems of miniature pigs may be magnified. These include hypoglycemia, idiopathic seizures, musculoskeletal deformities, heart disease, cleft palate, atresia ani, and reproductive problems such as dystocia and agalactia.

MANAGEMENT

Environment: PBPs are sensitive to extremes of heat and cold and should be provided a clean, dry, draft-free environment. Adults are usually comfortable in a temperature range of 65–75°F (18.3–23.9°C). Because pigs do not sweat, temperatures ≥85°F (29.4°C) are stressful to adults. Extended exposure to high temperatures combined with high humidity may be fatal to PBPs not acclimated to such an environment. Cooling methods for adult PBPs include moving air across the body, wetting the skin for evaporative cooling (more efficient as humidity decreases), providing shade, and resting on cool surfaces.

Newborn pigs are very susceptible to drafts and chilling and require an environmental temperature of ~90°F (32°C). Chilled pigs will pile on each other and shiver, and their hair will stand on end. A poor environment may cause neonates to become moribund and hypoglycemic (*see* MANAGEMENT OF THE NEONATE IN LARGE ANIMALS, p 2088) within 24–36 hr. Heat lamps or pads can be used to provide supplemental warmth, but their use should be monitored closely because of the electrocution risk from chewed cords; pigs that become too hot will spread out and pant.

Housing: PBPs may be housed outdoors or indoors (or both) but must be appropriately acclimated to the specific environmental situation.

PBPs housed outdoors should have a large pen (≥50 sq ft/pig) with a structure within to provide sleeping, feeding, and watering areas. Pigs will use dirt for elimination, and daily removal of feces and addition of fresh dirt to cover and absorb urine is required. Hay or straw may be added to partially satisfy the need to root. However, "rooted-up" pen ground should be filled in with fresh dirt from time to time. Fencing should be well secured in the ground to prevent it from being rooted up, but it should also be portable so that the entire pen can be moved periodically, giving access to fresh, clean dirt. The old pen dirt should then be smoothed out and left unused for several months before being used again. If pens are maintained on solid surfaces (eg, concrete pads), feces and urine should be removed daily, and fresh hay or straw provided as needed. Water dispensers must be secured to keep pigs from spilling the water by rooting or damaging the device by chewing.

PBPs housed indoors should have a particular area (eg, a laundry room), with an elimination area in one corner and a sleeping and eating area in another corner. A litter box with the side cut down to accommodate easy entry and exit may be used for elimination. Nontoxic material should be used for litter because pigs are curious and tend to chew on everything. A blanket may be provided to allow the pig to burrow under and partially satisfy the need to root while indoors; a box of dirt is another alternative.

Exercise: PBPs should be exercised whether kept outside or indoors. They may be trained to walk on a leash or released into exercise areas. Daily exercise is important not only for physical health but also to relieve boredom that may otherwise manifest as destructive chewing or rooting or as aggression. Even if the PBP does not exercise much when given the opportunity, the various stimuli from an outside environment appear to be beneficial to overall temperament. Many household and *garden plants are toxic to PBPs*, which are adventurous eaters (*see* p 3103).

Temperament: As healthy, neutered PBPs mature, they may become more aggressive and challenge other PBPs or people for status. Such challenges need to be addressed, or the pet may learn to use aggression to get what it wants. A combination of aversive techniques (eg, hand clapping, gruff vocalizations, stomping) and rewarding the PBP for positive behavior may help manage the problem. Failure to deter this unwanted behavior is a common reason why PBPs are placed in rescue operations or abandoned.

Vaccinations: Neutered PBPs should be vaccinated against erysipelas and tetanus. Tetanus toxoid is especially important in PBPs housed outside in contact with other species (eg, petting zoos). Leptospirosis vaccine (6-way) may also be considered, but there is a substantial risk of high fever after use. Vaccines are not specifically approved for PBPs, so those commercially available for domestic swine are substituted. Two initial vaccinations 3–4 wk apart are followed by boosters every 6 mo for erysipelas and every year for tetanus, or both boostered yearly at the time of annual physical examination. Breeding PBPs should be minimally vaccinated against erysipelas, leptospirosis (6-way), and parvovirus; they should be vaccinated twice, 3–4 wk apart, before breeding and before rebreeding or every 6–12 mo. Other vaccines should be used as exposure risk indicates. Routine vaccination against various pathogens not only minimizes sickness but helps prevent zoonotic disease and may satisfy requirements for pet licensure. Safety and efficacy are concerns when using commercial domestic swine vaccines in PBPs. Consideration should always be given to the amount of antigen per body weight that is injected, especially in small pigs. Excessive antigen administration may cause adverse reactions. No rabies vaccine is approved for use in PBPs because of the extremely low incidence of rabies in swine in the USA.

Parasite Control: External and internal parasites are possible health problems in PBPs, and the zoonotic potential of sarcoptic mange and roundworms should be considered when counseling owners. Fecal samples via fecal flotation may be evaluated in PBPs as early as 6 and 10 wk old for whipworms and roundworms, respectively. Dewormers, such as oral fenbendazole at 3 mg/kg/day for 3 days; ivermectin at 300 mcg/kg, SC; or doramectin at 300 mcg/kg, IM, should be used as indicated. Injectable ivermectin and doramectin are highly effective against sarcoptic mange, the most common external parasite in PBPs.

Dental Care: The eight needle teeth (four deciduous lateral incisors and four deciduous canines) of newborn PBPs should be trimmed to prevent injury to littermates and laceration of the sow's underline. Four permanent canine teeth erupt at ~5–7 mo of age and are first trimmed at or after 1 yr of age. Elongated permanent canine teeth may cause discomfort, malocclusion, and persistent chewing motion and salivation. In PBPs, the canine teeth grow continually and should be cut about once a year using obstetrical wire, mechanical saws, or other instruments. Sedation or anesthesia is required. Teeth should be cut as close as possible to the gum line without cutting the oral mucosa or lips; there should be no exposed root canal after cutting the canine teeth of any type of swine. Tetanus antitoxin (500–1,500 U, depending on PBP size) and antibacterials are usually administered. In PBPs properly vaccinated with tetanus toxoid, a tetanus antitoxin injection is unnecessary. Tartar buildup can be removed manually by instrument scraping at the same time the canine teeth are cut. Dental cleaners for small animals may be used with care, positioning the head of the PBP downward during use to prevent water aspiration.

Geriatric PBPs may have abscessed and/or exposed tooth roots; sedation (tiletamine-zolazepam 2.2 mg/kg, IM, in ham) and examination of the oral cavity with or without endoscopy is indicated if anorexia and/or bruxism are reported. Radiographs may be necessary to diagnose tooth root abscessation. Swelling followed by a draining tract at the angle of the mandible, especially in geriatric PBPs, indicates canine tooth abscessation. Removal is challenging even for skilled surgeons and may result in mandibular fractures. However, PBPs seem to recover well after tooth extraction followed by antibiotics and tetanus prophylaxis.

REPRODUCTION

Females: First estrus occurs as early as 3 mo of age in gilt piglets. The lack of estrus or a distended abdomen in a young gilt may be due to pregnancy if she has been exposed to littermate boars. If the female does not cycle, the abortifacient prostaglandin $F_2\alpha$, given as two injections (8 mg and 5 mg in a 25-kg pig) 12 hr apart, can be administered when corpora lutea have become susceptible to luteolysis after day 13 after estrus. Estrus should occur 3–7 days later.

Dystocia is of special concern in PBPs. Because the birth canal is too small to inspect for unborn pigs via palpation, radiography or ultrasonography may be indicated to reveal undelivered piglets. Oxytocin (5–10 U) may be used to aid delivery if the vaginal canal is patent. The decision to perform a cesarean section, if indicated, should be made promptly, before the sow becomes toxic and has friable uterine tissue and vessels. Cesarean section may be performed by several approaches, but the right flank approach has two advantages: the piglets nurse away from the incision, and gravity pulls the incision shut, minimizing the chance of dehiscence. Regardless of surgical approach, surviving piglets will probably require hand-raising.

Ovariohysterectomy in PBPs at 4–6 mo of age is ideal. Older female PBPs generally display irritable behavior for 2–3 days of estrus out of every 21 days of the estrous cycle. Performing an ovariohysterectomy during estrus in older PBPs is a formidable task because of the tremendous vasculature in the broad ligaments of the horns of the uterus; surgery should be delayed until ~7–10 days after estrus. A distal midline approach, as if performing a cystotomy, is routinely used for ovariohysterectomy. The uterine horns fold back and are located beside the body of the uterus with the ovaries. No ovarian ligament tearing is necessary as in dogs and cats. Penetration of the cervix by sutures should be avoided when ligating the uterine stump to prevent intermittent postsurgical hemorrhage from the vulva. A right flank approach may be used in extremely obese PBPs, in which wound dehiscence could be a complication. Isoflurane or sevoflurane anesthesia provides excellent muscle relaxation. (Malignant hyperthermia [*see* p 1027] has been reported only once in a PBP under isoflurane gas anesthesia, so it is thought to be rare in PBPs.) Hypothermia during and after surgery is an important concern. A baseline rectal temperature should be recorded at anesthesia induction, and normal body temperature should be maintained until recovery is complete. Injectable anesthetics such as xylazine plus tiletamine-zolazepam can delay normal thermoregulation for 5–6 hr after anesthesia. Because some PBPs may become apneic when placed in prolonged dorsal recumbency, intubation is preferred to masking; however, PBPs may be difficult to intubate, and prolonged efforts at intubation may cause laryngeal edema and postsurgical complications.

Early spaying also reduces the risk of ovarian cysts, uterine tumors, and cystic endometrial hyperplasia. An obviously distended abdomen is seen with large ovarian or uterine masses (≥20–30 lb). Vulvar hemorrhage may be a sign of uterine tumor and can be life-threatening. Although most ovarian or uterine masses can be surgically removed, some are so extensive and invasive that euthanasia is required.

Males: PBP boars retained for breeding should be kept in secure pens; they should not be kept as pets because of the unpredictable behavior of boars around other animals or people. Neutering is usually performed at 8–12 wk of age, using injectable or gas anesthesia. One protocol for injectable anesthesia is xylazine at 2.2 mg/kg, IM, followed by tiletamine-zolazepam at 6.6 mg/kg, IM, both injections in the hams. Determining whether both testicles are descended before surgery is important because cryptorchidism is seen in PBPs. An inguinal hernia is another possible complicating factor. The midline skin incision is made cranial to the scrotum, and structures such as the vas deferens and blood vessels are ligated and excised similar to the procedure in dogs. Both inguinal ring areas should be closed to prevent herniation. Removal of tunic, cremaster muscle, and extraneous subcutaneous tissue, followed by closure to obliterate empty space, help prevent seroma formation. At the time of castration, the preputial diverticulum or "scent gland" may be removed by eversion and excision to minimize the pooling and discharge of foul-smelling preputial fluid. Umbilical hernia may complicate removal. Early castration may interfere with the development of the preputial diverticulum, making its removal unnecessary, especially in PBPs kept outside. Tetanus antitoxin (if no current tetanus toxoid vaccination) and antibacterial injection are given after surgery of the reproductive tract.

FEEDING AND NUTRITION

Fresh water should be available at all times to prevent dehydration and salt toxicity (water deprivation). Balanced diets are essential to provide proper daily nutrients and prevent obesity. Starter, grower, and maintenance rations for PBPs are commercially available as crumbles or pellets. The recommended amount per body weight should be fed divided into at least two meals/day. Rations for commercial domestic swine, available in meal, crumble, or pellets, may also be used with professional veterinary guidance. Green leafy vegetables, alfalfa, and green grasses (but not weeds, because some are toxic) can be added to the ration to satisfy appetite. Fruits such as apples and grapes may be given in limited amounts. High-energy treats should be avoided because PBPs tend to become overweight.

Even when calorie intake is restricted, weight loss is difficult because the minimal amount of exercise possible in obese PBPs burns few calories. Lameness is another common factor limiting exercise capacity. Maintaining normal hoof length via trimming is important for mobility. Swimming is an alternative form of exercise for obese, lame PBPs, but acclimation and supervision is necessary.

Young weaned PBPs thrive best if adequate colostrum was consumed within the first 24 hr of life. PBPs deprived of colostrum easily succumb to diarrheal and septicemic disease. For early nutrition, commercial milk replacers are available, but 2%–3% pasteurized milk or powdered milk also can be used successfully. Approximately 1 oz every 4–6 hr should be fed from a bottle with a nipple until the pig is trained to drink the milk from a shallow bowl or pan; usually, this can be done in <24 hr. The volume fed should be increased as the pig grows but decreased if diarrhea occurs. Overeating diarrhea may be controlled with kaolin/pectin preparations given every 4 hr. Infectious diarrhea that may be from gram-negative bacteria (eg, *Escherichia coli*) should respond to parenteral or oral gentamicin or oral spectinomycin. The diet can be converted to solid feed by mixing a small amount with milk to make a gruel and gradually increasing the ratio of feed to milk (conversion to all feed in ~14 days). Increasing amounts of fresh water should be provided as the diet is converted.

Urolithiasis from triple phosphate crystalluria may occur in PBPs but can be prevented through addition of urinary acidifiers to the ration. At least one commercial PBP feed contains ammonium chloride, and feed additives containing ammonium chloride or citric acid are available. Owners may feed fruits or vitamin C in an attempt to acidify the urine. A constant source of clean, fresh water is also important to prevent the accumulation of triple phosphate crystals. Adding fruit juice to water may increase water consumption and help acidify the urine. Inadequate water consumption by sedentary PBPs in cool weather has been associated with urolithiasis.

DISEASES

Furnishing adequate housing, nutrition, and care will minimize disease in PBPs, as in other species. Many diseases of PBPs are similar to those of domestic commercial swine, although some are more common in PBPs.

Gastrointestinal System

Gastritis and gastric foreign bodies are common in PBPs because they are omnivorous and prone to ingest many types of objects. Keeping PBPs indoors where they are unable to root and restricting calorie intake to prevent obesity probably contribute to this continual search for food. Dividing the daily ration into two or more portions and furnishing low-calorie foods (eg, lettuce, cabbage, celery, carrots, or green grasses) may help satisfy appetite. If an ingested foreign body is small or pliable enough, it may pass through the GI tract and cause mild gastritis that is self-limiting or only requires antibiotic therapy. Larger objects may remain in the stomach or partially pass into the duodenum or a more distal part of the small intestine. Clinical signs such as vomiting and colic can be acute but may be more subtle and increase in intensity over several days or weeks. Radiographs may reveal obvious foreign material or delayed gastric emptying. CBCs may indicate infection but are usually not informative; serum enzyme and electrolyte panels may only reflect dehydration. Surgical correction is indicated but may not be successful if extensive necrosis of GI tissue is present. Fluid replacement and nutritional supplementation plus antibacterial therapy and tetanus prophylaxis are indicated in convalescing PBPs.

Lower GI obstruction due to bowel stricture occurs in geriatric PBPs. Anorexia, scant fecal production, and a bloated abdomen with massively distended intestines seen radiographically are typical. Sedation and endoscopic examination of the oral cavity, esophagus, and stomach are indicated to exclude other problems. Exploratory laparotomy and anastomosis with or without bowel resection is usually remedial.

Colibacillosis or *Escherichia coli* diarrhea is generally an important disease in young PBPs. Mortality may be high in piglets that have not ingested adequate colostrum in their first 24 hr of life. Older PBPs apparently develop resistance to colibacillosis. Diagnosis is through signalment, history, and fecal culture. Sanitation to minimize infective doses of pathogenic coliforms in the environment of young, nursing PBPs is important for prevention. Commercial swine vaccines to prevent colibacillosis are available but must be given to sows before farrowing to stimulate immunity and secretion of IgA into the milk. Treatment is based on in vitro antibacterial sensitivity testing, but antibiotics such as oral or injectable gentamicin or injectable ceftiofur are usually effective.

Enterocolitis from *Salmonella* Typhimurium infection can affect PBPs of any age, but it usually occurs after weaning. Sources of salmonellae include waste food from overturned garbage cans, exposure to carrier swine (such as the dam), or fecal material from other animal species. Mild to severe diarrhea with mucus and blood can result. Diagnosis is through signalment, history, and fecal culture or PCR. *Salmonella* spp are characteristically resistant to many antibiotics, so in vitro antibacterial sensitivity testing is important. Parenteral gentamicin at 2.2 mg/kg/day for 3 days may be effective in the interim. Untreated PBPs may die. Some recovered PBPs may develop rectal stricture after enterocolitis, resulting in megacolon and a distended abdomen. Subsequent straining to defecate can cause rectal prolapse. Surgical correction of the rectal prolapse will not correct the underlying problem. Owners should be advised that many *Salmonella* spp, including *S* Typhimurium, are zoonotic. Healthy PBPs may be tested via fecal culture or PCR to determine their salmonella status. Multiple tests are more accurate predictors than single tests. Vaccines available for commercial swine have not been used much in PBPs.

Bacteremia or septicemia after *S* Choleraesuis infection may also affect PBPs, usually after weaning. Sources of infection are similar to those of *S* Typhimurium. Mild to inapparent diarrhea followed by fever, lethargy, anorexia, cyanosis of extremities, recumbency, and death may ensue. Diagnosis, treatment, prevention, and zoonotic potential are similar to those of *S* Typhimurium; zoonosis is mainly a threat in immunocompromised people.

Constipation may be seen in PBPs; however, each normal bowel movement of a PBP is typically composed of one or more cylindrical formations made up of smaller, multiple fecal balls that may give the impression that the PBP is constipated. True constipation may occur due to low water intake in sedentary PBPs or to an actual disease. Careful evaluation is warranted before treatment is administered. Enemas may be contraindicated if there is pathology such as colitis. In simple constipation, fecal softeners or mild laxatives such as sodium sulfate or magnesium sulfate may be used. These should be given with food, if possible, because forced PO administration can result in aspiration pneumonia and death, especially with mineral oil. Encouraging increased water intake by flavoring with fruit juice or liquid gelatin may be helpful. Regular exercise is also beneficial to promote normal feces.

Rectal prolapse occurs due to straining from bowel irritation from diarrheal disease, rectal stricture after *S* Typhimurium enterocolitis or previous rectal prolapse repair, cystitis or urolithiasis, persistent coughing, dystocia, or possibly genetic predisposition. Small, uncomplicated, recent rectal prolapses may be repaired via anesthesia and purse-string closure of the rectum that allows for minimal passage of feces. Larger, complicated prolapses require surgical excision. Recurrence is less likely after surgery but is possible regardless of method of repair.

Lymphosarcoma, lymphoma, and carcinoma of the intestines occur in aged PBPs. Signs are vomiting, anorexia, melena, anemia, and chronic weight loss followed by death (or euthanasia). Confirmation is by postmortem histopathology.

Integumentary System

Dry, flaky skin with minimal to severe pruritus is seen in virtually all PBPs. Wiping down the skin with wet towels each week will remove the flakes. Moisturizing lotions (eg, aloe vera) also temporarily alleviate this problem. Fatty acid supplementation can be used as a more longterm remedy, but caution must be exercised not to promote obesity.

Sarcoptic mange is the most important ectoparasitic disease of PBPs. Intense pruritus and dermatitis are the basis for a presumptive diagnosis. In many cases, the owners have pruritic skin lesions on the arms or abdomen. Examination of skin scrapings (deep enough to contain some blood) from several sites usually confirms the diagnosis in advanced cases but may be negative in less advanced cases if very few mites are present. In young PBPs, the source of infestation is usually the dam; in older PBPs, the source is usually other infested pigs. Young PBPs isolated from other pigs and kept as pets may harbor mange mites as a subclinical problem until mite populations increase sufficiently to make the condition obvious. Treatment with ivermectin (300 mcg/kg, SC, repeated in 2 wk) or doramectin (300 mcg/kg, IM, repeated in 3 wk) is indicated. Recently acquired young PBPs should be given a routine preventive injection of either parasiticide when first presented for examination.

Melanoma is an important skin tumor in swine. Tumor removal and evaluation of metastatic potential through histopathology is important for prognosis. Spontaneous regression of melanomas, with subsequent depigmentation of the hair, skin, and iris, is occasionally seen in PBPs; affected swine usually have normal life spans.

Sunburn may develop in PBPs exposed to sudden, high-intensity sunlight. Skin lesions may or may not be obvious, but affected PBPs appear painful and seem to have hindlimb weakness or paresis. A sunburned PBP may be "down in the back legs" and show intense pain with vocalization. A thorough history is important for the diagnosis. Exposure to further sunlight should be prevented. Symptomatic treatment is remedial.

Bleeding back syndrome (dippity pig syndrome) is of unknown etiology. Signs are almost identical to those of sunburn (pigs dip their backs, vocalize, and show signs of extreme pain) but with no history of sun exposure. Circular, serum-oozing lesions of various sizes are seen on lumbar skin surfaces. Affected PBPs recover in several days with restricted activity with or without symptomatic treatment. The condition may recur in some animals.

Erysipelas, caused by *Erysipelothrix rhusiopathiae*, is a generalized bacterial infection that affects swine. For details on clinical signs, diagnosis, and treatment, *see* p 626.

Musculoskeletal System

Lameness due to lower back, hindlimb, or forelimb weakness is common in PBPs. Because of their conformation, PBPs are susceptible to muscle pulls, ligament damage, and fractures of the back and limbs. Because PBPs usually struggle against manual restraint (predisposing to injury), sedation or anesthesia is often used for procedures such as prolonged examination, radiography, foot trimming, blood collection, and dental work. Tiletamine-zolazepam at 2.2 mg/kg body weight, IM (in the ham), provides excellent analgesia and chemical restraint for these minor procedures; recovery, although smooth, is prolonged and requires careful monitoring. Gas anesthesia is also used and has the advantage of rapid recovery time. Fasting for 24 hr and withholding water for 4–6 hr before sedation or anesthesia is recommended.

PBPs with injuries to the back or limbs are usually treated with anti-inflammatory drugs, such as buffered aspirin with antacid, flunixin meglumine, or glucocorticoids (eg, dexamethasone). Polysulfated glycosaminoglycan and/or glucosamine/chondroitin sulfate products may be tried in nonresponsive cases.

Fractures of the distal humerus and elbow area and femur are common. These occur from jumps off furniture (distal humerus), dog bites (elbow area), restraint (elbow area and femur), equine kicks (femur), and other trauma. Repair via pins, screws, plates, and external devices successfully restores some range of motion if fractures are immobilized properly and any sepsis is controlled.

Infectious arthritis may affect the very young to older PBPs. Lameness with or without joint swelling in one or more limbs is the usual clinical finding. *Erysipelothrix rhusiopathiae*, *Streptococcus* spp, *Mycoplasma hyosynoviae*, *M hyorhinis*, *Staphylococcus* spp, and *Haemophilus parasuis* are possible causes. Treatment early in the disease course with an effective antimicrobial (eg, lincomycin at 11 mg/kg, bid for 3 days) may be effective. Treatment after chronic changes have occurred, antimicrobial ineffectiveness against the etiologic agent, or misdiagnosis are reasons for treatment failure and persistence of lameness. In chronic cases, pain management with anti-inflammatory drugs should be considered. Polyarthritis from neonatal infection of the navel may be due to various environmental bacteria, including *Pseudomonas* spp. If degenerative arthritis and joint fusion from chronic inflammation are present after polyarthritis, euthanasia may be warranted. Osteochondrosis may also be considered in shoulder, elbow, hip, and stifle lameness, but this condition is not common in slow-growing, light-muscled animals such as PBPs.

Overgrown and/or cracked hooves are a common cause of lameness. Regular exercise on abrasive surfaces (eg, concrete) will wear hoof ends and help keep them the appropriate length. In PBPs with overgrown, elongated hooves, normal yearly length can be maintained by routine yearly trimming under sedation or anesthesia. Hoof cracks can be caused by overgrown hooves. PBPs with cracked hooves may additionally require antiseptic cleaning with tamed iodine and systemic antimicrobial therapy (ceftiofur at 4.4 mg/kg/day for 3–10 days, or ampicillin at 11 mg/kg, PO, bid for 7–10 days).

Zygomycosis from *Mucor* spp infection has occurred in the distal hindlimb of a PBP. The large growth that encompassed the entire foot was composed of infected/abscessed tissue that involved bone. Amputation was remedial.

Tetanus may occur after wound contamination from dog bites, skin abrasions, oral cavity abrasions, or surgical procedures. Tetanus toxoid should be part of the routine vaccination schedule of PBPs at high risk of exposure. If there is no current tetanus toxoid vaccination, tetanus antitoxin (500–1,500 U, depending on body weight) should be administered IM in the neck after recovery from any surgery or dental procedure (eg, trimming of canine teeth). Treatment for tetanus is by massive doses of tetanus antitoxin and penicillin early in the disease, along with tranquilizers, isolation to minimize external stimuli, and supportive therapy.

Nervous System

Systemic bacterial infection can be caused by (in approximate decreasing order of importance) *Streptococcus suis* type 2, other *Streptococcus* spp, *Salmonella* Choleraesuis, *Haemophilus parasuis*, *Escherichia coli*, other gram-negative bacteria, and *Listeria monocytogenes*. CNS signs may include fever, depression, incoordination, staggering, postural abnormality, head tilt, circling, nystagmus, seizures, and death. PBPs are most commonly affected from birth through 4–6 mo of age. Treatment with the appropriate antibacterial therapy (eg, extra-label florfenicol, which penetrates the blood-brain barrier) in the early stages of infection is most effective; however, death may be the first clinical sign. Because *S suis* type 2 is a zoonotic disease agent, care should be exercised to prevent human infection when performing necropsies on pigs dying from suspected CNS disease.

Overheated PBPs may be depressed, inactive, and recumbent and show open-mouth breathing or panting with an initial fever followed by a subnormal and decreasing temperature. The prognosis is grave, but some overheated PBPs may respond to resting on a cool surface and cooling only the head with water for 10–15 min followed by packing ice bags around the head. If the temperature is still not controlled, cold-water enemas can be used while additional areas of the skin surface are packed in ice. Symptomatic treatment is continued as indicated.

Salt toxicity occurs after water deprivation for ≥36 hr followed by sudden rehydration or, less commonly, after prolonged consumption of high-salt foods. Affected PBPs may have seizures, walk aimlessly, or show other CNS signs such as blindness or postural abnormalities. Diagnosis in the affected live animal is confirmed by high levels of serum sodium, usually 160–183 mEq/dL (normal range 142–153 mEq/dL). Gradual rehydration and symptomatic treatment to counteract cerebral edema is indicated, but severely affected PBPs may only be stabilized to a vegetative and blind status. The histopathologic finding of eosinophilic infiltration into brain tissue is also diagnostic.

Seizure from unknown cause occurs in PBPs. Animals <1 yr old seem most susceptible. Frequency may range from 1–2 seizures per month to several per day. Infrequent seizures may require no preventive medication. Diazepam is used to control more frequent episodes. Phenobarbital in addition to diazepam may be required to control the most severe cases. Seizures may cease as the affected PBP ages.

Respiratory System

Atrophic rhinitis is an infectious disease of swine that initially causes sneezing, nasal discharge, tearing, and growth retardation. Younger PBPs are more commonly affected. For details on clinical signs, diagnosis, and treatment, *see* p 1465.

Pneumonia can be a very serious disease in PBPs because of their relatively small lung capacity. The most common cause of pneumonia is from initial *Mycoplasma hyopneumoniae* infection (*see* p 1467), which immunocompromises the lungs, followed by *Pasteurella multocida* infection. Young pigs contract these infectious agents from their dams or from mixing with infected pigs after weaning. Antibiotic treatment may be more effective if directed against *P multocida*, because this bacterium becomes the most important pathogen once coughing is present for several days. Vaccines available for *M hyopneumoniae* in domestic commercial swine have been used in young PBPs to prevent mycoplasmal pneumonia and subsequent *Pasteurella* pneumonia. Vaccination in older PBPs is probably unnecessary unless risk of exposure warrants continued use.

Actinobacillus pleuropneumoniae (*see* p 1469) causes a life-threatening pneumonia that may occur after infection from the sow or exposure to carrier animals. Signs range from coughing, fever, and lethargy to sudden death, depending on the serotype of *A pleuropneumoniae*. Prompt antibiotic treatment with penicillin or ceftiofur is indicated. Recovered PBPs usually have permanent tissue loss in affected lung areas and may have recurrent respiratory problems. Vaccines available for domestic commercial swine may be used in PBPs if there is an exposure risk.

Swine influenza (*see* p 1470) is an important viral pneumonia in PBPs that are taken to fairs, exhibitions, and petting zoos and exposed to other pig populations. It is usually self-limiting after 7–10 days but can be fatal. H1N1, H3N2, H1N2, and H2N3 are the most common strains in domestic swine. Multivalent vaccines available for domestic swine could be used in PBPs if indicated. Swine influenza is a zoonotic disease.

Urinary System

Cystitis and urolithiasis are common in PBPs. Signs include frequent urination or straining to urinate. Urinalysis, urine culture, CBC, serum chemistry, radiography, and ultrasonography are important diagnostic aids. A sterile urine sample for culture can be obtained via cystocentesis. Cystitis without triple phosphate crystalluria should respond to extended antibacterial therapy based on in vitro sensitivity testing. Acidification of the urine may minimize recurrence of infection. Nephritis can occur after cystitis as an ascending infection. Leptospirosis may be a primary cause of nephritis. Increased BUN and creatinine values may aid in the diagnosis of nephritis and kidney failure. A 6-way vaccine for leptospirosis is routinely given to breeding PBPs (*see* p 1930) but may also be considered for routine use in rescue operations where many PBPs are housed in close contact. Vaccination may possibly reduce renal shedding of leptospires should PBPs become chronically infected and, therefore, minimize transmission of this zoonotic disease.

In a PBP that is straining and unable to urinate, the bladder size should be reduced immediately by cystocentesis after sedation and radiography (plain or contrast) or ultrasonography to evaluate the location of urethral and bladder stones. If the blockage is in the urethra, cystotomy is recommended (both sexes) to identify and remove calculi in all possible locations. Calculi in the urethra of males may be removed by cutting through the sheath to expose the distal penis, catheterizing the urethra, and backflushing into the bladder. Calculi that cannot be removed by this method must be surgically removed by incising the urethra at the location of the blockage. However, scar tissue at the healed incision may also cause urethral obstruction. Suturing of the urethra is followed by cystotomy and bladder flushing to minimize recurrence and then by inspection for more calculi. The bladder is then closed, and a Foley catheter is inserted into the bladder, tunneled through the abdominal muscles, and sutured to the skin. Several days later, the Foley catheter is occluded, and the urethra is inspected to determine patency and urine flow; if not patent, the Foley catheter is opened again, and the process is repeated several days later. When the urethra becomes patent, the Foley catheter is removed. Although the urethra in females is short, blockage can still occur. Because urethral catheterization is difficult without endoscopy, a Foley catheter is inserted into the vagina and inflated, and a purse-string suture is placed at the vulva. Retrograde flushing through the urethral opening in the vaginal floor is attempted. A cystotomy is then performed to remove all possible calculi, followed by routine closure of the bladder. Foley catheter placement into the bladder may not be necessary. Further treatment includes antibiotic therapy and acidification of the urine. Despite these efforts, some affected PBPs do not recover and require euthanasia. Perineal urethrostomies are usually only temporarily successful because the surgical site becomes occluded by amorphous material or urethral polyps, and patency cannot be reestablished. However, surgical methods have been described to correct failed perineal urethrostomies in PBPs. Rupture of the bladder is a grave complication because normal bladder tone may not return even after stones have been removed and the bladder has been surgically repaired. Laser lithotripsy has been used to fracture urethral calculi not removable by flushing.

Routine urinalysis as part of an annual examination may enable early diagnosis and prevention of serious urinary tract disease in PBPs.

Psychogenic water consumption should be considered in PBPs (especially young PBPs) with polydipsia and polyuria. PBPs may develop a habit of drinking water and urinating frequently because of possible boredom or unknown causes. Cystitis and crystalluria should be eliminated as differential diagnoses. Measuring urine specific gravity before and after a 12-hr water fast will demonstrate whether the affected PBP is able to concentrate urine. Ability to concentrate urine indicates normal kidney function and helps exclude diabetes insipidus. Estimating the daily water intake and urine output will further aid the diagnosis of psychogenic water intake or establish that water consumption and urination are, in fact, normal. Relieving boredom may be helpful to change this behavior. Affected young PBPs typically outgrow this condition. If water is restricted and offered only with meals, care must be taken to prevent salt toxicity.

Chronic kidney failure is a common cause of death in geriatric PBPs. Lethargy, anorexia, dehydration, azotemia, ammonia breath odor, and low temperature are possible presenting signs. Symptomatic treatment such as rehydration and antibiotics (procaine penicillin 22,000 IU/kg/day, IM, for 3 days) may be at least temporarily helpful in less severe cases.

RABBITS

The European or Old World rabbit (*Oryctolagus cuniculus*) is the only genus of domestic rabbits. Wild rabbits and hares include cottontail rabbits (*Sylvilagus*) and the "true" hares or jackrabbits (*Lepus*). Rabbits have been bred for fur, meat, wool, exhibition, and for use as laboratory animals. The closest relative to the rabbit is the pika (*Ochotona princeps*), which lives in cold climates such as the Rocky Mountains. Rabbits are not rodents.

MANAGEMENT

Management of rabbits for meat, fur, or wool production is quite different from maintenance of a pet or house rabbit. The American Rabbit Breeders Association (www.arba.net) provides guidance for both production and pet rabbit care. The House Rabbit Society (www.rabbit.org) is another resource regarding pet rabbit care.

Restraint: Proper handling and restraint is important. Rabbits have powerful hindlimbs, which can kick out and lead to broken backs. Rabbits should never be held by the ears; they should be scruffed at the neck, and the body firmly supported at the rump. If they are not held properly and securely, fractures or luxations of lumbar vertebrae can easily follow struggling. If a rabbit appears to be very stressed or excited, a sedative may be indicated to avoid injuries caused by handling. Midazolam at 0.5–1 mg/kg, IM, is often enough to adequately sedate the rabbit for a thorough physical examination.

Physical Examination and Sample Collection: Most techniques for physical examination suitable for dogs and cats may be applied to rabbits. A thorough oral examination, including palpation of the face and bottom of the jaw, should be performed to evaluate dental health. An otoscope or a pediatric nasal speculum can assist visualization of the molars. Conscious rabbits will usually resist a full dental examination, and sedation or anesthesia is required. Sex can be determined by depressing the external genitalia to reveal a slit-like vulva in females or the penis in males. The testicles descend at 10–12 wk. Normal body temperature is 103.3°–104°F (39.6°–40°C). Body temperature <100.4°F or >105°F is cause for concern.

Blood can be collected from the cephalic vein, lateral saphenous vein, and the jugular vein. The lateral saphenous vein is easy to access when the rabbit is held and resting on someone's forearm, with the restrainer holding the leg above the stifle joint. The lateral saphenous vein runs across the lateral aspect of the tibia at the middle of the length of the bone. In larger rabbits (>3 kg), the ear veins can also be used. The auricular or marginal ear vein provides a site for venous administration or catheterization. Drugs should not be injected through the ear veins, because this can lead to phlebitis and subsequent ear sloughing. Only physiologic crystalloid fluids should be administered via the ear vein. The central artery can be accessed for direct blood pressure monitoring during anesthesia; no drugs should be injected into the central artery. The auricular vasculature is sensitive to temperature; having the rabbit warm (or at least having the ear warm) and applying a topical anesthetic cream greatly facilitate these procedures.

Clinical Pathology: Clinical pathology in rabbits varies from that in other domestic animals. The normal neutrophil:lymphocyte ratio is 1:1. The rabbit neutrophil is called a "pseudoeosinophil" or heterophil because of its red-staining cytoplasmic granules. Both the heterophil and the granules are smaller than the eosinophil and eosinophil red granules. Rabbits do not usually respond with a leukocytosis to an active infection. In case of stress, the ratio of the heterophils and lymphocytes changes toward a relative heterophilia without increasing the total WBC count. Many sick rabbits have hemoglobin and PCV values much lower than normal; this makes the PCV one of the best indicators of healthy or sick animals. Calcium metabolism in rabbits results in higher normal blood calcium levels (up to 16 mg/dL) and a wider range than in other animals, which can lead to an erroneous diagnosis of hypercalcemia. Rabbit urine ranges from yellow to brown or reddish. A dipstick can quickly differentiate normal rabbit urinary pigments from hematuria. Traces of glucose and protein are normal in rabbit urine.

Therapeutics: Very few products are licensed for use in rabbits, leading to extra-label use of drug therapies approved for use in other species. Particular caution must be exercised in use of antibiotics that suppress normal GI microflora and result in enteric dysbiosis and/or enterotoxemia. This has been called "antibiotic toxicity." Antibiotics contraindicated in rabbits include clindamycin, lincomycin, erythromycin, ampicillin, amoxicillin/clavulanic acid, and cephalosporins. The flea treatment fipronil is contraindicated in rabbits because of severe toxic reactions in some individuals. Supportive care for rabbits often includes aggressive IV fluid support. The maintenance fluid rate for rabbits (120 mL/kg/day) is much higher than that for dogs and cats. Hospitalized rabbits often require doubling of maintenance rates, or 10 mL/kg/hr. In addition to fluid support, pain control is also commonly needed. NSAIDs and opioids are often used in synergy. The dosage of meloxicam in rabbits is 1 mg/kg/day, which is also significantly higher than that in dogs and cats. Opioids such as oxymorphone or hydromorphine can readily be used and have not been shown to cause GI stasis. In most cases, additional force feeding is not required, and the rabbit should be offered food after fluid and pain management has been initiated. Syringe-assisted feeding can be offered to see whether the rabbit is interested in food intake. In rare cases in which the rabbit refuses to eat, eg, cases of severe hepatic lipidosis, active feeding is necessary; treatment may require aggressive nutritional support via syringe feeding, nasogastric tube (3–5 French), or pharyngostomy tube (soft esophagostomy tube designed for cats). The least invasive method is often the most successful approach. Various commercial products for assisted feeding of rabbits are available. Products are available for immediate critical care (eg, Emeraid®) as well as for longterm assisted feeding and to meet the needs of the recovering rabbit (eg, Recovery®, Recovery Plus®, Critical Care®).

Reproduction: Rabbit breeds of medium size are sexually mature at 4–4.5 mo, giant breeds at 6–9 mo, and small breeds (eg, the Polish Dwarf and Dutch) at 3.5–4 mo of age. The rabbit is an induced ovulator and, contrary to popular belief, has a cycle of mating receptivity; rabbits are receptive to mating ~14 of every 16 days. The degree of mating receptivity is indicated by the color of the vaginal orifice and by the amount of moisture on the labia. A doe is most receptive when the vagina is red and moist. Does that are not receptive have a whitish pink vaginal color with little or no moisture. Many breeders test mate the doe 10–16 days after breeding as a way to detect pregnancy, but this is unreliable. Palpation of the doe's abdomen for "grape-sized" embryos in the uterus is a much better technique to detect pregnancy. The best time to palpate is 12 days after breeding. Pseudopregnancy is common in rabbits and can follow any induced ovulation, the introduction of a male rabbit in the environment, or other stimuli.

A ratio of 1 buck to 10 does is common practice, but many commercial growers find that 1 buck to 20–25 does is more economical. Bucks can be used daily without decreasing fertility; more frequent use requires periods of rest. The doe should always be taken to the buck's cage for breeding. The breeding program should continue year round. Does that experience long periods of rest between litters tend to become obese and difficult to breed. Does constantly in gestation and lactation may become underweight, and their receptivity to the buck and fertility decrease dramatically. If breeding is delayed several weeks and the doe is given full feed, weight is quickly regained.

The gestation period is ~31–33 days. Does with a small litter (usually ≤4) seem to have a longer gestation period than does that produce larger litters. If a doe has not kindled by day 32 of gestation, oxytocin (1–2 IU) should be given to induce parturition; otherwise, a dead litter is almost always delivered sometime after day 34. Occasionally, pregnant does abort or resorb the fetuses because of nutritional deficiencies or disease.

Nest boxes should be added to the cages 28–29 days after breeding. If boxes are added too soon, the does foul the nests with urine and feces. A day or two before kindling, the doe pulls fur from her body and builds a nest in the nest box. The young are born naked, blind, and deaf. They begin to show hair on day 2–3 after birth, and their eyes and ears are open by day 10. Neonatal rabbits are unable to thermoregulate until about day 7. Rebreeding can occur any time after parturition, because the doe can conceive 24 hr after kindling. Some commercial growers use accelerated breeding schedules and rebreed 7–21 days after parturition, whereas most people raising rabbits for show or home use rebreed 35–42 days after parturition.

Most medium-sized female rabbits have 8–10 nipples, and many kindle 12–15 young. If a doe is unable to nurse all the kits effectively, kits may be fostered by removing them from the nest box during the first 3 days and giving them to a doe of approximately the same age with a smaller litter. If the fostered kits are mixed with the doe's own kits and covered with hair of the doe, they are generally accepted. Moving the larger kits to the new litter instead of the smaller kits increases the chance of success. Does nurse only once or twice daily. Kits nurse <3 min. Kits are weaned at ~4–5 wk of age.

Rearing Orphaned Kits: Kits can be hand-reared, but mortality is high. They should be kept warm, dry, and quiet. Kitten milk or goat milk replacer or a formula of ½ cup evaporated milk, ½ cup water, 1 egg yolk, and 1 tbsp corn syrup can be used. Feedings vary from ½ tsp to 2 tbsp, depending on the age of the kits. Kits should be fed only every 12 hr to avoid overfeeding and to mimic the natural feeding behavior of the doe. Cottontail kits start eating greens around day 15–18, whereas domestic rabbit kits are weaned when ~6 wk old.

Surgery: Preoperative fasting is not required or recommended. Rabbits cannot vomit. Additionally, rabbit stomachs are never empty, even after prolonged fasting. However, a short fast (1–2 hr) should be done to assure that the oral cavity is free of food. Premedication with butorphanol or diazepam/midazolam will reduce stress from preoperative handling. Premedication with atropine will be useful for only a short time, because many rabbits have an atropinase that clears the drug from the system rapidly. Instead, glycopyrrolate may be used to reduce bradycardia and upper airway and salivary secretions (0.01–0.1 mg/kg, IM or SC, or 0.01 mg/kg, IV). Isoflurane is recommended for general anesthesia, but premedication with a combination of an NSAID and an opiate (such as meloxicam at 1 mg/kg, PO, and butorphanol at 0.4 mg/kg, IV) can reduce the minimum alveolar concentration (MAC) of isoflurane from 2.5% to 2.3%. Lidocaine administered as a constant-rate infusion has also been shown to reduce the MAC of isoflurane (lidocaine can be given at a loading dose of 2 mg/kg, IV, followed by 100 mcg/kg/min).

The long and narrow pharynx and large tongue make rabbits difficult to intubate. Laryngospasm can be minimized by application of lidocaine on the epiglottis. There are several reported techniques to intubate rabbits; all require selection of the appropriate tube size and length to avoid tracheal injury. A pediatric laryngeal mask, uncuffed Cole, or cuffed Murphy eye type endotracheal tube (ET) can be used, but selecting the appropriate size (2–4 mm) is critical. The risk of tracheal injury increases with repeated intubation attempts, but ET cuff pressure, prolonged duration of intubation, and movement of the ET during mechanical ventilation and animal positioning for anesthesia seem to be more critical because of the vascular anatomy of the rabbit trachea. Rabbits are best intubated with visualization, using an endoscope or similar technology. Direct visualization of the epiglottis and ET placement can also be accomplished by using a laryngoscope with a Miller 0 blade, a rabbit oral specula, and cheek dilators. The glottis should be visualized using the endoscope, and the tube carefully advanced toward the glottis. The natural position of the epiglottis is behind the soft palate. The ET can be used to disengage the glottis from the soft palate, and then introduced into the glottis and down the trachea. Care must be taken to not damage the arytenoid cartilages when inserting the tube into the trachea, because these cartilages reduce the diameter of the glottis significantly and can be easily damaged by a larger-size tube. If no visual aid is available, the rabbit can be intubated blindly, but this procedure requires much skill and has the potential for iatrogenic trauma if not performed properly. In the classic blind technique, the rabbit is placed in a sternal position with the head held and the nose pointing at the ceiling. The ET is guided behind the incisors and to the larynx. The operator listens for the sounds of inspiration and expiration and times the advancement of the ET with maximal inspiration. A second technique involves placing the rabbit in lateral recumbency with the head dorsiflexed. The ET is advanced along the hard palate to the back of the throat until condensation can be seen within the lumen of the ET. The condensation is used to judge the cycles of inspiration and expiration, and the ET is advanced at maximal inspiration. Proper ET placement should be confirmed regardless of placement method. An alternative to intubation is a supraglottic airway device (V-gel®). A species-specific pharyngeal device is placed in the oral cavity and advanced caudally until it sets in place automatically. The device sits on top of the glottis and seals the surrounding structures, creating an airtight connection between the trachea and the tube.

Adequate general anesthesia can be achieved for a short procedure with injectable ketamine (25–50 mg/kg) in combination with a tranquilizer such as xylazine (5–10 mg/kg, IM). The combination of ketamine (10–20 mg/kg, IM) and dexmedetomidine (0.125–0.25 mg/kg, IM) provides adequate anesthesia; ~⅓ of the original dose can be repeated if anesthesia needs to be prolonged. Atipamezole can be given IM in equal volume to dexmedetomidine volume for reversal.

It is critical for rabbits to start eating postoperatively, and analgesic treatment for 1–2 days will help prevent inappetence. A rabbit in pain may chatter or grind its teeth while sitting in a hunched position. Analgesic treatment may include opioid drugs such as buprenorphine (0.01–0.05 mg/kg, SC, IM, or IV, bid-tid) or butorphanol (0.05–0.4 mg/kg, SC or IM, bid-tid), or NSAIDs such as carprofen (1.5 mg/kg, PO or SC, bid), flunixin (0.5–2 mg/kg/day, PO, deep IM, or IV, for no more than 3 days), or meloxicam (1 mg/kg/day, PO or SC). Tramadol used at 11 mg/kg, PO, causes no adverse effects and has been reported empirically to be effective in rabbits. However, a study showed that this dose does not achieve plasma levels that would be considered adequate in people. Prolonged opiate exposure has not been associated with GI stasis.

Postoperative supportive care is critical to a successful surgical outcome. Hay and water should be offered as soon as possible after surgery. Alfalfa hay can be used to improve appetite. Banana is favored as a treat by many rabbits. Hand feeding or syringe-assisted feeding is necessary if the rabbit does not eat on its own soon after the surgery. If the rabbit does not eat within 2–3 hr after surgery, the analgesic protocol should be reevaluated. The rabbit should be assisted fed until it refuses further food intake in each session.

Castration can reduce aggressive behavior and is suggested for house rabbits and group-housed rabbits. It has no advantage for meat-type rabbits. The testicles are lateral and anterior to the penis, as in marsupials and not as in most other placental mammals. Castration is performed using a closed technique or by an open technique with closure of the large superficial inguinal ring to prevent herniation.

Female pet rabbits should be spayed because of the high risk of uterine cancer. Rabbits have two uterine horns connected to the vagina by two separate cervices. The oviduct loops around and is much longer than in cats or dogs. Ovariohysterectomy is more complicated in older or multiparous rabbits because of the large amount of fat in the mesometrium. Postoperative adhesions are a common complication, which may be reduced by calcium-blocker treatment (verapamil, 200 mcg/kg, SC, tid for 3 days). To avoid adhesions, all blood clots should be removed before closing the abdomen, and the GI tract should not be handled at all. The use of spay hooks is not recommended in rabbits, because the intestinal loops are easily damaged; tissue forceps (eg, Adson-Brown) are a better choice.

Although the vast majority of trichobezoars can be managed medically with aggressive fluid therapy (10–12 mL/kg/hr) and appropriate pain medication (eg, oxymorphone), a small percentage of GI cases need to be surgically corrected. Surgery should usually be considered if the condition has not improved after 24 hr of aggressive medical therapy. When gastrotomies are performed, the stomach is elevated by stay sutures through a cranial celiotomy incision. An incision is made through the greater curvature of the stomach. It is important to remove stomach contents from the pyloric sphincter and to examine the stomach lining for abnormalities. A fine, absorbable monofilament suture should be used for closure of the stomach wall and incorporate, but not penetrate, the gastric mucosa. Pre- and postsurgical care should include fluids and antibiotic therapy.

Rabbits can chew out skin sutures; therefore, skin closure should be performed with a 4-0 absorbable synthetic suture with a cuticular-cuticular pattern. Tissue glue may be added to finish this closure. Rabbits tolerate staples.

Euthanasia: Rabbits may jump or scream when the traditional overdose of barbiturate is given in the marginal ear vein. Sedation with midazolam (5 mg/kg, IM or IV) or propofol (10 mg/kg, IV) is recommended before administration of the barbiturate. As a further precaution, euthanasia solution may be diluted 1:1 with saline to prevent a negative reaction and to reduce viscosity of the solution to facilitate a faster and smoother injection.

Other Management Techniques: Toenails on the hindlimbs may severely scratch unprotected arms of handlers. Nails should be trimmed every 1–2 mo. Declawing is not recommended, but some rabbits tolerate application of adhesive nail caps.

Some breeders tattoo or place ear tags on their rabbits for identification purposes. For show purposes, the right ear is reserved for registration marks applied by registrars of the American Rabbit Breeders Association. A tag placed in the anterior cartilaginous part of the ear, nearer to the head, is less likely to be pulled out.

HOUSING

Pet Rabbits: A rabbit hutch placed in the back yard, basement, or garage has been and continues to be traditional housing for rabbits. The hutch should be conveniently accessed for proper care of the rabbit, because diseases of neglect are common in rabbits abandoned in a hutch at the back of the yard. Care must be taken to prevent the hutch from being exposed to severe heat, because rabbits are prone to heat stroke. The flooring of the hutch should be covered with some type of soft padding to provide a comfortable resting spot. Sore hocks can lead to more problems if the rabbits are housed on wire or wooden flooring for long periods. Keeping the area around the hutch clean is important to avoid a large population of flies, which often lead to fly strike (myiasis) that is often fatal. There should be adequate ventilation and protection from dogs or other predators such as raccoons.

House Rabbits: In the natural setting, rabbits use a latrine system. This behavior can easily be exploited by providing a litter box. Rabbits usually readily accept a litterbox with little training. Rabbits have continuously growing teeth and need to chew on things to appropriately wear down the teeth. If no appropriate food material that requires significant chewing efforts (eg, hay) is offered, rabbits are likely to gnaw on various objects in the environment, such as furniture, curtains, carpeting, or electrical wiring, which is dangerous for the rabbit and creates a fire hazard. Rabbits should be confined to safe quarters when unsupervised.

Cages and Ancillary Equipment: Rabbits can gnaw, and caging should be constructed of durable materials. Cages should be easily sanitized and allow easy cleaning. All-wire cages with a minimum of 12-gauge wire (16-gauge recommended for cage floor to support the weight of the rabbit) are preferred. Aquariums are not appropriate housing for rabbits (or other small mammals) because of inadequate air circulation. The size of the cage depends on the size of the rabbit. Giant breeds (>12 lb) require a minimum of 30 × 36 in. to 36 × 48 in. Medium breeds (7–12 lb) require 24 × 30 in. to 30 × 36 in. Smaller breeds can be accommodated by 18 × 24 in. The cage should be tall enough to allow the rabbit to stand on its hindlimbs. The cage should be equipped with a feed hopper and a watering system. Feed hoppers are best constructed of sheet metal with holes or a screen in the bottom for removal of "fines" (small, broken feed particles). Rabbits drink more than other animals of similar size, and they should be offered ad lib potable water. Rabbits will consume significantly more water when water is offered from a dish versus a sipper bottle. Rabbits often chew on the watering valve and may eventually destroy it unless it is made of stainless steel or has a stainless centerpiece. If a water dish cannot be offered, water bottles with sipper tubes are a good alternative. However, food dishes are easily contaminated and should be washed and disinfected daily. A barren cage is inadequate; the cage environment should be enriched (eg, cage furniture, toys) to provide stimulation. Optimally, rabbits should be given run time outside of the cage daily.

Nest boxes should be constructed so that they can be easily placed in the cage and later removed for cleaning and disinfecting between litters. Disinfecting the nest box after cleaning and again just before placing it in the cage helps reduce incidence of disease. The box should be large enough to prevent crowding but small enough to keep the kits warm. A standard size nest box for medium-sized rabbits is 16 × 10 × 8 in. Wooden, metal, or plastic nest boxes with nesting material (eg, straw, hardwood shavings, CareFresh® bedding) serve well in either warm or cold weather. Rough edges such as splintering wood should be avoided, because they contribute to mastitis when does hop in and out of the nest box.

Pens: Pens should have a nonslip floor and may be bedded with straw or shredded paper covered with straw or hay to increase absorbency. Shavings or sawdust are not the best, because the scent is too powerful. Pen sides should be at least 4 ft high or high enough to allow the rabbit to stand erect on the hindlimbs.

Group Housing: When setting up group housing, compatibility is a major factor. Personalities should be evaluated for docility and aggressiveness. Strain influences personality. Rabbits that have grown up together are best, although adults may be so aggressive toward each other that serious fights occur. Neutering will improve compatibility. A period of adjacent proximity is prudent before group housing rabbits. Another factor to consider is stocking density. Floor space recommendations vary from 3.5 to 10 sq ft/rabbit to allow territory establishment. Others recommend 3.5 hop lengths per rabbit as a general rule. Regardless, group-housed rabbits should be provided escape and hiding places and should be frequently monitored.

Production Housing: Housing requirements for rabbits depend on climate. Minimal housing (an A-frame roof without sides) can be used in moderate climates, whereas a climate-controlled rabbitry may be necessary in hot or cold climates. Rabbitries should be located on nearly level ground and use well-drained soil or tile-drained pits for manure. Shade should be provided over as much of the rabbitry as possible. Rabbits are prone to heat stress. Although rabbits tolerate subzero temperatures when provided proper shelter, the optimal rabbit environment is 61°–72°F. Increased humidity levels should also be avoided, because they will increase the likelihood of heat stress and potentially dermatopathies. Good ventilation at all times is imperative.

Sanitation: Cleaning frequency depends of the type of facility or caging system. Rabbits typically choose a preferred latrine site, such as a corner of the cage. This normal behavior can be exploited during litterbox training. A strategically placed litterbox is readily accepted by most pet rabbits. Sanitation is especially important in rabbit production. Poor sanitation leads to disease and deaths; therefore, cleaning and sanitizing must be constant. Nest boxes must be disinfected between uses. Cages, feeders, and watering equipment should be sanitized periodically with an effective and inexpensive sanitizing solution such as diluted household chlorine bleach (1 oz/1 quart water) or other less corrosive disinfectants. Complete cleaning should be performed before housing new stock.

An active rabbitry constantly experiences a loose hair problem. Does pull hair from their bodies to make nests, and some of this hair becomes airborne. It sticks to almost any surface, including cages, ceilings, and lights, and must be removed periodically. The most effective ways to remove hair from cages are washing or using a propane torch or flame. Washing, brushing, sweeping, and vacuuming also are effective in other parts of the rabbitry. Pens or wire-floored cages should be brushed or hosed every 2 wk. An acid wash may be required to descale rabbit urine from solid floor pans.

Frequent manure removal is essential. Excess manure leads to unacceptable levels of ammonia in the air, which predisposes to respiratory disease. The manure can be composted in an efficient pit system.

NUTRITION

Rabbits are small herbivores with specialized feeding needs and digestive systems. They are selective eaters and choose nutrient-rich leaves and new plant shoots over mature plant material that is higher in fiber. Rabbits are therefore considered concentrate selectors, because they naturally pick and choose foods higher in energy density, which predisposes them to obesity in captivity. Anatomically, rabbits are nonruminant herbivores with an enlarged hindgut. The large cecum supports a population of microorganisms that uses nutrients not digested in the small intestine. Most of the bacterial population in the cecum is made up of the gram-positive *Bacteroides* sp. This makes the rabbit very sensitive to oral antibiotics; administration of oral antibiotics can disturb the *Bacteroides* population and lead to fatal GI upsets. Separation of digesta on the basis of particle size occurs in the hindgut. Peristaltic action rapidly moves large particles (>0.5 mm), primarily lignocellulose, through the colon and excretes them as hard fecal pellets. This is the "indigestible fiber" component of the diet. The clinical importance of a diet high in long particle length is to maintain the motility of the cecum and colon. This is why these fibers are sometimes referred to as "scratch factor," because they mechanically stimulate GI motility. Antiperistaltic action moves smaller particles (<0.3 mm) and soluble material into the cecum, where they undergo fermentation. This component of the diet is known as "digestible" or "fermentable" fiber. At intervals, the cecal contents are expelled as "soft feces" or cecotrophs and consumed by the rabbit directly from the anus. Cecotroph ingestion is highest when rabbits are fed a diet high in nondigestible fiber. This reingested material provides microbial protein, vitamins (including all the B vitamins needed), and small quantities of volatile fatty acids, which are essential in rabbit nutrition. However, because amino acids obtained in this manner make only a minor contribution to the rabbits' protein needs (particularly young, growing rabbits), the diet must supply the additional amino acids, although the requirements for essential amino acids in rabbits have not yet been defined.

Rabbits digest fiber poorly because of the selective separation and rapid excretion of large particles in the hindgut. A generous amount of dietary fiber (~15% crude fiber) is needed to promote intestinal motility and minimize intestinal disease. High-fiber intake can be provided by use of ad lib timothy hay (~30%–35% fiber). Fiber may also absorb bacterial toxins and eliminate them via the hard feces. Diets low in fiber promote an increased incidence of intestinal problems, eg, enterotoxemia. Carbohydrates will actually inhibit motilin release. Motilin is a polypeptide hormone secreted by cells of the duodenum and jejunum, which stimulates the GI smooth muscle. Excess starch can also be substrate for the proliferation of pathogenic bacteria such as *Clostridium spiroforme*, which produce a potent toxin. Cecum fermentation produces volatile fatty acids, which are responsible for 40% of the rabbits' calorie requirement. Volatile fatty acids also aid in the control of pathogenic organisms by helping to maintain the normal pH (6–7) in the cecum.

A dietary supply of vitamins A, D, and E is necessary. Bacteria in the gut synthesize B vitamins and vitamin K in adequate quantities; thus, dietary supplements are unnecessary. Disease and stress may increase the daily vitamin requirements. Feed preparation and storage must be done in a manner that will reduce losses from oxidation, which destroys vitamins A and E more readily than other vitamins. Diets containing ≥30% of alfalfa meal generally provide sufficient vitamin A. Levels of vitamin A in the diet must be >5,000 IU/kg and <75,000 IU/kg. Levels out of this range may cause abortion, resorbed litters, and fetal hydrocephalus. Vitamin E deficiency has been associated with infertility, muscular dystrophy, and fetal and neonatal death. Pet rabbit diets sold in pet stores or even in bulk at feed stores may not have adequate turnover, which may result in nutritional deficiency. Hay packaged for small mammals may have been sitting on the shelf for an extended period.

All the components of the basic diet (ie, protein, fiber, fat, and energy) should be managed in consideration of the life stage (growth, gestation, lactation, maintenance), breed, condition, and lifestyle of the rabbit. Ratios should meet the nutrient requirements of the National Research Council (*see* TABLE 21). Pelleted rabbit feeds provide good nutrition at reasonable cost. Fresh, clean water should always be available. Prolonged intake of typical commercial diets containing alfalfa meal by laboratory or pet rabbits kept for extended periods under maintenance conditions may lead to kidney damage and calcium carbonate deposits in the urinary tract. Ad lib timothy hay is usually recommended for the maintenance diet of adult rabbits. Reducing the calcium level to 0.4%–0.5% of the diet for nonlactating rabbits helps reduce these problems. This can be accomplished by feeding pelleted diets with a timothy hay base. Adult pet rabbits not intended for breeding should be fed a high-fiber pelleted diet, restricted to ¼ cup/5 lb body wt/day to prevent obesity and maintain GI health.

Production Rabbit Nutrition: Rabbits are efficient converters of poorly digestible materials to meat. Therefore, it is easy to overfeed or underfeed does and growing, adolescent rabbits (fryers). The amount to feed depends on the age of the fryers or on the stage of pregnancy or lactation of the does. A general rule in feeding fryers is to feed all that can be consumed in 20 hr, with the feed hopper empty ~4 hr/day. Does are usually fed ad lib once they kindle. The general practice is to bring does from restricted to full feed slowly during the first week of lactation. Does bred to kindle five times during the year generally have their feed restricted between litters; those bred intensively should be on full feed continually once they begin the first lactation.

BACTERIAL AND MYCOTIC DISEASES

Pasteurellosis

Pasteurellosis is common in domestic rabbits. It is highly contagious and transmitted primarily by direct contact, although aerosol transmission may also occur. The etiologic agent is *Pasteurella multocida*, a gram-negative, nonmotile coccobacillus. In conventional colonies, 30%–90% of apparently healthy rabbits may be asymptomatic carriers. This is important to consider when nasal cultures are collected, because not every positive result indicates a pathologic condition. To get a

TABLE 21 NUTRIENT REQUIREMENTS OF RABBITS

	Protein (%) Total	Protein (%) Digestible	Fat (%)	Fiber (%)	Digestible Carbohydrates (NFE,%)[a]	Total Digestible Nutrients (%)
Maintenance	12	9	1.5–2	14–20	40–45	50–60
Growth and finishing	16	12	2–4	14–16	45–50	60–70
Gestation	15	11	2–3	14–16	45–50	55–65
Lactation (with litter of 7–8)	17	13	2.5–3.5	12–14	45–50	65–75

[a] NFE = nitrogen-free extract

true representative culture of the nasal bacterial fauna, the rabbit needs to be heavily sedated or anesthetized and a deep nasal culture obtained by introducing the culture tip relatively far into the nasal opening. Several barrier colonies of laboratory rabbits have been established as *Pasteurella*-free.

Clinical Findings: Pasteurellosis presents with a variety of clinical symptoms, including rhinitis, pneumonia, abscesses, reproductive tract infections, torticollis, and septicemia. Rabbits may develop *Pasteurella* septicemia and die acutely without any clinical signs. Septicemia necropsy findings may reveal only congestion and petechial hemorrhages in multiple organs.

Rhinitis (snuffles or nasal catarrh) is an acute, subacute, or chronic inflammation of the mucous membranes of the air passages and lungs, induced primarily by *Pasteurella*, but *Pseudomonas*, *Bordetella bronchiseptica*, *Staphylococcus*, and *Streptococcus* have also been isolated. The initial sign is a thin, serous exudate from the nose and eyes that later becomes purulent. The fur on the inside of the front legs just above the paws may be matted and caked with dried exudate, or this area may be clean with thinned fur as a result of pawing at the nose. Infected rabbits usually sneeze and cough. In general, snuffles occurs when the resistance of the rabbit is low. Recovered rabbits are likely carriers. Pneumonia can ensue.

Pneumonia is common in domestic rabbits. Frequently, it is a secondary and complicating factor in the enteritis complex. The cause is typically *Pasteurella multocida*, but other bacteria such as *Klebsiella pneumoniae*, *Bordetella bronchiseptica*, *Staphylococcus aureus*, and pneumococci may be involved. Upper respiratory disease (snuffles, *see* above) is often a precursor of pneumonia. Inadequate ventilation, sanitation, and nesting material are predisposing factors. The number of cases of pneumonia is directly proportional to the level of ammonia in the cage, hutch, or rabbitry. Ventilation is of utmost importance to provide good air quality. Affected rabbits are anorectic, listless, dyspneic, and might have a fever. Treatment should include systemic antibiotics, optimally based on a culture and sensitivity, because of possible resistance to common pathogens. The rabbits are usually dehydrated, and supportive care with hydration and syringe feeding is often necessary as well. Topically administered ophthalmologic antibiotic products instilled into the nostril can also be beneficial. Necropsy reveals bronchopneumonia, pleuritis, pyothorax, or pericardial petechiae.

Otitis media or interna ("wry neck" or head tilt) results from infections with various agents. *Pasteurella multocida* was reported to be isolated from 97% of cases of otitis media, including clinical and subclinical cases. *Bordetella bronchiseptica* and staphylococci were also found in 5%–10% of cases. An accumulation of pus or fluid in the middle or inner ear causes the rabbit to twist its head, eg, "wry neck" or torticollis. However, not all rabbits with middle ear infections show torticollis. Longterm antibiotic treatment is required for drug penetration into the affected area. Antibiotic therapy may only prevent worsening of clinical signs, and the prognosis is guarded with medical therapy alone. Total ear canal ablation and bulla osteotomy are often indicated when medical management of otitis media and interna fails. Proper imaging of the ear lesions is indicated before surgery. Often, a CT scan of the head will help to identify the lesion and potentially help to differentiate otitis media/interna from intracranial disease in cases of torticollis (eg, *Encephalitozoon cuniculi* infection).

Conjunctivitis and dacryocystitis (weepy eye) is a common problem in rabbits. Predisposing factors include mechanical irritation, eyelid diseases, and dental disease. Conjunctivitis in rabbits may be associated with other disease processes, especially dacryocystitis. The most incriminated cause of conjunctivitis is *P multocida*; however, this may be only a secondary infection. Primary infections are less common than opportunistic infections. Transmission is by direct contact or fomites. Affected rabbits rub their eyes with their front feet. Bacterial conjunctivitis can be treated with topical chloramphenicol, ciprofloxacin, or gentamicin combined with systemic broad-spectrum antibiotic therapy if topical treatment alone is ineffective. Dacryocystitis and acquired nasal duct obstruction may arise from chronic rhinitis that travels up the nasolacrimal duct to the eye or occasionally from dental disease such as tooth root inflammation or abscessation. Treatment includes gentle flushing with saline of the duct through the nasolacrimal punctum, but care is warranted to not damage the nasolacrimal duct during flushing. Dacryocystorhinography or injection of contrast material into the lacrimal punctum will provide good radiographic detail of the duct throughout its course and show the site of obstruction. In long-standing cases of dacryocystitis and conjunctivitis, the punctum and segments of the nasolacrimal duct may progressively narrow and be replaced with scar tissue until they are irreversibly obstructed. This results in permanent epiphora, and owners should be advised accordingly. To relieve discomfort and inflammation associated with these conditions, the use of topical nonsteroidal anti-inflammatory ophthalmic preparations such as flurbiprofen can be considered. Systemic NSAIDs such as meloxicam should also be used.

Conjunctivitis also accompanies rabbitpox (*see* p 1951) and myxomatosis (*see* p 1950).

Subcutaneous and visceral **abscesses** caused by *Pasteurella* may be clinically silent for long periods and spontaneously rupture. When bucks penned together fight, their wounds frequently develop abscesses. Abscesses in rabbits are treated differently than abscesses in cats; rupture or drainage via Penrose is not the recommended course. Thick-walled abscesses should be surgically excised en bloc if possible. Open wounds should be debrided or curetted, marsupialized, and left to heal by second intention. Facial abscesses are often related to dental disease (*see* p 1954). Drainage of the abscess accompanied by systemic antibiotic therapy based on culture and sensitivity tests has been successful, although recurrence can be common.

Pasteurella can cause **genital infections**, but several other organisms also may be involved. The spirochete *Treponema paraluiscuniculi* is the causative agent of rabbit syphilis. Genital infections are manifest by an acute or subacute inflammation of the reproductive tract and most frequently are found in adults, more often in does than bucks. In the case of *Treponoma*, a severe conjunctivitis or dermatosis between the toes can also be a key clinical sign. If both horns of the uterus are affected, the does often become sterile; if only one horn is involved, a normal litter may develop in the other. The only sign of pyometra may be a thick, yellowish gray vaginal discharge. If bloody discharge from the vulva is observed and a large uterine horn can be palpated, uterine adenocarcinoma should be included in the differential diagnosis. Bucks may discharge pus from the urethra or have an enlarged testicle. Chronic infection of the prostate and seminal vesicles is likely, and because venereal transmission may ensue, it is best to cull the animal in a production rabbitry colony. Surgical removal of the infected reproductive organs in conjunction with antibiotic therapy is indicated for pet rabbits. The contaminated hutch and its equipment should be thoroughly disinfected.

Diagnosis: Diagnosis of pasteurellosis is based on clinical signs and isolation of *P multocida*. Carriers can be identified by an indirect fluorescent antibody test on nasal swabs. A technique that uses small, saline-moistened, pediatric nasopharyngeal swabs has proved superior to the standard, larger nasal swab. The swab is directed medially through the external nares past the turbinates and onto the dorsal surface of the soft palate; sedation is recommended. The swab is then retracted and can be used in the fluorescent antibody test or plated onto a culture medium. An ELISA test to detect antibodies against *P multocida* may also help detect carriers. PCR can discriminate between different isolates, but it is not commercially available. It is important to remember that *Pasteurella* can be sampled from a large percentage of clinically normal rabbits, and culture results must be interpreted carefully and in combination with the clinical signs and the antibiogram from sensitivity testing. Not every strain of *Pasteurella* is pathogenic.

Treatment and Control: Treatment is difficult and will most likely not eradicate the organism. Antibiotics seem to provide only temporary remission, and the next stress (eg, kindling) may cause relapse. Prolonged treatment for 6–8 wk is often needed. Many of the newer antibiotics are already ineffective because of an increase in resistant strains. Before treatment, a culture and sensitivity should be done to determine the best antibiotic to use. Very often, systemic antibiotic therapy can be augmented by local antibiotic therapy. Gentamicin ophthalmologic drugs instilled into the nostrils can be a significant aid to treat upper respiratory tract problems with systemic antibiotics. Fluoroquinolones are usually good drugs if no resistance has built up. Oral medication is usually well tolerated and without adverse effects. In case of unsatisfactory results, doxycycline can be added, because both drugs appear to have a synergistic effect. Sometimes, amikacin or azithromycin must be used based on culture results. Although medication in the drinking water is not recommended because of the tainting of the flavor and potential underdosing, this is sometimes the only possible route to treat animals on a larger scale. Enrofloxacin (200 mg/L of drinking water for 30 days) can be effective for upper respiratory *P multocida* infections. Procaine penicillin (60,000 IU/kg/day, SC, for 10–14 days) is also recommended for individual rabbits, but caution is warranted, because deaths from enterotoxemia can follow if the drug is accidentally given orally.

An effective intranasal vaccine is in development but not commercially available; therefore, the best method of control in large rabbitries is strict culling. Two methods to free a production colony of *Pasteurella* have been reported. The first involves culture and culling of positive animals; once the colony is *Pasteurella*-free, it must be maintained in isolation. In the second method, pregnant does past kindling are treated with enrofloxacin. While does remain *Pasteurella*-culture positive, the kits remain *Pasteurella*-culture negative. Carriers can be identified by an indirect fluorescent antibody test on nasal swabs.

Listeriosis

Listeriosis, a sporadic septicemic disease characterized by sudden deaths or abortions, is most common in does in advanced pregnancy. Poor husbandry and stress may be important in initiating the disease. Clinical signs are variable and nonspecific and include anorexia, depression, and weight loss. In contrast to the disease in cattle and sheep, listeriosis seldom affects the CNS in rabbits. The causal agent, *Listeria monocytogenes*, spreads via the blood to the liver, spleen, and gravid uterus. At necropsy, the liver consistently contains multiple, pinpoint, gray-white foci. Because diagnosis is rarely made premortem, treatment is seldom attempted. *L monocytogenes* can infect many animals, including people. It is difficult to isolate with normal methods, and special techniques are often required.

Intestinal Diseases

Intestinal disease is a major cause of death in young rabbits. Although most diarrheal diseases were once lumped together (as the enteritis complex) or simply called mucoid enteritis, specific diseases are being delineated. Diet, antibiotic treatment, and other factors create disturbances of the GI microflora and may predispose rabbits to dysbiosis and intestinal disease. For discussion of GI stasis due to hairballs, *see* p 1956.

Enterotoxemia: Enterotoxemia is a severe diarrheal disease, primarily of rabbits 4–8 wk old when naturally infected; it also can affect rabbits at all life stages if an inappropriate antibiotic is given orally. Signs are lethargy, rough coat, greenish brown fecal material covering the perineal area, and death within 48 hr. Often, a rabbit looks healthy in the evening and is dead the next morning. Necropsy reveals the typical lesions of enterotoxemia, ie, a fluid-distended intestine with hemorrhagic petechiae on the serosal surface. The primary causative agent is *Clostridium spiroforme*, which produces an iota toxin. Little is known about transmission of the organism; it is assumed to be a commensal normally present in low numbers. The type of diet seems to be a factor in development of the disease; enterotoxemia is seen less often when high-fiber diets are fed. Because most β-lactams, lincomycin, clindamycin, and erythromycin induce *Clostridium*-related (eg, *Clostridium difficile*) enterotoxemia because of their selective effect on normal, gram-positive bacteria, their oral use is contraindicated in rabbits. Enterotoxemia is a consideration for these antibiotic therapies. These diarrheas are remarkably similar to those that occur naturally (described above as enterotoxemia). Treatment of colony rabbits is seldom attempted because of the rapidity of death. However, when population size permits, cholestyramine has been used with promising results, both as a preventive and a treatment. Reducing stress of the young rabbits (weaning, etc) and ad lib feeding of hay or straw are helpful in prevention. Adding 250 ppm of copper sulfate to the diet of young rabbits also helps prevent enterotoxemia. Individual animal treatment for enterotoxemia should include aggressive fluid therapy and intensive supportive care. Monitoring of hydration status, body temperature, and heart rates is extremely important. There is little evidence that antibiotics are helpful. Prognosis for advanced cases is often poor. Diagnosis depends on history, signs, lesions, and demonstration of *C spiroforme*. Centrifugation of intestinal contents at 20,000 g for 15 min followed by culture of the supernatant-pellet interface will reveal the organism. For a definitive diagnosis, the presence of iota toxin in the supernatant of centrifuged cecal contents can be demonstrated by in vivo or in vitro assays.

Tyzzer Disease: Tyzzer disease (*see* p 199), caused by *Clostridium piliforme*, is characterized by profuse watery diarrhea, anorexia, dehydration, lethargy, staining of the hindquarters, and death within 1–3 days in weanling rabbits 6–12 wk old. Acute outbreaks have been associated with >90% mortality. Some rabbits may develop chronic infections that present clinically as a wasting disease. Infection occurs by ingestion and is associated with poor sanitation and stress. The lesions consist of necrotic enteritis along with multifocal necrosis in the liver and heart. Diagnosis is made histologically; special stains (eg, Giemsa or Warthin-Starry silver) show the characteristic intracellular bacterium. Culturing is impractical, because the bacterium does not grow on artificial media. Serologic tests are available from animal diagnostic laboratories. Tyzzer disease affects a wide spectrum of other species but has not been reported in people, although titers have been documented in pregnant women. Although antibiotics used in treatment of other animals have not been effective in rabbits, oxytetracycline has been of some value in limiting an outbreak. No vaccine is available. Aggressive disinfection and decontamination of the housing facility to reduce the presence of hardy spores is indicated with either 1% peracetic acid or 3% hypochlorite.

Colibacillosis: *Escherichia coli* as a cause of rabbit diarrhea has been confused by the circumstance that *E coli* often proliferate when rabbits develop diarrhea for any reason. Enteropathogenic strains of *E coli* (serotype O103) commonly express the *eae* gene, which codes for intimin, an outer membrane protein associated with the attaching and effacing lesions. Serotypes O15:H, O109:H2, O103:H2, O128, and O132 are also important. Healthy rabbits do not have *E coli* of any strain associated with their GI tract.

Two types of colibacillosis are seen in rabbits, depending on age. Rabbits 1–2 wk old develop a severe yellowish diarrhea that results in high mortality. It is common for entire litters to succumb to this disease. In weaned rabbits 4–6 wk old, a diarrheal disease very similar to that described for enterotoxemia is seen. The intestines are fluid filled, with petechial hemorrhages on the serosal surface, similar to the pathology described for both Tyzzer disease and enterotoxemia (*see* above). Death occurs in 5–14 days, or rabbits are left stunted and unthrifty. Diagnosis is made by isolating *E coli* on blood agar and then having the isolate biotyped or serotyped. Electron micrographs of *E coli* attached to the mucosa are also helpful. In severe cases, treatment is not successful; in mild cases, antibiotics may be effective. Severely affected rabbits should be culled, and facilities thoroughly sanitized. High-fiber diets appear to help prevent the disease in weaned rabbits.

Proliferative Enteropathy: Proliferative enteropathy caused by *Lawsonia intracellularis* has been reported to cause diarrhea in weanling rabbits. Clinical symptoms include diarrhea, depression, and dehydration, which resolve over 1–2 wk. Disease does not cause death unless associated with a dual infection with another enteropathogenic agent. Diagnosis is based on necropsy findings of a thickened and corrugated ileum and histologic identification of the rod-shaped to curved or spiral silver-staining organism in crypt enterocytes. The organism requires cell-containing media (enterocytes) for culture. Immunohistochemistry and PCR may be useful to identify *L intracellularis*. Isolation of sick animals and symptomatic treatment is advised. Chloramphenicol or florfenicol is the treatment of choice, but some rabbits appear sensitive to these antibiotics when given orally, so careful GI monitoring is required.

Mucoid Enteropathy: Mucoid enteropathy is a distinct diarrheal disease of rabbits, characterized by minimal inflammation, hypersecretion, and accumulation of mucus in the small and large intestines. The cause is unknown, and it may occur concurrent with other enteric diseases. Predisposing factors include dietary changes, dietary fiber <6% or >22%, antibiotic treatments, environmental stress, and challenges with other bacteria. Clinical signs are gelatinous or mucus-covered feces, anorexia, lethargy, subnormal temperature, dehydration, rough coat, and often a bloated abdomen due to excess water in the stomach. A firm, impacted cecum may be palpable. The perineal area is often covered with mucus and feces. Diagnosis is based on clinical signs and necropsy findings of gelatinous mucus in the colon. Rabbits may live for ~1 wk. Treatment is difficult and often unrewarding in severe cases, but intense fluid therapy, antibiotics, and analgesics should be tried. Prevention is the same as for any rabbit enteropathy by focusing on an adequate, fiber-rich diet.

Mastitis

(Blue breasts)

Mastitis is common in commercial rabbitries and is occasionally seen in smaller units but rarely in pet rabbits. Poor sanitation enhances spread throughout the rabbitry. Mastitis affects lactating does and may progress to a septicemia that rapidly kills the doe. Generally, it is caused by staphylococci, but streptococci and other bacteria have been isolated. Initially, the mammary glands become hot, reddened, and swollen. Later, they may become cyanotic, hence the common name, "blue bag." The doe will not eat but may crave water. Fever ≥105°F (40.5°C) is often noted. If antibiotic treatment is started early (the first day the doe goes off feed), the rabbit may be saved and damage limited to one or two mammary glands. If more than two glands are lost, keeping the doe may not be economical. Because penicillin often causes diarrhea in rabbits, does should be treated only after the pelleted ration has been replaced with hay or some other high-fiber diet (*see* p 1947). Kits should not be fostered to another doe, because they will spread the infection to the foster mother. Handrearing of infected young may be attempted but is difficult. The incidence of mastitis can be reduced if nest boxes are maintained without rough edges to the entrance, which can traumatize the teats when the doe jumps in and out of the nest box. It is essential for the nest box to be sanitized before and after use. Vaccines have not proved to be beneficial to prevent mastitis.

Treponematosis

(Vent disease, Syphilis, Spirochetosis)

Treponematosis, a specific venereal disease of domestic rabbits, is caused by the spirochete *Treponema paraluiscuniculi*. It is seen in both sexes and is transmitted by breeding and from the doe to offspring. Although closely related to the organism that causes human syphilis (*T pallidum*), *T paraluiscuniculi* is not transmissible to other domestic animals or people. The incubation period is 3–6 wk. Small vesicles or ulcers are formed, which ultimately become covered with a heavy scab. These lesions usually are confined to the genital region, but the lips and eyelids may be involved. Infected rabbits should not be bred. Diagnosis is based on the lesions and observation of the spirochete's corkscrew motility under darkfield microscopy. Serologic tests used to diagnose *T pallidum*, such as the VDRL slide test and the rapid-plasma regain card test, are widely available and can be used to diagnose *T paraluiscuniculi*. Hutch burn is a differential diagnosis.

Benzathine penicillin G, 42,000 IU/kg, SC, at weekly intervals for 3 wk, is necessary to eradicate treponematosis from a herd. Procaine penicillin (60,000 IU/kg/day, SC, for 7 days) is also recommended for individual rabbits. All rabbits must be treated even if no lesions are present. Lesions usually heal within 10–14 days, and recovered rabbits can be bred without danger of transmitting the infection.

Dermatophytosis

(Ringworm)

Clinical dermatophytosis commonly affects individual rabbits, but epizootics can also occur. Ringworm is generally associated with poor husbandry, poor nutrition, and other environmental stressors. The cause is most commonly *Trichophyton mentagrophytes* and occasionally *Microsporum canis*. Transmission is by direct contact. Fomites, such as hair brushes, that evade proper disinfection can play a significant role in spreading infection. Asymptomatic carriers are very common. The lesions usually appear first on the head and may spread to any area of the skin. Affected areas are circular, raised, reddened, and capped with white, bran-like, flaky material. A negative result with a Wood's lamp illumination does not exclude dermatophytosis, because all agents do not fluoresce. Hair plucked from the edge of the lesion may be cultured on special media, such as dermatophyte test media or Sabouraud's agar. A KOH skin scraping taken from the periphery of the lesion that reveals fungal forms confirms the diagnosis. Because rabbits with active infections are infectious for people and other animals, they should be either isolated and treated or euthanized. Griseofulvin at an individual dosage of 25 mg/kg body wt/day, PO, for 4 wk, or in the feed at 825 mg/kg of feed, is effective but not approved for use in rabbits; it should not be used in rabbits intended for human consumption. Griseofulvin may be teratogenic and should not be used in pregnant does. Topical antifungal creams containing itraconazole (5 mg/kg/day, PO, for 4–6 wk), clotrimazole, or miconazole may be effective extra-label treatments. For rabbitries, treatment with either 1% copper sulfate as a dip or 8 oz of MECA (metabolized chlorous acid/chlorine dioxide compound, 1:1:10 mix of base:activator: water) sprayed on six times in a 26-day period was shown to be effective.

Tularemia

Tularemia is rare in domestic rabbits, but wild rabbits and rodents are highly susceptible and have been involved in most epizootics. Up to 90% of human cases of tularemia are linked to wild lagomorph exposure. The etiologic agent, *Francisella tularensis*, is an aerobic nonmotile, gram-negative, pleomorphic, bipolar coccobacillus prevalent in the south central USA. It is highly infectious and passed through the skin, through the respiratory tract via aerosols, by ingestion, and via bloodsucking arthropods. Tularemia causes an acute fatal septicemia. Diagnosis is based on necropsy findings of septicemic bacterial disease with numerous small, bright-white hepatic foci, congestion, and enlargement of the liver and spleen. Treatment of the animal is not indicated. Tularemia is a reportable disease. *See also* p 692.

VIRAL DISEASES

Viruses are not important causes of clinical disease of rabbits in the USA but include the infectious fibromas, papillomatosis, rabbitpox, myxomatosis, and a herpesvirus infection (virus 3). Rotaviral enteritis also has been diagnosed in the USA and seems to contribute to the overall problem of intestinal disease in rabbits. Viral hemorrhagic disease is found in almost every country that raises rabbits except the USA. In April 2000, the USDA diagnosed rabbit calicivirus in a backyard facility in Iowa. Rapid response and cooperation between federal and state agencies contained this outbreak and eliminated the source of infection. The USA is currently considered free of rabbit hemorrhagic disease.

Myxomatosis

Myxomatosis is a fatal disease of all breeds of domesticated rabbits caused by myxoma virus, a member of the poxvirus group. Myxomatosis is called "big head" and is characterized by mucinous skin lesions or myxedema of the head. Wild rabbits such as the cottontail (*Sylvilagus*) and jackrabbits (*Lepus*) are quite resistant. Myxoma virus–infected *Sylvilagus* develop fibroma-like lesions similar to those caused by rabbit fibroma virus. All other mammals are refractory to the virus. Myxomatosis has a worldwide distribution. In the USA, *myxomatosis* is restricted largely to the coastal area of California and Oregon, where epidemics occur infrequently but sporadic cases are common. These areas correspond to the geographic distribution of the California brush rabbit (*S bachmani*), the reservoir of the infection. Losses in rabbitries may be 25%–90%. Transmission occurs via mosquitoes, fleas, biting flies, and direct contact.

The initial sign is conjunctivitis that rapidly becomes more marked and is accompanied by a milky ocular discharge. The rabbit is listless and anorectic, with a fever that frequently reaches 108°F (42°C). In acute outbreaks, some rabbits may die within 48 hr after signs appear. Those that survive become progressively depressed and develop a rough coat. The eyelids, nose, lips, and ears become edematous, which gives a swollen appearance to the head. In females, the vulva becomes inflamed and edematous; in males, the scrotum swells. A characteristic sign at this stage is drooping of the edematous ears. A purulent nasal discharge invariably appears, breathing becomes labored, and the rabbit goes into a coma just before death, which usually occurs within 1–2 wk after clinical signs appear. Occasionally, a rabbit survives for several weeks; in these cases, fibrotic nodules appear on the nose, ears, and forefeet. Rabbits inoculated experimentally with laboratory strains of the virus invariably develop small nodules at the point of injection after several days; similar nodules develop later on other parts of the body, particularly the ears.

Few characteristic gross lesions are found at necropsy in the acute form of the disease. The spleen is occasionally enlarged and is almost always devoid of lymphocytes when examined histologically. In rabbits that survive longer, subcutaneous edema and nodular skin tumors are seen. The seasonal incidence of the disease, clinical signs (especially the swollen genitalia), and high mortality are all of diagnostic significance. Large, eosinophilic, cytoplasmic inclusion bodies in the conjunctival epithelial cells are also helpful in diagnosis. Outside the USA, vaccination is an option and highly recommended in endemic areas.

An attenuated vaccine prepared from a myxomatosis virus has protected rabbits infected under both field and laboratory conditions. This vaccine is not available in the USA, and because there is no effective treatment, euthanasia and burying or burning of affected rabbits is indicated. Preventive measures include protecting rabbits from exposure to arthropod vectors.

Rabbit (Shope) Fibroma Virus

Shope fibromas are found under natural conditions only in cottontails, although domestic rabbits can be infected by inoculation of virus-containing material. Fibromas may be found in domestic rabbits in areas where they are endemic in wild rabbits and where husbandry practices allow contact with arthropod vectors.

A fibroma virus, a member of the pox-virus group, causes this tumor, which is found on the legs, feet, and ears. The earliest lesion is a slight thickening of the subcutaneous tissues, followed by development of a clearly demarcated soft swelling. These tumors may persist for several months before regressing, leaving the rabbit essentially normal. Intracytoplasmic inclusion bodies are seen when sections of the tumor are examined histologically. Because Shope fibromas are of little significance in domestic rabbits, no control measures have been developed.

Rabbitpox

Rabbitpox is an acute, generalized disease of laboratory rabbits (*Oryctolagus*) that apparently has not been recognized in wild rabbits (*Sylvilagus*). A few outbreaks have been reported in the USA since 1930. The causative virus is closely related to vaccinia virus, and some outbreaks may have been caused by a virulent strain of vaccinia. Pox lesions may be present on the skin. Most rabbits develop a fever and nasal discharge. The mortality rate varies but is always high. The most characteristic lesions seen at necropsy are a skin rash, subcutaneous edema, and edema of the mouth and other body openings. Because of the edematous condition, "poxless" rabbitpox may be confused with myxomatosis. The virus may be isolated or the infection diagnosed serologically by methods appropriate to vaccinia. (*See also* POX DISEASES, p 867.) Spread through a rabbitry is rapid, but rabbits inoculated with smallpox vaccine (vaccinia virus) are immune. Rabbitpox virus does not infect people.

Papillomatosis

Two types of infectious papillomas occur infrequently in domestic rabbits. The oral papilloma, caused by the rabbit oral papillomavirus, is the most important clinically. The lesions consist of small, grayish white, pedunculated nodules or warts on the undersurface of the tongue or floor of the mouth. The second type, caused by the cottontail (Shope) papillomavirus, is characterized by horny warts on the neck, shoulders, ears, or abdomen and is primarily a natural disease of cottontail rabbits. Arthropod vectors transmit the Shope papillomavirus; therefore, arthropod control could be used as means of disease prevention. The oral papillomavirus is distinct from the Shope papillomavirus (which is also distinct from the Shope fibroma virus). Skin tumors caused by the Shope papillomavirus never occur in the mouth. Neither type of papillomatosis is treated, and the condition usually resolves spontaneously over time.

Rotaviral Infection

Rotavirus has been isolated from rabbits with diarrhea in many different countries. In serologic studies of rabbit colonies around the world, almost 100% of the adult rabbits in some rabbitries were positive for rotavirus, demonstrating its widespread nature. Rotavirus is shed in the feces of infected rabbits and, therefore, is probably transmitted by the fecal-oral route. Young rabbits of weaning age are most susceptible. It is probable that rotavirus is only mildly pathogenic, but most rotavirus infections are complicated with pathogenic bacteria such as *Clostridium* spp or *E coli*. The mixed infection results in a much more deadly syndrome. There is no treatment, but the infection appears to be self-limiting if susceptible rabbits are not continually introduced into the population. Experimentally, the virus is shed for only 1 wk after inoculation. Therefore, cessation of breeding for 4–6 wk seems to allow the disease to run its course, because seropositive does do not infect their offspring.

Rabbit Calicivirus Disease

(Viral hemorrhagic disease)

Rabbit calicivirus disease was first reported in 1984 in the People's Republic of China, from whence it spread through the domestic and wild rabbit populations in continental Europe. The first report of the virus in the Western hemisphere was in Mexico City in 1988. Mexico successfully eradicated the virus by 1992. Outbreaks of rabbit calicivirus disease have since occurred in Australia (1995), New Zealand (1997), and Cuba (1997). In 1995, as a result of a laboratory accident in southern Australia, the virus escaped from quarantine and killed 10 million rabbits in 8 wk. Rabbit calicivirus disease was confirmed in a group of 27 rabbits in Iowa in April 2000 in the USA. The source of infection was not determined. The outbreak was contained, the virus eradicated, and the USA remains disease free. Rabbit calicivirus is a reportable disease in the USA.

Rabbit calicivirus disease is highly infectious in European rabbits (*Oryctolagus*), but cottontail rabbits and jackrabbits are not susceptible. People and other mammals are not affected. The calicivirus is highly contagious and can be transmitted by direct contact with infected rabbits or indirectly by fomites. Infection results in a peracute febrile disease causing hepatic necrosis, enteritis, and lymphoid necrosis, followed by massive coagulopathy and hemorrhages in multiple organs. Rabbits show few clinical signs and die within 6–24 hr of fever onset. Morbidity rate is often 100%, and mortality 60%–90%. A killed vaccine effectively reduced the incidence of rabbit calicivirus in Europe in the late 1980s. Rabbits are vaccinated at 10 wk, and annual boosters are recommended.

PARASITIC DISEASES

Coccidiosis

Coccidiosis is a common and worldwide protozoal disease of rabbits. Rabbits that recover frequently become carriers. There are two anatomic forms: hepatic, caused by *Eimeria stiedae*, and intestinal, caused by *E magna*, *E irresidua*, *E media*, *E perforans*, *E flavescens*, *E intestinalis*, or other *Eimeria* spp. Transmission of both the hepatic and intestinal forms is by ingestion of the sporulated oocysts, usually in contaminated feed or water.

Hepatic Coccidiosis: Severity of disease depends on the number of oocysts ingested. Young rabbits are most susceptible. Affected rabbits may be anorectic and have a rough coat. Hepatic coccidiosis is most often subclinical, but growing rabbits may not make normal gains. Infrequently, death may follow a short course. Rabbits usually succumb within 1 mo after a severe experimental exposure. At necropsy, small, yellowish white nodules are found throughout the hepatic parenchyma. In the early stages, they may be sharply demarcated, whereas in the later stages they coalesce. The early lesions have a milky content; older lesions may have a more cheese-like consistency. Microscopically, the nodules are composed of hypertrophied bile ducts or gallbladder. Diagnosis of this form of coccidiosis is based on the gross and microscopic changes, along with demonstration of the oocysts in the bile ducts. An impression smear of a lesion in the liver examined under light microscopy often reveals oocysts. The oocysts may also be demonstrated by fecal flotation. It is important not to confuse the oocysts with the normal yeast (*Cyniclomyces guttulatus*), which is commonly seen in fecal examinations.

Treatment is difficult, and control rather than cure is expected. Sulfaquinoxaline administered continuously in the drinking water (0.04% for 30 days) prevents clinical signs of hepatic coccidiosis in rabbits heavily exposed to *E stiedae*. However, it may not prevent the lesions. Sulfaquinoxaline may also be given in the feed at 0.025% for 20 days, or for 2 days out of every 8 days. A single oral dose of sulfadimethoxine at 50 mg/kg, followed by its inclusion in drinking water at 1 g/4 L for 9 days, was found to significantly reduce fecal oocyst count. Because feed-grade sulfaquinoxaline can be difficult to obtain, liquid sulfaquinoxaline is used more commonly. Withdrawal time is 10 days for rabbits used for food. Other coccidiostats that may prove to be effective include amprolium (9.6% in water or 0.5 mL/500 mL), salinomycin, diclazuril, and toltrazuril. A single oral dose of toltrazuril at 2.5 mg/kg or 5 mg/kg has also significantly reduced oocyst count. Treatment is best administered for a minimum of 5 days and repeated after 5 days. Rabbits treated successfully are immune to subsequent infections.

Treatment will not be successful unless a sanitation program is instituted simultaneously. Elimination of fecal-oral transmission of infective oocysts is achieved by preventing feed hoppers and water crocks from becoming contaminated with feces. Hutches should be kept dry and the accumulated feces removed frequently. Wire cage bottoms should be brushed daily with a wire brush to help break the life cycle of the protozoa. Ammonia (10%) solution is lethal to oocysts and is the best choice to disinfect cages or ancillary equipment exposed to fecal material.

Intestinal Coccidiosis: This form of coccidiosis can occur in rabbits receiving the best of care, as well as in rabbits raised under unsanitary conditions. Typically, infections are mild, and often no clinical signs are seen. In early infections, there are few lesions; later, the intestine may be thickened and pale. Good sanitation programs that can eliminate hepatic coccidiosis do not seem to eliminate intestinal coccidiosis. Intestinal coccidiosis is generally diagnosed by fecal flotation and microscopic identification of the oocysts (species). It is important to distinguish coccidian oocysts from the nonpathogenic yeast *Cyniclomyces guttulatus* that can also be found in large numbers. Treatment is similar to that for hepatic coccidiosis except that sulfaquinoxaline is given for 7 days and repeated after a 7-day interval.

Larval Worm Infection

Although adult tapeworm infections are rare in domestic rabbits, the discovery of larval tapeworm cysts on the serosal peritoneum is common. Rabbits are intermediate hosts for two species of canine tapeworm, *Taenia serialis* and *T pisiformis*. Although *T serialis* is rare in domestic rabbits, it is somewhat more common in wild ones. The larval stage of *T pisiformis*, a cysticercus, is found attached to the mesenteries. Before forming these fluid-filled cysts, the young larvae migrate through the liver, where they leave white, tortuous subcapsular tracts. Generally, there are no clinical signs, and diagnosis occurs at necropsy. Treatment is usually not attempted, but control is accomplished by restricting access of dogs (the final host of the tapeworm) to the area in which food and nesting material are stored. Mebendazole at 1 g/kg of feed (50 mg/kg) for 14 days is reported to be an effective treatment.

Baylisascaris procyonis has been reported in rabbits. Signs are similar to those induced by *Encephalitozoon cuniculi*. No treatment is available.

Ectoparasites

The ear mite *Psoroptes cuniculi* is a common parasite of rabbits worldwide. Mites irritate the lining of the ear and cause serum and thick brown crusts to accumulate, creating an "ear canker." Infested rabbits scratch at and shake their head and ears. They lose weight, fail to produce, and suffer secondary infections, which may damage the inner ear, reach the CNS, and result in torticollis (*see* p 1945). The brown crumbly exudate should never be removed in a conscious rabbit, because this is very painful. The crusts will slowly slough off as the mites die and the tissue underneath heals. The incidence is much lower when rabbits are housed in wire cages instead of solid cages. The mite is readily transmitted by direct contact. Rabbits should be treated systemically with any of the miticides approved for use in dogs and cats. A variety of injectable ivermectin treatment regimens effective against both fur and ear mites have been reported, with the dosage of ivermectin 200–400 mcg/kg, SC, two or three treatments 10–21 days apart. Mites may also be treated with selamectin (20 mg topically every 7 days has been effective).

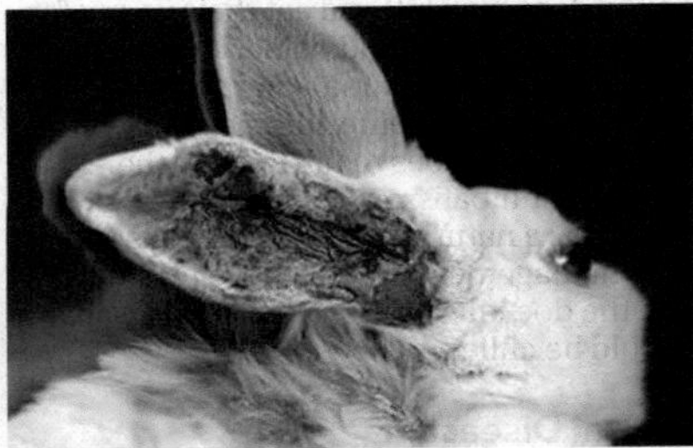

Gross lesions of *Psoroptes cuniculi* in a rabbit. *Courtesy of Dr. Louise Bauck.*

Fur mite infestations are common, and two genera, *Cheyletiella* and *Listrophorus*, are found worldwide. A number of different species of the genus *Cheyletiella* are found on rabbits. The most common in North America is *C parasitovorax*. The genus *Listrophorus* has but one species, *L gibbus*. These mites live on the surface of the skin and do not cause the intense pruritus seen with sarcoptic mange. Fur mite infestations usually are asymptomatic unless the rabbit becomes debilitated. *Cheyletiella* may be noticed as "dandruff." Scraping the dandruff onto a dark paper or background will demonstrate the "walking dandruff," as *Cheyletiella* is called. Transmission is by direct contact. Diagnosis is accomplished by skin scraping and light microscopy. *Cheyletiella* mites may cause a mild dermatitis in people, especially on the arms. Weekly dusting of animals and bedding with permethrin powder can control *Cheyletiella* mites.

Rabbits are rarely infested with either *Sarcoptes scabiei* or *Notoedres cati*. These mites burrow into the skin and lay eggs. The rabbits are extremely pruritic, and the parasites are difficult to eliminate on domestic rabbits. The condition is extremely contagious and can be transmitted to people.

Fleas of the *Ctenocephalides felis*, *C canis*, and *Pulex irritans* species can affect rabbits and many other animals. Imidacloprid is a flea adulticide; the feline dose should be divided in two or three spots to treat rabbits infested with fleas. Fipronil is contraindicated for use in rabbits because of potential toxicity. Flea collars are also not recommended. It is important to also treat every cat and dog in the house, because the original host is not usually the rabbit.

Encephalitozoonosis

Encephalitozoon cuniculi is a widespread protozoal (microsporidian) infection of rabbits and occasionally of mice, guinea pigs, rats, and dogs. Usually, no clinical signs are seen, but a few rabbits develop mild, chronic renal disease. Some develop brain lesions that may result in convulsions, tremors, or head tilt. Head tilt is often caused by bacterial infection with *Pasteurella multocida*; this can be difficult to distinguish from head tilt associated with *E cuniculi* infection, because both infections are common and can occur together. The mode of transmission is not definitively known, but the organism is shed in the urine and potentially can infect the fetus in utero. It seems to be mildly contagious in a rabbitry. At necropsy, the most significant macroscopic lesion is pitting of the kidneys. Microscopic lesions consist of focal granulomas and pseudocysts in the brain and kidneys. Sometimes a severe, focal, interstitial nephritis is seen. In some cases, an ocular manifestation is a key clinical presentation, and lesions range from phacoclastic uveitis to mature cataracts. Diagnosis is made by histologically identifying the lesions (pseudocysts) and observing the organisms when stained with Giemsa, Gram, or Goodpasture carbol fuchsin stains. Several serologic and skin tests are helpful in screening rabbits for antibodies to the organism, but positive serology only indicates past infection and does not confirm a diagnosis. Effective treatment has not been established. Some evidence suggests that oxibendazole or albendazole (20–30 mg/kg/day, PO, for 7–14 days, then 15 mg/kg/day, PO, for 30–60 days) or fenbendazole (20 mg/kg/day, PO, for 28 days) may be effective. Prevention entails good sanitation and possibly serologic screening of breeding stock with elimination of positive reactors. A differential diagnosis in rabbits with outdoor access is an aberrant migration of *Baylisascaris* spp into the nervous system. Encephalitozoonosis is an emerging disease of immunodeficient people.

Pinworms

Passalurus ambiguus, the rabbit pinworm, usually is not clinically significant but often is upsetting to owners. It is common in many rabbitries and is distributed worldwide. Transmission is by ingestion of contaminated food or water. The adult worm lives in the cecum or anterior colon. Diagnosis is made by observing the adults at necropsy or by finding the eggs during examination of the feces. Single treatments are not very effective, because the life cycle is direct and reinfection is common. Piperazine citrates in the water (3 g/L) for alternating 2-wk periods or fenbendazole (50 ppm in feed for 5 days) are effective treatments. Rabbit pinworms are not transmissible to people.

NONINFECTIOUS DISEASES

Broken Back

Fracture or dislocation of lumbar vertebrae with compression or severing of the spinal cord is common in both pet and commercial rabbits. The predisposition to a fractured back highlights the importance of adequate and proper restraint skills by the handler. If a rabbit struggles during restraint, it is often best to carefully release the grip and relax the rabbit instead of fighting against the forceful movements of the scared animal. Common signs include posterior paresis or paralysis and urinary and fecal incontinence due to loss of sphincter control. Initial signs of paralysis may resolve within 3–5 days as swelling around the cord diminishes. Supportive therapy includes anti-inflammatory medication to reduce damage from swelling. In acute cases, methylprednisolone sodium succinate might be beneficial. The rabbit should be hospitalized and medical treatment, including pain management, IV fluid therapy, nutritional support, and cage rest should be initiated; with this approach, the severe clinical signs of paraplegia can gradually resolve over 3 mo of conservative therapy. Although these cases may appear "hopeless," rabbits can improve to the point of being able to voluntarily move both hindlimbs and to ambulate by walking and hopping. Intense nursing and management are required.

Cannibalism

Young does may kill and eat their young for several reasons, including nervousness, neglect (failure to nurse), and severe cold. Dogs or predators entering a rabbitry often cause nervous does to kill and eat the young. Cannibalism of the dead young occurs as a natural, nest-cleaning instinct. If all management practices are proper and the doe kills two litters in a row, she should be culled.

Dental Disease

Dental disease may present as excess salivation (slobbers), teeth grinding, or anorexia. Oral examination and palpation along the ventral surface of the jaw should be a part of routine physical examinations of rabbits. Dental abscesses may develop as a consequence of foreign bodies (eg, plant material embedded between the tooth and gum), pulp exposure after tooth trimming, inappropriate diet, or other diseases. Dental abscesses also may appear as retrobulbar abscesses. Hence, a rabbit that presents for primarily ophthalmologic signs such as epiphora or exophthalmus should receive a full dental examination. Rabbit incisors may wear differently depending on diet, and a pelleted diet may predispose the rabbit to dental disease. Multiple teeth are commonly affected. A thorough oral examination under heavy sedation or full anesthesia and diagnostic radiographs are indicated. Often, a skull CT provides significantly more information because of the complexity of the lesions and the 3D structure of the head (which is difficult to fully image with plain radiographs).

Dental extractions may be accomplished using a fine-tipped dental elevator worked along the root to free the tooth. Incisors are curved and require use of a specialized rabbit incisor luxator or similar curved instrument for removal. Curettage of the alveolus to destroy the apical germinal tissue is required to prevent regrowth of the tooth. Regrowth is unlikely if the pulp remains in the extracted tooth, but follow-up radiographs in 2–3 mo will confirm successful extraction. After lavage, infected sockets can be filled with doxycycline periceutical gel or antibiotic-impregnated polymethyl methacrylate (PMMA) beads. PMMA beads are sometimes available from compounding pharmacies or can be self-manufactured. Care has to be taken to choose an antibiotic that is heat stabile (eg, gentamicin) in the beads. Other treatment options include leaving the surgical site open and marsupializing the skin to allow healing by secondary intention and to facilitate local antibiotic therapy. Antibiotics can be instilled into the open wound by eye drops or by packing the wound with antibiotic-impregnated gauze. Gingival tissues can be sutured closed if needed or can remain open to avoid development of an anaerobic environment. It is important to avoid any cutting of the teeth with wire cutters or even dental pliers. The pressure of such cutters can be transmitted through the tooth and fracture the whole tooth, which will result in further problems. An elongated tooth should always be drilled down by a dedicated dental burr. Defect treatment with calcium hydroxide paste results in tissue necrosis and is contraindicated.

Extraction of cheek teeth involves delicate elevation and luxation if the dental anatomy is normal. Extraction of multiple cheek teeth carries a very poor prognosis for recovery, although some pet rabbits do well with very few molars if the diet is suitably modified. Continued monitoring of the occlusal surface and followup adjustment is expected. Pain management and extended-duration (4 wk to months) systemic antibiotic therapy based on culture and sensitivity are indicated.

Dental Malocclusion: The incisors, premolars, and molars of rabbits grow throughout life. The normal length is maintained by the wearing action of opposing teeth. Malocclusion (mandibular prognathism, brachygnathism) probably is the most common inherited disease in rabbits and leads to overgrowth of incisors with resultant difficulty in eating and drinking. Dental trimming is often done with combined anesthesia of diazepam (1–5 mg/kg, IM) followed by or in combination with ketamine (10–20 mg/kg, IM), or a combination of ketamine and dexmeditomidine (*see* p 1939).

Occasionally, the cheek teeth overgrow and cause severe tongue or buccal lesions. Because malocclusion is generally considered to be inherited, rabbits with this condition should not be bred. However, young rabbits can damage their incisor teeth by pulling on the cage wire, which results in misalignment and possibly malocclusion as the teeth grow. This condition is difficult to differentiate from genetic malocclusion, and these rabbits should also be culled. Genetic malocclusion generally can be detected in rabbits 3–8 wk

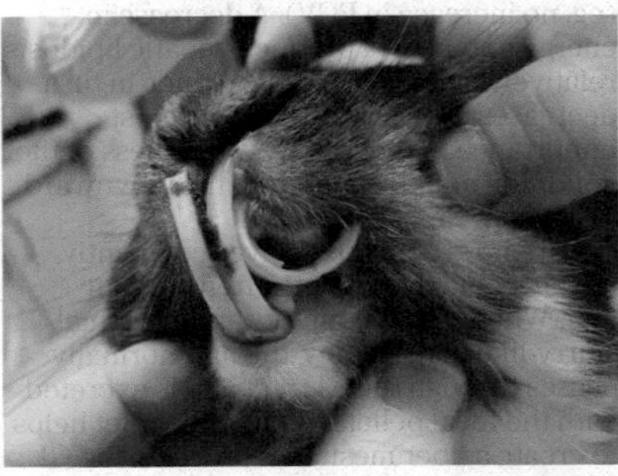

Severely overgrown incisor teeth in a rabbit. If younger animals, the cause (eg, brachygnathia) is often genetic. In older animals, the cheek teeth are often part of the problem. *Courtesy of Dr. Joerg Mayer.*

old. If incisors are suddenly overgrown in an adult rabbit, it is not enough to trim the incisors down. The problem commonly originates in the back of the mouth, and a full assessment of the cheek teeth is warranted. The dental procedure needs to be done under full anesthesia and with special equipment. Rabbit dentistry is very different from that in dogs and cats because of the differences in anatomy and physiology. Special training and literature about rabbit dentistry is readily available, and dental procedures in rabbits should be performed only by those with specific training.

Gastric Stasis, Hair Chewing, and Hairballs

The GI tract of the rabbit is similar to that of the horse, with an anatomy and physiology that often leads to clinical complications. One of the most frequent presentations is gastric stasis, which has a variety of causes, including stress and/or pain. The initial phase of the problem commonly goes unrecognized by the owner or untrained veterinarian. Because they are a prey species, rabbits do not overtly show signs of discomfort or pain and remain quiet and inactive. Rabbits are commonly presented in an advanced state of stasis that has already led to dehydration, pain, and hepatic lipidosis. Decreased food intake has a large impact on the health of rabbits and affects many other factors of homeostasis. When food intake is decreased, water intake is also commonly decreased. The GI contents lose the typical slurry-like consistency and become pasty. As the rabbit becomes dehydrated, water is absorbed from the GI tract into the vascular space, which masks the typical hematologic signs of dehydration (eg, no increase in PCV). A decrease in energy uptake will produce hepatic lipidosis relatively quickly in rabbits, which in turn decreases food intake. It is of utmost importance to realize the seriousness of the condition and to counteract the downward spiral.

Rabbits groom themselves constantly, so the stomach contents often contain hair. When the GI contents are of normal, slurry-like consistency, the hair normally passes through the GI tract and is excreted with the fecal pellets. A high-fiber diet helps to create a fiber mesh that prevents the GI contents from becoming too dense so that hair can more easily pass through the upper GI tract along with the mesh of fiber. Hair chewing is generally a result of low fiber in the diet and can be corrected by increasing the fiber or feeding hay along with the pellets. Adding magnesium oxide to the diet at 0.25% also may be helpful. In some cases, hair chewing is a result of boredom because of lack of fiber or chew substrate. Providing environmental enrichment often halts this behavior.

The hair becomes a problem only if excess amounts are consumed or if it accumulates in the stomach and blocks the pylorus. If this happens, the rabbit becomes anorectic, loses weight, and dies within 3–4 wk. Premortem diagnosis of pyloric obstruction can be difficult, because palpable hairballs can be an incidental finding and radiography is often nondiagnostic.

Once GI stasis affects the emptying of the stomach, gas accumulation creates further visceral distention and pain. The resulting decreased food intake and GI hypomotility cause an increased cecal pH and altered cecal microflora, creating cecal dysbiosis. Alterations in water and electrolyte balance result in systemic ketoacidosis and hepatic lipidosis. Gastric ulceration and even gastric rupture may occur.

The goals of treatment are to remove the obstruction, stimulate motility, restore GI microorganism balance, and relieve dehydration and anorexia. Most cases can be managed by aggressive fluid management (maintenance is 100–120 mL/kg/24 hr), with affected rabbits receiving double the rate of maintenance fluids (10 mL/kg/hr) IV. Pain medication (eg, oxymorphone 0.2 mg/kg every 4–6 hr) is essential to relieve the GI discomfort. With aggressive fluid and pain management, the rabbits usually feel better within 24 hr. Because the GI tract is either full or distended with contents, oral force feeding should be discouraged. Energy can be provided by adding dextrose to the IV fluids. Food should be available at all times and in different forms (eg, hay, vegetable matter, supportive care formula). Rabbits often start to eat on their own after they are properly hydrated and received analgesia for visceral pain. If the rabbit does not eat because of advanced stages of hepatic lipidosis, assist syringe feeding should be started. Once a true GI obstruction has been excluded, treatment can then include a motility stimulant such as metoclopramide (0.5 mg/kg, PO or SC, tid-qid) or cisapride (0.5 mg/kg, PO, bid-tid); however, this should not be started before hydration and pain management. Reestablishment of GI microflora may be assisted by probiotic treatment or cecotrophs from healthy rabbits.

Mineral oil and laxatives do not effectively remove the hair mass. Roughage (hay or straw) should be fed during the treatment to help carry the hair fibers through the GI tract and out with the feces. Surgical treatment should be considered only if medical management has not resulted in improvement.

Prevention of GI stasis is the best option and can be accomplished by providing a high-fiber diet, avoiding stress and obesity, providing environmental enrichment, and combing daily to remove loose hair. Rabbits also consume significantly more water when offered by bowl vs sipper bottle. Clinical research does not support routine doses of mineral oil, wetting agents, or proteolytic enzymes as effective preventives.

Heat Exhaustion

Rabbits are sensitive to heat. Hot, humid weather, along with poorly ventilated hutches or transport in poorly ventilated vehicles, may lead to the death of many rabbits, particularly pregnant does. Affected rabbits stretch out and breathe rapidly. Hutches should be constructed so that they can be sprinkled in hot, humid weather. Free access to cool water should be provided. When the environment can be controlled, optimal conditions are a temperature of 50°–70°F (15.5°–21°C) and a relative humidity of 40%–60%, with 10–20 air changes/hr. Wire cages are preferable to solid hutches. Treatment consists of immersing rabbits in cold water during the heat of the day, especially those that will kindle in the next day or two. Breeding bucks may lose a majority of viable sperm and might not breed successfully for several weeks until new sperm production replaces the sperm killed by thermal stress.

Hutch Burn

(Urine burn)

Prolonged irritation of the bladder mucosa with calcium sediment can cause a cystitis that can manifest in incontinence and soiled fur (*see* p 1959). A wet perianal area often causes additional problems such as fly strike and dermatitis. This condition is often referred to as hutch burn, Hutch burn is often confused with treponematosis and can be truly differentiated only by the absence of spirochetes on darkfield microscopy and by the lack of antibodies to *Treponema paraluiscuniculi*. It is caused by wet and dirty hutch floors and affects the anus and external genitalia. Also, rabbits that lack adequate sphincter control of the bladder constantly dribble urine and may be affected. The membranes of the anus and genital region become inflamed and chapped. The area soon becomes secondarily infected with opportunistic pathogenic bacteria. Brownish crusts cover the area, and a hemorrhagic, purulent exudate may be present. Keeping hutch floors clean and dry and applying nitrofurazone or an antibiotic ointment to the lesions hastens recovery.

Ketosis

(Pregnancy toxemia)

Ketosis is a rare disorder in rabbits that may result in death of does at or 1–2 days before kindling. The disease is more common in first-litter does. Predisposing factors include obesity and lack of exercise. The probable cause is starvation. Other signs are dullness of eyes, sluggishness, respiratory distress, prostration, and death. The most significant lesions are fatty liver and kidneys. The body mobilizes fat and transports it to the liver to be broken down for energy, thus the fatty liver. Diagnosis depends on a detailed history and physical examination and clinical signs. A key clinical sign is clear urine; the urine of healthy rabbits is usually cloudy. Injection of fluids that contain glucose and assisted syringe feeding may help correct the disease. Breeding young does early, before they become too fat, is also helpful. Hairballs in the stomach are often a factor in ketosis.

Moist Dermatitis

(Wet dewlap)

Female rabbits have a heavy fold of skin on the ventral aspect of the neck. As the rabbit drinks, this skin may become wet and soggy ("slobbers"), which leads to inflammation. Contributing factors include dental malocclusion, open water crocks, and damp bedding. The hair may slip, and the area may become infected or flyblown. The area often turns green if infected with *Pseudomonas* spp. Automatic watering systems with drinking valves generally prevent wet dewlaps. If open water receptacles are used, they should have small openings or be elevated. Once the area is infected, the hair should be clipped and antiseptic dusting powder applied. In severe cases, parenteral antibiotics and analgesics are necessary.

Ophthalmologic Disease

Corneal ulceration is the most common ophthalmic problem of rabbits. Rabbits appear predisposed to this condition for two main reasons: 1) the globe and surface of the cornea are significantly larger in rabbits than in most other domesticated pets, and 2) rabbits do not blink as frequently as other species, which leaves the cornea less moist. Many potential underlying issues should be excluded, although environmental causes and trauma are the most frequent causes. The cornea should be carefully protected during anesthetic procedures. The lack of tear production associated with keratoconjunctivitis sicca or dry eye may further increase the risk of corneal damage. Exophthalmia as a result of orbital or dental disease or facial paralysis associated with encephalitocytozoonosis can make blinking difficult and lead to corneal damage. Superficial ulcers can be treated with broad-spectrum ophthalmic antibiotic solutions. Treatment progress should be assessed in 1–2 days. Epithelial "lips" indicate a nonhealing ulcer. Such ulcers should be debrided after application of a topical anesthetic, followed by the same treatment as for a superficial ulcer. If the ulcer does not respond to topical treatment, collagen shields or even contact lenses have been used successfully. In severe cases, surgery and placement of a conjunctival pedicle graft may be required. Differential diagnoses of corneal lesions in rabbits include corneal occlusion (overgrowth of conjunctival tissue) and limbic or corneal dermoid (skin-like tissue in an abnormal location over the cornea). Hair may protrude from a limbic dermoid. These growths do not appear painful.

Pseudopterygium, an aberrant growth of conjunctival membrane tissue, is sometimes seen in rabbits. The cause is not known, and the condition is slowly progressive. The conjunctival membrane extends from the bulbar conjunctiva and slowly grows onto the cornea, giving the eye an opaque appearance. Surgical removal of the overgrown conjunctiva is straightforward but leads to recurrence. Daily administration of topical cyclosporine 0.2% in the affected eye might help slow down recurrence.

Phacoclastic uveitis secondary to *Encephalitozoon cuniculi* (*see* p 1954) has been recognized to present as iridal swelling and white or pink nodules on the iris. The nodules are bacterial iridal or corneal stromal abscesses and give the typical appearance of cotton candy in the anterior chamber. Spores replicating in the lens may result in cataract formation and even lens rupture, leading to a painful uveitis. Diagnosis is confirmed by presence of the organisms on histopathology of excised tissue or DNA probe on removed lens material. Treatment involves lens removal by phacoemulsification or enucleation. Spontaneous lens regeneration may occur. Prosthetic lens insertion is not recommended. The prognosis is guarded without surgery; glaucoma develops in most affected rabbits. Topical treatment includes NSAIDs and mydriatic and antibiotic medications. After starting topical medications, progress and intraocular pressure should be checked in 5–7 days. Monitoring should continue every 2–3 wk for the next 2 mo. Systemic therapy for *Encephalitozoon* should be started.

Inherited glaucoma is discussed below (*see* below).

Ulcerative Pododermatitis

(Sore hocks)

Ulcerative pododermatitis does not involve the hock but the plantar surface of the metatarsals and, less commonly, the volar surface of the metacarpal-phalangeal region. The cause is either pressure on the skin from bearing the body weight on wire-floored cages or trauma to the skin from stamping, with secondary infection of the necrotic skin. Several factors, including accumulation of urine-soaked feces, nervousness, posterior paralysis after a spinal cord injury, and the type of wire used, may influence development. Genetics are also involved. The Rex appears to be predisposed because of the lack of the longer guard hairs that usually act as a cushion over the predisposed area of the hock. Heavy-breed rabbits such as the Flemish Giant and the Checkered Giant are also susceptible. Affected rabbits sit in a peculiar position with their weight on their front feet; if all four feet are affected, they tiptoe when walking. Various debriding agents can be used to clean the lesion, followed by topical antibiotic treatment along with parenteral antibiotics. Radiographs exclude osteomyelitis with severe lesions. The rabbit must be removed from the cage or given a solid floor (board or mat) on which to sit or rest. Treatment is often difficult and time consuming, with application of bandages that need frequent changing. Low-level laser therapy has shown some benefits and is encouraged. Husbandry improvement should focus on providing soft, dust-free bedding. In many cases, weight management is also indicated. Because large feet and thick footpads are hereditary, selection of breeding stock for these traits has reduced the incidence of pododermatitis.

Urolithiasis

Urolithiasis is seen routinely in pet rabbits and occasionally in commercial rabbitries. It is generally suspected when hematuria is seen. (A dipstick can quickly exclude normal pigment causes of red urine.) The rabbit's calcium metabolism is significantly different from that in other vertebrates. Rabbits do not require vitamin D_3 to absorb calcium from the gut into the bloodstream. The vast majority of dietary calcium is readily absorbed into the bloodstream, leading to relatively higher blood calcium levels (up to 16 mg/dL [4 mmol/L] can be normal). Renal elimination of calcium is much higher in rabbits (as high as 60%) than in other vertebrates (2%–5%). This often gives the urine a cloudy appearance, which is normal. Feeding a calcium-rich diet for a prolonged time to a metabolically inactive rabbit (ie, not growing, pregnant, or lactating) can lead to an abnormal hypercalciuria, and calcium can precipitate out as bladder sludge or form uroliths. Small stones are often voided, but surgery is frequently needed to remove larger urinary stones. Uroliths are caused by calcium carbonate and triple phosphate crystals precipitating out of normal urine when the pH increases to 8.5–9.5. Normal rabbit urine has an average pH of 8.2. Several factors have been incriminated in urolithiasis, including nutritional imbalance (especially the calcium:phosphorus ratio), genetic predisposition, infection, inadequate water intake, and metabolic disorders. Short-term treatment involves surgically removing the uroliths, whereas longterm treatment focuses on reducing dietary calcium intake. Because alfalfa is high in calcium and one of the main dietary components of regular rabbit pellets, switching to timothy-based pellets and to grass or timothy hay and rolled oats helps to prevent recurrence.

Heritable Diseases

Hydrocephalus: Hydrocephalus, characterized by an enlarged head, is occasionally seen in neonatal rabbits. The top of the skull appears dome-shaped, and the fontanelle is wider than normal. Most affected rabbits are born dead; occasionally, they live for several weeks but generally exhibit neurologic signs. At necropsy, the brain is enlarged; on cut section, the ventricles are greatly enlarged and filled with CSF. The cause can either be genetic or result from dietary deficiency or excess of vitamin A. In the case of a dietary deficiency or hypervitaminosis, poor reproduction (low fertility, small litter size, abortion, etc) also is seen in the breeding herd. A correct assessment of vitamin A becomes critical in treatment, and both serum and liver should be analyzed. In deficiency, the serum level of vitamin A is below normal (2.6–4.2 IU/mL). In toxicosis, the serum level can be normal, but the concentration of vitamin A in the liver is very high (>4,000 IU/g). Treatment of the deficiency involves increasing the carotene content of the diet or adding a vitamin A supplement. Treatment of hypervitaminosis A requires reducing vitamin A in the diet. However, reducing the amount of vitamin A stored in the liver is extremely difficult. If the doe's reproduction has been impaired, replacing the doe is probably more cost-effective than trying to decrease the vitamin A level. Because genetic hydrocephalus appears to be inherited recessively, control requires culling both parents.

Buphthalmia (Blue Eye, Moon Eye, Infantile Glaucoma): Buphthalmia is an autosomal trait with incomplete penetrance that results in variable clinical severity. Intraocular pressures begin to rise as early as 3 mo. One or both eyes may be affected. Glaucoma can be treated medically (dorzolamide 2%; 1 drop tid) or by surgical enucleation. Affected rabbits should not be bred.

Splayleg: Splayleg is presumed to be an inherited disorder presenting with abduction of one or more legs as early as 3–4 wk of age. The right rear limb is most commonly affected, although the condition may be unilateral or bilateral. Hip dysplasia can occur during postnatal development among rabbits housed on slick nest boxes or flooring.

Neoplasia

By far, the most common tumor in rabbits is uterine adenocarcinoma. The incidence can be as high as 60% in intact does >3 yr old. The disease may present with multicentric tumors that involve both horns of the uterus. The masses can often be palpated as globular polypoid structures. The tumor often metastasizes to the liver, lungs, and other organs; cystic mastitis may develop concurrently. This disease is the primary reason to recommend spaying of nonbreeding female rabbits at the age of 4–6 mo. Lymphoma and other neoplastic disorders of lymphoid tissue are common tumors that occur in all ages of pet rabbits. Malignant lymphomas (lymphosarcoma) are relatively common and may occur in rabbits <2 yr old.

The manifestation can be extremely varied, ranging from ocular lesions, to skin, to leukemic forms. Lymphosarcoma presents with a tetrad of lesions, including enlarged kidneys, splenomegaly, hepatomegaly, and lymphadenopathy. Treatment of lymphoma can be attempted by chemotherapy, but prognosis is often poor due to the often aggressive form of the disease. Rabbits can be treated with "typical" chemotherapeutic agents, and adverse effects to these drugs appear less common than in other domesticated pets. Thymoma and thymic lymphoma are the most common mediastinal masses in rabbits. Differentiation between the two is difficult and usually requires a fine-needle aspirate or a biopsy of the chest mass. The typical clinical sign for a chest mass in rabbits is intermittent or permanent exophthalmos. Because of the impaired venous return from the head through the chest, the venous sinuses behind the globe expand and cause the exophthalmos. A chest radiograph to scan for masses should be performed in all rabbits with exophthalmos. The thymoma can sometimes be removed surgically relatively easily, because it does not involve other major structures in the chest cavity. In the case of thymic lymphoma, surgery is often less successful, because the structure is often not possible to be removed in toto. Radiation of the thorax has been described as an effective therapy, and animals have survived for years after the treatment. If no advanced therapy is an option, oral prednisolone has been used in a few cases with moderate success.

RATITES

Twelve species of birds are grouped as ratites, not including the order Tinamiformes. These include the ostrich, emu, rhea, cassowary, and kiwi. The ostrich, emu, and rhea are the ratite species primarily raised in production facilities, whereas all may be found in zoo collections. The ostrich originated in Africa and has been commercially raised since 1850 for feathers, meat, and hide products. The emu is native to Australia and has been raised for meat, oil, and leather in many countries around the world, including the USA. The South American rhea has been produced primarily for feathers.

Ostriches (*Struthio camelus*) are the largest members of the ratite group. Mature ostriches may stand 2.4–2.8 m tall and weigh up to 160 kg, although most are 65–130 kg. Males are black and white, females are brown.

Emus (*Dromaius novaehollandiae*) are second only to ostriches in size, measuring up to 2 m tall and weighing 18–48 kg. Female emus are typically larger than males. Both females and males have brown to gray-brown plumage with black feather shafts and tips. Emus are flightless but travel at a quick trot and can sprint at speeds up to 51 km/hr.

Rheas can reach 1.7 m in height and 40 kg in weight. They are native to South America and are divided into two species: the Greater Rheas (*Rhea americana*) include five subspecies, and the Lesser Rheas (*Rhea pennata*) include three subspecies. Similar to emus, rheas have brown to gray-brown feathers.

MANAGEMENT

Physical restraint of ratites is different for each. The ostrich's head can be caught by hand or hook, and a hood can be placed over the head. Once hooded, the ostrich's head should be maintained below the level of its body to restrict it from kicking its legs forward. An ostrich kick can seriously injure a handler and, once captured, the bird will quickly try to back up and kick anyone in front of its body. Because an ostrich will back up when its head is held, an assistant should be positioned behind the bird to push as the person holding its head leads the ostrich forward. Emus must be handled from behind, grasping the wings and lifting the bird slightly upward and back. The front of the bird should be avoided to prevent being injured by the claws on the feet, because, as with all ratites, emus will kick forward to try to escape. Rheas are handled much like emus. Some handlers use hoods to facilitate handling emus and rheas, although this technique is not as effective as it is with ostriches.

Juvenile birds from 4 mo to yearlings are best handled by slowly and calmly herding them into an enclosed barn. If they cannot see out of an enclosure and are crowded into a corner, they will often sit if not startled. When calmly herded into a confined area, young birds can easily be sexed, banded, and administered antiparasitic medication, and diagnostic samples (eg, blood) can be collected. If there is no enclosed area, portable panels with plywood or plastic applied can be used to herd the birds into the desired space.

Physical and Laboratory Examination: Before the bird is restrained, it should be examined from a distance while walking/running in its enclosure for conformation, gait, body condition, respiration rate and character, and behavior-related problems.

The enclosure should be inspected for fresh droppings and urine. Green urates may be an indication of hepatitis, whereas dry, hard fecal material is common in birds that are dehydrated or suffering from GI impaction. The droppings should be examined for tapeworm segments and collected for fecal flotation and direct parasite evaluation.

The eyes and sinuses are examined for any discharge or swelling, and the beak and oral cavity examined for any lesions. The neck is palpated, especially in the area of the thoracic inlet, for any swellings. Overall body condition should be noted and is determined by the epaxial muscle mass, rated on a scale of 1–5, with 1 being emaciated and 5 obese. The feathers and skin are examined for lesions and parasites. The thorax is auscultated, and heart rhythm and rate are determined. The abdomen is palpated from the ventriculus, which lies immediately caudal to the breastplate, to the proventriculus, located between the legs. The caudal abdomen is palpated and balloted for any evidence of coelomic fluid or retained eggs. Finally, a cloacal examination is performed to verify normal anatomy. When indicated, samples for microbial culture can be collected from the trachea, cloaca, and caudal oviduct, and blood can be collected for a CBC and serum chemistry panel. (For hematologic and serum biochemical reference ranges for ostriches, *see* TABLES 6 and 7, pp 3176 and 3178). Sodium heparin is the preferred anticoagulant for both the CBC and serum chemistry panel. A slide should be prepared immediately for cytologic evaluation.

Recommended sites for venipuncture and catheterization in ostriches and rheas are the cutaneous ulnar veins on the ventral side of the wings and the medial metatarsal veins. In emus, the jugular vein and medial metatarsal vein are the blood collection sites of choice. Venipuncture of the jugular vein is more difficult in ostriches because of their size and because sudden movement by the bird can result in lacerations and exsanguination. In debilitated ratites, catheterization (adults, 14-gauge, 13-cm catheter) of the jugular vein is easy and provides a readily accessible port to the vascular system. The right jugular vein is more developed than the left.

Anesthesia: Chemical restraint for handling and surgical procedures in ratites use typical veterinary drugs. Anesthesia may be induced in younger birds with isoflurane or sevoflurane using the same procedures as with small animals. Intubation for maintenance is recommended, but the cuff should not be inflated because of the possibility of pressure necrosis (birds have complete tracheal rings that do not expand with the tracheal cuff). Xylazine and ketamine combinations are commonly used for short procedures on induction, followed by intubation and gas anesthesia. Xylazine administered at 2.5 mg/kg, IV, followed, after sedative effect is noticed, by ketamine at 1 mg/kg, is an effective protocol. However, xylazine has significant cardiorespiratory depressant effects and should not be used in severely ill birds. Also, xylazine is not recommended as a premedication for inhalation anesthesia, because it may greatly enhance the cardiodepressant effects of gas anesthetic agents. Recovery may be smoother if diazepam is given at 0.2 mg/kg, IV or IM. Tiletamine/zolazepam is an induction alternative for ratites, dosed at 2–10 mg/kg, IM, or 1–3 mg/kg, IV, with the higher end of the dose range recommended for emus and rheas. Once the bird has been induced, padding should be placed under the body during the entire procedure to minimize neuropathy and myositis. Ostriches may develop peroneal nerve paralysis when placed in lateral recumbency, without padding, for <1 hr. Sternal recumbency does not appear to interfere with respiration while anesthetized, but the large body size of ratites may restrict their ability to breathe. Therefore, manual or mechanical respiration is recommended during general anesthesia to reduce the cardiorespiratory depressant effects of both gas anesthetic agents and physical compression of air sac volume. The neck should be straight and the head elevated slightly above the body during general anesthesia. Vital signs of ratites should be monitored while under anesthesia along with body temperature (esophageal) to maintain normothermia; intravenous access should be established for drug and fluid administration. During recovery, the bird should be placed in a dark, quiet, preferably padded enclosure in sternal recumbency. Wrapping the body with the legs immobilized under the animal while in sternal recumbency will often allow the bird to recover with minimal struggle.

Surgical Procedures: Surgical procedures in ratites generally are related to the GI tract, orthopedics, and trauma repair. Proventriculotomy for foreign body removal and impactions in ratite species is a common surgical procedure. In young birds, incisions should be made carefully, because the abdominal wall is very thin. To perform a proventriculotomy, the bird is positioned in right lateral recumbency with the left pelvic limb abducted and supported caudally in a stand. In ostriches, the ventriculus is located caudal to the proventriculus in the coelomic cavity; therefore, the surgical incision to access this part of the GI tract should be through a left paramedian approach beginning ~15 cm caudal to the keel. Yolk sac removal due to nonabsorption and/or infection is common. Egg retention in hens is addressed surgically, and often multiple eggs are removed. Orthopedic surgeries are addressed as in other species with pins, plates, and transfixation casting as needed for fracture repair. Laceration repair is performed as in other species. Upper esophageal tears from attempted hooking (capture) will often heal by second intention and, unless severe, do not require surgical repair.

As in all production animals, the cost of surgical correction of many conditions might be greater than the commercial value of the individual animal presented. Producers should be made aware of cost considerations.

Nutrition: To date, there has been little reliable research on ratite nutrition. The formulations of commercial diets available are based on studies in Africa and Australia, as well as extrapolations from available poultry information. Current trends are to feed 14%–20% protein from the time chicks hatch to 3 mo of age, reducing the protein level after 3 mo of age. Ostriches and rheas are hindgut fermenters and have the ability to digest fiber from a young age. For optimal health and production results, appropriate ratite feed formulated for ostriches, emus, and rheas is recommended. Ostriches, emus, and rheas have significantly different digestive systems and specific nutritional requirements for optimal growth, reproduction, and health. High-quality grass can be used as a grazing supplement for ostriches and rheas. Chicks allowed to hatch in the nest are coprophagous, eating feces from the parents for the first few weeks of life.

Vaccination: When indicated in a specific flock, autogenous bacterins for *Salmonella*, *Escherichia coli*, and clostridial diseases have been used; however, this is not a common practice, and these products may be difficult to obtain. For emus, equine encephalitis vaccination is recommended. Tissue-culture propagated, inactivated bivalent Eastern and Western equine encephalomyelitis (EEE, WEE) vaccine prepared and licensed for use in horses, and that may contain equine tetanus antitoxin, has effectively protected emus against EEE and WEE infection. A vaccination protocol is to administer IM an initial full equine dose at 6 wk of age, followed by booster vaccinations at 10 wk of age and at 5- and 6-mo intervals thereafter and before and after breeding season (April and September). A booster should be administered when EEE or WEE is identified within 10 miles of the production facility or before transfer to an endemic area. The recommended vaccine protocol (emus) for *Clostridium chauvoei* (blackleg) using the ruminant vaccine with or without tetanus antitoxin is to administer an initial vaccine at 2 mo of age, followed by a booster vaccination at 3 mo and then annually after the end of breeding season in April.

REPRODUCTION

Anatomy: All female ratites have a single left ovary and oviduct. The oviduct consists of 1) the infundibulum, where fertilization occurs; 2) the magnum, where the thick albumin is put on; 3) the isthmus, where the inner and outer shell membranes are added; 4) the uterus, where the shell is added; and 5) the vagina. The opening of the vagina into the cloaca is on the left side of the cloaca at the ten o'clock position.

The male ratite has two intra-abdominal testicles located near the kidneys. During the breeding season, the testicles increase 200%–300% in size. The rooster does not pro-

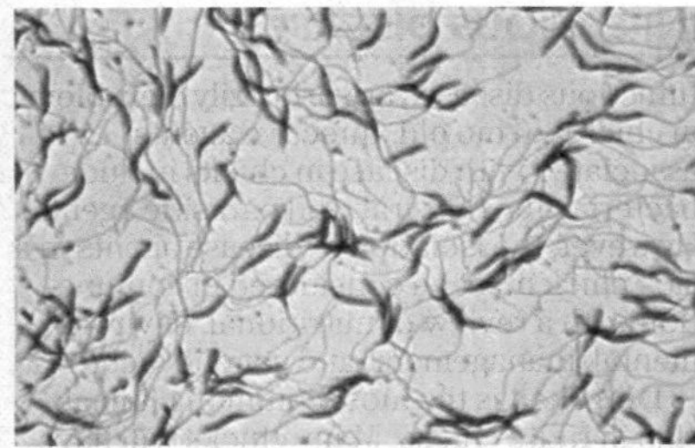

Ostrich semen. *Courtesy of Dr. Karen Hicks-Alldredge.*

duce sperm when not in season. Roosters in the ratite family all have a phallus that serves to transport semen from the ejaculatory ducts in the cloaca of the male to the cloaca of the female. The phallus is shaped differently in ostriches, emus, and rheas; however, the function is similar. All ratite phalluses have a dorsal groove through which the semen travels.

Breeding: Ostriches and rheas are long day breeders. The season is controlled by the photoperiod (length of daylight) as well as the ambient temperature; in North America, the breeding season is spring and summer. The emu is a short day breeder and lays in the late fall and winter. Once the breeding season has started, the cock and hen become reproductively active. The ostrich cock develops external "breeding" colors and begins to display; the hen begins to flutter. This behavior continues for days to weeks before egg laying begins. In general, females become reproductively active before the males. Therefore, early eggs are often infertile. This is also true for emus and rheas. Ostrich hens lay every other day during the proper season if the eggs are collected daily. In the wild, normal clutch sizes for ratites are 15 to 25 eggs, whereas 30 is average in a captive production facility. The range is from 0 to 167 consecutive eggs.

Hatching: If eggs are gathered and stored for "batch setting," they should be cooled, if possible, to 60°F (15.6°C). Physiologic zero—or the point at which the embryo stops developing—is 72°F (22.2°C). The egg is laid with the embryo in the 60,000 cell stage, and cooling the egg before incubation ensures that all cells develop in synchrony. In general, hatching eggs should not be washed if they are clean. If eggs are wet or dirty, they should be washed in a warm 110°F (43.3°C) disinfectant solution (eg, chlorhexidine, sodium hypochlorite, quaternary ammonia) before cooling.

Commercial incubation of eggs is performed in forced air incubators. Ostrich eggs generally are incubated at 97°F (36.1°C) for 40–42 days and moved to the hatcher at 40 days or when the chick "pips" (breaks the egg). Emu eggs are incubated at 97°–98°F (36.1°–36.7°C) for 54–58 days and moved to the hatcher at 50–52 days or at "pipping." Rhea eggs are incubated at 98°F (36.7°C) for 40 days and moved to the hatcher at 38 days or at "pipping." While temperature in the hatcher is the same as incubation, the humidity should be higher.

For optimal performance of hatchery operations, excellent basic management and biosecurity practices must be followed, including "all-in/all-out" management. Groups of newly hatched birds should be placed in an area of adequate space (to run and exercise their rapidly growing legs and bodies), heat, and ventilation, with fresh water and feed. Mixing groups of young birds should be avoided (to reduce stress) until chicks are at least 3 mo old.

Reproductive Diseases: Many diseases can result in reproductive failure, either through failure to produce eggs or through production of abnormal or contaminated eggs. Bacterial salpingitis or metritis is common. The etiologic agents vary, as does the severity of the infection. In mild cases, only the uterus or shell gland is affected (metritis), and clinical signs range from abnormal shells to no egg production at all. Infection may result from retrograde bacterial invasion (from breeding or uterine fatigue), extension of an airsacculitis, or perforation of the abdominal cavity by a foreign body. Affected hens generally have a history of erratic egg production, malformed or odoriferous eggs, or a sudden stop in production. On physical examination, temperature and respiration are variable, there may be a discharge below the cloaca, and hens may have a fetid odor. Affected hens have WBC counts ranging from 8,000 to >100,000/µL. Ultrasonography and radiology are useful to assess the amount and consistency of exudates in the oviduct. If a bacterial salpingitis is diagnosed through a caudal oviductal (vaginal) culture, subsequent treatment is based on organism isolation and sensitivity.

CHICK MANAGEMENT

The basic principles of animal husbandry and aviary management, including an "all-in/all-out" system of management, biosecurity of the flock and facility, and a stress-free environment, are inherent to successful ratite production. Generally, the level of identifiable infectious or contagious disease among chicks is low, and most clinical signs are produced by stress factors such as poor ventilation, overcrowding, excessively high ambient temperatures, overuse of antibiotics, improper incubation or hatching procedures, improper nutrition, and other management-related disease. When considering the sick chick, it is important to evaluate the population at risk and take appropriate steps to prevent spread of disease. This often means elimination of clinically ill chicks by appropriate quarantine or euthanasia. If an infectious disease is involved, treating the individual chick in its environment places the other birds within the group at risk.

Ratite chicks do well on a wide range of substrates (including sand, grass, alfalfa, or native pasture) if they are introduced to the substrate at hatch and have adequate space, ventilation, and sufficient feeders and waterers. Ostrich chicks up to 3 mo old grow best and have the fewest management-related diseases (eg, proventricular impaction, leg problems, and feather picking) if 100–133 sq ft of pen space per bird is available. Ostrich chicks do not do well when confined to concrete floored housing. Adequate exercise is an important consideration for normal leg growth and digestive function.

Musculoskeletal abnormalities of the coxofemoral joint, stifle joint, femur, and tibiotarsus are common physical problems of ratite chicks. Spraddle leg is an abnormality of the coxofemoral joints that prevents normal adduction of the limbs. Lack of exercise and excess weight due to edema at hatch or overfeeding are the main underlying causes of spraddle leg and progressive lateral rotation of the tibiotarsus and the tarsometatarsus. Limb musculoskeletal abnormalities are progressive and have an extremely poor prognosis; management practices must be in place to prevent their occurrence, including maintenance of an appropriate growth rate and provision of acceptable substrate and opportunity to exercise. Rolled toes are diagnosed more often in young ostriches and can be treated by splinting the affected toe(s) in a normal position.

INFECTIOUS DISEASES

Infectious diseases are primarily a problem in chicks <6 mo old. Infective agents associated with disease in chicks include bacterial, fungal, viral, and parasitic agents. However, the isolation of disease agents in a sick chick must be considered in conjunction with a review of nutritional, environmental, management, and genetic factors.

Diarrhea is the most common clinical sign in ratite chicks. Many chicks will have diarrhea when the yolk sac is absorbed and the chick starts eating well, at 8–12 days of age. If the chicks are alert and active, no treatment is needed. Chicks will also develop diarrhea after a sudden change in diet for which treatment with probiotics is indicated. Bacterial causes of diarrhea include *Escherichia coli*, *Salmonella* spp, *Pseudomonas* spp, *Campylobacter jejuni*, *Klebsiella* spp, *Clostridium perfringens*, *Clostridium colinum*, *Mycobacterium* spp (adults), *Streptococcus* spp, and *Staphylococcus* spp. The appropriate antibiotic should be determined by culture and subsequent microorganism isolation and sensitivity, and the source of bacteria identified (eg, barn, hatcher, inadequate hygiene, airborne vectors). Viral agents (suspected pathogens) that may cause diarrhea include paramyxovirus, reovirus, herpesvirus, birna-like virus, enterovirus, adenovirus, and coronavirus. Treatment for viral diarrhea is supportive only, and any potential source of the virus (eg, wild birds, infected hens, people) should be eliminated. GI obstruction is another cause of diarrhea; treatment is surgical, and any changes in environment or feed should be made slowly to prevent recurrence. In cases of fungal candidiasis, antibiotic treatment should be discontinued and a dry environment maintained. Although the pathogenicity of protozoa relating to diarrhea diagnosed in ostrich chicks is unknown, metronidazole is considered the treatment of choice. Enteritis may also be caused by management errors, including overmedication and excess electrolyte supplementation in drinking water during hot weather.

The incidence of **yolk sac infection and retention** generally is low in naturally hatched chicks. However, this condition often occurs when owners assist to hatch a chick or tie off the omphalomesenteric vessels and bandage the abdomen. The yolk sac may also be contaminated through the ostium at the ileal opening when absorption of the yolk material by the vitelline membrane (yolk sac lining) is delayed. Bacteria commonly isolated from the yolk sac are gram-negative; however, yolk sac retention secondary to noninfectious causes also occurs.

Poxvirus infections are more frequent in ostrich chicks and produce typical, crusty granulomatous lesions on the face, ears, and neck. Poxvirus is transmitted by insect vectors, primarily mosquitoes. The disease is self-limiting, and mortality is low. Vaccination of a flock during an outbreak with fowlpox vaccine may stop the spread of disease. The vaccine is a cutaneous fowlpox vaccine administered by dipping a large needle with reservoirs near the tip that allow inoculation when a puncture is made through the propatagium. Staphylococcal dermatitis occurs as a secondary problem in debilitated chicks, especially when external parasites disrupt the epithelial integrity.

Eastern equine encephalomyelitis can cause death in ostrich chicks as a fading chick syndrome and as a violent and fatal gastroenteritis in emus of all ages. Vaccination of emus for this disease is necessary in areas where the virus exists.

Avian influenza has been diagnosed in rheas and other ratite species. Routine testing for avian influenza is required for most intrastate shipments of ratites.

Parasitic Diseases

Protozoa: A number of intestinal protozoa, including *Hexamita*, *Giardia*, *Trichomonas* spp, *Cryptosporidium*, and *Toxoplasma* spp, have been isolated from ratite chicks. The pathogenicity of these parasites in all ratite species is unknown, and immunosuppression may be required for disease to develop. Metronidazole at 10 mg/kg, PO, bid, is recommended for protozoal parasite infections diagnosed in ratite species. Coccidiosis is common, and although not believed to be pathogenic, it can be treated with sulfa drugs. If coccidiosis is causing clinical signs (eg, diarrhea), the underlying immunosuppressive disease condition(s) must be diagnosed to effectively treat the protozoal disease.

Cestodes: The tapeworm *Houttuynia struthionis* is common in Africa but rarely diagnosed in the USA. The intermediate host is not known. Treatment is fenbendazole, PO, at 15 mg/kg/day for 5 days, used at regular intervals.

Nematodes: The wireworm *Libostrongylus douglassii* is the most economically significant GI parasite of ostriches. Mature worms and late larval stages live in the crypts of the glandular portion of the stomach. Diagnosis is based on finding trichostrongyloid-type eggs in the feces. The recommended treatment for the ostrich wireworm is ivermectin at 0.2 mg/kg or fenbendazole at 15 mg/kg. Another nematode with clinical significance for ratite species is *Baylisascaris* spp, which is transmitted from skunks or raccoons through feed. This neurotropic parasite causes CNS lesions and signs. Restricting exposure to raccoon and skunk feces is the best prevention. *Chandlerella quiscali* is a nematode identified in emus that results in cerebral larval migrans. The common grackle is the definitive host for *C quiscali*, and emus are exposed to the parasite through the bite of *Culicoides crepuscularis*. Birds infected with *C quiscali* develop profound torticollis and incoordination that leads to emaciation, scoliosis, and death. Ivermectin is the treatment of choice for *C quiscali* infections in emus.

Arthropods: Three types of arthropods can affect ratites: lice, ticks, and quill mites. Lice can be a problem, especially in ostriches. Biting lice (*Struthioliperurus struthionis*) cause skin and feather damage. Treatment with permethrin spray (poultry concentration) is effective, as is injectable ivermectin at 1 mL/110 lb, IM. Several species of ticks have been identified on ratite species; their main significance is as vectors of disease. Feather mites live in the vein on the underside of the feather and feed on blood. Ratite feather mites can be visualized as small, reddish, dust-like particles in the feather vein. Treatment for ticks and mites is ivermectin at 0.2 mg/kg at 30-day intervals.

DIGESTIVE SYSTEM DISORDERS

Impaction of the proventriculus and ingestion of foreign bodies are management-related problems. Chicks are at high risk of impaction for the first 2 wk after movement to a new environment, with or without a change in substrate or diet. Proventricular impactions are also diagnosed as a sequela of diseases involving ileus of the GI tract. Impactions with sand and concentrated feed can be managed medically with psyllium laxatives and supportive therapy. Impactions with forages or ingestions of foreign material (eg, hardware, rocks, jewelry, etc) require proventriculotomy surgery for removal and subsequent resolution of the problem.

Cloacal prolapses are common in young chicks. Frequently, the chick has diarrhea or an impaction within the GI tract that causes straining and subsequent prolapse of the cloaca. The prolapse is easily reduced and a purse-string suture is placed for 24–48 hr, making sure there is adequate room for the bird to defecate/urinate while the suture is in place.

Intestinal torsion or volvulus, primarily involving the colon, occurs in ostriches of all ages. It can present as a flock problem when the diet is suddenly changed, especially if the new diet has a high fiber content. Clinical signs include scant to no feces, slight diarrhea, abdominal enlargement, and vomiting. Abdominocentesis and radiographic imaging of the coelom are diagnostic. When an early diagnosis is achieved, surgical intervention is corrective but often not economically feasible.

MUSCULOSKELETAL DISORDERS

Exertional myopathy results from capture, transport, attack by predators, or fighting; it can occur in birds of all ages. Borderline nutritional deficiencies may exacerbate stress-related myopathy. Clinically, birds are often unable to stand but are otherwise bright, alert, and responsive. Fluid therapy to correct metabolic acidosis and to effect diuresis, combined with anti-inflammatory and antibiotic therapy to prevent clostridial disease, are indicated. Administration of vitamin E at 5 mg/kg, with or without selenium at 0.06 mg/kg, is recommended. If nutritional deficiencies are expected, correcting the diet by adding oral vitamin E to the diet or drinking water is indicated.

Various treatments, including slinging the bird to exercise the legs and swimming, have been tried for myositis secondary to overexertion or trauma. However, handling the bird in this manner is very stressful; it is preferable to allow the bird to sit until it can stand on its own, which may take up to 90 days. The prognosis remains guarded, even if the bird is alert and has a good appetite.

TOXICITIES

Many different disease toxicoses have been documented in ratites. Exogenously administered selenium has resulted in acute selenium toxicity in ostriches, leading to pulmonary edema and congestion. The feed additive monensin has been associated with myositis and malabsorption syndrome in ostriches and emus. Gossypol in commercial ostrich feed contaminated with cattle feed resulted in a malabsorption syndrome. Cantharidin from blister beetles has resulted in hemorrhagic gastritis and enteritis in emus. Young chicks are sensitive to insect stings, and death is common when chicks eat and are stung in the oral cavity by red ants or wasps. Nicotine from cigarette butts has resulted in CNS signs. Toxic plants that contain solanine (eg, silverleaf, nightshade) result in vomiting and diarrhea, whereas plants that contain high levels of nitrates result in dyspnea and CNS signs. Ammonia toxicity is seen in birds housed in poorly ventilated barns and results in clinical signs of corneal edema, epiphora, and dyspnea.

TRAUMA

Wing luxations and fractures can result from hauling or breeding accidents. Most cases of wing luxation are actually a radial paralysis rather than a true luxation of the joint. However, a true humeral luxation from the shoulder can occur. Treatment for both injuries is the same and involves taping the wings up over the back. Maintaining the wings in this position for 1–2 wk generally resolves the problem. Fractured wings, depending on the location of the fracture, can be repaired with a half-Kirschner apparatus or splints (or both). Occasionally, intramedullary pinning is required. With minor wing fractures in emus, taping may be sufficient to treat the injury.

Lacerations of the neck skin and musculature may involve the trachea and esophagus of ratites that are injured due to contact with fences. Primary closure of the trachea and esophagus in acute injuries is recommended. If the esophageal injury is old, the esophagus will often heal through secondary intention. With severe neck injuries, an esophagotomy tube, placed in the distal third of the cervical portion of the esophagus, may be required for alimentation.

Lower leg injuries commonly occur in ratites that contact cable fencing at a high rate of speed. Standard principles of wound management (*see* p 1701) should be applied, including debriding and bandaging the wound. If bone is exposed in a lower leg injury, radiographic imaging of the affected area, at weekly intervals, is recommended, because stress fractures and sequestra can occur. Often, the soft-tissue injury shows normal healing 3 wk after trauma, but the bird may still have a fracture of the tarsometatarsus. Luxation of the phalanges is common, especially if the bird's enclosure has icy or muddy areas. If the luxation is not treated promptly, casting the foot in a normal flexed position for 5–6 wk generally allows enough soft-tissue fibrosis and repair to maintain the luxated joint in place. When casting alone is unsuccessful, arthrodesis of the joint according to standard equine procedures can be performed.

REPTILES

The class Reptilia includes >8,000 species, but only a few dozen are likely to be encountered in general practice. All the Crocodilia, front-fanged poisonous snakes (but not all backed-fanged poisonous species) and both species of poisonous lizard (*Heloderma* spp) are considered to be dangerous animals and are usually covered by federal and/or state legislation. These species are not generally kept as pets and will therefore not be discussed here. The class Reptilia includes four orders: Crocodyla (crocodiles, alligators, gharials), Testudines (turtles and tortoises), Squamata (lizards and snakes), and Rhynchocephalia (tuataras).

Reptiles are vertebrates with organ systems similar to those of mammals. However, they are ectothermic and rely on environmental temperature and behavior to control their core body temperature. They possess both renal and hepatic portal circulations, and predominantly excrete ammonia, urea, or uric acid depending on their evolutionary adaptations. Their RBCs are nucleated, and their metabolic rates are lower than those of mammals. All reptiles exhibit ecdysis—a normal process by which the outer skin is periodically shed. Diurnal species require broad-spectrum light for vitamin D_3 synthesis and calcium homeostasis. Fertilization is internal, and females may produce eggs (oviparous) or live young (ovoviviparous).

Reptiles are not considered highly social creatures, and multiple-male groups can lead to intraspecies aggression. Single-male, multiple-female groupings can work well for certain species, but the solitary reptile is often the healthiest pet. The life span of many reptiles can exceed 10–20 yr, requiring a longterm commitment from owners.

Anatomy: Reptiles possess a common cloaca, which receives the lower GI, reproductive, and urinary tracts. In addition, lungs are simpler and composed of vascular pockets, more like a cavitated sponge than alveoli.

Lizards and chelonians are quadrupeds and have a familiar pentadactyl limb arrangement. Reptiles lack a true diaphragm; in many species, all organs are contained within a single coelomic cavity. Some lizards (eg, tegus and monitors) have thin postpulmonary and/or post-hepatic membranes that divide the coelom into compartments. Snakes' organs are distributed in a longitudinal arrangement. Boas and pythons are primitive snakes and have both left and right lungs; however, other snakes lack a developed left lung. Squamates have incomplete tracheal rings, and males have paired copulatory organs (hemipenes).

The chelonians are characterized by their shell, which comprises a dorsal carapace and ventral plastron. The internal organs are separated by two thin membranes. The heart is located within a cardiac membrane, while the lungs are dorsad and separated from the remaining viscera by a postpulmonary membrane (or septum horizontale). Chelonians have complete tracheal rings, and males have a single copulatory phallus.

Physiology: Reptiles rely on environmental temperature and behavior to maintain their body temperature within their preferred optimal temperature zone (POTZ). Within this species-specific POTZ, a reptile is able to achieve the preferred body temperature for specific metabolic activities, which may vary diurnally and seasonally and by age and gender. The metabolic rate of reptiles is lower than that of mammals and birds. Consequently the K constant to determine energy expenditure, nutritional requirements, and allometric drug doses is given by the equation BMR = K(body wt [in kg]$^{0.75}$), in which BMR = basal metabolic rate in Kcal/day and K = 10 (the energy constant for reptiles).

All snakes, lizards, and chelonians have a three-chambered heart (two atria and one ventricle), whereas crocodilians have a four-chambered heart. All reptiles have both pulmonary and systemic circulations (similar to mammals). In noncrocodilian reptiles, functional separation of venous and arterial blood is largely maintained via a muscular ridge within the ventricle. Peripheral blood cell types include erythrocytes, heterophils, eosinophils, basophils, lymphocytes, monocytes (including azurophils), and thrombocytes. Renal and hepatic portal circulations exist, and intra- and extracardiac vascular shunts may be present, especially in aquatic species.

Reptilian skin is usually heavily keratinized and protected by scales. The chelonian shell is composed of both dermal bone plates and keratinized epithelial scutes. Reptiles do not have extensive skin glands, and their skin is essentially dry. However, many male lizards have a series of pre-anal or femoral pores located cranial to the vent or along the craniomedial aspect of the hindlimbs. In some species, both sexes have these glands, but they are more pronounced in the male. Chromatophores are common and enable many species, most notably the Chamaeleonidae, to change color. Bony skin structures, osteoderms, are found in the crocodilians and some lizards. These structures may interfere with radiographic interpretations and surgery. Certain species of snakes have heat-sensitive receptors located around the maxilla that are used to locate prey. Skin characteristics (eg, crests, spines, dewlaps) are often used for species or gender identification in those species that exhibit dimorphic variation.

All reptiles shed their skin. The frequency of ecdysis depends on species, age, nutritional status, environmental temperature and humidity, reproductive status, parasite load, hormonal balance, bacterial/fungal skin disease, and skin damage. The entire process can take 7–14 days.

Reproduction: Most species require some form of conditioning before breeding (eg, hibernation, seasonal nocturnal cooling). Many species are sexually dimorphic. Male lizards are generally larger, have pre-anal or pre-femoral pores, have hemipenal bulges at the tail base, and often are more brightly colored. The gender of snakes is determined by probing for the hemipenes with a blunt, lubricated probe. In males, the probe will enter to a depth of 6–14 subcaudal scales, whereas in females it enters a cloacal gland only to a depth of 3–6 scales. Sexual dimorphism in chelonians is usually obvious in adults; males often have a concave plastron and a longer tail. Many reptiles, especially lizards and chelonians, are territorial and will fight conspecific males, causing severe injuries. In addition, overzealous and unrelenting males may ardently pursue females, causing repeated harassment. Fertilization is internal, and reproduction is either oviparous (egg production) or ovoviviparous (live bearing). Gender determination may be genetic (most snakes, many lizards) or related to incubation temperature (most chelonians, some lizards).

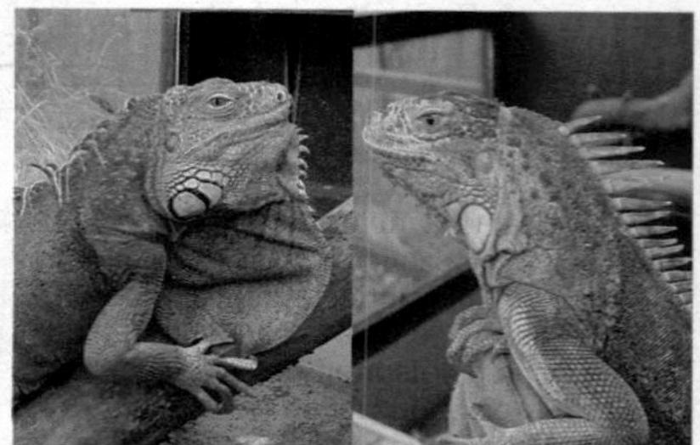

Green iguanas, male (left) displaying a larger dewlap and jowls than the female (right).
Courtesy of Dr. Stephen Divers.

MANAGEMENT

Veterinarians must not only be familiar with common reptile species and their management but also be able to extract clinically relevant husbandry information from the owner in a timely manner. The

TABLE 22 RECOMMENDED MINIMUM SPACE REQUIREMENTS FOR REPTILES

Reptile Group	Minimum Space Requirement
Tortoises and terrapins	$0.4\ m^2/0.1$ m carapace length
Purely aquatic chelonians	$0.25\ m^3/0.1$ m carapace length
Terrestrial lizards	$0.2\ m^2/0.1$ m total length
Arboreal lizards	$0.4\ m^3/0.1$ m total length
Boas and pythons	$0.6\ m^2$/meter of snake
Kingsnakes and rat snakes	$0.6\ m^2$/meter of snake
Whipsnakes and racers	$1.2\ m^2$/meter of snake
Arboreal snakes	$0.8\ m^3$/meter of snake

use of a history form can greatly facilitate this process and ensure that nothing is overlooked.

Species: Different species from different locations must not be mixed. Ideally, only a single species should be kept in any enclosure, and care must be exercised to avoid competition for resources such as food, basking areas, and retreats. In general, the solitary reptile pet is often the healthiest. Most nonbreeding pet snakes and aquatic turtles are best maintained as a single pet, because trauma while feeding is common in groups. Some lizards, notably the chameleons (*Chameleo* spp), are so territorial that isolation is often essential for longterm survival in captivity.

Enclosure: The size of the enclosure is important, and although many breeders and retailers may be able to intensively manage stock, pet owners should be advised on minimum enclosure sizes (*see* TABLE 22), the importance of providing the largest enclosure possible, and correct cage furniture. The type of enclosure (arboreal, terrestrial, subterranean, or aquatic) should be appropriate for the species (*see* TABLE 23).

Glass aquaria are commonly used, but the greater visualization perceived as an advantage to the owner may be stressful to the reptile. Glass is also a poor insulator, and greater heat loss may lead to dramatic temperature fluctuations. Even if the entire top of the enclosure is covered by mesh, ventilation may be severely hampered. Plastic or fiberglass enclosures are more expensive but more versatile.

Newspaper, artificial turf, and organic particulates (eg, bark chips) are suitable materials to line cages and vivaria, but they must be completely replaced regularly. Soil, sand, and natural leaf litter can also be used, but oven baking is recommended to sterilize before use. Gravel and pebbles are not recommended for terrestrial species, because they are difficult to clean and often ingested by reptiles. Other essential items include a water bowl (large enough for the reptile to bathe) and various retreats (eg, cardboard boxes, cork bark, shredded paper). Clean, secure branches are required for arboreal species. Soap and water is generally all that is required to clean cages, but bleach can be used as long as rinsing is thorough. Some cleansers (eg, phenolic disinfectants) are toxic. In certain areas, the climate may permit keeping reptiles in outdoor enclosures, which is highly desirable, although theft, predators, and wildlife carriers of disease should be considered.

Heating: A variety of heaters can be used, including incandescent bulbs, infrared ceramics, heating pads or mats, warming cables, tubular heaters, radiators, convector heaters, and natural sunlight radiation. Heaters of an appropriate size should be thermostat controlled, screened from the animals, and positioned toward one end of the enclosure to provide a thermal gradient. "Hot rocks" frequently result in burns in larger animals and should be avoided. Light bulbs cannot be used to provide nocturnal heat.

Environmental Lighting: All reptiles benefit from broad-spectrum lighting. However, UVB light (290–300 nm) is especially important for most diurnal lizards and chelonians for vitamin D_3 synthesis and calcium regulation. The best source of lighting is unfiltered sunlight. However, many artificial fluorescent strip-lights, compact fluorescent, and mercury halide bulbs are available. Almost every light marketed for reptiles has the term "broad" or "full" or "natural" on its packaging, creating confusion for veterinarians and owners alike. Appropriate lights must be labeled as providing UVB or, better still, be examined and tested using a spectrometer. Even suitable fluorescent lights must be placed relatively close to the reptile and replaced every 9–12 mo. Most transparent plastic and glass barriers filter out UVB wavelengths. A photoperiod of 12 hr/day is suitable for general maintenance.

Humidity: Humidity that is too high or low can create serious problems. Humidity is seldom directly controlled, although the advent of dedicated humidifiers and sprinkler systems makes this practical. Decreasing ventilation to maintain temperature and humidity is ill advised and frequently causes skin and respiratory disease.

Quarantine and Record Keeping: Although the incubation period of many reptile disorders is unknown, quarantine periods of 3–6 mo are recommended. Owners should also be encouraged to keep detailed records of any changes in husbandry or nutrition, breeding activity, in-contact animals, disease outbreaks, health issues, and previous treatments.

Nutrition: Species identification is essential to critically appraise captive

TABLE 23 IMPORTANT HUSBANDRY REQUIREMENTS FOR SELECTED REPTILES

Species	Habitat/Vivarium Type
Corn/rat snake	Terrestrial, scrubland
Boa constrictor	Terrestrial, rain forest (semi-arboreal/aquatic)
Ball python	Terrestrial, scrubland
Leopard gecko	Terrestrial, arid scrub
Green iguana	Arboreal, rain forest
Bearded dragon	Terrestrial, desert
Water dragon	Arboreal, rain forest
Savannah monitor	Terrestrial, arid scrub
Greek tortoise	Terrestrial, temperate to subtropical
Box tortoise	Terrestrial, temperate to subtropical
Leopard tortoise	Terrestrial, tropical
Red-footed tortoise	Terrestrial, tropical
Red-eared slider	Temperate to subtropical gravel bottom or bare, water depth 30 cm min, land area ⅓ of tank

[a] POTZ = preferred optimal temperature zone. Temperature requirements shown are air temperature gradients. In general, basking temperatures should be 5°C warmer, whereas at night these temperatures should fall by 5°C.

[b] BS = broad-spectrum lighting (UVB 290–300 nm) essential, NS = no special lighting requirements

[c] I or i = insectivorous, H or h = herbivorous, C or c = carnivorous; upper case indicates major food preference, lower case minor food preference.

[d] Humidity requirements are significantly greater during ecdysis.

diets (*see* TABLES 24 and 25). Rodent-eating carnivores such as most snakes present few problems as long as the rodent is recognizable to the snake as food. Obese rodents that have been frozen for prolonged periods may contain fewer nutrients. Feeding live rodents is not advised (and is illegal in some countries) because of the dangers of prey-induced trauma to sedate reptiles and the welfare implications for the live prey. Insectivorous reptiles can be well catered for with a variety of commercially available crickets, waxworms, tebos, locusts, mealworms, cockroaches, and flies. Feeding insects a nutritional diet high in calcium and dusting the insects with a high-calcium reptile supplement immediately before feeding is required to prevent deficiencies.

Providing herbivorous reptiles with a varied and nutritious diet can be difficult. Foods with a high calcium:phosphorus ratio should be selected with due regard given to the species-specific requirements for vegetables and fruits. Human nutrient databases can be useful (*see* http://ndb.nal.usda.gov for the USDA National Nutrient Database for Standard Reference). Calcium or vitamin D_3 deficiency (generally due to poor quality lighting and low-calcium diets) leads to secondary nutritional hyperparathyroidism in insectivores and herbivores. A variety of commercially available foods are available in moist, canned, and dry pellet forms. These may help provide a balanced diet, but they have not been critically evaluated.

Although some species will drink from a water bowl, others will only imbibe water droplets on plants and décor. Poor water quality has been implicated as a cause of stomatitis in snakes. Lack of appropriate water delivery has been implicated as a predisposing cause of renal disease in green iguanas. The advent of timer-controlled sprinkler systems makes regular water provision possible for many of these more fastidious drinkers.

See also NUTRITION: EXOTIC AND ZOO ANIMALS (REPTILES), p 2302.

TABLE 23 IMPORTANT HUSBANDRY REQUIREMENTS FOR SELECTED REPTILES *(continued)*

POTZ[a] (°C)	Humidity %	Lighting[b]	Hibernation	Diet[c]
25–30	30–70[d]	NS	Yes	C
28–31	70–95	NS	No	C
25–30	50–80	NS	No	C
25–30	20–30[d]	NS	No	I, c
29–33	60–85	BS	No	H
20–32	20–30[d]	BS	No	I, c, h
24–30	80–90	BS	No	I, c, h
25–32	20–40[d]	BS	No	C, i
20–26	30–50	BS	Yes	H, c
22–28	50–80	BS	Yes	H, I, c
25–30	30–50	BS	No	H, c
25–30	50–90	BS	No	H, c
24–28	Aquatic	BS	Possible	H, I, c

Physical Examination

The successful diagnosis and treatment of reptile diseases requires proper restraint and performance of a variety of clinical techniques. Although the principles are similar to those used for domestic animals, there are a number of reptile-specific peculiarities. It may be possible to observe calm specimens unrestrained, permitting an assessment of demeanor, locomotion, and obvious neurologic disorders such as lameness, paralysis, paresis, and head tilt. Observation of reptiles within their usual environment is particularly valuable and should be done whenever possible. Nervous or aggressive species are best restrained at all times using towels, snake hooks, clear plastic containers, and restraint tubes. Gauntlets severely reduce the clinician's tactile sensation but may be required when dealing with large lizards or small to medium-sized aggressive crocodilians. Careful consideration should be given to the safety of veterinary staff, zoo keepers, and private owners when dealing with large or otherwise potentially dangerous reptiles. In many cases, chemical agents can expedite procedures and considerably reduce risks to both the reptile and human handlers. Given the improvements in reptile anesthesia, even manageable reptiles may be preferentially sedated or anesthetized for procedures that would otherwise take longer to accomplish and cause unnecessary stress or discomfort to the animal. It is possible that sedatives and anesthetics may affect clinical pathologic results, especially hematology.

The decision to examine a potentially dangerous reptile should be made with due regard to legislative and safety requirements. No species of Chelonia is legally considered dangerous, but several species (eg, snapping turtles, *Chelydra* spp) have a ferocious bite that makes them a formidable opponent. In addition, the Convention on the International Trade of Endangered Species of Fauna and Flora (CITES) may also have implications for Appendix 1 and 2 reptiles kept as pets. Even some common pet species (eg, corn snake) may be illegal in some endemic areas, whereas native venomous snakes may be freely collected because they are considered "vermin."

The risks of reptile-borne zoonoses are probably no greater than for other animal groups, and basic personal hygiene after handling reptile patients will minimize these risks. The major zoonoses include *Salmonella*, *Pseudomonas*, *Mycobacterium*, *Cryptosporidium*, and *Rickettsia* spp and pentastomids (arachnid lung parasites). Major public concern centers on the commensal reptile *Salmonella* spp, and clinicians are advised to obtain a copy of the statement policy and client brochure on this subject produced by the Association of Reptilian and Amphibian Veterinarians (www.arav.org/special-topics/).

Every reptile must be accurately weighed; an accurate weight is important to avoid deaths associated with drug overdose, particularly anesthetics and aminoglycosides. In addition, serial weight measurements permit an appraisal of growth and captive management, response to treatment, and disease progression or resolution. Relating body weight to length and conformation gives an assessment of body condition. The snout-vent length of lizards and especially snakes is worth noting, because organ position and growth can be calculated as a result. Chelonian body condition relies on relating total weight to straight carapace length or body volume.

TABLE 24 COMPOSITION OF ANIMAL FOODS THAT MAY BE OFFERED TO REPTILES

Food Item	Dry Matter (%)	Protein (%)	Fat (%)
Mealworms (*Tenibrio*)	42.2	52.8	35
Superworms (*Zophoba*)	40.6	17.4	17.9
Locusts	31.2	61.7	19.4
Crickets	38.2	55.3	30.2
Earthworms	22	49.9	5.8
Waxworms	38.3	15.5	22.2
Chicken muscle	25.6	20.5	4.3
Egg, whole	25.2	12.3	10.9
Mice, 1–2 days old	—	—	—
Mice, adult	—	19.86	8.81

TABLE 25 COMPOSITION OF PLANT FOODS THAT MAY BE OFFERED TO REPTILES

Food Item	Dry Matter (%)	Protein (%)	Fat (%)
Alfalfa	—	15.5	37.1
Apple[a]	—	0.2	0.6
Banana[a]	29.3	1.1	0.3
Black currants	—	—	—
Blackberry	—	—	—
Broccoli	—	3.6	0.3
Cabbage	—	1.3	0.2
Carrots	10.1	0.7	—
Clover hay	—	11	1.9
Collard	—	—	—
Cranberries	—	—	—
Damsons	—	—	—
Dandelions	—	—	—
Endive	—	1.7	0.1

Transillumination of the coelom using a cold light source can be used to visualize the internal structures of small lizards and snakes and is particularly useful to confirm suspected impactions and foreign bodies. Care must be exercised if a hot light source (eg, incandescent spotlight) is used, because of the possibility of burns.

Auscultation of reptiles is difficult and often unrewarding. Electronic stethoscopes with moistened gauze between the shell or scales and the stethoscope diaphragm can be helpful. Doppler ultrasound is particularly useful to determine heart rates.

Snakes: The head of an aggressive snake or a snake of unknown disposition should be identified and restrained before opening the transportation bag to remove the animal. In general, the head of the snake is

TABLE 24 COMPOSITION OF ANIMAL FOODS THAT MAY BE OFFERED TO REPTILES *(continued)*

Energy (Kcal/g)	Calcium (%)	Phosphorus (%)	Ca:P Ratio
6.53	0.06	0.53	0.11
—	0.01	0.02	0.43
—	0.1	0.75	0.13
—	0.23	0.74	0.31
—	0.59	0.85	0.69
—	0.03	0.22	0.13
1.21	0.01	0.2	0.05
1.47	0.05	0.22	0.02
—	1.6	1.8	0.88
2.07	0.84	0.61	1.37

TABLE 25 COMPOSITION OF PLANT FOODS THAT MAY BE OFFERED TO REPTILES *(continued)*

Energy (Kcal/g)	Calcium (%)	Phosphorus (%)	Ca:P Ratio
3.94	1.29	0.21	6.14
0.57	0	0	0.57
0.79	0	0.02	0.25
—	0.06	0.04	1.4
—	0.06	0.02	2.62
—	0.1	0.06	1.49
—	0.04	0.03	1.22
0.23	0.04	0.02	2.29
—	1	0.2	5.0
—	0.2	0.07	2.76
—	0.01	0.01	1.36
—	0.02	0.01	1.5
—	0.18	0.07	2.4
—	0.08	0.03	2.67

TABLE 25 COMPOSITION OF PLANT FOODS THAT MAY BE OFFERED TO REPTILES *(continued)*

Food Item	Dry Matter (%)	Protein (%)	Fat (%)
Fennel	—	2.8	0.4
Fig	—	—	—
Grass (lawn)	33	2.4	1.2
Iceberg lettuce	—	1.2	2.5
Kale	—	—	—
Lemon	—	—	—
Lettuce[a]	4.1	1	0.4
Mustard cress	—	—	—
Orange	13.9	0.8	—
Parsley	—	—	—
Radish	—	—	—
Raspberry	—	—	—
Red currants	—	—	—
Spinach	—	3	0.3
Tomato[a]	6.6	0.9	trace
Turnip	—	1.1	0.9
Watercress	—	2.2	0.3
White grape[a]	20.7	0.6	trace

[a] The poor Ca:P ratio of these commonly used items may make them less suitable as a staple component of a reptile diet.

held behind the occiput using the thumb and middle finger to support the lateral aspects of the cranium. The index finger is placed on top of the head. The other hand is used to support the body. Restraining the snake's head in this manner supports the cranial-cervical junction, which, having only a single occiput, is prone to dislocation. When dealing with large boids, a second, third, or even fourth handler is required to support the body during the examination. It is usually safer and more convenient to sedate a large, pugnacious snake than to risk injury to the snake, owner, or staff.

Nonvenomous species should be supported using one or two hands, depending on size. Nervous or aggressive snakes can be restrained using plexiglass tubes or sedated before examination. The clinician should attempt to gauge muscle tone, proprioception, and mobility. Systemically ill serpents will often be limp, lack strength, and be less mobile. Head carriage, body posture, cloacal tone, proprioception, skin pinch, withdrawal, and papillary and righting reflexes can be used to assess neurologic function.

The entire integument, particularly the head and ventral scales, should be thoroughly examined for evidence of dysecdysis (poor shedding), trauma, parasitism (especially the common snake mite, *Ophionyssus natricis*, and ticks), and microbiologic infection. Any recently shed skin should also be examined, if available, for evidence of retained spectacles. Skin tenting and ridges may indicate cachexia ("poverty lines") or dehydration; ticks and mites may congregate in skin folds, infraorbital pits, nostrils, and corneal rims. The infraorbital pits (where present) and the nostrils should be free from discharges or retained skin. The eyes should be clear, unless ecdysis is imminent. The spectacles covering the eyes should be smooth; any wrinkles usually indicate the presence of

TABLE 25 COMPOSITION OF PLANT FOODS THAT MAY BE OFFERED TO REPTILES *(continued)*

Energy (Kcal/g)	Calcium (%)	Phosphorus (%)	Ca:P Ratio
—	0.1	0.05	1.96
—	0.28	0.09	3.04
1.58	0.1	0.09	1.1
0.14	0.03	0.02	1.34
—	0.17	0.06	2.9
—	0.11	0.01	9.17
0.12	0.02	0.02	0.85
—	0.06	0.06	1
0.35	0.04	0.02	1.71
—	0.2	0.13	1.53
—	0.04	0.02	1.63
—	0.04	0.02	1.41
—	0.03	0.03	1.2
—	0.09	0.05	1.69
0.14	0.01	0.02	0.62
—	0.05	0.01	2.89
—	0.22	0.05	4.23
0.63	0.01	0.02	0.86

a retained spectacle. The spectacle represents the transparent fused eyelids, and therefore the cornea is not normally exposed. The subspectacular fluid drains through a duct to the cranial roof of the maxilla. When blocked, the buildup of fluid causes a subspectacular swelling that often becomes infected. Damage to the underlying cornea can result in panophthalmitis and ocular swelling. Retrobulbar abscessation results in protrusion of a normal-sized globe. Other ocular pathologies can include uveitis, corneal lipidosis, and spectacular foreign bodies, including slivers of wood or other vivarium materials.

Working from cranial to caudal, the head and body are palpated for swellings, wounds, and other abnormalities. The position of any internal anomalies, noted as a distance from the snout and interpreted as a percentage of snout-vent length, enables an assessment of possible organ involvement. Recently fed snakes have a midbody swelling associated with the prey within the stomach; handling such individuals may well lead to regurgitation. Preovulatory follicles, eggs, feces, enlarged organs, and masses may be palpable. The cloaca can be examined using a dedicated otoscope or by digital palpation.

Examination of the oral cavity is often left until last, because many snakes object to such manipulation. However, even before the mouth is opened, the tongue should be seen flicking in and out of the labial notch with regularity. The mouth can be gently opened using a plastic or wooden spatula to permit an assessment of mucous membrane color and the buccal cavity for evidence of mucosal edema, ptyalism, hemorrhage, necrosis, and inspissated exudates. White deposits may indicate uric acid deposition due to visceral gout. The pharynx and glottis should be examined for hemorrhage, foreign bodies, parasites, and discharges. Open-mouth breathing is a reliable indicator of severe respiratory compromise. The patency of the internal nares and the state of the polyphyodontic teeth should be noted.

Lizards: Lizards vary considerably in size, strength, and temperament; therefore, a variety of handling techniques are required.

The tegus and monitors are renowned for their powerful bites, whereas other species, particularly the green iguana, are much more likely to use their claws and tail. The main problem when handling small lizards is restraining them before they flee. The lizard should be transported in a securely tied cloth bag, so that the position of the lizard can be identified and the lizard held before the bag is opened. Large lizards are best restrained with the forelimbs held laterally against their coelom and the hindlimbs held laterally against the tail base. The limbs should never be held over the spine, because fractures and dislocations can occur. Nervous lizards can be wrapped in a towel to aid restraint. Smaller lizards can be restrained around the pectoral girdle, holding the forelimbs against the coelom, although care is required not to impair respiratory movements. A lizard should never be grasped by the tail, because many species can drop the tail (autotomy) in an attempt to evade capture. Restricting the vision of a lizard (eg, a towel placed over the head) is often the simplest way to facilitate handling and examination. A useful restraint technique for iguanid or monitor lizards uses the vasovagal response: gentle digital pressure applied to both orbits causes many lizards to enter a state of stupor for up to 45 min (or until a painful or noisy stimulus is applied). This technique enables the mouth to be gently opened without the need for excessive force. If possible, the lizard should be observed unrestrained to check for neurologic problems. Calm lizards may be permitted to walk around the examination table or on the floor. However, if in any doubt, the lizard should be placed in a large plastic enclosure to prevent escape during observation.

The integument should be examined for parasites (essentially mites and ticks) and trauma due to fighting, mating, and burns. Lizards tend to shed their skin in stages. Classically, dysecdysis and skin retention occurs around the digits and tail, causing ischemic necrosis. Extensive skin folding and tenting may indicate cachexia and dehydration.

The head should be examined for abnormal conformation. The mouth can be opened using a blunt spatula or, in iguanas, by gently applying pressure to the dewlap. The buccal cavity and glottis should be examined thoroughly for evidence of trauma, infection, neoplasia, and edema, especially pharyngeal edema. The internal extent of any rostral abrasions should be evaluated. The nostrils, eyes, and tympanic scales should be clean and free of discharges. The presence of dry, white material around the nostrils of some iguanid lizards is normal, because some species excrete salt through specialized nasal glands. The rostrum should be examined for trauma, often caused by repeated attempts to escape from a poorly designed vivarium or to evade cagemates. The head, body, and limbs should be palpated for masses or swellings, which can be abscesses or metabolic bone disorders. Lizards suffering from severe hypocalcemia and hyperphosphatemia may exhibit periodic tremors and muscle fasciculations. The coelomic body cavity of most lizards can be gently palpated. Food and fecal material within the GI tract, fat bodies, liver, ova, and eggs are usually appreciable. Cystic calculi, fecoliths, enlarged kidneys, impactions, retained eggs or ova, and unusual coelomic masses may also be noted.

The cloaca should be free from fecal staining, with visual and digital examination considered routine. In the green iguana, renomegaly can be appreciated by digital cloacal palpation. The high incidence of dystocia necessitates a need to identify gender during examination. Many species of lizards are sexually dimorphic, although sexing juveniles can be difficult.

Tortoises, Turtles, and Terrapins: Small to medium-sized tortoises are not difficult to handle, although their strength and uncooperative nature can hinder examination. Patiently holding the tortoise with its head down will often persuade a shy individual to protrude the head from the shell. Placing the thumb and middle finger behind the occipital condyles prevents retraction of the head. However, with larger species, it may be physically impossible to prevent a strong individual from pulling free. In such cases, sedation or use of a neuromuscular blocking agent may be necessary. The more aggressive aquatic species should be held at the rear of the carapace. Some species (eg, snapping turtles) have long necks and an extremely powerful bite, necessitating great care. Certain species also have functional hinges at the front and/or back of the plastron, and care should be exercised not to trap a finger when the hinge closes.

Examination of the head should include the nostrils for any discharges and the beak for damage and overgrowth. The eyelids should be open and not obviously distended or inflamed, and the eyes should be clear and bright. Conjunctivitis, corneal ulceration, and opacities are frequent presentations. The tympanic scales should be examined for signs of swelling associated with aural abscessation. Applying steady distractive pressure to the maxilla and mandible can open the mouth, and a mouth gag can be inserted to prevent closure. Aggressive chelonians, generally aquatic species, often threaten by open-mouth displays, which provide a good opportunity to examine the buccal cavity with minimal handling. Mucus membrane coloration is normally pale; hyperemia may be associated with septicemia or toxemia. Icterus is rare but may occur with biliverdinemia due to severe liver disease. Pale deposits within the oral membranes may represent infection or urate tophi associated with visceral gout. The glottis is positioned at the back of the fleshy tongue and may be difficult to visualize; however, it is important to check for any inflammation and glottal discharges consistent with respiratory disease.

The integument should be free of damage. Subcutaneous swellings are usually abscesses. Aquatic species appear more susceptible to superficial and deep mycotic dermatitis, especially around the head, neck, and limbs. The withdrawn limbs can be extended from the shell of small to medium-sized chelonians by applying steady traction. Because the coelomic space within the shell is restricted, gently forcing the hindlimbs into the shell will often lead to partial protrusion of the forelimbs and head, and vice versa. A wedge or mouth gag can be used to prevent complete closure of a hinge. No chelonian will close a hinge on an extended limb. The integument should be examined for parasites (particularly ticks and flies), dysecdysis, trauma, and infection that may arise due to predator attacks. Aggressive conflicts and courting trauma must also be considered in the communal environment. Limb fractures are less common in chelonians than in other reptiles, but when they do occur they are often associated with rough handling and secondary nutritional hyperparathyroidism. Focal subcutaneous swellings are usually abscesses, but grossly swollen joints or limbs are more often cases of fracture, osteomyelitis, or septic arthritis.

The prefemoral fossae should be palpated with the chelonian held head-up. Gently rocking the animal may enable palpation of eggs, cystic calculi, or other coelomic masses. The shell should be examined for hardness, poor conformation, trauma, or infection. Soft, poorly mineralized shells are usually a result of secondary nutritional hyperparathyroidism resulting from dietary deficiencies of calcium, excess phosphorus, or a lack of full-spectrum lighting. Pyramiding of the shell appears to be more associated with inappropriate humidity than dietary imbalances. Shell infection may present as loosening and softening of the scutes with erythema, petechiae, purulent or caseous discharges, and a foul odor.

Prolapses through the vent are obvious, but it is necessary to determine the structure(s) involved. Prolapses may include cloacal tissue, shell gland, colon, bladder, or phallus. Internal examination using digital palpation and an endoscope is recommended.

Anesthesia and Analgesia

For some minor procedures (eg, blood sampling), simple restraint may be all that is required. This can be enhanced by temporary immobilization techniques such as dorsal recumbency, reduced light intensity, or gentle ocular pressure (vasovagal response). For more invasive and painful procedures, general anesthesia must be used. Although considerable anatomic, physiologic, and pharmacologic differences exist between reptiles, some general guidelines are applicable. The following is therefore intended as a practical approach, rather than an exhaustive review of reptile anesthesia.

Preanesthetic Assessment and Stabilization: All reptiles should be hospitalized and maintained at their preferred optimal temperature zone at all times to minimize physiologic disturbance, facilitate recovery, and maintain immunocompetence. Although hypothermia will reduce movement, it does not provide analgesia and is therefore unacceptable as a means of anesthesia on welfare grounds. It can also dramatically affect the pharmacokinetics of any drugs administered and greatly prolong recovery.

A full clinical examination should be performed and the animal accurately weighed, although this may not be practical or possible in some cases. The hydration status of all reptiles should be assessed, especially if debilitated or post-hibernation. For elective procedures (eg, neutering), underweight, dehydrated, or debilitated animals should be nursed for days, weeks, or months until their condition improves. For nonelective surgery, dehydration should be corrected before anesthesia. Even the most moribund egg-bound reptile will usually benefit from stabilization for 24–48 hr before surgery is performed. Reptiles that have not been stabilized before surgery tend to succumb intra- or postoperatively. Although oral fluids are least invasive to administer and provide the most physiologically normal method of rehydration, they are sufficient only for mildly dehydrated animals and are contraindicated immediately before surgery because of the risks associated with regurgitation. Intracoelomic fluids are more suitable, but uptake can take many hours and their use is problematic if coeliotomy or coelioscopy is planned. For dehydrated surgical candidates, IV or intraosseous fluid therapy should be administered before, during, and after surgery as necessary.

Reptiles should be fasted before all elective surgery to avoid the compression of lung(s) associated with large meals and potential regurgitation. Fasting depends on the feeding regimen of the reptile, but in general one feeding cycle should be skipped before surgery. Premedication with sedatives such as acepromazine and atropine is generally rare in reptiles, although midazolam has been advocated in large chelonians. However, presurgical administration of analgesics should be considered routine (*see* TABLE 26).

Anesthetic Induction: IV or intraosseous propofol provides a rapid, controlled mode of induction. It is relatively nontoxic, and there is reduced risk of thrombophlebi-

TABLE 26 ANALGESICS, SEDATIVES, AND ANESTHETICS USED IN REPTILES

Drug	Dose and Route	Comments
Morphine	1.5 mg/kg, IM, SC 10 mg/kg, IM, SC	Chelonians (red-eared sliders) Lizards (bearded dragons) Not analgesic for snakes. Causes pronounced respiratory depression in turtles.
Hydromorphone	0.5 mg/kg, IM, SC	Chelonians: appears to cause less respiratory depression than morphine
Tramadol	5 mg/kg/day, PO, SC; 10 mg/kg, PO, every 4 days	Chelonians (red-eared sliders); less respiratory depression than morphine
Butorphanol	20 mg/kg, SC	Snakes (cornsnakes) at high doses. Not analgesic for bearded dragons or red-eared sliders. May cause respiratory depression, and high-dose volume may be impractical. May be able to partially antagonize opiate agonists like morphine.
Meloxicam	0.2 mg/kg, IV, IM, SC, every 24–48 hr	
Ketamine	10–40 mg/kg, IM 40–60 mg/kg, IM	Sedation, prolonged hangover effects Deeper sedation but not sufficient for painful procedures and care in debilitated individuals
	Ketamine 10 mg/kg, combined with medetomidine 0.1–0.2 mg/kg (or dexmedetomidine 0.05–0.1 mg/kg) and morphine 1.5 mg/kg or hydromorphone 0.5 mg/kg, IM (or 50% dose, IV)	Deep sedation/anesthesia in many chelonians. Reversed using atipamezole (0.5 mg/kg, IM) and, if necessary, naloxone (0.2 mg/kg, IM)

TABLE 26 ANALGESICS, SEDATIVES, AND ANESTHETICS USED IN REPTILES *(continued)*

Drug	Dose and Route	Comments
Midazolam	2 mg/kg, IM	Premedication, or can be given with ketamine to increase sedative effects or promote similar effects at lower ketamine doses.
Dexmedetomidine	0.05–0.1 mg/kg, IV or IM	Often used in combination with ketamine and opiates as a sedative to light anesthetic. Useful when IV access is difficult.
Atipamezole	10 × mg dose of dexmedetomidine, IM	Used to reverse dexmedetomidine
Tiletamine/ zolazepam	3–12 mg/kg, IM	Tortoises, lizards, snakes. Low dose useful to facilitate intubation. Higher doses associated with prolonged recoveries.
Propofol	3–10 mg/kg, IV, intraosseous	Low dose rate for larger reptiles. Subanesthetic doses produce variable short-term sedation.
Alfaxalone	5–10 mg/kg, IV 10–20 mg/kg, IM	Similar effects to those of propofol IV, but higher doses effective IM. Larger IM dose volumes may warrant dividing into two or more injections.
Isoflurane	1%–5%	Routine gaseous agent; subanesthetic levels provide short-term sedation. Mask down or conscious (sedated) intubation possible in some species.
Sevoflurane	2%–7%	Very similar effects to those of isoflurane but recoveries appear to be faster. Preferred agent for critical or large reptiles.

tis if it is injected perivascularly. This is of particular concern, because IV access may be relatively difficult, especially in active animals undergoing elective procedures. Alfaxalone has been licensed in the USA; it is an excellent IV induction agent and is also effective when used IM.

If IV access is impractical or dangerous to attempt, IM agents can be used to induce sufficient chemical restraint for intubation. For IM injections in lizards and chelonians, the forelimb muscles are preferred, whereas for snakes, the epaxial muscles are used. An IM combination of ketamine, medetomidine (or dexmedetomidine), and morphine or hydromorphone has proved effective for a variety of chelonians; this can be readily reversed using atipamezole and, if necessary, naloxone or naltrexone.

Squamates can also be induced by inhalation agents in an induction chamber or by mask. However, breath holding tends to occur in turtles and crocodilians, which can respire anaerobically for prolonged periods. Induction may take 10–30 min in cooperative lizards and snakes. Intubation of conscious patients has been suggested after local lidocaine spray, but the adverse effects of increased stress and catecholamine release should always be considered. There is also the potential danger of being bitten.

Maintenance of Anesthesia: Isoflurane or sevoflurane are the agents of choice for maintenance of anesthesia. These volatile inhalation agents have faster modes of action, are more controllable, and facilitate faster recoveries than most alternatives. Furthermore, their lack of reliance on hepatic metabolism or renal excretion reduces the anesthetic risk to debilitated reptiles or those with questionable renal or hepatic function.

Intubation of reptiles is relatively simple. Small-gauge endotracheal tubes or catheters are easily inserted through the glottis immediately caudal to the tongue; this may be aided by forcing the tongue up and forward by pressing a finger into the intermandibular space from under the jaw. The reptilian glottis is actively dilated, and therefore its movement will often be abolished in anesthetized animals; a guiding stylet can be useful to facilitate endotracheal tube placement. The bifurcation of the trachea may be far craniad in some chelonians, and gaseous exchange has also been reported within the tracheal lung of some snakes; care should be taken to use a short endotracheal tube that is securely taped in position.

Noncrocodilian reptiles lack a diaphragm; skeletal intercostal muscles (Squamata) or limb movements (Chelonia) control breathing. The action of these muscles is abolished at a surgical plane of anesthesia, and intermittent positive-pressure ventilation is required. Ventilation rates should initially mirror preanesthesia evaluations and then be adjusted to maintain end-tidal capnography readings of 15–25 mmHg. Electrical ventilators enable precise control of ventilation rates and pressures.

Monitoring anesthesia in reptiles differs considerably from doing so in mammals. Palpebral and corneal reflexes are reliable in those species in which they can be elicited (ie, all chelonians, all crocodilians, most lizards, but no snakes). However, corneal reflexes are abolished at toxic doses, and pupillary diameter may bear little relation to the depth of anesthesia (unless fixed and dilated, which indicates excessive anesthetic depth or brain anoxia and death). Jaw tone and withdrawal reflexes (tongue, limb, or tail) are abolished only at a surgical plane of anesthesia. This also correlates with full loss of the righting reflex, loss of spontaneous movement, and complete muscle relaxation.

Heart rate may be monitored by auscultation or by visualization or palpation of the heart beat in most snakes and some lizards. Pulse oximetry, using either an esophageal or cloacal reflectance probe, is useful to monitor pulse rate and strength. Although the blood oxygen saturation (SpO_2) readings are often low and have not been validated for reptiles, monitoring the trend in SpO_2 is often helpful. Doppler ultrasonography can also be used over peripheral arteries or the heart. Blood gas estimations are often affected by intracardiac or pulmonary shunts, especially in aquatic species. However, end-tidal capnography has proved effective.

Toward the end of surgery, the anesthetic gas should be discontinued while maintaining ventilation for another 5–10 min to facilitate excretion. At this point, oxygen should be discontinued in favor of room air delivered by bag-valve mask to encourage spontaneous respiration.

Postoperative Support: Once it is breathing spontaneously, the reptile can be returned to an incubator or vivarium to fully recover. Continued monitoring is essential until righting reflexes return and the animal is ambulatory. Additional analgesia, fluid, and nutritional support should be provided as indicated.

Diagnostic Techniques

Radiology: Several anatomic differences make it difficult to obtain quality radiographs in reptiles. The relatively small size of most pet reptiles and the lack of diffuse body fat often produce images of poor contrast. Thick, highly keratinized scales, osteoderms, or shells can severely hinder the x-ray beam, necessitating greater power and a subsequent loss of fine soft-tissue detail.

Despite these difficulties, most high-capacity units can be set to produce quality radiographs of reptiles. High-detailed screen/film combinations (eg, mammography film) are essential to obtain sufficient detail and contrast, especially in smaller animals. Various agents can be used to improve contrast. Barium sulfate (30%) can be used for GI studies. Water-soluble iodine compounds such as iohexol can be used for GI, urogenital, and IV techniques. The injection of air into the coelom of a lizard can greatly improve the appreciation of preovulatory follicles.

Snakes: Snakes can be difficult to position and restrain for radiographic examinations unless anesthetized. If the purpose of the examination is simply to exclude radiodense foreign bodies, the snake may be allowed to coil in its natural position. If detailed examination of the skeletal, respiratory, and digestive system is desired, the snake must be extended. A plastic restraint tube can be used for this purpose; however, this may produce some radiographic artifact. In larger snakes, several films will be needed to radiograph the entire length of the body. Lateral views are best taken using horizontal beams to avoid displacement artifact of the viscera. However, standard laterals with the snake taped in lateral recumbency can be useful, especially when horizontal beams are not possible or safe to undertake. The interpretation of dorsoventral views are hindered by the spine and ribs but can still be useful when dealing with obvious lesions, including eggs and mineralized masses.

Lizards: Small lizards can often be restrained by taping them to the radiography film or table for a dorsoventral view. Placing cotton balls over the eyes, and wrapping them with self-adhesive tape will often produce a calm, motionless lizard. A dorsoventral view can help identify foreign bodies, intestinal impaction, or coelomic masses. A horizontal x-ray beam provides the best lateral imaging in lizards, especially when evaluating the respiratory system. The positioning for this view involves rotating the x-ray tube 90° and placing the film vertically behind the lizard. Elevating the body of the lizard on rolled towels or foam pads helps prevent superimposition of the limbs with the coelomic cavity. The positioning for, and interpretation of, crocodilian radiographs are similar to those used for lizards.

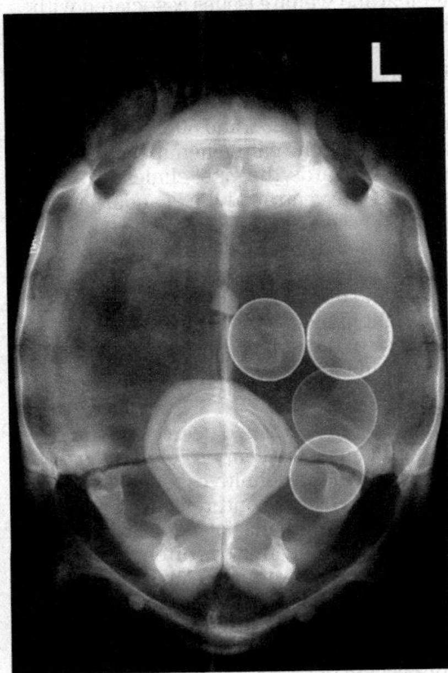

Radiograph of a Greek tortoise demonstrating several abnormal eggs, including one within the bladder and encased by uric acid, forming a large urolith. *Courtesy of Dr. Stephen Divers.*

Chelonians: Most chelonians are fairly easy to position and restrain. For vertical beam dorsoventral radiographs, most conscious animals will remain motionless long enough to permit exposure. Ideally, the head and limbs should be extended from the shell to reduce superimposition of the limb musculature on the coelomic viscera. More active animals can be restrained by taping them to the cassette or by placing them in a radiolucent container, although this should be avoided with smaller specimens (and lower exposures), because material artifacts may appear. For lateral horizontal beam radiographs, the chelonian is best placed on a central plastron stand to encourage extension of the limbs and head while the tortoise remains immobile. Both left and right lateral projections should be taken with the lateral edge of the shell touching (or as close as possible to) the cassette. The third basic coelomic view is the horizontal craniocaudal (or anterior-posterior) view. The chelonian is positioned on a central plastron stand, with the caudal edge of the carapace touching (or as close as possible to) the cassette; the head should be facing the x-ray tube and the beam centered on the midline of the cranial rim of the carapace. Radiology of the head and limbs requires exteriorization from the shell, usually under general anesthesia. The use of sandbags, foam, and tape aid positioning. Standard interpretation requires that both true lateral and dorsoventral views should be taken—even slight rotation makes interpretation more difficult.

Ultrasonography: A useful and often underrated technique, ultrasonography has gained popularity as a diagnostic technique for reptiles. It is particularly useful for examining tissue parenchyma, guiding biopsy needles, and, with color flow Doppler, investigating cardiac disease. Unfortunately, the equipment tends to be expensive, and several probes with small footprints are required, given the variation in reptile size and ultrasound applications. Ultrasound waves cannot penetrate through mineralized tissue or air and, therefore, ultrasonography has obvious limitations to investigate respiratory and GI diseases.

The giant species require a 5-MHz probe, whereas a 7.5-MHz probe suffices for most reptiles. When examining very small specimens (or for ultrasonography of eyes), a 10–20 MHz probe is more appropriate. Good contact and imaging generally require copious quantities of gel or a water bath. It is helpful to maintain the animal in a normal position or, failing that, at least appreciate the complications associated with organ displacement. Ultrasonography can be a useful adjunct to radiography, especially to assess the reproductive tract (evaluating ovarian activity and distinguishing between pre- and postovulatory egg stasis), liver and gallbladder, urinary system, soft-tissue masses, and heart. Ultrasonography has been used to guide liver biopsy, although iatrogenic trauma has been reported in snakes.

CT and MRI: CT offers excellent, high-resolution, detailed images. Potentially, it would be the diagnostic imaging technique of choice for the respiratory system and skeleton of reptiles. MRI produces primarily high-detailed images of soft-tissue structures and is useful to diagnose neurologic, hepatic, renal, and reproductive diseases in reptiles. Disadvantages of these techniques are the need for general anesthesia to completely eliminate motion, equipment availability, and cost.

Endoscopy: Endoscopy has proved to be a most useful diagnostic tool in reptile medicine, and given the small and delicate nature of many species, continued development of minimally invasive techniques is likely. Flexible endoscopes are useful for respiratory endoscopy in snakes or GI endoscopy in many species. The main disadvantage of the flexible, fiberoptic endoscope is the poorer image quality than for those obtained using rigid scopes of a similar diameter. However, the continued development of smaller videoscopes looks likely to redefine flexible endoscopy in reptiles. The compact body size of most pet reptiles, coupled with their coelomic body design, makes rigid endoscopy useful in many situations. Although equipment must be matched to size of the reptile, in general the 1.9-mm and 2.7-mm telescope and sheath systems work well for most pet species, enabling gas insufflation, fluid irrigation, and biopsy capability.

Insufflation is essential to provide the lens-organ distance required for visualization. For GI endoscopy, air and/or saline is used; for coelioscopy, medical grade CO_2 or saline is preferred. Coelomic pressures seldom need to be >5 mmHg. When performing endoscopy in small neonates or within a hollow viscus (eg, bladder, oviduct, cloaca, stomach), warmed sterile saline irrigation often provides better clarity than gas insufflation.

General anesthesia is recommended for all endoscopy procedures. Certain examinations (eg, buccal cavity and cloaca) may be possible in a conscious or sedated animal using a mouth gag or other appropriate restraint, but complete immobilization is preferred to avoid risking damage to patient, staff, or equipment. Anesthesia is mandatory for coelioscopy.

Blood Collection: Venipuncture is generally a blind technique in reptiles. Up to 0.5 mL/100 g may be safely collected from healthy reptiles, less in debilitated animals. There is a relative lack of hematologic or biochemical data for most reptiles. In addition, blood values can vary dramatically with species, environment, nutrition, age, breeding, and hibernation. Given this variability, published ranges may be of limited value. More reliance should be placed on establishing an individual's observed range and using serial sampling to monitor the progress of hematologic and biochemical changes. The use of a toenail clip to obtain blood may result in fecal or urate contamination, increased tissue enzymes, and hemogram and electrolyte changes due to the peripheral nature of the sample and the crushing artifact of collection. Of even greater concern are the ethical and welfare issues associated with toenail clipping.

The two common sites for venipuncture in snakes are the caudal vein and the heart. The caudal vein is accessed caudal to the cloaca, between 25% and 50% down the tail, and avoiding the paired hemipenes of males. In lizards, the most clinically useful vessel is the ventral midline caudal vein, best accessed 20%–80% down the tail. The most clinically useful vessels in chelonians appear to be the jugulars, subcarapacial sinus, and dorsal coccygeal veins. The left and right jugular veins are preferred because of the reduced risk of lymphatic contamination.

Necropsy: A detailed necropsy should be undertaken whenever possible, because it often provides a definitive diagnosis. When managing a disease outbreak in a population, elective euthanasia and necropsy of one or more individuals is often the most efficient and cost-effective means of diagnosis. Fresh necropsies can provide organ biopsies, blood, and other bodily fluids for laboratory examination. The submission of microbiology samples, especially bacteriology, from reptiles that have died and remained within a heated enclosure must, however, be interpreted with caution.

Surgery

In general, performing surgery on a reptile patient should be approached with the same principles as those used for domestic animals. However, there are some specific anatomic considerations, as well as unique aspects of patient preparation, positioning, and equipment. Only a basic discussion follows here, and consulting other sources on reptile anatomy, physiology, husbandry, anesthesia, and surgery, as well as domestic animal surgery literature, is essential before performing surgery on any reptile.

For truly giant reptiles, such as giant tortoises, the use of stronger, large animal instruments is recommended. For reptiles weighing 5–50 kg, most instruments used for small animals are appropriate. However, most pet reptiles weigh <1 kg, and microsurgical instruments are often required. These instruments are not miniaturized versions of standard instruments but rather balanced instruments with fine, small tips. Because microinstruments can be costly, ophthalmologic instruments can be useful alternatives. Plastic, self-retaining retractors can be adjusted to fit different sizes of incisions and do not compromise ventilation. Smaller versions of standard abdominal retractors can also be used but are significantly heavier. Eyelid retractors can be useful to retract coelomic incisions in small lizards and snakes. Epoxy resins or low-temperature veterinary acrylics are used for many chelonian plastron closures and shell repairs.

Rapidly absorbable suture materials are recommended for internal soft-tissue applications. For prolonged internal durability, polydioxanone or nylon are preferred. Poliglecaprone, monofilament nylon, and polydioxanone are favored for skin suturing, although wire may be necessary for giant tortoises or monitor lizards.

Because most reptile patients that require surgery are significantly smaller than mammalian patients, some degree of magnification is generally recommended. Headband or frame-mounted operating loupes (2–4 × magnification) with a dedicated halogen or xenon light source are affordable, versatile, comfortable, and simple to use. While operating, microscopy telescopes can provide magnification with selected rigid endoscopy systems.

A healthy reptile can generally tolerate 0.4–0.8 mL/100 g body wt of blood loss. Reptiles in need of surgery are often compromised, and diagnostic blood samples may have been collected before surgery. Therefore, the amount of blood a reptile can afford to lose during surgery may be considerably less. Careful consideration must be given to minimizing hemorrhage using cotton-tipped spears or applicators, vascular clips, and radiosurgery.

Patient positioning will depend on the species and the nature of the surgery. Consideration should be given to ensuring that head and neck position does not interfere with ventilation; avoiding excessive compression of the head, limbs, or coelom to prevent pressure necrosis, visceral rupture, or hypoventilation of the lungs; avoiding extreme and prolonged hyperextension or hyperflexion of any joint; and ensuring that the surgical site is easily accessible and does not require surgeon positioning that will result in fatigue. Sand-bags, bean-bags, foam supports, and adhesive tapes can be used to maintain patient position.

When reptile skin is incised, it tends to invert. Therefore, everting suture patterns (eg, horizontal mattress) are recommended to ensure opposition of tissue without future dysecdysis. The skin suture materials should be monofilament. Wire suture may be required for repairs involving shell or thickly keratinized skin containing osteoderms. Staples have also been advocated, because they cause mild eversion of the skin. Given the length of time it takes for reptile wounds to heal, sutures should not be removed until 6–8 wk after surgery.

The primary factors to consider postoperatively are analgesia and continued vigilance concerning hydration, temperature, nutrition, and hygiene. It is widely understood and accepted that reptiles can feel pain. Pain slows the healing process and depresses the normal function of the immune system in mammals. There is no evidence to suggest this process would not be similar in reptiles. Clinically, reptiles that receive postoperative analgesia appear to recover better than those that do not. The continuation of preemptive analgesia using opioids and/or NSAIDs should be a routine part of postoperative care.

Few drugs are approved by the FDA for use in reptiles. Medications can be given by a variety of routes, including PO, SC, IM, IV, intracardiac, intracoelomic, intraosseous, intrasynovial, or intratracheal injection. Certain drugs can be applied topically, given per cloaca, by inhalation (nebulization), or by direct intralesional administration. Because reptiles are ectotherms, temperatures outside the preferred optimal temperature zone (POTZ) can have profound influences on drug distribution, metabolism, excretion, and elimination half-life. Some therapeutic regimens state a fixed temperature at which the reptile should be held during treatment. If there are pharmacokinetic data on the drug, then the elimination of the drug will be known and constant. However, if this stated temperature is below or above the POTZ for the species being treated, then stress and debilitation may ensue. Even when the stated therapeutic temperature is within the POTZ for the species being treated, constant exposure to a fixed temperature is likely to be stressful.

Reptiles have a well-developed renal portal system; blood from the caudal half of the body passes through the kidneys before reaching the systemic venous circulation. Drugs injected into the caudal half of the body may have a significantly reduced half-life if excreted via tubular secretion. However, studies have demonstrated that these effects are unlikely to be clinically significant. Of potential concern is the caudal injection of nephrotoxic drugs that may reach renal tissue in high concentration. Also, the large bladder of chelonians may act as a drug reservoir and lead to a secondary therapeutic peak many hours after drug administration. The shell of tortoises, turtles, and terrapins is largely living tissue; therefore, all chelonian medication should be based on total body weight.

Drug Dosage and Allometric Scaling: Numerous pharmacokinetic studies have been published for reptiles, and these should be considered the most reliable source for information on drug dosages. When species-specific information is not available, it is possible to extrapolate from closely related species. If there are no pharmacokinetic data or reliable clinical experience for a particular species, it may be necessary to extrapolate pharmacokinetic data from other animals. Allometric scaling calculates the drug dose and dosing frequency using metabolic rate rather than body weight. The basic allometric equations are shown below, in which W = body weight (kg) and K = energy constant, which is 10 for reptiles. These equations can be used to calculate a dose and dose frequency for a species for which no data are available, by using pharmacokinetic data from a known species (control), whether another reptile or mammal or bird:

Minimum energy cost = $K(W^{0.75})$
Specific minimum energy cost = $K(W^{-0.25})$

Antimicrobials: Many bacterial infections in reptiles are caused by gram-negative bacteria, particularly *Pseudomonas*, *Aeromonas*, *Citrobacter*, *Klebsiella*, and *Proteus* spp. Bacterial resistance to many commonly used antibacterials is seen, and many gram-negative bacteria can have unexpected sensitivity to particular antibacterials; therefore, sampling for Gram stain, cytology, culture, and sensitivity testing should be done before starting therapy. Antibacterial therapy must usually be given while awaiting the results of bacterial sensitivity tests. In these circumstances, amikacin, ceftazidime, and enrofloxacin or ciprofloxacin are often preferred (see TABLE 27). In severe infections, amikacin may be combined with ampicillin or amoxicillin for respiratory tract infections or with ceftazidime for generalized or systemic infections. Chloramphenicol in combination with neomycin may be given for GI infections. Penicillin, metronidazole, lincomycin, or clindamycin can be used for anaerobic infections.

Fungal and yeast infections commonly occur in reptiles. GI and skin mycoses are particularly common in reptiles maintained on inappropriately longterm broad-spectrum antibacterials. Cutaneous mycoses can often be treated by debridement and topical application of antifungals. GI infections can be treated with nystatin, whereas systemic infections may require itraconazole or fluconazole. In cases of pulmonary mycoses, antifungal medication may be given by nebulization or intratracheal or intrapulmonary injection.

Herpesviruses can cause severe morbidity and mortality in chelonians. Acyclovir has been used with some success during the early stages.

Parasiticides: Parasiticides used commonly in reptiles are listed in TABLE 28. Parasiticide overdosage may lead to drug toxicity, which may be seen as neurologic signs, including seizures. Ivermectin is contraindicated in chelonians, and adverse reactions have been reported in some iguanid lizards, skinks, and indigo snakes. Milbemycin has been successfully used in box tortoises and terrapins, but it is recommended that ivermectins and milbemycins be avoided in all chelonians because safer alternatives are available. Permethrin is licensed for use in reptiles and appears safe and effective against mites and ticks.

TABLE 27 ANTIMICROBIAL DRUGS USED IN REPTILES

Drug	Dosage	Comments
Acyclovir	80 mg/kg/day, PO; topical cream 12 times daily	Antiviral
Amikacin	Corn snake: loading dose 1.7 mg/kg, IM, followed by 26 mcg/kg/hr via osmotic infusion-pump implant Gopher snake: initial dose 5 mg/kg, IM, then 2.5 mg/kg, IM, every 3 days Gopher tortoise: 5 mg/kg, IM, on alternate days American alligator (juvenile): 2.25 mg/kg, IM, every 3–4 days Ball python: 3.5 mg/kg, IM, every 4–5 days 50 mg/10 mL saline × 30 min nebulization bid	Maintain hydration
Amoxicillin	22 mg/kg, PO, bid 10 mg/kg/day, IM	Often ineffective unless given in combination with aminoglycosides
Amphotericin B	0.5–1 mg/kg, intracoelomic, IV, 1–3 days for 14–28 days	Aspergillosis; fluid therapy recommended
	Tortoise: 0.1 mg/kg/day, intrapulmonary, for 28 days 5 mg/150 mL saline for 1 hr of nebulization, bid for 7 days	Pulmonary candidiasis
Ampicillin	Most species: 10–20 mg/kg, SC, IM, 1–2 times/day Tortoises: 50 mg/kg, IM, bid	
Azithromycin	Ball python: 10 mg/kg, PO, every 3–7 days (3 days for skin infections, 5 days for respiratory tract, 7 days for liver and kidneys)	
Carbenicillin	200–400 mg/kg/day, IM	
Cephalexin	20–40 mg/kg, PO, bid	
Ceftazidime	20–40 mg/kg, SC, IM, IV, every 2–3 days	
Ceftiofur	Tortoises: 2.2–4 mg/kg/day, IM Snakes: 2.2 mg/kg, IM, on alternate days Lizards: 5 mg/kg/day, IM, SC	
Cefuroxime	100 mg/kg/day, IM, for 10 days at 30°C	
Chloramphenicol	Indigo snake: 50 mg/kg, IM, bid Midland water snakes: 50 mg/kg, IM, every 4 days Most species: 20–40 mg/kg, IM, once to twice daily	
Ciprofloxacin	10 mg/kg, PO, on alternate days	
Clarithromycin	Desert tortoise: 15 mg/kg, PO, every 2–3 days	*Mycoplasma*
Clindamycin	5 mg/kg, PO, bid	
Clotrimazole	Topical	Fungal dermatitis

TABLE 27 ANTIMICROBIAL DRUGS USED IN REPTILES *(continued)*

Drug	Dosage	Comments
Doxycycline	Most species: 5–10 mg/kg/day, PO Hermann's tortoise: 50 mg/kg, IM, then 25 mg/kg, every 3 days	
Enrofloxacin	Most species: 5-10 mg/kg/day, IM, PO	IM injection likely causes necrosis, and consideration should be given to single injection followed by oral administration
	Nasal flush 50 mg/250 mL sterile water; 1–3 mL/nares daily to every other day	
	Burmese python (juvenile): 10 mg/kg, IM, initial dosage, then 5 mg/kg, IM, every 48 hr. *Pseudomonas*: 10 mg/kg, IM, every 48 hr	IM injection likely causes necrosis, and consideration should be given to single injection followed by oral administration
	Hermann's tortoise: 10 mg/kg/day, IM	IM injection likely causes necrosis, and consideration should be given to single injection followed by oral administration
	Monitor lizards: 10 mg/kg, IM, every 5 days	
	Indian star tortoise: 5 mg/kg, IM, once to twice daily	IM injection likely causes necrosis, and consideration should be given to single injection followed by oral administration
	Crocodilians: 5 mg/kg IV every 2–3 days	
Fluconazole	Lizards: 5 mg/kg/day, PO	
	Sea turtles: 21 mg/kg, SC, once; then 10 mg/kg, SC, 5 days later	
Gentamicin	American alligator: 1.75 mg/kg, IM, every 3–4 days at 22°C	Maintain hydration, nephrotoxicity reported
	Painted turtle: 10 mg/kg, IM, on alternate days at 26°C	Maintain hydration, nephrotoxicity reported
	Red-eared terrapin: 6 mg/kg, IM, every 25 days	Maintain hydration, nephrotoxicity reported
	Gopher snake: 2.5 mg/kg, IM, every 3 days at 24°C	Maintain hydration, nephrotoxicity reported
Itraconazole	Chameleon: 5 mg/kg/day, PO	Fungal dermatitis
	Spiny lizard: 23.5 mg/kg/day, PO, for 3 days, with persistent drug concentration for 6 days	
	Snakes: 10 mg/kg/day, PO	
	Sea turtles: 5 mg/kg/day, PO, or 15 mg/kg, PO, every 72 hr	
Kanamycin	10 mg/kg/day, IM, at 24°C	Fluid therapy recommended

TABLE 27 ANTIMICROBIAL DRUGS USED IN REPTILES *(continued)*

Drug	Dosage	Comments
Ketoconazole	Crocodilians: 50 mg/kg/day, PO Most species: 15–30 mg/kg/day, PO, for 14–28 days	
Lincomycin	10 mg/kg/day, PO; 5 mg/kg, IM, once to twice daily	
Marbofloxacin	Ball python: 10 mg/kg, PO, every 48 hr	
Metronidazole	Bacterial infections, 20–50 mg/kg, PO, every 1–2 days	Maximal dose for tricolor snake, king snake, indigo snake, or Uracoan rattlesnake, is 40 mg/kg
Neomycin	10 mg/kg/day, PO	Oral only, not to be given systemically
Nystatin	Enteric fungal conditions in turtles: 100,000 U/kg/day, PO, for 10 days	
Oxytetracycline	Most species: 5–10 mg/kg/day, IM, PO	Pain, irritation, and inflammation at injection site
	American alligator: 10 mg/kg, IV, IM, every 4–5 days	Mycoplasmosis
Piperacillin	50–100 mg/kg, IM, every 12 days	Fluid therapy recommended
Polymixin B	Topical	Abrasions, wounds
Silver sulfadiazine	Topical every 24–72 hr	Broad spectrum for skin infections
Sulfamethoxydiazine	80 mg/kg, SC, IM, then 40 mg/kg/day, for 5–7 days	Coccidial infections
Tobramycin	Chelonians: 10 mg/kg, IM, every 1–2 days Most species: 2.5 mg/kg, IM, every 1–3 days	Potentially nephrotoxic, fluid therapy recommended
Tylosin	5 mg/kg/day, IM	Mycoplasmosis
Voriconazole	10 mg/kg, PO	

TABLE 28 PARASITICIDES USED IN REPTILES

Drug	Dosage	Parasite	Comments
	ENDOPARASITICIDES		
Fenbendazole	25–100 mg/kg, PO every 14 days for up to 4 treatments 50 mg/kg/day, PO, for 3–5 days	Roundworms, *Hexamita*	Can cause leukopenia
Ivermectin	200 mcg/kg, PO, IM, SC, repeat after 14 days		Not in chelonians; care in skinks and indigo snakes

TABLE 28 PARASITICIDES USED IN REPTILES *(continued)*

Drug	Dosage	Parasite	Comments
Levamisole	5–10 mg/kg, SC, intracoelomic, repeat after 14 days	Lungworms and other nematodes	Snakes, lizards, care in tortoises (use 5 mg/kg)
Mebendazole	20–25 mg/kg, PO, repeat after 14 days	Strongyles and ascarids	
Metronidazole	20–40 mg/kg, PO, every 1–2 days for 2–5 treatments	Protozoa	
Oxfendazole	68 mg/kg, PO, as a single dose	Nematodes	
Paromomycin	35–100 mg/kg/day, PO, for 28 days	Amoebas, cryptosporidia	Does not eliminate cryptosporidia
Ponazuril	Bearded dragons: 30 mg/kg, PO, every 2 days for two treatments	Coccidiosis	
Praziquantel	8 mg/kg, PO, SC, IM, repeat after 14 days and 28 days	Tapeworms, flukes	
Pyrantel	5 mg/kg, PO, repeat in 14 days	Nematodes	
Spiramycin	160 mg/kg/day for 10 days, then twice weekly for 3 mo	Snakes with cryptosporidiosis	May reduce clinical signs but does not clear infection
Toltrazuril	5–15 mg/kg, PO, repeat in 14 days 15 mg/kg, every 48 hr for 10 days; discontinue for 2 wk; repeat every 48 hr for 10 days, and repeat as necessary	Bearded dragons, coccidiosis Tortoises, intranuclear coccidiosis	Safety, efficacy, and pharmacokinetic data lacking
Trimethoprim-sulfa	30 mg/kg/day, PO, for 10–28 days	Coccidia	
ECTOPARASITICIDES			
Dichlorvos-impregnated strip	1 cm² of strip/30 cm³ vivarium for 28 days or 2.5 cm² of strip/25 cm³ vivarium for 2–3 days every week		Toxic, vivarium should be emptied; keep out of direct contact of animals
Fipronil	By spraying, every 7–10 days	Mites and ticks	
Ivermectin (10 mg/mL)	By spraying, 1–2 mL/L water every 7–10 days 200 mcg/kg, IM, every 7–14 days	Mites and ticks	Should not be used in chelonians; use care in skinks and indigo snakes
Permethrin (10%)	Topical spray	Mites and ticks	Licensed product available for reptiles in the USA

Other Medications: Dosages for medications used for a variety of other disorders of reptiles are listed in TABLE 29.

Fluid Therapy: Dehydration in reptiles is usually associated with prolonged anorexia and water loss, deprivation, or an inability to drink, rather than mixed electrolyte losses through frequent vomiting or diarrhea. Water balance in reptiles differs from that in mammals, because, per unit body weight, reptiles have a higher percentage of total body water (63.0%–74.4%) and a higher percentage of intracellular water (45.8%–58.0%). These values appear to be highest in freshwater species,

TABLE 29 MISCELLANEOUS DRUGS FOR REPTILES

Drug	Dosage	Condition
Allopurinol	20–25 mg/kg/day, PO	Gout, reduces uric acid production
Aluminium hydroxide	100 mg/kg, PO, every 12–24 hr	Reduces blood phosphorus levels
Aminophylline	2–4 mg/kg, IM	Respiratory disease when bronchodilation required
Argipressin (vasopressin)	0.01–1 mcg/kg	Egg binding (more potent than oxytocin)
Ascorbic acid	10–200 mg/kg, IM, as required	Ulcerative stomatitis
Calcitonin	1.5 units/kg, SC, tid 50 units/kg, IM, repeat after 2 wk	Hypercalcemia, fluid therapy also recommended Secondary hyperparathyroidism
Calcium gluconate (10 mg/mL)	100 mg/kg, IM, qid, or 400 mg/kg, IV, intraosseous, given over 24 hr	Hypocalcemia in iguanas; high phosphorus concentration may cause soft-tissue mineralization
Cimetidine	4 mg/kg, PO, tid-qid	Regurgitation, vomiting, gastritis, GI ulceration
Cisapride	0.5–2 mg/kg/day, PO	GI motility modification; not recommended to use with clarithromycin in tortoises
Cholecalciferol	100–1,000 units/kg, IM, as a single dose	Hypocalcemia, fibrous osteodystrophy in iguanas
Cyanocobalamin	50 mcg/kg, SC, IM	Appetite stimulation
Dexamethasone	30–150 mcg/kg, IM, IV, intraosseous	Inflammation, shock, beware of immunosuppression
Dinoprost (prostaglandin)	500 mcg/kg, IM, as a single dose	Egg binding in snakes
Doxapram	5–10 mg/kg, IV, intraosseous	Respiratory stimulation
Flunixin	100–500 mcg/kg, IM, IV, once to twice daily	Inflammation, pain
Furosemide	2–5 mg/kg, IM, IV, once to twice daily	Diuresis (effective despite lack of loop of Henle in reptiles)
Iodine	2–4 mg/kg, PO, every 7 days	Prophylaxis for goitrogenic diets
Iron	12 mg/kg, IM, every 7 days (alligators)	Anemia in alligators
Levothyroxine	20 mcg/kg, PO, on alternate days	Hypothyroidism in tortoises

TABLE 29 MISCELLANEOUS DRUGS FOR REPTILES *(continued)*

Drug	Dosage	Condition
Metoclopramide	60 mcg/kg/day, PO, for 7 days	Stimulation of gastric emptying in tortoises
Prednisolone	1–2 mg/kg, PO	Anti-inflammatory, reduction of nephrocalcinosis, beware of immunosuppression
Selenium	25–500 mcg/kg, IM	Deficiency in lizards
Sucralfate	0.5–1 g/kg, PO, tid-qid	Gastric irritation/ulceration
Thiamine	50–100 mg/kg, IM	Thiamine deficiency
Vitamin A	5,000 units/kg, PO, every 7 days	Hypovitaminosis A (iatrogenic hypervitaminosis A may result from repeated treatment)

lower in terrestrial reptiles, and lowest in marine reptiles, with the concentration of isotonic saline in nonmarine reptiles being 0.8%. This has led to the conclusion that normal 0.9% saline may be too concentrated for most reptiles. Balanced crystalloid fluids containing dextrose (260–290 mOsm/L) appear to be effective. As a general guide, maintenance requirements are about 5–15 mL/kg/day, and rehydration should proceed at 35–40 mL/kg/day, although in cases of shock, rates of 3–5 mL/kg/hr can be used for several hours.

In many instances, simply permitting a reptile to bathe in shallow, warm water within a vivarium maintained at the species-specific preferred optimal temperature zone will promote drinking. Such a method is acceptable when reptiles are able and willing to drink voluntarily. However, in many cases oral fluids must be delivered via a stomach tube. For oral rehydration, mammalian electrolyte solutions can be used but are best diluted by a further 10%–15% to produce a slightly hypotonic solution. Significant amounts of water may also be absorbed via the cloaca when chelonians (and possibly other species) bathe. Oral fluid therapy works well to provide maintenance requirements, rehydrate mildly dehydrated reptiles, and as a vehicle to give oral medications and food. For alert and active reptiles, this method is preferred because it facilitates GI activity, and fluids are rapidly absorbed when the reptile is maintained at correct temperatures. Repeated stomach tubing is stressful and can be difficult in strong chelonians; therefore, esophagostomy tubes are recommended for longterm oral therapy. Small fluid volumes can be given SC, but in moderate to severe cases, intracoelomic, IV, or intraosseous routes are favored.

Intracoelomic administration of fluids is faster, less stressful, and allows delivery of a larger volume than stomach tubing. Large volumes of intracoelomic fluid could compromise lung function and may be slowly absorbed; however, IV catheterization is not easy, and cut-down procedures are often required. In emergencies with larger snakes, it is possible to place an intracardiac catheter. Fluid infusion is best controlled by a syringe driver or infusion pump. If such devices are not available, the total daily fluid volume can be divided into three or four bolus injections, each given slowly over 10–20 min. IV catheters can usually be left in place for up to 72 hr; intracardiac catheters up to 24 hr. Intraosseous infusion is an easier technique in lizards, small crocodilians, and chelonians. The needle is directed into the medullary cavity of a long bone, and aspiration of marrow or radiography can verify correct positioning. Great care must be exercised when dealing with osteodystrophic lizards to avoid limb fractures. Infusion rates for IV and intraosseous administration are similar. As a general guide, 0.8–1.2 mL/kg/hr is suitable for rehydration purposes, but in cases of severe dehydration or shock or during surgery, 3–5 mL/kg/hr can be given for 2–3 hr.

Colloids are less frequently used in reptiles because much of the water loss is from the intracellular space rather than plasma, but they can be used in cases of acute hemorrhage. If severe hemorrhage occurs (ie, PCV <5%), whole blood may be given by IV and intraosseous routes. Cross-matching does not appear necessary, at least for a single transfusion. Ideally the donor and recipient are of the same species.

BACTERIAL DISEASES

Bacterial diseases are common in reptiles, with most infections caused by opportunistic agents that infect immunosuppressed hosts. A comprehensive approach is required to ensure the success of a therapeutic plan. It is important not only to determine the causative agent but also to correct predisposing factors. Appropriate therapy in the absence of appropriate husbandry and nutrition will ultimately fail.

Culture and sensitivity are recommended to determine appropriate therapy. Most bacterial infections involve gram-negative bacteria, many of which are considered commensal. Anaerobic infections are not uncommon, but organisms can be difficult to culture. Gram-positive bacteria on smears, in conjunction with a negative culture, may indicate an anaerobic infection. Alternatively, if a therapeutic choice was based on aerobic culture and sensitivity and response is poor, then the presence of an anaerobe should be considered.

Septicemia: A number of infectious conditions are similar in appearance, regardless of species. Septicemia is a common cause of death. The systemic disease may be preceded by trauma, local abscessation, parasitism, or environmental stress. *Aeromonas* and *Pseudomonas* spp are frequently isolated; the former may be transmitted by ectoparasites. Death may be peracute or follow a protracted course. Common terminal signs are respiratory distress, lethargy, convulsions, and incoordination. Petechiae may be found on the ventrum, and chelonians develop erythema of the plastron. Sanitation and husbandry can be significant factors in reducing outbreaks. Affected reptiles should be isolated, and antibiotic therapy initiated.

Septicemic Cutaneous Ulcerative Disease (SCUD): Classically, SCUD is a shell disease of aquatic turtles caused by *Citrobacter freundii*; however, various bacteria have been isolated from diseased skin and shell. *Serratia* spp may act synergistically by facilitating entry of *C freundii*. The scutes are pitted and may slough with an underlying purulent discharge. Anorexia, lethargy, and petechial hemorrhages on the shell and skin are seen; liver necrosis is also common. Systemic antibiotics are recommended. Good sanitation is paramount for prevention.

Another shell disease of turtles is caused by *Beneckea chitinovora*, a common infectious agent of crustaceans. Erythema and pitting of the shell with ulceration is seen. Septicemia is uncommon. Topical iodine is recommended in addition to antibiotics. The practice of feeding crayfish is often implicated in this condition and should be discouraged.

Ulcerative or Necrotic Dermatitis: Ulcerative dermatitis (scale rot) is seen in snakes and lizards kept in unhygienic conditions with excessive humidity and moisture. Moist, contaminated bedding allows bacterial and fungal growth that, when coupled with exposure to fecal degradation products, can predispose to small cutaneous erosions. Secondary infection with *Aeromonas* spp, *Pseudomonas* spp, and a number of other bacteria may result in septicemia and death if untreated. Erythema, necrosis, and ulceration of the dermis, and an exudative discharge are common. Although lesions are often sequelae of skin injuries, they more often develop from within, as is the case with classic necrotic dermatitis in the ball python. The disease can develop even when these animals are maintained under pristine conditions, so it is not simply a matter of excessive moisture and poor hygiene. The condition starts with hemorrhage into scales, followed by pustules that eventually lead to open and ulcerated lesions. Treatment with systemic antibiotics, topical antibiotic ointment, and excellent hygiene and husbandry are essential.

Blister disease has traditionally been considered a separate entity but is simply an early stage of ulcerative (necrotic) dermatitis. The cutaneous involvement is characterized by pustules or blisters that may resolve without development of ulcerative lesions if treatment is started early. A low-grade thermal injury may mimic blister disease because of the potential development of fluid-filled vesicles.

Abscesses: Focal infections caused by traumatic injuries, bite wounds, or poor husbandry are seen in all orders of reptiles. Subcutaneous abscesses are seen as nodules or swellings. Differential diagnoses include parasitic nodules, tumors, and hematomas. Isolates of the anaerobic organism *Peptostreptococcus* and of the aerobes *Pseudomonas*, *Aeromonas*, *Serratia*, *Salmonella*, *Micrococcus*,

Erysipelothrix, Citrobacter freundii, Morganella morganii, Proteus, Staphylococcus, Streptococcus, Escherichia coli, Klebsiella, and *Dermatophilus* have been recovered from reptilian abscesses, often in combinations. Small, localized abscesses should be completely excised to avoid recurrence, which is frequent. Larger abscesses should be marsupialized, followed by aggressive local wound treatment. The lining of the abscess must be aggressively scraped to remove as much material as possible. Appropriate systemic antibiotics may also be indicated but are seldom necessary after complete excision. Anaerobic bacteria are common in these lesions, and an appropriate antimicrobial agent (eg, metronidazole, ceftazidime, or a potentiated penicillin product) may need to be used or added to a current regimen.

Visceral abscessation may occur as a result of hematogenous infection. Abscesses of the female reproductive system are common and may result in coelomitis. Surgical intervention is indicated; systemic antibiotics alone are rarely, if ever, successful.

Subspectacle abscessation is seen in snakes, and conjunctivitis is seen in the other orders. Severity ranges from mild inflammation to panophthalmitis and may occur as a result of ascending infectious stomatitis (*see* below). Topical antibiotic ointments are used in turtles, lizards without spectacles, and crocodilians. In snakes and lizards with spectacles, drainage is achieved by surgically removing a small wedge from the spectacle and flushing the subspectacular space and lacrimal duct with an antibiotic solution (eg, gentamicin). Some affected reptiles, especially turtles, may need supplemental vitamin A.

Infectious Stomatitis: Infectious stomatitis is reported in snakes, lizards, and turtles and characterized early by petechiae in the oral cavity; caseous material develops along the dental arcade as the condition worsens. In severe cases, infection extends into the mandible and maxilla. *Aeromonas* and *Pseudomonas* spp, common oral inhabitants, are most frequently isolated, along with a variety of other gram-negative and gram-positive bacteria. Respiratory or GI infection may develop in poorly managed cases. Surgical debridement, irrigation with antiseptics, systemic antibiotics, and supportive therapy are indicated. In severe cases with ulceration or granuloma formation, aggressive surgery may be indicated. Vitamin supplementation, especially with vitamins A and C, has been advocated but does not always affect the disease course.

Pneumonia: Respiratory infections are common; the incidence can be influenced by respiratory or systemic parasitism, unfavorable environmental temperatures, unsanitary conditions, concurrent disease, malnutrition, and hypovitaminosis A. Open-mouth breathing, nasal discharge, and dyspnea are frequent signs. *Aeromonas* and *Pseudomonas* spp are frequently isolated, but many respiratory infections are mixed. Septicemia may develop in severe or prolonged cases. Treatment consists of improving husbandry and initiating systemic antibiotics. Nebulization therapy with antibiotics diluted in saline, in combination with acetylcysteine, has been used together with parenteral antibiotics. Reptiles with respiratory infections should be maintained at the mid to upper end of their preferred optimal temperature zone. Increased temperatures are important not only to stimulate the immune system but also to help mobilize respiratory secretions. Turtles often have an underlying vitamin A deficiency and require dietary correction. Many turtles treated for pneumonia do not improve completely until after treatment for vitamin A deficiency.

Mycoplasmosis: Mycoplasmosis is a known cause of rhinitis and upper respiratory tract disease in chelonians and polyserositis in crocodilians. In chelonians, the disease has been associated with population declines, and the disease is often chronic and/or intermittent. In American alligators, mycoplasmosis results in severe systemic disease and frequently death. A

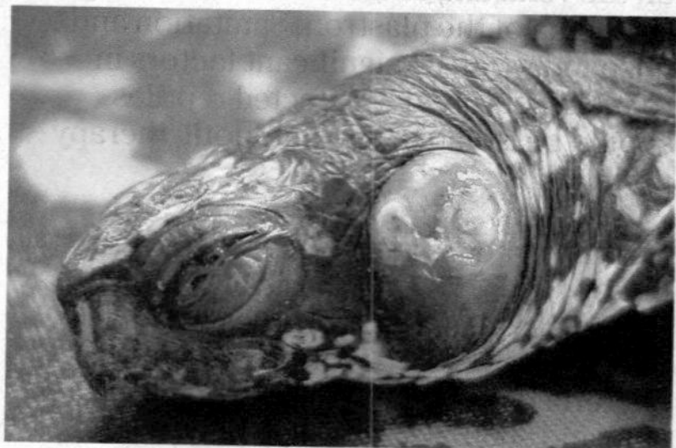

Aural abscesses represent middle ear infections in turtles and chelonians. In box turtles, these abscesses are commonly associated with vitamin A deficiencies. *Courtesy of Dr. Stephen Divers.*

variety of *Mycoplasma* species have been isolated. PCR and serologic diagnostic aids have been developed, and treatment using fluoroquinolones, clarithromycin, and oxytetracyline has been advocated.

Otitis: Ear infections occur frequently in turtles, especially box turtles and aquatic turtles. Marked swelling is seen at the tympanic membrane, and caseous material is present. *Proteus* spp, *Pseudomonas* spp, *Citrobacter* spp, *Morganella morganii*, *Enterobacter* spp, and other bacteria have been isolated. The tympanic membrane must be incised, and aggressive curettage of the area performed. Surgical removal of the abscess is usually curative as long as all infection is removed and the Eustachian tube is patent. The open area should be flushed with diluted povidone-iodine or a similar product for a few days to prevent premature closure and to keep the area clean. Systemic antibiotics are rarely required. Ear infections may be secondary to hypovitaminosis A; dietary supplementation of vitamin A may be beneficial.

Cloacitis: Often traumatic in origin, infectious cloacitis is characterized by edema and hemopurulent discharge. Cloacal calculi may form in vitamin or mineral imbalances and should be manually removed and followed by dietary correction. In pericloacal abscesses, the infection often migrates craniad. Ascending urinary or genital tract infections are common sequelae. Aggressive therapy, including surgical debridement, local wound treatment, and appropriate systemic antibiotics, is indicated. Fecal examinations should be performed to identify potential parasitic causes.

Spinal Osteopathy/Osteomyelitis: Although previously reported in the reptile literature as Paget disease, this condition is now thought to be a chronic bacterial osteomyelitis of the spine. Traditionally, Paget disease is characterized by repeated episodes of osteoclastic bone resorption and deposition, leading to dense, brittle bones. Commonly reported in snakes, these proliferative and progressive spinal lesions have been investigated and are thought to be associated with chronic bacterial infections, most commonly involving *Salmonella* spp in snakes. Diagnosis is by biopsy or blood culture. Longterm antibiotic therapy may be helpful, but the prognosis is guarded to poor.

Mycobacteriosis: Mycobacterial infections are often associated with chronic wasting in wild, imported reptiles and are seen as granulomatous lesions at necropsy. Chelonians generally exhibit pulmonary involvement, whereas lizards, snakes, and crocodilians commonly show visceral granulomas. The species isolated are *Mycobacterium ulcerans*, *M chelonae*, *M haemophilum*, and *M marinum*. All are cultured at reduced temperatures and may require long periods for growth. Rifampin and isoniazid are hepatotoxic, and the longterm administration required is unlikely to be safe. There are no reports of successful treatment.

***Salmonella* Arizonae and *Edwardsiella* Infection:** These bacteria have been isolated from clinically healthy reptiles. The zoonotic nature of these commensal organisms must be considered when handling or treating reptiles. Attempts to eliminate these microorganisms from reptiles and their eggs have been unsuccessful and are not recommended. Veterinarians and reptile owners should be aware of the informational brochures available from the Association of Reptile and Amphibian Veterinarians.

MYCOTIC DISEASES

Excessively high humidity, low environmental temperature, concurrent disease, malnutrition, and other stressors may predispose reptiles to development of various mycoses. Little is known about the pathogenesis of systemic mycoses, which can develop over a long period, but maintaining good sanitation and husbandry reduces the frequency of infection. *Aspergillus*, *Candida*, *Cladosporium*, *Metarhizium*, *Mucor*, *Paecilomyces*, *Penicillium* spp, and the *Chrysosporium* anamorph of *Nannizziopsis vriesii* are a few of the organisms associated with systemic disease. Reports of successful treatment of systemic mycoses in reptiles are few. Suggested treatments for deep fungal respiratory infections include amphotericin B, itraconazole, fluconazole, and voriconazole. For superficial or localized mycotic infections, surgical removal of the granuloma with local wound treatment is advised. *Basidiobolus* spp, pathogenic for mammals, are found in feces of healthy reptiles.

Dermatophytosis has been described in all orders of reptiles. *Geotrichum*, *Fusarium*, and *Trichosporon* are the genera most frequently isolated. In most cases, cutaneous injury precedes a secondary fungal infection. Chelonians with fungal infections of the shell can be treated by local debridement and topical application of Lugol solution or povidone-iodine. Exposure to ultraviolet light also may be beneficial.

Ulceration of GI tissues has been associated with infections by *Mucor* and *Fusarium* spp. Chronic visceral granulomatous disease of liver, kidneys, and spleen has been caused by *Metarhizium* and *Paecilomyces* spp. Few signs other than weight loss are seen before death. Animals may continue to feed until a few days before death.

The most frequent sites of mycotic infection are the skin and respiratory tract. *Metarhizium*, *Mucor*, and *Paecilomyces* spp are frequent isolates. *Aspergillus* and *Candida* spp have been isolated from pulmonary lesions of lizards and chelonians. Most infections involve granuloma or plaque formation with resultant signs of respiratory distress before death. Candidiasis in large snakes has been treated with nystatin (100,000 U, PO, for 10 days).

VIRAL DISEASES

Few viruses have been clearly proved as etiologic agents of disease in reptiles, but several have been linked strongly enough for them to be considered the causative agent until proved otherwise. A number of viral PCR and serology tests are available.

Inclusion Body Disease (IBD) of Boid Snakes: Boa constrictors and several species of pythons are most commonly affected by IBD, which was originally thought to be caused by a retrovirus but recently an arenavirus has been implicated. Boas are considered a more typical host because so many are infected, and they can harbor the virus for years with few to no clinical signs. Early signs, possibly precipitated by any factor causing immunosuppression, include a history of unthriftiness, anorexia, weight loss, secondary bacterial infections, poor wound healing, dermal necrosis, and regurgitation. In essence, IBD should be considered in every sick boa. Typical findings in the acute phase of the disease include leukocytosis and a normal chemistry panel. As the disease progresses, WBC counts tend to decline to subnormal levels. Blood chemistry results vary depending on how debilitated and dehydrated the boa becomes, but organ damage may occur. As the disease becomes chronic, some boas exhibit neurologic symptoms ranging from mild facial tics and abnormal tongue flicking to failure of the snake to right itself when placed in dorsal recumbency and severe seizures.

Pythons are thought to be a more abnormal host for the IBD virus, because the course of disease is more acute and neurologic symptoms more profound. Most pythons present with severe neurologic disease. Although the active disease can linger for months or more in boas, most pythons die within days or weeks of the onset of clinical signs.

Exposure to this retrovirus/arenavirus appears to be due to a transfer of body fluids. Breeding, fight wounds, fecal/oral contamination, and snake mites have been implicated as common ways of transfer. A tentative diagnosis is based on history and clinical signs. Blood work varies depending on the stage of the disease, but few diseases in snakes will cause such increased WBC counts in the early stages. On blood smears, inclusion bodies are frequently found in the cytoplasm of leukocytes. A definitive diagnosis is obtained via biopsy of internal tissues in which the characteristic eosinophilic inclusion bodies are found, eg, the liver, kidney, esophageal tonsils, and stomach.

IBD is not curable, and many owners choose euthanasia. However, individuals may elect to isolate their snakes and treat with supportive and palliative measures. It is essential to educate owners not to sell infected specimens or their offspring, because this has caused the disease to spread worldwide.

Retroviruses: Retroviruses have also been found in Russell vipers, corn snakes, and California kingsnakes in association with malignant tumors. A retrovirus isolated from a sarcoma in a Russell viper was designated as viper virus. A related virus was isolated in a corn snake from a rhabdomyosarcoma and designated cornsnake retrovirus.

Adenoviruses: Adenoviruses have been implicated in fatal hepatic or GI diseases in snakes (gaboon vipers, ball pythons, boa constrictors, rosy boas, and rat snakes), lizards (Jackson chameleons, savannah monitors, and bearded dragons), and crocodilians.

In bearded dragons, the route of transmission appears to be fecal/oral contamination. Clinical signs are more commonly noted in juvenile dragons but can affect adults, usually to a lesser extent. Signs are vague and include lethargy, weakness, weight loss, diarrhea, and sudden death. The morbidity is high in young bearded dragons, but survival is increased with supportive care. Fluid administration, force feeding, and antibiotics for secondary infections are useful.

Because the signs of disease in bearded dragons are vague and similar to those caused by coccidia and nutritional disorders, it is important to confirm the diagnosis. Characteristic intranuclear inclusion bodies are found in several internal organs, primarily the liver. When working with a large breeding group of lizards, it is practical to sacrifice a failing specimen to make a diagnosis. Premortem diagnosis can be accomplished by liver biopsy. Identification of adenovirus from fresh feces may be possible in the future.

Recovered lizards should be quarantined for at least 3 mo. Duration of viral shedding after recovery is unknown, so owners should be discouraged from selling or trading previously infected animals.

Herpesviruses: Herpesviruses have been isolated from freshwater turtles, tortoises, and green sea turtles. In freshwater turtles, the virus may be associated with hepatic necrosis. In tortoises, the virus may cause necrosis of oral mucosa accompanied by anorexia, regurgitation, and oral and ocular discharge. Treatment in tortoises includes isolation, supportive care, and application of 5% acyclovir to oral lesions. Oral acyclovir appeared to improve the lesions in a desert tortoise. Herpesvirus is diagnosed by the presence of intranuclear inclusion bodies and electron microscopic demonstration of viral particles.

Herpesvirus infection of farmed green sea turtles have been associated with gray patch disease and lung-eye-trachea disease, whereas fibropapillomas plague certain free-ranging populations. Gray patch disease (chelonian herpesvirus 1) causes epizootics of small, circular papular skin lesions that coalesce into patches and is associated with young turtles maintained in crowded, warmer, stressful situations. Biopsies of the skin reveal basophilic intranuclear inclusion bodies in epidermal cells; viral particles are noted in the cytoplasm by electron microscopy. There is no specific treatment, but reduction of crowding and stress appears to decrease the incidence. Lung-eye-trachea disease causes harsh respiratory sounds, with ulcerations and caseous debris over the globe and throughout the oropharynx and trachea. Buoyancy problems and high mortality are reported.

Fibropapillomatosis has been reported from free-ranging sea turtles, especially around Hawaii. The route of transmission is not known. The light gray to black masses range in size up to 20 cm in diameter. The location of the masses seems to dictate the severity of signs. Masses occurring on periocular tissue can obscure vision. Growths on the flippers can interfere with swimming and the ability to forage for food. Internal masses also are seen, primarily in the lungs, liver, kidneys, and GI tract. Diagnosis is made by characteristic lesions and histology. Treatment consists of surgical removal, with wide margins to help reduce recurrence. Some turtles recover spontaneously, whereas those with internal lesions usually perish. It is suspected that fibropapillomas are caused by a herpesvirus, and infected specimens should be isolated from healthy turtles.

Paramyxovirus: Paramyxovirus infections are more common in viperid snakes but have been reported in nonvenomous snakes as well. This highly contagious virus causes predominantly respiratory signs; transmission appears to be from respiratory secretions. Secondary bacterial infections are common because of the severe inflammation initiated by the virus, and it is not unusual to note nasal discharge, open-mouth breathing, caseated pus in the oral cavity, and labored breathing. Neurologic involvement, including tremors and opisthotonos, is occasionally noted.

Paramyxovirus should be suspected in any respiratory infection that does not respond to treatment with supportive care, antibiotics, and nebulization. Endoscopic biopsies and postmortem samples of lung can be submitted to detect viral particles by histology and electron microscopy. A hemagglutination inhibition test is available to measure antibodies against ophidian paramyxovirus in zoos and private collections; a positive titer should be used as a screening tool to help eliminate infected animals and prevent carriers from entering noninfected collections.

There is no specific treatment, but supportive care and antibiotics may prove useful. Affected specimens should be isolated and strict hygiene practices followed. Although a vaccine is under development, it is currently not effective.

West Nile Virus: West Nile virus has resulted in epizootic outbreaks in farmed alligators, with the virus causing multiorgan necrosis, heterophilic granulomas, heterophilic perivasculitis, and lymphoplasmacytic mengingoencephalitis. Very high viremia titers have been reported in various reptiles, suggesting that reptiles may play a role as an amplification host.

Papillomas: Viral particles appear to be transmitted from one European green lizard to another via bite wounds. The resulting papillomas are 2–20 mm in diameter and may be single or multiple. Although there are no signs in the initial phase, affected lizards may become lethargic and anorectic and die. Diagnosis involves detection of viral particles by electron microscopy. Treatment consists of surgical removal of single masses, although regrowth is common. Isolation of affected lizards is perhaps the only way to prevent spread.

A papilloma-type virus also appears to affect Bolivian side-neck turtles and appears as white, oval skin lesions distributed over the head. Ulcerative shell lesions are also seen, primarily on the plastron. Diagnosis is made by identifying viral particles on electron microscopy. Treatment is supportive and palliative, and affected animals should be isolated.

Iridoviruses: Iridoviruses have been reported in various chelonians, snakes, and lizards. An iridovirus was found in a Hermann's tortoise, which died without prior signs of disease. Progressive anemia in Australian geckos has been linked to an iridovirus. Clinical signs range from none to stomatitis, rhinitis, conjunctivitis, tracheitis, edema, and cutaneous abscessation. In some cases, the recovered iridoviruses have been closely related to amphibian ranaviruses. Although the clinical importance of several of these viruses remain unclear, iridoviruses deserve close attention, especially in chelonians.

Other Viruses: Many other viruses continue to be isolated from reptiles, but little information exists regarding disease, diagnosis, control, and treatment. Two nonpathogenic rhabdoviruses were isolated from *Ameiva* sp lizards. In addition to herpesviruses and adenoviruses, parvoviruses and picornaviruses have been found in the intestinal tract of snakes, but their exact role is unknown. A poxvirus-like virus has been isolated from circumscribed cutaneous lesions in a caiman and from dermal lesions in a tegu. A reovirus isolated from Chinese vipers was associated with death without prior signs of illness.

PARASITIC DISEASES

Ectoparasites: A limited number of ectoparasites are seen, except on wild and newly acquired reptiles. Mites are distributed worldwide, and most reptilian species are affected. Reduced vitality and, in heavy infestations, death due to anemia may occur. Skin of affected reptiles appears coarse, and dysecdysis is frequent. The common snake mite (*Ophionyssus natricis*) and lizard mite (*Hirstiella* spp) are generally <1.5 mm long and are often found around the eyes, gluttal folds, or any other indentation on the reptile. Mites may also be associated with mechanical transmission of *Aeromonas hydrophila*, a variety of other bacteria, rickettsial agents, and probably viruses. Mites are visible to the naked eye but are hard to see in small numbers. If mites are suspected, gently rubbing the reptile while it is standing over a piece of white paper will allow the mites to be seen after they have fallen off. Affected reptiles often spend an inordinate amount of time soaking to drown the mites. Examination of the water dish can reveal the drowned remains of many mites. The gluttal folds, involutions around the face, and the space between the eye and its orbit are favored areas and should be inspected carefully.

There are many methods of treatment; however, a permethrin is specifically licensed for use in reptiles, and ivermectin is also frequently effective in squamates.

Ticks are common on reptiles, and heavy infestations may result in anemia. Argasid ticks may cause paralysis, with muscle degeneration at the site of the bite. The transmission of green-lizard papilloma–associated virus, several hemogregarines, and the filarid worm *Macdonaldius oscheri* have been associated with ticks. Ticks can transmit *Ehrlichia ruminantium*, the cause of heartwater, and consequently the importation of African reptiles has been controlled. Ticks can be removed manually or by using permethrin spray. Systemic antibiotics are often indicated because of systemic infections associated with multiple cutaneous bite wounds and, potentially, with transmission of pathogenic bacteria.

Leeches have been found on the legs, head, neck, and in the oral cavity of a variety of turtles and crocodilians.

Chelonians frequently have cutaneous myiasis. Bot flies (including *Cuterebra* sp) create a cutaneous wound in which to lay their eggs, which hatch into bots that live in cyst-like structures until mature enough to leave the wound. These lesions are characterized as a lump under the skin; on closer inspection, they have an opening often lined by a black, crusted material. Treatment consists of slightly expanding the natural opening and manually removing the bot with a forceps. The wound is then flushed with povidone-iodine, chlorhexidine, etc, and an antibiotic ointment is instilled. Systemic antibiotics are indicated in reptiles that have multiple lesions. Cutaneous myiasis also occurs secondary to existing wounds, and maggots must be manually removed and the underlying lesion treated with topical and systemic antibiotics as needed. During heavy fly season, turtles often are housed indoors or with screens over their enclosures to offer some protection.

Ectoparasite infestations are best prevented by thorough screening and quarantine of all new animals entering a collection.

Helminths: The stress of captivity coupled with a closed environment predisposes to heavy burdens of parasites with direct life cycles. Every effort must be taken to rid reptiles of parasite burdens and the environment of intermediate hosts.

Pathogenic trematodes infect the vascular system of turtles and infect the oral cavity, respiratory system, renal tubules, and ureters of snakes. Chemotherapeutic agents have not effectively eliminated these parasites, although praziquantel has shown some promise.

Tapeworms are found in all orders of reptiles but are rare in crocodilians. Reptiles may act as the definitive, paratenic, or intermediate hosts for a large number of species. Although most species of tapeworms are generally nonpathogenic in wild reptiles, weight loss and death have been reported. The complex life cycle of cestodes and restricted geographic range of intermediate hosts limit the number of cases in captive reptiles. When present, proglottids may be found around the cloaca, or typical cestode ova may be isolated from feces. Treatment is with praziquantel, repeated in 2 wk. Plerocercoids of the genus *Spirometra* may be found as soft swellings in the subcutis. These larval stages may be removed surgically.

Nematodes are found in all orders of reptiles, and several genera are important. *Strongyloides* spp frequently inhabit the intestinal tract of reptiles; larvae are seen in the respiratory tract and respiratory exudate. In snakes, the larvae have been seen within granulomas distributed throughout the body wall, suggesting that the larvae may be able to penetrate the skin. Overwhelming parasitism is common when poor hygiene results in highly contaminated environments. *Rhabdias* and related species have been found in the lungs of a variety of snakes; embryonated ova may be found in the oral cavity and in lung aspirates. Embryonated ova and free larval forms may be seen in the feces. Larvae resembling *Rhabdias* also have been seen in the gingiva of snakes with stomatitis. Infections often are subclinical but may be associated with secondary bacterial pneumonia. In severe cases, death may result.

Stomach worms of the genus *Physaloptera* are seen in lizards. Gastric ulceration may occur in severe infections. Ova are elliptical and may be embryonated. Numerous snakes are infected by *Kalicephalus* spp. This hookworm, capable of transcutaneous infestation, prefers the upper GI tract and causes erosive lesions at sites of attachment. Ova are similar to those of *Physaloptera* spp. Large granulomas caused by the above species have also caused GI obstruction in snakes.

Ascarids frequently infect reptiles. Ova are similar to those of ascarids from mammalian hosts. Severe lesions and death may be seen in infected snakes. Clinically infected snakes frequently regurgitate partially digested food or adult nematodes and are anorectic. The major lesions are large granulomatous masses in the GI tract; they may abscess and perforate the intestinal wall.

Many other nematode species may be found in reptiles. Capillarid, trichurid, and oxyurid ova may be found on fecal examination. The nonpathogenic larval and oval forms of parasites of prey items (eg, *Syphacia obvelata*, the mouse pinworm) may be found when infected prey is consumed. Treatment should be attempted when evidence of parasitism is present.

Some larval forms of nematodes are suspected or confirmed to penetrate the skin (eg, *Strongyloides* and *Kalicephalus*), bypassing the oral reinfection route. The subtle nature of reinfection by this route often goes unnoticed until the reptile is overwhelmed by parasites. Close attention to the immediate removal of excreta and fastidious sanitation help reduce parasite burdens in captivity.

Dermal lesions caused by the spirurid worm *Dracunculus* spp may be seen. Numerous species of spirurids infect the mesentery, coelomic cavity, and blood vessels. These worms require a mechanical vector, so their incidence is reduced in captive-bred reptiles or in reptiles that have been in captivity longterm. Treatment consists of increasing the environmental temperature to 95°–98°F (35°–37°C) for 24–48 hr. However, some "cool-adapted" reptiles may not tolerate this treatment.

Pentastomes: Pentastomes are found in a wide variety of reptiles, with variable pathogenicity. Pentastomid infections are occasionally associated with pneumonic signs, but these primitive arthropods can inhabit any tissue, and symptoms will vary with their migration path and tissues responses. Pentastomes were initially found primarily in tropical poisonous snakes; however, as more necropsies on reptiles were performed, more were found. Necropsy results from 88 bearded dragons showed that 11 were infested with pentastomes. No truly effective treatment has been reported, but praziquantel at dosages of 8 mg/kg and ivermectin at 5–10 times normal dosages have been shown to reduce ova numbers being shed but have not eliminated the worms. The most novel approach has been to endoscopically locate and mechanically remove all the adult pentastomes. Recognition of pentastomal infestations is important, because these parasites are thought to present a zoonotic risk.

Protozoal Diseases: Numerous protozoans are found on reptiles; most are harmless commensals. The most serious protozoal pathogen of reptiles is *Entamoeba invadens*. Clinical signs are anorexia, weight loss, vomiting, mucoidal or hemorrhagic diarrhea, and death. Entamoebiasis may be epidemic in large snake collections. Herbivores appear less susceptible than carnivores; a number of reptiles that seldom become affected or

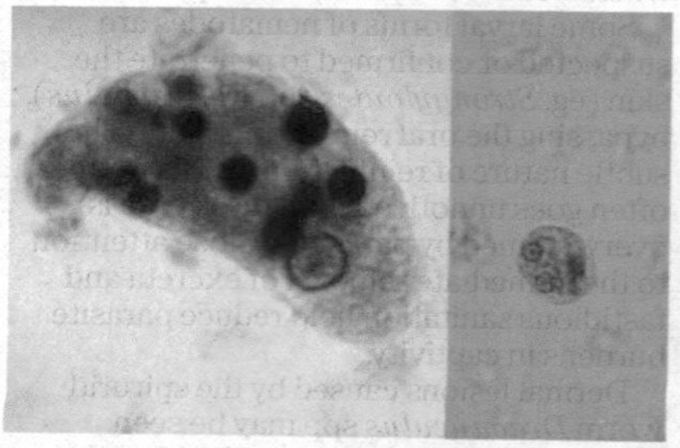

Entamoeba invadens trophozoite (left) and cyst (right) (1,000× oil immersion). *Courtesy of Dr. Stephen Divers.*

die can serve as carriers, including garter snakes, northern black racers, and box turtles. Although most turtles are resistant, the giant tortoises are susceptible. Other resistant groups include eastern king snakes, crocodiles, and cobras (possibly as an adaptation that allows them to eat snakes). Most boas, colubrids, elapids, vipers, and crotalids are highly susceptible. Transmission is by direct contact with the cyst form. Hepatic abscesses containing numerous *E invadens* trophozoites are common in chronic cases. At necropsy, gross lesions may extend from the stomach to the cloaca. The intestine shows areas of ulceration that tend to coalesce, caseous necrosis, edema, and hemorrhage. Multifocal abscesses in a swollen, friable liver are seen in the hepatic form. Identification of trophozoites or cysts in a wet preparation of fresh feces or tissue impressions, or in histologic sections, is diagnostic. Turtles and snakes should not be housed together.

E invadens is best treated with metronidazole. Tetracycline and paromomycin have been used but are considered ineffective against the hepatic form. Strict sanitation and hygiene measures should be observed.

Flagellates, especially *Hexamita* spp, have been reported to cause urinary tract disease in chelonians and intestinal disease in snakes. The "Giardia" seen in some cases of enteritis in snakes may actually be *Hexamita* or one of the relatively nonpathogenic flagellates that inhabit the intestinal tract of snakes. Differentiation between the species requires expertise, and special preservatives and stains are required to identify most of these organisms. Metronidazole has been used to treat flagellates. Indigo snakes, king snakes, and uracoan rattlers should be treated at the low end of this dosage range. Early studies with benzimidazoles are very encouraging and should also be considered as a viable therapy.

Several coccidial organisms have been reported: *Klossiella* from the kidney, *Isospora* from the gallbladder and intestine, and *Eimeria* from the gallbladder. The severity of disease varies with the coccidia and affected species. Because of their direct life cycle, these parasites can increase to tremendous numbers, especially in immunosuppressed reptiles. Oocysts are not fragile and can survive for weeks in a dessicated condition. Fastidious, daily cleanings are necessary to remove all feces and feces-contaminated food and water. Insects and other food items must be removed on a daily basis, because they are another source of contamination (eg, crickets may eat the oocysts while gathering fluid from the feces). Persistent treatment using sulfadimethoxine is required until infection is resolved, often taking 2–4 wk; success should be measured by serial fecal samples.

Trimethoprim-sulfa is another useful drug to treat coccidia. Care should be taken when using sulfa in reptiles with dehydration or renal compromise. If in doubt, a balanced electrolyte solution should be administered PO at appropriate dosages. Even under the best conditions, treatment will eliminate coccidia in only 50% of cases. Treatment resulting in a reduction of coccidia is still important, and coccidial numbers should be periodically monitored.

Plasmodial (malarial) organisms, as well as other intracellular blood protozoans, have been reported in reptiles. Their significance is unknown, and treatment is not considered necessary.

Cryptosporidiosis is frequently reported in association with postprandial regurgitation (snakes, *Cryptosporidium serpentes*), diarrhea (lizards, *Cryptosporidium saurophilum*), marked weight loss, and chronic debilitation. The organism affects the GI mucosa, resulting in marked thickening of the gastric rugae and loss of segmented motility. A mass in the gastric region is often, but not always, palpable in snakes, and contrast radiographs or endoscopic examination reveals rugal thickening. Many lizards, including Old World chameleons and savannah monitors, are affected primarily in the intestine. Mucosal thickening develops as a result of invasion by numerous cryptosporidial organisms. Diagnosis can be made using acid-fast stains on fresh feces or on the coating from regurgitated items or endoscopic gastric biopsies, which will identify the tiny oocysts. Although several treatments have been suggested, none (except for hyperimmune bovine colostrum) have been consistently effective. Intensive supportive care will often stabilize and help prolong the life of the affected reptile. Euthanasia is a valid option for infected reptiles. Cryptosporidiosis was previously considered a zoonotic disease; however, it now appears that the species commonly found in reptiles do not affect mammals.

ENVIRONMENTAL DISEASES AND TRAUMATIC INJURIES

Beak anomalies in chelonians inhibit feeding and are often associated with secondary nutritional hyperparathyroidism leading to hypocalcemia, distortion of the skull, and abnormal occlusion and wear. Increased levels of dietary protein may contribute to accelerated growth of these tissues, while a lack of abrasive food items limits natural wear in captivity. Treatment consists of trimming or grinding the beak into a more normal conformation. The condition usually recurs because of primary malocclusion, and longterm maintenance may be required.

Males of many species can be highly territorial and exhibit **aggression** toward other males or toward females during mating periods. Injuries to cagemates can be severe and are best avoided by separating animals at feeding and reducing the number of animals allowed in a breeding group. When separated individuals are placed together for breeding, they should be carefully monitored. If reptiles must be kept together, it is vital the enclosure is large enough to avoid competition for resources, especially basking areas, and retreats. Food and water is best placed in multiple locations to prevent dominant cohabitants from intimidating the others.

Fractures due to trauma are commonly seen in all species. They are often associated with secondary nutritional hyperparathyroidism in chelonians and lizards. Long bones may be repaired with lightweight external coaptation. A simple way of splinting the legs of lizards is to tape the injured leg to the body (front legs) or the tail (rear legs). These splints are tolerated well and protect the injured limb from further injury.

Injury to the spinal column must be assessed individually; when clear displacement is not evident, radiographic evaluation should be performed. Spinal injuries caudal to the vent may be tolerated, but injuries cranial to the vent frequently result in constipation and retention of urates, with variable limb movement. Environmental changes (eg, low branches, shallow water dish, nonabrasive substrates) and teaching the owner how to empty the cloacal content will allow the lizard to survive. Because these fractures are often secondary to secondary nutritional hyperparathyroidism, a thorough history of the reptile's husbandry may also reveal the need for nutritional changes.

Aggressive iguanids may frequently lash out with their tails and damage them against the vivarium glass or other furniture. Continual damage can lead to **ischemic necrosis** of the tail. Secondary infection may follow and progress to osteomyelitis. In some cases, septic emboli may lead to tail infection. In either scenario, tail amputation, in addition to investigation and correction of predisposing factors, is required. Radiography should precede surgery, because osteomyelitis may appear more cranial than the external lesion. Tail amputation in iguanids should be performed under anesthesia, taking advantage of the lizard's ability to perform autotomy. The tail is simply bent and twisted sharply to cause a fracture through a fracture plane. Muscle fibers are trimmed, but the tail is left unsutured to encourage regeneration. Clean postoperative conditions are essential, but antibiotics are not. Tail necrosis in reptiles that do not exhibit autotomy requires a more traditional surgical amputation with primary closure of the wound.

Burns are generally associated with unscreened incandescent lights or other heat sources. Fluid loss, dehydration, and septicemia are common sequelae. However, many can be treated by cleansing the site, applying antibiotic ointment, providing analgesics, and placing the reptile in a clean, dry environment. Silvadene cream is the preferred topical dressing, because it is water miscible and is effective against yeast and bacteria, including *Pseudomonas* spp. In uninfected burns, sterile skin protectants can be applied to the area to act as a "second skin." These products allow access to the water and help keep contaminants out. In severe burn cases, fluids are given to offset fluid losses, and systemic antibiotics are required to prevent secondary infection. Pain management and assisted feeding techniques may also be applied.

Traumatic injuries to turtles may result in fractures to the plastron, the carapace, or both. Repairs should be delayed in anything other than fresh wounds. Contaminated tissues should be gently debrided, flushed, and appropriately bandaged using a wet-to-dry technique. Holes in the bandages can be created to allow the legs to remain exposed. If obvious infection is present, samples should be submitted for microbiology before systemic antibiotics are started. Once stable, the wounds should be cleaned again, and the fractures realigned under general anesthesia and repaired using zip ties. These injuries also can be repaired using epoxy resin or a quick-setting, epoxy glue layered over fiberglass screen. Dental and orthopedic cements have also been used to stabilize fractured tissues. Healing is slow and may require 4–6 mo or longer.

Dysecdysis, or incomplete or inadequate skin shedding, may be caused by low humidity, ectoparasitism, nutritional deficiencies, infectious diseases, lack of suitable abrasive surfaces, or even decreased thyroid function. Often, eyecaps or annular bands on the tail or digits are retained. Eyecaps are best treated by application of an ophthalmic ointment bid for several days until they either fall off or can be grasped with a pair of fine forceps and carefully removed. Patience is advised—eyecaps should never be forced off because of the possibility of damaging the spectacle.

Recalcitrant, retained sheds are best treated by soaking the reptile in warm (77°–85°F [25°–29°C]) water for several hours and then pulling gently with a gauze sponge. A humidity chamber also works well and can be as simple as a 10-gal. aquarium with an undertank heater in which wet bath towels are placed. The top can be covered with a light cloth to increase humidity levels, but excessive heat must be avoided and can be relieved by allowing more ventilation if needed.

Prey-induced trauma, caused by live, uneaten invertebrate and vertebrate prey, can frequently cause severe trauma, with secondary infection and abscessation. Whenever possible, rodents that have been freshly killed or frozen and thawed should be offered to prevent injury to the reptile (dead prey should be discarded after 12 hr if uneaten). The feeding of live prey is illegal in many countries. Fresh bite wounds may be treated by cleansing with povidone-iodine (diluted 1:10). Parenteral antibiotics, based on results of culture and sensitivity tests, should be used. Untreated wounds frequently abscess and are seen as a soft or hard swelling. The abscess, including the fibrous capsule, should be removed surgically, and the defect sutured. Open or draining abscesses should be curetted, flushed with povidone-iodine, and parenteral antibiotics administered. Antibiotic ointments with proteolytic enzymes may be helpful. (*See also* ABSCESSES, p 1991.)

METABOLIC AND ENDOCRINE DISEASES

Gout: Gout is seen in all orders of reptiles; visceral and articular forms have been reported. Radiographs often reveal mineralized tophi in affected organs and joints. Primary visceral gout is the accumulation of urate microcrystals in organs secondary to a chronic hyperuricemia and is generally caused by excessive protein in the diet. Secondary visceral gout is due to chronic hyperuricemia from such causes as dehydration and renal insufficiency. Gout can be very debilitating, causing discomfort to the point that some reptiles refuse to move, eat, or drink.

Primary visceral gout is treated by correcting the diet. Secondary visceral gout is treated by attempting to correct the underlying problem, be it dehydration or renal disease. The prognosis is poor in advanced cases. Allopurinol is effective at reducing blood uric acid levels. Drug administration usually must be longterm, because signs typically recur if treatment is discontinued. Euthanasia must be considered in reptiles in which movement is painful and appetite becomes suppressed.

Metabolic Bone Diseases: **Secondary nutritional hyperparathyroidism** is the most common bone disease seen in reptile practice. It relates to poor diet (low calcium to phosphorus ratio, vitamin D_3 deficiency) or poor husbandry (lack of UVB light, inadequate thermal provision). Affected reptiles are generally rapidly growing herbivorous and insectivorous lizards and chelonians. Signs include anorexia; lethargy; an inability to walk normally; swollen/distorted mandible, maxilla, and/or long bones; limb and spinal pathologic fractures; cloacal prolapse; muscle fasciculations; and tetany. Diagnosis requires radiography to document generalized demineralization of the skeleton and low plasma levels of 25-dihydroxycholecalciferol. Findings in the late stages include hyperphosphatemia and low total and ionized calcium. Treatment of critical cases requires fluid therapy, nutritional support, and parenteral calcium therapy if hypocalcemic. Correction of the diet and husbandry are the mainstays of successful therapy.

Secondary renal hyperparathyroidism occurs in adult reptiles and is associated with hyperphosphatemia, soft-tissue calcification, osteodystrophy, and hypocalcemia. Provisional diagnosis generally rests on history, radiography, and plasma biochemistry, although a definitive diagnosis requires demonstration of reduced renal function (eg, iohexol clearance) and renal pathology (eg, renal biopsy).

Reports of **hypertrophic osteopathy** are uncommon and currently appear to be limited to lizards with extensive periosteal proliferation beginning in the distal long bones and progressing proximally. The pathogenesis is unknown, but theories include chronic anoxia, toxins, and vagal neurologic pathways.

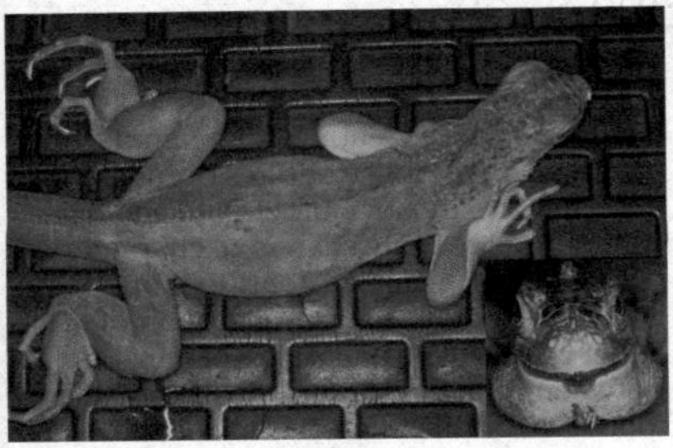

Secondary nutritional hyperparathyroidism in a green iguana. Note the swollen, fibrous long bones and maxilla (insert). *Courtesy of Dr. Stephen Divers.*

Miscellaneous Endocrine Disorders: Endocrine diseases are not often documented in reptiles. Diabetes mellitus has been reported in chelonians; glucosuria and hyperglycemia are the primary findings, and polyphagia may or may not be apparent. The etiology is often undetermined but has been associated with gastric neuroendocrine carcinomas in bearded dragons. Pancreatectomy in lizards may result in hypoglycemia, implying that other hormones, such as glucagon or somatotropin, may play a role in the pathogenesis of diabetes mellitus in reptiles.

Hypothyroidism and thyroid hyperplasia have been reported in Galapagos Islands tortoises. It has been speculated that high amounts of dietary iodine in the natural diet may play a significant role. Feeding goitrogenic foods to tortoises has been incriminated in development of this condition. The primary clinical sign is subcutaneous edema.

Hyperthyroidism has been reported in a female green iguana that presented with polyphagia, loss of the dorsal spines, hyperactivity, increased aggression, tachycardia, and a bilobate mass palpable anterior to the thoracic inlet. Surgical thyroidectomy returned the lizard to a euthyroid state.

REPRODUCTIVE DISEASES

Dystocia (Egg Retention): Sterilization is rarely performed in reptiles, and therefore reproductive disease remains a common presentation. In oviparous reptiles, eggs (demonstrating various degrees of shell mineralization) may be retained, whereas in (ovo)viviparous species unfertilized ova or fetuses may be seen. In some cases, abnormal and persistent preovulatory follicles may also be diagnosed as spherical masses that fail to ovulate or resorb. Dystocia is generally not an acute presentation as in mammals or birds, and reptiles may retain eggs/fetuses for weeks or even months after the normal timing of laying/birth. Coupled with imprecise details of copulation, this can often make the distinction between normal gravidity and dystocia difficult in otherwise clinically healthy reptiles. Certainly, severe metabolic disturbance and infection can exacerbate the issue. In general, a presumptive diagnosis can be achieved through palpation and diagnostic imaging, especially radiography and ultrasonography. Hematology and plasma biochemistry may also help identify inflammatory/infectious changes and metabolic disturbances, especially hypercalcemia.

Unless there is evidence of acute disease, medical management may be tried, although it frequently fails. Improvements in husbandry (especially provision of solitude and a suitable substrate), corrections of any metabolic disturbances, subcutaneous dilute oxytocin/vasotocin, and potentially prostaglandin (PGF_{2a} and PGE) may be helpful. In most cases, surgical ovariosalpingectomy is required (unless a valuable breeding animal) after medical stabilization.

Vent Prolapse: A variety of prolapses may be seen emanating from the vent of reptiles, including cloaca, colon, oviduct, hemipenes/phallus, and (if present) bladder. Common causes include dystocia, copulation trauma, cloacitis, bacterial/fungal/parasitic infection, metabolic disease (especially secondary hyperparathyroidism), cystic calculi, renal disease, neoplasia, or any space-occupying lesion within the coelom causing tenesmus. It is important to identify the prolapsed organ, because some (eg, phallus/hemipenes) can be amputated, whereas others (eg, cloaca, colon, bladder) cannot. The prolapse should be gently cleaned, and the application of hyperosmotics may help reduce swelling and facilitate replacement. However, it is also important to determine the cause to prevent recurrence.

Prolapses of the hemipenes and phallus can be amputated after induction of general anesthesia or intrathecal (caudal spinal) block; this will render the animal infertile. If the prolapsed tissue is viable and can be replaced, purse-string sutures of the vent should be avoided, because they tend to deform the vent and may interfere with the urogenital openings. In such cases, it is preferable to use a transcutaneous cloacopexy technique. If the tissue is not viable, then careful and detailed surgery is required when attempting debridement and resection-anastomosis of the cloaca, colon, or bladder and often necessitates both cloacal and coeliotomy approaches.

NEOPLASTIC DISEASES

Neoplasia is becoming increasingly common as captive reptile populations age, and it should always be included in the differential diagnosis of disease. In addition to spontaneously developing neoplastic diseases, tumors have been associated with parasitism and oncogenic viruses. Surgical or endoscopic biopsies are preferred for diagnosis. Techniques such as radiography, CT, MRI, ultrasonography, endoscopy, cytology, histopathology (biopsy), and viral isolation provide improved diagnostic capabilities. Once neoplasia is diagnosed, treatment protocols similar to those used in other animals could be considered.

RODENTS

The order Rodentia, with ~2,020 living species placed in 28 families (approximately half of all mammalian species), is the largest order of mammals. They are found worldwide except in Antarctica and on some oceanic islands. Ecologically, they are remarkably diverse. Some species spend their entire lives above the ground in the canopy of rainforests; others rarely emerge from beneath the ground. Some species are aquatic, whereas others are equally specialized for life in deserts. Many rodents are to some degree omnivorous; others are highly specialized, eating, for example, only a few species of invertebrates or fungi.

Despite their morphologic and ecologic diversity, all rodents share one characteristic: a highly specialized dentition for gnawing. Rodents have a single pair of upper and a single pair of lower incisors. Between each incisor and the first cheek tooth is a toothless interval called the diastema. The incisors are rootless and grow continuously. Enamel is deposited on the anterior and lateral incisor surfaces; the posterior incisor surface is dentin. During gnawing, as the incisors chisel against each other, they wear away the softer dentin, leaving a sharp enamel edge. This "self-sharpening" system is very effective and is one of the keys to the enormous ecologic success of rodents.

Using the incisors together to chisel away at a surface requires muscle that forcefully brings the lower jaw forward. The masseter muscle does this in rodents. Rodents are traditionally divided into three groups based on how the masseter attachments evolved: sciuromorphs (eg, squirrels, beavers), hystricomorphs (eg, New and Old World porcupines, guinea pigs, jerboas), and myomorphs (eg, New and Old World rats and mice, hamsters, gerbils, voles).

Most modern rodents have adapted to eat seeds, which links them to the evolution of modern grasses. All rodents evolved from shrewlike carnivorous or insectivorous ancestors and have since diverged into various families and subfamilies.

Despite the large number of rodents, only a few species are owned as pets. The common pet rodents are chinchillas, gerbils, guinea pigs, hamsters, mice, and rats. Less common pet rodents are African giant pouched rats, degus, prairie dogs, spiny mice, and voles.

As prey animals, rodents do not show obvious signs of pain or disease until near death. Consequently, sick rodents are often presented late in disease progression when the prognosis is more guarded. Dermatologic conditions make up 25% of rodent cases presented for small animal consultation. Traumatic injuries are also frequent and seen in rodents of all ages. Although some diseases are caused by shortcomings in husbandry, often rodents subjected to "benign neglect" live long, healthy lives. The adverse effects of overfeeding pet rodents are seen in the early development of many spontaneous tumors and degenerative diseases.

CHINCHILLAS

Chinchillas are slender-bodied, medium-size rodents with short forelimbs and long muscular hindlimbs that give the animal a rabbitlike appearance. The head, eyes, and ears are relatively large, and the bullae are greatly expanded. Chinchillas have long gestation periods and deliver fully furred young with open eyes.

In the wild, chinchillas live in relatively barren areas of the Andes of Northern Chile at elevations of 3,000–5,000 m. Chinchillas live in burrows or rock crevices but are well adapted for running. They dust bathe, are vegetarian, and are active throughout the year. They are gregarious, living in groups of several hundred. All domestic (USA) chinchillas are descendants of 13 individuals brought to the USA in 1927.

Biology

Chinchillas come in a variety of colors. The original chinchilla fur color in the wild was mottled yellow-gray. Through selective breeding, the most common color seen is dark blue grey (the dominant fur color). Other colors have emerged and include the dominant colors of beige, white, and ebony, and the recessive colors of sapphire, violet, charcoal, and velvet. Eye color may be black, pink, or red due to fur color genes.

TABLE 30 BIOLOGIC DATA OF PET RODENTS

	Chinchilla	Gerbil	Guinea Pig	Hamster	Mouse
Life span[a] (yr)	4–15	2.5–4	4–8	1–2	1–2
Adult male body wt (g)	400–500	45–130	800–1,600	85–140	20–30
Adult female body wt (g)	400–600	55–135	700–1,300	95–120	18–35
Sexual maturity (wk)	32–36	9–12	10–12	4–7	6–8
Gestation (days)	111	24–26	63–69	16	19–21
Litter size (average)	2	1–12	3–4	6–10	5–12
Weaning (days)	42–56[b]	21	30[b]	21–30	21–23

[a] Life span data is for typical life span range in pet rodents. Life spans exceeding these times have been recorded for rodents in research studies.

[b] Guinea pigs and chinchillas have precocious young that can eat some solid food at 7–14 days. Early weaning results in lower body wt and social maladaptation in later life.

Ten different sounds comprise the vocal repertoire of chinchillas, depending on the behavioral context. Different sounds are made during exploratory behavior, predator avoidance, sexual behavior, and social behavior, including social contact and agonistic (defensive and offensive) behavior. In addition, chinchillas can raise and lower the tones of the calls they make. All chinchillas have a similar cry that is used commonly from birth.

The female chinchilla has an estrous cycle of 38 days. Females are seasonally polyestrous, and the breeding season is November to May in the northern hemisphere. The gestation period averages 111 days. Generally, the female will have two litters a year with 1 to 6 young (average 2) per litter. Young become sexually mature at 8 mo of age. Chinchillas have a long life span, reported to be up to 20 yr.

Sexing chinchillas (and guinea pigs) can be difficult. In females, a vaginal closure membrane seals the vaginal orifice at all times except estrus and parturition. The vaginal orifice is U-shaped and situated between the anus and the mound-shaped urethral orifice. It is difficult to distinguish when closed and is indicated by a slightly raised, semicircular area. When its closure membrane covers the vaginal orifice, the urethral orifice can be mistaken as a genital opening. The well-developed clitoris of female chinchillas (and guinea pigs) can be manually extruded through the urethral orifice and mistaken for a penis. The vagina is open during estrus. During these times, the vaginal closure membrane dissolves and then repairs. During estrus, there is no vulval swelling. Instead, the perineum changes color, going from a dull pink to a deep red. The perineal color increases dramatically at the time of vaginal perforation and remains intense throughout most of the luteal phase of the estrous cycle.

Male chinchillas do not have a true scrotum. The testes are contained within the inguinal canal or abdomen, and two small, moveable scrotal sacs are next to the anus, into which the caudal epididymis can drop. The external appearance of the scrotal sacs is similar to the nonpendulous scrotum of pigs and cats. The penis is readily apparent below the anus, from which it is separated by an expanse of bare skin. The penis can be manually extruded 1–2 cm when flaccid. The tip of the erect penis extends to the level of the axilla, a distance of ~11 cm.

As with other rodents, the anogenital distance gives the best initial indication of the animal's sex. In males, the anogenital distance is greater. Extrusion of the penis from the urethral orifice will confirm the sex of the chinchilla, as long as the clitoris is not mistaken for a penis. There are two major differentiating features: the penis is significantly larger than the clitoris, and the extruded penis can be separated and distinguished from the prepuce (whereas the extruded clitoris tends to evaginate, and the clitoral prepuce is not apparent).

Husbandry

Chinchillas are very tolerant of cold but sensitive to heat. The ambient temperature range to which chinchillas are adapted is 65°–80°F (18.3°–26.7°C). Exposure to higher ambient temperatures, especially in the presence of high humidity, can result in heatstroke. A good general rule is to add the unit values of the temperature (Fahrenheit) and humidity, and consider any value >150 to be dangerous. For example, 85°F + 65% humidity = 150. Chinchillas will develop matted fur if kept in a warm (>80°F [26.7°C]), humid environment.

Chinchillas are easily housed in either wire mesh-bottom or solid-bottom cages, although solid-bottom cages are recommended for pregnant females about to have young. Wire mesh spacing in cages should be narrow, because tibial fractures commonly occur in young chinchillas that catch a hindleg in wide floor mesh grating. Chinchillas are shy animals and need a place to hide when in captivity. In the wild, chinchillas conceal themselves in rock crevices. Polyvinyl chloride (PVC) plumbing pipes, especially elbow, Y, and T sections, make ideal hiding places. The pipes should be 4–5 in. in diameter and are easy to sanitize by placing in a dishwasher.

Because chinchillas have a habit of dust bathing, a box containing a mixture of silver sand and Fuller's earth (9:1), 2–4 in. deep should be placed in the cage daily. Dust baths should be provided for ~30 min/day. If dust baths are left in the cage for long periods, they become soiled with feces. When chinchillas do not have access to a dust bath in captivity, the fur becomes matted from oily secretions. Dust bathing often causes irritation of the eyes, resulting in conjunctivitis without associated clinical signs of upper respiratory infection. Excessive dust bathing has been reported to result in pulmonary epithelial hyperplasia and granulomas.

Chinchillas have a high requirement for dietary fiber. Their diet should mainly consist of high-quality grass hay. Pelleted chinchilla diets are commercially available and should be used to supplement the diet. Guinea pig or rabbit pelleted diets have also been used successfully to supplement the diet. Like rabbits and guinea pigs, chinchillas produce two types of fecal pellets: one nitrogen-rich intended for cecotrophy, and one nitrogen-poor delivered as fecal pellets.

Urinary calculi, urolithiasis, metastatic renal calcification, and nephritis are reported occasionally. Calculi are typically composed of calcium carbonate. Such conditions are often associated with feeding a diet high in calcium and low in phosphorus, such as alfalfa hay.

Polygamous breeding colonies are common among chinchilla ranchers, and a system of individual female housing has been devised that allows a single male to serve 12 females. A variety of breeding techniques have been used successfully, and mating is facilitated by observing changes in the vaginal closure membrane and performing vaginal cytology. Pregnant females do not make a nest.

Chinchillas possess well developed and anatomically elaborate male accessory reproductive glands. The secretions from these glands form a hard plug that remains in the female tract after copulation. In chinchillas, the vesicular gland provides the bulk of the accessory gland secretions, and the fluid hardens or gels when mixed with prostatic secretions. A 2–3 in. long, 1-in. diameter, irregularly shaped, firm, waxy plug is often found in the female's cage after mating.

Physical Examination

The chinchilla's overall appearance and behavior should be noted. Sick chinchillas may show weight loss, hunched posture, abnormal gait, scruffy fur, or labored breathing. They may be lethargic or unresponsive to stimulation. Chinchillas should be handled calmly and gently to minimize stress. Docile, nonpregnant animals can be removed from a cage by grasping and lifting the base of the tail while using the opposite hand to support the body. Routine restraint can be accomplished by wrapping a towel around the body. Small chinchillas may be grasped gently around the thorax, taking care not to restrict breathing. Pregnant females should not be handled unless necessary. Pregnancy is detectable by palpation at 90 days gestation and may be determined by regular weighing. By day 42 of gestation, weight gain in pregnant chinchillas will increase rapidly.

A protective reaction in chinchillas known as fur slip results in the release of a large patch of fur, revealing smooth, clean skin underneath. It may also occur with improper handling, fighting, or situations that overexcite a chinchilla. The fur can take several months to regrow and frequently is a different shade. To prevent fur slip, chinchillas should always be handled gently with minimal stress.

Infectious Diseases

Nearly all significant reports on infectious diseases of chinchillas over the past 60 yr come from colonies of chinchillas raised for fur, and most reports of bacterial disease in colonies are ≥30 yr old. Reviews of chinchilla disease often give the false impression that these animals are highly susceptible to infectious disease. However, the incidence of infectious disease in pet chinchillas is low.

Bacterial Infections: Historically, *Pseudomonas aeruginosa* infections, yersiniosis, and listeriosis occurred frequently among fur-ranched chinchillas. Estimates of fur-ranched chinchilla numbers in the USA in 1954 were >100,000 animals. By the mid-1960s, these numbers were reduced significantly to only a few thousand. Reports since 1980 of yersiniosis and listeriosis in chinchillas come almost exclusively from fur-ranched chinchillas in Hungary, Poland, Slovakia, and Croatia. These four European countries supply almost 50% of the 200,000 chinchilla pelts produced annually worldwide.

Opportunistic bacterial infections in chinchillas can cause disease, localized either to one organ or as septicemia. Affected animals usually are immunocompromised by age, underlying disease, nutritional status, or husbandry-related factors (eg, poor hygiene, poor ventilation, contaminated feed). Members of the family Enterobacteriaceae and *P aeruginosa* have been associated with significant morbidity and mortality in chinchillas. However, Enterobacteriaceae and *P aeruginosa* can also be isolated from clinically healthy animals. Therefore, most of these organisms are not considered primary pathogens.

P aeruginosa infections in pet chinchillas and epizootic outbreaks in fur-ranched chinchillas are the most frequent bacterial diseases reported. Initially, the infection is usually localized to one organ and can be associated with conjunctivitis, enteritis, pneumonia, otitis media and interna, metritis, and abortion. As the infection progresses, systemic spread is common. An acute generalized form with septicemia and sudden death can occur. *P aeruginosa* can be part of the normal intestinal flora in healthy chinchillas and has been isolated from 40% of healthy chinchillas. Stress, concurrent disease, or contaminated drinking water predispose to infection and clinical disease. Conjunctivitis is a common initial sign of *Pseudomonas* infection in chinchillas. Anorexia, lethargy, and decreased fecal output often follow. Characteristic pathologic lesions are miliary necrosis in the internal parenchymal organs and a necrotizing typhlocolitis. Strains of *P aeruginosa* that are multidrug resistant have reduced antibiotic susceptibility and are highly virulent and widespread in chinchillas. Antimicrobial drug selection should be based on culture and susceptibility testing. Generally, *P aeruginosa* is susceptible to fluoroquinolones, third-generation cephalosporins, or aminoglycosides. Topical polymyxin B and gentamicin-containing formulations can be used for empiric treatment because of the low prevalence of isolates resistant to these drugs. Multicomponent *P aeruginosa* vaccines (formalin-killed bacteria, endotoxin-associated protein and/or toxoids) have been used in fur-ranched chinchillas with some success. However, they are not suitable for pet chinchillas because of their variable immunity against different *Pseudomonas* strains, limited immune response of 6–8 mo, and adverse reactions at the local injection site.

The causative agents of yersiniosis, *Yersinia pseudotuberculosis* and *Y enterocolitica* occur worldwide in areas of moderate and subtropical climate, and outbreaks in fur-ranched chinchillas are described. *Y enterocolitica* is the species most frequently isolated from chinchillas. Yersiniosis is an enteric disease that damages epithelium of the ileum, cecum, and colon, resulting in mucosal hemorrhage and ulceration. Lymphoid infiltration results in hypertrophy of Peyer's patches and mesenteric lymph nodes and necrotizing granulomas. Systemic spread results in granulomatous lesions in the lungs, spleen, and liver and death. A chinchilla-type strain of *Y enterocolitica* (biovar 3, antigens or serovar 1, 2a, 3) persists enzootically among chinchilla stock worldwide.

Listeriosis is common in fur-ranched chinchillas but has not been reported in pet chinchillas. The original scientists who described listeriosis in chinchillas claimed that chinchillas are highly susceptible to infection with *Listeria monocytogenes*. It has not been proved, but unfortunately, this claim is often repeated. *L monocytogenes* is an environmental bacterium capable of existing both as an animal pathogen and plant saprophyte. Most cases of listeriosis in animals arise from ingestion of contaminated food, and the disease is common in animals, including chinchillas, fed on silage. Listeriosis is a cecal disease in chinchillas with bloodborne dissemination. The main target organ is the liver, where the bacteria multiply inside hepatocytes. Early recruitment of polymorphonuclear cells lead to lysis of hepatocytes, bacterial release, septicemia, and, in surviving hosts, development of lung, brain, spleen, lymph node, and liver abscesses.

Other recorded infections in chinchillas include clostridial enterotoxemia, salmonellosis, and *Klebsiella* infection. Affected animals display nonspecific septicemic signs such as loss of appetite, respiratory distress, and diarrhea and die within a few days after onset of clinical signs. *Salmonella* epizootics characterized by gastroenteritis and abortion are reported in fur-ranched chinchillas. Case reports of *Salmonella* infection in pet chinchillas have been linked to the presence of pet reptiles or wild birds.

Viral Infections: There are no species-specific viral diseases described for chinchillas. Chinchillas are susceptible to human herpesvirus 1 (HSV-1) and may play a role as a temporary reservoir for human infections. Two case reports exist that describe spontaneous, herpeslike viral infection in chinchillas. Affected animals displayed conjunctivitis and subsequently showed neurologic signs of seizures, disorientation, recumbency, and apathy. Nonsuppurative meningitis and polioencephalitis with neuronal necrosis and intranuclear inclusion bodies were found on histologic examination. In addition, the eyes displayed ulcerative keratitis, uveitis, retinitis and retinal degeneration, and optic neuritis. The clinical signs, distribution of lesions, and the viral antigen suggest HSV-1 is a primary ocular infection with subsequent spread to the CNS in chinchillas.

Parasitic Infections: **Protozoa:** Historically, group-housed chinchillas in fur ranches and research colonies had a high prevalence of giardiasis. However, the role of *Giardia duodenalis* (synonym *G lamblia*) in causing disease in chinchillas is difficult to establish. *Giardia* is rarely found in fecal samples from wild chinchillas, and healthy chinchillas can harbor *G duodenalis* organisms in low numbers in the small intestine. Experimental infection of healthy chinchillas with *Giardia* cysts failed to induce clinical disease. Predisposing factors, such as stress and poor husbandry, are believed to cause an increase in parasite numbers, resulting in diarrhea and potentially death. Recently weaned animals seem prone to developing clinical signs. Signs of giardiasis in pet chinchillas can include a cyclic sequence of appetite loss and diarrhea, associated with declining body and fur condition. Chinchillas with giardiasis can be treated with metronidazole, albendazole, or fenbendazole. Whether these compounds eradicate *Giardia* cysts completely or only inhibit cyst production is unknown; therefore, treated animals may remain a source of chronic cyst shedding. To prevent reinfection, all animals in contact with infected individuals should be treated, and the environment should be thoroughly disinfected. Wooden cage interior parts such as resting boards should be discarded. *Giardia* cysts remain infectious for up to several weeks in a cool, humid environment.

Toxoplasmosis was commonly found in fur-ranched chinchillas but is now rarely seen. Necropsy lesions include hemorrhagic lungs, an enlarged spleen, and enlarged mesenteric lymph nodes. Chinchillas may also develop focal necrotic meningoencephalitis due to *Toxoplasma gondii*.

Other protozoan infections include *Eimeria chinchilla*, which is seen in fur-ranched chinchillas. Single case reports described in pet chinchillas include hepatic sarcocystosis, *Cryptosporidium* spp gastroenteritis, and *Frenkelia* spp meningitis.

Cestodes and Nematodes: Pet chinchillas have a low prevalence of nematode and cestode infections. Outbreaks of cerebral nematodiasis caused by the raccoon ascarid *Baylisascaris procyonis* are reported in chinchillas housed outside in high northern American climates. An orbital cyst due to *Taenia coenurus* has been reported in a pet chinchilla with exophthalmos.

Fungal Infections: There are two reports of *Histoplasma capsulatum* infection in chinchillas. At necropsy, there was pulmonary hemorrhage, bronchopneumonia, and pyogranulomatous splenitis and hepatitis, with the organism seen in numerous giant cells. *H capsulatum* was cultured from timothy hay used for food.

Dermatophytosis is uncommon in chinchillas. *Trichophyton mentagrophytes* is the dermatophyte most commonly isolated, although *Microsporum canis* and *M gypseum* have been incriminated in outbreaks of spontaneously occurring dermatophytosis. Infected chinchillas show small, scaly patches of alopecia on the nose, behind the ears, or on the forefeet. Lesions may appear on any part of the body, and in advanced cases a large circumscribed area of inflammation with scab formation occurs. Although most mycologic studies of chinchillas are based on animals with clinical signs, fungal cultures of fur-ranched chinchillas show a 5% incidence of *T mentagrophytes* in animals with normal skin and a 30% incidence in animals with fur damage.

Diagnosis of dermatophytosis is based on appearance of lesions and isolation of the causative agent by using dermatophyte test medium (DTM). Wood's lamp examination is rarely helpful, because most cases are caused by *T mentagrophytes*, which does not fluoresce under ultraviolet light. Treatment consists of either itraconazole (10 mg/kg/day, PO) or terbinafine (30–40 mg/kg/day, PO) for 4–8 wk. Dermatophytosis is contagious to people and other animals.

Metabolic and Nutritional Disorders

Systemic disease or painful conditions may result in secondary GI problems with nonspecific clinical signs such as anorexia, decreased fecal production, and lethargy. Identifying the underlying cause is critical to improve the outcome and reduce chance of recurrence. The initial diagnostic evaluation should consist of whole body radiographs, fecal parasite examination, fecal cytology, and fecal culture for enteric opportunistic pathogens (eg, *E coli*, *P aeruginosa*). Urinalysis, plasma biochemical analysis, and a CBC help to diagnose non-GI and coexisting metabolic disorders (eg, hepatic lipidosis, ketosis, renal disease) to determine prognosis and therapy. In addition to specific treatment for the primary underlying GI disorder, general treatment guidelines include replacing fluid deficits and maintaining normovolemia by parenteral and enteral fluid therapy, nutritional and caloric support, and analgesia (buprenorphine 0.03–0.05 mg/kg, SC, tid) if a painful condition is suspected.

Cheek tooth crown and root abnormalities are common in chinchillas. Abnormalities related to subclinical dental disease have been reported in one-third of apparently healthy chinchillas presented for routine physical examination. Nutritional (eg, less abrasive diet in captivity) and genetic causes have been proposed as predisposing factors for development of dental disease. Tooth elongation and its secondary complications, affecting the reserve or the clinical crown or both, are the underlying cause of most clinical signs. Chinchillas are often able to eat and maintain good body condition until severe complications such as soft-tissue trauma from sharp dental spikes or periodontal abscessation have developed. A history of reduced food intake, changed food preferences toward more easily chewed feed items, weight loss, reduced fecal output, saliva-stained skin and fur with crusting and alopecia of the perioral area, wetting and crusting of the chin ("slobbers") and forefeet, epiphora, poor fur condition, and fur chewing are indicative of dental disease. On clinical examination, palpable irregularities of the ventral borders of the mandible and overgrown or irregular occlusal surfaces of the incisor teeth may be found.

A thorough examination of the oral cavity under general anesthesia is required, because 50% of intraoral lesions can be missed when examining the mouth in a conscious chinchilla. Endoscopic-guided intraoral examination is the preferred method. Cheek teeth often show coronal elongation, formation of sharp spikes buccally on the edges of the occlusal surfaces, and widened interproximal coronal spaces containing feed and fur. Loss of tooth substance or brown discoloration of occlusal and interproximal tooth surfaces is often seen. Erosions of the buccal mucosa, gingival hyperplasia, and gingival pocketing are common secondary findings. Radiography is a helpful tool to check tooth position and overgrowth of the roots. CT scans of the skull are useful in early diagnosis of malocclusion.

The prognosis for chinchillas with dental disease depends on the severity of disease, the animal's general condition, and owner compliance. Repeated intraoral examinations and treatments under general anesthesia are necessary to control complications and to maintain an acceptable quality of life for the animal. Treatment consists of removing spikes, reducing elongated crowns, and removing impacted debris in gingival pockets. Instilling doxycycline gel in deep gingival and periodontal pockets reduces periodontal inflammation. Animals with significant periodontal infection can be treated with penicillin G benzathine (50,000 IU, SC, every 5 days). Extraction of cheek teeth should be limited to severely diseased and mobile cheek teeth. Analgesia is essential after any dental procedure (buprenorphine 0.03–0.05 mg/kg, SC, tid; meloxicam 0.3–0.5 mg/kg, PO or SC, once or twice daily). Chinchillas in advanced stages of dental disease should be fed soft, leafy grass hay, vegetables, moistened pellets, and "critical-care" formulas offered on a dish.

Chinchilla anatomy precludes the ability to vomit. Choking may be observed when the entrance to the trachea is occluded by a large piece of food or bedding or in postpartum females that eat their placentas. Aspiration of tiny particles from the foreign body can irritate the lower respiratory tract and precipitate a suffocating, edematous response leading to drooling, retching, coughing, and dyspnea as the chinchilla attempts to dislodge the foreign body. If untreated, choking may lead to asphyxiation and death. Megaesophagus, which leads to regurgitation and aspiration pneumonia, is described. Affected chinchillas show recurring pneumonia despite treatment. Contrast radiographs are used for diagnosis.

Gastric ulcers are common in young chinchillas and are frequently caused by feeding coarse, fibrous roughage or moldy feeds. Clinically affected animals may be anorectic or asymptomatic. Lesions may only be noted at necropsy, with gastric mucosal ulcers and erosions covered by thick, black fluid. Prevention includes decreasing dietary roughage and feeding a commercial pelleted diet.

Bloat, or tympany, can result from sudden dietary changes, especially overeating. Bloat has been reported in lactating females 2–3 wk postpartum and may be related to hypocalcemia. Gas production from the bacterial flora in static bowel loops rapidly accumulates within 2–4 hr. Affected animals are lethargic and dyspneic, with a painful, distended abdomen. They may roll or stretch while attempting to relieve their discomfort. Treatment may require passage of a stomach tube or paracentesis to relieve gas build-up. Lactating females may respond favorably to calcium gluconate administered IV slowly to effect.

Diarrhea and soft feces are common. Besides infectious causes (eg, parasites, bacteria), inappropriate feeding of fresh green feed high in simple carbohydrates or sudden changes in diet will result in dysbacteriosis and cause soft feces. Owners may describe feces smeared on the cage resting board and the presence of fecal-stained perianal fur. On clinical examination, the chinchilla may show no signs or, in severe cases, be anorectic, dehydrated, and depressed. Infectious causes are excluded based on the history and by appropriate diagnostic testing. Systemic parenteral antimicrobial therapy (enrofloxacin 10 mg/kg, SC, diluted bid) should be used to treat predominately gram-negative opportunistic pathogens in chinchillas with severe dysbacteriosis, when an infectious cause is suspected but unconfirmed, or when the animal is in a compromised general condition. Oral drug administration should be avoided, because absorption and effectiveness of oral drugs are decreased when GI function is abnormal. Once an animal is eating and GI function is improved, the oral route can be used. Intestinal secondary yeast overgrowth, caused by *Cyniclomyces guttulatus* (previously *Saccharomycopsis guttulata*) that lines the stomach, is often seen in chinchillas with soft feces. However, increased numbers of this yeast in chinchillas is considered secondary, rather than a cause, promoted by an underlying gastroenteric disease process.

Constipation is more common than diarrhea. Chinchillas may strain to defecate and produce no fecal pellets or have a reduced output of smaller, thin, hard fecal pellets that may be stained with blood. Abdominal palpation reveals firm cecal ingesta and a tense abdomen. Intestinal intussusception is a critical differential diagnosis for absence of fecal pellets. A sudden change in diet, an inappropriate diet of insufficient dietary fiber and roughage, or infectious causes can result in dysbacteriosis, gastroenteritis, ileus, and consequently constipation. Dehydration, anorexia, dental disease, and uterine compression in gravid females may also result in constipation. Chronic cases may lead to rectal prolapse, intestinal torsion, cecal impaction, or colonic flexure. To provide relief, the GI tract should be rehydrated. Enteral fluid therapy (100 mL/kg/day, PO, divided into 4–5 doses) will stimulate the gastrocecal reflex and rehydrate dehydrated ingesta. Chinchillas with abdominal pain may resist enteral fluid therapy, and buprenorphine (0.03–0.05 mg/kg, SC, tid) and parenteral fluid therapy will be required.

Pathologists often see fatty liver without clinical signs or other histologic lesions in routine necropsies of chinchillas. This is most likely due to prolonged anorexia before death.

A few cases of apparent type II diabetes mellitus have been described in overweight chinchillas. Clinical signs may include poor appetite, lethargy, and weight loss. Diagnosis is based on a history of polydipsia and polyuria, hyperglycemia (≥200 mg/dL), and glucosuria. Chinchillas and other hystricognath rodents (eg, guinea pigs, degus, tuco-tucos) are unusual in that their insulins exhibit a very low biologic potency relative to pig insulin, yet the receptor-binding affinity is significantly higher, indicating that the efficacy of their insulin on receptors is ~2-fold lower than that of pig insulin. Hypoglycemia is always a great risk when treating diabetes with recombinant human insulin or porcine insulin. Treatment involves reducing obesity and feeding a diet high in protein, low in fat, and high in complex carbohydrates.

Traumatic Injuries

The predator avoidance mechanism known as fur slip, in which a chinchilla releases a large patch of fur, thus enabling it to escape, should not be confused with the vice of fur chewing. Chinchillas may chew each other's fur, resulting in a moth-eaten coat. Clinically, hair loss is seen along the shoulders, flanks, sides, and paws. The affected areas appear darker because the underfur is exposed. Mothers often transmit the vice to offspring. The higher incidence of fur chewing in commercial herds may be evidence of maladapted displacement behavior. Some clinicians claim affected chinchillas suffer from malnutrition and chew their fur for dietary requirements. Multiple food factors are probably involved in this type of malnutrition, and the exact cause requires further dietary studies.

During breeding, bite wounds that abscess are often seen in group-housed animals. Culture of the abscesses often yields *Staphylococcus* spp. Female chinchillas are larger than males and more aggressive. They are highly selective in their choice of males for mating and will keep "unsuitable" males at bay by urination, kicking, and biting. Bite wounds often result in the loss of pieces of ears and toes. Older females commonly kill a young male housed in the same cage.

The chinchilla's large, delicate ear pinnae are easily traumatized, most often from bite wounds. Therapy includes cleaning the traumatized area and applying topical antibiotics. Suturing large ear lacerations is usually not effective and not recommended. If damage is severe, ear tissue may require significant debridement or partial surgical removal. Trauma can result in rapid hematoma development, with blood and serum filling the space between skin and cartilage. Hematomas should be lanced, and contents gently removed to avoid further damage to the ear. The skin over the hematoma must remain in contact with the underlying cartilage and should be immobilized by sutures if necessary.

Traumatic fractures of the tibia are commonly seen and associated with the animal catching its hindlimb in a cage bar. The tibia is a straight bone longer than the femur, with little soft-tissue covering; the fibula is virtually nonexistent. Tibial fractures are either transverse or short spiral and generally are associated with bony fragments. Tibias of chinchillas are thin and fragile, and surgical repair can be difficult; complications are common. Soft, padded bandages and lateral splints usually do not provide adequate stability for tibial fractures to heal. External fixation and intramedullary pins, alone or in combination, have been recommended for surgical stabilization of tibial fractures in chinchillas. Restricted exercise in a single-level enclosure, ideally without cage bars, is necessary. The prognosis for tibial fractures is guarded, and complications after surgical fixation are common and include bone-pin loosening and infection, nonunion, necrosis of the distal limb, and self-mutilation. Hindlimb amputation should be considered if surgical fracture stabilization fails or is not indicated. Chinchillas usually adapt very well after amputation.

Reproductive and Iatrogenic Disorders

In chinchillas, the fine structure of the interhemal membrane of the placental labyrinth is hemomonochorial, consisting of a single layer of syncytial trophoblasts. In this respect, the placental labyrinth is similar to that of the guinea pig, another hystricognath rodent. Female chinchillas may experience an unusual puerperal disorder of trophoblastic emboli, resulting in pulmonary embolism.

Chinchillas usually give birth early in the morning and only rarely after midnight. Dystocia is usually associated with the presentation of a single, oversized fetus or malpresentation of one or more kits. Uterine inertia has also been reported as a cause of dystocia. Chinchillas respond well to cesarean section.

Male chinchillas that groom excessively frequently produce small amounts of urine or strain to urinate; repeated cleaning of the penis may mean the animal has a fur ring. This is a ring of hair around the penis and under the prepuce that eventually stops the penis from going back into the prepuce. In severe cases, an engorged penis is seen protruding 4–5 cm from the prepuce, resulting in paraphimosis. This painful condition may cause urethral constriction and acute urinary retention. Chronic paraphimosis may culminate in infection and severe damage to the penis, affecting breeding ability. Getting fur from a female during copulation is the most common cause of fur ring. However, the fur may come from other males or the same animal, because the condition is also seen in group-housed and single-housed males not exposed to females. Males should be examined for fur rings at least four times a year; active stud males should be examined every few days. In some male chinchillas, the penis will hang out of the prepuce all the time and is not engorged. In these cases, the condition is not caused by fur-ring but by excitement brought on by separation from a mate or exhaustion because of too many females in the same cage. Fur rings can be cut or gently rolled off the penis after applying a sterile lubricant. Occasionally, sedation or anesthesia may be required to remove the fur ring.

Neoplastic Disorders

Despite a life span reported up to 20 years, references on neoplasia in chinchillas are rare. Postmortem examinations of 1,005 fur-ranched chinchillas before 1949 and another 1,000 fur-ranched chinchillas ranging in age from <6 mo to 11 yr between 1949 and 1952 did not list neoplasia as a cause of death. Between 1994 and 2003, 325 chinchillas were presented for clinical investigation at a major university veterinary hospital. Tumors were diagnosed in only three animals (1%). During the same period, the incidence of neoplasia was higher in rabbits and rodents than in chinchillas (guinea pigs, 7%; rats, 34%; and rabbits, 6%). Single reports of tumors in chinchillas include neuroblastoma, carcinoma, lipoma, hemangioma, malignant lymphoma, hepatic carcinoma, and lumbar osteosarcoma.

Miscellaneous Disorders

Age-related Disorders: Aged chinchillas may develop posterior cortical cataracts and asteroid hyalosis.

Cardiac Disease: Heart murmurs ranging from mild to moderate are often heard in young chinchillas. Reports of cardiac disease in chinchillas are scarce, and the significance of heart murmurs in young, clinically healthy chinchillas remains unknown. There have been anecdotal reports of cardiomyopathy, ventricular septal defect, and mitral and tricuspid valve insufficiencies. Echocardiography is used to differentiate innocent from pathologic murmurs.

Foot Disorders: Foot disorders predominantly affect the hind feet. Lesions can include hyperkeratosis and erythema; less commonly, deep infections or open lesions of the plantar aspect of the feet can develop. In mild cases, environmental improvements and application of glycerin or petroleum-based ointment often resolve the hyperkeratosis and erythema. In severe cases, lesions are surgically debrided, followed by open-wound management and bandaging until healing is complete.

Zoonotic Risk

The major zoonotic risk from chinchillas is potential transmission of *Giardia*. Studies have indicated the existence of seven genetic groups (or assemblages) within *Giardia*, two of which (A and B) are found in both people and animals, whereas the remaining five (C-G) are host-specific. Most chinchilla infections occur with assemblage B. However, genotyping within assemblages A and B of animal species *Giardia* to determine zoonotic potential has not been done. Therefore, *Giardia*-infected chinchillas could be a potential reservoir of zoonotic transmission.

GERBILS

Gerbils are also known as jirds or sand rats. The pet and laboratory gerbil is *Meriones unguiculates*, commonly known as the Mongolian gerbil. There are 14 species in the genus *Meriones*.

Externally, gerbils are quite ratlike. The head and body length is 95–180 mm, and tail length is 100–193 mm. The average weight is 50–55 g for females and 60 g for males. The covering of fur on the tail is short near the base and progressively longer toward the tip so that it is slightly bushy. Coloration of upper parts varies from pale, clear yellowish through sandy and gray. The sides of the body are generally lighter than the back.

Wild Mongolian gerbils are found in Mongolia, adjacent parts of southern Siberia and northern China, and Manchuria. Gerbils inhabit clay and sandy deserts, bush country, and arid steppes. They have a high degree of resistance to heat stress and dehydration. They are terrestrial, and wild Mongolian gerbils construct simple burrows (2–3 ft long) in soft soil where they spend most of their time.

Biology

Mongolian gerbils have several coat colors. The wild coat color is agouti and is controlled by an autosomal dominant gene. Sandy gerbils have a recessive color gene and show a yellow to ginger color on the dorsum and the typical creamy white belly of a wild-type Mongolian gerbil. The dorsal yellow hairs have short black tips and a light olive green base. A clear demarcation line between dorsal and ventral color is present. Black gerbils have an autosomal recessive gene; white albino gerbils with red eyes also have an autosomal recessive gene.

Gerbils have a large, ventral abdominal marking gland that is androgen dependent. It attains greater size in males and develops at an earlier age. The gland is used for territorial marking. Females mark their territory after parturition and become more aggressive.

The adrenal cortex produces nearly equal amounts of corticosterone and 19-hydroxy-corticosterone. When the gland weight is compared with body weight, the adrenal gland is ~3 times larger in gerbils than in rats. Gerbils have a high proportion of RBCs with polychromasia, basophilic stippling, and reticulocytosis.

Male gerbils attain sexual maturity by 70–84 days. Vaginal opening in females occurs between 40–60 days, followed by 30 days before sexual maturity occurs. Gerbils tend to pair bond, and when older females lose their mate, getting them to accept another is often impossible. Early-maturing females are more likely to breed successfully on first pairing, and the lifetime fecundity of early-maturing females is more than twice that of their late-maturing littermates. Two-thirds of the early-maturing females that do not reproduce after a first pairing will become pregnant after a second pairing, but only 10% of late-maturing females do so.

The gestation period of nonlactating gerbils is 24–26 days, but lactating females always have a prolonged gestation of 27 days. If females are bred in the postpartum period, implantation is delayed, and gestation can be as long as 48 days. Mean litter size ranges from 3 to 7 animals. Young gerbils suckle for ~21 days and begin to eat solid foods at 16 days. In general, day 25 is considered suitable for weaning. The normal life span of a gerbil is 2–3 yr.

Husbandry

The diet of wild Mongolian gerbils consists of green vegetation, roots, bulb seeds, cereals, fruits, and insects. They hoard food and are not normally coprophagic, unless diets lack adequate nutrient value. Gerbils thrive on commercially available pelleted rodent diets with 18%–20% protein but may have deficiency problems when fed primarily homemade diets, sunflower seeds, or table scraps, which lack specific nutrients. Sunflower seeds are high in fat and low in calcium. Pelleted chow (5 g/day) has been recommended to avoid obesity. Gerbils will develop high blood cholesterol concentrations on diets containing >4% fat. This is manifest as lipemia and is more pronounced in males.

Gerbils excrete little urine, and fecal pellets are hard and dry. Their cages require less frequent cleaning than other pet and laboratory rodents. Gerbils adapt to a wide range of ambient temperatures. Because they have a propensity to develop nasal dermatitis at relative humidities >50%, a low humidity is advisable.

Gerbils require sandbathing to keep their coats from becoming oily. The lipids have two sources: Harderian gland nasal excretions spread by autogrooming and sebaceous exudates from the skin. The consequences of lipid removal by sandbathing are multiple; it not only cleans and grooms the pelage but also deposits lipids on the substrate that act as olfactory signals. Sandbathing is usually completed within 5 min. Additionally, it has homeostatic consequences. Hair color lightens in Mongolian gerbils allowed to sandbathe. When sandbathing is prevented, accumulating hair lipids mat the pelage, and behavior changes. Sandbath-deprived gerbils increase their frequency of "sand rolls" (rolling onto their side or back and returning to their feet within 1 second), decrease grooming, and increase territorial marking (especially males).

Gerbils often stand erect on their hindlimbs, so it is important that cages have a solid bottom and that the floor-to-lid height is tall enough to allow for this behavior.

Pet gerbils kept in inferior cages painted with lead paint or that use alloys containing lead have a high potential to develop chronic lead toxicosis because of their gnawing behavior and the urine-concentrating ability of their kidneys. Chronically, gerbils become emaciated, livers are small and pigmented, and kidneys are small and pitted. Microscopically, acid-fast inclusions are noted in the proximal collecting tubules and hepatocytes.

Physical Examination

The gerbil's overall appearance and behavior, particularly in relation to its cagemates, should be noted. Sick animals are often isolated from others and may demonstrate weight loss, hunched posture, lethargy, rough fur, labored breathing, and a loss of exploratory behavior. Early signs of illness involve changes in the color, consistency, odor, and amount of urine and feces. The perineal area should be checked for fecal or urine stains or discharges from the vulva in females. Fecal samples may be taken for parasite detection and bacterial culture. The fur and skin should be examined for alopecia, fight wounds or other trauma, ectoparasites, and elasticity for evidence of dehydration. The oral cavity should be checked for overgrown teeth. Ears and eyes should be examined for discharges or inflammation. Feet should be examined for sores and overgrown or broken nails. The abdomen should be palpated for masses. Normal body temperature is 98°–102°F (37°–39°C). Respiratory rate or signs of labored breathing should be noted. The thorax can be auscultated with a pediatric stethoscope.

Gerbil tails are fragile, and only the base of the tail should be grasped during handling to avoid injury.

Infectious Diseases

Bacterial, Mycoplasmal, and Rickettsial Infections: "Facial eczema," "sore nose," and nasal dermatitis all describe a common skin condition seen in gerbils. Clinical lesions next to the external nares appear erythematous initially, progress to localized alopecia, and develop into an extensive moist dermatitis. The cause is believed to be increased Harderian gland secretion of porphyrins (similar to chromodacryorrhea in rats), which act as a primary skin irritant. Experimental Harderian gland–adenectomized gerbils do not develop nasal or facial lesions. Various staphylococcal species (*Staphylococcus aureus* and *S xylosus*) may act synergistically to produce the dermatitis. Stress factors such as environmental humidity >50% or overcrowding cause excessive Harderian gland secretion. Nasal dermatitis infection may extend to the maxillary sinuses. Affected gerbils develop anorexia, stop drinking water, lose weight, and die. The distribution and nature of the lesions are useful in diagnosis. Accumulated porphyrins will fluoresce under ultraviolet light (Wood's lamp). Routine bacteriology yields isolation of pathogenic staphylococci. Treatment includes carefully cleaning the skin lesions and use of topical (chloramphenicol 1% ophthalmic ointment, tid) or parenteral antibiotics (except streptomycin, which is fatal in gerbils). Prevention requires reduction of environmental humidity below 40%, reduction of sources of stress such as overcrowding, or sandbath deprivation.

Naturally occurring Tyzzer disease, an enterohepatic disease caused by the obligately intracellular bacterium *Clostridium piliforme*, is the most frequently described fatal infectious disease of gerbils. Common clinical and pathologic findings are sudden death or death after a short period of disease, and the presence of multiple foci of hepatic necrosis. Diarrhea and necrotic lesions in the intestinal tracts are variably present. The probable route of infection in naturally occurring infection is by mouth, because gerbils exposed to infected bedding will contract Tyzzer disease. Supportive fluids and prophylactic treatment with doxycycline (5 mg/kg, PO, bid for 7–10 days) or metronidazole (20 mg/kg, PO, bid for 7–10 days) are recommended to reduce mortality in cagemates. Because the bacteria form spores, the housing environment should be thoroughly sanitized and disinfected.

The Mongolian gerbil is susceptible to infection by *Helicobacter pylori*, which causes severe gastritis, gastric ulceration, and intestinal metaplasia. Gastric adenocarcinoma develops in approximately one-third of infected gerbils >15 mo old. *Clostridium difficile*–associated fatal enterotoxemia has been associated with treatment using nutritionally balanced triple-antibiotic wafers (containing amoxicillin, metronidazole, and bismuth) to eliminate naturally occurring *Helicobacter* infections. Affected animals are reported to die within 7 days of antibiotic treatment.

Viral Infections: Naturally occurring viral infections of gerbils are not reported.

Parasitic Infections: *Syphacia obvelata*, the mouse pinworm, and *Dentostomella translucida*, an oxyurid, are found in Mongolian gerbils. Pet store gerbils often are infected with mouse pinworms. *D translucida* is commonly found in the small intestine of both research and pet gerbils. There is an average of four parasites per animal, but no clinical manifestations of disease are associated with the infection.

Infections with dwarf tapeworms, *Hymenolepis diminuta* and *Rodentolepis* (formerly *Hymenolepis*) *nana*, are reported in pet gerbils. Dehydration and mucoid diarrhea are often presenting signs. *R nana* has a direct life cycle and may potentially infect people if ingested. Recommended treatment is niclosamide fed at 10 mg feed/100 g body wt for two 7-day periods separated by 1 wk. Also effective are thiabendazole (0.33% mixed in the feed for 7–14 days) or praziquantel (5–10 mg/kg, IM, SC, or PO, repeated in 10 days).

Historically, reports exist of pet gerbils infected with the tropical rat mite *Ornithonyssus bacoti* (*see* p 2030).

Fungal Infections: There have been no reports of naturally occurring or experimental dermatophyte infections in the Mongolian gerbil. Other fungal infections in *Meriones* spp are exceedingly rare.

Metabolic and Nutritional Disorders

Gerbils develop spontaneous, insidious periodontal disease after 6 mo on standard laboratory rodent diets. On the same diets, ~10% of the animals will become obese, and some will show decreased glucose tolerance, increased serum immunoreactive insulin, and diabetic changes in the pancreas and other organs.

Traumatic Injuries

Thin skin covers the tail of the gerbil. Unlike rats or mice, if a gerbil is picked up by the tip of its tail, the skin will often slip off, leaving a raw, exposed tail that eventually becomes necrotic and will shed. If the tail skin is lost, the bare tail must be surgically amputated where the skin ends.

Iatrogenic Conditions

A fatal syndrome of acute toxicity is produced in Mongolian gerbils after injection of penicillin-dihydrostreptomycin-procaine combination. The toxicity is due to the dihydrostreptomycin, and 50 mg will produce almost 100% mortality in adult gerbils. Approximately 20%–40% of gerbils develop reflex, stereotypic, epileptiform (clonic-tonic) seizures from ~2 mo of age. Animals seize in response to sensory stimulation and forced exploratory behavior, but the incidence and severity of their seizures are variable; the seizures generally pass in a few minutes, may be mild or severe, and have no lasting effects. Although the incidence and severity of seizures often decrease with age, certain subsets of adult gerbils do not improve with age but progressively become more severe. The susceptibility is seen in selectively bred lines but may occur in pet gerbils. Seizures can be suppressed in genetically predisposed gerbils if they are frequently stimulated by handling during the first 3 wk of life. Anticonvulsant therapy is unnecessary.

Cystic ovaries occur frequently in Mongolian gerbils. Cysts range in size from 1–50 mm in diameter. Removal of affected ovaries does not significantly affect reproductive performance.

Females with one ovary are slightly inferior in fertility compared with normal females; a general decline in fertility may be evident in older females.

Neoplasia

Major surveys of spontaneous neoplasia in laboratory colonies of Mongolian gerbils have been reported. A 25%–40% incidence of neoplasia in gerbils usually occurs after 2–3 yr of age. Squamous cell carcinoma of the sebaceous ventral marking gland in males and ovarian granulosa cell tumor in females account for 80% of tumors seen in animals >3 yr old. The ventral marking gland tumors invade locally and can metastasize to lymph nodes and lung. Adrenocortical tumors, cutaneous squamous cell carcinoma, malignant melanoma, and renal and splenic hemangiomas were the next most commonly reported tumors. Numerous other tumors, including duodenal and cecal adenocarcinoma, hepatic lymphangioma, hemangioma and cholangiocarcinoma, splenic and renal hemangioma, uterine leiomyoma and hemangiopericytoma, ovarian teratoma, testicular teratoma, and malignant melanoma, were also reported. However, the total incidence of these tumors was <5%.

Case reports of spontaneously occurring tumors in pet gerbils include infiltrative craniopharyngioma, histiocytic sarcoma, systemic mastocytosis, malignant melanoma, and astrocytoma.

Miscellaneous Disorders

Congenital Disorders: Ventricular septal heart disease is seen occasionally in newborn gerbils.

Age-related Disorders: In two separate reviews, the pathologic findings in aging Mongolian gerbil colonies have been reported. Besides neoplasia, there was a high incidence of chronic glomerulonephropathy and focal myocardial degeneration and fibrosis, especially in older male gerbils.

Mongolian gerbils have a remarkable propensity for development of aural cholesteatoma. They occur in 50% of gerbils > 2 yr old. Cholesteatomas in the ear canal displace the tympanum into the middle ear. Compression and secondary infection result in bone necrosis and inner ear destruction. Clinical signs include head tilt.

Zoonotic Risk

There are no specific reports of zoonotic disease transmitted by pet Mongolian gerbils, although pet gerbils infested with *Ornithonyssus sylviarum* (the northern fowl mite) and *Dermanyssus gallinae* (the chicken mite) have been the source of avian mite dermatitis in children. Avian mite infestation is a rare cause of pruritic dermatoses in people. The mites spend most of their life cycle on the avian host but may be transmitted to people by direct or indirect contact. The scarcity of reports may be a true reflection of the absence of zoonotic disease in gerbils or may reflect their low popularity as a pet rodent.

GUINEA PIGS

Guinea pigs, like chinchillas, are hystricognath rodents. They belong to the family Cavidae, which contains 14 species of animals commonly known as cavies and Patagonian hares (or maras). Four digits on the forepaw and three on the hindfoot characterize Cavidae.

A stocky build, large head, short legs, and unfurred, short ears characterize guinea pigs. Head and body length is 200–400 mm, there is no external tail, and weight is 500–1,500 g.

In South America, wild cavies inhabit rocky areas, savannas, forest edges, and swamps from Columbia and Venezuela southward to Brazil and northern Argentina. They live in groups of up to 10 individuals and inhabit burrows that they or other animals dig. They are most active at night, when they forage for a variety of plant materials. Domestication of the guinea pig began at least by 900 BCE and may have begun as early as 5,000 BCE.

Biology

The American Cavy Breeders Association recognizes 13 breeds that it divides into groups or varieties. The most common breed is the American cavy and was known originally as the English cavy. Self cavies are a group of solid-colored animals (eg, black, cream, red, lilac, beige, saffron, and chocolate). Nonselfs are a group made up of the coated breeds, the marked breeds, and the ticked or agouti breeds. The coated cavies include the Abyssinian, Rex, Longhaired varieties (Peruvians, Silkies, Shelties, Coronets, and Texels), Crested, Teddy, and Satins. The short, wire-haired Abyssinian may look unhealthy because its coat is arranged in whorls or rosettes, giving it a ruffled, untidy appearance. An undercoat and projecting guard hairs make up the normal fur coat of a cavy. The Rex has short guard hairs that do not appear above the level of the undercoat, the Satin breeds have an abnormal hair fiber that produces a sheen, and the Teddy breeds have a kinked or bent hair shaft that causes the coat to stand erect over the entire body. The marked group contains Dalmatian, tortoise shell, and Himalayan varieties. The term "variety" describes a color (eg, steel grey, tortoiseshell) that is not yet a recognized breed.

Several researchers have analyzed guinea pig calls and distinguish between 7 and 11 distinct sound patterns. Although different authors have given different names to each unique sound, there is general agreement on at least 7 sounds.

Lymphocytes are the predominant WBC in guinea pigs and range from 45%–80% of the WBC count. Many small lymphocytes are similar in size to erythrocytes. Large lymphocytes contain Kurloff bodies, large intracytoplasmic mucopolysaccharide inclusion bodies. Kurloff bodies are seen under normal conditions in guinea pigs and are estrogen dependent. Pregnant females may have 2%–5% lymphocytes with Kurloff bodies in their peripheral blood; they are present in large numbers in adult females, and numbers fluctuate with the stage of estrous cycle. There are few Kurloff bodies in adult males, and they are rarely seen in newborns.

Like chinchillas, guinea pigs share unusual reproductive physiologic characteristics of hystricomorph rodents. Female guinea pigs (or sows) have a pregnancy of 68 days (range 59–72 days) and an average estrous cycle length of 17 days (range 13–25 days). They have a vaginal closure membrane that is open at estrus and parturition but sealed during anestrus and pregnancy. Guinea pigs have an average of 4 young per litter, with a range of 1–13. The young (of both species) are born fully furred and well developed. Young guinea pigs usually nurse for 21 days, although they can survive on solid food alone after 5 days. Guinea pigs have only a single pair of inguinal nipples.

Male guinea pigs have pronounced penile styles or spicules on the glans penis. Young male guinea pigs reach puberty at ~3 mo of age and females at 2 mo. Guinea pigs live 6–8 yr.

Husbandry

As a species, guinea pigs are extremely adaptable to a great range of climates, although as individuals they are highly susceptible to variations in local temperature and humidity. Guinea pigs are nervous animals and may refuse to drink or eat for a period after any significant change in their location, feed, or husbandry. The effect of environmental changes on guinea pigs is minimal or nonexistent when two animals are kept together. If a sick guinea pig must be kept in hospital, housing a cagemate with the sick animal reduces stress.

Guinea pigs live in family units centered on an alpha male. Mature males, and especially strangers, will fight. However, two males raised together from a young age or a group of nonbreeding females will not encounter dominance problems. Social problems are diminished with castration and ovariohysterectomy, but learned behavior in adult males after castration may still make them antisocial.

Guinea pigs require a constant source of water that must be changed daily. They dirty their water bowls or sipper tubes with food when they drink. They do not lick sipper tubes without training, defecate indiscriminately, and are prone to sit in and soil their food bowls and sleeping areas. However, they are generally good eaters and not as fussy as rabbits.

Guinea pigs produce two types of fecal pellets: one nitrogen-rich intended for cecotrophy, and one nitrogen-poor delivered as fecal pellets. When food is continually available, ~40% of the feces are reingested, and 90% of this coprophagy occurs at night. However, when food is limited, guinea pigs ingest feces during parts of the day when food is unavailable.

Physical Examination

Guinea pigs are easy to hold and restrain. Although they do not bite, very young guinea pigs may nip. Healthy guinea pigs feel "dense" and are alert. Fatigue, lack of interest in surroundings, and light body weight are often general signs of illness. Sick guinea pigs may show evidence of weight loss, hunched posture, abnormal gait, drawn in abdomen, scruffy fur, or labored breathing. They may be lethargic or unresponsive to stimulation. Respiratory and GI conditions are most commonly encountered; thus, ocular or nasal discharges or diarrhea may be present. Feet should be examined for sores or broken nails. Teeth may sometimes overgrow and should be checked. However, the mouth is small, and examination of the oral cavity is difficult. Ears and eyes should be examined for discharges or inflammation, and the submandibular area should be examined for swellings.

Venipuncture can be difficult in guinea pigs because of the lack of obviously accessible peripheral veins. The lateral saphenous vein and the cephalic vein are useful to draw small amounts of blood. For large amounts of blood, the anterior vena cava can be used, with the guinea pig under anesthesia. This technique requires practice. If performed incorrectly, there is a risk of death associated with intrathoracic, pericardial, or pulmonary hemorrhage.

Infectious Diseases

Bacterial Infections: *Streptococcus equi* subsp *zooepidemicus* (previously *S zooepidemicus*) may be carried in the nasopharynx as a latent infection. Abrasions of the oral cavity (eg, molar malocclusion) allow bacteria to be transported to draining lymph nodes of the head and neck, causing suppurative lymphadenitis. Clinically, guinea pigs present with large, unilateral swellings in the neck. The affected animal is often in good flesh and shows no other signs of disease. The differential diagnosis should always include cavian leukemia. Treatment is surgical excision of the affected lymph nodes and systemic antibiotic treatment. Bacterial culture and antibiotic sensitivity should always be recommended. Streptococci are generally sensitive to chloramphenicol (50 mg/kg, PO, bid), and this antibiotic is "safe" to give systemically to guinea pigs. Alternative "safe" antibiotics are azithromycin (15–30 mg/kg/day, PO; discontinue if soft feces) and fluoroquinolones; however, bacterial resistance to these antibiotics is now frequently seen.

Streptococcus pneumoniae may be carried in nares as an inapparent infection. Predisposing factors for development of bacterial pneumonia are changes in environmental temperature, humidity, or ventilation. This always occurs in winter in guinea pigs kept outside. The young, old, and pregnant are the most susceptible. Clinical signs of pneumonia are dyspnea, wheezy breathing, sneezing, nasal discharge, and coughing. The affected guinea pig becomes depressed and anorectic. *S pneumoniae* infections are nearly always associated with middle ear infection and head tilt. Increased radiodensity of the affected tympanic bulla may be seen on radiographs. Because of limited antimicrobial sensitivity, chloramphenicol (50 mg/kg, PO, bid) is the recommended treatment. A major differential diagnosis for pneumonia is *Bordetella bronchiseptica* infection.

Rabbits may harbor *B bronchiseptica* in their respiratory tracts without developing disease. However, this organism is an aggressive pathogen in guinea pigs, causing pneumonia, conjunctivitis, otitis media, abortions, and stillbirths. The clinical signs include anorexia, inappetence, nasal and ocular discharge, dyspnea, and often sudden death (this could also include *S pneumoniae* and *S equi zooepidemicus*). Rabbits and guinea pigs should not be housed together as pets. Treatment is ciprofloxacin (10–20 mg/kg, PO, bid). *B bronchiseptica* possesses a β-lactamase and is resistant to many penicillins and cephalosporins and mostly resistant to trimethoprim-sulfamethoxazole. Most isolates are sensitive to doxycycline (2.5–5 mg/kg, PO, bid) and fluoroquinolones (marbofloxacin, 4 mg/kg/day, PO; ciprofloxacin, 10–20 mg/kg, PO, bid; enrofloxacin, 5–10 mg/kg, PO, bid for 14 days).

Salmonella infections were historically common in guinea pigs in research colonies. With present standards of husbandry, rodent control, and good quality feed, the disease rarely occurs. It is most likely seen when guinea pigs are kept outside and wild rodents have access to their feed. Disease is more often seen in young or stressed animals. Infection may be subclinical, and diarrhea is rarely present. Clinical signs include conjunctivitis, fever, lethargy, anorexia, rough fur, palpable hepatosplenomegaly, cervical lymphadenitis, and abortion in pregnant sows. Mortality is often high in epizootic outbreaks. If animals recover, organisms may be shed intermittently. Diagnosis is accomplished by isolating the organism from blood, ocular secretions, lymph nodes, or spleen. Because of zoonotic considerations and the potential for a carrier state, treatment is not recommended.

Chronic dermatitis (especially of the forepaws) is a common condition usually seen in obese guinea pigs housed on wire or abrasive floors. Poor sanitation is also a predisposing factor. The feet are swollen and hairless with ulcers and scabs 1–3 cm in diameter on the plantar surface. *Staphylococcus aureus* is the usual causative agent and probably enters the foot through a cutaneous wound. Awns and straw in the bedding can also cause foot punctures. The inflammation can progress to osteoarthritis and systemic amyloidosis secondary to chronic staphylococcal infection. Surgical treatment is often unsuccessful, because there is rarely an abscess to be excised or drained but rather a diffuse cellulitis that infiltrates surrounding tissue. Treatment involves housing the affected guinea pig on clean, dry, soft bedding, topical or parenteral administration of antibiotics, and foot bandages as needed. Unfortunately, the condition may not respond to therapy.

Chlamydial conjunctivitis is one of the most common causes of infectious conjunctivitis in guinea pigs. It is caused by *Chlamydia caviae*, an obligate intracellular bacterium. Clinical disease usually is found in young animals 4–8 wk old. Rhinitis, lower respiratory tract disease, and abortion can also occur. Concurrent bacterial infections can contribute to the respiratory symptoms. *C caviae* can rapidly spread through a breeding or research colony. The organism infects primarily the mucosal epithelium of the conjunctiva and, less frequently, the genital tract of guinea pigs. Asymptomatic infection can occur, but clinical disease most often results in mild inflammatory conjunctivitis with a slight, yellow-white discharge, conjunctival hyperemia, chemosis, and even severe conjunctivitis with profuse, purulent ocular exudate. Demonstration of intracytoplasmic inclusion bodies in Giemsa-stained conjunctival epithelial cells often confirms the diagnosis. The most sensitive and reliable method of diagnosis of chlamydiosis is PCR testing. Antichlamydial therapy with doxycycline (5 mg/kg, PO, bid for 10 days) is the treatment of choice and usually results in complete recovery. Guinea pigs develop short-lived immunity to *C caviae* and, after a short period, may be susceptible to reinfection.

Viral Infections: Adenovirus is species-specific for guinea pigs and may cause a primary respiratory pneumonia. The asymptomatic carrier state is thought to be common, but prevalence is unknown. Clinical disease, while rare, can be initiated by stress or inhalation anesthesia and occurs more often in immunocompromised, young, or aged animals. Morbidity is low, but animals usually die suddenly without clinical signs.

Other naturally occurring viral infections of guinea pigs such as cytomegalovirus and parainfluenza rarely cause detectable clinical disease. Serologic surveys indicate that guinea pigs will develop antibodies to rat and mouse pathogenic viruses but do not develop disease.

Parasitic Infestations: Mange, caused by the sarcoptid mite *Trixacarus caviae*, is a common disease. The clinical signs are dramatic: intense pruritus, widespread alopecia, and hyperkeratosis. *T caviae* is transmitted through direct animal-to-animal contact from sow to weanlings during feeding, and through contact with infested cage material such as bedding. The mites may be capable of existing subclinically, becoming active with stressors (such as shipping or pregnancy), immunosuppression, or other underlying diseases. In affected animals that exhibit hematologic changes such as heterophilia, monocytosis, eosinophilia, and basophilia, vigorous scratching may trigger convulsive seizures. The seizures are controlled by diazepam (1–2 mg/kg, IM, as needed). The clinical presumptive diagnosis should be confirmed with several skin scrapings, usually revealing a massive *T caviae* infestation. Treatment involves ivermectin (0.4–0.5 mg/kg, SC, repeated 2–3 times at intervals of 7–10 days), or spot-on dermal treatment with either selamectin (15 mg/kg for <800 g body wt; 30 mg/kg for >800 g body wt). The guinea pig should also have a whole body washing with fipronil repeated twice at intervals of 7–10 days. Fipronil should not be used when open skin wounds are present.

Other ectoparasitic diseases are infrequent in guinea pigs. Infestation with the fur mite *Chirodiscoides caviae* may result in pruritus and alopecia along the posterior trunk of the body, while underlying skin is relatively unaffected. Subclinical cases may be asymptomatic. Treatment is with selamectin (15 mg/kg for <800 g body wt, 30 mg/kg for >800 g body wt) administered twice at 2-wk intervals.

Lice infestation with either *Gyropus ovalis* or *Gliricola porcelli* is usually asymptomatic but in severe cases may lead to pruritus, alopecia, and flaky skin surfaces around the neck and ears. Lice may be observed directly on hair shafts with a magnifying glass. A single application of 0.05 mL of a topical solution containing 10% imidacloprid and 1% moxidectin is an effective treatment for lice infestations in guinea pigs. Prevention is aimed at improving sanitary conditions in the animal's environment.

Fungal Infections: Dermatophytosis is common in guinea pigs, and natural infection is always associated with *Trichophyton mentagrophytes* var *mentagrophytes*. Lesions typically begin as broken hairs and circular, scaly alopecia initially occurring at the tip of the nose, which spreads to the periocular, forehead, and pinnal areas. In severe cases, the dorsal sacrolumbar area is also affected, but the limbs and ventrum are usually spared. Pruritus is usually minimal or absent. Some animals have more inflammatory lesions characterized by erythema, follicular papules, pustules, crusts, pruritus, and occasional scarring. High temperature and humidity may contribute to a more severe infection.

T mentagrophytes can be isolated from the skin and fur in up to 15% of clinically normal guinea pigs. Guinea pigs can be tested for dermatophytes by using a new toothbrush to comb all parts of the hair coat and impress the bristles onto dermatophyte test medium (DTM) in several sites. In a healthy animal, dermatophytosis is generally a self-limiting disease, with full resolution after development of an appropriate cell-mediated immune response. In immunocompetent animals, this usually takes 100 days. Nevertheless, treatment is recommended because it will accelerate resolution of lesions caused by dermatophytes, thereby minimizing the time course of the infection and minimizing the potential for spread to other animals or people. Whenever possible, curing the infection in the pet, while simultaneously decontaminating the environment, is desirable. Environmental control should be performed every 14 days with enilconazole (0.2%) or concentrated chlorine laundry bleach (1:10) solutions.

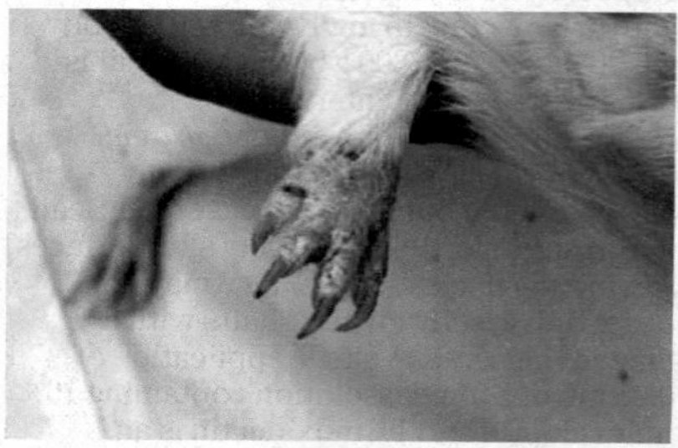

Ringworm (*Trichophyton*) in a guinea pig. Dermatophyte infections on guinea pigs are often located on the face, back, or front feet. *Courtesy of Dr. Louise Bauck.*

Treatment is systemic therapy with or without topical treatment. Spot-on treatment products should not be used alone, because they may predispose individuals to chronic subclinical infection. Rather, whole-body shampooing, dipping, or rinsing with topical antifungal agents in conjunction with systemic therapy is preferred. For topical therapy, either enilconazole (0.2% at a dilution of 1:70) or miconazole shampoo (with or without chlorhexidine), once or twice weekly, can be used. Enilconazole is licensed for use as an environmental disinfectant and is used off-label in treatment of dermatophytosis. Systemic therapy is either itraconazole (10 mg/kg/day, PO) or terbinafine (30–40 mg/kg/day, PO) for 4–8 wk. Lesions may resolve in 2–3 wk, but antifungal therapy should be continued until two DTM cultures are negative, with a 2-wk interval between cultures. Often, dermatophyte infections of the skin require 2–3 mo of therapy.

Metabolic and Nutritional Disorders

Guinea pigs of all ages require a dietary source of vitamin C. The stability of vitamin C in diets varies with composition of the diet, storage temperature, and humidity. The feed content of vitamin C is reduced by dampness, heat, and light. In fortified diets, approximately half of the initial vitamin C may be oxidized and lost 90 days after the diet has been mixed and stored at temperatures >22°C (71.6°F). Water in an open container may lose up to 50% of its vitamin C content in 24 hr. Aqueous solutions of vitamin C will more rapidly deteriorate in metal, hard water, or heat and are more stable in neutral to alkaline solutions.

Clinical signs of hypovitaminosis C include diarrhea, alopecia, and pain (from joints); animals are thin and unkempt. Petechiae on mucous membranes are not always seen, although hematuria may be present. Guinea pigs will show signs of vitamin C deficiency within 2 wk if it is not provided. Serum hypercholesterolemia (>60 mg/dL) and hypertriglyceridemia (>30 mg/dL) is seen in vitamin C–deficient guinea pigs after an overnight fast. Guinea pigs need ~10 mg vitamin C/kg body wt daily for maintenance and 30 mg vitamin C/kg body wt daily for pregnancy. Vegetables high in vitamin C include red or green capsicums, tomatoes, spinach, and asparagus.

Metastatic calcification occurs most often in guinea pigs >1 yr old. Clinically, animals present with muscle stiffness and failure to thrive. Mineralization may be confined to soft tissues around elbows and ribs. Mineral deposition may also be more widespread, involving lungs, heart, aorta, liver, kidneys, uterus, and sclera. Dietary factors such as a low-magnesium and high-phosphorus diet, and high calcium and/or high vitamin D intake have been implicated. Feeding commercial, high-quality guinea pig diets has reduced the incidence seen in laboratory colonies.

There are two other, similar syndromes in guinea pigs that affect either the skeletal muscles (muscular dystrophy) or the myocardium and skeletal muscles (muscular degeneration and mineralization). These two conditions are associated with a vitamin E/selenium deficiency. A separate, incidental finding of multifocal mineralization of individual muscle fibers may be seen in major muscles of hindlimbs. Affected animals are often asymptomatic.

Spontaneous diabetes mellitus is common in guinea pigs. The clinical manifestations are mild or variable. Guinea pigs show polydipsia and weight loss while maintaining a good appetite. Hematology and urinalysis show glycosuria, hyperglycemia, and high serum triglyceride levels; ketonemia and ketonuria are not seen. Exogenous insulin is not required for survival.

Reproductive and Iatrogenic Disorders

Multiple cysts are often present on ovaries of females >1 yr old. The cysts contain clear, serous fluid and may reach 2–4 cm in diameter. Cysts may be unilateral or bilateral. Clinically, ovarian cysts are associated with reduced reproductive performance, cystic endometrial hyperplasia, mucometra, endometritis, and alopecia. Radiography and ultrasonography should be performed, especially if an abdominal mass is palpable. Diagnosis of the disease by plain radiography is difficult because of the similar opacity of ovarian cysts and abdominal neoplasms. Abdominal ultrasound allows differentiation by imaging the inner structure of the ovarian cyst. Treatment is laparotomy and surgical removal of the ovary and cyst. Differential diagnoses include splenic, uterine, and ovarian tumors.

Although the clinical signs are similar, there are two recognized forms of pregnancy toxemia: the fasting/metabolic form and the toxic form. Both occur in late pregnancy. Affected sows show depression, acidosis, ketosis, proteinuria, ketonuria, and a lowered urinary pH (from ~9 to 5–6).

Metabolic pregnancy toxemia occurs in obese sows, especially females in their first or second pregnancy. The disease is caused by a reduced carbohydrate intake and mobilization of fat as a source of energy. Changes in feeding routine and stress may precipitate the crisis. Clinically, the sow stops eating and is initially depressed, then becomes comatose and usually dies within 5–6 days. Treatment is rarely successful in advanced cases. Aggressive treatment is necessary and involves administration of 5% glucose solution either IV or SC and/or propylene glycol orally, nutritional supplementation, and cesarean section. Sows in late pregnancy can be given water within which a small amount of glucose has been dissolved as a preventive measure.

The circulatory or preeclampsia form of pregnancy toxemia is due to uteroplacental ischemia. The gravid uterus compresses the aorta, resulting in significant reduction of blood flow to the uterine vessels. Placental necrosis, hemorrhage, ketosis, and death follow. If suspected, emergency cesarean section and/or ovariohysterectomy are required to save the sow's life.

Guinea pigs have a high perinatal mortality. Dystocia and stillbirths are related to large fetuses, subclinical ketosis, and fusion of the symphysis pubis. If females are first bred after 6 mo of age, the symphysis pubis often fuses and does not separate during parturition. Many stillbirths are often seen in primiparous females. Pregnancy lasts 59–72 days (average 63 days). If a female strains continually for >20 min or fails to produce young after 2 hr of intermittent straining, dystocia may be occurring. Careful examination of the cervix is necessary to assess how much separation of the symphysis pubis is present. There should be at least the width of the index finger to permit passage of the fetus. If adequate separation has occurred, oxytocin (1–2 units, IM) can be given. If the fetus is stuck, or parturition does not begin within 15 min of giving oxytocin, performing a cesarean section is necessary. The uterus should be opened close to the bifurcation of the horns. The guinea pig has a bicornuate uterus with one cervix.

Neoplasia

Spontaneous tumors are relatively uncommon in guinea pigs and are usually seen in animals >3 yr old. Trichofolliculoma, a benign tumor of the hair follicle epithelium, is the most common skin tumor of guinea pigs. The tumor presents as a slow-growing, oval mass varying in diameter from 0.5–7 cm and located predominantly in the subcutis of the dorsal lumbar or sacral region, or in the lateral femoral and lateral thoracic area. Males are affected twice as frequently as females. The average age of affected animals is 3 yr. Epidermoid cysts arising from hair follicles are often associated with these tumors or may arise independently. Ulcerating tumors and ruptured cysts discharge caseous material. Treatment of trichofolliculomas and epidermoid cysts is surgical excision.

Tumors of the reproductive tract represent 25% of spontaneous tumors in guinea pigs. Most are ovarian and uterine tumors, although mammary adenocarcinoma is seen in both male and female guinea pigs. The prevalence of mammary tumors in males is higher than in other species.

Miscellaneous Disorders

Antibiotic Toxicity: The lethal sensitivity of guinea pigs to antibiotic therapy cannot be overemphasized. Antibiotics reported to cause enterotoxemia are penicillin, ampicillin (amoxicillin), bacitracin, erythromycin, spiramycin, streptomycin, lincomycin, clindamycin, vancomycin, and tetracycline. Topical antibiotics have also caused fatal enterotoxemia. The following therapeutic dosages of antibiotics have been used clinically in guinea pigs (*see* TABLE 31).

Trimethoprim-sulfamethoxazole, chloramphenicol, and enrofloxacin are safe to use in guinea pigs. Narrow-spectrum antibiotics with antibacterial activity against gram-positive bacteria should be avoided; the cause of death is a decreased gram-positive bacterial flora and increased gram-negative flora, with related bacteremia/septicemia. Paradoxically, clostridial overgrowth (*Clostridium difficile*) has also been identified. *C difficile* is a pathogenic organism, not normally recoverable from intestinal contents.

Treatment for antibiotic toxicity is primarily supportive. The antibiotics should be stopped immediately, fluid therapy (IV or intraosseous) should be administered, and analgesics should be provided to prevent abdominal discomfort. High-fiber diets should be syringe fed to prevent ileus. Cholestyramine (1 g in 10 mL water, tid, for 5–10 days), an ion exchange resin, has been used experimentally to bind clostridial toxins in clindamycin-induced enterotoxemia. If the enterotoxemia is severe, the condition is life-threatening and the prognosis guarded.

Age-related Disorders: Urolithiasis is a common problem in older guinea pigs, especially females, because of the proximity of the urethral orifice to the anus and the high risk of infection with fecal contaminants like *E coli*. However, it may be seen in guinea pigs of both sexes and all ages. Clinical signs include dysuria, crying when attempting to urinate, and occasionally hematuria. Diagnosis is by abdominal radiology. The calculi are radiopaque and usually composed of calcium carbonate or calcium phosphate; calculi can also be composed of calcium oxalate. Obstructive urolithiasis, hydroureter, hydronephrosis, and possible concurrent septicemia can develop if the problem is not treated.

In addition to sex and age, diet may be related to urolithiasis. Foods high in calcium, eg, alfalfa hay, may result in a high

TABLE 31 ANTIBIOTIC DOSAGES FOR USE IN GUINEA PIGS

Antibiotic	Dosage
Azithromycin	15–30 mg/kg/day, PO (discontinue if soft feces occur)
Ceftiofur	1 mg/kg/day, IM (for pneumonia)
Cephaloridine	12.5 mg/kg, IM, once to three times daily for 5–14 days
Chloramphenicol	30–50 mg/kg, PO, SC, or IM, bid
Ciprofloxacin	10–20 mg/kg, PO, bid
Doxycycline	2.5–5 mg/kg, PO, bid
Enrofloxacin	5–10 mg/kg, PO or IM, bid
Gentamicin	6 mg/kg/day, SC (use cautiously)
Metronidazole	10–40 mg/kg/day, PO
Trimethoprim-sulfamethoxazole	30–50 mg/kg, PO, bid

dietary calcium:phosphorus ratio. Urinary ascorbate, if present at a high concentration, increases stone formation in guinea pigs given high-calcium or high-oxalate diets. This may be both beneficial and deleterious, ie, needing to give enough vitamin C to prevent scurvy but not increase stone formation.

Surgical removal is standard treatment. However, it is often complicated by exuberant inflammatory reactions to suture material. Prophylactically, potassium citrate/citric acid can be given as an inhibitor of crystal formation in urine. Citrate is not administered for its urine-acidifying effect as it is in dogs and cats, but because of its ability to bind calcium into water-soluble calcium citrate.

Dental Disease: The clinical signs and treatment of malocclusion in guinea pigs are almost identical to those in rabbits, except premolar teeth are more commonly affected (*see* p 1955).

Alopecia: Alopecia develops to a degree in all guinea pigs in late pregnancy (60–70 days) and during nursing. It results from reduced anabolism of maternal skin associated with fetal growth. Hair loss usually begins on the back and progresses bilaterally on the flanks and ventral abdomen. Nursing guinea pigs may worsen the condition by pulling hair from their mothers. The alopecia resolves slowly either after parturition or when the sow stops nursing.

Thinning hair is common in young animals at weaning. It is associated with a period of transition in which coarse guard hairs of the adult coat are developing and neonatal fur is being lost. Ear chewing and barbering are seen in group-housed guinea pigs that develop a social hierarchy. Often younger animals of lower rank develop hair loss from fur chewing by dominant older members. The hair loss is characterized by an irregular, almost stepwise pattern. Treatment involves separation of the aggressive animal(s).

Single-housed guinea pigs that become bored may inflict self-barbering. In these cases, areas the animal cannot reach such as the head, neck, and anterior shoulders are not affected. Changing the guinea pig's environment and providing large amounts of fresh hay often prevent boredom and stop this vice.

Bilateral, symmetric alopecia may be seen in older females with ovarian cysts. Other differential diagnoses for alopecia are mite infections and dermatophytosis.

Sebaceous glands are abundant along the dorsal surface of guinea pigs and around the anal orifice. The circumanal region contains a large accumulation of sebaceous glands. The sebaceous glands are testosterone dependent, and in adult males, excessive accumulation of sebaceous secretions occurs in the skin around the base of the spine and the folds of the circumanal and genital region. In areas covered by fur, the hair becomes thick, matted, and greasy. These folds can be periodically cleaned with surgical alcohol or a gel hand cleanser to preclude infection and unpleasant smell.

Zoonotic Risk

Pet guinea pigs carrying dermatophytes are a zoonotic risk for their owners, especially children, who are often the only affected members of a household. Risk factors for human dermatophytosis are young guinea pigs and recent acquisition of a new guinea pig. When treating ringworm in guinea pigs, environmental treatment should also be recommended to the owners, with special attention given to the bedding and clothing of people in contact with infected or carrier animals. Contagious material may persist in the owner's clothing and bedding and is a common reason for a pet's relapse after an initial response.

HAMSTERS

The most common pet and research hamster is the golden or Syrian hamster (*Mesocricetus auratus*). All Syrian hamsters in captivity appear to have originated from a litter of eight hamsters collected near Aleppo in Syria in 1930. Four of the animals escaped, a male killed one female, and only one male and two females remained. From these three animals, litters were raised that were distributed to Europe and the USA for research and subsequently as pets. In 1971, an additional 12 Syrian hamsters were captured in the field by farmers and imported to the USA.

Syrian hamsters have a head and body length of 170–180 mm and tail length of 12 mm. They range in weight from 110–140 g, and females are larger than males. Wild Syrian hamsters have a light, reddish brown dorsal coat, and the underparts are white. The skin of Syrian hamsters is very loose.

Other species now common as pets are the dwarf hamsters such as the Djungarian (*Phodopus sungorus*) and Roborovsky (*P roborovskii*) hamsters. They are small (<100 g body wt), have a docile disposition, do not attempt to bite or run away, thrive in captivity, and make good pets. This discussion primarily deals with diseases of the Syrian hamster.

Biology

At least 20 mutations affecting coat color in Syrian hamsters are known. Most are simple recessive traits, four are dominant, and two are sex-linked. Five mutations affect the fur, giving rise to long hair (also known as "teddy bear" hamsters), rex, and satin coats. Length of hair in the longhaired Syrian hamster is influenced by testosterone. Longhaired males from the age of sexual maturity have significantly longer hair than females or castrated males, which display fluffy, shorter hair.

Syrian hamsters possess paired, flank organs in the costovertebral area that are androgen dependent and consist of sebaceous glands, pigmented cells, and terminal hairs. They are larger and heavily pigmented in males and used for territorial marking. All hamsters possess enormous cheek pouches that open inside the lips, extend well back of the shoulders, and when filled with food more than double the width of the animal's head and shoulders.

Adult male Syrian hamsters develop large adrenal glands due to enlargement of the zona reticularis, which is three times the size of that in female hamsters. Like gerbils, Syrian hamsters have a high proportion of erythrocytes with polychromasia.

Female Syrian hamsters are heavier than males and generally are aggressive toward other hamsters. Nonestrous females can behave especially aggressively toward young males and may kill them. The 4-day estrous cycle is characterized by a copious postovulatory discharge on the last day. The discharge is creamy white and has a distinctive odor; it fills the vagina and usually extrudes through the vaginal orifice. Its stringy nature is distinctive, and if touched it can be drawn out as a thread of about 4–6 in. length. Estrus lasts ~1 day, and the gestation period is 16–19 days. The litter size ranges from 2 to 16, with an average of 9. Cannibalism of young accounts for nearly all preweaning mortality. Cold ambient temperatures (<10°C [50°F]), lean diets, and low body weight during pregnancy increase cannibalism. Disturbing the mother by handling the young or nest, and not providing adequate nesting material, warmth, food, or water, often results in cannibalism. Syrian hamsters are prolific breeders, and there may be 3–5 litters/yr. The young are weaned at 20 days and capable of reproducing at 7–8 wk. The life span of Syrian hamsters is 2–3 yr.

Husbandry

In the wild, Syrian hamsters live on dry rocky steppes or brushy slopes. They construct shallow burrows. Deep bedding that is appropriate for burrowing is recommended. Cages with at least 40–80 cm of bedding enhance the welfare of Syrian hamsters.

Wild Syrian hamsters are omnivorous, eating many kinds of green vegetation, seeds, fruit, and meat. Exposure to cold stimulates hamsters to gather food, and they will often hibernate at temperatures <5°C (41°F). Syrian hamsters do not fatten before hibernation and will starve unless they waken periodically to eat. Hibernating animals remain sensitive to external stimuli and are usually aroused if handled. Syrian hamsters have prominent depositions of brown fat beneath and between the shoulder blades, in the axilla, and in the neck and perirenal areas.

Syrian hamsters are active chewers and skillful at escaping from their cages. Glass water tubes are contraindicated for Syrian hamsters, because they will readily bite through glass. Stainless steel sipper tubes close to the floor are recommended. Because Syrian hamsters have broad muzzles that often prevent them eating from feed hoppers, feed pellets are placed on the floor of their cage. Hamsters are naturally coprophagic.

Physical Examination

The animal's overall appearance and behavior, particularly in relation to its cagemates, should be noted. Sick animals are often isolated from others and may show weight loss, hunched posture, lethargy, rough fur, labored breathing, and a loss of exploratory behavior. Early signs of disease involve changes in the color, consistency, odor, and volume of urine and feces. The perineal area should be checked for fecal or urine stains or discharges from the vulva in females. Fecal samples may be taken for parasite detection and bacterial culture. The fur and skin should be examined for alopecia, fight wounds or other trauma, and ectoparasites. The oral cavity should be checked for overgrown teeth or impacted cheek pouches. Ears should be examined for discharges or inflammation and eyes for discharges or conjunctivitis. Feet should be examined for sores and overgrown or broken nails. The abdomen should be palpated for masses.

Syrian hamsters are not normally aggressive but can be provoked if suddenly startled, awakened, or roughly handled. It may be easier to scoop Syrian hamsters up in a small container rather than pick them up directly. Their highly elastic skin should be grasped sufficiently to prevent the animal from biting.

Infectious Diseases

Bacterial Infections: Diarrhea may occur in Syrian hamsters of any age and is known as "wet tail," although this euphemism is frequently used to describe the disease in young hamsters. Proliferative ileitis is the most significant intestinal disease of 3- to 10-wk old Syrian hamsters and results in high mortality. It is caused by the intracellular bacterium *Lawsonia intracellularis*. Treatment involves correcting life-threatening electrolyte imbalance and dehydration, administering antibiotics, and force feeding. Several antibiotic treatments are recommended, including doxycycline (5–10 mg/kg, PO, bid for 5–7 days), enrofloxacin (10 mg/kg, PO or IM, bid for 5–7 days), and trimethoprim-sulfamethoxazole (30 mg/kg, PO, bid for 5–7 days). Symptomatic treatment with bismuth subsalicylate may be given if diarrhea persists. Replacement electrolyte and glucose solutions should be given orally, and electrolyte fluid replacement such as saline or lactated Ringer's solution should be given at a dosage of 20 mL/100 g body wt once daily. Sequelae of proliferative ileitis in surviving Syrian hamsters may include eventual obstruction, intussusception, or rectal prolapse.

Diarrhea in adult Syrian hamsters is associated with *Clostridium difficile* enterotoxemia and, as in guinea pigs, may occur 3–5 days after administration of antibiotics such as penicillin, lincomycin, or bacitracin.

Tyzzer disease due to *Clostridium piliforme* is seen in Syrian hamsters and is usually precipitated by stress such as overcrowding, high environmental temperature and humidity, heavy internal and external parasite load, and nutritionally inadequate diets. *C piliforme* is opportunistic in immunosuppressed animals and not seen in immunocompetent animals.

Bacterial pseudomycetoma has been described in several dwarf hamsters. The treatment is excision.

Viral Infections: Hamster polyoma virus (HaPV) is the cause of epizootic lymphoma in young Syrian hamsters and epitheliomas in older enzootically infected hamsters. When first introduced into a naive population of breeding Syrian hamsters, HaPV results in an epizootic of lymphoma, with an incidence as high as 80%. Lymphomas often arise in the mesentery but can arise in the axillary and cervical lymph nodes. Once enzootic in a hamster population, the occurrence of lymphoma declines to a much lower level. Enzootically infected Syrian hamsters develop HaPV skin tumors rather than lymphoma. HaPV lymphoma–affected Syrian hamsters appear thin, often with palpable masses in the abdomen. Often, they have demodectic mange due to either *Demodex criceti* or *D aurati*.

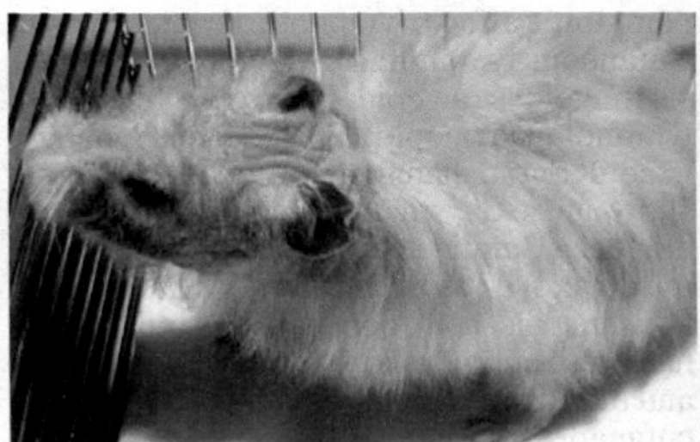

Gross lesions of *Demodex* infection in a hamster. Note the characteristic hair loss on the head and neck. *Courtesy of Dr. Louise Bauck.*

Parasitic Infections: Fecal smears of Syrian hamsters are abundant in protozoan organisms. However, their role in enteric disease is speculative, because similar protozoa are found in comparable numbers in both healthy and diseased animals.

Demodex criceti and *D aurati* are occasionally found on hamsters. Clinical signs consist of mild to moderate alopecia, pruritus, and erythema generally on the dorsal region of the body, the hindlimbs, and face. Additionally, crusts and scaling may be found on physical examination. Skin scrapings confirm the presence of a large number of *Demodex* spp in various stages of development. Treatment consists of a combination of 1% selenium sulfide shampoo and topical application of selamectin (15 mg/kg, applied once). Hamsters that do not respond to treatment or relapse often have serious underlying disease and typically die within 3 mo. Historically, reports exist of pet hamsters infected with the tropical rat mite *Ornithonyssus bacoti* (*see* p 2030).

Fungal Infections: Spontaneously occurring dermatophytosis is extremely rare in Syrian hamsters.

Neoplasia

In older Syrian hamsters, lymphoma is the most frequently observed neoplasm of the hematopoietic system. It is multicentric and commonly affects lymphatic organs. Cutaneous lymphoma, resembling mycosis fungoides (an epidermotropic T-cell lymphoma in people), is seen occasionally in adult Syrian hamsters. Affected animals show anorexia, weight loss, and patchy alopecia. Cutaneous lymphoma can be misdiagnosed as hyperadrenocorticism (Cushing disease), because affected hamsters initially show patchy alopecia and dermal hyperpigmentation. However, cutaneous lymphoma shows rapid progression of the disease, with mean time from presentation to euthanasia ~10 wk. Adenomas of the adrenal gland are common in Syrian hamsters, but few reports exist of confirmed clinical Cushing disease in hamsters.

Melanomas, not only of the flank organ but also of the skin, are frequently reported in Syrian hamsters. There is a striking 10:1 male:female melanoma ratio.

Djungarian hamsters showed a high prevalence of neoplastic disease (5 times greater than Syrian hamsters), and most tumors are integumental (eg, mammary tumors, atypical fibromas, and papillomas).

Miscellaneous Disorders

Age-related Disorders: Atrial thrombosis occurs in aging Syrian hamsters with an incidence of up to 70%. Most thromboses develop in the left atrium secondary to heart failure and lead to a consumptive coagulopathy. Although the incidence does not differ between the sexes near the end of their respective life spans, atrial thrombosis occurs on average at a younger age in females (13.5 mo) than in males (21.5 mo). Aged Syrian hamsters present with clinical signs of cardiomyopathy such as hyperpnea, tachycardia, and cyanosis. In untreated Syrian hamsters, death usually follows within a week after these signs are evident. The incidence of atrial thrombosis is influenced by the endocrine status of the animal, especially by the amount of circulating androgens. Thus, the castration of male Syrian hamsters is linked to an increase in the prevalence of atrial thrombosis.

Weight loss is seen in older Syrian hamsters and often associated with hepatic and renal amyloidosis. It is the principal cause of death in longterm research studies. Females have a higher incidence (80% among hamsters >18 mo old), increased severity, and earlier age of onset of amyloidosis than males. There is a correlation between social stress induced by crowding and amyloidosis in laboratory Syrian hamsters. Not surprisingly, it is infrequently reported in pet Syrian hamsters, in which overcrowding is not a problem.

Degenerative renal disease also occurs more frequently in older female Syrian hamsters. Affected kidneys are pale and granular. Microscopically, glomerular changes vary from thickening of the basement membrane to glomerular obliteration. Amyloid deposition occurs frequently as a concurrent event.

Polycystic liver disease is seen in Syrian hamsters >1 yr old. The lesions are due to developmental defects of the bile duct and are not associated with clinical signs. At necropsy, numerous thin-walled cysts may be seen.

Zoonotic Risk

Syrian hamsters have a reputation as carriers of lymphocytic choriomeningitis virus (LMCV), a rodent-borne virus that can cause substantial neurologic disease, particularly among prenatal and immunocompromised people. The common house mouse, *Mus musculus*, is the natural host and principal reservoir of LCMV. People are typically infected through close proximity to wild mice and their droppings. However, three of the largest outbreaks of LCMV infection in the USA were attributable to hamsters obtained from a single supplier in the late 1970s. More recently, individual cases of LCMV infection have been epidemiologically linked to hamsters among organ transplant recipients. Although the risk of hamsters transmitting LCMV to the general population may be overstated, a German survey of persons in contact with pet hamsters confirmed an increased risk of LCMV infection, especially in city dwellers, younger age groups, and females. Transplacental infection occurs in the fetus of women who develop viremia during the first and second trimesters. The virus acts as a neuroteratogen, causing chorioretinopathy, hydrocephalus, microcephalus, lissencephaly, and potentially fetal death. The relative risk posed by hamsters should be considered among transplant recipients and pregnant women, because infected animals may remain clinically unaffected by LCMV and can transmit the virus for at least 8 mo. When apparent, LCMV infection in hamsters is characterized by wasting. Early signs are decreased activity and appetite and unkempt coat. Later signs include weight loss, hunched posture, blepharitis, convulsions, and eventually death.

MICE AND RATS AS PETS

Mice and rats are not as common as pets as other rodents. They are used extensively in research and, consequently, a separate section on mice and rats as laboratory animals follows below (*see* p 2032). Although a great deal of information has been accumulated on wild and laboratory rodents, very little of this information pertains to pet rodents.

The prevalence and type of mouse and rat diseases seen in clinical practice are quite different from those seen in a research setting. The diagnosis and treatment of pet mice and rats involves evaluation and care of an individual animal from a household, not the health management of rodents from a research colony. Most problems in mice and rats are dermatopathies, respiratory infections, and neoplasia.

Biology

Male rats are sexually mature by 6–10 wk; female rats are sexually mature by 8–12 wk. The breeding life of both male and female rats is 9–12 mo. Estrous cycle length in female rats is 4–5 days, and estrus lasts 10–20 hr. Female rats ovulate ~10–20 eggs. Gestation lasts 21–23 days; pseudopregnancy from sterile matings lasts 12 days. Rats have an average litter size of 8–18 pups. Weaning takes place at ~21 days.

Both male and female mice are sexually mature by 6–8 wk and have a breeding life of 9 mo. Estrous cycle length in female mice is 4–5 days, and estrus lasts 10–20 hr. Female mice ovulate ~6–10 eggs. Gestation lasts 19–21 days; pseudopregnancy from sterile matings lasts 12 days. Mice have an average litter size of 5–12 pups. Weaning takes place at ~21 days.

Male mice and rats produce a small amount of sperm daily at puberty (eg, 40–50 days in a rat). It is not until 75–100 days (10–14 wk) in rats that optimal sperm production and reserve occur. Male rodents show a constant libido after sexual maturity; in contrast, females are receptive to copulation only during estrus. Males cannot fertilize females until 6–8 wk after reaching puberty.

The average life span of mice is 18–24 mo and of rats 18–36 mo. Restricting dietary calories without compromising overall nutrition results in increased life span. Obesity in pet rats and mice is common, and calorie-restricted pets live significantly longer lives.

Husbandry

The best cages are made of a material that is easy to clean and deodorize and is indestructible to rodent chewing or digging in the corners. The cage floor can be solid but should be waterproof and easy to clean. Wire mesh floors should be avoided, because rats and mice can trap their feet and especially hindlimbs in the openings, resulting in fractures and injuries.

Animal cage bedding is described based on its use (eg, contact, noncontact, and enrichment bedding) or the material from which it is made (eg, wood-based [chips, shavings, peelings, wood-wool and sawdust], paper-based [cotton and pulp fiber, recycled paper], corn [husks and cobs], cellulose, and vermiculite). The purpose of bedding is to keep animals dry and clean. Pet owners generally choose bedding based on cost and availability, whereas laboratory veterinarians choose bedding based on cost and water-holding capacity. Some pet bedding contains lemon and chlorophyll to give it a pleasant scent. This type of bedding irritates pet rodents, and the coloring agents can stain the coat of white rats or mice. Traditionally, owners prefer paper and softwood chips, such as pine or aspen, to straw because it requires fewer bedding changes. Cedar and other wood chip shavings reduce ectoparasite problems and have a pleasant scent. However, such bedding is not recommended, because it emits toxic aromatic hydrocarbons that increase the incidence of cancer in animals and cause mouse and rat pup mortality.

Owners must combine frequent bedding changes with good husbandry such as regular cage cleaning, low animal density, and low environmental temperature and humidity. This will reduce toxic or odor-causing gases such as ammonia from building up, because urease-positive bacteria in the feces act to break down urea in the urine. Aquariums are not suitable cages for rats and mice because of inadequate air circulation and subsequent buildup of ammonia. Environmental temperature and relative humidity can depend on husbandry and housing design and can differ considerably between the cage and room. Factors that contribute to variation in temperature and humidity include cage material and construction, number of animals per cage, frequency of bedding changes, and bedding type.

Size and manipulability of bedding material are the main determinants of mice and rats' choices. Mice and rats avoid bedding consisting of small particles, whereas they prefer bedding consisting of large, fibrous particles. When exposed to different types of nesting materials such as paper strips, cornhusks, sawdust, and wood materials (shavings, peelings, and chips), rats choose long strips of soft paper. Rats also select opaque or semiopaque nest boxes to transparent nest boxes. Mice show no preference between paper and wood-derived materials but show a clear preference for materials that they can manipulate such as paper tissues, string, and wood materials (shavings, peelings, and chips). Many mice will combine two preferred nesting materials to make complex nests. Mice typically dislike wire-bottomed cages; however, both male and female mice will spend more time in a wire-bottomed cage with nesting material, despite the grid floor that they usually avoid.

In environmentally enriched cages with hollow tubes, mice have no overwhelming group preference for shape, opacity, or openness of tubes and prefer to sleep in sawdust when it is available. Mice will sleep in hollow tubes only after the sawdust is removed; they use short, wide tubes more frequently than long or short narrow tubes.

Mice and rats are optimally maintained at temperatures of 64°–79°F (18°–26°C). Relative humidity should also be controlled but not nearly as narrowly as temperature. An acceptable range of relative humidity is 30%–70%. Both temperature and humidity regulation are important to prevent ringtail and exacerbation of respiratory disease. Avascular necrosis of the tail, or ringtail, occurs primarily in young rats in low-humidity environments. Excess heat and humidity cause heat stroke and indirectly cause decompensation of chronic respiratory disease, resulting in death.

Mouse and rat owners should check water bottles daily. If mice are deprived of water for only a short time and experience dramatic fluctuations in the surrounding temperature, especially >99°F (37°C), they die. In contrast, healthy rats tolerate water deprivation and temperature fluctuations better. They can live for 7 days without water, in temperatures between 64°–79°F (18°–26°C), although they may lose up to 65% of their body weight.

Minimal space allocations of 23 sq in. (58 sq cm) are recommended for individual rats weighing ≤200 g, and 60 sq in. (152 sq cm) for rats weighing ≥500 g. For mice, minimal space allocations of 15 sq in (38 sq cm) for individual mice weighing >25 g are recommended. These are small surface areas, and veterinarians should advocate that owners provide larger space for their pets.

Most rodent enrichment studies focus on modifying the area inside the enclosure rather than the size of an enclosure. However, rats prefer larger cages, and experimental studies suggest rats should have a larger space that allows sharing of the environment with up to four other rats.

The minimum recommended height of cages should take into account typical postures of rats and mice. This includes the animal standing fully erect on its hindlegs, and vertical movements such as stretching upward and possibly climbing. Consequently, minimal cage heights of 12–15 in. (30–38 cm) for rats and 7–8 in. (18–20 cm) for mice are recommended.

Environmental enrichment is important for both mice and rats. For example, suspended cloth hammocks are popular with rats, and suspended (plastic or stainless steel) shower hooks fitted into one another can make a swinging chain. Rats will use more enrichment devices than mice, but they usually stop using the devices after 3–4 days. Rotation of enrichment toys and introduction of novel devices excite their curiosity. Food treats are also valuable enrichment items. These can range from simple, inexpensive treats such as a daily piece of a breakfast cereal to formulated nutritious or calorie-free treats. Rats also love chocolate, and it is not toxic when fed in small amounts. Pet rodents accustomed to handling will eat food treats out of the owner's hand. This daily routine can allow owners to detect subtle changes in the pet's behavior. Sick rodents effectively hide signs of disease. Sick rats do not show the same interest in their daily treat, and this can alert the owner early to disease when it is still treatable and/or reversible.

Housing male and female rodents together will result in mating and subsequent litters. Mice and rats experience postparturient estrus, and fertilization can occur. However, implantation of the resulting blastocysts is delayed during lactation and occurs at weaning, ensuring that the next litter is not born until the earlier one has been weaned. Female mice become sexually mature at 6–8 wk of age, and female rats are sexually mature by 10 wk of age. Unless opposite-sex rodents housed together are separated or neutered, having a new litter every 3–5 wk is possible.

Rats and mice are omnivores and will eat food of both plant and animal origin. In the wild, rats and mice will eat a wide variety of seeds, grains, and other plant material as well as invertebrates, small vertebrates, and carrion. Their ability to scavenge partly accounts for their successful colonization of diverse geographic regions.

Formulated pelleted diets for laboratory rodents are convenient and nutritionally balanced diets for early life and reproduction. However, laboratory rodent diets are relatively high in fat and low in fiber, and when provided ad libitum, they cause obesity. Consequently, the amount of pelleted diet owners provide daily should be limited. Diets formulated specifically for pet rodents are now commercially available. Owners should supplement their pet's diet with feeds high in fiber such as vegetables, limited amounts of fruit, and occasional treats.

Coprophagy is a normal behavior in rats and mice. It is an inherent behavior, because it is seen in germ-free rodents purposely bred for research. Unlike rabbits, which eat cecal feces from their anus, mice and rats eat fecal pellets on the floor of their caging. The amount of feces eaten varies between rodents, their age and physiologic status (eg, coprophagy increases in pregnancy), and the diet fed. On a nutritionally complete diet, rats will eat ~10% of their feces. When rats are housed together, they ingest each other's feces. The unique odor of a colony is due in part to ingestion of feces, and the group scent enables distinction between members and nonmembers. Mice engage in coprophagy ~6 times/day. Growing mice show vigorous coprophagous activity, eating 13 pellets/day. However, it gradually decreases to 1½ pellets at 2 yr of age.

Owners should house different species of rodents separately to prevent interspecies disease transmission. For example, rats carry *Streptobacillus moniliformis* (see p 2418), a cause of fatal septicemia in mice, as part of the normal nasopharyngeal bacterial flora. Rodents of the same species should be housed in such a way to protect vulnerable animals from more aggressive members of their group. This includes separating young animals from older ones. Female rodents are generally compatible when housed in the same cage, unless one female has lived much of its life alone. Male rats are generally compatible, especially if raised together. However, owners should never house strange male rats in the same cage together because they will fight. Male mice generally fight if housed together, unless they are littermates raised together without females present. Male mice are best housed singly or with female mice.

Rats are social animals, and grooming is a socially affiliative behavior. Singly housed rats may develop isolated-rat stress syndrome if left alone without human contact and environmental enrichment. Isolation-reared rats will experience fighting, physical injuries, and weight loss when placed into a colony of socially experienced rats. Young rats should be housed together to develop social affiliation. Singly housed rats should not be put together. Owners should be advised to encourage enrichment and human contact with pet rats.

Physical Examination

Observing the condition of the rodent's living quarters provides useful information. Information obtained from a physical examination is often limited because of the mouse or rat's size. Activity of the rat, condition of grooming, and the presence of a head tilt or discharges in the cage should be noted. If dyspnea or depression is seen, extreme care should be used when handling the animal, because it is probably very sick and could die from the stress of a physical examination.

Pet rodents that have been frequently and gently handled usually require only minimal restraint. Less cooperative animals need to be more firmly restrained, and use of a towel or even heavy gloves may be required. Weight measurement is essential to calculate appropriate dosages of medications and provides an opportunity to gauge the rodent's temperament before beginning the actual physical examination.

The head, ears, eyes, and nose should be examined for discharges, and the oral cavity for dentition. Lymph nodes and glands of the head can be observed for size and palpated for consistency. Assessment of the head is probably the most time-consuming part of the examination. The abdomen can be palpated for consistency and the presence of unusual masses. Animals should not be squeezed too vigorously, because overzealous palpation can result in visceral rupture. The anogenital region should be examined for discharges and staining of the fur or skin. When a rodent is picked up, it generally urinates and defecates. A dipstick should be ready to perform an immediate urinalysis; feces can be caught in a small tube and examined later. The limbs should be palpated for tenderness or fractures, with special attention given to the paws, noting the length of the nails and condition of the footpads.

Respirations and heart rate in mice and rats are rapid and, therefore, difficult to measure. Instead, signs of dyspnea should be noted. Some respiratory infections, such as mycoplasmosis, are clinically silent. These diseases can be better heard than seen; abnormal sounds called "snuffling" in rats and "chattering" in mice are noticeable without a stethoscope.

Infectious Diseases

Bacterial Infections: Rats are the natural host of the bacterium *Streptobacillus moniliformis*. It is a commensal organism of the nasopharyngeal flora and does not cause disease in rats. However, individuals bitten by rats may become infected with *S moniliformis* and develop rat bite fever, a potentially fatal disease (*see* p 2418). Mice housed with rats will become infected with *S moniliformis* and develop fatal septicemia characterized by polyarthritis, cervical lymphadenitis, pneumonia, and splenomegaly.

Respiratory disease caused by infectious agents is the most common health problem in rats. Three major respiratory pathogens cause overt clinical disease: *Mycoplasma pulmonis*, *Streptococcus pneumoniae*, and *Corynebacterium kutscheri*. Other organisms such as Sendai virus (a paramyxovirus), pneumonia virus of mice (a paramyxovirus), rat respiratory virus (a hantavirus), cilia-associated respiratory (CAR) bacillus, and *Haemophilus* species are minor respiratory pathogens that rarely cause overt clinical disease by themselves. However, the minor respiratory pathogens interact synergistically as copathogens with the major respiratory pathogens to produce two major clinical syndromes: chronic respiratory disease (CRD) and bacterial pneumonia.

CRD is the best-understood multifactorial respiratory infection in rats. *M pulmonis* is the major component of CRD, and the disease is also known as murine respiratory mycoplasmosis. Rats with CRD rarely live >2 yr. Clinical signs are highly variable. Initial infection commonly occurs without any clinical signs; early signs involve both the upper and lower respiratory tracts and may include snuffling, nasal discharge, polypnea, weight loss, hunched posture, ruffled coat, head tilt, and red tears. Dyspnea, the primary presenting complaint, is caused by ciliostasis, subsequent buildup of lysozyme-rich inflammatory exudate in airways, bronchiectasis, and bronchiolectasis from inflammatory damage to bronchiolar membranes. Chronic disease often includes middle ear infection (via the eustachian tube). Antibiotic therapy may alleviate clinical signs but does not eliminate the infection. Enrofloxacin (10 mg/kg) and doxycycline (5–10 mg/kg) given orally bid for 14 days often alleviates severe clinical signs. Additional treatments such as daily nebulization therapy with 7% hypertonic saline to break down the mucus biofilm in respiratory passages, bronchodilators (theophylline 10 mg/kg, bid) to improve airway patency, and reducing ammonia levels in cages by daily removal of bedding and use of clean paper will ameliorate the disease. Chronic low dose doxycycline (5–10 mg/kg/day, PO) helps to prevent acute relapses. The doxycycline is both bactericidal for mycoplasma organisms and has a marked immunomodulatory effect on the chronic airway inflammation.

The most important aspect of CRD for clinicians is that respiratory mycoplasmosis varies greatly in disease expression because of environmental, host, and organism factors that influence the host-pathogen relationship. Examples of such factors include intracage ammonia levels; concurrent Sendai virus, coronavirus (sialodacryoadenitis virus), pneumonia virus of mice, rat respiratory virus, and/or CAR bacillus infection; the genetic susceptibility of the host; the virulence of the *Mycoplasma* strain; and vitamin A or E deficiency. Although CRD is rarely seen in laboratory rats, most pet rats have CRD to some degree. One survey of pet ratteries in the northwest USA showed virtually all (95%) were positive for CAR-bacillus and *M pulmonis*, and approximately half were positive for other viral respiratory agents.

Bacterial pneumonia is nearly always caused by *S pneumoniae*, but seldom in the absence of some combination involving *M pulmonis*, Sendai virus, or CAR bacillus. Infection with *C kutscheri* also results in pneumonia but only in conjunction with debilitation or immunosuppression. In pet rats, immunosuppression can result from diabetes, neoplasia, or dietary deficiencies. *C kutscheri* pneumonia is rare in pet rats. Pneumonia caused by *S pneumoniae* can be of sudden onset. Young rats are more severely affected than older ones, and often the only sign they exhibit is sudden death. Mature rats may demonstrate dyspnea, snuffling, and abdominal breathing. A purulent exudate may be seen around the nares and on the front paws from wiping of the nostrils. A tentative diagnosis is based on identification of numerous gram-positive diplococci on a Gram stain of the exudate or in a sample submitted for cytologic examination. Severe bacteremia is an important consequence of advanced disease and results in multiorgan abscesses and infarction. Treatment is amoxicillin/clavulanic acid (13.75 mg/kg, PO, bid) or β-lactamase–resistant penicillins such as cloxacillin, oxacillin, and dicloxacillin, which can all be administered orally or parenterally.

Ulcerative dermatitis caused by *Staphylococcus aureus* infection results from self-trauma associated with fur mite infestation or, more commonly, from scratching of the skin over an inflamed salivary gland. Rats have a remarkable ability to resist infection with *S aureus*. Treatment consists of clipping the toenails of the hindpaws, cleaning the ulcerated skin, and applying a topical antibiotic. Systemic treatment is rarely necessary.

The two most common causes of clinical respiratory disease in mice are Sendai virus and *M pulmonis* infection. Sendai virus is associated with an acute respiratory infection in which mice display chattering and mild respiratory distress. Neonates and weanlings may die. Adults generally recover within 2 mo. When the disease expression exceeds this pattern, the cause is most likely concurrent mycoplasmal infection. *M pulmonis* is the cause of chronic pneumonia, suppurative rhinitis, and occasionally otitis media. Chattering and dyspnea are caused by accumulations of purulent exudate in inflamed and thickened nasal passages. Survivors often develop chronic bronchopneumonia, bronchiectasis, and pulmonary abscesses. Antibiotic therapy may alleviate clinical signs but does not eliminate the infection.

Viral Infections: Viral diseases of mice and rats are common. However, most diseases are subclinical and important only in laboratory animals in which they have the potential to have a significant effect on research.

Sialodacryoadenitis virus, a coronavirus, causes inflammation and edema of the cervical salivary glands in rats. Owners of infected rats often describe their pets as having mumps. Sialodacryoadenitis virus infection is highly contagious. It initially causes rhinitis followed by epithelial necrosis and inflammatory swelling of the salivary and lacrimal glands. Cervical lymph nodes also become enlarged. There is no treatment for this disease. Glandular healing follows within 7–10 days, and clinical signs subside within 30 days, with minimal residual lesions remaining. During acute inflammation, affected rats are at high risk of anesthesia-related mortality because of the decreased diameter of the upper respiratory tract lumen. Ocular lesions such as conjunctivitis, keratitis, corneal ulcers, synechia, and hyphema can develop secondary to lacrimal dysfunction. The eye lesions usually resolve but occasionally progress to chronic keratitis and megaglobus.

Parasitic Infections:

Protozoa: Endoparasites are relatively common in mice. However, only two parasites regularly encountered in the digestive tract, the protozoan parasites *Spironucleus muris* and *Giardia muris*, are considered pathogenic, even though they are not associated with clinical signs in immunocompetent hosts. Diagnosis is based on demonstration of characteristic trophozoites in wet mounts of fresh intestinal contents or feces. Treatment is metronidazole (10–40 mg/kg/day, PO, or 0.04%–0.1% drinking water solution for 14 days), but it does not completely eliminate the infection.

Nematodes: Pinworms are ubiquitous and considered nonpathogenic in mice. Two are commonly encountered: *Syphacia obvelata* and *Aspicularis tetraptera*. Often, the only indication of pinworm infestation is rectal prolapse due to straining. To establish a diagnosis of *S obvelata* infestation, a clear cellophane tape impression of the perianal skin can be made. Adult *S obvelata* females deposit ova around the anus. *A tetraptera* does not deposit its ova in this area, and fecal smear or flotation is required to confirm a diagnosis. Ivermectin (2 mg/kg, PO, given twice at a 10-day interval) eliminates pinworms from mice. The recommended label dosage for mice with ectoparasites (0.2 mg/kg, given twice at a 10-day interval) does not eliminate pinworms.

Mites: Most infectious causes of alopecia and dermatitis in mice are associated with fur mites. Generalized thinning of the hair, especially on difficult-to-groom areas such as the head and trunk, is seen. The coat often has a greasy appearance and, in cases of heavy infestation, noticeable pruritus and self-inflicted dermal ulceration may occur. Three mites are commonly seen: *Myobia musculi*, *Myocoptes musculinus*, and *Radfordia affinis*. *M musculi* is the most clinically significant mouse mite. Infestations are usually caused by more than one species. Mites are spread by direct contact with infected mice or infested bedding. Diagnosis is based on identification of adult mites, nymphs, or eggs on hair shafts with the use of a hand lens or stereoscopic microscope. Adults and nymphs appear pearly white and elongate; eggs are oval and can be seen attached to the base of hairs or inside mature females. Mite infestations are treated with ivermectin (0.2 mg/kg, SC or PO, twice at 10-day intervals). Alternatively, a few drops of ivermectin solution (diluted to 1:100 in equal parts of water and propylene glycol for three treatments) can be placed on the mouse's head to allow spread by grooming and ingestion.

Ectoparasitic infestation is less common in rats than in mice. Occasionally, the fur mite *Radfordia ensifera* is seen. Although *R ensifera* infestation produces few ill effects, heavy infestation may lead to self-trauma and ulcerative dermatitis.

Ornithonyssus bacoti, the tropical rat mite or red mite, is a bloodsucking parasitic mite primarily found in wild rats such as the brown rat (*Rattus norvegicus*) or the black roof rat (*Rattus rattus*). It has a wide host range and occasionally infects pet hamsters, gerbils, rats, and mice living in very old buildings or when building construction or renovations disturb colonies of wild rodents that had been on the premises and acting as hosts. *O bacoti* can survive for long periods in the environment and travel considerable distances in search of new hosts. If it does not find a suitable rodent host, it will feed on people. Its common name is a misnomer, because it is found worldwide in tropical and temperate climates. Mites appear white before feeding and become red-brown after engorgement. Heavy infestations on pet rodents resemble fine sawdust within the fur. *O bacoti* typically does not cause clinical signs in pet rodents, but heavy infestations cause anemia, debility, weakness, pruritus, and death in small rodents. As well as causing discomfort, the mite is a vector for the rodent filarial nematode *Litomosoides carinii* and a potential vector of several human pathogens. Most infestations occur in late spring or early summer when fledglings are leaving the nest and the mites are searching for another food source. Infestation of *O bacoti* is eliminated by a combination of bathing and treating the host animal with selamectin (15 mg/kg, one topical treatment), elimination of commensal rodent reservoirs, and insecticide treatment of the pet's cage (permethrin-impregnated cotton balls 7.4% placed inside the cage weekly for 6 wk) and environment (fipronil spray or synthetic pyrethroids).

Fungal Infections: Dermatophytosis is uncommon in pet mice and rats. It is caused by *Trichophyton mentagrophytes*. Lesions, when present, are most common on the face, head, neck, and tail. The lesions have a scurfy appearance, with patchy areas of alopecia and variable degrees of erythema and crusting. Pruritus is usually minimal to absent, and the lesions do not fluoresce under a Wood's lamp. *T mentagrophytes* can be isolated from the fur of clinically normal mice but is rare in rats.

Neoplasia

The most common subcutaneous tumor in rats is fibroadenoma of the mammary glands. The distribution of the mammary tissue is extensive, and the tumors can develop anywhere from the neck to inguinal region. Tumors can reach 8–10 cm in diameter and are seen in both males and females. The surgical technique for tumor removal is straightforward, and survival after mastectomy has been reported to be good if the tumor is benign. The prevalence of mammary tumors, as well as that of pituitary tumors, is significantly lower in ovariectomized rats than in sexually intact rats. However, the recurrence of fibroadenomas is common in uninvolved mammary tissue, and often several surgeries are needed.

In contrast, mammary tumors in mice are nearly always malignant and often are not amenable to surgical removal. The most common spontaneous tumors associated with the skin are mammary adenocarcinomas, followed by fibrosarcomas. The incidence of mammary tumors varies according to the mouse strain and the presence or absence of mouse mammary tumor viruses; the incidence is as high as 70% in some strains. In wild and outbred mice, the incidence of fibrosarcomas is 1%–6%.

Subcutaneous tumors are nearly always malignant and often have ulcerated by the time a diagnosis is made. Tumors can be treated by surgical excision, but the chance of recurrence is high and the prognosis is poor.

Miscellaneous and Iatrogenic Disorders

Dental Overgrowth: Dental problems are commonly seen in pet mice and rats because of their continually erupting teeth. Overgrown incisors are seen most frequently in rats and mice, in contrast with molar occlusion seen in guinea pigs and chinchillas. Overgrowth is easily treated with a high-speed drill that cuts through the overgrown incisors without splitting or splintering them, leaving a clean, smooth surface. Cutting the teeth with rongeurs does not produce good longterm results, and problems may arise. The incisor may fracture longitudinally; the fracture may reach the apex and cause the animal discomfort. Bacteria can enter the fractured tooth, track down to the apex, and cause an apical abscess. Extraction of the incisors is an alternative to trimming; however, this procedure is difficult because of the incisors' long roots.

Age-related Disorders: Chronic progressive nephrosis is a common age-related disease in rats. The kidneys are enlarged, pale, and have a pitted, mottled surface that often contains pinpoint cysts. Lesions consist of a progressive glomerulosclerosis and widespread tubulointerstitial disease, primarily involving the proximal convoluted tubule. Proteinuria often is >10 mg/day. The disease occurs earlier and is of greater severity in males than in females. Dietary factors appear to have an important role in the progression of renal disease. Caloric restriction, the feeding of low-protein diets (4%–7%), and limiting the source of dietary protein reduce the incidence and severity of the disease. Treatment is supportive and involves feeding a low-protein diet.

Avascular necrosis of the tail, or ringtail, is seen primarily in young rats, and occasionally in young mice, kept in low-humidity environments. If ringtail is diagnosed, treatment involves amputation of the tail below the necrotic annular constriction.

Skin Disease in Mice: Most of the diseases seen in pet mice are associated with the skin and represent >25% of all cases. Behavioral disorders, husbandry-related problems, microbiologic/parasitic infections, and idiopathic skin diseases are seen. Behavioral, husbandry-related, and infectious causes of skin disease are relatively straightforward to diagnose and treat. However, many skin diseases characterized by chronic or ulcerated skin (often secondarily colonized by bacteria) are diagnosed as idiopathic. This group is commonly unresponsive to treatment, topical or systemic, and affected mice are often euthanized.

Barbering and fighting are manifestations of social dominance, a form of behavior relating to the social rank and dominance status of an individual mouse in a group. Barbering is a unique condition seen in group-housed mice in which the dominant mouse nibbles off the whiskers and hair around the muzzle and eyes of cagemates. There are no other lesions, and only one mouse, the dominant individual, retains all of its fur. Removal of the dominant mouse stops barbering; frequently, however, another mouse assumes the dominant role. Barbering is often seen in female mice caged together. Male mice, except littermates raised together from birth, are more likely to fight, often very savagely, and inflict severe bite wounds on one another, especially over the rump, tail, and shoulders.

Mechanical abrasion resulting from self-trauma on cage equipment is a form of husbandry-related alopecia. Small patches of alopecia appear on the lateral surfaces of the muzzle. They result from chafing on metal feeders, poorly constructed watering device openings, and metal cage tops. Unlike barbering, dermatitis may also be associated with alopecia. Treatment consists of replacing the poorly constructed equipment with nonabrading equipment. Individually housed mice can display aberrant stereotypic behavior such as polydipsia and bar chewing that results in mechanical abrasion and alopecia. In these cases with one mouse, replacing the cage equipment does not help. Instead, environmental enrichment toys such as running wheels or hollow tubes should be provided. Nursing mice often have ventral abdominal and thoracic alopecia; this is normal and is nearly always associated with the extensive distribution of mammary glands.

Sometimes a pet mouse presents with clinical signs of mite infestation but no evidence of mites or known history of recent exposure to other animals. Biopsy samples may be useful in these cases to distinguish active acariasis from dermal hypersensitivity to mites or other allergens such as timber chip bedding. Dermal hypersensitivity is well described in certain inbred strains of mice and is characterized by severe pruritus, the presence of fine dandruff all over the body, and occasionally ulcerative dermatitis.

Idiopathic skin disease is characterized by ulcerative dermatitis with pruritus in mice that are negative for primary ectoparasitic, bacterial, or mycotic infections. Histopathologic examination and immunofluorescent microscopy of selected inbred strains of mice have revealed an underlying vasculitis attributed to immune complex deposition on dermal vessels. Dietary factors and dysregulated fatty acid metabolism have been implicated in the development of the ulcerative dermatitis in these mice. This common disease of mice of a C57BL6 background is caused by an underlying immune-mediated vasculitis, and the severity appears to be modulated by dietary fat and vitamin E content. Topical treatment twice daily with 0.2% cyclosporine in 2% lidocaine gel supplemented with gentamicin at 50 mcg/mL results in either complete healing or near-complete healing of the ulcerated skin, regardless of the size of the skin ulceration.

Skin swellings in mice are usually tumors or abscesses. Needle biopsy often reveals the nature of the contents and allows diagnosis. Three opportunistic pathogens, *Staphylococcus aureus*, *Pasteurella pneumotropica*, and *Streptococcus pyogenes*, are isolated frequently and can cause abscesses in other organs. Antibiotic therapy with penicillins or cephalosporins, concurrent with drainage and debridement of the abscess, is effective.

Chromodacryorrhea in Rats: The Harderian glands of rats are located behind the eyes and secrete porphyrins that are increased in response to stress and disease, coloring the tears red. When porphyrin-enriched tear fluid dries around the eyes and external nares, it resembles crusts of blood. Owners often describe their rats as hemorrhaging from the eyes and nose. The porphyrins can be readily differentiated from blood with a Wood's lamp, because they fluoresce under ultraviolet light. Although chromodacryorrhea is not pathologic, it is a consequence of acute-onset stress such as that caused by pain, illness, or restraint. It usually indicates a chronic underlying disease.

Zoonotic Risk

As rats have become popular as pets, children now account for >50% of the cases of rat bite fever (RBF) in the USA; 14% of RBF cases in children involved exposure to a rat at school. RBF manifests as a bacteremia and septicemia characterized by fever, chills, myalgia, arthralgia, headache, and vomiting. A petechial rash develops over the extremities, in particular the palms and soles, but sometimes is present all over the body. The incubation period is 3–10 days (average 5 days). Infants and children may experience severe diarrhea resulting in weight loss. Mortality occurs in 7%–13% of untreated patients. After infection, a polyarthritis develops in 50%–70% of patients. Prognosis is good with treatment with parenteral penicillin early in the disease. Fatalities are associated with late reporting or late recognition of the disease. The nonspecific initial presentation combined with difficulties in culturing *Streptococcus moniliformis* produce a significant risk of delay or failure in diagnosis. Rats are not recommended as pets for children. Adults with pet rats should practice regular handwashing and avoid hand-to-mouth contact when handling rats or cleaning rat cages.

There are sporadic but persistent reports of cases of *Ornithonyssus bacoti* dermatitis from pet rodents that manifests as an erythematous papular rash. It often excoriates because of intense pruritus. Occasionally, vesicles, urticarial plaques, diffuse erythema, or hemorrhage are seen. Affected areas of the skin are those usually covered by clothing (such as arms and trunk), with the face and webs of fingers usually spared. There is considerable evidence that *O bacoti* carry and have the potential to transmit several human pathogens. Experiments have shown that *O bacoti* transmits *Rickettsia akari* (rickettsialpox), *Yersinia pestis* (plague), Coxsackie virus, *Francisella tularensis* (tularemia), and *Trypanosoma cruzi* (Chagas' disease). Researchers have also documented *O bacoti* specimens with *Coxiella burnetii* (Q fever), hantavirus, *Borrelia* spp (Lyme disease), *Bartonella* spp, and *Rickettsia* spp.

Mice are inapparent carriers of dermatophytes, and pet mice are a zoonotic risk for their owners, especially children.

MICE AND RATS AS LABORATORY ANIMALS

Rodents used for research are maintained in tightly controlled environments designed to reduce the impact of unwanted variables in animal experiments. Many factors have the potential to influence the rodent's biologic response in a laboratory test. Besides a description of the experiment, research journals often require a description of the research rodent's source, microbiologic status, and environment (eg, feed, water, temperature, humidity, light exposure) in the materials and methods section. Environmental conditions, husbandry procedures, and animals must be similar if research data generated from one laboratory is to be judged based on reproducibility and thus validation. If variables such as feed, housing, rodent genetic background and disease-free or microbiologic status are not properly controlled, then experimental results can be of limited use or even worthless. Although complete elimination of variables in animal experiments is not possible, many factors that contribute to variation can be significantly reduced or eliminated. One of the most important variables is the effect of infectious agents on research mice and rats.

Few infectious agents found in laboratory mice and rats today cause overt, clinical disease. Distinguishing between infection and disease is critical to interpreting the microbiologic status of laboratory animals. Infection indicates the presence of microorganisms, which may be pathogens, opportunists, or commensals, of which the last two are most numerous. Clinical disease does not need to be present for microorganisms to affect research. Animals that appear normal and healthy may be unsuitable as research subjects because of the unobservable but significant local or systemic effects of viruses, bacteria, and parasites with which they may be infected.

Knowledge of the varied and unwanted effects of natural pathogens in laboratory rodents has steadily increased over the past 130 years of conducting animal research. The historic struggle against pathogens of laboratory rodents is often divided into three periods. The first (1880–1950) was when mice and rats became common research animals. Many of these original stocks harbored a variety of natural, or indigenous, pathogens. During this period, improvements were made in sanitation, nutrition, environmental control, and other aspects of animal husbandry. The result was a great reduction in the range and prevalence of pathogens found in laboratory rodents. The second period (1950–1980) was one of gnotobiotic derivation, when cesarean rederivation was used to replace infected stock with uninfected offspring. Full-term fetuses were removed from an infected mother and transferred to a germ-free environment and foster care. This procedure was successful in eliminating many pathogens not transmissible in utero, eg, endoparasites, most bacteria, and some viruses. The third period (1980– present) has been one of eradicating indigenous rodent viruses. The reduction in known viruses infecting rodents was accomplished through serologic testing of animals for antibodies to specific pathogens. Antibody-positive colonies were subsequently eliminated or cesarean-rederived.

Most modern research animal facilities incorporate some form of health monitoring into their animal care program (*see* TABLE 32). Since the 1980s, it has been based on serology, although molecular methods of detection (eg, PCR) are rapidly increasing in use. The laboratories that perform serologic assays primarily test groups of research rodents or their samples. The well-being of the animal colony is more important than the well-being of an individual animal, and laboratory animal medicine is effectively a type of "herd medicine." Although health monitoring is costly, it results in significant longterm savings, because researchers can use fewer animals and the animals' daily care is not as labor intensive. Health monitoring allows laboratory animal veterinarians to check the health status of a colony, inform researchers of their animals' pathogen status, prevent entry of pathogens into the facility by screening animals received from unknown sources, and promptly deal with the presence of unexpected infectious agents in rodents. Undetected infection makes laboratory animals unfit for research and renders experimental data unreliable. It is more cost-effective to prevent entry of infectious agents into a facility or to detect and eliminate them early than to discard months of research data.

TABLE 32 INFECTIOUS AGENTS COMMONLY TESTED FOR IN LABORATORY RODENTS

Test	Agent	Description	Species
		PROTOZOA	
E cun	*Encephalitozoon cuniculi*	A sporozoan parasite of rabbits and rodents	Mice, rats
		BACTERIA	
C pil	*Clostridium piliforme*	Agent of Tyzzer disease	Mice, rats

TABLE 32 INFECTIOUS AGENTS COMMONLY TESTED FOR IN LABORATORY RODENTS *(continued)*

Test	Agent	Description	Species
CARB	Cilia-associated–respiratory bacillus	A bacterial respiratory pathogen of rodents and rabbits	Mice, rats
M pul	*Mycoplasma pulmonis*	Agent of mouse and rat pulmonary mycoplasmosis	Mice, rats
	VIRUSES		
ECT	Ectromelia	A mouse poxvirus	Mice
TH-1	Toolan's H-1 virus	A rat parvovirus	Rats
	Hantaan virus	A zoonotic hantavirus of rats; several types (HPS, NED) exist throughout world	Rats
K-virus	Mouse pneumonitis virus	A mouse papovavirus	Mice
KRV	Kilham rat virus	A rat parvovirus	Rats
LCM	Lymphocytic choriomeningitis virus	A zoonotic arenavirus	Mice, rats
LDEV	Lactate dehydrogenase–elevating virus	A mouse arterivirus	Mice
MAD1 (FL)	Rodent adenovirus strain 1	Mouse adenovirus, rodent adenovirus strain 1 (FL)	Mice, rats
MAD2 (K87)	Rodent adenovirus strain 2	Mouse adenovirus, rodent adenovirus strain 2 (K87)	Mice
MCMV	Mouse cytomegalovirus	A mouse herpesvirus	Mice
MHV	Mouse hepatitis virus	A mouse coronavirus	Mice
MNV	Murine norovirus	A mouse calicivirus	Mice
MPV	Mouse parvovirus	A mouse parvovirus	Mice
MTV	Mouse thymic virus	A mouse herpesvirus	Mice
MVM (MMV)	Minute virus of mice	A mouse parvovirus	Mice
PolyVM	Polyoma virus of mice	A mouse papovavirus	Mice
PVM	Pneumonia virus of mice	A rodent pneumovirus	Mice, rats
SDAV	Sialodacryoadenitis virus	A rat coronavirus	Rats
Reo3	Reovirus type 3	A rodent reovirus	Mice, rats
SenV	Sendai virus	A type 1 paramyxovirus	Mice, rats
RTV	Rat theilovirus	A rat picornavirus	Rats
TMEV (GDVII)	Theiler murine encephalomyelitis virus	Mouse poliovirus, strain GDVII	Mice

SUGAR GLIDERS

Sugar gliders (*Petaurus breviceps*) are small, nocturnal marsupials native to Australia, Indonesia, and New Guinea that live in eucalyptus and acacia forests. They belong to the family Petauridae, which includes the wrist-winged gliders. Gliders in this family possess a gliding membrane (patagium) that runs from the wrist of the forelimb to the ankle of the hindlimb and that allows them to glide as far as 50 m and forage for food using less energy. They use their tails as stabilizing rudders that enable them to change direction easily. The second and third toes on their hindfeet are fused to form a "grooming comb" that helps them clean their fur. Females are seasonally polyestrous and have a double vagina, two uteri, and a pouch containing four teats; they often have twin births. After 16 days of gestation, the young (joeys), each weighing only 0.2 g, migrate to the pouch to develop further and finally leave the pouch after 70–74 days. They remain in the nest until 110–120 days of age, when they are weaned. They stay with the colony until 7–10 mo old. Males have a forked penis (to match the female's double vagina) and a pendulous scrotum containing two testicles. Males do not urinate from the forked end of the penis but from the proximal end. Both males and females have paracloacal scent glands adjacent to the vent (the cloacal opening or common opening of urinary, reproductive, and GI tracts) with which they mark territory and each other, and males also have frontal scent glands on their foreheads and glands on their throats and chests. Sparse fur and an oily discharge are normal on the frontal and sternal glands of post-pubescent males. These glands give both sexes a musky odor.

Forked penis of a male sugar glider. *Courtesy of Dr. Laurie Hess.*

Sugar gliders have large, protruding, widely spaced eyes, giving them a wide field of vision, especially at night. Their ears move independently and are highly sensitive to sound. They also have a great sense of smell to locate food, sense predators, and recognize both their territory and their colony-mates. Wild gliders have gray fur and a central black stripe dorsally on their heads; domesticated gliders may look similar to the wild type but also come in several color variations. Sugar gliders are polygamous, territorial, and live in colonies of 5 to 12 individuals with a dominant male. They sleep in tree hollows by day and between foraging trips at night. They tolerate a wide range of environmental temperatures and go into torpor to conserve energy in very cold conditions. Sugar gliders are omnivorous and feed on sugar-rich plant and insect exudates (sap, gum, nectar, manna, pollen) and invertebrates as a source of protein. They are hindgut fermenters and possess a well-developed cecum that utilizes bacterial fermentation to break down complex polysaccharides contained in gum. *See also* TABLE 33, which summarizes important biologic and physiologic data for sugar gliders.

Physical Examination: For a full clinical examination, anesthesia with isoflurane via face mask may be required if gliders are very stressed or biting. More docile animals may be examined while wrapped in a small towel and cupped in the palm of the hand. Gliders inside fabric bags or pouches may be partially exposed, one body part at a time, for examination. Because gliders are nocturnal, it may be best to schedule clinical examinations earlier in the day when they are less active. If possible, the animal should be first observed moving in its cage to assess posture, coordination, and demeanor. If the glider is anesthetized, cloacal temperature, heart rate, and respiration rate can be recorded, and the heart and lungs assessed with a pediatric stethoscope. The fur and skin should be examined for ectoparasites, traumatic injury, fur loss, and degree of hydration; the oral cavity for broken teeth, dental abscesses, or tartar build up; and the eyes

TABLE 33 SELECTED PHYSIOLOGIC DATA FOR SUGAR GLIDERS

Life span	9–12 yr
Adult male body wt	100–160 g
Adult female body wt	80–135 g
Respiratory rate	16–40/min
Heart rate	200–300 bpm
Body temperature	97.3°F (36.3°C)
Thermoneutral zone	80°–88°F (27°–31°C)
Food consumption	15%–20% body wt/day
Dentition	Diprotodont
Dental formula	2(I 3/1-2 C 1/0 P 3/3 M 4/4)
Puberty	8–12 mo in females, 12–15 mo in males
Estrous cycle	29 days
Gestation period	15–17 days
Litter size	2 (81%)
Birth weight	0.2 g
Pouch emergence	70–74 days
Weaning	110–120 days

and ears for any abnormalities. The cloacal area should be examined, and the penis of males extruded. The abdomen should be palpated, and the pouch in females examined. Major joints should also be palpated, and digits and toenails checked for evidence of trauma.

Diagnostic and Treatment Techniques: If animals are dehydrated, isotonic fluids up to 10% of body wt can be administered SC over the shoulder region. Care should be taken not to induce edema to the patagium. Fluids also may be administered intraosseously in the proximal femur or tibia. SC injections may be given in the same area that SC fluids are administered. IM injections may be given in the epaxial muscles of the neck and dorsal thorax. IV injections are very difficult to perform but may be accomplished in cephalic or lateral saphenous veins in an anesthetized glider.

Radiographs generally require the glider be anesthetized for proper positioning. Pulmonary diseases are easiest to detect with radiographs. Feces may be easily sampled and checked annually with a fecal float and direct smear for parasites; animals with diarrhea should have their feces cultured and tested for appropriate antibiotic sensitivity.

Blood Collection, Hematology, and Biochemistry: Reference ranges for sugar gliders are presented in TABLE 34. Chemical restraint, essential to allow blood collection, is most safely achieved with isoflurane/oxygen administered via mask and T-piece. To assist in making clinical diagnoses, blood samples may be obtained from the cranial vena cava, jugular vein, medial tibial artery, or lateral tail vein. Blood volumes of up to 1% of body wt can be collected; typically 0.5–1 mL is obtained. To access the cranial vena cava, a 27- or 25-gauge needle on an insulin syringe may be inserted in the thoracic inlet just lateral to the manubrium, with the needle directed at a 30° angle from midline toward the opposite hindleg. The vena cava is not visualized directly during venipuncture but is accessed blindly using the manubrium as a palpable landmark. The jugular vein can be visualized if the hair is clipped and the vein is forced to fill by applying gentle digital pressure at the thoracic inlet; it sits midway between the point of the shoulder and the mandibular ramus. The needle can be bent at its base to facilitate venipuncture at this site. The medial tibial artery, which runs very superficially just distal and medial to the stifle joint, is easier to access and can be sampled with a 27- or 25-gauge needle and 0.5–1 mL syringe.

Pressure after sampling is required to prevent hematoma formation. The size of the lateral tail vein is most suited to skin prick and droplet collection into capillary tubes. Small blood samples (0.25 mL) may also be obtained from the cephalic, lateral saphenous, femoral, and ventral coccygeal veins with a 27-gauge needle on an insulin syringe.

Anesthesia and Surgery: Anesthesia in sugar gliders should be approached the same way it is in other small mammals. Gliders ideally should be fasted for at least 4 hr preoperatively. Preoperative analgesics, sedatives to reduce preoperative stress, and local and gas anesthetics all may be used. Care must be taken to keep gliders warm during surgery to ensure rapid recovery. Gliders undergoing surgeries that last >1 hr or that require intra-abdominal access should be administered fluids intraosseously (in the femur or tibia) throughout the procedure if IV access is impossible because of small size. Shorter, simple

TABLE 34 SELECTED HEMATOLOGIC AND SERUM BIOCHEMICAL VALUES FOR SUGAR GLIDERS

	Conventional (USA) Units	SI Units
HEMATOLOGY		
Hemoglobin	13–15 g/dL	130–150 g/L
Hematocrit	45%–53%	0.45–0.53 L/L
RBCs	5.1–7.2 × 10^6/μL	5.1–7.2 × 10^{12}/L
Mean corpuscular Hgb concentration	30–33 g/dL	300–330 g/L
Mean corpuscular Hgb	18.2–20.6 pg	18.2–20.6 pg
WBCs	5–12.2 × 10^3/μL	5–12.2 × 10^9/L
Neutrophils	1.5–3 × 10^3/μL	1.5–3 × 10^9/L
Lymphocytes	2.8–9.2 × 10^3/μL	2.8–9.2 × 10^9/L
Monocytes	0.06–0.2 × 10^3/μL	0.06–0.2 × 10^9/L
Eosinophils	0.02–0.14 × 10^3/μL	0.02–0.14 × 10^9/L
Basophils	0	0
Plasma proteins	5.6–6.9 g/dL	56–69 g/L
Albumin	3–3.5 g/dL	30–35 g/L
Globulin	2.2–3.6 g/dL	22–36 g/L
BIOCHEMISTRY		
ALT	50–106 U/L	50–106 U/L
AST	46–179 U/L	46–179 U/L
Calcium	6.9–8.4 mg/dL	1.7–2.1 mmol/L
CK	210–589 U/L	210–589 U/L
Creatinine	0.2–0.5 mg/dL	17.7–44.2 μmol/L
Glucose	130–183 mg/dL	7.2–10 mmol/L
Phosphorus	3.8–4.4 mg/dL	1.2–1.4 mmol/L
Potassium	3.3–5.9 mEq/L	3.3–5.9 mmol/L
Sodium	135–145 mEq/L	135–145 mmol/L
Urea	18–24 mg/dL	6.4–8.6 mmol/L

procedures may necessitate only SC fluids. Commonly used preanesthetics include atropine or glycopyrrolate, midazolam, and either butorphanol or buprenorphine. Local anesthetic injections of a 50:50 mixture of 2% lidocaine with 5% bupivicaine may be used to infiltrate the incision site to help reduce the chance of postoperative self-mutilation. To facilitate castration, this mixture may be diluted with sterile water and infused into the base of the scrotal stalk nearest to the abdomen, while a low concentration of gas anesthetic is administered. Both isoflurane and sevoflurane may be administered via small face mask or via a large face mask used as an induction chamber. For surgery, gliders may be maintained on gas anesthesia with a face mask or intubated with a 1-mm Cook endotracheal tube threaded with a stylet.

During surgery, blood loss should be monitored carefully; use of radiosurgery may help minimize bleeding. Because sugar gliders tend to chew incisions after surgery, ideally subcuticular sutures and skin glue should be used to close skin incisions. Analgesics should be administered before surgery to minimize pain immediately after surgery. Gliders should recover from surgery in temperature-controlled incubators.

Orchiectomy and scrotal ablation are commonly performed on male sugar gliders to prevent breeding and decrease sexual frustration. Hair is clipped around the base of the scrotal sac and stalk, and the skin is cleaned without alcohol so as not to lower body temperature. A local anesthetic is administered at the base of the stalk, and with the glider under gas anesthesia, the incision is made over the scrotal stalk ~2–3 mm from the body wall. The spermatic cords are exposed by blunt dissection and are clamped and ligated with 5-0 polydioxanone suture or cut and cauterized with radiosurgery. The scrotal sac containing the testicles and distal spermatic cord is then removed, and the ligated stalk can be sutured to the abdominal wall fascia to prevent herniation. The skin is then closed with tissue glue. Standard ovariohysterectomy is not routinely performed because of the internal position of the female reproductive organs, which are difficult to access beneath the pouch. With ovariohysterectomy, the area around the pouch is clipped and scrubbed in a routine manner, and a 1–2 mm incision is made paramedian to the pouch. The linea alba is bluntly dissected and incised, and the bladder is exteriorized from the incision to reveal the ovaries beneath. The ovarian arteries are ligated, as is the uterus proximally to the lateral vaginal canals. After resection of both ovaries and uteri, the linea is closed, and the skin is sutured subcuticularly and closed with skin glue. Distal penile amputation is another common surgery. Sexually frustrated males may self-mutilate the distal end of their penises or develop paraphimosis. Because males urinate only from the proximal end, the distal, forked segment may be safely amputated. Other surgeries performed in sugar gliders include cystotomy to remove uroliths, urethrostomy to alleviate urinary tract obstruction from uroliths in males, and surgical removal of impacted paracloacal glands. The skin over impacted glands is infiltrated with a small volume of local anesthetic and incised; the gland is bluntly dissected and removed without rupturing it. The blood vessel supplying the gland may be ligated with 5-0 or 6-0 polydioxanone or cut and cauterized with radiosurgery. The skin is closed with tissue glue.

Drug Dosages: Very few pharmacologic studies have been performed in sugar gliders, and most published drug dosages have been extrapolated from those determined for cats, ferrets, and hedgehogs. For drugs and dosages commonly used in sugar gliders, *see* TABLE 35.

Nutrition and Housing: Ideally, sugar gliders should be maintained as a group with one male and a number of females. If breeding occurs, the young should be removed soon after weaning, or violent attempts to disperse them may occur. Because sugar gliders are arboreal (tree-dwelling), a large cage (ideally of PVC-coated stainless steel) is best for nocturnal climbing. As large a cage as possible should be provided with a minimum size of 36 × 24 × 36 in. Bar spacing should not be more than 1 × 0.5 in. wide, or feet and heads may become entrapped. Caging containing vertical bars should be avoided, because vertical bars do not facilitate climbing. A wooden nest box (made for birds) or a fabric pouch positioned high up in the cage should be provided for hiding and sleeping. Cages should contain numerous branches (commercially available for bird cages) and horizontal shelves to promote climbing. Swings and chew toys made for birds are ideal for gliders to play with. Exercise wheels containing smooth interiors (so as not to entrap toes) should be provided for physical and mental stimulation. The cage bottom may be covered with newspaper or other

TABLE 35 COMMONLY USED DRUGS IN SUGAR GLIDERS

Drug	Dosage	Considerations
	ANTIBIOTICS	
Amoxicillin	30 mg/kg, PO or IM, once daily or divided bid	For dermatitis
Amoxicillin-clavulanic acid	12.5 mg/kg/day, PO	Broad-spectrum against anaerobes and aerobes
Cephalexin	30 mg/kg/day, PO	
Enrofloxacin	2.5–5 mg/kg, PO or IM, once or twice daily	Potential tissue necrosis when injected
Gentamicin	1.5–2.5 mg/kg, SC, IM, IV, bid	Nephrotoxic
Metronidazole	25 mg/kg/day, PO	
Penicillin	22,000–25,000 IU/kg, once or twice daily	
Sulfadimethoxine	5–10 mg/kg, PO, once or twice daily	Ensure hydrated
Trimethoprim/sulfa	10–20 mg/kg, PO, once or twice daily	
	ANTIPARASITICS	
Carbaryl 5% powder	Topically or in cage	Use small amounts to treat ectoparasites
Fenbendazole	20–50 mg/kg/day, PO, × 3 days	For roundworms, hookworms, whipworms, tapeworms
Ivermectin	0.2 mg/kg, PO, SC; repeat in 14 days	For roundworms, hookworms, whipworms, mites
Metronidazole	25 mg/kg/day × 3 days; repeat in 14 days	For intestinal protozoa
Piperazine	100 mg/kg, PO	
Pyrethrin powder	Topically	For ectoparasites
Selamectin	6–8 mg/kg, topically; repeat in 30 days	For ectoparasites
	ANTIFUNGALS	
Itraconazole	5–10 mg/kg, PO, bid	
Nystatin	5,000 IU/kg, tid × 3 days	For *Candida*
	ANALGESICS	
Acepromazine/butorphanol	1.7 mg/kg/1.7 mg/kg, PO	Postoperative analgesic and sedative to decrease self-mutilation of incision
Buprenorphine	0.01–0.03 mg/kg, PO or SC, bid	
Butorphanol	0.1–0.5 mg/kg, SC or IM, every 6–8 hr	
Meloxicam	0.1–0.2 mg/kg/day, PO or SC	Anti-inflammatory

TABLE 35 COMMONLY USED DRUGS IN SUGAR GLIDERS *(continued)*

Drug	Dosage	Considerations
	PREANESTHETICS	
Atropine	0.02–0.04 mg/kg, IM, SC, IV	To lessen intraoperative secretions
Glycopyrrolate	0.01–0.02 mg/kg, IM, SC, IV	To lessen intraoperative secretions
	ANESTHETICS	
Diazepam	0.5–2 mg/kg, PO, IM, IV	Sedative, anticonvulsant
Isoflurane	1%–5%	Via face mask or intubation
Ketamine	30–50 mg/kg, IM	
Ketamine/medetomidine	2–3 mg/kg/0.05-0.1 mg/kg, IM	Immobilization
Ketamine/midazolam	10–20 mg/kg/0.35–0.5 mg/kg, IM	Give ketamine 10 min after midazolam
Midazolam	0.25–0.5 mg/kg, IM or IV	Sedative, anxiolytic
Sevoflurane	1%–5%	Via face mask or intubation; possible toxicity, use cautiously
	CARDIAC DRUGS	
Enalapril	0.22–0.44 mg/kg/day, PO	
Furosemide	1–4 mg/kg, SC or IM, every 6–12 hr	Diuretic
	GI DRUGS	
Cisapride	0.25 mg/kg, PO, once to three times a day	GI motility enhancer
Metaclopramide	0.05–0.1 mg/kg, PO, bid–qid	GI motility enhancer
	HORMONES	
Calcitonin	50–100 IU/kg, SC or IM	Helps mobilize calcium
Prednisolone	0.1-0.2 mg/kg/day, PO, SC, IM	Corticosteroid
	VITAMINS	
Calcium glubionate	150 mg/kg/day, PO	Calcium supplement
Vitamin A	500–5,000 IU/kg, IM, once	For dermatitis
Vitamin E	25–100 IU/glider/day	
Vitamin K	2 mg/kg, SC, every 1–3 days	Intestinal and liver disease

recycled paper product that is nontoxic if ingested. Several food and water bowls should be provided throughout the cage, with designated areas for eating, drinking, exercising, and hiding.

The recommended diet for captive sugar gliders includes calcium-loaded insects (crickets, mealworms, waxworms, cockroaches, moths) to promote dental health, as well as a daily nectar/sap substitute (eg, fructose/sucrose/glucose or honey diluted to 10% with water). Nectar should account for ~50% of the diet. Several nectar substitutes are commercially available, including Gliderade nectar supplement (Exotic Pet Nutrition Company, Newport

News, VA), acacia gum powder, and nectar diets meant for lory birds. Other protein sources in addition to insects include eggs, lean meat, newborn mice, and commercial pelleted diets meant for sugar gliders. Commercial diets or homemade insectivore or omnivore mixes should be provided in addition to live food, with insects and pelleted food accounting for nearly 50% of the total diet. Fruits, nuts, and vegetables should be offered only in moderation (<10% of total diet), because many fruits and vegetables lack essential vitamins, minerals, and protein and contain mostly water. Several commercial diets and recipes for homemade diets are available; no single diet studied has yet proved to be ideal for captive sugar gliders. Traditionally, before the availability of commercial pelleted diets, a homemade formula called Leadbeater's mixture was fed successfully in addition to insects, fruits, and vegetables. The mixture contains 150 mL of warm water mixed with 150 mL of honey, one hard-boiled shelled egg, one teaspoon of multivitamin/mineral supplement, and 25 g of high-protein dry human infant cereal. An alternative to the homemade Leadbeater's diet is commercially available High Protein Wombaroo Diet (Wombaroo Food Products, Glen Osmond, South Australia), a powdered protein supplement that is mixed with water before feeding. In addition, if not provided in the diet, a multivitamin and mineral supplement with calcium should be sprinkled on food daily. Food should be offered in the evening, when sugar gliders are active, on an elevated platform, because gliders feel more secure eating up high, as they would in trees in the wild. Sugar gliders are generally robust in captivity when proper husbandry practices are followed; however, nutritional deficiencies, especially of calcium and protein, are commonly seen in captive gliders fed inappropriately. Obesity also is common in gliders fed excessive amounts of treats high in fat and protein and not provided with the opportunity to exercise. Iron storage disease, in which excessive dietary iron accumulates in the liver (hemochromatosis), spleen, and other tissues, has been reported in captive gliders and may be associated with wild gliders' evolutionary adaptation to extract limited iron available in natural diets. Hepatocellular toxic changes and cirrhosis from iron deposition may lead to death, unless the disease is caught and treated early with chelation and supportive care.

DISEASES AND SYNDROMES

Bacterial Diseases: Sugar gliders are susceptible to infection with common bacteria, including *Pasteurella multocida* (commonly contracted from pet rabbits), staphylococci, streptococci, *Mycobacterium* sp (especially in skin), *Klebsiella* sp, and *Clostridium*. Clinical signs may be nonspecific, with depression, loss of appetite, and weight loss being the most readily detected. Bacterial infections in gliders may present as opportunistic skin infections associated with trauma or may result in sepsis from other underlying primary diseases. Although sugar gliders are hindgut fermenters, broad-spectrum antibiotic therapy is well tolerated, probably because diets fed in captivity are digestible without fermentation. Injectable, long-acting penicillin with clavulanic acid is an appropriate first-line antibiotic. If indicated by culture and sensitivity or by failure to respond to first-line treatment, chloramphenicol and enrofloxacin are also well tolerated in this species. Injections can be given IM into the epaxial muscles or SC over the shoulders. Palatable oral medications may also be administered.

Protozoal Disease: Toxoplasmosis is a common and serious disease of marsupials, typically presenting with neurologic signs. Gliders may be infected with toxoplasmosis oocysts found in cat feces. Care should be taken to avoid cat feces coming in contact with the bedding or food of sugar gliders. Prevention is more successful than treatment. Coccidia may also cause severe, sometimes fatal diarrhea in young gliders and may be contracted via fecal-oral transmission from other species.

Parasitic Diseases: Internal parasites rarely cause disease in captive gliders, but giardiasis and cryptosporidiosis have been seen in captive animals. Strongyle eggs also have been seen on fecal flotation. Internal parasites reported to infect sugar gliders include nematodes of the genus *Parastrongyloides* and *Paraustrostrongylus* and a liver trematode of the genus *Athesmia*. Wild sugar glider nests generally contain a range of host-specific mites and fleas, but ectoparasites are uncommon in captivity. Dusting with pyrethrin or carbaryl powder (50 g/kg) has controlled fleas and mites. Both the nest and the animal should be treated. Selamectin also has been used to treat ectoparasites on sugar gliders. Ivermectin and fenbendazole have been used to treat GI parasites.

Nutritional Osteodystrophy: Pet sugar gliders maintained on a mainly fruit diet with few gut-loaded insects or other protein sources are very susceptible to nutritional osteodystrophy (nutritional secondary hyperparathyroidism). This condition results from an imbalance in dietary calcium, phosphorus, and vitamin D and manifests clinically as a posterior paresis progressing to hindlimb paralysis, muscle tremors, pathologic bone fractures, and sometimes, in advanced cases, seizures. Chronic malnutrition can lead to increased liver and kidney values, hypoproteinemia, and anemia. Radiography reveals osteoporosis of the vertebral column, pelvis, and long bones in particular. Measurement of ionized blood calcium typically demonstrates a low ionized calcium level. Treatment involves cage rest; administration of calcium, vitamin D_3, and fluids; assisted feeding; and correction of the diet. Seizuring gliders should be given diazepam IV, ideally, or if not possible, IM, intraosseously, or intrarectally, to stop seizures. Severely affected gliders may be given calcitonin to decrease calcium resorption from bone once calcium supplementation has normalized plasma calcium levels. Severe skeletal (especially spinal) deformities may not be reversible.

Dental Disease: Sugar gliders consuming large amounts of soft, sugary foods are prone to tartar buildup and periodontal disease. Tartar may be scaled off under anesthesia. Advanced periodontal disease or traumatic tooth fracture may lead to tooth decay and exposed roots, necessitating extraction and treatment with antibiotics, analgesics, NSAIDs, and antiseptic mouthwash (either made for cats and dogs or fruit-flavored for children). Unlike rodent teeth, sugar glider teeth do not grow continuously or require trimming.

Diarrhea: Potential causes of diarrhea in sugar gliders include bacterial infection (from *Escherichia coli*, *Clostridium* sp, and other bacteria), GI parasites, malnutrition, stress, and metabolic disease (such as liver or kidney disorders). Sugar gliders with diarrhea should have a fecal analysis for parasites, fecal bacterial culture and Gram stain, blood testing (CBC and chemistry panel), and possibly radiographs. Gliders with diarrhea should be given supportive care with fluids, supplemental feeding, and drug therapy, as dictated by the cause of the GI signs. Rectal and cloacal prolapse can occur in gliders secondary to diarrhea and straining and is more common in malnourished animals. The prolapsed tissue must be cleaned, checked for necrotic areas (which must be removed if present), and replaced once the glider is anesthetized. Vertical mattress sutures may be placed next to the vent to help prevent recurrence, and the glider should be given postoperative analgesics, antibiotics, and NSAIDs.

Urinary Tract Disorders: Sugar gliders can develop cystitis, crystalluria, and urolithiasis. They may show hematuria, stranguria, and dysuria. Affected gliders should have a urinalysis and urine culture and sensitivity testing and should be properly hydrated. Antibiotics should be administered based on results of culture and sensitivity testing. Cystotomy may be required to remove uroliths. Male gliders may develop urinary tract obstruction from uroliths and require urethrostomy if cystocentesis and flushing of the distal urethra do not relieve the obstruction. These gliders should receive analgesics, antibiotics, fluids, and NSAIDs. Sugar gliders with renal failure may show weakness, polyuria, and polydypsia and should be treated with standard treatment used in other mammals for renal disease.

Neurologic Disease: Causes of neurologic signs in pet sugar gliders include nutritional secondary hyperparathyroidism, bacterial meningitis, toxoplasmosis, traumatic brain injury, otitis media/interna, encephalitis from aberrant CNS migration of *Baylisascaris procyonis*, and encephalomalacia from hypovitaminosis E. Gliders exhibiting neurologic signs should undergo a full evaluation, including blood testing (CBC and chemistry), fecal testing for parasites, radiographs, and CT scanning plus CSF analysis, if indicated. Prognosis in many of these cases is poor.

Neoplasia: Gliders are prone to neoplastic disease in old age. Hepatocellular tumors and lymphoid neoplasia are common, as is mammary gland adenocarcinoma. Cutaneous melanoma, scent gland tumors, bronchogenic carcinoma, and chondrosarcoma of the jaw also have been reported. A soft-tissue carcinoma associated with a microchip implant was reported in a mahogany glider (*Petaurus gracilis*). A malignant testicular interstitial cell tumor in a mahogany glider was managed by hemicastration. Transitional cell carcinoma with squamous differentiation was noted pericloacally in a 10-yr-old male sugar glider.

Miscellaneous Disorders: Sugar gliders may develop cardiomyopathy/myocarditis, cataracts in juveniles (possibly associated with nutritionally imbalanced handfeeding formula, hyperglycemia, and hypovitaminosis A), cloacitis/vaginitis (females), irregularity of ear margins/crusting of pinnae from ear mite infections, and retrobulbar abscesses associated with facial bite wounds in competing males. These syndromes are treated with medications and surgical procedures, when indicated, similarly to those used in other mammals with these conditions.

Behavior: Sugar gliders live in colonies in the wild and are very social. Thus, they should be kept in captivity in groups of two or more. Gliders love to crawl into pockets or pouches, where they feel safe and more relaxed. Behavioral disorders can develop in sugar gliders housed alone, with incompatible mates, or in inappropriate cages. When housed singly, not given enough social stimulation, or not provided with a nest box or pouch in which to hide or enough room to exercise, they may self-mutilate their fur and skin, develop stereotypic behaviors, or become aggressive. Anxious gliders will overgroom, causing fur loss, particularly at the tail base. Anorexia, polyphagia, polydipsia, coprophagia, cannibalism, and pacing are also seen in stressed gliders. Sexually mature male sugar gliders without access to females may self-mutilate the tail base, limbs, scrotum, penis, or perineum and may develop paraphimosis, in which the penis remains extruded from the cloaca and becomes traumatized and devitalized, necessitating amputation. These gliders should receive pain relievers, antibiotics, and possibly antidepressants, plus an Elizabethan collar, to enable healing. At least 2 hr per day, preferentially at night, when they are awake, must be spent with pet gliders for proper socialization.

Zoonoses: Diseases that may infect sugar gliders, such as salmonellosis, giardiasis, leptospirosis, clostridiosis, and toxoplasmosis, are potentially zoonotic. Sugar gliders are best handled wrapped in a small towel, because they may bite and scratch, and although they are small, their lower incisors, which are designed to bite through tree bark, may inflict significant damage. Biting and scratching can be avoided by gentle handling and proper socialization. All ocular, nasal, GI, and genitourinary discharges should be treated as potentially infectious.

TASMANIAN DEVILS

The Tasmanian devil is the largest marsupial carnivore in existence, currently restricted to the island-state of Tasmania, Australia. Devils have black fur, and white flashes on the chest and rump may be present. They are sexually dimorphic, with males having a thicker neck and broader head than females. Males typically weigh 9–12 kg (up to 14 kg), and females 6–8 kg (up to 9 kg). Devils are mainly nocturnal and hide during the day in rock dens, log cavities, or underground burrows made by other animals. They live up to 6 yr in the wild and 9 yr in captivity. Devils are nonterritorial and generally live within an area of 10 km^2. They can occupy a wide range of habitats, from dry sclerophyll forest, open eucalypt environment, and coastal woodland, to pasture and agricultural areas where carrion (from domestic livestock and macropod populations) is abundant. Devils are specialist carrion feeders but will hunt prey, particularly those weakened by disease, injury, or old age. Wallabies, wombats, and sheep are the usual source of carrion, but other dead domestic livestock, roadkill, and 1080-poisoned wildlife are also consumed. The proportion of hunting to scavenging is unknown. Female devils are facultative polyestrus with up to three estrous cycles within a breeding season, each cycle ~60 days apart. They are polyovular (up to 114 oocytes per ovulation) and may give birth to up to 40 embryos. Mating peaks over late February to the end of March and, as is typical for marsupials, females give birth to highly undeveloped young ~3 wk after mating. Females have a rear-facing pouch, with four teats in the pouch cavity, limiting the maximum total offspring raised per year to four. The young are carried in the pouch until they are 4–5 mo old, weaned at 5–8 mo, and become independent at 10–12 mo. Sexual maturity is reached at 2 yr of age for both females and males, although females have been confirmed to reproduce as young as 1 yr old.

Physical Examination and General Anesthesia: Wild Tasmanian devils can be restrained and examined in a hessian sack by an experienced handler. Devils have an exceptionally strong bite for their body size, and handling conscious animals must only be done by or attempted in the presence of experienced personnel.

The handler sits on the ground and locates and holds the devil's muzzle closed from outside the sack. The devil is then positioned between the handler's legs, with the devil facing outward and head uppermost. The head and face are gently revealed with one side of the sack left covering the devil's eyes. The handler then moves the free hand directly onto the muzzle, continuing to hold it closed, and the teeth/mouth can be examined to estimate age of the devil by lifting the upper lip. The mouth can be opened for intraoral examination. It is important to visualize all aspects of the oral cavity, including under the tongue, for signs of tumors. Normal lymph nodes are not palpable in devils; therefore, subcutaneous masses should be considered suspicious. If a blood sample is required, the devil is positioned as described, ie, facing away from the handler. An assistant can collect up to 12 mL of blood from the jugular vein. The jugular vein is not visible or palpable; to locate it, the index finger of one hand palpates the groove immediately cranial to the clavicle and just lateral to the sternohyoideus muscle. The finger pulls the skin distally and, with the other hand, a 21-gauge needle is inserted 0.2–0.5 cm into the groove while applying negative pressure to the syringe. Gentle digital pressure is applied to the venipuncture site after blood collection is complete. The devil can then be placed back into the sack, with the head facing up and away from the handler, so the tail, cloaca, and pouch can be examined.

Devils bred in captivity or brought to captivity before 2 yr of age are generally not amenable to handling, so general anesthesia is required for examination. These animals can be trapped in their enclosure and transferred to a hessian sack or picked up by the tail base and transferred to the sack. Anesthesia can be induced by using a mask on the devil through the sack. Isofluorane has been used successfully. Ideally, the devil's muzzle is positioned in a corner of the sack to facilitate mask placement. The sack should be secured around the devil to prevent excessive movement and escape from the mask. Devils are induced in 2–3 min and then removed from the sack. A pulse oximeter can be attached to the ear to monitor heart rate and peripheral oxygen saturation. For quick procedures such as physical examination and blood collection, a mask is sufficient to maintain anesthesia. For longer procedures, an endotracheal tube (5–5.5 Fr) is indicated. The devil's larynx is narrow, and a laryngoscope is essential. Local anesthetic must be applied to prevent laryngospasm before intubation. As the devil starts to recover from anesthesia, it is placed back in the sack and observed until it is fully awake and ready to be returned to its enclosure.

Proliferative Lesions: Tasmanian devils are prone to developing proliferative lesions, the most common being devil facial tumor disease (DFTD). Cell proliferations (benign and malignant) affecting skin and adnexa, and endocrine and lymphoreticular tissues (eg, squamous cell carcinomas, lymphosarcomas, adenocarcinomas) are commonly seen at necropsy in adult and senile captive devils. In older captive devils (≥5 yr old), mammary and anal gland tumors are the most common.

Devil Facial Tumor Disease: Devil facial tumor disease (DFTD) is a malignant infectious tumor first observed in 1996. As a result of >70% of the population having succumbed to DFTD, devils have been listed as an endangered species. The prevalent characteristic of DFTD, as the name suggests, is the presence of tumor(s) on the facial area. Tumors are also found inside the mouth (gingival mucosa, hard palate, lips) and on the head and neck. Rarely, DFTD tumors may be found on the rump or other areas of the body, but these are thought to be metastatic tumors rather than primary. More than one tumor is often

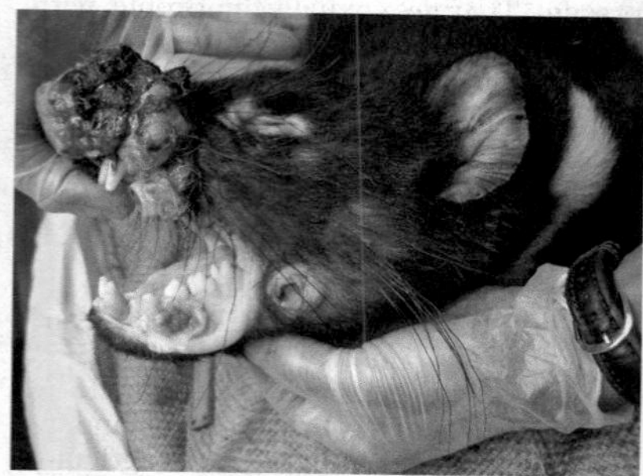

Tasmanian devil with extensive ulcerated tumors on the muzzle and nose. Devil facial tumor disease nodules can be seen also on the lower left gum and left cheek. *Courtesy of Dr. Alexandre Kreiss.*

seen, and tumors on the same devil often vary considerably in size and appearance. The tumors often ulcerate and display epithelium break up, necrosis, exudation, and bacterial contamination. Most devils affected with DFTD show signs of metastases (65% of cases in a study of 91 affected devils), principally to the regional lymph nodes but also to the lungs and spleen.

The most remarkable characteristic of DFTD is its transmissible nature, a concept supported by several independent lines of research. The tumor is of Schwann cell origin and is transmitted by biting. Devils with tumors in the oral cavity have free tumor cells "coating" the canine teeth. The tumor cells are transplanted when a bite wound penetrates the subcutaneous tissue or mucosa of the next devil. The most common bite site in devils is the head, which, therefore, is where almost all DFTD tumors are present. The incubation period is unknown but is estimated to be 3–15 mo. Most devils die within 6 mo of a tumor becoming grossly visible. Death results from starvation, depending on the size and location of the tumor, or from metastatic disease. No evidence of this disease in other species has been found.

No preclinical diagnostic test is available. The tumor cells have a characteristic and consistent karyotype, showing loss of three autosomes, loss of both sex chromosomes, and addition of four marker chromosomes. Histologically, DFTD tumors share the same morphologic features as a high-grade malignant tumor composed of diffuse sheets of small, rounded to polygonal shaped cells with ovoid hyperchromatic nuclei. Mitotic figures are frequent, and eccentrically located nuclei result in a plasmacytoid appearance. Tumor cells might appear cohesive and epithelioid in appearance and form elongated trabecular and solid alveolar structures. The gold standard diagnostic test for DFTD tumors is immune-staining with periaxin. It is common for devils to develop other cell proliferations, which must be differentiated from DFTD.

There is currently no known treatment for DFTD; vincristine and doxorubicin have been tried without tumor reduction, and to date surgery has not been successful. Radiation therapy has not been assessed. Research into a vaccine is underway.

The only other tumor transmitted by direct cell implantation is the canine transmissible venereal tumor (CTVT, see p 1408) of dogs. Although CTVT is generally a benign tumor, it shares the same immune-escape mechanism as DFTD; the tumor cells "down regulate" major histocompatibility complex (MHC) molecules on the cell surface, so that antigen presenting cells do not recognize the tumor cells. In dogs, the immune system might overcome this by producing cytokines and "forcing" the tumor cells to express MHC and become targets for cytotoxic T cells.

Cutaneous Lymphoma: This lymphoid skin tumor has been recently seen in both captive and wild caught devils, affecting predominantly older females. No etiologic agent has been implicated. It can present as a localized erythematous lesion, mainly in the limbs and ventral part of the body, or as a generalized alopecic and exudative form. This condition progresses over several months. There is no known treatment.

Parasitic Diseases: Tasmanian devils are susceptible to both *Demodex* sp infection and the sarcoptiform *Diabolicoptes sarcophilus*. The latter is common and can be treated with ivermectin 200 mcg/kg, SC, every 4 wk for 3–4 mo. Wild Tasmanian devils often harbor the dasyurid-specific flea *Uropsylla tasmanica*. This unusual flea has all stages of its life cycle on the host. The larva is commonly found embedded in the subcutis of the tail, limbs, or ventral area. Adult fleas are less common.

The two most common GI parasites are the nematode *Baylisascaris tasmaniensis* and the cestode *Anoplotaenia dasyuri*. If the cestode burden appears excessive in captive devils (visible proglottids on feces), they can be treated with praziquantel (5 mg/kg, SC).

Spinal Cord Degeneration: A common condition in aged (≥5 yr old), captive Tasmanian devils has been described as a degenerative leukoencephalopathy and myelopathy. It manifests by a progressive swaying of the hindlegs, eventually worsening to paresis and paralysis in several months. Histologically, it is characterized by axonopathy and vacuolation of the spinal cord. Intervertebral disc disease is a common finding. There is no known treatment.

Zoonotic Concerns: *Trichinella pseudospiralis* appears to be endemic in the Tasmanian devil population, with no known human cases to date derived from devils. Devils also harbor *Salmonella* species in the feces.

ZOO ANIMALS

The physical health as well as the social and behavioral well-being of zoo animals depends on enclosure design, nutrition, husbandry, management, group social structure, behavioral enrichment, and good medical and surgical care. Naturalistic enclosures with soil and vegetation are appealing to the public and more stimulating for the animals, but they present challenges for both sanitation and parasite control programs and may complicate restraint procedures. Mixed species exhibits may increase risk of disease transmission between species and can result in interspecific aggression if appropriate choices are not made.

This chapter provides a general discussion of management practices, preventive medicine, clinical care programs, and some of the more commonly encountered disorders in zoo animals. For more specific information, refer to other chapters within this section (eg, *see* AMPHIBIANS, p 1734; MARINE MAMMALS, p 1856; LLAMAS AND ALPACAS, p 1844; RATITES, p 1960; NONHUMAN PRIMATES, p 1876; REPTILES, p 1967; and VACCINATION OF EXOTIC MAMMALS, p 2054). For more information on nutrition, *see* NUTRITION: EXOTIC AND ZOO ANIMALS, p 2287.

MANAGEMENT

Husbandry: The animal's exhibit should approximate its natural environment and enhance the visual experience for zoo visitors. Many healthy mammals and birds can tolerate a fairly wide temperature range if given access to shade and water in hot weather and to a dry, draft-free shelter with a warm spot and ample food to meet increased energy requirements in cold weather. It is essential to ensure that each animal has access to the protected environment and that one dominant individual does not exclude others from shelter, food, or water; such exclusion can result in frostbite or even death due to exposure. Feed receptacles should be designed to avoid fecal contamination and be easy to clean.

With large numbers of birds or mammals, and especially in mixed species exhibits, several watering and feeding stations should be established at appropriate heights *to reduce territorial conflicts* that may result in injuries or deaths. The timing of feedings is important. In many species, it is best to feed small amounts throughout the day to stimulate activity; this is beneficial for the animal and results in a better display. Food can also be used to attract an animal to an area where it can be more easily and safely examined or treated.

Reproduction: The biology and social behavior of animals must be understood to promote reproduction. Species should be maintained alone, in pairs, or in groups, depending on their established social systems. For example, in mixed species groups of Artiodactyla, it is possible to establish species estrous cycles through a variety of techniques, including monitoring hormone levels in the urine and feces. Monitoring reproductive cycles may be used to determine when to introduce and remove breeding males, with males of other species rotated to coincide with the estrous periods of the females of each species. This may also reduce injuries from interaction between breeding males. At parturition, the males of some species should be removed for several weeks to prevent attacks on the postpartum females or their offspring. In colder climates, males should be introduced at a time that will allow births to occur during warm weather.

Artificial reproductive technologies such as artificial insemination, in vitro fertilization, and embryo transfer have been successfully used in diverse zoo species. These efforts have made a significant difference in some endangered species breeding programs (eg, black-footed ferret). However, success requires substantial investment of resources (financial, personnel, etc) to determine basic parameters of reproductive cycles and responses to pharmacologic manipulation.

An emerging management priority in maintenance of zoologic collections is the need for selective reproduction. Indiscriminate reproduction is unethical and carries the potential for overproduction that exceeds the capacity of the exhibit, the zoo, or other zoos to appropriately house the progeny. Overly successful breeding programs carry a risk of limiting resources that could compromise other captive propagation programs. Regional cooperative breeding programs such as Species Survival Plans should be followed. Management is aimed at ensuring genetic diversity of the species into the future. Contraceptive efforts in zoos are multifaceted and include permanent techniques (castration, vasectomy, ovariohysterectomy, tubal ligation), as well as reversible ones such as separation of the sexes, administration of birth control pills, hormonal implants, gonadotropin-releasing hormone agonists, and oral or injectable progestins. Reversible contraception can also be used to control timing of reproductive cycles. There is ongoing work with immunocontraception through administration of porcine zona pellucida vaccines. The Association of Zoos and Aquaria Wildlife Contraception Center is a good source of up-to-date information on contraception techniques.

PREVENTIVE MEDICINE

The foundation of a medical program for zoo animals is preventive medicine. Preventive medical programs should be adaptive and include attention to individual specimens as well as the herd, troop, or flock. Components of the program include quarantine of new arrivals, periodic fecal examinations and treatments for parasites, booster vaccinations, health screening procedures, nutrition evaluation, necropsy examination of deceased specimens, and a comprehensive pest control program. Animals should be evaluated to ensure their health complies with local, state, and federal health requirements before shipment to other zoos or before release in managed reintroduction programs. Preshipment evaluations can also be used as an opportunity to assess the overall health status of the group in which the animal has been living.

Quarantine: Animals entering a collection must undergo quarantine. Quarantine facilities should be designed to allow handling of animals and proper cleaning and sanitizing of enclosures. Shipping crates should be cleaned and disinfected before they leave the quarantine area, and the crates' contents disposed of appropriately. Quarantine facilities require barriers against ingress of potential vectors and vermin. Separate keepers who are skilled at recognizing signs of stress and disease and who will carefully monitor feed intake and fecal characteristics should care for quarantined animals.

Quarantine entry should be strictly controlled. Only essential personnel should be allowed into the quarantine facility. Individuals leaving the quarantine facility should not return to other animal areas without showering and changing clothing. The duration of quarantine should be appropriate to ensure that infectious diseases are not introduced into the permanent collection when the quarantined animals are released to exhibits. Quarantine facilities should follow the "all-in/all-out" principle, ie, if additional animals are added to an ongoing quarantine, the quarantine period should be restarted.

During quarantine, animals should receive appropriate vaccinations and diagnostic testing (eg, tuberculosis, heartworm). They should be examined and treated for ecto- and endoparasites and screened for enteric bacterial pathogens. Before release, animals should receive physical and laboratory examinations, which may include radiographs, serology, hematology, and clinical chemistries. Serum should be frozen for future reference and possible epidemiologic studies. All procedures and results should be recorded in each individual animal's medical record, which is an essential component of the medical program. Each animal should also be identified by some permanent method (eg, tattoo, tag, band, eartag, transponder) to ensure future identification.

When new animals are introduced to enclosures, caution and forethought are necessary to prevent self-induced trauma. Visual barriers, eg, suspending canvasses from fences or enclosure walls or obscuring glass with soap to provide a visual cue, are standard management steps to protect newly introduced specimens from accidents during acclimation to a new exhibit.

Parasite Control: Like domestic animals, zoo animals are vulnerable to a wide variety of ecto- and endoparasites, and similar drugs are used for treatment. Care must be exercised in the choice of medications because of species-specific sensitivities to some drugs. Young animals and those stressed by shipment, disease, or injury are the most likely to be adversely affected by parasites. At these times, commensal parasites (especially protozoa) can cause disease. Acute diarrhea can result from massive infections of coccidia, *Trichomonas*, *Giardia*, or *Balantidium* spp. Amebiasis, which is fairly common in primates and reptiles, can be fatal in a compromised animal. Intestinal parasites may be a major, continuous problem in species kept in naturalistic exhibits or on dirt substrate or pasture, especially in young, newly introduced, or stressed individuals. Of most concern are parasites with direct life cycles. Incorporating anthelmintics directly into the feed is helpful. As in domestic species, anthelmintic resistance may develop and necessitate rotating medication. Parasites with indirect life cycles are less frequently a problem if the exhibit area is free of intermediate hosts.

Vaccination: Vaccination programs for carnivores, nonhuman primates, equids, artiodactylids, and birds should be developed. Vaccination of zoo carnivores is essential because of their susceptibility to various diseases such as feline panleukopenia, feline rhinotracheitis, feline calicivirus, rabies, canine distemper, and canine parvovirus. (*See also* VACCINATION OF EXOTIC MAMMALS, p 2054). Previously, only killed virus vaccines were recommended, but recent studies have shown that some modified-live vaccines are safe for use in select species. Further studies are required, because some modified-live vaccines (especially canine distemper) can result in fatal disease in certain species. A canarypox-vectored recombinant canine distemper vaccine has proved safe for use in those species susceptible to modified-live virus vaccine-induced disease. Appropriateness of rabies vaccination depends on the circumstances of each collection. If indicated in rabies-endemic areas for protection of individual animals, only a killed rabies vaccine should be used. The decision to vaccinate zoo animals for less common diseases for which a vaccine is available should be made on an individual basis. Recombinant and subunit vaccines are being developed for a variety of infectious diseases for domestic animals. Extra-label use of vaccines should be done with caution until safety and efficacy studies have been completed for zoologic species.

Necropsy: All dead animals should be necropsied. This should include gross and histopathologic evaluation of tissue and viral, bacterial, or fungal cultures when appropriate. Tissues should also be saved for potential future examinations. A thorough pathology examination allows evaluation of medical, management, and nutritional programs. It is also valuable in identifying problems requiring immediate action to safeguard the health of the collection. Variations in anatomy should be recorded, because such observations may aid in future diagnostic procedures or therapy in the species.

Pest Control: A successful control program is continual and requires a concerted effort by zoo staff to minimize harborage and food for pests, in addition to the use of mechanical and chemical control methods. Choice of agent, method of use, and storage may minimize zoo animals' access to pesticides and the risk of secondary poisoning. Common zoo pests may serve as important disease vectors. For example, cockroaches are intermediate hosts for GI parasites of primates and birds; rodents can harbor and spread *Listeria*, *Salmonella*, and *Leptospira* spp and *Francisella tularensis*. Wild and feral carnivores such as foxes, raccoons, and domestic dogs and cats can devastate animal collections through predatory attacks and may be important vectors for viral diseases such as rabies, parvovirus, and canine distemper. Raccoons may also transmit *Baylisascaris* parasites, which can cause larval migration, resulting in fatal neuropathy in some species. Pigeons, geese, ducks, and starlings are potential reservoirs for avian diseases; they consume or contaminate animal food and deposit droppings everywhere. Arthropod vectors can transmit pathogens such as West Nile virus.

Nutrition: Some zoos have either a staff nutritionist or a nutritional consultant on contract. Zoos that do not should have some degree of veterinary oversight of diets and diet changes. This is especially true for addition of native or exotic plant species to the diet as browse for either enrichment or as an integral part of the diet. Protocols should be developed for diet formulation, diet changes, and addition of plant material to the diet.

CLINICAL CARE PROGRAMS

The mainstay of the zoo medical program is a qualified and dedicated keeper staff. The keepers know the individual animals under their care and observe them daily. They are the first to recognize abnormalities such as anorexia, inactivity, abnormal feces, or changes in behavior that may reflect early medical problems. Overzealous reporting of observations is preferable to indifference. Because many zoo animals, especially prey species, instinctively conceal overt signs of illness until the disease process is well advanced, it is necessary to make keepers aware of the significance of what may seem to be trivial changes. Past associations with the veterinarian may arouse some animals' responses to the veterinarian's presence, which will mask subtle changes noticeable to keepers.

Once a diagnosis is made, the treatment of zoo animals is similar to that of domestic species except in the method of drug administration and restraint. A comparative medical approach is generally most successful and involves application of medical or surgical information about diseases affecting free-ranging animals, related domestic animals, or people. Frequently, other veterinary experts or human medical or dental specialists are consulted for advice or assistance with complicated medical or surgical cases. Knowledge of comparative anatomy, physiology, behavior, nutrition, pathology, and taxonomy is useful. Attention must be paid to both individual and population health.

Unless medical conditions dictate otherwise, it is often preferable to leave an animal under treatment at its home exhibit where it can maintain contact with its conspecifics and keepers. This can also prevent disruptions in social hierarchies, which may cause difficulties with reintroductions to an established group.

Behavioral Training: An active behavioral training program enables improved health care. Through positive reinforcement, amphibians, reptiles, birds, and mammals in zoo settings have been trained to perform behaviors on command that facilitate accomplishment of various management or medical procedures. Management behaviors include shifting on and off exhibit, onto scales, and into restraint devices or shipping containers. Medical procedures include urine collection, venipuncture, IM injection, tuberculin testing, ultrasonographic examination, and rectal or vaginal examination. Often, these behaviors are incorporated into behavioral and environmental enrichment programs. Enrichment programs are designed to encourage animals to display more of their normal behavioral repertoire, eg, increasing opportunities for foraging or social interaction, which allows animals to spend their time more as they would in nature.

Protected contact, a management system for elephants, uses positive reinforcement to encourage the elephant to present appropriate body parts through openings in a wall. Procedures such as venipuncture from the ear, foot trimming, reproductive evaluation, artificial insemination, and trunk washes are routinely performed using protected contact. This system provides safety for personnel working with elephants and gives the elephant a degree of choice.

Physical Restraint: Most zoo animals resent being handled and resist manual restraint. Struggling with an animal to administer treatment may do more harm than can be offset by treatment. Physical restraint is indicated in some species for minor manipulation or close observation. Restraint devices (squeeze cages) or chute systems are frequently used for species that are large, dangerous, or difficult to handle. Many procedures can be performed on unanesthetized animals so confined, including limited physical examinations, tuberculin testing, administration of injections or anesthetics, collection of blood samples, trimming malformed claws or overgrown hooves, and application of topical medications.

Although the dimensions and construction of these devices vary, some operate by movement of one wall to restrain the animal against the other. Openings are provided to allow safe access to the animal. Many restraint devices for hoofstock are designed with a "V" shape; once the animal enters, the floor is lowered and the animal's body is restrained by the "V" with its feet suspended off the ground. Whenever possible, animals should be trained to enter or be enticed, rather than forced, into the restraint device. Ideally, these facilities should be designed as part of the animal's regular quarters and located in an area where the animal is normally shifted as part of the daily routine. Exhibits should contain nest boxes or restraint pens equipped with doors that operate remotely to confine the animal. From these areas, the animal can be transferred to a restraint device, anesthetic chamber, or shipping container. Weighing facilities are essential.

Small mammals and birds may be caught and restrained in long-handled hoop nets. These nets must be deep enough that the animal can be confined in the blind end, with the upper part of the net twisted to prevent escape.

Personnel participating in capture or restraint procedures must understand their role and be aware of the behavioral characteristics and physical abilities of animals. This is essential to ensure safety of both animals and personnel. Heavy gloves protect handlers from teeth and claws when animals are manually held after capture. Care must be used to avoid excessive pressure on animals, because gloves hinder both dexterity and the perception of the amount of pressure being exerted. Gloves are also difficult to clean and can be a fomite for transmitting infectious agents.

Diagnostic Techniques: The fundamental diagnostic technique is a good history and thorough visual and physical examination (often requiring anesthesia). Ease of sample collection for laboratory testing (CBC, biochemical profile, serology, cytology); fecal examination for parasites; urine for urinalysis; and aerobic, anaerobic, fungal, and viral culture depends on species anatomic differences. Radiography and ultrasonography are commonly done. Endoscopy, laparoscopy, and minimally invasive surgery are used when indicated, with use of CT and MRI becoming more common. Virtually any technique used for other species can be modified for use in zoo species.

Drug Administration: Few drugs are approved for use in zoo species, but extra-label drug use laws allow drugs to be legally used in species for which they are not licensed. Providing quality medical care to zoo animals requires that medications be used without documented therapeutic benefit, dosage, treatment schedule, contraindication, and toxicity data in these species. Whenever possible, drug administration should be based on pharmacokinetic data. If appropriate data are not available, extrapolation from what is known about these parameters in other species using metabolic scaling is necessary. Appropriate dosage is necessary if therapy is to be beneficial, especially with drugs that have the potential for organ toxicity. Antibiotic, antifungal, and analgesic treatments, as well as anesthetic dosages, are becoming less empirical because of increasing species-specific knowledge resulting from pharmacokinetics studies in zoo species. When using a drug on a group of animals for the first time, it is often wise to initially administer it to just one or two individuals. If no adverse effects are seen, the rest of the group can then be treated.

Drug administration can be challenging. Oral medication has the advantage of minimal disturbance to the animal, but ensuring adequate individual intake may be a problem, especially when animals are housed in a group. Mixing the medication with favorite foods or treats is helpful. Oral antibiotics in hoofstock and other species can disrupt normal bacterial flora and lead to GI problems. Oral sedative or anesthetic administration can result in variable onset, duration, and depth of effect because of inadequate consumption or delayed absorption. IM injections with a hand syringe can be difficult unless a restraint device or other means of physical restraint is used. Remote IM injections may be made by firing a projectile syringe from a dart gun. However, these injections may be painful and add the trauma of dart impact and injection, especially when delivering large volumes (eg, 10 mL) over long distances (50 m). Problems can be minimized through careful selection of the most appropriate drug and drug concentration, as well as the type of dart gun for the intended use. In addition, practice with projectile darts is mandatory before their use. Marksmanship and familiarity with the weapon are essential—such weapons in the hands of a novice can be fatal. Other less traumatic methods of IM injection, over shorter distance, include syringe poles or blow guns. Through behavioral training, it is also possible to administer IM injections through voluntary participation of the animal. IV therapy is generally restricted to anesthetized animals or those maintained in restraint devices or small enclosures for the duration of treatment.

Anesthesia: Safe anesthesia of zoo animals is of special concern. Many procedures routinely accomplished on domestic animals with minimal restraint require anesthesia of zoologic species for the welfare and safety of both zoo animals and personnel. Before anesthesia of a zoo animal, the veterinarian should be familiar with the species and choice of anesthetic agent. Anesthesia records for the individual, other specimens of the same species in the collection, or published references for the species should be reviewed. Consultation with someone knowledgeable in the field is advised, because there are large differences in effective drugs and dosages in the diversity of species in a zoologic practice. An anesthetic plan should be developed for each anesthetic episode; the plan should include the anesthetic drugs and doses to be used, other needed pharmaceuticals (eg, emergency drugs, analgesics, anthelmintics, vaccines), monitoring equipment, and any other special equipment to perform the procedure at hand.

Many factors influence an animal's response to anesthetic drugs, including age, sex, stage of reproductive cycle, general nutritional status, and most especially mental state before drug administration. Variations may be marked between species as well as individuals and between different collections of the same species. An excited animal usually requires more drug and, once anesthetized, has a greater tendency to develop capture myopathy secondary to hyperthermia, respiratory depression, and acidosis. Capture myopathy can also occur in manually restrained animals and is more common in ungulates or long-legged birds (*see* p 2884). Monitoring of anesthetized animals may include heart and respiratory rates, temperature, ECG, oxygenation (measured by blood gas determination or pulse oximetry), ventilation (measured by blood gas determination or end-tidal CO_2), and blood pressure (measured directly or by oscillometric techniques). Attention must be paid at all times to appropriate positioning and padding of anesthetized animals and extremes of environmental conditions to prevent secondary complications.

The nature of an enclosure in which animals are to be anesthetized should be carefully considered before initiation of an anesthetic episode to minimize complications. For example, prey species that are darted may startle and hit fences or other barriers. In herd situations, the herd members may attack and injure or kill the darted animal as anesthetic induction begins (eg, ataxia).

Xylazine, detomidine, or medetomidine (α_2-adrenoreceptor agonists) used alone produce adequate sedation in some ungulates, mainly bovids, to allow some manipulative procedures. The sedative effects can be antagonized by administration of yohimbine, tolazoline, or atipamezole. α_2-Agonists should not be used as the sole anesthetic agent in dangerous carnivores, because the animals may appear sedated but can respond aggressively when stimulated. Peripheral vasoconstriction caused by these agents alone or in combination with other drugs can lead to significant hypertension, so blood pressure should be monitored. Peripheral vasoconstriction may also interfere with monitoring pulse oximetry and can make venipuncture more difficult.

The cyclohexamine ketamine (either alone or in combination with tranquilizers or sedatives such as xylazine or medetomidine) is a common anesthetic for small to medium-sized mammals, especially carnivores, primates, and some ungulates. A concentrated ketamine preparation (200 mg/mL) can be obtained from compounding pharmacies, with a resultant decrease in the required injection volume. Combining ketamine with a sedative or tranquilizer speeds induction, minimizes excitement, increases muscle relaxation, and provides a smoother anesthetic induction and recovery than using ketamine alone. The ability to reverse the sedative effects of xylazine or medetomidine with the antagonists yohimbine, tolazoline, or atipamezole enables the use of a lower ketamine dosage and a more complete and rapid reversal after the procedure has been completed.

Tiletamine-zolazepam, a dissociative anesthetic-tranquilizer combination, is relatively safe in most species, has a rapid induction, and can be concentrated to 200 mg/mL to allow a small delivery volume. It is commonly used for anesthesia of carnivores and primates. However, a disadvantage of this drug combination is that no complete antagonist exists; therefore, recoveries can be longer than with other combinations that can be completely reversed.

The rapid onset and short duration of anesthesia induced by the sedative-hypnotic propofol renders it particularly attractive for use in zoo species. However, because of the necessity for IV administration, its use is limited to species such as reptiles, birds, and small mammals that can safely be manually restrained for drug administration. It is also useful as an adjunct anesthetic agent in large mammals first immobilized with another drug combination.

The potent opioids etorphine, carfentanil, and thiofentanil, alone or in combination with other agents (eg, azaparone, acepromazine, xylazine, detomidine), have been used extensively for anesthesia of ungulates, elephants, and rhinoceros. The antagonist of choice for these opioids is naltrexone, a pure narcotic antagonist, which induces complete reversal when given at 100 mg of naltrexone per mg of opioid. The reversal dosage of naltrexone can be given IV or IM, and in species prone to renarcotization after reversal, additional naltrexone may be administered SC. It can also be given IM 6–8 hr later by remote delivery to prevent renarcotization when the animal is not being observed. Accidental exposure of people to ultrapotent narcotic analgesics is quite dangerous. Therefore, they should be used only by trained, experienced personnel, and only after development of accidental exposure protocols.

Various drug combinations (using ketamine, telazol, medetomidine, detomidine, butorphanol, midazolam, diazepam, or xylazine) have been developed for specific species and purposes. Administration to novel species should be undertaken with care.

Isoflurane has become the inhalation anesthetic of choice for small mammals, birds, and reptiles. It is also used as a supplement to an injectable anesthetic or as an anesthetic maintenance agent to prolong anesthesia in virtually all species. Isoflurane is safe and potent and has minimal adverse effects, short induction, and quick recovery periods. Sevoflurane has the advantage of even shorter induction and recovery periods and may be preferred over isoflurane in some species. Small animals can be induced with a face mask or placed in an anesthetic chamber. Inhalation anesthesia can be maintained or supplemented using a face mask, nasal cannulae, or intratracheal intubation, depending on the species and anesthetic plane.

Regulatory Issues: Collection, transport, and exhibition of wild animals requires compliance with local, state, and federal laws. Permits may be necessary to maintain these species. Institutions in the USA must comply with appropriate rules and regulations such as those of the USDA, United States Fish and Wildlife Service, National Oceanographic and Atmospheric Administration, and National Marine Fisheries Service. Some specific health requirements in the USA include compliance with the USDA's Animal Welfare Act and CDC regulations governing importation of primates and maintenance of colonies of captive bats. The Drug Enforcement Agency governs the purchase and use of controlled substances in the USA. Specific regulatory rules and regulations may dictate management of certain species. As an example, in the USA, the USDA requires that elephants have three negative trunk wash cultures for tuberculosis during a 12-mo period, collected on separate days, preferably during a 7-day period.

Zoonoses: Many human infectious and parasitic diseases are of animal origin, ie, are zoonotic. Free-ranging and captive wild animals may harbor zoonotic diseases that pose a potential health risk for those who work with these animals. Reptiles are commonly asymptomatic carriers of *Salmonella* spp. Avian species may be infected with *Chlamydia* spp. Tuberculosis infections in mammals, especially primates, ungulates, and elephants, can be transmitted from people or harbored and shed by animals to infect zoo staff. Many enteric bacterial or parasitic pathogens of primates can be transmitted to people. Bats may be a source of *Histoplasma* spp or rabies. Carnivorous species of reptiles, birds, and mammals that consume uncooked meat-based commercial diets or whole prey may develop an asymptomatic *Salmonella* carrier state. Numerous zoo species, as well as feral domestic or native species on zoo grounds, may harbor *Leptospira* spp, *Baylisascaris*, etc. Recognition of these zoonotic diseases and institution of procedures to minimize the disease risk to zoo staff and the visiting public are important components of a zoologic practice. An occupational health program should be developed for personnel coming in contact with collection animals. Personal protective equipment (eg, disposable gowns, gloves, face shields) should be used as required by zoo personnel. Frequent hand washing is also recommended. (*See also* ZOONOSES, p 2414.)

COMMON DISORDERS AND PROCEDURES

In general, the disease processes and treatments of zoo species are similar to those of domestic pets, agricultural species, laboratory animals, or people. Commonly encountered medical problems include acute or chronic gastroenteritis, traumatic injuries (bite or gore wounds, lacerations, fractures, luxations), localized (abscess or cellulitis) or generalized (septicemia) bacterial infections, parasitic infestations, obstetric problems, lameness, arthritis, and GI foreign bodies.

Avian *Aspergillus* infection generally results in chronic respiratory tract disease (*see* p 1901). Affected birds may exhibit weight loss, markedly increased WBC counts, and in later stages, dyspnea. Death can also occur peracutely if there is a localized aspergilloma that occludes the trachea or in cases of fungal septicemia. Necropsy generally demonstrates extensive fungal granulomas in the air sac and lungs. Species that are more sensitive to *Aspergillus* infections are penguins, pheasants, and waterfowl. Treatment is generally unrewarding because of the advanced state of infection when diagnosed but can include oral (flucytosine or itraconazole), IV (amphotericin B), or nebulized (enilconazole) antifungal medications.

Infectious pododermatitis (bumblefoot) is a common disorder of birds. It can be either unilateral or bilateral and is characterized by lameness, inflammation, and swelling of the footpad due to localized bacterial infection. Sequelae of infection can include chronic pododermatitis, septicemia, or amyloidosis. It can occur due to injury, infection, inappropriate substrate, obesity, or unilateral limb problems (trauma, arthritis) that result in excess and abnormal weight bearing on the contralateral foot. Treatment includes correction of the primary problem, local and systemic antibiotic and symptomatic treatment, and in more advanced cases, surgery.

Avian mycobacteriosis is a chronic problem in many bird collections, and control measures are difficult, because premortem tests are unreliable (*see* TUBERCULOSIS, p 2869). Aggressive sanitation of the infected enclosures and culling of infected and exposed birds may help limit disease dissemination but will not eliminate it. Marsupials and young primates may also develop infection when exposed to infected birds or contaminated environments (such as in a mixed species exhibit). The disease in marsupials can manifest by development of lung or bone lesions and is resistant to most therapies. The disease in primates is often benign but may result in nonspecific tuberculin test responses.

Prevention of flight in birds is accomplished by amputating one wing just distal to the radiocarpal joint (pinion) or less commonly by performing a tenectomy and fusing the radiocarpal joint. Pinioning of young birds soon after hatching is easier and more successful. The appropriateness of performing this procedure on birds is controversial. (*See also* ROUTINE GROOMING PROCEDURES, p 1888 et seq.)

Bone fractures are repaired with splints, casts, surgical fixation, or a combination of these methods. Because maintaining a splint on a zoo animal can be difficult, rigid internal fixation or an external fixater are preferable. For best results, fixation should be rigid, strong, and require minimal postoperative care. Because casts must be left in place for 6–8 wk, freedom of movement and a minimum of discomfort must be assured. Newer lightweight, strong, waterproof, fiberglass casting material is especially useful.

Mammalian tuberculosis still occasionally occurs in zoo collections, and routine screening of primates, hoofstock, elephants, and keeper staff is indicated (*see* p 687). Interpretation of intradermal tuberculin tests can be problematic in nondomestic species because of the occurrence of nonspecific responses. When a test is suspicious or positive, a complete health evaluation should be performed, including additional tests such as radiographs and gastric and bronchial lavage for mycobacterial cytology and culture. Diagnostic immunologic tests are available for zoo bovids and cervids and include lymphocyte stimulation tests and ELISA. Other tests under development include antigen 85 and γ-interferon testing. The incidence of elephant-to-human transmission of tuberculosis has increased in recent years. Most cases of tuberculosis in elephants is caused by *Mycobacterium tuberculosis*; however other species, including *M bovis*, have caused clinical disease in elephants. Asian elephants are more frequently infected than African elephants. Clinical signs are nonspecific and usually present only in advanced cases; they include chronic weight loss, anorexia, weakness, exercise intolerance, discharge from the trunk, cough, and dyspnea. Definitive diagnosis is by culture. Screening by serologic testing, including immunochromatographic (lateral flow), multi-antigen print immunoassay, and dual path platform test, are not confirmatory and are not used as definitive regulatory tests. The USDA has established testing and treatment protocols for captive elephants in the USA.

Hoof and nail trims are necessary when overgrowth occurs and are most often required in ruminants, equids, elephants, rhinoceros, and larger carnivores. These procedures should be conducted on a regular basis to avoid excessive overgrowth. On occasion, the services of an equine farrier are used for more complicated cases such as when an equid has foundered. Elephant foot care is especially important to prevent chronic musculoskeletal problems and can usually be accomplished in an awake elephant through training. Many other species require chemical immobilization for foot care.

Mandibular osteomyelitis (lumpy jaw) is a common problem of small ruminants and macropods (wallabies and kangaroos). It can occur secondary to coarse feed, oral trauma, or dental disease. Animals generally present with localized facial swelling and a foul oral odor or discharge. Treatment consists of lancing the abscess, debriding infected bone, removing affected teeth if indicated by radiographs, and treating with systemic antibiotics.

Dentistry in zoo animals presents unique problems. The roots of canine teeth in primates and carnivores are more extensive than the exposed crown. Simple traction and rotation cannot remove such teeth intact; dislodging with a dental elevator is essential. A small electric drill or bone chisel is used to remove a section of alveolar bone around the root. Root canals are indicated when a large canine tooth is fractured and viable pulp exposure occurs. Specialized long dental instruments are required to remove the nerve tissue from these elongated canals. The incisor teeth of rodents, such as beavers, porcupines, and capybaras, grow continually; unless these animals are supplied with coarse feed or logs to gnaw on, their incisors grow excessively and interfere with their ability to feed. Periodontal disease in zoo animals is treated by routine cleaning (under general anesthesia) and by providing adequate chewing substances to supplement the soft, prepared diets fed to many zoo animals.

Because of excellent management, husbandry, nutrition, and veterinary care, many zoo animals live to advanced ages. Care of **geriatric specimens** is becoming increasingly common, including such disorders as diabetes, heart failure, chronic arthritis, and neoplasia. The same diagnostic and therapeutic principles of management of these disorders in people or domestic animals may be successfully applied to the care of affected zoo animals.

Elephant endotheliotropic herpesvirus infection (EEHV) is one of the most significant disease threats to captive elephants. Several virus types that cause disease have been described, although viral latency is common. EEHV primarily causes acute hemorrhagic disease, mostly in young Asian elephants (*Elaphas maximus*) with a mortality rate of up to 85%. Clinical signs are predominately nonspecific and include lethargy, anorexia, mild colic, and tachycardia. There is often edema of the head, neck, trunk, and thoracic limbs. Cyanosis of the tip of the tongue that progresses caudally and hemorrhage of the tongue and oral ulcers are also seen. Antemortem diagnosis is currently made by PCR analysis of whole blood. Early, aggressive treatment with antiviral agents (famciclovir or ganciclovir) with good supportive care has decreased the mortality rate since 2009.

Since the emergence of **West Nile virus** in the USA in 1999, it has been detected in 22 orders of birds, 8 orders of mammals, and 2 orders of reptiles. Mammals showing clinical infections in zoos include alpacas, sheep, reindeer, harbor seals, Indian rhinoceroses, a polar bear, a wolf and several domestic canids, a Barbary macaque, white-tailed deer, and a killer whale. Clinical signs have also been seen in alligators.

Highly pathogenic avian influenza (HPAI) is a threat to zoo bird collections. Zoos should develop HPAI response plans and establish a dialogue with state and national agricultural regulatory agencies to mitigate the impact of HPAI on zoo collections.

VACCINATION OF EXOTIC MAMMALS

Exotic mammals are susceptible to many of the same infectious diseases that affect domestic mammals. However, vaccination of these species is often extra-label, because vaccines are tested and approved for use only in domestic species. Vaccination protocols recommended for exotic mammals are therefore based on limited published information, anecdotal experience, and relative risk of disease to the species from the infectious agent or vaccination itself. Reports of lack of seroconversion, antibody production, sustained protection, and induction of the disease resulting in morbidity and mortality in a variety of species, particularly for rabies and distemper, are common after vaccination of exotic mammals. Regardless, vaccination should be considered in captive wildlife and conservation programs based on a number of factors. Many diseases preventable by vaccination such as canine distemper virus, canine parvovirus, feline calicivirus, feline panleukopenia virus, and rabies virus have caused population declines or reduced host fitness in critically endangered mammals. Certainly, infectious disease outbreaks in small numbers of highly genetically valuable individuals can disastrously affect conservation projects. Unfortunately, the biology of many of these preventable diseases (incubation period, transmissibility, etc) in exotic mammals is often unknown. Captivity may enhance the risk of acquiring disease based on food sources, exposure to rodents and other disease hosts, and an unknown degree of exposure of other zoo animals, which is unlikely to occur in nature. Thus, due consideration of protection of captive nondomestic species, even those destined for release to the wild, is warranted. Core vaccines are designated as those that protect captive animals from life-threatening, globally distributed diseases. The determination of protection has largely been based on studies in domestic species; nonetheless, based on current knowledge, these vaccines deserve full consideration for inclusion into vaccination regimens for captive exotic mammals.

Individual animal safety dictates that inactivated or recombinant viral or bacterial vaccines are preferable to modified-live virus (MLV) vaccines, which have the potential to cause disease in exotic mammals and abortions in hoofstock. However, in select species, especially Old World apes, MLV vaccines have received sufficient use to warrant consideration based on the serious risk of morbidity and mortality. Use of MLV vaccines for rabies and distemper are generally contraindicated in exotic mammals. In particular, use of MLV distemper vaccines in exotic mammals may result in postvaccinal myelitis or distemper. Recently developed canary pox–vectored vaccines are the current vaccine of choice for distemper and appear both safe and efficacious. The following concepts should be considered before extra-label use of a vaccine in an exotic animal. Possession of the animal should be legal per state community and other applicable laws. Informed consent of the owner and discussion of the availability or lack of safety and efficacy trials associated with the use of this vaccine in the animal should be documented in the medical record. Use of product and vaccination procedures with record of previous success such as those used or recommended in zoo (Association of Zoos and Aquariums or American Association of Zoo Veterinarians) protocols, and those with publications supporting their safety and efficacy in the species, should be considered. Vaccination may be foregone in the face of lack of data to support that a certain disease occurs, despite antibody presence, in some species.

Vaccination protocols developed for exotic mammals should be determined with respect to number of animals, husbandry, relative value of animal and offspring, pregnancy, species susceptibility to a disease, likelihood of encountering disease, disease prevalence in the surrounding locality, ability to obtain useful products, information of reported or anecdotal benefits or disadvantages with usage of a vaccine in that species, housing and vector control programs, and zoonotic and infectious potential of the disease. As in domestic species, animals that are febrile or have other clinical signs of illness should not be vaccinated. Because a full vaccine dose is required to elicit a satisfactory immune response, remote vaccine administration should be weighed against anesthetic and disease risk. Some nondomestic mammals and their recommended vaccination protocols (eg, cervids, rodents, lagomorphs, camelids) are reviewed elsewhere in the Manual, and the reader should refer to the relevant chapters. In domestic mammals, young animals have differing vaccine schedules than those presented in TABLE 36 based on waning maternal antibodies. Consideration of the provided references and consultation with experts in zoo medicine and exotic mammal husbandry are recommended to develop vaccination protocols. Specific vaccine protocols should be developed for neonates. For apes, a youngster vaccination schedule, based on the human schedule, should include the killed polio series and *Haemophilus* vaccination (*see* www.cdc.gov/vaccines/schedules/index.html).

Although titer determinations may be useful for evaluation of vaccination in exotic mammals, the lack of antibodies does not equate to lack of immune response. This method quantifies only the humoral immune response, not the cell-mediated aspect, and protective titer levels for exotic mammals have not been evaluated or established. Examples of titers that may be assessed include rabies, distemper, parvovirus, and leptospires, as well as the encephalitic viruses and many viruses affecting nonhuman primates that also affect people. Yearly and preshipment viral titers, which vary based on species, are recommended for all primates. Titers change based on natural disease exposure, independent of vaccination, may or may not confer protection from disease, and may also wane quickly, despite repeated exposure.

Bovine Herpesvirus 1: Inactivated and attenuated-live vaccines for infectious bovine rhinotracheitis and infectious pustular vulvovaginitis are available. Vaccines may not prevent infection but reduce clinical signs and significantly reduce shedding of field virus. Use of the inactivated vaccine in exotic hoofstock may be preferred, because abortions and initiation of disease in vaccinated hoofstock have not been adequately studied.

Canine Distemper: Most, if not all of the Carnivora, including canids, procyonids, mustelids, and the viverrids, are considered susceptible to canine distemper virus (CDV); the susceptibility of most Ursidae and Hyenidae is unknown. Giant and red pandas are an important exception among the ursids and appear quite susceptible; canine distemper vaccination has been specifically evaluated in and is recommended for use in this species. Large felids, particularly tigers and lions, also appear susceptible to disease, which in exotic mammals manifests primarily in the neurologic form. CDV is considered a core vaccination in captive canids and should also be considered in captive exotic felids with a history of disease in the collection. Many species of small carnivores have developed vaccine-induced distemper after receiving an MLV vaccine. The recombinant canary pox–vectored subunit distemper vaccine, which causes appropriate serologic titers and appears safe and effective, is now recommended for use in susceptible exotic mammals. Generally recommended vaccination regimens for young animals incorporate an initial vaccination after weaning with a 1-mo booster followed by yearly revaccination. Vaccination of

TABLE 36 VACCINATIONS RECOMMENDED FOR EXOTIC MAMMALS

Animal Group	Disease or Vaccine	Vaccine Type[a]	Vaccination Frequency
Primates (especially Pongidae): monkey, ape	Poliomyelitis	MLV	Annual
	Measles	MLV	Annual
	Mumps	MLV	Annual
	Rubella	MLV	Annual
	DPT[b] or tetanus	K	Annual
Canidae: fox, wolf, coyote, wild dog	Canine distemper	Vectored, MLV[d]	Annual
	Canine adenovirus 2	MLV	Annual
	Canine parvovirus	K	Annual
	Canine parainfluenza	MLV	Annual
	Leptospira bacterin-CI[c]	K	Annual
Felidae: exotic cats	Feline panleukopenia	K/MLV[d]	Annual
	Feline rhinotracheitis	K/MLV	Annual
	Feline caliciviruses	K/MLV	Annual
Mustelidae/Viverridae/ Procyonidae: raccoon, skunk, ferret, coati, genet, otter, weasel, mink, kinkajou	Canine distemper	K/MLV, Vectored[d]	Annual
	Feline panleukopenia	K/MLV	Annual
	Canine adenovirus 2 bacterin-CI	K/MLV	Annual
	Leptospira bacterin-CI	K	Annual
Ursidae: bear	Canine adenovirus 2	K	Annual
	Leptospira bacterin-CI	K	Annual
Hyaenidae: hyena, aardwolf	Canine distemper[e]	K/MLV	Annual
	Feline panleukopenia[e]	K/MLV	Annual
Artiodactyla/ Ruminantia: deer, sheep, cattle, goat, antelope, camelids	BVD[f] (in endemic areas)	K	Annual
	8-way *Clostridium* bacterin	K	Annual
	5-way *Leptospira* bacterin	K	Annual or every 6 mo
	Parainfluenza 3	MLV	Annual
Perissodactyla Equidae: ass, zebra	Tetanus	K	Annual
	EEE[g]	K	Annual
	WEE[h]	K	Annual

TABLE 36 VACCINATIONS RECOMMENDED FOR EXOTIC MAMMALS *(continued)*

Animal Group	Disease or Vaccine	Vaccine Type[a]	Vaccination Frequency
	Equine rhinopneumonitis	K	Every 4 mo
	West Nile virus	K, DNA	Annual
	Influenza	K	Annual
Suidae/Tayassuidae: pigs, peccaries	5-way *Leptospira* bacterin	K	Annual
	Erysipelas bacterin	K	Annual

[a] MLV = modified live virus; K = killed

[b] DPT = diptheria, pertussis, and tetanus

[c] Canicola or Icterohaemorrhagiae

[d] Not ferret origin; recombinant canarypox origin preferred

[e] Controversial; some believe hyaenids are not susceptible

[f] BVD = bovine viral diarrhea

[g] EEE = Eastern equine encephalomyelitis

[h] WEE = Western equine encephalomyelitis

free-living animals should be carefully considered, because vaccine efficacy is unknown for many nontarget species, and animals may have recovered from or be incubating disease, rendering vaccination a poor use of resources.

Canine Parvovirus and Feline Panleukopenia: Canine parvovirus, raccoon parvovirus, and feline panleukopenia virus are closely related antigenically and pathogenetically. Canidae, Felidae, most Mustelidae, Procyonidae, and Viverridae are considered susceptible to one or more of these parvoviruses. Binturongs are susceptible to feline panleukopenia, and vaccination is recommended. Vaccinations that protect from feline panleukopenia are considered core vaccines in exotic felids, while those that protect from canine parvovirus are core vaccine for canids. Based on insufficient attenuation of MLV vaccines for some species, only inactivated vaccines of tissue or tissue-culture origin are recommended for use in exotic mammals. Vaccine and dosage regimen have been empirically determined but should adhere to label directions, with boosters recommended at 2 wk, 6 mo, and then annually. Based on reports of vaccine reaction associated with MLV combinations of canine distemper, canine adenovirus 2, canine parainfluenza, and canine parvovirus, multivalent vaccination with killed feline panleukopenia, feline rhinotracheitis, and feline calicivirus is preferred for use in exotic mammals.

Equine Encephalomyelitis: Because nondomestic equids are susceptible to equine encephalomyelitis, vaccination should follow guidelines for domestic equids in endemic areas. Inactivated trivalent (Eastern, Western, Venezuelan) or bivalent (Eastern, Western) vaccine, or a combination of these with tetanus toxoid, are administered according to manufacturer instructions. Initial immunization is two doses, 1–2 wk apart with annual revaccination. Although susceptibility of tapir species is unknown, a similar vaccination regimen has been recommended in this species. The susceptibility of exotic equids to West Nile virus is unclear, but zebra, tapir, and related species are often vaccinated for West Nile virus; efficacy and safety of the inactivated equine (more commonly used) or the DNA West Nile virus vaccination in these species is unknown.

Equine Herpesvirus 1 Infection: Equine herpesvirus 1 (EHV-1) can cause abortion in exotic equids; killed virus vaccination is recommended, because adequacy of attenuation in MLV vaccines is unknown for nontarget species. Vaccination of foals should begin at 4 mo, with boosters at 4-mo intervals up to 1 yr. Mares must be vaccinated often to provide protection from abortion, because EHV-1 natural protective immunity after infection lasts only 4 mo.

Erysipelas: The bacterium *Erysipelothrix rhusiopathiae* is pathogenic for the Tayassuidae, nondomestic Suidae, cetaceans, and pinnepeds. Erysipelas bacterin can be administered with the standard regimen to nondomestic swine and peccaries (*see* p 2817). Despite the importance of preventing erysipelas in marine mammals, there is no bacterin designed specifically for these animals. Vaccination of cetaceans and pinnepeds is controversial, but a subunit vaccine has been investigated in dolphins (*see also* BACTERIAL DISEASES OF MARINE MAMMALS, p 1861). In facilities where captive cetaceans are vaccinated, extra-label bacterins are used to prevent erysipelas outbreak. Based on vaccine breaks, the necessity of bacterin culture and sensitivity testing before revaccination, and the risks of fatal anaphylaxis, sterile abscessation, tissue reaction, and animal immobilization, some facilities have reduced vaccination to one-time administration, even though antibody titers fall below the presumed effective level. Booster at 6 mo and annual revaccination are recommended to maintain protective antibody titers. Because disease appears less common and vaccination is not without significant risk of morbidity and mortality while protective efficacy remains unknown, vaccination is not routinely recommended in pinnepeds.

Feline Caliciviruses: Exotic felids are susceptible to feline caliciviruses, and some strains may cause serious morbidity and mortality. This is considered a core vaccine in exotic felids. Vaccines are often combined into a multivalent formulation, and vaccine regimens are as for feline rhinotracheitis.

Feline Herpesvirus Rhinotracheitis: Feline viral rhinotracheitis is a serious disease threat in exotic Felidae and is considered a core vaccine. Available vaccines, inactivated, subunit, and MLV, are combined with feline calicivirus and are usually in multivalent formulations with other pathogens (eg, feline panleukopenia). A single dose should be administered at weaning, with monthly boosters until 4 mo of age and annually thereafter. In domestic cats, vaccination provides reasonable disease protection but does prevent infection or viral latency. Vaccinated cats can be infected; however, clinical signs and viral shedding are reduced.

Infectious Canine Hepatitis (Canine Adenovirus 1): All Canidae and binturong, a viverrid, are susceptible; Ursidae may also be susceptible. In foxes, the disease is called fox encephalitis due to a predominant neurotropism and neurologic signs. Canine adenovirus (CAV) is a core vaccination for captive canids. Because a killed vaccine is not commercially available, multivalent MLV vaccines containing canine distemper and CAV-1 or CAV-2 are often administered. Based on the close antigenic relationship of CAV-1 and CAV-2, vaccination with either virus provides cross-protection. CAV-2 is thought less likely to cause postvaccinal reactions, such as corneal opacity and hemorrhagic and necrotizing hepatitis (vaccine-induced adenoviral hepatitis). However, administration of CAV-2 MLV vaccine to a maned wolf (*Chrysocyon brachyurus*) has resulted in vaccine-induced adenoviral hepatitis. Therefore, vaccination recommendations for this species are limited to canine distemper virus, canine parvovirus, and rabies; vaccination with MLV CAV-2 is contraindicated in this species. For other canids, recommended vaccine regimens are a single dose of the multivalent vaccine at weaning, with monthly boosters until 4 mo of age followed by annual revaccination.

Canine Influenza Virus: Canine influenza virus vaccination for domestic carnivores is considered noncore. However, if a collection has a history of canine influenza or is located in an endemic area, vaccination may be considered. Vaccination may also be considered for great apes, as well as for contact staff on a yearly basis before flu season. Equine influenza vaccine is administered to nondomestic equids in some zoos.

Leptospirosis: Leptospirosis occurs sporadically in exotic Canidae, Procyonidae, Viverridae, Ursidae, Mustelidae, Suidae, primates, Tayassuidae, and in Cervidae and other ruminants of the families Bovidae, Artiodactyla, Perisodactyla, Proboscidae, Camelidae, Giraffidae, etc. Vaccination of domestic carnivores with *Leptospira* bacterins is considered noncore. However, if a collection has a history of or is in an endemic area for leptospirosis, vaccination should be considered with bacterins that contain immunogens against *Leptospira interrogans* serovars Canicola and Icterohaemorrhagiae. Carnivores are vaccinated with a 1- or 2-mL dose, IM or SC, at 6–8 wk of age, repeated in 14 days. Boosters are given every 6 mo. Hoofed animals are immunized with 5 mL of pentavalent bacterin IM; annual or preferably semiannual boosters are recommended. Vaccination does not necessarily prevent shedding of the causal organism(s).

Ruminants, pigs, and peccaries are immunized with pentavalent bacterins that contain the serovars Pomona, Hardjo, Icterohaemorrhagiae, Canicola, and Grippotyphosa. Hoofstock should have an initial vaccination with a booster 4–8 wk later (as per label instructions); booster vaccination is essential, because leptospirosis vaccines are killed vaccines. At a minimum, hoofstock should be revaccinated yearly approximately 6–8 wk before the breeding season. However, because protective titers can wane within a year, a semiannual vaccination schedule may be instituted if leptospirosis is an issue or occurs in valuable breeding stock. Vaccination does not necessarily prevent shedding of the causal organism(s).

Measles, Mumps, and Rubella: Pongidae are often immunized against measles, mumps, and rubella at 2–3 mo of age and annually thereafter with 0.5 mL of MLV human vaccine injected SC. This vaccination is also recommended for monkeys. New World monkeys are more resistant than Old World monkeys, but mortality is high when infected. Vaccine administration in other primates is optional, depending on colony-specific concerns. Vaccination of susceptible populations of nonhuman primates (>6 mo old) should be considered when contact with people cannot be adequately controlled (eg, nonhuman primates as pets). Annual booster doses are given.

Parainfluenza 3: Exotic sheep and goats are susceptible to pneumonia caused by parainfluenza 3 (PI-3) and *Mannheimia haemolytica*. Modified-live virus PI-3 vaccines, particularly those administered intranasally are useful to reduce the incidence of pneumonia in lambs. Vaccine is administered at 3–4 mo of age, 1 mL per nostril, and repeated 3–4 wk before anticipated shipment and annually thereafter.

Poliomyelitis: Primates, particularly the Pongidae (great apes) are susceptible to poliomyelitis. Oral trivalent MLV poliomyelitis vaccine is preferred to parenteral inactivated vaccine because of ease of administration. A single human dose (0.5 mL) is given PO on a sugar cube after 6 mo of age and annually thereafter. Vaccinated animals should be isolated from unvaccinated primates (including people) for 1 mo after inoculation.

Rabies: All exotic mammals are susceptible to rabies (*see* p 1302). Vaccination is considered core for felids and canids in endemic areas and recommended for mammals in zoos in areas where incidence of rabies in free-living wildlife is high. However, the efficacy of parenteral rabies vaccination of exotic mammals has not been established, and no commercially available vaccine is licensed for use in free-living animals. Use of rabies vaccines in these species is extra-label and is not considered protective in the event of a bite. Based on the potential for human rabies exposure, keeping wild-caught carnivores as pets should be discouraged and is illegal in many jurisdictions. Wild-caught animals such as foxes, raccoons, and skunks may have been exposed to the virus when quite young and may incubate disease for a prolonged period (>1 yr), rendering a short observation period inadequate. The National Association of State Public Health Veterinarians recommends that wild-caught animals with public contact (eg, in zoos) should be quarantined for at least 180 days.

When vaccination is considered necessary, only killed-virus vaccine should be used, and it should be administered via deep IM injection. MLV rabies vaccine licensed for use in domestic species should never be used in exotic animals, because such vaccines are often insufficiently attenuated and may produce clinical rabies and death. Several inactivated vaccines prepared of nervous tissue (eg, murine, ovine, or caprine) or tissue culture have been found satisfactory in terms of safety and immunogenicity, the latter based on limited tests that demonstrated adequate antibody responses in some exotic carnivores. The human diploid cell-line origin killed-virus vaccines appear to have the best immunogenicity in domestic species. Young animals are vaccinated at 3–4 mo of age, and vaccinations must be repeated annually. Vaccination for rabies of bats in captivity is done at some institutions; MLV vaccination of bats incubating the rabies virus may hasten the disease course and result in death (as occurs in people). Use of oral bait vaccination for control of rabies in wildlife continues in several countries; this vaccination is not intended for use in captive, single animals.

Clostridial Diseases: Primates, exotic Equidae, Proboscidae (elephants), Pongidae, Cervidae (deer), camelids, and exotic sheep and goats should be immunized against tetanus. Although the susceptibility of tapirs to tetanus has not been documented, vaccination is recommended. Exotic Equidae and elephants are vaccinated on the same schedule as domestic horses; primary immunization at 3–4 mo of age consists of two IM injections of tetanus toxoid, 1 mo apart. A single booster dose is given annually.

Pongidae are often vaccinated against tetanus using the diphtheria, tetanus toxoid, and phase 1 pertussis (DPT) vaccines intended for use in human children or monovalent human tetanus toxoid. Monovalent tetanus toxoid is preferred, because pertussis and diptheria are not considered health risks for nonhuman primates. However, susceptibility of these diseases likely varies in primates, because olive baboons were recently found to develop clinical signs of pertussis and a strong anamnestic response. Primary immunization consists of 0.5 mL of vaccine injected IM on three occasions at 3-mo intervals, with a booster dose 1 yr after the third injection. Thereafter, booster immunizations of 0.5 mL of diphtheria-tetanus toxoid or tetanus toxoid alone are given every 3–5 yr or after potential exposure due to injury.

In exotic hoofstock, the need for clostridial vaccines depends on animal husbandry and density, environment, and local disease circumstances. If vaccination is warranted, vaccines should be given according to manufacturers' recommendations for hoofstock. Multivalent clostridial vaccines are available for prophylaxis; tetanus antitoxin can be used if tetanus is a concern. Pregnant animals should be vaccinated 4–8 wk before parturition to increase specific colostral immunoglobulins. Neonates can be vaccinated at 4 and 8 wk of age with *Clostridium perfringens* type C and D. Exotic sheep, goats, and cervids are sometimes vaccinated beginning at 10–12 wk of age with multivalent clostridial bacterin-toxoids containing immunogens for *Clostridium tetani*, *C perfringens* (types B, C, D), *C septicum*, *C chauvoei*, *C novyi*, *C sordellii*, and *C haemolyticum* in areas of high exposure risk. The initial dose is 5 mL followed in 6 wk by a 2-mL dose, administered SC. A 2-mL booster dose should be given annually.

Miscellaneous: A number of infectious diseases, including bovine viral diarrhea (BVD), bluetongue, malignant catarrhal fever, epizootic hemorrhagic disease of deer, anthrax, encephalomyocarditis virus, cowpox, and brucellosis, may appear as serious local problems but are not widespread in zoos. Unfortunately, satisfactory vaccines for many infectious diseases are not available for exotic animals. Inactivated BVD vaccines are recommended in situations in which BVD has been a problem. Annual vaccination with one standard bovine dose IM should begin at 3 mo of age. Satisfactory vaccines for bluetongue, epizootic hemorrhagic disease, malignant catarrhal fever, and encephalomyocarditis virus are not currently available in the USA. In contrast, a number of vaccines are available for extra-label use in exotic mammals, which may not be efficacious or necessary. These noncore vaccines for domestic carnivores include feline leukemia virus, feline immunodeficiency virus, *Chlamydia felis*, feline infectious peritonitis, feline *Giardia* vaccine, coronavirus, and Lyme disease. If a collection has a history of these diseases or is in an area endemic for disease, vaccination may be considered. Anthrax vaccine has been administered to cheetah (*Acinonyx jubatus*) and black rhinoceros (*Diceros bicornis*) without apparent ill effect, and conference of protective immunity in some with a single booster was recommended. Vaccination of valuable animals could be considered in the event of an outbreak. Brucellosis affects both free-living and captive marine mammals, with minimal apparent zoonotic potential. No vaccination or other control methods for brucellosis are established for these or other exotic mammal species in captivity. Vaccination programs for free-living bison and cervids are controversial. Although the MLV vaccine effectively prevents future abortions and the transmission of brucellosis, it does not protect from infection or seroconversion, may induce abortions in pregnant animals, and is infectious to people. The reemergence of brucellosis worldwide and an increasing incidence of human disease underscore the need for new and improved brucellosis vaccines. The vaccinia, cowpox, and smallpox (variola) viruses are closely related pox viruses that may have all evolved from a single ancestral virus. Cowpox virus has caused morbidity and mortality in canids, felids, equids, elephant, rhino, camelids, viverrids, rodents, primates, and hoofstock; zoonotic disease has been reported. Vaccinia titers have been documented in free-living nonhuman primates in South America. The CDC currently limits distribution of vaccinia vaccine to health care and bioindustrial laboratory workers with exposure risk.

MANAGEMENT AND NUTRITION

HEALTH-MANAGEMENT INTERACTION

MANAGEMENT OF REPRODUCTION

NUTRITION

MANAGEMENT AND NUTRITION INTRODUCTION

Almost all domesticated animals rely on their caretakers to maintain their health and well-being, to provide appropriate nutrition, and to meet behavioral needs and any special physiologic requirements. The success of proper management and nutrition is especially important to agricultural species that must sustain growth and production. Genetic advancement has led to continual increases in productivity that place similar continual pressure on animal husbandry management to ensure it does not limit animal health, well-being, or productivity.

Proper management and nutrition are also central to the prevention and control of infectious and noninfectious diseases.

Infectious diseases occur after colonization of an animal by microbes (eg, a bacterium, virus, rickettsia, parasite), but simple infection by a microorganism is not usually sufficient for disease to develop. Environmental and host factors influence whether the animal will develop clinical or subclinical disease or have impaired productivity. Management has a substantial impact on environmental and host conditions that contribute to disease susceptibility.

Eradication and exclusion of specific organism(s) that cause disease is the only certain way to prevent infectious disease. This is usually impractical or impossible for many common diseases of agricultural animals. As a result, it becomes necessary to control rather than to prevent infectious disease by reducing circumstances that favor the presence or the spread of the infectious agent, by mitigating environmental circumstances that contribute to development of disease once animals have become infected, and by minimizing circumstances that increase host susceptibility. Circumstances that contribute to the development of a disease are called risk factors, and they can be related to the microbe, the environment, or the host. Identifying and mitigating the impact of risk factors is the goal of a management strategy to prevent specific diseases and to maintain productivity.

A multifaceted approach to disease prevention and control through management practices is particularly important when dealing with many of the common infectious and noninfectious diseases seen in food animal production systems (eg, enzootic pneumonia in calves and piglets, neonatal diarrhea, bovine respiratory disease complex of feedlot cattle, infectious infertility in swine and cattle, metabolic disease in dairy cows) as well as in companion animals (eg, respiratory disease in catteries, kennel cough in canine boarding facilities, infertility and viral respiratory disease in horses). Many of these diseases are difficult to control without an integrated approach, because they either have a complex etiology involving the interaction of multiple microbes or are caused by pathogens for which there are no reliable treatments or effective specific preventive measures.

Prevention and control of these diseases is best achieved by implementing management practices to mitigate recognized risk factors for infection, disease development, and impaired productivity. Often, these are general management recommendations that are not targeted at specific infectious organisms. Effective control may also require implementation of management practices to address risk factors unique to particular pathogens and diseases.

The need to identify and implement multifaceted management strategies that will maintain health and enhance productivity is likely to increase in animal agriculture. This need for new strategies is driven by competitive and economic forces within the industry and by pressure for change from interested parties outside agriculture. Identifying and implementing these management changes requires collaborative efforts of all groups working in livestock production, including veterinarians, animal scientists, and nutritionists, with consideration of economic and other forces acting on producers.

All of agriculture, but particularly animal agriculture, is under pressure from consumer and special interest groups to address concerns arising from some industry practices. These concerns include potential links between agricultural practices and antimicrobial resistance in human pathogens, relationships between environmental contamination and intensive animal production, the role of agricultural management practices in reducing the risks of foodborne illnesses and risks of exposure to zoonotic pathogens, and the impact of agricultural practices on animal welfare. Even though there may be no conclusive evidence linking livestock production to these public health and public interest issues, livestock production management will likely change in response to the perception of such links. Any changes in current practices will require development of new approaches to maintain animal health and production, which will require a substantial investment in research and education.

Increasingly, livestock production must ensure that management practices are implemented at the farm level as part of the industry-wide system to maintain the safety and wholesomeness of the food supply. Validated on-farm food safety programs are often based on Hazard Analysis and Critical Control Point (HACCP) principles. They emphasize that all stages of the food production chain have a role in ensuring food quality and safety. Developing, implementing, and auditing these management programs are essential to maintain consumer confidence. These programs require implementation and documentation of management practices that reduce the risk of physical, chemical, or microbial hazards entering the human food supply through production practices on farms.

Animal agriculture is also under pressure from within the industry to better protect the industry itself. Well-publicized outbreaks of disease such as bluetongue, Schmallenberg virus, avian influenza, and transmissible spongiform encephalopathies in several species (eg, bovine spongiform encephalopathy, scrapie, chronic wasting disease) have focused the industry's attention on biosecurity as a disease prevention and control strategy. Biosecurity is a set of management practices that aims to prevent the introduction of infectious or other disease-causing agents and/or to prevent the further spread of agents that are introduced or are already present (*see also* below). Biosecurity programs can be implemented at a room, building, farm, regional, or national level. Similar to disease prevention programs, biosecurity programs often comprise a set of general practices and sets of management practices targeted at specific pathogens.

Nutritional management is a subcategory of animal management. Proper nutrition is essential to health and productivity. Nutrition also plays a role in susceptibility to disease (eg, feline lower urinary tract disease) as well as in medical management of certain diseases (eg, diabetes in dogs and cats, equine metabolic syndrome, ketosis and hypocalcemia in dairy cattle). Rations/diets must be formulated to provide for basic physiologic needs (eg, energy, protein, fats, carbohydrates, vitamins, minerals) and to ensure optimal growth and productivity. Proper ration formulation considers age, sex, breed, physical activity, and lactation and gestational status.

Nutritionally related diseases include diseases associated with a nutritional excess (eg, direct toxic effect, digestive upset), nutritional deficiency (either primary or secondary), or nutritional imbalance. In animal agriculture, health and production are also heavily influenced by feeding management in addition to ration formulation. Feed preparation and delivery are often as important in ensuring animal health and productivity as the actual nutritional value of the ration itself. Inadequacies in nutritional delivery can directly cause disease (eg, ruminal acidosis, laminitis) or increase susceptibility to disease (eg, *Clostridium perfringens* enterotoxemia).

Nutritionally related diseases in companion animals also include both conditions of excess (eg, developmental orthopedic disease in dogs related to excess calcium and energy) and of deficiency (eg, blindness in cats related to taurine deficiency).

Feeds and feeding management can also influence animal health if feeding results in exposure to physical hazards (eg, sharp objects), chemicals (eg, mycotoxins, toxic plants), allergens (eg, dust mites, mold spores), or microbes (eg, molds, *Salmonella* spp). Feeding and waste management practices are also important to prevent and control infectious disease spread through fecal-oral transmission (eg, salmonellosis, neosporosis, paratuberculosis, toxoplasmosis).

BIOSECURITY

The tenets of biosecurity have been long recognized by veterinarians. However, throughout the past decades, interest in biosecurity as a scientific discipline has surged because of 1) disease outbreaks that have threatened to devastate agricultural economies, and 2) bioterrorism. In fact, the meaning of the term biosecurity and the structure and focus of biosecurity programs have evolved throughout time to more accurately reflect the scientific community's evolving perception of disease as well as the needs of the consumer, the veterinary profession, and producers and owners.

In modern animal medicine, biosecurity is probably best defined as "all procedures implemented to reduce the risk and consequence of infection with a disease-causing agent." This broad definition recognizes that disease is a complex interaction between the host, the disease-causing agent, and the environment. Biosecurity can be considered in terms of individual animals or populations of animals (flocks or herds), economic entities (production facilities or companies), or geographic regions (counties, states, countries, or continents), thus facilitating compartmentalization for trade purposes. Importantly, it addresses strategies for both disease prevention (eradication) and control (limiting the consequence of infection).

Benefits of an effective biosecurity program include optimized animal health and welfare and, in the case of food animal medicine, improved productivity and end-product value, as well as safe regional/international trade. Although implementation of a comprehensive biosecurity plan or program has obvious benefits, allocation of resources must be economically (food animals) or emotionally (companion animals) justified. Unless a disease poses a specific risk to human health or animal welfare, its mere presence in an individual animal or population of animals is not significant. Intervention strategies are consequently chosen based on both their economic and biologic efficiency.

A dynamic and integrated epidemiologic and economic analysis is required to determine and quantify the negative effect of a disease challenge, and the anticipated positive response to the proposed intervention strategy. Such integrated analysis has become significantly more important in intensive production systems.

The economic impact of disease can be difficult to assess. This is particularly so in intensive production systems in which economic return is governed by not only animal productivity but also product quality. In addition, the consequential loss from disease challenge is, at best, only partially recoverable. Using the cost of disease to justify intervention overemphasizes the consequence of inaction, and it is useful only in justifying intervention strategies directed at preventing disease challenge.

PRINCIPLES OF BIOSECURITY

Disease control and prevention relies on the interrelated processes of bioexclusion, surveillance, and biocontainment. Prevention of disease is costly, difficult, and time consuming and is primarily directed at preventing epidemic or exotic diseases. It invariably involves eradication of disease-causing agents from a population of animals or geographic area. In contrast, control programs are less demanding and primarily focus on limiting endemic diseases to tolerable levels within a population of animals or geographic area. Although preventing exposure to disease-causing agents remains an objective of control strategies, strategies are primarily focused on limiting the consequence of disease.

Disease Prevention: Disease prevention depends on 1) stringent bioexclusion to avoid contact between the disease-causing agent and the host, 2) early detection of a breach in biosecurity through vigilant surveillance, and 3) rapid implementation of a ruthless biocontainment policy. This is feasible only if there is an effective means of detecting infection; containing the infection through slaughter, clean-out, and disinfection; and preventing dissemination of the disease-causing agent. Eradication is reserved for those diseases that pose a dire public health threat, that have a devastating effect on animal performance, or that severely compromise end-product quality.

Disease Control: In disease control strategies, the emphasis shifts from preventing disease to reducing its consequence or economic impact. Prevalence data are now used primarily to assess the level of protection and challenge, not merely the presence or absence of disease. Although biosecurity still relies on principles of prevention, disease-control programs focus more on limiting the extent and consequence of exposure. Many biosecurity measures aimed at preventing or eradicating epidemic disease also produce beneficial by-products, such as establishment of a firm foundation for control of erosive/endemic diseases and enhancement of host resistance through immunization.

Disease Management and Disease Determinants: Disease-risk management must be an integral part of any animal management program. Economic analysis is a critical step in biosecurity plan design, because resource allocation must be aligned with risk. The success of a disease control program depends on the ability to identify and subsequently address risk of infection. Disease risk in a population is characterized by the probability of point infection and subsequent spread. Aggregate risk is the sum of each individual risk of adverse health effects in an exposed population. The spread and consequence of point infection is influenced by several factors referred to as disease determinants.

Because infectious disease is the result of a complex interaction between several factors, any factor that influences the risk and consequence of disease challenge is a disease determinant. Disease determinants have traditionally been classified as primary or secondary; intrinsic or extrinsic; and host-, agent-, or environment associated. In intensive production units, the housing environment, agent, and host determinants are largely under the control of the manager/caretaker, who thus has the greatest influence on disease determinants.

Risk Assessment: Risk assessment is used to estimate the probability of exposure to an agent, the probability that exposure will cause infection and disease, the probability that disease will spread, and the consequence of such spread. Statistical techniques such as the chi-square test can be used to assess whether a specific factor/process is correlated with disease, but these provide no estimate of the degree of disease risk. The measure of association most frequently used to assess risk magnitude is the risk ratio (probability of disease given exposure divided by the probability of disease given no exposure).

Disease control begins with evaluating each part of the production process as a risk factor for infection. On a basic level, risk of infection equals the probability of each event causing infection multiplied by the number of times each event occurs. But estimating the degree of risk requires analysis of many other factors, including host resistance and the dose/virulence of the organism.

As a first step to limit health risk, a biosecurity program should critically assess the necessity of all events or processes that potentially carry risk, and only crucial ones should be allowed. Limiting the potential for infection within crucial events is focused on improving host resistance or reducing the challenge dose or virulence of the infecting organism.

Host Resistance: Immune efficiency is the key factor governing host resistance. A healthy animal produces an appropriate immune response sufficient to combat infection and its impact on productivity. Conversely, a response that is either excessive or insufficient will adversely affect well-being and performance. Resistance varies among individuals primarily due to genetic differences that typically follow a Poisson distribution.

Immunosuppression reduces both individual and herd/flock immunity. The weakest members of a population will be most negatively impacted by individual stressors (eg, disease or poor nutrition), which have a cumulative impact on immunity. Such highly susceptible animals tend to skew the resistance curve to the right, resulting in a dramatic decline in flock/herd immunity.

Host resistance, challenge dose, and organism virulence determine whether an infectious challenge results in disease. Dose is the number of organisms to which an individual animal is exposed, and virulence is the inherent capability of the agent to infect (infectivity) and cause disease (pathogenicity) within the host. The traditional measure of infectivity is the infective dose 50 (ID_{50}), which is defined as the dose required to infect 50% of the animals in a specific population.

When designing a health program, it is important to remember that the ID_{50} represents more than a measure of disease virulence. It is more factually the dose required to infect the least resistant animal within the population. This is because the risk of a challenge exposure increases once one animal in a population becomes infected or diseased. Agent replication increases the risk of exposure by increasing the dose and (possibly) virulence of the agent, with each new infection escalating the risk further until even relatively resistant animals become at risk.

Epidemiology: *See also* BASIC PRINCIPLES OF EPIDEMIOLOGY, p 2397. Effective biosecurity requires an understanding of the causal relations between exposure and disease, because the prevalence and consequence of any infectious disease involves a complex interaction between several disease determinants. The epidemiology and relative risk for each disease should be assessed to determine the best way to allocate resources for effective control procedures. Furthermore, epidemiologic statistics can be used to determine the best way to limit current and future financial risk. Several important epidemiologic factors need to be considered (below).

Source of Infection: In addition to identifying those animals that have become infected, other variables, which are associated with the relative importance of a particular source, should be assessed, including the shedding pattern, host range, mode of transmission, and farming practices.

Transmission: Disease transmission within a population is influenced by direct contact with infected animals, as well as by indirect exposure from contaminated objects (fomites). These forms of horizontal transmission influence the rate and extent of transmission within and among groups. This is in contrast to vertical transmission between parent and offspring. Vertical transmission may result from direct contamination or (in some cases) from transovarial transmission of disease-causing agents within the embryo itself.

Spread: Disease spread is influenced by factors such as incubation period, replication rate, resilience, and virulence of the disease agent. These factors influence spread within the population as well as disease course (acute, subacute, chronic) within individuals. For example, disease spread is accelerated by a resilient organism with a short incubation period and high replication/shed rate.

Susceptibility and Predisposition: For an effective control program, it is important to know the range (species, breed, type) of susceptible hosts. Furthermore, host, agent, and environmental factors can predispose animals to infection or disease. For example, environmental stress can compromise immune function.

Prevalence: Disease prevalence is directly proportional to the risk of challenge. Endemic diseases are difficult to prevent, whereas diseases that are exotic (ie, not normally present) or epidemic in nature are easier to track, contain, and eradicate.

Morbidity and Mortality: Morbidity refers to the animals in a population showing signs of disease at particular times. Diseases that spread rapidly typically have a high morbidity rate (percent). Mortality rate represents the percentage of animals in a population expected to die during a particular disease outbreak.

Recovery: Disease recovery is influenced by many factors (ie, disease determinants).

THE THREE LEVELS OF BIOSECURITY

A comprehensive biosecurity program should represent a hierarchy of conceptual, structural, and procedural components directed at preventing infectious disease transmission within and across farms, companies, facilities, regions, countries, and continents. Avoidance is the most effective way to prevent disease transmission involved with animal ownership or production. But given that all movement of animals within or across groups/borders involves risk of contact, biosecurity measures are needed to reduce unavoidable risk.

Conceptual Biosecurity: This primary level of biosecurity revolves around the location of animal facilities and their various components. The most effective way to limit risk is physical isolation, making this a primary consideration when siting new confinement facilities or farms. Facilities/farms should not be located next to public roads, especially when the area has a high density of animal facilities. Similar isolation methods include limiting the use of common vehicles and facilities, limiting access by personnel not directly involved with the operation, and controlling the spread of disease by vermin, wild animals, and wind.

Structural Biosecurity: This secondary level of biosecurity deals with physical factors such as farm layout, perimeter fencing, drainage, number/location of changing rooms, and housing design. Long-range planning and programming is important and should consider on-site movement of vehicles, equipment, and animals; traffic patterns; and feed delivery/storage.

Procedural Biosecurity: This tertiary level deals with routine procedures to prevent introduction (bioexclusion) and spread (biocontainment) of infection within a facility. These activities should be constantly reviewed and quickly adjusted as needed in response to emergencies.

DEVELOPING A BIOSECURITY PROGRAM

Biosecurity programs consist of bioexclusion, surveillance, and biocontainment.

Bioexclusion

The primary focus of bioexclusion is to limit the level of exposure to disease-causing agents below the threshold for infection or colonization. This requires a systematic approach to preventing pathogen movement across physical or imaginary barriers (protection zones), so as to eliminate or decrease the number of disease-causing organisms within the animal's environment. Sound epidemiologic principles should be used to establish zone boundaries while making use of existing physical/geographic barriers.

Global Perspective: The global nature of the animal industry results in daily shipment of animals and animal products throughout the world. This trade is regulated by the World Organization for Animal Health (OIE), and such commerce must comply with OIE regulations, including those pertaining to farm-level control measures.

Country Perspective: To control spread of disease, the OIE aids in the establishment of international agreement on animal and plant sanitary (SPS) measures. Such an agreement within the World Trade Organization establishes common definitions and describes OIE in-house procedures for dealing with international trade disputes. This treaty has also established guidelines and principles governing the transparent, objective, and defensible assessment of risk. More specifically, import risk analysis provides importing countries with an objective and defensible assessment of the disease risks associated with importation of such items as animals, animal products, biologic products, genetic material, feedstuffs, and pathologic material.

Region or State Perspective: To account for the difficulties in controlling the disease status and management practices of animal populations across the vast expanse of large countries (eg, the USA), the Terrestrial Code makes allowance for zoning and compartmentalization. The code defines subpopulations based on animal health status, allowing member countries to limit damaging trade effects associated with disease outbreaks, without exposing the importing country to risk from disease spread. There are also "compartments" based on biosecurity procedures and "zones" based on geography. The requirements to establish these subpopulations vary based on disease specifics and the requirements of the trading partners, and they are best decided before disease outbreak. Factors such as disease epidemiology, environmental influences, natural/artificial boundaries, surveillance and monitoring, and applicable biosecurity measures (eg, movement controls and husbandry) are of particular interest. To establish local zones/compartments, the veterinary services of an exporting country must clearly define subpopulations as stipulated in the Code. Relevant claims must be reported to the veterinary services of an importing country and supported by official, detailed documentation.

Zone borders are based on natural, artificial, or legal boundaries, making them relatively easy to establish and officially communicate. Compartments based on biosecurity procedures are more difficult to define. The requirements for a compartment include defining adequate biosecurity plans, operating procedures, and management practices that are well documented (including documentation of compliance). This process involves developing a partnership and clearly stipulated responsibilities between animal owners and the appropriate veterinary authority.

Requirements of biosecurity plans include adequate and robust disease surveillance, animal identification, and traceability. This necessitates detailed records for factors such as animal movement and production, feed sources, sources of replacement stock, disease surveillance (including morbidity and mortality), vaccination and medication history, personnel training, and visitor logs. Risk mitigation also requires that the plan be regularly audited, reviewed, and adjusted as needed.

Company Perspective: For purposes of biosecurity, companies operate as compartments within a country, state, or region. Minimal requirements of international trade require that companies conform to international standards, thereby meeting OIE requirements. As compartments within the biosecurity rubric, each trading company, region, state, or country should classify prescribed OIE diseases according to expected prevalence; design, document, and implement a biosecurity plan to prevent/control these diseases; and provide proof of plan compliance. This biosecurity plan forms the basis for all disease prevention, diagnosis, and control strategies. The plan should identify potential pathways for disease introduction/spread within the company and describe the measures being (or that will be) taken to minimize risk as prescribed within the OIE Terrestrial Code.

Primary Control Zone—Animal Confinement Facility: Bioexclusion begins at the animal confinement facility, which is the smallest epidemiologic unit within the company. The animals within this facility share a common environment, common management practices, and similar likelihood of pathogen exposure. The boundaries of these facilities represent well-defined barriers to entry and an ideal place for implementation of critical control procedures. Every crossing of the facility perimeter should be considered an "event" with potential for pathogen transfer or disease risk.

Reducing the risk from such events requires an "all-in, all-out" strategy. Thorough cleaning, decontamination, and chemical disinfection should be performed when the facility is empty. Once animals arrive, the focus shifts to limiting the number of events (in-house perimeter crossings), as well as the probability of pathogen transmission and infection during unavoidable events.

Secondary Control Zone—Farm or Site: The next zone/compartment in the disease-control hierarchy is the farm or site. In this case, the epidemiologic unit is the farm rather than the containment facility. There is a defined boundary surrounding the farm, and the farm animals share a common environment with common management practices, thereby sharing a common likelihood of exposure to pathogens from nearby containment facilities.

The farm/site establishes real (eg, fence) or imaginary boundaries that serve as access points to the secondary control zone, which is a critical zone for disease control. From a biosecurity standpoint, the site is considered "closed" if the farmer/producer enforces full biosecurity with no uncontrolled access after disinfection. The site is considered "open" if general biosecurity is enforced at the start of transfer/depletion, with access granted only to necessary vehicular traffic. The site is "fully open" if routine control is enforced from the point of last animal removal. Sites involved in an outbreak should remain closed until the responsible veterinarian declares them clean.

Tertiary Control Zone – Complex:

Groups of animals that share a communal animal handling facility (ie, a complex) constitute a tertiary control zone. The complex represents its own epidemiologic unit, because sites/farms within it share facilities such as feed mills and processing plants. Production processes within the complex (eg, rearing farms and grow-out farms) similarly constitute separate epidemiologic units. All the defined areas may represent tertiary control zones for biosecurity purposes. Tertiary zones are seldom fenced, so access boundaries are typically imaginary.

As a cost-effectiveness measure, tertiary zones are often established around high-value sectors of the operation, such as the valuable stock used in breeding operations. To reduce transmission risk, critical control points such as transit facilities can be established beyond the site perimeter. At these points, procedures such as showering, changing into protective clothing, and transfer to site/zone-dedicated transport significantly reduce the probability of disease transmission onto the site.

Surveillance

The terms monitoring and surveillance are both used to describe ongoing data collection to estimate disease prevalence and severity in a population. However, a monitoring program is typically geared toward collecting statistically reliable prevalence data that can be used to track trends in disease incidence and severity over time. A surveillance program is based on prevalence data from a readily available sample of the population, with the goal being timely action to correct perceived increases in disease incidence. The importance of these programs increases when remote management-control is needed to keep up with increases in herd/flock size and production.

When catastrophic outbreaks require eradication, the surveillance program should be focused toward detecting source cases, allowing implementation of biocontainment through quarantine and slaughter. For situations in which eradication is not required, collection of prevalence data should be adjusted so as to differentiate background variation from effects of disease.

The data collection system should be designed so as to provide insightful and epidemiologically informative disease indicators. During design, it is good to keep in mind the need for important parameters (eg, sample size) that can be used to calculate other animal-health estimates, such as prevalence, incidence, morbidity, mortality, and herd/flock immunity (as indicated by antibody titers, farm production records, etc). In the absence of random sampling, such statistical estimates cannot be taken as absolutely accurate but may serve as adequate markers of the need for intervention.

For purposes of disease eradication and trade, it may be necessary to demonstrate freedom from infection in the country, zone, or compartment/company. Although there may be no obvious evidence of infection in the population, it is impossible to definitively prove freedom from infection unless a perfect (100% sensitive/specific) test is used to examine every member of the population. In this situation, the surveillance system should be able to statistically estimate to an acceptable level of confidence that infection is below a specified prevalence level.

As part of health tracking, individuals should be monitored for disease at regular intervals. Any change in prevalence suggests a change in incidence that may require corrective action to prevent disease spread. The frequency at which animals are monitored depends on disease epidemiology and the level of biocontainment (eg, need for quarantine or slaughter). Factors such as latent period, mode of transmission (eg, vertical or horizontal), potential for animal dispersion and tracking, and test sensitivity are important considerations.

Biocontainment

Biocontainment strategies reduce the consequence of disease challenge by limiting the opportunity for challenge (bioexclusion), enhancing resistance (immunization), and preventing spread (quarantine). When eradication is required, quarantine is usually followed by emergency slaughter. Control measures are routinely applied for endemic diseases but more sporadically for epidemic outbreaks.

The term quarantine refers to the practice of enforced isolation of animals exposed to infectious agents, as well as the place in which these animals are isolated and the time period of isolation. Quarantine is routinely required when live animals or their products are imported. To avoid disease entry into a country, region, zone, compartment, or population, potentially infectious animals/material must be isolated until they have been shown to be disease free.

Enforced isolation is the first biocontainment step when potentially infected animals are brought to a production setting. Movement within or through the control area is restricted and monitored. The size/nature of the control zone depends on disease risk but usually involves a containment facility, farm, site, or complex within a particular company. The control zone may be expanded to a 2-mile radius for diseases of national/regional importance.

Disease monitoring is used to establish the extent of an outbreak, first within the quarantine zone and then in a well-defined surrounding contact zone. The relevant veterinary authority assumes control in cases of foreign/notifiable disease. All vested parties (eg, countries, states, regions, companies, owners) should prearrange an emergency response plan sufficient to address relevant details of containment and eradication.

Chemoprophylaxis and Vaccination: Medication may be added to feed or water to reduce disease risk. Vaccination is commonly used to reduce the risk and/or consequence of infection among exposed individuals or populations. The main purpose of immunization is to prevent clinical illness by raising the ID_{50} of the population. Vaccinations can be used to protect individuals from disease or to protect the next generation by limiting direct vertical transmission and enhancing maternal antibody transfer.

HANDLING DISEASE OUTBREAKS

Feed and water consumption and production should be carefully monitored at all times, as well as the typical sounds and behaviors of individual animals. Any deviation from normal indicates the possibility of infectious disease, and immediate action should be taken to prevent inadvertent spread of infection. Initial steps include setting up a quarantine of the pen, building, farm unit area, or entire farm, depending on its design and programming; designating separate caretakers for affected animals; and checking and examining sick animals last.

Owners should seek professional diagnostic assistance, rather than trying to hide some disease because of possible public recrimination. Veterinarians and caretakers can and should help dispel this apprehension by maintaining high ethical standards and refraining from discussing one producer's problems with others. Yet, there comes a time when all producers must be apprised of a problem. Service workers visiting affected animals should wear protective footwear and clothing when they enter the facility, and no other farm should be visited without adequate decontamination.

It is important to reach a diagnosis as soon as possible. The nature of the disease will determine the course of action. Although it is not always possible to treat a disease or stop its deleterious effects, identifying primary and contributing diseases is important to plan effectively for the future. Veterinarians should be aware of the owner's economic plight and render advice and assistance as quickly as information is available or a judgment can be made.

In addition to causing serious economic and emotional loss, some diseases are hazardous for people. When zoonotic conditions are suspected or diagnosed, extra precautions must be taken to prevent infection of attending personnel. Notifiable diseases require that appropriate government authorities be alerted and that all in-contact personnel be carefully tracked and assessed. In some regions, certain diseases must be reported immediately to the state animal disease control authorities so that proper investigation and action can be taken to protect the affected industry.

Every effort should be taken to ensure appropriate nursing care, which plays a key role in improving the outcome of a disease outbreak. Therapeutic medication should be used only after the problem has been diagnosed and recommended/prescribed by the veterinarian. Therapy is not a sustainable method of disease control and should not be considered an ongoing part of any biosecurity program. The flock response to medication merely provides the time necessary to investigate, design, and implement further control measures to avert additional need for therapeutic medication. No drugs should be given until a diagnosis is made and a veterinarian consulted.

Sick animals should not be moved or handled until they have recovered/stopped shedding the disease-causing agent, unless the move is to a more favorable environment as part of therapy. It is important to consider that some healthy carriers may remain among apparently recovered animals.

CLONING OF DOMESTIC ANIMALS

The basic concept of cloning via nuclear transfer is that the nucleus of a cell, taken from a tissue sample of a donor individual, is transferred to an enucleated oocyte, and then the oocyte is stimulated to develop into an embryo. The embryo thus produced has the same genotype as the original donor individual.

TECHNICAL ASPECTS OF CLONING

Cells recovered from early embryos, up to the morula stage, work efficiently as donor cells for cloning. Cloning from embryonic cells was conducted successfully for more than a decade before the birth of the first mammal produced via nuclear transfer using adult somatic cells ("Dolly," a sheep reported by the Roslin Institute, Scotland, in 1997).

The most common tissue used for cloning from adult animals is subcutaneous connective tissue. The tissue is minced and cultured in vitro. Outgrowing fibroblasts are harvested and replated (passaged) in new dishes to continue proliferation until millions of cells have been produced. These are then typically cryopreserved for future use.

Mature oocytes from the same or closely related species are required for the nuclear transfer. The genetic value of the oocytes is not important, although their mitochondrial makeup may be, because the resulting clone will carry the mitochondria of the host oocyte (*see* below). Oocytes are typically recovered from slaughterhouse material and then matured in vitro, although in some species, meiotically mature oocytes (from preovulatory follicles or from the oviduct after ovulation) are collected.

Nuclear transfer is typically performed using a microscope with micromanipulators. The chromosomes of the oocyte are removed, creating an enucleated oocyte, or ooplast. The somatic cell used for cloning must be synchronized to early in the cell cycle (before DNA synthesis). The somatic cell is combined with the ooplast, either by membrane fusion using an electric pulse or by direct injection of the donor cell into the ooplast via micromanipulation.

The recombined oocyte, now containing the nucleus of the donor cell, is treated to mimic the activation signal of fertilization, which stimulates it to develop into an embryo. After activation, the developing embryo may be transferred surgically to the oviduct of a recipient female or may be cultured in vitro to a stage at which it can be transferred to the uterus transcervically (nonsurgically), as for standard embryo transfer.

Health and Phenotype of the Cloned Animal:

Health and Phenotype of the Cloned Animal: Several factors influence the health and phenotype of the cloned individual, including epigenetic effects, mitochondrial DNA, uterine and postnatal environment, mutations, and individual variation.

Epigenetic Effects: After nuclear transfer, the ooplast must reprogram the DNA from the somatic cell so that it functions like that of a zygote. This is controlled largely by methylation and demethylation of bases in the DNA and by modification of the histones, the proteins around which the DNA is wrapped. Controlling the transcription of DNA in this manner, without altering the structure of the DNA itself, is termed epigenetic control. The oocyte must reprogram the DNA of the donor cell initially at the time of cloning, and then maintain the normal patterns of epigenetic modification through the different stages of development. The amount and accuracy of reprogramming of the donor DNA is probably the major reason for success or failure of fetal development in cloning. Minor changes in epigenetic status may not affect the general health of the cloned individual but may still cause it to vary in phenotype from the donor animal. A visible example of this is seen in the first cloned cat, CC. CC expresses only brown coat color, whereas her genetic donor expresses both orange and brown (eg, calico). Because the X chromosome carries the gene for coat color in cats, this indicates that in CC, X chromosome inactivation is not random; rather, the same X chromosome is inactivated in all cells, presumably because of failure to reactivate the inactive X at the time of cloning.

Epigenetic effects may also influence the phenotype of the nuclear transfer–derived animal after birth; eg, an animal with growth-factor genes transcribed at high levels may grow larger than its cloned sibling with less active genes, even though the actual number and makeup of the genes are the same. However, it has been shown in all species studied that major epigenetic anomalies are not passed on to the offspring of clones because of resetting of epigenetic status during sperm and oocyte development.

Mitochondrial DNA: The nuclear transfer embryo will have the nuclear DNA of the genetic donor but have the mitochondrial DNA of the recipient oocyte. A small number of mitochondria from the donor cell may also be present, but proportionately few. The impact of the source of mitochondria, or a mixture of mitochondria, on the traits of the progeny is currently unknown. Because mitochondria are the source of energy for the cell, differences in mitochondria could potentially have an effect on production, stamina, or other physical or behavioral traits.

The heterogeneous mitochondria present in a female produced by nuclear transfer will be passed down to the female's offspring, because they will be present in her oocytes. However, although sperm from a male produced by nuclear transfer will carry the heterogeneous mitochondria, these mitochondria will be eliminated after the sperm fertilize an egg, so a male clone can be considered to produce progeny that are genetically identical to those that the original donor animal would have produced.

Environment: Uterine size and health; milk production of the dam; nutritional, exercise, and training programs; and handling to which the neonate is exposed may all influence the animal as an adult. For example, the cloned cat, CC, is outgoing and gregarious, whereas her genetic donor was reserved. However, the genetic donor was a research cat, raised in a cage and unused to attention, whereas CC was raised with an overabundance of attention and stimulation.

Mutations: Genetic mutations are potentially more likely in cloned animals, because cultured cells are used as the DNA source. The donor cells are grown and passaged in vitro, and this is associated with an increasing number of chromosomal abnormalities with increasing passages. However, cells with chromosomal abnormalities are unlikely to produce viable embryos.

Individual Variation: Cell differentiation occurs in cascades, as differentiation of one cell type affects the status of the cells around it. During development, cell multiplication and apoptosis occur in response to many environmental and internal stimuli. Thus, random individual variations will occur in the makeup of tissues, even in individuals of the same genetic background. A visual example of this is in the markings of cloned animals; individuals cloned from the same cell line tend to have white in similar places, but the markings can vary dramatically in size and shape.

STATUS OF CLONING DOMESTIC ANIMALS

Live young have been produced by nuclear transfer in all major domestic mammalian species: cats, dogs, horses, cattle, goats, sheep, and pigs. Cloning in cats appears to be repeatably successful; oocytes may be obtained using tissue recovered from clinical ovariohysterectomies. Interspecies cloning of closely related nondomestic cat species using domestic cat oocytes has produced live young.

Cloning in dogs is complicated by several factors. Mature canine oocytes must be obtained from the oviduct after ovulation, because effective methods for in vitro maturation of canine oocytes have not been developed; additionally, bitches are in estrus only about once every 6 mo, so oocyte availability is low and synchronization of recipients is problematic. Cloning in horses results in a low blastocyst development rate (3%–10%), but viability after transfer is among the highest reported; ~30% of transferred embryos produce live foals, and postnatal survival is high (>85%).

Cloning in food animal species is facilitated by the ready availability of oocytes from slaughterhouse tissue. Cloning in sheep and cattle is inefficient (5%–15% of transferred embryos result in live young), and 30%–50% of live neonates die by 4 yr of age. Cloning in sheep and cattle is associated with frequent placental abnormalities, especially low numbers of atypically large cotyledons. There is a high incidence of large offspring syndrome in cloned calves and lambs (ie, fetal overgrowth with related abnormalities) and, in live calves, of transient metabolic abnormalities such as hypoglycemia or poor renal function. Cloning in goats has similar efficiency in production of live young per embryo transferred, but cloned kids tend to have greater viability. Goat oocytes are typically obtained by follicle aspiration ex vivo, and this may increase viability of resulting clones. In pigs, 1%–5% of transferred recombined oocytes produce live young, but cloning is made practicable by the ready availability of large numbers of oocytes and the ability to transfer hundreds of recombined oocytes to the oviducts of a single recipient. Cloned piglets are generally healthy; they have a higher than normal incidence of stillbirth and of some abnormalities but do not develop large offspring syndrome.

RATIONALE FOR CLONING

Companion animals may be cloned for emotional reasons or as models for endangered species. Horses are cloned mainly to allow continued production of offspring from individuals with valuable genotypes or to retain a genetic type (eg, geldings that are exceptional performers). Cloning of farm animals may be performed for agricultural or biomedical applications. Agricultural applications include production of animals with valuable production traits, such as high-producing dairy cows, animals with superior carcass quality at slaughter, or production of additional sires of an established valuable genotype.

Biomedical applications of cloning are largely related to the ability to perform nuclear transfer using a cell line that is genetically altered (transgenic) and, thus, to produce an animal with those characteristics. Biomedical applications include generation of animals of specific genotypes as disease models, animals carrying genes for the production of medically important proteins that may be harvested from the milk or tissues, and animals having genetically altered organs (of low immunogenicity) for transplantation to people.

CONTROVERSIES

Ethical concerns about cloning may be broadly divided into two categories: concern about the effect of cloning on animal and human welfare, and objection to the principle of cloning, ie, to producing an animal by a means other than fertilization.

Currently, cloning is associated with an increase in animal suffering when compared with production of animals by standard breeding methods. This is due to surgeries performed to obtain oocytes or transfer embryos, pregnancy losses, sickness and death of neonates, low-level abnormalities in surviving young, and possible distress from disease in animals produced as disease models. These concerns are somewhat mitigated by the fact that most of these findings are not unique to cloning; they are also associated with other procedures that have been generally accepted as worthwhile, such as in vitro fertilization and embryo production, oocyte transfer, and embryo transfer. In addition, the accepted normal fate of many species being cloned is to be housed for maximal production and then be slaughtered and eaten. A compelling argument for cloning is that the potential benefits of the procedure to the understanding of life processes and animal disease, to human health, and to food production outweigh the cost of the procedure in terms of animal welfare.

Additional concerns rest with the effect of cloning on the entire animal population, most commonly related to the genetic variation of the species. This is a legitimate concern in some species and uses, such as in dairy cattle, in which one bull may sire thousands of offspring. However, this is more related to the technology of semen freezing and distribution than to the fact that a bull itself was cloned. In companion animals, it is improbable that the very few pets likely to be cloned will have an effect on the population in general. In horses, cloning may in fact increase genetic variation, because a major proposed use is to clone geldings that have been found to be superior competitors, thus rescuing genetic types that would otherwise have been lost.

Concerns about human health focus mainly on consumption of food produced from cloned animals. After years of study, the FDA and the European Food Safety Authority have concluded that consumption of meat or milk from cloned animals poses no public health risk. Therefore, remaining concerns about consumption of food from cloned animals is likely based more on principle than on actual potential for harm. Because cloning is used to produce transgenic animals, many perceived concerns regarding cloning are actually concerns about transgenic animals, which present a completely different set of potential hazards to animal and human health and the environment. European nations have relaxed their position on use of cloned animals and their progeny in the food chain based on the lack of evidence of a human health risk and the difficulty in establishing a tracing or labeling system to identify such meat when coming from outside countries.

A key ethical question regarding the principle of producing animals by cloning is whether this technique is violating some moral prohibition, ie, that people are "playing God" by producing embryos without using fertilization. Similar questions have arisen with each new reproductive technique that has been developed; however, many people feel that cloning is a special case. This general moral aversion of the public to the concept of cloning is enhanced by the portrayal of cloning as a malevolent force in science fiction books and films.

Counter-arguments to these moral concerns are that cloning occurs in nature in the form of identical twins; that people have been producing plants and animals by "unnatural" means from the first time they planted a seed in a new area or bred a cow to a selected bull, and that this is simply a new development in the same line. Embryonic cloning was being performed for more than 10 years before the birth of Dolly with essentially no public attention, and even the birth of two lambs cloned from cultured cells of embryonic origin, announced a year before Dolly, had no public impact. Thus, it appears that the main moral issue of public concern is not the production of embryos without fertilization, but the production of embryos from cells of an existing, known animal.

Arguments against cloning of companion animals have focused on the cost of producing a clone—tens to hundreds of thousands of dollars—when millions of unwanted dogs and cats are killed each year. However, people currently buy purebred dogs and cats for thousands of dollars when they could get animals for no or low cost. American culture supports the concept that people can spend their own money on whatever they wish.

A related argument is that cloning turns animals into a commodity or an object, rather than a sentient being, and that producing an animal in this way shows a lack of respect for the animal as an individual. However, animals have been bought and sold since they were domesticated; currently semen and embryos are frozen, shipped across the country, and used to produce desired young. Cloning does not seem to offer any unique distinction in this area.

Commercialization of cloning brings with it the possibility of fraud and of preying on the emotions of bereaved pet owners. Cloning companies should state clearly that the technique will produce another individual with the same genetics as the original animal; it does not "resurrect" an animal. The best simile to draw is to that of an identical twin born later in time; just as with naturally occurring identical twins, they will be very similar but also different in many ways.

COMPLEMENTARY AND ALTERNATIVE VETERINARY MEDICINE

Complementary and alternative veterinary medicine (CAVM) as defined in 2001 by the American Veterinary Medical Association, is "...a heterogeneous group of preventive, diagnostic, and therapeutic philosophies and practices. The theoretical bases and techniques of CAVM may diverge from veterinary medicine routinely taught in North American veterinary medical schools or may differ from current scientific knowledge, or both." Although some of the myriad approaches have been used to treat animals for centuries, many have not. Instead, they have been extrapolated from human approaches without first undergoing assessment for safety and effectiveness in nonhuman animals.

Despite the popularity of CAVM among some segments of the public, along with intensive promotion by certain groups, much remains unknown regarding the true therapeutic utility of many aspects of CAVM. Thus, to gain a legitimate foothold in modern medicine, CAVM must demonstrate a rational mechanism of action and withstand scientific scrutiny.

The diversity of approaches that constitute CAM range from the well-studied to the bizarre and baseless. Certain treatments, such as homeopathy, lack biologic plausibility. Others require belief systems more consistent with faith-based healing than medicine. Much of the material published regarding CAM promotes unreliable and potentially dangerous advice. CAM providers cannot always provide a scientific basis and critical perspective for what they practice.

The responsibility for protecting and benefiting veterinary patients remains with the scientifically educated clinician. Veterinarians who consider referring patients for CAVM or practice modalities have a responsibility to distinguish tried-and-true from too-good-to-be-true. This is accomplished by conducting well-designed scientific trials to investigate relevant clinical questions and by regularly reviewing the medical literature to reassess which modalities have accumulated independently confirmed data. Even if a certain clinical application has not yet received research scrutiny, studies showing a plausible and unique mechanism of action, as well as a safety record, can help support a rational decision about whether to recommend it.

Although numerous modalities and treatments are associated with CAVM, the ones discussed below are some of the more well known or considered for veterinary use.

ACUPUNCTURE

Acupuncture refers to a method of inserting thin, sterile, solid needles into specific sites on the body. Its myriad applications span analgesia to treatment of organ dysfunction, neurologic abnormalities, myofascial restriction, immune disorders, and many other conditions. Although most think of needles when they hear the term, acupuncture actually incorporates an array of interventions intended to either augment the needle's effects or obviate the need for needling altogether. Such interventions include electrical stimulation (ie, electroacupuncture); moxibustion (in which a smoldering herb heats the acupuncture point or embedded needle); low-level laser stimulation (laser puncture); pressing techniques (acupressure); and injection of vitamins, saline, or other solutions into sites (aquapuncture).

Practitioners of "traditional Chinese medicine" (TCM) adhere to principles developed in prescientific times, replete with mistaken interpretations about organ functions and suffused with metaphors such as "wind invasion" and "spleen damp heat" instead of modern medical knowledge.

Although the roots of Chinese medicine can be traced as far back as the Han dynasty (206 BCE to 220 CE) or earlier, the field of TCM as adopted by many veterinarians is recent. TCM was updated and compiled by order of Chairman Mao Tse Tung in the mid-twentieth century. Confronted with widespread epidemics and too few Western-trained physicians, Mao sought a revised and simplified compilation of Chinese medical theories that would help address the public health needs of the ailing masses. He also eventually found it helpful to promote quintessentially Chinese approaches as a matter of national pride. Subsequently, he marketed TCM to Western doctors. An unfortunate mixing of western metaphysics with TCM transformed acupuncture into a pseudoscientific "energy medicine" practice that disavows science and its true underlying actions of neuromodulation and connective tissue effects. Making matters worse, TCM practitioners cling to dubious diagnostic techniques such as tongue diagnosis and pulse diagnosis. No research supports the validity or reliability of these techniques, even for people for whom these practices were developed.

Fortunately, decades of scientific research on its mechanisms and indications now make it possible to practice acupuncture and related techniques without metaphors or belief systems. Patients receive diagnoses based on modern medical methods and informed palpation. Needling is regarded as a means of afferent stimulation that engenders modulation of central, peripheral, and autonomic nervous system function, as well as signal initiation and transfer among associated connective tissue structures. Objective outcomes can be measured and assessed through scientific research, as results from rigorous, controlled trials lend further sophistication and insights into treatment plans and physiologic outcomes, respectively.

Mechanisms of Action: The belief among TCM practitioners that acupuncture works by moving invisible energies began with a mistranslation of the Chinese word "qi" into energy in the 1930s. A French bankteller working in China, Georges Soulié de Morant, strongly believed that "energies" formed the basis of healing. For lack of a better word, Soulié de Morant translated the term "qi" into "energy." Thus began the misplaced notion in the West that acupuncture moved "energy." In reality, the term "qi" referred to dissolved gases and nutrients that circulated throughout the vascular system. Given that acupuncture was originally a blood-letting technique, this explains the correspondence between acupuncture channels and blood vessels. Over time, as needles became thinner and more refined, acupuncturists ceased bleeding patients. By the 1950s, Chinese scientists began accepting that the effects they found in patients occurred as a result of the nerves being stimulated near the former blood vessel targets. Today, the term "neuromodulation" has been accepted by scientific acupuncturists around the world as explaining the basis for acupuncture's effects.

Research findings from physiologic studies show that acupuncture needles, or other devices, affect afferent nerve fibers in the skin, subcutaneous tissue, fascia, muscle, tendons, vascular walls, or periosteum, purportedly eliciting local or peripheral reflexes that have beneficial effects on the body.

Several explanations exist for how acupuncture reduces pain. Some assert that acupuncture interrupts nociceptive transmission at the level of the spinal cord, producing spinal segmental analgesia, or that acupuncture alters the processing and perception of pain centrally. Others have suggested that any pain-relieving effects may be more simply attributed to placebo effects, distraction, a diffuse noxious stimulus, or psychologic alteration of the perception of pain. Various neurotransmitter and neuroendocrine responses have been associated with acupuncture. Specific parameters important for optimal effects in acupuncture are emerging as research defines how treatment design impacts clinical outcomes. For example, targeting specific dermatomes corresponding to local pathology rather than remote sites leads to greater improvements in pain control, physical activity, and sleep quality. Frequency and duration of stimulus also influence the analgesic response. Mounting evidence reveals a multiplicity of mechanisms and clinical benefits from acupuncture. Research is expanding regarding the clinically relevant benefits that acupuncture confers on many problems, including those of inflammatory, musculoskeletal, neuropathic, neoplastic, or visceral origin.

Indications: Acupuncture holds value for treatment of acute and chronic pain, neurologic dysfunction, musculoskeletal disorders, GI motility disorders, circulatory problems and insufficiency, immune dysfunction, reproductive disorders, and the negative sequelae of conventional cancer treatment.

Contraindications: Acupuncture has a strong safety profile, and few contraindications exist. Although pregnancy is often considered a contraindication, based on concern that acupuncture might affect hormone levels or uterine innervation, evidence of serious adverse effects is lacking, even in late pregnancy. Coagulopathies or immune compromise might represent contraindications if needling leads to excessive bleeding or local infection, respectively.

Acupuncture may be contraindicated if an animal cannot remain still enough to perform needling safely. High levels of anxiety, fear, or aggression could counteract health-promoting autonomic changes generated by acupuncture. In such cases, efforts to calm the animal may be warranted.

Some TCM-based acupuncture practitioners may claim that cancer is a contraindication for acupuncture, although no evidence exists to support their claims that unseen energies emanate from the point into the tumor and incite growth. The belief that acupuncture will encourage cancer metastasis because it can augment circulation is similarly unfounded; however, there is also no proof that acupuncture itself fights cancer.

Adverse Effects: Acupuncture provided by medically educated professionals such as veterinarians results in few adverse effects and is generally considered safe. The risks of invading a major organ or vessel with a needle are limited as long as the practitioner remains aware of the patient's anatomy. Extreme negative reactions to a needle may indicate that it has entered a nerve; in those cases, the needle should be withdrawn. Handlers of horses have been injured when horses have kicked during acupuncture treatment. Needle ingestion by the patient appears to constitute the most frequent concern in animals, although there are no published reports of injury. Adverse reactions that have been reported in people include fainting, skin infections, and hepatitis; such reactions have not been reported in animals.

Controversies: The fundamental tenets of energy-based acupuncture remain unproved. No evidence indicates that invisible meridians or qi energies exist. Due to the limited number of clinical studies in acupuncture for veterinary patients and the current disavowal of the scientific basis of acupuncture by TCM practitioners, acupuncture has not been recognized as a specialty by the American Board of Veterinary Specialties.

Gold bead implantation, the process of intentionally inserting small bits of metal into the body as a type of "permanent acupuncture," resembles a Japanese technique in which acupuncturists buried acupuncture needles into tissue and cut them off at the surface, leaving a lifelong implant.

The medical literature contains cases in which acupuncture needle fragments or implants have migrated to the spinal cord, peritoneal cavity, heart, stomach, liver, breast, brain, bladder, kidney, and colon. In animals, radiographic evidence has shown that implants can migrate long distances, eg, from the hip to the thoracolumbar region or abdominal wall. Embedding ferromagnetic objects in tissue may compromise the quality of computerized scans such as CT and MRI, causing artifacts and obscuring diagnoses. So far, no studies of gold bead implantation justify the risks of migration and artifact-laden imaging studies.

Additional adverse effects of implants include activation of mast cells, argyria, contact dermatitis, and gold-induced myelotoxicity.

MANUAL THERAPY

Manual therapy is a general term that refers to treatment approaches involving the hands (such as massage or chiropractic). Treatments done with the hands may also be instrument-assisted. Although manual therapies are most commonly used for the treatment of somatic pain or other musculoskeletal maladies, other indications may include lymphedema, immunosuppression, or visceral discomfort.

Massage techniques vary widely, ranging from the traditional kneading and stroking to deep tissue work requiring concerted pressure. The most commonly researched technique is Swedish massage, also known as classic muscular massage. Swedish massage incorporates several maneuvers, including effleurage (stroking and gliding), tapotment (percussion), petrissage (kneading), and friction massage. Effleurage involves tissue compression. Tapotment vibrates tissue, petrissage stretches adherent fibrous tissue, and friction lengthens connective tissue to reduce contractures. Massage techniques are multicultural and share similarities; for example, Swedish massage has similarities to the Chinese manual therapy technique Tui Na. Other massage techniques include German connective tissue massage and Rolfing, a strong and sometimes painful form of "deep tissue" massage introduced in the USA. "Medical massage" addresses specific diagnoses with soft-tissue techniques, with the goal of treating certain conditions. It differs from relaxation massage in its "manual medicine" approach, ie, using the hands to help heal conditions seen in practice.

Manual therapy frequently targets the spine. When people speak about "animal chiropractic," "veterinary manual therapy," or "animal adjusting," they are usually referring to forceful maneuvers directed to the back or neck in an effort to alleviate pain or, more generally, spinal dysfunction. Some interventions are borrowed from the human chiropractic field and incorporate mechanical devices known as adjusting tools or activators. When used, this hand-held device, which resembles a metal syringe with a rubber knob at the end, delivers a rapid "thump" to the patient, roughly mimicking the action of a person applying a thumb thrust to the body. More violent and less sophisticated methods applied to horses incorporate mallets and blocks of wood intended to "drive protruding spines into line"; all such methods have, as yet, failed to demonstrate therapeutic utility in animals.

Mechanisms of Action: Massage focuses on soft-tissue elements—namely, muscles and the enveloping fascia. Benefits such as stress and blood pressure reduction, normalized gastric motility, immune regulation, and amelioration of depression may share a common mechanism of action. That is, the neuromodulatory and homeostatic effects of massage likely pertain to parasympathetic nervous system stimulation.

Evidence now supports use of massage as an aid to muscle recovery after exercise or injury, a means to improved circulation, and a way to bolster immune function. It also addresses GI motility dysfunction and neonatal issues such as failure to thrive. Massage also can improve lymphatic drainage in cases of lymphedema, although the effects may be transient.

In contrast to massage, the rapid thrusts in chiropractic have many theoretical—but no proven—mechanism(s) of action. The lack of current knowledge tends to be extrapolated into speculation, and chiropractic theories may be presented as fact. Claims are made that chiropractic manipulation activates muscle spindles, Golgi tendon organs, joint capsule mechanoreceptors, and receptors in the skin, and that simultaneous firing of multiple types of receptors modifies CNS activity, blunting nociception and normalizing muscle tone, joint mobility, and sympathetic nervous system activity. However, there is inadequate basic science data to substantiate any of these claims. No chiropractic technique has been shown to be superior to another; little chiropractic research has been done in veterinary patients.

Indications: For massage and chiropractic in veterinary patients, indications may include neck or back pain or stiffness, inability to sit straight, reduced flexibility, muscle spasms, poor performance, difficulty going up or down stairs, inability to walk or run in a straight line, and abnormal tail carriage. However, there are no data from well-designed scientific trials to support the utility of such interventions in dogs, cats, or horses. The evidence for massage in human babies and adults suggests support for including this approach in animals with stress, pain, arthritis, sluggish digestion, or spinal cord injury.

Contraindications: Because adverse events of complementary therapies are underreported, the true range and incidence of risks from massage remain unknown. Patients who are especially fragile or ill generally require briefer and gentler treatments with less digital pressure and compression. Soft-tissue techniques would not be applied directly over areas of infection, acute inflammation, tumor, recent surgical procedures, or thrombosis. Similarly, massage may not be ideal in areas of acute inflammation, skin infection, bone fracture, burn, deep vein thrombosis, or cancer.

Contraindications for chiropractic might include conditions that weaken bone or other structural elements such that applying a thrust to a vulnerable spine or limb could lead to serious injury. Examples of deossifying or destabilizing conditions include hyperadrenocorticism, neoplasia, secondary renal hyperparathyroidism, degenerative joint disease, and disk disease. Some animal chiropractors have advocated chiropractic for a gamut of problems, including idiopathic lameness, intervertebral disc disease, Wobbler syndrome/cervical vertebral insufficiency, spondylosis, cauda equina syndrome, urinary incontinence, neuropathies, postsurgical rehabilitation, trauma, and organ pathology. However, many of these may actually constitute contraindications. One research-based human CAM reference places joint hypermobility, arthritis, and neurologic problems from disc disease under the heading of contraindications to chiropractic, along with cancer, infectious disease, fractures, clotting disorders, osteopenia, and osteoporosis.

Adverse Effects: Excessive pressure from massage and forceful thrusts from chiropractic both have the potential to injure organs, vessels, neural tissue, or bones. Deep massage of the abdomen may damage organs (rupture/bleeding) and nerves (from direct pressure onto nerves); intense pressure could dislodge a stent or catheter or embolize thrombi. With chiropractic manipulation, thrusts are not always innocuous. A heavy-handed individual can seriously harm or even kill an animal. Even milder thrusts may injure animals weakened by age, joint pathology, osteopenia, or neoplasia.

Injuries from chiropractic usually result from trauma to the spinal cord or brain arising from impacted blood vessels, discs, or nervous tissue. Human neurologic and neurosurgical reports have revealed an association between stroke and upper cervical manipulation. In addition to high velocity techniques, deep massage or other pressing techniques in the suboccipital region have damaged vessels and caused neurologic impairment and death. Although rare, stroke from cervical chiropractic manipulation of human patients is well recognized and likely occurs more often than is reported. The mechanism of injury typically involves arterial dissection or spasm.

A study of human patients with neck pain showed that 25% of patients reported increased neck pain or stiffness after chiropractic treatment, and adverse reactions were more likely to follow higher force techniques. The study concluded that because high-force techniques failed to demonstrate superior effectiveness to low-force maneuvers, chiropractors should consider conservative manipulative procedures. Especially in geriatric or otherwise fragile animals, manual therapy techniques from the soft-tissue therapy repertoire constitute safer approaches than forceful, high-velocity techniques.

Controversies: From a mechanical standpoint, extrapolating human chiropractic theories to animals raises questions. Biomechanical forces on the spine of a quadruped differ from those in bipeds. Furthermore, the vertebrae of horses are the size of a human fist and are surrounded by muscle, tendon, and ligament layers several inches thick, leading to questions as to whether equine vertebrae can be manipulated at all.

Claims that spinal joints or other bones move "out of place" have not been substantiated. Even if such lesions exist, the diagnostic measures commonly used to detect them are not reproducible or reliable. The overall utility of manipulative therapy for the treatment of a condition (including its most common indication, musculoskeletal pain) has not been established.

Finally, additional controversy arises from the fact that manual therapies may be delivered by nonveterinarians. Manual therapies pose potential risks; when they are practiced by overzealous therapists with insufficient education about anatomy and pathology, the risk of injury to the patient or the practitioner increases. Lack of familiarity with animal behavior, zoonotic illness, and proper restraint techniques can pose risks to the therapist or bystanders. Furthermore, nonprofessionals may not have suitable liability insurance for such incidents.

State laws may or may not allow nonveterinarians to treat animals. Some may allow a human chiropractor or massage therapist to treat nonhumans but require a certain level of supervision by a veterinarian. Because state laws differ, veterinarians should check into the legal framework that allows or specifically disallows this form of care by nonveterinarians before referring or delegating care to them.

LASER THERAPY

The term "laser" originated as an acronym that describes its process, ie, light amplification of stimulated emission of radiation. Like acupuncture and massage, laser therapy lessens pain, relaxes muscles, and improves circulation. It accomplishes this by altering the physiology of cells and tissue by means of light (photons) instead of an acupuncture needle or manual pressure. Therefore, treatment effectiveness and the types of responses seen depend heavily on if and how light enters living tissue.

Mechanisms of Action: For tissue to absorb light and alter its physiology, a photochemical or photobiologic event must occur. Ideally, this event would take place within the target tissue(s), whether it be skin, muscle, fascia, nerves, vessels, bones, and/or joints. A "photoacceptor" molecule, also known as a "chromophore," responds to light by initiating a series of physiologic responses that engender healing and improved tissue homeostasis. When a chromophore (such as cytochrome c oxidase in the mitochrondria respiratory chain) absorbs a photon from laser-treated tissue, an electron within the chromophore becomes excited and jumps from a low- to a higher-energy orbit. This increased electron energy provides the impetus for the system to perform cellular activities geared toward growth and repair.

The effects of laser on mitochondria, cells, and tissue is called "photobiomodulation." This collective process encompasses not only the effects of lasers but also those of light-emitting diodes (LEDs) and other light sources. Light therapy also causes vasodilation by relaxing endothelial smooth muscle, likely through nitric oxide mechanisms. Vasodilation improves tissue oxygenation and supports the migration of immune cells into tissue, further aiding recovery.

Treatment Parameters: Many factors impact how light influences tissue, including its power, wavelength, strength, pulse characteristics, tissue contact, and the nature of its beam. As indicated above, photobiomodulation entails changes at the subcellular, cellular, and tissular levels. Within the mitochondria, activated photons engender increases in production of ATP, modulation of reactive oxygen species, and induction of transcription factors. These factors encourage cell proliferation and migration, normalized cytokine levels, enhanced production of growth factors, modulated levels of inflammatory mediators, and improved oxygenation of tissue.

Power and Dose: The term "low level laser therapy" (LLLT) refers to the use of light at much lower levels than those used for tissue ablation or photocoagulation. Newer, high-powered therapy devices that deliver power similar to surgical lasers (but with a less concentrated beam) no longer constitute LLLT. Some even heat tissue, meaning that the term "cold laser" is also inaccurate.

The specific dose(s) of laser required to heal tissue and treat pain remains unclear. Calculating actual joules of energy delivered requires calculations of considerable complexity. Fortunately, a wide range of doses shows benefit for people and experimental animals, despite the wide variety in size, color, and hair coat.

Wavelength: Most therapy units use red or near infrared light, from 600 nm to 1070 nm. This range constitutes the "optical window" wherein effective absorption into tissue is maximal. That said, units with green, blue, and violet light (~400 nm range) are becoming more popular. Visible light ranges from 390 to 760 nm, progressing from violet to blue, green, yellow, orange, and red at 600 nm.

The types and depth of tissue that respond to light therapy depend on the wavelength delivered. Certain molecules, such as melanin and hemoglobin, preferentially absorb light in the 600 nm range. To reach deeper tissues, wavelengths (810 nm, 980 nm) that absorb less in superficial tissue can be used, leaving more light to reach for deeper sites such as bone, the brain, and internal organs.

Certain laser therapy units emit two or more beams to target a variety of tissues.

Laser beams differ from other types of light therapy, including LEDs, by being monochromatic (existing within a narrow band of wavelengths), coherent (tightly aligned), and collimated (photons travel in parallel). The more light scatters within tissue, the less intense the biologic impact, which may or may not be the desired outcome. However, debate continues about the relative value and differences between laser light and LEDs.

Pulsed Therapy: It remains unclear whether pulsed wave or continous wave treatment is preferable for certain conditions. Pulsing reduces tissue warming, which is especially important to deliver light to deeper tissue; this requires more power to provide adequate energy supply to the deep tissue target(s). Furthermore, pulsing limits damage to nerves and surrounding tissue.

Pulsing may also improve tissue responses by resonating with a fundamental frequency to which cells innately respond, commonly exhibited by neural structures.

Indications: For more than half a century, scientists have recognized the potential for photomedicine approaches to reduce inflammation, pain, and swelling, as well as to speed wound healing. More recently, medical researchers have uncovered additional benefits pertaining to serious conditions, such as myocardial infarction, spinal cord injury, traumatic brain injury, and stroke. Additional applications include alleviation of pain, trigger point pathology, and joint dysfunction.

Contraindications: Contraindications to direct laser treatment include carcinoma, thyroid gland, active hemorrhage, and autonomic nerve centers. Laser therapy should be avoided in patients in which immune stimulation is not desired, including those with lymphoma or on immunosuppressant medications. In immature patients, higher powered laser therapy devices may stimulate premature closure of epiphyses. Thus, caution is warranted over long bones in animals <1 yr old.

Adverse Effects: Properly used, laser therapy appears to be very safe. However, higher powered lasers run the risk of inducing thermal burns when improperly used. Tattoos, when lasered, can cause intense pain due to the high amount of light absorption by deposited pigment. Questions remain about the ability of laser therapy to stimulate neoplastic growth and, if so, at what wavelength(s) and power(s).

Laser light can damage the retina, whether reflected off shiny surfaces or shown directly into the eye. Laser goggles protect against indirect exposure but not against direct. One should never look into the applicator of a laser therapy device.

Laser light longer than 760 nm is invisible to the human eye. As such, unless a treatment applicator produces a visible finder beam or audible signal, the practitioner will not know when the laser is emitting light. This could cause inadvertent eye exposure and retinal damage. It also could cause confusion about where the beam is pointing. For this reason, infrared laser devices that lack a clear indicator of when the beam is on pose potential safety hazards.

Drug Interactions: The immunostimulatory effects of laser therapy may counteract immunosuppressive actions of certain medications. In addition, photosensitizing agents such as hypericin in St. John's wort may augment the dermatologic impact of laser light.

Controversies: The main controversies surrounding laser therapy involve questions and unproven claims related to pulsed therapy, the advantage of low- or high-powered units, and the longterm safety of high-powered treatment.

HERBAL MEDICINE

Herbal (botanical) medicine involves the practice of prescribing plant products, or products derived directly from plants, for the treatment of disease. Herbal medicine has survived since prehistoric times, in part because, until recently, there were no effective alternatives. Some plants do contain biologically active ingredients, and some pharmaceuticals in widespread use today are identical to, or derivatives of, bioactive constituents of historic folk remedies. Indeed, herbal and botanical sources form the origin of as much as 30% of all modern pharmaceuticals.

Evidential support concerning use of plant products in veterinary patients is scarce and ranges from effective and safe to ineffective and risky. However, the methodologic quality of primary studies on herbal medicines for many species is generally poor. Trials usually lack firm endpoints, and periods of observation are usually short; the clinical relevance of the observed effects is not always clear. In addition, data that directly compare herbal remedies with well-established pharmaceutical products are often not available. However, as the database on herbs continues to grow, veterinarians seeking to prescribe natural, plant-based compounds should inspect the latest scientific literature for information on the compound or product of interest.

Making a rational decision about an herbal product requires knowledge of its active ingredients, its safety and adverse effects, and whether the herb has been shown to be as good as or better than pharmaceutical products available for the same purpose. This information is incomplete or unavailable for most herbal products. In addition, there are no standards or quality control testing of the products regularly recommended for animals. Risk versus benefit questions must be considered for products with unclear constituents and unknown active ingredients.

Preparations: Botanical products come in a variety of preparations intended either for ingestion or external application. They may be fresh, dried, or freeze-dried; extracted and preserved in oil, alcohol, or water; and delivered as liquids, capsules, pills, poultices, or powders. Other forms of plant-derived substances include essential oils—volatile, rapidly evaporating oils obtained from the leaves, stems, flowers, seeds, or roots of a plant, commonly used in aromatherapy or massage.

Philosophical or Cultural Approaches: The philosophical approach of the practitioner tends to dictate the type(s) of herbs prescribed. For example, North American botanical medicine evolved from European and Native American traditions relies more on pharmacologic actions than on folklore and metaphysics. In comparison, traditional Chinese veterinary medical (TCVM) herbology considers the supposed "energetic" nature of herbs. Western herbal prescribing practices incorporate physical examination findings akin to standard medical assessments, whereas TCVM recommendations depend heavily on the appearance of the tongue and the feel of the pulse. Instead of considering the pharmacologic effects of plants, TCVM practitioners rely on prescientific metaphors to describe the mechanisms of action of products prescribed. This, by definition, leaves them unaware of the actual biochemical processes occurring and is inconsistent with modern medical principles and ethics.

Mechanisms of Action: As aforementioned, herbs are plant-based drugs. However, they differ from pharmaceuticals by having a multiplicity of active, inactive, and unknown constituents with additive, synergistic, and/or balancing properties. The medicinal effects of herbs may vary from batch to batch as growing, harvesting, processing, and storage conditions change from year to year. These factors highlight the challenges of not only characterizing but also anticipating patient responses to plant-based prescriptions.

Indications: Herbalists recommend herbs for a wide range of disorders. For some conditions, the effects of plant-based drugs rival those of pharmaceuticals. There is evidence of effectiveness of botanical medicine for conditions ranging from digestive ailments to inflammatory conditions and immune support. Many herbs exhibit anticancer and antioxidant benefits. Veterinarians should consult the latest publications in medical literature to assess the strength of research for a condition in question, because the field and evidential support for a variety of conditions is growing rapidly.

Contraindications: Contraindications to the use of herbal products are mostly empirical and depend on the health status of the animal and the putative actions of the herb(s) under consideration. Situations warranting special caution include pregnancy, presurgical states in which the antiplatelet actions of plants interfere with coagulation, and cancer. That is, unforeseen herb-drug interactions could interfere with conventional care and cause unexpected results.

Adverse Effects: Rightly or wrongly, most herbal medicines are generally considered safe. However, because of the lack of manufacturing standards, quality control, and known effects in veterinary patients, herbal medicines probably present a greater risk of adverse effects and interactions than any other CAVM therapy. Harmful effects of herbs arise from intrinsic toxicity of the plant, herb-drug or herb-herb interactions, contaminants introduced during processing (eg, heavy metals, microbial contaminants, chemical toxins, or pesticides), intentionally added adulterants (eg, pharmaceuticals), or inappropriate prescribing. Examples of especially risky herbs with known toxicities include those containing pyrrolizidine alkaloids (eg, comfrey and chaparral); natural flea treatments made from pennyroyal, known to be lethal for small animals; and skin treatments containing tea tree (melaleuca) oil, which can cause severe neurologic manifestations and hepatotoxicity in cats if absorbed or consumed in sufficient concentrations. For many herbal poisonings, no antidote exists, making death from "natural" treatments such as herbs frustrating. Many Chinese mixtures have toxic components; their amount may be kept "secret" by the manufacturer as a proprietary ingredient. Substances such as strychnine (a neurotoxin) and aconite (a cardiotoxin) are not uncommon and pose particular risks to veterinary patients. The unwillingness of manufacturers to appropriately label bottles with the amounts of these toxic constituents raises the danger to patients and public health.

Controversies: Before the development of modern pharmaceuticals, botanical-based treatments for veterinary patients were common, as evidenced by veterinary texts of the 19th and early 20th centuries. However, significant differences exist between historical and current use of these products. In the past, herbal products were used as treatment because underlying disease conditions had yet to be identified. Treatment "success" reflected elimination (or spontaneous resolution) of the problem. Because the underlying pathology was either vague or completely unknown, diseases with similar signs could not be differentiated. Veterinarians had few other approaches from which to choose. These factors make it exceedingly difficult to objectively evaluate the true utility of historically used herbal remedies; they also *highlight* the imprudence of placing undue faith in the prescribing practices of the past to determine treatments today.

Animal-based ingredients such as testes, penis, placenta, and horn found in Chinese "herbal" medicines harbor potential for zoonotic disease transmission. In addition to health concerns, animal-derived products in Chinese herbs contribute significantly to animal mistreatment and the endangerment of certain species. The unknown benefits of most mammal or insect ingredients currently do not appear to justify administering these agents to veterinary patients.

NUTRACEUTICALS AND DIETARY SUPPLEMENTS

Nutraceuticals comprise foods, or extracts from foods, that supposedly confer medicinal benefits. Nutraceuticals have become popular with the veterinary community; worldwide estimates of sales approach $100 billion. Such economic success has, for the most part, not been accompanied by scientific evidence of efficacy. As with herbs, a broad and continually expanding spectrum of nutraceuticals exists, but the mechanisms of action, indications, contraindications, adverse effects, and evidential support vary with the product and species. It is beyond the scope of this brief summary to discuss specific nutraceutical products.

One type of nutraceutical in particular warrants mention. "Glandulars," "tissue extracts," or other scientific-sounding equivalent names purportedly improve the health of animals in which the same glands or tissues have become dysfunctional. Although these products are not FDA approved for veterinary usage, veterinary glandulars and related supplements are heavily promoted in the lay animal health literature. Their usage began in the USA during the late 19th century when the practice arose of giving fresh thyroid glands to patients as treatment for hypothyroidism. Subsequently, tissues and extracts from other organs (ovary, adrenal, testis, thymus, brain, etc) became popular treatments. Once standardized medications and hormonal replacements became available, medical practitioners largely ceased prescribing glandular derivatives because medication offered more reliable effects without the unpredictable hormonal effects of extracts and concentrates. The use of raw bovine pancreas in some dogs with exocrine pancreatic insufficiency is a notable exception. Of specific concern with spinal cord and brain "glandulars" is the potential for these CNS derivatives to transmit spongiform encephalopathy.

HOMEOPATHY

Homeopathy, a form of practice initiated in the late 18th century by the German physician Samuel Hahnemann, refers to treatment of disease with sometimes extreme dilutions of substances that in undiluted form might cause symptoms of that same disease; these substances supposedly promote healing. The substances are said to possess vital healing energies that are unchanged, or even strengthened, through the dilution process. Homeopathic remedies usually consist of lactose pills or liquids.

No known, or even credible, mechanism of action exists by which extremely dilute homeopathic preparations might have a therapeutic effect. Controlled studies have demonstrated that the homeopathic "provings"—sessions in which individuals record the symptoms caused by ingestion of the remedies—cannot distinguish between homeopathic dilutions and placebo. Indeed, no study has been able to distinguish homeopathic remedies from control solutions, by any method of analysis. As a result, most authorities consider that any clinical effects obtained from homeopathic remedies are actually placebo effects.

Indications: Although largely unsupported by research, homeopaths typically feel that their remedies can be prescribed for most medical conditions, including cancer. Reported veterinary uses have included inappropriate urination in cats; babesiosis, atopic dermatitis, idiopathic epilepsy, and paroxysmal tachycardia in dogs; fattening of, stillbirths, and diarrhea in pigs; postpartum fertility, mastitis, anestrus, and control of ticks in cattle; diarrhea in calves; salmonellosis in broiler chickens; and helminth parasitism in sheep.

Contraindications: Conditions for which regular medical treatment would provide a more meaningful diagnosis and effective treatment, and for which delay of proper care could prove injurious, should not be treated by homeopathy. Adjunctive homeopathic remedies, which may be prescribed as "complementary" treatments to more conventional therapies, have been shown to be no different from placebo in improving the quality of life of children with mild to moderate asthma when prescribed in addition to conventional treatment in primary care.

Adverse Effects: Chances of homeopathic remedies causing direct toxicities are slight, given their extreme dilution. Homeopathic literature does describe a situation involving a transient worsening of signs called a symptom aggravation or healing "crisis." Homeopaths may regard this as a treatment breakthrough and sign of impending improvement.

Some practitioners advocate giving homeopathic "vaccines" or nosodes instead of conventional vaccines to avoid perceived health risks of standard vaccines. However, homeopathic vaccines have consistently failed to provide reliable protection against infectious agents in scientific studies of both people and animals.

Controversies: A preponderance of evidence indicates that effects of homeopathy cannot be distinguished from placebo. Therefore, the question remains whether it is ethical or misleading to offer an ineffective treatment to patients and their caregivers. The unscientific premise of homeopathy calls into question its legitimacy as a medical treatment.

MANAGEMENT OF THE NEONATE

LARGE ANIMALS

Appropriate management in the peripartum period can substantially reduce morbidity and mortality for large animal dams and their offspring. As much as 5% of foals, 5%–10% of calves, and 10%–15% of the annual lamb crops die before weaning in the USA, with 50%–70% of neonatal mortality occurring in the first 3 days of life. A key aspect of managing the large animal dam includes appropriate nutrition and body conditioning in the pre- and postpartum periods to reduce the risk of pregnancy-related diseases such as pregnancy toxemia, hypocalcemia, and vaginal prolapse; as well as to optimize hygiene, colostrum quality, and fetal and neonatal growth. Appropriate anthelmintic therapy and vaccination of the dam several weeks before parturition will further protect dam and offspring from subsequent disease.

Particular conditions affecting large animal neonates in the immediate postpartum period include prematurity, failure of passive transfer, sepsis, perinatal asphyxia, predation, mismothering, meconium impaction, and various congenital diseases. Substantial losses can occur in flock or herd situations, and altering problematic aspects of management can therefore be of great benefit. Generally, equine and camelid neonates can be managed more intensively than neonatal calves, pigs, or lambs because of economic considerations. However, rapid assessment and appropriate management of all large animal neonates in the immediate postpartum period can substantially reduce the need for intensive and expensive measures in any species.

Growth rates of neonates are particularly rapid during the first month of life. For example, the average Thoroughbred foal is born at ~68% of its mature height and 10%–11% of adult weight, with an average weight gain of 1.5–1.7 kg/day. Regular monitoring of weight gain can thus be a practical aid in determining healthy growth and development. Foals that lack maturity can display a spectrum of clinical and clinicopathologic abnormalities that include short silky hair coat, "floppy" ears, incomplete ossification of the tarsal and carpal bones, hyperextended fetlock joints, domed forehead, abnormal temperature regulation (normal to low body temperature), depressed mentation, weakness, poor suckle reflex, and respiratory dysfunction.

See also NEONATAL INTENSIVE CARE AND EMERGENCIES IN FOALS, p 1708, and DIARRHEA IN NEONATAL RUMINANTS, p 275.

FAILURE OF PASSIVE TRANSFER

Large animal neonates are born with limited energy reserves and are considered immunocompetent but immunologically naive at birth (ie, agammaglobulinemic). Thus, ensuring the provision of good-quality colostrum by the dam and adequate colostrum intake by the neonate are critical influences on neonatal survival. Good-quality colostrum tends to be sticky, yellow, and thick with a specific gravity of >1.060 in mares. All factors that might compromise colostrum quality, volume, and delivery to the neonate should be recognized; these include maternal factors (disease during gestation, premature lactation, maiden dam), delivery factors (abnormal parturition, placental abnormalities), and neonatal factors (prematurity, dysmaturity, maternal rejection, multiple birth, or any other condition limiting neonatal mobility and strength). Manually stripping the teats of the dam to remove wax plugs and to check for the presence of colostrum may facilitate successful nursing attempts. The neonate should be examined for any obvious congenital problems that may inhibit the ability to stand or to nurse effectively, including signs of prematurity, musculoskeletal abnormalities, and cleft palate (and in crias, choanal atresia).

Healthy foals begin sucking colostrum within 1–2 hr after birth, and maternal antibodies are detectable in the foal's blood within 6 hr. Although adequacy of passive transfer of immunoglobulin is generally assessed at 18–48 hr, neonates at high risk of failure of passive transfer (FPT) and/or sepsis may be tested as early as 6–12 hr after birth. Weak or abnormal neonates that do not stand or nurse successfully within 2–4 hr should be supplemented with colostrum early (commonly tube or bottle fed). A 50-kg foal requires a minimum 1.5–2 L (ideally 5%–12% of body wt) of good-quality colostrum (~70–75 g of IgG), fed over multiple feedings in the first 12–18 hr after birth. Colostrum of other species has been used (such as cow colostrum for foals, crias, kids, and lambs) but will not necessarily provide pathogen-specific immunity. Commercial colostrum substitutes have similar limitations and may increase the risk of adverse immunologic reactions if a subsequent plasma transfusion is needed. Oral administration of colostrum or colostral substitutes has only minimal benefit in neonates >18–24 hr after birth because of the limited capacity of the neonatal small intestine to absorb macromolecules.

Complete FPT in foals is defined as a serum IgG concentration of <400 mg/dL at 24 hr of age, with partial FPT being associated with a serum IgG concentration of 400–800 mg/dL. Healthy, vigorous foals with complete FPT (<400 mg/dL) and high-risk foals with partial or complete FPT (IgG ≤800 mg/dL) should receive equine plasma (IV) that contains an IgG concentration of >1,200 mg/dL. The average IgG concentration in 1 L of equine plasma will typically increase the serum IgG concentration of a 50-kg foal by 200–300 mg/dL; therefore, 2–4 L of plasma may be necessary to achieve a final serum IgG concentration of >800 mg/dL in a foal with complete FPT (initial IgG <200 mg/dL).

Frozen plasma should be thawed and warmed slowly to room temperature using warm water, and subsequently administered slowly through an aseptically placed jugular catheter, using an appropriate blood filter set. Initially, plasma is administered at 0.5 mL/kg over 10–20 min (~20–30 mL to an average foal) while monitoring for transfusion reactions. Clinical signs of transfusion reactions may include muscle fasciculation, increased heart or respiratory rates, fever, respiratory distress, laryngeal swelling, abdominal pain, pale mucous membranes, or collapse. If no adverse reactions are observed during the initial slow infusion, the remainder of the transfusion may be administered at rates up to 40 mL/kg over 60–90 min (eg, 2 L throughout 60 min for a 50-kg foal).

Although serum IgG is measured less commonly in ruminants, concentrations >1,600 mg/dL are ideal. Serum total protein may also be used as a rough estimate of colostral transfer in ruminants and should exceed 5–5.5 g/dL. An IgG concentration >1,000 mg/dL is considered adequate in neonatal camelids. Administration of camelid plasma (either IV or IP) is an acceptable treatment of FPT in llamas and alpacas, although IP administration should be limited to vigorous neonates, to minimize the risk of secondary complications.

SEPSIS IN FOALS

Sepsis is a clinical syndrome defined by the development of a systemic inflammatory response syndrome (SIRS) in response to proven or suspected infection. The condition implies an extensive, whole body insult after invasion of bacteria into tissue or a body fluid or cavity. The presence of viable bacteria in the bloodstream is termed bacteremia. Sepsis and SIRS are two of the most common problems of equine neonates, while bacterial infection accounts for nearly one-third of all foal mortality.

Etiology and Pathogenesis: Gram-negative bacteria, particularly Enterobacteriaceae with a predominance of *Escherichia coli*, remain the most common isolates (60%–70%) from neonatal foals with sepsis. However, the prevalence of gram-positive bacteria has increased throughout time, and blood cultures remain important in diagnosis and treatment. Common gram-negative pathogens include *E coli*, *Klebsiella* spp, *Enterobacter* spp, *Actinobacillus* spp, *Salmonella* spp, and *Pseudomonas* spp. Approximately 25%–40% of infections also involve gram-positive bacteria, with *Streptococcus* spp being the predominant isolate. Anaerobic pathogens, especially *Clostridium* spp, are reported in <5% of systemic neonatal infections. The routes of entry for these bacteria may include the placenta, umbilicus, and respiratory and GI tracts.

All sepsis syndromes (eg, sepsis, severe sepsis, septic shock, multiple organ dysfunction) have a common pathogenesis that also includes endotoxemia related to gram-negative infections. Endotoxins stimulate macrophages to release an array of cytokines (eg, IL-6, IL-1, TNF-α) and activate pro-inflammatory enzymes (eg, phospholipase A_2). Together, these factors lead to signs of inflammation (fever, vasodilation, myocardial depression), impaired microcirculation, capillary leak, and intravascular coagulation. Sepsis initially triggers a procoagulant state, which may lead to disseminated intravascular coagulation and secondary consumptive coagulopathy. A variety of other pathogen-derived molecules can set off similar host responses. Thus, toxic shock syndromes resulting from streptococcal or *Staphylococcus aureus* infection are hyperinflammatory septic syndromes that closely resemble diseases characterized by endotoxemia.

A variety of immunologic and management factors predispose foals to sepsis. Although foals can respond immunologically in utero to bacterial or viral infections, their ability to do so is less than that of adults. Deficits in the physiologic response to infectious agents in neonates relate to reduced chemotaxis and killing capacity of neonatal neutrophils, the presence of antigenically naive T cells, and a decreased concentration and impaired function of monocytes. However, the major risk factor for sepsis in foals is failure to receive an adequate quality or quantity of colostral antibodies. If colostrum intake is insufficient and IgG levels remain low, the foal is not only deprived of specific antibody protection, but neutrophil function is also seriously impaired. Other factors that influence disease incidence include unsanitary environmental conditions, low gestational age of the foal (prematurity or immaturity), poor health and condition of the dam, difficulty of parturition, and the presence of new pathogens in the environment against which the mare has no antibodies.

Clinical Findings and Lesions: The clinical presentation of sepsis depends on the duration of illness, the integrity of the host immune system, the affected body systems, and the severity and route of infection. Frequently affected organ systems include the umbilical remnants, and CNS, respiratory, cardiovascular, musculoskeletal, renal, ophthalmic, hepatobiliary, and GI organs. In the early stages of sepsis, clinical signs are often vague and nonspecific, with affected neonates merely displaying some degree of depression and lethargy. Owners report that foals appear to lie down more than usual. The mare's udder is often distended with milk, indicating that the foal is not nursing at a normal frequency.

Clinical signs can progress to a complete loss of suckle reflex, hyperemic mucous membranes with a rapid capillary refill time due to peripheral vasodilation, tachycardia, and potentially early petechiae related to capillary leak. In the advanced stage of illness, when the infection overwhelms the host's immune system and compensatory responses, septic shock ensues. Affected foals are severely depressed, recumbent, and hypovolemic, which manifests as cold extremities, thready pulse, and poor capillary refill time. Foals may be hyper- or hypothermic, tachycardic, or bradycardic. In the face of sepsis, bacteria spread hematogenously to various organs, manifesting as respiratory distress, pneumonia, diarrhea, uveitis, meningitis, osteomyelitis, or septic arthritis. Dysfunction of two or more organs is termed multiple organ dysfunction syndrome.

Hypoglycemia commonly accompanies systemic infection and is associated with bacterial consumption and reduced glycogen reserves. Severely hypoglycemic foals may be unable to rise and show depression, convulsions, and eventually death. Furthermore, clinical signs suggestive of relative adrenal insufficiency have been identified in animals with prolonged sepsis. Primary relative adrenal insufficiency can occur after a direct insult to the adrenal glands (hemorrhage or adrenal ischemia), whereas chronic, illness-induced stress may exhaust the adrenal reserve and deplete the production of cortisol. Septic neonatal foals are often neutropenic with a high ratio of band (immature) to segmented neutrophils. The neutrophils may exhibit toxic changes, which are highly suggestive of sepsis. Fibrinogen levels >600 mg/dL in a foal <24 hr old are indicative of an in-utero infection. Other chemistry abnormalities may include azotemia due to inadequate renal perfusion or perinatal asphyxia, and increased bilirubin secondary to endotoxin damage to the liver. A high anion gap (>20 mEq/L), hyperlactatemia, hypoxemia, hypercapnia, and a mixed respiratory and metabolic acidosis may be present with arterial blood gas analysis.

Diagnosis: Currently, there is no ideal diagnostic tool to detect early sepsis. However, a scoring system has been developed for neonatal foals to establish the likelihood of neonatal infection and aid the identification of sepsis at a treatable stage. This "sepsis score" incorporates a combination of historical, clinical, and laboratory variables and may also serve as an indicator of whole body insult, SIRS, or multiple organ dysfunction. However, the specific definition criteria for both SIRS and sepsis are most rigorously validated in people and have been conceptually applied to equine neonates only recently. Based on pediatric human and general veterinary guidelines, SIRS may be clinically defined by the presence of at least two of the following five clinical criteria, one of which must be abnormal temperature or leukocyte count: 1) core temperature below or above the normal range for the animal's age; 2) tachycardia, defined as a mean heart rate >2 standard deviations (SD) above normal for the animal's age in the absence of external stimulus, chronic drugs, or painful stimuli; 3) bradycardia, defined as a mean heart rate below the normal range for the animal's age, in the absence of external vagal stimulus, β-blocker drugs, or congenital heart disease; 4) mean respiratory rate >2 SD above normal for age, or animals undergoing mechanical ventilation for an acute process not related to general anesthesia or underlying neuromuscular disease; 5) leukocyte count increased or depressed for age (not secondary to chemotherapy-induced leukopenia) or >10% immature neutrophils. Infection itself may be suspected or proven (by positive culture, tissue stain, or PCR) and caused by any pathogen, or refer to a clinical syndrome associated with a high probability of infection. Evidence of infection includes positive findings from clinical examination, imaging, or laboratory tests (eg, WBCs in a normally sterile body fluid, perforated viscus, chest radiograph consistent with pneumonia). Ultimately, sepsis refers to the presence of SIRS with suspected or proven infection.

Depending on the specific organ systems involved, an umbilical, abdominal, and synovial ultrasound examination; arterial blood gas analysis; arthrocentesis; cerebrospinal centesis; and chest, abdominal, and distal limb radiographs are indicated. Advanced diagnostic imaging techniques (eg, CT of the distal limbs in foals with septic arthritis) may also help with prognosis.

Serum IgG levels should be measured in any questionably sick neonate to eliminate inadequate transfer of passive immunity as a risk factor for sepsis. IgG levels <200 mg/dL indicate complete failure of passive transfer of maternal antibodies, whereas IgG levels >800 mg/dL are considered normal.

A positive blood culture confirms the presence of bacteremia in septic foals, but a negative culture does not exclude the possibility of infection. Differential diagnoses include neonatal encephalopathy (*see* p 2094), hypoglycemia, hypothermia, neonatal isoerythrolysis (*see* p 11), white muscle disease (*see* p 1172), prematurity or immaturity, neonatal pneumonia, and uroperitoneum (*see* p 1506).

Treatment, Control, and Prevention: Foals suspected of being septic should be placed on broad-spectrum antibiotics active against both gram-positive and gram-negative organisms. Penicillin (22,000 IU/kg, IV, qid) in combination with amikacin sulfate (20–25 mg/kg/day, IV) provides good initial coverage until culture results are available. Metronidazole (10–15 mg/kg, PO or IV, tid) may be necessary if an anaerobic infection (eg, *Clostridium*) is suspected. A third-generation cephalosporin (eg, ceftiofur, 4.4–6 mg/kg, IV, bid-qid) may also be used as a broad-spectrum agent in foals with renal compromise. Cefpodoxime proxetil (10 mg/kg, bid-qid) has been recommended for treatment of bacterial infections in equine neonates. Cefepime (11 mg/kg, IV, tid) is a fourth-generation cephalosporin with enhanced antibacterial activity.

Early goal-directed IV fluid therapy is needed to restore tissue perfusion, attenuate the cytokine response, and reverse cellular injury. Volume expansion should be achieved using a balanced electrolyte solution (crystalloid) or plasma (colloid). Immunologic support in the form of IV plasma transfusion (1–2 L) is also indicated to raise the IgG level to >800 mg/dL. Fluid resuscitation is aimed at normalizing specific cardiovascular variables (central venous pressure, mean arterial pressure, urine output, and central venous oxygen saturation), while improving clinical parameters. Severe septic shock may require initial fluid rates of 40–80 mL/kg/hr. Because many foals are hypoglycemic, slower continuous infusions of 2.5%–5% dextrose-containing solution should be administered simultaneously with rehydration fluids.

Treatment with hyperimmune antiendotoxin serum may be considered in foals with endotoxemia. Antiprostaglandin drugs have been found to counteract several of the clinical and hemodynamic changes associated with endotoxemia and septic shock. Low doses of flunixin meglumine (0.25 mg/kg, IV, tid-qid) may help reduce signs of endotoxemia. Additionally, administration of low doses of polymyxin B (6,000 IU/kg, diluted in 300–500 mL of saline, slowly IV) is an investigational treatment used to neutralize systemic endotoxin.

Nutritional support is important, because sepsis creates a catabolic state in foals. If the foal is not nursing adequately, it should be fed mare's milk or a mare milk substitute at 15%–25% of its body weight throughout each 24-hr period. An indwelling nasogastric tube should be placed in foals with a decreased suckle reflex. Parenteral nutrition may also be helpful to provide adequate nutrients in the face of GI dysfunction. Administration of gastric protectants (eg, ranitidine, cimetidine, omeprazole) has been proposed as an adjunct therapy in sick neonates.

System-specific therapy includes lavage of septic joints with sterile fluids, regional limb perfusion, and nasal oxygen support (2–10 L/min) or ventilation for foals with respiratory failure or central hypoventilation. Corneal ulceration may be treated with low doses of topical atropine (although it may cause ileus), NSAIDs, and broad-spectrum topical antimicrobials. Entropion generally requires mattress sutures of the lower eyelid. Surgical removal of infected umbilical remnants may be indicated.

Prognosis: Recovery from neonatal sepsis depends on the severity and manifestation of the infection. Currently reported survival rates are 50%–81% in referral centers, depending on the underlying disease. Severe neonatal pulmonary disease has been associated with a higher mortality (35%–50%). Early recognition and intensive treatment of neonatal sepsis improves the outcome, although an average of 1–4 wk of intensive care should be expected. If the foal survives the initial problems, it has the potential of becoming a healthy and useful adult. One report documented that surviving bacteremic Thoroughbred foals were as likely to start races as their siblings, although their earnings were lower. The latter retrospective case series (n=423) further identified that odds of survival were negatively associated with age at admission, band neutrophil count, and serum creatinine concentration, and positively associated with rectal temperature, neutrophil count, and arterial blood pH. Additionally, in a recent prospective multicenter study, septic foals had increased odds of nonsurvival for each 1 mmol/L increase in L-lactate concentration at admission.

SPECIFIC CLINICAL MANIFESTATIONS OF SEPSIS

Neonatal Pneumonia

See also ENZOOTIC PNEUMONIA OF CALVES AND SHIPPING FEVER PNEUMONIA, p 1431, and ACUTE BRONCHOINTERSTITIAL PNEUMONIA IN FOALS, p 1452.

Hematogenous infection of the lung occurs in association with sepsis, which may be acquired in utero from placental infection or perinatally through environmental contamination (eg, omphalitis, omphalophlebitis), and is more common in neonates with failure of passive transfer (FTP). *Escherichia coli*, *Klebsiella* spp, *Actinobacillus equuli*, *Salmonella* spp, and *Streptococcus* spp are some of the more common bacteria involved in neonatal pneumonia in foals. Descending respiratory infections may be related to inhalation pneumonia (transmission of viral, bacterial, or fungal airborne pathogens), aspiration of infected amniotic fluid due to placental infection, aspiration of gastric reflux, iatrogenic aspiration (oil, medication, oral supplements), and aspiration of milk and meconium. Aspiration of meconium occurs in utero in foals that experience fetal distress.

Early in life, localizing clinical signs of lung infection may be absent even in the presence of extensive disease. Dyspnea may be seen in severely affected foals and manifest as an increase in respiratory rate, effort, or thoraco-abdominal asynchrony (paradoxical breathing). However, signs of respiratory distress and hypoxemia are frequently vague. Even some severely hypoxemic foals may show only restlessness or considerable resistance/struggling during handling or restraint. Auscultation of the lung fields in newborn foals can be very misleading. Fluid sounds are normal immediately after birth, as are crackles due to simple atelectasis of the "down" lung during lateral recumbency. Conversely, foals with significant pneumonia can have minimal abnormal findings on auscultation. Mucous membranes should be examined for color, moisture, injected vessels, and the presence of cyanosis (which likely indicates severe hypoxemia with a PaO_2 <40 mmHg). Additionally, weakness, depression, anorexia, weak or absent suckle reflex, dehydration, and fever may be noted in foals with respiratory disease. Cough and nasal discharge are usually absent in the early stages of neonatal pneumonia. Apparent signs of lung dysfunction may also be associated with nonrespiratory conditions such as metabolic derangements (eg, severe acidosis), pain, abdominal crisis, fever, high environmental temperatures, or excitement.

Diagnosis: Thoracic radiographs are often essential to establish the presence of respiratory disease and determine the type and extent of lung involvement in neonates. Arterial blood gas analysis is preferentially used to assess the degree of hypoxemia and hypercarbia. The more common arterial blood sampling sites in neonatal foals include the dorsal metatarsal artery, the brachial artery on the medial aspect of the elbow, the carotid artery, and the transverse facial artery. Thoracic ultrasonography may further identify the presence and location (affected side) of peripheral lung consolidation, pleural effusion, and abscesses in foals with pneumonia.

Treatment: Broad-spectrum antibiotic treatment of septic pneumonia should be initiated before culture results are available and is targeted toward the most common pathogenic bacteria (*see* above). Additionally, intranasal oxygen therapy and cardiovascular support (including goal-directed fluid therapy) are essential in treatment of compromised foals. Specific respiratory support may further include judicious suctioning, coupage, bronchodilators (eg, albuterol inhalants), and mucolytic agents. Recumbent foals should be maintained in a sternal position to limit positional atelectasis.

Omphalitis, Omphalophlebitis, and Patent Urachus

A patent urachus is the most common umbilical abnormality in neonatal foals. Diagnosis may be based on visual appearance (urine dripping from the umbilicus) or on umbilical ultrasound examination, which can also exclude umbilical infections. Clinical signs of infection may include discharge, pain, and heat and swelling of the umbilicus, although some infections of deeper structures may only be confirmed via ultrasound. The normal equine umbilical stump is usually <18 mm in diameter at 24 hr of age, and it decreases to <15 mm at 7 days of age. The umbilical vein (as it courses cranially to the liver) should be <10 mm in diameter at 24 hr after birth and is slightly smaller than the arteries, which can be followed via ultrasound as they course caudally on either side of the bladder. Ultrasonographic abnormalities consistent with omphalitis or omphalophlebitis in foals include enlargement of the vessels beyond normal limits, asymmetry of arteries with enlargement, abscessation of stump or single vessel, gas shadowing indicative of an anaerobic infection, edema of structures, and hematoma formation.

Treatment and Prognosis: A congenital patent urachus and many milder cases of patent urachus secondary to omphalitis may respond to local therapy (chemical cautery with silver nitrate, topical procaine penicillin G, and thermocautery) and systemic antimicrobials. However, caution must be used not to place caustic agents further than 1 cm into the stump, because ensuing tissue necrosis may predispose to further bacterial infection. Treatment of umbilical infections may include both medical (longterm systemic antimicrobials) and surgical options (umbilical resection). Foals that should be referred to surgery include those with substantial abscessation or venous involvement that extends as far as the liver. Mixed infections are likely, and common isolates include gram-negative bacteria (eg, *E coli*, *Klebsiella*, and *Enterococcus*), gram-positive organisms (especially β-hemolytic *Streptococcus*), and anaerobes (including *Bacteroides* and *Clostridium*), similar to organisms identified in generalized neonatal sepsis.

Overall survival rate with appropriate treatment is reported as 87%. However, severe concurrent disease such as secondary hepatic abscessation, sepsis, or multiple joint arthritis are suggestive of a poorer outcome. Septic peritonitis or uroperitoneum are considered rare complications. Umbilical infections are generally less common in neonatal camelids than in neonatal foals.

Prevention: After an uncomplicated birth, it is ideal to allow the umbilical cord to break spontaneously when the dam rises. In foals, the cord is narrowest at ~5 cm from the body wall, which is the natural separation (break) point. If the cord has to be manually separated, it is best to provide steady traction on the cord while supporting the foal's abdomen at the umbilicus. Sharp transection of the cord with a clamp or ligature prevents retraction of the umbilical structures and may be associated with a greater incidence of subsequent umbilical complications. However, excessive hemorrhage can be addressed by transient ligation with umbilical tape or a clamp. After birth, 1% iodine or 0.5% chlorhexidine solution (preferred) should be applied 2–4 times daily to the umbilical stump until the umbilical remnant is dry.

Neonatal Uveitis

Neonatal sepsis may initiate intraocular seeding or endogenous inflammation due to uveal tissue injury. Secondary ocular infection as well as endotoxemia, free radical formation, tissue hypoxia, and alterations in pH may trigger vascular damage at a cellular level and induce clinical uveitis. Various chemical mediators, including histamine, serotonin, plasmin, kinins, complement, and arachidonic acid derivatives mediate acute vascular changes. The ensuing increase in vascular permeability of the blood-ocular barrier allows cellular components, fluid, and plasma proteins to escape into the surrounding extravascular uveal stroma (edema), ocular fluid compartments (aqueous flare, plasmoid vitreous), and subretinal space (retinal detachment). Congenital and acquired adnexal disease, prolonged lateral recumbency, dehydration, and a decreased menace response in the neonate may also induce a reflex-mediated uveitis due to corneal trauma. Reflex-mediated uveitis is generally transient and leaves the uveal tract unaltered once the corneal insult resolves.

Clinical signs of **anterior uveitis** are more evident and generally consist of conjunctival hyperemia, ciliary flush, corneal edema, aqueous flare, hyperemia and swelling of the iris, miosis, and a decrease in intraocular pressure. Signs of ocular pain, blepharospasm, increased lacrimation, and photophobia are variable, whereas hyphema, hypopyon, and intraocular fibrin deposition are seen in cases of severe inflammation. Intraocular fibrin formation occurs due to egress of essential clotting factors into the aqueous and vitreous humor during uveal inflammation. Furthermore, the regulation of fibrinolysis is altered in endotoxemic animals. A prolonged increase in the activity of plasminogen activator inhibitor may favor coagulation and impede intraocular fibrinolysis.

Acute **posterior uveitis** is often overlooked if unaccompanied by apparent changes in the anterior chamber. Retinal vascular congestion, hemorrhage, edema, cellular infiltration, or retinal detachment may be seen. The vitreous also tends to appear hazy, with blurring of fundus details, due to cellular infiltration and proteinaceous debris. The type of inflammatory cell reaction is generally classified as neutrophilic (suppurative), granulomatous, or lymphocytic-plasmacytic. Neutrophilic inflammation is an acute response to bacterial infection and sepsis, although intraocular bacteria may not be present. Neutrophils can accumulate in the anterior chamber in the form of hypopyon, which is often sterile and thus indicative of inflammation rather than local infection. Proteases released from neutrophils may also induce corneal endothelial damage, thereby resulting in corneal edema. Lymphocytic-plasmacytic inflammation is often suggestive of an immune-mediated reaction and indicates some type of chronicity.

Septic Arthritis

See SEPTIC ARTHRITIS, p 1062.

NEONATAL ENCEPHALOPATHY

(Neonatal maladjustment syndrome, Hypoxic ischemic encephalopathy, Barker, Wanderer, Dummy)

Neonatal encephalopathy (NE) is a common, noninfectious CNS disorder of neonatal foals, resulting in clinical signs such as lethargy, inappropriate behavior, seizures, and other neurologic deficits. The condition is associated with the broader syndrome of **perinatal asphyxia syndrome**, which is believed to result from unrecognized in-utero or peripartum hypoxia, and can injure multiple organ systems. In this context, asphyxia is caused by impaired oxygen delivery to cells, most often resulting from a combination of hypoxemia or anemia (leading to decreased blood oxygen content), and ischemia (decreased blood perfusion).

Pathogenesis and Risk Factors: Species-specific information on the pathogenesis of NE in foals is exceedingly scarce and mostly extrapolated from nonequine species. Primary neuronal cell death may be related to cellular hypoxia, energy failure, and cellular membrane depolarization, whereas delayed neuronal cell death is associated with reperfusion injury (oxidative stress), excitotoxicity, accumulation of intracellular calcium, activation of numerous enzymes and pathways, cytotoxic actions of activated microglia, inflammation, and apoptosis. In this context, excessive activation of glutamatergic neurotransmission (ie, excitatory amino acids and neurotransmitters), increased production of reactive oxygen and nitrogen species, as well as fetal systemic inflammatory responses with production of pro-inflammatory cytokines (eg, IL-1, IL-6, TNF-α) may all contribute to cell injury and/or death.

Risk factors for perinatal asphyxia may include maternal (eg, respiratory disease, endotoxemia, hemorrhage/anemia, surgery/cesarean delivery), placental (eg, bacterial, fungal- or endophyte-associated placentitis, chronic or acute premature uteroplacental separation), and fetal causes (eg, twinning, congenital abnormalities, dystocia, meconium aspiration, sepsis, prematurity, dysmaturity). Fetal and maternal factors are those that induce hypotension or reduced tissue oxygenation, whereas placental pathology will impair uteroplacental perfusion. Areas of chronic placental separations may thus lead to chronic hypoxia of the fetus. However, the most acute cause of perinatal asphyxia is complete premature placental separation at birth ("red bag" delivery).

Clinical Findings: CNS signs are most prominent in cases of perinatal asphyxia, but renal, cardiac, GI, and pulmonary systems may also be affected. A detailed, systematic examination of foals with NE is therefore warranted. Renal compromise of foals with NE may present as anuria or oliguria, whereas GI effects of perinatal asphyxia may include colic, transient ileus, meconium impaction, gastric ulcers, gastric reflux, bloat, diarrhea, and necrotizing enterocolitis. Cardiac arrhythmias, edema, poor cardiac output, and systemic hypotension may result from hypoxia of the myocardium. A decrease in pulmonary perfusion may impair surfactant production and lead to ventilation-perfusion mismatch and secondary pulmonary atelectasis. Hepatic and endocrine dysfunction may also be seen. For example, perinatal asphyxia syndrome may cause lower T_3 and T_4 concentrations in affected foals than in age-matched healthy control subjects.

The neurologic signs of foals with NE are variable and may include weakness (hypotonia), mental depression (stupor, somnolence, difficult to arouse, coma), seizure activity, tremors, and hypertonia. Seizures are relatively common and may range from mildly abnormal movement of the face and jaw to generalized seizures with recumbency and paddling. Other clinical signs include an inability to find the udder, loss of suckle reflex, loss of affinity for the dam, loss of recognition of the environment, abnormal vocalization (hence "barker foals"), dysphagia, weak tongue tone or persistent tongue protrusion, central blindness, opisthotonos, irregular respiratory pattern (apnea, abnormally slow respiratory rate), and proprioceptive deficits. Clinical signs can be asymmetric and may include a head tilt, circling, and asymmetric pupillary reflexes. Foals may appear healthy at birth but often exhibit CNS abnormalities within hours of delivery or by 1–2 days of age. Affected foals are usually afebrile unless secondary infection or sepsis occurs.

Diagnosis: Diagnosis is based on compatible clinical findings and exclusion of differential diagnoses. A history of dystocia, premature placental separation, or placentitis may support a diagnosis of NE. The foal's CBC is usually unremarkable unless sepsis is present. A serum chemistry may also be normal but often indicates organ dysfunction secondary to hypoxic or cytokine-mediated injury. For example, a markedly increased CK concentration may correlate with a recent hypoxic-ischemic muscle insult, whereas an increased GGT concentration can accompany hepatic injury. Transient or spurious hypercreatininemia may indicate adverse maternal and/or placental conditions, or suggest ingestion of creatinine-rich fetal fluids in neonatal foals experiencing periods of peripartum asphyxia. Creatinine in affected foals decreases by >50% within 24 hr of standard neonatal support and generally normalizes within 72 hr. However, if creatinine values remain high, then renal dysfunction must be considered. Hypoxemia, hypercarbia (due to respiratory depression), acidemia, and hypocalcemia may also be seen in foals with NE. CSF may be normal or show an increased RBC count and protein concentration. CNS necrosis, edema, and hemorrhage are found in some cases at necropsy; however, these findings are inconsistent.

Differential diagnoses for NE include bacterial meningitis, equine herpesvirus 1 infection, metabolic abnormalities (eg, hypoglycemia, electrolyte derangements), acid-base disturbances, kernicterus subsequent to massive hemolysis (ie, neonatal isoerythrolysis), brain or spinal trauma, congenital defects (eg, hydrocephalus, hydranencephaly), and nutritional myodegeneration (white muscle disease).

Treatment and Prognosis: Treatment of NE is primarily supportive. Maintenance of adequate blood pressure and perfusion is vital for supporting cerebral blood flow and avoiding further ischemic injury. This can be accomplished by cautiously administered, goal-directed IV fluid therapy and inotrope or vasopressor support, if needed, while avoiding hypertension. Mild hypothermia, use of barbiturates, and mild hypercapnia have been suggested to decrease cerebral metabolic rate and preserve energy. Because foals have minimal energy reserves, IV glucose administration may be necessary to maintain normal blood glucose concentrations. If the foal is unable to nurse, nutrition can be supplied via an indwelling nasogastric tube. Total parenteral nutrition is indicated in foals with GI dysfunction.

Mannitol (0.25–1 g/kg, IV, as 20% solution over 20 min every 12–24 hr) has been used to reduce cerebral edema. Anticonvulsants (phenobarbital 2–10 mg/kg, IV, bid; diazepam 0.1–0.4 mg/kg, IV, as needed; midazolam 0.04–0.1 mg/kg, IV, as needed or 0.02–0.06 mg/kg/hr constant-rate infusion) are implemented to treat seizures that can otherwise increase cerebral oxygen consumption and contribute to ongoing injury. Self-trauma during seizures should be limited by providing a protected or padded environment. Trauma to the eye and corneal ulceration is particularly common; the eyes should therefore be monitored closely and treatment implemented if necessary. In recumbent foals, ophthalmic lubricants may be used to reduce the incidence of corneal injury.

Magnesium sulfate supplementation administered as a constant-rate infusion (0.05 mg/kg/hr, IV, loading dose, then 0.025 mg/kg/hr maintenance) has been suggested to block the release of glutamate, whereas antioxidants such as vitamins E (5,000 IU/day, PO) and C (100 mg/kg/day, IV or PO) can be administered along with thiamine (10 mg/kg slowly IV or SC every 12–24 hr) to support cellular metabolism. DMSO 10% solution (0.5 g/kg, IV) has been used as a free radical scavenger. Allopurinol (44 mg/kg, PO, within the first 4 hr), a xanthine oxidase inhibitor, can also be administered to decrease free radicals, whereas pentoxifylline (10 mg/kg, PO, bid) may inhibit TNF-α production in foals with NE.

Most foals with NE will benefit from intranasal administration of humidified oxygen (3–5 L/min), whereas mechanical ventilation may be required in cases of severe respiratory depression. Doxapram (0.02–0.05 mg/kg/hr constant-rate infusion) and caffeine (10 mg/kg, PO or per rectum loading dose, then 2.5 mg/kg as needed) may be used as a central respiratory stimulant. Availability of hyperbaric oxygen therapy is limited, but it has also been used to treat NE in foals. Foals with NE appear to be predisposed to sepsis. Whether this is due to an underlying infectious process, impaired immune function, or increased exposure to pathogens (ie, indiscriminant nursing behavior) is unclear. In addition, foals neurologically abnormal at birth often fail to nurse and commonly have failure of passive transfer of immunity (*see* p 819). For these reasons, broad-spectrum antimicrobials, plasma transfusion, and anti-inflammatory management are commonly indicated.

Most foals with NE have a good to very good prognosis. In uncomplicated cases, the reported survival rate is 70%–75%, with complete recovery in most cases. Sepsis and related complications adversely affect the prognosis. Foals that remain comatose or difficult to arouse, show no improvement in neurologic function during the first 5 days of life, or demonstrate severe, recurrent seizures have a guarded to poor prognosis.

MECONIUM IMPACTION

Meconium is the earliest feces of newborn foals. It is composed of intestinal secretions, swallowed amniotic fluid, and cellular debris; it has a sticky, caramelized appearance. Most foals pass their meconium within the first 9–12 hr of life. If sufficient quantities of meconium are not evacuated, meconium impaction can lead to clinical signs of colonic obstruction, which usually manifest in the first 12–96 hr. These signs may include abdominal pain (colic), tachypnea and tachycardia, tail "swishing," restlessness, straining to defecate, and abdominal (gas) distention. Published reports suggest that meconium impaction may be more likely in foals born after >340 days of gestation and in colts. Meconium can usually be identified either by plain or contrast abdominal radiography or ultrasonography, or by careful digital rectal examination with adequate restraint or sedation. On radiographs, meconium often appears as granular contents in the ascending or descending colon, with fluid- or gas-distended intestine proximal to the obstruction.

Treatment: Many cases of meconium impaction respond to medical therapy, including judicious use of analgesics, IV fluid therapy, oral laxatives (4–8 oz mineral oil administered via a nasogastric tube; 1–2 oz milk of magnesia), and enemas as the mainstay of therapy. Warm-water liquid detergent (eg, Palmolive®) enemas (½ teaspoon liquid detergent added to 500 mL water) are preferred, although commercial phosphate (Fleet®) enemas can also be used (repeated administration may increase risk of phosphate toxicity). Acetylcysteine retention enemas may also be highly effective, because acetylcysteine is hypothesized to cleave disulfide bonds in the mucoprotein molecules of meconium, which decreases its overall tenacity. A 4% acetylcysteine solution is made by adding 20 g of baking soda and 8 g of acetylcysteine to 200 mL of water. A 30-french Foley catheter with a 30-mL balloon is inserted ~2.5–5 cm into the rectum, and the balloon is slowly inflated to occlude the rectum. Subsequently, 100–200 mL of the 4% acetylcysteine solution is administered by gravity flow and retained for 30–45 min. If needed, treatment can be repeated in 12 hr. Occasionally, repeated enemas can result in significant mucosal irritation and persistent straining beyond the resolution of the meconium impaction, thereby confounding the assessment of treatment success.

Surgical intervention should be considered if medical therapy is unsuccessful, especially in the face of persistent pain unresponsive to analgesics, persistent tachycardia, progressive abdominal enlargement, or increased peritoneal fluid protein and/or nucleated cell count.

The prognosis of uncomplicated meconium impaction is generally considered good to excellent.

SMALL ANIMALS

Average reported canine and feline neonatal mortality rates (greatest during the first week of life) vary, ranging from 9%-26%. Prudent veterinary intervention in the prenatal, parturient, and postpartum periods can increase neonatal survival by controlling or eliminating factors that contribute to puppy morbidity and mortality. Poor prepartum condition of the dam, dystocia, congenital malformations, genetic defects, injury, environmental exposure, malnutrition, parasitism, and infectious disease all contribute to neonatal morbidity and mortality. Optimal husbandry impacts neonatal survival favorably by managing labor and delivery to reduce stillbirths, controlling parasitism and reducing infectious disease, preventing injury and environmental exposure, and optimizing nutrition of the dam and neonates. Proper genetic screening for selection of breeding animals minimizes inherited congenital defects.

Immediate Postpartum Resuscitation: Optimal neonatal resuscitation (if needed after birth or cesarean section) involves the same "ABC's" as any cardiopulmonary resuscitation. Prompt clearing of airways

("A") by gentle suction with a bulb syringe, and then drying and stimulation of the neonate to promote respiration ("B") and to avoid chilling are performed. Neonates should not be swung to clear airways because of the potential for cerebral hemorrhage from concussion. The use of doxapram as a respiratory stimulant is unlikely to improve hypoxemia associated with hypoventilation and is not recommended. Spontaneous breathing and vocalization at birth are positively associated with survival through 7 days of age. Intervention for resuscitation of neonates after vaginal delivery should be done if the dam's actions do not stimulate respiration, vocalization, and movement within 1 min of birth.

Cardiopulmonary resuscitation for neonates that do not breathe spontaneously is challenging yet potentially rewarding. Ventilatory support should include constant flow O_2 delivery by facemask. If this is ineffective after 1 min, positive pressure with a snugly fitting mask or endotracheal intubation and rebreathing bag (using a 2-mm endotracheal tube or a 12- to 16-gauge IV catheter) is advised. Cardiac stimulation ("C") should follow ventilatory support, because myocardial hypoxemia is the most common cause of bradycardia or asystole. Direct transthoracic cardiac compressions are advised as the first step; epinephrine is the drug of choice for cardiac arrest/standstill (0.2 mg/kg, administered best by the IV or intraosseous route). Venous access in neonates is challenging; the single umbilical vein is one possibility. The proximal humerus, proximal femur, and proximomedial tibia offer intraosseous sites for drug administration. Atropine is not advised in neonatal resuscitation. The mechanism of bradycardia is hypoxemia-induced myocardial depression rather than vagal mediation, and anticholinergic-induced tachycardia can actually exacerbate myocardial oxygen deficits.

Chilled neonates may not respond to resuscitation. Body temperature drops rapidly when a neonate is damp. Keeping the neonate warm is important during resuscitation and in the immediate postpartum period. During resuscitation, placing the chilled neonate's trunk into a warm water bath (95°–99°F) can improve response. Working under a heat lamp or within a Bair hugger warming device is helpful. After resuscitation, neonates should be placed in a warm box (a styrofoam picnic box with ventilation holes is ideal) with warm bedding until they can be left with their dam. Neonates delivered by cesarean section should be left with the dam only after she is fully recovered from anesthesia and exhibiting good maternal behavior; otherwise, nursing should be directly monitored and permitted every 2 hr.

Neonates lack glucose reserves and have minimal capacity for gluconeogenesis. Providing energy during or just after prolonged resuscitation efforts becomes critical. Clinical hypoglycemia (blood glucose levels <30–40 mg/dL) can be treated with dextrose solution IV or intraosseously, at a dosage of 0.5–1 g/kg (0.0005–0.001 g/g body wt) using a 5%–10% solution, or a dosage of 2–4 mL/kg (0.002–0.004 mL/g body wt) of a 10% dextrose solution. A 500-g neonate would get 1–2 mL. Single administration of parenteral glucose is adequate if the hypoglycemic puppy can then be fed or nurses. If a neonate is too weak to nurse or suckle, 0.05–1 mL of warmed 5% dextrose can be administered orally by stomach tube every 15–30 min until the neonate is capable of suckling. If colostrum can be acquired from the dam, it can be administered in the same way. Dextrose solution (50%) should be applied to the mucous membranes only because of the potential for phlebitis if administered IV; however, circulation must be adequate for absorption from the mucosa. Neonates administered dextrose should be monitored for hyperglycemia because of immature metabolic regulatory mechanisms.

When to Stop Resuscitation: Resuscitation may be stopped when there has been no response after 15–20 min of effort (continued agonal respiration, bradycardia) or when a serious congenital defect has been detected (cleft palate, loud murmur, gastroschisis, large omphalocele, large fontanel).

Husbandry in the First Days of Life:

After resuscitation or within the first 24 hr of a natural delivery, a complete physical examination should be performed. Lack of cleft palate, a normal umbilicus, and functional urethral and anal openings should be established. A fontanelle, if present, should be small. The oral cavity, hair coat, limbs, umbilicus, and urogenital structures should be visually inspected. The mucous membranes should be pink and moist, a suckle reflex present, the coat full and clean, and the urethra and anus patent. A normal umbilicus is dry without surrounding erythema. The thorax should be ausculted; vesicular breath sounds and a lack of murmur are normal. The abdomen should be pliant and not painful. A normal neonate will squirm and vocalize when examined, and nurse and sleep quietly when returned to the dam. Healthy neonates will attempt to right themselves and orient by rooting toward their dam. Neonates are highly susceptible to environmental stress, infection, and malnutrition. Proper husbandry is critical and should include daily examination of each neonate for vigor and recording of weight.

Warmth: Puppies and kittens lack thermoregulatory mechanisms until 4 wk of age; thus, the ambient temperature must be high enough to facilitate maintenance of a body temperature of at least 97°F (36°C). Hypothermia negatively impacts immunity, nursing, and digestion. Exogenous heat should be supplied, best in the form of an overhead heat lamp. Heating pads run the risk of burning neonates incapable of moving away from excessively hot surfaces.

Chilled neonates must be rewarmed slowly (30 min) to avoid peripheral vasodilation and dehydration. Tube feeding should be delayed until the neonate is euthermic. Hypothermia induces ileus, and regurgitation and aspiration can result.

Immunity: Incompletely developed immune systems during the first 10 days of life make neonates vulnerable to systemic infection (most commonly bacterial and viral). Puppies must ingest adequate colostrum promptly after birth to acquire passive immunity. The intestinal absorption of IgG generally ceases by 24 hr after parturition. Colostrum-deprived kittens given adult cat serum at a dosage of 150 mL/kg, SC or IP, developed serum IgG levels comparable to those of suckling littermates. However, colostrum-deprived puppies given 40 mL/kg of adult dog serum orally and parentally did not match IgG levels of suckling littermates. Neonates should be encouraged to suckle promptly after resuscitation is completed; this usually necessitates close monitoring after a cesarean section, because the dam has not fully recovered from anesthesia. Maternal instincts (protecting, retrieving, grooming, nursing) usually return within 24 hr.

The umbilicus of neonates should be trimmed 1 cm from the abdominal wall, ligated, and treated with 2% tincture of iodine immediately after birth to reduce contamination and prevent ascent of bacteria into the peritoneal cavity (omphalitis-peritonitis).

Neonatal bacterial septicemia can cause rapid deterioration and result in death if not recognized and treated promptly. Predisposing factors include endometritis in the dam, a prolonged delivery/dystocia, feeding of replacement formulas, the use of ampicillin, stress, low birth weight (<350 g for a medium-size breed dog), and chilling with body temperature <96°F. The organisms most frequently associated with septicemia are *Escherichia coli*, streptococci, staphylococci, and *Klebsiella* spp. Premortem diagnosis can be challenging, because sudden death may preclude recognition of clinical signs. Commonly, a decrease in weight gain, failure to suckle, hematuria, persistent diarrhea, unusual vocalization, abdominal distention and pain, and sloughing of the extremities indicate septicemia may be present. Prompt therapy with broad-spectrum, bactericidal antibiotics; improved nutrition via supported nursing, tube feeding, or bottle feeding; maintenance of body temperature; and appropriate fluid replacement are indicated. The third-generation cephalosporin ceftiofur sodium is an appropriate choice for neonatal septicemia, because it alters normal intestinal flora minimally and is usually effective against the causative organisms. Ceftiofur sodium should be administered at a dosage of 2.5 mg/kg, SC, bid, for no longer than 5 days. Because neonates <48 hr old have reduced thrombin levels, presumptive therapy with vitamin K_1 at 0.5–2.5 mg/kg can be used (0.01–1 mg/neonate, SC) if a coagulopathy is suspected (umbilical bleeding, hematuria, epistaxis).

Nutrition: Neonates have minimal body fat reserves and limited metabolic capacity to generate glucose from precursors. Glycogen stores are depleted shortly after birth, making adequate nourishment from nursing vital. Even minimal fasting can result in hypoglycemia. Hypoglycemia can also result from endotoxemia, septicemia, portosys-

TABLE 1 NORMAL RECTAL TEMPERATURE OF SMALL ANIMAL NEONATES

Period	Normal Rectal Temperature
Wk 1	95°–99°F (35°–37.2°C)
Wk 2–3	97°–100°F (36.1°–37.8°C)
At weaning	99°–101°F (37.2°–38.3°C)

TABLE 2 ENVIRONMENTAL WARMTH REQUIRED FOR SMALL ANIMAL NEONATES

Period	Temperature
Wk 1	84°–89°F (28.9°–31.7°C)
Wk 2–3	80°F (26.7°C)
Wk 4	69°–75°F (20.6°–23.9°C)
Wk 5	69°F (20.6°C)

temic shunts, and glycogen storage abnormalities. Oral fluid and glucose replacement may be preferable if the neonate has an adequate swallowing reflex and is not clinically compromised. The neonatal caloric requirement is 133 cal/kg/day during the first week of life, 155 cal/kg/day for the second, 175–198 cal/kg/day for the third, and 220 cal/kg/day for the fourth. Commercially manufactured milk replacement formulas are usually superior to homemade versions, but none is equal to the dam's milk. The use of milk obtained from the dam can be considered and is superior if available. An osmotic diarrhea (usually yellow, curdled fecal appearance) can result from overfeeding formula, necessitating diluting the product 50% with water or a balanced crystalloid solution. Neonates should gain weight steadily from the first day after birth (a transient mild loss from birth weight is acceptable on day 1), with puppies gaining 1–3 g/day/lb (2.2 kg) of anticipated adult weight and kittens 50–100 g/wk. Neonatal weights should be recorded daily for the first 2 wk, then every 3 days until 1 mo old. Healthy, well-nourished neonates are quiet and sleep when not nursing. The normal neonatal weight gain is an increase of 5%–10% body wt/day.

Neonatal Anesthesia: Anesthesia of the neonate may be necessitated by an emergency or for an elective procedure. The distribution and metabolism of drugs are different in neonates than in adults. Neonates have decreased protein binding and increased permeability of the blood-brain barrier. Decreased protein binding is due to lower albumin levels with a lower affinity for drugs. Neonates have higher body water content and lower fat content than adults. This results in a greater initial volume of distribution for some drugs. In most neonates, the ability to metabolize drugs (via conjugation, hydrolysis, oxidation, and reduction) is reduced, as is renal clearance mechanisms. Nephrogenesis in puppies is not complete until the third week of life; the outer cortical nephrons are the last ones to become fully functional. The ability of the neonatal kidney to produce a concentrated urine is less than that of the adult, and so fluid balance is more labile in neonates. The differences in neonatal respiratory function mean that inhaled agents will have a more rapid onset and recovery. Neonates have immature central and peripheral nervous systems and immature neuromuscular junctions, such that less general/local anesthetic is required to produce anesthesia/local block than in adults.

Fluid support is indicated with neonates, but fluid overload is simply because of the capacity of the fluid lines used for larger animals. To avoid this problem, tubing with a much smaller internal diameter should be used. Care must also be taken to ensure that the lines do not contain any air, because these very small patients may still have communication between the left and right atrium, making it possible for IV air to result in coronary or cerebral emboli.

Core body temperature should be monitored, and hypothermia treated as soon as possible. A supplemental source of heat should be available (circulating water blanket or warm air blanket) to prevent hypothermia, because many of the anesthetic drugs eliminate the ability of the neonate to thermoregulate, and neonates are more prone to hypothermia than adults. Premedication with an anticholinergic is acceptable and usually sufficient by itself. Most neonates tolerate a simple mask induction with an inhalant such as isoflurane or sevoflurane. Propofol can be used as an induction drug in young animals. Maintenance by mask avoids the potential for trauma during intubation in tiny neonates, but less control of the airway is achieved.

During anesthesia of neonates, supporting and monitoring cardiopulmonary function is especially important. Cardiac output in neonates depends on heart rate; preventing bradycardia is more important than in adults. Monitoring blood pressure is also important. If hypotension is detected or tissue perfusion judged inadequate, treatment should be instituted. Initial therapy should include reducing the amount of anesthetic, if possible, and increasing the rate of fluid administration. If these treatments are ineffective, it is probably better to use a positive inotrope/chronotrope than a peripheral vasoconstrictor to try to increase blood pressure (unless it is very low, and a vasoconstrictor is needed to raise the pressure long enough to allow other therapies to work). Dopamine has been shown to increase blood pressure in puppies <10 days old at 5–10 mcg/kg/min but has little effect on heart rate or cardiac output. Dobutamine appears to have little effect at clinical doses.

CARE OF ORPHANED NATIVE BIRDS AND MAMMALS

If an orphaned bird or mammal is found, further information should be sought before attempting wildlife rehabilitation. Specialized books about hand-rearing wild and domestic mammals and birds and the National Wildlife Rehabilitators Association Web site (www.nwrawildlife.org) are valuable resources. The following is a general overview, and all species require more information for a full course of captive care. Correct species and age identification is crucial for determination of behavioral considerations, weaning diets, and adult fate. It is illegal to keep most species of North American wild animals as pets. Permits are required, even by veterinarians, to care for most wild species beyond initial medical care. The USA Fish and Wildlife Service and state natural resource agencies should be contacted for applicable rules. Injured limbs of wild animals should never be amputated without consultation with regulatory agencies, because permanent captive placement for disabled wildlife may be difficult to find. Euthanasia should be considered when injury resolution will result in a disabled, unreleasable animal. When hand-rearing for wild release, infants should be raised with conspecifics to avoid human imprinting, using techniques that avoid habituation. Wild infants must be isolated from domestic animals.

The first step is to determine whether young are truly orphaned. If chicks are returned to nests or mammals are left alone *and monitored from afar*, the parent may return and resume care. Human handling does not preclude most parents accepting returned offspring. Neonatal wildlife, especially unidentified species, have the best chance of survival if kept warm and taken to local wildlife rehabilitation centers. Skunks, raccoons, foxes, and bats should only be rehabilitated by professionals because of potential zoonotic diseases. Marine mammals and seabirds require specialized care facilities (*see* p 1856).

All neonates require physical examination and assessment of hydration, body temperature, and weight. Warmth, hydration, and energy are critical. Because most orphans initially cannot maintain or regulate their body temperature, supplemental heat should be provided with heating pads, hot water bottles, incandescent light bulbs, or brooders. A heat gradient for ambulatory young allows orphans to select their own comfort zone. Thermal support of altricial species must be closely regulated. Most placental mammals and birds have normal body temperatures warmer than that of people, and should feel warm to the human hand. Maintaining humidity of 50%–70% in housing reduces dehydration, and insulating orphans from direct heat prevents burns. Hypothermic orphans should be warmed until body temperature is near normal and administered warm fluids to maintain hydration or correct deficits. Once the infant is warmed and well hydrated, species-appropriate diets can be fed to provide energy. Initial feedings should be conservatively sized and dilute until it has been determined that the infant's excretory systems are functioning. Infants of most species have a stomach or crop capacity of ~50 mL/kg. Overfeeding may result in aspiration pneumonia or diarrhea. Once infants are stabilized, the advice of a permitted rehabilitator should be obtained.

Hair, feathers, skin, and eyes should be kept free of spilled food or excreta, and foods maintained hygienically. Nests/housing should be cleaned regularly and secured against vermin. Treatment for ecto- and endoparasites or fly strike may be necessary. Products deemed safe for infants of domestic species should be used, and an exotic animal formulary consulted for dosing information.

Metabolic bone disease may develop quickly in wild orphans fed inadequate diets. Corvids, other passerines, herons, egrets, shorebirds, raptors, opossums, and canids are especially susceptible, including when transitioned off formulas onto inadequately supplemented animal protein diets before skeletal maturity. Ground meat or poultry must be supplemented with calcium carbonate at 5 g/ 0.5 kg of meat.

Growing chicks require a dietary ratio of elemental calcium:phosphorus of ~2:1 by weight.

Birds

Nest replacements should be constructed so as to provide nonambulatory chicks with a comfortable upright posture with the head elevated and legs underneath the body. Housing chicks on flat surfaces may result in splayed legs. Fractured bones are considered life-threatening injuries because of the requirement of functionality for release. Trauma to soft tissues can be minimized by stabilizing fractures promptly. Elbow, carpus, spine, stifle, and hock fractures or luxations carry a poor prognosis for release. Mid-shaft long-bone fractures often heal well. Humerus and femur fractures heal best with a simple intramedullary pin, and pinning may be successful even in extremely young or small-bodied chicks. Minimally restrictive splints and wraps for other fractures result in fastest recovery and release. Chicks should be allowed to use stabilized, fractured limbs as normally as possible during recovery. Stable callus formation occurs in 5–7 days in nestling passerines and in 10–21 days in larger-bodied species, well before radiographic changes occur. Some species form joint contractures easily and require physical therapy after the fracture and then continuing intermittently for return to function. Chicks may heal rapidly from seemingly severe soft-tissue injuries. Lacerations should have primary closure to minimize time in captivity and reduce adverse effects on growing plumage. Antibiotic therapy against gram-negative bacteria is advisable for predator-injured chicks; it should be continued until wounds have completely healed. Meloxicam and butorphanol are commonly used for pain. Chicks with head injuries may recover well; changes in neurologic signs can be used as prognostic indicators while giving supportive care. Beak or jaw injuries must resolve with beak tips well aligned to ensure ability to forage normally after release.

Nearly all North American bird species feed vertebrate or invertebrate prey to their chicks. Milk and bread, hamburger, condensed milk, or uncooked rice should not be fed. Soaked dog kibble and monkey biscuits are inadequate for most species. All species require 8–12 hr uninterrupted sleep. Self-feeding requires daylight-level lighting in diurnal species. All growing chicks should gain weight every day, so weight should be monitored closely.

Altricial Species: Chicks should be warmed to normal body temperature, hydrated until droppings are produced, and then fed. Tiny, unfeathered chicks require environments as warm as 100°F (37.8°C); larger-feathered chicks do well initially in temperatures of 90°–95°F (32.2°–35°C). Overheated chicks may hold perpetual open-mouthed postures, droop heads over nest edges, and cease producing droppings if dehydrated. Not all species gape/beg (swifts, nightjars). Some species stop begging when full (corvids); some do not and may dangerously overeat (finches, goldfinches). Crops should empty between feeds; not all species have crops (insectivores, owls). Hatchlings require more water than older chicks. Common problems that cause lack of gaping include too cold, hot, weak, or dehydrated; untreated illness or injury; and misidentified species. Overfeeding may cause droppings that appear as undigested diet.

Higher protein/fat, lower carbohydrate diets are desirable for most species. Puréed, high-quality kitten or ferret kibble is an acceptable temporary food for most altricial chicks, supplemented with elemental calcium at 150 mg/kg/day, PO, until on a balanced diet. Puréed, skinned prey animals (quail or adult mice, including bones and organs, minus feet and heads) form an adequate diet for many species. Bone fragments must be completely pulverized to avoid GI trauma. A diet of thawed-frozen prey requires vitamin supplementation. Vitamin E and thiamine supplementation is necessary for species ingesting frozen-thawed fish. Feeding prey frozen >6 mo should be avoided. Vitamin A may be inadequate in insect prey, and deficiency may occur if prey are fed with viscera removed. Pinky mice, insects, and small-bodied fish often contain inadequate calcium for growing birds; hence, supplementation is necessary.

Songbirds and Woodpeckers: A simple hand-feeding diet consists of 1 cup (116 g) Purina Pro-Plan® kitten kibble, 1.25–1.5 cup (300–360 mL) water, 2 tbsp (14 g) powdered egg white, 750 mg calcium from $CaCO_3$, and ½ tsp (1.4 g) Avi-Era® powdered avian vitamins. Do not delete or substitute ingredients haphazardly, soak kibble and blend until smooth, and feed with appropriately sized syringe. For hatchlings/nestlings, feed 50 mL/kg every 20–45 min (by age)

12–14 hr/day (16 hr/day for insectivores). For fledglings, hand-feed 50 mL/kg every 1–2 hr, 12 hr/day, offering appropriate self-feeding diet.

Hummingbirds: A temporary diet consists of 1 part water to 6 parts table sugar or 5% dextrose, fed every 20 min. This diet does not meet hummingbird chick nutrient requirements. These chicks should be transferred to an experienced caretaker immediately. Sugar water should not be spilled on the bird.

Doves and Pigeons: Commercial diets for hatchlings are Roudybush™ Squab Diet and Lafeber's® Emeraid® Carnivore; for nestlings/fledglings, Kaytee® Exact® Hand Feeding Formula. Crop capacity is 100–120 mL/kg. Birds should be fed when crop empties, 12–14 hr/day, every 1–2 hr until eyes open and then every 3 hr until ambulating and ingesting seed. Palpating the crop before each feeding will assess self-feeding and prevent overfilling.

Raptors: Hatchlings can be fed small pieces of warm, water-dipped meat every 2 hr, 12 hr/day, with blunt-tipped forceps; tiny bone pieces can be included by day 3 after hatch, and casting material (skin/hair) by day 5. The crop should empty between meals. Most species will pick up chopped prey from a dish by day 14. Feeding with a puppet parent can be done once the eyes open.

Herons and Egrets: Thawed-frozen fish (5–20 g, sliced diagonally if larger), live insects, or thawed-frozen chopped mice, should be offered hourly until self-feeding, then several times daily. Hatchlings may require force feeding; older chicks may eat from a dish. Using a feeding puppet reduces habituation.

Precocial Species: Once warm and secure, many species drink and eat independently. Solitude stresses chicks; a mirror, small stuffed animals, clean feather duster, or chicks of closely related species can be companions. Uncommon species and debilitated hatchlings require professional rehabilitative care for a positive outcome. Placing pebbles in water dishes may prevent quail/ducklings from drowning. Hatchling quail/killdeer require habitat brooders kept at 95°–100°F (35°–37.8°C).

Shorebirds (Killdeer, Sandpipers, Avocets): Live, fresh-frozen, and freeze-dried small invertebrate prey (tubifex worms, brine shrimp, mosquito larvae, tiny krill, small freshly shed mealworms, fly larvae, or cichlid mini-pellets) should be offered in shallow water at least four times daily.

Waterfowl (Geese, Ducks, Swans): Natural duckweed or watercress, small invertebrates, crushed hard-boiled egg, small minnows, and waterfowl starter (Mazuri®) should be offered. Access to shallow water should be controlled; chicks must be able to easily exit water to warm under a heat source. Chicks may lose waterproofing and become chilled if plumage becomes contaminated with food or droppings.

Gamebirds (Pheasants, Quail, Turkeys): Soaked puppy kibble, small-bodied invertebrates, small clumps of grass or weeds with soil, or commercial gamebird starter can be offered.

Mammals

Hypothermia and dehydration must be corrected before feeding neonate mammals. Hairless neonates require ambient temperatures of 85°–90°F (29.4°–32.2°C), while haired infants may be housed at cooler temperatures depending on maturity and body condition. Once warm and hydrated, milk replacer should be introduced using this regimen: 100% oral electrolyte solution, gradually increasing the strength of milk replacer in one to several feedings to ¼ strength, then ½, then ¾, and finally to full strength. During this process, if the neonate develops digestive upset (vomiting, diarrhea, bloating), feeding should return to the last well-tolerated ratio. Overfeeding or sudden diet changes may cause bloating or diarrhea. Neonates need to be stimulated to eliminate by gently stroking the perineal area with warm moist gauze or tissue. Dorsal side up is normal nursing posture; infants should not be put on their backs to feed. The environment should be quiet.

Fawns: Fawns should be raised in groups with minimal human contact and kept away from dogs. Newborn to 2-day-old fawns should be fed colostrum, such as Colostrx®, for the first 24–48 hr. After reconstitution, one 454-g package can be administered via bottle or stomach tube over 8–10 hr (5 meals/day, 30–40 mL/kg). Acceptable milk replacers include Fox Valley® Milk Replacer, lamb's milk replacer, or goat's milk. Fawns 2–7 days old should be fed four times daily, gradually increasing volume to 50 mL/kg. From 8 to 14 days of age, up to 300 mL should be fed, reaching a goal of 300 mL, tid. From 2 to 4 wk, the amount should be increased to 460 mL, tid, adding solid food (eg, goat chow, calf manna, and alfalfa hay). Indigenous natural browse should always be available. By 7 wk, fawns should be eating solid food and fed one 480 mL bottle daily. By 8–10 wk, fawns should eat solid food exclusively.

Squirrels: For squirrels, syringe-feeding is preferred; Catac® nipples work well. Eastern gray and fox squirrel neonates should be fed every 2 hr until 2 wk old. From 2 to 3 wk, feeding should be every 3 hr, eight times/day. At 4 wk, the late-night feed is eliminated. At 5–6 wk, feedings are reduced to five and then to four times/day, at 7–8 wk to three times/day, and at 10 wk to once a day. Weight should be monitored daily, and the squirrel fed 50 mL/kg initially, gradually increasing to 70 mL/kg by 3 wk. Acceptable milk replacers (ratios by volume) include 2:3 Fox Valley® 32/40:water, or 1:½:2 Esbilac®, MultiMilk®, and water. When eyes are open and squirrels are ambulatory, natural foods and rodent block can be offered; fruit should be strictly limited. Ground squirrels wean at 6 wk old, and Western gray squirrels at 12 wk.

Rabbits and Hares: Neonatal rabbit stomachs hold 100–125 mL/kg. Healthy neonates should be fed twice a day, although feedings up to four times a day may be needed. Use of a slip-tip syringe is preferred. If suckling response is poor, meals should be tube fed, with the volume reduced by 30% and an extra feeding to ensure adequate intake. Acceptable milk replacers (ratios by volume) include 2:1 parts KMR® powder:water (with pinch of acidophilus) or 1:1 parts Esbilac® powder:water. When the eyes open, a variety of chopped leafy greens and grass (orchard, timothy, or oat) hay should be provided. Because hares are precocial (born furred with eyes open), forage should be offered immediately in addition to milk replacer. Fruits and high-sugar vegetables (eg, carrots) should be avoided.

Opossums: Infant opossums weighing <20 g have a poor prognosis. Infants weighing 20–35 g should be fed 50 mL/kg, six times a day; those weighing 40–100 g, 50–60 mL/kg, five times a day. An acceptable milk replacer (ratio by volume) is 1:½:2 parts Esbilac®, MultiMilk®, and water. Tube-feeding is preferred, and a size 3.5 French red rubber catheter measured to the caudal rib may be used. If syringe feeding, a cut smoothed tomcat catheter can be attached to the syringe and the infant fed drop-wise. When eyes open (~45 g), infants can be taught to lap formula from a shallow dish. When infants weigh ~60 g and are walking, kitten kibble soaked in Esbilac® can be offered. Once the infant is eating soaked kibble (~80–100 g), 10% other natural food items (crickets, worms, chopped mice, local fruits, high-calcium vegetables) can be introduced. Most opossums self-feed by the time they weigh 100–120 g. Adequate calcium intake must be ensured to prevent metabolic bone disease.

Raccoons: Gloves should always be worn when handling raccoons. Raccoons are the definitive hosts for *Baylisascaris procyonis*, a roundworm parasite that may be transmitted to people or other animals, primarily via feces, and result in sometimes fatal infection. Raccoons also may carry rabies.

Newborns weigh 60–75 g with eyes and ears sealed. Incubators are necessary until weight is >500 g. The preferred milk replacer is KMR® or Zoologic® 42/25 (1:2.25 parts powder:water). Infants should be fed via 8 French gavage tube, or drop by drop into the mouth (using a cut smoothed tomcat catheter attached to a syringe) until they are stronger and/or eyes are open. Over-feeding should be avoided. The stomach should be plump but not taut. Four Paws™ large squirrel nipple on a 6-mL syringe may be used. Infants should be stimulated to urinate/defecate after each feed until they eliminate without stimulation. Infants should be weighed daily, and fed 50 mL/kg, six times a day, until they weigh 200 g. They can then be fed using a preemie nipple on a bottle or from a dish at the rate of 42.5 mL/kg, five times/day, until they weigh 500 g. At a weight of 400 g, if infants are strong enough and their eyes are open, in addition to the milk replacer, "mush" made of soaked puppy chow, high-protein baby cereal, and KMR® powder (with water added to create oatmeal consistency) can be offered. At 500 g, one of four feeds should be mush in a dish. At 850 g, small bits of cut fruit and soaked puppy chow should be added, decreasing milk replacer to three times a day. As the infants mature, hard puppy chow, prey items (mice, fish), egg, and 10% fruits and vegetables can be offered and formula feeds reduced.

PAIN ASSESSMENT AND MANAGEMENT

Pain delays recovery, impacts negatively on patient well-being, and can affect the client-veterinarian relationship. Behaviors suggestive of pain are routinely used to diagnose injuries and diseases, guide therapy, and provide prognostic information. Obvious signs of pain alert owners and veterinarians of a problem with the animal. Certainly, there is nothing novel about considering pain clinically relevant in the overall evaluation of an animal. What is relatively new is our understanding of the complexity of pain and the emphasis on ethical and medical obligations to treat pain in animals. Although limited survey data and anecdotal evidence suggest that the management of pain is receiving more attention in veterinary medicine than before, the assessment, prevention, and treatment of pain has yet to become an integral part of every physical examination and treatment plan.

PAIN PERCEPTION

Pain serves a protective role that alerts an individual to injury from the environment or from within. Based on current knowledge, all vertebrates, and some invertebrates, experience pain in response to actual or potential tissue damage. Many types of pain are encountered, with the most common being acute, chronic, cancer, and neuropathic. Acute pain is sudden in onset and can be severe. However, it disappears when the stimulus is removed or in a short period of time, and it tends to be self-limiting. Acute pain has a biologic function, because it serves as a warning that something is wrong while leading to protective behavioral changes. Acute pain is a symptom of disease, whereas chronic pain in and of itself, is a disease of altered neuroprocessing. Chronic pain lasts for several weeks to months and persists beyond the expected healing time. Chronic pain does not serve a biologic function and imposes severe detrimental stresses. Cancer pain is the result of primary tumor growth, metastatic disease, or the toxic effects of chemotherapy and radiation. Cancer pain can be acute, *chronic, or intermittent* and is related to the disease itself or the treatment. Neuropathic pain originates from injury or after injury of the peripheral or central nervous systems, such as trauma (eg, amputation and crushing injury), vascular injury (eg, thromboembolic disease), endocrinopathy (eg, diabetes mellitus), or infection (eg, post-herpetic neuralgia), possibly associated with motor, sensory, or autonomic deficits.

For an animal to experience pain, nociceptive information must be sent to higher centers in the CNS to be integrated, modulated, and interpreted into the conscious perception of pain. Noxious stimuli (heat, cold, mechanical, chemical) activate free sensory nerve endings known as nociceptors. A-δ and C-fibers transmit sensory information from nociceptors to the dorsal horn of the spinal cord, which directs and modulates input from the periphery and higher centers. Nociceptive information arriving in the dorsal horn of the spinal cord may activate motor neurons responsible for the reflex responses to noxious stimuli (such as withdrawing a limb). Importantly, nociceptive sensory input may be amplified or inhibited by spinal interneurons and glial cells.

Sensory information is relayed to higher centers in the CNS along a variety of pathways that differ according to species. In general, nociceptive information ascends the spinal cord along superficial and deep pathways to the brain stem with connections to the thalamus, reticular formation (responsible for level of arousal), and limbic system (responsible for emotions). From these areas of the brain, nociceptive information is relayed to the cortex, where it is perceived as pain. Activity in spinal nociceptive pathways is strongly influenced by descending antinociceptive systems that originate in the brain stem. Endogenous antinociceptive neurotransmitters (eg, endorphin, enkephalin, dynorphin, serotonin, and norepinephrine) inhibit the transmission of nociceptive information in the spinal cord and brain.

The neuroanatomic components of the nociceptive/pain pathways and pain-suppressing systems can change in response to sustained sensory input. Peripheral sensitization of nociceptors and central sensitization of nociceptive pathways in the dorsal horn, spinal cord, and brain can develop as a result of extensive tissue trauma or nerve injury. The process of peripheral and central sensitization has been termed "wind-up" and refers to the neuroanatomic changes (plasticity) that result in heightened or exaggerated pain states. Additionally, these exaggerated pain states often do not respond to conventional analgesic therapy. The use of opioids is especially limited, likely because of a down regulation of opioid receptors, a phenomenon that has been reported in the dorsal root ganglion and the dorsal horn. Thus, changes in the CNS in response to repeated and sustained nociceptive input (ie, pain) complicate the clinical management of pain.

RECOGNITION AND ASSESSMENT OF PAIN IN ANIMALS

Pain is a complex, multidimensional experience with sensory and affective elements. All mammals process the neuroanatomic and neuropharmacologic components involved in transduction, transmission, and perception of noxious stimuli; therefore, it is expected that animals experience pain even if they cannot exactly perceive or communicate it in the same way people do. Recognizing pain in animals is not intuitive, particularly for those unfamiliar with normal species-specific or individual behaviors. In recent years, there has been an increased focus on determining and measuring such specific pain behaviors. These efforts should improve recognition and treatment of pain in animals as validated pain assessment tools are developed. Nevertheless, the accurate assessment of pain in animals remains a subjective and challenging undertaking. Numerous factors complicate evaluation of pain in animals. Veterinary pain scales should consider the following characteristics: species, breed, environment and rearing conditions, age, gender, origin of pain (eg, trauma, surgery, pathology), body region affected (eg, abdominal pain, musculoskeletal pain), type of pain (eg, acute, chronic), and pain intensity. Any pain scale or methodology used for pain assessment must be able to distinguish individual sensitivities. Differences in pain tolerance have been demonstrated experimentally in people and animals and play an important role in the clinical management of pain. For example, the existence of a lower threshold for pain in an individual does not obviate the necessity of treatment, nor does a particularly stoic nature.

There is no "gold standard" to assess pain in animals. Many scoring methods that include physiologic and behavioral variables have been published, but few have been validated. Most veterinary pain scales rely on the recognition and/or interpretation of some behavior and are subject to some degree of variability among observers. Pain scales based on the presence or absence of species-specific behaviors, and that minimize the interpretation of those behaviors, are likely to be more accurate than generic scales that rely heavily on subjective assessment and interpretation. All current methods used to measure pain in animals are prone to errors of under- or overestimation. Even if the amount of pain is correctly estimated, determining how well the individual animal is coping with pain may be difficult. This is particularly true if the animal is removed from its normal environment. Assessment systems must also consider the different types and sources of pain, such as acute versus chronic or neuropathic pain and visceral pain versus somatic pain. Finally, all current methods assess the effects of physical pain; none has been designed to evaluate mental or psychological dimensions of pain in animals.

Physiologic parameters (eg, changes in heart rate, respiratory rate, arterial blood pressure, pupil dilation) may be used to assess responses to an acute noxious (painful) stimulus, particularly during anesthesia, and to assess pain in some clinical situations (eg, horses with acute colic pain). However, physiologic measurements often do not differentiate between animals that have undergone surgery and are experiencing pain and those that did not undergo surgery. Likewise, animals experiencing chronic pain may have normal physiologic parameters. Lack of change in physiologic responses should not be construed to mean there is no pain if other clinical signs suggest otherwise. Physiologic parameters are not specific enough to differentiate pain from other stressors such as anxiety, fear, or physiologic responses to metabolic conditions (eg, anemia).

Lack of familiarity with normal behaviors typical of a particular species or breed makes recognition of pain-induced behaviors difficult or impossible. **Behavioral changes** indicative of pain may be too subtle or take too long to recognize under routine clinical situations in both large and small animals. Sporadic observation of animal behavior may not reveal signs of pain. Except in the most severe circumstances, signs of pain may be "masked" by behavior that is stereotypical of the species being observed. For instance, dogs may wag their tails and greet observers despite being in pain. Flock animals, such as sheep, may be startled when an observer approaches and attempt to conceal signs of pain by staying bunched up with the rest of the flock. Behavioral changes indicating pain may not be what we expect. A cat sitting quietly in the back of the cage after surgery may be in pain; however, pain would not be recognized if the caregiver expects to see more active signs of pain such as pacing, agitation, or vocalization. Because it is difficult to detect sudden behavior changes, recent research has focused more on sudden changes in facial expressions. The mouse and rodent grimace scale appears to offer a means to assess postoperative pain in mice and rats as effectively as manual behavioral-based scoring, without the limitation of such schemes in the latter.

In general, responses to acute surgical and traumatic pain are likely to be more marked and readily recognizable than clinical signs associated with chronic pain. Often, clinical criteria used to assess chronic pain (eg, lack of activity, lack of grooming, decreased appetite, weight loss) are not specific signs of pain and point only to an underlying problem in need of further diagnosis. A significant time commitment is required in the diagnosis and formulation of a treatment plan for animals in chronic pain. Observations by owners are essential to detect more subtle signs of chronic pain in animals, such as changes in attitude or interaction with family members or members of the herd or flock. The Helsinki Chronic Pain Index and the Canine Brief Pain Inventory are owner-completed questionnaires designed to quantify the severity and impact of chronic pain in companion dogs. They have been validated for canine osteoarthritis. The Canine Brief Pain Inventory, which is based on the human Brief Pain Inventory, also has been validated for canine bone cancer. A thorough history and physical examination are integral to the evaluation. Evaluating the degree of lameness and sensitivity to manipulation are also critically important when assessing chronic orthopedic pain and pain of spinal origin. A comprehensive neurologic examination must be included for complete assessment and accurate diagnosis of any chronic pain syndrome. Lastly, response to therapy, such as increased activity after administering an NSAID, may provide important diagnostic information regarding the role of pain in behavioral changes.

Cancer pain may have components of acute pain (eg, expansion of a tumor or secondary responses to surgical, radiation, or chemotherapy treatment), chronic pain, and neuropathic pain (eg, nerve entrapment). Thus, assessment of cancer pain requires methods capable of detecting behavioral changes associated with both acute and chronic pain.

PAIN ALLEVIATION

Acute perioperative, traumatic, and disease-related (eg, cancer, pancreatitis, pleuritis, otitis externa) pain is generally treated pharmacologically with one or more analgesics. The optimal drug or drug combinations are determined principally by the anticipated severity of pain, health status, and available drugs for the given species. The more extensive the tissue trauma or disease-induced tissue damage is, the greater the need to use analgesics from more than one drug class (multimodal or balanced analgesia). Multimodal analgesia maximizes the beneficial analgesic effects of multiple drugs through additive or synergistic interactions while minimizing adverse drug effects by lowering the dose of any individual drug.

A perioperative approach to managing surgically induced pain should be used,

TABLE 3 SELECTED ANALGESICS FOR USE IN DOGS AND CATS

Class	Drug	Pain Category	Dosage (mg/kg)	
			Dogs	**Cats**
Opioids				
Agonists	Morphine	Moderate to severe	0.1–2	0.1–0.5
	Hydromorphone	Moderate to severe	0.05–0.2	0.025–0.2
	Oxymorphone	Moderate to severe	0.05–0.2	0.025–0.1
	Methadone	Moderate to severe	0.1–1	0.1–0.5

beginning with the administration of an analgesic before surgery (preemptive analgesia) and continuing with appropriate analgesia throughout the intraoperative period. Three days is a useful guideline for the duration of analgesic therapy after acute surgical pain. Depending on multiple factors (eg, procedure performed, rehabilitation plan, species, breed), some animals require a shorter duration of therapy, whereas other animals require analgesia for longer periods. Aggressive analgesic therapy of several days' duration should be tapered rather than stopped abruptly. As-needed dosing schedules are less effective than scheduled analgesic dosing to treat pain. As-needed protocols require the animal to demonstrate overt pain behaviors to the extent they are recognized by the veterinarian and/or owner. Aggressive prevention and management of acute pain often prevents wind-up of the nociceptive pathways, hastens return to normal function, and decreases the risk of development of chronic pain syndromes.

Minimizing stress and ensuring that overall care and husbandry are in accordance with the needs of the animal improve pain management. Proper housing conditions, nutritional support, and interaction with other animals and/or people should be optimal for the given species and breed. For example, separating a sheep from the flock for pain management may be quite stressful, whereas separating a companion animal from other animals may not be stressful, provided there is sufficient interaction with human caregivers.

Appropriate analgesia after surgery or trauma allows animals to rest. For example, dogs and cats often sleep but should be arousable after surgery if their pain is controlled. The use of pain as a means of restraint (ie, to prevent the animal from injuring a surgical site) is inappropriate; many efficacious chemical and physical restraint modalities are available.

Managing painful and distressed animals requires a combination of good nursing care, nonpharmacologic methods (eg, bandaging, ice packs or heat, physical therapy), and pharmacologic methods. Pharmacologic methods available for the treatment of acute pain may include opioids, NSAIDs, corticosteroids, local anesthetics, α_2-agonists, and N-methyl-D-aspartate (NMDA) receptor antagonists such as ketamine. Many animals benefit from the management of anxiety. Acepromazine is an effective anxiolytic in small animals but should be used only after appropriate analgesics have been administered. Acepromazine does not have analgesic properties and is not reversible.

ANALGESIC PHARMACOLOGY

Opioids: Opioids continue to be the cornerstone of effective pain treatment in veterinary medicine. The opioids are a diverse group of naturally occurring and synthetic drugs used primarily for their analgesic activity. Despite some well-known adverse effects and disadvantages, opioids are the most effective analgesics available for the systemic treatment of acute pain in many species, particularly dogs and cats. Opioid receptors are part of a large superfamily of membrane-bound receptors that are coupled to G proteins. Each opioid receptor has a unique distribution in the brain, spinal card, and periphery. Opioids combine reversibly with these receptors and alter the transmission and perception of pain. In addition to analgesia, opioids can induce other CNS effects that include sedation, euphoria, dysphoria, and excitement. The clinical

TABLE 3 SELECTED ANALGESICS FOR USE IN DOGS AND CATS *(continued)*

Route	Dose Interval (hr)	Epidural[a] (mg/kg)	Constant-rate Infusion (mg/kg/hr)
IV, SC, IM	4–6	0.1–0.2	0.05–0.2
IV, SC, IM	2–4		0.01–0.03
IV, SC, IM	2–4	0.05	
IV, SC, IM	4–6		

(continued)

TABLE 3 SELECTED ANALGESICS FOR USE IN DOGS AND CATS *(continued)*

Class	Drug	Pain Category	Dosage (mg/kg) Dogs	Dosage (mg/kg) Cats
	Fentanyl	Moderate to severe	0.005-0.01	0.0025–0.005
	Meperidine	Mild to moderate	3–10	3–5
	Codeine	Mild to moderate	0.5–2	0.5–2
	Codeine 60 mg/ acetaminophen 300 mg	Mild to moderate	1–2 (codeine)	Contraindicated
	Hydrocodone	Moderate	0.5	Reliable dosages not established
Agonist-antagonist	Butorphanol	Mild (good visceral analgesia)	0.1–0.5	0.1–0.5
Partial agonist	Buprenorphine	Mild to moderate	0.005–0.02	0.01–0.03
Opioid-like	Tramadol	Mild to moderate	5–10	1–4
α_2-Adrenergic agonists	Xylazine	Sedative/analgesic, emetic effects in cats	0.05-1	0.1–1
	Medetomidine	Sedation longer than anesthesia	0.001–0.02	0.001–0.01
	Dexmedetomidine		0.001–0.015	0.0025–0.02
NMDA receptor antagonists	Ketamine	Adjunctive pain control	0.1–1	0.1–1
	Amantadine	Adjunct drug for chronic/neuropathic pain	3–5	3–5
Calcium channel blocker	Gabapentin	Adjunct drug for chronic/cancer/ neuropathic pain	5–15	2.5–20
NK1 receptor antagonist	Maropitant	Visceral pain	2	1
Muscle relaxant	Methocarbamol	Intervertebral disc disease	15–20	

[a]Preservative-free formulations recommended.

effects of opioids vary between the mu opioid receptor agonists (eg, morphine, hydromorphone), partial mu agonists (ie, *buprenorphine*), and agonist-antagonists (eg, butorphanol). Species and individual differences in the response to opioids are marked, necessitating the careful selection of opioid and adjustment of dose for different species. For example, a 30-kg dog may receive a preoperative dose of morphine (15–30 mg) that is similar to that for a 500-kg horse. Likewise, although butorphanol is widely used as an effective analgesic in horses, its use as an analgesic in small animals is falling out of favor because of its expense, relatively poor

TABLE 3 SELECTED ANALGESICS FOR USE IN DOGS AND CATS *(continued)*

Route	Dose Interval (hr)	Epidural[a] (mg/kg)	Constant-rate Infusion (mg/kg/hr)
IV	15–20 min	0.004	0.002–0.05
SC, IM	1–2		
PO	6–8		
PO	6–8		
PO	6–12		
IV, SC, IM	1–2 (sedation up to 4)	0.25	0.14–0.4
IV, SC, IM, buccal (cats)	6–12	0.005–0.03	0.001–0.005
PO	6–8		
IV, SC, IM		0.02–0.025	
IV, SC, IM			0.001 (loading dose), 0.001–0.003
IV, SC, IM			0.001–0.003
SC, IM, PO	4–6		0.5 (loading dose), intraoperative 0.01–0.02, postoperative 0.002–0.01
PO	Once daily		
PO	6–8		
PO	Once daily		
PO	6–8		

somatic analgesic effect, and short duration of action. The clinical effect of an opioid depends on additional patient factors, including the presence or absence of pain, health status of the animal, concurrent drugs administered (eg, tranquilizers), and individual sensitivity to opioids.

Recent information regarding the peripheral endogenous opioid system (PEOS) has presented a unique opportunity to use the powerful analgesic effect of opiates while minimizing untoward systemic effects. The PEOS includes peripheral opioid receptors (POR) and peripheral leukocyte-derived opioids

(PLDO): endomorphins, endorphins, enkephalins, and dynorphins. To activate the PEOS, tissue must have sufficient numbers of leukocytes able to secrete PLDO as well as functional POR in sufficient numbers. Inflammation due to tissue damage results in accumulation of PLDO-secreting leukocytes at the site of injury. Inflammation also increases the number and efficiency of POR. These receptors, inactive under normal conditions and expressed on primary sensory neurons, are synthesized in the dorsal root ganglion and transported distally to peripheral sensory nerve endings due to tissue injury and inflammation. Experimental trials and clinical studies show that peripheral opiates are effective, particularly in the presence of inflammation. For example, preservative-free morphine has been instilled into canine and equine joints after arthroscopy or arthrotomy.

Nonsteroidal Anti-inflammatory Drugs and Corticosteroids: NSAIDs are useful adjuncts in the treatment of postsurgical pain in a variety of species, because they block prostaglandin synthesis mediated by inhibition of cyclooxygenase (COX). Decreasing inflammation after surgery or trauma can greatly improve analgesia. Inflammation is a key component in both peripheral and central sensitization leading to wind-up. Early and aggressive control of wind-up is critical in the prevention of chronic pain syndromes. NSAIDs appear to confer synergism when used in combination with opioids and may demonstrate an opioid-sparing effect. Significant advantages of NSAIDs include availability, a relatively long duration of action, low cost, and relative ease of administration. Lack of CNS alteration (sedation or dysphoria) make NSAIDs ideal for treating acute and chronic pain in animals. Careful patient selection is critical.

Although a number of NSAIDs have been approved for use in dogs and horses, only meloxicam and robenacoxib are FDA approved for use in cats in the USA. Meloxicam is approved for a single dose and robenacoxib for up to 3 days. As with all analgesic agents, special attention to drug withdrawal times is necessary when using NSAIDs in production animals.

Corticosteroids also reduce inflammation and provide analgesia. Depending on the product, they are administered PO, IV, IM, SC, and intra-articularly. Corticosteroids are used less frequently in the postoperative period because of the potential to decrease immune function and because of other well-known adverse effects (eg, polyphagia, polydipsia, polyuria) after repeated dosing. However, they are used occasionally in chronic pain syndromes, including PO for degenerative disc disease in dogs and intra-articularly for unresponsive osteoarthritis. Corticosteroids and NSAIDs should not be administered concurrently.

For pharmacology of NSAIDs and corticosteroids, *see* p 2707.

α_2-Agonists: Xylazine, medetomidine, dexmedetomidine, detomidine, and romifidine are potent analgesics. α_2-Agonists are used in large animals for standing restraint and provide both analgesia and sedation, although there is evidence to suggest that sedation lasts longer than analgesia. Combination therapy with α_2-agonists and opioids induces profound analgesia and sedation that is additive or synergistic as compared with the effects of either drug alone in both large and small animals. The mechanism of action is through G protein–coupled receptors. Alpha 2_A and alpha 2_C receptors mediate analgesia. α_2-Agonists are used as part of multimodal analgesia in the perioperative period in many species. α_2-Receptors play an important role in the modulation of pain by the CNS. α_2-Agonists may be used to induce analgesia when administered as anesthetic premedications (preemptive analgesia), as a constant-rate infusion intraoperatively, and to supplement postoperative analgesia. In general, postoperative doses of α_2-agonists are considerably lower than would be required preoperatively.

Caution is advised to prevent excessive sedation and concomitant ataxia, particularly in large animals. Furthermore, even at relatively low doses, these agents cause profound reductions in cardiac output and may cause significant arrhythmia in all species. Ruminants in particular require lower doses, and arterial hypoxemia and pulmonary edema have been described in sheep. Careful patient selection is warranted.

Xylazine, medetomidine, and dexmedetomidine (the pure s-enantiomer of the racemic medetomidine) may be reversed in small animals after surgery to hasten recovery and minimize cardiopulmonary depression. Once reversed, however, these drugs provide no analgesia.

Ketamine: Ketamine has long been known to provide excellent somatic analgesia but rather poor visceral analgesia. Interest in ketamine has increased because of its role in preventing sensitization of central nociceptive pathways. Ketamine is an antagonist at the NMDA receptors in the spinal cord and brain. Inhibition of the NMDA receptors prevents or decreases central sensitization (wind-up) in laboratory animals and people. Ketamine may be incorporated into the anesthetic protocol either as a bolus or a constant-rate infusion to prevent development of exaggerated or chronic pain states.

Other Analgesic Agents: **Tramadol**, a synthetic codeine analogue, is a weak mu opioid receptor agonist. In addition to opioid activity, it inhibits neuronal reuptake of norepinephrine and 5-hydroxytryptamine (serotonin) and may facilitate serotonin release. It is recommended for acute and chronic pain of moderate to severe intensity. Because of its inhibitory effects on serotonin uptake, tramadol should not be used in animals that may have received monoamine oxidase inhibitors such as selegiline, in animals on selective serotonin reuptake inhibitors, or in animals with a recent history of seizure activity. In people, the principal active metabolite (O-desmethyl tramadol, M1) is more active at mu receptors than the parent drug. Cats produce significant amounts of M1, whereas dogs produce minimal amounts. Oral bioavailability is 93% in cats but only 65% in dogs. Dogs eliminate and clear tramadol more rapidly than cats. The dosing interval must be adjusted in cats. Adverse effects include decreased seizure thresholds, nausea/vomiting, and in some animals, altered behavior.

There are few clinical studies examining the use of tramadol in animals. However, it has been shown to reduce minimum alveolar concentration of sevoflurane in cats and is reported to have an analgesic effect after ovariohysterectomy similar to that of morphine in dogs. Tramadol may be used alone to treat mild pain and adjunctively in a multimodal plan to treat moderate to severe pain.

Gabapentin was originally developed and licensed as a human anticonvulsant agent and has been approved by the FDA since 1993. Reports of its antihyperalgesic effects in rodent experimental pain models and case reports involving human patients suffering from neuropathic pain suggest increasing evidence for its use in neuropathic pain. The mechanism of action appears to be voltage-dependent Ca^{2+} channel blocker, and it may increase central inhibition or reduce the synthesis of glutamate, even though it does not appear to interact directly with NMDA receptors. Adverse effects are usually mild and self-limiting (drowsiness, fatigue, and weight gain with chronic administration).

Amantadine, an antiviral agent developed to inhibit the replication of influenza A in human patients, has efficacy in the treatment of drug-induced extrapyramidal effects and in treatment of Parkinson disease. It exerts its analgesic effects through antagonism of NMDA receptors. Amantadine seems most efficacious in the management of chronic neuropathic pain with signs of hyperalgesia and allodynia. Animals suffering from opioid tolerance may also benefit. A 2008 study demonstrated improved activity in dogs with NSAID-refractory osteoarthritis when amantadine was added to meloxicam.

Acetaminophen is not approved for use in animals but has been used effectively for the treatment of breakthrough pain in dogs at a dosage of 10–15 mg/kg, bid, for as long as 5 consecutive days. The exact mechanism of action is unclear, although recent evidence suggests indirect activation of the cannabinoid CB(1) receptor. The so-called COX-3, splice variant of COX-1, has been suggested as an additional mechanism for acetaminophen in dogs. Acetaminophen is not considered a classic NSAID partly because of its low anti-inflammatory action; as such, the risk of thrombocytopenia, bleeding, and GI adverse effects is minimal. Hepatopathy is of concern, and routine serum chemistry evaluation is warranted. Acetaminophen should not be used in cats because of inadequate cytochrome P_{450}–dependent hydroxylation (glucuronidation) and subsequent fatal methemoglobinemia.

Maropitant is a potent selective neurokinin (NK1) receptor antagonist that acts in the CNS by inhibiting substance P, the key neurotransmitter involved in vomiting. It provides visceral analgesia for conditions such as pancreatitis, cholangitis, and painful GI disorders.

LOCAL AND REGIONAL ANALGESIC TECHNIQUES

Local and regional anesthetic techniques are used extensively in large animals for a variety of minor and major surgical procedures. Local anesthetics are used in small animals much less frequently and primarily to facilitate suturing of minor lacerations. Because of the relative ease and safety of inducing general anesthesia in small animals, local and regional anesthetic techniques are often overlooked. Nevertheless, these techniques provide an excellent alternative to general anesthesia for select cases and are being used increasingly in conjunction with general anesthesia to improve postoperative analgesia. Local anesthetics used before surgery may decrease the requirement for potent injectable and/or inhalant general anesthetics.

Conduction blockade of nerve fibers by local anesthetics is related to the size of the nerve, amount of myelination, and frequency of activity. Small sensory and autonomic fibers tend to be anesthetized before larger motor and proprioceptive fibers. Nerves that are repetitively stimulated are more sensitive to local anesthetics than resting nerves. The most commonly used agents are lidocaine, mepivacaine, bupivacaine, and ropivacaine.

Lidocaine, the prototype aminoamide local anesthetic, decreases minimum alveolar concentration of isoflurane in a variety of species. It also has the potential to decrease ileus in horses after general anesthesia and is used commonly as an adjunct in colic surgery. This has become the theoretical basis for its systemic use as an analgesic agent. Constant-rate infusion of lidocaine has been advocated for pain management in a number of species; notably, a number of combination analgesic protocols (eg, morphine, lidocaine, ketamine [known as MLK]) have been developed for dogs. The use of constant-rate infusion lidocaine during anesthesia is not recommended for cats because of their increased sensitivity and its negative cardiovascular effects.

Lidocaine transdermal patches have been developed for the treatment of neuropathic pain in people. Systemic absorption of lidocaine in dogs and cats has been reported to be minimal, while local tissue concentration is reported to be as much as 100 times greater than plasma concentration. The low systemic absorption rate coupled with high local lidocaine concentrations on the skin support the safe use of lidocaine patches in dogs and cats. These patches appear to result in a differential blockade, preserving sensory function of the skin and motor function of regional muscles while inducing analgesia at the site for as long as 72 hr. However, further clinical efficacy studies are warranted. Patches must be applied close to the site of pain, and toxicity is of concern if the patch is orally ingested.

EMLA cream, a eutectic mixture of 2.5% lidocaine and 2.5% prilocaine, has been used to decrease venipuncture pain in children and has been evaluated for use in dogs, cats, rabbits, horses, and pigs. Significant results are not achieved until the cream has been in place for 60–90 min beneath an occlusive dressing. Nonclinical methemoglobinemia, lasting as long as 24 hr, has been reported in children. Repeated dosing of neonatal or small animals should be done cautiously.

Bupivacaine is the preferred drug for postoperative analgesia because of its relatively long duration of action (~3–8 hr). Bupivacaine (0.25–0.75%), with or without epinephrine, is administered in a dosage not to exceed 3 mg/kg (dogs) for line or ring blocks of an incision, ring blocks before declaw in cats (epinephrine-containing solutions should not be used for distal extremity ring blocks), intercostal nerve blocks and intrapleural local anesthesia (diluted to twice the volume) after a thoracotomy or the management of pain associated with pancreatitis, proximal nerve infiltration during limb amputations, regional anesthesia in which a nerve proximal to the surgical site is targeted, tissue infiltration for lateral ear resections, and local blocks of facial nerves (maxillary, infraorbital, mental, and mandibular). Bupivacaine is frequently administered into the epidural space at the lumbosacral space for pelvic limb and perianal procedures. Bupivacaine is cardiotoxic if administered IV.

Ropivacaine is a long-lasting amide-type local anesthetic. Its duration is similar to that of bupivacaine, but it has lower potential to induce cardiovascular and CNS toxicity.

Topical capsaicin, the active component in chili peppers, has been used extensively to treat pain associated with diabetic neuropathy, post-herpetic neuralgia, and osteoarthritis in people. Capsaicin binds to the TRPV1 receptor on nonmyelinated primary afferent pain fibers, causing increased firing through the release of substance P. With repeat application, desensitization occurs due to degeneration of these pain fibers with resultant hypoalgesia. Reinnervation occurs when use is discontinued. No controlled studies have been published in veterinary species; however, one study using intrathecal resinferatoxin, a potent analogue of capsaicin, reported encouraging results for palliative treatment of pain in a canine osteosarcoma model. The benefits of these TRPV1 ligands include specific loss of pain sensation without concomitant loss of motor and nonpain sensation.

CHRONIC PAIN

The treatment of chronic pain relies on pharmacologic and nonpharmacologic methods. Commonly treated chronic pain syndromes include osteoarthritis, nonsurgical intervertebral disc disease, and laminitis. Some chronic pain responds to drugs used to treat acute pain, such as opioids and NSAIDs; however, other types of chronic pain require the addition of novel drugs such as gabapentin, tramadol, acetaminophen, and amantadine. Regardless of the cause or the species, chronic pain is itself a dynamic disease process requiring careful assessment and frequent reassessment. Therapy is rarely monomodal, and adjustments in therapy are necessary over time.

The nonpharmacologic treatment of chronic pain depends on the underlying cause and the species. Among these therapies are acupuncture, rehabilitation, nutraceutical supplements, low-level laser, massage, transcutaneous electric nerve stimulation, and herbal supplements. The body of literature critically examining these is relatively small. (*See also* COMPLEMENTARY AND ALTERNATIVE VETERINARY MEDICINE, p 2078).

Osteoarthritis Pain: Osteoarthritis is the most common reason for persistent pain in people, dogs, cats, and horses. The nonpharmacologic goals to manage osteoarthritis pain include increasing mobility, limiting disease progression, and possibly facilitating tissue repair within the joint. Weight control or reduction and mild to moderate daily exercise are beneficial. Excessive and strenuous exercise should be avoided, because it may further strain the joints and exacerbate pain, thus limiting the ability to exercise routinely. Providing warmth during cold and damp weather and extra bedding or padding may also improve comfort. Surgical removal of bone fragments and osteochondritic lesions and the restoration of joint stability is often necessary to slow the progression of disease and reduce pain. Joint replacement or arthrodesis may be indicated in severe cases. Orthotic bracing may be beneficial in small animals when surgical intervention is not appropriate. A number of studies using chondroprotective agents such as polysulfated glycosaminoglycans, chondroitin sulfate, glucosamine, and hyaluronic acid suggest a benefit through stimulation of cartilage matrix synthesis and inhibition of enzymatic degradation of cartilage. However, the efficacy of these agents may vary with specific product used, route of administration, and underlying conformational, pathologic, and neurologic issues. Recent work in regenerative medicine, including the use of autologous adult stem cells, may prove highly effective as well. Finally, acupuncture and rehabilitation therapy have been used to treat chronic osteoarthritis pain in a number of veterinary species with promising results.

Cancer Pain: Cancer pain presents a unique clinical challenge. Components of cancer pain are tumorigenic (tumor-related products), inflammatory, and neuropathic. Similar to other forms of chronic pain, it does not always respond adequately to common therapies. Opioids remain a cornerstone of treatment and are usually one part of a multimodal plan. Other analgesics include NSAIDs, tramadol, acetaminophen (in dogs), and amantadine for its ability to decrease wind-up. An opioid and an NSAID are routinely used in combination because of their synergistic analgesic effect. Recently, bisphosphonates have been used to treat osteolytic pain associated with bony metastasis. Pamidronate is the synthetic analogue of inorganic pyrophosphate. It has proved useful in pain palliation because of its ability to adsorb to bone mineral matrix, inhibit pathologic lysis induced by osteoclasts, and delay progression of bony metastatic lesions.

Similar to all chronic pain syndromes, cancer pain management requires frequent assessment and reassessment combined with appropriate adjustments in therapy.

STRAY VOLTAGE IN ANIMAL HOUSING

The term stray voltage describes a special case of voltage developed on the grounded-neutral system of a farm and is defined as <10 volts (measured as the root-mean-square value of 50 or 60 Hz alternating voltage, Vrms) between two points that can be contacted simultaneously by an animal (animal contact voltage). The grounding and neutral systems on a farm or in a home wiring system should be properly bonded to ensure electrical safety. As a result, some level of voltage between the grounded-neutral system and the earth (neutral-to-earth voltage) is always present as a normal consequence of the operation of properly installed electrical equipment. The term stray voltage is often applied incorrectly to other electrical phenomena such as electric fields, magnetic fields, electric current flowing in the earth (earth currents), or electric current flowing on a grounding conductor (ground currents). Electric currents flowing in the earth or on grounded metal objects will affect animals only if sufficient animal contact voltage is developed.

If stray voltage reaches sufficient levels, animals coming into contact with grounded devices may receive a mild electric shock that can cause a behavioral response. At voltage levels that are just perceptible to the animal, behaviors indicative of perception (eg, flinches) may result, with little change in normal routines. At higher exposure levels, avoidance behaviors may result. Contact voltages <10 Vrms are not lethal to farm animals or people. If neutral-to-earth voltages >10 Vrms are measured on a farm, the safety of the farm wiring system should be carefully evaluated by a competent electrician.

Animals respond to the current flowing through their bodies. Ohms law describes the relationship between voltage exposure and current conducted through an animal: current = voltage / resistance or amps = volts / ohms

This simple relationship has been a source of much confusion and resulting controversy. Ohm's law indicates that if the voltage across animal contact points is increased, the current flowing through the animal will increase. If the resistance of the circuit is increased, the current flowing through the animal will decrease. The current measurement used in most studies is the milliamp (mA) or 1/1,000th of an amp. Applying Ohm's law to a circuit with contact voltage of 1 Vrms across a resistance of 500 ohms results in current flow of 2 mA.

In most situations, cows are less sensitive to current and more sensitive to voltage than are people. While the resistance of bovine and human tissues is similar, the contact resistance is often lower for cows than for people, particularly in wet environments. The resistance of a cow's body plus the contact resistance with the floor is estimated as 500 ohms for a cow standing on a wet floor. Cows standing on a dry surface typically have body plus contact resistance of ≥1,000 ohms. Cows standing or lying on dry bedding have a resistance many times higher than this. The resistance of a person can be as low as 1,000 ohms for wet hand-foot contact to >10,000 ohms for dry hand-foot contact. The contact voltage to produce sensation can therefore be higher for people than for cows, depending on the conditions of the contact points. The standard measurement circuit used for field investigations uses a 500-ohm "shunt" resistor to simulate the combined resistance of a cow's body plus a conservative (lowest or worst case) estimate of the resistance of the two contact points (cow + contact resistance).

A great deal of research on the effects of stray voltage on dairy cows has been conducted throughout the past 50 yr. The most sensitive cows (<1%) begin to react to 60 Hz electrical current of 2 mA (measured as the root-mean-square average, or rms) applied from muzzle to hooves or from hoof to hoof. This corresponds to a contact voltage level of ~1 Vrms in wet locations or >2 Vrms in dry locations. Numerous studies have documented that avoidance behaviors occur at exposure levels well above this first behavioral reaction threshold. As the current dose increases above 2 mA, an increasing percentage of cows show mild behavioral responses, and some cows start to show avoidance behaviors. The median avoidance threshold for 60 Hz current flowing through a cow is ~8 mA (or 4 Vrms contact voltage in wet locations and >8 Vrms in dry locations). Even when the threshold is exceeded, all cows do not respond behaviorally all the time, nor do they exhibit the same signs; however, as the voltage increases, signs in the herd become more widespread and uniform. Cows have resumed normal behaviors within 1 day of removal of aversive voltage and current levels.

The only studies that have documented reduced water or feed intake in cows had both sufficient current applied to cause aversion and forced exposures (ie, cows could not eat or drink without being exposed to aversive voltage and current). It is typical for voltage levels to vary considerably through the normal daily operation of electrical equipment on a farm. Decreased feed and/or water intake will result only if current exposure levels at watering and feeding locations are sufficient to produce aversion at these locations and they occur often enough to interfere with drinking and eating behaviors. If an aversive current occurs only a few times per day, it is not likely to have an adverse effect on cow behavior. The more often aversive current exposures occur in areas critical to drinking or feeding, the more likely it is to affect the cows.

Studies investigating the effects of high-frequency or short-duration transient voltages on cows clearly indicate that as the duration of a current pulse gets shorter (or the frequency increases), more voltage and current is required to cause behavioral responses. The main cause of short-duration electric pulses on farms is improperly installed electric fences and electrified crowd gates. These devices are designed to produce a powerful electric impulse that is used to control animal behavior. Improper installation of these devices can cause these pulses to appear in unintended areas on the farm. The other common source of high-frequency events is a switching transient that occurs when electric equipment is turned on or off. These high-frequency pulses decay quickly and do not travel far from their source, and it is extremely rare for them to reach problematic exposure levels.

Research suggests that swine respond to voltage/current exposure in a way similar to that of cows. Behavioral modification in swine has been seen above 60 Hz exposures of ~5 Vrms, with avoidance behaviors at exposures >8 Vrms. The body plus contact resistance for swine appears to be somewhat higher than for cows, and 1,000 ohms appears to be a conservative value for measurement purposes. Ewes have been shown to avoid electrified feed bowls when 60 Hz exposure levels exceed 5.5 Vrms, whereas lambs showed this same preferential behavior when exposure levels exceeded 5 Vrms. Exposures to voltages as high as 18 Vrms had no effect on hens' production and behavior. This is likely because of the very high electrical resistance of poultry, which has been documented to be between 350,000 and 544,000 ohms.

Clinical Findings: A wide variety of behavioral signs have been reported in cows exposed to voltage and current. No one sign is pathognomonic, however, because these behaviors can also be caused by other factors in the animal environment. The only way to determine whether stray voltage is a potential cause of abnormal behaviors is to perform electric testing.

The direct effects of stray voltage can range from mild behavioral reactions indicative of sensation to intense behavioral responses indicative of pain. The severity of response depends on the amount of electric current flowing through the animal's body, the pathway it takes through the body, and the sensitivity of the individual animal. The indirect effects of these behaviors can vary considerably depending on the specifics of the contact location, level of current flow, body pathway, frequency of occurrence, and many other factors related to the daily activities of animals. All of the documented effects of excessive voltage exposure have been behaviorally mediated.

Results of studies to investigate direct physiologic effects that may be produced at levels both above and below those required to produce behavioral responses have shown that blood cortisol concentrations and other stress hormones do not increase at levels below behavioral response levels. Increases in stress-related hormones have been documented in some, but not all, cows at voltage/current exposures substantially higher than the threshold required for behavioral modification. A large body of research clearly indicates that at levels of voltage exposure typically used as regulatory limits (1 volt at cow contact locations, or 2 mA of current flow through a cow) will not result in increased somatic cell counts or incidence of mastitis.

Diagnosis: Several common situations are of concern in animal environments, including 1) changes in drinking behavior, such as decreased number of drinks of water per day and increased length of time per drink; 2) avoidance of locations that may result in reduced feed or water intake; and 3) difficulty of moving or handling animals in some areas. If these behaviors are seen, electric testing indicating cow contact exposure in excess of 4 mA (2 Vrms in wet locations with a 500 ohm cow + contact resistor, or 4 Vrms in dry locations with a 1,000 ohm cow + contact resistor) is necessary to confirm a stray voltage diagnosis. Signs in pigs, ewes, and poultry are similar, although threshold response levels are higher than for cows.

It is critically important to use a realistic value of animal resistance to relate voltage exposures to the level of current conducted through an animal and the resulting effects on nerve stimulation, sensation, and behavioral reaction. A competent field investigation will include voltage measurements at cow contact locations both with an appropriate "shunt" resistor (cow contact voltage) and without a shunt resistor (open circuit voltage). The shunt resistor is meant to represent the resistance of the body resistance of a cow plus the contact resistance representative of the exposure location. Both animal-contact and open circuit voltage measurements are required to determine the "source resistance" of the electric parts of the circuit. Note that source resistance is different from the cow contact resistance and can be used as a diagnostic to determine the voltage source.

Animal-contact voltage levels should be monitored at different times of the day and on different days to represent the normal operating conditions of the farm electrical system. Point-to-reference ground measurements can be useful for diagnostic purposes. A reference ground can be established with a copper-clad rod driven into the ground at least 25 ft (8.5 m) from any part of the grounding network on the farm. The other contact point is typically the ground-neutral interconnection in the barn service entrance panel or some other part of the grounded-neutral system. Cow contact measurements are typically ½ to ⅓ of point-to-reference voltage levels.

Long, insulated meter leads (6–10 ft [2–3 m]) facilitate measurements on the farm and give a reasonable estimate of power frequency (60 Hz and 50 Hz) events but introduce considerable noise to higher frequency measurements. The measurement of high frequency events requires proper equipment and careful measurement technique. Details on measurement techniques are available through electric power suppliers and extension publications.

Prevention and Control: Off-farm sources of stray voltage are most often related to improper function of the grounded-neutral system of the electric utility. On-farm sources of stray voltage are most often due to wiring systems that do not meet wiring codes and standards. Deficiencies may include loose or corroded connections; ground faults (shorts); undersized wiring; or wiring damaged by animals, accidents, moisture, or corrosion.

The first step in a competent stray voltage investigation is to determine the source of neutral-to-earth voltage. Faults or electric code violations that could pose an electrocution hazard should be corrected immediately to protect both animals and people. If stray voltage levels are excessive, a competent electrician should assess the situation to determine the most practical, safe, and efficient way to reduce neutral-to-earth voltage. Equipotential planes are required at critical animal contact locations in animal confinement facilities and effectively eliminate contact voltage even if substantial levels of neutral-to-earth voltage are present.

VENTILATION

Ventilation is often associated with respiratory health of animals; the quality of the air that animals breathe directly influences animal health and disease. Ventilation, directly and indirectly, impacts many other aspects of animal health as well. Good ventilation in the lying area of lactating animals helps bedding stay dry, a factor in favor of good mammary health. Good ventilation along alleys helps to keep walking surfaces dry, which contributes to healthy feet. Good ventilation may lead to greater productivity, eg, maintaining air movement in the eating area makes animals more comfortable, especially important during hot weather as an aid to maintaining dry matter intake. A comfortable, well-ventilated lying area encourages animals to lie down, an important contribution to many aspects of animal health.

During ventilation, outside air is brought into a barn where it collects moisture, heat, and other contaminants. Air is then exhausted to the outside. To determine ventilation rates, the focus is on the moisture content of the air, measured by relative humidity.

AIR QUALITY

Air quality is not easily defined. It is related to ventilation and the absence (or presence) of contaminants in the air. For animals, good air quality generally implies that the ambient air causes no harmful effects on the animals in the space. Ambient air contains varying amounts of water vapor. Moisture in the air becomes a problem when it exceeds the relative humidity range of 60%–75% preferred for animals; above this level, it is considered to be an air contaminant. Other contaminants may include pathogens, harmful gases, dust, and undesirable odors. Concern arises from the concentration of a contaminant above some predetermined level rather than the mere presence of the contaminant itself.

Numerous viral pathogens known to survive in aerosols are apparently spread by the airborne route. Two factors can be significant in the relationship between microbial aerosols and disease incidence: 1) the survival time of the aerosolized pathogen, and 2) the total number of pathogens per volume of air (ie, concentration). Survival is influenced by conditions of the ambient air; conditions of the ambient air and concentration are related to ventilating air.

Relative humidity is the most important factor influencing pathogen survival and concentration, but its effects vary greatly between pathogens—some survive best in humid conditions, others survive best in dry air. Maintaining a relative humidity in the range of 60%–75% apparently results in the shortest survival time for the greatest number of potential pathogens. Ventilation is used to remove moisture from an animal space with the intention of maintaining relative humidity in this range. Inside air is diluted with outside air, reducing moisture levels. Continuous replacement of contaminated air with fresh, outside air is also the most effective way to reduce the concentration of aerosol pathogens.

Most likely, reducing the concentration of any air contaminant, including gases and dust, is important to reducing its detrimental effect. For example, ammonia is produced by the decay of feces and urine and is probably the most significant air pollutant in cattle barns. Allowed to accumulate, ammonia's irritating effects on the respiratory epithelium appear to directly reduce the number of ciliated cells and thus decrease the efficiency of mucociliary transport.

THE DILUTION EFFECT OF VENTILATION

Dilution reduces heat and concentrations of moisture, as well as concentrations of airborne disease organisms, harmful gases and dust, and undesirable odors. The dilution rate of ventilation is often expressed in air changes per unit time. For example, a ventilation rate of 4 air changes/hr implies that the entire volume of the ventilated space is replaced 4 times every hour. In fact, some of the air may bypass the occupied zone in the barn, depending on geometry of the space, design of diffusers controlling inlet air, etc. Therefore, the effectiveness of ventilation is not 100% but perhaps approaches 65%. Ventilation effectiveness becomes important to the actual dilution achieved by a particular rate of ventilation (ie, to the ability of ventilating air to reduce the concentrations of contaminants in the animal space). For a ventilation effectiveness of 1.0, one air change would achieve a complete change of air in the space, yielding a 100% reduction in contaminant levels (if the condition of the outside air is considered to be the reference standard). But if ventilation effectiveness is only 0.65, one air change will reduce contaminant levels by only 65%. As ventilation effectiveness diminishes, the ventilation rate required to achieve a certain air change rate increases.

When ventilation is reduced below recommended levels—usually in a misguided effort in cold climates to warm the barn using animal heat—less moisture is removed. Sometimes the consequences of the resulting moisture buildup and lack of proper ventilation (eg, condensation) are masked by insulating the barn, using a greenhouse effect, providing supplemental heat, or dehumidifying the inside air. For example, adding heat to the air reduces relative humidity, without the need for air exchange. It is quite possible to maintain substantial quantities of moisture in the air and, if accompanied by heating, keep the relative humidity within an acceptable range. If relative humidity is the only measure of air quality, it may be deemed to be satisfactory. However, even though excess moisture may not be apparent, the reduced dilution does result in increased concentrations of airborne disease organisms, harmful gases and dust, and undesirable odors. If these increases are ignored, animal health problems are inevitable. In addition, heating of barns is rarely economical in cold climates.

COLD WEATHER VENTILATION

A minimal ventilation rate is required in animal housing in cold weather, regardless of outside temperature. This minimal rate is necessary whether the barn is designed to be a warm barn or a cold barn in winter. In addition, the minimal ventilation should be continuous to maintain concentrations of contaminants in the air at minimal levels. The minimal rate depends on outside weather, design conditions, animal factors (number, type, age, and size), and whether the barn is intended to be cold or warm.

Barn Categories and Winter Temperatures

Barn environments can be categorized according to temperatures maintained in the barn in winter. The particular environment, based on desired indoor temperature, must be established before ventilation system design can begin. In **cold barns**, indoor temperatures are allowed to fluctuate with outdoor temperatures. Ventilation is sufficient to maintain indoor temperatures within 3°–6°C of outdoor temperatures. Ventilation is largely unregulated, except to adjust for seasonal changes. In general, a cold barn with natural ventilation has no insulation, an open ridge and eaves, and sidewalls and endwalls that open. Providing an open ridge along with open eaves has long been recognized as a way to use a stack effect to cause air exchange, especially to control moisture in winter. Indoor temperatures are expected to be a few degrees warmer than outdoor air temperature because of the heat given off by the animals being housed. Current recommendations call for providing a ridge opening of 5 cm per 3 m of barn width and equivalent open area divided between the two eaves. Raised ridge caps are to be avoided. Their performance is unpredictable because of local wind patterns, which often channel winds into the structure and increase the entry of snow and rain. The combination of the open ridge and eaves should be viewed as the sole source of ventilation only during the most severe winter weather, ie, during periods when temperatures reach the lowest levels or times when conditions are especially windy or stormy. During all other times in winter, additional ventilation should be provided.

Warm barns are well insulated and, by necessity, have well-controlled ventilation systems. These barns are designed to provide a relatively uniform environment throughout the winter. Tie stall barns for dairy cows (indoor temperatures at least above freezing) and farrowing and nursery barns for swine (indoor temperatures 25°–30°C) are examples of this type of housing. Keys to success include ventilating fans and controls chosen to match the needs of the animals being housed, a well-insulated building, supplemental heating (if required), and a ventilation system that is well managed and regulated to compensate for changing outside climatic conditions.

Some barns do not fit into either the warm or cold category. **In-between or modified environment barns** usually have indoor temperatures in winter above freezing. These buildings have some insulation, perhaps only under the roof, and are naturally ventilated (usually with an open ridge, eaves, and sidewalls). Unfortunately, even though a minimal ventilation rate is always necessary, ventilation openings may be closed or blocked during extreme weather to keep manure from freezing and for other reasons. This practice can result in inside temperatures rising 10°–20°C above the outside temperature, significantly higher than the 3°–6°C temperature difference limit considered acceptable for cold barns. This alone can create problems because of excess moisture buildup and a high relative humidity. Even more seriously, openings remain closed or blocked after severe weather conditions have passed. As a consequence, blocked ventilation openings restrict airflow during less severe conditions, resulting in underventilation and poor environmental conditions. A properly designed and managed in-between barn is more like a warm barn, in terms of both design and operation, than a cold barn. Thus, to avoid problems, the design and management of in-between barns should follow the guidelines for a warm barn.

Consequences of Mismanaged Ventilation in Winter

Underventilation in winter is one of the most serious threats to the environment of animals. Both improper design and improper management of the ventilation may compromise animal health. In colder climates, problems are most likely during winter, spring, and fall, especially during rainy weather and warmer days coupled with cold nights.

Reduced Dilution of Ambient Air:

Adjusting ventilation for severe winter weather and not readjusting to allow increased ventilation for milder winter weather appears to be a major reason for air quality problems in barns in winter. This is especially true for cold barns with manually controlled natural ventilation. For example, ventilation openings are closed in anticipation of a windy, cold, blustery night, but are not opened the next day when, although the temperature may still be cold, the wind subsides and the sun shines. The lack of wind reduces ventilation and thus air exchange and the positive effects of dilution.

Sometimes, good ventilation system management does call for openings to be reduced. For example, a slot inlet in a mechanically ventilated tie stall barn may be adjusted, or fabric may be placed over an open sidewall to match the lower ventilation rate in winter. All openings should never be covered, however, because this leaves no means of air exchange for moisture control.

Building Components Affected by Poor Ventilation: In addition to adversely affecting the animal environment, the design and operation of naturally ventilated barns also influence moisture-related deterioration in wood members and metal fasteners. In naturally ventilated dairy free-stall barns in Michigan, where air exchange in winter was defeated by blocking ventilation openings, average wood moisture contents >30% dry basis (capable of supporting wood decay and corrosion in metal fasteners) were found after 2–3 mo of cold weather operation. Moreover, restricted air movement in these barns inhibited drying and allowed wood moisture content to remain high even during warm weather. Warm, moist conditions favor growth of mold, bacteria, and decay fungi and accelerate metal corrosion. The presence of insulation under the roofing in these barns fostered the situation. In barns in which design details and management efforts allowed optimal air exchange rates, increases in moisture were minimal. Even if free water from precipitation and condensation caused slightly increased moisture contents, adequate air exchange, especially during warm weather, promoted drying of wood truss components so that deterioration was not a problem.

WARM WEATHER VENTILATION

In barns with natural ventilation, the combination of the open ridge and eaves is the source of ventilation during the most severe winter weather, ie, during periods when temperatures reach the lowest levels or times when conditions are especially windy or stormy. During all other times in winter, however, additional ventilation must be provided. Typically, doorways are left open, portions of the end wall sections of the gable roof may be left uncovered, or sidewalls away from prevailing winter winds may be left open for this purpose. Then, as temperatures rise into spring and summer, sidewalls and end walls are fully opened. As a general rule, too much ventilation is preferred over too little.

Hot, muggy summer weather is one of the most critical times for animal health, comfort, and productivity. For barns with natural ventilation, completely open sidewalls and end walls allow wind to blow through the animal zone for heat stress reduction. However, when winds are calm, providing adequate air movement to avoid heat stress is difficult. Supplemental cooling can be provided in several ways. Fans are commonly used to increase air movement. The increased air velocity over the skin increases the rate at which animals are able to dissipate excess body heat. Two other methods rely on evaporative cooling to either cool the air around the animals or wet the animal's skin and allow body heat to evaporate the water. However, water should be added to the animals' environment only if ample air movement is present.

Barns with mechanical ventilation require staged fans to provide ventilation ranging from the minimal continuous rate, through an intermediate rate for spring and fall, to a high rate for summer. An air exchange rate of 60 air changes/hr is considered the absolute minimum for summer. Often, ventilation rates of 90–120 air changes/hr are provided for hot weather.

HEALTH-MANAGEMENT INTERACTION: BEEF CATTLE

BEEF CATTLE BREEDING HERDS

Several managerial practices increase productivity within cow-calf herds when they can be implemented economically and practically. These practices are mostly associated with reproduction, because improvements in herd fertility generally offer potential for increased profitability in cow-calf operations. They include a restricted breeding season, identification of the optimal calving season, a good heifer replacement program, heifer reproductive tract scoring, proper nutrition, good herd health, bull breeding soundness examinations, crossbreeding, and maintaining good records. Other management practices associated with increased beef herd profitability include decreasing unit cost of production, use of growth promotants in calves, internal and external parasite control, improved calf management, management-intensive grazing, preconditioning of calves, and having a marketing plan.

REPRODUCTION

In most regions of the world, there is an optimal period for females to calve, suckle, and rebreed. This period is mostly related to nutritional opportunity, although other environmental factors such as cold or heat stress and parasite populations may play a role. Producers have traditionally aimed for females to calve during this optimal period because they tend to breed back faster, and their calves are more likely to thrive, than females that calve at less opportune times. Benefits of restricted breeding seasons (65–80 days) include enhanced production potential, favorable environmental factors, a concentrated calving season and more homogeneous calf crop to sell, increased opportunities to perform prebreeding management procedures and monitor nutrition, improved female replacement and culling procedures, and the ability to detect problems early, using herd pregnancy diagnosis and breeding season evaluation. (*See also* MANAGEMENT OF REPRODUCTION: CATTLE, p 2171.)

Pregnancy Testing: The longterm goal is to develop a beef herd of uniform, low-maintenance cows that thrive in their given environment. This goal is strengthened by having a restricted breeding season in which open cows are culled from the herd. Often, these cows are too big, produce too much milk, or lack inherent fertility compared with cows that are pregnant year after year. In herds that are years away from this goal, instead of simply calling cows pregnant or open, cows should be sorted by projected calving date and body condition score (BCS). The herd pregnancy diagnosis represents an important starting point for beef herd diagnostics and advice and is a pivotal component for informed decision making. It allows analysis of group patterns for problem solving (breeding soundness evaluation, *see* below), as well as sorting of animals into groups for specific purposes such as strategic feeding, calving supervision, culling, or rebreeding. Herd pregnancy diagnosis facilitates the selection of replacement females and culling for infertility.

Breeding Soundness Evaluation: Reproductive performance is influenced by many factors, including sire fertility, herd health aspects, and opportunities to mate. Breeding soundness evaluation is a technique to assess the reproductive performance of the cow herd. It includes obtaining relevant information, analysis and interpretation, and recommendations for improvement. One measure of reproductive performance is the number of bred females that actually raise a live calf. Other valuable information may be obtained from an analysis of the distribution of pregnancies (and calvings) that resulted from a particular breeding season. This distribution may be studied on the basis of timing (eg, 21-day estrus periods), breeding groups, female age or parity, nutritional opportunity (eg, BCS), etc. Such analyses provide the basis for evaluation of either the breeding or calving season. For evaluation of the breeding season, good records must be obtained at the time of pregnancy testing for the subsequent analysis to be valid.

Because reproductive performance is an important economic trait in the cow herd, the reproductive capabilities of breeding bulls assume great importance. The best assurance that a bull is likely to be fertile is a successful breeding soundness evaluation (*see* BREEDING SOUNDNESS EXAMINATION OF THE MALE, p 2230). A rule of thumb for bulls is that they can breed ~1 cow/mo of age in a breeding season of 65–80 days. For example, a 38-mo-old bull that passes his breeding soundness examination should be able to breed 38 cows in 65–80 days. This rule can be applied to bulls approximately 14–50 mo old, with 50 cows per bull being the maximum.

CULL COW SELECTION AND MANAGEMENT

Culling of cattle in a beef operation usually implies removing those that cannot meet or maintain performance and economic criteria for the herd. Other reasons may include physical or temperament problems in animals, as well as judicious culling during periods of environmental hardship or economic necessity. The judicious removal of nonperforming females is also important to maintain or improve herd fertility. However, the assumption that cull cows are necessarily infertile may not always be correct; recent surveys indicate that ~43% of cull cows in the USA are pregnant at the time of culling. All "open" females are not necessarily infertile. Identification of appropriate candidates for culling is critical and should be an important component of pregnancy testing.

NUTRITIONAL MANAGEMENT

Nutrition is the most important limiting factor of beef herd reproductive performance. An understanding of the principles underlying the nutritional management of breeding females is necessary, including a working knowledge of the different energy measuring systems commonly used and their applications for different classes of animals, activities, and feedstuffs. (*See* NUTRITION: CATTLE, p 2248.) Increasing stocking rate tends to cause increased gain per unit land area but can result in decreased gain per animal. The key is to have these two factors in balance so that pasture land is optimally grazed and gain per animal is adequate. Overgrazed pasture is detrimental to the environment and can severely reduce gain per animal.

Nutritional requirements vary throughout the year. The most critical periods for reproduction are immediately precalving, when fetal growth is maximal along with lactation preparation, and early postcalving, when maximal lactation is combined with the need for rebreeding. (*See also* MANAGEMENT OF REPRODUCTION: CATTLE, p 2171.)

Environmental conditions can strongly influence the nutritional requirements and intake of cattle. For example, cold weather increases energy needs, whereas hot or inclement weather can reduce foraging opportunity. The quality and quantity of range forage varies greatly throughout the year and between years, influenced by moisture, soil fertility, plant species, and grazing pressure. Seasonal changes in the nutrient density of rangeland forages are mainly associated with the degree of plant maturity. In general, the greatest nutritional value of plants develops before maturity. Good nutritional management involves matching, as far as possible, the nutrient requirements of cows and nutrient density of the pasture by careful consideration of factors such as the types of animals involved, stocking rates, plant species available, season of grazing, fertilization, and grazing methods used.

Body Condition Score: Accurate and timely determination of the nutritional status of grazing animals represents a challenge for beef producers, because many variables can influence a cow's response to a given level of nutrition. The use of a BCS is an effective indirect method to determine nutritional status in breeding females. The BCS represents a subjective assessment of body fat (or energy reserves) that is strongly related to female reproductive performance. BCS, and changes in BCS, appear to be more reliable indicators of nutritional status than is body weight or changes in body weight, which can vary with gut fill and pregnancy status. In addition, BCS can often be assessed more conveniently than body weight can be measured. BCS is both repeatable and accurate in experienced hands. It is best done through visual appraisal, reinforced by palpation of body regions most likely to demonstrate fat deposits. Group observations of BCS made from a distance when animals are in the pasture or paddock are less accurate than those made when animals are nearby in the pen or chute.

BCS varies throughout the year and should be monitored regularly. In the 1–9 BCS system widely used in North America, the reference standard for beef females is a BCS of 5, which represents an average, moderately fleshed cow that is neither fat nor thin. However, the BCS for optimal female efficiency varies with breed and operation and may be higher or lower. In general, cows should calve when they are between condition scores 5–6 (heifers 6–7) and then regain the weight lost at calving and gain slightly until breeding. It generally takes ~2 mo to gain 1 score (75–100 lb [34.1–45.5 kg]) for nonlactating cows under pasture conditions. Care should be taken not to rely on averages, because these can mask variations that might adversely affect herd fertility.

Whereas BCS at calving has been long proved to impact reproductive success, recent studies have demonstrated that an increasing BCS from after calving to breeding is just as important or can be more important than precalving BCS in terms of herd fertility. The concept of increasing BCS just before breeding is especially true of yearling heifers. These heifers are often developed on more of a feedlot type ration during the winter and then turned out to pasture at breeding time. This causes a decrease in available energy, which can significantly decrease first-service conception rate. Solutions to this are to feed a lower energy ration during the development stage and to add additional energy to the diet after pasture turn-out.

The BCS of females at calving can provide much information about their rebreeding prospects. However, assessment of BCS at this time provides a relatively short length of time in which to meet targets if cows are too thin. Assessment of BCS in females at breeding should provide the most accurate prediction of herd fertility, because it is done just before the predictive event. The disadvantage is that there is no opportunity to correct significant shortfalls in time to affect the current breeding season. Assessment of BCS at the time of pregnancy checking has the advantage of not requiring a separate animal handling. It also allows considerable time to remedy obvious deficiencies before calving and subsequent rebreeding. The disadvantage is that, although it can provide clues to explain current pregnancy patterns, it is again too late to remedy them. The ideal time to assign BCS to cows is ~2–3 mo precalving. This gives ample time to move cows to an optimal precalving BCS, because BCS at calving is highly correlated to herd fertility. It is best if someone other than the owner (eg, veterinarian, extension specialist, etc) does the BCS evaluation of the herd, because the owner sees the cows every day and is less likely to see changes.

HEALTH AND PRODUCTION MANAGEMENT PROGRAM

A cost-effective herd health and production management program is essential for the economic viability of cow-calf operations. Such programs vary by region, relative economics, perceptions, and opportunity. A good herd health program manages risk of disease and lowered productivity at a number of levels, including considerations of biosecurity, nutrition, and the judicious use of biologics and parasiticides.

One starting point for such a program is to identify current production losses by comparing the performance of the particular herd with relevant standards, eg, from regional or national surveys, which can also provide an economic estimate of losses.

The major disease risks for a given herd, along with appropriate preventive measures, should be established in consultation with herd owners. The best times for herd intervention must be identified. These often coincide with other managerial tasks and can be synchronized to minimize herd disruption and labor costs. One approach is to devise a herd-health "calendar" in which the health events are coordinated with major operational events. Interventions for a particular herd vary based on factors such as available labor, normal herd working dates, calf weaning dates, calf management practices, and previous disease problems.

VACCINATIONS

Prebreeding vaccinations should be completed ~4 wk before the start of breeding and should be based on local patterns of disease and state and national requirements. Replacement females should be vaccinated with the same vaccines given to mature females before breeding.

Precalving vaccinations are intended to protect the newborn calf through colostral transfer. The most common immunizations are those that offer protection against some of the infectious causes of diarrhea in neonatal calves. Others are based on local patterns of disease. Many of these vaccines have variable results when used in field conditions and should not be used in substitution of excellent management practices.

Preweaning is an important intervention that can help prepare calves for the stress of weaning and reduce the possibility that such stress will compromise the efficacy of biologicals. Common vaccinations include those against the clostridials and bovine respiratory disease complex (BRD). A broad-spectrum anthelmintic should also be given at this time, because calves that have been on pasture have almost certainly been exposed to internal parasites. At weaning, a second vaccination should be given for those products recommending two injections. Modified-live virus (MLV) products should be given at this stage. Another clostridial vaccination is not indicated if calves were previously vaccinated at working and preweaning. For areas where brucellosis is under regulatory control, heifers should be vaccinated appropriately within the age ranges stipulated.

Bulls should receive the same vaccines as the cow-calf herd, with some exceptions. Bulls should not be vaccinated for brucellosis. Also, the trichomoniasis vaccine currently approved for use in the USA is not approved for bulls. Caution is advised with MLV infectious bovine rhinotracheitis vaccines, because this virus may recrudesce in bulls and be shed in semen; the manufacturer's technical services veterinarian should always be asked if this is a concern. Also, if MLV infectious bovine rhinotracheitis vaccine is used, semen shipment to other countries may be jeopardized.

CALF MANAGEMENT

Management of the calving season is critical to optimize the weaned calf crop. Research indicates that 57% of mortality is seen in the first 24 hr and 75% within 7 days of birth. In addition, there are significant risk factors for increased calf morbidity at the time of calving that can lead to increased mortality and decreased calf performance. Factors to consider in calving management include dystocia management (of primary concern in first-calf heifers), calving environment (including ambient temperature), passive transfer, and cow-calf pair management. (*See* MANAGEMENT OF REPRODUCTION: CATTLE, p 2171.) A visit to the farm or ranch ~4 wk before the onset of the calving season provides the opportunity to evaluate the preparations made by the producer and to recommend any changes.

Keeping records on calving ease and morbidity and mortality incidence allows for analysis of risks and risk groups and detection of any increased incidence of disease. At least one additional visit should be made to the farm 2–3 wk after calving has begun to assess the management and environment. Morbidity and mortality incidence levels may be established; if these are exceeded, the herd health veterinarian should be called and an investigation begun.

The most common cause of calf morbidity in the neonatal period is diarrhea (*see* p 275). It is sometimes not possible and many times not important to differentiate diarrheas associated with different etiologic agents, especially when diarrhea occurs in the 7- to 14-day range. Control for pathogenic agents of neonatal diarrhea involves segregation of sick animals from the healthy nursery to decrease environmental contamination and transmission. In addition, *Escherichia coli* and *Salmonella* control involves biosecurity rules to prevent the purchase and introduction of new calves or cows during the calving season. Sick calves should be isolated quickly to prevent further environmental contamination. Once the environment is contaminated, moist, cool conditions allow survival of infectious agents for an extended period. Cryptosporidia are especially suited to survival in the environment, and prevention of contamination in the healthy nursery is critical. Commercial vaccines for rotavirus, coronavirus, *E coli*, and *Clostridium perfringens* types B and C may be given to cows and heifers before calving to increase levels of specific immunoglobulins in colostrum. An initial vaccination and booster followed by a yearly booster is generally required. If a booster vaccination is needed, it should be given at least 2 wk and not more than 6 wk before calving. Clinical trial data are not consistent; some trials report no effect, whereas others report significant decreases in morbidity. Vaccination may be a useful adjunct to proper management in controlling neonatal diarrhea, but the key is environmental control.

An excellent environmental control program is the "Sandhills calving system" developed at the University of Nebraska. In this system, pregnant cows are wintered in an area separate from the calving area. When the first cow calves or is about to calve, the entire herd is moved to the first calving pasture. Cows stay here for 2 wk; after this time, all cows with calves stay on pasture 1 while all cows yet to calve move to pasture 2. After 1 wk on pasture 2, all cows with calves stay and all pregnant cows move to pasture 3. This continues for the next 6 wk. Cow-calf pairs can be combined when the youngest calf in the group is 4 wk old and at low risk of diarrhea. This system assures that each calf is born into a clean environment, so disease transmission is minimal to nonexistent. Herds that had severe morbidity and mortality from scours before using the system may have almost no health concerns after its adoption.

In this and in all calving systems, heifers should be wintered and calved separately from adult cows, because heifers have lower immunity to pathogens than cows.

Castration and Dehorning: Castration of male calves in early life (before 3 mo of age) is less stressful to calves than castration performed later, when testicular size is dramatically increased. A number of methods may be used, including the open surgical technique, the use of rubber rings, and the Burdizzo method. Calves castrated surgically initially exhibit more agitation than calves castrated with rubber rings, but both groups resume normal behavior soon after the operation. Dehorning early in life is also less stressful than when performed later, when horns have increased in size. Horns are mostly a problem for the feeding period (ie, horned calves require more bunk space), and they may cause bruising in penmates. Such problems are best managed by polled breeding or early dehorning.

Identification: Individual identification of cows and calves allows for selection based on performance as well as for tracing the animal to its herd of origin to track or contain disease. Plastic ear tags are the most commonly used method of individual identification. Branding as a method of herd identification is coming under increasing scrutiny for product quality and animal welfare reasons. Commercial products are currently on the market that allow individual electronic identification. Such initiatives may eventually replace current identification systems.

Vaccinations: Vaccines are available for viral and bacterial respiratory pathogens. Residual passive immunity in young calves may limit the detectable antibody response to vaccination at an early age, but use of MLV infectious bovine rhinotracheitis and bovine viral diarrhea vaccines stimulates a significant cell-mediated immune response in calves with residual passive immunity to these diseases. Specific age recommendations for initial vaccination are made by vaccine manufacturers. Calves vaccinated at branding time or pasture turn-out may be sensitized to the antigens and respond with an anamnestic response when given another vaccine at arrival in the feedlot. Recommended vaccination programs include clostridial and viral respiratory vaccination at the time of branding. A number of "value-added" calf programs have been initiated, some of which require a vaccination program at branding time. Pneumonia incidence is typically low during the summer grazing periods, making clinical effectiveness of a vaccination program against respiratory disease difficult to demonstrate. Primary sensitization to increase subsequent vaccination response before weaning may be the major benefit of such a vaccination program. A repeat vaccination against viral respiratory agents is often administered to calves before weaning. Vaccination for *Mannheimia* has been recommended for inclusion in some preweaning or weaning vaccination programs as well.

Infectious keratoconjunctivitis (*see* p 512) can be a significant problem in suckling calves, and control can be difficult. Vaccination has shown variable results. Challenge with a homologous strain after vaccination may provide some level of control, but challenge with a heterologous strain creates little protection.

Implant Strategies: Use of hormonal implants as a management practice for suckling calves may increase weaning weights by 3%–5%. Optimal response is seen in healthy calves with adequate nutrition. Heifers kept for breeding should not be implanted if <45 days old, and bulls should never be implanted. (*See* p 2758.)

Parasite Control: Egg burdens of calves are typically low at spring branding but may rise significantly by midsummer. Deworming of cows in late spring may lead to increased weaning weights in calves. Studies examining the effects of deworming calves only at branding have been few, and results were inconsistent—some showed positive effects, whereas others found no effect. Deworming of calves in addition to cows in late spring appears to confer minimal additional benefit. External parasites of cattle are estimated to be an important cause of economic loss as well. Studies have generally shown a weight gain of 10–20 lb in suckling calves when fly control is provided. The most common method of fly control is the use of insecticide-impregnated ear tags. With the widespread use of pyrethroid insecticides in ear tags, emerging resistance has become a problem, so rotating to organophosphate or endosulfan tags can be helpful. Insecticide sprays and back rubbers can also be effective (and less expensive), but cattle must be forced to use them.

Nutrition: Suckling beef calves are generally not supplemented during the summer grazing period, when milk and an increasing intake of forage provide their diet. Deficiency of trace minerals may be a concern in some areas. Proper nutrition of the herd before calving should provide the calf with adequate reserves at birth. Subsequent supplementation is difficult, however, because trace mineral mix intake in calves is sporadic at best. Creep feeding may increase the reliability of intake, but it is an expensive substitute for available forage, and the response is highly variable. Creep feeding for 3–4 wk before weaning may be an effective way to reduce stress and disease at weaning. (*See also* NUTRITIONAL REQUIREMENTS OF BEEF CATTLE, p 2248.)

Weaning: Weaning is stressful because the calf is removed from its dam and has to adjust to a different diet and environment; population density is increased, leading to potential for increased disease exposure and transmission. Management procedures should aim to minimize stress to calves while ensuring they are in sound condition nutritionally and immunologically. Castration and dehorning should be performed well before weaning. Completion of vaccination, deworming, and implant procedures before weaning allows calves to be weaned without handling.

Early weaning of beef calves at 90–150 days of age may create more efficient use of feed resources by directly supplementing calves to maintain weight gain rather than supplementing cows to produce milk. Weaning times as early as 30–60 days can increase reproductive performance of cows and heifers. Cows and heifers cycle and rebreed earlier in the calving season, and pregnancy rates are higher in a limited breeding season after early weaning. Nutritional needs of the weaned calves must be met carefully to ensure acceptable health and performance. Weaning this early should be done only in an emergency situation to salvage the reproductive future of cows in extremely thin (BCS <4) condition at calving. The goal is to prevent this situation through strategies that improve precalving BCS (*see* p 2120). Weaning at 150–170 days of age decreases lactational stress on cows when forage resources are limited and improves cow condition. Reproductive performance in the breeding season is not affected by weaning at this time. When forage resources are limited, weaning calves to decrease the nutritional requirements of the cows allows them to regain condition before winter with less or no supplementation. It is more efficient to wean the calves and feed them directly than to feed the cows more to increase milk production late in lactation.

REPLACEMENT HEIFERS

Replacement heifer development programs generally begin at weaning as the heifers begin preparation for their initial breeding season. However, decisions relating to use of hormonal growth-promoting implant programs (*see* p 2758) for replacements must be made beginning at the working of calves at 2–3 mo of age. Reimplanting heifers intended for breeding at weaning, or after 6 mo of age, is not recommended. Heifers that calve at 22–24 mo of age have increased lifetime production compared with heifers that calve first at 30–36 mo of age.

Heifer Selection: Selection of replacement heifer prospects begins at weaning, when heifers are typically 6–8 mo old, and is based on birth date, genetics, frame score, disposition, weaning weight and ratio, and dam production records. Selection of heifers born early in the calving season leads to replacement heifers that are older and heavier at the start of the breeding season. Heifers should be evaluated for structural soundness, and unacceptable conformation should disqualify a heifer as a replacement prospect. Age-adjusted frame scores can be used to estimate the mature size of prospects. These scores provide an objective method of selecting replacements to maintain a consistent cow size suitable for the environment and feed resources.

Once potential replacement heifers are selected, a nutrition and vaccination program should be instituted in preparation for breeding. If heifers are to calve at 22–23 mo of age, they must be bred at 13–14 mo of age. For optimal fertility, heifers should weigh ~53%–65% of their mature body weight by this time. The ration must be balanced to provide the required rate of gain to meet the target goal of 53%–65% of mature body weight in the time available. Specific requirements vary with the weight and breed of the heifers and the amount of time available before breeding. (*See also* NUTRITION: CATTLE, p 2248.)

Considerable research on the most cost-effective target weight for breeding heifers has shown that it is almost always below the previous recommendation of 65% of mature body weight. Instead of a goal of the maximum number of heifers conceiving, a better goal may be to have a slightly lower percentage of heifers bred at a cost that is significantly lower than developing heifers to breed at 65% of mature body weight.

Vaccination: The vaccination program for replacement heifers should provide optimal protection from reproductive diseases and should include vaccination for infectious bovine rhinotracheitis (IBR) and bovine viral diarrhea (BVD) types 1 and 2. Depending on the local disease risk, vaccinations for *Brucella*, *Leptospira*, *Trichomonas*, and *Campylobacter* may also be indicated. *Brucella* vaccination is performed according to state or regional regulations. Modified-live vaccines for IBR and BVD give the broadest immunity to strain differences and should be given twice to ensure a high level of immunity. Some evidence suggests that modified-live BVD and IBR vaccines may transiently infect the ovary and cause decreased fertility. For this reason, vaccination should be done ≥1 mo before breeding. Vaccination of heifers with *Trichomonas* vaccine increases calving rate and decreases duration of infection in infected herds but does not prevent infection. A vaccine for trichomoniasis may be useful in infected herds or in herds at high risk of infection, but it may not be economic in low-risk herds.

Management: Heifers should be adequately developed at the time of first breeding, and their management during gestation must ensure their continued growth. Pregnant heifers should be separated from the main cow herd at the time of pregnancy testing and maintained separately until reentry into the breeding herd as animals move to pasture. Undernutrition during pregnancy in first-calf heifers can lead to an increased incidence of dystocia because of lack of weight and size, weakness at the time of parturition, insufficient colostrum, weak calves at birth, and a high incidence of prolonged postpartum anestrus, which leads to a high percentage of nonpregnant animals that will need to be culled. Thus, pregnant heifers should be fed and managed separately from cows and should be on a higher plane of nutrition than cows. Such management may slightly increase calf birth weight but will not increase dystocia scores if heifers calve in BCS 6–7. Heifers are ideally bred 2–3 wk before cows, and they should always be bred for a shorter period of time (~42 days) to ensure that those with the highest inherent fertility are retained in the herd. This also ensures that any increase in the postpartum anestrus period after their first, perhaps difficult, calving does not compromise their chances for cycling and rebreeding with the main cow herd.

GENERAL HEALTH MANAGEMENT CONSIDERATIONS

The greatest risk for initial introduction of many infectious diseases into a herd is the addition of subclinically infected animals, although some risk is also attributable to wildlife carriers. Potential sources of infection may be seen with herd additions, or through intentional or inadvertent movements and contacts. Herds may be classified as "closed" or "open," based on their potential for pathogen exposure. (*See also* BIOSECURITY, p 2068.) Closed herds restrict the introduction of animals and vehicles from livestock sources as well as contact with other herds and animals. Open herds have a higher risk of introducing pathogens through such practices as introduction of purchased replacements (especially from commingled sale groups), purchase of bulls, direct introduction of high-risk stocker calves (especially into high population densities), and mingling of animals of different backgrounds, through either cooperative breeding programs or poor herd biosecurity.

In general, all purchased or introduced animals should be separated from the home herd for a reasonable observation period (eg, 4 wk); these animals should undergo the same health procedures as the home herd. It is prudent to obtain animals from herds in which the herd health history is known and to have a record of vaccinations and treatments. Before purchasing animals, buyers should be sure that herds have tested negative for paratuberculosis and are free of persistently infected BVD, tuberculosis, and brucellosis. If the herd is free of diseases such as bovine leukosis and anaplasmosis, purchasing only animals from other herds negative for these diseases is vitally important. Pubertal bulls should be tested for trichomoniasis and vibriosis when indicated. For artificial insemination (AI) programs, semen should be used only if it was processed by an approved AI center with a comprehensive health program for minimizing the risk of transmission of venereal (and other) diseases through frozen semen.

BEEF FEEDLOTS

In beef feedlots, young growing cattle are fed a high-energy diet to produce marketable beef at a low cost of gain. Depending on the starting body weight and age of the cattle, the period of feeding varies from 60 days to 12 mo. The success of a modern feedlot depends on excellent management, a favorable economic climate, and relative freedom from unfortunate events such as disease epidemics or unexpected increases in costs (eg, feed) or decreases in the price received for the final product. The concept of disease should include all of the identifiable factors that cause suboptimal performance: inadequacies in feeds and feeding systems, the purchase of undesirable types of cattle, and clinical and subclinical disease.

The feedlot veterinarian is responsible for maintaining optimal animal health through the following activities: 1) Making regularly scheduled visits to the feedlot. The frequency of visits depends on the size of the feedlot, the time of year, the expertise of the feedlot personnel, whether animals have recently arrived, and the degree to which the veterinarian is contractually responsible for the total animal health program. 2) Being available for emergency visits to the feedlot when disease epidemics are seen. 3) Performing necropsies during visits and training feedlot personnel to do necropsies at other times. 4) Examining sick animals to ensure that reasonably accurate diagnoses are being made and rational therapy is being given according to established treatment protocol. 5) Regularly examining, analyzing, and interpreting animal health and production data and making recommendations in a written report. The effectiveness of detection of sick animals, based on response and relapse rates and case fatality rates, should be determined, and the effectiveness of the processing program for new arrivals, which includes the vaccines used and the medications given, should be examined and analyzed regularly. 6) Selecting and prescribing all drugs used in the feedlot, giving specific advice about the use of drugs, and establishing a drug residue-avoidance program. 7) Discussing overall animal health and production performance with the feedlot manager and other consultants, setting animal health and production goals, and monitoring achievement. 8) Comparing the feedlot with other operations. The veterinarian should produce a monthly report that compares processing costs, treatment costs, and death loss by arrival weight and days on feed.

When the consulting veterinarian is not readily available, a local practitioner can serve as a valuable resource for the feedlot. Serving as part of the feedlot's health care team, the local veterinarian can make significant contributions to the animal health program.

ECONOMIC IMPACT OF DISEASE

Disease may cause economic loss in feedlots through mortality, treatment cost, or effects on productivity. The impact of clinical and subclinical disease on production efficiency and economic returns may be greater than the losses associated with mortality. A thorough understanding of the impact of disease on animal performance and economic loss is essential to make cost-effective recommendations to feedlot managers. The costs associated with death loss, chronically ill cattle marketed prematurely at a discount, and treatment are obvious and easy to calculate. Hidden costs, such as reduced performance and lower carcass quality, are often overlooked.

Treatment costs are another source of economic loss. Factors influencing the average cost include the morbidity rate, retreatment rate, cost of the drug(s), combination versus single antimicrobial therapy, whether adjunct therapy is used, labor, and feedlot markup on the products used. The morbidity rate has the strongest influence on the average treatment cost for all cattle in the pen. When metaphylaxis is used to manage bovine respiratory tract disease, it must be added to the total medical cost for the pen.

IMPLEMENTING A FEEDLOT MEDICINE PROGRAM

Regular Inspection: Regular inspection of all areas of the feedlot should be included in a feedlot health service. Credit for keen observation and a job well done along with recommendations for improvement in animal husbandry should be noted and recorded for discussion with personnel. Attention should be given particularly to the delivery of feed and water, the general well-being of cattle, and any unusual characteristics of each feeding pen. Many feedlot health problems can be prevented with excellent management.

Disease Surveillance: Continued disease surveillance through regular necropsy examination of all dead cattle and regular observations of sick cattle are necessary. In colder climates, carcasses may freeze solid before the veterinarian is available. Conversely, in warmer climates, carcasses may decompose beyond usefulness. When distance prevents the consulting veterinarian from performing a necropsy on every animal that dies, a more accessible veterinarian may be employed. In many cases, feedlot personnel can be trained to recognize common postmortem lesions, take digital photographs of such lesions and send them to the consulting veterinarian, and collect tissues for potential analysis.

A key to management of disease in feedlots is a fast and accurate diagnosis. This requires a good surveillance system, a systematic plan to search for sick animals, appropriate facilities for examination and treatment, accurate identification of animals, and appropriate laboratory facilities, especially a necropsy service. Emphasis is placed on training and supervising feedlot employees in the detection and early treatment of sick cattle. Employees, particularly any personnel responsible for checking the cattle pens for sick cattle, should be given regular instruction in the clinical signs of common diseases. These include anorexia, depression, lameness or abnormal gait, stiff movement, coughing, nasal and ocular discharge, increased breathing rate, crusted muzzle, sunken eyes, rough hair coat, loose or very firm feces, abnormal abdominal fill, and straining. Cattle with these or other signs of illness are examined more closely in the hospital area and, if necessary, treated. In some feedlots, treated cattle are immediately returned to their original pens, whereas in others cattle are kept in hospital pens until they recover. Most animals that do not recover or that relapse after the first treatment are re-treated, although this decision depends on the nature of the disease and the economics involved. If an animal becomes chronically ill and chances of recovery are slim, it should be sold for slaughter if this is a viable option (after the appropriate withdrawal time) or, in the case of a calf, euthanized.

Pens from which sick animals are taken should be closely observed. A potential epidemic must be identified early so that pen-level intervention can be considered.

Despite its importance, pen surveillance is not highly reliable for the detection of sick feedlot animals, particularly calves in the first week after arrival. It is difficult to distinguish tired, gaunt calves that may have been weaned a few days earlier from calves in the early stage of acute, undifferentiated respiratory disease. As many as 50% of animals pulled from a pen of recently arrived calves will not show clinical signs of respiratory disease based on measurement of body temperature and a cursory clinical examination.

Treatment Protocols: The veterinarian must specify procedures for the clinical management of sick cattle and provide a standard protocol that outlines specific treatments for disease syndromes, including drug dosages, treatment intervals, routes of administration, and withdrawal times. The protocol should be followed strictly by all personnel so that the success or failure of therapy can be evaluated accurately and that chances of creating food safety hazards are zero. The effectiveness of the treatment protocol should be evaluated regularly by determination of the response rates for the various treatment regimens. Failure to develop and implement appropriate treatment protocols often leads to the use of many different drugs indiscriminately, which then leads to excessive treatment costs and often an increase in the case fatality rate.

FEEDLOT RECORDS

Records are essential to monitor the incidence of disease, response to treatment, and production performance, and they should be analyzed regularly by the veterinarian, nutritionist, and feedlot manager. They can be maintained by hand or by using commercially available computer software. The necessary input records include the lot description, processing record, lot update, sale information, animal identification, and feed and animal health product purchases. The necessary output records include the numbers of animals pulled from each pen daily, from which an epidemic curve can be drawn; the treatment response report according to pen or drug used; the percentage of pulled animals that had a fever, which is an indication of how many are probably affected with an acute respiratory disease rather than a noninfectious disease such as grain overload; the daily mortality report, which should include the list of animals that died, along with their arrival dates, the dates of treatment, and the causes of death; a case abstract of the treatment history of each individual animal; and a close-out summary, which includes all production costs, the health and production performance of the lot or pen of cattle (including morbidity, mortality, ratio of feed conversion to body weight gain, average daily gain), the costs of gain per unit of gain, the number of days on feed, and the profit or loss.

Individual Treatment Record: Each animal treated should be individually identified, if this was not done on entry, and the information recorded on the treatment report. Treatment personnel should record the feeding pen, lot number, body temperature, body weight, disease suspected, treatment given, and location of the animal after treatment (eg, which hospital pen). The severity of the illness should be assessed to properly evaluate response to treatment. Late treatment in advanced stages of disease, particularly respiratory disease, is a major cause of failure to respond, even when the treatment of choice is instituted.

A report is filled out for each animal treated, and all subsequent treatments are recorded. The updated reports are retrieved for animals that relapse or die. The cumulative information on the report can be used to decide whether an animal should be culled for chronic or recurring illnesses that are refractory to treatment, to decide on alternative treatments, to explain reasons for death, and to evaluate the effectiveness of the treatments recommended. Some feedlots record animals that are removed from the pen but sent back untreated because they did not meet the temperature criterion in the case definition for a given disease. This information can be of value if the animal is removed again or dies.

Daily Morbidity and Mortality Record: This record contains the number of treated cattle by pen and lot number, the disease diagnosed, and the date. It provides both the manager and the veterinarian with a rapid assessment of the location of disease problems in the feedlot. It contains information on the number of animals removed and the number not treated and then classifies those treated according to diagnosis and whether they are a relapse or new case. By using this report in conjunction with an inventory report showing filling dates and numbers added to the pen on those dates, it is possible to generate epidemic curves.

Morbidity and Treatment Analysis Record: This aggregation of data summarizes the morbidity rate, the relapse rate, and the death rate for a lot or pen of cattle. It is especially important as a tool to evaluate the overall effectiveness of the treatment program for various diseases; the relapse rates and death rates are compared with goals set for the feedlot and with standards published in the literature. The disposition summary alerts the feedlot manager and consulting veterinarian when the results are highly positive, so this feedback can be relayed to all employees to acknowledge their hard work, and when the chronic or culling rates are abnormally high, so that appropriate changes can be made.

Mortality Analysis: The causes of death as determined by necropsy should be summarized on a regular basis. A mortality analysis includes the number of days the animal was in the feedlot, any observed premonitory signs, and treatment (diagnosis, drug used, and when treated). The pen location of the animal in the feedlot at the time of death should also be considered.

Feedlot Performance Summary: Most feedlots complete a close-out summary for each group of cattle that have been finished and marketed. The performance record and feeding summary sections include average daily gain, total feed consumption, feed conversion ratios and cost per unit of body weight gain, mortality rates, culling rate, and medical costs. The financial summary provides the profit or loss on an individual and lot basis. If cattle are marketed on a grid basis with rewards for certain carcass characteristics, this information is also included.

VACCINATION PROTOCOLS

An important component of feedlot health programs is the planning of vaccination programs. Vaccination schedules vary depending on the prevalence of disease both in the feedlot area and in the area from which the cattle originated. The vaccines used and the vaccination schedule should be based on the expected incidence of the disease, the cost of the disease when it is seen, the cost of the preventive procedure (vaccine plus labor), the field efficacy of the vaccine, and other available control procedures.

NUTRITIONAL ADVICE

Feedlots frequently consult a qualified nutritionist to assist in the formulation of cost-effective diets. The veterinarian should communicate with the nutritionist regarding the composition of the diets and any changes being planned. Most of the emphasis in feedlot nutrition has been on the development of cost-effective diets that support an optimal growth rate without any deleterious effects. Considerable information is available on the nutrient requirements for feedlot cattle and on the feeds and feeding systems used. (*See also* NUTRITION: BEEF CATTLE, p 2248.)

Nutritional deficiency diseases are uncommon in feedlot cattle, because cattle usually receive a diet that contains the nutrients required for maintenance and promotion of rapid growth. Diets prepared according to published standards should meet all the requirements under most conditions. Specific nutrient deficiencies are extremely rare; however, such a situation may be seen in a small farm feedlot that prepares its own diet with little or no attention to the necessity for supplementation of homegrown feeds. Although only a few nutritional diseases may affect a well-managed feedlot, these diseases may cause large economic losses when they develop. They include carbohydrate engorgement (grain overload or D-lactic acidosis), feedlot bloat or ruminal tympany, and feeding errors (ie, accidental incorporation of an excessive amount of a feed additive, such as monensin or urea, or sudden unintended changes in the ingredient composition of the diet).

DISEASE EPIDEMICS

In spite of good management, unexpected disease epidemics are seen in feedlot cattle. When feeding accidents occur, many animals can be affected suddenly, ie, within 1–2 days. In outbreaks of acute infectious diseases, such as infectious bovine rhinotracheitis, pneumonic pasteurellosis, or *Histophilus* meningoencephalitis, the first few cases are followed by a steady increase in the morbidity rate for several days and then a decline as the outbreak subsides 10–14 days after the index case.

In some cases, the diagnosis may be obvious (eg, carbohydrate engorgement caused by a feeding error). In other cases (eg, infectious diseases of the respiratory tract), the diagnosis may not be readily obvious, and a detailed epidemiologic, clinical, and laboratory investigation may be required. A complete investigation may require specialists from several disciplines. Every effort should be made to determine the specific source of the disease. The investigation should include a general description of the problem, a complete history of the disease outbreak (including details and date of index case, total number of sick animals, treatments, case fatality rate, population mortality rate, and vaccination history), and clinical examination of several affected animals (with appropriate samples) as well as necropsies. After the diagnosis is determined, the rationale for treatment is outlined. When outbreaks of infectious disease are encountered, the intensity of surveillance must be increased to detect new cases in the early stages of disease when response to treatment is usually good.

All of the details of the outbreak should be listed in chronologic order and then analyzed. Correlations can be made between exposure factors and the development of new cases during the course of the outbreak. Often, epidemiologic determinants that explain disease occurrence can be identified and the information used to control future episodes. A detailed report of the outbreak, outlining the conclusion and recommendations, should be prepared by the veterinarian and nutritionist and submitted to the owner.

CONTROL AND PREVENTION OF DISEASE IN FEEDLOT CATTLE

Control and prevention of disease in feedlot cattle depends on purchasing healthy animals; providing a transportation system that minimizes stress, a comfortable feedlot pen environment, and an adequate feeding system; establishing a good surveillance system; and judiciously using vaccines and, when necessary, antimicrobial agents.

Feedlot Facilities

One of the most important considerations in the construction of a feedlot is good drainage. The pens and alleyways should be well drained and easily accessible for scraping the ground surface as necessary. Good drainage requires a 6% slope. To avoid overstocking, each animal should be provided with 18 m^2 of space in well-drained land and with 9 m^2 in a paved lot.

Cattle need protection from wind, rain, snow, excessive heat, and excessive sunshine. Trees are planted as windbreaks, and buildings and fences are placed so the wind is not deflected into feeding areas or sheds. An open-front shed provides protection from winter storms and hot summer sun. Each animal needs ~1–1.5 m^2 of cover. The shed should be open to the south or southeast, and the front should be high enough so the sun strikes the ground at the back on the shortest day of the winter. The back of the shed should be ≥2.5 m high. A covered feed bunk protects feed from weather damage and affords cattle added comfort when eating. Feed remains dry and palatable, and waste is reduced. Shades to provide relief from extreme summer heat are useful in feedlots where this is a major concern during the year.

Environmental concerns about feedlot operations have greatly increased in recent years. Stricter environmental laws require that all feedlot waste and run-off be contained in approved lagoon systems. Pollution prevention plans must be on file with the appropriate government agency. Monitoring, testing, and record-keeping requirements vary from country to country as well as regionally. In addition, foodborne illnesses, particularly those caused by *Escherichia coli* O157:H7 and *Salmonella*, have forced the meat-packing industry to change the way beef carcasses are processed. The packing industry has placed pressure on feedlots to provide animals that are as clean as possible.

Transportation of Cattle

Transportation or shipping of cattle has long been associated with increased bovine respiratory disease (BRD) in the feedlot, hence the term "shipping fever." With current improvements in transportation, however, there is no correlation between the distance cattle are shipped and the risk of fatal fibrinous pneumonia in the feedlot. Factors such as weaning, level of immunity, commingling, and other stressors appear more important in the risk of BRD than distance shipped.

Cattle can lose considerable weight within the first 24–48 hr after weaning, during shipment, and after deprivation of feed and water. This loss in body weight (known as shrink) varies from a minimum of 4% in cattle deprived of feed and water for 24 hr to up to 9% in animals transported long distances over a period of 2–4 days or in unweaned, high-risk, lightweight calves. Most of the fluid and electrolyte loss can be restored within a few days if the animals begin to eat and drink normally, but some studies show as few as 35% of high-risk calves consume an appreciable amount of feed the first 24 hr in the lot. Shrink >7% has been associated with increased health problems. The total loss in body weight may not be restored for as long as 3 wk in some highly stressed calves.

Transportation equipment and facilities should meet local standards and be able to transport cattle comfortably regardless of the season of the year. Some countries prohibit the transport of cattle over a certain length of time without unloading for rest, feed, and water. On arrival at their destination, cattle should be examined carefully for evidence of clinical disease or injury. Provision of fresh hay, a small amount of starter feed, and water can help detect those that are anorectic and require closer examination. This is particularly important if unexpected delays in transportation have occurred that increase the level of stress in the animals.

Cattle Purchase and Introduction to a Feedlot

Infectious diseases of the respiratory tract are major causes of morbidity and mortality during the first 30–45 days after arrival in the feedlot. Digestive diseases, especially carbohydrate engorgement, in cattle placed on a high-energy diet within 30 days after arrival in the feedlot are a major potential threat but can be controlled. The acute respiratory disease complex (*see* p 1431) is more difficult to control in feedlot cattle, even under good management conditions.

The major objective on arrival at the feedlot is to get the cattle onto a high-energy diet—which will result in rapid growth—as soon as possible, usually within 21 days, while minimizing the morbidity and mortality associated with acute respiratory disease, other common infections, and digestive diseases associated with adjustments to high-energy diets.

Preimmunization and Preconditioning

Preconditioning is the preparation of feeder calves for marketing, shipment, and the feedlot environment; it may include vaccinations, castration, and training calves to eat and drink in pens. The concept of preconditioning is based in part on immunologic and nutritional principles. Preimmunization, or vaccination of calves 2–3 wk before shipment from the ranch to the feedlot, was the basis of preconditioning. In addition to vaccination, more recent efforts have been directed toward increasing the number of days weaned before movement and improving management procedures on the ranch, such as genetic selection and nutrition, that assist calves in making an easier transition to the feedlot.

In the USA, preconditioning has been defined by the following elements: 1) weaning at least 30 days before sale, 2) training to eat from a feed bunk and to drink from a tank, 3) parasite treatment, 4) vaccination for blackleg, malignant edema, parainfluenza 3, infectious bovine rhinotracheitis, bovine viral diarrhea (some programs also call for vaccination against *Mannheimia haemolytica*, *Pasteurella multocida*, and/or *Histophilus somni*), 5) castration and dehorning with wounds healed, 6) identification with an ear tag, and 7) sale through special auctions. When preconditioned calves are placed in a feedlot, they usually begin to eat and drink on arrival; if they have not been subjected to unusual stressors, the incidence of disease is minimal. However, daily surveillance is still necessary to identify cases of illness. Because these cattle generally go onto feed more easily than calves that have not been preconditioned, care must be taken not to increase intake too quickly and cause digestive concerns.

When preconditioning is examined on a partial budget basis, the cost effectiveness for the cow-calf producer is generally quite favorable. Calves can gain 2–3 lb/day at a very low cost of gain while not getting fat. The health program "bonus" can add \$3–\$8/100 lb to the price when calves are sold at large, special preconditioned sales, but the primary financial reward to the cow-calf producer is in the form of added weight sold at a low cost of gain.

Backgrounding is a variation of preconditioning in which recently weaned calves are grown to heavier weights, usually in a smaller feedlot. The principal objective is to prepare these cattle to adjust to a high-energy finishing ration in a feedlot with minimal problems. This is achieved by feeding the calves a growth diet that yields rapid, efficient body weight gains without fattening. The spectrum of diseases seen in backgrounding operations during the first

45 days after arrival of the calves depends on whether the calves were preimmunized, preconditioned, or obtained from several different sources with no preconditioning. Infectious diseases of the respiratory tract (eg, BRD) and of the digestive tract (coccidiosis) account for most of the losses.

Recently arrived cattle of unknown backgrounds (eg, those from auction markets) require extra surveillance and care. After a 24-hr rest, these cattle should be vaccinated and some need to be castrated, dehorned, and treated for internal and external parasites. Nonpreconditioned, stressed cattle of unknown backgrounds should be watched closely for signs of BRD for ≥3 wk after arrival. On their starter ration, the cattle are limit-fed good-quality roughage along with a quantity of a highly palatable, nutrient-dense concentrate ration. They are checked carefully at least twice daily for evidence of illness, and sick cattle are identified and treated. Once the animals are determined to be healthy and the common infectious diseases are not a problem, they can be moved up to finishing diets.

Vaccination against certain respiratory diseases at 24 hr after arrival is standard practice for most feedlot and backgrounding operations. Vaccination should be limited to those products that actually reduce losses resulting from respiratory disease. The use of metaphylactic antimicrobials against respiratory disease may be necessary in high-risk, nonpreconditioned calves. Numerous studies show a financial benefit to using metaphylactic antibiotics on high-risk calves, because BRD morbidity and mortality can be greatly reduced.

Regardless of the system used, soon after arrival the cattle should be weighed, examined for evidence of illness, and treated if necessary. Some feedlots administer antimicrobials to all calves considered to be at high risk of acute respiratory disease. If the illness appears different from the usual case of respiratory disease, diagnosis by a veterinarian should be sought at the earliest possible time. Close examination and surveillance are desirable for groups of cattle with a history of unusual stress. The youngest and smallest cattle often need special attention, and it may be necessary to separate them from older cattle. A reliable history of vaccination, vitamin injections, implants, and anthelmintic administration would be useful but is usually not available. The major objective during the first few days is to avoid unnecessary stress and get most cattle consuming the starter ration.

Depending on the condition of the cattle, it may be difficult during the first few days after arrival to easily distinguish sick cattle from healthy cattle, and careful clinical surveillance every few hours may be necessary. Observations at the time of feeding often reveal anorectic animals that should be pulled from the pen and examined.

Processing Procedures

Identification: Each animal must be identified immediately, preferably with a color-coded and numbered plastic ear tag that is easily visible from a distance. In many feedlots, each animal is not identified individually but instead receives a tag with a lot number (group) or pen number. Systems are now in place that individually identify animals with tags that can be read electronically from a distance of 8–10 in. Information maintained on individual animals through this technology may include performance, vaccination, and treatment history. These tags remain on the animal until slaughter, at which time the identification from the ear tag can be transferred to the overhead trolley system.

Measurement of Body Temperature: On arrival, some animals may be affected with acute disease but show no obvious clinical signs. Others may appear fatigued and gaunt but are not affected with clinical disease. Identifying animals with acute infectious disease that should be treated early to minimize mortality can be difficult. The body temperature of high-risk cattle (eg, unweaned calves, calves from auctions, or calves transported long distances over several days) is often measured at processing. Animals with a body temperature >104°F (40°C) may be treated with an antimicrobial. Treated animals may be tagged and noted in the individual animal database, or the total number of animals treated (total amount of drug administered) in a group or pen may be recorded.

Vaccination: The value of vaccinating feedlot cattle for common infectious diseases, particularly those of the respiratory tract, has been controversial since the vaccines were introduced. Nevertheless, a wide variety of vaccines are used in feedlot health programs.

Vaccines are available for the following diseases or infections of feedlot cattle: infectious bovine rhinotracheitis, pneumonic pasteurellosis, parainfluenza 3 virus infection, bovine respiratory syncytial virus infection, *Histophilus somni* disease complex, bovine viral diarrhea types 1 and 2, and clostridial disease. The vaccines available for clostridial diseases are highly effective. The number of clostridial antigens to be used (2- to 8-way) depends on local prevalence of clostridial diseases, including blackleg (*Clostridium chauvoei*), malignant edema (*C septicum*), bacillary hemoglobinuria (*C novyi*, type D [*haemolyticum*]), infectious hepatitis (*C novyi*, type B), tetanus (*C tetani*), and enterotoxemia (*C perfringens* types B, C, and D). Leptospirosis (*Leptospira* serovars Hardjo, Pomona, Grippotyphosa, Canicola, and Icterohaemorrhagiae) bacterins are also used in some situations.

A basic vaccination schedule for receiving calves should include a viral respiratory vaccine plus a clostridial vaccine. Additional vaccines should be included only if two criteria can be met: the disease is enough of a risk that prevention is necessary (eg, leptospirosis in some areas), and data are available to support the use of vaccines to prevent disease.

Castration and Dehorning: These surgical procedures are best performed well ahead of entry to the feedlot, but invariably there will be bulls and horned cattle offered for sale. When to castrate and dehorn these mismanaged cattle is quite controversial, with studies showing that performing surgery at initial processing 24 hr after arrival was superior to delaying these procedures.

Anthelmintics and Insecticides: Anthelmintics and insecticides are administered according to local conditions. Most incoming cattle will have been exposed to internal parasites, and appropriate deworming methods should be implemented. Young cattle raised on small farms in which the stocking rate on pasture is high may harbor helminths. Young cattle may also be affected by chronic verminous pneumonia caused by *Dictyocaulus viviparus*. Most young cattle will be infected with coccidia, and having an appropriate anticoccidial agent in the feed is necessary.

Growth-promoting Agents: Growth-promoting agents (*see* p 2758) increase growth rate of animals without being used themselves to provide nutrients for growth. They are generally administered in small amounts—often via implants or in feed—to alter metabolism so the animal increases body tissues and grows more rapidly. They include antibacterials, antimicrobials, steroids (eg, estrogens, androgens), and ionophores. They promote changes in composition, conformation, mature weight, or efficiency of growth, along with changes in the rate of live weight gain.

BEEF QUALITY ASSURANCE AND BEEF SAFETY PROGRAMS

The purpose of a beef quality assurance (BQA) program is to identify and avoid areas in the feedlot where quality or safety defects can be seen. The goal of the BQA program is to assure the consumer that all cattle shipped from a feedlot are healthy, wholesome, and safe and that their management has met all government and industry standards.

The feedlot must be able to document all steps of production. Critical points in production must be monitored to ensure no residue violations or carcass defects. These critical points include, but are not limited to, incoming cattle, product and commodities, cattle handling, and evaluation of outgoing cattle. There is a built-in margin of safety for withdrawal times in the feedlot industry, because most withdrawal times for animal health products are shorter than the feeding periods. Feedlot personnel must be aware of situations that create high risk of residues. Nonperforming cattle could have organ damage, which could prevent normal clearance of a drug product, causing violative residues even after the preslaughter withdrawal time has elapsed.

The BQA program is based on the principles of the Hazard Analysis of Critical Control Points (HACCP) system. Each production step should be evaluated for potential quality or safety defects, including bacterial contamination, which can cause infectious disease in cattle or employees; chemical usage/contamination, which can lead to violative residues; and physical damage, such as injection site damage, bruising, or broken needles in animal tissues. The analysis should include sanitation standard operating procedures (eg, finding ways to prevent or minimize fecal-oral contamination).

All relevant government regulations on feedstuffs, feed additives, and medications (including route of administration and withdrawal times) must be closely followed. Extra-label drug use must be prescribed only by the herd health veterinarian. All owners of cattle treated with medications administered extra-label must comply with prescribed, extended withdrawal times that have been set by the herd health veterinarian under the guidelines of a valid veterinarian-client-patient relationship. The Food Animal Residue Avoidance Databank is the primary resource to determine the preslaughter withdrawal time when an animal has been treated in an extra-label manner.

Record Keeping: All records should be kept for ≥2 yr after cattle have been shipped from the feedlot. If a violative residue is found in any cattle shipped for slaughter, the feedlot must make applicable records available to the appropriate government agencies. The source and cause of violative residue should be determined and corrective action taken to prevent reoccurrence.

Individual Records: Treatment records should be maintained for all cattle treated individually. This can be done using handwritten records or a computerized record system. Essential information includes the individual animal identification, treatment date(s), diagnosis, drug administered, serial/lot number, dosage used, approximate weight of animal, route and location of administration, and earliest date the animal could clear the preslaughter withdrawal period. The treatment history of cattle with chronic medical problems, or of those that have a poor, unexplained growth rate, should be scrutinized carefully. In many cases, residue screening, such as the live animal swab test, is advisable. Residue screening should be performed under the supervision of the herd health veterinarian. The results of such testing determine whether an animal can be released for shipment.

Group Records: All animals treated as part of a group (processing or mass medication) should be identified by group or lot, and the treatment information should be recorded. Records should include the animal lot or group identification, product used, serial/lot number of the product, date treated, dosage used, route and location of administration, and withdrawal information. A preslaughter withdrawal time is assigned to the entire pen. Recording treatments under this system assumes that every animal in the lot or group received the treatment. The health records of cattle shipped to slaughter should be checked by feedlot personnel to ensure that treated animals have cleared the appropriate withdrawal times. All pesticides should be used in accordance with label directions, and their use and withdrawal time should be recorded.

Treatment Protocol Book: The herd health veterinarian should provide a treatment protocol book specific to the feedlot operation. It should be reviewed regularly and updated at least every 90 days. One copy should be kept at the treatment facility and another copy should be maintained in the feedlot office. A written treatment protocol and current prescriptions are important documents the feedlot must have if there is a government inspection of the feedlot facilities, drug usage procedures, and residue avoidance plans. It also provides written guidelines for animal health programs, thus minimizing chances of mistakes or misunderstandings.

Culling of Feedlot Cattle

Culling may be done at any point between examination of the cattle on arrival and a few weeks later, before the cattle are placed on a high-energy diet. Diseases that justify culling include chronic unthriftiness and inappetence of undetermined etiology, chronic laminitis, chronic lameness caused by footrot, chronic bloat, chronic pneumonia, acute and chronic pulmonary abscess, and bovine viral diarrhea. Each of these diseases leads to unthriftiness, and a clinical examination is necessary for diagnosis.

Animal Welfare in Feedlots

Good feedlot design is important to ensure animal comfort. Handling facilities must be modern and efficient and must not induce animal attendants to be cruel to animals when they are being moved from one location to another; excessive force should not be used to get the animals to move. The feedlot personnel must be educated in the techniques of low-stress cattle handling and recognition of signs of pain and discomfort associated with certain illnesses.

The veterinarian should emphasize good feedlot design and equipment that will ensure comfort for the animals and minimize pain and stress associated with handling procedures. The veterinarian must also be a vigilant guardian, denouncing inhumane practices and encouraging sound animal welfare management. (*See also* ANIMAL WELFARE, p 1579.)

DEVELOPMENT OF ANTIMICROBIAL-RESISTANT BACTERIA IN FEEDLOT CATTLE

The use of antimicrobials in feedlot cattle, as in all food animal species, has come under increased scrutiny because of concerns about the potential transfer of resistant zoonotic pathogens to people and also transfer of resistant genetic determinants to human pathogens. A pathogen of concern related to resistance in cattle is *Salmonella* spp. Transfer of *Escherichia coli* O157:H7 through the food chain, while a valid zoonotic disease concern, is not related to an issue of resistance. The American Association of Bovine Practitioners publishes *Prudent Drug Usage Guidelines*, which provides guidelines for antimicrobial usage in cattle feedlot operations.

HEALTH-MANAGEMENT INTERACTION: DAIRY CATTLE

The dairy industry is in a period of economic volatility of historic proportions. An era of modest fluctuation in milk and feed pricing in the late 1990s to the early 2000s was followed by increases in milk prices not seen before. The period of high dairy profitability in early 2008 was soon dampened because of substantial increases in production costs as a result of high fuel and feed costs as the USA government encouraged crop farmers to produce corn for ethanol distillation. Since then, milk prices have rebounded and dropped several times, although not to the same extent. USA dairy product exports have also fluctuated widely, contributing significantly to milk price volatility and overall profitability. As of early 2014, some 15% of USA dairy products are exported, milk prices are at an all-time high, and feed prices are somewhat lower.

THE MODERN DAIRY INDUSTRY

The structure of the dairy industry in developed countries has continued to evolve as production efficiency has risen. Industry consolidation is the norm, with reduced herd numbers, increased herd sizes, and adoption of specialized management practices that encourage higher productivity.

In the past, most dairy cows were housed in stall-barn facilities designed to maximize operator comfort. Today, free-stall facilities are built to maximize natural ventilation and cow comfort. Historically, barns were often placed in sheltered locations, whereas today they are usually located in open fields or on hilltops to ensure adequate airflow. The type of milking facility is also evolving; whereas in 2007, 49.2% of operations reported using tie-stall or stanchion milking facilities, almost 75% of cows are now milked in parlors, reflecting the fact that most large herds are housed in free-stall or open facilities (and milked in parlors). Most parlors are highly mechanized and designed to minimize the amount of labor required, and economics dictate that milking proceed nearly around the clock to maximize the return on investment.

Milk quality is traditionally defined by the somatic cell count (SCC) and bacterial count in prepasteurized bulk tank milk. In all developed nations, regulatory officials set allowable maximums for SCC. Since 1986, limits for SCC and bacteria have been gradually lowered. The current upper limit for the bulk tank SCC is 750,000 in the USA and 500,000 cells/mL in Canada. The SCC maximum in the EU is 400,000 cells/mL using geometric means as the basis for calculation.

Artificial insemination (through the commercial distribution of frozen semen) is the preferred method of reproductive management in most dairy operations. In fact, 45% of USA dairy operators in 1996 reported that no breeding bulls were present on their farms. The use of genetically elite sires has contributed to increases of >150 kg/yr in genetic merit for milk production. Declining fertility has accompanied advancements in genetic merit. Dairy farms commonly record herd conception rates of <40%. Technologies such as embryo transfer, rapid hormonal assays, controlled breeding programs that use reproductive hormones, and ultrasonography are used increasingly on modern dairy farms.

Nutritional research also has advanced rapidly, especially in areas such as rumen physiology and lipid metabolism (*see* NUTRITION: DAIRY CATTLE, p 2265). Lactating dairy cows are generally fed either a component-based ration (forages and grain are fed separately) or a total mixed ration (TMR, forages and grain are mixed and fed together). The basis of a successful nutritional program is the determination of nutrient content of the ration ingredients through laboratory testing, formulation of nutritionally sound diets, and assurance of adequate intake of required nutrients through feed bunk management. Maintaining a stable, healthy rumen environment is difficult with component-based feeding systems. TMR diets are generally based on mixing stored forages (in North America, usually alfalfa hay or haylage and corn silage) with grains (such as high-moisture corn or soybeans) and byproducts such as cottonseed or locally available commodities such as citrus pulp, brewers grains, or bakery waste. On larger farms, cows are often grouped and fed diets specifically formulated to meet their production and metabolic needs. Many farms use professional nutritionists to formulate rations.

Most producers raise their own replacement animals, but an increasing number of large dairy farms contract with specialized heifer growing operations. In the USA, >60% of newborn heifer calves are hand-fed colostrum within the first 24 hr of life to ensure adequate intake of immunoglobulins. The feeding of waste milk from cows undergoing antibiotic treatment or with mastitis is economical but may transmit infectious diseases to the calf. To decrease the potential for disease transmission, some producers pasteurize waste milk (15% of all calves in 2007) or feed milk replacer (>70% of calves in 2007). The amount of milk fed to heifers (typically 8%–10% of body wt at birth) has typically been restricted to encourage consumption of high-protein calf starters, with a goal of early rumen development and weaning by 8–10 wk of age. However, calf health was found to improve when calves were fed more milk than this, and current practice recommends that calves be fed an increasing amount of milk—up to 12%–15% of body wt after the first week of age (10–11 L/day). Holstein heifers are now heavier and taller at the withers than in published standards recommended from years past. The goal of efficient Holstein heifer-raising programs in North America is for heifers to calve at a weight of 550 kg at 22.5–25 mo of age. Various health management programs are used to reach this goal, including deworming and the use of oral coccidiostats, supplemental selenium, and ionophores.

ANIMAL AND HERD PRODUCTIVITY

The productivity of an individual cow is the sum of the value of the milk she produces, the value of her offspring, and her individual market value when she leaves the herd. Many factors influence individual cow productivity, which is also based on longevity and the proportion of the cow's lifetime spent producing milk. Nonproductive periods include the period from birth until first parturition and dry periods before subsequent calvings. Heifers must be managed to reach appropriate breeding size by 13–15 mo of age to maximize lifetime production.

Milk yield is related to stage of lactation. Milk yield increases rapidly after calving, reaches a plateau 40–60 days after calving, and then declines at a rate of 5%–10%/mo. The rate of decline is lower in first-parity animals than in older cows. Good reproductive management ensures that the largest proportion of a cow's total lifetime production is spent during early high-producing stages of lactation rather than late, lower-producing periods. Milk yield increases with age and parity until about the sixth lactation; these cows may produce up to 25% more milk volume than first lactation cows. Health disorders or other management problems that reduce longevity have a negative impact on productivity.

Nutritional Management

In most dairy herds, nutritional management is the most important determinant of herd productivity. The relationship between nutrition and productivity begins at birth. The feeding system must deliver the necessary nutrients to each cow at the correct stage of lactation to maintain optimal productivity.

Research has documented the importance of the ration fed to cows in the transition during the 2–3 wk before calving. Dry cows are fed a diet relatively low in carbohydrates and protein and high in fiber, reflecting the low nutrient demands of the nonlactating cow. The transition period ration must allow the rumen to adapt to the lower-forage, more nutrient-dense lactating ration. Further, the stresses associated with moving animals to the transition pen and of calving itself tend to reduce feed consumption at this critical time. Reduced feed intake in the transition period is associated with excessive weight loss, reduced peak milk production, and an increased incidence of postpartum diseases such as metritis, retained placenta, ketosis, displaced abomasum, and fatty liver. Research has documented the benefits of monitoring postpartum cattle for excessive energy mobilization by measuring blood β-hydroxybutyric acid, one of the ketone bodies.

Rations for lactating cows must strike a balance between providing high levels of energy and protein to support high milk production and maintaining optimal rumen health and motility. Subacute rumen acidosis (SARA) is a common condition resulting from excessive fermentable carbohydrates, inadequate fiber of adequate length, or a combination of the two. Health effects of SARA include digestive upsets and diarrhea, reduced feed consumption and milk production, reduced butterfat content of milk, ulceration of rumen epithelium, liver abscessation, and a series of foot problems related to subclinical laminitis.

The choice of a feeding system is associated with herd size and production level. Three general types of feeding systems are used currently by dairy farmers: total mixed ration (TMR), component feeding, and management-intensive grazing. Each of these systems, when implemented correctly, can deliver adequate nutrients for a highly productive dairy herd. Each system has its own inherent challenges in achieving optimal productivity.

The use of TMR feeding systems has increased as more herds have adopted free-stall or dry-lot housing. TMR diets have several advantages: cows consume the desired proportion of forages, risk of digestive upset is reduced, feed efficiency is increased, byproduct feeds may be used, accuracy of diet formulation is higher, and labor needs are reduced. The performance of herds using TMR diets can be lowered by errors in ration formulation and feed delivery. An oft-quoted statement illustrates the challenges of TMR feeding. There are three rations for a dairy herd: the ration on paper as formulated by the nutritionist, the ration fed to the cows, and the ration the cows actually consume. Some common errors include inadequate or nonexistent forage testing, variation in forage dry matter, variation in dry-matter intakes, overmixing of diets that reduces effective fiber length, errors or imprecision in the mixing of the ration, and overfeeding or underfeeding energy to late-lactation cattle. When TMR are fed, feeding mistakes are often spread across the entire group or herd. Health management programs of herds that receive TMR diets should include systems to monitor the adequacy of the ration formulation and delivery.

Component-fed herds receive grain and forage separately. Advocates of component feeding emphasize the ability to meet the production and metabolic needs of individual cows throughout their production cycle. The primary disadvantage of component feeding systems is that the cow receives concentrates separate from forages, enabling ingestion of these concentrates in a single feeding, leading to rumen acidosis and indigestion.

Management-intensive grazing systems can be used to meet the needs of modern dairy cows. In some regions of the world (eg, New Zealand and Australia), pasture-based systems are the predominant method of feeding dairy cattle. In these truly pastoral systems, nutrition frequently limits productivity because of significant annual variation in growing conditions. However, the economic model in such a system emphasizes low costs of production rather than maximal productivity. In other areas such as Britain and the northeastern USA, rotational grazing is used to provide for the forage requirements of lactating cattle during the spring and summer months, and supplemental concentrates and corn silage are fed to achieve high milk production. In both situations, seasonal calving is practiced to match rainy or spring season pasture conditions with the energy needs of early lactation cows. Attention to reproductive management is therefore critical for herds that attempt to breed all cows within a defined period. Production management programs for herds using management-intensive grazing systems must include programs to control bloat, hypomagnesemia, and copper and selenium deficiency. Pastured cattle may walk considerable distances to harvest forages. Therefore, a system to monitor and minimize lameness must be included in the health delivery system.

Reproductive Management

Artificial insemination (AI) using semen from genetically superior sires is the most important factor leading to increased productivity in the dairy industry, accounting for at least 150 kg increased annual production since its inception. Even today, the genetic potential for milk production greatly exceeds the actual milk yield achieved on most farms. Reproductive disorders are the most common and costly reasons for premature culling of dairy cows (*see* MANAGEMENT OF REPRODUCTION: CATTLE, p 2171). In conventional dairy herds in which calving occurs throughout the year, suboptimal reproductive management leads to the failure of cows to conceive in a timely fashion, or at all. Cows remaining open longer reduce productivity in the following ways: 1) Open cows spend more time in late lactation, with lower milk production. 2) Cows taking longer to conceive may dry off sooner, leading to longer dry periods. 3) Risk of culling increases greatly in cows remaining open >300 days after calving. 4) Fewer replacement heifers are available. 5) Higher labor and treatment costs are associated with prolonged efforts to synchronize and breed open cows.

Successful AI requires that cows be inseminated during estrus in a narrow range of optimal fertility, and that the semen be thawed properly, transported quickly to the cow, and deposited in the appropriate area of the reproductive tract. The most important factor affecting the success of an AI program is the detection of estrus: recent data from the USA indicate that fewer than 40% of estrus periods were detected in lactating dairy cattle. Efforts to improve heat detection using estrus synchronization and artificial detection aids have been largely unsuccessful and are hampered by the reduced duration and intensity of estrus exhibited by modern USA Holsteins, and by the increasing size of farms making estrus observation more difficult. Because heat detection rates are so low, some dairy managers have returned to extensive use of natural service sires to ensure that cows conceive promptly. In these herds, breeding soundness examinations and bull management programs should be included to ensure continued herd productivity. (*See also* BREEDING SOUNDNESS EXAMINATION OF BULLS, p 2231.) However, the problems associated with natural service include reduced genetic improvement of offspring; costs associated with purchase, raising, and feeding bulls; damage to facilities; and danger to people.

Researchers in Wisconsin and Florida have developed hormonal synchronization protocols that allow timed insemination to be performed with acceptable conception rates. These programs have been widely adopted and have enabled herds to dramatically increase the number of pregnant cows throughout defined time periods. Many of the injections and the inseminations can be scheduled on a weekly basis, leading to more efficient use of labor.

Replacement Management

Herd productivity can be profoundly affected by the success of the replacement program. The cost of raising heifers is a significant proportion of the overall cost of production; a replacement animal does not begin to earn a profit until midway through her second lactation. A wide range of mortality rates (5%–25%) is reported for replacement animals. The highest morbidity and mortality rates on dairy farms generally are seen before weaning. The most significant causes of preweaning death are infectious diseases of the digestive and respiratory systems. These disorders can be controlled by well-designed health management procedures that define the care and housing of the dam during the periparturient period, the calving process, feeding adequate quantities of high-quality colostrum, and the application of proper preventive measures (including sound nutritional programs) for newborn calves.

Delayed age at first calving reduces dairy productivity by increasing the need for replacement animals and increasing the costs of raising the replacements because of longer feeding periods. Heifers should be 23–25 mo old at first calving, which means they should conceive when 14–16 mo old. Adequate nutrition is important to ensure that heifers are fertile and cycling at this stage and that continued growth occurs so that heifers are large enough at calving to limit dystocia and maximize mammary development and lactation.

Herd Size, Composition, and Culling

There is a well-demonstrated relationship between productivity and herd size. One reason for this is the greater willingness for larger operations to adopt production-enhancing technologies. Government policies can also substantially influence herd size (eg, countries with supply management systems effectively limit the annual income a farm can achieve from the sale of milk). The amount and productivity of pasture can influence the size of herds that use grazing. In these herds, productivity is determined by balancing the ability of the pasture to produce nutrients against the ability of the cows to produce milk. The size of both grazing and confinement herds are increasingly affected by competing demands for land.

The proportion of the herd producing milk versus the nonproductive stock (dry cows, calves, heifers, and bulls) has an effect on total herd productivity. Herd composition is the result of a number of interrelated management decisions, such as culling policy, rate of reproductive success, rate of disease, replacement management, and longterm goals regarding herd size. The ability of a herd manager to cull animals can have a significant impact on herd composition. When numerous replacement heifers are available, culling may intensify, leading to a younger herd with improved genetic potential for future milk production. In countries such as the USA, where herd production is not limited, longterm plans regarding expansion often influence herd composition. In some growing or start-up herds, only nonlactating cattle are purchased to reduce the risk of purchasing animals with infectious diseases such as contagious mastitis or bovine viral diarrhea. These herds often consist of a high proportion of first-lactation animals.

Decisions regarding cow removal can significantly impact productivity of the dairy herd. Culling rates vary between herds and may be related to disease rates or disease control programs. Fertility, mastitis, and lameness are common reasons for cow removal. Culling is an important aspect of controlling other diseases such as bovine tuberculosis, brucellosis, paratuberculosis, and chronic mastitis caused by some contagious mastitis pathogens.

Environmental Conditions

Even with optimal housing situations, herd productivity can be affected by environmental conditions. High-producing cows have higher dry-matter intake, generate more internal heat, and are less tolerant of high ambient temperature. Weather conditions that combine high ambient temperature and high humidity without periods of cooling generally depress dry-matter intake and reduce milk yield. The increased concentration of dairy farming in regions that experience considerable periods of high temperatures (eg, southwestern USA) has resulted in more seasonal variation in milk output.

Farmers have adopted a variety of systems to combat heat stress. New facilities are constructed with large, open sides and ends (often >4.3 m high) and use fans and sprinkler systems to keep cows comfortable. Older, enclosed facilities can be retrofitted with tunnel ventilation systems to provide adequate air movement. (*See also* VENTILATION, p 2116.)

Drying Off and Dry Cow Management

Risk factors for most postpartum diseases of dairy cows are present during the dry period, with clinical signs of disease becoming evident after calving. Diseases such as hypocalcemia (milk fever), hypomagnesemia, udder edema, ketosis, displaced abomasum, and mastitis often begin during the dry period. Dairy health management programs focus on many preventive practices such as vaccination, hoof care, and nutritional monitoring during this period.

The length of the dry period influences milk yield in the subsequent lactation. The recommended dry period is 6–8 wk. Dry periods of <40 days reduce milk yield in the following lactation. Dry periods that are too long may lead to excessive weight gain and reduced production efficiency. Both short and long dry periods are most common when breeding dates are uncertain because of either bull breeding or inaccurate (or missing) reproductive records.

INTERACTIONS BETWEEN HEALTH AND PRODUCTION

An important factor that influences dairy herd productivity is the amount and type of disease in the herd. The basis of disease control programs includes knowledge of the frequency of disease, information about the biologic effect of disease, and information on the effectiveness of control procedures.

Most studies report incidence rates of only common, easily diagnosed clinical diseases such as mastitis, lameness, milk fever, retained placenta, or displaced abomasum. The frequency of subclinical disease is much more difficult to discern. The cost to obtain subclinical disease information is inflated by the need to use screening tests (eg, culture or somatic cell counts [SCC] for mastitis, fecal culture or ELISA for paratuberculosis) for diagnosis. The lack of repeated testing leads to the reporting of prevalence rather than incidence for many subclinical diseases. Estimates of the frequency of sporadic or endemic infectious diseases (such as listeriosis, infectious bovine rhinotracheitis, or leptospirosis) are also sparse. There is zero tolerance for some diseases that have serious consequences for public health. The diagnosis of even one case of bovine spongiform encephalopathy, brucellosis, rabies, or tuberculosis in areas thought to be free of those conditions is cause for immediate action.

Influence of Disease on Productivity

Increased culling, reduced milk or protein yield, increased adult cow mortality, and reduced reproductive efficiency are all potential results of disease in adult cows. Milk production is often profoundly reduced in cows with clinical disease. The duration of acute clinical syndromes is often short, but the effects of the disease may persist throughout the entire lactation. Early lactation is the highest risk period for many diseases. Disease during early lactation may reduce peak milk yields and therefore contribute to lower total lactational yields. Through advances in animal husbandry and health management programs, many farms have minimized clinical syndromes associated with infectious and metabolic disease.

Although epidemics of clinical syndromes still are seen, the nature of disease has changed on many dairy farms. The trend toward larger units and shrinking profit margins has encouraged a shift toward optimizing herd or group productivity through reduction of subclinical diseases, such as ketosis, mastitis, acidosis, and laminitis, which can have a major impact on productivity.

Infectious disease still represents a major source of loss to dairy industries worldwide. In Britain, outbreaks of foot and mouth disease (as well as bovine spongiform encephalopathy) are dramatic examples of the disastrous effects of infectious diseases on productivity. Other serious infectious diseases such as tuberculosis, brucellosis, bluetongue, and vesicular stomatitis continue to affect livestock around the world. In North America, more common infectious diseases that must be actively controlled include the contagious mastitis pathogens *Mycoplasma bovis*, *Staphylococcus aureus*, and *Streptococcus agalactiae*; bovine viral diarrhea; salmonellosis; paratuberculosis; and pneumonia. Excellent control programs have been developed for most of these diseases, but their adoption is quite variable.

The effects of disease on productivity can be direct (such as mastitis causing a profound reduction in milk yield) or indirect (lameness leading to reduced feed intake, thus causing reduced milk yield). Diseases occurring in early lactation can also cause cascading effects that ultimately reduce productivity. For example, periparturient disorders often are seen as a complex, and cows diagnosed with parturient paresis are at increased risk of retained placenta, complicated ketosis, and mastitis. Cows with dystocia and retained placenta are at increased risk of metritis. Subclinical ketosis leads to increased risk of displaced abomasum and reduced milk production. The best documented direct effect is the effect of mastitis on milk yield. A single case of clinical mastitis can result in a milk yield loss of 300–400 kg/lactation, with variations ranging from negligible to 1,050 kg. Mastitis during early lactation is associated with higher losses (450–550 kg) than cases seen later in lactation. (*See also* MASTITIS IN CATTLE, p 1358.)

Losses resulting from subclinical disease are often considerable. The best described relationship between subclinical disease and productivity is the effect of subclinical mastitis on milk yield. Each 2-fold increase in SCC >50,000 cells/mL caused a loss of 0.4 kg milk/day in primiparous cows and 0.6 kg milk/day in multiparous cows. Total lactational milk yields were estimated to be reduced by 80 kg for primiparous cows and 120 kg for multiparous cows for each 2-fold increase in the geometric mean SCC >50,000 cells/mL. Other subclinical diseases (eg, paratuberculosis) have also been related to reduced productivity.

Diseases that delay or prohibit conception have a negative effect on herd productivity by prolonging the time cows spend in lower-producing stages of lactation, by reducing the number of offspring for replacements or for sale, and by increasing the likelihood the animal will be culled prematurely. Several diseases have been associated with decreased conception rates. The likelihood of conception was reduced by 14%, 15%, and 21% for cows that experienced retained placenta, metritis, or ovarian cysts, respectively. Mastitis, metritis, and ovarian cysts reduced the likelihood of cattle being bred for the first time. Postpartum diseases that prolong negative energy balance in early lactation also have a negative effect on reproductive performance through alterations in hormonal activities.

The effect of disease on longevity has been investigated. A large proportion of cow culling is considered involuntary (driven by disease, injury, or death) rather than for reasons of low production. The premature removal of a cow from the herd reduces lifetime milk yield. Reproductive failure and mastitis are consistently recorded as the top two reasons for culling.

THE HEALTH MANAGEMENT PROGRAM

The goal of health management programs is to ensure the optimal care and well-being of dairy cattle and to reduce losses in productivity caused by disease and management errors. The health management program is generally developed cooperatively by the herd veterinarian and the dairy producer based on comparisons of herd performance with predetermined performance goals. The structure of health management programs is unique to each farm but is typically keyed to the scheduled veterinary herd visits that combine routine reproductive examinations, review of selected herd performance records, and decisions and actions related to specific herd management issues.

Scheduled Farm Visits

The frequency of scheduled veterinarian visits is somewhat dependent on herd size. In herds of <100 cows, one or two cows calve every week and a single, scheduled monthly visit is probably appropriate. These herds may have more unscheduled visits for examination of sick cows than herds visited more regularly. Larger herds in which cows are calving daily warrant more frequent visits, and weekly scheduled visits are not uncommon for herds of >200 cows. A trend on extremely large dairy farms (>2,000 cows) is employment of a full-time staff veterinarian to oversee and direct day-to-day issues regarding health and performance. The frequency of scheduled herd visits for grass-based seasonal dairy operations varies depending on the herd's stage of lactation. More frequent visits are necessary in early lactation and during the breeding period.

Activities at herd visits fall into four general categories: provision of individual animal health care and emergency services, scheduled technical activities, scheduled analytic and training activities, and provision of quality control programs. The frequency of individual activities varies.

Individual Health Care and Emergency Services: The examination and treatment of individual animals is an important activity during scheduled dairy visits. Frequent herd visits allow practitioners to examine cows early in the course of disease when the likelihood of successful treatment is higher. Routine visits also allow veterinarians to monitor the outcome of treatments and modify treatment protocols as needed. Ideally, monitoring programs include a system to detect cows not performing as expected. Special attention should be paid to the highest-risk cows, including frequent observation of animals during the periparturient period. Some farms have adopted a system that includes routine daily monitoring of body temperature and rumen activity of cows during the first 7 days after calving. Animals that fall outside normal limits are treated according to predefined criteria or detained for examination by the herd veterinarian. All treatments administered to dairy cows should be recorded in treatment logs (either computerized or handwritten) to ensure adherence to proper meat and milk withholding periods. The frequency of unscheduled visits for emergency medical services usually diminishes in herds that have adopted a health and production management program.

Scheduled, Traditional, and Technical Activities: Routine reproductive examinations account for much of the veterinarian's time during scheduled herd visits. Attaining reproductive success is an essential determinant of herd productivity. For a description of reproductive programs, *see* p 2171. The end point of reproductive examinations should be to identify nonpregnant cows that can be returned to the breeding program and to generate data that can be used to determine the success or failure of breeding programs. The implementation, success, and cost-effectiveness of scheduled breeding programs should be reviewed frequently.

On smaller farms, it is often customary for the veterinarian to perform routine individual animal treatments (such as IV injections), prophylactic activities (such as vaccinations), and some technical tasks (such as dehorning calves) during scheduled herd visits. It is appropriate for the veterinarian, or a technician under the veterinarian's supervision, to perform these tasks, because the farm staff may not perform them often enough to become technically proficient. On larger farms, these tasks must often be performed on a daily basis; in this case, farm employees should be trained to accomplish these tasks.

Scheduled Analytic and Training Activities: Conducting scheduled or unscheduled technical activities will not be effective unless a system exists to capture the results of the activities and allow for analysis and ongoing revision. The structure of the health and production management program must include time for the farmer and the herd veterinarian to analyze and discuss herd management issues. In herds that depend on hired personnel to implement designated tasks, time must be scheduled to observe and effectively train personnel ultimately responsible for performing the activities. Development of standard operating procedures is one method to ensure that agreed-on practices are implemented.

Treatment protocols are used to define standard treatments for common diseases on dairy farms and should be used when multiple people have responsibility for administering antibiotic treatments to dairy cattle or when extra-label drug use is prescribed. They also provide a mechanism for increased communication about treatment plans between the veterinarian and producer.

The avoidance of residues in food products is a major responsibility of dairy practitioners. Increased scrutiny regarding antimicrobial use in food-producing animals has arisen because of concern about the development of antimicrobial resistance in foodborne pathogens. Although the level of detected antibiotic residues in meat and milk products is extremely low, antibiotic residues in bulk milk and carcasses are seen occasionally. In the USA, contamination of bulk milk is rare because of an effective surveillance system based on rapid testing for selected antimicrobial agents of every load of raw milk. Milk contaminated with antibiotics is discarded, and the producer is fined.

The requirements for extra-label drug use in the USA have been defined by regulatory officials under the Animal Medicinal Drug Use Clarification Act and should be closely followed. The American Association of Bovine Practitioners has responded to societal and regulatory concerns about the use of antimicrobial agents by adopting recommendations for the prudent and judicious use of antimicrobial agents in dairy cattle. In response to concerns about the development of antimicrobial resistance in human medicine, the FDA is requesting that drug manufacturers begin the process of eliminating the labeling and use of certain antimicrobials for production purposes (to increase feed efficiency or weight gain). Specifically, antimicrobials of importance to human medicine will no longer be permitted to be provided in feed or water solely for production purposes, and no new antimicrobials will be approved for production purposes, although they can be approved for use in feed or water for treatment or prevention of disease. For producers to use an antimicrobial in feed or water, they must receive a feed directive from their veterinarian (essentially a prescription); over-the-counter sales of antimicrobials for use in feed or water will no longer be allowed. *See also* THE VETERINARY FEED DIRECTIVE, p 2634.

Some dairy practitioners function as the nutritional specialists for the dairy farms they serve. They may collect feed samples for nutrient analysis, formulate rations, and advise the farmer regarding crop and harvesting conditions. These veterinarians often devote a considerable amount of their professional time to nutritional management. Other farms employ a professional nutritionist or use a nutritionist employed by a feed company or local cooperative to formulate the rations and submit feed samples for nutrient analysis. Regardless of the source of the dairy's nutrition program, the veterinarian can perform an essential oversight function simply by observing body condition and general health in cows in certain high-risk areas (periparturient and high milk production), monitoring the incidence of nutrition-related diseases such as parturient hypocalcemia and displaced abomasum, and ensuring that the diet described on paper is adequately formulated and delivered to the cows. Assessing pasture conditions by periodic inspection of pasture is an important component of managing the nutritional program of herds that use management-intensive grazing. These quality control activities should be conducted routinely as part of the health and production management program.

Quality Control Programs

Quality control refers to activities that ensure consistency in performing key management processes. Vital management areas for most herds include nutritional management, milking management, and young-stock programs. Some farms may also develop quality control processes for environment and housing and farm-specific management of breeding bulls.

Milking management should be a standard element of quality control programs. Tasks such as observing the milking routine and scoring the condition of teats should be performed at least quarterly. A scheduled system of routine screening for mastitis pathogens can be implemented as part of the milking management program. The veterinarian can teach farm personnel how to perform the California Mastitis Test as part of a surveillance program. Animals routinely screened may include cows at dry off, fresh cows and heifers, and newly purchased cows. Milk samples can be collected and submitted for culture from quarters that show positive reactions.

Newborn calves and replacement heifers are often housed separately from lactating cows and may not be observed routinely by the herd veterinarian. However, routine surveillance of critical management issues such as adequate delivery of colostrum to calves and growth rates of replacement heifers can be done as part of scheduled herd visits. The environment of dairy cattle can have considerable influence on health and productivity. Some veterinarians routinely schedule "walkabouts" through the housing areas to assess factors related to animal comfort and hygiene. Udder cleanliness, hoof and hock lesions, and respiratory disease are often determined by housing conditions. Herd walkabouts should include areas often ignored, such as dry-cow and heifer housing.

Performance Targets

Performance targets reflect herd standards of performance that are perceived as indicators of successful herd management. They are useful as comparison values for herd performance and as a starting point to initiate discussions about potential areas for improvement. To use a performance target, it is necessary for a herd to have a record system that allows for generation of comparable herd indices. In many instances, performance targets have been calculated as arithmetic averages, which are useful indicators of herd performance when the contributing data (such as milk, fat, and protein yields) are normally distributed and have a reasonable degree of variation. However, many reproductive indices and values such as SCCs are not distributed normally, and erroneous conclusions about herd performance may be made if averages alone are used to make management decisions. Appropriate frequency distributions are more useful for these types of data.

Key indicators for performance targets should be defined. The monitoring system should specify the indices used, the animals included, and the time interval to reassess progress made toward reaching each target. Typical performance indicators include milk production, reproductive performance, milk quality, replacement management, cow removal, animal health, and special reports (*see* TABLE 4). Performance targets should be reviewed at appropriate intervals with realistic expectations regarding the amount of time it takes to effect change in an index. For example, management actions taken to reduce days to first calving would require ≥9–10 mo to become apparent. A more timely value such as age at conception would more rapidly reflect current management changes.

TABLE 4 EXAMPLES OF ACTIVITIES FOR ROUTINE MONITORING[a]

Cow Monitoring	Environment Monitoring	Records Monitoring
Body condition	Stalls and bedding	Milk production
Rumen fill	Barn climate	Milk quality features
Feces consistency	Milking method	Roughage analysis
Undigested fraction in feces	Milking parlor condition	Drinking water quality
Teat end callosity	Pasture management	Sire evaluations
Lesions of udder/teat/skin	Grass harvesting (silage)	Soil analysis
Clinical disease cases	Maize harvesting (silage)	Artificial insemination records
Reproductive examinations	Floor design and maintenance	Disease and drug records
Ectoparasites	Ration formulation	Farm economics report
Locomotion and claw score	Feeding management	Slaughter findings
Young stock growth	Hygiene practices	Laboratory findings

[a]From Noordhuizen JP, Dairy herd health and production management practice in Europe: state of the art. Proc 23rd World Buiatrics Congress, Quebec, Canada, 2004.

Record Keeping

A system of unique individual cow identification is a prerequisite for a successful health management program. The most common methods of animal identification are ear tags, collars, and branding. Increasingly, farms are using electronic identification via transponders on ankle bands or neck straps. At a minimum, data must be recorded on birth, breeding, and calving dates and periodic milk yield. Under ideal circumstances, summarized data should be available for the nutritional program, disease occurrence, and financial performance.

Record analysis is a necessary component of the health management cycle. Most or all dairy herd improvement (DHI) systems allow for electronic access to performance data, and various computerized systems for herd management are used throughout the industry. Most monitoring systems can be characterized broadly as one of the following: 1) manual (handwritten) card systems, 2) on-farm computer programs, 3) DHI, or 4) DHI and on-farm computer. Regardless of the type of system used, it should be easy to use and relevant to the day-to-day operations of the dairy.

One important function of record systems is the generation of "action" lists (due to calve, due to dry, etc). This function is critical in large herds in which cattle are not individually known by the animal handlers and can be overlooked easily. Most systems also provide for a minimal level of herd analysis, such as the generation of timely performance reports for production, reproduction, and disease. Some programs can also generate statistics. The record-keeping system should allow the producer and veterinarian to understand and modify the formulas used to generate herd performance indices. For parameters and values used to monitor herd health and production, *see* TABLE 5.

The veterinarian should ensure that collected data are used in a timely manner. Accurate data collection is most likely when the producer is using the data frequently and understands its value. The validity of data generated from both manual and automated data collection systems should be reviewed and critically assessed. Unusual results and deviations from normal performance targets should be challenged. The producer and the veterinarian should agree on defined actions based on the herd status and goals. Actions are generally diagnostic, preventive, or treatment oriented. Typical activities might include listing animals for routine herd fertility or illness examinations, or selecting cows to obtain milk samples for culture, to vaccinate, to consider culling, to breed, to receive body condition scoring, or to receive treatments.

TABLE 5 PARAMETERS USEFUL TO MONITOR HEALTH AND PRODUCTION OF DAIRY HERDS

Parameter	Goal
Adult Cow Disease	
Average percent of herd lame	<25%
Metritis/endometritis incidence	<5%–25%
Subclinical ketosis (>1.2 mmol/L)	<10%
Clinical ketosis	<2%
Left displaced abomasum	<3%–5%
Milk fever	<3% of adult cows calving per month
Retained fetal membranes	<3% of cows calving per month
Cut point for ruminal acidosis	pH <5.5
Clinical mastitis monthly incidence	<3% of lactating herd
Culling and Death Loss	
Annual average overall cull rate	35%
Annual average selective cull rate	>15%

(continued)

TABLE 5 PARAMETERS USEFUL TO MONITOR HEALTH AND PRODUCTION OF DAIRY HERDS *(continued)*

Parameter	Goal
Annual death loss	<10%
Annual disease and injury culling	<5%
Annual reproductive cull rate	5%–10%
% Removed <60 days in milk (lactation = 1)	<4%
% Removed <60 days in milk (lactation >1)	<6%
Udder Health and Milk Quality	
SCC legal limit	750,000 cells/mL
SCC farm goal	<150,000 cells/mL (or adjust for a dairy)
Standard plate count legal limit	100,000 CFU/mL
Standard plate count farm goal	2,000–4,000 CFU/mL
Preliminary incubation count	2,000–6,000 CFU/mL
Bulk Tank Cultures - Bacterium	
Streptococcus agalactiae	0 CFU/mL
Staphylococcus aureus	<50 CFU/mL
Staphylococcus spp	<1,000 CFU/mL
Mycoplasma spp	0 CFU/mL
Environmental streptococci	<1,000 CFU/mL
Coliforms	<500 CFU/mL
General Reproductive	**Standard**
Average days open	100–110 (ideally low 100's to achieve 12-mo calving)
Average gestation	283 days
Calving interval	13.5 mo
Average days in milk	200
Percentage of cows <90 days in milk	25%
Percentage of cows 90–180 days in milk	25%
Voluntary waiting period (VWP)	50–60 days for cows; 80–90 days for heifers
Days in milk at first breeding	Goal: VWP + 11 days
First service conception rate	40%
Heat detection	Goal overall >50% (national average <40%)
Intervals between breedings	18–24 days for 65% of cows
Length of estrous cycle	18–24 days
Overall conception rate	>35%
Services per conception	2
Definition of pregnancy rate	Heat detection rate × conception rate (21-day interval)

(continued)

TABLE 5 PARAMETERS USEFUL TO MONITOR HEALTH AND PRODUCTION OF DAIRY HERDS *(continued)*

Parameter	Goal
First cycle pregnancy rate	>30%
Percent pregnant by three cycles	>50%
Overall pregnancy rate	>20%
Percent of herd pregnant	50%
Pregnancy Diagnosis	
When to do pregnancy checks	>40 days after being bred
Ability to locate amnion	42–65 days
"Membrane slip"	Day 30 to term
Ability to locate fetus	65–95 days
Placentomes present	After 3 mo of gestation
Ability to sex fetus	After 60–70 days of gestation
"Placentomes"	Day 70 to term
By amnion size (days)	
35	7 mm (½ finger)
42	15 mm (1 finger)
48	35 mm (2 fingers)
53	55 mm (3 fingers)
58	75 mm (4 fingers)
62	90 mm (palm)
65	105 mm (hand)
By fetal crown-nose length (days)	
70	1.5 cm (1 finger)
80	3.5 cm (2 fingers)
90	5.5 cm (3 fingers)
100	7.5 cm (4 fingers)
110	9 cm (palm)
120	10.5 cm (hand)
Postpartum Involution	
Lochia (normal)	
Day 1–2	Bright red blood, thick mucus, little smell
Day 3–7	Dark red, thin, odor not foul but objectionable
Day 7–14	Progressively less red to white to translucent, thicker, smell improves
Entire uterus palpable	2 wk
Full reduction in size	40–45 days
Epithelialization complete	40–45 days

(continued)

TABLE 5 PARAMETERS USEFUL TO MONITOR HEALTH AND PRODUCTION OF DAIRY HERDS *(continued)*

Parameter	Goal
Occurrence of endometritis	>26 days after calving
Full uterine involution	40–45 days postpartum
Abortion	
Normal embryonic loss (<50 days)	<10%
Average rate of early embryonic loss	15%
Normal rate of abortion	3%
Major infectious abortion agents	Bovine viral diarrhea, mycotic, leptospirosis, *Neospora*
Noninfectious causes	
Heat stress	>90°C, 80% relative humidity
Toxins	Nitrates: methemoglobinemia
Plants	Locoweed, snakeweed, pine needles, lupine
Urea	Excess rumen degradable protein or nonprotein nitrogen; milk urea nitrogen 10–14 mg/dL

Investigations of Health and Production Problems

Even on the best managed farms, unexpected health and production problems arise. Surveillance programs incorporated in health and production management programs should detect problems early, before considerable financial damage has occurred. Systems to investigate herd outbreaks have been described. Epidemiologic concepts of disease investigation are useful to identify risk factors and to stimulate corrective action.

HEALTH-MANAGEMENT INTERACTION: GOATS

Management of goats depends on the type (eg, dairy, pygmy, meat, mohair, or cashmere) and the reasons for which they are kept (eg, companionship or commercial enterprise). However, all are ruminants, and the basic principles of livestock husbandry are applicable. Dairy goats and pygmies are often raised intensively, with most of the feed being brought to the animals. Meat goats and fiber goats are usually raised extensively, with most of the diet coming from browse and occasionally from high-quality pasture at times of highest nutritional need, such as the last 6 wk of gestation and the first 18 mo of life. A pregnant Angora doe without adequate energy and protein continues to grow mohair, even if stressed until she aborts.

Of all farm animals, goats have the strongest social hierarchy; thus, adequate feeder space or pasture should be provided so the dominant animals cannot guard feed and prevent others from eating. The amount of floor space available per doe affects the amount of aggressive behavior. A goat can become so subordinated to its penmates that it does not eat and loses condition. This behavioral component must be considered in cases of wasting goats. To maximize longevity and to avoid fighting injuries, adult males should be fed and housed individually, especially during the breeding season when fighting increases. If group penned, bucks should be kept together and given time to get to know each other before breeding season begins. Introducing a new buck to a pen of existing bucks during breeding season may result in injury or death.

Goats are adventurous and are natural climbers, and efforts to control them are necessary. The ultimate control would be high-tensile, electric fences; goats stand and push on other fences and can be very destructive. Hazards that might contribute to broken legs and strangulations should be removed. Tethering goats is potentially dangerous, because they are vulnerable to dog attacks; also, if two goats are chained too close to each other, one might strangle. Chafing of ropes too tight on the neck can lead to deep abrasions and tetanus. Because goats chew on painted surfaces, lead poisoning is a potential hazard in old barns. An efficient layout of pens, easy access to well-designed feeders, and effective control of movement minimize management-related problems.

It is extremely difficult to keep goats' feet, urine, and feces out of many types of grain feeders, hay racks, and waterers. Goats often refuse to eat soiled feed or water, hay that has fallen on the floor, and grain contaminated with urine or feces. Design of hay feeders is critical to reduce feed wastage. Many dairy and pygmy goats are bedded on wasted hay, but this practice may lead to an increase in parasitism. Wet bedding contributes to development of coccidiosis in kids and staphylococcal impetigo on the udder, commonly but erroneously known as "goatpox." Under similar conditions, joint-ill (*see* p 1094) and navel infections of the newborn are likely. Separate, dry, well-bedded pens should be maintained for kidding. In certain areas, kids are susceptible to white muscle disease (*see* p 1095), which can be controlled by dietary selenium supplementation or by injection of vitamin E/selenium to the pregnant doe and/or newborn. Concerns about abortions associated with vitamin E/selenium injection in ewes have prompted caution about parenteral injection in pregnant does, and oral supplementation may be preferred.

Housing of goats affects disease patterns. Angoras in the southern and western USA are usually given access to shelter only during severe storms or for a few weeks after the twice-yearly shearing, without which they may die of cold weather stress. Goats in the northern USA are housed in the winter, perhaps more for the owners' comfort than for optimal health of the goats. Combinations of manure packs, overhead hay-mows, or noninsulated ceilings lead to dampness and ammonia buildup, especially if the barn is closed tightly. Warm, wet, poorly ventilated barns are conducive to development of neonatal navel infections, mastitis, enteritis, pneumonia, and coccidiosis. Caseous lymphadenitis (the disease known as "abscesses"), caused by *Corynebacterium pseudotuberculosis (ovis)*, spreads rapidly in closely confined goats (*see* p 63). The slow-growing, nonpainful lymph node abscesses eventually rupture and contaminate the feeders, walls, and other animals. Keyhole-style feeders and head catches on milking stands are prime sources of transmission, because they promote rupture of abscesses on the head and neck. The infection is spread by contact with the pus, and the organism can penetrate intact skin. Isolating affected goats, preferably culling them, and preventing environmental contamination is important. A commercial vaccine approved for goats is available, and autogenous bacterins have been used to decrease the incidence of these abscesses. Intensive management of adult goats may promote horizontal transmission of the virus that causes caprine arthritis and encephalitis (CAE, *see* p 747).

Mature bucks develop a powerful, characteristic odor that is most intense in the breeding season, and personnel are reluctant to handle them. This often leads to neglect of feet, failure to recognize heavy parasite loads, or loss of body condition. The sebaceous glands on top of the head can be removed surgically at any age or can be cauterized at the time of disbudding; however, this does not render the buck totally odorless. Does are attracted by this smell and may refuse to be bred by a descented buck if there is an odoriferous one nearby; therefore, the glands should not be removed inadvertently at the time of disbudding if male kids are to be kept for breeding. The habit of urinating on the face, beard, and forelegs also contributes to buck odor and often leads to ulcerating sores in cold weather. During the breeding season, most bucks lose weight, although this is not necessarily due to breeding too many does. Many bucks lose weight when housed close to does in heat, even when breeding is not allowed. One management strategy is to ensure that bucks are in prime physical condition before the breeding season.

In the European dairy breeds, the genetically homozygous polled doe usually is anatomically an intersex and, therefore, infertile. Aberrations vary from a slightly enlarged clitoris visible only after puberty, to a buck-like conformation with a scrotum, penis (often shortened), and ovotestes. Some phenotypically male pseudohermaphrodites show male libido with breeding activity. Because these animals are infertile, early recognition and culling is advisable. Some homozygous polled males may be able to sire kids, but these bucks are likely to develop sperm granulomas as they mature and should be culled rather than used for breeding. Most owners reduce the incidence of homozygous polled animals by never mating two polled animals. While most intersex goats are polled, similar anatomic aberrations are seen occasionally in horned goats. These would most probably be chimeras (freemartins), the result of anastomoses developing in utero between males and females. Such chimeras in goats are rare (considering the high frequency of twins) when compared with cattle.

For foot care, *see* p 1092.

PERINATAL MANAGEMENT

Common problems in does are extra teats, double teats, and fish-tail teats with double orifices. In cattle, extra teats can be removed with impunity, but in dairy goats there is often a functional milk gland behind the spare teat, and removal of abnormal teats is discouraged.

Newborn goats must be fed colostrum, and if caprine arthritis and encephalitis (CAE) is a problem, heat treatment is essential for control. Later, kids can be fed (in decreasing order of desirability) goat's milk, goat-milk replacer, lamb-milk replacer, or cow's milk. Any fresh milk fed should be pasteurized or from stock known to be free of CAE virus, mycoplasmas, and paratuberculosis. Newborn goats should be fed at 10%–12% of their body wt per day. Kids should be provided sufficient milk or replacer at regular intervals to achieve normal growth.

Kids should have access to hay and a grain-based creep feed as early as 1 wk of age. They can be weaned when they are readily eating solid feed as most of the diet; this varies from early weaning at 6 wk of age until weaning as late as 12 wk of age. Weaning may be delayed in some goat operations because there is no commercial outlet for doe's milk, so it is fed to kids.

Dairy goat doe kids of European breeds should be disbudded at 5–7 days of age. Bucks of the European breeds should be disbudded 2 days earlier to maximally inhibit horn growth or subsequent development of abnormal regrowth (scurs). Horns may develop more slowly in Nubian, Nigerian Dwarf, and Pygmy does, but disbudding before 2 wk of age is preferred to decrease pain during the procedure and to prevent scur development. Hot-iron disbudding is the method of choice, using either a restraint box and nerve block, or general anesthesia. Excessive applications of the hot iron can lead to brain damage or subsequent death. Disbudding kids with caustic paste is not recommended.

Angora goats in range operations are not disbudded because the horns are thought to be helpful against predators, and because owners handle the goats by their horns. When goats are housed in winter, disbudding is advantageous, because it reduces trauma and prevents accidents in which goats are trapped by their horns in feeders and fence lines. Pygmies can be disbudded according to the owner's preference; it is not a cause for disqualification or discrimination in the show ring in the USA. Dairy goats generally are disbudded, and horned animals usually are barred from the show ring in the USA. Tetanus can be seen after disbudding or castration and, as a precaution, antitoxin can be administered at disbudding.

Dairy goats and pygmy bucks are castrated in the first few weeks; Angoras are castrated later, after they have attained good horn growth. In males to be kept as pets, castration should be delayed to allow maximal urethral development, which reduces the likelihood of urolithiasis (*see* p 1502). To improve their desirability as pets, wethers should have the scent glands, located caudomedially to the horn base, removed during disbudding.

NUTRITION

Dairy goats should be fed similarly to dairy cattle (*see* p 2308 and *see* p 2265). A good-quality hay, preferably alfalfa, should be the basis of the ration, and a 14%–16% protein concentrate should be fed as a supplement during lactation. Silage is not commonly fed to goats because of the lack of mechanical equipment. Overfeeding grain to pregnant does in late lactation is a common problem that may lead to increased levels of internal fat deposition in the abdomen and result in pregnancy toxemia and dystocia.

To increase salt consumption, loose trace mineral salt (TMS) should be fed rather than block salt. The choice of salt should be based on the mineral content of available feeds in that specific area. Goats are highly susceptible to copper deficiency and, unlike sheep, fairly resistant to copper toxicity. Therefore, cattle TMS, rather than sheep salt with no copper, should be offered unless the soils or water source are known to have high levels of copper. Goats raised for fiber may require supplementation of sulfur for proper fiber production.

Pet wethers fed substantial amounts of grain are prone to develop urinary calculi. Management practices that decrease the incidence of urolithiasis include reducing grain consumption, adding ammonium chloride to the diet, keeping the calcium:phosphorus ratio ~2:1, and keeping the magnesium level low. Perineal urethrostomy can be used as a salvage operation for commercial goats with urolithiasis but is not recommended for pet goats, because recurrences of obstruction and urethral scarring necessitate euthanasia for many. The surgical interventions of choice for pet goats are surgical tube cystotomy or bladder marsupialization. To encourage water consumption, clean, loose TMS should be fed, and clean, fresh water available ad lib. To increase water consumption, especially for high-yielding does, water should be fresh and warm in winter, and fresh and cool in summer.

COMMON DISEASES

Goats harbor several species of **coccidia** but not all exhibit clinical coccidiosis (*see* p 207). Adult goats shed coccidia in feces, contaminate the environment, and infect the newborn. As infection pressure builds up in the pens, morbidity in kids born later increases. Signs include diarrhea or pasty feces, loss of condition, general frailness, and failure to grow. In peracute cases, kids may die without clinical signs. Rotating all the kids through one or two pens is dangerous. To help prevent coccidiosis in artificially reared dairy goats, the kids should be put in small, age-matched groups in outside, portable pens that are moved to clean ground periodically. Eradication is not feasible, but infection can be controlled through good management practices. Coccidiostats added to the water or feed are adjuncts to a management control program and not substitutes. Chronic coccidiosis is one of the main causes of poor growth in kids and is responsible for the uneconomical practice of delaying breeding for a year until the goat has reached adequate size (70 lb [32 kg] for dairy breeds). In Angora goats kept extensively, the problem is seen at weaning, when the kids are kept in smaller lots and fed supplement on the ground.

In pastured and free-ranging goats, **helminthiasis** can assume great clinical significance. GI nematodiasis, liver fluke infestation, and lungworm infections all may be seen. Age-related resistance to parasitism in goats is weak relative to that in other ruminants. Although most common in yearlings during their first season on pasture, clinical parasitism may be seen in adults as well. Poor growth, weight loss, diarrhea, a scruffy hair coat, signs of anemia, and intermandibular edema (bottle jaw) may be seen with GI parasitism or liver fluke disease. *Haemonchus contortus* infection has emerged as a major constraint in the expanding meat goat industry in the southeastern USA. Persistent coughing in late summer and autumn is the usual presentation of lungworms; secondary bacterial pneumonia with fever is a common sequela. Parasitism is insidious on hobby farms, where the problem may not exist for several years and then suddenly explodes as goat numbers continue to increase and facilities become overstocked. Tapeworm proglottids are often noted in goat feces by owners. Although tapeworms are not generally considered to be of clinical importance, their discovery can be used to review the subject of helminthiasis with owners and develop an overall parasite control program (*see* p 312).

Clostridium perfringens type D can be fatal, and it is not always associated with the classic "change in quality and quantity of feed." In problem herds, vaccination every 4–6 mo may be necessary, because goats may not maintain protective immunity as long as sheep or cattle when given the same commercial vaccines. Vaccination prevents the acute death syndrome, but occasionally even vaccinated goats may develop acute enteritis. Affected goats develop severe diarrhea and profound depression; milk yield drops abruptly. Death may result in 24 hr. Treatment involves administration of antitoxin, analgesics, fluid therapy, correction of acidosis, and antibiotics.

Vaccination for **contagious ecthyma** (sore mouth, *see* p 866) is not indicated unless the disease exists on the premises. The main problems with infected kids are difficulty in nursing, spreading lesions to the does' udders or the assistants' hands, and attendance at goat shows being disallowed. Live virus vaccine is used by scarifying the skin (eg, inside the thighs or under the tail) and painting on the vaccine. Both natural lesions and those resulting from vaccination may last as long as 4 wk, but after the scabs have dropped off, the goats can go to shows.

Chronic wasting is seen quite frequently; it is not a single disease but a syndrome. Generally, if a goat is well fed, kept in a stress-free environment, and has good teeth and a low parasite load, it should thrive and produce. If it does not, and begins "wasting," it should be culled immediately. The major causes of chronic wasting include poor nutrition, parasitism, dental problems, paratuberculosis, internal visceral abscesses due to *Corynebacterium pseudotuberculosis* (*ovis*) or *Trueperella pyogenes*, locomotor problems (particularly arthritis due to retrovirus infection [CAE virus]), and chronic hidden infections such as metritis, peritonitis, or pneumonia. Tumors are occasionally diagnosed in older goats. These diseases are rarely treatable, and many are contagious; this is the basis for the strict culling policy, which is vital to the overall productivity of a herd.

Paratuberculosis in goats differs from that in cattle (*see* p 762); gross postmortem lesions are less pronounced, and profuse diarrhea occurs less commonly in goats until right before death. Consequently, many cases may go undiagnosed until necropsy. The ileocecal node is the most rewarding tissue for bacteriologic culture and histopathology. Diagnostic testing for caprine paratuberculosis includes agar gel immunodiffusion, pooled liquid fecal culture, direct fecal PCR, and ELISA. The control program for paratuberculosis in goats is similar to that in cattle.

Caprine arthritis and encephalitis (CAE, *see* p 747) virus has emerged as an important infectious agent of intensively raised dairy goats, but all breeds of goats are susceptible to this retrovirus. CAE infection in goats can manifest in numerous ways: subclinical, persistent infection; a progressive paresis of young goats 2–12 mo old; agalactia with a firm, noninflamed udder at parturition in bred females; or an arthritic condition with pain and swollen joints in adults. A chronic, progressive interstitial pneumonia or a wasting syndrome may also be seen in adults. CAE infection has been considered primarily to be spread from dam to offspring through virus-laden colostrum and milk, and control programs have been aimed at separating the newborns from the adult population and feeding heat-treated colostrum and pasteurized milk. Infection may persist in herds in which this is practiced due to horizontal transmission between adults. Regular testing and rigorous culling of all seropositive goats, or strict segregation of seropositive and seronegative goats, must be practiced if disease eradication is the goal.

For mastitis in goats, *see* p 1367.

HEALTH-MANAGEMENT INTERACTION: HORSES

Proper management can reduce the incidence of many disease conditions in horses. Informed management of the environment and diet, routine foot and dental care, and adherence to an appropriate deworming and vaccination program form the basis of a preventive health program. Client education is important for compliance; owners are more likely to follow recommended changes in husbandry programs once they appreciate the advantages. Diet manipulation reduces the incidence of certain types of colic and exercise-induced myopathies, good dental care improves feed utilization, minimizing exposure to barn dusts and molds reduces the risk of recurrent airway obstruction (chronic obstructive pulmonary disease), and individually designed deworming and vaccination programs reduce morbidity and mortality due to parasitism and infectious disease. Owners should be aware of the normal vital signs and proper movement of a healthy horse, so that they will be better able to recognize when a health problem such as pneumonia, colic, or lameness develops. New modalities for prevention and treatment are always evolving. In addition, the use of complementary or alternative medicine such as acupuncture, acupressure, chiropractic procedures, photomodulation, and massage has grown in equine care (*see* COMPLEMENTARY AND ALTERNATIVE VETERINARY MEDICINE, p 2078). Knowledgeable owners working with a veterinarian and a farrier can result in a productive and pleasant life for every horse.

HOUSING

Stabled horses are exposed to numerous respiratory and GI pathogens, including viruses, bacteria, mold spores, dust mites, and parasites. Stable environments affect disease transmission in terms of air quality and ventilation, population density, and general cleanliness. Barns should be constructed to optimize ventilation and light, minimize exposure to dust and molds, provide temperature regulation, facilitate cleaning and disinfection, and provide ample space for each horse. Windows and skylights provide sunlight and natural ventilation. Sunlight is a potent killer of many bacteria and viruses; it also promotes coat shedding and regular estrous cycles. Eight air changes per hour is considered adequate ventilation for temperate climates and average humidity. (*See also* VENTILATION, p 2116.) Ceiling or wall-mounted fans can be used to increase air circulation on hot, humid days. Stall doors open at the top or made of heavy mesh screening provide better ventilation. Stalls should have nonslip flooring and walls or partitions that prevent direct contact between horses in adjacent stalls. Suggested stall dimensions for adult horses and for mares with foals are 3.6 × 3.6 m and 5 × 5 m, respectively. Doorways should be at least 2.4 m high × 1.2 m wide.

Recurrent airway obstruction (chronic obstructive pulmonary disease [see p 1455]), and noninfectious inflammatory airway disease are associated with airway hypersensitivity to environmental allergens and irritants and exposure to organic dust. The most commonly incriminated allergens are fungal spores and pollens, but barn dust is also rich in dust from shavings, sawdust, manure, hay, animal hair and dander, silica from dirt in indoor arenas, and endotoxin. The amount of air contaminants increases with the dustiness of the barn, bedding, and forage. Management techniques that help prevent this condition include substituting wood chips, peat moss, or shredded paper for dusty straw bedding; avoiding dusty concentrates; using shallow rather than deep feed containers; and soaking hay before feeding at ground level. Air quality can be improved further if bedding and feed are not stored above the stalls. Riding areas and the dust they generate should be situated away from stalls to reduce exposure to dust.

Feeds should be stored in dry containers to reduce contamination with molds and animal excreta. Moldy hay and silage feeding have been associated with cases of equine botulism. Opossum feces can transmit infective sporocysts of *Sarcocystis neurona*, the causative agent of equine protozoal myeloencephalitis (*see* p 1309). Contamination of feeds by deer urine has been incriminated in the spread of certain strains of *Leptospira* (*see* p 652).

Regular disinfection of stables and feed and water buckets helps reduce persistence of infectious agents in the environment. Organic debris inactivates most chemical disinfectants; therefore, disinfection should begin with physical cleaning (ie, hosing, scrubbing) of all surfaces followed by chemical disinfection. Phenols, quaternary ammonium compounds, and chlorine are the most commonly used disinfectants. (*See also* ANTISEPTICS AND DISINFECTANTS, p 2738.)

To further reduce spread of infectious disease, stalls should have walls or partitions to prevent direct contact between horses in adjacent stalls. Pregnant mares, mares with foals, and weanlings should be kept separate from yearlings and adult horses. Ideally, new arrivals should be isolated from the resident horse population for 30 days to reduce introduction of contagious respiratory diseases, including respiratory viruses (eg, equine influenza virus and equine herpesviruses 1 and 4) and bacterial infections (eg, *Streptococcus equi*). Alcohol-based hand sanitizer gels are very effective against most infectious respiratory viruses and bacteria. Wall-mounted hand gel dispensers can be placed strategically throughout barns and tack rooms to improve hand hygiene and to reduce transfer of infectious diseases.

PASTURE

Horses should have ample time on good quality pasture. The opportunity to graze and exercise improves condition, prevents boredom-related behaviors (eg, cribbing and weaving), and reduces the risk of large-intestinal impactions. Grazing on grass also helps reduce the incidence of gastric ulcers. Reducing the time spent in poorly ventilated barns reduces exposure to many inhalant allergens incriminated in development of recurrent airway obstruction. Access to good forage provides a natural source of vitamins and fiber. If horses are fed in groups, sufficient space should be allowed to minimize competition and to ensure that even the most submissive horse has access to an adequate diet. Feeding hay and grain in elevated feeders off the ground reduces ingestion of sand, infective parasite eggs, and animal excreta.

Safe, durable fencing should be used for pastures and paddocks to reduce the risk of self-trauma. Double fencing between paddocks minimizes transmission of contagious disease between horses. Overcrowding should be avoided. Overgrazed pastures, which result from overstocking, lead to extremes in ground conditions (eg, dust or mud), contribute to increased parasite burdens, and favor overgrowth of potentially toxic plants.

Excessive dust increases the risk of respiratory infections among young horses by inhalation of soil saprophytes, such as *Rhodococcus equi* (*see* p 1451). The risk of this potentially fatal bacterial pneumonia on farms where the disease is enzootic can be reduced by minimizing exposure of young (<4 mo old), susceptible foals to aerosolized *R equi* using environmental control strategies such as decreasing dust formation on pastures and paddocks, housing foals in well-ventilated areas, rotating pastures, reducing the size of mare-foal bands, irrigating and planting dirt areas with grass, and removing feces frequently from stalls, paddocks, indoor arenas, and pastures. Breeding mares earlier in the season to ensure foaling during colder weather may reduce the number of susceptible foals exposed to dry, dusty summer conditions. On farms where *R equi* is endemic and foal morbidity and mortality rates are high despite attempts at pasture management, the incidence of disease can be reduced with preventive administration of 1 L of hyperimmune plasma containing high concentrations of antibodies against *R equi* to newborn foals within the first week of life, followed by a second dose 25 days later.

Overstocking in barns and pastures favors outbreaks of other contagious respiratory infections caused by viral and bacterial pathogens spread between horses via aerosolization of respiratory tract secretions. Enteric infections with *Clostridium difficile* and *C perfringens* can become endemic on some farms. An increased incidence of *Clostridium* diarrhea in newborn foals has been associated with foaling on dirt, gravel, or sand surfaces, and with stall confinement or limited turnout on dry lots during the first 3 days of life.

Whenever possible, horses should not be pastured on sandy soils, because sand ingestion during grazing predisposes to colonic and rectal sand impaction, chronic diarrhea, and weight loss. If sandy pastures are unavoidable, the risk of sand colic can be reduced by feeding psyllium at regular intervals and by providing trace mineralized salt with equal parts of bone meal.

Horses grazing on pastures near water may be at increased risk of contracting certain diseases such as Potomac horse fever, caused by *Neorickettsia risticii* and disseminated by aquatic insects and snails (*see* p 283). Pastures and paddocks should be kept free of standing or stagnant water to reduce the breeding grounds for mosquitoes carrying infectious equine viral pathogens, including West Nile virus and Eastern and Western equine encephalomyelitis viruses (*see* p 1291).

NUTRITION

During the last 20–30 yr, there has been an increased awareness of equine nutrition and its importance to the health of the horse. (*See also* NUTRITION: HORSES, p 2312). In every stage of life, nutrition is the foundation for equine health and longevity. The dietary needs of a horse change as it goes through each life stage. The great varieties of commercial feeds on the market attest to the recognition of different diets for different life stages. Horses must be provided with an adequate supply of energy, protein, vitamins, and minerals and have access to fresh, clean water.

Adequate fresh water intake is essential for every horse. Storage tanks, troughs, or pails should be placed so the horse can reach in comfortably. Because most horses are reluctant to put their head in a trough or pail below eye level, the water level should be kept high. If water levels get too low, many horses will refuse to drink. The optimal temperature for drinking water is 68°–78°F (20°–26°C). Horses will reduce water intake if the water temperature is too cold or too warm. When daytime temperatures exceed 100°F (38°C), water in exposed pipes or hoses will be dangerously hot and should not be used for drinking or bathing.

The nutrient energy requirement of the horse depends on its level of activity, the energy content of the diet, and the capacity of the animal's digestive system. The size and weight of the newborn foal is influenced by the nutrition of the pregnant mare. Horses fed for rapid body and skeletal growth may develop bone abnormalities or be more prone to lameness conditions. A balanced diet should be fed according to the desired rate of gain within the sound parameters of good health. The best measure of growth in a young horse is weight, and the best description of size of a horse is a combination of height and weight. A high correlation between the measure of the heart girth and body weight in the horse has been reported. In young, growing horses, monthly measurements are helpful to monitor growth changes.

There are several reasons to know the weight of horses. Many feeding requirements are based on percentages of the horse's weight. Most feed recommendations are stated in the amount of feed (in pounds or kilograms) the horse should receive based on body weight. In young horses, "developmental orthopedic disease," although a multifactorial condition, can be related to rapid growth or imbalances in energy, protein, and minerals (*see* p 1148). The proper balance of protein, calcium, phosphorus, zinc, and copper is important in supporting healthy endochondral ossification and in stabilizing bone collagen and elastin synthesis. The amount of nutrients required in the diet for normal bone development are dictated by rate of growth. Excessive energy intake contributes to osteochondrosis by decreasing bone density and cortical thickness.

Deficiency of protein must be severe to interfere with endochondral ossification. Rapidly increasing protein intake may produce faster bone growth; however, if the diet lacks adequate minerals to support this increased growth, altered endochondral ossification can be seen. Calcium and phosphorus balance affect bone density, rate of growth, and cartilage thickness. Inadequate amounts of copper and zinc have been associated with an increased incidence of osteochondrosis and osteodysgenesis.

Some of the most common mistakes made when feeding young horses include feeding excessive grain and leafy legumes (eg, alfalfa, which results in too high an energy intake), feeding a diet with too little zinc or copper to support rate of growth, and feeding a diet with an improper calcium:phosphorus ratio. Cereal grains and grass forages are low in calcium, phosphorus, protein, and lysine. Excess energy from cereal grains may be more detrimental than excess energy from grass forages; one reason may be that energy from grain is derived from starch, whereas energy from grass forage comes from microbial production of volatile fatty acids. Starch, but not volatile fatty acids, stimulates insulin secretion, which has been implicated in stimulating hormone changes that contribute to osteochondrosis.

Older horses often have dental problems that compromise feed intake and mastication. Extruded or soft pelleted feeds are ideal. Hay should be good quality, leafy, and easy to chew. The most variable dietary requirement for any horse is energy. A certain amount of energy is required for maintenance and daily activity. Metabolic demands are increased for such activities as growing, performance activity, or lactation. In some activities, such as racing, jumping, or polo, the energy requirement may be increased by as much as 100%.

Diet manipulation can help treat, control, and prevent other disease conditions. Horses with recurrent airway obstruction should be fed as dust-free a feed as possible. Adding water or oil to grains decreases dust. Hay should be thoroughly soaked and fed close to the ground. If complete pelleted feeds are fed, hay can be removed completely from the diet. On sandy soils, hay should be fed off the ground to reduce sand ingestion. Dietary management can be used to reduce the risk of gastric ulcers. Alfalfa hay, with its high calcium and protein concentration, acts as a buffering antacid and has a protective effect on the nonglandular squamous mucosa. Small hay meals fed frequently or access to pasture also reduces the risk of gastric ulceration.

Nutritional management for Quarter horses with hyperkalemic periodic paralysis (*see* p 1047) is focused on decreasing dietary intake of potassium and increasing renal potassium losses. Dietary manipulation includes avoiding high-potassium feeds such as alfalfa hay, brome grass, canola oil, soybean meal or oil, and sugar or beet molasses and replacing them with timothy or bermuda grass, beet pulp, and grains such as oats, corn, wheat, or barley. Affected horses should be exercised regularly and have access to pasture.

Heavily muscled breeds of horses, including Quarter horses, draft horses, and Warmbloods, are prone to myopathies associated with increased muscle glycogen stores and polysaccharide storage inclusions in type II muscle fibers. Successful management of this condition, known as polysaccharide storage myopathy, focuses on increasing the fat content of the diet and eliminating or reducing grain intake. (*See also* MYOPATHIES IN HORSES, p 1176.)

Management practices to reduce the risk of impaction include ad lib access to fresh water, adequate exercise, good quality feed, and good dental care. If impaction has been a problem, poorly digestible feeds (eg, mature forages) should be replaced with low-fiber, highly digestible forages (eg, growing grass or legume hays). A complete pelleted or extruded feed helps maintain soft feces.

Grazing lush pastures or consuming large amounts of legume hay and the development of laminitis have long been associated. Anecdotal observations indicate that pasture-associated laminitis occurs at times of rapid grass growth (eg, spring and early summer and in the fall after rainfall) that favor accumulation of certain carbohydrates such as fructans, starches, and sugars. Some horses and ponies may be more susceptible to pasture-associated laminitis because of genetic predisposition and other metabolic factors, including obesity, peripheral insulin resistance, and hyperinsulinemia. Strategies to reduce the risk of laminitis focus on limiting the intake of nonstructural carbohydrates such as fructans from pasture and other feedstuffs.

Horses and ponies with a history of recurrent laminitis should have limited pasture access during periods of rapid grass growth, such as spring and early summer. Nonstructural carbohydrate content also tends to increase during the morning, reaches maximal values in the afternoon, and then declines overnight. Therefore, a popular recommendation is to turn "susceptible" individuals out on pasture overnight or during the early morning and to remove them from pasture by mid-morning. Stemmy, mature pastures should be avoided, because mature grasses may contain more fructans. Turning susceptible individuals onto pasture that has been exposed to low temperatures in conjunction with bright sunlight (eg, as in the fall after a flush of growth followed by cool sunny days) should be avoided, because colder temperatures reduce grass growth and result in concentration of the fructan.

If feeding forage, lush legume hays should be avoided, because they tend to have higher nonstructural carbohydrate content. Soaking hay before feeding may help reduce the amount of fructans being fed. Grain and sweet feeds should be avoided.

The terms mature, senior, and geriatric refer to horses that have completed their growth cycle. However, because aging is a continuous process, there is no discrete age range for each category. Improved methods of overall care, management, and diet have enabled horses to live into their 20s or 30s. This increased longevity means they are used in a variety of leisure or competitive activities well into their teens or 20s. Good management of still-active older horses means recognition and evaluation of conditions that occur with age (eg, arthritis, hyperadrenocorticism, gastric ulcers, laminitis, navicular disease, kidney or liver dysfunction), followed by therapeutic management and special dietary considerations. Horses with arthritis require a balanced diet with adequate minerals. In horses prone to hyperadrenocorticism, the use of fat-supplemented feeds with highly digestible fiber and reduced starch and sugar intake is important. Horses with liver or kidney conditions should not be fed legume hays and fat-supplemented feeds. Horses confined to stalls most of the time are more prone to intestinal problems and development of undesirable behaviors.

FOOT CARE

Hoof care is essential for good mobility and comfort of the horse. "No hoof, no horse" is a common expression as true today as it was 200 yr ago. Proper trimming at regular intervals will result in good hoof and leg balance. Conditions such as hoof cracks, thrush, and white line disease can be recognized early and treated properly. All horse owners should learn to recognize the initial signs of laminitis so that treatment can be started as soon as possible. In young foals, weanlings, and yearlings, frequent hoof trimming will assure proper weight bearing and bone alignment. A balanced foot early in a horse's life will also help to avoid potential lameness and alleviate injuries later in life. For a horse to perform to the best of its ability, it must be sound (free from pain). Soundness is an aspect of health and is more than the absence of lameness. A sound horse can better meet the demands of physical and mental activity. (*See also* LAMENESS IN HORSES, p 1096.)

DENTAL CARE

Regular dental care is essential for the comfort and longevity of the horse. The upper jaw of the horse is wider than the lower jaw, which results in very efficient crushing of food particles. The chewing surface of the teeth are at an angle of 10–15 degrees to each other. The grinding action of the molar teeth tend to produce sharp points on the outside of the upper molars and on the lingual aspect of the lower molars. Floating to balance the arcade is required for general maintenance of the horse's teeth. Irregularities are most common in the incisor and molar teeth of mature and geriatric horses. The mouth of the horse changes throughout life, but the greatest changes occur from ages 2–5; therefore, semiannual or annual treatment is important. Sharp points and uneven wear can cause problems not initially considered to be tooth related; eg, the horse may be prone to mouth ulcers, choke, gastric ulcers, back pain, or erratic head carriage when the bit is in the mouth. Behavior problems may be a result of long, sharp teeth, an uneven arcade, or abscesses in the teeth or gums. Complete oral examination, including visualization of the premolars and molars, requires sedation, a speculum, and good lighting. Motorized dental instruments and carbide float blades have made equine dental care more precise as well as more comfortable for the horse. Age determination of horses has traditionally been done by examining the incisor arcade. Although not an exact science, it is a useful tool for those with experience. (*See also* DENTISTRY IN LARGE ANIMALS, p 175.)

PARASITE CONTROL

Control of internal parasites is a cornerstone of equine management and a continual endeavor. Control programs should be tailored to each farm situation and require a cooperative program between the horse owner and the veterinarian. The principal internal parasites of horses are nematodes. Unfortunately, many species of adult cyathostomes have developed resistance to standard doses of the benzimidazoles and the tetrahydropyrimidines. Among intensively managed horse populations, treatment with macrocyclic lactones (eg, ivermectin, moxidectin) does not suppress strongyle egg counts for as long as previously expected. Among foals, weanlings, and even yearlings, there are increasing reports of ascarids becoming resistant to ivermectin and moxidectin. (*See also* GASTROINTESTINAL PARASITES OF HORSES, p 315, and ANTHELMINTICS, p 2637.)

A program of anthelmintic resistance involves multiple parasites and multiple drug classes, and must consider horses of all ages. No single parasite control program is ideal for all horses. Age of the horse, population density, region of the country, climate, method of confinement (eg, stall or pasture), and pasture size and quality can affect the choice of parasite control programs. As horses age, they develop resistance to reinfection with certain parasites, such as *Strongyloides westeri* and *Parascaris equorum*. Resistance to most strongyles is incomplete. Although anthelmintics are the primary method of parasite control, other factors such as pasture management and stable environment are also important.

The parasites of greatest concern in horses are large strongyles, small strongyles, roundworms, pinworms, stomach bots, and tapeworms. GI parasites can cause acute medical problems as well as chronic debilitation. They may be responsible for diarrhea, intestinal impactions or irritation (colic), and poor performance. The result can be slow growth in young horses, poor performance, acute bouts of colic, and death in severe instances. The migrating ascarids (*Parascaris equorum*) are the primary cause of pulmonary inflammation and intestinal rupture in foals and weanlings. The control of large strongyles with improved anthelmintics has allowed the small strongyles (cyathostomes) to become a greater problem. Reports of tapeworms have also increased.

The three methods of diagnosis of parasites are direct examination of feces, concentrations of worm eggs by flotation, and culture of feces for infective larva. The direct examination method is quick but not always accurate. The flotation method for parasite egg concentration is more accurate to determine the type and number of parasites. The culture method is more suitable for laboratory use and research purposes. The effectiveness of any parasite control program can be evaluated by fecal examination. The fecal examination should be done before administration of a particular dewormer and then again 14 days later. The amount of decreases in egg population will determine the effectiveness of the dewormer. Parasite egg counts that remain high after use of a particular dewormer indicate the presence of resistance and a need to change the control program.

The three major classes of anthelmintics available for parasite control in horses are the avermectins, benzimidazoles, and pyrantels. The avermectins have a broad range of activity, are safe and effective at low doses, and control adult and migrating larval nematodes. Deworming of mares immediately after foaling lessens the foal's exposure to parasites in the mare's manure. Avermectins are not effective against tapeworms; however, the combination of ivermectin with praziquantel is effective against tapeworms as well as large and small strongyles, ascarids, pinworms, and bots. The benzimidazoles (oxibendazole, fenbendazole, and oxfendazole) are effective against most nematodes but not against encysted small strongyles or tapeworms. The pyrantels are effective against large and small strongyles, ascarids, and pinworms. Pyrantels kill nematode parasites slowly. Pyrantel is available as a paste (single dose), and as a tartrate salt that can be used as a daily dewormer mixed in the feed; it is effective against tapeworms but not bots. The avermectins are effective against bot larva and are recommended in the fall after the botfly season.

A fourth class of anthelmintics, the isoquinolines, contains praziquantel, a narrow-spectrum drug approved for horses as a cestocide. Praziquantel is available in combination with either ivermectin or moxidectin.

To slow the development of drug-resistant parasites, the focus of most parasite control programs is to reduce selection pressure for resistance by customizing deworming protocols for the farm and individual horses. This strategy includes identifying horses most susceptible to parasites (ie, the high egg shredders) and maximizing refugia (those parasites not exposed to drug selection pressure) by reducing the overall number of anthelmintic treatments administered and by monitoring the efficacy of different classes of dewormers using the fecal egg count reduction test. An effective deworming protocol for horses should incorporate a cestocide (eg, a praziquantel-containing product or a double dose of pyrantel pamoate) and a boticide (eg, ivermectin or moxidectin) once or twice a year to control tapeworms and bots, respectively, and a larvicidal dose of anthelmintic effective against encysted cyanthostomes (eg, fenbendazole 10 mg/kg/day, PO, for 5 days, or a single dose of moxidectin) during early winter months in northern climates or during early summer in warmer climates. Foals should be maintained on a regular deworming schedule every 60 days that includes anthelmintics safe and effective against ascarids. Treatments effective against other nematodes (including encysted cyathostomes) and cestodes should be included in the deworming protocols for foals during the first year of life.

Effective deworming programs should also include one or more of the following nonchemical methods of parasite control: 1) Avoid overstocking and overgrazing pastures. 2) Keep pasture roughs mowed to a height of 3–8 in. 3) During hot, dry weather, harrow or rake pastures to disperse manure piles and expose larvae to sun. Rest the pasture at least 3–4 wk after harrowing. 4) Cross-graze pastures with other species. Cattle, sheep, and goats serve as biological vacuums for equine parasites. 5) Make at least one cutting of hay off some pastures to help reduce the parasite burden. 6) Plant an annual crop such as winter wheat. 7) Feed hay and grain in raised containers and not directly on the ground. 8) Remove manure from stalls, paddocks, and pastures every 24–72 hr before strongyle eggs have a chance to hatch and develop into infective larvae (5–7 days during optimal conditions). 9) Clean water sources regularly to prevent fecal contamination. 10) Quarantine new arrivals and perform fecal examinations. Use a larvicidal treatment before turning out new arrivals on pastures. 11) Use fecal egg counts, performed at the proper times, to identify and monitor high, medium, and low strongyle egg shedders, to monitor the efficacy of anthelmintics being used, and to evaluate new arrivals. 12) Compost manure. Properly composted manure will kill strongyle larvae and many ascarid eggs.

VACCINATION PROGRAM

The goal of vaccination is to develop and maintain both individual and herd immunity against infectious diseases. Commercial vaccines are available for rabies, encephalomyelitis (Eastern, Western, and Venezuelan), tetanus, influenza, equine herpesviruses 1 and 4, botulism, equine ehrlichiosis (Potomac horse fever), equine viral arteritis, rotavirus, West Nile virus, and *Streptococcus equi* (strangles). Vaccination programs are formulated based on the animal's age, use, and level of exposure. Broodmare vaccination is important to provide active immunity for the mare and passive immunity for the foal via transfer of colostral antibodies. Vaccination guidelines for foals have been modified because of the interference of maternal antibodies with the initial vaccination response. Sources such as the American Association of Equine Practitioners can provide the most current equine vaccination recommendations for horses in the USA.

The following vaccination recommendations assume that foals are born to vaccinated mares and have absorbed adequate colostral antibodies with IgG levels >800 mg/dL.

Foals with failure of passive antibody transfer (ie, IgG levels <200 mg/dL) and/or foals born to unvaccinated mares can receive their initial vaccination for equine herpesvirus 1 and 4, tetanus, and Eastern and Western equine encephalomyelitis beginning at 3–4 mo of age, followed by a second dose 4–6 wk later and a third dose at 10–12 mo of age. These foals can receive their first dose of rabies vaccine at 3–4 mo of age, followed by a booster at 12 mo. Influenza vaccination can be started at 6 mo of age. Foals born to mares that have never been exposed to or vaccinated against West Nile virus can receive their first vaccination at 3–5 mo of age.

Tetanus: *Clostridium tetani* is present in all parts of the world. Tetanus occurs most commonly when wounds become contaminated with the organism from the soil. Vaccination is recommended for all horses and ponies on an annual basis. A horse with an unknown vaccination status that sustains an injury should receive a dose of tetanus antitoxin along with a dose of tetanus toxoid. A second dose of toxoid should be given 4 wk later. Foals from vaccinated mares should be given a three-dose series at 6, 7, and 9 mo of age. Foals from unvaccinated mares should receive tetanus toxoid at 3, 4, and 6 mo of age. Whenever a vaccinated horse experiences a serious wound, a tetanus booster may be indicated.

Equine Herpesvirus 1 and 4 (Rhinopneumonitis): Two types of equine herpesviruses vaccine are available, EHV-1 and EHV-4. The EHV-1 virus is the primary cause of abortion and neurologic disease in horses. The EHV-4 virus is the primary cause of respiratory infections, especially in young horses. The control of rhinopneumonitis is by a combination of vaccination and good management practices. To prevent abortion, a killed EHV-1 vaccine should be administered to pregnant mares at 3, 5, 7, and 9 mo of gestation. Respiratory disease is best prevented using a combination vaccine of EHV-1 and EHV-4. There is no evidence that vaccination protects against the neurologic form of the disease. Vaccine recommendations for foals are three doses every 4 wk starting at 6 mo of age, and a booster at 1 yr of age. Pleasure and performance horses should be vaccinated every 3–6 mo, depending on the risk of exposure. Broodmares should have an EHV-4 vaccination 2–4 wk before foaling to ensure the availability of colostral immunity.

Encephalitis: Eastern equine encephalitis (EEE) virus has a wide distribution. This includes the eastern USA, Central and South America, and eastern Canada. In the USA, EEE is seen primarily in the southeastern states but has been reported in all states east of the Mississippi River. EEE in horses is nearly always fatal regardless of treatment. Infected horses usually become comatose, seizure, and die in 36–48 hr.

The virus of Western equine encephalitis (WEE) is primarily located in the western USA. In recent years, reports of WEE have not been common, probably as a result of adequate vaccination programs. The virus is not as pathogenic as EEE, and animals infected with WEE have a greater chance of survival. Mortality is usually 50%.

Venezuelan equine encephalitis (VEE) virus causes outbreaks of disease in horses in Mexico, Central and South America, and occasionally the southern USA. The VEE vaccine is a single vaccine or in combination with EEE and WEE. Its need is limited to those horses traveling to or located in endemic areas.

West Nile virus (WNV) disease is considered a zoonotic disease similar to the encephalitis viruses. The bird population allows for maintenance of the virus, which is then transmitted by mosquitoes to both people and horses. There is very little risk of disease from any infected horses. Vaccination protocols for broodmares, foals, and adult horses are the same as those for Eastern and Western encephalitis. Combination vaccines that include EEE, WEE, and WNV are available.

Influenza: Influenza is one of the most frequent causes of viral respiratory disease in horses and is highly contagious among susceptible horses. Therefore, vaccination is recommended for all foals, broodmares, and horses at risk of exposure, usually as a result of showing, racing, or shipping. Young foals from vaccinated mares, because of maternal antibodies, should be vaccinated at 9, 10, and 12 mo of age. Foals from unvaccinated mares should be vaccinated earlier. The intranasal vaccine can be used every 6 mo in young, susceptible performance horses 2–4 yr old. A vaccination is recommended every 6 mo for horses exposed to other horses at equine events.

Rabies: Signs of rabies include the inability to eat or drink, disorientation, and incoordination. Rabies is fatal, and also poses a health risk to those who handle infected horses. Prevention in horses is primarily via vaccination. Broodmares should be vaccinated 4–6 wk before foaling. Foals from vaccinated mares should be vaccinated at 6 and 7 mo of age and again at 12 mo of age. Foals from unvaccinated mares should be vaccinated at 3, 4, and 12 mo of age. All adult horses should be vaccinated annually.

Potomac Horse Fever: Potomac horse fever (equine monocytic ehrlichiosis, equine ehrlichial colitis) is caused by *Neorickettsia risticii*. Vaccination is recommended in endemic areas, such as near freshwater streams, rivers, ponds, and heavily irrigated pastures. Annual boosters in the spring are recommended. Pregnant mares should receive a booster before foaling. Although the vaccine may lessen the impact of the disease, it appears not to prevent abortion in pregnant mares.

Botulism: Equine botulism is mostly seen in the Mid-Atlantic area of the United States, but the disease has also been reported worldwide. In the USA, the most common types are B and C botulism, although type A has been reported in the western USA. The spores of *Colostridium botulinum* are found in the soil and are resistant to light, drying, and heat. The Type B vaccine gives good protection in adult horses. Adult horses and broodmares in areas where botulism is a potential hazard should receive initially three doses at 30-day intervals and then annual boosters. Foals from vaccinated mares in endemic areas should be vaccinated at 2, 3, and 4 mo of age, because colostral immunity does not always occur. Foals from unvaccinated mares should be vaccinated at 2, 4, and 8 wk of age. The use of Type B vaccine in areas where Type C occurs has uncertain results.

***Streptococcus equi* Infection:** *Streptococcus equi* infection (equine strangles, equine distemper) can be highly contagious. Use of the IM or intranasal vaccine is recommended only in those situations or on premises where the disease has been a problem. The IM vaccine involves three injections administered 2–4 wk apart, starting at 4 mo of age in foals, with a booster at 12 mo of age. If the intranasal vaccine is used, vaccination can begin at 6–9 mo of age, with a second dose given 3–4 wk later and a third dose administered at 12 mo of age. Adult horses, if in potential disease situations, should receive an annual vaccination. Broodmares on endemic farms should receive an annual booster using the IM vaccine 4–6 wk before foaling. Because of the increased risk of inducing immune-mediated purpura hemorrhagica, horses with titers to the SeM surface protein of *S equi* in excess of 1:1,600 may not need to be vaccinated.

Rotavirus: Foal diarrhea as a result of rotavirus infection can be a severe problem on some breeding farms. Single cases or a farm outbreak can occur. Therefore, pregnant mares should be vaccinated IM at 8, 9, and 10 mo of gestation. This will increase the amount of colostral immunoglobulins. It is a vaccine for use in particular situations or areas of high endemicity.

Equine Infectious Anemia: In the acute state, equine infectious anemia (swamp fever) causes severe RBC destruction and anemia. Once infected, a horse can become a carrier for life and is a threat to other horses. The virus is transmitted by bloodsucking insects. Currently, the disease is uncommon, and most horse owners are aware of its dire consequences. A simple blood test, the Coggins test, is available to detect infected horses. A horse that tests positive cannot cross state lines and is required to be maintained in strict isolation for life. For horses participating in equine activities or being transported across state lines, proof of a negative Coggins test is required. Annual testing of every horse is recommended. No vaccine is available.

PERINATAL MARE AND FOAL CARE

Pregnant mares need adequate daily exercise in a paddock or pasture, and any horses kept together should be compatible, which helps to reduce stress. Vaccinations and deworming should be done before the mare is bred, with no vaccinations given during the first 90 days of gestation. In general, except for rhinopneumonitis and possibly botulism, all vaccinations should be avoided until 30 days before foaling. Thirty days before foaling, the mare should receive vaccinations for Eastern, Western, and West Nile encephalitis, as well as for tetanus.

For the first 7 or 8 mo of gestation, the routine diet of pasture or hay and concentrate to maintain good body condition is all that is necessary. Mares too thin at foaling will not milk well, and mares too fat are subject to developing laminitis or have foaling difficulties. During the last 3 mo of gestation, the mare should be on a gradual, increasing plane of nutrition. The size of the fetus increases significantly during the last trimester, and the mare's weight can be expected to increase. During this time, the mare should be on good-quality legume or grass hay and a concentrate ration of 12%–14% protein. A mare weighing 1,000–1,200 pounds (454–544 kg) can be expected to gain 150–200 pounds during the last trimester with the proper diet. A body condition score of 6.5–7.5 is ideal for most pregnant mares at foaling.

The mare should be checked for the presence of a Caslick's operation of the vulva, which should be opened if present. The foaling process is continuous, with labor divided into three stages. Stage 1 may be 1–4 hr as uterine contractions increase in strength and frequency. Stage 2 is the actual delivery of the foal, which takes 5–15 min unless there are complications. Stage 3 is the passage of the fetal membranes, which should occur within a 3-hr period. If the membranes are retained for >3 hr, then veterinary treatment is necessary because severe sepsis or laminitis can result. Some mares may exhibit abdominal pain after foaling, and low-dose analgesics may be helpful. The normal placenta will weigh ~10–12 pounds (4.5–5.4 kg) or ~10% of the foal's birth weight.

The mare should be dewormed within 48 hr after foaling to reduce exposure of the foal to parasites. In 90% of foalings, the newborn foal is usually sternal within 1 hr, stands within 2 hr, and nurses within 3 hr. The foaling stall should be at least 14 × 14 feet (4.3 × 4.3 m); a double stall 12 × 20 feet (3.7 × 6.1 m) is more satisfactory. The stall should be bedded with straw or short stem hay. Wood shavings are less desirable because of the possibility of the shavings entering the foal's nostrils or mouth and also contaminating the mare's birth canal. The newborn foal's umbilicus should be dipped in a dilute solution of chlorhexidine (0.5%) or povidone-iodine (1%) several times a day for 2–3 days.

The passage of meconium can be facilitated by use of an enema (warm soapy water, or a commercial sodium-phosphate enema can be used once). Many foals will not nurse satisfactorily or with vigor until the meconium has passed.

Foals have no immunity at birth and acquire it through ingestion of colostrum. Absorption of colostral antibodies occurs within the first 24 hr of life. Ideally, when ~12 hr old, the foal should have a complete veterinary physical examination, including temperature, heart and lung auscultation, and examination for cleft palate, fractured ribs, or entropion. Evaluation of the foal's IgG level is most important. If the foal's serum level is <800 mg/dL, an IV transfusion of plasma is necessary.

Foals should be monitored closely during the first 7 days of life. A healthy foal can become critically ill in a matter of hours. The mare and foal should remain in the box stall for 24–48 hr until the foal is strong enough to follow the mare at a trot or gallop. Then the pair can be turned out in a small area for exercise, which is essential. Haltering and handling the foal during the first week of life will set the stage for the animal's behavior in the future. Mares that reject their foals usually do so right after birth. This is more common in primiparous mares and requires intense supervision.

HEALTH-MANAGEMENT INTERACTION: PIGS

Disease in pork production is generally caused by multiple factors. Microbial pathogens are rarely the sole cause of a health problem on a pig farm. Clinical disease is usually the interaction of a pathogen with errors in management and a variety of contributing influences such as environment and host factors. Many pathogens are endemic in the swine population and yet some farms suffer heavy losses from disease, whereas the impact on other farms is much less because of management differences.

Management and Economic Considerations: Economic considerations influence all decisions regarding health care on pig farms. Health management and *disease prevention* programs tend to be prioritized based on financial return, although other important considerations include animal welfare, food safety, and risk management. Pigs are omnivores extremely well suited to convert low-cost feedstuffs (often including waste products) into meat. Pigs efficiently convert feed to muscle while growing at a rapid rate. In addition, their fecundity is remarkable. Female pigs reach sexual maturity, breed, and produce a litter of ≥10 piglets at ~1 year of age and then continue to produce litters 2.5 times per year.

Health management plays a key role in profitable farming enterprises. Profit is based on maximizing income and minimizing costs. Income is a function of the price received per kg of pork produced times the total amount of pork produced. Therefore, aspects of health management that ensure good reproductive performance and consistent pig numbers at all stages of production and rapid growth contribute to a steady, high income. Production parameters, such as pigs produced per sow per year and measures of throughput, should be carefully monitored to ensure the farm is achieving a high level of productivity. At the same time, production costs must be evaluated to assess the health or profitability of a swine operation. Because feed costs are well over half the cost of production, health management initiatives to reduce feed costs or improve feed efficiency tend to be areas of high priority. Some of the most economically important swine diseases may present with little in the way of clinical signs. For example, porcine proliferative enteropathy (*Lawsonia intracellularis* infection, *see* p 299) might cause thickening of the bowel and reduced feed efficiency without signs of diarrhea or obvious illness, but the cost of the resulting increase in feed consumption likely makes this disease a high priority with regard to a health management program. Cost-benefit of programs should be evaluated to avoid spending so much to reduce the risk of the disease that it outweighs the benefits in improved performance. Therefore, a producer might choose to ignore a management protocol directed at disease control to save money longterm; however, this decision may change with time and circumstances, so medication and vaccine programs, for example, should be constantly assessed.

Production Records: The use of production records is an essential part of a herd health program. Records are used to assess performance and identify areas of concern. When a general issue is identified, records also can be used to help pinpoint the problem as well as assess whether the intervention strategy was successful. Records can be used to set targets and motivate staff to achieve these targets as well as help the veterinarian develop partial budget scenarios to justify health care expenses.

In breeding herds, the parameter most commonly used to assess overall herd performance is average number of pigs weaned per sow per year. On many North American farms, this number is ≥25; some producers achieve a number >30. When this number is lower than the target, it is useful to examine the specific components of the parameter to determine the source of the problem. Pigs weaned per sow per year is a product of "pigs weaned per sow per litter" and "number of litters per sow per year." With a 3-wk lactation, it is possible to achieve ~2.5 litters per sow per year. If the number of litters per sow per year is low, it may be because of a poor farrowing rate (sows bred but failing to farrow; generally 80%–85% is achievable) or it may be because of prebreeding problems such as a long weaning-to-breeding interval (<7 days is typical). A low number of litters per sow per year will probably lead the herd veterinarian to investigate the breeding management; in contrast, if litters per sow per year is close to 2.5 but pigs weaned per sow per year is low, the veterinarian can begin to investigate the farrowing room to determine why litter size at weaning is low (10 pigs per litter is commonly achieved, but this number is increasing because of larger litter sizes being born). The cause of low numbers weaned may be because of small litters being born or a high preweaning mortality.

Record analysis can be used to focus attention so that resources can be concentrated on solving a specific problem. In the post-weaning until market period, the main production records include mortality, growth rate, and feed efficiency. Because feed cost contributes substantially to the cost of producing a market hog, measuring feed consumption and monitoring feed costs are extremely important. During the early growing period, pigs are extremely efficient in using feed to produce muscle. Feed:gain ratios of 1.5:1 or better are expected during the nursery phase (3–10 wk of age). As the pig approaches market age, metabolism changes and the pig begins to produce more fat, which shifts the feed:gain ratio so that >3 kg of feed is needed to produce 1 kg of gain. Overall through the grower-finisher phase, most herds achieve a feed:gain ratio of better than 3:1. Mortality records throughout the production stage are possibly the most useful parameter to identify a health problem. In general, preweaning mortality of ≥10% can be achieved on most farms, with nursery mortality of 3%–4% and grower-finisher mortality of 2%–3% achievable.

Herd Size and Disease Challenge: As in most agricultural businesses, pig farming has an economy of scale; hence, pig farms have grown larger and larger over the past few decades, with a trend toward vertical integration in the industry. The management of health issues in large populations requires a major focus on biosecurity (*see* p 2068). Great efforts are warranted to keep new diseases from entering an immunologically naive population, in addition to programs to restrict the spread of endemic diseases within the herd and especially between one production stage and another. The general strategy to prevent outbreaks of clinical disease is to minimize the level of pathogen challenge while maximizing herd and individual immunity. Poor management might result in a population of pigs with naive immune systems encountering novel pathogens, or in stress leading to a weakened immune system in vulnerable pigs. Alternatively, management errors might result in an overwhelming pathogen challenge in the case of an endemic disease or the entry of a new pathogen into a population of pigs without specific immunity.

One of the most effective management techniques to minimize the challenge from endemic diseases and possibly to eliminate a disease from a swine operation is the use of all-in/all-out pig flow through the various production stages. Commonly a group of sows are moved together into a clean and disinfected farrowing room, and later their piglets are weaned and the sows moved out as a group; all the weanling pigs enter a clean, empty nursery possibly on a separate site from the sow herd. Similarly, the pigs leave the nursery as a group and enter a clean, empty grower-finisher barn, possibly at a different site. This type of flow reduces the chance of endemic disease continuing to cycle in the population.

In summary, many pig diseases are controlled by this combined strategy of minimizing disease challenge and maximizing individual and herd immunity. For example, the common methods used to prevent neonatal diarrhea caused by enterotoxigenic *Escherichia coli* (ETEC) include all-in/all-out farrowing room management, the use of slatted flooring constructed of nonporous material that is easily cleaned, and washing and disinfection protocols to ensure minimal bacteria will be present in the environment to challenge the newborn piglets. At the same time, it is common practice to vaccinate the sows against ETEC before farrowing so they have high levels of specific immunoglobulins present in colostrum and milk to provide passive immunity to the piglets. In addition, it is necessary to ensure the piglets receive these immunoglobulins, so steps such as cross-fostering are important. Disease can occur if either the challenge becomes too great or the immune protection waivers, so both approaches are important and complementary.

Because herd size is often very large, ensuring that the population as a whole has immunity and that pockets of naive animals are not present within the herd can be a challenge. A subpopulation of susceptible animals is likely to act as a reservoir for endemic diseases. This is particularly true for viral diseases for which vaccination is not very effective. For example, it is a common practice to purposely infect all sows in a herd with porcine reproductive and respiratory syndrome (PRRS) virus (*see* p 729) using a live field strain of the virus and at the same time closing the herd to new introduction if the herd is experiencing an outbreak of PRRS. The goal of such a program is to expose all the sows to the PRRS virus so that the entire herd develops immunity. When all the sows are immune, they will pass antibodies and not the virus in colostrum to the piglets. In this way, PRRS can be eliminated from the herd.

Health Strategies: Health strategies can be divided into three categories. First, there are strategies designed to live with endemic diseases. Generally, these are caused by pathogens that survive in the environment and are too difficult to eliminate, or they are ubiquitous organisms that generally cause little problem. The former are handled by maximizing immunity and minimizing the challenge, as outlined above. In the latter, disease flare-ups are often triggered by environmental-management deficiencies, which if corrected will restore the healthy state in the herd. Second, some pathogens can be eliminated. For example, *Sarcoptes scabiei* var *suis* can be eliminated from a herd using the strategic administration of agents such as ivermectin and doramectin. Alternatively, diseases such as transmissible gastroenteritis and PRRS can be eliminated from a herd by closing the herd to new introductions and purposely exposing all animals to the disease to create herd immunity. It is usually desirable in the longterm to eliminate the diseases, if possible and if it results in savings from reduced routine medication or vaccination. Third, there are strategies to prevent pathogens from entering the herd. As herd size has increased, the emphasis in maintaining the population of animals free of certain diseases has increased in importance. Some key components of a biosecurity program include careful management of replacement stock with quarantine and monitoring; preventing entry of rodents, birds, and other animals; precautions to prevent disease transfer from trucks and fomites; and the restricted entry of people (*See also* BIOSECURITY, 2068).

Vaccination and Disease Status: Vaccination is a key health management tool to enhance individual and herd immunity. Commercial vaccines are available for most of the important swine diseases, and when commercial vaccines are not available, autogenous vaccine may be a possibility. Generally, only a small number of vaccines are used in most herds. The decision to use a vaccine depends on a number of factors and needs to be assessed and frequently reassessed on an individual herd basis. To use all of the available vaccines would be cost prohibitive. Criteria used to decide which vaccines to incorporate into a herd vaccination program include cost (including labor) and efficacy of the vaccine, cost of the disease or possibly the risk of the disease occurring in the herd, and availability of alternative measures that might be more useful than vaccination. On many farms, gilts and sows are vaccinated before breeding to protect from reproductive failure caused by *Leptospira* sp, *Erysipelothrix rhusiopathiae*, and parvovirus infection. It is also common practice on many farms to vaccinate sows during gestation with an enterotoxigenic *E coli* vaccine to boost antibodies in the colostrum and milk to protect piglets from diarrhea via passive immunity. Common vaccines given to weaned pigs include porcine circovirus and *Mycoplasma hyopneumoniae*. Several other vaccines warrant important consideration for most farms, including *L intracellularis*, swine influenza virus, and PRRS virus.

The decision to vaccinate for a particular pathogen or develop specific control strategies sometimes depends on whether the disease is present on the farm. Knowing the disease status of a herd is an important consideration for a number of reasons. For example, it is critical if two sources of pigs need to be mixed or sources of replacement stock need to be chosen. To know what diseases are present in a herd, monitoring needs to be regularly performed and multiple sources of information incorporated into the assessment. On herd visits, animal inspection can identify clinical signs of disease. Pigs that are scratching may cast suspicion that mange is present in the herd. The presence of coughing and sneezing might prompt further investigation of respiratory diseases. It is common practice to euthanize and conduct postmortem examinations on unthrifty pigs to screen for the presence of diseases such as enzootic pneumonia or ileitis. Analysis of blood or oral fluid from a representative sample of animals to monitor for disease is an important part of herd health evaluations. In addition, production records and drug use records can help to assess health status. Another information source may be abattoir reports, or if possible following pigs through the slaughterhouse floor and assessing lesions such as milk spots on liver that indicate roundworm migration.

Herd Visit and Facility Inspection: The herd visit is also important to determine possible housing-environmental-management shortcomings. Animal inspection may reveal signs of stress or mismanagement affecting animal welfare and productivity. Behavioral vices such as tail biting may indicate underlying environmental problems such as crowding, or insufficient resources such as waterers or feeding space. A facility inspection should spot damaged penning and flooring that could lead to injury. Air quality, room temperature, and presence of drafts can all be assessed. Stocking density is possibly the most obvious potential stressor that should be investigated during a herd visit. Published guidelines for space requirements are being used more and more in animal welfare audits. Space requirements (*see* TABLE 6) vary according to age and weight of pigs as well as for flooring type and other considerations such as season, ventilation or cooling systems, and group size. Investigation of disease outbreaks may require a team approach, with a veterinarian interacting with experts in nutrition, building design or engineering, and other fields to determine the triggering factors. The longterm solution to a disease problem often depends on a change in management.

TABLE 6 SPACE RECOMMENDATIONS FOR GROWING PIGS

Production Stage	Body Weight	Space Allowance
Nursery	Weaning to 27 kg (30 lb)	0.16–0.23 m^2 (1.7–2.5 ft^2)
Grower	27–68 kg (30–100 lb)	0.28–0.56 m^2 (3–6 ft^2)
Finisher	68 kg (150 lb) to market wt	0.74–0.84 m^2 (8–9 ft^2)

Adapted from Zimmerman JJ, et al (eds), *Diseases of Swine*, 10th ed. 2012.

HEALTH-MANAGEMENT INTERACTION: SHEEP

Sheep and goats were first domesticated around 8,000 BC, making them the first of the domesticated food animals. Sheep are extremely adaptable and found all over the world, particularly in arid areas that do not support other types of livestock. Because sheep are raised in various environments, specific breeds have been developed to meet the needs of the environment and people. More than 100 breeds have been recorded. Different production systems are used in various areas of the world. Extensive year-round grazing, with large flocks (>1,000 sheep) and minimal sheep handling, is the typical system of sheep management where the climate and area to graze allow. Systems in New Zealand, South Africa, and Australia, where forage is available throughout the year, are prime examples of this type of management. Confinement and intensive feeding during the winter months, with access to range land pasture for the rest of the year, is a common system of large sheep flocks in parts of Europe, the UK, the western USA, and other countries that have snow and inclement weather seasonally.

Intensively managed smaller flocks can be found around the world, with sheep kept for milking, natural colored wool, purebred breeding stock, sale of lambs for home freezer trade, and hobby flocks on small acreages. Small flocks of breeding stock or hobby and pet flocks are common in the more developed areas of the world, particularly the USA and Canada.

Shepherding small flocks of sheep and goats along roadsides and common grazing areas is a typical management system in the Middle East, Asia, and Mexico.

EXTENSIVE GRAZING SYSTEMS

Veterinary services for sheep are typically not readily available in the poorer areas of the world unless provided by governments to satisfy exports to other countries. Where veterinary services are available, private practitioners are mostly called upon by extensive grazers that confine their sheep *during the colder periods of the year* for feeding. Veterinarians are often needed to manage lambing problems such as scours/diarrhea outbreaks, baby lamb mortalities, and other major disease outbreaks. Because predation from coyotes, wild cats, bears, wild pigs, wolves, dingos, etc (depending on the country), usually accounts for the major losses during the rest of the year, private practitioners are generally not a part of flock health and management programs in these systems. However, extensive management systems often use government or university veterinary extension education and services where provided.

Veterinarians can use a request to solve a current problem from such a producer to also educate and advise on flock health. This is more common in extensive grazing units in which sheep are confined during the winter months and so are available for handling and examination. Abortion, still births, weak lambs, and open ewes require accurate diagnosis, and management of these problems can evolve into development of a vaccination program, breeding soundness examinations for rams, looking at mineral and protein supplementation programs, and other preventive programs.

Baby lamb deaths require formal diagnostic aid, which can be used to develop preventive programs for *Escherichia coli*, coccidia, *Mannheimia*, white muscle disease, and navel ill. Starvation deaths should lead to examining ewe body condition, preparturient supplementation, mastitis control, and lambing management in general.

Some knowledge of range land nutrition, including toxicities and deficiencies common to the area, feed costs, labor problems, and markets, in addition to knowledge of sheep diseases, is very helpful when giving advice and providing preventive programs and management changes to extensive grazing producers. The aim is to increase net farm income rather than just control disease. Although the diagnosis, treatment, and control of disease are important, an overall management change that will contribute to longterm profitability may be far more important. Net income per hectare/acre should be the major consideration of any recommended change.

A flock health plan, tailored to the specific needs of a large producer, should include: 1) a good mineral/nutritional supplementation program (after determining any deficiencies); 2) control of external parasites (internal parasites may not be a problem on arid ground but that should be determined); 3) prevention of diseases for which cost-effective vaccines are available; 4) methods to prevent introduction of contagious diseases, such as sore mouth/scab, caseous lymphadenitis, footrot, epididymitis/brucellosis, and Johne disease; and 5) improvement of the number of lambs weaned per ewe bred, with enhanced ewe and ram fertility and reduced lamb mortalities (may be related to nutritional program).

In most sheep operations, wool is not the major source of income, so the economic outcome from an outbreak of disease or a serious nutritional problem is usually obvious. However, in operations in which wool is the predominant source of income, a moderate parasite burden or nutritional deficiencies can cause ill-thrift, reduced kilograms of wool shorn per head, and reduced fiber diameter. The latter outcome may result in a more valuable fleece and thus, no reduction of income. In this situation, reduced health of the ewes may not be obvious. A ewe that does not conceive or aborts in the first 3 mo of pregnancy will produce more wool than a ewe that rears a lamb, because a ewe rearing a lamb has a higher nutritional requirement and produces less wool than a dry ewe. However, in most places, the price of lamb, somewhat influenced by pelt price, is worth far more than that of the wool.

In some areas of the world, veterinarians may be able to go beyond a flock health program by developing a comprehensive flock management advisory service. This service would adopt a whole farm approach that considers the physical and financial resources of the farm/ranch and the interaction of livestock production with other activities such as cropping and pasture production. The stocking rate, type of stock run, timing of husbandry procedures, marketing strategies, and risk management should be reviewed as part of the program. A financial analysis of the farm as a business and preparation of farm budgets and gross margin analyses is a key part of most programs. However, this type of service has not been readily adopted by producers in most places, and most veterinarians do not have the expertise.

SUMMER GRAZING WITH WINTER CONFINEMENT (INTENSIVE MANAGEMENT)

These types of sheep enterprises tend to use veterinary services the most. Smaller backyard producers may use veterinarians to perform procedures such as vaccinating, docking/tailing, castrating, and hoof trimming as well as to treat sick animals. However, larger producers in many countries often perform these routine procedures themselves, using veterinarians for such things as cesarean sections and help with disease control.

Wool production is usually a minor concern on the smaller production units; the number/pounds/kilos of lambs marketed per ewe joined/bred is the major determinant of economic return. The greatest potential loss is caused by neonatal lamb mortality, resulting from abortion, mismothering, starvation, and hypothermia. Second to that may be lack of growth weight due to internal and external parasites, protein deficiency, and lack of highly digestible and palatable feed for young lambs. Intensive management and good sanitation at lambing will reduce this loss. Labor-intensive lambing systems; intensive care of young lambs; and diagnosis, treatment, and occasional surgery of individual sheep may be justified by the value of the animals. However, preventive medicine programs are greatly needed in these management situations to prevent the numerous husbandry-related diseases associated with higher stocking rates. Attention to pastoral-related disease is important in the summer (ie, internal parasite control) and in the winter for problems related to closer confinement, winter nutrition, and lambing problems.

In these types of production situations, record keeping becomes critically important for improvement. Animals must be individually identified so that the production of each can be monitored. Some countries/regions, such as the UK, the European Union, Australia, Canada, and the USA mandate individual animal identification for disease tracking.

Lambs should be identified at birth, usually with a unique ear tag. The identification number, date of birth, dam, type of birth (single, twin, etc), sex, and remarks such as "weak," "required help birthing," etc, are recorded. Recording birth weight is also desirable. Thus, scales, one appropriate for baby lambs and another to weigh market-size lambs, are an important tool to determine productivity.

Lambs should be weighed again at 50–60 days and 100–120 days, which indicates some measure of the milking ability of the ewe (60-day weight) and genetics of the lamb (120-day weight). Comparisons of the lambs' rate of gain and twinning are two measures that can then be used to cull the ewe flock. It often is the thinnest ewe that turns out to be the best producer, and the fattest ewe the poorest. This is a relatively basic record keeping system in which other criteria can be assessed if desired.

In Australia, computer-based programs are used to compare animals within a flock as well as to compare flocks with other flocks on the plan. The USA sheep industry offers a similar plan (the National Sheep Improvement Plan), to which any producer can subscribe.

Feed and labor are always the largest annual expense for livestock producers, particularly for winter-fed or intensively fed sheep and lambs. Producers and their families usually provide the labor for smaller flocks, making feed the largest out-of-pocket cost. Therefore, nutritional management is of major importance. Veterinarians with knowledge of nutrition and mineral management can be extremely helpful, because feed imbalances can be costly.

Feedlot lamb feeding and management is also an area in which veterinary services can be very useful, providing least-cost rations and preventing major nutritional diseases such as acidosis, urolithiasis (*see* p 1502), rectal prolapse, type D enterotoxemia (pulpy kidney disease, *see* p 610), and polioencephalomalacia (*see* p 1281) and stress-related diseases such as pneumonia (*see* p 1472).

SHEPHERDING

Veterinary services to the small, shepherded sheep and goat flocks in the Middle East and Asia are primarily concerned with controlling clinical diseases and improving the survival rate of young lambs and kids. The restricted availability and low nutritional value of feed limit productivity. Sheep and goats are kept primarily as a source of meat and milk for the owner's family and for sale as a source of cash income. Veterinary care is often provided by government programs and is directed toward control of specific contagious and zoonotic diseases. Even though the value of animals in the flock is often high relative to the income of the owner, the funds available to invest in veterinary services are limited. Thus, private veterinary care is seldom used, even if available, despite the fact that the death or severe ill health of a few animals can have a major impact on both the productivity of the flock and the well-being of the owner.

In Asia, the system of land use is often complex, with sheep and goats integrated with other grazing animals or grazing around the fringes of a more productive cropping or plantation enterprise. This may also be true in the Middle East, or sheep and goats may graze poorly productive arid areas that will support little else. In either case, opportunities for major changes to the management system are limited.

ORGANIC SHEEP PRODUCTION

Public demand is moving animal-based production toward organic systems. The standards required to allow an organic label for sheep products, although allegedly making the product safer for the consumer, do not tend to promote animal health. They prohibit the use of antibiotics, chemotherapeutics, and parasiticides ("chemicals"); therefore, organic producers cannot use preventive or therapeutic medications and rather must rely on "natural" or home remedies with questionable effects but no withdrawal times. This forces them to manage for disease prevention rather than use labeled medicines with known withdrawal times. These standards are often aspirational rather than practical and can lead to health issues and welfare concerns in organic flocks, even those that have excellent management systems dedicated to this approach. Veterinarians can be extremely helpful in this type of production system.

Organic flocks should be established from known health-status flocks that are free of testable and eradicable diseases such as orf/sore mouth, *Corynebacterium pseudotuberculosis* (cheesy gland, caseous lymphadenitis), *Brucella ovis* (ram epididymitis), footrot, maedi/ovine progressive pneumonia, scrapie, Johne disease, and chlamydial and *Campylobacter* abortion. Flocks should be maintained as closed flocks as much as practical, and new genetic stock should be sourced from known health-status flocks. New stock must be quarantined and thoroughly examined and tested before introduction to the flock and its pastures. Preventing entry of disease is critical, necessitating a high degree of biosecurity (*see* p 2068).

Parasitic gastroenteritis can be of particular concern in organic sheep production. In addition, although the regulations of some countries allow judicious use of anthelmintics and antiparasiticides, others do not. Management plans must include methods to avoid or reduce parasitic larval intake. Grazing crop aftermaths, using mixed-species rotational grazing, attention to stocking rates, drylotting, and using pastures for hay and grazing only after a good freeze for a season, can all be used to limit internal parasites. Other strategies that have been suggested include grazing plants that may reduce GI parasitism such as chicory, sanfoin, birdsfoot trefoil, and the use of copper oxide needles. Breeding and selecting for genetic resistance is definitely a viable option and not too difficult using the help of individual fecal egg counts.

DISORDERS ASSOCIATED WITH MANAGEMENT PRACTICES

Management practices, particularly feeding practices, can be the primary determinant of cases or outbreaks of infectious or metabolic disease in all flocks of sheep.

Pregnancy toxemia (*see* p 1021) may be seen in late-pregnant ewes bearing multiple fetuses subjected to a falling plane of nutrition, specifically energy. It is associated with simple starvation, ewes too fat in early pregnancy, ewes too fat in late pregnancy and that voluntarily reduce feed intake, poor quality feed, and ewes subjected to stress in late-pregnancy (eg, trailing or transport, or severe environmental changes). Ewes rarely survive after showing signs of pregnancy toxemia, even with excellent veterinary care, and it is difficult to stop losses even after interceding with adequate feed.

Hypocalcemia (*see* p 991) is seen in pregnant ewes or ewes in early lactation subjected to a period of temporary starvation or to feeds particularly low in calcium, especially ewes with multiple fetuses, as a result of decreased food intake in late pregnancy. It is also seen in feeder lambs on a grain-based ration without adequate mineral supplementation, and during drought conditions. Calcium deficiency can be confused with pregnancy toxemia and is often a part of the pregnancy toxemia syndrome. Fortunately, pure calcium deficiency can be easily treated and rectified, saving the ewe and her pregnancy.

Hypomagnesemia (*see* p 995) may be seen during a period of temporary starvation in late pregnancy or early lactation, and also after movement of lactating ewes to lush spring growth pasture (especially green cereal crops). As with hypocalcemia, this condition is easily treated and rectified if properly diagnosed.

Dermatophilosis (*see* p 858) is associated with poor shearing practices leading to shearing cuts, particularly in areas that still use dipping vats for ectoparasite control (this practice has largely disappeared since the advent of the avermectin parasiticides). Sheep in long wool at times of high rainfall tend to be at higher risk of infection, and some sheep are also genetically predisposed.

Caseous lymphadenitis (*see* p 63) may be associated with shearing by not separating infected or discharging sheep before shearing, not shearing affected sheep last, not changing blades and disinfecting shears after cutting into an abscess, dipping in contaminated dip, and by close confinement of infected sheep with noninfected sheep after shearing and at other times.

Other means of spreading this very contagious disease is the use of feed bunks or working chutes where the organism (*Corynebacterium pseudotuberculosis*) has been smeared on slats or railings by sheep with draining abscesses. The organism can survive for up to a year in the environment. It can be controlled by vaccination.

This disease is responsible for huge economic losses in North America due to the rejection or trimming of large parts of carcasses of affected animals when slaughtered.

Enterotoxemia (*Clostridium perfringens* type D infection, *see* p 610) is seen in weaned, unvaccinated lambs on a rising plane of nutrition high in carbohydrates, as when moved to better pasture or following a "flush" in pasture growth, particularly cereal grains and in feeder lambs fed grain. It generally causes a "sudden death" syndrome and can be confused with acidosis. These animals are found dead and even if found alive can rarely be saved. There is an enterotoxemia antiserum, which if administered early, can be used for treatment. The vaccine is very effective.

Acidosis is seen in adults and lambs exposed suddenly to a higher carbohydrate diet than normal and is often confused with enterotoxemia. It is seen commonly when late-pregnancy ewes are started on grain, when feedlot self-feeders run out of feed for more than a few hours, and when children not properly instructed in correct feeding of animals perform feeding chores.

***C perfringens* type C infection** is generally a suckling lamb disease seen in very young single lambs suckling ewes that produce an overabundance of milk or in a lamb after its twin dies. It is also seen in artificially reared orphan "bummer" lambs that have not had sufficient colostrum. The disease can be prevented by vaccinating ewes close to parturition with enterotoxemia C and D vaccine to provide antibodies in their colostrum; saving frozen colostrum from vaccinated ewes, does, or cows for administration to lambs that received no colostrum; or giving those lambs injections of enterotoxemia antiserum.

Malignant edema (*see* p 604) and **blackleg** (*see* p 602) may follow wounds (eg, improper shearing, vaccination). However, these are clostridial diseases not commonly seen in sheep.

Tetanus (*see* p 611) may also be seen in unvaccinated sheep and lambs after a wound associated with procedures such as castration, docking (tailing), shearing, or vaccination performed in contaminated yards/corrals. Tetanus has been specifically associated with the use of elastrator (castrating) bands to remove tails and testicles of young lambs. Vaccinating ewes with a *C tetani*–containing vaccine shortly before lambing will prevent the disease for up to 60 days of age if the lambs receive their dams' colostrum.

Black disease (*see* p 603) is caused by *C novyi* type D. Sudden death is a hallmark of this disease seen among unvaccinated grazing sheep on pastures with wet areas that support the snail that is the intermediate host of *Fasciola hepatica*. The organism, which produces a potent toxin, colonizes the necrotic areas of the liver caused by the migrating flukes on their way to the gallbladder.

C novyi is also the cause of "big head" in rams, in which necrotic and anaerobic tissue on the head caused by the head butting of unvaccinated fighting rams becomes infected with the anaerobic clostridial organisms. Black disease and big head can be prevented by vaccinating.

Navel ill (*E coli* and *Erysipelas* arthritis) (*see* p 625) are associated with navel infections of lambs born in muddy or dirty areas and that have not had their navels dipped in 7% iodine at birth. These two infections are often confused with one another and are usually seen around 3 wk of age, although simmering infections can exacerbate later. Other causes may be contaminated dip or poor hygiene at docking/tailing or castration.

Poor lambing management and sanitation of the lambing area can result in significant economic loss due to varied problems ranging from baby lambs dying of hypothermia-related hypoglycemia, starvation due to mismothering or ewes with mastitis, and sudden death due to overwhelming coccidial infection at 3 wk of age. Lambs that get little or no colostrum for whatever reason are at significant risk of succumbing to disease because of the lack of passive immunity even after weaning. Diseases particularly common to lambs lacking passive immunity are *E coli* scours, septicemias, navel ill, coccidia, pneumonia, tetanus, enterotoxemia, sore mouth, and arthritis.

Coccidiosis can cause a sudden death syndrome at 21 days of age if the infecting dose was large enough. Otherwise, the disease is characterized by the area around a young lamb's tail smeared with diarrhea. If not treated, the diarrhea can turn bloody after a time and the lamb can dehydrate and die. The lambs' environment or the dam's contaminated teats is the source of the infections; most adults carry small to moderate amounts with no signs. Lambs, too, can carry moderate infections and show only lack of vigor and weight gain. Coccidia is the most common cause of poor-doing lambs and significant loss to the producer.

Coccidiosis can be controlled by keeping the lambs' area clean and dry and by treating ewes before lambing with a coccidostat. Feeding coccidiostats in feed accessible only to the lambs such as decoquinolate, amprolium, lasalocid, or monesin further controls the disease. It is treated with sulfonamides.

Ovine posthitis (pizzle rot) is seen in merino wethers on high-protein pasture and in breeding rams kept in corrals or paddocks, particularly with moist areas where the animals prefer to lie during hot periods of the day. Ammonium salts in the urine are broken down by soil organisms contaminating the wool around the prepuce, and the resultant NH_4 causes erosions and scabbing of the preputial orifice. It can interfere with breeding because of pain and discomfort. Clipping wool around the preputial opening, keeping animals in dry paddocks, and reducing protein in the diet will help eliminate the problem.

Actinobacillosis (*see* p 589) is seen in sheep grazing on abrasive, thorny pasture.

For disease risks associated with **pasture or with specific plants** (eg, bloat, polioencephalomalacia, hemolytic anemia, esophageal obstruction, enterotoxemia in sheep, and goiter in the lambs born to ewes grazing *Brassica* spp), *see* POISONOUS PLANTS, p 3103. For the risk of nutritional deficiency or toxic disease associated with formulated feeds, *see* NUTRITION: SHEEP, p 2345.

HEALTH-MANAGEMENT INTERACTION: SMALL ANIMALS

Proper management to prevent and control disease has historically been a higher priority in production animal medicine than in small animal medicine. However, appropriate management is just as important for small animals, whether their environment is that of a single or multiple-pet household or a more intensive housing situation such as a kennel or cattery.

Responsible pet ownership must be emphasized to all those owning and considering owning pets. Areas of client education that should be emphasized include the following: 1) routine care and grooming, 2) preventive health care, 3) parasite control, 4) nutrition, 5) household hazards, and 6) housing requirements and environmental factors.

Routine care and grooming not only help maintain pet health but also allow identification of health problems early in the course of disease. Compared with disease in people, disease in animals is generally identified at a later stage. Close observation of pets allows for evaluation of changes in appetite, thirst, urination, defecation, ambulation, and general behavior. Any changes may suggest the need for a more thorough examination and possible intervention. Special attention should be given to hair coat, skin, ears, eyes, and teeth. Anal sac impaction and overgrowth of nails are common problems.

Preventive health care in small animals primarily involves vaccination and parasite prevention. Vaccines are available for a variety of infectious diseases in dogs, including distemper, parvovirus, hepatitis, leptospirosis, tracheobronchitis, rabies, Lyme disease, and coronavirus. Vaccines available against infectious diseases in cats include those for panleukopenia, rhinotracheitis, calicivirus, rabies, feline infectious peritonitis (FIP), and feline leukemia virus (FeLV).

Vaccination schedules vary but generally require an initial vaccination at 6–8 wk of age, followed by additional vaccinations at 3-wk intervals until the animal is 4–5 mo old. After this, most vaccines are given annually. Rabies vaccination is dictated by state law or local jurisdiction. First-time vaccination for diseases other than rabies in adult animals should include an initial vaccination followed by at least one booster.

In the past, there has been some question concerning the overvaccination or hyperimmunization of both dogs and cats. Vaccine-associated sarcomas, specifically fibrosarcoma, have been an increasing problem in cats (*see* p 955). The etiology of this tumor is not completely understood, but it appears at vaccination sites of rabies and FeLV vaccines. In dogs, there has been some correlation between vaccination and immune-mediated disorders such as immune-mediated hemolytic anemia.

Current canine vaccination guidelines, published in 2011 by the American Animal Hospital Association, identify core and noncore vaccines. Core vaccines include distemper, parvovirus, and adenovirus-2. A killed rabies vaccine is also core and is available as a 1-yr and 3-yr product. The specific vaccine schedule is 8 wk, 12 wk, and 16 wk of age. The first booster should be given no later than 1 yr after the final vaccine dose of the initial series. Subsequent boosters should be administered every 3 yr. Current feline vaccination guidelines, published in 2013 by the American Association of Feline Practitioners, suggest vaccination for panleukopenia, herpesvirus 1, calicivirus, and feline leukemia virus (FeLV). Additional vaccines may be suggested depending on risk of exposure, eg, indoor versus outdoor or cattery situations. Current recommendations for vaccination sites also follow the guidelines of the American Association for Feline Practitioners. This protocol can also be used for dogs. The guidelines suggest that cats be vaccinated in an area amenable to surgical resection, ie, distal limbs rather than torso. Vaccines for feline panleukopenia virus, feline herpesvirus 1, and feline calicivirus are administered below the right elbow. FeLV vaccines are given below the left stifle, and rabies vaccines below the right stifle. Vaccinating dogs and cats less frequently has also been suggested. A triannual vaccination protocol for vaccines other than rabies has been adopted at many institutions. It is also recommended to reserve vaccines for certain diseases such as FeLV, Lyme disease, leptospirosis, feline immunodeficiency virus, and FIP for at-risk animals.

Other preventive health care measures may include castration or ovariohysterectomy, and annual veterinary examinations. The current trend in preventive health care is to emphasize an annual examination separate from visits for vaccination. The preventive health visits allow the veterinarian to see the animal frequently and detect disease at an earlier stage.

Parasite control continues to be important. The primary endoparasites include GI parasites such as roundworms, whipworms, and tapeworms (*see* p 412, et seq). Heartworm disease (*see* p 127), an important clinical entity in both dogs and cats, is preventable with prophylactic therapy. Although a treatment is currently available for heartworm disease in dogs, no safe or acceptable treatment is available for cats. The American Heartworm Association provides treatment guidelines for canine and feline heartworm disease. The primary ectoparasites include fleas, ticks, and mites. Both oral and topical products are available for flea control in dogs and cats. Another important aspect of parasite control includes prevention of zoonotic diseases such as visceral larva migrans and toxoplasmosis. *Bartonella* may also be an important vector-borne disease affecting people.

Nutrition is an important and often overlooked aspect of pet ownership. Most pet foods on the market have been formulated based on significant research and development. Specialty diets are available (both over-the-counter and from veterinarians, including prescription diets) for young, growing, and geriatric pets, as well as for specific disease processes. Overfeeding and oversupplementation may lead to numerous problems, and feeding of table scraps should be kept to a minimum. (*See also* NUTRITION: SMALL ANIMALS, p 2354.)

Water quality should not be overlooked, especially in rural areas and in kennels and catteries. Fresh water should be available ad lib.

Household hazards provide a variety of dangers to dogs and cats. Potential hazards include electrical cords, lead-based paint, cleaning supplies, antifreeze (*see* p 3046), houseplants (*see* p 3103), insecticides (*see* p 3058), prescription drugs (*see* p 3032), illicit and abused drugs (*see* p 3038), alcoholic beverages, chocolate (*see* p 2966), artificial sweeteners (xylitol, *see* p 2698), sewing needles, fish hooks, and many others. (*See also* HOUSEHOLD HAZARDS, p 3000.) Elements of house design, such as steep stairs, slippery floors, open windows, etc, may also be hazardous.

Housing requirements and environmental factors are an important consideration for pets. For companion animals sharing an owner's home, concerns are generally limited. However, outdoor housing must provide cover from direct sunlight, shelter from excessive wind and extreme temperatures, adequate ventilation, and an adequate supply of fresh water. These factors are critical in kennels and catteries. Drainage must be appropriate for proper sanitation, and surfaces must be suitable for cleaning and disinfection. Hazardous environmental conditions can result in hyperthermia, sunburn, dehydration, hypothermia, or frostbite. Housing must also be safe and keep pets away from dangers such as other animals, motor vehicles, and malicious mischief. If animals are restrained by a leash or a chain, care should be taken that self-trauma cannot be inflicted. Some municipalities have introduced chain laws to prevent this type of injury.

Miscellaneous considerations include obedience training, which may help reduce aggressive interactions with other animals and people.

Traveling with pets is another important consideration. If crossing state lines, a health certificate should be issued. When international travel is planned, owners should be advised to become familiar with the appropriate health, quarantine, agriculture, and customs requirements. Transport of animals by airlines is under the jurisdiction of the specific airline company, but a veterinarian should be consulted and a health certificate issued. Animals should not be allowed to ride unrestrained in motor vehicles and should never be allowed to ride in the back of open vehicles such as pick-up trucks. Motion sickness (*see* p 1267) and anxiety are common problems in dogs and cats when traveling. The phenothiazine tranquilizer acepromazine may be beneficial in this situation, and antihistamine therapy such as diphenhydramine may be useful. Maropitant citrate is also approved for treatment of motion sickness.

The potential disease-management interaction between pets and owners is important in prevention of **zoonotic diseases**, especially when pets are owned by immunocompromised people. Pet owners with human immunodeficiency virus or those being treated with chemotherapy or other immunosuppressive agents can safely own animals but should consult both their veterinarian and physician. Most animal-associated infections, including those due to *Toxoplasma gondii*, *Cryptosporidium*, *Salmonella*, and *Campylobacter*, appear to be acquired by immunosuppressed individuals from sources other than exposure to animals. The possible exception may be *Bartonella* or cat scratch disease. Because the risk of zoonotic transmission is low, animals pose minimal risk to immunocompromised people if basic precautions are followed. Precautions include avoiding the cleaning of litter boxes or using gloves when doing so, avoiding dog feces, avoiding young or unhealthy pets in favor of healthy or adult pets, having sick animals evaluated by a veterinarian, not allowing cats to hunt, not feeding pets undercooked meat, and preventing coprophagy or access to garbage.

MANAGEMENT OF REPRODUCTION: CATTLE

Dairy and beef producers should strive to increase reproductive efficiency as a key driver of economic efficiency in the sector. Reproductive efficiency, or "pregnancy rate," is defined as the proportion of cows eligible to be bred that become pregnant during an estrous cycle (or approximately 21 days), and which determines the calving to conception interval at the end of the voluntary waiting period. As pregnancy rate increases in dairy herds, the calving to conception interval decreases, and the herd status becomes, on average, less "days in milk" (DIM). This has the effect of increasing the potential amount of milk produced per day of herd lifetime, because yield classically declines at 0.3% per day after peak lactation production. A major and realistic goal of every beef cow/calf operator should be to raise or market 85 calves per 100 cows every year. Greater reproductive efficiency also reduces the number of cows culled for reproductive failure; collectively, these changes increase herd income.

Reproductive performance in both beef cow/calf and dairy operations can be improved by the following: 1) properly identifying and managing animals to carry out reproductive programs; 2) keeping records that enable determination of important herd indices, such as percent calf crop, pregnancy rate, length of calving season, culling rates, calf morbidity and mortality, breeding efficiency of bulls, and performance and production information; 3) meeting the nutritional requirements of various classes of livestock in the herd, emphasizing nutritional needs and cost efficiencies; 4) establishing a breeding program for heifer replacements and cows; 5) practicing sire selection and reproductive management; 6) adopting a vaccination/immunization program for the cow/calf herd, bulls, and calves; 7) evaluating reproductive failure and abortions; 8) providing adequate facilities; and 9) ensuring that the calf is well cared for at birth and receives adequate colostrum.

NUTRITION

Nutrition is one of the most important management factors in reaching calf crop goals and in attaining a short calving season every year in beef breeding herds. The limiting nutrient related to reproduction in beef and dairy cattle is usually energy; although dairy cattle are usually fed rations that supply adequate energy during lactation, genetic drivers for milk production inevitably lead to a period of some negative energy balance postpartum. The level of energy and body condition before calving primarily influences when a beef cow returns to estrus, whereas level of energy after calving primarily influences subsequent conception. Feed requirements vary during the reproductive cycle (*see* p 2248).

There are four periods of beef cow nutrient requirements, and generally three for dairy cows. **Period 1** is the interval from calving to breeding; it is ~70–90 days and is the period of greatest nutritional demand. The dairy cow is at maximal milk production and recovering from the stress of parturition. During this period, she is expected to be ready to breed.

Period 2 is the interval from rebreeding to weaning the beef calf; it is ~120–150 days in beef cows. Periods 2 and 3 overlap in dairy cows and are not as easily separated as in beef cattle. The beef cow should gain weight while still milking. Although some dairy cows maintain body weight, many high producers continue to lose weight during this period.

Period 3 is from weaning to 50 days before calving; it lasts ~100 days and is the period of least nutritional demand. The beef cow has only to maintain her condition and continue fetal development. The dairy cow should be managed to gain or lose body weight during the last months of lactation to achieve target body condition ready to enter the stable dry period.

Period 4 is a critical stage and is the 50 days before calving; it is during this time that 75% of fetal growth occurs. Cows are usually not lactating during this "dry period." Cow condition at calving is critical to rebreeding; the onset of estrus after calving is delayed in cows that lose weight or are thin and not gaining during late pregnancy.

Dairy cows are usually fed (*see* p 2265) for optimal milk production throughout their 305-day lactation. It is assumed they will lose weight during heavy lactation (the early months) and regain the loss during the remainder of lactation. Dairy cows should not be overfed during the dry period because of a genetic predisposition to sacrifice body condition to maximize milk production through insulin resistance. This leads to the increased probability of metabolic diseases, eg, type II ketosis and fatty liver disease (*see* p 1024 and *see* p 1018), during early lactation as insulin resistance leads to excessive fat mobilization from adipose tissue storage and overwhelms the capacity of lipoprotein transport mechanisms in the bovine liver to transport and metabolize lipid. In addition, dairy cows should be fed to minimize the incidence of calving-related disorders (eg, dystocia, hypocalcemia, and retained fetal membranes), including control of dietary cation-anion balance (DCAB), which have a negative effect on fertility and health postpartum.

The amount of cow feed required per pound or kg of calf weaned is fairly constant, although larger cows require more feed for maintenance than smaller cows. Cows that give more milk require more feed, generally with a higher level of protein. Increased milk is produced at the expense of reproduction when feed is not adequate to meet all needs.

The protein requirement of young growing stock and heavy-milking cows is often a limiting factor, while mature dry cows are often overfed protein. Heifers must be fed adequately from weaning to breeding if they are to calve at 2 yr of age; this target is critical for herd economics, because before this point the absence of beef calf or milk for sale represents significant investment and risk.

To provide the essential nutrient requirements during various stages of the reproductive cycle, major forages and homegrown cereals should be analyzed to monitor nutrient content and actual value. Variation in amounts of trace minerals is common between and within different geographic areas. Globally, different systems are used to determine energy levels of the ration, such as the metabolizable protein (MP) or "Feed into Milk" (FiM) models or the Total Digestible Nutrient System and the California Net Energy System. All are commonly used, and application should be tailored to fit the individual operation.

Even within nutritional need categories, cattle benefit from feeding and handling in subgroups: lightweight heifers at weaning need to gain more than heavier heifers to reach puberty by breeding season; first-calf heifers require special attention from both an energy and competition standpoint if they are expected to breed and conceive at the proper time. These heifers are still growing, as well as lactating, and they may not have the rumen capacity to meet postcalving energy needs on forage alone. Monitoring of growth rates is important to achieve successful rearing targets. Supplemental feeding of both high-energy and high-protein feeds to first-calf heifers may be required for optimal reproductive potential. Calves from first-calf beef heifers may be weaned 30–40 days earlier than calves from cows in the main herd to allow the heifer more time to grow and recover from demands associated with lactation.

Thin, old, and small cows may not compete favorably with heavier cows within the same herd and often benefit from being fed as a separate subgroup.

Lactating dairy cattle are usually fed according to milk production. They may be fed concentrate on an individual basis or divided into groups according to milk production and fed an appropriate total mixed ration.

BREEDING PROGRAM FOR HEIFER REPLACEMENTS AND COWS

If a cow is to calve consistently, she must deliver her first calf early. Puberty is a function of breed, age, and weight. Beef heifers that are bred at 13–15 mo and calve at 22–24 mo have two advantages: they get closer attention from herdspeople by calving before the main herd starts to calve, and subsequently they have the extra time needed to rebreed with the mature cow herd. For heifers to breed at 14 mo, they should have attained at least 65%–75% of their projected mature weight; therefore, adequate nutrition is of major importance. The breeding season for virgin beef heifers should start 3 wk before that of the main cow herd. The above considerations do not apply to dairy cattle, which calve throughout the year; however, scheduling heifer calvings at the start of a seasonal calving dairy herd such as in New Zealand or Ireland represents an opportunity to "reset" the calving pattern. Lifetime profit of dairy replacement heifers is maximized when heifers calve at 23–25 mo of age. Thus, to maintain genetic progress and maximize profitability, heifer breeding strategies on dairy operations should include artificial insemination (AI) that results in attainment of pregnancy to allow calving at ~24 mo of age.

To compensate for the greater attrition rate usually seen with virgin heifers, a greater number should be bred than is needed to maintain or increase herd numbers, eg, 150%.

Irregularities of Estrus and Anestrus

Breeding will not occur if the cow is anestrous, or if estrus is undetected. Genuine anestrus is not common in dairy cows but is more common in postpartum beef cows in below target body condition. Anestrus, subestrus, or irregular estrous cycles in cows may result from a number of factors, including poor management or nutrition, disease, injury, or disturbances in endocrine functions. One of the most important management factors in artificially bred herds is failure to detect or observe estrus. The average duration of estrus is 18 hr, but in many cows it is appreciably shorter. A systematic program for detection of estrus is important if cows are to be bred at the right time. A producer must be familiar with signs of estrus. Aids in estrus detection that are valuable adjuncts to the heat-detection program include chalk marks on the tailhead, chemically or electronically activated devices attached to the tailhead of the cow that reveal when other cows have mounted, and a vaginal probe that measures the electrical conductivity of the vaginal mucus. Accidental access of bulls to cows and failure to keep proper breeding records often result in apparent anestrus because of pregnancy without a service history.

Although genuine anestrus is generally not common in dairy cows, "subestrus" with poor estrous expression or irregular estrous cycles in cows may result from a number of factors, including poor management or nutrition, disease, injury, or disturbances in endocrine functions. In many dairy herds, detection of estrus for AI is inefficient, because not all cows are identified in estrus because of human error, attenuated expression of estrus in high-producing cows, and adverse responses to heat stress. Systematic breeding programs for AI at a predetermined time (ie, timed AI [TAI]), without the need for estrus detection, coupled with early rebreeding of nonpregnant cows are successful options for reproductive management of lactating dairy cows. These systems optimize pregnancy rate by synchronizing follicle development, regression of the corpus luteum (CL), and precise induction of ovulation to provide a fixed TAI. Incorporation of TAI in dairy herd reproductive management programs reduces labor requirements for detection of estrus while improving overall reproductive performance and maximizing profit.

Silent heat refers to normal follicular development and ovulation without evident signs of estrus. Its frequency decreases as lactation progresses, so that incidence is low by 4 mo postpartum. Cows with true silent heats may be detected only through rectal palpation or ultrasound of the ovaries, via accelerometers/activity meters, or the use of progesterone assay in milk or plasma.

Cyclic changes occur in the ovary over 18–24 days. These changes generally can be recognized and the time of the cycle estimated, particularly in the 3–4 days before ovulation, at the time of ovulation, or 3–4 days after ovulation. The CL regresses 3–4 days before the onset of estrus; it becomes smaller in size and changes from a diestrous, liver-like consistency to one more fibrous. Estrus is evidenced by the presence of a palpable follicle, an absent or regressed CL, and firm uterine tone. The vaginal mucosa is edematous, the cervix is relaxed and hyperemic, and a variable amount of clear serous mucus is frequently seen at the vulva, which is puffy and swollen. The immediate postovulatory period is characterized by blood in the mucous discharge and an ovary with a corpus hemorrhagicum, which on palpation is recognized as a soft area (5–15 mm in diameter) in the ovary. The CL is detectable by day 4–5 as a small and somewhat softer structure than the mature CL, which reaches maximal size by day 7.

The examiner can sometimes predict the next estrus from previous observations around estrus, and the cow can be watched closely at the next anticipated estrus. The primary behavioral sign of estrus—standing to be mounted—is the accurate predictor of ovulation. In cows that are approaching ovulation, the appropriate time can be estimated, and the cow bred on secondary signs such as mounting other cows; however, breeding on secondary signs may be associated with wide variation in time to ovulation. Aged gametes (either semen or oocytes) are associated with reduced embryo viability.

Regimens have therefore been developed for administration of prostaglandins (PGs) and their analogues alongside other products to synchronize estrus and to reduce dependence on estrus detection. Prostaglandins are effective only if a cow has a functional CL. A range of synchronization options are in common use, including double prostaglandin regimens, GnRH and prostaglandin protocols, and regimens that use combinations of GnRH and prostaglandin alongside intravaginal progesterone-releasing devices. For estrus synchronization, the prostaglandin or its analogue is administered to all cows. In those in days 6–18 of the cycle, the CL will regress and estrus will occur in 2–7 days. The others may either have been in estrus recently or will be in a few days. Eleven days later, all cows will be between days 6 and 18 of their cycle, and prostaglandin is administered a second time. Most cows will be in estrus in 3–4 days and will ovulate in 4–5 days. Breeding is done either on signs of estrus or fixed time. Cystic ovary disease (*see* p 1354) may be responsible for irregularities of the estrous cycle, eg, follicular cysts (anestrus, nymphomania, and shortened cycles) and luteal cysts (anestrus).

Under certain circumstances, ovaries are nonfunctional. They can be recognized as smooth, small, bean-shaped structures on a single examination, or reveal no activity or change after several examinations over a period of 3 wk. The most common causes are low total energy intake during late winter or droughty summer pastures, and excessive loss of body weight in lactating dairy cows postpartum.

The stress of chronic or severe disease, injury, or ovarian tumors may interrupt ovarian activity and result in anestrus. Congenital defects, such as freemartinism and ovarian hypoplasia, result in estrual failure. Inactive ovaries are treated by correcting the basic cause; they usually do not respond to gonadotropin or steroid hormone treatment.

BULL REPRODUCTIVE MANAGEMENT

A desirable goal for beef producers is a 95% calf crop delivered within 45–65 days, with an optimal weaning weight obtained at the most efficient cost. Bull selection, management, and evaluation of performance are integral aspects of beef improvement. The bull can affect calving percentage as well as quality of calves. The use of performance-tested bulls (beef and dairy) is recommended for both natural breeding and artificial insemination.

A disease control program for bulls should include the following procedures: 1) Before use, bulls should be checked for brucellosis, tuberculosis, trichomoniasis, and paratuberculosis (ie, from a herd free of paratuberculosis). Bulls previously used in other herds, particularly herds in which disease status is not known, may spread diseases, particularly campylobacteriosis and trichomoniasis. Prophylactic sheath-washing with antibiotics may reduce the risk of *Campylobacter* transmission. 2) Depending on prevailing health status and market requirements, bulls should be vaccinated against infectious bovine rhinotracheitis, bovine viral diarrhea, clostridia, *Haemophilus*, campylobacteriosis, and leptospirosis if available. Vaccines should be administered around puberty, at 6 mo and 1 yr of age, and then annually, 1 mo before the breeding season. 3) Breeding soundness examinations should be performed annually at the most economically advantageous time for the producer (usually 1 mo before the breeding season).

All bulls should be on the premises 2 mo before the breeding season to allow them to adapt to the environment. Isolation of all new additions to the herd (bulls or cows) is recommended for proper adaptation and preparation. A breeding soundness examination consisting of a thorough physical examination, including internal and external genitalia, measurement of scrotal circumference, and microscopic examination of semen for sperm motility and morphology, should be conducted ~1 mo before the breeding season. Opportunities are emerging for more objective methods of semen evaluation to be used alongside standard microscopy, such as computer-assisted semen analysis (CASA) for motility and flow cytometry to assess morphologic defects. (*See also* BREEDING SOUNDNESS EXAMINATION OF BULLS, p 2231.)

During the breeding season, the bull should be watched closely for mating behavior. The standard recommendation is 25 cows per bull. There are significant variations in this ratio, depending on the breeding soundness and libido of individual bulls, differences in terrain, and length of breeding season.

The weight loss that develops in bulls during the breeding season should be restored during the off-period, but overconditioning should be avoided.

BREEDING

The breeding program may use either artificial insemination (AI) or natural service. AI has been commercially available for >60 yr; it is widely used in dairy cattle but is used much less in beef cattle because of handling and labor costs. AI offers a selection of bulls with known genetic potential, such as measured by estimated breeding values (EBVs) for traits such as ease of calving or growth rates. When nutrition and heat detection are properly managed, satisfactory results are obtained. Failure to detect estrus is the major reason for unsuccessful AI. When cows are properly inseminated with good-quality semen at the proper time, 50%–60% may conceive on first service, the same percentage on second service.

Embryo transfer (*see* p 2239) is frequently used to increase the number of progeny from the most valuable beef and dairy cows. Sexing of semen has been adapted to commercial field usage and is increasingly used. Sexing of embryos is becoming more readily available and practical for field usage, and some cloning techniques are emerging in availability.

Heifers should be bred according to size and age at puberty; at first breeding they should be 65%–70% of their projected mature body weight, with dairy heifers achieving >125 cm withers height at this stage. Selection of bulls to be used for natural service should be based on likely size of the calf at birth; the bull's own birth weight (not his adult weight) is a useful guide, but genetic proofs such as EBVs are vital.

Heat synchronization of heifers and cows is possible, but such programs depend on adequate management and cooperation. Also, sufficient skilled labor to breed and assist during calving is essential.

Artificial Insemination (AI)

In cattle, AI is used primarily for genetic improvement of livestock and to facilitate high health replacement strategies. The worldwide adoption of AI for genetic improvement in dairy cattle was made possible by development of a progeny test system and subsequent use of milk production records as an objective measure of performance on which to select superior bulls, techniques for freezing semen, and liquid nitrogen storage refrigerators.

The development of objective systems such as EBVs to measure economic traits in beef cattle (eg, growth rate, carcass conformation and composition, efficiency of feed conversion) and thus the more accurate selection of sires, as well as control of the estrous cycle, is leading to an increase in use of AI in beef cattle.

Processing of frozen semen is a highly specialized technique. Attention to detail at each step is important to maintain semen quality. The freezability of semen varies among bulls. However, semen of high motility and morphology quality generally freezes well. Best results are obtained when semen is processed in a properly equipped laboratory by experienced staff at an AI center.

Collection and Handling of the Semen Sample: (*See also* BREEDING SOUNDNESS EXAMINATION OF THE MALE, p 2230.) Semen is collected using an artificial vagina or by electroejaculation (electrical stimulation of the seminal vesicles and ampullae). As long as the sample is of high quality, freezability and fertility should be normal. These techniques should not be used if the bull is unable to naturally service a cow for reasons that could be genetic.

Most AI in cattle today is performed with frozen semen. Frozen semen may be maintained for years; extenders permit more insemination doses to be processed from one collection of semen, maintain the fertility of the semen longer, protect the spermatozoa from sudden temperature or pH change, and prolong viability. Semen is usually extended with citrate-buffered egg yolk or heat-treated skim milk plus glycerol, sugars, enzymes, and antibiotics. Final extension is designed to package 0.25 mL or 0.5 mL of semen containing 20–30 million spermatozoa at time of freezing.

Extenders are often divided into fraction A and fraction B. The initial extension of semen is done with fraction A at the same temperature, eg, 86°F (30°C). The extended semen is then cooled to 41°F (5°C) over 40–50 min, or more slowly. Holding the extended semen at this temperature for 3–4 hr enables the antibiotics in fraction A to complete their action before being inhibited by the cryoprotectant glycerol. Fraction B contains a cryoprotectant such as ethylene glycol or glycerol (eg, 14%) and is added at 5°C in equal quantity to the extended semen. Each AI center has its own standard extenders and processing procedures. Glycerol (11%–13%) may be used with milk-based diluents. Before freezing, semen should be stored for 4–18 hr at 5°C.

For freezing, bull semen is usually packaged in appropriately identified plastic straws (0.25 or 0.5 mL). Optimal freezing rates are known for many cell types, and spermatozoa can withstand a wide range of rates. In practice, extended semen is frozen in liquid nitrogen vapor before being plunged into liquid nitrogen at –320°F (–196°C). Storage in liquid nitrogen tanks is safe for ≥20 yr, and semen is transported in such tanks. The level of liquid nitrogen in tanks must be monitored to avoid semen losses, which is seen when the tanks become defective or when liquid nitrogen gradually evaporates.

Because spermatozoa do not survive for long after thawing, the semen should be used immediately. Thawing is best done as quickly as possible without damaging the semen by overheating. In practice, straws may be thawed in warm water (95°–98°F [35°–36.5°C]) for ≥30 sec and immediately placed in the cow's reproductive tract. Recommendations by the AI center that processed the semen should be followed.

Insemination Technique: The rectovaginal method is used almost exclusively. After thoroughly cleaning the external genitalia with disposable toweling, one gloved hand is introduced into the rectum and grasps the cervix. The insemination pipette is introduced through the vulva and vagina to the external cervical os. By manipulating the cervix, along with light cranial pressure on the pipette, the pipette is advanced through the annular rings of the cervix to the junction of the internal cervical os and the body of the uterus. The semen should be expelled slowly (5 sec) to avoid sperm loss. If insemination records and consistency of the cervical mucus suggest possible pregnancy, the pipette should be advanced less than one-half of the way through the cervix, and the semen expelled. The optimal time to inseminate is between the last half of standing estrus and 6 hr thereafter, which is described as the "AM/PM rule," in that cows observed beginning standing heat in the morning should be inseminated that afternoon, etc.

If fertility problems arise when AI is being used, the semen should be investigated, although many factors other than semen are involved in attaining high fertility. Motility after thawing is an important criterion. An adequate number of motile spermatozoa at the time of insemination is critical. Morphologic examination also helps assess the role of semen in infertility cases. Comparisons within herds of diagnosable pregnancies resulting from the suspect semen and from semen from other bulls may be useful. Estrus detection continues to be the most important factor that influences AI efficiency. This factor should be investigated first, and inseminator proficiency second. The latter includes an evaluation of thawing temperature, time of thawing in relation to actual insemination, temperature changes from thawing to insemination, site and speed of semen deposition, and sanitary procedures. If semen is purchased from a reputable supplier, it is unusual for the cause of the infertility to be poor-quality semen, although transport and storage factors should be considered.

PREGNANCY DETERMINATION

Pregnancy determination is recommended to maximize breeding efficiency. In beef herds, the breeding season (natural service or AI) is ideally fixed at a length of 60–70 days. This gives the average cow two or three services to conceive. Cows that are not pregnant or were bred late should be identified; if kept in the herd, they will calve later in the season. Maintenance costs are significant, although they vary widely by farm and by year.

Pregnancy determination of beef cows should be done shortly after the breeding season is over (eg, 45–60 days); if the breeding season starts June 1 and ends early in August, it can be done during late September while the cows still have plenty of flesh from summer pasture. It is then possible to profitably market nonpregnant cows before expensive winter feeding starts. When excessive returns are noted or bull performance issues are suspected, early pregnancy determination by ultrasound 50 days after the start of the breeding season can be invaluable. A target of 65% of cows should be pregnant to the first cycle in beef herds, and so by 50 days this can be measured as pregnancy determination success 30 days after breeding. Supplementary AI or new bull power can be implemented with poor success, alongside further investigation.

Dairy cows should be examined to determine their pregnancy status and if found open can be synchronized into estrus with prostaglandin $F_2\alpha$, or timed AI. In cows that are open or that have not been detected in heat, the decision on which hormones to use to induce estrus is based on evaluating the ovaries for CL, follicles, and ovarian cysts. The most common method to determine pregnancy and evaluate ovaries is transrectal palpation and, increasingly, the use of ultrasonography. Ultrasonography may have the following advantages: 1) Nonpregnant cows can be found earlier (28–32 days after breeding), and diagnostic information on the status of the ovaries and uterus can be obtained. 2) The viability of the embryo or fetus can be assessed, eg, by visualization of a fetal heart beat. 3) Twins are more readily detected. 4) Sex of the fetus can be determined. 5) Age of the conceptus can be estimated more accurately. 6) The producer can be shown the conceptus, which could be reassuring in herd cases of embryonic losses.

Other herd health examinations should be considered while the cows are being checked for pregnancy. These include an accurate evaluation of body condition, the reproductive tract, teats and udder, feet and legs, teeth, and early neoplastic eye lesions. Vaccinations, internal and external parasite control, and processing of beef calves also can be done at this time.

EMBRYONIC DEATH, ABORTION, AND ABNORMAL FETAL DEVELOPMENT

Pregnancy may be terminated prematurely, resulting in abortion due to death of the conceptus or failure of the uterine environment to support the fetus. Abnormal fetal development may result in abortion or in a calf that dies soon after birth. Many cases of bovine abortion are not diagnosed. (*See also* ABORTION IN LARGE ANIMALS, p 1333.)

Etiology: Viruses, bacteria (including rickettsia and chlamydiae), molds, protozoa, or other infectious agents may attack the placenta or the fetus, or both. Some of these microorganisms reach the uterus hematogenously; others (such as venereal infections) are contracted during mating.

Infectious abortion may be sporadic or a herd problem. Herd problems usually are associated with significant losses and may be caused by infectious bovine rhinotracheitis, bovine viral diarrhea, brucellosis, leptospirosis (various serotypes), campylobacteriosis, trichomoniasis, anaplasmosis, ureaplasmas, mycoplasmas, and others not yet identified.

Mycotic abortion usually is caused by *Aspergillus* or *Mucor* spp, which reach the uterus hematogenously and cause abortion in late gestation. In many of these fetuses, the skin is not affected; in others, ringworm-like lesions are seen. The placenta frequently is severely affected with necrosis of the cotyledons and thickening of the intercotyledonary areas. Diagnosis is based on identification of the fungus through culture of the fetal or placental tissues, histologic examination of these tissues, or direct examination of cotyledons after clearing with potassium hydroxide solution. These abortions are almost always sporadic, and the only means of control is to reduce exposure to the fungi.

Sporadic losses may result from *Listeria* sp (a bacterium occasionally present in silage when pH is >7); miscellaneous bacteria such as *Haemophilus* sp, *Trueperella pyogenes*, *Staphylococcus aureus*, *Bacillus cereus*, *Pasteurella multocida*, *Pseudomonas aeruginosa*, *Streptococcus bovis*, *Chlamydia* sp, and others; or viruses (eg, bluetongue).

Noninfectious causes of abortion are numerous; the most common include 1) recessive or lethal genes (or both) such as cervical vertebral malformation, hydrocephalus, osteopetrosis ("marble bone" disease), arthrogryposis ("crooked calf" syndrome), and several others, some not fully identified; 2) toxins (eg, excessive nitrates from feed or water), certain pine needles, poisonous plants (eg, lupine, locoweed), or mycotoxins (moldy feeds); 3) hormonal imbalances in the pregnant dam; 4) injuries affecting the pregnant cow; and 5) nutritional deficiencies, particularly of vitamin A, vitamin E or selenium (or both), iodine, and manganese.

Heat stress in cattle can cause early embryonic death and lower the herd pregnancy rate. The mechanism by which heat stress affects embryonic survival is complex. Heat stress can disrupt early embryonic development. Effects of heat stress on embryonic survival decrease as embryos advance in development. Heat stress at day 1 or days 1–3 after breeding reduces embryonic survival. In contrast, heat stress of superovulated cows at day 3, 5, or 7 after estrus did not affect embryonic development in one study.

Diagnosis: Accurate diagnoses of reproductive loss contribute to the cumulative herd history and provide criteria to evaluate the impact on herd performance and the need for implementation of preventive measures. Laboratory assistance is needed in most cases. Carefully selected, properly preserved, quality specimens should be submitted to a diagnostic laboratory for analysis. Even with these, the exact cause of an abortion may not be detected, especially if it is noninfectious. Laboratory diagnosis of abortion may include serology and examination of the fetus and placenta. However, a definitive diagnosis of bovine abortion remains challenging because, in many cases, the causative agent may have challenged a cow months previously and may no longer be present when abortion occurs.

Defective newborn calves can be recognized only by a thorough examination and sometimes only after some time has passed.

Prevention and Control: Several factors are critical to prevent and control abortion and development of defective calves. Measurement and management of herd health status and planning to control infectious disease risk with appropriate boundary and purchased stock biosecurity alongside vaccination programs are essential. A balanced nutritional program helps control losses associated with mineral or vitamin deficiencies and poor-quality feeds, including moldy grains and forages. Genetic selection and accurate record-keeping help to detect and eliminate bloodlines that prove to be carriers of recessive or lethal genes. Appropriate housing and handling facilities decrease the incidence of accidents and provide an environment conducive to health. The cattle producer and veterinarian should work together to assess the herd's reproductive performance, tailor a vaccination program to the herd's specific needs, and diagnose and control potential herd problems.

For successful abatement of heat stress, the environment of the cow must be modified to maintain the cow within a normal temperature range of 101.3°–102.8°F (38.5°–39.3°C). Common approaches include providing shade (to intercept solar radiation) and fans or sprinklers to promote evaporative cooling. Tactically avoiding breeding at hottest times of the year may be advisable.

Infectious diseases in a herd can disrupt and reduce reproductive efficiency by causing embryonic or fetal death, abortion, or illness and death of neonates. A complete vaccination program will not eliminate reproductive problems but may prevent or reduce losses associated with specific infections (*see* TABLES 7 and 8).

CALVING MANAGEMENT

Dystocia is expected to occur in ~10%–15% of first-calf heifers and in 3%–5% of mature cattle. Although dystocia cannot be eliminated from a herd, the incidence can be

TABLE 7 VACCINATION/IMMUNIZATION PROGRAM TO PROTECT AGAINST PREPARTUM DISEASES OF THE BREEDING HERD

	Disease	When to Vaccinate/Immunize
Heifers	Brucellosis	Calfhood
	IBR[a], BVD[b]	Before weaning and before breeding
	Campylobacteriosis, leptospirosis, trichomoniasis	Before breeding
Cows	IBR, BVD	May booster early before breeding
	Campylobacteriosis, leptospirosis, trichomoniasis	Each year, before breeding
Bulls	IBR, BVD	Calfhood and booster before first breeding
	Campylobacteriosis, leptospirosis	Each year, before breeding

[a] Infectious bovine rhinotracheitis

[b] Bovine viral diarrhea

TABLE 8 VACCINATION/IMMUNIZATION PROGRAM TO PROTECT AGAINST DISEASES OF THE NEONATAL CALF

	Disease	When to Vaccinate/ Immunize
Heifers and cows	Rotaviruses and coronaviruses, *Escherichia coli* bacterins, clostridial bacterins	As on label
Calves	Rotaviruses and coronaviruses (if indicated)	As on label

greatly reduced by management decisions made before the breeding season and during gestation.

Nutrition: Heifers and cows should maintain body condition before calving, but overconditioning causes excess fat deposition in the udder and results in lower milk production. Excessive fat deposition in the pelvis also may result in dystocia. Good body condition aids in calving ease, early return to cyclicity in beef cows, and also milk production. There is a balance to achieve between avoiding excessive condition, which leads to dystocia, and insufficient condition, which leads to postcalving subestrus/anestrus.

Calving Facilities: Dedicated calving facilities may be needed in many herds. They should be in good repair and functional before the calving season starts. Weather conditions, geographic differences, and local experience usually dictate how much attention and individual care calves will need immediately after birth. The calving environment (eg, calving sheds, small pastures) must be clean, dry, and protected from the weather. A clean area to handle dystocia problems is also needed. Calving in a clean area, separated from the rest of the herd, helps to reduce calfhood diseases, particularly diarrhea (scours) and Johne's disease. In large herds, several small calving pastures that allow regular rotation may help to reduce buildup of disease-causing organisms. When calving stalls are used during inclement weather, they should be cleaned and disinfected between calvings.

Calving: Close observation of labor is necessary to determine when or whether a delivery should be assisted. Labor is divided into three stages. Stage 1 begins with uterine contractions and dilation of the cervix and ends with passage of the amnion and part of the fetus into the vagina. Stage 1 may last 1–24 hr, with 1–4 hr being normal. Stage 2 is characterized by abdominal contractions due to the fetus in the vaginal canal and ends with expulsion of the fetus through the vulva. Birth should be expected within 1–4 hr for heifers. A mature cow should calve in <3 hr if the presentation of the calf is normal; if no progress is seen within 1 hr, assistance may be required. Disruption of labor may occur with inappropriate intervention or social group stresses. "Just in time" calving strategies are based around the need to minimize social group changes at the point of calving, because these social changes are associated with challenges to dry-matter feed intake. Stage 3 is expulsion of the fetal membranes and initiation of uterine involution. Expulsion of the fetal membranes normally occurs within 12 hr after parturition.

Feeding preparturient cows in the late morning (11 AM–noon) and again at night (9:30–10 PM) encourages cows to calve during the day (7 AM–7 PM), when a problem is more likely to be identified and assistance more likely to be available.

Parturition is often difficult for both fetus and dam. Many factors influence the degree of difficulty, including breed, age, nutrition, and pelvic area of the dam; breed and genotype of the sire; gestation length; and sex, size, position, and presentation of the fetus. Some, though not all, of these factors are directly influenced by management.

When dystocia (*see* below) develops, survival of both dam and calf depends on proper assistance. This requires identification of the problem, proper facilities, and adequate help. A delay in assisting may mean the loss of the calf or injury and even death of the cow. However, it is important to allow sufficient time for the dam to dilate before applying traction. Before assisting the delivery, the position of the fetus must be determined accurately, and any abnormal presentation corrected. If the calf is simply too large to pass through the birth canal without danger to the cow or calf, a cesarean section or other surgical assistance may be necessary.

Management After Calving: Muddy lots, crowding, filth, chilling, and inclement weather make the calf more vulnerable to disease organisms and may result in sickness and possibly death for both dam and calf. Provision of adequate trough space, ie, 1 m per fresh cow, and lying space in bedded yards, ie, 1.25 m^2/1,000 kg milk yield, are key factors for freshly calved dairy cows to maximize feed intake and minimize risk of poor hygiene on udder health. (*See also* HEALTH-MANAGEMENT INTERACTION: CATTLE, p 2119, and MANAGEMENT OF THE NEONATE, p 2087.)

Passive Transfer: Calves receive immunity passively from the dam through ingestion of colostrum. The calf's immune system is immature at birth and depends on acquisition of passive immunity for disease protection in early life. Immunoglobulins (IgG and IgM) and lymphocytes are absorbed directly across the gut into the calf's circulation to provide immunity. The ability of the gut to absorb these large molecules and cells is a transient phenomenon; gut closure is complete by 24 hr, and absorption has decreased significantly by 6–8 hr of age. Ingestion of adequate amounts of quality colostrum as early as possible after birth is important for calf survival and growth. Calves with failure of passive transfer (FPT) are 3–9 times more likely to become sick before weaning, and 5 times more likely to die before weaning than calves with adequate passive transfer.

Minimizing the incidence of FPT should emphasize dystocia management, proper nutrition, and intervention for calves at high risk of FPT. Cows that have dystocia should be milked out immediately, and the calf actively fed colostrum to ensure ingestion. Calves should consume 3-4 L as soon as possible after calving by nasogastric tube as necessary. Cows with poor udder conformation or mastitis should be milked, and the colostrum fed to the calf to ensure timely intake. Colostrum supplements may not prove adequate, as shown in controlled clinical trials, to increase serum IgG levels. Vaccination of the cow with pathogens causing enteric disease in calves before calving may be a useful adjunct to good overall management in reducing morbidity. Hygienic management of colostrum is vital to effective absorption, and either careful pasteurization or cooling of lidded containers should be considered.

DYSTOCIA MANAGEMENT

Dystocia management must begin with proper heifer development. Fetopelvic disproportion is a major contributing cause of dystocia. Calf birth weight, the size of the pelvic area of the dam, and the interrelationships of these two factors are major determinants of dystocia. The weight of the calf is a function of genetic and environmental factors. Genetic factors include sex, length of gestation, breed, heterosis, inbreeding, and genotype. Nongenetic factors include age and parity of the dam, nutrition of the dam during various phases of gestation, and environmental temperature. Efforts to manage the dystocia rate and moderate its effects should focus on replacement heifer development, sire selection using EBVs for calving ease, and early dystocia intervention.

Replacement Heifer Development: Dystocia rates in beef heifers may not be controlled by nutritional restriction during late pregnancy. On the contrary, the loss of 0.5 kg/day during the last trimester of pregnancy in beef heifers is associated with weak labor, increased dystocia rate, reduced calf growth rate, prolonged postpartum anestrus, reduced pregnancy rate, and increased morbidity and mortality. It is recommended that heifers be fed to allow modest rates of gain (0.5 kg/day) during late pregnancy. Protein malnutrition in late pregnancy has been associated with weak calf syndrome and may be a factor contributing to neonatal mortality.

Measurement of the pelvic area of the dam to predict dystocia is sometimes used as a criterion for selection of replacement heifers, even though pelvic area alone explains only a small proportion of the variability in dystocia. Pelvic area measurements before the breeding season or at the time of pregnancy examination have been used to estimate the pelvic area before calving. Those heifers with a small pelvic area before the breeding season may then be culled or selectively mated to easy calving bulls, and those with a small pelvic area at the time of pregnancy examination may be aborted, culled, or identified for careful observation at calving. Some evidence suggests that culling heifers with the narrowest pelvic width may be more effective than culling based on pelvic area; however, such "pelvimetry" measurements may only detect the outlier animals in this multifactorial condition.

Sire Selection: A combination of culling heifers with small pelvic areas and using bulls that sire calves with small birth weights may reduce dystocia significantly. Using only the sires' birth weight to control calf birth weight and dystocia is not effective. A large number of nongenetic influences affect birth weight, such as age of the dam, environment, and birth type. The ability to identify sires appropriate for use on replacement heifers has advanced significantly.

The use of estimated breeding values (EBVs) or expected progeny differences (EPDs) for birth weight is more effective than using only sire birth weight in selecting for acceptable birth weights. EPDs are reported in the units of the trait they reflect (eg, pounds for birth weight). Along with each EPD is reported an accuracy ranging from 0 to 1. Higher accuracies indicate a higher level of confidence that the stated EPD truly reflects the bull's effect. EPDs most effectively help compare bulls rather than identify the specific effect a bull will have on a herd. For example, a bull with a birth weight EPD of 4.0 would be expected to sire calves 6 lb heavier on average than a bull with a birth weight EPD of –2.0 when bred to the same group of heifers. An attempt should be made to identify bulls with good calving ease EBV figures and low birth-weight EPD for use on heifers while maintaining at least moderate weaning and yearling weight EPD. This is best achieved by the use of AI sires with high accuracy EPD. EPD can be calculated on yearling bulls with no progeny, but the accuracy is low. Until recently, EPDs were useful only in comparisons within breeds; however, methods for across-breed EPDs have now been developed. This is of particular use in selecting bulls to control dystocia in crossbreeding programs. Two recent innovations in the use of EBVs/EPDs for management of dystocia are the calving ease EPD and the maternal calving ease EPD. Calving ease EPD is related to birth weight EPD but may predict calving ease more effectively. Maternal calving ease is a measure of the effect of the maternal grandsire and the ease with which a bull's daughters will calve.

As the birth weight of the calf increases, the incidence of dystocia often also increases. Calving difficulty is higher for male than female calves. Abnormal presentations of the calf accounted for 22% of dystocias and 4% of all births in one study. Most dystocias are seen in primiparous 2-yr-old heifers, and the frequency decreases with increasing age and weight of the cow. Some studies have suggested that cows that previously experienced dystocia are more likely to do so again. Environmental effects may also have an effect on calf birth weight and dystocia. Cold weather may increase birth weights and subsequently increase the incidence of dystocia.

Appropriately Early Intervention: Despite the best efforts to avoid dystocia, some cases will be seen. Early intervention minimizes the effects of dystocia on calves; however, heifers especially may require significant time to dilate to point of delivery. Heifers should be monitored regularly and provided with assistance promptly if stage II labor is prolonged (eg, 1 hr). Producers need to identify the level of dystocia and growth that is economically acceptable and select a bull to match. They must be well trained to intervene appropriately in dystocia and recognize when to call the veterinarian. A general rule is that if a heifer has not made significant progress in delivering her calf within 30 min, it is time to get help.

COW–CALF PAIR MANAGEMENT

Cows and heifers should be moved from winter grounds to calving grounds 2–3 wk before calving season begins. They should be sorted into groups based on estimated calving date. This date can be determined at the time of pregnancy examination, when cows and heifers are grouped based on estimated duration of gestation. Separation of the herd into groups allows more concentrated observation of a smaller number of cows or heifers that are more likely to calve and potentially need help.

Cows and heifers should be observed to ensure they accept and mother their calves. Heifers especially are at risk of calf rejection, which increases the risk of calf disease. If heifers do not accept their calves and allow nursing within a short time, they should be brought into the calving barn and restrained to allow the calf to suck. Heifers that experience dystocia and human assistance are at increased risk of rejecting their calves. Cows or heifers that experience difficulty in calving or mothering should be moved to the calving barn for assistance and monitoring. Pairs entering the calving barn are at increased risk of disease because of dystocia, mismothering, hypothermia, and exposure to a higher population density. Once a pair enters the calving barn, they should not go to the general nursery pasture but to a separate high-risk nursery. Calves in the high-risk nursery can be monitored more closely for morbidity and treated promptly. Segregation of these high-risk calves also avoids exposure of the rest of the herd. Consideration should be given to management of infectious diseases such as Johnes disease by segregating higher-risk cows from lower-risk cows throughout this calving management period.

Once cows or heifers have calved, the pair should be moved out of the calving area to a nursery pasture within 24 hr. When the pair has bonded and passive transfer has occurred, movement to a nursery with decreased population density minimizes infection rates. Sick calves in the healthy nursery pasture should be removed and brought to the barn for treatment if necessary and placed in a morbidity nursery. Infectious agents can multiply in clinically ill calves and cause high levels of environmental contamination. The morbidity nursery may be combined with the high-risk nursery, but this increases exposure of the high-risk calves to pathogens. Ill calves should not be returned to the general nursery area. Treatment equipment should be disinfected thoroughly between calves to avoid transfer of infectious agents from calf to calf.

MANAGEMENT OF REPRODUCTION: GOATS

PUBERTY AND ESTRUS

Goats are spontaneously ovulating, seasonally polyestrous animals with peak sexual activity occurring in the fall when day length is decreasing. Factors that affect onset and length of the breeding season include geographic location (latitude and climate, specifically), breed, social structure, and photoperiod. In temperate regions, the natural breeding season is mostly restricted to the fall and winter to allow for kidding in the spring and summer, when nutritional conditions are adequate. Under tropical and subtropical conditions, where temperature and photoperiod are less variable, certain breeds can have an extended breeding period if appropriate resources are available to allow for kidding year-round. The average duration of the goat estrous cycle is 21 days but can vary with different breeds or environment. A relatively high frequency of short cycles is characteristic of goats and tend to occur in young does, at the onset of the breeding season, and with prostaglandin induction of ovulation. Longer cycles may be seen later in the season.

The average duration of standing estrus is 36 hr but can range from 24–48 hr depending on age, breed, season, and presence of a male. Breed-specific estrus duration has been reported for Mossi (20 hr), Angora (22 hr), Creole (27 hr), French Alpine (31 hr), Boer (37 hr), and Matou (58 hr) breeds. Estrus detection is based on behavioral signs, bleating, flagging of the tail, reddened vulva, vaginal discharge (which causes the tail hairs to stick together), and occasional "riding" by other does, although this last sign is far less common than in cattle. Goats can show overt signs of estrus while pregnant, and although natural service will not interfere with pregnancy, these does should not be artificially inseminated. Ovulation can occur anytime from 9–72 hr after the onset of estrus, typically toward the end of standing estrus. The ovulation rate varies based on breed, season, and nutrition. Angora goats typically have a single ovulation but may have two if sufficient nutrition is available. The average ovulation rate has been reported to be 1.7 eggs per doe in Boer goats and 1.5 in Maure goats. "Focused feeding," in which a nutritional boost is supplied in a short period of time, has enhanced reproductive efficiency in ruminants without affecting body condition. Also known as both "acute" or "immediate nutrient" effect, this practice leads to a positive energy balance, which increases leptin and insulin concentrations, enhances glucose uptake, and is positively associated with increased folliculogenesis and increased ovulation rate. Supplementation with β-carotene, a vitamin A and retinoid precursor, at 50 mg/goat/day has been shown to produce this effect in does.

The onset of puberty typically occurs at 6–8 mo of age but varies depending on the season of birth, breed, nutritional status, and presence of a male. Pygmy goats and does of larger breeds may reach puberty as early as 3 mo old; however, breeding should be delayed until the animal has reached at least 60% of its mature body weight to allow for higher conception rates and safer parturition. Larger goat breeds (eg, Nubian, LaMancha, Boer, and Saanen) can be safely bred at ~70 lb (32 kg). Angora kids should weigh a minimum of 27 kg and are frequently not bred until they are 1½–2½ yr old. Puberty in well-grown bucks can be seen as early as 4 mo.

BREEDING SOUNDNESS EXAMINATION

The external genitalia of does should be examined for abnormalities such as an enlarged clitoris, hypotrophic vulva, or increased urogenital distance that suggest intersex, a condition common in homozygous polled females, especially in Alpine, Saanen, and Toggenburg breeds. Intersex goats are sterile and should be culled. Occasionally, a doe has a shortened vagina and no cervix, and segmental aplasia of various parts of the tract can occur. A speculum can be used to examine the walls of the vagina, vestibules, and cervix to search for lesions in does with fertility issues. Transabdominal and/or transrectal ultrasonography can be used to examine the uterus and ovaries for cysts, pseudopregnancy, or other abnormalities. In cases of valuable breeding does, surgical laparoscopy or laparotomy may be used to check for causes of infertility such as oviductal blockage, tumors, adhesions, or segmental aplasia that may not be visible on speculum examination or ultrasonography.

A thorough physical examination of the buck before the breeding season is important to determine the ability of the buck to safely mount and breed a doe. Bucks should have a body condition score of 3–3.5 (out of 5) and be structurally sound with no visible foot or leg abnormalities. The buck should be in overall good health, because anemia due to heavy parasite infections and chronic debilitating diseases, such as pneumonia, can lead to loss of libido. Any degree of foot abnormalities, from overgrown hooves to severe laminitis, may cause the bucks to be reluctant to mount and should be treated appropriately. Bucks with caprine arthritis-encephalitis virus infection (*see* p 747) may have painful, enlarged stifles, and if they are even able to mount, are usually reluctant to ejaculate because of pain.

A complete assessment of the reproductive organs should be performed and include an evaluation of the penis and prepuce. The buck is set on his rump, and the shoulders pushed down to curve the spine convexly; this makes it easier to protrude the penis. Shearing wounds (especially in Angoras), prior balanoposthitis, and old fly-strike wounds and scarring around the prepuce may make protrusion of the penis impossible. Prior amputation of the urethral process to prevent obstruction by a calculus has no apparent deleterious effect on breeding ability. Although cryptorchidism is rare, a thorough reproductive examination in a young breeding buck should include confirmation that both testicles have descended. The scrotum should be evaluated for size, lesions, or other signs of injury. Testicular hypoplasia occurs in only ~2% of intact bucks and is mostly associated with intersex condition, but it may also be a manifestation of malnutrition. As in other species, scrotal circumference is positively correlated with semen production capacity and should be >25 cm in mature bucks (>14 mo old). Scrotal circumference can vary by season and decrease by as many as 3 cm outside the breeding season. Because scrotal circumference and body weight are positively correlated in bucks, scrotal circumference measurements are of minimal value before 14 mo of age.

The testicles and epididymis should be symmetrical and firm on palpation. Any asymmetry or changes in tone may indicate infection or injury and will likely adversely affect fertility. Orchitis and epididymitis are both rare, occurring in ~1% of breeding bucks, and affected bucks should be tested for *Brucella melitensis*, because bred does are at risk of stillbirths and abortions. Other causes of orchitis and epididymitis are of minimal concerns for transmission; however, treatments are generally unrewarding. Caseous lymphadenitis (*see* p 63), spermatic granuloma, and calcification of the testicles (which also may be due to *Corynebacterium pseudotuberculosis* infection) all reduce or eliminate the buck's fertility, and infected bucks should be culled. In extreme cases, ultrasound may be used to determine whether one or both testicles are affected and if hemi-castration is an option.

Evaluation of semen quality is another important part of the breeding soundness examination. Semen can be collected either by use of an artificial vagina or with an electroejaculator. The former yields a higher quality sample but requires the presence of a doe in heat to perform. Electroejaculation is more convenient and, thus, used more commonly. Once semen is obtained, it should be maintained at 37°C (98.6°F) and evaluated as quickly as possible. Grossly, the semen should be cloudy, white, and free of urine, blood, pus, or dirt. Occasionally, semen will be an off-yellow color and may be normal but should be examined more closely for urine contamination. The semen should be evaluated microscopically for motility, morphology, and presence of WBCs. Gross motility can be measured by placing a drop of undiluted semen on a warmed slide and evaluating on low-magnification. A satisfactory sample should exhibit anywhere from general oscillation to vigorous swirling. Sporadic oscillation to no motility at all indicates poor semen viability. Individual and progressive motility should also be measured by diluting the semen with an isotonic diluent (eg, 0.9% saline) and evaluating microscopically. Sperm cells should be counted to determine a percentage of progressively motile sperm, with a minimum of 30% being acceptable. Sperm morphology should also be assessed microscopically, with a minimum of 70% normal being acceptable. (*See also* BREEDING SOUNDNESS EXAMINATION OF THE MALE, p 2234.)

BREEDING

Natural service is the easiest and most common breeding system. Most hobby operations have a low doe:buck ratio (5:1) because of multiple breeds and different bloodlines. Bucks have a strong libido and can breed far more does than this, although as they get older, and especially during the off-season, they are less efficient.

Artificial insemination (AI) is increasingly being used by goat producers, because it allows for both dissemination of valuable genetics and control of sexually transmitted diseases. Proper heat detection and/or hormonal synchronization of the estrous cycle is essential and may lead to increased labor and costs. Ovulation in does occurs toward the end of standing estrus; therefore, insemination must occur around this time to be effective. The AM:PM rule is generally used: if the doe is first noticed to be in standing heat in the morning, AI should be performed in the evening (or vice versa). However, breed-specific estrus durations should be considered when deciding the best time to inseminate. Vaginal (pericervical deposition) or cervical (intracervical deposition) insemination techniques are inexpensive and easy to perform and can result in acceptable pregnancy rates if fresh semen is used. However, if frozen semen is used, transcervical or laparoscopic intrauterine insemination techniques must be used, which are more expensive and require more skilled personnel. Frozen semen in 0.25–0.5 mL straws may be purchased directly from buck owners or custom collectors.

Semen can be collected for AI in an artificial vagina or with an electroejaculator. Most bucks will mount a doe in estrus and ejaculate; with training they can ejaculate year round and even mount wethers. Older bucks are often reluctant to breed does that have had estrus induced outside the normal breeding season; therefore, collections are more successful when young bucks are used. The optimal sperm concentrations depend on the individual buck and production settings but should be ~200–400 million/mL to account for an approximate 50% death and damage rate during semen processing and thawing. There is no legislation or industry-wide standard in North America that governs the collection, processing, and sale of frozen semen, but country-specific legislations should be reviewed and followed before exporting semen.

Embryo transfer allows for dissemination of valuable female genetics. Its application in goats is somewhat limited because of the variable response of does to superovulation techniques. Control of the estrous cycle is crucial to ensure adequate timing for induction of superovulation, which is achieved by treating with commercially available follicle-stimulating hormone (FSH) products. Laparoscopic insemination of semen is recommended to confirm that superovulation occurred (via visualization of multiple corpora lutea) and to allow for the greatest conception rate. Embryo retrieval can be achieved surgically, laparoscopically, or transcervically, with surgical techniques providing the highest recovery rates. Embryos can then either be transferred immediately via laparoscopic or surgical techniques into synchronized does or frozen in liquid nitrogen.

INDUCTION OF ESTRUS

Estrus can be induced in several ways, depending on the time of year and the relationship to the doe's natural breeding season. Out-of-season breeding is of interest to dairy goat owners, because it reduces seasonal fluctuation in the herd's milk production. In meat production systems, increasing conception rates and litter sizes are important and can be manipulated using hormone therapy.

The sudden introduction of an odoriferous buck often advances the onset of cycling by a few weeks, and the does also may show some synchronization. The buck should be housed well away from the does (out of their sight and smell) for ≥3 wk before introduction. Even if the whole group does not cycle, this method can get a few to conceive in the theoretically out-of-season period.

Providing 20 hr of light per day in January and February (northern USA), with a sudden return to available daylight on

March 1, will bring goats into estrus several weeks later. In this system, it is more difficult for the owner to pick out the does that are in estrus; consequently, running a young, vigorous buck with the does gives the highest conception rate. If a portion of the herd is artificially synchronized, some of the remaining does also may come into estrus.

The Animal Medicinal Drug Use Clarification Act of 1994 (AMDUCA) places limits on extra-label drug usage in food-producing animals in the USA and restricts extra-label use to animals that are suffering or in danger of death. Under AMDUCA, pharmaceuticals cannot be used to alter reproduction for production purposes, and the following comments about manipulating reproduction are provided for use in countries outside the USA.

If the corpus luteum is functional, a synthetic $PGF_2\alpha$ analogue will induce estrus; however, this is not effective during anestrus. Additionally, it may provoke short cycles that tend to be seen normally at the beginning of the season. Melatonin implants may also be used to produce short-day effects and induce sexual activity in both does and bucks.

Progestagen treatment, followed by administration of FSH or pregnant mare serum gonadotropin (PMSG), will cause out-of-season estrous activity. Good conception rates can be achieved with this system, and fixed-time insemination is feasible, but these products (FSH and PMSG) are not approved for use in goats. Progestagen treatment can be in the form of injections with an oily base every 3 days, impregnated vaginal sponges (eg, flurogestone acetate or methyl acetoxyprogesterone), norgestomet implants, oral administration of melengestrol acetate, or a controlled intravaginal drug-releasing device, or CIDR (which is a form of progestagen-impregnated silastic for vaginal use). A commercial product marketed for use in swine containing both PMSG and human chorionic gonadotropin will also cause does to cycle outside the normal breeding season when administered at the end of progestagen treatment.

PREGNANCY DETERMINATION

Pregnancy determination can be performed using real-time ultrasonography and is very accurate with a skilled operator. Transabdominal ultrasound is quick and reliable and can detect pregnancy as early as 25 days, with the fetal heart beat detectable by day 27. Transrectal ultrasound is more difficult and time consuming but can diagnose pregnancy as early as 20 days. The accuracy of transabdominal ultrasound to differentiate the presence of a single fetus from multiples varies from 45%–55% (possibly higher with skilled operators). It is extremely difficult to accurately differentiate between twins, triplets, and quadruplets using ultrasound at any time during gestation. Fetal sexing may be performed by skilled ultrasonographers between days 55 and 70 of gestation and is more accurate in singles versus multiples. Routine radiography can be used to detect pregnancy with 100% accuracy after day 70 and can detect the number of kids after day 75.

Progesterone concentrations can be measured in milk or serum, but samples must be collected precisely one cycle after the doe was bred. Whereas low progesterone levels can confirm a nonpregnant status, high progesterone is not a positive pregnancy test, because it cannot differentiate between midcycle, true pregnancy, or false pregnancy. Plasma progesterone levels in pregnant does have been reported to be higher in triplets versus twins versus single fetuses at 84–21 days before kidding. The estrone sulfate test, performed on plasma, milk, or urine, is another way to determine pregnancy. Between 15 and 20 days after conception, the level of estrone sulfate, a conjugated estrogen produced by the conceptus, increases substantially and stays increased throughout pregnancy. Higher concentrations of estrone sulfate have been reported in does carrying twins or triplets than those bearing a single fetus. Abortion, fetal death, or resorption causes the estrone sulfate level to drop; therefore, the test also is a useful measure of fetal viability. Pregnancy-specific protein B (PSP-B), also known as pregnancy-associated glycoprotein, is produced by the placenta and can be detected in serum or plasma of pregnant does by ELISA at least 30 days after breeding.

Precocious milking is common in heavy-milking strains of goats. It can be seen in a virgin doe or during the first pregnancy. Therefore, udder development is no guarantee of pregnancy.

Hydrometra, or pseudopregnancy, is well documented in goats, although its cause is largely unknown. Aseptic fluid accumulates within the uterus and is accompanied by high peripheral concentrations of progesterone due to a failure of luteolysis. It can be both shorter or longer than a true pregnancy and occurs in 3%–30% of dairy herds.

Approximately 50% of pseudopregnancies occur as a result of early embryonic death at ≤40 days of gestation. An additional mechanism involves spontaneous persistence of the corpus luteum, which occurs more commonly in older goats, does bred out of the natural breeding season, or after induced ovulation. In some cases, ovarian cysts may also be present; therefore, it is recommended to always treat for both. Usually, the udder enlarges, but true filling does not occur. The doe may show behavioral signs of impending parturition, possibly even calling or searching for the nonexistent kid. The diagnosis can be made by excluding pregnancy coupled with the presence of clinical signs. This condition can be treated with prostaglandin to lyse the corpus luteum, and does may be able to conceive again if diagnosed and treated early. However, if the condition persists or recurs, the chances of future conception decline. For commercial dairy herds, this can produce moderate to severe economic losses.

Goats tend to have a high incidence of abortion, with chlamydiosis (*Chlamydia psittaci*) and toxoplasmosis (*Toxoplasma gondii*) being commonly identified causes in the USA (*see* ABORTION IN GOATS, p 1340). In cases of abortion, the fetus and placenta should be submitted to a diagnostic laboratory to exclude infectious causes. Paired serum samples should be obtained from the doe and saved in case serology is indicated. A thorough history, including nutrition and any recent changes in husbandry, should be taken.

PREGNANCY

Gestation length is 145–155 days (average 150 days) and can be affected by breed, litter weight, environment, and parity. Generally, first-kidding does have one or two kids, and in subsequent kiddings, triplets and quadruplets are not uncommon, especially in large, well-fed, heavy milkers. Quintuplets and sextuplets are rare. Progesterone production for maintenance of pregnancy is entirely dependent on the corpus luteum, with a drastic decline in progesterone occurring 12–24 hr before kidding. Induction of parturition is a useful technique to increase survival in dairy goat kids and to catch and separate kids from dams before they suckle in herds with control programs for caprine arthritis *encephalitis virus and mycoplasma.* Induction with synthetic $PGF_2\alpha$ analogues such as cloprostenol (125 mg) or dinoprost tromethamine (10 mg) usually results in delivery of kids ~30–35 hr after injection, whereas dexamethasone (20 mg) requires ~48 hr to induce kidding. Viability of multiple fetuses may be compromised if parturition is induced before day 144.

Pregnancy toxemia in goats is similar to that in sheep (*see* p 1021). It occurs during the final 6 wk of pregnancy and is more common in overconditioned does and in does pregnant with multiple kids. It is caused by reduced feed intake coupled with high energy demand, leading to ketosis. Treatment depends on severity of the condition and can range from dietary modification with oral administration of propylene glycol to intensive supportive care with administration of IV fluids with dextrose, insulin, and pregnancy induction. Vitamin B_{12} may also be administered as an appetite stimulant. Lactational ketosis is similar and occurs within the first 3 wk of lactation in high-producing dairy goat breeds; clinical signs include irritability, anorexia, reduced milk production, and weight loss. Treatments include IV glucose, oral glucose, and/or oral propylene glycol, depending on severity. Hypocalcemia or milk fever (*see* p 991) is seen in high-producing, older (>3 yr) dairy goats, but not nearly so frequently, nor as severely, as in cattle. Treatment includes IV administration of calcium gluconate or calcium borogluconate solution.

Vaginal prolapse is fairly common (*see* p 1390) in does and is believed to have a hereditary component. It may intermittently occur during late pregnancy due to increased intra-abdominal pressure. If complete vaginal prolapse occurs, intervention is required to prevent injury, infection, or dystocia. Owners should be advised that vaginal prolapses will recur with each pregnancy, so they can decide whether to cull the animal.

PARTURITION

Parturition tends to be uneventful in goats, with the incidence of dystocia <5%. If the doe has been in active labor for 30 min with no progress, assistance is likely required. Most kids present cranially, in dorsosacral position, with limbs extended. If kids present caudally, which is more common in twins, triplets, and quadruplets than singletons, assistance for delivery is more likely to be required. The most common cause of dystocia is when two or more kids present at the same time; other causes include malposition, fetomaternal mismatch, failure of cervical dilation (ringwomb), vaginal prolapse, uterine torsion, and uterine inertia. Most dystocias can be corrected by repositioning kids and providing lubrication and traction. However, in more severe cases, fetotomy or cesarean section may be indicated. Extreme care must be exerted when assisting with kidding to prevent uterine tears, which can be diagnosed on palpation of the uterus after the dystocia. Small tears can be treated by hastening involution of the uterus with oxytocin administration. Larger tears may require surgical intervention to minimize excessive bleeding and peritonitis. Systemic antibiotics, anti-inflammatory drugs, and a clostridial vaccine booster should be provided after a prolonged dystocia.

Retained placenta (not passed 12 hr after parturition) is uncommon in goats and is usually associated with selenium deficiency, the birth of a mummified or rotten fetus, or a difficult delivery. It can be treated by gentle traction or hormone therapy to facilitate expulsion, but diagnosis and treatment of the underlying cause will usually solve the problem. Metritis is almost always a sequela of retained placenta, and systemic antibiotics are warranted. Clostridial organisms (*Clostridium tetani* and *C perfringens*) may colonize the uterus, resulting in a frequently fatal toxemia that requires aggressive supportive care, antibiotics, and antitoxin therapy. Less severe causes of metritis may lead to a chronic endometritis and cause infertility if not treated.

Uterine prolapse is uncommon in goats but may occur after dystocia. Treatment is similar to that in other species, and prognosis is good if recognized and treated early.

In extremely cold weather, newborn kids should be dried (especially the ears) to prevent frostbite. Heat lamps are not necessary if the kids are dry, well fed, and out of a draft. Kids born in intensive systems should have their navels dipped in tincture of iodine to prevent infection. Angora, pygmy, and meat kids are typically raised on the dam. Dairy goat kids often are removed at birth and, after receiving colostrum, fed from a bottle or nipple-pail.

MANAGEMENT OF REPRODUCTION: HORSES

REPRODUCTIVE CYCLE

Nearly all mares are seasonally polyestrous and cycle when the length of daylight is long. Anestrus is seen during the winter when daylight length is short. During anestrus, the uterus is flaccid, and the ovaries are inactive with no significant follicles or corpora lutea. The cervix may be closed but not firm and tight, or it may be thin, short, and dilated. As the length of daylight increases, mares undergo a vernal transition and the ovaries become active, with numerous large (>25 mm) follicles. The cervix and uterus have minimal tone. Mares have three or four prolonged intervals of estrus (periods of sexual receptivity to the stallion) during the vernal transition, but ovulation does not occur. The end of vernal transition is marked by a surge of luteinizing hormone and subsequent ovulation. After this ovulation, the first 21-day interovulatory period of that breeding season occurs and a regular estrous cycle is established.

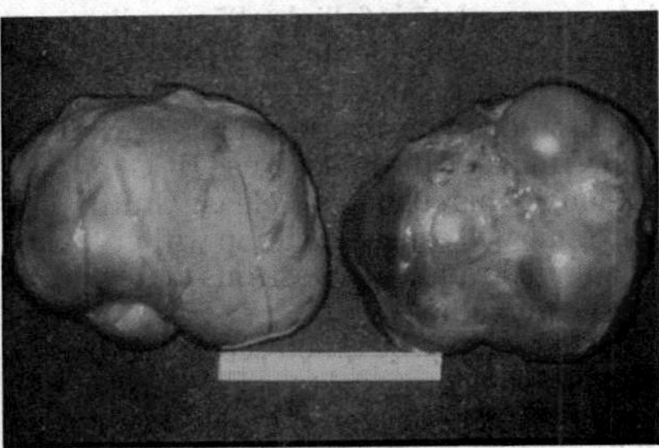

During the vernal transition, the mare's ovaries will enlarge and contain numerous large (>25 mm) follicles but no luteal structures. *Courtesy of Dr. Patricia Sertich.*

Although the mare continues to ovulate regularly every 21 days throughout the breeding season, the length of estrus varies, ranging from 2–8 days, and the length of diestrus varies accordingly to maintain a 21-day interval. Early in the breeding season, estrus tends to be longer, whereas around the summer solstice the mare may be sexually receptive for only 2–3 days.

Mares have two follicular waves each cycle. The first wave of follicular development occurs during diestrus, and these follicles become atretic. The second wave occurs after luteolysis and is associated with estrus. Early in estrus, the endometrial folds of the uterus are edematous, but the edema wanes as ovulation approaches. Usually, one follicle becomes dominant and ovulates when it is ≥30 mm in diameter. The dominant follicle enlarges and then softens just before ovulation. The oocyte is released through the ovulation fossa. A corpus hemorrhagicum and subsequent corpus luteum form and produce progesterone, which stimulates closure of the cervix and an increase in uterine tone. This corpus luteum will be mature and become responsive to prostaglandin in ~5 days. If pregnancy is not established, luteolysis occurs at 14 days, and the mare returns to estrus and continues to cycle.

Artificial Manipulation of Photoperiod: After winter anestrus and the vernal transition, cyclicity naturally starts sometime in the spring, when breeding can begin. Because changes in the mare's genital tract are seen in response to the length of daylight, the onset of ovulation and subsequent regular estrous cycles—and thus, the onset of the breeding season—can be hastened by exposing the mare to 16 hr of light per day; 8–10 wk are required for mares to respond. If the breeding season is scheduled to begin February 15, mares should be exposed to daily supplemental artificial lighting starting on December 1. Mares need to experience a natural photoperiod of decreasing length of daylight in the fall. Mares can then be abruptly exposed to 16 hr of light each day, or the supplemental light can be gradually increased to a 16-hr day throughout 60 days. In an abrupt lighting program, mares living in natural daylight are exposed to supplemental light from ~4:30 pm until 11:00 pm daily. In a less expensive, energy conserving, stepwise program, mares can be exposed to 3 hr of supplemental light in the evening the first week of December, and then the supplemental light is increased by 30 min each week until mares are exposed to 16 hr of light each day. An automatic timer aids compliance and saves on labor.

The supplemental light must be added at dusk; light added in the morning before dawn is not effective. A minimum of 10 foot-candles (107 lux) of incandescent or fluorescent light is necessary. The amount of light should allow one to comfortably read newsprint. Mares can be stimulated individually in a stall or as a group in a lighted paddock.

Manipulation of Ovarian Activity: Ovarian activity is frequently manipulated by administration of hormones to facilitate scheduling of breeding appointments and to limit the number of breedings per estrus. Breedings should be spaced for stallions with large books of mares so that semen use is optimized. Geographic locations and transportation constraints may also necessitate scheduled breedings. Many situations can benefit from an ovulation control program. (*See also* HORMONAL CONTROL OF ESTRUS, p 2244.)

Administration of prostaglandin ($PGF_2\alpha$), IM, to a mare in diestrus causes luteolysis and allows a follicle to mature and ovulate. The corpus luteum must be 5–14 days old to respond to $PGF_2\alpha$. The mare will come into estrus 2–5 days after administration of $PGF_2\alpha$. Time to ovulation is variable (3–10 days) and depends on the stage of the mare's current follicular wave and on the size and character of follicles at the time of $PGF_2\alpha$ administration. It is recommended that the mare's ovaries be examined by palpation and ultrasonography at the time of $PGF_2\alpha$ administration to optimize the prediction of ovulation.

Dinoprost, a naturally occurring $PGF_2\alpha$ (1 mg/45.5 kg, IM), may cause transient adverse effects such as lowered body temperature, increased heart and respiratory rates, sweating, muscle cramping, colic, ataxia, and weakness. Signs are seen within 15 min and usually subside within 1 hr. Synthetic preparations, eg, cloprostenol sodium (0.55 mcg/kg, IM), have fewer adverse effects.

Human chorionic gonadotropin (HCG) 2,500–5,000 IU, IV or IM, has been administered (off-label use) to hasten ovulation of a dominant follicle during estrus. If the mare has a preovulatory follicle ≥35 mm diameter, ovulation occurs within 36–48 hr after administration. An FDA-approved preparation of deslorelin acetate is available and eliminates the need to use HCG off-label. This sustained-release GnRH analogue will cause ovulation within 48 hr of administration to an estrous mare with a 30–40 mm follicle.

Ovulation can be timed accurately using the following protocol (not FDA approved): On days 1–10, 10 mg of estradiol 17-β and 150 mg of progesterone are administered IM. On day 10, dinoprost (1 mg/45.5 kg, IM) is also administered. On day 16, mares come into estrus, and insemination should be performed on day 19 or 20. Most (85%)

mares ovulate on day 20, 21, or 22. This regimen is effective at any time in cycling mares except when a large, dominant follicle <48 hr from ovulation is present. If a mature follicle is present, the protocol should not begin until after ovulation.

Altrenogest is a synthetic progestin that suppresses the receptive sexual behavior of estrus. Altrenogest is administered at 0.44 mg/kg, PO by dose syringe or top-dressed on feed for 12–15 days. Estrus occurs 4–5 days after treatment ends, with variable timing of ovulation (8–15 days). Although altrenogest effectively suppresses estrus (sexual receptive behavior), it does not consistently control the time interval to ovulation.

Estrus Detection: Frequent palpation and ultrasonography of the genital tract, excellent record keeping, and administration of hormones allow veterinarians to intensively monitor and manipulate a mare's estrous cycle. But breeding management can be optimized if a good estrus detection program is in place. A mare detected in estrus will prompt the breeding farm manager to examine and prepare the mare for breeding. Estrus may be the first indication that a pregnant mare has experienced early embryonic death or an abortion.

The mare should be presented to a stallion (teaser) daily or every other day during the breeding season, and the mare's behavioral response accurately interpreted and recorded. Mares in estrus raise their tail, squat, urinate, evert the vulvar lips to expose the clitoris, and ultimately tolerate copulation. Mares in diestrus usually squeal, kick, bite, and reject the stallion's advances. Adequate exposure to and contact with the teaser may be needed to elicit the mare's response; a mare with a dominant follicle may initially not appear receptive because of nervousness or inexperience. Some mares with foals by their side may not exhibit estrus to the teaser because of their protective nature. The mare's behavior when teased should be consistent with the findings on examination of the genital tract. Response to teasing can determine whether estrus has begun and indicate when a mare should be palpated and bred. Failure to return to estrus 2–3 wk after breeding may suggest that the mare is pregnant.

Mares in seasonal anestrus may remain passive in the presence of a stallion.

Some anestrus mares will be receptive when confronted by a stallion and will tolerate a stallion's sexual advances. This tolerance seems to be due to a lack of progesterone, similar to the tolerance seen in an ovariectomized mare when used as a stimulus for semen collection from a stallion.

Mares normally have three or four prolonged periods (7–14 days) of sexual receptivity during the vernal transition before the first ovulation of the breeding season occurs. Similar long periods of sexual receptivity occur during the autumnal transition between the breeding season and winter anestrus.

BREEDING SOUNDNESS EXAMINATION OF THE MARE

A comprehensive reproductive evaluation is recommended for the mare that has unknown or questionable fertility. Abnormalities can be diagnosed and appropriate therapy instituted to correct any problem before breeding is scheduled. A coordinated plan of management should be developed based on the mare's history of reproductive performance, previous treatments, examination findings, laboratory test results, and intended use.

Theriogenologists typically examine mares for breeding soundness before purchase or breeding or when a mare is barren. A complete breeding soundness examination includes examination of the external genitalia and mammary gland, palpation and ultrasonography per rectum of the internal genitalia, manual and visual vaginal examination (vaginoscopy), aerobic culture of an endometrial swab/sample, cytologic evaluation of an endometrial swab/sample, and histologic evaluation of an endometrial biopsy sample.

In the case of a young, healthy, maiden mare, palpation and ultrasonography per rectum to determine the presence of a uterus of normal size and consistency, normal active ovaries, and functional cervix may suffice. Perineal conformation should be evaluated. A manual vaginal examination should be performed to confirm the hymen is patent. If there is evidence of pneumovagina or vaginitis, commonly present in slim, fit, racing fillies, an endometrial swab and biopsy are indicated.

In postpartum mares, palpation and ultrasonography per rectum are required to evaluate uterine involution. A manual vaginal examination should be performed to ascertain whether the reproductive tract was traumatized during foaling. Thorough evaluation of the cervix requires direct manual palpation per vagina of the cervix after foal heat ovulation when the mare is in diestrus and under progesterone stimulation. Mares that had foaling problems (eg, dystocia, retained placenta) require a more extensive evaluation. All postpartum mares have a transient endometritis during uterine involution; therefore, uterine swab and biopsy typically provide more useful information if delayed for ≥3 wk after parturition.

Barren mares require a complete breeding soundness examination. Occasionally, hysteroscopy, endocrine assay, or a karyotype may provide additional information.

Signalment and History: A standard breeding soundness examination form to record examination findings can be helpful in ensuring all areas are covered during the examination. The horse should be accurately identified.

Determination of stage of reproductive cycle and estrous cycle is essential for proper evaluation and interpretation of laboratory test results. The history should include previous length and character of estrus, breedings and their results, therapy, and specific reproductive problems. In particular, histologic findings of an endometrial biopsy sample reflect the stage of the mare's reproductive cycle and any recent intrauterine activities (breeding, treatment, foaling). Regardless of the history, the mare's nonpregnant status should be confirmed before performing any procedures (eg, endometrial swab, endometrial biopsy, direct manual cervical palpation) that would compromise an existing pregnancy (*see* p 2194).

Restraint: The mare can be restrained in hand, in stocks, or placed against a stall wall with the hindquarters positioned in a doorway. For fractious mares, a twitch may provide short-term restraint to allow completion of the examination. For the occasional situation in which the temperament of the mare poses risk of injury to the mare or examiner, chemical restraint may be used. A combination of acepromazine (0.02 mg/kg) and xylazine (0.3–0.5 mg/kg) administered IV works well for short procedures. If possible, the external genitalia should be evaluated before tranquilizers are administered, because the drug's use will alter the tone and competency of the perineum.

Physical Examination: The mare's tail *should be wrapped* and tied to one side. The tail and inner thighs should be examined for the presence of dried exudate indicative of genital infection or urine staining that may be associated with urine pooling or incontinence. The size and shape of the clitoris should be assessed. A mare with an excessively large clitoris may have been androgenized either by excessive exogenous hormone administration during pregnancy or by endogenous hormones in an intersex condition (male pseudohermaphrodite). Normal vulvar lips have good tone and apposition and form the first barrier of the uterus against environmental contaminants. The vulvar lips should be parted to determine the competency of the vestibulovaginal fold. If air readily aspirates into the vagina, the mare may be prone to pneumovagina and may require a vulvoplasty (Caslick operation).

For per rectum procedures, the examiner, wearing a clean examination sleeve with water-soluble lubricant, must first empty the rectum of feces. Palpation and ultrasonography per rectum permit assessment of the internal genital tract. Each part of the genital tract should be systematically palpated. Typically, a real-time 5–10 MHz linear ultrasound probe, which produces a rectangular, cross-sectional image of the structure scanned, is used for ultrasonographic examinations of the reproductive tract. Ovarian size and character as well as the presence of an ovulation fossa should be noted. Anechoic follicles should be measured and counted, and the presence of a hyperechoic corpus luteum recorded. Normal oviducts are not routinely examined because their small size prevents palpation and imaging.

The size, shape, and contents of the uterus should be recorded. The mare's uterus is T-shaped with the horns perpendicular to the body of the uterus. It is suspended in the pelvic canal by the broad ligament, which is attached dorsally to the sublumbar region. Ultrasonography permits accurate assessment and measurement of the uterine horns. The size and character of any anechoic endometrial cysts should be recorded for reference so their presence will not be confused with a conceptus during subsequent early pregnancy examinations.

The uterus has several endometrial folds that increase the surface area of the uterine lumen. The endometrial folds should be carefully assessed during palpation per rectum by "slipping" the folds through the examiner's fingers along the entire length of each horn. The character of the uterus changes during the estrous cycle. During estrus, the endometrial folds become edematous, causing the uterine horns to have alternating areas of hypo- and hyperechogenicity when a cross-section is viewed ultrasonographically. As estrus progresses, the edema in the endometrial folds wanes so that it is minimal by the time of ovulation. After ovulation and development of the corpus luteum, the uterus is stimulated by progesterone, uterine tone increases, and the endometrial folds are no longer edematous. After 14–18 days of gestation, the endometrial folds are not readily palpable because of the gradual but marked increase in uterine wall thickness.

The length, width, and tone of the cervix are palpable per rectum; however, complete evaluation of the cervix requires direct palpation per vagina (*see* p 2193). A cervical evaluation also serves as a bioassay, because the cervix changes in response to the steroid hormone status of the mare. During anestrus, ovarian steroid serum concentrations are low, and the cervix is either short, thin, and open or closed but readily opened. After the first ovulation of the season and during subsequent periods of diestrus, serum progesterone concentrations are increased and the cervix is closed, with a long cylindrical shape. During estrus, serum progesterone concentrations are low, and estrogen concentrations are high; the cervix is relaxed and edematous. Visual (speculum) vaginal examination will allow further assessment of the character of the cervix.

Urine in the vagina (urovagina) may be seen sporadically or be a chronic problem. Mares with urovagina may have an abnormal voiding pattern, and the endometrium may show histologic evidence of chronic irritation. The neck of the bladder can be used to indicate the caudal boundary of the vagina during ultrasonography. The vagina can be imaged dorsal to the bladder and examined for any accumulation of echogenic fluid caudal to the cervix. A definitive diagnosis of urovagina requires direct observation of urine in the vagina via vaginoscopy.

Endometrial Swab: Before an endometrial swab is taken, the nonpregnant status of the mare must be confirmed because the swabbing could lead to termination of a pregnancy (*see* p 2194). The perineum is cleansed with povidone-iodine scrub, rinsed, and dried. The operator dons a sterile sleeve or clean examination sleeve with the hand encased in a sterile glove. A water-soluble lubricant free of bacteriostatic chemicals is placed on the back of the hand and lower arm. When obtaining an endometrial swab sample, the vestibule, vagina, and cervix must be passed. Care must be taken to avoid contamination of the swab by microorganisms in the structures caudal to the uterus that would hinder accurate interpretation of the culture results.

A double-guarded occluded uterine swab is gently guided through the cranial end of the cervix. Once inside the uterine body, the inner guard is advanced from the outer guard, and the swab is exposed to the uterine lumen for 30–60 sec. The swab tip is withdrawn into the inner guard, which is then withdrawn into the outer guard before the entire swabbing instrument is removed from the uterine body. The swab tip is carefully placed into a transport system, which is vital to maintain viability of the organisms from the time of sample collection until aerobic culture in the laboratory. Stuart's carrier medium may maintain microorganisms for as long as 72 hr if stored at ambient temperature. A second endometrial sample may be taken immediately after the first or simultaneously with a uterine swab or cytology brush. This sample is then evaluated cytologically by rolling it onto a glass microscope slide, fixing and staining with a Romanowsky-type stain, and viewing it microscopically for evidence of neutrophils, debris, and microorganisms.

A low-volume uterine lavage can be performed in mares with negative culture results despite obvious clinical signs of endometritis. Sterile saline (60–150 mL) is infused into the uterus using a closed system with a small uterine catheter. Oxytocin (20 IU, IV) is administered to enhance uterine evacuation. The effluent is collected by gravity flow into a sterile centrifuge tube and then centrifuged. The pellet is then swabbed, placed into transport media, and submitted for aerobic culture. A second swab can be made of the pellet for cytologic examination after staining.

Most laboratories streak the swabs on 5% sheep blood agar for general growth and on MacConkey's agar for growth of gram-negative organisms, after which cultures are aerobically incubated at 37°C (98.6°F).

Organisms commonly isolated that are associated with endometritis include β-hemolytic streptococci (90% *Streptococcus zooepidemicus*, 10% *S equisimilis*), *Escherichia coli*, *Pseudomonas* (65% *P aeruginosa*), and *Klebsiella pneumoniae*. Organisms isolated that are commonly suspected to be contaminants include α-hemolytic streptococci, *Actinobacillus equuli*, *Salmonella enteritidis*, *Pasteurella*-like species, and *Staphylococcus*, *Enterobacter*, *Acinetobacter*, *Proteus*, *Citrobacter*, *Alcaligenes*, and *Aeromonas* spp.

In most cases, the mixed growth of a few miscellaneous microorganisms is not significant. A heavy growth of any microorganism should be considered significant unless obvious contamination has occurred. Clinical signs must be correlated with culture results to determine clinical significance and to develop a therapeutic plan. Isolation of an organism transmitted venereally, such as *Taylorella equigenitalis* (requires a special culture system) and certain strains of *Pseudomonas* and *Klebsiella* spp, is considered a significant finding. Occasionally, microorganisms causing a pyometra may not be detected on aerobic culture, because products of the inflammatory reaction prohibit their growth.

Aerobic culture results of the endometrial swab should be used as a diagnostic adjunct and not as the sole determinant in diagnosing a uterine infection. A positive culture result must be accompanied by evidence of inflammation for the diagnosis of endometritis to be made. Mares exhibiting clinical signs of infection (uterine fluid as seen on ultrasonographic examination per rectum, tail matting or uterine discharge, and the presence of inflammatory cells seen on a stained smear from a uterine sample) with a positive endometrial swab are likely to have endometritis. Inflammation seen on histologic evaluation of the endometrium confirms the diagnosis of endometritis. In these cases, the culture results are useful in determining the sensitivity of the causative microorganism and developing an antimicrobial treatment plan.

The following antibiotics (*see* TABLE 9) have been used for daily (3–7 days) uterine infusion by diluting with sterile saline to an infusion volume of 60–100 mL. Systemic administration of antibiotics may be considered if the microorganism, management situation, and ease of treatment indicate. Two doses of long-acting ceftiofur crystalline free acid (6.6 mg/kg, IM) can be administered 96 hr apart for adequate serum concentration for 10 days, which may be an efficacious treatment for endometritis due to *S zooepidemicus*.

Endometrial Biopsy: An endometrial biopsy sample is usually obtained immediately after the endometrial samples have been procured. It should be kept in mind that manipulation of the endometrium can quickly cause a neutrophilic response in the endometrium. Preparation for biopsy is the same as for taking a swab (*see* above). The basket of the biopsy instrument should be kept closed during positioning to prevent accidental procurement of vagina, cervix, or examination glove. The instrument is manually guided with the gloved hand through the caudal genital tract into the uterine lumen. While keeping the instrument in place within the uterus with the nongloved (external) hand, the gloved hand is carefully withdrawn from the genital tract and inserted into the rectum to allow positioning of the basket of the biopsy instrument at the ventral luminal surface of the base of a uterine horn. The instrument jaws are then opened, the uterine wall is pressed into the side of the basket, and the jaws are closed. The jaws should be kept closed while the instrument is withdrawn from the genital tract. The tissue should be gently teased from the basket and placed into Bouin's fixative. If the sample will not

TABLE 9 INTRAUTERINE ANTIBIOTICS FOR USE IN MARES

Antibiotic	Intrauterine Dose
Penicillin (sodium or potassium salt)	5 million U
Ampicillin	1–3 g
Ticarcillin	3–6 g
Ticarcillin with clavulanic acid	3–6 g
Carbenicillin	2–5 g
Gentamicin sulfate diluted with 20 mL sodium bicarbonate and 20 mL saline	1 g
Amikacin sulfate	1–2 g
Ceftiofur sodium	1 g
Clotrimazole	400–700 mg

be processed within a few days, it should be transferred into 70% ethanol or 10% formalin.

It is not unusual for a small amount of uterine bleeding to occur after biopsy. The biopsy procedure is not detrimental to fertility, and a mare can conceive from a breeding that occurred during an estrus when biopsy was performed.

Histologic evaluation of the endometrium provides prognostic information about the mare's ability to carry a foal to term. The luminal contents may indicate the presence of uterine fluid or exudate. Epithelial cell height is related to hormone status; cells are cuboidal during anestrus and low to tall columnar during the breeding season. Transepithelial cells may indicate active inflammation. The pattern, character, and location of inflammation indicate the chronicity of response—neutrophils indicate an acute reaction, and lymphocytes and plasma cells indicate a chronic reaction. Focal or diffuse cellular distribution pattern, frequency of inflammatory cells, and degree of infiltration (slight to severe) relate to severity of inflammation. Histologic evidence of significant inflammation, combined with a report of growth of microorganisms from aerobic culture of endometrial swab and the presence of clinical signs of infection (uterine fluid, uterine discharge), support the decision that an endometrium would benefit from therapy to decrease inflammation.

Knowledge of the pattern of distribution and severity of periglandular fibrosis is prognostically useful. Fibrosis surrounding groups of glands ("fibrotic nest") is thought to be more clinically significant than fibrosis of individual glands. Periglandular fibrosis may interfere with endometrial gland function and may be a factor causing early embryonic death. Glandular distention normally develops during pregnancy, but widespread cystic glandular distention in the nonpregnant mare is undesirable. Cystic glandular distention is often associated with periglandular fibrosis and may result from an accumulation of gland secretions proximal to the occlusion of the endometrial gland by periglandular fibrosis.

Endometria are classified in four categories that attempt to predict ability to carry a foal to term. **Category I** indicates no significant changes are present in the endometrium, and no treatment is required. The estimated foaling rate is 80%–90%. An endometrium with any notable periglandular fibrosis cannot be classified as Category I. **Category II** is a broad category that includes most mares. It has been divided into **Category IIA**, for mares with less severe changes, and **Category IIB**, for mares with more severe changes. The estimated foaling rate is 50%–80% in mares with Category IIA endometria and 10%–50% in mares with Category IIB endometria. Often, therapy may improve the state of the endometrium by reducing inflammation, cystic glandular distention, and lymphatic lacunae. Improvement in the endometrium may allow for better classification at a later date. There is no effective treatment to decrease the severity of periglandular fibrosis. **Category III** is the poorest classification, and these endometria have widespread, severe changes that include periglandular fibrosis or inflammation. A widespread pattern of distribution of slight to moderate changes may be more deleterious than more severe changes that are infrequent and only involve individual glands. The estimated foaling rate of a Category III endometrium is <10%.

During interpretation of the findings on histologic evaluation of an endometrial biopsy sample, the extent of normal, unaffected endometrium is more significant than the presence of any particular lesion. In barren mares with a Category I or IIA endometrium, other reproductive abnormalities or poor breeding management should be investigated as the cause of infertility.

Vaginal Examination: The perineum is cleansed, rinsed, and dried before the visual vaginal examination via speculum. The vulvar lips are separated, and the speculum is advanced cranially at a dorsal angle so as to pass over and through the transverse (vestibulovaginal) fold of the vagina. Resistance against the speculum by this fold of tissue indicates good tone and function. A bright light is necessary to adequately view the cervix and vaginal wall. The character of the cervix reflects the hormonal status of the mare. As the speculum is being withdrawn, it should be noted whether the vestibulovaginal fold occludes the vagina. The competency of the vestibulovaginal fold is important, because it forms the second barrier for the uterus against external contaminants.

Thorough evaluation of the completeness and competency of the cervix can be accomplished only by direct palpation per vagina while the mare is under progesterone stimulation (ie, cervix closed). The cervix forms the third barrier for the uterus against external contaminants.

PREGNANCY DETERMINATION

The schedule for determination of pregnancy varies among breeding farms. One schedule is as follows: 1) days 14–18—check for pregnancy and twins; if open, mare can be rebred on days 19–20; 2) days 25–30—evaluate normal embryo development (heartbeat present at 24–25 days), recheck for twins; 3) days 40–60—evaluate normal fetal development; 4) fall check—confirm mare is still pregnant.

Palpation Per Rectum: The pregnant cervix should be tightly closed and elongated with a prominent portio vaginalis 14–21 days after ovulation. Uterine tone increases and the uterine wall thickens so that by 14–18 days, the endometrial folds can no longer be readily palpated per rectum.

The conceptus develops in a recognizable pattern of size and shape, allowing estimation of age based on palpable characteristics. In maiden and barren mares, at 25–28 days of gestation, a careful, experienced examiner may be able to feel the embryonic vesicle ventrally at the base of one uterine horn, as a bulge 3.5 cm in diameter. At 30 days, the uterine horns are small with pronounced tone, and the conceptus can be felt as a ventral bulge 4 cm in diameter and positioned at the base of the gravid uterine horn. The uterine wall is thin over the expanding conceptus. At 42–45 days, the conceptus occupies about half of the gravid uterine horn and is 5–7 cm in diameter. By 48–50 days, the enlargement of the conceptus begins to involve the uterine body and is 6–8 cm in diameter and 8–10 cm long.

At 60 days, nearly the entire gravid horn and half of the uterine body is occupied by conceptus, but the nongravid horn remains small with considerable tone. The 60-day conceptus is 8–10 cm in diameter and 12–15 cm long. After 85 days, the turgidity of the conceptus decreases so that the fetus becomes palpable. At 90 days, the conceptus fills the entire uterus, and the cranial portion of the uterus may extend over the brim of the pelvis into the abdominal cavity.

After 100–120 days of gestation, the gravid uterus is positioned cranial to the pelvic brim in the abdominal cavity. The ovaries are positioned cranially and ventrally and closer together because of the downward traction exerted by the enlarging uterus on the broad ligament. After 150 days of gestation, the ovaries are not routinely felt per rectum. During midgestation, the gravid uterus may be difficult to reach, because it is positioned ventrally in the abdomen. But as the conceptus/gravid uterus enlarges, its dorsal surface comes back into reach in late gestation. One should always confirm that two uterine horns with palpable endometrial folds cannot be identified in the pelvic canal before making a midterm pregnancy diagnosis.

Ultrasonography: The spherical shape of the equine embryo and the characteristic pattern of development of the fetal membranes permit accurate estimation of stage of gestation by ultrasonography until 45 days after ovulation. The embryo may first be imaged in the uterus with a 5–10 MHz linear transducer at 9–10 days as a round anechoic yolk sac 4 mm in diameter. The spherical conceptus moves throughout the lumen of the uterine horns and uterine body from day 6–16. The early conceptus is seen to have a bright white (echogenic) line on the dorsal and sometimes the ventral aspect of its image that is called a specular reflector, which is an artifact seen when the ultrasound beam strikes the wide, smooth surface of the conceptus at a 90° angle. This specular reflector, embryonic motility, and linear growth rate may help differentiate an early (<16 day), motile embryo from some uterine cysts.

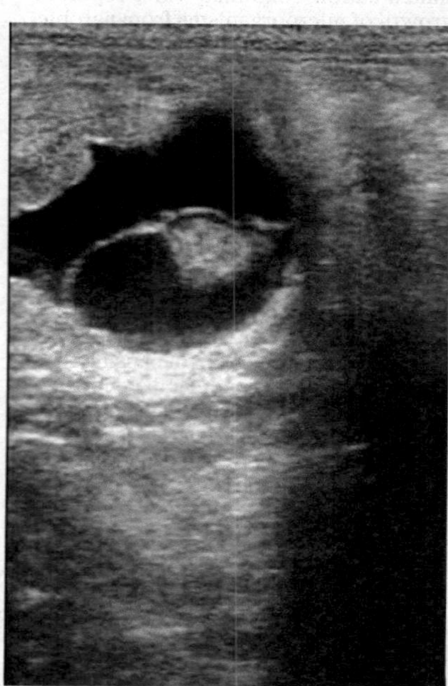

Sonogram of 29-day conceptus in a mare. The dorsal anechoic yolk sac is nearly equal in size to developing ventral allantoic cavity. *Courtesy of Dr. Patricia Sertich.*

At day 17–18, the conceptus has a characteristic "guitar-pick" shape. At day 21, the embryo proper can be seen in the ventral aspect of the yolk sac, and by 24 days the allantoic cavity is visible as an anechoic compartment ventral to the embryo proper. At day 25, a heart beat should be present in the embryo proper. As the allantoic cavity enlarges, the yolk sac comprises a decreasing proportion of the conceptus. The position of the allantois and relative sizes of the developing allantoic cavity and the regressing yolk sac can indicate the stage of gestation between days 24 and 45. At 30 days, the allantoic cavity occupies approximately one-half of the conceptus, so that the size of the yolk sac is equal to that of the allantoic cavity. At 45 days, the only visible fluid cavity is the allantoic cavity, and the fetus appears to be suspended from the dorsal wall of the uterus by its umbilical cord and is positioned in dorsal recumbency.

Endocrine Tests: Cells from the chorionic girdle of the conceptus invade the endometrium to form endometrial cups that produce equine chorionic gonadotropin (eCG). Increased serum concentrations of eCG 40–120 days after ovulation indicate the presence of endometrial cups. Concentrations of eCG may remain increased until 120 days, even if fetal death occurs (false-positive). A false-negative result will be obtained if eCG assay is used as a pregnancy test in a pregnant mare before 40 or after 120 days of gestation.

Estrone sulfate is produced by the fetus and is a good indicator of fetal viability. Plasma and urine concentrations of estrone sulfate are increased after 60 days and 150 days, respectively, of pregnancy. Either endocrine assay can be used properly as a pregnancy test only if the breeding and ovulation dates are known.

PARASITE CONTROL DURING PREGNANCY

Most anthelmintics are safe for use throughout pregnancy, but precautions and contraindications on package inserts should be heeded. In general, anthelmintics should not be administered to mares during the first 60 days of gestation (organogenesis). Parasite control programs should be tailored to meet the particular farm needs. *See also* GASTROINTESTINAL PARASITES OF HORSES, p 315, and ANTHELMINTICS, p 2637. Pregnant mares should be administered ivermectin or a benzimidazole 1–3 days before foaling to prevent lactogenic transmission of *Strongyloides westeri*, which can cause diarrhea in young foals.

VACCINATIONS

Vaccination programs should follow a continuous, year-round schedule based on local health problems. Vaccination against rhinopneumonitis should be performed at 5, 7, and 9 mo of gestation. Vaccines that require annual boosters should be administered 4–6 wk before the mare's due date to stimulate the dam to produce antibodies that will be transferred to the foal via the colostrum (*see* TABLE 10). Detailed information regarding current vaccination recommendations is available on the AAEP website (www.aaep.org). Colostrum should be ingested in the first 24 hr of life to effectively provide passive transfer of immunoglobulins.

ABORTION

See also ABORTION IN HORSES, p 1343. Twin pregnancy is the most common noninfectious cause of abortion in mares. In most cases, uterine capacity and subsequent placentation are inadequate to support two fetuses to term. Although twins may spontaneously reduce to a viable singleton early in gestation (<60 days), visible abortions tend to be seen after 7–9 mo. Premonitory clinical signs of impending abortion may be only premature mammary gland development. Fetal membranes should always be examined for large avillous areas typically located between the twin conceptuses.

Because of the risk of abortion and dystocia in a mare carrying twins, if twins are detected by ultrasonography per rectum at <30 days, reduction to one embryo by manual crushing per rectum is recommended. Between 30–60 days of gestation, transvaginal aspiration of one conceptus may result in a viable singleton. At approximately 60 days of gestation, one fetus may be eliminated by cervical dislocation. After 110 days of gestation, one twin may be reduced by intracardiac injection of potassium chloride guided by transabdominal ultrasonography. Success rates vary depending on the procedure performed, the experience of the veterinarian, and the character of the pregnancy. Pregnancy should be monitored repeatedly by ultrasonography after twin reduction.

The most common cause of viral abortion in mares is equine rhinopneumonitis, which is caused by equine herpesvirus 1 (EHV-1). These abortions occur predominantly in the last trimester and usually are not associated

TABLE 10 EXAMPLE OF VACCINATION SCHEDULE FOR BROODMARES

Vaccine	Schedule
Equine rhinopneumonitis (inactivated)	EHV-1 at 5, 7, and 9 mo of gestation; EHV-1/EHV-4 4–6 wk before due date
Tetanus (toxoid)	4–6 wk before due date
Equine influenza	4–6 wk before due date; if unvaccinated, initially administer two doses at 4–6 wk intervals and then a third dose 4–6 wk before due date
Eastern and Western equine encephalomyelitis	Usually administered to mares in late spring or early summer before onset of insect season; initially administer two doses at a 4–6 wk interval; 4–6 wk before due date
Rabies	4–6 wk before due date
Botulism (toxoid)	Initially three doses at 4–6 wk intervals, then annual booster 4–6 wk before due date
West Nile virus	Initially two doses at a 4–6 wk interval; 4–6 wk before due date
Rotaviral diarrhea	8, 9, and 10 mo of gestation
Equine viral arteritis (modified-live virus)	A negative titer should be documented by a USDA-approved laboratory before vaccination; pregnant mares should not be vaccinated; open mares should be vaccinated before breeding to a positive stallion that is shedding the virus; vaccinated horses must be isolated for 3 wk after vaccination; annual boosters recommended; positive titers may cause problems if mare is to be exported or bred on certain farms. (Stallions should also be vaccinated 3 mo before breeding.)
Equine monocytic ehrlichiosis (Potomac horse fever)	Initially administer two doses at a 3–4 mo interval; 4–6 wk before due date

with a respiratory infection. All pregnant mares should be vaccinated against EHV-1 at 5, 7, and 9 mo of gestation.

The equine arteritis virus can cause equine viral arteritis (EVA) abortion. An EVA-seronegative mare scheduled to be bred to an EVA-positive stallion that is shedding the arteritis virus in the semen should be vaccinated before breeding. Horses must be isolated for 3 wk after EVA vaccination. Mares should not be vaccinated against EVA during pregnancy.

Sporadic abortions due to placentitis can be caused by bacterial and mycotic infections of the placenta. These are predominantly ascending infections acquired through the caudal genital tract but may also be focal or diffuse. Bacteria involved include *Streptococcus zooepidemicus*, *Escherichia coli*, *Klebsiella pneumoniae*, *Pseudomonas aeruginosa*, *Staphylococcus aureus*, *Rhodococcus equi*, and *Actinobacillus equuli*. Mycotic organisms include *Mucor* and *Aspergillus* spp. Efforts to reduce the incidence of these abortions should include good breeding hygiene, treatment of genital disease before breeding, maintaining good body condition throughout pregnancy, and vulvoplasty (Caslick operation) to prevent pneumovagina. Mares at risk of placentitis should be examined by ultrasonography per rectum periodically during late gestation for evidence of genital infection and placental abnormalities as evidenced by uterine discharge and increased uteroplacental thickness.

Any aborted fetus and fetal membranes should promptly be submitted fresh or cooled (never frozen) to a diagnostic laboratory to determine the cause of the abortion.

PARTURITION

The pregnant mare should be taken to the foaling location 3–4 wk before the expected foaling date to enhance immunity against pathogens present in the environment. Antibodies will be sequestered in colostrum for passive immunity in the newborn. Quality of colostrum will be improved by administering booster vaccinations 4–6 wk before the mare's due date (*see also* VACCINATIONS, p 2195).

Foaling box stalls should be large (at least 3.5 × 3 × 3.5 m). The foaling area should have good ventilation and be well bedded with clean, dry straw. The walls should be solidly constructed and free of sharp edges. Mares may benefit from foaling outdoors on turf, weather permitting. Regardless of location, the mare should be observed without disturbance.

Evaluation of the premonitory signs of parturition is useful but does not permit precise prediction of the time of delivery. The mammary gland starts developing 3–6 wk before foaling and distends with colostrum in most mares 2–3 days before parturition. Colostrum may drip from the teats and dry to form a waxy material at each teat orifice. This "waxing" develops in ~95% of mares 6–48 hr before foaling, but in some cases, it is not seen at all or it may precede parturition by many days. Before the mare foals, the calcium and potassium content of udder secretions increase, and the sodium content decreases. Water hardness chemical tests have been used to measure these in mammary gland secretions to predict parturition.

If a mare has had a vulvoplasty (Caslick operation) during pregnancy, it is necessary that an episiotomy be performed ~2 wk before parturition.

Stages of Parturition: It is critical to understand the normal progression of events during parturition. Abnormal events can then be identified and intervention provided as needed. Parturition is divided into three stages.

Stage I is characterized by signs of abdominal discomfort and restlessness due to uterine contractions. Patches of sweat on the flank and behind the elbows usually appear a few hours before foaling. The uterine contractions increase in frequency and intensity, causing the fetus to engage into the cervix and pelvic canal. The fetus rotates from a dorsopubic to a dorsosacral position before expulsion. Mares may roll during the first stage, which is thought to facilitate rotation of the fetus.

Increasing pressure in the uterus causes the chorioallantois to protrude through the internal os of the cervix. The chorion over the cervix is smooth—it does not have microvilli and is referred to as the cervical star. The chorioallantois usually ruptures at the cervical star, and the release of the tea-colored allantoic fluid marks the end of the first stage of parturition. In lay terminology, this event is referred to as the mare "breaking her water."

Stage II starts with the rupture of the chorioallantois and ends when the fetus is expelled. Second stage labor usually lasts 15–30 min. When the fetus engages the cervix, the Ferguson reflex occurs and stimulates the mare to have abdominal contractions. The allantoic fluid lubricates the canal, facilitating expulsion of the amnion and fetus. Vaginal distention causes release of oxytocin and further myometrial and abdominal contractions. The amnion appears at the vulvar lips as a whitish, fluid-filled membrane. The straining efforts of the mare consist of three to four strong contractions, followed by a short period of rest. During the actual expulsion of the foal, the mare usually assumes lateral recumbency with all four limbs extended.

The foal is normally delivered in an anterior, longitudinal presentation and dorsosacral position with the head, neck, and forelimbs extended. One front hoof of the foal usually precedes the other hoof by ~15 cm, facilitating passage of the elbows and shoulders through the pelvic canal. The foal is usually born with the umbilical cord intact and covered by the amnion, which is ruptured by movements of the mare or foal. If amnion remains over the foal's nose, an attendant should remove it to prevent suffocation. If left undisturbed, the mare may lie for some time with the foal's hindlimbs in the vagina. If the foal has not been delivered within 30 min of the rupture of the chorioallantois and release of the allantoic fluid, obstetric intervention is indicated.

Stage III involves expulsion of the fetal membranes. Normally, fetal membrane passage occurs rapidly (within 3 hr) after delivery of the foal. The weight of the amnion and cord may help the chorion separate from the endometrium. Progressive traction by the amnion and moderate uterine contractions originating at the tip of the horn cause complete separation of the chorioallantois, which may become inverted during the process. The mare may stand with the amnion hanging from the vulva at the level of the hocks or below. If the mare kicks at the hanging membranes, endangering the foal, the exposed membranes should be tied in knots to shorten the length to above the hocks.

If the fetal membranes have not been passed by 3 hr after parturition, oxytocin

(20 IU, IV or IM) should be administered at 15- to 30-min intervals until membranes pass. If fetal membranes are still retained at 8 hr after foaling, therapy for retained placenta should be instituted (*see* p 1381).

Premature Separation of the Placenta: Normally, the translucent white amnion appears first at the vulvar lips during the expulsion stage of labor. Premature separation of the placenta is characterized by the appearance of the bright red, velvety, intact chorioallantois between the vulvar lips before the foal is delivered. The presence of the chorion at the vulvar lips indicates that it has separated from the endometrium before the foal is able to breathe spontaneously. The chorioallantois must immediately be ruptured and the foal manually delivered, or the foal will asphyxiate. The severity and duration of hypoxia that results determines the severity of neurologic abnormalities displayed by the foal (peripartum asphyxia or hypoxic ischemic encephalopathy [see p 2094]).

DYSTOCIA

Most causes of dystocia in the mare are due to abnormal presentation, position, or posture. A dead or compromised fetus often is not properly positioned in the pelvic canal. Dystocia due to fetal–maternal disproportion or primary uterine inertia is rare in mares. A vaginal examination should be performed if the foal is not delivered within 30 min after rupture of the chorioallantois or if second-stage labor does not begin after >4 hr of obvious first-stage labor.

The initial examination may be performed in the standing mare. The perineum should be cleansed with povidone-iodine scrub and rinsed well with water. Efforts should be made to maintain hygiene at all times. A diagnosis of the presentation, position, and posture must be made, and a plan formulated to mutate the fetus into an anterior longitudinal, dorsosacral position with head, neck, and front limbs extended. Copious amounts of clean lubricant will ease mutations and fetal expulsion. Excessive mechanical or manual traction should be avoided. Length of time spent on manipulations and any progress should be noted. Once the fetus is properly presented and positioned in the pelvic canal, if it *cannot* be delivered using traction exerted by two strong adults, the diagnosis should be reconsidered and plan of action altered. Compassion for the foaling mare must be considered in case management decisions.

Sedation can be provided by administration of xylazine (0.5–1 mg/kg, IV) and butorphanol (0.01–0.02 mg/kg, IV). If abdominal straining prevents adequate vaginal examination and fetal mutation, epidural anesthesia may be administered using xylazine (0.17 mg/kg) and lidocaine (0.22 mg/kg) diluted to a total volume of 8 mL.

The front legs of the fetus should be identified and extended out the vulva. Obstetrical chains should be applied with one loop of the chain at the distal metacarpus and a second loop around the pastern to decrease trauma to the fetlock joint. The chains will aid manipulation and assist the application of traction. Once the head is exposed and the neck extended, it may be possible to intubate the fetus and administer low-flow oxygen using a portable oxygen tank or ventilate with a resuscitator (bag-valve mask). Proper rotation of the fetus may be facilitated by the mare getting up and down. After confirming that the fetus is in the proper orientation, manual traction can be applied, initially dorsally and then caudally. Once the foal's chest is exposed, traction should be applied in a ventral caudal direction. Traction should be applied intermittently in rhythm with the mare's abdominal contractions.

After the foal is delivered, an internal examination of the genital tract per vagina should be performed to identify any lacerations in the mare's genital tract or the presence of a twin. A few low doses of oxytocin (5–10 IU, IV or IM) can be administered every 15–20 min to stimulate passage of the fetal membranes and uterine evacuation. Repair of primary perineal lacerations usually can be delayed until after foal heat, but the dorsal aspect of the vulvar lips should be temporarily sutured if pneumovagina/pneumometra develops.

Controlled Vaginal Delivery: If resolution of the dystocia seems challenging or not possible in the standing mare because of the mare's straining or the orientation of the fetus, a controlled vaginal delivery should be considered. This is performed in an anesthetized mare. Field anesthesia can be accomplished by first heavily sedating with xylazine (1 mg/kg, IV) followed by diazepam (0.05–0.1 mg/kg, IV) and ketamine (2.2–2.5 mg/kg, IV). If gas anesthesia is available, routine induction and maintenance by inhalation will provide longer working time and greater relaxation. If general anesthesia and a controlled vaginal delivery are likely, epidural anesthesia should not be done. The mare's hindquarters are hoisted to allow the GI tract to move cranially in the abdomen, providing space to more readily perform fetal manipulations. It is prudent for managers of large breeding farms to have a designated location on the farm where a mare could be anesthetized and its hindquarters elevated (hobbles, winch, front end loader readily available) to hasten resolution of a dystocia.

Cesarean Section: If vaginal delivery attempts fail, the mare's value justifies it, and surgical facilities are available, a decision should rapidly be made to deliver the foal by cesarean section to spare the mare's caudal genital tract from further trauma. Treatment for retained placenta should be initiated immediately after surgery. Barring complications, mares can usually be rebred 60 days after cesarean section.

Fetotomy: If surgical facilities are not available or the economic situation prevents referral to a surgical facility, a fetotomy may allow delivery of the fetus. In the mare, fetotomy is usually recommended only if fetal expulsion can be accomplished after one or two cuts. Care should be taken to avoid damage to the mare's cervix and pelvic canal. Treatment for retained placenta should be initiated immediately after fetal delivery.

EXAMINATION OF THE FETAL MEMBRANES

Normally, the membranes are ruptured by the foal over the avillous cervical star region of the chorioallantois. The chorion (red velvety surface) and allantois (shiny surface containing many blood vessels) should be examined. Normally, the chorionic surface color ranges from red to brownish red. Patches of discolored, thick, exudate-covered chorioallantois at the cervical star or between the two horns may indicate an ascending or focal placentitis, respectively. The fetal membranes should be examined for completeness, paying particular attention to the presence of the edematous gravid horn tip and puckered nongravid horn tip.

The amnion has a white translucent appearance and may contain many blood vessels near the umbilical cord. Small, pale amniotic plaques can normally be seen along the umbilical cord.

Fetal and neonatal foal deaths may be associated with pathologic changes present in the fetal membranes. Typically, the fetal membranes weigh ~10%–11% of the foal's body weight. Placentitis or placental edema may increase the weight of the membranes. Integrity of the junction between the fetal and maternal components of the placenta is essential for normal fetal development. The mare has a diffuse microcotyledonary, epitheliochorial, nondeciduate type of placentation, which directly reflects the presence of abnormalities in the endometrium.

Retained Fetal Membranes: Fetal membranes that are not expelled within 3 hr of parturition are considered to be retained. Fetal membrane retention may be complete, but commonly only the nongravid horn is retained. If the typically puckered nongravid tip is not observed, it is assumed to be retained. If any membranes are hanging from the vulva of a postpartum mare, the amnion and cord should not be cut and removed, because their weight provides tension thought to enhance placental separation and expulsion. Fetal membranes not passed within 3–10 hr are considered to be pathologic and can lead to metritis, endotoxemia, and subsequently laminitis with fatal results. Accordingly, it is prudent to treat the condition as potentially

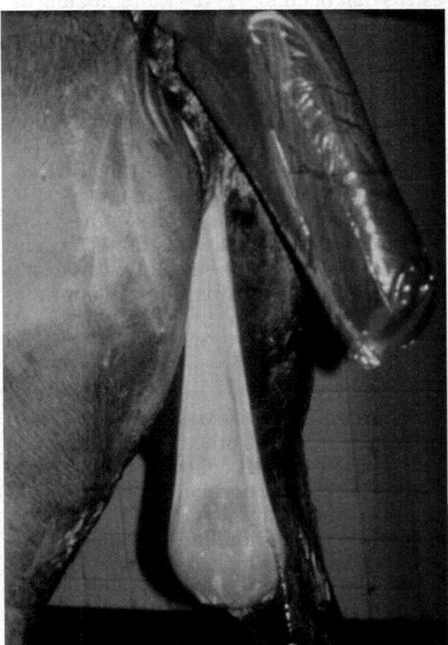

If membranes are seen hanging from the vulva in a mare that foaled>3 hr prior, the mare is considered to have retained fetal membranes. *Courtesy of Dr. Patricia Sertich.*

serious. If dystocia or traumatic uterine manipulation has occurred, aggressive treatment for retained membranes should be instituted immediately after parturition.

For early (3–8 hr) retention, 10–20 IU oxytocin can be repeatedly administered IV or IM every 30 min until the fetal membranes have passed. The dose of oxytocin should be decreased if the mare shows severe signs of colic or discomfort. Milking or sucking also stimulates endogenous release of oxytocin. Mares that retain fetal membranes >8 hr should be administered broad-spectrum antibiotics, such as potassium penicillin (22,000–44,000 IU/kg, IV, qid), gentamicin (2.2 mg/kg, IV, qid), or flunixin meglumine (0.25–0.5 mg/kg, IV, tid).

THE EARLY POSTPARTUM PERIOD

Uterine involution is characterized by expulsion of the fetal membranes and contraction of the uterus, cervix, and broad ligaments to normal nongravid dimensions. To achieve maximal reproductive efficiency, a broodmare must produce a foal every year. Horses have an average gestation length of ~340 days. Therefore, to maintain a 12-mo foaling interval, the mare must be bred again within 25 days of foaling. Mares can be bred on "foal heat," which is the first postpartum estrus that occurs 5–11 days after foaling in most mares. However, mares that experienced dystocia or retained membranes and metritis should not be bred on foal heat. Foal heat pregnancy rates are higher for mares bred after 10 days postpartum.

The fertility of the first breeding may be increased if breeding is delayed and $PGF_{2}\alpha$ (dinoprost, 1 mg/45.5 kg, IM, or cloprostenol, 0.55 mcg/kg, IM) administered ~5 days after the foal heat (first) ovulation. The mare can then be bred at the ensuing estrus just before the second postpartum ovulation.

BREEDING SOUNDNESS EXAMINATION OF THE STALLION

See also BREEDING SOUNDNESS EXAMINATION OF THE MALE, p 2230. The breeding soundness examination should begin with a thorough history, including information regarding libido, mating ability, number of mares bred, pregnancy rates, prior illness or injury, and any medications administered. A general physical examination should be performed, noting lameness (particularly of the back and hindlimbs) and heritable conditions that may affect breeding ability or desirability as a sire. The penis and prepuce should be free of lesions. The testes and epididymides should be evaluated for size, shape, and consistency. The testes should be freely movable within the scrotum and have a total scrotal width >8 cm. The length (L), width (W), and height (H) of the testicles can be determined using calipers or ultrasonography to calculate the volume of each testicle using the equation: $0.523 (L \times W \times H) =$ testicular volume. The stallion's daily sperm output (DSO) can then be predicted by the equation: total testicular volume $\times 0.024 - 0.76 =$ DSO. The internal genitalia, inguinal rings, and aorta and iliac vessels are evaluated by palpation and ultrasonography per rectum. For semen collection and evaluation techniques and criteria considered for determination of breeding soundness classifications, *see* p 2230.

Swabs of the external genital tract (penile fossa and the urethra before and after ejaculation) can be obtained and submitted for aerobic culture to detect the presence of possible pathogens. If consistent heavy growth of potential pathogens such as *Pseudomonas aeruginosa*, *Klebsiella pneumoniae*, or *Streptococcus zooepidemicus* is seen on aerobic culture of swabs of the penile fossa or urethra and there is a history of repeated infection in mares bred, it may be necessary to breed by artificial insemination using semen extender containing an appropriate antibiotic to which the isolated organism is sensitive. If natural service is required, semen extender containing that antibiotic may be infused into the mare's uterus before servicing.

Stallions found to have an overgrowth of *P aeruginosa* on the external genitalia (penis, prepuce) may benefit from a once-daily rinse of the penis and prepuce using a dilute acid solution prepared by mixing 10 mL 38% HCl (concentrated) with 4 L of water. Rinsing should be repeated daily until *P aeruginosa* is no longer isolated. Stagnant water should be removed from the stallion's environment.

If a heavy growth of *K pneumoniae* is isolated from the stallion's penis and prepuce, a daily rinse of the penis and prepuce may be considered using a dilute bleach solution prepared by mixing 45 mL 5.25% sodium hypochlorite (bleach) with 4 L of water. This rinsing should be performed daily for 1–2 wk and then discontinued for 4 days, after which swabs should be taken from the penile fossa and preputial fold for aerobic culture. Treatment can be repeated if needed. Stagnant water and sawdust bedding should be eliminated from the stallion's environment.

If *Taylorella equigenitalis* is present, the stallion should not be used for breeding (*see* p 1371). The isolation of *T equigenitalis* requires special culture conditions; the organism will not grow in routine aerobic cultures. Stallions with lesions of coital exanthema (*see* p 1357) should not be used for breeding until skin ulcers are completely healed.

BREEDING

Natural Service: Mares are commonly bred by natural service. The proper time to breed is determined by teasing, palpation, and ultrasonography per rectum, which permits detection of estrus and the presence of a dominant follicle. Estrous mares should be bred when a follicle >30–35 mm is present or beginning on day 2–3 of estrus and every other day until ovulation occurs or the mare goes out of heat. Mares ovulate 0–48 hr before the end of estrus. Breeding should take place before ovulation. Ovulation can be induced by administration of deslorelin if the mare has a dominant follicle. (*See also* MANIPULATION OF OVARIAN ACTIVITY, p 2188.)

A tail wrap should be applied on the mare, and the perineum cleansed. The stallion's penis should be rinsed with water before breeding to remove smegma and to minimize contamination of the mare's reproductive tract. The mare should be slowly introduced to the stallion and teased until obvious signs of receptivity (tail raise, abduction of hindlegs, eversion of vulvar lips, urination) are displayed. A nose twitch may be used for additional restraint but may interfere with the mare's expression of sexual receptivity. For breeding, the stallion should be fitted with a well-adjusted halter with large rings that allow the chain shank to freely slide. During breeding, the stallion should be controlled adequately to prevent injury to the mare. After breeding, the penis can be rinsed with warm water to reduce contamination from the mare's genital tract.

Artificial Insemination: Semen is obtained using an artificial vagina; motility, morphology, and concentration of sperm are determined; and the number of morphologically normal, progressively motile sperm is calculated. Semen extender containing an antibiotic is then slowly added to semen to improve sperm survival. The temperature of the semen extender should be similar to the temperature of the semen at the time of dilution. A commonly used semen extender is glucose skim milk extender (made with 4.9 g glucose, 2.4 g instant nonfat dry milk, and 100 mL sterile distilled water). One of the following antibiotics can be added: piperacillin 100 mg (1 mg/mL); ticarcillin 100 mg (1 mg/mL); reagent grade gentamicin, which must be buffered with 2 mL 8.4% $NaHCO_3$, 100 mg (1 mg/mL); or amikacin sulfate 100 mg (1 mg/mL). Effective proprietary semen extenders are also available commercially.

The mare is prepared for insemination by application of a tail wrap and cleansing of the perineum. If soap is used, it should be rinsed thoroughly to remove any residue. Mares should be inseminated with at least 250–500 $\times 10^6$ progressively motile, morphologically normal spermatozoa before ovulation. Insemination is accomplished by depositing the semen into the body of the uterus using a sterile, plastic insemination pipette. Disposable sterile equipment is recommended to prevent contamination. Normal sperm can be expected to remain viable in the mare's reproductive tract for at least 48 hr. Mares should be examined by palpation and ultrasonography per rectum to confirm that ovulation occurs. Stallion semen can be extended, cooled to 4°C, and packaged for transport in a commercial transport device. If semen from fertile stallions is properly handled, good pregnancy rates can be achieved when the semen is used up to 48 hr later.

MANAGEMENT OF REPRODUCTION: PIGS

Management of commercial swine breeding herds involves a thorough understanding of reproductive physiology, genetics, nutrition, immunology, disease control, environment, and other factors. (*See also* ABORTION IN PIGS, p 1341.) The closed-herd concept, which emphasizes preventive medicine strategies along with herd protection, minimizes the risk of disease loss when combined with intensive management, sound nutrition, and genetic selection. The breeding program should be evaluated at specified intervals to ensure that progress in both efficiency and productivity is being made. Several efficiency/production parameters to review when analyzing herd reproductive performance are shown in TABLE 11. The postweaning performance of a breeding herd's offspring can be measured through assessment of such parameters as feed conversion ratio, average daily gain, total days to market, and postweaning death loss.

Problems on a swine farm can have a single cause or be caused by a combination of genetic, nutritional, environmental, health, and management factors. When investigating a herd problem, the practitioner can best benefit from remaining focused on the herd and not individual animals. Accurate, up-to-date records are essential when investigating a herd problem. When analyzing a herd and its records, a certain percentage of "abnormal" animals and/or reproductive problems are to be expected.

SOW AND GILT MANAGEMENT

Selection: Gilt selection for genetic improvement should be indexed based on such categories as growth rate, disease status, sexual development, reproductive history (including dam's performance as to wean-to-service and wean-to-estrus intervals, litter size, milking ability, and pigs weaned), structure/conformation, and underline (including teat number [7 pair] and placement). Of potential replacements, up to 30%–40% may be culled, with most eliminated because of problems with structure/conformation, teat issues, and genital defects. Prepubertal gilts are usually fed a sex-specific ration ad lib until they reach market weight (250–275 lb [113–125 kg]) or are 5–6 mo old. At that time, selected animals are then moved into gilt development, where they are fed a diet formulated

TABLE 11 REPRODUCTIVE BENCHMARKING INDICES USED IN COMMERCIAL SWINE HERDS

Reproductive Index	Target	Intervention Level
Wean-to-estrus interval (95% in estrus by 10 days postweaning)	<7 days	>9 days
Wean-to-service interval	≤5 days	>7 days
Repeat services at 21 (± 2) days	<8.5%	>11%
Abnormal returns to service (25–37 days)	<3%	>5%
Multiple matings (if not using fixed timed insemination)	>89%	<86%
Abortions	<1.5%	>2.5%
Not-in-pig	1%	2%
Farrowing rate	>86%	<82%
Total piglets born/litter	>12.5	<12
Live piglets born/litter	>11.5	<11
Stillbirths	<6%	>8%
Mummies	<1.5%	>3%
Litter scatter (≤8 pigs/litter)	<12%	>15%
Pigs weaned/litter	>10.4	<9.5
Preweaning mortality	<13%	>18%
Litters/mated female/year	>2.3	<2.2
Pigs weaned/mated female/year	>24	<22
Nonproductive sow days (without gilt pool)	<40	>50
Culling rate	30%–50%	<30% and >50%

specifically for introduction into the breeding herd and are exposed to boars to stimulate estrus cyclicity.

Disease Precautions: Porcine reproductive and respiratory syndrome (PRRS), parvovirus, porcine circovirus type 2, porcine epidemic diarrhea virus, pseudorabies (Aujeszky disease), Japanese encephalitis, influenza, brucellosis, chlamydiosis, leptospirosis, and other infectious diseases can directly or indirectly affect reproductive performance depending on animal age at infection and stage of gestation. The reproductive herd (gilts, sows, and boars) should be vaccinated, at a minimum, against leptospirosis, parvovirus, and erysipelas. Brought-in gilts should be isolated for a minimum of 45–60 days, during which visual observation and serial testing (ie, serology, oral fluids) for exposure to undesirable infectious diseases should be done. To minimize the number of days for introduction of these gilts into the breeding herd, the latter portion of the isolation period can be used for acclimatization to the herd's resident pathogens through the introduction of cull sows, internal grow-finish hogs, and manure exchange and/or feedback. This natural exposure to endemic herd pathogens can provide essential protection against diseases such as PRRS, parvovirus, and influenza.

Puberty: Early puberty is desirable to decrease production costs and is considered a good indicator of reproductive capability. Onset of puberty depends on a variety of factors, including genotype, liveweight, nutritional status, season, and management (including exposure to the boar). Exposure to a sexually mature boar, also known as the "boar effect," is the most influential of all management factors. The boar effect is strongest when females are exposed to the sight, sound, touch, and smell of a mature boar, and it decreases as the number of senses stimulated by the boar decrease. Consequently, the boar effect is greatest with direct contact using a mature, sterile boar. Exposure of peripubertal gilts (5–6 mo old) to a mature boar for 10–15 min/day appears to provide an adequate stimulus. Along with the boar effect, other management tools to manipulate the onset of puberty include select crossbreeding, housing changes (eg, confinement to outside pens and vice versa), and forming new groups by mixing gilts from different pens of similar health status.

Strict culling criteria should be established for the gilt pool. Gilts in which first visible estrus does not occur by 136 kg body wt and 210 days of age should be culled. Initial estrus in gilts may be weak, so a robust estrus detection program with experienced personnel is essential. Some producers may elect to use exogenous hormones to bring these reproductively inefficient gilts into estrus; if this is the case, the progeny should not be kept for breeding herd replacements. Gilts that have been serviced for two or three consecutive estrous cycles and do not conceive should also be culled.

Timing of estrus can be controlled by adding a progestagen to the feed (eg, altrenogest at 15–20 mg/day for 14–18 days). Estrus will be seen in gilts 4–9 days after the last feeding and with appropriate boar exposure. This allows estrus in gilts to be synchronized with that of a batch of weaned sows or formation of a group of gilts that will farrow together. Prostaglandins can also be used as an abortifacient to synchronize estrus when administered after day 12 and before day 55 of gestation; females generally come into heat 4–7 days later. The cost-benefit of these programs should be assessed before implementation.

BOAR MANAGEMENT

Male fertility in the breeding program more often than not receives too little attention in herd health programs. As with other food animal species, boars should be examined for breeding soundness before use in a breeding program, whenever they show lack of libido or inability to copulate, or if an increased number of females bred by the boar return to estrus ~3 wk later. At a minimum, a breeding soundness evaluation should include a history, general physical examination (including genital examination), a semen evaluation, and a behavior evaluation (*see* p 2237).

Selection: When selecting a boar for a breeding program, factors such as origination from a specific disease-free herd, performance, soundness and conformation, age of puberty, and other pertinent parameters related to reproduction should be considered. All boars that are to be used in a breeding program should, at a minimum, be seronegative for brucellosis, porcine reproductive and respiratory syndrome, and pseudorabies (Aujeszky disease). Additionally, all boars should be isolated and acclimatized for at least 45–60 days and be tested/retested for diseases naive to the herd before introduction into the herd. If involved in the selection process, boars from large litters (>10 piglets) that reach puberty early (5½–6 mo) tend to produce highly productive daughters who also reach puberty at an early age. Performance parameters such as feed efficiency, backfat, and average daily gain are also highly heritable.

Skeletal conformation and examination for current or potential locomotor dysfunction should be assessed. Any unsoundness that may interfere with the boar's ability to approach, mount, and successfully breed/ejaculate should be determined. Acute or chronic musculoskeletal conditions may elicit pain that causes the boar to appear uninterested in mounting. Boars are usually selected as breeding prospects at 3–6 mo. The genetic background of the boar should be consistent with the intended use. Selection of boars with heritable defects such as umbilical or inguinal hernias, cryptorchidism, rectal prolapse, and poor underlines can be avoided by careful analysis of the source herd production records.

History: A complete history should include the age and origin of the boar, source herd health, immunizations, previous disease problems and treatments, exposure to other animals and premises, as well as the time spent in isolation and exposure to the present premises and its breeding animals. It should also include, if available, a description of the boar's previous libido, mating behavior, conception rates, litter size, and performance of relatives and other boars in the herd. For young boars, observations of sexual behavior may be useful.

Physical and Genital Examinations: A general physical examination should be part of every fertility evaluation. Attention should be given to body condition and conformation, including the back and legs, and locomotor function. Osteomalacia, osteoarthrosis, and arthritis, which may result in lameness and reluctance to mount or bear weight on the rear legs, are serious problems.

The testicles, epididymides, and scrotum should be examined and palpated for size, symmetry (<1 cm difference in diameter), consistency, and pathologic changes. An appreciation of normal testicular consistency is necessary to detect subtle changes. The penis and prepuce should be examined for abnormalities during semen collection. Testicular size is directly correlated with genotype, age, and weight of boars between 142–282 days of age and 185–375 lb (84–171 kg) body wt. Testicular size increases until ~18 mo of age; testicular growth and sperm numbers increase at the greatest rate between 5 and 12 mo of age. Because age and testicular weight are important identifiers of early sexual development, boars should be ≥8 mo old before use in a breeding program.

The testicles can be affected by diseases (eg, brucellosis, actinobacillosis) and are vulnerable to trauma by handlers or other animals or as a result of improperly designed or maintained facilities. They should contain no nodules or soft masses. The initial reaction of testicles to trauma or infection is swelling; if untreated, the longterm result is testicular atrophy, identified by increased firmness and loss of resiliency. Asymmetry, as a result of unilateral atrophy, is potentially deleterious to fertility, and semen evaluation may reveal azoospermia, oligospermia, asthenospermia, or morphologic changes indicative of testicular damage.

Behavioral Evaluation and Semen Collection: Collection allows evaluation of libido and ability to mate and ejaculate; in addition, it provides a sample ejaculate. Precopulatory behavior involves visual and olfactory stimulation. The boar grunts or barks rhythmically, chomps jaws, salivates, and typically engages in head-to-head contact with the sow or dummy, followed by nuzzling her flanks to test for voluntary immobilization. These activities should be observed, because aberrant sexual behavior may result in infertility. Constant head mounting is a common problem with inexperienced boars.

Poor libido is likely caused by behavioral rather than endocrinologic problems. Fighting and domination by older boars and sows can inhibit libido in young boars. Breed and strain differences are also seen; the tendency to be timid, nervous, and nonaggressive can be influenced by selection in a breed over several generations and can result in boars with poor libido. Pain from genital lesions or musculoskeletal problems can have a strong negative effect. Libido can also be impaired by an unfamiliar environment, the presence of a feared person, or distractions such as available feed.

Once the boar has mounted, erection and protrusion of the penis occur as the boar searches for the vulva. Close observation is necessary to notice injuries and lesions of the penis as well as improper erection.

Congenital and genetic problems include incomplete erection, penile hypoplasia, masturbation into the diverticulum (ie, "balling up"), and persistent frenulum.

There are basically two methods of semen collection in the boar—the gloved-hand method and electroejaculation. A third method using a water-jacketed artificial vagina is no longer in common use. Although satisfactory ejaculates can be obtained using either the gloved-hand or electroejaculation methods, the gloved-hand method is preferable because it is simpler and reproductive behavior can be simultaneously assessed. The boar is allowed to mount an estrous female or collection dummy and attempt to copulate. Boars used for artificial insemination are usually trained from the onset to mount a collection dummy. The boar should then be approached quietly from the rear without being touched or frightened. Preputial fluids are first evacuated by massaging the prepuce to prevent contamination of the ejaculate. The back of the gloved hand is then placed against the ventral abdomen of the boar just cranial to the preputial orifice, and the penis is allowed to thrust into the gloved hand. Digital pressure is applied to the distal 3–6 cm of the penis. If properly stimulated, the boar will fully extend the penis and become very quiet. This is followed immediately by ejaculation. Once the tip of the penis is firmly in the hand and ejaculation has begun, it continues for ≥3–7 min. If the boar dismounts when the attempt is made to grasp the penis, he should be allowed to make several false mounts until he is aggressively attempting intromission again. Most experienced boar trainers achieve a >96% success rate in training boars to mount a dummy and to ejaculate.

A nervous boar may not allow the penis to be locked into the hand, even after several attempts. Semen can be collected from many such boars by allowing them to achieve natural intromission and lock the penis into the sow's cervix to begin the ejaculation, then quickly retrieving the penis and locking it into the hand. The boar will continue to ejaculate, and the major portion of the ejaculate can be collected.

A prewarmed (37°C) thermos or styrofoam cup is a convenient and economical collection vessel. The pre-sperm fraction, consisting of 5–15 mL of fluid, is usually ejaculated first and allowed to fall on the ground (ie, it is not collected). The boar then usually ejaculates a small amount of gel, which is filtered out of the ejaculate by a double layer of coarse gauze (placed over the mouth of the collection receptacle), because it coagulates into a semisolid mass that can interfere with subsequent evaluation of semen quality. The boar then ejaculates the milky to cream-colored, sperm-rich fraction. The final, sperm-poor fraction contains the largest volume of fluid and gel. Care should be taken to let the boar complete the ejaculation, voluntarily withdraw the penis from the hand, and dismount. Some boars will go through two or more complete ejaculations before voluntarily dismounting.

Semen collection by electroejaculation is done only on an anesthetized boar. An injectable anesthetic that will allow for 15–30 min of general anesthesia is recommended. The rectum is cleaned out using a lubricated hand, and a lubricated rectal probe is inserted. The penis is then exteriorized with the aid of Bozeman sponge forceps and grasped with a surgical sponge wrapped around the penis 5–10 cm distal to the glans penis. Electrostimulation of the boar is performed as in the bull or ram, with the ejaculate collected in a clear, plastic bag that envelops the glans penis.

Semen Evaluation: Standard tests used to evaluate boar semen include sperm motility, morphology, concentration, total numbers, and ejaculate volume. The ejaculate should be protected from changes in temperature, osmotic pressure, and pH during handling and analysis. All equipment and materials that come into contact with semen should be warmed to 35°–39°C.

Sperm motility should be evaluated as soon as possible after collection. Estimating sperm motility in an ejaculate by examining the mass activity or swirl motion of a drop of semen on a slide is of limited value and is not recommended. Gross sperm motility is best estimated on prepared samples in which a monolayer of individual sperm can be visualized using light microscopy. To do this, a 5–10 μL drop of semen is placed on a prewarmed slide and overlaid with a coverglass. Sample motility is then subjectively estimated to the nearest 5% by viewing several random fields under 20× magnification.

Sperm morphology can be a valuable indicator of fertility potential, especially in those ejaculates with a high percentage of abnormal sperm. When using bright-light microscopy, stained slides are necessary to provide adequate contrast to evaluate sperm morphology. When using higher resolution microscopy (ie, phase-contrast, differential interference contrast), glutaraldehyde or buffered formalin preserved samples can be used. A minimum of 100 (preferably 200) sperm should be assessed for morphology of the head, midpiece, and principal piece (ie, the tail distal to the midpiece). Sperm can be categorized into three groups: normal, sperm with abnormal heads, and sperm with abnormal tails (midpiece, principal piece, including cytoplasmic droplets). Samples with a high number of sperm defects can be examined further, and abnormalities classified as major and minor defects. Acrosome morphology should also be assessed if possible.

Several techniques are available to determine sperm concentration in a filtered boar ejaculate. A crude, subjective, qualitative estimation of sperm concentration can be done by assessing visual opacity of a raw ejaculate, either by direct examination or with the aid of a Karras spermiodensimeter. Analytical determination of sperm concentration can be performed by measuring opacity via a calibrated (spectro) photometer on a diluted semen sample. It is essential that the photometer be calibrated for boar semen. Even with a calibrated photometer, estimates of sperm numbers may be ±30% from that of the actual concentration; this can be attributed, in part, to improper technique, human error, and/or the inherent opacity of the secretions of the accessory sex glands present in the boar ejaculate. Photometric readings can also be inaccurate if the reading is outside the calibration curve or optimal operating range. A second, more direct method to measure sperm concentration is with a hemocytometer or counting chamber. In this method, concentration can be determined by diluting a portion of the filtered ejaculate to a 1:200 ratio—most easily done using a Unopette® system. The hemocytometer should be charged, and the charged unit allowed to set for 5 min, so that the sperm settle into one visual field. Using microscopy, a sperm count is performed and calculated as normally done for RBC determination. Determining sperm concentration using a counting chamber is tedious and time consuming, making its use on a routine basis impractical in most commercial operations.

After calculating sperm concentration/mL, total sperm numbers in an ejaculate can be calculated by multiplying sperm concentration with the total volume (in mL) of the gel-free ejaculate. Ejaculate volume can be measured by using a warmed measuring apparatus (eg, graduated cylinder, disposable plastic measuring cups) or by measuring the weight of the ejaculate (with 1 g equivalent to 1 mL). More frequently, computer-automated semen analysis systems are being used to objectively determine sperm motility, sperm morphology, and sperm concentration.

Interpretation of Findings: Semen values can be affected by frequency of boar use, age, environment, disease, level of nutrition, genotype, and method of sperm cell fixation. Therefore, boars that do not have acceptable semen values are not necessarily subfertile or infertile. Spermiograms can change dramatically over a short period of time, and boars should not be culled on the evaluation of a single ejaculate. Breed differences in onset of puberty, libido, mating ability, and conception rate have been seen.

Environment can affect fertility over a short period of time, primarily because of disturbances in the thermoregulation of the testes. Boars exposed to cold or hot environmental temperatures may have abnormal spermiograms for ≥7 wk after the insult. Severe exposure may result in abnormal spermiograms for a longer time or may even lead to permanent spermatogenic disruption. Any disease that increases body temperature, and thus disrupts thermoregulation of the testes, also has the potential to cause temporary sub- or infertility.

Guidelines for Boar Evaluation:

Ideally, libido, mating ability, semen quality (*see* TABLE 12), and breeding results (conception rate and litter size) should be considered. The duration of spermatogenesis and spermatozoal maturation is ~51 days in the boar. If a boar produces an ejaculate of low or marginal quality when examined in vitro, additional ejaculates should be assessed at 1- to 2-wk intervals to ascertain whether quality has improved over time. Boars with spermiograms that do not improve over 2–3 mo are unlikely to ever improve. Boars with azoospermia on two complete ejaculates or that are unable to achieve complete erection should be culled immediately. Those that have penile lesions or blood in the semen should be sexually rested for ≥2–3 wk and reevaluated. For boars with persistent frenulum or that habitually masturbate in the diverticulum, surgical correction is recommended; however, the progeny should not be kept for breeding, because these conditions are most likely heritable. All results of the fertility examination must be considered in relation to age, disease history, environmental stress, prior breeding usage, mating system, and the techniques of semen collection and handling.

TABLE 12 SUGGESTED MINIMUM SPERMIOGRAM VALUES FOR BREEDING BOARS

Parameter	Natural Service	Artificial Insemination
Color	Opaque to white (vulvar discharge)	Opaque to white
Total sperm numbers	$>35 \times 10^9$ sperm/ejaculate	$>35 \times 10^9$ sperm/ejaculate
Gross motility (raw)	>60%	>70%
Abnormal morphology (including cytoplasmic droplets)	<25%	<20%–25%
Cytoplasmic droplets (both proximal and distal)	<15%	<15%–20%

BREEDING MANAGEMENT

Estrus: Sows and gilts are nonseasonal and polyestrous, with the estrous cycle lasting 18–24 (average 21) days. Sows are behaviorally anestrous during pregnancy. Ovulatory estrus usually is not seen during lactation except under conditions of group rearing, high feed levels, or boar contact. Partial weaning or gonadotropin treatment can induce estrus during lactation, but the results are inconsistent and not economical. Normal uterine physiology is reestablished by 20–25 days postpartum. Most sows exhibit estrus 3–7 days after weaning. Estrus in gilts and postweaning anestrous sows can be initiated with exogenous hormones. However, these hormones circumvent natural selection for reproductive efficiency, and this should be kept in mind when they are used in breeding management programs. Exogenous hormones should not be used as a long-term solution to address reproductive inefficiency in a herd.

Estrus lasts ~36–48 hr in gilts and ≥48–72 hr in sows. Time to estrus after weaning and duration of estrus in sows can be influenced by length of lactation, nutrition, body condition, genetics, and other management practices (*see* TABLE 13). Estrus is characterized by behavioral (eg, mounting, fence walking, vocalizing, tilted ears, kyphosis) and sometimes physical (eg, vulvar swelling, vaginal discharge) changes. Ovulation generally occurs in mid to late estrus. During ovulation, ~15–24 ova are released over a 1- to 4-hr period. Ovulation rate increases over the first four parities, so that the fourth to sixth litters tend to be the largest in number. Ovulation rate can decrease when gilts or sows are undernourished. Most gilts are on full feed, thereby averting the adverse affects of undernourishment on early reproductive performance. In countries in which gilts are not routinely provided full feed, increasing energy intake for 10 days before estrus (ie, "flushing") is performed. This has optimized ovulation rate under these circumstances. To prevent undernourishment in recently weaned sows, an energy-dense diet should be fed until after estrus and breeding.

Behavioral changes are most pronounced when the sow or gilt is exposed directly to the sight, sound, odor, and attention (nuzzling and grunting) of a mature boar. A sow or gilt in standing heat normally assumes a rigid, immobile, receptive stance when exposed to a boar. Physical changes such as vulvar swelling and discharge are often unreliable; they do, however, appear to be more marked in gilts than sows and commonly develop 2–3 days before estrus. The ultimate criterion of estrus is either standing to the boar or a positive response to the "riding test" (an attendant applies pressure with the hands in the loin area, then gently sits on the pig's back to elicit the standing reaction); this test is best conducted in the presence of a boar (eg, in an adjacent pen) or, as an alternative, after exposing the sow to a synthetic boar-odor aerosol or taint rag.

Anestrus is a common problem. Failure to detect estrus must be distinguished from true cases of ovarian inactivity. First-litter and early-weaned sows are particularly vulnerable to postweaning anestrus. The primiparous sow must support her own growth as well as maintenance and lactation demands, while her feed intake capacity is not yet fully developed. This problem can be avoided by breeding only gilts in good condition; not overfeeding during the first gestation; and encouraging energy intake

TABLE 13 FACTORS AFFECTING OVARIAN ACTIVITY OF PIGS

	Stage of Breeding Affected		
Proven or Suspected Factors	**Puberty**	**After Weaning**	**After Service**
Insufficient male stimulation	+[a]	+	–[b]
Housing and social environment	+	+	–
High ambient temperature	+	+	+
Season of year (summer/fall)	+	+	+
Photoperiod	+	?[c]	–
Genotype	+	+	–
Nutrition	+	+	+
Short lactation	–	+	–
Large litter reared	–	+	–

Adapted, with permission, from Meredith MJ, *Pig News and Information* 5, 1984, published by CAB International, Wallingford, Oxon, UK.

[a] Effect has been demonstrated

[b] No evidence for effect

[c] Effect uncertain

during the first lactation by frequent feeding of high-density diets, wet feeding, and avoiding high temperatures in the farrowing rooms. Management practices such as segregated early weaning, modified medicated early weaning, and medicated early weaning recommend weaning as early as 10 days postpartum; postweaning anestrus is not an uncommon sequela of these management techniques. General guidelines to minimize the negative effect of early weaning on sow reproduction recommend weaning at no less than 14–16 days into lactation for primiparous sows, at no less than 12–14 days into lactation for sows on their second litter, and at no less than 9–11 days into lactation for sows on their third or subsequent litters.

Hormonal Control of the Estrous Cycle: Estrous synchronization may be achieved by synchronized weaning of lactating sows; estrus occurs 4–10 days later. Administration of a commercially available combination of 400 IU of equine chorionic gonadotropin (eCG) and 200 IU of human chorionic gonadotropin (hCG) per 5 mL dose given as a single IM injection within 12 hr after weaning tightens the *synchronization*, and estrus occurs 4–5 days after weaning. This eCG and hCG combination also induces estrus in gilts with delayed puberty and in sows with postweaning anestrus.

Fixed-time insemination protocols continue to gain interest in the swine industry. Current recommendations call for the use of progestins to prime the gilt before administration of a GnRH analogue. With sows, a GnRH analogue is administered 83–96 hr after weaning. Breeding of both gilts and sows is then performed 20–33 hr after GnRH administration (depending on product and route of administration).

Exogenous prostaglandin induces luteolysis of the corpus luteum only after day 12 of the estrous cycle and, therefore, is not a practical agent for estrous cycle control; however, estrus may be synchronized by induction of abortion in sows pregnant >15 days by administration of $PGF_{2}\alpha$ (15 mg, IM, then 10 mg, IM, 12 hr later) or an equivalent analogue. Estrus may also be synchronized by feeding altrenogest (15–20 mg, PO, daily for 14–18 days), with estrus being observed 4–9 days after the last dose with appropriate boar exposure. Combination eCG and hCG may be given on the day of progestagen withdrawal to better synchronize estrus.

Breeding: The three methods of breeding are pen mating (boar run with females), hand mating (supervised natural mating), and artificial insemination (AI). Pen mating is generally found on smaller operations and works best in a pen of pigs in various stages of the estrous cycle. Pen mating with a group of recently weaned sows is less desirable, because their estrous cycles may occur close together and lead to overuse of the boar. In hand mating, the female is usually mated two or three times during estrus, with the first service on the first day of standing estrus, and subsequent matings at 24-hr intervals; confirmed matings should be recorded. Many commercial producers breed the sow or gilt once daily as long as she will accept the boar. The use of two different boars may increase the number of pigs per litter but may mask infertility in one of the boars.

In AI programs, heat detection is performed either twice or once per day. If heat detection is performed twice per day, gilts should be inseminated twice, 8–12 hr after the onset of standing heat and again 12–16 hr later. Sows should be inseminated 24 hr after onset of standing heat and again 18–24 hr later. If heat detection is performed once per day, gilts should be inseminated within 4 hr and sows within 12–16 hr from when they were first seen in standing heat. A second insemination should be performed as described above for those animals that remain in standing heat.

Timing of AI may need to be modified based on a particular farm's availability of labor, building design, or herd genetics. Some experienced users of AI obtain satisfactory results in gilts with a timed, single insemination; however, performing two inseminations is more common. Inseminations can be performed using either single-sire (sourced from one boar) or pooled (sourced from multiple [three to six] boar ejaculates) extended semen. In general, single-sire matings are performed when particular genetic (ie, breeding or show animals) offspring are desired, whereas matings with pooled semen are used as a means to produce market hog offspring. Minimum suggested values for extended semen used within 72 hr after collection are provided in TABLE 14. Total sperm numbers in a dose of semen depend on quality and storage time of the semen.

Boars should not be overused (*see* TABLE 15). If sows are weaned in groups, a boar-to-sow ratio of 1:4 for mature boars and 1:2 for young boars is recommended. In hand mating, a mature boar should be used for ≤2 breedings/day. When using natural service, a boar-to-sow ratio of 1:15–1:25 (average 1:17 or 18) is usually needed. When using AI, the boar-to-sow ratio can be increased to 1:150–1:400.

Pregnancy: Sperm cells reach the oviducts within 30 min of mating, and fertilization can occur within 2–6 hr. Fertilization rates approach 100% in sows, but embryo mortality up to 30%–40% accounts for the usual litter size of 10–16 pigs. Embryos enter the uterus ~48–60 hr after ovulation. Embryos hatch from the zona pellucida and form blastocysts 144 hr after ovulation. Maternal recognition of pregnancy (embryos secreting estradiol) occurs by day 10–14 of gestation, with intrauterine migration and distribution of embryos. Embryo attachment begins by day 13–14, with implantation complete by day 40; a minimum of four embryos must be present at this time for pregnancy to continue. Skeletal mineralization develops by day 35, with fetuses immunocompetent by day 70–75. Fetal deaths that occur after day 35 can result in expulsion or retention of recognizable piglets. Retained dead fetuses in this sterile environment become mummified and are usually expelled at the time of farrowing. The average gestation length is 114 ± 2 days and is somewhat shortened in sows with large litters.

TABLE 14 MINIMUM SUGGESTED VALUES OF EXTENDED PORCINE SEMEN FOR USE IN AN ARTIFICIAL INSEMINATION PROGRAM

Semen Variable	Value
Gross sperm motility	≥70%
Normal sperm morphology	≥75%
Sperm concentration	25 to 65 × 10^6 sperm/mL
Dose volume (cervical deposition)	≥70 mL
Microbial content	No significant aerobic growth
Arrival temperature	15°–19°C

TABLE 15 SUGGESTED GUIDELINES FOR BOAR USAGE BASED ON BREEDING PROGRAM

Artificial Insemination		Natural Mating		
Boar Age (mo)	**Semen Collection Frequency[a]**	**Matings/day**	**Matings/wk**	**Pen-breeding (females/mo)**
6–8	1 time/wk	1	4	<8
8–12	1–2 times/wk	1	5–7	8–10
>13	≥4 times/2 wk	2 (spaced)	8–10	10–12

Adapted from Althouse GC. *Animal Health and Production Compendium*, 2002, by CAB International, Wallingford, Oxon, UK.

[a] Depends on boar libido

Embryos are at greatest risk of dying during the first 30 days, and efforts should be directed toward avoiding stresses to the sow (eg, overfeeding, heat, handling or moving, immunization) during this critical period. Pregnancies of <16 days are especially sensitive to heat stress. Avoiding exposure to outside animals reduces disease risk. Feed intake should be reduced to the limit feeding level of 4–5 lb (~2 kg) immediately after breeding to avoid embryo loss due to high energy intake. Farrowing less than five piglets is indicative of embryo death after the time of attachment.

To increase colostral antibodies, the gilt or sow should be immunized during the last 6 wk of gestation. An immunization program may include vaccination against *Escherichia coli*, atrophic rhinitis, and erysipelas, and provision of any other vaccines appropriate for the disease situation on the individual farm.

Pregnancy Determination: Several techniques are available for pregnancy determination (*see* TABLE 16). Pregnancy is most commonly diagnosed by noting that the female does not return to estrus in 18–25 days; this is 75%–85% accurate. Ultrasonography is another popular technique, and three types can be used: pulse echo (A-mode), Doppler, and real-time. Pulse echo or amplitude depth involves emitting ultrasonic waves from a hand-held transducer placed on the skin in the flank area. Reflected waves from a fluid-filled area (ie, developing conceptus or fetus) are picked up by the transducer and converted into either an audible or visual signal. Doppler ultrasonography detects changes in sound frequency (fluid movement) using an audible signal; movements indicative of pregnancy include blood flow in middle uterine or umbilical arteries, fetal heartbeat, and fetal movements. Real-time ultrasonography involves visualization of a 2-dimensional image of scanned tissues directly under the transducer. Ultrasonographic techniques are generally used at 22–75 days to determine pregnancy, with real-time ultrasonography being used as early as 18 days after breeding. Although uncommonly used for this purpose, rectal palpation can be performed to confirm pregnancy at >30 days gestation. The examiner palpates for fremitus, size, and position of the middle (medial) uterine artery in relation to the external iliac artery. The tone and tension of the cervix and weight and contents of the uterus can also be used to help confirm pregnancy. Other techniques such as hormonal assays (eg, estrone glucuronide, progesterone, prostaglandin) and vaginal biopsy can be used but are not economically feasible.

Parturition: The preparturient period involves restlessness and nest building the last 24 hr. Mammary glands become turgid, and the secretion changes from serous to milk as parturition approaches. Parturition is initiated by increased cortisol levels, which also stimulate release of prostaglandin (PG) $F_2\alpha$ from the uterus. $PGF_2\alpha$ causes luteolysis of the corpora lutea and release of relaxin, which causes relaxation of the birth canal and cervix. Oxytocin is released from the pituitary gland, which causes uterine contractions and onset of labor. Piglets are usually delivered at frequent intervals (10–15 min; 5–45 min range). Uterine horn evacuation is random.

The stillbirth rate usually is 5%–10%; intra-uterine deaths are due to infection, incorrect position in the uterine horn during delivery, or anoxia. Anoxia is seen

TABLE 16 COMMON TESTS FOR DETECTION OF PREGNANCY IN PIGS

Technique	Test Type	Application of Test After Breeding (Accuracy)
Estrus detection	Indirect	Daily testing 18–25 days (75%–85%) and through gestation (98%)
External physical signs	Indirect	>55 days (gilts); >84 days (sows)
Rectal palpation (sows)	Indirect	30 days (94%), >60 days (100%)
Ultrasonography		
A-mode	Indirect	30–75 days (95%)
Doppler	Direct/Indirect	≥35 days (>85%)
Real-time (B-mode)	Direct	≥22 days (>95%)

when the umbilical cord ruptures or becomes constricted because of the extreme length of the uterine horn, or when there is a delay in transit along the birth canal. Stillborn and weak piglets also may be due to low temperatures in the farrowing house or low Hgb levels (<9 g/dL) in the sow. Any increase in the time interval between pigs born (eg, due to exhaustion, atony of the uterus, or dystocia) increases the chance of injury or death to the piglets still in the uterus. Piglets are born in both cranial (60%) and caudal (40%) presentation. Assistance can be provided in the form of oxytocin injections (10–30 IU) and manual removal of piglets. Walking the sow for a few moments also can be helpful. The number of pigs born alive can be increased by approximately one per sow if an attendant is present to assist delivery (*see* below). Passage of the fetal membranes should occur within 4 hr of delivering the last piglet.

Farrowing can be induced by IM injection of 10–15 mg of natural $PGF_2\alpha$ or equivalent dose of synthetic analogues. Farrowing generally occurs 18–36 hr later (most within 22–32 hr) in 80%–90% of sows when $PGF_2\alpha$ is given at or after 112–113 days gestation. Induction can be used so that most farrowings occur during normal working hours, avoiding evenings, weekends, and holidays. Good records are essential, and average days of gestation for the sow herd and individual breeding dates for each sow must be known. $PGF_2\alpha$ must be used within 72 hr of the expected farrowing date to prevent an increase in stillbirths. The slightly premature piglets require good environmental conditions, particularly in cold weather. Farrowings may be concentrated into an even shorter period by injecting 20 IU of oxytocin IM 15–24 hr after the $PGF_2\alpha$ injection. This shortens the interval to parturition but can be accompanied by an increase in dystocia. Successful farrowing can also be induced by giving a single vulvomucosal injection of 5–10 IU of oxytocin.

Incidence of dystocia is low (1%–2%) in sows. As with all polytocous species, uterine inertia accounts for most dystocia in swine. Other causes include fetal malposition, obstruction of the birth canal, deviation of the uterus, fetopelvic disproportion, and maternal excitement. A thorough digital examination of the birth canal is prerequisite to therapeutic intervention. Medical therapy for unobstructive dystocia may include use of an ecbolic agent (oxytocin at 20–30 IU every 30 min, up to three times). Administration of injectable calcium may be warranted if uterine inertia is suspected.

Lactation peaks at 3–4 wk postpartum. Sows that have been on an 8-wk lactation produce 400–700 lb of milk. Poor lactation is a significant cause of impaired productivity in pigs (*see* POSTPARTUM DYSGALACTIA SYNDROME, p 1373).

Preweaning Mortality: Supervised farrowing alone can help to reduce piglet mortality, because it minimizes stillbirths, facilitates access of piglets to needed warmth, allows for observation of nursing activity, and prevents crushing and cannibalism. Other management techniques available to reduce piglet mortality include cross-fostering, split-suckling, well-designed farrowing crates and pens, prepartum vaccination of sows, appropriate feeding programs for lactating sows, and cleanliness.

MANAGEMENT OF REPRODUCTION: SHEEP

When establishing a flock health management program for reproduction, it is important to remember these points: 1) Sheep are short-day polyestrous breeders, ie, estrus occurs in response to shortening day length. 2) The ovulatory season tends to be in the autumn and early winter months; the anovulatory season in the late winter, spring, and early summer months; and the transition season in the late summer months. 3) There is tremendous breed-to-breed variation in prolificacy and length of the ovulatory season.

REPRODUCTIVE PHYSIOLOGY

Ewes are seasonally polyestrous, cycling every 16–17 days during the breeding season. The major environmental factor controlling the estrous cycle is the photoperiod. Decreasing photoperiod after the summer solstice causes secretion of melatonin, which triggers the hypothalamus to produce gonadotropin-releasing hormone. Geographic location and environmental temperatures also modify the length of anestrus, as does the breed of sheep. Fine-wool breeds (eg, Rambouillet, Merino), tropical breeds, and Dorsets have a shorter anestrous period than other breeds such as the Suffolk, Hampshire, Border Leicester, and Columbia. Regardless of this breed-related variation in the length of the breeding season, all breeds are most fertile in the autumn, and anestrus is an unlikely problem associated with regular annual mating.

The duration of estrus (~30 hr) is influenced by the breed and age of the ewe, the onset of puberty, the presence of the male, and the season. Estrous periods that occur in the autumn are longer and more intense, and maiden ewes have a shorter and less intense estrus than mature ewes. The optimal time to mate ewes (naturally or artificially) is in the first half of the estrous period, or 12–18 hr after the onset of estrus. Ewes show no overt signs of estrus, and heat detection requires the presence of a ram, a teaser ram (made infertile by either vasectomy or epididymectomy), or a testosterone- or estrogen-treated wether.

The age of puberty of ewe lambs varies greatly and is influenced by breed, nutrition, presence of the ram, and season of birth. Well-grown ewe lambs with a body condition score of 3–3.5, particularly of the meat breeds, can be mated at 7–8 mo of age and 70% of mature body wt. Two exceptions exist: lambs born in the autumn to a spring breeding will reach puberty in the spring and be less fertile to an induced estrus, and some breeds of sheep are slow maturing (eg, range breeds) and may not be fertile at 7–8 mo of age. However, breeding ewe lambs early is encouraged; ewes that breed as lambs are able to produce more lamb crops in their lifetime than those bred as 2-yr-olds.

Ewe lambs should be separated from ram lambs by 5 mo of age to avoid unwanted pregnancies, and from all market lambs to avoid overconditioning from a diet too high in energy. Overconditioned ewe lambs are less fertile and produce less milk than those fed to achieve a body condition score of 3.

Follicle development and ovulation rates are major determinants of fertility. Ovulation rate is a polygenic trait showing marked breed difference; heritability estimates are moderate (0.3%–0.5%). Although by selecting replacement animals born as twins or triplets will slowly increase prolificacy within a flock, using more maternal breeds is recommended because their offspring will also have desirable traits of better mothering and milk production.

Nutritional supplementation starting a few weeks before mating ("flushing") may result in higher ovulation rates if the ewes are not in good body condition (score <3). Ewes already in good fit will have a similar ovulation rate and will not respond further to flushing. The diet should be balanced for protein (not >14% crude protein) and have a good availability of energy. High levels of soluble protein can cause early embryonic death through increased urea nitrogen levels in the blood. Overfeeding of energy to ewes in good body condition can cause decreased fertility.

Estrus Induction in Acyclic Ewes:

Estrus and ovulation can be induced in anestrous ewes by the introduction of rams (ram effect) or by treatment with exogenous progestagen or equine chorionic gonadotropin (eCG), or through the effects of melatonin either by manipulating the photoperiod in housed sheep or through the use of exogenous melatonin in the feed or as an implant. (*See also* HORMONAL CONTROL OF ESTRUS, p 2244.) Factors affecting fertility after estrus induction include breed, season, lactation, nutritional status, and postpartum period, as well as the ewe's dry/suckling status, ram to ewe ratio, time of ram introduction, mating by natural or artificial insemination, and number of inseminations (one or two).

The sudden introduction of novel rams or teasers ("ram effect") to anestrous ewes can induce the onset of ovarian cyclicity during the transition season, most often 4–6 wk before the onset of the ovulatory season in seasonal breeds; however, it works poorly to synchronize estrus once the ewes have started to cycle. Responding ewes commonly ovulate within 48 hr of ram introduction but usually are not receptive, ie, the estrus is silent. In ewes with a silent estrus, ovulation is followed by the formation of either a normal or a short-lived (5–6 days) corpus luteum (CL). After regression of a normal CL, most ewes display estrus (~19 days after ram introduction). After regression of a short-lived CL, ewes ovulate without displaying estrus and commonly form a normal CL. Regression of this CL results in estrus (~25 days after ram introduction). This gives two peaks of breeding activity and very good synchronization of estrus without the use of exogenous hormones.

Acyclic, seasonally anestrous ewes can be induced into estrus and ovulation with exogenous melatonin. Ewes are given melatonin 6 wk before joining and are isolated from rams during that period. The joining period should cover two complete estrous cycles (35 days). Exogenous melatonin is more successful toward the end of the seasonal anestrous period, ie, transition period. This product is not commercially available in many countries. A similar effect can be obtained by manipulating the photoperiod under management programs in which the ewes and rams are in confinement housing. Usually starting in late autumn up to the winter solstice, ewes are exposed to artificial light, usually 16 hr/day for 8–12 wk. At the end of this period (eg, mid-winter), the length of light exposure is reduced to 8 hr/day. This may require darkening windows to reduce exogenous light sources and completing barn chores during only those 8 hr to avoid using lights during the dark period. After 6–8 wk, ewes will start to cycle. If the rams are housed under similar conditions, scrotal circumference and breeding capacity will increase.

Estrus Induction/Synchronization: Estrus induction in acyclic ewes requires exposure to exogenous progestagen for a minimum of 5 days; most programs use 7 days. The progestagen used may be either natural progesterone delivered intravaginally in a controlled intravaginal drug-releasing device (CIDR), or melengestrol acetate (MGA) fed at 12-hr intervals at a dose of 0.125 mg/head. Ovulation and subsequent fertility is usually poor unless eCG is given at removal of the progestagen; usually 500 IU is administered. If ewes are cycling, then either the progestagen exposure needs to be sufficiently long to outlast any CLs present on the ovaries. This is usually 11–14 days. Use of eCG at progestagen removal time is optional (200–400 IU) and is generally not necessary during the ovulatory season if artificial insemination is not being used. Shorter exposures in cycling ewes can be used if prostaglandin (PG) $F_2\alpha$ or its analogues is administered either at, or 12–24 hr before, pessary or CIDR removal. Estrous cyclic ewes can also be synchronized by two injections of $PGF_2\alpha$ or its analogues 8–11 days apart, although fertility is poorer than with progestagen programs. Estrus commonly is seen 1–3 days after progestagen removal, with a shorter interval during the autumn or with the use of CIDRs, or within 3 days of the second $PGF_2\alpha$ injection.

Ram Management: Before a program is set up, the veterinarian should be sure sufficient numbers of rams are available for the program and that the rams are fertile. During the normal ovulatory season and without synchronization, a ram to ewe ratio of 1:40 is usually sufficient, although if the rams are young, or the environment is rough, then the number of ewes per ram should be lowered. This is also true if estrus is synchronized, in which case the ram to ewe ratio should be ~1:10 to 15. When breeding out of season, ram fertility is usually lower, and if estrus is synchronized the ram to ewe ratio should be ~1:5 to 7.

MEASURING REPRODUCTIVE PERFORMANCE

Reproductive performance is measured by several parameters. The most commonly used ones are the proportion of ewes exposed or mated to the ram that lamb (the measure of fertility), the proportion of lambs born (alive and dead) per ewe lambing (also called drop rate and a measure of prolificacy), and age at first lambing. Also often measured are lambs tail-docked per ewe lambing (lambs marked); lambing percentage (number of lambs born per ewe exposed to the ram); and weaning percentage (percentage of lambs weaned per ewe exposed to the ram), although the latter is more of an economic measure. To measure lamb losses, it is preferable to calculate stillbirth rates and preweaning mortality rates as a proportion of lambs born and lambs born alive, respectively.

Goals for reproductive performance vary tremendously between different sheep-raising systems and must be matched with the management system and constraints. Extensive range flocks that produce primarily wool (eg, the Australian Merino) may seek only flock replacement so that lambing rates of <90%, 1 lamb born/ewe lambing, and <0.8 lambs weaned/ewe lambing are considered acceptable. Ewes are traditionally not expected to lamb until 2 yr of age. Conversely, flocks that produce primarily meat under conditions that require the feeding of stored feeds (eg, where growing seasons are short) and/or housing for a significant proportion of the year must have much better fecundity and lamb weaning percentages to be economically viable. Age at first lambing should be 12–14 mo, and a ewe should raise at least 1.8 or more likely 2 lambs/yr. Fertility rates during the ovulatory season should be 95%–100% in ewes and 90% in ewe lambs.

Producers seeking to further increase ewe production and to reach the more lucrative lamb meat markets also practice accelerated lambing in which ewes lamb every 8 mo (ie, three lambings in 2 years) or every 7.2 mo (the Cornell Star system, *see* p 2216). Both of these systems require that ewes breed during the anovulatory and transition season, as well as the ovulatory season. However, in most of the world, autumn breeding with spring lambing is the predominant reproduction management system, which coincides with optimal grass production for the lambs and lactating ewes, regardless of the desired prolificacy of the management system.

FACTORS AFFECTING REPRODUCTIVE PERFORMANCE

Reasons for reproductive failure in the ewe and ram are numerous. Performance must be considered in light of the management system and genetics of the breed. If targets are not being met, the following can be used as a guideline to investigate contributing factors.

Breed: Breed selection can greatly influence reproductive performance, particularly prolificacy and age at first lambing. Sheep breeds around the world are very diverse in performance, and it is advisable to be familiar with the traits of some of the more popular ones. Terminal sire breeds such as Suffolk, Hampshire, and Texel are often used to obtain rapid growth and muscling. Traditionally, these breeds are only moderately to lowly prolific and so are not preferred in the ewe flock except to produce replacement terminal sire rams. Maternal breeds should possess the following characteristics: fertile, prolific, easy lambing with good maternal instincts (eg, bonding), high milk production, longevity, suitable for the environment (eg, grassland, confinement, hilly country), and for some management systems, long ovulatory seasons. Within each geographic region and production system, specific breeds tend to be more commonly used. Some of the more popular maternal breeds in northeastern North America are the Finnish Landrace, Romanov, and Polled Dorset. In western USA, range breeds are more popular.

Some regions commonly use a crossbred sheep that includes traits from several breeds. In a crossbreeding system, maternal heterosis is used to improve performance, ie, the offspring (the F1 generation) possess traits that are better than the average of their parents, also known as hybrid vigor. A well-known example is the British "mule" sheep in which ewes of a hill breed (eg, Scottish Blackface) that possess the traits of hardiness and good mothering but are not prolific are crossed with a ram of a lowland prolific heavy-milking breed (eg, Bluefaced Leicester). The resultant F1 ewe is a prolific, heavy-milking mother with longevity and hardiness. No ram lambs are retained for breeding. These ewes are then bred to a terminal sire (eg, Suffolk or Texel). The offspring of this mating–a terminal cross–gain well and have good carcass characteristics.

Composite breeds are the result of a planned crossbreeding program coupled with stringent selection based on preselected production traits. The more successful are phenotypically stable and are considered new breeds. In the USA, the Polypay, a composite of the Finnish Landrace, Targhee, Dorset, and Rambouillet, is very prolific and hardy and has excellent wool production. The Rideau sheep, developed in Canada, is a composite of Finnish Landrace, Dorset, Suffolk, and East Friesian. These ewes are very prolific, heavy milkers, and excellent mothers and are frequently used in accelerated lambing programs. Other examples of popular composites include the Katahdin (North American haired sheep), Dorper (South Africa and North America), Coopworth (New Zealand and Australia), Corriedale (New Zealand), and British Milk Sheep (UK and Canada).

Reproductive Failure of the Ram: Rams may fail to mate the ewes, even when the ewes are in estrus, or mating may occur but pregnancy does not ensue. Possible reasons are numerous. For failure to mate, these include: 1) The ewes are being mated but the marking harness or crayon is not functioning properly. 2) The ram lacks libido because it is ill with another disease, is too thin, is too old, it is during the anovulatory period, or the weather is too hot. 3) The ram is reluctant to breed, perhaps because of the pain of infectious balanoposthitis (pizzle rot), contagious ecthyma of the penis or prepuce, or because it is lame and cannot mount comfortably. 4) The ram may be inexperienced and has not been "taught" how to breed by observing a more experienced ram. 5) The ram may not be able to cope properly with the environment, eg, a barn-raised ram turned out to mountainous pasture. 6) Too few rams are available to breed the ewes (ram to ewe ratio) for the type of ram (age, experience), conditions (paddock vs range), time of year (ovulatory vs anovulatory), or synchronization programs. 7) Rams may have behavioral issues such as inter-ram aggression, shy rams, or rams "falling in love" with or disliking specific ewes.

Mating not followed by pregnancy may present as ewes being marked repeatedly, a spread-out lambing period, and/or poor prolificacy in the ewes. Many of the reasons for failure to mate can also influence failure to achieve pregnancy. Additional reasons for lack of pregnancy after mating include impaired fertility due to disease such as *Brucella ovis* infection, chorioptic mange of the scrotum, infertility after a fever, or other causes of orchitis and/or epididymitis; impaired fertility due to mechanical reasons such as excessive heat or cold, inguinal hernia, or injury from fighting; impaired fertility due to environmental hormone disrupters (eg, phytoestrogenic plants); inadequate testicular circumference because of age, season, genetics, or disease; abnormalities of the penis due to a congenital defect or trauma; and sperm abnormalities.

Reproductive Failure of the Ewe: As with the ram, ewes may fail to be mated, or be mated but do not become pregnant. In addition, the ewe may not maintain the pregnancy or have decreased prolificacy. Again, the possible reasons are numerous. Ewes may not be mated because of the following: 1) The ewe may already be pregnant. 2) It may be anovulatory season, which is longer in ewe lambs. 3) The ewe lamb may be prepubertal, influenced by growth (nutrition) and breed. 4) If a synchronization/estrus induction program is used, there could be a fatal error in the program, eg, loss of CIDR, too low dose of eCG, or improper MGA feeding program. 5) Phytoestrogens or specific mycotoxins may temporarily or permanently suppress estrus. 6) Ewes may be too thin, lactating, or recently weaned. 7) Ewe lambs that are overfed postpubertally may not cycle. 8) Ewes may display behavior such as dominating the ram or being shy, particularly maiden ewes. 9) There may be a freemartin/pseudohermaphrodite condition.

Ewes may not conceive or maintain pregnancy because of the following: 1) The synchronization program is not correct, eg, rams are joined too early with the ewes before they are in estrus or too low a dose of eCG is given and ovulation does not occur. 2) There is pathology of the reproductive tract. 3) Early embryonic death occurs, which can be due to a number of issues, eg, selenium deficiency, specific abortion disease (eg, border disease, toxoplasmosis, chlamydiosis), stress, heat shock in early pregnancy, or high levels of soluble protein in the feed leading to high urea nitrogen levels in the blood. 4) Abortion (mid to late term), if not observed, may also present as failure to conceive or maintain pregnancy.

Reasons for poor prolificacy in ewes that become pregnant include insufficient energy at breeding when in poor body condition (low body condition score), very young or very old age, anovulatory or transition season, insufficient dose of eCG, early embryonic death (*see* above), and genetics.

BREEDING PROGRAMS

The most common breeding program is annual lambing in which autumn-mated ewes lamb in the spring. However, to produce lambs for more lucrative markets, ewes are bred in early autumn or late summer to lamb in winter (eg, January for the Easter lamb market in March or April) or bred in late spring to lamb in autumn (eg,

September for the Christmas lamb market). This requires the use of programs that advance the ovulatory season into the late summer (ram effect, melatonin) or induce estrus during the anovulatory period in the spring (progestagens in the form of CIDR devices or MGA; photoperiod manipulation). However, producers whose flocks lamb out of season rarely adhere to an annual breeding program, because overall production is generally too low to account for the increased costs associated with lambs born in the winter or autumn; instead, these producers adopt an accelerated program to take advantage of the ewe's ability to lamb more than once per year.

The two most popular accelerated lambing programs are the "3 lambings in 2 years" (3 in 2) and the Cornell Star system. The former requires the producer to manage two flocks that lamb every 8 mo (January, May, and September), alternating the first and second flocks. For example, in the northern hemisphere, over 24 mo, a ewe would be bred in the ovulatory season to lamb in the spring (December to lamb in May), then the transition season to lamb in the winter (August to lamb in January, and then the anovulatory season to lamb in the autumn (April to lamb in September). If the ewe was found to be open at pregnancy scanning ~50 days after breeding, it could be "slipped" to the other flock and reexposed to the ram. To be successful, breeding exposures would need to be short to shorten the lambing interval, and lambs would need to be weaned by 2 mo of age to allow breeding back.

The Cornell Star system is similar but more tightly controlled. Ewes lamb every 7.2 mo instead of every 8 mo. This means a ewe can lamb five times in 3 yr. Length of exposure to the ram, time for ewes to wean lambs and be rebred, lambing, and lactation are all very short.

Although the benefits of these programs are considerable in terms of increased productivity and access to lucrative lamb markets, they require a high level of management to work well. Poor flock fertility tends to create a system heavily weighted to spring lambing, because ewes bred in the late spring that do not conceive are rebred in the autumn when more naturally fertile. Disease control programs must be very well managed; there is little "down time" in the barns or pastures for cleanup of contaminated environments. In addition, ewe nutrition must be such that body condition scores do not get too low during lactation, because there is no opportunity for ewes to regain weight after weaning and before breeding. Breeds that are naturally fertile out of season (eg, Dorset, Merino) have an advantage in these systems.

Accelerated lambing systems are commonly used in northeastern USA and Canada and are becoming more common in South Africa and New Zealand. However, the increased revenue from extra market lambs sold into higher value markets must be carefully weighed against the increased input costs such as feed availability, labor, and housing (for winter lambing).

PREGNANCY DETERMINATION

Accurate determination of pregnancy facilitates differential ewe management by allowing the separation of multiple pregnant ewes for supplementary feed and lambing supervision and the culling of nonpregnant ewes. Procedures for diagnosis of pregnancy can involve detection of ewes that do not return to estrus (nonmarking by ram or teaser fitted with harness and crayon); transabdominal, real-time ultrasonographic scanning; rectoabdominal palpation (from 70 days); abdominal palpation (from 100 days); measurement of plasma progesterone concentrations 18 days after mating (detectable progesterone levels indicate an active CL); and laparoscopy (from 30 days). Real-time ultrasonography is a rapid, highly sensitive and very specific test for pregnancy diagnosis of ewes (and does). For detection of early pregnancy (eg, 20–40 days), it is done most accurately transrectally. When imaging is done later in pregnancy, the ultrasonographic transducer is placed in the woolless area of both flanks and the beam directed forward and upward toward the last rib on the opposite side. It is possible to examine, at low cost, 100–150 ewes/hr and to accurately diagnose single and multiple fetuses.

PRENATAL LOSSES

In healthy sheep, fetal losses after pregnancy diagnosis is performed are normally low, ie, <2%. However, embryo loss can be surprisingly high without an apparent problem at lambing (up to 30% of conceptions). Embryo death before day 12 does not disturb the normal cycle length, whereas embryo death after this time increases cycle length and may appear as repeat marking and a stretched-out lambing period. Pathologic levels of embryo loss are due to issues mentioned previously, but some losses occur in healthy ewes, with higher levels in more prolific breeds.

Fetal loss in the second and third trimester is generally low in healthy flocks. However, when it is abnormally high and due to a pathologic process, it may appear as an observed abortion, abnormal discharge during pregnancy, open ewes at lambing, stillbirth, early neonatal mortality, or all of the above. Causes are most often infectious but may also be nutritional deficiencies or toxins. The most commonly diagnosed causes of abortion are *Chlamydia abortus*, *Campylobacter jejuni*, *Campylobacter fetus fetus*, *Toxoplasma gondii*, border disease virus, *Coxiella burnetii*, Cache Valley virus, *Salmonella* Abortusovis and other salmonellae, iodine deficiency, selenium deficiency, and some plant toxins (eg, locoweed). Abortion rates of 25%–30% are not unusual in these outbreaks, but in general an abortion rate >5% is considered abnormal and should be investigated.

RAM MANAGEMENT

To achieve maximal fertility, rams should be physically examined for reproductive fitness to detect any abnormalities that may limit mating. (*See also* BREEDING SOUNDNESS EXAMINATION OF RAMS, p 2233.) The scrotum and its contents and the penis and prepuce must be carefully examined. The size and symmetry of both testes and epididymides should be assessed, and both testes should be firmly palpated for consistency and resilience. Any palpable lesions, particularly of the epididymis, should be considered potentially contagious (eg, *Brucella ovis* and *Histophilus somni/Actinobacillus seminis*). Appropriate tests should be performed to establish a flock diagnosis to initiate a test and eradicate program for infected rams. Semen can be collected and evaluated to screen potential sires, particularly in single-sire mating systems. All screening procedures should be done 6–8 wk before mating to allow management changes of the ram team or purchase of replacements for defective rams.

Supplementary feeding of the rams can be started 6 wk before joining. High-protein grains, particularly lupines, increase both testicular size and the number of cells in the germinal layers of the testicle, resulting in increased sperm production. However, dietary protein levels >14% have been associated with infectious balanoposthitis due to *Corynebacterium renale* (*see* p 1372, also called pizzle rot).

Mating activity can be monitored by using a breeding harness on the rams and changing the crayon color every 14–17 days. When fewer than expected ewes are marked, poor ram libido, insufficient number of rams to breed the ewe flock, or anestrus is suspected. When ewes are serially marked with different colors, conception failure or early embryonic death is suspected.

The ram to ewe ratio varies with breed, maturity of ram, and whether synchronization or induction of estrus is being practiced. Ratios of 1:40 are common in farm flocks, but excellent fertility can be achieved with a lower ratio if rams from prolific breeds are used (eg, Finnish Landrace). For ram effect, the ratio should be 1:20; for estrus synchronization, 1:10 to 15 (in season); and for estrus induction (out of season), 1:5 to 1:7.

Length of ram exposure during the ovulatory season should be limited to two or three cycles so as to tighten the lambing period to optimize lambing management and lamb survival. Excellent fertility can be achieved with a breeding exposure of 35–42 days (2–2 ½ cycles). Poor fertility indicates an issue with the breeding management. Flock dispersion should be avoided at mating, but normal handling should not affect mating. Because younger ewes have a shorter, less intense estrous period, they are better mated separately from older ewes with experienced, although not necessarily older, rams.

Collection of Semen: The artificial vagina is used most commonly for collection of ram semen. It is prepared for collection by the introduction of warm water (100°–130°F [40°–55°C]) and air between the outer casing and soft inner sleeve, lubrication with petrolatum in the end where intromission of the penis occurs, and attachment of a graduated collecting glass at the opposite end. Rams quickly learn to mount a restrained ewe, and intromission and ejaculation are extremely rapid.

The second method of semen collection is by electroejaculation, for which the ram may be restrained on its side. The lubricated bipolar electrode is inserted into the rectum. The withdrawn penis is held with a piece of gauze to facilitate insertion of the glans into a 10- to 15-mm diameter graduated collecting tube. Ejaculation usually occurs after a few short electrical stimulations; "stripping" of the urethra may be helpful when expulsion of semen seems incomplete. Electroejaculation is less reliable than the artificial vagina; specimens vary in quality and can be contaminated with urine.

The volume of semen collected with the artificial vagina is 0.5–1.8 mL, and the concentration of the spermatozoa is 2.5–6 × 10^9/mL. Semen obtained by electroejaculation generally is of larger volume but lower concentration.

Evaluation of Semen: Immediately after collection, the semen is assessed for contamination, volume, concentration of spermatozoa, and sperm motility (wave motion and sperm progression).

Extension of Semen: Semen can be processed by extending or diluting, packaging, and storing. Semen may be extended 5-fold, depending on the initial concentration, the processing and storage method, and whether the semen will be used fresh, chilled, or frozen-thawed. Most semen extenders or diluents are based on Tris, egg yolk, and additional cryoprotectants such as glycerol. Commercial extender concentrates contain cryoprotectants and require the addition of egg yolk and double-distilled water. These extenders can be used for either fresh or frozen semen.

Extenders for fresh and chilled semen include whole, skimmed, or reconstituted cow's milk that has been heated to 92°–95°C for 8–10 min in a water bath to inactivate toxic factors, egg yolk/glucose/citrate (15% egg yolk, 0.8% glucose [anhydrous], 2.8% sodium citrate dihydrate in glass-distilled water). The addition of Tris or glycerol improves the sperm survival of frozen-thawed semen. The reconstitution of frozen-thawed semen with fresh seminal plasma improves its fertilizing ability when used for intracervical insemination but not for intrauterine insemination. The number of motile spermatozoa and the volume of an insemination dose for the ewe depends on the site of insemination and the method of processing. For vaginal insemination, 0.3–0.5 mL with 300 million motile spermatozoa is used; for cervical insemination, 0.05–0.2 mL is used with 100, 150, and 180 million spermatozoa of fresh, liquid-stored, and frozen-thawed semen, respectively. Intrauterine insemination by laparoscopy requires 0.08–0.25 mL (with a total of 20 million motile spermatozoa) into each uterine horn.

Storage of Semen: Ram semen may be stored for up to 24 hr by cooling the extended semen to 2°–5°C over 90–120 min and by holding at this temperature. Fertility decreases rapidly and is low by 48 hr.

Freezing and storage of ram semen in 0.25–0.3 mL, three-dose pellets or in 0.25 mL, single-dose synthetic straws at liquid nitrogen temperature (196°C) is successful in maintaining sperm viability, but there may be a range in motility after thawing and in fertility between rams or processing batches. Use of frozen-thawed semen may result in lambing rates of 50% with cervical insemination and 50%–80% with intrauterine insemination.

Freeze-thawing reduces the numbers of motile sperm. Chilling results in membrane changes that reduce the longevity of sperm. The membrane changes are similar to capacitation and acrosome reactions, and affected sperm are thus ready to fertilize oocytes. Fresh seminal plasma mitigates the effects of some of the capacitation changes.

ARTIFICIAL INSEMINATION

The optimal time for insemination with nonfrozen semen is 12–18 hr after the onset of estrus. When estrus has been synchronized or induced using progestagens and gonadotropins and/or ram effect, most ewes are in estrus within 36–48 hr and ovulate at ~60 hr. Insemination should be done 48–58 hr after pessary removal for cervical insemination, or 48–60 hr for intrauterine insemination with frozen-thawed semen, with highest conception at ~53–54 hr.

Extended fresh or chilled semen can be placed into the vagina or cervix, and extended fresh, chilled, or frozen-thawed semen can be placed into the uterus. Frozen-thawed semen reconstituted with fresh seminal plasma can be placed into the cervix with conception rates >50%.

Vaginal Insemination: An artificial insemination pipette with a 1–2 mL syringe attached is placed deep into the vagina. This method is quick and involves minimal restraint of the ewe. For cervical insemination, the ewe is restrained to limit movement and to present the hindquarters at a convenient height for easy access to the vagina. After cleaning the vulvar region, the cervix is located with the aid of a speculum and suitable illumination, and the insemination made as deeply as possible into the cervical canal. A long, thin inseminating tube with attached syringe or a semiautomatic inseminating device can be used. The relatively long, tortuous, and firm-walled cervical canal of the ewe usually precludes penetration by the tube for >1 cm. In old, multiparous ewes with cervical tissue distortion, the difficulty increases, and the semen is deposited into the posterior folds of the cervix. In periparturient ewes, the cervix may be fully penetrated. In maiden ewes, in which insertion of the speculum and dilation of the vagina can cause injury, the semen should be deposited in the anterior vagina.

Intrauterine Laparoscopic Insemination: Food and water should be withheld from the ewe for ~12 hr. Ewes should be sedated with 1.5–2 mg xylazine, IM, and placed in cradles that restrain and invert them, first in dorsal recumbency for preparation of the abdomen. Local anesthetic may be injected SC at two sites (~4 cm on each side of the ventral midline and ~6 cm anterior to the udder). The cradle is then raised at the posterior end so that the ewe is tilted at ~45° with the lateral abdomen presented to the operator. The anesthetized sites allow for entrance of two trocars and cannulae; carbon dioxide is insufflated through the first cannula to distend the abdomen. The laparoscope is inserted through the near cannula, the uterine horns are visualized, and a glass or plastic inseminating pipette or sheathed inseminating gun is inserted through the second cannula. Semen is deposited into the lumen of the uterus. Conception rates are similar if semen is deposited into one or both horns of the uterus.

MANAGEMENT OF REPRODUCTION: SMALL ANIMALS

BREEDING SOUNDNESS EXAMINATION

Female: The breeding soundness examination should begin with a thorough reproductive and medical history, including information on previous cycles (onset and regularity), breeding management (past and intended), outcome of any breeding(s), and relevant family history, as well as routine medical information (diet, medications, environment, health status). A thorough physical examination, with particular attention given to the genitalia and mammary glands, should be performed. Vestibulovaginal defects (strictures) should be excluded by digital examination. Evaluation of the mammary glands should include inspection of the nipples for normal anatomy. Screening for hereditary defects common to the breed should be advised, which may require techniques such as radiography (eg, elbow dysplasia), ultrasonography (eg, renal dysplasia), ophthalmoscopy (eg, cataract), specific DNA testing (eg, progressive rod-cone degeneration), as well as the physical examination (eg, patellar luxation).

Digital vaginal examination and vaginoscopy of the bitch may detect strictures or other defects of the vulva or vagina that may hinder copulation or whelping. Vaginal strictures are more commonly congenital than acquired and may be in the form of either a septate strand or a circumferential band. They most commonly form at the vestibulovaginal junction, cranial to the urethral papilla. The heritability of such defects is unknown. Strictures of the vagina or vestibule are not uncommon in the bitch and usually prevent normal copulation, but if pregnancy ensues from mating without a tie or from artificial insemination, dystocia can result. Septate strands can be easily resected surgically, but circumferential strictures are difficult to resolve without episiotomy and major revision, and tend to reform. Elective artificial insemination and cesarean section may be preferable if the bitch has outstanding breeding potential.

Routine vaginal cultures are not advised because the vagina normally harbors a wide variety of bacteria, including β-hemolytic streptococci and *Mycoplasma* spp. Bitches should be screened for brucellosis before each estrus when breeding is planned. A negative *Brucella canis* screening test is reliable; positive results warrant further specific (eg, agar gel immunodiffusion [AGID]) serologic evaluation, culture, or PCR, because false-positives are common. Clinicians should contact their commercial laboratory or veterinary school for updated screening protocols. Queens should be screened for feline leukemia virus and feline immunodeficiency virus as medically indicated. Bitches and queens >5 yr old should also have their general health assessed by performing a CBC, serum chemistries, and a urinalysis.

Before an anticipated breeding, females should be in optimal body condition to improve conception rate and whelping outcome. Breeders commonly skip cycles between breedings; this is not optimal husbandry because the inevitable exposure to estrogen (queen) and progesterone (bitch, sometimes queen) during the estrous cycle promotes cystic endometrial hyperplasia and may result in pyometra. Bitches and queens kept in optimal health can be bred sequentially and should be ovariohysterectomized or ovariectomized when no further breedings are planned. Proper nutrition and exercise strategies for pregnancy and lactation should be outlined.

Bitches should be currently vaccinated for core infectious diseases (canine distemper, parvovirus, adenovirus 2, and rabies). Other noncore vaccinations should be administered only according to good medical practice (appropriate for the dog's age, health status, home and travel environment, and lifestyle). Queens should similarly be vaccinated appropriately (based on duration of immunity recommendations) for feline distemper, rhinotracheitis, and calicivirus. Vaccination against rabies virus, feline leukemia virus, and other noncore diseases should be done when indicated by good medical practice, based on risk factors associated with the cat's age and husbandry. Unnecessary revaccination of bitches and queens before breeding is not advised, because little improvement in immunity can be expected and adverse effects may be seen. Vaccination during pregnancy is advised only when prior vaccination status is lacking or unknown, and risk of exposure is high (eg, a shelter). In that case, the use of recombinant core vaccines is optimal.

The use of preventive medication for heartworm disease and internal and external parasite control (according to manufacturers' recommendations) during pregnancy and lactation is advised. Appropriate isolation of the pregnant female during the last half of pregnancy for infectious disease prevention is important (eg, avoiding exposure to canine herpesvirus in the bitch and upper respiratory infections in the queen). Client education concerning normal whelping and queening events and about the timely identification of dystocias is essential. Fetal and uterine monitoring systems developed for routine use in the bitch and queen improve neonatal survival with reduced morbidity and mortality for the dam.

Male: The breeding soundness examination for males should begin with a thorough reproductive and general health history, including past and intended breeding management, outcome of any breedings already performed, relevant family history, as well as routine general history (diet, medication, environment, and health status). Screening for relevant heritable defects of concern for the breed should be advised.

A thorough physical examination should be performed, with particular attention given to the genitalia. The penis should be fully extruded from the prepuce and examined. This may require sedation in toms. If hair accumulates around the base of the feline penis, it can prevent copulation and should be removed. Prostate size and symmetry should be assessed in dogs by simultaneous abdominal and rectal palpation or with ultrasonography; this is not generally necessary in cats because prostate disease is rare. Palpable abnormalities (pain or asymmetry) or semen abnormalities always warrant ultrasonographic evaluation of the prostate and further clinical testing as indicated (eg, urinalysis, cytology, culture). The testes and epididymi should be palpated carefully for symmetry and normalcy—abnormalities again warrant ultrasonographic evaluation. The scrotum should be evaluated for evidence of dermatitis or trauma, which can impact fertility. A small amount of mucoid discharge at the preputial opening is normal in dogs. (*See also* REPRODUCTIVE DISEASES OF THE MALE SMALL ANIMAL, p 1400.)

Cryptorchidism, a common genital defect in males, is diagnosed if either or both testes are not present in the scrotum at puberty; testicles normally descend into the scrotum by 6–16 wk of age. Descent as late as 10 mo has been documented in dogs. Unilateral cryptorchidism does not result in infertility. In dogs, cryptorchidism is hereditary, and affected animals should not be bred. Both late descent and failure of descent are heritable. Both parents of affected individuals should be implicated as carriers. Because retained testes have a higher incidence of neoplasia and torsion, bilateral orchiectomy is recommended. Attempts at inducing descent with medical therapy with gonadotropins or testosterone have been unsuccessful and are not ethical. Orchiopexy is also considered unethical. Failure of one testis to develop (true monorchidism) may be seen in dogs but is rare. Serum luteinizing hormone (LH) levels are high (>1 ng/mL) if a dog or cat is completely neutered.

A persistent penile frenulum prevents protrusion of the penis from the prepuce and thus copulation. Treatment is surgical. Deviation of the penis is uncommon; these animals require assistance in breeding or may be bred via artificial insemination. Hypospadias prevents normal sperm transport from the testes to the glans penis and is easily detected by physical examination. Small defects may close spontaneously, but some type of reconstructive surgery involving urethrostomy and penile amputation is usually necessary. Phimosis can be caused by stenosis of the preputial opening, which may be congenital or result from chronic inflammation (trauma or bacterial dermatitis). Any underlying cause should be treated and then, if necessary, the opening enlarged surgically.

Semen Evaluation: Ideally, a complete semen evaluation should be performed in male dogs intended for breeding and repeated at least annually in active stud dogs. Semen is readily collected from most dogs by manual stimulation; the presence of a teaser (estrual) bitch is advised to optimize results by improving libido. All equipment (artificial vagina, collecting tubes, pipettes, slides, and coverslips) should be room to body temperature, dry, and free of water and contaminants such as chemical disinfectants. The canine ejaculate consists of three fractions—the first and third are of prostatic origin, while the second is sperm-rich. Sperm production is related to testicular size, so large dogs should produce higher sperm counts than small dogs.

Semen evaluation should include an assessment of libido, total sperm count per ejaculate (normal in dogs is 200–400+ million), sperm motility (normal >90% progressively motile, with moderate to fast speed), and morphology (>90% normal). The sperm count (sperm/mL) is usually determined with a hemocytometer or by spectrophotometry. Sperm per ejaculate is calculated by multiplying the sperm count by the volume of semen collected. Motility is evaluated in an unstained sample as soon as the sample is collected, ideally using clean slides prewarmed on a slide warmer. Several commercially available stains are suitable for morphology examination; eosin-nigrosin and Giemsa stains are used most commonly.

An adequate amount of the third fraction should be collected to ensure that the entire sperm-rich fraction has been acquired and to permit evaluation of the prostatic component, which should be clear (free of urine and cellular contamination). Subfertility or infertility should never be diagnosed based on one collection. If the sample is azoospermic, semen alkaline phosphatase can be measured in the ejaculate to assess whether the ejaculate was complete, because it is an epididymal marker. Levels >5,000 mcg/dL indicate the ejaculate included the second, normally sperm-rich fraction. Levels <5,000 mcg/dL indicate either bilateral obstructive disease or libido problems preventing the release of the second fraction. Sperm function is not assessed with routine semen evaluation. Acrosomal evaluation requires special techniques that are not usually commercially available.

Collection of semen for evaluation is difficult in toms, unless the cat has been trained to ejaculate into an artificial vagina or electroejaculation equipment is available. Cats can be trained to ejaculate with manual stimulation in some instances, but training can take weeks to months. Chemical ejaculation using urethral catheterization under dexmedetomidine sedation or by fine needle aspiration of the testes for sperm cytology has been described. Nonspecific methods of evaluating a tom for spermatogenesis include evaluation of urine for sperm and collecting a vaginal wash from the queen immediately after copulation.

Sperm disappear from the vagina within 1–2 hr of copulation. Warm saline (0.05–1 mL) is flushed into the vagina of the queen and aspirated, the sample is centrifuged, and the sediment examined (new methylene blue or routine hematologic stains are adequate). Breeding a questionable tom to a proven queen may be the most practical way to assess his fertility. Adequate coital contact to induce ovulation should be confirmed by measuring progesterone levels in the queen 1–2 wk after breeding.

BREEDING MANAGEMENT

Dogs

Bitches may be bred naturally or also artificially inseminated using fresh, chilled, or frozen-thawed semen. The practice of ovulation timing has become increasingly desirable to breeders. Owners of popular stud dogs commonly permit a limited number of breedings (usually two) and may need to prioritize bitches based on their timing. Owners of bitches wish to minimize travel time to the stud dog facility. Boarding of bitches in season can be reduced with recognition of their fertile period. The use of extended and chilled semen and frozen semen, or subfertile stud dogs, necessitates ovulation timing for optimal conception. Proper ovulation timing permits accurate evaluation of gestational length and is essential in the evaluation of apparent infertility in bitches. In addition, litter size is optimal with properly timed breedings.

Sound knowledge of the canine reproductive cycle is essential. (*See also* REPRODUCTIVE DISEASES OF THE FEMALE SMALL ANIMAL, p 1393.) Individual bitches may vary from normal, be presented at variable times during their estrous cycle for evaluation, and sometimes exhibit pathologic variations in cycles. Each of these scenarios requires veterinary interpretation. The normal canine reproductive cycle can be divided into four phases, each having characteristic behavioral, physical, and endocrinologic patterns, although considerable variation exists. Bitches with normal estrous cycles but unexpected patterns must be differentiated from those with true abnormalities. Detection of individual variation within the normal range of events in a fertile bitch can be crucial to breeding management. Evaluation of the estrous cycle for true abnormalities is an important part of the evaluation of an apparently infertile bitch.

The interestrous interval is normally 4–13 mo, with 7 mo the average. The **anestrus** phase of the estrous cycle is marked by ovarian inactivity, uterine involution, and endometrial repair. An anestrous bitch neither attracts nor is receptive to male dogs. No overt vulvar discharge is present, and the vulva is small. Vaginal cytology is predominated by small parabasal cells, with occasional neutrophils and small numbers of mixed bacteria. The endoscopic appearance of vaginal mucosal folds is flat, thin, and red.

The physiologic controls terminating anestrus are not well understood, but the deterioration of luteal function and the decline of prolactin secretion seem to be prerequisites. The termination of anestrus is marked by an increase in the pulsatile secretion of pituitary gonadotropins, follicle stimulating hormone (FSH), and luteinizing hormone (LH), induced by gonadotropin-releasing hormone (GnRH). Hypothalamic GnRH secretion is itself pulsatile, its intermittent secretion is a physiologic requirement of gonadotropin release. Mean levels of FSH are moderately increased, and those of LH slightly increased, during anestrus. At late anestrus, the pulsatile release of LH increases, causing the proestrous folliculogenesis. Estrogen levels are basal (2–10 pg/mL) and progesterone levels at nadir (<1 ng/mL) in late anestrus. Anestrus normally lasts 1–6 mo.

During **proestrus**, the bitch attracts male dogs but is still not receptive to breeding, although she may become more playful. A serosanguineous to hemorrhagic vulvar discharge of uterine origin is present, and the vulva is mildly enlarged. Vaginal cytology shows a progressive shift from small parabasal cells to small and large intermediate cells, superficial-intermediate cells, and finally superficial (cornified) epithelial cells, reflecting the degree of estrogen influence. RBCs are usually, but not invariably, present. The vaginal mucosal folds appear edematous, pink, and round. FSH and LH levels are low during most of proestrus, rising during the preovulatory surge. Estrogen rises from basal anestrous levels (2–10 pg/mL) to peak levels (50–100 pg/mL) at late proestrus, while progesterone remains at basal levels (<1 ng/mL) until rising at the LH surge (2–4 ng/mL). Proestrus lasts from 2 or 3 days to 3 wk, with 9 days average. The follicular phase of the ovarian cycle coincides with proestrus and very early estrus.

During **estrus**, the healthy bitch displays receptive or passive behavior, enabling breeding. This behavior correlates with decreasing estrogen levels and increasing progesterone levels. Serosanguineous to hemorrhagic vulvar discharge may diminish to variable degrees. Vulvar edema tends to be maximal. Vaginal cytology remains predominated by superficial cells; RBCs tend to decrease but may persist throughout. Vaginal mucosal folds become progressively wrinkled (crenulated) in conjunction with ovulation and oocyte maturation. Estrogen levels decrease markedly after the LH peak to variable levels, while progesterone levels steadily increase (usually 4–10 ng/mL at ovulation), marking the luteal phase of the ovarian cycle. Estrus lasts 3 days to 3 wk, with an average of 9 days. Estrous behavior may precede or follow the LH peak—its duration is variable and may not coincide precisely with the fertile period. Primary oocytes ovulate 2–3 days after the LH peak, and oocyte maturation is seen 2–3 days later; the life span of secondary oocytes is 2–3 days.

During **diestrus**, the healthy bitch becomes refractory to breeding, with diminishing attraction of male dogs. Vulvar discharge diminishes, and edema slowly resolves. Vaginal cytology is abruptly altered by the reappearance of parabasal epithelial cells and frequently neutrophils. The appearance of vaginal mucosal folds becomes flattened and flaccid. Estrogen levels are variably low, and progesterone levels steadily rise to a peak of 15–80 ng/mL before progressively declining in late diestrus. Progesterone secretion depends on both pituitary LH and prolactin secretion. Proliferation of the endometrium and quiescence of the myometrium develop under the influence of increased progesterone levels.

Diestrus usually lasts 2–3 mo in the absence of pregnancy. Parturition terminates pregnancy 64–66 days after the LH peak. Prolactin levels increase in a reciprocal fashion to falling progesterone levels at the termination of diestrus or gestation, reaching much higher levels in the pregnant state. Mammary ductal and glandular tissues increase in response to prolactin levels.

Estrogen, LH, and progesterone are important in ovulation timing. All may be assessed as part of a reproductive evaluation.

Estrogen: Increased estrogen causes an increased turnover rate of vaginal epithelial cells, resulting in the progressive cornification seen on vaginal cytology. Progressive edema of the vaginal mucosa also develops and can be visualized with endoscopic examination. Estrogen assays are performed by many commercial laboratories; however, the information is of little value for ovulation timing because peak estrogen levels vary from bitch to bitch, and even relative changes do not correlate to ovulation or the fertile period. Estrogen is best assessed by serial vaginal cytologies and vaginoscopy. Estrogen levels do not indicate the fertile period, because ovulation is triggered by the LH surge and not an estrogen peak.

Examination of the cells on the surface of the vaginal epithelium can provide information about the stage of the estrous cycle. Proper technique is important so that the cells obtained are representative of the hormonal changes occurring. The sample should be collected from the cranial vagina; cells from the clitoral fossa, vestibule, or caudal vagina are not as indicative of the stage of the cycle. Under the influence of rising estrogen levels, the number of layers composing the vaginal epithelium increases dramatically, presumably to provide protection to the mucosa during copulation. As estrogen rises during proestrus, the maturation rate of the epithelial cells increases, as does the number of keratinized, cornified epithelial cells seen on a vaginal smear. Full cornification continues throughout estrus until the "diestral shift" occurs 7–10 days after the LH surge, signifying the first day of diestrus. The vaginal smear then changes abruptly, with appearance of neutrophils and epithelial cells changing from full cornification to 40%–60% immature (parabasal and intermediate) cells over the next 24–36 hr. If vaginal cytology is performed until the diestral shift is seen, the LH surge, ovulation, and the fertile period can be analyzed retrospectively.

Luteinizing Hormone: At the end of the follicular phase of the estrous cycle, a marked increase in LH over usual baseline values develops over 24–48 hr, followed by a return to baseline values. This surge is thought to occur in response to the decline in estrogen levels and increase in progesterone levels. The LH surge triggers ovulation, making it the central endocrinologic event in the reproductive cycle of the bitch.

Daily serial measurement of LH to identify the exact date of the LH surge is an accurate diagnostic tool to time breedings. Affordable semiquantitative in-house kits are available to measure serum LH levels in dogs and to identify the preovulatory LH surge and thus the time of ovulation and the true fertile period. Blood samples must be drawn daily (at approximately the same time) for LH testing, because the LH surge may last only 24 hr in many bitches. The kits can be subject to variable interpretation, so the same person should run the tests if possible. Progesterone testing should always be performed concurrently in case the LH surge is missed.

Progesterone: Progesterone levels begin to rise at approximately the time of the LH surge (before ovulation). Rising progesterone acts synergistically with declining estrogen to reduce edema of the vulva and vagina, which can be seen on vaginoscopic examination. Other observable clinical signs are minimal. Serial blood samples performed every 2 days may identify the initial rise in progesterone (usually >2 ng/mL), which indicates that the LH surge has occurred. Progesterone can be assayed by radioimmunoassay at most veterinary commercial laboratories. Several in-house semiquantitative kits are also available.

No single absolute value of progesterone correlates to any particular stage of the cycle. Progesterone varies from 0.8–3 ng/mL at the point of the LH surge, from 1–8 ng/mL at ovulation, and from 4–20+ ng/mL during the fertile period. However, if accurate serial quantitative progesterone assays are obtained, the LH surge may be estimated as the day a distinct increase in progesterone level is seen. Although this is not as accurate as actual identification of the LH surge by assay, estimation by progesterone levels is still very useful and is often more widely available and convenient.

When timing breeding using semiquantitative in-clinic progesterone assays, only a range of progesterone is obtained, which makes it difficult to accurately identify the day of the initial rise in progesterone or the true fertile period. Technical problems with these kits have also been seen. Therefore, these assays should be used only for routine breedings in which a wider margin of error is acceptable. A gemeral guideline is that when progesterone is >2 ng/mL, breeding should begin. Optimal ovulation timing should use quantitative progesterone assays from commercial laboratories (the cost difference is minimal). Regardless of which assay is used, an additional test should always be performed 2–4 days after the first rise is detected to indicate that the cycle has progressed as expected, a functional corpus luteum has been formed, and ovulation has occurred.

Use of Hormonal Evaluation to Time Breeding: Owners of breeding animals should be advised to notify their veterinarian when they first notice that a bitch for which timing is planned is in season, based on vaginal discharge or vulvar swelling/attraction to males. Even the most astute owner may not notice the true onset of proestrus for a few days. Early proestrus should be documented with vaginal cytology (<50% cornification/superficial cells). A baseline progesterone level (usually 0–1 ng/mL) might be informative if the true onset of the cycle is unknown. Vaginal cytology should be performed every 2 days until cornification progresses significantly, usually >70% superficial cells. At that point, serial hormonal assays should begin. For routine breedings, progesterone testing may be done every other day until a rise in progesterone >2 ng/mL is identified. The day of the initial rise in progesterone >2 ng/mL is identified as "day 0." Breedings are advised on days 2, 4, and 6.

When increased accuracy of ovulation timing is necessary (eg, frozen or chilled semen breedings, infertility cases, breedings with subfertile stud dogs), daily LH testing is recommended. Once the LH surge is identified, breeding days may be planned. The day of the LH surge is also "day 0." It is useful to perform vaginal cytology every 2–3 days until cornification is complete (generally >80%–90% superficial cells). This maximal cornification usually develops before the fertile period and continues until the onset of diestrus, which is usually a few days after the end of the fertile period. Vaginal cytology may be continued until the diestral shift is identified, which gives a retrospective evaluation of the breeding just completed. In addition, at least one progesterone assay should be performed after day 0 is identified to document that levels continue to rise. This illustrates sustained corpus luteum function and strongly suggests that an ovulatory cycle has occurred.

Insemination with extended, chilled semen should be done on days 4 and 6, or 3 and 5, after day 0. The days chosen can depend on overnight shipping possibilities and the schedules of all involved parties. Frozen semen breedings should be done on day 5 or 6.

Vaginoscopy may be performed throughout the cycle as an adjunct to vaginal cytology and hormonal assays, especially when evaluating an unusual cycle. Behavior and other observations should also be made. Ovulation timing is most accurate when information from several tests is pooled (vaginal cytologies, vaginoscopy, and progesterone or LH tests).

Artificial Insemination: Artificial insemination is becoming more common in canine reproduction, permitting the use of shipped semen, assistance for geriatric or subfertile males, coverage of dominant females, and advanced reproductive technology such as intrauterine deposition of semen. Insemination may be performed with fresh, chilled, or frozen semen. All instruments should be clean and free of any chemical contamination. After semen has been collected and evaluated (*see* p 2221), it can be deposited in the cranial vagina of the bitch using a rigid insemination pipette of appropriate length, or into the uterus via transcervical catheterization. Access to the uterus via laparoscopy or laparotomy is less desirable because of invasiveness.

Semen (the second fraction) may be diluted with extenders and chilled for later or distant use (within 48 hr), or extended and frozen in liquid nitrogen (in straws or pellets) for longterm storage. Phosphate-buffered egg yolk diluent or Tris-buffered diluent is used most often; several commercial extenders are available. A drop of chilled semen should be warmed for evaluation before use. Frozen semen should be thawed as directed by the cryopreservation center, evaluated, and immediately inseminated. Dogs should be screened for *Brucella canis* when semen is collected for cryopreservation.

Cats

The queen should be taken to the tom when showing signs of estrus. The breeding area should be familiar to the tom, quiet, and have good footing and a minimum of interference, while permitting observation. The courtship should not be interrupted unless there is concern for the safety of either cat. Toms have been known to mate to the point of physical exhaustion, but queens normally go through a period of rolling and grooming after a breeding and may not let the tom remount for some time.

Because ovulation is induced by vaginal-cervical stimulation, multiple breedings over 2–3 days are advised. Periods of separation between matings prevent exhaustion and diminish the chances of fighting. The stress of transportation may affect reproductive functions in nervous queens. Evaluation for pregnancy can be performed 21–30 days after breeding by abdominal palpation and ultrasonography.

MANIPULATION OF THE ESTROUS CYCLE

The estrous cycles of dogs and cats are not as easily manipulated as in other species. Most protocols are not based on controlled studies, so manipulation of the estrous cycle in valuable breeding individuals is not advised. Although onset of a particular cycle may be delayed, return to normal cycling is highly variable. Induction of estrus is possible in late anestrus bitches by using prolactin inhibitors (eg, bromocriptine, cabergoline).

Ovariohysterectomy or ovariectomy is the best method to prevent estrus in the bitch and queen. Longterm suppression of estrus by using androgens is not advised, because it is not documented to be safe in breeding bitches. Common adverse effects are breakthrough proestrus, clitoral hypertrophy, vaginitis (especially in prepubertal bitches), increased activity of skin sebaceous glands, mild epiphora, and alterations in hepatic function studies. After treatment is discontinued, return to estrus is ~70–90 days but variable. Conception rates are reportedly normal by the second cycle after treatment. If given to pregnant bitches, synthetic androgens induce severe developmental anomalies in the urogenital system of female puppies. The safety and efficacy of injectable testosterone, as is practiced commonly in racing Greyhounds, has not been supported by controlled studies and is not advised. Androgens should not be given to cats.

The use of megestrol acetate, a synthetic progestagen, is not advised in breeding females because of the increased risk of cystic endometrial hyperplasia and pyometra, as well as other adverse effects (eg, mammary hyperplasia and neoplasia, hyperglycemia secondary to insulin resistance, and rebound hyperprolactinemia and lactation).

Suppression (and induction) of estrous cycles by the use of synthetic GnRH implants has been described in the bitch; it can be successful, but the products are not universally available. Estrus induction in the bitch can be accomplished with oral prolactin inhibitors (cabergoline 2.5–5 mcg/kg/day); anestrus of at least 2 mo duration must precede induction.

Ovulation can be induced in estrual queens physically or, more reliably, hormonally to produce a luteal phase (diestrus or metestrus) of ~45 days. Physical methods include mating with a vasectomized tom (very effective) or inserting a sterile swab or glass rod into the vagina. The latter should be performed repeatedly for best results. Hormonal methods include administration of human chorionic gonadotropin at 500 IU/cat or GnRH at 25 mcg/cat. Both are given IM, once daily for 2 days.

PREGNANCY DETERMINATION

Fertilization occurs in the oviducts in both the bitch and queen. Implantation of zygotes in the uterus occurs at ~18 days in the bitch and 14 days in the queen. This is accompanied by the formation of small swellings along the uterine horns (deciduomata) by ~21 days. These are palpable, assuming the animal is cooperative, at this time. Fetal growth is rapid during early pregnancy, and these swellings double in diameter every 7 days. After day 35–38, they become indistinct, and palpation becomes difficult until late pregnancy when fetal heads and rumps are palpable as firm, nodular structures in the ventral posterior abdomen. A commercial relaxin assay, specific and sensitive for pregnancy diagnosis in the bitch after 30 days gestation, is available.

Although the fetal skeleton begins to calcify as early as day 28, it is not detectable by routine radiography until approximately day 42–45 and is quite prominent by day 47–48. Radiography at this time is not teratogenic. Late gestational radiography (>55 days) is the best method to determine litter size. Fetal dentition becomes visible at term, and its appearance can be used to confirm fetal develpment adequate for an elective cesarean section when ovulation

TABLE 17 GESTATIONAL AGE IN DOGS AND CATS

Dogs: Gestational Age ± 3 days		Cats: Gestational Age ± 2 days
<40 days	*>40 days*	*>40 days*
(6 × GSD[a]) + 20	(15 × BP[b]) + 20	25 × BP + 3
(3 × CRL[c]) + 27	(7 × BD[d]) + 29	11 × BD + 21
	(6 × HD) + (3 × BD) + 30	
Days before parturition = 64–66 minus gestational age		Days before parturition = 61 minus gestational age

[a] Gestational sac diameter (cm)
[b] Biparietal diameter (cm)
[c] Crown rump length (cm)
[d] Body diameter at the liver (cm)

timing is not available and breeding dates are vague or spread over many days.

Ultrasonography is also useful in pregnancy determination and permits evaluation of fetal viability. Ultrasonography is best performed at 25–35 days gestation. Before 21 days, "false-negative" results are seen. Doppler-type instruments allow one to "hear" the fetal heart, which beats 2–3 times faster than that of the dam. Placental sounds may also be heard. Ultrasonography is especially helpful in differentiating pregnancy from other causes of uterine distention (eg, hydrometra, pyometra, mucometra). Ultrasonographic measurements can be used to calculate gestational age (*see* TABLE 17).

Gestational age in cats can also be determined by the following formula:

mean litter crown rump length (in cm) = 0.2423 × gestational age – 4.2165

PREVENTION OR TERMINATION OF PREGNANCY

Unplanned and unwanted mating of cats and dogs is a common concern. Pregnancy can be completely prevented or terminated by ovariohysterectomy. Sixty percent of misbred bitches do not conceive, so confirmation of an undesired pregnancy is advised before proceeding. Postcoital douches are of no value in preventing unwanted pregnancy. Although injectable estrogens, when administered appropriately, can prevent pregnancy, their use involves great risk of serious adverse effects, including pyometra and potentially fatal bone marrow suppression, and they are not advised. If used, they must be administered soon after copulation, before potentially fertilized ova reach the uterus. Oral estrogens given during diestrus greatly increase the risk of pyometra, are unreliable in terminating pregnancy, and are not advised.

Safe and effective termination of pregnancy is possible in both the bitch and queen by administration of prostaglandin $F_2\alpha$ (natural hormone) at 0.1 mg/kg, SC, tid for 48 hr followed by 0.2 mg/kg, SC, tid to effect (until all fetuses are evacuated as confirmed by ultrasonography). Treatment times can reach 14 days. In the bitch, treatment time can be reduced (usually by 48 hr) by the concurrent administration of prostaglandin E (misoprostol) intravaginally at 1–3 mcg/kg/day. The adverse effects of prostaglandins at this dosage (panting, trembling, nausea, and diarrhea) are mild and transient. The therapeutic window for prostaglandins is narrow, and doses should be calculated carefully. Synthetic prostaglandins (cloprostenol 1–3 mcg/kg every 12–24 hr to effect) more specifically target the myometrium, causing fewer systemic adverse effects, and are currently preferred.

Pregnancy can also be reliably terminated in the bitch by administration of dexamethasone at 0.2 mg/kg, PO, bid to effect. The owner should be informed of the adverse effects of corticosteroid administration (eg, panting, polyuria, polydipsia).

Combination drug protocols (cabergoline 5 mcg/kg, PO, divided every 24 hr for as long as 10 days, cloprostenol 1 mcg/kg given SC twice at ~28 and 32 days after the LH surge) have been reported to terminate pregnancy reliably with minimal adverse effects, shortest treatment times, and greatest sucess rates; their cost and need for compounding are disadvantages.

Antiprogestins (aglepristone) are safe and effective abortifacients; availability remains problematic.

WHELPING AND QUEENING

Normal gestation in the bitch is 56–58 days from the first day of diestrus, or 64–66 days from the initial rise in progesterone from baseline (generally >2 ng/mL), or 58–72 days from the first instance that the bitch permitted breeding. Parturition in the queen occurs 64–66 days from the LH surge triggered by copulation.

Predicting length of gestation without prior ovulation timing is difficult because of the disparity between estrual behavior and the actual time of conception in the bitch, and the length of time semen can remain viable in the reproductive tract (often ≥7 days). Breeding dates and conception dates do not correlate closely enough to permit accurate prediction of whelping dates. Additionally, clinical signs of term pregnancy are not specific—radiographic appearance of fetal skeletal mineralization varies at term, and fetal size varies with breed and litter size. A drop in rectal temperature to a mean of 98.8°F (range 98.1°–100.0°F) (37.1°C [range 36.7°-37.8°C]) is seen in most bitches 8–24 hr before whelping. Breed, parity, and litter size can also influence gestational length. Subtle signs of impending delivery include relaxation of the perineum, mammary engorgement, and a change in the appearance of the gravid abdomen, but these changes are not sensitive or specific. Because there is no means to effectively manage prematurely born puppies, premature intervention in the whelping process is undesirable. Likewise, an excessively conservative approach resulting in intrauterine fetal death is undesirable as well.

Bitches typically enter stage I labor within 24 hr of a decline in serum progesterone to <2–5 ng/mL, which develops in conjunction with increased circulating prostaglandins and is commonly associated with a transient drop in body temperature (<99°F [37.2°C]). Monitoring serial progesterone levels for impending labor is problematic because in-house kits enabling rapid results are inherently inaccurate between 2 and 5 ng/mL. Commercial laboratories offering quantitative progesterone by radioimmunoassay or hemiluminescence typically have a 12–24 hr turnaround time, which is not rapid enough to make decisions about immediate obstetric intervention. Progesterone levels can drop rapidly in a matter of hours. If progesterone is <2 ng/mL, gestation is likely at term and labor pending. Clearly, it is beneficial to obtain information about ovulation timing, minimally by determining the onset of cytologic diestrus, to evaluate length of gestation at term.

A predictable and safe way to induce successful parturition in the bitch and queen has not been developed.

LABOR AND DELIVERY

Normal Labor: Stage I labor in the bitch and queen normally lasts 12–24 hr, during which time the myometrial contractions of the uterus increase in frequency and strength and the cervix dilates. No abdominal efforts (visible contractions) are evident during stage I labor. Bitches and queens may exhibit changes in disposition and behavior during stage I labor, becoming reclusive, restless, and nesting intermittently, often refusing to eat and sometimes vomiting. Panting and trembling may be seen. Vaginal discharge is clear and watery.

Normal stage II labor is marked by visible abdominal efforts, which are accompanied by myometrial contractions that culminate in the delivery of a neonate. Typically, these efforts should not last >1–2 hr between puppies or kittens, although great variation exists. The entire delivery can take 1 to >24 hr; however, normal labor is associated with shorter total delivery time and intervals between neonates. Vaginal discharge can be clear, serous to hemorrhagic, or green (uteroverdin). Typically, bitches and queens continue to nest between deliveries and may nurse and groom neonates intermittently. Anorexia, panting, and trembling are common.

Stage III labor is defined as the delivery of the placenta. Bitches and queens typically vacillate between stages II and III of labor until the delivery is complete. During normal labor, all fetuses and placentae are delivered vaginally, although they may not be delivered together in every instance.

Dystocia: Dystocia results from maternal factors (uterine inertia, pelvic canal anomalies), fetal factors (oversize, malposition, malposture, anomalies), or a combination of both. Clinically, uterine inertia developing after the delivery of one or more neonates (secondary inertia) is the most common cause of dystocia.

Dystocia can be objectively diagnosed if uterine contractility is inappropriate (generally infrequent, weak myometrial contractions) for the stage of labor, or if excessive fetal stress results from labor. Subjectively, dystocia is diagnosed if stage I labor is not initiated at term, if stage I labor is >24 hr without progression to stage II, if stage II labor does not produce a vaginal delivery within 1–4 hr, if fetal or maternal stress is excessive, if moribund or stillborn neonates are seen, or if stage II labor does not result in the completion of deliveries in a timely manner (within 12–24 hr).

Uterine and fetal monitors can be used to detect and monitor labor and to manage dystocia. Unresponsive uterine inertia, obstructive dystocia, aberrant uterine contractions, or progressive fetal distress without response to medical management are indications for cesarean section.

Medical management includes administration of calcium gluconate and oxytocin based on the results of monitoring. Drugs are given only after 8–12 hr of an established contraction pattern (stage I labor) as detected by the uterine monitor and only if inertia is detected when stage II labor is anticipated. Premature administration of drugs results in suboptimal response.

Generally, the administration of calcium increases the strength of myometrial contractions, while oxytocin increases the frequency. Calcium gluconate (10% solution, 1 mL/22 kg body wt bid-qid) is given when uterine contractions are ineffective or weak. It can be given SC, avoiding the potential for cardiac irritability associated with IV administration. Oxytocin (0.5–2 U in bitches; 0.25–1 U in queens) is given when uterine contractions are less frequent than expected for the stage of labor. The most effective time for treatment is when uterine inertia begins to develop, before the contractions stop completely. High doses of oxytocin saturate the receptor sites and make it ineffective as a uterotonic. If fetal stress is evident (persistent bradycardia) and response to medications is poor, cesarean section is indicated.

POSTPARTUM CARE

Palpation and, if necessary, radiography should be used to determine that all puppies or kittens have been delivered. The routine postpartum administration of oxytoxin or antibiotics is unnecessary in healthy dams with nursing neonates, unless the placenta has been retained. The dam's body temperature and the character of the postpartum discharge or lochia and milk should be monitored. Normally, the lochia is dark red to black and is heavy for the first few days after parturition. It is not necessary that the dam consume the placentas. Disinfection of the neonatal umbilicus with tincture of iodine helps prevent bacterial contamination.

The neonate should be weighed accurately as soon as it is dry and then twice daily for the first week. Any weight loss beyond the first 24 hr indicates a potential problem and should be given immediate attention (eg, supplemental feeding, assisted nursing, evaluation for sepsis). Neonates should gain 10% of their body weight daily.

PERIPARTURIENT PROBLEMS

Bitches and queens should deliver in a familiar area where they will not be disturbed. Unfamiliar surroundings or strangers may impede delivery, interfere with milk letdown, or adversely affect maternal instincts. This is especially true in young or primiparous animals. The dam's apprehension or nervousness may subside in a few hours, but in the meantime the neonates must receive colostrum and be kept warm; nursing should be closely supervised. The use of acepromazine at low dosages (0.01 mg/kg, PO, bid-tid) can effectively relax nervous dams and does not sedate neonates detectably nor interfere with milk production.

A nervous dam may ignore the neonates or give them excess attention. She may lick and bite at the umbilical stump, causing hemorrhage or damage to the abdominal wall that may lead to evisceration. Excess grooming of the neonate may prevent it from nursing. If the dam's maternal instincts fail, she may assume sternal recumbency and not allow nursing, or leave the neonates unattended. It is not unusual for the dam to pick up the pups and to rearrange them in the box, especially after delivery of each pup; however, she should then assume the normal nursing position.

The principal metabolic disease associated with pregnancy is puerperal hypocalcemia (*see* p 992). It is rare in cats and most common in dogs weighing <20 kg, exacerbated by improper perinatal nutrition (excessive calcium/phosphorus supplementation or an imbalanced prenatal diet).

Common inflammatory diseases in the postpartum period include metritis and mastitis. Retention of a placenta or its remnants could lead to metritis. Signs include continued straining as if in labor, the presence of a fusiform mass associated with the uterus (best identified by ultrasonographic evaluation), abnormal vulvar discharge, fever, and lethargy as the infection develops. If given within 24 hr of labor, oxytocin may cause passage of the placenta; if oxytocin is ineffective, prostaglandin $F_2\alpha$ (0.1 mg/kg, SC, every

12–24 hr) or cloprostenol (1–3 mcg/kg, SC, every 12–24 hr to effect) can usually induce passage of the placenta.

Mastitis (*see* p 1396) is more common in bitches than in queens. The bacteria associated with mastitis tend to be coliforms or *Staphylococcus* spp. Galactostasis can predispose bitches to mastitis, as can excessive human manipulation of the mammary glands. Mammary glands should be observed to ensure that all are being nursed.

Significant postpartum uterine hemorrhage is rare. Oxytocin (<24 hr postpartum) and prostaglandins can be administered if the uterus is healthy; ovariohysterectomy must be performed if hemorrhage is unabated and significant (ie, causing blood loss anemia). Screening for an underlying coagulopathy and appropriate therapy should be undertaken.

Uterine subinvolution results in hemorrhagic spotting for >12–16 wk (the normal period of involution in the bitch). Treatment is unnecessary unless blood loss is significant, because the condition resolves spontaneously. Future fertility is unaffected.

Agalactia (other than that caused by severe illness) is uncommon in dogs and cats. Determination that lactation is adequate should be performed before elective cesarean section. If an emergency cesarean section is required, regardless of the status of lactation, intervention is indicated (*see* below). Bitches and queens with inadequate lactation at term should be thoroughly evaluated for metabolic or inflammatory disorders (metritis, eclampsia, mastitis), nutritional and hydration status, or periparturient pain, and treated appropriately. Evaluation of a hemogram, serum chemistries, vaginal discharge, and ultrasonographic evaluation of the uterus may be required. The normal presence of colostrum (typically not copious) should not be confused with agalactia. The level of neonatal contentment and daily weight gain (after the first 24 hr) indicates adequate lactation. Milk letdown is promoted by oxytocin release, a reflex triggered by nursing; therefore, neonates must spend adequate time suckling. Disruption of the pituitary-ovarian-mammary gland axis can result in idiopathic agalactia. Agalactia can be associated with premature delivery of neonates. Iatrogenic agalactia can result from progesterone supplementation during gestation and should be avoided unless essential.

Because estrogen promotes lactogenesis, the adequacy of mammary development should be assessed before removal of the ovaries at cesarean section. Ovariohysterectomy should not have a negative effect on bitches and queens with adequate lactogenesis at term. If this is seen, a genetic component may be involved.

Lactation can be stimulated if treatment is prompt. Mini-dose oxytocin (0.5–2 U/dose, SC, every 2 hr) should be administered. The neonates should be removed from the dam before each injection and returned 10 min later. The neonates should be supplemented adequately to ensure survival, but not excessively, so that they will suckle vigorously. Mammary glands should be gently hand stripped if suckling is not vigorous. Concurrent administration of metoclopramide (0.1–0.2 mg/kg, SC, tid-qid) promotes prolactin release. Acepromazine at mild tranquilization dosages may also facilitate milk letdown. Therapy should continue until lactation is adequate, usually 12–24 hr later.

INFERTILITY

The most common cause of infertility in dogs and cats is related to husbandry problems. Breeding with a proven fertile male must occur at the optimal time for the female. Infectious, anatomic, metabolic, and functional problems associated with infertility are seen less frequently. (*See also* INFERTILITY, p 1328.)

The only confirmed infectious cause of infertility in the bitch is brucellosis (*see* p 1402). This highly contagious disease caused by *Brucella canis* results in abortion and infertility in bitches and infertility in males. A rapid slide agglutination test (RSAT) kit to detect serum antibodies is commercially available. If the RSAT is negative, the bitch is presumed to be *Brucella*-free; if positive, further confirmatory laboratory testing is indicated (eg, AGID, PCR, 2-mercapto-ethanol RSAT).

In cats, infectious causes of infertility include toxoplasmosis, feline leukemia virus infection, feline infectious peritonitis, and feline viral rhinotracheitis. These may cause abortion, neonatal death, fetal resorption, and apparent infertility.

Anatomic causes of infertility include acquired and congenital problems. Fibrosis of the oviducts or uterine horns, probably a result of inflammation after infection or trauma, leads to infertility. Diagnosis is via laparotomy with dye studies. There is no reliable treatment, although microsurgery may be attempted. Similarly, bilateral obstruction of the sperm ducts can cause azoospermia and infertility. High environmental temperature and excessive conditioning resulting in increased body temperature can induce either temporary or permanent azoospermia. Kennel or cattery management should allow for breeding males to remain cool during the summer. Scrotal dermatitis can have the same result. Disorders of sexual differentiation result in infertility (eg, hermaphroditism, pseudohermaphroditism).

Metabolic causes of infertility, other than in severely ill individuals, are rare. Hypothyroidism has no effect on male libido or semen quality. Hypothyroid bitches might not cycle or have increased abortion rates, or neonatal survival may be poor.

Estrous cycle abnormalities can cause infertility. Prolonged anestrus may be congenital or acquired. Some large breeds of dogs may not have their first estrus until they are ≥2 yr old, and some individuals and some breeds typically have only one estrous cycle each year. Congenital forms of anestrus may be due to lack of function of the hypothalamic-pituitary axis or ovarian dysgenesis.

The diagnosis of congenital anestrus is based on the age of the animal and exclusion of all other possible causes (including chromosomal defects, endocrine disorders, and previous oophorectomy). Because cyclicity in queens is determined by photoperiod, lighting conditions should be appropriate for several months before congenital anestrus is diagnosed and exogenous hormones are administered. One reported method to induce estrus in cats is FSH at 2 mg/cat, IM, once daily until signs of estrus appear (not administered for >5 days).

Acquired anestrus may result from previous oophorectomy, exogenous hormonal treatment (including glucocorticoids), profound hypothyroidism, or ovarian disease (cysts or neoplasia). Diagnosis is based on history, physical examination, biochemical evaluation, ultrasonography, and laparotomy.

Prolonged estrus may be caused by ovarian cysts that produce estrogen, functional ovarian tumors, or exogenous estrogens (including human transdermal hormone replacement therapy). Exogenous hormones should be discontinued. Laparotomy with histopathology is usually indicated, because medical attempts at inducing ovulation (human chorionic gonadotropin, FSH, GnRH) are usually unrewarding. Prolonged diestrus can result from luteal cysts in the ovary. Medical manipulation with prostaglandins is usually unrewarding, and ovariectomy with histopathology is indicated.

Prostatitis can be subclinical or contribute to subfertility and infertility in dogs. Benign prostatic hyperplasia does not affect fertility.

Testicular neoplasia, commonly producing estrogen, usually causes infertility. Castration of the affected testis may allow the other testis to regain its ability to produce sperm, but the prognosis is guarded.

BREEDING SOUNDNESS EXAMINATION OF THE MALE

The breeding soundness examination (BSE) involves a complete and systematic evaluation of the reproductive potential of a given male, including mating ability and libido, general physical examination and inspection of the genital organs, and assessment of sperm production and quality. The BSE is not a direct evaluation of fertility: this can be confirmed only by successful production of offspring after breeding a fertile female. The specific male animal must be properly identified, and a detailed history is important because sub- or infertile males might require more exhaustive evaluation. The evaluation of mating ability and libido is possible only when collecting semen via artificial vagina or manual stimulation in the presence of a female in estrus. Therefore, mating ability is seldom evaluated in bulls and rams for routine BSE in which semen is typically collected via electroejaculation.

The components of semen quality evaluation are: 1) semen volume and sperm concentration, which allow for the calculation of the total number of sperm in the ejaculate; 2) sperm motility, including gross motility (ruminants only) and percent individual sperm motility (total and progressive) of a diluted sample; and 3) the percent morphologically normal sperm. A Romanowsky-stained cytology sample also allows for evaluation of red (hemospermia) or white (pyospermia) blood cells in the ejaculate. When collecting semen from ruminants via electroejaculation, the sperm production potential is estimated by measuring scrotal circumference. Scrotal circumference is correlated with daily sperm output and therefore the serving capacity of a bull or ram (ie, number of females he can settle in a limited time).

After the BSE is complete, the male is classified as a satisfactory, questionable, or unsatisfactory prospective breeder. An animal with physical defects that may be inherited (including cryptorchidism) should be declared unsatisfactory. Guidelines for the BSE in each domestic species are included in the following species-specific discussions.

Spermatogonial Stem Cells and Prospects for Preservation of Male Fertility: Spermatogonial stem cells (SSCs) are stem cells located against the basement membrane of the seminiferous tubules. As such, they can regenerate themselves but also give rise to daughter cells that follow the replication and differentiation path toward the generation of mature sperm. Of particular interest is that SSCs are present throughout the life of a given male and hence may provide an avenue to preserve or even restore male fertility.

Although much work is still needed for SSCs to become a reality in the management of male infertility, these cells have been isolated and partially characterized in boars, bulls, tom cats, and stallions. Most knowledge derives from studies in the mouse, in which SSCs can be cultured indefinitely, cryopreserved, genetically modified, and transplanted into the testes of sterile recipient mice for generation of mature sperm cells. Studies are underway to pursue these goals in domestic species. In the future, SSCs may be used to preserve fertility in valuable domestic species as well as in their endangered wild counterparts (eg, felids). Moreover, SSCs could also become an integral tool in the assessment of male fertility or ability to restore fertility in a given male. In addition, and given some of the advances in assisted reproductive technologies in domestic species, it is feasible that SSCs could be differentiated into haploid germ cells in vitro for intracytoplasmic sperm injection and the generation of offspring from valuable azoospermic males.

BULLS

In bulls, assessment of libido is often not possible during a routine breeding soundness examination (BSE). However, if possible, the bull should be observed serving cows to allow assessment of his desire to breed, ease of mounting, ability to achieve erection and extend the penis, and presence of penile deviation or other abnormalities that may prevent successful service. Libido and serving capacity tests (scoring the number of services achieved during a set time that a bull is in a pen with a restrained cow) have been devised but are time consuming and difficult to standardize under field conditions. In addition, the results are difficult to interpret in light of the variety of stocking conditions used, eg, single versus multiple bulls or small paddocks versus large ranges.

BSE forms have been developed and should be used to ensure the systematic completion of the examination and accurate reporting of results. The bull should be restrained in a chute for the examination. Body condition should be scored, and a general physical examination conducted with special attention paid to the feet, legs, eyes, and sheath. The inguinal rings and internal genitalia should be palpated per rectum to detect any abnormalities, eg, seminal vesiculitis. The scrotum should be palpated to evaluate the testes, epididymides, spermatic cords, and scrotal skin. The testes should be symmetrical in size, smooth, resilient, and freely movable within the scrotum. Cryptorchidism is considered an undesirable heritable trait and renders a bull unsatisfactory for breeding even though his semen quality might be acceptable. In ruminants, the epididymides run caudomedially along the testes in a dorsoventral orientation, with the tail most ventrad. The epididymis should have no palpable masses. The measurement of scrotal circumference (SC) is considered a reliable predictor of paired testis weight, which in turn provides an accurate estimate of daily sperm production and quality. The SC should be measured at its maximal diameter, and size depends greatly on bull age and breed. As a general rule, SC should be ≥30 cm for bulls <15 mo old, 31 cm for bulls 16–18 mo, 32 cm for bulls 19–21 mo, 33 cm for bulls 22–23 mo, and 34 cm for bulls ≥2 yr old. However, readers should consult the latest published breed-specific average SC measures.

Although not used routinely in practice, additional techniques to evaluate the scrotal contents include thermography and ultrasonography. Bull testes must be 2°–6°C (35.6°–42.8°F) cooler than core body temperature for optimal sperm production, and increases in scrotal temperature negatively affect semen quality. Infrared thermography can be used to evaluate scrotal temperature, which should yield a left to right symmetry with a 6° to 4°C (42.8° to 39.2°F) temperature gradient from top to bottom. Abnormal thermograms are almost always associated with poor sperm quality and have been correlated with decreased pregnancy rates. Conversely, evaluation of the testes by ultrasonography does not appear to improve the predictive value of standard evaluation techniques (physical examination, palpation, SC measurement, sperm evaluation). Therefore, it appears that the value of ultrasonography as a tool in BSE in bulls rests on assessment and characterization of grossly detectable lesions of the testes.

For the purpose of a routine BSE, semen is most often collected via electroejaculation; semen can be collected with an artificial vagina (AV) in bulls trained to use one (eg, those in bull studs). The penis usually extends during electroejaculation and should be examined at that time for any abnormalities. If it is not extended during electroejaculation, it should be gently exteriorized for examination by grasping the glans with a cotton gauze and, if necessary, by putting pressure on the sigmoid flexure immediately caudal to the scrotum. Preputial wash samples may be taken for isolation and culture of *Campylobacter fetus venerealis* (using Clark's medium) or *Tritrichomonas foetus* (using Diamond's medium or a commercially available diagnostic medium kit), in particular when investigating subfertility in bulls ≥4 yr old.

The electroejaculator consists of a rectal probe that has a series of linear banded electrodes connected to a variable current and voltage source. The bull is restrained in a chute, the rectum is emptied, and the entire lubricated probe is inserted rectally with the electrodes oriented ventrally. A hand-operated rheostat permits intermittent pulses of current to be given as the voltage is gradually increased. The response varies considerably, but it is common to use 2- to 4-sec pulses repeated at 5- to 7-sec intervals. After a variable number of such stimulations, erection and protrusion of the penis may be seen, followed by a flow of seminal fluid, or the bull may ejaculate into the sheath without protruding the penis. The semen may be collected by any convenient method; typically a rubber AV cone inserted within a plastic cylinder attached to an 18-in. handle, with a test tube attached to the cone, is used. In some bulls, ejaculation is seen only after a final series of momentary pulses at 1- to 2-sec intervals. Older bulls usually require a higher voltage for ejaculation. In some large bulls, the probe may not reach the correct areas for stimulation; having two or more probe sizes is recommended if BSEs are to be done on a variety of sizes of bulls. The semen collected via electroejaculation is not representative of a full ejaculate in regard to volume and concentration, and thus the sperm production potential of the bull is based on the evaluation of SC. Conversely, sperm quality (motility and morphology) does not differ from that in an ejaculate collected with an AV.

If an AV is to be used, bulls are induced to mount a teaser animal (eg, restrained steer, cow, or phantom), and the erect penis is directed into the AV by the collector as the bull mounts. In preparing the AV, the temperature, which is a critical factor in stimulating ejaculation, is maintained at 105°–107°F (40.5°–42°C). Temperatures up to 118°F (48°C) may assist collections in untrained bulls. The AV should be lubricated with nonspermicidal jelly. The typical volume of an ejaculate is 4–8 mL, and the concentration 1–1.5 billion sperm/mL. A semen sample can be collected from some bulls by transrectal massage of the accessory sex glands. With this technique, erection seldom occurs. After the rectum is completely emptied, the vesicular glands are massaged with a backward motion until a few mL of fluid drop from the sheath. The ampullae are then massaged, and an assistant collects the semen as for electroejaculation. This method is not always successful, and the quality of the semen emission is usually lower than the ejaculate collected by the other two methods.

Sperm concentration, ejaculate volume, and the total number of sperm in the ejaculate are evaluated only if the sample has been collected with an AV. The semen sample should be evaluated immediately for sperm motility. The materials that contact the sperm should be at the same temperature as the sperm (to avoid temperature shock), clean, dry, and nontoxic. Motility evaluation is best when the temperature of the semen is either maintained at ~37°C (~98.6°F) during the short time before it is evaluated, or when the semen is gently warmed to 37°C before evaluation. Both gross motility ("swirl pattern") in the semen and motility of individual spermatozoa should be assessed; individual motility is the more accurate measure and should be used for classification of the bull.

Gross motility is a function of sperm concentration and individual sperm motility and is evaluated in an undiluted drop of semen placed on a slide without a coverslip and examined at low power (~100×). The intensity of wave motion may be classified into four categories: very good—intense swirling, rapid dark and light waves; good—slower swirling, waves not as intense; fair—slow movement with fewer waves; or poor—very little or no swirl activity. Individual motility is assessed in a sample diluted with warmed saline or semen extender. A drop of diluted sperm is placed on a slide, covered with a coverslip, and examined at 200–400×. The proportion of sperm that are moving progressively across the field of view is estimated by finding multiple groups of ~10 sperm and estimating how many sperm are progressive versus how many are not.

The environments in which BSE are done are variable, and there is a high chance of temperature shock to sperm before they may be evaluated. Therefore, >30% individual progressive motility, or fair gross motility, is considered acceptable. If the examination is performed under optimal conditions, some associations (eg, the Canadian Bovine Practitioners Association) recommend a minimum of 60% motility for a bull to be classified as a satisfactory potential breeder.

Visual estimates of sperm motility are considered appropriate for bull classification in field BSEs. However, in commercial artificial insemination centers, sperm motion evaluation is performed using computer-assisted sperm analysis (CASA), which provides more objective values as well as specific measures not only of percent motile sperm but also of velocities and the track followed by each sperm. For instance, the combination of measures such as beat cross frequency, linearity, average path velocity, straightness, and curvilinear velocity have been correlated with bull fertility. Moreover, some of the motion measures evaluated by CASA such as curvilinear velocity, straightness, and linearity correlate with sperm function such as the acquisition of hyperactivated motility.

The presence of cells other than spermatozoa in the sample should be investigated while estimating motility. RBCs, WBCs, and excess numbers of round epithelial cells and developing forms of spermatozoa may indicate a genital tract abnormality. Careful evaluation of the tract, especially the internal genitalia, may indicate the source of WBCs. The most common cause is seminal vesiculitis. Round, immature germ cells and spermatozoa with proximal cytoplasmic droplets may indicate immaturity or, alternatively, testicular degeneration. For a better assessment of the types of cells present in semen, staining an air-dried smear of fresh semen with Romanowski stain is recommended. This simple technique can provide critical information, in particular when cells other than mature sperm are present in the sample.

A sample of the semen should be fixed in a buffered formaldehyde saline solution to evaluate sperm morphology. This is best done with the fixed, unstained sperm examined under high power (1,000×) using a phase-contrast microscope. At least 100 sperm should be counted, and the proportion of sperm showing different types of abnormalities noted. However, the only number used in the evaluation of the bull is the proportion of normal sperm, which should be >70%. Sperm plasma integrity, which is required for sperm function, can be assessed with the use of a vital stain such as eosin. Eosin penetrates cells with a disrupted sperm membrane, which appear pink on evaluation under light microscopy, in contrast to live cells, which do not stain. Eosin is often combined with nigrosin, which provides a dark background that allows better observation of live/dead sperm cells. An eosin-nigrosin–stained smear can also be used to assess sperm morphology, although it is considered less reliable than using phase-contrast microscopy of an unstained wet preparation. Other, more sophisticated measures of sperm function are not used routinely in cattle BSEs, although they may become more common in referral and artificial insemination centers. Such tests may include combinations of fluorescent probes and flow cytometry to assess membrane integrity, mitochondrial function, or sperm chromatin integrity, and functional assays such as ability of sperm to undergo in vitro capacitation, zona binding, and/or homologous in vitro fertilization.

Bulls are classified as "satisfactory potential breeders" if they have no physical abnormalities that would prevent breeding and if they meet the minimal qualifications for SC, sperm motility, and sperm morphology. Bulls that do not meet these criteria are classified as "unsatisfactory potential breeders" or, if the results are marginal or questionable, they are considered "classification deferred" and a retest should be recommended.

RAMS

In rams, the breeding soundness examination (BSE) is performed much as for bulls, using an electroejaculator with a smaller (ram) probe. Body score is classified as 1–2, questionable (underconditioned); 3–4, satisfactory; and 5, questionable (overconditioned). Any major abnormalities of the external genitalia or lumps or irregularities of the testes or epididymides render the ram unsatisfactory. Epididymal masses are commonly found to be sperm granulomas caused by infection with *Brucella ovis*, which is a major cause of reproductive loss in sheep. *B ovis* may also be associated with testicular atrophy. Scrotal circumference should be ≥28 cm for rams 8–14 mo old (>36 cm is exceptional) and ≥32 cm for rams >14 mo old (>40 cm is exceptional). Scrotal circumference lower than satisfactory is questionable. Motility of individual spermatozoa is evaluated as for bulls, with >70% progressive motility being exceptional, >30% satisfactory, 10%–30% questionable, and 0% unsatisfactory. The percentage of morphologically normal sperm should be >50%; between 30% and 50% is questionable, and <30% unsatisfactory; >80% normal sperm is exceptional. Presence of >5 WBCs per high power field is questionable (WBCs are correlated with *B ovis* infection). An ELISA test for *B ovis* should be done on range rams and rams >9 mo old. A positive test renders the ram unsatisfactory. Suspect tests should be repeated. (*See also* RAM MANAGEMENT, p 2217.)

Any ram with one unsatisfactory rating in any parameter is classified "unsatisfactory"; a ram with a questionable rating in any parameter is "questionable." For a ram to be classified exceptional, he must have exceptional ratings in scrotal circumference, sperm motility, and sperm morphology. All other rams are considered "satisfactory."

BUCKS

Breeding soundness examination in bucks has not been detailed to the extent that it has in rams. The testes should be palpated carefully. *Brucella ovis* infection is rare, but sperm granulomas are frequently related to the polled condition; these are most often found in the head of the epididymis. Cryptorchidism is also common and heritable; as in other species, cryptorchid bucks should not be used for breeding. Testicular degeneration is a common cause of fertility loss in older bucks. Semen is collected using an artificial vagina (AV); bucks are easily trained for this method and do not tolerate an electroejaculator. An electroejaculator might be used only if the buck is sedated. Parameters for semen evaluation are similar to those for rams. Because the ejaculate is typically collected with an AV, sperm production may be measured rather than estimated from scrotal circumference. Semen volume should be 0.5–2 mL, and concentration 1.5–4 billion sperm/mL.

STALLIONS

Given the high economic value of some stallions and the willingness to breed horses based more on their competitive potential than on their breeding soundness, many resources and expensive tests are sometimes used to evaluate breeding soundness, and especially to assess sperm function in those stallions proven subfertile after their first breeding season or displaying potential defects after a routine breeding soundness examination (BSE). Classically, a complete BSE of the stallion has comprised a history, general physical examination, examination of the external and internal genitalia, culture of urethral and possibly penile swabs, and collection and evaluation of at least two ejaculates collected 1 hr apart for total sperm number, sperm motility, and sperm morphology.

The history should include the stallion's prior fertility and type of management used for breeding. If <10 mares were bred, individual mare fertility should be considered if pregnancy rates were low. If the stallion has been racing or training recently, he may have been receiving anabolic steroids or other drugs. Stallions recently retired from a performance career may be evaluated again in 3–6 mo if they fail the initial BSE.

During the physical examination, the stallion should be evaluated for general body condition and the presence of any conditions that might interfere with breeding. Genetically inherited defects, including parrot mouth and cataracts, render the stallion unfit for breeding. Blindness, lameness or ataxia, penile paralysis, or other defects that prevent the stallion from breeding also render him unsatisfactory as a breeding prospect. Recent evidence supports cryptorchidism as a potentially inherited defect in horses, thus rendering the stallion an unsatisfactory prospective breeder.

Scrotal palpation should be performed and may be done after the first ejaculation when the stallion may be more relaxed. Total scrotal width should measure >8 cm (preferably >9 cm), as assessed with a blunt caliper across both testes together. The testes should be firm, resilient, and homogeneous on palpation. The epididymides run dorsally along the testes, in a craniocaudal orientation, with the tail most caudad. The tail of the epididymis is easily palpable, whereas the body and head of the epididymis tend to blend with the dorsal surface of the testis. Rotation of one testis 180° (the tail of the epididymis being palpated on the cranial aspect of the testis; also called torsion of the spermatic cord) is common and has no clinical significance in healthy stallions.

Ultrasonography is also commonly used to evaluate scrotal contents and to take individual measurements of each testis. A portable console fitted with a linear 5 MHz transducer typically used for reproductive evaluation of mares can be used. The testes should have a homogeneous echoic appearance; a cross or longitudinal section of a central vein that runs along the longitudinal aspect of the testis starting at the cranial pole is a hallmark of the normal equine testis and should not be confused with pathology. The tail of the epididymis and spermatic cord display a homogeneous "cheesecloth-like" appearance; asymmetric dilations of the vessels of the spermatic cord may be consistent with varicose veins and may or may not affect blood flow and testis function. Measurements of the width (W), height (H), and length (L) of each testis can be used to calculate testis volume and to estimate expected daily sperm output by applying the following formulas: testis volume = (W × H × L) × 0.5233 for each testis; daily sperm output = (0.024 × testis volume) – 0.76, in which testis volume is the total volume, or the sum of volume for both testes.

The penis is usually examined while it is washed before the first semen collection. The penis can vary in size with no effect on fertility. It should be freely distensible from the sheath without lesions. Of the internal genitalia of the stallion, the ampullae, vesicular glands, and lobes of the prostate gland are palpable per rectum. The vesicular glands are difficult to palpate unless the stallion is first teased to a mare in estrus to stimulate filling of the glandular lumina with fluid. The bulbourethral glands are covered by muscle, making it impossible to palpate their structure. Transrectal ultrasonography can be used to more thoroughly evaluate each of the accessory sex glands and pelvic urethra. Because of the danger inherent in adequately restraining a stallion, some veterinarians perform a transrectal examination only if deemed necessary because of an abnormal finding on the remainder of the examination, such as blood or pus in the ejaculate. When performing palpation per rectum on a stallion, the internal inguinal rings should also be palpated to determine their size and presence of any abnormalities. They are felt as flaps of peritoneum that form pockets in the abdominal lining at the 3 o'clock and 9 o'clock locations at the entrance of the pelvis.

Semen is collected from the stallion using an artificial vagina (AV) filled with water at ~50°C (~122°F), which typically cools to 42°–45°C (107.6°–113°F) by the time of collection; some stallions might be accustomed to higher AV temperatures (50°–55°C [122°–131°F]) for adequate stimulation, but the internal temperature of the AV should not exceed 55°C (131°F) at the time of semen collection. The stallion is teased to an estrous (or ovariectomized) mare; once an erection is achieved, the penis is washed with warm water and blotted dry with a paper towel. If the penile skin is suspected to harbor potentially transmissible bacteria (eg, *Klebsiella pneumoniae* or *Pseudomonas aeruginosa*), a culture swab of the sheath and fossa glandis should be obtained before the penile area is washed and rinsed for semen collection. Smegma can fill the dorsal urethral diverticulum, located dorsal to the urethral process, and harden to form a "bean." This can cause irritation and swelling and should be removed. After the penis is washed and dried, a swab sample of the distal urethra is obtained. The stallion is then allowed to mount the mare or phantom (breeding dummy), and the semen is collected by diverting the penis into the AV. A second swab sample is taken from the distal urethra immediately after ejaculation. The stallion should be given 1 hr of rest before the second ejaculate is collected.

The culture results of the urethral swab samples can be difficult to interpret. Prewash penile cultures usually show moderate to heavy growth of mixed bacteria. Preejaculate urethral swabs also may reveal growth of a mixed bacterial population. Growth of *Pseudomonas* or *Klebsiella* may indicate that the penis has been colonized by these organisms; in the USA these are the only bacteria (besides *Taylorella equigenitalis*, the cause of contagious equine metritis, *see* p 1371) that, in some cases, may be passed to mares and cause endometritis. The postejaculate urethral swab should yield less bacterial growth, because the urethra has been "washed" by the ejaculate. High numbers of bacteria, especially of a single species, on the postejaculate swab may indicate infection of the internal genitalia, most commonly the urethra and/or seminal vesicles.

The ejaculate should be evaluated for gross appearance, volume, sperm concentration, sperm motility, percentage of morphologically normal sperm, and percentages of specific spermatozoal morphologic abnormalities. The ejaculate should be free of pus, urine, or blood. The normal ejaculate may contain gel, a viscous, clear to cloudy material, that originates from the seminal vesicles and forms the third and last fraction of the ejaculate. Because it is ejected last, the gel fraction can be removed by having an in-line filter at the mouth of the collection bottle in the AV (preferred), or alternatively, by pouring the ejaculate through a milk filter once in the laboratory.

The analysis of the semen is done on the gel-free (sperm-rich) fraction. Concentration may be determined using a hemocytometer or a properly calibrated photometric instrument. Several instruments specially designed for this purpose are commercially available. Sperm motility and morphology evaluations are performed as described for the bull (*see* p 2231); however, the sperm concentration is much lower in stallions (typically 100–400 million/mL), so only individual sperm motility is evaluated. Assessment of motility should be performed with both raw semen and semen diluted with a good quality extender. Semen should be warmed to 35°–37°C (95°–98.6°F) before assessing spermatozoal motility.

Notably, conventional measures of sperm quality correlate only moderately with fertility, and variations in the percentages of motile/progressively motile and morphologically normal sperm account for only 20% of the total variation in fertility. Given the limitations of standard sperm tests in predicting fertility or identifying subfertile stallions, other sperm tests have been evaluated and may be applied for stallion BSEs performed in referral centers. While not necessarily providing a better correlation with fertility, CASA offers a more objective and complete assessment of sperm motion characteristics. As in bulls, certain changes in different motion parameters, namely increases in curvilinear velocity and decreases in linearity and straightness, correlate with the acquisition of hyperactivated motility, which has been recently characterized in stallions. In addition, computer-assisted sperm head morphometry (shape) assessment has been suggested as a useful adjunctive test to predict stallion fertility. Membrane integrity can be easily evaluated via eosin-nigrosin staining (as in bulls), and the hypoosmotic swelling test or ability of sperm to swell to establish an osmotic equilibrium with a hypoosmotic surrounding medium may also hold some value for sperm membrane evaluation; however, a direct correlation with fertility has not been established. Fluorescent probes such as rhodamine 123 or JC-1 in conjunction with flow cytometry have also been used to evaluate mitochondrial potential and hence integrity. In addition, the combination of these with other fluorescent stains offers the advantage of concomitantly evaluating viability and chromatin integrity in a large number of sperm. In this regard, the sperm structure chromatin assay, which assesses sperm chromatin stability, has been thoroughly researched in stallions and moderately correlated with fertility. It is a good adjunctive test for stallions in which routine laboratory test results do not correlate with subfertility or infertility. Finally, true tests of sperm function (ie, ability to fertilize an oocyte) have been restricted because of the inability to capacitate stallion sperm in vitro or to perform in vitro fertilization in this species. Recent advances in this area may permit the application of these assays for more meaningful evaluation of stallion sperm.

In addition to assessing sperm quality, once two ejaculates have been collected, the total number of spermatozoa in each is calculated as volume (gel-free) × concentration.

The total number of sperm in the second ejaculate of two collected 1 hr apart is considered a rough estimate of the daily sperm output for that stallion (ie, ejaculates are considered to be representative if the second ejaculate contains about half the number of sperm as the first). The second ejaculate should have about the same, or a slightly higher, percentage of morphologically normal sperm, as well as the same or better motility than the first. If sperm numbers or quality differ from this guideline, then either prolonged sperm storage in the excurrent ducts has occurred (*see* below), or one of the ejaculates was not complete, and a third ejaculate should be obtained. The third ejaculate should have about half as many sperm as the second ejaculate, and the same or better morphology and motility. A third ejaculate may also be collected if the sperm evaluation does not appear to agree with the total scrotal width (eg, high sperm numbers from a stallion with small testes) or the calculated daily sperm output. Prolonged storage of sperm in the excurrent ducts results in high numbers in the initial ejaculate, but these sperm may have poor motility and morphology.

Some stallions with extreme sperm storage require daily collection for 7–10 days before representative ejaculates are obtained (sperm evaluation results are consistent on successive collections). In extreme cases, sperm may accumulate in the ampullae and inspissate, causing blockage of the ductuli deferentiae. This may result in no sperm or few sperm, typically with detached heads, present in the ejaculate. Multiple attempts at collection may be necessary before the blockage is cleared. Relief of the blockage is typically evident by the ejaculation of very large numbers of dead sperm with detached heads.

In cases of severe ampullary blockage or in stallions with ejaculatory problems, attempts at semen collection might initially yield only clear seminal fluid. In such instances, it might be warranted to differentiate between these problems and azoospermia (ie, lack of sperm production) before successive semen collection attempts. For this purpose, collected seminal fluid can be submitted for determination of alkaline phosphatase levels. Because alkaline phosphatase concentrations are high in epididymal fluid, a value <100 U/L is consistent with blockage or ejaculation failure, whereas a value >1,000 U/L is consistent with collection of epididymal fluid and thus true azoospermia.

In a satisfactory potential breeding stallion, sperm numbers after >5 days of sexual rest should be ≥8–10 billion in the first ejaculate and ≥4 billion in the second ejaculate. Total spermatozoal motility should be ≥65%, and progressive motility ≥50%. At least 50% of the sperm should be morphologically normal. A stallion is considered satisfactory if it produces at least 1 billion progressively motile and morphologically normal sperm in the second (or third) ejaculate of two (or three) collected 1 hr apart.

Stallions are classified as "satisfactory," "questionable," or "unsatisfactory" potential breeders based on the results of the above detailed examination. However, classification can be somewhat subjective, and an excellent finding in one category can balance a marginal finding in another. Satisfactory potential breeders should achieve a seasonal pregnancy rate of >80% when bred to 50 mares by natural breeding or to 120 mares by artificial insemination under normal management conditions. Questionable potential breeders may experience difficulty in doing the above. Typically, stallions are placed in this category if a problem is detected that might resolve over time with or without treatment; thus, a recheck is recommended within 6–12 mo. Unsatisfactory breeders have problems that may profoundly reduce their fertility or have undesirable heritable traits that may be transmissible to their offspring. Some stallions may be used to inseminate a percentage of mares with cooled-transported semen. Under these circumstances, longevity of spermatozoal motility should be tested using commercial semen containers before a decision is rendered regarding fertility potential.

BOARS

In postpubertal boars, testes should be symmetric (<1 cm difference), with each testis having a minimum length and width of 8 and 5 cm, respectively. Semen is collected with the boar mounted on a phantom or an estrous sow. As the penis is extruded, the tip (incorporating the coiled part) is grasped with a gloved hand and compressed; this stimulates full erection and ejaculation. The opening of the urethra is ~1 cm proximal to the tip of the glans, and care must be taken not to block it while applying digital pressure. The volume of semen is high, and ejaculation occurs over a long period, so semen is usually collected into an insulated container to maintain a relatively constant temperature. A filter or opened gauze sponge is fastened across the opening of the container to filter out gel and debris. Normal semen values for the boar are volume, 50–500 mL; sperm concentration, $>50 \times 10^6$/mL; progressive motility, >70%; total sperm per ejaculate, $>60 \times 10^9$; and percentage of morphologically normal sperm, >80%.

DOGS

A complete breeding soundness examination (BSE) in dogs consists of a history, physical examination, semen evaluation, and testing for *Brucella canis*. If infertility is suggested from the history, it should be established that adequate breeding management was practiced and that bitches had normal fertility when bred to other dogs. The time sequence of litters sired and bitches that did not conceive should be recorded, as should any recent illness during or before the time the bitches were bred. These should be assessed to determine whether the infertility may be transient (eg, fever can adversely affect semen production for >60 days after the initial insult).

A general physical examination should be performed. Dogs with abnormalities such as severe joint disease or spinal problems may not be able to mount. Endocrinopathies such as hyperadrenocorticism or hypothyroidism may reduce fertility; these may be associated with abnormalities in weight or hair coat. The penis and prepuce should be examined; problems such as persistent frenulum, growths, or swelling due to balanoposthitis may prevent normal intromission. Abrasions or lacerations on the penis may bleed during breeding, and blood may be seen in the semen.

The prostate should be digitally palpated per rectum. The most common prostatic problem in mature (>5 yr old) intact dogs is benign prostatic hyperplasia (BPH); the prostate appears uniformly enlarged and is not painful on palpation per rectum. Dogs with BPH might be asymptomatic or have a history of hematuria and/or hemospermia or rectal tenesmus. In dogs with clinical signs, the treatment of choice is castration, although breeding dogs can be treated medically with 5α-reductase inhibitors, which prevent the conversion of testosterone to dihydrotestosterone. Treatment is important, because affected dogs are predisposed to developing prostatitis. Ultrasonography has become a common adjunctive tool for prostate evaluation in dogs, allowing for accurate measurements and assessment of the gland's echotexture for identification of potential pathologies, in which case a fine needle or biopsy instrument can be guided to sample a lesion.

The scrotum, testes, and epididymides should be palpated. Small, soft testes are usually associated with poor semen quality; greatly enlarged testes suggest orchitis or epididymitis. Lumps suggesting neoplasia may also be palpable. Scrotal abnormalities such as dermatitis may adversely affect semen quality by decreasing scrotal thermoregulation. Length, width, and height of testes should be measured with blunt calipers; these measurements are often of value for future comparison in cases of suspected testicular degeneration. Additionally, total scrotal width is highly correlated with body wt and an estimate of the dog's sperm production potential. Ultrasonographic examination of the scrotal contents is valuable not only to obtain more accurate measurements but also to evaluate for the presence of testicular or epididymal masses, which may not always be readily palpable in the early stages of a pathologic process.

Semen collection is performed with the dog on good footing (eg, a rug) rather than on a slippery surface or table. Care should be taken not to intimidate the dog; thus, any general examination procedures are best performed after semen collection. Semen may be collected in the absence of a bitch (although sperm numbers may be lower), but the presence of a bitch is preferable, especially for inexperienced dogs. The pheromone methyl paraben may be helpful for collection in the absence of a bitch; some veterinarians freeze swabs of estrous bitch urine or vaginal secretions for this purpose, but the reaction of male dogs is variable.

A collecting cone such as the liner of a bull artificial vagina, lubricated with sterile nonspermicidal lubricant or petroleum jelly and attached to a test tube, can be used. The penile sheath is gently pulled back, and the cone is slipped over the penis. As soon as the bulbus glandis is exteriorized from the sheath and is within the cone, the penis is grasped through the cone, immediately caudal to the bulbus. Constant pressure is maintained caudal to the bulbus, and erection and eventually ejaculation should be achieved. Contact of the penis with the lubricated cone typically stimulates the dog to thrust into the cone, and the penis is compressed through the cone caudal to the bulbus as described above. Semen may also be collected with the gloved hand technique, by stimulating the dog's penis within the prepuce until a partial erection is achieved; the prepuce is then slid caudally, behind the bulbus glandis, and steady pressure is applied as with the cone technique until the dog ejaculates. A cup or tube fitted with a funnel is held over the tip of the penis to collect the ejaculate. Some breeders simply use a plastic bag held over the penis to collect semen.

The first (prostatic, clear) fraction and the second (sperm-rich, cloudy) fraction should be collected. After these fractions are ejaculated, close inspection of the collection tube should demonstrate that clear (prostatic) fluid is starting to layer on the cloudy second fraction; at this point, the collection may be stopped. The dog may continue to ejaculate prostatic fluid for up to 10 min before the erection subsides. The sheath should be examined after the penis is retracted to ensure that the penis is situated normally within the sheath and that no hair is caught within the sheath. Residual protrusion may occur if the sheath rolls inward as the penis retracts.

Semen evaluation consists of determination of appearance, volume, concentration, motility, and percent morphologically normal sperm. Yellow, brown, or red samples may indicate the presence of blood or urine in the ejaculate. The volume is variable, depending on how much prostatic fluid was collected and the size of the dog; it ranges from <2 to >20 mL but is typically ~5 mL. Sperm motility should be evaluated immediately using warmed equipment; this should yield >70% progressively motile spermatozoa. Sperm morphology is determined as for bulls (*see* p 2231). At least 80% of the sperm should be morphologically normal. The concentration is determined using a hemocytometer. To do this, the sperm is diluted at 1:100, and the number of sperm in the large central square (made up of 25 smaller squares) on the hemocytometer is counted. The number of sperm counted × 10^6 is the concentration of spermatozoa/mL. The total number of sperm in the ejaculate is calculated as volume × concentration. Total sperm number in the ejaculate ranges from 400 × 10^6 to >1,000 × 10^6 and is correlated with body wt; as a general rule, a dog should produce ~10 × 10^6 sperm/lb body wt.

Every dog investigated for infertility should be screened for *Brucella canis*. (*See also* BRUCELLOSIS IN DOGS, p 1402.)

Sperm quality may be normal or abnormal, or no sperm may be seen in the ejaculate. Infertility is rare in dogs with a normal sperm evaluation and, if seen, the history should be reviewed for mismanagement or bitch infertility. The presence of WBCs or RBCs in the ejaculate suggests inflammation of the tract, most commonly prostatitis; culture of prostatic fluid and appropriate treatment may help fertility. If sperm quality is abnormal, the history should again be reviewed to determine whether the dog has been sick recently or has received any drugs, especially anabolic steroids. Other recognized causes of abnormal sperm quality include inflammation of the scrotum or other factors that may be causing a high scrotal temperature, testicular neoplasia (ultrasonography of the testes is recommended because many neoplasms of the testes are not palpable), trauma to the area of the scrotum, or brucellosis. However, most cases of low sperm quality in dogs are idiopathic.

The dog's pituitary status can be investigated but is usually unrevealing. Luteinizing hormone and follicle-stimulating hormone are typically normal to high in dogs with abnormal semen quality, because the degenerating testes are not able to provide the feedback mechanism to the pituitary. Because abnormal sperm quality may be induced by a recent transient disease or exposure to toxins, and spermatogenesis might resume, collections should be repeated about every 3 mo for ~1 yr before a definitive prognosis for breeding can be given.

Azoospermia is relatively common in dogs. It may be due to failure of the dog's testes to produce sperm, or to failure of the sperm to exit the testes because of epididymal blockage or incomplete ejaculation. As in stallions, the ejaculate may be tested for the presence of alkaline phosphatase, which is secreted by the epididymis. A high value (5,000–40,000 IU/L) indicates fluid from the epididymis was collected and thus is consistent with true azoospermia. Low values (<5,000 IU/L) suggest epididymal blockage or ejaculation failure; semen collections should be repeated, using a strong stimulus such as a bitch in estrus. A cystocentesis should be performed after semen collection to determine whether retrograde ejaculation is occurring; swab samples of the vagina of a bitch after natural mating may also be performed to determine whether the dog is not ejaculating because of aversion to manual collection. Careful palpation and ultrasonographic examination should be performed to detect any abnormality of the epididymides or spermatic cords, such as absence (epididymal aplasia) or blockage of the epididymis.

A dog is considered "satisfactory" if all the above findings are within normal limits and the dog is seronegative for *B canis*. Breeding dogs should be retested annually for *B canis*. As in other species, "questionable" dogs are those with a condition that might resolve over time (eg, recent febrile episode with temporary testicular degeneration, BPH), whereas a dog with an untreatable condition or an inherited disorder is classified as "unsatisfactory" for breeding.

EMBRYO TRANSFER IN FARM ANIMALS

Embryo transfer has proved to be a powerful technology in genetic improvement of farm animals, primarily to propagate the genes of females of superior pedigree. In cattle, particularly in the dairy industry, breeding programs have been developed to promote genetic progress by strategic use of elite females through multiple ovulation embryo transfer (MOET) programs. In addition to conventional methods to produce embryos available for transfer, new technologies that produce embryos after cloning by somatic cell transfer or transgenesis are available but not widely used commercially.

Embryo transfer protocols have also been extensively used in research critical to understand several areas of biology and medicine, such as fetal-maternal interactions, models of human and animal diseases, production of transgenic animals to produce therapeutic proteins for people, etc. However, this discussion is restricted to the principles and methods currently used in commercial embryo transfer of farm animals. Except in horses, embryo transfer programs in most mammals include administration of drugs that superovulate females to allow the probability that multiple embryos are collected per procedure. Globally, it was reported in 2012 that 699,586 bovine embryos were collected from superovulated cows, and 443,533 bovine embryos were produced via in vitro fertilization procedures.

CATTLE

Although collection of a single embryo is occasionally done in cattle, the vast majority of embryo transfers in cattle are programmed after a hormonal treatment to superovulate donor cows and to maximize recovery of embryos during the collection procedure. In cattle, there are two generally accepted methods of superovulation. One method consists of administering a single IM injection (2,000–2,500 IU) of equine chorionic gonadotropin (eCG), typically on day 10 of the estrous cycle (in which day 0 is defined as the day cows are observed in estrus), followed 2–3 days later by two injections of prostaglandin $F_2\alpha$ (dinoprost or cloprostenol) 12–24 hr apart. The other commonly used method is to administer follicle-stimulating hormone (FSH). The superovulatory response induced by eCG treatment is often greater than that induced by FSH; however, more embryos of transferable (good) quality are produced on average after FSH treatment. For this reason, FSH has become the method of choice of superovulating cows for commercial use. The two most commonly used commercial FSH preparations are made from porcine pituitary extracts and contain some contamination with luteinizing hormone (LH). Whereas high amounts of LH in FSH preparations may interfere with optimal superovulatory response, it is believed that a low level of LH contamination does not interfere and may even be needed for superovulation.

Although some good results have been reported with a single administration, FSH is typically administered (IM) over 4–5 consecutive days, twice daily in decreasing doses. Both commercial FSH preparations can be diluted into 20 mL of saline solution and given over 4–5 days. A typical 4-day FSH treatment protocol is as follows: day 1, 4 mL bid; day 2, 3 mL bid; day 3, 2 mL bid; day 4, 1 mL bid (total volume = 20 mL). FSH treatments typically begin on day 10 after estrus. On the third or fourth day of FSH treatment, a luteolytic injection of $PGF_2\alpha$ is given and repeated 12 hr later. Estrus can be expected 36–48 hr later, and the artificial insemination can be scheduled based on the observed heat (12 and 24 hr after onset of estrus) or by appointment (72, 84, and 96 hr after the administration of $PGF_2\alpha$) that is accompanied by administration of an agent to induce ovulation, human chorionic gonadotropin or gonadotropin releasing hormone (GnRH). Many variations of methods to increase the efficiency of superovulation programs in cattle exist. For example, the induction of a new follicle wave before gonadotropin treatments is desirable to increase the ovary response to superovulatory treatments. Injections of estradiol or GnRH, or transvaginal aspiration (follicle ablation) of the dominant follicle (known as dominant follicle removal [DFR]) are examples of approaches to induce a new follicle wave. A new follicle wave emerges 4, 2, or 1–2 days after treatments with estradiol, GnRH, or DFR, respectively. Responses to gonadotropin treatments to induce superovulation are best when treatments are started when the follicle wave emerges. These treatments aim to promote a more uniform follicle recruitment and growth that ultimately may result in more viable embryos per procedure. In the USA and many other countries, the use of estrogen preparations is not approved for use in reproduction.

Management of recipients can be done after observation of natural estrus or based on synchronization protocols. In either scenario, a luteolytic dose of $PGF_2\alpha$ is given ~12 hr before the first treatment of $PGF_2\alpha$ of donor cows. Recipient cows ovulating on the same day as donor cows are preferred for embryo transfer, but asynchrony of ±1 day has produced pregnancy rates comparable to those of perfectly synchronized recipients. It is expected that 75%–90% will respond to the superovulation treatment, but 20%–30% of flushed cows do not produce embryos of transferable quality. Among those cows that successfully respond to the FSH treatment, the variability in producing good quality embryos is very good (from 0 to >20 per flush). On average, a production of 5–7 embryos of good quality per embryo collection is considered a good commercial outcome.

Embryo collection is done on day 7 of the cycle when uterine stage embryos (morula and blastocysts) are expected to be recovered. Before the embryo collection, the donor cow is palpated and the ovarian response to the superovulation treatment assessed manually by determining the number of palpable corpora lutea in the ovaries. The procedure to collect the embryos from the uterus (flush) involves the following steps: 1) An epidural with 5–7 mL of lidocaine is given. 2) The perineum is carefully washed with hand soap or an antiseptic scrub (chlorhexidine or iodine); depending on the animal and cervical size, a 12–24 French Foley-type catheter placed over a metal rod (stylet) is introduced in the vagina as the palpating arm is placed in the rectum to manipulate it through the cervix. 3) Once inside the uterus, the catheter is advanced beyond the uterine body until it is located at the first third of one of the uterine horns; the rod inside the catheter is then withdrawn and the cuff is inflated with 15–20 mL of air, depending on the size of the uterine horn, which varies with breed, age, parity, etc. 4) Each uterine horn is then flushed with commercially available, complete, and ready-to-use flushing media; these embryo flushing solutions also contain antibiotics and bovine serum albumin as a source of protein. Some commercial preparations of complete flush media also contain surfactants to minimize the formation of foam and bubbles in the embryo search dish. In the past, the flush media had to be prepared for each collection and consisted primarily of Dulbecco's phosphate buffered saline with added antibiotics and 1% fetal/calf bovine serum (or alternatively, 0.1% bovine serum albumin); around the world, many flushes are still prepared in this manner. 5) The uterine horn may be lavaged by repeated small volume (25–50 mL) infusions of flush media that are allowed to drain into an embryo filter. Alternatively, the uterine horn may be flushed continuously; 1–2 L of flush media is used to flush a cow uterus. 6) After the flush is completed, the cuff is deflated and the contents of the catheter are carefully allowed to flow into the embryo filter located at the end of the outflow tubing. 7) The embryo filter is then taken to the laboratory, and its contents are dispensed into a search dish with grid and visualized using a stereoscope (dissecting microscope) at 10× magnification.

All embryos are transferred to a clean dish (with wells) containing holding media similar in composition to the flush media except for a higher concentration of bovine fetal/calf serum (10%–20%) or bovine serum albumin (0.4%). As with flush media, complete holding media are also available commercially. Embryos are then visualized at a higher magnification (40–60×) and classified according to their morphology, stage of development (unfertilized oocytes, early morula, tight morula, blastocyst, expanded blastocyst, hatched blastocyst, etc), and quality (excellent, good, fair, poor, degenerate). The quality score is based on morphologic assessment of the physical integrity of embryos and morphologic characteristics according to the stage of embryonic development, compaction status, color of cytoplasm, areas of cellular degeneration, number of extruded blastomeres, size of perivitelline space, and the size and sphericity of the embryo.

Only embryos classified as fair, good, or excellent should be transferred. Embryos are kept in holding media after being "washed" at least three times. Embryo washing is performed by transferring embryos into different, clean wells containing holding media. This procedure, recommended by the International Embryo Transfer Society, aids in removing cellular debris and potential pathogens adhered to the zona pellucida. Embryos are kept in holding media at room temperature until they are transferred to recipients or prepared for freezing, bisection ("splitting"), or determination of gender by embryo sexing. Alternatively, embryos can be refrigerated in transfer medium for up to 24 hr with no appreciable loss of viability. Splitting embryos into identical halves by microsurgery is practiced by a few commercial embryo transfer teams. The number of embryos to be transferred can be doubled with only a minor reduction in pregnancy rates. However, techniques to freeze manipulated embryos require improvement.

Since 1978, the current preferred and most common method to transfer cattle embryos into synchronized recipients is via nonsurgical techniques. The embryo is loaded into a small plastic straw (0.25 mL) fitted into a specialized (Cassou-type) insemination "gun." The embryo transfer gun is then placed into the vagina protected by a disposable sterile cover sheath to prevent contamination of the tip of the gun with potential perineal and vaginal contaminants. The gun is passed through the cervix, aided by palpation per rectum, and advanced into the uterine horn ipsilateral to the corpus luteum. The contents of the straw are then deposited as cranial as possible into the uterine horn with care to avoid prolonged and unnecessary manipulation. After direct transfer of single fresh embryos, 60%–70% of recipients are expected to become pregnant; transfer of two embryos may result in pregnancy rates as high as 90%. A significant proportion of bovine embryo transfers are made with frozen-thawed embryos (~46%) and, with good management, pregnancy rates routinely are >50%. Under the same management conditions and well-trained staff, the pregnancy rate of frozen-thawed embryos is expected to be 10% lower than that derived from transfers of fresh bovine embryos. Although increased pregnancy rates may be obtained with transfer of multiple embryos, the risk of dystocia and retention of fetal membranes associated with twin pregnancies and the increased probability of producing freemartin calves preclude widespread use of this approach. The use of sexed semen in embryo transfer programs is considered economically viable, especially if attention is given to inseminate donor cows with sperm numbers comparable to those used in artificial inseminations with conventional nonsorted semen.

SHEEP AND GOATS

The amount of embryo transfers done in small ruminants are a fraction of those recorded for cattle. Globally, almost 900,000 embryo transfers were reported for cattle in 2012, while only 12,458 were reported for sheep and 1,013 for goats. In addition to commercial and market factors limiting the production of embryos in small ruminants, current embryo transfer techniques in sheep and goats almost exclusively consist of surgical and/or laparoscopic methods for embryo collection and transfer.

Donor and recipients are synchronized using progestagens with an injection of $PGF_2\alpha$ given on the day the intravaginal progestagen device is inserted. Because of the additional superovulation hormonal treatment donor females receive, recipients come into estrus earlier than donor ewes and does; therefore, the progestagen source (typically an intravaginal device) in recipients is removed 12 hr before it is removed in donors.

FSH is commonly used to superovulate small ruminants. As in cattle, FSH is commonly administered twice daily in a series of decreasing doses administered over 3 days (eg, day 1 = 5 and 5 mg; day 2 = 3 and 3 mg; day 3 = 2 and 2 mg). On the last day of FSH treatment, the progestagen source is removed and a luteolytic injection of $PGF_2\alpha$ given. Estrus is typically detected by vasectomized bucks/rams; artificial insemination should take place 12–24 hr after estrus is detected or 45–50 hr after progestagen removal. Intracervical or transcervical artificial insemination is difficult and requires advanced training and practice. Increased pregnancy rates are obtained by laparoscopic artificial insemination, because it allows the semen to be deposited in the cranial aspect of the uterine horns.

Surgical embryo collection is still very common, but laparoscopic and nonsurgical transcervical catheterization procedures are consistently improving and yielding good results, albeit still lower than those obtained with surgical methods. Embryos are collected 7–8 days after estrus.

PIGS

Embryo collection and transfer in pigs is not yet done commercially or as intensively as in ruminants. Until recently, embryo transfer in pigs was primarily performed for research purposes. In 2012, Canada, France, and Ireland were the only countries to report the commercial collection and transfer of 2,478 swine embryos. Owing to the high ovulatory rate in sows, superovulation treatment may or may not be used in embryo transfer procedures. Embryo collection can be done soon after a genetically valuable sow is slaughtered and the reproductive tract is collected for embryo retrieval. Surgical collection of embryos is also performed using ventral laparotomy of the caudal abdomen. Most embryo transfers are performed using surgical techniques (abdominal ventral laparotomy under general anesthesia). Recently, nonsurgical techniques to collect and transfer porcine embryos have been developed and proved successful, but they require specialized equipment and highly skilled individuals. Embryos are typically collected 4–7 days after ovulation. Current pregnancy rates with nonsurgical techniques remain lower than those obtained after surgical embryo transfers. Embryos should not be transferred to the uterine body, because this results in low pregnancy rates. The transfer of 16–22 embryos per recipient is recommended to achieve optimal pregnancy rates.

HORSES

Embryo transfer in the equine industry has been primarily used to obtain offspring from mares with restricted reproductive potential (mares with undiagnosed subfertility, uterine pathologies, or simply older mares) or from performance mares that must remain nonpregnant to continue to compete. Most breed associations allow the registration of foals born by embryo transfer, and an increasing number now allow the registration of multiple foals born in the same year. Because of this recent increased acceptance by breed registries, many horse breeders have obtained several foals in one breeding season from a single donor mare.

Superovulating mares with a purified form of equine follicle-stimulating hormone extract preparation (eFSH) to increase ovulation and embryo recovery rates is no longer commonly done commercially. Difficulties with manufacturing suitable gonadotropins and the variable response of mares to FSH stimulation have precluded widespread commercial use of this approach to produce equine embryos. It was thought that the low embryo recovery rate in mares ovulating >4 follicles/ovary could be attributed to an inability of the ovarian fossa to accommodate multiple ovulations in that area, or alternatively, excessive response to the FSH stimulation could result in dysmatured oocytes.

A recent advance in embryo transfer technologies in commercial settings has been the possibility of producing in vitro equine embryos using intracytoplasmic sperm injection (ICSI). Frozen semen from deceased stallions can be efficiently used to produce in vitro embryos by using only a portion of a frozen semen straw to provide sperm for the ICSI procedure. The number of ICSI-derived equine embryos is expected to continue to increase sharply during the next few years.

The horse embryo is notoriously challenging to cryopreserve, probably owing to its relatively large diameter and the presence of an embryonic capsule that limits interaction between cryoprotectant agents and the embryo. Embryos of morula or early blastocyst stage (<6.5 days after ovulation) are preferable for cryopreserving, because after thawing, older embryos have invariably low morphologic quality that results in poor pregnancy rates. A vitrification media for horse embryos is commercially available, and acceptable pregnancy rates varying from 40%–60% have been reported. Successful cryopreservation of expanded equine blastocysts also has been reported for embryos that had their blastoceles collapsed after embryo biopsy procedures.

Because one of two embryos are typically recovered from the donor mare, it is important that breeding soundness evaluations are done for both donor and recipients. Daily ultrasonography of the uterus and ovaries of donor and potential recipient mares during estrus provide critical information about the time of ovulation, which is essential for determining the day of ovulation and day of embryo collection and to assist in the selection of qualified recipient candidates for embryo transfer.

Nonsurgical techniques are currently used to collect and transfer horse embryos. Embryo collection is usually performed on day 7 or 8 (day 0 = ovulation). The use of good standard techniques generally yields a recovery rate of ~75%; this rate can be as high as 90% for young maiden or fertile mares or as low as 10%–20% in subfertile mares. Before embryo collection, palpation per rectum and ultrasonography are performed mainly to document the presence of the corpus luteum, the degree of cervical tone, and absence of any fluid in the uterus. Mild soap or povidone-iodine scrub can be used to wash the perineal region, followed by a thorough rinsing with clean water.

Sedation is not used in most cases, but it may be needed when working with uncooperative mares. Acepromazine should be avoided, because it may cause relaxation of the uterus and potentially impair fluid recovery or manipulation of the reproductive tract during flushing of the uterus; sedation with an α_2-agonist (eg, xylazine, detomidine) is preferred. Embryo collection is performed using a routine transcervical uterine lavage procedure, using a silicone catheter with an inflatable cuff. Using sterile technique, the silicone catheter (28–34 in. long, French size 28–37, depending on the size of the reproductive tract of the mare) is introduced through the cervix into the uterus, and then the balloon is inflated (typically 60–80 mL) with air or collection medium; the catheter is then gently pulled back so the cuff seals the internal cervical os. Complete flush media with antibiotics, surfactant, and bovine serum albumin is available commercially and ready to use. Alternatively, as with cattle, flush media can be prepared with Dulbecco's phosphate-buffered saline and 1%–5% fetal bovine serum; 1–2 L are infused into the uterus and then allowed to flow back into a graduated cylinder or plastic bucket to measure the recovered volume. Once the uterus is filled, it can be gently manipulated per rectum to aid the recovery of fluid. An embryo filter equipped with a 75-micron mesh is usually connected to the end of the outflow tubing to yield ~40–60 mL of fluid. In some cases, an injection of oxytocin (10 IU) may be given to minimize the retention of a large amount of flush media in the uterus. The recovered fluid should be clear and free of significant amount of debris and blood. Nearly 100% of the fluid used to lavage the uterus should be recovered. A total of 4–8 L of flush media is used to complete the embryo collection procedure (flush). If retention of fluid is suspected or if the outflow of media is interrupted, transrectal ultrasonography may be used to assess the presence of intraluminal fluid. A common cause of interrupted outflow drainage of flush media results from placing the tip of the catheter intracervically and not in the body of the uterus: the media easily flow into the uterus but not outward.

Once the flush is completed, the remaining fluid in the filter is searched in a sterile dish with grid under a magnification of 15× using a stereomicroscope. Once the embryo is found, it is transferred to a well in a sterile tissue culture dish containing holding media (commercial, ready-to-use with 0.4% albumin or made with Dulbecco's phosphate-buffered saline plus 10%–20% fetal bovine serum). The embryo should be washed at least 3 times by transferring into two other wells previously filled with holding media. Embryo manipulation is done with a 0.25-mL straw connected to a tuberculin syringe with a 16-gauge needle, a 0.5-mL straw directly connected to a tuberculin syringe, or a capillary pipette (20 μL) attached to a tuberculin syringe. After being washed, the embryo should be transferred to a recipient mare (within 1 hr) or prepared for short storage and transportation. The stage of the embryo (morula, early, or expanded blastocyst) and quality (1, best; 5, dead) should be recorded.

Although surgical transfer of equine embryos was once thought to yield higher pregnancy rates than nonsurgical transfer techniques, the latter are now the preferred method to transfer horse embryos. Recipient mares should be reproductively sound and in good body condition and health. Synchronization of ovulation should be maximized by hormonal manipulation of the estrous cycle and daily transrectal ultrasonography. Good pregnancy rates result from using recipients that have ovulated from 1 day before the donor to 3 days after the donor. In addition, progestagens such as altrenogest may be used until the day of pregnancy examination 4–5 days after the transfer (~12–13 days of gestation).

The nonsurgical embryo transfer is performed using transcervical catheterization. Plastic straws, 0.25 or 0.5 mL, are used to load the embryo; the column of medium containing the embryo should be surrounded by two small columns of air, which are in turn surrounded by two columns of medium. The straw loaded with the embryo is fitted into an embryo transfer "gun." Embryo transfer sheaths with side delivery can minimize embryo damage during the transfer procedure.

Preparation for Short Storage and Transport: Horse breeders without an adequate number of recipients and veterinarians with modest investment in equipment can collect embryos and prepare them for short storage and transport to a centralized embryo transfer facility. Pregnancy rates do not appear to differ from those obtained with fresh embryos, especially if embryos are shipped counter-to-counter on the same day they are collected. Embryos are routinely shipped in commercially available holding media that are ready-to-use preparations containing 0.4% bovine serum albumin and antibiotics. The embryo is placed into a 2-mL polypropylene cryotube vial or a 5-mL snap-cap tube that contains the holding media. The tube with the embryo is then placed into a semen shipping container designed to cool and transport horse semen. The container is preferably shipped to an embryo transfer facility on the same day the collection is performed using an airline carrier (counter-to-counter) or processed for overnight delivery using a commercial carrier.

HORMONAL CONTROL OF ESTRUS

Hormones are commonly used to manipulate the estrous cycle. The major indications for hormonal control of estrus are to induce luteolysis, induce ovulation of a mature follicle, suppress estrus, induce cyclicity in anestrous animals, and superovulate cyclic animals. Effective treatments for these manipulations vary among species. A number of treatments currently lack regulatory approval; label instructions should be followed.

HORSES

Estrous behavior may be undesirable in performance horses and can be suppressed in mares by administration of progestagens, either progesterone in oil (150–300 mg/day, IM) or altrenogest (0.44 mg/kg/day, PO). In the past, oral progestagen was preferable because of muscle irritation from the injectable preparation. However, progesterone in a biorelease vehicle is available by prescription from a compounding pharmacy. This preparation (1.5 g, IM) is administered once every 7–10 days. Treatment with progestagens for 15 days during the late transition season can advance the first ovulation of the year by ~10 days. Although these preparations suppress estrous behavior, they may not effectively suppress follicle growth and ovulation in cyclic mares.

Ovulation may be synchronized in mares by administration of progesterone in oil (150 mg) and estradiol 17β in oil (10 mg/day, IM, for 10 days) with prostaglandin $F_2\alpha$ ($PGF_2\alpha$; 10 mg, IM) administered on the tenth day. Progesterone plus estradiol in a biorelease vehicle is also available by prescription from a compounding pharmacy. Mares should come into estrus ~3 days after the end of treatment, and 85% of mares ovulate 9–13 days after the end of treatment.

Estrus may be induced in diestrous mares (having a corpus luteum that is 5 or more days postovulation) by treatment with $PGF_2\alpha$ (10 mg, IM) or cloprostenol (250 mcg, IM) to lyse the corpus luteum. Mares should return to estrus in ~3 days and ovulate an average of 9–10 days after prostaglandin treatment. The time to ovulation is variable, however, depending on the size of the largest follicle on the ovary at the time of prostaglandin administration. $PGF_2\alpha$ causes numerous transient adverse effects in horses, including sweating, colic, and trembling. Greatly reduced doses of cloprostenol (25 mcg) also effectively induce luteolysis in mares while virtually eliminating the unwanted adverse effects of $PGF_2\alpha$. However, although widely used in mares, cloprostenol is labeled only for use in cattle. Prostaglandin causes luteolysis of a mature corpus luteum and so does not induce estrus in anestrous mares.

Behavioral estrus may be induced in anestrous or ovariectomized mares by administration of estradiol 17β in oil (1–10 mg, IM) or estradiol cypionate (0.5 mg, IM). Mares should show estrus 12–24 hr after injection. This estrus is not associated with follicular growth and is not fertile. Treatment with estradiol cypionate is longlasting, but repeated or high doses may cause aggressive or defensive behavior when the mare is approached by a stallion. Treatment with estrogen in the presence of progesterone (eg, in a cyclic mare in diestrus) will not induce estrous behavior.

Ovulation may be induced in mares with mature preovulatory follicles (>33 mm diameter) by administration of human chorionic gonadotropin (hCG), 2,500 IU, IV; by administration of a deslorelin implant, 2.2 mg, SC; or by administration of deslorelin, 1–2 mg, IM, in a biorelease vehicle. Ovulation is seen in 85% of mares within 48 hr, typically 36–42 hr after hCG or injectable deslorelin treatment or 40–44 hr after treatment with a deslorelin implant. Repeated use of hCG over a long period is associated with antibody formation and may decrease response to treatment; this has not been seen with deslorelin. Use of deslorelin in implant form has been associated with periods of anestrus in treated mares, especially if the corpus luteum of ovulation is lysed with prostaglandin. For this reason, many veterinarians remove the implant after ovulation is seen; this is easily performed if the implant is placed in the vulvar mucosa.

Mares do not superovulate in response to equine chorionic gonadotropin (eCG), and they do not respond well to follicle-stimulating hormone (FSH) derived from other species, but they may be superovulated (average of three to four follicles ovulated) by treatment with equine FSH (no longer commercially available in the USA). GnRH given at 2–20 mcg/hr (by infusion pump) throughout ~10 days induced normal follicular growth and ovulation in anestrous mares; the larger dose induces superovulation (average of three follicles). Cyclicity has also been induced in anestrous mares by treatment with 200 mcg GnRH every 6 hr, 500 mcg GnRH every 12 hr, or by administration of a GnRH agonist, buserelin (10 mcg, SC), every 12 hr plus hCG (2,500 IU, IV) once a follicle has reached 35 mm in diameter. The dopamine receptor antagonist domperidone (1.1 mg/kg/day, PO) alone or in combination with GnRH (250 mcg, SC, qid) has also been used to stimulate follicular development in mares with quiescent ovaries.

CATTLE

In cows, ovulation may be synchronized with a progestagen and estrogen combination treatment, a two-dose prostaglandin regimen, or a GnRH and prostaglandin combination. Administration of $PGF_2\alpha$ (25 mg, IM) or prostaglandin analogue (cloprostenol at 500 mcg, IM) to cows with a corpus luteum from 5 days after ovulation results in estrus in ~2–5 days. Two prostaglandin injections given 12–14 days apart synchronize estrus and ovulation in most cows. Time to estrus is more variable than with progesterone suppression, so insemination should be based on detection of estrus. Ovulation may also be synchronized by administration of GnRH, 100 mcg, IM (day 0), followed by prostaglandin treatment on day 7 and a second GnRH treatment on day 9. Cows should be inseminated 0–20 hr after the second GnRH treatment. This GnRH and $PGF_2\alpha$ protocol is termed "ovsynch." There are many variations on this protocol, using additional steroids, prostaglandin, or GnRH treatments, that may increase the degree of synchrony or pregnancy rates after artificial insemination.

A progesterone-releasing intravaginal device (PRID) consists of micronized progesterone distributed homogeneously in an inert silicone rubber coated onto a cylindrical stainless spiral coil. The PRID is maintained in the vagina for 7 days, and a luteolytic dose of $PGF_2\alpha$ is administered 1 day before or at "pull-out" day. There are no milk or meat withdrawal requirements. In noncycling animals, an injection of equine chorionic gonadotropin (eCG) is administered when the PRID is removed.

A controlled intravaginal drug-release (CIDR) device may also be used for estrus synchronization. A CIDR is an intravaginal device constructed of a progesterone-impregnated medical silicone elastomere molded into a T-shape. It is labeled for estrus synchronization in beef and dairy cattle. Cows are administered GnRH, and concomitantly a CIDR is inserted and maintained for 7 days. At the time of removal, cows receive an injection of $PGF_2\alpha$. Cows can be inseminated, with or without another GnRH injection, 48–72 hr after $PGF_2\alpha$ injection. The most effective synchronization treatment, an IM injection of a combination of 5 mg estradiol valerate and 3 mg norgestomet, with an ear implant of 3 mg norgestomet left in for 9 days, is no longer commercially available in the USA because of the ban on the use of estrogens in food animals. Note that all estrus synchronization protocols are less effective in *Bos indicus* cattle and *B indicus* crossbreds than in *Bos taurus* cattle.

Melengestrol acetate (MGA) is a steroidal progestagen used as a feed additive to promote growth and suppress estrus in heifers. MGA is used at a dosage of 0.5 mg/head/day for 14 days for estrus synchronization. Fertility after this treatment is low, and females should not be bred. This protocol could be improved by administering $PGF_2\alpha$ 17 days after the last feed containing MGA. The fertility of this estrus is reestablished.

Ovulation may be induced in cows with mature follicles (10–15 mm diameter) by treatment with GnRH at 100–250 mcg, IM; luteinizing hormone (LH) at 25 mg, IM; or hCG at 5,000–10,000 IU, IM. Because the endogenous LH peak develops at the onset of estrus, this administration will not speed the time of ovulation in estrous cows but may be used to ensure luteinization in cows with histories of cystic ovarian disease or to induce ovulation in anestrous postpartum cows.

Superovulation may be achieved in cows by treatment with eCG (not currently commercially available in the USA) in mid-diestrus followed by prostaglandin-induced luteolysis 2–3 days later, or by treatment with FSH (potencies differ, refer to label instructions), typically IM, bid for 4–5 days, at a decreasing or constant dose with administration of prostaglandin (25–35 mg, IM) usually on day 3 or 4 of treatment. FSH treatment is discontinued at the onset of estrus.

GOATS AND SHEEP

In cycling goats, luteolysis may be induced by administration of $PGF_2\alpha$ (2.5–5 mg, IM) or cloprostenol (62.5–125 mcg, IM) as early as day 3. In sheep, $PGF_2\alpha$ (≥15 mg) or cloprostenol (125 mcg) is effective after day 5 of the cycle (estrus is day 0). Estrus may be synchronized by two doses of prostaglandin, 11–13 days apart in does or 7–9 days apart in ewes. Estrus may also be synchronized in cyclic or anestrous does and ewes by administration of progestagens; impregnated intravaginal sponges (medroxyprogesterone or fluorgestone) have been the most widely used agents for control of ovulation but are not currently available for clinical use in the USA. In small ruminants, a controlled internal drug release (CIDR) intravaginal plastic device impregnated with progesterone (300 mg) can also be used. The CIDR is maintained in the vagina for 7 days, and a luteolytic dose of $PGF_2\alpha$ administered 1 day before or at device removal. The estrus response is high within 72–84 hr. A portion of a bovine norgestomet ear implant (1.5-mg/goat) or injection of progesterone in oil (10 mg/day, IM) has also been effective. In sheep and goats, the ear implant is placed subcutaneously near the base of the ear or the base of the tail and then removed 7–9 days later. Progestagen treatment is administered for 10–14 days in sheep and for 14–21 days in goats. Ewes should be joined with rams the day after cessation of treatment; does return to heat on the second or third day after treatment ends. Injection of equine chorionic gonadotropin (eCG; 100–500 IU) at the end of treatment increases synchronization of ovulation or ovulation rate. Alternatively, in does, progestagens may be given for 11 days with eCG and prostaglandin administered on day 9, and fixed-time insemination performed on days 12 and 13. In regimens involving treatments other than prostaglandin alone, fertility may be reduced on the first estrus after treatment in ewes but not in does. During the nonbreeding season, melatonin implants (18 mg) induce fertile estrus 50–70 days after implant insertion. Better results are obtained when melatonin implants are inserted early or during the transitional period. The implant is biodegradable and does not need to be removed. Estrus synchronization may be improved by using an estrus synchronization protocol at the end of implant action. During the nonbreeding season, a source of gonadotropin is also required. The most common gonadotropin used is eCG, administered at the end of a progestagen treatment (or 24 hr before device removal). The dose of eCG depends on the season, breed, age, and postpartum interval, among other factors. A high eCG dose is characterized by superovulation, low fertility, shortened estrous cycles, pregnancy loss, and problems with multiple lambs or kids. The repetitive use of eCG has produced antibodies against eCG in certain sheep and goats, resulting in modification in the time of ovulation and consequent reduction of fertility when artificial insemination at a fixed time is done.

PIGS

In pigs, estrus synchronization may be easily achieved by synchronized weaning of lactating sows; estrus is seen 4–10 days later. Administration IM of a commercially available combination of equine chorionic gonadotropin (eCG; 400 IU) and human chorionic gonadotropin (hCG; 200 IU), per 5 mL dose, given as a single injection within 12 hr after weaning, tightens the synchronization, and estrus is seen 4–5 days after weaning. This eCG and hCG combination also induces estrus in gilts with delayed puberty and in sows with postweaning anestrus. Exogenous prostaglandin induces luteolysis of the porcine corpus luteum only after day 12 of the estrous cycle and, therefore, is not a practical agent for estrous cycle control; however, estrus may be synchronized by induction of abortion in sows pregnant >15 days by administration of $PGF_{2}\alpha$ (15 mg, IM, then 10 mg, IM, 12 hr later) or cloprostenol (1 mg, followed 24 hr later by 0.5 mg); sows return to estrus 4–10 days after treatment. Oral altrenogest (15–20 mg/day, PO, for 14–18 days) may be used for estrus synchronization and for improvement of farrowing rate and litter size in mature sows. In lactating sows, one daily dose of altrenogest from the day of weaning until 5 days before the planned breeding day is also effective and results in estrus 4–9 days after completion of treatment. Estrus may also be synchronized by using bovine norgestomet implants (one implant followed by addition of a second implant 9 days later) removed 19 days after initiation of treatment; neither treatment is currently approved in the USA for swine. Combination eCG and hCG may be given on the day of progestagen withdrawal to better synchronize estrus.

DOGS

In bitches, estrus suppression, for no more than 24 mo, can be accomplished by administration of mibolerone (an androgen, 30–180 mcg/day, PO, depending on the weight of the bitch). To be effective, treatment must be started at least 30 days before estrus. Estrus is variable but typically develops soon after cessation of treatment; fertility should be normal by the second estrus after treatment. If the bitch has already entered proestrus, the progestagen megestrol acetate (2.2 mg/kg/day, PO, for 8 days) may be used to stop the cycle. Administration must start in the first 3 days of proestrus (vulvar bleeding). The next estrus usually develops 4–6 wk earlier than expected. To delay estrus, treatment with megestrol acetate (0.55 mg/kg/day, PO, for 32 days) is begun in late anestrus (up to a few weeks before estrus is expected). After treatment, estrus is seen in 2–9 mo (typically 5–6 mo), and fertility is not affected.

Neither mibolerone nor megestrol acetate is recommended for use in bitches on their first estrus or in bitches primarily used for breeding. Adverse effects of progestins such as megestrol acetate include cystic endometrial hyperplasia and pyometra; longterm treatment may result in obesity, diabetes mellitus, and neoplasia of the uterus and mammary glands. Mibolerone may cause skin, vaginal, and clitoral changes.

Clinical use of deslorelin for estrus suppression is under investigation. Extended-release implants of deslorelin can suppress estrus for >1 yr in bitches without apparent adverse effects and with full return to fertility.

Estrus induction in bitches remains problematic, and none of the drugs presented below are approved for this use in the USA. Many methods have been proposed, but repeatability is low and fertility of the induced estrus is variable. Estrus induction in the bitch before endometrial involution is complete (135 days after the most recent estrus) can result in reduced fertility. The dopamine agonists cabergoline (5 mcg/kg/day, PO, until 2 days after onset of proestrus), metergoline (0.56–1.2 mg/kg, IM, every third day until proestrus), and bromocryptine (0.3 mg/bitch for 3 days followed by 0.6–2.5 mg per bitch for 3–6 days after onset of proestrus) are reported to induce fertile estrus in most bitches. Average length of treatment was 16–19 days. Two notable adverse effects of dopamine agonist treatment in the bitch are vomiting and coat color changes.

Use of deslorelin implants may also be effective for induction of estrus but has been associated with low progesterone values during diestrus and, subsequently, prolonged estrus suppression. Removal of the implant 10 days after insertion may overcome this problem. Induction of estrus with GnRH analogues continues to be investigated. Synchronous estrus using whole (2.1 mg) or half (1.05 mg) deslorelin implants after termination of diestrus with $PGF_{2}\alpha$ has been reported. The $PGF_{2}\alpha$ protocol started with a low dosage (50 mcg/kg, SC, bid) on the first day, followed by a moderate dosage (100 mcg/kg, SC, bid) on the second day, and then a full dosage (250 mcg/kg, SC, bid) for 5 days. Encouraging results have also been reported using a single 1.5-mg IM injection of a sustained-release formulation of deslorelin marketed for use in mares.

The most widely studied gonadotropin for estrus induction in canids is equine chorionic gonadotropin (eCG), which is available in the USA only in a porcine product that contains a combination of 80 IU eCG and 40 IU hCG/mL. A single 5-mL injection of this product was highly effective for inducing proestrus in 89.5% of treated bitches, but ovulation rate was poor. However, whelping rates of 50%–84% have also been reported when eCG and hCG were used to induce estrus in bitches.

CATS

Megestrol acetate may be used to suppress estrus in queens by treating with 5 mg/cat daily for 3 days, then 2.5–5 mg once weekly for a maximum of 10 wk. Administration of megestrol acetate to queens is an extra-label use of the drug, and informed consent should be obtained from the owners. The queen should be allowed an estrus before resuming therapy. Mibolerone is also not approved for use in queens (because of hepato-toxicity) but is effective at 50 mcg/cat/day, PO. Longterm deslorelin implants have also suppressed estrus in cats, but the length of suppression is variable. Estrus may be induced in queens with follicle-stimulating hormone (FSH), 2 mg, IM, the first day, then 0.5–1 mg, IM, daily for 4 additional days. Recommended doses of human chorionic gonadotropin (hCG) range from 25 to 500 IU. The higher doses are more effective at inducing ovulation but may also result in oocyte degeneration. For queens with anovulation or for queens undergoing artificial insemination, ovulation of mature follicles (present on day 2 of estrus) may be induced by treatment with hCG at 250 IU, IM, or GnRH at 25 mcg, IM. Ovulation is reported to occur 25–27 hr after hCG administration to queens.

NUTRITION: BEEF CATTLE

NUTRITIONAL REQUIREMENTS

Beef cattle production, whether on range, improved pasture, or in the feedlot, is most economic when feedstuffs are used effectively. Young growing grass or other high-quality pasture crops usually supply ample nutrients, such that mature and young growing cattle can consume sufficient good-quality mixed pasture (grasses and legumes) for normal growth and maintenance. However, mature pasture, crop residues, or forage crops harvested in a manner that results in shattering, leaching, or spoilage may be so reduced in nutritive value (particularly energy, protein, phosphorus, and provitamin A or β-carotene) that they are suitable only in a maintenance ration for adult cattle. Such feedstuffs should be supplemented if used for any other purposes.

The mineral content of forages is influenced by the corresponding mineral levels in the soil and by excess levels of some minerals that reduce the availability of others. Mature forages also may be lower in mineral content, especially phosphorus. Normally, supplemental minerals are supplied in a free-choice mineral mix or force-fed in the total mixed ration.

Certain nutrients are required by beef cattle in the daily ration, whereas others can be stored in the body. When body stores of a nutrient are high, eg, vitamin A, dietary supplementation is unnecessary until such stores are depleted. However, it may be difficult to determine when body stores have been depleted until advanced signs of deficiency start to appear.

The following are dietary requirements for maintenance, growth, finishing, reproduction, and lactation in beef cattle.

Water: Water, although not considered a nutrient per se, is required for regulation of body temperature, as well as for growth, reproduction, lactation, digestion, metabolism, excretion, hydrolysis of nutrients, transportation of nutrients and waste in the body, joint lubrication, plus many more functions. Restricting water intake results in impaired performance. An animal will expire more quickly from a water deficiency than from a deficiency of any nutrient.

Because feeds themselves contain water, and the metabolism of ingested feeds releases water (called metabolic water), not all of the animal's water needs have to be met by drinking water. Thirst is the result of need, and animals drink to meet this need. The need for water results from an increase in the electrolyte concentration in the body fluids, which activates the thirst mechanism.

Many factors, including temperature and body weight, affect water consumption in cattle. An 800-lb (364-kg) heifer at an environmental temperature of 4.4°C (40°F) can be expected to consume 6.3 gal. (23 L) per day; at 21°C (70°F), this will increase to 9.2 gal. (34.8 L). At the same 4.4°C temperature, a 400-lb (182-kg) heifer will consume ~4 gal. (15.1 L). Note that water consumption and body weight are not correlated by a straight-line relationship. A 900-lb (409-kg) lactating cow at the 4.4°C temperature will consume 11.4 gal. (43.1 L) per day.

Energy: Productive animals need essentially two types of energy. Energy of maintenance is that needed to maintain respiration, circulation, digestion, etc. Therefore, in calculating total energy needs, the net energy for maintenance, or NE_m, must be considered. The energy required for growth and reproduction is called the net energy for production, or NE_g. It is the amount of energy intake deposited as muscle and/or fat in animals gaining weight. (*See* TABLES 18–22.)

Except for preruminant calves, beef cattle can meet their maintenance energy requirements from roughages of reasonably good quality (green, leafy, fine-stemmed, free of mold and weeds). A shortage of energy may exist on overstocked pastures, with inadequate feed allowance or poor-quality forages, or during a drought. For production, additional energy from concentrates or co-product feeds may be necessary, especially when forages of fair to poor quality are consumed.

Especially in cold weather, roughages of varying quality may have similar maintenance energy values. Heat released during digestion and assimilation—called "heat increment"—contributes to the maintenance of body temperature for wintering stock.

Protein: Protein requirements currently are evaluated as metabolizable protein, which is interchangeable with absorbed protein. Metabolizable protein defines the protein more nearly as that which is available to the animal for maintenance and production. It is defined as the combination of the true protein absorbed by the intestine, supplied by microbial synthesized protein plus undegraded intake protein (UIP). The latter often has been called "bypass" protein.

Energy deficiency due to low feed intake or intake of poor quality feed is the most common deficiency that limits growth, development in heifers and bulls, milk production, and reproduction, with protein deficiency being the next most common. Protein deficiency of long duration eventually depresses appetite, with eventual weight loss and unthriftiness, even when ample energy is available.

Feedstuffs vary greatly in protein digestibility. For example, the protein of common grains and most protein supplements is ~75%–85% digestible, that of alfalfa hay ~70%, and that of grass hays usually

TABLE 18 MEAN NUTRIENT CONTENT OF FEEDS COMMONLY USED IN BEEF CATTLE DIETS[a]

Feedstuff	DE (Mcal/kg)	ME (Mcal/kg)	NE_m (Mcal/kg)	NE_g (Mcal/kg)	TDNs (%)
Alfalfa *(Medicago sativa)*					
Fresh	2.73	2.24	1.38	0.80	62
Fresh, late vegetative	2.91	2.39	1.51	0.92	66
Fresh, full bloom	2.22	1.81	0.97	0.42	50
Hay	2.65	2.17	1.31	0.74	60
Hay, sun-cured, early bloom	2.65	2.17	1.31	0.74	60
Hay, sun-cured, mid bloom	2.56	2.10	1.24	0.68	58
Hay, sun-cured, full bloom	2.43	1.99	1.14	0.58	55
Silage	2.78	2.28	1.41	0.83	63
Barley *(Hordeum vulgare)*					
Grain	3.84	3.03	2.06	1.40	88
Silage	2.65	2.17	1.31	0.74	60
Beet pulp, dried	3.26	2.68	1.76	1.14	74
Bermuda grass *(Cynodon dactylon)*					
Fresh	2.82	2.31	1.44	0.86	64
Hay, sun-cured	2.16	1.77	0.93	0.39	49
Brewer's grains, dried	2.39	2.39	1.51	0.91	66
Citrus pulp, dried	3.62	2.96	2.00	1.35	82
Corn *(Zea mays indentata)*					
Distiller's grains, dried	3.88	3.18	2.18	1.50	90
Gluten feed	3.53	2.89	1.94	1.30	80
Grain, cracked	3.92	3.25	2.24	1.55	90
Silage, well-eared	3.17	2.60	1.69	1.08	72
Cotton *(Gossypium spp)*					
Seed	3.97	3.25	2.24	1.55	90
Meal	3.31	2.71	1.79	1.16	75
Molasses, cane	3.17	2.60	1.70	1.08	72
Oats	3.40	2.78	1.85	1.22	77
Sorghum (*Sorghum bicolor*), grain	3.62	2.96	2.00	1.35	82

TABLE 18 MEAN NUTRIENT CONTENT OF FEEDS COMMONLY USED IN BEEF CATTLE DIETS[a] *(continued)*

Crude Protein (%)	Crude Fiber (%)	Ash (%)	NDF (%)	ADF (%)	Ca (%)	P (%)	Dry Matter (%)
Alfalfa *(Medicago sativa)*							
18.9	26.5	10.5	47.1	36.8	1.29	0.26	23.4
22.2	24.2	10.2	30.9	24.0	1.71	0.30	23.2
19.3	30.4	10.9	4.79	3.7	1.19	0.26	23.8
18.6	26.1	8.6	43.9	33.8	1.40	0.28	90.6
19.9	28.5	9.2	39.3	31.9	1.63	0.21	90.5
18.7	28.0	8.5	47.1	36.7	1.37	0.22	91.0
17.0	30.1	7.8	48.8	38.7	1.19	0.24	90.9
19.5	25.4	9.5	47.5	37.5	1.32	0.31	44.2
Barley *(Hordeum vulgare)*							
13.2	3.37	2.4	18.1	5.8	0.05	0.35	88.1
11.9	2.92	8.3	56.8	33.9	0.52	0.29	37.1
9.8	20.0	5.3	44.6	27.5	0.68	0.10	91.0
Bermuda grass *(Cynodon dactylon)*							
12.6	28.4	8.1	73.3	36.8	0.49	0.27	30.3
7.8	2.7	76.6	—	—	38.3	8.0	93.0
29.2	7.8	4.18	48.7	31.2	0.29	0.70	90.2
6.7	12.8	6.6	23.0	23.0	1.88	0.18	91.1
Corn *(Zea mays indentata)*							
30.4	6.9	4.6	46.0	21.3	0.26	0.83	90.3
23.8	7.5	6.9	36.2	12.7	0.07	0.95	90.0
9.8	2.3	1.5	10.8	3.3	0.03	0.32	90.0
8.7	19.5	3.6	46.0	26.6	0.25	0.22	34.6
Cotton *(Gossypium spp)*							
24.4	25.6	4.2	51.6	41.8	0.17	0.52	89.4
46.1	13.2	7.0	28.9	17.9	0.20	1.16	90.2
5.8	0.5	13.3	—	0.4	1.00	0.10	74.3
13.6	12.0	3.3	29.3	14.0	0.01	0.41	89.2
12.6	2.76	1.9	16.1	6.4	0.04	0.34	90.0

(continued)

TABLE 18 MEAN NUTRIENT CONTENT OF FEEDS COMMONLY USED IN BEEF CATTLE DIETS[a] *(continued)*

Feedstuff	DE (Mcal/kg)	ME (Mcal/kg)	NE_m (Mcal/kg)	NE_g (Mcal/kg)	TDNs (%)
Soybeans (*Glycine max*), meal	3.70	3.04	2.06	1.40	84
Wheat *(Triticum aestivum)*					
Wheat bran	3.09	2.53	1.63	1.03	70
Fresh, early vegetative	3.22	2.64	1.73	1.11	73

[a] Dry-matter basis; DE, digestible energy; ME, metabolizable energy; NE_m, net energy for maintenance; NE_g, net energy for gain; TDNs, total digestible nutrients; NDF, neutral detergent fiber; ADF, acid detergent fiber.

Adapted, with permission, from *Nutrient Requirements of Beef Cattle*, 2000, National Academy of Sciences, National Academy Press, Washington, DC.

35%–50%. The protein of low-quality feeds, such as weathered grass hay, range grass, or cottonseed hulls, is digested poorly. Thus, even though total protein intake may appear to be adequate, metabolizable protein might be deficient.

A lack of protein in the diet adversely affects the microbial protein production in the rumen, which in turn reduces the utilization of low-protein feeds. Thus, much of the potential nutritive value of roughages (especially energy) may be lost if protein levels are inadequate.

Urea and other sources of nonprotein nitrogen (NPN) are used commonly in commercial protein supplements to supply one-third or more of the total nitrogen requirement. Such products are broken down readily by the ruminal microbial protein to ammonia and then synthesized to high-quality microbial protein. The use of NPN needs available sources of ample phosphorus, trace minerals, sulfur, and soluble carbohydrates for the microbial synthesis of utilizable protein. The amount of crude protein (% N × 6.25) supplied by NPN must be stated on the feed tag accompanying commercial supplements. Toxicity is not a serious problem when urea is fed at recommended levels and mixed thoroughly with the other ingredients of the ration. However, rapid ingestion of urea at levels >20 g/100 lb (45 kg) body wt may lead to toxicity (*see* p 3043). Several urea-molasses liquid supplements, containing as much as 10% urea, currently are self-fed to beef cattle. Caution should be exercised when cattle are started on such supplements.

Minerals: Qualitatively, beef cattle require the same mineral elements as do dairy cattle; however, the relative quantities of the several minerals are different (*see* TABLE 23, p 2262). The minerals most apt to be deficient in beef cattle diets are sodium (as salt), calcium, phosphorus, magnesium, zinc, copper, and selenium. In some areas, including the interior of the USA, iodine may be deficient in diets for pregnant cows; likewise, there are regional deficiencies (probably reflecting soil deficiencies) of several trace minerals, including copper, cobalt, and selenium. However, there are areas where some mineral elements (eg, selenium, molybdenum) are present at toxic levels. Attempts have been made to correct natural soil deficiencies for trace minerals by soil fertilization practices. Thus, it is implied that a beef producer needs to know the mineral and trace mineral content of the feedstuffs used in cattle rations. A general approach to prevent such deficiencies is to feed a commercial salt mineral mix developed for the geographic location of the herd.

The **salt** (NaCl) requirement for beef cattle is quite low (0.2% of the dry matter); however, there appears to be a satiety factor involved—almost all animals appear to seek out salt if it is not readily available. Range cattle may consume 2–2.5 lb (1 kg) salt/head/mo when forage is succulent but about half that amount when forage is mature and drier. When salt is added to a free-choice protein feed to limit intake, beef cows might consume >1 lb salt/day over long periods of time

TABLE 18 MEAN NUTRIENT CONTENT OF FEEDS COMMONLY USED IN BEEF CATTLE DIETS[a] *(continued)*

Crude Protein (%)	Crude Fiber (%)	Ash (%)	NDF (%)	ADF (%)	Ca (%)	P (%)	Dry Matter (%)
51.8	5.4	6.9	10.3	7.0	0.46	0.73	90.9
Wheat *(Triticum aestivum)*							
17.4	11.3	6.6	42.8	14.0	0.14	1.27	89
27.4	17.4	13.3	46.2	28.4	0.42	0.40	22.2

without adverse effects if they have plenty of drinking water. Signs of a salt deficiency are rather nonspecific and include pica and reduced feed intake, growth, and milk production.

Calcium is the most abundant mineral element in the body; ~98% functions as a structural component of bones and teeth. The remaining 2% is distributed in extracellular fluids and soft tissues and is involved in such vital functions as blood clotting, membrane permeability, muscle contraction, transmission of nerve impulses, cardiac regulation, secretion of certain hormones, and activation and stabilization of certain enzymes. Most roughages are relatively good sources of calcium. Cereal hays and silages and such crop residues are relatively low in calcium. Although leguminous roughages are excellent sources of calcium, even nonlegume roughages may supply adequate calcium for maintenance of beef cattle. When cattle are fed such roughages produced on low-calcium soils, or when finishing cattle are fed high-grain diets with limited nonlegume roughage, a calcium deficiency may develop. Because lactating beef cows do not produce nearly the amount of milk that dairy cattle do, their calcium requirement is much less. Nevertheless, it is sound management to provide a free-choice salt mineral mixture tailored to the environment and production class of the grazing cattle. Salt should always be mixed with mineral, because salt drives intake. Cows have almost zero "nutritional wisdom," ie, they do not seek out feedstuffs or minerals when they are deficient, with the exception being sodium, so adding mineral to the salt generally improves intake among cattle with free-choice access to the mineral mix.

The total ration should provide a calcium: phosphorus ratio of 1.2 to 2:1, with cows at minimum of 1.2:1 and feedlot steers at minimum of 2:1. Wider ratios appear to be tolerated if the minimum requirements for each mineral element are met and if adequate vitamin D (exposure to sunlight) is available. Range cattle should be provided a mineral supplement that has as much or more phosphorus than calcium, because green forage is many times higher in calcium. Research has shown that intake among cattle receiving free-choice mineral mix is highly variable. One study showed that 14%–15% of cows with free-choice access to mineral in block or loose form consumed zero mineral. The only time cattle should be offered mineral free choice is when they are grazing and no other feed is being fed. If cows are consuming any other feed, the salt and mineral should be mixed with the ration so all cattle will ingest the prescribed amount of mineral.

Approximately 80% of the **phosphorus** in the body is found in the bones and teeth, with the remainder distributed among the soft tissues. Phosphorus may be deficient in some beef cattle rations, because roughages often are low in phosphorus. Furthermore, as forage plants mature, their phosphorus content declines, making mature and weathered forages a poor source. Phosphorus has been described as the most prevalent mineral deficiency for grazing cattle worldwide. Most natural protein supplements are fairly good sources of phosphorus. Because adequate phosphorus is critical for optimal performance of beef cattle, including growth, reproduction, and lactation, a phosphorus supplementation program is recommended using either a free-choice mineral mixture or direct

TABLE 19 NUTRIENT REQUIREMENTS OF PREGNANT REPLACEMENT BEEF COWS[a]

	Months Since Conception								
	1	2	3	4	5	6	7	8	9
NE_m required (Mcal/day)									
Maintenance	5.98	6.14	6.30	6.46	6.61	6.77	6.92	7.07	7.23
Growth	2.29	2.36	2.42	2.48	2.54	2.59	2.65	2.71	2.77
Pregnancy	0.03	0.07	0.16	0.32	0.64	1.18	2.08	3.44	5.37
Total	8.31	8.57	8.87	9.26	9.79	10.55	11.65	13.23	15.37
MP required (g/day)									
Maintenance	295	303	311	319	326	334	342	349	357
Growth	118	119	119	119	119	117	115	113	110
Pregnancy	2	4	7	18	27	50	88	151	251
Total	415	425	437	457	472	501	545	613	718
Calcium required (g/day)									
Maintenance	10	11	11	11	12	12	12	13	13
Growth	9	9	9	8	8	8	8	8	8
Pregnancy	0	0	0	0	0	0	12	12	12
Total	19	19	20	20	20	20	33	33	33
Phosphorus required (g/day)									
Maintenance	8	8	8	9	9	9	10	10	10
Growth	4	4	3	3	3	3	3	3	3
Pregnancy	0	0	0	0	0	0	7	7	7
Total	12	12	12	12	12	13	20	20	20
Average daily gain (kg/day)									
Growth	0.39	0.39	0.39	0.39	0.39	0.39	0.39	0.39	0.39
Pregnancy	0.03	0.05	0.08	0.12	0.19	0.28	0.40	0.57	0.77
Total	0.42	0.44	0.47	0.51	0.58	0.67	0.79	0.96	1.16
Body wt (kg)									
Shrunk body	332	343	355	367	379	391	403	415	426
Gravid uterus mass	1	3	4	7	12	19	29	44	64
Total (kg)	333	346	359	374	391	410	432	459	490
Total (lb)	733	761	790	823	860	902	950	1,010	1,078

[a] Mature weight, 533 kg (1,173 lb); calf birth weight, 40 kg (88 lb); age at breeding, 15 mo; breed code Angus; *see* TABLE 18 for abbreviations. The concentration of vitamin A in all diets should be 2,200 IU/kg (1,000 IU/lb) of dry matter.

Adapted, with permission, from *Nutrient Requirements of Beef Cattle*, 2000, National Academy of Sciences, National Academy Press, Washington, DC.

supplementation in the diet. In a phosphorus deficiency, reduced growth and efficiency of feed conversion, decreased appetite, impaired reproduction, reduced milk production, and weak, fragile bones can be expected. There does not appear to be any advantage to feeding more phosphorus than is recommended. Furthermore, feeding excess phosphorus contributes to increased environmental pollution. Good sources of supplemental phosphorus include steamed bone meal, mono- and dicalcium phosphate, defluorinated rock phosphate, and phosphoric acid. Corn co-products like corn gluten and distillers grains with solubles are also high in phosphorus. Because most grains are relatively good sources of phosphorus, feedlot cattle rarely suffer a phosphorus deficiency, although phytic acid chelation of phosphorus in grains may render up to one-half of it unavailable—especially for monogastric animals such as swine and poultry.

Magnesium maintains electrical potentials across nerve endings. In a deficiency, the lack of control of muscles is obvious. However, normally deficiencies are not anticipated. A magnesium deficiency in calves results in excitability, anorexia, hyperemia, convulsions, frothing at the mouth, and salivation, but such a condition is uncommon. Usually, a magnesium deficiency is seen in the spring in more mature grazing cattle under field conditions (ie, grass tetany, *see* p 996). The initial signs are nervousness, reduced feed intake, and muscular twitching about the face and ears. Animals are uncoordinated and walk with a stiff gait. In advanced stages, affected cows fall to the ground, convulse, and die shortly after. A blood sample from affected cows would show a serum magnesium level of <2 mg/dL, with a corresponding calcium deficiency. This condition is sufficiently prevalent that many beef cow herd managers supplement in the spring with magnesium oxide at 28–56 g/head/day. Beef cows generally do not like magnesium oxide; dilution by mixing it with ground corn or incorporating it into a free-choice liquid supplement improves acceptability.

Potassium is the major cation in intracellular fluid and is important in acid-base balance; it is involved in regulation of osmotic pressure, water balance, muscle contractions, nerve impulse transmission, and several enzymatic reactions. Potassium deficiencies normally are not anticipated in cattle diets because most forages are good sources, containing 1%–4%. In fact, the high potassium content of spring pasture grass is one of the highest risk factors for grass tetany (*see* p 996). A potassium deficiency might be anticipated when diets extremely high in grain are fed (eg, in finishing cattle), because grains may contain <0.5% potassium. A marginal to deficient level of potassium in growing and finishing cattle results in decreased feed intake and rate of gain. However, this effect is subtle and probably would not be noticed other than by the very experienced cattle feeder. Body stores of potassium are small, and a deficiency may develop rapidly. It is good practice to supplement rations for growing and finishing cattle such that they will contain >0.6% potassium on a dry-matter basis.

Copper and **cobalt** deficiencies are likely more widespread than previously thought. Cobalt functions as a component of vitamin B_{12}. Cattle do not depend on dietary vitamin B_{12}, because ruminal microorganisms can synthesize it from dietary cobalt. In cattle, therefore, a cobalt deficiency is a relative vitamin B_{12} deficiency, and such cattle show weight loss, poor immune function, unthriftiness, fatty degeneration of the liver, and pale skin and mucosa. Copper functions as an essential component of many enzyme systems, including those that involve the production of blood components. Recommended levels of cobalt and copper should be provided in the diet, either by supplementation of the total mixed ration or as part of the free-choice mineral mix or supplemental mix.

Iodine is an integral part of thyroxine and, as such, is largely responsible for control of many metabolic functions. Typically, coastal regions subjected to iodine-carrying winds off the ocean have abundant supplies of iodine; however, in inland soils (in the USA, especially between the Allegheny and Rocky mountains), the soil generally does not have sufficient iodine to meet most livestock needs. Iodine requirements in cattle can be met adequately by feeding stabilized iodized salt.

Selenium is part of the enzyme glutathione peroxidase, which catalyzes the reduction of hydrogen peroxide and lipid hydroperoxides, thus preventing oxidative damage to the body tissues. White muscle disease in calves (*see* p 1172), characterized by degeneration and necrosis of skeletal and heart muscles, is the result of a selenium deficiency. Vitamin E plays a role in preventing such conditions. Other signs of a selenium deficiency include unthriftiness, weight loss, reduced immune response, and decreased reproductive performance. Selenium can be included in mineral mixes at a level up to 120 ppm so that cattle intake is 3 mg/head/day.

TABLE 20 NUTRIENT REQUIREMENTS OF BEEF COWS[a]

	Months Since Calving				
	1	2	3	4	5
NE_m required (Mcal/day)					
Maintenance	10.25	10.25	10.25	10.25	10.25
Lactation	4.78	5.74	5.17	4.13	3.10
Pregnancy	0	0	0.01	0.03	0.07
Total	15.03	15.99	15.43	14.41	13.42
MP required (g/day)[b]					
Maintenance	422	422	422	422	422
Lactation	349	418	376	301	226
Pregnancy	0	0	1	2	4
Total (g)	771	840	799	725	652
Total (lb)	1.7	1.9	1.8	1.6	1.4
Calcium required (g/day)[b]					
Maintenance	16	16	16	16	16
Lactation	16	20	18	14	11
Pregnancy	0	0	0	0	0
Total	32	36	34	30	27
Phosphorus required (g/day)[b]					
Maintenance	13	13	13	13	13
Lactation	9	11	10	8	6
Pregnancy	0	0	0	0	0
Total	22	24	23	21	19
Gain in weight from pregnancy/day[b]					
Grams	0	0	20	30	50
Pounds	0	0	0.04	0.07	0.11
Milk production/day					
Kilograms	6.7	8.0	7.2	5.8	4.3
Pounds	14.7	17.6	15.8	12.8	9.5
Weight of conceptus					
Kilograms	0	0	1	1	3
Pounds	0	0	2	2	7

[a] Mature weight, 533 kg (1,172 lb); calf birth weight, 40 kg (88 lb); age at calving, 60 mo; peak milk, 8 kg (17.6 lb); age of calf at weaning, 30 wk; breed code Angus; milk protein, 3.4%; calving interval, 12 mo; *see* TABLE 18 for abbreviations. Crystalline vitamin A should be added at a level of 2,200 IU/kg (1,000 IU/lb) dry matter feed.

[b] No allowance made for gain because these are mature cows.

Adapted, with permission, from *Nutrient Requirements of Beef Cattle*, 2000, National Academy of Sciences, National Academy Press, Washington, DC.

TABLE 20 NUTRIENT REQUIREMENTS OF BEEF COWS[a] *(continued)*

Months Since Calving						
6	**7**	**8**	**9**	**10**	**11**	**12**
10.25	8.54	8.54	8.54	8.54	8.54	8.54
2.23	0	0	0	0	0	0
0.16	0.32	0.64	1.18	2.08	3.44	5.37
12.64	8.87	9.18	9.72	10.62	11.98	13.91
422	422	422	422	422	422	422
163	0	0	0	0	0	0
7	14	27	50	88	151	251
592	436	449	472	510	573	673
1.3	1.0	1.0	1.0	1.1	1.3	1.5
16	16	16	16	16	16	16
8	0	0	0	0	0	0
0	0	0	0	12	12	12
24	16	16	16	28	28	28
13	13	13	13	13	13	13
4	0	0	0	0	0	0
0	0	0	0	5	5	5
17	13	13	13	18	18	18
80	120	190	280	400	570	770
0.18	0.26	0.42	0.62	0.88	1.25	1.70
3.1	0	0	0	0	0	0
6.8	0	0	0	0	0	0
4	7	12	19	29	44	64
9	15	26	42	64	97	141

Vitamins: Although cattle probably have a metabolic requirement for all the known vitamins, dietary sources of vitamins C and K and the B-vitamin complex are not necessary in all but the very young. Vitamin K and the B vitamins are synthesized in sufficient amounts by the ruminal microflora, and vitamin C is synthesized in the tissues of all cattle. However, if rumen function is impaired, as by starvation, nutrient deficiencies, or excessive levels of antimicrobials, synthesis of these vitamins may be impaired.

TABLE 21 NUTRIENT REQUIREMENTS OF GROWING AND FINISHING BEEF CATTLE[a]

Body Weight in kg (lb)	200 (440)	250 (550)
MAINTENANCE REQUIREMENT		
NE_m (Mcal/day)	4.1	4.84
MP (g/day)	202	239
Calcium (g/day)	6	8
Phosphorus (g/day)	5	6
GROWTH REQUIREMENT (AVERAGE DAILY GAIN IN KG [LB])		
NE_g required for gain (Mcal/day)		
0.5 (1.1)	1.27	1.50
1.0 (2.2)	2.72	3.21
1.5 (3.3)	4.24	5.01
2.0 (4.4)	5.81	6.87
2.5 (5.5)	7.42	8.78
MP required for gain (g/day)		
0.5 (1.1)	154	155
1.0 (2.2)	299	300
1.5 (3.3)	441	440
2.0 (4.4)	580	577
2.5 (5.5)	718	721
Calcium required for gain (g/day)		
0.5 (1.1)	14	13
1.0 (2.2)	27	25
1.5 (3.3)	39	36
2.0 (4.4)	52	47
2.5 (5.5)	64	59
Phosphorus required for gain (g/day)		
0.5 (1.1)	6	5
1.0 (2.2)	11	10
1.5 (3.3)	16	15
2.0 (4.4)	21	19
2.5 (5.5)	26	24

[a] Weight at small marbling, 533 kg (1,173); weight range, breed code Angus; *see* TABLE 18 for abbreviations. The concentration of vitamin A in all diets for finishing steers and heifers is 2,200 IU/kg (1,000 IU/lb) dry diet.

Adapted, with permission, from *Nutrient Requirements of Beef Cattle*, 2000, National Academy of Sciences, National Academy Press, Washington, DC.

TABLE 21 NUTRIENT REQUIREMENTS OF GROWING AND FINISHING BEEF CATTLE[a] *(continued)*

300 (660)	350 (770)	400 (880)	450 (990)
MAINTENANCE REQUIREMENT			
5.55	6.23	6.89	7.52
274	307	340	371
9	11	12	14
7	8	10	11
GROWTH REQUIREMENT (AVERAGE DAILY GAIN IN KG [LB])			
1.72	1.93	2.14	2.33
3.68	4.13	4.57	4.99
5.74	6.45	7.13	7.79
7.88	8.84	9.77	10.68
10.06	11.29	12.48	13.64
158	157	145	133
303	298	272	246
442	432	391	352
577	561	505	451
710	687	616	547
12	11	10	9
23	21	19	17
33	30	27	25
43	39	35	32
53	48	43	38
5	4	4	4
9	8	8	7
13	12	11	10
18	16	14	13
22	19	17	15

Vitamin A can be synthesized from β-carotene contained in feedstuffs such as green forages and yellow corn. However, this ability varies among breeds; Holstein cattle perhaps are the most efficient converters of carotenes, whereas some of the beef breeds are much less efficient. Therefore, providing supplemental vitamin A to beef cattle should be considered. Vitamin A is one of the few vitamins that cattle store in their livers—as much as a 6-mo supply. Cattle on a diet deficient in

TABLE 22 NUTRIENT REQUIREMENTS OF GROWING BEEF BULLS[a]

Body Weight in kg (lb)	300 (660)	400 (880)
MAINTENANCE REQUIREMENT		
NE_m (Mcal/day)	6.38	7.92
MP (g/day)	274	340
Calcium (g/day)	9	12
Phosphorus (g/day)	7	10
GROWTH REQUIREMENT (AVERAGE DAILY GAIN IN KG [LB])		
NE_g required for gain (Mcal/day)		
0.5 (1.1)	1.72	2.13
1.0 (2.2)	3.68	4.56
1.5 (3.3)	5.74	7.12
2.0 (4.4)	7.87	9.76
2.5 (5.5)	10.05	12.47
MP required for gain (g/day)		
0.5 (1.1)	158	145
1.0 (2.2)	303	272
1.5 (3.3)	442	392
2.0 (4.4)	577	506
2.5 (5.5)	710	617
Calcium required for gain (g/day)		
0.5 (1.1)	12	10
1.0 (2.2)	23	19
1.5 (3.3)	33	27
2.0 (4.4)	43	35
2.5 (5.5)	53	43
Phosphorus required for gain (g/day)		
0.5 (1.1)	5	4
1.0 (2.2)	9	8
1.5 (3.3)	13	11
2.0 (4.4)	18	14
2.5 (5.5)	22	17

[a] Weight at maturity, 890 kg (1,958 lb); breed code Angus; *see* TABLE 18 for abbreviations. Vitamin A should be added at a level of 2,200 IU/kg (1,000 IU/lb) feed dry matter.

Adapted, with permission, from *Nutrient Requirements of Beef Cattle*, 2000, National Academy of Sciences, National Academy Press, Washington, DC.

TABLE 22 NUTRIENT REQUIREMENTS OF GROWING BEEF BULLS[a] *(continued)*

500 (1,100)	600 (1,320)	700 (1,540)	800 (1,760)
MAINTENANCE REQUIREMENT			
9.36	10.73	12.05	13.32
402	461	517	572
15	19	22	25
12	14	17	19
GROWTH REQUIREMENT (AVERAGE DAILY GAIN IN KG [LB])			
2.52	2.89	3.25	3.59
5.39	6.18	6.94	7.67
8.42	9.65	10.83	11.97
11.54	13.23	14.85	16.41
14.74	16.90	18.97	20.97
122	100	78	58
222	175	130	86
314	241	170	102
400	299	202	109
481	352	228	109
9	7	6	4
16	12	9	6
22	17	12	7
28	21	14	8
34	25	16	8
3	3	2	2
6	5	4	2
9	7	5	3
11	8	6	3
14	10	6	3

vitamin A may not begin to show signs for several weeks. Newborn calves, which have small stores of vitamin A, depend on colostrum and milk to meet their needs. If the dam is fed a ration low in carotene or vitamin A during gestation (eg, in winter), severe deficiency signs may become apparent in the young suckling calf within 2–4 wk of birth, while the dam may appear healthy.

It is sound practice to provide 2–5 lb (1–2 kg) of early-cut, good-quality legume or grass hay in the daily ration of stocker cattle and pregnant cows to prevent

TABLE 23 REQUIREMENTS AND MAXIMUM TOLERABLE LEVELS OF MINERALS FOR BEEF CATTLE[a]

	Requirement			
Mineral	Growing and Finishing	Gestation	Early Lactation	Maximum Tolerable Level
Chlorine (%)	—	—	—	—
Chromium (mg/kg)	—	—	—	1,000
Cobalt (mg/kg)	0.10	0.10	0.10	10
Copper (mg/kg)	10	10	10	100
Iodine (mg/kg)	0.50	0.50	0.50	50
Iron (mg/kg)	50	50	50	1,000
Magnesium (%)	0.10	0.12	0.20	0.40
Manganese (mg/kg)	20	40	40	1,000
Molybdenum (mg/kg)	—	—	—	5
Nickel (mg/kg)	—	—	—	50
Potassium (%)	0.60	0.60	0.70	3
Selenium (mg/kg)	0.10	0.10	0.10	2
Sodium (%)	0.06–0.08	0.06–0.08	0.10	—
Sulfur (%)	0.15	0.15	0.15	0.40
Zinc (mg/kg)	30	30	30	500

[a] Requirements for calcium and phosphorus are listed in the preceding nutrient requirement tables.

Adapted, with permission, from *Nutrient Requirements of Beef Cattle*, 2000, National Academy of Sciences, National Academy Press, Washington, DC.

vitamin A deficiency. Most commercial protein and mineral supplements are fortified with dry, stabilized vitamin A. The daily requirements for beef cattle appear to be ~5 mg of carotene or 2,000 IU of vitamin A/100 lb (45 kg) body wt; lactating cows may require twice this amount to maintain high vitamin levels in the milk.

Vitamin A deficiency under feedlot conditions can cause considerable loss to cattle feeders, especially if high-concentrate and corn silage rations low in carotene have been fed. Destruction of carotene during hay storage or in the GI tract, or the failure of beef cattle to convert carotene to vitamin A efficiently, may increase the need for supplemental vitamin A. Growing and finishing steers and heifers fed low-carotene diets for several months require 2,200 IU of vitamin A/kg of air-dry ration. Commercial vitamin A supplements are not expensive and should be used when such rations are fed and any danger of a deficiency exists. An alternative way to supply supplemental vitamin A is by IM injection: studies show that an extremely high dose (6 million U) would be needed to supply adequate vitamin A for 7 mo. As with all vitamins and minerals, a steady supply in the diet is the ideal method for supplementation.

Vitamin D deficiency is comparatively rare in beef cattle, because they are usually outside in direct sunlight or fed sun-cured roughage. In northern latitudes during long winters, or in show calves kept in the barn or turned out only at night, a deficiency is possible. The ultraviolet rays of sunlight convert provitamin D found in the skin of animals (7-dehydrocholesterol) or in harvested plants (ergosterol) to active vitamin D. Direct exposure to sunlight, consumption of sun-cured feed, or supplementary vitamin D (300 IU/45 kg body wt) prevent a deficiency.

For the interrelationships of vitamin E and selenium in reproduction and in the etiology of various myopathies and the predisposition of a relative thiamine (vitamin B_1) deficiency, *see* NUTRITIONAL MYOPATHIES, p 1172. (*See also* POLIOENCEPHALOMALACIA, p 1281.)

FEEDING AND NUTRITIONAL MANAGEMENT

Feeds for beef cattle vary widely in quality, palatability, and essential nutrient content (*see* TABLE 18). To be most effective, any supplement must be patterned to fit the kind and quality of roughage available. Chemical analyses of roughages are very useful to determine their nutrient deficiencies and adequacies. Under certain systems of management, beef cattle are wintered on low-quality roughages and thus may not receive the recommended nutrients for optimal performance. If heifers are fed low-quality roughages during winter, they will produce inadequate quality and quantity of colostrum, take longer to deliver their calves, and have poor rebreeding rates. This can be prevented by ensuring that heifers are fed a balanced ration that will allow them to calve in body condition score 6.5–7 (0–9 scale). Cattle should always be fed an adequate ration that allows them to thrive in their given environment. (*See* TABLES 19–22.)

Feeding and nutritional management for three systems of beef production are discussed separately. (*See* BEEF CATTLE BREEDING HERDS, p 2119.)

The Breeding Herd

In many areas, producers follow a late winter/early spring calving program (February to May in the USA), depending on the available feed, growth of early pasture, and prevailing climate. Fall calving has become more prevalent, particularly in the south. Wintering the lactating cow presents a much greater nutritional problem than does wintering the pregnant, nonlactating cow. Spring-born calves commonly are weaned at 6–7 mo, and their dams bred back while on pasture. Heifers may be bred to calve first as 2-yr-olds (22–25 mo) if good winter feeding is practiced to ensure adequate development. Heifers should weigh 55%–60% of mature body wt at breeding time and should be fed well thereafter to allow for continued growth, good milk production, and prompt rebreeding.

Mature cows have greater body reserves and lower nutrient requirements than heifers; therefore, they can be wintered on rations of poorer quality. Their ration should provide a minimum of 8% total or crude protein in the dry matter; if it does not, then 1–2 lb (0.5–1 kg) of a 20%–30% protein supplement or its equivalent should be fed daily. A mineral mix and salt should be provided. Cows should calve in body condition score 5.5–6 (0–9 scale).

Under profitable systems of management, a mature beef cow should maintain her weight from fall to fall. Lactation requires more nutrients than gestation. However, feeding beef cows more than is necessary for satisfactory production, such as is frequently done in purebred herds and show herds, is also undesirable. Large accumulations of body fat may lead to lowered conception rates, difficult calving, a lower calf crop, and a shorter life span for the cow.

A system of "creep feeding" can be practiced in which suckling calves are allowed access to a grain mixture in a self-feeder in an enclosure or to high-quality forage in an adjacent pasture where only calves have access. A creep-feed mixture of high-fiber co-product feeds such as corn gluten, dry distiller's grains, and soyhulls can be combined with a salt-vitamin-mineral mix to provide a palatable ration for the calves. The mixture should be rather large particles to prevent dustiness. A commercial 14%–16% protein creep feed may be used as an alternative.

Growing bull calves should also receive a balanced ration. Young bulls should not be fed large amounts of starch, with gains of 2.5–3.5 lb (1.1–1.6 kg) per day being very adequate. Yearling bulls grown on extremely high energy diets are more likely to have disease issues and reduced longevity in the breeding herd. Mature bulls commonly are wintered in the same manner as the cow herd, with a greater feed allowance during the late winter. In highly fitted show bulls, a gradual reduction in the ration and much exercise are needed before they will be in suitable shape and condition for pasture breeding. Breeding stock should have adequate nutrients in their ration and be gaining weight before and during the breeding season. Deficiency of several nutrients, especially carotene, phosphorus, energy, and protein, reduces fertility. These nutrients should be present in adequate amounts in the ration at least 6–8 wk before breeding.

Stocker Cattle

It is common practice to feed calves and yearlings to make moderate gains in winter, with faster and less expensive gains on summer pasture. Such cattle may be sold as feeders in the spring or finished out in dry lot the following fall. The cost of winter gain on harvested feeds invariably is higher than summer gain on pasture; hence, it is advisable to winter cattle so as to make the greatest possible gains on pasture. To maintain good health, weanling calves should gain >1 lb (0.5 kg)/day. Two pounds

(1 kg) of grain plus 1–2 lb (0.5–1 kg) of protein supplement are recommended in addition to nonlegume roughage. If legume roughage is fed, no protein supplement is needed. Older cattle, particularly if they enter the winter in fleshy condition, may just maintain their weight. A free-choice mineral mixture with trace mineralized salt should be supplied. Limited amounts of grain fed to yearling cattle on pasture during the late summer may increase their market value.

Finishing Cattle

This phase of beef production consists of full feeding of grain with limited amounts of roughage until market weight and finish are reached. Older cattle may reach finish weight on pasture alone (or with only a few pounds of grain/day) or after 60–90 days in the feedlot on high-grain rations to improve market grade and to remove any yellow tinges from their body fat (due to stored carotene from pasture forage). Weanling calves can be shipped directly to the feedlot and fed finishing rations for 150–250 days, whereas yearlings require ~150 days. Grain consumption of cattle on full-feed is ~2–2.5 lb/100 lb (1 kg/45 kg) body wt. Roughage consumption usually is limited to approximately one-fourth to one-third of the total concentrate consumption after cattle are on full-feed. Cattle consume ~3% of their body wt/day when self-fed mixed rations. For calves, ~1.5–2 lb (<1 kg) of a 33% protein supplement is required daily for best gains and market grades when nonlegume roughage is fed.

The grain (concentrate) allowance for finishing cattle should be increased gradually over 2–3 wk from the time they are started on a finishing program to get them on full feed. Feeding too much grain to finishing cattle too rapidly can lead to lactic acidosis or founder (*see* p 225).

PERFORMANCE MODIFIERS

See also GROWTH PROMOTANTS AND PRODUCTION ENHANCERS, p 2758.

There are three groups of performance modifiers used in beef cattle production: hormone-like growth enhancers; ruminal chemistry modifiers, which alter volatile fatty acid production in the rumen; and β-agonists, which increase muscle.

Hormone-like growth enhancers for finishing beef cattle have been used for almost 70 yr. There are many implant choices, and the specific implant protocol needs to be tailored to the cattle genetics, nutrition, and marketing plan. The average increase in daily gain due to the use of effective implants is ~0.23 kg (0.5 lb)/day, and the improvement in the feed to gain ratio is 0.56 kg feed/kg gain.

Ionophores are antibiotics that alter the chemistry of the rumen by altering the rumen microflora to produce increased proportions of propionic acid and decreased proportions of acetic and butyric acids. These three acids, called volatile fatty acids (VFAs), are the products of ruminal fermentation and can be absorbed from the digestive tract of the cow and used as energy sources. Because propionic acid releases more energy per unit weight to the host cow upon oxidation than do the other two VFAs, it is important in beef cattle production.

In modern feedlot diets, ionophores improve feed efficiency by 2.5%–3.5%, decrease dry matter intake 3%, and increase average daily gain (ADG) 2.5%. A more dramatic improvement in ADG is seen in cattle fed ionophores on high-roughage diets than in cattle fed high-energy diets. This is explained by energy availability between the two systems. On high-energy diets, cattle eat until they meet energy requirements; thus, ionophores help them derive more energy per unit of ingested feed, and they eat less. On high-roughage diets, which have less energy per unit weight, cattle consume feed until the rumen will hold no more. In grazing or high forage feeding systems, if ionophores are fed, these cattle derive more energy per unit of feed consumed, and thus gain more. Additional benefits of feeding ionophores include improving the consistency of feed intake in cattle fed high-grain diets, thus reducing the incidence of ruminal acidosis along with control of coccidiosis.

β-Agonists are the newest of the performance modifiers used in feedlot operations. These feed additives are absorbed in the blood and distributed to muscle tissue, where they bind to specific β receptors. Their action results in increased protein synthesis, which results in increased muscle fiber size. The β-agonist ractopamine is fed for the final 28–42 days before slaughter, whereas zilpaterol is fed for the final 20-40 days before slaughter. Performance improvements of β-agonists include live slaughter wt 18–22 lbs, hot carcass wt 20–30 lbs, ADG (during β-agonist feeding period of 20–42 days) 8.5%–30%, feed efficiency (during β-agonist feeding period of 20–42 days) 12.5%–31%, and dressing percentage 0–1.5 units.

β-agonists can increase muscle shear force and reduce the percentage of cattle that grade prime and high choice, so use in cattle with low genetic potential for tenderness and/or marbling may be less advantageous.

NUTRITION: DAIRY CATTLE

NUTRITIONAL REQUIREMENTS

During lactation, dairy cows have very high nutritional requirements relative to most other species (*see* TABLE 24). Meeting these requirements, especially for energy and protein, is challenging. Diets must have sufficient nutrient concentrations to support production and metabolic health, while also supporting rumen health and the efficiency of fermentative digestion.

Feed Intake

Under nearly all practical management conditions, dairy cows and growing dairy heifers are fed ad lib. Thus, voluntary feed intake is the major limitation to nutrient supply in dairy cattle. Feed intake is usually characterized as dry matter intake (DMI) to compare diets of variable moisture concentrations. DMI is affected by both animal and feed factors. Body size, milk production, and stage of lactation or gestation are the major animal factors. At peak DMI, daily DMI of high-producing cows may be 5% of body wt, and even higher in extremely high-producing cows. More typical peak DMI values are in the range of 3.5%–4% of body wt. In mature cows, DMI as a percentage of body weight is lowest during the nonlactating, or dry, period. In most cows, DMI declines to its lowest rate in the last 2–3 wk of gestation. Typical DMI during this period is <2% of body wt/day, with intake rates depressed more in fat cows than in thin ones. Feed intake during this period has an important relationship to postpartum health, with low DMI and associated prepartum negative energy balance increasing the risk of postpartum disease. After calving, DMI increases as milk production increases; however, the rate of increase in feed consumption is such that energy intake lags behind energy requirements for the first several weeks of lactation. Milk production and associated energy requirements generally peak around 6–10 wk into lactation, whereas DMI usually does not peak until 12–14 wk into lactation. This lag in DMI relative to energy requirements creates a period of negative energy balance in early lactation. Cows are at greater risk of metabolic disease during this period than at other times during their lactation cycle. Management and nutritional strategies should be designed to maximize DMI through the period of late gestation and early lactation.

Feed factors also affect DMI. Total ration moisture concentrations >50% generally decrease DMI, although this may be related more to fermentation characteristics than to moisture per se, because high-moisture feeds for dairy cattle are typically from fermented (ensiled) sources. Rations high (>30%) in neutral detergent fiber (NDF) may also limit feed intake, although the degree to which this occurs is related to the source of NDF. Environment also affects feed intake with temperatures above the thermal neutral zone (>20°C [68°F]), resulting in reduced DMI. Monitoring DMI, when possible, is a useful tool in diagnosing nutritional problems in diets of dairy cows.

Carbohydrates

Energy requirements for lactating dairy cows are met primarily by carbohydrate fractions of the diet. These consist of fibrous and nonfibrous carbohydrates. Fibrous carbohydrate proportions are generally measured as NDF and expressed as a percentage of dry matter. Nonfiber carbohydrate (NFC) proportions are calculated by subtracting the proportions (as dry matter) of NDF, crude protein, fat, and ash from 100%. Nonfiber carbohydrates primarily consist of sugars and fructans, starch, organic acids, and pectin. In fermented feeds, fermentation acids also contribute to the NFC fraction. The sum of sugars and starch is referred to as nonstructural carbohydrate (NSC), which should not be confused with NFC. Balancing fiber and NFC fractions to optimize energy intake and rumen health is a challenging aspect of dairy nutrition.

In general, fiber in the diet supports rumen health. Fiber in the rumen, especially fiber from forage sources that have not been finely chopped or ground, maintains rumen distention, which stimulates motility, cud chewing, and salivary flow. These actions affect the rumen environment favorably by stimulating the endogenous production of salivary buffers and a high rate of fluid movement through the rumen. Salivary buffers maintain rumen pH in a desirable range, while high fluid flow rates increase the efficiency of microbial energy and protein yield. Fiber, however, delivers less

TABLE 24 FEEDING GUIDELINES FOR LARGE-BREED DAIRY CATTLE[a]

	Dry (Far off)	Close (Close up)
Body wt, lb (kg)	1,500 (675)	1,500 (675)
DMI, lb (kg/day)	32 (14)	22 (10)
Milk, lb[b] (kg/day)		
CP (%)[c]	9.9	12.4
RDP (%)	7.7	9.6
RUP (%)	2.2	2.8
MP (%)	6.0	8.0
NE_L, Mcal/lb (Mcal/kg)	0.60 (1.32)	0.65 (1.43)
ME, Mcal/lb (Mcal/kg)		
NDF (%)	40	35
ADF (%)	30	25
NFC (%)	30	34
Calcium (%)	0.44	0.48
Phosphorus (%)	0.22	0.26
Magnesium (%)	0.11	0.40
Chlorine (%)	0.13	0.20
Sodium (%)	0.10	0.14
Potassium (%)	0.51	0.62
Sulfur (%)	0.20	0.20
Vitamin A (IU/day)	80,300	83,270
Vitamin D (IU/day)	21,900	22,700
Vitamin E (IU/day)	1,168	1,200

Adapted, with permission, from *Nutrient Requirements of Dairy Cattle*, 2001, National Academy of Sciences, National Academy Press, Washington, DC.

[a] DMI, dry matter intake; CP, crude protein; RDP, rumen degradable protein; RUP, rumen undegraded protein; MP, metabolizable protein; NE_L, net energy lactation; ME, metabolizable energy; NDF, neutral detergent fiber; ADF, acid detergent fiber; NFC, non-fiber carbohydrate. Trace mineral added to ration (expressed as ppm): cobalt: 0.11; copper 10–18; iodine: 0.3–0.4; iron: 13–130; manganese: 14–24; selenium: 0.30; zinc: 22–70.

[b] Milk components: 3.5% fat, 3.0% true protein, and 4.8% lactose.

[c] All concentration values are on a dry-matter basis.

[d] These cows will lose body weight (values >0.82 not feasible).

dietary energy than NFC. Fiber is generally less fermentable in the rumen than NFC, and rumen fermentation is the major mechanism by which energy is provided, both for the animal and the rumen microbes. Therefore, diets with high NDF concentrations promote rumen health but provide relatively less energy than diets high in NFC.

To increase the energy supply, dietary NDF concentrations are usually reduced by adding starch and other sources of NFC.

TABLE 24 FEEDING GUIDELINES FOR LARGE-BREED DAIRY CATTLE[a] *(continued)*

Cows				Heifers (age in mo)			
Fresh	**Early**	**Mid**	**Late**	**6**	**12**	**18**	**24 (Close up)**
1,500 (675)	1,500 (675)	1,500 (675)	1,500 (675)	440 (200)	660 (300)	1,000 (450)	1,375 (625)
34 (15)	66 (30)	52 (24)	45 (20)	11 (5)	16 (7)	25 (11)	23 (10)
77 (35)	120 (55)	77 (35)	55 (25)				
19.5	16.7	15.2	14.1	12.3	11.4	8.8	15.0
10.5	9.8	9.7	9.5	9.4	9.5	8.8	10.1
9.0	6.9	5.5	4.6	2.9	1.9	0.004	4.9
13.8	11.6	10.2	9.2	7.2	7.0	5.3	9.7
1.01[d] (2.22)	0.73 (1.61)	0.67 (1.47)	0.62 (1.36)	—	—	—	0.72 (1.58)
				0.93 (2.05)	1.03 (2.27)	0.82 (1.80)	
30	28	30	32	30	32	33	35
21	19	21	24	20	22	24	25
35	38	35	32	35	30	25	34
0.79	0.60	0.61	0.62	0.41	0.41	0.37	0.40
0.42	0.38	0.35	0.32	0.28	0.23	0.18	0.23
0.29	0.21	0.19	0.18	0.11	0.11	0.08	0.40
0.20	0.29	0.26	0.24	0.11	0.12	0.10	0.20
0.34	0.22	0.23	0.22	0.08	0.08	0.07	0.14
1.24	1.07	1.04	1.00	0.47	0.48	0.46	0.55
0.20	0.20	0.20	0.20	0.20	0.20	0.20	0.20
75,000	75,000	75,000	75,000	24,000	24,000	36,000	75,000
21,000	21,000	21,000	21,000	6,000	9,000	13,500	20,000
545	545	545	545	240	240	360	1,200

This increases the rate and extent of rumen fermentation, which leads to greater energy availability. Increased ruminal fermentation also leads to the increased production of volatile fatty acids, which tends to lower rumen pH. At rumen pH values <6.2, fiber digestion is reduced; at values ≤5.5, fiber digestion is severely diminished, feed intake may be reduced, and rumen health is generally compromised. There is a reciprocal relationship between NFC and NDF proportions, so the adverse effects of high dietary NFC may be especially evident as cud chewing and salivary flow may be simultaneously diminished because of reductions in dietary NDF.

Recommended minimum NDF concentrations depend on the source and physical effectiveness of the NDF and the dietary concentration of NFC. Fiber from forage sources is, in general, more effective at stimulating salivation and cud chewing than is fiber from nonforage sources. Thus, one variable in the assessment of dietary NDF adequacy is the proportion of NDF coming from forages. Minimum NDF concentrations in the diets for high-producing cows are 25%–30%. When fiber sources from forage make up ≥75% of the NDF, then total NDF concentrations in the lower end of this range may be acceptable (*see* TABLE 25). When a smaller portion of total NDF is derived from

TABLE 25 RECOMMENDED MINIMUM NDF CONCENTRATIONS BASED ON PROPORTION OF NDF COMING FROM FORAGE SOURCES[a]

NDF from Forage (% of Dietary Dry Matter)	NDF from Forage (% of NDF)	Minimum Total NDF (% of Dietary Dry Matter)
19	75	25
18	66	27
17	58	29

[a] Reprinted with permission from the National Academies Press, copyright 2001, National Academy of Sciences. As the proportion of neutral detergent fiber (NDF) from forage sources decreases, the minimum requirement for total NDF increases. These represent minimum requirements; diets with higher NDF concentrations present no problem and are generally appropriate for animals with relatively low energy requirements.

forage sources, then total NDF concentrations should be in the upper end of this range. Maximum recommended NFC concentrations are 38%–44%. Diets with higher NFC concentrations will benefit from higher proportions of NDF coming from forage sources. These recommendations must be viewed as broad guidelines rather than strict rules. Factors including the total fermentability of the diet as well as the fermentability of

TABLE 26 DRY MATTER, ENERGY, CRUDE PROTEIN, FIBER, AND NON-FIBER CARBOHYDRATE CONCENTRATIONS OF SOME FEEDSTUFFS COMMONLY FED TO DAIRY CATTLE[a]

	Dry Matter (%)	Metabolizable Energy (Mcal/kg)	Net Energy for Lactation (Mcal/kg)
Ground shell corn	88	3.12	2.01
Corn silage	35	2.33	1.45
Pasture	20	2.46	1.54
Hay (cool-season grasses)	84	2.02	1.23
Hay crop silage (cool-season grasses)	42	1.92	1.16
Grass-legume mix hay	85	2.07	1.25
Grass-legume mix hay crop silage	44	1.96	1.23
Legume hay	84	2.09	1.28
Legume hay crop silage	43	2.01	1.22
Oats (rolled)	90	2.78	1.77
Sorghum silage	29	1.85	1.11
Soybean meal (solvent extracted, 44% CP)	89	3.31	2.13
Cotton seeds	90	2.91	1.94
Dried distillers grains with solubles	90	3.03	1.97
Corn and cob meal	89.2	2.91	1.86

[a] Reprinted with permission from the National Academies Press, copyright 2001, National Academy of Sciences. Energy values are estimated based on a consumption rate 3 times the rate of consumption at maintenance. These are representative values intended primarily for relative comparison among feeds. Analyzed values of actual feed samples will vary substantially, especially among forages.

the NDF influence the NDF requirement. Diets with highly fermentable NDF sources require higher total concentrations of NDF but provide more energy per mass unit of NDF than diets with less fermentable NDF. Feeding management schemes such as totally mixed rations result in lower minimum NDF concentrations than feeding dietary components individually (*see* p 2265).

Energy

Dietary energy is usually measured in megacalories (Mcal) or megajoules (MJ). When the energy in a given feedstuff is expressed in terms of the Mcal or MJ actually available for metabolism, heat production, or storage in the animal, the term metabolizable energy (ME) is used. The efficiency of utilization of ME varies based on the physiologic functions supported, which include body maintenance, growth, and lactation. The net energy (NE) system takes into account the differences in efficiency of ME utilization for each of these processes and assigns a separate NE value to individual feedstuffs based on each of these energy-requiring processes, ie, body maintenance, growth, and lactation. Thus, in the USA, in which the NE system is typically used, energy values of feedstuffs for ruminants are expressed as NE for maintenance (NE_M), NE for gain (NE_G), and NE for lactation (NE_L). This system is cumbersome and nonintuitive and has many computational disadvantages compared with alternative systems based directly on ME. However, the NE system has the major advantage of more equitably comparing the energy values of forages to concentrates when used in ruminant diets. TABLE 26 has typical values for ME, NE_L, NE_M, and NE_G, for some feedstuffs commonly fed to dairy

TABLE 26 DRY MATTER, ENERGY, CRUDE PROTEIN, FIBER, AND NON-FIBER CARBOHYDRATE CONCENTRATIONS OF SOME FEEDSTUFFS COMMONLY FED TO DAIRY CATTLE[a] *(continued)*

Net Energy for Maintenance (Mcal/kg)	Net Energy for Gain (Mcal/kg)	Neutral Detergent Fiber (%)	Non-fiber Carbohydrate (%)	Crude Protein (%)
2.16	1.48	9.5	75.47	9.4
1.57	0.97	45	40	8.8
1.67	1.06	45.8	19.6	26
1.33	0.75	58	21.6	13
1.25	0.68	58	18.2	17
1.35	0.77	50.8	23.8	18.4
1.32	0.74	50.4	21.5	19
1.38	0.8	43	27.3	20.8
1.32	0.74	43	25.1	22
1.9	1.26	30	50.2	13.2
1.18	0.62	61	21.9	9.1
2.29	1.59	15	27.6	49.9
1.96	1.31	50.3	5.1	23.5
2.07	1.41	39	24.4	30
2	1.35	21.5	65.2	8.6

cows. The values in these and other published tables are estimates of the energy delivered to lactating cows consuming feed at three times the maintenance consumption rate, ie, three times more feed than they would consume were they not in production. The listed values are typical averages for the feeds; the actual values for individual feeds may vary considerably, especially for forages. Laboratory analyses of feeds and forages are always advisable for both comparative evaluation and ration balancing. Values for ME and NE cannot be measured directly by typical laboratory analyses. These and any other energy values on a laboratory report are estimates, usually based on formulas with acid detergent fiber concentration as the primary independent variable. Many contemporary computer programs for ration evaluation or balancing in dairy cows do not rely on laboratory estimates of feed energy concentrations. Rather, they estimate the contributions of individual feeds to the energy supply based on feed characteristics, intake rates, and estimated rates of passage through the rumen. Such programs are frequently referred to as "models." When using programs of this type, the estimated energy values of individual feeds will diminish with increasing rates of feed intake.

In the USA, energy requirements of adult dairy cows are typically expressed in terms of NE_l. This applies to pregnant dry cows as well as lactating animals. Maintenance requirements for mature cows of various mature body weights are given in TABLE 27. Energy requirements per kg of milk produced at various milk fat concentrations are given in TABLE 28.

The required dietary energy concentration is a function of the energy requirement and the feed intake rate. Calculated requirements for dietary energy concentration typically are very high in early lactation because the rate of milk production is high relative to the feed intake rate. However, the ration energy density concentrations required to meet the energy requirement of cows in very early lactation may be too high to be compatible with adequate dietary fiber concentrations (*see* p 2265). In general, diets with energy concentrations >1.71–1.76 Mcal/kg do not contain adequate fiber to support good rumen health and function. Thus, dairy cows in early lactation typically cannot meet their energy requirements and are expected to lose weight. During the first 3 wk of lactation, dairy cows commonly have rates of negative energy balance in the range of −5 to −10 Mcal/day. The risk of metabolic disease increases with the degree of negative energy balance, although there is great variability among individual cows in the capacity to adapt to negative energy balance without incurring metabolic disease. Feed intake, rather than milk production, is generally the most limiting factor influencing energy balance in early lactation dairy cows. Thus, nutritional management strategies that result in rapid increases in feed intake rates after calving are the most beneficial in terms of both cow health and productivity.

TABLE 27 MAINTENANCE ENERGY REQUIREMENTS FOR COWS OF VARIOUS BODY WEIGHTS

Body Weight (kg)	Daily Energy Requirement (Mcal NE_L/day)
400	7.16
450	7.82
500	8.46
550	9.09
600	9.70
650	10.30
700	10.89
750	11.47
800	12.03

TABLE 28 DIETARY NET ENERGY REQUIREMENT FOR MILK PRODUCTION

Milk Fat Concentration (%)	Dietary Energy Requirement/day/kg Milk Produced (Mcal NE_L)
3.5	0.70
4	0.75
4.5	0.80
5	0.84
5.5	0.89
6	0.94
6.5	0.99

Fats

Supplemental fats can be added to increase energy concentration. Fat concentrations in typical dairy diets without supplemental fat are usually low, ~2.5% of dry matter. Supplemental fats may be added to attain a total ration fat concentration of ~6% of dry matter. Fats in ruminant diets can induce undesirable metabolic effects, both within the rumen microbial population and within the animal. Ramifications of these effects include reduced fiber digestion, indigestion and poor rumen health, and suppression of milk fat concentration. The major benefit of supplemental fat in ruminant diets is that dietary energy concentration can be increased without increasing the NFC concentration.

Fats may be supplemented from vegetable sources such as oil seeds, animal sources such as tallow, and specialty fat sources that are manufactured to be rumen inert, ie, not interact with the metabolism of rumen microbes. Supplemental fats from vegetable sources generally have a relatively high proportion of unsaturated fatty acids. Unsaturated fats adversely affect rumen microbial activity. In addition, these fatty acids are extensively converted to saturated fatty acids in the rumen. When fed in excessive dietary concentration, intermediate products from the saturation process may escape the rumen and be absorbed by intestinal digestion. Some of these products are trans-fatty acids, some of which directly suppress mammary butterfat synthesis. Supplemental fats from animal sources are more saturated and thus less detrimental to microbial activity and less apt to result in suppression of butterfat synthesis. Rumen-inert fats are designed to have little or no effect on rumen microbial activity and mammary butterfat synthesis. In general, when supplementing fats to dairy diets, up to 400 g (~2% of diet dry matter) may be added as vegetable fats, particularly if the fats are added as oil seeds, which tend to be less detrimental than free oils. An additional 200–400 g may be added from highly saturated or preferably rumen-inert sources, generally not to exceed a total of 6.5% fat in the total dietary dry matter.

Protein

The protein requirements of lactating dairy cows are high because of the demand for amino acids for milk protein synthesis. Two systems of describing the dietary protein supply and requirements for dairy cows are in general use: the crude protein system and the metabolizable protein system. The crude protein system considers only the total amount of dietary protein, or protein equivalent from nonprotein nitrogen sources. Crude protein values are based on the measurement of total dietary nitrogen and the assumption that protein is 16% nitrogen. The crude protein system is relatively simple to use and has provided a traditional means of formulating dairy cow rations. TABLE 29 provides general guidelines for the required crude protein concentration of diets for large- and small-breed dairy cattle at various levels of production. It can be used for general evaluations of the protein adequacy of dairy diets. The metabolizable protein (MP) system is more complex than the crude protein system, and it was developed in recognition of the fact that not all crude protein provided to cows may be available for absorption as amino acids.

MP refers to amino acids absorbed from the small intestine and available for metabolism. MP in ruminants is derived from two sources: microbial protein synthesized in the rumen and dietary

TABLE 29 RECOMMENDED MINIMUM DIETARY PROTEIN CONCENTRATIONS FOR DAIRY COWS AT VARIOUS LEVELS OF PRODUCTION[a]

	Dietary Protein Requirements (% of Dry Matter)			
	Large-breed Cows		Small-breed Cows	
Milk Production (kg/day)	Crude Protein[b]	Metabolizable Protein[c]	Crude Protein	Metabolizable Protein
18			15.0	12.9
23			16.4	13.1
27	14.5	11.0	17.5	13.3
32	15.0	11.2	18.4	13.3
36	15.8	11.5	19.0	13.3
40	16.5	11.7		
45	17.3	11.9		
50	17.8	12.0		
55	18.3	12.1		

[a] This table is intended to provide a general reference for initial evaluations of dairy diets, not a standard against which rations are balanced. Calculation of dietary metabolizable protein concentrations generally requires specialized software.

[b] Crude protein requirements were generated by Spartan Dairy 3.0 (Michigan State University), assuming a mature cow in mid lactation.

[c] Metabolizable protein requirements were generated by the Nutrient Requirements of Dairy Cattle Computer Program that accompanies *Nutrient Requirements of Dairy Cattle*, 2001, National Academy of Sciences, National Academy Press, Washington, DC.

proteins that escape rumen degradation. Protein escaping rumen degradation is referred to as rumen undegraded protein (RUP), while protein that is broken down in the rumen is referred to as rumen degraded protein (RDP). Both sources are important and must be considered in diet evaluation and formulation.

RUP passes unaltered through the rumen and forms a direct source of protein for intestinal digestion and amino acid absorption. Nitrogen from RDP, in contrast, must be incorporated into newly synthesized microbial protein before it will provide amino acids available for intestinal absorption. The efficiency with which RDP is recovered as microbial protein depends on the growth rate of the rumen microbes, which in turn depends on the supply of fermentable energy sources in the rumen. Thus, diets with sufficient RDP and relatively high energy concentrations will result in high yields of microbial protein, which will become available for intestinal digestion and absorption as MP. Calculations that balance dairy diets for MP must consider the complex interrelations among fermentable energy sources, RUP, and RDP.

In general, specialized software, commercially available, is necessary to formulate dairy diets using the MP system. Even with such software, many variables must be estimated with uncertainty. Therefore, calculations of MP supply must be recognized to be approximations.

Dietary ingredients vary in their proportion of RUP and RDP. In general, feeds with high moisture and high protein concentrations, eg, legume silages, will have a high proportion of RDP. In contrast, feeds that have been processed and especially those that have undergone drying will have relatively high proportions of RUP. The proportions of RUP and RDP in diets and individual ingredients are not fixed but can vary somewhat depending on intake rate. At high rates of feed intake, the rate of feed passage through the rumen is high; thus, there is less opportunity for rumen protein degradation than with the same feeds at lower intake rates. Therefore, on the same diet, RUP proportions are higher in animals with high rates of feed intake than in those with low rates of feed intake. Animals most likely to benefit from supplements selected for high RUP proportions are those with relatively

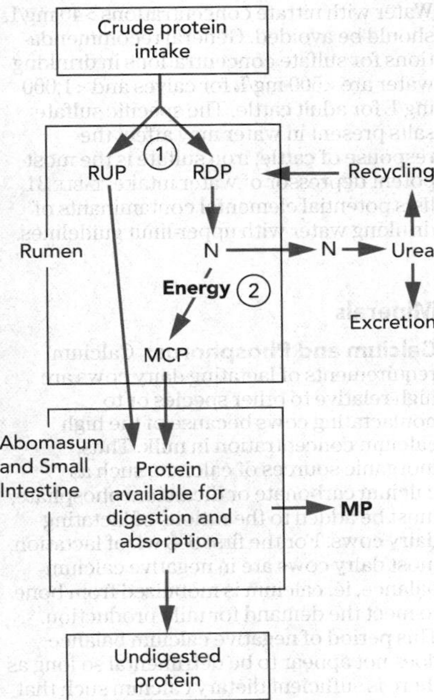

The relationship of dietary protein intake to metabolizable protein supply. The two branch points (indicated by 1 and 2) constitute the major variables relating the dietary crude protein supply to the metabolizable protein supply. The first branch point represents the proportion of protein that is degraded in the rumen. This branch point is influenced by inherent properties of the protein and the rate of ingesta passage through the rumen. The second branch point represents the proportion of nitrogen from degraded protein that is recaptured as microbial protein. This is influenced by the microbial growth rate, which depends on the supply of rumen available energy. Nitrogen that is not recaptured as microbial protein is absorbed from the rumen as ammonia and converted to urea by the liver. Some urea is recycled back to the rumen, but a large portion is excreted in urine. RUP, rumen undegraded protein; RDP, rumen degraded protein; N, nitrogen; MCP, metabolizable crude protein; MP, metabolizable protein.

high protein requirements and relatively low rates of feed intake. Cows in very early lactation and young, rapidly growing heifers are the primary examples. Supplements formulated for high RUP proportions are commonly known as rumen bypass protein supplements; however, even with these types of supplements, some portion of the protein is degraded in the rumen.

Along with overall protein requirements, dairy cows, as all other animals, have specific amino acid requirements. However, evaluating dairy cow diets relative to amino acid requirements is more difficult than making similar evaluations of diets for monogastric animals. This is because the amino acid supply for dairy cows and other ruminants is a combination of the amino acids provided by the microbial protein and the RUP. Microbial protein has an excellent amino acid profile, and diets with a large supply of microbial protein typically meet amino acid requirements if MP requirements are met. In some cases, however, high-producing dairy cows may benefit from the selection of RUP sources with specific amino acid profiles, or from adding rumen-protected forms of specific amino acids. Software is available that estimates the amino acid supply for dairy cows on different diets. The first limiting amino acids in typical dairy cow diets are lysine and methionine. With typical feedstuffs, if the MP requirement is met and the dietary lysine:methionine ratio is ~3:1, then the amino acid requirements for milk production are probably being optimized.

Water

The availability of high-quality water for ad lib consumption is critical. Insufficient water intake leads immediately to reduced feed intake and milk production. Water requirements of dairy cows are related to milk production, DMI, ration dry matter concentration, salt or sodium intake, and ambient temperature. Various formulas have been devised to predict water requirements. Two formulas to estimate water consumption of lactating dairy cows are as follows:

$$FWI = 12.3 + 2.15 \times DMI + 0.73 \times milk$$

$$FWI = 15.99 + 1.58 \times DMI + 0.9 \times milk + 0.05 \times Na + 1.2 \times minimum\ temperature$$

Note: FWI is free water intake (water consumed by drinking rather than in feed), DMI is in kg/day, milk is in kg/day, Na is in g/day, and temperature is in °C. Water consumed as part of the diet contributes to the total water requirements; thus, diets with higher moisture concentrations result in lower FWI.

Providing adequate access to water is critical to encourage maximal water intake. Water should be placed near feed sources and in milking parlor return alleys, because most water is consumed in association with feeding or after milking. For water troughs, a minimum of 5 cm of length per cow at a height of 90 cm is recommended. One water cup per 10 cows is recommended when cows are housed in groups and given water via drinking cups or fountains. Individual cow water intake rates are 4–15 L/min. Many cows may drink simultaneously, especially right after milking, so trough volumes and drinking cup flow rates should be great enough that water availability is not limited during times of peak demand. Water troughs and drinking cups should be cleaned frequently and positioned to avoid fecal contamination.

Poor water quality may result in reduced water consumption, with resultant decreases in feed consumption and milk production. Several factors determine water quality. Total dissolved solids (TDSs), also referred to as total soluble salts, is a major factor that refers to the total amount of inorganic solute in the water. TDS is generally expressed in units of mg/L or parts per million (ppm) which are numerically equivalent values (*see* TABLE 30). TDS is not equivalent to water hardness, which is a measure of the amount of calcium and magnesium in water. Water hardness has not been shown to affect dairy cow performance.

Other inorganic contaminants that affect water quality include nitrates, sulfates, and trace minerals. Concentrations of nitrate (expressed as nitrate nitrogen) <10 mg/L are safe for ruminants. At concentrations >20 mg/L, cattle may be at risk, especially if nitrate concentrations in the feed are high. Water with nitrate concentrations >40 mg/L should be avoided. General recommendations for sulfate concentrations in drinking water are <500 mg/L for calves and <1,000 mg/L for adult cattle. The specific sulfate salts present in water may affect the response of cattle; iron sulfate is the most potent depressor of water intake. TABLE 31 lists potential elemental contaminants of drinking water with upper-limit guidelines.

Minerals

Calcium and Phosphorus: Calcium requirements of lactating dairy cows are high relative to other species or to nonlactating cows because of the high calcium concentration in milk. Thus, inorganic sources of calcium, such as calcium carbonate or dicalcium phosphate, must be added to the rations of lactating dairy cows. For the first 6–8 wk of lactation, most dairy cows are in negative calcium balance, ie, calcium is mobilized from bone to meet the demand for milk production. This period of negative calcium balance does not appear to be detrimental so long as there is sufficient dietary calcium such that bone reserves can be replenished in later lactation. The availability of dietary calcium for absorption varies with dietary source. Dietary calcium from inorganic sources is generally absorbed with greater efficiency than that from organic sources. Furthermore, cows in negative calcium balance absorb calcium more efficiently than cows in positive calcium balance.

TABLE 30 GUIDELINES FOR TOTAL SOLUBLE SALTS (TOTAL DISSOLVED SOLIDS) IN DRINKING WATER FOR CATTLE

Total Soluble Salts (mg/L)	Comments
<1,000	Safe and should pose no health problems.
1,000–2,999	Generally safe but may cause a mild temporary diarrhea in animals not accustomed to the water.
3,000–4,999	Water may be refused when first offered to animals or cause temporary diarrhea. Animal performance may be less than optimum because water intake is not maximized.
5,000–6,999	Pregnant or lactating animals should not drink such water. May be offered with reasonable safety to animals when maximum performance is not required.
≥7,000	These waters should not be offered to cattle. Health problems and/or poor production will result.

TABLE 31 CONCENTRATIONS OF POTENTIALLY TOXIC NUTRIENTS AND CONTAMINANTS IN DRINKING WATER GENERALLY CONSIDERED SAFE FOR CATTLE

Element	Upper-limit Guideline (mg/L or ppm)
Aluminum	0.5
Arsenic	0.05
Boron	5.0
Cadmium	0.005
Chromium	0.1
Cobalt	1.0
Copper	1.0
Fluorine	2.0
Lead	0.015
Manganese	0.05
Mercury	0.01
Nickel	0.25
Selenium	0.05
Vanadium	0.1
Zinc	5.0

When calculating calcium requirements, newer nutritional models take into account the variability in calcium availability from different sources. This availability generally ranges from 75%–85% for inorganic calcium supplements to a low of 30% for forage sources of calcium. This approach makes it difficult to generate general recommendations for total dietary calcium concentrations across various diets. Generally, diets with large portions of forage from legume sources will have minimum calcium concentration requirements in the range of 0.71%–0.75%, while diets with forages from primarily grass (including corn silage) sources will have minimum calcium concentration requirements in the range of 0.42%–0.47%.

Two approaches are taken with respect to the calcium supply for dry cows, each with the objective of preventing milk fever, or parturient paresis (*see* p 988). One approach is to place cows in a calcium-deficient state during the last 2–3 wk of gestation; the rationale is to stimulate parathyroid hormone secretion and skeletal calcium mobilization before calving. This makes calcium homeostatic mechanisms more responsive at the time of parturition, allowing cows to maintain serum calcium concentrations during lactation. This approach requires diets with calcium concentrations near 0.3% of dry matter. Such diets are difficult to formulate with available feedstuffs while still meeting other nutritional requirements. Another approach is to feed an acidifying diet, usually referred to as a diet with a low or negative dietary cation-anion difference (DCAD). The low-calcium diet approach is not additive with the DCAD approach to milk fever prevention. When low-DCAD diets are fed, total dietary calcium concentrations should be near 0.9%, which is substantially greater than the requirement for a dry cow on a conventional diet.

Phosphorus nutrition for lactating dairy cows has dynamics similar to those of calcium. The efficiency of phosphorus absorption is affected by physiologic state and dietary source. As is the case with calcium, most dairy cows in early lactation are in negative phosphorus balance. Phosphorus mobilized from bone early in lactation is replaced during later lactation when feed intakes are higher. Young animals and animals in negative phosphorus balance absorb phosphorus more efficiently than do older animals or animals in positive phosphorus balance. Phosphorus from inorganic sources is more available than that from organic feed sources.

Judiciously balancing diets to meet, but not exceed, phosphorus requirements is important for dairy cow performance and environmental stewardship. Excess phosphorus excreted in feces is one of the major pollutant risks associated with livestock production. Newer nutritional models account for variation in phosphorus availability from different sources, but there is less variation in availability among phosphorus sources than among calcium sources. In general, concentrates when fed to ruminants have a phosphorus availability of 70%, and forages close to 64%. Inorganic mineral supplements are usually rated at 75%–80% availability, but rock phosphate is very low, ~30%. Total dietary phosphorus concentration requirements for most dairy diets will be in the range of 0.35%–0.4%, and for dry cows, 0.3%–0.35%. Phosphorus supplementation for dry cows is seldom necessary.

The dietary calcium:phosphorus ratio is not of particular importance in ruminants. Ratios from 7:1 to 1:1 are acceptable, so long as the total amount of each element meets the dietary requirements.

Serum concentrations of calcium and inorganic phosphorus are of value in assessing the short-term homeostasis of these minerals but of little value in assessing longterm nutritional status. Bone ash concentrations are the best way to assess longterm calcium and phosphorus nutritional status.

Other Macrominerals: Other macrominerals required in dairy cow diets include sodium, potassium, chloride, magnesium, and sulfur. Of these, **sodium** generally needs to be supplemented, typically as sodium chloride or common salt. Insufficient dietary sodium results in reduced feed intake with subsequent reductions in animal performance. Signs of severe salt deficiency include licking and chewing on fences and other environmental objects, urine drinking, and general ill thrift. Milk production is reduced within 1–2 wk of removing supplemental salt from the diets of lactating cows. Completely withholding salt from dry cow diets in an effort to prevent udder edema at calving is not a good practice. Maintenance requirements for sodium in nonlactating cows are estimated at 1.5 g/100 kg body wt/day, with gestation requirements estimated at an additional 1.4 g/day after 190 days of gestation. For large-breed dairy cows, this results in a sodium requirement of ~9–10 g/day. Unsupplemented dry cow diets seldom provide sodium at >3 g/day. Therefore, daily supplementation of dry cow diets with a minimum of 6–7 g of sodium per day (~15–16 g of salt) is important. Additional salt is necessary during heat stress. Although salt should be supplemented to dry cows in required amounts, excessive salt supplementation is unnecessary and may contribute to udder edema at calving.

Supplemental **magnesium** may need to be fed with diets containing high proportions of grass forages, especially those consisting of rapidly growing pasture grasses. Such forages typically have low magnesium concentrations as well as high concentrations of potassium and organic acids, which interfere with the availability of dietary magnesium. Magnesium oxide is the typical magnesium supplement in ruminant diets.

Dairy cattle, like other animals, have no dietary requirement for inorganic **sulfur**. The dietary requirement for sulfur reflects only the dietary requirement for sulfur-containing amino acids. In ruminants, rumen microbes can synthesize sulfur-containing amino acids from nonprotein sources of nitrogen and sulfur. Dairy cow diets most likely to require supplemental sulfur are those with low protein concentrations and those with supplemental nonprotein nitrogen. In general, a nitrogen:sulfur ratio of 15:1 is recommended in ruminant diets.

Recommended dietary concentrations for typical dairy cow diets are: sodium (0.23%), chloride (0.29%), potassium (1.1%), magnesium (0.21%), and sulfur (0.21%).

Trace Minerals: The trace minerals typically supplemented or measured in dairy cow diets include cobalt, copper, iron, manganese, selenium, iodine, and zinc. Of these, selenium and copper are the trace minerals most likely to be deficient. Several areas of North America, Europe, and other continents are characterized by growing conditions that result in feeds with low selenium concentrations. In these areas, livestock feeds need to be supplemented with selenium. Sources of supplemental selenium include sodium selenite, sodium selenate, and selenomethionine. The latter source is typically referred to as organic selenium.

Selenium deficiency is known to cause myopathies in calves, which may affect cardiac or skeletal muscle (ie, white muscle disease, *see* p 1172). In adult cattle, selenium deficiency appears to suppress immune function and especially neutrophil function. It also increases the risk of retained placenta, although feeding selenium in excess of requirements does not prevent this condition. Dietary selenium requirements in dairy cattle are estimated at 0.1–0.3 mg/kg diet dry matter. In the USA, 0.3 mg/kg dry matter is the maximum legal concentration of supplemental selenium in dairy cattle diets.

The selenium status of cattle can be accurately assessed from blood or serum concentrations. Whole blood concentrations of 120–250 ng/mL or serum concentrations of 70–100 ng/mL in adult cattle indicate adequate selenium status.

Recommended dietary **copper** concentrations in cattle diets are 10–15 mg/kg diet dry matter; however, the dietary copper requirement depends greatly on the concentration of interfering substances. These include primarily sulfur and molybdenum, but iron, zinc, and calcium may also interfere with copper availability. The adsorption efficiency for dietary copper in ruminants is normally quite low, 4%–5%. However, with increasing concentrations of dietary sulfur and/or molybdenum, absorption efficiency may be reduced to ≤1%.

Copper deficiency is characterized by loss of hair pigmentation, loss of hair around the eyes, anemia, and general ill thrift and suppressed immunity. In severe cases, persistent diarrhea may also occur.

The copper status of cattle can be assessed from liver or serum copper concentrations. Liver concentrations <20 mg/kg dry tissue or serum concentrations <0.5 mcg/mL indicate copper deficiency. Because the liver is a physiologic storage site for copper, copper concentrations in the liver will be reduced before serum concentrations.

Dietary **manganese** deficiencies in dairy cattle are less common than deficiencies of copper or selenium. Signs include poor growth and skeletal deformities in newborn calves and reproductive abnormalities, including anestrus, in adult cows. Recently recommended dietary manganese concentrations for cattle are 15–25 mg/kg; previous recommendations have been as high as 40 mg/kg dry matter.

Recommended **zinc** concentrations in the diets of dairy cattle and calves are 23–63 mg/kg dry matter. Signs of zinc deficiency include reduced feed intake and general ill thrift. Parakeratosis, particularly around the nostrils and lower legs, and weakening of the hoof horn are signs of prolonged zinc deficiency. Normal concentrations of serum zinc are 0.7–1.3 mcg/mL. Concentrations <0.4 mcg/mL are considered deficient.

Iron deficiency is extremely rare in adult cattle, because iron is ubiquitous in the environment and the endogenous concentrations of iron in most feedstuffs will more than meet requirements. Signs of iron deficiency are primarily anemia and low serum iron concentrations. Adequate serum iron concentrations are 110–150 mcg/dL. However, these concentrations drop quickly in the presence of inflammatory disease, and such changes in serum iron concentrations should not be interpreted as being due to a dietary deficiency. Suckling calves are the only group of cattle generally at risk of iron deficiency and to which supplemental iron need be provided.

Iodine deficiency occurs with some frequency in cattle and is primarily manifest by goiters in newborn calves. The required dietary iodine concentration is generally ~0.2 mg/kg of dietary dry matter. However, dietary iodine concentrations of 0.6 mg/kg are recommended as a safety factor because of the potential presence of goitrogenic substances in common protein supplements.

Vitamins

Vitamin A: Preformed vitamin A, or retinol, does not exist in any plant material, so there is no vitamin A in natural diets for dairy cattle. Vitamin A activity from natural sources comes primarily from β-carotene, which is found in plants and is particularly abundant in fresh forages. β-carotene is labile; its concentrations in forages are not constant but diminish with time in storage. Therefore, measurement of β-carotene concentrations in feeds is not practical and seldom done. Recommended vitamin A consumption rates for various classes of cattle are based on providing supplemental vitamin A, which is derived from commercial sources: for adult cows (lactating and dry)—110 IU/kg body wt, which is ~4,400 IU/kg dry diet; for growing heifers—80 IU/kg body wt, which is ~2,500 IU/kg dry diet. Conditions that can increase dietary vitamin A requirements in adult cows include low forage diets, high corn silage diets, poor quality forages, and infection.

The vitamin A status of cattle may be assessed via serum or hepatic vitamin A concentrations. The liver stores vitamin A for release during periods of insufficient dietary intake, thus making liver the ideal tissue for nutritional assessment. For adult cattle receiving diets with recommended supplemental vitamin A concentrations, hepatic vitamin A concentrations are 300–1,100 mg/kg dry tissue (expressed as retinol). Clinical signs of vitamin A deficiency do not occur until these reserves have been substantially depleted. Adequate serum vitamin A concentrations in adult cattle are 225–500 ng/mL, with values usually dropping to ~150 ng/mL within 1 wk of calving.

Calves are born with low body stores of vitamin A and depend on colostrum consumption to supply hepatic vitamin A stores. The NRC recommends dietary vitamin A concentrations for young calves at ~9,000 IU/kg diet dry matter. Most milk replacer diets have substantially higher concentrations of vitamin A, possibly because vitamin A requirements may be increased by infectious diseases, especially those affecting the respiratory or enteric epithelium.

Vitamin A deficiency is associated initially with night blindness followed by poor growth, poor hair coats, and suppressed immunity. In adult cattle, vitamin A deficiency is associated with retained placentas and impaired fertility.

Vitamin D: Vitamin D is necessary for the absorption and metabolism of calcium and phosphorus. Recent research suggests that vitamin D may also be necessary for immune cell function. Vitamin D_3 (cholecalciferol) can be formed by the solar irradiation of skin or vitamin D_2 by the solar irradiation of forages. However, reliance on natural vitamin D formation is considered unreliable, and vitamin D requirements are based on recommendations for supplement addition to diets. The recommended rate of vitamin D supplementation for adult dairy cows is 30 IU/kg body wt, which would be supplied by diets with ~1,000 IU/kg dry matter.

Vitamin D status can be assessed via blood serum concentrations of 25-hydroxy-cholecalciferol. Adequate values are 20–50 ng/mL, with concentrations <5 ng/mL indicating deficiency.

Vitamin E: Vitamin E is present in relatively high concentrations in fresh forages. Thus, cattle receiving pasture or fresh-cut forages may require little vitamin E supplement. In contrast, vitamin E *degrades in stored forages, so dairy cattle* on typical confinement-reared diets require supplemental vitamin E.

Vitamin E functions to protect cellular membranes from oxidative damage. Clinical manifestations of deficiency include nutritional myopathy (white muscle disease, *see* p 1172) in young calves and diseases in older cattle including retained placenta and increased susceptibility to environmental mastitis.

Recommended rates of vitamin E intake vary based on gestation stage: terminal dry period—1.8 IU/kg body wt, which is ~90 IU/kg dry matter; lactation—0.8 IU/kg body wt, which is ~30 IU/kg dry matter. Much higher concentrations are occasionally supplemented when environmental mastitis is a particular problem. Vitamin E is essentially nontoxic, and there is little risk of oversupplementation.

Vitamin E supplements may be natural or synthetic. Natural sources of vitamin E are derived from plant oils and are designated *RRR*-α-tocopherol or D-α-tocopherol, based on stereoisomer characteristics of their chemical structure. Synthetic supplements are designated all *rac*-α-tocopherol, or DL-α-tocopherol. The natural-source supplements appear to have much greater biologic activity.

Blood serum vitamin E concentrations may be used to assess vitamin E status in dairy cattle. Serum concentrations of 2–4 mcg/mL are generally adequate. However, in addition to vitamin E nutritional status, these concentrations are influenced by the total concentration of serum lipid, with higher serum lipid concentrations resulting in higher vitamin E concentrations. Serum lipids are generally low in late gestation and high in the period of peak feed intake. To compensate for this fluctuation, serum vitamin E concentrations are sometimes expressed as a ratio, with some serum lipid component, such as cholesterol or triglyceride, used as the denominator.

Other Vitamins: Most ruminant diets provide adequate amounts of vitamin K and the B vitamins, either through natural feedstuffs or synthesis by microbial activity in the rumen. Thus, there are no recommended dietary concentrations of these vitamins for ruminants.

FEEDING AND NUTRITIONAL MANAGEMENT

Three general types of nutritional management systems are typically used in dairy production: confinement systems with totally mixed rations (TMRs), confinement systems in which concentrates and forages are fed separately, and pasture-based systems.

Totally Mixed Rations

TMRs have all dietary components included in a single uniform mixture. TMRs have the nutritional advantage over other types of feeding systems, in that fiber and nonfiber ration components are delivered in uniform proportions throughout the feeding period. This minimizes fluctuations in rumen pH and promotes healthy rumen conditions, even at relatively high rates of energy intake.

Adequate management of TMR systems requires a means of accurately weighing each component of the mixture and a mixer capable of incorporating forages and concentrates into a uniform product. Several types of suitable mixers with self-contained weighing devices are available commercially. Many mixers are limited in their capacity to mix long-stemmed forage into the diet, thus limiting the use of dry hay in TMR diets. This means that maintaining particle size adequate to deliver sufficient effective fiber can be a challenge with TMR diets. Limiting the duration of the mixing process helps maintain sufficient effective fiber if silages have adequate particle length initially and the particles are not further comminuted during the mixing process. Sieves to monitor particle size in TMR mixes are available commercially. *See* TABLE 32 for recommended particle size distribution in TMR mixes, based on a popular sieving system.

Frequent monitoring of dry-matter concentrations of moist feeds is particularly important in the management of TMR diets. This is because diets are formulated based on the nutrient concentrations of the feeds on a dry-matter basis, but the ingredients are mixed based on their moist weight. Therefore, accurate dry-matter concentration values are critical to ensure the nutrient profile of the final diet is as intended. Routine analysis of the TMR mixture for major nutrient fractions, such as moisture or fiber, is useful in assuring that the ingredient nutrient profiles and proportions are consistent with the intended diet formulation and are stable over time.

Management of feed delivery and availability is another important aspect in the use of TMR mixes. Cattle should have continuous or nearly continuous access to feed. Adequate bunk space is important, with recommendations for optimal linear space usually 45–60 cm/animal. Bunks should be cleaned daily, and the orts weighed so that daily feed intake for the group may be calculated. To assure optimal feed availability, orts should be 2%–4% of the total amount fed. Particle length of the orts should be measured to assure that sorting of the feed, which usually results in large particles being left behind, is not occurring.

For effective use of TMR diets, cows must be separated into feeding groups: minimally, a lactating and a nonlactating group, and optimally, two or more lactating cow groups and two dry cow groups. One dry cow group should comprise those cows in the first 4–6 wk of the dry period, and the other those in the 2–4 wk before calving. Diets for lactating cow groups should be formulated with a lead factor, meaning the diet should be balanced for more milk production than the average of the group. This is to ensure that the nutrient requirements of the higher-producing cows in the group are met. Optimal lead factors depend on the number of feeding groups and their stage of lactation. When two groups of lactating cows are used, feeding for >20% of the average production is frequently recommended.

Unmixed or Component-fed Rations

Confinement feeding systems in which concentrates are fed separately from forages are traditional in many areas of the world. Advantages of this system relative to the

TABLE 32 PARTICLE SIZE RECOMMENDATIONS FOR TOTALLY MIXED RATIONS[a]

	Pore Size[b] (cm)	Particle Size (cm)	Percentage by Weight
Upper sieve	1.9	>1.9	2–8
Middle sieve	0.79	0.77–1.9	30–50
Lower sieve	0.13	0.18–0.77	30–50
Bottom pan		<0.18	≤20

[a] Based on the use of the Penn State Particle Separator. Data from J. Heinrichs and P. Kononoff, Pennsylvania State University.

[b] Pores are square, so the largest opening is the diagonal.

TMR system include the lack of need for specialized mixing and feed delivery equipment and the ability to adjust concentrate feeding amounts to the needs of individual animals. A major disadvantage is that starch and other nonfiber carbohydrates are generally provided in a small number of meals per day, typically at milking time. Thus, there is the possibility for large fluctuations in rumen pH, which may impair fiber digestion and contribute to poor rumen health. Systems have been developed to avoid large concentrate meals. These include computer-delivered diets in which cows are electronically identified and a computerized feeding apparatus delivers small, individually programmed meals throughout the day.

In addition to the potential for fluctuations in rumen pH, another disadvantage of component feeding systems is the inability to monitor forage intake. This is because there is no direct need to weigh the amount of forage offered if it is not being mixed with other diet components. Thus, there is no means to accurately adjust concentrate intake to match fluctuations in forage consumption. This becomes a particular problem in hot weather during which forage consumption may be reduced substantially while concentrate consumption is less affected. This leads to alterations in the intended proportions of fiber and nonfiber carbohydrates in the diets.

Pasture-based Feeding Systems

Modern means of pasture management have evolved to optimize use of forage resources in pasture systems. Such systems require intensive management of pasture for optimal dry-matter and nutrient yields and for optimal feeding and nutrition of high-producing modern dairy cows. To achieve these objectives, paddocks must be rotated frequently, so forages are consumed at an optimal stage of growth and overgrazing does not occur. Pastures are typically divided into paddocks via the use of easily moved electric fences. Cattle are rotated through paddocks as forages reach stages of growth optimal for both dry-matter yields and nutrient composition.

From a nutritional standpoint, the three major challenges of pasture-based dairy systems are maintaining favorable rumen fermentation conditions, maintaining adequate dry matter intake, and meeting energy and protein requirements. Managing *rumen health* and dietary fiber adequacy can be as challenging with pasture-based systems as with other dairy feeding systems. Lush, rapidly growing pasture grasses with high energy and protein density typically have low NDF concentrations. Thus, rumen fermentation conditions, particularly pH, may be a problem. Supplementing the pasture with dry forages to maintain adequate effective fiber concentrations is frequently necessary.

Dry matter consumption in pasture systems may limit nutrient intake because maximal consumption rates are lower than in confinement systems. This will limit energy intake, thus requiring supplemental energy sources to be fed to achieve high milk production. Milk production rates in unsupplemented pasture feeding situations are seldom >25 kg/day. Energy supplements may include starches such as cereal grains or highly fermentable fiber sources such as grain byproducts. Protein, and particularly sources of RUP, may also need to be supplemented. Protein concentrations in pasture grasses may be high but are generally highly rumen degradable.

FEEDING YOUNG CALVES

To assure adequate passive transfer of antibodies, all calves should receive at least 2 L of high-quality colostrum within 6 hr of birth. Colostrum feeding should continue until calves are 3 days old, but the initial feeding of colostrum is critical for passive transfer of immunity.

Traditional System of Replacement Dairy Calf Feeding

After the period of colostrum feeding, the traditional nutritional strategy for raising dairy replacement calves has been to minimize liquid feed consumption, maximize solid feed consumption, stimulate early rumen development, and wean calves at a relatively young age (usually 4–8 wk). Although growth rates are less than maximal, feed costs are minimal. In addition, the risk of enteric disease after weaning is less than during the liquid feeding period, making early weaning beneficial in the management of enteric disease.

Under this system, targeted rates of gain for calves of the large dairy breeds are ~400–600 g/day for the first 3–4 wk of life. This requires a dry-matter intake of 600–750 g/day; ~450 g of this is supplied from liquid feed, which equates to ~4 L of milk or reconstituted milk replacer/day for calves weighing 40–50 kg at birth. This amount should be divided between at least two feedings/day. The remaining dry matter should come from a high-quality calf starter, which is a concentrate mixture specially prepared for young calves. As calves grow, the amount of liquid feed/day remains constant, and increases in growth rate are accounted for by increases in calf starter consumption.

Liquid feeds for young calves include milk, waste milk, excess colostrum, and milk replacers. Milk and excess colostrum can be high-quality feeds for suckling calves, but adequate biosecurity precautions, such as pasteurization and screening of cows for chronic infectious diseases such as bovine leukosis and Johne's disease, need to be in place.

Milk replacers are designed to mimic bovine milk and thus contain a source of protein, fat, and carbohydrate. Protein concentrations in milk replacers vary from 18% to as much as 30% on a dry-matter basis but typically are 20%–25%. Protein sources in milk replacers vary and may substantially affect the quality of the replacer. Proteins derived from milk sources, such as whey protein isolate, delactosed whey, dried skim milk, and casein, are generally excellent sources of protein, but the quality of even these protein sources may be affected by processing methods. Other animal proteins such as plasma proteins also may be of good quality. Plant protein sources vary in their acceptability, particularly for calves <3 wk old. Appropriately processed plant proteins may be acceptable but are generally less desirable than animal proteins for calves <3 wk old. Plant proteins acceptable for use in milk replacers include soy protein isolate and soy protein concentrate; these proteins may be processed to reduce antigenicity and to remove antinutritional factors such as trypsin inhibitor. The degree of processing varies by manufacturer, and not all milk replacers containing these protein sources are of equal quality. Unprocessed soy flour is an unacceptable protein source for milk replacers.

Fat concentrations in milk replacers vary from 10% to as high as 30%, with most in the range of 15%–20%. Fat sources usually contain some coconut oil and major contributions from tallow, choice white grease, or lard. Lecithin and/or monoglycerides are usually added as emulsifying agents. Fat concentration substantially influences the energy concentration of milk replacer. In cold climates in which high energy consumption is critical for young calves, fat concentration should be ≥15%. The drawback of higher fat concentrations is that the rate of starter consumption is reduced as replacer fat concentrations increase.

Early introduction of solid feed is important for replacement calf rearing. Solid feed stimulates rumen development. Calves are born with small, nonfunctional rumens, and rapid rumen development is critical for early weaning. Rumen maturation is stimulated by the presence of fermentation products, particularly butyric acid. Thus, introduction of highly fermentable substrate into the diet is important to rumen development. High-quality calf starters are composed of highly fermentable carbohydrates in a mixture that is coarse in texture, contains few fine or powdery particles, and has a relatively high fiber concentration (~12%–15% NDF). The crude protein concentration should be ~18%–24% on a dry-matter basis. Calves should not be fed hay before weaning. Hay consumption may actually impede rumen development, because hay is less fermentable than concentrate.

A critical factor in stimulating starter consumption is the availability of fresh water. Calves should have readily available fresh water. Water consumption will vary greatly by calf but may be >4 L/day in addition to milk or milk replacer.

Feeding Calves in Cold Weather

The lower limit of the thermoneutral zone for calves between birth and 3 wk of age is 20° C and for calves >3 wk old, 10° C. Maintenance energy requirements increase as temperatures fall below these values. To compensate for these increased energy requirements, milk replacers with fat concentrations ≥15% should be fed in cold weather. Furthermore, the amount of dry powder should be increased by 50 g/day for each incremental decline of 5° C below the thermoneutral zone. For example, if calves <3 wk old are receiving milk replacer powder at 450 g/day at ≥20° C, the amount should be increased to 650 g/day at 0° C and to 900 g/day at –25° C. The dry powder should be reconstituted with proportionate increases in the amount of water. Feeding this amount of liquid frequently requires more than two feedings per day. In addition to milk or milk replacer, fresh water should be made available at least twice per day.

Feeding Calves with Enteric Disease

Diarrhea is a common condition in young calves and frequently results in life-threatening dehydration. Electrolyte solutions administered orally can be beneficial in supporting hydration and successfully treating calves with diarrhea. To help control and correct dehydration, it may be necessary to reduce milk or milk replacer feeding for a brief period after the onset of diarrhea. Nutritionally, however, the objective is for calves being treated for diarrhea to be back receiving milk or milk replacer as soon as possible. With appropriate use of oral electrolytes, milk or milk replacer feeding should be reinstituted within 12–24 hr after the onset of diarrhea. Electrolyte solutions can be fed along with milk or milk replacer. Supporting the calf with adequate nutrition speeds restoration of the gut epithelium and generally improves calf health and immunity.

FEEDING CALVES FROM WEANING THROUGH MATURATION

After weaning, calves should receive free-choice calf starter until 3 mo old. If hay is fed during this period, it should be of excellent quality and fed in limited amounts. Energy requirements for adequate growth in calves 3–15 mo old may be derived largely from good quality forage. Meeting protein requirements during this period is challenging, because protein requirements are high relative to energy requirements. This is because in replacement heifers, lean body weight gain is preferred over fattening. For sample diets for large-breed dairy heifers 3–15 mo old, *see* TABLE 33. The crude protein concentrations of these example diets are high, because there is excess RDP. If rumen bypass (high RUP) ingredients were included, the crude protein concentrations could be lower and still meet the metabolizable protein requirements. However, such RUP concentrations would be difficult to achieve without inclusion of animal-protein products or specially processed protein supplements. Diets such as those in these examples would best be delivered as TMR.

Heifers of appropriate body weight become sexually mature at ~15 mo old and should be bred at that time. After breeding, requirements for protein and energy during gestation may be met with good quality forages. In general, the feeding of corn silage during this period should be limited to no more than one-half of the diet dry matter, preferably less. This it to prevent fattening, which increases disease risk at calving.

Optimal growth rates of dairy heifers between 2 mo of age and conception are important for dairy herd profitability. Insufficient growth rates result in either an older age at first calving, which increases the cost of heifer rearing, or smaller dams at first calving, which limits milk production and conception rates during the first lactation. Conversely, excessive growth rates, especially those associated primarily with fattening, can adversely affect subsequent milk production and also increase the risk of metabolic problems at calving. Target growth rates between weaning and conception should be 700–900 g/day. As growth rates increase within this range, the proportion of crude protein and RUP in the diet needs to be

TABLE 33 EXAMPLE DIETARY CHARACTERISTICS FOR GROWING REPLACEMENT HEIFERS

	Body Wt (kg)			
	100	150	200	250
DMI (kg/day)	3.1	4.2	5.2	6.1
Concentrates (% of dry matter)	40	20	5	0
Forage (% of dry matter)	60	80	95	100
Crude protein (% of dry matter)	21	20	18.5	18.4
Metabolizable protein (% of dry matter)	11.7	9.6	8.5	7.7
RUP (% of CP)	32%	28%	22%	21%
RDP (% of CP)	68%	72%	78%	79%
ME (Mcal/kg)	2.5	2.4	2.2	2.2

Based on requirements generated by the computer program that accompanies *Nutrient Requirements of Dairy Cattle*, 2001, National Academy of Sciences, National Academy Press, Washington, DC. The crude protein requirements of animals <150 kg are relatively high and could be reduced by the use of protein sources with higher RUP proportions. DMI, dry matter intake; RUP, rumen undegradable protein; RDP, rumen degradable protein; ME, metabolizable energy.

increased to support greater lean body gain and prevent fattening. Weight and height should be measured periodically to check that growth rates and frame development are as intended. The growth response of heifers to apparently similar diets varies greatly among farms, making the monitoring of growth rates particularly important. For target body weight values at a range of age increments for heifers of various mature body sizes, *see* TABLE 34.

The different dietary requirements of calves at various ages dictate that they be kept in separate pens based on their age and size. Calves between weaning and 5 mo old should be kept in groups of six or less. Older calves may be kept in larger groups, but animal size should be fairly uniform.

ACCELERATED CALF-REARING PROGRAMS

In accelerated calf rearing programs, larger quantities of liquid feeds are fed during the preweaning period, and larger proportions of concentrates are fed during the growing period. Weaning is later, and solid feed

TABLE 34 RECOMMENDED BODY WEIGHTS FOR HEIFERS OF DIFFERENT AGES

Heifer Age (mo)	Approximate Target Body Wt (kg)			
	% of Mature Body Weight	Small Breeds	Medium Breeds	Large Breeds
Birth	6.2	28	34	47
1	9.1	41	50	68
2	12.3	55	68	92
3	16.2	73	89	122
4	20.0	90	110	150
5	23.7	107	130	178
6	27.5	124	151	206
7	31.2	140	172	234
8	35.0	158	193	263
9	38.9	175	214	291
10	42.5	191	234	319
11	46.3	208	255	347
12	49.9	224	274	374
13	53.7	242	295	403
14	57.4	258	316	430
15	61.1	275	336	458
16	64.7	291	356	485
17	68.5	308	377	513
18	72.2	325	397	541
19	76.0	342	418	570
20	79.6	358	438	597
21	83.3	375	458	625
22	87.1	392	479	653
23	90.8	409	499	681

consumption is delayed (relative to traditional programs). After weaning, forage is not offered until heifers are >3 mo old. Dietary protein concentrations during the pre- and postweaning periods are increased (relative to traditional programs) to assure adequate lean gain and to avoid excessive fattening. Rates of gain can be as high as 1 kg/day, with heifers entering the milking herd at 22–23 mo old. Close monitoring is necessary to assure that heifers have adequate frame development and do not become excessively fat.

FEED ADDITIVES

Many non-nutrient feed additives are marketed and approved for use in dairy cattle (*see* TABLE 35).

NUTRITION AND DISEASE

Nutrition has a large effect on the occurrence and severity of many diseases of dairy cattle. *See* TABLE 36 for brief descriptions of nutritionally associated diseases, disease signs, etc.

TABLE 35 FEED ADDITIVES INCLUDED FOR NON-NUTRIENT BENEFITS

Additive	Effect	Feeding Rate
HIGH PROBABILITY OF POSITIVE ECONOMIC RETURN IN GENERAL FEEDING SITUATIONS		
Rumensin	Increased feed efficiency, improved energy metabolism	200–400 mg/day
Sodium bicarbonate and other buffers	Improved feed consumption, stabilization of rumen pH, increased butterfat production	0.75% of dry matter
Yeast culture	Improved feed consumption, improved fiber digestion	Variable, consult manufacturer directions
HIGH PROBABILITY OF POSITIVE ECONOMIC RETURN IN SPECIFIC PROBLEM SITUATIONS		
Strong anion additives for prepartum diets	Improved calcium homeostasis, milk fever prevention	Variable, calculate DCAD[a], monitor urine pH and dry-matter intake, late gestation only
Propylene glycol	Improved energy metabolism, ketosis prevention	300–500 mL/day, late gestation and early lactation only
Niacin	Improved lipid metabolism, improved rumen fermentation, increased feed efficiency and milk component concentrations	6 g/day, include protected and unprotected sources
Mycotoxin neutralizers	Many products available; effectiveness best demonstrated against aflatoxin; effectiveness against trichothecene toxins including DON[b] or vomitoxin needs further evaluation.	Variable, consult manufacturer instructions
Protected choline	Improved lipid metabolism, fatty liver and ketosis prevention	15 g/day, late gestation and early lactation only

[a] DCAD (dietary cation-anion difference)

[b] DON (deoxynivalenol)

TABLE 36 DISEASES OR CLINICAL SIGNS IN DAIRY CATTLE THAT MAY BE RELATED TO DIETARY CHARACTERISTICS OR NUTRITIONAL DEFICIENCIES

Sign	Possible Nutrient or Dietary Involvement
Abortion (*see* p 1333)	Deficiencies of trace minerals or vitamins, especially selenium, vitamin A, or vitamin E
Anemia (*see* p 7)	Possible copper or cobalt deficiency in adult cattle; iron deficiency in young calves (unlikely in adult cattle)
Blindness and night blindness	May be an initial isolated sign of polioencephalomalacia; may be associated with vitamin A deficiency, with or without signs of corneal opacity
Bloat (*see* p 227)	Consumption of legume pastures or finely ground, high-starch diets (such as are frequently fed to feedlot cattle) are predisposing; cattle not acclimated to these diets are particularly susceptible
CNS signs	Incoordination, blindness, nystagmus, thrashing, and opisthotonos may be associated with polioencephalomalacia; high-starch diets with microbial inactivation of thiamine and high-sulfur diets such as those associated with heavy feeding of distiller's grains and solubles
Congenital defects	Deficiencies of vitamin A, manganese, or copper
Convulsions	Sign of vitamin A deficiency, particularly if they occur intermittently interspersed with periods of normal activity in growing calves; should be differentiated from nervous coccidiosis
Cystic ovaries (*see* p 1354)	Energy insufficiency and associated subclinical ketosis in early lactation are predisposing; vitamin E and selenium deficiency speculated to contribute
Diarrhea	Numerous dietary factors, including abrupt changes in diet, especially those associated with increases in dietary nonfiber carbohydrates and dietary rumen fermentability; lush rapidly growing pasture and increased dietary protein or salt concentrations
Displaced abomasum (*see* p 238)	Both metabolic and nutritional causes; feeding should be to prevent ketosis and stimulate high dry-matter intakes; both pre- and postpartum diets are important in management
Dyspnea	Atypical interstitial pneumonia associated with movement of cattle from poor pasture to lush pasture; associated with ruminal conversion of tryptophan to 3-methyl indole
Fatty liver (*see* p 1018)	Overfattening in late lactation or during the dry period accompanied by poor feed intake in late gestation and early lactation
Hypomagnesemic tetany (*see* p 996)	Functional and absolute magnesium deficiency; risk increases with consumption of lush pasture grasses, especially with high potassium concentrations
Inappetence (off feed)	Many nutritional deficiencies (protein, mineral, vitamin) eventually result in reduced feed intake
Incoordination	Blind staggers associated with chronic selenium intoxication; demyelinization associated with copper deficiency
Infertility	Energy is the most clearly associated nutrient; insufficiencies of carotene or manganese may affect ovarian function

(*continued*)

TABLE 36 DISEASES OR CLINICAL SIGNS IN DAIRY CATTLE THAT MAY BE RELATED TO DIETARY CHARACTERISTICS OR NUTRITIONAL DEFICIENCIES *(continued)*

Sign	Possible Nutrient or Dietary Involvement
Ketosis (*see* p 1024)	Excessive lipid mobilization and insufficient gluconeogenesis; overfattening in late gestation and insufficient feed intake in early lactation are the primary nutritional influences
Laminitis (*see* p 1082)	Chronic or acute laminitis and their sequelae are thought to result from diets with high concentrations of nonfiber carbohydrates
Milk fever (parturient paresis, *see* p 988)	Caused by failure of calcium homeostasis rather than dietary calcium deficiency; control by feeding low-calcium diets or acidifying diets prepartum
Pica and dirt eating	Common causes are not well determined; sodium deficiency, potentially phosphorus deficiency, low-fiber diets implicated
Polioencephalomalacia (*see* p 1281)	Associated with either ruminal destruction of thiamine or with ruminal production of hydrogen sulfide associated with high-sulfur diets; more common in feedlot than dairy cattle
Retained fetal membranes (*see* p 1381)	Deficiencies of selenium, vitamin A, or vitamin E, but adding these nutrients to adequate diets will not reduce incidence; metabolic problems associated with prepartum negative energy balance may also be predisposing
Rickets and osteomalacia (*see* p 1051)	Insufficient calcium, phosphorus, or vitamin D consumption
Rumen acidosis, acute clinical	Usually associated with major errors or inconsistencies in feed delivery in which high starch intake occurs in cattle unaccustomed to such diets; associated with formation of lactic acid in the rumen with severe drops in rumen pH
Rumen acidosis, chronic subclinical (*see* p 225)	Associated with lactation diets with high nonfiber carbohydrate concentrations and low fiber concentrations; also associated with high rumen concentrations of volatile fatty acids and rumen pH values ≤5.2
Skin problems	Problems such as dull, brittle hair coats, hypotrichia, easily depilated hair, hyperkeratosis, thin skin, and poor healing may be associated with nutritional problems; deficiencies of vitamin A and zinc, generalized protein-calorie malnutrition
Sudden death	Deficiencies of vitamins A or E, selenium, or copper
Suppressed immunity	Generalized immunosuppression, including both cellular and humoral immunity, may occur due to malnutrition; specific nutrient deficiencies include vitamin A, vitamin E, zinc, copper, and selenium; also generalized protein-calorie malnutrition
Toxicities	Many toxicities associated with feedborne toxicants; including nitrates, cyanide, many mycotoxins, toxic plants
Urolithiasis (*see* p 1502)	Diets with high phosphorus and low fiber concentrations
Wasting and failure to thrive	Signs of many nutritional deficiencies, as well as of chronic diseases such as internal parasitism; cobalt deficiency is a well-documented cause of ill thrift in cattle; protein-calorie malnutrition should always be evaluated
White muscle disease (*see* p 1172)	Dietary deficiency of selenium or vitamin E

NUTRITION: EXOTIC AND ZOO ANIMALS

The field of zoo and exotic animal nutrition continues to make advances that result in better diets. Exotic animal nutritionists in zoos and in the feed industry are studying problems and generating information on proper nutritional management for many species.

All animals require nutrients and energy in a metabolizable form. The nutrients and energy must be properly balanced and in the correct form to accommodate particular tastes, digestive systems, and feeding methods. For example, large psittacines typically use their feet to hold food, whereas other species obtain or position food using other appendages (or they do not manipulate food). If a commercial extruded food is fed, the pieces must be large enough for the bird to grasp easily. Diets for exotic and zoo animals have been developed by considering food habits in the wild, oral and GI tract morphology, nutrient requirements established for domestic and laboratory animals and people, nutritional research on exotic species, and practical experience. The ultimate criteria to evaluate the suitability of a diet for a given species are growth, reproductive success, and longevity.

The minimum nutrient requirements established by the National Research Council (NRC) for domestic and laboratory animals can be useful starting points in setting target nutrient levels for an exotic species. For example, the Nutrient Requirements of Small Ruminants, published by the NRC in 2007, contains nutritional information on cervids (white-tailed deer, red deer, wapiti, and caribou) and camelids (llamas and alpacas).

For many exotic species that have closely related domestic counterparts, diets can be formulated to contain nutrients that would meet the requirements established for ungulates, mustelids, canids, felids, rodents, primates, lagomorphs, gallinaceous and anseriform birds, and fish. However, nutrient requirements established by the NRC should be used only as guidelines, because the goals of livestock producers in feeding their animals include rapid and efficient gain and high milk yield or egg production—goals that differ from the goals in zoo animal management. In zoos and other exotic animal collections, a maintenance diet should be fed in general, although a breeding or other specific diet may be needed sometimes, depending on the animal and circumstances.

Although the NRC requirements are less directly applicable to other species, they can still serve as a useful general reference to evaluate the nutritional adequacy for most birds and mammals. The formulation and evaluation of diets for reptiles and amphibians is even more difficult, because there are no domestic animal models and because metabolic rates of poikilothermic animals fluctuate with changes in ambient temperature. Once the nutrient concentrations for the diet have been established, the types and amounts of foodstuffs, methods of presentation, and feeding frequencies should be selected based on the physical and behavioral attributes of the species.

All food should be of good quality. Spoiled or moldy foods, or foods stored for long periods (eg, >1 yr for most bagged feeds and 6–12 mo for most frozen foods) should not be fed. The practice of "topping off" the feed bowl daily or every other day should be discouraged, because uneaten food on the bottom can spoil. Food and water dishes should be thoroughly cleaned before adding food or water. Clean, fresh water should always be available to nonmarine species. Trace mineral salt blocks, bricks, or "spools" are commonly offered to ungulates, psittacine birds, and some rodents.

Cafeteria-style feeding is strongly discouraged, because captive animals rarely select a balanced diet if given a wide selection of foods. Usually, a nutritionally complete commercial product or in-house mixture that cannot be sorted should comprise the bulk of the diet, with components such as meat, fruit, and seeds comprising only a small percentage. Pelleted diets are especially important with psittacines, to avoid self-selection of calcium-deficient seeds.

To improve consumption of pelleted diets, feeding should be done in the morning, with the other food items offered during the day. All diet items to be fed should be weighed, and the actual intake recorded.

Muscle and organ meat, fruit, most grains and seeds, and most insects are poor sources of calcium, and excess consumption can result in calcium deficiency. Calcium gut-loading diets containing at least 12%–15% calcium should be fed to insects.

Dusting with a balanced calcium-phosphorus powder is also a possibility; however, it is doubtful this can add enough calcium to the diet. Other sources of calcium include oyster shell, cuttle bone, and ground calcium carbonate tablets.

Obesity is more common than inadequate nutrient intake. Ungulates, primates, and carnivores can rapidly become overweight when excess amounts of a high-quality diet are offered, particularly when activity is limited. In some birds (eg, ratites, waterfowl), rapid growth rates increase the incidence of leg and wing problems. Both adult and growing animals should be routinely weighed to monitor changes. If weighing four times a year is not possible, a body score index should be performed.

If a dietary change is contemplated because of suspected nutrient imbalances, deficiencies, or toxicities, the diet currently fed should first be computer-analyzed to assess nutrient concentrations. Ingredient or nutrient changes can then be made based on correcting a suspected or confirmed health problem. For captive, exotic animals, establishing and maintaining dietary histories can be particularly helpful in health assessment. Activity patterns of individuals are also important (eg, atherosclerosis is relatively common in obese birds).

Nutritional Supplements: The use of nutritional supplements is popular among animal caretakers. Although many keepers and pet owners use nutritionally complete feeds that require no supplementation, supplements are still often provided. The nutrient content of the current diet should be established or estimated first to determine whether any supplement is needed or whether a supplement should be discontinued. Unfortunately, diets are rarely evaluated first to determine which nutrients (if any) are unbalanced.

If a nutrient is deficient in a diet, a specific supplement in a specific amount should be recommended. Excessive supplementation of some nutrients (eg, some fat-soluble vitamins, selenium, copper) can be just as harmful as not enough because of toxicity and nutrient imbalance. Diets consisting primarily of grain products and cultivated fruits and vegetables may need micronutrient supplementation; however, supplements vary widely in their composition.

Water: Water intake should be assessed routinely but especially in animals with compromised renal function, in lizards or birds prone to gout, and in animals under conditions of high temperature or low humidity in which evaporative losses can be expected. The salt content of water should be known, because some species are less tolerant than others. Animals fed dry feeds (pellets, extrusions, hay, etc) require more water than those fed succulent feeds. Potable water should be available ad lib.

Many animals in the wild consume much of their water in the foods they eat. When low-moisture foods are consumed (pellets, extrusions, etc), some animals, depending on how water is presented, may not maintain adequate hydration. Many free-ranging small and tropical lizards receive water from foods and from licking drops that accumulate after rainfall. When in captivity, they frequently do not drink readily from containers. In nature, birds of prey do not drink; however, in captivity, they do drink sometimes, depending on the circumstances, so clean drinking water must be available at all times.

Humidity may be especially important to maintain hydration of many reptiles, especially tropical species. Daily misting with warm water is an important source of hydration for some lizards that may not be observed drinking standing water. Eye lesions in semiaquatic turtles (eg, box turtles) and some tortoises may be the result of low environmental humidity (or possibly upper respiratory tract disease) and not vitamin A deficiency. Conjunctivitis may respond better to supportive antibiotic therapy and higher humidity than to supplemental vitamin A. Dietary histories may be especially important in such cases, because many captive turtles are fed commercial food, which is mostly cat food high in vitamin A.

For a discussion of nutrition for orphaned animals, *see* p 2100.

BIRDS

The exact nutritional requirements for most species of birds are still unknown. The exceptions are birds raised for food or other products, such as poultry, ducks, ostriches, and pheasants. Avian diets for many species are extrapolated from the *Nutrient Requirements of Poultry* published by the NRC.

PSITTACINES

The pet bird population consists largely of psittacine species, primarily passerines and other genera such as those that include toucans. Psittacines eat mainly a plant-based diet and can be classified overall as florivores. The content of the diet—fruit, nectar, seeds, or a combination—varies by species. Some species ingest a percentage of insects or carrion. Although requirements and dietary sensitivities vary among psittacine species, the pelleted and extruded diets that have been produced for parrots have tremendously improved the nutritional intake and subsequent health and quality of life of these birds. However, pelleted diets differ in content and quality and must be evaluated individually. Extruded pellets in different shapes and sizes are available for maintenance and breeding purposes. Many pellets contain omega-3 fatty acids as well as probiotics.

Psittacine nutrition has been the focus of research throughout the past several decades. Several myths of psittacine nutrition have been debunked during this period. Grit, while probably necessary for some passerines and Columbiformes to aid in mechanical digestion, is not needed by psittacines. If seeds are consumed by psittacines, they are hulled before ingestion. Monkey chow biscuits are nutritionally incomplete, and some brands tend to harbor bacteria or promote excessive gram-negative bacterial growth when included in bird diets. Strictly seed diets, regardless of supplementation, are suboptimal for psittacine species. Deficiencies of vitamin A, protein (the amino acids lysine and methionine, in particular), calcium, and other nutrients are seen in most psittacine species on seed-based diets. Conversely, excessive vitamins, such as vitamin A, are added to some pelleted diets, which can have equally detrimental effects.

Protein: Protein (amino acid) requirements of psittacines have not been well established. The amino acid deficiencies most consistently noted in psittacine birds on seed-based and table-food diets are lysine and methionine. Fiber content must always be considered when determining dietary protein requirements, because increased fiber causes increased fecal protein "loss." Birds with low-fiber, more readily digestible diets (such as nectar-feeding lories and lorikeets) may do well on diets with easily digestible protein levels as low as 3%–5%. Adult maintenance levels of protein for budgerigars and cockatiels (7%–12%) are lower than those for African Grey parrots (10%–15%). Protein requirements for growth and for egg-laying hens are higher than maintenance levels in all birds. Periods of heavy molt also greatly increase protein requirements, particularly the need for the sulfur-containing amino acid cysteine, because feathers average 25% of the total body protein content of birds.

Excessively high dietary protein has the potential to cause renal insufficiency and gout in birds with preexisting renal impairment or a genetic predisposition to gout. Cockatiels with no preexisting renal disease have been shown to tolerate extremely high dietary protein levels (up to 70%) with no renal impairment. A genetic predisposition to renal disease/gout has been documented in some strains of poultry and may be seen in other avian species.

Sudden, dramatic increases in dietary protein may overload the kidneys, producing hyperuricemia and visceral gout. When increased dietary protein is indicated, it should be increased gradually to avoid renal damage.

Fat: Dietary fat provides essential fatty acids, energy, and hormone precursors. It also contributes to egg yolk formation and aids in absorption of fat-soluble vitamins. Diets should contain 5%–12% fat, depending on the species, the general condition of the psittacines, and the physiologic stage and brood condition. At least 1% of the dry diet should consist of PUFA (eg, linoleic acid). Excessive dietary fat leads to obesity, metabolic diseases, cardiac disease, and atherosclerosis (*see also* PET BIRDS, p 1885). The fat requirements of psittacines for reproduction are generally lower than those of poultry, because the psittacines' altricial young do not require the same quantity of fatty acids as do the precocial young of chickens. However, diets that are borderline deficient often manifest as problems in either the psittacine hen or the chicks during reproduction.

Vitamins: Vitamin A is necessary for vision, reproduction, immunologic integrity, and growth, and for the maintenance of epithelial cells in respiratory, GI, and renal tissues. Vitamin A deficiency has historically been noted in psittacines on all-seed diets, so supplementation is commonly recommended. However, indiscriminate supplementation leads to vitamin A toxicosis, as well as to decreased absorption of other fat-soluble vitamins and carotenoids. In nature, psittacines do not consume vitamin A but obtain vitamin A precursors such as carotenoids from various plants. Pelleted diets should contain vitamin A at levels of 5,000–8,000 IU/kg of feed. Higher amounts should be avoided. The source of vitamin A added to bird feed is not regulated, and significant quality control issues have been documented.

Ideally, a quality pelleted diet for psittacines will contain multiple carotenoids and other vitamin A precursors, with a minimum level of vitamin A.

Some **carotenoids** in birds are precursors for the body's formation of vitamin A. Carotenoids also act as antioxidants and are necessary in some species (such as canaries and flamingos) for feather pigmentation.

The primary function of **vitamin D** is to increase absorption of calcium and phosphorus. Vitamin D can be obtained either directly from the diet or from UVB (285–315 nm) light exposure. Vitamin D deficiency is probably rare in nature because of exposure to sunlight. Birds living in polar conditions get their vitamin D during the winter by consuming diets with high amounts of vitamin D (eg, fish, plankton). In the absence of natural sunlight, the minimum oral vitamin D requirement for African Greys is likely to be 500–1,000 IU/kg.

Vitamin D deficiency may be caused by dietary deficiency or lack of exposure to UVB radiation. Limited studies have shown that species variation in psittacines for UVB light requirements exist. Unfortunately, many birds are housed totally indoors, and owners often mistakenly assume either that the birds do not need direct sunlight or that the sunlight the birds receive through glass will supply UVB radiation. Owners of pet birds should be encouraged to expose their bird to direct sunlight (with appropriate cautions regarding excessive heat) or to purchase and properly use UVB bulbs. However, pet bird owners must consider that the further away from the equator, the less UVB is generated, especially in late autumn, winter, and early spring. Some research indicates that UVA and/or UVB can affect vitamin D synthesis in some bird species, the finding of food, well-being, and feather colors. However, more research is needed to determine how much UVA and/or UVB is needed for each bird species.

Vitamin D toxicity is caused by excessive supplementation. Some psittacine species, notably macaws, are sensitive to excessive dietary vitamin D and may develop soft-tissue calcification and renal failure. Toxic levels for psittacines have not been established, but levels that may be toxic for poultry begin at 2,800 IU/kg of feed.

For discussion of **vitamin E**, *see* p 2291.

PASSERINES

The order Passeriformes contains >5,000 species of birds and includes frugivorous, carnivorous, insectivorous, and granivorous species. Most passerines maintained as pets (finches and canaries) have historically been fed primarily seed and are considered florivorous to granivorous. Commercial seed mixtures for canaries often contain a mixture of canary, rape, niger, hemp, linseed, and oats. Most of these commercially available seed mixtures are deficient in numerous vitamins and amino acids. The fat-soluble vitamins A, D_3, E, and K are generally low, the calcium:phosphorus ratio is poor, and the amino acids lysine and methionine are insufficient. High amounts of fat in seed-based diets can lead to obesity and to nutritional disorders in the offered food (eg, calcium and vitamin deficiency, as well as an amino acid disorder).

Egg food (hard-boiled egg–based soft food with added vitamins and minerals) has traditionally been fed by canary breeders during the reproductive season, with soaked seed added to increase acceptance. Extruded pellets, such as organic pellets or pellet-based mash, which contains balanced nutrients, are offered by many breeders as a nutritionally consistent alternative. Pellets are fed for maintenance or breeding purposes. Extruded pellets fed for breeding contain 18%–22% crude protein as well as a limited amount of fat (5%–8%), compared with the high amounts of fat in seeds.

Soluble grit (ie, oyster shell, cuttlebone) should be provided to canaries and finches. Sprouts, fruits, and vegetables may be psychologically stimulating and enhance breeding in these passerines.

Plumage colors in canaries partially depend on the pigments in the diet. For example, red-colored canaries are fed canthaxanthins before breeding season. Carotenoids vary in their bioavailability, and there are species differences in the types of carotenoids absorbed and metabolized.

COLUMBIFORMES

(Pigeons and doves)

Most pigeons are either primarily granivorous or frugivorous, with some invertebrates also consumed. Seed-eating pigeons and doves can be fed commercial pigeon pellets (2 mm). These pellets should be comparable in composition to that listed in the NRC requirement of growing chickens 6–12 wk old. Alternatively, psittacine small pellets and mash are accepted by most Columbiformes but, depending on the composition, may have to be supplemented.

Columbiforme parents feed their young with crop milk, which is produced from desquamated epithelial cells and glandular secretions of the crop. Crop milk is rich in fat and protein, devoid of carbohydrates, has a low pH, and contains several *Lactobacillus* species. Seed-eating pigeons switch in 3–5 days from crop milk production to feeding their young mostly regurgitated seed. Frugivorous pigeon squabs (eg, crowned pigeons) rely on crop milk for at least 30 days.

RAPTORS

Raptors include birds of prey from many genera. Most medium to large raptors consume whole vertebrate prey. Commonly fed items include mice, rats, day-old chicks, quail, and pigeons. Kestrels generally consume insects. Fish are the natural diet of piscivorous raptors such as ospreys and sea eagles. If fish is fed, thiamine supplementation (30–35 mg/kg feed) as well as vitamin E (100 mg/kg) is advised.

Commercial diets for birds of prey are available and consist mostly of a mash of several different prey items with a specific amount of vitamins and minerals.

Small raptors (100–200 g) eat as much as 20%–25% of their body wt/day; raptors weighing 200–800 g eat 15%, raptors weighing 800–7,000 g eat 6%–10%, and raptors >7,000 g eat 3.5% of their body wt/day. Captive raptors should be weighed regularly, and food volume adjusted as needed to prevent emaciation as well as obesity. If weighing is not possible, the breast-comb can be checked: if sharp, the animal is emaciated; if fat, it is obese.

The best food for birds of prey is mice and rats; however, day-old chicks and other whole birds or mammal species also are an adequate feed. The egg yolk of day-old chicks should not be removed when fed, because it contains a considerable amount of vitamins and minerals. It is advised not to feed animals from the wild (eg, rats, pigeons, rabbits) because of potential diseases, toxins, and poisonings.

Although whole prey, including their organs, should be a complete nutrient sufficient feed, it is advised to add a small amount of a balanced vitamin and mineral supplement, especially when the birds are under stress. Prey with relatively large bones must be avoided because of obstructions in the gizzard, which prevent casting. Birds <12 days old should not be fed too many bones, because they cannot digest them, and metabolic bone diseases can result. Metabolic bone diseases can also result when a chick is growing too fast. Birds of prey should not be fed before travelling. If an organ meat–based diet is fed, vitamins and minerals should be supplemented; calcium supplementation should be 10 g of calcium carbonate/kg of fresh meat.

PISCIVOROUS BIRDS

Penguins, pelicans, and other fish-eating species in the wild feed primarily on fish, crustaceans, and squid. These food sources vary in their fatty acid, vitamin, and carbohydrate contents. In captivity, squid, smelt, herring, mackerel, and whiting fish are commonly available. One of the most important aspects of feeding piscivorous birds is fish quality (*see* p 2297). It is advised to feed several fish species, although in some cases one species of fish has been fed for a lifetime. Captive seabirds develop strong preferences for a particular fish if it is fed exclusively for prolonged periods, which can lead to both nutritional deficiencies and inanition if the feeder fish becomes unavailable.

Supplements commonly given to captive penguins include vitamins A, D, B_1, and E. The need for these and the quantity that must be supplemented depends on the quality and content of the primary diet. Supplements can be added to the fish as tablets, as a gel, or as a liquid to be injected in the fish.

Dietary salt (NaCl; 0.5–1 g salt/bird/day) is often provided to birds in freshwater exhibits to help maintain proper functioning of the salt glands.

Thiamine: The process of thawing fish in running water depletes them of water-soluble vitamins. Additionally, several fish species contain thiaminase, leading to thiamine (B_1) deficiency during the defrosting process.

Supplementation of thiamine is recommended at 30–35 mg/kg fish, daily.

Vitamin E: Most fish are deficient in vitamin E. Clinical signs of vitamin E deficiency in piscivorous birds include weakness and inability to stand or hold the wings in normal posture. Severe generalized myopathy with muscle atrophy, degeneration and necrosis, and replacement with fibrous connective tissue can occur with chronic pronounced vitamin E deficiency. Supplementation with 100 IU vitamin E/kg fish has been proposed. However, oversupplementation (vitamin E at 500–10,500 IU/kg food) may result in decreased growth and coagulation disorders, possibly from creating vitamin K deficiency rather than directly from vitamin E toxicity.

Hand feeding of species and individuals of concern will ensure that each bird receives the proper amount of food and supplement. Some piscivorous species will accept commercial bird-of-prey diets, trout pellets, and/or mice in the diet, as well as fish.

WATERFOWL

The order Anseriformes includes ducks, geese, and swans. These waterfowl vary from strictly herbivorous (swans, most geese, most ducks) to highly piscivorous (marine ducks, mergansers). Commercial duck or game-bird pellets should contain 14%–17% protein and 3%–6% fat with an adequate vitamin mineral supplement. During breeding season, the amount of protein can be increased to 16%–18%. In winter in colder areas, more fat can be added by adding 20% of corn to the diet. Piscivorous waterfowl consume mostly a fish-based pellet containing 25%–40% protein and 5%–10% fat. Some breeders prefer to feed a "sinking" or "floating" waterfowl pellet in the water. However, pellets fed in water should not be allowed to dissolve before consumption.

Swans and geese are fed the same diet as herbivorous ducks. Although waterfowl can live on only nutrient adequate pellets, usually some lettuce is also fed.

Diets of only lettuce and corn, which are unfortunately often provided, lead to protein and multiple vitamin deficiencies. These often manifest as poor plumage, swollen joints, and pododermatitis.

As is true for most bird species, young waterfowl should be fed starter pellets with higher fat (5%–8%) and protein (16%–20%) content. However, excessively rapid growth of large waterfowl must be avoided to prevent bone and joint deformities, such as angel wing and perosis.

GALLINACEOUS BIRDS

Many gallinaceous birds are omnivorous. Commercial diets for domestic fowl, domestic turkeys, and Japanese quail are available. During nonbreeding periods, a maintenance diet can be offered two or three times daily and generally should contain <20% crude protein. During the breeding season, food should be offered free choice and contain a higher protein content (20%–25% crude protein).

Most quail are primarily seed-eaters and are easy to feed. Some Old World quail species are insectivorous and must be provided a diet with specific protein requirements. Peafowl in general (*Pavo* spp) consume invertebrates, mollusks, beetle larvae, and in the case of the Indian blue peafowl, even the venomous cobra. Other gallinaceous birds consume almost exclusively vegetable material. The tragopans (*Tragopan* spp), some pheasants (*Syrmaticus* spp), and several species of grouse are largely vegetarian. Tragopans consume sprouts, grasses, mosses, berries, and a few insects. In captivity, tragopans can be fed lucerne, grasses, cucumbers, apples, and different kinds of berries. Grouse are noted for their ability to feed on plants containing quinones, which are not consumed by other animals. Captive grouse should receive natural foods or at least large amounts of leaves, grass, and berries supplemented with a limited quantity of pellets and grain. Feeding these largely herbivorous species with game bird or domestic fowl commercial diets will result in suboptimal fertility and health.

Coccidiostats are added to some poultry feeds. Monensin is commonly used and is toxic for guinea fowl. All gallinaceous birds should have access to grit. Poultry pellets generally contain adequate calcium and vitamins, and additional supplementation should be done only when a deficiency exists.

RATITES

See also RATITES, p 1960.

Ratites are flightless birds and do not require the high-energy diets of flighted birds. Ostriches, rheas, and emus consume low-quality roughage in nature, which is fermented in their intestinal tract. The nutritional requirements of juveniles are much higher in protein and calcium than those of adults. Breeders have even higher calcium requirements (*see* TABLE 37).

In most parts of the world, the commercial breeding market for ratites is declining; however, in some areas significant numbers of ostriches and nandus are being kept. Ratite production for meat and leather has necessitated the development of diets to maximize growth and minimize cost. Bringing an animal to market in minimal time is financially advantageous, but excessively rapid growth can lead to angular deformities of the legs.

Cassowaries are rainforest ratites and are primarily frugivorous. They are not raised commercially, and their nutritional requirements are not documented. Adult birds often consume 3–5 kg of food/day. Diets fed in zoos include fruits and vegetables such as bananas, apples, tomatoes, papaya, watermelon, grapes, mangoes, plums, nectarines, cherries, kiwi fruit, figs, sweet potatoes, and carrots. These are commonly supplemented with animal protein (eg, day-old chicks, mice, dry dog food).

MYNAHS

Mynah birds of the family Sturnidae are omnivorous. Preferred food items in the wild include fruits, a variety of insects, and small reptiles and amphibians. In captivity, a low-iron pelleted diet to prevent iron storage disease (≤100 ppm iron) and fruit are generally fed. Fruits high in vitamin C should be avoided, because these facilitate iron absorption.

During breeding, insects such as mealworms are preferred by the parents for feeding their young. Calcium gut-loading or dusting of insects with calcium powder will help prevent hypocalcemia in the chicks.

TOUCANS

In nature, toucans (*Ramphastos* spp) eat mostly fruit but also consume insects, rodents, and invertebrates. Like mynahs, toucans are susceptible to iron storage disease. Their basic diet should be a low-iron pellet with a variety of fruits (apples, banana, grapes) offered daily. If the bird picks the fruit preferentially over the large toucan pellets, the pellets can either be crushed, or very small low-iron pellets can be mixed with the fruit, so the pellets adhere to the fruit and are ingested. These long-beaked birds may have difficulty drinking water and may become dehydrated if not provided a large enough drinking pan.

MANAGING AVIAN ZOOLOGICAL COLLECTIONS

When working with large zoological collections containing disparate species, a team approach is critical to improve nutrition for multiple species. The keepers' experience regarding the birds' habits and preferences, combined with input from the curator, veterinarian, and outside nutritional consultants are all necessary. Input from other institutions where a given species has a history of longevity and successful reproduction can be invaluable. In large collections, decreasing waste, spoilage, overfeeding, and excessively time-consuming diet preparation must be considered along with improvement of the birds' nutritional intake.

MAMMALS

HANDREARING ZOO MAMMALS

Successful nutrition of handreared mammals requires 1) selecting a formula that will support adequate growth and not cause GI upset; 2) offering it at proper intervals, in proper amounts, and in the proper way to ensure acceptance and prevent overfeeding, underfeeding, or aspiration into the lungs; and 3) keeping all feeding utensils clean and disinfected. If success is judged in terms of survival and not in comparison with maternal-raised growth and health, most precocial species maintained in captive collections have been handreared successfully. Handrearing more altricial species (eg, marsupials, rodents, rabbits) is generally less successful unless the young have been dam-raised to a more advanced stage.

Whenever possible, data on milk composition and handrearing case histories should be consulted before attempting to bottle-raise a species for the first time. Extensive books with general information on handrearing birds and handrearing wild

TABLE 37 SELECTED NUTRITIONAL REQUIREMENTS FOR RATITE PRODUCTION[a]

Diet	Age (mo)	Estimated Body Wt (kg)	Crude Protein (%)	Calcium (%)	Fiber (%)
Pre-starter	0–2	0.8–10.5	25	1.2–1.5	—
Starter	2–4	11–28	21.5	1.2–1.5	>4
Grower	4–6	29–52	17	1.2–1.5	>4
Finisher	6–10	53–90	13.5	0.9–1.0	—
Post-finisher	10–20	91–110	8.5	0.9–1.0	—
Maintenance	Mature	—	8.0	0.9–1.0	6
Breeder	Laying	—	14	2.0–2.5	8

[a] Portions reprinted with permission of Spix Publishing, Donnelly R., *Clinical Avian Medicine*, 2006.

and domestic mammals are available. However, most milk composition data are not available for most species, and some of the published data are of dubious value. Lactose content of milk varies widely between different species.

Animals (eg, pinnipeds, rabbits) that normally consume milk low in lactose generally produce little lactase and often develop severe GI problems and diarrhea when fed a high-lactose milk, eg, bovine. Similarly, adding sucrose to milk formulas is often contraindicated, because many neonates produce little sucrase. Many species have been raised using diluted evaporated milk or commercial calf, lamb, foal, or doe milk replacers (eg, most ungulates), commercial dog milk replacer (eg, canids, procyonids, bears, bats, edentates, mustelids, rabbits, rodents), commercial cat milk replacer (eg, felids), human infant formulas in general (eg, most primates), and soy-based human infant formulas in particular (eg, rabbits, some marsupials). In some cases, these basic formulas can be modified to better suit the needs of a particular species by adding ingredients such as egg yolk, butterfat, cream, and casein. Supplementation with vitamin and mineral products may be warranted. Some companies offer a range of products with different amounts of protein and fat, so the desired amount of protein or fat can be provided in the formula. *See* TABLE 38.

It is preferred that some species (eg, ungulates, marsupials, mink) receive colostrum within 12–48 hr of birth to acquire immunoglobulins necessary for survival. Including some colostrum in the diet of ungulates for up to 2–3 wk after birth may provide additional local gut protection. Colostrum from domestic cows has proved satisfactory for many exotic ruminants and can be stored frozen. When colostrum is fed, the best way to do so is to offer it from the dam or from a similar species from the same stable. Studies suggest that conspecific serum, collected aseptically, can be given PO or SC as a substitute for colostrum.

Frequency of feeding and the amount fed depends on natural nursing behavior, formula composition, and the desired rate of gain as well as practical labor restrictions. The stomach capacity of most species can be estimated at 50 mL/kg. Overfilling the stomach leads to GI upset, decreased transit time, and diarrhea. Daily intake, as a rule, should not exceed 20% body wt/day and should be divided into frequent feedings that do not exceed 35–40 mL/kg. In general, most newborns should be fed every 2–4 hr, and daily metabolizable energy intake (kcal) should be ~$210 \times$ body wt $(kg)^{0.75}$. Appetite, condition of feces, and general health should be monitored closely. Pulmonary aspiration is the main problem during bottle feeding. Body weights should be recorded at frequent intervals. Smaller, more altricial species often must be fed by stomach tube.

See also CARE OF ORPHANED NATIVE BIRDS AND MAMMALS, p 2100.

BATS

Captive insectivorous bats frequently are fed diets consisting primarily of mealworms. Crickets, fruit flies, blowfly larvae, and other insects also are commonly offered. Because insects typically are low in calcium, they should be maintained on a

TABLE 38 NUTRIENT REQUIREMENTS FOR HANDREARING SELECTED ZOO MAMMALS

		% of Dry Matter		
Animal	**Dry Matter**	**Protein**	**Fat**	**Carbohydrates/ Lactose**
Horses, rhinos	8–12	15–20	2–15	59–75
Primates	2–14	7–15	25–35	50–60
Elephants, ruminants, pigs	12–23	21–27	30–45	20–37
Rodents, carnivores, deer	18–34	28–42	32–55	5–25
Rabbits, bears	30–40	25–45	40–50	5–10
Seals	41–61	10–20	74–82	0–2
Marsupials	23–28	—	—	1

calcium-enriched diet so that the bat will consume the insect's high-calcium gut contents. A suitable mealworm diet can be formulated using 35% wheat middlings, 35% ground dry dog or cat food, and 30% ground calcium carbonate, which should be fed at least 3 days. Gels containing water and a calcium solution can also be fed. Frugivorous bats should be fed a diet that contains a low amount of iron to prevent iron storage disease. The diet could contain a low-iron pellet for birds mixed with apples, bananas, and oranges.

Often, captive insectivorous bats must be fed by hand when flying insects are not available. Some bats can be trained to accept insects from a food dish by being placed directly on the live food.

Many insectivorous bats can be maintained successfully in captivity using artificial liquid or solid diets (*see* TABLE 39). Liquid diet can be placed in shallow plastic trays positioned near wire or branches for the bats to land on and hang from while feeding. Leftover liquid diet should be replaced daily. Solid diets usually include bananas as the major ingredient. Additional ingredients frequently offered include papaya, apple, pear, melon, grape, and cooked carrot and sweet potato. Canned cat or dog food, chopped eggs, and mealworms also have been fed with the fruit.

TABLE 39 DIETS OF SELECTED MAMMALS

Freshwater Otter Diet	**Percent (%)**
Ground horse or cow meat	38
Ground beef heart	20
Ground dry cat food	13
Beet pulp	2.9
Mirra-Coat®	1.9
Calcium carbonate	0.8
Poultry fat	4.9
Water	16.9
Lactose	0.04
Yogurt	0.72
Mineral-vitamin mix	0.84
All ingredients should be combined in a large mixer, divided into daily portions, and frozen. Lactose for lactobacilli can be added in yogurt to help maintain freshness. Lactose and yogurt are optional.	
Liquid Diet for Bats	**Percent (%)**
Dry mix:	
Mixed baby cereal	20.7
Wheat germ	4
Nonfat dried milk powder	9
Calcium caseinate	15.8
Sugar	45.5
Protein supplement (casein-based)	3
Mineral-vitamin mix	2
The dry mix (100 g) should be mixed with canned peach nectar (540 mL), water (260 mL), and corn oil (6 mL), and fed with peeled bananas.	

(continued)

TABLE 39 DIETS OF SELECTED MAMMALS *(continued)*

Large Herbivore Pellet for Grazers	Percent (%)
Wheat middlings	30
Alfalfa hay, sun-cured, ground (16% crude protein)	22
Corn grain, ground	19.1
Soybean meal without hulls (48% crude protein)	11.4
Alfalfa meal, dehydrated (17% crude protein)	10
Sugarcane molasses	5
Soybean oil	1
Phosphorus supplement	0.8
Sodium chloride	0.5
Mineral premix[a]	0.1
Vitamin premix[b]	0.1
Calculated composition (dry-matter basis): 89% dry matter, 19% crude protein, 4.3% fat, 16% acid detergent fiber, 12% crude fiber, 0.75% calcium, 0.7% phosphorus	

[a] Mineral premix (mg/kg of premix): 75,000 Zn, 50,000 Fe, 30,000 Mn, 10,000 Cu, 800 I, 200 Se, and 100 Co

[b] Vitamin premix (per kg of premix): 5,000,000 IU vitamin A, 400,000 IU vitamin D_3, 200,000 mg vitamin E, 500,000 mg choline, 40,000 mg niacin, 20,000 mg pantothenic acid, 4,000 mg riboflavin, 20 mg vitamin B_{12}

CARNIVORES

Most zoos in the USA use nutritionally complete commercial diets to feed exotic felids, canids, mustelids, and viverrids rather than attempt to prepare diets in-house. In other parts of the world, a whole or partial carcass (eg, of cows or horses) may regularly be fed. Other prey animals, such as rabbit and chicken, are also regularly offered. A supplement containing at a minimum calcium, vitamin A, iodine, taurine, and some B vitamins should be added to the meat diet. Feeding a complete mixed diet greatly reduces incidence of nutritional problems in captive exotic carnivores; however, such a diet regularly causes fecal problems. Most commercial diets are based on horsemeat and its byproducts, but diets based on beef and poultry are also available. Typical lesser ingredients include fish meal, soybean meal, beet pulp, and ground corn, as well as mineral and vitamin supplements.

Exotic feline diets are usually higher than canine diets in fat, protein, and vitamin A. A diet suitable for most cat species contains 45%–50% protein, 30%–35% fat, 3%–4% crude fiber, 1.2%–1.5% calcium, 1%–1.2% phosphorus, and 20,000–40,000 IU of vitamin A/kg diet (dry-matter basis). Apparently, exotic cats, like domestic cats, are unable to convert carotene to vitamin A, tryptophan to niacin, and linoleic acid to arachidonic acid. They also probably cannot synthesize adequate taurine (a taurine deficiency has been reported in leopards) and would be susceptible to ammonia toxicity if fed an arginine-deficient diet. Therefore, these nutrients should be considered dietary essentials for all felids.

Frozen and canned cat foods usually are more palatable than dry ones to exotic cats. Many zoos prefer to use frozen diets over canned products, because generally they are less expensive and large quantities are easier to feed. The soft, hamburger-like consistency of commercial diets can result in excess calculus deposits and periodontal disease if hard or unprocessed items are not also provided. All cats fed a soft diet should receive bones with some meat intact twice weekly. Horse or beef shank bones are suitable for large cat species; oxtails, rib bones, or whole rodents can be used for smaller cats. Mice, rats, and chicks are frequently included in the diets of smaller cats. Rodents, poultry, fish, and organ and chunk muscle meats can be offered as occasional treat items to administer medication or to stimulate appetite, but generally they are not required as dietary staples for large cats fed commercial diets.

Canids can be fed frozen, canned, or dry canine diets. Although most canids are less particular than cats, frozen and canned foods are generally preferred over dry ones. Bones should be included in the diet when soft foods are fed. Canids can also be fed meat, with the right amount of vitamins and minerals added, varied with small prey animals like rats, mice, rabbits, and chicken. Small amounts of fruits and vegetables can be included in the diets of foxes and coyotes.

Most mustelids and viverrids do well on frozen feline diets or canned cat foods; a meat-based diet supplemented with the right amount of vitamins and minerals is also appropriate. Many species readily accept small amounts of fruits, vegetables, and cooked egg. Mice, fish, and chicks can be offered as occasional treat items and to stimulate appetite and activity. Rib bones can be given twice weekly to promote dental health. Canned foods may be more palatable but are not recommended as a base diet, because ferrets may not be able to eat enough to meet their needs for calories and protein. *See* TABLE 39 for a diet used successfully for freshwater otter species.

Procyonids can be fed diets similar to those offered to small canids, or an adequate meat diet can be fed. Feeding a good-quality dry dog food along with apple, banana, and carrot is satisfactory for raccoons and helps minimize obesity problems that commonly result when frozen or canned diets are fed. The red or lesser panda has been maintained successfully on commercial high-fiber primate biscuits and bamboo. The herbivorous food habits of the giant panda require large amounts of bamboo supplemented with high-fiber primate biscuits.

Bears can be fed meat supplemented with vitamins and minerals, frozen canine diet, dry dog food, fish, and commercial omnivore biscuits. Polar and Kodiak bears do well on a diet of 25% frozen canine diet, 25% fish (eg, smelt), 15% dry dog food, 15% omnivore biscuits, 10% bread, and 10% apples. Commercial diets formulated especially for polar bears are available. Other bear species can be fed less fish and more omnivore biscuits, bread, and produce. Bananas and green vegetables can be included in the diet of sun, sloth, spectacled, and black bears. Food intake of captive bears varies widely with the season. Intakes generally are maximal during summer and early fall and minimal during winter. It is advisable to feed extra cod oil (0.5–1 L) to polar bears before their hibernation starts.

INSECTIVORES, EDENTATES, AND AARDVARKS

Most shrews, hedgehogs, tenrecs, and moles can be fed frozen cat food supplemented with mealworms, earthworms, crickets, and mouse pups. Ground meat fortified with minerals and vitamins, canned dog food, cooked egg, and small amounts of fruits and vegetables also are readily accepted by many species. Bacterial hazards have been associated with the feeding of raw, meat-based diets to some species. Carnivorous and insectivorous small mammals appear particularly susceptible, and septicemia and deaths have been reported. Canned, meat-based products are a safer alternative.

Armadillos will eat frozen feline diet, moistened dry cat food, canned dog food, or ground meat fortified with minerals and vitamins. Milk, chopped egg, cooked sweet potato, diced banana, and other fruits also are consumed. Vitamin K supplementation of armadillos has been recommended to help prevent hemorrhages: 5 mg of menadione sodium bisulfite/kg dry diet should be adequate. Sloths can digest fiber, but if they are kept in an environment that is too cold, their digestion rate will be very slow. Their diet should consist of a mixture of primate and high-fiber primate diets and some green, diced vegetables and preferred leaves. Food pans should be placed in such a way that the animal can hang from a perch while feeding.

In captivity, aardvarks, lesser anteaters, and giant anteaters readily accept semiliquid diets instead of termites, ants, and other natural foods. Artificial diets typically consist of milk, water, ground meat, and/or meat-based product such as frozen feline diet, mink chow or dry dog food, hard-boiled egg, protein powder, baby cereal, and a mineral-vitamin supplement. All ingredients are mixed in a blender to the consistency of a thick gruel. For adult giant anteaters, a commercial diet is available. Loose feces may develop when a semiliquid diet is fed. If this occurs, milk and water can be withdrawn gradually from the formula. As a precaution, vitamin K often is added to all edentate diets.

MARINE MAMMALS

See also MARINE MAMMALS, p 1856.

Fish are the primary food of captive marine mammals except for the herbivorous sirenians. The purchase and subsequent proper storage and handling of high-quality fish are the most important aspects of feeding cetaceans and pinnipeds.

On receipt, fish should always be inspected for quality. The following are useful for evaluation: 1) The boxes should be checked to see whether catch dates are indicated. 2) Overall appearance of the fish should be good. 3) Gills should be red (light pink gills indicate considerable time may have elapsed before the fish were frozen after being caught). 4) Eyes should not be sunken, indicating dehydration. 5) Flesh of thawed fish should be firm, skin should be intact and not discolored, and there should not be a bad odor. 6) There should not be excess water and blood pooled on the bottom of frozen cases, which indicates the fish have thawed and been refrozen. 7) Ideally, the lenses of frozen fish should be cloudy, which indicates the fish have been properly stored at or below –30°C before purchase (higher temperatures often result in clear lenses).

To minimize peroxidative damage and nutrient destruction, fish should be stored at or below –25°C. Most fish species should not be stored >6 mo if at all possible. A maximum of 3–4 mo is recommended for fatty fish such as mackerel; lean fish such as smelt may remain in good condition for up to 9 mo. Ideally, fish should be thawed overnight under refrigeration. If this is not possible, thawing at room temperature is preferable to thawing in water, which can cause significant nutrient leaching. Thawing temperature should not be >10°C. Individually quick frozen fish are preferred by many zoos, because proper quantities can be thawed without waste.

As a general rule, marine mammals should be given marine fish. Composition of marine fishes can vary greatly between species and even within species depending on age, season, and catch location. Fish that have been used successfully include Atlantic and Pacific herring; Atlantic, Pacific, and Spanish mackerel; bluerunner; capelin; and anadromous smelt. Squid are readily consumed by many pinnipeds, and clams can be included in walrus diets. No commercial substitute for fish has been developed that will be accepted by cetaceans, but such products have been used with some success for pinnipeds. The regular diet of any marine mammal should consist of two or more fish species to help ensure a balanced diet. It is not recommended to feed fish that are threatened in the wild. For example, Marine Stewardship Council (MSC) fish can be fed.

Thiamine should be added (at 30–35 mg/kg fish, as fed daily) to any marine mammal feeding program because of the possibility of thiamine destruction by thiaminases found in several fish species. Supplemental vitamin E helps compensate for oxidative destruction of natural vitamin E in fish during storage and helps protect against the deleterious effects of peroxides formed in stored fish. Oily fish such as mackerel, which are high in unsaturated fatty acids, are particularly susceptible to vitamin E destruction and peroxidative damage. Vitamin E at 100 IU/kg fish, as fed per day, is generally recommended whenever fish are fed.

Although subject to some debate, salt (NaCl) supplementation of pinnipeds maintained in freshwater is sometimes recommended to prevent hyponatremia; 3 g salt/kg fish should be adequate. Although supplemental vitamin C is frequently given to captive cetaceans, there is no conclusive evidence it is beneficial. Evidence indicates hepatic vitamin A levels in captive dolphins are often much lower than in their wild counterparts. Although specific recommendations cannot be made, vitamin A supplementation of some captive cetacean diets may be desirable.

Food intake in marine mammals varies considerably, depending on fat content of fish, water temperature, and activity. Performing Atlantic bottlenose dolphins generally eat 7–10 kg fish/day. Adult seals and sea lions consume ~5%–8% of their body wt in fish/day. Captive sirenians can be maintained on a diet of lettuce, cabbage, alfalfa, and aquatic plants (eg, water hyacinth).

MARSUPIALS

Most didelphid marsupials can be fed dry or canned dog or cat food. Smaller species can be fed canned primate diet. Hard-boiled egg, green vegetables, carrot, sweet potato, apple, and banana can also be offered. Dasyurids (eg, marsupial “mice,” native cats, Tasmanian devils) and bandicoots can be fed canned or frozen feline diet. In addition, crickets, mealworms, and mouse pups can be given to smaller species; larger species can be given mice and shank or rib bones. Wombats and the larger macropod marsupials can be fed a combination of large herbivore pellets, rabbit pellets, or special kangaroo pellets. Rat kangaroos will eat a combination of mouse pellets and rabbit pellets. To prevent lumpy jaw, the diet of marsupials should contain at least 200 mg of vitamin E and 0.2 mg of selenium/kg dry matter.

Green vegetables, carrot, sweet potato, apple, and banana can be offered to all herbivorous and omnivorous marsupials. For herbivores, greens and vegetables should be added in limited amounts; these marsupials should be fed a good-quality hay that has not too long stems. Currently, captive koalas can be fed successfully only on leaves of certain species of eucalyptus. Special pellets for koalas are being tested and may be available in the future.

PRIMATES

In general, primates can be fed a diet based on commercial monkey biscuits or canned primate diet. Marmosets should be fed a marmoset diet. Moderate amounts of assorted carrot, sweet potato, apple, banana, and orange also can be offered; however, it is advised to feed greens and green vegetables, which are more comparable to the natural diet. Monkey biscuits and the canned products should comprise 20% of the dry-matter intake of gorilla and orangutan diets; fruits and treat items should comprise ≤20%. Green vegetables and browse should be at least 40% of the diet, depending on the species.

Feeding only greens and vegetables, with vitamin and mineral supplements, is being tested in several species of primates. Diets should be developed and offered in such a way that enrichment is supported.

Dietary crude protein ranges for Pongidae such as gorillas are 14%–16% and for New World primates such as pinches 18%–22%. The unsaturated fatty acid composition should be at least 2.5% (⅔ n-6 fatty acids). Neutral detergent fiber in the dry matter ranges from at least 10% in macaques, to 10% in marmosets, 30% in Howlers and langurs, and 20% in lemurs, chimpanzees, and gorillas. Acid detergent fiber ranges from 5% in macaques, to 5% in marmoset and tamarins, 10% in lemurs and Pongidae, and 15% in Howler and langur diets. For all primates, the diet should contain 0.8% calcium and 0.6% phosphorus. Primate diets should contain 5,000–8,000 IU vitamin A and 800–1,500 IU vitamin D, except diets for squirrel monkeys and marmoset/tamarin should contain 2,400 IU vitamin D. The vitamin C level should be at least 200 mg/kg dry matter. The maintenance metabolic rate (kcal/day) is for Pongidae (gorillas, orangutans), 3,621; baboons, 1,099–1,324; langurs, 632–637; Rhesus macaques, 567–1146; marmoset, 31–76; and tamarin, 57–105. Obesity should be prevented; therefore, it is important to weigh animals regularly or to perform body condition scoring.

Monkey biscuits containing high-quality protein (18%–22.5% crude protein) should be fed to New World primates to ensure that their higher protein requirements are met. Regular monkey biscuits can be fed to Old World species depending on other components in the diet, although many larger Old World species such as gibbons, orangutans, chimpanzees, and gorillas also need high-fiber products. Laboratory primate biscuits are typically formulated with very low fiber levels (eg, 5%). Because many of the natural foods consumed by these species appear to contain very high fiber levels (eg, >20%), increasing the dietary fiber intakes of larger primate species is widely practiced. High-fiber biscuits should comprise at least 50% of the dietary dry matter, and browse should be at least 40% of the diet fed. Most of the time, however, these amounts are not available, and greens and vegetables can be a replacement for the browse.

Cultivated fruits should be used sparingly for great apes and leaf-eating species because, compared with cultivated green vegetables, they are typically high in sugars and simple carbohydrates and low in protein and calcium. Monkey biscuits can be made more palatable for some species by soaking them in water or fruit juice. To prevent leaching of nutrients, the biscuits should be placed in a thin film of liquid so that the liquid is drawn up into the biscuit.

Other items commonly included in primate diets include hard-boiled egg (if cholesterol is not a concern), yogurt, and bread. Grapes, raisins, peanuts, crickets, and mealworms are treat items well liked by most species. However, these items should be fed two or three times a week at the most, not every day. The energy amount of these enrichment items should not exceed 5%–10% of the energy consumed by the animal.

Mouse pups are favored items for many smaller primates. However, callitrichid hepatitis in tamarins and marmosets has been associated with the feeding of newborn mice infected with lymphocytic choriomeningitis virus. Most zoos have discontinued the feeding of mouse pups to these New World primates. Sunflower seeds, instant rice, cracked corn, and shredded coconut can be scattered around the exhibit or holding areas to promote foraging activity. The amount of energy used for these enrichment feeds should not exceed 5%–10% of planned dietary energy. Hay should be provided for nesting materials and diversion, and it can act as a foraging substrate.

Many zoos offer meat to their great apes; although meat is often relished by the animals, there is no evidence it is necessary if the diet is properly balanced. Because hypercholesterolemia is seen in many captive gorillas, the feeding of meat may be contraindicated. For most primates, meals should be offered at least twice daily. Smaller species may benefit from even more frequent feedings.

New World primates use vitamin D_2 poorly. It is particularly important that these species receive an adequate source of stabilized vitamin D_3 (cholecalciferol) in their diet if they are not exposed daily to direct sunlight. Marmosets require up to four times the amount of vitamin D_3 required by other New World primates. Because of potential vitamin D toxicity, commercial marmoset diets should be fed only to marmosets. In noncommercial mixtures for smaller primates (mixtures of cut apples, bananas, and cereal products with vitamins and minerals added), vitamin D_3 should be included; however, care should be taken to prevent vitamin D toxicity.

Several cases of rickets in some Old World species at weaning have been reported. This may be because barred, outdoor primate exhibits have been replaced with indoor, albeit more naturalistic, exhibits. Although most free-ranging primate species probably satisfy their requirement for vitamin D by exposure to ultraviolet B (UVB) from sunlight, captive animals may rely entirely on a dietary source. Infants at weaning appear to be particularly at risk because milk levels of vitamin D are probably quite low, and many foods the young begin to eat are not fortified with this vitamin. Exposing the infant or juvenile to natural sunlight may be the best solution, because assuring that a dietary supplement is consumed by a young primate may not be possible.

The amount of UVB from sunlight is the highest in and around the equator; in regions at latitudes farther away from the sun the amount of radiated UVB, particularly in autumn, winter, and spring, is not enough. Lights that emit energy in the UVB range can be practical for use with primates, provided precautions are taken to prevent the primates from being able to touch the UVB lamp.

All primates require a source of vitamin C, which is added to commercial monkey biscuits. Most of the time, stable vitamin C is added to the pellet, meaning it will not undergo significant destruction within 6 mo of milling. Supplementation is done, because the amount of vitamin C consumed via green vegetables, oranges, multiple vitamins, chocolate, fruit juice, or fruit-juice powders may not be sufficient.

Members of the subfamily Colobinae are perhaps the greatest challenge in proper feeding of captive primates. Pregastric fermentation, similar to that in ruminants, occurs in the complex stomach of these species. In the wild, leaves and high-fiber fruits and nuts form a major part of the diet of most colobines. Therefore, natural diets are high in fiber, and animals spend much time foraging. Offering a rich, rapidly consumable diet of monkey biscuits and fruit (easily digestible sugars and starches) in captivity presents a situation quite different from that typically found in the wild, and it may frequently cause GI problems. In addition, some evidence suggests that a high percentage of colobus monkeys may be sensitive to starch and gluten.

Commercial, preferably gluten-free, high-fiber monkey biscuits (25%–50% neutral detergent fiber and up to 15%–35% acid detergent fiber) have been developed to feed captive colobines. A diet consisting of 30% of a palatable high-fiber biscuit and ≥70% green vegetables and fresh browse is recommended for most colobines. Only a high-fiber primate biscuit and browse is the preferable food for colobines. If the biscuit is not readily accepted, adding a limited amount of applesauce or banana flavor can increase palatability. Also, alfalfa pellets and a good-quality alfalfa hay can be provided in limited quantities. If a gluten-sensitive enteropathy is suspected, any product that contains wheat, barley, rye, or oats should be removed from the diet. In colobines, dietary changes always should be made gradually to allow their gastric microflora time to adapt.

RODENTS AND LAGOMORPHS

Most rodent and lagomorph species do well on diets based on commercial laboratory rodent pellets or rabbit pellets. Rabbits, hares, pikas, marmots, and prairie dogs can be maintained on rabbit pellets, alfalfa or grass hay, and a limited amount of assorted vegetables. Most other sciurids can be fed rat pellets and a limited mixture of sunflower seeds, millet, corn, and rolled oats. Ground squirrels can also be offered a limited amount of green leafy vegetables, carrot, and apple. Most murids, cricetids, gophers, dormice, and jerboas do well on rat pellets; for smaller species, mouse pellets, a seed and grain mix, green leafy vegetables, carrot, and apple can be fed.

Hay should be made available to voles and lemmings. Captive voles may be difficult to manage unless a high-fiber rabbit pellet is used. Muskrats, agoutis, and capybaras will eat a combination of rat and rabbit pellets along with alfalfa hay, carrot, and apple. Porcupines can be fed rat pellets, rabbit pellets, and dry dog food in equal portions along with some apple, carrot, and bread; evergreen (willow) branches should be made available whenever possible. It is also advised to provide bones for gnawing. Beavers will eat a combination of rabbit pellets, large herbivore pellets, and dry dog food, regularly augmented with willow, poplar, aspen, or alder branches.

Guinea pigs can be offered commercial guinea-pig pellets, which are rabbit pellets with vitamin C added, along with greens and carrot. Although guinea pigs and cavies are the only rodents known to require a dietary source of vitamin C, lagomorphs and rodents may benefit from it.

SUBUNGULATES AND UNGULATES

Hay comprises the bulk of the diet for most ungulates in captivity and should be available for most of the day rather than fed at intervals as meals. In general, a leafy legume hay, eg, alfalfa, should be used for species that are primarily browsers (eg, Giraffidae, Cervidae, sitatunga, bongo, duiker, tapir), whereas a good-quality grass hay is satisfactory for most grazers or bulk feeders (eg, zebra, elephant, bison, buffalo, wildebeest, camel). Legume hays are higher in nitrogen and calcium and, if of good quality, are more digestible than grass hays. Hay should be leafy and green, free of mold, dirt, excess weeds, and other foreign matter, and should not be overmature. Several zoos are test-feeding hay and alfalfa silage. In general, palatability is good.

Hay analysis can be very useful to evaluate quality and design proper feeding programs. "Poor" hay will have a good fiber percentage, but the protein quality can be low and poor, and the mineral status, especially of calcium, can be too low. Low levels of calcium can cause poor bone calcification and also affect the calcium level in the blood, which can cause birth problems.

Precautions should be taken if feeding silage products. If the silage was not processed or stored properly or contaminated by animal or meat products, it may contain fungi or bacteria (eg, *Clostridium botulinum*) that can produce lethal toxins.

In addition to hay, a pelleted diet that contains protein, minerals, and vitamins in concentrations adequate to meet the needs of domestic species and those wild species for which data are available (eg, white-tailed deer) should be offered. *See* TABLE 39 for composition of a sample pellet for large herbivores. In the frequent situation in which animals are fed as a group rather than as individuals, it is preferable to use a pelleted diet that is not excessively high in digestible energy (~3 kcal DE/g dry matter is suggested) and that contains sufficient fiber to support proper rumen or colon function. This precaution reduces the possibility of untoward effects (eg, rumen acidosis, colic, obesity) caused by overconsumption of concentrates. Depending on the nutritional status of the animal, ~0.5–1.5 kg should be fed per animal. Overfeeding can result in obesity. Animals should be weighed regularly, or body condition scoring performed.

A specialized pellet with high amounts of neutral detergent fiber (NDF) and acid detergent fiber (ADF) is recommended for browsers (eg, giraffe, kudu, okapi, reindeer), and a pellet with moderate amounts of NDF and ADF is recommended for grazers (eg, elephant, bison, banteng, addax antelope). The intermediate feeding animals should get an equal mix of the browser and grazer pellets. Preferably, the diet of browsers should consist of equal parts of browser pellets, good palatable alfalfa, and browse. Diets for grazers and browsers should contain high amounts of vitamin E and biotin to prevent muscle dystrophy and hoof problems.

A pellet size of 3⁄16 in. is satisfactory for most artiodactyls, whereas a pellet or cube size of ½ in. (~13 mm) helps minimize waste when fed to larger perissodactyls and subungulates. Commercial cattle products should not be fed to zoo herbivores because of palatability problems and low vitamin E levels, and some products may contain nonprotein nitrogen sources such as urea that are not tolerated by hindgut-fermenting species (eg, equids). Also, the amount of easily digestible energy may be high, leading to obesity. Tapirs should get a mixture of grazer and browser pellets combined with some greens, alfalfa, and browse.

In general, most large ungulates (>250 kg) consume 1.5%–2% of their weight in dry matter daily. Smaller species (<250 kg) generally consume 2%–4%. Offering a pelleted diet at 10%–15% of the dry-matter intake is adequate for most grazers if good-quality hay is fed. The amount of minerals and vitamins should be balanced in the pellets in such a way that the total diet (including greens, browse, and hay) should be adequate. When hay quality declines, or for more delicate species, the percentage of high-fiber pellets should be increased. Ungulates and subungulates should always have salt blocks available, preferably with a balanced vitamin and mineral supplement. However, excessive licking can become a neurotic behavior and should be prevented.

Elephants should receive extra calcium, because mostly poor hay with a low level of calcium is fed. Because of the sensitivity to hemosiderosis, black rhinos should be fed a diet with a low level of iron (<100 mg/kg dry matter). Browse can contain significant amounts of iron; however, rose leaves contain low amounts. It is speculated that other ungulate species may also get hemosiderosis. It is advised that all ungulates be exposed to UVB from sunlight, because it has been suggested that oral supplementation of vitamin D in some cases is not sufficient (elephant, kudu).

Hay should be fed from a rack rather than off the ground for most species (elephants are an exception). Hay racks should be located at eye level for tall browsers such as giraffes and gerenuks. Pellets can be offered from a covered trough or (rubber) feed pans. Regularly feeding the pelleted diet in an animal's holding area can facilitate close observation and easy capture. If possible, animals should be fed separately to ensure that each individual receives a similar amount of food. If feeding separately is not possible, at least two widely separated feeding stations may be necessary to reduce conflict and to ensure that subordinate animals obtain their share of food.

In addition to hay and pelleted diet, assorted fruits and vegetables often are fed to exotic ungulates. For most species, these items usually are not necessary except as an occasional treat; the amount should be limited to <10% of the total diet. The exception might be for those species that regularly feed on fruits and succulents in the wild. It may be advisable to include some greens and vegetables (~0.5 kg/100 kg body wt) in the diet of species such as okapi, duikers, dik diks, bongo, and tapirs. Fresh, frozen, or dried browse is consumed avidly by most captive ungulates and subungulates and should be offered to browsers if possible ad lib, because it improves rumen function.

REPTILES

See also REPTILES, p 1967.

Appropriate husbandry of reptiles is as important as providing adequate nutrients. Photoperiod, temperature, humidity, substrate, and cage "furniture" can affect feeding behavior and, thus, nutrient intake. Temperature and humidity gradients within a reptile enclosure allow the animal to select warm, dry spots or cooler, moist areas. Competition for preferred sites and for food pans in an enclosure with multiple animals should also be assessed. Sufficient numbers of warm spots, UVB exposure spots, and food pans should be available for all animals within an enclosure. Visual barriers may be useful to reduce competition for preferred sites or food dishes.

Prey such as rabbits, rats, or mice should come from commercial breeding centers and be offered dead to prevent injury to the reptile and for welfare reasons of the offered prey. Although it is not common, prey have been known to attack predators and can inflict serious bites. Offering dead prey can also reduce the chance of injury to the predator caused by striking the walls of the enclosure. However, some reptiles may initially need the stimulation of live prey, particularly if they are not adapted to captivity. The possibility of disease or parasite transmission from prey to predator should be considered.

Vertebrate prey should be fed nutritionally complete diets appropriate for the species (eg, mouse diet, rabbit diet, rat diet, etc). The nutrient content of the prey depends on what it is fed (eg, mice raised on a diet deficient in vitamin A have decreased liver storage of this essential nutrient). Additionally, if frozen mice or rats are routinely used to feed carnivorous reptiles, freezer storage conditions should be optimal (eg, ≤6 mo and in thick, plastic bags to retard deterioration). Methods of thawing that minimize water loss are also important. Because many carnivorous reptiles rely on their prey not only as sources of nutrients but also as sources of water, the state of hydration of the prey can be very important.

Familiarity with a species' food habits in the wild is essential if appropriate foods and nutrient levels are to be offered. Common practice has been to offer two or more different prey species, because differences in nutrient content exist among vertebrate and invertebrate prey. Reduced dependence on a single food or prey species is also desirable, because some prey items may be periodically difficult to obtain. Dependence on a single prey item is frequently seen in snakes and may be unavoidable.

Many commercial diets for reptiles are marketed. Products for carnivorous, herbivorous, and omnivorous reptiles are now available in frozen, freeze-dried, canned, extruded, pelleted, or sausage forms. Acceptability may be better when the commercial diets are offered to reptiles when they are young. Appropriately formulated, manufactured diets for reptiles are a potentially simpler and more economical alternative to feeding fresh produce or live prey. However, some of these diets may not be formulated rationally, and frequently little information concerning micronutrient concentrations is provided by the manufacturers. When selecting a commercial product, the buyer should obtain accurate information about product formulation and specific nutrient concentrations. Unfortunately, little controlled research has been conducted on nutrient requirements of reptiles, and claims of product superiority may not have a scientific justification.

Herbivorous reptile pellets should make up 25%–50% of the diet of herbivorous reptiles. Animals should be fed 1%–4% of their body weight on a dry-matter basis. Vegetables with a low amount of oxalate should be fed to prevent kidney stones. A good quality grass hay or a so-called herbs-hay should be fed. No more than 50% of the diet should consist of fresh greens, fruits, and vegetables. The amount of fruit should be no more than 5%. In Europe, often herbs and dandelions are fed to herbivorous reptiles. Fresh, clean water must be available at all times.

See TABLE 40 for recommended nutrient concentrations for reptiles.

TABLE 40 RECOMMENDED NUTRIENT CONCENTRATIONS FOR REPTILES

	Concentration[a]		
Nutrient[b]	**Carnivorous Reptiles**	**Omnivorous Reptiles**	**Herbivorous Reptiles**
Crude protein[c]	30%–50%	20%–25%	18%–22%
Fat		3%–6%	
Crude fiber		20%–35%	
Arginine	1.0%	1.8%	
Isoleucine	0.5%	1.3%	
Lysine	0.8%	1.5%	
Methionine	0.4%	0.4%	
Methionine + cysteine	0.75%	0.75%	
Threonine	0.7%	1.0%	
Tryptophan	0.15%	0.3%	
Linoleic acid[d]	1.0%	1.0%	
Calcium	0.8%–1.1%	1.0%–1.5%	1.4%–2.0%
Phosphorus	0.5%–0.9%	0.6%–0.9%	0.8%–1.0%
Potassium	0.4%–0.6%	0.4%–0.6%	
Sodium	0.2%	0.2%	
Magnesium	0.04%	0.2%	
Manganese	5 ppm	150 ppm	
Zinc	50 ppm	130 ppm	
Iron	60–80 ppm	200 ppm	

(continued)

TABLE 40 RECOMMENDED NUTRIENT CONCENTRATIONS FOR REPTILES *(continued)*

Nutrient[b]	Concentration[a]		
	Carnivorous Reptiles	Omnivorous Reptiles	Herbivorous Reptiles
Copper	5–8 ppm	15 ppm	
Iodine	0.3–0.6 ppm	0.4 ppm	
Selenium	0.3 ppm	0.3 ppm	
Riboflavin	2–4 ppm	8 ppm	
Pantothenic acid	10 ppm	60 ppm	
Niacin	10–40 ppm	100 ppm	
Vitamin B_{12}	0.020 ppm	0.025 ppm	
Choline	1,250–2,400 ppm	3,500 ppm	
Biotin	70–100 ppb	400 ppb	
Folacin	200–800 ppb	6,000 ppb	
Thiamine[e]	1–5 ppm	5 ppm	
Pyridoxine	1–4 ppm	10 ppm	
Vitamin A[f]	5,000–10,000 IU/kg	15,000 IU/kg	
Cholecalciferol (vitamin D_3)[g]	500–1,000 IU/kg	500–1,000 IU/kg	
Vitamin E[h]	200 IU/kg	200 IU/kg	

[a] Nutrient concentrations are recommended minimums for carnivorous reptiles and averages for omnivorous reptiles.

[b] Nutrient levels expressed on a dry-matter basis.

[c] Taurine requirements have not been determined for reptiles (the requirement for cats is 400–500 mg of taurine/kg dry diet).

[d] A dietary source of arachidonic acid at 200 mg/kg dry diet may be necessary.

[e] Thiamine concentrations should be increased to 10–20 mg/kg if frozen, thawed fish constitute >25% of the diet offered.

[f] A source of preformed vitamin A may be required because it is not known if reptiles can convert carotenes to retinol (vitamin A), although it is likely that herbivorous reptiles can.

[g] Requirements for vitamin D may be partially or totally satisfied by exposure to sunlight or appropriate sources of artificial ultraviolet light. These suggested concentrations are not sufficient to prevent signs of vitamin D deficiency in green iguanas.

[h] 300 IU/kg dry matter is advisable if the diet is high in fat, especially unsaturated fat.

Ulcerative Stomatitis: Vitamin C synthesis has been reported in many reptile species. It has been suggested that ulcerative stomatitis seen in snakes and lizards may be associated with a vitamin C deficiency, although there is no supportive evidence. In controlled studies with garter snakes (*Thamnophis* sp) fed supplemental vitamin C, tissue levels and body stores remained stable, although synthesis by the snakes was reduced.

Gout: Although most reptiles excrete nitrogen primarily as uric acid, aquatic reptiles typically excrete excess nitrogen as urea or ammonia. The relative proportions of various nitrogenous wastes may depend on the amount and composition of feed, frequency of feeding, and state of hydration. The excessive precipitation of urate crystals in joints, kidneys, or other organs (gout) can be a common condition in some species of captive reptiles. The etiology is not clear, but it is commonly thought that diets high in protein may predispose reptiles to gout. Impaired renal function and dehydration have also been suggested as possible causes.

If poor-quality protein is fed (unbalanced amino acids) or when tissue is catabolized for energy, uric acid excretion increases. Although gout in some reptiles is associated with increased circulating levels, postprandial transient increases in circulating uric acid may be seen in some species and confound the diagnosis. Assuring an adequate state of hydration in a susceptible animal may help prevent uric acid precipitation in joints and organs. Feeding diets low in protein to carnivorous reptiles is unwise, because they are adapted to feeding on high-protein prey.

Vitamin D and Ultraviolet Light: Most vertebrates can either absorb vitamin D from the diet or synthesize it in the skin from 7-dehydrocholesterol using energy from ultraviolet (UVB) light of certain wavelengths (290–315 nm) in a temperature-dependent reaction. Thus, vitamin D is required in the diet only when endogenous synthesis is inadequate, as develops when animals are not exposed to UV light of appropriate wavelengths.

Many captive basking species appear susceptible to rickets or osteomalacia. Bone fractures, soft-tissue mineralization, renal complications, and tetany can develop. Reptiles frequently show few premonitory signs, although lethargy, inappetence, and reluctance to move are commonly reported. Serum calcium concentrations may not be diagnostically useful. Although blood levels of vitamin D can be measured, normal values for most species are not known. Supplementation with injectable calcium and vitamin D may provide some short-term relief. However, exposure to UV light, or lack of it, may be an important, yet often overlooked, factor in the differential diagnosis. Complicating the diagnosis may be soft-tissue mineralization, seen radiographically or at necropsy.

In green iguanas, metastatic calcification may not result from vitamin D toxicity. Iguanas with both fractured bones and extremely low or undetectable levels of circulating 25-hydroxycholecalciferol also had calcified soft tissues. The etiology of the metastatic calcification is not understood and is contrary to conventional understanding of the signs of vitamin D deficiency and toxicity in domestic species. Dietary sources of vitamin D may not be sufficient to prevent rickets and osteomalacia. Diets with as much as 3,000 IU vitamin D_3/kg did not prevent bone fractures and cortical thinning in green iguanas. Bulbs emitting UVB placed over the lizards at ~12–18 in. for 12 hr/day appeared to reverse the signs in the least severely affected lizards.

Because some lizards seek a warm spot to increase body temperature, placement of a warming bulb, usually incandescent, adjacent to a UVB bulb helps ensure adequate exposure to UVB light. Exposure to unfiltered natural sunlight, depending on latitude, during warmer months and use of UVB bulbs during the rest of the year usually eliminate the risk of bone disease caused by insufficient absorption of calcium (due to a vitamin D deficiency).

Some lizard species may be unable to absorb sufficient dietary vitamin D_3, although the reason is poorly understood. New World primates are believed to have exceptionally high dietary requirements for vitamin D, which may be related to lower numbers of vitamin D cellular receptors than are present in Old World primates. Similar metabolic differences may exist in some basking lizard species, although this has not been established. UVB bulbs are sold in pet stores, but label claims may not be reliable.

UVB Lighting: Three types of UVB lighting are on the market: fluorescent tubes, compact fluorescent lamps, and mercury lamps. Fluorescent tubes supply a diffuse light with a low amount of visible light. Heat radiation is low, and the UVB gradient is fairly uniform. The light from fluorescent tubes resembles more or less the natural UVB in the shade of a sunny day spread over a relatively large area. Compact fluorescent lamps provide a more intensive UVB gradient focused on a small area. These lamps are characterized by fairly low intensity visible light and little heat. Mercury lamps (vapor spot and narrow spots) produce an intensive UVB gradient on a smaller area, producing heat and an intense light.

Mercury lamps can become very hot. Reptiles must be prevented from getting burned during UVB basking. It is important to recognize that when a UVB lamp is added to a terrarium, the emission of UVB drops with the square of the distance; this explains the low exposure level of UVB at the level of the reptile when the lamp has been hung too high.

The radiation of UVB declines during the lighting time. In general, UVB lamps should be replaced once a year. However, it is best to regularly measure the amount of UVB with meters used in the artificial sunbath industry. A "D3 Yield Index" that compares the vitamin D_3–producing ability of the lamp with the sun is under development.

How long and how much exposure to UVB is needed in reptiles is not exactly known. In general, reptiles that need UVB must be exposed to 30 min to 2 hr of UVB each day. However, there can be exceptions. For example, bearded dragons do not develop metabolic bone diseases if they are exposed only a few times a week to UVB for a limited time.

Enlisting the assistance of a specialist is advised, because there is no ideal UV bulb (*see* p 1969).

CROCODILIANS

Captive alligators and crocodiles are usually fed a combination of rodents, poultry, fish, and meat-based diets. A varied diet is recommended. Diets consisting primarily of fish should include three or more different species of fish and should be supplemented with 30–35 mg of thiamine and 100 IU vitamin E/kg of fish, as fed. Signs of vitamin E deficiency (eg, steatitis) have been reported in crocodilians fed fish inadequately supplemented with vitamin E. Although previously reported otherwise, alligators can digest some carbohydrate; however, the total carbohydrate in the diet should not exceed 20%. Commercial, dry alligator diets are being marketed, largely to reduce the cost and to improve nutrient intakes of farmed alligators; their use is still uncommon in zoos.

SNAKES

Snakes feed almost exclusively on vertebrate or invertebrate prey. A few species are specialized egg feeders. Most boids, pythons, vipers, colubrids, crotalids, and elapids are fed mouse pups, mice, chicks, hamsters, rats, guinea pigs, chickens, ducks, or rabbits. Frozen, thawed prey are usually used in zoos; thawing under refrigeration is recommended. After thawing, prey should not be fed cold but at room temperature, or preferably warmer. Some species (eg, king cobra, hognose snake, garter snake) feed primarily on other poikilotherms in the wild. Some of these species can be switched, at least in part, to homeothermic prey, which is often more available and less expensive.

Minced prey is sometimes fed in agar, gel, or sausage form. Advantages include the ability to formulate and feed a nutritionally complete diet, to add a balanced vitamin and mineral mixture, and, if needed, to add antibiotics or coccidiostats. Mostly a complete diet is fed in a sausage; however, tests are also being done with gel feeding to reptiles.

The scent of preferred foods can be rubbed on the new item. Alternatively, the preferred foods can be inserted into, or attached to, the new food. Anoles, yellow rat snakes, frogs, and smelt, depending on natural feeding habits, can be fed when homeotherms are not accepted. Prey size is usually proportional to snake size and should not be much larger in diameter than the snake's head. Snakes that are routinely handled can be fed in a separate tank to reduce biting. To reduce the chance of regurgitation, snakes should not be handled for 3 days after feeding.

Most species should be fed every 1–2 wk. Some large, less active snakes may typically go 6 wk between feedings. Force-feeding should be used only if necessary. Animals can be force-fed whole prey lubricated with egg white by gently inserting the food a few inches down the throat using forceps. Tube feeding is also possible using ground (homogenized) prey.

TURTLES

Many freshwater turtles in the wild eat primarily animal matter but also consume some plant material. Some species may be carnivorous when young and shift to omnivorous or herbivorous feeding patterns as adults. Most aquatic turtles cannot be considered strict carnivores, because they consume at least some plant material. Commercially available turtle feeds are available from many manufacturers, although nutrient content can vary widely. These products are usually manufactured as extruded or pelleted diets and are typically 30%–50% protein. Such diets may be appropriate for carnivorous and omnivorous turtles, although the more omnivorous species would benefit from the addition of some fruits or vegetables.

A sample diet for carnivorous and omnivorous turtles consists of the following feed items: water (272 g), gelatin (unsweetened or dry, 34 g), corn oil (11 g), spinach (23 g), cooked sweet potato (23 g), Vionate® (a vitamin/mineral supplement, 5 g), trout pellets (50 g), and vitamin E at 50 IU/g (1 g). This diet contains on a dry-matter basis 47% protein, 14% fat, 1.5% calcium, 0.55% phosphorus, vitamin A at 10,000 IU/kg, vitamin D_3 at 1,000 IU/kg, vitamin E at 279 IU/kg, and vitamin C at 280 mg/kg.

TORTOISES

Tortoises are herbivorous and, like herbivorous lizards (*see* below), must consume plant material to maintain healthy gut physiology. Microbial fermentation of plant fiber can be a significant source of nutrients for tortoises. Diets of tortoises in the wild often contain >15% protein (dry-matter basis) in plant materials consumed, because natural vegetative materials are usually high in protein in the pre-seed stage, although a part of that protein is indigestible. Although small tortoises consuming pelleted diets can use plant fiber effectively, they should be fed more frequently than larger animals. Small and large tortoises can be maintained on appropriately formulated, extruded, pelleted, or coarsely ground tortoise diets.

Larger tortoises, such as Aldabra or Galapagos tortoises, can consume grass or alfalfa hay along with a complete pelleted food formulated for tortoises or exotic herbivores. Hay should be cut short, because the mouth shape of these tortoises makes it impossible for them to chew long hay. A vegetable mix consisting of broccoli, green beans, leafy greens (eg, romaine, green leaf lettuce, endive), kale, and shredded carrots may be fed as a supplement to a formulated tortoise diet. Such mixes contain adequate protein, calcium, and micronutrients; only limited vitamin and mineral supplements should be added. Cultivated fruits are typically poorer sources of protein, calcium, and micronutrients and, if fed in significant amounts, vitamins and minerals should be added. Some herpetologists offer oyster shell and pea gravel to tortoises, because "mining" activity has been seen in free-ranging animals.

Shell deformities in tortoises have been thought to result from rapid growth associated with consumption of high-protein diets. Humidity and temperature also may influence shell deformation.

LIZARDS

The feeding patterns of lizards are extremely diverse. Lizards may be insectivorous (eg, day and leopard gecko, whiptail lizard, anole, chameleon), carnivorous (eg, varanids such as monitor lizard, Gila monster, Mexican beaded lizard), omnivorous (eg, many iguanid and agamid species), or herbivorous (eg, iguanid species, prehensile-tailed skink).

Insectivorous lizards in captivity are usually fed diets of mealworm larvae or crickets. Because calcium concentrations in these, and in most insects, are extremely low (0.03%–0.3% calcium with 0.8%–0.9% phosphorus), the inverse calcium:phosphorus ratio must be corrected before the insects are fed to lizards. A diet with a balanced vitamin and mineral mixture and containing 12% calcium as calcium carbonate can be fed to crickets or mealworm larvae 3 days before the insect is fed to the lizard. However, this diet should not be used to maintain a cricket colony. Within 2 days of feeding the high-calcium diet, the gut of the insect is filled with calcium, raising the calcium concentration of the insect to ~0.8%–0.9% and resulting in a calcium:phosphorus ratio of ~1.2:1. A satisfactory high-calcium diet for crickets can be inexpensively made by using 29% wheat middlings, 10% corn meal, 40% ground dry cat or dog food, and 21% ground oyster shell or calcium carbonate (*see also* BATS, p 2294, for mealworm diet). Larger insectivorous lizards may also consume mouse pups and earthworms.

Carnivorous lizards may be offered mouse or rat pups, adult mice and rats, chickens, and eggs. The size of prey should be appropriate for the lizard species. Omnivorous lizards are usually fed a combination of foods, including insects, vertebrate prey, and a chopped vegetable mixture (*see* TORTOISES, p 2307, for vegetable mix). Most lizards should be fed daily (juveniles and small species) or at least every other day. Large carnivorous species should be fed once or twice a week.

Herbivorous lizards are adapted to ferment plant fiber in enlarged hindguts. The microbes in the cecum and colon digest plant fiber that the lizard could not otherwise use. As with tortoises, herbivorous lizards should be fed plant-based diets to assure healthy gut function. The use of insects, vertebrate prey, or diets high in fruits is not advised, because these feeds are low in fiber and are inappropriate for herbivores. Diets for lizards may be commercial preparations formulated for herbivorous reptiles, or vegetable mixes (*see* p 2307).

FISH

Knowledge of fish nutrition is increasing, but it has been mostly focused on commercial fish and not on specific fish held in cold or warm freshwater or seawater tanks. Pellets and flakes are available; some claim to be especially developed for specific species, but detailed nutritional information is not always available. Pellets fed in water should not be allowed to dissolve before eating to prevent pollution of the water.

Marine fish can be herbivorous, carnivorous, or omnivorous. Grazing or herbivorous fish eat plant materials from the rocks of the sea and need more fiber than carnivorous fish. This can be accomplished by feeding plant material in a basket in the water or by feeding an herbivorous fish pellet. Carnivorous fish should be fed a diet with high amounts of protein and fat, which can be a pellet or different fish species. Nonpelleted food for fishes can consist of artemia, algae, squid, herring, mackerel, whiting, sprat, bream, and shrimp. It is important to know the origin of the food, because threatened fish or fish harvested in areas or ways that negatively affect the environment should not be fed. Moreover, the fish should not be contaminated with heavy metals or organic components such as PCB and DDT.

Vitamins should be added to fish diets, including vitamins E and B_1 and stabilized vitamin C. Iodine should be added to prevent struma in sharks and rays. Some zoos also add glucans. Vitamins and minerals can be injected into the fed fish. Alternatively, tablets can be added just behind the gills of the fed fish.

Fish products or pellets should contain the right amount and type of feed. Regularly checking whether the fish are too fat or too thin is an important factor in proper feeding. In a mixed exhibit, the feeder should ensure that all fish get the right amount and type of food. If possible, sharks should be fed individually.

See also NUTRITIONAL DISEASES OF FISH, p 1798.

NUTRITION: GOATS

Although goats and sheep have several similarities, their nutrient requirements differ in several ways. Goats exhibit significant differences from sheep in grazing habits, physical activities, feed selection, milk composition, carcass composition, and metabolic disorders. Goats browse more than sheep, whereas sheep tend to be true grazers. Still, many of the principles useful for sheep feeding and nutrition are applicable for goats. The basic assessment for nutritional well-being should be body condition or body fat covering. Goats in good flesh, or with normal fat stores, are usually being fed a diet with adequate energy and to a lesser extent, protein. (*See also* NUTRITION: SHEEP, p 2345.)

NUTRITIONAL REQUIREMENTS

Water: Goats should be provided unlimited access to fresh, clean, nonstagnant sources of freely accessible water. Goats are among the most efficient of domestic animals in their use of water; however, only ~10% of body water loss may prove fatal. They appear to be less subject to high temperature stress than other species of domestic livestock. In addition to a lesser need for body water evaporation to maintain comfort in hot climates, goats can conserve body losses of water by decreasing losses in urine and feces. Factors affecting water intake in goats include lactation, environmental temperature, water content of forage consumed, amount of exercise, stage of production (growth, maintenance, lactation, etc), and salt and mineral content of the diet. Goats grazing lush pastures may consume much lower quantities of water than those feeding on dry hay. Still, it is imperative to allow free access to water for all goats regardless of age, breed, purpose, stage of life cycle, or environment.

Energy: Energy limitations may result from inadequate feed intake or from poor diet quality; excessive water content of the feedstuffs also may become a limiting factor. Energy requirements are affected by age, body size, body condition, stage of production (growth, maintenance, pregnancy, and lactation), and concurrent medical conditions (eg, parasitism, dental disease, arthritis). Energy requirements also may be affected by the environment, hair growth, activity, and relationship with other nutrients in the diet. Increased temperature, humidity, sunshine, and wind velocity may decrease energy requirements. Shearing mohair from Angora goats and pashmina from Cashmere goats decreases insulation and results in increased energy needs (at least in colder environments).

Goats exhibit a wide range of grazing activity, ranging from light activity for goats under intensive management, through moderate activity on semiarid land, to high activity for goats grazing on sparsely vegetated grassland and on mountainous pastures that necessitate long-distance travel daily.

The best assessment of energy intake adequacy in goats is proper body condition or fat covering the loin, brisket, inner thigh, and ribs. Using herd/individual medical record systems, a standardized body condition score (1–5, with 1 being extremely thin, to 5 being extremely obese) should be used to monitor body fat changes and make less subjective decisions with respect to longterm dietary energy adequacy. If animals are parasite- and disease-free, yet underconditioned, then they are usually being fed an energy-deficient diet; the reverse is true for obese animals. The energy values required for growth and lactation are very comparable to the numbers used for sheep and cattle, respectively. Therefore, sheep nutrition principles from an energy standpoint will probably suffice when dealing with all classes of goats, except for lactating dairy goats.

Protein: Protein is required for most normal functions of the body, including maintenance, growth, reproduction, lactation, and hair production. Protein deficiencies in the diet deplete stores in the blood, liver, and muscles and predispose animals to a variety of serious and even fatal ailments. Feed intake and dietary digestibility are reduced if dietary crude protein is <6%, further compounding an energy-protein deficiency; thus, for maintenance of mature, healthy animals, the diet should have a minimum of 7% crude protein. Dietary crude protein requirements are higher for growth, gestation, and lactation.

Most forages contain adequate amounts of dietary protein for maintenance, but lactating, growing, sick, or debilitated animals may require diets fortified with legumes or protein supplements (eg, soybean meal, cottonseed meal, etc). Feeding adequate to slightly greater amounts of protein than required appears to aid in the control (both resistance and resilience) of internal nematode parasites.

Minerals: Requirements for minerals have not been established definitively for goats at either maintenance or production levels. Research has been conducted with goats in mineral metabolism studies, especially with calcium and phosphorus. In general, these data support assumptions that several mineral requirements for goats are similar to those for sheep. (For detailed nutrient requirements for goats, refer to the most current *Nutrient Requirements of Small Ruminants*, published by the National Research Council [www.nap.edu].) Feeding to meet the goat's needs will maximize its production, reproduction, and immune system. The addition of specific minerals (phosphorus for dry winter forages, selenium in deficient areas, etc) to salt (NaCl), preferably in granular form and offered free choice, helps prevent most mineral deficiencies and improves performance.

Calcium requirements are generally met under grazing conditions with either Angora or meat-type goats, but levels should be checked in high-producing dairy goats because a deficiency can lead to reduced milk production. Adequate levels of calcium for lactating goats are necessary to prevent parturient paresis (milk fever). In browsing or grain-fed goats, the addition of a calcium supplement (dicalcium phosphate, limestone, etc) to the feed or to a salt or trace mineral–salt mixture usually meets calcium requirements. Legumes (eg, clover, alfalfa, kudzu) are also good sources of calcium.

Phosphorus deficiency results in slowed growth, unthrifty appearance, and occasionally a depraved appetite. Goats can maintain milk production on phosphorus-deficient diets for several weeks by using phosphorus from body reserves, but during long periods of phosphorus deficiency, milk production was shown to decline by 60%. The calcium:phosphorus ratio should be maintained between 1:1 and 2:1, preferably 1.2–1.5:1 in goats because of their predisposition for urinary calculi. Phosphorus deficiency in grazing goats is more likely than a calcium deficiency. In cases of struvite calculi, the ratio should be maintained at 2:1.

Magnesium deficiency is associated with hypomagnesemic tetany (grass tetany), but ordinarily this condition is less common in grazing goats than it is in cattle. Goats do have marginal ability to compensate for low magnesium by decreasing the amount of magnesium they excrete. Both urinary excretion and milk production are reduced in a magnesium deficiency.

Salt (NaCl) is usually recognized as a necessary dietary component but is often forgotten. Goats may consume more salt than is required when it is offered ad lib; this does not present a nutritional problem but may depress feed and water intakes in some arid areas where salt content of the drinking water is quite high. Salt formulations are used as carriers for trace minerals, because goats have a clear drive for sodium intake.

Potassium has an important role in metabolism. However, forages generally are quite rich in potassium, so a deficiency in grazing goats is extremely rare. Marginal potassium intake is seen only in heavily lactating does fed diets composed predominately of cereal grains. Excessive potassium intake (particularly in late gestation) may be associated with hypocalcemia in dairy goats. If hypocalcemia is a herd problem, attention should be paid to reducing or monitoring potassium-rich feedstuffs (eg, alfalfa).

Iron deficiency is seldom seen in mature grazing goats. Such deficiency might be seen in young kids because of their minimal stores at birth, plus the low iron content of the dam's milk. This is more commonly seen in kids fed in complete confinement and heavily parasitized animals. Iron deficiency can be prevented by access to pasture or a good quality trace mineral salt containing iron. In severe cases, and for kids reared in confinement, iron dextran injections at 2- to 3-wk intervals (150 mg, IM) for the first few months may be curative. In the cases of mixed iron/selenium deficiencies, caution should be used when injecting iron dextrans until the selenium deficiency is also corrected.

Iodine deficiency in the soil, and in the crops produced thereon, is seen in some areas of the USA. Therefore, iodine should be provided in stabilized salt. Conditional iodine deficiency may develop with normal to marginal iodine intake in goats consuming goitrogenous plants. Marked deficiency of iodine results in an enlarged thyroid; poor growth; small, weak kids at birth; and poor reproductive ability.

Zinc deficiency results in parakeratosis, stiffness of joints, smaller testicles, and lowered libido. A minimal level of 10 ppm of zinc in the diet, or a trace mineral salt mixture of 0.5%–2% zinc, prevents deficiencies. Excessive dietary calcium (alfalfa) may increase the likelihood of zinc deficiency in goats.

Copper deficiency may result in microcytic anemia, poor production, lighter or faded hair color, poor fiber quality, infertility, poor health and slowed growth, some forms of metabolic bone disease, diarrhea, and possibly a greater susceptibility to internal parasites. Copper deficiency in a diet may be caused by inadequate copper intake, a lowered copper-molybdenum ratio, or excessive dietary sulfur. Goats appear to be much more resistant to copper toxicity than sheep.

Selenium deficiency in the diet is usually associated with nutritional muscular dystrophy, retained placentas and metritis, poor growth, weak or premature kids, and mastitis.

Vitamins: Recommendations for vitamin requirements of goats are even more sparse than for mineral requirements. At best, almost all vitamin recommendations for goats must be based on those for sheep (*see* p 2345).

HERBAGE AND BROWSE UTILIZATION

In contrast to other farm animals, except llamas, goats prefer shrubs and tree leaves, whether deciduous or evergreen. Because of this preference, goats have been used to control encroaching shrub-type growth in pastures. Goats consume approximately the same weight of forage as do sheep of similar size. Goats tend to select highly digestible portions of most forages and show a preference to browse along fence lines and rough areas. Goats usually perform on improved pastures and prefer browse to grass (a diet of >80% browse).

Browse (leaves and twigs of trees and shrubs) generally contain higher levels of crude protein and phosphorus during their growing season than do grasses. However, some palatable browse species are limited in value because of one or more inhibitors that may bind or otherwise prevent use of nutrients contained in the plants. One such inhibitor is lignification of woody twigs and tree leaves, which physically binds (or encapsulates) the desirable nutrients. Certain oils (terpene-based compounds) are present in relatively high concentrations in some range shrubs and apparently inhibit growth of rumen bacteria. High concentrations of tannins are present in certain browse plants and depress digestion of feedstuffs by binding enzymes or by inhibiting enzymatic activity. Excessive tannins may also increase sulfur requirements, which may be more critical for hair-producing goats. However, in spite of these potential problems, when given the opportunity to choose, goats appear to be able to select more digestible and beneficial browse. Grazing or browsing tannin-containing plants may help control many species of internal nematode parasites.

For sample rations for kids and goats, *see* TABLE 41.

TABLE 41 SAMPLE RATIONS FOR GOATS[a]

For a 30-kg (66-lb) goat in a nonproductive state, minimal activity, maintenance only:
Chickpea straw 630 g (1.4 lb)
Alfalfa, fresh 95 g (0.20 lb)
For a 50-kg (110-lb) goat in a nonproductive state, minimal activity, maintenance only:
Wheat straw 716 g (1.6 lb)
Alexandrian clover, fresh 333 g (0.73 lb)
For a 20-kg (44-lb) kid gaining 50 g/day, minimal activity:
Alfalfa hay, full bloom 80 g (0.18 lb)
Corn grain 360 g (0.79 lb)
For a 30-kg (66-lb) kid gaining 150 g/day (0.33 lb):
Chickpea straw 500 g (1.1 lb)
Corn grain 400 g (0.88 lb)
Linseed meal 65 g
For a 40-kg (88-lb) doe in late gestation with minimal activity:
Johnsongrass hay 960 g (2.11 lb)
Sorghum grain 350 g (0.77 lb)
For a 70-kg (154-lb) doe producing 5 kg (11 lb) of milk testing 3.5% butterfat:
Corn silage (dough stage) 1,000 g (2.2 lb)
Alfalfa hay, full bloom 500 g (1.1 lb)
Corn grain 1,365 g (3.00 lb)
Soybean meal 280 g (0.62 lb)

[a] Dry-matter basis

NUTRITIONAL DISEASES

Enterotoxemia: This feed-related malady causes almost sudden death due to a toxin produced by *Clostridium perfringens* type D and sometimes type C. The organism appears to be widespread in nature. Under conditions of high carbohydrate consumption or high intake of immature succulent forage, the causative bacteria multiply rapidly and produce an ε toxin that increases intestinal permeability. (*See also* ENTEROTOXEMIAS, p 609.) Some cases of enterotoxemia are seen in goats, usually those fed diets with high concentrations of carbohydrates. Diarrhea, depression, lack of coordination, digestive upsets, coma, and death may be seen after excessive carbohydrate feeding of both baby kids and mature goats. The best method to prevent enterotoxemia in stable-fed goats is frequent, small-volume feeding of milk, grain, and forage. Large meals fed once a day should be avoided. Acute indigestion and a rumen pH of <4.8 indicates lactic acidosis, which can lead to the secondary complication of enterotoxemia.

Polioencephalomalacia: Clinical signs include disorientation, dullness, aimless wandering, loss of appetite, circling, progressive cortical blindness, extensor spasms, and occasionally head pressing. Some animals become recumbent and may eventually die without treatment. Diets that produce a low rumen pH or that are high in grain and low in forages predispose ruminants to polioencephalomalacia. Such dietary conditions can result in depressed production of thiamine, the production of thiamine antimetabolites, or the production of thiaminases in the rumen.

Affected animals can usually be treated successfully with thiamine (200–500 mg, IV, IM, or SC). Although response is dramatic and almost immediate, if significant brain damage has occurred, animals rarely return to a satisfactory level of production. Therefore, prompt treatment is critical.

The diet should be modified to reduce grain and increase forage intake. During times of stress, or when predisposing diets are unavoidable, the inclusion of thiamine mononitrate in the diet may aid in prevention. (*See also* POLIOENCEPHALOMALACIA, p 1281.)

Pregnancy Toxemia: Seen in late pregnancy, pregnancy toxemia is much more common in dams carrying multiple fetuses. Clinical features include abnormally increased blood levels of ketone bodies with concurrent hypoglycemia. Affected animals exhibit many of the signs described for enterotoxemia (*see* above). During late gestation, the developing fetuses have high demands for glucose; in an attempt to meet the glucose needs, the dam begins to metabolize adipose tissue (fat). The ability of the liver to metabolize this extra fat load is compromised, with a subsequent increase in the release of ketone bodies into the bloodstream. Signs include depression, dullness, opisthotonos, and eventually death.

In early stages of the disease, when signs first appear, a drench of 200–300 mL of propylene glycol or glycerol can be used as an energy source for the dam to prevent so much body fat from being metabolized. However, the administration of glucose (5% dextrose or 50–120 mL of 23% calcium borogluconate solution into a liter of 5% dextrose IV) is the treatment of choice.

Prevention should be aimed at maintaining a proper body condition score, identifying females with twins and triplets and feeding accordingly, reducing the incidence of chronic disease, shearing long-fibered does in late gestation, and possibly including niacin (1 g/day in the diet during late gestation) in the diet. Ensuring adequate winter feedstuffs while monitoring body condition changes throughout gestation will help reduce the incidence of this condition. (*See also* PREGNANCY TOXEMIA IN EWES AND DOES, p 1021.)

Urinary Calculi: Calculi result from mineral deposits in the urinary tract. Difficult and painful urination is evidenced by straining, slow urination, stomping of the feet, and kicking at the area of the penis. Blockage of the flow of urine generally is seen only in intact or castrated males. The blockage may rupture the urinary bladder, resulting in a condition known as water-belly, and cause death. It is common when diets with high concentrations of cereal grains are fed (feedlot lambs, pet goats, etc). Affected animals excrete an alkaline urine that has a high phosphorus content.

The incidence of urinary struvite calculi can be reduced by lowering phosphorus consumption to minimal levels and maintaining a calcium:phosphorus ratio >2:1 (with the phosphorus content <0.45% of the diet). The use of anionic salts such as ammonium chloride (0.5% of the complete diet), dietary tetracycline, adequate vitamin A (or β-carotene) intake, increased dietary intake of NaCl, reducing grain intake, minimizing use of pelleted cereal grains, and ensuring an adequate source of fresh, clean, palatable water free choice have proved beneficial. Affected animals drenched with ammonium chloride (7–14 g/day for 3–5 days) may show a good response. In range sheep and goats, the disease is associated with consumption of forages having a high silica content. (*See also* NONINFECTIOUS DISEASES OF THE URINARY SYSTEM IN LARGE ANIMALS, p 1502.)

White Muscle Disease: White muscle disease is caused by low levels of selenium and possibly vitamin E. It seems to develop less frequently in goats than in sheep. Signs include stiffness (especially in the hindquarters), tucked-up rear flanks, arched backs, pneumonia, and acute death. On necropsy, white striations are found in cardiac, diaphragmatic, and skeletal muscles. Levels of AST and lactic dehydrogenase are increased, indicating muscle damage. Blood levels of the selenium-containing glutathione peroxidase are reduced. (*See also* NUTRITIONAL MYODEGENERATION, p 1172.)

NUTRITION: HORSES

Horses are maintained for a much longer time than most farm animals and have more varied uses as athletes and service and companion animals. Feeding programs, therefore, must sustain a long, productive, and athletic life. The feeding recommendations given below are based on both practical experience and scientific research. Detailed recommendations can be found in *Nutrient Requirements of Horses*, 6th Ed, published in 2007 by the National Research Council (NRC).

NUTRITIONAL REQUIREMENTS

Horses can use hay and other roughages as nutrient sources much more efficiently than other nonruminants such as poultry or pigs, although utilization is less efficient than in ruminants. Traditionally, it was stated that a good source of roughage should comprise at least 50% of the total equine ration by weight. Current recommendations are that horses receive at least 1.5%–2% of their body weight in forage or forage substitutes such as hay cubes or other high-fiber source daily. The average maximum daily dry matter intake is 2.5%–3% body wt (although some breeds and age groups, notably ponies and weanlings, can exceed those maximums if on good pastures); therefore, forage or forage substitutes should be the major components of an equine ration. The main sites of fermentation in horses are in the cecum and large colons, where products of microbial fermentation, such as volatile fatty acids, amino acids, and vitamins, are also absorbed. Microbial fermentation also occurs in the stomach and small intestine to lesser degrees, depending on the type of feed. Enzymatic digestion of carbohydrates, protein, and fats occurs only in the duodenum and jejunum. Any of these nutrient sources that escape small-intestinal digestion/absorption are passed on for microbial degradation in the large intestine, where their fermentation will alter pH and microbial activity, both acutely and longterm.

Water: Water requirements depend largely on environmental conditions, amount of work or physical activity being performed, type and amount of feed, and physiologic status of the horse. The minimal maintenance daily water requirement of a sedentary adult horse in a thermoneutral environment is 5 L/100 kg body wt/day, assuming the horse is consuming at least 1.5% of its body wt in feed dry matter. However, a 500-kg horse will usually drink 21–29 L of water per day when fed a mixed hay/grain ration or pasture. If fed only dry hay, water intake will almost double. Lactation or sweat losses also increase the needs by 50%–200%. A 500-kg horse exercising for 1 hr in a hot environment will need to drink 72–92 L of water to replace sweat and evaporative losses. Lactating mares need 12–14 L per 100 kg body wt to sustain good health and milk production.

Unlimited free access to clean water is usually recommended, although horses can easily adapt to only periodic access throughout the day if the amounts offered during the watering sessions are not limited. Inadequate water access will reduce feed intake and increase the incidence of impaction colic, anhidrosis, and other metabolic disorders.

Energy: Energy requirements may be classified into those needed for maintenance, growth, pregnancy, lactation, and work. Equations to estimate energy requirements at any state of performance or production have been derived primarily from studies of light horse breeds (*see* TABLES 42 and 43). However, the need for energy differs considerably among individuals; some horses require much greater amounts of feed than others ("hard keepers"), and others are much more efficient at feed digestion/utilization ("easy keepers"). Digestibility of feedstuffs also often differs significantly from published values. Therefore, the caloric recommendations provided herein should be considered only a starting point to determine the actual energy needs of a given horse.

Amounts fed should be adjusted to maintain a body condition score between 4 and 6 (*see* TABLE 44). Emaciated and very thin horses have decreased stress and cold tolerance and increased susceptibility to infections. Obese horses have decreased tolerance of exercise and heat, increased risk of laminitis and lipoma strangulation colic, and if fasted, hyperlipidemia and hypertriglyceridemia. Obesity is also associated with insulin resistance and glucose intolerance.

Maintenance: For maintenance of body weight and to support normal activity, the daily digestible energy (DE) requirement (in Mcal) of the nonworking adult horse in good body condition is estimated to be on average 33.3 kcal/kg body wt, with a minimum requirement of 30.3 kcal/kg for easy keepers or draft/warmblood types of horses and 36.3 kcal/kg for hard keeper adult horses. For obese or emaciated horses, the estimated ideal body weight in kg should be used in the equation rather than current body weight. For weight gain, it is estimated that 1 unit of change in body condition score takes 16–20 kg body wt gain and that each kg of gain requires 20 Mcal DE above maintenance requirements. Caloric intake in obese horses should not be restricted severely for prolonged periods of time because of the risk of hyperlipidemia, especially in ponies and donkeys.

Cold weather increases the energy requirement by 0.00082 Mcal DE/kg body wt for each degree Celsius drop below the

TABLE 42 ESTIMATED DAILY NUTRIENT REQUIREMENTS OF GROWING HORSES AND PONIES

			Daily Nutrients Per Animal[a]				
Age (mo)	Body Weight (kg)	Daily Gain (kg)	Digestible Energy (Mcal)	Crude Protein (g)	Ca (g)	P (g)	Vitamin A[b] (IU)
ADULT WEIGHT 200 KG (PONIES)							
4	67	0.34	5.3	268	15.6	8.7	3,000
6	86	0.29	6.2	270	15.5	8.6	3,900
12	128	0.18	7.5	338	15.1	8.4	5,800
18	155	0.11	7.7	320	14.8	8.2	7,000
24	172	0.07	7.5	308	14.7	8.1	7,700
ADULT WEIGHT 500 KG (AVERAGE HORSES)							
4	168	0.84	13.3	669	39.1	21.7	7,600
6	216	0.72	15.5	676	38.6	21.5	9,700
12	321	0.45	18.8	846	37.7	20.9	14,500
18	387	0.29	19.2	799	37.0	20.6	17,400
24	365	0.18	18.7	770	36.7	20.4	19,300
ADULT WEIGHT 900 KG (DRAFT HORSES)							
4	303	1.52	23.9	1,204	70.3	39.1	13,600
6	389	1.30	28.0	1,217	69.5	38.7	17,500
12	578	0.82	33.8	1,522	67.8	37.7	26,000
18	697	0.51	34.6	1,438	66.7	37.1	31,400
24	773	0.324	39.2	1,492	66.0	36.7	34,800

[a] Assumes good-quality forage with or without additional concentrates. Maximal daily intake is estimated to be 2.5%–3% body wt in dry matter.

[b] One mg of β-carotene equals 400 IU of vitamin A for the horse.

Adapted from *Nutrient Requirements of Horses*, 2007, National Academy of Sciences, National Academy Press, Washington, DC.

lower critical temperature (LCT) of the animal. However, the LCT of cold-adapted adult horses in Canada was estimated to be –15°C, whereas donkeys acclimatized to summer temperatures in Nevada had an LCT of 26°C. Wind, precipitation, and body condition also affect LCT. Therefore, LCT must be estimated based on regional average temperatures and conditions and perhaps type of horse. For example, draft breeds with thick hair coats would tolerate lower temperatures than a thin-haired, *thin-skinned* Thoroughbred.

Growth: For growth, the daily DE requirement of light horse breeds is estimated to be maintenance DE Mcal/day = $(56.5X^{-0.145})/1{,}000$ times body wt in kg plus the caloric requirements for growth = $(1.99 + 1.21X - (0.021X^2) \times ADG$, using the above equation(s) for the maintenance DE, and X as the age in months and ADG as the desired average daily gain in kg. This equation will give an estimate of caloric requirements; intakes should be adjusted to maintain body condition scores of 5 or 6 in growing horses. Warmblood, draft, and draft-cross breeds may require 10%–20% less than calculated by the equations above to sustain rapid growth and avoid obesity.

Pregnancy and Lactation: During pregnancy, if the mare is not exercised or exposed to extreme weather conditions,

TABLE 43 ESTIMATED AVERAGE DAILY NUTRIENT REQUIREMENTS OF MATURE HORSES AND PONIES

Body Weight (kg)	Daily Nutrients Per Animal[a]					Daily Milk Production (kg)
	Digestible Energy (Mcal)	Crude Protein (g)	Ca (g)	P (g)	Vitamin A[b] (IU)	
MAINTENANCE						
200	6.7	252	8	6	6,000	—
500	16.7	630	20	14	15,000	—
900	30.0	1,134	36	25.2	27,000	—
LAST 90 DAYS OF GESTATION						
214–226	7.7–8.6	319–357	14.4	10.5	12,000	—
500	19.2–21.4	797–893	36	26.3	30,000	—
600	34.6–38.5	1,434–1,607	64.8	47.3	54,000	—
LACTATING MARES, FIRST 3 MO						
200	12.2–12.7	587–614	22.4–23.6	14.4–15.3	12,000	6.0–6.5
500	30.6–31.7	1,468–1,535	55.9–59.0	36.0–38.3	30,000	15.0–16.3
900	52.4–54.4	2,642–2,763	100.6–106.4	64.9–68.9	54,000	26.91–29.3
LACTATING MARES, 3 MO TO WEANING						
200	10.9–12.2	506–587	15.0–22.4	9.3–10.5	12,000	4.4–6.0
500	27.2–30.6	1,265–1,468	37.4–55.9	23.2–36.0	30,000	10.9–14.9
900	46.3–52.5	2,277–2,642	67.4–100.6	41.8–64.9	54,000	19.6–26.9

[a] Assumes good-quality forage with or without additional concentrates. Maximal daily intake is estimated to be 2.5%–3.0% body wt in dry matter. Ranges are given for requirements that change with time of pregnancy/lactation.

[b] One mg of β-carotene equals 400 IU of vitamin A for the horse.

Adapted from *Nutrient Requirements of Horses*, 2007, National Academy of Sciences, National Academy Press, Washington, DC

maintenance DE intakes are usually adequate until the last 90 days of gestation. Energy requirements during months 9, 10, and 11 of gestation are estimated by multiplying estimated maintenance requirements by 1.11, 1.13, and 1.20, respectively. Voluntary intake of roughage decreases as the fetus gets larger, and it may be necessary to increase the energy density of the ration by using supplemental concentrates in late pregnancy.

To support lactation, the NRC has estimated that 792 kcal of DE/kg of milk produced per day (see TABLE 43) should be added to the increased (36.3 kcal/kg body wt) maintenance needs. Lactating light horses (eg, Thoroughbred, Quarter horses) maintained body weight when fed 28–31 Mcal DE/day. Draft mares may require as much as 43 Mcal/day. However, this recommended level of energy intake has increased body weight gain in lactating

TABLE 44 BODY CONDITION SCORES FOR HORSES

Score		Description
1	Emaciated	Spinous processes, ribs, tailhead, tuber coxae, and ischii prominent. Bone structure of neck, withers, and shoulders easily visible. No fat palpable over lumbar vertebral transverse processes.
2	Very thin	Slight fat covering spinous processes and tailhead. Transverse processes slightly rounded. Ribs, tailhead, and tuber coxae and ischii prominent. Bone structure of neck, withers, and shoulders faintly discernible.
3	Thin	Fat buildup halfway on spinous process and tailhead; both prominent, but individual vertebrae in tailhead not visible. Transverse processes cannot be felt. Slight fat buildup over ribs and tuber coxae but easily visible. Tuber ischii not discernible. Withers, neck, and shoulder accentuated, but bone structure not visible.
4	Lean	Slight ridge visible over loin, faint outline of ribs visible. Tailhead prominence depends on conformation, but fat palpable around it. Tuber coxae not visible. Withers, shoulder, and neck not obviously thin.
5	Moderate	Loin is flat (no crease or ridge). Ribs not visible but easily felt. Fat around tailhead is spongy, withers rounded over spinous process, and shoulders and neck blend smoothly into body.
6	Moderately fleshy	May have slight crease down loin, ribs barely palpable with light pressure, and fat around tailhead soft. Some fat palpable on side of withers, neck, and behind shoulder.
7	Fleshy	May have crease down loin, and ribs difficult to feel. Fat deposited along withers, behind shoulder, and along neck.
8	Fat	Crease down loin. Ribs very difficult to feel; fat around tailhead very soft. Fat filling area over withers and behind shoulder with noticeable thickening of neck.
9	Obese	Obvious crease down loin. Patchy fat deposits over ribs. Fat bulging around tailhead, along withers, behind shoulders, and along neck. Flank filled with fat (no abdominal tuck).

pony mares, indicating that it may exceed the needs of some breeds or individuals. The mare's body condition should be evaluated on a regular basis and maintained in the range of 5 to 7 using the body condition scores of 1 to 9 (described above) throughout pregnancy and lactation. Mares should be maintaining or gaining in condition to optimize reproductive success during the breeding season, even if lactating at the same time.

Work: The energy requirements of work are influenced by many factors, including type of work, condition and training of the horse, fatigue, environmental temperature, and skill of the rider or driver. As the duration of exercise increases and level of activity is maintained, the DE requirement per unit of time worked actually decreases. For these reasons, DE recommendations for various activities of light horses (*see* TABLE 45) should be adjusted to meet individual needs and to maintain body condition scores between 4 and 6 for optimal athletic performance.

Protein and Amino Acids: Although some amino acid synthesis and absorption occurs in the cecum and large intestine, it is not sufficient to meet the amino acid needs of growing, working, or lactating horses; therefore, the protein quality of the feed provided to these classes of horses is important. Weanlings require 2.1 g, and yearlings 1.9 g, of lysine/Mcal DE/day. Requirements for other dietary amino acids have not been well established; however, the crude protein recommendations given

TABLE 45 ENERGY REQUIREMENTS OF WORK FOR LIGHT HORSES[a] AND DESIRABLE BODY CONDITION SCORES

Activity	DE (Mcal/day)	Body Condition Score
Idle (maintenance)	0.033 × body wt (kg)	4–6
Halter competition, pleasure trail riding	1.20 × DE for maintenance	5–6
Performance/show (park, English, and Western pleasure, youth activity), equestrian instruction	1.4 × DE for maintenance	5–6
Ranch work, frequent strenuous show (cutting and roping, barrel racing), endurance trail ride, lower level 3-day event (hunt course, stadium jumping, dressage), polo	1.60 × DE for maintenance	4–5
Race training, elite 3-day event	1.9 × DE for maintenance	4–5

[a] 200–600 kg body wt

in TABLES 42 and 43 should be adequate if good quality forages and concentrates are used in the ration. The amino acid balance in alfalfa and other legumes such as soybeans appears to be better than that found in cereal grains or some grass hays. This should be considered when formulating rations, especially for rapidly growing young horses.

Growing horses have a higher need for protein (14%–16% of total ration) than mature horses (8%–10% of total ration). Aged horses (>20 yr old) may require protein intakes equivalent to those for young, growing horses to maintain body condition; however, hepatic and renal function should be assessed before increasing the protein intake of old horses. Fetal growth during the last third of pregnancy increases protein requirements somewhat (10%–11% of total ration), and lactation increases requirements still further (12%–14% of total ration). Work apparently does not significantly increase the protein requirement, provided that the ratio of crude protein to DE in the diet remains constant and the increased energy requirements are met.

Minerals: Because the skeleton is of such fundamental importance to performance of the horse, calcium and phosphorus requirements deserve careful attention (TABLES 42 and 43). Excessive intakes of certain minerals may be as harmful as deficiencies; therefore, mineral supplements should complement the composition of the basic ration. For example, if the horse is consuming mostly roughage with little or no grain, phosphorus is more likely to be in short supply, especially for growth, than calcium. However, if more grain than roughage is being fed, a deficit of calcium is much more common. The total mineral contribution and availability from all parts of the ration (forages and roughages, concentrates, and all supplements) should be considered when evaluating the mineral intake. However, aside from actual feeding trials, no suitable test for availability of dietary minerals exists. Blood concentrations do not reflect dietary intake adequately for any of the macrominerals, especially calcium.

Calcium and Phosphorus: Requirements for calcium and phosphorus are much greater during growth than for maintenance of mature animals. The last third of pregnancy and lactation also appreciably increase the requirement. Aged horses (>20 yr old) may require more phosphorus than is required for adult maintenance (0.3%–0.4% of total ration). Excess calcium intake (>1% of total ration) should be avoided in aged horses, especially if renal function is reduced.

For all horses, the calcium:phosphorus ratio should be maintained at >1:1. A desirable ratio is ~1.5:1, although if adequate phosphorus is fed, foals can apparently tolerate a ratio of up to 3:1 and young adult horses a ratio even higher. Work does not appreciably increase calcium or phosphorus requirements as a portion of diet.

Salt: Salt (NaCl) requirements are markedly influenced by sweat losses. It is recommended that horse rations contain 1.6–1.8 g salt/kg feed dry matter, although there are limited data on the precise requirements. Sweat losses may cause NaCl losses >30 g (1 oz) in only 1–2 hr of hard work, and feed concentrations of salt for working horses are recommended to be at least 3.6 g NaCl/kg feed dry matter. The upper limit for salt inclusion in the ration of even hard-working horses is recommended at 6% of the total ration. However, NaCl is the only mineral for which horses are known to have true "nutritional wisdom." Horses voluntarily seek out and consume salt in amounts to meet their daily needs if given the opportunity. Salt or salt blocks should be available free choice. Supplemental salt may be provided by oral dosing or added to feed or water in addition to free-choice salt to replace acute losses during hard work, but prolonged, excessive, forced supplementation will enhance excretion, which will reduce the ability to adjust to acute losses in the future. Forced oral administration of concentrated salt pastes (electrolytes) to dehydrated horses can cause abdominal malaise. Some horses, usually those confined to stalls, will ingest excessive amounts of salt, possibly due to restricted feed intake and/or boredom. This will not cause health problems as long as adequate water is available, although it will increase water intake and urination. Salt poisoning is unlikely unless a deprived horse is suddenly allowed free access to salt, or if water is not available to horses force-fed salt (eg, electrolyte mixtures given PO during competitions). Excessive salt content of feed or water will limit voluntary intakes, precluding toxicity but putting the horse at risk of energy deficits.

The most satisfactory method to provide supplemental calcium, phosphorus, and salt is to furnish a mixture of one-third trace mineral or plain salt and two-thirds dicalcium phosphate free choice. Trace mineral salt blocks do not contain additional calcium or phosphorus.

Magnesium: The daily magnesium requirement for maintenance has been estimated at 0.015 g/kg body wt based on limited studies. Working horses are estimated to require 0.019 to 0.03 g/kg body wt for light to strenuous exercise, respectively, due to sweat losses. The requirements for growth have not been well established but have been estimated to be 0.07% of the total ration. Most feeds used for horses contain 0.1%–0.3% magnesium. Although deficiencies are unlikely, hypomagnesemic tetany has been reported in lactating mares and stressed horses. The upper limit of recommended intake is estimated to be 0.3% of ration dry matter based on data from other species, but adult horses have been fed rations with higher magnesium content without apparent adverse effects. Anecdotally, high magnesium intake has a pharmacologic calming effect on horses, but large doses of magnesium sulfate (ie, Epsom salts) are also laxative.

Potassium: The recommended potassium intake for maintenance in adult horses is 0.05 g/kg body wt. Most roughages contain >1% potassium, and a ration containing ≥50% roughage provides more than sufficient potassium for maintenance animals. Working horses, lactating mares, and horses receiving diuretics need higher potassium intakes because of sweat, milk, and urinary losses. Hard work may increase intake needs by a factor of 1.8. It has been proposed that rations fed to hard working horses should provide 4.5 g potassium/Mcal DE. Potassium chloride is the most common salt used to supplement rations. However, upper safe limits have not been established, and although excesses are usually efficiently excreted by the kidneys in healthy horses, acute hyperkalemia caused by the rapid absorption of concentrated salt mixtures can induce potentially fatal cardiac arrhythmias. Forced oral supplementation with large doses of potassium salts should be avoided, even in hard working horses.

Iodine: Iodized salts used in salt blocks or commercial feeds easily fulfill the dietary iodine requirement (estimated to be 0.35 mg/kg feed dry matter), as do forages grown in iodine replete soils. Late pregnant mares may require slightly higher intakes (0.4 mg/kg feed dry matter), but iodine toxicity has been noted in pregnant mares consuming as little as 40 mg of iodine/day. Goiter due to excess iodine intake has been well documented in both mares and their foals, and several cases were associated with large amounts of dried seaweed (kelp) in the diet. Except in regions where the soils are known to be severely iodine deficient, iodine supplementation should not be necessary for horses.

Copper: The dietary copper requirement for horses is probably 8–10 ppm, although many commercial concentrates formulated for horses contain >20 ppm. The presence of 1–3 ppm of molybdenum in forages, which interferes with copper utilization in ruminants, does not cause problems in horses. However, excessive iron supplementation (fairly common, especially in performance horses [see below]) may inhibit adequate absorption. Copper deficiency may cause osteochondritis dissecans in young, growing horses and is associated with a higher risk of aortic or uterine artery rupture in adults. Copper deficits may also cause hypochromic microcytic anemia and pigmentation loss. Horses are extremely tolerant of copper intakes that would be fatal to sheep. However, excessively high copper intakes potentially reduce the absorption and utilization of selenium and iron, and should be avoided.

Iron: The dietary maintenance requirement for iron is estimated to be 40 mg/kg feed dry matter. For rapidly growing foals and pregnant and lactating mares, the requirement is estimated to be 50 mg/kg feed dry matter. Virtually all commercial concentrates formulated for horses and most forages contain iron well in excess of the recommended concentrations. Only horses with chronic blood loss (eg, parasitism) should be considered to be at risk of iron deficiency. Excess iron intake potentially interferes with copper utilization. The presence of anemia (low PCV or red cell volume) alone is not sufficient indication for iron supplementation in horses.

Zinc: The zinc requirement is estimated to be 40 mg/kg feed dry matter, although there is evidence that this recommendation may be as much as twice the actual requirement to prevent signs of deficiency in most horses. This mineral is relatively innocuous, and intakes several times the requirement are considered safe, although intakes >1,000 ppm have induced copper deficiency and developmental orthopedic disease in young horses.

Selenium: The dietary requirement for selenium is estimated to be 0.1 mg/kg feed dry matter in most regions. However, there are regions of the world (including the lower Great Lakes, the Pacific northwest, the Atlantic coast, and Florida in the USA, as well as parts of New Zealand) where soils are profoundly deficient in this important but potentially very toxic trace mineral. In other areas (including parts of Colorado, Wyoming, and North and South Dakota), forages may contain 5–40 ppm of selenium, which is sufficient to produce clinical signs of toxicity (*see* p 3085). Exercise increases glutathione peroxidase (selenium-containing enzyme) activity and may increase need for supplementation in heavily exercised horses. No more than 0.002 mg/kg body wt should be supplemented on a daily basis; toxicity has been seen with as little as 5 mg selenium/kg feed dry matter.

Other Minerals: The requirement for **sulfur** in horses is not established. However, sulfur-containing amino acids (methionine) and vitamins (biotin) are essential for healthy hoof growth. If the protein requirement is met, the sulfur intake of horses is usually ~0.15% dry-matter intake—a concentration apparently adequate for most individuals. Sulfur deficits may contribute to poor hoof quality.

The dietary requirement for **cobalt** is apparently <0.05 ppm. It is incorporated into vitamin B_{12} by microorganisms in the cecum and colon and, therefore, is an essential nutrient per se only if exogenous sources of B_{12} are not incorporated into the ration. The upper limit of intake is estimated to be 25 mg/kg feed dry matter based on data from other species.

Manganese requirements for horses have not been well established; amounts found in the usual forages (40–140 mg/kg dry matter) are considered sufficient.

Rock phosphates, when used as mineral supplements for horses, should contain <0.1% **fluorine**. Fluorine intake should not exceed 40 mg/kg feed dry matter. Excessive ingestion can result in fluorosis, although horses are more resistant to fluorine excesses than are ruminants.

Although **molybdenum** is an essential cofactor for xanthine oxidase activity, no quantitative requirement for horses has been demonstrated. Excessive levels (>15 mg/kg feed dry matter) may interfere with copper utilization.

Vitamins:

Vitamin A: The vitamin A requirement of horses can be met by β-carotene, a naturally occurring precursor, or by active forms of the vitamin (eg, retinol). Fresh green forages and good-quality hays are excellent sources of carotene, as are corn and carrots. It is estimated that 1 mg of β-carotene is equivalent to ~400 IU of active vitamin A. However, because of oxidation, the carotene content of forages decreases with storage, and hays stored >1 yr may not furnish sufficient vitamin A activity. Horses consuming fresh green forage for 3–4 mo of the year usually have sufficient stores of active forms of vitamin A in the liver to maintain adequate plasma concentrations for an additional 3–6 mo. Rations for all classes of horses should provide a minimum of 30 IU active vitamin A/kg body wt (whether as β-carotene or an active synthetic form such as retinyl acetate). Prolonged feeding of excess retinyl or retinol compounds (>10 times recommended amounts) may cause bone fragility, bone exostoses, skin lesions, and birth defects such as cleft palate and microphthalmia (based on data from both horses and other species). The proposed upper safe concentration for chronic administration is 16,000 IU of the active form of the vitamin per kg feed dry matter. There is no known toxicity associated with β-carotene in horses.

Vitamin D: Horses exposed to ≥4 hr of sunlight per day or that consume sun-cured hay do not have dietary requirements for vitamin D. For horses deprived of sunlight, suggested dietary vitamin D_3 concentrations are 800–1,000 IU/kg feed dry matter for early growth and 500 IU/kg feed dry matter for later growth and other life stages. Vitamin D toxicity is characterized by general weakness; loss of body weight; calcification of the blood vessels, heart, and other soft tissues; and bone abnormalities. Dietary excesses as small as 10 times the recommended amounts may be toxic and are aggravated by excessive calcium intake.

Vitamin E: No minimal requirement for vitamin E has been established. However, it has been established that selenium and vitamin E work together to prevent nutritional muscular dystrophy (white muscle disease, *see* p 1095), equine degenerative myeloencephalopathy, and equine motor neuron disease. Evidence of vitamin E deficiency is most likely to appear in foals nursing mares on dry winter pasture or horses fed only low-quality hay unsupplemented with commercial concentrates. Horses forced to exert great physical effort and/or fed high-fat (>5%) rations may have increased needs for vitamin E. However, if selenium intakes are adequate, it is likely that 50 IU vitamin E/kg feed dry matter is adequate for most stages of the life cycle and moderate activity. Supplementation with 500–1,000 IU vitamin E may be necessary for horses working hard and/or fed high-fat (>7%) rations. Excessive supplementation (>5,000 IU/day for an average adult horse) results in decreased vitamin A absorption and should be avoided.

Vitamin K: Vitamin K is synthesized by the microorganisms of the cecum and colon in sufficient quantities to meet the normal requirements of horses. However, consumption of moldy sweet clover hay may induce vitamin K–dependent coagulation deficits (*see* p 3156). The synthetic form of vitamin K (menadione) is nephrotoxic if administered parenterally to dehydrated horses.

Ascorbic Acid: Mature horses synthesize adequate amounts of ascorbic acid for maintenance from glucose in the liver. Some horses may need supplemental ascorbic acid (0.01 g/kg body wt/day) during periods of severe physical or psychologic stress, eg, prolonged transportation or weaning. Oral availability is variable. Ascorbyl palmitate is reportedly more readily absorbed than ascorbic acid or ascorbyl stearate. Prolonged supplementation to nonstressed horses may reduce endogenous synthesis and/or enhance excretion, resulting in deficiencies if supplementation is abruptly discontinued.

Thiamine: Although thiamine is synthesized in the cecum and colon by bacteria and ~25% of this may be absorbed, thiamine deficiency has been reported in horses fed poor-quality hay and grain. Although not necessarily a minimum value, 3 mg thiamine/kg ration dry matter has maintained peak food consumption, normal gains, and normal blood thiamine concentrations in skeletal muscle in young horses. As much as 5 mg/kg feed dry matter may be necessary for horses exercising strenuously, although verifiable deficits have not been recorded. Occasionally, horses are poisoned by consuming plants that contain thiaminases, which results in acute deficits (*see* p 3089).

Riboflavin: Riboflavin deficits have not been documented in horses. Previous correlations with low riboflavin intake and recurrent uveitis in horses have not been substantiated. However, there is no evidence of toxic effects as a result of supplementing this water-soluble vitamin, and daily intakes of 0.04 mg riboflavin/kg body wt are recommended.

Vitamin B_{12}: Intestinal synthesis of vitamin B_{12} is probably adequate to meet ordinary needs, provided there is sufficient cobalt in the diet. Deficiencies of cobalt in horses have not been reported. Vitamin B_{12} is absorbed from the cecum, and feeding a ration essentially devoid of vitamin B_{12} for 11 mo had no effect on the normal hematology or apparent health of adult horses. Vitamin B_{12} injected parenterally into racehorses and foals is rapidly and nearly completely excreted via bile into the feces.

Niacin: Niacin is synthesized by the bacterial flora of the cecum and colon and is synthesized in the liver from tryptophan. There is no known dietary requirement for niacin in healthy horses.

Other Vitamins: **Folacin, biotin, pantothenic acid, and vitamin B_6** probably are synthesized in adequate quantities in the normal equine intestine. However, biotin supplementation (15–25 mg/day) has been documented to improve hoof quality in adult horses with soft, shelly hoofwalls.

FEEDING PRACTICES

Ideally, horses should be given free access to hay and/or pasture forages with salt and water ad lib. Horses should not be offered >0.5% of their body weight in high starch/sugar grain-based concentrates (eg, textured grain, pellets, or extruded feed) in a single feeding. More than this in a single meal reduces digestive efficiency and predisposes to problems such as gastric ulcers, insulin resistance, laminitis, and colic. If large amounts of grain-based concentrates are being fed (>0.4% body wt/day), the total amount offered daily should be divided into two or more feedings. Most horses fed good-quality forages require little to no concentrate supplementation. Exceptions are hard-working horses or those with limited access to good-quality forage (<2% body wt in feed dry matter).

It has been well documented that feeding >50% of the total ration in the form of grain-based concentrates increases the risk of colic and laminitis in adult horses. High starch/sugar intake also has been correlated to increased incidence of insulin resistance in both adult and young growing horses. Large (>0.25% body wt) meals of grain-based concentrates should not be offered <1 hr before strenuous exercise, transport, or other stress, or to exhausted horses with poor gut motility.

Because horses are particularly sensitive to toxins found in spoiled feeds, all grains and roughages offered should be of good quality and free of mold. Grains should be stored at a moisture content of <13%. In warm, humid areas, mold inhibitors may help reduce feed spoilage. In contrast, excessively dry, dusty feeds tend to initiate or aggravate respiratory problems. Dampening or soaking such feeds in water before feeding can help alleviate this problem.

Feeds

Pasture: Good pasture provides both an excellent source of nutrients and the opportunity to exercise. The pasture should be kept as free of weeds as possible by regular mowing or clipping. A legume-grass mixture offers the advantages of good nutrient supply, persistence, and durability. Ideal mixes vary with region, and local recommendations from specialists should be followed. However, some forages should not be used for horse pastures. Alsike clover (*Trifolium hybridum*) and kleingrass (*Panicum coloratum*) are potentially hepatotoxic to horses, and Johnson grass (*Sorghum halepense*) and Sudan grass (*S sudanense*) contain cyanogenic glycosides. Buffel (*Cenchrus* spp), panic (*Panicum* spp), pangola (*Digitaria decumbens*), kikuyu (*Pennisetum* spp), and *Setaria* spp grasses all contain potentially harmful concentrations of oxalates. None of these forage species should be used for horse pastures.

In sandy areas, horses should be provided with supplemental hay when pasture is short (ie, overgrazed) to prevent sand ingestion and subsequent colic. The hay should be offered in feeders or on a platform to reduce sand ingestion. The use of psyllium products to enhance the elimination of sand from the equine GI tract can be expensive, and efficacy has not been well documented. Supplemental hay is also recommended in any situation when the pasture is limited in quality (lots of weeds, undesirable weeds) or quantity to avoid weed ingestion and preserve the pasture cover.

Hay: Common types of hay used to feed horses include both grass hays, such as timothy, brome, coastal Bermuda, or orchard, and legumes such as alfalfa or clover. Legume-grass mixtures are generally high-yielding and contain considerably more protein, minerals, and vitamins than do grasses alone. However, they may be more difficult to cure in a warm, humid climate and more prone to mold. Coastal Bermuda grass has been associated with an increased risk of impaction colic, especially when harvested late. Alfalfa may be contaminated with blister beetles and also tends to be more allergenic than grass hays or clover. Oat hay has been used in some regions and, if properly harvested and baled, is roughly equivalent to good-quality grass hays. Teff grasses are used in some regions of the world but may be deficient in calcium and should be used with caution (or only if an accurate nutrient analysis is done), especially for growing, pregnant, or lactating horses.

The form in which harvested forages are provided to horses is of concern. High-moisture haylages and silages made from whole corn plants should be used with caution as forage sources for horses because of the risk of molds. Moldy corn silage especially can cause fatal leukoencephalomalacia. Feeding large round bales of hay in pastures can be economically advantageous if feeders that reduce waste are used, but it has been documented to increase the risk of botulism. Cubed or chopped forages are often recommended as substitutes for long-stem hay or pasture and for horses that have trouble chewing. Forage-based cubes may need to be soaked in water to decrease the risk of choke, at least initially.

Concentrates and Other Supplements: Concentrates include all grains and byproduct feeds high in energy and/or protein (eg, wheat bran, soybean meal, rice bran). Processing grains before feeding is often desirable to improve nutrient availability. However, cracked or rolled grains are more susceptible to mold. Because of differences in density, grains should be measured by weight, not volume.

Oats, one of the most traditional grains for horses, may be fed whole, rolled, or crimped. Processing increases the bulk 20%–30% and improves digestibility by ~10%. "Hulled" or "naked" oats are more energy dense than regular oats and should be introduced slowly to reduce the risk of founder or colic.

Barley is a good grain for horses. It is higher in energy than regular oats but lower than corn. It may be fed as the only grain to horses that have a high energy need. Barley should be rolled or crimped to improve digestibility. Palatability, however, is not as high as that of oats or corn.

Corn (maize) is a high-energy feed, useful for horses that are working hard or in need of extra weight gain. However, the starch in corn is less digestible than that of oats and can more easily bypass small-intestinal digestion, resulting in colic and/or laminitis if suddenly fed in large amounts. To maximize digestibility, shelled corn may be cracked or rolled, but the moisture level should be low enough to avoid spoilage during storage. Moldy corn can cause fatal leukoencephalomalacia.

Sorghum grain (milo) and **wheat** should be fed with care. These grains must be cracked or rolled if fed to horses. They are not commonly used in horse rations.

Other concentrate sources of energy/protein used in various regions of the world include dried peas (Great Britain), sugar cane pulp (Brazil), fava beans (Middle East), and bread (note that additives such as sesame or chocolate might cause positive drug-test reactions).

Other Supplements: **Wheat bran** and **rice bran** are byproduct supplements commonly fed to horses. However, both are very high in phosphorus (>1.2%), and the proper calcium:phosphorus ratio should be maintained when any form of bran is added to the diet. Wheat bran is not laxative, contrary to popular belief, but is extremely palatable to horses and often used as a wet "mash" to increase water intake or mask the flavor of other supplements. Because of its high phosphorus content, wheat bran is not recommended as a major or daily component of the ration unless the calcium intake is carefully balanced. Rice bran is a high-fat product added to rations of horses that need extra calories. Many rice bran products have added calcium to offset the high phosphorus content but still are designed to be fed in only limited (<1 kg/day) amounts.

Beet pulp, a byproduct of the sugar beet industry, is added to horse rations as both a source of calories and fiber. It contains moderate amounts of calcium and protein and can be safely fed on a daily basis in larger amounts than the bran products. Shredded beet pulp usually should be soaked in water before feeding to horses. Beet pulp pellets do not require presoaking and are often included in concentrate mixes.

Edible oils and fats may be added to rations to increase the energy density. Normal horse rations contain only 3%–4% fat, but horses can easily tolerate up to 10% fat if it is introduced slowly and they are given 3–4 wk to fully adapt to the change. Corn and vegetable oils are commonly used. Edible oils should be introduced slowly to the ration to avoid diarrhea. Although highly digestible, animal fat is not commonly used in horse rations.

Soybean meal is a palatable protein supplement with good amino acid balance for use in concentrate mixes. It may be fed when pastures or hay are low in protein and are of poor quality or when protein requirements are greatest, such as during early growth or lactation. **Linseed meal** or **cottonseed meal** should not be used as a protein supplement for young, growing horses because of their low lysine content, but they are adequate for adult horses.

Cane molasses is frequently added to grain mixtures (sweet feeds). It is highly palatable, minimizes separation of "fines," and reduces dustiness of concentrate mixtures. It is also high in potassium. The readily fermentable carbohydrates and moisture that cane molasses contains may increase mold growth in hot weather and freeze solid in cold winter weather. High sugar/starch (>30% nonstructural carbohydrate) rations have been documented to induce relative insulin resistance in horses and are associated with increased incidence of vices such as wind sucking and wood chewing.

Limestone of a high grade (38% calcium) may be used as a supplemental source of calcium. When both supplemental calcium and phosphorus are needed, dicalcium phosphate, steamed bone meal, or defluorinated rock phosphate is recommended. Dicalcium phosphate is particularly good because the cost per unit of phosphorus is low, the elements are quite available, and it is fairly palatable.

Salt (NaCl) should be provided in a block or in granular form free choice to all horses. Salt content of forages in some regions (notably the southwestern USA) and many commercial feeds may reduce the need for supplemental salt but, because of variable losses in sweat, exact needs are hard to estimate. Horses, if given the opportunity, will voluntarily consume sufficient salt to meet their longterm needs for maintenance, even in hot climates. For maintenance, in horses that do not have high mineral needs, trace mineralized salt that contains added iodine, iron, copper, cobalt, manganese, zinc, and selenium is often used. The need for these additional minerals varies with the locality.

Exercise- and/or heat-induced sweat losses can cause acute sodium/chloride/potassium deficits that must be replaced more rapidly than voluntary homeostatic mechanisms can accommodate. It is common in these circumstances (eg, performance horses) to give oral electrolyte drenches before, during, and/or after strenuous activities.

Feeding Rates

Individual differences in the need for energy and nutrients and gross variations in nutrient contents of feedstuffs make it difficult to generalize about the amount of feed to provide. The amounts given in TABLES 46 and 47 can be used as guidelines, but body condition should be monitored and amounts adjusted accordingly. The maximal dry matter intake in 24 hr is only 3%–3.5% of a horse's body wt, and many horses voluntarily consume <2.5% of their body wt in dry matter in 24 hr. Feed intake should therefore be monitored.

The need for concentrate supplementation while on pasture depends on pasture quality but is more important for young horses and lactating mares. If the pasture is of good to excellent quality, no supplementation other than water and salt are needed by most adult horses at maintenance or in light work. It is desirable to creep-feed nursing foals at the rate of 0.5%–1% body wt with concentrates formulated specifically for growth. Good-quality hay may be needed even when on pasture, especially in winter.

Forage-based total mixed rations and "complete" feeds,which may have concentrates added, have been developed for horses. These can be textured, pelleted, cubed, or extruded products. They have the advantage of uniform quality, complete control over nutrient intake, suitability for horses with bad teeth, less dustiness (which reduces respiratory problems), and reduced bulk for storage and transport. Disadvantages include an increased risk of choke and increased wood chewing, especially with the pelleted and extruded feeds fed as the sole source of nutrition. Most, however, are sufficiently high calorie that they need to be limit fed (<2.5% body wt/day). Wood chewing and boredom can be minimized by feeding long-stem hay with these products or by dividing the total daily allotment into multiple small feedings. Damage to stables and fences can be reduced by treating wood with foul-tasting substances or by covering or replacing wood with metal in vulnerable areas.

NUTRITIONAL DISEASES

Reports of uncomplicated nutrient deficiencies in horses are rare. The nutrients most likely to be deficient are caloric sources, protein, calcium, phosphorus, copper, sodium chloride, and selenium, depending on age and type of horse and geographic area. Signs of deficiency are frequently nonspecific, and diagnosis may be complicated by deficiencies of several nutrients simultaneously. The consequences of increased susceptibility to parasitism and bacterial infections may be superimposed over still other clinical signs. Simple excesses are more common. Nutrients most commonly given in excess of needs, leading

TABLE 46 RECOMMENDED NUTRIENT CONCENTRATIONS IN RATIONS[a] FOR HORSES AND PONIES

	Digestible Energy (Mcal/kg)	Crude Protein (%)	Ca (%)	P (%)	Vitamin A (IU/kg)[d]
Mature horses and ponies, maintenance	1.80	7.2	0.21	0.15	1,650
Mares, last 90 days of gestation	2.15	9.5	0.41	0.31	3,280
Lactating mares, first 3 mo	2.35	12.0	0.47	0.30	2,480
Lactating mares, 3 mo to weaning	2.20	10.0	0.33	0.20	2,720
Stallions, breeding season	2.15	8.6	0.26	0.19	2,370
Creep fed	2.80	16.0	0.65	0.35	1,800
Foal (3 mo old)	2.70	14.0	0.65	0.35	1,500
Weanling (6 mo old)	2.60	13.1	0.55	0.30	1,680
Yearling (12 mo old)	2.50	11.3	0.40	0.22	1,950
Long yearling (18 mo old)	2.35	10.4	0.32	0.18	2,050
2-yr-old (light training)	2.40	10.1	0.31	0.17	2,380
Mature working horses					
Light work[f]	2.20	8.8	0.27	0.19	2,420
Moderate work[g]	2.40	9.4	0.28	0.22	2,140
Intense work[h]	2.55	10.3	0.31	0.23	1,760

[a] 90% dry matter

[b] Good quality legume-grass hay; DE = digestible energy

[c] Grass hay

[d] One mg of β-carotene equals 400 IU of vitamin A for the horse.

[e] Concentrate containing 3.2 Mcal DE/kg; A or B refers to suitable concentrates (*see* TABLE 47).

[f] Western pleasure, bridle path hack, equitation

[g] Ranch work, roping, cutting, barrel racing, jumping

[h] Race training, polo

Adapted, with permission, from *Nutrient Requirements of Horses*, 1989, National Academy of Sciences, National Academy Press, Washington, DC.

to toxicity or induced deficits of other nutrients, are energy, phosphorus, iron, copper, selenium, and vitamin A.

Energy Deficiency: Many nonspecific changes found in horses with caloric deficiency can result from inadequate intake, maldigestion, or malabsorption. Weight loss is the cardinal sign of inadequate energy intake. In partial or complete starvation, most internal organs exhibit some atrophy. The brain is least affected, but the size of the gonads may be strikingly decreased, and estrus may be delayed. The immune system is adversely affected, resulting in increased risk of viral diseases. The young skeleton is extremely sensitive, and growth slows or may completely stop. A decrease in adipose tissue is an early and conspicuous sign and is seen not only in the subcutis but also in the mesentery; around the kidneys, uterus, and testes; and in the retroperitoneum. Low-fat

TABLE 46 RECOMMENDED NUTRIENT CONCENTRATIONS IN RATIONS[a] FOR HORSES AND PONIES *(continued)*

Example Diet Proportions			
Hay Containing 2.0 Mcal DE/kg[b]		Hay Containing 1.8 Mcal DE/kg[c]	
Concentrate (%)[e]	Roughage (%)	Concentrate (%)[e]	Roughage (%)
0	100	0	100
20B	80	25A	75
40A	60	50A	50
30B	70	40A	60
25A	75	30A	70
70A	30		
50A	50	70A	30
50A	50	60A	40
40B	60	50A	50
30B	70	40B	60
40B	60	50B	50
0–25B	75	25B	75
40B	60	50B	50
50B	50	60B	40

content of long bone marrow is a good indicator of prolonged inanition. The ability to perform work is impaired, and endogenous nitrogen losses increase as muscle proteins are metabolized for energy, causing muscle wasting.

Energy Excess: Overfeeding high-calorie feeds results in obesity in horses and may contribute to developmental orthopedic disease in growing horses. However, some horses, especially those that are sedentary, can become obese on only good-quality hay or pasture. Obesity increases the risk of laminitis (presumably associated with relative insulin resistance) and colic, due to strangulation of the small intestine by pedunculated mesenteric lipomas. Obese horses and ponies have reduced heat and exercise tolerance.

Protein Deficiency: A deficiency of dietary protein maybe caused by either inadequate intake of high-quality protein or lack of a specific essential amino acid. The effects of deficiency are generally nonspecific, and many of the signs do not differ from the effects of partial or total caloric restriction. In general, the horse will have poor-quality hair and hoof growth, weight loss, and inappetence. In addition, there may be decreased formation of Hgb, RBCs, and plasma proteins. Milk production is decreased in lactating mares. The following liver enzymes have shown decreased activity: pyruvic oxidase, succinoxidase, succinic acid dehydrogenase, D-amino acid oxidase, DPN-cytochrome C reductase, and uricase. Corneal vascularization and lens degeneration have been noted. Antibody formation is also impaired.

Mineral Deficiencies and Excesses:

Nutritional Secondary Hyperparathyroidism (Bighead, Bran disease): Horses of all ages fed grass hay or pasture and supplemented with large amounts of

TABLE 47 CONCENTRATES SATISFACTORY FOR USE WITH HAYS AS INDICATED IN TABLE 46

Ingredient[a]	Formula A	Formula B
Corn[b] or sorghum grain, rolled or cracked	45	55
Oats[b], rolled or crimped	24	24
Soybean meal (44% crude protein)	20	10
Cane molasses[c]	8	8
Limestone (34% Ca)	0.5	0.5
Calcium phosphate, monobasic (16% Ca, 22% P)	1.5	1.5
Trace mineral salt[d]	1	1
	100%	100%
Analysis		
Digestible energy (Mcal/kg)	3.2	3.2
Crude protein (%)	16	12
Digestible protein (%)	12	8.5
Calcium (%)	0.60	0.58
Phosphorus (%)	0.67	0.62

[a] Except for the cane molasses, all figures are on a 90% dry-matter basis.

[b] Barley may be used to replace the corn or sorghum and the oats, by using weights of barley equal to the combined weights of the grains replaced.

[c] Cane molasses is not an essential part of a concentrate mixture, but it may help to minimize separation of "fines" and reduce dustiness.

[d] Providing NaCl, Fe, Cu, Mn, Co, I, Zn, and Se (from sodium selenite) to provide 0.2 mg selenium/kg concentrate.

grain-based concentrates or wheat bran are most likely to develop relative or absolute calcium deficiencies leading to nutritional secondary hyperparathyroidism. Excess phosphorus intake (Ca:P ratio <1) causes the same clinical signs. Blood concentrations of calcium do not reflect intake because of homeostatic mechanisms, although blood inorganic phosphorus may be increased because of mobilization of bone mineral content. Serum alkaline phosphatase activity is usually increased, and clotting time may be prolonged slightly. Young, growing bone is frequently rachitic and brittle. Fractures may be common and heal poorly. Swelling and softening of the facial bones and alternating limb lameness are frequently reported. (*See also* OSTEOMALACIA, p 1052.)

Phosphorus Deficiency: Phosphorus deficiency is most likely in horses being fed *poor-quality grass hay or pasture without* grain. Serum inorganic phosphorus concentrations may be decreased, and serum alkaline phosphatase activity increased. Occasionally, serum calcium levels may be increased. An insidious shifting lameness may be seen. Bone changes resemble those described for calcium deficiency. Affected horses may start to consume large quantities of soil or exhibit other manifestations of pica before other clinical signs are apparent.

Salt Deficiency: Horses are most likely to develop signs of salt (NaCl) deficiency when worked hard in hot weather. Sweat and urinary losses are appreciable. Horses deprived of salt tire easily, stop sweating, and exhibit muscle spasms if exercised strenuously. Hemoconcentration and acidosis may be expected. Anorexia and pica may be evident in chronic deprivation, although these are not specific signs of salt deficiency. In lactating mares, milk production seriously declines. Polyuria and polydipsia secondary to renal medullary washout may be seen in prolonged deficits.

Potassium: Chronic dietary deficiency of potassium results in a decreased rate of growth, anorexia, and perhaps hypokalemia.

However, most forages contain more than sufficient potassium for the average horse. Acute deficits due to sweat losses are more likely and may cause muscle tremors, cardiac arrhythmias, and weakness. Excess potassium intake, especially if given as a bolus PO or IV, also will induce cardiac arrhythmias such as atrial fibrillation.

Magnesium: Foals fed a purified diet containing magnesium at 8 mg/kg (3.6 mg/lb) exhibited hypomagnesemia, nervousness, muscular tremors, and ataxia followed by collapse, with increased respiratory rates, sweating, convulsive paddling, and death after a few weeks. However, most commonly used feeds contain magnesium well in excess of the 70–100 mg/kg dry ration currently recommended. Oversupplementation of this mineral is more likely. Although the effects of excessive magnesium intake in horses have not been determined, based on data from other species, it may cause clinical signs of calcium deficiency.

Iron: Iron deficiency may be secondary to parasitism or chronic blood loss and results in microcytic, hypochromic anemia. However, it is highly unlikely that even anemic horses are iron deficient. Iron excess interferes with copper metabolism and also causes microcytic, hypochromic anemia. Blood transferrin concentrations are the most reliable method to determine the iron status of a horse.

Zinc: Zinc deficiency in foals causes reduced growth rate, anorexia, cutaneous lesions on the lower extremities, alopecia, decreased blood levels of zinc, and decreased serum alkaline phosphatase activity. Excesses (>1,000 ppm) were associated with developmental orthopedic disease in young horses. The effects of excesses or deficits of zinc have not been documented in adult horses.

Copper: An apparent relationship between low blood copper concentrations and uterine artery rupture in aged parturient mares suggests reduced copper absorption with age or reduced ability to mobilize copper stores. Dietary deficiency may cause aortic aneurysm, contracted tendons, and improper cartilage formation in growing foals. Excessive copper intake may interfere with selenium and/or iron metabolism.

Selenium: Selenium deficiency results in reduced serum selenium, increased AST activity, white muscle disease, and perhaps rhabdomyolysis in working horses. (*See also* NUTRITIONAL MYOPATHIES, p 1185.) Selenium excesses of as little as 5 ppm in the ration cause loss of mane and tail hairs and sloughing of the distal portion of the hoof.

Vitamins: A **vitamin A** deficiency may develop if dried, poor-quality roughage is fed for a prolonged period. If body stores of vitamin A are high, signs may not appear for several months. The deficiency is characterized by nyctalopia, lacrimation, keratinization of the cornea, susceptibility to pneumonia, abscesses of the sublingual gland, incoordination, impaired reproduction, capricious appetite, and progressive weakness. Hooves are frequently deformed, with the horny layer unevenly laid down and unusually brittle. Metaplasia of the intestinal mucosa and achlorhydria have been reported. Genitourinary mucosal metaplasia may be expected. Bone remodeling is defective. The foramina do not enlarge properly during early growth, and skeletal deformities are evident. The latter may be seen in foals of vitamin A–deficient mares.

Vitamin E is very labile and quickly lost with storage in both hays and commercial feeds. It is an important antioxidant, and deficiency has been reported to be associated with an increased incidence of rhabdomyolysis, impaired immune function, reproductive failure, and ocular lesions. Some prolonged, aggressive antibiotic treatments, such as recommended for equine protozoal myelitis, have also been reported to induce vitamin E deficits. Fresh forages, however, are excellent sources of vitamin E, and horses with free access to good pasture rarely need supplementation.

If sun-cured hay is consumed or the horse is exposed to sunlight, it is doubtful a **vitamin D** deficiency will develop. Prolonged confinement of young horses offered only limited amounts of sun-cured hay may result in reduced bone calcification, stiff and swollen joints, stiffness of gait, irritability, and reduced serum calcium and phosphorus. Clinical signs are easily reversible with supplementation or exposure to sunlight.

Signs of experimental **thiamine** deficiency include anorexia, weight loss, incoordination, decreased blood thiamine, and increased blood pyruvate. At necropsy, the heart is dilated. Similar signs have been seen in bracken fern poisoning (*see* p 3089). Under normal circumstances, the natural diet plus synthesis by microorganisms in the gut probably meet the need for thiamine. However, needs may be increased by stress.

Although natural feeds plus synthesis within the gut normally provide adequate **riboflavin**, limited evidence indicates an occasional deficiency when the diet is of poor quality. The first sign of acute deficiency is catarrhal conjunctivitis in one or both eyes, accompanied by photophobia and lacrimation. The retina, lens, and ocular fluids may deteriorate gradually and result in impaired vision or blindness. Equine recurrent uveitis (*see* p 508) has been linked to riboflavin deficiency but may be a sequela of leptospirosis or onchocerciasis.

The normal feedstuffs of horses generally contain very little **vitamin B_{12}**. However, horses can synthesize this vitamin in the gut, from which it is absorbed.

FEEDING THE SICK HORSE

Nutrition is an important part of the management and treatment of sick horses. Stresses (eg, surgery, severe orthopedic problems, or infection) can significantly increase caloric needs due to an increase in catabolism. In addition, anorexia or dysphagia can lead to inadequate intake of the proper nutrients. The consequences of not providing proper nutrition include impairment of the immune system, delayed wound and fracture healing, hypoproteinemia, muscle wasting, and weakness. Generally, supportive nutritional therapy should be considered if an adult horse has been hypophagic for ≥3 days. Neonatal foals require some energy source within 24 hr of decreased intake.

The order of nutrient priorities is water, energy, electrolytes, and protein. Some water-soluble vitamins are poorly stored in the body and should be supplemented. The basal energy requirement (BER) in kcal/day can be calculated by the following formula: BER = 70 (body wt in kg)$^{0.75}$. For example, BER is ~6,800 kcal/day for a 450-kg horse and 1,300 kcal/day for a 50-kg foal. Severe illness or trauma (eg, barn fire burns) significantly increase these needs.

There are several methods to provide nutritional support to a sick horse. The simplest method is to encourage the horse to eat on its own. Unusual feed preferences may be seen. Offering a variety of feeds and letting the horse choose can best determine what is most palatable to the animal. Many horses will eat fresh, green grass even though they refuse other feeds. Alfalfa hay is more palatable than grass hays. Whole oats and sweet-feed mixtures of rolled grains and molasses are the most appetizing of grains. Bran mashes are usually palatable, but the addition of molasses, applesauce, and salt may increase their acceptance in anorectic horses.

When horses experience pain or fever, analgesics can improve food intake; NSAIDs, such as dipyrone, flunixin meglumine, meclofenamic acid, and phenylbutazone, can be used. Prolonged use of phenylbutazone should be avoided because of the adverse effects of gastric and small-intestinal ulceration and renal papillary necrosis.

Tube feeding is a second way to provide nutrition to horses that will not (or cannot) eat voluntarily. A normal stomach tube may be passed several times a day or may be sutured to the nostril and left as an indwelling feeding tube. This is an effective method to provide nutrients to sick neonates. It is also an inexpensive method to replace fluid and electrolyte losses. Enteral nutritional supplements used in human medicine are particularly useful to provide sufficient caloric intake to adult horses. These products have a known caloric content, which facilitates calculation of the animal's needs. Soaking a complete pelleted feed in water can make a slurry for tube feeding; however, when feeding a slurry in this manner, the stomach tube may clog with feedstuff.

The third method to provide energy and protein to sick horses is through use of total or partial parenteral nutrition (TPN or PPN). Fluid administration (IV) can maintain hydration in horses unable either to drink or absorb fluids. Common replacement solutions include sodium chloride, lactated Ringer's, and 5% dextrose. The nutritional value of these fluids is insignificant. Fat and amino acid solutions are also available. The components of parenteral nutrition are glucose, amino acids, lipid, trace minerals, and multivitamins. The resultant solution is hypertonic and is delivered by constant infusion through a jugular catheter. Delivery is optimized through use of a fluid pump. Blood and urine glucose should be monitored twice daily to regulate the rate of infusion. TPN is costly and requires intensive care and monitoring, which limits its usefulness in adult horses.

Nutrition for Specific Diseases/ Problems: Horses with **recurrent airway obstruction** (*see* p 1455) are frequently sensitive to the dust and molds found in normal hay. They often improve when hay is removed from their diet and they are placed on a complete ration that is pelleted or contains a roughage source such as beet pulp. They do best on pasture. Another source of dust-free roughage is haylage.

Diarrhea in horses is primarily a colonic disease. Traditionally, affected horses are fed less grain and more hay. This increase in dietary fiber can bind water and may result in better formed feces. If weight loss is a concurrent problem, it may be better to maintain grain intake. Grain is digested mainly in the small intestine, and hay in the large intestine. Unless the small intestine is also affected, feeding grain helps maintain body mass. (*See also* COLIC IN HORSES, p 248, and INTESTINAL DISEASES IN HORSES AND FOALS, p 281.)

The role of nutrition in horses with **hepatic disease** (*see* p 329) is to provide adequate energy, thus easing the liver's role in energy production and decreasing the amount of metabolic waste to which the liver is exposed. Parenteral or enteral glucose administration may be important as an energy source in anorectic horses. In horses that are eating, cereal grains should provide adequate carbohydrates. Corn is the grain of choice because of its low-protein, high-carbohydrate content. High-protein feeds, such as alfalfa hay, should be avoided.

Horses excrete significant amounts of calcium in their urine. In cases of **renal disease**, low-protein, low-calcium diets should be fed. Corn and grass hay are the feeds of choice.

FEEDING THE AGED HORSE AND THE ORPHAN FOAL

Aged horses often lose weight because of dental wear. Their teeth lose the grinding surface, which results in poor mastication of food. Aged horses also may have reduced protein, fiber, and phosphorus digestion. Feeding a moistened, complete pelleted ration designed for aged horses may improve the horse's well-being.

If an **orphan foal** has not received colostrum from its dam, it must receive either colostrum from another mare or frozen-stored colostrum within 24 hr of birth—preferably within the first 3–12 hr. Antibody-rich plasma-replacement products for IV administration are available but are expensive and provide protection of questionable duration.

A nurse mare, preferably with a good disposition, is best for the overall care of an orphan foal. The amnion and/or placenta of a mare who has lost a newborn foal can be placed over the orphan foal to increase the mare's acceptance of the foal. The mare and foal should not be left unattended until the mare has accepted the orphan; physical or chemical restraint of the mare may be required initially and repeated on several occasions before she will accept the new foal.

If a nurse mare is not available, a lactating dairy goat (positioned on a stand or bale of hay or straw) may serve as an alternative. Constant monitoring is necessary, because the foal should be fed every 4 hr.

Artificial mare's milk diets and goat's milk have also been used successfully to feed orphan foals. Foals should be fed every 1–2 hr for the first 1–2 days of life, then every 2–4 hr for the next 2 wk at the rate of 250–500 mL per feeding, using a warmed milk container and an artificial nipple. Of the various artificial nipples available, those designed for use by lambs are best suited for foals. The feeding intervals may be lengthened gradually after 2 wk; however, the amount per feeding also should be increased so that the foal consumes 10%–15% of its body wt/day.

A foal should be encouraged to drink freshly prepared milk out of a bucket, ad lib, early in life. After 1 mo, the foal can be encouraged to eat grain mixes (with ≥18% crude protein designed for growing foals) and good-quality hay in addition to the milk or milk replacer. The foal can be weaned off the milk replacer at 3 mo of age. Fresh water should be available to the foal at all times from birth. (*See also* PERINATAL MARE AND FOAL CARE, p 2159.)

NUTRITION: PIGS

NUTRITIONAL REQUIREMENTS

Pigs require a number of essential nutrients to meet their needs for maintenance, growth, reproduction, lactation, and other functions. The National Research Council (NRC), in its publication, *Nutrient Requirements of Swine* (updated in 2012), provides estimates of the amounts of these nutrients for various classes of swine under average conditions. However, factors such as genetic variation, environment, availability of nutrients in feedstuffs, disease levels, and other stressors may increase the needed level of some nutrients for optimal performance and reproduction.

The NRC uses a modeling approach to take some of these factors into consideration in its estimates of requirements for energy, amino acids, calcium, and phosphorus, but requirements for other minerals and vitamins are estimated strictly from empirical data.

Although the NRC addresses factors such as lean growth rate, gender, energy density of the diet, environmental temperature, crowding, parity, stage of gestation, and various measures of sow productivity when estimating nutrient requirements, nutritionists, feed manufacturers, veterinarians, or swine producers may wish to include higher levels of certain nutrients than those listed by the NRC to ensure adequate intake of nutrients and for insurance purposes. Any negative effects from oversupplementing diets are generally minimal except in cases of extreme imbalance.

Swine require six general classes of nutrients: water, carbohydrates, fats, protein (amino acids), minerals, and vitamins. Energy, although not a specific nutrient, is an important nutritional component and is primarily derived from the oxidation of carbohydrates and fats. In addition, amino acids (from protein) that exceed the animal's requirements for maintenance and tissue protein synthesis provide energy when their carbon skeletons are oxidized. Antibiotics, chemotherapeutic agents, microbial supplements (prebiotics and probiotics), enzymes, and other feed additives are often added to swine diets to increase the rate and efficiency of gain, to improve digestibility, and for other purposes, but they are not considered nutrients.

The NRC estimates of nutrient requirements for various body weight groups of pigs from 5–135 kg body wt, expressed as dietary concentrations, are shown in TABLE 48. Requirements for gestating and lactating sows, expressed as dietary concentrations, are shown in TABLE 49. The dietary concentrations listed in the NRC tables are based on a given amount of feed intake; if intake is less than the amount listed, the dietary concentration may need to be increased to ensure an adequate daily intake of the nutrients.

TABLE 48 DIETARY NUTRIENT REQUIREMENTS OF GROWING PIGS ALLOWED AD LIB FEED (90% DRY MATTER)[a,b,c]

	Body Weight (kg)						
	5–7	7–11	11–25	25–50	50–75	75–100	100–135
NE content of diet (kcal/kg)[d]	2,448	2,448	2,412	2,475	2,475	2,475	2,475
DE content of diet (kcal/kg)[d]	3,542	3,542	3,490	3,402	3,402	3,402	3,402
ME content of diet (kcal/kg)[d]	3,400	3,400	3,350	3,300	3,300	3,300	3,300
Estimated ME intake (kcal/day)	904	1,592	3,033	4,959	6,989	8,265	9,196
Estimated feed intake + wastage (g/day)[e]	280	493	953	1,582	2,229	2,636	2,933
Body wt gain (g/day)	210	335	585	758	900	917	867
Body protein deposition (g/day)	–	–	–	128	147	141	122
AMINO ACIDS, TOTAL (%)[f]							
Arginine	0.75	0.68	0.62	0.50	0.44	0.38	0.32
Histidine	0.58	0.53	0.48	0.39	0.34	0.30	0.25
Isoleucine	0.88	0.79	0.73	0.59	0.52	0.45	0.39
Leucine	1.71	1.54	1.41	1.13	0.98	0.85	0.71

TABLE 48 DIETARY NUTRIENT REQUIREMENTS OF GROWING PIGS ALLOWED AD LIB FEED (90% DRY MATTER)[a,b,c] *(continued)*

	Body Weight (kg)						
	5–7	7–11	11–25	25–50	50–75	75–100	100–135
Lysine	1.70	1.53	1.40	1.12	0.97	0.84	0.71
Methionine	0.49	0.44	0.40	0.32	0.28	0.25	0.21
Methionine + cystine	0.96	0.87	0.79	0.65	0.57	0.50	0.43
Phenylalanine	1.01	0.91	0.83	0.68	0.59	0.51	0.43
Phenylalanine + tyrosine	1.60	1.44	1.32	1.08	0.94	0.82	0.70
Threonine	1.05	0.95	0.87	0.72	0.64	0.56	0.49
Tryptophan	0.28	0.25	0.23	0.19	0.17	0.15	0.13
Valine	1.10	1.00	0.91	0.75	0.65	0.57	0.49
Approximate crude protein[g]	24–26	22–24	21–23	19.3	17.1	15.2	13.4
MINERALS							
Calcium (%)	0.85	0.80	0.70	0.66	0.59	0.52	0.46
Phosphorus, total (%)[h]	0.70	0.65	0.60	0.56	0.52	0.47	0.43
STTD phosphorus (%)[h]	0.45	0.40	0.33	0.31	0.27	0.24	0.21
ATTD phosphorus (%)[h]	0.41	0.36	0.29	0.26	0.23	0.21	0.18
Sodium (%)	0.40	0.35	0.28	0.10	0.10	0.10	0.10
Chlorine (%)	0.50	0.45	0.32	0.08	0.08	0.08	0.08
Magnesium (%)	0.04	0.04	0.04	0.04	0.04	0.04	0.04
Potassium (%)	0.30	0.28	0.26	0.23	0.19	0.17	0.17
Copper (ppm)	6.00	6.00	5.00	4.00	3.50	3.00	3.00
Iodine (ppm)	0.14	0.14	0.14	0.14	0.14	0.14	0.14
Iron (ppm)	100	100	100	60	50	40	40
Manganese (ppm)	4.00	4.00	3.00	2.00	2.00	2.00	2.00
Selenium (ppm)	0.30	0.30	0.25	0.20	0.15	0.15	0.15
Zinc (ppm)	100	100	80	60	50	50	50
VITAMINS AND FATTY ACIDS							
Vitamin A (IU/kg)[i]	2,200	2,200	1,750	1,300	1,300	1,300	1,300
Vitamin D (IU/kg)[i]	220	220	200	150	150	150	150
Vitamin E (IU/kg)[i]	16	16	11	11	11	11	11
Vitamin K (menadione, mg/kg)	0.50	0.50	0.50	0.50	0.50	0.50	0.50
Biotin (mg/kg)	0.08	0.05	0.05	0.05	0.05	0.05	0.05
Choline (g/kg)	0.60	0.50	0.40	0.30	0.30	0.30	0.30
Folacin (mg/kg)	0.30	0.30	0.30	0.30	0.30	0.30	0.30

TABLE 48 DIETARY NUTRIENT REQUIREMENTS OF GROWING PIGS ALLOWED AD LIB FEED (90% DRY MATTER)[a,b,c] *(continued)*

	Body Weight (kg)						
	5–7	7–11	11–25	25–50	50–75	75–100	100–135
Niacin, available (mg/kg)[j]	30.00	30.00	30.00	30.00	30.00	30.00	30.00
Pantothenic acid (mg/kg)	12.00	10.00	9.00	8.00	7.00	7.00	7.00
Riboflavin (mg/kg)	4.00	3.50	3.00	2.50	2.00	2.00	2.00
Thiamine (mg/kg)	1.50	1.00	1.00	1.00	1.00	1.00	1.00
Vitamin B_6 (mg/kg)	7.00	7.00	3.00	1.00	1.00	1.00	1.00
Vitamin B_{12} (mcg/kg)	20.00	17.50	15.00	10.00	5.00	5.00	5.00
Linoleic acid (%)	0.10	0.10	0.10	0.10	0.10	0.10	0.10

[a] Adapted, with permission, from *Nutrient Requirements of Swine* (2012), National Research Council, National Academies Press, Washington, DC.

[b] Estimates of nutrient requirements are for the midpoint of the weight range as determined by the NRC growth model for pigs of mixed gender (1:1 ratio of barrows and gilts) with high-medium lean growth rate (mean whole body-protein deposition of 135 g/day) from 25–125 kg body wt.

[c] Estimates of amino acid, calcium, and phosphorus requirements differ for barrows, gilts, and intact boars, for pigs with differing lean growth rates, for pigs fed ractopamine, and for boars immunized against gonadotropin-releasing hormone. For additional information, see *Nutrient Requirements of Swine* (2012), National Research Council, National Academies Press, Washington, DC.

[d] NE = net energy, DE = digestible energy, ME = metabolizable energy. Dietary energy contents relate to corn and soybean meal–based diets. DE and ME are calculated from NE.

[e] Assumes 5% feed wastage.

[f] Total amino acid requirements apply to corn-soybean meal—based diets. For 5- to 25-kg pigs, lysine percentages are estimated from empirical data, and the other amino acids are based on the ratios of amino acids to lysine based on amino acid requirements for maintenance and growth. The requirements for 25- to 135-kg pigs are estimated from the NRC growth model.

[g] The calculated crude protein levels are based on corn-soybean meal diets containing 0.1% supplemental lysine and 3% minerals and vitamins. In addition, specialty ingredients (lactose, dried whey, dried blood plasma, dried blood cells, etc) are included in diets for 5–11 kg pigs.

[h] STTD = standardized total tract digestible, ATTD = apparent total tract digestible, ATTD phosphorus and total phosphorus requirements apply to corn and soybean meal–based diets.

[i] Conversions: 1 IU vitamin A = 0.30 mcg retinol or 0.344 mcg retinyl acetate; 1 IU vitamin D_2 or D_3 = 0.025 mcg cholecalciferol; 1 IU vitamin E = 0.67 mg of D-α-tocopherol or 1 mg of DL-α-tocopherol acetate.

[j] The niacin in corn, grain sorghum, wheat, and barley is unavailable. Similarly, the niacin in by-products made from these cereal grains is poorly available unless the by-products have undergone fermentation or wet-milling process.

Water: Pigs should have free and convenient access to water, beginning before weaning. The amount required varies with age, type of feed, environmental temperature, status of lactation, fever, high urinary output (as from high salt or protein intake), or diarrhea. Normally, growing pigs consume ~2–3 kg of water for every kg of dry feed. Lactating sows consume more water because of the high water content of the milk they produce. Water restriction reduces performance and milk production and may result in death if the restriction is severe.

Water quality is important. Water should be relatively free of microbial contamination; if not, chlorination may be necessary. Excessive minerals in water may create problems. Water should have <1,000 ppm of total dissolved solids (TDS). Higher levels of TDS (2,000–5,000 ppm) can cause diarrhea or temporary water refusal, TDS levels of

5,000–7,000 should be avoided for breeding animals, and TDS levels >7,000 ppm are unfit for pigs. Pigs tolerate moderate levels of sulfates in water, but high levels (>3,000 ppm) of sulfates should be avoided.

Energy: Energy requirements are expressed as kilocalories (kcal) of digestible energy (DE), metabolizable energy (ME), or net energy (NE). DE and ME values are used most commonly, but

TABLE 49 REPRODUCTIVE MEASURES AND DIETARY NUTRIENT REQUIREMENTS OF GESTATING AND LACTATING SOWS[a,b]

	Gestation				Lactation (21-day)	
Reproductive Measures						
Parity	1		3		1	2+
Body weight at breeding (kg)	140		185		–	–
Anticipated gestation weight gain (kg)	65.0		52.2		–	–
Anticipated litter size	12.5		13.5		–	–
Day of gestation	**0–90**	**90–115**	**0–90**	**90–115**	–	–
Body weight postfarrowing (kg)	–	–	–	–	175	210
Litter size	–	–	–	–	11	11.5
Daily weight gain of nursing pigs (g)	–	–	–	–	230	230
Nutrient Requirements						
NE content of diet (kcal/kg)[c]	2,518	2,518	2,518	2,518	2,518	2,518
DE content of diet (kcal/kg)[c]	3,388	3,388	3,388	3,388	3,388	3,388
ME content of diet (kcal/kg)[c]	3,300	3,300	3,300	3,300	3,300	3,300
Estimated ME intake (kcal/day)	6,678	7,932	6,928	8,182	18,700	20,700
Estimated feed intake (g/day) + wastage[d]	2,130	2,530	2,210	2,610	5,950	6,610
Body wt gain (g/day)	578	543	472	408	–	–
Body wt loss (21-day lactation, kg)	–	–	–	–	7.7	5.8
AMINO ACIDS, TOTAL (%)[e]						
Arginine	0.32	0.42	0.23	0.32	0.50	0.48
Histidine	0.22	0.27	0.16	0.20	0.37	0.36
Isoleucine	0.36	0.43	0.27	0.33	0.52	0.50
Leucine	0.55	0.75	0.41	0.59	1.05	1.01
Lysine	0.61	0.80	0.45	0.62	0.93	0.90

(continued)

TABLE 49 REPRODUCTIVE MEASURES AND DIETARY NUTRIENT REQUIREMENTS OF GESTATING AND LACTATING SOWS[a,b] *(continued)*

	Gestation				Lactation (21-day)	
Day of gestation	0–90	90–115	0–90	90–115	–	–
Methionine	0.18	0.23	0.13	0.18	0.25	0.24
Methionine + cystine	0.41	0.54	0.32	0.44	0.51	0.49
Phenylalanine	0.34	0.44	0.25	0.35	0.51	0. 49
Phenylalanine + tyrosine	0.61	0.79	0.46	0.62	1.07	1.03
Threonine	0.46	0.58	0.37	0.48	0.62	0.60
Tryptophan	0.11	0.15	0.09	0.13	0.18	0.17
Valine	0.45	0.58	0.34	0.46	0.81	0.78
Approximate crude protein[f]	11.9	14.7	9.6	12.0	16.6	16.1
MINERALS						
Calcium (%)	0.61	0.83	0.49	0.72	0.71	0. 68
Phosphorus, total (%)[g]	0.49	0.62	0.41	0.55	0.62	0. 60
STTD phosphorus (%)[g]	0.27	0.36	0.21	0.31	0.36	0. 34
ATTD phosphorus (%)[g]	0.23	0.31	0.18	0.27	0.31	0. 29
Sodium (%)	0.15	0.15	0.15	0.15	0.20	0. 20
Chlorine (%)	0.12	0.12	0.12	0.12	0.16	0. 16
Magnesium (%)	0.06	0.06	0.06	0.06	0.06	0. 06
Potassium (%)	0.20	0.20	0.20	0.20	0.20	0. 20
Copper (ppm)	10.00	10	10	10	20	20
Iodine (ppm)	0.14	0.14	0.14	0.14	0.14	0. 14
Iron (ppm)	80	80	80	80	80	80
Manganese (ppm)	25	25	25	25	25	25
Selenium (ppm)	0.15	0.15	0.15	0.15	0.15	0. 15
Zinc (ppm)	100	100	100	100	100	100
VITAMINS AND FATTY ACIDS						
Vitamin A (IU/kg)[h]	4,000	4,000	4,000	4,000	2,000	2, 000
Vitamin D (IU/kg)[h]	800	800	800	800	800	800
Vitamin E (IU/kg)[h]	44	44	44	44	44	44
Vitamin K (menadione, mg/kg)	0.50	0.50	0.50	0.50	0.50	0.50
Biotin (mg/kg)	0.20	0.20	0.20	0.20	0.20	0.20
Choline (g/kg)	1.25	1.25	1.25	1.25	1.00	1.00
Folacin (mg/kg)	1.30	1.30	1.30	1.30	1.30	1.30
Niacin, available (mg/kg)[i]	*10*	*10*	10	10	10	10
Pantothenic acid (mg/kg)	12	12	12	12	12	12
Riboflavin (mg/kg)	3.75	3.75	3.75	3.75	3.75	3.75

(continued)

TABLE 49 REPRODUCTIVE MEASURES AND DIETARY NUTRIENT REQUIREMENTS OF GESTATING AND LACTATING SOWS[a,b] *(continued)*

	Gestation				Lactation (21-day)	
Day of gestation	0–90	90–115	0–90	90–115	–	–
Thiamine (mg/kg)	1.00	1.00	1.00	1.00	1.00	1.00
Vitamin B_6 (mg/kg)	1.00	1.00	1.00	1.00	1.00	1.00
Vitamin B_{12} (mcg/kg)	15	15	15	15	15	15
Linoleic acid (%)	0.10	0.10	0.10	0.10	0.10	0.10

[a] Adapted, with permission, from *Nutrient Requirements of Swine* (2012), National Research Council, National Academies Press, Washington, DC.

[b] Estimates of amino acid, calcium, and phosphorus requirements during gestation differ for parity 1, 2, 3, and 4+ sows, stage of gestation, body weight at breeding, anticipated litter size, and other factors. Requirements for these nutrients during lactation differ for parity 1 and 2+ sows, body weight after farrowing, litter size, and other factors. For additional information, see *Nutrient Requirements of Swine* (2012), National Research Council, National Academies Press, Washington, DC.

[c] NE = net energy, DE = digestible energy, ME = metabolizable energy. Dietary energy contents related to corn and soybean meal–based diets. DE and ME are calculated from NE.

[d] Assumes 5% feed wastage.

[e] Total amino acid requirements apply to corn-soybean meal–based diets.

[f] The calculated crude protein levels are based on corn-soybean meal diets containing 0.1% supplemental lysine and 3% minerals and vitamins.

[g] STTD = standardized total tract digestible, ATTD = apparent total tract digestible, ATTD phosphorus and total phosphorus requirements apply to corn and soybean meal–based diets.

[h] Conversions: 1 IU vitamin A = 0.30 mcg retinol or 0.344 mcg retinyl acetate; 1 IU vitamin D_2 or D_3 = 0.025 mcg cholecalciferol; 1 IU vitamin E = 0.67 mg of D-α-tocopherol or 1 mg of DL-α-tocopherol acetate.

[i] The niacin in corn, grain sorghum, wheat, and barley is unavailable. Similarly, the niacin in by-products made from these cereal grains is poorly available unless the by-products have undergone fermentation or wet-milling process.

there is a trend in the industry to formulate diets on the basis of NE. The NRC determines energy requirements on the basis of NE, and then DE and ME are estimated from NE. Energy requirements of pigs are influenced by their weight (which influences the maintenance requirement), their genetic capacity for lean tissue growth or milk production, and the environmental temperature at which they are housed. The amount of feed consumed by growing pigs allowed to consume feed ad lib is controlled principally by the energy content of the diet. If the energy density of the diet is increased by including supplemental fat, voluntary feed consumption decreases. Pigs fed such a diet generally will gain faster, and efficiency of gain will improve, but carcass fat may increase. If the diet contains excessive amounts of fiber (>5%–7%) without commensurate increases in fat, the rate—and especially the efficiency—of gain are decreased.

Protein and Amino Acids: Amino acids, normally supplied by dietary protein, are required for maintenance, muscle growth, development of fetuses and supporting tissues in gestating sows, and milk production in lactating sows. Of the 22 amino acids, 12 are synthesized by the animal; the other 10 must be provided in the diet for normal growth. The 10 dietary essential amino acids for swine are arginine, histidine, isoleucine, leucine, lysine, methionine, phenylalanine, threonine, tryptophan, and valine. Cystine and tyrosine can meet a portion of the requirement for methionine and phenylalanine, respectively. The percentages of crude protein listed in TABLES 48 and 49 provide the required levels of lysine (the first limiting amino acid) and sufficient amounts of the other essential amino acids in diets consisting of corn and soybean meal. The dietary lysine requirement during the early starter phase is quite high (1.70%) but decreases to 1.53% and 1.40% during the middle and final starter phases, respectively. The requirement continues to decrease throughout the growing-finishing stage from 1.12% during the early growing phase to 0.71% during late finishing.

The amino acids of greatest practical importance in diet formulation (ie, those most likely to be at deficient levels) are lysine, tryptophan, threonine, and methionine. Corn, the basic grain in most swine diets, is markedly deficient in lysine and tryptophan. The other principal grains for pigs (grain sorghum, barley, and wheat) are low in lysine and threonine. The first limiting amino acid in soybean meal is methionine, but sufficient amounts are provided when soybean meal is combined with cereal grains into a complete diet that meets the lysine requirement. An exception might be in young pigs that consume diets with high levels of soybean meal or diets containing dried blood products low in the sulfur-amino acids.

Milk protein is well balanced in essential amino acids but usually is too expensive to be used in swine diets, except for very young pigs. Dried whey, commonly used in starter diets, contains protein with an excellent profile of amino acids, but the total protein content of whey is low. Diets based on corn and animal-protein byproducts (eg, meat meal, meat and bone meal) are inferior to corn-soybean meal diets, but they can be improved significantly by adding tryptophan or supplements that are good sources of tryptophan. Animal proteins are also good sources of minerals and B-complex vitamins.

Diets formulated for early weaned pigs that contain high levels of dried animal plasma or dried blood cells may be deficient in methionine. However, high levels of methionine can depress growth, so methionine should not be added indiscriminately to diets. Supplemental valine may be of value in corn-soybean meal diets fed to lactating sows, but it is still too expensive to be considered as a dietary supplement.

Lysine is generally the first limiting amino acid in almost all practical diets, so if diets are formulated on a lysine basis, the other amino acid requirements should be met. However, caution must be exercised when a crystalline lysine supplement is included in the diet to meet a portion of the pig's lysine requirement. A general rule of thumb is that crude protein content can be reduced by 2 percentage points and the diet supplemented with 0.15% lysine (0.19% lysine•HCl). However, greater reductions in dietary protein coupled with additional lysine may result in deficiencies of tryptophan, *threonine, and/or methionine* unless they are also supplemented.

It is quite common today to formulate swine diets based on the concept of "ideal" protein; ie, to express essential amino acid requirements as a percent of the lysine requirement. Additionally, it is becoming more popular to formulate swine diets on the basis of standardized (or true) or apparent digestible amino acids. This method is particularly advantageous when substantial amounts of byproduct feeds are included in the diet.

Minerals: These nutritional elements have many important functions in the body. The dietary requirements for the essential macro- and trace minerals are listed in TABLES 48 and 49.

Calcium and Phosphorus: Although used primarily in skeletal growth, calcium and phosphorus play important metabolic roles in the body and are essential for all stages of growth, gestation, and lactation. The NRC estimates requirements of 0.66% calcium and 0.56% total phosphorus for growing pigs of 25–50 kg body wt. The requirements are higher for younger pigs and lower for finishing pigs, but the ratios of calcium:phosphorus are approximately the same for all weight groups. These levels are adequate for maximal growth (rate and efficiency of gain), but they do not allow for maximal bone mineralization. Generally, maximal bone ash and strength can be achieved by including 0.1%–0.15% additional calcium and phosphorus in the diet.

For gestating and lactating sows, calcium and phosphorus requirements are influenced by stage of gestation (the first 90 days versus the final 25 days of gestation), parity, milk production, and other factors (*see* TABLE 49). The higher requirements during late gestation are attributed to rapid development of the fetuses. Swine producers may choose to feed slightly higher levels to sows to ensure adequacy of these minerals and to prevent posterior paralysis in heavy milking sows. The calcium and phosphorus requirements listed are based on daily feed intakes of 4.7–5.7 lb (2.1–2.6 kg) during gestation and 13.1–14.6 lb (5.9–6.6 kg) during lactation (these amounts include 5% wastage). If less feed is consumed per day, the percentages of calcium and phosphorus may need to be adjusted upward.

The ratio of total calcium:total phosphorus should be kept between 1.25:1 and 1:1 for maximal utilization of both minerals. A wide calcium:phosphorus ratio reduces phosphorus absorption, especially if the diet is marginal in phosphorus. The ratio is less critical if the diet contains excess phosphorus. When based on digestible phosphorus, the ideal ratio of calcium to digestible phosphorus is between 2:1 and 2.5:1.

Most of the phosphorus in cereal grains and oilseed meals is in the form of phytic acid (organically bound phosphorus) and is poorly available to pigs, whereas the phosphorus in protein sources of animal origin, such as meat meal, meat and bone meal, and fish meal, is in inorganic form and is highly available to pigs. Even in cereal grains, availability of phosphorus varies. For example, the phosphorus in corn is only 10%–20% available, whereas the phosphorus in wheat is 50% available. Therefore, swine diets should be formulated on an "available phosphorus" basis to ensure that the phosphorus requirement is met. The NRC publication expresses the digestible phosphorus requirements as apparent total tract digestible (ATTD) and standardized total tract digestible (STTD) phosphorus. ATTD phosphorus represents the phosphorus digested, and STTD phosphorus is the digestible phosphorus corrected for endogenous phosphorus excretions.

Phosphorus supplements such as monocalcium or dicalcium phosphate, defluorinated phosphate, and steamed bone meal are excellent sources of highly available phosphorus. These supplements also are good sources of calcium. Ground limestone also is an excellent source of calcium.

Phosphorus is considered a potential environmental pollutant, so many swine producers feed diets with less excess phosphorus than in the past to reduce phosphorus excretion. Supplemental phytase, an enzyme that degrades some of the phytic acid in feedstuffs, is commonly added to diets to further reduce phosphorus excretion. The general recommendation is that dietary calcium and phosphorus can both be reduced by 0.05%–0.1% when ≥500 units of phytase per kg of diet are included.

Sodium and Chloride: These minerals are provided by common salt, which contains 40% sodium and 60% chloride. The recommended level of salt is 0.25% in growing and finishing diets, 0.5–0.75% in starter diets, and 0.5% in sow diets. These levels should provide ample sodium and chloride to meet the animal's requirements. Animal, fish, and milk byproducts can contribute some of the sodium and chloride requirement.

Potassium, Magnesium, and Sulfur: Practical diets contain ample amounts of these minerals from the grain and protein sources, and supplemental sources are not needed. Magnesium oxide supplementation has been used to prevent cannibalism, but controlled studies do not support this practice.

Iron and Copper: These minerals are involved in many enzyme systems. Both are necessary for formation of Hgb and, therefore, for prevention of nutritional anemia. Because the amount of iron in milk is very low, suckling pigs should receive supplemental iron, preferably by IM injection of 100–200 mg in the form of iron dextran, iron dextrin, or gleptoferron during the first 3 days of life (*see also* IRON TOXICITY IN NEWBORN PIGS, p 3077). Giving oral or injectable iron and copper to sows will not increase piglet stores at birth nor will it increase the iron in colostrum and milk sufficiently to prevent anemia in neonatal pigs. High levels of iron in lactation feed results in iron-rich sow feces that pigs can obtain from the pen. Iron can also be supplied by mixing ferric ammonium citrate with water in a piglet waterer or by frequently placing a mixture of iron sulfate and a carrier, such as ground corn, on the floor of the farrowing stall.

The copper requirement for growing pigs is low (3–6 ppm) but higher for sows. The estimated copper requirement of 5 ppm for sows in the previous NRC publication was increased to 10 ppm for gestation and 20 ppm for lactation in the 2012 edition.

Copper at pharmaceutical levels in the diet (100–250 mg/kg) is an effective growth stimulant for weanling and growing pigs. The action of copper at high levels appears to be independent of, and additive to, the growth-stimulating effect of antibiotics. Copper sulfate at high levels in the diet results in very dark-colored feces. Also, high copper diets result in marked increases in the copper content of excreted manure.

Iodine: The thyroid gland uses iodine to produce thyroxine, which affects cell activity and metabolic rate. The iodine requirement of all classes of pigs is 0.14 mg/kg of diet. Stabilized iodized salt contains 0.007% iodine; when fed at sufficient levels to meet the salt requirement, it will also meet the iodine needs of pigs.

Manganese: Although essential for normal reproduction and growth, the quantitative requirement for manganese is not well defined. Manganese at 2–4 mg/kg in the diet is adequate for growth, but a higher level (25 mg/kg) is needed by sows during gestation and lactation.

Zinc: Zinc is an important trace mineral with many biologic functions. Grain-soybean meal diets must contain supplemental zinc to prevent parakeratosis (*see* p 975).

Higher levels of zinc may be needed when dietary calcium is excessive, especially in diets typically high in phytic acid such as corn-soybean meal diets. Pharmacologic levels of zinc (1,500–3,000 mg/kg) as zinc oxide have consistently been found to increase pig performance during the postweaning period. In some instances, high levels of zinc oxide have been reported to reduce the incidence and severity of postweaning diarrhea. Responses to zinc oxide and antibiotics seem to be additive in nature, much like the responses to high copper and antibiotics; however, there is no advantage to including high copper and high zinc in the same diet. Similar to copper, high levels of dietary zinc cause increased zinc content in the excreted manure. For sows, the estimated zinc requirement was increased from 50 ppm in the previous NRC publication to 100 ppm in the 2012 edition.

Selenium: The selenium content of soils and, ultimately, crops is quite variable. In the USA, areas west of the Mississippi River generally contain higher amounts of selenium, whereas areas east of the river tend to yield crops deficient in selenium. Under most practical conditions, 0.2–0.3 mg of added selenium/kg of diet should meet the requirements. This trace mineral is regulated by the FDA, and the maximal amount of selenium that can be added to swine diets is 0.3 mg/kg.

Chromium: This trace mineral, which is a cofactor with insulin, is required by pigs, but the quantitative requirement has not been established. In some studies, chromium at a supplemental level of 200 mcg/kg (ppb) improved carcass leanness in finishing pigs and improved reproductive performance in gestating sows, but these effects have been somewhat inconsistent.

Cobalt: Cobalt is present in the vitamin B_{12} molecule and has no benefit when added to swine diets in the elemental form.

Vitamins: These micronutrients serve many important roles in the body. The estimated requirements for the essential vitamins are given in TABLES 48 and 49.

Vitamin A: This fat-soluble vitamin is essential for vision, reproduction, growth and maintenance of epithelial tissue, and mucous secretions. Vitamin A is found as carotenoid precursors in green plant material and yellow corn. β-Carotene is the *most active form of the* various carotenes. Unfortunately, only about one-fourth of the total carotene in yellow corn is in the form of β-carotene. The NRC suggests that for pigs, 1 mg of chemically determined carotene in corn or a corn-soybean mixture is equal to 267 IU of vitamin A.

The use of stabilized vitamin A is common in manufactured feeds and in vitamin supplements or premixes. Concentrates containing natural vitamin A (fish oils most often) may be used to fortify diets. Green forage, dehydrated alfalfa meal, and high-quality legume hays are also good sources of β-carotene. Both natural vitamin A and β-carotene are easily destroyed by air, light, high temperatures, rancid fats, organic acids, and certain mineral elements. For these reasons, natural feedstuffs probably should not be entirely relied on as sources of vitamin A, especially because synthetic vitamin A is very inexpensive. An international unit of vitamin A is equivalent to 0.30 mcg of retinol or 0.344 mcg of retinyl acetate.

Vitamin D: This antirachitic, fat-soluble vitamin is necessary for proper bone growth and ossification. Vitamin D occurs as the precursor sterols, ergocalciferol (vitamin D_2) and cholecalciferol (vitamin D_3), which are converted to active vitamin D by UV radiation. Although pigs can use vitamin D_2 (irradiated plant sterol) or vitamin D_3 (irradiated animal sterol), they seem to preferentially use D_3. Some of the vitamin D requirement can be met by exposing pigs to direct sunlight for a short period each day. Sources of vitamin D include irradiated yeast, sun-cured hays, activated plant or animal sterols, fish oils, and vitamin premixes. For this vitamin, 1 IU is equivalent to 0.025 mg of cholecalciferol. The estimated vitamin D requirement of 200 IU/kg for gestating and lactating sows was increased to 800 IU/kg in the 2012 NRC publication.

Vitamin E: This fat-soluble vitamin serves as a natural antioxidant in feedstuffs. There are eight naturally occurring forms of vitamin E, but D-α-tocopherol has the greatest biologic activity. Vitamin E is required by pigs of all ages and is closely interrelated with selenium. The vitamin E requirement is 11–16 IU/kg of diet for growing pigs and 44 IU/kg for sows. Some nutritionists recommend higher dietary levels for sows in the eastern corn belt of the USA, where selenium levels in feeds are likely to be low. Vitamin E supplementation can only partially obviate a selenium deficiency.

Green forage, legume hays and meals, cereal grains, and especially the germ of cereal grains contain appreciable amounts of vitamin E. Activity of vitamin E is reduced in feedstuffs when exposed to heat, high-moisture conditions, rancid fat, organic acids, and high levels of certain trace elements. One IU of vitamin E activity is equivalent to 0.67 mg of D-α-tocopherol or 1 mg of DL-α-tocopherol acetate.

Vitamin K: This fat-soluble vitamin is necessary to maintain normal blood clotting. The requirement for vitamin K is low, 0.5 mg/kg of diet. Bacterial synthesis of the vitamin and subsequent absorption, directly or by coprophagy, generally will meet the requirement for pigs. Although rare, hemorrhages have been reported in newborn as well as growing pigs, so supplemental vitamin K is recommended at 2 mg/kg of diet as a preventive measure. Generally, hemorrhaging problems can be traced back to the feeding of diets with moldy grain or other ingredients that contain molds.

Riboflavin: This water-soluble vitamin is a constituent of two important enzyme systems involved with carbohydrate, protein, and fat metabolism. Swine diets are normally deficient in this vitamin, and the crystalline form is included in premixes. Natural sources include green forage, milk byproducts, brewer's yeast, legume meals, and some fermentation and distillery by-products.

Niacin (Nicotinic acid): Niacin is a component of coenzymes involved with metabolism of carbohydrates, fats, and protein. Pigs can convert excess tryptophan to niacin, but the conversion is inefficient. The niacin in most cereal grains is completely unavailable to pigs. Swine diets are normally deficient in this vitamin, and the crystalline form is included in premixes. Natural sources of niacin include fish and animal byproducts, brewer's yeast, and distiller's solubles. Based on recent research, the NRC increased the niacin requirement to 30 ppm during all phases of growth.

Pantothenic Acid: This vitamin is a component of coenzyme A, an important enzyme in energy metabolism. Swine diets are deficient in this vitamin, and the crystalline salt, D-calcium pantothenate, is included in vitamin premixes. Natural sources of pantothenic acid include green forage, legume meals, milk products, brewer's yeast, fish solubles, and certain other byproducts.

Vitamin B_{12}: This vitamin, also called cyanocobalamin, contains cobalt and has numerous important metabolic functions. Feedstuffs of plant origin are devoid of this vitamin, but animal products are good sources. Although some intestinal synthesis of this vitamin occurs, vitamin B_{12} is generally included in vitamin premixes for swine.

Thiamine: This vitamin has important roles in the body, but it is of little practical significance for swine because grains and other feed ingredients supply ample amounts to meet the requirement in pigs.

Vitamin B_6: A group of compounds called the pyridoxines have vitamin B_6 activity and are important in amino acid metabolism. They are present in plentiful quantities in the natural feed ingredients usually fed to pigs. The requirement for vitamin B_6 in young pigs (5–25 kg) was increased by 3–4 fold in the 2012 NRC publication compared with the previous edition.

Choline: Choline is essential for the normal functioning of all tissues. Pigs can synthesize some choline from methionine in the diet. Sufficient choline is found in the natural dietary ingredients to meet the requirements of growing pigs. However, in some studies, choline supplemented at 440–800 mg/kg of diet increased litter size in gilts and sows. Natural sources of choline include fish solubles, fish meal, soybean meal, liver meal, brewer's yeast, and meat meal. Choline chloride, which is 75% choline, is the common form of supplemental choline used in feeds. If choline is added as a supplement to sow diets, it should not be combined with other vitamins in a premix, especially if trace minerals are present, because choline chloride is hygroscopic and destroys some of the activity of vitamin A and other less stable vitamins.

Biotin: This vitamin is present in a highly available form in corn and soybean meal, but the biotin in grain sorghum, oats, barley, and wheat is less available to pigs. There is evidence that when these latter cereal grains are fed to swine, especially breeding animals, biotin may be marginal or deficient. Reproductive performance in sows has been found to improve with biotin additions. Although not as clear, there is evidence that reproductive performance also is improved with addition of biotin to corn-soybean meal diets. In some instances, biotin supplementation decreased footpad lesions in adult pigs. For insurance, biotin supplementation is recommended, especially for sow diets. Raw eggs should not be fed to pigs because egg white contains avidin, a protein that complexes with biotin and renders it unavailable.

Folacin: This group of compounds has folic acid activity. Sufficient folacin is present in natural feedstuffs to meet the requirement for growth, but some studies have shown a benefit in litter size when folic acid was added to sow diets.

Ascorbic Acid (Vitamin C): Pigs are thought to synthesize this vitamin at a rapid enough rate to meet their needs under normal conditions. However, a few studies have shown benefits in performance of early-weaned pigs under stressful conditions when this vitamin was added to the diet.

Fatty Acids: Linoleic acid, arachidonic acid, and probably other long-chain, polyunsaturated fatty acids are required by pigs. However, the longer chain fatty acids can be synthesized in vivo from linoleic acid, so linoleic acid is considered the dietary essential fatty acid. The NRC estimates the linoleic acid requirement at 0.1% for growing and breeding swine. The requirement is generally met by the fat present in natural dietary ingredients. The oil in corn is a rich source of linoleic acid.

FEEDING LEVELS AND PRACTICES

Performance of weanling, growing, and finishing pigs; gestating sows; and lactating sows and their nursing pigs is related to both the quality of the diet and the amount consumed on a daily basis. Knowing the amount of feed animals consume is important in the overall feeding management process. Weanling, growing, and finishing pigs are ordinarily allowed to consume feed ad lib, and the amount consumed is affected by the energy density of the diet, environmental temperature, gender, and feed quality (eg, absence of molds), as well as a host of other management factors such as feeder design, crowding, etc.

Growing-Finishing Pigs: Daily feed intakes of various weight classes of growing-finishing pigs fed a diet containing 3,300 kcal of ME/kg (typical of a corn-soybean meal diet) as estimated by the NRC growth model are shown in TABLE 48. These intake levels represent an average for barrows and gilts. Feed intakes will be slightly higher for barrows and slightly less for gilts weighing 50–135 kg. Preventing overcrowding and cooling pigs with automatic water sprayers during hot weather help to alleviate reduced feed intake. These intake levels can be used as a guide to project total feed requirements or prescribe in-feed medication.

Gestating Gilts and Sows: For gestating gilts and sows, the NRC estimates that a feeding level of approximately 4.7–4.9 lb/day (2.1–2.2 kg/day) during the first 90 days of gestation and 5.6–5.7 lb/day (2.5–2.6 kg/day) for the final 25 days to farrowing of a corn-soybean meal diet (3,300 kcal ME/kg) provides sufficient energy for maintenance; some lean and fat tissue accretion (particularly in gilts); and the energy needs of the developing fetuses, placenta, and other supporting tissues (*see* TABLE 49). Mature sows do not need more energy than that required for maintenance and some increase in body weight. If gestation diets contain oats, alfalfa meal, or other energy diluents, higher feeding levels will be needed to meet the sow's daily energy requirement. Attempts to limit voluntary feed intake during gestation by allowing ad lib access to extremely high-fiber diets has not been successful; invariably, excess weight gain occurs.

Producers should adjust the feeding level of pregnant gilts and sows to keep them in good condition. Excess body condition at the end of gestation is often associated with reduced feed intake during lactation and sometimes results in reduced litter size, greater incidence of dystocia, more pig overlay, and a greater incidence of postpartum dysgalactia syndrome (*see* p 1373). Poor body condition results in a greater incidence of shoulder sores in sows, lower birth weights, and thin sows at weaning with delayed return to postweaning estrus (or even anestrus). Litter size at the subsequent farrowing can also be negatively affected if sows are in poor condition at breeding.

The amino acid requirements of first-litter gilts are higher than those for sows. Both gilts and sows require higher levels of dietary amino acids during the latter stage of gestation than in the initial 90 days of gestation. (*See* TABLE 49.)

Lactating Gilts and Sows: The NRC estimates that lactating gilts and sows nursing 11–11.5 pigs that gain 240 g/day during a 21-day lactation require 13.1–14.6 lb (6.0–6.6 kg) of feed (3,300 kcal of ME/kg) daily to meet their energy requirements (*see* TABLE 49). The amount of energy and feed depends on number of pigs nursed, weight gain of the pigs (both of these factors influence milk production), and weight loss of the sow. High-energy diets should be fed ad lib to sows during lactation, or sows should be hand-fed all they will consume three times daily. Proper temperature regulation in the farrowing room and the use of drip-coolers during hot weather help to alleviate low feed intake.

If feed intake is too low, sows will lose excessive weight during lactation (*see* p 2340). If this is a problem, including 3%–6% fat in the lactation diet or top-dressing the lactation feed with additional fat should be considered. If problems persist, more energy during the final 3–6 wk of pregnancy may be helpful.

Diets high in protein and amino acids should be fed to prolific sows nursing large litters to maximize milk production and to prevent excessive weight loss of the sow. Such sows may require diets containing 16%–18% or more crude protein (minimum of 0.9% lysine). If energy intake is sufficient, high-protein lactation diets will minimize or even eliminate weight loss in sows during lactation.

Major Feed Ingredients

A fundamental principle of the economics of pork production is to feed the most economical cereal grains and to correct the deficiencies by supplementation with good-quality protein sources, minerals, and vitamins. Dependable mineral and vitamin premixes or complete manufactured supplements are commercially available. Fortified corn-soybean meal diets are very popular in pig operations, but other cereals and protein sources can be used.

Corn (maize) is by far the most widely used grain for feeding pigs in the USA. It is very palatable and high in energy but relatively low in crude protein. In addition, corn is deficient in lysine, tryptophan, threonine, and several other essential amino acids, as well as vitamins and minerals.

Grain sorghum is a major energy source for pigs in western and southwestern USA. The protein content is variable depending on factors such as variety, whether the crop was grown on irrigated or dry land, amount of fertilizer used, and other environmental factors. In general, grain sorghum can be substituted for corn on an equal-weight basis, but because the ME value is slightly lower than that of corn, a poorer feed conversion should be expected.

Wheat has about the same energy content as corn and contains 2%–3% more protein and 0.05%–0.1% more lysine than corn. Wheat can be substituted for corn on either an equal-weight basis or on a lysine basis, but not on a crude protein basis or it will result in a lysine deficiency. Wheat can constitute all of the grain in a swine diet. The two main types of wheat grown in the USA, hard red winter and soft red winter, have equivalent nutritional value.

Barley has ~85%–90% of the feeding value of corn, even though it usually contains 2%–3% more protein. Scabby barley should not be fed to pigs.

Oats have a relatively low energy content and, therefore, should not account for >20%–25% of the cereal grain in the diet. Generally, when oats are included in the diet, the rate and efficiency of gain should be expected to decline. Rolled oats groats are sometimes used in starter diets because of their excellent palatability.

Cereal grains should be ground or rolled to maximize their feeding value. Corn and grain sorghum should be reduced to a medium-fine particle size (550–600 microns). Wheat should be ground more coarsely (650–700 microns) to prevent pasting. Fine grinding improves feed conversion, but excessive reduction in particle size may lead to an increased incidence of gastric ulcers. Pelleting of diets may result in a small improvement in gain and especially feed efficiency. In general, the benefit is greatest with pelleted diets that contain high levels of fiber, such as barley-based diets. Cereal grains should be as free as possible from mycotoxins. Aflatoxins, vomitoxin, zearalenone, fumonisins, and other mycotoxins can reduce animal performance, depending on level in the feed, and can especially cause reproductive problems in breeding animals.

Soybean meal accounts for >90% of the supplemental protein fed to pigs in the USA. It is very palatable and has an excellent amino acid profile that complements the amino acid pattern in cereal grains. Ground, full-fat soybeans can also be fed to swine but only after they are heated (by extrusion or roasting) to inactivate the trypsin inhibitors and other heat-labile antinutritional factors.

Canola meal also is an excellent protein source. Low-gossypol cottonseed meal (<100 ppm free gossypol), peanut meal, sunflower meal, and other oilseed-based meals can be used in swine feed but generally not as the sole source of supplemental protein because of the lower lysine content of their protein. Animal protein sources such as meat meal, meat and bone meal, or fish meal can supply a portion of the supplemental protein in swine diets.

Distillers dried grains with solubles (DDGS) is a byproduct that has received a lot of attention in recent years because of the increased number of ethanol plants that use corn to produce ethanol for fuel. This byproduct is an excellent and generally economical feed ingredient for swine. Although DDGS has essentially no starch and considerably more fiber than corn, it is considerably higher in fat (corn oil); hence, the ME content of DDGS containing 9%–12% fat is similar to that of corn. Recently, some ethanol plants extract a portion of the oil from the solubles before adding the solubles back to the dried grains. This results in a "low-fat" DDGS, generally 5%–9% fat, which has slightly less ME than conventional DDGS. Further removal of fat, called "de-oiled DDGS" (<5% fat) has substantially less ME than either of the other types of DDGS, so it has a lower feeding value. DDGS is also higher in protein than corn, but the quality of protein (ie, balance of amino acids), like corn protein, is poor.

A considerable amount of research has been done with DDGS in recent years. Diets containing 20%–25% DDGS are well utilized by pigs, but when high levels (>30%) of DDGS are fed in finishing diets, body fat of pigs becomes more unsaturated, as evidenced by higher iodine values. This results in softer, more flexible bellies that are more difficult to process into bacon slices. To overcome this problem, producers should consider either removing DDGS from the late finishing diet or reducing the level of DDGS to 10% during the final 3–4 wk of the finishing period.

Feeding Management of Sows and Litters

Gestation diets adequate in all nutrients should be fed to sows to produce healthy, vigorous pigs. Sows should be fed so that they are in good body condition at farrowing—not too fat or too thin. Thin sows tend to farrow smaller pigs that have a poorer chance of survival than larger, more vigorous pigs. After farrowing, the sow should be returned to full feed as soon as possible. Constipation in sows is generally not a problem if the sow is eating well. Wheat bran or dried beet pulp can be included in the farrowing diet at 5%–10% if constipation is a problem, or chemical laxatives such as potassium chloride or magnesium sulfate can be included in the diet at 0.75%–1%.

Newly farrowed pigs should be checked to ensure that each has nursed. If necessary, milk flow may be stimulated by giving oxytocin. If the sow is slow in coming into milk, weak pigs may benefit from receiving artificial milk, but success depends on good management and sanitation. Nutritional anemia should be prevented by giving an iron injection before 3 days of age or by other means discussed previously. Pigs from large litters may be transferred to sows with smaller litters after they receive colostrum; however, the transfer should be done within the first 24 hr after birth. A palatable pig starter diet should be provided beginning at 2–3 wk if pigs are weaned later than 3 wk of age. (*See also* HEALTH-MANAGEMENT INTERACTION: PIGS, p 2160, and MANAGEMENT OF REPRODUCTION: PIGS, p 2201.)

Feeding Management of Weanling Pigs

Pigs weaned at an early age (3–4 wk) perform best if fed a complex starter diet for 1–2 wk after weaning. Typically, the starter diet contains dried whey and/or lactose, dried blood products, and a high level of lysine. Some producers use a medicated early weaning program or segregated early weaning program to produce healthier pigs. This entails weaning at 10–16 days of age and requires excellent nutritional management. Such diets should contain even higher levels of lysine as well as high levels of lactose (as the sugar or from dried whey) and 3%–7% dried animal plasma. A gradual transition should eventually be made to less expensive starter diets and then to corn-soybean meal diets.

The nutritional needs of growing-finishing pigs are best met by a full-feeding program. Limit-feeding reduces the rate and efficiency of gain but may improve carcass quality of finishing pigs. Proper design and adjustment of self-feeders is necessary to prevent feed wastage or restricted growth.

Growth Stimulants

For many years, antibiotics and other chemotherapeutic agents have commonly been added to swine diets to promote growth and feed efficiency, reduce mortality and morbidity, and improve health. The greatest response to these growth enhancing agents is in young pigs, with lesser responses as pigs progress in age and weight. The levels of antibiotics fed and drug withdrawal requirements should be in accordance with manufacturers' recommendations and legal restrictions. (*See also* GROWTH PROMOTANTS AND PRODUCTION ENHANCERS, p 2758.)

The antibiotics approved as feed additives for swine include bacitracin methylene disalicylate, bacitracin zinc, bambermycins, chlortetracycline, lincomycin, neomycin, oxytetracycline, penicillin, tiamulin, tylosin, and virginiamycin. Chemotherapeutic agents include carbadox, roxarsone, sulfamethazine, and sulfathiazole. Several of these are approved only in combination with certain other additives. Apramycin also is approved for use as a water medication. Also, pharmaceutical levels of zinc (1,500–3,000 ppm) as zinc oxide, or copper (100–250 ppm) as copper sulfate or tribasic copper chloride are effective growth stimulants in young pigs.

However, FDA action has changed how antibiotics can be used. According to Final Guidance 213 and the Veterinary Feed Directive (VFD) rule, antimicrobials medically important in human medicine (this includes all of the antimicrobials approved for swine except carbadox, bacitracin, and bambermycins) previously used at subtherapeutic levels for production purposes (improved growth and efficiency) are no longer allowed for that purpose. Instead, they are allowed only for disease prevention and only under veterinary supervision and oversight. This regulation applies to antibiotics used in feed or water. Companies that produce those antimicrobials are asked to voluntarily remove the production improvement claim on their product labels. These products will no longer be available to producers on an "over-the-counter" basis; they will only be available on a VFD basis.

Microbials that are directly fed (once referred to as probiotics), such as live cultures of *Lactobacillus acidophilus*, *Streptococcus faecium*, and *Saccharomyces cerevisiae*, have been evaluated as possible substitutes for antibiotics, but controlled studies have not shown consistent, beneficial responses from their inclusion. In some instances, inclusion of specific sugars (mannanoligosaccharides, fructooligosaccharides [also called prebiotics]) have shown promise as possible alternatives to antibiotics for young pigs, but growth responses are less consistent and of lower magnitude than from the inclusion of antibiotics. The direct-fed microbials and oligosaccharides are thought to encourage growth of desirable microorganisms in the GI tract, such as lactobacilli species and bifidobacteria that partially displace some of the less desirable microorganisms, including some pathogenic microbes.

Certain "repartitioning agents" have been tested with finishing swine and found to be very effective in improving growth rate, feed conversion, and carcass leanness. Examples are β-agonists, such as ractopamine and porcine somatotropin. As of 2015, ractopamine is the only such agent approved for use in pigs in the USA. These agents affect nutrient requirements, in particular by increasing the dietary requirements for amino acids.

NUTRITIONAL DISEASES

Diagnosis of nutritional deficiencies by observation is difficult. Quite often, the clinical signs are the result of a complex of mismanagement and infectious diseases, including parasitism, as well as malnutrition. For most nutritional deficiencies, the signs are not specific, eg, poor appetite, reduced growth, and unthriftiness. Deficiency of a single nutrient may bring about inanition, and the subsequent starvation may cause multiple deficiencies. Then, too, a nutritional deficiency may exist without the appearance of definite signs. In the field, the deficiency may be only slight or borderline, which makes diagnosis difficult.

Diagnosis of a deficiency by observing the response to nutritional therapy is not always clear, particularly for longterm deficiencies, the lesions of which may be irreversible. A nutritional deficiency should be diagnosed positively only after observance of several of the expected clinical signs and a careful review of the dietary, disease, and management history of the animals.

Protein Deficiency: Protein deficiency, which may result from suboptimal feed intake or a deficiency of one or more of the essential amino acids, causes reduced gains, poor feed conversion, and fatter carcasses in growing and finishing pigs. In lactating sows, milk production is reduced, excess weight loss occurs, and sows may fail to exhibit postweaning estrus or have delayed return to estrus. For optimal use of protein, all essential amino acids must be liberated during digestion at rates commensurate with needs. Therefore, protein supplements should not be handfed at infrequent intervals but should be mixed with the grain or be available at all times with grain on a free-choice basis.

No evidence has been presented to support the theory of "protein poisoning" in pigs. Diets containing as much as 35%–50% protein were found to be laxative and less efficiently used, but no toxic effects were noted.

Fat Deficiency: Certain long-chain polyunsaturated fatty acids are essential for swine. Linoleic acid is essential in the diet and is used to produce longer-chain fatty acids that are probably also essential. A linoleic acid deficiency induces hair loss, scaly dermatitis, skin necrosis on the neck and shoulders, and an unthrifty appearance in growing pigs. Conventional swine diets generally contain adequate fat from the natural ingredients to furnish ample amounts of essential fatty acids.

Mineral Deficiency: Deficiencies of **calcium** or **phosphorus** result in rickets (*see* p 1051) in growing pigs and osteomalacia (*see* p 1052) in mature pigs. Signs include deformity and bending of long bones and lameness in young pigs, and fractures and posterior paralysis (a result of fractures in the lumbar region) in older pigs. Sows that produce high levels of milk and nurse large litters are particularly susceptible to posterior paralysis toward the end of lactation or after weaning if dietary calcium or phosphorus is deficient. These signs can also result from a deficiency of vitamin D, but phosphorus deficiency is the most common cause.

Pigs fed diets low in **salt** (NaCl) grow poorly and inefficiently, largely because of a marked reduction in feed intake. Although not specific for salt deficiency, poor hair and skin condition may also develop. There have been reports of salt-deficient pigs attempting to consume urine of other pigs.

Sows fed diets deficient in **iodine** produce hairless pigs that are weak or stillborn. With a borderline deficiency, the newborn pigs may be weak only at birth, but their thyroids are enlarged and have histologic abnormalities. (*See also* NON-NEOPLASTIC ENLARGEMENT OF THE THYROID GLAND, p 558.) Some feedstuffs (including soybeans and soybean meal) contain goitrogens that may cause marginal goiter if iodine is not included in the diet. Iodized salt at recommended levels prevents this deficiency.

Deficiencies of **iron** and **copper** reduce the rate of Hgb formation and produce typical nutritional anemia. Signs of nutritional anemia in suckling pigs include low Hgb and RBC count, pale mucous membranes, enlarged heart, skin edema about the neck and shoulders, listlessness, and spastic breathing (thumps). Iron deficiency is more common than copper deficiency and is most common in nursing pigs that do not receive an iron injection or oral iron early in life.

A *deficiency of* **zinc** *results in* parakeratosis (*see* p 975) in growing pigs, particularly when fed diets high in phytic acid (or phytate, the primary form of phosphorus in cereal grains and oilseed meals) and more than the recommended amount of calcium. The exact mode of action of zinc in the prevention of parakeratosis is not known.

Deficiencies of **selenium** and/or **vitamin E** can cause sudden death of young, rapidly growing pigs (*see* p 1174). In addition, selenium/vitamin E deficiency in nursing pigs makes them more susceptible to iron toxicosis from iron injections (*see* p 3077.)

Vitamin Deficiency: Most commercial diets are fortified with vitamins, and vitamin premixes are readily available for farm-mixed feeds, so deficiencies are less common than they were years ago. Deficiency of **vitamin A** results in disturbances of the eyes and the epithelial tissues of the respiratory, reproductive, nervous, urinary, and digestive systems. Reproduction is impaired in sows, and they may farrow blind, eyeless, weak, or malformed pigs. Herniation of the spinal cord in fetal pigs is reported as a unique sign of vitamin A deficiency in pregnant sows. Growing pigs deficient in vitamin A show incoordination and develop night blindness and respiratory disorders. Vitamin A deficiency is rare because of the ability of the liver to store this vitamin.

Signs of **vitamin D** deficiency include rickets, stiffness, weak and bent bones, and posterior paralysis. These signs are indistinguishable from those of a calcium or phosphorus deficiency (*see* above).

Vitamin E deficiency can result in poor reproduction and impaired immune system. Many of the signs of vitamin E deficiency are similar to those of selenium deficiency (*see* above).

Pigs deficient in **vitamin K** have prolonged blood clotting time and may die from hemorrhages. Certain components in moldy feed can interfere with vitamin K synthesis. Also, excessive levels of dietary calcium interfere with vitamin K activity, causing these signs.

In pigs deficient in **riboflavin**, reproduction is impaired; postpubertal gilts fail to cycle but show no other clinical signs. Deficient sows are anorectic and farrow dead pigs 4–16 days prematurely. The stillborn pigs have very little hair, often are partially resorbed, and may have enlarged forelegs. Growing pigs fed diets low in riboflavin gain weight slowly and have a poor appetite, a rough coat, an exudate on the skin, and possibly cataracts.

Pigs deficient in **niacin** have inflammatory lesions of the digestive tract and exhibit diarrhea, weight loss, rough skin and coat, and dermatitis on the ears. Intestinal conditions can be due to niacin deficiency or bacterial infection. Deficient pigs respond readily to niacin therapy and, although not a cure for infectious enteritis, adequate dietary niacin probably allows the pig to maintain its resistance to bacterial invasion.

Growing pigs and pregnant sows develop a typical "goose-stepping" gait, ataxia, and a noninfectious bloody diarrhea when maintained on diets deficient in **pantothenic acid**. When the deficiency becomes severe, anorexia develops.

Pigs with a **choline** deficiency exhibit incoordination and an abnormal shoulder conformation. At necropsy, they may have fatty livers and usually show kidney damage. Sows deficient in choline have reduced litter size and may give birth to spraddle-legged pigs.

Biotin deficiency includes excessive hair loss, skin ulcerations and dermatitis, exudates around the eyes, inflammation of the mucous membranes of the mouth, transverse cracking of the hooves, and cracking or bleeding of the footpads.

Neonatal pigs fed synthetic diets low in **vitamin B_{12}** show hyperirritability, voice failure, and pain and incoordination in the hindquarters. Histologic examination of the bone marrow reveals an impaired hematopoietic system. Fatty livers are also noted at necropsy.

NUTRITION: SHEEP

The economical and efficient production of sheep for meat, wool, show and/or pets is contingent on proper feeding, husbandry practices, and health care. All of these are influenced by dietary intake. Maintenance of breeding animals, a high percentage of the lamb crop weaned, growth of lambs, optimal weaning weights, and a heavy fleece weight and fleece quality are important to efficiency. The nutritional requirements for maintenance, reproduction, growth, finishing, and wool production are complex because sheep are maintained under a wide variety of environmental conditions; however, attempts should be made to ensure each production unit or individual sheep has adequate nutrient intake to be healthy and productive.

NUTRITIONAL REQUIREMENTS

An adequate diet for optimal growth and production must include water, energy (carbohydrates and fats), proteins, minerals, and vitamins. Under field conditions of particular stress, additional nutrients may be needed. (For detailed nutrient requirements for sheep, refer to the most current *Nutrient Requirements of Small Ruminants*, published by the National Research Council [www.nap.edu].)

Water: A clean, fresh, easily accessible source of water should be available at all times. As a minimum requirement in temperate environments, the usual recommendations are ~1 gal. (3.8 L) of water/day for ewes on dry feed in winter, 1½ gal./day for ewes nursing lambs, and ½ gal./day for finishing lambs. In many range areas, water is the limiting nutrient; even when present, it may be unpotable because of filth or high mineral content. For best production, all sheep should have their water availability monitored daily during all weather conditions. However, the cost of supplying water often makes it economical to water range sheep every other day. When soft snow is available, range sheep do not need additional water except when dry feeds such as alfalfa hay and pellets are fed. If the snow is crusted with ice, the crust should be broken to allow access. Still, when possible, sheep should have unlimited access to fresh, clean water.

Energy: Because so much of the diet can depend on grass and forage that is either sparse or of poor quality, the provision of adequate energy is important. Poor-quality forage, even in abundance, may not provide sufficient available energy for maintenance and production. The energy requirement of ewes is greatest during the first 8–10 wk of lactation. Because milk production declines after this period and the lambs have begun foraging, the requirement of the ewe is then reduced to prelambing levels. The easiest way to assess energy adequacy in sheep is to perform and record body condition using an objective 1–5 scoring system, with 1 being extremely thin and 5 being extremely obese.

The body condition score is determined by palpating the amount of fat covering on the spinous processes and transverse processes in the lumbar region. Most healthy productive ewes will have a score of 2–3.5. Sheep with a score of 1–2 should be examined and fed to attain a higher score, whereas those with a score >3.5 should be fed less. Dietary changes should be done slowly, and abrupt reduction in total energy intake should always be avoided, particularly in middle to late gestation.

Protein: Good-quality forage and pasture generally provide adequate protein for mature sheep. However, sheep do not digest poor-quality protein as efficiently as do cattle, and there are instances when a protein supplement should be fed with mature grass and hay, or when on winter range. Therefore, a minimum of 7% dietary crude protein is needed for maintenance in most sheep. Protein requirements depend on the stage of production (growth, gestation, lactation, etc) and the presence of certain diseases (internal nematode parasites, dental disease, etc). If available forages are unable to supply adequate dietary crude protein, protein supplements, such as oilseed meals (cottonseed meal, soybean meal) or commercially blended supplements should be fed to meet nutrient requirements. Protein should be fed to meet, but not exceed, requirements. Excess protein feeding can be beneficial in cases of excessive internal parasite burdens but result in increased production costs and may result in higher incidences of diseases (eg, heat stress, pizzle rot).

Sheep can convert nonprotein nitrogen (such as urea, ammonium phosphate, and biuret) into protein in the rumen but possibly less efficiently than beef cattle. This source of nitrogen can provide at least a part of the necessary supplemental nitrogen in high-energy diets with a nitrogen:sulfur ratio of 10:1. In lamb-finishing diets, the inclusion of alfalfa, approved growth stimulants, and a source of fermentable carbohydrates (eg, ground corn, ground milo) enhance nitrogen utilization.

Minerals: Sheep require the major minerals sodium, chlorine, calcium, phosphorus, magnesium, sulfur, potassium, and trace minerals, including cobalt, copper, iodine, iron, manganese, molybdenum, zinc, and selenium. Trace mineralized salt provides an economical way to prevent deficiencies of sodium, chlorine, iodine, manganese, cobalt, copper, iron, and zinc. Selenium should be included in rations, mineral mixtures, or other supplements in deficient areas. Sheep diets usually contain sufficient potassium, iron, magnesium, sulfur, and manganese. Of the trace minerals, iodine, cobalt, and copper status in ewes are best assessed via analysis of liver biopsy tissue. Zinc adequacy can be assessed from the careful collection of nonhemolyzed blood placed in trace element–free collection tubes. Selenium status is easily assessed by collection of whole, preferably heparinized, blood.

Salt: In the USA, except on certain alkaline areas of the western range and along the seacoast, sheep should be provided with ad lib salt (sodium chloride). Sheep need salt to remain thrifty, make economical gains, lactate, and reproduce. Mature sheep will consume ~0.02 lb (9 g) of salt daily, and lambs half this amount. Range operators commonly provide 0.5–0.75 lb (225–350 g) of salt/ewe/mo. Salt as 0.2%–0.5% of the dietary dry matter is usually adequate.

Calcium and Phosphorus: In plants, generally the leafy parts are relatively high in calcium and low in phosphorus, whereas the reverse is true of the seeds. Legumes, in general, have a higher calcium content than grasses. As grasses mature, phosphorus is transferred to the seed (grain). Furthermore, the phosphorus content of the plant is influenced markedly by the availability of phosphorus in the soil. Therefore, low-quality pasture devoid of legumes and range plants tends to be naturally low in phosphorus, particularly as the forage matures and the seeds fall.

Sheep subsisting on mature, brown, summer forage and winter range sometimes develop a phosphorus deficiency. Sheep kept on such forages or fed low-quality hay with no grain should be provided a phosphorus supplement (ie, defluorinated rock phosphate) added to a salt-trace mineral mixture. Because most forages have a relatively high calcium content, particularly if there is a mixture of legumes, diets usually meet maintenance requirements for this element. However, when corn silage or other feeds from the cereal grains are fed exclusively, ground limestone should be fed daily at the rate of 0.02–0.03 lb (9–14 g).

Sheep seem to be able to tolerate wide calcium:phosphorus ratios as long as their diets contain more calcium than phosphorus. However, an excess of phosphorus may be conducive to development of urinary calculi or osteodystrophy. A calcium: phosphorus ratio of 1.5:1 is appropriate for feedlot lambs. For pregnant ewes, the diet should contain ≥0.18% and, for lactating ewes, ≥0.27%. A content of 0.2%–0.4% calcium is considered adequate, as long as the ratio is maintained between 1:1 and 2:1.

Iodine: Occasionally, the iodine requirements of sheep are not met in the natural diet and thus iodine supplements must be fed. Goitrogenic substances are found in many types of plants (eg, *Brassica* spp) and interfere with the use of iodine by the thyroid. Regions naturally deficient are found throughout the western USA, in the Great Lakes area, and in other parts of the world. A deficiency of iodine (manifested as goiter in the adult and as lack of wool and/or goiter in lambs) can be prevented by feeding stabilized iodized salt to pregnant ewes. The young of iodine-deficient ewes may be aborted, stillborn, or born with goiters. Diets containing iodine at 0.2%–0.8% ppm are usually sufficient, depending on the animals' level of production (maintenance/ growth, lactation, etc).

Cobalt: Sheep require ~0.1 ppm of cobalt in their diet. Cobalt-deficient soils are found in North America but are relatively rare compared with other parts of the world. Normally, legumes have a higher content than grasses. Because cobalt levels of the feedstuffs are seldom known, a good practice is to feed trace mineralized salt that contains cobalt.

Copper: Pregnant ewes require ~5 mg of copper (Cu) daily, which is the amount provided when the forage contains ≥5 ppm. However, the amount of copper in the diet necessary to prevent copper deficiency is influenced by the intake of other dietary constituents, notably molybdenum (Mo), inorganic sulfate, and iron. High intake of molybdenum in the presence of adequate sulfate increases copper requirements. Because sheep are more susceptible than cattle to copper toxicity, care must be taken to avoid excessive copper intake (*see* p 3073). Toxicity may be produced in lambs being fed diets with 10–20 ppm of copper, particularly if the Cu:Mo ratio is >10:1. The Cu:Mo ratio should be maintained between 5:1 and 10:1.

Selenium: Selenium is effective in at least partially controlling nutritional muscular dystrophy. Areas east of the Mississippi River and in the northwestern USA appear to be low in selenium. The dietary requirement is ~0.3 ppm. Providing selenium-containing mineral mixture may prevent selenium deficiency if animals are allowed free access. Levels of 7–10 ppm or higher may be toxic.

Zinc: Growing lambs require ~30 ppm of zinc in the diet on a dry-matter basis. The requirement for normal testicular development is somewhat higher. Classic zinc deficiency (parakeratosis) is more common in other small ruminants (goats), but is occasionally encountered in sheep, particularly if fed excessive quantities of dietary calcium (legumes).

Vitamins: Sheep diets usually contain an ample supply of vitamins A (provitamin A), D, and E. Under certain circumstances, however, supplements may be needed. The B vitamins and vitamin K are synthesized by the rumen microorganisms and, under practical conditions, supplements are unnecessary. However, polioencephalomalacia can be seen and is due to aberrations in ruminal thiamine metabolism, secondary to altered ruminal pH and/or microflora content. Vitamin C is synthesized in the tissues of sheep. On diets rich in carotene, such as high-quality pasture or green hays, sheep can store large quantities of vitamin A in the liver, often sufficient to meet their requirements for as long as 6 mo.

Vitamin D_2 is derived from sun-cured forage, and vitamin D_3 from exposure of the skin to ultraviolet light. When exposure of the skin to sunshine is reduced by prolonged cloudy weather or confinement rearing, and when the vitamin D_2 content of the diet is low, the amount supplied may be inadequate. The requirement for vitamin D is increased when the amounts of either calcium or phosphorus in the diet are low or when the ratio between them is wide. But such dietary modification should be done cautiously, because vitamin D toxicity is a severe syndrome. Fast-growing lambs kept in sheds away from direct sunlight or maintained on green feeds (high carotene) during the winter months (low irradiation) may have impaired bone formation and show other signs of vitamin D deficiency. Normally, sheep on pasture seldom need vitamin D supplements.

The major sources of vitamin E in the natural diet of sheep are green feeds and the germ of seeds. Because vitamin E is poorly stored in the body, a daily intake is needed. When ewes are being fed poor-quality hay or forage, supplemental vitamin E may result in improved production, lamb weaning weights, and colostrum quality. Vitamin E deficiency in young lambs may contribute to nutritional muscular dystrophy if selenium intake is low.

FEEDING PRACTICES

Feeding Farm Sheep

Sheep make excellent use of high-quality roughage stored either as hay or low-moisture, grass-legume silage or occasionally chopped green feed. Good-quality hay or stored forage is a highly productive feed; poor-quality forage, no matter how much is available, is suitable only for maintenance. Hay quality is determined primarily by the following: 1) its composition, eg, a mixture of grasses and legumes such as brome/alfalfa or bluegrass/clover; 2) the stage of maturity when cut, eg, the grass before heading and alfalfa before one-tenth bloom; 3) method and speed of harvesting because they affect loss of leaf, bleaching by sun, and leaching by rain; and 4) spoilage and loss during storage and feeding. In general, the same factors influence the quality of silage. Complete analysis of cut-stored forages enhances the utilization of these feedstuffs and allows for the most efficient use of supplemental grains and minerals.

Feeding Ewes

The period from weaning to breeding of ewes is critical if a high twinning rate is desired. Ewes should not be allowed to become excessively fat but should make daily gains from weaning to breeding. The rate of gain depends on the desired weight but should be ~60%–70% of projected mature weight at breeding and 80%–90% of projected mature weight at lambing. If pasture production is inadequate, ewes may be confined and fed high-quality hay and a small amount of grain if necessary. Breeding while grazing legume pastures (eg, sage, white clovers) may tend to depress the size of the lamb crop, lowering the intake of certain feedstuffs. After mating, ewes can be maintained on pasture, thus allowing feed to be conserved for other times of the year. Good pasture for this period allows the ewes to enter the winter feeding period in good condition. When pasture is unavailable, an appropriate ration should be formulated (*see* TABLE 50).

During the last 6–8 wk of pregnancy, growth of the fetus is rapid. This is a critical period nutritionally, particularly for ewes carrying more than one fetus. Beginning 6–8 wk before lambing, the plane of nutrition should be increased gradually and continued without interruption until after lambing. The amount offered depends on the condition or fat covering of the ewes and quality of the forage. If ewes are in fair to good condition, 0.5–0.75 lb (225–350 g) daily is usually sufficient. The roughage content of the ration should provide all the protein required for all nonlactating ewes. If necessary, the ewes may be classified according to age, condition, and number of fetuses and divided into groups for different treatment.

Lactating Ewes: Succulent pasture furnishes adequate energy, protein, vitamins, and minerals for ewes and lambs;

TABLE 50 RATIONS FOR PREGNANT EWES UP TO 6 WK BEFORE LAMBING

	Ration No.			
Feed	1	2	3	4
	lb (kg)	lb (kg)	lb (kg)	lb (kg)
Legume hay, such as alfalfa, clover, or lespedeza	3–4.5 (1.36–2.04)	1.5–2 (0.68–0.91)	—	—
Corn or sorghum silage	—	4–5 (1.81–2.27)	—	—
Legume grass, low-moisture silage (50%)	—	—	6–8 (2.72–3.63)	—
Cottonseed, soybean, linseed, or peanut meal (90%); limestone (10%)	—	—	—	0.25 (0.112)
Minerals[a]	ad lib	ad lib	ad lib	ad lib

[a] Mineral mix: 2 parts dicalcium phosphate to 1 part trace mineralized salt

TABLE 51 GRAIN MIXTURE FOR PREGNANT EWES

Feed	Mixture No. 1	2	3	4
	%	%	%	%
Whole barley, corn, or wheat	60	75	75	50
Whole oats	30	—	25	50
Beet pulp, dried	—	25	—	—
Wheat bran	10	—	—	—

no added grain is necessary. When pasture is not being used (confinement rearing), ewes should be fed one of the rations outlined for pregnant ewes in TABLE 50, and 1–1.5 lb (450–675 g) of one of the grain mixtures in TABLE 51. Ewes should have access to a mixture of trace mineralized salt and dicalcium phosphate. Ewes with twin or triplet lambs should be separated from those with single lambs and fed more concentrates (grain) and/or better-quality forages. Ewes nursing twin lambs produce 20%–40% more milk than those with singles. Under confinement rearing or accelerated lambing, lambs are commonly weaned at 2 mo of age. The ewe's milk production declines rapidly after this period, and creep feed is more efficiently converted into weight gains when fed to lambs than to the ewe.

Feeding Lambs

From ~2 wk of age, lambs should have free access to creep feed. Where pasture is limited, they should be creep-fed for 1–2 mo until adequate forages are available. If pasture will not be available until the lambs are 3–4 mo old, they can be finished in a dry lot. The grain used should be ground coarse or rolled, but as the feeding period progresses, whole grains may be used. Small amounts of fresh, clean grain should be slowly introduced to the lambs' diet. The amount of grain is increased gradually until the lambs are on full feed.

Feeding lambs from birth to market in a dry lot, together with early weaning at 2–3 mo of age, has become more popular throughout the USA. A complete diet of hay, grain, and vitamin-mineral supplement is ground, mixed, and either fed as is or pressed into pellets 3⁄16- or 3⁄8-in. (5–10 mm) long. Such lambs usually reach market weight in 3½–4 mo. *See also* TABLE 52 for examples of creep rations used in dry lot feeding.

Rearing Lambs on Milk Replacer: Orphaned lambs, extras, triplets, or those from poor-milking ewes can be raised on milk replacers to improve productivity. Such lambs should receive 10%–20% of their body wt in colostrum divided into multiple feedings within 18–24 hr of birth. If ewe colostrum is unavailable, a frozen, pooled supply from several cows can be used. Milk replacers designed specifically for lambs are available and contain ~30% fat, 25% protein, and a high level of antibiotic. Under certain conditions, it may be advisable to inject orphaned lambs with vitamins A, D, and E and selenium. In handrearing systems, ewe milk replacers are preferable; however, good quality replacers designed for calves may be fed to lambs. When mixing milk replacers, care should be taken to ensure that the powder and water are properly mixed into a suspension. Feeding small quantities throughout numerous feedings helps reduce the incidence of bloat and/or diarrhea. Milk replacers should be fed at 10%–20% of the lamb's body wt, divided into 4–6 feedings/day during the first week of life. The number of feedings can be reduced over time to twice a day by 3–4 wk of age.

Multiple-nipple pails or containers can be used. Cold milk replacer can be used by older lambs who nurse more often. By 9–10 days of age, lambs should be given water in addition to the milk if a creep ration is offered. They can be weaned abruptly at 4–5 wk of age if consumption of creep feed and water intake is at a reasonable level.

Finishing Feeder Lambs: Lambs should be preconditioned before they leave the producer's property. This includes starting on feed, vaccinating, worming, and under some conditions, shearing. If this is not done, the lambs should be rested for several days and fed dry, average-quality hay after arrival at the feedlot. *See also* TABLE 53 for some recommended formulas for finishing lambs.

TABLE 52 CREEP RATIONS FOR SUCKLING AND EARLY-WEANED LAMBS

Feed	Mixture No.			
	1	2	3	4
	%	%	%	%
Alfalfa hay, leafy ground	25	30	40	—
Dehydrated alfalfa leaf meal	53.5	—	20	48
Corn, shelled	—	—	—	35
Corn or wheat	—	55	—	—
Oats or barley	—	—	20	—
Soybean, linseed, or cottonseed meal	19	10	10	10
Molasses	—	3.5	8.5	5.5
Bone meal or dicalcium phosphate	1	1	1	1
Limestone	1	—	1	—
Trace mineralized salt	0.5	0.5	0.5	0.5
Antibiotic	—	—	0.002	0.002

There is no best method or diet for finishing lambs. They may be finished on good to excellent quality forage (alfalfa, wheat) with no supplemental grain. They may be started on pasture or crop residue and moved to grain feeding systems as the forage is used up. When fed in a dry lot, they are usually allowed free access to feed-

TABLE 53 RECOMMENDED FORMULAS FOR FINISHING LAMBS[a]

Feed	Starter 10-day Period		High Roughage			
	Loose	Pelleted	Loose	Pelleted	High Concentrate	Corn Silage
Grain (corn, barley, or milo)[b]	500	200	780	400	1,500	540
Alfalfa hay	1,280	1,700	1,000	1,400	200	
Molasses	100	100	100			
Oilseed meal	100		100			100
Urea					45	
Beet pulp			200	200		
Silage						1,350
Limestone	10				35	10
Trace mineralized salt	10		20	20	35	
Antibiotic (g)	50	20	20	10	20	10
Vitamin A (*IU/ton*)						1,000,000

[a] Lb/ton or kg/metric ton; feeder lambs should have ~14% crude protein in rations (dry basis).

[b] Wheat can be substituted for other grains, but a period of time should be allowed for adaptation.

stuffs. These diets may be completely pelleted, ground and mixed, a mixture of ground forage (alfalfa) pellets and grain, and/or high-concentrate type. Self-feeding usually results in maximal feed intake and gain, and labor costs may be reduced. Hand-feeding can be mechanized with an auger system or self-unloading wagon. It involves feeding at regular intervals so that the lambs consume all the feed before more feed is offered. Feed consumption and gain can be controlled. When used, corn silage should be hand-fed to minimize spoilage.

Producers who feed lambs year-round, or feed heavy lambs, usually prefer to place the lambs on full feed as soon as possible (10–14 days). Lambs can be started safely on self-fed, ground, or pelleted diets containing 60%–70% hay. Within 2 wk, the hay can be reduced to 30%–40% when the ration is not pelleted. Other roughages such as cottonseed hulls or silage can be used in a similar manner.

Corn, sorghum, or alfalfa silage can replace about half the hay with hand-feeding, but finish and yield will be decreased to some extent. *See also* TABLE 52 for rations that can be used in self-feeding. Corn, barley, milo, wheat, or a mixture of these are used; 0.5% salt and 0.5% bone meal or equivalent should be added to the grain. Pelleting of rations for finishing lambs is beneficial when low-grade roughages or high-roughage rations are used. Caution should be used when feeding large amounts of wheat; lambs not adapted to it are more apt to develop acute indigestion than if fed grains such as corn, sorghum, or barley.

Mineral supplements, including salt, should be offered separately whether or not they are included in the grain mixture. Approved growth stimulants usually increase growth rate 10%–15% and feed efficiency 8%–10% but may decrease carcass quality.

Feeding Mature Breeding Rams

Mature breeding rams should be grazed on pasture when available, or fed rations 1, 2, or 3 according to TABLE 50. If rams are in a thrifty condition at breeding time and the ewes are on a good flushing pasture, it should not be necessary to grain-feed the rams while with the ewes. Rams should be maintained at a good body condition (3–3.5 on a 1–5 scale) before the breeding season.

Feeding Range Sheep

The condition of the sheep, the amount and kind of forage on the range, and the climatic conditions determine the kind and amount of supplement to feed. Supplements usually consist of high-protein pellets or cottonseed meal and salt, medium-protein pellets, low-protein pellets or corn, alfalfa hay, and minerals. When the diets of sheep on the western winter range are supplemented properly, the lamb crop can be increased 10%–15% and wool production increased by ~1 lb (400–500 g) per ewe.

One recommended practice is to feed ~0.25 lb (115 g) of high-protein (36%) supplement or 0.33–0.5 lb (150–225 g) of medium-protein (24%) pellets ~3 wk before and during the breeding season, during extremely cold weather, and for ~1 mo before green feed starts in the spring. In addition, small lambs, small yearling ewes, old ewes with poor teeth, and thin ewes should be separated from the main flock and fed one of the above supplements from approximately December 1 (northern hemisphere) until shearing time. In many instances, the old ewes, lambs, and yearlings from more than one band can be maintained in a flock for special dietary supplementation.

When sheep are unable to obtain a full ration of forage because of deep snow or other weather conditions, 1–3 lb (450–1,350 g) of alfalfa hay and 0.2–0.3 lb (90–150 g) of a low-protein pellet mixture or corn should be fed (*see* TABLE 54). If alfalfa hay is not available, 0.5–1 lb (225–450 g) per head of a low-protein pellet mixture should be fed daily for emergency feeding periods.

Deficiencies of Range Forages: Deficiencies most apt to be seen among range forages are protein, energy, salt, and phosphorus. These are most prevalent as the forages approach maturity or are dormant, and they may appear singly or in combination. Range sheep often travel long distances and are exposed to cold weather, resulting in higher energy requirements. Protein supplements (soybean or cottonseed meal, alfalfa pellets, etc) increase digestibility and use of poor-quality forages. When possible, the inclusion of a phosphorus supplement (eg, dicalcium phosphate, monocalcium phosphate, defluorinated rock phosphate) to a salt or trace mineral salt mixture may greatly improve productivity.

Most ranges used for winter grazing are considered adequate in carotene, because many species of browse furnish as much carotene as sun-cured alfalfa hay. However, when sheep are required to graze dry grass ranges for >6 mo without intermittent periods of green feed, vitamin A supplements are recommended. The addition of 45–50 IU of vitamin A/kg/day improves

TABLE 54 PATTERN FOR RANGE SUPPLEMENTS FOR SHEEP

Supplement			Proportions of Individual Feeds (%)			
				Recommended Amount of Protein		
Group	Subgroup	Feedstuff	Suggested Maximum	High	Medium	Low
Energy feeds	Grains	Barley	75		33	57.5
		Corn	60	5	10	15
		Wheat	60			
		Milo	60			
		Oats	15			
		Screenings No. 1	10			
	Mill feeds	Wheat mixed feed	10			
		Shorts	10			
		Molasses	15	5	5	10
		Beet pulp	10			10
Protein supplements	30%–40% Protein feeds	Cottonseed meal	75	62.5	32.5	5
		Linseed meal	25			
		Soybean meal	75	10	10	
		Peanut meal	25			
	20%–30% Protein feeds	Corn gluten feed	15			
		Corn distiller's dried grains	10			
		Wheat distiller's grains	10			
		Brewer's dried grains	5			
		Safflower meal	25			
		Cull beans	15			
Mineral supplements		Bone meal or defluorinated phosphate		4	3	2
		Dicalcium phosphate		1	0.5	0.5
		Disodium phosphate				
		Monocalcium phosphate				
		Monosodium phosphate				
		Salt or trace mineralized salt				
Vitamin supplements		Dehydrated alfalfa meal	20	12.5	6	
		Sun-cured alfalfa meal	20			
		Vitamin A and carotene concentrates				
Total				100	100	100

(continued)

TABLE 54 PATTERN FOR RANGE SUPPLEMENTS FOR SHEEP *(continued)*

Supplement			Proportions of Individual Feeds (%)			
				Recommended Amount of Protein		
Group	Subgroup	Feedstuff	Suggested Maximum	High	Medium	Low
Suggested composition						
Total crude protein (%)				36	24	12
Phosphorus (%)				1.5	1	0.5
Carotene (mg/kg)				35	17	—
Rate of feeding (g/day)—ewes				115	150–225	90–450

productivity in cases of extended consumption (>2 mo) of dry or weathered forages.

Mineral Mixtures: On the range, portable mineral boxes are convenient for sheep. One of these mineral mixtures should be fed free choice. A salt and dicalcium phosphate or phosphorus supplement (defluorinated rock phosphate) can be used if there are no iodine or trace-mineral deficiencies. Iodized salt is substituted for regular salt when an iodine deficiency exists, and trace mineralized salt is substituted if deficiencies of trace minerals are present.

Under winter range conditions, the amount of phosphorus supplement that should be added to range pellets varies with the type of range forage available, the rate of feeding, and the ingredients used in the pellets. It is suggested that 36%, 24%, and 12% protein pellets contain 1.5%, 1%, and 0.5% phosphorus, respectively. When feeding supplemental protein, 36% protein pellets should be fed at the rate of 0.25 lb (115 g) per head daily, the 24% protein pellets at 0.33–0.5 lb (150–225 g), and the 12% protein pellets at 0.2–0.5 lb (90–225 g), together with alfalfa or clover hay. Care should be taken when adding supplemental phosphorus and magnesium to the diet of rams or whethers, because this is associated with urolithiasis.

NUTRITIONAL DISEASES

Nutritional diseases in sheep are for the most part the same as those seen in goats (*see* NUTRITION: GOATS, p 2308).

Enterotoxemia: This feed-related malady causes almost sudden death in sheep due to a toxin produced by *Clostridium perfringens* type D and sometimes type C. The organism appears to be widespread in nature. Under conditions of high carbohydrate consumption or high intake of immature succulent forage, the causative bacteria multiply rapidly and produce an ε toxin that increases intestinal permeability. Protection of lambs is possible by vaccinating twice at least 10 days apart with *C perfringens* type D toxoid or by administering antitoxin at birth. (*See also* ENTEROTOXEMIAS, p 609.)

White Muscle Disease: White muscle disease is caused by low levels of selenium and possibly vitamin E. Signs include stiffness (especially in the hindquarters), tucked-up rear flanks, arched backs, pneumonia, and acute death. On necropsy, white striations are found in cardiac, diaphragmatic, and skeletal muscles. Levels of AST and lactic dehydrogenase are increased, indicating muscle damage. Blood levels of the selenium-containing glutathione peroxidase are reduced. Although several feedstuffs are fairly rich in selenium and vitamin E, it may be a good management practice in deficient areas to inject lambs shortly after birth with a preparation of vitamin E and selenium designed for parenteral use. The use of a selenium and/or vitamin E supplemented trace mineral mixture (up to 90 ppm) as the only source of salt fed may be useful as a preventive measure. (*See also* NUTRITIONAL MYOPATHIES IN RUMINANTS AND PIGS, p 1172.)

NUTRITION: SMALL ANIMALS

Domestic dogs and cats are both members of the order Carnivora. Observations of feral canids indicate that their feeding habits are broad and include various parts of plants as well as both small and large prey. By comparison, cats do not show omnivorous feeding behaviors and have a requirement for specific animal-derived sources of nutrients, such as preformed vitamin A, arachidonic acid, and taurine. As a result, dogs are classified nutritionally as omnivores, while cats are classified as true carnivores.

Using appropriate feeding practices is one of the most important components of maintaining companion animal health. Nutritional management is also important as an integral part of both preventive health care and treatment protocols for medical and surgical patients, and ignoring nutritional needs can often be more detrimental to a dog or cat than the illness or injury for which it is being treated. Feeding an appropriately formulated and tested complete and balanced commercial diet is the simplest way to meet the nutritional requirements of dogs or cats. Numerous products are available, and many are formulated for specific life stages. However, dogs and cats can thrive eating a variety of commercial or appropriately formulated home-prepared foods.

Despite the wide availability of commercially complete and balanced diets for dogs and cats, malnutrition still occurs. Malnutrition is defined as an imbalance of nutrients and includes both nutrient deficiencies and nutrient excesses. In recent years, obesity has become the most common nutritional disorder encountered in small animal medicine. Obesity is a serious medical condition that can lead to a variety of related health problems as well as shortened life span.

Body weight in combination with body condition score (BCS) is used in many species to provide an estimate of nutritional adequacy and can help determine ideal body weight. BCS is a semiquantitative assessment of body composition that ranges from cachectic to severely obese. Physical examination, visual observation, and palpation are used to assign a BCS.

Two BCS systems exist for dogs and cats, a 5-point system and a 9-point system (*see* TABLE 55). In a 9-point system, each unit increase in BCS above ideal represents body weight ~10%–15% greater than ideal body weight. For example, a dog or cat with a BCS of 7 is approximately 20%–30% heavier than its ideal weight.

Parameters used to assess BCS include evaluation of fat cover over the ribs, down the topline (waist), around the tailbase, and ventrally along the abdomen (abdominal tuck in front of hind legs). It is important to use both a visual assessment and palpation to assign a BCS (*see* TABLE 56).

NUTRITIONAL REQUIREMENTS AND RELATED DISEASES

Dogs are a biologically diverse species, with normal body weight of 4–80 kg (2–175 lb). Normal birth weight of pups depends on breed type (120–550 g). The first 2 wk of a puppy's life is spent eating, seeking warmth, and sleeping. External food sources beyond bitch's milk are rarely needed, unless the bitch cannot produce enough milk or the puppy is orphaned. In these cases, the puppy must be handreared. Growth rates of puppies are rapid for the first 5 mo; in this period, pups gain an average of 2–4 g/day/kg of their anticipated adult weight. The growth rate begins to plateau after 6 mo, and growth may be completed by 8–12 mo

TABLE 55 BODY CONDITION SCORE SCALES[a] FOR DOGS AND CATS

Body Condition	5-Point Scale	9-Point Scale
Very thin	1	1
Ideal weight	3	4–5 (dogs); 5 (cats)
Obese	5	9

[a] The scale used should be noted in the record (eg, BCS = 4/5 or BCS = 4/9).

TABLE 56 PARAMETERS USED TO ASSESS BODY CONDITION SCORE

Body Condition	Ribs	Overhead View	Side View	Tail Base
Very thin	Ribs easily felt with no fat cover; prominent visibility of individual ribs in dogs with short hair coats	Accentuated hourglass shape	Severe abdominal tuck	Bones are raised with no tissue between the skin and bone
Ideal	Ribs easily felt with slight fat cover; individual ribs not visible	Lumbar waist well-proportioned	Abdominal tuck present	Smooth contour but bones can be felt under a thin layer of fat
Obese	Ribs difficult to feel under thick fat cover	Lumbar waist not visible	No abdominal tuck; fat hangs from abdomen	Thickened and difficult to feel under prominent layer of fat; dimple may be visible at tail base

of age in small and medium breeds and by 10–16 mo in large and giant breeds.

By comparison, the average mature body weight of domestic cats is 3.2 kg (7 lb) for toms and 2.8 kg (6 lb) for queens. Normal birth weight of kittens is 90–100 g. The growth rate is exceptionally rapid for the first 3–4 mo, and kittens gain 50–100 g/wk. The growth rate begins to plateau at 150–160 days of age, and growth is usually completed within 200–220 days.

Dogs and cats require specific dietary nutrient concentrations based on their life stage. The Association of American Feed Control Officials (AAFCO) publishes dog and cat nutrient profiles for adult maintenance and reproduction (*see* TABLES 57 and 58). The National Research Council (NRC) also publishes nutrient profiles for dogs and cats for various life stages, most recently in 2006 (*see* TABLES 59 and 60). Both AAFCO and NRC list minimum nutrient requirements and maximum nutrient requirements for nutrients with potential toxicity.

In developed countries, nutritional diseases are rarely seen in dogs and cats, especially when they are fed good quality, commercial, complete and balanced diets. Nutritional problems occur most commonly when dogs and cats are fed imbalanced homemade diets, when cats are fed diets formulated for dogs, or when dogs or cats are fed certain human foods. Dog or cat foods or homemade diets derived from a single food item are inadequate. For example, feeding predominantly meat or even an exclusive hamburger and rice diet to dogs or cats can induce calcium deficiency and secondary hyperparathyroidism. Raw, freshwater fish contain thiamine antagonists and can induce thiamine deficiency when fed to cats. Feeding liver can induce vitamin A toxicity in both dogs and cats.

Cats have some dietary requirements that are different from those of dogs and can develop nutritional deficiencies when fed diets formulated to meet the nutritional needs of dogs. For example, unlike dogs, cats require dietary sources of vitamin A, arachidonic acid, and taurine. Cats also require higher quantities of fat and protein than dogs, as well as of the amino acid arginine and the vitamins niacin and pyridoxine (vitamin B_6). Cats lack the enzyme glucokinase, which unfortunately has led some to believe that cats cannot digest dietary carbohydrates. Cats produce the enzyme hexakinase, which allows them to digest and use properly processed dietary carbohydrates.

Well-intentioned owners occasionally cause problems by feeding dogs and cats certain human foods. For example, raisins and grapes contain an unknown substance that is toxic to dogs and can cause kidney damage. Chocolate contains theobromine and much smaller amounts of caffeine, both of which are methylxanthines. Dogs and cats metabolize theobromine much more slowly than people. Initial signs of toxicity include GI signs, such as vomiting and diarrhea. This can progress to polyuria, muscle tremors, cardiac arrhythmias,

TABLE 57 AAFCO NUTRIENT REQUIREMENTS FOR DOGS[a]

Nutrient	Growth and Reproduction Minimum	Adult Maintenance	
		Minimum	Maximum
Protein (%)	22.0	18.0	
Arginine (%)	0.62	0.51	
Histidine (%)	0.22	0.18	
Isoleucine (%)	0.45	0.37	
Leucine (%)	0.72	0.59	
Lysine (%)	0.77	0.63	
Methionine + cystine (%)	0.53	0.43	
Phenylalanine + tyrosine (%)	0.89	0.73	
Threonine (%)	0.58	0.48	
Tryptophan (%)	0.20	0.16	
Valine (%)	0.48	0.39	
Fat (%)	8.0	5.0	
Linoleic acid (%)	1.0	1.0	
Minerals			
Calcium (%)	1.0	0.6	2.5
Phosphorus (%)	0.8	0.5	1.6
Ca:P ratio	1:1	1:1	2:1
Potassium (%)	0.6	0.6	
Sodium (%)	0.3	0.06	
Chloride (%)	0.45	0.09	
Magnesium (%)	0.04	0.04	0.3
Iron (mg/kg)	80	80	3,000
Copper (mg/kg)	7.3	7.3	250
Manganese (mg/kg)	5.0	5.0	
Zinc (mg/kg)	120	120	1,000
Iodine (mg/kg)	1.5	1.5	50
Selenium (mg/kg)	0.11	0.11	2
Vitamins			
Vitamin A (IU/kg)	5,000	5,000	250,000
Vitamin D (IU/kg)	500	500	5,000
Vitamin E (IU/kg)	50	50	1,000
Thiamine (mg/kg)	1.0	1.0	
Riboflavin (mg/kg)	2.2	2.2	
Pantothenic acid (mg/kg)	10	10	
Niacin (mg/kg)	11.4	11.4	

(continued)

TABLE 57 AAFCO NUTRIENT REQUIREMENTS FOR DOGS[a] *(continued)*

Nutrient	Growth and Reproduction Minimum	Adult Maintenance	
		Minimum	Maximum
Pyridoxine (mg/kg)	1.0	1.0	
Folic acid (mg/kg)	0.18	0.18	
Vitamin B_{12} (mg/kg)	0.022	0.022	
Choline (mg/kg)	1,200	1,200	

[a] Nutrient requirements are indicated on a dry-matter basis. These AAFCO nutrient profiles for dog foods presume an energy density of 3.5 kcal ME/g dry matter. Rations >4 kcal/g should be corrected for energy density.

TABLE 58 AAFCO NUTRIENT REQUIREMENTS FOR CATS[a]

Nutrient	Growth and Reproduction Minimum	Adult Maintenance	
		Minimum	Maximum
Protein (%)	30.0	26.0	
Arginine (%)	1.25	1.04	
Histidine (%)	0.31	0.31	
Isoleucine (%)	0.52	0.52	
Leucine (%)	1.25	1.25	
Lysine (%)	1.20	0.83	
Methionine + cystine (%)	1.10	1.10	
Methionine (%)	0.62	0.62	1.5
Phenylalanine + tyrosine (%)	0.88	0.88	
Phenylalanine (%)	0.42	0.42	
Taurine (extruded, %)	0.10	0.10	
Taurine (canned, %)	0.20	0.20	
Threonine (%)	0.73	0.73	
Tryptophan (%)	0.25	0.16	
Valine (%)	0.62	0.62	
Fat (%)	9.0	9.0	
Linoleic acid (%)	0.5	0.5	
Arachidonic acid (%)	0.02	0.02	
Minerals			
Calcium (%)	1.0	0.6	
Phosphorus (%)	0.8	0.5	
Potassium (%)	0.6	0.6	
Sodium (%)	0.2	0.2	
Chloride (%)	0.3	0.3	

(continued)

TABLE 58 AAFCO NUTRIENT REQUIREMENTS FOR CATS[a] *(continued)*

Nutrient	Growth and Reproduction Minimum	Adult Maintenance	
		Minimum	Maximum
Magnesium (%)	0.08	0.04	
Iron (mg/kg)	80	80	
Copper (mg/kg)	5	5	
Iodine (mg/kg)	0.35	0.35	
Zinc (mg/kg)	75	75	2,000
Manganese (mg/kg)	7.5	7.5	
Selenium (mg/kg)	0.1	0.1	
Vitamins			
Vitamin A (IU/kg)	9,000	5,000	750,000
Vitamin D (IU/kg)	750	500	10,000
Vitamin E (IU/kg)	30	30	
Vitamin K (mg/kg)	0.1	0.1	
Thiamine (mg/kg)	5.0	5.0	
Riboflavin (mg/kg)	4.0	4.0	
Pyridoxine (mg/kg)	4.0	4.0	
Niacin (mg/kg)	60	60	
Pantothenic acid (mg/kg)	5.0	5.0	
Folic acid (mg/kg)	0.8	0.8	
Biotin (mg/kg)	0.07	0.07	
Vitamin B_{12} (mg/kg)	0.02	0.02	
Choline (mg/kg)	2,400	2,400	

[a] Nutrient requirements are indicated on a dry-matter basis. These AAFCO nutrient profiles for cat foods presume an energy density of 4 kcal ME/g dry matter. Rations >4.5 kcal/g should be corrected for energy density.

TABLE 59 2006 NRC NUTRIENT REQUIREMENTS FOR ADULT DOGS (MAINTENANCE)[a]

Nutrient (Amount/1,000 kcal ME)[b]	Minimum	Maximum	Recommended Allowance
Protein (g)	20		25
Arginine (g)	0.70		0.88
Histidine (g)	0.37		0.48
Isoleucine (g)	0.75		0.95
Leucine (g)	1.35		1.70
Lysine (g)	0.70		0.88
Methionine (g)	0.65		0.83
Methionine + cystine (g)	1.30		1.63
Phenylalanine (g)	0.90		1.13

(continued)

TABLE 59 2006 NRC NUTRIENT REQUIREMENTS FOR ADULT DOGS (MAINTENANCE)[a] *(continued)*

Nutrient (Amount/1,000 kcal ME)[b]	Minimum	Maximum	Recommended Allowance
Phenylalanine + tyrosine (g)	1.48		1.85
Threonine (g)	0.85		1.08
Tryptophan (g)	0.28		0.35
Valine (g)	0.98		1.23
Fat (g)		82.5	13.8
Linoleic acid (g)		16.3	2.8
α-Linolenic acid (g)			0.11
Eicosapentaenoic + docosahexaenoic acid (g)		2.8	0.11
Minerals			
Calcium (g)	0.50		1.0
Phosphorus (g)		0.5	0.75
Potassium (g)			1.0
Sodium (g)	75		200
Chloride (mg)			300
Magnesium (mg)	45		150
Iron (mg)			7.5
Copper (mg)			1.5
Manganese (mg)			1.2
Zinc (mg)			15
Iodine (mcg)	175		220
Selenium (mcg)			87.5
Vitamins			
Vitamin A (retinol equivalents)		16,000	379
Cholecalciferol (mcg)		20	3.4
Vitamin E (α-tocopherol, mg)			7.5
Vitamin K (menadione, mg)			0.41
Thiamine (mg)			0.56
Riboflavin (mg)	1.05		1.3
Pantothenic acid (mg)			3.75
Niacin (mg)			4.25
Pyridoxine (mg)			0.375
Folic acid (mcg)			67.5
Vitamin B_{12} (mcg)			8.75
Choline (mg)			425

[a] Reprinted with permission from the National Academies Press, copyright 2006, National Academy of Sciences.

[b] ME = metabolizable energy

TABLE 60 2006 NRC NUTRIENT REQUIREMENTS FOR PUPPIES AFTER WEANING[a]

Nutrient (Amount/1,000 kcal ME)[b]	Minimum	Maximum	Recommended Allowance
	PROTEIN, GROWING PUPPIES 4–14 WK OLD		
Protein (g)	45		56.3
Arginine (g)	1.58		1.98
Histidine (g)	0.78		0.98
Isoleucine (g)	1.30		1.63
Leucine (g)	2.58		3.22
Lysine (g)	1.75	>20	2.20
Methionine (g)	0.70		0.88
Methionine + cystine (g)	1.40		1.75
Phenylalanine (g)	1.30		1.63
Phenylalanine + tyrosine (g)	2.60		3.25
Threonine (g)	1.63		2.03
Tryptophan (g)	0.45		0.58
Valine (g)	1.35		1.70
	PROTEIN, GROWING PUPPIES ≥14 WK OLD		
Protein (g)	35		43.8
Arginine (g)	1.33		1.65
Histidine (g)	0.50		0.63
Isoleucine (g)	1.00		1.25
Leucine (g)	1.63		2.05
Lysine (g)	1.40		1.75
Methionine (g)	0.53		0.65
Methionine + cystine (g)	1.05		1.33
Phenylalanine (g)	1.00		1.25
Phenylalanine + tyrosine (g)	2.00		2.50
Threonine (g)	1.25		1.58
Tryptophan (g)	0.35		0.45
Valine (g)	1.13		1.40
	FAT, MINERALS, AND VITAMINS, ALL PUPPIES		
Fat (g)		330	21.3
Linoleic acid (g)		65	3.3
α-Linolenic acid (g)			0.2
Arachidonic acid (g)			0.08
Eicosapentaenoic + docosahexaenoic acid (g)		11	0.13

(continued)

TABLE 60 2006 NRC NUTRIENT REQUIREMENTS FOR PUPPIES AFTER WEANING[a] *(continued)*

Nutrient (Amount/1,000 kcal ME)[b]	Minimum	Maximum	Recommended Allowance
Minerals			
Calcium (g)	2.0	18	3.0
Phosphorus (g)			2.5
Potassium (g)			1.1
Sodium (mg)			550
Chloride (mg)			720
Magnesium (mg)	45		100
Iron (mg)	18		22
Copper (mg)			2.7
Manganese (mg)			1.4
Zinc (mg)	10		25
Iodine (mcg)			220
Selenium (mcg)	52.5		87.5
Vitamins			
Vitamin A (retinol equivalents)		3,750	379
Cholecalciferol (mcg)		20	3.4
Vitamin E (α-tocopherol, mg)			7.5
Vitamin K (menadione, mg)			0.41
Thiamine (mg)			0.34
Riboflavin (mg)	1.05		1.32
Pantothenic acid (mg)			3.75
Niacin (mg)			4.25
Pyridoxine (mg)			0.375
Folic acid (mcg)			68
Vitamin B_{12} (mcg)			8.75
Choline (mg)			425

[a] Reprinted with permission from the National Academies Press, copyright 2006, National Academy of Sciences.

[b] ME = metabolizable energy

seizures, and death. Macadamia nuts are also potentially toxic to dogs and cats and can cause weakness, depression, vomiting, ataxia, muscle tremors, hyperthermia, and tachycardia. As few as six macadamia nuts can be toxic to dogs. Onions and garlic contain thiosulfate, which can cause oxidative damage to RBCs and result in anemia. Onions are more toxic than garlic. Guatemalan avocados contain a substance called persin, which can cause dyspnea, pulmonary edema, and pleural and pericardial effusion in goats and possibly dogs. Food high in fat, such as chicken skin, can result in some dogs developing pancreatitis. Broccoli toxicity has been reported to occur in dairy cattle, but it is a poorly documented problem in dogs and cats. Sugar-free foods containing xylitol can cause liver damage in dogs. Raw food diets

TABLE 61 2006 NRC NUTRIENT REQUIREMENTS FOR ADULT CATS (MAINTENANCE)[a]

Nutrient (Amount/1,000 kcal ME)[b]	Minimum	Maximum	Recommended Allowance
Protein (g)	40		50
Arginine (g)			1.93
Histidine (g)			0.65
Isoleucine (g)			1.08
Leucine (g)			2.55
Lysine (g)	0.68		0.85
Methionine (g)	0.34		0.43
Methionine + cystine (g)	0.68		0.85
Phenylalanine (g)			1.00
Phenylalanine + tyrosine (g)			3.83
Threonine (g)			1.30
Tryptophan (g)			0.33
Valine (g)			1.28
Taurine (g)	0.080		0.10
Fat (g)		82.5	22.5
Linoleic acid (g)		13.8	1.4
Arachidonic acid (g)		0.5	0.015
Eicosapentaenoic + docosahexaenoic acid (g)			0.025
Minerals			
Calcium (g)	0.40		0.72
Phosphorus (g)	0.35		0.64
Potassium (g)			1.3
Sodium (mg)	160		170
Chloride (mg)			240
Magnesium (mg)	50		100
Iron (mg)			20
Copper (mg)			1.2
Manganese (mg)			1.2
Zinc (mg)			18.5
Iodine (mcg)	320		350
Selenium (mcg)			75
Vitamins			
Vitamin A (retinol *equivalents*)		25,000	250
Cholecalciferol (mcg)		188	1.75

(continued)

TABLE 61 2006 NRC NUTRIENT REQUIREMENTS FOR ADULT CATS (MAINTENANCE)[a] *(continued)*

Nutrient (Amount/1,000 kcal ME)[b]	Minimum	Maximum	Recommended Allowance
Vitamin E (α-tocopherol, mg)			10
Vitamin K (menadione, mg)			0.25
Thiamine (mg)			1.40
Riboflavin (mg)			1.0
Pantothenic acid (mg)	1.15		1.44
Niacin (mg)			10.0
Pyridoxine (mg)	0.5		0.625
Folic acid (mcg)	150		188
Vitamin B_{12} (mcg)			5.6
Choline (mg)	510		637

[a] Reprinted with permission from the National Academies Press, copyright 2006, National Academy of Sciences.

[b] ME = metabolizable energy

TABLE 62 2006 NRC NUTRIENT REQUIREMENTS FOR KITTENS AFTER WEANING[a]

Nutrient (Amount/1,000 kcal ME)[b]	Minimum	Maximum	Recommended Allowance
Protein (g)	45		56.3
Arginine (g)	1.93	8.75	2.4
Histidine (g)	0.65	>5.5	0.83
Isoleucine (g)	1.08	>21.7	1.4
Leucine (g)	2.55	>21.7	3.2
Lysine (g)	1.70	>14.5	2.1
Methionine (g)	0.88	3.25	1.1
Methionine + cystine (g)	1.75		2.2
Phenylalanine (g)	1.00	>7.25	1.3
Phenylalanine + tyrosine (g)	3.83	17	4.8
Threonine (g)	1.30	>12.7	1.6
Tryptophan (g)	0.33	4.25	0.40
Valine (g)	1.28	>21.7	1.6
Glutamic acid (g)		18.8	
Taurine (g)	0.080	>2.22	0.10
Fat (g)		82.5	22.5
Linoleic acid (g)		13.8	1.4

(continued)

TABLE 62 2006 NRC NUTRIENT REQUIREMENTS FOR KITTENS AFTER WEANING[a] *(continued)*

Nutrient (Amount/1,000 kcal ME)[b]	Minimum	Maximum	Recommended Allowance
α-Linolenic acid (g)			0.05
Arachidonic acid (g)			0.05
Eicosapentaenoic + docosahexaenoic acid (g)			0.025
Minerals			
Calcium (g)	1.3		2.0
Phosphorus (g)	1.2		1.8
Potassium (g)	0.67		1.0
Sodium (mg)	310		350
Chloride (mg)	190		225
Magnesium (mg)	40		100
Iron (mg)	17		20
Copper (mg)	1.1		2.1
Manganese (mg)			1.2
Zinc (mg)	12.5		18.5
Iodine (mcg)			450
Selenium (mcg)	30		75
Vitamins			
Vitamin A (retinol equivalents)		20,000	250
Cholecalciferol (mcg)	0.70	188	1.4
Vitamin E (α-tocopherol, mg)			9.4
Vitamin K (menadione, mg)			0.25
Thiamine (mg)	1.1		1.40
Riboflavin (mg)			1.0
Pantothenic acid (mg)	1.15		1.43
Niacin (mg)			10
Pyridoxine (mg)	0.5		0.625
Folic acid (mcg)	150		188
Vitamin B_{12} (mcg)			5.6
Choline (mg)	510		637

[a] Reprinted with permission from the National Academies Press, copyright 2006, National Academy of Sciences.

[b] ME = metabolizable energy

TABLE 63 DAILY MAINTENANCE ENERGY REQUIREMENTS FOR DOGS AND CATS

Animal	MER[a] (kcal/day)
Healthy adult dogs	
Intact	1.8 × RER[b]
Neutered	1.6 × RER
Obese prone	1.4 × RER
Healthy puppies	
<4 mo old	3 × RER
>4 mo old	2 × RER
Healthy adult cats	
Intact	1.4 × RER
Neutered	1.2 × RER
Obese prone	1.0 × RER
Healthy kittens	2.5 × RER[c]

[a] MER = maintenance energy requirement

[b] RER = resting energy requirement

[c] Kittens can alternatively be fed free choice

(*see* p 2375) are also not recommended for dogs and cats. Raw meat products may contain pathogens. (*See also* FOOD HAZARDS, p 2964.)

Nutrient deficiencies have also been seen in dogs and cats fed "natural," "organic," or "vegetarian" diets produced by owners with good intentions. Many published recipes have been only crudely balanced by computer, if at all, using nutrient averages. In addition, most homemade diets do not undergo the scrutiny and rigorous testing applied to commercial complete and balanced diets. If pet owners wish to feed their pets homemade diets, the diets should be prepared and cooked using recipes formulated by a veterinary nutritionist.

Some nutritional diseases are seen secondary to other pathologic conditions or anorexia, or both. Owner neglect is also a frequent contributing factor in malnutrition.

Energy: The most useful measure of energy for nutritional purposes is metabolizable energy (ME), which is defined as that portion of the total energy of a diet that is retained within the body. It is typically measured in calories or joules. The caloric content of pets foods is usually expressed in kilocalories (kcal), which is 1,000 calories. Dogs and cats require sufficient energy to allow for optimal use of proteins and to maintain optimal body weight and condition through growth, maintenance, activity, pregnancy, and lactation.

Energy requirements for dogs and cats are not a linear function of body weight. Recent evidence indicates that dogs maintained in households require fewer calories per day than dogs kept in kennels, but considerable variability exists. Breed differences also affect caloric needs independent of body size, eg, Newfoundlands appear to require fewer calories/day than Great Danes. Other factors that determine daily energy needs include activity level, life stage, percent lean body mass, age, and environment. Even when specific formulas are used, any given animal may require as much as 30% more or less of the calculated amount. Consequently, general recommendations may need to be modified within this 30% range, and body condition scoring should be regularly performed.

The precise ME values for many dog food ingredients have not been experimentally determined and are often estimated using those for other monogastric species (such as pigs) or calculated using Atwater physiologic fuel values modified for use with typical dog food ingredients. Likewise, the precise ME values for many cats are not known, although it is believed that the factors used for dogs may apply. The modified Atwater ME values for dogs are 3.5 kcal/g for carbohydrate and protein and 8.5 kcal/g of fat. The impact of various environmental temperatures is described in the recent NRC publication on nutrient requirements of dogs and cats and has been documented under certain conditions. For example, energy requirements increased from 120 to 205 kcal/kg$^{0.75}$ in Huskies as ambient temperatures decreased from 14°C in summer to –20°C in winter. Effects of environmental temperature are not well characterized in cats, because most of the research was done under thermoneutral (68°–72°F [20°–22°C]) conditions. However, unacclimatized adult cats increased their daily caloric intakes nearly 2-fold when environmental temperatures of 23°C and 0°C were studied.

Caloric Requirements: Energy requirements are quite variable among dogs and cats. Animals with the same body weight can have 3-fold variation in daily kcal requirements, which are affected by age, neutering status, physiologic status (growth, gestation, lactation, etc), physical activity, environmental temperature, and any underlying abnormalities. Any recommendations for kcal requirements are only starting points and may need to be modified based on the response of the individual dog or cat.

Many formulas are available to calculate caloric requirements for dogs and cats. A simple method for healthy dogs and cats starts with calculating the resting energy requirement (RER). The RER is the energy requirement for a healthy but fed animal, at rest in a thermoneutral environment. It includes energy expended for recovery from physical activity and feeding. There is an exponential and a linear formula for calculating RER. The exponential formula (RER = 70 [body wt in kg$^{0.75}$]) can be used for animals of any body weight, whereas the linear formula (RER = 30 × [body wt in kg] + 70) is restricted for use in animals that weigh >2 kg and <45 kg.

The maintenance energy requirement (MER) is the energy requirement of a moderately active animal in a thermoneutral environment. It includes energy needed to obtain, digest, and absorb food in amounts to maintain body weight, as well as energy for spontaneous activity. The *formulas to calculate MER take into* account age and neuter status.

Formulas for daily maintenance energy requirements (kcal/day) are listed in TABLE 63.

Nutrient Classifications

The six classes of nutrients are water, protein, fat, carbohydrates, vitamins, and minerals. Only protein, fat, and carbohydrate provide energy; vitamins, minerals, and water do not.

Water: Water is the most important nutrient; a lack of water can lead to death in a matter of days. Clean, fresh water should be available at all times. Multiple water sources encourage consumption. This is particularly important in cats, which often do not drink a lot of water.

Several approaches have been used to estimate daily water needs. There are general guidelines for daily fluid requirements in dogs and cats, but individual variations exist. The quantity of water required depends on a number of different factors, including the animal's diet, environment, activity level, and health status. The moisture content of canned pet foods varies from 60% to >87%. Dry pet foods contain 3%–11% water, and semimoist foods contain 25%–35% water. As a result, dogs and cats consuming predominantly canned food generally drink less water than those consuming predominantly dry diets.

In a thermoneutral environment, most mammalian species need ~44–66 mL/kg body wt. Another approach considers that water needs appear to be highly associated with the amount of food consumed. In this case, daily maintenance fluid requirements in mL should equal the animal's MER in kcal of ME. A third technique sets daily water intake as 2–3 times the dietary dry matter intake. When provided ample amounts of water, healthy animals can effectively self-regulate their intake. Water deficiency can be seen as a result of poor husbandry or disease. Dehydration is a serious problem in many different disorders, including those of the GI, respiratory, and urinary systems.

Protein: Protein is required to increase and renew the nitrogenous components of the body. A primary function of dietary protein is as a source of essential amino acids and nitrogen for the synthesis of nonessential amino acids. Amino acids supply both nitrogen for the synthesis of all other nitrogenous compounds and energy when catabolized. Ten amino acids are essential in the diet of dogs: arginine, histidine, isoleucine, leucine, lysine, methionine, phenylalanine, threonine, tryptophan, and valine. Cats have a dietary requirement for an additional amino acid, taurine. Other nonessential amino acids may become conditionally essential when an animal has an underlying disorder that either interferes with synthesis of the amino acid or results in its excessive consumption or loss.

Protein requirements of dogs and cats vary with age, activity level, temperament, life stage, health status, and protein quality of the diet. Most commercial dog foods contain a combination of plant- and animal-based proteins, with protein digestibilities of 75%–90%. Digestibility is less for plant protein ingredients, protein of poor biologic value, and for poor-quality diets. If excessive heat is used in processing, proteins can become chemically unavailable for digestion and absorption; however, these are not the types of temperatures typically used to produce commercial pet foods.

Healthy adult dogs need a minimum of 2.62 g of protein of high biologic value per kg metabolic body wt (ie, $BW_{kg}^{0.75}$)/day (NRC guidelines). Healthy puppies 4–14 wk old and >14 wk old need a minimum of 9.7 g and 12.5 g of protein of high biologic value per kg metabolic body wt/day, respectively. The cat has a higher protein requirement than most species, and healthy adult cats need a minimum of 3.97 g of protein of high biologic value per kg metabolic body wt/day. Healthy kittens need a minimum of 9.4 g of protein of high biologic value per kg metabolic body wt/day. The biologic value of a protein is related to the number and types of essential amino acids it contains and to its digestibility and metabolizability. The higher the biologic value of a protein, the less protein is needed in the diet to supply the essential amino acid requirements. Egg has been given the highest biologic value, and organ and skeletal meats have a higher biologic value than plant-based proteins.

General guidelines for dietary protein requirements in dogs and cats exist, but requirements vary depending on the digestibility of the protein in the diet. If an animal is consuming a diet containing predominantly plant protein sources, protein requirements may be higher than if the animal is consuming a diet containing predominantly animal protein sources. The dietary requirement for protein in healthy adult dogs is satisfied when the dog's metabolic need for amino acids and nitrogen is satisfied. Optimal diets for growing puppies should contain a minimum of 22% protein as dry matter (AAFCO guidelines) or 45 g protein/1,000 kcal ME for puppies 4–14 wk old and 35 g protein/1,000 kcal ME for puppies >14 wk old (NRC guidelines). Adult dogs require a minimum of 18% protein as dry matter (AAFCO guidelines) or ~20 g protein/1,000 kcal of ME required (NRC guidelines).

Optimal diets for growing kittens should contain at least 24%–28% ME as protein or 30% protein as dry matter (AAFCO guidelines) or 45 g protein/1,000 kcal ME (NRC guidelines). Optimal diets for adult cats should contain ~20% ME as protein or 26% protein as dry matter (AAFCO guidelines or 40 g protein/1,000 kcal ME (NRC guidelines). Growing kittens are more sensitive to the quality of dietary protein and amino acid balance than are adult cats. Protein suitable for cats must supply >500 mg of taurine/kg diet dry matter. Unless synthetic essential amino acids are added, some animal protein is necessary in the diet to prevent taurine depletion and development of feline central retinal degeneration or dilated cardiomyopathy.

Without sufficient energy from dietary fat or carbohydrate, dietary protein ordinarily used for growth or maintenance of body functions is less efficiently converted to energy. Too little high biologic protein in the diet, relative to the energy density, can cause an apparent protein deficiency.

Signs produced by protein deficiency or an improper protein:calorie ratio may include any or all of the following: reduced growth rates in puppies and kittens, anemia, weight loss, skeletal muscle atrophy, dull unkempt hair coat, anorexia, reproductive problems, persistent unresponsive parasitism or low-grade microbial infection, impaired protection via vaccination, rapid weight loss after injury or during disease, and failure to respond properly to treatment of injury or disease. High protein intakes per se do not cause skeletal abnormalities in dogs (including osteochondrosis in large breeds) or renal insufficiency later in life in dogs or cats.

Fats: Dietary fat consists mainly of triglyceride with varying amounts of free fatty acids and glycerol. Lipids can either be simple (triglycerides, wax) or complex (containing many other elements).

Triglycerides are divided into short, medium, and long chain based on the number of carbon atoms in the fatty acid chain. Essential fatty acids are long-chain fatty acids that cannot be synthesized in the body; most fatty acids consumed in the diet are long-chain fatty acids. Most nutrients consumed are digested and absorbed in the small intestines, where they then enter the blood supply via the portal vein and are delivered to the liver. When long-chain fatty acids are consumed, they are digested and absorbed into the small-intestinal epithelial cells; however, they are not transported directly into the blood supply but rather enter the lymphatics first. There are conflicting studies regarding the fate of dietary medium-chain fatty acids. Most studies suggest that medium-chain fatty acids do not require initial transport in the lymphatics and instead can be absorbed from the intestines directly into the blood supply via the portal vein.

Fatty acids are either saturated, indicating there are no double bonds, or unsaturated, indicating there are one or more double bonds. Fatty acids that contain more than one double bond are called polyunsaturated fatty acids (PUFA). PUFA are designated as either omega-3, omega-6, or omega-9 fatty acids, depending on the location of the first double bond. The more double bonds a fatty acid contains, the more prone it is to rancidity if not properly preserved. Saturated fatty acids are used primarily for energy in the body, whereas unsaturated fatty acids are found in cell membranes and blood lipoproteins.

Dietary fatty acid profiles are reflected in the fatty acid composition of tissues and cell membranes. In general, as the fat content of a diet increases, so does the caloric density and palatability, which promotes excess calorie consumption and obesity. Fat is a concentrated source of energy, yielding ~2.25 times the ME (as an equal dry-weight portion) of soluble carbohydrate or protein. The addition of too much dietary fat relative to other nutrients may result in excessive energy intake and subsequent suboptimal intakes of protein, minerals, and vitamins.

Dietary fats also facilitate the absorption, storage, and transport of the fat-soluble vitamins (A, D, E, and K). They are also a source of essential fatty acids (EFA), which maintain functional integrity of cell membranes and are precursors of prostaglandins and leukotrienes.

Dietary fats, especially the unsaturated variety, require a protective (natural or synthetic preservatives) antioxidation system. If antioxidant protection from a natural preservative system (eg, vitamin C or mixed tocopherols) or from synthetic preservatives (eg, BHA, BHT, ethoxyquin) in the diet is insufficient, dietary and body polyunsaturated fats become oxidized and lead to steatitis. Rancid fats in the diet can also result in fat-soluble vitamin deficiency.

Dietary fat requirements vary with age and species. Optimal diets for growing puppies should contain a minimum 8% fat as dry matter (AAFCO guidelines) or 5.9 g of fat per kg metabolic body wt/day (NRC guidelines) or 21.3 g fat/1,000 kcal ME (NRC guidelines). Optimal diets for adult dogs should contain a minimum 5% fat as dry matter (AAFCO guidelines) or 1.3 g of fat per kg metabolic body wt/day (NRC guidelines) or 10 g fat/1,000 kcal ME (NRC guidelines). Optimal diets for growing kittens and adult cats should contain a minimum 9% fat as dry matter (AAFCO guidelines), 4.7 g of fat per kg metabolic body wt/day for kittens, 4.7 g of fat per kg metabolic body wt/day for kittens, 2.2 g of fat per kg metabolic body wt/day for adult cats (NRC guidelines), or 22.5 g fat/1,000 kcal ME for growing kittens and adult cats (NRC guidelines).

Dogs and cats have a dietary requirement for specific EFA, including linoleic acid, an unsaturated EFA found in appreciable amounts in corn and soy oil. Cats also have a dietary requirement for another unsaturated EFA, arachidonic acid. Unlike dogs, cats cannot readily convert linoleic to arachidonic acid, which must be obtained from animal sources. Recommendations for dietary intake of both linoleic acid and arachidonic acid are ~5 g and 0.2 g/kg diet, respectively, for kittens and adult cats. Both linoleic acid and arachidonic acid are omega-6 fatty acids.

Recent studies suggest that α-linolenic acid (an omega-3 fatty acid) is also essential in dogs and possibly in cats. This omega-3 fatty acid is found primarily in flaxseed oils. The amount of dietary α-linolenic acid needed likely depends on the linoleic acid content. Although the required amounts of this omega-3 fatty acid are presently unknown, current minimal recommendations include 0.8 g/kg diet of α-linoleic acid when linoleic acid is 13 g/kg diet (dry-matter basis) for puppies and 0.44 g/kg diet of α-linoleic acid when linoleic acid is 11 g/kg diet (dry-matter basis) for adults. In addition, the longer chain omega-3 fatty acid, docosahexaenoic acid (DHA), may be conditionally essential for normal neurologic growth and development of puppies and kittens. Puppies fed diets containing DHA perform better in learning experiments and are easier to train than puppies fed diets without DHA. Eicosapentaenoic acid (EPA) is another longer chain omega-3 fatty acid that has been shown to be beneficial in the diet for treatment of certain skin, renal, and GI conditions, as well as cancer, arthritis, and hyperlipidemia. These longer chain omega-3 fatty acids are found primarily in marine sources of lipids. Very little α-linolenic acid gets converted to DHA/EPA in dogs and cats. Therefore, when choosing omega-3 fatty acids to treat certain medical conditions, it is best to choose marine sources. NRC recommends a level of 0.025 g/1,000 kcal ME of a combination of DHA and EPA for both kittens and adult cats. NRC recommends levels of DHA and EPA in the diet of 0.13 g/1,000 kcal ME for puppies and 0.11 g/1,000 kcal ME for adult dogs.

Most commercial adult dog foods typically contain 5%–15% fat (dry-matter basis). Puppy diets usually contain 8%–20% fat (dry-matter basis). One reason for this wide range of fat content is the purpose of the diet; work, stress, growth, and lactation require higher levels than maintenance. As much as 60% of the calories in a cat's diet may come from fat, although diets that contain 8%–40% fat (dry-matter basis) have also been fed successfully. Because fat can add considerably more calories to a finished diet, the amount of protein relative to energy must be balanced appropriately to the life stage and typical intakes expected for an animal's size and needs.

EFA deficiencies are extremely rare in dogs and cats fed properly preserved complete and balanced diets formulated according to AAFCO profiles. Deficiencies of EFA induce one or several signs, such as a dry, scaly, lusterless coat; inactivity; or reproductive disorders such as anestrus, testicular underdevelopment, or lack of libido. Fatty acid supplements are often recommended for dogs with dry, flaky skin and dull coats, but underlying metabolic conditions should always be evaluated first.

Carbohydrates and Crude Fiber:

Carbohydrates in pet foods include low- and high-molecular-weight sugars, starches, and various cell wall and storage nonstarch polysaccharides or dietary fibers. The four carbohydrate groups functionally are absorbable (eg, monosaccharides such as glucose, galactose, and fructose), digestible (eg, disaccharides, some oligosaccharides), fermentable (eg, lactose, some oligosaccharides), and poorly fermentable (eg, fibers such as cellulose, which is an insoluble fiber).

Although there is no minimum dietary requirement for simple carbohydrates or starches for dogs and cats, certain tissues, such as the brain and RBCs, require glucose for energy. If inadequate amounts of dietary carbohydrates are available, the body will synthesize glucose from glucogenic amino acids and glycerol. Cats normally use glucogenic amino acids and glycerol to synthesize glucose, which is one reason why cats are classified as true carnivores. However, dogs usually synthesize glucose from dietary carbohydrates. The use of dietary protein to synthesize energy in dogs diverts amino acids away from functions such as synthesis of nonessential amino acids and building muscle. Carbohydrates can become conditionally essential when energy needs are high, such as during growth, gestation, and lactation. Different carbohydrate sources have varying physiologic effects. In cats, carbohydrates apparently are not essential in the diet when ample protein and fats supply glucogenic amino acids and glycerol. However, properly cooked nonfibrous carbohydrates are utilized well by both cats and dogs. In both dogs and cats, if starches are not cooked, they are poorly digested and may result in flatulence or diarrhea. Except for the occasional case of lactose or sucrose intolerance, most cooked carbohydrates are well tolerated in both dogs and cats.

Fiber: Fiber is defined as the edible parts of plants or analogous carbohydrates that are resistant to digestion and absorption in the small intestine and have complete or partial fermentation in the large intestine. Although there is no dietary requirement for fiber in dogs and cats, there are health benefits of having certain fiber sources in the diet. Fiber is resistant to hydrolysis by mammalian digestive secretions but is not an inert traveler through the GI tract. Increased levels of fiber in diets increase fecal output, normalize transit time, alter colonic microflora and fermentation patterns, alter glucose absorption and insulin kinetics, and, at high levels, can depress diet digestibility.

The diverse nature of fiber has led to numerous classification methods. One way fiber is classified is based on its solubility. Soluble fibers have greater water-holding capacity than insoluble fibers. Fiber sources such as beet pulp, cellulose, and rice bran have low solubilities, while gum arabic, methylcellulose, and inulin have high solubility. Psyllium contains both low-soluble and high-soluble fiber. Although the classification of fiber based on its solubility is still used, fiber is better classified based on its rate of fermentability. Fermentation is defined as the capacity of fiber breakdown by intestinal bacteria, and this definition more accurately assesses the potential benefits of fiber in the GI tract. Fermentation of fiber produces the short-chain fatty acids acetate, propionate, and butyrate. Short-chain fatty acids have numerous benefits, including supplying energy to the large-intestinal epithelial cells, stimulating intestinal sodium and water absorption, and lowering the pH in the large intestines—an environment that favors survival of beneficial bacteria in the GI tract.

Conversely, fermentation also produces less desirable substances such as gases, ammonia, and phenols. Highly fermentable fibers are rapidly metabolized by intestinal bacteria and produce large amounts of gas that can result in cramping and diarrhea. Production of less desirable fermentation products can be minimized by using a moderately fermentable fiber source; examples include beet pulp, inulin, and psyllium. Beet pulp provides good fecal quality in dogs without affecting other nutrient digestibility when included at ≤7.5% (dry-matter basis).

Dietary fermentable fiber also functions as a prebiotic in dogs and cats. Prebiotics are defined as nondigestible food ingredients that selectively stimulate the growth or activity of beneficial bacteria in the intestines, such as *Bifidobacterium* and *Lactobacillus*. They also inhibit the survival and colonization of pathogenic bacteria. The beneficial bacteria produce short-chain fatty acids and some nutrients (eg, some B vitamins and vitamin K). Beneficial bacteria also function as immunomodulators and reduce liver toxins (eg, blood amine and ammonia).

Dietary fructooligosaccharides (FOS) and mannanoligosaccharides (MOS) also promote the survival and growth of beneficial bacteria in the GI tract. FOS are nondigestible oligosaccharides consisting of chains of fructose molecules. Dietary sources of FOS include beet pulp, psyllium, and chicory. Beneficial bacteria are able to use FOS as a metabolic fuel, whereas pathogenic bacteria cannot. FOS also enhance the effectiveness of the GI immune system. MOS are similar to FOS, except the predominant sugar molecule in MOS is mannose instead of fructose. Dietary sources of MOS include natural fibers found in yeast cells. MOS use a different mechanism than FOS to inhibit the growth of harmful bacteria. Pathogenic bacteria attach to the intestinal wall using finger-like projections called fimbriae. Fimbriae bind to specific mannose residues on intestinal cells. Fimbriated mannose-specific pathogens can also bind to MOS instead of adhering to the intestinal epithelium, and harmful bacteria are then excreted in the feces.

Several chemical methods are used to determine the fiber level of a food; all extract the components of fiber to different degrees, which results in different estimates of fiber level for the same feedstuff. Crude fiber, which is what is listed on pet food labels, quantifies insoluble dietary fiber, which is primarily cellulose, some lignin, and a small amount of hemicellulose. However, it does not measure a large portion of insoluble dietary fiber, nor any of the soluble dietary fiber. Therefore, crude fiber is not an accurate measure of total dietary fiber. The physiologic effects of fiber are not uniform across all fiber types, and relying solely on fiber content listed on pet food labels does not accurately reflect either fiber content and fiber types in commercial pet foods, or the physiologic effects from a diet.

Vitamins: Most commercial dog and cat foods are fortified with vitamins to levels that exceed minimal requirements. There is no AAFCO dietary requirement for vitamin C for dogs and cats, because they are able to synthesize it in the liver. Although dogs and cats can synthesize vitamin C in levels sufficient to prevent signs of deficiency, supplementation may provide additional health benefits because vitamin C functions as a free radical scavenger and an antioxidant in the body.

There is also no AAFCO dietary requirement for vitamin K for dogs and cats, because intestinal bacteria are able to synthesize it. However, any condition that alters the intestinal microflora, such as antibiotic therapy, may result in vitamin K deficiency. As a result, NRC recommends vitamin K at 0.33 mg/1,000 kcal ME in puppies, at 0.45 mg/1,000 kcal ME in adult dogs, and at 0.25 mg/1,000 kcal ME in kittens and adult cats.

Deficiencies of fat-soluble vitamins (A, D, and E in dogs; A, D, E, and K in cats) and some of the 11 water-soluble B-complex vitamins have been produced experimentally. Water-soluble vitamins are usually readily excreted if excess amounts are consumed and are thought to be far less likely to cause toxicity or adverse effects when ingested in megadoses. Vitamin B_{12} is the only water-soluble vitamin stored in the liver, and dogs may have a 2- to 5-yr depot. Fat-soluble vitamins (except for vitamin K in cats) are stored to an appreciable extent in the body, and when vitamins A and D are ingested in large amounts (10–100 times daily requirement) throughout a period of months, toxic reactions may be seen. Only clinically relevant vitamin-related imbalances are described below.

Vitamin A: Excessive consumption of liver can lead to hypervitaminosis A and may produce skeletal lesions, including deforming cervical spondylosis, ankylosis of vertebrae and large joints, osseocartilagenous hyperplasia, osteoporosis, inhibited collagen synthesis, decreased chrondrogenesis in growth plates of growing dogs, and narrowed intervertebral foramina.

Unlike most other mammals, cats cannot convert β-carotene to vitamin A, because they lack the intestinal dioxygenase enzyme necessary for β-carotene cleavage. Therefore, cats require a preformed source in their diet, such as that supplied by liver, fish liver oils, or synthetic vitamin A.

Signs of a vitamin A deficiency in cats are similar to those in other species, except that classic xerophthalmia, follicular hyperkeratosis, and retinal degeneration are rarely seen and usually are associated with concomitant protein deficiency. Nonetheless, cats fed diets deficient in vitamin A exhibited conjunctivitis, xerosis with keratitis and corneal vascularization, retinal degeneration, photophobia, and slowed pupillary response to light. Certain of these alterations also result from the retinal degeneration that is seen in taurine deprivation.

Hypovitaminosis A in cats may exhaust vitamin A reserves of the kidneys and liver; affect reproduction to cause stillbirths, congenital anomalies (hydrocephaly, blindness, hairlessness, deafness, ataxia, cerebellar dysplasia, intestinal hernia), and resorption of fetuses; and cause the same changes in epithelial cells noted in other animals. Squamous metaplasia of the respiratory tract, conjunctiva, endometrium, and salivary glands has been noted. Changes such as subpleural cysts lined by keratinizing squamous epithelium and extensive infectious sequelae are frequent in the lungs and are occasionally noted in the conjunctiva and salivary glands. Focal dysplasia of pancreatic acinar tissue and marked hypoplasia of seminiferous tubules, depletion of adrenal lipid, and focal atrophy of the skin have been reported. Borderline deficiency is more common, especially in chronic ill health.

Retinol at 9,000 IU/kg of diet should meet dietary needs for vitamin A during gestation and lactation and exceed the needs of growing kittens. *See* TABLES 58, 61, and 62 for dietary levels of vitamin A and other nutrients recommended by AAFCO and NRC.

Vitamin D: Vitamin D deficiency results in rickets in young animals and osteomalacia in adult animals. Classic signs of rickets are rare in puppies and kittens and most often are seen when homemade diets are fed without supplementation. Rickets has been reported in kittens fed diets deficient in vitamin D, even though dietary amounts of calcium and phosphorus were normal. In rickets, serum calcium and phosphorus are decreased or low normal with a corresponding high parathyroid hormone level; bone mineralization is decreased, and the metaphyseal areas are enlarged. Osteomalacia rarely causes clinical signs in dogs or cats. Hypervitaminosis D causes hypercalcemia and hyperphosphatemia with irreversible soft-tissue calcification of the kidney tubules, heart valves, and large-vessel walls. Death in dogs is either related to chronic renal failure or acutely due to a massive aortic rupture. Death in cats is related to chronic renal failure.

Vitamin E: In cats, steatitis results from a diet high in PUFA, particularly from marine fish oils when these are not protected with added antioxidants. Kittens or adult cats develop anorexia and muscular degeneration; depot fat becomes discolored by brown or orange ceroid pigments. Lesions are seen in cardiac and skeletal muscles and are similar to those described in other species.

Thiamine: Thiamine deficiency generally does not develop in cats fed properly prepared, commercial, complete, and balanced diets. Thiaminase, which tends to be high in uncooked freshwater fish, can produce a deficiency by rapid destruction of dietary thiamine. Although canned commercial cat foods may contain fish, the heat associated with canning is sufficient to destroy thiaminase. Destruction of thiamine has also resulted from treatment of food with sulfur dioxide or overheating during drying or canning, but deficiencies are now rare.

Thiamine-deficient cats develop anorexia, an unkempt coat, a hunched position, and with time, convulsions that become more severe, leading later to prostration and death. At necropsy, small petechiae may be found in the cerebrum and midbrain. Diagnosis can be confirmed in the early stages by giving 100–250 mg thiamine, PO or IM, bid for several days. Recovery occurs in minutes to hours but, if the diet is not supplemented after this treatment, relapse can be expected. Thiamine deficiency may cause a number of other neurologic disorders, including impairment of labyrinthine righting reactions, seen as head ventroflexion and loss of the ability to maintain equilibrium when moving or jumping; impairment of the pupillary light reflex; and dysfunction of the cerebellum, suggested by asynergia, ataxia, and dysmetria.

Minerals: Minerals can be classified into three major categories: macrominerals (sodium, potassium, calcium, phosphorus, magnesium) required in gram amounts/day, trace minerals of known importance (iron, zinc, copper, iodine, fluorine, selenium, chromium) required in mg or mcg amounts/day, and other trace minerals important in laboratory animals but that have an unclear role in companion animal nutrition (cobalt, molybdenum, cadmium, arsenic, silicon, vanadium, nickel, lead, tin). A balanced amount of the necessary dietary minerals in relation to the energy density of the diet is important. As intake of a mineral exceeds the requirement, an excessive amount may be absorbed, or a large amount of the unabsorbed mineral may prevent intestinal absorption of other minerals in adequate amounts. Indiscriminate mineral supplementation should be avoided because of the likelihood of causing a mineral imbalance.

Mineral deficiency is rare in well-balanced diets. Manipulation of dietary intake of calcium, phosphorus, sodium, magnesium (dogs and cats), and copper (dogs) for therapeutic effect is common. Limited evidence exists for the recommendations of dietary mineral requirements for cats in TABLES 61 and 62; many are based on the mineral content of successfully fed diets.

Macrominerals: Calcium and phosphorus deficiencies are uncommon in well-balanced growth diets. Exceptions may include high-meat diets high in phosphorus and low in calcium and diets high in phytates, which inhibit absorption of trace minerals. In dogs and cats, the requirements for dietary calcium and phosphorus are increased over maintenance during growth, pregnancy, and lactation. In dogs, the optimal calcium:phosphorus ratio should be ~1.2–1.4:1; however, minimum and maximum ratios by AAFCO are 1:1 to 2.1:1. Less phosphorus is absorbed at the higher ratios, so an appropriate balance of these two minerals is necessary. Also, insufficient supplies of calcium or excess phosphorus decrease calcium absorption and result in irritability, hyperesthesia, and loss of muscle tone, with temporary or permanent paralysis associated with nutritional secondary hyperparathyroidism. Skeletal demineralization, particularly of the pelvis and vertebral bodies, develops with calcium deficiency. By the time there is a pathologic fracture and the condition can be confirmed *radiographically*, bone demineralization is severe. Often, there is a history of feeding a diet composed almost entirely of meat, liver, fish, or poultry.

Excess intakes of calcium are more problematic for growing (weaning to 1 yr) large- and giant-breed dogs. Excessive supplementation (>3% calcium [dry-matter basis]) causes more severe signs of osteochondrosis and decreased skeletal remodeling in young, rapidly growing large-breed dogs than in dogs fed diets with lower dietary calcium (1%–3% [dry-matter basis]). The clinical signs of lameness, pain, and decreased mobility have not been reported in small-breed dogs or more slowly growing breeds fed the higher calcium amounts.

Magnesium is an essential cofactor of many intercellular metabolic enzyme pathways and is rarely deficient in complete and balanced diets. However, when calcium or phosphorus supplementation is excessive, insoluble and indigestible mineral complexes form within the intestine and may decrease magnesium absorption. Clinical signs of magnesium deficiency in puppies are depression, lethargy, and muscle weakness. Excessive magnesium is excreted in the urine. In cats, there is evidence that magnesium concentrations >0.3% (dry-matter basis) may be detrimental if the diet is too alkaline.

Trace Minerals: Iodine deficiency is rare when complete and balanced diets are fed but may be seen when high-meat diets are used (dogs and cats) or when diets contain saltwater fish (cats). Kittens with iodine deficiency show signs of hyperthyroidism in the early stages, with increased excitability, followed later by hypothyroidism and lethargy. Abnormal calcium metabolism, alopecia, and fetal resorption have been reported. The condition can be confirmed by thyroid size (>12 mg/100 g body wt) and histopathology at necropsy. The cause of hyperthyroidism that develops in older cats with increased blood thyroxine and triiodothyronine is unknown.

Iron and copper found in most meats are used efficiently, and nutritional deficiencies are rare except in animals fed a diet composed almost entirely of milk or vegetables. Deficiency of iron or copper is marked by a microcytic, hypochromic anemia and, often, by a reddish tinge to the hair in a white-haired animal.

Deficiency of zinc results in emesis, keratitis, achromotrichia, retarded growth, and emaciation. Decreased zinc availability has been noted in canine diets containing excessive levels of phytate, which emphasizes the value of feeding trial tests over laboratory nutrient analyses of pet foods.

Manganese toxicity has been reported to produce albinism in some Siamese cats; a deficiency of manganese in other species results in bone dyscrasia.

DOG AND CAT FOODS

Pet Food Labels

Current regulations require that all labels of pet foods manufactured and sold in the USA must contain the following items: 1) product name, 2) net weight of the product, 3) name and address of the manufacturer, 4) guaranteed analysis, 5) list of ingredients, 6) the words "dog or cat food" (intended animal species), 7) statement of nutritional adequacy, and 8) feeding guidelines. The AAFCO has also adopted an amendment that will require all pet food labels to contain information on the calorie content of the diet, expressed both in kcal ME/kg and per familiar household unit (eg, cups, cans).

The product name is the primary means by which a specific pet food is identified. The way ingredients are listed in the product name may also indicate the percentage of that ingredient present in the product, eg, using the term "beef" in the product name requires that beef ingredients must be at least 70% of the total product or ≥95% of the total weight of all ingredients, excluding water. Using the term "beef dinner," "beef entree," or "beef platter," etc, implies that beef must be at least 10% of the total product, and at least 25% but not more than 95% of the total weight of all ingredients, excluding water. Using the term "with beef" means at least 3% of the total product must be beef, and using the term "beef flavor" implies that there is only enough beef in the product to be detected by taste (<3%).

The product weight must be listed on the front of the pet food label within the bottom third of the principal display panel.

Guaranteed Analysis: This part of the label lists the minimal amounts of crude protein and crude fat and the maximal amounts of water and crude fiber on an as-fed (not dry-matter) basis. This analysis does not specify the actual amount of protein, fat, water, and fiber in the product. Instead, it indicates the legal minimums of protein and fat and the legal maximums of water and crude fiber content contained in the product. A laboratory proximate analysis lists the actual nutrient concentrations in the food, and two foods that have identical guaranteed analyses may have very different proximate analyses. A guaranteed analysis for protein may list a minimal level of 25%, while the product may (and usually does) contain >25%. A certain variance above or below a minimum or maximum should be expected. Consequently, whenever possible, the manufacturer's average nutrient profile should be used to evaluate a food.

Direct product comparisons made between like (similar water content) products (ie, dry vs dry, or canned vs canned) are generally valid. However, comparisons across different food types should be made on a dry-matter or caloric basis. As a general rule, dry-food analyses can be converted to a dry-matter basis by simply adding 10% to the as-is value, because most dry foods contain ~10% water (eg, a dry-food protein content of 25% on an as-fed basis is equal to 27.5% dry-matter basis). Canned food analyses can be converted to a dry-matter basis by simply multiplying by 4, because most canned foods contain ~75% water (ie, a canned-food protein content of 6% on an as-fed basis is equal to 24% dry-matter basis). Alternatively, the approximate percent dry matter of a nutrient in a product can be calculated from the information in the guaranteed analysis. First, dry matter in the diet is calculated by subtracting the moisture level from 100%. Next, the percent of the nutrient of interest on a dry-matter basis is calculated using the following equation:

(% nutrient [as fed]/% dry matter in diet) × 100 = ~% of nutrient (dry matter)

Ingredient List: In the USA, all pet foods sold must be registered with state feed control officials and must contain approved ingredients generally regarded as safe, unless they are for specialized purposes such as the amelioration or prevention of disease. Such foods are considered to be drugs and must be approved by the FDA.

Ingredients are listed in descending order of weight, on an as-fed basis, in the food. Although a food ingredient (eg, chicken) may be listed first, if that ingredient is 75% moisture, it will contribute a much smaller percentage of total nutrients to the food dry matter. In addition, an ingredient such as corn may be listed by individual types, eg, flaked corn, ground corn, screened corn, kibbled corn, etc. In this case, the total corn amount may be a significant amount of the total food dry matter, but when presented as individual types, each type appears lower on the ingredient list. This is referred to as ingredient splitting.

No reference to quality or grade of an ingredient is allowed to be listed; therefore, it is difficult to evaluate a product solely on the basis of the ingredient list. The value of this list is limited to determining the sources of the proteins and carbohydrates for dogs or cats. This kind of information is useful when evaluating animals experiencing an adverse reaction to a food, possibly due to an allergy or intolerance to one or more ingredient sources such as beef, wheat, etc.

Product formulations can be either fixed or open. In a fixed formula, combinations of ingredients and nutrient profiles do not change regardless of fluctuating market prices of the ingredients. In an open formula, ingredients, and possibly actual nutrient profiles, change depending on availability and market prices. Most commercial complete and balanced diets have a fixed formulation.

Statement of Nutritional Adequacy: This statement indicates how the food was tested (feeding versus laboratory analysis or formulation) and for which life stage the food is intended. AAFCO recognizes only four life stages: growth, maintenance, gestation, and lactation. The term "all life stages" is frequently used on a label and indicates that the product has been either formulated or tested for growth. By default, it is anticipated that such a food would also pass a maintenance protocol, because testing a food for growth generally includes gestation and lactation. There are no AAFCO-approved nutrient profiles for geriatric, senior, or weight loss stages.

The statement "complete and balanced" indicates the product contains all nutrients presently known to be required by dogs or cats and that these nutrients are properly balanced to the energy density of the diet. The "complete and balanced" claim must be substantiated by successfully completing AAFCO feeding trials, or the food must contain at least the minimal amount of each nutrient recommended by AAFCO. There are cautions "against the use of these requirements (levels) without demonstration of nutrient availability" because some of the requirements are based on studies in which the nutrients were supplied as purified ingredients and, therefore, are not representative of ingredients used in commercial pet foods. Laboratory analysis does not address the issue of bioavailability. Supplements, snacks, treat products (ie, those intended for intermittent or supplemental feeding), and therapeutic or dietary products (ie, those intended for use under the direction of a veterinarian) are exempted from AAFCO testing.

Feeding Guidelines: These must be expressed in common terms, such as "feed (weight/unit of product) per body wt of dog or cat." They are general recommendations at best, and body weight and body condition must be monitored to prevent over- or underfeeding.

Pet Food Product Types

Commercial dog and cat foods are available in three principal forms: canned, dry, and semimoist. The classifications used depend on the processing method and water content more than on the ingredient content or nutrient profile. Complete and balanced commercial dog and cat diets are formulated to provide adequate quantities of each required nutrient without an intolerable excess of any nutrient. Supplementation of particular nutrients to commercially produced complete and balanced dog and cat foods should be done carefully and only with appropriate justification. Dog foods are not satisfactory for cats because most dog foods are lower in protein, often do not contain assured concentrations of taurine, and are not designed to produce a urinary pH of <6.5 (which helps prevent the crystallization of struvite or magnesium-ammonium-phosphate in the feline urinary tract. (*See also* FELINE LOWER URINARY TRACT DISEASE, p 2383.)

Dry Food: This is the most popular category of pet food in the USA and some other countries. Dry foods generally contain ~90% dry matter and 10% water. Approximately 95% of dry dog and cat foods are extruded, ie, they are made by combining and cooking ingredients (grains, meat and meat byproducts, fats, minerals, and vitamins), then forcing the mixture through a die. During cooking and extrusion, a temperature of ~150°C (~302°F) converts the starches into a form more easily digested, destroys toxins and inhibitory substances, and flash sterilizes the product. The food is then enrobed with fat and/or digest (material derived from controlled degradation of animal tissues, eg, chicken digest) during drying to increase palatability.

Advantages of dry food include a lower cost than canned or soft-moist food, and refrigeration of unused portions is not needed. Certain types of dry food may also provide beneficial massage of the teeth and gums to help decrease periodontal disease (although unless specifically formulated to deter it, remain mainly ineffective in dogs for this purpose).

Canned Food: Canned dog and cat foods contain 68%–78% water and 22%–32% dry matter. Many of the same ingredients are used in canned pet foods as in dry-extruded types but usually not at the same levels of inclusion. Given their high moisture content, canned foods typically contain higher amounts of fresh or frozen meat, poultry, or fish products and animal byproducts. Many canned pet foods contain textured proteins derived from grains, such as wheat or soy. These materials function as meat analogues, having a physical structure similar to that of meat and high nutritional quality. The use of meat in combination with some of the textured proteins not only controls costs but can improve the overall nutritional profile of the final product.

Canned pet food processing begins with blending meat or meat analogues and fat ingredients with water and dry ingredients, such as vitamins and minerals, for proper nutrient content. The mixture is blended and sometimes ground to produce a fine slurry, depending on product profile. After cans are filled, they are sealed and retorted (a heat and pressure-cooking process that also sterilizes the contents), assuring destruction of foodborne pathogens. Advantages of canned food include a long shelf life in a durable container and high palatability. However, canned food is more expensive than dry food.

Soft-moist Food: Soft-moist dog and cat foods contain 25%–40% water and 60%–75% dry matter. They do not require refrigeration and are preserved using humectants—substances that bind water so that it is unavailable for bacteria and mold growth and assure shelf life. They include simple sugars (usually sucrose), sorbitol, propylene glycol, and salts. Many soft-moist foods are acidified using phosphoric, malic, or hydrochloric acid to further retard spoilage. Advantages of soft-moist foods include convenience, high energy digestibility, and palatability. However, soft-moist food is more expensive than dry food.

Home-cooked Diets: Dogs can be successfully maintained on properly formulated home-cooked diets; this is much more difficult in cats. Advantages of home-cooked diets include the use of fresh, high-quality ingredients chosen by the owner. Disadvantages include preparation time, variable quality control and diet consistency, higher cost, and the difficulty in formulating and preparing a nutritionally complete and balanced diet. It is most difficult to formulate a nutritionally complete and balanced diet with sufficient nutrient density in a small volume of food that is palatable for cats. Many home-cooked diets result in foods that are high in protein and caloric density and have inappropriate calcium:phosphorus ratios and inadequate levels of calcium, copper, iodine, fat-soluble vitamins, and several of the B vitamins. Many published recipes for feline diets have very high ash or mineral levels because of the extent of synthetic nutrient supplementation required. If owners choose to feed a home-cooked diet, they should use a recipe formulated by a veterinary nutritionist (vs found on the Internet). It is also important to realize that no home-cooked diets have undergone the testing and research used to formulate complete and balanced commercial pet foods.

Raw Meat–based Diets: Raw meat–based diets have received a lot of attention in recent years. The controversy, lack of good data, and paucity of high-quality research make it difficult for veterinarians to make informed recommendations to pet owners regarding this feeding practice. However, the American Animal Hospital Association, the American Veterinary Medical Association, and the Canadian Veterinary Medicial Association have all developed statements discouraging the feeding of raw or undercooked animal-source protein to dogs and cats. In addition, in 2010, the Delta Society's Pet Partners Program initiated a policy precluding animals eating raw meat–based diets from participating in the Therapy Animal Program.

There are two main types of raw meat–based diets: home-prepared and commercial. In addition, a variety of raw dried or freeze-dried pet treats fall under this category. Home-prepared diets include a variety of feeding regimens, including BARF (Bone and Raw Food or Biologically Appropriate Raw Food), the Ultimate Diet, and the Volhard Diet. Commercial raw meat–based diets most commonly are fresh, frozen, pasteurized, or freeze-dried. Some of these commercial diets are formulated to meet AAFCO nutrient profiles, but many are not.

One of the biggest areas of controversy surrounding these types of diets are the safety of these diets to not only the pets consuming them, but to the pet owners and others who are exposed to the animals consuming them. Even if owners purchase meat meant for human consumption to produce home-prepared diets, there is no assurance these ingredients are free of pathogens and safe to consume uncooked. Raw chicken is a common source of *Salmonella*, and it is estimated that 21%–44% of chicken purchased from retail locations meant for human consumption throughout North America is contaminated with *Salmonella*. Even if a pet owner takes precautions while handling and preparing these diets, it has been shown that after consumption of a single meal contaminated with *Salmonella*, 44% of dogs shed *Salmonella* in their feces for as long as 7 days, and none of these dogs was symptomatic for *Salmonella* infection. *Salmonella* contamination rates for beef and pork intended for human consumption are estimated to range from 3.5%–4%; however, beef and pork are a source of other potential pathogens, including the pathogenic strain of *E coli* O157:H7. *Campylobacter* spp is estimated to be present in 29%–74% of chicken, and *Listeria* spp is estimated to be present in 15%–34% of chicken and 25%–52% of beef and pork. In two separate studies, consumption of raw meat was shown to significantly increase the seroprevalence rate of *Toxoplasma gondii* in cats.

Some commercial raw meat–based diets are frozen or freeze-dried; however, neither freezing nor freeze-drying destroys all the potential pathogens in these products. Some commercial raw meat–based diet manufacturers now use high-pressure pasteurization in an attempt to reduce the risk of pathogens. Although this process can reduce the numbers of many pathogens, it usually does not completely eliminate them, and bacteria and viruses vary in their susceptibility to this process. Commercial pet foods have also been recalled in recent years because of contamination from *Salmonella*; however, considering the number of commercially available pet food products, the percentage of products affected is relatively small compared with the number of raw meat–based diets affected.

Another concern, particularly of home-prepared raw meat–based diets, is nutrient imbalances. In a European study that evaluated 95 homemade raw meat–based diets being fed to dogs, 60% had major nutritional imbalances. There have been a number of case reports pertaining to the development of vitamin D–dependent rickets type I and nutritional secondary hyperparathyroidism associated with dogs being fed raw meat–based diets. Other concerns regarding the practice of feeding raw meat and bones to dogs and cats is the risk associated with esophageal and intestinal foreign bodies and perforation. Feeding raw bones has also been associated with slab fractures and other dental problems in dogs.

Proponents of raw diets often cite that raw meat–based diets are the evolutionary diet of dogs and cats and that domestic dogs and cats have never evolved into being able to digest and absorb commercial pet foods. However, a recent report shows that dogs have 36 regions of the genome that differ from that of wolves, and 10 of these regions play a critical role in starch digestion and fat metabolism. Therefore, the genetic makeup of domestic dogs and cats is not the same as that of wolves. Proponents of raw diets also cite that cooking destroys essential enzymes needed for digestion. While a small amount of protein is destroyed during cooking, and enzymes are proteins, there is no evidence that animals or people require these exogenous sources of enzymes. In addition, many of these enzymes are destroyed in the highly acidic environment in the stomach and never reach the small intestines, where most nutrients are absorbed.

Finally, veterinarians must also consider the potential legal implications of recommending raw meat–based diets. While zoonotic risks can be associated with feeding both commercial and home-prepared diets, if a pet owner, for example, develops a *Salmonella* infection from feeding a contaminated commercial diet, the pet food manufacturer is generally at risk of legal action. However, veterinarians who recommend home-prepared raw meat–based diets are potentially liable if an owner becomes sick from preparing these diets or as a result of pets shedding pathogens in their feces.

FEEDING PRACTICES

Domestication and use of dogs and cats as companions may have modified eating patterns of these animals to varying extents. Easier access to food and consistency of food quality has led to increased food consumption and the possibility of decreased energy expenditure overall. Hence, there is greater risk of obesity. At the same time, longevity of companion animals has also increased and, along with it, the emergence of other chronic progressive diseases such as osteoarthritis, cancer, and immune and cognitive disorders. Healthy dogs and cats eat a variety of foods. During a 24-hr period, most dogs will eat 1–3 meals, whereas most cats will eat frequent small meals, as many as 18 a day.

Although odor, consistency, taste, and learned dietary habits determine which foods a dog will eat, most dogs are indiscriminate eaters. Finicky, begging dogs have learned such behaviors. Likewise, odor, consistency, taste, and learned dietary habits determine which foods a cat prefers, but how much a cat will eat is affected by factors such as noises, lights, food containers, the presence or absence of people or other animals (including other cats), physiologic state, and disease. Cats can and will refuse to eat to the point of starving themselves under stressful conditions. These cats are at risk of developing hepatic lipidosis, which can be fatal if not treated early and aggressively.

Some dogs and cats have adequate appetite controls and maintain an optimal body condition, even with dietary changes. By contrast, other dogs and cats overeat, consume excessive calories, and become obese. The thickness of the fat layer over the rib cage and pelvic bones is a good indicator of obesity, as is regular body condition scoring over time (*see* TABLES 55 and 56).

Dietary modifications are required by changes in life stage, environment, body weight and condition, and disease. Energy density varies from 2,500 to >5,000 kcal/kg dry matter for dog foods and from 3,000 to >5,000 kcal/kg dry matter for cat foods. Therefore, general feeding recommendations cannot be given for all dogs and cats on any particular food. Instead, feeding recommendations should be individualized. The best feeding method is one that maintains optimal body weight and condition, bearing in mind that disease conditions may require dietary changes.

When a dietary change is necessary, it should not be done abruptly. New food should be introduced gradually throughout 5–7 days. Also, it is better to offer slightly less than the calculated new food amount. Overindulgence and abrupt changes are frequently the inciting cause of GI disorders that may ultimately lead to diet refusal. In dogs, the new food should be introduced slowly by replacing 25% more of the old food every day or two until the new diet makes up the entire amount fed. Cats can easily become habituated to a particular food and may resist any dietary change. In cats, new food should also be introduced slowly. Some cats have definitive preferences for dry food, whereas others prefer the same food moistened or canned.

If the dog or cat is to be switched from a canned to a dry diet, it may be useful to moisten the product by adding sufficient warm water, and the food can be warmed to release odors and flavors that encourage consumption. Dry-matter digestibilities are 60%–90% for dog food and 75%–90% for cat food because of ingredient quality, crude-fiber content, processing, and level of intake. Small, formed, brown feces suggest high nutrient digestion and absorption, while large volumes of pale feces indicate less dietary utilization.

Maintenance: After a dog has reached ~90% of its expected adult weight, a diet less nutrient dense than the growth diet is recommended. The dietary goal is to maintain optimal body weight and condition for that particular dog. Some adult dogs can be fed free choice, but most cannot without becoming obese. The best feeding regimen to use in most adult dogs to prevent obesity is portion-controlled feeding, eg, feeding two premeasured meals at regular times each day. Most dogs will eat all their food immediately, but some dogs will graze throughout the day.

Many owners feed treats and snacks, which are often an important aspect of the human-animal bond. Complete and balanced treat products that use low-fat, high-fiber ingredients are available. However, most treats are not complete and balanced; therefore, to prevent nutrient deficiencies, the total daily amount of treats should be <10% of the total caloric intake. Nutritional supplements are not required and, in fact, may be harmful. In an animal prone to obesity, the caloric content of all treats fed should be considered in an effort to match energy intake to expenditure. Regular assessment of the animal's body condition helps ensure minimal weight gain beyond optimal adult values throughout life.

Most inactive, neutered adult cats can be fed a reduced fat diet (9% dry-matter basis) ad lib, but increasing the insoluble fiber content may be necessary in some animals to satisfy hunger. Cats exposed to variations in temperature (eg, cats that remain outdoors year-round or at night) may eat more during the winter. The need for a different nutritional profile in older cats versus middle-aged cats may be necessary. Middle-aged cats are at increased risk of developing obesity, whereas older cats often have a difficult time keeping weight on. The ability of older cats to digest protein and fat is often less than that of younger and middle-aged cats. Therefore, it is important to feed a diet with highly digestible protein and fat sources. The quantity of these nutrients in the diet may also have to be modified (usually increased) to compensate for impaired protein and fat digestion. However, depending on activity level, feeding a food with a different fat and fiber content (increased or decreased as needed) may be required to maintain optimal body weight and condition.

Growth and Reproduction in Dogs: Growth, pregnancy, and lactation greatly increase nutrient demands over those of maintenance. Growth diets have increased nutrient density, digestibility, and bioavailability to provide nutrients necessary in a smaller volume of food. Supplementation of calcium, phosphorus, and vitamin D beyond amounts present in complete and balanced diets designed for growth and reproduction is rarely necessary and may be contraindicated.

Growth: Overfeeding during growth increases growth rate. This is not desirable, because it is incompatible with proper skeletal development and also contributes to obesity later in life. Feeding methods for growing puppies should be individualized for the puppy and owner. General recommendations are that puppies between weaning and 6 mo of age should be fed three times a day; puppies 6–12 mo old should be fed twice daily. Large- and giant-breed puppies should be fed complete and balanced growth diets that have been tested in feeding trials and that contain calcium, fat, and protein at levels closer to the minimums stated by AAFCO. Small-breed puppies may have to be fed more than three times a day using a tested diet that contains calcium, fat, and protein at levels greater than the minimums stated by AAFCO.

Only limited data have been published with respect to breed growth curves. Nonetheless, a slow growth rate is preferable to a fast growth rate. Weight gains should be closely monitored (weekly), and feeding recommendations adjusted such that the puppy gains a small amount of weight each week. When growing large-breed puppies were fed 50%–70% of their littermate's ad lib intake, adult height, length, and bone or muscle mass were not stunted; only total body fat was affected. It is difficult to stunt the growth of a puppy being fed a complete and balanced growth diet that has passed an approved AAFCO feeding trial using meal feeding of an appropriate amount for 2–3 times/day.

Gestation: Feeding recommendations for pregnant bitches through the first *two-thirds* of gestation are the same as those for maintenance. A common mistake is to overfeed during early gestation and to underfeed during lactation. In the last third of gestation, the total amount of food offered should be increased at least 20%–30% over the amount for maintenance. Growth diets are often used during gestation because of their higher energy density and smooth transition after parturition to support lactation.

Lactation: Depending on litter size, lactating bitches often require energy levels 2–4 times those of maintenance to avoid excessive loss of body condition. Ad lib feeding using a complete and balanced growth diet containing 10%–20% fat (dry-matter basis) that has passed an approved AAFCO feeding trial is recommended to maintain lactation and to permit optimal body weight and condition to be required by weaning. If a bitch loses significant body condition during lactation, the fat content of the diet should be increased to 20%–30% fat (dry-matter basis), and she should be fed ad lib.

Growth and Reproduction in Cats: One of the most important differences between queens and bitches is that pregnant queens exhibit a linear increase in weight (fetal growth) throughout pregnancy. As a result, pregnant queens need to consume more calories almost immediately after becoming pregnant. In contrast, fetal growth is minimal during the first two trimesters of pregnancy in the bitch, and caloric intake does not generally have to be increased until sometime between the end of the second trimester and the beginning of the third trimester.

Because queens tend to lose weight during lactation regardless of diet fed, it has been assumed that net tissue reserves should increase somewhat in preparation for lactation. A growth diet for kittens that contains 10%–35% fat, 30%–40% protein, and low (<5%) fiber (dry-matter basis) should be fed. Growing kittens and pregnant and lactating queens can be fed ad lib or several times a day to meet their daily needs. During the latter third of gestation, the amount of food and level of nutrient intake normally increases an average of 25%, although energy intakes for cats during pregnancy have been estimated to be as much as 40% greater than for maintenance. Some queens may eat less early in gestation and immediately before parturition; such changes are of concern only if prolonged. Queens require 2–3 times the normal food intake during lactation, depending on litter size. Supplementing an already balanced diet is not necessary and should be discouraged.

Geriatric Dogs and Cats: Older dogs and cats may not be as efficient in metabolizing dietary protein than younger animals. They may actually require more dietary protein than their younger counterparts to maintain protein reserves and maximize protein turnover rates. In addition, decreased fat digestion occurs with age in cats, so geriatric cats may actually require a higher-fat diet than their younger counterparts. In contrast, some dogs and cats begin old age considerably overweight, whereas others may show some loss of condition. Feeding an appropriate food with a different nutrient profile with respect to energy, fat, or fiber content (increased or decreased) may be needed to maintain optimal body weight and condition. Geriatric dogs and cats should be monitored in a preventive health program that includes periodic assessments of body weight and condition. The incidence of chronic degenerative organ disease increases with age, and early diagnosis fosters earlier treatment and more effective nutritional management.

Work or Stress: The caloric needs of working or stressed dogs may exceed the levels of a maintenance diet, depending on the animal and extent of work performed. Most diets designed for work or stress have increased levels of animal fats, with the other nutrients appropriately balanced to the increased energy density. At extreme levels of stress (eg, an Alaskan sled dog requiring 10,000 kcal/day), many recommend not only increasing the percent ME from fat but also from protein, while minimizing the contribution of carbohydrate.

Any daily feeding recommendation should be considered an estimate or starting point and should be modified based on continual evaluation of the dog's weight and condition, skin and coat, performance, and general attitude. Feeding a smaller amount of the daily ration (eg, ⅓ of the daily amount) before beginning a work shift is recommended with the remainder being fed thereafter. Plenty of fresh water should be available, and opportunities to stop work for a water break should be scheduled in any daily work routine for these dogs.

NUTRITION IN DISEASE MANAGEMENT

Nutrition is an important part of disease management, even though few disorders can be cured solely with diet. The interaction between illness, health, and nutritional status is multifactorial and complex. The nutritional requirements of many sick dogs and cats are qualitatively the same as those of healthy ones; however, they differ in the amounts required—certain nutrients may be needed in greater amounts or may need to be restricted.

Adverse Reaction to Foods: Food reactions are classified using specific terminology. An adverse reaction to a food is a clinically abnormal response to any type of food ingested. Food intolerance is a type of adverse reaction that does not involve the immune system, eg, food poisoning. A food allergy is a type of adverse reaction that does involve the immune system, eg, colitis or atopic dermatitis. (*See also* FOOD ALLERGY, p 855, and LOCALIZED ANAPHYLACTIC REACTIONS, p 824.)

Dogs and cats with food allergy usually have GI signs (eg, vomiting or diarrhea, or both) or a pruritic skin condition, especially in the regions of the ears, rear, and feet. The prevalence of true food allergies is very small. Some dogs and cats with nonseasonal pruritus are having an adverse reaction to food. Unfortunately, food allergy cannot be differentiated from food intolerance, and skin testing for food allergies is unreliable. Blood tests are also an unreliable way to diagnose food allergies in dogs and cats. Hence, given all the possible etiologies and limited diagnostics available, any animal suspected of having an adverse reaction to food should undergo a food trial. The length of time needed for a food trial depends on the condition being managed. Food trials for adverse reactions to food associated with clinical signs involving the GI tract should continue for ≥2 wk, whereas food trials for clinical signs involving dermatologic conditions should continue for ≥10–12 wk.

During a food trial, the only item fed should be a diet containing a single novel protein source or a hydrolyzed protein diet. A careful dietary history must be obtained from the pet owner before selecting the type of diet. If the owner elects to feed a commercially prepared food, several products are available for dogs that use single novel protein sources (eg, kangaroo, venison, rabbit, duck, or fish). Commercially available diets available for cats use protein sources consisting of rabbit, duck, venison, and lamb. Fish is not a novel option for most cats, and there is a possible, but yet unclear, relationship between adverse food reactions in cats fed foods containing scombroid fish and histamine content. Most importantly, the formulation of whatever product or diet is fed must be fixed to ensure that the ingredient composition is consistent from batch to batch. These products are more expensive not only because of their unique and limited sources of protein but also because of the quality control procedures required to ensure fixed formulations and to eliminate cross-contamination with previous production batches of different foods.

A newer alternative diet commercially available for use in dogs and cats with suspected adverse reactions to food is a hydrolyzed protein diet. Protein is the most common nutrient associated with adverse reactions to food, because it is needed to bridge two IgE molecules together to cause the release of histamine. The protein in hydrolyzed diets is broken down into smaller peptide fragments that are too short to bridge two IgE molecules. Although these diets are helpful in many dogs and cats with adverse reactions to food, they are expensive, and some animals with allergies to the protein sources in these diets will still react to the typical hydrolyzed protein diet. Therefore, a novel protein diet is often tried first; if clinical signs do not resolve, then a hydrolyzed protein diet can be used.

Simplified homemade diets are also possible using the same protein sources suggested above (or other ingredient sources the owner wants to test). Homemade diets actually allow for a wider selection of source ingredients. Beef, wheat, and dairy products should be discouraged for use as a protein source in dogs, and beef, fish, and dairy products should be discouraged for use in cats, because animals have likely been exposed to these sources if previously fed foods with an open formulation. The basic recipe should closely resemble "complete and balanced," but single sources of protein can be sequentially tested and replaced. The owner is responsible for quality control and consistency and must be willing to make such a diet for ≥2 wk for GI conditions and ≥10–12 wk for dermatologic conditions. On average, there is no price advantage in making a homemade diet over using commercially prepared foods. Formulating a homemade diet containing hydrolyzed protein is both very difficult and expensive.

The trial diet should be exclusively fed for the recommended length of time, and all treats, snacks, and table foods eliminated unless they are made of the exact same ingredients as the trial diet or contain a hydrolyzed protein source. All chewable medications and supplements must be eliminated from the trial diet, because most contain the same protein and additive ingredients as pet foods and treats. Other therapies such as hyposensitization and flea control are necessary in animals with concurrent disease. Testing various suspect ingredients by reintroducing them to the diet one at a time followed by recurrence of clinical signs is affirmation of an adverse reaction to that ingredient. Dietary ingredients reintroduced may reproduce clinical signs as early as 12 hr after ingestion but can take as long as 10 days. Lifelong treatment is dietary avoidance, which may be difficult if the offending ingredients are not positively identified.

Anemia: Iron or copper deficiency (or both) is the major cause of hypochromic, microcytic anemia. A folic acid and B_{12} (cobalamin) deficiency also produces anemia. Most commercial diets have more than required amounts of iron, copper, and vitamins; therefore, secondary causes such as inadequate food intake, malabsorption, hemorrhage, or heavy parasite infection should be investigated. Feeding an unbalanced homemade diet may also result in anemia.

Rarely can severe iron deficiency be corrected with diet alone, and feeding large quantities of liver in an attempt to correct iron deficiency is usually ineffective and can result in vitamin A toxicosis. Most animals require a supplemental source of iron administered either PO or IM to correct severe iron deficiency and, depending on the underlying cause, may need to continue receiving a supplemental source of iron indefinitely. If the underlying cause of iron deficiency is related to hemorrhage, parasitism, consuming an unbalanced diet, or consuming too little of a complete and balanced diet, once the underlying cause is eliminated and the iron deficiency is corrected, longterm supplemental iron may not be necessary.

Folic acid and vitamin B_{12} are necessary to support normal cell division, and treatment for vitamin B_{12} deficiency usually requires parenteral administration of vitamin B_{12}. Vitamin B_{12} deficiency develops most commonly from intestinal malabsorption; however, it can also result from short-gut syndrome. Vitamin B_{12} absorption in the GI tract is limited to the ileum, and surgical removal of large portions of the ileum may result in the need for lifelong parenteral B_{12} supplementation.

Anorexia: Partial anorexia is seen when the animal is eating some food but not enough to provide at least 30 kcal/kg body wt in dogs and 40 kcal/kg body wt in cats.

Complete anorexia occurs when the animal does not consume any food for ~3 days.

Anorexia (partial or complete) accompanies many underlying disorders, including drug reactions or reactions to environmental changes. Pain may also be a significant contributor to anorexia, and in most cases when the pain is adequately controlled, the anorexia resolves. Learned food aversions may also contribute to anorexia. This occurs most commonly when animals are started on a therapeutic diet while they are ill, eg, offering a therapeutic diet to manage renal failure while the animal is still in a uremic crisis. Food aversions can also occur as a result of force-feeding. Obviously, therapeutic diets do not help if they are not consumed. Eating some of a diet that is less than optimal is better than none of the "right" one. Assuming that an animal will eat a therapeutic diet when it gets hungry enough is inappropriate, and allowing an animal to starve in an attempt to stimulate its appetite is never recommended. If a particular diet is refused, an alternative(s) should be tried until one that the animal will eat is identified. Anorectic dogs and cats can sometimes be persuaded to eat by adding highly flavored substances to the diet (eg, animal fat, meat drippings, fish [fish juices or oils for cats]) or by hand-feeding. If these are not successful, nutritional support intervention may be necessary.

Nutritional support can be provided by either enteral or parenteral routes. Unless there is a contraindication to using the gut, enteral support is usually preferred over parenteral support. Enteral support is more physiologic, cheaper, and safer than parenteral support. In addition, more dietary options are available for enteral support than for parenteral support.

Many options for feeding tubes are available, including esophagostomy tubes, nasogastric or nasoesophageal tubes, gastrostomy tubes, and jejunostomy tubes. Both esophagostomy tubes and nasogastric or nasoesophageal tubes can be placed without the need for any specialized equipment. Nasogastric tubes are used more commonly for short durations (1–7 days) or when sedation or anesthesia are contraindicated. Esophagostomy tubes and gastric tubes are more commonly used when nutritional support is required for longer durations (weeks or months). Dogs and cats can be maintained at home with tube feedings (except in the case of jejunostomy tubes) after the procedure has been accepted by the animal and fully explained to the owner and if the frequency of feeding is something the owner can reasonably manage and the animal can tolerate.

It is advisable to take a stepwise approach to reintroduction of calories, and multiple small meals are often tolerated better than large meals. Vomiting, diarrhea, or refeeding syndrome can be a consequence of being too aggressive with reintroduction of calories. The size of the tube determines what dietary options can be used. Sizes 5 or 8 French tubes usually limit feeding to liquid enteral diets. Larger esophagostomy or gastrostomy tubes can also accommodate critical care diets and blenderized therapeutic diets. If use of a feeding tube is contraindicated or a tube cannot be placed, dogs and cats can be maintained by IV solutions that provide adequate calories, protein, electrolytes, B vitamins, and selected trace minerals until access to the small intestine is possible. Unfortunately, the parenteral route is more expensive and is associated with a higher incidence of complications, including catheter problems, infection, and electrolyte abnormalities.

Cachexia: Cachexia is most commonly associated with cases of neoplasia or chronic renal or cardiac disease. Cachexia appears to be a response to increased catabolism with either normal or decreased appetite. The deterioration of the animal's condition clearly indicates that nutritional requirements are not being met, and the dietary goal is to increase the caloric density and palatability of the food while meeting the animal's requirements for protein and other nutrients. The usual management of cachexia is to feed smaller amounts of a more calorically dense (ie, higher fat content), complete and balanced diet more frequently (3–6 meals/day). The form of food (dry or canned) that the dog or cat prefers should be fed. Tube feeding and partial or complete parenteral nutritional support (*see* above) should also be considered if the dog or cat continues to lose weight and condition.

Diarrhea: Diarrhea can result from numerous GI diseases and can also occur secondary to disease outside the GI tract. Primary causes of GI disease are numerous and include adverse reaction to food, infections (bacterial, parasitic, fungal, and viral), inflammatory bowel disease, neoplasia, and toxin- or drug-induced. Certain breeds of dogs are predisposed to GI disease. German Shepherds are at increased risk of developing antibiotic-responsive diarrhea (formerly known as small-intestinal bacterial overgrowth),

TABLE 64 CHARACTERISTICS OF SMALL-BOWEL AND LARGE-BOWEL DIARRHEA

Characteristics	Small Bowel	Large Bowel
Blood in feces	Melena	Hematochezia
Fecal quality	Loose, watery "cow-pie"	Loose to semiformed
Fecal volume	Large quantities	Small quantities
Frequency of defecation	Normal to increased	Increased
Mucus in feces	Absent	Usually present
Tenesmus	Absent	Usually present
Urgency	Absent	Usually present
Weight loss	May be present	Rare

Doberman Pinschers and Rottweilers are at increased risk of parvoviral enteritis, and Yorkshire Terriers are at increased risk of lymphangiectasia.

Clinical signs associated with diarrhea are different in small-bowel versus large-bowel diarrhea (*see* TABLE 64). Dietary recommendations may vary depending on where the diarrhea is localized and the underlying cause.

Animals with small-bowel diarrhea usually benefit from a highly digestible diet, whereas those with large-bowel diarrhea often benefit from prebiotics (*see* p 2369). Small, frequent meals (3–6/day) should be offered. Probiotics are an additional tool available for management of small- or large-bowel diarrhea. Probiotics are defined as nutritional supplements containing live, viable, beneficial bacteria in sufficient numbers to provide a health benefit. Not all probiotics are created equal—a probiotic effective in one species may be ineffective in another. Probiotic bacteria provide many of the same benefits to the host as prebiotics. Synbiotics are a mixture of prebiotics and probiotics in which the prebiotic increases the survival of and nourishes the probiotic bacteria. Although clinical studies of probiotics in dogs and cats are limited, probiotics have been helpful in numerous causes of diarrhea.

Constipation: Constipation results from impaired peristalsis or increased water absorption from the large intestine. The objective of dietary management is to provide a balanced diet with increased amounts of insoluble fiber (10%–25% dry-matter basis to effect) or moderately fermentable fiber in dogs or a highly digestible balanced diet containing prebiotics in cats. Constipated cats tend to do poorly on diets supplemented with insoluble fiber. Animals should be fed 2–4 times/day. In dogs, adding canned pumpkin or psyllium to the diet is also sometimes effective in mild cases of constipation.

Congestive Heart Failure (CHF): One objective in managing CHF is to reduce water retention; restricting sodium intake and lowering sodium levels encourage diuresis. Typical commercial dog and cat foods have a sodium content of 0.45%–0.9% (450–900 mg sodium/100 g diet dry matter). Dietary sodium restriction is classified as mild (400 mg sodium/100 g diet dry matter) to severe (240 mg sodium/100 g diet dry matter). In view of these values, commercial dog and cat diets cannot even be classified as mild sodium restriction. Therefore, commercially prepared low-sodium diets or recipes that use low-sodium foods must be substituted. Sodium restriction often requires a special diet, although some manufacturers provide veterinary therapeutic diets for heart disorders. When using a home-prepared diet, all processed meats, cheeses, bread, heart, kidney, liver, salted fats, whole eggs, and snack foods should be avoided. Foods reasonably low in sodium include beef, rabbit, chicken, horsemeat, lamb, freshwater fish, oatmeal, corn, and rice.

Failed cardiac contractility may contribute to CHF, and taurine supplementation should be used to exclude a possible depletion of this amino acid in cardiac muscle. Both dogs and cats can develop dilated cardiomyopathy secondary to taurine deficiency. Some breeds of dogs with dilated cardiomyopathy may respond favorably to carnitine supplementation, which has also been beneficial in some breeds of dogs with CHF (including Boxers and Cocker Spaniels), in dogs with cystine or urate urolithiasis, and in dogs consuming a protein-restricted diet. Because obesity can be a contributing factor in CHF, a weight management program is needed in obese animals in addition to sodium restriction. In some instances, edema may give the appearance of obesity and mask emaciation. The edema should first be resolved, so that body weight and condition can be evaluated. If the animal is underweight, the food intake should be increased or the caloric content of the diet increased. If renal failure is also present, protein and phosphorus intake must be restricted.

Diabetes Mellitus (DM): Most DM in dogs is type I (insulin dependent) due to immune-mediated destruction of pancreatic islet cells (*see* p 579). Although insulin sensitivity remains high in most diabetic dogs, no residual insulin production is left in the pancreas, and exogenous insulin therapy is required. Some dogs develop DM as a result of chronic pancreatitis causing widespread destruction of both endocrine and exocrine pancreatic tissue. Obesity does not appear to be a risk factor for developing DM in dogs, although obese dogs can have insulin resistance. Type 2 DM has not been reported in dogs, although some dogs may develop diestrus-associated diabetes that results in insulin resistance secondary to progesterone production. Remission of diabetes is possible when dogs are spayed or diestrus ends.

Some diabetic dogs have concurrent diseases, such as hyperadrenocorticism, and they may be very difficult to regulate if the hyperadrenocorticism remains untreated. Underlying urinary tract infection can also result in poor regulation and insulin resistance until the infection is cured. For diabetic dogs receiving insulin therapy, the nutritional requirements of any concurrent disease may take precedence over the dietary therapy for diabetes. Dietary recommendations for diabetic dogs without concurrent disease include feeding a diet that contains a moderate amount of a blend of soluble and insoluble fiber (3.5 g/100 kcal), such as a mixture of beet pulp and cellulose. Independent of the type of diet chosen, dietary intake should be consistent from day to day. Diabetic dogs usually require insulin twice a day, and it is recommended that dogs be fed first to ensure they eat before administering insulin.

Cats most commonly develop type 2 DM, although some cats may develop type 1, often secondary to chronic pancreatitis. The most common risk factors for DM in cats are obesity and increasing age. Most of these cats develop amyloid-mediated destruction of pancreatic islets. Although residual insulin capacity remains in most type 2 diabetic cats, insulin resistance is a characteristic of this form of DM.

Feline DM is similar to type 2 DM in people, and the main goals of therapy for diabetic cats are to control excess body weight and maintain optimal body condition, to reduce postprandial hyperglycemia and glucose toxicity, and to stimulate endogenous insulin secretion. Transient DM occurs in ~20% of diabetic cats, and these cats go into spontaneous remission usually within 1–4 mo after starting therapy for DM. The most likely reason for this is that untreated diabetic cats may develop glucose toxicity, and hyperglycemia decreases pancreatic β-cell function. When the cat is treated for DM and hyperglycemia is controlled, the glucose toxicity interfering with pancreatic islet cell function is removed.

Traditionally, diabetic cats have been fed fiber-supplemented diets similar to those recommended for diabetic dogs, and some cats have done well. However, more recently it has been shown that feeding diabetic cats a diet high in protein (>45% of calories) and low in carbohydrates (<20% of calories) improves glucose regulation and increases incidence of spontaneous remission. Nonetheless, some diabetic cats may have concurrent diseases for which the dietary management takes precedent.

Feline Lower Urinary Tract Disease (FLUTD): FLUTD (*see* p 1531) has many possible underlying causes, including urolithiasis, urethral plugs, urinary tract infection, neoplasia, neurologic abnormalities, feline idiopathic cystitis (FIC), and anatomic defects, The underlying cause of FLUTD must be determined, because treatment for one cause may be contraindicated for other causes. The most common cause of FLUTD is FIC, followed by urolithiasis. Urethral plugs are most commonly composed of either mucus or mucus and struvite crystals. Urinary tract infections in cats without renal failure or diabetes mellitus is uncommon.

Urine dilution appears to be helpful in the treatment of FIC, because it decreases the concentration of substances in the urine that may be irritating to the bladder mucosa. Numerous ways to dilute urine have been investigated in cats, but one of the safest and most effective is to feed a canned-food diet. Other dietary modifications have been used to dilute urine, including sodium supplementation. Although sodium-supplemented diets are helpful in cats with FIC, they are contraindicated in cats with underlying renal disease. Highly acidic diets are not recommended, because highly acidic urine may increase sensory nerve fiber transmission in the bladder and increase pain perception. Regardless of treatment, clinical signs of FIC usually spontaneously resolve in 2–7 days. Unfortunately, FIC recurs within 12 mo in approximately half of the cats that experience spontaneous remission, and multiple recurrences are possible.

The two most common uroliths in the lower urinary tract of cats are magnesium ammonium phosphate (struvite) and calcium oxalate, although other mineral types are possible. Dietary management varies depending on the specific mineral composition of the urolith; however, regardless of composition, diluting the urine is important. Medical dissolution is an option for struvite uroliths but not for calcium oxalate uroliths. Producing a dilute urine reduces the concentration of minerals and crystals that form uroliths. Feeding a canned-food diet and encouraging water intake, eg, with water fountains, are safe and simple ways to dilute urine. Three major pet food companies have formulated diets for cats to manage both struvite and calcium oxalate. Two of these diets have high levels of sodium and, therefore, are contraindicated in cats with underlying renal disease. Diets reduce risk factors for developing uroliths but unfortunately do not prevent recurrence, which is common for calcium oxalate.

Fever: Fever increases energy requirements because of increased metabolic activity—a 1°F (0.5°C) rise causes an increase in caloric need of ~7 kcal/kg body wt/day. A highly palatable diet should be fed in quantities that can be consumed easily, and the caloric content should be increased by feeding a higher fat diet, if such a diet is not contraindicated. Because animals with fever generally have a decreased appetite, offering smaller meals more frequently with personal attention and encouragement may help stimulate intake. Feeding a feline growth diet or a calorically dense recovery-type diet also increases protein and energy intake in smaller feedings.

Gastric Dilatation (Bloat): Currently, there is little evidence to suggest that certain specific nutrients in the diet, such as soy protein, lead to the development of gastric dilatation in susceptible dogs (*see* p 384). The most common risk factors for developing gastric dilatation and volvulus (GDV) include breed risks (ie, large breeds with a deep chest), eating only one meal/day, elevated feeding bowls, and vigorous exercise 1 hr before or 2 hr after eating. Prophylactic gastropexy has been shown to prevent GDV if performed at the time of elective surgical neutering, and owners of high-risk breeds should be so advised. Other recommendations to prevent GDV include feeding multiple small meals/day and avoiding vigorous exercise before and after eating.

Head Trauma, Burns, and Respiratory Diseases: It is unknown whether the metabolic effects and energy expenditure in dogs and cats with severe head trauma, burns with ≥50% loss of skin, or prolonged dyspnea are the same as those in people with similar conditions. However, it is a reasonable supposition. The brain is one of the most metabolically active tissues; thus, providing aggressive nutritional support early is essential. Head trauma significantly alters neurologic control of metabolic rate, which is usually increased. Burns and other causes of significant areas of skin loss increase heat and water loss to the environment, thereby increasing energy needs. Increased respiratory rate and dyspnea are deceptively intense work that also result in increased energy needs. If a dog or cat is in an oxygen cage for >1 day, nutritional support (feeding IV or via feeding tube) should be instituted.

Brain trauma, burns, and sepsis are all conditions with high metabolic demands, and the amount of energy needed varies among animals. In all cases, energy is provided minimally at 30 kcal/kg body wt (dogs) or 40 kcal/kg body wt (cats) and increased in increments of 5 kcal/kg as the condition progresses and if weight loss is apparent. The energy source should be predominantly fat (60%–90% calories from fat, 10%–40% from glucose), because the body metabolism is predominantly lipolytic under these conditions, with the liver utilizing fat better than glucose during response to burns or trauma. Protein intake must also be matched with the energy intake to avoid net protein and muscle catabolism. Food that is 30%–45% protein and 25%–30% fat (dry-matter basis) and that is complete and balanced for all other nutrients should be fed using tube feeding. Human baby foods are not suitable for this purpose. These nutritional goals can also be met by parenteral (IV) nutrition, remembering that enteral and parenteral support are not mutually exclusive.

Hepatic Disease: Dietary recommendations for dogs vary depending on the underlying cause and severity of liver dysfunction, and care must be taken to avoid overwhelming the metabolic capacity of the liver. In contrast, it is equally important not to unnecessarily restrict protein intake, because protein requirements are as high or higher in dogs with liver disease than in dogs without liver disease. Therefore, in dogs without encephalopathy, providing adequate intake of energy and a high-quality protein is essential to ensure a positive protein and energy balance and enable hepatic regeneration. Dietary antioxidants, such as vitamins C and E, as well as taurine, may also help minimize oxidative damage. Dietary copper restriction is recommended in dogs with documented increased copper levels in the liver.

In dogs with hepatic encephalopathy, reduced levels of high-quality protein may be necessary to reduce the accumulation of ammonia and other hepatic toxins. Soluble fiber or moderately fermentable fiber is helpful; colonic fermentation of these fibers produces short-chain fatty acids, which reduce both the intraluminal pH of the colon and the absorption of ammonia. Short-chain fatty acids also increase the blood supply to the colon and the amount of ammonia transported into the colon.

Frequent feeding of small meals (4–6/day) lowers the amount of nutrients or metabolites that require hepatic processing at a single time, thereby imposing less metabolic demand on the liver. Animals with liver disorders are frequently anorectic. Thus, food consumption and body weight and condition should be monitored.

Feline hepatic lipidosis is the most common liver disease in cats. It usually occurs in obese cats that are anorectic. This life-threatening condition requires aggressive nutritional support to reverse the changes in the liver. Most cats require a feeding tube. Energy-dense, high-protein diets, such as critical care diets, are usually selected for cats without encephalopathy. A step-wise reintroduction to calories is necessary to prevent complications, such as vomiting or electrolyte abnormalities. Hypokalemia is the most frequent electrolyte abnormality, and it can be exacerbated by too aggressive reintroduction to calories. Carnitine supplementation is also beneficial. Fluid needs must be met, and parenteral fluid support may be needed in many cats, at least initially. In encephalopathic cats with hepatic lipidosis, dietary protein may need to be restricted but should not be severely so. These cats usually have protein malnutrition secondary to anorexia, and providing too little dietary protein can interfere with hepatic repair and regeneration.

See also HEPATIC DISEASE IN SMALL ANIMALS, p 429.

Hyperlipidemia in Dogs: Hyperlipidemia in dogs can be primary or secondary to hypothyroidism, pancreatitis, hepatic disease, diabetes mellitus, nephrotic syndrome, hyperadrenocorticism, or high-fat diets. Hyperlipidemia is present when blood lipids are increased with or without gross lipemia and probably results from abnormalities in the synthesis or use of plasma lipoproteins. In primary hyperlipidemia, the abnormalities can be familial and might be genetic, as has been suggested in Miniature Schnauzers. Some dogs with hyperlipidemia are asymptomatic. Clinically affected dogs may have recurrent seizures, depression, recurrent pancreatitis, vomiting, acute blindness, corneal opacity, and xanthogranulomas.

The goal of dietary management is to decrease the digestion and absorption of fat by feeding a diet restricted in fat (<10% dry-matter basis). The use of fish oil capsule supplements at a dosage of 1 g/4.5 kg body wt either once a day or in divided doses, depending on the number of capsules needed, helps reduce serum triglyceride concentrations. Although fish oil supplements generally do not return serum triglycerides to normal values, partial reduction is believed to mitigate the risk of pancreatitis or other problems related to marked increases of this lipid.

Malabsorption and Maldigestion in Dogs: Diseases of the small intestine and pancreas often lead to a vague clinical syndrome characterized by weight loss, vomiting, diarrhea (with or without steatorrhea), and changes in appetite. In such cases, a highly digestible diet low in fiber (0–5%), moderate in fat (10%–15%) and protein (20%–25%), and containing carbohydrate from noncereal byproduct sources is recommended. Supplemental water-soluble vitamins should also be used. Malabsorption and maldigestion are often secondary to other underlying GI disease, such as inflammatory bowel disease. Appropriate management of the underlying disease may reverse malabsorption and maldigestion. Exocrine pancreatic insufficiency (EPI) is one of the most common causes of malabsorption/maldigestion in dogs. Certain breeds of dogs, eg, German Shepherds, are at increased risk of developing EPI. EPI can also result from severe or chronic pancreatitis. In EPI, supplementation with a powdered enzyme supplement, mixed with the food a few minutes before feeding, should be considered. Parenteral administration of vitamin B_{12} (cobalamin) is also required in some animals with EPI, especially cats. (*See also* MALABSORPTION SYNDROMES IN SMALL ANIMALS, p 400.)

Obesity: Obesity is the most common nutritional health problem in dogs and cats, and obesity-associated health risks continue to increase. Obesity is the excessive accumulation of adipose tissue—for dogs and cats, >20% above ideal body weight. Dogs and cats 10%–20% above ideal body weight are considered overweight. It is estimated that 24%–44% of dogs and 25%–30% of cats seen by veterinarians are overweight or obese, and ~50% of dogs 5–10 yr old are overweight or obese.

Obesity occurs when energy intake exceeds energy expenditure. Risk factors for developing obesity include 1) lack of exercise, 2) breed predisposition (breeds with an increased risk include Labrador Retrievers, Miniature Schnauzers, Dachshunds, Shetland Sheepdogs, Cocker Spaniels, Beagles, Basset Hounds, and Cairn Terriers), 3) increasing age (metabolic rate decreases with age as lean muscle mass decreases and fat mass increases, 4) neutering, 5) certain endocrine disorders, and 6) certain drugs, such as corticosteroids and phenobarbital.

Health problems associated with obesity include decreased life expectancy, impaired quality of life, chronic inflammation, pulmonary and cardiovascular problems, exercise and heat intolerance, joint and musculoskeletal problems (eg, arthritis), compromised immune function, pancreatitis (dogs), diabetes mellitus and hepatic lipidosis (cats), and increased morbidity and mortality during and after anesthesia.

Adipose tissue was long considered metabolically inert, and its primary role in disease was attributed to stress on the joints caused by increased weight bearing and increased workload on the heart. However, it is now known that *adipose tissue is not* inert, but rather a major endocrine organ that produces hormones and protein factors and signals called adipokines. The expression, production, and release of many adipokines are increased in obesity, which results in persistent, low-grade inflammation and increased oxidative stress that plays a role in many chronic diseases, such as osteoarthritis and diabetes mellitus.

Treatment for obesity should include both short- and longterm goals. Short-term goals are to lose weight and reach an ideal body condition score. Longterm goals are to maintain ideal body condition score. Both of these goals require modification of behaviors that resulted in the dog or cat becoming overweight. Recommendations for lifestyle changes should be done in the context of maintaining the owner-animal bond. If this is ignored, owner compliance is unlikely.

The most successful weight loss programs include a combination of caloric restriction and exercise. The first step is to obtain a thorough diet history, followed by calculating the caloric intake appropriate to induce weight loss. Determining 60% of MER for dogs and 70% of MER for cats is one way to calculate starting caloric intake for a weight management program. Regardless of the formula used, the calculated caloric intake is only a starting point and may require modification based on response.

The next step is to decide on a diet for the weight loss program. Maintenance diets are generally not recommended for weight loss programs, because they are formulated to meet the nutritional needs of moderately active adults. Restricting caloric intake using maintenance diets may result in inadequate intake of some nutrients. Therapeutic weight loss diets are formulated to be restricted in calories while providing other nutrients in appropriate amounts. Adequate protein levels are important in any weight loss diet chosen. Most diets formulated for weight loss also have increased levels of dietary fiber. It is better to divide total daily caloric intake into multiple meals rather than one large meal. If giving treats is an important owner-pet interaction, providing the owner with low-calorie treat options is important. Most treats are not complete and balanced, so they should be restricted to <10% of the total caloric intake to avoid causing nutrient imbalances.

The next step is to decide on a rate of weight loss: a reasonable goal is loss of ~1% of body wt/wk. If the animal is losing weight at a slower rate than that chosen but is doing well otherwise and the owner is satisfied, then it may be best to allow weight loss to continue at the slower rate. The animal's weight should be monitored every 2 wk and the program modified if needed based on response. Any weight loss is good weight loss, and celebrating successes with the owner helps maintain motivation.

Obese cats undergoing weight loss are at increased risk of developing hepatic lipidosis. Cats must continue to consume adequate calories and nutrients. If a cat does not like the weight loss diet chosen, then an alternative should be found. Starvation is never a safe or humane way to cause weight loss.

Pancreatitis in Dogs: The goal in treating pancreatitis is to minimize stimulation of the exocrine function of the pancreas until inflammation has decreased. Often, the dog has multiple episodes of vomiting. A standard treatment is nothing per os (NPO) until vomiting ceases, which can last 3–15 days. Antibiotic, fluid, and electrolyte therapy during NPO treatment is essential, and IV nutritional support (total parenteral nutrition) should be instituted if NPO therapy continues for ≥3 days. Adult and young dogs can be nutritionally maintained by IV parenteral solutions that provide adequate calories, protein, electrolytes, B vitamins, and selected trace minerals until oral feeding is possible. If the dog appears painful or uncomfortable, medications to manage pain as well as plasma transfusions should be administered.

Unfortunately, total parenteral nutrition does not provide any nutrients to the enterocytes, and atrophy of the gut occurs as in starvation. The amino acid glutamine provides ~40% of the energy needs to the small-intestinal epithelial cells; it can be provided orally in very small quantities every 8 hr to provide some nutrition for the enterocytes.

When oral feeding can be resumed, a commercially prepared, easily digestible diet that has moderate fiber (10%–15% dry-matter basis) and is low in fat (5%–10%) can be fed in small, frequent meals (3–6 times/day). Because recurrent episodes of pancreatitis are common, feeding a complete and balanced low-fat diet is recommended for longterm management. Obesity and hyperlipidemia are common concurrent problems and should be investigated and resolved.

Parvovirus Enteritis in Dogs: Parvovirus enteritis is most common in puppies 6–24 wk old. It is extremely infrequent in adult dogs. It is characterized by vomiting, diarrhea (often bloody), and weight loss. Severe cases can result in sepsis and disseminated intravascular coagulation. IV fluids, antiemetics, and antibiotic therapy are important. Fluid rates must be sufficient to account for maintenance needs as well as ongoing losses. Crystalloid therapy or plasma transfusions may be necessary in hypoalbuminemic dogs. Food and water are usually withheld until vomiting ceases. Severe cases may require total parenteral nutrition. Once vomiting has ceased, small amounts of water are offered first. If there is no vomiting, then small amounts of an easily digestible diet should be fed until the dog recovers. (*See also* CANINE PARVOVIRUS, p 373.)

Chronic Kidney Disease (CKD): Numerous metabolic abnormalities that may alter an animal's nutritional status develop in progressive renal failure. These include impaired clearance of nitrogenous products of protein metabolism; impaired regulation of sodium, potassium, and phosphorus; acidosis; impaired vitamin D metabolism; and often anorexia. The objective of dietary management in renal failure is to lessen the metabolic demands on the kidneys and to diminish metabolic end-products that cannot be readily excreted. The first consideration is to ensure normal water homeostasis. Regardless of whether the animal is polyuric, oliguric, or anuric, water should always be readily available. In addition, dietary management remains the mainstay of therapy for animals with CKD. Therapeutic renal diets are formulated to address many of the metabolic abnormalities associated with CKD. Any therapeutic renal diet should be phosphorus restricted, supplemented with omega-3 fatty acids (EPA/DHA) that come from fish oil, alkalinizing, supplemented with B vitamins, and in cats supplemented with potassium. In addition, feeding moderately fermentable fiber can facilitate enteric dialysis and provide a nonrenal route of urea excretion. Newer research has also shown the benefits of antioxidants in the management of CKD in dogs. The rate of decline of glomerular filtration rate by use of both dietary omega-3 fatty acids and antioxidants were additive. In addition, research in dogs is also showing that higher protein levels than what are typically used in most therapeutic renal diets is beneficial as long as the diets are phosphorus restricted. Energy should be supplied primarily via feeding relatively more digestible fat and carbohydrates.

The criteria used (eg, serum creatinine concentration, BUN) to define when dietary modifications should be made are under debate. However, it is easier to change the diet when the animal is feeling reasonably well than when it is anorectic. There is good evidence that animals with International

Renal Interest Society (IRIS) Stage 3 and 4 CKD benefit from dietary management, and there is likely to be benefit in changing the diet early in the course of renal disease, such as that associated with IRIS Stage 2 CKD. Additional symptomatic and supportive care, such as H_2-blockers, antiemetics, medications to treat hypertension, intestinal phosphate binders, calcitriol, erythropoietin, and potassium gluconate (in cats) may be necessary as the disease advances.

Urolithiasis in Dogs: The most common mineral composition for uroliths in dogs are primarily struvite (magnesium-ammonium-phosphate) and calcium oxalate, followed by urate and cysteine. Regardless of the type of stone, diluting the urine (eg, by encouraging water consumption) is warranted.

Struvite stones are more common in females than males. Most struvite stones in dogs are induced by infection with urease-producing bacteria. Although diet can be used to try to dissolve these stones, the most important therapy is to treat the urinary tract infection. Struvite stones can be medically dissolved, after which calculolytic therapeutic diets are usually unnecessary. Preventing a recurrence of the urinary tract infection and prompt treatment of a recurrence are important.

Calcium oxalate stones are not amenable to medical dissolution and must be removed through voiding, urohydropropulsion, surgery, or laser lithotripsy in symptomatic dogs. Two approaches are used for dietary management: 1) feeding an alkalinizing, protein-restricted diet low in oxalate, or 2) feeding a diet supplemented with sodium to encourage water consumption and production of dilute urine. Despite dietary management, the recurrence rate is high (33% in the first year and 50% by the third year).

Urate uroliths can occur in cases of liver disease, most commonly portosystemic shunts. However, two breeds of dogs, Dalmatians and English Bulldogs, are predisposed to developing urate uroliths without overt liver dysfunction. Medical dissolution is an option and consists of using a protein-restricted diet low in purines and alkalinizing the urine in combination with treatment with allopurinol, a xanthine oxidase inhibitor. The use of low-dose allopurinol as a strategy to prevent recurrences is discouraged. Instead, water should be added to the diet in the maximal amount the dog can tolerate without needing to urinate overnight. Recurrence rates are high, especially in dogs 1–6 yr old; however, this stone type becomes much easier to manage once the dogs reach middle age.

Cystine urolithiasis is due to a renal tubular defect. It is most common in Dachshunds, English Bulldogs, French Bulldogs, and Newfoundlands. Medical dissolution is an option using dietary management and thiola. However, protein-restricted diets should be used with caution, because some of these dogs also have aminoaciduria and carnitinuria. (*See also* UROLITHIASIS IN SMALL ANIMALS, p 1525.)

Steatitis in Cats: Steatitis (pansteatitis, yellow fat disease) is seen most often in kittens fed exclusively large amounts of unsaturated fatty acids, oily fish such as tuna or mackerel (packed in oil not water), diets that do not have an appropriate balance of antioxidants relative to polyunsaturated fats, or diets that have gone rancid. Clinical signs are anorexia, fever, pain over the thorax and abdomen, neutrophilia, and subcutaneous nodules of necrotic fat. Cats with steatitis should be fed diets restricted in polyunsaturated fatty acids (monounsatu rated and saturated fats are permitted) and given vitamin E supplementation at 10–20 mg, bid for 5–7 days. The diet of choice is a commercial food to which vitamin E (α-tocopherol) or other antioxidants have been added.

PUBLIC HEALTH

PUBLIC HEALTH PRIMER

Although only a minority of veterinarians report primary public health employment, virtually all veterinarians contribute to the overall public health effort. According to the World Health Organization, "health is a state of complete physical, mental and social well-being and not merely the absence of disease or infirmity." Public health can be defined as the totality of all evidence-based public and private efforts that preserve and promote health and prevent disease, disability, and death. The concept of **One Health** is the collaborative effort of multiple health science professions, together with their related disciplines and institutions—working locally, nationally, and globally—to attain optimal health for people, domestic animals, wildlife, plants, and our environment.

One Health can be thought of as having three major subcomponents: basic sciences, clinical medicine, and public health. Major components of public health include population health, community health, mental health, environmental/ecological health, and occupational/recreational health. The differentiating variables among these components are the dynamics of the population(s), changing social/health behaviors, and, perhaps most importantly, the selection of the population to study/surveil. A relevant, frequently debated question is the definition of the "environment." Typically, it is equated with the "physical" environment and implies all influences other than social, economic, cultural, and genetic. An additional underlying theme in One Health is the economic environment in which it (and all professions that contribute to it) is pursued. Therefore, an understanding of basic economics is key to understanding the most practical application of (and opportunity for) One Health in a particular community, country, or region.

Public Health Practitioners: A generally accepted definition of a public health practitioner does not exist. However, for practical purposes, any health professional who sees and acts beyond the single patient is functioning in a public health capacity. Most typically, this includes physicians, veterinarians, dentists, nurses, epidemiologists, laboratorians, industrial hygienists, public health inspectors, and regulatory agency administrators. Allied health professionals, including optometrists, physician assistants, psychologists, pharmacists, entomologists, etc, also contribute according to the scope of their respective practices. No medical profession exists in a vacuum.

Many public health practitioners possess specific training, and various board-certifying bodies, accrediting entities, and professional societies bolster this training by requiring experience and fostering collaboration. These include the American College of Preventive Medicine, the American College of Veterinary Preventive Medicine, the American Public Health Association, the American Society of Public Health, and the Association of State and Territorial Health Officials.

Several overarching public health organizations have jointly developed a set of core competencies that reflect skills appropriate to the effective delivery of public health services. Core competencies are divided into the following eight domains: 1) analytic/assessment skills, 2) policy development/program planning skills, 3) communication skills, 4) cultural competency skills, 5) community dimensions of practice skills, 6) public health sciences skills, 7) financial planning and management skills, and 8) leadership and systems thinking skills.

PUBLIC HEALTH AGENCIES

In the USA, responsibilities and authorities for health services are spread across federal, state, and local levels of government. In addition, certain nongovernmental organizations perform critical functions regarding the provision and influence of public health policies.

Federal Level: The Constitution contains no legal basis for the provision of health care to the general population. Therefore, as per the Tenth Amendment, this responsibility automatically falls to the states. When the federal government directly influences national health care issues, it generally does so under the auspices of the Constitution's Interstate Commerce Clause, which gives Congress the power "to regulate commerce with foreign nations, and among the several states, and with the Indian tribes." The federal government also significantly influences health care issues in an indirect fashion through the provision of federal funds. Commonly, funds allocated to state and local governments for health issues are contingent on that entity participating in national programs such as disease reporting and adhering to national health goals and standards.

The Department of Health and Human Services (DHHS) is the primary public health agency at the federal level and serves to assess the general health of the nation, establish national goals and policies, and direct federal efforts in support of the states. Major public health–oriented components of DHHS include the Agency for Healthcare Research and Quality (AHRQ), the Agency for Toxic Substances and Disease Registry (ATSDR), the Centers for Disease Control and Prevention (CDC), the Food and Drug Administration (FDA), the Health Resources and Services Administration (HRSA), the Indian Health Service (IHS), the National Institutes of Health (NIH), and the Substance Abuse and Mental Health Services Administration (SAMHSA).

Other federal departments with significant equities in national health care and public health responsibilities include 1) Department of Agriculture (USDA), which is responsible for meat inspection and disease prevention and control; 2) Department of Defense (DoD), which is responsible for health care policies and provision of health care for active duty members, family members, and retirees; 3) Department of Homeland Security (DHS), which is responsible for disaster planning and response; 4) Department of the Interior (DoI), which operates the National Park Service (public health and disease outbreak investigations on National Park lands), the Bureau of Indian Affairs (treaty obligations to tribes, including provision of health care and environmental health infrastructure projects), and the Bureau of Reclamation (provides potable drinking water and agricultural irrigation water to much of the western USA); 5) Department of Veteran Affairs (VA), which is responsible for health care policies and provision of health care for qualified veterans, and administers significant civilian medical education systems; and 6) Environmental Protection Agency (EPA), which sets and enforces national environmental health standards.

State Level: The state is the primary public health legal authority. Although specific activities and delegations may vary from state to state, state public health responsibilities generally include the following: 1) collection and maintenance of vital health data, 2) maternal and child health, 3) diagnostic and public health laboratories, 4) statewide nutrition programs, 5) regulation of health facilities (including nursing homes), 6) environmental health programs (eg, safe drinking water, waste treatment), 7) state Medicaid program, and 8) regulation and licensing of medical professionals (eg, veterinarians, physicians, dentists, etc).

Local Level: Local public health agencies are structured and empowered to provide services where they are most effective—at the community level. These services may be primary or delegated from the state level and commonly include the following: 1) immunizations not covered under private insurance systems, 2) disease surveillance and investigation, 3) communicable disease control, 4) inspection and licensing of food establishments, 5) public health screening programs, 6) tobacco control programs, 7) disaster preparedness and response, and 8) care for the underserved, indigent, and disabled.

Nongovernmental Organizations (NGOs): An NGO is any nonprofit, voluntary citizens group organized on a local, national, or international level. Task-oriented and staffed by individuals sharing common interests, NGOs perform a variety of service and humanitarian functions. Functions of health-oriented NGOs may include raising citizen concerns to governments, advocating and monitoring health policies, and encouraging political participation through public information dissemination. NGOs that exist and act domestically (and overseas in some cases) in the public health sector include the American Red Cross, the American Cancer Association, the American Lung Association, the CDC Foundation, Heifer International, the March of Dimes, and the Bill and Melinda Gates Foundation.

ROLE OF THE VETERINARIAN IN PUBLIC HEALTH/ONE HEALTH

Most veterinarians contribute, directly or indirectly, to public health goals and outcomes. Veterinary public health contributions can be categorized into six core domains, described below.

Diagnosis, Surveillance, Epidemiology, Control, Prevention, and Elimination of Zoonotic Diseases: Most private veterinary practitioners contribute to public health during routine practice. Both large and small animal practitioners become skilled diagnosticians for acute and chronic diseases of animals that may affect the owners and their families and the surrounding communities. Specific examples of public health activities include performing routine health examinations, maintaining immunization regimens, implementing parasite control programs, advising on the risks of animal contact for immunocompromised individuals, facilitating the use of guide and service dogs for people with disabilities, and promoting the benefits of the human-animal bond for the disabled and elderly, as well as war veterans and others suffering from post-traumatic stress disorder. Communities are best served when veterinarians approach collective health issues with a "herd health" perspective, applying relevant epidemiologic principles. In addition to these direct services, veterinary practitioners report disease events and trends to state public health and regulatory agencies, collaborate with human medical counterparts on zoonotic diseases, and advise local health boards and commissions. These relationships would not exist if not for the inextricable link between animal and human health.

In addition to managing direct zoonotic diseases in animals, veterinarians also diagnose, investigate, and control indirect zoonoses and non-zoonotic communicable diseases that affect human health. Examples include West Nile disease and coccidioidomycosis among pet animals, and bovine leukosis, foot and mouth disease, fowlpox, and many other diseases that affect the food supply, the national economy, and the livelihood of the nation's farmers.

Many factors contribute to the increasing vulnerability of livestock to infectious disease. These include increasing intensity and concentration of production agriculture, genetic convergence of many food-producing species, accessibility of livestock to external contact (despite rigorous biosecurity measures), scale and frequency of animal transport (domestic and international), increasing size of feedlots, lack of immunity to foreign animal diseases, the relatively porous nature of national borders, and the significant shortage of trained foreign animal disease diagnosticians and epidemiologists. Although many significant diseases transmitted by food-producing animals (eg, brucellosis, tuberculosis, coxiellosis/Q fever, etc) have been eradicated or controlled in North America and Europe by pasteurization and inspections at slaughter, still many others are seemingly ubiquitous (eg, listeriosis, salmonellosis, staphylococcosis, etc) and cause a significant fraction of the national burden of foodborne morbidity and mortality. Each year in the USA, there are reported approximately 20,000 foodborne illnesses, 4,200 hospitalizations, and 80 deaths, most of which are caused by pathogens of animal origin.

Management of Health Aspects of Laboratory Animal Facilities and Diagnostic Laboratories: The challenges of recognizing resurgent infectious diseases and developing novel therapeutics have placed unprecedented emphasis on managing and maintaining laboratory animal colonies for research and diagnostic efforts. Providing these services both successfully and humanely falls to the veterinarians in these institutions. Because few nations have the individual capacity to provide these services internally, increasing emphasis is being placed on international collaboration and reference centers, many of which focus on zoonotic diseases and comparative medicine. Because most outbreaks of zoonotic disease occur in tropical regions devoid of local surveillance and diagnostic and response capacity, the role of these international collaboration and reference centers likely will expand, requiring larger numbers of trained, experienced veterinary personnel.

Biomedical Research: Building on the information from public health surveillance, research institutions must follow with a greater understanding of the interactions between hosts, parasites, vectors, pathogens, and the environment. Establishing a causal link between human and animal disease relies on such research efforts, often through some combination of molecular studies, mathematical theory, and experimental epidemiology, using either field or laboratory research. As highlighted by the World Health Organization, research of endemic and resurgent zoonoses is often handicapped by a lack of basic knowledge of host-parasite interactions. For many zoonotic species, even the route of transmission to people remains uncertain. In some cases, the molecular biology of the agents in human and animal hosts may be very different. For example, there are major research efforts aimed toward the identification of virulence factors for *E coli* O157:H7 and the reasons for their differential expressions in people and cattle.

Health Education and Extension: Although training new veterinary practitioners and disseminating new capabilities to those already in practice falls largely on the nation's academic (especially land-grant) institutions, virtually all veterinarians help educate the public on the threat of infectious and noninfectious diseases. At the collegiate level, this will increasingly involve multidisciplinary relationships between schools of medicine, veterinary medicine, sociology, and basic sciences.

Enabling appropriate knowledge and awareness among the public requires a skillful blend of risk perception and risk awareness, especially because community stakeholders play significant roles in risk resolution. Most epidemiologists are employed by governmental or industrial stakeholders that have not historically been viewed as valid proxies for the public. This represents an important opportunity, perhaps responsibility, for veterinary practitioners to remain knowledgeable about disease threats and credible sources of that knowledge for their communities.

Production and Control of Biologic Products and Medical Devices: Ensuring that animal drugs, vaccines, and devices are safe and efficacious is a shared responsibility between the FDA, the USDA, and the EPA. In general, the FDA, specifically the Center for Veterinary Medicine, regulates animal drugs, animal feeds, and veterinary devices, whereas the USDA regulates animal vaccines and biologics. Specific to pesticides, FDA regulates certain flea and tick products for animals, whereas the EPA regulates others. Within each of these governmental agencies, veterinarians serve to encourage the development of novel products and, at the same time, protect the consumers of those products from false or misleading claims.

Another important function regarding biologic agents is the regulation of their storage, use, and transfer. Because of inherent virulence and transmissibility, access to many disease pathogens, termed **select agents**, has increasingly been limited to legitimate facilities for legitimate uses. The Federal Select Agent Program is jointly administered by the CDC and the USDA's Animal and Plant Health Inspection Service (APHIS). This effort oversees the possession, use, and transfer of certain biologic agents and toxins that have the potential to pose a severe threat to the public, to animal or plant health, or to animal or plant products.

Government/Legislative Activity: Significant numbers of veterinarians are employed at various levels of state and federal government. More than 3,000 veterinarians are employed at the federal level, nearly two-thirds of which are with the USDA. Other federal agencies employing large numbers of veterinarians include the DoD (Army and Air Force) and DHHS (CDC, FDA, and NIH). Public health programs comprise the vast majority of these opportunities, with direct animal care being a minor fraction. Examples include oversight of food safety inspection programs, disease surveillance and outbreak investigation, laboratory animal care, biomedical research, and public health program management and leadership.

At the state level, each department of agriculture typically has a State Veterinarian who is responsible for protecting the livestock, poultry, and aquaculture industries directly, and the public indirectly, through the prevention, early detection, containment, and eradication of economically important livestock, poultry, and fish diseases that, in many cases, are transmissible to people. The State Veterinarian regulates the importation, transportation, and processing of animals and is responsible for the control and eradication of poultry and livestock diseases, regulation of fish farming, and emergency response programs. Welfare of farm animals is monitored, and when necessary, the Office of the State Veterinarian conducts investigations and prosecutions relating to cases of cruelty to animals.

Currently, 41 states and territories employ veterinarians in their state health departments as State Public Health Veterinarians (SPHVs). SPHVs generally work in zoonotic disease control and prevention, directly focusing on protecting public health. They typically are located in health department divisions of epidemiology, toxicology, or environmental health.

A final category of governmental activity is legislative; a relatively small number of veterinarians serve at various levels to promulgate laws, rules, and regulations that serve to protect public health, domestic preparedness, and national defense. Veterinarians serve in the United States House of Representatives, in senior leadership positions of several United States Cabinet-level departments (including USDA, DHHS, DoD, and DHS), and as legislative liaisons for professional associations such as the AVMA. They are assisted in their legislative efforts by the communicative action of practicing veterinarians across the nation. It is through this pathway that ideas and issues are effectively transmitted to legislators and translated into improved legal and policy outcomes.

SIGNIFICANT NATIONAL PUBLIC HEALTH ACHIEVEMENTS

During the 20th century, the health and life expectancy of Americans improved dramatically. Since 1900, the average life span of people in the USA has increased by 30 yr, largely attributable to advances in public health. To commemorate these advances, the CDC named the following as the Ten Great Public Health Achievements, 1900–1999: vaccination, motor vehicle safety, safer workplaces, control of infectious diseases, mortality decline from coronary heart disease and stroke, safer and healthier foods, healthier mothers and babies, family planning, fluoridation of drinking water, and recognition of tobacco as a health hazard.

To further commemorate national advances in public health and to specifically highlight the veterinary public health contribution to the overall effort, the following were named as the Ten Great Veterinary Public Health Achievements–United States, 1901–2000.

1) Eradication of animal disease: Largely attributable to national programmatic efforts involving local, state, and federal veterinarians, the following diseases were declared eliminated from animal populations within the USA: contagious pleuropneumonia (1892), fowl plague (1929), foot-and-mouth disease (1929), glanders (1934), dourine (1942), cattle tick fever (1943), vesicular exanthema of swine (1959), screwworm myiasis (1959), sheep scabies (1973), exotic Newcastle disease (1974), and classical swine fever (hog cholera, 1978).

2) Laboratory animal science: The first professor of laboratory animal science in the USA was Dr. Carl Schlotthauer, appointed in 1945 at the University of Minnesota. Dr. Charles Griffin oversaw the development of pathogen-free animal colonies at the New York State Board of Health Laboratories from 1919 to 1954. Other veterinary pioneers in laboratory animal medicine included Dr. William Thorp at the National Institutes of Health, Dr. James Steele at the CDC, and Dr. Karl Meyer at the University of California at San Francisco.

3) Infectious disease control: In 1900, tuberculosis was the leading cause of death in people in the USA and commonly resulted in malformations in the bones of children. Of this disease burden, 40%–50% was reported to be bovine in origin, as the result of drinking unpasteurized milk. Constant public health (Pasteurized Milk Ordinance; FDA) and veterinary disease control (USDA eradication program) measures have eliminated this route of transmission in the USA. The early 1900s also saw the discovery of the etiologic agents for many prevalent animal diseases. Among these were African horse sickness (1900), rinderpest (1902), sheeppox (1902), rabies (1903), hog cholera (1903), and the first discovery of a viral cause of a cancer, fowl leukosis (1908). On a broader scale, the first cancer-preventing vaccines, which are to protect against Marek disease and feline leukemia virus, were developed by veterinarians and are contributing to development of human applications.

4) Livestock herd health and production optimization: Dr. C.L. Cole, who was at the North Central Experiment Station at Grand Rapids, Minnesota, was the first to demonstrate that large numbers of cows could be bred successfully by artificial insemination (1937–1938). The first calf sired by artificial insemination of frozen semen was born in 1953. A 10-year dairy production study published in the late 1940s noted that among the many benefits of annual physical examinations for dairy cattle was an average increase in milk production of 40%. More recently, widespread application of preventive medicine and environmental health best practices serve to maximize dairy cow health and comfort, all but eliminating milk as a source of foodborne illness. Moreover, annual milk production increased from 5,000 to 21,000 lb per cow.

5) Food safety (human): Although the 1904 publication of Upton Sinclair's provocative book *The Jungle* led to the dismissal of Dr. Daniel E. Salmon from the fledging Bureau of Animal Industry, the resultant public furor successfully reinvigorated his mission and facilitated the promulgation of the Meat Inspection Act of 1906. Dr. Salmon's contribution to foodborne disease control was considered so valuable that the *Salmonella* spp were named for him. In 1900, the first local community instituted routine microbiologic examination of milk. In 1908, Chicago required pasteurization of dairy products and, in 1948, Michigan was the first state to require milk pasteurization. In the 1920s, veterinarians also accomplished the basic work in developing the USPHS (FDA) Pasteurized Milk Ordinance and Code. Although slow to achieve industry acceptance, irradiation of food has substantial beneficial effects on the safety and quality of many foodstuffs. Previously approved for items such as spices, fruits, vegetables, and poultry, ionizing radiation was approved for use in 1999 to reduce bacterial loads on frozen raw meat and meat by-products.

6) Recognition and enhancement of the human-animal bond: Throughout recorded history, mankind has partnered and benefited from association with domesticated animals. The dairy cow is recognized as the "foster mother of the human race," and the horse, ox, donkey, camel, water buffalo, reindeer, and yak have provided mankind with our primary

transport and tractor power for thousands of years. Indeed, the histories of all animals, including people, cannot be dissociated. That symbiotic partnership, perhaps the cornerstone of veterinary medicine, became the life work of Dr. Leo Bustad, who once stated, "One cannot have a healthy community without a strong human-animal bond." An enhanced understanding of that inextricable bond has led to relationships between people and animals, including guide dogs for the vision and hearing impaired and military working dogs and dolphins. Further, the positive physical and psychological benefits of human-animal relationships, such as the lowering of blood pressure and as companions for older, ill, and traumatized people, have been described.

7) Border inspection/surveillance: The USDA has primary responsibility for preventing the introduction or reintroduction of foreign animal diseases into the USA. The Herculean proportions of this task are exemplified by the fact that before free trade, the USA imported 1.9 million cattle, 700,000 swine, and about 28 million birds annually. Inspecting representative samples of these animals and their by-products is the direct or indirect task of USDA veterinarians. This effort has been greatly aided since 1954 by the USDA Foreign Animal Disease Diagnostic Laboratory on Plum Island, New York, which provides valuable research toward the prevention and control of these biologically and economically devastating diseases. Similarly, veterinarians employed by DHHS/CDC's Division of Global Migration and Quarantine and the U.S. Fish and Wildlife Service (Department of the Interior) oversee programs to control importation of nonhuman primates, vector species, and potentially dangerous or injurious wildlife species.

8) Surgery and medicine: Regional anesthesia via the spinal route was first introduced in the USA at the 1926 AVMA meeting. Dr. Otto Stader developed the first steel pin method for external fracture fixation. In the 1950s, Dr. H. A. Gorman developed the first prosthetic hip joint, and Dr. F. L. Earl discovered the tranquilizing effects of reserpine.

9) Uniformed services veterinary medicine: In 1916, with the establishment of the United States Army Veterinary Corps, the USA was the last of the industrialized countries to commission a corps of military veterinarians. During World War II, army veterinarians were credited with providing higher quality rations for troops, as well as more space for armaments on cargo ships by thoroughly trimming meat products and freezing them in compact containers. Dr. Robert A. Whitney, Jr. (USPHS) served as Deputy Surgeon General and later as the Acting Surgeon General in 1993. Today, veterinarians in the U.S. Army, Air Force, and Public Health Service contribute substantially to military and civilian public health missions, such as human and animal disease control, occupational health, food safety, medical research, deployment health surveillance, and biologic warfare/terrorism defense.

10) Integration with public health practitioners: Under the leadership of Dr. Karl Meyer, an early architect of veterinary public health, the Hooper Foundation of Medical Research became a leading institute for the study of comparative medicine and zoonotic diseases. Additionally, he developed the original curriculum for the University of California School of Public Health. One of the many important achievements by Dr. James H. Steele was the status elevation of veterinarians in the USPHS from sanitarians to veterinary medical officers. Dr. Calvin Schwabe's seminal work, *Veterinary Medicine and Human Health* (1964), provides one of the most concrete examples of this integration.

NATIONAL PUBLIC HEALTH INDICATORS

Unfortunately, there are no direct measurements of public health in a population. Therefore, it is difficult to compare overarching changes over time or against other populations, except with surrogates such as surveillance for specific diseases/events and specific population attributes. Accepted among many public health officials is some combination of the following national health indicators: 1) life expectancy at birth (years)—the average number of years that a newborn could expect to live, if he or she were to pass through life exposed to the sex- and age-specific death rates prevailing at the time of his or her birth; 2) infant mortality rate (per 1,000 live births)—the probability of a child born in a specific year dying before reaching the age of 1 yr; 3) age-standardized mortality rate (number/unit population)—a weighted average of the age-specific (ages 30–70) mortality rates per 100,000 persons, in which the weights are the proportions of persons in the corresponding age groups of the WHO standard population; 4) childhood immunization rate (%)—the percentage of children (19–35 mo old) who have received the recommended combined vaccine series; 5) annual population growth rate (%)—average exponential rate of annual growth of the population over a given time period; 6) density of physicians (number/unit population)—number of medical doctors (physicians), including generalist and specialist practitioners, per 10,000 persons; 7) gross national income per capita ($USD)—total annual purchasing power, standardized to the US dollar; 8) government expenditure on health as a percentage of total government expenditure (%); 9) per capita total expenditure on health ($USD); 10) population median age (years); 11) obesity (%)—adults (>20 yr old) who have a body mass index (BMI) ≥30 kg/m^2.

ESSENTIAL PUBLIC HEALTH FUNCTIONS

Under the auspices of DHHS, the USPHS developed (and adopted in 1994) the following ten essential public health functions to assist state and local health agencies achieve their mission of promoting physical and mental health and preventing disease, injury, and disability.

1) Monitor health status to identify community health problems. A generally accepted definition of public health surveillance is "the ongoing systematic collection, analysis, interpretation, and dissemination of outcome-specific data essential to the planning, implementation, and evaluation of public health practice." Without this type of activity over time, baseline data cannot be analyzed for adverse events and trends.

2) Diagnose and investigate health problems and health hazards in the community. As an adjunct to surveillance, public health agencies conduct targeted screening programs and/or surveys to detect problems and hazards in the community. When detected, they are investigated to determine their magnitude, and results are used to inform public education and prevention efforts.

3) Inform, educate, and empower people about health issues. Once priorities have been established through surveillance, detection, and investigation, educational activities that promote improved health should be disseminated.

4) Mobilize community partnerships to identify and solve health problems. Public health agencies at all levels can mobilize community partnerships to solve health problems. Of particular importance is identification of potential stakeholders who can contribute to or benefit from public health interventions.

5) Develop policies and plans that support individual and community health efforts. Policies and laws can effectively modify human behavior and reduce negative health outcomes. Examples include limiting access to high-calorie beverages in school-age children and "dram shop liability" to discourage overconsumption of alcoholic beverages in public establishments.

6) Enforce laws and regulations that protect health and ensure safety. The existence of policies and laws is not enough; compliance must be enforced to ensure the overall safety and health of the community. Ongoing assessment and education efforts are undertaken to ensure that these policies and laws remain relevant and known to the public.

7) Link people to needed personal health services and assure the provision of health care when otherwise unavailable. Having access to care when it is needed is important in helping individuals prevent and avoid unfavorable health outcomes and medical costs. Components of these efforts are undertaken at the local, state, and federal levels to provide a coordinated system of health care.

8) Assure a competent public health and personal health care workforce. Competent health care workers provide care more effectively and efficiently than those less competent. This is facilitated by licensing and credentialing processes, incorporating core public health competencies into personnel systems, and adopting continual quality improvement opportunities for public health workforce members.

9) Evaluate effectiveness, accessibility, and quality of personal and population-based health services. Given scarce resources, it is imperative to assess whether programs and policies achieve intended outcomes. Cost-effectiveness analyses have been proposed as one strategy to inform policymakers on how best to allocate health care resources.

10) Support/sponsor research for new insights and innovative solutions to health problems. From the evidence-based results of coordinated research programs, health and health care problems can be better understood and improved over time.

PUBLIC HEALTH FOCI OF PREVENTION

When considering opportunities and methods to address health problems, three stages of prevention are generally recognized:

1) Primary prevention—focuses on avoiding development of a disease by preventing

it before exposure. Examples of primary prevention strategies include immunization programs, health education, and smoking cessation interventions. Because disease is largely avoided by these strategies, primary prevention is generally regarded as the most cost-effective form of prevention.

2) Secondary prevention—focuses on early disease detection and intervention, ideally before the onset of clinical signs. Examples include screening programs against various forms of cancer (eg, breast, colon, prostate, etc), postexposure rabies prophylaxis, tuberculosis skin tests, and infectious disease contact investigations.

3) Tertiary prevention—focuses on the treatment and rehabilitation of individuals with disease(s). Examples include antimicrobial therapies, hypertension drugs, and heart attack and stroke rehabilitation. Because this stage focuses its efforts after a disease is established, tertiary prevention has proved the most expensive form of prevention.

BASIC PRINCIPLES OF EPIDEMIOLOGY

The definition of epidemiology is "the study of disease in populations and of factors that determine its occurrence over time." The purpose is to describe and identify opportunities for intervention. Epidemiology is concerned with the distribution and determinants of health and disease, morbidity, injury, disability, and mortality in populations. For veterinary epidemiology, this intervention is to enhance not only health but also productivity. **Distribution** implies that diseases and other health outcomes do not occur randomly in populations; **determinants** are any factors that cause a change in a health condition or other defined characteristic; **morbidity** is illness due to a specific disease or health condition; **mortality** is death due to a specific disease or health condition; and the **population at risk** can be people, animals, or plants.

Epidemiology is applied in many areas of public health practice. Among the most salient are to observe historical health trends to make useful projections into the future, discover (diagnose) current health and disease burden in a population, identify specific causes and risk factors of disease, differentiate between natural and intentional events (eg, bioterrorism), describe the natural history of a particular disease, compare various treatment and prevention products/techniques, assess the impact/efficiency/cost/outcome of interventions, prioritize intervention strategies, and provide foundation for public policy.

Epidemiologic Terms and Concepts

The **natural history** of a disease in a population, sometimes termed the disease's ecology, refers to the course of the disease from its beginning to its final clinical endpoints. The natural history begins before infection (prepathogenesis period) when the agent simply exists in the environment, includes the factors that affect its incidence and distribution, and concludes with either its disappearance or persistence (endemnicity) in that environment. Although knowledge of the complete natural history is not absolutely necessary for treatment and control of disease in a population, it does facilitate the most effective interventions.

An important epidemiologic concept is that neither health nor disease occurs randomly throughout populations. Innumerable factors influence the temporal waxing and waning of disease. A disease is considered **endemic** when it is constantly present within a given geographic area. For instance, animal rabies is endemic in the USA. An **epidemic** occurs when a disease occurs in larger numbers than expected in a given population and geographic area. Raccoon rabies was epidemic throughout the eastern USA for much of the 1980s and 1990s. A subset of an epidemic is an **outbreak**, when the higher disease occurrence occurs in a smaller geographic area and shorter period of time. Finally, a **pandemic** occurs when an epidemic becomes global in scope (eg, influenza, HIV/AIDS).

The **population at risk** is an extremely important concept in epidemiology and includes members of the overall population who are capable of developing the disease or condition being studied. This concept seems simple at first, but misinterpretations can lead to erroneous study results and conclusions. As a simple example, a study of testicular cancer among residents in a population should not include women in the population at risk (frequently expressed as the "denominator" in an epidemiologic ratio).

A **ratio** is the value obtained from dividing one quantity by another (X/Y). The numerator and denominator may be independent of each other. In fact, in epidemiology, the term ratio is applied when the numerator is not a subset of the denominator. For example, in a class of veterinary students in which 88 are female and 14 are male, the sex ratio of female students to male students is 88/14, or 6.3 to 1.

A **proportion** is a type of ratio in which the numerator is part of the denominator (A/[A + B]). Therefore, they are not independent. For example, suppose that, among domestic dogs testing positive for internal parasites in Glendale, Arizona, 889 were male and 643 were female. The proportion of female dogs among those found to have parasite infections would be 643/(889 + 643), or 0.42.

A **rate** is another type of ratio in which the denominator involves the passage of time. This is important in epidemiology, because rates can be used to measure the speed of a disease event or to make epidemiologic comparisons between populations over time. Rates are typically expressed as a measure of the frequency with which an event occurs in a defined population in a defined time (eg, the number of foodborne *Salmonella* infections per 100,000 people annually in the USA).

Incidence is a measure of the new occurrence of a disease event (eg, illness or death) within a defined time period in a specified population. Two essential components are the number of new cases and the period of time in which those new cases appear. In an example regarding the class of veterinary students, if 13 of them developed influenza over the course of 3 mo (one quarter), the incidence would be 13 cases per quarter.

An **incidence rate** takes the population at risk into account. In the previous example, the incidence rate would be 13 cases per quarter/102 students, or 0.127 cases per quarter per student. Incidence rates are usually expressed by a multiplier that makes the number easier to conceptualize and compare. In this example, the multiplier would be 100, and the incidence rate would be 12.7 cases per quarter per 100 students (or 12.7%). An **attack rate** is an incidence rate; however, the period of susceptibility is very short (usually confined to a single outbreak).

A similar concept to incidence is **prevalence**. Prevalence (synonymous with "point prevalence") is the total number of cases that exist at a particular point in time in a particular population at risk. Again using the influenza example from above, if 7 students had influenza at the same time during the academic quarter, the prevalence would be 7/102 or 0.069 cases per class (or 6.9%).

Measures of disease burden typically describe illness and death outcomes as **morbidity** and **mortality**, respectively. Morbidity is the measure of illness in a population, and numbers and rates are calculated in a similar fashion as with *incidence and prevalence. Mortality* is the corresponding measure of death in a population and can be applied to death from general (nonspecific) causes or from a specific disease. In the latter case, cause-specific mortality is expressed as the **case fatality rate**, which is the number of deaths due to a particular disease occurring among individuals afflicted with that disease in a given time period. In another example, consider a large veterinary practice in the southwest USA that frequently sees dogs with coccidioidomycosis. The practice diagnosed 542 clinical cases in a particular year, 83 of which died from the disease in the course of that year. The month in which the most cases were diagnosed was September, in which 97 cases were diagnosed. Further, at a single point in time (perhaps based on the results of a serosurvey of dogs in the practice area), 237 dogs of 6,821 dogs with active records in the practice had the disease. In this scenario, the prevalence of coccidioidomycosis at the time of the serosurvey would be 237/6,821 or 0.035 (3.5%); the incidence in September would be 97 cases, and the incidence rate would be 97/6,821 or 0.014 (1.4%). Finally, the annual mortality rate due to coccidioidomycosis would be 83/6,821 or 0.013 (1.3%), and the case fatality rate would be 83/542 or 0.153 (or 15.3%).

Public health surveillance is defined as the ongoing systematic collection, analysis, interpretation, and dissemination of outcome-specific data essential to the planning, implementation, and evaluation of public health practice. In epidemiology, health surveillance is accomplished in either passive or active systems. **Passive surveillance** occurs when individual health care providers or diagnostic laboratories send periodic reports to the public health agency. Because this reporting is voluntary (sometimes referred to as being "pushed" to health agencies), passive surveillance tends to underreport disease, especially in diseases with low morbidity and mortality. Passive surveillance is useful for longterm trend analysis (if reporting criteria remain consistent) and is much less expensive than active surveillance. An example of passive surveillance is the system of officially notifiable diseases routinely reported to CDC by select health departments across the USA. **Active surveillance**, in contrast, occurs when an epidemiologist or public health agency seeks specific data from individual health care providers or laboratories. In this case, the data are "pulled" by the requestor, usually during emerging diseases or significant changes in disease incidence. Active surveillance is usually much more expensive and labor intensive; it typically is limited to short-term analyses of high-impact events. An example is the 1-yr surveillance conducted by CDC of the rapid increase in incidence of coccidioidomycosis among people in Arizona in 2007–2008.

Descriptive Epidemiology

Given that neither health nor disease is equally distributed throughout a population, epidemiologists use various methods to study and describe their occurrence. In descriptive epidemiology, diseases are classified according to the variables of person, place, and time.

Person: Who is affected by this disease? This is relevant, because certain variables may highlight changes in disease status and can be used to focus additional studies and interventions. Common person variables include age, sex, race, socioeconomic status, marital status, religion, smoker/nonsmoker, etc. In the case of animals, equivalent variables may include species, breed, reproductive status (eg, intact vs neutered, pregnant vs nonpregnant), function (eg, meat/milk/fiber production, race horse vs working horse vs pleasure horse, companion dog vs military working dog), and wild/feral vs domesticated (cats).

Place: Where does this disease occur? Place variables commonly illustrate geographic differences in the occurrence of a particular disease. Focused studies can help epidemiologists to determine why those differences have occurred and to identify specific risk factors. Common place variables include comparisons across national, state, and municipal boundaries and between urban and rural communities. For animal populations, "place" may refer to housing (eg, indoors vs outdoors, pen number or stall) or type of herd management (eg, intensive feedlot confinement vs extensive grazing). Place may also relate to risk of exposure to infectious animals at sale barns or during shipment or to external factors such as severe weather and natural disasters.

Time: When and over what time period (hours, days, weeks, day vs night) does this disease occur? Time variables are important to describe when disease occurs in relation to various factors of potential exposure and vulnerability. In animals, time may refer to milking shift, breeding season, lambing/calving season, at weaning, during shipment, on arrival at the feedlot, dry vs wet season, etc. Common time variables include secular trends (changes over long periods of time), seasonal/cyclic periods, and specific points in time (eg, outbreaks, epidemics, clusters, etc).

When a particular disease is observed relative to the variables of person, place, and time, it is often systematically described to facilitate more in-depth study. These systematic descriptions commonly take the form of case reports, case series, or cross-sectional studies.

Case reports are accounts of single or a few noteworthy health-related incidents (eg, an epidemiologic description of a case of human rabies).

Case series are listings of a larger number of cases, usually presented consecutively (eg, a characterization of dog bite incidents in a population of veterinarians and/or technicians over time). Case series articles are useful for comparing variables of person, place, or time as they appear to affect the occurrence of a particular disease.

Cross-sectional studies are one-time assessments of the incidence or prevalence of a disease in a defined population, which is usually selected at random from a larger population at risk (eg, a serosurvey of veterinarians for the presence of antibodies to *Bartonella henselae* organisms to determine risk factors and for cat scratch disease). Cross-sectional studies are especially useful in forming hypotheses to be addressed by follow-on analytic studies.

Two main types of bias in descriptive epidemiology are **selection bias** and **observation bias**. Selection bias results from the identification of subjects/cases from a subset that is not representative of the entire population at risk. A nonmedical example of selection bias would occur in a voter survey, intended to predict the outcome of a political election, but drawn from a sample of voters from either high- or low-income status, neither of which would be representative of the overall voting population. Observation bias arises from systematic differences in the method of obtaining information from subjects/cases. Consider a study comparing library usage between students at two universities. Significant differences might result if students from one university were queried over the phone regarding library visits, whereas students at the other university were directly observed for actual usage. In general, bias in descriptive studies is not as prevalent or significant as bias in analytical studies.

In summary, descriptive epidemiology serves to describe the occurrence of disease in a population. Descriptive methods are commonly applied to little-known diseases; they use preexisting data, address the questions of who/where/when, and identify potential associations for more in-depth analytical studies.

Analytical Epidemiology

Analytical studies are applied to study the etiology of disease, to identify a causal relationship between exposures and health outcomes. They are typically used when insights of a particular health issue are available, commonly from previous descriptive studies. In evaluating the causality of disease associations, analytical studies address the question of "why" as opposed to the "person/place/time" of descriptive studies.

Once potential associations have been observed between those who have a particular disease and those who do not, further investigations are undertaken to determine causality and identify effective interventions. The first step in an analytic study is to form some conjecture regarding observed exposures and health outcomes. In analytical studies, this conjecture is termed the **null hypothesis**, meaning that the default assumption is that there is no association between the exposure in question and the disease outcome. Note that this assumption of no association is made even though the epidemiologist often thinks that some association actually exists. Once the null hypothesis is generated, studies are designed to test it and either reject it (by finding that some association actually does exist between exposure and disease outcome) or accept it (by finding that no association exists).

Analytical epidemiology is accomplished through either observational studies or interventional studies. In the former, the investigator does not control the exposure between the groups under study and typically cannot randomly assign subjects to study groups.

Observational Studies:

Ecologic Studies: The unit under study is a group of people or animals versus an individual. The group has no size limitation but must be able to be defined. For instance, the group could be a kennel of dogs, a class of veterinary students, or the citizens of an entire country. Once defined, the group is analyzed against some exposure to see what outcome(s) ensue. Examples of ecologic studies include Dr. John Snow's analysis of the association between the incidence of cholera in London and where people obtained their drinking water, an analysis of how tobacco taxes affect tobacco usage, and an analysis of certain occupations for resultant hearing loss.

Ecologic studies have several advantages over other types of observational studies. They are relatively quick, easy, and inexpensive. Individual data are not necessary, only aggregate data for the group(s) under study. Finally, they are useful in generating information about the overall context of health, especially how it is affected by variables such as demographics, geography, and the social environment.

Ecologic studies also have several disadvantages. First, the measurement of many exposures is imprecise, especially of large groups in which the influence(s) of those exposures is difficult to define or not equally exerted. This phenomenon of unequal variable exertion results in another potential drawback to ecologic studies. Known as ecologic fallacy, it is described by "associations observed at the group level do not necessarily hold true at the individual level." As an example, one could determine that the average IQ of a class of veterinary students is above average (which, by definition, would be 100). If a particular student was randomly selected from that class, could it be inferred that that student's IQ was above 100? The answer is no, because of the difference between average and median. If the class had only a few people above average, but these students were significantly above average, and the rest of the students were only slightly below average, the distribution would be skewed toward a higher IQ when, in actuality, many members of the class would be below average.

Cohort Studies: In this type of study, a group of individuals (termed a cohort) is observed over time for changes in health outcomes.

When the period of the study is from the present into the future, the study is a **prospective cohort study**. In this case, the cohort is assumed to share a particular exposure and is followed over time to document the occurrence of new instances of a particular disease or outcome. Obviously, each member of the cohort must not have the disease or outcome at the beginning of the study. One of the most famous medical prospective cohort studies is the Framingham Heart Study. Researchers began the study in 1948 by recruiting 5,209 men and women, 30–62 yr old, from the town of Framingham, Massachusetts. Since that time, they have accomplished extensive serial physical examinations and surveys relating to the development of cardiovascular disease.

The major advantage of the prospective cohort study is that many different exposures can be considered and analyzed for influencing the outcome under study. Disadvantages include the high cost in terms of money and time during the period of the study and the inability to study very rare diseases or health outcomes unless the cohort is extremely large.

When the period of the study is from the past to the present, the study is a **retrospective cohort study**. The methodology is very similar to that of the prospective cohort study, except that all the events (exposures and outcomes) have already occurred; the investigator is merely looking back rather than forward. Retrospective studies are conceived after some individuals have already developed the outcomes of interest. The investigators jump back in time to identify a cohort of individuals at a point in time before they developed the outcomes of interest, and try to establish their exposure status at that point in time. They then determine whether the subject subsequently developed the outcomes of interest. If so, they can analyze the exposure(s) that may have contributed to those outcomes.

Retrospective cohort studies have several advantages over prospective cohort studies. They typically take less time and are less expensive. Additionally, they can address rare outcomes, because the cases are selected after having already developed the disease or outcome. Disadvantages include a potentially high possibility of selection bias, the fact that individuals may have difficulty recalling certain exposures (termed **recall bias**), and the requirement for the existence of medical and/or exposure records.

Regardless of being retrospective or prospective, the measure of association of all cohort studies is the **relative risk** (RR). Relative risk is calculated by dividing the incidence rate of the disease or outcome in the exposed individuals by the incidence rate in the unexposed individuals. An RR of 1 means there is no difference in risk between the two groups. An RR <1 means that the outcome is less likely to occur in the exposed group than in the unexposed group. Conversely, an RR >1 means the outcome is more likely to occur in the exposed group than in the unexposed group. Consider an example in which the incidence of prostate cancer among neutered male dogs was found to be 1.37%, and the incidence in intact male dogs was 0.36%. In this case, the relative risk would be 1.37/0.36 or 3.8. This could be stated as "Neutered male dogs would be nearly four times as likely as intact male dogs to develop prostate cancer."

Case-Control Studies: In this type of study, subjects are selected as either having a particular outcome (cases) or not having the outcome (controls). They are then compared in a retrospective way to identify differences in their exposures that might explain the differences in outcomes. Ideally, cases and controls should be as similar as possible in all characteristics except the outcome in order to make the comparisons simpler and more meaningful. That is why some investigators "match" cases and controls. In one notable example, a very large case-control study in 1950 studied people with lung cancer and demonstrated a very positive association between smoking and lung cancer. Although it did not prove causality alone, it was instrumental in the U.S. Surgeon General's now-standard warnings.

Case-control studies have several advantages. They are inherently retrospective, so they are relatively quick and inexpensive. Because the cases have already been identified, they are appropriate for studying rare diseases and examining multiple exposures. Disadvantages include the fact that, like cohort studies, they are prone to selection, recall, and observer bias. Additionally, their application is limited to the study of one outcome.

The most common measurement of association in case-control studies is the odds ratio. The **odds ratio** (OR) represents the odds that an outcome will occur from a particular exposure, compared with the odds of the outcome occurring in the absence of that exposure. ORs are calculated using a 2 × 2 frequency table (TABLE 1).

TABLE 1 CALCULATING AN ODDS RATIO

		Outcome Status	
		+	–
Exposure Status	+	a	b
	–	c	d

a = Number of exposed cases
b = Number of exposed non-cases
c = Number of unexposed cases
d = Number of unexposed non-cases

$$OR = \frac{a/c}{b/d} = \frac{ad}{bc}$$

An OR of 1 means the exposure did not affect the odds of the outcome. An OR >1 means the exposure is associated with a higher odds of the outcome, and an OR <1 means the exposure is associated with a lower odds of the outcome. Although a higher OR indicates a stronger association between exposure and outcome, it does not necessarily imply statistical significance and, by itself, is not enough to prove causality.

Interventional Studies: The other category of studies that comprise analytical epidemiology are interventional studies. In contrast to observational studies, the investigator using an interventional approach can intentionally change some form of exposure between several groups to determine differences in outcome(s). In medical research, these exposures typically include interventions such as vaccines, therapeutic drugs, surgical techniques, or medical devices. The results of interventional studies can be very powerful in proving causality or identifying efficacy of various interventions. Interventional studies typically take one of two forms, either a randomized controlled (clinical) trial or a nonrandomized (community) trial.

Randomized Controlled (Clinical) Trials: In this type of study, participants are selected from a population and randomly assigned to one of two groups, one being the study group and the other being the control group. Study groups receive the intervention, and the controls do not.

Bias can be introduced in such a trial when either the participants or the investigator know which participants are in which group. This bias can be alleviated in one of two ways. First, in a single-blinded design, the participants are unaware whether they are in the study group or the control group. Additionally, in a double-blinded design, neither the investigator nor the participants are aware of the group assignments.

A major advantage of randomized controlled clinical trials is an inherently high validity for identifying differences in therapeutic efficacy of various interventions. Perhaps the major disadvantage is the high potential for ethical implications if an intervention with great potential benefit is intentionally withheld from the control group (eg, the historic Tuskegee Syphilis Study). For this reason, it can be very difficult to legally use human participants in many such trials. Additionally, this type of study is not usually applicable for discovering disease etiologies; observational studies are much better suited for this purpose.

Nonrandomized (Community) Trials: In this type of study, the units are groups (or communities) of participants assigned to treatment or control conditions. Although the communities may be selected at random, the individuals within them obviously are not. These studies are commonly undertaken to assess the quality and effectiveness of educational programs, behavioral changes, or mass interventions such as water fluoridation.

Bias

Bias is defined as the systematic deviation of results or inferences from truth. Bias is extremely difficult to completely avoid when undertaking scientific study. Therefore, studies are designed in ways that minimize the sources and effects of bias. Examples of bias are described below.

The Hawthorne effect: Participants in a study may act or behave differently because they know they are being studied. In 1924–1932, workers at the Hawthorne Works (an electric company near Chicago) were studied to see whether productivity was greater depending on how much light was provided at work. Results showed that productivity increased during the course of the study regardless of the changes in light; the workers just performed better because of the attention. When the study ended, productivity went back to prestudy levels.

Recall bias: Cases and controls may remember an exposure differently (and non-randomly). Usually, cases remember exposures more clearly than controls.

Selection bias: This occurs when selected controls are not representative of the population from which the cases were selected. In other words, there is an important characteristic of the controls that make them different from the general population. An example is the healthy worker effect, which refers to the phenomenon that employed groups have lower mortality than the general population. Therefore, if the study groups are comprised of differing fractions of employed and unemployed people, the results may very well be skewed.

Observer bias: The investigator, having knowledge of the outcome(s), might record exposures differently between cases and controls.

Confounding: In epidemiologic studies, a confounder is a variable that is not considered in the study design but is associated with the exposure and exerts an effect on the outcome. Confounders can either produce a false association between variables or mask a true association between variables. An example of the former was a spurious conclusion drawn from a study of the relationship between alcohol consumption and heart disease. In the study, it was concluded that alcohol consumption was significantly associated with heart disease. Smoking was later identified as a confounder, because smoking was correlated both with alcohol consumption and also with heart disease. When corrected for the effects of this confounder, no association was found between alcohol consumption and heart disease.

Error

When analyzing results of an epidemiologic study, there are two categorical types of error when either accepting or rejecting the null hypothesis.

Type I error, also known as a **false positive**, is when the null hypothesis is rejected when it actually should have been accepted. In other words, this is the error of accepting an alternative hypothesis (the real hypothesis of interest) when the results can actually be attributed to chance. Type I error (which can never be zero) is generally reported as the **P value**. In scientific studies, the most common *P* value is .05, which means an error of <5% of detecting an association between a variable and an outcome is acceptable.

Type II error, also known as a **false negative**, is when the null hypothesis is accepted when it actually should have been rejected. In other words, the study did not have adequate power to detect an association between a variable and an outcome when the association actually existed.

Variable Associations and Causality

In epidemiology, variables are either associated or they are not. If the variables are not associated, there is no relationship; they are independent. If the variables are associated, that relationship can be either positive or negative. If two variables are positively associated, the values of both variables increase or decrease together. If they are negatively associated, the value of one variable increases when the other decreases. Finally, if an association exists (positive or negative), it is either causal or noncausal related to the outcome.

When two variables are associated, it is sometimes obvious as to whether it is causal. Consider the relationship between animal bites and rabies; we know they are causally associated. However, in most epidemiologic studies, the relationship between variables (such as exposure and outcome) is much more difficult to ascertain and requires more extensive analysis. Several sets of systematic criteria for determining causality have been proposed: 1) Strength—Although a small association does not mean that there is not a causal effect, the larger the association, the more likely that it is causal. 2) Consistency—Repeatedly similar findings observed by different persons in different places with different samples strengthen the likelihood of a causal effect. 3) Specificity—Causation is more likely in a very specific population at a specific site and disease with no other likely explanation. The more specific the association between an exposure and an outcome, the higher the probability of causation. 4) Temporality—The outcome must occur after the exposure. 5) Biological gradient—Greater exposure generally results in greater incidence of the outcome. However, in some cases, the mere presence of the exposure, without regard to its magnitude, can trigger the effect. In yet other cases, an inverse relationship is observed when greater exposure of a protective factor leads to lower incidence of outcomes. 6) Plausibility—A rational, explainable mechanism between cause and effect is helpful (but may be limited by current knowledge). 7) Coherence—Agreement between epidemiologic and laboratory findings increases the likelihood of a causal effect. 8) Analogy—The effect of similar associations between other variables of exposure and outcome may be considered.

Sensitivity and Specificity

Veterinary practitioners use many diagnostic tests to determine what may be wrong with an animal and how it may be treated. The diagnostician must realize that these tests are fallible and that results are usually only close approximations of "truth." We can assume that an animal either has a medical condition or does not; however, no tests are 100% sensitive and specific. That is, no test can eliminate the potential for false-positive and false-negative results. However, there are methods to interpret test results to reduce their inherent fallibility. Those tests or diagnostic procedures known to produce the absolute best results are termed "gold standard" tests. It is against these gold standards that newer, usually faster and more convenient, tests are measured in terms of sensitivity and specificity.

Sensitivity is the probability of a positive test result when the disease is actually present. A sensitive test is "positive in disease" and minimizes false-negative results, thus minimizing type II error. **Specificity**, in contrast, is the probability of a negative test result in the absence of disease, thereby correctly classifying an individual as disease-free (regarding that particular condition). A specific test is "negative in health" and minimizes false-positive results, thus minimizing type I error. To calculate the sensitivity and specificity of a test, consider the following 2 × 2 table (*see* TABLE 2).

Sensitivity and specificity are inversely proportional, ie, when one increases, the other decreases. Therefore, the accuracy of a test is a trade-off between each of these parameters. **Screening tests** tend to have higher sensitivity and lower specificity, because the purpose of such a test is to detect the maximum number of individuals with the particular disease condition. A negative test result, therefore, strongly implies that disease is absent, whereas a positive result may require additional, confirmatory testing. For that reason, positive tests are often followed up with a **confirmatory test** that displays higher specificity to identify which positive results are true and which are false. Given the high specificity of confirmatory tests, a positive result strongly implies that disease is present.

In clinical medicine, two additional diagnostic test parameters are relevant. The **positive predictive value** (PPV) of a test is the probability of a patient actually having the disease condition when the test is positive. PPV is calculated as true positives divided by the sum of the true positives and the false positives: a/(a + b). False-negative test results do not affect the PPV. Therefore, if the PPV of a test is 100%, the validity of a negative test result is still unknown.

The **negative predictive value** (NPV) is the probability of a patient not having the disease condition when the test is negative. NPV is calculated as true negatives divided by the sum of the true negatives and the false negatives: d/(c + d). False-positive test results do not affect the NPV. Therefore, if a test was reported to have an NPV of 100%, the validity of a positive test result is still unknown.

PPV and NPV are clinically relevant, because they are directly related to the prevalence of disease. For diseases of high prevalence, the PPV of a test will be high and the NPV will be low. For rarer diseases, the opposite will be true, ie, the PPV will be low and the NPV will be high. For these reasons, the assumed prevalence of a disease must be taken into account when interpreting diagnostic test results.

Disease Outbreak Investigation

Public health officials investigate disease outbreaks to control them, to prevent additional illnesses, and to learn how to prevent similar outbreaks from happening in the future. Whether an outbreak is foodborne in origin or from another infectious source, the methodology is similar. The following steps in investigating disease outbreaks are used by the CDC: prepare for field work, confirm the existence of an outbreak, verify the

TABLE 2 CALCULATING TEST SENSITIVITY AND SPECIFICITY

		Gold Standard		
		Disease Present	**Disease Absent**	**Total**
Test Result	Positive	a	b	a+b
	Negative	c	d	c+d
	Total	a+c	b+d	

a = True positives; the test has correctly diagnosed the disease

b = False positives; the test is positive but disease is absent

c = False negatives; the test is negative but disease is present

d = True negatives; the test correctly diagnosed the absence of disease

Sensitivity is the true positives divided by the sum of the true positives and the false negatives: a/(a +c)

Specificity is the true negatives divided by the sum of the true negatives and the false positives: d/(b + d)

diagnosis, establish a working case definition, engage in systematic case finding, apply descriptive epidemiology, develop and test hypotheses (analytical epidemiology), implement control measures, and communicate findings.

Although these steps are accomplished in a systematic fashion, they frequently overlap or occur concurrently. For example, establishing a working case definition typically begins while the diagnosis is in the process of being verified and continues through the initial process of systematic case finding.

Establishing a working case definition is the method by which public health officials define what individuals are included as official cases in the outbreak and illustrate the boundaries of the outbreak. An effective case definition is critical because it may be confusing, especially in the absence of definitive diagnostics, to differentiate between actual disease cases and those ill from other causes. The case definition defines a case in terms of person, place, and time. Person criteria typically include vulnerability factors such as age, sex, signs/symptoms, or attendance at certain meals or public functions. Place criteria usually include a geographic boundary such as a state or local area, a school class, or a particular restaurant. Time parameters may be after an implicated meal (if foodborne) or other types of exposures. Case definitions are usually based on either clinical signs or diagnostic test results. The former is more subjective than the latter but can be just as effective, especially in field epidemiologic conditions. As the investigation ensues and more information becomes available, it may be necessary to revise the case definition. However, this is done judiciously, because changes to the case definition result in changes to the epidemic curve.

The **epidemic (epi) curve** shows progression of an outbreak over time. The horizontal axis represents the date when an individual became ill, also called the date of onset. The vertical axis is the number of individuals who became ill on each date. These are updated as new data come in and thus are subject to change. The epi curve is complex and may be limited by information deficiencies and inaccurate case definitions. Despite these potential limitations, detailed information regarding the dates and numbers of reported cases is visually useful. Moreover, in addition to the magnitude and duration of the outbreak, the shape of the curve can show useful information regarding the nature of the outbreak.

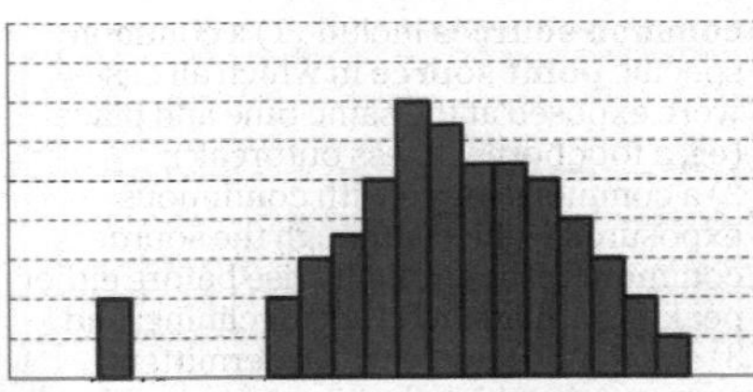

Epidemic curve common point source. *Courtesy of Dr. Donald L. Noah.*

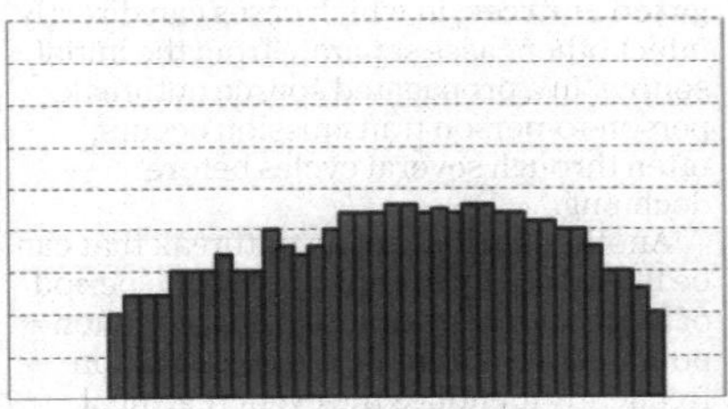

Epidemic curve common continuous source. *Courtesy of Dr. Donald L. Noah.*

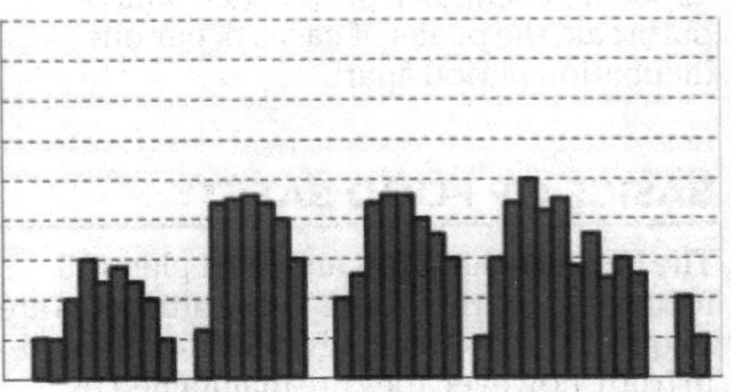

Epidemic curve common intermittent source. *Courtesy of Dr. Donald L. Noah.*

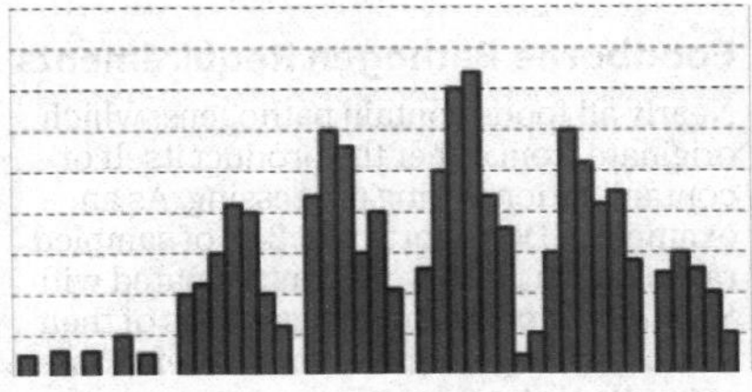

Epidemic curve propagated source. *Courtesy of Dr. Donald L. Noah.*

The overall shape of the epi curve can give clues to the type of exposure that resulted in the outbreak. Typical epi curves from

common sources include 1) a common specific **point source** in which all cases were exposed at the same time and place (eg, a foodborne illness outbreak); 2) a common source with continuous exposure in which although the source is common, cases gradually rise before either peaking or plateauing and declining; and 3) a common source with intermittent exposure in which the peaks occur at irregular times corresponding to the earlier exposures. In addition to outbreaks having common sources, they can have **propagated sources**, in which cases can directly infect other cases separate from the initial source. In a propagated source outbreak, person-to-person transmission occurs, often through several cycles before declining.

Another attribute of an outbreak that can be illustrated by the epi curve is the period of incubation. For example, in a common point source outbreak, the investigation frequently identifies the event (eg, meal, social gathering, etc) when the exposure occurred. In this case, the peak of cases occur one incubation period after the exposure event. In a propagated source outbreak, the peaks of cases occur one incubation period apart.

BASICS OF FOOD SAFETY

The USA has the safest and most plentiful food supply in the world. These attributes are frequently and mistakenly taken for granted. In truth, however, they are maintained by motivations such as increases in production efficiency, reductions in market uncertainty, and the goal of higher profits.

Foodborne Pathogen Requirements

Nearly all foods contain pathogens, which originate from either the product itself or contamination during processing. As an example, CDC reports that 24% of sampled raw chicken parts were contaminated with *Salmonella* organisms. Regardless of their source, pathogens have common environmental/nutritional requirements, each of which presents various control opportunities. The acronym FAT TOM can aid in learning these common requirements.

Food (some source of energy): Controlling this requirement is perhaps the most difficult because, as the nutrient content of the food is reduced, the quality and usefulness is similarly reduced. However, certain methods of processing and preserving serve to limit microbial access to nutrient sources. Nearly all foods are washed, rinsed, sifted, sorted, or trimmed during processing, which serves to limit the initial level of contamination. Additionally, simple packaging increases the shelf life of many foods and prevents contamination from the environment and other food items.

Acidity (measured by pH): The optimal pH range for microbial growth is 4.6–7.5. Therefore, for items such as bottled sauces/condiments and pickled foods, a common and effective preservation technique is to lower the pH (acidify) of the item below 4.6. Conversely, some food products (eg, fish, olives, eggs) can be processed with sodium hydroxide (lye) to raise the pH above this range.

Temperature: The optimal temperature range for many foodborne pathogens is 40°F–140°F. For this reason, prepared foods are held in this range for as little time as possible. As a general rule, 4 hr is considered the maximal time in this danger zone to limit microbial growth.

Time: Bacteria require time to propagate to the point of being infective and virulent. In general, 4 hr is considered the maximal time period in the temperature danger zone in retail food establishments.

Oxygen: Most foodborne pathogens are aerobic in nature, ie, they require oxygen for multiplication. Oxygen also facilitates the spoilage process. Techniques that limit available oxygen include drying, canning, bottling, vacuum packaging, adding antioxidants, and modifying the storage atmosphere by replacing oxygen with an inert gas such as nitrogen or carbon dioxide. An added benefit to a modified/controlled atmosphere is that it slows the ripening process and can extend the shelf life of many fruits and vegetables by months.

Moisture: Foods lower in water activity are more resistant to the growth of many foodborne pathogens. By definition, the water activity (aw) of water is 1. Foods with an aw <0.85 are considered generally safer than foods with a higher aw. Techniques that lower the water activity of foods include drying, dehydrating, freezing, salt/sugar curing, and pickling.

Food Processing and Preservation

Virtually all foods are processed to some degree. Examples of minimal processing techniques include washing, peeling, slicing, juicing, freezing, drying, fermenting, and pasteurizing. More extensive processing techniques include baking, frying, smoking, toasting, puffing, shredding, flavoring, coloring, and fortifying. Regardless of the degree, foods are processed for the purposes of preservation, safety, variety, convenience, nutritional enhancement, and increased marketability. Although these processing techniques have resulted in a safer and more plentiful supply, health concerns about food processing have been raised because of certain attributes of processed foods, such as added sugar, sodium, saturated/trans fats, refined grains, low fiber content, and their conducive nature toward unhealthy behaviors. Moreover, processing techniques such as grinding increase the surface area of foods, as in the case of hamburger, which renders them more capable of supporting the growth of pathogenic microorganisms.

In the 1960s, the National Aeronautics and Space Administration (NASA) asked the U.S. Army and the Pillsbury Company to develop safe foods for manned space flights. In a novel approach, Pillsbury required contractors to identify "critical failure areas" and eliminate them from the production system. This systematic approach became known as the Hazard Analysis Critical Control Point (HACCP) process. The underlying principle of HACCP, which focuses on health safety issues rather than quality issues, is to prevent the hazards during processing rather than merely inspecting the end product. Since that time, HACCP has been mandated by FDA and USDA for many food production sectors and also has been implemented in the cosmetics and pharmaceutical industries.

The HACCP process consists of the following seven principles: 1) Conduct a hazard analysis, ie, determine the hazards and preventive measures that could be applied to prevent them. 2) Identify critical control points, ie, any point, step, or procedure in a food manufacturing process at which controls can be applied. 3) Establish critical limits for each critical control point, ie, the maximum or minimum value to which a physical, biologic, or chemical hazard must be controlled at a critical control point. 4) Establish critical control point monitoring requirements, which are necessary to ensure that the process is under control at that point. 5) Establish corrective actions, or actions that must be taken when monitoring indicates a deviation from an established critical limit. 6) Establish procedures to ensure the HACCP system is working as intended, ie, validate the specific HACCP plan. 7) Establish record keeping procedures; each plant must maintain records of the entire process, as well as records to verify the plan.

The primary purposes of food preservation are to inhibit the growth of pathogenic microorganisms and to retard organic degradation such as oxidative rancidity. Many processes involve the use of multiple techniques. In addition to extending the shelf life of food products, the quality and acceptability of many food products, such as cheese, yogurt, and pickled onions, are actually enhanced by the preservation process. These purposes are attained through one or more actions of the preservation process. They include reducing the existing pathogen load, altering the pH and temperature, lowering the oxygen content, reducing the water available for microbial growth, and providing a physical barrier to contamination.

Traditional food preservation techniques, aimed toward one or more of the above purposes, include the following: drying (reduces water necessary for microbial growth), refrigeration (slows microbial growth and enzymatic activity), freezing (preserves food for longer periods), salt or sugar curing (reduces water [especially in meats and fruit]), smoking (coats foods with natural antimicrobials), pickling and brining (reduces both aw and pH), canning and bottling (reduces oxygen and provides physical barrier to contamination), jellying (cooking in a medium that cools to form a gel [eg, aspic]; reduces aw), jugging (meats stewed in earthenware jugs or casseroles), burying (reduces aw, oxygen, light, temperature, and pH), and fermenting (adds beneficial microbes that successfully compete with pathogens; also lowers pH and adds alcohol).

More modern food preservation techniques are listed below.

1) Pasteurization is used mainly for dairy products and other liquid foods, and it can reduce microorganisms by 99.999%. In a "high temperature, short time" process, the product is held at 161°F for 15 sec. In an "ultra-high temperature" process, pasteurization is achieved after reaching 275°F for 2 sec. In a less conventional technique, home pasteurization involves holding the product at 145°F for 30 min. Finally, an "extended shelf life" process combines heating with filtration.

2) Vacuum packaging is usually in air-tight bags or bottles.

3) Additives typically involve the addition of antimicrobials to limit the growth of microorganisms or antioxidants to inhibit

Food irradiation radura. Since 1986, all food treated with irradiation must display this radura.

spoilage. Common antimicrobials include calcium propionate, sodium nitrate, sodium nitrite, disodium EDTA, and various sulfites. Common antioxidants include butylated hydroxyanisole (BHA), butylated hydroxytoluene (BHT), ascorbic acid (vitamin C), and tocopherol (vitamin E).

4) Irradiation, which is commonly termed "cold pasteurization," involves exposing the product to low-dose ionizing gamma rays from a radioactive source such as cesium (Cs-137) or cobalt (Co-60). The process does not render the food radioactive but results in the killing of nearly all surface pathogens. Commonly used for products such as spices and fruits, food irradiation is endorsed by the World Health Organization and approved by the FDA. Since 1986, all food treated with irradiation must display the radura.

5) Pulsed electric field electroporation consists of brief pulses of a strong electric field that enlarges cell membrane pores, which kills microorganisms. It is commonly used for fruit juices.

6) Modified atmosphere replaces oxygen with an inert gas such as nitrogen or carbon dioxide. It is commonly used for salads, grains, apples, bananas, and fish.

7) Nonthermal plasma treats food surfaces with "flame" of helium or nitrogen.

8) High pressurization reduces microorganisms while retaining freshness. It is commonly used for deli meats and guacamole.

9) Biopreservation is the addition of beneficial microbes such as *Lactobacillus* to compete with pathogens.

10) "Hurdle" technology combines multiple techniques to produce additive benefits. An example of placing multiple hurdles in such a combination might involve high temperature and salt curing during processing, addition of antioxidants before packaging, and low temperature during storage and transportation.

INCIDENCE AND IMPACT OF FOODBORNE DISEASES

The global burden of foodborne diseases is difficult to assess, because no overarching estimation has yet been performed. The World Health Organization has initiated this process but reports that efforts are limited by regional lack of funding, public health infrastructure, and political will. However, despite specific data, the burden seems obvious; diarrheal diseases, many of which are foodborne in origin, kill approximately 1.9 million children worldwide.

In the USA, the foodborne diseases are not generally reportable, so their burden likely is significantly underestimated. Contributing to this underestimation is that many foodborne illnesses lack the severity, duration, and specific diagnosis required for definitive identification and intervention. Recent estimates by the CDC indicate that foodborne pathogens cause approximately 9.6 million illnesses, 57,500 hospitalizations, and 1,500 deaths each year in the USA.

In an effort to maintain awareness of foodborne disease events and trends, CDC conducts the Foodborne Diseases Active Surveillance Network (FoodNet), which monitors the incidence of nine foodborne pathogens in ten USA cities, covering approximately 15% of the American population (*see* TABLE 3).

CDC reports that this epidemiologic situation has not changed appreciably since 2006, suggesting that there are gaps in the current food safety system and a need for better, more effective interventions.

Factors in Emerging Foodborne Illness Trends

Pathogenic organisms that contaminate food and result in foodborne illness are dynamic in that they adapt to new foods, processes, and human behaviors. The following categorical factors contribute to foodborne illness trends.

Human Demographics and Behavior: The proportion of the USA population that is immunocompromised is increasing because of factors such as advancing age, underlying disease, and therapeutic drug regimens. Additionally, people consume more fresh fruits and vegetables, which may be more contaminated than processed or prepared foods, and consume an increasing number of meals outside the home. Finally, "organic" foods have not been shown to be microbiologically safer and in some cases may even increase the risk from certain foodborne pathogens.

Technologies Within the Food Industry: Increasing concentration and vertical integration of many food produc-

TABLE 3 FOODBORNE PATHOGENS IN TEN USA CITIES

Pathogen	Incidence of Illness per 100,000 Population
Salmonella	15.19
Campylobacter	13.82
Shigella	4.82
Cryptosporidium	2.48
Shigatoxin-producing *E coli*	2.32
Vibrio	0.51
Yersinia	0.36
Listeria	0.26
Cyclospora	0.03

tion sectors have resulted in foods of higher quality and greater consistency but with certain inherent vulnerabilities. Foods (and constituent ingredients) are transported in larger batch sizes, over longer distances, and are processed into an increasing number of end products. This means that refrigeration breakdowns and cross-contamination incidents can result in more widespread effects of food recalls and illness outbreaks.

International Travel and Commerce: The concept of "traveler's diarrhea" is expanding because, increasingly, bulk food shipments cross international borders at least as often as people. Therefore, foodborne illnesses acquired from foreign foods can be contracted without leaving home. Additionally, when people travel, they frequently take cultural foods with them to share with extended family. Despite prohibitions against such importation practices, ~4,000 pounds of meat products are confiscated from travelers each month from Haiti to the USA. Undoubtedly, this represents only a fraction of the amount actually crossing the border.

Microbial Adaptation: Foodborne pathogens have inexorably adapted to traditional preservation techniques. Others may even be selected by various techniques. Finally, antimicrobial resistance patterns change constantly, requiring correspondingly dynamic interventions.

Economic Development and Land Use: USDA reports a continuing decrease in the number of farms in the USA, with the average number of livestock animals on remaining farms increasing. This concentrates the number of animals that may be affected, both by contagious pathogens and by interventions such as quarantines and depopulation efforts. Increases in ocean water temperature have been associated with increases in the number and scope of foodborne illnesses from certain seafood products such as oysters.

Lack of Food Safety Education: Health classes at the intermediate and high school levels rarely, if ever, cover food safety in favor of topics such as sexually transmitted diseases, drug abuse, and teen pregnancy. With the increasing fraction of two-worker and single-parent homes, time demands may also preclude education of children in food safety principles and further contribute to the lack of awareness.

ROLE OF FOOD ANIMAL VETERINARIANS IN CONTROL OF FOODBORNE PATHOGENS

Veterinarians in food animal practice and government service contribute significantly to the safety of the food supply. These roles can be categorized by stage of production (eg, antemortem, postmortem, and general).

Antemortem activities include assurance of animal welfare, zoonotic disease recognition and prevention, inspection of preslaughter animals, and antibiotic residue testing.

Postmortem activities include carcass inspection and tissue residue determination.

General activities begin with herd health programs, including disease treatment and prevention, husbandry/handling/environmental advice, reproductive efficiency, vaccination regimens, nutrition, stress reduction, commodity group protocols (eg, Beef Quality Assurance), and biosecurity and biocontainment plans. In addition to herd health, other important activities include appropriate/judicious use of antimicrobials, disease surveillance, illness/outbreak/epidemic investigation and mitigation, vaccination against specific high-consequence or high-prevalence pathogens (eg, *E coli* O157:H7 and *Salmonella*), collaboration with other health professionals (One Health), food facility inspection (eg, production, retail, storage), import/export examinations, health department leadership, public health (risk) communication, food supply after disasters, and research into safer food production processes.

FOOD SAFETY REGULATION

In the USA, food safety is a shared responsibility at various governmental and private levels. Federal departments and agencies have regulatory authority over virtually all food products. State and local governments typically are responsible for sanitary inspections of restaurants and food preparation sites. Food industry sectors have internal quality control procedures to ensure both safe products and adherence to regulatory requirements. Finally, informed consumers are charged with the safe storage, preparation, and service of privately obtained foods.

At the federal level, responsibilities are shared between Congress, various regulatory agencies, and the court system. Congress enacts statutes that give agencies authority to regulate food safety and enforce those regulations. Typically, these *statutes* are specific in identifying individual agencies but broad in allowing discretion in how those agencies exercise their authority. Finally, the courts review challenges to statutes, regulations, and enforcement actions.

Department of Agriculture: The Department of Agriculture consists of the Food Safety and Inspection Service (FSIS) and the Animal and Plant Health Inspection Service (APHIS). The FSIS is the primary food regulatory agency within USDA, domestic and imported (and employs most of the veterinarians in federal service). FSIS responsibilities include inspecting food animals for disease before and after slaughter; inspecting meat and poultry slaughter and processing plants; inspecting domestic and imported meat and poultry products (raw and processed); inspecting processed egg products (liquid, dried, and frozen but not eggs in shells); analyzing food products for microbial, chemical, and toxicologic agents; seeking voluntary recalls of unsafe meat and poultry products; conducting and sponsoring research on meat and poultry safety, and educating industry and consumers on safe food handling practices.

APHIS is responsible for livestock production and transport (preslaughter); inspection and quarantine at U.S. Ports of Entry; and veterinary services, including surveillance and disease control/eradication programs, as well as representing USA animal agriculture internationally.

Department of Health and Human Services (DHHS): The Food and Drug Administration (FDA) and the Centers for Disease Control and Prevention (CDC) are within DHHS.

The FDA is the primary food regulatory agency within DHHS. It is responsible for domestic and imported food sold in interstate commerce, including shell eggs (but not meat and poultry), bottled water, wine beverages <7% alcohol, livestock feeds, veterinary drugs, infant formulas, and dietary supplements; adulteration and misbranding of foods, drugs, and cosmetics; inspection of food production establishments and warehouses for contamination by microbial, chemical, and toxicologic agents; and HACCP programs for seafood products and fruit/vegetable juices. The FDA also works with industry to recall unsafe food products, as well as conducts research and educates industry and consumers.

The CDC investigates foodborne illness outbreaks (in conjunction with states), maintains nationwide disease surveillance (FoodNet), develops and advocates for public health policies, conducts research and educational programs in foodborne illness, and trains state and local food safety personnel.

The CDC also operates the Division of Global Migration and Quarantine, which is the enforcement authority for International Health Regulations. This Division investigates deaths and disease outbreaks on all international vessels (commercial and cruise ships and aircraft) and is responsible for quarantine stations at major international ports of entry to intercept/destroy smuggled bushmeat, vector species, and other contraband of public health concern.

In addition, the CDC operates the Cruise Ship Inspection Service, which is an enforcement authority responsible for sanitary inspection of cruise ships.

Department of Defense: The DoD is responsible for emergency food supplies, research activities on military food rations (many civilian applications), and approves food and water sources for all military bases.

Department of Homeland Security: The DHS prevents terrorist attacks on USA soil (to include foodborne, crop, livestock) and ostensibly has primary authority during attack and response phases.

Department of Commerce: The DoC is responsible for management of living marine resources, including fisheries.

Environmental Protection Agency: The EPA has authority over pesticides, herbicides, and fungicides. The EPA determines the safety of pesticides and sets tolerance levels in foods, regulates toxic substances to prevent entry into food and the environment, and establishes and enforces safe drinking water standards.

PUBLIC HEALTH LAW

The U.S. Constitution makes no specific provision for health or public health. Therefore, in accordance with the Tenth Amendment, these powers are reserved by the states. However, a salient exemption from this federal exclusion is represented by the concept of legal preemption. Rooted in the "Supremacy Clause" of the Constitution (Article VI), preemption occurs when a state law is invalidated after being determined to conflict with a federal law. In the absence of a federal declaration of emergency, federal preemption is rare; one example is the federally enacted Airline Smoking Ban.

Primary Sources of State Public Health Authority

Police Power: Authority of "police power" usually is invoked to protect the common good. Not synonymous with criminal enforcement, this authority establishes means by which a community promulgates and enforces self-protective measures. Examples include regulation of health care professionals and facilities; establishment of health and safety standards; quarantine, health, and inspection laws to limit the spread of infectious diseases; mandatory vaccination programs; age restrictions for drinking alcohol and purchasing tobacco products; and requirements for speed limits, seatbelts, and helmets.

***Parens Patriae* Power:** This is the power of the state to serve as guardian of persons under legal disability. Examples include juveniles and the insane.

State Constitutional Power: These authorities are granted under each individual state constitution (varies by state).

After the terrorist attacks of September 11, 2001, the "Amerithrax" attacks, natural disasters such as Hurricane Katrina, the severe acute respiratory syndrome (SARS) outbreak, and pandemic influenza, the federal government strengthened its legal preparedness for all types of public health emergencies. These activities addressed a variety of concerns related to emergency declarations, quarantine and isolation, licensure and liability of health care workers, and mutual aid.

Selected General Federal Emergency Legal Authorities

Homeland Security Act of 2002: This Act merged 22 disparate agencies and organizations into the new Department of Homeland Security (DHS), including the U.S. Coast Guard and the Federal Emergency Management Agency (FEMA). The Act charged DHS with securing the nation against terrorist attacks and carrying out the functions of all transferred entities, including acting as a focal point regarding natural and manmade crises and emergency planning.

Robert T. Stafford Disaster Relief and Emergency Assistance Act of 1988: The Stafford Act authorizes the President to declare a "major disaster" or "emergency" in response to an event (or threat) that overwhelms state or local government resources. Declaration under the Act triggers access to federal technical, financial, logistical, and other assistance to state and local governments. The governor of an affected state must first respond to the disaster and execute the state's emergency plan before requesting that the President declare a major disaster or emergency, and the governor must certify that the magnitude of the emergency exceeds the state's capability. As of 2013, tribal leaders can also request a Stafford Act declaration from the President. The President may declare an emergency without the request of a governor or tribal leader if the emergency involves "federal primary responsibility" (such as an event occurring on federal property, eg, the bombing of the Murrah Federal Building in 1995).

National Emergencies Act: This Act authorizes the President to declare a "national emergency." The declaration of emergency must specify the powers or authorities made available by virtue of the declaration.

Emergency Management Assistance Compact (EMAC) of 1996: Enacted by every state, this agreement facilitates resource sharing among member states during an emergency. A governor's declaration of emergency and request for assistance triggers EMAC for the requesting state. An assisting state then responds to the request by providing the needed resources. Further, EMAC establishes that the requesting state is responsible for compensating the assisting state for any expenses incurred.

Public Health Service Act: Originally enacted in 1944, this Act has been amended several times to facilitate various types of responses, listed below.

Public Health Emergencies: Authorizes the Secretary of DHHS to determine that a public health emergency exists if "1) a disease or disorder presents a public health emergency; or 2) a public health emergency, including significant outbreaks of infectious diseases or bioterrorist attacks, otherwise exists."

General Grant of Authority for Cooperation: This grant states that the Secretary of DHHS shall assist states and local authorities to prevent and suppress communicable diseases and to help state and local authorities enforce quarantine regulations.

Strategic National Stockpile: The Stockpile (including drugs, vaccines, biologic products, medical devices, and other supplies) is maintained by the Secretary of DHHS, in collaboration with Director of the CDC, and in coordination with the Secretary of DHS, to provide for the emergency health security of the USA. The Secretary may deploy stockpile assets in response to an actual or potential public health emergency to protect public health or safety, or as required by the Secretary of DHS.

Bioterrorism Preparedness and Response Act of 2002: This Act amends the Public Health Service Act to "improve the ability of the United States to prevent, prepare for, and respond to bioterrorism and other public health emergencies." The Act requires the Secretary of DHHS to "develop and implement" a coordinated strategy in the form of a national preparedness plan.

Regulations to Control Communicable Diseases: Regulations to control communicable diseases authorize the Secretary of DHHS to make and enforce regulations "to prevent the introduction, transmission, or spread of communicable diseases" into the USA from foreign countries or from one state into another. These regulations also authorize the apprehension, detention, examination, and conditional release of individuals with certain communicable diseases that are specified in an executive order of the President.

Executive Order 13295 (Amended): Revised List of Quarantinable Communicable Diseases: This Executive Order identifies the nine communicable diseases (cholera, diphtheria, infectious tuberculosis, plague, smallpox, yellow fever, viral hemorrhagic fevers, severe acute respiratory syndrome [SARS], and pandemic influenza), for which an individual can be apprehended, detained, examined, or conditionally released by federal public health authorities.

Interstate Quarantine (42 CFR, Part 70): This allows the CDC Director to take measures to prevent the spread of communicable diseases from one state into another, including in the event the Director determines that the measures taken by the health authorities of a state are insufficient to prevent such spread of communicable disease.

Pandemic and All-Hazards Preparedness Act of 2006: This Act identifies the Secretary of DHHS as the lead federal official for public health emergency preparedness and response. It also provides new authorities to develop countermeasures, establishes mechanisms and grants to continue strengthening state and local public health security infrastructure, and addresses surge capacity by placing the National Disaster Medical System under the purview of DHHS.

Social Security Act: Authority to Waive Requirements During National Emergencies: This authorizes the Secretary of DHHS to waive or modify certain requirements of Medicare, Medicaid, and the State Children's Health Insurance Program during certain emergencies.

Public Readiness and Emergency Preparedness Act of 2005: This Act authorizes the Secretary of DHHS to issue a declaration that provides immunity from tort liability for claims of loss (except willful misconduct) caused by, arising out of, relating to, or resulting from administration or use of countermeasures to diseases, threats, and conditions determined by the Secretary to constitute a present or credible risk of a future public health emergency.

Emergency Use Authorization: The Secretary of DHHS may, based on the request of the Secretary of either DHS, DoD, or DHS, declare that circumstances exist to justify an Emergency Use Authorization (EUA) for an unapproved drug, device, or biologic product, or for an unapproved use of an approved drug, device, or biologic product.

Pandemic and All-Hazards Preparedness Reauthorization Act of 2013: This Act established streamlined mechanisms to facilitate certain medical countermeasure preparedness and response activities without having to issue an EUA (which can be a time- and resource-intensive process). These new authorities are focused toward medical products against chemical, biologic, radiologic, and nuclear emergencies.

Volunteer Protection Act of 1997: This Act supports and promotes the activities of organizations that rely on volunteers by providing the volunteers some protections from liability for economic damages for activities relating to the work of the organizations. Under the Act, to be found not liable for the injury caused by a negligent act or omission of the volunteer, the volunteer must have been acting within the scope of his or her responsibilities in the nonprofit or government agency. The volunteer must have appropriate licensure or certification if required for the volunteer's duties; he or she must not have acted with gross negligence, reckless disregard, willful or criminal misconduct, or flagrant indifference; and the injury cannot have occurred while the volunteer was intoxicated.

***Posse Comitatus* Act of 1878:** This Act generally prohibits the use of federal military personnel in a law enforcement capacity within the USA unless authorized by the U.S. Constitution or an act of Congress. Certain exceptions exist, such as when the Department of Defense aids the Department of Justice in responding to an emergency situation involving a weapon of mass destruction.

Insurrection Act of 1807: This Act grants authority to the President to call the National Guard into federal service in the event of an insurrection in any state or if a state fails to uphold the constitutional rights of its citizens.

ZOOEYIA

Zooeyia is defined as "the positive inverse of zoonosis" and represents the innumerable benefits that stem from human interaction with animals. (*See also* THE HUMAN-ANIMAL BOND, p 1575.) Too often, that interaction focuses on negative issues such as disease and injury rather than on the positive contributions to our physical, mental, and social well-being. These contributions are manifested at both the individual and community levels. Documented individual benefits of interaction with animals include increased physical activity, smoking cessation, hypertension control, reduced anxiety, and treatment of post-traumatic stress disorder. Interaction with domestic animals contributes at the community level by facilitating social interaction, promoting a sense of safety, enhancing the "give and take" communication between neighbors and fellow pet owners, and perhaps even lowering overall health care costs.

ZOONOSES

Zoonotic diseases present challenges not only to veterinarians but also to all professions concerned with public health. Cooperation between veterinarians and public health physicians has been an important factor in zoonosis control programs. An example of this collaboration is the eradication of bovine tuberculosis, first in Denmark, Sweden, Finland, and Norway, and then in the USA, Canada, and other countries. Unfortunately, some zoonoses that are well controlled in developed nations, such as bovine and porcine brucellosis, bovine tuberculosis, and rabies, remain major problems in the developing world. Diseases can also reemerge in areas where they have been eradicated. Newly recognized zoonotic organisms such as Hendra and Nipah viruses are emerging, and many other zoonoses remain a constant concern.

The occurrence of a pathogen in both people and animals does not always mean it is a significant zoonosis. Some diseases are acquired from the environment, and transmission between animal or human hosts is either absent, or occurs very rarely and under unusual conditions. These are considered infections common to people and animals rather than true zoonoses. Histoplasmosis, blastomycosis, and coccidioidomycosis, for example, are acquired by inhaling the microconidia of soil fungi, but the organisms exist as yeasts in tissues. Some agents, such as *Candida* spp, are widespread commensals in healthy people and animals and can cause disease when the host becomes debilitated. Although such organisms might be transmitted from animals to people, this transfer has little epidemiologic significance. In some cases, organisms were once thought to be zoonotic, but current knowledge, particularly the use of genetic techniques, has changed that perception. For example, *Streptococcus agalactiae* was once thought to be acquired from animals, but most strains in people are now known to be distinct from animal strains. There are also some organisms (eg, simian foamy viruses) that can be transmitted from animals to people, but with no currently known consequences.

PATHOGENS AND HOST SPECIES

Zoonotic diseases can be caused by bacteria, viruses, fungi, parasites, or prions. Because organisms are more readily transmitted between closely related hosts, most of these agents are pathogens of mammals. A particularly large number of diseases are shared by people and nonhuman primates. Birds, reptiles, amphibians, fish, and invertebrates can also be sources of infection (*see* TABLE 4). Many of the zoonotic agents in poikilotherms are parasitic, but these species can also carry zoonotic bacteria and viruses including *Salmonella*, West Nile virus, and opportunistic *Mycobacterium* spp. People are incidental hosts for many zoonoses; however, some agents have both human and animal reservoirs. In some cases, animal reservoirs have been revealed after a disease was controlled in people. Yellow fever, for example, is known to have a zoonotic jungle cycle in nonhuman primates, as well as an urban cycle maintained in people. Wildlife is increasingly recognized as a reservoir for zoonoses, including some that were thought to be strictly livestock pathogens. Reverse zoonoses are caused by human pathogens transmitted *to animals*. In some cases, these agents can later infect people. For example, *Mycobacterium tuberculosis*, the agent of human tuberculosis, can colonize the bovine udder and be shed in milk.

TRANSMISSION BETWEEN ANIMALS AND PEOPLE

Zoonotic pathogens can be acquired during close contact with an animal, generally through inhalation, ingestion, or other mechanisms resulting in the contamination of mucous membranes, damaged skin, or in some cases, intact skin. Sources of organisms include body fluids, secretions and excretions, and lesions. Unprotected contact with tissues during necropsies often carries a high risk of transmission. Aerosols are occasionally involved, particularly in confined spaces. Fomites can transmit some agents; the likelihood of this route correlates with the organism's persistence in the environment. Some organisms are spread by ingestion of contaminated food or water and may infect large numbers of people. Sources of zoonotic pathogens in foodborne disease include undercooked meat or other animal tissues (including seafood and invertebrates), unpasteurized milk and dairy products, and contaminated vegetables. Insect vectors, serving as either biologic or mechanical vectors, are important in transmitting some organisms.

The risk of acquiring a zoonosis can be affected by many factors, including the susceptibility of the host (*see* p 2415), the potential route(s) of transmission, the number of organisms shed by the animal, and the ability of the agent to cross species barriers. Some pathogens, such as *Bacillus anthracis*, readily infect people with appropriate exposure; others are uncommon zoonoses even when exposure is frequent. Certain occupations or activities can significantly increase the probability of exposure. Contact with soil during gardening or childhood play carries a risk of infection with pathogens that reside temporarily or permanently in the soil, such as *Toxocara* spp or *Sporothrix schenckii*. Veterinary practice, agricultural activities, and pet ownership are obvious hazards. Dogs, cats, livestock, or birds may also bring wildlife pathogens into closer proximity to people. The animal can be infected directly with the agent, either clinically or subclinically, or it may act as a transport host for infected arthropods such as ticks. Nontraditional pets have a relatively high probability of being infected with zoonotic agents, especially when captured directly from the wild. During an outbreak of monkeypox in the USA, the virus spread from exotic African rodents, imported as pets, to pet prairie dogs and then to people. Activities that bring people into closer contact with wildlife, including hunting, fishing, and camping, can result in exposure to organisms carried in wild animals (eg, *Francisella tularensis*, *Yersinia pestis*, and *Leptospira* spp) or transmitted by arthropod vectors (eg, *Borrelia burgdorferi* and West Nile virus). Hunters, in particular, may contact pathogens in animal tissues during butchering. The growing popularity of ecotourism has resulted in human exposure to some exotic wildlife diseases. The prevalence of other zoonoses may be linked to cultural practices such as eating raw fish, gastropods, or mollusks. Knowledge of a person's leisure and vocational activities, travel, and pet ownership can sometimes raise the index of suspicion for zoonoses that are uncommon in urban populations.

Once a zoonotic disease has been acquired by a person, it can sometimes be transmitted from person to person. The risk varies with the specific disease, the agent's ability to spread readily in people, and the routes of transmission. Often, the people most at risk are health care workers and close family members. However, diseases such as plague have the potential to spread widely in human populations under some conditions. Some zoonotic diseases are not contagious during casual contact but can be spread by transfusion or organ transplantation, or from mother to fetus in utero. A particularly wide variety of agents, from encysted parasites to latent viruses, are potentially transferable in organs. Agents that were well controlled in the organ donor can be reactivated in the recipient, who is immunosuppressed by drugs taken to prevent rejection. Transfusion can also bypass normal barriers if the agent is found in the blood at the time of the donation. The bovine spongiform encephalopathy agent, for example, is ordinarily transmitted from host to host only by ingestion of tissues, but it can be acquired in transfused blood.

ROLE OF IMMUNOSUPPRESSION

The spectrum of zoonotic illness varies from skin eruptions or mild, self-limiting infections easily misdiagnosed as human influenza to serious, life-threatening disease. Some zoonoses can affect healthy people, whereas others are primarily found in individuals with debilitating illnesses and other conditions that compromise immunity. Zoonoses that are mild or asymptomatic in healthy hosts can be serious illnesses or have unusual presentations in those who are immunocompromised. In some cases, a suppressed immune response may also slow diagnosis if common tests rely on serology.

Primary immunodeficiencies, which are congenital defects, may affect humoral or cell-mediated immunity, or both. Some primary immunodeficiencies increase susceptibility to a single category of pathogens, while others broadly suppress defenses. Some may remain unnoticed except as an unusual susceptibility to certain illnesses, whereas others are obvious from infancy. Secondary immunodeficiencies can be caused by any acquired condition that compromises the immune system. Examples include splenectomy, diseases that affect metabolism (eg, diabetes), illnesses such as cancer that result in generalized debilitation, and infections such as malaria or AIDS. Some illnesses, such as chronic lung disease, can increase susceptibility by affecting innate (nonspecific) defenses. Injuries and burns can compromise the skin defenses that prevent pathogens from entering the body, as can indwelling catheters and implanted medical devices. Drugs can suppress immunity as an intended effect (eg, drugs used to treat autoimmune diseases or prevent rejection in organ transplant patients) or as an adverse effect. Some drugs used in cancer chemotherapy are highly immunosuppressive. (*See also* IMMUNOLOGIC DISEASES, p 817.)

Physiologic states can also affect immunity. The immune system is relatively immature in newborns and young children, and it declines in older adults. Pregnancy may result in risks to the mother, the fetus, or both. For example, in some geographic locations, the case fatality rate for hepatitis E is ~1% in the general population but may reach 20% among pregnant women. Other pathogens, such as *Toxoplasma gondii*, may severely damage the fetus while remaining mild in the mother.

EMERGENCE AND REEMERGENCE OF ZOONOTIC DISEASES

Emerging diseases are commonly defined as illnesses that have increased in incidence during the past two decades or are likely to increase in the near future. Many of these diseases are zoonotic. A zoonotic disease can emerge as the result of increased human contact with the animal host(s), animal tissues, vectors, or environmental sources of the pathogens. It may also result from an increased prevalence of the agent in domesticated or wild animals or in vectors. Many currently emerging and reemerging diseases have reservoirs in wildlife and/or are foodborne.

Factors that can cause emergence include altered human demographics or behavior, ranging from societal upheavals that cause people to leave urban areas to simple changes in food preferences. For example, the popularity of prewashed greens can facilitate some outbreaks of *E coli* O157:H7. Breakdowns in public health measures such as sanitation and vaccination also increase the spread of disease. Changing land use patterns may alter the number of reservoir hosts, increase the incidence of infection in these animals, encourage genetic changes in the pathogen (eg, recombination with other strains), or bring animal hosts or disease vectors into closer contact with people. Because many mosquitoes preferentially breed along the edges of forests rather than deep among the trees, deforestation can increase populations of these species. Degradation of their natural habitats, as well as the ready availability of food near human dwellings, can encourage wildlife to move into suburban areas. The growth of the human population also exerts pressures that ultimately result in increased contact with wildlife. Climate change can be a factor in disease emergence, particularly for arthropodborne pathogens such as *Rickettsia* spp. A warmer climate not only allows vectors to survive the winter but also permits a longer transmission season. Climate changes may also favor some non-arthropodborne diseases; for example, increased rainfall has been linked to outbreaks of plague in some areas.

Technologic and industrial changes in food production can contribute to disease emergence by increasing the concentration, movement, and mixing of animals. Long-distance transport has been associated with increased shedding of enteric pathogens, including *Salmonella*. Decreased genetic diversity may eliminate species, breeds, or individuals with innate resistance to a disease. The development of large-scale farms and food-processing facilities has led to the exposure of greater numbers of people to a contaminated food source. Increased mobility of people, animals, and goods allows diseases to spread quickly. Viruses that formerly died out after affecting small numbers of animals and/or people can now find many susceptible hosts within a short period. The SARS coronavirus spread to 30 countries on 6 continents within months of the initial outbreak. Occasionally, the pathogen itself may become more virulent or better adapted to people, or it may undergo changes that affect transmission patterns. More virulent strains of the West Nile virus have emerged since the 1980s, and a new variant, which can replicate more rapidly in mosquitoes, has become established in North America.

Some diseases are emerging not because they are more common but because they are better recognized. Increased recognition can result from improved diagnostic techniques, increased use of laboratories for identification of specific pathogens, and better awareness among physicians. Some spotted fever *Rickettsia* spp are emerging, in part, because the increased use of molecular techniques facilitates their identification. Marburg virus, once thought to be a very rare and less virulent relative of ebolaviruses, was recently found to have caused hemorrhagic disease in workers at one African mine since the 1980s or earlier. This focus of bat-transmitted infections was only recognized when highly fatal outbreaks affected hundreds of people in the Democratic Republic of the Congo in 1998–2000.

Increased human susceptibility has contributed to the emergence or recognition of some opportunistic pathogens. The number of immunocompromised people has been increased by factors such as the AIDS epidemic, the success of organ transplantation programs, and the improved survival of those with primary and secondary immunodeficiencies. Modern medicine also allows more people, many of whom develop chronic conditions, to survive to an advanced age.

TREATMENT

The treatment of zoonotic and nonzoonotic diseases of animals is similar; however, treatments that prolong the shedding of zoonotic organisms should be avoided unless there are overriding considerations. For example, antibiotic treatment is usually contraindicated in uncomplicated *Salmonella*-associated diarrhea, because these drugs may prolong shedding of this organism. Conversely, animals that carry zoonotic organisms may sometimes be treated to reduce human exposure, even when the infection is subclinical or expected to be self-limiting, such as a minor skin lesion caused by dermatophytes. During treatment of zoonotic diseases, every precaution should be taken to prevent human infection. Professional judgment is required to determine whether to keep the animal in its home environment or isolate it in a hospital ward. Factors to consider include the potential severity of the disease in people, the susceptibility of individuals in the household, and the ability of human caregiver(s) to effectively perform barrier nursing, sanitation, and hygiene protocols. The owner should always be informed if treatment is not certain to eliminate the pathogen, which could then persist in a latent or chronic, subclinical form. Zoonotic concerns may dictate euthanasia of the animal, especially when the disease is likely to be fatal.

People who may have contracted a zoonotic disease should be referred to their physician for diagnosis and treatment. The physician should be given any information necessary to facilitate diagnosis, particularly if the disease is unusual and would not ordinarily be among the differential diagnoses. Simultaneous elimination of the pathogen from both animal and human hosts is ideal, to prevent it from cycling between the hosts. Public health authorities must be contacted when a reportable zoonotic disease (eg, rabies) is found in an animal.

PREVENTION

People can be protected from some zoonoses by eliminating the pathogen from its animal reservoir(s). In some countries, livestock diseases such as bovine and porcine brucellosis and bovine tuberculosis have been eradicated, and the prevalence of *Salmonella* in poultry has been significantly reduced. Vaccination (eg, rabies), treatment of clinical cases, flea and tick control, periodic testing for enteric parasites or other pathogens, and other disease control measures in domestic animals can also protect people. Human vaccines are available for a few diseases, and arthropod control measures decrease the risk of vectorborne infections.

Foodborne zoonoses can often be interrupted by using good sanitation and hygiene during food preparation, eliminating cross-contamination of foods, cooking all foods of animal origin (including invertebrates such as mollusks and snails) to safe temperatures, and thoroughly washing vegetables shortly before eating. Prions cannot be destroyed by cooking; meat inspection and elimination of the pathogen from animals remain the only ways to reduce the risks from these agents. Modern water treatment procedures eliminate most waterborne zoonoses. Where such facilities are unavailable, drinking water should be boiled, filtered, or otherwise treated to remove pathogens. Accidental ingestion of lake or stream water should be avoided. The contamination of irrigation water used for agriculture has become an increasing concern with the rise of pathogens such as enterohemorrhagic *Escherichia coli* (eg, *E coli* O157:H7). Measures such as composting livestock manure before spreading it on fields may lower the risks from this source. However, post-harvest procedures to eliminate contamination are also critical.

It is often difficult to avoid diseases acquired from the environment. However, measures to eliminate skin contact with soil, such as wearing gloves when gardening and avoiding dust inhalation, are helpful.

During contact with apparently healthy animals, good hygiene (including hand washing) is an important preventive measure. Hand washing is particularly important before eating or any other hand-to-mouth contact. In fairs, petting zoos, or other environments where the public may contact animals, hand-washing facilities should be provided, and eating or drinking in the animal areas should be discouraged. Children <5 yr old should be supervised closely; their immune systems are generally more vulnerable to pathogens, they are less likely to follow sanitary precautions, and they are more likely to engage in risky behaviors such as tasting dirt. Detailed zoonosis control programs for various types of facilities have been published.

Protective measures in veterinary hospitals include barrier precautions (including gloves, protective outerwear, and other personal protective equipment as appropriate), good hygiene, sanitation and disinfection, appropriate disposal of infectious material, and use of isolation units for animals with known zoonoses.

Prevention in Immunocompromised Populations: Counseling immunocompromised owners must strike a balance between awareness of the risks from zoonoses and acknowledgement of the human-animal bond and the psychologic benefits of animal companionship. If the person chooses to have a pet, the veterinarian can help make that decision as safe as possible. Topics to discuss include the risks from feeding raw meat or eggs, the prevention of garbage eating and coprophagia in dogs, the importance of flea and tick control, and the dangers of allowing cats and dogs to hunt. Pets should not be allowed to drink nonpotable water, including water from lakes or streams and water from toilet bowls. Claws should be kept clipped short to reduce the risk of scratches, and rough play that might encourage biting or scratching should be avoided. Regular and thorough cleaning of bedding and cages prevents the accumulation of debris that can shelter microorganisms. Owners should be counseled to avoid any direct contact with feces, as well as to practice excellent hygiene when handling the pet. The litter box should be cleaned daily, preferably by a household member who is not immunocompromised, to reduce the risk of toxoplasmosis. Similarly, cleaning aquariums carries the risk of exposure to *Mycobacterium marinum* and is best done by a healthy individual. Regular veterinary visits, with periodic screening for intestinal parasites and/or other zoonotic pathogens as appropriate, are essential for all pets. Pets that develop diarrhea or other diseases should be brought in promptly for diagnosis.

Any new pet should be examined by a veterinarian to ensure it is not carrying intestinal parasites, mites, dermatophytes, or other zoonotic pathogens. A healthy, unstressed adult dog or cat with a known history and no recent exposure to environments with high concentrations of pathogens is preferable to a puppy or kitten. Immunocompromised persons should avoid contact with reptiles, baby chicks, or ducklings, all of which may shed *Salmonella*. Some amphibians and exotic mammalian pets may also have a higher likelihood of carrying *Salmonella*. Avoidance of strays, wildlife, nonhuman primates, and animals with diarrhea or any other illness is particularly important. It is also prudent to stay away from animals in fairs, petting zoos, farms, schools, and

TABLE 4 GLOBAL ZOONOSES[a]

Disease	Causative Organism	Animals Involved
	BACTERIAL DISEASES	
Actinomycosis (*see* p 590)	*Actinomyces bovis* and other species in animals may affect people, but most human infections are caused by commensals of people, especially *Actinomyces israelii*	Mammals
Anthrax (*see* p 593)	*Bacillus anthracis*	Mainly in cattle, sheep, goats, horses, wild herbivorous animals; virtually all mammals and some birds are susceptible to high dose

similar settings, and to take additional precautions if avoidance is impractical.

Veterinarians have a vital role in educating immunocompromised owners on the risks from zoonotic diseases, as well as the steps that can be taken to decrease risk. Educational materials such as signs and brochures may prompt owners to ask for advice. Educational materials can also be used to warn pregnant women of the risks from toxoplasmosis and other zoonotic pathogens, or to remind owners that their veterinarian can provide help with safe pet selection and zoonosis prevention in households with children. Guidelines on zoonosis prevention for therapy animals used in hospitals and convalescent homes have also been published.

ZOONOTIC DISEASES

TABLE 4 lists zoonotic bacterial, viral, fungal, and parasitic diseases, grouped by category. Many proven zoonoses, including some diseases that are rare in people, organisms that are maintained primarily in people, some primate diseases, and diseases caused by fish and reptile toxins have been omitted. The table is intended to give a general clinical picture of each disease; current medical texts or review articles should be consulted for a more complete description. Clinical signs are listed; asymptomatic infections can also be assumed to occur in most cases. An indication of the mortality rate among healthy individuals has been provided for many infections. However, there is almost always a chance of death whenever lesions can become generalized, vital organs may be affected, secondary infections occur, and/or the patient is immunosuppressed. The mortality rate is often influenced by the availability of medical care, and it is generally lower when advanced medical support is available. The risk of death from some bacterial diseases with high mortality rates can be nearly eliminated with prompt antibiotic treatment.

If a disease is known to have unusual manifestations or to be particularly common and/or severe in immunocompromised people, this has been noted. In addition to these diseases, many pathogens can cause more severe disease and/or unusual signs in immunocompromised patients. Information on the geographic range of an organism should be taken as a rough guide. The precise ranges of many pathogens have not been completely determined. Organisms may also expand their range or be eradicated from areas where they were once abundant. In this table, "worldwide" indicates those organisms that are widespread and found on all major continents, although they may absent from some areas (eg, polar regions or some islands). In some cases, organisms indicated as being present on a continent may nevertheless have a limited distribution.

TABLE 4 GLOBAL ZOONOSES[a] *(continued)*

Known Distribution	Probable Means of Spread to People	Clinical Manifestations in People
	BACTERIAL DISEASES	
Worldwide; very rare in people	Probably contact; actinomycosis usually disseminates from endogenous human flora	Granulomas, abscesses, skin lesions; chronic bronchopneumonia; abdominal mass that may mimic a tumor; endocarditis; sepsis
Worldwide but distribution is focal; common in Africa, Asia, South America, Middle East, parts of Europe	Occupational contact exposure (abraded skin, mechanical transmission by biting flies, other routes); ingestion/foodborne, rarely airborne	Early signs vary with route of inoculation; papule to ulcerative skin lesions; mild to severe gastroenteritis ± hematemesis, bloody diarrhea, ascites (abdominal GI form); sore throat, dysphagia, fever, neck swelling, mouth lesions (oropharyngeal GI form); pneumonia; all may progress to sepsis, meningitis; untreated cases fatal in 5%–20% (cutaneous) to 100% (inhalation)

(continued)

TABLE 4 GLOBAL ZOONOSES[a] *(continued)*

Disease	Causative Organism	Animals Involved
	BACTERIAL DISEASES (continued)	
Arcobacter infections	*Arcobacter butzleri*, *A cryaerophilus*, *A skirrowii*, possibly others	Poultry, cattle, pigs, sheep, horses, shellfish; some studies detected these organisms in dogs and/or cats
Bordetellosis (*see* p 1464 and p 1491)	*Bordetella bronchiseptica*	Dogs, rabbits, cats, pigs, guinea pigs, other mammals
Borreliosis (*see* p 659)		
—Lyme disease	*Borrelia burgdorferi* sensu lato complex (*B burgdorferi* sensu stricto, *B garinii*, *B afzelii*, *B spielmanii*, *B japonica*)	Wild rodents, insectivores, hedgehogs, hares, other mammals; birds are reservoirs for agent; deer are hosts for tick vector only (blood meals)
—Tickborne relapsing fever	*B recurrentis*, *B crocidurae*, *B turicatae*, *B hermsii*, *B persica*, *B hispanica*, others; some species such as *B duttoni* are human pathogens and not zoonotic	Wild rodents, insectivores, possibly birds
—Southern tick-associated rash illness	Etiology uncertain; various *Borrelia* spp suggested	
Brucellosis (*see* p 1348 and p 1402)	*Brucella abortus*	Cattle, bison, water buffalo, African buffalo, elk, deer, sheep, goats, camels, South American camelids; other mammalian spillover hosts
	B melitensis	Goats, sheep, camels; other mammalian spillover hosts
	B suis biovars 1–4; biovar 5 has not been reported in people	Swine and wild pigs (biovars 1, 2, 3), European hares (biovar 2), reindeer and caribou (biovar 4); *B suis* also in some other mammals

TABLE 4 GLOBAL ZOONOSES[a] *(continued)*

Known Distribution	Probable Means of Spread to People	Clinical Manifestations in People
	BACTERIAL DISEASES (continued)	
Worldwide	Ingestion of contaminated water, undercooked meat (especially poultry) has been suggested	Gastroenteritis; bacteremia, mainly in patients with chronic illnesses; endocarditis, peritonitis; emerging and incompletely understood
Worldwide; uncommon in people	Exposure to saliva or sputum, aerosols	Sinusitis, bronchitis, pertussis-like illness; pneumonia and disseminated disease (eg, endocarditis, peritonitis, meningitis), usually in immunocompromised; wound infection
Agents exist worldwide where *Ixodes* ticks are found; human cases have been reported in North America, Europe, Australia, parts of Asia, Amazon region of South America	*Ixodes* spp bites	Nonspecific febrile illness early; target skin lesions in many; may progress to arthritis, neurologic, cardiac, and/ or skin signs (acrodermatitis chronica atrophicans); syndromes may vary with infecting agent
Africa, Asia, Europe, Americas; species varies with region	Tick bites (mainly *Ornithodoros* spp)	High fever, malaise, headache, myalgia, chills; neurologic signs or abortion possible; recurring episodes, often milder, after a symptom-free period; death in 2%–5%
USA; most cases in southeast	Tick bite (*Amblyomma americanum*)	Resembles Lyme disease
Once worldwide, now eradicated from domestic animals in some countries or regions; reservoirs in wildlife in some disease-free areas	Ingestion (especially unpasteurized dairy products or undercooked meat), contact with mucous membranes and broken skin; strain 19 vaccine	Extremely variable, subacute and undulant to sepsis; often nonspecific febrile illness with drenching sweats early; arthritis, spondylitis, epididymo-orchitis, endocarditis, neurologic, other syndromes if chronic; case fatality 5% in untreated
Asia, Africa, Middle East, Mexico, Central and South America, some parts of Europe	Ingestion (including unpasteurized dairy products or undercooked meat), contact with mucous membranes and broken skin; Rev 1 vaccine	As above; this species highly pathogenic for people
Biovars 1 and 3 worldwide in swine-raising regions except eradicated or nearly eradicated from domestic pigs in some countries; biovar 2 in wild boar in Europe; biovar 4 in Arctic	Ingestion, direct contact with mucous membranes and broken skin	As above

(continued)

TABLE 4 GLOBAL ZOONOSES[a] *(continued)*

Disease	Causative Organism	Animals Involved
BACTERIAL DISEASES (continued)		
Brucellosis *(continued)*	*B canis*	Dogs; evidence of infection in wild canids including coyotes, foxes
	B pinnipedialis and *B ceti*	Marine mammals
Campylobacter enteritis (*see* p 191)	*C jejuni*, *C coli*, occasionally other species; some strains of *C jejuni* seem to have broader host ranges than others	Poultry, cattle, swine, dogs, cats, rodents, other mammals, wild birds
Campylobacter fetus infection	*C fetus* subsp *fetus* (most cases), *C fetus* subsp *testudinum* (proposed name); possibly *C fetus* subsp *venerealis*	*C fetus* subsp *fetus* and *C* subsp *venerealis* in cattle, sheep, goats; *C fetus* subsp *testudinum* in reptiles
Capnocytophaga infection	*C canimorsus*, *C cynodegmi*	Dogs, cats
Cat scratch disease	*Bartonella henselae*; *B clarridgeiae* and other *Bartonella* species also implicated rarely in cat scratch disease or other conditions (eg, endocarditis)	Cats and other felids; other *Bartonella* spp in canids, rodents, rabbits, other animals
Chlamydiosis (*see also* PSITTACOSIS, p 2428)	*Chlamydia (Chlamydophila) abortus*, *C felis*	*C abortus* in sheep, goats, cattle, other mammals; *C felis* in cats
Clostridial diseases (*see* p 601)	*Clostridium difficile*; some ribotypes found in animals have been implicated as potential zoonoses	Ribotypes from some calves, pigs, dogs are identical to some ribotypes found in people

TABLE 4 GLOBAL ZOONOSES[a] *(continued)*

Known Distribution	Probable Means of Spread to People	Clinical Manifestations in People
	BACTERIAL DISEASES (continued)	
Worldwide; rare in people	Probably via ingestion or contact with mucous membranes, broken skin; close contact, especially with animals that recently aborted or gave birth	Probably as above
Atlantic, Arctic, and Pacific oceans; Mediterranean sea	Laboratory exposure; sources of other infections unknown (possibly contact with animals or exposure to seawater); rare or underdiagnosed in people	Few cases known: mild to severe febrile illness, similar to that caused by other *Brucella* spp; neurobrucellosis with headache and chronic neurologic signs; spinal osteomyelitis
Worldwide	Foodborne (especially poultry and other meats, unpasteurized dairy products); waterborne; contact with infected animals (fecal/oral)	Gastroenteritis from mild cases to fulminating or relapsing colitis; occasional sequelae such as reactive arthritis; occasionally, other syndromes, including sepsis
Worldwide	Probably direct contact or ingestion; often unknown	Opportunist; sepsis, meningitis, endocarditis, abscesses, other systemic infections in elderly, immunocompromised, or infants; abortions, preterm births in pregnant women, neonatal sepsis; gastroenteritis not prominent in most cases
Probably worldwide	Bites or scratches	Fever, localized infections to bacteremia or sepsis, endocarditis, meningitis; often in immunocompromised or elderly
Worldwide	Often associated with scratches, bites, especially from cats; potential for other exposures to broken skin via saliva; exposure of conjunctiva	Lymphadenopathy (may be absent in elderly), fever, malaise, skin lesions at inoculation site in immunocompetent, usually self-limiting with complications (eg, endocarditis, neuroretinitis, neurologic disease) uncommon; inoculation into eye results in conjunctivitis ± ocular granuloma and local lymphadenopathy; risk of bacteremia, disseminated disease, bacillary angiomatosis in immunosuppressed
C felis worldwide; *C abortus* in most sheep-raising areas but not Australia or New Zealand	Contact with animals; *C abortus* probably contact with pregnant or aborting ruminants	*C abortus*: abortions, septicemia; *C felis* suspected agent of keratoconjunctivitis, also implicated in other conditions (controversial)
Worldwide	Possible zoonosis; from contact or ingestion in contaminated meat; also from environment and contact with infected people	Gastroenteritis, varying in severity from diarrhea to fulminant colitis, usually in conjunction with antibiotic use

(continued)

TABLE 4 GLOBAL ZOONOSES[a] *(continued)*

Disease	Causative Organism	Animals Involved
	BACTERIAL DISEASES (continued)	
Clostridial diseases *(continued)*	*Clostridium perfringens*, type A (most common), C, or D; environmental or endogenous source, with some potential for zoonotic transmission	Domestic and wild animals, people
Corynebacterium ulcerans and *C pseudotuberculosis* infections	*C ulcerans*, *C pseudotuberculosis*	*C ulcerans* in cattle, pigs, small ruminants, dogs, cats, ferrets, other domestic and wild animals; *C pseudotuberculosis* in sheep, goats, cattle, horses, camelids, other mammals
Dermatophilosis (*see* p 858)	*Dermatophilus congolensis*	Cattle, horses, deer, sheep, goats, other mammals
Enterohemorrhagic *Escherichia coli* infections[b]	*E coli* O157:H7; also implicated are types O157:H, and members of serogroups O26, O103, O104, O111, O145, and others	Especially cattle, sheep; also goats, bison, deer, pigs, other species of mammals, birds
Erysipeloid (*see* p 625)	*Erysipelothrix rhusiopathiae*	Swine, sheep, cattle, rodents, marine mammals; many other domestic and wild mammals and marsupials, birds (including poultry), reptiles, fish, mollusks, crustaceans
Glanders (*see* p 706)	*Burkholderia mallei*	Equids are reservoirs; felids, many other domesticated and wild mammals also susceptible
Helicobacter infection	*H pullorum*, *H suis*, other species suspected as zoonoses	Poultry (*H pullorum*), rodents (*H pullorum* and other species), pigs (*H suis*), dogs (*H canis*), many other mammals

TABLE 4 GLOBAL ZOONOSES[a] (*continued*)

Known Distribution	Probable Means of Spread to People	Clinical Manifestations in People
	BACTERIAL DISEASES (continued)	
Worldwide	Foodborne (usually type A); nonfood-associated intestinal infection; wound contaminant, usually environmental; may be endogenous in debilitated from GI or urogenital tract	Foodborne gastroenteritis, usually brief, self-limited except in debilitated; nonfood-related intestinal infection with prolonged diarrhea, sometimes bloody, mainly in elderly after antibiotics; life-threatening necrotic enteritis, often in debilitated; gas gangrene, sepsis; necrotic enteritis, gas gangrene, sepsis are fatal if not treated
Probably worldwide; uncommon in people but may be increasing	Direct contact, consumption of unpasteurized milk products	Acute upper respiratory illness with sinusitis, sore throat, tonsillitis, or more severe pharyngitis resembling diphtheria (pseudomembranous pharyngitis); cardiorespiratory complications possible; peritonitis; isolated skin infection; some cases serious or fatal
Worldwide, especially in warmer regions	Usually direct contact with lesions; mechanical transmission on arthropod vectors, fomites possible	Pustular desquamative dermatitis, other skin lesions
Worldwide	Ingestion of undercooked meat (especially ground beef), vegetables or water contaminated with feces; direct contact with feces or contaminated soil	Diarrhea or hemorrhagic colitis; up to 15% of patients with hemorrhagic colitis progress to hemolytic uremic syndrome (HUS); case fatality rate for HUS is 3%–5%, higher in some populations (eg, 5%–10% in children, up to 50% in elderly)
Worldwide	Contact with animal products; via skin, usually after scratch or puncture wound; contaminated soil (survives for weeks to months)	Localized cellulitis, usually self-limiting, often on hands; generalized skin lesions (uncommon); arthritis, often in finger joints near skin lesion; endocarditis (with high mortality, 38%); generalization with sepsis, other syndromes uncommon and often in immunocompromised
Middle East, Asia, Africa and South America	Contact with infected animals, tissues through broken skin, mucous membrane; ingestion; inhalation	Mucous membrane or skin lesions; pneumonia and pulmonary abscess; sepsis; chronic abscesses, nodules, ulcers in many organs, weight loss, lymphadenopathy; case fatality rate varies with form, but >95% in untreated septicemia
	Uncertain; possibly ingestion of undercooked meat or direct contact	Gastroenteritis or diarrhea, liver disease; bacteremia in immunosuppressed patients

(*continued*)

TABLE 4 GLOBAL ZOONOSES[a] *(continued)*

Disease	Causative Organism	Animals Involved
	BACTERIAL DISEASES (continued)	
Leprosy (*see* p 692)	*Mycobacterium leprae*	Armadillos; nonhuman primates (rare)
Leptospirosis (*see* p 646)	*Leptospira* spp	Domestic and wild animals; reservoir hosts include rodents, dogs, cattle, pigs, farmed red deer, others
Listeriosis (*see* p 656)	*Listeria monocytogenes* (types most often associated with disease are ½a, ½b, 4b), *Listeria ivanovii* (rare)	Numerous mammals, birds, fish, crustaceans
Melioidosis (Pseudoglanders, *see* p 661)	*Burkholderia pseudomallei* (other species of soil-associated *Burkholderia*, such as *B oklahomensis* sp *nov* in North America, rarely linked to human infections)	Sheep, goats, swine; occasional cases in many other terrestrial and aquatic mammals; also reptiles, some birds including parrots, tropical fish
Methicillin-resistant *Staphylococcus aureus* (MRSA) infections	*S aureus* that carry *mecA* gene; some strains maintained in animals (eg, livestock-associated CC398), other strains mainly in people but animals can become carriers	Pigs (major reservoirs for livestock-associated strain CC398, also carry ST9); cats, dogs mainly acquire strains from people; MRSA also reported in other mammals, including horses, cattle; birds, including poultry, psittacines; turtles
Mycobacteriosis (*see* p 687)	*Mycobacterium avium* complex	Many species of mammals, some birds

TABLE 4 GLOBAL ZOONOSES[a] *(continued)*

Known Distribution	Probable Means of Spread to People	Clinical Manifestations in People
	BACTERIAL DISEASES (continued)	
Armadillos in parts of southern USA, Mexico, South America; nonhuman primates in Africa, possibly other locations; only human reservoirs in other areas	Transmission of animal leprosy to people likely	Various skin lesions, sensory nerve lesions and deficits, nasal mucosal lesions; mild, self-limiting to progressive destruction
Worldwide	Occupational and recreational exposure, or exposure to rodent-contaminated material in urban locations; especially skin, mucous membrane contact with contaminated urine, infected fetuses, or reproductive fluids; water- and foodborne	Asymptomatic to severe, sometimes biphasic; nonspecific febrile illness followed by aseptic meningitis or icteric form (especially liver, kidney, CNS involvement, hemorrhages possible); pulmonary hemorrhage and edema, other syndromes; uveitis can be sequela; case fatality rate varies with syndrome (uncommon in aseptic meningitis, 5%–15% in icteric form, 30%–60% in severe pulmonary form)
Worldwide	Foodborne, especially unpasteurized dairy products, raw meat and fish, vegetables, processed foods contaminated after processing; ingestion of contaminated water, soil; direct contact with infected animals; nosocomial in hospitals, institutions	Acute, self-limited febrile gastroenteritis or mild, flu-like illness; ocular disease, conjunctivitis; abortion, premature or septicemic newborn if infected during pregnancy; meningitis, meningoencephalitis, septicemia in elderly, immunosuppressed, and infants; papular or pustular rash ± fever, chills in healthy adults after handling infected fetuses
Asia, Africa, Australia, South America, Middle East, Caribbean	Wound infection, inhalation, and ingestion; organisms live in soil and surface water; most cases are acquired from environment, but direct transmission from animals is possible	Mimics many other diseases; acute localized infections, including skin lesions, cellulitis, abscesses, corneal ulcers; pulmonary disease, septicemia, internal organ abscesses; often occurs in immunocompromised; case fatality rate varies with form, >90% in untreated septicemia
Worldwide; can be reverse zoonosis or zoonosis; major strains in animals can vary with region	Usually by direct contact (typically with asymptomatic carrier animals); other routes also described; can be nosocomial in hospitals	Opportunist; localized skin and soft-tissue infections, invasive disease including septicemia, toxic shock syndrome; mortality varies with syndrome and success in finding antibiotic
Worldwide	Environmental, mainly from water, and/or soil; infection common to people and animals	Soft-tissue and bone infections; cervical lymphadenitis; pulmonary disease, often in immunocompromised or those with preexisting lung conditions; disseminated in immunocompromised, especially AIDS patients with uncontrolled disease

(continued)

TABLE 4 GLOBAL ZOONOSES[a] *(continued)*

Disease	Causative Organism	Animals Involved
	BACTERIAL DISEASES (continued)	
Mycobacteriosis *(continued)*	*M avium paratuberculosis*	Cattle, sheep, goats, camelids, deer, other ruminants; rabbits and other nonruminants; corvids
	Mycobacteria other than tuberculosis (includes *M simiae, M kansasii, M xenopi, M scrofulaceum, M szulgai, M chelonae, M marinum, M ulcerans*, others)	Cattle, other ruminants; swine, cats, dogs, koalas, other mammals, amphibians, reptiles (uncommon), fish; predominant *Mycobacterium* spp vary with host
Mycoplasma infections	*Mycoplasma* spp	Livestock, nonhuman primates, marine mammals, cats, dogs, rodents, other mammals
Pasteurellosis (*see* p 765 and p 1944)	*Pasteurella multocida* and other species	Many species of domestic and wild animals, including dogs, cats, livestock, rabbits, birds
Plague (*see* p 677)	*Yersinia pestis*	Rodents (eg, squirrels, prairie dogs, rats) and lagomorphs (pikas in Asia) are main reservoir; many mammals can be incidental hosts; cats and wild felids especially susceptible
Psittacosis and ornithosis (*see* p 2808)	*Chlamydia (Chlamydophila) psittaci*	Psittacine birds (especially parakeets, cockatiels), pigeons, turkeys, ducks, geese, and other domestic or wild birds; mammalian strains of *C psittaci* also exist (zoonotic potential still undetermined)
Rat bite fever	*Streptobacillus moniliformis*	Rodents; might also be transmitted by carnivores (eg, dogs, cats, ferrets), which are probably infected or transiently colonized from rodents
	Spirillum minus	Rodents; might also be transmitted by carnivores, which are probably infected or transiently colonized from rodents

TABLE 4 GLOBAL ZOONOSES[a] *(continued)*

Known Distribution	Probable Means of Spread to People	Clinical Manifestations in People
	BACTERIAL DISEASES (continued)	
Worldwide	Ingestion; accidental injection of vaccine	Postulated involvement in Crohn's disease after ingestion (controversial); severe local reaction if vaccine accidentally injected
Worldwide; distribution varies with the organism	Environmental, from water and/or soil	Same syndromes as *M avium* complex; some organisms tend to be associated with certain syndromes (eg, *M marinum*, *M ulcerans*, with ulcerative or nodular dermatitis)
Worldwide; zoonotic infections rare	Direct contact; bites; wound contamination, including accidental inoculation	Asymptomatic carriage; cellulitis; other syndromes, including respiratory disease, septic arthritis, septicemia have been reported, especially in immunocompromised
Worldwide	Wounds, scratches, bites, close contact with mucus membranes	Wound infections, cellulitis most common; other syndromes possible, including osteomyelitis, septic arthritis, sepsis, meningitis, respiratory disease; systemic conditions more common in immunocompromised
Foci in North and South America, Asia, Middle East, and Africa	Flea bites, aerosols, handling infected animals or tissues (contact with broken skin or mucous membranes), bites or scratches, eating uncooked infected tissues	Febrile flu-like syndrome with swollen, very painful draining lymph node(s) (buboes); pneumonia; sepsis can occur in either bubonic or pneumonic form; case fatality rate in untreated 40%–70% (bubonic) to 100% (pneumonic); < 5% mortality if bubonic form treated early
Worldwide	Inhalation of respiratory secretions or dried guano	Influenza-like febrile illness with nonproductive cough that may progress to pneumonia; complications, including endocarditis, myocarditis, meningoencephalitis, hepatitis, glomerulonephritis, and other organ dysfunction; sepsis; some cases fatal if untreated, <1% with treatment
Probably worldwide	Bites and scratches; handling or kissing a rodent, exposure to rodent urine; can be waterborne or foodborne	Fever, severe myalgia and joint pain, headache, rash, sometimes GI signs; complications, including polyarthritis (usually but not always sterile), hepatitis, endocarditis, focal abscesses, sepsis possible if untreated; overall case fatality rate 10%–13% if untreated
Organism is common only in Asia	Mainly bites and scratches	As above, but indurated, often ulcerated lesion at inoculation site; can relapse; some (minority) may have distinctive rash (large violaceous or reddish macules); polyarthritis is rare; overall case fatality rate 7%–10% if untreated

(continued)

TABLE 4 GLOBAL ZOONOSES[a] (*continued*)

Disease	Causative Organism	Animals Involved
	BACTERIAL DISEASES (continued)	
Salmonellosis (*see* p 195)	*Salmonella enterica* and *S bongori* (>2,500 serovars)	Widespread in mammals, birds, reptiles, amphibians, including domestic species; also in crustaceans; higher-risk pets for human exposure may include reptiles, amphibians, young poultry, some exotic mammals
Streptococcal infections	*Streptococcus* spp, including *S suis*, *S equi zooepidemicus*, *S canis*, *S iniae*, possibly others	*S suis* in swine; *S equi zooepidemicus* in horses; *S canis* in dogs, cats; *S iniae* in fish; each species can also be found in other animals
Tuberculosis (*see also* MYCOBACTERIOSIS, p 2426, p 2869, and p 687)	*Mycobacterium bovis*	Cattle, bison, African buffalo, cervids, brushtail opossums, badgers, kudu can be reservoirs; swine and many other mammals can be spillover hosts
	Mycobacterium caprae	Mainly goats, also infects other ruminants; can occur in other mammals, including pigs, horses, cervids, camels, carnivores
	Mycobacterium microti	Rodents thought to be reservoir; can occur in domestic animals, including cats, dogs, ferrets, livestock
Tularemia (*see* p 692)	*Francisella tularensis* subsp *tularensis* more virulent, *F tularensis* subsp *holarctica* (*F tularensis* type B) less virulent, *F tularensis* subsp *mediasiatica*, *F tularensis* subsp *novicida*	Rabbits, rodents, cats, sheep, other mammals, birds, reptiles, fish; often in wild animals
Vibriosis	*Vibrio parahaemolyticus*	Marine and estuarine shellfish, fish; also environmental in aquatic environments

TABLE 4 GLOBAL ZOONOSES[a] *(continued)*

Known Distribution	Probable Means of Spread to People	Clinical Manifestations in People
	BACTERIAL DISEASES (continued)	
Worldwide	Foodborne infection or fecal-oral; some cases of occupational and recreational exposure	Gastroenteritis to sepsis; focal infections possible; especially severe in the elderly, young children, or immunocompromised
Worldwide	Ingestion, especially of unpasteurized dairy products, pork; direct contact often through broken skin; the human pathogen *S pyogenes* can also colonize bovine udder and be transmitted in milk	Skin and soft-tissue infections; pharyngitis; other conditions, including pneumonia, meningitis, arthritis, endocarditis, streptococcal toxic shock syndrome, sepsis
Once worldwide, now eradicated or rare in some countries	Ingestion (unpasteurized dairy products, undercooked meat including bushmeat), inhalation, contamination of breaks in the skin	Skin lesions, cervical lymphadenitis (scrofula), pulmonary disease; genitourinary disease; can affect bones and joints, meninges; gastroenteritis
Reported mainly in Europe	Thought to be ingestion or direct contact with livestock, similarly to *M bovis*	Extrapulmonary conditions, including skin lesions, meningitis, lymphadenitis, pericarditis, urinary, dissemination; also pulmonary disease
Appears to be rare human zoonosis		Most reported cases have been pulmonary; can also cause extrapulmonary disease
F tularensis subsp *tularensis* almost exclusively in North America; *F tularensis* subsp *holarctica* in North America, Europe, Asia; *F tularensis* subsp *mediasiatica* in Central Asia; *F tularensis* subsp *novicida* reported in North America, Australia, Spain	Contact with mucous membranes, broken skin; insect bites (tabanids, mosquitoes, hard ticks); fomites; ingestion in food or water; inhalation	Nonspecific febrile illness, lymphadenitis; ulcerative skin lesions, exudative pharyngitis and stomatitis, conjunctivitis, gastroenteritis, respiratory signs or pneumonia, sepsis; case fatality rate 5% (localized disease, untreated) to >50% (untreated typhoidal form or severe respiratory disease)
Worldwide	Ingestion; wound infections	Gastroenteritis; dysentery (especially in some geographic regions); wound infections (mild to severe, including necrotizing fasciitis); sepsis; severe wound infections and sepsis usually in immunocompromised or those with liver disease (case fatality rate for sepsis 29%)

(continued)

TABLE 4 GLOBAL ZOONOSES[a] *(continued)*

Disease	Causative Organism	Animals Involved
	BACTERIAL DISEASES (continued)	
Vibriosis *(continued)*	*V vulnificus*	Marine shellfish, crustaceans (eg, shrimp), fish; also environmental in aquatic environments
	V cholerae O1/O139 (epidemic strains)	Oysters, crabs, shrimp, mussels; most cases acquired from people
	V cholerae non-O1/O139 (nonepidemic strains)	Oysters, other seafood; also environmental in aquatic environments
Yersiniosis	*Yersinia pseudotuberculosis*	Many species of mammals, including swine, dogs, cats, rodents, wild mammals, birds
	Y enterocolitica; not all serotypes are pathogenic	Many domestic and wild mammals, including rodents; some birds, reptiles, amphibians; zoonotic serotypes most common in pigs (major zoonotic source), pathogenic types also occur in dogs, cats
	RICKETTSIAL DISEASES	
Human ewingii ehrlichiosis (formerly granulocytic ehrlichiosis)	*Ehrlichia ewingii*	Dogs, deer proposed
Human monocytic ehrlichiosis (*see* p 803)	*Ehrlichia chaffeensis*	Deer are probably major reservoir in North America, dogs and other canids, lemurs, other mammals can also be infected

TABLE 4 GLOBAL ZOONOSES[a] *(continued)*

Known Distribution	Probable Means of Spread to People	Clinical Manifestations in People
	BACTERIAL DISEASES (continued)	
Worldwide; human cases have been reported in North America, Europe, Asia	Ingestion (often raw oysters); wound infection from water or handling hosts	Wound infections from mild, self-limited lesions, bullae to cellulitis, myositis; necrotizing fasciitis; gastroenteritis; sepsis, usually in immunocompromised or those with liver disease, other debilitating illnesses; case fatality rate for sepsis >50%, and up to 25% for wound infections
Rare/absent to epidemic in different regions; one focus along USA Gulf Coast in shellfish	Ingestion	Mild to severe, voluminous diarrhea, vomiting, dehydration; severe cases fatal if untreated, but low mortality if treated
Worldwide	Ingestion; wound infection	Gastroenteritis, usually mild and self-limited; wound infections; septicemia, usually in immunosuppressed or those with liver disease (case fatality rate for sepsis 47%–60% or higher)
Agent probably worldwide; prevalence may vary between regions	Ingestion of contaminated water, food (including meat [especially pork], vegetables); fecal-oral (animal contact); dog bite (rare)	Gastroenteritis (enterocolitis); pseudoappendicitis (with mesenteric lymphadenitis, terminal ileitis, fever, abdominal pain); severe GI bleeding possible in some cases of colitis; pharyngitis; sequelae may include erythema nodosum, reactive arthritis; sepsis, especially in elderly or immunocompromised
Worldwide; prevalence of human disease may vary between regions (commonly reported in Europe)	Ingestion	Gastroenteritis with watery diarrhea especially in young children, bloody feces uncommon; pseudoappendicitis; sequelae may include erythema nodosum, reactive arthritis; sepsis, other syndromes
	RICKETTSIAL DISEASES	
Southeastern and south central USA; has been detected in South America	Ticks, including *Amblyomma americanum*	Few cases described; fever, headache, malaise, myalgia, nausea, vomiting; many patients were immunosuppressed
North America; also reported in South America, Asia, and Africa	Ticks, including *Amblyomma americanum*	Asymptomatic to nonspecific febrile illness; rash in many pediatric cases, some adults; may progress to prolonged fever, renal failure, respiratory distress, hemorrhages, cardiomyopathy, neurologic signs, multiorgan failure; more severe in immunosuppressed, elderly; estimated case fatality rate 2%–3%

(continued)

TABLE 4 GLOBAL ZOONOSES[a] *(continued)*

Disease	Causative Organism	Animals Involved
RICKETTSIAL DISEASES (continued)		
Human granulocytic anaplasmosis (formerly human granulocytic ehrlichiosis)	*Anaplasma phagocytophilum* (formerly *Ehrlichia phagocytophilum* and *E equi*)	Wild rodents, deer may be reservoirs in North America; livestock, wild ungulates, wild rodents may be reservoirs in Europe; many other animals (eg, equids, ruminants, dogs, cats, birds) can also be infected
Infection by other *Ehrlichia* species	*E canis*, *E muris*–like organism implicated rarely in human illness	Dogs and other canids thought to be reservoirs for *E canis*, might also occur in felids; rodents may be reservoirs for *E muris*
Q fever (Query fever, *see* p 623)	*Coxiella burnetii*	Sheep, cattle, goats, cats, dogs, rodents, other mammals, birds, ticks
Sennetsu fever	*Neorickettsia sennetsu*	Uncertain, possibly fish
Spotted fever group of *Rickettsia*		
—African tick bite fever	*R africae*	Ungulates
—Mediterranean spotted fever; Boutonneuse fever; Tick bite fever;	*R conorii* subsp *conorii*	Dogs, rabbits implicated as reservoirs; other animals can be infected
—Israeli spotted fever, Astrakhan spotted fever, Indian tick typhus	*R conorii* subsp *israelensis* (Israeli spotted fever), *R conorii* subsp *caspia* (Astrakhan spotted fever), *R conorii* subsp *indica* (Indian tick typhus)	Reservoir hosts uncertain
—*Fleaborne* spotted fever; Cat flea typhus	*R felis* (synonym ELB agent)	Unknown; dogs have been suggested as possible amplifying hosts

TABLE 4 GLOBAL ZOONOSES[a] *(continued)*

Known Distribution	Probable Means of Spread to People	Clinical Manifestations in People
	RICKETTSIAL DISEASES (continued)	
Worldwide	Tick bites (*Ixodes* spp)	Resembles human monocytic ehrlichiosis; often asymptomatic to mild in immunocompetent; rash uncommon; estimated case fatality rate <1%
E canis worldwide; *E muris* Eastern Europe to Asia; *E muris*–like organism in North America	Ticks (*E canis* transmitted by *Rhipicephalus sanguineus*, *E muris* by *Haemaphysalis flava* and *Ixodes persulcatus* complex)	Rare cases of febrile illness, in both healthy and immunosuppressed
Worldwide	Mainly airborne; exposure to placenta, birth tissues, animal excreta; occasionally ingestion (including unpasteurized milk); tickborne infections probably rare or nonexistent in people	Febrile influenza-like illness; atypical pneumonia, hepatitis, endocarditis in some; possible pregnancy complications; overall case fatality rate 1%–2% if untreated
Japan, Malaysia, Laos, possibly other Asian countries	Thought to be ingestion of raw fish	Relatively mild, nonspecific, febrile illness, resembles infectious mononucleosis
Sub-Saharan Africa, eastern Caribbean	Bite of infected tick (mainly *Amblyomma hebraeum*, *A variegatum*, also *A lepidum*, possibly *Rhipicephalus decoloratus*, *Rhipicephalus appendiculatus*)	Nonspecific febrile illness; painful regional lymphadenopathy in many; eschars often multiple; nuchal myalgia; sometimes sparse maculopapular and/or vesicular rash; deaths do not seem to occur
Europe, especially Mediterranean; cases reported in sub-Saharan Africa	Bite of infected ticks (mainly *Rhipicephalus sanguineus*, also others), crushing tick	Nonspecific febrile illness; eschar (typically single) may or may not be present; rash, often maculopapular, in most; life-threatening disseminated disease or neurologic signs possible but uncommon; case fatality rate 1%–3% if untreated
Israeli spotted fever in Middle East, reported in Europe; Astrakhan spotted fever in Russia, Kazakhstan; Indian tick typhus in Asia (Indian subcontinent)	Bite of infected ticks (mainly *Rhipicephalus* spp), crushing tick	Astrakhan spotted fever and Indian tick typhus resemble Mediterranean spotted fever, but Israeli spotted fever may be more severe
North and South America, Europe, Asia, Africa, probably worldwide	Flea bites; mainly associated with *Ctenocephalides felis* (cat flea), also infects *C canis* and other fleas	Few clinical cases have been described but resembles other spotted fevers; febrile illness; rash in most; eschar may be uncommon; most cases seem to be mild but CNS involvement, pneumonia possible

(continued)

TABLE 4 GLOBAL ZOONOSES[a] *(continued)*

Disease	Causative Organism	Animals Involved
	RICKETTSIAL DISEASES (continued)	
—Queensland tick typhus	*R australis*	Bandicoots, rodents
—Rickettsial pox	*R akari*	Mice; also rats, Korean voles
—*Rickettsia parkeri* rickettsiosis	*R parkeri*	
—Rocky Mountain spotted fever (*see* p 806)	*R rickettsii*	Rodents, rabbits, opossums, and other small mammals might amplify; dogs can be infected
—Tickborne lymphadenopathy; *Dermacentor* necrosis-erythema-lymphadenopathy	*R slovaca*, *R raoultii*	Uncertain; wild boar may be involved
—Other tickborne species in spotted fever group	*R sibirica*, *R japonica*, *R helvetica*, *R honei*, *R heilongjiangensis*, *R aeschlimannii*, *R massiliae*, *R monacensi*, *R amblyommii*, others	Various vertebrates
Typhus group of *Rickettsia*		
—Murine typhus; Fleaborne typhus	*R typhi* (formerly *R mooseri*)	Rats are major reservoir; cats, opossums, possibly dogs, other species in peridomestic cycle

TABLE 4 GLOBAL ZOONOSES[a] *(continued)*

Known Distribution	Probable Means of Spread to People	Clinical Manifestations in People
	RICKETTSIAL DISEASES (continued)	
Australia	Bite of infected *Ixodes* tick, especially *I holocyclus*, *I tasmani*	Febrile illness, eschar may be present, rash (either maculopapular or vesicular) in most; mild in most, but serious disseminated disease, complications, death possible
Organism may be cosmopolitan; human cases seem to be uncommon	Bite of infected rodent mites, *Liponyssoides sanguineus*	Eschar (single) in most; febrile illness; maculopapular rash progresses to vesicular, pustular, resembles chickenpox; self-limiting
North America, detected in parts of South America	Bite of infected ticks, *Amblyomma maculatum*; also found in other *Amblyomma* spp	Resembles Rocky Mountain spotted fever (RMSF) but seems to be milder in most cases; differs from RMSF in that eschars occur in most cases (may be multiple), petechial rash does not seem to be characteristic
Western hemisphere	Bite of infected ticks, especially *Dermacentor variabilis*, *D andersoni* (*D variabilis* in USA); *Amblyomma cajennense*, *A aureolatum* in South America; *Rhipicephalus sanguineus* in Arizona, Mexico, and South America; also from crushing tick	Moderate to severe febrile illness; macular to generalized petechial rash; edema in some; usually no eschar; neurologic, pulmonary, hemorrhagic, and kidney signs in some; sepsis; gangrene; case fatality rate 15%–30% or higher (up to 85%) if untreated, ~3% or less with treatment in North America but higher in parts of Brazil
Europe to Central Asia	Bites of infected ticks; *R slovaca* especially in *Dermacentor marginatus*, *D reticulatus*; *R raoultii* in *Rhipicephalus pumilio*, *D nuttalli*, other *Dermacentor* spp	Eschar, local lymphadenopathy; localized alopecia at bite site; mild illness, fever and rash uncommon; no deaths reported
Worldwide; distribution varies by species	Bites of ixodid ticks; specific vector varies by species	Inoculation site eschar (most); febrile illness with headache, myalgia, sometimes other signs; rash; local lymphadenopathy (some species); major signs, risk of complications, severity vary with species of *Rickettsia*
Worldwide, especially warmer regions	Infected rodent fleas, usually via flea feces; cat fleas seem to be involved in some cycles	Fever, severe headache, central rash (not always observed); other signs, including arthralgia, cough, nausea/vomiting in some; mortality rate 4% without treatment

(continued)

TABLE 4 GLOBAL ZOONOSES[a] (continued)

Disease	Causative Organism	Animals Involved
RICKETTSIAL DISEASES (continued)		
—Scrub typhus; Chigger-borne rickettsiosis	*Orientia tsutsugamushi* and related species	Rodents, insectivores
—Typhus	*R prowazekii*	Flying squirrels
FUNGAL DISEASES		
Aspergillosis; Allergic bronchopulmonary aspergillosis (*see* p 2901)	*Aspergillus* spp	Birds and mammals
Blastomycosis (*see* p 634)	*Blastomyces dermatitidis*	Dogs, cats, horses, marine mammals, other mammals
Coccidioidomycosis (*see* p 637)	*Coccidioides immitis*, *C posadasii*	Cattle, sheep, horses, llamas, dogs, many other mammals
Cryptococcosis (*see* p 637)	*Cryptococcus neoformans* var *grubii*, *C neoformans* var *neoformans*, *C gattii*	Birds including pigeons, psittacines (mainly grows in guano; temporary colonization of intestinal tract also possible); clinical cases in cats, other mammals

TABLE 4 GLOBAL ZOONOSES[a] (continued)

Known Distribution	Probable Means of Spread to People	Clinical Manifestations in People
	RICKETTSIAL DISEASES (continued)	
Asia, Australia, islands of southwestern Pacific Ocean; cases are usually concentrated regionally in "typhus islands"	Bite of infected larval trombiculid mites (chiggers)	Eschar in some; rash, headache, fever, painful lymphadenopathy, body aches, interstitial pneumonitis, GI signs; pneumonia, neurologic signs or cardiac complications in some; mild to severe; convalescence prolonged; case fatality rate up to 30%–50% if untreated
Eastern USA	Squirrel lice or fleas suspected	Nonspecific febrile illness, rash; GI signs in some; sepsis possible; appears to be somewhat milder than nonzoonotic typhus, which has a mortality rate of 20%–60% if untreated
	FUNGAL DISEASES	
Worldwide	Environmental exposure (decaying vegetation or grains); infection common to people and animals, insignificant as zoonosis	Allergic respiratory signs, especially in people with certain respiratory conditions or immunodeficiencies; allergic sinusitis; pneumonia sometimes with dissemination in immunocompromised (can be fatal); chronic pulmonary disease ± aspergilloma (fungus ball); localized infections of other organs, tissues
Distribution in environment uncertain; clinical cases focal; locally acquired cases reported in parts of North America, Africa, Middle East, India	Environmental exposure, organism is most common in moist soil; infection common in people and animals; also reported rarely by animal exposure	Acute to chronic pulmonary disease; skin or bone lesions; meningitis, other syndromes, disseminated disease possible; course mild to severe, some cases fatal
Especially southwestern USA, Mexico, Central and South America; in arid or semiarid foci; some cases might be acquired outside usual foci	Principally environmental exposure (inhalation of arthrospores), including fungal cultures; infection common in people and animals, one unusual case reported after necropsy of horse with disseminated disease	Self-limited, febrile, flu-like illness, sometimes with cough, chest pain in healthy host; serious, possibly life-threatening pulmonary disease or disseminated infection with cutaneous/subcutaneous lesions, persistent meningitis or osteomyelitis, especially in immunocompromised
Worldwide	Principally environmental exposure, especially pigeon nests for *C neoformans*, trees for *C gattii*; via inhalation or through the skin; infection common in people and animals, insignificant as zoonosis	Respiratory signs, mild to severe, often self-limiting in healthy host but more likely to be severe in immunocompromised; dissemination with CNS disease, ocular signs, other syndromes, most often in immunocompromised; skin lesions, either localized from inoculation (uncommon) or from disseminated disease

(continued)

TABLE 4 GLOBAL ZOONOSES[a] *(continued)*

Disease	Causative Organism	Animals Involved
	FUNGAL DISEASES (continued)	
Histoplasmosis (*see* p 639)	*Histoplasma capsulatum* var *capsulatum*	Dogs, cats, bats, cattle, sheep, horses, many other domestic and wild mammals, birds
	H capsulatum var *duboisii*	As above
Malassezia infection	*Malassezia* spp	Dogs, cats, other animals
Ringworm (Dermatophytosis, *see* p 872)	*Microsporum* and *Trichophyton* spp	Dogs, cats, hedgehogs, cattle, sheep, goats, horses, rodents, other mammals, birds, very rarely reptiles
Sporotrichosis (*see* p 644)	*Sporothrix schenckii*	Cats, other mammals, birds
	PARASITIC DISEASES—PROTOZOANS	
Babesiosis (*see* p 21)	*Babesia microti* complex, *B duncani* (formerly WA-1), and other species	Rodents, insectivores, lagomorphs, some other mammals; reservoirs uncertain for some species
	B divergens	Cattle; *B divergens* or closely related organism in farmed reindeer, wild cervids
	B bovis; uncertain zoonosis; some historical cases were probably *B divergens*	Cattle, water buffalo, African buffalo, possibly other species

TABLE 4 GLOBAL ZOONOSES[a] *(continued)*

Known Distribution	Probable Means of Spread to People	Clinical Manifestations in People
FUNGAL DISEASES (continued)		
Worldwide; clinical cases often cluster in regional foci	Principally environmental exposure, avian or bat feces encourage growth of organism; infection common in people and animals; insignificant as zoonosis	Flu-like, febrile illness, usually self-limiting in healthy hosts; skin lesions; chronic pulmonary disease, usually with preexisting lung disease; dissemination in very young, elderly, immunocompromised
Africa	As above	Usually skin and subcutaneous lesions, osteolytic bone lesions but can disseminate
Worldwide	Exposure to symptomatic animals; normal levels on skin not thought to be a significant risk	Dermatitis; zoonotic strains might be implicated in fungemia in preterm neonates, other immunocompromised
Worldwide	Direct skin/hair contact with infected animals, fomites	Skin and hair lesions, usually pruritic; rare skin dissemination in immunocompromised
Worldwide; epizootics in cats in South America	Primarily environmental in vegetation, wood, soil; inoculation from environment in penetrating wounds (splinters, bites, pecks), skin contact with lesions, especially in cats; bites, scratches, other close contact implicated during feline epidemics; inhalation rare	Papules, pustules, nodules, ulcerative skin lesions, may follow course of draining lymphatics; mucosa can be affected; extracutaneous involvement, especially bones, joints; disseminated disease (including meningitis) can be seen in immunocompromised; acute or chronic pulmonary disease resembling tuberculosis after inhalation, especially with underlying lung disease (rare)
PARASITIC DISEASES—PROTOZOANS		
Babesia spp worldwide in wild animals, many agents not identified to species; human illness due to *B microti* complex reported in North America (most), Europe, Asia, Australia	Bite of infected *Ixodes* ticks for *B microti*	Many immunocompetent patients may have mild to moderate flu-like, febrile illness; mild to severe hemolytic anemia, especially severe in immunocompromised and elderly; respiratory, hepatic, renal, and other organ dysfunction; recurrent or chronic infection may develop; dual infection with *B burgdorferi* may worsen both diseases; death possible in severe cases
Europe, possibly North Africa; similar organisms might be present in North America; reported in Asia (China)	Tick bites (*Ixodes ricinus*)	Usually in splenectomized; acute, severe hemolysis; persistent high fever, headache, myalgia, abdominal pain, sometimes GI signs; shock and renal failure; cases progress rapidly; usually fatal if untreated; milder flu-like cases have been reported in immunocompetent patients
Africa, Asia, Central and South America, Mexico, Australia, parts of Europe	Tick bites (*Rhipicephalus microplus* and *R annulatus*)	

(continued)

TABLE 4 GLOBAL ZOONOSES[a] *(continued)*

Disease	Causative Organism	Animals Involved
PARASITIC DISEASES—PROTOZOANS (continued)		
Balantidiasis	*Balantidium coli* and related species	Swine, rats, nonhuman primates, other animals
Chagas' disease (American trypanosomiasis, *see* p 38)	*Trypanosoma cruzi*	Opossums, lagomorphs, rodents, armadillos, dogs, cats, other wild and domestic mammals
Cryptosporidiosis (*see* p 209)	*Cryptosporidium parvum, C canis, C felis, C meleagridis, C cuniculus, C viatorum, C muris,* and other species (*C hominis* and likely some genotypes of *C parvum* are adapted mainly to people)	Cattle and other ruminants, dogs, cats, rabbits, other domestic and wild mammals, birds, reptiles, fish
Giardiasis (*see* p 211)	*Giardia intestinalis,* also known as *G duodenalis* (formerly *G lamblia*); only some genotypes seem to have zoonotic potential	Many domestic and wild mammals, including dogs, cats, ruminants, aquatic mammals such as beavers
Leishmaniosis —Visceral (Kalaazar; *see* p 800)	*Leishmania infantum*	Wild canids and dogs are primary reservoirs, also in other mammals
—Cutaneous and mucocutaneous	*L tropica* complex (except *L tropica,* which is maintained in people), *L braziliensis* complex, *L mexicana* complex, others	Dogs (*L peruviana*), rodents, various wild mammals act as reservoir hosts; other mammals can be infected

TABLE 4 GLOBAL ZOONOSES[a] *(continued)*

Known Distribution	Probable Means of Spread to People	Clinical Manifestations in People
	PARASITIC DISEASES—PROTOZOANS (continued)	
Worldwide	Ingestion, especially of water contaminated with feces	Asymptomatic to mucoid, bloody feces; intestinal hemorrhage and perforation possible; rare extraintestinal cases
Western hemisphere—southern USA, Mexico, Central and South America	Fecal material of reduviid bug in family Triatomidae contaminates bite wounds, abrasions, or mucous membranes; ingestion in contaminated food	Acute disease—erratic fever, adenopathy, headache, myalgia, hepatosplenomegaly, swelling at inoculation site and eyelid; myocarditis or encephalitis in some; worse in immunocompromised Chronic form (in 10%–30% of patients)—cardiomyopathy, megaesophagus, megacolon, other forms; reported annual mortality rate in chronic form 0.2%–19% (higher rates from studies that include only cardiac patients)
Worldwide	Fecal-oral; ingestion of contaminated food and water; inhalation	Self-limiting gastroenteritis in healthy; can be cholera-like and persistent in immunocompromised, with weight loss, wasting; cholecystitis; respiratory signs, pancreatitis, other syndromes mainly in immunosuppressed
Worldwide	Ingestion of water and less often food; direct fecal-oral (hands or fomites)	Gastroenteritis, may be persistent
Asia, South America, Caribbean, Africa, the Middle East, Europe (Mediterranean spreading north), North America	Bite of sand flies *Phlebotomus* and *Lutzomyia* spp	Undulating fever, hepatosplenomegaly; some have cough, diarrhea, lymphadenopathy, weight loss, petechiae or hemorrhages on mucous membranes, nodular lesions or darkening of skin; pancytopenia; mild cases with only a few signs may resolve on their own, but most other cases fatal if untreated
Mediterranean, Asia, Africa, Middle East, Mexico to South America, Caribbean; localized focus in USA (Texas and Oklahoma)	As above	Papules to ulcers or nodules on skin ± mucous membranes; single or multiple lesions; localized or disseminated; may persist or recur; atypical forms in immunosuppressed; cutaneous form rarely fatal, mucocutaneous form can be disfiguring and may be fatal if pharynx affected

(continued)

TABLE 4 GLOBAL ZOONOSES[a] (*continued*)

Disease	Causative Organism	Animals Involved
PARASITIC DISEASES—PROTOZOANS (continued)		
Malaria of nonhuman primates	Nonhuman primate–associated *Plasmodium* spp, *P knowlesi*, rarely *P cynomolgi*, others also potential zoonoses	Old and New World monkeys, apes
Microsporidiosis	Microsporidia of *Enterocytozoon bieneusi*, *Encephalitozoon cuniculi*, *E intestinalis*, *E hellem*, others; both zoonotic and anthroponotic transmission reported for some agents	Widespread in vertebrates, including primates, rabbits, rodents, dogs, cats, cattle, pigs, goats, birds, fish; also in invertebrates
Rhinosporidiosis (*see* p 644)	*Rhinosporidium seeberi*; some strains may be host specific	Natural hosts thought to be fish and amphibians; also found in various mammals, including horses, cattle, mules, dogs, and cats; birds
Sarcocystosis (Sarcosporidiosis, *see* p 1058)	*Sarcocystis suihominis*, also called *S meischeriana*	People, nonhuman primates are definitive hosts; swine are intermediate host
	S hominis, also called *S fusiformis*	People, nonhuman primates are definitive hosts; cattle are intermediate host
	Sarcocystis spp; *S nesbitti* may be one cause	People are intermediate host; species of *Sarcocystis* and definitive host(s) are often unknown; definitive host for *S nesbitti* thought to be snakes
Toxoplasmosis (*see* p 685)	*Toxoplasma gondii*	Felidae, including domestic cats, are definitive hosts; essentially all other mammals (including livestock) and birds thought to be susceptible as intermediate hosts
Trypanosomiasis (African sleeping sickness, *see* p 35)	*Trypanosoma brucei*; *T brucei rhodesiense* is zoonotic; *T brucei gambiense* is primarily a human pathogen, although some animals (eg, pigs) can be infected and might serve as minor reservoirs	*T brucei rhodesiense* reservoirs may include cattle, sheep, antelope, hyenas, lions, other wildlife, people; also isolated from other mammals

TABLE 4 GLOBAL ZOONOSES[a] *(continued)*

Known Distribution	Probable Means of Spread to People	Clinical Manifestations in People
PARASITIC DISEASES—PROTOZOANS (continued)		
P knowlesi in Asia; other species exist in Central and South America, Asia, Africa	Bite of anopheline mosquitoes	Febrile episodes with chills; headache, myalgia, malaise, cough, nausea, vomiting, and other symptoms in some; cases range from mild, self-limiting to fatal (3% case fatality rate for *P knowlesi*)
Worldwide	Fecal-oral; direct contact; ingestion of contaminated food or water; aerosols; possibly vector-transmitted	Keratitis; acute diarrhea (traveler's diarrhea); chronic diarrhea in immunocompromised; may disseminate to systemic disease with variable symptoms in immunocompromised
Worldwide, especially in tropics; endemic in South America, Asia, and Africa	Environmental exposure, probably water	Nasal and other mucous membrane masses and polyps (mainly nose, nasopharynx, eye); may cause obstruction; rare disseminated disease with osteolytic lesions or affecting viscera; rare skin and subcutaneous lesions
Worldwide	Ingestion of raw pork	Gastroenteritis, usually mild, or asymptomatic
Worldwide	Ingestion of raw beef	Gastroenteritis, usually mild or asymptomatic
Worldwide; symptomatic cases mainly in Asia, probably because of distribution of definitive host	Assumed to be ingestion of oocysts shed in feces of definitive host(s) or sporocysts	Main syndrome is myositis, acute and self-limited to chronic, moderately severe; also cough, arthralgia, transient pruritic rashes, headache, malaise, lymphadenopathy in some
Worldwide	Ingestion of oocysts shed in feces of infected cats (including contaminated soil, food, water) or ingestion of tissue cysts in undercooked meat or unpasteurized milk	Lymphadenopathy or mild, febrile, flu-like syndrome or uveitis in immunocompetent, nonpregnant host; often severe in immunocompromised, with neurologic disease, chorioretinitis, myocarditis, pneumonitis, or disseminated disease; infection of fetus may result in CNS damage or generalized infection; abortions and stillbirths
Africa; common below the Sahara desert	Bite of infected tsetse fly (*Glossina* spp)	Painful chancre at bite site in some patients; intermittent fever, headache, adenopathy, rash, arthralgia; neurologic signs such as somnolence, seizures; cardiac complications possible; *gambiense* disease may last years; *rhodesiense* disease acute, may last weeks to months; both usually fatal without treatment

(continued)

TABLE 4 GLOBAL ZOONOSES[a] *(continued)*

Disease	Causative Organism	Animals Involved
	PARASITIC DISEASES—TREMATODES (FLUKES)	
Clonorchiasis	*Clonorchis sinensis* (Chinese liver fluke)	Dogs, cats, swine, rats, other mammals are definitive hosts; fish (and snails) are intermediate hosts
Dicrocoeliasis	*Dicrocoelium dendriticum*, possibly *D hospes* (lancet flukes)	Ruminants, especially sheep, goats, cattle, occasionally other domestic and wild mammals are definitive hosts; land snails (first) and ants (second) are intermediate hosts
Echinostomiasis	*Echinostoma revolutum*, *E ilocanum*, *E hortense*, and other *Echinostoma* spp; *Echinochasmus japonicus* and other members of Echinostomatidae can also be zoonotic	Cats, dogs, rodents, pigs, other mammals; birds, including poultry, are definitive hosts; fish, shellfish, tadpoles, snails are intermediate hosts
Fascioliasis	*Fasciola hepatica*	Cattle, sheep, water buffalo, horses, rabbits, other herbivores are definitive hosts; snails are intermediate hosts
	F gigantica	Cattle, buffalo, goats, sheep, zebras, other mammals are definitive hosts; snails are intermediate hosts
Fasciolopsiasis	*Fasciolopsis buski*	Swine, people are definitive hosts; snails are intermediate hosts
Gastrodiscoidiasis	*Gastrodiscoides hominis*; uncertain whether people and swine carry the same strains	Swine, people, nonhuman primates, rodents, other mammals are definitive hosts; snails are intermediate hosts
Heterophyiasis	*Heterophyes* spp, *Haplorchis* spp, other heterophids	Cats, dogs, foxes, wolves, cattle, other mammals, fish-eating birds are definitive hosts (host varies with species of parasite); fish (and snails) are intermediate hosts
Metagonimiasis	*Metagonimus yokogawai*, *M miyatai*, *M takahashii*, and other *Metagonimus* spp	Cats, dogs, rats, other fish-eating mammals, possibly birds are definitive hosts; fish (and snails) are intermediate hosts

TABLE 4 GLOBAL ZOONOSES[a] *(continued)*

Known Distribution	Probable Means of Spread to People	Clinical Manifestations in People
PARASITIC DISEASES—TREMATODES (FLUKES) (continued)		
Asia	Ingestion of undercooked infected freshwater fish or shrimp containing encysted larvae	Cholecystitis symptoms, indigestion, diarrhea, mild fever; chronic infections associated with cirrhosis, pancreatitis, or cholangiocarcinoma
D dendriticum on all major continents (may be focal); *D hospes* in Africa south of Sahara desert	Ingestion of infected ants	Abdominal discomfort, flatulent indigestion; occasionally GI signs (diarrhea, constipation, vomiting, pain); weight loss, fatigue; biliary obstruction, cholangitis, hepatomegaly, or acute urticaria possible
Most human cases in Asia, Western Pacific; this group of parasites is widely distributed, including Europe, Americas, Middle East	Ingestion of undercooked fish, shellfish, snails, or amphibians (frogs)	Abdominal discomfort; diarrhea, especially in heavy infestation; malnutrition, anemia, edema may occur, especially in children; intestinal perforation has been reported
Worldwide or nearly worldwide; previously thought to be mainly in temperate areas but may be more widely distributed	Ingestion of contaminated greens, eg, watercress, or water that contains metacercariae	Gastroenteritis, hepatomegaly, fever, urticaria possible acutely; biliary colic and obstructive jaundice in chronic cases; aberrant migration with extrahepatic signs (eg, pulmonary infiltrates, neurologic signs, lymphadenopathy, skin lesions or subcutaneous swelling) in some
Thought to occur mainly in tropical areas: Africa, Asia, Middle East, and western Pacific	As above	Signs resemble fascioliasis caused by *F hepatica*
Asian pig-raising regions	Ingestion of aquatic vegetables or contaminated drinking water containing metacercariae	Often asymptomatic; gastroenteritis; intestinal bleeding, obstruction, or perforation possible; facial, abdominal, extremity edema may occur
Asia (including the Philippines), also reported in Africa, Volga delta in Russia	Possibly ingestion of water or aquatic plants	Mild diarrhea if high parasite burden
Middle East (especially Nile delta), Turkey, Asia	Ingestion of undercooked fish containing encysted larvae	Diarrhea with mucus, colicky pain; heart or CNS involvement possible; severity of signs may vary with species
Human illness mainly in Asia, also reported in Siberia; parasites have been found in Europe	Ingestion of undercooked freshwater fish containing encysted larvae	Diarrhea with mucus, anorexia, mild epigastric pain or abdominal cramps; malabsorption, weight loss if high parasite burden

(continued)

TABLE 4 GLOBAL ZOONOSES[a] *(continued)*

Disease	Causative Organism	Animals Involved
PARASITIC DISEASES—TREMATODES (FLUKES) (continued)		
Metorchiasis	*Metorchis conjunctus*, Canadian liver fluke	Dogs, foxes and other canids, cats, raccoons, muskrats, mink, other fish-eating mammals are definitive hosts; fish (and snails) are intermediate hosts
Nanophyetiasis	*Troglotrema salmincola* (also called *Nanophyetus salmincola*)	Raccoons, foxes, dogs, cats, skunks, and other fish-eating mammals and birds are definitive hosts; salmonid and some non-salmonid fish (and snails) are intermediate hosts
Opisthorchiasis	*Opisthorchis felineus* (cat liver fluke)	Cats, dogs, foxes, swine, seals, other fish-eating mammals are definitive hosts; fish (and snails) are intermediate hosts
	O viverrini (small liver fluke); zoonotic transmission can occur, but people are important hosts	People, dogs, cats, rats, pigs, fish-eating mammals are definitive hosts; fish and snails are intermediate hosts
	Amphimerus pseudofelineus	Various mammals, birds, reptiles are definitive hosts; fish suspected as intermediate hosts
Paragonimiasis (Lung fluke disease)	*Paragonimus westermani*, *P heterotremus*, *P africanus*, *P mexicanus*, and other species	Dogs, cats, swine, wild carnivores, opossums, and other mammals are definitive hosts; snails and freshwater crustaceans are intermediate hosts; wild boars, sheep, goats, rabbits, birds, other animals are paratenic hosts
Schistosomiasis, intestinal and hepatic	*Schistosoma japonicum*	Many mammals, including cattle, water buffalo (important host in Asia), swine, dogs, cats, deer, horses, nonhuman primates, and rodents, are definitive hosts; snails are intermediate hosts

TABLE 4 GLOBAL ZOONOSES[a] *(continued)*

Known Distribution	Probable Means of Spread to People	Clinical Manifestations in People
PARASITIC DISEASES—TREMATODES (FLUKES) (continued)		
North America; human infection rare	Ingestion of undercooked freshwater fish containing encysted larvae	Fever, abdominal pain (mainly epigastric), anorexia during acute stage; effects of chronic infection uncertain
North America along Pacific coast, Russia	Ingestion of undercooked fish or roe	Mild gastroenteritis
Europe, Kazakhstan, Russia, Ukraine	Ingestion of undercooked freshwater fish containing encysted larvae	Acute febrile illness with arthralgia, lymphadenopathy, skin rash; suppurative cholangitis and liver abscess in subacute, chronic stages; possible increased risk of cholangiocarcinoma
Southeast Asia	Ingestion of undercooked freshwater fish containing encysted larvae	Upper abdominal pain, diarrhea, fever, jaundice possible acutely; chronic infections with cirrhosis, pancreatitis, high incidence of cholangiocarcinoma
North and South America	Undetermined but probably ingestion of undercooked fish	
Flukes are worldwide (distribution varies with species); most human infections in Asia, Africa, tropical America	Ingestion of undercooked, infected freshwater crustaceans (crabs, crayfish); metacercariae on contaminated hands, fomites after preparing crustaceans, or undercooked meat from paratenic hosts such as wild boars	Chills, fever possible during migration to lungs; pulmonary disease resembling tuberculosis with cough, blood-tinged sputum; abdominal form with dull pain, tenderness, possibly diarrhea; less often, neurologic signs, migratory skin nodules, other organ-specific symptoms; predominant signs vary with species of fluke
Asia	Penetration of unbroken skin by cercariae from infected snails in water	Acute disease can include urticarial rash, mild signs, isolated pulmonary signs, or Katayama syndrome (occurs especially after first infection; febrile illness, sometimes with cough, diarrhea, abdominal pain, hepatosplenomegaly, and/or rash/urticaria); apparent clinical recovery may be followed by chronic intestinal schistosomiasis with abdominal pain/discomfort, diarrhea ± blood; chronic hepatic schistosomiasis with hepatosplenomegaly followed by liver fibrosis, ascites, portal hypertension with hematemesis and/or melena, portocaval shunting with pulmonary signs; ectopic parasites can cause seizures, paralysis, meningoencephalitis; intestinal and hepatic lesions tend to progress rapidly; death can occur

(continued)

TABLE 4 GLOBAL ZOONOSES[a] (continued)

Disease	Causative Organism	Animals Involved
PARASITIC DISEASES—TREMATODES (FLUKES) (continued)		
Schistosomiasis, intestinal and hepatic (*continued*)	*S mansoni*	People, nonhuman primates are major reservoir (definitive) hosts; also in rodents, insectivores, cattle, dogs; snails are intermediate hosts
	S mattheei; *S bovis* and *S margrebowiei* might also be zoonotic	Definitive hosts are artiodactylid ruminants (cattle, sheep, goats, waterbuck, wildebeest, antelope, buffalo), also found in nonhuman primates; snails are intermediate hosts
	S mekongi	People are reservoir (definitive) hosts; also found in dogs, pigs; snails are intermediate hosts
	S intercalatum, *S guineensis*	Primarily people, rodents may also be definitive hosts; some other mammals, including nonhuman primates, susceptible to infection; snails are intermediate hosts
Schistosomiasis, urinary	*S haematobium*	People are main reservoir (definitive host); occasionally infects nonhuman primates, pigs, buffalo, sheep, rodents, or other mammals; snails are intermediate hosts
Swimmer's itch (Cercarial dermatitis)	Schistosome cercariae from *Schistosoma* spp (mammals); *Gigantobilharzia*, *Trichobilharzia*, and *Austrobilharzia* spp (birds)	Birds, mammals are definitive hosts; snails are intermediate hosts
PARASITIC DISEASES—CESTODES (TAPEWORMS)		
Bertielliasis	*Bertiella studeri*, *B mucronata*	Nonhuman primates are usual hosts; other mammals, including dogs, people can be infected
Coenuriasis (Coenurosis)	*Taenia multiceps*	Definitive hosts are canids; intermediate hosts are sheep, other herbivores
	T serialis	Definitive hosts are canids; intermediate hosts are lagomorphs, rodents, occasionally other mammals

TABLE 4 GLOBAL ZOONOSES[a] (*continued*)

Known Distribution	Probable Means of Spread to People	Clinical Manifestations in People
PARASITIC DISEASES—TREMATODES (FLUKES) (continued)		
Africa, Middle East, South America, Caribbean	Penetration of unbroken skin by cercariae from infected snails in water	Acute disease in some; intestinal (most often) and/or hepatic schistosomiasis similar to *S japonicum* but not as rapidly progressive; glomerulonephritis a possible complication; ectopic CNS parasites tend to cause transverse myelitis; also causes genital schistosomiasis with reproductive problems; death can occur
Southern Africa; seems to be rare in people, and some infections may have been misidentified	Penetration of unbroken skin by cercariae from infected snails in water	Suggested agent in intestinal and hepatic schistosomiasis
Southeast Asia	Penetration of unbroken skin by cercariae from infected snails in water	Acute disease absent or very rare; intestinal and hepatic schistosomiasis; death can occur
Africa	Penetration of unbroken skin by cercariae from infected snails in water	Intestinal schistosomiasis only, often mild or asymptomatic; occasionally bloody feces, diarrhea
Africa (including Madagascar, Mauritius), the Middle East	Penetration of unbroken skin by cercariae from infected snails in water	Acute disease in some; chronic disease—hematuria, dysuria, kidney failure; calcification of bladder wall, ureter, and bladder can lead to bladder cancer; ectopic CNS parasites tend to cause transverse myelitis; genital schistosomiasis; death can occur
Worldwide	Penetration of unbroken skin by cercariae from infected snails in fresh- and saltwater	Self-limiting urticaria, pruritus, rash; fever, local lymph node swelling possible in some cases
PARASITIC DISEASES—CESTODES (TAPEWORMS)		
Asia, South America, Africa; can occur in imported primates in other areas	Ingestion of infected oribatid mites in food	Most cases asymptomatic; abdominal pain, vomiting, diarrhea, constipation, weight loss
Worldwide in scattered foci; mainly reported from Europe, Asia	Ingestion of tapeworm eggs in canine feces, may be via water, vegetables, soil	Painless skin swelling; possible CNS involvement (signs of mass lesion in brain) or larva in eye
Africa, Europe, North America, Australia; rare in people	As above	Painless skin swelling; also in muscles and retroperitoneally; CNS involvement possible

(*continued*)

TABLE 4 GLOBAL ZOONOSES[a] *(continued)*

Disease	Causative Organism	Animals Involved
PARASITIC DISEASES—CESTODES (TAPEWORMS) (continued)		
Coenuriasis (Coenurosis) *(continued)*	*T brauni*	Definitive hosts are canids; intermediate hosts are gerbils, wild rodents, also people
Cysticercosis	*Taenia solium* (*see also* Taeniasis)	People are definitive hosts; swine, other mammals are intermediate hosts (people can be both definitive and intermediate hosts)
	T crassiceps	Foxes, also other canids and carnivores, including dogs, are definitive hosts; rodents, insectivores, rabbits, occasionally other mammals are intermediate hosts
Diphyllobothriasis (Fish tapeworm infection)	*Diphyllobothrium latum* (*Dibothriocephalus latus*), *D nihonkaiense*, *D pacificum*, *D dendriticum*, and other *Diphyllobothrium* spp	Dogs, bears, seals, sea lions, gulls, and other fish-eating mammals and birds are definitive hosts; freshwater or marine fish (and copepods) are intermediate hosts
Dipylidiasis (Dog tapeworm infection)	*Dipylidium caninum*	Dogs, cats, wild canids, some other wild carnivores are definitive hosts; fleas are intermediate hosts
Echinococcosis	*Echinococcus granulosus* sensu lato	Dogs, other canids, hyenas are definitive hosts; sheep, goats, cattle, water buffalo, swine, camels, cervids, rodents, other mammals, or marsupials are intermediate or aberrant hosts; strains of parasite can be adapted to different intermediate hosts
	E multilocularis	Foxes and other wild canids and felids are usual definitive hosts, but parasite can also mature in dogs, cats; intermediate hosts are usually rodents, insectivores, some other mammals
	E oligarthrus	Wild felids are definitive hosts, can mature in cats; agouti, pacas, spiny rats are intermediate hosts
	E vogeli	Bush dogs are usual definitive host, can mature in other canids, including dogs; pacas, agouti, nutria, nonhuman primates, and other mammals can be intermediate hosts
Hymenolepiasis	*Hymenolepis nana* (dwarf tapeworm); most human infections probably transmitted from people, but zoonoses possible	People, nonhuman primates, rodents are definitive hosts; insects, including fleas, flour beetles, cereal beetles are intermediate hosts

TABLE 4 GLOBAL ZOONOSES[a] *(continued)*

Known Distribution	Probable Means of Spread to People	Clinical Manifestations in People
PARASITIC DISEASES—CESTODES (TAPEWORMS) (continued)		
Africa	As above	Most often in subcutaneous tissues (skin swelling) or eye, also CNS
Worldwide where swine are reared; most cases seen in Africa, Asia, Central and South America	Ingestion of eggs (including autoinfection from adult parasite in human intestine)	Inflammation in CNS caused by death of small larva or growth to large size (often years after infection); can cause seizures, other CNS signs; less often in eye or heart; massive numbers in muscles can also be symptomatic
North America, Europe, Asia, and other areas where foxes are present	Ingestion of eggs	Tissue invasion (mainly subcutaneous, muscle), ocular; one paravertebral pseudohematoma with local bleeding, one CNS larva; many but not all cases in immunocompromised
Worldwide; distribution of species varies	Ingestion of undercooked infected fish	Usually asymptomatic; may cause mild abdominal distress, diarrhea (chronic relapsing diarrhea possible in some cases)
Worldwide; uncommonly reported in people	Ingestion of dog or cat fleas	Usually in children; asymptomatic or mild abdominal distress, diarrhea; proglottids in feces resemble cucumber seeds
Worldwide, strains differ in distribution	Ingestion of tapeworm eggs in food or water, to mouth on hands; eggs stick to fur and hands	Cause space-occupying lesions of organs, especially lung, liver, also other organs, rarely CNS; cyst grows slowly, can cause death if untreated; rupture can cause allergic reactions, dissemination of cysts
North America (mainly Canada to north central USA), northern and central Eurasia	Ingestion of tapeworm eggs in food or water, to mouth on hands; eggs stick to fur and hands	Usually involves liver with mass lesions, occasionally lung or CNS; primary lesion can metastasize to many organs; without treatment, 70%–100% cases are fatal
Central and South America; rare in people	Ingestion of tapeworm eggs in food or water, to mouth on hands; eggs stick to fur and hands	Has been seen in a variety of internal organs, eyes
Central and South America	Ingestion of tapeworm eggs in food or water, to mouth on hands; eggs stick to fur and hands	Usually involves liver, may invade adjacent tissues; mortality high in advanced cases, even with treatment (22% in one study)
Worldwide	Accidental ingestion of tapeworm eggs or infected insects; autoinfection possible	Mainly in children; mild abdominal distress, decreased appetite, irritability are most common; weight loss, flatulence, diarrhea possible

(continued)

TABLE 4 GLOBAL ZOONOSES[a] *(continued)*

Disease	Causative Organism	Animals Involved
PARASITIC DISEASES—CESTODES (TAPEWORMS) (continued)		
Hymenolepiasis *(continued)*	*H diminuta* (mouse tapeworm, rat tapeworm)	Rats, mice are definitive hosts; insects, including fleas and cereal beetles are intermediate hosts
Inermicapsifer infection	*Inermicapsifer* spp	Rodents, people are definitive hosts in Africa; people may be exclusive host outside Africa
Raillietina infection	*R celebensis*, *R demerariensis*; most *Raillietina* spp have not been reported in people	Rodents, nonhuman primates are definitive hosts for *R celebensis*, *R demerariensis*; other species in birds, mammals; arthropods, including ants, are intermediate hosts
Sparganosis	*Spirometra* spp (pseudophyllidean tapeworms, second larval stage)	Dogs, cats, wild canids and felids are definitive hosts; copepods are first intermediate host; fish, frogs, reptiles are second intermediate hosts; primates, pigs, weasels, rodents, insectivores, other mammals, birds are paratenic hosts
Taeniasis		
—Asian taeniasis	*Taenia asiatica* (also called *T taiwanensis*, *T saginata asiatica*	Domestic and wild pigs, occasionally cattle, goats, monkeys are intermediate hosts; people are definitive hosts
—Beef tapeworm disease	*T saginata*	Cattle, water buffalo, llamas, reindeer, camels, other domestic and wild ruminants are intermediate hosts; people are definitive host
—Pork tapeworm disease; cysticercosis and neurocysticercosis	*T solium*	People are definitive host; swine, occasionally other mammals, including people, are intermediate hosts
PARASITIC DISEASES—NEMATODES (ROUNDWORMS)		
Angiostrongyliasis	*Angiostrongylus costaricensis*, also called *Parastrongylus costaricensis*	Cotton rats and other rodents are definitive hosts; slugs are intermediate hosts

TABLE 4 GLOBAL ZOONOSES[a] (continued)

Known Distribution	Probable Means of Spread to People	Clinical Manifestations in People
PARASITIC DISEASES—CESTODES (TAPEWORMS) (continued)		
Worldwide	Ingestion of infected insects in food	Mild abdominal symptoms of short duration
Africa, southeast Asia, tropical America	Probably ingestion of infected arthropods	Mild abdominal symptoms, if any
R demerariensis in tropical America (human cases mainly Ecuador, Cuba, Guyana, Honduras); *R celebensis* in Asia, Australia, Africa	Probably ingestion of infected arthropods in food	Vague discomfort, many cases asymptomatic; gastroenteritis, possibly other signs; mainly in children
Worldwide; human cases most common in Asia	Ingestion of infected cyclops (in water) or undercooked intermediate or paratenic host; application of contaminated tissues to skin (eg, as poultice)	Nodular, itchy skin lesions that can migrate; conjunctival and eyelid lesions; urticaria, painful edema; other organ involvement, including CNS, eye
Asia	Ingestion of undercooked animal products, usually visceral organs such as liver and lung	Vague abdominal complaints and proglottid passage; anal pruritus; possible that ingestion of eggs may be followed by larval migration and disseminated disease (uncertain/controversial)
Worldwide	Ingestion of undercooked meat containing larvae	Mild abdominal discomfort and proglottid passage; gravid proglottids may travel to ectopic sites and cause symptoms; eggs do not cause disseminated disease
Worldwide where swine are reared; most cases seen in Africa, Asia, Central and South America	Ingestion of undercooked pork containing larvae causes taeniasis; ingestion of eggs (including autoinfection from adult worm in intestine) causes cysticercosis	Adult stage in intestine (taeniasis) mild or asymptomatic; cysticercosis usually asymptomatic for years until cysticercus becomes large or death of small cysticerci result in inflammation in CNS (seizures, other CNS signs) or infrequently in eye or heart; massive numbers in muscles can also be symptomatic
PARASITIC DISEASES—NEMATODES (ROUNDWORMS)		
Mainly in Central and South America, Caribbean parasite has also been reported in North America	Accidental ingestion of slugs or possibly plants contaminated by their secretions	Acute abdominal angiostrongyliasis; severe pain resembles appendicitis, especially in children; rarely, more insidious disease with liver involvement; complications can include intestinal ischemia, perforation; fatalities possible

(continued)

TABLE 4 GLOBAL ZOONOSES[a] *(continued)*

Disease	Causative Organism	Animals Involved
PARASITIC DISEASES—NEMATODES (ROUNDWORMS) (continued)		
Angiostrongyliasis *(continued)*	*Angiostrongylus cantonensis*, also called *Parastrongylus cantonensis*	Rodents (rats, including *Rattus* and *Bandicota* spp) are definitive hosts; snails, slugs are intermediate hosts; land planarians, crustaceans (crabs, shrimp, prawns), amphibians, fish, reptiles are paratenic hosts
Anisakiasis	*Anisakis, Pseudoterranova*, and *Contracaecum* spp	Marine mammals (cetaceans and pinnipeds) and fish-eating birds are definitive hosts; fish, crustaceans, and cephalopod mollusks are intermediate or paratenic hosts
Ascariasis	*Ascaris suum*; potentially zoonotic (controversial)	Pigs, also reported occasionally in other mammals, including nonhuman primates, sheep, cattle
Capillariasis		
—Hepatic capillariasis	*Capillaria hepatica* (also called *Calodium hepaticum*)	Rodents major host, also in many other wild and domestic mammals
—Intestinal capillariasis	*C philippinensis* (also called *Paracapillaria philippinensis*)	Aquatic birds, people can be definitive hosts; freshwater fish are intermediate host
—Pulmonary capillariasis	*C aerophila* (also called *Eucoleus aerophilus*)	Dogs, cats, other carnivores
Dioctophymosis (Giant kidney worm infection)	*Dioctophyma renale*	Mink, dogs, and other carnivores are definitive hosts; annelids are intermediate hosts; frogs, fish are paratenic hosts
Dracunculiasis (Guinea worm infection)	*Dracunculus medinensis*; people are most important host but possible role for zoonotic transmission in some locations	People, nonhuman primates are definitive hosts; infections have also been reported in animals, but parasite identification sometimes uncertain; domestic animals not thought to maintain parasite but possible exceptions (eg, dogs in Chad); copepods are intermediate hosts
Filariasis		
—Dirofilariasis	*Dirofilaria immitis*	Dogs, cats, other mammals especially carnivores, mustelids, primates are definitive hosts (mainly patent in dogs and wild canids); mosquitoes are intermediate hosts

TABLE 4 GLOBAL ZOONOSES[a] *(continued)*

Known Distribution	Probable Means of Spread to People	Clinical Manifestations in People
PARASITIC DISEASES—NEMATODES (ROUNDWORMS) (continued)		
Originated in Asia, spread to many other regions, mainly tropics, including Americas, Caribbean, Middle East, Australia	Ingestion of raw/undercooked intermediate or paratenic host (or accidental ingestion on vegetables); possibly ingestion of plants contaminated by secretions of intermediate host	Eosinophilic meningitis or meningoencephalitis, spinal cord involvement; ocular involvement with decreased vision; transient abdominal pain, pruritus in some; most cases relatively mild and self-limiting, but some fatal
Worldwide but many cases in northern Asia and western Europe	Ingestion of undercooked marine fish, squid, octopus	Gastroenteritis with upper quadrant pain; parasite usually in stomach; small-intestinal infections unusual but can occur; colon, esophagus rarely involved; oropharyngeal worm can cause hematemesis, cough; urticaria and other allergic signs after ingestion of live or dead worms
Worldwide, prevalence varies	Ingestion of eggs from environment (shed in feces)	Visceral larva migrans (respiratory signs, fever during larval migration); GI signs
Worldwide in scattered foci	Ingestion of embryonated eggs in soil	Acute or subacute hepatitis with marked eosinophilia; subclinical to fatal
Philippines, Thailand, also reported occasionally in other parts of Asia, Middle East, Cuba	Ingestion of undercooked infected fish	Enteropathy with protein loss and malabsorption; diarrhea, abdominal pain; weight loss can be severe; death possible
Worldwide; rare in people	Accidental ingestion of infective eggs in soil or contaminated food	Fever, cough, bronchospasm, bronchitis, dyspnea; can mimic bronchial carcinoma
Worldwide; rare in people	Ingestion of infected fish, frog, or annelid	Renal colic, hematuria, pyuria, ureteral obstruction, various kidney complications can be fatal; subcutaneous nodule
Asia (mainly Indian subcontinent) and Africa	Ingestion of infected cyclops in water	No symptoms until just before larviposition (~1 yr); papule to vesicular skin lesion to ulcer that opens in water to reveal worm; allergic reaction common at this time, and secondary infection may occur
Worldwide	Bite of infected mosquitoes	Fever, cough acutely, larvae result in infarct or coin lesion in the lungs; often asymptomatic; rarely involves eye or other body sites

(continued)

TABLE 4 GLOBAL ZOONOSES[a] *(continued)*

Disease	Causative Organism	Animals Involved
PARASITIC DISEASES—NEMATODES (ROUNDWORMS) (continued)		
Dirofilariasis *(continued)*	*D tenuis*, *D repens*, rarely other species	*D tenuis* in raccoons; *D repens* mainly patent in dogs and some wild canids (eg, foxes); also infects cats but not usually patent
—Malayan filariasis	*Brugia malayi*; subperiodic form is of uncertain origin, thought to be zoonotic or maintained in both animals and people; periodic form is exclusive to people	Cats, wild felids, pangolins, other carnivores, nonhuman primates susceptible
Filariasis caused by other *Brugia* species	*Brugia* spp other than *B malayi*, including *B pahangi*	Various domestic and wild mammals, including dogs and cats, are definitive hosts
Gnathostomiasis	*Gnathostoma spinigerum*, *G binucleatum*, and some other *Gnathostoma* spp	Dogs, cats, wild carnivores are definitive hosts (*G doloresi* and *G hispidum* in pigs and wild boars); copepods, freshwater fish, eels, frogs, snakes, chickens, snails, pigs are intermediate or paratenic hosts
Gongylonemiasis	*Gongylonema pulchrum*	Ruminants, domestic and wild swine, other mammals, birds are definitive hosts; coprophagous insects (eg, beetles, cockroaches) are intermediate hosts
Larva migrans, cutaneous (*see also* GNATHOSTOMIASIS, above)	*Ancylostoma braziliense*, *A caninum*, *A ceylanicum*, *Uncinaria stenocephala*	Cats, dogs, wild carnivores are definitive hosts
	Bunostomum phlebotomum	Cattle
	Strongyloides stercoralis and other *Strongyloides* spp found in animals	*S stercoralis* in dogs, cats, primates, including people; other species in swine, sheep, goats, cattle, horses, raccoons, and other domestic and wild mammals

TABLE 4 GLOBAL ZOONOSES[a] *(continued)*

Known Distribution	Probable Means of Spread to People	Clinical Manifestations in People
PARASITIC DISEASES—NEMATODES (ROUNDWORMS) (continued)		
D tenuis in North America; *D repens* in Asia, Europe, Africa	Bite of infected mosquitoes	Subcutaneous nodule or submucosal swelling, some migratory and/or painful; subconjunctival (rarely intraocular); internal location (mainly lung but also brain, other organs) possible
Asia; subperiodic form limited to peninsular Malaysia, Thailand, and parts of Indonesia, Vietnam, and the Philippines in swamp-forest environments	Bite of infected mosquitoes, *Mansonia* spp mainly associated with subperiodic form	Lymphatic filariasis: recurrent painful lymphadenitis, lymphangitis, often preceded by prodromal illness with malaise or urticaria; may progress to elephantiasis, usually of legs; hypersensitivity syndrome with cough, chest pain, asthmatic attacks especially at night
Asia, Africa, Americas	Mosquitoes	Occasional zoonotic infections (eg, cutaneous nodules, granuloma in lymph nodes)
Worldwide; most human cases from Asia; emerging along Pacific coast of Mexico, Ecuador, Peru, Argentina	Ingestion of undercooked fish, poultry, or other intermediate or paratenic host, drinking water contaminated with copepods containing larvae; handling meat that contains larvae	Fever, malaise, gastroenteritis, urticaria, soon after ingestion; migratory skin lesions (intermittent swelling, often painful or pruritic, or linear erythematous lesions) after weeks to years; may involve viscera, eye, or CNS; CNS involvement can be fatal or result in permanent damage with reported case fatality rates of 7%–25%
Worldwide; rare in people	Ingestion of infected beetles, probably on vegetables; possible inhalation of small beetles	Movement of parasite in submucosa of mouth is sensed; local irritation; pharyngitis, stomatitis possible
Worldwide; distribution varies with the species	Contact with infective larvae that penetrate skin, usually via soil	Itchy, serpiginous, migrating skin lesions; papules, nonspecific dermatitis, vesicles; wheezing, cough, and urticaria may occur; myositis or ocular lesions possible; eosinophilic enteritis after ingestion of *A caninum*; *A ceylanicum* can also become patent in intestine, causing GI signs, anemia
Temperate regions	As above	As above
Worldwide, more common in tropics and subtropics	Contact with infective larvae that penetrate skin, from soil or direct contact with feces; autoinfection possible with *S stercoralis*	Larva currens (linear, serpiginous urticarial inflammation, often rapidly progressive); *S stercoralis* may also mature in intestine, causing enteritis and other signs (*see* below)

(continued)

TABLE 4 GLOBAL ZOONOSES[a] *(continued)*

Disease	Causative Organism	Animals Involved
PARASITIC DISEASES—NEMATODES (ROUNDWORMS) (continued)		
Larva migrans, visceral (*see also* ANGIOSTRONGYLIASIS, p 2454, and ANISAKIASIS, p 2456)	*Toxocara canis*, *T cati*, possibly others	Dogs and wild canids (*T canis*), cats and wild felids (*T cati*) are definitive hosts; many species can be paratenic hosts
	Baylisascaris procyonis, possibly other species of *Bayliscascaris*	Raccoons, kinkajous are definitive hosts; dogs can be definitive or intermediate host; many mammals (including people), marsupials, and birds are intermediate or paratenic hosts
Oesophagostomiasis, Ternidensiasis	*Oesophagostomum* spp, *Ternidens deminutus*; zoonotic potential may vary with parasite species/strain and geographic area	Primates, including people
Onchocercosis	*Onchocerca gutturosa*, *O cervicalis*, *O jakutensis*, *O dewittei japonica*, *O reticulata*, *O lupi*, others	Definitive hosts include cattle, horses, cervids, wild boars, dogs and other canids, camels, other species
Strongyloidiasis	*Strongyloides stercoralis*; most human infections thought to be from strains adapted to people; frequency of maturation of canine *S stercoralis* in people undetermined, thought to be rare	*S stercoralis* in dogs, cats, foxes, primates, including people
	S fuelleborni	Primates, including people
Thelaziasis (Eyeworms)	*Thelazia callipaedia*, *T californiensis*, possibly *T rhodesii*	Definitive hosts are dogs and other canids, cats (*T callipaedia*); dogs, wild mammals, occasionally cats (*T californiensis*); flies are intermediate hosts
Trichinosis (Trichinellosis)	*Trichinella spiralis* and subspecies, *T nativa*, *T britovi*, *T nelsoni*, *T pseudospiralis*, possibly others	Main reservoir may be wild carnivores (foxes, badgers, wolves, lynx), omnivores (bears, boars); also in any mammal that eats (or is fed) meat, including domestic swine, rodents, cats, dogs, horses, marine mammals; also birds (*T pseudospiralis*); *T zimbabwensis* (zoonotic potential unknown) can infect reptiles

TABLE 4 GLOBAL ZOONOSES[a] *(continued)*

Known Distribution	Probable Means of Spread to People	Clinical Manifestations in People
PARASITIC DISEASES—NEMATODES (ROUNDWORMS) (continued)		
Worldwide	Ingestion of embryonated eggs shed in feces of dogs and cats; via soil, water, food, fomites	Fever, wheezing cough, upper abdominal discomfort; other symptoms, including neurologic signs, skin rashes also possible; may wax and wane for months; eye involvement (ocular migrans) may resemble retinoblastoma
North America, Europe, Japan	Accidental ingestion of embryonated eggs in soil, water, or fecal-contaminated material	Nonspecific signs, including fever, lethargy; hepatomegaly, pneumonitis, parasitic meningoencephalitis (may be fatal in infants, young children), ocular disease; other syndromes, including cardiac disease
Parasites found in Africa, Asia, South America; human cases mainly reported in Africa	Ingestion of infective larvae in soil, often in food or water	Abdominal pain and one or more masses ± mild fever; intestinal obstruction or abscessation possible; multinodular form (less common) with abdominal pain, persistent diarrhea, weight loss; rarely ectopic in omentum, liver, or skin
Distribution varies with species	Probably transmitted by black flies (Diptera: Simuliidae), possibly other vectors	Ocular disease, subcutaneous nodules
S stercoralis worldwide; more common in tropical and subtropical climates	Contact with infective larvae that penetrate skin, in soil or direct contact with feces; autoinfection possible	Frequently asymptomatic in healthy; possible larva currens (*see* LARVA MIGRANS, p 2458); respiratory signs in some (cough to bronchopneumonia), especially in elderly, immunocompromised; abdominal pain, diarrhea, sometimes with periodic urticarial or maculopapular rash; disseminated strongyloidiasis, neurologic complications, septicemia, and death may occur in immunocompromised
Africa, Asia, and in captive primates in other areas	As above	Associated with abdominal pain, occasional diarrhea, not well studied
T callipaedia in Asia, Europe; *T californiensis* in North America (western USA); rarely in people	Flies release parasite larvae on conjunctiva	Conjunctivitis; corneal scarring, opacity in chronic cases
Worldwide, especially in temperate regions; some species are limited in their distribution	Ingestion of undercooked pork, horse meat, game, and other tissues containing viable cysts	Gastroenteritis in some; followed by fever, headache, severe myalgia, facial swelling (especially eyelids); ocular pain, rashes, or pruritus possible; pneumonitis, CNS, or myocardial involvement can occur; inapparent to fatal

(continued)

TABLE 4 GLOBAL ZOONOSES[a] (continued)

Disease	Causative Organism	Animals Involved
PARASITIC DISEASES—NEMATODES (ROUNDWORMS) (continued)		
Trichostrongyliasis	*Trichostrongylus* spp	Cattle, sheep, other domestic and wild ruminants, sometimes other mammals
Trichuriasis (Whipworm infection)	*Trichuris suis*, possibly *T vulpis* and other species; main species in people is *T trichiura*, but zoonotic infections are unusual	*T vulpis* in canids; *T suis* in domestic and wild swine
PARASITIC DISEASES—ACANTHOCEPHALANS		
Acanthocephaliasis, Macracanthorhynchosis	*Macracanthorhynchus hirudinaceus* and other species	Hosts vary with parasite species; definitive hosts include domestic and wild pigs, rodents, muskrats, arctic foxes, dogs, sea otters, other terrestrial and marine mammals; intermediate hosts are beetles, cockroaches, crustaceans; fish are paratenic hosts
PARASITIC DISEASES—ANNELIDS (LEECHES)		
Hirudiniasis (internal)	*Limnatis nilotica* and other aquatic leeches	Cattle, buffalo, other domestic and wild mammals, probably frogs
ARTHROPOD DISEASES		
Acariasis (Mange)	Mites of *Sarcoptes*, *Cheyletiella*, *Dermanyssus*, and *Ornithonyssus* spp, *Notoedres cati*, *Trixacarus caviae*, *Liponyssoides sanguineus*; possibly others (uncommon)	Mammals and birds
Myiasis	*Cochliomyia hominivorax* and *Chrysomya bezziana* (screwworms)	Mammals; rare in birds
	Cordylobia anthropophaga, rarely *C rodhaini* (Tumbu flies)	Mammals, often found in dogs, rodents

TABLE 4 GLOBAL ZOONOSES[a] (*continued*)

Known Distribution	Probable Means of Spread to People	Clinical Manifestations in People
PARASITIC DISEASES—NEMATODES (ROUNDWORMS) (continued)		
Worldwide	Ingestion of infective larvae on vegetables or in contaminated water, soil	Asymptomatic or mild gastroenteritis
Worldwide, especially warm, humid climates	Ingestion of embryonated eggs on plant foods, water, or in soil	*T suis* can colonize people, who develop GI signs; rare larva migrans or intestinal infections suggested from *T vulpis* (controversial identification)
PARASITIC DISEASES—ACANTHOCEPHALANS		
Worldwide	Ingestion of infected beetles, other intermediate hosts, or fish	Gastroenteritis, may lead to gut perforation or intestinal obstruction; some cases asymptomatic
PARASITIC DISEASES—ANNELIDS (LEECHES)		
Africa, Asia, southern Europe, Middle East	Drinking unfiltered water (leech enters nares or mouth), wading in deep water (enters genitourinary tract)	Attaches to nasopharynx, pharynx, esophagus, occasionally deeper in respiratory tract, or in genitourinary tract; pressure and/or pain at attachment site; bleeding (eg, hemoptysis, hematemesis, epistaxis, vaginal bleeding), anemia (can be severe); other signs depend on location
ARTHROPOD DISEASES		
Worldwide	Contact with infected animals, fomites	Itchy skin lesions
C hominivorax in South America, Caribbean; *C bezziana* in Asia, Africa, Middle East	Flies lay eggs on host, larvae enter wounds (as small as a tick bite), mucous membranes	Painful, pruritic, foul-smelling, enlarging dermal and subdermal wounds or nodules, often with serosanguineous discharge; some infestations in cavities, including nasal cavity; larvae can invade living tissue, locally destructive (including bone, eye, sinuses, or cranial cavity); can be fatal if untreated
Africa, Middle East; also reported in Mediterranean region of Europe	Larvae from environment invade unbroken skin	Furuncular swelling at site of invasion, often feet; fever, malaise, focal lymphadenopathy possible

(*continued*)

TABLE 4 GLOBAL ZOONOSES[a] *(continued)*

Disease	Causative Organism	Animals Involved
ARTHROPOD DISEASES (continued)		
Myiasis *(continued)*	*Cuterebra* spp	Rodents, lagomorphs, occasionally other mammals
	Dermatobia hominis (human botfly)	Mammals, some birds
	Gasterophilus spp (equine botfly)	Equids, occasionally other mammals
	Hypoderma lineatum, *H bovis* (warbles), and other *Hypoderma* spp	*H bovis* and *H lineatum* in cattle, sometimes other mammals; other species primarily parasites of deer, caribou, or yaks
	Oestrus ovis, *Rhinoestrus purpureus*	*O ovis* mainly in sheep, goats, also other mammals; *R purpureus* mainly in equids
	Wohlfahrtia spp, *Wohlfahrtia vigil*, *W magnifica*	*W vigil* in rabbits, rodents, mink, foxes, dogs, and other carnivores, other mammals; *W magnifica* in sheep, cattle, dogs, other mammals, some birds, especially geese
Pentastomid infections	*Armillifer* spp (tongue worms)	Definitive hosts are snakes; intermediate hosts are rodents and other wild animals

TABLE 4 GLOBAL ZOONOSES[a] *(continued)*

Known Distribution	Probable Means of Spread to People	Clinical Manifestations in People
ARTHROPOD DISEASES (continued)		
North America	Larvae from vegetation enter host in natural cavities or invade intact skin	Subcutaneous furunculoid nodule(s); creeping skin eruption (uncommon); ocular lesions; rarely larvae might be found in upper respiratory tract
South and Central America, Mexico	Eggs carried by other insects (eg, mosquitoes); larvae hatch and penetrate skin of mammalian host when insect lands	Nonmigratory larvae in furuncles; episodes of pain, intense pruritus, sometimes with lymphangitis or lymphadenitis; can invade eyelids, eye sockets, mouth, especially in children
Worldwide	Accidental exposure to larvae	Serpiginous, pruritic red stripes on skin resembling cutaneous larva migrans; very rarely might reach stomach (nausea, vomiting)
North America, Europe, Asia; species distribution varies	Eggs laid on host, larvae invade skin	Usually subcutaneous (slowly moving furuncles that can appear and disappear) or similar to cutaneous larva migrans; endophthalmia uncommon; *H lineatum* may also cause an eosinophilic syndrome with fever, muscle pain, sometimes respiratory, cardiac, or neurologic signs
O ovis worldwide, usually in warmer climates; *R purpureus* in Asia, Africa, Europe	Larvae are deposited in nares, conjunctiva, occasionally lips/mouth by adult fly	Conjunctival form, with lacrimation and sensation of irritating foreign body in eye, ocular destruction rare; nasal form with localized pain or pruritus, congestion, headache; also reported in pharynx (inflammation, vomiting, dysphagia), rarely ear; usually self-limiting (except inside eye), because larvae cannot develop beyond first stage in people
W vigil in North America; *W magnifica* in Europe (mainly Mediterranean), north Africa, Asia	Larvae deposited on host or nearby, penetrate lesions (both agents) or intact skin (*W vigil*) and natural orifices	*W vigil* causes subcutaneous abscesses, furuncles; *W magnifica* has been reported from skin, eye, vulva, ear, orotracheal region
Africa, Asia	Ingestion, via water or vegetables contaminated with eggs (from feces or saliva of snakes); undercooked snake meat; contaminated hands, fomites after handling snake meat	Usually asymptomatic; large numbers of parasites can cause multifocal abscesses, masses, or obstruction of ducts in internal organs; symptoms vary with location; death rare

(continued)

TABLE 4 GLOBAL ZOONOSES[a] *(continued)*

Disease	Causative Organism	Animals Involved
	ARTHROPOD DISEASES (continued)	
Pentastomid infections *(continued)*	*Linguatula serrata*	Definitive hosts are dogs and other canids, felids; intermediate hosts are herbivores (especially sheep, goats, lagomorphs) and people
Tick paralysis (*see* p 1314)	More than 40 species of ticks are capable of causing this disease; *Dermacentor andersoni*, *D variabilis* most common in North America	Various animals carry ticks
Tunga infections	*Tunga penetrans* (sand fleas, jiggers)	People, dogs, pigs, other mammals
	VIRAL DISEASES	
Alkhurma virus infection	Alkhurma virus (family Flaviviirdae, genus *Flavivirus*); may be a variant or strain of Kyasanur Forest virus	Sheep, goats, camels
Barmah Forest virus infection; epidemic polyarthritis	Barmah Forest virus (family Togaviridae, genus *Alphavirus*)	Natural hosts unknown; horses, brushtail possums may be hosts
Buffalopox virus infection	Vaccinia virus, Buffalopox virus strain (family Poxviridae, genus *Orthopoxvirus*)	Water buffalo, cattle
California encephalitis virus serogroup (California serogroup) infections	California encephalitis virus serogroup (family Bunyaviridae, genus *Orthobunyavirus*); includes California, La Crosse, Tahyna, Inkoo, Jamestown Canyon, Morro Bay, Snowshoe hare, Guaroa, Lumbo, Chatanga, and other viruses	Many wild and domestic mammals

TABLE 4 GLOBAL ZOONOSES[a] *(continued)*

Known Distribution	Probable Means of Spread to People	Clinical Manifestations in People
	ARTHROPOD DISEASES (continued)	
Worldwide	Ingestion of water or vegetables contaminated with eggs (from feces, saliva, or nasal discharge of definitive host); ingestion of larvae in undercooked liver or lymph nodes from intermediate hosts	Ingestion of eggs—usually asymptomatic; ocular or pulmonary signs, abdominal pain, icterus, and other symptoms possible from invasion of internal organs Ingestion of larvae—throat irritation, pain; edema, congestion of nasopharynx may cause dyspnea, difficulty swallowing; most severe cases are probably in people who have been sensitized
Worldwide	Tick attachment	Ascending flaccid paralysis, may be preceded by prodromal flu-like illness (malaise, weakness); can cause respiratory paralysis, also paresthesia; ends when tick is removed
Africa, Central and South America, Caribbean, south Asia	Skin contact with contaminated soil	Penetration of skin and burrowing result in pain and itching around discrete sores, often on feet; may be secondarily infected
	VIRAL DISEASES	
Middle East, mainly reported in Saudi Arabia, also Egypt	Ticks (*Ornithodoros* and *Hyalomma* spp); direct contact with animal meat via broken skin or ingestion of unpasteurized camel milk linked to some cases	Febrile illness, often with GI signs (eg, vomiting, abdominal pain); encephalitic/neurologic and hemorrhagic signs in some; case fatality up to 25% in early reports, recently <1%
Australia	Mosquito bites; *Culex annulirostris* and *Aedes* spp implicated	Resembles disease caused by Ross River virus (*see* p 2478) but seems to persist longterm in fewer patients, rash more common
Indian subcontinent (south Asia), Egypt, Indonesia	Skin contact with infected animals, often when milking	Pox skin lesions mainly on hands, face, legs, buttocks; occasionally lymphadenopathy, fever, malaise
North and South America, Europe, Africa, Asia; possibly worldwide; distribution of each virus varies	Mosquito bites	Syndromes, severity vary with the virus; flu-like illness, meningitis, or encephalitis common with North American viruses

(continued)

TABLE 4 GLOBAL ZOONOSES[a] *(continued)*

Disease	Causative Organism	Animals Involved
	VIRAL DISEASES (continued)	
—La Crosse encephalitis	La Crosse virus (California encephalitis virus serogroup)	Chipmunks, squirrels are major amplifying hosts; rabbits, foxes, and other mammals can be infected
—Tahyna fever	Tahyna virus (California encephalitis virus serogroup)	Hares, rabbits, rodents, hedgehogs, and other mammals
Camelpox	Camelpox virus	Old World camelids, possibly other species
Chikungunya virus infection	Chikungunya virus (family Togaviridae, genus *Alphavirus*)	Sylvatic cycle in nonhuman primates, possibly rodents in Africa; virus thought to be maintained in people in Asia, but sylvatic cycle may also exist
Colorado tick fever	Colorado tick fever virus (family Reoviridae, genus *Coltivurus*; Salmon River virus and California hare coltivirus may be variants	Rodents; also found in porcupines, lagomorphs, deer, elk, and other mammals
Contagious ecthyma (Orf, *see* p 866)	Orf virus (family Poxviridae, genus *Parapoxvirus*)	Sheep, goats, camelids, reindeer, wild ungulates; rare cases in dogs
Cowpox (*see* p 868)	Cowpox virus (family Poxviridae, genus *Orthopoxvirus*)	Rodents are usual reservoir host; also in domestic and wild cats, occasionally cattle, other mammals

TABLE 4 GLOBAL ZOONOSES[a] *(continued)*

Known Distribution	Probable Means of Spread to People	Clinical Manifestations in People
VIRAL DISEASES (continued)		
North America	Mosquito bites	Many cases mild and flu-like; meningitis or encephalitis with seizures, paralysis, and focal neurologic signs possible; most cases in children; estimated case fatality rate <1% in cases with encephalitis
Europe, Asia, Africa	Mosquito bites (culicine and anopheles)	Influenza-like illness, sometimes including GI signs; arthritis or respiratory signs, including broncho-pneumonia in some; meningitis possible; most often in children; does not appear to cause fatal disease
Middle East, Asia, Africa, possibly other areas; human cases recently described in India in camel handlers, rare unconfirmed cases suggested in other locations	Direct contact	Skin lesions similar to cowpox, variola virus infections
Asia, Africa	Mosquito bites (especially *Aedes* spp)	Febrile illness, may have rash and/or GI signs; arthralgia, especially in small joints, and myalgia prominent, may persist for months; myocarditis, neurologic signs, hemorrhages reported in a few cases
Rocky Mountain region of North America	Tick bites (primary vector is *Dermacentor andersoni*)	Nonspecific febrile illness; pharyngitis, rash, or GI signs possible; biphasic or triphasic in some; complications (eg, neurologic signs, hemorrhages, pericarditis, myocarditis, orchitis) uncommon but can occur in severe cases; deaths rare
Worldwide	Occupational exposure via contact with broken skin (both live animals and meat processing)	Papule(s) that umbilicate and ulcerate, usually on hands; dissemination rare; large lesions refractory to treatment can be seen in immunosuppressed
Parts of Europe and Asia	Contact exposure via broken skin, bites, scratches	Papules, vesicles that become pustular, to ulcerative nodules, scars; single or multiple lesions, often on hands; regional adenopathy and malaise, flu-like symptoms in some; lesions remain localized in healthy people; more extensive or generalized disease may be seen in children, people with eczema, immunocompromised; severe cases can involve respiratory mucosa; rare fatal cases (eg, complications of encephalitis)

(continued)

TABLE 4 GLOBAL ZOONOSES[a] (continued)

Disease	Causative Organism	Animals Involved
VIRAL DISEASES (continued)		
Crimean-Congo hemorrhagic fever (*see* p 751)	Crimean-Congo hemorrhagic fever virus (family Bunyaviridae, genus *Nairovirus*)	Cattle, rodents, sheep, goats, hares, other mammals, some birds
Eastern equine encephalomyelitis (*see* p 1291)	Eastern equine encephalomyelitis virus (family Togaviridae, genus *Alphavirus*); North American lineage 1 strains more virulent than South American lineages	Birds are principal reservoir hosts in North America, snakes might have role in overwintering virus; rodents, marsupials might be reservoir hosts in South America; clinical cases seen in equids and occasionally other mammals and birds; mammals are almost always dead-end hosts
Ebola hemorrhagic fever	Zaire ebolavirus, Sudan ebolavirus, Ivory Coast ebolavirus, Bundibugyo ebolavirus (family Filoviridae, genus *Ebolavirus*); Reston ebolavirus does not seem to affect people	Bats are reservoir hosts for Zaire ebolavirus and suspected reservoir hosts for others; primates, duikers, possibly other mammals can be infected
Encephalomyocarditis	Encephalomyocarditis virus (family Picornaviridae, genus *Cardiovirus*); thought to be zoonotic	Rodents may be reservoir hosts; also in swine, nonhuman primates, elephants, other mammals, and wild birds
Foot-and-mouth disease (*see* p 629)	Foot-and-mouth disease virus (family Picornaviridae, genus *Aphthovirus*, types A, O, C, SAT 1, SAT 2, SAT 3, and Asia 1)	Cattle, swine, sheep, goats, other cloven-hoofed animals (Artiodactyla), a few mammals in other orders
Hantaviral diseases		
—Hantaviral pulmonary syndrome	Sin Nombre, Black Creek Canal, Bayou, Andes, Bermejo, Choclo, Araraquara, *Juquitiba*, Laguna Negra, and Castelo dos Sonhosviruses, others (family Bunyaviridae, genus *Hantavirus*)	Rodents; each virus tends to be associated with a single reservoir host
—Hemorrhagic fever with renal syndrome	Hantaan virus, Dobrava virus, Puumala virus, Seoul virus, Saaremaa virus, others (family Bunyaviridae, genus *Hantavirus*)	Rodents; each virus tends to be associated with a single reservoir host, but Seoul virus is carried by both *Rattus norvegicus* and *R rattus*

TABLE 4 GLOBAL ZOONOSES[a] *(continued)*

Known Distribution	Probable Means of Spread to People	Clinical Manifestations in People
VIRAL DISEASES (continued)		
Africa, Middle East, central Asia, southeastern Europe; appears to be spreading	Tick bites, especially *Hyalomma* but also *Rhipicephalus*, *Dermacentor*, other species; skin contact with animal or human blood or tissues or crushed ticks; ingestion of unpasteurized milk	Fever, headache, pharyngitis, abdominal symptoms, petechial rash, hemorrhage, hepatitis, other organ involvement in some cases; very severe in pregnant women; case fatality rate 3%–50%, varies with region
Western hemisphere	Mosquito bites; *Culiseta melanura* important in maintenance cycle in birds in North America; various mosquito species (*Aedes*, *Coquillettidia*, *Culex*) can transmit to people	Nonspecific febrile illness may be followed by severe encephalitis, especially with North American lineage; neurologic sequelae common after encephalitis; case fatality rate 30%–70% with North American lineage; more severe in infants and elderly
Africa	Contact with infected tissues (especially nonhuman primates and duikers); probable transmission from bats in caves	Initially nonspecific febrile illness; maculopapular rash with desquamation; mild to severe bleeding tendency develops a few days after onset; mortality rate 36%–90%, varies with isolate
Worldwide in animals	Uncertain	Nonspecific febrile illness, sometimes with GI signs, and/or decreased reflexes have been reported in adults, with recovery within several days; CNS signs, including paralysis, have been reported in children
Asia, Africa, Middle East, South America	Contact exposure, often in laboratories or other high concentrations of virus	People may become temporary nasal carriers of virus but do not usually become ill; mild influenza-like disease with vesicular lesions occurs very rarely
North and South America	Aerosols from rodent excretions and secretions; contact with broken skin and mucous membranes; rodent bites	Prodromal stage with nonspecific febrile illness; followed by respiratory failure, cardiac abnormalities; hemorrhagic signs possible with South American viruses; significant kidney disease uncommon; mortality rate varies with the virus, but can reach 40%–60%
Europe, Asia; Seoul virus is worldwide	Aerosols from rodent excretions and secretions; contact with broken skin and mucous membranes; rodent bites	Prodromal stage with abrupt onset of fever, headache, back pain, sometimes petechiae, GI signs (may be severe); followed by hypotension, renal signs to renal failure with oliguria; hemorrhage, other syndromes in some; mortality rate varies with the virus, from <1% (Puumala virus) to 10%–15% (Hantaan virus)

(continued)

TABLE 4 GLOBAL ZOONOSES[a] (*continued*)

Disease	Causative Organism	Animals Involved
VIRAL DISEASES (continued)		
Hendra virus infection (*see* p 707)	Hendra virus (family Paramyxoviridae, genus *Henipavirus*)	Fruit bats are normal reservoir host; horses can be infected
Hepatitis E	Hepatitis E virus, mammalian isolates (family Hepeviridae, genus *Hepevirus*); genotypes 3 and 4 zoonotic; genotypes 1 and 2 maintained in people	People; animals, including swine, wild boar, deer, rabbits, ferrets, rats, mongoose, others; swine and probably other hosts are reservoirs for human infections
Herpes B virus disease	Cercopithecine herpesvirus 1 (McHV, Herpesvirus simiae, B virus) (family Herpesviridae, genus *Simplexvirus*)	Carried in genus *Macaca* (Old World macaques), with lifelong latency and potential for periodic shedding after infection; other nonhuman primates susceptible; cell cultures
Influenza virus infections		
—Avian influenza	Influenza A virus (family Orthomyxoviridae, genus *Influenzavirus A*); avian influenza viruses; many severe human cases linked to Asian lineage H5N1 highly pathogenic avian influenza (HPAI) viruses, but other viruses also cause illness	Avian influenza viruses in wild and domestic birds, especially poultry; uncommon in mammals
—Swine influenza	Influenza A virus (family Orthomyxoviridae, genus *Influenzavirus A*); swine influenza viruses	Usually in pigs; also turkeys; can infect mink, ferrets
Japanese encephalitis (Japanese B encephalitis)	Japanese encephalitis virus (family Flaviviridae, genus *Flavivirus*)	Swine, wild birds are important maintenance hosts; horses ill but epidemiologically unimportant in amplification; other mammals, reptiles, amphibians may be infected, usually asymptomatically
Kyasanur Forest disease	Kyasanur Forest virus (family Flaviviridae, genus *Flavivirus*)	Rodents, shrews, other small mammals might be reservoirs (uncertain); affects monkeys; possible infections in other mammals, birds

TABLE 4 GLOBAL ZOONOSES[a] *(continued)*

Known Distribution	Probable Means of Spread to People	Clinical Manifestations in People
	VIRAL DISEASES (continued)	
Australia	Direct contact with infected animals (all human cases have been linked with horses) or contaminated tissues	Respiratory infection, encephalitis (including recurrent encephalitis); few cases described but several were fatal
Worldwide; human and zoonotic genotypes may differ in prevalence between areas	Fecal-oral spread; consumption of raw or undercooked meat and liver; waterborne, contact with animal reservoirs	Mild, self-limiting hepatitis to liver failure, more severe in pregnancy and can result in abortion, death of newborn, premature birth; usually acute, but can be chronic in organ-transplant patients; case fatality rate <1% to 4% in general population, up to 20% in pregnant
Worldwide, can be common, especially in closed groups of macaques; human cases rare	Monkey bites and scratches, contamination of mucous membranes with infected saliva, secretions	Influenza-like symptoms; vesicular skin lesions, pain, or itching around wound, followed by severe encephalitis with seizures, paralysis, coma; 85% mortality rate
Worldwide, distribution of strains varies	Usually by contact with infected poultry; avian viruses may be shed in respiratory secretions and feces	Avian influenza viruses can cause conjunctivitis, human influenza-like illness, or severe disease with multiorgan dysfunction, death; severity of disease varies with influenza strain
Worldwide	Usually by contact with infected animals; swine influenza viruses occur in respiratory secretions	Seems to resemble human influenza; severity of disease varies; fatal cases have been reported uncommonly
Asia, Australia, Papua New Guinea, Pacific islands from Japan to the Philippines	Mosquito bites (*Culex tritaeniorhynchus* important in maintenance cycle, other *Culex* and *Aedes* spp can transmit); also through broken skin or mucous membranes after direct contact with infected tissues	Fever, chills, myalgia, severe headache, GI symptoms; can progress to severe encephalitis; neurologic sequelae very common in survivors of encephalitis; case fatality rate 15%–30%
India	Tick bites (especially *Haemaphysalis spinigera*, also others)	Nonspecific febrile illness; course may be biphasic; hemorrhagic signs (eg, ecchymoses, purpura, petechiae, GI bleeding, epistaxis) and/or neurologic signs possible in second stage; prolonged convalescence in many; case fatality rate ~3%

(continued)

TABLE 4 GLOBAL ZOONOSES[a] *(continued)*

Disease	Causative Organism	Animals Involved
VIRAL DISEASES (continued)		
Lassa fever	Lassa virus (family Arenaviridae, genus *Arenavirus*)	Wild rodents, usually multimammate mouse
Louping ill (Ovine encephalomyelitis, *see* p 1299)	Louping ill virus (family Flaviviridae, genus *Flavivirus*)	Sheep, goats, also in llamas, cattle, horses, other domestic and wild mammals, grouse, ptarmigan
Lymphocytic choriomeningitis	Lymphocytic choriomeningitis virus (family Arenaviridae, genus *Arenavirus*)	Reservoir mainly house mouse; can be maintained in some other mice, hamster populations; also infects guinea pigs, chinchillas, rats, nonhuman primates, some other mammals
Marburg hemorrhagic fever	Marburg virus (family Filoviridae, genus *Marburgvirus*)	Bats are reservoir hosts; primates can be infected
Menangle virus infection	Menangle virus (family Paramyxoviridae)	Fruit bats are normal reservoir host; pigs can also be reservoir
Middle East respiratory syndrome (MERS)	MERS coronavirus	Unknown reservoir host, possibly bats; source of infection for people uncertain, camels implicated
Milker's nodules (Pseudocowpox, *see* p 868)	Pseudocowpox virus (family Poxviridae, genus *Parapoxvirus*)	Cattle
Monkeypox	Monkeypox virus (family Poxviridae, genus *Orthopoxvirus*); Congo Basin clade causes more severe illness than West African clade	Nonhuman primates, some wild and pet rodents, including Gambian rats, dormice, prairie dogs, African squirrels, some other mammals such as opossums; full host range uncertain

TABLE 4 **GLOBAL ZOONOSES**[a] *(continued)*

Known Distribution	Probable Means of Spread to People	Clinical Manifestations in People
	VIRAL DISEASES (continued)	
West Africa	Contact with rodent excretions, secretions, or tissues; aerosols	Gradual onset of nonspecific febrile illness, may be followed by chest pain, cough, GI signs, hepatitis; severe swelling of head and neck, hypotension/ shock can develop; pleural/pericardial effusions; hemorrhagic syndrome less common; overall mortality rate 1% in endemic areas; case fatality rate 20% among hospitalized patients
UK, Northern Ireland; also reported in Norway, Spain; uncommon in people	Tick bites (*Ixodes ricinus*); aerosol exposure in laboratory, contamination of skin wounds, contact with infected animals; possibly ingestion of milk	Biphasic influenza-like illness, sometimes followed by meningitis or meningoencephalitis, paralysis, joint pain in second phase; not usually fatal
Worldwide	Contact with host excretions and secretions; bites; possibly ingestion	Ranges from mild flu-like illness to biphasic with meningitis in second phase; complications (eg, arthritis, parotitis, orchitis) possible; can cause congenital defects (CNS defects, chorioretinitis, and other ocular lesions) or abortion; rarely fatal in immunocompetent (overall case fatality rate <1%)
Africa	Contact with infected tissues (especially nonhuman primates); probable transmission from bats in caves	Initially nonspecific febrile illness; maculopapular rash with desquamation; hepatitis; mild to severe bleeding tendency develops a few days after onset; mortality rate 20%–88%, varies with isolate
Australia	Close direct contact with tissues, amniotic fluid or blood of pigs reported in human cases	Severe illness with fever, severe headache, myalgia, lymphadenopathy, drenching sweats, macular rash
Middle East		Pneumonia, more likely in people with coexisting illness or immunosuppression but also in healthy; ~50% of known cases were fatal
Worldwide	Skin contact (especially broken skin) with lesions on cow's udder or mouth of calf; also from fomites	Papular to nodular red skin lesions; self-limiting
West and central Africa	Contact with lesions, blood or body fluids, fomites; bites; aerosols during close contact	Smallpox-like disease; flu-like symptoms followed by maculopapular rash, which develops into vesicles, pustules, scabs; lymphadenopathy prominent; respiratory signs, encephalitis possible; case fatality rate varies with strain, <1% to 10%–17% or higher; milder in those vaccinated for smallpox

(continued)

TABLE 4 GLOBAL ZOONOSES[a] (continued)

Disease	Causative Organism	Animals Involved
VIRAL DISEASES (continued)		
Murray Valley encephalitis	Murray Valley encephalitis virus (family Flaviviridae, genus *Flavivirus*)	Wild water birds
Newcastle disease	Newcastle disease virus/ Avian paramyxovirus 1 (family Paramyxoviridae, genus *Avulavirus*)	Domestic and wild birds
New World hemorrhagic fever (Argentinean, Bolivian, Venezuelan and Brazilian hemorrhagic fevers [HF])	Arenaviruses in Tacaribe complex (family Arenaviridae, genus *Arenavirus*): Juin virus (Argentine HF), Machupo virus (Bolivian HF), Guanarito virus (Venezuelan HF), Sabiá virus (Brazilian HF), Chapare virus; possibly others	Rodents
Nipah virus infection (*see* p 721)	Nipah virus (family Paramyxoviridae, genus *Henipavirus*)	Fruit bats are normal reservoir; swine can be reservoir; occasionally in other mammals (spillover hosts)
Omsk hemorrhagic fever	Omsk hemorrhagic fever virus (family Flaviviridae, genus *Flavivirus*)	Voles, muskrats; also found in other animals
Powassan virus encephalitis	Powassan virus (family Flaviviridae, genus *Flavivirus*); two closely related lineages in different reservoirs	Rodents (groundhog, squirrels, mice) and other small mammals thought to be reservoirs

TABLE 4 GLOBAL ZOONOSES[a] *(continued)*

Known Distribution	Probable Means of Spread to People	Clinical Manifestations in People
	VIRAL DISEASES (continued)	
Australia, New Guinea	Mosquito bites (*Culex annulirostris*)	Asymptomatic or mild nonspecific febrile illness in majority; encephalitis, often with neurologic sequelae, or poliomyelitis-like flaccid paralysis in small number of patients; case fatality rate 15%–30% in encephalitic form
Mildly virulent (lentogenic, mesogenic strains) are found worldwide; highly virulent (velogenic) strains found in Asia, the Middle East, Africa, Central and South America, parts of Mexico; also in cormorants in USA	Occupational exposure, usually after contact with large amounts of virus	Highly virulent (velogenic) strains can cause self-limiting conjunctivitis, possibly other syndromes
South America, related viruses might exist among rodents in Mexico	Viruses found in rodent excretions, secretions, tissues; inhalation of aerosolized virus or direct contact with mucous membranes or broken skin	Gradual onset of nonspecific signs, including myalgia, headache, and fever; may develop petechial or ecchymotic hemorrhages, bleeding, CNS signs, hypotension/shock; case fatality rate in untreated Bolivian hemorrhagic fever 5%–30%, untreated Argentine hemorrhagic fever 15%–30%
Malaysia, Bangladesh, and Northern India; virus is probably endemic in southeast Asia, but outbreaks seem to cluster in certain geographic areas	Direct contact with infected pigs or contaminated tissue; direct or indirect (eg, contaminated fruit juice) bat-to-human transmission	Initial signs flu-like with fever, headache, myalgia, sometimes vomiting; encephalitis and meningitis; respiratory disease, including acute respiratory distress syndromes in some; septicemia; other complications in severely ill; case fatality rate 33%–75%
Siberia	Tick bites (*Dermacentor* spp); direct contact with body fluids or carcasses of muskrats and possibly other animal hosts	Biphasic febrile illness with headache, GI signs, ± hemorrhages (nose, gums, lungs, uterus); CNS signs in minority of patients; mortality rate <3%
North America, eastern Russia	*Ixodes* spp ticks, also found in *Dermacentor andersoni*	Nonspecific febrile illness; may progress to neurologic signs, which may be severe; some cases fatal

(continued)

TABLE 4 GLOBAL ZOONOSES[a] *(continued)*

Disease	Causative Organism	Animals Involved
VIRAL DISEASES (continued)		
Rabies and rabies-related infections (*see* p 1302)	Lyssaviruses: rabies virus (family Rhabdoviridae, genus *Lyssavirus*) and the related lyssaviruses, Duvenhage virus, Mokola virus, Australian bat lyssavirus, European bat lyssaviruses 1 and 2, Irkut virus, possibly others	Wild and domestic canids, Mustelidae, Viverridae, Procyonidae, and order Chiroptera (bats) are important reservoir hosts; all mammals are susceptible; bats are reservoir hosts for Duvenhage virus, Australian bat lyssavirus, and European bat lyssaviruses; Mokola virus carried in rodents and shrews
Rift Valley fever (*see* p 768)	Rift Valley fever virus (family Bunyaviridae, genus *Flavivirus*)	Sheep, goats, cattle, buffalo, African buffalo, camels, nonhuman primates; squirrels and other rodents; puppies and kittens
Ross River virus infection, Ross River fever; epidemic polyarthritis	Ross River virus (family Togaviridae, genus *Alphavirus*)	Marsupials, including wallaby, brushtail possum, might be natural hosts; dusky rat also proposed; people, horses, ruminants, pigs, rabbits, other mammals (minor hosts) may also be a source of virus during epidemics
St. Louis encephalitis	St. Louis encephalitis virus (family Flaviviridae, genus *Flavivirus*)	Wild birds, domestic fowl; rodents, bats, other mammals might also maintain viruses in South America
Severe acute respiratory syndrome (SARS)	SARS coronavirus (family Coronaviridae, genus *Coronavirus*)	Bats are thought to be reservoir hosts; can also infect palm civets, raccoon dogs, cats, pigs, ferrets, rodents, nonhuman primates, other mammals
Sindbis virus disease	Sindbis virus (family Togaviridae, genus *Alphavirus*)	Birds (passeriforms suspected as main reservoirs/amplifying hosts); occasionally found in other vertebrates
Tanapox	Tanapox virus (family Poxviridae, genus *Yatapoxvirus*); Yaba-like disease virus may be a variant of tanapox virus	Nonhuman primates

TABLE 4 GLOBAL ZOONOSES[a] *(continued)*

Known Distribution	Probable Means of Spread to People	Clinical Manifestations in People
	VIRAL DISEASES (continued)	
Rabies is worldwide with some exceptions: completely absent from some islands; countries also considered rabies-free if no cases in people or domestic animals for 2 yr; rabies-related lyssaviruses found only in Eastern Hemisphere (distribution varies)	Bites of diseased animals; aerosols in closed environments	Paresthesias or pain at bite site; nonspecific prodromal signs such as fever, myalgia, malaise; mood changes progress to paresthesias, paresis, seizures, and many other neurologic signs; survival in clinical cases thought to be very rare
Africa, foci on Arabian peninsula, Indian subcontinent	Mosquito bites (*Aedes* spp and *Culex tritaeniorynchus*); contact with tissues	Influenza-like febrile illness in most; complications, including hemorrhagic fever, meningoencephalitis in <5%; ocular disease in 1%–10%; other syndromes include acute renal failure or thrombosis; death uncommon except with hemorrhagic syndrome
Australia, South Pacific Islands	Mosquito bites (especially *Culex annulirostris* and *Aedes* spp)	Mild fever, arthralgia ± arthritis, headache, rash; small joints most affected but large joints can also be involved; arthralgia, myalgia, lethargy may persist for months
Western hemisphere	Mosquito bites (*Culex tarsalis*, *C pipiens-quinquefasciatus* complex, *C nigripalpus*, also reported in other genera)	Flu-like illness sometimes followed by meningitis or encephalitis, focal neurologic signs, dysuria; more severe in elderly and those with debilitating diseases; case fatality rate of 5%–20% reported in epidemics
China, southeast Asia	Contamination of mucous membranes with respiratory droplets or virus on fomites; possibly aerosol transmission	Fever, myalgia, headache, diarrhea, cough; viral pneumonia with rapid deterioration; case fatality rate 15%
Virus widespread in Eastern hemisphere; human cases tend to occur in limited geographic regions	Mosquito bites; *Culex* and *Culiseta*, also others	Fever, arthritis, rash, prominent myalgia; nausea, vomiting, mild jaundice in some; joint pain can persist for months; seems to be mild or asymptomatic in most children; no fatal cases reported
Asia, Africa, and in monkey colonies	Direct contact through broken skin; mosquitoes suspected to be vector in Africa	Nonspecific febrile illness and papulovesicular or nodular lesions (lesions may be pruritic or tender), often on extremities; more than one or two skin lesions uncommon

(continued)

TABLE 4 GLOBAL ZOONOSES[a] (continued)

Disease	Causative Organism	Animals Involved
VIRAL DISEASES (continued)		
Tickborne encephalitis (Far eastern tickborne encephalitis, Russian spring-summer encephalitis, Central European tickborne encephalitis)	Tickborne encephalitis virus (TBEV) (family Flaviviridae, genus *Flavivirus*); three subtypes: European (TBEV-Eu [least virulent]), Siberian (TBEV-Sib), Far Eastern (TBEV-FE)	Small mammals especially rodents; also in goats, sheep, dogs, and other mammals; birds
Usutu virus infections	Usutu virus (family Flaviviridae, genus *Flavivirus*)	Birds
Vaccinia-related poxviruses	Vaccinia or vaccinia-like viruses (family Poxviridae, genus *Orthopoxvirus*) of uncertain origin	Reservoir uncertain; found in wild rodents, cattle, horses, nonhuman primates
Venezuelan equine encephalomyelitis	Venezuelan equine encephalitis virus (family Togaviridae, genus *Alphavirus*)	Enzootic subtypes maintained in rodents, other small mammals, bats; epizootic subtypes amplified in equids; occasionally in other mammals and birds
Vesicular stomatitis	Vesicular stomatitis Indiana virus, vesicular stomatitis New Jersey virus, vesicular stomatitis Alagoas virus, and Cocal virus (family Rhadboviridae, genus *Vesiculovirus*)	Swine, cattle, horses; occasionally in South American camelids, sheep, and goats; also rodents; serologic evidence of infection in many wild mammals, especially bats
Wesselsbron fever	Wesselsbron virus (family Flaviviridae, genus *Flavivirus*)	Ruminants, especially sheep, goats; also evidence of infection in other mammals, including lemurs; can infect birds
West Nile fever and neuroinvasive disease (*see* p 1291)	West Nile virus (family Flaviviridae, genus *Flavivirus*); lineage 1 and lineage 2 viruses are both pathogenic	Birds are primary reservoir hosts; also affects horses, other mammals, alligators, possibly other reptiles and amphibians

TABLE 4 GLOBAL ZOONOSES[a] *(continued)*

Known Distribution	Probable Means of Spread to People	Clinical Manifestations in People
VIRAL DISEASES (continued)		
Eurasia; TBEV-Eu mainly Europe to former USSR; TBEV-FE mainly Asia to former USSR; TBEV-Sib mainly in Siberia	Tick bites (mainly *Ixodes ricinus* and *I persculatus*; also other species); may be ingested in milk	Often biphasic, with flu-like febrile illness in initial stage; neurologic signs from mild meningitis to severe encephalitis in some; myelitis or flaccid poliomyelitis-like paralysis (usually arms, shoulders, levator muscles of head); possibility of chronic and progressive forms, especially with TBEV-Sib; case fatality rate <2% (TBEV-Eu), 2%–3% (TBEV-Sib); case fatality rate 20%–30% in TBEV-FE may be based on severe cases
Africa, Europe	Mosquito bites (*Culex* spp)	Very few cases identified: fever with rash, fever with jaundice, or meningoencephalitis
Appear to be endemic in Brazil	Direct contact	Pox skin lesions (papules, pustules, ulcerative nodules), may be accompanied by fever, lymphadenopathy
Western hemisphere; enzootic strains Florida to South America; epizootic strains emerge in South America, spread	Mosquito bites (*Aedes*, *Culex*, and *Psorophora* spp); exposure to aerosolized debris from infected laboratory rodents; laboratory accidents	Most have nonspecific febrile illness, can be followed by neurologic signs; <5% children, <1% adults progress to encephalitis with case fatality rate of 10%–35% (highest rates in children <5 yr old)
North and South America; most likely not endemic north of Mexico but sporadic outbreaks	Contact with animals or in laboratory, probably also from insect bites, including mosquitoes and biting flies (*Phlebotomus* spp, *Lutzomyia* spp, and black flies)	Usually asymptomatic; may develop acute, febrile, flu-like illness; vesicles can be found in mouth, pharynx, or inoculation site (eg, hands); self-limiting
Southern Africa, southeast Asia	Mosquito bites (mainly *Aedes* spp, possibly others); also by contact with contaminated material	Nonspecific febrile illness ± maculopapular rash or ocular signs in some; few cases described but seems to be self-limiting
Eastern and Western hemisphere	Mosquito bites (primarily *Culex univittatus*, *Culex* spp); also by handling infected birds or reptiles or their tissues	Nonspecific febrile illness, occasionally with rash; some cases progress to encephalitis, meningitis, and/or acute flaccid paralysis that resembles poliomyelitis; occasionally other syndromes; worse in elderly and immunocompromised; case fatality rate ~10% in all patients with neurologic disease, but higher in elderly

TABLE 4 GLOBAL ZOONOSES[a] *(continued)*

Disease	Causative Organism	Animals Involved
	VIRAL DISEASES (continued)	
Western equine encephalomyelitis (*see* p 1291)	Western equine encephalomyelitis virus (family Togaviridae, genus *Alphavirus*)	Birds are reservoir hosts, may also cycle in jackrabbits, rodents; equids, other mammals are incidental hosts; virus also found in reptiles, amphibians
Yellow fever	Yellow fever virus (family Flaviviridae, genus *Flavivirus*); only jungle cycle is zoonotic (people are reservoir for urban cycle)	Nonhuman primates
	PRION DISEASE	
Variant Creutzfeldt-Jakob disease	Bovine spongiform encephalopathy prion	Cattle are most important host; also infects other ruminants, cats and other felids, lemurs

[a] Many proven zoonoses, including some relatively rare arthropodborne viral infections and helminth infections, have been omitted, as well as those diseases caused by fish and reptile toxins.

[b] Enterotoxigenic, enteroinvasive, enteropathogenic, and enteroaggressive strains are not considered zoonotic.

TABLE 4 GLOBAL ZOONOSES[a] *(continued)*

Known Distribution	Probable Means of Spread to People	Clinical Manifestations in People
VIRAL DISEASES (continued)		
Americas	Mosquito bites (*Aedes*, *Culex*, and *Ochlerotatus* spp); *Culex tarsalis* important in maintenance cycle in birds	Nonspecific febrile illness may be followed by encephalitis in infants and children, uncommonly in adults; case fatality rate 3%–4%
South America, Africa	Mosquito bites (*Haemagogus* spp and *Sabethes* spp in jungle cycles in South America, *Aedes* spp in jungle cycles in Africa)	Nonspecific, mild to severe febrile illness followed by liver and renal failure in some; hemorrhages (eg, epistaxis, hematemesis, melena, uterine hemorrhage) and often jaundice in severe cases; cases with hemorrhages often fatal
PRION DISEASE		
Most cases in the UK but also in many other countries	Ingestion of bovine products, especially those contaminated with CNS tissues	Neurodegenerative disorder similar to sporadic Creutzfeldt-Jakob disease but often in younger patients and progresses more rapidly; always fatal

PHARMACOLOGY

SYSTEMIC PHARMACOTHERAPEUTICS

CHEMOTHERAPEUTICS

PHARMACOLOGY INTRODUCTION

Once a diagnosis has been made and medical treatment is deemed necessary, safe and effective pharmacologic agents that exert the appropriate actions should be selected. A dosing regimen should be individualized for each patient. In addition to the route, which often is based on drug availability or convenience, a number of factors should be considered when designing a dosing regimen. These include host considerations that may alter the response to or disposition of the drugs. Adjustment in route, dose, or interval may be indicated based on host and drug factors. For antimicrobial drugs, *microbial factors*, including resistance, also should be considered. Finally, particularly for food animals, public health, environmental implications, and regulatory constraints must be considered.

EXTRA-LABEL DRUG USE, COMPOUNDED DRUGS, AND GENERIC DRUGS

A **new animal drug (NAD)** is "any drug intended for use in animals other than man...not generally recognized as safe and effective for the use under the conditions prescribed, recommended, or suggested in the labeling of the drug." A drug's label includes the label on the product itself as well as any accompanying material in or on the package, including the package insert.

To use an NAD in a legal manner, veterinarians must adhere to the specifications noted on the label. Otherwise, the drug is being used in an **extra-label** manner. Extra-label drug use, whether actual or intended, occurs when the drug is used in a manner not in accordance with approved label directions. This includes but is not limited to a different dosage, interval, route, indication, or species.

In 1994, Congress passed the Animal Medicinal Drug Use Clarification Act (AMDUCA), which legalized extra-label drug use by veterinarians as long as specific criteria or restrictions are met. Most restrictions are largely applicable to extra-label drug use in food animals. For both food and nonfood animals, a valid **veterinary-client-patient relationship** must exist. For food animals, in the absence of a drug labeled for the intended use, extra-label drug use might involve drugs approved for use in other food animals, approved for use in nonfood animals, or approved for use in people. Restrictions regarding extra-label drug use of nonfood animal and human drugs are progressively restrictive. Extra-label drug use in food animals is permitted only by or under the supervision of a veterinarian, is allowed only for therapeutic purposes (ie, the animal's health is suffering or threatened), is not allowed when the drug is administered in feed, is not permitted if it results in violative food residues or any residues that may present a risk to public health, and is not allowed if specifically prohibited by the FDA.

Drugs specifically prohibited in food animals by the FDA as of May 2015 include chloramphenicol, clenbuterol, diethylstilbestrol, dimetridazole, ipronidazole, other nitroimadazoles, furazolidone, nitrofurazone, sulfonamide drugs in lactating dairy cattle (except for those specifically approved), fluoroquinolones, aglycopeptides (eg, vancomycin), phenylbutazone in female dairy cattle ≥20 mo old, cephalosporins (except cephapirin) in cattle, swine, chickens, or turkeys for disease prevention, and amantadine or neuraminidase inhibitor classes of drugs used to treat influenza A in poultry and ducks.

Use of a **compounded preparation** also constitutes extra-label drug use. However, a major distinction is that a compounded preparation undergoes no regulatory assessment or approval. Conditions under which compounding is legal also are specified in the AMDUCA. Compounding includes any manipulation of the drug beyond that stipulated on the label. Guidelines regarding the compounding of pharmaceuticals under the direction of a veterinarian are delineated in Compliance Policy Guideline 7125.40. Among the greatest concerns of the FDA regarding compounded products is compounding intended to circumvent the drug approval process, resulting in mass marketing of products that have had little or no quality control to ensure purity, potency, and stability. The FDA considers a compounded product to be an adulterated, ie, unapproved, new animal drug and thus a violation. Conditions under which compounding is not subject to regulatory actions include a legitimate practice (pharmacy or veterinary; includes licensure), operation within the conformity of state law, for pharmacists in response to a prescription, and for veterinarians operating within a valid veterinary-client-patient relationship. Compounding of human drugs and, very occasionally, bulk drugs into appropriate dosage forms may be acceptable in certain circumstances. A legitimate medical need must be identified (eg, health or life of the animal is threatened or suffering may occur). Additionally, there must be no marketed, approved animal or human drug, regardless of whether it is used as labeled or in an extra-label fashion, that may be substituted for the compounded agent. Occasionally, other rare circumstances may be considered. In 2013, Congress passed the Drug Quality and Security Act that, among other things, increases regulation of compounding in human medicine. However, this Act does not cover compounding of animal products, and Congress is examining further actions to more effectively regulate such compounding.

Pharmacists often can dispense an equivalent, less expensive, nonproprietary (generic) drug without prescriber approval. An exception occurs if a state has a mandatory substitution law or if the brand name product is dispensed along with a "dispensed as written" order. **Generic products** must not only contain the same active ingredient as the proprietary drug but also meet bioequivalence standards. Generics may be pharmaceutically equivalent but may not be therapeutically equivalent. Substitutions of generic drugs for proprietary drugs are recommended only for those drugs shown to be therapeutically equivalent. Those human drugs tested by the FDA and found to be therapeutically equivalent are listed in *Approved Drug Products with Therapeutic Equivalence Evaluations*, otherwise known as the "Orange Book." However, status of a generic drug is relevant only for the approved species and, as such, therapeutic equivalence of a human generic drug does not apply to extra-label use of that drug in an animal.

Although AMDUCA legalizes extra-label drug use in the USA, selected states or other countries may have additional or complementary regulatory or legal restrictions. In all instances, it is important to read carefully the label instructions for use of specific drugs.

DISPOSITION AND FATE OF DRUGS

The goal of drug therapy is to achieve a pharmacologic response. The magnitude of the pharmacodynamic response to a drug generally reflects the number of receptors with which the drug interacts (drug-receptor theory). Because tissue drug concentrations generally parallel tissue concentrations, the ideal dose will result in plasma drug concentrations in a "therapeutic range." This population statistic is defined by a maximum drug concentration, above which the risk of adverse events (eg, toxicity) increases, and a minimum drug concentration, below which therapeutic failure may result. Plasma drug concentrations generally fluctuate during a dosing interval, because they are impacted by four drug movements acting simultaneously on the drug: **absorption** from the site of nonintravenous administration into the plasma, **distribution** into tissues and then back into plasma, where the drug can then be eliminated from the body either by **metabolism** or **excretion** of parent drug and/or metabolites. Many factors influence each of these four drug movements (ADME) and thus the time course of plasma drug concentrations after a dose is administered by any route. Understanding these factors, in turn, is important to individualizing drug therapy for the patient, because dosing regimens are modified to adjust for physiologic (eg, species, breed, gender, age), pharmacologic (eg, drug-drug or drug-diet interactions), and pathologic (eg, renal, hepatic, or cardiac disease) influences on drug disposition. Pharmacokinetics is the science that mathematically describes the time course of plasma drug concentrations after administration of a dose, ie, the result of ADME on plasma drug concentrations.

Passage of Drugs Across Cellular Membranes

Each of the drug movements generally relies on the drug passing through cell membranes (transcellular). Membrane barriers may be composed of several layers of cells (eg, skin, vagina, cornea, placenta) or a single layer of cells (eg, enterocytes, renal tubular epithelial cells), or they may consist only of a boundary less than one cell in thickness (eg, hepatic sinusoids). Multilayered tissues each may present different types of barriers, eg, skin is protected by the dense stratum corneum, which is absent in mucous membranes. Not all drugs must pass through cell membranes; paracellular movement between cells increasingly is an important movement for some drugs, eg, in the GI tract.

Drugs and other molecules cross cellular membranes by several processes. Methods by which drugs move include bulk flow (eg, movement with blood, glomerular filtration), passive diffusion, carrier-mediated transport (ie, active or facilitated transport), and pinocytosis. Of these, passive diffusion is most important for movement of drug molecules and other xenobiotics (foreign chemicals), as well as many endogenous compounds.

The rate at which a drug passively diffuses through membranes is influenced by several factors, the most important of which is the concentration gradient of diffusible (eg, dissolved) drug across the membrane. However, other host and drug factors influence the rate and extent of passive diffusion. Host factors that increase diffusion include permeability and surface area of the membrane; thickness of the membrane negatively impacts diffusion. Drug characteristics that influence diffusion include molecular weight, lipophilicity, and degree of ionization. Most drugs are "small molecules" (<900 daltons), but diffusibility is more likely to occur for drugs <500 daltons. Drugs must be sufficiently lipid soluble (lipophilic) to pass through some level of cell membrane lipid bilayer to reach most drug receptors. The lipid-to-water partition coefficient describes the distribution (ratio) of a drug (concentration) in a lipid compared with water media. The distribution coefficient also takes into account ionization.

Many drugs are weak organic acids or bases. At physiologic pH, they tend to be partially ionized (dissociated) and partially nonionized (undissociated); the ratio of the respective forms depends on the dissociation constant (pK_a) of the drug, ie, the pH at which the drug is present in equal concentration in ionized and nonionized forms, and the pH of the solution in which the drug is dissolved. Only nonionized fraction diffuses through lipid membranes. Distribution across any membrane of a drug with any given pK_a reflects the degree of ionization and thus environmental pH on each side of the membrane. The Henderson Hasselbach equation predicts the ratio of ionized vs nonionized drug. In general, weak acids are nonionized in acidic compared with alkaline environments, and weak bases are nonionized in alkaline compared with acidic environments. The more similar the environmental pH is to that of the pK_a of a weak acid or base, the more nonionized is the drug and the more likely it will diffuse. As long as the ratio of nonionized to ionized drug is ≥0.01, the drug is considered diffusible.

Not all drugs must pass through cell membranes to reach their receptor. Aqueous pores in lipoproteinaceous biologic membranes offer a means of xenobiotic movement through the membrane for predominantly aqueous soluble drugs. Lipid-insoluble (water-soluble) compounds pass easily through these pores and to a lesser degree directly through the membrane. A hydrostatic or osmotic pressure difference across a membrane facilitates movement by promoting water flow through the aqueous pores. Bulk fluid movement carries or "drags" solute molecules through the pores as long as the solute molecules are smaller than the aqueous channels.

Several specialized transfer processes account for the passage of certain organic ions and other large lipid-insoluble substances across biologic membranes. Active transport, facilitated diffusion, and exchange diffusion are three distinct types of carrier-mediated systems used to move specific substances across cellular membranes. The highly selective carrier-mediated systems are principally used for transporting nutrients and natural substrates across biologic membranes. Among the mechanisms of active transport are transport proteins that move compounds, including drugs, into or out of cells. Transport proteins are located at portals of entry (eg, enterocytes of the GI tract or sinusoidal hepatic cells) or "sanctuary" tissues (eg, brain, CSF, placenta, prostate, eyes, or testicles), where they attempt to ensure that xenobiotics do not enter the protected tissue. As such, transport proteins are able to influence each drug movement (absorption, distribution, metabolism, and excretion). The most well known of the transport proteins is the ATP-binding cassette superfamily of efflux transporters, which includes P-glycoprotein, the multidrug resistance protein. Substrates for P-glycoprotein include both xenobiotics and dietary components. Additional transport proteins carry cations, anions, or organic compounds. Competition for transport increases oral absorption or distribution of one of the competing molecules.

Pinocytosis is an important transport process in mammalian cells, particularly intestinal epithelial cells and renal tubular cells. Drugs that exist in solution as molecular aggregates have large molecular masses themselves or that are bound to macromolecules may be transferred across membranes by pinocytosis.

Drug Absorption

Absorption from the GI Tract: Many factors influence orally administered drugs. Before absorption, orally administered drugs must disintegrate and then dissolve; dissolution often is the rate-limiting factor in oral drug absorption. Drugs may be formulated by manufacturers to result in extended (occurring throughout the GI tract) or delayed absorption. Often, release kinetics of these drugs limit extrapolation of dosing regimens from one species to another. Once an orally administered drug has dissolved, multiple factors influence its absorption. Drug characteristics include molecular size, lipophilicity, and drug pK_a. Drug pK_a is particularly important in the GI tract, because environmental pH is markedly variable among the different regions or compartments. Host factors (in addition to environmental pH) determining oral absorption include epithelial permeability, GI motility, surface area (being greatest in the small intestine, which is the major site of drug absorption), transport and metabolizing proteins, and GI blood (which maintains the concentration gradient) and lymphatic flow. Epithelial permeability is influenced by disease. Additionally, in those species in which colostrum absorption is important, epithelial permeability is much greater. GI motility is important because it influences mixing of luminal contents, which is necessary for dissolved drug to come into contact with absorptive surfaces. Gastric motility determines gastric emptying, which in turn influences the rate of drug absorption. Changes in GI blood flow have minimal impact on drug absorption, because although GI blood flow maintains the concentration gradient necessary for passive diffusion, it is rarely the rate-limiting factor. Both efflux transport proteins (eg, P-glycoprotein) and drug-metabolizing enzymes located in the GI epithelium can markedly decrease drug absorption, contributing to a "first-pass effect." These proteins are subject to clinically relevant drug interactions and are likely to differ among physiologic influences (eg, species, gender, age). A drug entering the portal circulation will be exposed to hepatocytes before reaching systemic circulation. If a large proportion of the drug (>75%) is removed or extracted as it passes through the liver, the oral bioavailability of the drug will be markedly reduced, also resulting in a "first-pass effect." For such drugs, the oral dose is proportionately higher than the parenteral dose. Food can markedly alter oral absorption of drugs by either diluting it, or more importantly, binding to it so that it is not absorbed.

Absorption from Topical Administration: Drugs may be absorbed through the skin after topical application; however, the stratum corneum presents an effective barrier to transdermal movement of most drugs into circulation. As such, many drugs are absorbed after paracellular rather than transcellular movement. Intact skin allows the passage of small lipophilic substances but efficiently retards the diffusion of water-soluble molecules in most cases. Lipid-insoluble drugs generally penetrate the skin slowly compared with their rates of absorption through other body membranes. Absorption of drugs through the skin may be enhanced by heat, moisture, or disruption of the stratum corneum. Occlusive dressings increase heat and moisture; transdermal patches also disrupt the stratum corneum. Smaller molecules are more conducive to transdermal drug delivery. Different transdermal systems have been developed with the intent of systemic drug delivery. Certain solvents (eg, dimethyl sulfoxide [DMSO]) may facilitate the penetration of drugs through the skin. Damaged, inflamed, or hyperemic skin allows many drugs to penetrate the dermal barrier much more readily. For example, drugs administered transdermally as pluronic lecithin or other gels presumably penetrate the stratum corneum because it is disrupted, becoming more permeable. The same principles that govern the absorption of drugs through the skin also apply to the application of topical preparations on epithelial surfaces. In contrast to skin, mucosal epithelium has no stratum corneum, facilitating drug absorption. An advantage of the buccal mucosa is that a drug avoids first-pass metabolism.

Absorption from Tracheobronchial Surfaces and Alveoli: Because volatile and gaseous anesthetics have relatively high lipid-to-water partition coefficients and generally are rather small molecules, they diffuse practically instantaneously into the blood in the alveolar capillaries. In contrast, for drugs administered as aerosols, particles containing drugs can be deposited on the mucosal surface of the bronchi or bronchioles, or even in the alveoli, with the site influenced by particle size and breathing rate and depth. Whether or not the drug is absorbed from these sites depends on the characteristics previously described.

Absorption from Injection Delivery Sites: After nonintravenous injection, diffusible drug molecules traverse the capillary wall by a combination of diffusion and filtration. Diffusion is the predominant mode of transfer for lipid-soluble molecules, small lipid-insoluble molecules, and ions. Because most capillaries are fenestrated, all drugs, whether lipid-soluble or not, cross the capillary wall at rates that are extremely rapid compared with their rates across other body membranes. In fact, the movement of most drug molecules in various tissues is limited only by the rate of blood flow rather than by the capillary wall. However, endothelial cells of sanctuaries, such as the blood-brain or CSF barrier, retina, and testicles, have tight intercellular junctions, thus restricting movement of drugs.

Aqueous solutions of drugs are usually absorbed from an IM injection site within 10–30 min, provided blood flow is unimpaired. Faster or slower absorption is possible, depending on the concentration and lipid solubility of the drug, vascularity (including number of vessels and state of vasoconstriction), the volume of injection, the osmolality of the solution, and other pharmaceutical factors. Substances with molecular weights >20,000 daltons are principally taken up into the lymphatics.

Absorption of drugs from subcutaneous tissues is influenced by the same factors that determine the rate of absorption from IM sites. Some drugs are absorbed as rapidly from subcutaneous tissues as from muscle, although absorption from injection sites in subcutaneous fat is always significantly delayed.

Increasing blood supply to the injection site by heating, massage, or exercise hastens the rate of dissemination and absorption.

The rate of absorption of an injected drug may be prolonged in a number of ways, including immobilization of the site, local cooling, a tourniquet, incorporation of a vasoconstrictor, an oil base, and implant pellets and insoluble "depot" preparations. Among these depot preparations are drugs that are converted to less soluble esters, which must be released by esterases (eg, procaine and benzathine esters of penicillin or acetate esters of steroids) or less soluble complexes (eg, protamine zinc insulin), or that are administered as insoluble microcrystalline suspensions (eg, methylprednisolone acetate).

Bioavailability

Bioavailability refers to the extent to which a drug is absorbed into the body and thus is available to act on its intended target site. A drug is considered 100% bioavailable (F=1) when given intravenously (although pulmonary metabolism may make this not entirely true). Bioavailability of a particular route or formulation is the ratio of the area under the plasma drug concentration versus time curve (AUC) of the drug when the drug is given via that route or as that preparation to the AUC when the drug is given intravenously at the same dosage (in mg/kg):

$$F = AUC_{non\text{-}IV}/AUC_{IV}$$

The equation must be adjusted for dosage when appropriate:

$$F = (AUC_{non\text{-}IV}) \times (dose_{IV})/(AUC_{IV}) \times (dose_{non\text{-}IV})$$

Two products are considered bioequivalent if they result in the same rate and extent of absorption. Rate of absorption is reflected as the maximum plasma drug concentration (C_{max}) and the time (T_{max}) that C_{max} occurs. Thus, two drugs are bioequivalent if their AUC, C_{max}, and T_{max} do not significantly differ. Two different preparations or routes of administration may be equally bioavailable but not bioequivalent. Generic drugs must be demonstrated to be bioequivalent.

Once a drug reaches the systemic circulation, all other drug movements (distribution, metabolism, and excretion) will be the same regardless of the route or preparation. However, in some instances, absorption may be so slow (eg, delayed or extended-release formulation, absorption impacted by food) that it limits the rate at which the drug is eliminated (metabolized and/or excreted) from the body.

Drug Distribution

After absorption into the bloodstream, drugs are disseminated to all parts of the body. Occasionally, the drug molecule may be so large (>65,000 daltons) or so highly bound to plasma proteins that it remains in the intravascular space after IV administration. Compounds that permeate freely through cell membranes become distributed, in time, throughout the body water to both extracellular and intracellular fluids, with the extent depending on drug chemistry. Substances that pass readily through and between capillary endothelial cells, but do not penetrate other cell membranes, are distributed into the extracellular fluid space. Drugs may also undergo redistribution in the body after initial high levels are achieved in tissues that have a rich vascular supply, eg, the brain. As the plasma concentration falls, the drug readily diffuses back into the circulation to be quickly redistributed to other tissues with high blood-flow rates, such as the muscles; over time, the drug also becomes deposited in lipid-rich tissues with poor blood supplies, such as the fat depots. Most drugs are not distributed equally throughout the body but tend to accumulate in certain specific tissues or fluids. The general principles that govern the passage and distribution of drugs across cellular membranes (*see* p 2492) are applicable to drug distribution. Basic drugs tend to accumulate in tissues and fluids with pH values lower than the pK_a of the drug; conversely, acidic drugs concentrate in regions of higher pH, provided the free drug is sufficiently lipid soluble to penetrate the membranes that separate the compartments. Even small differences in pH across boundary membranes, such as those that exist between plasma (pH 7.4) and other tissues such as CSF (pH 7.3), milk (pH 6.5–6.8), renal tubular fluid (pH 5–8), and inflamed tissue (pH 6–7) can lead to unequal distribution of drugs, referred to as "ion-trapping." Only freely diffusible and unbound drug molecules are generally able to pass from one compartment to another. However, some drugs are transported by carrier-mediated systems across certain cellular membranes, which leads to higher concentrations on one side than the other. Examples of such nonspecific transport mechanisms are found in renal tubular epithelial cells, hepatocytes, and the choroid plexus. Among the transport proteins, genetic differences in P-glycoprotein profoundly impact drug movement, particularly at portals of xenobiotic entry or sanctuaries.

Passive diffusion of drugs from capillaries to tissues may be limited by binding to plasma proteins. The most important is albumin, although the globulins and, especially, α-1 acid glycoprotein (for bases) may also play a significant role. In general, protein binding is considered clinically relevant if ≥80%. For such drugs, factors influencing binding can impact drug disposition. These include plasma pH, concentration of plasma proteins, concentration of the drug, or the presence of a competing agent with a greater affinity for the limited number of binding sites. For example, a potentially toxic compound (such as most NSAIDs) may be 98% bound, but if for any reason it becomes only 96% bound, then the concentration of the free active drug that becomes available in the plasma is doubled, with potentially harmful consequences. The concentration of a drug administered in overdose may exceed the binding capacity of the plasma protein and lead to an excess of free drug, which can diffuse into various target tissues and produce exaggerated effects. Other reasons the fraction of unbound drug might increase include hypoalbuminemia and competition with other highly protein-bound drugs. The degree of protein binding of a drug cannot be extrapolated among the species, but in most species, NSAIDs, antifungal imidazoles, and doxycycline are examples of highly protein-bound drugs. More rapid clearance of the now unbound drug may mitigate the impact of higher drug concentrations.

Dissociation of a drug from plasma proteins also influences elimination from the body in that those drugs more tightly bound tend to have much longer elimination half-lives, because they are released gradually from the plasma protein reservoir (eg, cefovecin or long-acting sulfonamides).

Most unbound drugs distribute easily from capillaries to extracellular fluid. However, only the more lipid-soluble drugs can distribute to all tissues because of the presence of physiologic barriers presented by "sanctuaries" (eg, blood-brain, placental, and mammary barriers). For the CNS, drugs may gain access through either the capillary circulation (blood-brain barrier) or the CSF (also a blood barrier). Drugs penetrate into the cortex more rapidly than into white matter, probably because of the greater delivery rate of drug via the bloodstream to the tissue.

The pharmacologic factors and consequences of the diverse rates of entry of different drugs into the CNS are clinically relevant in that *water-soluble, ionized* drugs are less likely to enter the CNS, whereas drugs with low ionization, low plasma-protein binding, and a fairly high lipid-water partition coefficient penetrate more rapidly. Inflammation, presented by for example meningoencephalitis, can substantially alter the permeability of the blood-brain barrier. In general, direct injection into the CSF is undesirable because of the risk of unexpected effects.

In pregnant animals, the degree of placentation may determine the extent of a placental barrier. Nutrients such as glucose, amino acids, minerals, and even some vitamins are actively transported across the placenta. The passage of drugs across the placenta is largely by lipid diffusion, and the factors discussed above play a role. The distribution of drugs within the fetus follows essentially the same pattern as in the adult, with some differences with respect to the volumes of drug distribution, plasma-protein binding, blood circulation, and greater permeability of interceding membranous barriers. Drugs that are potentially teratogenic should be avoided, particularly in early gestation.

The mammary gland epithelium, like other biologic membranes, acts as a lipid barrier, and many drugs readily diffuse from the plasma into milk. The pH of normal milk varies, being 6.5–6.8 in goats and cows. As such, weak bases tend to accumulate in milk. Drugs delivered by intramammary infusion can diffuse into plasma to a greater or lesser degree by the same processes noted earlier.

Once a drug is distributed into tissues, binding to macromolecules such as protein components of cells or fluids, dissolution in adipose tissue, formation of nondiffusible complexes in tissues such as bone, incorporation into specific storage granules, or binding to selective sites in tissues all impede movement of drugs back into plasma and account for differences in the cellular and organ distribution of particular drugs.

Drug Metabolism

Drugs that are lipid soluble will be passively reabsorbed as urine concentrates in the kidney unless they are converted by enzymatic processes to water-soluble drugs. This is accomplished by drug metabolism. Metabolism and subsequent excretion of drugs together comprise drug "elimination" from the body. Most drug metabolism occurs in the smooth endoplasmic reticulum of the liver. Metabolism generally consists of two phases: Phase I induces a chemical change (most frequently oxidation, but also reduction) that renders the drug more conducive to phase II. Phase II is a conjugative or synthetic addition of a large, polar molecule that renders the drug water soluble and amenable to renal excretion.

Four possible sequelae follow phase I metabolism: 1) inactivation (eg, most NSAIDs); 2) activation from a "pro-drug" to the active form of the drug (eg, enalapril to enalaprilat); 3) modification of activity, ie, formation of active metabolites that may be characterized by activity greater than (eg, tramadol), less than (eg, diazepam), or equal to that of the parent compound; and 4) formation of toxic metabolites, which is generally due to direct cell damage (eg, acetaminophen). In some instances the toxic metabolite acts as an antigen, causing immune-mediated toxicity (eg, sulfonamides). Because phase II drug metabolism almost exclusively inactivates drugs (the notable exception being some acetylated and methylated drugs), it often protects the organ of metabolism from drug-induced toxicity. This is particularly true with the addition of glutathione, which scavenges oxygen radicals; in the face of drug toxicity, *N*-acetylcysteine will increase intracellular glutathione. Multiple isoforms of phase II drug-metabolizing enzymes exist. Glucuronide (the addition of which is catalyzed by glucuronide transferase) is the most common phase II reaction; cats are deficient in some, but not all, glucuronyl transferases. Other important phase II enzymes include sulfation (deficient in swine), acetylation (deficient in dogs), and methylation. Amino acid conjugations are particularly important in avian species.

Phase I drug metabolism is largely, but not exclusively, accomplished by heme-containing enzymes referred to as cytochrome P450 (CYP450). More than 20 superfamilies have been identified, with some being specific for some drug or drug classes but others characterized by broad substrate specificity. Among the major superfamilies are CYP3A, which in people has been demonstrated to be responsible for the larger proportion of drug metabolism. Others important to drug metabolism are CYP2C and CYP2D. CYP enzymes are responsible for synthesis (eg, adrenal steroids, fatty acids) and metabolism of many endogenous compounds.

Drug metabolism has largely been considered to be negligible in early life, with neonates being less able to eliminate lipid-soluble drugs than adults; dosing intervals should be prolonged in such instances. However, evidence is emerging that some pediatric animals may have increased rather than decreased metabolic capacity for some drugs compared with adults. In those instances in which metabolic capacity has been demonstrated to be less, postnatal development in the liver appears to be biphasic, consisting of a rapid and nearly linear increase in activity during the first 3–4 wk, followed by slower development up to the tenth week postpartum. In older animals, decreases in hepatic mass, hepatic blood flow, and drug-metabolizing enzyme activity should lead to longer dosing intervals, and for drugs characterized by first-pass metabolism, to lower oral doses.

Many disease states impair the normal activity of the hepatic drug-metabolizing enzyme systems, which in turn decreases clearance and thus prolongs the half-lives of many drugs. Hepatotoxicity, acute hepatitis, or other extensive liver lesions invariably depress enzyme activity. Evidence of decreased plasma albumin as a result of hepatic disease generally indicates that hepatic drug metabolism will likewise be decreased. Hypothyroidism tends to decrease, and hyperthyroidism increase drug-metabolizing enzyme activity.

Pharmacogenomics refers to the study of the genetic basis for differential response to drugs. Differences in the duration of action of drugs in various species frequently can be attributed to differences in their rates of biotransformation. Species variations in drug metabolism are common. CYP450 3A4 is responsible for the broadest substrate activity in people, but this may not be true in animals and certainly may vary among species.

Differences in content and activity of CYP enzymes among ages, genders, and species are likely to play a role in differences to response to drugs. Polymorphisms among the breeds can result in "poor" versus "efficient" metabolizers, with the former predisposed to drug toxicity because of decreased metabolism. Such variants for certain enzymes have been described in people as being responsible for potentially lethal differences in drug metabolism.

Several other factors impact the rate and extent of drug metabolism. Drug interactions may reflect induction (eg, phenobarbital, rifampin, griseofulvin) or inhibition (eg, chloramphenicol, cimetidine, imidazole antifungals) of CYP enzymes, with the impact varying among isoenzymes and the sequelae of drug metabolism. Nutritional state and disease (especially hepatic disease) can also impact drug metabolism. The liver is not the only site of CYP450 activity, with sanctuaries and portals of entry being examples of sites where CYP activity can alter several aspects of ADME.

In addition to differences in CYP450 enzymes, differential handling of enantiomers is increasingly recognized among species. Enantiomers are mirror images of drug molecules that result when groups of atoms rotate around a center or "chiral" carbon. Generally, such compounds are sold as racemic mixtures (50:50 of each isomer); however, the body frequently handles each stereoisomer differentially, with differences also being seen among species. Many cardiac drugs and NSAIDs exist as racemic mixtures of enantiomers. This must be remembered when either dosages or withdrawal times are extrapolated from one species to another. However, some drugs are sold only as one isomer or the other, with the name often reflecting as such (eg, levetiracetam, dexmedetomidine, esomeprazole). Species differences have been better documented for phase II metabolism. Among the more important phase II reactions and the species in which the reactions are deficient are glucuronidation (cats), glutathione transferase (important for scavenging potentially toxic metabolites), sulfation (swine), and acetylation (dogs).

Drug Excretion

The body can clear itself of drugs either by metabolism or excretion. Excretion irreversibly removes drugs or metabolites from the body. The kidneys are the principal organ of excretion, but the liver, GI tract, and lungs also may play important roles. Milk, saliva, and sweat are usually of less importance, although the presence of an active drug in milk may affect nursing young and contributes to milk discard times.

Renal excretion of foreign compounds is accomplished either by glomerular filtration, passive diffusion into and out (eg, resorption) of the tubular lumen, and carrier-mediated secretion (eg, active transport or facilitated diffusion).

Among the more important factors determining renal excretion is renal blood flow, which in turn is influenced by cardiac output. Glomerular filtration in particular, but also carrier-mediated transport, is influenced by changes in cardiac output. Drugs that impact renal blood flow (eg, angiotensin-converting enzyme inhibitors) can also impact renal clearance.

Only unbound molecules <66,000 daltons *are readily filtered through* the glomerular membranes into the tubular lumen. Most active tubular secretion of drugs into tubules (renal exertion) occurs in the proximal convoluted tubule. Binding to plasma proteins usually does not hinder tubular excretion of drugs. Transport proteins exist for weak acids (anions), bases (cations), or organic compounds. Most (passive) reabsorption of nonionized, lipid-soluble drugs occurs as urine is concentrated in the distal and collecting tubules. Acidification or alkalinization of the urine may alter the rate of excretion of some drugs because of ion trapping in the tubular fluid.

Concurrent administration of either acidic or basic drugs that are substrates for carrier-mediated secretion processes prolongs the elimination of the drug that has the lesser affinity for the carrier sites, thus increasing its duration of action.

Among the more important factors impacting renal excretion is renal or cardiac disease. Decreased renal blood flow will result in a proportional decrease in renal excretion. However, renal disease may also be accompanied by changes in the metabolic capacity of the kidneys and production of toxins that will compete with drug for protein-binding sites. Changes in acid-base balance may also influence urine pH.

Drugs and their metabolites may also be excreted either passively or actively by hepatocytes into the bile canaliculi and, ultimately, into the duodenum in the bile. Generally, biliary excretion occurs for drugs with molecular weights that exceed 600 daltons. Biliary excretion is a relatively slow process. Further, many drugs excreted in bile as glucuronide conjugates may become unconjugated by intestinal microflora. Released drug can be reabsorbed into the systemic circulation, resulting in "enterohepatic circulation." Such recirculation often accounts for prolonged half-lives of drugs that are primarily excreted in bile. Impairment of the excretory functions of the hepatocytes or obstruction of bile flow due to any cause interferes with the biliary excretion of drugs. Dose or interval should then be adjusted accordingly.

The other routes of excretion are of lesser clinical importance. Many drugs are excreted in the feces either because of limited oral absorption or diffusion directly into the GI tract. The ruminoreticulum can act as a drug reservoir because of ion trapping or can remove a drug because of microbial metabolism. The tracheobronchial tree also may be a potential avenue of excretion, as is alveolar elimination of inhalant anesthetics. The main factors governing elimination by this route are the same as those determining the uptake of inhalant anesthetics—the concentrations in plasma and alveolar air and the blood/gas partition coefficient. The mammary and salivary glands excrete drugs by nonionic passive diffusion. The salivary route of excretion is important in ruminants because they secrete such voluminous amounts of alkaline saliva, although such drugs are likely to enter the GI tract.

PHARMACOKINETICS

Predicting how a drug behaves in the body can be accomplished through mathematical modeling of the time course of the drug in the body, or pharmacokinetics. Simplistically, pharmacokinetics describe what the body does to the drug, whereas pharmacodynamics describe what the drug does to the body. Pharmacokinetics are determined by following changes in plasma drug concentrations after a dose of the drug is administered at least via the desired route and ideally also after IV administration (100% bioavailability). The time course of plasma drug concentrations is mathematically "modeled" such that physiologic events impacting the changes in drug concentration might be determined. Most pharmacokinetic studies are conducted in healthy animals, yet dosing regimens should be individualized to adjust for physiologic (age, gender, species, and breed), pharmacologic (drug interactions), or pathologic (eg, renal or hepatic disease) differences or for animals receiving multiple drugs.

The pharmacodynamic response to a drug generally reflects the number of receptors with which the drug interacts (drug-receptor theory). In most instances, tissue drug concentrations parallel plasma drug concentrations.

After intravenous administration, the most relevant pharmacokinetic parameters that describe a drug and provide a basis for the dosing regimen are the apparent volume of distribution and the plasma clearance, both of which determine the elimination rate constant and elimination half-life. Additional parameters include the distribution rate constant and half-life and, if the drug is also given orally, the *absorption rate constant* and half-life.

After a drug is administered by rapid IV (eg, bolus) injection, the drug will be immediately distributed to the "central" vascular compartment, which includes highly perfused organs. Also immediately, plasma drug concentrations decline for two reasons: distribution of drug from plasma into tissues and back, and elimination from the body because of irreversible removal (ie, metabolism or excretion). As such, the decline in plasma drug concentrations initially is rapid, but once distribution reaches a "pseudo" equilibrium such that the amount of drug moving into tissues equals that moving back into plasma, plasma drug concentration will decline only because of elimination from the body (metabolism and excretion). Each drug movement is "first order," meaning a constant fraction or percentage (rather than amount) moves per unit time. As such, the time course of the drug in plasma must be plotted semilogarithmically (y = log plasma drug concentration, x = time). The result will be a decline in plasma drug concentrations that can be "fitted" by two lines: the first line, representing distribution and elimination, which declines very rapidly (steep slope), followed by a second "terminal" line, with a flatter slope because it represents elimination only. If the terminal line is drawn back to the y-axis, the Y intercept represents the plasma drug concentration after distribution has reached pseudoequilibrium ("B"). The slope of this terminal line is the elimination "rate constant," k_{el}, and from it is derived the elimination half-life, $t_{1/2}$. The line that describes distribution also is characterized by a Y intercept (the drug concentration in the "central" compartment, or "A") and a "distribution" rate constant (often referred to as α or k_d); it is from this rate constant that a distribution half-life can be determined. Once the curve is mathematically described by slopes and Y intercepts, given any time (t) point after the drug is administered, the amount of drug in the body or the plasma drug concentration (C_p) can then be predicted (C_p) = $Ae^{-at} + Be^{-kt}$ in which e is the natural log. From this data, clinically relevant parameters that influence the dosing regimen are then determined.

Apparent Volume of Distribution

If both the dose (mg/kg) and the drug concentration in plasma (the Y intercept of the terminal component of the plasma drug concentration [PDC] versus time curve, or "B") are known, then an "apparent" volume of distribution can be calculated from V_d = dose/PDC. This theoretical volume describes the volume to which the drug must be distributed if the concentration in plasma represents the concentration throughout the body (ie, distribution has reached equilibrium). The term "apparent" underscores the fact that where the drug is distributed cannot be determined from V_d; only that it goes *somewhere*. The pharmacokinetic measure used to indicate the pattern of distribution of a drug in plasma and in the different tissues, as well as the size of the compartment into which a drug would seem to have distributed in relation to its concentration in plasma, is known as the apparent volume of distribution (V_d). It is usually reported as liters per kilogram (L/kg) and is determined by measuring peak plasma drug concentrations after distribution has reached equilibrium for a drug administered IV. That concentration is compared with the IV dose that was given: V_d = dose/PDC. For example, if 12 mg/kg of phenobarbital is given, and the resulting PDC after distribution has occurred is 20 mg/L, then the apparent volume to which phenobarbital is distributed (V_d) = (12 mg/kg/20 mg/L) or 0.6 L/kg.

The V_d is useful for three reasons. First, and perhaps most importantly, it can be used to calculate a dose if the target PDC is known: dose = $V_d \times$ target PDC. For example, if the V_d of phenobarbital is 0.6 L/kg, and the target concentration of phenobarbital in a drug-naive animal is 10 mg/L, the IV dose would be 10 mg/L × 0.6 L/kg or 6 mg/kg. Second, if the PDC at any time after the dose is known, the V_d can be used to calculate how much drug is left in the body. Finally, the V_d can be used to predict the relative ability of the drug to distribute to different body compartments: if the drug is limited to the extracellular compartment (interstitial fluid, plasma), as is typical of water-soluble drugs, this represents 20%–30% of the body weight, and the V_d of such a drug should be <0.3 L/kg. Lipid-soluble drugs are generally able to penetrate cell membranes and thus are distributed to both extracellular and intracellular fluid, which represents ~60% of the body weight. Such drugs are generally characterized by a V_d >0.6 L/kg. Some drugs are limited to the plasma compartment and do not distribute well. An example would be a drug very tightly bound to plasma proteins; for such drugs, the V_d approximates the size of the blood compartment, or >0.1 L/kg. However, as the drug is freed from the protein, it will leave the plasma compartment and distribute into tissues. Many drugs are characterized by a V_d that exceeds the body weight of the animal (ie, >1 L/kg). For example, the mean digoxin V_d in dogs is 13 L/kg. This points out that the basis to determine V_d is PDC: if the drug leaves the plasma, regardless of where it goes, the V_d will increase. For digoxin, the drug binds to cardiac tissue; however, this is known only because follow-up studies demonstrated as such.

The V_d of a drug is usually constant over a wide dose range for a given species. However, a number of clinically significant factors can influence the V_d, including age (larger in neonates and pediatrics, smaller in geriatrics); functional status of the kidneys (decreased with dehydration), liver (increased with edema), and heart; fluid accumulations; concentration of plasma proteins (influencing unbound drug only); acid-base status (particularly if ion trapping causes the drug to accumulate in tissues); inflammatory processes or necrosis; and any other causes for alteration in the degree of plasma-protein binding.

Drug Clearance

As soon as a drug reaches the systemic circulation, it immediately begins to be cleared from plasma. Clearance is the volume of blood from which a drug is irreversibly eliminated, or cleared. Plasma is most commonly sampled; however, plasma clearance represents the sum clearances by all organs. If the drug is cleared by only a single organ, then plasma clearance is the clearance of that organ. Clearance is a volume and, as such, its units are volume/mass/time (eg, mL/kg/min). An alternative definition of clearance is the volume of plasma that would contain the amount of drug excreted per unit time; this definition demonstrates the link between volume of distribution (V_d) and clearance: if the elimination rate constant is known, it describes the fraction of the V_d cleared and, together, they can be used to calculate clearance (CL) from the PDC vs time curve: CL = $V_d \times k_{el}$/time (min). As such, like V_d, CL directly influences k_{el}, ie, rate at which drug is eliminated from the body: as CL increases, k_{el} becomes more steep. Clearance is independent of the V_d of a drug and thus the concentration of drug in the blood; no matter how much drug is in the blood, the same volume will be cleared per unit time.

The two major organs responsible for clearance are the liver and kidneys. Once a drug is metabolized, it is irreversibly eliminated from the body. Its metabolites, however, must be excreted (usually by the kidneys). Hepatic clearance is defined as the volume of plasma totally cleared per unit time as blood passes through the liver. The rate of hepatic clearance depends on drug delivery to the liver, ie, blood flow (Q) and the extraction (E) ratio of the drug, or fraction of the drug removed as it passes through the liver. Extraction, in turn, is determined by the intrinsic clearance (metabolic capacity) of the liver. Drugs cleared by the liver fall into two major categories.

"Flow-limited" drugs are extracted so rapidly that Q becomes the limiting factor of hepatic clearance. Binding to plasma proteins will not influence clearance of such drugs. In contrast, the rate-limiting step of "capacity-limited" drugs is intrinsic clearance, ie, the metabolic capacity of the liver. For such drugs, binding to serum proteins will decrease the rate of clearance. As such, highly protein-bound drugs are referred to as "capacity limited, binding sensitive" as opposed to drugs not highly protein bound and thus "capacity limited, binding insensitive."

Hepatic disease differentially impacts flow- and capacity-limited drugs. Hepatic clearance of flow-limited drugs will markedly decrease with changes in hepatic flow such as might occur with portosystemic shunting. When administered orally, such drugs are normally characterized by a high first-pass metabolism and reduced oral bioavailability. With portosystemic shunting, oral bioavailability can markedly increase and, as such, oral doses must be decreased in proportion to the shunted blood. Changes in hepatic mass and function will impact capacity-limited drugs. In general, if liver disease has negatively impacted serum albumin and BUN, the intrinsic metabolic capacity of the liver is also likely to be negatively impacted. However, if protein-binding decreases for a highly protein-bound drug such that more of the drug is unbound, hepatic clearance may not be as negatively impacted.

Renal clearance is defined as the volume of plasma totally cleared of a drug per unit time (eg,1 min) during passage through the kidneys. The renal clearance of drugs depends primarily on renal blood flow but also is impacted by urine pH, extent of plasma-protein binding, urine concentrating ability, and concomitant use of certain drugs. Serum creatinine or serum creatinine clearance can be used to assess changes in renal clearance as renal function declines. Either the dose or interval can be proportionately modified. For drugs with a short half-life, intervals are more appropriately prolonged (compared with decreasing dose) as serum creatinine increases; for drugs that accumulate because of a long half-life, the dose or interval might be proportionately decreased or prolonged, respectively.

Elimination Rate Constant: Among the most commonly cited pharmacokinetic parameters is the elimination half-life. It is derived from the elimination rate constant, k_{el}, which is the slope of the terminal, or elimination, component of the PDC vs time curve. A "hybrid" parameter, k_{el} is impacted by both CL and V_d. CL determines the decline in PDC; thus, the greater the volume of drug cleared, the steeper the slope, or k_{el}. The impact of V_d on half-life reflects its effect on PDC: a larger V_d means less drug is in the volume of blood cleared by the liver or kidneys. As such, the rate of elimination declines as V_d increases, resulting in an inverse relationship. The elimination half-life of a drug is the time that lapses as PDC declines by 50%. It is calculated from the slope of the line k_{el}: $t_{1/2} = 0.693/k_{el}$. The relationship between k_{el} and half-life reflects the fact that half-life becomes run of the slope (t_2-t_1) as C_1 declines by 50% (ie, $C_1/C_2 = 2$). The natural log of 2 = 0.693. Because $t_{1/2}$ is the inverse of k_{el}, then $t_{1/2}$ is directly proportional to V_d (larger V_d results in a longer half-life) and inversely proportional to CL. Note that CL and V_d can be profoundly altered, yet $t_{1/2}$ may not change. For example, in an animal dehydrated because of renal dysfunction, CL may be decreased by 50%, doubling $t_{1/2}$. However, if the animal is markedly dehydrated, then V_d will decrease because of contraction of extracellular fluid volume. Because more drug is in each mL of blood cleared by the kidney, the same amount of drug may be eliminated, and as such k_{el} or $t_{1/2}$ may not change.

The elimination half-life determines the time to steady-state (*see* below) and the time for a drug to be eliminated from the body once drug administration is discontinued. Once a drug is discontinued, 50% of the drug is eliminated in one half-life, 75% in the second (half of 50%), 87.5% in the third, and so on. For practical purposes, most drug is eliminated by 3–5 half-lives. The $t_{1/2}$ along with tolerances determines withdrawal or milk discard times in food animals. The relationship between dosing interval and elimination half-life also determines whether a drug will fluctuate or accumulate during a dosing interval.

Single-dose Concentration Curves After Extravascular Administration: When a drug is administered by an extravascular route, plasma drug concentrations rise until a peak or maximum drug concentration (C_{max}) is reached. Once the drug enters circulation, it is subjected immediately and simultaneously to distribution, metabolism, and excretion. The plasma drug concentration vs time curve after extravascular administration has an additional Y intercept and slope, with the slope reflecting the rate constant of absorption, k_a. The absorption half-life is the time that elapses as 50% of the drug is absorbed into the system. Absorption generally is sufficiently slow that drug distribution is generally "masked" by the absorption phase. As such, as plasma drug concentrations decline after C_{max} is reached, the slope generally reflects k_{el}.

The term "bioavailability" is used to express the rate and extent of absorption of a drug (*see* above).

Steady State Plasma Concentration (Repeated Administration or Constant IV Infusion): In some cases, the desired therapeutic effect of a drug is produced with a single dose. However, to achieve a satisfactory response, it is frequently necessary to maintain drug concentrations in the therapeutic range for a longer time. Rather than administering large doses, which could result in potentially toxic plasma drug concentrations, multiple dosing occurs at regular, safer intervals. For drugs with a very short half-life, the drug may be administered through a catheter as a constant-rate infusion, which is essentially continuous IV delivery. The rate of administration depends on the amount of fluctuation in drug concentration that can occur during a dosing interval, which in turn is determined by the relationship between $t_{1/2}$ and the dosing interval, T.

If a drug is administered at an interval substantively longer than its half-life, most of the drug will be eliminated during each dosing interval. As such, little drug remains with the subsequent dose, and plasma drug concentrations will fluctuate (C_{max} to C_{min}) during the dosing interval. For example, if a drug with a 4-hr half-life is administered every 12 hr, 87.5% of the drug will be eliminated during each dosing interval. With each dose, there is a risk of drug concentrations becoming subtherapeutic; increasing the dose will result in a small increase in C_{min} but may substantially increase C_{max}, thus increasing the risk of toxicity. A more appropriate response would be to decrease the dosing interval. However, this may be necessary only if drug efficacy depends on the presence of the drug. For example, this degree of fluctuation may be acceptable for a concentration-dependent antimicrobial. However, if the drug is an anticonvulsant, the risk of seizures increases just before the next dose. If the drug is time-dependent, drug concentrations may drop below the minimum inhibitory concentration of the infecting microbe. In contrast to drugs with a short half-life, drugs with a long half-life compared with the dosing interval will accumulate with each dose, because much of the drug remains in the body when the next dose is given. Such drugs will begin to accumulate with the first dose and will continue to do so until a "steady state" equilibrium is reached such that the amount of drug eliminated during each dosing interval is equivalent to the amount of drug administered during that same interval. The accumulation ratio describes the magnitude of increase of either C_{max} or C_{min} at steady state compared with the first dose. The longer the half-life compared with the dosing interval, the greater the accumulation ratio. The time to steady state, regardless of the drug or dose is 3–5 drug elimination half-lives. However, administration must occur with the same preparation at the same dosing regimen. In such cases, 50% of the plateau or steady-state concentration will be reached in one $t_{1/2}$, 75% at two $t_{1/2}$, 87.6% at three $t_{1/2}$, and 93.6% at four $t_{1/2}$. As with drug elimination, for practical purposes, steady state is achieved by 3–5 half-lives. Response to the drug, whether efficacy or toxicity, cannot be assessed until steady state is reached. Because the amount of drug in the body is large compared with each dose, manipulating plasma drug concentrations for such drugs is difficult, because changes require dosing for 3–5 half-lives at the new dose.

If the time to reach steady state, and thus time to therapeutic effect, is unacceptable, steady-state plasma drug concentrations may be achieved more rapidly by administration of a loading dose or doses (dose = V_d × target concentration; if the drug is given orally, dose = (V_d/F) × target concentration. However, the drug is not at steady state but only at steady state concentrations. If the maintenance dose does not maintain what the loading dose achieved, then as steady state at the maintenance dose is reached, plasma drug concentrations may increase to toxicity or decline to a subtherapeutic concentration. Drugs with very short half-lives are often administered by constant-rate infusions in animals in critical condition; in such cases, the interval is infinitely short compared with the half-life, and the drug will accumulate until steady state is reached. The rate of infusion (mcg/kg/min) is equal to the CL (mL/min/kg) × target concentration (mcg/mL); a loading dose should be given if the time to steady state is unacceptably long.

DRUG ACTION AND PHARMACODYNAMICS

Pharmacodynamics is the study of the biochemical and physiologic effects of drugs and their mechanisms of action on the body or on microorganisms and other parasites within or on the body. It considers both drug action, which refers to the initial consequence of a drug-receptor interaction, and drug effect, which refers to the subsequent effects. The drug action of digoxin, for example, is inhibition of membrane Na^+/K^+-ATPase; the drug effect is augmentation of cardiac contractility. In this example, the clinical response might comprise improved exercise tolerance.

Not all drugs exert their pharmacologic actions via receptor-mediated mechanisms. The action of some drugs—including inhalation anesthetic agents, osmotic diuretics, purgatives, antiseptics, antacids, chelating agents, and urinary acidifying and alkalinizing agents—is attributed to their chemical action or physicochemical properties. Certain cancer and antiviral chemotherapeutic agents, which are analogues of pyrimidine and purine bases, elicit their effects when they are incorporated into nucleic acids and serve as substrates for DNA or RNA synthesis. The effect of most drugs, however, results from their interactions with receptors. These interactions and the resulting conformational changes in the receptor initiate biochemical and physiologic changes that characterize the drug's response.

Drug Concentration and Effect

Drug therapy is intended to result in a particular pharmacologic response of desired intensity and duration while avoiding adverse drug reactions. The relationship between the administered dose and the clinical response has been investigated for some drugs using a pharmacokinetic/pharmacodynamic (PK/PD) modeling approach, which is generally based on the plasma concentration-response relationship. For other drugs, a simpler relationship between the concentration and effect in an idealized in vitro system is modeled mathematically to conceptualize receptor occupancy and drug response. The model assumes that the drug interacts reversibly with its receptor and produces an effect proportional to the number of receptors occupied, up to a maximal effect when all receptors are occupied. The reaction scheme for the model is:

$$\text{Drug (D)} + \text{Receptor (R)} \underset{k_1}{\overset{k_2}{\leftrightarrow}} \text{DR} \rightarrow \text{Effect}$$

in which k_2 and k_1 are rate constants.

The relationship between effect and the concentration of free drug for the model is given by the Hill equation, which can be written as:

$$E = \frac{E_{max} \times C}{EC_{50} + C}$$

in which E is the effect observed at concentration C, E_{max} is the maximal response that can be produced by the drug (efficacy), EC_{50} is the concentration of drug that produces 50% of maximal effect (potency), and the Hill coefficient n is the slope of the $\log_{10}$ concentration-effect relationship (sensitivity).

The above equation describes a rectangular hyperbola when response (y-axis) is plotted against concentration (x-axis). However, dose- or concentration-response data is generally plotted as drug effect (y-axis) against $\log_{10}$ dose or concentration (x-axis). The transformation yields a sigmoidal curve that allows the potency of different drugs to be readily compared. In addition, the effect of drugs used at therapeutic concentrations commonly falls on the portion of the sigmoidal curve that is approximately linear, ie, between 20% and 80% of maximal effect. This makes for easier interpretation of the plotted data.

Agonists and Antagonists

An **agonist** is a drug that binds to receptors and thereby alters (stabilizes) the proportion of receptors in the active conformation, resulting in a biologic response. A full agonist results in a maximal response by occupying all or a fraction of receptors. A partial agonist results in less than a maximal response even when the drug occupies all of the receptors.

There are four types of drug antagonism. **Chemical antagonism** involves chemical interaction between a drug and either a chemical or another drug leading to a reduced or nil response. **Physiologic antagonism** occurs when two drugs acting on different receptors and pathways exert opposing actions on the same physiologic system. **Pharmacokinetic antagonism** is the result of one drug suppressing the effect of a second drug by reducing its absorption, altering its distribution, or increasing its rate of elimination. **Pharmacologic antagonism** occurs when the antagonist inhibits the effect of a full or partial agonist by acting on the same pathway but not necessarily on the same receptor.

Pharmacologic antagonists comprise three subcategories. A **reversible competitive antagonist** results in inhibition that can be overcome by increasing the concentration of agonist. The presence of a reversible competitive antagonist causes a parallel rightward shift of the log concentration-effect curve of the agonist without altering E_{max} or EC_{50}. An **irreversible competitive antagonist** also involves competition between agonist and antagonist for the same receptors, but stronger binding forces prevent the effect of the antagonist being fully reversed, even at high agonist concentrations. The presence of an irreversible competitive antagonist causes a rightward shift of the log concentration-effect curve of the agonist that generally displays decreased slope and reduced maximum effect. A **noncompetitive antagonist** inhibits agonist activity by blocking one of the sequential reactions between receptor activation and the pharmacologic response. Noncompetitive antagonism is generally reversible but can be irreversible. Noncompetitive antagonists and irreversible competitive antagonists cause similar perturbations in the log concentration-effect curve of agonists. Isolated tissue experiments are used to distinguish the two subcategories, because noncompetitive antagonists are generally reversible.

Agonists, but not antagonists, elicit an effect even when they bind to the same site on the same receptor. An explanation is provided by both structural and functional studies, which indicate that receptors exist in at least two conformations, active and inactive, and these are in equilibrium. Because agonists have a higher affinity for the receptor's active conformation, agonists drive the equilibrium to the active state, thereby activating the receptor. Conversely, antagonists have a higher affinity for the receptor's inactive conformation and push the equilibrium to the inactive state, producing no effect.

The concept of **spare receptors** explains a maximum response being achieved when only a fraction of the total number of receptors is occupied. For example, an action potential and maximal twitch of muscle fibers is elicited when 0.13% of the total number of receptors at a skeletal neuromuscular junction is simultaneously activated. From a functional perspective, spare receptors are significant, because they increase both the sensitivity and speed of a tissue's responsiveness to a ligand.

Structure–Activity Relationships

Structure-activity relationships are exploited in drug design, because small changes in chemical structure can produce profound changes in potency. For example, the substitution of a proton by a methyl group accounts for codeine being ~1,000 times less potent than morphine in its action on opioid receptors.

Signal Transduction and Drug Action

Most receptors are proteins. The best characterized of these are regulatory proteins, enzymes, transport proteins, and structural proteins. Nucleic acids are also important drug receptors, particularly for cancer chemotherapeutic agents.

The receptors for several neurotransmitters modulate the opening and closing of ion channels through ligand gating or voltage gating. The nicotinic acetylcholine receptor is an example of a ligand-gated receptor; it allows Na^+ to flow down its concentration gradient into cells, resulting in depolarization. Most clinically useful neuromuscular blocking drugs compete with acetylcholine for the receptor but do not initiate ion-channel opening. Other ligand-gated ion channels include the CNS receptors for the excitatory amino acids (glutamate and aspartate), the inhibitory amino acids (γ-aminobutyric acid [GABA] and glycine), and certain serotonin (5-HT3) receptors. The sodium channel receptor is an example of a voltage-gated receptor; these are present in the membranes of excitable nerve, cardiac, and skeletal muscle cells. In the resting state, the Na^+/K^+-ATPase pump in these cells maintains an intracellular Na^+ concentration much lower than that in the extracellular environment. Membrane depolarization causes channel opening and a transient influx of Na^+ ions, followed by inactivation and return to the resting state. The action of local anesthetics is due to their direct interaction with voltage-gated Na^+ channels.

Many transmembrane receptors are linked to guanosine triphosphate binding proteins, which activate second messenger systems. Two important second messenger systems are cyclic adenosine monophosphate (cAMP) and the phosphoinositides. In cAMP second messenger systems, binding of the ligand to the receptor increases or decreases adenylyl cyclase activity, which in turn regulates the formation of cAMP from adenosine triphosphate. The activation of protein kinase A by cAMP results in the phosphorylation of proteins and a physiologic effect. From a therapeutic standpoint, drug binding to β-adrenergic, histamine H_2, or dopamine D_1 receptors activates adenylyl cyclase, whereas binding to muscarinic M_2, α_2-adrenergic, dopamine

D_2, opiate μ and δ, adenosine A_1, or GABA type B receptors inhibits adenylyl cyclase. In phosphoinositide second messenger systems, membrane phosphatidylinositol 4,5-biphosphate is hydrolyzed to 1,4,5-trisphosphate (IP3) and 1,2-diacylglycerol (DAG) by activation of phospholipase C. Both IP3 and DAG activate kinases, and in the case of IP3, this involves the mobilization of calcium from intracellular stores. The action of numerous drugs is due to their interaction with receptors that rely on these second messengers, which include α_1-adrenergic, muscarinic M_1 or M_2, serotonin 5-HT2, and thyrotropin-releasing hormone receptors.

Protein tyrosine kinase receptors are generally transmembrane enzymes that phosphorylate proteins exclusively on tyrosine residues, rather than on serine or threonine residues. They include endocrine hormone receptors for insulin and receptors for several growth hormones.

Intracellular receptors mediate the action of hormones such as glucocorticoids, estrogen, and thyroid hormone and related drugs. The hormones, which regulate gene expression in the nucleus, are lipophilic and freely diffuse through the cell membrane to reach the receptor. Glucocorticoid receptors reside predominantly in the cytoplasm in an inactive form until they bind to the glucocorticoid steroid ligand. This results in receptor activation and translocation to the nucleus, where the receptor interacts with specific DNA sequences. Unlike glucocorticoid receptors, the receptors for estrogen and thyroid hormone reside in the nucleus.

Intracellular receptors are also important in mediating the action of antimicrobial drugs, including the penicillins, sulfonamides, trimethoprim, aminoglycosides, phenicols, macrolides, and fluoroquinolones. The mechanisms of action include inhibition of bacterial protein synthesis, inhibition of cell wall synthesis, inhibition of enzymatic activity, alteration of cell membrane permeability, and blockade of specific biochemical pathways.

Receptor-mediated mechanisms of action of several classes of anthelmintics are well understood. For example, the benzimidazoles and pro-benzimidazoles bind to nematode tubulin, preventing its polymerization during microtubular assembly and thus disrupting cell division. Depletion of ATP as the result of salicylanilides uncoupling oxidative phosphorylation and the inhibition of enzymes in the glycolytic pathway by benzene sulfonamides are other examples. Several classes of anthelmintics interfere with neurotransmission in parasites. A case in point is macrocyclic lactones, which potentiate inhibitory neurotransmission via GABA and glutamate-gated chlorine channels (*see* ANTHELMINTICS, p 2647).

Drug Dose and Clinical Response

To make rational therapeutic decisions, it is necessary to understand the fundamental concepts linking drug doses to concentrations to clinical responses. The concentration-response relationships for drugs may be graded or quantal. A **graded concentration-response curve** can be constructed for responses measured on a continuous scale, eg, heart rate. Graded concentration-response curves relate the intensity of response to the size of the dose and, hence, are useful to characterize the actions of drugs. A **quantal concentration-response curve** can be constructed for drugs that elicit an all-or-none response, eg, presence or absence of convulsions. For most drugs, the doses required to produce a specified quantal effect in a population are log normally distributed, so that the frequency distribution of responses plotted against log dose is a gaussian normal distribution curve. The percentage of the population requiring a particular dose to exhibit the effect can be determined from this curve. When these data are plotted as a cumulative frequency distribution, a sigmoidal dose-response curve is generated.

The **equilibrium dissociation constant of the receptor-drug complex, K_D,** is the ratio of rate constants for the reverse (k_2) and forward (k_1) reaction between the drug and receptor and the drug-receptor complex (*see* p 2503). K_D is also the drug concentration at which receptor occupancy is half of maximum. Drugs with a high K_D (low affinity) dissociate rapidly from receptors; conversely, drugs with a low K_D (high affinity) dissociate slowly from receptors. These effects impact the rate at which biologic responses end.

Potency refers to the concentration (EC_{50}) or dose (ED_{50}) of a drug required to produce 50% of the drug's maximal effect as depicted by a graded dose-response curve. EC_{50} equals K_D when there is a linear relationship between occupancy and response. Often, signal amplification occurs between receptor occupancy and response, which results in the EC_{50} for response being much less (ie, positioned to the left on the x-axis of the log dose-response curve) than K_D for receptor occupancy. Potency depends on both the affinity of a drug for its receptor and the efficiency with which drug-receptor interaction is coupled to response. The dose of drug required to produce an effect is inversely related to potency. In general, low potency is important only if it results in a need to administer the drug in large doses that are impractical. Quantal dose-response curves provide information on the potency of drugs that is different from the information derived from graded dose-response curves. In a quantal dose-response relationship, the ED_{50} is the dose at which 50% of individuals exhibit the specified quantal effect.

The **median inhibitory concentration**, or IC_{50}, is the concentration of an antagonist that reduces a specified response to 50% of the maximal possible effect.

Efficacy (also referred to as intrinsic activity) of a drug is the ability of the drug to elicit a response when it binds to the receptor. As discussed above, conformational changes in receptors as a result of drug occupancy initiate biochemical and physiologic events that characterize the drug's response. In some tissues, agonists demonstrating high efficacy can result in a maximal effect, even when only a small fraction of the receptors is occupied (the concept of spare receptors is discussed above).

Selectivity refers to a drug's ability to preferentially produce a particular effect and is related to the structural specificity of drug binding to receptors. For example, cyclooxygenase-2 (COX-2) preferential NSAIDs demonstrate partial specificity for COX-2, the inducible enzyme formed at sites of inflammation. By comparison, COX-2 selective NSAIDs are without significant effect on COX-1, the constitutive enzyme that performs a range of physiologic functions. For certain drugs, selectivity is species dependent. For example, *S*(+)-carprofen is COX-2 selective in dogs and cats, nonselective of COX-1 and COX-2 in horses, and COX-2 preferential in calves.

Specificity of drug action relates to the number of different mechanisms involved. Examples of specific drugs include atropine (a muscarinic receptor antagonist), salbutamol (a β_2-adrenoceptor agonist), and cimetidine (an H_2-receptor antagonist). By contrast, nonspecific drugs result in drug effects through several mechanisms of action. For example, phenothiazine causes blockade of D_2-dopamine receptors, α-adrenergic receptors, and muscarinic receptors.

The **affinity** of a drug for a receptor describes how avidly the drug binds to the receptor (ie, the K_D). The chemical forces in drug-receptor interactions include electrostatic forces, van der Waal forces, and the forces associated with hydrogen bonds and hydrophobic bonds. Variation in the strength of these forces, and therefore the thermal energy in the system, determines the degree of association and dissociation of the drug and the receptor. Covalent binding of drug to receptor (exemplified by fluoroquinolones acting on bacteria) leads to formation of an irreversible link.

The **therapeutic index** of a drug is the ratio of the dose that results in an undesired effect to the dose that results in a desired effect. The therapeutic index of a drug is usually defined as the ratio of LD_{50} to ED_{50} (median lethal and median effective doses, respectively, in 50% of individuals), which indicates how selective the drug is in eliciting its desired effect. Values of LD_{50} and ED_{50} for this purpose are derived from quantal dose-response curves generated in animal studies.

The information obtained from dose- and concentration-response curves is critically important when choosing between drugs and when determining the dose to administer. A drug is chosen largely on the basis of its clinical effectiveness for a particular therapeutic indication. In this context, the drug concentration at the receptor (determined by the pharmacokinetic properties of the drug) and the efficacy of the drug-receptor complex are the primary determinants of a drug's clinical effectiveness. The administered dose of a drug, by comparison, depends to a greater extent on potency than on maximal efficacy.

The maximal efficacy of the drug-receptor complex to result in a graded effect is E_{max} or I_{max} on a graded dose-response curve. E_{max} or I_{max} is derived from a quantitative dose-response relationship for a single animal and varies among individuals. The extrapolation of this value of E_{max} to a clinical case is only an estimate, but it facilitates a comparison of the maximal efficacy of drugs that result in a specified effect by identical receptors. A drug's potency (ie, EC_{50}, ED_{50}, or IC_{50}) obtained from either graded or quantal dose-response curves is used to determine the dose that should be administered. The slope of the graded dose-response curve (n in the Hill equation, p 2507) provides information concerning the dose range over which a drug elicits its effect. Other information concerning the selectivity of drug action and the therapeutic index is also obtained from the graded dose-response curve. When quantal effects are being considered, information concerning pharmacologic potency, selectivity of drug action, the margin of safety, and the potential variability of responsiveness among individuals is obtained from quantal dose-response curves.

Pharmacodynamics of Antimicrobial Drugs

The approach used to investigate the pharmacodynamics of antimicrobial drugs (and parasiticides) differs from that of other veterinary drugs on account of the need to address target pathogens that have structure, biochemistry, and capacity for replication which are markedly dissimilar to those of their mammalian host. The individual drugs within each group of antimicrobial drugs differ in potency and in antimicrobial spectrum of activity. The minimum inhibitory concentration (MIC), which is the lowest concentration of drug that completely inhibits bacterial growth, is determined in vitro as a measure of susceptibility of bacterial species and strains to a given drug. Importantly, the MIC_{50} provides a measure of potency, EC_{50}.

Other surrogate markers of bacteriologic effect exist and include the minimum bactericidal concentration (MBC), which is the concentration of antimicrobial drug that produces a 3-log-unit or 99.9% reduction in bacterial count, postantibiotic effect, sub-MIC postantibiotic effect, and time-kill data. More recently, the application of PK/PD principles to antimicrobial drug action has led to PK/PD integration and PK/PD modeling. **PK/PD integration** brings together data from PK and PD studies. The surrogate PK/PD index that best correlates with efficacy for a given drug is selected based on the drug's killing mechanism, namely concentration dependent, time dependent, or codependent (ie, both time and concentration determine outcome). The PK/PD index selected for aminoglycosides, which act by concentration-dependent killing mechanisms, is C_{max}/MIC ratio (C_{max} is the maximum plasma concentration after administration of a drug by a nonvascular route); for β-lactams, which act by time-dependent killing mechanisms, it is T>MIC (T is the time for which plasma concentration exceeds MIC, expressed as a percentage of the dosage interval); and for fluoroquinolones, which act by concentration-dependent killing mechanisms, AUC/MIC ratio (AUC is the area under the plasma drug concentration-time curve) is selected. The objective of **PK/PD modeling** is to define the three key pharmacodynamic properties that define any drug, namely E_{max} or I_{max} (efficacy); EC_{50} (or EC_{80} or EC_{90}) (potency); and slope (n) in the Hill equation, which indicates sensitivity and selectivity. PK/PD modeling permits breakpoint values to achieve a bacteriostatic or bactericidal effect, or bacterial eradication to be computed, which are used to optimize efficacy and minimize resistance.

Time-effect Relationships: The ability of drugs to reach the receptor is determined by pharmacokinetic parameters that characterize the absorption, distribution, and clearance of a drug. There may not be a simple temporal correlation between plasma concentration of a drug and its therapeutic effect. Plotting plasma concentrations (x-axis) versus therapeutic effect (y-axis) in chronologic order displays the data as a loop for some drugs. This phenomenon is referred to as hysteresis in the concentration-effect relationship. The effect of most drugs lag behind the plasma concentration. This results in a counterclockwise hysteresis loop. For example, the NSAID robenicoxib has prolonged local effects after blood concentrations have decreased below effective levels. A clockwise hysteresis loop is observed for cocaine and pseudoephedrine when tachyphylaxis develops (*see* below). The temporal correlation between plasma concentration and therapeutic effect also varies for the different classes of antagonists. For instance, the extent and duration of action of a competitive antagonist depends on its concentration in plasma, which depends (in part) on its rate of elimination. This requires that the dose be adjusted accordingly to maintain plasma concentrations in the therapeutic range. By contrast, the duration of action of an irreversible antagonist is relatively independent of its rate of elimination and, therefore, plasma concentration, and more dependent on the rate of turnover of receptor molecules.

Down-regulation and Up-regulation of Receptors: The density of most receptors is not constant with time, which has important therapeutic implications. Down-regulation of receptors may occur as a result of continual stimulation by an agonist and manifests as the development of tachyphylaxis, which demonstrates a clockwise hysteresis loop in the concentration-effect relationship. Conversely, additional receptors can be synthesized in response to chronic receptor antagonism—a phenomenon known as up-regulation.

Because more receptors are now available, a hyperreactive response occurs when the cell is exposed to an agonist.

ROUTES OF ADMINISTRATION AND DOSAGE FORMS

A diverse range of dosage forms and delivery systems has been developed to provide for the care and welfare of animals. The development of dosage forms draws on the discipline of biopharmaceutics, which integrates an understanding of formulations, dissolution, stability, and controlled release (pharmaceutics); absorption, distribution, metabolism, and excretion (pharmacokinetics, PK); concentration-effect relationships and drug-receptor interactions (pharmacodynamics, PD); and treatment of the disease state (therapeutics). Formulation of a dosage form typically involves combining an active ingredient and one or more excipients; the resultant dosage form determines the route of administration and the clinical efficacy and safety of the drug. Optimization of drug doses is also critical to achieving clinical efficacy and safety. Increasingly, a PK/PD model that describes the drug response is the basis of dose optimization. The PK and PD phases are linked by the premise that free drug in the systemic circulation is in equilibrium with the receptors. The PD phase generally involves interaction of the drug with a receptor, which triggers post-receptor events and eventually leads to a drug effect (*see* p 2503).

Drug delivery strategies for veterinary formulations are complicated by the diversity of species and breeds treated, the wide range in body sizes, different husbandry practices, seasonal variations, cost constraints associated with the value of the animal being treated, the persistence of residues in food and fiber (*see* p 2518), and the level of convenience, among other factors. Innovative solutions have been developed to meet many of these challenges (eg, the convenient dosing option offered by topical spot-on formulations to treat external and internal parasites on dogs and cats, the microencapsulation of NSAIDs as a way to mask taste when these agents are added to the rations of horses). The anatomy of the GI tract of ruminants presents unique opportunities for controlled-release drug delivery systems, and many such systems are on the market. For example, controlled-release boluses have been developed to deliver antimicrobials, anthelmintics, production enhancers, nutritional supplements, and other drugs.

Oral Route of Administration and Dosage Forms

The oral route of administration is frequently used in both companion and food animals. In dogs and cats, tablets, capsules, solutions, and suspensions are administered orally; pastes are also applied to the forelimbs of cats from which they are licked and ingested. In horses, solutions and suspensions are administered by nasogastric tubes, pastes are applied to the tongue, and granules are added to rations for ingestion. The oral route of administration is the most widely used in cattle, pigs, and poultry. Formulations range from premixes and drinking water additives to licks, pastes, drenches, tablets, capsules, and boluses. Oral dosage forms are usually intended for systemic effects resulting from drug absorption from the GI tract; however, some oral suspensions, eg, kaolin, are intended to produce local effects, and these are not absorbed. Disadvantages of the oral route of administration include the relatively slow onset of action, the possibilities of irregular absorption, the destruction of acid-labile drugs in the stomach, and the unsuitability of this route for many high-molecular-weight drugs. Oral dosage forms require careful pharmaceutical formulation.

Oral dosage forms comprise liquids (solutions, suspensions, emulsions, elixirs, and syrups), semisolids (pastes), and solids (tablets, capsules, powders, granules, premixes, and medicated blocks). These dosage forms together with examples of modified-release delivery systems for ruminants are discussed below.

A **solution** is a mixture of two or more components that form a single phase that is homogeneous down to the molecular level. Solutions offer several advantages over other dosage forms. Compared with solid dosage forms, solutions are absorbed faster and generally cause less irritation of the GI mucosa. Moreover, phase separation on storage is not a concern with solutions, as it may be for suspensions and emulsions. The disadvantages of solutions include susceptibility to microbial contamination and the hydrolysis in aqueous solution of susceptible active ingredients. In addition, the taste of some drugs is more unpleasant when in solution. A range of additives is used in the formulation of oral solutions, including buffers, flavors, antioxidants, and preservatives. Oral solutions provide a convenient means of drug administration to neonates and young animals.

A **suspension** is a coarse dispersion of insoluble drug particles, generally with a diameter >1 µm, in a liquid (usually aqueous) medium. Suspensions are useful to administer insoluble or poorly soluble drugs or when the presence of a finely divided form of the material in the GI tract is required. An example of the latter is the treatment of "frothy bloat" with dimethyl polysiloxanes, which relies on a dispersion of finely divided silica in the forestomach of ruminants. The taste of most drugs is less noticeable in suspension than in solution, because the drug is less soluble in suspension. Particle size is an important determinant of the dissolution rate and bioavailability of drugs in suspension. In addition to the excipients described above for solutions, suspensions include surfactants and thickening agents. Surfactants wet the solid particles, thereby ensuring the particles disperse readily throughout the liquid. Thickening agents reduce the rate at which particles settle to the bottom of the container. Some settling is acceptable, provided the sediment can be readily dispersed when the container is shaken. Redispersion of the suspension may not be achievable if the sediment has packed closely to form a hard mass, a process known as "caking."

An **emulsion** is a system consisting of two immiscible liquid phases, one of which is dispersed throughout the other in the form of fine droplets; droplet diameter generally ranges from 0.1–100 µm. The two phases of an emulsion are known as the dispersed phase and the continuous phase. Emulsions are inherently unstable and are stabilized through the use of an emulsifying agent, which prevents coalescence of the dispersed droplets. Creaming, as occurs with milk, also occurs with pharmaceutical emulsions. However, it is not a serious problem because a uniform dispersion returns upon shaking. Creaming is, nonetheless, undesirable because it is associated with an increased likelihood of the droplets coalescing and the emulsion "breaking." Other additives include buffers, antioxidants, and preservatives. Emulsions for oral administration are usually oil (the active ingredient) in water, and they facilitate the administration of oily substances such as castor oil or liquid paraffin in a more palatable form.

An **elixir** is a sweetened, usually hydroalcoholic solution of a bitter or nauseous drug intended for oral administration. The hydroalcoholic character of elixirs allows, within limits, both water-soluble and alcohol-soluble medicinal substances to be maintained in solution. The proportion of alcohol in elixirs varies widely, a characteristic used to advantage to solubilize medicinal agents. If the active ingredient is sensitive to moisture, it may be formulated as a flavored powder or granulation and reconstituted in water immediately before oral administration. Nonmedicated elixirs are used as the vehicles for pharmaceutical formulations.

A **syrup** is a concentrated aqueous solution of sugar or a sugar substitute with or without flavoring agents and a water-soluble drug. Sucrose is the most frequently used sugar, and syrups usually contain 60%–80%. Syrups may also contain cosolvents, solubilizing agents, thickeners, or stabilizers. Nonmedicated syrups are used as vehicles for water-soluble drugs.

A **paste** is a two-component semisolid in which drug is dispersed as a powder in an aqueous or fatty base. The particle size of the active ingredient in pastes can be as large as 100 µm. The vehicle containing the drug may be water; a polyhydroxy liquid such as glycerin, propylene glycol, or polyethylene glycol; a vegetable oil; or a mineral oil. Other formulation excipients include thickening agents, cosolvents, adsorbents, humectants, and preservatives. The thickening agent may be a naturally occurring material such as acacia or tragacanth, or a synthetic or chemically modified derivative such as xanthum gum or hydroxypropylmethyl cellulose. The degree of cohesiveness, plasticity, and syringeability of pastes is attributed to the thickening agent. It may be necessary to include a cosolvent to increase the solubility of the drug. Syneresis of pastes is a form of instability in which the solid and liquid components of the formulation separate over time; it is prevented by including an adsorbent such as microcrystalline cellulose. A humectant (eg, glycerin or propylene glycol) is used to prevent the paste that collects at the nozzle of the dispenser from forming a hard crust. Microbial growth in the formulation is inhibited using a preservative. It is critical that pastes have a pleasant taste or are tasteless and are able to be used throughout a wide temperature range. Pastes are a popular dosage form to treat cats and horses and can be easily and safely administered by owners.

A **tablet** consists of one or more active ingredients and numerous excipients and may be a conventional tablet that is swallowed whole, a chewable tablet, or a modified-release tablet (these are commonly referred to as modified-release boluses when the unit size is large). Conventional and chewable tablets are used to administer drugs to dogs and cats, whereas modified-release boluses are administered to cattle, sheep, and goats. The physical and chemical stability of tablets is generally better than that of liquid dosage forms. The main disadvantages of tablets are a relatively slow onset of action because of the need to pass into the intestine and then undergo disintegration and dissolution before absorption across the gut wall, the low bioavailability of poorly water-soluble drugs or poorly absorbed drugs, and the local irritation of the GI mucosa that some drugs may cause.

A **capsule** is an oral dosage form usually made from gelatin and filled with an active ingredient and excipients. Two common capsule types are available: hard gelatin capsules for solid-fill formulations, and soft gelatin capsules for liquid-fill or semisolid-fill formulations. Soft gelatin capsules are suitable to formulate poorly water-soluble drugs because they afford good drug release and absorption by the GI tract. Gelatin capsules are frequently more expensive than tablets but have some advantages. For example, particle size is rarely altered during capsule manufacture, and capsules mask the taste and odor of the active ingredient and protect photolabile ingredients.

A **powder** is a formulation in which a drug powder is mixed with other powdered excipients to produce a final product for oral administration. Powders have better chemical stability than liquids and dissolve faster than tablets or capsules because disintegration is not an issue. This translates into faster absorption for those drugs characterized by dissolution rate-limited absorption. Unpleasant tastes can be more pronounced with powders than with other dosage forms and can be a particular concern with in-feed powders, leading to variable ingestion of the desired dose. Moreover, sick animals often eat less and are therefore not amenable to treatment with in-feed powder formulations. Drug powders are principally used prophylactically in feed or formulated as a soluble powder for addition to drinking water or milk replacer. Powders have also been formulated with emulsifying agents to facilitate their administration as liquid drenches.

A **granule** is a dosage form consisting of powder particles that have been aggregated to form a larger mass, usually 2–4 mm in diameter. Granulation overcomes segregation of the different particle sizes during storage and/or dose administration, the latter being a potential source of inaccurate dosing. Granules and powders generally behave similarly; however, granules must deaggregate before dissolution and absorption.

A **premix** is a solid dosage form in which an active ingredient, such as a coccidiostat, production enhancer, or nutritional supplement, is formulated with excipients. Premix products are mixed homogeneously with feed at rates (when expressed on an active ingredient basis) that range from a few milligrams to ~200 g/ton of feed. They are administered to poultry, pigs, and ruminants. The density, particle size, and geometry of the premix particles should match as closely as possible those of the feed in which the premix will be incorporated to facilitate uniform mixing. Issues such as instability, electrostatic charge, and hygroscopicity must also be addressed. The excipients present in premix formulations include carriers, liquid binders, diluents, anticaking agents, and antidust agents. Carriers, such as wheat middlings, soybean mill run, and rice hulls, bind active ingredients to their surfaces and are important in attaining uniform mixing of the active ingredient. A liquid binding agent, such as a vegetable oil, should be included in the formulation whenever a carrier is used. Diluents increase the bulk of premix formulations, but unlike carriers, they do not bind the active ingredients. Examples of diluents include ground limestone, dicalcium phosphate, dextrose, and kaolin. Caking in a premix formulation may be caused by hygroscopic ingredients and is addressed by adding small amounts of anticaking agents such as calcium silicate, silicon dioxide, and hydrophobic starch. The dust associated with powdered premix formulations can have serious implications for both operator safety and economic losses and is reduced by including a vegetable oil or light mineral oil in the formulation. An alternative approach to overcoming dust is to granulate the premix formulation.

A **medicated block** is a compressed feed material that contains an active ingredient, such as a drug, anthelmintic, surfactant (for bloat prevention), or a nutritional supplement, and is commonly packaged in a cardboard box to feed to livestock. Ruminants typically have free access to the medicated block over several days, and variable consumption may be problematic. This concern is addressed by ensuring the active ingredient is nontoxic, stable, palatable, and preferably of low solubility. In addition, excipients in the formulation modulate consumption by altering the palatability and/or the hardness of the medicated block. For example, molasses increases palatability, and sodium chloride decreases it. Additionally, the incorporation of a binder such as lignin sulfonate in blocks manufactured by compression, or magnesium oxide in blocks manufactured by chemical reaction, increases hardness. The hygroscopic nature of molasses in a formulation may also impact the hardness of medicated blocks and is addressed by using appropriate packaging.

Oral Modified-release Delivery Systems for Ruminants

Several modified-release delivery systems have been developed that take advantage of the unique anatomy of the ruminant forestomach. Prominent among these systems are intraruminal boluses, which contain a range of active ingredients including parasiticides, nutritional supplements, antibloat agents, and production enhancers. They are administered using a balling gun. Most of the commercially available intraruminal boluses are continuous-release devices that rely on erosion, diffusion from a reservoir, dissolution of a dispersed matrix, or an osmotic "driver" to release the active ingredient. The pay-out period for intraruminal boluses is commonly >100 days. Regurgitation during rumination is prevented by the bolus having a density of ~3 g/cm^3 or a variable geometry.

Other types of oral modified-release delivery systems are also available for ruminants. For example, sustained-release boluses that deliver sulfonamides throughout a period of ~72 hr are available to treat cattle. In addition, sustained-release boluses containing methoprene or diflubenzuron are approved for the control of manure-breeding flies in cattle.

The intraruminal devices to supplement ruminants with selenium, cobalt, or copper include soluble glass boluses and intraruminal pellets. Boluses of soluble glass containing selenium, cobalt, and copper are available for cattle and sheep. Because glass is susceptible to sudden changes in temperature, glass boluses should be at least 15°–20°C at the time of administration to avoid fracturing, which in turn may lead to regurgitation. Glass boluses are designed to dissolve in ruminal fluids, thereby releasing the incorporated elements. The composition of the glass determines the solubility of the bolus, with an increase in the ratio of monovalent to divalent cations resulting in an increase in solubility. The glass boluses are retained in the rumen for up to 9 mo.

Intraruminal pellets containing selenium or cobalt are available for sheep. Selenium or cobalt is released throughout a period of ~3 yr from the pellet matrix, which consists of compressed iron grit. When selenium or cobalt intraruminal pellets are administered alone, a "grinder" is usually coadministered to prevent the formation of calcium phosphate coatings on the surface of the pellets.

Copper capsules, which contain oxidized copper wire particles encapsulated in gelatin, are available for adult sheep and goats. After oral administration, the gelatin capsule dissolves in the rumen and releases the particles of copper oxide. The particles progress to the abomasum, where some are trapped in the mucosal folds and release copper.

Parenteral Route of Administration and Dosage Forms

A drug given parenterally is one given by a route other than the mouth (topical dosage forms are considered separately). The three main parenteral routes of drug administration are IV, IM, and SC, and in all cases administration is usually via a hollow needle. Injectable preparations are usually sterile solutions or suspensions of drug in water or other suitable physiologically acceptable vehicles. Volumes delivered can range from milliliter to liter quantities. The time of onset of action for IV administration is seconds, and for IM and SC injections is minutes. Depot injectable preparations achieve prolonged release and maintain therapeutic concentrations of drug throughout 2–5 days. The bioavailability of a drug, particularly from prolonged-release formulations, can be influenced by the location of the IM injection site. SC implants and pellets also achieve prolonged release of drug. A number of recombinant proteins and peptides are orally inactive and must be given by the parenteral route. Specialized dosage forms, usually for parenteral administration, are required for vaccines. In food animals, intramammary infusions and intravaginal devices are administered by the parenteral route.

Parenteral dosage forms and delivery systems include injectables (ie, solutions, suspensions, emulsions, and dry powders for reconstitution), intramammary infusions, intravaginal delivery systems, and implants. These dosage forms and delivery systems as well as the special considerations relating to intra-articular injections, recombinant proteins and peptides, and vaccines are discussed below.

A **solution** for injection is a mixture of two or more components that form a single phase that is homogeneous down to the molecular level. "Water for injection" is the most widely used solvent for parenteral formulations. However, a nonaqueous solvent or a mixed aqueous/nonaqueous solvent system may be necessary to stabilize drugs that are readily hydrolyzed by water or to improve solubility. A range of excipients may be included in parenteral solutions, including antioxidants, antimicrobial agents, buffers, chelating agents, inert gases, and substances to adjust tonicity. Antioxidants maintain product stability by being preferentially oxidized over the shelf life of the product. Antimicrobial preservatives inhibit the growth of any microbes accidentally introduced when doses are being withdrawn from multiple-dose bottles, and they act as adjuncts in aseptic processing of products. Buffers are necessary to maintain both solubility of the active ingredient and stability of the product. Chelating agents are added to complex and thereby inactivate metals, including copper, iron, and zinc, which generally catalyze oxidative degradation of drugs. Inert gases are used to displace the air in solutions and enhance product integrity of oxygen-sensitive drugs. Isotonicity of the formulation is achieved by including a tonicity-adjusting agent. Failing to adjust the tonicity of the solution can result in the hemolysis or crenation of erythrocytes when hypotonic or hypertonic solutions, respectively, are given IV in quantities >100 mL. Injectable formulations must be sterile and free of pyrogens. Pyrogenic substances are primarily lipid polysaccharides derived from microorganisms, with those produced by gram-negative bacilli generally being most potent. Injectable solutions are very commonly used, and aqueous solutions given IM result in immediate drug absorption, provided precipitation at the injection site does not occur.

A **suspension** for injection consists of insoluble solid particles dispersed in a liquid medium, with the solid particles accounting for 0.5%–30% of the suspension. The vehicle may be aqueous, oil, or both. Caking of injectable suspensions is minimized through the production of flocculated systems, comprising clusters of particles (flocs) held together in a loose, open structure. Excipients in injectable suspensions include antimicrobial preservatives, surfactants, dispersing or suspending agents, and buffers. Surfactants wet the suspended powders and provide acceptable syringeability while suspending agents modify the viscosity of the formulation. The ease of injection and the availability of the drug in depot therapy are affected by the viscosity of the suspension and the particle size of the suspended drug. These systems afford enhanced stability to active ingredients that are prone to hydrolysis in aqueous solutions. Injectable suspensions are commonly used. Compared with that of injectable solutions, the rate of drug absorption of injectable suspensions is prolonged, because additional time is required for disintegration and dissolution of the suspended drug particles. The slower release of drug from an oily suspension compared with that of an aqueous suspension is attributed to the additional time taken by drug particles suspended in an oil depot to reach the oil/water boundary and become wetted before dissolving in tissue fluids.

An **emulsion** for injection is a heterogeneous dispersion of one immiscible liquid in another; it relies on an emulsifying agent for stability. Parenteral emulsions are rare, because it is seldom necessary to achieve an emulsion for drug administration. Untoward physiologic effects after IV administration may occur, including emboli in blood vessels if the droplets are >1 μm in diameter. Formulation options for injectable emulsions are also severely restricted, because suitable stabilizers and emulsifiers are very limited. Examples of parenteral emulsions include oil-in-water, sustained-release depot preparations (given IM), and water-in-oil emulsions of allergenic extracts (given SC).

A **dry powder** for parenteral administration is reconstituted as a solution or as a suspension immediately before injection. The principal advantage of this dosage form is that it overcomes the problem of instability in solution. Proteins and other materials that are extremely heat sensitive cannot be dried in pharmaceutical driers. Rather, freeze-drying, or lyophilization, is used to produce a porous powder that reconstitutes readily.

Intramammary infusion products to treat mastitis are available for lactating and nonlactating (dry) cows. Lactating cow intramammary infusions should demonstrate fast and even distribution of the drug and a low degree of binding to udder tissue. These properties result in lower concentrations of drug residues in the milk. In contrast, it is desirable for nonlactating cow formulations to demonstrate prolonged drug release and a high degree of binding to mammary secretions and udder tissues. Particle size is particularly important, because it affects both the rate of release of the active ingredient and irritancy to the udder tissue. Drug particle size in nonlactating intramammary formulations is usually smaller than in those for lactating cows, which is critical to reduce irritancy during prolonged retention in the udder. Thickening agents are added to modify the rate of release of the suspended particles from oil formulations, and antioxidants are commonly incorporated to prevent rancidity. Mastitis infusion products are often terminally sterilized by irradiation.

Intravaginal delivery systems include controlled internal drug-release (CIDR) devices, progesterone-releasing intravaginal devices (PRIDs), and vaginal sponges. These systems are used for estrus synchronization in sheep, goats, and cattle. Silicone is used in the manufacture of the T-shaped CIDR device and the coil-shaped PRID, whereas intravaginal sponges are made from polyurethane. The active ingredients in these systems are synthetic or natural hormones such as progesterone, methylacetoxy progesterone, fluorogestone acetate, or estradiol benzoate. An applicator consisting of a speculum and a separate plunger is used to insert sponges into the vaginal cavities of sheep and goats, and PRIDs into the vaginal cavities of cattle. A different type of applicator is used to insert CIDR devices into the vaginal cavities of sheep, goats, and cattle. Retention in the vagina depends on either the wings (CIDR device) or the entire device (sponges and PRIDs) expanding. With all three devices, gentle pressure is exerted on the vaginal wall. Retention of the device is >95%.

Most **implants** used in veterinary medicine are compressed tablets or dispersed matrix systems in which the drug is uniformly dispersed within a nondegradable polymer. Drug release from dispersed matrix systems involves dissolution of the drug into the polymer, followed by diffusion of the drug through the polymer and partitioning from the surface of the polymer into the surrounding aqueous environment. Implants are available to increase weight gain and feed conversion efficiency in food animals. These implants are typically prepared in a manner similar to tablets. One controlled-release implant consists of a cylindrical core of silicone, surrounded by an outer layer of estradiol-loaded silicone. A range of implants is available to enhance reproductive performance in breeding animals. These include ear implants containing norgestomet dispersed in polyethylene methacrylate or silicone, a biocompatible tablet implant containing deslorelin (a GnRH agonist) for use in mares that does not require removal, and a sustained-release pellet of melatonin, which is implanted in the ear of ewes to enhance breeding performance. Testosterone pellets are available to implant in the ears of wethers at doses of 70–100 mg every 3 mo for the prevention of ulcerative posthitis.

Special Dosage Form Considerations with Intra-articular Injections: The dosage forms used in intra-articular administration are sterile aqueous solutions. In horses, the two most common reasons for intra-articular injections are to anesthetize or "block" a joint during a lameness examination and to treat noninfectious inflammatory joint diseases such as synovitis and capsulitis. Drugs, including glucocorticoids, pentosan polysulfate sodium, and hyaluronic acid, are administered intra-articularly in inflammatory joint disease. The intra-articular administration of glucocorticoids avoids the adverse effects associated with large systemic doses. In dogs, hyaluronate sodium is administered by intra-articular injection for adjunctive treatment of synovitis.

Special Dosage Form Considerations with Recombinant Proteins and Peptides: Recombinant proteins and peptides are used in some countries to increase feed conversion efficiency and milk production in cattle (bovine growth hormone), increase feed conversion efficiency and produce leaner carcasses in pigs (porcine growth hormone), for the chemical shearing of sheep (epidermal growth factor), to reduce the incidence of skeletal weaknesses leading to leg injuries in horses (equine growth hormone), and for other uses. Recombinant proteins and peptides have been formulated as solutions, lyophilized powders, implants, and microparticles. The chemical and physical instability of recombinant proteins and peptides is a special consideration during formulation development. The major causes of chemical instability are proteolysis, deamidation, oxidation, and racemization. Causes of physical instability are aggregation, precipitation, denaturation, and adsorption to surfaces. A range of strategies has been reported to stabilize formulations containing recombinant proteins and peptides, including the choice of carrier vehicle (eg, oleaginous vehicles), the use of lyophilization excipients, the use of stabilizers such as sugars and detergents, chemical modification of the proteins and peptides, and the use of site-directed mutagenesis to synthesize more stable proteins.

Special Dosage Form Considerations with Live Vaccines, Inactivated and Subunit Vaccines, and DNA Vaccines: The organisms in live vaccines are subjected to freeze drying and, less commonly, to deep freezing at or below –70°C. To maintain the viability of organisms under these conditions, formulations include complex mixtures of proteins, peptides or amino acids, sugars, and mineral salts. The viability of organisms is additionally protected using stabilizers such as lactose or other saccharides, skim milk, and serum.

Formulations used for inactivated and subunit vaccines consist of antigen(s), adjuvants, stabilizers, and preservatives (in the case of multiple-dose products). Inactivating agents such as phenol, thiomersal, and formaldehyde are used to kill the virus or bacteria without destroying the critical integrity of the antigens necessary to induce a protective immune response. Adjuvants enhance the immunogenicity of antigens by stimulating the immune system and prolonging antigen release. In this respect, aluminum hydroxide, aluminum phosphate, and oil emulsions are generally preferred to confer antibody-mediated immunity, whereas saponin, quil A, and immunity-stimulating complexes are preferred to confer cell-mediated immunity.

Plasmid DNA vectors have been used to express antigens in vivo to generate immune responses. Two delivery systems for DNA vaccines have been reported. In one system, the segment of DNA is coated with gold and administered to the patient using a "gene gun." The other delivery system uses a viral vector or plasmid to carry the DNA segment into the patient.

Topical Route of Administration and Dosage Forms

The topical route of administration is used for local treatment of skin, control of external and internal parasites, and transdermal delivery of therapeutic agents. Drugs applied to the skin for local effect include *antiseptics, antifungals, anti-inflammatory agents,* and skin emollients. The rate of drug release from ointments, creams, and pastes is principally determined by the semisolid base used. In dogs and cats, an extensive range of topical formulations is used in the control of fleas, lice, mites, and ticks. These include insecticidal and acaracidal soaps, foams, shampoos, sprays, and rinses. Also available are topical delivery systems such as spot-on formulations and flea and tick collars and medallions. In food animals, a diverse range of topical dosage forms and delivery systems are used to control external parasites. For example, most pour-on formulations, plunge and shower dip concentrates, and jetting fluids are suspension concentrates or emulsifiable concentrates. In addition, many pour-on formulations display endectocidal activity in cattle. The efficacious systemic concentrations attained with these preparations result from the animal's licking behavior and, to a lesser extent, percutaneous absorption of the active ingredient. Numerous methods are used to apply parasiticides to farm animals (*see* below). A special consideration relating to the use of topical dosage forms is the potential for residues in wool and mohair to occur. The topical route of administration is also used to deliver therapeutic agents systemically. Transdermal patches, for instance, are used to deliver analgesics to the systemic circulation.

The topical dosage forms available to treat animals include solids (dusting powders), semisolids (creams, ointments, pastes, and gels), and liquids (solutions, suspension concentrates, suspoemulsions, emulsifiable concentrates, paints, and tinctures). These dosage forms as well as the specialized topical dosage forms and delivery systems for transdermal drug delivery and parasite control are discussed below.

A **dusting powder** is a finely divided insoluble powder containing ingredients such as talc, zinc oxide, or starch. Coarse powders often have a gritty feel, whereas powders containing particles that are <20 μm in all dimensions have a smooth feel. Some dusting powders absorb moisture, which discourages bacterial growth. Others are used for their lubricant properties. The use of dusting powders is indicated on skin folds and contraindicated on wet surfaces, because caking is likely to result.

A **cream** is a semisolid emulsion formulated for application to the skin or mucous membranes. Droplet diameter in topical emulsions generally ranges from 0.1–100 μm. Cream emulsions are most commonly oil-in-water but may be water-in-oil. The former readily rub into the skin (hence the term "vanishing" cream) and are removed by licking and washing.

By comparison, water-in-oil emulsions are emollient and cleansing. Water-in-oil emulsions are also less greasy and spread more readily than ointments, and they soothe inflamed skin as a consequence of the water in the formulation evaporating.

An **ointment** is a greasy, semisolid preparation that contains dissolved or dispersed drug. A range of ointment bases is used, including hydrocarbons, vegetable oils, silicones, absorption bases consisting of a mixture of hydrocarbons and lanolin, emulsifying bases consisting of a mixture of hydrocarbons and an emulsifying agent, and water-soluble bases. Ointment bases influence topical drug bioavailability via two mechanisms. First, their occlusive properties are responsible for hydrating the stratum corneum, which enhances the flux of drug across the skin. Second, they affect drug dissolution within the ointment and drug partitioning from the ointment into the skin. Ointments are effective emollients because of their occlusive nature. They are indicated for chronic, dry lesions and contraindicated in exudative lesions.

A **paste** for topical use is a stiff preparation containing a high proportion of finely powdered solids such as starch, zinc oxide, calcium carbonate, and talc. Pastes are less greasy than ointments, because much of the fluid hydrocarbon fraction is absorbed onto the solid particles; they are also less occlusive than ointments. Pastes are indicated for ulcerated lesions.

A **gel** is a nongreasy, semisolid, aqueous solution. The semisolid properties are due to a polymer imparting a continuous structure to the hydrophilic liquid. The polymers used include natural gums such as tragacanth, pectin, and agar; semisynthetic materials such as methylcellulose, hydroxymethylcellulose, and carboxymethylcellulose; and synthetic polymers such as carbopol. Medicaments are generally well released from gels, which are easily washed off on account of their water miscibility.

A **solution** for topical use is a mixture of two or more components that form a single phase down to the molecular level. Topical solutions include eye drops, ear drops, and lotions. Eye drops are sterile liquids that contain a range of drugs, including local anesthetics, antibiotics, anti-inflammatory agents, and drugs acting on the autonomic nervous system of the eye. They are instilled onto the eyeball or within the conjunctival sac. Ear drops are solutions of drugs such as antibiotics, insecticides, or anti-inflammatory agents. The vehicle may be water, glycerol, propylene glycol, or alcohol/water mixtures. They are applied to the external auditory canal.

A **lotion** is usually an aqueous solution (or suspension) for application to inflamed, ulcerated skin. Lotions cool the skin by evaporation of solvents, leaving a film of dry powder. Lotions are suitable for use on hairy areas and for lesions with minor exudation and ulceration.

A **suspension concentrate** for topical use is a mixture of insoluble, solid active ingredients, which are typically at high concentrations, in water or oil. Suspension concentrate formulations are generally water-based; the water-insoluble active ingredients and inert ingredients are of very small particle size (0.1–5 μm). Other formulation additives include suspending agents, surfactants, and other excipients to ensure the production of a shelf-stable, pourable product. Surfactants wet, disperse, and stabilize the solid particles in the continuous phase, prevent flocculation, and prevent changes in particle size. Thickening agents are included to increase the viscosity of the formulation, thereby overcoming sedimentation of the suspended particles and affording good longterm stability. Suspension concentrates are used topically as pour-ons, plunge and shower dip concentrates, and jetting fluids.

A **suspoemulsion** combines the elements of an emulsion and a suspension, allowing active ingredients with widely varying physical properties to be formulated in a single product. Typically, a suspoemulsion contains one or more solvent-soluble active ingredients in an emulsion phase, combined with one or more low solubility active ingredients in a continuous aqueous suspension phase.

After dilution, an **emulsifiable concentrate** for topical use produces a two-phase system involving two immiscible liquids, a dispersed phase, consisting of fine oil droplets ranging in size from 0.5 μm to several hundred microns, and a continuous phase. Addition of an emulsifiable concentrate formulation to water results in the formation of an emulsion, which relies on surface-active agents concentrating at the oil/water interface. Active ingredients that are soluble in water-immiscible organic solvents are frequently formulated as emulsifiable concentrates. The flocculation of oil droplets in emulsifiable concentrate formulations leads to a layer of cream that can be readily dispersed by mild agitation, whereas the coalescence of droplets leads to the inversion or "breaking" of the emulsion. Water with a high content of Ca^{2+} and/or Mg^{2+} reacts with anionic surfactants in the emulsifiable concentrate formulation; this affects both spontaneity of emulsification and stability. Zinc sulfate, used as a dip additive to minimize the spread of dermatophilosis in sheep, also adversely affects emulsions.

A **flank paint** comprises an antifoaming agent such as a detergent or mineral oil and is used to prevent pasture bloating in cattle. A flank paint is applied to the flanks of animals, from where it is licked off and ingested. Bloat, or ruminal tympany, refers to excessive accumulation of gas in the rumen. Frothy bloat commonly develops in cattle on pasture, particularly those grazing lush, leguminous pastures. Frothing of rumen ingesta occurs when the viscosity of the fluid is increased. Froth obstructs the cardia of the stomach, preventing the eructation of excessive gas produced in the rumen. Antifoaming agents reduce the stability of the froth by lowering the viscosity of the fluid ingesta.

A **tincture** for topical application uses a vehicle containing 15%–80% alcohol, requiring the preparation to be tightly stoppered and not exposed to high temperatures. In addition to alcohol, tinctures may contain cosolvents, stabilizers, and solubilizers. Iodine tincture is a topical anti-infective that contains 44%–50% alcohol. The reddish brown color of iodine tincture produces skin staining that delineates treated skin. Friar's balsam is compound benzoin tincture and is used to protect and toughen ulcerated or fissured skin.

Specialized Topical Dosage Forms and Delivery Systems for Transdermal Drug Delivery: A **transdermal delivery gel** consists of a vehicle, most commonly pluronic lecithin organogel (PLO gel), which delivers drug via the transdermal route to the bloodstream. The micellar composition of PLO gel enhances skin penetration of the pharmaceutical agent present in the formulation. PLO gel is generally well tolerated and is nontoxic if ingested. However, not all drugs are suitable for transdermal application, and there are relatively few studies of the bioavailability of drugs from compounded transdermal gels. Transdermal gels are used to deliver drugs to treat several diseases in dogs and cats, including undesirable behavior, cardiac disease, and hyperthyroidism. The dose is applied to the inner surface of the pinnae, thereby offering ease of administration, especially in cats.

A **transdermal delivery patch** typically consists of a drug incorporated into a reservoir, a protective backing layer, a rate-limiting release membrane, and an adhesive layer to secure the patch to the skin. The physicochemical properties of a drug suitable for transdermal delivery ideally include low molecular weight (<500 daltons), high potency, water solubility (to facilitate movement of the drug out of the reservoir and to allow passage through the epidermal and dermal layers of the skin), and lipid solubility (to permit penetration of the stratum corneum of the skin). Fentanyl, a synthetic opioid agonist, is delivered by transdermal patch in dogs, cats, and horses.

Specialized Topical Dosage Forms, Delivery Systems, and Application Methods for Parasite Control: The control of internal and external parasites of companion and food-producing animals has led to development of specialized dosage forms, delivery systems, and application methods unique to veterinary medicine.

A **spot-on formulation** is a solution of active ingredient(s) that typically contains a cosolvent and a spreading agent. The active ingredients in spot-on products for flea, GI parasite, or heartworm control in dogs and cats include fipronil, imidacloprid, selamectin, pyriproxyfen, ivermectin, and moxidectin. Spot-on formulations are also available to control lice in cattle. The physicochemical properties of the active ingredient(s) are important determinants of topical or transdermal behavior. Topical activity against ectoparasites depends to some extent on the active ingredient spreading, mixing with the sebum coating the skin and hair, and forming depots in the pilosebaceous units. The mechanism of percutaneous drug absorption varies between species and is not completely understood. However, low molecular weight and a high lipid/water partition coefficient tend to favor passage of the drug through the skin.

Backliner products for sheep consist of pour-on and spray-on formulations for the control of lice and sheep blowflies. Sheep lousicides include synthetic pyrethroids, organophosphates, and insect growth regulators. These products are formulated for pour-on application within 24 hr after shearing (ie, off-shears) or spray-on application (in short-wool sheep with wool growth <6 wk, and in long-wool sheep with wool growth >6 wk). Their efficacy against lice depends on topical activity and not on percutaneous absorption of the active ingredient into the bloodstream. Translocation of the pesticide from the application site to remote sites at concentrations lethal to lice is critical to the efficacy of these products and, in the case of pour-on applications, is facilitated by the increased secretion of wool grease that occurs at shearing.

The active ingredients in sheep blowfly products include insect growth regulators, synthetic pyrethroids, and organophosphates. After their topical application, sheep blowfly larvicides form follicular depots and subsequently translocate as a coating on new wool growing out of the follicles.

Hand-jetting of long-wool sheep (wool growth >6 wk) is done to control lice, keds, mites, and sheep blowflies. The pesticides used include rotenone, synthetic pyrethroids, organophosphates, insect growth regulators, and macrocyclic lactones. Hand-jetting involves the use of a handpiece (or wand) to "rake" a pesticide solution into the wool along the dorsal midline and sometimes into the breech, crutch, and poll. The solution is applied under pressure and penetrates to the skin.

Some **pour-on products** on the market are formulated to deliver an active ingredient percutaneously. The macrocyclic lactones ivermectin, moxidectin, doramectin, and eprinomectin are formulated as pour-on preparations for application to cattle. These formulations are usually solutions or emulsifiable concentrates for dilution with water before use. The principal route of percutaneous absorption for most drugs in people is the intercellular pathway, making the intercellular lipid matrix the primary barrier to absorption. However, this may not be the case in species in which the emulsifying properties of skin secretions and the large numbers of follicles and glands per unit surface area must be considered (eg, cattle and sheep). Ionized solutes, for example, are reported to cross the skin of animals via shunt pathways (sweat ducts, follicles). Pour-on products are formulated to spread without run-off when applied to the skin and to be resistant to rain. The formulation also facilitates the partitioning of the drug out of the vehicle and into the skin and transport of the drug across the skin. The control of these processes is critical, because some drug is required to remain at the skin if the drug is to be active against external parasites that are not blood sucking. In addition, too rapid passage of drug through the skin may result in unacceptable chemical residues in tissues or milk.

The **plunge dipping** of sheep and cattle for external parasites requires a dipping vat, which may be a portable unit or a permanent in-ground structure shielded from direct sunlight by roofing. A draining pen located at the exit of the vat allows dip wash that drains off treated animals to return to the vat. Dip chemicals are usually formulated as aqueous solutions, emulsifiable concentrates, or suspension concentrates, all of which are diluted with water before use. The high costs associated with plunge dipping relate principally to the costs of chemicals for charging large vats, labor, and the disposal of the hazardous wastes. Plunge dips must be managed properly and the pesticide maintained at the concentration recommended by the manufacturer. Dipping of sheep and cattle is associated with "stripping" of the active ingredient from the dip wash (eg, pesticide loss from the dip wash occurring at a greater rate than water loss) and is categorized as mechanical or chemical. In the case of sheep, mechanical stripping results from the fleece acting as a sieve toward the active ingredient, with the degree of filtration being primarily determined by particle size. Chemical stripping is due to the preferential absorption of pesticide by the fleece. To counteract stripping, a complex dip management regimen that involves reinforcement and "topping-up" is used. Reinforcement refers to the addition of undiluted chemical product to the dip without the addition of water, whereas topping-up refers to the addition of water and undiluted chemical product to the dip vat to return the volume to the starting level. Proper dip management also minimizes contamination of the dip with organic matter. This requires that the race leading to the vat is constructed of concrete or slats to remove dirt from the animals' feet and that animals be held in a yard overnight before dipping, during which time they are offered water but no feed.

Hand spraying generally results in uneven coverage of animals and is considered an inefficient method of application. By comparison, recirculating and nonrecirculating **spray races** facilitate whole body spraying and wet cattle to the skin. The situation with sheep is different—the very short contact time in a spray race limits the uptake of insecticide, which means the fleece seldom becomes saturated. Because of this, spray races should be used as an adjunct to shower or plunge dipping of sheep.

Shower dips are less labor intensive than plunge dips and are cheaper to operate. A typical shower dip consists of a sump containing the dip wash, a pump, and a showering pen constructed with a concrete floor and fitted with rotating and fixed nozzles. There are two types of shower dips: a conventional shower dip in which the sump volume is periodically maintained by adding fresh dip wash, and a constant replenishment shower dip in which a small-volume sump is continually filled from a large-volume supply tank to maintain dip levels. Proper dip management requires attention to the factors described above for plunge dipping. In addition, all equipment must be functioning properly for the fleece to become saturated. Sheep should not be dipped (by either the plunge or shower method) until shearing wounds have healed to avoid clostridial infections or caseous lymphadenitis caused by *Corynebacterium pseudotuberculosis*. Moreover, the correct use of bacteriostats is recommended to prevent post-dipping lameness caused by *Erysipelothrix insidiosa*.

Insecticidal collars are plasticized polymer resins impregnated with an active ingredient. Collars for the control of ticks and fleas on dogs and cats release the active ingredient as a vapor, a dust, or a liquid, depending on the physicochemical properties of the chemical. Volatile liquid insecticides such as dichlorvos or naled are used in vapor-release collars. The insecticide distributes through the collar matrix as a vapor before being released. Powdered insecticides such as phosmet, stirofos, carbaryl, and propoxur are used in dust-release collars. Translocation of the active ingredient within the collar matrix leads to deposits forming at the surface; distribution of the insecticide to the animal depends on the animal's physical activity. Nonvolatile liquid insecticides such as chlorfenvinphos or diazinon are used in liquid-release collars. The active ingredient distributes as a liquid in the collar matrix and to the surface, where it is released. The animal's activity plus the dissolution of lipophilic insecticides in skin secretions are important factors in translocation of the insecticide from the collar to the animal.

Two types of insecticide-releasing **ear tags** to control flies on cattle are available. One is constructed from a polymer that provides structural support and acts as a release rate-controlling matrix. The other is a membrane-based ear tag that consists of an insecticidal reservoir with a relatively impermeable backing on one side and a rate-controlling membrane on the other. Both types rely on the animal's ear and head movements and grooming to transfer insecticide from the surface of the ear tag to the animal's skin or to other animals.

Back rubbers typically consist of burlap supported across lanes, gateways, or areas where cattle congregate. Back rubbers are charged by soaking thoroughly in oil-containing pesticide, typically a synthetic pyrethroid, an organophosphate, or a combination of the two. The oil retards evaporation of the insecticide and enhances adherence to the animal's coat.

Dust bags facilitate the self-treatment of cattle to control flies and lice. They are constructed of an inner porous bag containing the active ingredient, which is commonly a synthetic pyrethroid or an organophosphate, and an outer weather-proof skirt. Dust bags are hung in lanes or gateways so that passing cattle brush against them and receive a topical application of pesticide.

Inhaled Dosage Forms and Delivery Systems

Inhalational anesthetics are critical in management of anesthesia. Currently, enflurane, halothane, isoflurane, methoxyflurane, and nitrous oxide are the most commonly used inhaled anesthetic agents. These agents are usually delivered to animals in a carrier gas that includes oxygen, using an anesthetic machine fitted with one or more vaporizers and a patient breathing circuit.

Inhalational therapy of airway disease is used to deliver high concentrations of drugs to the lungs while avoiding or minimizing systemic adverse effects. To be delivered into the airways, a drug must be presented as an aerosol, either as solid particles or liquid droplets in air. Particle or droplet size largely determines the extent to which the drug penetrates the alveoli. Particles too small or too large for optimal delivery into alveolar sacs are either exhaled or deposited on larger bronchial airways. Compared with delivery by the oral or parenteral routes, the onset of pharmacologic action of inhaled agents is faster and the doses administered smaller, thereby reducing the potential incidence of adverse systemic effects. The delivery systems used for inhalational therapy of airway disease in animals are nebulizers and metered-dose inhalers. In the poultry industry, inhalation of aerosolized vaccines is a common way to immunize flocks of birds.

CHEMICAL RESIDUES IN FOOD AND FIBER

Veterinary drugs and pesticides are used routinely in animal production to manage diseases and control parasites, and crop protection chemicals are used in production of animal feeds. It is possible, therefore, for foodstuffs of animal origin to be adulterated with residues of veterinary drugs and pesticides, and for animal fibers to be contaminated with residues of ectoparasiticides. Veterinarians must consider the implications of both possibilities when providing for the health and welfare of animals. First, animals and animal products destined for human consumption must not contain residues of drugs or pesticides that exceed legally permitted concentrations. Second, pesticide residues in fiber have potential implications for public health, occupational health and safety, and environmental safety.

Chemical Residues in Foodstuffs of Animal Origin

Chemical residues can be found in animal tissues, milk, honey, or eggs after administration of veterinary drugs and medicated premixes, application of pesticides to animals, or consumption of stockfeeds previously treated with agricultural chemicals.

Residues Resulting from Veterinary Drugs, Medicated Feeds, or Application of Pesticides: Extensive regulatory and monitoring systems have been established to ensure that chemical residues in food do not constitute an unacceptable health risk. The premarket approval process undertaken by regulatory authorities for new veterinary drugs and medicated feeds evaluates the quality, safety, and efficacy of these products. For veterinary medicines intended for administration to food-producing animals, an additional consideration is the safety of edible tissues and products (milk, honey, eggs) derived from treated animals. Regulatory authorities establish maximum residue limits (MRLs) or tolerances and set withdrawal times that ensure residues of the active constituent will not exceed the MRL when the label instructions for the product are followed.

Residue programs consist of two principal activities: monitoring and surveillance. Residue-monitoring programs randomly sample food commodities from animals. Samples are assayed for residues of specific veterinary drugs, pesticides, and environmental contaminants, and the residues are assessed for compliance with the applicable MRL or environmental standard. The number of samples taken for monitoring purposes typically provides a 95% probability of detecting at least one violation when 1% of the animal population contains residues above the MRL. Surveillance programs, by comparison, take samples from animals suspected of having violative residues on the basis of clinical signs or herd history. Food from animals identified with violative residues of veterinary drugs or pesticides do not enter the food chain.

Residue monitoring is also a trade requirement, either mandatory or as an expectation, of importing countries allowing market access to food products derived from animals. Compliance with the national standards of importing countries becomes more difficult when the health standards, regulatory policies, and MRL-setting approaches of the exporting country and importing country differ. The situation is further exacerbated when patterns of use differ across countries or when the minor status of a disease or pest in a country does not warrant product registration, in which case MRLs are unlikely to be established.

Regulatory authorities undertake premarket approval assessments of applications in support of new veterinary drugs and medicated feeds. These assessments consider scientific data submitted by the sponsor. In the case of veterinary medicines proposed for use in food-producing animals, the data must demonstrate the safety of any residues remaining in the edible tissues or products from treated animals. These data describe the compound's toxicology, metabolism, pharmacokinetics, residue depletion, and dietary exposure. The key parameters derived in the safety and residue evaluations are defined below.

The **acceptable daily intake (ADI)** is the amount of a veterinary drug, expressed on a body weight basis, that can be ingested daily over a lifetime without an appreciable risk to human health. The ADI is established based on a review of animal studies on toxicologic, pharmacologic, or microbiologic effects as appropriate. Conservative safety factors are built into the ADI.

The **safe concentration** is the maximal allowable concentration of total residues of toxicologic concern in edible tissue. The safe concentration is calculated from the ADI and considers the weight of an average person and the amount of meat, milk, honey, or eggs consumed daily by a high-consuming individual.

An **MRL,** or **tolerance**, is the maximal concentration of residue resulting from the use of a veterinary drug (expressed in mg/kg or mcg/kg on a fresh-weight basis) that is legally permitted as acceptable in or on a food. It is based on the type and amount of residue considered to be without any toxicologic hazard for human health as expressed by the ADI. Other relevant public health risks and aspects relating to food technology, good practice in the use of veterinary drugs, and analytical methodologies are also considered when establishing the MRL.

The **marker residue** is the parent drug, its metabolites, or any combination of these, with a known relationship to the concentration of the total residue in the last tissue to deplete to the safe concentration. When the marker residue in the target tissue has depleted to the MRL, the total residue will have depleted to the safe concentration in all edible tissues.

The **target tissue** is the edible tissue with residues that deplete to a concentration below the MRL at a slower rate than that in other edible tissues. It is considered suitable for monitoring compliance with the MRL of each edible tissue from a treated animal. The target tissue is frequently liver or kidney for the purpose of domestic monitoring, and muscle or fat for monitoring meat or carcasses in international trade.

The **withdrawal time** is the period of time between the last administration of a drug and the detection of residues of that drug to levels below the MRL in food from a treated animal. Compliance with the preslaughter withdrawal time ensures the total residues deplete to below the safe concentration, and the marker residue depletes to below the MRL. Failure to observe the correct withdrawal time is the most common cause of violative residues of veterinary drugs in food.

Regulatory authorities determine withdrawal times based on residue depletion data that has been generated using healthy animals representative of those typically treated with the specific product. The drug formulation used in these trials is identical to the market formulation, which is administered at the maximal label rate. The withdrawal time is usually determined statistically, taking into account variability among animals in drug disposition.

Unlike an MRL, which applies to a veterinary drug regardless of the dosage form, route of administration, or dosage regimen, the withdrawal time stated in the product labeling applies only to that *particular formulation* when administered by the recommended route and in accordance with the dosage regimen. Altering any of these factors modifies the pharmacokinetic behavior of the drug in the animal and invalidates the stated withdrawal time. In addition, a range of physiologic and pathologic factors may modify the drug's disposition in the animal and prolong drug elimination.

In the USA, some veterinary or human drugs can be used extra-label (off-label) in food-producing animals under the Animal Medicinal Drug Use Clarification Act, provided certain conditions are met (more information can be obtained on the FDA website, www.fda.gov). Veterinarians must be mindful, however, that the extra-label use of a small number of veterinary drugs is prohibited by the FDA. Extra-label use refers to use in a species not included in the product labeling or at a dosage rate higher than that stated in the product labeling. For drugs used in this manner, data are inadequate to demonstrate the safety of food products derived from the treated animal. An understanding of pharmacokinetic principles allows extended withdrawal times to be estimated both when veterinary drugs are used in an extra-label manner and in situations that may lead to changes in the kinetic behavior of a drug in an individual animal. The pharmacokinetic principles involved as well as two relevant practical examples that demonstrate such occurrences are discussed below.

The elimination **half-life** is the time required for the concentration of a drug to be reduced by 50%. Therefore, 99.9% of an administered dose is eliminated over 10 half-lives. In food-producing animals, the residues of drugs with longer terminal elimination half-lives take longer to deplete to below the MRL. The pharmacokinetic behavior of the drug determines whether the elimination half-life in tissues will exceed the elimination half-life in plasma. In food-producing animals, the terminal elimination half-life for the slow elimination phase, or γ phase, of the residue concentration versus time profile determines the withdrawal time. Half-life is determined by both clearance (Cl) and volume of distribution (Vd) as shown by the relationship:

$$t_{1/2} = 0.693 \times \frac{Vd}{Cl}$$

Clearance is the blood volume cleared of drug per unit time and refers to the irreversible elimination of a drug from the body. The principal organs of elimination are the liver and kidneys; organ clearance is related to blood flow and the efficiency of drug removal. To determine hepatic clearance, for example:

$$Cl_H = Q_H \times E_H$$

in which Q = blood flow and E = the extraction ratio. Factors that affect hepatic clearance include hepatic function, hepatic microsomal enzyme activity, and hepatic blood flow.

Volume of distribution relates the amount of drug in the body to the concentration of drug in plasma. For a drug administered IV, the relationship is:

$$Vd = \frac{\text{amount of drug in body (dose)}}{\text{concentration } (C_{max})}$$

Vd is a characteristic property of the drug rather than the biologic system. A drug confined to the vascular compartment has a minimal value of Vd equal to plasma volume. Factors influencing Vd include the size of the drug molecule, lipid solubility, drug pKa, and tissue blood flow. Certain disease states effect changes in the Vd of a drug, particularly changes in drug binding.

If it is necessary to administer a drug to a healthy animal at twice the recommended rate, the elimination half-life of the drug is unchanged. Assuming the pharmacokinetic behavior of the drug demonstrates first-order kinetics, which is generally the case, doubling the administered dose will increase the depletion time by one half-life. Thus, the withdrawal time should be extended by one half-life to arrive at the same concentration as observed for the recommended rate. However, if a drug is administered to an unhealthy animal with impaired drug excretion in which clearance is reduced by 50%, it can be seen from the relationship for half-life shown above that reducing clearance by 50% will double the half-life. Accordingly, the withdrawal time should be doubled to arrive at the same concentration as seen in an animal with a fully functional excretory system.

The predicted result should always be verified using a rapid-screening test. The detection of residues is likely to signal that the withdrawal time should be extended and the rapid-screening test repeated.

Residues Resulting from Consumption of Stockfeeds Treated with Agricultural Chemicals: The use of agricultural chemicals can result in residues in crops and pastures that are subsequently consumed by animals. During drought conditions, the feeding of potentially contaminated crop byproducts, such as stubbles and fodder, and processed fractions, including grape marc, citrus pulp, fruit pomace, and cannery wastes, is likely to become more prevalent. In all cases, chemical residues may result in the edible tissues, milk, honey, or eggs derived from these animals.

For approved uses of crop protection chemicals that are likely to result in dietary exposure of food-producing animals, regulatory authorities establish animal commodity MRLs. The approach adopted for establishing these MRLs is fundamentally different from the one that applies to veterinary drugs. Animal transfer studies, which allow determination of the relationship between the level of chemical in the animal diet and the concentration of residue found in edible tissues, milk, honey, and eggs, are pivotal in determining MRLs. MRLs for animal tissues, milk, honey, and eggs are established at concentrations that cover the highest residues expected to be found from the estimated livestock dietary exposure. Human dietary exposure assessments are also performed to verify that food complying with MRLs is safe for consumption. In animal production systems, compliance with animal commodity MRLs relies on adherence to a stipulated period to allow residues in the crop to deplete before it is fed to animals, a stipulated period to allow residues in the animal to deplete before slaughter, or a combination of both.

Chemical Residues in Animal Fibers

From an economic standpoint, the major animal fibers are wool and mohair. Although this discussion primarily focuses on pesticide residues in wool, many of the concepts apply equally to mohair.

Flies, lice, keds, and mites adversely affect wool production and have animal welfare implications for the sheep industry. Ectoparasiticides have been the mainstay to manage infestations of these parasites in sheep flocks for many years. Two important manifestations of chemical application to sheep are the emergence of resistant strains of parasites and the contamination of wool with pesticide residues. These two factors are linked, because the application of pesticides to resistant strains of flies or lice increases the likelihood of treatment failure and the need to re-treat later in the wool-growing season. Higher residues in both the wool on treated sheep and in harvested fleeces are possible consequences. Nonetheless, late-season applications are justified in some situations on animal health and welfare or economic grounds. In view of community health and safety expectations and changing environmental standards, wool producers are seeking ways to manage external parasites on sheep that rely less on chemicals. Integrated pest management (IPM) approaches may involve various husbandry options, such as shearing and crutching to combat flystrike; genetic improvements, such as selecting against animals susceptible to fleece rot and flystrike; biologic and environmental controls, such as the use of fly traps; and the selective use of chemicals.

Pesticide residues in wool are influenced by many factors, including the chemical and formulation used, the method of application, the rate and timing of the chemical application, and the length of wool at the time of application. (*See also* ROUTES OF ADMINISTRATION AND DOSAGE FORMS, p 2508.) The product types and chemical groups commonly used in the management of flies and lice on sheep include off-shears backline or spray-on products containing insect growth regulators (IGRs), organophosphate pesticides (OPs), and synthetic pyrethroid pesticides; short-wool plunge or shower dips that use IGRs, magnesium fluorosilicate, OPs, and spinosad; long-wool backline or spray-on products containing IGRs; and long-wool jetting products containing IGRs, macrocyclic lactones, OPs, or spinosad. Wool producers must ensure that pesticides are applied in accordance with the label directions. With some chemicals, application to sheep with >6 wk wool growth results in unacceptably high residues remaining in wool to the next shearing. Repeat applications of pesticides may also result in higher wool residues at the next shearing, and backline products commonly leave higher residues at the site of application.

Although the use of sheep ectoparasiticides can result in significant chemical residues on treated wool, any risk to public health is successfully mitigated by the following steps. First, scouring removes residual pesticide from processed wool destined for the manufacture of woolen garments. Second, in the case of lanolin used in pharmaceuticals and cosmetics and as nipple emollients by nursing mothers, any residual pesticide associated with the wax component is removed during refining of the lanolin. Additional assurance regarding the quality of low-pesticide grades of lanolin is provided by compliance with the applicable regulatory standards.

With respect to occupational health and safety, residual pesticide in wool wax poses a hazard to shearers and other wool handlers during wool harvesting. For instance, nervous disorders and dermal irritation have allegedly occurred in shearers after shearing sheep treated with certain OPs and synthetic pyrethroid pesticides, respectively. In addition, long-wool backline applications of synthetic pyrethroid pesticides can result in residue concentrations at the tips of backline staples high enough to cause dermal erythema in shearers and wool handlers. In Australia, such occupational health risks are managed by prescribing a sheep rehandling period in the product labeling. The sheep rehandling period is the time that must elapse between the application of the ectoparasiticide and safely handling the treated animal. If sheep must be handled during the rehandling period, personal protective equipment should be used.

Chemical residues on treated wool may pose a risk to the environment when effluent is discharged during processing (eg, into rivers). This concern has led to the enactment of legislation to protect the environment. For some pesticides, environmental quality standards at concentrations that will not harm the most sensitive organisms in aquatic ecosystems have been established. In the EU, textile products are subject to eco-label requirements. In Australia, environmental risks posed by residues of ectoparasiticides on treated wool are mitigated by assigning a wool-harvesting interval (also referred to as a wool withholding period). The wool-harvesting interval is the time that must elapse before treated sheep may be shorn, ensuring that harvested wool meets the prescribed environmental residue limits.

The depletion of pesticide residues in wool has been mathematically modeled to predict the likely consequences of treatments at different times during the wool-growing season and to determine how late a pesticide may be applied to sheep without resulting in excessive residues at shearing. Modeling is a useful tool to determine wool-harvesting intervals and to help wool producers choose a pesticide and method of application. Test kits to quantify pesticide residues in wool are also available.

NANOTECHNOLOGY

Nanotechnology is a new enabling technology with the potential to revolutionize animal health. A nanomaterial has been defined as a material engineered to be <100 nm in one or more dimensions. A nanometer is one one-billionth of a meter; to put the nanoscale into perspective, a human hair is ~80,000 nm in diameter. Chemicals at the nanoscale display physical and chemical behaviors that can differ markedly from those of the bulk chemical (eg, in optical properties, conductivity, or electromagnetism). These behaviors are attributed to a combination of the small size, chemical composition, physicochemical properties, and surface structures of nanomaterials. Of major importance to the development of nanotechnologies for animal health will be a thoughtful, thorough, and balanced assessment of the benefits and risks involved. Risks can originate from any novel hazards of nanomaterials, the distribution profiles of nanomaterials in animals, the exposure of people to nanomaterials, and the toxicity and fate of nanomaterials in the environment. Additional challenges relate to the detection and analysis of nanomaterials.

This discussion focuses on the application of nanotechnology in the delivery of veterinary drugs and vaccines, a field predicted to expand. Many of the benefits of nanotechnology in drug delivery are the result of improved apparent solubility or stability or both; an increased concentration of drug at the site of action (increased efficacy); a decreased concentration of drug at locations in the body remote from the site of action (reduced systemic toxicity); and modified pharmacokinetics, including controlled release.

There are numerous "drivers" of nanotechnology-based drug delivery. Pharmaceutical considerations are one such driver (*see* drug nanocrystals, below); another is the need for veterinary nanomedicines that overcome problems refractory to conventional therapy. One objective of "smart" drug delivery is to target specific sites. This strategy allows the use of smaller quantities of drug than would otherwise be possible. The passive targeting of intravenously administered drug, for example, depends on the enhanced permeability and retention (EPR) effect, a phenomenon whereby nanoparticles extravasate at sites of increased vascular permeability, such as tumors, infections, and areas of inflammation, and then accumulate at these sites. Surface modification of nanoparticles is used to prolong the circulation time and enhance the EPR effect. For example, coating nanoparticles with the hydrophilic substance polyethylene glycol lessens opsonization through a steric effect, thereby reducing the subsequent uptake of nanoparticles by the reticuloendothelial system. Conversely, uncoated nanoparticles are rapidly phagocytosed, a process used to advantage to treat intracellular parasites and infections located in phagocytic cells. In a separate process known as active drug targeting, nanoparticles with targeting moieties (eg, antibodies, ligands) attached to their surfaces are able to bind to specific tissues or cell types. Similarly, magnetic nanoparticles under the influence of an alternating magnetic field transport drugs to their sites of action. Individualized and targeted drug therapy across animal species is an extension of the "smart" drug delivery concept. With this approach, miniature sensing and delivery devices, some with embedded PK/PD algorithms or using nanodelivery platforms that provide local feedback on delivery mechanisms, are envisioned. Also envisioned are nanoscale devices with the capability to detect and treat an infection, nutrient deficiency, or other health problem before symptoms are evident. In the case of antibiotics, the envisioned system would use less drug, thereby relieving concerns surrounding the potential development of antibiotic-resistant strains of bacteria and thus increasing food safety for consumers. Exciting advancements in the field of vaccine delivery are also being made (*see* vaccine delivery and vaccine adjuvants, below).

The ratio of surface area to volume of a **drug nanocrystal** is orders of magnitude greater than that of its microscale or macroscale drug counterpart. Poorly water soluble drugs with a bioavailability that is dissolution-rate limited demonstrate markedly improved bioavailability when administered in a nanoform. Another advantage is that drug nanocrystals demonstrate reduced variability in bioavailability for the fed and fasted states. Nanosized drug crystals are produced either by top-down technology, in which micronized particles are subjected to milling or grinding, or by bottom-up technology involving nanoprecipitation.

Drugs and proteins conjugated to polymers such as polyethylene glycol degrade more slowly than do drugs or proteins alone. As a consequence, conjugates remain in the circulation longer than the parent drug or protein. A prolonged circulation time allows for less frequent administration and results in increased extravasation of drug due to the EPR effect and, consequently, a higher drug concentration at the site of action.

Dendrimers are highly branched polymers consisting of an initiator core; interior layers composed of repeating units; and terminal moieties that can be functionalized to modify solubility, miscibility, and reactivity of the resulting macromolecule. From a drug-carrying perspective, dendrimers are relatively new. High loadings of drug can be incorporated into the dendrimer core or attached to the terminal moieties on the dendrimer surface.

Dendrimers are particularly attractive for ocular, pulmonary, and oral drug delivery.

Polyplexes are complexes of polymers and DNA with promising benefits for gene therapy.

Polymeric micelles comprise an internal zone known as the "core" and an external zone known as the "shell" formed by amphiphilic block copolymers such as poly(propylene oxide), poly(L-amino acids), and poly(esters). The advantages of polymeric micelles for drug delivery include solubilization of poorly soluble molecules and sustained drug release due to drug encapsulation protecting the drug from degradation and metabolism. Polymeric micelles can also enhance the delivery of drugs to desired biologic sites, thereby improving therapeutic efficacy and attentuating unwanted adverse effects.

Liposomes are self-assembled vesicles that possess a central aqueous cavity surrounded by a lipid membrane formed by a concentric bilayer(s) (also known as a lamella[e]). When liposomes come in contact with biologic cells, they tend to unravel and merge with the membrane of the cell, releasing their payload of drugs or other agents. Liposomes can be designed to achieve various functions, including the protection of the active ingredient from degradation in the GI tract, the transport of drugs to sites of action, and prolongation of the residence time of the active ingredient in vivo.

Solid lipid nanoparticles are synthesized from solid lipids. These nanoparticles demonstrate excellent physical stability and protect the incorporated drug from chemical degradation; however, low drug loading capacity is a disadvantage. Studies suggest it will be possible to develop a range of dosage forms, allowing solid lipid nanoparticles to be delivered by most routes of administration.

Polymeric nanoparticles consist of two main forms: polymeric nanocapsules and polymeric nanospheres. Polymeric nanocapsules can be prepared from natural and synthetic materials such as chitosan and poly(lactide-co-glycolide), respectively. From a drug delivery perspective, polymeric nanocapsules demonstrate a high drug loading capacity and facilitate increased drug bioavailability and controlled drug release. Other applications of polymeric nanocapsules include the detection, diagnosis, and treatment of disease, and imaging. Polymeric nanospheres differ from polymeric nanocapsules, because drug is physically and uniformly dispersed in a dense polymeric matrix with the former.

Magnetic nanoparticles have two therapeutic applications: drug delivery and therapeutic hyperthermia. The former application involves drug-coated magnetic nanoparticles that are generally >50 nm in size. After IV administration, these nanoparticles are directed to the site of drug action using a magnetic field. Subsequent retention of the nanoparticles at the site of action is also achieved using a magnetic field, and this facilitates localized drug release. By comparison, magnetic nanoparticles for therapeutic hyperthermia are smaller in size (~5 nm). Hyperthermia via hysteresis energy loss results when an external alternating magnetic field is applied to the magnetic nanoparticles. A typical outcome of therapeutic hyperthermia is tumor cell necrosis.

An example of a nanotechnology-based device for **vaccine delivery** is the Nanopatch®, used in people to deliver vaccines dermally. The Nanopatch® is a silicon wafer the size of a postage stamp with thousands of projections (>20,000/cm^3), each of which is ~100 μm long and with a tip diameter of ~1 μm. The tips of the projections are dry coated with vaccine at the nanoscale; hence, there is no requirement for refrigeration of the vaccine during storage and transport. When the device is applied to a patient's skin, the projections protrude into the wet cellular environment below the skin surface; on wetting, the vaccine is delivered in <2 min. Only one one-hundredth of the dose delivered conventionally by a needle and syringe is administered to achieve a comparable immunologic response, which is consistent with skin having more immune cells than muscle.

Nanotechnology-based vaccines may decrease unwanted inflammatory response. For example, studies have shown that the delivery of 50 nm ovalbumin adjuvant coupled to polystyrene nanobeads to sheep do not cause inflammatory reactions at the injection site. This outcome is thought to be attributed to the fact that adjuvants at the nanoscale mimic the size of viruses, which are well tolerated by cells.

Nanoclays have numerous applications, including the delivery of agrochemicals and the control of blue-green algae in waterways, and many potential applications in human and veterinary medicine. For example, nanobiohybrids are nanoclay hosts with various biologic materials such as DNA intercalated between the layers that have potential applications in gene therapy. The nanobiohybrid host system is comprised of magnesium-aluminum layered double hydroxides wherein the positive charge of the sheets of magnesium and aluminum hydroxides is balanced by the negative charge of hydrated anions. Through ion exchange, the interlayer anions can be replaced with negatively charged biomolecules such as DNA. After delivery to a biologic system, nanobiohybrids are phagocytosed, and the biologic material released from the inorganic host either by dissolution of the inorganic host in the acidic environment of lysosomes or through reverse ion-exchange within the cellular fluids.

Gold nanomaterial is biocompatible, and when formulated as gold nanoparticles it is used in the diagnosis and treatment of diseases such as cancer. For therapeutic purposes, gold nanoparticles are coated with disease-specific surface moieties and a hydrophilic substance such as polyethylene glycol to prolong circulation time. Near infrared irradiation is used to visualize and destroy gold-targeted cancer cells by optical hyperthermia.

Carbon nanotubes are being investigated as nanovector systems. These nanomaterials have a high optical absorbance at infrared frequencies and may in the future be used in a similar manner to gold nanoshells. The possible longterm toxicity of carbon nanotubes due to bioaccumulation is currently under investigation.

Quantum dots are luminescent semiconductor crystals with unique optical properties, including high-level fluorescence, long-term stability, simultaneous detection of multiple signals, and tunable emission spectra. In the future, they may be used as a multifunctional therapeutic for lymph node mapping, identification of molecular targets, photodynamic therapy, drug delivery, and surgical oncology. Quantum dots with cadmium selenium/zinc sulfide cores with sizes ranging from 13–24 nm emit different narrow wavelengths of detectable light. This capability would allow detection of heterogenous tumors by coating quantum dots of different core sizes, and therefore emitting different wavelengths of light, with different cancer-specific antibodies to help understand optimal tumor therapy. The in vitro toxicity associated with the core of quantum dots (eg, cadmium selenium) can generally be overcome by coating the core with other metals such as zinc sulfide or adding a protective hydrophilic coating (eg, polyethylene glycol). Further research is necessary to evaluate the longterm stability of quantum dots in vivo, which is a major barrier to clinical translation.

Increased bioavailability as well as improvements in targeted and controlled delivery of existing drugs and their application through nanotechnology should improve ease of administration and safety and efficacy profiles for both animals and people.

SYSTEMIC PHARMACOTHERAPEUTICS OF THE CARDIOVASCULAR SYSTEM

See also PRINCIPLES OF THERAPY OF CARDIOVASCULAR DISEASE, p 74, MANAGEMENT OF HEART FAILURE, p 103, and FLUID THERAPY, p 1675.

See table 1 for a listing of commonly used cardiovascular drugs and dosages. *See also* p 2625.

DIURETICS

Diuretics are the cornerstone of therapy in management of animals with congestive heart failure (CHF) characterized by cardiogenic pulmonary edema, pleural effusion, ascites, or a combination of these signs. Three classes of diuretics are used to treat CHF in dogs and cats: loop diuretics, thiazide diuretics, and potassium-sparing diuretics. They differ in their relative potency and mechanisms of action. The loop diuretics are the most potent and have a high ceiling, enabling them to be used in a dose-dependent way to treat mild to life-threatening CHF. Additionally, they can be administered orally or parenterally. Thiazide diuretics are mild to moderate in potency. They are typically used in conjunction with a loop diuretic (eg, furosemide) in animals with severe refractory CHF. Historically, the use of potassium-sparing diuretics (eg, spironolactone) has been reserved for those animals that have right heart failure or have become hypokalemic secondary to the use of other diuretics, or for those animals refractory to other agents.

TABLE 1 COMMONLY USED CARDIOVASCULAR DRUGS AND DOSAGES

Drug	Dosage
Amiodarone	Dog: 8–10 mg/kg, PO, every 12–24 hr for 7–10 days, then reduce to 4–6 mg/kg/day for longterm treatment
Amlodipine	Dog: 0.1–0.2 mg/kg, PO, bid; or 0.2–0.4 mg/kg/day, PO Cat: 0.625–1.25 mg/cat, PO, once to twice daily
Aspirin (antiplatelet dosage)	Dog: 5–10 mg/kg, PO, every 1–2 days Cat: 1–2 mg/kg/day, PO; or ¼ of an 81-mg tablet/cat, PO, every 3 days (or twice per week)
Atenolol	Dog: 0.2–1 mg/kg, PO, bid Cat: 1–2.5 mg/kg, PO, bid; or 6.25–12.5 mg/cat, bid
Benazepril	Dog: 0.25–0.5 mg/kg, PO, once to twice daily Cat: 0.25–0.5 mg/kg, PO, bid; or 0.5 mg/kg/day, PO
Clopidogrel	Dog: loading dose for rapid onset of action (90 min) 10 mg/kg, PO (once); 1–2 mg/kg/day, PO, longterm Cat: ¼ of a 75-mg tablet (18.75 mg)/day/cat, PO
Diltiazem	Dog: 0.5–2 mg/kg, PO, tid (standard formulation); 1–4 mg/kg, PO, bid (sustained release) Cat: 7.5 mg/cat, PO, tid (standard formulation); 3–6 mg/cat, PO, once to twice daily (sustained release)
Dobutamine	Dog: 2.5–15 mcg/kg/min, CRI[a]
Enalapril	Dog: 0.25–0.5 mg/kg, PO, bid Cat: 0.25–0.5 mg/kg, PO, bid; or 0.5 mg/kg/day, PO
Furosemide	Dog: 2–4 mg/kg, IV, IM, SC, every 1–6 hr; 0.25–1 mg/kg/hr, CRI; or 1–5 mg/kg, PO, bid-tid Cat: 0.5–2 mg/kg, IV, IM, SC, every 1–8 hr; 0.25–0.6 mg/kg/hr, CRI; or 1–2 mg/kg, PO, once to twice daily
Heparin	Dog: 100–200 U/kg, SC, tid-qid (unfractionated) Dog and cat: 100–200 IU/kg, SC, once to twice daily (low molecular weight)
Hydralazine	Dog: 0.5–3 mg/kg, PO, bid
Lidocaine	Dog: 2–4 mg/kg, IV; 25–75 mcg/kg/min, CRI
Mexiletine	Dog: 4–6 mg/kg, PO, tid
Nitroglycerin ointment 2% (1 in. = 15 mg)	Dog: 4–12 mg, topically, bid (maximum 15 mg/dog/dose) Cat: 2–4 mg/cat, topically, tid-qid for 1–2 days
Pimobendan	Dog, cat: 0.25–0.3 mg/kg, PO, bid
Procainamide	Dog: 4–6 mg/kg, PO, every 2–4 hr (regular formulation); 10–20 mg/kg, PO, tid (sustained release); 2–25 mg/kg, slow IV bolus to effect, or CRI at 25–40 mcg/kg/min
Quinidine sulfate	Dog: 5–10 mg/kg, IV, qid; or 6–20 mg/kg, PO, tid-qid
Quinidine gluconate	Dog: 6–20 mg/kg, IM, qid; or 6–20 mg/kg, PO, tid-qid

TABLE 1 COMMONLY USED CARDIOVASCULAR DRUGS AND DOSAGES *(continued)*

Drug	Dosage
Sildenafil	Dog: 1–3 mg/kg, PO, bid-tid
Sotalol	Dog, cat: 1–2.5 mg/kg, PO, bid
Spironolactone	Dog: 1–2 mg/kg, PO, bid; or 2 mg/kg/day, PO
	Cat: 1–2 mg/kg, PO, once to twice daily
Torsemide	Dog: 0.25–0.4 mg/kg, PO, once to twice daily

[a] CRI = constant-rate infusion

All diuretics share a similar adverse effect profile, including electrolyte and acid-base disturbances, dehydration, and prerenal and renal azotemia. The relative risk of azotemia is increased when a diuretic is used concurrently with an angiotensin-converting enzyme (ACE) inhibitor and/or an NSAID or other potential renal toxin. Diuretics may also increase the risk of digoxin toxicity. In addition, diuretic resistance can develop with longterm treatment. The most common electrolyte and acid-base abnormalities include hypokalemia, hyponatremia, hypomagnesemia, and metabolic alkalosis. These effects are potentiated by the use of more than one diuretic (sequential nephron blockade), concurrent hyporexia/anorexia, and the use of higher doses. Typically, potential adverse effects are more severe in cats than in dogs.

Numerous factors determine the response to diuretic therapy. These include the potency of the drug, the dosage administered, the duration of action of the drug, the route of administration, renal blood flow, glomerular filtration rate, and nephron function. The plasma concentration depends on the route of administration (IV administration will produce a higher concentration than PO administration) and the dose. The duration of effect will also determine the total diuretic effect produced in a certain time period.

Animals with CHF may become refractory to furosemide because of decreased delivery of the drug to the nephron as a result of reduced renal blood flow or hormonal stimulus for sodium and water retention. Therefore, strategies to increase renal blood flow and/or plasma concentration may ameliorate diuretic resistance.

Furosemide

Furosemide is a loop diuretic and the most commonly used diuretic to treat CHF in dogs and cats. Torsemide is another loop diuretic that is ~10 times as potent and has a longer duration of action than furosemide with a similar adverse effect profile. However, current clinical experience with torsemide is far less than that of furosemide; thus, furosemide remains the diuretic of choice in dogs and cats with CHF.

Preparations and Disposition: Furosemide is available in oral (tablets, suspensions) and parenteral formulations. Compounded liquids (from tablets) may be better tolerated in cats than the commercially available, alcohol-based, 1% syrup.

All loop diuretics inhibit sodium, potassium, and chloride reabsorption in the thick portion of the ascending loop of Henle, leading to inhibition of sodium and commensurate water reabsorption in the nephron. Furosemide diuresis results in enhanced excretion of sodium, chloride, potassium, hydrogen, calcium, magnesium, and possibly phosphate. Chloride excretion is equal to or exceeds sodium excretion. Enhanced hydrogen ion excretion without a concomitant increase in bicarbonate excretion can result in metabolic alkalosis. Despite the increase in net acid excretion, urinary pH falls slightly after furosemide administration, while urine specific gravity is generally reduced to approximately 1.006–1.020.

In addition to its diuretic effects, furosemide acts as a mild systemic venodilator, decreasing systemic venous pressure before diuresis occurs, especially after IV administration. Furosemide decreases renal vascular resistance. Thus, it acutely increases renal blood flow (~50%) without changing glomerular filtration rate.

Furosemide is highly protein bound (86%–91%). The ratio of kidney to plasma concentration is 5:1. A small amount of furosemide (1%–14%) is metabolized to a glucuronide derivative in dogs, but this metabolism does not occur in the liver. In dogs, ~45% of furosemide is excreted in the bile and 55% in the urine. After IV administration, furosemide has an elimination half-life of ~1 hr, and its onset of action is within 5 min; peak effects occur within 30 min, and duration of effect is 2–3 hr. Approximately 50% of the drug is cleared from the body within the first 30 min, 90% within the first 2 hr, and almost all is eliminated within 3 hr.

Furosemide is rapidly but incompletely absorbed after PO administration with a bioavailability of 40%–50%. The terminal half-life after administration PO is biexponential. The initial phase has a half-life of ~30 min, with the second phase half-life of ~7 hr. The initial disposition phase has the most effect on plasma concentration, with concentration decreasing from therapeutic to subtherapeutic within 4–6 hr of PO administration. After PO administration, onset of action occurs within 60 min, peak effects occur within 1–2 hr, and duration of effect is ~6 hr. In healthy dogs, a dose of furosemide given at 2.5 mg/kg, IM, results in maximal natriuresis (beyond that dose there is no further increase in sodium excretion). This occurs at a plasma concentration of ~0.8 mcg/mL. Because the diuretic effect of furosemide depends on its hematogenous delivery to the kidneys, animals with decreased renal blood flow (eg, those with heart failure) need a higher plasma concentration (higher dose) to produce the same effect observed in healthy dogs. This is achieved by administering higher oral doses or by administering the drug IV.

Cats are more sensitive to furosemide than dogs. Clinically, cats commonly require no more than 1–2 mg/kg, PO, once to twice daily for longterm treatment of pulmonary edema. However, higher dosages may be needed in cats with severe heart failure because of reduced renal blood flow.

Drug Interactions and Toxicity: Drug interactions and adverse effects/toxicities are typically those described for diuretics as a class. However, some special considerations for furosemide bear mentioning. Furosemide has the potential for ototoxicity. When administered as the sole agent, furosemide in dosages >20 mg/kg, IV, can result in loss of hearing in dogs. Dosages of 50–100 mg/kg result in profound loss of hearing. Furosemide can also potentiate the ototoxic and nephrotoxic effects of other drugs such as the aminoglycosides.

Clinical Use: For treatment of life-threatening cardiogenic pulmonary edema in dogs, parenteral dosages of 2–4 mg/kg, every 1–6 hr, IV, IM, or SC in dogs and 0.5–2 mg/kg, every 1–8 hr, IV, IM, or SC in cats are typically used. Dosing intervals depend on the response to therapy; initially, boluses can be given every 1–2 hr and decreased to every 4–8 hr in dogs, and given every 2 hr and decreased to every 6–8 hr in cats. Alternatively, a constant-rate infusion (CRI) of 0.25–1 mg/kg/hr in dogs or 0.25–0.6 mg/kg/hr in cats could be used. Bolus administration and CRI for treatment of life-threatening pulmonary edema is tapered over 12–24 hr as clinical signs resolve. Typical starting dosages for longterm management of CHF in dogs are 2 mg/kg, PO, bid, with a range of 1–5 mg/kg, PO, bid-tid, and in cats are 1 mg/kg/day, PO, with a range of 1–2 mg/kg, PO, once to twice daily to a maximum total daily dose of 4–6 mg/kg.

Furosemide should be stored at 15°–30°C and protected from light. Parenteral formulations having a yellow color have degraded and should not be used. Furosemide tablets that have been exposed to light may be discolored and should not be used. Furosemide injection can be mixed with 0.9% saline or Ringer's solution. A precipitate may form if the injection is mixed with strongly acidic solutions such as those containing ascorbic acid, tetracycline, adrenaline (epinephrine), or noradrenaline (norepinephrine). Furosemide injection should not be mixed with lidocaine, alkaloids, antihistamines, or morphine.

Thiazide Diuretics

The thiazides act primarily by reducing membrane permeability to sodium and chloride in the distal convoluted tubule. They promote potassium loss at this site and produce large increases in urine sodium concentration but only mild to moderate increases in urine volume. The thiazides are ineffective when renal blood flow is low, which may explain their lack of efficacy as a sole agent in animals with severe heart failure.

Preparations and Disposition: Hydrochlorothiazide is available in tablet form. In dogs, thiazides are well absorbed after oral administration. Hydrochlorothiazide has an onset of action within 2 hr, peaks at 4 hr, and lasts 12 hr.

Drug Interactions and Toxicity: Drug interactions include a decrease in efficacy of anticoagulants and insulin and an increase in efficacy of digoxin, loop diuretics, vitamin D, and some anesthetics. Thiazide diuretics are also reported to prolong the half-life of quinidine.

The most common adverse effects of thiazide diuretics are electrolyte disturbances. Thiazide diuretics are potassium wasting, and when combined with loop diuretics, the likelihood of adverse effects such as azotemia and hypokalemia are increased. They may also increase calcium reabsorption and thus lead to hypercalcemia. Adverse effects, including renal failure, can be minimized when hydrochlorothiazide is added to chronic CHF treatment protocols that include high-dose furosemide by reducing the total daily dose of furosemide by approximately 25%–50% and starting at the lower end of the monotherapy dosage range for hydrochlorothiazide (2 mg/kg, PO, bid).

Clinical Use: Compared with that of furosemide, the relative potency of thiazide diuretics is low in dogs and cats when used as monotherapy; thus, they are rarely used as first-line diuretics in these species. Thiazides are primarily used in dogs that have developed furosemide resistance and are commonly referred to as rescue diuretics in dogs. The typical monotherapy dosage for hydrochlorothiazide in dogs is 2–4 mg/kg, PO, bid. When hydrochlorothiazide is added to furosemide, the initial dosage should be 2 mg/kg, PO, bid. The typical monotherapy dosage for hydrochlorothiazide in cats is 0.5–2 mg/kg, PO, once to twice daily.

Potassium-sparing Diuretics

This class of diuretics acts by inhibiting the action of aldosterone on distal tubular cells or by blocking sodium reabsorption in the latter regions of the distal tubule and collecting tubules, exerting a mild diuretic effect compared with that of furosemide. Spironolactone is structurally similar to aldosterone and binds competitively to aldosterone-binding sites in the distal tubule. Because of its aldosterone antagonism, spironolactone is also considered an inhibitor of the renin-angiotensin aldosterone system (RAAS) and thus a neuroendocrine modulator. Spironolactone is the most commonly used potassium-sparing diuretic in veterinary medicine.

Preparations and Disposition: Spironolactone is available as a tablet for oral administration. It is highly protein-bound, metabolized by the liver, and excreted by the kidneys. Peak diuresis occurs as late as 2–3 days after administration.

Drug Interactions and Toxicity: Potential toxicities include hyperkalemia, which may be exacerbated by concurrent therapy with an ACE inhibitor, especially if furosemide is not also administered. Facial excoriation has been reported in cats, but initial reports may overestimate the frequency.

Clinical Use: In dogs with CHF, particularly those with ascites secondary to right heart failure, an increased plasma aldosterone concentration may be present, and the effect of these diuretics may be enhanced. However, potassium-sparing diuretics are weak diuretics when used alone and thus should never be used as sole agents in animals with heart failure. When potassium-sparing diuretics are administered with other diuretics such as furosemide, potassium loss is decreased, which may be beneficial. Recent studies suggest that adding spironolactone to chronic CHF treatment in dogs may improve survival. The increasing use of spironolactone in veterinary medicine is related to these potential cardioprotective/antifibrotic effects and not its diuretic effect per se. The dosage of spironolactone for diuretic use is 2–4 mg/kg/day. Lower dosages (0.5–1 mg/kg, bid) may be considered for inhibition of the RAAS. Typical dosages for adjunctive treatment of CHF in dogs are 1–2 mg/kg, PO, bid, or 2 mg/kg/day, PO; similar dosages are used for a cardioprotective indication in dogs. Typical dosages for adjunctive treatment of CHF in cats are 1–2 mg/kg, PO, once to twice daily.

POSITIVE INOTROPES

Positive inotropes increase the strength of cardiac muscle contraction by increasing the quantity of intracellular calcium available for binding by muscle proteins, by increasing the sensitivity of contractile proteins to calcium, or a combination of both (eg, pimobendan). This, in turn, augments contractile protein interaction in the myocardial cell. Intracellular calcium can be increased by altering the Na^+/Ca^{2+} exchange pump, by increasing production of cyclic adenosine monophosphate (cAMP) via stimulation of adenylate cyclase, or by decreasing degradation of cAMP via inhibition of phosphodiesterases.

Cardiac Glycosides

The probable mechanism of action for the modest inotropic effect of digoxin is inhibition of the membrane-bound Na^+/K^+-ATPase pump; when this occurs, Na^+ increases in the cell, the exchange of Na^+ for Ca^{2+} via the Na^+/Ca^{2+} exchange pump is augmented, and there is a small increase in calcium influx. The increased intracellular calcium in turn leads to increased release of Ca^{2+} from the sarcoplasmic reticulum and increased contractility of the cardiac muscle. However, because these changes are modest, digoxin does not result in significant inotropy, and the availability of more potent oral positive inotropes has superseded its use for this indication.

Digoxin also has a combination of both proarrhythmic and antiarrhythmic properties. The alterations in the ratio of intracellular and extracellular electrolytes caused by digoxin can result in increased automaticity and cardiac arrhythmias. Negative chronotropic effects are due to decreased conduction velocity in the atrioventricular (AV) node via increased parasympathetic tone, as well as direct effects that help slow AV nodal conduction and prolong the AV nodal cell refractory period. Digoxin also has parasympathomimetic effects on the sinoatrial node and atria. In addition, it potentiates vagal (cholinergic) activity in the heart. The changes in conduction can lead to AV nodal blockade and reductions in heart rate (ventricular response rate) when digoxin is used to treat supraventricular arrhythmias, including atrial fibrillation. However, digoxin is rarely efficacious as a single agent for this indication. Digoxin has a narrow therapeutic window, and at toxic levels it can directly slow sinus nodal activity due to increased sensitivity to acetylcholine. Because the atria are sensitive to acetylcholine, atrial conduction is also enhanced in the diseased heart, which can then lead to atrial arrhythmias. Digoxin is believed to improve vascular baroreceptor responsiveness, thereby minimizing sympathetic activation in heart failure states. This is accomplished via decreasing plasma catecholamine concentrations, which affect both sympathetic nerve activity and plasma renin activity, thereby minimizing sympathetic activation. In this way, digoxin may be considered to be a neuromodulator. Lastly, digoxin also has been reported to have a mild diuretic effect via the Na^+/K^+ ATPase pumps present in the renal tubular epithelial cells.

Preparations and Disposition: The oral form of digoxin is the most widely used preparation. Other preparations are available but not used routinely in veterinary medicine.

Absorption of oral digoxin is variable; ~60% of the tablet formulation is absorbed. With little hepatic metabolism, almost all the absorbed drug reaches the vasculature. Absorption is slowed by food. Digoxin is distributed slowly and concentrated in cardiac tissues, and ~25% is bound to plasma proteins. It is primarily eliminated unchanged via the kidneys (15% is metabolized and excreted via the liver); its half-life (~23–39 hr in dogs, and extremely variable in cats) is strongly influenced by renal function. Steady state is reached after ~5 half-lives, and maintenance doses should theoretically achieve a therapeutic serum concentration within 2–4 days.

Drug Interactions and Toxicity: A number of medications can increase plasma digoxin concentrations, including aspirin, quinidine, chloramphenicol, aminoglycosides (eg, neomycin), amiodarone, anticholinergics, diltiazem, esmolol, flecainide, tetracycline, and spironolactone. Furosemide, hydrochlorothiazide, amphotericin B, and glucocorticoids deplete body potassium and thus potentiate digitalis intoxication and proarrhythmic effects. Administration of β-adrenergic agonists (eg, dobutamine) also increases the risk of proarrhythmia. Longterm administration of phenobarbital may decrease digoxin concentrations by increasing clearance. Calcium channel blockers and β-blockers will potentiate action on the AV node conduction, increasing risk of AV block.

Toxic effects with digitalis glycosides are common and can be lethal. Cats are more sensitive to digoxin than dogs. Probably the most frequent cause of toxicity is inadvertent overdosing. The potential for toxicity is increased with hypokalemia and azotemia. The likelihood and severity of toxicity are related to the severity of cardiac disease. Other factors that would require dosage adjustment to prevent toxicity include renal failure (azotemia), hypothyroidism, decreased muscle mass (a significant amount of digoxin is bound to skeletal muscle), ascites, hypercalcemia, and myocardial failure leading to reduced renal blood flow. Signs of toxicity relate to the GI system (most common adverse effects) or CNS, or manifest as arrhythmias, with digitalis capable of inducing any type of cardiac arrhythmia. GI signs of toxicity include diarrhea, anorexia, and nausea and vomiting due to direct stimulation of the chemoreceptor trigger zone. Frequently, these are the earliest indications of toxicity. Neurologic effects include malaise and drowsiness. Digoxin toxicity can be diagnosed (and avoided) by monitoring plasma drug concentrations. Treatment of intoxication includes discontinuing therapy with digitalis and potassium-depleting diuretics and administering phenytoin (blocks AV nodal effects of digitalis), lidocaine (for ventricular arrhythmias), and if indicated, potassium (preferably PO). Atropine may be useful to treat both clinically significant sinus bradycardia and second- or third-degree heart block induced by cholinergic augmentation. Arrhythmias, clinical signs, and electrolyte abnormalities should be treated as clinically indicated on a case-by-case basis.

Clinical Use: In general, the availability of other medications with similar activities and more favorable risk-benefit ratios with respect to toxicity have dramatically reduced the clinical use of digoxin in dogs. Digoxin is rarely if ever used in cats for any indication. Current typical clinical indications in dogs are for adjunctive (in combination with another antiarrhythmic) treatment of supraventricular arrhythmias such as atrial fibrillation or flutter, as part of management of chronic, advanced, or refractory CHF, or to treat vasovagal syncope.

Maintenance dosages are 0.003–0.011 mg/kg, PO, bid, for dogs, and 0.005–0.01 mg/kg, PO, every 24–48 hr for cats. In general, initial dosages should be at the lower end of the range and rounded down, and then titrated up, if needed, based on measurement of serum digoxin levels (target serum concentrations 0.8–1.2 ng/mL 8–12 hr after administration). Toxicity can occur even in animals that have levels in the therapeutic range. Levels should be monitored 3–5 days after initial treatment (8–12 hours after administration) and every 6 mo thereafter or sooner if signs of toxicity develop. Digoxin dosages should be calculated based on lean body weight and reduced in obese or cachectic animals and in the presence of ascites. Known electrolyte disorders should be corrected before digitalis glycosides are administered.

Phosphodiesterase Inhibitors

Phosphodiesterase (PDE) inhibitors, also known as inodilators, block the breakdown of cAMP and therefore increase intracellular cAMP concentrations. The result is an increase in myocardial contractility and peripheral vasodilation. Methylxanthine derivatives have been classified as PDE inhibitors, but this is controversial. Of the methylxanthines, theophylline is the most cardiopotent. In addition to their cardiac effects, methylxanthines have significant CNS, renal, and smooth muscle effects, including on bronchial smooth muscle. The use of methylxanthines in cardiac disease is limited to conditions that would benefit from bronchodilation.

Pimobendan is a benzimidazole pyridazinone derivative and is a positive inotrope and balanced systemic arterial and venous dilator. In failing hearts, it exerts positive inotropic effects primarily through sensitization of the cardiac contractile apparatus to intracellular calcium. As a PDE 3 inhibitor, pimobendan can potentially increase intracellular calcium concentration and myocardial oxygen consumption. However, the cardiac PDE effects of pimobendan are reportedly minimal at pharmacologic doses in dogs with heart disease, which is a major advantage relative to other inotropic PDE inhibitors such as milrinone. PDE 3 inhibitors such as pimobendan result in balanced vasodilation (combination of venous and arterial dilation) leading to a reduction of both cardiac preload and afterload. In addition, pimobendan may have some direct endothelial-derived vasodilatory effects. The significance of alterations in proinflammatory cytokine concentrations such as tumor necrosis factor-β and interleukins 1β and 6 on the progression of heart failure has been documented in many forms of heart disease. Maladaptive alterations in these cytokine concentrations are associated with increased morbidity and mortality, and pimobendan has demonstrated beneficial modulation of several such cytokines in various models of heart failure. Pimobendan reportedly may have some platelet inhibitory effect in dogs and cats, but the clinical significance of this is not yet clear. Lastly, PDE 3 inhibition in cardiomyocytes leads to more rapid relaxation; thus, pimobendan can also be considered to be a positive lusiotrope.

In dogs, pimobendan is extensively metabolized, and both the parent drug and active metabolite are >90% bound to plasma protein. The steady state volume of distribution of pimobendan is 2.6 L/kg, and the terminal elimination half-lives of pimobendan and its active metabolite are 0.5 and 2 hr, respectively. Oral bioavailability is reduced by food until steady state is reached in a few days. Consequently, pimobendan should be administered on an empty stomach at least 1 hr before feeding for maximal effects when starting therapy. Hemodynamic effects after PO administration on an empty stomach peak in 1 hr and last 8–12 hr; therefore, pimobendan can provide rapid short-term support to dogs with acute or decompensated heart failure. IV preparations are available in some countries.

Pimobendan is approved for treatment of CHF due to dilated cardiomyopathy (DCM) and chronic degenerative mitral valvular disease (DMVD) in dogs. It has also been shown to prolong symptom-free survival in Doberman Pinschers with occult DCM. Pimobendan has an excellent safety profile, and clinical data suggest that it is safe when administered concomitantly with other medications commonly used in treatment of canine CHF. Reported adverse effects are minimal, but the main one is GI intolerance of the chewable tablet formulation. Pimobendan is contraindicated in dogs with known outflow tract obstruction (eg, subaortic stenosis). Pimobendan is not approved for use in cats. A number of retrospective studies in cats, using dosages similar to those used in dogs, suggest it is well tolerated, but there is no definitive proof of efficacy.

The mechanism of action of the bipyridine derivatives **amrinone** and **milrinone** is probably inhibition of PDE and increased levels of intracellular cAMP. Both amrinone and milrinone are available for IV administration and are suitable only for short-term management of CHF. However, with the wide availability and known efficacy of pimobendan, these medications have fallen out of favor for treatment of CHF.

β-Adrenergic Agonists

These drugs cause a positive inotropic effect by activating β-receptors with subsequent stimulation of adenylate cyclase and increased cAMP.

Dopamine is an endogenous catecholamine precursor with selective β_1 activity. However, it also stimulates release of norepinephrine. At low doses, it stimulates renal dopaminergic receptors, which causes increased renal blood flow and diuresis. It is rapidly metabolized by the body and has a half-life of <2 min. Dopamine is available as a solution, which is further diluted with saline or dextrose. It is administered IV, usually by CRI (1–15 mcg/kg/min). Cardiac arrhythmias may develop due to β-adrenergic activity. *Indications include* cardiogenic or endotoxic shock and oliguria. In cardiogenic shock, infusion of equal concentrations of dopamine and dobutamine may afford more advantages than either drug alone. Both medications should be titrated up slowly while monitoring for arrhythmias, blood pressure, and clinical response to treatment. Dopamine is contraindicated in the face of ventricular arrhythmias and when a pheochromocytoma is suspected. Care should be used in the setting of aortic stenosis. If the animal has recently taken a monoamine oxidase inhibitor, the rate of dopamine metabolism by the tissue will fall and the dosage should be reduced to one-tenth of usual.

Dobutamine is a synthetic drug similar to dopamine, but it does not cause release of norepinephrine and therefore has minimal effects other than β_1 activity. Dobutamine is a more effective positive inotrope than dopamine with less chronotropic effects, although it does not dilate the renal vascular bed. Its plasma half-life is ~2 min. Dobutamine is prepared as a solution to be diluted with 5% dextrose or normal saline. When compared with dopamine, dobutamine is the preferred β-adrenergic agonist for short-term therapy of refractory CHF when pimobendan alone is not successful or insufficient. Dobutamine causes an immediate increase in blood pressure due to increased cardiac output. It is given as a CRI at 2–15 mcg/kg/min; heart rate, blood pressure, and cardiac output should be monitored. In cats, dobutamine has a longer half-life and causes CNS stimulation, so lower infusion rates (0.5–10 mcg/kg/min) should be used. It is rarely indicated in cats.

Compared with other inotropic drugs, **epinephrine** , with its β_1 and β_2 effects, causes the greatest increase in the rate of energy usage and myocardial oxygen demand. This increase in oxygen need may be detrimental to the failing heart. Epinephrine also causes vasoconstriction and bronchodilation. Epinephrine is rapidly metabolized in the GI tract and is not effective after administration PO. Absorption is more rapid after IM versus SC administration. Epinephrine is available in several preparations and is effective after IV, pulmonary, and nasal administration. However, because of the decreased efficiency of cardiac work, epinephrine is not used as a positive inotropic agent but rather for emergency therapy of cardiac arrest and anaphylactic shock. Ventricular arrhythmias should be expected and are a contraindication to using epinephrine except in life-threatening situations.

Isoproterenol is a nonspecific β-agonist that, like epinephrine, increases myocardial oxygen demand. Tachycardia and the potential for other arrhythmias excludes its use in a cardiac patient except for short-term therapy of bradyarrhythmias (eg, AV block). It is typically used as a CRI to effect based on the heart rate desired.

ANGIOTENSIN-CONVERTING ENZYME INHIBITORS

Angiotensin-converting enzyme (ACE) inhibitors are widely used to treat chronic CHF in dogs and cats. In the pathogenesis of CHF, the proteolytic enzyme renin is released by the kidneys and acts on angiotensinogen, which is produced by the liver and distributed in the blood, to produce angiotensin I. The formation of angiotensin II from angiotensin I occurs through the action of ACE. Angiotensin II causes retention of Na^+ and water, in part through stimulation of the synthesis and release of aldosterone by the adrenal cortex. Angiotensin II also causes vasoconstriction, thus increasing systemic vascular resistance. ACE also results in degradation of bradykinin and, thus, ACE inhibitors lead to increased levels of bradykinin that contribute to their vasodilatory effects. By inhibiting the formation of angiotensin II, ACE inhibitors prevent vasoconstriction and reduce retention of Na^+ and water in animals with CHF. ACE inhibitors are balanced vasodilators, reducing both preload and afterload. The effects during CHF include decreased vascular resistance and cardiac filling pressures and increased cardiac output and exercise tolerance. However, ACE inhibitors have only a mild effect on afterload reduction and should not be used as monotherapy in animals with severe systemic hypertension (>160 mmHg).

Preparations and Disposition: Enalapril and benazepril are widely used ACE inhibitors and are available in a variety of tablet sizes for oral administration. Compared with enalapril and benazepril, captopril has a greater propensity for GI adverse effects and a shorter half-life in dogs, necessitating more frequent dosing; thus, its use has fallen out of favor. A wide variety of other ACE inhibitors (eg, lisonopril, ramipril) are sometimes used in veterinary medicine. Choice in part is often related to drug availability, cost, and availability of canine and feline pharmacokinetic and pharmacodynamic data.

After absorption from the GI tract, enalapril is converted in the liver to the active metabolite enalaprilat. Oral bioavailability is ~60%. Serum concentration of enalaprilat peaks in 3–4 hr. The half-life is ~11 hr, and effects last 12–14 hr, indicating the need for dosing intervals of every 12 hr if 24-hr suppression of ACE is desired. Excretion of enalapril and enalaprilat is primarily renal; therefore, the half-life of enalapril/enalaprilat is increased in animals with severe CHF (reduced renal perfusion) or renal failure, and dose reduction may be warranted.

Like enalapril, benazepril is a prodrug converted to its main active metabolite benazeprilat in the liver. Benazepril is well absorbed in dogs, and oral bioavailability increases by ~35% with repeated dosing. After administration of oral benazepril, benazeprilat concentration peaks in plasma within 1–3 hr and is rapidly distributed. Benazeprilat is excreted approximately equally in the bile and urine in dogs. The terminal half-life is ~3.5 hr. This combined excretion may allow better dosing control in animals with preexisting renal insufficiency; however, benazepril is no more renal protective than any other ACE inhibitor at equipotent doses. When benazepril is administered longterm, dosages from 0.25–1 mg/kg produce indistinguishable effects at the time of peak effect (2 hr after PO administration) and at trough effect (24 hr after PO administration); thus, dosing intervals may be as long as 24 hr, but benazepril is often dosed every 12 hr to ensure continuous ACE throughout the day.

Drug Interactions and Toxicity: Hypotension may develop with concurrent use of ACE inhibitors and other vasodilators (eg, amlodipine) or diuretics. Concurrent use of potassium-sparing diuretics (eg, spironolactone) may cause hyperkalemia. Enalapril and benazepril appear safe when used concomitantly with furosemide, pimobendan, digoxin, antiarrhythmics, β-blockers, bronchodilators, and cough suppressants. However, it has been suggested that concurrent use of NSAIDs may increase risk of adverse effects.

ACE inhibitors have a good safety profile and have been used safely in combination with other cardiovascular drugs (including diuretics and pimobendan). However, azotemia may develop, and monitoring of BUN and creatinine (with possible dosage adjustments) is warranted. This possible complication is the result of the partial loss of renal autoregulation of blood flow mediated by angiotensin II. Other possible, albeit rare, adverse effects include GI disturbances (anorexia, vomiting, diarrhea), syncope due to hypotension, weakness, and ataxia. Preexisting renal disease and dehydration increase the risk of adverse effects; thus, animals with these predisposing conditions should be monitored closely. Cough is a common adverse effect of this class of drugs in people but is not a recognized problem in dogs or cats.

Clinical Use: ACE inhibitors are indicated in treatment of CHF in dogs and cats stemming from a wide variety of diseases. However, there is no proof that ACE inhibitors may delay the onset of CHF in asymptomatic animals with cardiac disease. ACE inhibitors are also frequently used (typically in combination with other arterial dilators) to manage systemic hypertension in dogs and cats. Somewhat paradoxically, ACE inhibitors such as benazepril have been shown to be beneficial in treatment of some forms of renal disease. Enalapril is approved in the USA to treat CHF secondary to DCM and MMVD in dogs. Benazepril is approved in several countries other than the USA to treat CHF in dogs.

The recommended dosage of enalapril and benazepril for treatment of CHF in dogs is 0.25–0.5 mg/kg, PO, once to twice daily. However, based on the half-life, if continuous ACE inhibition is desired and well tolerated, then a 12-hr dosing interval is recommended. The recommended dosage for adjunctive treatment of CHF in cats is 0.25–0.5 mg/kg, PO, bid, or 0.5 mg/kg/day, PO. Similar doses are used when enalapril or benazepril is used to treat systemic hypertension. However, enalapril and benazepril have only modest arterial vasodilatory effects and should not be used as monotherapy in animals with severe systemic hypertension (systolic blood pressure >160–180 mmHg). In general, regardless of clinical indication, starting at the lower dose range and increasing to maximal dose with monitoring of renal function, serum potassium, and systemic blood pressure is recommended. Higher doses of benazepril, if tolerated, may be indicated to treat some forms of renal disease (eg, protein-losing glomerulopathy).

VASOACTIVE DRUGS

Vasodilator drugs can be categorized as afterload reducers or preload reducers. Afterload is reduced by dilation of arterioles (ie, resistance vessels), whereas preload is reduced by dilation of veins (ie, capacitance vessels). Arterial dilators are used in *treatment of* systemic hypertension in dogs and cats and as adjunctive treatment for CHF in dogs, particularly when CHF is secondary to degenerative mitral valve disease.

Arterial Dilators

Hydralazine is an arteriolar vasodilator, the mechanism of action of which is not clearly elucidated. It directly relaxes the vascular smooth muscle in systemic arterioles by inhibiting calcium fluxes into the cell or by increasing local prostacyclin concentrations. Hydralazine has no effect on systemic venous tone. It is bound to smooth muscle, which results in a biologic half-life longer than plasma half-life. Hydralazine is well absorbed after administration PO but (in people) is subject to first-pass metabolism. The incidence of toxicity caused by hydralazine may be significant and related to its potency as an arterial dilator leading to hypotension. The potency of hydralazine can be both beneficial and detrimental: it results in good to profound improvement in most animals in which it is indicated, but it can also result in systemic hypotension. The effective dosage range in dogs is 0.5–3 mg/kg, PO, bid. This dose must be titrated, starting with a low dose and titrating up to an effective clinical endpoint while monitoring for hypotension. Doses may need to be even lower when hydralazine is combined with other drugs that have arterial dilatory effects.

Calcium channel blockers as a class are considered vasodilators, but individual agents have different relative potencies and additional effects. Calcium channel blockers are also class IV antiarrhythmics, negative inotropes (an adverse property), and positive lusitropes (drugs that improve relaxation of cardiomyocytes).

Amlodipine primarily affects the calcium channels in the small arterioles, leading to arterial dilation. Amlodipine is the only calcium channel blocker used in veterinary medicine that has potent arterial dilatory effects with negligible effects on inotropy and conduction. The effects of amlodipine are similar to those of hydralazine, and it is used for similar indications in dogs and cats. Amlodipine appears to be better tolerated by the GI tract. The effective dosage range in dogs is 0.1–0.2 mg/kg, PO, bid, or 0.2–0.4 mg/kg/day, PO. The effective dosage range in cats is 0.625–1.25 mg/cat, PO, once to twice daily. This dose must be titrated, starting with a low dose and titrating up to an effective clinical endpoint while monitoring for hypotension. Doses may need to be even lower when amlodipine is combined with other drugs that have arterial dilatory effects. In resistant systemic hypertension, doses at the higher end of the range are needed. In

CHF in dogs, initial dosages should be at the lower end of the range and titrated to effect with appropriate monitoring. Gingival hyperplasia has been reported as an adverse effect of amlodipine in dogs and cats.

Arterial and Venous Dilators

(Mixed dilators)

Organic nitrates and nitrites relax both arterial and venous vascular smooth muscle through a complex series of events. At low concentrations, which are generally used clinically, venous dilation predominates, and net systemic vascular resistance is usually not affected. Pharmacologic effects occur rapidly. First-pass metabolism limits the use of these drugs to IV, sublingual, and topical (ointment) administration. Tolerance is a problem with sustained administration.

Nitroglycerin, an organic nitrate, relaxes vascular smooth muscle. However, the dosage of nitroglycerin used clinically results in predominantly venous dilation and preload reduction. Nitroglycerin is indicated for acute (emergency) adjunctive treatment of CHF in dogs and cats; however, efficacy for this indication in these species is anecdotal. It is available for IV and sublingual use and as an ointment. The 2% ointment preparation (1 in. = 15 mg) is the most commonly used; it is applied to the hairless portion of the animal's skin (abdomen or ear). The dosage in dogs is 4–12 mg, topically, bid (maximum of 15 mg/dog per dose) for 1–2 days, and in cats, 2–4 mg/cat, topically, every 6–8 hr for 1–2 days. The most prevalent adverse effect involves accidental exposure of veterinary personnel, which can be avoided by careful application and labeling of application sites.

Nitroprusside is one of the most potent vasodilators available. It is an organic nitrate and reduces preload (venous dilation) and afterload (arterial dilation) in a dose-dependent manner. Advantages of nitroprusside include potency, rapid onset of action, and short half-life. The main disadvantage is that it must be administered by CRI (1–10 mcg/kg/min, IV), with appropriate, typically invasive, blood pressure monitoring. Nitroprusside is indicated in dogs for emergency reduction of blood pressure in a hypertensive crisis and for immediate afterload reduction (severe, life-threatening CHF). Nitroprusside should only be used for 48–72 hr because of buildup of its toxic metabolite, cyanide.

Prazosin is an α_1-adrenergic receptor blocker and thus considered to be a mixed vasodilator. It is effective when given PO, but tolerance develops rapidly. It also undergoes significant first-pass metabolism. Prazosin is rarely used clinically in small animals to treat primary cardiac disease. The dosage in dogs and cats is 0.5–2 mg per animal, PO, bid-tid, or 0.07 mg/kg, PO, bid-tid.

Phosphodiesterase 5 Inhibitor

Sildenafil is an orally active phosphodiesterase 5 inhibitor. Phosphodiesterase 5 (PDE 5) is found in a relatively high concentration in the lungs and the corpus cavernosum of the penis. In dogs, pulmonary hypertension is a clinically important disease with high morbidity and mortality rates; it is typically a sequela of another disease process and thus requires a balanced therapeutic approach that targets the underlying etiology as well as palliation of clinical signs. An important goal of therapy is to reduce pulmonary artery resistance. Conventional systemic arteriolar dilators have no preferential effect on pulmonary vasculature and thus have no benefit and may worsen clinical signs attributable to pulmonary hypertension. Inhibition of PDE 5 in the small arterioles of the lung leads to dilation that is more significant than dilation of the systemic arterioles. In people with pulmonary hypertension, PDE 5 inhibitors improve both exercise tolerance and quality of life. Sildenafil has been used in dogs for adjunctive treatment of clinical signs related to pulmonary hypertension secondary to a variety of etiologies; proof of efficacy remains predominantly anecdotal, although it does appear to be safe and well tolerated for this indication.

The typical starting dosage in dogs is 1 mg/kg PO, tid, or 1–2 mg/kg, PO, bid. The reported dosage range is 1–3 mg/kg, PO, bid-tid. Efficacy may be potentiated with coadministration of L-arginine at 250–500 mg/dog, PO, bid. Adverse effects of sildenafil appear to be rare in dogs, but anecdotally systemic hypotension is possible. There are no reported drug interactions, and published reports have documented use of sildenafil in dogs in combination with many other medications, including conventional heart failure medications (eg, diuretics, ACE inhibitors, pimobendan), with no recognized adverse effects.

ANTIARRHYTHMICS

Antiarrhythmics are typically classified according to their predominant electrophysiologic effect on myocardial cells.

However, the electrophysiologic effects of some agents span more than one class, and some have ancillary properties unrelated to their antiarrhythmic effects. However, this classification scheme typically does not aid in selection of an antiarrhythmic for a specific clinical indication (eg, ventricular vs supraventricular arrhythmias). Many antiarrhythmics have never been used with any frequency in veterinary medicine (and are not covered here). In addition, many of these agents (in particular the class I medications) have fallen out of favor for treatment of arrhythmias in people, and as a consequence their availability and costs are becoming problematic.

Class I Drugs

Class I agents comprise the group of agents generally known as "membrane-stabilizing drugs" such as quinidine, procainamide, and lidocaine. These agents work by selectively blocking a proportion of the fast sodium channels in cardiomyocytes, leading to depression of phase 0 of the action potential and subsequent reductions in conduction velocity. These agents are often subdivided into three subclasses (A, B, and C) based on their concurrent effects on repolarization; however, this has little clinical relevance.

Class IA Drugs: Class IA drugs used in veterinary medicine include quinidine and procainamide.

Quinidine is related to the antimalarial drug quinine. In addition to its membrane-stabilizing properties inherent to Class I agents, it also has indirect, antivagal ("atropine-like") effects in the atria. It has efficacy against supraventricular and ventricular arrhythmias. Its main indication in veterinary medicine is to treat atrial fibrillation. It has the potential to convert atrial fibrillation to sinus rhythm and is used for this indication in horses. In dogs, it is used to facilitate synchronized cardioversion of atrial fibrillation. It is not typically used for rate control of chronic atrial fibrillation in dogs or horses, or to treat ventricular arrhythmias. The sulfate preparation of quinidine is absorbed rapidly after administration PO. The gluconate form is absorbed more slowly. It can be given IM but is painful. Although 90% of quinidine is protein-bound, distribution is rapid to most tissues. The half-life varies among species and is ~6 hr in dogs and ~8 hr in horses.

Dosages of quinidine sulfate are as follows: in dogs, 5–10 mg/kg, IV, qid, or 6–20 mg/kg, PO, tid-qid; and in horses, 22 mg/kg, PO, every 2 hr. Dosages of quinidine gluconate are in dogs, 6–20 mg/kg, IM, qid, or 6–20 mg/kg, PO, tid-qid; and in horses, 1–1.5 mg/kg, IV, every 5–10 min. Individualized therapy is necessary because of significant pharmacodynamic variation among animals and the potential for toxicity. Cardiotoxicity can manifest in the form of ventricular arrhythmias. The atropine-like effects of quinidine may result in increased impulse conduction through the AV node to the ventricles and paradoxical acceleration in ventricular response in animals with atrial fibrillation. Quinidine, particularly in the sulfate form, can cause vasodilation and GI adverse effects (25% of dogs). In horses, swelling of the nasal mucosa, urticarial wheals, and laminitis are other potential adverse effects. The most important clinical problem limiting use of quinidine is exacerbation of heart failure after administration, likely as a consequence of its negative inotropic effects. In general, quinidine use should be avoided in dogs with severe myocardial failure or in dogs that have, or have had, heart failure. Quinidine should not be used in cats. Monitoring the ECG and serum quinidine concentration can reduce the likelihood of adverse effects.

Procainamide effects are similar to those of quinidine. However, its effects on the autonomic nervous system are significantly weaker (less antivagal effect). Procainamide has efficacy against ventricular and supraventricular arrhythmias and has been used for both indications in dogs. It is often used parenterally in combination with lidocaine to treat life-threatening ventricular arrhythmias. The parenteral formulation has also been used to treat supraventricular arrhythmias, including conversion of recent onset atrial fibrillation. The oral formulation is useful to treat ventricular arrhythmias and supraventricular arrhythmias secondary to accessory pathways. It has little efficacy in longterm management of atrial fibrillation. Procainamide is rapidly and almost completely absorbed after administration PO. Only ~20% is protein bound. Procainamide is extensively biotransformed by the liver to metabolites that are generally inactive in dogs. Both oral ("regular" and sustained-release) and parenteral formulations (IV and IM administration) are available. The "regular" formulation necessitates dosing every 4 hr for maintenance in dogs, severely limiting its use for longterm treatment. The sustained-release product has fallen out of favor in people, limiting its availability; it is not currently available in the USA.

Procainamide is dosed in dogs at 2 mg/kg, slow IV bolus, to a maximum cumulative dose of 25 mg/kg over 10–15 min, continuing if needed as a CRI at 25–40 mcg/kg/min or at 10–20 mg/kg, tid-qid, IM or SC. The oral (regular) formulation is dosed at 4–6 mg/kg, PO, every 2–4 hr (maintenance dose every 4 hr), and the sustained-release formulation at 10–20 mg/kg, PO, tid.

Toxicities include hypotension and AV block (IV administration only), proarrhythmia (longterm administration), alteration in coat color (longterm administration), and GI disturbances with the oral formulations.

Class IB Drugs: Class IB drugs used in veterinary medicine include lidocaine, mexiletine, tocainide, and phenytoin.

Lidocaine is used predominantly for acute treatment of ventricular arrhythmias. It has no efficacy against supraventricular arrhythmias and minimal effects on the autonomic nervous system. It is ideal for acute treatment because it has a rapid onset of action and short half-life (~1 hr in a dog) and is effective and safe. The short half-life facilitates rapid changes in serum concentrations and, therefore, titration to effect. Lidocaine is extensively metabolized by the liver; thus, hepatic disease and reduced hepatic blood flow can prolong the half-life. Hypokalemia seriously impairs the efficacy of lidocaine. Lidocaine is available only as a parenteral formulation for IV administration. It should not be infused through the same catheter or line as other medications. The typical clinical approach in dogs is to administer 2 mg/kg, IV boluses over ~1 min to effect (slowing the ventricular arrhythmia or conversion to sinus rhythm) or to a cumulative dose of 8 mg/kg over ~30 min. Given the very short half-life, repeat boluses or a CRI (25–75 mcg/kg/min) is needed to maintain rhythm control. Lidocaine is rarely indicated in cats, because clinically significant or life-threatening ventricular arrhythmias are rare in this species. The dosage in cats is 0.1–0.4 mg/kg, IV bolus over ~1 min, then increase to a total dose of 0.25–1 mg/kg, IV slowly, if no response. This can be followed by a CRI (10–20 mcg/kg/min). Lidocaine has few undesirable effects. Toxicity is manifest in dogs primarily as GI and CNS signs. Drowsiness or agitation may progress to muscle twitching and convulsions at higher plasma concentrations. Hypotension may develop if the IV bolus is given too rapidly. In cats, which are more susceptible to toxicity, cardiac suppression and CNS excitation may be seen.

Mexiletine is an oral analogue of lidocaine used to treat ventricular arrhythmias in dogs. It is rarely used as monotherapy for ventricular arrhythmias. It is most often an adjunctive treatment in severe, chronic ventricular arrhythmias not well controlled by sotalol alone or in dogs that do not tolerate sotalol. It has fallen out of favor for treatment of people; thus, its availability is limited and cost is increasing. It should be administered at its lowest effective dose with food to limit toxicity. Common adverse effects include anorexia, vomiting, tremors, and hepatic toxicity. Hepatic enzymes should be evaluated before treatment and periodically (approximately every 6 mo) during chronic treatment as well as any time GI disturbances develop during treatment. The dosage in dogs is 4–6 mg/kg, PO, tid.

Tocainide is an analogue of lidocaine used to treat ventricular arrhythmias in dogs. Similar to mexiletine, it is rarely used as monotherapy for ventricular arrhythmias. It is most often an add-on treatment of choice for severe chronic ventricular arrhythmias not well controlled by sotalol alone, in dogs that do not tolerate sotalol, or if mexiletine is not available or cost prohibitive. It has fallen out of favor for treatment of people; thus, its availability is limited and cost is increasing. Potential adverse effects include CNS and GI disturbances (35% of dogs), hypotension, bradycardia, tachycardia, other arrhythmias, and progressive corneal edema. Because of these adverse effects, use of tocainide is limited if other efficacious agents are available. Tocainide has been used in dogs at 15–20 mg/kg, PO, tid.

Phenytoin has a limited spectrum of antiarrhythmic activity. Its primary use is in management of digitalis-induced arrhythmias, because it abolishes digitalis-induced abnormal automaticity. The recommended dosage in dogs is 30 mg/kg, PO, tid, or 10 mg/kg, IV, over 5 min.

Class IC Drugs: Examples of drugs in this class include encainide, flecainide, and propafenone. These drugs are not typically used in veterinary medicine.

Class II Drugs

Class II antiarrhythmic drugs are the β-adrenergic receptor blocking agents. β-Blockers are classified as nonselective (block both β_1 and β_2 receptors) or selective (block predominantly β_1 receptors). As a class, all β-blockers are dose-dependent negative inotropes and chronotropes. Although characterized as class II antiarrhythmic agents, β-adrenergic blockers are used for a variety of indications in veterinary medicine, including control of inappropriate or undesirable sinus tachycardia, treatment of ventricular and supraventricular arrhythmias, management of chronic hypertension in dogs and cats, and palliation of adverse effects of uncontrolled hyperthyroidism in cats and pheochromocytoma in dogs. They are well recognized for their cardioprotective effects in people with heart failure, leading to improved survival. Data and experience supporting this indication in veterinary medicine is lacking in dogs and cats, and the relative risks of initiation of a β-blocker in the face of heart failure should not be ignored. The earliest generation of this class was nonselective, blocking both β_1 and β_2 receptors (eg, propranolol). Subsequent generations became selective β_1-receptor blockers in an attempt to limit the adverse effects associated with β_2-receptor blockade (eg, atenolol). Third-generation β-blockers (eg, carvedilol) were developed to be more complete adrenergic blockers and are β_1, β_2, and α_1-receptor blockers. Carvedilol may also have some important antioxidant effects that have contributed to its proven efficacy for treatment of heart failure in people.

Propranolol, the prototype, is competitive and nonselective, blocking both β_1 and β_2 receptors. The dosage in dogs is 0.2–1 mg/kg, PO, tid (titrate dose to effect) and in cats is 0.4–1.2 mg/kg (2.5–5 mg/cat), PO, tid. Use of propranolol should be avoided in dogs and cats with evidence of primary respiratory disease (eg, asthma).

Atenolol is a β_1-selective blocking agent and is the most commonly used β-blocker in veterinary medicine. Because it is β_1-selective, it has less potential to cause or contribute to bronchospasm in predisposed dogs and cats, although the β_1-selectivity is likely limited or absent at high doses. The dosage in dogs is 0.2–1 mg/kg, PO, bid, and in cats 1–2.5 mg/kg, PO, bid, or 6.25–12.5 mg/cat, PO, bid. Some references suggest cats can be dosed every 24 hr, but most cardiologists believe that continuous β-blockade (the clinical target) is not possible with daily dosing. In both dogs and cats, titrating up gradually is required, especially if atenolol is initiated in the face of active or stable CHF or in DCM. In general, dogs and cats without CHF and normal systolic function can tolerate higher initial and target dosages. Abrupt discontinuation should be avoided; if cessation is indicated, titrating down gradually is recommended. If CHF develops in an animal receiving atenolol, the dosage may need to be reduced and the drug eventually discontinued, but unless the CHF is life-threatening, abrupt cessation should still be avoided. Potential adverse effects are dose related and more likely if underlying systolic function is present. Adverse effects include myocardial depression, bradycardia (sinus and AV block), and hypotension.

Carvedilol is a third-generation β-blocker that has a more complete adrenergic blocking spectrum. Carvedilol blocks β_1, β_2, and α_1 receptors and has some ancillary antioxidant effects. It is routinely used in treatment of heart failure in people. Its oral bioavailability is highly variable in dogs. Carvedilol has been mainly evaluated in veterinary medicine for its potential survival benefits in canine DCM and cardiovascular disease with and without CHF, but experience to date is limited and thus it is not routinely used for this indication. If β-blockers are used for this indication, the general rule of thumb is to never initiate in the face of active heart failure (pulmonary edema), start low (initial dose), go slow (and titrate up), and aim high (target dose tolerated). The initial dosage in dogs is 0.15–0.25 mg/kg, PO, bid, titrated up by increasing the dose ~25% every 2 wk while monitoring for clinical signs suggestive of decompensation. The target dosage is 1 mg/kg, PO, every 2 hr (if tolerated). Higher target doses may be tolerated in dogs concurrently receiving pimobendan and in dogs with cardiovascular disease (vs those with DCM).

Class III Drugs

The predominant electrophysiologic effect of class III drugs is potassium channel blockade leading to prolongation of the cardiac action potential and its refractory period. The two drugs in this class commonly used in veterinary medicine are sotalol and amiodarone.

Sotalol is an oral class III drug with nonselective β-blocking activity. Sotalol is the most commonly used longterm treatment for hemodynamically significant ventricular arrhythmias in dogs and cats. It is often used as monotherapy for this indication but can be combined with mexiletine if rhythm control is suboptimal with sotalol alone. It has some efficacy in treatment of atrial fibrillation (rate control), but it is not as efficacious as other agents and is not commonly used for this indication. Sotalol is safe and well tolerated and is often used in combination with other drugs commonly used to treat heart disease and heart failure, including ACE inhibitors, furosemide, spironolactone, and pimobendan. Because it has β-blocking effects, it should not be combined with other β-blockers (eg, atenolol) or other negative inotropes (eg, diltiazem). In addition, it should not be combined with another class III agent (eg, amiodarone). The dosage in dogs and cats is 1–2.5 mg/kg, PO, bid. It should be used with caution and at the lower end of the dosage range in patients with CHF or DCM or when combined with mexiletine. In this situation, titrating up (dosage increases every 10–14 days) to a higher target dose may be attempted if lower doses are not efficacious. Dogs and cats with normal systolic function can tolerate higher initial and target doses. Possible adverse effects include negative inotropy, bradyarrhythmia (sinus and AV block), and proarrhythmia.

Amiodarone is a class III drug with a variety of other properties. Its predominant electrophysiologic effect is to prolong the refractory period of atrial and ventricular myocardium and the AV junction. In addition, it has class I effects (sodium channel–blocking properties), some class II effects (β- and α-receptor blockade), and some class IV effects (calcium channel blockade). Amiodarone is used to treat life-threatening ventricular arrhythmias (rhythm control) and atrial fibrillation (rate control) in dogs refractory to other, more common treatments. In some cases, it is used because of its effectiveness in treatment of both ventricular and supraventricular arrhythmias. It is rarely used as a first-line drug.

Amiodarone has unusual pharmacokinetics. After repeated administration in dogs, it has a long half-life of 3.2 days, with myocardial concentrations reaching 15 times that of plasma. The long half-life suggests a long time is needed to produce a significant effect once treatment is initiated as well as for effects to end if treatment is discontinued. However, some clinical effect appears to occur within hours of PO administration, especially if a higher loading dose is used, which is likely a consequence of the large and variable number of metabolites.

Amiodarone is often used in combination with other drugs commonly used to treat heart disease and heart failure, including ACE inhibitors, furosemide, spironolactone, and pimobendan. Because it has β-blocking effects it should not be combined with other β-blockers (eg, atenolol) or other negative inotropes (eg, diltiazem). In addition, it should not be combined with another class III agent (eg, sotalol). Amiodarone has a number of known common adverse effects that limit its longterm (>6 mo) use clinically. Adverse effects seem to be related to dose and duration of treatment and include significant increases in liver enzymes, GI signs, thyroid dysfunction, blood dyscrasias (neutropenia), and proarrhythmia. The liver effects seem to be the most common adverse effect encountered clinically and are typically reversible after cessation of therapy. The oral dosage in dogs is 8–10 mg/kg, PO, once to twice daily for 7–10 days, and then decreased to 4–6 mg/kg/day for longterm treatment; the parenteral dosage in dogs is 2–5 mg/kg, IV, infused over 30–60 min. Formulations preserved with polysorbate 80 should not be used IV because of risk of anaphylactoid reaction and angioedema.

Class IV Drugs

The predominant electrophysiologic effect of class IV antiarrhythmic drugs is blockade of the slow calcium channels in cardiac cells and vascular smooth muscle. The two drugs in this class commonly used in veterinary medicine are diltiazem and amlodipine. The relative affinity of a drug in this class for cardiac versus vascular tissue determines its predominant effect. Amlodipine (*see* p 2534) is most active in vascular smooth muscle, where it causes vasodilation and is thus considered to be a vasodilator. Diltiazem is most active in cardiac cells.

Diltiazem blocks entry of calcium into cardiomyocytes during the action potential, leading to a dose-dependent reduction in calcium release from the sarcoplasmic reticulum, limiting the availability of calcium to the contractile apparatus, and resulting in negative inotropy and positive lusitropy. It also blocks calcium channels in the specialized conduction tissue in the heart, on which automaticity of intrinsic pacemaker cells and AV conduction depend for normal function. Blockade of these calcium channels can therefore slow heart rate and AV conduction. Diltiazem is therefore typically indicated for treatment of atrial fibrillation (rate control) and other supraventricular arrhythmias in dogs and cats. Another historical indication is for treatment of feline hypertrophic cardiomyopathy. However, limited practicality in combination with its unconfirmed efficacy for feline hypertrophic cardiomyopathy has caused diltiazem to fall into disfavor for this indication. Diltiazem has no effect on ventricular arrhythmias.

The dosage in dogs is 0.05–0.2 mg/kg, IV, over 5 min, which can be repeated to a cumulative dose of 0.3 mg/kg, after which the dog should be reassessed or an oral formulation initiated. In dogs, the dosage of the standard oral formulation is 0.5–2 mg/kg, PO, tid, and of the sustained-release formulation 1–4 mg/kg, PO, bid. In cats, the dosage of the standard oral formulation is 7.5 mg/cat, PO, tid, and of the sustained-release formulation 30–60 mg/cat, PO, once to twice daily. Initial doses should be at the lower end of the dose range and titrated up to a clinically effective dose. Blood pressure and heart rate and rhythm should be monitored during IV administration. Dogs and cats without CHF and with normal systolic function can tolerate higher initial and target dosages. The sustained-release formulation cannot be made into suspensions but can be reformulated into lower-dose capsules.

Possible adverse effects include systemic hypotension, negative inotropy and bradycardia (sinus or AV block), and exacerbation of CHF. GI signs are the common noncardiac adverse effect and are more common in cats, especially with sustained-release preparations. Diltiazem is often used in combination with other drugs commonly used to treat heart disease and heart failure, including ACE inhibitors, furosemide, spironolactone, and pimobendan. Because diltiazem is a negative inotrope and chronotrope, it should not be administered concurrently with a β-blocker.

Amlodipine is selective for calcium-channel blockade in vascular smooth muscle, with minimal effects on cardiac calcium transport. Amlodipine is recommended for hypertension in cats and dogs.

DRUGS ACTING ON THE BLOOD OR BLOOD-FORMING ORGANS

Hematinics

Anemia can be treated pharmacologically by providing components needed for RBC production, including hemoglobin synthesis, and by stimulating bone marrow formation of RBCs.

Vitamin B_{12} is essential for DNA synthesis. Deficiency causes inhibited nuclear maturation and division. RBC maturation arrest in the bone marrow leads to megaloblastic or pernicious anemia. Vitamin B_{12}, a porphyrin-like compound consisting of a ring structure that contains centrally located cobalt, is derived from the diet and microbial synthesis in the GI tract. However, except for ruminants, microbial production occurs in the large intestine, from which vitamin B_{12} is not readily absorbed. Dietary deficiency of B_{12} is rare; deficiency usually results from poor absorption from the GI tract.

Vitamin B_{12} absorption is complex and depends on gastric acid, pepsin, and intrinsic factor secreted from gastric parietal cells or pancreatic duct cells. Intrinsic factor binds to and protects vitamin B_{12} from digestion. In this form, B_{12} binds to highly specific receptor sites in the brush border of the ileum, where it enters enterocytes by pinocytosis. Interference with its absorption in the ileum results in continuous depletion, although many months of defective absorption are necessary before deficiency develops. Vitamin B_{12} is bound in the plasma to transcobalamin. It is stored in large quantities in the liver and slowly released as needed. It is excreted into the bile but undergoes enterohepatic cycling.

Vitamin B_{12} (dogs: 100–200 mcg/day, PO or SC; cats: 50–100 mcg/day, PO or SC) is available in oral and parenteral preparations of cyanocobalamin. There are no significant toxicities associated with therapy. Indications for therapy are limited to cases of vitamin B_{12} malabsorption, such as ileectomy, gastrectomy, or deficiency malabsorption syndromes (eg, exocrine pancreatic insufficiency). Chronic administration of H_2-receptor blockers (cimetidine, ranitidine, famotidine) can also lead to vitamin B_{12} deficiency, because an acid environment is necessary for its absorption.

Folic acid is needed for DNA and RNA synthesis. Anemia associated with folic acid deficiency is characterized as megaloblastic. Sources of folic acid in the diet include yeast, liver, kidney, and green vegetables, although it can also be formed by microbes. Folic acid is stored in the liver but not as avidly as vitamin B_{12}. Because folic acid is destroyed by catabolic processes every day, serum levels decrease rapidly in the presence of deficient diets. Absorption of folic acid is not as sensitive as that of vitamin B_{12}, although jejunal pathology can result in folate deficiency.

Folic acid (dogs: 5 mg/day, PO; cats: 2.5 mg/day, PO) is available in both oral and parenteral formulations. Significant toxicity is not associated with therapy. Indications for therapy include inadequate intake due to administration of selected drugs (eg, methotrexate, potentiated sulfa drugs, some anticonvulsants [eg, primidone and phenytoin]), liver disease, malabsorption, or other chronic debilitating diseases.

Iron is necessary for hemoglobin formation. It is available in the diet either as a heme form, which is a small percentage of the total but readily absorbed, or a nonheme form. Absorption of the nonheme form is profoundly affected by diet. Iron is absorbed from the proximal jejunum, where it immediately combines in the enterocyte to the globulin transferrin. It is transported in the plasma in this form, but the binding is loose and iron can be easily transferred to tissues. Iron enters cells via specific receptors that interact with transferrin. In the cell, iron combines with the protein apoferritin to become ferritin, the soluble form of iron storage. Smaller quantities are also stored as the insoluble hemosiderin; the amount of this storage form increases when the total amount of iron in the body is much more than apoferritin can accommodate. There is no mechanism for the excretion of iron other than via the GI tract. GI elimination occurs by exfoliation of enterocytes containing iron, biliary elimination, and elimination of dietary iron that has not been absorbed.

Indications for iron therapy are limited to treatment or prevention of iron deficiency (eg, blood loss, pregnancy). Iron is available in both oral and parenteral preparations. Oral preparations should be ferrous salts, such as sulfate (dogs: 100–300 mg/day; cats: 50–100 mg/day), gluconate, and fumarate. Therapy can be continued for several months to replenish body iron stores. Response to iron therapy can be assessed by monitoring circulating hemoglobin concentrations. Adverse effects are dose-related. Parenteral preparations are indicated for initial treatment of iron deficiency or if oral preparations cannot be tolerated or are not feasible (eg, in neonatal pigs). Iron dextrans can be given as a single IM injection (100 mg) at 2–4 days of age in newborn piglets. Toxicity may be seen and is manifest as pale skin, bloody diarrhea, and shock (*see* p 3077). When efficacy of parenteral preparations is compared, dextran complexes and hydrogenated dextrans are more effective than dextrins. Hemoglobin formation requires pyridoxine and the trace elements copper and cobalt (necessary for B_{12} synthesis by ruminal microflora). "Shotgun" preparations contain a combination of hematinic agents; the efficacy of such products is questionable. As with any hematinic preparation, provision of these compounds will be ineffective if the nutritional status of the animal is poor.

Epoetin alfa is the synthetic form of the human glycoprotein erythropoietin (ERP). Epoetin alfa is indicated in treatment of anemia associated with chronic renal failure in dogs and cats. The initial dosage is 100 U/kg, SC, 3 times/wk for 4 mo, while monitoring PCV, followed by a maintenance dosage of 75–100 U/kg, SC, 2–3 times/wk. The most significant adverse effects in dogs and cats are development of antibodies to ERP, resistance to treatment, and worsening of anemia. Other potential adverse effects include iron deficiency, hypertension, fever, local cellulitis, arthralgia, mucocutaneous ulcers, polycythemia, and CNS disturbances (seizures).

Anabolic steroids are compounds structurally related to testosterone that have similar protein-anabolic activity but minimal androgenic effects, such as masculinization. As part of their anabolic activity, these compounds increase the circulating RBC mass and possibly granulocytic mass. Clinical indications for use of anabolic steroids include chronic, nonregenerative anemias. Response to therapy is variable, and the time to clinical improvement is long, frequently ≥3 mo. The proposed mechanisms of action include increased ERP production via ERP-stimulating factor, differentiation of stem cells into ERP-stimulating factor-sensitive cells (eg, hemocytoblasts), and direct stimulation of erythroid-progenitor cells. The effect of anabolic steroids requires adequate ERP levels and sufficient cells in the bone marrow. Thus, the effectiveness of anabolic steroids in treating anemia may be limited, depending on the cause.

Anabolic steroids can be divided into two categories depending on the presence or absence of an alkyl group at the 17-carbon position. They are available as oral and parenteral preparations, including oil-based products intended for slow release. The absorption and disposition of anabolic steroids depend on the type of preparation and the animal species. Most are eliminated after hepatic metabolism. The alkylated products are more effectively absorbed when given PO and are more effective stimulants of bone marrow. Alkylated anabolic steroids include oxymetholone (dogs and cats: 1–5 mg/kg, PO, every 18–24 hr). Nonalkylated anabolic steroids include nandrolone decanoate (dogs: 1–1.5 mg/kg/wk, IM; cats: 1 mg/kg/wk, IM; horse: 1 mg/kg, IM, once every 4 wk). Boldenone undecylenate is approved for horses at 1.1 mg/kg, IM, every 3 wk. Adverse effects of anabolic steroids include sodium and water retention, virilization, and hepatotoxicity. The alkylated products are more hepatotoxic than the nonalkylated products, particularly in cats. Cholestatic liver damage develops early and can be significant but frequently is reversible.

Hemostatics

Lyophilized concentrates of one or more clotting factors are available as topical or local hemostatics. Most act to provide an artificial factor or structural matrix that facilitates control of capillary bleeding. An intact hemostatic mechanism is necessary. These absorbable products are indicated for capillary oozing from small, superficial vessels. Concentrated factors include thromboplastin, thrombin (available as a powder, solution, or sponge), collagen, and fibrinogen. Artificial matrices include fibrin foam, absorbable gelatin sponge, and oxidized cellulose.

Astringents act locally by precipitating proteins. These agents do not penetrate tissues and, thus, are restricted to surface cells. They can be damaging to surrounding tissues. Examples include ferric sulfate, silver nitrate, and tannic acid.

Epinephrine and **norepinephrine** are hemostatics by virtue of their vasoconstrictive effects. They may be included in topical medications to decrease blood flow to the tissues, or applied intranasally in tampons to decrease epistaxis.

Systemic hemostatics include fresh blood or blood components administered to animals that have a coagulation factor deficiency. Examples include fresh plasma, fresh frozen plasma, cryoprecipitate, and platelet-rich plasma.

Vitamin K is a hemostatic only in instances of vitamin K deficiency. It is necessary for hepatic synthesis of coagulation factors II, VII, IX, and X. The principal indication is treatment of rodenticide toxicity, moldy sweet clover poisoning (dicumarol), and sulfaquinoxaline toxicity.

Vitamin K_1 (phytonadione) is a plant form of vitamin K that is safer and more effective with more rapid restoration of coagulation factors than other analogues such as vitamin K_3 (menadione). The preferred routes to administer phytonadione are SC and PO, although it can be given by slow IV (anaphylactic reactions have been reported) or IM injections. After IM administration, bleeding may occur at the injection site. The dosage regimen selected depends on the nature of the anticoagulant toxicity. Vitamin K_1 must be given as long as the anticoagulant is present in the body at toxic levels; this duration varies depending on the rodenticide. Second-generation coumarin derivatives or indanediones are potent and *have long half-lives.* Several weeks of vitamin K_1 therapy may be necessary after ingestion of these long-acting rodenticides. Coagulation status should be monitored during therapy. The lag period after administration of phytonadione and synthesis of new clotting factors is 6–12 hr.

Desmopressin is a synthetic analogue of vasopressin and is used to treat diabetes insipidus. In animals with von Willebrand disease, desmopressin transiently increases von Willebrand factor and shortens bleeding time. It may be useful in dogs with von Willebrand disease (0.4 mcg/kg, SC; 1 mcg/kg, IV, diluted in 20 mL of saline and given over 10 min), to permit surgical procedures or control capillary bleeding.

Anticoagulants

Anticoagulants interfere either directly or indirectly with the clotting cascade.

Heparin is a heterogeneous mixture of sulfated (anionic) mucopolysaccharides named because of its initial discovery in high concentrations in the liver. It is prepared from porcine intestinal mucosa and bovine lung. It acts indirectly to facilitate endogenous anticoagulants, specifically antithrombin III and heparin cofactor II. These molecules form stable complexes with (and thus inactivate) clotting factors, especially thrombin. Heparin is released in its active form after inactivation of the clotting factor and thus can interact with other molecules. The effect is greater with low concentrations of heparin. Heparin is also antithrombotic due to binding to endothelial cell walls, thus impairing platelet aggregation and adhesion.

Clinical indications for heparin therapy include the prevention or treatment of venous or pulmonary embolism and embolization associated with atrial fibrillation. It is also used as an anticoagulant for diagnostic use and blood transfusions. Heparin is used in conjunction with blood and/or plasma to treat disseminated intravascular coagulation (DIC) and other hypercoagulable conditions. It has also been used to clear hyperlipidemia.

Heparin is available as a sodium or calcium salt. Absorption and distribution of heparin are limited by the large size and polarity of the molecule. Oral absorption is poor; hence, it is a parenteral anticoagulant. Although anticoagulant activity is first order, half-life of the drug is dose-dependent, steady-state concentrations are difficult to achieve, and pharmacokinetics vary among individuals. Heparin is metabolized by heparinase in the liver and by reticuloendothelial cells. Metabolites of heparinase activity are excreted in the urine. The half-life is prolonged in renal or hepatic failure.

Heparin can be given IV (either intermittently or as a constant infusion) or SC. Deep SC or intrafat injection prolongs persistence of therapeutic concentrations. Large hematomas can develop after deep IM injection. High-dose heparin therapy (dogs: 150–250 U/kg, SC, tid; cats: 250–375 U/kg, SC, bid) has been recommended for established thromboembolism. Lower dosages (dogs and cats: 75 U/kg, SC, tid; horses: 25–100 U/kg, SC, tid) are indicated in management of DIC. Blood coagulation times (eg, activated partial thromboplastin time) should be monitored during therapy. Adverse effects and toxicities of heparin are limited to potential hemorrhage and, because heparin is a foreign protein, possible allergic reactions. Heparin is contraindicated in bleeding animals and in DIC unless replacement blood or plasma therapy is also given.

Low-molecular-weight heparins (LMWHs, eg, dalteparin and enoxaparin) are alternatives to "unfractionated heparin" and are used extensively in people as anticoagulants for various thromboembolic conditions. LMWHs differ from heparin in that the molecular weights are approximately one-tenth that of heparin, dosing can be once to twice daily in people, there is no need to monitor activated partial thromboplastin time, the risk of bleeding and thrombocytopenia is smaller, and the effect on thrombin is less than that of heparin. LMWHs target antifactor Xa activity. Limited efficacy, safety, and dosing data are available to guide use in veterinary medicine. However, a suggested dosage regimen for dalteparin in dogs and cats is 100–200 IU/kg, SC, once to twice daily, and a suggested dosage regimen for enoxaparin in dogs and cats is 1–2 mg/kg, SC, bid, while monitoring prothrombin time. Individual responses to LMWHs appear to be quite variable in cats.

Vitamin K antagonists (oral anticoagulants) differ from heparin primarily in their duration of activity and magnitude of effect. Their primary importance has been because of their toxic rather than therapeutic effects. Therapeutic indications include oral longterm treatment and prevention of recurrence of thrombotic conditions (eg, aortic or pulmonary thromboembolism and venous thrombosis) in cats, dogs, and horses.

There are several groups of vitamin K antagonists. They interfere with the hepatic synthesis of vitamin K–dependent clotting factors by blocking the reduction of vitamin K epoxide after clotting factor synthesis, thus effectively reducing the concentration of vitamin K. Their anticoagulant activity (and therefore therapeutic or toxic effect) is delayed for 8–12 hr after administration or accidental ingestion because of the persistence of factors synthesized before administration. Factor VII has the shortest half-life and is the first factor to become deficient.

The vitamin K antagonists are rapidly and completely absorbed after administration PO. Levels peak in 1 hr. They are almost totally protein bound in plasma, and their volume of distribution is limited to the plasma volume. They are metabolized by the liver to primary metabolites and then conjugated to glucuronides. They undergo an enterohepatic cycle. A variety of factors can increase the activity of these drugs, including hypoproteinemia, antimicrobial therapy, hepatic disease, hypermetabolic states, pregnancy, and the nephrotic syndrome. The potential for drug interactions is significant. Because they are highly protein bound, they can be displaced by other drugs that are protein bound (eg, acetylsalicylic acid and phenylbutazone), and their anticoagulant effects can be increased to the point of toxicity. Drug interactions also are seen with other antihemostatics.

Warfarin sodium is the most commonly used therapeutic preparation. The dosage is 0.1–0.2 mg/kg/day, PO, for dogs and cats, and 0.067–0.167 mg/kg/day, PO, for horses. Toxicity, manifest as hemorrhage, is a major concern with vitamin K antagonists. Coagulation times (particularly prothrombin time), CBCs, and clinical evidence of bleeding (eg, occult blood in feces and urine) must be monitored carefully during warfarin therapy.

Fibrinolytic agents increase the activity of plasmin (fibrinolysin), the endogenous compound responsible for dissolving clots. The inactive precursor of plasmin is plasminogen, which exists in two forms: plasma soluble form and fibrin (clot) bound form. Streptokinase and streptodornase are synthesized by streptococci and activate both forms of plasminogen. They are used locally as a powder, infusion, or irrigation in treatment of selected chronic wounds (eg, burns, ulcers, chronic eczemas, ear hematomas, otitis externa, osteomyelitis, chronic sinusitis, or other chronic lesions) that have not responded to other therapy. Tissue-type plasminogen activator (tPA) preferentially activates the fibrin-bound form of plasminogen. Unlike parenterally administered streptokinase, tPA does not induce a systemic proteolytic state. Selective clot lysis occurs without increasing circulating plasmin; thus, tPA has a lower risk of bleeding than does parenteral streptokinase. Although tPA has been used to treat aortic thromboembolism in cats (0.25–1 mg/kg/hr, IV, for a total dosage of 1–10 mg/kg), both the risk of death due to reperfusion (and release of toxic metabolites) and the expense of this genetically engineered product may limit its use.

Antithrombotic drugs affect platelet activity, which is normally controlled by substances (such as prostaglandins) generated both outside and within the platelet. Platelet activity can be modulated by interacting with these substances. NSAIDs inhibit the formation of cyclooxygenase, the enzyme responsible for synthesis of prostaglandin products from arachidonic acid that has been released into cells and platelets. The formation of all prostaglandins is inhibited, including that of thromboxane, a potent platelet aggregator and vasoconstrictor. In addition to its inhibitory effects on cyclooxygenase, aspirin irreversibly acetylates thromboxane synthetase, the specific enzyme responsible for synthesis of thromboxane. Aspirin is a potent inhibitor of platelet activity; new platelets must be generated before the effects of aspirin on platelet activity disappear. At higher dosages, aspirin inhibits prostacyclin, a prostaglandin product that counteracts the thrombogenic effects of thromboxane. Thus, aspirin must be used cautiously for antiplatelet effects. The antiplatelet dosage for dogs is 5–10 mg/kg, PO, every 24–48 hr, and for cats 80 mg, PO, every 48–72 hr. Clopidogrel is an antithrombotic agent used in small animals in treatment of autoimmune hemolytic anemia and in cats with aortic/pulmonary thromboembolism.

SYSTEMIC PHARMACOTHERAPEUTICS OF THE DIGESTIVE SYSTEM

See also PRINCIPLES OF THERAPY OF GI DISEASE, p 161.

THE MONOGASTRIC DIGESTIVE SYSTEM

DRUGS AFFECTING APPETITE

Disorders of appetite are very common in veterinary patients. Obesity from overfeeding is common in companion animals and is best managed by educating the owner and regulating the animal's diet. Anorexia is a common clinical problem seen with many systemic diseases, which exacerbates disease-induced catabolism. In the anorexic animal that does not respond to coaxing with small quantities of highly palatable foods, drug therapy may be used to stimulate appetite. The effect of specific drugs on food intake can involve hunger, satiety, or enhancement of the positive evaluation of taste.

Appetite Suppression: **Dirlotapide** is a microsomal triglyceride transfer protein (MTP) inhibitor developed specifically for weight loss in dogs. MTP catalyzes the assembly of triglyceride-rich apolipoprotein B–containing lipoproteins to form chylomicrons in the intestinal mucosa and very low-density lipoproteins in the liver. After oral administration, dirlotapide has in vivo selectivity for intestinal MTP. The mechanism of weight loss action is not completely understood, but dirlotapide appears to reduce fat absorption and send a satiety signal from lipid-filled enterocytes. Dirlotapide also decreases appetite in a dose-dependent manner, probably via increased release of peptide YY into the circulation. The decrease in food intake is responsible for most of the weight reduction effect.

Dirlotapide is available systemically, but absorption in dogs is highly variable. Absorbed dirlotapide is metabolized in the liver; parent drug and metabolites are secreted in the bile, with potential for enterohepatic circulation. Although blood concentrations do not directly correlate with effectiveness (effectiveness has been linked to drug concentrations in the gut), they seem to correlate with systemic toxicity.

Dirlotapide is available as a 5 mg/mL solution for oral administration. The dosage is adjusted according to the weight loss of each individual dog. The initial dosage of 0.5 mg/kg is doubled after 14 days and then adjusted monthly; the maximum permitted daily dosage is 1 mg/kg, although dosages as high as 10 mg/kg have been administered to dogs without severe adverse effects in safety studies. Dirlotapide can be used without changing the dog's current feeding or exercise regimens, but food intake should be monitored during weight stabilization to establish feeding and exercise routines that will minimize weight gain after treatment. Anorexia, emesis, and loose feces occur in some dogs. The incidence of emesis generally increases with dose and decreases with treatment time. Increases in hepatic transaminase activity were seen in dogs treated with >1.5 mg/kg/day but were not associated with clinical signs or histopathologic evidence of hepatic degeneration or necrosis.

Dirlotapide should not be used in cats. It increases the risk of hepatic lipidosis during weight loss in obese cats. Dirlotapide is not recommended for use in dogs currently receiving longterm glucocorticoid therapy or in dogs with liver disease. In people, adverse reactions associated with ingesting dirlotapide include abdominal distention, abdominal pain, diarrhea, flatulence, headache, increased serum transaminases, nausea, and vomiting.

Appetite Stimulation: **Anabolic steroids** are synthetic derivatives of testosterone that have enhanced anabolic effects with reduced androgenic effects. Anabolic steroids do not directly affect hunger, satiety, or sensory perception of food. Instead, they antagonize the catabolic effect of glucocorticoids and the negative nitrogen balance associated with surgery, illness, trauma, and aging. In all cases, improved nitrogen balance depends on adequate protein/calorie intake and treatment of the underlying disease. Anabolic steroids stimulate hematopoiesis, appetite, and weight gain. Adverse effects of anabolic steroid therapy include hepatotoxicity, masculinization, and early closure of bony epiphyses in young animals. Anabolic steroids are contraindicated in animals with congestive heart failure because of sodium and water retention. Because of human abuse potential, anabolic steroids are controlled substances. Although once (in)famous for abuse in people and horses, stanozolol and boldenone undecylenate are no longer marketed by veterinary pharmaceutical companies in North America. Currently, any anabolic product for veterinary use can only be obtained from a compounding pharmacy. Use of anabolic steroids in performance horses is prohibited by most equine sport organizations, and detection times can be >2 mo.

Glucocorticoids increase gluconeogenesis and antagonize insulin for an overall hyperglycemic effect. Appetite is stimulated by the steroid-induced euphoria. Continued use of glucocorticoids has catabolic effects because skeletal muscle and collagen proteins are broken down to provide the precursors for gluconeogenesis.

When used as anxiolytics, the **benzodiazepines** (BZD) became well known for their appetite stimulation effects independent of their anxiolytic activity. Stereospecific binding of a BZD to GABA A receptors in the parabrachial nucleus produces a strong dose-dependent (ie, voracious) increase in food consumption. Hunger level and degree of satiety has no effect on BZD-induced food intake. So, it appears that the BZDs do not modulate hunger or satiety directly but act specifically to enhance taste and other sensory characteristics of food. By manipulating the stereospecificity of the

TABLE 2 DRUGS USED TO STIMULATE APPETITE

Drug	Dosage
Diazepam	Cats: 0.005–0.4 mg/kg, IV
Oxazepam	Cats: 2 mg, PO, bid
Cyproheptadine	Cats: 1–4 mg, PO, bid
Mirtazapine	Cats: 3.75 mg/cat (¼ of a 15-mg tablet), PO, every 3 days
	Dogs: ¼ of a 15-mg tablet for dogs <7 kg, ½ of a 15-mg tablet for dogs 8–15 kg, 15 mg for dogs 16–30 kg, 30 mg for dogs >30 kg; no higher than 30 mg per dog
Megestrol acetate	Dogs: 0.5-1 mg/kg/day, PO
Prednisone/prednisolone	1 mg/kg, PO, every other day

BZD drugs, appetite-selective partial agonist compounds have been developed that have actions disassociated from the other major effects of full agonists (eg, amnesia, sedation, incoordination, anxiolysis). Likewise, inverse agonists of the BZD receptors reduce food consumption. BZD receptor antagonists block the appetite-simulating effects of the full or partial agonists, as well as the appetite-suppressive effects of the inverse agonists. So, there is a bidirectional control of food intake mediated by a common subset of BZD receptors. Levels of food intake, ranging from voracious consumption at one extreme to complete anorexia at the other, with every level in between, can be achieved by the relative concentration of agonists and inverse agonists binding to those BZD receptors specifically involved in the control of appetite. **Diazepam** is an appetite stimulant when administered IV to cats. If responsive, cats begin eating within a few seconds of IV administration, so palatable food should be available before injection. **Oxazepam**, a metabolite of diazepam, can be given orally to cats. Diazepam is the more effective appetite stimulant but also causes a greater sedative effect than oxazepam.

Cyproheptadine is an antihistamine with serotonin-antagonist action used clinically in cats as an appetite stimulant. It acts as a 5-HT2 receptor antagonist. The lateral hypothalamus normally excretes endogenous opiates, which stimulate eating. The release of these endogenous opiates is inhibited by serotonin and cholecystokinin release, thus inhibiting eating. Cats are very sensitive to changes in serotonin concentrations, so serotonin antagonists are very potent in cats. CNS excitement and aggressive behavior may occur in some cats.

Mirtazapine is an antidepressant used to treat moderate to severe depression in people. Mirtazapine is not a serotonin or norepinephrine reuptake inhibitor (SSRIs such as fluoxetine are noted to decrease appetite). It is an antagonist of presynaptic α_2-adrenergic autoreceptors and heteroreceptors on both norepinephrine and serotonin (5-HT) presynaptic axons, plus is a potent antagonist of postsynaptic 5-HT2 and 5-HT3 receptors. This mechanism of action maintains equivalent antidepressant efficacy but minimizes many of the adverse effects common to both tricyclic antidepressants and SSRIs. Because of its unique pharmacologic profile, mirtazapine usually does not cause anticholinergic effects, serotonin-related adverse effects, or adrenergic adverse effects (orthostatic hypotension and sexual dysfunction). Antihistaminic drowsiness is a common effect. Mirtazapine is used for disease conditions in which inappetance and nausea go together, such as in the treatment of GI disease or liver or kidney disease. Mirtazapine can also be used to alleviate the nausea and appetite loss that accompanies chemotherapy. α-Adrenergic receptors in the chemoreceptor trigger zone are important in inducing emesis in cats. Clinically, mirtazapine is an effective appetite stimulant and antiemetic for cats with chronic kidney disease and appears to be a useful adjunct in nutritional management of these cats. There is little pharmacokinetic information on mirtazapine in dogs and cats, but mirtazapine shows sexual effects in hepatic metabolism in people, so it is likely there is similar variation in metabolism in dogs and cats and the potential for variation in efficacy.

Mirtazapine is typically given once a day to dogs and twice a week to cats. It should be used with caution in dogs and cats with severe liver or kidney disease, because mirtazapine clearance will be reduced. In cats and small dogs, it is difficult to reduce the dose, because the smallest tablet manufactured cannot be accurately cut much smaller than the regular dosing schedule allows. In this situation, a compounding pharmacy could be employed to create a lower dose, or the dosing schedule can be extended. This is especially important for cats with liver disease.

Megestrol acetate is a synthetic progestin. It has significant antiestrogen and glucocorticoid activity, with resulting adrenal suppression. It is used to stimulate appetite and promote weight gain in people with cancer and cachexia (related to acquired immunodeficiency syndrome) and may have a similar effect in anorectic cats and dogs. Megestrol acetate is contraindicated in pregnant animals and in animals with uterine disease, diabetes mellitus, or mammary neoplasia. In cats, megestrol acetate can induce a profound adrenocortical suppression, adrenal atrophy, and diabetes mellitus, which may or may not be reversible. Toxicity is less of a problem in dogs.

Other drugs used as appetite stimulants include **B vitamins** and **glucocorticoids**. B vitamin preparations are administered orally and parenterally to debilitated animals, especially horses, to promote appetite. Glucocorticoids increase gluconeogenesis and antagonize insulin for an overall hyperglycemic effect. Appetite is stimulated by the steroid-induced euphoria. Continued use of glucocorticoids results in catabolic effects, as skeletal muscle and collage proteins are broken down to provide the precursors for gluconeogenesis.

DRUGS TO CONTROL OR STIMULATE VOMITING

Animals possess an arsenal of special abilities for survival, many of which are used for food consumption. Ingesting food can lead to exposure of internal organs to possible food-related disorders, including viral and bacterial infection, toxins, and allergens. Smell and taste are not always effective in determining the quality of food, so nausea, vomiting, and diarrhea are additional mechanisms of defense of the GI system.

Humorally mediated emesis results from emetogenic substances in the systemic circulation that activate the chemoreceptor trigger zone (CRTZ) in the area postrema. The CRTZ lies outside the blood-brain barrier. Neurally mediated emesis results from activation of an afferent neural pathway typically coming from the abdominal viscera and synapsing at one or more nuclei in the emetic center. Most pharmacologic interventions focus on the humoral pathway of emesis, based on neurotransmitter interactions at the CRTZ. The neural pathway has received less emphasis, even though it is a much more important pathway.

Nausea is an aversive experience that often accompanies emesis; it is a distinct perception, different from pain or stress. Nausea is more difficult to treat than emesis using antiemetic drugs. This became apparent with the excellent control of drug-induced emesis from cancer chemotherapy, but human patients still experience nausea. This suggests that nausea and vomiting are separate physiologic processes.

Motion-induced emesis appears to have a very early evolutionary origin, because it is present in most animal models of emesis. Motion sickness is thought to result from sensory conflict regarding the body's position in space, yet there is no satisfactory theory as to why people and animals have this mechanism in the first place.

Nausea and vomiting, as defense systems of the GI tract, by necessity must have a low threshold for activation. Cats are well known for their tendency to vomit, particularly when attempting to dislodge hairballs from the throat or upper GI tract. Chronic vomiting in cats may indicate underlying thyroid, liver, or kidney dysfunction and should be investigated. Dogs also vomit often (frequently after eating grass) and often eat their own vomit.

Neurotransmitters of Emesis: Acetylcholine (muscarinic receptors) and substance P (NK-1 receptors) act on the emetic center. The CRTZ is stimulated by dopamine (D2 receptors), α_2-adrenergic drugs (NE receptors), serotonin (5-HT3 receptors), acetylcholine (M1 receptors), enkephalins, and histamine (H1 and H2 receptors).

α-Adrenergic receptors in the CRTZ are important in inducing emesis in cats. α_2-Adrenergic agonists (eg, xylazine) are more potent emetics in cats than in dogs. 5-HT1A antagonists (eg, buspirone) and α_2-adrenergic antagonists (eg, acepromazine, yohimbine, mirtazapine) suppress vomiting in cats.

CRTZ D2 dopamine receptors are not as important in mediating humoral emesis in cats as they are in dogs. Apomorphine, a D2 dopamine receptor agonist is a more reliable emetic in dogs than cats, and D2 dopamine receptor antagonists (eg, metoclopramide) are not very effective antiemetic drugs in cats.

Histamine H1 and H2 receptors are found in the CRTZ of dogs but not cats. Histamine is a potent emetic in dogs but not cats, and H1 antagonists (eg, diphenhydramine) are ineffective for motion sickness in cats.

Muscarinic M1 receptors are found in the vestibular apparatus of cats. Mixed M1/M2 antagonists (eg, atropine) inhibit motion sickness in cats.

Substance P binds to NK-1 receptors, which are found in the gut and the emetic center of the CNS. Substance P induces emesis, and selective substance P antagonists (eg, maropitant) are potent antiemetics in both dogs and cats with a broad spectrum of activity against a variety of emetic stimuli.

Emetic Drugs: Emetic drugs are usually administered in emergency situations after ingestion of a toxin (*see* TABLE 3). They generally remove <80% of the stomach contents. The most reliable emetic drugs act centrally to stimulate the vomiting center, either directly or via the CRTZ.

Apomorphine is an opioid drug that acts as a potent central dopamine agonist to directly stimulate the CRTZ. Therefore, it is less effective in cats than in dogs. It can be administered PO, IV, or SC; the IM route is not as effective. It can also be applied directly to conjunctival and gingival

TABLE 3 EMETIC DRUGS

Drug	Dosage
Apomorphine	Dogs: 4 mg/kg, PO; 0.02 mg/kg, IV; 0.3 mg/kg, SC; 0.25 mg in the conjunctival sac
Xylazine	Cats: 0.4–0.5 mg/kg, IV or IM
Hydrogen peroxide	Dogs: 5–10 mL, PO

membranes, using the tablet formulation, which can easily be removed once emesis is initiated. Vomiting usually occurs in 5–10 min. Although apomorphine directly stimulates the CRTZ, it has a depressant effect on the emetic center. Therefore, if the first dose does not induce emesis, additional doses are not helpful. Because the vestibular apparatus may also be involved in apomorphine-induced vomiting, sedate and motionless animals will not vomit as readily as active animals. Excitement that results from apomorphine in cats can be treated with the opioid antagonist naloxone.

Xylazine is an α_2-adrenergic agonist used primarily for its sedative and analgesic action. It is a reliable emetic, particularly in cats, in which it stimulates the CRTZ. Because xylazine can produce profound sedation and hypotension, animals should be closely monitored after administration.

Hydrogen peroxide (3%) applied to the back of the pharynx stimulates vomiting via the ninth cranial nerve. Small doses (5–10 mL) of hydrogen peroxide can be administered via oral syringe until emesis occurs. It should be administered cautiously, especially in cats, because aspiration of hydrogen peroxide foam causes severe aspiration pneumonia. When small amounts are administered, 3% hydrogen peroxide is relatively nontoxic. Stronger concentrations (eg, hair dye peroxide) are more toxic.

Other products have been used but are not recommended to induce emesis in dogs and cats. **Syrup of ipecac** is no longer recommended for "home use" in people or animals. The active ingredient is emetine, a toxic alkaloid, which produces vomiting by acting as a stomach irritant. If repeated use fails to induce emesis, then gastric lavage is necessary to remove the emetine to prevent additional toxicosis. Although sometimes suggested, **sodium chloride (salt)** and ***powdered mustard*** *should not* be used. Mustard is rarely effective and can be inhaled and cause lung damage, whereas salt toxicity can easily occur if overdosed and can result in fatal cerebral edema.

Antiemetic Drugs: Protracted vomiting is physically exhausting and can cause dehydration, acid-base and electrolyte disturbances, and aspiration pneumonia. Antiemetic drugs are used to control excessive vomiting once an etiologic diagnosis has been made, to prevent motion sickness and psychogenic vomiting, and to control emesis from radiation and chemotherapy (*see* TABLE 4). Antiemetics may act peripherally to reduce afferent input from receptors or to inhibit efferent components of the vomiting reflex response. They may also act centrally to block stimulation of the CRTZ and emetic center.

The **phenothiazine tranquilizers** are α_2-adrenergic antagonists and antagonize the CNS stimulatory effects of dopamine and decrease vomiting from a variety of causes, including motion sickness in cats. These drugs also have antihistaminic and weak anticholinergic action. Phenothiazine tranquilizers used as antiemetics include acepromazine, chlorpromazine, and prochlorperazine. Potential adverse effects include hypotension due to α-adrenergic blockade, excessive sedation, extrapyramidal signs, and a lowering of the seizure threshold in animals with epilepsy. Extrapyramidal signs can be counteracted with an antihistamine (eg, diphenhydramine).

The **anticholinergic drugs** block cholinergic afferent pathways from the GI tract and the vestibular system to the vomiting center. Alone, they are less effective than the other emetics. Aminopentamide is approved for use in dogs and cats in the USA as an injectable formulation and oral tablets. It should be more efficacious in the treatment of motion sickness in cats than in dogs, because muscarinic M1 receptors are found in the vestibular apparatus of cats. Aminopentamide has low efficacy for other causes of vomiting.

The **antihistamines** can block both cholinergic and histaminic nerve transmission responsible for transmission of the vestibular stimulus to the vomiting center of

TABLE 4 ANTIEMETIC DRUGS

Drug	Dosage
Acepromazine	0.025–0.2 mg/kg, IV, IM, SC, maximum 3 mg; 1–3 mg/kg, PO
Chlorpromazine	0.5 mg/kg, IV, IM, SC, tid-qid
Prochlorperazine	0.1 mg/kg, IM, tid-qid; 1 mg/kg, PO, bid
Aminopentamide	0.022 mg/kg, PO, SC, or IM, bid-tid
Dimenhydrinate	4–8 mg/kg, PO, tid
Diphenhydramine	2–4 mg/kg, PO, tid
Butorphanol	0.2–0.4 mg/kg, IM, once to twice daily
Metoclopramide	0.1–0.5 mg/kg, IM, SC, or PO, tid; 0.01–0.02 mg/kg/hr, IV infusion
Ondansetron	0.1–0.2 mg/kg, PO, once to twice daily; 0.1–0.15 mg/kg, IV, bid-tid
Granisetron	0.5–1 mg/kg, PO, bid; 0.1–0.15 mg/kg, IV, bid-tid
Dolasetron	0.6–1 mg/kg/day, IV
Maropitant	2 mg/kg, PO or 1 mg/kg/day, SC, for up to 5 days (acute vomiting); 8 mg/kg/day, PO, for up to 2 days (motion sickness)

dogs. The commonly used histamine (H1) blocking drugs are diphenhydramine and dimenhydrinate (diphenhydramine plus 8-chlorotheophylline). They may cause mild sedation, especially diphenhydramine, but paradoxical CNS stimulation may also occur, presumably from anticholinergic effects.

Metoclopramide exerts its antiemetic effects via three mechanisms. At low doses, it inhibits dopaminergic transmission in the CNS, whereas at high doses, it inhibits serotonin receptors in the CRTZ. Peripherally, metoclopramide increases gastric and upper duodenal emptying. Metoclopramide is a useful antiemetic for dogs. Because CRTZ D2 dopamine receptors are not very important in mediating humoral emesis in cats, metoclopramide is less effective in cats than in dogs. It is used to control emesis induced by chemotherapy, nausea and vomiting associated with delayed gastric emptying, reflux gastritis, and viral enteritis. There is tremendous individual variability in metoclopramide pharmacokinetics, and oral bioavailability is only ~50% because of a significant first-pass effect. At high doses or with rapid IV administration, metoclopramide causes CNS excitement by dopamine antagonism (similar to the phenothiazine tranquilizers). Extrapyramidal signs can be counteracted with an antihistamine such as diphenhydramine. Metoclopramide should not be administered if a GI obstruction or perforation is suspected.

The **serotonin antagonists** ondansetron, granisetron, and dolasetron are specific inhibitors of serotonin subtype 3 receptors in the CRTZ. These receptors are located peripherally on vagal nerve terminals and centrally in the area postrema of the brain. Cytotoxic drugs and radiation damage the GI mucosa, causing release of serotonin. These are the most effective antiemetics used in people undergoing radiation and chemotherapy, and they have been used in cats and dogs receiving chemotherapy. Although very effective at controlling vomiting associated with chemotherapy and drug-induced vomiting, these drugs do not prevent or relieve nausea, which may be more debilitating than vomiting. They are not effective for emesis caused by motion sickness. All serotonin subtype 3 antagonists have been associated with prolongation of the QT interval in people. Adverse effects of dolasetron include ECG changes (PR and QT prolongation, QRS widening) caused by dolasetron metabolites that block sodium channels.

Butorphanol is an effective antiemetic for dogs receiving cisplatin chemotherapy. It causes only mild sedation. It is believed to exert its antiemetic effect directly on the vomiting center.

Maropitant is a neurokinin 1 (NK-1) receptor antagonist approved to treat and prevent emesis in dogs and cats. Substance P is a regulatory peptide that binds to the NK-1 receptors and induces emesis. NK-1 receptor antagonists are believed to provide antiemetic activity by suppressing activity at the nucleus of the solitary tract, where vagal afferents from the GI tract converge with inputs from the CRTZ and other regions of the brain involved in the control and initiation of emesis. Despite its selectivity for the NK-1 receptor, maropitant blocks apomorphine, cisplatin, and syrup of ipecac–induced vomiting in dogs, which suggests that activation of the nucleus of the solitary tract is a final common step in the initiation of emesis. Despite being very effective antiemetics in people, NK-1 receptor antagonists have little effect on chemotherapy-associated nausea in people or hydromorphone-induced nausea in dogs.

Maropitant injectable is approved for vomiting in cats ≥16 wk old and acute vomiting in dogs ≥8 wk old at 1 mg/kg/day. Maropitant tablets are approved for acute vomiting in dogs ≥8 wk old (2 mg/kg), and to prevent vomiting due to motion sickness in dogs ≥16 wk older (8 mg/kg). Dogs should not be fed for 1 hr before giving maropitant. The best time to give maropitant is 2 hr before travelling, with a small amount of food. The tablets should not be wrapped tightly in fatty food such as cheese or meat, because this may keep the tablets from dissolving and delay the effect of maropitant.

Adverse effects are rare with maropitant, but the most common ones are excessive drooling, lethargy, lack of appetite, and diarrhea. Maropitant injections may also cause a stinging sensation; this can be minimized by keeping the injectable solution refrigerated and, once the drug is drawn up, injecting right away at the refrigerated temperature. A few dogs may vomit after treatment. Giving maropitant with a small amount of food will help avoid this.

THERAPY OF GASTROINTESTINAL ULCERS

GI ulceration is a common problem in small and large animals, in association with physiologic stress (endogenous cortisol), dietary management, or as a sequela of administration of ulcerogenic drugs (*see* p 393 and *see* p 218). *Helicobacter* organisms, the most frequent cause of ulcers in people, appear to be involved in some cases of gastritis in animals (*see* p 394). Antiulcerative drugs include antagonists that interact with stimulatory receptors (histamine H_2-receptor antagonists, muscarinic receptor antagonists, and gastrin receptor antagonists), agonists that interact with inhibitory receptors (somatostatin and prostaglandin E analogues), and irreversible inhibitors of H^+/K^+-ATPase (proton pump inhibitors). Antiulcerative drugs are listed in TABLE 5.

TABLE 5 ANTIULCERATIVE DRUGS

Drug	Dosage
Antacids	2–10 mL, PO, every 2–4 hr
Sucralfate	Cats: 250 mg, bid-tid
	Dogs: 500 mg to 1 g, tid-qid
	Foals: 1–2 g, qid
Cimetidine	Dogs: 5–10 mg/kg, PO, qid
	Horses: 4 mg/kg, IV, bid; 18 mg/kg, PO, bid
Ranitidine	Dogs: 0.5 mg/kg, PO, SC, or IV, bid
	Horses: 1.3 mg/kg, IV, bid; 11 mg/kg, PO, bid
Famotidine	Dogs: 0.5–1 mg/kg/day, PO or IV
	Horses: 0.4 mg/kg, IV, bid; 3 mg/kg, PO, bid
Omeprazole	Dogs: 0.5–1 mg/kg/day, PO
	Horses: 4 mg/kg/day, PO, for treatment; 2 mg/kg/day, PO, to prevent recurrence
Misoprostol	Dogs: 2–5 mcg/kg, PO, tid-qid

Antacids: The common antacids are bases of aluminum, magnesium, or calcium (aluminum hydroxide, magnesium oxide or hydroxide, and calcium carbonate). These drugs neutralize stomach acid to form water and a neutral salt. They are usually not absorbed systemically. In addition to their acid-neutralizing ability, antacids decrease pepsin activity, binding to bile acids in the stomach and stimulating local prostaglandin (PGE_1) production. Over-the-counter antacid preparations are combinations of magnesium hydroxide and aluminum hydroxide; such combinations optimize the buffering capabilities of each compound and balance the constipating effect (from aluminum hydroxide) and the laxative effect (from magnesium hydroxide). Up to 20% of the magnesium can be absorbed after administration PO and can cause hypermagnesemia in animals with renal insufficiency. Antacids frequently interfere with the GI absorption of concurrently administered drugs (eg, digoxin, tetracyclines, fluoroquinolones). Aluminum-containing antacids impair absorption of phosphate. Because they are difficult to administer and require frequent dosing, they are not as popular as newer therapies.

Sucralfate: Sucralfate is an antiulcerative drug that has a cytoprotective effect on GI mucosa. It disassociates in the acid environment of the stomach to sucrose octasulfate and aluminum hydroxide. Sucrose octasulfate polymerizes to a viscous, sticky substance that creates a protective effect by binding to ulcerated mucosa. This prevents "back diffusion" of hydrogen ions, inactivates pepsin, and adsorbs bile acid. In addition, sucralfate increases the mucosal synthesis of prostaglandins, which have a cytoprotective role. Because sucralfate is not absorbed, it causes virtually no adverse effects. Dosage regimens are extrapolated from human dosages. Although sucralfate is frequently administered to horses and small animals as an ulcer preventive, there is little evidence of efficacy in animals, and it may prevent the absorption of truly useful drugs. Animals in renal failure may have increased aluminum absorption.

H_2-Receptor Antagonists: **Cimetidine**, **ranitidine**, and **famotidine** are the commonly used H_2-receptor antagonists. Ranitidine is 3–13 times as potent on a molar basis as cimetidine in inhibiting gastric acid secretion. Famotidine is 20–150 times as potent as cimetidine. In people, food tends to delay the absorption of cimetidine, has minimal effect on ranitidine, and slightly enhances absorption of famotidine. Some evidence suggests that cimetidine strengthens the gastric mucosal defenses against ulceration and enhances cytoprotection. Cimetidine reduces the metabolism of other drugs (warfarin, phenytoin, lidocaine, metronidazole, theophylline) by inhibiting hepatic microsomal enzyme systems. Ranitidine interacts differently than cimetidine and only minimally (10%) inhibits hepatic metabolism of some drugs. Famotidine seems to have no effect on metabolism of other drugs. Antacids should be given 1 hr before or after cimetidine to avoid interactions. Famotidine may be given with antacids; ranitidine may be given with low doses of antacids. Sucralfate may alter absorption of cimetidine and ranitidine.

Cimetidine suppresses gastric acid secretion in dogs for 3–5 hr. Because ranitidine has a longer elimination half-life, it suppresses acid for up to 8 hr and it may be administered less frequently. Famotidine can be administered once a day. Oral bioavailability in horses for these drugs is only 10%–30%, so large oral doses must be administered.

Proton Pump Inhibitors: Proton pump inhibitors (PPIs) irreversibly block the H^+/K^+-ATPase proton pump of the gastric parietal cell. They are given in an inactive form, which is neutrally charged (lipophilic) and readily crosses cell membranes into intracellular compartments (like the parietal cell canaliculus) that have acidic environments. The inactive drug is protonated, rearranges into its active form, and irreversibly binds to and deactivates the proton pump. The most widely used PPI is **omeprazole**. In dogs and horses, a single dose of omeprazole inhibits acid secretion for 3–4 days, despite a relatively short plasma half-life. This is because of accumulation of the drug in parietal cell canaliculi and the irreversible nature of proton pump inhibition. A specific equine product has been developed, because oral bioavailability of the human omeprazole formulation or compounded formulations is poor in horses. Although ulcers in horses will heal while on omeprazole therapy, they tend to recur once therapy is discontinued. Human formulations are used in dogs and cats. In people, adverse effects from suppression of gastric acid secretion include hypergastrinemia, which causes mucosal cell hyperplasia, hypertrophy of the gastric rugae, and eventually development of carcinoids. It has also been associated with acute renal failure and disorders of calcium homeostasis, including fractures associated with longterm use. Studies in rodents show that PPIs can exacerbate NSAID-induced intestinal damage from significant shifts in enteric microbial populations. Prevention or reversal of this dysbiosis may be an important clinical consideration for reducing the incidence and severity of NSAID enteropathy. Therefore, omeprazole is contraindicated for chronic therapy. Omeprazole is also a microsomal enzyme inhibitor (to a similar extent as cimetidine). For animals that cannot receive oral medications, IV injectable formulations approved for people (pantoprazole and esomeprazole) can be considered for use.

Acid Rebound: Acid rebound is an increase in gastric acid secretion above pretreatment levels after discontinuation of antiulcer therapy. Rebound is reported after the use of histamine H_2-receptor antagonists and PPIs and is thought to be due to increased serum gastrin and/or upregulation of the H_2-receptors. An increased gastrin level, or hypergastrinemia, is a secondary effect that occurs during chronic inhibition of gastric acid secretion, such as with longterm antiulcer therapy. Gastrin is the primary regulator of gastric acid secretion, which is mediated by histamine released by the enterochromaffin-like (ECL) cell. Increased plasma gastrin stimulates and upregulates ECL cells to produce and release more histamine to stimulate parietal cells. In addition, an increase in parietal cell mass may occur with the chronic use of H_2-blockers or PPIs, and this may be an additional mechanism for increased acid secretion that occurs after discontinuation of therapy.

Misoprostol: Misoprostol is a synthetic prostaglandin E_1 analogue used in dogs to reduce the risk of GI ulcers induced by chronic NSAID therapy. Misoprostol suppresses gastric acid secretion by inhibiting the activation of histamine-sensitive adenylate cyclase. It has a cytoprotective effect from stimulation of bicarbonate and mucus secretion, increased mucosal blood flow, decreased vascular permeability, and increased cellular proliferation and migration. Misoprostol is clinically effective in preventing GI bleeding and ulceration from NSAID therapy but not from methylprednisolone sodium succinate, and it is less efficacious than H_2-receptor antagonists or PPIs for treatment of ulcers. Adverse effects of misoprostol are mainly limited to diarrhea and flatulence. Magnesium-containing antacids may aggravate the diarrhea. Misoprostol is contraindicated in pregnant dogs, because it can induce abortion.

DRUGS USED IN TREATMENT OF DIARRHEA

Therapy for diarrhea includes fluids, electrolyte replacement, maintenance of acid/base balance, and control of discomfort. Antiparasitic drugs or dietary therapy can also play an important role in treatment of some types of diarrhea. Additional therapy may include intestinal protectants, motility modifiers, antimicrobials, anti-inflammatory drugs, and antitoxins (*see* TABLE 6).

TABLE 6 ANTIDIARRHEAL DRUGS

Drug	Dosage
Kaolin-pectin	1–2 mL/kg, PO, qid
Activated charcoal	2–8 g/kg, PO
Bismuth subsalicylate	1–3 mL/kg/day in divided doses, PO
Aminopentamide	0.1–0.4 mg, IM, SC, or PO, bid
Isopropamide	0.2–1 mg/kg, PO, bid
Propantheline	0.25–0.5 mg/kg, PO, bid-tid
Paregoric	0.06 mg/kg, PO, tid
Diphenoxylate	0.05–0.1 mg/kg, PO, qid
Loperamide	0.08 mg/kg, PO, tid-qid

Mucosal Protectants and Adsorbents: **Kaolin-pectin** formulations are popular for symptomatic therapy of diarrhea. Kaolin is a form of aluminum silicate, and pectin is a carbohydrate extracted from the rind of citrus fruits. The manufacturers claim that kaolin-pectin acts as a demulcent and adsorbent in the treatment of diarrhea. This action is claimed to be related to the binding of bacterial toxins (endotoxins and enterotoxins) in the GI tract. However, clinical studies have not demonstrated any benefit from administration of kaolin-pectin. It may change the consistency of the feces but neither decreases the fluid or electrolyte loss nor shortens the duration of illness. Nevertheless, it is often administered to small animals, foals, calves, lambs, and kids. Kaolin-pectin products may adsorb or bind other drugs administered PO and reduce bioavailability.

Activated charcoal is derived from wood, peat, coconut, or pecan shells. The material is heated and treated in such a way that many large pores are formed, which dramatically increases the internal surface area. Activated charcoal is available in a variety of pore sizes. The formulations sold for drug and toxicant adsorption typically have pore sizes of 10–20 Å. Activated charcoal is very effective for adsorbing bacterial enterotoxins and endotoxins that cause some types of diarrhea. It also adsorbs many drugs and toxins and prevents GI absorption, so it is a common nonspecific treatment for intoxications. Activated charcoal is not absorbed, so overdose is not a problem.

Although other "mucosal protectants" have questionable efficacy, **bismuth subsalicylate** is considered by many human gastroenterologists to be the symptomatic treatment of choice for acute diarrhea. Its efficacy has been proved in controlled clinical trials in people with acute diarrhea (enterotoxigenic *Escherichia coli* or "traveller's diarrhea"). Bismuth adsorbs bacterial enterotoxins and endotoxins and has a GI protective effect. The salicylate component has antiprostaglandin activity. Practically all of the salicylate is absorbed systemically when administered to dogs and cats. Some animals may dislike the taste of bismuth subsalicylate, and owners should be warned that it will turn the feces black. This may interfere with evaluating the feces for hemorrhage. Salicylate toxicosis is possible, especially in cats.

Motility-modifying Drugs: **Anticholinergic drugs** are common ingredients in antidiarrheal preparations, because they significantly decrease intestinal motility and secretions. Their parasympatholytic effects decrease segmental and propulsive intestinal smooth muscle contractions and relax spasms of smooth muscle. Although they do not alter the course of the disease, anticholinergic drugs decrease the urgency associated with some forms of diarrhea in small animals, the amount of fluid secreted into the intestine, and abdominal cramping associated with hypermotility. Because few of the types of diarrhea seen in animals can be classified as "hypermotile," use of anticholinergic drugs is limited in veterinary medicine. Intestinal motility is already impaired in many animals with diarrhea, and these drugs may actually worsen the diarrhea. The anticholinergic drugs also have profound systemic pharmacologic effects. If they are administered in sufficient doses to affect intestinal motility, possible adverse effects include severe ileus, xerostomia, urine retention, cycloplegia, tachycardia, and CNS excitement. Chronic administration may lead to serious intestinal atony.

Atropine is the best known anticholinergic drug, but because it has many other systemic effects, it is not ordinarily used for an antidiarrheal effect. To avoid CNS excitement, quaternary amines such as aminopentamide, isopropamide, and propantheline are preferred, because they do not cross the blood-brain barrier readily.

Hyoscine butylbromide is an antispasmodic and anticholinergic drug that relaxes the smooth muscle of the GI tract. It is approved for treatment of uncomplicated, spasmodic colic in horses. Initial relief of colic pain is seen within 5–10 minutes, with a duration of action of 3–4 hr. Because of its parasympatholytic effects, it causes transient tachycardia; therefore, heart rate monitoring is not an effective indicator of response to treatment for up to 30 min after treatment. It will also decrease gut sounds for 30 min after administration. Rectal relaxation will also make rectal palpation easier. It may also be beneficial in cases of choke, and it will relieve acute bronchoconstriction in horses with recurrent airway obstruction. Hyoscine butylbromide can be administered concurrently with NSAIDs and sedatives.

Opiates have both antisecretory and antimotility effects by action on the μ (mu) and δ (delta) receptors of the GI tract. They decrease propulsive intestinal contractions and increase segmentation for an overall constipating effect. They also increase GI sphincter tone. There is some evidence that opiates inhibit colonic motor activity in horses. In addition to affecting motility, opiates stimulate absorption of fluid, electrolytes, and glucose. Their effects on secretory diarrhea are probably related to inhibition of calcium influx and decreased calmodulin activity. They are frequently used for treatment of diarrhea in dogs, but their use in cats is controversial because they may cause excitement. The constipating effects of morphine and codeine have been known for many years, but they are not used clinically as antidiarrheal drugs. Paregoric is a tincture of opium product and a controlled substance (5 mL of paregoric corresponds to ~2 mg of morphine). Diphenoxylate and loperamide are two synthetic opiates that have specific action on the GI tract without causing other systemic effects. They have been used in small animals and large animal neonates. Diphenoxylate is a controlled substance in a formulation that contains atropine to discourage abuse; at therapeutic doses, there is no effect from the atropine. Opiates can have potent effects on the GI tract and should be used cautiously. Loperamide is available over-the-counter.

Loperamide should not be used in dog breeds known to be sensitive to ivermectin (Collies, Australian Shepherds, Old English Sheepdogs) without genetic testing. These dogs may have a gene mutation (ABCB-1 gene deletion) that causes a functional defect in P-glycoprotein, which controls drug movement in many tissues. In people and genetically normal dogs, large doses of loperamide do not cause the typical CNS effects of opioids, because loperamide does not achieve high concentrations within the CNS because of P-glycoprotein–mediated efflux of loperamide. Dogs with the ABCB-1 gene deletion show signs of ptyalism, panting, ataxia, and recumbency at doses of loperamide that do not affect healthy dogs. These drugs are contraindicated in infectious diarrhea, because slowing GI transit time may increase the absorption of bacterial toxins. In dogs, constipation and bloat are the most common adverse effects. Potentially, paralytic ileus, toxic megacolon, pancreatitis, and CNS effects can develop, especially in cats.

Antimicrobial Therapy: The efficacy of antimicrobials in the therapy of diarrhea is unknown or unproved in most clinical situations. In most cases of diarrhea in small animals, a bacterial *etiology is not identified*. In large animals, antimicrobial therapy has not been shown to alter the course of bacterial enteritis, and in some cases, is thought to perpetuate the disease by producing "carrier" animals (eg, salmonellosis). Nonabsorbed antimicrobials are frequently combined with motility modifiers, adsorbents, and intestinal protectants in some preparations. Many of these combinations are irrational. Antimicrobials frequently are a treatment for diarrhea in animals, but there are few conditions that have a known etiology for which antimicrobial therapy is indicated. *Campylobacter* enteritis, from infection with *Campylobacter jejuni*, is seen in cats and dogs and can be zoonotic. Treatment alleviates clinical signs, but animals usually remain carriers. Suggested antimicrobial therapy includes erythromycin, enrofloxacin, clindamycin, tylosin, tetracycline, or chloramphenicol. Intestinal bacterial overgrowth is usually due to *Escherichia coli* or *Clostridium* spp, so therapy is initiated with an oral drug effective in the GI lumen with anaerobic activity (eg, metronidazole, amoxicillin, ampicillin, tylosin, or clindamycin). Equine monocytic ehrlichiosis (*see* p 283) is caused by the rickettsial organism *Neorickettsia (Ehrlichia) risticii* but clinically resembles salmonellosis. Treatment of choice is IV oxytetracycline. Oral doxycycline can be used in mildly affected horses.

Enteritis from a variety of pathogens is common in young animals. When integrity of the intestinal mucosa is lost, septicemia or endotoxemia is likely. Signs of sepsis include severe bloody diarrhea, fever, scleral injection, dehydration, and alteration in the leukogram (early leukopenia in endotoxic shock, followed by leukocytosis). If septicemia or endotoxemia is suspected, systemic antimicrobials are warranted along with NSAIDs. Neonates with diarrhea deteriorate rapidly before culture and sensitivity results are available. Therefore, broad-spectrum antimicrobial therapy should be initiated. Suggested antimicrobials (depending on species) include fluoroquinolones, a penicillin or cephalosporin plus an aminoglycoside (gentamicin, amikacin), ampicillin or amoxicillin, tetracyclines, potentiated sulfonamides, chloramphenicol, or florfenicol. In septic animals, GI absorption is likely to be altered, so parenteral administration is preferred.

Nonsteroidal Anti-inflammatory Drugs (NSAIDs): The antiprostaglandin activity of NSAIDs may be beneficial with some types of diarrhea and may be important in treatment of septicemia or endotoxemia. Prostaglandins are important intracellular messengers for stimulating hypersecretion by the intestinal mucosa, possibly by stimulating an increase in cAMP. Antiprostaglandin drugs may directly inhibit fluid and electrolyte hypersecretion by the intestinal cells. NSAIDs should be administered cautiously, because they have adverse GI, hepatic, and renal effects.

DRUGS USED IN TREATMENT OF CHRONIC COLITIS

The specific cause of chronic colitis in animals is frequently unknown; therefore, it is difficult to prescribe a specific treatment for the underlying disorder (*see* TABLE 7). Colitis is often classified as plasmacytic/ lymphocytic, eosinophilic, histiocytic, or granulomatous. The goal of colitis therapy is to restore normal intestinal motility and to relieve inflammation, spasm, or ulceration. In small animals, dietary therapy is a major component of therapy for chronic colitis (*see* p 377).

Sulfasalazine is composed of sulfapyridine and 5-aminosalicylic acid (mesalamine) joined by an azo bond. The bond is broken by bacteria in the colon to release the two drugs. The sulfonamide component is absorbed into the circulation, whereas the salicylic acid component is active locally in the GI tract. Less than half of the salicylate component is absorbed systemically. Clinical efficacy appears to be primarily due to the anti-inflammatory effect of the salicylate component. There is evidence for antilipoxygenase activity, decreased interleukin-1, decreased prostaglandin synthesis, and oxygen radical scavenging activity. Sulfasalazine is commonly used in small animals in the therapy of ulcerative or idiopathic colitis or of plasmacytic-lymphocytic colitis once dietary causes have been excluded.

Because the salicylate component is only minimally absorbed, its systemic effects are minimal. The sulfonamide component may cause keratoconjunctivitis sicca in dogs, and the salicylate component may cause toxicity in cats. Dosage recommendations for sulfasalazine vary widely, and the dosage is gradually reduced after an initial response. New products have been developed to overcome the difficulty of the 5-aminosalicylic acid reaching the colon and the systemic adverse effects. Mesalamine is a pH-sensitive, coated 5-aminosalicylic acid. The polymer coating prevents release of the active drug until it reaches the colon. Olsalazine consists of two molecules of 5-aminosalicylic acid joined together by an azo bond. Mesalamine is also available as an enema. Rectal administration allows delivery of active drug to the colon. It appears useful in dogs with chemotherapy-induced hemorrhagic colitis or with idiopathic distal proctitis. It may also be useful in dogs with perianal fistulas.

Tylosin is a macrolide antimicrobial used successfully in some animals with colitis. It is commonly administered on a chronic basis as an alternative to sulfasalazine therapy. The mechanism of action is unknown, but it is suspected that its activity against mycoplasmas, spirochetes, and chlamydiae is important. Best results are attained when the powdered form, labeled for use in swine, is mixed with food or added to water. Some animals may find the bitter taste unpalatable.

Metronidazole has fair efficacy against *Giardia*, and it is also efficacious in some cases of diarrhea in which giardiasis was not definitively diagnosed. It is suspected that this efficacy is related to the activity of metronidazole against anaerobic

TABLE 7 DRUGS USED FOR CHRONIC COLITIS

Drug	Dosage
Sulfasalazine	10–30 mg/kg, PO, bid-tid
Tylosin	40–80 mg/kg/day
Metronidazole	10–30 mg/kg, PO, once to three times daily
Prednisone	2–4 mg/kg, PO, every other day
Budesonide	3 mg/m^2/day, PO
Raw linseed oil	1 oz/day in the feed
Azathioprine	50 mg/m^2, PO, daily for 2 wk, then every other day
Chlorambucil	2 mg/m^2, PO, every other day

bacteria. Metronidazole also has an immunosuppressive effect on the GI mucosa by decreasing the cell-mediated response. Adverse neurologic effects have been reported in dogs and cats treated with metronidazole. Diazepam appears effective for treatment of neurotoxicity.

The efficacy of **glucocorticoids** for treating colitis is probably related to their anti-inflammatory and immunosuppressive capabilities. Some cases of colitis may be due to autoantibodies and T lymphocytes directed against colonic epithelial cells. Glucocorticoids suppress the immune reaction and are used when biopsy results suggest eosinophilic or plasmacytic-lymphocytic colitis. They are used in dogs, cats, and horses, often when all other forms of therapy have failed. Immunosuppressive doses of oral prednisone or dexamethasone are usually administered and slowly tapered to every-other-day therapy with the lowest effective dose.

Budesonide is a glucocorticoid used in people to treat asthma, rhinitis, and inflammatory bowel disease. Budesonide has a high affinity for glucocorticoid receptors, high hepatic clearance, and high local and low systemic activity compared with prednisone or dexamethasone. The human formulation of budesonide consists of coated granules with a matrix of ethyl cellulose to target release into the lumen of the ileum or ascending colon. It is not known whether the human budesonide formulation provides release in the same anatomic site in dogs, but it appears clinically effective in some dogs.

N-3 fatty acids have been suggested for therapy in people with ulcerative colitis or Crohn disease. The addition of n-3 fatty acids to the diet makes fewer n-6 fatty acids available for the arachidonic acid cascade. Several formulations are available for small animals, and raw linseed oil may be added to horses' grain for this effect.

Potent immunosuppressive drugs such as **azathioprine** are used to manage some forms of colitis. Azathioprine is metabolized to 6-mercaptopurine, which is immunosuppressive by interfering with nucleic acid synthesis and by impairing lymphocyte proliferation. It may take several weeks or months of therapy for azathioprine to become maximally effective. Cats particularly should be monitored for adverse effects, including myelosuppression, hepatic disease, and acute pancreatic necrosis. Chlorambucil has been used in place of azathioprine in some difficult or refractory cases of feline inflammatory bowel disease. It is too expensive to use in all but very small dogs.

GASTROINTESTINAL PROKINETIC DRUGS

Prokinetic drugs increase the movement of ingested material through the GI tract (*see* TABLE 8). They are useful in the treatment of motility disorders, because they induce coordinated motility patterns. Unfortunately, some prokinetic drugs may produce a number of serious adverse effects that complicate their use.

The enteric nervous system of the GI tract can function independently of the CNS to control bowel function. Because there are no nerve fibers that actually penetrate the intestinal epithelium, the enteric nervous system uses enteroendocrine cells such as the enterochromaffin cells as sensory transducers. More than 95% of the body's serotonin is located in the GI tract, and >90% of that store is in the enterochromaffin cells scattered in the enteric epithelium from the stomach to the colon. The remaining serotonin is located in the enteric nervous system, where 5-HT acts as a neurotransmitter. From the enterochromaffin cells, serotonin is secreted into the lamina propria in high concentrations, which overflow into the portal circulation and intestinal lumen. The effect of serotonin on intestinal activity is coordinated by 5-HT receptor subtypes. The 5-HT1P receptor initiates peristaltic and secretory reflexes, and so far no drugs have been developed to target this specific receptor. The 5-HT3 receptor activates extrinsic sensory nerves and is responsible for the sensation of nausea and induction of vomiting from visceral hypersensitivity. Therefore, specific 5-HT3 antagonists such as ondansetron and granisetron are very effective for treatment of vomiting seen with chemotherapy. Stimulation of the 5-HT4 receptor increases the presynaptic release of acetylcholine and calcitonin gene-related peptide, thereby enhancing neurotransmission. This enhancement promotes propulsive peristaltic and secretory reflexes. Specific 5-HT4 agonists such as cisapride enhance neurotransmission and depend on natural stimuli to evoke peristaltic and secretory reflexes. This makes these drugs very well tolerated, because they do not induce perpetual or excessive motility. It is also the reason for the limitations of these drugs, because they are not effective if enteric nerves have degenerated or become nonfunctional (as in cats with end-stage megacolon).

Metoclopramide is a central dopaminergic antagonist and peripheral 5-HT3 receptor antagonist and 5-HT4 receptor agonist with GI and CNS effects. In the

TABLE 8 PROKINETIC DRUGS

Drug	Dosage
Metoclopramide	Dogs and cats: 0.2–0.5 mg/kg, PO or SC, tid; 0.01–0.02 mg/kg/hr, IV infusion
	Horses: 0.125–0.25 mg/kg, diluted in 500 mL of polyionic solution and administered IV over 60 min
Domperidone	0.1–0.5 mg/kg, IM; 0.5–1 mg/kg, PO
Cisapride	Dogs: 0.1 mg/kg, PO, tid
	Cats: 2.5 mg/cat, tid for cats <5 kg, and 5 mg/cat for cats >5 kg
Erythromycin	0.5–1 mg/kg, PO, bid-tid
Ranitidine	1–2 mg/kg, PO, bid
Nitazidine	2.5–5 mg/kg, PO, bid
Lidocaine	Horses: 1.3 mg/kg, IV, as a bolus followed by a constant-rate infusion of 0.05 mg/kg/min

upper GI tract, metoclopramide increases both acetylcholine release from neurons and cholinergic receptor sensitivity to acetylcholine. Metoclopramide stimulates and coordinates esophageal, gastric, pyloric, and duodenal motor activity. It increases lower esophageal sphincter tone and stimulates gastric contractions, while relaxing the pylorus and duodenum. Inadequate cholinergic activity is incriminated in many GI motility disorders; therefore, metoclopramide should be most effective in diseases in which normal motility is diminished or impaired. Metoclopramide speeds gastric emptying of liquids but may slow the emptying of solids. It is effective in treating postoperative ileus in dogs, which is characterized by decreased GI myoelectric activity and motility. Metoclopramide has little or no effect on colonic motility.

Metoclopramide is primarily indicated for relief of vomiting associated with chemotherapy in dogs, as an antiemetic for dogs with parvoviral enteritis, and for treatment of gastroesophageal reflux and postoperative ileus. GI obstruction, such as intussusception in puppies with parvoviral enteritis, must be excluded before initiating metoclopramide therapy. Its prokinetic action is negated by narcotic analgesics and anticholinergic drugs, such as atropine. Drugs that dissolve or are absorbed in the stomach, such as digoxin, may have reduced absorption. Bioavailability may be increased for drugs absorbed in the small intestine. Because of accelerated food absorption, metoclopramide therapy may increase the insulin dose required in animals with diabetes.

Metoclopramide readily crosses the blood-brain barrier, where dopamine antagonism at the CRTZ produces an antiemetic effect. However, dopamine antagonism in the striatum causes adverse effects known collectively as extrapyramidal signs, which include involuntary muscle spasms, motor restlessness, and inappropriate aggression. Concurrent use of phenothiazine and butyrophenone tranquilizers should be avoided, because they also have central antidopaminergic activity, which increases the potential for extrapyramidal reactions. If recognized in time, the extrapyramidal signs can be reversed by restoring an appropriate dopamine: acetylcholine balance with the anticholinergic action of an antihistamine, such as diphenhydramine hydrochloride given IV at a dosage of 1 mg/kg.

Cisapride is chemically related to metoclopramide, but unlike metoclopramide, it does not cross the blood-brain barrier or have antidopaminergic effects. Therefore, it does not have antiemetic action or cause extrapyramidal effects (extreme CNS stimulation). Cisapride is a serotonin 5-HT4 agonist with some 5-HT3 antagonist activity, so it enhances the release of acetylcholine from postganglionic nerve endings of the myenteric plexus and antagonizes the inhibitory action of serotonin (5-HT3) on the myenteric plexus, resulting in increased GI motility and increased heart rate. Cisapride is more potent and has broader prokinetic activity than metoclopramide, increasing the motility of the colon, as well as that of the esophagus, stomach, and small intestine.

Cisapride is especially useful in animals that experience neurologic effects from metoclopramide. Cisapride is very useful in managing gastric stasis, idiopathic constipation, and postoperative ileus in dogs and cats. Cisapride may be especially useful in managing chronic constipation in cats with megacolon; in many cases, it alleviates or delays the need for subtotal colectomy. Cisapride is also useful in managing cats with hairball problems and in dogs with idiopathic megaesophagus that continue to regurgitate frequently despite a carefully managed, elevated feeding program. In comparative studies of GI motility in people and animals, cisapride is clearly superior to other treatments.

Initially, the only adverse effects reported in people were increased defecation, headache, abdominal pain, and cramping and flatulence; cisapride appeared to be well tolerated in animals. As cisapride became widely used in management of gastroesophageal reflux in people, cases of heart rhythm disorders and deaths were reported to the FDA. These cardiac problems in people were highly associated with concurrent drug therapy or specific underlying conditions. In veterinary medicine, adverse reactions to clinical use of cisapride have not been reported. Cisapride for animals can only be obtained through compounding veterinary pharmacies.

Domperidone is a peripheral dopamine receptor antagonist that has been marketed outside the USA since 1978. It is available in Canada as a 10-mg tablet. Currently, it is available in the USA only as an investigational new drug (1% oral domperidone gel) to treat agalactia in mares due to fescue toxicosis. Domperidone regulates the motility of gastric and small-intestinal smooth muscle and has some effect on esophageal motility. It appears to have very little physiologic effect in the colon. It has antiemetic activity from dopaminergic blockade in the CRTZ. But because very little domperidone crosses the blood-brain barrier, reports of extrapyramidal reactions are rare; however, if a reaction occurs, the treatment is the same as for reactions to metoclopramide. Domperidone failed to enhance gastric emptying in healthy dogs in one study. In other studies, however, domperidone was superior to metoclopramide in stimulating antral contractions in dogs but not cats, and it improved antroduodenal coordination in dogs. Because of its favorable safety profile, domperidone appears to be an attractive alternative to metoclopramide.

Macrolide antibiotics, including erythromycin and clarithromycin, are motilin receptor agonists. They also appear to stimulate cholinergic and noncholinergic neuronal pathways to stimulate motility. At microbially ineffective doses, some macrolide antibiotics stimulate migrating motility complexes and antegrade peristalsis in the proximal GI tract. Erythromycin has been effective in the treatment of gastroparesis in human patients in whom metoclopramide or domperidone was ineffective. Erythromycin increases the gastric emptying rate in healthy dogs, but large food chunks may enter the small intestine and be inadequately digested. Erythromycin induces contractions from the stomach to the terminal ileum and proximal colon, but the colon contractions do not appear to result in propulsive motility. Therefore, erythromycin is unlikely to benefit patients with colonic motility disorders.

Human pharmacokinetic studies indicate that erythromycin suspension is the ideal dosage form for administration of erythromycin as a prokinetic agent. Other macrolide antibiotics have prokinetic activity with fewer adverse effects than erythromycin and may be suitable for use in small animals. Both erythromycin and clarithromycin are metabolized by the hepatic cytochrome P450 enzyme system and inhibit the hepatic metabolism of other drugs, including theophylline, cyclosporine, and cisapride. Nonantibiotic derivatives of erythromycin are being developed as prokinetic agents.

Ranitidine and **nizatidine** are histamine H_2-receptor antagonists that are prokinetics in addition to inhibiting gastric acid secretion in dogs and rats. Their prokinetic activity is due to acetylcholinesterase inhibition, with the greatest activity in the proximal GI tract. Cimetidine and famotidine are not acetylcholinesterase inhibitors and do not have prokinetic effects. Ranitidine and nizatidine stimulate GI motility by increasing the amount of acetylcholinesterase available to bind smooth muscle muscarinic cholinergic receptors. They also stimulate colonic smooth muscle contraction in cats through a cholinergic mechanism.

Ranitidine causes less interference with cytochrome P450 metabolism of other drugs than does cimetidine, and nizatidine does not affect hepatic microsomal enzyme activity, so both drugs have a wide margin of safety.

IV **lidocaine** is used in the treatment of postoperative ileus in people and has been shown to be useful in treating ileus and proximal duodenitis-jejunitis in horses. It is thought to suppress firing of primary afferent neurons, as well as to have anti-inflammatory properties and direct stimulatory effects on smooth muscle. It is also thought to suppress the primary afferent neurons from firing, as well as have anti-inflammatory properties and direct stimulatory effects on smooth muscle. Most horses respond within 12 hr of starting an infusion.

CATHARTIC AND LAXATIVE DRUGS

Cathartics and laxatives increase the motility of the intestine or increase the bulk of feces. The dosages for all of these drugs are highly empirical and usually extracted from human dosages (*see* TABLE 9). Clinically, these drugs are administered to increase passage of gut contents associated with intestinal impaction, to cleanse the bowel before radiography or endoscopy, to eliminate toxins from the GI tract, and to soften feces after intestinal or anal surgery.

Stimulant Cathartics: Stimulant (irritant) cathartics appear to stimulate intestinal motility via an irritant effect on the mucosa or stimulation of intramural nerve plexi. They also activate secretory mechanisms, provoking fluid accumulation in the GI lumen. These drugs can have potent effects, and excessive fluid and electrolyte loss can result. They act directly or indirectly (if a metabolic conversion is necessary before the compound is active).

Emodin is an irritant glycoside that is an active ingredient in several products. Its action is limited to the large intestine, and it may take 4–6 hr for an effect to be seen. Repeat doses should be avoided in horses because of the long latent period and risk of severe superpurgation. The naturally occurring emodins (eg, senna) are found in human formulations.

Vegetable oils are indirect-acting cathartics. They are hydrolyzed by pancreatic lipase in the small intestine to irritating fatty acids. Castor oil is a potent cathartic. It is hydrolyzed to release ricinoleic acid, which causes increased water secretion in the small intestine. Raw linseed oil (cooked linseed oil is toxic) is hydrolyzed to release linoleates, which are less irritating than ricinoleic acid. In smaller daily doses, linseed oil is a mild lubricant laxative and a source of fatty acids for horses.

Senna and **bisacodyl** are stimulant cathartics that affect the large intestine and are found in many over-the-counter human laxative formulations.

TABLE 9 CATHARTIC AND LAXATIVE DRUGS

Drug	Dosage
Castor oil	Dogs: 5–25 mL, PO Foals: 25–50 mL, PO
Bisacodyl	Dogs: 5–20 mg, PO, once to twice daily Cats: 2.5–5 mg, PO, once to twice daily
Magnesium sulfate (Epsom salts)	Dogs: 5–25 g, PO Cats: 2–5 g, PO Horses: 30–100 g, PO
Magnesium hydroxide (milk of magnesia)	Dogs: 5–10 mL, PO Cats: 2–6 mL, PO Horses: 1–4 L, PO
Lactulose	Dogs: 5–15 mL, PO, tid Cats: 2–3 mL, PO, tid
Docusate sodium, docusate calcium, docusate potassium	Dogs and cats: 2 mg/kg/day, PO Horses: 10–20 mg/kg in 2 L water

Hyperosmotic Cathartics: These drugs are poorly absorbed from the GI tract and draw fluid into the intestine by osmosis. The fluid content of the feces increases, which causes intestinal distention and promotes peristalsis. Although hyperosmotic cathartics are relatively safe, overdoses can cause excessive fluid loss and dehydration, so adequate water intake must be assured. Examples of hyperosmotic cathartics include magnesium salts, sodium salts, and sugar alcohols.

Magnesium salts are frequently used PO as saline purgatives. Normally, only 20% of the magnesium is systemically absorbed and eliminated by the kidneys. If absorption is excessive or renal elimination is impaired, then severe hypermagnesemia and metabolic alkalosis may develop.

Sodium salts can be given PO as saline cathartics but are more commonly administered as sodium biphosphate or sodium phosphate enemas. These should not be used in cats because fatal hyperphosphatemia, hypocalcemia, and hypernatremia may result.

Sugar alcohols, such as mannitol and sorbitol, are poorly absorbed and fermented in the terminal ileum and large intestine. Lactulose is a synthetic disaccharide fermented in the large intestine to produce acetic, lactic, and other organic acids that have an osmotic effect. Lactulose is used to treat chronic constipation in cats with megacolon. It is also used in the management of hepatic encephalopathy, in which acidification of the large intestine promotes formation of nonabsorbable ammonium ions and quaternary amines, thereby reducing the need for detoxification by the liver.

Polyethylene glycol (PEG3350) is a large molecular weight, water-soluble polymer used widely in people as a bulking and softening agent for treatment of constipation. It is not metabolized by the intestinal bacterial flora and is minimally absorbed by the intestines. It forms hydrogen bonds with 100 molecules of water per molecule, creating high osmotic pressures within the bowel lumen. The osmotic pressure prevents absorption of water out of the lumen. It is relatively free of adverse effects. PEG3350 is readily available in a powder form, which can be added to a dog or cat's regular food. It can also be administered as a solution via nasogastric tube. Unlike fiber laxatives, it does not cause bloating or gas.

Hydrophilic Colloids ("Bulk Laxatives"): The bulk laxatives use fiber to draw water in to the bowel. Fiber is made up of several different compounds, all of which are carbohydrates. The term "fiber" is used to describe the "insoluble carbohydrates" that resist enzymatic digestion in the small intestine. Found in the cell walls of plants and grains, the most common fibers are cellulose, hemicellulose, pectin, gums, and resistant starches. Almost all carbohydrate sources contain some fiber. Some of the most common sources of fiber in pet foods include rice hulls, corn and corn byproducts, soybean hulls, beet pulp, bran, peanut hulls, and pectin. Adding fiber to a diet improves colon health, helps with weight management, and helps with diarrhea, constipation, and diabetes mellitus. Many commercial brands of pet food are available in a high-fiber formula. Bulk laxatives may cause bloating and flatulence. Contrary to popular belief, bran mashes do not cause a laxative effect in horses. In cats with megacolon, high-fiber diets are used initially to help manage constipation when there is still some normal colonic motility. But once the colonic innervation has deteriorated, the diet may need to be switched to a low-residue diet with aggressive laxative treatment.

Lubricant Laxatives: These act by coating the surface of the feces with a water-immiscible film and by increasing the water content of the feces to provide a lubricant action. Lubricant laxatives usually contain mineral oil or white petroleum. Chronic use may reduce intestinal absorption of fat-soluble vitamins and cause a granulomatous enteritis. Mineral oil is very commonly used in horses and cattle, and commercial products are available to promote passage of hairballs in cats.

Fecal Softeners (Surfactants): Docusate sodium, docusate calcium, and docusate potassium are salts that decrease surface tension and allow water to accumulate in the feces. Docusate also increases cAMP in colonic mucosal cells, which increases ion secretion and fluid permeability. Usually considered very safe, concentrations of dioctyl sodium sulfosuccinate (DSS) ranging from 3–5 times the recommended dosage produced severe diarrhea, rapid dehydration, and death in horses. DSS should not be administered concurrently with mineral oil; soaps are formed and oil absorption is increased.

DRUGS AFFECTING DIGESTIVE FUNCTIONS

Pancrealipase contains the pancreatic enzymes lipase, amylase, and protease. It is derived from the pancreatic tissues of swine. These enzymes help digest and absorb fats, proteins, and carbohydrates. Pancrealipase is used to treat dogs and cats with exocrine pancreatic insufficiency. Several formulations are available, including oral capsules, tablets, and delayed-release capsules and tablets. The powdered forms can be added to food, and the dosage adjusted to maintain normal feces. Antacids may diminish the efficacy of pancrealipase, whereas H_2-receptor antagonists may increase the amount of pancrealipase that reaches the duodenum.

Ursodiol, also known as ursodeoxycholic acid, is a naturally occurring bile acid. It suppresses hepatic synthesis and secretion of cholesterol and decreases intestinal absorption of cholesterol. Reducing cholesterol saturation allows solubilization of cholesterol-containing gallstones. Ursodiol also increases bile flow and reduces the hepatotoxic effect of bile salts by decreasing their detergent action. In small animals, ursodiol may be useful in treatment of cholesterol-containing gallstones, idiopathic hepatic lipidosis, and chronic active hepatitis. The dosage in dogs and cats is 15 mg/kg/day, PO.

***S*-Adenosylmethionine (SAMe)** is an endogenous molecule synthesized by cells throughout the body. Formed from the amino acid methionine and ATP, SAMe is an essential part of three major biochemical pathways: transmethylation, transsulfuration, and aminopropylation. Deficiency of SAMe is associated with cellular derangements in hepatocytes, and there is evidence that a SAMe deficiency may contribute to abnormalities of cellular structure and function in many body tissues, including the liver. Exogenous administration of SAMe appears to improve hepatocellular function in in vivo and in vitro studies without cytotoxicity or significant adverse effects. SAMe increases hepatic glutathione levels in cats and dogs. Glutathione is a potent antioxidant that protects hepatic cells from toxins and death. The daily dosage is 18 mg/kg, rounded to the nearest size of enteric-coated tablet, and given on an empty stomach.

Milk thistle is used as a natural remedy for diseases of the liver and biliary tract. Silymarin is the active extract and contains flavonignans that reportedly act as antioxidants, scavenging free radicals and inhibiting lipid peroxidation. Several controlled clinical trials have demonstrated the benefits of milk thistle in human patients with acute or chronic liver disease. A veterinary formulation has been approved in the USA for dogs and cats.

THE RUMINANT DIGESTIVE SYSTEM

Other than the forestomachs (rumen, reticulum, omasum), the components of the ruminant GI tract are similar to those of monogastric mammals, and the use of pharmacologic agents to treat diseases of the glandular stomach (abomasum) and intestine follows principles common to both monogastric and ruminant species. Ruminants differ significantly from other mammals in that much of their feed undergoes microbial predigestion in the forestomachs, chiefly in the rumen and reticulum. There is also postgastric fermentation in the cecum and colon, but this is much less important than in some other herbivores, eg, horses.

Ruminoreticular motility or fermentation is depressed in many conditions, including improper feeding (overload or deficiency of specific nutrients), lack of water, infectious diseases, intoxications, lesions of any part of the upper GI tract, metabolic states (eg, hypocalcemia), or reduced flow of alkaline saliva that allows pH to fall and the microbial population to be altered to an extent that is harmful to the animal. (*See also* DISEASES OF THE RUMINANT FORESTOMACH, p 221 et seq.)

The primary objectives of pharmacotherapy are to remove the cause and to promote the return of normal digestive function by meeting or reestablishing the requirements for optimal ruminoreticular function as quickly as possible. This may include any of the following: 1) ensuring an appropriate substrate for microbial fermentation; 2) providing any cofactors (eg, phosphorus, sulfur) necessary for microbial fermentative processes; 3) removing any soluble end-products, undigested solid residues, and gas; 4) maintaining continual flow culture of ruminal microorganisms; 5) ensuring that the contents of the ruminoreticulum are fluid; 6) maintaining optimal intraruminal pH (generally between 6 and 7); and 7) promoting active ruminoreticular activity.

DRUGS FOR SPECIFIC PURPOSES

Esophageal Obstruction: Esophageal obstruction due to a foreign body (*see* p 215) leads to severe discomfort and acute free-gas bloat. Physical removal of the object may be hampered by marked spasm of the surrounding muscle. Specific spasmolytic drugs such as acepromazine may be used (0.05–0.1 mg/kg, IV, IM, or SC in cattle). Alternatively, the moderate sedative and muscle relaxant effects of a low dose of xylazine (0.05 mg/kg, IM in cattle) or detomidine (0.02–0.05 mg/kg, IM in cattle) may aid removal of obstructions. None of these compounds has been approved by the FDA for use in cattle.

Ruminotorics: Agents and mixtures that promote forestomach function (fermentation and motility) are known as ruminotorics. Formulations that contain glucogenic substrates, minerals, cofactors, and bitters (eg, nux vomica) have limited application in current therapy of ruminoreticular indigestion. Generally, restoration of the normal ruminoreticular environment using a physiologic approach is much more satisfactory.

Oral administration of specific alkalinizing or acidifying agents should not be routinely undertaken in cases of indigestion. Magnesium oxide or magnesium hydroxide are strongly alkalinizing agents able to substantially increase rumen pH and thus create a hostile environment for rumen protozoa. These compounds, when given at label dose to dairy cattle, result in significant decrease in rumen fermentation and a decrease in number of rumen protozoa. Therefore, these compounds should only be administered to cattle with a confirmed diagnosis of grain overload.

Mineral oil (1–2 L) or dioctyl sodium sulfosuccinate (DSS, 90–120 mL in 1–2 L of water) administered PO or via nasogastric tube followed by gentle ruminal massage can help promote the dissolution and passage of impacted fibrous ruminal omasal or abomasal contents. DSS can markedly depress rumen protozoa; thus, ruminal transfaunation should follow use of this agent if ruminal hypomotility continues.

Ruminal Fluid Transfer: Fresh ruminal fluid is considered to be the best available "ruminotoric," because it contains viable ruminal bacteria (1×10^8–10^{11}/mL) and protozoa (1×10^5–10^6/mL) as well as many useful fermentation factors (volatile fatty acids, microbial protein, minerals, vitamins, buffers). Strained fresh ruminal juice (at least 3 L, but 8–16 L is ideal in cattle; sheep require ~1 L) given PO or by tube is indicated in cases of ruminoreticular stasis. Ruminal fluid can be aspirated through a stomach tube from the ruminoreticulum of healthy animals using an extractor pump or by siphoning, or it can be collected at slaughterhouses. A rumen-cannulated donor animal is particularly convenient. It is best for the donor to be on a ration similar to that of the recipient, because the ruminal microflora will then be more appropriately adapted. Provided the initiating condition or lesion is responding favorably, improvement almost invariably follows the reestablishment of normal ruminal microflora, with consequent normalization of the fermentation process and ruminoreticular motility. When the ruminoreticular contents are putrified, ingesta must first be removed before transfer of fresh ruminal fluid. This can be accomplished using a large-bore stomach tube or by performing a rumenotomy. Acetic acid (vinegar, 4–10 L, PO) can be administered to cattle with putrefaction of the rumen associated with high rumen pH.

Antifoaming Agents: Therapeutic approaches to the control of acute frothy bloat involve administration of antifoaming agents to reduce foam stability and to promote release of free gas, which is then promptly eructated. (*See also* BLOAT IN RUMINANTS, p 227.)

Acute frothy bloat in cattle should be treated with poloxalene, which may be administered as a drench or by stomach tube (25–50 g). Frothy bloat can be prevented by administering poloxalene as a top dressing to feed (1 g/45 kg body wt/day) or in a molasses block (1.5 g/45 kg body wt/day). Polymerized methyl silicone (3.3% emulsion [cattle: 30–60 mL; sheep: 7–15 mL]) may be used in a similar manner as poloxalene, although direct intraruminal injection via a needle or cannula may be more satisfactory in this case. Administration of docusate sodium in emulsified soybean oil (6–12 fl oz containing 240 mg/mL) or administration of vegetable oils alone, such as peanut oil, sunflower oil, or soybean oil (cattle: 60 mL; sheep: 10–15 mL), also relieves acute frothy bloat when given PO. The incidence of frothy bloat in feedlot cattle may be reduced by including ionophores (such as monensin) either in the ration or administering as controlled-release capsules.

Ruminoreticular Antacids: Ruminal alkalinizing agents are principally used to treat ruminal lactic acidosis (pH <5.5) due to grain engorgement or soluble carbohydrate overload. (*See also* GRAIN OVERLOAD IN RUMINANTS, p 222.) The resultant systemic dehydration and acidosis necessitate immediate correction of fluid and electrolyte balance and restoration of a viable microbial population. Often, the latter involves removal of ruminoreticular contents and replacement with fresh ruminoreticular fluid. Antacids that may be given PO, bid-tid, include magnesium hydroxide (cattle:

100–300 g; sheep: 10–30 g) and magnesium carbonate (cattle: 10–80 g; sheep: 1–8 g). Antacids should be mixed in ~10 L of warm water to ensure adequate dispersion through the ruminoreticular contents. Administration PO of activated charcoal (2 g/kg) is believed to protect the ruminoreticular mucosa from further injury by inactivating toxins. Oral administration of sodium bicarbonate (baking soda), either as powder dissolved in water or commercially available solutions prepared for IV infusion, rapidly neutralize the rumen pH but are accompanied by rapid release of large amounts of CO_2. Because of decreased rumen motility in ruminants with acute rumen acidosis, these animals are at increased risk of developing potentially life-threatening free gas bloat.

Ruminoreticular Acidifying Agents: Ruminal acidifying agents are used to treat ruminal stasis or simple indigestion as well as acute ammonia poisoning. In ruminal stasis, the intraruminal pH often increases to >7.5 because of the constant inflow of bicarbonate-rich saliva in the absence of active ruminal fermentation and formation of volatile fatty acids. In acute ammonia intoxication, the increased intraruminal pH increases the activity of urease and facilitates the absorption of free ammonia (pK_a of ammonium is 9.1). Administration of weak acids in cold water returns the pH of ruminoreticular content toward physiologic levels, promotes the uptake of volatile fatty acids, depresses the absorption of ammonia, and inhibits excessive urease activity. Acetic acid (4%–5%) or vinegar (cattle: 4–8 L; sheep: 250–500 mL) is the most common acidifying agent used.

Modulators of Ruminoreticular Motility: The use of motility modifiers in cattle is controversial, because evidence-based data demonstrating clinical efficacy are scarce. Several diseases, including paralytic ileus, cecal dilatation, and abomasal displacement, are accompanied by GI tract motility disorders. Pharmacologic motility modification may hasten recovery in some cases. However, in most instances, the most effective strategy to reestablish motility is correction of the underlying disorder (hypocalcemia, endotoxemia, alkalemia, obstruction, or organ displacement) followed by restoration of the normal ruminoreticular environment through transfaunation. Furthermore, conditioned responses to the presence of feed and feeding itself are physiologic means by which ruminoreticular motility can be notably enhanced.

Motility modifiers are categorized based on their mechanism of action. These can be cholinergics (parasympathomimetics), adrenergics, antidopaminergics, serotonergics, motilin agonists, opioid receptor blockers, or sodium channel blockers (lidocaine).

The use of parasympathomimetic agents (eg, neostigmine, physostigmine, bethanechol) is seldom appropriate. These drugs have cholinergic effects, which are potentially hazardous. Neostigmine (cattle: 0.02 mg/kg, SC; sheep: 0.01–0.02 mg/kg, SC) generally produces the fewest adverse effects but tends to increase frequency, rather than strength, of ruminoreticular contractions. Neostigmine given as a constant-rate IV infusion (87.5 mg in 10 L of sodium-glucose infusion at 2 drops/sec) has been used to treat cecal dilatation/dislocation. However, the stimulatory effect of neostigmine is not always reliable, and some inhibition of motility can be seen. This may be due to the adrenergic component associated with ganglion stimulation by cholinergic agents.

Bethanechol (0.07 mg/kg, SC, tid for 2 days) has been used to treat spontaneous cecal dilatation without torsion. Potential adverse effects include salivation and diarrhea. Recommendations involving neostigmine and bethanechol have not been confirmed in randomized, controlled experiments. Neither compound has been approved by the FDA for use in cattle. Parasympathomimetics are sometimes used in practice to conservatively treat left displaced abomasum in cows, although the literature indicates that use of these compounds is of no value for this purpose.

N-butylscopolammonium bromide (nonlactating adult cattle: 0.2 mg/kg, IM or IV; calves: 0.4 mg/kg, IM or IV) is a parasympatholytic agent approved for the control of diarrhea in cattle in some European countries. The commercial formulation is combined with an NSAID, metamizole (nonlactating adult cattle: 25 mg/kg, IM or IV; calves: 50 mg/kg, IM or IV). Administration of N-butylscopolammonium bromide (80 mg/cow) in combination with dipyrone has been proposed as a conservative treatment of spontaneously occurring right-side displacement of the abomasum in cattle. However, this has not been demonstrated in randomized, controlled studies. N-butylscopolammonium bromide is not approved by the FDA, and the use of dipyrone in food animals in the USA is prohibited.

Atropine (0.04 mg/kg, IV) has been found to mitigate abomasal contractions for 1–3 hr.

Atropine sulfate (0.5 mg/kg, IV) administered 5 min before placement of a reticular magnet is suggested to prevent magnet loss into the cranial sac of the rumen. Atropine (40 mg/cow as a 1% solution, SC) is also used to determine disruption of forestomach motility in cattle suspected to have vagal indigestion. An increase of >16% in heart rate 15 min after atropine administration is considered indicative of severe disruption of forestomach motility.

Xylazine hydrochloride (0.2 mg/kg, IV) administered 5 min before placement of a reticular magnet may prevent loss into the cranial sac of the rumen but will also result in deep sedation of the animal and thus is unlikely to be of any practical use. Xylazine-induced atony of the reticulorumen may be reversed by pretreatment with tolazoline (0.5 mg/kg, IV), atipamezole hydrochloride (0.08 mg/kg), or yohimbine (0.2 mg/kg, IV). Adverse effects of xylazine in cattle include bradycardia, hypothermia, salivation, diuresis, ruminal bloat, and aspiration pneumonia. Neither xylazine nor its antidotes have been approved by the FDA for use in cattle.

Metoclopramide (cattle: 0.15 mg/kg, IM; sheep: 0.023–0.045 mg/kg) has cholinergic and antidopaminergic effects but does not appear to increase the myoelectric activity of the pyloric antrum in either species. However, metoclopramide at 0.5 mg/kg given IM or IV to goats has been shown to increase myoelectric activity of the pyloric antrum but not the body of the abomasum. Because metoclopramide can cross the blood-brain barrier, restlessness and excitement are potential adverse effects. Metoclopramide has not been approved by the FDA for use in cattle.

Erythromycin lactobionate is a macrolide antimicrobial that increases gut myoelectric activity by binding to motilin receptors in intestinal smooth muscle cells. In cows, erythromycin (0.1 mg/kg, IV, or 1 mg/kg, IM) was found to increase myoelectrical activity in the abomasum and duodenum for >2 hr. This effect was increased to 6–8 hr when erythromycin was administered in polyethylene glycol at 10 mg/kg, IM. Erythromycin is approved by the FDA only for treatment of shipping fever, pneumonia, footrot, and metritis at 2.2 mg/kg, IM. Deep IM injection in muscles of the neck is recommended because of the risk of pain, swelling, and tissue blemishes at the injection site.

The prokinetic serotoninergic drug cisapride (cattle: 0.08 mg/kg) is widely used in equine medicine, yet significant prokinetic effects have not been conclusively demonstrated in ruminants. Furthermore, definitive clinical and experimental data to support the use of opioids or lidocaine in ruminants have not been published.

DRUG DISPOSITION IN THE RUMINORETICULUM

Morphologic and functional characteristics of the ruminoreticulum that make it suitable for fermentative digestion of plant material also affect the activity, distribution, and absorption of many drugs, particularly when given PO. The anaerobic and reductive environment of the ruminoreticulum and the presence of many microbial enzymes result in inactivation of drugs such as trimethoprim and cardiac glycosides. Slow and inefficient mixing of drugs in the large volume of the ruminoreticular fluid delays attainment of uniform concentrations throughout the multiphasic ingesta and retards absorption from the ruminoreticulum. Absorption is also affected by the polarity and ionization status of the drug, which is determined by the pK_a of the drug and the pH of the ruminoreticular fluid. The latter depends on the diet and the relative contributions of alkaline saliva and acidic ruminoreticular fluid. Aside from the many effects that the ruminoreticular environment can have on the activity and disposition of drugs, the drugs themselves may have unintended effects on ruminoreticular function. In particular, broad-spectrum antibacterial agents and antiprotozoal agents can disrupt the normal balance of microflora in the ruminoreticulum.

These factors affecting the activity and disposition of drugs in the ruminoreticulum, together with the possible effects of drugs on ruminoreticular function, complicate oral administration of drugs to ruminants. In young animals, these undesirable effects can be avoided by making use of the esophageal groove reflex. This reflex, which is elicited by receptors in the mouth and pharynx, is well developed in suckling neonates but becomes less reliable in older animals. After ~24 mo in cattle and ~18 mo in sheep, provoked reticular groove closure is often irregular, incomplete, or absent.

Ruminoreticular morphology and function has less influence on drug disposition in neonatal ruminants than in adults. At birth, the forestomachs are underdeveloped, and the newborn ruminant is essentially monogastric. Drugs that are usually destroyed in the ruminoreticulum of adults (eg, trimethoprim) may be well absorbed during the first 2–3 wk of life. This developmental pattern depends on the period between birth and initiation of a roughage diet and exposure to microbes in the environment.

SYSTEMIC PHARMACOTHERAPEUTICS OF THE EYE

See also OPHTHALMOLOGY, p 488.

The anatomy of the eye presents unique opportunities for topical and/or systemic medical treatment of neural tissue. Like the brain, the eye has protective barriers from the vascular system. The blood-ocular barriers (ie, the blood-aqueous and blood-retinal barriers) allow the eye to control entry of inflammatory cells, protein, and low-molecular-weight compounds from the systemic circulation.

The **blood-aqueous barrier** is a function of the iris and ciliary body epithelium. In the iris, the capillary endothelium is not fenestrated, but there are tight junctions. In the ciliary body, there are tight connections between the apical ends of the nonpigmented epithelial cells. Breakdown of this barrier results in entry of protein and cells into the anterior chamber and is seen as aqueous flare or plasmoid aqueous. The **blood-retinal barrier** is composed of two layers: an endothelial and epithelial portion. The endothelial part is composed of the endothelium of the retinal capillaries, which are also nonfenestrated. The epithelial portion is the retinal pigment epithelium. When treating the eye via the systemic circulation, these barriers can limit the entry and amount of medications into the eye, especially highly water-soluble compounds. They are less effective in the face of inflammation, and many drugs gain increased access to the intraocular structures when the eye is inflamed. The time required for drugs to reach their peak concentrations in the eye depends highly on the physicochemical properties of the particular drug.

The presence of barriers such as the iris, ciliary body, and lens, as well as normal movement of aqueous humor through the pupil and out the trabecular and uveoscleral meshwork can further limit the distribution of drugs. Several enzymes are present in the cornea and ciliary body. These can metabolize drugs to inactive metabolites before and after the compound reaches the anterior chamber. Drugs predominantly leave the anterior chamber with the aqueous humor via the corneal trabecular and/or uveoscleral meshwork, although small amounts may move posteriorly into the vitreous.

ROUTES OF ADMINISTRATION

The three primary methods of delivery of ocular medications to the eye are topical, local ocular (ie, subconjunctival, intravitreal, retrobulbar, intracameral), and systemic. The most appropriate method of administration depends on the area of the eye to be medicated. The conjunctiva, cornea, anterior chamber, and iris usually respond well to topical therapy. The eyelids can be treated with topical therapy but more frequently require systemic therapy. The posterior segment always requires systemic therapy, because most topical medications do not penetrate to the posterior segment. Retrobulbar and orbital tissues are treated systemically.

Subconjunctival or sub-Tenon's therapy, although not a true form of systemic medication administration, has the potential to increase both drug absorption and contact time. Medications both leak onto the cornea from the entry hole of injection and diffuse through the sclera into the globe. Drugs with low solubility such as corticosteroids may provide a repository of drug lasting days to weeks. Appropriate amounts of medication must be used. Large amounts, especially of long-acting salts, can cause a significant inflammatory reaction. For sub-Tenon's injections, 0.5 mL per site is usually safe and effective in small animals, and ≤1 mL can be used in large animals such as horses and cows.

Retrobulbar medications are used infrequently for therapeutics. In cattle, the retrobulbar tissues can be anesthetized with local anesthetic (lidocaine/bupivicaine) for enucleation using either a Peterson block (15–20 mL) or a 4-point block of the orbit (5–10 mL/site). Whenever any medication is placed into the orbit, extreme care must be taken to ensure that the medication is not inadvertently injected into a blood vessel, the optic nerve, or one of the orbital foramen. Retrobulbar injection has a high risk of adverse effects and should not be used unless the clinician is experienced and the animal is appropriately restrained.

Systemic medication is required for posterior segment therapy and to complement topical therapy for the anterior segment. The blood-ocular barriers can limit absorption of less lipophilic drugs, but inflammation will initially allow greater drug concentrations to reach the site. As the eye starts to heal, these barriers will again become more effective and can limit further drug penetration. This should be considered when treating posterior segment disease, eg, blastomycosis in small animals with hydrophilic drugs such as itraconazole.

After topical administration, up to 80% of the applied drug(s) is absorbed systemically across the highly vascularized nasopharyngeal mucosa. Because absorption via this route bypasses the liver, there is not the large first-pass metabolism seen after oral administration. Depending on the drugs used, this can result in systemic adverse effects. Topically applied β-blockers used in the treatment of glaucoma can cause heart block, atrial tachycardia, congestive heart failure, bronchospasm, dyspnea, and decreased exercise tolerance. These drugs should be used very carefully in older animals or in animals with cardiac or respiratory disease. Cushing syndrome can be easily induced in small or medium-sized dogs with chronic use of potent topical steroids.

LOCAL ANESTHETICS

Parenterally, local nerve blocks are an excellent aid for routine ocular evaluation and diagnostic procedures in horses. The auriculopalpebral block is the most helpful block to limit blepharospasm during examination. This procedure blocks some of the motor nerves of the upper eyelid and enables the examiner to control the horse's upper eyelid. The auriculopalpebral nerve is a branch of the facial nerve and can be palpated as it runs across the superior margin of the zygomatic arch. To block sensory input, a supraorbital nerve block or a ring block is used. The supraorbital nerve is a branch of the frontal nerve that traverses the supraorbital foramen of the upper orbit. If placed correctly, a dose of 1–2 mL of lidocaine is usually sufficient to block either the auriculopalpebral or supraorbital nerve. The block is usually effective within 3–5 min and can last up to 2–3 hr.

The same principles are used in food animals, such as cattle, in which both a retrobulbar and ring block may be used. A correctly placed retrobulbar block will block cranial nerves II, III, IV, the ophthalmic branch of V, and VI. The ring block is needed to inhibit sensory input from the skin around the eye.

TREATMENT OF INFECTIOUS DISEASE

Feline Herpesvirus Keratitis and Conjunctivitis: Systemic antiviral drugs to treat feline ocular herpesvirus are needed only in circumstances when topical antiviral therapy is not effective. Famciclovir (the prodrug of penciclovir) at 15–30 mg/kg, PO, bid-tid for 10–14 days (or empirically at 31.25 mg/kitten or small cat, or 62.5 mg/cat, bid for 2 wk) is the drug of choice for treatment and longterm management. Acyclovir has also been used at 200 mg, PO, bid-tid, although repeated dosing can cause systemic toxicity and is not recommended as first-line treatment. Previously, lifelong oral L-lysine (250–500 mg/day) was recommended to help prevent or reduce the severity of recurrent feline herpesvirus infections. However, recent work has shown that oral L-lysine can actually exacerbate feline herpesvirus infections. Recombinant human α-interferon (5–25 U/day, PO and topically) has also been recommended and may work by inhibiting replication of herpesvirus and enhancing macrophage activation and lymphocyte-mediated cytotoxicity.

Feline Chlamydial Conjunctivitis: Feline conjunctivitis caused by *Chlamydia felis* (*see* p 506) that is nonresponsive to topical tetracycline therapy can be treated with oral doxycycline (10 mg/kg/day, or 5 mg/kg, bid). To avoid esophageal strictures, animals should be treated with 3–5 mL of oral fluid after dosing to ensure the tablets pass into the stomach. All cats in the household should be treated for at least 4 wk, or for 2 wk after clinical signs have resolved. To avoid issues associated with tetracycline use in pregnant queens or young cats, systemic macrolides such as erythromycin (15–25 mg/kg, PO, bid, or 10–15 mg/kg, PO, tid for 3–4 wk) or azithromycin (10–15 mg/kg/day, PO, for 3–5 days then twice weekly for 3 wk) are also effective. Alternatively, potentiated amoxicillin (12.5–25 mg/kg, bid for 3 wk) can be used. If signs recur after treatment ceases, therapy should be continued for an additional 4–5 wk.

Feline Toxoplasmosis: Many cases of feline anterior uveitis with increasing *Toxoplasma gondii* titers, as shown by serology and anterior chamber centesis, remain undiagnosed. Chorioretinitis is often the most common presentation. Treatment is clindamycin at 8–17 mg/kg, PO, tid, or 10–12.5 mg/kg, PO, bid for 3–4 wk, in association with topical corticosteroids

(0.5%–1% prednisolone acetate or 0.01% dexamethasone alcohol tid-qid) and topical atropine for mydriasis. Adverse effects of clindamycin include anorexia, vomiting, and diarrhea, mainly at the higher doses. Other systemic antibiotics less frequently used include the synergistic combination of sulfonamides (sulfadiazine, sulfamethazine, sulfamerazine, 100 mg/kg/day, PO) and pyrimethamine (2 mg/kg/day, PO) for 1–2 wk. Adverse effects include gastric upsets and bone marrow suppression. Frequent hematologic monitoring is recommended if therapy is to last >2 wk.

Feline and Canine Rickettsial Infection: Anterior and posterior uveitis and chorioretinitis secondary to infection with *Ehrlichia* or *Rickettsia* spp (*see* p 803) is common. Tetracyclines (doxycycline at 5–10 mg/kg, once to twice daily for dogs, and 10 mg/kg, bid, for cats, for 14–21 days) are the drugs of choice and have excellent intraocular penetration. In a dog from an area associated with rickettsial disease, it is rational to empirically treat uveitis with doxycycline pending serology. Enrofloxacin (3 mg/kg, PO, bid for 7 days) can also be used, although care should be taken not to exceed the dosage associated with retinal toxicity in cats (>5 mg/kg/day). Chloramphenicol is not recommended, because it directly interferes with heme and bone marrow synthesis. Appropriate topical and systemic NSAID therapy is also recommended to control ocular inflammation. When the intraocular inflammation is severe or there is a serous retinal detachment, short-term (2–7 days) corticosteroids (0.25–0.5 mg/kg, PO, once to twice daily) may be used concurrently 24–48 hr after the start of oral antibiotic therapy. Animals can regain some vision after reattachment of the retina; the amount depends on the duration of the detachment and degree of inflammation.

Canine and Feline Ocular Mycoses: Dogs and cats diagnosed with ocular mycoses require systemic treatment. Along with systemic antifungals, topical and systemic anti-inflammatories and topical mydriatics/cycloplegics are needed to control the secondary and potentially blinding intraocular inflammation.

Blastomycosis (*see* p 634) is more common in dogs than cats. Up to 40% have ocular signs, usually anterior uveitis. Treatment options include parenteral amphotericin B deoxycholate or PO or IV triazoles. In dogs, itraconazole is used at 5 mg/kg, PO, bid for 5 days, then continued at 5 mg/kg/day, PO, for a minimum of 60 days or 1 mo after all signs of the disease have resolved. Adverse effects include anorexia, which is associated with liver toxicity. Cats can be treated with 10 mg/kg/day or 5 mg/kg, bid; however, there are few published cases of successful treatment in cats. Ketoconazole may also be used to treat blastomycosis, but because the onset of effect is so slow, other triazoles should be used initially. Amphotericin B deoxycholate is also effective but is nephrotoxic. The dosage (dogs: 0.5 mg/kg, IV; cats: 0.25 mg/kg, IV) is given three times weekly until the animal becomes azotemic or a cumulative dose of 4–6 mg/kg in dogs or 4 mg/kg in cats is reached. Amphotericin B lipid complex used at the same or a slightly higher dosage is less nephrotoxic.

The predominant lesion of histoplasmosis (*see* p 639) is granulomatous choroiditis, but anterior uveitis, retinal detachment, and optic neuritis can be present. Treatment options are itraconazole (10 mg/kg, PO) or fluconazole (2.5–5 mg/kg, PO) once to twice daily for 4–6 mo, or amphotericin B deoxycholate (0.25–0.5 mg/kg, IV, every 48 hr) until a cumulative dose of 5–10 mg/kg (dogs) or 4–8 mg/kg (cats) is reached. Because of its lipophilic nature and ability to cross the blood-ocular barriers, fluconazole is recommended for use in ocular disease, although animals have also had complete resolution when treated with the more hydrophilic triazole itraconazole.

Ocular signs are present in 15% of cryptococcosis (*see* p 637) cases and are more common in cats than in dogs. Treatment can be with amphotericin B deoxycholate (0.1–0.5 mg/kg, IV, three times per wk) alone or in combination with flucytosine (30–75 mg/kg, bid-qid for up to 9 mo). Ketoconazole, itraconazole, and fluconazole are also effective. In cats, ketoconazole is administered PO at either 5–10 mg/kg, bid, or 10–20 mg/kg/day for 6–10 mo. If toxicity occurs, the dosage can be changed to 50 mg/kg/cat, PO, every other day. In dogs, dosages are either 5–15 mg/kg, PO, bid, or 30 mg/kg/day, PO, for 6–10 mo. Systemic absorption from the GI tract is significantly enhanced by food. Adverse effects of ketoconazole include anorexia, diarrhea, vomiting, and increased liver enzymes. Because of poor CNS penetration, ketoconazole is not recommended for use as the sole agent in ocular cryptococcosis. Itraconazole (cats: 5–10 mg/kg, PO, bid, or 20 mg/kg/day, PO) is less likely to cause adverse effects than ketoconazole, and its GI tract bioavailability is enhanced by fatty food. Like ketoconazole, its hydrophilic nature leads to poor distribution into the

CNS, but it has been successful in treating CNS and ocular cryptococcosis. Adverse effects are mainly associated with the GI tract (anorexia and vomiting), but liver disease can also develop. Liver enzymes (ALT) should be monitored every 2 wk for the first month of treatment and monthly thereafter. Fluconazole is more lipophilic and has better bioavailability than itraconazole. It also penetrates the CNS better (60%–80% of serum levels) and causes fewer adverse effects than itraconazole. The dosage for cats and dogs is 5–15 mg/kg, PO, once to twice daily for 6–10 mo.

Ocular coccidioidomycosis (*see* p 637) is more common in dogs than in cats. Ocular involvement requires systemic treatment with ketoconazole (dogs: 15–20 mg/kg, PO, bid; cats: 15–20 mg/kg, PO, once to twice daily), although there is poor CNS and ocular penetration. Ketoconazole can be toxic in cats, so itraconazole (5–10 mg/kg/day, PO) would be a safer choice. Treatment is for 3–6 mo or longer, and relapses are common. Amphotericin B deoxycholate can also be used (0.4–0.5 mg/kg, IV, every 48–72 hr) until a cumulative dose of 8–11 mg/kg is reached.

Over the past 10 yr, a number of newer triazoles (voriconazole, ravuconazole [both fluconazole derivatives], and posaconazole [an itraconazole derivative]) with broader spectrum of activity against systemic mycoses (including those resistant to other azoles) have become available. Information on their clinical usage is limited and mostly published as pharmacokinetic studies or individual case reports. Doses have been extrapolated from their use and preclinical toxicology trials in people, and using these doses must be done carefully. Because posaconazole is primarily metabolized in most species by glucuronidation, care needs to be taken with the dose and duration, especially in cats. Voriconazole is predominantly hepatically metabolized, and in toxicology trials, chronic usage at 12 mg/kg for 6–12 months caused hepatotoxicosis. Very limited information is available on the use of ravuconazole in dogs and cats. The current literature should be reviewed before using any of these compounds.

Infectious Keratoconjunctivitis: Treatment of infectious keratoconjunctivitis (*see* p 512) associated with *Moraxella bovis* in cattle is improved with use of systemic antibiotics. Oxytetracycline and florfenicol are the two most commonly used. Two doses of parenteral long-acting oxytetracycline (20 mg/kg, IM or SC) 48–72 hr apart is effective, although care should be taken using tetracyclines in endemic anaplasmosis areas. Florfenicol, at a single dose of 40 mg/kg, SC, or two doses of 20 mg/kg, IM, 48 hr apart, is also effective. The organism is also sensitive to trimethoprim-sulfonamide (15–30 mg/kg, IM or IV, once to twice daily) or a single SC dose of tilmicosin (5–10 mg/kg), ceftiofur (6.6 mg/kg), or tulathromycin (2.5 mg/kg). *M bovis* is resistant to systemic macrolides, lincosamides, and often penicillins.

Chlamydial keratoconjunctivitis in sheep and goats and nonchlamydial keratoconjunctivitis caused by *Mycoplasma* spp in goats can be treated with systemic antibiotics in addition to topical therapy. These include oxytetracycline (6–11 mg/kg, IV or IM), florfenicol (20 mg/kg, IM or SC), tylosin (10 mg/kg, IM), erythromycin base (2.2–15 mg/kg, IM, once to twice daily), or tilmicosin (10 mg/kg, IM). Most animals are treated with a single dose because of management issues involved in treating flock outbreaks.

Penetrating Trauma: All penetrating wounds of the eye should be considered infected, and animals should be treated promptly with systemic broad-spectrum bactericidal antibiotics. For dogs and cats, oral amoxicillin-clavulanic acid (10–20 mg/kg, bid) is appropriate. When feasible, culture and sensitivity and cytology performed on anterior chamber centesis samples best guide appropriate antibiotic selection. Treatment should continue for a minimum of 14–21 days. In horses, the combination of systemic penicillin G procaine (22,000–44,000 U/kg, IM, bid) and gentamicin (6.6 mg/kg/day, IM or IV) is an appropriate choice.

In all cases, intensive systemic NSAIDs (flunixin 0.5–1 mg/kg, IV or PO, once to twice daily; ketoprofen 1.1–2.2 mg/kg/day, PO or IV) are warranted to control the severe inflammation usually associated with these injuries. Because treatment duration in these cases extends beyond label recommendations of 5 days, an appropriate H_2-blocker (ranitidine, famotidine) or proton pump inhibitor (omeprazole) should be used prophylactically to prevent gastric ulceration. When inflammation is also associated with leakage of lens material into the anterior chamber, the only treatment to control the inflammation is removal of the lens.

TREATMENT OF INTRAOCULAR INFLAMMATION

Many infectious and noninfectious diseases cause intraocular inflammation. Unless inflammation is controlled early, irreversible damage and blindness may result.

Topical and systemic corticosteroids and NSAIDs are used to control inflammation, depending on the cause. Care should be taken when using longterm treatment. Adrenocortical suppression can develop, and animals must be weaned off treatment slowly after the inflammation has resolved. In all species, control of noninfectious intraocular inflammation involves use of high initial doses of systemic corticosteroids (prednisone 1–2 mg/kg) in combination with topical corticosteroids (0.5% or 1% prednisolone acetate or 0.1% dexamethasone alcohol, tid-qid). Some cases of infectious disease (eg, rickettsial infections) can be treated with low doses of systemic corticosteroids but only after antibiotic therapy has been started for 24–48 hr. Topical steroids can be started at the same time as systemic antibiotic therapy. If the cause of intraocular inflammation is unknown, a combination of topical corticosteroids and systemic NSAIDs is also appropriate. Use of H_2-blockers or proton pump inhibitors should be considered when starting therapy; GI, liver, and renal parameters should be routinely monitored.

Canine Immune-mediated Disease: Immune-mediated ocular disease is not uncommon in dogs. This can include episcleritis, nodular granulomatous episclerokeratitis (often seen in Collies as a raised granulomatous lesion involving the episclera and third eyelid and infiltrating into the cornea), and extraocular muscle myositis. In addition to infectious anterior and posterior uveitis, immune-mediated uveitis (uveodermatologic syndrome) associated with an immune reaction to melanin is seen in a number of breeds, more commonly those of Arctic origin.

These diseases can be treated with either combined topical and oral corticosteroids (prednisone, 0.5–1 mg/kg, bid) or a lower corticosteroid dose in combination with another immunosuppressive drug. This could be oral azathioprine (1.5–2 mg/kg/day, reducing the dose after 3–5 days), mycophenolate mofetil (7–20 mg/kg, bid for 3–4 wk, then reducing the dose to 10 mg/kg/day), or cyclosporine (5 mg/kg, bid for 2 wk, decreasing to daily if clinical improvement). An alternative treatment for episcleritis in dogs >10 kg is niacinamide (500 mg, PO) and tetracycline (500 mg, PO), tid, decreasing to once to twice daily once improvement occurs.

Many cases of immune-mediated ocular disease can be kept in remission with either azathioprine, 1–2 mg/kg, PO, every 3–7 days for 1–8 mo; mycophenolate mofetil, 10 mg/kg every day or every other day; or cyclosporine 5 mg/kg daily, every other day, or once weekly with or without concurrent low-dose prednisone or prednisolone. Adverse effects of azathioprine include pancreatitis, liver disease, and bone marrow suppression. Frequent hematology and serum biochemistry monitoring is recommended. There are fewer adverse effects with mycophenolate and cyclosporine. These are mainly related to the GI tract and include anorexia, vomiting, and diarrhea. In uveodermatologic syndrome, recurrence is common and prognosis for longterm control is only fair. Many animals become blind from secondary glaucoma associated with the chronic uveitis and/or retinal detachment and degeneration.

Canine Optic Neuritis: Inflammation of the optic nerve is more common in dogs than in other species. It can be caused by infection (eg, distemper, systemic mycoses), neoplasia, contiguous inflammation, or granulomatous infiltration (reticulosis/granulomatous encephalomyelitis). Systemic corticosteroids (prednisone, 1–2 mg/kg, PO) for extended periods (often weeks) are used in an attempt to retain vision. Granulomatous encephalomyelitis is responsive to early treatment with systemic corticosteroids.

Damage to the optic nerve as a result of trauma is treated with systemic corticosteroids at similar dose rates as above. Prognosis depends on the degree of damage.

Equine Uveitis: The principles of anti-inflammatory treatment for equine uveitis (*see* p 508) are very similar regardless of the initiating cause. In acute uveitis, systemic NSAIDs (flunixin meglumine, 0.25–1 mg/kg, IV or PO, bid) are used in conjunction with topical and/or subconjunctival corticosteroids to control the intraocular inflammation. Phenylbutazone does not seem to be as effective in the initial treatment of equine uveitis. Horses are often treated with high doses of NSAIDs for longer than label recommendations (often 7–10 days); once the uveitis is controlled, the dose is slowly tapered over 2–3 wk. Concurrent gastric protection with either an H_2-blocker (ranitidine, 6.6 mg/kg, PO, tid, or 1 mg/kg, IV, tid; or famotidine, 0.23–0.35 mg/kg, IV, bid-tid, or 1.88–2.8 mg/kg, PO, bid-tid) or a proton pump inhibitor (omeprazole, 4 mg/kg/day, PO) is recommended. Renal function should be monitored, and extreme care taken if the horse is also being treated with gentamicin. Oral aspirin (25 mg/kg/day) has been used longterm to help prevent recurrence in horses diagnosed with equine recurrent uveitis. Suprachoroidal cyclosporine implants are now more commonly used for longterm management (up to 3 yr).

Equine Optic Neuritis: Trauma to the poll in horses associated with rearing and hitting objects or falling over backward can result in sudden blindness. This is associated with overextension or shearing of the optic nerve within the optic canal secondary to movement of the brain in the skull. Treatment is systemic anti-inflammatory agents, usually NSAIDs at higher dosages (flunixin meglumine, 0.5–1.1 mg/kg, IV or PO) and for longer than label recommendations. Prophylactic use of H_2-blockers or a proton pump inhibitor is recommended. In addition, dimethyl sulfoxide (DMSO; 1 g/kg, IV as a 20% solution in saline or 5% dextrose in water given daily for 3 days, then every other day for 6 days) can be used. When given IV, DMSO can cause hemolysis and hemoglobinuria. Prognosis is poor for any return of vision if there has been no improvement after 72 hr.

TREATMENT OF MISCELLANEOUS FELINE CONDITIONS

Feline Eosinophilic Keratitis: Eosinophilic keratitis is associated with infiltration of eosinophils into the feline cornea. It may be an unusual immune response to latent feline herpesvirus. Treatment with topical steroids usually is sufficient, but some cases do not respond. Oral megestrol acetate (0.5 mg/kg/day until a response is noted, then 1.25 mg, PO, 2–3 times weekly as required) helps to improve or resolve the corneal inflammation via an unknown mechanism. However, its use is associated with adverse effects such as diabetes mellitus, adrenocortical suppression, and uterine hyperplasia, and this drug should be used with extreme caution. Megestrol acetate can also be dangerous to women handling the pills.

Feline Hypertensive Retinopathy: Older cats can present with sudden blindness due to serous retinal detachments secondary to systemic hypertension, or less commonly hyperthyroidism. Treatment is with the calcium channel blocker amlodipine (0.625 mg/cat once to twice daily; some cats may require 1.25 mg/cat, bid) and systemic corticosteroids (prednisone, 0.5–1 mg/kg, PO) to help control the posterior inflammation. Retinas can reattach once blood pressure returns to the normal range. At least 50% of cats will regain some clinical vision if treated early. Cats should be rechecked 1 wk after starting therapy, and blood pressure regularly monitored. Adverse effects of amlodipine are uncommon but include azotemia, lethargy, hypokalemia, and tachycardia.

TREATMENT OF GLAUCOMA

Topical medications, such as prostaglandins, miotics, β-blocking adrenergics, and topical carbonic anhydrase inhibitors, are the primary drugs for treatment of glaucoma (*see* p 497), but these are often supplemented with systemic drugs.

Osmotic Diuretics: In the emergency treatment of acute glaucoma, intraocular pressure must be reduced urgently. This is done pharmacologically using osmotic diuretics such as mannitol or glycerol in combination with other topical and systemic drugs. Osmotic diuretics are large-molecular-weight molecules that increase the osmotic pressure of plasma relative to the aqueous and vitreous. Most of the water in the eye is in the vitreous. Dehydration of the vitreous allows the lens and iris to move posteriorly, opening the iridocorneal angle. The other effect is to decrease formation of aqueous humor. Mannitol is given (1–1.5 g/kg, IV over 20–30 min), with the effect peaking in 2–3 hr and lasting up to 5 hr. Mannitol is not metabolized and thus can be used in diabetic animals. Glycerol (1–2 g/kg, PO) can be used but is unpalatable, and most dogs vomit. With both drugs, water should be withheld for 3–5 hr, and the animal should be given regular opportunities to urinate. Kidney and cardiac function should be checked before treatment, and cardiac function monitored during treatment. Mannitol can be used again within 8–12 hr if initial control of intraocular pressure is not maintained; longterm control is unlikely if intraocular pressures do not stay within the normal range after two treatments.

Carbonic Anhydrase Inhibitors: Oral carbonic anhydrase inhibitors are also used to treat and manage acute glaucoma. These inhibit the enzyme carbonic anhydrase in the nonpigmented ciliary epithelium responsible for catalyzing the following reaction: $CO_2 + H_2O \leftarrow$ carbonic anhydrase $\rightarrow H_2CO_3 \leftrightarrow H^+ + HCO_3^-$

The bicarbonate and sodium ions are actively transported into the anterior chamber, leading to passive movement of water. This mechanism produces 40%–60% of aqueous humor. Drugs used include methazolamide (2–4 mg/kg, PO, bid-tid), acetazolamide (5–8 mg/kg, PO, bid-tid), and dichlorphenamide (2–4 mg/kg, PO, bid-tid). Methazolamide is the drug of choice.

Maximal effect occurs 3–6 hr after administration. The most common adverse effect is a metabolic acidosis that causes panting. Other effects can include vomiting, diarrhea, and hypokalemia. Acetazolamide commonly causes anorexia. Potassium supplementation can be given with potassium bicarbonate or citrate (1–2 g/day) added to the food. Cats are more sensitive than dogs to the adverse effects of these drugs and need careful monitoring. In general, systemic carbonic anhydrase inhibitors are not recommended for use in cats.

SYSTEMIC PHARMACOTHERAPEUTICS OF THE INTEGUMENTARY SYSTEM

See also PRINCIPLES OF TOPICAL THERAPY, p 844.

Drugs that may be used in the integumentary system fall into several therapeutic categories: antimicrobials (antibacterials, antifungals), antiparasitics, NSAIDs, immunomodulators, hormones, psychotropic agents, and vitamin and mineral supplements.

Several factors may contribute to the development of the particular clinical presentation. Each factor should be identified and treated for therapy to succeed. For example, recurrent otitis may have a primary underlying skin disease but be complicated by both predisposing and perpetuating factors. Further, successful treatment of skin disease may require longterm or lifelong therapy and is frequently a matter of successful control rather than "cure."

ANTIBACTERIALS

Most canine skin infections are caused by coagulase-positive *Staphylococcus pseudintermedius* (formerly *S intermedius*), which commonly produce β-lactamase. Other staphylococcal species have been described, including *S aureus*, *S schleiferi*, and *S hyicus*. There does not appear to be any difference in the disease patterns or clinical signs produced by the different species, although species-specific differences in antimicrobial resistance profiles have been seen in North America, with *S pseudintermedius* and *S aureus* showing more resistance than *S schleiferi coagulans*. Species identification requires molecular techniques such as PCR detection of species-specific thermonuclease genes (*nuc*) or 16S rDNA sequencing, because phenotypic differentiation is unreliable.

Occasionally, *Proteus* spp, *Pseudomonas* spp, and *Escherichia coli* are secondary invaders of the dermis. *Pasteurella multocida* and β-hemolytic streptococci are the most common bacteria isolated from the epidermis of cats. *Actinomycetes* and mycobacteria are rare opportunistic invaders in dogs and cats. Bactericidal drugs expected to be effective against these bacteria should be used when treating the first occurrence of pyoderma in an animal.

Bacterial skin disease in large animals may be caused by *Dermatophilus congolensis*, staphylococci, *Corynebacterium* spp, *Actinomyces*, and rarely *Bacillus* spp or *Pseudomonas* spp. Draining tracts or abscesses in the skin of sheep or goats may be caused by *Corynebacterium pseudotuberculosis*. *Fusobacterium* spp and *Bacteroides* spp are the primary invaders in interdigital necrobacillosis (footrot). The spirochete *Borrelia suilla* is a secondary invader of skin lesions caused by sarcoptic mange or ear biting in swine. Clostridial diseases in cattle and erysipelas in swine are disorders that involve the integumentary system and cause serious economic losses.

Methicillin resistance (a marker for resistance to all β-lactam antibiotics, including penicillins, cephalosporins, and carbapenems) is the most important mechanism of resistance in staphylococci; the reported incidence of antimicrobial-resistant bacteria has increased markedly over the past 5–10 yr, although this varies depending on the geographic location. For example, a 2010 Japanese study reported the incidence of methicillin-resistant *S pseudintermedius* (MRSP) at 66.7%. Many methicillin-resistant isolates are also multidrug resistant (resistant to more than three classes of antibiotics), which makes clinical management, particularly empirical therapy, more difficult. Before the increase in incidence of resistant strains, if the exudative cytology showed the presence of an active infection with coccoid organisms, empirical antibiotic treatment could begin. The rise of antimicrobial resistance has led to the development of guidelines by several organizations (British Veterinary Association [www.bva.co.uk], Federation of European Companion Animal Veterinary Associations [www.fecava.org], International Society for Companion Animal Infectious Disease [www.iscaid.org]) on the appropriate use of antibiotics for case management. (*See* TABLE 10.)

Empiric therapy may still be appropriate in the case of first-time or previously untreated superficial infections in which positive exudative cytology (with coccoid bacteria) has been established. The following may be used as first-line antimicrobials: cephalexin, cephadroxil, amoxicillin-clavulanate, trimethoprim-sulfas, lincosamides, and cefovecin (if owner compliance is consid-

TABLE 10 DOSAGES OF ANTISTAPHYLOCOCCAL ANTIBIOTICS

Drug	Dosage
CEPHALOSPORINS	
Cephalexin	20–30 mg/kg, bid, PO
Cephadroxil	Dogs: 20 mg/kg, bid, PO
	Cats: 20 mg/kg/day, PO
Cefaclor	10–25 mg/kg, bid, PO
Cefovecin	8 mg/kg, SC, every 14 days
Cefpodoxime	5–10 mg/kg/day, PO
PENICILLINS	
Amoxicillin-clavulanate	13.75 mg/kg, bid, PO
Oxacillin	22 mg/kg, tid, PO
FLUOROQUINOLONES	
Enrofloxacin	5 mg/kg/day, PO
Marbofloxacin	2 mg/kg/day, PO
Orbifloxacin	2.5 mg/kg/day, PO
Difloxacin	5 mg/kg/day, PO
Pradofloxacin	3 mg/kg/day, PO
SULFONAMIDES	
Trimethoprim-sulfadiazine	15–30 mg/kg, bid, PO
Trimethoprim-sulfamethoxazole	15–30 mg/kg, bid, PO
MACROLIDES	
Erythromycin	15–30 mg/kg, tid, PO
Clindamycin	Dogs: 10–20 mg/kg, bid, PO
	Cats: 12.5–25 mg/kg, bid, PO
Azithromycin	10 mg/kg/day, PO
OTHERS	
Lincomycin	10–20 mg/kg, bid, PO
Chloramphenicol	50 mg/kg, tid, PO
Rifampin	5–10 mg/kg, once or twice daily, PO

ered an issue). Culture and sensitivity testing should be performed in any of the following circumstances: infections that have not responded to appropriate empiric therapy, presence of deep infections (nodules, hemorrhagic bullae, draining tracts), rod-shaped or unusual organisms on cytology, recurrent or relapsing infection, history of previous courses (particularly multiple) of antibiotic therapy, nonhealing wounds, recent potential exposure of owner or affected animal to methicillin-resistant staphylococci in health care environments, or history of prior MRSP infections. Second-line antimicrobials should be used only if there is no sensitivity to first-line antimicrobials on culture and sensitivity testing. These antibiotics are not appropriate for empiric therapy and include cefovecin (except when owner compliance is an issue), cefpodoxime, and fluoroquinolones (difloxacin, enrofloxacin, marbofloxacin, orbifloxacin, pradofloxacin). Third-line antimicrobials should be used only in cases in which there is evidence of sensitivity, no sensitivity to first or second-line antimicrobials, and topical antiseptics are not feasible or effective. Third-line antimicrobials include aminoglycosides, azithromycin, chloramphenicol, clarithromycin, imipenem, rifampin, and ticarcillin. With the increase in methicillin- and multidrug-resistant strains of staphylococci, the use of topical antiseptics has increased. They can be used as sole therapy for mild to moderate superficial infections and can reduce the treatment duration in more severe infections. There is little evidence that even multidrug-resistant staphylococci are not susceptible to topical antiseptics.

Duration of therapy varies with the type of infection present but should continue until the clinical lesions have resolved and cytology is normal. In general, superficial infections should be treated for 7 days beyond surface healing (commonly 3–4 wk); deep infections should be treated 7–21 days beyond resolution, which may require treatment durations of 8–12 wk if continued improvement is seen. Clinical resolution of MRSP infections may take longer than methicillin-susceptible *S pseudintermedius* infections, but this is most likely due to infection chronicity and secondary changes of the skin rather than to any inherent virulence of the bacterial strain.

The potential for serious adverse effects when using either chloramphenicol or rifampin should be understood. Chloramphenicol can cause a dose-dependent bone marrow suppression (cats more sensitive), although GI irritation, inappetence, and weight loss are the most common. Rifampin may cause hepatic enzyme induction and increase in hepatic enzyme activity, particularly alkaline phosphatase. Some dogs may develop a fatal hepatotoxicity. Other adverse effects include GI upset, hemolytic anemia, thrombocytopenia, and orange discoloration of body fluids. Liver enzymes should be monitored at least every 2 wk for the duration of therapy.

ANTIFUNGALS

The antifungal drugs used most commonly to treat integumentary diseases are listed in TABLE 11.

Griseofulvin: Griseofulvin has a very low solubility in water; GI absorption is variable and incomplete with the micronized form. Absorption may be enhanced by administration with a fat-containing meal or by formulations using polyethylene glycol or very small particles (micronization). The ultramicronized form is nearly 100% absorbed.

Griseofulvin is concentrated in skin (the highest concentration is in the stratum corneum), hair, nails, fat, skeletal muscle, and liver and can be found in the stratum corneum within 4 hr of dosing. It is also secreted in sweat and is deposited in keratinocytes and remains tightly bound during differentiation, so new skin growth is the first to be clear of infection. It is effective only against dermatophytes, eg, *Microsporum*, *Trichophyton*, and *Epidermophyton*.

In dogs, adverse effects (eg, vomiting, diarrhea) and increased liver enzymes predominate. In cats, anemia, leukopenia, vomiting, diarrhea, depression, pruritus, fever, and ataxia have been described. Bone marrow suppression (usually manifest as neutropenia) may occur idiosyncratically, especially in feline immunodeficiency virus (FIV)-positive cats and in kittens. FIV status should be determined before use, and griseofulvin avoided in kittens <8 wk old. The reactions may be more common and severe in Persian, Himalayan, Siamese, and Abyssinian cats. Teratogenicity is a major problem in all species.

Hemograms should be collected every 2 wk and close observation maintained. Leukopenia is more common in FIV-positive cats, so screening should be done before initiating treatment.

Ketoconazole: Ketoconazole is a synthetic, broad-spectrum antifungal drug belonging to the imidazole family. It is a potent inhibitor of ergosterol (a main membrane lipid of fungi) synthesis. Fungal

TABLE 11 DOSAGES OF ANTIFUNGAL MEDICATIONS

Drug	Dosage
Griseofulvin	
Microsize	25–60 mg/kg, PO, bid
Ultramicrosize	2.5–15 mg/kg, PO, bid
Ketoconazole	10 mg/kg/day, PO; 20 mg/kg, PO, every 48 hr
Itraconazole	5–10 mg/kg/day, PO
Fluconazole	10–20 mg/kg, PO, bid
Amphotericin B	Dogs: 0.25–0.75 mg/kg, IV, 3 times/wk to total cumulative dose of 4–8 mg/kg or until azotemia develops
	Cats: 0.1–0.25 mg/kg, IV, 3 times/wk to cumulative dose of 4–6 mg/kg
Flucytosine	25–50 mg/kg, PO, tid-qid
Terbinafine	10–30 mg/kg/day, PO
Potassium iodine	Dogs: 40 mg/kg, PO, once or twice daily with food
	Cats: 20 mg/kg, PO, once or twice daily with food

cells are thus unable to maintain the integrity of plasma membranes, which leads to cell wall rupture. Because the therapeutic effect of ketoconazole is delayed, amphotericin B is often used in combination for cases of serious systemic disease.

For dermatophytosis, ketoconazole is active against *Trichophyton verrucosum*, *T equinum*, *T mentagrophytes*, *Microsporum canis*, and *M nanum*. It is also active against the yeast *Malassezia pachydermatis* and *Cryptococcus neoformans* and is normally used at 10 mg/kg/day, PO. For candidiasis, the dosage is 10 mg/kg/day, PO, for 6–8 wk. In some chronic cases, a maintenance dosage of 2.5–5 mg/kg can be used. Coccidioidomycosis responds better to ketoconazole than to amphotericin B in many instances, with a minimal treatment period of 12 mo in animals with disseminated disease. Blastomycosis, histoplasmosis, and cryptococcosis may be treated with a combination of ketoconazole and amphotericin B (the combination is not more effective than the latter alone, but there are fewer nephrotoxic signs). For blastomycosis, a 4–6 mg/kg total dose of amphotericin B is combined with ketoconazole (20 mg/kg/day in dogs, and 10 mg/kg/day in cats). For histoplasmosis, amphotericin B (2–4 mg/kg total dose) is combined with ketoconazole (20 mg/kg/day in dogs, and 10 mg/kg/day in cats).

Ketoconazole inhibits cortisol synthesis and has been used to treat canine hyperadrenocorticism at 10 mg/kg/day. If the cortisol level is still above resting levels after 10 days, the dosage may be increased to 15 mg/kg/day.

Ketoconazole requires an acidic environment for optimal absorption, so H_2-blockers or antacids should not be administered concurrently.

In dogs, the most common adverse effects are inappetence, vomiting, pruritus, alopecia, and reversible lightening of the hair coat. Anorexia may be reduced by administering the dose with food. Cats appear to be more sensitive to ketoconazole. Clinical signs of toxicity include anorexia, fever, depression, diarrhea, and increased liver enzymes. Dosages >10 mg/kg/day are rarely given. Hepatotoxicity (cholangiohepatitis and increased liver enzymes) has also been reported.

Itraconazole: The primary antifungal mechanism of action of itraconazole seems to be the same as that of ketoconazole; however, it has a greater potency, decreased toxicity, and a wider spectrum of activity. Even at high dosages, it does not alter hormone levels in rats, dogs, or people. Itraconazole should be administered with food; the concurrent administration of antacids, H_2-blockers, and cholinergics is contraindicated.

Itraconazole is effective against dermatophytes, *Candida*, *Cryptococcus*, *Histoplasma*, *Blastomyces*, and *Sporothrix* spp, and the protozoans *Leishmania* and *Trypanosoma*. For dermatophytosis in dogs, the dosage is 5 mg/kg/day. For systemic mycoses, the dosage is 5–10 mg/kg/day, but the addition of amphotericin should be considered in rapidly progressing infections. For treatment of dermatophytosis and systemic mycoses in cats, the dosage is 10 mg/kg/day.

A severe, dose-related ulcerative dermatitis (due to vasculitis) has been seen in 5%–10% of dogs given itraconazole in doses of 10 mg/kg. If the condition is identified early, drug withdrawal leads to resolution; if not recognized early, severe, extensive necrosis and sloughing can develop.

Fluconazole: Fluconazole is a fungistatic triazole compound with a mode of action similar to that of ketoconazole. However, it does not affect mammalian hormone synthesis. Because of its small molecular size and low lipophilicity, it may be more useful in treating CNS mycoses.

Fluconazole is effective against superficial dermatophytes and *Candida*, *Cryptococcus*, *Histoplasma*, and *Blastomyces* spp. The dosage is 2.5–10 mg/kg/day in dogs. Cats with cryptococcosis can be given 2.5–10 mg/kg, bid.

Fluconazole has had limited use in small animals. In people, it can cause occasional GI adverse effects (eg, vomiting, diarrhea, anorexia, nausea).

Amphotericin B: Amphotericin is a lipophilic polyene from *Streptomyces nodosus* that binds to sterols (especially ergosterol), causing increased permeability and leakage of nutrients and electrolytes. It is poorly absorbed from the GI tract and must be given parenterally. IV administration gives good penetration, except into muscle, bone, eye, or synovial fluid.

Amphotericin B is used in progressive or disseminated deep mycosis. It may be combined with flucytosine or minocycline for treatment of *Candida* and *Cryptococcus*. Rifampin potentiates the effect of amphotericin on *Aspergillus* (which is usually resistant against amphotericin alone), *Candida*, and *Histoplasma*.

Amphotericin B is insoluble in water and is prepared as an IV solution by forming a colloidal dispersion with sodium deoxycholate. Because it is inactivated by sunlight, it should be stored in the dark. Dilution with large volumes of 5% glucose (10 mg amphotericin B/100 mL fluid) is recommended to reduce nephrotoxicity. The dilution should be given over 2–6 hr. If a bolus is given in 10–60 mL of dextrose (via a butterfly catheter), supplemental fluid diuresis is helpful. Amphotericin B is given at 0.15–0.5 mg/kg every 48 hr until a total cumulative dose of 4–12 mg/kg is reached. Renal toxic effects are monitored by electrolytes or urinalysis at least weekly (urinalysis detects toxicity earlier than biochemistry); BUN, creatinine, PCV, and total plasma proteins should be checked before the administration of each dose. Monthly maintenance therapy is recommended to avoid relapses.

The major adverse effect seen with amphotericin B is nephrotoxicity—most dogs incur some kidney damage. The damage is not correlated with either total dose or duration of therapy. The causes of toxicity include vasoconstriction, impaired acid excretion, and direct tubular injury. Cats are more sensitive, so lower doses are recommended. Adverse effects such as fever, nausea, and vomiting are less severe if diphenhydramine (0.5 mg/kg, IV), aspirin (10 mg/kg, PO), or hydrocortisone sodium succinate (0.5 mg/kg, IV) is given before administration of amphotericin B.

Flucytosine: This fluorinated pyrimidine was developed as an antineoplastic agent. It interferes with RNA metabolism and protein synthesis in fungal cells. It is well absorbed and enters the CNS in high concentrations. Most of the drug is excreted unchanged in the urine.

Flucytosine is effective against *Cryptococcus neoformans*, *Candida*, and other yeasts but has little or no effect on other fungi. Resistance develops frequently; thus, it is given in combination with amphotericin B. It is used almost exclusively for treatment of cryptococcosis. The dosage in dogs and cats is 25–50 mg/kg, tid-qid.

GI tract disturbances (vomiting, diarrhea, anorexia), bone marrow suppression (anemia, leukopenia, thrombocytopenia), and cutaneous eruption (depigmentation, ulceration, exudation, and crust formation) are the most common adverse effects.

Terbinafine: Terbinafine is an allylamine compound that interferes with fungal sterol biosynthesis at an early stage, causing deficiency of ergosterol, intracellular accumulation of squalene, and fungal cell death. It achieves high concentrations in hair follicles, hair, sebum-rich skin, nail plates, and nails. In people, levels exceeding the minimum inhibitory concentration may be found for up to 3 wk after treatment has ended. There are anecdotal reports of its use against *Trichophyton*, *Microsporum*, and *Epidermophyton*, as well as *Malassezia* dermatitis. The dosage in cats is 10–30 mg/kg/day. In people, rare cases of hepatic toxicity are seen, along with GI tract signs (eg, nausea, vomiting, diarrhea) and skin signs (eg, urticaria, itch, erythema).

Systemic Iodine: The mechanism of action of systemic iodine is unknown; no fungicidal effects are seen in vitro. It is used in small animals for sporotrichosis; in cattle for actinomycosis and actinobacillosis; and in horses for mycetomas, zygomycosis, and *Sporothrix schenckii*. Dogs are treated with potassium iodide 40 mg/kg, PO, bid; cats with potassium iodide 20 mg/kg, PO, once to twice daily; cattle with sodium iodide 60 mg/kg, IV, weekly; and horses (sporotrichosis) with sodium iodide, 40 mg/kg/day, IV, for 2–5 days, followed by potassium iodide, 2 mg/kg/day, PO, for 60 days.

In small animals, vomiting, diarrhea, depression, and inappetence (especially in cats) may develop. Ocular and nasal discharge, scaling, and a dry hair coat also may be seen in dogs. In large animals, seromucoid discharge, lacrimation, cough, variable appetite, joint pain, and seborrhea sicca with partial alopecia may develop. Systemic iodine may also cause abortion and should not be used in pregnant or lactating animals.

ANTIPARASITICS

Ivermectin: Ivermectin is an avermectin and a fermentation product of *Streptomyces avermitilis* (*see also* MACROCYCLIC LACTONES, p 2647). It acts as a GABA agonist, causing paralysis in susceptible arthropods and nematodes. It is used in small animals for treatment of *Sarcoptes scabiei*, *Otodectes cynotis*, *Cheyletiella blakei*, *C yasguri*, and *Demodex canis*; in cattle for psoroptic mange, lice, and *Hypoderma* larvae; in horses for equine filarial dermatitis from *Onchocerca cervicalis*; and in swine for *Sarcoptes scabiei*.

In small animals, all use for skin conditions is extra-label in the USA. For *Demodex*, the dosage is 0.3–0.6 mg/kg/day, PO, until two negative skin scrapings 1 mo apart. For *Sarcoptes*, *Otodectes*, and *Cheyletiella*, the dosage is 0.3 mg/kg, PO, repeated in 2 wk. In cattle, 0.2 mg/kg is given as a single SC injection for *Psoroptes* and lice. In horses, 0.2 mg/kg, PO, kills microfilariae but not adult *Onchocerca cervicalis*, so relapse may be noted within 2 mo of treatment. In swine, the dosage is 0.3 mg/kg, SC, repeated in 2 wk, or 0.1–0.2 mg/kg in feed for 7 days.

In mammals, GABA is found only in the CNS and does not readily cross the blood-brain barrier. At least 10 times the normal dose of ivermectin is needed for toxic reactions. Ataxia, depression, and visual impairment develop in horses given 2 mg/kg, PO. In cattle, 4 mg/kg by drench or 8 mg/kg, SC, leads to listlessness and ataxia; 30 mg/kg induces ataxia in swine.

Some dog breeds (Collies, Shetland Sheepdogs, Old English Sheepdogs, Australian Collies, and their crosses) have an abnormality in the blood-brain barrier associated with a mutation of the multiple drug resistance gene MDR1, which allows increased ivermectin into the CNS and results in toxicity. Dogs that are homozygous for the mutation produce a severely truncated P-glycoprotein (<10% of the normal amino acid sequence) and will develop ivermectin toxicity at any of the dosages used to treat demodicosis. The critical point seems to be 120–150 mcg/kg, at which transient, nonfatal clinical signs (mydriasis, ataxia, tremors) are seen. At higher dosages, collapse, coma, and respiratory collapse may develop. Similar idiosyncratic reactions may develop in any breed, so a gradually increasing dose (daily progression of 50, 100, 150, 200, then 300 mcg/kg) should be given to identify susceptible individuals. Administration should be stopped if any adverse effects are seen. One cat treated with 4 mg of the oral paste (~70 mcg/kg) showed ataxia, blindness, tremors, and mydriasis, with retinal atrophy in one eye 10 hr later.

Milbemycin: Milbemycin is derived from fermentation products of *Streptomyces hygroscopicus* and, like ivermectin, acts as a GABA agonist but with a wider spectrum of activity against intestinal parasites. It has been used extra-label in dogs to treat nasal mites, scabies, and generalized demodicosis. No adverse effects have been seen in ivermectin-sensitive breeds. The dosage in dogs is 1–2 mg/kg every 7 days for 3–5 treatments for nasal mites and scabies and 1–2 mg/kg/day for *Demodex*.

Moxidectin: Moxidectin belongs to the milbemycin class of compounds. It is registered for heartworm control (*Dirofilaria immitis*) but has also been used extra-label for treatment of *Otodectes* and demodicosis in dogs. In cattle, it is used to treat lice (*Linognathus vituli*, *Solenopotes capillatus*, *Bovicola bovis*), mites (*Psoroptes*, *Chorioptes bovis*), ticks (*Boophilus microplus*), and fly warbles and grubs (*Hypoderma bovis*, *Hypoderma lineatum*). In sheep, it is used for *Psorobia ovis* infestation. The dosage is 0.2–0.4 mg/kg/day, PO, in dogs and 0.2 mg/kg in cattle and sheep.

Selamectin: This semisynthetic macrocyclic lactone is applied topically but acts systemically. It is effective against *Ctenocephalides* spp (both adults and larvae), *Sarcoptes scabiei*, *Otodectes cynotis*, and *Dermacentor variabilis*. The dosage in dogs and cats is 6 mg/kg, applied topically.

Lufenuron: Lufenuron is an insect growth regulator that inhibits the synthesis of chitin, a critical component of insect exoskeletons. It is taken up by adult fleas while feeding. While it has no effect on adult fleas, it prevents development of the intermediate stages of the flea life cycle (ie, eggs, larvae, pupae). It is effective against *Ctenocephalides* spp in dogs and cats at a dosage of 10 mg/kg, PO, once a month. Chitin is also a component in the fungal cell wall of dermatophytes. An initial study showed efficacy of lufenuron in treating small animal dermatophytosis; however, additional studies have failed to show efficacy.

Nitenpyram: Nitenpyram inhibits the nicotinic acetylcholine receptor. It is used to treat *Ctenocephalides* spp in dogs and cats at a dosage of 1 mg/kg, PO. Nitenpyram has a short half-life and kills fleas on the animal within 30 min of administration. It is toxic to fleas for only 24–48 hr and is normally used in combination with an insect growth regulator to provide continuous flea control.

Spinosad: Spinosad stimulates the nicotinic acetycholine receptor, which causes activation of motor neurons and results in involuntary muscle contractions and tremors, leading to paralysis and death of the insect. It is used to treat *Ctenophalides* spp in dogs at a dosage of 31–70 mg/kg monthly and in cats at a dosage of 50–90 mg/kg monthly. It may trigger severe signs of ivermectin toxicity if administered concurrently with extra-label, high-dose ivermectin.

Indoxacarb: Indoxacarb blocks sodium channels in the insect to cause paralysis and death. It is effective against *Ctenophalides* spp, both adults and larvae, and is applied as a spot-on topically, once a month.

Cythioate: Cythioate is an organophosphate that kills via anticholinesterase activity. It is indicated for *Ctenocephalides* spp infestations at a dosage of 3 mg/kg, PO, twice weekly (dogs) or 1.5 mg/kg, PO, twice weekly (cats). Although effective blood levels are maintained for <12 hr, serum cholinesterase activity may be decreased for >1 mo after dosing.

Sodium Stibogluonate: Sodium stiboglucoante is used for treatment of cutaneous leishmaniasis, either as a sole therapy or in combination with allopurinol, paromomycin, or pentamidine. The exact mode of action is unknown, but it is believed to interfere with energy metabolism in *Leishmania* amastigotes. Dosage in dogs is 30–50 mg/kg/day, IV or SC, for 3–4 wk. If adverse effects occur (musculoskeletal pain, increase in liver transaminases, pancreatitis, myocardial injury, hemolytic anemia, leukopenia, renal dysfunction), the dose may be administered every other day for longer periods. Note that IV administration should be over 5 min to minimize cardiotoxicity.

ANTIHISTAMINES

Antihistamines block either H_1 or H_2 receptors. H_1 receptors are responsible for pruritus, increased vascular permeability, release of inflammatory mediators, and attraction of inflammatory cells. H_1 blockers act by competing with histamine for H_1-receptor sites on effector cells (they do not block release of histamine but can antagonize its effects). They also have anticholinergic, sedative, and local anesthetic effects and vary greatly in their potency, dosage, incidence of adverse effects, and cost.

Second-generation H_1 blockers (eg, terfenadine, cetirazine, loratadine, astemazole) are less likely to cross the blood-brain barrier, or they have a low affinity for brain compared with peripheral H_1 receptors. They have not proved useful to date in controlling pruritus in small animals. Responses to antihistamines vary considerably, and several trials may be necessary to find one effective for an animal (*see* TABLE 12). Antihistamines may act synergistically with NSAIDs, glucocorticoids, or fatty acid supplements and may allow dosages of these agents to be reduced in some cases.

First-generation antihistamines may cause drowsiness or GI signs (eg, vomiting, diarrhea). Overdoses may cause CNS hyperexcitability and may be fatal. Anticholinergic properties lead to hypertension (and thus contraindicated in cardiac patients), dry mouth, blurred vision (contraindicated in glaucoma), and urinary retention. Hydroxyzine is teratogenic. They may also stimulate appetite (particularly cyproheptadine).

Second-generation antihistamines are cardiotoxic at high doses. High doses of terfenadine and astemizole lead to

TABLE 12 ANTIHISTAMINE DOSAGES

Drug	Dosage
Diphenhydramine	2–4 mg/kg, bid-tid
Hydroxyzine	0.5–2 mg/kg, tid-qid
Clorpheniramine	Cats: 2–4 mg, bid Dogs <20 kg: 4 mg, tid Dogs >20 kg: 8 mg, tid; 0.25–0.5 mg/kg, tid
Cyproheptadine	0.25–0.5 mg/kg, tid; 1.1 mg/kg, bid
Terfenadine	5 mg/kg, bid
Clemastine	Cats: 0.05 mg/kg, bid Dogs: 0.1 mg/kg, bid
Trimeprazine	1 mg/kg, bid
Cetirizine	Dogs: 1 mg/kg or 10–20 mg per dog, once or twice daily Cats: 1 mg/kg or 5 mg per cat, once or twice daily
Fexofenadine	Dogs: 2–5 mg/kg, once or twice daily Cats: 10–15 mg per cat, once or twice daily

prolonged QT intervals and arrhythmias (eg, ventricular tachycardia, cardiac arrest). Cardiotoxicity has been reported only as a result of overdose in animals with impaired hepatic metabolism.

ESSENTIAL FATTY ACIDS

Fatty acids are essential components of cell membranes and are an integral component of the intercellular barrier in the stratum corneum. Essential fatty acids cannot be synthesized and therefore must be supplied in the diet. The essential fatty acids most important for homeostasis of the skin in dogs and cats are linoleic acid and linolenic acid. The anti-inflammatory properties of fatty acids are thought to be due to competitive inhibition of arachidonic acid metabolism, leading to a reduction in inflammatory leukotriene and prostaglandin synthesis and activity, and to the formation of metabolic byproducts of normal fatty acid metabolism that have direct anti-inflammatory properties.

Essential fatty acids are indicated for pruritic inflammatory diseases (eg, allergies, feline eosinophilic granuloma), crusting diseases (eg, discoid lupus erythematosus), and onychodystrophy. Many commercial products are available and may be used at the manufacturers' recommended dose. Lack of response to one product does not preclude response to another, and increasing the dose to several times the label recommendation can help in some cases. Approximately 20% of dogs and 50% of cats with allergic pruritus will show some improvement. There are few adverse effects; however, pancreatitis has rarely been reported. Large doses may also cause weight gain or diarrhea.

HORMONAL THERAPY

Glucocorticoids: Glucocorticoids have profound effects on nearly all cell types and organ systems, particularly immunologic and inflammatory activity. They may be used in either an anti-inflammatory or immunosuppressive capacity, depending on the dosage selected. Glucocorticoids are used for hypersensitivity dermatoses, contact dermatitis, immune-mediated diseases (eg, pemphigus, pemphigoid, lupus erythematosus), and neoplasia (eg, mast cell tumor, lymphoma). Glucocorticoids may be classified according to their duration of effect and relative potency (*see* TABLE 13). They may be administered PO, IV, IM, or SC.

The anti-inflammatory dosage of prednisolone is 0.5–1 mg/kg/day in dogs (severe cases may require 2 mg/kg/day) and 1–2 mg/kg/day in cats. This dosage is given for an induction period of 5–7 days and then reduced to the lowest possible maintenance dosage (ideally 0.25 mg/kg, every 48–72 hr

TABLE 13 GLUCOCORTICOIDS

Drug	Relative Potency	Duration of Effect
Hydrocortisone (cortisol)	1	<12 hr
Prednisolone	4	12–36 hr
Prednisone	4	12–36 hr
Methylprednisolone	5	12–36 hr
Triamcinolone	5	12–36 hr
Flumethasone	15–30	36–48 hr
Betamethasone	25	>48 hr
Dexamethasone	30	>48 hr

or lower in dogs). Maintenance doses must be given ≥48 hr apart to minimize adrenal suppression and chronic adverse effects. The immunosuppressive dosage of prednisolone is 2.2 mg/kg/day in dogs (up to 6.6 mg/kg/day may be required in severe disease) and 4.4 mg/kg/day in cats.

The induction period is generally longer (10–20 days) than with anti-inflammatory dosing but is then gradually tapered in a stepwise fashion to an alternate-day dosing regimen once there is evidence of disease remission. Treatment should never be stopped abruptly, because of the risk of inducing signs of hypoadrenocorticism. If relapse occurs during the tapering process, the dose is increased to at least one step above the point at which the relapse occurred and tapered again if possible. In many cases, therapy may be withdrawn entirely without relapse, whereas others require lifelong treatment.

Administration PO is preferred, because dosing can be more closely regulated and physiologic processes are disrupted less than with repositol forms. In some cases, difficulties with animal handling or owner adherence may require injectable therapy. This is normally satisfactory for acute, short-term disease that does not require repeated administration (eg, a single injection of methylprednisolone acetate alters adrenocortical function in dogs for up to 10 wk).

Adverse effects include polyuria, polydipsia, polyphagia, weight gain, increased susceptibility to infection, GI ulceration, pancreatitis, osteoporosis, hyperglycemia, steroid myopathy, and calcinosis cutis. The extent and severity of adverse effects are related to the dose, duration, and type of glucocorticoid used, along with individual animal sensitivity. The most commonly encountered infections are urinary tract infections, pyoderma, and pulmonary infections. Urinary tract infections may develop in many animals on longterm glucocorticoid therapy (68% in one study), and these animals may show no clinical signs of the infection. Urine should be cultured for bacterial growth every 3–6 mo in all animals on longterm therapy.

Progressive hepatocellular swelling due to glycogen accumulation may develop during glucocorticoid therapy. Alkaline phosphatase (ALP), ALT, and γ-glutamyl transferase all show progressive increases. In dogs, the initial ALP increase is due to hepatic ALP but later is due to a cortisone isoenzyme.

Most injectable forms are labeled for IM use; however, they are commonly given SC. Local areas of alopecia, pigmentation, and epidermal and dermal atrophy may be seen with SC injection.

Thyroid Hormone: Thyroid hormones are indicated as replacement therapy for primary, secondary, and tertiary hypothyroidism. Most cases of canine hypothyroidism are primary in nature and are due to autoimmune destruction of the thyroid gland. Drug-induced low hormone levels or "euthyroid sick syndrome" are not indications for supplementation with thyroid hormones.

Synthetic levothyroxine (T_4) is the drug of choice for canine hypothyroidism. Most dogs respond clinically to a dosage of 0.02 mg/kg, bid. Insufficient serum levels after 4–6 wk of treatment or lack of a clinical response after 12 wk are indications to increase the dose. Synthetic liothyronine (T_3) may be used for those rare animals that cannot convert T_4 to T_3. It should not be used for routine treatment of hypothyroidism, because it bypasses the normal cellular regulatory pathways and has a short half-life. Dosage is 4–6 mcg/kg, PO, bid-tid. Crude preparations from thyroid tissue and synthetic thyroid hormone combinations that mimic the T_4:T_3 ratio in people should not be used in animals.

Signs of thyrotoxicosis in cats and dogs are rare. They include polyuria, polydipsia, nervousness, aggressiveness, panting, diarrhea, tachycardia, pyrexia, and pruritus. Complications in dogs are usually related to concurrent cardiac or adrenal insufficiencies. In animals with a marginal cardiac reserve, T_4 medication should be initiated at one-fourth the recommended dosage and gradually increased to full dosage over a 1-mo period.

Trilostane: Trilostane is a hormonally inactive, steroid competitive inhibitor of the adrenal enzyme 3β-hydroxysteroid dehydrogenase. It is used in treatment of pituitary-dependent hyperadrenocorticism. It inhibits the production of progesterone and 17-hydroxyprogestrone and their end products, including adrenal, gonadal, and placental hormones. However, the inhibition of adrenal steroidogenesis occurs at lower doses than those required to inhibit steroid hormone synthesis in other organs. The recommended starting dosage for dogs is 2–10 mg/kg/day, PO, but this may be increased or decreased, based on periodic adrenocorticotropic hormone (ACTH) stimulation test results (performed 3–8 hr after trilostane administration). If the post-ACTH plasma cortisol concentration is <20 nmol/L, trilostane administration should be stopped for 48–72 hr and the ACTH stimulation test repeated. If the post-ACTH plasma cortisol concentration is 20–200 nmol/L, the dosage should not be altered. If the post-ACTH plasma cortisol concentration is >200 nmol/L, the dosage should be increased.

Adverse effects include depression, ataxia, hypersalivation, vomiting, muscle tremors, and skin changes. Sudden death has been reported in a small number of cases. Iatrogenic hypoadrenocorticism can occur but is generally reversible. Because of its inhibition of placental hormones, trilostane is contraindicated in pregnant and nursing animals and in any animals intended for breeding. Serial biochemical, electrolyte, and hematologic analyses and ACTH stimulation tests should be performed to monitor hepatic and renal function before treatment and at 10 days, 4 wk, 12 wk, and every 3–6 mo thereafter.

Mitotane (o,p′DDD): o,p′DDD is a chlorinated hydrocarbon with potent adrenocorticolytic effects causing selective necrosis of the zona fasciculata and zona reticularis and partial or complete necrosis of the zona glomerulosa. It is used to treat pituitary-dependent hyperadrenocorticism. Before starting therapy, food intake (amount), time taken to eat, and the 24-hr water intake should be recorded to determine a baseline. Once this has been established, a loading dose is administered daily (25 mg/kg, bid) until the animal becomes lethargic, water intake drops, appetite is reduced, or the animal has other GI adverse effects (vomiting, diarrhea) or after 5 days of administration. An ACTH stimulation test should be performed to confirm whether adequate suppression of the adrenals has been achieved.

Most dogs respond to o,p′DDD therapy at the initial loading dose within 5–10 days, and the decision to change to maintenance therapy should be based on clinical signs (reduced appetite and water intake) and ACTH stimulation test results. Dogs with a post-ACTH plasma cortisol concentration <25 nmol/L should receive no medication for 2 wk and should then be treated with 25 mg/kg/wk divided into 2 or 3 doses. Dogs with a post-ACTH plasma cortisol concentration of 25–125 nmol/L should receive 25 mg/kg/wk in 2 or 3 doses, and dogs with a post-ACTH cortisol concentration >125 nmol/L should receive 50 mg/kg/wk.

During maintenance therapy, an ACTH stimulation test should be performed after 1 mo and then every 3–4 mo. If the post-ACTH plasma cortisol concentration is <25 nmol/L, the dose of o,p′DDD should be reduced; if the concentration exceeds 125 nmol/L, the dose should be increased, usually by about 20%–25% weekly. Although most dogs are stable on maintenance therapy, their adrenal reserve may not be adequate to handle major stress (physiologic or psychologic). In these cases, o,p′DDD administration should be discontinued and replaced with glucocorticoids (0.2 mg/kg/day, PO, tapered) during this period.

Adverse effects are relatively common, particularly in cases of o,p′DDD overdose. These include signs of hypoadrenocorticism, eg, weakness, ataxia, depression, vomiting, diarrhea, and inappetence. Biochemical and hematologic analysis may be unremarkable despite systemic illness. Treatment includes lowering the dose or ceasing administration of o,p′DDD and supplementing with glucocorticoids. Clinical improvement is usually seen within 1–6 hr. Iatrogenic hypoadrenocorticism is the most serious adverse effect and may develop at any time during maintenance treatment. Administration of o,p′DDD should be stopped and appropriate supplementation with glucocorticoids and mineralocorticoids started. Other rare CNS adverse effects include ataxia, apparent blindness, circling, and head pressing.

Progesterones: The two most commonly used forms of progesterone are megestrol acetate and medroxyprogesterone acetate. Megestrol acetate has a quick onset of action and potent glucocorticoid and slight mineralocorticoid activity, and it may be given PO. Medroxyprogesterone acetate is antiestrogenic and has significant glucocorticoid activity. Neutered male and female cats with bilateral alopecia suspected to be caused by sex hormone imbalances may respond to treatment. The dosage of megestrol acetate is 2.5–5 mg/cat, PO, every 48 hr, decreasing to every 1–2 wk for maintenance. Medroxyprogesterone acetate is given at a dosage of 50–100 mg/cat, IM, and may be repeated in 3–6 mo.

Progestagens should be avoided whenever possible because of adverse effects; severe, prolonged adrenocortical suppression is seen even with low doses. Diabetes mellitus has been reported in cats treated with megestrol acetate. Decreased spermatogenesis, pyometra, increased levels of growth hormone with acromegaly, mammary gland hyperplasia and tumors, and behavioral changes may be seen.

Growth Hormone: Growth hormone (somatotropin) is a polypeptide produced by the anterior pituitary that acts either directly on target tissues or indirectly through insulin-like growth factors (somatomedins) produced by the liver (*see also* THE PITUITARY GLAND, p 542). It is necessary for hair growth and for development of elastin fibers in the skin. It is used to treat growth hormone–responsive alopecia in dogs. Either bovine, porcine, or human growth hormone (0.1 IU/kg, 3 times/wk for 4–6 wk) is effective. Hair usually regrows in 2–3 mo, and remission may last from 6 mo to 3 yr. Growth hormone is diabetogenic, and dogs can develop transient or permanent diabetes mellitus during therapy. Weekly monitoring of blood glucose before and during therapy is recommended.

Sex Hormones: Several syndromes in dogs and cats have been attributed to imbalances of sex hormones; however, the etiopathogenesis of these disorders is generally poorly documented. Hypoestrogenism in spayed female dogs, hypoandrogenism in male dogs, and feline acquired symmetric alopecia may respond to sex-hormone therapy. Dosages for sex-hormone replacement therapy are empirical. Hypoestrogenism in spayed female dogs may be treated with diethylstilbestrol (0.02 mg/kg/day for 3 wk of every month until hair regrows or for a maximum total dose of 1 mg/dog). After hair regrows, the maintenance dosage should be given 1–2 times/wk. An alternative protocol is to treat every other day or twice weekly until a response is seen. Hair regrowth should be evident in 3–4 wk, with a complete response within 4 mo. Exogenous estrogen can cause bone marrow hypoplasia, so a CBC and platelet count should be performed weekly during therapy. Other potential adverse effects include induction of estrus, hepatotoxicity, nymphomania, abortion, pyometra, or prostatic hyperplasia. Cats are highly sensitive to estrogens, and a total dose of 10 mg of diethylstilbestrol can be lethal.

Hypoandrogenism of male dogs may be treated with methyltestosterone, 0.5–1 mg/kg, PO, up to a total maximal dose of 30 mg every 48 hr. Alternatively, testosterone proprionate can be given IM once weekly at dosages of 0.5–1 mg/kg, or every 4–16 wk at 2 mg/kg. Complications include aggressive behavior, greasy hair coat, prostatic hypertrophy, and hepatotoxicity. Liver function should be evaluated before treatment and monthly during therapy.

Repositol testosterone, 12 mg/cat, IM, may be given once for treatment of feline acquired symmetric alopecia or may be combined with a low dose of diethylstilbestrol, 0.625 mg/cat, IM, or with a low dose of estradiol, 0.5 mg/cat, IM. Hepatobiliary disease has been reported in cats given testosterone.

Melatonin: Melatonin is produced in the pineal gland and is involved in the control of photoperiod-dependent molting of some mammals. Secretion is inversely related to daylight length and is highest during the winter. Various canine hair-growth disorders including recurrent flank alopecia, pattern baldness, and excessive tricholemmal keratinization have improved with melatonin supplementation. Recurrent flank alopecia may be treated with 36-mg SC implants. Oral melatonin is also available; an empirical dosage of 3–6 mg/dog, tid-qid, has been used successfully.

IMMUNOMODULATORS

Immunostimulants

Immunostimulation is used to enhance a deficient immunologic response; however, animals that appear to benefit from these agents are not severely immunosuppressed. The most common use of immunostimulants in dogs is for chronic, recurrent staphylococcal pyoderma. For primary therapy, immunomodulatory bacterins should not be substituted for antibiotics; they should be used concurrently with an appropriate antibiotic until the infection has been resolved. The immunomodulator is then continued and success judged on the time to and severity of any infection relapse. They are clearly helpful as adjunct agents or for maintenance therapy for some dogs with recurrent pyoderma but have no benefit in other cases.

Staphage lysate is a preparation of *Staphylococcus aureus* and polyvalent staphylococcus bacteriophage. When given concurrently with antibiotics, staphage lysate (0.5 mL, SC, twice weekly, or 1 mL, SC, weekly) has improved the response of dogs with superficial staphylococcal pyoderma compared with antibiotics alone. The mechanism of action is believed to be stimulation of T lymphocytes and activation of phagocytic cells. Deficient IgM levels—but not IgA or IgG levels—may be normalized with treatment.

S aureus bacterin-toxoid, used for prevention of staphylococcal mastitis in cattle, has been used with some success in cases of canine bacterial hypersensitivity. Various treatment protocols have been advocated. One schedule consists of 0.1 mL, intradermally, daily for 5 days, then weekly for 1 mo, then at monthly intervals. At corresponding times, doses given SC increase from 0.15 mL to 1.9 mL. Local swelling at the injection site, fever, and malaise are common adverse effects in dogs.

Propionibacterium acnes bacterin is labeled for use in dogs (0.25–2 mL, IV, 1–2 times/wk) and appears to have some benefit as adjunct treatment for recurrent pyoderma.

Many other immunostimulants have been described for use; however, responses in dermatologic disorders have been equivocal.

Immunosuppressants

Glucocorticoids: Glucocorticoids are the immunosuppressive agents most commonly used to treat immune-mediated skin disease (*see* p 827). A range of other immunosuppressants may be used either concurrently with glucocorticoids or alone for the treatment of various immune-mediated dermatoses, including systemic lupus erythematosus (SLE), pemphigus complex, bullous pemphigoid, and vasculitis.

Azathioprine: Azathioprine is converted to 6-mercaptopurine in the liver. It competes with purines in the synthesis of nucleic acids and prevents proliferation of rapidly dividing cells. It is used for treatment of pemphigus disorders, bullous pemphigoid and SLE in dogs, ocular inflammation in the uveodermatologic syndrome, and histiocytomas. There is a 3- to 5-wk lag period before its effects are evident, so it is often initially combined with glucocorticoids. The dosage is 2.2 mg/kg (50 mg/m^2), daily for 2 wk, and then reduced to every 48 hr. In dogs, it may be used in combination with metronidazole (10 mg/kg/day) for perianal furunculosis, although surgery may be necessary to remove residual scarring.

GI adverse effects (vomiting, diarrhea) may be avoided by administering with food or lowering the dose. Bone marrow suppression may also develop. All three cell lines can be affected, but leukopenia is the most common. The CBC should be monitored every 2 wk during induction and at least every 4 mo during maintenance therapy. Acute pancreatitis and hepatotoxicity has been reported in dogs. Azathioprine is contraindicated in cats because of rapid, lethal bone marrow suppression.

Cyclophosphamide: Cyclophosphamide is an alkylating agent used to treat a wide variety of cancers, especially lymphoreticular neoplasms, and is usually given in combination with other drugs. It may also be used short-term in severe cases of SLE, rheumatoid arthritis, pemphigus complex, and vasculitis. The dosage for immunosuppression is 1.5–2.5 mg/kg, every 48 hr. The dose should be given in the morning so that it does not remain in the bladder overnight. Because most animals treated with cyclophosphamide also receive corticosteroids, polyuria induced by the steroids may be somewhat protective. The potential for hemorrhagic cystitis and bladder fibrosis limits the use of cyclophosphamide to no more than 3–4 mo. GI tract toxicity, bone marrow suppression, alopecia, infertility, and teratogenic effects may also be seen.

Chlorambucil: Chlorambucil is an alkylating agent similar to cyclophosphamide. However, it is slower acting and the least toxic of the group. It may be used for treatment of immune complex diseases in which azathioprine or cyclophosphamide are not tolerated, and it may be given to cats. The dosage is 0.1–0.2 mg/kg/day, reduced to every other day once a response is seen. It is mostly used in combination with glucocorticoids but can be used with azathioprine in dogs only in particularly refractory cases. It may also be used to replace cyclophosphamide if hemorrhagic cystitis develops. Adverse effects are rare and include bone marrow suppression (which generally develops within 7–14 days of starting treatment and resolves in 7–14 days), GI irritation, and seizures. Delayed hair regrowth has been reported in shaved dogs.

Crysotherapy: Gold salts have anti-inflammatory, antirheumatic, immunomodulating, and antimicrobial (in vitro) effects. Parenteral and oral forms are available. Aurothiomalate is given parenterally. It is absorbed rapidly and reaches peak levels in 4–6 hr. Rising serum values are noted for 5–10 wk. Beneficial effects are seen 6–12 wk after the start of treatment. The oral form is auranofin. Only 25% is absorbed, and lower and more predictable plasma concentrations are found. The half-life is ~21 days, but the retention and tissue accumulation are only 1% (parenteral gold 30%). Results with this compound are equivocal in dogs. Gold salts are indicated for canine and feline pemphigus unresponsive to glucocorticoids and feline plasma cell pododermatitis.

Routine protocols start with a test dose IM (1 mg if <10 kg body wt, 5 mg if >10 kg body wt). The next week a second test dose is given IM (2 or 10 mg), and if no adverse reactions are seen, treatment continues at 1 mg/kg, IM, weekly until remission. Once in remission, the dose is given every 2 wk and may later be reduced to monthly injections. Occasionally, a higher dosage (1.5–2 mg/kg) may be required to induce remission. Treatment effects are not seen for 6–12 wk, so other medications (commonly glucocorticoids) must be given at therapeutic doses during this time. Gold salts should not be administered with other cytotoxic drugs because of the increased risk of toxic reactions. Adverse effects include allergic reactions (skin eruption, oral reactions), nephrotoxicity, and bone marrow suppression. Toxic epidermal necrolysis has been reported in dogs starting gold therapy immediately after azathioprine, so a 4-wk washout period is recommended in these cases.

Cyclosporine: Cyclosporine impairs the proliferation of activated T cells by inhibiting transcription of interleukin-2, gene activation, and RNA transcription. This early inhibition of T cells also leads to reduced production of other cytokines, mast cells, and eosinophils, and inhibition of mononuclear cells, antigen presentation, histamine release from mast cells, neutrophil adherence, natural killer cell activity, and B-cell growth and differentiation.

Cyclosporine is used for treatment of atopic dermatitis and anal furunculosis. Extra-label use for the treatment of immune-mediated disorders (pemphigus, SLE) and epitheliotropic lymphoma has been less successful. Response has been good when used for sebaceous adenitis. The dosage for atopic dermatitis in dogs is 5 mg/kg/day for 30 days, after which the dose may be reduced to alternate-day or even third-day dosing in some animals. The dosage for anal furunculosis is 7.5 mg/kg/day. The dosage for feline atopic dermatitis is 7 mg/kg/day for 30 days and then reduced to 7 mg/kg alternate-day dosing.

Adverse effects include GI signs (nausea, vomiting, soft feces, diarrhea), gingival hypertrophy, hirsutism, and papillomatosis (which generally decreases when the dose is decreased). Drugs that inhibit cytochrome P450 (eg, ketoconazole) potentiate cyclosporine toxicity significantly. If ketoconazole (10 mg/kg, bid) is also administered to animals with anal furunculosis, the dosage of cyclosporine can be reduced to 1 mg/kg, bid. This induction dose is maintained for 4 wk and then reduced if the response is adequate or adverse effects (vomiting, lethargy) develop.

Oclacitinib: Oclacitinib is a Janus kinase (JAK) inhibitor and exerts its action through the inhibition of a variety of pruritogenic cytokines (eg, IL-31) and pro-inflammatory cytokines dependent on JAK 1 or JAK 3 enzyme activity. However, it may also exert effects on other cytokines (eg, involved in host defense or hematopoiesis) with the potential for adverse effects.

It is rapidly absorbed and reaches peak plasma concentrations within 1 hr, leading to rapid onset of clinical effect. It is indicated for the treatment of pruritus associated with allergic dermatitis in dogs at a dosage of 0.4–0.6 mg/kg, bid, for 2 wk and then reduced to once daily administration for maintenance therapy. In a double-blind, placebo-controlled study for treatment of atopic dermatitis, the treatment success was 66% in reducing pruritus and 49% for Canine Atopic Dermatitis Extent and Severity Index (CADESI) scores.

Sulfones: Dapsone is an anti-inflammatory, antibacterial sulfone that inhibits neutrophil chemotaxis and adhesion to basement membrane zone antibodies, degranulation of mast cells, action of lysosomal enzymes, and activation of the alternative complement pathway. Dapsone also inhibits synthesis of IgG, IgA, and prostaglandins, as well as T-cell responses. Although it is used for a variety of diseases characterized by accumulation of neutrophils in people, the results are more equivocal in dogs. However, it has been used for pemphigus foliaceus and erythematosus, subcorneal pustular dermatosis, leukocytoclastic vasculitis, and IgA dermatosis. The dosage is 1 mg/kg, tid (dogs only) for 2–4 wk or until a response is seen, then every 24–48 hr. Longterm therapy is not recommended. Mild anemia or severe leukopenia, blood dyscrasias, hepatotoxicity, or skin reactions may develop. Animals should be monitored by CBC, urinalysis, BUN, and ALT every 2 wk during induction. Cats are particularly sensitive to toxicity, and a dosage of 1 mg/kg/day is recommended. Concurrent use may allow the dosage of glucocorticoids to be reduced.

Tetracycline and Niacinamide: Although the precise mechanism of action is unknown, tetracyclines may inhibit in vitro lymphocyte blastogenic transformation and antibody production, activation of complement (component C3), prostaglandin synthesis, lipases and collagenases, and suppress leukocyte chemotaxis in vitro and in vivo. Niacinamide blocks IgE-induced histamine release, inhibits phosphodiesterases, and decreases protease release by leukocytes. The combination is indicated for discoid lupus erythematosus and pemphigus erythematosus. These diseases are characterized by leukocyte chemotaxis secondary to complement activation by antigen-antibody complexes and by release of proteases. Dogs weighing >10 kg are given 500 mg of each drug tid. If a clinical response is seen, the frequency may be decreased to once or twice daily. Vomiting, diarrhea, and anorexia are the most common adverse effects.

Pentoxifylline: Pentoxifylline results in a range of immunologic and rheologic effects, including increases in RBC and WBC deformability; decreases in RBC and platelet aggregation, leukocyte endothelial adherence, natural killer cell activity, neutrophil degranulation, and production of monocyte TNF-α, IL-1, IL-4, and IL-12; and inhibition of T- and B-cell activation. It has been used in limited numbers of animals for a variety of conditions, including vasculitis, canine familial dermatomyositis, ulcerative dermatitis of Shetland Sheepdogs and Collies, rabies vaccine–induced ischemic alopecia, ear margin dermatosis, contact allergy, and atopic dermatitis. The dosage is 10 mg/kg, bid-tid. Once a response is seen, the dosage may be tapered to once or twice daily. GI-related adverse effects have been reported (eg, nausea, vomiting).

PSYCHOTROPIC AGENTS

Psychotropic drugs have been used extra-label for treatment of feline psychogenic alopecia and canine acral lick dermatitis, syndromes characterized by excessive self-licking (*see also* ABNORMAL REPETITIVE BEHAVIORS IN DOGS, p 1561, and FELINE COMPULSIVE DISORDERS, p 1574). Classes of drugs used include antidepressants, antipsychotics, opiate antagonists, anxiolytics, and mood stabilizers (*see* table 14).

Sedation is the most common adverse effect of diazepam. It is also an appetite stimulant in cats. Idiosyncratic fatal hepatic necrosis has been reported in several cats treated for as little as 8–14 days. Tricyclic antidepressants are potent H_1 blockers in addition to inhibiting uptake of serotonin and norepinephrine. These drugs can induce cardiac arrhythmias and lower the seizure threshold. Other adverse effects include dry mouth, hypersalivation, vomiting, constipation, urinary retention, ataxia, disorientation, depression, and anorexia. Tricyclic antidepressants should not be used concurrently with monoamine oxidase inhibitors, including amitraz dips for demodicosis. Dosages should be tapered slowly when discontinued.

VITAMINS AND MINERALS

Retinoids: Naturally occurring and synthetic compounds with vitamin A activity include retinol, retinoic acid, and retinol derivatives or analogues. At the molecular level, retinoids are important in regulation of proliferation, growth, differentiation, and maintenance of epithelial tissues. Retinoids also affect proteases, biosynthesis of mucopolysaccharides, prostaglandins, cellular adhesion, cellular communication, and immunity. They prevent tumor promotion by inhibition of ornithine decarboxylase, a key enzyme for cell proliferation and differentiation. Vitamin A (1,000 IU/kg) has been used for follicular keratosis in cats. However, the

TABLE 14 PSYCHOTROPIC DRUGS USED FOR SKIN DISORDERS

Drug	Dosage
	ANTIDEPRESSANTS
Clomipramine	Dogs: 1–3 mg/kg, bid Cats: 0.5–1.5 mg/kg/day
Amitriptyline	1–3 mg/kg, bid
Doxepin	0.5–2 mg/kg, bid
Fluoxetine	1 mg/kg/day
	ANXIOLYTICS
Diazepam	1–2 mg/kg, bid
Phenobarbital	0.5–2.2 mg/kg, bid; 15 mg/cat, twice weekly
Hydroxyzine	2.2 mg/kg, tid
	OPIATE ANTAGONISTS
Naltrexone	2.2 mg/kg/day

retinoids used most commonly are isotretinoin (13-cis-retinoic acid) and etretinate (no longer available but replaced with acitretin, a metabolically active metabolite of etretinate).

Isotretinoin is indicated for Schnauzer comedone syndrome, ichthyosis, feline acne, sebaceous adenitis, epitheliotropic lymphoma, keratoacanthoma, and sebaceous gland hyperplasias and adenomas. The dosage is 1–3 mg/kg/day. Adverse effects include conjunctivitis, mucocutaneous drying, alopecia, pruritus, hyperactivity, vomiting, and diarrhea. In dogs, blood chemistry increases not normally associated with clinical disease include plasma cholesterol, triglycerides, ALT, AST, and alkaline phosphatase. Rarely, keratoconjunctivitis sicca may develop in dogs. Conjunctivitis, anorexia, diarrhea, and vomiting are the major adverse effects in cats. All retinoids are potent teratogens, and teratogenicity may persist for up to 2 yr after treatment with etretinate because the half-life is ~100 days. Skeletal abnormalities that may be seen with longterm therapy, including premature closure of the epiphyses in growing animals, cortical hyperostosis, periosteal calcification, and long-bone demineralization, are less common with etretinate than with isotretinoin. Monitoring during longterm therapy should include complete physical examinations and serum chemistry profiles at monthly intervals for the first 3–4 mo and then every 4–6 mo.

Zinc: Zinc is an important factor of many enzyme systems and is necessary for maintenance of growth, metabolism, normal reproduction, and hormonal regulation. It is essential for keratinization and immune function. Zinc supplementation is given in cases of insufficient intestinal absorption, including deficiency syndrome I (Siberian Huskies, Alaskan Malamutes) and syndrome II (rapidly growing dogs on zinc-deficient diets). Dietary deficiency may be either absolute or relative—diets high in phytates or minerals may inhibit zinc absorption. For syndrome I, zinc supplementation is given as elemental zinc 1 mg/kg/day, PO (zinc sulfate 10 mg/kg, zinc gluconate 5 mg/kg, or zinc methionine 1.7 mg/kg). Supplementation is typically lifelong. If the response is insufficient after 4 wk, the dose should be increased by 50%. Low-dose corticosteroids may also enhance zinc absorption through induction of metallothionein in some nonresponsive cases. Animals with syndrome II normally respond to correction of the diet with resolution within 2–6 wk, although supplementation speeds this process.

Hereditary zinc deficiency associated with deficient intestinal absorption has also been reported in Friesian, Danish Black Pied, and Shorthorn cattle. There is a rapid response to zinc oxide given at 0.5 g/day, PO, or zinc sulfate at 2 g, PO, given weekly. Response to zinc supplementation is usually rapid (a few days) except for cases of achromotrichia, which requires several weeks for resolution.

SYSTEMIC PHARMACOTHERAPEUTICS OF THE MUSCULAR SYSTEM

Drugs that affect skeletal muscle function fall into several therapeutic categories. Some are used during surgical procedures to produce paralysis (neuromuscular blocking agents); others reduce spasticity (skeletal muscle relaxants) associated with various neurologic and musculoskeletal conditions. In addition, several therapeutic agents influence metabolic and other processes in skeletal muscle, including the nutrients required for normal muscle function used to prevent or mitigate degenerative muscular conditions. For example, selenium and vitamin E are used to prevent or treat muscular dystrophies such as white muscle disease (*see* p 1172). The steroidal, nonsteroidal, and various other anti-inflammatory agents (eg, dimethyl sulfoxide) are also commonly used to treat acute and chronic inflammatory conditions involving skeletal muscle. Anabolic steroids promote muscle growth and development and are administered in selected cases in which serious muscle deterioration has developed as a complication of a primary disease syndrome.

The clinical pharmacology of the neuromuscular blocking agents, skeletal muscle relaxants, and anabolic steroids are discussed below. (For anti-inflammatory agents, *see* p 2707.)

NEUROMUSCULAR BLOCKING AGENTS

The peripherally acting skeletal muscle relaxants characteristically interfere with the transmission of impulses from motor nerves to skeletal muscle fibers at the neuromuscular junction, thus reducing or abolishing motor activity. The skeletal muscle paralysis that ensues is not associated with depression of the CNS. Animals are fully conscious throughout the period of immobilization unless an anesthetic or hypnotic agent is administered concurrently.

Neuromuscular transmission can be modified either at the axonal membrane (prejunctional blockade) or at the cholinergic receptors in the sarcolemma (postjunctional blockade).

There are no clinically useful drugs that act prejunctionally, but a number of important substances can impair the synthesis, storage, and release of acetylcholine, thus resulting in prejunctional blockade at the motor endplate and consequently paralysis. Examples of prejunctional blocking agents include biotoxins, electrolytes, local anesthetics or other drugs, and antibiotics. **Biotoxins** include black widow spider venom, which depletes acetylcholine stores; botulinum toxin, which decreases acetylcholine release; tetradotoxin from the puffer fish and saxitoxin from shellfish, which block Na^+-conducting channels; and grayanotoxin found in rhododendrons, which facilitates excessive Na^+ entry through the sarcolemma, leading to constant depolarization of the membrane. **Electrolytes** include excess Mg^{2+}, which inhibits release of acetylcholine from the axon and uncouples the excitation-contraction process by competing with Ca^{2+}; and depleted Ca^{2+} levels, which decrease release of acetylcholine and impairment of excitation-contraction coupling. **Local anesthetics** in high concentration can stabilize membranes by blocking both Na^+ and K^+ channels; **hemicholinium** can inhibit synthesis of acetylcholine by blocking choline uptake into the nerve. **Antibiotics**, such as the aminoglycosides, polymyxins, tetracyclines, and lincosamides, appear to act by decreasing the availability of Ca^{2+} at membrane-binding sites on the axonal terminal and perhaps by reducing the sensitivity of the nicotinic receptors to acetylcholine.

Postjunctional blocking agents are used clinically and act either by blocking the nicotinic receptors in a competitive fashion (nondepolarizing agents) or by interacting with these receptors in a manner that does not allow the membrane to repolarize so that paralysis results (depolarizing agents). The mechanisms involved in the latter case are not fully understood. All of the neuromuscular blocking agents are structurally similar to acetylcholine (actually two molecules linked end-to-end). The depolarizing agents are usually simple linear structures, and the nondepolarizing agents are more complex bulky molecules. With a single exception (vecuronium), all have a quaternary nitrogen in their structure, which makes these drugs poorly lipid soluble.

Competitive Nondepolarizing Agents: The members of this group of peripherally acting skeletal muscle relaxants are often referred to as curarizing agents because of their relationships with the curare alkaloids that were first used clinically. The currently available drugs, which interact with nicotinic cholinergic receptors on skeletal muscle cells and render them inaccessible to the transmitter function of acetylcholine (and thus produce a flaccid paralysis) include tubocurarine, metocurine (dimethyltubocurarine), gallamine, pancuronium, alcuronium, atracurium, vecuronium, and fazadinium.

In general, nondepolarizing muscle relaxants are not absorbed from the GI tract and must be administered parenterally, usually IV. Plasma-protein binding is insignificant, and there is rapid equilibration but only within the extracellular fluid. The blood-brain and blood-placental barriers are rarely crossed. Tubocurarine, metocurine, and gallamine are not biotransformed to any extent and are excreted unchanged, principally in the urine but sometimes in bile. The other members of the group undergo metabolic transformation to some degree, and the metabolites are excreted by both renal and biliary routes in most instances. The elimination half-lives at standard dosages are 60–100 min, and the duration of paralysis is 30–60 min, except in the case of atracurium and vecuronium, which have shorter actions of ~20–30 min.

After IV administration of these agents, the skeletal muscles become totally flaccid and nonresponsive to neuronal stimulation. Muscles capable of rapid movement, such as those of the eye, are paralyzed before the larger muscles of the head and neck, which are followed by those of the limbs and body. Lastly, the diaphragm becomes paralyzed, and respiration ceases. If ventilation is controlled (tracheal intubation and positive-pressure ventilation), there are no adverse effects, and full recovery ensues in reverse order, with the diaphragm regaining function first. All of the currently used nondepolarizing muscle relaxants have cardiovascular effects, many of which are mediated by autonomic and histamine receptors. Tubocurarine and, to a much lesser extent, metocurine result in hypotension, which probably results from the liberation of histamine and, in larger doses, from ganglionic blockade. Premedication with an antihistamine reduces tubocurarine-induced hypotension. Pancuronium causes a moderate increase in heart rate and, to a lesser degree, cardiac output. Gallamine increases heart rate by both a vagolytic action and sympathetic stimulation.

A number of agents can potentiate the activity of neuromuscular blockers. These include other peripherally acting skeletal muscle relaxants, inhalant anesthetics (halothane, methoxyflurane), antibiotics (aminoglycosides, polymyxins, tetracyclines, and lincosamides), and various other drugs (quinidine, procaine, lidocaine, diazepam, and barbiturates). Several states, such as hyper- and hypomagnesemia, hypokalemia, acidosis, and hypothermia, also prolong the action of this group of drugs. Animals with myasthenia gravis are much more susceptible to the action of muscle relaxants.

Indications for the use of nondepolarizing neuromuscular blocking agents include muscle relaxation of the operative field, hypoxemic animals resisting mechanical ventilation, tracheal intubation, animals with unstable cardiovascular function that require anesthesia but cannot tolerate cardiac depression, cesarean section in toxic or high-risk animals, epileptiform convulsions not controllable with usual anticonvulsant agents, tetanus, strychnine poisoning, shivering animals in which the metabolic demand for oxygen should be reduced, and capture of certain exotic species (eg, gallamine used for immobilization of crocodiles). Animals should always be carefully monitored when under the influence of neuromuscular blocking drugs, and support of ventilation is essential.

The action of the competitive relaxants can be reversed by anticholinesterase drugs, especially neostigmine, after the administration of atropine, which eliminates excessive muscarinic responses. This attribute is a great advantage for this group of peripherally acting muscle relaxants.

The selection of dose rates (*see* TABLE 15) serves only as general guidelines for the use of competitive blocking agents.

Depolarizing Agents: Succinylcholine (suxamethonium) is the only commonly used, peripherally acting muscle relaxant that is a depolarizing agent. Decamethonium, the other member of the group, is rarely used clinically.

Depolarizing blocking drugs occupy the postjunctional cholinergic receptors and, by mechanisms that remain obscure, elicit prolonged depolarization of the endplate region. This prevents the synaptic membrane from completely repolarizing, thus rendering the motor endplate unresponsive to the normal action of acetylcholine. Characteristically, succinylcholine elicits transient muscle fasciculations before causing neuromuscular paralysis. The onset of action of succinylcholine is rapid after IV injection (20–50 sec), and the duration of the effect is usually 5–10 min in most species. Succinylcholine is rapidly hydrolyzed by pseudocholinesterases in the plasma and liver in most species, but substantial genetic differences exist.

TABLE 15 COMPETITIVE NONDEPOLARIZING AGENTS AND ANTAGONISTS

Drug	Dosage
NONDEPOLARIZING AGENTS	
Tubocurarine chloride	Horses: ≤0.22–0.25 mg/kg , IV
	Dogs, cats: ≤0.4 mg/kg, IV
Gallamine triethiodide	All species (except pigs): 0.8–1 mg/kg, IV
Pancuronium bromide	Dogs, cats: 0.6 mg/kg, IV
Alcuronium chloride	Dogs, cats: 0.1 mg/kg, IV
Atracurium besylate	Dogs, cats: 0.5 mg/kg, IV
ANTAGONISTS	
Neostigmine	0.04 mg/kg, with atropine at 0.04 mg/kg, IV
Pyridostigmine	0.2–0.25 mg/kg, with atropine at 0.04 mg/kg, IV
Edrophonium	0.125 mg/kg, IV

Other pharmacologic effects are associated with the depolarizing muscle relaxants. After IV administration of succinylcholine, transient muscle fasciculations are usually evident, although general anesthesia tends to attenuate them. Succinylcholine-induced cardiac arrhythmias are many and varied. Succinylcholine stimulates all autonomic cholinergic receptors—both nicotinic and muscarinic. Sudden hyperkalemia may be precipitated by succinylcholine, and muscle pain is seen with the use of succinylcholine in the absence of anesthesia. After recovery from succinylcholine-induced muscle paralysis, muscle damage and even myoglobinuria can develop. Malignant hyperthermia (*see* p 1027) or clinical signs related to this syndrome may also follow the use of succinylcholine in susceptible animals.

Factors that can alter the activity of competitive blocking agents (*see* p 2586) can also affect the action of succinylcholine. In addition, previous (within 1 mo) or concurrent use of organophosphate anthelmintics or external parasiticides can have a significant impact on the recovery time from succinylcholine immobilization because of prolonged inhibition of the pseudocholinesterase enzyme systems. A genetically mediated deficiency of pseudocholinesterases also has been identified in certain strains of sheep. Cattle are much more susceptible to the effects of succinylcholine than other species.

The indications for the clinical use of *succinylcholine* are similar to those for the nondepolarizing agents. However, it must be emphasized that succinylcholine should *never* be used as an agent for euthanasia or for immobilization for castration without local or general analgesia. The use of succinylcholine for game-cropping procedures is also highly undesirable.

No antagonists are available to reverse the action of the depolarizing muscle relaxants. Continued positive-pressure ventilation until recovery occurs is the only therapy in cases of overdosage.

The IV dose rates for succinylcholine by species are as follows: horses: 0.125–0.20 mg/kg (~8 min recumbency); cattle: 0.012–0.02 mg/kg (~15 min recumbency); dogs: 0.22–1.1 mg/kg (~15–20 min paralysis); and cats: 0.22–1.1 mg/kg (~3–5 min paralysis).

SKELETAL MUSCLE RELAXANTS

Muscle spasticity is a characteristic of many clinical conditions, including trauma, myositis, muscular and ligamentous sprains and strains, intervertebral disc disease, tetanus, strychnine poisoning, neurologic disorders, and exertional rhabdomyolysis. An increase in tonic stretch reflexes originates from the CNS with involvement of descending pathways and results in hyperexcitability of motor neurons in the spinal cord. Drug therapy (*see* TABLE 16) alleviates muscle spasms by modifying the stretch reflex arc or by interfering with the excitation-coupling process in the muscle itself. Centrally acting muscle relaxants block interneuronal pathways in the spinal cord and in the midbrain reticular activating system. Some drugs also have sedative effects, which are beneficial to animals that are anxious or in pain. The hydantoin derivatives have a direct action on muscle.

Methocarbamol is a centrally acting muscle relaxant chemically related to guaifenesin. Its exact mechanism of action is unknown, and it has no direct relaxant effect on striated muscle, nerve fibers, or the motor endplate. It also has a sedative effect. In dogs, cats, and horses, methocarbamol is indicated as adjunct therapy of acute inflammatory and traumatic conditions of skeletal muscle and to reduce muscle spasms. Because methocarbamol is a CNS depressant, it should not be given with other drugs that depress the CNS. Overdosage is generally characterized by CNS depression, but emesis (small animals), salivation, weakness, and ataxia may be seen.

Guaifenesin (glyceryl guaiacolate) is a centrally acting muscle relaxant believed to depress or block nerve impulse transmission at the internuncial neuron level of the subcortical areas of the brain, brain stem, and spinal cord. It also has mild analgesic and sedative actions. Guaifenesin is given IV to induce muscle relaxation as an adjunct to anesthesia for short procedures. It relaxes both laryngeal and pharyngeal muscles, allowing easier intubation, but has little effect on diaphragm and respiratory function. It may cause transient increases in cardiac rate and decreases in blood pressure. It is also used in treatment of horses with exertional rhabdomyolysis and in dogs with strychnine intoxication. Overdose results in apneustic breathing, nystagmus, hypotension, and contradictory muscle rigidity. Treatment of overdose is supportive until the drug is cleared to nontoxic levels.

Benzodiazepines, such as diazepam, affect polysynaptic reflexes at the supraspinal level, act as a spinal cord depressant at the interneuronal level, and inhibit presynaptic acetylcholine release. Clinically, diazepam is used as an adjunct to anesthesia, in management of clinical signs of tetanus, and in treatment of functional urethral obstruction and urethral sphincter hypertonus in cats.

Dantrolene, a hydantoin derivative, is structurally and pharmacologically different from other skeletal muscle relaxants. Dantrolene has a direct action on muscle, probably by interfering with the release of calcium from the sarcoplasmic reticulum. It has no discernible effects on respiratory and cardiac function but can cause dizziness and sedation. In veterinary medicine, dantrolene is used to treat malignant hyperthermia in various species, porcine stress syndrome, equine postanesthetic myositis, and equine exertional rhabdomyolysis (*see* p 1027 and p 1202).

Phenytoin is a hydantoin derivative, primarily used as an anticonvulsant in people. Phenytoin has shown efficacy in some horses susceptible to exertional rhabdomyolysis. Phenytoin may alter the function of neurotransmitters at the neuromuscular junction, the release of calcium from the sarcoplasmic reticulum, and sodium flux at the sarcolemma. Dosages are adjusted in horses to maintain serum concentrations of 5–10 mcg/mL.

Baclofen is a centrally acting skeletal muscle relaxant used to control spasticity and pain in people with multiple sclerosis and spinal disorders. Baclofen is structurally similar to the inhibitory neurotransmitter gamma-aminobutyric acid (GABA). It acts as a GABA receptor B agonist to reduce calcium

TABLE 16 SKELETAL MUSCLE RELAXANTS

Drug	Dosage
Methocarbamol	Dogs, cats: 44 mg/kg, IV, up to 330 mg/kg/day for tetanus or strychnine poisoning; 132 mg/kg/day, PO, divided bid-tid
	Horses: 4.4–5.5 mg/kg, IV
Guaifenesin	Dogs: 44–88 mg/kg, IV
	Horses, ruminants: 66–132 mg/kg, IV
Diazepam	Cats: 2–5 mg, PO, tid, for urethral obstruction
Dantrolene	Horses: 15–25 mg/kg, slow IV, qid; 2 mg/kg/day, PO, for prevention of exertional rhabdomyolysis
	Swine: 3.5 mg/kg, IV
Phenytoin	Horses: 6–8 mg/kg/day, PO, increase by 1 mg/kg every 3 days until rhabdomyolysis is prevented or the horse appears sedated

influx into presynaptic nerve terminals, thereby decreasing the amount of excitatory neurotransmitters released by primary afferent neurons in the spinal cord and brain. This results in reduced muscle tone as well as pain associated with spasticity. Because of a very narrow safety margin, baclofen has limited use in veterinary medicine. It has been used to treat dogs with tetanus and to reduce urethral resistance in treatment of urinary retention. Baclofen transiently inhibits lower esophageal sphincter relaxation in dogs and theoretically is of benefit in the treatment of gastroesophageal reflux disease. Baclofen is not recommended for use in cats. Even at therapeutic doses, dogs may show clinical signs of vomiting, depression, and vocalization. With overdose, the severity of CNS signs can be substantial and may include dysphoria, lateral recumbency, or coma. Treatment of baclofen toxicity should include rapid and aggressive decontamination, along with intensive supportive treatment. Management of affected dogs may require positive-pressure ventilation as a result of severe obtundation, respiratory depression, and respiratory arrest or hypoventilation. Cyproheptadine, a serotonin antagonist, may be given orally or rectally as needed to reduce vocalization or disorientation. IV lipid emulsion has been useful to treat some dogs with baclofen toxicity.

ANABOLIC STEROIDS

Anabolic steroids are synthetic derivatives of testosterone with enhanced anabolic activity and reduced androgenic activity. Testosterone or its derivatives diffuse through cell membranes of target organs and combine with specific receptor proteins in the cytoplasm. The receptor-hormone migrates into the cell nucleus and binds to nuclear chromatin, stimulating the production of specific messenger RNA. The messenger RNA then regulates the enzyme synthesis responsible for the physiologic activity of the anabolic steroid.

Anabolic steroids stimulate and maintain a positive nitrogen balance by reducing renal elimination of nitrogen, sodium, potassium, chloride, and calcium. Production of myosin, sarcoplasm, and myofibrillar protein is enhanced. Anabolic steroids promote appetite, weight gain, and improved mental attitude, so they are used to reverse debilitation associated with surgery, trauma, illness, glucocorticoid-induced catabolism, and aging. In all cases, improved well-being depends on adequate intake of protein and calories and on treatment of the underlying disease.

Anabolic steroids have a variety of undesirable effects. They induce androgenic effects, such as increased libido in males and abnormal sexual behavior in females, along with adverse reproductive effects, including azoospermia, anestrus, testicular atrophy, and clitoral hypertrophy. They promote edema formation due to sodium and water retention. Icterus can develop due to intrahepatic cholestasis. Anabolic steroids can induce epiphyseal plate closure, thereby retarding growth. Anabolic steroids are used in treatment of debilitated animals; however, they are often misused to gain a competitive advantage in performance animals. Approved veterinary formulations are no longer marketed in North America. Currently, any anabolic product for veterinary use (aside from bovine ear implants) can be obtained only from a compounding pharmacy. Use of anabolic steroids in performance horses is prohibited by most equine sport organizations, and drug detection times can be >2 mo.

SYSTEMIC PHARMACOTHERAPEUTICS OF THE NERVOUS SYSTEM

Drugs used to modify or treat disorders of the nervous system fall into several categories: anticonvulsants or antiepileptic drugs (AEDs), tranquilizers, sedatives, analgesics, and psychotropic agents. *See also* PRINCIPLES OF THERAPY OF NEUROLOGIC DISEASE, p 1220, ANALGESIC PHARMACOLOGY, p 2107, and PRINCIPLES OF PHARMACOLOGIC AND NATURAL TREATMENT FOR BEHAVIORAL PROBLEMS, p 1543.

ANTICONVULSANTS OR ANTIEPILEPTIC DRUGS

Anticonvulsants or antiepileptic drugs (AEDs) are used to stop an ongoing seizure or to decrease the frequency or severity of anticipated future seizures. During a seizure episode or status epilepticus, the route of administration for AEDs is IV (*see* TABLE 17). For longterm maintenance, the oral route is preferred, although absorption may be limited or variable depending on the drug used (*see* TABLE 18). SC or IM injections are seldom used because of the variability in drug absorption.

ANTIEPILEPTIC DRUGS USED TO STOP ONGOING SEIZURE ACTIVITY

In status epilepticus, treatment is essential to prevent death from hyperthermia, acidosis, hypoperfusion, and hypoxia. Because diazepam has a rapid onset of action that prevents the spread of the seizure, it is usually the drug of choice to control status epilepticus and stop seizures in small and large animals.

Foals and Horses

Diazepam in horses has a long elimination half-life (7–22 hr). In foals, the dosage is 0.05–0.4 mg/kg, slowly IV (or about 5–20 mg/dose); higher doses can be fatal to neonates. For seizures in adult horses, diazepam can be given at 25–50 mg/horse, IV. To prevent further seizures after initial diazepam injection, IV phenobarbital may be started as a follow up at 12–20 mg/kg, IV over 20 min, and then maintained at a dosage of 6.65–9 mg/kg over 20 min, bid or tid. If sedation occurs, the dose should be reduced. Alternatively, treatment of seizures in foals can be initiated with phenytoin at 5–10 mg/kg, IV or PO, with subsequent treatments of 1–5 mg/kg, IV, IM, or PO, every 2–4 hr for 12 hr and later maintained with oral phenytoin at 2.83–16.43 mg/kg, tid, although erratic plasma concentrations may limit usefulness. The dose may need to be reduced if sedation occurs.

TABLE 17 DRUGS USED FOR TREATMENT OF STATUS EPILEPTICUS

Drug	Species and Dosage
Diazepam	Dogs, cats: 0.5–2 mg/kg, IV bolus; can be repeated 2–3 times at intervals of 5–10 min; CRI[a] 0.5–2 mg/kg/hr
	Foals: 0.05–0.4 mg/kg, IV slowly
	Adult horses: 25–50 mg/horse, IV
	Ruminants: 0.5–1.5 mg/kg, IV or IM
Midazolam	Dogs, cats: 0.2 mg/kg, IV bolus; can be repeated 2–3 times at intervals of 5–10 min; CRI 0.05-0.5 mg/kg/hr
Phenobarbital	Dogs, cats: For those not already on maintenance phenobarbital, loading dose of 15 mg/kg, slowly IV. Alternatively, 3–6 mg/kg, IV or IM, every 15–30 min until a total dosage of 20 mg/kg is reached. In an animal already receiving maintenance phenobarbital, a single 3 mg/kg bolus, IV or IM, CRI 3–10 mg/hr to effect.
	Foals, adult horses: loading dose of 12–20 mg/kg, IV over 20 min, then 6.65–9 mg/kg, IV over 20 min every 8–12 hr
Sodium pentobarbital	Dogs, cats: 2–15 mg/kg, IV, to effect to stop motor activity
	Foals, adult horses: 2–4 mg/kg, IV to effect
Levetiracetam	Dogs: 20–60 mg/kg, IV; can be repeated at 8-hr intervals
Propofol	Dogs, cats: 2.5–4 mg/kg, IV, to effect to stop motor activity; CRI 0.1–0.3 mg/kg/min to effect
Phenytoin	Dogs: 2–5 mg/kg as slow IV infusion
	Foals, adult horses: 5–10 mg/kg, IV followed by 1–5 mg/kg, IV, IM, or PO, every 2–4 hr until seizures stop and maintenance dose started

[a] CRI = constant-rate infusion

TABLE 18 ANTIEPILEPTIC DRUGS

Drug	Dosage and Frequency	Half-life
FIRST-LINE MAINTENANCE ANTIEPILEPTIC DRUGS		
Phenobarbital	Dogs: 2–4 mg/kg, PO, bid (starting dose); up to 10 mg/kg, bid	40–90 hr (Beagles 25–38 hr)
	Cats: 2–4 mg/kg, PO, bid (starting dose)	34–43 hr
	Horses: 3–5 mg/kg/day, PO, as a starting dose; up to 11 mg/kg/day, PO	18 hr
	Foals: as above	13 hr
	Ruminants: 11 mg/kg/day, PO	
Bromide (potassium salt)	Dogs, cats: 20–40 mg/kg, PO, once daily or divided bid if GI upset. Caution using bromide in cats (see comments). Dogs: loading dose 400–600 mg/kg, PO divided into 4 doses, given over 1–4 days Horses: 90 mg/kg/day, PO	Dogs: 20–46 days Cats: 10 days Horses: 5 days
Bromide (sodium salt)	17–30 mg/kg, PO, once daily or divided bid if GI upset. The dose of sodium bromide is less than that of potassium bromide to account for the higher bromide content.	
Diazepam	Cats: 0.25–0.5 mg/kg, PO, bid-tid	Cats:15–20 hr
SECOND-LINE (ADD-ON) ANTIEPILEPTIC DRUGS FOR DOGS		
Clonazepam	Dogs: 0.1–0.5 mg/kg, PO, bid-tid	1.5–3 hr
Clorazepate	Dogs: 0.5–1 mg/kg, PO, tid	5–6 hr
Felbamate	Dogs: 15 mg/kg, PO, tid; increase by 15 mg/kg biweekly until seizures controlled; maximal (toxic) dosage 300 mg/kg	5–6 hr

TABLE 18 ANTIEPILEPTIC DRUGS *(continued)*

Time to Steady State	Therapeutic Level	Adverse Effects/Comments
FIRST-LINE MAINTENANCE ANTIEPILEPTIC DRUGS		
		Adjust dosage in all species by monitoring serum levels and seizure diary.
10–24 days	15–45 mcg/mL (66–200 μmol/L), preferably keep values within 20–35 mcg/mL (85–150 μmol/L)	Sedation, polydipsia, induces P450 system, increase in alkaline phosphatase common; liver failure is possible but uncommon.
	10–30 mcg/mL	Liver enzymes do not typically increase in cats.
	10–40 mcg/mL (43–175 μmol/L)	
Dogs: 100–200 days Cats: 6 wk	Bromide alone: 1–3 mg/mL (15–20 μmol/L) Bromide/phenobarbital combined: 1–2 mg/mL	Sedation, weakness, polydipsia, vomiting, polyphagia, skin rash. Reduce dose with renal insufficiency. High chloride intake increases bromide elimination. Chloride content of diet should be stable. Use with extreme caution in cats and monitor with thoracic radiographs because bronchial/asthmatic signs may be fatal in cats.
		See potassium bromide comments.
		While oral diazepam is not effective as maintenance AED in dogs, it can be used in cats as a maintenance AED. Sedation and liver failure are potential problems in cats.
SECOND-LINE (ADD-ON) ANTIEPILEPTIC DRUGS FOR DOGS		
	22–77 ng/mL	Extremely potent benzodiazepine; sedation; withdrawal signs if drug stopped abruptly.
1–2 days	20–75 mcg/L	15 times less potent than clonazepam; sedation; withdrawal seizures. Can increase phenobarbital concentration.
1 day	125–250 μmol/L[a]	Nervousness, keratoconjunctivitis sicca, mild thrombocytopenia, leukopenia; induces P450 system; liver disease. Use with care with other potentially hepatotoxic drugs.

(continued)

TABLE 18 ANTIEPILEPTIC DRUGS *(continued)*

Drug	Dosage and Frequency	Half-life
Gabapentin	Dogs: 10 mg/kg, PO, tid; up to 30–60 mg/kg, tid	3–4 hr
Levetiracetam	Dogs: 20 mg/kg, PO, tid	4–10 hr
Topiramate	Dogs: 5–10 mg/kg/day, PO, bid	2–4 hr
Valproic acid	Dogs: 10–60 mg/kg, PO, tid	90–120 min
Zonisamide	Dogs: 5 mg/kg/day, PO, bid, if phenobarbital is not concurrently given; 10 mg/kg, PO, bid if phenobarbital is concurrently administered.	15–20 hr

[a] Therapeutic range established for people

Other ways to control ongoing seizure activity include sodium pentobarbital (2–4 mg/kg, IV to effect), a mixture of 12% chloral hydrate and 6% magnesium sulfate at a rate not exceeding 30 mL/min to avoid excessive depression, or a mixture of 44–88 mg/kg of 5% guaifenesin and 2.2–6.6 mg/kg thiamyal, given IV to effect. Horses with seizures induced by toxins or adverse drug effect (eg, xylazine) can be treated with diazepam (0.1–0.15 mg/kg, IV). If cerebral edema is suspected, *see* PRINCIPLES OF THERAPY OF THE NERVOUS SYSTEM, p 1220.

Ruminants

Diazepam has been used at 0.5–1.5 mg/kg, IM or IV. In sheep and goats, pentobarbital at 20–30 mg/kg can be used IV to effect to induce anesthesia. The duration of effect is 5–30 min.

Dogs and Cats

A variety of drugs can be used to stop seizures in dogs and cats.

Benzodiazepines: Diazepam is the most common benzodiazepine used in dogs and cats to reduce motor activity and permit placement of an IV catheter. When used as an IV bolus (0.5–2 mg/kg), the dose may be repeated up to three times at intervals of 5–10 min. However if seizures occur after the second or third bolus, a constant-rate infusion (CRI) of diazepam at 0.5–2 mg/kg/hr may be more effective (especially if titrated based on seizure control and sedation level), and IV phenobarbital should be started as a preventive (*see* p 2595). When diazepam is used as a CRI, it should be mixed with 5% dextrose or 0.9% saline. It should not be mixed with lactated Ringer's solution, because the calcium may cause precipitation of the diazepam. Because plastic will absorb diazepam, it should not be left in plastic syringes or IV sets for prolonged intervals. When diazepam is administered as a CRI, it is thought that the initial pass-through in the IV set saturates the surface of the tubing such that there is no further absorption. If IV access is not possible in dogs, diazepam can be administered rectally at 0.5–2 mg/kg (2 mg/kg if the dog is receiving phenobarbital) or intranasally at 0.5 mg/kg. Rectal diazepam has been recommended as an at-home emergency treatment for some dogs that have clusters of seizures; it can be administered up to three times in a 24-hr period by owners.

Other benzodiazepines that can be used in dogs to stop seizure activity are

TABLE 18 ANTIEPILEPTIC DRUGS *(continued)*

Time to Steady State	Therapeutic Level	Adverse Effects/Comments
<24 hr	4–16 mg/L[a] (70–120 μmol/L)	Sedation, dizziness, ataxia, fatigue, diarrhea; reduce dose with renal dysfunction.
2–3 days	35–120 μmol/L[a]	Restlessness, vomiting, ataxia at dosages >400 mg/kg/day
3–5 days	2–25 mg/L (15–60 μmol/L)[a]	GI upset, irritability
<24 hr		Probably ineffective due to very short half-life; liver, alopecia, and pancreatitis; vomiting usually avoided by giving drug with food.
3–4 days	10–40 mg/L (45–180 μmol/L)	Sedation, ataxia, loss of appetite. Potential adverse effects (eg, keratoconjunctivitis sicca, bone marrow dyscrasia, hepatopathy, vasculitis, and metabolic acidosis) could occur because of sulfonamide base.

clonazepam (0.05–0.2 mg/kg, IV; the IV form of the drug may not be available in the USA), lorazepam (0.2 mg/kg, every 4–6 hr), and midazolam (0.2 mg/kg, IV or IM; CRI dose 0.05–0.5 mg/kg/hr).

Barbiturates: Phenobarbital is often used in status epilepticus cases to prevent further seizure activity. For animals not already on maintenance phenobarbital, a loading dose of 15 mg/kg, slow IV or IM, can be used. Alternatively, 3–6 mg/kg, IV or IM, can be administered every 15–30 min to attain the desired serum concentration; serum level increases by ~5 mcg/mL for every 3 mg/kg dose of phenobarbital. It is usually not necessary to exceed a total dose of 20 mg/kg. If injectable phenobarbital is effective in preventing or controlling seizures, an oral maintenance dose may be initiated, with the plan to decrease or stop injectable anticonvulsant infusions within the following 24 hr. Caution is necessary when administering both diazepam and phenobarbital, because a potentiation of their effects increases the risk of respiratory and cardiovascular collapse.

Propofol is a short-acting IV hypnotic anesthetic agent that may have anticonvulsant activity because it is GABA-mimetic, stabilizing GABA-inhibitory neurotransmitter sites. After IV administration, propofol rapidly crosses the blood-brain barrier and usually has an onset of action of <1 min. However, the duration of action after a single bolus is only ~2–5 min. When used as a single dose (2.5–4 mg/kg, IV) in dogs and cats, ~25% of the calculated dose is administered every 30 sec until the desired effect is reached. If seizures recur after 1–2 injections, a propofol CRI (0.05–0.2 up to 0.4 mg/kg/min) can be used if definitive airway control and hemodynamic support are available and if the animal can be closely monitored. During IV injection, seizure-like signs of excitement, paddling, nystagmus, muscle twitching, and opisthotonos may sometimes be seen.

Sodium pentobarbital is generally reserved for treatment of uncontrollable status epilepticus in dogs and cats, especially when diazepam and phenobarbital have failed (*see* TABLE 17). In these species, it is administered at 2–15 mg/kg to effect for anesthesia. Pentobarbital is a respiratory depressant, so respiratory assistance must be readily available. The drug is irritating if administered perivascularly or subcutaneously. As the animal recovers from the drug's effects, excitement may occur, which can be mistaken for seizure activity.

Inhalation Anesthesia: In some cases, inhalation anesthesia is necessary to control or stop seizure activity. This requires constant monitoring and mechanical ventilation.

Alternative Methods to Stop a Seizure: Phenytoin at 2–5 mg/kg has been used as a slow IV infusion in dogs to stop a seizure. Ocular compression (application of digital pressure to one or both eyes) may be beneficial via stimulation of the vagus nerve. An implantable pacemaker device that delivers repetitive stimulation to the left cervical vagus nerve has been investigated in dogs and may be of benefit in some epileptic animals. Acupuncture points KID 1 and/or GV 26 might also be of benefit.

MAINTENANCE ANTICONVULSANT OR ANTIEPILEPTIC THERAPY

The decision to start maintenance anticonvulsant or antiepileptic therapy should be based on the frequency and severity of the seizures, the age of onset, the likely cause(s) of the seizures, and the results of diagnostic testing. In general, a maintenance antiepileptic drug (AED) should be considered in animals that have had more than one or two seizures within a 6-mo period (assuming these seizures were not caused by repeated toxin exposure) or in animals that have had more than one seizure of unknown cause on any particular day. A maintenance AED should also be considered if the first seizure episode is protracted or severe, or during an episode of status epilepticus (as a followup to emergency treatment, *see* p 2591).

Treatment should begin with a single drug at the minimal required level for effect. Owners should keep a calendar to document the frequency and pattern of seizures as a guide for treatment strategy. This calendar, in conjunction with serum AED levels, can be used as a guide for dosage and drug treatment changes. If seizure control is unsatisfactory, the drug level should be checked. If the level is not within the middle of the therapeutic range, the dose should be increased before adding or switching to a new drug. Doses may be doubled in early stages and increased by 25%–50% in later stages. Monotherapy is preferred, but if the drug level is well into the middle or high therapeutic range, it may be necessary to consider the addition of another AED. To discontinue any AED, except bromide, the dose of the drug should be tapered gradually over a few weeks to avoid precipitating a seizure. Tapering phenobarbital is crucial, because it is addictive and can result in withdrawal seizures if stopped abruptly.

Maintenance Antiepileptic Drugs (Anticonvulsants)

In dogs, phenobarbital and bromide are considered first-line maintenance AEDs, but levetiracetam and zonisamide are often used as well. In cats, phenobarbital is the usual first choice, but levetiracetam and zonisamide are becoming more acceptable; diazepam is an alternative choice. In ruminants, phenobarbital is the first choice; in horses, both bromide and phenobarbital have been used.

Phenobarbital: Phenobarbital has a long record of safety, efficacy, low cost, and convenience in regard to monitoring serum concentrations. For longterm maintenance in cats and dogs, phenobarbital may be given at 2–4 mg/kg/day, PO, bid. In all species, it takes ~2 wk to approach a steady-state plasma concentration, because oral absorption is extremely variable and the half-life is long. Drug levels are monitored 2 wk after initiation of therapy, 2 wk after any dosage change, and usually every 6–12 mo once seizure control is achieved. Serum therapeutic concentrations are 15–45 mcg/mL. The dosage should be adjusted on the basis of serum level and the history of seizure control. Tolerance to phenobarbital therapy may develop in dogs treated continually for months to years and may result in decreased seizure control; however, an increase (25%) in the dose usually will result in improved seizure control.

Phenobarbital causes physical dependence, and thus abrupt withdrawal may cause "barbiturate withdrawal" seizures. Hepatotoxicity and liver failure in dogs have been associated with high serum concentrations (>35 mcg/mL), necessitating the serum level checks every 6–12 mo. Adverse effects such as sedation, polydipsia, polyuria, and polyphagia are common but may decrease within the first few weeks. Other, less common adverse effects are idiosyncratic hyperexcitability, dermatitis, anemia, neutropenia, thrombocytopenia, gingival hyperplasia, and osteomalacia. Phenobarbital has also been used to treat episodic dyscontrol syndrome (rage) in dogs when seizure activity is demonstrable via electroencephalogram recordings.

Oral phenobarbital has been used in ruminants at 11 mg/kg/day and in horses at 3–11 mg/kg/day. Serum concentrations should be checked periodically.

Bromide: Bromide appears to stabilize neuronal cell membranes by interfering with chloride transport across cell membranes and by potentiating the effect of GABA via hyperpolarizing membranes. Bromide (potassium or sodium salt) can be used as a first-choice AED in dogs with epilepsy, as an adjunctive AED in dogs with refractory seizure disorders, or for dogs that have unacceptable adverse effects related to phenobarbital or other AEDs. In countries where bromide is not available as a pharmaceutical formulation (USA), an analytical grade may be obtained from a chemical supply company, although caution is recommended in handling and packaging. Bromide can be formulated into a solution of various concentrations (100 mg/mL, 200 mg/mL, 250 mg/mL are convenient ones) or into tablets or capsules.

The elimination half-life is extremely long (24 days) in dogs; therefore, it takes ~4 mo to achieve steady state kinetics. Bromide is renally eliminated and thus should not be used in dogs with renal dysfunction without careful monitoring. If azotemia is present, a different AED can be used, or the initial bromide dose can be reduced by half and serum concentrations monitored. Because it does not undergo hepatic metabolism, bromide is useful in dogs with liver disease.

As adjunct therapy with phenobarbital, potassium bromide can be administered at 20–40 mg/kg/day, PO, either as one dose or divided into two or more doses; the sodium bromide dosage is slightly lower at 17–30 mg/kg/day, PO. When bromide is used as the sole treatment for epilepsy in dogs, higher dosages (50–80 mg/kg/day) may be necessary. Dogs on a high salt diet may require dosages of 50–80 mg/kg/day to maintain adequate serum concentrations, because high chloride intake increases bromide loss in the urine and lowers serum bromide concentrations. Many laboratory assays cannot distinguish between serum bromide and chloride ions, so serum chloride values may be reported as falsely high.

Because a daily maintenance dose may take 4 mo to reach steady state serum concentration, there are situations (eg, severe seizures, seizures that occur on a monthly basis, the need to rapidly switch from phenobarbital to bromide because of phenobarbital toxicity) when a loading dose of bromide should be administered. An oral loading dosage of 400–600 mg/kg of bromide is divided into four doses and given with food over a 1- to 4-day period. Smaller doses, such as 50 mg/kg, bid for 4–6 days, may reduce adverse effects (eg, nausea and vomiting) caused by rapid increase in serum bromide concentrations. The regular maintenance dose can be started at the same time as the loading dose or immediately afterward. The loading dose regimen can be discontinued if the dog becomes too sedated, or smaller divided daily doses can be tried. A serum sample can be submitted within 2 wk after loading to determine whether a therapeutic level has been reached. (If cost is an issue, however, a sample is best checked in 4 mo when steady-state concentrations have been reached.) The therapeutic range for bromide is 1–2 mg/mL (10–20 mmol/L) with concurrent phenobarbital treatment, or 1–3 mg/mL (10–30 mmol/L) for bromide as a monotherapy. However, the dosing regimen needs to be tailored for each animal; the upper end of the therapeutic range is only limited by adverse effects of bromide.

Bromide is generally well tolerated by dogs, but potential adverse effects include bitter taste, gastric irritation, nausea (particularly with the potassium form), polyuria, polydipsia, polyphagia, sedation, ataxia, and pancreatitis. It should be administered with food; the amount and type of food given should be kept constant, because variable dietary salt content will affect the elimination of bromide via the kidneys. Bromide therapy must be titrated to the individual animal based on careful therapeutic drug monitoring and careful monitoring by the owner for early signs of toxicity. Reports of hindlimb weakness should be investigated as potential bromide toxicosis by measuring serum bromide concentration and discontinuing bromide for several days to see whether the weakness improves. Severe bromide toxicosis (bromism) is characterized by lethargy, disorientation, delirium, and ataxia progressing to quadriplegia and coma. Bromide toxicity can be seen at any concentration in an unusually sensitive dog, but it is rare when bromide is used alone and when serum concentrations are <1.5 mg/mL (15 mmol/L). When used in combination with phenobarbital, bromide toxicity can be seen at concentrations of 2–3 mg/mL (20–30 mmol/L). Severe signs of toxicity are easily treated by IV administration of 0.9% sodium chloride, which promotes renal excretion of the bromide ion.

Bromide is an effective maintenance AED in cats, but the incidence of adverse effects does not warrant its routine use unless there is no other choice. Approximately 25%–50% of cats administered bromide developed signs of bronchial disease characterized by a cough and marked pulmonary infiltrates seen on radiographs. In some cases, the asthmatic changes were fatal, but in most cases the signs resolved after discontinuation of bromide.

Bromide has been used in horses as a maintenance AED, but there are no published studies on its clinical efficacy. Pharmacokinetic studies have suggested that a loading dose of potassium bromide of 120 mg/kg/day over 5 days and maintenance dosages of ~90–100 mg/kg/day will likely result in effective serum bromide concentrations.

Primidone: Primidone is a barbiturate that has three metabolites: phenobarbital, primidone, and phenylethylmalonamide. The phenobarbital metabolite is likely the major functional one, and there may not be an advantage to using primidone over phenobarbital. Nevertheless, one report indicated that dogs with seizures that are not well controlled with phenobarbital may respond better to primidone (eg, psychomotor seizures). The initial dosage (dogs only) is 5–15 mg/kg/day in three divided doses, increased over time to a maximum of 35 mg/kg/day. Effective serum levels are determined by the serum level of phenobarbital (15–45 mcg/mL). If primidone is switched to phenobarbital, one grain of phenobarbital can be substituted for 250 mg primidone.

Primidone may be more likely to cause hepatotoxicity than phenobarbital, and it has been associated with hepatic necrosis and lipidosis and bile canaliculi obstruction. ALT, serum alkaline phosphatase, and/or bile acids should be monitored. Other adverse effects and signs of overdosage are similar to those of phenobarbital.

Primidone is not recommended for use in cats because of toxicity concerns. However, preliminary studies suggest primidone at 40 mg/kg/day for 90 days may be acceptable in cats.

Diazepam: Diazepam is not suitable for oral maintenance therapy in dogs, because it is absorbed poorly, has a short half-life of 2.5–3.2 hr, and tolerance to its anticonvulsant effects develops rapidly. However, cats not only have a longer half-life (15–20 hr) than dogs but also do not develop a tolerance to the anticonvulsant effects. Thus, diazepam can be used as a maintenance treatment in cats, with dosages ranging from 0.25–0.5 mg/kg, PO, bid-tid. Acute hepatic failure has been reported in cats given diazepam for behavioral problems; thus, a pretreatment chemistry profile should be evaluated before using diazepam, and cats should be watched closely during the first 2 wk of use.

Newer or Adjunctive Anticonvulsants

Levetiracetam: This pyrrolidine-based anticonvulsant has an unknown mechanism of action. It has been used as an adjunct AED for dogs and cats and is occasionally used as monotherapy. In dogs, it has excellent oral bioavailability, does not appear to undergo hepatic metabolism, is primarily excreted unchanged in the urine, and has a half-life of ~4 hr. It appears very safe with no to few adverse effects (ataxia, sedation, vomiting) reported at the routine dosage ranges. Levetiracetam is initially administered at 20 mg/kg, PO, tid, in dogs; 10–20 mg/kg, PO, tid, in cats. If adverse effects occur, the dosage should be reduced to 20 mg/kg, bid, and increased to 20 mg/kg, tid, gradually. Studies suggest that 60% of dogs respond initially; however, after 4–8 mo, there is a loss of effect in ⅔ of previous responders because of development of tolerance. In dogs, the dosage can be increased every 2 wk in increments of 20 mg/kg if therapeutic benefit has not been noted. Adverse effects of salivation, restlessness, vomiting, and ataxia at dosages >400 mg/kg/day have been seen experimentally in dogs but resolved within 24 hr of discontinuing the drug. Therapeutic monitoring is generally not necessary when using this drug, and there does not appear to be a correlation between serum drug concentration and therapeutic efficacy. An IV formulation can be used in status epilepticus.

Zonisamide: This sulfonamide-based anticonvulsant restricts the propagation and spread of seizures and suppresses epileptogenic focus activity. It has been used as first-line AED as well as an adjunct AED in dogs not adequately controlled by phenobarbital and bromide. Although some of it is metabolized by the P450 enzyme system, much is excreted unchanged in the urine. Dogs receiving concurrent drug therapy known to induce hepatic microsomal enzymes (ie, phenobarbital) require nearly twice the dosage of zonisamide to achieve and maintain serum concentrations than dogs receiving zonisamide alone. Thus, the dose of zonisamide in dogs receiving phenobarbital is 10 mg/kg, PO, bid. In dogs not on drugs that induce hepatic microsomal enzymes, the dosage is 5 mg/kg, PO, bid. The dosage in cats has varied from 5 mg/kg, PO, bid, to 5–10 mg/kg/day, PO. The recommended therapeutic range is 10–40 mg/mL; trough concentrations can be measured ~7–10 days after initiating treatment or altering the dosage. The adverse effects are usually mild, such as transient ataxia, loss of appetite, lethargy, and vomiting. Although the drug appears safe, owners should be warned that because of the sulfonamide base, potential adverse effects (eg, keratoconjunctivitis sicca, bone marrow dyscrasia, hepatopathy, vasculitis, and metabolic acidosis) could occur. A nonfatal hepatopathy in a dog was attributed to zonisamide.

Gabapentin: This synthetic analogue of the inhibitory neurotransmitter γ-aminobutyric acid (GABA) inhibits seizure activity via multiple mechanisms, including inhibition of neuronal sodium channels and potentiation of the release and action of GABA. It is well absorbed in dogs after oral administration and undergoes both hepatic and renal metabolism. In dogs, the initial dosage is 10–15 mg/kg, PO, tid. Higher dosages (30–60 mg/kg, PO, tid-qid) may be necessary but can produce sedation and ataxia. If excessive sedation occurs, a lower dose should be used initially and gradually increased. Therapeutic monitoring is not usually necessary with this drug. No drug interactions have been reported. Gabapentin has been used in cats at 5–10 mg/kg, bid-tid.

Felbamate: Felbamate is a dicarbamate AED that exerts its anticonvulsant effects through multiple mechanisms, including potentiating GABA-mediated neuronal inhibition, inhibiting voltage-sensitive neuronal calcium and sodium channels, and blocking N-methyl-D-aspartate–mediated neuronal excitation. It is primarily (70%) renally excreted in dogs, with the remainder of the drug undergoing hepatic metabolism. The recommended initial dosage is 15 mg/kg, PO, tid, but the dose can be increased every 14–21 days in increments of 15 mg/kg if therapeutic benefit has not been noted. The principle advantage of felbamate is a lack of sedation, and adverse effects are reportedly rare. Potential adverse effects are hepatotoxicity, reversible myelosuppression, generalized tremors, and possibly keratoconjunctivitis sicca; regular monitoring for anemia and liver dysfunction in dogs is recommended. In people, felbamate has been associated with aplastic anemia and liver toxicity. There is no clinical information on use of felbamate in cats.

Valproic Acid: Valproic acid (10–60 mg/kg, tid) has been used as an adjunct to phenobarbital and primidone in dogs with refractory seizures. It has also been used to treat aggressive behavior problems (*see* p 2601). Common adverse effects include transient GI distress, alopecia, sedation, and vomiting. Hepatic failure is rare. Use of valproic acid in dogs is limited because of rapid metabolism.

Clonazepam: Clonazepam, unlike diazepam, can be used in dogs for oral maintenance therapy, because anticonvulsant tolerance develops less rapidly, the saturability of its metabolism reduces the elimination rate at therapeutic concentrations, and because it is more highly absorbed orally (particularly in micronized formulations). For maintenance therapy in dogs, it may be used alone at 0.5 mg/kg, tid, but it is best used as an adjunct to phenobarbital at dosages of 0.1–0.5 mg/kg/day. Diarrhea sometimes develops with clonazepam, but this may be avoided by starting with once daily dosing and increasing the frequency to three times daily over a period of several days.

Carbamazepine: Carbamazepine is not recommended for use in dogs because of a rapid induction of hepatic enzymes that eliminate the drug quickly. Although plasma concentrations declined rapidly in dogs on a 1-wk regimen of 30 mg/kg, tid, one case report described adequate seizure control despite undetectable drug concentrations in plasma, possibly due either to an active metabolite or to a highly sensitive drug reaction. Carbamazepine has been used to treat aggressive behavior problems in cats (*see* p 2601).

Clorazepate Dipotassium: Clorazepate dipotassium (0.5–1 g/kg, tid) has been proposed as an adjunct to phenobarbital treatment in dogs. Severe withdrawal symptoms, even lethal seizures, may appear after abrupt discontinuation of chronic clorazepate treatment, in spite of the relatively low tolerance liability of clorazepate. Administration of phenobarbital alters the deposition of clorazepate such that the amount of nordiazepam in circulation during each dose interval is significantly reduced. Adequate control of seizures in epileptic dogs, therefore, may require higher dosages of clorazepate when coadministered with phenobarbital. However, clorazepate may increase phenobarbital concentrations, resulting in adverse effects.

Phenytoin: Phenytoin (diphenylhydantoin) is no longer recommended for maintenance use in dogs, cats, or foals because of undesirable pharmacokinetic properties. Its metabolism is too rapid in dogs, which reduces its effectiveness, and too slow in cats, which increases the risk of toxicity (salivation, vomiting, weight loss). In foals, phenytoin has erratic plasma concentrations. It may still be used in status epilepticus in dogs as a slow IV injection of 2–5 mg/kg.

Mephenytoin: Mephenytoin, although related to phenytoin, has been effective in dogs (10 mg/kg, tid) because of a slower rate of elimination. It may be combined with phenobarbital or bromide. Adverse effects consist of sedation only, but periodic hematologic monitoring is advised, because blood dyscrasia and hepatotoxicity are reported in people.

Topiramate: Topiramate is a newer AED that is well tolerated by people and increasingly used for neuropathic pain. In one report, it was listed as an adjunct AED for dogs, but its effectiveness is not yet known. Because the elimination half-life is short in dogs (2–4 hr), it is probably not an effective anticonvulsant, but a dosage of 5–10 mg/kg, bid, has been suggested. There have been no clinical studies to date, and only limited information is currently available.

TRANQUILIZERS, SEDATIVES, AND ANALGESICS

Tranquilization reduces anxiety and induces a sense of tranquility without drowsiness. Drug-induced sedation has a more profound effect and produces drowsiness and hypnosis. Analgesia is the reduction of pain, which according to a drug's effect, may be more pronounced in either the viscera or the musculoskeletal system (*see* p 2104). Many drugs cannot be categorized by only

TABLE 19 TRANQUILIZERS AND SEDATIVES WITHOUT ANALGESIC EFFECTS

Drug	Dosage		
	Dogs	Cats	Ferrets
BENZODIAZEPINES			
Diazepam	1 mg/kg, IV or PO	1 mg/kg, IV	2 mg/kg, IM
Midazolam	0.2–0.4 mg/kg, IV or IM	0.2–0.4 mg/kg, IV or IM	
BUTYROPHENONE			
Azaperone			
PHENOTHIAZINES			
Acepromazine maleate	0.05–0.1 mg/kg, IV, IM, or SC; 0.55–2.2 mg/kg, PO, tid-qid	0.11–0.22 mg/kg, IV, IM, or SC; 1.1–2.2 mg/kg, PO, bid-tid	0.1–0.25 mg/kg, IM or SC
Chlorpromazine hydrochloride	0.55–4.4 mg/kg, IV; 1.1–6.6 mg/kg, IM; 3.2 mg/kg, PO, tid-qid as needed	1–2 mg/kg, IV or IM, bid	
Promazine hydrochloride	2–6 mg/kg, IV, IM, or PO, tid-qid	2–4.4 mg/kg, IV, IM, or PO, tid-qid	
Triflupromazine hydrochloride	1.1–2.2 mg/kg, IV; 2.2–4.4 mg/kg, IM	4.4–8.8 mg/kg, IM	

one pharmacologic effect, ie, as tranquilizers, sedatives, or analgesics. For example, many psychotropic drugs can either tranquilize or sedate according to the dose administered, and many sedatives are also analgesics. Also, drugs classified as tranquilizers, sedatives, and/or analgesics may have additional effects (eg, behavioral modification, antiemesis).

For drugs commonly used in various species for tranquilization, sedation, or analgesia, *see* TABLES 19 and 20. Drugs that have some of these effects but are used mainly for other properties (eg, as antispasmodics, antiemetics, or preanesthetics) are not listed. Single-use doses are emphasized because many situations require only a brief duration of effect, but frequency of administration is also provided for drugs likely to be used for multiple-dose therapy. The dosages listed serve only as a general guideline and apply to the use of each drug alone, not to a combination for anesthesia or neuroleptanalgesia. No reference is made to schedule restrictions, extra-label use, or precautions in the use of these drugs; the product label and referenced texts should be consulted for information on the pharmacology and alternative applications of each drug.

PSYCHOTROPIC AGENTS

Anxiolytics, antipsychotics, antidepressants, and mood stabilizers used to treat human behavioral disorders are being used more commonly in veterinary medicine as adjuncts to behavioral modification therapy (*see also* PRINCIPLES OF PHARMACOLOGIC AND NATURAL TREATMENT FOR BEHAVIORAL PROBLEMS, p 1543). Few veterinary clinical studies have been reported, and guidelines for veterinary use are grounded on therapeutic applications in human medicine.

Anxiolytics

Anxiolytics, including the benzodiazepines and an azapirone (buspirone), have been

TABLE 19 TRANQUILIZERS AND SEDATIVES WITHOUT ANALGESIC EFFECTS *(continued)*

Dosage			
Rabbits	**Horses**	**Cattle**	**Pigs**
	BENZODIAZEPINES		
1–5 mg/kg, IV, IM; 2–10 mg/kg, IM or IP	0.05–0.4 mg/kg, IV	0.5–1.5 mg/kg, IV	0.5–10 mg/kg, IM; 0.5–1.5 mg/kg, IV
2 mg/kg, IM or IV			
	BUTYROPHENONE		
	0.4–0.8 mg/kg, IM		2.2 mg/kg, IM
	PHENOTHIAZINES		
1–5 mg/kg, IM	0.04–0.1 mg/kg/day, IV, IM, SC, or PO	0.05–0.1 mg/kg, IV, IM, or SC	0.1–0.2 mg/kg, IV, IM, or SC
3 mg/kg, IV or IM (may produce myositis)			0.5–4 mg/kg, IM
	0.4–1 mg/kg, IV or IM; 1–2 mg/kg, PO	0.4–1 mg/kg, IV or IM; 1.6–2.8 mg/kg, PO	0.4–1 mg/kg, IV or IM
	0.22–0.33 mg/kg, IV or IM (maximum 100 mg/horse/day)		

TABLE 20 ANALGESICS

Drug	Dosage		
	Dogs	Cats	Ferrets
OPIOID ANALGESICS[a]			
Buprenorphine	0.01–0.02 mg/kg, SC, bid	0.01–0.03 mg/kg, SC or IM, bid	0.01–0.03 mg/kg, IV, IM, or SC, bid-tid
Butorphanol tartrate	0.2–0.4 mg/kg, IM or SC; 0.55 mg/kg, PO, every 6–12 hr	0.1–0.2 mg/kg, IV; 0.2–0.4 mg/kg, IM or SC, every 4 hr	0.05–0.4 mg/kg, IM, every 4–6 hr
Medetomidine	0.002–0.03 mg/kg, IM, IV, or SC	0.002–0.03 mg/kg, IM, IV, or SC	
Meperidine hydrochloride	2–10 mg/kg, IM or SC, every 2 hr	2–5 mg/kg, IM or SC, every 2 hr	2–5 mg/kg, IM or SC, every 2–4 hr
Morphine sulfate	0.22–0.88 mg/kg, IM, IV slowly, or SC, every 4–6 hr as needed	0.1 mg/kg, IM or SC, as needed	0.5–5 mg/kg, IM or SC, qid
Nalbuphine	0.5–2 mg/kg, SC, every 4–8 hr	1.5–3 mg/kg, IV, every 3 hr	
Oxymorphone hydrochloride	0.05–0.1 mg/kg, IV, IM, or SC, every 1–3 hr	0.025–0.05 mg/kg, IV, IM, or SC	0.05–0.2 mg/kg, IV or IM, bid-qid
Pentazocine lactate	2–3 mg/kg, IM, every 4 hr; 15 mg/kg, PO, tid		5–10 mg/kg, SC or IM, every 4 hr
NONOPIOID SEDATIVE ANALGESICS			
Xylazine hydrochloride	0.5–1 mg/kg, IV; 1–2 mg/kg, IM or SC	0.5–1 mg/kg, IV; 1–2 mg/kg, IM or SC	1 mg/kg, IM or SC
Detomidine			
NONPSYCHOTROPIC ANALGESICS			
Acetaminophen	15 mg/kg, PO, qid as needed	Contraindicated	
Aspirin	10–25 mg/kg, PO, bid	10 mg/kg, PO, every 48 hr	0.5–20 mg/kg, PO, once to three times daily
Carprofen	4 mg/kg/day, IV or SC	4 mg/kg/day, IV or SC	
Dipyrone	28 mg/kg, IV, IM, SC, or PO, tid	28 mg/kg, IV, IM, SC, or PO, tid	
Flunixin meglumine	1–2 mg/kg/day, PO, IV, or IM, up to 3 days; use of flunixin meglumine in dogs has decreased since the introduction of other NSAIDs with higher therapeutic indexes.	Use of flunixin meglumine in cats has decreased since the introduction of other NSAIDs with higher therapeutic indexes.	0.5–2 mg/kg, SC, once to twice daily

TABLE 20 ANALGESICS *(continued)*

Dosage			
Rabbits	**Horses**	**Cattle**	**Pigs**
	OPIOID ANALGESICS[a]		
0.02–0.05 mg/kg, SC, IM, or IV, bid			0.005–0.02 mg/kg, IM or IV, bid-qid
0.1–0.5 mg/kg, IV, every 4 hr	0.05–0.1 mg/kg, IV, IM, or SC	Adult: 20–30 mg, IV, jugular	0.1–0.3 mg/kg, IM
5–10 mg/kg, IM or SC, every 2–3 hr	0.2–0.4 mg/kg, IV; 1–3 mg/kg, IM or SC	500 mg/cow, IV slowly, IM or SC	1–2 mg/kg, IM or IV
2–5 mg/kg, SC or IM, every 2–4 hr	0.2 mg/kg, IV; 0.2–0.4 mg/kg, IM		0.2–1 mg/kg, IM, every 4 hr
1–2 mg/kg, IV, every 4 hr			
0.1–0.2 mg/kg, IM, every 2–4 hr	0.02–0.03 mg/kg, IV or IM		0.075 mg/kg, IM
10–20 mg/kg, SC or IM, every 4 hr; 5 mg/kg, IV, every 2–4 hr	0.33 mg/kg, IV		2–5 mg/kg, IM, every 4 hr
	NONOPIOID SEDATIVE ANALGESICS		
	0.1–1 mg/kg, IV; 0.5–1 mg/kg, IM or SC	0.05–0.1 mg/kg, IV; 0.1–0.2 mg/kg, IM	2 mg/kg, IM
	0.02–0.04 mg/kg, IV or IM		
	NONPSYCHOTROPIC ANALGESICS		
5–20 mg/kg/day, PO	30–47.5 mg/kg, PO, bid-qid	26 mg/kg, IV; 100–124 mg/kg, PO, bid	10–20 mg/kg, PO, every 4 hr as needed
1.5 mg/kg, PO, bid	0.7 mg/kg/day, IV, IM, or SC	0.7 mg/kg/day, IV, IM, or SC	
	5–10 g/horse, IV or IM, tid as needed	50 mg/kg, IV, IM, or SC	50 mg/kg, IV, IM, or SC
1.1 mg/kg, SC or IM, bid	1–2.2 mg/kg, IV; 2.2 mg/kg/day, IM or PO	1.1–2.2 mg/kg, IM or PO, once to three times daily	1–2 mg/kg/day, IV or IM

TABLE 20 ANALGESICS *(continued)*

	Dosage		
Drug	**Dogs**	**Cats**	**Ferrets**
Ketoprofen	2 mg/kg/day, SC, IM, or IV, up to 3 days; 1 mg/kg/day, PO, up to 5 days	1 mg/kg/day, SC up to 3 days, or PO up to 5 days	
Meclofenamic acid	2.2 mg/kg/day, PO	2.2 mg/kg/day, PO	
Phenylbutazone	15–22 mg/kg, PO; 15 mg/kg, IV, bid-tid (maximum 0.8 g/dog/day or 44 mg/kg/day); use of phenylbutazone in dogs has decreased since the introduction of other NSAIDs with better safety margins.	15 mg/kg, IV, tid; 10–14 mg/kg, PO, bid; use of phenylbutazone in cats has decreased since the introduction of other NSAIDs with better safety margins.	

[a] Recommended dosages of opiates may produce excitement in cats and horses.

used to treat generalized anxiety and panic disorder in dogs and cats, as well as urine spraying in cats. Benzodiazepines, such as diazepam, alprazolam, oxazepam, and clorazepate, act by binding to γ-amino butyric acid (GABA) receptors and enhancing GABA-mediated chloride influx. They may cause sedation and muscle relaxation; dependence and withdrawal signs also can occur.

Diazepam has been recommended to alleviate fear-related behaviors in dogs and social anxiety and urine spraying in cats. However, benzodiazepines may not alleviate fear-related aggression in certain animals but instead may cause a paradoxical increase in such behaviors. Although diazepam has been reported to diminish urine spraying in cats, most cats resume spraying when the drug is withdrawn. There have been rare reports of hepatic failure within 3–5 days of starting diazepam in cats.

Oxazepam (dogs 0.2–0.5 mg/kg, PO, once to twice daily; cats 1–2.5 mg/cat, PO, bid) and alprazolam have been used to treat fears and phobias in both dogs and cats. In addition, alprazolam has been used to treat night-time anxiety in dogs (0.01–0.1 mg/kg, PO) and refractory housesoiling in cats (0.1 mg/kg or 0.125–0.25 mg [total dose] per cat, PO, bid-tid). Clorazepate has been used to treat anxiety in cats (1.75–3.75 mg/cat, PO, once to twice daily). Diazepam, clonazepam, and clorazepate dipotassium also have anticonvulsant properties.

Buspirone differs from the benzodiazepines in pharmacologic properties (ie, it blocks serotonin pre- and postsynaptically and acts as a dopamine agonist), onset of action (delayed onset of 7–30 days), and lack of sedative effect. Buspirone appears to offer no greater control for anxiety-related behaviors than the benzodiazepines, but it helps treat urine spraying in cats at 2.5–7.5 mg/cat.

Antipsychotics

Antipsychotics are classified as low-potency agents (acepromazine, chlorpromazine, and thioridazine hydrochloride) and high-potency agents (haloperidol, fluphenazine, trifluoperazine hydrochloride, prochlorperazine, thiothixene, risperidone). Low-potency agents require larger doses and produce more sedation, more anticholinergic adverse effects, and cardiovascular effects, but they have a lower incidence of extrapyramidal adverse effects (parkinsonism, dystonia, dyskinesia, and akathisia) than the high-potency agents. All the antipsychotics are used for nonselective tranquilization and diminishing behavioral arousal. Acepromazine is commonly used for infrequent anxietal episodes, but it may induce a paradoxical hyperactivity in some dogs and cats. In one report, a dog with aberrant behavior (tail chewing, growling, snapping, barking) was controlled with thioridazine at 1.1 mg/kg.

TABLE 20 ANALGESICS *(continued)*

Dosage			
Rabbits	**Horses**	**Cattle**	**Pigs**
3 mg/kg, IM	2.2 mg/kg/day, IV	2.2 mg/kg, IV; 3 mg/kg/day, IM	
	2.2 mg/kg/day, PO		
	4.4 mg/kg, PO, bid on day 1; 2.2 mg/kg, PO, bid for 4 days; 2.2 mg/kg, PO, daily or every other day	2–5 mg/kg, IV; 4–8 mg/kg, PO	2–5 mg/kg, IV; 4–8 mg/kg, PO

Mood-stabilizing Drugs

Mood-stabilizing drugs (lithium, carbamazepine, and valproic acid) are unrelated chemical compounds used in human medicine to treat bipolar disorder, impulsivity, emotional reactivity, and aggression. Carbamazepine and valproic acid are also antiepileptic drugs. Carbamazepine has been used in cats (25 mg/cat, PO, bid) to decrease fear-related aggression against people, but it may paradoxically increase aggression against conspecifics. Lithium is excreted unmetabolized via the urine. Serum concentration monitoring is necessary because of its narrow therapeutic index (recommended range: 0.8–1.2 mEq/L). Adverse effects include polyuria, polydipsia, memory problems, weight gain, and diarrhea. In one report, lithium (75 mg total dose, bid) was used to treat owner-directed aggression and psychotic behavior (random air-snapping, pawing) in a Cocker Spaniel.

Antidepressants

Antidepressants are classified as tricyclic compounds (tertiary amines, secondary amines), selective serotonin reuptake inhibitors, and atypical antidepressants. They can be used to treat behavioral disorders, including obsessive-compulsive behaviors, stereotypies, aggression, and inappropriate elimination. The mode of action is to block reuptake of serotonin and/or norepinephrine or to reduce neurotransmitter turnover. All have a lag time until a behavioral effect is seen.

The **tricyclic antidepressants** include amitriptyline, imipramine, clomipramine, and doxepin. Case reports indicate that treatment success for behavioral disorders is highly variable among drugs within the same chemical class. The antihistaminic effect of these agents may be a useful adjunct in controlling pruritus due to atopy and food allergies. Adverse effects include vomiting, diarrhea, hyperexcitability, sedation, arrhythmias including tachycardia, orthostatic hypotension, mydriasis, reduced lacrimation and salivation, urine retention, constipation, and weight gain. Widening of the QRS complex on an ECG has been used as an early indication of toxicity. It may take 7–30 days for drugs to be effective. Amitriptyline hydrochloride has been used in dogs at 1–2 mg/kg for separation anxiety, anxiety-related aggression, urination due to submission or excitement, and allergy-related pruritus, and in cats at 0.5–1 mg/kg for urine marking and hypervocalization. Imipramine hydrochloride has been used in dogs at 2.2–4.4 mg/kg, bid-tid, for urination due to submission or excitement. Clomipramine hydrochloride has been used in dogs at 1–3 mg/kg to reduce lick behavior for canine lick granuloma and for stereotypies such as circling and tail chasing, and in cats at 0.5 mg/kg. In some countries, it is approved for treatment of separation anxiety in dogs. Doxepine has been used in dogs at 3–5 mg/kg.

Selective serotonin reuptake inhibitors, including fluoxetine, sertraline, and paroxetine, have been used to treat psychogenic alopecia, allergy-related pruritus, owner-directed aggression, fearful behaviors, obsessive-compulsive behaviors, and urine marking. It may take 7–30 days for these drugs to be effective. The most common adverse effects are changes in appetite and GI signs, although seizures have been reported. These drugs inhibit liver P450 enzymes, so drug interactions are possible. Dosages for fluoxetine are 1 mg/kg/day, PO, for dogs, and 0.5–1 mg/kg/day, PO, for cats.

Other Agents and Hormones

Monoamine oxidase inhibitors, such as selegiline, are used for cognitive impairment in aging dogs. The use of progestin hormones to treat behavioral problems is currently considered a "last resort" therapy because of the risk of adverse effects. In castrated and intact male dogs, megestrol acetate has been used to treat aggression, urine marking, and roaming. Likewise, in neutered male cats, megestrol acetate can reduce spraying, but potential adverse effects of inducing diabetes mellitus, mammary gland hyperplasia and adenocarcinoma, and bone marrow suppression make it risky to use. Medroxyprogesterone acetate, an injectable, long-acting progestin, has been used to treat aggression, urine marking, and roaming; however, it is rarely used because of the risk of adverse effects and availability of other, safer behavioral drugs.

SYSTEMIC PHARMACOTHERAPEUTICS OF THE REPRODUCTIVE SYSTEM

See also PRINCIPLES OF THERAPY OF THE REPRODUCTIVE SYSTEM, p 1328.

Drugs used to regulate or control the reproductive system are often naturally occurring hormones or chemical modifications of hormones. **Gonadotropin-releasing hormone** (GnRH) and its analogues are used for treatment of ovarian cysts and for control of ovarian follicular dynamics in cattle, for estrus induction (by pulsatile administration) in mares and bitches, and for stimulation of testicular function (eg, in testing for cryptorchidism). Implants of GnRH analogues (eg, deslorelin) are effective for induction of estrus and ovulation in mares and bitches and, in higher doses over a prolonged period, are useful for contraception in male and female animals (such as dogs) by mediating longterm (≥12 mo) reversible infertility caused by downregulation of GnRH receptors.

Follicle-stimulating hormone (FSH), usually extracted from animal pituitary glands, stimulates follicular growth and estrogen production in females and spermatogenesis in males. It is used for superovulation of several domestic species. It has also found application in induction of fertile estrus in bitches and queens. Prolonged FSH use or higher doses can *cause adverse effects* such as cystic endometrial hyperplasia and follicular cysts.

Human chorionic gonadotropin (hCG), which exerts mainly luteinizing hormone–like effects in domestic animals, is used for stimulation of gonads (as a test for cryptorchidism and also for treatment of ovarian cysts in cattle or dogs). It is also used to cause ovulation of mature ovarian follicles in cows or mares in controlled-breeding programs. hCG is given parenterally; plasma levels peak in ~6 hr. It is primarily distributed to the ovaries in females and the testes in males, although some is also distributed to the renal proximal tubules.

Equine chorionic gonadotropin (eCG) has FSH activity in most species and is used to induce ovarian follicular growth, both for superovulation and for estrus induction. (*See also* HORMONAL CONTROL OF ESTRUS, p 2244, and MANAGEMENT OF REPRODUCTION: CATTLE, p 2171 et seq.)

Estradiol esters (eg, valerate, cypionate, or propionate) have a longer duration of action than the parent compound. These compounds are used in bitches, mares, and cows for induction or enhancement of fertile estrus or for induction of estrous behavior; treatment of urinary incontinence in bitches; and for antitumor activity in prostatic and perianal tumors. Availability of these compounds and restrictions on their use vary by country. Estrogenic therapy may cause bone marrow suppression and potentially fatal aplastic anemia in dogs and cats; its use is also associated with development of cystic endometrial hyperplasia in these species, and it may have teratogenic effects in pregnant animals. Because of these potential complications, estrogens are no longer recommended for termination of pregnancy in cases of mismating.

The nonsteroidal synthetic compound **diethylstilbestrol** also has estrogenic activity; its use is prohibited in food animals in the USA. Estrogen antagonists, such as tamoxifen, have been proposed for treatment of metastatic mammary carcinoma in dogs.

Progesterone and **synthetic progestins** are used for suppression or postponement of estrus in bitches and queens. They have also been used in behavior modification and to treat dermatologic disorders. Progesterone supplementation is used to support pregnancies regarded as at risk (eg, in pregnant mares with potentially endotoxemic conditions) and in horses or dogs with demonstrated hypoluteoidism. Adverse effects of progestin administration in small animals include induction of cystic endometrial hyperplasia, adrenocortical suppression, induction or exacerbation of diabetes mellitus, and mammary gland development. Mifepristone (a progesterone-receptor antagonist) has been used experimentally as a canine abortifacient; epostane, a progesterone-synthesis inhibitor, also terminates canine pregnancy.

Testosterone is used for estrus suppression (particularly in racing Greyhounds). Mibolerone, a weak androgenic steroid, is used to prevent estrus in bitches. It should not be used in Bedlington Terriers or cats, and it may exacerbate perianal tumors. After PO administration, mibolerone is absorbed from the intestine, metabolized in the liver, and excreted in the urine and feces. Chronic administration of testosterone may cause testicular degeneration in male animals. Finasteride, a 5α-reductase inhibitor, prevents the conversion of testosterone to 5α-dihydrotestosterone, the active androgen in male accessory sex glands. It is useful in the treatment of benign prostatic hyperplasia of dogs (0.1–0.5 mg/kg/day, PO). Flutamide blocks dihydrotestosterone receptors and is used for the same purpose. Chemical modifications of testosterone potentiate its anabolic actions while minimizing virilizing effects. These compounds (eg, boldenone undecylenate, stanozolol, nandrolone decanoate) are used for their anabolic effects in convalescing or athletic animals. Protracted use may cause at least temporary infertility in both sexes.

Prostaglandin $F_2\alpha$ and its analogues are used mainly for their luteolytic effects to induce predictable onset of estrus (or synchronization of estrus) in a variety of species. They may also be used for termination of pregnancy either alone or in combination with corticosteroids (cattle, sheep) or dopaminergic agents (dogs). These compounds also cause marked uterine contractions, which may be useful for expulsion of uterine contents in pathologic conditions (eg, pyometra).

Oxytocin is used to promote milk letdown, to treat agalactia, as an adjunctive treatment of mastitis, and to cause contraction of the uterus either to induce (or supplement) labor or to enhance postpartum uterine contraction and expulsion of uterine fluid or fetal membranes. It is administered parenterally (IV, IM, or SC). Oxytocin may be given intranasally, but absorption can be erratic. Uterine relaxation is caused by β_2-mimetic agents, such as clenbuterol. Such agents have been used to postpone parturition (to reduce obstetrical complications in heifers) and to facilitate obstetric manipulations in large domestic animals. Clenbuterol use in food-producing animals is illegal in the USA.

Dopaminergic agents, such as bromocryptine or cabergoline, cause decreased serum prolactin concentrations. They are useful in treatment of pseudopregnancy in dogs (bromocryptine at 10 mcg/kg, PO, for 10 days, or at 30 mcg/kg for 16 days) and as an adjunct to $PGF_2\alpha$ in terminating pregnancy, although not approved in the USA for this use. Prolactin is luteotrophic in some species, including dogs.

Dopamine antagonists, such as sulpiride, have shown promise in the manipulation of seasonal breeding species—their use hastens the onset of estrous cycles in mares in the spring.

In the UK and New Zealand, **melatonin** is labeled for use in sheep (and goats in New Zealand) to improve early breeding and ovulation rates. It is available as an 18-mg SC implant; combined with exposure to rams, its use is associated with hastened onset of the breeding season and increased prolificacy.

Glucocorticoids, especially the C-16 substituted steroids dexamethasone, betamethasone, and flumethasone, are used for induction of parturition in ruminants (eg, dexamethasone 20–30 mg, IM, given within 2 wk of normal term). Their therapeutic administration may inadvertently lead to abortion. Xylazine and other α_2-adrenergic agents cause myometrial contraction that may harm the fetus or impede obstetrical manipulations.

EFFECT OF REPRODUCTIVE THERAPY ON THE FETUS OR NEONATE

An important component of reproductive pharmacology encompasses the effect of treatment on the fetus or neonate of medication administered to pregnant or lactating dams that are nursing. Many factors influence the ability of a drug to cross the placenta, including placental architecture of the particular species, but in general, drugs that are lipid-soluble, nonionized, and of low molecular weight can be expected to cross the placenta readily. Among antimicrobials, aminoglycosides are associated with nephrotoxicity and ototoxicity in the fetus, fluoroquinolones may affect developing cartilage, and tetracyclines affect bone and tooth development. Teratogenicity has been associated with use of the antifungal agents griseofulvin and ketoconazole in pregnant animals. All cancer chemotherapeutic agents are potentially harmful to developing fetuses. Glucocorticoids may induce palatoschisis or other defects in puppies.

Any administration of medication to lactating animals requires consideration of the excretion of the drug or its metabolites in milk and of the effects on suckling neonates. Milk produced for human consumption must be free of potentially harmful residues, and all relevant laws and regulations regarding usage and appropriate withdrawal times should be followed.

SYSTEMIC PHARMACOTHERAPEUTICS OF THE RESPIRATORY SYSTEM

See also PRINCIPLES OF THERAPY OF RESPIRATORY DISEASE, p 1416.

Drugs used to treat respiratory tract diseases fall into several categories: antitussives, bronchodilators, anti-inflammatories, expectorants, decongestants, and respiratory stimulants. In addition, antimicrobials and antifungals are important in the therapy of many respiratory diseases.

ANTITUSSIVE DRUGS

A **cough** is a sudden, explosive exhalation of air that functions to clear material from the airways. Coughing is one way in which the lungs and airways are protected from inhaled particles. Coughing sometimes brings up sputum (also called phlegm), a mixture of mucus, debris, and cells expelled from the lungs. The cough reflex has both sensory (afferent) and motor (efferent) pathways. The internal laryngeal nerve carries the sensory information away from the area above the glottis in the trachea to the cough center located in the medulla oblongata via the vagus nerve. Stimulation of this area by dust or foreign particles produces a cough to remove the foreign material from the respiratory tract before it reaches the lungs. Mucus production in the bronchi is an airway defense mechanism, and it increases with inflammation and infection. In dogs and cats, coughing occurs because of a primary disease process, such as *Bordetella bronchiseptica* infection ("kennel cough") or chronic bronchitis in dogs, or feline asthma or heartworm-associated respiratory disease in cats. In most cases, addressing the primary disease will resolve the cough. Antitussive therapy is symptomatic and is primarily for the comfort of the animal and the owner. Most antitussive drugs are opiates or opioids that directly suppress the cough center in the medulla oblongata (*see* TABLE 21). The antitussive effect does not appear to be related to the binding of traditional opiate receptors (mu and kappa). For example, dextromethorphan is an opioid derivative with good antitussive activity, but it does not have activity at opiate receptors and is not analgesic or addictive.

Morphine is an effective antitussive at doses lower than those that produce analgesia and sedation. It is not commonly used for antitussive activity because of adverse effects and the potential for abuse and addiction. Morphine has poor oral bioavailability due to a significant first-pass effect by the liver.

Codeine is methylmorphine; methylation of morphine significantly improves the oral bioavailability by reducing the first-pass effect. Codeine phosphate and codeine sulfate are found in many

TABLE 21 ANTITUSSIVE DRUGS

Drug	Dosage
Codeine	Dogs: 1–2 mg/kg, PO, bid-qid
Hydrocodone	Dogs: 0.25 mg/kg, PO, bid-qid
Butorphanol	Dogs: 0.055–0.11 mg/kg, SC, bid-qid, or 0.55–1.1 mg/kg, PO, bid-qid Cats: 0.1–0.4 mg/kg, SC, bid-qid

preparations, including tablets, liquids, and syrups. Codeine has analgesic effects that are about one-tenth that of morphine, but its antitussive potency is about equal to that of morphine. The adverse effects of codeine are significantly less than those seen with morphine at antitussive doses. Toxicity (especially in cats) is exhibited as excitement, muscular spasms, convulsions, respiratory depression, sedation, and constipation. Codeine should not be used after GI tract surgery because of its effects on intestinal motility. The potential for addiction and abuse of codeine is considerably lower than that for morphine.

Hydrocodone is chemically and pharmacologically similar to codeine but more potent. It is combined with an anticholinergic drug (homatropine) to discourage abuse by people. It can be prescribed for small animals but should be used with caution in cats.

Dextromethorphan is technically not considered an opiate, because it does not bind to traditional opiate receptors and is not addictive or analgesic. It is the D-isomer of levorphanol. The L-isomer of levorphanol has addictive and analgesic properties. Although it is recommended anecdotally to treat cough, a pharmacokinetic study in dogs demonstrated a short elimination half-life, rapid clearance, and poor oral bioavailability, making its use as an orally administered cough suppressant in dogs questionable.

Butorphanol, an opioid agonist-antagonist, is used as an analgesic and antitussive in dogs. As an antitussive in dogs, butorphanol is 4 times more potent than morphine and 100 times more potent than codeine. At antitussive dosages, it may produce considerable sedation in dogs. Because butorphanol has poor bioavailability, the oral dose in dogs is 10 times the SC dose. In cats, butorphanol is primarily used as an injectable analgesic. In some cats, it may cause pain on injection, as well as mydriasis, disorientation, swallowing/licking, and sedation.

SPECIES APPROACH TO INFLAMMATORY AIRWAY DISEASE

Dogs, cats, horses, and people develop spontaneous bronchoconstriction associated with airway inflammation and characterized by chronic cough and wheeze. Attacks of airway obstruction are induced by exposure of susceptible animals to antigens (typically hay dust, molds, and pollens). Effective therapy of allergic airway disease is species dependent because of the inflammatory mediators involved in bronchoconstriction. The pathogenesis of feline asthma differs from allergic airway disease in other species in that cats are exceptionally responsive to serotonin (5-hydroxytryptamine). Serotonin, which is released from degranulating mast cells, appears to be the major mediator of allergen-induced bronchoconstriction in cats. Cats also appear to suffer from chronic bronchitis, similar in clinical presentation to feline asthma; the main feature that differentiates these two conditions is the lack of bronchoconstriction in chronic bronchitis. In dogs, chronic bronchitis is an inflammatory, chronic pulmonary disease that results in cough and can lead to exercise intolerance and respiratory distress but is typically not characterized by severe bronchoconstriction. In horses, there are two clinical syndromes of airway inflammation. Recurrent airway obstruction, or "heaves," is an inflammatory, obstructive airway disease clinically evident in middle-aged horses. Inflammatory airway disease is a low-grade inflammation of the small airways that is a common cause of poor performance in young to middle-aged, athletic horses. Inflammatory airway disease is typically not treated in ruminants or swine.

The goals of therapy for inflammatory airway disease are to prevent recurrent exacerbations of airway obstruction and reduce emergency visits and expenses, to provide optimal chronic anti-inflammatory therapy with minimal or no adverse effects, to maintain (near) "normal" pulmonary function, and to meet the owner's expectations of quality of life for their animal.

SYSTEMIC THERAPY OF INFLAMMATORY AIRWAY DISEASE

β-Adrenergic Receptor Agonists:

The β-adrenergic receptor agonists have beneficial effects in treatment of bronchoconstrictive respiratory tract diseases (*see* TABLE 22). Bronchial smooth muscle is innervated by β_2-adrenergic receptors. Stimulation of these receptors leads to increased activity of the enzyme adenylate cyclase, increased cAMP, and relaxation of bronchial smooth muscle. Stimulation of β receptors on mast cells decreases the release of inflammatory mediators from mast cells, but other inflammatory cells are not suppressed. There is some evidence that β-adrenergic receptor agonists increase mucociliary clearance in the respiratory tract. The β-adrenergic receptor agonists should be used with caution in animals with preexisting cardiac disease, diabetes mellitus, hyperthyroidism, hypertension, or seizure disorders, or that are being treated with digoxin, tricyclic antidepressants, or monoamine oxidase inhibitors.

Epinephrine (adrenaline) stimulates α and β receptors, resulting in pronounced vasopressive and cardiac effects in addition to bronchodilation. Epinephrine is reserved for emergency treatment of life-threatening bronchoconstriction (eg, anaphylaxis). The nonspecific stimulation of other receptors and its short duration of action make it unsuitable for longterm use. Epinephrine is available as a 1 mg/mL solution. Its onset of action is immediate, and the duration of effect is 1–3 hr.

Isoproterenol is a potent β-receptor agonist. It is selective for β receptors, but cardiac (β_1) effects make it unsuitable for longterm use. It is administered by inhalation or injection and has a short duration of action (<1 hr). For emergency relief of bronchoconstriction in horses, it is given by slow IV solution at a dilution of 0.2 mg/50 mL of saline. Administration is discontinued when the heart rate doubles.

Terbutaline is a β_2-receptor agonist similar to isoproterenol but longer acting (6–8 hr). It may be available in some countries as an injectable solution, powder inhaler, or oral syrup and tablets. For cats with feline asthma that experience frequent, severe bronchoconstrictive episodes despite chronic glucocorticoid therapy, injectable terbutaline can be dispensed to owners with instructions to administer 0.01 mg/kg, SC, to treat episodes of bronchoconstriction at home. An increase in the cat's heart rate to 240 bpm and a 50% decrease in respiratory rate indicates a positive effect. Terbutaline also can be given as chronic oral therapy at 0.625 mg/cat, bid (¼ of a 2.5-mg tablet). It should not be used in cats with hypertrophic cardiomyopathy or glaucoma, in which β_2-receptor stimulation would be detrimental.

Albuterol (salbutamol) is similar to terbutaline and may be used systemically in

TABLE 22 β-ADRENERGIC RECEPTOR AGONIST DRUGS

Drug	Dosage
Epinephrine	Dogs: 0.05–0.5 mg, intratracheally or IV
	Cats: 0.1 mg, IV or IM
	Large animals: 0.1 mg/kg, IV, SC, or IM
Isoproterenol	Dogs: 0.1–0.2 mg, IM or SC, qid
	Cats: 4–6 mcg, IM, every 30 min as needed
	Horses: 0.4 mcg/kg, IV (diluted)
Terbutaline	Dogs, cats: 0.1 mg/kg, SC, every 4 hr, or 0.03 mg/kg, PO, tid
	Horses: 0.0033 mg/kg, IV, or 0.2–0.6 mg/kg, PO, bid
Albuterol	Dogs: 0.05 mg/kg, PO, tid
	Horses: 8 mcg/kg, PO, bid
Clenbuterol	Horses: 0.8–3.2 mcg/kg, PO, bid

dogs and horses. Oral syrup, oral tablets, and oral extended-release tablets are available, but albuterol is more commonly used as inhalation therapy.

Clenbuterol is used in the treatment of recurrent airway obstruction in horses; it is not used in dogs and cats. It is available as an oral syrup and may be available as an injectable solution for IV injection in some countries. Results of efficacy studies for bronchoconstriction have been conflicting, but clenbuterol appears to significantly increase mucociliary transport in horses with the disorder. The dosage is increased gradually until a satisfactory clinical response is seen. If there is no response at the highest recommended dose, the horse is considered to have irreversible bronchospasm. It should not be administered chronically to horses with recurrent airway obstruction without concurrent anti-inflammatory therapy. The most common adverse effects of clenbuterol are tachycardia and muscle tremors. Clenbuterol inhibits uterine contractions, so it should be used during late pregnancy only if this effect is desired for obstetric manipulations. Clenbuterol is also a repartitioning agent; it directs nutrients away from adipose tissue and toward muscle. The result is increased carcass weight, increased ratio of muscle to fat, and increased feed efficiency. Because there is a significant human health risk from clenbuterol residues, it is banned in food animals in most countries and should not be used in horses that will be sent to slaughter.

Methylxanthines: The methylxanthines, particularly theophylline, are bronchodilators (*see* TABLE 23). Once the mainstay of human asthma therapy, theophylline has a high incidence of adverse effects, and its use has diminished with the development of metered-dose or disk inhalers for local drug delivery. The methylxanthines have a variety of pharmacologic effects on various organ systems, including bronchial smooth muscle relaxation, CNS stimulation, mild diuresis, and mild cardiac stimulation.

The respiratory effects of methylxanthines are the result of several cellular mechanisms. Antagonism of adenosine is currently thought to be the most important action. Adenosine induces bronchoconstriction in asthmatic animals and antagonizes adenylate cyclase. Adenylate cyclase is responsible for the synthesis of cAMP, which controls bronchial smooth muscle relaxation and inhibits the release of inflammatory mediators from mast cells. Methylxanthines also inhibit phosphodiesterase, which further increases intracellular cAMP. They also inhibit calcium mobilization in smooth muscle, inhibit prostaglandin production, augment the release of catecholamines from storage granules, and increase the availability of calcium to contractile proteins of the heart and

TABLE 23 METHYLXANTHINE BRONCHODILATORS

Drug	Dosage
Theophylline (parenteral)	Dogs: 10 mg/kg, IV (slow) or IM Horses: 15 mg/kg, IV (slow)
Theophylline (oral)	Dogs: 5–7 mg/kg, PO, tid Cats: 3 mg/kg, PO, bid Horses: 10–15 mg/kg, PO, bid
Theophylline (extended-release tablets)	Dogs: 20 mg/kg/day, PO Cats: 25 mg/kg/day, PO Horses: 15 mg/kg/day, PO
Aminophylline (parenteral)	Dogs: 10 mg/kg, IV (slow) Cats: 5 mg/kg, IV (slow) Horses: 5 mg/kg, IV (slow)
Aminophylline (oral)	Dogs: 10 mg/kg, PO, tid Cats: 5 mg/kg, PO, bid Horses: 15 mg/kg, PO, bid

diaphragm. In addition to promoting bronchial smooth muscle relaxation, methylxanthines decrease the release of inflammatory mediators from mast cells and increase mucociliary transport.

Theophylline is available in several formulations, including injectable, aqueous solutions, elixirs, tablets, and capsules. Theophylline base is poorly soluble in water and often results in GI irritation when administered PO. Aminophylline is a theophylline salt that is 78%–86% theophylline. It is more water soluble and results in less GI irritation. Other theophylline salts, such as oxtriphylline (a choline salt), are available, and their theophylline content must be considered when developing a drug dosage regimen.

Several sustained-release formulations of theophylline are suitable for use in dogs and cats and may be administered less frequently than the regular formulations. After oral administration, theophylline is rapidly and completely absorbed. Therapeutic plasma concentrations, extrapolated from people, are 5–20 mcg/mL. Animals are sensitive to high concentrations of theophylline, especially after rapid IV administration, and toxicity may be seen with concentrations <20 mcg/mL. Theophylline tablets may become trapped in bezoars (such as hairballs in cats), and continued absorption can result in toxicity. Cardiac arrhythmias, CNS excitement, tremors, convulsions, and GI irritation may be seen. Theophylline undergoes enterohepatic recirculation, so activated charcoal is recommended if clinical signs are present, no matter how long after the drug was administered. Theophylline metabolism is inhibited by erythromycin, cimetidine, propranolol, enrofloxacin, and marbofloxacin; concomitant therapy can result in theophylline toxicity. Theophylline metabolism is induced by rifampin and phenobarbital, which may necessitate increasing the dose of theophylline.

Theophylline is used to treat both cardiac and respiratory diseases in dogs and cats. Theophylline is also used in management of intrathoracic collapsing trachea and various forms of canine bronchitis, but it is less effective than glucocorticoids such as prednisone. Theophylline or aminophylline was used in horses in the management of recurrent airway obstruction, but efficacy was often poor and use of these drugs has been replaced by β-agonist bronchodilators delivered by metered-dose inhalers.

Anticholinergic Drugs: The anticholinergic (parasympatholytic) drugs are effective bronchodilators that reduce the sensitivity of irritant receptors and inhibit vagally mediated cholinergic smooth muscle tone in the respiratory tract. Cholinergic stimulation causes bronchoconstriction; asthmatic individuals appear to have excessive stimulation of cholinergic receptors.

Atropine is primarily used as a preanesthetic to prevent bradycardia and reduce airway secretions, and as emergency therapy of dyspneic animals with organophosphate intoxication. Atropine is also used for bronchodilation in horses; a low IV dose (0.014 mg/kg) is more effective and less toxic than IV theophylline. A test dose of 0.022 mg/kg may also be used to determine prognosis in horses with recurrent airway obstruction; if pulmonary function does not improve with a test dose of atropine, successful management with bronchodilators is unlikely. Atropine should be used with caution, because even low doses may cause tachycardia, ileus, neurologic derangement, and blurred vision in horses.

Glycopyrrolate is twice as potent as atropine in people and does not cross the blood-brain barrier. Its onset of action is slower than atropine, but its duration of effect is longer. Information about use in horses is sparse, but doses of 2–3 mg can be given IM, bid-tid.

N-butylscopolammonium bromide is an anticholinergic drug approved to relieve spasmodic colic in horses. Unlike atropine, N-butylscopolammonium bromide does not cross the blood-brain barrier. Adverse effects are minimal and include transient tachycardia, decreased borborygmi, and transient pupillary dilatation. In horses with recurrent airway obstruction challenged with moldy hay, N-butylscopolammonium bromide was a potent bronchodilator, with maximum relief occurring 10 min after IV administration. The bronchodilatory effect is short lived, dissipating within 1 hr of drug administration.

Glucocorticoids: The glucocorticoids inhibit the release of inflammatory mediators from macrophages and eosinophils but do not inhibit the release of granules from mast cells. Glucocorticoids decrease synthesis of prostaglandins, leukotrienes, and platelet-activating factor, which play important roles in the pathophysiology of respiratory tract inflammation. Studies suggest glucocorticoids enhance the action of adrenergic agonists on α_2-receptors in the bronchial smooth muscle. Because of immunosuppressive effects, glucocorticoids are generally avoided in infectious respiratory diseases.

For severe attacks of canine bronchitis, feline asthma, or recurrent airway obstruction, parenteral injection of glucocorticoids usually provides rapid relief. For chronic therapy in dogs, oral prednisone is usually the drug of choice. Prednisone is a prodrug; it is metabolized by the liver to the active drug prednisolone. Pharmacokinetic studies have shown poor oral bioavailability of prednisone in cats and horses. Therefore, it is preferable to administer prednisolone to these species. In dogs, a typical anti-inflammatory dosage is 0.5–1 mg/kg, with chronic therapy on an every-other-day basis. A similar dose of prednisolone can be used in cats; if prednisone is used, higher doses may be necessary. Cats are somewhat resistant to the effects of glucocorticoids, and dosages of prednisone of 1 mg/kg/day may be necessary for chronic therapy of feline asthma. Alternatively, 20 mg of methylprednisolone acetate can be administered IM to asthmatic cats every 3 wk. For emergency treatment of dyspneic cats, a shock dose of an IV glucocorticoid (prednisone sodium succinate, 5–10 mg/kg; or dexamethasone sodium phosphate, 1–2 mg/kg) should be used. It is common for clinical signs to resolve in cats with feline asthma or chronic bronchitis that are treated with oral glucocorticoids despite persistent lower airway inflammation, so therapy should be tapered very carefully. Although prednisolone can be administered to horses, the small tablet sizes available make it inconvenient, so equine formulations of oral dexamethasone (10 mg/450 kg) are recommended. The injectable formulation of dexamethasone can be given IV to horses with acute bronchoconstriction and dyspnea. Flumethasone or isoflupredone may also be used in horses. Isoflupredone is as effective as dexamethasone in the treatment of recurrent airway obstruction in horses, but as in cattle, it is associated with hypokalemia.

Cyproheptadine: Because of the role of serotonin in allergen-induced bronchoconstriction in cats, the serotonin antagonist/antihistamine cyproheptadine (2 mg, PO, once to twice daily) may be used as an adjunct to glucocorticoids and bronchodilators to block bronchoconstriction in chronically asthmatic cats. In experimental models of feline asthma, cyproheptadine decreased airway hyperreactivity but did not significantly decrease eosinophilic airway inflammation. However, pharmacokinetic studies of cyproheptadine suggest that some cats may require doses as high as 8 mg to reach therapeutic concentrations. Because of its long elimination half-life (12 hr), cyproheptadine requires several days to reach steady-state concentrations, and 4–7 days may be needed to see clinical effects. Serotonin antagonism in the appetite center stimulates appetite, so weight gain may be a problem. Lethargy, depression, and increased appetite may occur within 24 hr of initiating therapy.

Antimicrobial Therapy: Antimicrobial therapy may or may not be necessary in treatment of airway inflammatory diseases. Antimicrobial therapy should be started for cats with tracheobronchial cultures suggestive of a true bacterial infection or those positive for *Mycoplasma*. *Mycoplasma* spp can be isolated from healthy dogs but are not found in healthy cats. Doxycycline, azithromycin, and fluoroquinolones treat *Mycoplasma* infections effectively. Secondary bacterial infection from *Streptococcus zooepidemicus* may exacerbate inflammatory airway disease in horses and can easily be treated with penicillin, ceftiofur, or a trimethoprim/sulfonamide.

INHALATION THERAPY OF AIRWAY DISEASE

The current approach to management of inflammatory airway disease is through inhalation therapy with nebulizers or metered-dose inhalers (MDIs). With inhalation therapy, high drug concentrations are delivered directly to the lungs via nebulizers or MDIs, and systemic adverse effects are avoided or minimized. The onset of action for inhaled bronchodilators and anti-inflammatory drugs is substantially shorter than that of oral or parenteral formulations. Nebulizers have long been used in animals, but the overall efficiency of drug delivery is low, and the equipment is cumbersome and inconvenient for owners. Administration of medications via MDIs is commonplace in treatment of human asthma and seems to benefit management of animals as well. Human MDIs are designed to provide optimal lung delivery after actuation during a slow, deep inhalation. However, this is impossible to control in animals. The addition of spacers enables MDIs to be used in animals. Spacers decrease the amount of drug deposited in the oropharynx (up to 80% of the actuated dose with the MDI alone), thereby reducing systemic drug absorption. Drugs available in MDI formulations include β_2-agonists, glucocorticoids, ipratropium bromide, cromolyn sodium, and nedocromil. Each product delivers a set amount of drug per actuation (puff). In the USA, MDIs are labeled according to the amount of drug delivered at the mouthpiece, whereas in Canada and the EU they are labeled according to the amount of drug delivered from the valve. MDIs are color-coded to aid identification. Even in human medicine, the relative potencies, risks of adverse effects, and optimal dose of the different inhaled asthma medications remain unclear. Unfortunately, some drugs that would be useful in veterinary patients are not available in MDIs; dry powder inhalers are not suitable for use in animals. Clinical use of MDI medications in asthmatic cats, dogs with chronic bronchitis, and horses with recurrent airway obstruction is promising but mostly anecdotal, and clinical trials are needed to determine the most efficacious therapies.

Spacers: MDIs (eg, OptiChamber™, AeroChamber®) used in human patients may be modified for use in dogs and cats, and small animal–specific spacers are available (eg, AeroKat™, AeroDawg™, Feline Breathe Easy™, Nebulair™). The OptiChamber™ must be modified with a suitable face mask, such as the type used to "mask" cats for anesthesia. The AeroChamber is available with a variety of face masks intended for infants, children, and adults that will conform to a variety of veterinary patients. The Nebulair and Feline Breathe Easy spacers are valveless, so the actuation must occur with the mask applied to the face of the animal. The AeroKat and AeroDawg are equipped with "flapper" valves so the dog or cat can be visualized breathing in the medication. MDIs were originally used in horses via the Aeromask™, but the mask is bulky and rather expensive. The Aerohippus™ is similar to the AeroKat and AeroDawg, with a large, bell-shaped cone that fits over a horse's nostril. It also has a valve indicator.

β_2-Agonists: Short-acting β_2-agonists such as **albuterol (salbutamol)** in MDIs are the medications of choice to treat acute exacerbations of bronchoconstriction, because they relax smooth muscle and promptly increase airflow. Although effective for *symptomatic relief*, β_2-agonists do not control inflammation. Airway obstruction may persist despite appropriate use of inhalant bronchodilators because of bronchial wall edema and airway mucus plugging. In general, β_2-agonists are extremely safe for use in animals when used as needed for bronchoconstriction. Toxicity typically requires a large overdose, such as when dogs chew on and puncture the inhaler, receiving a very large dose at one time (there are 200 doses in an albuterol/salbutamol inhaler). Massive overdose may induce severe tachycardia and hypokalemia, which, in turn, lead to extreme weakness, incoordination, and potentially cardiac standstill. Other less serious signs include dilated pupils, severe agitation and hyperactivity, hypertension, and vomiting.

Albuterol (salbutamol) is the medication of choice in all species for inhalation therapy of acute airway obstruction. It relaxes smooth muscle and increases airflow within minutes of administration; effects last 3–6 hr. Although effective for symptomatic relief, the β_2-agonists do not control inflammation, and monotherapy may exacerbate asthma and increase morbidity and mortality. Racemic albuterol (R, S albuterol) is the most commonly prescribed short-acting β_2-agonist and is composed of a 1:1 mixture of (R)-albuterol (the R enantiomer) and (S)-albuterol (the S enantiomer). The R-enantiomer has bronchodilatory and anti-inflammatory effects, and the S-enantiomer paradoxically is associated with increased airway hyperreactivity and pro-inflammatory effects. The paradoxical exacerbation of asthma with regular use of inhaled racemic albuterol in people is thought to be linked to preferential accumulation of S-albuterol in the lung, which has a much slower metabolism than R-albuterol. Neutrophilic airway inflammation in healthy cats was induced when receiving treatment with albuterol containing the S-enantiomer. These data suggest that the form of albuterol commonly prescribed to asthmatic cats can actually cause inflammation in "healthy" cats without preexisting airway disease. The S-enantiomer also exacerbates eosinophilic airway inflammation in experimentally asthmatic cats. This increase in airway inflammation associated with use of albuterol can be attenuated by concurrent use of glucocorticoids. Proper control of the underlying inflammation should reduce albuterol use to an as-needed only basis. One actuation (100 mcg Canada; 90 mcg USA) of albuterol can be administered for relief of bronchoconstriction as needed until clinical signs resolve.

Salmeterol is a long-acting β_2-agonist; its onset of action is slow (15–30 min), but its duration of action is >12 hr. The long duration of action is due to diffusion into the plasma membrane of the pulmonary cells followed by slow release from the cells to interact with β_2 receptors. It is not recommended for use in acute bronchoconstriction, but daily use with glucocorticoids provides better control of symptoms than simply increasing the glucocorticoid dose. It is not available in an MDI in all countries, and the dry powder inhaler is not suitable for animal use.

Other β_2-agonists that may be available in MDIs include isoproterenol, fenoterol, formoterol, and terbutaline. Isoproterenol was commonly used to treat asthma before the more widespread use of albuterol, which has more selective effects on the airways. In Europe, an epidemic of deaths due to cardiotoxicity from overuse of isoproterenol inhalers led to withdrawal of the products. North American products have clear warning labels regarding the potential toxicity.

Glucocorticoids: Inhaled glucocorticoids are the most potent inhaled anti-inflammatory drugs available. In people, early intervention with inhaled glucocorticoids improves asthma control, normalizes lung function, and may prevent irreversible airway damage. The potential risk of adverse effects is well balanced by their efficacy in management of chronic inflammation. Oral candidiasis (thrush), dysphonia, and reflex cough and bronchospasm are the most common adverse effects in people; all of these effects are reduced by use of a spacer. The risk of systemic adverse effects, such as suppression of the hypothalamic-pituitary axis, is less than with oral prednisone therapy. Inhaled glucocorticoid formulations include fluticasone, beclomethasone, flunisolide, and triamcinolone. Currently, fluticasone is considered the most potent formulation with the longest duration of action and is the most commonly used inhaled glucocorticoid in veterinary patients.

Ipratropium Bromide: Ipratropium bromide is a quaternary derivative of atropine that lacks its adverse effects and is available in an MDI (500 mcg/actuation), alone or in combination with albuterol. In people with asthma, ipratropium bromide is used as an additional reliever medication to reverse bronchoconstriction when inhaled short-acting β_2-agonists do not provide enough relief. Its anticholinergic action also decreases mucous secretions. In an experimental model of feline asthma, longterm antigen sensitization caused an augmented muscarinic receptor response to acetylcholine. Modulation of muscarinic receptors with anticholinergic drugs may be useful to treat asthmatic cats. Ipratropium has shown efficacy for recurrent airway obstruction in horses. It is not well absorbed after inhalation, so it does not cause systemic anticholinergic effects.

Cromolyn Sodium and Nedocromil: Cromolyn sodium and nedocromil sodium are chloride-channel blockers that modulate mast cell–mediator release and eosinophil recruitment. They are both available in MDIs. Cromolyn sodium and nedocromil sodium have strong human safety profiles, but nedocromil sodium has been reported to have a broader spectrum of efficacy. In people, the clinical response to these drugs is less predictable than the response to glucocorticoids. There are no published reports of the use of cromolyn or nedocromil in asthmatic cats or dogs with bronchitis; however, pretreatment with nedocromil sodium aerosols attenuated viral-induced airway inflammation in Beagle puppies. Further investigation of these drugs in asthmatic cats seems warranted given the sensitivity of this species to serotonin released from degranulating mast cells.

Lidocaine: Lidocaine, commonly used as a local anesthetic and antiarrhythmic agent, is used as a steroid-sparing treatment in human asthma. Initially used topically to prevent cough during bronchoscopic procedures, lidocaine, administered via nebulization, is effective for intractable cough and asthma by inhibition of eosinophil-active cytokines. Nebulization provides direct drug delivery to the lung, with minimal systemic drug absorption and few adverse effects. Nebulized lidocaine reduced airway hyperresponsiveness in experimentally asthmatic cats but did not affect airway eosinophilia, so it probably should be combined with glucocorticoids in management of feline asthma.

Suggested Treatment Regimens: For emergency management of dyspnea in cats and dogs, 2–4 puffs of albuterol should be given every 5 min until clinical signs resolve. Additional therapy may include oxygen and an IV dose of a rapid-acting glucocorticoid.

Current recommendations for therapy of feline asthma and canine bronchitis are to use albuterol only as needed for bronchodilation and fluticasone bid. For initial therapy of moderately affected animals, a 5-day course of oral prednisone (or prednisolone) at 1 mg/kg may be helpful. Severely affected animals may require 1 mg/kg of prednisone (or prednisolone) every other day. Adjunctive therapy with other inhaled or orally administered anti-inflammatories and bronchodilators may be useful in some animals. Therapy must be individualized for each animal.

For horses with recurrent airway obstruction, environmental management and a combination of bronchodilator and anti-inflammatory therapy is recommended. Current recommendations are to use 500 mcg of albuterol every 2 hr as needed and fluticasone at 2–4 mcg/kg bid. Beclomethasone has also been used at 1–3 mcg/kg, bid, but it causes more adrenal suppression in horses than fluticasone at these doses.

EXPECTORANTS AND MUCOLYTIC DRUGS

Expectorants and mucolytic drugs are used to increase the output of bronchial secretions, enhance the clearance of bronchial exudate, and promote a productive cough. Saline expectorants are promoted to stimulate bronchial mucous secretions via a vagally mediated reflex action on the gastric mucosa. However, there are no well-designed studies that support these claims. Examples of these drugs include ammonium chloride, ammonium carbonate, potassium iodide, calcium iodide, and ethylenediamine dihydroiodide. Iodine-containing products should not be administered to pregnant, hyperthyroid, or milk-producing animals.

Direct stimulants of respiratory secretions include the volatile oils, such as eucalyptus oil and oil of lemon. They are believed to directly increase respiratory tract secretions. Their efficacy in animals is unknown.

Guaifenesin (glyceryl guaiacolate) is a centrally acting muscle relaxant that may also have an expectorant effect. It may stimulate bronchial secretions via vagal pathways. The volume and viscosity of bronchial secretions does not change, but particle clearance from the airways may accelerate. It is a common component of human cold remedies in combination with dextromethorphan.

***N*-acetylcysteine** is available as a 10% solution that can be nebulized. Its mucolytic effect is the result of the exposed sulfhydryl groups on the compound, which interact with disulfide bonds on mucoprotein. Acetylcysteine helps to break down respiratory mucus and enhance clearance. It may also increase the levels of glutathione, which is a scavenger of oxygen-free radicals. Aerosolization of acetylcysteine can cause reflex bronchoconstriction due to irritant receptor stimulation, so its use should be preceded by bronchodilator therapy.

Dembrexine is a phenolic benzylamine available in some countries for respiratory disease in horses. The proposed effect is through an alteration of the constituents and viscosity of abnormal respiratory mucus and an improved efficiency of respiratory clearance mechanisms. It also has an antitussive action and enhances concentrations of antibiotics in lung secretions. It is supplied as a powder that is sprinkled on the feed at a dosage of 0.33 mg/kg, bid.

DECONGESTANTS

Decongestants are commonly used in people to treat allergic rhinitis, but they are rarely used for this purpose in animals. The α-adrenergic agonist drugs cause local vasoconstriction in mucous membranes, which reduces swelling and edema. They are used topically as nasal decongestants in allergic and viral rhinitis, or systemically in combination with antihistamines as respiratory tract decongestants. Antihistamines are effective for treatment of allergic rhinitis in people when combined with the α-adrenergic agonist drugs, but their effectiveness in animals has not been demonstrated. The topical α-adrenergic agonist drugs act within minutes with few adverse effects, but extended use may cause rebound hyperemia and mucosal damage. Systemic administration can result in hypertension, cardiac stimulation, urinary retention, CNS stimulation, and mydriasis. Systemic administration of antihistamines often causes sedation.

RESPIRATORY STIMULANTS

Doxapram stimulates the medullary respiratory center and the chemoreceptors of the carotid artery and aorta to increase tidal volume. Other portions of the CNS are stimulated only when high doses are administered. Doxapram is used primarily in emergency situations during anesthesia or to decrease the respiratory depressant effects of opiates and barbiturates. Recommended dosages are 1–5 mg/kg, IV, in dogs and cats, or 1–2 drops under the tongue of apneic neonates. In adult horses, the dosage is 0.5–1 mg/kg, IV, while foals are dosed carefully at 0.02–0.05 mg/kg/hr, IV.

SYSTEMIC PHARMACOTHERAPEUTICS OF THE URINARY SYSTEM

See also PRINCIPLES OF THERAPY OF URINARY DISEASE, p 1496.

BACTERIAL URINARY TRACT INFECTIONS

Bacterial urinary tract infections (UTIs) typically result from normal skin and GI tract flora ascending the urinary tract and overcoming the normal urinary tract defenses that prevent colonization. Bacterial UTI is the most common infectious disease of dogs, affecting 14% of all dogs during their lifetime. Although UTIs are uncommon in young cats, the incidence of UTI is much higher in older cats, which may be more susceptible to infection because of diminished host defenses secondary to aging or concomitant disease (such as diabetes mellitus, renal failure, or hyperthyroidism). Approximately two-thirds of those cats also have some degree of renal failure. Bacterial UTIs in ruminants are associated with catheterization or parturition in females and as both a cause and consequence of urolithiasis in males. In horses, UTIs are uncommon and typically associated with bladder paralysis, urolithiasis, or urethral damage.

Unlike human patients, veterinary patients are often asymptomatic, and the UTI may be an incidental finding. The consequences of untreated UTI include lower urinary tract dysfunction, urolithiasis, prostatitis, infertility, septicemia, and pyelonephritis with scarring and eventual kidney failure. Coagulase-positive staphylococci are involved in the formation of struvite ($MgNH_4PO_4$) calculi in dogs. In intact male dogs, UTI frequently extends to the prostate gland. Because of the blood-prostate barrier, it is difficult to eradicate bacteria from the prostate, and the urinary tract may be reinfected after appropriate treatment, causing a systemic bacteremia, infecting the rest of the reproductive tract, or causing an abscess within the prostate.

Large, retrospective studies have documented the most common species of uropathogens in dogs and cats, with *Escherichia coli* being the single most common pathogen in both acute and recurrent UTIs. The other common pathogens include *Staphylococcus*, *Proteus*, *Streptococcus*, *Klebsiella*, and *Pseudomonas* spp. In UTIs in horses, *E coli*, *Streptococcus*, and *Enterococcus* spp predominate, whereas *Corynebacterium renale* and *E coli* are the most common pathogens in ruminants. In immunocompromised animals, funguria from *Candida* spp may occur.

Antimicrobials are the cornerstone of UTI therapy, and many animals with recurring UTIs are managed empirically with repeated courses (*see* TABLE 24). This approach fails if the underlying pathophysiology predisposing the animal to the UTI is not addressed; as well, it encourages emergence of resistant bacteria. With chronic UTI from highly resistant bacteria, therapeutic options are extremely limited.

Antimicrobial Therapy: Urine culture is the "gold standard" for diagnosis of UTI. Indications to perform urine culture include visualization of bacteria during urine sediment examination, evidence of pyuria, dilute urine (<1.013 SG), immunosuppression, and diabetes mellitus or hyperadrenocorticism. Antimicrobial susceptibility testing should be done with complicated or recurrent cases of UTIs, immunosuppressed animals, animals recently catheterized, or animals treated with antimicrobials within the preceding 3 wk (because of selection for antimicrobial resistance). In addition, culture and susceptibility testing should be performed in cases that do not respond within 7 days of therapy for UTI or in cases associated with multiple pathogens.

High urine concentrations of antimicrobials are correlated with efficacy in treatment of uncomplicated cystitis. But in complicated cases and in pyelonephritis, tissue concentrations may be equally important. Most antimicrobials undergo renal elimination to a great extent, so urine concentrations may be up to 100 times peak plasma concentrations. Drug excretion through the kidney involves various processes such as secretion and/or reabsorption in different parts of the nephron, depending on the molecular structure of the drug, its pK_a, the pH in the tubular fluid, and degree of protein binding. The flow of urine through the urinary tract is part of the defense against invading pathogens, because the flow of fluid rinses the

TABLE 24 DRUGS COMMONLY USED TO TREAT URINARY TRACT INFECTIONS IN SMALL ANIMALS

Drug	Suggested Dosage	Typical Antimicrobial Activity
Amoxicillin	11 mg/kg, PO, bid-tid	Staphylococci, streptococci, enterococci, *Proteus*, some *E coli*
Ampicillin	25 mg/kg, PO, tid	Staphylococci, streptococci, enterococci, *Proteus*, some *E coli*
Amoxicillin-clavulanic acid	25 mg/kg, PO, tid	Staphylococci, streptococci, enterococci, *Proteus*, some *E coli*
Cephalexin/ cefadroxil	20–30 mg/kg, PO, bid-tid	Staphylococci, streptococci, *Proteus*, *E coli*, *Klebsiella*
Cefovecin	8 mg/kg, SC, every 14 days	*Proteus*, *E coli*
Cefpodoxime	5–10 mg/kg/day, PO	*Proteus*, *E coli*
Ceftiofur	2 mg/kg/day, SC	*Proteus*, *E coli*
Chloramphenicol	Dogs: 25–50 mg/kg, PO, bid-tid Cats: 50 mg/cat, PO, q 12 h	Staphylococci, streptococci, enterococci, *E coli*
Doxycycline	5 mg/kg, PO, bid	Streptococci, some activity against *E coli*, staphylococci, and enterococci at high urine concentrations
Enrofloxacin, orbifloxacin, marbofloxacin, pradofloxacin (cats only)	2.5–10 mg/kg/day, PO	Staphylococci, *E coli*, *Proteus*, *Klebsiella*, *Pseudomonas*, *Enterobacter*
Gentamicin	4–6 mg/kg/day, SC	Staphylococci, some streptococci, some enterococci, *E coli*, *Proteus*, *Klebsiella*, *Pseudomonas*, *Enterobacter*
Nitrofurantoin	5 mg/kg, PO, tid	Staphylococci, some streptococci, enterococci, *E coli*, *Klebsiella*, *Enterobacter*
Tetracycline	18 mg/kg, PO, tid	Streptococci, some activity against *E coli*, staphylococci, and enterococci at high urine concentrations
Trimethoprim-sulfa	15 mg/kg, PO, bid	Streptococci, staphylococci, *E coli*, *Proteus*, some activity against *Klebsiella*

epithelial linings. High urine antimicrobial concentrations are important for eradication of bacteria in the urine, but for infection of the bladder wall or renal tissue it is necessary to use antimicrobials that have active concentrations in the tissues. Serum or plasma concentrations are useful surrogate markers for antimicrobial concentrations in the renal or bladder tissues.

In addition to having the appropriate antimicrobial activity and achieving effective concentrations in urine, the selected antimicrobial should be easy for owners to administer, have few adverse effects, and be relatively inexpensive. Once urine culture and sensitivity results are known, the bacterial minimum inhibitory concentration (MIC) can be compared with the mean urinary concentration of the drug and an appropriate antimicrobial chosen.

Amoxicillin and **ampicillin** are bactericidal and relatively nontoxic, with a spectrum of antibacterial activity greater than that of penicillin G. They have excellent activity against staphylococci, streptococci, enterococci, and *Proteus*, and may achieve urinary concentrations high enough to be effective against *E coli* and *Klebsiella*. *Pseudomonas* and *Enterobacter* are resistant. Amoxicillin is more bioavailable in dogs and cats (better absorbed from the GI tract) than ampicillin, hence the lower dosage. Absorption of ampicillin is also affected by feeding, so therapeutic success may be easier to achieve with amoxicillin. As penicillins, they are weak acids with a low volume of distribution, so they do not achieve therapeutic concentrations in prostatic fluid.

Amoxicillin-clavulanic acid has an increased spectrum of activity against gram-negative bacteria because of the presence of clavulanic acid. Clavulanic acid irreversibly binds to β-lactamases, allowing the amoxicillin fraction to interact with the bacterial pathogen. This combination usually has excellent bactericidal activity against β-lactamase–producing staphylococci, *E coli*, and *Klebsiella*. *Pseudomonas* and *Enterobacter* remain resistant. However, clavulanic acid undergoes some hepatic metabolism and excretion, so much of the antimicrobial activity in the bladder may be due to the high concentrations of amoxicillin achieved in urine. Thus, despite an unfavorable susceptibility report for amoxicillin, clinically amoxicillin alone may be as effective as amoxicillin-clavulanic acid to treat UTIs.

Cefadroxil and **cephalexin** are first-generation cephalosporins. Cefadroxil is a veterinary-labeled suspension product, whereas cephalexin is available in both human and veterinary formulations as tablets, paste, or suspension products. Like the penicillins, they are bactericidal, acidic drugs with a low volume of distribution and are relatively nontoxic. Vomiting and other GI signs may occur in dogs and cats treated with cephalosporins. Cephalosporins have greater stability to β-lactamases than penicillins, so they have greater activity against staphylococci and gram-negative bacteria. They have excellent activity against *Staphylococcus* spp, *Streptococcus* spp, *E coli*, *Proteus*, and *Klebsiella*. *Pseudomonas*, enterococci, and *Enterobacter* are resistant.

Cefovecin is an injectable, third-generation cephalosporin approved for treatment of dogs with a UTI due to *E coli* or *Proteus*. In cats, it is only approved for skin infections but may be used in an extra-label manner for UTIs. With SC dosing, therapeutic concentrations are achieved for 14 days, making this an attractive treatment choice for fractious animals.

Cefpodoxime is an oral, third-generation cephalosporin approved for use in dogs for skin infections (wounds and abscesses), but it is used extra-label for treatment of canine UTI. Cefpodoxime has a relatively long half-life in dogs, so it is dosed once daily.

Ceftiofur is an injectable cephalosporin approved for respiratory disease in horses, swine, and cattle and for treatment of canine UTI caused by *E coli* and *Proteus*. Ceftiofur has pharmacokinetic properties very different from those of other cephalosporins. After injection, ceftiofur is immediately metabolized to desfuroylceftiofur, which has different antimicrobial activity than the parent compound. Desfuroylceftiofur has equivalent activity to ceftiofur against *E coli* (MIC 4 mcg/mL) but is much less active against *Staphylococcus* spp and has variable activity against *Proteus* (MIC 0.5–16 mcg/mL). Because of the instability of desfuroylceftiofur, microbiology services use a ceftiofur disk when performing susceptibility testing, so a false expectation of therapeutic efficacy may result for some pathogens. *Pseudomonas*, enterococci, and *Enterobacter* spp are resistant to ceftiofur and desfuroylceftiofur. Ceftiofur is associated with a duration- and dose-related thrombocytopenia and anemia in dogs, which would not be expected with the recommended dosage regimen.

Chloramphenicol has a high volume of distribution, and high tissue concentrations can be achieved, including in the prostate of male dogs and cats. It is active against a wide range of gram-positive and many gram-negative bacteria, against which it is usually bacteriostatic. Chloramphenicol is typically active against enterococci, staphylococci, streptococci, *E coli*, *Klebsiella*, and *Proteus*. *Pseudomonas* are resistant. North American isolates of methicillin-resistant *Staphylococcus aureus* and *Staphylococcus pseudintermedius* are typically susceptible. Well known for causing idiosyncratic (non-dose-dependent) anemia in people and dose-dependent bone marrow suppression in animals, its use in both human and veterinary medicine is increasing because of resistance to other antimicrobial drugs.

Enrofloxacin, orbifloxacin, and **marbofloxacin** are all fluoroquinolones approved to treat UTIs in dogs; although all are used in cats, only some are approved for this use. **Pradofloxacin** is only approved for skin infections in cats in North America, but it is approved for treatment of UTI in dogs in Europe and is used to treat feline UTI. The fluoroquinolones are bactericidal, amphoteric drugs. They possess acidic and basic properties but are very lipid soluble at physiologic pH (pH 6–8) and thus have a high volume of distribution. All fluoroquinolones usually have excellent activity against staphylococci and gram-negative bacteria, but they may have variable activity against streptococci and enterococci. The therapeutic advantages of these drugs are their gram-negative antimicrobial activity and high degree of lipid solubility. They are the only orally administered antimicrobials effective against *Pseudomonas*. Therefore, fluoroquinolones should be reserved for UTIs that involve gram-negative bacteria, especially *Pseudomonas*, and for UTIs in intact male dogs and cats because of their excellent penetration into the prostate gland and activity in abscesses. They are concentration-dependent killers with a long postadministration effect, so once daily, high-dose therapy for a relatively short duration of treatment is effective.

Fluoroquinolones should be avoided for chronic, low-dose therapy, because this encourages emergence of resistant bacteria that are cross-resistant to other antimicrobial drugs as well. Cases that involve *Pseudomonas* should be carefully investigated for underlying pathology, which must corrected if at all possible. Once *Pseudomonas* spp become resistant to the fluoroquinolones, there are no other convenient therapeutic options.

Gentamicin and the other aminoglycosides are very large, polar (water-soluble) molecules, so they have a low volume of distribution and do not penetrate the blood-prostate barrier. They are not absorbed orally and must be given by SC, IM, or IV injection. The aminoglycosides have a similar spectrum of activity to that of the fluoroquinolones, but their use for UTI is limited because of the necessity of parenteral injections and the risk of toxicity with anything but short-term use. Like the fluoroquinolones, the aminoglycosides are concentration dependent, bactericidal killers with a long postadministration effect, so once-daily therapy of short duration is effective and minimizes the risk of nephrotoxicity. They can be considered for in-hospital or outpatient treatment of UTI due to fluoroquinolone-resistant pathogens; however, the importance of identifying and correcting underlying pathology must be emphasized.

Nitrofurantoin is a *human product available* as tablets, capsules, and a pediatric suspension. It is not commonly used in veterinary medicine. It is typically used only for treatment of UTI in people, because it has a very low volume of distribution, and therapeutic concentrations are attained only in urine. It is considered a carcinogen, so it is banned for use in food-producing animals, but its use in small animals is increasing with the rising rates of antimicrobial resistance to veterinary antimicrobials. Nitrofurantoin is used for infections caused by *E coli*, enterococci, staphylococci, *Klebsiella* spp, and *Enterobacter* spp. It is increasingly indicated for treatment of UTIs caused by multidrug-resistant bacteria, which are otherwise difficult to treat using conventional veterinary antimicrobial agents. The pharmacokinetics and adverse effect profile of nitrofurantoin have not been investigated in dogs, cats, or horses, and the need for multiple daily dosing makes it inconvenient for owners.

Tetracyclines are bacteriostatic, amphoteric drugs with a high volume of distribution. Tetracyclines are broad-spectrum antimicrobials, but because of plasmid-mediated resistance, susceptibility is variable in staphylococci, enterococci, *Enterobacter*, *E coli*, *Klebsiella*, and *Proteus*. In most tissues, *Pseudomonas* spp are resistant. However, the tetracyclines are excreted unchanged in urine, so high urinary concentrations may result in therapeutic efficacy. **Doxycycline** is a very lipid-soluble tetracycline better tolerated in cats and reaches therapeutic concentrations in the prostate, so it may be useful for some UTIs. Doxycycline may also be effective to treat methicillin-resistant staphylococcal UTIs. If capsules are administered, it is critical to have the animal drink afterward to ensure passage into the stomach. If capsules remain in the esophagus, severe local necrosis with subsequent esophageal stricture can occur.

Trimethoprim-sulfonamides (TMP-sulfas) are combinations of two very different drugs that act synergistically on different steps in the bacterial folic acid pathway. Trimethoprim is a bacteriostatic, basic drug with a high volume of distribution and a short elimination half-life, whereas the sulfonamides are bacteriostatic, acidic drugs with a medium volume of distribution and long half-lives (ranging from 6 to >24 hr). These drugs are formulated in a 1:5 ratio of TMP to sulfa, although the optimal bactericidal concentration is a ratio of 1:20 TMP:sulfa. Microbiology services use the 1:20 ratio in susceptibility testing; however, the widely varying pharmacokinetic properties of this drug combination make it difficult to determine a therapeutic regimen that achieves the 1:20

ratio at the infection site. Although the combination does penetrate the blood-prostate barrier, sulfa drugs are ineffective in purulent material because of freely available para-aminobenzoic acid from dead neutrophils. The combination of TMP-sulfa is synergistic and bactericidal against staphylococci, streptococci, *E coli*, and *Proteus*. Activity against enterococci and *Klebsiella* is variable, and *Pseudomonas* is resistant. TMP-sulfas are associated with a number of adverse effects, and chronic low-dose therapy may result in bone marrow suppression and keratoconjunctivitis sicca in dogs.

Dosage Regimens for UTI: Currently, the duration of therapy for UTI is controversial. Although animals are routinely treated with antimicrobial drugs for 10–14 days, shorter duration antimicrobial regimens are routinely prescribed in human patients, including single-dose fluoroquinolone therapy. A clinical comparison of 3 days of therapy with a once-daily high dose of enrofloxacin with 2 wk of twice daily amoxicillin-clavulanic acid showed equivalence in the treatment of simple UTI in dogs. However, further studies are needed to determine the optimal dosage regimens for different classes of antimicrobials, and it is inappropriate to use fluoroquinolones as first-line therapy for simple UTIs. Animals with complicated UTI may require longer courses of therapy, and underlying pathology must be addressed. Chronic complicated cases of UTI, pyelonephritis, and prostatitis may require antimicrobial treatment for 4–6 wk, with the risk of selecting for antimicrobial resistance. A follow-up urine culture should be performed after 4–7 days of therapy to determine efficacy. If the same or a different pathogen is seen, then an alternative therapy should be chosen and the culture repeated again after 4–7 days. Urine should also be cultured 7–10 days after completing antimicrobial therapy to determine whether the UTI has resolved or recurred.

Managing Multiple Episodes of UTI: In dogs and cats, if UTI occurs only once or twice yearly, each episode may be treated as an acute, uncomplicated UTI. If episodes occur more often, and predisposing causes of UTI cannot be identified or corrected, chronic low-dose therapy may be necessary. Low antimicrobial concentrations in the urine may interfere with fimbriae production by some pathogens and prevent their adhesion to the uroepithelium. In dogs, recurrent UTIs are due to a different strain or species of bacteria ~80% of the time; therefore, antimicrobial culture and susceptibility is still indicated. Antimicrobial therapy should be started as previously described and when urine culture is negative, continued daily at ⅓ the total daily dose. The antimicrobial should be administered last thing at night to ensure that the bladder contains urine with a high antimicrobial concentration for as long as possible.

Appropriate antimicrobials for chronic, low-dose therapy include amoxicillin, ampicillin, amoxicillin-clavulanic acid, doxycycline, cephalexin, cefadroxil, and nitrofurantoin. A trimethoprim-sulfonamide can be used, but folate supplementation should be provided (15 mg/kg, bid) to prevent bone marrow suppression; there is also the risk of keratoconjunctivitis sicca developing with longterm use. Although attractive for owner convenience, third-generation cephalosporins such as cefpodoxime and cefovecin and fluoroquinolones should not be used for longterm therapy. During longterm therapy, urine culture should be repeated every 4–6 wk. As long as the culture is negative, therapy is continued for 6 mo. If bacteriuria occurs, the infection is treated as an acute episode with an appropriate antimicrobial. After 6 mo of bacteria-free urine, the longterm, low-dose antimicrobial therapy may be discontinued, and many animals will not have additional recurrences. In some cases, longterm therapy may be continued for years in animals that continue to have recurrent UTIs.

Therapeutic Failures: Treatment failures may be due to poor owner compliance, inappropriate choice of antimicrobials, inappropriate dose or duration of treatment, antimicrobial resistance, superinfection, or an underlying predisposing cause (eg, urolithiasis, neoplasia, urachal diverticula). If treatment for a simple or complicated UTI fails, a thorough evaluation should be performed to determine and, when possible, address the cause of failure. When faced with a therapeutic failure, the practitioner must consider whether the UTI is due to a relapse or a reinfection. Relapses due to infection by uropathogens with enhanced intrinsic virulence occur with what should be effective antimicrobial therapy. Strains of uropathogenic *E coli* have a number of virulence mechanisms that enable them to invade, survive, and multiply within the uroepithelium. The sequestration of uropathogenic *E coli* within the bladder uroepithelium presents a great therapeutic challenge in both human and veterinary patients. There is no clear consensus in the human medical literature about how to approach these recurrent and persistent UTIs.

Antimicrobial Resistance in Uropathogens: Acquired resistance to antimicrobials by uropathogens is of great concern in both human and veterinary medicine. The prevalence of multidrug resistance in uropathogens is increasing, particularly in infections in dogs and cats. Extended-spectrum β-lactamase genes are increasingly identified in *E coli* isolates from companion animals. Increases in the occurrence of fluoroquionolone-resistant *E coli* in dogs have been widely reported. Because the mechanism of resistance to fluoroquinolones frequently involves efflux pumps, it also conveys multidrug resistance. Fluoroquinolone resistance is also increasing in other uropathogens, including enterococci, *Proteus mirabilis*, and *Staphylococcus pseudintermedius* isolates. Methicillin-resistant staphylococci have been identified in cases of canine UTI. There is increasing evidence that animals are an important reservoir of antimicrobial-resistant bacteria causing infections in people. Enterococci isolated from canine UTIs have been associated with several different resistant phenotypes, with most exhibiting resistance to three or more antimicrobials. One *Enterococcus faecium* isolate displayed high-level resistance to vancomycin and gentamicin. Sequence analysis suggested that resistance was due to gene exchange between human and canine enterococci. The use of "last resort" human antimicrobials in veterinary patients with resistant infections is controversial. Vancomycin, imipenem-cilastatin, meropenem, fosfomycin, quinupristin-dalfopristin, and tigecycline should not be used routinely in treatment of UTI in animals. Nonantimicrobial control of infection should be considered whenever feasible. Custom-made vaccines, cranberry juice/extract, probiotics and adherence/colonization inhibitors, and establishment of asymptomatic bacteriuria may help preserve the efficacy of antimicrobials.

FUNGAL URINARY TRACT INFECTIONS

Although uncommon, most fungal UTIs in dogs and cats are caused by *Candida* spp. Finding *Candida* organisms in the urine may indicate sample contamination; however, finding *Candida* organisms in two serial urine samples collected by cystocentesis is consistent with infection and warrants culture and definitive identification. Treatment includes eliminating potential predisposing factors (eg, excessive endogenous or exogenous corticosteroids, urinary catheters) and administering antifungal drugs with or without urinary alkalinization. Fluconazole is the antifungal drug of choice for treatment of candidal cystitis. The dosage in cats is 50 mg/cat, PO, once to twice daily, and in dogs is 2.5–5 mg/kg/day, PO, divided bid. The duration of treatment needed to eliminate infection is unknown but may be as short as 7 days.

BACTERIAL PROSTATITIS

Bacterial prostatitis is a common prostate disease in sexually intact male dogs and may be seen in intact male cats. It can develop as an acutely fulminating systemic disorder or, most commonly, as a chronic problem associated with recurrent UTIs. Care should be taken when rectally palpating an acutely infected prostate, because septicemia/endotoxemia can occur. Most, if not all, sexually intact male dogs with UTI also have infectious prostatitis. The prostate gland is uniquely different from the rest of the urinary tract because of the acidity of the prostate glands, leading to a decreasing pH gradient from the blood through the tissue to the acinar glands. The distribution of antimicrobials in the prostatic tissue as well as in the prostatic secretions depends completely on the local pH (6.4) and the pK_a of the drugs. For alkaline drugs, a high degree of ionic trapping leads to high antimicrobial concentrations in the tissue and secretions, whereas the acidic drugs such as the β-lactam antimicrobials do not reach concentrations equivalent to plasma concentrations. The choice of antimicrobial for treatment should be based on culture and susceptibility results, and on the ability of the drug to penetrate the blood-prostate barrier. Ideal antimicrobials should be very lipid-soluble, basic, and not highly protein-bound. Fluoroquinolones are the best empirical choice for *E coli* infections, whereas chloramphenicol, doxycycline, or trimethoprim-sulfas can otherwise be considered with favorable culture and susceptibility results. Antimicrobial therapy may need to be continued for up to 2 mo, which may promote emergence of antimicrobial resistance. Chronic bacterial prostatitis may be difficult to cure. Neutering the dog may increase the likelihood of successful therapy and prevent recurrence.

DIURETICS

Diuretics are used to remove inappropriate water volume in animals with edema or volume overload, correct specific ion imbalances, and reduce blood pressure and pulmonary capillary wedge pressure (*see* TABLE 25). They are classified by their mechanism of action as loop diuretics, carbonic anhydrase inhibitors, thiazides, osmotic diuretics, and potassium-sparing diuretics. The efficacy and use of each class of diuretic depends on the mechanism and site of action. Patterns of electrolyte excretion vary between classes, whereas maximal response is the same within a class. Therefore, if one drug within a class is ineffective, a different drug from the same class will likely be ineffective as well. Combining diuretics from different classes can lead to additive and potentially synergistic effects. *See also* p 2525.

Furosemide: Furosemide is a sulfonamide derivative and the most commonly administered diuretic in veterinary medicine. Furosemide is a loop diuretic; it inhibits the reabsorption of sodium and chloride in the thick, ascending loop of Henle, resulting in loss of sodium, chloride, and water into the urine. Furosemide induces beneficial hemodynamic effects before the onset of diuresis. Vasodilation increases renal blood flow, thereby increasing renal perfusion and lessening fluid retention. It appears that renal vasodilation depends on the local synthesis of prostaglandins.

The elimination half-life of furosemide is short in most animals (~15 min). The effect peaks 30 min after IV administration and 1–2 hr after PO administration. The duration of diuretic action is 2 and 6 hr after IV and PO administration, respectively. Furosemide is highly protein bound (91%–97%), almost totally to albumin. It is cleared through the kidneys by renal tubular secretion. Bioavailability of oral furosemide is low (only 50% is absorbed).

Furosemide is usually dosed to effect. For acute, short-term therapy, single IV, IM, or SC doses of 4–6 mg/kg are given. The major adverse effect from acute administration of large doses is acute intravascular volume reduction, which worsens cardiac output and hypotension and may precipitate acute renal failure. Chronic therapy in cats and some dogs can be accomplished by therapy every second or third day. Higher than normal doses of furosemide may be required in animals with renal disease due to functional abnormalities of the renal tubule and binding of furosemide to protein in the urine. If escalating doses of furosemide are required to control fluid retention, adding other types of volume-modifying medications, such as a potassium-sparing diuretic or an angiontensin-converting enzyme (ACE) inhibitor, may help avoid adverse effects.

Furosemide therapy is associated with a number of adverse effects. By nature of its mechanism of action, it causes dehydration, volume depletion, hypokalemia, and hyponatremia, which may be excessive and detrimental. Furosemide's most important drug interaction is with the digitalis glycosides digoxin and digitoxin. The hypokalemia induced by furosemide diuresis potentiates digitalis toxicity. As long as animals continue to eat, hypokalemia does not usually develop. Hypokalemia also predisposes animals to

TABLE 25 DOSAGES OF DIURETICS

Drug	Dosage
Furosemide	4–6 mg/kg IV, IM, or SC, as needed for acute therapy
	Dogs: 2–4 mg/kg, PO, once to three times daily
	Cats:1–2 mg/kg, PO, once or twice daily
	Large animals: 0.5–1 mg/kg/day, IV or IM
Hydrochlorothiazide	Dogs and cats: 2–4 mg/kg, PO, once or twice daily
Chlorothiazide	Dogs and cats: 20–40 mg/kg, PO, once or twice daily
Spironolactone	Dogs: 2–4 mg/kg, PO, bid
Mannitol	0.25–0.5 g/kg, IV
Dimethyl sulfoxide	Large animals: 1 g/kg, IV or via nasogastric tube

hyponatremia by enhancing antidiuretic hormone secretion and the exchange of sodium ions for lost intracellular potassium ions. Concurrent administration of NSAIDs may interfere with furosemide's prostaglandin-controlled renal vasodilation and reduce the diuretic effect. Furosemide-induced dehydration of airway secretions may exacerbate respiratory disease.

Thiazide Diuretics: The thiazide diuretics, **hydrochlorothiazide** and **chlorothiazide**, are not as potent as furosemide and thus are infrequently used in veterinary medicine. The thiazides act on the proximal portion of the distal convoluted tubule to inhibit sodium resorption and promote potassium excretion. They may be administered to animals that cannot tolerate a potent loop diuretic such as furosemide. They should not be administered to azotemic animals, because they decrease renal blood flow. Because the thiazides act on a different site of the renal tubule than other diuretics, they may be combined with a loop diuretic or potassium-sparing diuretic for treatment of refractory fluid retention. Adverse effects are electrolyte and fluid balance disturbances, similar to furosemide. Thiazides decrease renal excretion of calcium, so they should not be used in hypercalcemic animals.

Potassium-sparing Diuretics: Potassium-sparing diuretics include **spironolactone**, **amiloride**, and **triamterene**. Spironolactone is the one most frequently used in veterinary medicine and is a competitive antagonist of aldosterone. Aldosterone is increased in animals with congestive heart failure when the renin-angiotensin system is activated in response to hyponatremia, hyperkalemia, and reductions in blood pressure or cardiac output. Aldosterone is responsible for increasing sodium and chloride reabsorption and potassium and calcium excretion from renal tubules. Spironolactone competes with aldosterone at its receptor site, causing a mild diuresis and potassium retention. Spironolactone is well absorbed after administration PO, especially if given with food. It is highly protein bound (>90%) and extensively metabolized by the liver to the active metabolite, canrenone. It is primarily eliminated by the kidneys. The onset of action for spironolactone is slow, and effects do not peak for 2–3 days. Spironolactone is not recommended as monotherapy but can be added to furosemide or thiazide therapy to treat cases of refractory heart failure. Because of the potential for hyperkalemia, spironolactone should not be administered concurrently with potassium supplements. It has been shown to be safe when used at low doses with concurrent ACE inhibitor therapy.

Carbonic Anhydrase Inhibitors: Carbonic anhydrase inhibitors act in the proximal tubule to noncompetitively and reversibly inhibit carbonic anhydrase, which decreases the formation of carbonic acid from carbon dioxide and water. Reduced formation of carbonic acid results in fewer hydrogen ions within proximal tubule cells. Because hydrogen ions are normally exchanged with sodium ions from the tubule lumen, more sodium is available to combine with urinary bicarbonate. Diuresis occurs when water is excreted with sodium bicarbonate. As bicarbonate is eliminated, systemic acidosis results. Because intracellular potassium can substitute for hydrogen ions in the sodium resorption step, carbonic anhydrase inhibitors also enhance potassium excretion.

Osmotic Diuretics: Osmotic diuretics include **mannitol**, **dimethyl sulfoxide (DMSO)**, **urea**, **glycerol**, and **isosorbide**. Mannitol is commonly used in small animals but is expensive for use in adult large animals, so DMSO is often used in its place. Mannitol acts as a protectant against further renal tubular damage and initiates an osmotic diuresis. The initial dosage is 0.25–0.5 g/kg, given IV over 3–5 min. A response should be noted within 20–30 min. If a response is seen, the dose can be repeated every 6–8 hr, or a constant-rate infusion of 2–5 mL/min of a 5%–10% solution can be given. The total daily dosage should not exceed 2 g/kg. If diuresis is not seen, the initial dose can be repeated up to a total dosage of 1.5–2 g/kg. However, repeated doses usually are not more effective and increase the likelihood of complications (eg, edema).

DMSO is an oxygen-derived free radical scavenger and an osmotic diuretic. It is used in large animals to treat inflammatory and edematous conditions. It is a very potent solvent that can penetrate intact skin and carry other chemicals along with it. It penetrates all body tissues and produces an odor that many people cannot tolerate. The dosage is 1 g/kg, IV or via nasogastric tube, as a 10% solution diluted in 5% dextrose or lactated Ringer's solution (higher concentrations can cause intravascular hemolysis).

DOPAMINE

Dopamine, an adrenergic neurotransmitter with specific receptors in the renal vasculature, is frequently used to combat reductions in renal blood flow that may contribute to acute renal failure. It also increases glomerular filtration and sodium excretion. Dopamine has a very short half-life and is administered as a constant-rate infusion of 2–5 mcg/kg/min. Higher dosages cause tachycardia, cardiac arrhythmias, and peripheral vasoconstriction. Animals that do not produce urine with dopamine alone may respond to a combination of dopamine and furosemide. Dopamine is given as above, and furosemide is given at 1 mg/kg/hr, by IV bolus. If no improvement occurs within 6 hr, conversion is unlikely, and infusion should be discontinued. Dialysis (hemodialysis or peritoneal dialysis) may be required to maintain these animals.

GLOMERULAR DISEASE

Angiotensin-converting enzyme (ACE) inhibitors may be beneficial in management of dogs and cats with chronic renal failure (CRF). Renal disease progresses to CRF as a consequence of functional adaptations of the remaining nephrons, including glomerular hyperperfusion and hypertension controlled by angiotensin II. These responses initially enhance nephron filtration capacity and compensate for the decrease of glomerular filtration rate but are detrimental in the longterm and cause further nephron loss. Administration of ACE inhibitors lowers glomerular pressure by decreasing systemic blood pressure and locally inhibiting angiotensin II. In animals with CRF, ACE inhibitors may decrease proteinuria caused by changes in glomerular membrane permeability and selectivity from mechanical injury induced by glomerular hypertension, potentially slowing disease progression. ACE inhibitors also tend to increase appetite and body weight in animals with renal failure. **Enalapril** is used in dogs at a dosage of 0.5 mg/kg, PO, once or twice daily; **benazepril** is used in cats at a dosage of 0.5–1 mg/kg/day, PO.

Dimethyl sulfoxide (DMSO) has been used in dogs with amyloidosis with variable results. It is given at a dosage of 80 mg/kg/day, divided tid, and given as a 10% solution either PO or SC. Thromboembolism and systemic hypertension are frequent complications of glomerular diseases in dogs, and to a lesser extent in cats, and should be managed as the need arises. Thromboembolism may be prevented by giving aspirin at 0.5–5 mg/kg bid, to high-risk animals such as those with serum albumin <2 g/dL, plasma fibrinogen >400 mg/dL, or plasma antithrombin III activity <70%.

DIABETES INSIPIDUS

Nephrogenic diabetes insipidus is a physiologic condition in which the kidneys fail to concentrate urine despite adequate amounts of antidiuretic hormone (ADH). Central, or pituitary-dependent, diabetes insipidus develops when there is a lack of ADH production. Animals with central diabetes insipidus can be given **desmopressin acetate**. The nasal spray formulation can be used, with 1–4 drops administered into the conjunctival sac once or twice daily. Alternatively, the parenteral form can be given at 0.5–2 mcg, SC, once or twice daily. **Thiazide diuretics** may reduce polyuria by 30%–50% in animals with nephrogenic or central diabetes insipidus. Inhibition of sodium resorption in the ascending loop of Henle leads to decreased total body sodium and contraction of the extracellular fluid volume. The net effect is to increase sodium and water resorption in the proximal renal tubule. Chlorothiazide is given at 20–40 mg/kg, PO, bid.

CONTROLLING URINE pH

The ideal urine pH should be 7.0–7.5 in dogs and 6.3–6.6 in cats. If the urine pH remains below these values after diet modification, **potassium citrate** at 80–150 mg/kg/day, PO, divided bid-tid, can be given to increase the pH. **Ammonium chloride** (200 mg/kg/day, PO, divided tid) and **DL-methionine** (1,000–1,500 mg/cat/day, PO) are the urinary acidifiers of choice. Chronic urine acidification, and ensuing acidosis, can be harmful and should not be instituted without complete evaluation of the animal.

CYSTINE-BINDING AGENTS

Cystinuria, with subsequent cystine urolith formation, results from an inherited disorder of renal tubular transport. Cystine stones are dissolved by dietary modification, urinary alkalinization or neutralization, and the use of cystine-binding agents. Urinary alkalinization or neutralization is accomplished as described above. **Tiopronin** at 15 mg/kg, PO, bid, or **D-penicillamine** at 15 mg/kg, PO, bid, given with food, are both cystine-binding agents. Tiopronin has fewer adverse effects and is the recommended choice. Both agents can cause Coombs'-positive anemia, thrombocytopenia, increased liver enzyme activity, glomerulonephritis, lymphadenopathy, cutaneous hypersensitivity, and delayed wound healing. Penicillamine also causes vomiting. Once stones are dissolved, a prevention protocol can be instituted. Dietary modification with or without urinary alkalinization may be all that is needed to prevent stone formation; however, tiopronin may also be needed if uroliths recur.

URINARY INCONTINENCE

Urinary incontinence is most commonly caused by urethral sphincter incompetence. It is most common in large breed, spayed female dogs (11%–20% incidence) but may be seen in intact females, male dogs, and cats. Estradiol-17β concentrations decrease after ovariohysterectomy in bitches, resulting in deterioration of urethral closure within 3–6 mo. Currently, there are no approved drugs to treat incontinence in animals, and most of the human products traditionally used have been removed from the market because of toxicity concerns. Some estrogen compounds and α-adrenergic drugs may still be available to veterinarians through compounding pharmacies (*see* TABLE 26).

Diethylstilbestrol (DES) is a nonsteroidal estrogen derivative that closely resembles the natural estrogen, estradiol. Because it is inexpensive and infrequently administered, it is the first choice to treat urinary incontinence in female dogs. It is orally bioavailable and reaches peak plasma concentrations in 1 hr in dogs; it has an elimination half-life of 24 hr because of enterohepatic recirculation. Estrogens sensitize the urethral sphincter to α-adrenergic stimulation; therefore, DES therapy is synergistic with α-adrenergic drugs. DES is given as a daily loading dose for 7–10 days and then reduced to once weekly dosing, if possible, to avoid toxicity. Treated dogs are susceptible to bone marrow suppression from estrogen, typified by early thrombocytopenia and potentially fatal aplastic anemia. Hematopoietic toxicity is rarely seen in cats. Other adverse effects seen in dogs include alopecia, cystic ovaries, cystic endometrial hyperplasia, pyometra, prolonged estrus, and infertility. When used once weekly in spayed female dogs, adverse effects from DES are rare.

α-Adrenergic agonists such as phenylpropanolamine (PPA), ephedrine, pseudoephedrine, and phenylephrine act directly on smooth muscle receptors to increase urethral tone and maximal urethral closure pressure. Although often more clinically effective than DES, their action is short lived, usually requiring dosing bid-tid. Of this class of drugs, PPA is the most effective and results in fewer cardiovascular adverse effects. Previously available in over-the-counter cold medications and appetite suppressants, it was withdrawn from the human market because of toxicity associated with overuse as a diet aid. Ephedrine, pseudoephedrine, or phenylephrine may be tried but are less efficacious than PPA. Adverse effects of α-adrenergic drugs include excitability, restlessness, hypertension, and anorexia.

In male dogs, testosterone injections are used to treat urinary incontinence but are generally less effective than estrogen therapy in female dogs.

TABLE 26 DRUGS USED TO TREAT URINARY INCONTINENCE

Drug	Dosage
Diethylstilbestrol	Dogs: 0.1–1 mg/dog, PO, q 24 h, for 5–7 days
Phenylpropanolamine	Dogs: 1.5–2 mg/kg, PO, once to three times daily
Ephedrine	Dogs: 1.2 mg/kg, PO, bid-tid
	Cats: 2–4 mg/kg, PO, bid-tid
Pseudoephedrine	Dogs >25 kg: 30 mg/dog, PO, tid
	Dogs <25 kg: 15 mg/dog, PO, tid
Testosterone propionate	Dogs: 2.2 mg/kg, IM, every 2–3 days
Testosterone cypionate	Dogs: 2.2 mg/kg, IM, every 30–60 days

URINE RETENTION

Disorders of micturition characterized by urine retention and a distended bladder are usually caused by hypocontractility of the bladder or by urethral obstruction. Prolonged bladder distention leads to breakdown of the tight junctions between detrusor muscle cells of the bladder, which prevents normal depolarization and contraction of the detrusor muscles.

An adrenergic antagonist may be indicated when manual expression or voluntary voiding is nonproductive because urethral sphincter tone is excessive, as is often the case in cats after relief of obstruction. **Phenoxybenzamine**, an irreversible antagonist, has been used with some success. The dosage for dogs or cats is 0.25 mg/kg, PO, bid.

Diazepam is a benzodiazepine anxiolytic that is also a central muscle relaxant. Dosages sufficient to allow for urethral relaxation may also cause sedation. The dosage in dogs is 0.2 mg/kg, PO, tid, and in cats is 0.5 mg/kg, IV. Diazepam given PO may cause idiosyncratic acute hepatic necrosis in cats.

In animals with detrusor hyporeflexia or bladder atony, **bethanechol chloride** may be of some benefit. This cholinergic agonist stimulates the initiation of detrusor muscle contraction. The dosage for dogs is 5–25 mg/dog, PO, tid, and for cats is 2.5–7.5 mg/cat, PO, tid.

CHEMOTHERAPEUTICS INTRODUCTION

Treatment with any chemotherapeutic agent involves an understanding of the complex interrelationships among the host animal, the infecting pathogen, and the drug, the interactions of which comprise the chemotherapeutic triangle. The advent of resistance places further emphasis on consideration of these factors when selecting a dosing regimen. That the FDA struggles to identify the most reasonable way to approve antimicrobials while maintaining high standards of proof of efficacy and safety as well as clinician flexibility in the design of dosing regimens is a testament to the complex host, drug, and microbial interactions associated with infections.

Chemotherapy is the use of chemical agents in treatment or control of disease. However, the term is most often used in the context of controlling harmful pathogens through their chemical destruction. As such,

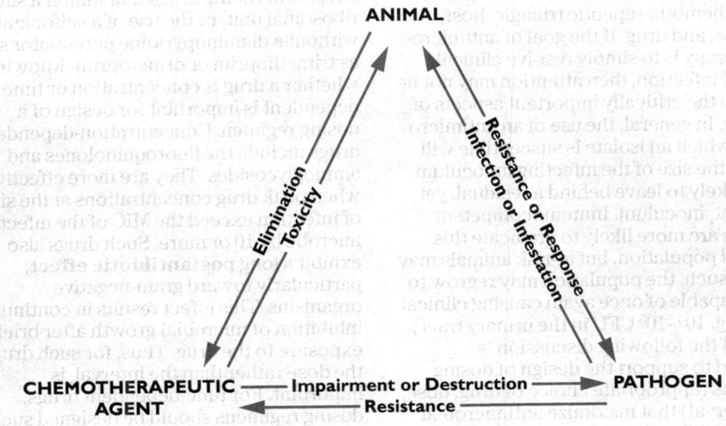

Chemotherapeutic triangle

the chemotherapeutic armamentarium includes antibacterial, antiviral, antifungal, antiparasitic, and antineoplastic compounds.

Chemotherapeutic agents may be selectively toxic to invade micro- or macroorganisms, but in many cases, they can also result in adverse effects in the host. This is particularly true when the infecting pathogen is eukaryotic (eg, fungal organisms, cancer cells) versus prokaryotic (eg, bacterial). To avoid toxic manifestations, particularly for drugs targeting eukaryotes, the dose rate often becomes critical; additionally, the clinical condition of the animal and concurrently administered drugs can be responsible for adverse events.

This discussion of chemotherapeutic agents focuses on infecting bacterial pathogens; fungal and viral pathogens are discussed in their respective chapters. Any time a drug is used with the intent to kill the target, multiple factors impact therapeutic success. The most obvious is that the target organism will implement mechanisms whereby it can avoid harm, the most notable being resistance mechanisms. However, microbes in particular are associated with numerous virulence factors and other mechanisms for self-protection, often also making the host sick at the same time. Likewise, host factors, which seemingly should help the host fend off infection, can become detrimental to therapeutic success. For most infections, a functional immune system is paramount to therapeutic success. Drug factors also influence therapeutic success, most notably because drugs must be able to penetrate any body tissue to successfully kill the microbe. These include the interactions between the three points of the chemotherapeutic triangle: host, microbe, and drug. If the goal of antimicrobial therapy is to simply resolve clinical signs of infection, then attention may not be given to the critically important aspects of therapy. In general, the use of an antimicrobial to which an isolate is susceptible will reduce the size of the infecting innoculum but is likely to leave behind a residual, yet resistant, inoculum. Immunocompetent animals are more likely to eradicate this residual population, but at-risk animals may not. As such, the population may regrow to a size capable of once again causing clinical signs (eg, 10^3–10^5 CFU in the urinary tract). Much of the following discussion is intended to support the design of dosing regimens (appropriate choice of drug, dose, and interval) that maximize antimicrobial efficacy while minimizing the risk of emergent antimicrobial resistance.

ANTIMICROBIAL DRUG FACTORS

Mechanism of Action

Understanding the mechanism of action (MOA) of antibacterial agents is important for several reasons. The MOA determines whether the antibacterial action is likely to be bactericidal or bacteriostatic, and whether the relationship between plasma drug concentration (PDC) and organism minimum inhibitory concentration (MIC) is concentration dependent or time dependent. Further, MOA often is related to the mechanism(s) by which resistance emerges. For some antimicrobials, the MOA also relates to the mechanism(s) of toxicity. Finally, if combination therapy is to be considered, drugs with MOAs that complement one another should be chosen.

The major MOA of antimicrobial agents, with examples of each type, are as follows (*see also* ANTIBACTERIAL AGENTS, p 2652): 1) inhibition of cell wall synthesis: β-lactams (penicillins, cephalosporins, and cephamycins), glycopeptides (vancomycin), bacitracin, fosfomycin; 2) impairment of cell membrane function: polymyxin B, colistin; 3) inhibition of protein synthesis through binding either to a single (tetracyclines, chloramphenicol, macrolides, lincosamides) or both (aminoglycosides) ribosomal subunits; 4) inhibition of DNA synthesis and replication: novobiocin, quinolones, metronidazole; 5) inhibition of DNA-dependent RNA polymerase: rifamycins; and 6) inhibition of folic acid and consequently DNA synthesis: sulfonamides, trimethoprim.

Most mechanisms will result in killing (rather than static) efficacy, with notable exceptions being drugs that inhibit a single ribosomal unit, or the use of a sulfonamide without a diaminopyridine potentiator such as trimethoprim or ormetoprim. Knowing whether a drug is concentration or time dependent is important for design of a dosing regimen. Concentration-dependent drugs include the fluoroquinolones and aminoglycosides. They are more effective when peak drug concentrations at the site of infection exceed the MIC of the infecting microbe by 10 or more. Such drugs also exhibit a long **postantibiotic effect**, particularly toward gram-negative organisms. This effect results in continued inhibition of microbial growth after brief exposure to the drug. Thus, for such drugs, the dose rather than the interval, is important. For time-dependent drugs, dosing regimens should be designed such that drug concentrations remain above the MIC for most of the dosing interval. For such drugs, the dose may need to be increased to surpass the MIC of the organisms, but the interval should be designed to maintain the concentrations. Examples of time-dependent drugs include the β-lactams, "bacteriostatic" drugs, and the sulfonamides. Designing a convenient dose for time-dependent drugs with very short-half lives is difficult. For example, most penicillins have an elimination half-life of ~1–2 hr, and as such, the majority (~90%) will be eliminated in 3–6 hr (for amoxicillin, ~4 hr). As such, dosing regimens should be at least every 8, if not every 6, hr. Choosing a drug with a longer half-life, if the isolate is sufficiently susceptible, is more prudent. Some drugs are both concentration and time dependent; eg, efficacy of the fluoroquinolones can be enhanced by adding a second dose in the face of treatment of an organism with a high, yet susceptible, MIC.

Drug Disposition

Drug disposition (absorption, distribution, metabolism, and excretion) of antimicrobials can impact therapeutic efficacy and should influence the design of the dosing regimen. Most antimicrobials are administered orally. Exceptions include those destroyed by GI acidity (eg, some β-lactams, and particularly penicillins) or microbes (ie, ruminants) and those insufficiently unstable for oral preparation. Food can impact absorption of some drugs, most notably tetracyclines (except doxycycline) and the fluoroquinolones (rate but not extent impacted). A drug that has a very high oral bioavailability in one species cannot be assumed to have a similarly high oral bioavailability in another. For example, the oral bioavailability of ciprofloxacin is good in people but fair or negligible in dogs and horses. Most antimicrobials must potentially reach any body tissues. Antimicrobials that have a distribution limited to extracellular fluid, ie, "water-soluble" drugs, include the β-lactams, fosfomycin, aminoglycosides, and some members of the sulfonamides and tetracyclines. Lipid-soluble drugs distribute to total body water and include the fluoroquinolones, macrolides, clindamycin, many sulfonamides, and doxycycline or minocycline. In general, drugs that are water soluble distribute well to extracellular fluid of most organs, but there are exceptions. For example, only ~30% of amoxicillin reaches tracheobronchial secretions, and distribution into sanctuaries is limited. Doses of such drugs should be increased, particularly for susceptible isolates with MICs approaching the breakpoint. Lipid-soluble drugs, in contrast, distribute to total body water and, therefore, are better able to reach intracellular organisms or infections in sanctuaries. Some drugs are characterized by volumes of distribution that exceed 1 L/kg, indicating the drug accumulates or becomes trapped at some sites. Few antimicrobials appear to be tightly bound to plasma proteins. Exceptions include doxycycline, minocycline, and cefovecin. For cefovecin, its tight binding to circulating albumin accounts for its very long half-life. Several antimicrobials undergo hepatic metabolism, with some drugs (eg, ceftiofur, enrofloxacin) metabolized to an active metabolite that can contribute substantively to antimicrobial activity. Some drugs undergo substantive to exclusive excretion in the bile, including the macrolides, minocycline (and some of doxycycline), and clindamycin. For such drugs, care must be taken in those species that have a GI microflora subject to antimicrobial disruption; use for urinary tract infections should be avoided. Many drugs are excreted renally and subsequently concentrated in the urine, including β-lactams, aminoglycosides, most fluoroquinolones, and several tetracyclines.

Adverse Effects and Toxicity

Toxicity is associated with harm in the animal and thus is discriminated from adverse effects, although such effects are rarely life threatening. Because bacteria are prokaryotic, most antimicrobials do not interact with eukaryotic host targets. As such, mechanisms of antimicrobial toxicity are generally not related to mechanisms of antibacterial action. An exception is drugs that target microbial cell membranes (polymixins), the use of which is generally limited to topical administration. Additionally, mammalian mitochondrial topoisomerases are subject to damage by fluorinated quinolones, resulting in a diversity of adverse effects. Drugs that disrupt microbial flora may be lethal to some species, particularly hindgut fermenters (horses, rabbits). The release of endotoxin when treating a large, gram-negative inoculum may be problematic for some drugs (especially penicillins), particularly in horses. Several classes of antimicrobials exhibit toxicity unrelated to their (known) mechanism of action. For example, the aminoglycosides are nephrotoxic because they are actively accumulated in and eventually disrupt renal tubular cells, and selected fluoroquinolones cause retinal degeneration in cats due to phototoxicity in the retina. Chloramphenicol is associated with irreversible bone marrow suppression in people, because it is converted to a toxic metabolite. Drug interactions might contribute to some adverse effects as well. For example, chloramphenicol is a marked inhibitor of drug-metabolizing enzymes, and its use with potentially toxic drugs metabolized by the liver should be avoided. Selected fluoroquinolones inhibit selected drug-metabolizing enzymes. Macrolides as a class may compete for both P-glycoprotein and thus impact all aspects of drug movement, as well as inhibit some drug-metabolizing enzymes.

Virulence and Resistance

Antimicrobial resistance is a common reason for therapeutic failure. Resistance is a natural response to exposure to toxins, including antimicrobials. However, although resistance is not desirable in an infecting pathogen, resistance by itself, including multidrug resistance (MDR), is not the problem. Rather, it is the virulent organism that causes harm to the animal. Acquisition of virulence factors or genes necessary for survival in a hostile environment is responsible for illness. A virulent, MDR organism is particularly problematic.

Bacterial resistance to drugs can be either inherent or acquired. Genes coding inherent resistance are present in all strains of an organism, with expression independent of antimicrobial exposure. The "spectrum" of antimicrobial drugs reflects inherent resistance. For example, bacterial wall–defective variants (such as L-forms, spheroblasts, and protoplasts) are resistant to cell-wall inhibitors. Conversely, cell-wall access to some drugs is prevented because of impermeability reflecting very small porins in selected gram-negative bacteria (eg, *Pseudomonas aeruginosa*).

In contrast to inherent resistance, acquired resistance occurs only in selected strains of an organism, usually emerging in response to exposure to an antimicrobial. Genes for resistance can be acquired either spontaneously due to mutations or through sharing of genetic material via plasmids or transposons. Mutations most commonly occur by chance, with the likelihood that at least one CFU in any given population being resistant to any chosen drug increasing as the population reaches 10^7 CFU. Because the mutation is transmitted to daughter cells, it will remain in the population genome ("vertical" resistance). Selection pressure causes less susceptible isolates to succumb to the drug, resulting in a residual population that expresses resistance to the drug even though exposure has been discontinued. However, with time, mutated bacteria, which are often physiologically impaired, also will disappear. Generally, mutations confer resistance only to the drug or drug class, and mutated cells may be less virulent. There are exceptions, with fluorinated quinolones being an example of a mutation that emerges in the presence of the drug and targets multiple drugs. This reflects their MOA, which results in damaged DNA. Subsequent mutations include those that alter regulators of efflux pumps. A marked increase in efflux activity results in MDR.

Acquired resistance also can be shared horizontally by transfer from one organism to another. Such resistance emerges in response to the presence of the drug. Shared resistance occurs rapidly, often during the course of therapy and often resulting in the transmission of multiple genes targeting multiple drugs. Transfer via plasmids is the most recognized mechanism of shared resistance. Plasmids are composed of extrachromosomal DNA, ie, DNA not vital to cell function. Plasmids are replicons, meaning they are capable of replicating autonomously in the host. Multiple mechanisms exist whereby plasmids can enter a bacterial cell.

Transformation, which occurs in only a limited number of bacteria, is accomplished by passage of naked DNA from donor to recipient. Transduction involves transfer via a bacteriophage that inserts itself into recipient bacteria. Phage-mediated transduction occurs in some gram-positive (especially *Staphylococcus aureus*) as well as gram-negative species. The most common method is conjugation in which DNA passes from the donor cell to the recipient via a bridge formed during direct cell-to-cell contact. This is the most sophisticated form of transmission, because the donor must have the necessary surface appendage (sex pilus) to form the bridge that is coded for by a resistance transfer factor on the plasmid. A single CFU may contain multiple plasmids, each of which in turn may carry multiple genes conferring resistance to multiple drugs. Among the disadvantages of plasmid-mediated resistance is the ease of sharing between gram-negative organisms and less commonly between gram-positive organisms; transfer can also occur between gram-positive and gram-negative organisms. Although plasmid-mediated resistance can occur rapidly, plasmids are generally shed by the bacterium once the drug is no longer present.

Among the mechanisms whereby genetic sequences can be transferred between extrachromosomal (plasmid) and chromosomal DNA is the transposon, which is a DNA sequence that can change position in a genome. Transposons can carry chromosomal DNA from one bacterial cell to a plasmid and back. These transpositional sequences may be carried on gene cassettes. Integrons are gene-capturing systems found in plasmids, chromosomes, and transposons. Integrons can carry genes imparting antimicrobial resistance; generally, such resistance impacts multiple drugs. Once incorporated into chromosomal or plasmid DNA, the genes are subsequently expressed or disseminated even further. Problematically, in addition to resistance genes, these cassettes may also include virulence factors. This is exemplified in certain strains of methicillin-resistant *Staphylococcus aureus* (MRSA), which reflects acquisition of the *mec* gene, encoding for a mutated penicillin-binding protein-2, which prevents binding by any β-lactam drug.

Infection by MRSA has transitioned from hospital acquired, occurring only in the immunocompromised, to community acquired because of acquisition of a virulence gene that facilitates infectivity. Acquired resistance primarily reflects three major cellular mechanisms: 1) Intracellular drug concentrations can be reduced. Multiple mechanisms can accomplish this. Drug movement into the microbial cell can be prevented by decreasing porin number or size or, more commonly, by transporting the drug out of the cell through efflux transport pumps located in the cell membrane. These mechanisms result in resistance to multiple drug classes. 2) Microbes can produce enzymes that destroy certain drugs or drug classes. This mechanism generally targets only a single drug class. Examples include β-lactamases and enzymes that target fosfomycin, aminoglycosides, or phenicols. These enzymes can be expressed constitutively, or on exposure to the drug, induced such that expression is increased. In general, the addition of larger R groups on the drug molecule sterically hinders the ability of destructive enzymes from reaching the vulnerable site of the drug molecule. 3) Microbes can acquire mutations that change the target such that it no longer binds to the drug. Examples include mutated penicillin-binding proteins that confer methicillin resistance to staphylococci, mutations in DNA gyrases that confer resistance to fluoroquinolones, or mutations in ribosomal subunits that confer resistance to various ribosomal inhibitors. Mutations also generally cause single-drug resistance.

Other less common methods include the presence of alternative metabolic pathways that circumvent the effect of the drug (eg, sulfonamides) or increased synthesis of a key metabolic intermediate that would thus require higher concentrations of the drug (eg, para-aminobenzoic acid in sulfonamide resistance).

Acquired resistance will be clinically manifested as an increase in the MIC of the isolate to the drug in question. Notably, resistance can emerge in an isolate that yet remains susceptible if the increase in MIC has not exceeded the MIC breakpoints determined for that drug. For recurrent infections, identifying the underlying cause is likely to be paramount to avoiding antimicrobial resistance, including MDR. Among the clinically relevant gram-negative isolates developing MDR are *E coli* and *Klebsiella*. Gram-positive organisms developing MDR include MRSA and its canine and feline counterpart, methicillin-resistant *S pseudintermedius* (MRSI). Enterococcus is another gram-positive isolate for which MDR is both natural and emerging. *Clostridium difficile* is an example of an obligate anaerobic organism for which MDR is clinically important.

Antimicrobial Resistance and the Veterinarian: Two major aspects of antimicrobial use are of particular concern to veterinarians: the likelihood of causing a pathogenic organism to become resistant to current antimicrobial therapy and the likelihood of commensal organisms, regardless of location in the body, becoming resistant to future antimicrobial therapy. Although designing the dosing regimen such that all infecting organisms are killed will minimize the risk of acquired resistance in the patient, any and all antimicrobial use contributes to global concerns regarding antimicrobial resistance. Historically, veterinary use of antimicrobials has focused on agricultural (eg, food-animal) applications. Yet, the concern is shifting to also include use in companion animals, particularly with greater awareness of the risk of transfer of resistant commensal organisms between pets and people.

The role of antimicrobial therapy in the advent of antimicrobial resistance is well recognized. Minimizing the risk of emerging resistance might be approached based on following the "3 Ds": decontamination, de-escalation, and designing a dosing regimen.

Decontamination decreases the spread of potentially resistant microbes and includes attentiveness to hygiene not only in the hospital but also in the home environment.

De-escalation includes avoiding inappropriate or unnecessary systemic antimicrobial use. For example, the use of low levels of antibiotics (as in animal feeds) or improper dosing regimens may lead to a high incidence of acquired resistance in a given population; as such, this practice increasingly is coming under critical scrutiny. Identifying the need to treat with systemic antimicrobials is among the most important questions to be addressed. Clinical signs consistent with infection (fever, inflammation, pain, neutrophilia) are not diagnostic of infection. The presence of bacteria does not necessarily indicate that systemic antimicrobial therapy is indicated. Bacteria may reflect normal flora, which must be distinguished from pathogenic microbes. If in a culture, this may reflect a poorly collected sample. Single rather than multiple (three or more) organisms is more indicative of a pathogen. The extent of growth may be used to support infection; for example, the presence of bacteria in urine collected by cystocentesis is not considered an infection unless >1,000–100,000 CFUs are present. Presence of infection alone does not justify systemic treatment with antimicrobials. For example, despite approval of antimicrobials to treat feline abscesses, most might be better managed by local treatment. Asymptomatic bacteriuria might be more wisely not treated with systemic antimicrobials until clinical signs become evident; nonvirulent organisms may be acting as commensals, preventing infection with more virulent pathogens. The use of topical therapy should be considered when possible; not only can much higher concentrations be achieved at the site of infection, the systemic impact of antimicrobials on microbiota can be minimized.

De-escalation might also reflect shorter duration of therapy. Identifying the most appropriate duration can be problematic. Short-term therapy at high doses and short intervals should be sufficient to kill the infecting microbe, negating the need for longer duration therapy at lower concentrations or shorter intervals that might facilitate resistance. However, for slower growing organisms or nonhealing tissues, longer durations might be prudent. The longterm use of antimicrobials for infections associated with an underlying cause is particularly problematic. Resistance is more likely in these animals, particularly if dosing regimens are (inadvertently) designed for promotion rather than for avoidance of resistance. Data are just beginning to emerge in veterinary medicine indicating that shorter duration of appropriately designed dosing regimens can be just as effective as longer-term therapy.

De-escalation also might be accomplished by initiating therapy with a higher-tier drug and switching to a lower-tier drug as soon as possible. Reasons that an antimicrobial might be considered a higher-tier drug, with use supported by culture and susceptibility data, versus a lower-tier drug, which might be used empirically, include the following: spectrum, with more narrow-spectrum drugs being reserved for problematic infection (eg, aminoglycosides and gram-negative infections, vancomycin and MRSA), safety, mechanisms of resistance that will emerge should therapy fail (eg, drugs causing emergence of extended-spectrum β-lactamases or MDR), and importance to human health (eg, vancomycin, linezolids, fosfomycin, etc).

Designing the dosing regimen should be approached such that the entire infecting inoculum is killed by the chosen antimicrobial. It may be among the most difficult "D" to implement, because it requires not only understanding the relationship between plasma or tissue drug concentrations and the MIC of the infecting microbe but also being willing to modify routine recommended dosing regimens as needed for individual patients. This requires delineation of host, microbial, and drug factors that might impact antimicrobial therapy, either negatively or positively. Even if a microbe is historically considered "susceptible," the amount of drug required to effectively inhibit its growth is likely to be greater now than it was when the drug was originally approved. Successful treatment of infection (ie, resolution of clinical signs) does not avoid the advent of resistance. In healthy, immunocompetent animals, adequate reduction of pathogen inoculum might be sufficient for the host to overcome residual microbial growth, whereas in an animal at risk, this residual growth may emerge as a resistant population after an initial response. The more "at risk" the animal is in being unable to overcome a residual resistant inoculum, the more important that dosing regimens be designed to kill the microbes. "Dead bugs don't mutate" should be the guiding impetus for antimicrobial use.

Designing appropriate dosing regimens requires the following: 1) The pathogen(s) should be identified and characterized, including antimicrobial susceptibility, so that the drug matches the organism as closely as possible, narrowing the spectrum of drug used. The role of culture and susceptibility testing in selecting the drug and designing the dosing regimen is becoming increasingly important. With notable exceptions, the ability to predict infecting pathogens is limited. Exceptions include respiratory tract infections in food animals, pyoderma in dogs and, with limitations, urinary tract infections in dogs and cats. However, for urinary tract infections, *E coli* is a cause in only 50% of cases. The more complicated the infection, the less likely it is that the infecting pathogen can be predicted. Likewise, even if the correct pathogen is identified, predicting susceptibility in all but the most uncomplicated infections is likely to be limited. This is true both historically and in the individual patient. Even historically "susceptible" organisms are characterized by higher MIC. For example, only 50% of clinical *E coli* collected from dogs or cats are susceptible to amoxicillin. If the animal has previously received antimicrobials, patterns of assumed susceptibility may no longer be relevant for that animal. 2) Once drugs to which the isolates are susceptible are identified, one that is more likely to penetrate the infected tissue should be chosen. This includes taking into consideration host and microbial responses to infection. Often, this requires that the drug be lipid soluble. A variety of host and microbial factors contribute to antimicrobial failure by presenting barriers to drug penetration. Debris (eg, inflammatory materials, necrotic tissue, foreign bodies) and biofilm or reduced blood flow and hypoxia contribute to failure. The organism is intracellular in location and able to avoid detrimental effects by phagocytic cells. Even urinary tract infections may present several barriers. Simply choosing a drug that is renally excreted may not be adequate. Renal function may not be normal, such that urine (and drug) is not concentrated. Bacteria are in the urine and also inside uroepithelial cells. Particularly with chronic infections, the microbes may be protected by biofilm and in a state of quiescence such that they are less susceptible to many antimicrobial drugs.

Other factors must be considered when designing the dosing regimen. Immunocompromise as a result of disease, malnutrition, or concurrent drug therapy, or local immunocompromise caused by invasive procedures may contribute to failure. The more "at risk" the animal is in being unable to overcome a residual resistant inoculum, the more important that dosing regimens be designed to kill the microbes (ie, "dead bugs don't mutate"). Because dosing regimens should be designed to kill, bactericidal drugs should be chosen whenever possible. Bactericidal drugs include β-lactams (penicillins and cephalosporins), fluoroquinolones, aminoglycosides, and potentiated (not single) sulfonamides. Tetracyclines, chloramphenicol, macrolides (eg, azithromycin), and lincosamides (eg, clindamycin) are bacteriostatic. However, the distinction between "cidal" and "static" is based on in vitro conditions and may not reflect what occurs in the animal. In general, however, it is easier to achieve killing concentrations of a bactericidal than of a bacteriostatic drug.

Special Considerations for Food Animal Veterinarians: The use of antibiotics in food animals, including use as growth promotants, contributes to the transfer of resistance genes among bacteria and ultimately from food animals to people. Additionally, contamination of food with resistant pathogenic bacteria during the processing of food is a concern. Carcasses may be contaminated at slaughter and processing, and subsequent improper handling or cooking of the product may lead to infection in people. The development of resistant pathogenic bacteria in poultry treated with fluoroquinolones has been documented. Infection of the human population is of particular concern, because the bacterial resistance created in the animal after veterinary use of a drug or drug class may result in resistance to human drugs of the same class. Whereas the organism developing resistance might be nonpathogenic, transfer of the resistance gene to other bacteria in the human GI tract may result in a pathogenic organism becoming resistant and ultimately in therapeutic failure in people. When selecting drug therapies for food animals, veterinarians must be aware of the potential for resistance. Use of antibacterial drugs should be in the context of a valid veterinarian-client-patient relationship. Selection should be based on all information available (clinical findings, experience, laboratory data, physical examination findings, culture and sensitivity data). Pathogens should be identified, and drugs with the narrowest spectrum of activity with known effectiveness against the pathogen should be used. Client education is important to prevent unnecessary use of antibacterial agents (such as using "leftover" antibacterial drugs to treat a new occurrence of disease), to advise on proper withdrawal guidelines of any prescribed drugs, and to ensure that drugs of the proper classes are administered at proper doses and through appropriate routes.

The Veterinary Feed Directive (VFD): In June 2015, the FDA released the final version of the VFD rule. The VFD amends the Animal Drug Availability Act of 1996 (21 CFR Part 558), and it delineates the FDA's strategy to promote the judicious use of antimicrobials in food animals. A VFD drug (which includes prescription drugs and over-the-counter drugs as a third potential category) is defined as "a drug intended for use in or on animal feed." The drug may be an approved new animal drug. A veterinary feed directive, or order, is the written statement issued by a licensed veterinarian, in the course of practice, that orders the use of the VFD drug, or combination VFD drug, in or on animal feed. A VFD order can only be issued under the supervision of a licensed veterinarian, and issuing veterinarians can only do so within the framework of a valid veterinary-client-patient relationship as defined by the state in which the issuing veterinarian is licensed and practicing (or federal definition in the absence of a state definition of a veterinary-client-patient relationship). The rule describes the federal process to authorize VFD drugs, which must be subject to a new animal drug approval, and to establish an antimicrobial considered medically necessary as a VFD drug. The rule further defines two categories of VFD drugs: category I, which is not associated with a withdrawal time, and category II, which requires some withdrawal time in at least one species in which the product is approved. Mixing of category II medicated feeds requires a medicated feed mill license. Guidelines by the FDA delineate the specific information that should be included on the VFD. These guidelines indicate that extra-label use of a medicated feed is not permitted.

DOSING REGIMENS

The design of a dosing regimen begins with an assessment of the *minimal inhibitory* concentration (MIC) of the antibacterial agent for a particular pathogen. Depending on the antimicrobial, plasma or tissue drug concentrations should either markedly exceed the MIC by 10- to 12-fold (for concentration [sometimes referred to as dose-dependent antimicrobials], such as the aminoglycosides and the fluorinated quinolones) or be above the MIC (T>MIC) for most (50%–75%) of the dosing interval (time-dependent antibiotics, such as cell-wall inhibitors [β-lactams, fosfomycin, vancomycin], sulfonamides, and most "bacteriostatic" drugs). To compensate for drug disposition to tissue sites and the effect of host factors on antibiotics, dosages for most drugs should result in plasma drug concentrations several times higher than the calculated concentration-dependent or time-dependent MIC in the infected tissues or fluids. For dose-dependent drugs, efficacy is enhanced by increasing the dose; for time-dependent drugs, therapeutic efficacy is enhanced by increasing the dose and shortening the dosing interval or by choosing a drug with a long half-life.

In today's infectious disease environment, appropriate design of a dosing regimen should depend not on labeled doses, but rather on access to information regarding the current pharmacodynamics of the infecting microbe (ie, MIC from the pathogen cultured from the patient, or the MIC_{90} of a sample population of the pathogen collected from the target animal) and the pharmacokinetics of that drug in the target species. Appropriate pharmacokinetic parameters on which the dosing regimen should be designed include maximum plasma concentration, or C_{max}, for concentration-dependent drugs, and C_{max} and drug elimination half-life for time-dependent drugs. Supportive information for design of dosing regimens often can be found in the literature. For example, if the MIC of a *Pseudomonas aeruginosa* isolate for amikacin (a concentration-dependent drug) is 4 mcg/mL, the dose should be selected so that peak plasma drug concentrations achieve 40–48 mcg/mL. Ideally, tissue concentrations should be that high as well. As such, the dose should be adjusted further if the drug does not penetrate the tissue well in the presence of marked inflammatory debris. Cephalexin is a time-dependent drug. If *Staphylococcus pseudintermedius* cultured from a skin biopsy in a dog has an MIC of 2 mcg/mL, then the dosing regimen should be selected to assure that drug concentrations are >2 mcg/mL for at least 50%–75% (and ideally 100%) of the dosing interval. The half-life of cephalexin is ~3 hr in dogs. Using data reported in the literature for dogs, an oral dosage of cephalexin at 22 mg/kg will achieve a C_{max} of 25 mcg/mL.

In one half-life, concentrations (mcg/mL) will decline to 12.5; in the second, to 6.25, in the third to 3.125, with concentrations below target by the fourth half-life, or 6 hr. Thus, three elimination half-lives, or 9 hr, can elapse before the target MIC is reached, and the next dose should occur by 9 hr. Shortening the interval is generally more cost-effective than increasing the dose of time-dependent drugs, particularly for drugs with a short half-life—for each half-life to be added to the T>MIC, the dose must be doubled. Amoxicillin (with or without clavulanic acid) has been an extremely popular lower-tier drug used for urinary tract and soft-tissue infections. For the latter, at 10 mg/kg, the drug achieves a concentration of ~5 mcg/mL in plasma. At an MIC of 2 mcg/mL, only one half-life can lapse. The half-life of amoxicillin is only 1–1.5 hr, indicating that dosing should occur every 3 hr. As such, amoxicillin may not be an appropriate choice for soft-tissue infections, and if used, it should be dosed at least every 8 hr, if not more often. However, because it is excreted in the urine, it is a good first choice to treat uncomplicated urinary tract infections, as long as urine is retained in the bladder.

The integration of pharmacokinetics and pharmacodynamics can also be accomplished based on package insert information of more recently approved drugs. For example, for concentration-dependent drugs, the C_{max} should be at least 10 × the MIC_{90} of the target microorganism for that drug. For time-dependent drugs, plasma drug concentrations should be above the MIC_{90} of the infecting microbe for ≥50% of the dosing interval.

REQUIREMENTS FOR SUCCESSFUL ANTIMICROBIAL THERAPY

Clinical Diagnosis: Successful chemotherapy usually requires a specific diagnosis, even though a reasonable preliminary diagnosis is often all that is possible, at least initially. The presence of bacteria requiring systemic therapy should be confirmed as much as possible; fever, inflammation, and leukocytosis are supportive of but not diagnostic for bacterial infection.

Microbiologic Diagnosis: Treatment should be aimed at a specific pathogen whenever feasible. Care must be taken when predicting the infecting pathogen based on historic data, because often such data did not discriminate between commensal and pathogen. The use of cytology should not be overlooked. Examination of a direct smear stained with Wright's or Gram's stain may help to establish the types of pathogens involved (gram-positive or gram-negative rods or cocci) and direct initial antibacterial therapy. However, even if the pathogen is correctly identified, the ability to predict the susceptibility pattern of the infecting pathogen has markedly decreased in recent years. If the animal has not been previously exposed to antimicrobials, it is safer to assume that standard expected susceptibility patterns for first-tier drugs (eg, amoxicillin with or without clavulanic acid for *E coli* or cephalexin for *Staphylococcus pseudintermedius*) may be relevant. However, if exposure to antimicrobials has previously occurred, eg, because of recurrence of the current infection, treatment of a different infection, or even exposure to antimicrobials through another household member, culture and susceptibility testing might be prudent. Under field conditions, culture and susceptibility testing may be difficult to accomplish. Use of an antibiogram, either generated locally for the practice or based on national data, might help identify current susceptibility patterns. Antibiograms reflect current population susceptibility patterns. Package insert data or recent literature may also help select a drug based on population MIC statistics; such data can also be useful for design of dosing regimens. Even in the event of culture submission, empirical antimicrobial therapy may need to be initiated before susceptibility data are received. If susceptibility data indicate the isolate is resistant, therapy should not change if the animal has responded to the chosen drug. Reculture might be important after therapy has been completed. If the animal has not responded, the data collected before treatment may no longer accurately predict the infecting population because the drug may have changed susceptibility patterns.

Culture and Susceptibility Testing: Isolation and characterization of the causative pathogen, susceptibility testing, and determination of the MIC provide a sound foundation from which to select the antimicrobial drug and the dosage regimen. However, culture and susceptibility data are only as good as how the sample was collected, handled, and tested. Samples must be collected without contamination. Free catch urines, swabs from endotracheal tubes, culture of drain tubes, and swabs from the surface of a contaminated wound are all examples of unacceptable culture samples. Swabs are less than ideal; not only is the temptation to collect a contaminated sample greater, but the swab itself can be inhibitory to growth. Whenever possible, a tissue or fluid sample is preferred, with handling of the sample left to the laboratory. Equally important is proper refrigeration. For example, with a reproduction rate as short as 20 min, *E coli* in an unrefrigerated urine sample can rapidly grow from 10^1 to $>10^5$ CFUs, thus transitioning from no infection to infection while overgrowing the true pathogens. The laboratory must also be selected carefully; it should follow guidelines promulgated by the Clinical Laboratory Standards Institute (CLSI), use veterinary rather than human materials, and be directed by a veterinary clinical microbiologist.

Of the culture and susceptibility procedures routinely used by laboratories, tube (or micro) dilution procedures are preferred to agar gel procedures, because they can provide a minimum inhibitory concentration (MIC) of the drug toward an isolate of the infecting organism that has been cultured from the animal. The MIC can be used to not only select the drug but also to design the dosing regimen. Some key points regarding susceptibility testing may facilitate interpretation. The S (susceptible), I (intermediate), or R (resistant) indicator accompanying each MIC is determined by comparing the MIC of the isolate to MIC "breakpoints" determined by CLSI. An isolate with an MIC below the breakpoint established for each drug is considered "S," versus an isolate with an MIC at or above the breakpoint, which is considered "R." Although the actual concentrations tested for all drugs are generally the same, the range tested varies for each drug, as do the breakpoints. For example, for enrofloxacin, tested concentrations generally range from 0.5 to 2 mcg/mL; for amikacin, from 4 to 32 mcg/mL; and for ticarcillin, from 16 to 128 mcg/mL. The current susceptible and resistant CLSI breakpoints (mcg/mL), respectively, established for each drug are <0.5 and >4 for enrofloxacin, and <4 and >64 for amikacin. These breakpoints are followed by any laboratory in the USA that follows CLSI protocols or guidelines. That the concentrations differ for each drug, reflects, in part, the different drug concentrations achieved in plasma (and thus tissues) for each drug when administered at recommended dosing regimens. Because the concentrations tested and achieved in the animal vary for each drug, an MIC of 0.25 mcg/mL for enrofloxacin should not be interpreted as being better than an MIC of 2 mcg/mL for amikacin. The drug to which the isolate is most susceptible to, based on susceptibility data, is the drug with the MIC most below the C_{max} achieved in the animal at the recommended dose. However, this may not necessarily be the best drug to treat the infection, based on other host, microbial, and drug factors. Finally, just because an isolate has been indicated as "S" on a culture report does not mean the isolate has not developed some level of resistance. Rather, particularly for commonly used drugs, MIC for a specific isolate may be approaching the CLSI breakpoint. Therefore, it is still considered "S," despite it having developed some level of resistance. Therefore, doses for antimicrobials ideally should err on the side of higher doses (concentration- or time-dependent drugs) or shorter intervals (time-dependent drugs); the more at risk the animal is for therapy to fail, with development of a recurrent, resistant infection, the more important the design of the dosing regimen.

In addition, data from even appropriately collected samples tested under ideal conditions remain subject to limitations. Testing cannot take into account the impact of distribution to the site of infection, host factors such as inflammation, or microbial factors, including the size of the inoculum. These and other factors may indicate a need to modify the dosing regimen to assure adequate concentrations at the site of infection. Lipid-soluble drugs may become increasingly important as infection becomes more complex. Most antimicrobials are lipid soluble, with the β-lactams (penicillins, cephalosporins) being common exceptions.

COMBINATION THERAPY

Treatment with antimicrobial combinations may be necessary in certain cases. The administration of two or more agents may be beneficial in the following situations: 1) to treat mixed bacterial infections in which the organisms are not susceptible to a common agent, 2) to achieve synergistic antimicrobial activity against particularly resistant strains (eg, *Pseudomonas aeruginosa*), or 3) to reduce the risk of or overcome bacterial resistance. In general, combination therapy is most appropriate with a mixed infection or when an empirical selection must be made in a life-threatening situation.

Additive or synergistic effects are seen when antibacterial agents are used in combination. Prime examples are the combination of clavulanic acid with amoxicillin or ticarcillin (or sulbactam with ampicillin), in which the first agent prevents β-lactamase destruction of the second agent, or the combination of a diaminopyrimidine such as trimethoprim or ormetoprim with a sulfonamide. Antibacterial antagonism may also emerge, sometimes with serious consequences. Generally, bacteriostatic agents act in an additive fashion with one another, whereas bactericidal agents are often synergistic when combined. However, the effects of several bactericidal antibiotics are substantially impaired by simultaneous use of drugs that impair microbial growth or "bacteriostatic" drugs (eg, most ribosomal inhibitors). This is a general guideline only; many exceptions are known, and confounding factors also play a role. Classification of antimicrobials as bactericidal or bacteriostatic can also be misleading, because "bactericidal" drugs can be rendered bacteriostatic if sufficient drug concentrations are not achieved at the site of infection. However, in general, the following common antimicrobials at MIC concentrations are likely to be bactericidal: penicillins, cephalosporins, aminoglycosides, trimethoprim/sulfonamides ("potentiated"), metronidazole, quinolones, rifampin, and glycopeptides. The following antimicrobials at usual concentrations are generally bacteriostatic: tetracyclines, the phenicols (eg, chloramphenicol, florfenicol), macrolides, lincosamides, spectinomycin, and the sulfonamides (nonpotentiated).

Ideally, antimicrobial selection should be based on different mechanisms of action and on complementary spectra of activity. β-Lactams are often selected, because their action may facilitate movement of other drugs through the damaged cell wall into the microbe. Examples of combination therapy for mixed infections include the use of clindamycin, metronidazole, or the semisynthetic penicillins for their anaerobic coverage in combination with aminoglycosides for their gram-negative efficacy. Synergism against certain bacterial pathogens frequently can be achieved with combinations of penicillins or cephalosporins and aminoglycosides. The combined use of trimethoprim with selected sulfonamides or clavulanic acid with other β-lactams are other examples of synergistic effects.

ANTHELMINTICS

Many highly effective and selective anthelmintics are available, but such compounds must be used correctly, judiciously, and with consideration of the parasite/host interaction to obtain a favorable clinical response, accomplish good control, and minimize selection for anthelmintic resistance. Any decrease or increase of the recommended dose rate must always be discouraged. Underdosing is likely to result in lowered efficacy and possibly increased pressure for development of resistance. Overdosing may result in toxicity without necessarily increasing product efficacy.

Most anthelmintics generally have a wide margin of safety, considerable activity against immature (larval) and mature stages of helminths, and a broad spectrum of activity. Nonetheless, the usefulness of any anthelmintic is limited by the intrinsic efficacy of the drug itself, its mechanism of action, its pharmacokinetic properties, characteristics of the host animal (eg, operation of the esophageal groove reflex), and characteristics of the parasite (eg, its location in the body, its degree of hypobiosis, susceptibility of the life stage, or susceptibility to the anthelmintic).

There are several classes of anthelmintics: benzimidazoles and probenzimidazoles, salicylanilides and substituted phenols, imidazothiazoles, tetrahydropyrimidines, organophosphates, macrocyclic lactones and, more recently introduced, the amino-acetonitrile derivatives, the cyclic octadepsipeptides, and the spiroindoles. Although it may be thought that chemotherapeutic control of helminth infections is currently satisfactory, selection for parasite resistance is an increasing concern.

MECHANISMS OF ACTION

Anthelmintics must be selectively toxic to the parasite. This is usually achieved either by inhibiting metabolic processes that are vital to the parasite but not vital to or absent in the host, or by inherent pharmacokinetic properties of the compound that cause the parasite to be exposed to higher concentrations of the anthelmintic than are the host cells. While the precise mode of action of many anthelmintics is not fully understood, the sites of action and biochemical mechanisms of many of them are generally known. Parasitic helminths must maintain an appropriate feeding site, and nematodes and trematodes must actively ingest and move food through their digestive tracts to maintain an appropriate energy state; this and reproductive processes require proper neuromuscular coordination. Parasites must also maintain homeostasis despite host immune reactions. The pharmacologic basis of the treatment for helminths generally involves interference with the integrity of parasite cells, neuromuscular coordination, or protective mechanisms against host immunity, which lead to starvation, paralysis, and expulsion or digestion of the parasite.

Cellular Integrity: Several classes of anthelmintics impair cell structure, integrity, or metabolism: 1) inhibitors of tubulin polymerization—benzimidazoles and probenzimidazoles (which are metabolized in vivo to active benzimidazoles and thus act in the same manner); 2) uncouplers of oxidative phosphorylation—salicylanilides and substituted phenols; and 3) inhibitors of enzymes in the glycolytic pathway—clorsulon.

The benzimidazoles inhibit tubulin polymerization; it is believed that the other observed effects, including inhibition of cellular transport and energy metabolism, are consequences of the depolymerization of microtubules. Inhibition of these secondary events appears to play an essential role in the lethal effect on worms. Benzimidazoles progressively deplete energy reserves and inhibit excretion of waste products and protective factors from parasite cells; therefore, an important factor in their efficacy is prolongation of contact time between drug and parasite. Cross-resistance can exist among all members of this group, because they act on the same receptor protein, β-tubulin, which is altered in resistant organisms such that none of the benzimidazoles can bind to the receptor with high affinity.

Uncoupling of oxidative phosphorylation processes has been demonstrated for the salicylanilides and substituted phenols, which are mainly fasciolicides. These compounds act as protonophores, allowing hydrogen ions to leak through the inner mitochondrial membrane. Although isolated nematode mitochondria are susceptible, many fasciolicides are ineffective against nematodes in vivo, apparently due to a lack of drug uptake. Exceptions are the hematophagous nematodes, eg, *Haemonchus* and *Bunostomum*.

Clorsulon is rapidly absorbed into the bloodstream. When *Fasciola hepatica* ingest it (in plasma and bound to RBCs), they are killed because glycolysis is inhibited and cellular energy production is disrupted.

Neuromuscular Coordination: Interference with this process may occur by inhibiting the breakdown or by mimicking or enhancing the action of neurotransmitters. The result is paralysis of the parasite. Either spastic or flaccid paralysis of an intestinal helminth allows it to be expelled by the normal peristaltic action of the host. Specific categories include drugs that act via a presynaptic latrophilin receptor (emodepside), various nicotinic acetylcholine receptors (agonists: imidazothiazoles, tetrahydropyrimidines; allosteric modulator: monepantel; antagonist: spiroindoles), glutamate-gated chloride channels (avermectins, milbemycins), GABA-gated chloride channels (piperazine), or via inhibition of acetylcholinesterases (coumaphos, naphthalophos).

Organophosphates inhibit many enzymes, especially acetylcholinesterase, by phosphorylating esterification sites. This phosphorylation blocks cholinergic nerve transmission in the parasite, resulting in spastic paralysis. The susceptibility of cholinesterases by host and parasite varies, as does the susceptibility of these different species to organophosphates.

The imidazothiazoles are nicotinic anthelmintics that act as agonists at nicotinic acetylcholine receptors of nematodes. Their anthelmintic activity is mainly attributed to their ganglion-stimulant (cholinomimetic) activity, whereby they stimulate ganglion-like structures in somatic muscle cells of nematodes. This stimulation first results in sustained muscle contractions, followed by a neuromuscular depolarizing blockade resulting in paralysis. Hexamethonium, a ganglionic blocker, inhibits the action of levamisole.

Monepantel, the only commercially available amino-acetonitrile derivative, is a direct agonist of the mptl-1 channel, which is a homomeric channel belonging to the DEG-3 family of nicotinic acetylcholine receptors. Binding of monepantel to the receptor results in a constant, uncontrolled flux of ions and finally in a depolarization of muscle cells, leading to irreversible paralysis of the nematodes. These receptors are unique in that they are found only in nematodes.

Derquantel, a semisynthetic member of the spiroindole class of anthelmintics, is an antagonist of B-subtype nicotinic acetylcholine receptors located at the nematode neuromuscular junction; it inhibits 45-pS channels, leading to a flaccid paralysis of nematodes.

Piperazine acts to block neuromuscular transmission in the parasite by hyperpolarizing the nerve membrane, which leads to flaccid paralysis. It also blocks succinate production by the worm. The parasites, paralyzed and depleted of energy, are expelled by peristalsis.

The macrocyclic lactones act by binding to glutamate-gated chloride channel receptors in nematode and arthropod nerve cells. This causes the channel to open, allowing an influx of chloride ions. Different chloride channel subunits may show variable sensitivity to macrocyclic lactones and different sites of expression, which could account for the paralytic effects of macrocyclic lactones on different neuromuscular systems at different concentrations. The macrocyclic lactones paralyze the pharynx, the body wall, and the uterine muscles of nematodes. Paralysis (flaccid) of body wall muscle may be critical for rapid expulsion, even though paralysis of pharyngeal muscle is more sensitive. As the macrocyclic lactone concentration decreases, motility may be regained, but paralysis of the pharynx and resultant inhibition of feeding may last longer than body muscle paralysis and contribute to worm deaths. None of the macrocyclic lactones are active against cestodes or trematodes, presumably because these parasites do not have a receptor at a glutamate-gated chloride channel.

Emodepside acts presynaptically at the neuromuscular junction, where it attaches to a latrophilin-like receptor. This receptor belongs to the group of so-called G-protein coupled receptors. Stimulation of the latrophilin-like receptor by emodepside activates a signal transduction cascade via Gq-protein and phospholipase C, causing an increase in intracellular calcium and diacylglycerol levels. At the end of the signal transduction cascade, vesicles containing inhibitory neuropeptide fuse with presynaptic membranes. After fusion of these membranes, inhibitory neuropeptides may be released into the synaptic cleft to then stimulate a postsynaptic receptor. Recent findings indicate that a second emodepside target is the calcium-activated potassium channel slo-1. Binding to the latrophilin receptor and the slo-1 ion channel leads to inhibition of pharyngeal pumping, paralysis, and death.

The mode of action of praziquantel is not certain, but it rapidly causes tegumental damage and paralytic muscular contraction of cestodes, followed by their death and expulsion.

PHARMACOKINETICS

After administration, anthelmintics are usually absorbed into the bloodstream and transported to different parts of the body, including the liver, where they may be metabolized and eventually excreted in the feces and urine. The disposition of anthelmintics throughout the body is considerably more complex than can be described by a set of pharmacokinetic parameters in the peripheral circulation. Improved drug performance requires knowledge of drug behavior in the multicompartmental system, including the complex interaction between formulation and route of administration, physicochemical properties of the compound, and physiology of the compartment into which the drug is distributed.

Although many helminth parasites reside in the lumen or close to the mucosa, others live at sites such as the liver and lungs; for action against these, absorption of drug from the GI tract, injection site, or skin is essential. Intestinal parasites come in contact not only with the unabsorbed drug passing through the GI tract but also with the absorbed fraction in the blood as they feed on the intestinal mucosa, and with any that is recycled into the gut. This is an important aspect of efficacy of many of the benzimidazoles.

The pharmacokinetics of an anthelmintic, its rate of metabolism and excretion, and its safety profile determine the length of the withdrawal time; this period can vary among species and can also be affected by route of administration and dose. The usual site of metabolism of anthelmintics is the liver, where oxidation and cleavage reactions commonly occur.

Benzimidazoles and Probenzimidazoles: With a few exceptions, eg, albendazole, oxfendazole, and triclabendazole, only limited amounts of any of the benzimidazoles are absorbed from the GI tract of the host. The limited absorption is probably related to the poor water solubility of these drugs. The little absorption that occurs is generally rapid, 2–7 hr after dosing with flubendazole and 6–30 hr after dosing with albendazole, fenbendazole, and oxfendazole, depending on the species. Many of the benzimidazoles and their metabolites re-enter the GI tract by passive diffusion, but the biliary route is the most important pathway for secretion and recycling of benzimidazoles in the GI tract.

A number of benzimidazoles (eg, febantel, thiophanate, netobimin) exist in the form of prodrugs that must be metabolized in the body to the biologically active benzimidazole carbamate nucleus. Febantel is hydrolyzed to the active metabolite fenbendazole, and netobimin undergoes processes of reduction, cyclization, and oxidation to yield albendazole sulfoxide. Benzimidazole sulfoxides such as oxfendazole and albendazole sulfoxide bind poorly to parasite β-tubulin and probably act as prodrugs for fenbendazole and albendazole, respectively. The thiometabolites have high affinity for helminth tubulin.

Metabolism of the benzimidazoles is variable and may alter their activity; eg, albendazole is rapidly and reversibly oxidized to its sulfoxide form. The sulfoxide may be irreversibly oxidized to its sulfone, which is significantly less active than the sulfoxide. Similarly, fenbendazole and oxfendazole (fenbendazole sulfoxide) are interchangeable, but the oxidation product fenbendazole sulfone is less active and is not reduced back to the sulfoxide or thio metabolites.

In ruminants, the benzimidazoles are most effective if deposited into the rumen. Administration directly into the abomasum, via the esophageal groove, may shorten the duration for drug absorption and increase the rate of excretion in the feces, which may reduce efficacy. For example, immediate arrival of oxfendazole in the abomasum after dosing reduces its efficacy from 91% to 45% against thiabendazole-resistant strains of *Haemonchus contortus*. The rumen acts as a drug reservoir from which plasma concentrations can be sustained, slowing the passage of unabsorbed drug through the GI tract.

Imidazothiazoles: The absorption and excretion of levamisole is rapid and not affected by the route of administration or ruminal bypass, because it is highly soluble. In cattle, blood concentrations of levamisole peak <1 hr after SC administration. These concentrations decline rapidly; 90% of the total dose is excreted in 24 hr, largely in the urine.

Tetrahydropyrimidines: Pyrantel tartrate (or citrate) is well absorbed by pigs and dogs, less well by ruminants. The pamoate salt (synonym embonate) of pyrantel is poorly soluble in water; this offers the advantage of reduced absorption from the gut and allows the drug to reach and be effective against parasites in the large intestine, which makes it useful in horses and dogs. Metabolism of pyrantel is rapid, and the metabolites are excreted rapidly in the urine (40% of the dose in dogs); some unchanged drug is excreted in the feces (principally in ruminants). Blood concentrations usually peak 4–6 hr after PO administration.

Morantel is the methyl ester analogue of pyrantel and, in ruminants, it tends to be safer and more effective than pyrantel. It is absorbed rapidly from the upper small intestine of sheep and metabolized rapidly in the liver; ~17% of the initial dose is excreted in the urine as metabolites within 96 hr after dosing.

Macrocyclic Lactones: Macrocyclic lactones are hydrophobic, an important characteristic of this class of anthelmintics. Regardless of their route of administration, macrocyclic lactones are distributed throughout the body and some concentrate in adipose tissue. Liver tissue contains the highest residue for the longest, reflecting the route of elimination. Although the magnitude of lipophilicity differs among chemical types, the limited vascularization and slow turnover rate of body fat and the slow rate of release or exchange of drug from these lipid reserves can prolong the residence of drug in the peripheral plasma. Ivermectin is arguably the least lipophilic macrocyclic lactone, with the possible exception of eprinomectin. Moxidectin is ~100 times more lipophilic than ivermectin. Doramectin is less lipophilic than moxidectin but more than ivermectin or eprinomectin.

Ivermectin was the first commercially available macrocyclic lactone and has been the most extensively studied. When given IV, ivermectin has an elimination half-life of 32–178 hr, depending on species. Despite the higher dose rate of the injectable formulation in pigs (300 mcg/kg) compared with that of cattle (200 mcg/kg), the maximum concentration (C_{max}) and area under the curve (AUC) in peripheral plasma in pigs are about one-third those in cattle. Although the elimination half-life after SC and IV administration of ivermectin is of similar duration, slow absorption from the injection site may broaden the concentration-time profile, with C_{max} in peripheral plasma of cattle occurring as late as 96 hr. The C_{max} and AUC in pigs and goats are considerably lower than those in cattle, horses, and sheep. Pigs, and possibly goats, may metabolize ivermectin faster than other species.

In ruminants, the macrocyclic lactones are, like benzimidazoles, most effective if deposited directly into the rumen. A 3- to 4-fold decrease in C_{max} and AUC of ivermectin after intra-abomasal compared with intraruminal administration has been reported. Significantly, time to maximal concentration of ivermectin was reduced from 23 hr to 4 hr with the former route of delivery.

Concentrations of ivermectin are high in digesta sampled from the distal intestine, indicating that biliary secretion is an important pathway for clearance of macrocyclic lactones. This pathway also has been conclusively demonstrated for clearance of benzimidazole compounds. The extended high concentration in bile is influenced by prolonged exchange of drug from lipid reserves and the enterohepatic recycling of biliary compounds through the portal and biliary pools. The macrocyclic lactones are primarily excreted in the feces, the remainder (<10%) in the urine. The more lipophilic macrocyclic lactones are also excreted in milk.

Salicylanilides and Substituted Phenols: Secretion via the liver and bile is especially important for drugs active against adult *Fasciola* spp. The fasciolicidal effects of salicylanilides (such as rafoxanide) in sheep depend on persistence of the drug in plasma, which influences their transport throughout the body and rate of elimination. Closantel, rafoxanide, and oxyclozanide have long terminal half-lives in sheep (14.5, 16.6, and 6.4 days, respectively), which are related to the high plasma-protein binding (>99%) of these three drugs. Residues in liver are detectable for weeks after administration. Associated with persistence, however, is the need for longer withholding periods. Oxyclozanide also is bound to plasma protein and then metabolized in the liver to the anthelmintically active glucuronide and excreted in high concentration in the bile duct, where it encounters the mature flukes.

Immature flukes in the liver parenchyma ingest mainly liver cells, which contain little anthelmintic; plasma-protein binding limits entry of the drug into the tissue cells. As the flukes grow and migrate through the liver, they cause extensive hemorrhaging and come into contact with anthelmintic bound to plasma protein. When they reach the bile ducts, they are in the main excretory channels for the active metabolites of the fasciolicides and are exposed to toxic concentrations. This may explain why mature flukes are more vulnerable to most fasciolicides than immature ones. The higher concentrations of fasciolicides and their metabolites in feces than in urine suggest that the bile ducts are their main excretory pathways.

It is important to understand the pharmacokinetics of prescribed anthelmintics. For example, nitroxynil has good efficacy against *F hepatica* in cattle and sheep and against *H contortus*, but because rumen bacteria metabolize and destroy the activity of nitroxynil, it must be injected.

Amino-acetonitrile Derivatives: After PO administration, monepantel is quickly absorbed into the bloodstream and metabolized to a major extent within 4 hr into monepantel sulfone. The sulfone expresses in vitro anthelmintic activity similar to that of the parent molecule and is responsible for the anthelmintic effect in animals, because 95 % of the administered dose is metabolized into the sulfone. The C_{max} of monepantel sulfone was 4 fold-higher compared with that measured for the parent compound. After PO administration in sheep of the recommended dosage of 2.5 mg/kg, the elimination half-life of the sulfone metabolite in plasma was 48.7 hr, with a mean residence time of 79.3 hr. Approximately 27% of the administered dose is excreted through the feces in the form of the sulfone derivative. The remaining amount is further metabolized and partly excreted through urine (up to 30% of the administered dose). In addition to the sulfone, the parent monepantel contributes to the anthelmintic activity against abomasal nematodes, because the concentration of the parent monepantel is considerably higher in the abomasum than in plasma.

Cyclic Octadepsipeptides: Studies in rats have been done to assess the general distribution, metabolism, and excretion patterns of emodepside after PO and IV administration. Bioavailability after PO administration is ~50%. Emodepside is distributed throughout the whole organism, but highest concentrations are found in fat tissues, where it forms a deposit that is slowly released. Emodepside is excreted predominantly via the bile and then eliminated in the feces. Approximately half of the administered dose is excreted within the first 24 hr. The elimination half-life after both PO and IV administration is 39–51 hr. Approximately 45%–56% of the administered dose is excreted unchanged, the rest in the form of inactive metabolites. After topical administration in cats, emodepside is absorbed slowly into the bloodstream. Maximum plasma levels are reached 2–3 days after treatment. Absorption after PO administration in dogs is higher if administered to fed animals.

Spiroindoles: Pharmacokinetics demonstrate that after a single oral administration, maximum concentrations of derquantel were reached at 4.2 hr. The terminal half-life of derquantel was 9.3 hr, and the absolute bioavailability was 56.3%. Metabolism of derquantel is extensive and complex. Derquantel undergoes biotransformation to a large number of metabolites over a short time and, as a result, extensive variation in metabolites has been found in tissues and over time periods.

Praziquantel: Praziquantel is rapidly and almost completely absorbed from the GI tract. After absorption, praziquantel is distributed to all organs; it is believed to re-enter the intestinal lumen via the mucosa and bile in dogs. Praziquantel is rapidly hydroxylated into inactive forms in the liver and secreted in bile. It has a wide safety margin.

WITHHOLDING PERIODS

Most anthelmintics have withholding periods if milk or meat from treated animals is intended for human consumption; the specific requirements for each must be observed. Of the benzimidazoles, thiabendazole is absorbed and excreted most quickly; fenbendazole, oxfendazole, and albendazole are absorbed and excreted over a longer period, which necessitates withholding periods of 8–14 days before slaughtering for meat and 3–5 days before milking for human consumption. Other members of the group have withholding periods between these extremes, but withholding periods are longer for bolus formulations.

A similar relationship between the rate of metabolism and activity against immature parasites also exists with certain fasciolicides. Closantel, rafoxanide, and nitroxynil bind more strongly to blood proteins than does oxyclozanide, and therefore remain in the blood for longer periods. While this greater persistence is associated with greater activity against immature liver flukes, the withholding period for slaughter is also longer: 21–77 days for closantel, rafoxanide, and nitroxynil, compared with 3–14 days for oxyclozanide. The low plasma-protein binding of diamfenetide, coupled with the rapid excretion of its active metabolite, necessitates only a short withdrawal time. Similarly, withholding periods for milk vary widely. Closantel and nitroxynil cannot be used in lactating animals when milk is intended for human consumption, whereas oxyclozanide has a withdrawal time of only 60 hr.

Levamisole and morantel are rapidly excreted; thus, withholding periods for meat are short, and frequently there is no, or only a short, withholding period for milk. However, in some countries, levamisole cannot be used in lactating animals when milk is intended for human consumption.

Ivermectin and doramectin are excreted in milk and are not recommended when milk is intended for human consumption. Commensurate with the long period of activity of macrocyclic lactones, ivermectin, abamectin, doramectin, and moxidectin have significant withholding periods before slaughter (eg, 35 days), which vary with the formulations and local regulations. Residual concentrations of moxidectin in milk after topical administration are below threshold limits, resulting in no milk withholding period in many countries. The chemical structure of the macrocyclic lactone molecule has been manipulated to change the milk partitioning coefficients in lactating dairy animals. For example, only 0.1% of the total dose of eprinumectin is eliminated in the milk, resulting in no withholding period for milk worldwide.

Monepantel has a withdrawal period of 7–14 days for meat and is not approved for use in lactating animals producing milk for human consumption.

In combination with abamectin, derquantel has a withholding period of 14 days for meat and is not approved for use in lactating animals producing milk for human consumption.

SAFETY

Most anthelmintics have wide safety margins, ie, the dosage that can be given to an animal before adverse effects are induced is much higher than the dosage recommended for use. The wide safety margin of benzimidazoles is because of their greater selective affinity for parasitic β-tubulin than for mammalian tissues. Nonetheless, this selective toxicity is not absolute; some toxic effects based on antimitotic activity (teratogenicity or embryotoxicity) can occur in some target species, and some benzimidazoles, depending on the dose rate, are contraindicated in early pregnancy.

The safety index (SI) is not as wide for levamisole (SI = 4–6), nor for most of the chemicals active against liver flukes (SI = 3–6). Mammalian toxicity with levamisole is seen more often than with benzimidazoles, although toxic signs are unusual unless the normal therapeutic dosage is exceeded. Levamisole toxicity in the host animal is largely an extension of its antiparasitic effect, ie, cholinergic-type signs of salivation, muscle tremors, ataxia, urination, defecation, and collapse. In fatal levamisole poisoning, the immediate cause of death is asphyxia due to respiratory failure. Atropine sulfate can alleviate such signs. Levamisole may cause some inflammation at the site of SC injection, but usually this is transient. Toxicity increases if other anticholinergic drugs (eg, organophosphates) are given at the same time.

Because of their low absorption from the gut, tetrahydropyrimidines have a high safety margin. Adverse effects (vomiting in dogs and cats) are rare. Toxicity increases when other cholinergic drugs (eg, levamisole, organophosphates) are used simultaneously.

The margin of safety for organophosphates is generally less than that of the benzimidazoles, and strict attention to dosage is necessary. Generally, their toxicity is additive; thus, concurrent use of other cholinesterase-inhibiting drugs should be avoided. Atropine and 2-PAM are used as antidotes to organophosphate toxicity (*see also* p 3064). Organophosphates also can be hazardous to people. Being lipid soluble, they are readily absorbed through unbroken skin. Sprays, collars, and washes of organophosphates used for small animals can present significant hazards to young infants after ingestion, inhalation, or transcutaneous absorption.

Mammals are generally not adversely affected by macrocyclic lactones. The SI for the macrocyclic lactones is typically wide, but both abamectin and moxidectin are contraindicated in calves and foals <4 mo old, respectively, because of narrow safety margins in these classes of stock. Otherwise, single administration at ~10 times and multiple administration at 3 times the recommended therapeutic dose levels do not have any secondary effects on healthy host animals.

Mammalian safety appears to depend on P-glycoprotein activity in the blood-brain barrier. A P-glycoprotein deficiency in certain animals decreases the ability to pump avermectins, milbemycins, and other drugs across cell membranes. The net effect is an increase in systemic bioavailability, because animals deficient in P-glycoprotein are not able to actively pump the macrocyclic lactones out of the CNS or efficiently process these drugs. This decreases the ability to redistribute, metabolize, and excrete macrocyclic lactones, as well as antineoplastic drugs, opioids, acepromazine, digoxin, and ondansetron, resulting in toxicity with what would be considered normal doses in most animals. There have been cases of CNS depression in cattle breeds (Murray Grey) and in individual dogs of multiple breeds, but these were first recognized in purebred and crossbred Collies. Nervous signs (idiosyncratic reactions), including depression, muscle weakness, blindness, coma, and death, were seen when high doses were administered.

Because salicylanilides, substituted phenols, and aromatic amides are general uncouplers of oxidative phosphorylation, their SIs are lower than those of many other anthelmintics. Nonetheless, they are safe if used as directed. Adverse effects are most commonly seen in animals that are severely stressed, in poor condition nutritionally or metabolically, or have severe parasitic infections. Mild anorexia and unformed feces may be seen after treatment at recommended dosages. High dosages may cause blindness, hyperthermia, convulsions, and death—classic signs of uncoupled phosphorylation.

The amino-acetonitrile derivatives target a nematode-specific receptor that is absent in mammals and other organisms. Because of this specific mode of action, monepantel has a very favorable safety profile. Monepantel has been administered to lambs in doses up to 30 times higher than the recommended dose without any adverse effects. In addition, repeated oral administration of monepantel at three times the recommended dose every 5 days over an entire reproductive cycle was not associated with any treatment-related adverse effects on the reproductive performance of rams or ewes or on the viability of their offspring, and it was systemically very well tolerated.

Emodepside appears to be of low acute toxicity in a variety of laboratory animal species and by a variety of routes. Although overt signs of toxicity include depressed neurologic and respiratory function, they occur only at dose rates far in excess of the recommended therapeutic dose in cats.

Repeated treatment at three times the therapeutic dose was tolerated in pregnant and lactating dams/queens, so adverse effects on reproductive function of the dams and/or kitten health are not anticipated when the product is administered at the recommended treatment dose. Safety in dogs was established only for puppies ≥12 wk old.

The combination of derquantel and abamectin did not result in any adverse clinical effects in ewes and lambs under field conditions, other than a commonly reported, mild, transient coughing.

RESISTANCE

The development of nematode and trematode resistance to various groups of anthelmintics is a major problem. Compared with development of antibiotic resistance in bacteria, resistance to anthelmintics in nematodes has been slower to develop under field conditions. However, resistance is becoming widespread, because relatively few chemically dissimilar groups of anthelmintics have been introduced over the past several decades. Most of the commonly used anthelmintics belong to one of three chemical classes, benzimidazoles, imidazothiazoles, and macrocyclic lactones, within which all individual compounds act in a similar fashion. Thus, resistance to one particular compound may be accompanied by resistance to other members of the group (ie, side-resistance).

In nematodes of small ruminants, and especially in *Haemonchus contortus*, resistance to all classes of broad-spectrum anthelmintics has reached serious levels in many parts of the world. Resistance also has been found in *Trichostrongylus* spp, *Cooperia* spp, and *Teladorsagia* spp in sheep and goats. Reports of multiple resistance to most major classes of anthelmintics are increasing. Recently, resistance to monepantel has occurred in the field (New Zealand) in at least two nematode species (*Teladorsagia circumcincta* and *Trichostrongylus colubriformis*) after being administered on 17 separate occasions to different stock classes and in <2 yr of the product first being used on the farm.

Resistance to benzimidazoles is widespread in cyathostome nematodes of horses. *Parascaris equorum* resistance to macrocyclic lactones (ivermectin and moxidectin) has been reported in many countries. Macrocyclic lactone resistance in cyathostomes is only occasionally suspected, however, and the problem is still not considered to be serious.

There are limited reports of resistance against levamisole, pyrantel, and benzimidazoles in *Oesophogostomum dentatum* in pigs.

Multidrug (benzimidazoles and macrocyclic lactones) resistance in cattle nematodes has been documented on farms in New Zealand, the Americas, and Europe, and this will probably become more widespread. In most cases of resistance against macrocyclic lactones, *Cooperia* spp were identified as the resistant worm species, but macrocyclic lactone resistance is also emerging in *Ostertagia ostertagi*. The full extent of anthelmintic resistance in cattle nematodes is unknown.

The development of significant levels of resistance seems to require successive generations of helminths exposed to the same class of anthelmintic. However, evidence suggests that genes for resistance are invariably present, at a low frequency, for any given anthelmintic. Selection for resistance simply requires the preferential killing of the susceptible parasites and survival of the parasites with the resistance genes. Side-resistance is frequently seen between members of the benzimidazole group because of their similar mechanisms of action; control of benzimidazole-resistant parasites by levamisole can be expected because of its different mode of action. Although there is no evidence for cross-resistance between levamisole and benzimidazoles, this does not mean that worms resistant to both kinds of drugs will not evolve if both types of anthelmintics are used frequently. Nematodes resistant to levamisole are cross-resistant to morantel because of the similarities of their mechanisms of action. When resistance to the recommended dose rate of an avermectin appears in some species of nematodes, a milbemycin, at its recommended dose rate, may still be effective. However, there is side-resistance among the avermectins and the milbemycins, which are within the same class of anthelmintics, and continued use of either subgroup will select for macrocyclic lactone resistance.

Recently, it was demonstrated in *Haemonchus contortus* and *Onchocerca volvulus* that macrocyclic lactone anthelmintics can affect β-tubulin, although no mechanistic explanation for this has been published. However, it suggests that macrocyclic lactone use may select for benzimidazole resistance, because benzimidazole resistance appears to be largely due to a single polymorphism being selected. However, benzimidazole resistance was widely reported before the commercial use of macrocyclic lactones. Ivermectin resistance has usually been reported in areas of the world where benzimidazole resistance is already widespread. In using anthelmintic combinations or rotations, consideration should be given to the genetic interactions in the parasite between benzimidazole and macrocyclic lactone anthelmintics in terms of selection for the alleles that confer benzimidazole resistance.

Every exposure of a target parasite to an anthelmintic exerts some selection pressure for development of resistance. Therefore, management practices designed to reduce exposure to parasites and to minimize the frequency of anthelmintic use should be recommended. The development of an anthelmintic resistance problem may theoretically be delayed by rotating chemicals with different modes of action annually between dosing seasons. Drug combinations may be another appropriate choice, provided the anthelmintics used in the combination are both effective and select for different resistance mechanisms.

In parasite control, economic benefit is best obtained by careful management practices. Planned (or targeted) treatment of a whole flock or herd should be based on the biology, ecology, and epidemiology of the parasite(s), with particular reference to climatic conditions. There is a trend among parasitologists to recommend replacing current practice for worm control involving repeated dosing of whole groups of animals with "targeted selective treatments" in which only individual animals showing clinical signs or reduced productivity are given drugs.

BENZIMIDAZOLES

The benzimidazoles are a large chemical family used to treat nematode and trematode infections in domestic animals. They also have limited activity against cestodes. However, with the widespread development of resistance and the availability of more efficient and easier to administer compounds, their use has decreased in ruminants. They are characterized by a broad spectrum of activity against roundworms (nematodes), an ovicidal effect, and a wide safety margin. Those of interest are mebendazole, flubendazole, fenbendazole, oxfendazole, oxibendazole, albendazole, albendazole sulfoxide, thiabendazole, thiophanate, febantel, netobimin, and triclabendazole. Netobimin, albendazole, and triclabendazole are also active against liver flukes; however, unlike all the other benzimidazoles, triclabendazole has no activity against roundworms. Because most benzimidazoles are sparingly soluble in water, they are generally given PO as a suspension, paste, or bolus, although topical formulations have also been developed. Differences in the rate and extent of absorption from the GI tract depend on such factors as species, dosage, formulation, solubility, and operation of the esophageal groove reflex. Flubendazole and fenbendazole are also available as an oral suspension or emulsion for application through drinking water, for administration to pigs and chickens.

The most effective of the group are those with the longest half-life, such as oxfendazole, fenbendazole, albendazole, and their prodrugs, because they are not rapidly metabolized to inactive products. Effective concentrations are maintained for an extended period in the plasma and gut, which increases efficacy against immature and arrested larvae and adult nematodes, including lungworms.

They are more effective in ruminants and horses, in which their rate of passage is slowed by the rumen or cecum. Because the nature of their antiparasitic action depends on prolongation of contact time, repeated (2–3 times) PO administration of a full dose at 12-hr intervals increases their efficacy, even against benzimidazole-resistant worms. In addition, a reduced feed intake, which reduces the flow rate of digesta, increases the availability of benzimidazoles.

In the case of oxfendazole, and probably other benzimidazoles, the major route of exposure is biliary metabolites, followed by enterohepatic recycling of the drug after absorption from the small and large intestine. Worms in the mucosa of the small intestine may be exposed to more recycled anthelmintic than to drug contained in the passing ingesta in the GI tract.

Ruminants: In ruminants, PO treatment with the benzimidazoles removes most of the major adult GI parasites and many of the larval stages. The relative rates of oxidation in the liver and reduction in the GI tract vary between cattle and sheep, with the metabolism and excretion of benzimidazole compounds being more extensive in cattle than in sheep. Consequently, the systemic anthelmintic activity of most benzimidazoles is greater in sheep than in cattle, and dose rates in cattle are often higher than those in sheep. Albendazole, fenbendazole, oxfendazole, and febantel are active against inhibited fourth-stage larvae of *Ostertagia* spp; however, inconsistent efficacy has been reported. Efficacy against *Dictyocaulus viviparus* has also been noted for these insoluble benzimidazoles. Oxfendazole, albendazole, and febantel are minimally teratogenic in sheep, whereas fenbendazole, mebendazole, and oxibendazole are not. An oxfendazole pulse-release bolus for intraruminal use has been developed for cattle in Europe; five or six therapeutic doses of oxfendazole (750 or 1,250 mg/tablet) are released approximately every 3 wk in the rumen. A sustained-release fenbendazole bolus is also available for cattle in some European countries; it contains 12 g fenbendazole and has a continual release profile of >140 days. An albendazole slow-release capsule has been marketed in Europe and Australasia for small ruminants. This device contains 3.85 g of albendazole and delivers a daily dose of 36.7 mg for 105 days. It is an efficient device to control benzimidazole-susceptible nematodes. It may also prevent infection with benzimidazole-resistant larvae but does not reduce existing infections.

In cattle and sheep, triclabendazole at 10 mg/kg, PO, is highly effective against immature *Fasciola hepatica* in the liver parenchyma and against the mature stage in the bile ducts. Albendazole and netobimin at 20 mg/kg are active against mature *F hepatica*; the other benzimidazoles and probenzimidazoles used for nematode control have only a marginal efficacy against liver flukes. Because of the lack of efficacy against the immature stages, only triclabendazole is indicated for treatment of acute fascioliosis. However, triclabendazole resistance has been reported in several countries. Triclabendazole is not approved for use in ruminants in the USA.

Benzimidazoles also have some anthelmintic activity against *Moniezia* spp in sheep and cattle.

Horses: In horses, the benzimidazoles are characterized by effective removal (90%–100%) of almost all mature strongyles, but third- and fourth-stage larvae are more difficult to eliminate. High levels and repeated administration may be necessary for extra-intestinal migrating stages of large strongyles and for small-strongyle larvae embedded or encysted in the wall of the intestine. However, widespread resistance to benzimidazoles in cyathostome nematodes of horses limits their usage. Repeated doses are thought to be advantageous, because the lethal effect of benzimidazoles is a slow process—hence, their recent incorporation into feed supplements. Ascarid removal in horses varies with various members of the benzimidazole group. Activity against *Strongyloides westeri* varies also, but *Oxyuris equi* is usually removed by any of the benzimidazoles at the recommended dose.

Swine: Benzimidazoles (eg, fenbendazole, flubendazole) show high efficacy against both adult and immature stages of *Ascaris suum*. Benzimidazoles are also highly effective against most other swine nematodes.

Dogs and Cats: In dogs and cats, mebendazole, fenbendazole, febantel, oxfendazole, oxibendazole, and flubendazole are used for treatment of roundworms, hookworms, and tapeworms. However, treatment must be given for 3 days.

Birds: Mebendazole, flubendazole, and fenbendazole can be used effectively against nematodes of the GI and respiratory tracts of birds.

IMIDAZOTHIAZOLES

The anthelmintic activity of tetramisole, a racemic mixture, resides in the L-isomer, levamisole. It is commonly used in cattle, sheep, pigs, goats, and poultry to treat nematode infections; it has no activity against flukes and tapeworms. It is normally administered PO or SC, and efficacy is generally considered equivalent with either route. Topical preparations for cattle have been developed.

Levamisole acts on the roundworm nervous system and is not ovicidal. Its broad spectrum of activity, ease of use (being water soluble), reasonable safety margin, and lack of teratogenic effects have allowed it to be used successfully. Because of its mechanism of action, the peak blood concentration is more relevant to its antiparasitic activity than the duration of concentration. Levamisole resistance appears to be associated with a loss of cholinergic receptors. Levamisole has immunostimulant effects at dosage rates higher than those used for anthelmintic activity, and it has been used in people and to a limited extent in other animals in several diseases.

Ruminants: In ruminants, levamisole (pour-on, injectable, and oral formulations) is highly effective against the common adult GI nematodes and lungworms and many larval stages. It lacks efficacy against arrested larvae, such as those of *Ostertagia ostertagi*. Levamisole slow-release boluses are available in some countries and contain 22.05 mg levamisole. They release 2.5 mg during the first 24 hr and the remainder over a 60-day period.

Swine: Levamisole (injectable and oral formulations) is highly effective against both adult and immatures stages of *Ascaris suum*. Levamisole is also highly effective against other adult swine nematodes, except for *Trichuris suis*.

Dogs: In some countries, levamisole is available as an oral formulation for treatment of *Toxocara canis* infections.

Birds: In poultry, levamisole is mainly used to remove ascarid infections. Because it is water soluble, it is available as an oral formulation for administration through drinking water.

TETRAHYDROPYRIMIDINES

Pyrantel was first introduced as a broad-spectrum anthelmintic against GI nematodes of sheep and has also been used in cattle, horses, dogs, cats, and pigs. It is available as a citrate, tartrate, embonate, or pamoate salt.

Aqueous solutions are subject to isomerization on exposure to light, with a resultant loss in potency; therefore, suspensions should be kept out of direct sunlight. It is not recommended for use in severely debilitated animals because of its levamisole-type pharmacologic action.

Pyrantel is used PO as a suspension, paste, drench, or tablets. Both pyrantel and morantel are effective against adult gut worms and larval stages that dwell in the lumen or on the mucosal surface.

Ruminants: Pyrantel tartrate is effective as a broad-spectrum anthelmintic in ruminants; however, its activity is mainly limited to the adult GI nematodes.

Horses: Pyrantel is effective against adult ascarids, large and small strongyles, and pinworms. At double the recommended dose, it has limited activity against the ileocecal tapeworm *Anoplocephala perfoliata*.

Swine: Pyrantel tartrate is used in swine to treat *Ascaris* and *Oesophagostomum*.

Dogs and Cats: Pyrantel pamoate or embonate is effective against the common GI nematodes, except for whipworms. Oxantel, a phenol analogue of pyrantel, is combined with pyrantel in some anthelmintic preparations for dogs (and people) to increase activity against whipworms.

MACROCYCLIC LACTONES

The macrocyclic lactones (avermectins and milbemycins) are products or chemical derivatives of soil microorganisms belonging to the genus *Streptomyces*. The avermectins in commercial use are ivermectin, abamectin, doramectin, eprinomectin, and selamectin. Commercially available milbemycins are milbemycin oxime and moxidectin. The macrocyclic lactones have a potent, broad antiparasitic spectrum at low dose levels. They are active against many immature nematodes (including hypobiotic larvae) and arthropods. The published literature contains reports of use to treat infections of >300 species of endo- and ectoparasites in a wide range of hosts. Moreover, a single therapeutic dose can persist in concentrations sufficient to be effective against new nematode infections for prolonged periods after treatment.

The macrocyclic lactones are well absorbed when administered PO or parenterally; the pour-on formulations exhibit greater variability. Regardless of the route of administration, macrocyclic lactones are extensively distributed throughout the body and concentrate particularly in adipose tissue. However, the route of administration and formulation may affect the drug pharmacokinetics. The residence time of macrocyclic lactones administered SC may also be influenced by the body condition of the animal.

Effective levels are reached in the GI system, lungs, and skin regardless of the route of administration. There is, however, a very complex interaction between pharmacokinetic compartments and the quantitative and qualitative availability of drug/metabolite in one compartment. For example, the association of macrocyclic lactones with digesta affects absorption; systemic availability and elimination of ivermectin given PO may differ significantly with feed quantity or composition in sheep. Also, the practice of feed withdrawal before PO treatment broadens the pharmacokinetic profile, significantly increasing anthelmintic efficacy.

Environmental Effects

Although there has long been concern over the use of chemical additives in livestock feed (eg, potential consequences of insect-free manure), the effects on nontarget dung insects and dung dispersal primarily became a concern with the macrocyclic lactones. The commercially available macrocyclic lactones are primarily excreted in the feces, and a broad range of insecticidal activities has been observed against dung-inhabiting insect species.

Extensive fate and effects studies have been conducted with the macrocyclic lactones, with most data reported for ivermectin. Ivermectin in feces or soil degrades at a slow but significant rate. In a northern hemisphere winter environment, decomposition is slow (half-life of 91–217 days); when exposed to an outdoor summer environment, ivermectin in soil has a half-life of 7–14 days.

Although macrocyclic lactones are highly toxic to some species of aquatic organisms, their tight soil-binding mitigates against aquatic exposure via run-off or leaching. Macrocyclic lactones have little adverse effect on freshwater algae and virtually none on germination or growth of plants; however, residues in animal feces have the potential to affect arthropod development in a variety of ways. The larvae of cyclorrhaphous Diptera are generally more sensitive to ivermectin and other macrocyclic lactones than are Coleopteran larvae. Mature adult Coleoptera are usually unaffected by macrocyclic lactone residues found in dung, probably because they are exposed to less macrocyclic lactone residue than their bulk-feeding larvae. Overall, the commercially available milbemycins appear to be less harmful to fly and beetle larvae tested than the avermectins. There is no evidence that ivermectin residues exert any direct effect on the development or survival of earthworms; however, effects on other dung-feeding organisms, in particular fly and beetle larvae, may disturb the processes of succession.

Although macrocyclic lactones have the potential to disrupt the ecology of dung fauna if given in persistent formulations or sustained-release devices, there is no evidence for longterm adverse effects of macrocyclic lactone residues on the degradation of dung pats or on the accumulation of dung on pasture. In most husbandry systems, a large proportion of the feces will not contain residues of macrocyclic lactones, thus providing a *large reservoir* of safe habitat for dung insects. Therefore, it is unlikely that use of macrocyclic lactones will have a significant ecotoxicologic impact on a global or regional scale.

Persistent Efficacy

A single therapeutic dose of an avermectin can persist in concentrations sufficient to be effective against susceptible nematode infections for prolonged periods. The clinical significance of prolonged efficacy is important. Sustained availability protects animals from reinfection by some nematode (and arthropod) species for several weeks, which helps control pests that intermittently or constantly challenge livestock. Large variations in the persistent efficacy of a particular macrocyclic lactone against a particular worm species have been reported. Potential reasons for these variable results include study design and host- and parasite-related factors. Persistent efficacy has been investigated mainly against the three major cattle nematodes *Ostertagia ostertagi*, *Cooperia oncophora*, and *Dictyocaulus viviparus*, and the sheep nematodes *Haemonchus contortus* and *Teladorsagia circumcincta*. The duration of persistent efficacy varies according to the macrocyclic lactone and formulation used and may be (excluding specific long-acting formulations) 14–45 days for *Ostertagia*, 0–35 days for *Cooperia*, and 21–42 days for *Dictyocaulus*. The persistent efficacy of oral moxidectin (2–5 wk) gives it a special role in control of haemonchosis and *T circumcincta* in sheep and in resistance development.

Cattle: Ivermectin, eprinomectin, abamectin, doramectin, and moxidectin are variously available as PO, SC, and pour-on formulations for use in cattle. The SC and PO formulations are given at 0.2 mg/kg, whereas the pour-on formulation is used at 0.5 mg/kg. Topical administration (ie, pour-on formulations) is more convenient but results are more variable between animals than when administration is SC or PO. Grooming behavior of cattle has a major influence on the plasma disposition of topical macrocyclic lactones. Undesirable subtherapeutic concentrations in both treated and untreated cattle may contribute to development of drug resistance.

An oil-based, long-acting formulation of ivermectin (3.15% w/v ivermectin) is available in Brazil and most Latin American and African countries. One low-volume SC dose (1 mL/50 kg, equivalent to ivermectin at 630 mcg/kg) effectively treats and prophylactically controls many internal and external parasites of cattle for up to 77 days. A long-acting parenteral formulation for moxidectin has also been developed. The injectable solution (1 mg/kg, SC, behind the ear) is an oil-based formulation containing 10% moxidectin; it is registered in Latin America, Australasia, and some European countries. In controlled studies, the periods of protection against some nematode infections using this long-acting moxidectin formulation were 90–150 days according to the species. Recently, a long-acting injectable formulation of eprinomectin (1 mg/kg, SC, in front of the shoulder) was registered for use in cattle. Treatment provides persistent parasite control for 100–150 days, depending on parasite species.

The macrocyclic lactones have a very high (>98%) efficacy against all stages (including inhibited forms) of the common cattle nematodes. The least susceptible nematodes are *Cooperia* and *Nematodirus* spp. Because of their high potency and elimination through milk, the macrocyclic lactones are not recommended for use in animals that produce milk for human consumption. Eprinomectin and moxidectin pour-ons are exceptions and have no milk withdrawal time in many countries.

A wide range of effective chemoprophylactic systems has been developed to prevent outbreaks of parasitic gastroenteritis and control infections in first-season grazing calves. Strategic anthelmintic medication during the first half of the grazing season, using carefully timed administration of macrocyclic lactones, has proved to be highly effective in western Europe for the control of GI nematodes of grazing calves during their first year. Because of differences in management, pasture infectivity, and climate, it is difficult to identify which program is most effective. Any chemoprophylactic program should be beneficial, as long as it is adapted to the epidemiologic situation and farm management.

Small Ruminants: Ivermectin, doramectin, and moxidectin are variously available as PO, SC, and IM formulations for use in small ruminants. As for cattle, the macrocyclic lactones have a very high (>98%) efficacy against all stages, including inactive forms, of the common sheep and goat nematodes. However, because of management practices leading to selection for resistance to macrocyclic lactones among nematodes of small ruminants, mainly in the southern hemisphere, their use is more problematic (*see* p 2644). Although moxidectin, at its recommended dose rate, can initially be effective against some parasite strains resistant to ivermectin, there is side-resistance between the avermectins and the milbemycins, so this efficacy is temporary. Oral moxidectin has a persistent efficacy of up to 5 wk for *Haemonchus contortus* and *Teladorsagia circumcincta*. Ivermectin controlled-release capsules have been used by sheep producers. The delivery rate, maintained for 100 days, is 0.8 mg ivermectin/day for sheep 20–40 kg in weight and 1.6 mg/day for sheep weighing 41–80 kg.

Swine: In pigs, ivermectin and doramectin are given at 0.3 mg/kg body wt, SC, or ivermectin is given in feed for 7 days at 0.1 mg/kg body wt/day for the treatment of all adult and larval stages of the common swine parasites, including the kidney worm *Stephanurus*. The exception is *Trichuris suis*, in which efficacy is ~80%.

Horses: Ivermectin and moxidectin are the two most common macrocyclic lactones available for use in horses. In certain regions, abamectin is also available. Ivermectin and abamectin are used in horses at a dosage of 200 mcg/kg, whereas moxidectin is used at 400 mcg/kg. Ivermectin, abamectin, and moxidectin are effective against a broad range of adult and migrating larval stages of nematode (including large and small strongyles) and arthropod (*Gasterophilus* spp) parasites. The only reported difference in efficacy of the two products is that at therapeutic dosages, ivermectin has not shown significant efficacy against the arrested stages and intramucosal developing stages of the cyathostomes, and moxidectin appears less potent against stomach bots (*Gasterophilus* spp). The persistence of moxidectin in circulation can provide horses with 2–3 wk of protection from infective cyathostome larvae. Moxidectin and ivermectin may not be the drugs of choice to treat infections with *Parascaris equorum* because of emerging resistance.

Dogs and Cats: Ivermectin, selamectin, moxidectin, and milbemycin oxime may be used in dogs for the prevention of heartworm disease and control of GI roundworms. Many canine parasites are susceptible to ivermectin at the dosages used in other animals; however, because some dogs are adversely affected at these levels, ivermectin is used in dogs at 6 mcg/kg body wt, PO, given at 1-mo intervals, to prevent development of *Dirofilaria immitis*, the cause of heartworm disease. At higher dosages (>100 mcg/kg), some Collies and individual dogs of other breeds are adversely affected by ivermectin. At a dosage of 0.5 mg/kg, PO, milbemycin oxime is used for prevention of heartworm infection and for treatment of hookworms, ascarids, and whipworms in dogs. Moxidectin is also effective for prevention of heartworm infection at a dose rate of 3 mcg/kg, PO. The safety of milbemycin and moxidectin in dogs, including those sensitive to macrocyclic lactones, appears to be similar to that of ivermectin.

Selamectin, an avermectin monosaccharide, and moxidectin are available in topical formulations. Selamectin and moxidectin are also true endectocides at their recommended dosages, because their activity encompasses common intestinal nematodes (eg, *Toxocara*), heartworms, and external parasites (fleas, biting lice, and mites).

Other Species: Ivermectin and other avermectin/milbemycin compounds have been used extensively as antiparasitic agents in a wide variety of exotic pets, including ferrets, rabbits, rodents, birds, and reptiles. Although the activity of these compounds was first established in laboratory animal parasite systems, their use in rodents and other exotic pets is extra-label, and treatment protocols are often established through empirical clinical experience rather than controlled studies.

SALICYLANILIDES, SUBSTITUTED PHENOLS, AND AROMATIC AMIDE

The members of this chemical grouping include salicylanilides (brotianide, clioxanide, closantel, niclosamide, oxyclozanide, rafoxanide), substituted phenols (bithionol, disophenol, hexachlorophene, niclofolan, menichlopholan, nitroxynil), and the aromatic amide diamfenetide (diamphenethide). All members of these groups are active mainly against adult stages of liver flukes. They are used extensively against fasciolosis and haemonchosis in sheep and cattle. Diamfenetide is unique in that it has exceptionally high activity against the youngest immature stages of the liver fluke in sheep, with a diminution of activity as the flukes mature. The lowered efficacy of a number of the salicylanilides and substituted phenols against immature flukes may be due to the high protein binding of these drugs in the blood. A number of these compounds, however, appear to have activity against 6-wk-old flukes in cattle and sheep, by affecting them either at the time of administration or, more likely, by persisting in blood until the flukes start to ingest blood and become exposed to higher drug concentrations. They are all given PO, except nitroxynil, which is typically given SC.

Niclosamide is used PO to treat cestode infections (*Dipylidium caninum* and *Taenia* spp) in dogs.

PRAZIQUANTEL AND EPSIPRANTEL

Praziquantel and epsiprantel are closely related analogues that have high efficacy against cestode parasites at relatively low dose rates but no effect on nematodes.

Praziquantel PO is highly effective against cestodes of ruminants (eg, *Moniezia* spp, *Stilesia*), horses (*Anoplocephala perfoliata*), dogs, cats, and poultry. The PO (5 mg/kg), SC (5.8 mg/kg), or spot-on (cats, 12 mg/kg) administration of praziquantel in dogs and cats is 100% effective against *Dipylidium caninum*, *Taenia* spp, and *Echinococcus* spp (both adult and immature forms). Praziquantel at a dosage of 40 mg/kg is also effective against *Schistosoma* infections in cattle (and people).

Epsiprantel at 5 mg/kg is used specifically to treat the common tapeworms of dogs and cats, including adult *E granulosus*.

AMINO-ACETONITRILE DERIVATIVES

Amino-acetonitrile derivatives are a class of synthetic compounds with high activity against GI nematodes, including isolates resistant to all other commercially available broad-spectrum anthelmintic classes, because of their novel mode of action. Efficacy studies have shown that monepantel (2.5 mg/kg, PO) effectively controls adult and L4 stages of ruminant nematodes, including strains that are resistant or multidrug resistant to the other currently available broad-spectrum anthelmintic classes.

CYCLIC OCTADEPSIPEPTIDES

Emodepside has demonstrated anthelmintic activity in studies conducted in sheep, cattle, horses, and dogs directed against trichostrongyles, roundworms, hookworms, whipworms, large and small strongyles, and lungworms. Emodepside has been shown to possess resistance-breaking properties against certain ivermectin-, benzimidazole-, and levamisole-resistant nematode strains in sheep and an ivermectin-resistant nematode isolate in cattle. Emodepside is currently available in some countries in combination with praziquantel (for treatment of cestode infections) as a topical formulation (3 mg/kg) for the treatment of ascarids and hookworms in cats (including larval stages) and as an oral formulation (1 mg/kg) for the treatment of ascarids, hookworms, and *Trichuris* in dogs (including larval stages). For dogs, emodepside is also available in combination with toltrazuril as an oral suspension for coccidia and GI nematode control.

SPIROINDOLES

Derquantel has been approved as a combination anthelmintic product with abamectin. By adding abamectin to derquantel, the spectrum of parasite species against which this combination exhibits ≥95% efficacy is significantly increased. At the dose rate selected for the combination product, derquantel has excellent anthelmintic activity against the adult and L4 stages of *Trichostrongylus* spp and *Nematodirus* spp and the adult stage of *Haemonchus* spp, and has demonstrated variable efficacy against *Teladorsagia circumcincta* and the L4 stages of *H contortus*.

MISCELLANEOUS ANTHELMINTICS

Piperazine is rapidly absorbed from the GI tract, and piperazine base can be detected in the urine as early as 30 min after administration. The excretion rate is maximal at 1–8 hr, and excretion is practically complete within 24 hr. The spectrum of activity of piperazine is largely against ascarid parasites in all animal species (including people). The safety margin is wide.

Diethylcarbamazine (DEC), a derivative of piperazine, also acts to paralyze nematodes by interfering with nerve function. Historically, DEC was widely used for heartworm prevention in dogs. It was given *daily* PO throughout the mosquito season to prevent patent infections. Before DEC use, dogs must first be cleared of adult heartworms and microfilariae to avoid an often fatal reaction. DEC has also been used to treat prepatent *Dictyocaulus viviparus* infections (*see* LUNGWORM INFECTION, p 1421) in cattle, although it is relatively ineffective against the adult worms. It is routinely given IM at 22 mg/kg body wt for 3 consecutive days, although it is reported that one injection at 44 mg/kg provides better relief of clinical signs.

Clorsulon is a sulfonamide given PO as a suspension for infections with (mainly) adult liver flukes in sheep and cattle and as a SC injection for cattle, in combination with ivermectin. In plasma, clorsulon is bound to protein and, when ingested by liver flukes, inhibits enzymes of the glycolytic pathway. Clorsulon has a wide safety margin and is licensed for use in some countries (eg, Australia, Europe) in lactating dairy cows producing milk for human consumption. It is not licensed in the USA.

Bunamidine is an anticestodal compound. It is used in small animals and is most effective if given after fasting. It is absorbed and metabolized in the liver and leads to digestion of tapeworms in the gut of the host. Vomiting and mild diarrhea may be seen, and exercise or excitement should be avoided in dogs soon after administration.

Nitroscanate, like the substituted phenols, probably acts by uncoupling oxidative phosphorylation. It is used in small animals against *Toxocara*, *Toxascaris*, *Taenia*, *Dipylidium*, *Ancylostoma*, *Uncinaria*, and *Echinococcus* spp. Vomiting occasionally occurs after treatment.

A number of organophosphates have been used as anthelmintics; however, because of their relative toxicity, limited efficacy against immature stages, narrow margin of safety, and contamination of the environment through fecal excretion, their use has declined. Dichlorvos is used as an anthelmintic in horses, pigs, dogs, and cats; trichlorfon in horses against bots, ascarids, and oxyurids; and coumaphos, crufomate, haloxon, and naphthalophos in ruminants. Because of its high volatility, dichlorvos is a particularly versatile organophosphate that can be incorporated as a plasticizer in vinyl resin pellets; it is released slowly from the inert pellets as they pass through the GI tract, providing a therapeutic concentration along the tract. Dichlorvos is particularly useful in pigs against all major adult nematodes and was one of the first broad-spectrum anthelmintics to be used in this species. There is little or no activity against larval migrating nematodes.

COMBINATION ANTHELMINTICS

The principle that combinations of chemotherapeutic agents benefit animals by maintaining drug efficacy in the presence of resistance has been repeatedly demonstrated for diverse pathogens and builds on knowledge gained from insecticide, pesticide, and herbicide use. Also, combinations of anthelmintics are being used more and more. According to the recent guidelines of the World Association for the Advancement of Veterinary Parasitology, there are three main reasons to use fixed-dose combinations of anthelmintics:

1) To cover the desired breadth of spectrum. For example, derquantel (spiroindole class) has been approved for use in some countries as a combination anthelmintic product with abamectin (macrocyclic lactone class). The combination exhibits ≥95% efficacy against a significantly increased spectrum of parasite species.

2) To minimize (delay) the development and spread of resistance to new and existing anthelmintic classes. Mathematical simulation studies have demonstrated that the full benefit of combination anthelmintic product therapy is realized when initial resistance-allele frequencies are low, and that the likelihood of resistance occurring to a combination anthelmintic product will increase with increasing resistance-allele frequency to its individual constituent actives.

3) To overcome existing species-specific resistance profiles. The wide use of anthelmintic combinations, often necessitated by the very high frequency of resistance to one or more available constituent actives when used alone, has revealed no issues of special concern with the routine use of such products.

Three primary areas of concern are apparent with fixed-dose commercial anthelmintic combination products, viz, drug-drug interactions (safety and efficacy implications of pharmacokinetics and pharmacodynamics), common mechanisms of resistance, and best-practice management to ensure appropriate use for sustainability of parasite control with the products.

ANTIBACTERIAL AGENTS

β-LACTAM ANTIBIOTICS

β-Lactam antibiotics, named after the active chemical component of the drug (the 4-membered β-lactam ring), include the 6-membered ring–structured penicillins, monobactams, and carbapenems; and the 7-membered ring–structured cephalosporins and cephamycins. In addition to their chemical structure, the major difference between these two subclasses of β-lactams is their susceptibility to β-lactamase destruction, with the cephalosporins, in general, being more resistant.

Antimicrobial Activity

Mode of Action: β-Lactams impair the development of bacterial cell walls by interfering with transpeptidase enzymes responsible for the formation of the cross-links between peptidoglycan strands. These enzymes are associated with a group of proteins in both gram-positive and gram-negative bacteria called the penicillin-binding proteins (PBPs). At least nine different PBPs comprise the cell wall; different β-lactam antibiotics may target different PBPs, accounting for differences in spectrum and resistance. During bacterial cell growth, while the peptidoglycan structure is being formed, autolysins continually cleave cell wall lattices, in anticipation of providing acceptor sites for new strands of bacterial cell synthesis. Normal bacterial growth depends on a balance between cell wall autolysis and synthesis. The β-lactam drug mimics the PBP substrate, thus inhibiting the PBP and thus cell wall synthesis. In the face of continued autolysin activity, the cell wall becomes deformed. The cell, which is generally hypertonic compared with its environment, is no longer impermeable to the flow of small molecules and is susceptible to osmotic lysis. The effect of the β-lactams when present in sufficient concentrations is generally bactericidal toward most bacteria (an exception is in listeriosis for which penicillins are bacteriostatic and cephalosporins are ineffective). However, at subinhibitory concentrations, β-lactam antibiotics do exert residual effects on bacterial structure and function that, in turn, promote host-mediated cell death.

Some bacterial isolates, when treated with inhibitors of cell-wall synthesis, undergo inhibition of growth but not lysis at usual concentrations. These "tolerant" organisms are defective in their production or use of autolytic enzymes and can survive exposure to β-lactam antibiotics. Clinically, relapses and failures in serious infections due to tolerant organisms may be prevented by the frequently synergistic effect of the aminoglycosides with β-lactam antibiotics. As with other bactericidal drugs, β-lactams are most effective during the log phase of growth. In any bacterial population, a few organisms will always be quiescent. Because the β-lactams are active against only growing bacteria, the static organisms are unaffected and may persist. These "persisters" may then develop normally after the antibiotic is removed.

β-Lactam antibiotics have little influence on formed bacterial cell walls, and even susceptible organisms must be actively multiplying or growing. β-Lactams are most active during the logarithmic phase of bacterial growth. They also tend to be somewhat more active in a slightly acidic environment (pH 5.5–6.5), perhaps because of enhanced membrane penetration. They also are likely to be less effective in the presence of hypertonic tissues.

Efficacy of the β-lactams is related to the time that plasma or tissue drug concentrations exceed the minimum inhibitory concentration (MIC) of the infecting organism (T >MIC). Generally, concentrations should remain above the MIC for approximately 25% (carbapenems) to100% (amoxicillin) of the dosing interval.

Bacterial Resistance: Only microorganisms that have cell walls are susceptible to the action of β-lactam antibiotics. Within this range of bacteria, resistance to β-lactams is well recognized and takes a number of forms.

Permeability Barrier: In gram-positive organisms, capsular materials may hinder access to the cytoplasmic membrane, but this rarely limits the diffusion of the cell-wall inhibitors. Gram-negative bacteria have a restricting sieving mechanism (porins) in their outer membranes (external cell wall), which reduces the penetration of several types of antibiotics. Different species of gram-negative bacteria exhibit varying permeability barriers to β-lactam antibiotics, and these impair access of the antibiotics to the membrane-associated binding proteins. For example, the permeability barrier of *Haemophilus influenzae* is readily crossed by β-lactam antibiotics, *Escherichia coli* presents a greater obstacle to these agents, and the outer membranes of *Pseudomonas aeruginosa* are penetrated with great difficulty by most β-lactam compounds. Penicillins, aminopenicillins, first- and second-generation cephalosporins, and selected other β-lactams cannot penetrate the outer membrane of *P aeruginosa*. In addition, porins are frequently associated with efflux proteins that effectively remove drug that has successfully penetrated the lipopolysaccharide covering of gram-negative organisms.

The chemical nature of β-lactams (penicillins, cephalosporins, and the β-lactamase inhibitors), as well as their concentration gradients, also greatly influence their penetration of bacteria to their targets at the surface of the cytoplasmic membrane, giving rise to the differences between antibacterial spectra of the various classes of penicillin. β-Lactams are often used in combination with other antibiotics that disrupt the integrity of the membranes and thereby facilitate access by β-lactams. The genetic loci controlling permeability generally have been considered to be chromosomally located, but they also may be plasmid-specified genes.

β-Lactamase Resistance: The most important mechanism of bacterial resistance to β-lactam antibiotics is enzymatic inactivation by β-lactamases by cleavage of the 4-member β-lactam ring. Cleavage results in the inability of the drugs to bind to the target PBPs. There currently are >800 different β-lactamases, representing six major classes, with the enzyme varying with the organism and drugs targeted varying with the enzyme. The increase in the number of enzymes reflects, in part, pressure brought with the increasingly widespread use of β-lactams and the continued manipulation of the drugs in an attempt to circumvent bacterial β-lactamase production. For example, the addition of larger R groups on the β-lactam structure rendered cephalosporins to be resistant to penicillinases. However, cephalosporinases emerged with continued use of first-generation cephalosporins. Second- and third-generation cephalosporins reflect modifications, including larger R groups that hindered β-lactamase access to the β-lactam ring. Inhibitors of β-lactamases (clavulanic acid, sulbactam) were added to minimize penicillin destruction. As a result, newer β-lactamases emerged. Approval and use of third-generation cephalosporins have been associated with emergence of extended-spectrum β-lactamases (ESBLs), particularly by *E coli*, *Klebsiella*, and *Proteus*, that target third-generation cephalosporins (but not cephamycins such as cefoxitin). In contrast, carbapenems (imipenem and meropenem) are not subject to ESBLs that target third-generation cephalosporins, but they are subjected to carbapenemases. β-Lactamases do not discriminate among the drugs within class, meaning both human and veterinary drugs will be targeted. Interestingly, clavulanic acid is not susceptible to ESBLs; susceptibility data indicating resistance to cephalosporins but susceptibility to amoxicillin-clavulanic acid indicates ESBL formation.

β-Lactamases are produced by both gram-positive (*Staphylococcus aureus*, *S epidermidis*, *S pseudintermedius* but generally not enterococci) and gram-negative organisms. Some of these enzymes are active exclusively against penicillins, others are principally active against cephalosporins, and several types hydrolyze both equally. The type and concentration of β-lactamases are also specific to bacterial species. Gram-positive β-lactamases generally are excreted into the external environment as exoenzymes, produced in large quantity, plasmid mediated (single determinant), usually inducible (rarely constitutive), unable to initiate self-transmission (rely principally on transduction), and are active primarily against penicillins. Staphylococcal strains are the main gram-positive bacteria in which β-lactamase resistance develops, often very quickly. Gram-negative β-lactamases generally are heterogeneous (wide range), retained within the periplasmic space, produced in small quantity, often constitutive (less often inducible), able to initiate self-transmission (conjugation mechanisms), and active against both penicillins and cephalosporins. The impact of β-lactamase protectors such as clavulanic acid may not be as positive for treatment of gram-negative versus gram-positive organisms. Gram-negative bacteria capable of resistance as a result of β-lactamase production include *Escherichia*, *Haemophilus*, *Klebsiella*, *Pasteurella*, *Proteus*, *Pseudomonas*, and *Salmonella* spp; resistance may take longer to develop in some of these strains.

Specific Bacterial-binding Proteins: Resistance to β-lactam antimicrobial agents can be acquired by alterations in the PBP targets of these drugs. A loss or decrease in affinity of crucial PBP can lead to a significant increase in resistance to β-lactams. For example, resistance of enterococci to cephalosporins appears to reflect the lack of affinity of a PBP to this subclass of drugs. Changes in PBP-2 of *Staphylococcus* spp render the organism resistant to all β-lactams. Methicillin resistance in *Staphylococcus* spp reflects acquisition of the *mec* gene, which results in a mutation in PBP-2. As such, no β-lactam can bind to this protein, resulting in resistance to all β-lactam drugs. Problematically, genes conferring methicillin resistance may be accompanied by genes conferring multidrug resistance.

Cell Wall–deficient Microbes: Organisms that have no cell wall, such as *Mycoplasma*, are intrinsically resistant to β-lactams. A phenotypic form of resistance can occur when spheroplasts (incomplete cell wall) or protoplasts (absence of cell wall) are present. These so-called "L-forms" must be present in a hyperosmotic environment (eg, the renal medulla) to survive; otherwise, they will lyse. The clinical significance of this form of resistance is unclear.

PENICILLINS

The penicillins are among the earliest classes of antibacterial drugs. Penicillins are divided into subclasses based on chemical structure (eg, penicillins, monobactams, and carbapenems), spectrum (narrow, broad, or extended), source (natural, semisynthetic, or synthetic), and susceptibility to β-lactamase destruction. Manipulation of some drugs has improved the spectrum, resistance to β-lactamase destruction, or clinical pharmacologic characteristics that enhance efficacy.

Classes by Spectrum

All penicillins are ineffective toward cell wall–deficient microorganisms such as *Mycoplasma* or *Chlamydia* spp.

Narrow-spectrum β-Lactamase–sensitive Penicillins: This group includes naturally occurring penicillin G (benzylpenicillin) in its various pharmaceutical forms and a few biosynthetic acid-stable penicillins intended for oral use (penicillin V [phenoxymethyl-penicillin] and phenethicillin). Penicillins in this class are active against many gram-positive but only a limited number of gram-negative bacteria. These drugs are also effective against anaerobic organisms. They are, however, susceptible to β-lactamase (penicillinase) hydrolysis.

Penicillin G and its oral congeners (eg, penicillin V) are active against both aerobic and anaerobic gram-positive bacteria and, with a few exceptions (*Haemophilus* and *Neisseria* spp and strains of *Bacteroides* other than *B fragilis*), are inactive against gram-negative organisms at usual concentrations. Organisms usually sensitive in vitro to penicillin G include streptococci, penicillin-sensitive staphylococci, *Trueperella (Arcanobacterium) pyogenes*, *Clostridium* spp, *Erysipelothrix rhusiopathiae*, *Actinomyces bovis*, *Leptospira* Canicola, *Bacillus anthracis*, *Fusiformis nodosus*, and *Nocardia* spp.

Broad-spectrum β-Lactamase–sensitive Penicillins: Penicillins in this class are derived semisynthetically and are active against many gram-positive and gram-negative bacteria. However, they are readily destroyed by the β-lactamases (produced by many bacteria). Many members of the group are acid stable and are administered either PO or parenterally. Of those used in veterinary medicine, aminopenicillins, eg, ampicillin and amoxicillin (which may also be produced naturally), are the best known. Several ampicillin precursors more completely absorbed from the GI tract also belong to this class (eg, hetacillin, pivampicillin, talampicillin).

A large number of gram-positive and gram-negative bacteria (but not β-lactamase–producing strains) are sensitive to the semisynthetic broad-spectrum penicillins (ampicillin and amoxicillin). Susceptible genera include *Staphylococcus*, *Streptococcus*, *Trueperella*, *Clostridium*, *Escherichia*, *Klebsiella*, *Shigella*, *Salmonella*, *Proteus*, and *Pasteurella*. Although bacterial resistance is widespread, the combination of β-lactamase inhibitors and broad-spectrum penicillins markedly enhances the spectrum and efficacy against both gram-positive and gram-negative pathogens. Clavulanate-potentiated amoxicillin is an excellent example of such a synergistic association.

Mecillinam is less active than ampicillin against gram-positive bacteria but is highly active against many intestinal organisms (except *Proteus* spp) that do not produce β-lactamases.

Broad-spectrum β-Lactamase–sensitive Penicillins with Extended Spectra: Several semisynthetic broad-spectrum penicillins are also active against *Pseudomonas aeruginosa*, certain *Proteus* spp, and even strains of *Klebsiella*, *Shigella*, and *Enterobacter* spp in certain cases. Examples of this class include carboxypenicillins (carbenicillin, its acid-stable indanyl ester, and ticarcillin), ureido-penicillins (azlocillin and mezlocillin), and piperazine penicillins (piperacillin).

The anti-*Pseudomonas* and other extended-spectrum penicillins are active against most of the usual penicillin-sensitive bacteria. They often have a degree of β-lactamase resistance and are usually active against one or more characteristic penicillin-resistant organisms. Yet, as a class, they remain susceptible to destruction by β-lactamases. Examples include the use of carbenicillin, ticarcillin, and piperacillin against *P aeruginosa* and several *Proteus* strains, and the use of piperacillin against *P aeruginosa*, several *Shigella* and *Proteus* strains, and some *Citrobacter* and *Enterobacter* spp. *Streptococcus faecalis* is often resistant to these new extended-spectrum penicillins. Imipenem and meropenem are relatively resistant to β-lactamase destruction. Their spectrum includes a wide variety of aerobic and anaerobic microorganisms, including most strains of *Pseudomonas*, streptococci, enterococci, staphylococci, and *Listeria*. Anaerobes, including *Bacteroides fragilis*, are highly susceptible.

β-Lactamase–protected Penicillins: Several naturally occurring and semisynthetic compounds can inhibit many of the β-lactamase enzymes produced by penicillin-resistant bacteria. When used in combination with broad- or extended-spectrum penicillins, there is a notable synergistic effect because the active penicillin is protected from enzymatic hydrolysis—and thus is fully active against a wide variety of previously resistant bacteria. Examples of this chemotherapeutic approach include clavulanate-potentiated amoxicillin and ticarcillin as well as sulbactam-potentiated ampicillin and tazobactam-potentiated piperacillin.

Narrow-spectrum β-Lactamase–resistant Penicillins: This group, through substitution on the penicillin nucleus (6-aminopenicillanic acid), is refractory to a greater or lesser degree to the effects of various β-lactamase enzymes produced by resistant gram-positive organisms, particularly *Staphylococcus aureus*. However, penicillins in this class are not as active against many gram-positive bacteria as penicillin G and are inactive against almost all gram-negative bacteria. Acid-stable members of this group may be given orally and include isoxazolyl penicillins, such as oxacillin, cloxacillin, dicloxacillin, and flucloxacillin. Methicillin and nafcillin are available as parenteral preparations. Temocillin is a semisynthetic penicillin that is β-lactamase stable but also active against nearly all isolates of gram-negative bacteria except *Pseudomonas* spp.

The semisynthetic β-lactamase–resistant penicillins, such as oxacillin, cloxacillin, floxacillin, and nafcillin, have spectra similar to those noted above (although often at higher MIC) but also include many of the β-lactamase–producing strains of staphylococci (especially *S aureus* and *S epidermidis*).

Carbapenems: Imipenem and meropenem are among the most active drugs against a wide variety of bacteria. Imipenem is derived from a compound produced by *Streptomyces cattleya*. Aztreonam is a related (monobactam) compound but differs from other β-lactams in that it has a second ring that is not fused to the β-lactam ring.

General Properties

Structure-activity Relationships: The penicillins, particularly the β-lactam ring, are somewhat unstable, being sensitive to heat, light, extremes in pH, heavy metals, and oxidizing and reducing agents. Also, they often deteriorate in aqueous solution and require reconstitution with a diluent just before injection. Penicillins are poorly soluble, weak organic acids administered parenterally either as suspensions in water or oil or as water-soluble salts. For example, sodium or potassium salts of penicillin G are highly water soluble and are absorbed rapidly from injection sites, whereas organic esters in microsuspension such as procaine penicillin G or benzathine penicillin G are gradually absorbed over 1–3 (or even more) days, respectively. The trihydrate forms of the semisynthetic penicillins have greater aqueous solubility than the parent compounds and are usually preferred for both parenteral and oral use.

The β-lactam nucleus that characterizes penicillins, when cleaved by a β-lactamase enzyme (penicillinase), produces penicilloic acid derivatives that are inactive but may act as the antigenic determinants for penicillin hypersensitivity. Modification of the 6-aminopenicillanic acid nucleus, either by biosynthetic or semisynthetic means, has produced the array of penicillins used clinically. These differ in their antibacterial spectra, pharmacokinetic characteristics, and susceptibility to microbial enzymatic degradation.

Pharmacokinetic Features

The pharmacokinetics of the many penicillins differ substantially. The general guidelines below emphasize singularly significant aspects.

Absorption: Most penicillins in aqueous solution are rapidly absorbed from parenteral sites. Absorption is delayed when the inorganic penicillin salts are suspended in vegetable oil vehicles or when the sparingly soluble repository organic salts (eg, procaine penicillin G and benzathine penicillin G) are administered parenterally. Although prolonged absorption results in longer persistence of plasma and tissue drug concentrations, peak concentrations may not be sufficiently high to be effective against organisms unless MICs are low. The penicillin G repositol salts should never be injected IV. Only selected penicillins are acid stable and can be administered PO at standard doses. Absorption from the upper GI tract differs markedly in amount and rate among the various penicillins. Penicillin V must be given at high oral doses. The aminopenicillins are orally bioavailable, although food impairs the absorption of ampicillin. Paracellular (as opposed to transcellular) transport may play a major role in oral absorption. The indanyl form of carbenicillin is orally bioavailable, but effective concentrations are likely to be achieved only in the urine. Serum concentrations of penicillins generally peak within 2 hr of PO administration. Penicillins may also be absorbed after intrauterine infusion. There is no information regarding bioavailability of human generic products when used off-label in veterinary patients.

Distribution: After absorption, penicillins are widely distributed in body fluids and tissues. The volume of distribution tends to reflect extracellular compartmentalization, although some penicillins (including carbapenems) penetrate tissues quite well. Potentially therapeutic concentrations of the various penicillins are generally found in the liver, bile, kidneys, intestines, muscle, and lungs, but only very low concentrations are found in poorly perfused areas such as the cornea, bronchial secretions, cartilage, and bone. The diethylamino salt of penicillin G produces particularly high concentrations in pulmonary tissue. The penicillins usually do not readily cross the normal blood-brain, placental, mammary, or prostatic barriers unless massive doses are given or inflammation is present. Penicillins may be substrates for P-glycoprotein efflux from the CNS. Selected penicillins are able to penetrate nonchronic abscesses and pleural, peritoneal, or synovial fluids. Penicillins are reversibly and loosely bound to plasma proteins. The extent of this binding varies with particular penicillins and their concentration, eg, ampicillin is usually ~20% bound, and cloxacillin may be ~80% bound. Pregnancy increases the volume of distribution, which has the effect of lowering the concentration of drug produced by a given dose.

Biotransformation: Penicillins are generally excreted unchanged, but fractions of a given dose may undergo metabolic transformations by unknown mechanisms (usually <20% metabolized). Penicilloic acid derivatives that are formed tend to be allergenic.

Excretion: Most (60%–90%) of a parenterally administered penicillin is eliminated in the urine within a short time (eg, up to 90% of penicillin G within 6 hr), which results in high concentrations in urine. Approximately 20% of renal excretion occurs by glomerular filtration and ~80% by active tubular secretion—a process that may be deliberately inhibited (to prolong effective concentrations in the body) by probenecid and other weak organic acids. Anuria may increase the half-life of penicillin G (normally ~30 min) to 10 hr. The biliary route also may be a major excretory pathway for the broad-spectrum semisynthetic penicillins. Clearance is considerably lower in neonates than in adults. Penicillins are also eliminated in milk, although often only in trace amounts in the normal udder, and may persist for up to 90 hr. Penicillin residues in milk also have been found after intrauterine infusion.

Pharmacokinetic Values: Selected pharmacokinetic values for some penicillins in a few species are listed in TABLE 27. Penicillins, in general, have very short elimination half-lives, which is problematic for time-dependent drugs. For example, ~90% of amoxicillin will be eliminated within 4 hr in dogs, suggesting that an 8-hr dosing interval is appropriate. Formulations that prolong absorption after IM administration are appropriate for time-dependent drugs, assuming peak concentrations surpass the MIC of the infecting microbes. Dosage modifications may be necessary because of age or disease. However, the general safety of β-lactams may negate the need for dose adjustment in all but profound renal disease.

Therapeutic Indications and Dose Rates

The penicillins are commonly used to treat or prevent local and systemic infections caused by susceptible bacteria. Several acute infectious disease syndromes are specifically responsive. Because of their synergistic interaction with other antimicrobials, they are often used as part of combination therapy. Penicillins also are used topically in the eye and ear as well as on the skin; intramammary administration is common for treatment or prevention of bovine mastitis. Amoxicillin with or without clavulanic acid is among the first-choice antimicrobials for treatment of canine or feline urinary tract infections.

A selection of general dosages for some penicillins is listed in TABLE 28. The dose rate and frequency should be adjusted as indicated by changes in MICs in target antimicrobial populations, and as necessary

TABLE 27 ELIMINATION, DISTRIBUTION, AND CLEARANCE OF PENICILLINS

Penicillin	Species	Elimination Half-life (min)	Volume of Distribution (mL/kg)	Clearance (mL/kg/min)
Penicillin G	Dogs	30	156	3.6
	Horses	38	301	5.5
Ampicillin	Dogs	48	270	3.9
Amoxicillin	Cattle	84	493	4.0
Ticarcillin	Dogs	48	347	4.9

TABLE 28 DOSAGES OF PENICILLINS

Penicillin	Dosage, Route, and Frequency
Sodium penicillin G	10,000–20,000 IU/kg, IV or IM, qid
Potassium penicillin G	25,000 IU/kg, PO, qid
Procaine penicillin G	10,000–30,000 IU/kg, IM or SC, once to twice daily
Benzathine penicillin G	10,000–40,000 IU/kg, IM (horses) or SC (cattle), every 48–72 hr
Penicillin V	15,000 IU/kg or 8–10 mg/kg, PO, tid-qid
Cloxacillin	10–25 mg/kg, IM or PO, qid
Ampicillin	5–10 mg/kg, IV, IM, or SC, bid-tid; 10–25 mg/kg, PO, bid-qid
Amoxicillin	4–10 mg/kg, IM, once to twice daily; 10–20 mg/kg, PO, bid-qid (dogs)
Sodium carbenicillin	10–20 mg/kg, IV or IM, bid-qid
Potassium clavulanate:amoxicillin (1:4)	10–20 mg/kg (amoxicillin) and 2.5–5 mg/kg (clavulanate), PO, bid-qid
Probenecid (prolongs blood concentrations of penicillins that have short plasma half-lives or that are costly)	1–2 mg/1,000 IU penicillin G (dogs), PO, qid
Amoxicillin-clavulanic acid	10–20 mg/kg, PO, bid-qid
Imepenem	1–7 mg/kg, IV or IM, bid-tid
Meropenem	12–24 mg/kg, IV or SC, bid-tid
Ticarcillin (with or without clavulanic acid)	40–110 mg/kg, IM or IV, tid-qid

to achieve and maintain an appropriate T>MIC for circumstances presented in the individual animal.

Special Clinical Concerns

Adverse Effects and Toxicity: Organ toxicity is rare. Hypersensitivity reactions to penicillin as a hapten reflects, in part, formation of penicillinoic acid. Hypersensitivity (particularly in cattle) includes skin reactions, angioedema, drug fever, serum sickness, vasculitis, eosinophilia, and anaphylaxis. Cross-sensitivity among penicillins is well recognized. Intrathecal administration may result in convulsions. Guinea pigs, chinchillas, birds, snakes, and turtles are sensitive to procaine penicillin. The use of broad-spectrum penicillins may lead to superinfection, and GI disturbances may occur after PO administration of ampicillin. Potassium penicillin G should be administered IV with some caution, especially if hyperkalemia is present. The sodium salt of penicillin G may also contribute to the sodium load in congestive heart failure.

Interactions: Active renal tubular secretion is delayed in the presence of selected organic ions, including salicylates, phenylbutazone, sulfonamides, and other weak acids. Gut-active penicillins potentiate the action of anticoagulants by depressing vitamin K production by gut flora. Absorption of ampicillin is impaired by the presence of food. β-lactams in general interact chemically with the aminoglycosides and should not be mixed in vitro. Ampicillin and penicillin G are incompatible with many other drugs and solutions and should not be mixed.

Effects on Laboratory Tests: Laboratory determinations may be altered, depending on the penicillin used. Alkaline phosphatase, AST, ALT, and eosinophil count may be increased. A false-positive Coombs' test may also result after penicillin therapy. A positive test for urine glucose and protein is also possible. Procaine is detectable in the urine of horses for several days after administration of procaine penicillin; withdrawal time before competition may be up to 6 days.

Drug Withdrawal and Milk Discard Times: Regulatory requirements for withdrawal times for food animals and milk discard times vary among countries. These must be followed carefully to prevent food residues and consequent public health implications. The times listed in TABLE 29 serve only as general guidelines.

CEPHALOSPORINS AND CEPHAMYCINS

The cephalosporins, and the closely related cephamycins, are similar to penicillins in several respects, sharing pharmacologic group features.

Classes and Antibacterial Spectra

Cephalosporins include cephamycins, the latter of which differ from other cephalosporins in that they contain a 7-alpha-methoxy group, which imparts resistance to extended-spectrum β-lactamases.. The early cephalosporins differed mainly with respect to pharmacokinetic characteristics. Whereas penicillins were classified based on source (natural versus semisynthetic) and spectra, cephalosporins are classified by generations (1–4). Later generations are more resistant to β-lactam destruction and are often characterized by extended but variable spectra.

First-generation Cephalosporins: This group includes cephalothin (no longer marketed in the USA), cephaloridine, cephapirin, cefazolin, cephalexin, cephradine, and cefadroxil. Cephalosporins in this group are usually quite active against many gram-positive bacteria but are only moderately active against gram-negative organisms. They are ineffective against enterococci. Susceptible gram-negative bacteria include *Escherichia coli* and *Proteus*, *Klebsiella*, *Salmonella*, *Shigella*, and *Enterobacter* spp. Cefazolin is more effective against *E coli* than cephalexin, the latter of which is minimally susceptible. Although generally less susceptible to β-lactamase destruction than penicillins, they are susceptible to cephalosporinases. They are not as effective against anaerobes as are the penicillins.

Second-generation Cephalosporins: This group includes cefamandole, cefoxitin (a cephamycin), cefotiam, cefachlor, cefuroxime, and ceforanide. These agents are generally active against both gram-positive and gram-negative bacteria. Moreover, they are relatively resistant to β-lactamases compared with first-generation drugs. They are ineffective against enterococci, *Pseudomonas aeruginosa* (with the frequent exception of cefoxitin), *Actinobacter* spp, and many obligate anaerobes (again, cefoxitin is an exception).

Third- and Fourth-generation Cephalosporins: The third-generation cephalosporins include ceftiofur, ceftriaxone, cefsulodin, cefotaxime, cefoperazone, moxalactam (not a true cephalosporin), and

TABLE 29 DRUG WITHDRAWAL AND MILK DISCARD TIMES OF PENICILLINS

Penicillin[a]	Species	Withdrawal Time (days)	Milk Discard Time (days)
Procaine penicillin G	Cattle	10 (at label dosage) 30 (at 20,000 IU/kg, bid)	3
	Sheep	9	
	Pigs	7	
Benzathine penicillin G	Cattle	30	
Ampicillin	Cattle	6	
	Preruminant calves	15	
Amoxicillin	Cattle	30	2

[a] All administered IM

several others, including cefpodoxime and cefovecin, approved for use in dogs and for use in dogs and cats, respectively. Cefepime is a fourth-generation cephalosporin. The spectrum of third- and fourth-generation cephalosporins varies and should be confirmed based on culture and susceptibility testing before use. The spectrum of veterinary third-generation cephalosporins should not be considered extended in that efficacy often does not include *Pseudomonas* or other problematic coliforms. Ceftiofur has been specifically approved for use in cattle with bronchopneumonia, especially if caused by *Mannheimia haemolytica* or *Pasteurella multocida*. Although it is approved for use in dogs to treat urinary tract infections (injectable), other more convenient drugs are generally used. Cefpodoxime and cefovecin are particularly effective against *Staphylococcus pseudintermedius*, while retaining fair efficacy toward gram-negative organisms such as *E coli*, *Klebsiella*, and *Proteus*. Some drugs approved for use in people have only moderate activity against gram-positive bacteria (again, enterococci are resistant) but have extensive activity against a wide variety of gram-negative bacteria, including *Pseudomonas* spp, *Proteus vulgaris*, *Enterobacter* spp, and *Citrobacter* spp (eg, cefotaxime, ceftazidime). Third- and fourth-generation cephalosporins were designed to be increasingly resistant to β-lactamases. However, differences in chemical structure have been overcome by the formation of extended-spectrum β-lactamases that target third- and fourth-generation drugs (but not, as a general rule, cephamycins). Ceftiofur is a third-generation cephalosporin with a gram-negative spectrum that is more similar to that of first-generation cephalosporins.

General Properties

The physical and chemical properties of the cephalosporins are similar to those of the penicillins, although the cephalosporins are somewhat more stable to pH and temperature changes. Cephalosporins are weak acids derived from 7-aminocephalosporanic acid. They are used either as the free base form for PO administration (if acid stable) or as sodium salts in aqueous solution for parenteral delivery (sodium salt of cephalothin contains 2.4 mEq sodium/g). Cephalosporins also contain a β-lactam nucleus susceptible to β-lactamase (cephalosporinase) hydrolysis. These β-lactamases may or may not also target penicillins. Modifications of the 7-aminocephalosporanic acid nucleus and substitutions on the sidechains by semisynthetic means have produced differences among cephalosporins in antibacterial spectra, β-lactamase sensitivities, and pharmacokinetics.

Antimicrobial Activity

Bacterial Resistance: Resistance to the cephalosporins includes mechanisms described in general for β-lactams (*see p 2652*). Cephalosporins generally are stable against the plasmid-mediated β-lactamases produced by gram-positive bacteria such as *Staphylococcus aureus*. Several types of inducible β-lactamases produced by gram-negative organisms may be mediated by either plasmids or chromosomally and may hydrolyze either or both penicillins and cephalosporins (cross-resistance). Second- and particularly third-generation cephalosporins have greater stability against gram-negative β-lactamases. However, third- and fourth-generation drugs are susceptible to extended-spectrum β-lactamases, the presence of which on susceptibility testing is indicated based on resistance to these drugs but susceptibility to clavulanic acid.

Pharmacokinetic Features

Limited information regarding the pharmacokinetics of cephalosporins in animals is available.

Absorption: Only a few cephalosporins are acid stable and thus effective when administered PO (eg, cephalexin, cephradine, cefadroxil, cefpodoxime, and cefachlor). They are usually well absorbed, and bioavailability values are 75%–90%. There is no information regarding bioavailability of human generic products when used off-label in veterinary patients. The others are administered either IV or IM, with plasma concentrations peaking ~30 min after injection. Ceftiofur is available in a sustained-release form; its duration of action is extended by administration at the base of the ear in food animals.

Distribution: Cephalosporins are distributed into most body fluids and tissues, including kidneys, lungs, joints, bone, soft tissues, and the biliary tract, but in general, the volume of distribution is <0.3 L/kg. However, poor penetration into the CSF, even in inflammation, is a notable feature of the standard cephalosporins. Cephalosporins are substrates for

P-glycoprotein efflux from the CNS. The third-generation cephalosporins (eg, moxalactam) may achieve good penetration into the CSF. The degree of plasma-protein binding is variable (eg, 20% for cefadroxil and 80% for cefazolin). The high degree of protein binding of cefovecin (90% dogs, 99% cats) contributes to its long elimination half-life (5.5 days in dogs, 6.9 days in cats). However, drug concentrations in transudate remain above the MIC_{90} of both *Staphylococcus intermedius* and *E coli* for up to 14 days. Third- or fourth-generation cephalosporins are often able to penetrate the blood-brain barrier and are frequently indicated in bacterial meningitis caused by susceptible pathogens.

Biotransformation: Several cephalosporins (such as cephalothin, cephapirin, ceftiofur, cephacetrile, and cefotaxime) are actively deacetylated, primarily in the liver but also in other tissues. The deacetylated derivatives are much less active, with the exception of ceftiofur. Ceftiofur is metabolized to several active metabolites, including an acetylated metabolite, that can contribute significantly to efficacy. Few of the other cephalosporins are metabolized to any appreciable extent.

Excretion: Most cephalosporins, including cefpodoxime and cefovecin, are renally excreted. Tubular secretion predominates, although glomerular filtration is important in some cases (cephalexin and cefazolin). In renal failure, dosages might be reduced, although the need for doing so is not clear. Biliary elimination of the newer cephalosporins (eg, cefoperazone) may be significant. Generally, these β-lactam antibiotics maintain effective blood concentrations for only 6–8 hr. Exceptions include ceftiofur, cefpodoxime, and cefovecin.

Pharmacokinetic Values: Plasma half-lives of cephalosporins are quite variable, being as short as 30–120 min, but generally are longer than those of penicillins. For example, the half-life of the approved cephalexin product in dogs is 7.3 hr (9 hr if given with food). Third-generation cephalosporins tend to have longer plasma half-lives in people, but this is not always the case in other animals—substantial species differences exist. A selection of pharmacokinetic values for cephalosporins is listed in TABLE 30 to serve as a guide. Dosage modifications are often required in hepatic and renal disease.

Therapeutic Indications and Dose Rates

First-generation cephalosporins have proved useful, particularly for infections involving *Staphylococcus* spp (eg, oral cephalexin for dermatitis) and for surgical prophylaxis (eg, cefazolin). However, their efficacy appears to be declining because of emerging resistance, including methicillin-resistant organisms. Ceftiofur is approved for use in a variety of food animals. It is approved for bovine respiratory disease principally caused by *Pasteurella* spp and in urinary tract infections in dogs. Use of ceftiofur for treatment of soft-tissue infections in dogs is not recommended, because proper dosages and safety have not

TABLE 30 ELIMINATION, DISTRIBUTION, AND CLEARANCE OF CEPHALOSPORINS

Cephalosporin	Species	Elimination Half-life (min)	Volume of Distribution (mL/kg)	Clearance (mL/kg/min)
Cefazolin	Horses	45	188	5.5
Cefotaxime	Sheep	25	134	9.0
Cefpodoxime	Dog	300	150	
Cefovecin	Dog	5.5 days	90	
Cephalexin	Dogs	7.3–9 hr	—	—
Cefadroxil	Dogs	120	—	—
	Cats	150–180	—	—
Ceftiofur	Cattle	~360	—	—

been documented. Cefpodoxime (PO) and cefovecin (SC) also have been approved for use in dogs and in dogs and cats, respectively. Cephalosporins are particularly useful to treat infections of soft tissue and bone due to bacteria that are resistant to other commonly used antibiotics. Cefazolin (IV) has been used prophylactically 1 hr before surgery. More than most penicillins, cephalosporins may penetrate tissues and fluids sufficiently (CSF being an exception for most) to be effective in management of osteomyelitis, prostatitis, and arthritis. Oral cephalosporins can be effective in management of urinary tract infections, except those due to *Pseudomonas aeruginosa*. Cephalexin should be anticipated to be ineffective against *E coli*. Cephapirin benzathine is used for dry-cow therapy, and cephapirin sodium is used to treat mastitis. Except for cephapirin, extra-label use of cephalosporins is banned in major food animal species.

A selection of general dosages for some cephalosporins is listed in TABLE 31. The dose rate and frequency should be adjusted as needed for the individual animal.

Special Clinical Concerns

Adverse Effects and Toxicity: The approved cephalosporins are relatively nontoxic. IM injections can be painful, and repeated IV administration may lead to local phlebitis. Nausea, vomiting, and diarrhea may occasionally be seen. Hypersensitivity reactions of several forms have been seen, with cross-reactivity to penicillin allergies possible. Superinfection may arise with the use of cephalosporins, and *Pseudomonas* or *Candida* spp are likely opportunistic pathogens.

Interactions: In vitro incompatibilities are quite common for cephalosporin and cephamycin preparations; an exception exists when mixing with weak bases such as aminoglycosides. Potential pharmacokinetic interactions are similar to those of the penicillin group.

Effects on Laboratory Tests: Several laboratory determinations may be altered by the cephalosporins. Alkaline phosphatase, AST, ALT, lactate dehydrogenase, and BUN may be increased. A false-positive Coombs' test and a false-positive urine glucose may occur. Hypernatremia may be caused by the sodium salts of various cephalosporins.

Drug Withdrawal and Milk Discard Times:

Although prolonged tissue residues for most cephalosporins are not anticipated, withdrawal times are not available for most of the cephalosporins because they are not approved for use in food animals in most countries (*see* TABLE 32). An exception exists for ceftiofur, the withdrawal time of which varies with the product.

AMINOGLYCOSIDES

(Aminocyclitols)

Aminoglycosides are mostly bactericidal drugs that share chemical, antimicrobial, pharmacologic, and toxic characteristics.

Classes

Narrow-spectrum Aminoglycosides: Included in this group are streptomycin and dihydrostreptomycin, which are mainly active against aerobic, gram-negative bacteria.

TABLE 31 DOSAGES OF CEPHALOSPORINS

Cephalosporin[a]	Dosage, Route, and Frequency
Cephalexin	20–60 mg/kg, PO, bid-tid
Cephapirin	30 mg/kg, IM or IV, every 4–6 hr
Cefazolin	20–25 mg/kg, IM or IV, tid-qid
Cefpodoxime	8 mg/kg, SC, every 14 days
Cefovecin	5–10 mg/kg, PO, once to twice daily
Cephalexin	10–30 mg/kg, PO, tid-qid
Cefadroxil	22 mg/kg, PO, bid
Ceftiofur	1.1–2.2 mg/kg/day, IM

[a] All for use in small animals, except ceftiofur, which is for use in cattle.

TABLE 32 DRUG WITHDRAWAL AND MILK DISCARD TIMES OF CEPHALOSPORINS

Cephalosporin	Withdrawal Time	Milk Discard Time
Ceftiofur	2–16 days, depending on formulation	
Sodium cephapirin (intramammary)	4 days before slaughter	4 days
Benzathine cephapirin (dry-cow treatment)	42 days after latest infusion	3 days after calving—milk not used for food

Expanded-spectrum Aminoglycosides: Neomycin, framycetin (neomycin B), paromomycin (aminosidine), and kanamycin have broader spectra than streptomycin that includes many gram-negative aerobic bacteria, as well as synergistic activity toward selected gram-positive organisms. Gentamicin, tobramycin, amikacin (synthesized from kanamycin), sisomicin, and netilmicin are aminoglycosides with extended spectra that include *Pseudomonas aeruginosa*.

Miscellaneous Aminoglycoside Antibiotics: The chemical structure of apramycin differs somewhat from that of the typical aminoglycosides but is similar enough to be included in this class. The structure of spectinomycin is unusual, but it is fairly comparable to other aminocyclitols with regard to its mechanism of action and antibacterial spectrum.

General Properties

Chemically, the aminoglycoside antibiotics are characterized by an aminocyclitol group, with aminosugars attached to the aminocyclitol ring in glycosidic linkage. Because of minor differences in the position of substitutions on the molecules, there may be several forms of a single aminoglycoside. For example, gentamicin is a complex of gentamicins C_1 and C_2, and neomycin is a mixture of neomycins B and C and fradiomycin. The amino groups contribute to the basic nature of this class of antibiotics, and the hydroxyl groups on the sugar moieties contribute to high aqueous solubility and poor lipid solubility. If these hydroxyl groups are removed (eg, tobramycin), antibiotic activity is markedly increased. Differences in the substitutions on the basic ring structures within the various aminoglycosides account for the relatively minor differences in antimicrobial spectra, patterns of resistance, and toxicities. Aminoglycosides are typically quite stable. When the water solubility of an aminoglycoside is marginal, it is usually the sulfate salt that is used for PO or parenteral administration. The pK_as of these drugs are generally between 8 and 10, and as a result, they tend to be ionized at physiologic pH, which may limit drug movement, particularly in acidic environments.

Antimicrobial Activity

Mode of Action: Aminoglycosides are more effective against rapidly multiplying organisms, and they affect and ultimately destroy bacteria by several mechanisms. They need only a short contact with bacteria to kill them and, as such, are concentration dependent in their actions. Their main site of action is the membrane-associated bacterial ribosome through which they interfere with protein synthesis. To reach the ribosome, they must first cross the lipopolysaccharide (LPS) covering (gram-negative organisms), the bacterial cell wall, and finally the cell membrane. Because of the polarity of these compounds, a specialized active transport process is required.

The first concentration-dependent step requires binding of the cationic aminoglycoside to anionic components in the cell membrane. The subsequent steps are energy dependent and involve the transport of the polar, highly charged cationic aminoglycoside across the cytoplasmic membrane, followed by interaction with the ribosomes. The driving force for this transfer is probably the membrane potential. These processes are much more efficient if the energy used is aerobically generated. The efficacy of the aminoglycosides is markedly curtailed in an anaerobic environment. Aminoglycosides are associated with a postantibiotic effect in a number of bacteria, principally gram-negative (eg, *E coli*, *Klebsiella pneumoniae*, *P aeruginosa*).

The effect generally lasts 2–8 hr after exposure and allows for dosing intervals longer than the half-lives of the drugs.

Several features of these mechanisms are of clinical significance: 1) The antibacterial activity of the aminoglycosides depends on an effective concentration of antibiotic outside the cell. 2) Anaerobic bacteria and induced mutants are generally resistant, because they lack appropriate transport systems. 3) With low oxygen tension, as in hypoxic tissues, transfer into bacteria is diminished. 4) Divalent cations (eg, calcium and magnesium) located in the LPS, cell wall, or membrane can interfere with transport into bacteria because they can combine with the specific anionic sites and exclude the cationic aminoglycosides. 5) Passive movement of aminoglycosides across bacterial cell membranes is facilitated by an alkaline pH; a low pH may increase membrane resistance more than 100-fold. 6) Changes in osmolality also can alter the uptake of aminoglycosides. 7) Some aminoglycosides are transported more efficiently than others and thus tend to have greater antibacterial activity. 8) Synergism is common when aminoglycosides and β-lactam antibiotics (penicillins and cephalosporins) are used in combination. The cell-wall injury induced by the β-lactam compounds allows increased uptake of the aminoglycoside by the bacteria because of easier accessibility to the bacterial cell membrane.

The intracellular site of action of the aminoglycosides is the ribosome, which is irreversibly bound by aminoglycosides, particularly at the 30 S but also the 50 S subunits (which comprise the 70 S subunit). Variability occurs between aminoglycosides with respect to their affinity and degree of binding. The number of steps in protein synthesis that are affected also varies. Spectinomycin cannot induce misreading of the mRNA and often is not bactericidal, in contrast to the other bactericidal members. However, at low concentrations, all aminoglycosides may be only bacteriostatic.

A cell-membrane effect also occurs with aminoglycosides. The functional integrity of the bacterial cell membrane is lost during the late phase of the transport process, and high concentrations of aminoglycosides may cause nonspecific membrane toxicity, even to the point of bacterial cell lysis.

Efficacy of aminoglycosides is enhanced if peak plasma or tissue drug concentrations exceed MIC by 10–12 times. Once-daily dosing has been used to enhance both efficacy and safety.

Bacterial Resistance: Several mechanisms of resistance to the aminoglycoside antibiotics have been described. These may be plasmid or chromosomally mediated.

Impaired transport across the cell membrane is an inherent mechanism of nonplasmid-mediated resistance that occurs in anaerobic bacteria (eg, *Bacteroides fragilis* and *Clostridium perfringens*), because the transport process is active and oxygen-dependent. Facultative anaerobes (eg, enterobacteria and *Staphylococcus aureus*) are more resistant to the aminoglycosides when in an anaerobic environment. Impaired transport can be induced by exposure to sublethal concentrations of these antibiotics. Examples include streptomycin resistance among strains of *P aeruginosa*, low-level aminoglycoside resistance among enterococci, and gentamicin resistance in *Streptococcus faecalis*.

Impaired ribosomal binding may not be a clinically important form of single-step resistance, because generally the drugs bind to multiple sites on the ribosomes. Exceptions include *E coli* strains in which a single-step mutation prevents the binding of streptomycin to the ribosome. The same mechanism has been described in *P aeruginosa*.

Enzymatic modification of aminoglycosides may be either plasmid-encoded or chromosomally mediated. Enzymes occur in both gram-negative and gram-positive bacteria. More than 50 enzymes have been identified, with three major types, each including several subclasses: acetylating enzymes (acetyltransferases), adenylating enzymes (nucleotidyltransferases), and phosphorylating enzymes (phosphotransferases). The susceptibility of each aminoglycoside to specific enzymatic attack varies among each subclass. Although cross-resistance is common, there are differences in susceptibility patterns. Chemical modification stabilizes the drug, which decreases susceptibility to enzymatic destruction. For example, chemically modified kanamycin yields amikacin, which is more resistant to enzymatic hydrolysis.

Other mechanisms of resistance include 1) increased concentration of divalent cations (especially Ca^{2+} and Mg^{2+}), which act to repel ionized drug from the microbe, and 2) increased production by *P aeruginosa* mutants of the outer cell membrane protein, H1, resulting in resistance to gentamicin. Note that efficacy will be reduced in the presence of decreased pH (eg, acidic urine or abscesses), which increases resistance to relatively high concentrations of aminoglycosides.

Antibacterial Spectra: Streptomycin and dihydrostreptomycin (no longer available in the USA) are characterized by narrow spectra, and efficacy is limited by bacterial resistance. Gram-negative bacilli are still susceptible, including strains of *Actinomyces bovis*, *Pasteurella* spp, *E coli*, *Salmonella* spp, *Campylobacter fetus*, *Leptospira* spp, and *Brucella* spp. *Mycobacterium tuberculosis* is also sensitive to streptomycin.

The spectra of neomycin, framycetin, and kanamycin are broader, with clinical use targeting gram-negative organisms, including *E coli* and *Salmonella*, *Klebsiella*, *Enterobacter*, *Proteus*, and *Acinetobacter* spp. Aminoglycosides with spectra that include *Pseudomonas aeruginosa* (gentamicin, tobramycin, amikacin, sisomicin, and netilmicin) are also often highly effective against a wide variety of aerobic bacteria. Because of their efficacy against *P aeruginosa*, aminoglycosides might be considered higher-tier drugs. Selected staphylococci are susceptible, but treatment should be based on synergistic effects, ie, combination with other antimicrobials (eg, β-lactams). With such combination therapy, generally low doses of aminoglycosides are used. Because oxygen is necessary for active transport of drug into the microbe, caution is recommended when treating facultative anaerobes in a low-oxygen environment. Obligate anaerobic bacteria and fungi are not appreciably affected; streptococci are usually only moderately sensitive or quite resistant.

Pharmacokinetic Features

The pharmacokinetic features of the aminoglycosides are similar in most species.

Absorption: Aminoglycosides are poorly absorbed (usually <10%) from the healthy GI tract. However, permeability may be increased in the neonate and in the presence of enteritis and other pathologic changes, allowing absorption to be significantly greater. In the presence of renal failure, toxic (trough) concentrations may accumulate. Aminoglycosides can be administered slowly by bolus IV injection or SC or IM routes. Absorption from IM injection sites is rapid and nearly complete (>90% availability), except in severely hypotensive animals. Blood concentrations usually peak within 30–90 min after IM administration. Absorption after SC injection may be protracted. Absorption after IP administration can be rapid and substantial. Short dosing intervals, including continuous infusions, are contraindicated for all aminoglycosides. Once-daily therapy is indicated for safety considerations. Serum concentrations of aminoglycosides may reach bactericidal levels after repeated intrauterine infusion, particularly in endometritis.

Distribution: Aminoglycosides are polar at physiologic pH, limiting distribution to extracellular fluids, with minimal penetration into most tissues. Exceptions include the renal cortex of the kidneys and the endolymph of the inner ear, sites at which aminoglycosides increasingly accumulate as ionization increases. The extracellular fluid compartment normally approximates 25% of body weight, but this volume can change substantially, which leads to indirectly proportional changes in the concentration of an aminoglycoside. For example, extracellular fluid space contracts with dehydration and during gram-negative sepsis, causing concentrations to increase, whereas the distribution volume of aminoglycosides increases with congestive heart failure or ascites, causing concentrations to decrease. Concentrations tend to be lower in neonates, which have a large extracellular fluid compartment relative to body weight. Aminoglycosides are not appreciably bound to plasma proteins (usually <20%). Therapeutic concentrations (~10 times the MIC of the infecting microbe) can be achieved in the synovial, pleural, and even peritoneal fluids, especially if inflammation is present. However, effective concentrations are not reached in CSF, ocular fluids, milk, intestinal fluids, or prostatic secretions. Fetal tissue and amniotic fluid concentrations are very low in most species.

Biotransformation, Excretion, and Pharmacokinetic Values: The aminoglycosides are excreted unchanged in the urine by glomerular filtration, with 80%–90% of administered drug recoverable from the urine within 24 hr of IM administration. A variable fraction of filtered aminoglycoside is absorbed onto the brush border of the proximal tubule and loop of Henle cells. Binding is facilitated by ionization. After binding, the drug is transported into the cell, sequestered in lysosomes. Rupture of lysozymes results in release into the cytosol. Excessive accumulation (mainly in the renal cortex) leads to a characteristic tubular cell necrosis. Glomerular filtration rates differ between species and are often less in neonates, which may explain the greater sensitivity to aminoglycosides in newborn foals and puppies.

Elimination varies with glomerular filtration changes associated with cardiovascular and renal function, age, fever, and several other factors. Half-life also will vary directly and proportionately with the volume of the extracellular fluid compartment. The aminoglycosides have relatively short plasma half-lives (~1 hr in carnivores and 2–3 hr in herbivores). The elimination kinetics often follow a three-compartment model, indicating a "deep" compartment that reflects binding of drug in the renal tubular cell. Approximately 90% of the injected drug, including that within therapeutic concentrations, is excreted unchanged through the kidneys during the β phase of elimination. The remaining deep or γ phase is excreted over a protracted period, probably due to the gradual release of the antibiotic from renal intracellular binding sites (terminal elimination half-life often 20–200 hr). Concentrations in plasma during this phase are generally below what would be considered therapeutic. The limited selection of pharmacokinetic values for two typical aminoglycosides (*see* TABLE 33) serves as a basis for any required dosage modifications that may be necessary because of age or renal insufficiency. The best way to alter a dosage regimen of aminoglycosides is to monitor plasma concentrations to assure that 10 times the MIC is achieved at peak concentrations, and concentrations less than target (generally <2 mcg/mL) are achieved before the next dose ("trough" concentrations).

Therapeutic Indications and Dose Rates

Despite their potential to cause nephrotoxicity, the aminoglycosides are commonly used to control local and systemic infections caused by susceptible aerobic bacteria (generally gram-negative). Several aminoglycosides are used topically in the ears and eyes and via intrauterine infusion to treat endometritis. Aminoglycosides occasionally may be infused into the udder to treat mastitis. In general, because of their concentration dependency and potential for

TABLE 33 ELIMINATION, DISTRIBUTION, AND CLEARANCE OF AMINOGLYCOSIDES

Aminoglycoside	Species	Elimination Half-life (min)	Volume of Distribution (mL/kg)	Clearance (mL/kg/min)
Gentamicin	Dogs	75	335	3.10
	Horses	110	190	1.23
	Foals	200	300	1.04
Amikacin	Dogs	60	300	3.50
	Horses	45	207	0.75
	Sheep	115	200	0.70

TABLE 34 DOSAGES OF AMINOGLYCOSIDES

Aminoglycoside	Dosage, Route, and Frequency
Gentamicin	6–12 mg/kg/day, IM or SC
Kanamycin	25–30 mg/kg/day, IM or SC
Streptomycin/dihydrostreptomycin	15–25 mg/kg/day, IM or SC
Amikacin	15–22 mg/kg/day, IM or SC
Netilmicin	6–12 mg/kg/day, IM or SC
Neomycin	15 mg/kg, PO, once to twice daily
	0.5–1 g/day/quarter (intramammary)

nephrotoxicity, aminoglycosides are administered once daily (same total daily dose; "high" dose), thus minimizing the risk of nephrotoxicity. If used at lower doses for synergistic activity against gram-positive organisms, such as staphylococci, lower doses (30%–50% of the higher dose) might be given at more frequent intervals.

A selection of general dosages for some aminoglycosides is listed in TABLE 34. The dose rate and frequency should be adjusted as needed for the individual animal.

If monitoring, two time points (a peak and a second sample 4 hr later) is ideal such that an extrapolated peak concentration can be determined, along with an elimination half-life. The peak should be collected after distribution into tissues is complete, or ~1 hr. The "trough" in this scenario should be collected 2–3 half-lives later (eg, 4–6 hr after dosing) such that concentrations will still be detectable. If a single sample is collected to determine safety, a trough concentration (just before the next dose) is indicated. Trough concentrations generally should be <2 mcg/mL. For efficacy, a 1.5–2 hr peak concentration might be collected; peak concentrations should be 10–12 times the MIC of the infecting organism. For renal function, both a peak and detectable trough (taken well before the next dose, because concentrations may not otherwise be detectable) are indicated so that a half-life, and, if IV administration is used, clearance might be calculated. As a precaution, the following general guidelines may be followed in cases of renal failure in which plasma creatinine values are increased (*see* TABLE 35).

The treatment interval should be increased in neonates (especially puppies and foals), in renal failure, and in obese animals. Doses may be increased in neonates or pediatric animals, in which the volume of distribution is greater than in adults, and in animals with edema, hydrothorax, or ascites, provided their renal function is unimpaired.

Special Clinical Concerns

Adverse Effects and Toxicity:

Ototoxicity, neuromuscular blockade, and nephrotoxicity are reported most frequently; these effects may vary with the aminoglycoside and dose or interval used, but all members of the group are potentially toxic. Nephrotoxicity is of major concern and may result in renal failure due to acute tubular necrosis with secondary interstitial damage. Aminoglycosides accumulate in proximal tubular epithelial cells, where they are sequestered in lysosomes and interact with ribosomes, mitochondria, and other intracellular constituents to cause cell injury. The greater the ionization (eg, the more the amine groups and the lower the pH), the greater the active uptake. Kidneys must have a drug-free period to eliminate accumulated drugs. As such, persistence of aminoglycosides in plasma and thus urine is likely to predispose the tubular cells to toxicity, and the risk may by reduced by allowing plasma drug concentrations to drop below recommended concentrations (generally 1–2 mcg/mL) before the next dose. Nonoliguric renal failure is the usual observation; it is generally reversible if damage is not sufficiently extensive to harm the basement membrane, although recovery may be prolonged.

Renal function should be monitored during therapy; however, no indicator of renal disease is sufficiently sensitive to prevent continued damage once nephrotoxicity is detected. Polyuria, decreased urine osmolality, enzymuria, proteinuria, cylindruria, and increased fractional sodium excretion are indicative of aminoglycoside nephrotoxicity. Later, BUN and creatinine concentrations may be increased. Early changes or evidence of nephrotoxicity can

TABLE 35 DOSAGE MODIFICATIONS OF AMINOGLYCOSIDES IN RENAL FAILURE

Increase in Normal Serum or Plasma Creatinine (mg/dL)	Dose and Dosage Interval
<1	Full dose at usual dosage interval
2-fold increase	Full dose at usual dosage interval or increased to 50% plus usual dosing interval (eg, 36 hr)
3- to 4-fold increase	Full dose, doubling usual dosage interval
>4-fold increase	Aminoglycosides contraindicated

be detected in 3–5 days, with more overt signs in 7–10 days. Several factors predispose to aminoglycoside nephrotoxicosis, including age (with young [especially the newborn foal] and old animals being sensitive), compromised renal function, total dose, duration of treatment, dehydration and hypovolemia, aciduria, acidosis, hypomagnesemia, severe sepsis or endotoxemia, concurrent administration of furosemide, and exposure to other potential nephrotoxins (eg, methoxyflurane, amphotericin B, cisplatinum, and perhaps some cephalosporins). In renal insufficiency, generally the interval between doses is prolonged (rather than reducing the dose) to minimize toxicity, while avoiding a negative impact on efficacy. Dosing in the morning may decrease toxicity in diurnal animals. The risk of toxicity is less in alkaline urine. Nephroactive drugs, including those that alter renal vascular response (eg, autoregulation) should be avoided or used cautiously (eg, NSAIDs, diuretics). Treatment with *N*-acetylcysteine should be considered (*see* ototoxicity, below).

Aminoglycosides can cause ototoxicity, which may manifest as either auditory or vestibular dysfunction. Binding or damage to mitochondria plays a prominent role in ototoxicity. Vestibular injury leads to nystagmus, incoordination, and loss of the righting reflex. The lesion is often irreversible, although physiologic adaptation can occur. Ototoxicity is not unusual in people, but relevance to veterinary patients is not clear. Cats are particularly sensitive to the toxic vestibular effects, although occurrence at therapeutic concentrations after systemic administration is unlikely. However, aminoglycosides should not be administered topically into the ear unless the tympanic membrane is intact. Hearing impairment reflects permanent damage and loss of the hair cells in the organ of Corti. Loss of high-frequency hearing is followed by deafness, which may not be complete if sufficiently low doses or durations were used. Aminoglycosides should be avoided in working dogs that depend on hearing (eg, guide dogs). Factors increasing the risk of vestibular and cochlear damage are the same as for nephrotoxicity but also include preexisting acoustic or vestibular impairment and concurrent treatment with potentially ototoxic drugs. The ototoxic potential is greatest for gentamicin, sisomicin, and neomycin, and least for netilmicin. In people, treatment with *N*-acetylcysteine has deceased the risk of aminoglycoside ototoxicity.

All aminoglycosides, when administered in doses that result in high plasma concentrations, have been associated with muscle weakness and respiratory arrest attributable to neuromuscular blockade. The effect is more pronounced when aminoglycosides are used with other drugs that cause neuromuscular blockade and with gas anesthetics. Neomycin, kanamycin, amikacin, gentamicin, and tobramycin are listed in order of most to least potent for these neuromuscular effects. The effect is due to the chelation of calcium and competitive inhibition of the prejunctional release of acetylcholine in most instances (there are some differences among aminoglycosides). The blockade is antagonized by calcium gluconate and somewhat less consistently by neostigmine.

CNS disturbances rarely include convulsions or collapse after rapid IV administration. Other adverse effects include superinfection when used topically or PO, a malabsorption syndrome due to attenuation of intestinal villous function when used PO in neonates, occasional hypersensitivity reactions, contact dermatitis, cardiovascular depression, and inhibition of some WBC functions (eg, neutrophil migration and chemotaxis and even bactericidal activity at high concentrations).

Interactions: Enhanced nephrotoxicity may become evident with concurrent administration of aminoglycosides and other potentially nephroactive (such as diuretics) or nephrotoxic (such as NSAIDs) agents. Neuromuscular blockade is more likely when aminoglycosides are administered at the same time as skeletal muscle relaxants and gas anesthetics. Aminoglycoside ototoxicity is enhanced by the loop-acting diuretics, especially furosemide. Cardiovascular depression may be aggravated by aminoglycosides when administered to animals under halothane anesthesia. High concentrations of carbenicillin, ticarcillin, and piperacillin inactivate aminoglycosides because of direct interactions both in vitro and in vivo in the presence of renal failure. Synergistic interactions that enhance antibacterial efficacy have been documented when aminoglycosides are administered with other antimicrobials, particularly β-lactams.

Effects on Laboratory Tests: BUN, serum creatinine, serum transaminases, and alkaline phosphatase values may be increased. Proteinuria is a significant laboratory finding.

Drug Withdrawal and Milk Discard Times: Note that withdrawal times do not exist for drugs not approved for used in food animals. Regulatory requirements for withdrawal times for food animals and milk discard times vary among countries. These must be followed carefully to prevent food residues and consequent public health implications. The times listed serve only as general guidelines (*see* TABLE 36).

Miscellaneous Aminocyclitol Antibiotics

Apramycin (administered orally) is used to control enteric gram-negative infections, particularly *E coli* and salmonellae in calves and piglets. It also is active against *Proteus*, *Klebsiella*, *Brachyspira*, and *Mycoplasma* spp. There is little cross-resistance within the aminoglycosides, and plasmid-mediated resistance is yet to be confirmed. Apramycin is poorly absorbed after administration PO (<10%). It is rapidly absorbed from parenteral injection sites. Plasma concentrations peak within 1–2 hr of IM administration. Apramycin distributes only into the extracellular fluid and is excreted unchanged in the urine (95% within 4 days). The elimination half-life in calves is ~4–5 hr. Apramycin is toxic in cats but considered safe in most other species (3–6 times the recommended oral dose rarely produces toxicity). The oral dose rate is 20–40 mg/kg/day, for 5 days. The parenteral dose rate is 20 mg/kg, bid. The withdrawal time in pigs and calves (in Europe) is 28 days after oral use.

The structure of spectinomycin differs from that of the aminoglycosides, but it also binds to bacterial ribosomes and interferes with protein synthesis. However, the effect is bacteriostatic rather than bactericidal. Spectinomycin can be inactivated by an enzyme coded for by an R factor, but mutant resistance due to diminished ribosomal binding is perhaps more common. It is active against several strains of streptococci, a wide range of gram-negative bacteria, and *Mycoplasma* spp; most *Chlamydia* spp are resistant. It is poorly absorbed from the GI tract but is rapidly absorbed after IM administration, with blood concentrations peaking within 1 hr. Like aminoglycosides, spectinomycin penetrates tissues rather poorly and distributes principally into extracellular fluid. Metabolic transformation of spectinomycin is limited, and 80% can be recovered unchanged in the urine over 24–48 hr; ~75% is eliminated by glomerular filtration in ~4 hr. At usual doses, no major toxic reactions have been reported. It is administered both PO at 20 mg/kg, bid, and IM at 5–10 mg/kg, bid. Withdrawal time for pigs is usually ~3 wk.

QUINOLONES, INCLUDING FLUOROQUINOLONES

Quinolone carboxylic acid derivatives are synthetic antimicrobial agents. Nalidixic acid and its congener oxolinic acid have been used for treatment of urinary tract infections for years, whereas flumequine has been used successfully in several countries to control intestinal infections in livestock. Many broad-spectrum antimicrobial agents have been produced by modification of the various 4-quinolone ring structures.

Classes

Known generically as quinolones or 4-quinolones, these drugs are derived from several closely related ring structures that have certain common features. Examples of the quinolone carboxylic acids and species in which they are approved are presented in TABLE 37. Nalidixic acid, considered a first-generation drug, is the earliest of the quinolones. In general, subsequent generations are based on spectrum, but this

TABLE 36 DRUG WITHDRAWAL AND MILK DISCARD TIMES OF AMINOGLYCOSIDES

Route	Approximate Withdrawal Time (days)
Oral	20–30 (3 for neonatal pigs)
Parenteral	100–200 (40 for neonatal pigs [often not approved for food animals])
Udder infusion	2–3[a] (often not approved for food animals)

[a] Milk discard time

often reflects similar changes in chemical structure. Subsequent drugs contain a fluorine group and, as such, are referred to as fluoroquinolones. Most veterinary drugs and many human drugs, including ciprofloxacin, are considered second generation. Pradofloxacin is an example of a later-generation drug approved for use in cats (USA) or dogs and cats (European Union).

General Properties

Within the diversity of their various ring structures, the quinolones have a number of common functional groups essential for their antimicrobial activity. For example, the quinolone nucleus contains a carboxylic acid group at position 3 and an exocyclic oxygen at position 4 (hence the term 4-quinolones), which are believed to be the active DNA-gyrase binding sites. Various modifications have produced compounds with differing physical, chemical, pharmacokinetic, and antimicrobial properties. For example, the side chain attached to the nitrogen at position 1 affects potency. Replacement of the ethyl group at this position with a bulkier group (eg, the cyclopropyl group of ciprofloxacin and similar drugs) enhances gram-negative and positive spectra. Addition of a fluorine atom at position 6 profoundly enhances the gram-positive spectrum, whereas the addition of a (heterocyclic nitrogen-containing) piperazyl ring at position 7 enhances bacterial penetration and potency, including toward *Pseudomonas aeruginosa*. Substitutions on the piperazyl (eg, ofloxacin and its L isomer, levofloxacin; sparfloxacin) enhance gram-positive penetration, whereas substitutions at position 8 enhance anaerobic activity (eg, sparfloxacin, pradofloxacin, moxifloxacin). If the substitution is with a methoxy group (rather than a halogen), the risk of phototoxicity is reduced.

The quinolones are amphoteric and, with a few exceptions, generally exhibit poor water solubility at pH 6–8. Although the impact on therapeutic efficacy is not clear, they appear to act as weak bases in that they are much less effective in acidic than in nonacidic urine pH. In concentrated acidic urine, some quinolones form needle-shaped crystals, although this apparently has not been reported with clinical use. Liquid formulations of various quinolones for PO or parenteral administration usually contain freely soluble salts in stable aqueous solutions. Solid formulations (eg, tablets, capsules, or boluses) contain the active ingredient either in its betaine form or, occasionally, as the hydrochloride salt.

Antimicrobial Activity

Mode of Action: The quinolones inhibit bacterial enzyme topoisomerases, including topoisomerase II (otherwise known as DNA gyrase) and topoisomerase IV. Bacterial DNA supercoils and then uncoils during replication. Supercoiling requires transient nicks that are subsequently sealed after DNA polymerase passes. Topoisomerase II allows for single strand nicks in the DNA that support coiling and uncoiling. Topoisomerase IV supports disentanglement of DNA as chromosomes separate. Inhibition of topoisomerases reduces supercoiling, resulting in disruption of the spatial arrangement of DNA, and reduces DNA repair. Mammalian topoisomerase

TABLE 37 QUINOLONES AND SPECIES APPROVALS IN THE USA

Quinolone	Species
Ciprofloxacin	Dogs, cats
Danofloxacin	Dogs, cattle
Difloxacin	Dogs
Enrofloxacin	Dogs, cats, cattle, swine
Marbofloxacin	Dogs, cats
Norfloxacin	Dogs, cats
Orbifloxacin	Dogs, cats
Pradofloxacin	Cats
Sarafloxicin	Voluntarily withdrawn

enzymes fundamentally differ from bacterial gyrase and are not susceptible to quinolone inhibition. The quinolones are usually bactericidal; susceptible organisms lose viability within 20 min of exposure to optimal concentrations of the newer fluoroquinolones. Typically, clearing of cytoplasm at the periphery of the affected bacterium is followed by lysis, rendering bacteria recognizable only as "ghosts."

Quinolones are associated with a postantibiotic effect in a number of bacteria, principally gram-negative (eg, *E coli*, *Klebsiella pneumoniae*, *P aeruginosa*). The effect generally lasts 4–8 hr after exposure.

Efficacy of the fluorinated quinolones depends on concentrations in plasma that exceed the MIC of the infecting organism by 10- to 12-fold. As such, the drugs are concentration dependent. However, efficacy also is correlated to the magnitude of the area under the inhibitory curve (AUC:MIC); as such, efficacy also takes into account elimination half-life.

The fluoroquinolones can have significant antibacterial activity at extraordinarily low concentrations, although efficacy toward some organisms (eg, *E coli*) is bimodal: some isolates are very susceptible (MIC <0.01–0.5 mcg/mL), whereas the MIC for a significant number of other isolates is very high (>64 mcg/mL). In general, MIC for most susceptible microbes, including *E coli*, *Klebsiella*, *Proteus*, *P aeruginosa*, and *Staphylococcus* have increased since the approval of the quinolones in the early 1990s.

Bacterial Resistance: Chromosomal mutational resistance to the original fluoroquinolones was considered to be low in frequency, and plasmid-mediated resistance nonexistent. However, resistance is increasingly being recognized, indicating that therapy based on culture and susceptibility is prudent. In general, cross-resistance should be anticipated among the more closely related members of this class.

Gram-negative bacteria more commonly target DNA gyrase; emerging resistance is more often associated with changes in the GyrA compared to the GyrB subunit. In contrast, the primary target of gram-positive organisms tends to be topoisomerase IV, with resistance mechanisms targeting it, followed by changes in DNA gyrase. Use of the drug selects for resistance. High-level resistance (3–4 times the breakpoint MIC) generally reflects a second-step mutation that leads to changes in the amino acid sequence of subsequent topoisomerase targets. However, even with this second step of resistance, MIC are often below the resistant breakpoint range on which susceptibility testing is based. With the second increase in MIC, mutations in efflux pump regulators also emerge, causing marked increase in expression. As a result, high-level, multidrug resistance emerges.

Another mechanism of resistance is the combined effect of increased efflux pumps and decreased porins that act in concert to reduce intracellular concentrations. Virulence of refractory mutants may not diminish.

Note that if resistance does emerge to one fluoroquinolone, it is likely to impact all fluoroquinolones. However, resistance may be slower to emerge to newer drugs, including gemifloxacin, trovafloxacin, gatifloxacin, or pradofloxacin, because of larger side chains that facilitate binding to either DNA gyrase or topoisomerase IV.

Antimicrobial Spectra: The fluoroquinolones are active against a wide range of gram-negative organisms and several gram-positive aerobes. This includes *E coli*, *Salmonella*, *Klebsiella*, *Enterobacter*, *Proteus*, and generally *Pseudomonas aeruginosa*. The fluoroquinolones are active against intracellular pathogens, including, eg, *Brucella* spp. Quinolones also have significant activity against *Mycoplasma* and *Chlamydia* spp. Obligate anaerobes tend to be resistant to most quinolones, as are most enterococci (previously group D *Streptococcus* spp (*Enterococcus faecalis* and *Enterococcus faecium*). *Nocardia* and atypical mycobacteria may also be susceptible.

The newer third- and fourth-generation fluorinated quinolones, such as pradofloxacin, are often characterized by an effective anaerobic spectrum.

A synergistic effect has been demonstrated in vitro between quinolones and β-lactams, aminoglycosides, clindamycin, and metronidazole.

Pharmacokinetic Features

Among the few quinolones that have been studied to any degree in domestic animals, pharmacokinetic differences can markedly differ. Because of the physicochemical nature of the group, this is to be expected. A general overview follows, but some diversity should be anticipated.

Absorption: Quinolones are commonly administered PO, although forms of enrofloxacin and ciprofloxacin are available for IV, IM, and SC (enrofloxacin) administration. Absorption into the blood after IM or SC delivery is rapid; after administration PO, blood concentrations usually peak within 1–3 hr. Bioavailability is often >80% for most quinolones, except for ciprofloxacin and in ruminants with functional forestomachs, in which bioavailability may be as low as 0–20%. The presence of food may delay absorption in monogastric animals, which may impact efficacy. The bioavailability of ciprofloxacin after administration PO in dogs is variable and can be as little as 40%; it is 0–20% in cats and horses. Marbofloxacin oral bioavailability is almost 100%.

Distribution: With few exceptions, the quinolones penetrate all tissues well and quickly. Particularly high concentrations are found in organs of elimination (kidneys, liver, and bile), but concentrations found in prostatic fluid, bone, endometrium, and CSF are also quite notable. Most quinolones also cross the placental barrier. The apparent volume of distribution of most quinolones is large. The degree of plasma-protein binding is extremely variable, from ~10% for norfloxacin to 30% for enrofloxacin in dogs and >90% for nalidixic acid. Fluorinated quinolones as a group accumulate in phagocytic WBCs.

Biotransformation: Some quinolones are eliminated unchanged (eg, ofloxacin), some are partially metabolized (eg, ciprofloxacin, enrofloxacin), and a few are completely degraded. Metabolites are sometimes active; enrofloxacin is de-ethylated to form ciprofloxacin. Characteristically, phase I reactions result in a number of primary metabolites (up to six have been described for some quinolones) that retain some antibacterial action. Conjugation with glucuronic acid then ensues, followed by excretion. In contrast, only ~10% of marbofloxacin is metabolized.

Excretion: Renal excretion is the major route of elimination for most quinolones. Both glomerular filtration and tubular secretion are involved. Urine concentrations are often high for 24 hr after administration, and crystals may form in concentrated acidic urine. The clinical significance of this finding is unclear. In renal failure, clearance is impaired, and reductions in dose rates are essential. Biliary excretion of parent drug, as well as conjugates, is an important route of elimination in some cases (eg, ciprofloxacin, marbofloxacin, difloxacin, pefloxacin, nalidixic acid). Quinolones appear in the milk of lactating animals, often at high concentrations that persist for some time.

Pharmacokinetic Values: The clearance and volume of distributions of the drugs vary among species, resulting in differences in plasma half-lives. Plasma concentrations attained are usually directly proportional to the dose administered but also vary with volume of distribution and oral bioavailability. Package inserts should be consulted for C_{max} for those drugs approved for use in the target species.

Therapeutic Indications and Dose Rates

Quinolones are indicated for the treatment of local and systemic infections caused by susceptible microorganisms, particularly against deep-seated infections and intracellular pathogens. Therapeutic success has been obtained in respiratory, intestinal, urinary, and skin infections, as well as in bacterial prostatitis, meningoencephalitis, osteomyelitis, and arthritis.

TABLE 38 PHARMACOKINETICS OF SELECTED FLUOROQUINOLONES

Drug	Species	Elimination Half-life (hr)	Volume of Distribution (L/kg)	Clearance (mL/min/kg)
Enrofloxacin	Cats	7		4.3
	Dogs	4.4	3.7	11
	Mares	4–7	2	0.5–4
Marbofloxacin	*Dogs*	12	2	1.5
Orbifloxacin	Cats	4.5	1.3	
	Dogs	5.4	1.2	

Because of their lipid solubility and ability to accumulate in phagocytic WBCs, quinolones should be considered for use in infections located in tough to penetrate tissues. Therapeutic failure is likely to result with multidrug-resistant organisms; this coupled with their emerging adverse events should cause these drugs to be considered second tier for dogs and cats.

A selection of general dosages for some quinolones is listed in TABLE 39. The dose rate and frequency should be adjusted as needed for the individual animal and the MIC of the infecting organisms. Plasma drug concentrations should approximate 10 times the MIC of the infecting microbe. Higher doses are encouraged unless mitigating circumstances preclude the increase; in such instances, unless the MIC is very low, alternative antimicrobials might be considered. In dogs and cats, use ideally is based on culture and susceptibility testing when possible. Extra-label use of fluoroquinolones is prohibited in food animals.

Special Clinical Concerns

Adverse Effects and Toxicity:

Although adverse effects with the older quinolones (nalidixic and oxolinic acids) were relatively common, the newer ones seem to be well tolerated. However, several adverse effects can limit use in selected species. Retinal degeneration may occur acutely in cats, with the risk greatest for enrofloxacin; because these drugs are concentration dependent, enrofloxacin probably should not be used in cats. The presence of renal disease may increase this risk. Pradofloxacin may be the least retinotoxic, followed by marbofloxacin and orbifloxacin, but each of these appears to be safe in cats at doses that would be necessary to achieve targeted C_{max}:MIC ratios for susceptible organisms. The mechanism is not known. Quinolones tend to be neurotoxic, and convulsions can occur at high doses. Vomiting and diarrhea rarely develop with fluoroquinolones. Dermal reactions and photosensitization have been described in people, but the occurrence seems low. Hemolytic anemia has also been seen. Administering large doses of quinolones for any length of time during pregnancy has resulted in embryonic loss and maternal toxicity. Because high prolonged dosages in growing dogs have produced cartilaginous erosions leading to permanent lameness, excessive use of quinolones should be avoided in immature animals. Quinolone administration in horses has not yet been extensively studied, but there is some indication that damage to the cartilage in weightbearing joints may be seen.

In 2008, the FDA added a "black-box" warning for seven fluoroquinolones that increased the risk of tendinitis and a tendon rupture.

An emerging toxicity associated with fluoroquinolones is mitotoxicity, ie, damage to mitochondrial topoisomerase or other mitochondrial structures. Mitochondrial effects may not emerge until some time after fluoroquinolone therapy is instituted.

TABLE 39 DOSAGES OF QUINOLONES

Quinolone[a]	Species	Dosage, Route, and Frequency
Nalidixic acid	Cats, dogs	3 mg/kg, PO, qid
Enrofloxacin	Dogs	5–20 mg/kg, PO, once to twice daily
		2.5 mg/kg, SC, once, then PO
	Beef cattle (not veal or dairy)	7.5–12.5 mg/kg, SC, once
		2.5–5 mg/kg/day, SC
	Pigs	2.5–5 mg/kg/day, PO or IM
	Preruminant calves	2.5–5 mg/kg/day, PO or SC
Marbofloxacin	Cats, dogs	2.75–5.5 mg/kg/day, PO
Difloxacin	Dogs	5–10 mg/kg/day, PO
Orbifloxacin	Cats, dogs	2.5–7.5 mg/kg/day, PO
Pradofloxacin	Cats	7.5 mg/kg/day, PO

[a] Extra-label use of fluorinated quinolones in food-producing animals is prohibited in the USA.

Although the entirety of the clinical impact of this toxicity is not known, nor its relevance to veterinary medicine, adverse events ranging from neurologic to musculoskeletal to cardiovascular may ultimately be attributed to this effect.

Interactions: The fluorinated quinolones may be involved in a number of drug interactions. Antacids or other drugs containing multivalent cations and sucralfate appear to interfere with the GI absorption of the quinolones. Nitrofurantoin impairs the efficacy of quinolones if used concurrently for urinary tract infections. Quinolones inhibit the biotransformation of methylxanthines, with theophylline being the most clinically relevant, but also including caffeine and theobromine. This is a class effect, with the risk varying among the fluoroquinolones in people. A similar ranking of risk is not available for veterinary medicine. In people, cyclosporine concentrations may also be increased by concurrent administration with fluoroquinolones, leading to prolonged and potentially toxic plasma concentrations.

Effects on Laboratory Tests: AST, ALT, alkaline phosphatase, and BUN may be increased. Urine glucose may be altered, and urinalysis may reveal needle-shaped crystals.

SULFONAMIDES AND SULFONAMIDE COMBINATIONS

Sulfonamides are the oldest and remain among the most widely used antibacterial agents in veterinary medicine, chiefly because of low cost and their relative efficacy in some common bacterial diseases. The synergistic action of sulfonamides with specific diaminopyrimidines renders these drugs much more effective than sulfonamides alone.

Classes

The many available sulfonamides and sulfonamide derivatives can be categorized into several types, based mainly on their indications and duration of action in the body. Probably the most common classification is based on water versus lipid solubility or duration of effect. Although there are many sulfonamide antimicrobials, only a few are used clinically in animals.

Standard Use Sulfonamides: In most species, members of this large group are administered 1–4 times/day, depending on the drug, to control systemic infections caused by susceptible bacteria. In some instances, administration of the sulfonamide can be less frequent if the drug is eliminated slowly in the species being treated. Sulfonamides included in this class, depending on the species, are sulfathiazole, sulfamethazine (sulfadimidine), sulfamerazine, sulfadiazine, sulfapyridine, sulfabromomethazine, sulfaethoxypyridazine, sulfamethoxypyridazine, sulfadimethoxine, and sulfachlorpyridazine.

Highly Soluble Sulfonamides Used for Urinary Tract Infections: A few very water-soluble sulfonamides, eg, sulfisoxazole (sulfafurazole) and sulfasomidine, are rapidly excreted via the urinary tract (>90% in 24 hr) mostly in an unchanged form; because of this, they are primarily used to treat urinary tract infections.

Poorly Soluble Sulfonamides Used for Intestinal Infections: Some sulfonamide derivatives, such as sulfaguanidine, are so insoluble that they are not absorbed from the GI tract (<5%). Phthalylsulfathiazole and succinylsulfathiazole undergo bacterial hydrolysis in the lower GI tract with the consequent release of active sulfathiazole. Salicylazosulfapyridine (sulfasalazine) is also hydrolyzed in the large intestine to sulfapyridine and 5-aminosalicylic acid, an anti-inflammatory agent that might be used for management of ulcerative colitis in dogs.

Potentiated Sulfonamides: A group of **diaminopyrimidines** (trimethoprim, methoprim, ormetoprim, aditoprim, pyrimethamine) inhibit dihydrofolate reductase in bacteria and protozoa far more efficiently than in mammalian cells. Used alone, these agents are not particularly effective against bacteria, and resistance develops rapidly. However, when combined with sulfonamides, a sequential blockade of microbial enzyme systems occurs with bactericidal consequences. Examples of such potentiated sulfonamide preparations include trimethoprim/sulfadiazine (co-trimazine), trimethoprim/sulfamethoxazole (co-trimoxazole), trimethoprim/sulfadoxine (co-trimoxine), and ormetoprim/sulfadimethoxine. Sulfonamides are used in combination with pyrimethamine to treat protozoal diseases such as leishmaniasis and toxoplasmosis. (*See also* TABLE 41, p 2679.)

Topical Sulfonamides: Several sulfonamides are used topically for specific purposes. Sulfacetamide is not highly efficacious but is occasionally used to treat ophthalmic infections. Mafenide and silver sulfadiazine are used on burn wounds to prevent invasion by many gram-negative and gram-positive organisms. Sulfathiazole is commonly included in wound powders for the same purpose.

General Properties

The sulfonamides are derivatives of sulfanilamide, which is the nucleus common to all. The addition or substitution of various functional groups to the amido group or in which various substitutions on other amino groups result in compounds with varying physical, chemical, pharmacologic, and antibacterial properties. Although amphoteric, sulfonamides generally behave as weak organic acids and are much more soluble in alkaline aqueous solutions than in acidic solutions. Those of therapeutic interest have pK_a values of 4.8–8.6. Water-soluble sodium or disodium salts are used for parenteral administration. Such solutions are highly alkaline, somewhat unstable, and readily precipitate with the addition of polyionic electrolytes. In a mixture of sulfonamides (eg, the sulfapyrimidine group), each component drug has its own solubility; therefore, a combination of sulfonamides is more water soluble than a single drug at the same total concentration. This is the basis of triple sulfonamide mixtures used clinically. The N-4 acetylated sulfonamides, except for the sulfapyrimidine group (sulfamethazine, sulfamerazine, sulfadiazine), are less water soluble than their nonacetylated forms. This has bearing in the development of sulfonamide crystalluria. The highly insoluble sulfonamides (phthalylsulfathiazole and succinylsulfathiazole) are retained in the lumen of the GI tract for prolonged periods and are known as "gut-active" sulfonamides. Trimethoprim and ormetoprim are basic drugs.

Antimicrobial Activity

Mode of Action: The sulfonamides are structural analogues of para-aminobenzoic acid (PABA) and competitively inhibit dihydropterate synthetase, an enzyme that facilitates PABA as a substrate for the synthesis of dihydrofolic acid (folic acid). Dihydrofolate is a precursor for formation of tetrahydrofolate (folinic acid), an essential component of the coenzymes responsible for single carbon metabolism in cells. Sulfonamides are antimetabolites that substitute for PABA, resulting in blockade of several enzymes needed for the biogenesis of purine bases and other metabolic reactions necessary for formation of RNA. Protein synthesis, metabolic processes, and inhibition of growth and replication occur in organisms that cannot use preformed (eg, dietary) folate. The effect is bacteriostatic, although a bactericidal action is evident at the high concentrations that may be found in urine. Diaminopyrimidines such as trimethoprim inhibit dihydrofolate reductase, which is further into the folic acid synthesis pathway. The combination of a sulfonamide and a diaminopyrimidine results in synergistic, bactericidal actions on susceptible organisms; as such, the combination is referred to as a "potentiated" sulfonamide.

The optimal ratio in vitro for the combination of trimethoprim or ormetoprim and a sulfonamide depends on the type of microorganism but is usually ~1:20. However, the commercially available preparations use a ratio of 1:5 because of pharmacokinetic considerations that presumably result in the optimal ratio at the site of infection.

Sulfonamides are most effective in the early stages of acute infections when organisms are rapidly multiplying. They are not active against quiescent bacteria. Typically, there is a latent period before the effects of sulfonamide therapy become evident. This lag period occurs because the bacteria use existing stores of folic acid, folinic acid, purines, thymidine, and amino acids. Once these stores are depleted, bacteriostasis occurs. Bacterial growth can resume when the concentration of PABA increases or when the level of sulfonamide falls below an enzyme-inhibitory concentration. Because of the bacteriostatic nature of sulfonamides, adequate cellular and humoral defense mechanisms are critical for successful sulfonamide therapy when used as sole agents. Even potentiated sulfonamides, which are bactericidal, are time dependent in their antibacterial efficacy.

Although all of the sulfonamides have the same mechanism of action, differences are evident with respect to activity, pharmacokinetic fate, and even antimicrobial spectrum at usual concentrations. The differences are due to the variety of physiochemical characteristics seen among the sulfonamides.

The efficacy of sulfonamides can be reduced radically by excess PABA, folic acid, thymine, purine, methionine, plasma, blood, albumin, tissue autolysates, and endogenous protein-degradation products.

Bacterial Resistance: Resistance to sulfonamides is both chromosomally and plasmid mediated. Altered proteins such that affinity is reduced appears to be the most common mechanism of resistance. For example, in staphylococci, chromosomally mediated resistance reflects mutations in genes encoding for dihydropterate synthetase and plasmid-mediated resistance reflects mutations in dihydrofolate reductases, with the latter causing high-level resistance to trimethoprim. Staphylococci may have acquired some mechanisms of sulfonamide resistance from enterococci. Because sulfonamides act in a competitive fashion, overproduction of PABA can also preclude inhibition of dihydropterate synthetase. Alternate pathways of folic acid synthesis may also contribute to low-level resistance. Cross-resistance between sulfonamides is common. Resistance emerges gradually and is widespread in many animal populations. Plasmid-mediated sulfonamide resistance in intestinal gram-negative bacteria is often linked with ampicillin and tetracycline resistance.

Antimicrobial Spectra: The spectrum of all sulfonamides is generally the same. Sulfonamides inhibit both gram-positive and gram-negative bacteria, *Nocardia*, *Actinomyces* spp, and some protozoa such as coccidia and *Toxoplasma* spp. More active sulfonamides may include several species of *Streptococcus*, *Staphylococcus*, *Salmonella*, *Pasteurella*, and even *Escherichia coli* in their spectra. Strains of *Pseudomonas*, *Klebsiella*, *Proteus*, *Clostridium*, and *Leptospira* spp are most often highly resistant, as are rickettsiae, mycoplasmas, and most *Chlamydia*.

Pharmacokinetic Features

There are notable differences among the many sulfonamides with respect to their pharmacokinetic fate in the various species. The standard classification of short-, medium-, and long-acting sulfonamides used in human therapeutics is usually inappropriate in veterinary medicine because of species differences in disposition and elimination.

Absorption: Sulfonamides may be administered PO, IV, IP, IM, intrauterine, or topically, depending on the specific preparation. Except for the poorly absorbed sulfonamides intended for local treatment of intestinal infections, most are rapidly and completely absorbed from the GI tract of monogastric animals. Absorption from the ruminoreticulum is delayed, especially if ruminal stasis is present. Therapeutic doses of sulfonamides are usually administered PO except in acute life-threatening infections when IV infusions are used to establish adequate blood concentrations as rapidly as possible. Sulfonamides are frequently added to drinking water or feed either for therapeutic purposes or to improve feed efficiency. A few highly water-soluble preparations may be injected IM (eg, sodium sulfadimethoxine) or IP (some irritation of the peritoneum can be seen). Absorption is rapid from these parenteral sites. Generally, sulfonamide solutions are too alkaline for routine parenteral use.

Trimethoprim is rapidly absorbed after administration PO (plasma concentrations peak in ~2–4 hr) except in ruminants, in which it tends to be trapped in the ruminoreticulum and appears to undergo a degree of microbial degradation.

Absorption occurs readily from parenteral injection sites; effective antibacterial concentrations are reached in <1 hr, and peak concentrations in ~4 hr.

Distribution: Sulfonamides are distributed throughout all body tissues. The distribution pattern depends on the ionization state of the sulfonamide, the vascularity of specific tissues, the presence of specific barriers to sulfonamide diffusion, and the fraction of the administered dose bound to plasma proteins. The unbound drug fraction is freely diffusible. Sulfonamides are bound to plasma proteins to a greater or lesser extent, and concentrations in pleural, peritoneal, synovial, and ocular fluids may be 50%–90% of that in blood. Sulfadiazine is ≥90% bound to plasma proteins. Concentrations in the kidneys exceed plasma concentrations, and those in the skin, liver, and lungs are only slightly less than the corresponding plasma concentrations. Concentrations in muscle and bone are ~50% of those in the plasma, and those in the CSF may be 20%–80% of blood concentrations, depending on the particular sulfonamide. Low concentrations are found in adipose tissue. After parenteral administration, sulfamethazine is found in jejunal and colonic contents at about the same concentration as in blood. Passive diffusion into milk also occurs; although the concentrations achieved are usually inadequate to control infections, sulfonamide residues may be detected in milk. Trimethoprim and ormetoprim are basic drugs that tend to accumulate in more acidic environments such as acidic urine, milk, and ruminal fluid.

Trimethoprim diffuses extensively into tissues and body fluids. Tissue concentrations are often higher than the corresponding plasma concentrations, especially in lungs, liver, and kidneys. Approximately 30%–60% of trimethoprim is bound to plasma proteins. The extent of metabolic transformation of trimethoprim has not yet been established, although there is a suggestion that hepatic biotransformation can be extensive, at least in ruminants. This may not be the case in all species; >50% of a dose is excreted unchanged in many instances. Trimethoprim is largely excreted in the urine by glomerular filtration and tubular secretion. A substantial amount may also be found in the feces. Concentrations in milk are often 1–3.5 times higher than those in plasma.

Biotransformation: Sulfonamides are usually extensively metabolized, mainly by several oxidative pathways, acetylation, and conjugation with sulfate or glucuronic acid. Species differences are marked in this regard. The acetylated, hydroxylated, and conjugated forms have little antibacterial activity. Acetylation (poorly developed in dogs) reduces the solubility of most sulfonamides except for the sulfapyrimidine group. The hydroxylated and conjugated forms are less likely to precipitate in urine.

Excretion: Most sulfonamides are excreted primarily in the urine. Bile, feces, milk, and sweat are excretory routes of lesser significance. Glomerular filtration, active tubular secretion, and tubular reabsorption are the main processes involved. The proportion reabsorbed is influenced by the inherent lipid solubility of individual sulfonamides and their metabolites and by urinary pH. Urinary pH, renal clearance, and the concentration and solubility of the respective sulfonamides and their metabolites determine whether solubilities are exceeded and crystals precipitate. This can be prevented by alkalinizing the urine, increasing fluid intake, reducing dose rates in renal insufficiency, and using triple-sulfonamide or sulfonamide-diaminopyrimidine combinations.

Pharmacokinetic Values: There are great differences between the pharmacokinetic values of various sulfonamides in animals, and extrapolation of these values is rarely appropriate; for example, the plasma half-life of sulfadiazine is 10.1 hr in cattle and 2.9 hr in pigs. The recommended dose rates and frequencies reflect this disparity in elimination kinetics.

The plasma half-life of trimethoprim is quite prolonged in most species; effective concentrations may be maintained for >12 hr, with the result that the frequency of administration is usually 12–24 hr. The elimination rates of trimethoprim in sheep seem to be much shorter than in monogastric species.

Therapeutic Indications and Dose Rates

The sulfonamides are commonly used to treat or prevent acute systemic or local infections. Disease syndromes treated with sulfonamides include actinobacillosis, coccidiosis, mastitis, metritis, colibacillosis, pododermatitis, polyarthritis, respiratory infections, and toxoplasmosis.

Sulfonamides are more effective when administered early in the course of a disease. Chronic infections, particularly with large amounts of exudate or tissue debris present, often are not responsive. In severe infections, the initial dose should be administered IV to reduce the lag time between dose and effect. For drugs with a long elimination half-life, the initial dose should be double the maintenance dose. Adequate drinking water should be available at all times, and urine output monitored. A course of treatment should not exceed 7 days under usual circumstances. If a favorable response is seen within 72 hr, treatment should be continued for 48 hr after remission to prevent relapse and the emergence of resistance. The ability to mount an immune response must be intact for successful sulfonamide therapy.

A selection of general dosages for some sulfonamides is listed in TABLE 40. The dose rate and frequency should be adjusted as needed for the individual animal.

Special Clinical Concerns

Adverse Effects and Toxicity: Adverse reactions to sulfonamides may be due to hypersensitivity or direct toxic effects. Possible hypersensitivity reactions include urticaria, angioedema, anaphylaxis, skin rashes, drug fever, polyarthritis, hemolytic anemia, and agranulocytosis. Keratitis sicca is a recognized adverse effect. The allergic response targets, in part, metabolites of the aryl amine of sulfonamides. Because dogs are deficient in acetylation, they may be at risk of increased formation of phase I metabolites associated with adverse effects.

TABLE 40 DOSAGES OF SULFONAMIDES

Sulfonamide	Species	Dosage, Route, and Frequency
Sulfathiazole	Horses	66 mg/kg, PO, tid
	Cattle, sheep, pigs	66 mg/kg, PO, every 4 hr
Sulfamethazine	Cattle	220 mg/kg/day, PO or IV (initial dose; half for subsequent doses)
Sulfadiazine	All	50 mg/kg, PO, bid
Sulfadimethoxine	All	55 mg/kg/day, PO (initial dose; half for subsequent doses)
Sulfaethoxypyridazine	Cattle	55 mg/kg/day, PO
	Pigs	110 mg/kg/day, PO (initial dose, half for subsequent doses)
Sulfapyridine	Cattle	132 mg/kg, PO, bid (initial dose, half for subsequent doses)
Succinylsulfathiazole	All	160 mg/kg, PO, bid (initial dose; half for subsequent doses)

Crystalluria with hematuria, and even tubular obstruction, is not common in veterinary medicine. Acute toxic manifestations may be seen after too rapid IV administration or if an excessive dose is injected. Clinical signs include muscle weakness, ataxia, blindness, and collapse. GI disturbances, in addition to nausea and vomiting, may occur when sulfonamide concentrations are sufficiently high in the tract to disturb normal microfloral balance and vitamin B synthesis. Sulfonamides depress the cellulolytic function of ruminal microflora, but the effect is usually transient (unless excessively high concentrations are reached). Several adverse effects have been reported after prolonged treatment, including bone marrow depression (aplastic anemia, granulocytopenia, thrombocytopenia), hepatitis and icterus, peripheral neuritis and myelin degeneration in the spinal cord and peripheral nerves, photosensitization, stomatitis, conjunctivitis, and keratitis sicca. Mild follicular thyroid hyperplasia may be associated with prolonged administration of sulfonamides in sensitive species such as dogs, and reversible hypothyroidism can be induced after treatment with high doses in dogs. Several sulfonamides can lead to decreased egg production and growth. Topically, the sulfonamides retard healing of uncontaminated wounds.

Up to 10 times the recommended dose of trimethoprim has been given with no adverse effects. Prolonged administration of trimethoprim at reasonably high concentrations leads to maturation defects in hematopoiesis due to impaired folinic acid synthesis. This effect is readily reversible by supplementation with folinic acid.

Interactions: Sulfonamide solutions are incompatible with calcium- or other polyionic-containing fluids as well as many other preparations. Sulfonamides may be displaced from their plasma-protein-binding sites by other acidic drugs with higher binding affinities. Antacids tend to inhibit the GI absorption of sulfonamides. Alkalinization of the urine promotes sulfonamide excretion, and urinary acidification increases the risk of crystalluria. Some sulfonamides act as microsomal enzyme inhibitors, which may lead to toxic manifestations of concurrently administered drugs such as phenytoin.

Effects on Laboratory Tests: Bilirubin, BUN, bromsulphthalein (BSP®), eosinophils, methemoglobin, AST, and ALT may be increased. Platelet, RBC, and WBC counts are often decreased. Urinalysis may show a change in color, glucose, porphyrins, and urobilinogen. Sulfonamide crystals may also be found.

Regulatory Considerations and Drug Withdrawal and Milk Discard Times: Sulfonamides are among the drugs for which extra-label use restrictions exist in lactating dairy cattle. Currently allowable drugs are sulfadimethoxine, sulfabro-

TABLE 41 DOSAGES OF POTENTIATED SULFONAMIDES

Combination Sulfonamide	Dosage, Route, and Frequency
Trimethoprim/sulfadiazine	15–60 mg/kg/day, PO, IV, or IM
Ormetoprim/sulfadimethoxine	55 mg/kg/day, PO (initial dose; half for subsequent doses)

TABLE 42 DRUG WITHDRAWAL AND MILK DISCARD TIMES OF SULFONAMIDES

Sulfonamide	Species	Withdrawal Time (days)	Milk Discard Time (hr)
Sulfamethazine	Cattle	10[a]	96
	Pigs	14	
Sulfabromethazine	Cattle	10	96
Triple sulfonamide solution[b]	Cattle	10	96
Sulfadimethoxidine	Cattle	7	60

[a] 28 days for slow-release bolus

[b] 8% sodium sulfamethazine, 8% sodium sulfapyridine, 8% sodium sulfathiazole

methazine, and sulfathoxypyridazine. In addition, sulfonamide residues, particularly in swine and poultry, continue to be a focus of detection. Because of adverse effects in people, including allergic reactions, attention must be made to withdrawal times. Regulatory requirements for withdrawal times for food animals and milk discard times vary among countries and may change. These must be followed carefully to prevent food residues and consequent public health implications. There are some prohibitions on use of sulfonamides in the USA, including use in dairy cattle. The times listed in TABLE 42 serve only as general guidelines.

TETRACYCLINES

The tetracyclines are broad-spectrum antibiotics with similar antimicrobial features, but they differ somewhat from one another in terms of their spectra and pharmacokinetic disposition.

Classes

There are three naturally occurring tetracyclines (oxytetracycline, chlortetracycline, and demethylchlortetracycline) and several that are derived semisynthetically (tetracycline, rolitetracycline, methacycline, minocycline, doxycycline, lymecycline, etc). Elimination times permit a further classification into short-acting (tetracycline, oxytetracycline, chlortetracycline), intermediate-acting (demethylchlortetracycline and methacycline), and long-acting (doxycycline and minocycline). The newest class of tetracycline-related antimicrobials are the glycylcyclines, represented by tigecycline, which contains a bulky side chain compared with minocycline.

General Properties

All of the tetracycline derivatives are crystalline, yellowish, amphoteric substances that, in aqueous solution, form salts with both acids and bases. They characteristically fluoresce when exposed to ultraviolet light. The most common salt form is the hydrochloride, except for doxycycline, which is available as doxycycline hyclate or monohydrate. The tetracyclines are stable as dry powders but not in aqueous solution, particularly at higher pH ranges (7–8.5). Preparations for parenteral administration must be carefully formulated, often in propylene glycol or polyvinyl pyrrolidone with additional dispersing agents, to provide stable solutions. Tetracyclines form poorly soluble chelates with bivalent and trivalent cations, particularly calcium, magnesium, aluminum, and iron. Doxycycline and minocycline exhibit the greatest liposolubility and better penetration of bacteria such as *Staphylococcus aureus* than does the group

TABLE 43 DRUG WITHDRAWAL AND MILK DISCARD TIMES OF POTENTIATED SULFONAMIDES

Combination Sulfonamide	Withdrawal Time (days)	Milk Discard Time (days)
Trimethoprim/ sulfadiazine	3	7
Trimethoprim/ sulfadoxine	5 (PO), 28 (parenteral)	

as a whole. This may contribute to their efficacy in treatment of gingival diseases that may be associated with bacterial glycocalyx. Tigecycline is a glycylcycline derivative of minocycline; its large side chain decreases the risk of resistance.

Antimicrobial Activity

Mode of Action: The antimicrobial activity of tetracyclines reflects reversible binding to the bacterial 30S ribosomal subunit, and specifically at the aminoacyl-tRNA acceptor ("A") site on the mRNA ribosomal complex, thus preventing ribosomal translation. This effect also is evident in mammalian cells, although microbial cells are selectively more susceptible because of the greater concentrations seen. Tetracyclines enter microorganisms in part by diffusion and in part by an energy-dependent, carrier-mediated system responsible for the high concentrations achieved in susceptible bacteria. The tetracyclines are generally bacteriostatic, and a responsive host-defense system is essential for their successful use. At high concentrations, as may be attained in urine, they become bactericidal because the organisms seem to lose the functional integrity of the cytoplasmic membrane. Tetracyclines are more effective against multiplying microorganisms and tend to be more active at a pH of 6–6.5. Antibacterial efficacy is described as time dependent.

Bacterial Resistance: The most common mechanism by which microbes become resistant to tetracyclines is decreased accumulation of drug into previously susceptible organisms. Two mechanisms include 1) impaired uptake into bacteria, which occurs in mutant strains that do not have the necessary transport system, and 2) the much more common plasmid- or transposon-mediated acquisition of active efflux pumps. The genomes for these capabilities may be transferred either by transduction (as in *Staphylococcus aureus*) or by conjugation (as in many enterobacteria). A second mechanism of resistance is the production of a "protective" protein that acts by either preventing binding, dislodging the bound drug, or altering the negative impact of binding on ribosomal function. Among the tetracyclines, tigecycline is characterized by less resistance due to efflux or ribosomal protection. Rarely, tetracyclines can be destroyed by acetylation. Resistance develops slowly in a multistep fashion but is widespread because of the extensive use of low concentrations of tetracyclines.

Antimicrobial Spectra: All tetracyclines are about equally active and typically have about the same broad spectrum, which comprises both aerobic and anaerobic gram-positive and gram-negative bacteria, mycoplasmas, rickettsiae, chlamydiae, and even some protozoa (amebae). Tetracyclines generally are the drug of choice to treat rickettsiae and mycoplasma. Among the susceptible organisms is *Wolbachia*, a rickettsial-like intracellular endosymbiont of nematodes, including *Dirofilaria immitis*. Strains of *Pseudomonas aeruginosa*, *Proteus*, *Serratia*, *Klebsiella*, and *Trueperella* spp frequently are resistant, as are many pathogenic *Escherichia coli* isolates. Even though there is general cross-resistance among tetracyclines, doxycycline and minocycline usually are more effective against staphylococci.

Pharmacokinetic Features

Absorption: After usual oral dosage, tetracyclines are absorbed primarily in the upper small intestine, and effective blood concentrations are reached in 2–4 hr. GI absorption can be impaired by sodium bicarbonate, aluminum hydroxide, magnesium hydroxide, iron, calcium salts, and (except for the lipid-soluble tetracyclines doxycycline and minocycline) milk and milk products. Oral bioavailability, however, can vary markedly among drugs, with chlortetracycline being the least and doxycycline the most orally bioavailable. Tetracyclines at therapeutic concentrations should not be administered PO to ruminants: they are poorly absorbed and can substantially depress ruminal microfloral activity. Specially buffered tetracycline solutions can be administered IM and IV. Through chemical manipulation (especially choice of carrier and high magnesium content), the absorption of oxytetracycline from IM sites may be delayed, which produces a long-acting effect. Tetracyclines can also be absorbed from the uterus and udder, although plasma concentrations remain low.

Distribution: Tetracyclines distribute rapidly and extensively in the body, particularly after parenteral administration. They enter almost all tissues and body fluids; high concentrations are found in the kidneys, liver, bile, lungs, spleen, and bone. Lower concentrations are found in serosal fluids, synovia, CSF, ascitic fluid, prostatic fluid, and vitreous humor. The more lipid-soluble tetracyclines (doxycycline and minocycline) readily penetrate tissues such as the blood-brain barrier, and CSF concentrations reach ~30% of the plasma concentrations. Doxycycline is the most extensively distributed. Because tetracyclines tend to chelate calcium ions (less so for doxycycline), they are deposited irreversibly in the growing bones and in dentin and enamel of unerupted teeth of young animals, or even the fetus if transplacental passage occurs (*see* p 2658). Drug bound in this fashion is pharmacologically inactive. Tetracyclines are bound to plasma proteins to varying degrees (eg, oxytetracycline, 30%; tetracycline, 60%; doxycycline, 90%).

Biotransformation: Biotransformation of the tetracyclines seems to be limited in most domestic animals, and generally about one-third of a given dose is excreted unchanged. Rolitetracycline is metabolized to tetracycline. Doxycycline and minocycline may be more extensively biotransformed than other tetracyclines (up to 40% of a given dose).

Excretion: Tetracyclines are excreted via the kidneys (glomerular filtration) and the GI tract (biliary elimination and directly). Generally 50%–80% of a given dose is recoverable from the urine, although several factors may influence renal elimination, including age, route of administration, urine pH, glomerular filtration rate, renal disease, and the particular tetracycline used. Biliary elimination is always significant, commonly being ~10%–20%, even with parenteral administration. Doxycycline appears to be eliminated through feces predominantly through intestinal cells, rather than bile. Only ~16% of an IV dose of doxycycline is eliminated unchanged in the urine of dogs. A portion of doxycycline is also renally excreted in active form in some species. For minocycline, bile appears to be the major route of excretion. Tetracyclines are also eliminated in milk; concentrations peak 6 hr after a parenteral dose, and traces are still present up to 48 hr later. Concentrations in milk usually attain ~50%–60% of the plasma concentration and are often higher in mastitic milk. Tetracyclines also are excreted in saliva and tears.

Pharmacokinetic Values: The plasma half-lives of tetracyclines are 6–12 hr and can be longer depending on age (slower elimination in animals <1 mo old), disease, and the tetracycline itself (*see* TABLE 44). In large animals, daily injections of standard dosages usually are sufficient to maintain effective inhibitory concentrations. Long-acting formulations of oxytetracycline, when injected IM, generally produce plasma concentrations >0.5 mcg/mL for ~72 hr. Tetracyclines usually are administered PO bid-tid (every 12–24 hr for doxycycline and minocycline).

Therapeutic Indications and Dose Rates

The tetracyclines are used to treat both systemic and local infections. However, resistance and their bacteriostatic nature suggest caution with empirical use for bacterial infections, particularly in dogs and cats. Specific conditions include infectious keratoconjunctivitis in cattle, chlamydiosis, heartwater, anaplasmosis, actinomycosis, actinobacillosis, nocardiosis (especially minocycline), ehrlichiosis (especially doxycycline), *Wolbachia*, eperythrozoonosis, and haemobartonellosis. Minocycline and doxycycline are often effective to a somewhat lesser degree against resistant strains of *Staphylococcus aureus*.

In addition to antimicrobial chemotherapy, the tetracyclines are used for other purposes. As additives in animal feeds, they serve as growth promoters. Because of the affinity of tetracyclines for bones, teeth, and necrotic tissue, they can be used to delineate tumors by fluorescence.

TABLE 44 ELIMINATION, DISTRIBUTION, AND CLEARANCE OF TETRACYCLINES

Tetracycline	Species	Elimination Half-life (hr)	Volume of Distribution (mL/kg)	Clearance (mL/kg/min)
Oxytetracycline	Dogs	6	3,000	4.23
	Calves (<3 mo old)	10–13	1,500–2,400	3.45
	Cattle	7–10	800–1,000	3.33
	Horses	8–10	1,100	2.89
Minocycline	Dogs	7	2,000	3.21
Doxycycline	Dogs	7–10	930	1.7
	Cats	5	340	1.0
	Horses	9		

Demethylchlortetracycline has been used to inhibit the action of antidiuretic hormone in cases of excessive water retention. Because of either their metalloproteinase-inhibiting effects or their binding of calcium, they are used to "stretch" flexor digital tendons in neonatal foals. Finally, they are being used to reduce the risk of adverse events and to enhance killing of adult heartworms and/or microfilaria before adulticide therapy.

A selection of general dosages for some tetracyclines is listed in TABLE 45. The dose rate and frequency should be adjusted as needed for the individual animal.

Special Clinical Concerns

Adverse Effects and Toxicity: Because several diverse effects may result from administration of tetracyclines, caution should be exercised. Superinfection by nonsusceptible pathogens such as fungi, yeasts, and resistant bacteria is always a possibility when broad-spectrum antibiotics are used. This may lead to GI disturbances after either PO or parenteral administration or to "persistent infection" when they are applied topically (eg, in the ear). Severe and even fatal diarrhea can occur in horses receiving tetracyclines, especially if the animals are severely stressed or critically ill.

High doses administered PO to ruminants seriously disrupt microfloral activity in the ruminoreticulum, eventually producing stasis. Elimination of the gut flora in monogastric animals reduces the synthesis and availability of the B vitamins and vitamin K from the large intestine. With prolonged therapy, vitamin supplementation is a useful precaution.

Tetracyclines chelate calcium in teeth and bones; they become incorporated into these structures, inhibit calcification (eg, hypoplastic dental enamel), and cause yellowish then brownish discoloration. At extremely high concentrations, the healing processes in fractured bones is impaired.

Rapid IV injection of a tetracycline can result in hypotension and sudden collapse. This appears to be related to the ability of the tetracyclines to chelate ionized calcium, although a depressant effect by the propylene glycol carrier itself may also be involved. This effect can be avoided by slow infusion of the drug (>5 min) or by pretreatment with IV calcium gluconate.

The IV administration of undiluted propylene glycol–based preparations leads to intravascular hemolysis, which results in hemoglobinuria and possibly other reactions such as hypotension, ataxia, and CNS depression.

Because tetracyclines interfere with protein synthesis even in host cells and therefore tend to be catabolic, an increase in BUN can be expected. The combined use of glucocorticoids and tetracyclines often leads to a significant weight loss, particularly in anorectic animals.

Hepatotoxic effects due to large doses of tetracyclines have been reported in pregnant women and in other animals. The mortality rate is high.

The tetracyclines are also potentially nephrotoxic and are contraindicated (except for doxycycline) in renal insufficiency. Fatal renal failure has been reported in septicemic and endotoxemic cattle given high doses of oxytetracycline. The administration of expired tetracycline

TABLE 45 DOSAGES OF TETRACYCLINES

Tetracycline	Species	Dosage, Route, and Frequency
Tetracycline	Cats, dogs	7 mg/kg, IM or IV, bid
		20 mg/kg, PO, tid
Oxytetracycline	Cats, dogs	7 mg/kg, IM or IV, bid
		20 mg/kg, PO, tid
	Cattle, sheep, pigs	5–10 mg/kg/day, IM or IV
	Calves, foals, lambs, piglets	10–20 mg/kg, PO, bid-tid
	Horses	5 mg/kg, IV, once to twice daily
Doxycycline	Dogs	5–10 mg/kg/day, PO
		5 mg/kg/day, IV
	Before heartworm adulticide therapy	10 mg/kg, PO, bid, for 30 days

products may lead to acute tubular nephrosis.

Swelling, necrosis, and yellow discoloration at the injection site almost inevitably are seen. Phototoxic dermatitis may occur in people treated with demethylchlortetracycline and other analogues, but this reaction is rare in other animals. Hypersensitivity reactions occur; for example, cats may develop a "drug fever" reaction, often accompanied by vomiting, diarrhea, depression, inappetence, fever, and eosinophilia.

The tetracyclines can inhibit WBC chemotaxis and phagocytosis when present in high concentrations at sites of infection. This clearly hinders normal host defense mechanisms and compounds the bacteriostatic activity of tetracyclines. The use of immunosuppressive drugs such as glucocorticoids impairs immunocompetence even further.

Doxycycline administered in tablets has been associated with esophageal erosion in cats. The incidence is reduced if administration is followed by a 5-mL volume of fluid. Doxycycline may be associated with GI upset; this might be reduced by administering the drug with food.

Interactions: Absorption of tetracyclines from the GI tract is decreased by milk and milk products (except for doxycycline and minocycline), antacids, kaolin, and iron preparations. Tetracyclines gradually lose activity when diluted in infusion fluids and exposed to ultraviolet light. Vitamins of the B-complex group, especially riboflavin, hasten this loss of activity in infusion fluids. Tetracyclines also bind to the calcium ions in Ringer's solution.

Methoxyflurane anesthesia combined with tetracycline therapy may be nephrotoxic. Microsomal enzyme inducers such as phenobarbital and phenytoin may shorten the plasma half-lives of minocycline and doxycycline. Except for minocycline and doxycycline, the presence of food can substantially delay absorption of tetracyclines from the GI tract. The tetracyclines are less active in alkaline urine, and urine acidification can increase their antimicrobial efficacy.

Effects on Laboratory Tests: Tetracyclines may increase amylase, BUN, bromsulphthalein (BSP®), eosinophil count, AST, and ALT. Tetracyclines used in combination with diuretics are often associated with a marked rise in BUN. Cholesterol, glucose, potassium, and prothrombin time may be decreased. A false-positive urine glucose test is also possible.

Drug Withdrawal and Milk Discard Times: Regulatory requirements for withdrawal times for food animals and milk discard times vary among countries. These must be followed carefully to prevent food residues and consequent public health implications. The withdrawal times listed in TABLE 46 serve only as general guidelines.

PHENICOLS

Chloramphenicol is a highly effective and well-tolerated broad-spectrum antibiotic. However, because it causes blood

TABLE 46 DRUG WITHDRAWAL AND MILK DISCARD TIMES OF TETRACYCLINES

Tetracycline	Species	Withdrawal Time (days)
Oxytetracycline[a]	Cattle	15–22
	Pigs	22
	Poultry	5
Oxytetracycline (long-acting)[a]	Cattle	28
Chlortetracycline	Cattle	10
	Pigs	1–7

[a] Not for use in lactating dairy cows

dyscrasias, it is prohibited for use in food-producing animals in several countries, including the USA and Canada. Thiamphenicol is less effective but safer than chloramphenicol; florfenicol, a thiamphenicol derivative, is significantly more active in vitro than chloramphenicol against many pathogenic strains of bacteria. Florfenicol is approved for use in cattle.

General Properties

Chloramphenicol is a relatively simple neutral nitrobenzene derivative with a bitter taste. It is highly lipid soluble and is used either as the free base or in ester forms (eg, the neutral-tasting palmitate for administration PO and the water-soluble sodium succinate for parenteral injection). Chloramphenicol is a relatively stable compound and is unaffected by boiling, provided that a pH of 9 is not exceeded. The nitrophenol group of chloramphenicol is replaced by a methyl sulfonyl group for thiamphenicol and florfenicol; florfenicol also contains a fluorine molecule. These structural changes improve efficacy, reduce toxicity, and for florfenicol, the fluorine molecule reduces bacterial resistance.

Antimicrobial Activity

Mode of Action: The phenicols inhibit microbial protein synthesis by binding to the 50S subunit of the 70S ribosome and impairing peptidyl transferase activity. Because peptide-bond formation is inhibited, peptides cannot elongate. The effect is usually bacteriostatic but, at high concentrations, chloramphenicol may be bactericidal for some species. Protein synthesis is inhibited in both prokaryotic and eukaryotic (mitochondrial) ribosomes.

Bacterial Resistance: Resistance against chloramphenicol develops slowly and in a stepwise fashion. In clinical bacterial isolates, high-level plasmid-mediated resistance reflects the production of chloramphenicol acetyltransferase (encoded for by the *cat* gene) and results in acetylation of the molecule, which can no longer bind to the ribosome. Other inactivating enzymes also may be involved. In resistant gram-negative bacteria, chloramphenicol acetyltransferase is a constitutive enzyme; in gram-positive organisms, the enzyme is inducible. The fluorine atom of florfenicol prevents acetylation, thus enhancing the efficacy of this drug. In *Pseudomonas aeruginosa* and in strains of *Proteus* and *Klebsiella* spp, resistance is also nonenzymatic and is based on an inducible permeability block that is both chromosomal and plasmid-mediated. Reduced permeability contributes to low level resistance. Very rarely, resistance may reflect altered ribosomal subunit structure and binding. Resistance to chloramphenicol often develops together with resistance to tetracycline, erythromycin, streptomycin, ampicillin, and other antibiotics because of multiple genes being carried on the same plasmid.

Antimicrobial Spectra: Many genera of gram-positive and gram-negative bacteria and several anaerobes such as *Bacteroides fragilis*, as well as *Rickettsia* and *Chlamydia* spp are susceptible. Chloramphenicol is notable for its anaerobic spectrum. Of special note is the efficacy against many *Salmonella* spp but the resistance of most strains of *P aeruginosa*.

Pharmacokinetic Features

Absorption: Absorption occurs promptly and rapidly from the upper GI tract when chloramphenicol base is administered PO to nonruminant animals. Blood concentrations usually are maximal in 1–3 hr. Because ruminal microflora readily reduce the nitro group, chloramphenicol is inactivated in the ruminoreticulum and is not available for absorption. The larger ester forms of chloramphenicol require hydrolysis by lipases to release the antibiotic for absorption from the GI tract; thus, the systemic availability of chloramphenicol is delayed when the palmitate and other ester preparations are used. Generic inequivalence has been seen with oral dosage forms. The presence of food and intestinal protectants does not interfere with absorption of chloramphenicol, although drugs that depress GI motility do. Florfenicol is rapidly absorbed after administration PO, although milk interferes with absorption.

Chloramphenicol sodium succinate may be injected both IV and IM. However, hydrolysis is required in the body because only free chloramphenicol base is active. The kinetics of this hydrolysis reaction may be slow and incomplete, with considerable individual and species variability. The absorption of chloramphenicol base itself from IM injection sites is notably restricted. For example, in horses, the therapeutic blood concentration of 5 mg/mL is achieved at a dosage of 50 mg/kg body wt, IM, after only 6–8 hr. Chloramphenicol base is absorbed after IP injection. Florfenicol is available as an injectable solution intended for IM use.

Distribution: Approximately 40%–60% of chloramphenicol in plasma is reversibly bound to albumin, and the free fraction readily diffuses into almost all tissues (including the brain); highest concentrations are reached in the kidneys, liver, and bile. Substantial concentrations (~50% of plasma values) are also reached in many body fluids such as the CSF and aqueous humor. Milk concentrations are ~50% those of plasma but may be higher in mastitis. Transplacental diffusion is seen in all species, with concentrations of ~75% being reached in the fetus as compared with the dam. Chloramphenicol does not attain effective concentrations in normal synovial fluid but does so in septic arthritis. The blood-prostate barrier is an exception to the extensive intracorporeal distribution of chloramphenicol, and concentrations in the inflamed prostate are low to nil. Approximately 15%–20% of peak serum concentrations are seen within abscesses. Florfenicol also penetrates most body tissues, although penetration of CSF and aqueous humor is less than that of chloramphenicol. Florfenicol does penetrate the milk of lactating cows.

Biotransformation: Unlike many other antibacterial agents, chloramphenicol undergoes extensive hepatic metabolism. Although some nitroreduction and other phase I reactions occur, free chloramphenicol is biotransformed primarily by glucuronide conjugation. Urinary products after administration of chloramphenicol sodium succinate include inactive forms, mainly the unhydrolyzed sodium succinate and the glucuronide; only 5%–15% appears as biologically active chloramphenicol.

There are several clinical concerns with respect to the biotransformation of chloramphenicol. In cats, a characteristic genetic deficiency in glucuronyl transferase activity leads to plasma half-lives that are often considerably longer than those in other species (eg, cats, 5.1 hr; ponies, 54 min), and dosages need to be adjusted accordingly. Phase I metabolism may also be deficient in cats. Very young animals frequently do not have full microsomal enzyme capabilities, and the plasma half-lives of chloramphenicol in the young (<4 wk old) of many species are often much longer than those of adults. Foals appear to be a notable exception to this generalization. Liver disease also prevents chloramphenicol from undergoing normal metabolic degradation, and active antibiotic accumulates in the body.

Excretion: The principal route of excretion of parent drug (minor) and glucuronide is renal. Free chloramphenicol and the chloramphenicol sodium succinate dosage form undergo glomerular filtration (5%–10%), whereas the glucuronide metabolite is eliminated by tubular secretion (90%–95%). Only 5%–15% of chloramphenicol is present in the urine in the active, unchanged form. The biliary route also plays a part in excretion, but enterohepatic cycling is often pronounced, and usually only a small amount of chloramphenicol is recoverable in feces. Enterohepatic cycling prolongs blood concentrations to some degree in herbivores.

Pharmacokinetic Values: The plasma half-life of chloramphenicol varies among species and depends on age in some species. The specific volumes of distribution usually reflect the extensive diffusion into tissues (*see* TABLE 47). Dose rates and frequencies are typically adjusted for the species and age of the animal. Florfenicol is eliminated by the kidneys.

TABLE 47 ELIMINATION AND DISTRIBUTION OF CHLORAMPHENICOL AND FLORFENICOL

Drug	Species	Elimination Half-life (hr)	Volume of Distribution (mL/kg)
Chloramphenicol	Cats	5.1	2,360
	Dogs	4.2	1,700
	Calves (<1 wk old)	5.0	1,080
	Cattle	3.0	1,580
	Horses	0.9	950
Florfenicol	Cattle	18.3	700

Therapeutic Indications and Dose Rates

Chloramphenicol is used to treat both systemic and local infections. Salmonellosis and *Bacteroides* sepsis have been specific indications, but use of chloramphenicol has decreased in the absence of an easily accessible, commercially available, approved preparation. Florfenicol is approved for use in treatment of bovine respiratory disease.

General dosages for chloramphenicol and florfenicol are listed in TABLE 48. The dose rate and frequency should be adjusted as needed for the individual animal.

Special Clinical Concerns

Adverse Effects and Toxicity: In people, chloramphenicol (but not florfenicol) can produce two distinctive syndromes of bone marrow suppression. One form is characterized by nonregenerative anemia (with or without thrombocytopenia or leukopenia), increased serum iron, bone marrow hypocellularity, cytoplasmic vacuolization of blast cells and lymphocytes, and maturation arrest of erythroid and myeloid precursors. This suppression is dose-dependent and reversible. Daily doses of 50 mg/kg for 3 wk can produce similar effects in cats. Milder hematologic effects are evident in dogs at much higher daily dosages (225 mg/kg). Such blood dyscrasias may also be seen in susceptible neonatal animals given standard adult doses of chloramphenicol. This toxic effect is postulated to be due to interference with mRNA and protein synthesis in rapidly multiplying cells.

The second form of bone marrow suppression is an irreversible aplastic anemia that is not related to dose or duration and may appear after the drug has been discontinued. Peripheral blood showing pancytopenia may be associated with hypoplastic or aplastic bone marrow. The incidence is ~1:25,000–40,000. The aplastic anemia appears to reflect lack of the nitro group and, as such, does not cause aplastic anemia. Because tissue residues in food animals might induce aplastic anemia in people, use of chloramphenicol in food animals is prohibited in the USA and several other countries. A form of aplastic anemia, apparently a type of hypersensitivity reaction to chloramphenicol, has been recognized in dogs and cats.

GI disturbances can develop in all nonruminant animals treated with oral chloramphenicol. Use in neonatal calves leads to a malabsorption syndrome associated with ultrastructural and functional changes of the small-intestinal enterocytes. Anorexia and depression have been seen in cats treated for >1 wk.

Because chloramphenicol can suppress anamnestic immune responses, animals should not be vaccinated while being treated with this antibiotic. Because of the ability of chloramphenicol to inhibit protein synthesis, excessive topical application on wounds may delay healing.

In both male and female rats, chloramphenicol has adversely affected the structure and functions of the gonads. In large animals, adverse signs are most often associated with propylene glycol–based preparations that, when infused rapidly IV, may result in collapse, hemolysis, and death.

Notwithstanding the severity of the chloramphenicol-associated adverse effects noted above, chloramphenicol is relatively safe, provided overdosage is avoided, courses of therapy are limited to 1 wk, the dose is reduced for newborn animals and

TABLE 48 DOSAGES OF CHLORAMPHENICOL AND FLORFENICOL

Drug	Species	Dosage, Route, and Frequency
Chloramphenicol	Cats	45–60 mg/kg, PO, IV, or IM, bid
	Dogs	45–60 mg/kg, PO, IV, or IM, tid-qid
	Horses	50 mg/kg, PO, tid-qid, or IV, every 2–4 hr
Florfenicol	Cattle	20 mg/kg, IM, repeated in 48 hr

for animals with impaired liver function, and there is no evidence of a preexisting bone marrow depression.

Interactions: Chloramphenicol is a potent noncompetitive microsomal enzyme inhibitor that can substantially prolong the duration of action of several drugs administered concurrently. Frank toxic effects are likely if administration is repeated. Examples of such drugs include pentobarbital, codeine, phenobarbital, phenytoin, NSAIDs, and coumarins.

In combination with sulfamethoxypyridazine, chloramphenicol can cause hepatic damage. Chloramphenicol also delays the response of anemia to iron, folic acid, and vitamin B_{12}. It interferes with the actions of many bactericidal drugs, such as the penicillins, cephalosporins, and aminoglycosides, and such combinations should not be used under most circumstances. Aqueous solutions of chloramphenicol sodium succinate should not be mixed with other preparations before administration because of a high incidence of incompatibility.

Chloramphenicol should not be administered concurrently with other antibacterial agents that bind to the 50S ribosomal subunit (eg, the macrolides and lincosamides).

Effects on Laboratory Tests: Chloramphenicol may cause increased alkaline phosphatase concentrations and prothrombin times. WBC and thrombocyte counts may be decreased. Anemia becomes evident in extreme cases. A false glucosuria test is possible.

Drug Withdrawal and Milk Discard Times: The use of chloramphenicol in food animals is prohibited in several countries including the USA; in others, withdrawal times vary considerably and may be as long as 2 wk. Withdrawal time for florfenicol is 28 days. Florfenicol should not be used in dairy cattle ≤20 mo old, veal calves, calves <1 mo old, or calves on an all-milk diet.

MACROLIDES

The macrolide antibiotics typically have a large lactone ring in their structure and are much more effective against gram-positive than gram-negative bacteria. They are also active against mycoplasmas and some rickettsiae. (*See also* POLYENE MACROLIDE ANTIBIOTICS, p 2698.)

Classes

Macrolides fall into three classes, depending on the size of the macrocyclic lactone ring. None of the 12-membered ring group is used clinically. Erythromycin and the closely related oleandomycin and troleandomycin belong to the 14-membered ring group. Azithromycin (synthesized from erythromycin) and gamithromycin are 15-ring members, a subclass referred to as azalides. Of the 16-membered ring group, spiramycin, josamycin, tylosin, and tilmicosin (synthesized from tylosin), are used clinically. Tulathromycin contains three amine rings and is classified as a triamilide. Ketolides, which include tylosin and spiramycin, are closely related macrolides.

General Properties

A macrolide is actually a complex mixture of closely related antibiotics that differ from one another with respect to the chemical substitutions on the various carbon atoms in the structure and in the aminosugars and neutral sugars. For example, erythromycin is mostly erythromycin A, but B, C, D, and E forms may also be included in the preparation.

The macrolide antibiotics are colorless, crystalline substances. They contain a dimethylamino group, which makes them basic. Although they are poorly water soluble, they do dissolve in more polar organic solvents. Macrolides are often inactivated in basic (pH >10) as well as acidic environments (pH <4 for erythromycin). The multiple functional groups make it possible for them to undergo a large number of chemical reactions. More stable ester forms, eg, acetylates, estolates, lactobionate, succinates, propionates, and stearates, are commonly used in pharmaceutical preparations.

Antimicrobial Activity

Mode of Action: The antimicrobial mechanism seems to be the same for all of the macrolides. They interfere with protein synthesis by reversibly binding to the 50S subunit of the ribosome. They appear to bind at the donor site, thus preventing the translocation necessary to keep the peptide chain growing. The effect is essentially confined to rapidly dividing bacteria and mycoplasmas. Macrolides are regarded as being bacteriostatic but demonstrate bactericidal activity at high concentrations. Macrolides are significantly more active at higher pH ranges (7.8–8). Macrolides are considered to be time dependent in terms of antimicrobial efficacy.

The macrolides appear to have immunomodulatory effects useful to treat respiratory infections, in particular, those associated with *Pseudomonas aeruginosa*, based on efficacy at doses (concentrations) considered ineffective against susceptible bacteria.

Bacterial Resistance: Lack of cell wall permeability renders most gram-negative organisms inherently resistant to macrolides. There are a few exceptions, and gram-negative forms without cell walls are usually susceptible. Resistance to macrolides in gram-positive organisms results from alterations in ribosomal structure (target site methylation or mutation) and loss of macrolide affinity. Post-translational methylation results in cross-resistance to lincosamides and streptogramins. Macrolide resistance may be intrinsic or plasmid-mediated and constitutive or inducible; it may develop rapidly (erythromycin) or slowly (tylosin) and generally results in cross-resistance between macrolides. Efflux from cells is a second important mechanism of resistance for some members of this class, as is, less frequently, drug inactivation.

Antimicrobial Spectra: Macrolides are active against most aerobic and anaerobic gram-positive bacteria, although there is considerable variation as to potency and activity. In general, macrolides are not active against gram-negative bacteria, but some strains of *Pasteurella*, *Haemophilus*, and *Neisseria* spp may be sensitive. Exceptions include tilmicosin, gamithromycin, and tulathromycin, for which the spectra are characterized as broader and include *Mannheimia haemolytica* and *Pasteurella multocida*, as well as the above-mentioned gram-negative bacteria. *Helicobacter* also is generally included in the spectrum. Azithromycin, derived from erythromycin, includes *Bordetella* in its spectrum. *Bacteroides fragilis* strains are moderately susceptible to macrolides. Macrolides are active against atypical mycobacteria, *Mycobacterium*, *Mycoplasma*, *Chlamydia*, and *Rickettsia* spp but not against protozoa or fungi. In vitro synergism is seen with cefamandole (against *B fragilis*), ampicillin (against *Nocardia asteroides*), and rifampin (against *Rhodococcus equi*).

Pharmacokinetic Features

Absorption: Macrolides are readily absorbed from the GI tract if not inactivated by gastric acid. Oral preparations are often enteric-coated, or stable salts or esters (such as stearate, lactobionate, glucoheptate, propionate, and ethylsuccinate) are used. Plasma concentrations peak within 1–2 hr in most cases, although absorption patterns may be erratic because of the presence of food and may depend on the salt or ester used. Absorption from the ruminoreticulum is usually delayed and is unreliable. Erythromycin and tylosin may also be administered IV or IM. Tilmicosin, gamithromycin, and tulathromycin are administered SC, except in swine, for which an oral tilmicosin preparation is available. Absorption after injection is rapid, but pain and swelling can develop at the injection sites.

Distribution: Macrolides become widely distributed in tissues, and concentrations are about the same as in plasma, or even higher in some instances. They actually accumulate within many cells, including macrophages, in which they may be ≥20 times the plasma concentration. WBCs will then facilitate distribution to the site of inflammation. This accumulation accounts in part for the long dosing interval that characterizes some macrolides (eg, tilmicosin). With spiramycin, the tissue concentrations remain especially high, even though plasma concentrations are rather low. Macrolides tend to concentrate in the spleen, liver, kidneys, and particularly the lungs. They enter pleural and ascitic fluids and concentrate in the eye but do not distribute to the eye or the CSF (only 2%–13% of plasma concentration unless the meninges are inflamed). They concentrate in the bile and milk. Up to 75% of the dose is bound to plasma proteins, and they bind to α1-acid glycoproteins rather than to albumin.

Biotransformation: Metabolic inactivation of the macrolides is usually extensive, but the relative proportion depends on the route of administration and the particular antibiotic. After administration PO, 80% of an erythromycin dose undergoes metabolic inactivation, whereas tylosin appears to be eliminated in an active form.

Excretion: Macrolide antibiotics and their metabolites are excreted mainly in bile (>60%) and often undergo enterohepatic cycling. Urinary clearance may be slow and variable (often <10%) but may represent a more significant route of elimination after parenteral administration. For example, in people, 14% of azithromycin and 20%–40% of clarithromycin is excreted unchanged in urine. The concentration of macrolides in milk often is several times greater than in plasma, especially in mastitis.

Pharmacokinetic Values: Macrolides tend to be characterized by high oral bioavailability, but this is variable among species, drugs, and salts. For example, oral bioavailability for tylosin is 0.35 for the tartrate salt versus 0.14 for the phosphate. For azithromycin, oral bioavailability is 39% in foals 6–10 wk old, 59% in cats, and 97% in dogs. The accumulation of macrolides among different tissues contributes to the large volume of distribution (for azithromycin 12 L/kg in dogs, 23 L/kg in cats, 22 L/kg in foals 6–10 wk old) and long elimination half-life (for azithromycin, 29 hr in dogs, 35 hr in cats, and 20 hr in foals). For tulathromycin, the elimination half-life is 65 hr in calves and 69 hr in pigs 2–3 mo old. Because of these long half-lives, time to steady state may be prolonged, and a loading dose may be indicated for multiple dosing. Tylosin, however, is an exception, with a volume of distribution approximating 1 L/kg and a half-life of 1–2 hr. Another exception is azithromycin, which has a half-life in cats that varies among tissues, reaching >72 hr for some. Effective plasma inhibitory concentrations are maintained for ~8 hr after administration PO and for ~12–24 hr after IM injection. Dosage frequencies are commonly 2–3 times/day, PO, or 1–2 times/day, parenterally.

Therapeutic Indications and Dose Rates

The macrolides are used to treat both systemic and local infections. They are often regarded as alternatives to penicillins for treatment of streptococcal and staphylococcal infections. General indications include upper respiratory tract infections, bronchopneumonia, bacterial enteritis, metritis, pyodermatitis, urinary tract infections, arthritis, and others. Macrolides are indicated for treatment of *Rhodococcus* respiratory tract infections in foals. Formulations to treat mastitis are also available and often have the advantage of a short withholding time for milk. Tilmicosin, gamithromycin, and tulathromycin are approved for use in treatment of bovine respiratory diseases associated with *Mannheimia haemolytica*, *Pasteurella multocida*, and *Histophilus somni*. In swine, tilmicosin phosphate is added to feed or water for control of swine respiratory disease.

A selection of general dosages for some macrolides is listed in TABLE 49. The dose rate and frequency should be adjusted as needed for the individual animal.

Special Clinical Concerns

Adverse Effects and Toxicity: Toxicity and adverse effects are uncommon for most macrolides (except tilmicosin), although pain and swelling may develop at injection sites. Hypersensitivity reactions have occasionally been seen. Erythromycin estolate may be hepatotoxic and cause cholestasis; it may also induce vomiting and diarrhea, particularly when high doses are administered. Horses are sensitive to macrolide-induced GI disturbances that can be serious and even fatal. In pigs, tylosin may cause edema of the rectal mucosa, mild anal protrusion with diarrhea, and anal erythema and pruritus. After 5 mg/kg/day, dogs had a greater tendency to develop ventricular tachycardia and fibrillation during acute myocardial ischemia. Tilmicosin is characterized by cardiac toxicity (tachycardia and decreased contractility). Parenteral (but not oral) administration should be avoided in swine, and extra-label use should be avoided. Cattle have died after IV injection of tilmicosin, and human injury is possible after accidental exposure.

Interactions: Macrolide antibiotics probably should not be used with chloramphenicol or the lincosamides, because they may compete for the same 50S ribosomal binding site, although the in vivo significance of this potential interaction is unclear. Activity of macrolides is depressed in acidic environments. Macrolide preparations for

TABLE 49 DOSAGES OF MACROLIDES

Macrolide	Species	Dosage, Route, and Frequency
Erythromycin	Cattle	8–15 mg/kg, IM, once to twice daily
	Cats	15 mg/kg, PO, tid
	Foals	25 mg/kg, IM, tid
Tylosin	Cattle	10–20 mg/kg, IM, once to twice daily
	Pigs	10 mg/kg, IM, once to twice daily
		7–10 mg/kg, PO, tid
	Cats	10 mg/kg, IM, bid
Tilmicosin	Cattle	10 mg/kg, SC, once
Tulathromycin	Cattle	2.5 mg/kg, SC, once
	Swine	2.5 mg/kg, IM, once
Gamithromycin	Cattle	6 mg/kg, SC, once
Azithromycin	Dogs	5–10 mg/kg, PO, once to twice daily

parenteral administration are incompatible with many other pharmaceutical preparations. Erythromycin and troleandomycin and other macrolides are microsomal enzyme inhibitors that depress CYP3A4 (in people) and thus the metabolism of many drugs. Macrolides also are substrates for and potentially potent inhibitors of P-glycoprotein efflux pumps.

Effects on Laboratory Tests: Alkaline phosphatase, bilirubin, bromsulphthalein (BSP®), total WBC count, eosinophil count, AST, and ALT may increase. Cholesterol concentrations may decrease.

Drug Withdrawal and Milk Discard Times: Regulatory requirements for withdrawal times and milk discard times vary among countries. These should be followed carefully to prevent food residues and consequent public health implications. The withdrawal times listed in TABLE 50 serve only as general guidelines. Tilmicosin is characterized by a 28-day withdrawal time and should not be used in any species other than adult cattle (but not in dairy cows >20 mo old).

STREPTOGRAMINS

The streptogramin antibiotics include two distinct groups. Group A contain a 23-membered unsaturated ring with lactone and peptide bonds, and group B are depsipeptides (lactone-cyclized peptides). These antibiotics are included in the macrolide-lincosamide-streptogramin (MLS) group. However, whereas the individual A and B components act in a bacteriostatic fashion when used as sole agents, together the affinity for the ribosome is enhanced, causing them to be bactericidal. Streptogramins include virginiamycin. Streptogramins are used to treat vancomycin-resistant staphylococci and *Enterococcus faecium*.

LINCOSAMIDES

General Properties

Lincosamides are derivatives of an amino acid and a sulfur-containing octose. They are monobasic and more stable in salt forms (hydrochlorides and phosphates).

Antimicrobial Activity

Mode of Action: Lincomycin and clindamycin bind exclusively to the 50S subunit of bacterial ribosomes and suppress protein synthesis. Lincosamides, macrolides, and chloramphenicol, although not structurally related, seem to act at this same site. The lincosamides are bacteriostatic or bactericidal depending on the concentration. Activity is enhanced at an alkaline pH. Efficacy is considered time dependent.

Bacterial Resistance: Lincosamides are generally ineffective against facultative anaerobic (but not anaerobic) gram-negative bacteria. Resistance to lincosamides appears slowly, perhaps as a result of

TABLE 50 DRUG WITHDRAWAL AND MILK DISCARD TIMES OF MACROLIDES

Macrolide	Species	Withdrawal Time (days)	Milk Discard Time (hr)
Erythromycin	Cattle	14	36–72
	Pigs	7	
Tylosin	Cattle	21	96
	Pigs	14	
Tilmicosin	Cattle	28	0
Tulathromycin	Cattle	18	
	Swine	5	
Gamithromycin	Cattle	63[a]	

[a] EU withdrawal; withdrawal period for USA (35 days) pending; withdrawal period for Canada is 49 days.

chromosomal mutation. Plasmid-mediated resistance has been found in strains of *Bacteroides fragilis*. Resistance appears to be due to plasmid or chromosomally mediated post-transcriptional methylation of the 50S ribosomal subunit. Cross-resistance occurs with macrolides and streptogramins. Other mechanisms include increased activation of an efflux pump and destruction of the drug.

Antimicrobial Spectra: Lincomycin has a limited spectrum against aerobic pathogens but a fairly broad spectrum against anaerobes. Clindamycin is a more active analogue with somewhat different pharmacokinetic patterns. Many gram-positive cocci, except for enterococci, and *Mycoplasma* are inhibited by lincosamides, but most gram-negative organisms are resistant. Clindamycin is less effective toward ureaplasmas. *Bacteroides* spp and other anaerobes are usually susceptible. *Clostridium difficile* strains appear to be regularly resistant.

Pharmacokinetic Features

Absorption: Lincomycin is incompletely absorbed from the GI tract, especially if administered soon after feeding; plasma concentrations peak within 2–4 hr. Absorption from IM injection sites is good; plasma concentrations peak in 1–2 hr. Approximately 90% of an oral dose of clindamycin is absorbed, and effective plasma concentrations are achieved more rapidly than with lincomycin. Absorption is not significantly affected by the ingestion of food. Clindamycin palmitate is used PO, and clindamycin phosphate IM; the latter reaches peak plasma concentration in 1–3 hr.

Distribution: Lincosamides are widely distributed in many fluids and tissues, including bone, but significant concentrations are not attained in the CSF even when the meninges are inflamed. They diffuse across the placenta in many species. Approximately 90% of clindamycin is bound to plasma proteins. It also accumulates in polymorphonuclear WBCs and alveolar macrophages such that concentrations exceed those of plasma 50-fold. Clindamycin is able to penetrate glycocalyx, such as that associated with dental tartar.

Biotransformation: After administration PO, ~50% of a dose of lincomycin and 80%–90% of a dose of clindamycin are metabolically altered in the liver. Metabolites often retain activity. Liver disease impairs the biotransformation of lincosamides.

Excretion: Unchanged antibiotic and several metabolites may be excreted in bile and urine. In people, as little as 10% of clindamycin is excreted in the urine. The proportions depend on the route of administration. Concentrations remain high in the feces for some days, and growth of sensitive microorganisms in the large intestine may be suppressed for up to 2 wk. Milk is also an important excretory route.

Pharmacokinetic Values: The elimination half-life of lincosamides is frequently >3 hr, and the apparent volume of distribution is >1 L/kg. They are usually administered bid. In dogs, clindamycin has an elimination half-life of 3.9 hr and a volume of distribution of 1.4 L/kg.

Therapeutic Indications and Dose Rates

The lincosamides are indicated for infections caused by susceptible gram-positive organisms, particularly streptococci and staphylococci, and for those caused by anaerobic pathogens. Clindamycin is approved for use in cats and dogs for treatment of infected wounds, abscesses, and dental infections. Clindamycin has also been used to treat selected protozoal diseases, including toxoplasmosis, but usually in combination with other antimicrobials.

A selection of general dosages for some lincosamides is listed in TABLE 51. The dose rate and frequency should be adjusted as needed for the individual animal.

Special Clinical Concerns

Adverse Effects and Toxicity: No serious organ toxicity has been reported, but GI disturbances do occur. Clindamycin-induced pseudomembranous enterocolitis (caused by toxigenic *Clostridium difficile*) or disruption of GI flora is a serious adverse reaction in a number of species and can be lethal; thus, clindamycin is contraindicated for use in some in horses, guinea pigs, hamsters, rabbits, chinchillas, and ruminants. Lincosamides are contraindicated in horses, because severe and even fatal colitis may develop. Skeletal muscle paralysis may be seen at high concentrations. Hypersensitivity reactions occasionally are seen. Lincosamides should not be used in neonates because of their limited ability to metabolize drugs.

Interactions: Lincosamides have additive neuromuscular effects with anesthetic agents and skeletal muscle relaxants. Kaolin-pectin prevents their absorption from the GI tract. They should not be combined with bactericidal agents or with the macrolides.

Effects on Laboratory Tests: Alkaline phosphatase, AST, and ALT may be increased.

Drug Withdrawal Times: In several countries, there is a 2-day withdrawal time for pigs.

MISCELLANEOUS ANTIMICROBIAL AGENTS

A number of antimicrobial agents are used periodically for several diverse purposes. Several of these are discussed below.

POLYMYXINS

This group of polypeptide antibiotics includes polymyxin B and polymyxin E, or colistin. Because of toxicity, these drugs are most commonly used topically, or PO for treatment of intestinal infections. Colistimethate is a form of colistin intended for parenteral administration. Polymyxins are bactericidal; they interact strongly with phospholipids in bacterial cell membranes and radically disrupt their permeability and function. The polymyxins are more effective against gram-negative than gram-positive bacteria. Their rather narrow spectrum includes *Enterobacter*, *Klebsiella*, *Salmonella*, *Pasteurella*, *Bordetella*, *Shigella*, *Pseudomonas* spp, and *Escherichia coli*. Most *Proteus* or *Neisseria* spp are not susceptible. Although intrinsic bacterial resistance to polymyxins is recognized, resistance is uncommon and is chromosome-dependent only. Polymyxins act synergistically when combined with potentiated sulfonamides, tetracyclines,

TABLE 51 DOSAGES OF LINCOSAMIDES

Lincosamide	Species	Dosage, Route, and Frequency
Lincomycin	Cattle	10 mg/kg, IM, bid
	Pigs	10 mg/kg, IM, bid 7 mg/kg, in-feed
	Dogs	20 mg/kg/day, PO
	Cats	10 mg/kg, IM, bid 25 mg/kg, PO, bid
Clindamycin	Dogs, cats	5–10 mg/kg, PO, bid

and some other antibacterials; they also reduce the activity of endotoxins in body fluids and may be beneficial in endotoxemia. Their action is inhibited by divalent cations, unsaturated fatty acids, and quaternary ammonium compounds.

Polymyxins are not absorbed after PO or topical administration; plasma concentrations peak ~2 hr after parenteral administration. Blood concentrations usually are low, because polymyxins bind to cell membranes as well as tissue debris and purulent exudates. The polymixins undergo renal elimination mostly as degradation products, and their plasma half-lives are 3–6 hr. They are notably nephrotoxic and neurotoxic and, as such, systemic therapy at antimicrobial doses should be avoided. Neuromuscular blockade can be seen at higher concentrations. Intense pain at sites of injection and hypersensitivity reactions also can be expected. Polymyxin B is a potent histamine releaser. The main indication for parenteral use of polymyxins is life-threatening infection due to gram-negative bacilli or *Pseudomonas* spp that are resistant to other drugs. Polymyxins are also used PO against susceptible intestinal infections. Anti-endotoxin binding activity is an additional therapy via slow IV bolus. Topical application is common, eg, for otitis externa.

Recommended dose rates for polymyxins vary considerably. A general guideline is 20,000 U/kg, PO, bid; 5,000 U/kg, IM, bid; 50,000–100,000 U by intramammary infusion; 100,000 U intrauterine in cattle. IV administration of polymyxins is potentially dangerous.

BACITRACINS

Bacitracins are branched, cyclic, decapeptide antibiotics. Bacitracin A is the most active of the group and the main component of the commercial bacitracin preparations used either topically or PO. These antibiotics are bactericidal. They interfere with cell membrane function, suppress cell wall formation by preventing the formation of peptidoglycan strands, and inhibit protein synthesis. Bactericidal activity requires the presence of divalent cations, such as zinc.

The spectrum of bacitracins is described as broad, but it is used primarily to treat gram-positive infections. Resistance is rare. Bacitracins are often used in combination with neomycin and polymyxins to enhance the antibacterial spectrum.

Bacitracins are not appreciably absorbed from the GI tract and are not used systemically because of their pronounced nephrotoxicity. However, they are used locally in wound powders and ointments, dermatologic preparations, eye and ear ointments, and as feed additives in swine and poultry rations for growth promotion. In antibiotic-associated pseudomembranous colitis caused by *Clostridium difficile* cytotoxin, bacitracin (given PO) is considered an alternative to vancomycin. Hypersensitivity reactions to bacitracins are seen occasionally.

GLYCOPEPTIDES

Vancomycin is a complex glycopeptide that binds to precursors of the peptidoglycan layer in bacterial cell walls. This effect prevents cell wall synthesis and produces a rapid bactericidal effect in dividing bacteria. Its efficacy is time dependent. Vancomycin is active against most gram-positive bacteria but is not effective against gram-negative cells because of their large size and poor penetrability. Resistance to vancomycin does not readily develop. The drug is widely distributed in the body. Excretion (in active form) is via the kidneys; in renal insufficiency, striking accumulations may develop. The plasma half-life in dogs is 2–3 hr. The only indication for use of parenteral vancomycin is serious infection due to methicillin-resistant *Staphylococcus aureus*. Although poorly absorbed, oral vancomycin is used to treat antibiotic-associated enterocolitis, especially if caused by *Clostridium difficile*. Febrile reactions and thrombophlebitis (because of tissue irritation) at injection sites may be seen. Hypersensitivity reactions are seen infrequently. Ototoxicity and nephrotoxicity were fairly common in the past but are rare today because of fewer impurities in the final form.

FOSFOMYCIN

Fosfomycin, a phosphonic acid that contains a carbon-phosphorus bond, is a natural antibiotic produced by *Streptomyces fradiae*. It is a phosphoenolpyruvate analogue that irreversibly inhibits phosphoenolpyruvate transferase, an enzyme that catalyzes the first step of peptidoglycan synthesis of microbial cell walls. Its in vitro spectrum is broad, with potential efficacy toward isolates expressing multidrug resistance, including *Escherichia coli* and methicillin-resistant staphylococci. As a cell wall inhibitor, fosfomycin is bactericidal when present at the site of infection at therapeutic concentrations. Cell wall inhibition is time dependent, but fosfomycin also exhibits a concentration-dependent effect. Resistance to fosfomycin is uncommon and reflects the FosX or FosA enzyme, which hydrolyzes the drug. The gene for this protein is chromosomally mediated. When resistance occurs, it generally is not associated with multidrug resistance. Studies in people have demonstrated that fosfomycin distributes well to soft tissues, reaching therapeutic breakpoints. Adverse effects of fosfomycin appear to be limited to diarrhea. Approved for human use in the USA as the tromethamine salt, its indication is as a one time (or up to 3 days) treatment of uncomplicated urinary tract infections in people. Fosfomycin has been added to the World Health Organization's list of critically important drugs. Accordingly, its use should be reserved, along with other critically important drugs, to situations in which lower-tier drugs are no longer appropriate.

NOVOBIOCIN SODIUM

Novobiocin is a narrow-spectrum antibiotic that may be bacteriostatic or bactericidal at higher concentrations. It is active mostly against gram-positive bacteria but also against a few gram-negative bacteria. There is a synergistic effect with tetracyclines. Many species of bacteria can develop resistance to novobiocin. Adverse reactions are quite frequent after administration. Its main use is in combination with other agents for treatment of bovine mastitis.

TIAMULIN FUMARATE

Tiamulin hydrogen fumarate is a semisynthetic derivative of pleuromutilin. Tiamulin is active against gram-positive bacteria, mycoplasmas, and anaerobes, including *Brachyspira hyodysenteriae*. It is also clinically effective in treatment of swine dysentery and mycoplasmal arthritis. Tiamulin is well absorbed when administered PO. The dosage is 8.8 mg/kg/day for 3–5 days, in either food or water. The parenteral dosage for mycoplasmal pneumonia in pigs is 15 mg/kg. In poultry, tiamulin interferes with monensin and salinomycin metabolism, and if the drugs are fed together, they become toxic. Generally, however, tiamulin has few adverse effects.

IONOPHORES

Ionophores are lipid-soluble molecules that transport ions across lipid cell membranes. The subsequent disruption of cell membrane permeability results in antibacterial effects. Monensin is an ionophore antibiotic derived from *Streptomyces* that forms complexes with monovalent cations, including sodium and potassium. The complexes are transported in a nonpolar manner across the bacterial cell membrane. As such, it acts as an Na^+/H^+ antiporter. Monensin blocks intracellular protein transport, resulting in antibacterial and antimalarial effects. Monensin is used extensively in the beef and dairy industries in feed to prevent coccidiosis and improve feed efficiency. Monensin also increases the production of propionic acid and thus prevents bloat.

RIFAMYCINS

Several semisynthetic derivatives (rifamycin SV, rifampin [rifampicin], rifamide) of natural rifamycins have been used as extended-spectrum antibiotics. Rifamycins interfere with the synthesis of RNA in microorganisms by binding to subunits of sensitive DNA-dependent RNA polymerase. They are active against gram-positive organisms, some mycobacteria, a few strains of gram-negative bacteria (mostly cocci; bacilli are more resistant), some anaerobes, and chlamydiae. At high concentrations, they are also active against several viruses. Fungal and yeast infections resistant to rifampin alone often respond when a rifamycin is added to an antifungal agent (eg, amphotericin B). Resistance to rifamycins may develop rapidly as a 1-step process. For this reason, they should be administered in combination with other antimicrobials, such as penicillins, erythromycin, miconazole, and amphotericin B.

The primary use of the rifamycins in people has been to treat tuberculosis. Rifampin has been used in foals to control *Rhodococcus equi* pneumonia. Because rifamycins penetrate tissues and cells to a substantial degree, they are particularly effective against intracellular organisms. Rifampin is readily but incompletely (~40%) absorbed from the GI tract, and plasma concentrations peak within 2–4 hr. Concurrent feeding may reduce or delay absorption. Rifampin may also be administered IM or IV. Approximately 75%–80% of rifampin is bound to plasma proteins. It is widely distributed in body tissues and fluids because of its high lipid solubility. Rifampin is biotransformed to several metabolites, some of which are active, and is primarily excreted in bile (used for cholangitis in people) and to a lesser degree in urine. Enterohepatic cycling of the parent drug and its main metabolite (desacetylrifampin) commonly occurs. The elimination half-life of rifampin is dose dependent: in horses, it is ~6 hr; in dogs, ~8 hr. The plasma half-life progressively shortens by ~40% during the first 2 wk of treatment because of the induction of hepatic microsomal enzymes; conversely, it is increased with hepatic dysfunction.

Rifampin is usually well tolerated and produces few adverse effects. GI disturbances and abnormalities in liver function (icterus) have been reported in people. Hypersensitivity reactions can also result from rifampin administration, and renal failure is a possible consequence when intermittent dosage schedules are followed. Partial, reversible immunosuppression of lymphocytes develops. Urine, feces, saliva, sputum, sweat, and tears are often colored red-orange by rifampin and its metabolites. CNS depression after IV administration and temporary inappetence are seen in horses. The dose range for rifampin in horses is 10–25 mg/kg/day, PO or parenterally.

NITROFURANS

Nitrofurans are synthetic chemotherapeutic agents with a broad antimicrobial spectrum; they are active against both gram-positive and gram-negative bacteria, including *Salmonella* and *Giardia* spp, trichomonads, amebae, and some coccidial species. However, when compared with other antimicrobial chemotherapeutic agents, their potency is not of particular note. The nitrofurans appear to inhibit a number of microbial enzyme systems, including those involved in carbohydrate metabolism, and they also block the initiation of translation. However, their basic mechanism of action has not yet been clarified. Their primary action is bacteriostatic, but at high doses they are also bactericidal. They are much more active in acidic environments (pH 5.5 is optimal for nitrofurantoin activity). Resistant mutants are rare, and clinical resistance emerges slowly. Among themselves, nitrofurans show complete cross-resistance, but there is no cross-resistance with any other antibacterial agents.

Because of very slight water solubility, the nitrofurans are used either PO or topically. No nitrofuran is effective systemically. They are either not absorbed at all from the GI tract or are so rapidly eliminated that they reach inhibitory concentrations only in the urine. Toxic signs seen with excessive doses of nitrofuran derivatives include CNS involvement (excitement, tremors, convulsions, peripheral neuritis), GI disturbances, poor weight gain, and depression of spermatogenesis. Various hypersensitivity reactions can also be seen. Some nitrofurans are carcinogenic, and their future use is in doubt.

Nitrofurans are among the drugs for which extra-label use is prohibited in food animals in the USA.

Nitrofurantoin

The mechanism of action of nitrofurantoin is unique. It is reduced by bacterial flavoproteins to reactive intermediates that inhibit bacterial ribosomes and other macromolecules. Protein synthesis, aerobic energy metabolism, DNA and RNA synthesis, and cell wall synthesis are inhibited. Nitrofurantoin is bactericidal in urine at therapeutic doses. Resistance is rare. Nitrofurantoin is used to treat urinary tract infections caused by susceptible bacteria, such as *Escherichia coli*, *Staphylococcus aureus*, *Streptococcus pyogenes*, and *Aerobacter aerogenes*. *Proteus* spp, *Pseudomonas aeruginosa*, and *Streptococcus faecalis* are usually resistant. After administration PO, nitrofurantoin is rapidly and completely absorbed (the macrocrystal form takes longer) and is swiftly eliminated by the kidneys, mainly by tubular secretion (~40% in the unchanged form). Serum concentrations are low, and little unbound drug is available for diffusion into the tissues. The plasma half-life is only ~20 min. Nitrofurantoin is concentrated in acid urine. When the pH reaches ~5, the drug becomes supersaturated without precipitation, and its antibacterial action is maximal. Nitrofurantoin can be administered PO or parenterally. The dosage for dogs and cats is 4.4 mg/kg, PO, tid for 4–10 days. Adverse effects are not common at usual dosages, but nausea, vomiting, and diarrhea can develop. CNS disorders have been seen, and polyneuropathy is a serious effect seen in people. Animals with decreased renal function have a predisposition for polyneuritis. Various manifestations of hypersensitivity reactions can be seen. Yellow discoloration of teeth occasionally has been reported in very young animals.

Nitrofurazone

Nitrofurazone is only slightly soluble in water but, in general, corresponds to nitrofurantoin in terms of its mechanism of action, antimicrobial spectrum, potency, and physicochemical characteristics. Its main indications include the treatment of bovine mastitis, bovine metritis, and wounds. However, pus, blood, and milk reduce the antibacterial activity. Nitrofurazone is also used as a feed additive (0.05%) to control intestinal bacterial and coccidial infections. The withdrawal time for nitrofurazone in pigs is 5 days.

Furazolidone

This is a nitrofuran with a wide range of antimicrobial activity that includes *Clostridium*, *Salmonella*, *Shigella*, *Staphylococcus* and *Streptococcus* spp, and *E coli*. It is also active against *Eimeria* and *Histomonas* spp. It is usually administered PO to treat intestinal infections but may also be applied topically. The usual oral dose of furazolidone in calves is 10–12 mg/kg, bid for 5–7 days. Caution should be exercised when treating small calves (eg, Jersey breed) to avoid excessive dose rates, lest neurotoxicity result; signs include head tremors, ataxia, visual impairment, and convulsions.

Miscellaneous Nitrofurans

Nifuraldezone, like furazolidone, is used to control bacterial enteritis in calves. Nifurprazine is used only topically as an antibacterial agent. Furaltadone is used both PO to prevent intestinal infections and directly into the teat to treat mastitis.

NITROIMIDAZOLES

The 5-nitroimidazoles are a group of drugs that have both antiprotozoal and antibacterial activity. Nitroimidazoles with activity against trichomonads and amebae include metronidazole, tinidazole, nimorazole, flunidazole, and ronidazole. Metronidazole and nimorazole are effective in treatment of giardiasis, whereas dimetridazole, ipronidazole, and ronidazole control histomoniasis in poultry. Several nitroimidazoles have activity against trypanosomes. Metronidazole, ronidazole, and other nitroimidazoles are active against anaerobic bacteria. Metronidazole is the compound that has been the most studied and is discussed as the prototype of the group. Extra-label use of nitroimidazoles is prohibited in food animals in the USA.

Metronidazole

Metronidazole has been used for many years in therapeutic management of trichomoniasis, giardiasis, and amebiasis. It is active against obligate anaerobic bacteria. It is not active against facultative anaerobes, obligate aerobes, or microaerophilic bacteria other than *Campylobacter fetus*. At concentrations readily attained in serum after PO or parenteral administration, metronidazole is active against *Bacteroides fragilis*, *B melaninogenicus*, *Fusobacterium* spp, and *Clostridium perfringens* and other *Clostridium* spp. It is generally less active against nonsporeforming, gram-positive bacilli such as *Actinomyces*, *Propionibacterium*, *Bifidobacterium*, and *Eubacterium* spp. Metronidazole is also somewhat less active against gram-positive cocci such as *Peptostreptococcus* and *Peptococcus* spp, but the less sensitive strains are usually not obligate anaerobes.

Metronidazole is bactericidal at concentrations equal to or slightly higher than the minimal inhibitory concentration. The precise mode of action is unclear, but reduction in an anaerobic environment yields a compound that then binds to DNA, causing loss of the helical structure, strand breakage, and impairment of DNA function. Only susceptible organisms (bacteria and protozoa) appear to be capable of metabolizing the drug.

The pharmacokinetic pattern of metronidazole generally follows that expected of a highly lipid-soluble basic drug. It is readily but variably absorbed from the GI tract (bioavailability 60%–100%), with serum concentrations peaking within 1–2 hr, and becomes widely distributed in all tissues. Metronidazole penetrates the blood-brain barrier and also attains therapeutic concentrations in abscesses and in empyema fluid. It is only slightly bound to plasma proteins. Biotransformation is quite extensive, and parent drug and metabolites are excreted by both the renal and biliary routes. The elimination half-life in dogs is ~4.5 hr, and in horses, 1.5–3.3 hr.

The principal clinical indications for metronidazole include the treatment of specific protozoal infections (amebiasis, trichomoniasis, giardiasis, and balantidiasis) and anaerobic bacterial infections such as those that may be seen in abdominal abscesses, peritonitis, empyema, genital tract infections, periodontitis, otitis media, osteitis, arthritis, and meningitis, and in necrotic tissue. Metronidazole has been successfully used to prevent infection after colonic surgery. Nitroimidazoles also act as radiosensitizers, and metronidazole has been used as an adjunct to the radiotherapy of solid tumors.

Adverse effects are not commonly associated with metronidazole. High doses may induce signs of neurotoxicity in dogs, such as tremors, muscle spasms, ataxia, and even convulsions. Reversible bone marrow depression has been reported. The drug should not be used in pregnant animals, particularly during the first trimester, although the evidence for carcinogenicity and mutagenicity is still tenuous. Metronidazole may produce a reddish brown discoloration of the urine due to unidentified pigments.

Recommended dose rates for metronidazole in dogs are 44 mg/kg, PO, followed by 22 mg/kg, qid, for anaerobic infections; 25 mg/kg, PO, bid, for giardiasis; and 66 mg/kg/day, PO, for trichomoniasis. Courses of therapy are generally 5–7 days. Both PO and IV preparations are available.

HYDROXYQUINOLINES

The 8-hydroxyquinolines are a group of synthetic compounds with antibacterial, antifungal, and antiprotozoal activity. The best-known compounds of this class are iodochlorhydroxyquin (clioquinol), diiodohydroxyquin (iodoquinol), broxyquinoline, and hydroxyquinoline. Because they are not absorbed from the GI tract to any degree, their main use has been to treat intestinal infections caused by bacteria or protozoa (such as *Giardia*). Hydroxyquinolines are also used topically for skin infections caused by bacteria and fungi. Hydroxyquinolines are potentially neurotoxic when used for prolonged periods. The dose for a 455-kg horse is 10 g/day, PO, using a decreasing dosage regimen to discontinue medication.

ANTIFUNGAL AGENTS

Pathogenic fungi affecting animals are eukaryotes, generally existing as either filamentous molds (hyphal forms) or intracellular yeasts. Fungal organisms are characterized by a low invasiveness and virulence. Factors that contribute to fungal infection include necrotic tissue, a moist environment, and immunosuppression. Fungal infections can be primarily superficial and irritating (eg, dermatophytosis) or systemic and life threatening (eg, blastomycosis, cryptococcosis, histoplasmosis, coccidioidomycosis). *See also* DERMATOPHYTOSIS, p 872, and FUNGAL INFECTIONS, p 632. Clinically relevant dimorphic fungi grow as yeast-like forms in a host but as molds in vitro at room temperature; they include *Candida* spp, *Blastomyces dermatitidis*, *Coccidioides immitis*, *Histoplasma capsulatum*, *Sporothrix schenckii*, and *Rhinosporidium*.

Several factors can lead to therapeutic failure or relapse after antifungal therapy. Drug access to fungal targets is often compromised. Host inflammatory response may be the first barrier, followed by location in sanctuaries (brain, eye, etc) as a second barrier for some infections, and the organisms themselves as a third barrier. The fungal cell wall is rigid and contains chitin, which along with polysaccharides, acts as a barrier to drug penetration. The cell membrane contains sterols such as ergosterol, which influences the efficacy and potential resistance to some drugs. *Cryptococcus* and occasionally *Sporothrix schenckii* produce an external coating or slime layer that encapsulates the cells and causes them to adhere and clump together. Finally, regarding drug access, most infections are located inside host cells, the lipid membrane of which can present a final barrier.

Discontinuing therapy after clinical signs have resolved but before infection is eradicated also leads to therapeutic failure. Therapy should extend well beyond clinical cure. Once drugs reach the site of action, therapeutic success is impeded by the nature of fungal infections. Fungal growth is slow, yet most antifungal drugs work better in rapidly growing organisms. Likewise, most antifungal agents are fungistatic in action, with clearance of infection largely dependent on host response. As such, the duration of therapy is long, and the "get in quick, hit hard, and get out quick" recommendation for antibacterial therapy is not appropriate for antifungal therapy; care must be taken to not discontinue therapy too early. However, longer duration of therapy contributes to another common cause of therapeutic failure: host toxicity. Because both the antifungal target organism and the host cells are eukaryotic, the cellular targets of fungal organisms are often similar to the host structures. Therefore, as a class, antifungal drugs tend to be more toxic than antibacterial drugs, and the number of antifungal drugs approved for use are markedly fewer than the number of antibacterial drugs. Drugs that can be used locally (including topically) or characterized by distribution to sites of infection (eg, liposomal products) may decrease this risk. The slow growth that characterizes fungal infections means that acquired resistance occurs less commonly than in bacterial infections. Therapeutic failure may also reflect the inability of the immunocompromised host to overcome residual fungal populations inhibited by the drug; those antifungals that are also (positive) immunomodulators may be more effective.

A number of serious systemic fungal diseases are well recognized in several parts of the world (*see* p 632). Antifungal agents have greatly reduced previously recorded human mortality rates due to systemic mycoses. A relatively narrow selection of drugs is used in these cases.

POLYENE MACROLIDE ANTIBIOTICS

Amphotericin B is the model polyene macrolide antibiotic and is the sole member of this class used systemically. Polyene antifungal antibiotics are large molecules, consisting of a long polyene, lipid-soluble component and a markedly hydrophilic component. Amphotericin B acts as both a weak base and a weak acid, and as such is amphoteric. The polyene macrolides have been isolated from various strains of bacteria; amphotericin B is an antibiotic product of *Streptomyces nodosus*. Amphotericin B, nystatin, and pimaricin (natamycin) are the only polyene macrolide antibiotics used in veterinary medicine. The polyenes are poorly soluble in water and the common organic solvents. They are reasonably soluble in highly polar solvents such as dimethylformamide and dimethyl sulfoxide. In combination with bile salts, such as sodium deoxycholate, amphotericin B is readily soluble (micellar suspension) in 5% glucose. This colloidal preparation has been used for IV infusion. The polyenes are unstable in aqueous, acidic, or alkaline media but in the dry state, in the absence of heat and light, they remain stable for indefinite periods. They should be administered parenterally (diluted in 5% dextrose) as freshly prepared aqueous suspensions. Lack of stability indicates that labeled expiration dates should be adhered to once the product is diluted. Amphotericin B is also prepared as liposomal and lipid-based preparations, enhancing its safety without loss of efficacy.

Antifungal Activity

Mode of Action: The polyenes bind to sterol components in the phospholipid-sterol membranes of fungal cells to form complexes that induce physical changes in the membrane. The number of conjugated bonds and the molecular size of a particular polyene macrolide influence its affinity for different sterols in fungal cell membranes. Amphotericin B has a greater affinity for fungal ergosterol, the major sterol in fungal membranes, than for eukaryotic (host) cell membrane cholesterol. The long polyene structure causes the formation of channels in the fungal cell membrane. The resultant loss of membrane permeability results in the loss of critically important molecules. Potassium ion efflux from the fungal cell and hydrogen ion influx cause internal acidification and a halt in enzymatic functions. Sugars and amino acids also eventually leak from an arrested cell. Fungistatic effects are most often evident at usual polyene concentrations. High drug concentrations and pH values between 6.0 and 7.3 in the surrounding medium may lead to fungicidal rather than fungistatic action.

In addition to these direct effects on susceptible yeasts and fungi, evidence suggests that amphotericin B may also act as an immunopotentiator (both humoral and cell mediated), thus enhancing the host's ability to overcome mycotic infections.

Fungal Resistance: Polyene macrolides are inherently resistant to dermatophytes. Acquired resistance to the polyene antifungal macrolides is rare both clinically and in vitro. *Pythium*, a pseudofungus, is less susceptible, because it contains limited ergosterol in its cell membranes. Resistance has been documented for *Candida* spp, which are among the more rapidly growing fungal organisms. In general, resistance develops slowly and does not reach high levels, even after prolonged treatment.

Antifungal Spectra: The polyene antibiotics have broad antifungal activity against organisms ranging from yeasts to filamentous fungi and from saprophytic to pathogenic fungi, but there are great differences between the susceptibilities of the various species and strains of fungi. They are ineffective against dermatophytes. In vitro susceptibilities (both resistant and highly susceptible) do not always correlate well with the clinical response, which suggests that host factors may also play a role. Many algae and some protozoa

(*Leishmania*, *Trypanosoma*, *Trichomonas*, and *Entamoeba* spp) are sensitive to the polyenes, but these compounds have no significant activity against bacteria, actinomycetes, viruses, or animal cells. Amphotericin B is effective against yeasts (eg, *Candida* spp, *Rhodotorula* spp, *Cryptococcus neoformans*), dimorphic fungi (eg, *Histoplasma capsulatum*, *Blastomyces dermatitidis*, *Coccidioides immitis*), dermatophytes (eg, *Trichophyton*, *Microsporum*, and *Epidermophyton* spp), and molds. It also has been used successfully to treat disseminated sporotrichosis, pythiosis, and zygomycosis, although it may not always be effective. Nystatin is mainly used to treat mucocutaneous candidiasis, but it is effective against other yeasts and fungi. The antimicrobial activity of pimaricin is similar to that of nystatin, although it is mainly used for local treatment of candidiasis, trichomoniasis, and mycotic keratitis.

Preparations: Amphotericin B is available as an IV solution complexed to bile acids but also as several different preparations complexed to lipid mixtures. Because reticuloendothelial cells phagocytize the lipid component, directed delivery to the site of fungal infection is facilitated, reducing renal exposure. Prolonged antifungal activity (compared with nonliposomal preparations) has been documented.

Pharmacokinetic Features

Absorption: The polyene macrolide antibiotics are poorly absorbed from the GI tract. Amphotericin B is usually administered IV or topically and occasionally locally, intrathecally, or intraocularly. Nystatin and piramycin are mostly applied topically. Nystatin is given PO to treat intestinal candidiasis. Absorption is minimal from sites of local application.

Distribution: Amphotericin B is widely distributed in the body after IV infusion. It associates with cholesterol in host cell membranes throughout the body and is subsequently released slowly into the circulation. Penetration into the CSF, saliva, aqueous humor, vitreous humor, and hemodialysis solutions is generally poor. Amphotericin B becomes highly bound to plasma lipoproteins (~95%). Complexing amphotericin B with various lipid-based products alters the distribution.

Biotransformation and Excretion: The disposition of amphotericin B is not well described in companion animals. Approximately 5% of a total daily dose of amphotericin B is excreted unchanged in the urine. Over a 2-wk period, ~20% of the drug may be recovered in the urine. The hepatobiliary system accounts for 20%–30% of excretion. The fate of the remainder of amphotericin B is unknown.

Pharmacokinetics: Amphotericin B has a biphasic elimination pattern. The initial phase lasts 24 hr, during which levels fall rapidly (70% for plasma and 50% for urine). The second elimination phase has a 15-day half-life, during which plasma concentrations decline very slowly. Amphotericin B is usually infused IV, every 48–72 hr, until the total cumulative dosage has been reached. The disposition of the various lipid-complexed amphotericin B products is variable. Because of its small size, AmBisome® is characterized by the slowest uptake by reticuloendothelial cells and thus the highest plasma drug concentrations of amphotericin B. However, the amount of free versus complexed amphotericin B is not clear. AmBisome also was able to achieve CNS concentrations and was associated with the least nephrotoxicity in human studies. AmBisome has been studied in Beagles. Achievable amphotericin concentrations were much higher at equivalent doses of AmBisome compared with other products; further, dogs were able to well tolerate 4 mg/kg for 30 days. Amphotericin concentrations accumulate with multiple dosing when administered as AmBisome.

Therapeutic Indications and Dose Rates

Amphotericin B is used principally to treat systemic mycotic infections. Despite its ability to cause nephrotoxicity (*see* p 2702), amphotericin B remains a commonly used antifungal agent because of its effectiveness. Multiple approaches to delivery have been described in an attempt to minimize nephrotoxicity. In addition, dosing continues until a maximal cumulative dose is reached, with the amount varying with the fungal organism. Nystatin is primarily indicated for treatment of mucocutaneous (skin, oropharynx, vagina) or intestinal candidiasis; pimaricin is mainly used in therapeutic management of mycotic keratitis.

General dosages for some polyene macrolide antibiotics are listed in TABLE 52. The dose rate and frequency should be adjusted as needed for the individual animal.

TABLE 52 DOSAGES OF POLYENE MACROLIDE ANTIBIOTICS

Polyene Macrolide	Dosage, Route, and Frequency
Amphotericin B (0.1 mg/mL in 5% dextrose)	0.1–1 mg/kg, given IV slowly, 3 times/wk Total dose: 4–11 mg/kg
Amphotericin B lipid complex injection (Abelcet®)	1–3 mg/kg, IV, every other day or 3 times/wk Total dose: 12–24 mg/kg
Amphotericin B liposome (AmBisome®)	3–4 mg/kg, IV, every other day or 3 times/wk Total dose: 12–30 mg/kg
Nystatin	50,000–150,000 U, PO, tid (dogs)
Pimaricin (5% ophthalmic solution)	1 drop, instilled into the eye, every 1–2 hr

Special Clinical Concerns

Adverse Effects and Toxicity: Oral administration of nystatin can lead to anorexia and GI disturbances. The IV infusion of amphotericin B can cause an anaphylactoid reaction due to direct mast cell degranulation. A pre-test dose is recommended to detect this reaction, and pretreatment with H_1 antihistamines and short-acting glucocorticoids may be appropriate. Thrombophlebitis may occur with perivascular leakage. The primary toxicity associated with amphotericin B is nephrotoxicity. Within 15 min of IV administration of amphotericin B, renal arterial vasoconstriction occurs and lasts for 4–6 hr. This leads to diminished renal blood flow and glomerular filtration. Because amphotericin B binds to the cholesterol component in the membranes of the distal renal tubules, a change in permeability occurs in these cells, leading to polyuria, polydipsia, concentration defects, and acidification abnormalities. The net result is a distal renal tubular acidosis syndrome. The metabolic acidosis leads to bone buffering, the excessive release of calcium into the circulation, and ultimately nephrocalcinosis due to calcium precipitation in the acidic environment of the distal tubules. Almost every animal treated with amphotericin B develops some degree of renal impairment, which may become permanent depending on the total cumulative dose.

The administration of amphotericin B can lead to a number of other adverse effects, including anorexia, nausea, vomiting, hypersensitivity reactions, drug fever, normocytic normochromic anemia, cardiac arrhythmias (and even arrest), hepatic dysfunction, CNS signs, and thrombophlebitis at the injection site.

A number of adjuvant therapies are used to minimize adverse events of amphotericin B. Pretreatment with antiemetic and antihistaminic agents prevents the nausea, vomiting, and hypersensitivity reactions. Giving corticosteroids IV also limits severe hypersensitivity reactions. Mannitol (1 g/kg, IV) with each dose of amphotericin B, and sodium bicarbonate (2 mEq/kg, IV or PO, daily) may help prevent acidification defects, metabolic acidosis, and azotemia; however, clinical evidence of efficacy has not been proved. Saralasin (6–12 mcg/kg/min, IV) and dopamine (7 mcg/kg/min, IV) infusions have prevented oliguria and azotemia induced by amphotericin B in dogs. Administering IV fluids or furosemide before amphotericin B prevents pronounced decreases in renal blood flow and glomerular filtration rate. Newer preparations in which amphotericin B is mixed with lipid or liposomal vehicles (particularly liposomes) are safer and have maintained efficacy.

Interactions: Amphotericin B may be combined with other antimicrobial agents with synergistic results. This often allows both the total dose of amphotericin B and the length of therapy to be decreased. Examples include combinations of 5-flucytosine and amphotericin B for treatment of cryptococcal meningitis, minocycline and amphotericin B for coccidioidomycosis, and imidazole and amphotericin B for several systemic mycotic infections. Rifampin may also potentiate the antifungal activity of amphotericin B.

Drugs that should be avoided during amphotericin B therapy include aminoglycosides (nephrotoxicity), digitalis drugs (increased toxicity), curarizing agents (neuromuscular blockade), mineralocorticoids (hypokalemia), thiazide diuretics (hypokalemia, hyponatremia), antineoplastic drugs (cytotoxicity), and cyclosporine (nephrotoxicity).

Effects on Laboratory Tests: Treatment with polyene macrolide antibiotics increases plasma bilirubin, CK, AST, ALT, BUN, eosinophil count, and urine protein, and decreases plasma potassium and platelet count.

IMIDAZOLES

Imidazoles may have antibacterial, antifungal, antiprotozoal, and anthelmintic activity. Several distinct phenylimidazoles are therapeutically useful antifungal agents with wide spectra against yeasts and filamentous fungi responsible for either superficial or systemic infections. The anthelmintic thiabendazole is also an imidazole with antifungal properties. Clotrimazole, miconazole, econazole, ketoconazole, itraconazole, and fluconazole are the most clinically important members of this group. Posaconazole and voriconazole are among the newer drugs; voriconazole is approved for use in people to treat aspergillosis.

Imidazoles generally are poorly soluble in water but can be dissolved in organic solvents such as chloroform, propylene glycol, and polyethoxylated castor oil (preparation for IV use but dangerous in dogs). An exception is fluconazole. Imidazoles are weak dibasic agents. Alterations in side-chain structure determine antifungal activity as well as the degree of toxicity.

Antifungal Activity

Mode of Action: Imidazoles alter the cell membrane permeability of susceptible yeasts and fungi by blocking the synthesis of ergosterol (demethylation of lanosterol is inhibited), the primary cell sterol of fungi. The enzyme targeted is a fungal cytochrome (CYP450). Other enzyme systems are also impaired, such as those required for fatty acid synthesis. Because of the drug-induced changes of oxidative and peroxidative enzyme activities, toxic concentrations of hydrogen peroxide develop intracellularly. The overall effect is cell membrane and internal organelle disruption and cell death. The cholesterol in host cells is not affected by the imidazoles, although some drugs impair synthesis of selected steroids and drug-metabolizing enzymes in the host. Because imidazoles impair synthesis, a lag time to efficacy occurs. This lag time may be prolonged because of the long half-life of these drugs.

Fungal Resistance: Sensitivity to the imidazoles varies greatly between various strains of yeasts and fungi, but neither natural nor acquired resistance appears to be prevalent.

Antimicrobial Spectra: The antifungal imidazoles also have some antibacterial action but are rarely used for this purpose. Miconazole has a wide antifungal spectrum against most fungi and yeasts of veterinary interest. Sensitive organisms include *Blastomyces dermatitidis*, *Paracoccidioides brasiliensis*, *Histoplasma capsulatum*, *Candida* spp, *Coccidioides immitis*, *Cryptococcus neoformans*, and *Aspergillus fumigatus*. Some *Aspergillus* and *Madurella* spp are only marginally sensitive.

Ketoconazole has an antifungal spectrum similar to that of miconazole, but it is more effective against *C immitis* and some other yeasts and fungi. Itraconazole and fluconazole are the most active of the antifungal imidazoles. Their spectrum includes dimorphic fungal organisms and dermatophytes. They are also effective against some cases of aspergillosis (60%–70%) and cutaneous sporotrichosis. Clotrimazole and econazole are used for superficial mycoses (dermatophytosis and candidiasis); econazole also has been used for oculomycosis. Thiabendazole is effective against *Aspergillus* and *Penicillium* spp, but its use has largely been replaced by the more effective imidazoles. Voriconazole is approved for human use in treatment of *Aspergillus* but is effective against many other fungal organisms.Posaconazole may be more effective than itraconazole or fluconazole but may be associated with more adverse effects.

Pharmacokinetic Features

Absorption and Distribution: The imidazoles are rapidly but sometimes erratically absorbed from the GI tract; plasma levels peak within 2 hr after administration PO. Fluconazole is an exception, being close to 100% bioavailable after administration PO. Except for fluconazole, an acidic environment is required for dissolution of the imidazoles, and a decrease in gastric acidity can reduce bioavailability after administration PO. The rate of absorption appears to be increased when the drug is given with meals, but reports are conflicting. Because oral bioavailability can be very poor with noncommercial imidazole products, caution is recommended with compounded products, and monitoring is recommended if a compounded preparation is used.

Imidazoles appear to be widely distributed in the body, with detectable concentrations in saliva, milk, and cerumen. CSF penetration is poor except for fluconazole, which reaches 50%–90% of plasma concentrations. Most imidazoles (except fluconazole) are highly protein bound in the circulation (>95%), most to albumin. The highest concentrations of imidazoles are found in the liver, adrenal glands, lungs, and kidneys.

Biotransformation and Excretion: Hepatic metabolism is the primary route of elimination. Metabolism of ketoconazole and most other imidazoles by oxidative pathways is extensive. Only ~2%–4% of a dose administered PO appears unchanged in the urine. Itraconazole is metabolized to an active metabolite that may contribute significantly to antimicrobial activity. The biliary route is the major excretory pathway (>80%); ~20% of the metabolites are eliminated in the urine. Fluconazole (in people) is eliminated (≥90%) unchanged in the urine. The kinetics of voriconazole have not yet been evaluated in animals.

Pharmacokinetics: The rate of elimination of ketoconazole appears to be dose dependent—the greater the dose, the longer the elimination half-life. There is also a biphasic elimination pattern, with rapid elimination in the first 1–2 hr, then a slower decline over the next 6–9 hr. Ketoconazole is usually administered bid. The half-life of itraconazole is longer (up to 48 hr in cats), thus allowing treatment once to twice daily. Because of the long half-life and mechanism of action (impaired synthesis of the fungal cell membrane), time to efficacy may take longer than drugs that have more rapid actions (such as amphotericin B).

Therapeutic Indications and Dose Rates

The imidazoles are used to treat systemic fungal diseases, dermatophyte infections that have not responded to griseofulvin or topical therapy, *Malassezia* infection in dogs, aspergillosis, and sporotrichosis in animals that cannot tolerate or do not respond to sodium iodide. For serious infections, combination with amphotericin B is strongly recommended. Among the imidazoles, fluconazole may be more likely to distribute into tissues that are tough to penetrate. Both itraconazole and fluconazole are generally preferred to other imidazoles for treatment of systemic fungal infections, including aspergillosis and sporotrichosis. Topically applied imidazoles (clotrimazole, miconazole, econazole) are used for local dermatophytosis. Thiabendazole is included in some otic preparations for treatment of yeast infections.

Enilconazole is an imidazole that can be applied topically for treatment of dermatophytosis and aspergillosis. It has been used safely in cats, dogs, cattle, horses, and chickens and is prepared as a 0.2% solution for treatment of fungal skin infections. When infused into the nasal turbinates of dogs with aspergillosis, enilconazole treated and prevented the recurrence of fungal disease. When applied topically to dog and cat hairs, enilconazole inhibits fungal growth in 2 rather than 4–8 treatments, as is necessary with other topically administered antifungal agents.

General dosages for the antifungal imidazoles are listed in TABLE 53. The dose rate and frequency should be adjusted as needed for the individual animal.

Special Clinical Concerns

Adverse Effects and Toxicity: The imidazoles given PO result in few adverse effects, but nausea, vomiting, and hepatic dysfunction can develop. Ketoconazole in particular is associated with hepatotoxicity, especially in cats. Because imidazoles also inhibit CYP450 associated with steroid synthesis, as a result, sex steroids, including testosterone and adrenal steroid (cortisol),

TABLE 53 DOSAGES OF IMIDAZOLES

Imidazole	Dosage, Route, and Frequency
Enilconazole	10 mg/kg in 5–10 mL, bid for 7–14 days
Fluconazole	5–10 mg/kg, PO, once to twice daily
Itraconazole	5–10 mg/kg, PO, once to twice daily
Ketoconazole	5–20 mg/kg, PO, bid (dogs)
Thiabendazole	44 mg/kg/day, PO, or 22 mg/kg, PO, bid

metabolism is inhibited. Adrenal responsiveness to adrenocorticotropic hormone (ACTH) will be decreased, particularly with ketoconazole. Reproductive disorders related to ketoconazole administration may be seen in dogs. Voriconazole is associated with a number of adverse effects in people, including vision disturbances.

Interactions: Imidazoles, in general, inhibit the metabolism of many drugs. Although ketoconazole has the broadest inhibitory effects, fluconazole followed by itraconazole also inhibit metabolism. Concurrent administration of these drugs with other drugs metabolized by the liver and potentially toxic should be done only with extreme caution. Imidazoles also are substrates for P-glycoprotein transport protein and may compete with other substrates, causing higher concentrations. Many of the substrates for P-glycoprotein are also substrates for CYP450. Rifampin, which is a P-glycoprotein substrate, decreases serum ketoconazole because of microsomal enzyme induction. The absorption of the imidazoles, except for that of fluconazole, is inhibited by concurrent administration of cimetidine, ranitidine, anticholinergic agents, or gastric antacids. The risk of hepatotoxicity is increased if ketoconazole and griseofulvin are administered together. Imidazoles might be used concurrently with other antifungals to facilitate synergistic efficacy.

Effects on Laboratory Tests: Treatment with imidazoles increases AST, ALT, plasma bilirubin, and plasma cholesterol. Adrenal responsiveness is altered.

FLUCYTOSINE

Flucytosine (5-fluorocytosine) is a fluorinated pyrimidine related to fluorouracil that was initially developed as an antineoplastic agent. It should be stored in airtight containers protected from light. Solutions for infusion are unstable and should be stored at 15°–20°C. Usually, it is given PO in capsules.

Antifungal Activity

Mode of Action: Flucytosine is converted by cytosine deaminase in fungal cells to fluorouracil, which then interferes with RNA and protein synthesis. Fluorouracil is metabolized to 5-fluorodeoxyuridylic acid, an inhibitor of thymidylate synthetase. DNA synthesis is then halted. Mammalian cells do not convert large amounts of flucytosine to fluorouracil and, thus, are not affected at usual dosage levels.

Fungal Resistance: Resistance to flucytosine can develop rapidly even during the course of treatment; this precludes its use as the sole treatment for mycotic infections. The mechanisms of resistance are not completely understood.

Antifungal Spectra: The following are the main organisms usually sensitive to flucytosine: *Cryptococcus neoformans*, *Candida albicans*, other *Candida* spp, *Torulopsis glabrata*, *Sporothrix schenckii*, *Aspergillus* spp, and agents of chromoblastomycosis (*Phialophora*, *Cladosporium*). The other fungi responsible for systemic mycoses and dermatophytes are resistant to flucytosine.

Pharmacokinetic Features

Absorption and Distribution: Flucytosine is rapidly and well absorbed from the GI tract, with plasma levels peaking in 1–2 hr in animals that have received the drug for several days. The drug is widely distributed in the body, with a volume of distribution approximating the total body water. Flucytosine is minimally bound to plasma proteins. There is excellent penetration into body fluids such as the CSF, synovial fluids, and aqueous humor.

Biotransformation and Excretion: Nearly all (85%–95%) of an oral dose is excreted unchanged. Flucytosine is principally excreted by glomerular filtration (>80%). The clearance of flucytosine is approximately equivalent to that of creatinine. In renal failure, elimination of flucytosine is markedly impaired.

Pharmacokinetics: With normal renal function, the plasma half-life of flucytosine is usually 2–4 hr but may be up to 200 hr with oliguria. Serum levels of 50–100 mcg/mL are usually in the therapeutic range.

Therapeutic Indications and Dose Rates

The more common indications for flucytosine include cryptococcal meningitis, used together with amphotericin B (~30% of isolates develop resistance during the course of treatment); candidiasis (~90% of isolates are usually sensitive); aspergillosis (some strains are sensitive at <5 mcg/mL); chromomycosis (some strains are very sensitive); and sporotrichosis (some cases may respond).

General dosages for flucytosine are 25–50 mg/kg and 30–40 mg/kg, PO, tid-qid in dogs and cats, respectively. The dose rate and frequency should be adjusted as needed for the individual animal. Dosage modification is essential in renal failure. Flucytosine serum levels should be monitored if possible.

Special Clinical Concerns

Adverse Effects and Toxicity: Flucytosine is often well tolerated over long periods, but toxic effects may be seen when serum levels are high (>100 mcg/mL). These include GI signs (nausea, vomiting, diarrhea) and reversible hepatic and hematologic effects (increased liver enzymes, anemia, neutropenia, thrombocytopenia). In dogs, erythemic and alopecic dermatitis may be seen but subsides when the drug is discontinued.

Interactions: There is synergistic antifungal activity between amphotericin B and ketoconazole, and the combination may retard the emergence of strains resistant to flucytosine. The renal effects of amphotericin B prolong elimination of flucytosine. If flucytosine is used together with immunosuppressive drugs, severe depression of bone marrow function is possible.

Effects on Laboratory Tests: Treatment with flucytosine increases alkaline phosphatase, AST, ALT, and other liver leakage enzymes, and decreases RBC, WBC, and platelet counts.

GRISEOFULVIN

Griseofulvin is a systemic antifungal agent effective against the common dermatophytes. It is practically insoluble in water and only slightly soluble in most organic solvents. Particle sizes of griseofulvin vary from 2.7 µm (ultramicrosized) to 10 µm (microsized).

Antifungal Activity

Mode of Action: Dermatophytes concentrate griseofulvin through an energy-dependent process. Griseofulvin *then disrupts the* mitotic spindle by interacting with the polymerized microtubules in susceptible dermatophytes. This leads to production of multinucleate fungal cells. The inhibition of nucleic acid synthesis and the formation of hyphal cell wall material also may be involved. The result is distortion, irregular swelling, and spiral curling of the hyphae. Griseofulvin is fungistatic rather than fungicidal, except in young active cells.

Fungal Resistance: Dermatophytes can be made resistant to griseofulvin in vitro.

Antifungal Spectra: Griseofulvin is active against *Microsporum, Epidermophyton*, and *Trichophyton* spp. It has no effect on bacteria (including *Actinomyces* and *Nocardia* spp), other fungi, or yeasts.

Pharmacokinetic Features

Absorption: Plasma levels peak ~4 hr after administration PO, but absorption from the GI tract continues over a prolonged period. Absorption is highly variable and influenced by a number of factors. The rates of disaggregation and dissolution in the GI tract limit the bioavailability of griseofulvin; thus, microsized and ultramicrosized particles are usually used. High-fat meals, margarine, or propylene glycol significantly enhance GI absorption of griseofulvin and are indicated if the microsized particles are used.

Distribution: Griseofulvin is deposited in keratin precursor cells within 4–8 hr of administration PO. Sweat and transdermal fluid loss appear to play an important role in griseofulvin transfer in the stratum corneum. When these cells differentiate, griseofulvin remains bound and persists in keratin, making it resistant to fungal invasion. For this reason, new growth of hair, nails, or horn is the first to become free of fungal infection. As the fungus-containing keratin is shed, it is replaced by normal skin and hair. Only a small fraction of a dose of griseofulvin remains in the body fluids or tissues.

Biotransformation and Pharmacokinetics: Depending on the species, 10%–50% of a griseofulvin dose is excreted almost exclusively as metabolites in the urine, and the remainder in the feces for ~4–5 days after administration. The elimination half-life of griseofulvin is ~24 hr in several species. The drug can be detected in 48–72 hr at the base level of the skin, in 6–12 days in the lower quarter, and in 2–19 days in the middle section of the horny layer.

Therapeutic Indications and Dose Rates

Griseofulvin is used for dermatophyte infections in dogs, cats, calves, horses, and other domestic and exotic animal species. Most dermatophytes are sensitive, but certain species present greater therapeutic challenges than others. Several may require higher dose rates for satisfactory control.

General dosages for griseofulvin are listed in TABLE 54. The dose rate and frequency should be adjusted as needed for the individual animal.

Special Clinical Concerns

Adverse Effects and Toxicity: Adverse effects induced by griseofulvin are rare. Nausea, vomiting, and diarrhea have been seen. Hepatotoxicity has also been reported. Animals with impaired liver function should not be given griseofulvin, because its biotransformation will be reduced and toxic levels may be reached. Idiosyncratic (Type B or Type II adverse reaction) toxicity in cats has been reported. Clinical signs are neurologic, GI, and hematologic. Griseofulvin is contraindicated in pregnant animals (especially mares and queens) because it is teratogenic.

Interactions: Lipids increase GI absorption of griseofulvin. Barbiturates decrease its absorption and antifungal activity. Griseofulvin is a microsomal enzyme inducer and promotes the biotransformation of many concurrently administered drugs. The combined use of ketoconazole and griseofulvin may lead to hepatotoxicity.

Effects on Laboratory Tests: Treatment with griseofulvin increases alkaline phosphatase, AST, and ALT. Proteinuria may be detected.

ALLYLAMINES

The allylamines include terbinafine, naftifine, and the much older thiocarbamate tolnaftate. Their mechanism is competitive inhibition of squalene epoxidase, blocking conversion of squalene to lanosterol, leading to squaline accumulation and ergosterol depletion in the cell membrane. Terbinafine has a much higher affinity for fungal than for mammalian squaline epoxidase. Avid uptake of terbinafine into body fat and epidermis presumably enhances treatment for dermatophytes of superficial yeast pathogens of the skin. However, data are emerging to potentially support its use for systemic fungal infections. Terbinafine is also active against yeasts (eg, *Blastomyces dermatitidis*, *Cryptococcus neoformans*, *Sporothrix schenckii*, *Histoplasma capsulatum*, *Candida*, and *Pityrosporum* spp). Terbinafine increasingly is used in combination with other antifungal drugs to enhance efficacy. Effects are fungicidal. The allylamines appear to be more efficacious than griseofulvin for treatment of dermatophyte infections. Efficacy has also been demonstrated against *S schenckii* and *Aspergillus*. Terbinafine may enhance efficacy of other antifungal drugs for a variety of fungal disorders and pythiosis. In contrast to terbinafine, tolnaftate is limited to treatment of dermatophytes. Resistance to the allylamines is rare, but the drugs potentially can be affected by multidrug resistance efflux mechanisms. Terbinafine, available in oral and topical preparations, is well absorbed (80% in people) after PO administration. Fat facilitates absorption. High concentrations occur in the stratum corneum, sebum, and hair. Terbinafine is metabolized by the liver in people; the elimination half-life is sufficiently long to allow once-daily administration, with steady state not occurring for 10–14 days in people. Adverse effects of terbinafine after PO administration are limited to GI and skin signs; hepatobiliary dysfunction is a rare adverse event. Because inhibition of ergosterol synthesis occurs at a step before cytochrome P450 involvement, the allylamines do not affect steroid synthesis as do the imidazoles.

TABLE 54 DOSAGES OF GRISEOFULVIN

Species	Dosage, Route, and Frequency
Dogs, cats	Microsized: 10–30 (up to 130) mg/kg/day, PO, or divided bid-tid Ultramicrosized: 5–10 (up to 50) mg/kg/day, PO
Horses, cattle	5–10 mg/kg/day, PO, for 3–6 wk, or longer if required

IODIDES

Sodium and potassium iodide have both been used to treat selected bacterial, actinomycete, and fungal infections, although sodium iodide is preferred. The in vivo effects of iodides against fungal cells are not well understood. Iodide is readily absorbed from the GI tract and distributes freely into the extracellular fluid and glandular secretions. Iodide concentrates in the thyroid gland (50 times corresponding plasma level) and to a much lesser degree in salivary, lacrimal, and tracheobronchial glands. Longterm use at high levels leads to accumulation in the body and to iodinism.

Clinical signs of iodinism include lacrimation, salivation, increased respiratory secretions, coughing, inappetence, dry scaly skin, and tachycardia. Cardiomyopathy has been reported in cats. Host defense systems, such as decreased immunoglobulin production and reduced phagocytic ability of leukocytes, are also impaired. Iodinism may also lead to abortion and infertility.

Sodium iodide has been used successfully to treat cutaneous and cutaneous/lymphadenitis forms of sporotrichosis; attempts to control various other mycotic infections with iodides yield equivocal results.

The dosage for sodium iodide (20% solution) is 44 mg/kg/day, PO, for dogs, and 22 mg/kg/day, PO, for cats. The dosage for horses is 125 mL of 20% sodium iodide solution, IV, daily for 3 days, then 30 g, PO, daily for 30 days after clinical remission. The dosage rate for treating actinomycosis and actinobacillosis in cattle is 66 mg/kg, by slow IV, repeated weekly. Potassium iodide should never be injected IV.

TOPICAL ANTIFUNGAL AGENTS

A number of agents that have antifungal activity are applied topically, either on the skin, in the ear or eye, or on mucous membranes (buccal, nasal, vaginal) to control superficial mycotic infections. Concurrent systemic therapy with griseofulvin is often helpful for therapeutic management of dermatophyte infections. The hair should be clipped from affected areas and the nails trimmed to fully expose the lesions before antifungal preparations are applied. Bathing the animal may also be helpful. Isolation or restricted movement of infected animals is wise, especially when dealing with zoonotic fungi.

Preparations may be used in the form of solutions, lotions, sprays, powders, creams, or ointments for dermal application, or in the form of irrigant solutions, ointments, tablets, or suppositories for intravaginal use. The concentration of active principle in these preparations varies and depends on the activity of the specific agent.

The clinical response to local antifungal agents is unpredictable. Resistance to many of the available drugs is common. Spread of infection and reinfection add to the difficulty of controlling superficial infections. Perseverance is often an essential element of therapy.

Some topical antifungal agents that have been used with success in various conditions and species include iodine preparations (tincture of iodine, potassium iodide, iodophors), copper preparations (copper sulfate, copper naphthenate, cuprimyxin), sulfur preparations (monosulfiram, benzoyl disulfide), phenols (phenol, thymol), fatty acids and salts (propionates, undecylenates), organic acids (benzoic acid, salicylic acids), dyes (crystal [gentian] violet, carbolfuchsin), hydroxyquinolines (iodochlorhydroxyquin), nitrofurans (nitrofuroxine, nitrofurfurylmethyl ether), imidazoles (miconazole, tioconazole, clotrimazole, econazole, thiabendazole), polyene antibiotics (amphotericin B, nystatin, pimaricin, candicidin, hachimycin), allylamines (naftifine, terbinafine), thiocarbamates (tolnaftate), and miscellaneous agents (acrisorcin, haloprogin, ciclopirox, olamine, dichlorophen, hexetidine, chlorphenesin, triacetin, polynoxylin, amorolfine).

Amorolfine is a topical antifungal agent used to treat onychomycosis and dermatophytosis. It is prepared as a cream or nail lacquer. Amorolfine is a morpholine derivative that appears to interfere with the synthesis of sterols essential for the functioning of fungal cell membranes. In vitro, activity has been shown against some yeasts and dimorphic, dematiaceous, and filamentous fungi (*Blastomyces dermatitidis*, *Candida* spp, *Histoplasma capsulatum*, *Sporothrix schenckii*, and *Aspergillus* spp). Despite its in vitro activity, amorolfine is inactive when given systemically and thus is limited to topical use in treatment of superficial infections. Its role in treatment of fungal infection in animals is not clear.

ANTI-INFLAMMATORY AGENTS

Inflammation is the complex pathophysiologic response of vascularized tissue to injury. The injury may result from various stimuli, including thermal, chemical, or physical damage; ischemia; infectious agents; antigen-antibody interactions; and other biologic processes. After tissue injury, the process of tissue healing includes three distinct phases: an inflammatory phase, a repair phase, and a remodeling phase. The desired outcome of the inflammatory response is isolation and elimination of the injurious agent to prepare for the repair of tissue damage at the site of injury and restoration of function. Finally, new tissue formed during the repair phase (eg, scar tissue) may be remodeled over several months.

PATHOPHYSIOLOGY OF INFLAMMATION

The initial inflammation phase consists of three subphases: acute, subacute, and chronic (or proliferative). The acute phase typically lasts 1–3 days and is characterized by the five classic clinical signs: heat, redness, swelling, pain, and loss of function. The subacute phase may last from 3–4 days to ~1 mo and corresponds to a cleaning phase required before the repair phase. If the subacute phase is not resolved within ~1 mo, then inflammation is said to become chronic and can last for several months. Tissue can degenerate and, in the locomotor system, chronic inflammation may lead to tearing and rupture. Alternatively, after the subacute inflammatory phase, tissue can repair and be strengthened during the remodeling phase.

From a mechanistic point of view, the acute response to tissue injury occurs in the microcirculation at the site of injury. Initially, there is a transient constriction of arterioles; however, within several minutes, chemical mediators released at the site relax arteriolar smooth muscle, leading to vasodilation and increased capillary permeability. Protein-rich fluid then exudes from capillaries into the interstitial space. This fluid contains many of the components of plasma including albumin, fibrinogen, kinins, complement, and immunoglobulins that mediate the inflammatory response.

The subacute phase is characterized by movement of phagocytic cells to the site of injury. In response to adhesion, molecules released from activated endothelial cells, leukocytes, platelets, and erythrocytes in injured vessels become sticky and adhere to the endothelial cell surfaces. Polymorphonuclear leukocytes such as neutrophils are the first cells to infiltrate the site of injury. Basophils and eosinophils are more prevalent in allergic reactions or parasitic infections. As inflammation continues, macrophages predominate, actively removing damaged cells or tissue. If the cause of injury is eliminated, the subacute phase of inflammation may be followed by a period of tissue repair. Blood clots are removed by fibrinolysis, and damaged tissues are regenerated or replaced with fibroblasts, collagen, or endothelial cells. During the remodeling phase, the new collagen laid down during the repair phase (mainly type III) is progressively replaced by type I collagen to adapt to the original tissue. However, if inflammation becomes chronic, further tissue destruction and/or fibrosis occurs.

CHEMICAL MEDIATORS OF INFLAMMATION

Biochemical mediators released during inflammation intensify and propagate the inflammatory response (*see* TABLE 55). These mediators are soluble, diffusible molecules that can act locally and systemically. Mediators derived from plasma include complement and complement-derived peptides and kinins. Released via the classic or alternative pathways of the complement cascade, **complement-derived peptides** (C3a, C3b, and C5a) increase vascular permeability, cause smooth muscle contraction, activate leukocytes, and induce mast-cell degranulation. C5a is a potent chemotactic factor for neutrophils and mononuclear phagocytes. The kinins are also important inflammatory mediators. The most important kinin is **bradykinin**, which increases vascular permeability and vasodilation and, importantly, activates phospholipase A_2 (PLA_2) to liberate arachidonic acid (AA). Bradykinin is also a major mediator involved in the pain response.

Other mediators are derived from injured tissue cells or leukocytes recruited to the site of inflammation. Mast cells, platelets,

TABLE 55 ACTIONS OF INFLAMMATORY MEDIATORS

Action	Mediators[a]
Vasodilation, increased vascular permeability	Histamine, serotonin, bradykinin, C3a, C5a, LTC_4, LTD_4, PGI_2, PGE_2, PGD_2, PGF_2, activated Hageman factor, kinonogen fragments, fibrinopeptides
Vasoconstriction	TXA_2, LTB_4, LTC_4, LTD_4, C5a
Smooth muscle contraction	C3a, C5a, histamine, LTB_4, LTC_4, LTD_4, TXA_2, serotonin, PAF, bradykinin
Mast cell degranulation	C5a, C3a
Stem cell proliferation	IL-3, G-CSF, GM-CSF, M-CSF
Chemotaxis	C5a, LTB_4, IL-8, PAF, 5-HETE, histamine, others
Lysosomal granule release	C5a, IL-8, PAF
Phagocytosis	C3b, iC3b
Platelet aggregation	TXA_2, PAF
Endothelial cell stickiness	IL-1, TNF-α, LTB_4
Granuloma formation	IL-1, TNF-α
Pain	PGE_2, bradykinin, histamine, serotonin
Fever	IL-1, IL-6, TNF-α, PGE_2

[a] C = complement, LT = leukotriene, PG = prostaglandin, TX = thromboxane, PAF = platelet activating factor, IL = interleukin, CSF = colony stimulating factor, HETE = hydroxyeicosatetranoate, TNF = tumor necrosis factor

and basophils produce the vasoactive amines serotonin and histamine. **Histamine** causes arteriolar dilation, increased capillary permeability, contraction of nonvascular smooth muscle, and eosinophil chemotaxis and can stimulate nociceptors responsible for the pain response. Its release is stimulated by the complement components C3a and C5a and by lysosomal proteins released from neutrophils. Histamine activity is mediated through the activation of one of four specific histamine receptors, designated H_1, H_2, H_3, or H_4, in target cells. Most histamine-induced vascular effects are mediated by H_1 receptors. H_2 receptors mediate some vascular effects but are more important for their role in histamine-induced gastric secretion. Less is understood about the role of H_3 receptors, which may be localized to the CNS. H_4 receptors are located on cells of hematopoietic origin, and H_4 antagonists are promising drug candidates to treat *inflammatory conditions* involving mast cells and eosinophils (allergic conditions). **Serotonin** (5-hydroxytryptamine) is a vasoactive mediator similar to histamine found in mast cells and platelets in the GI tract and CNS. Serotonin also increases vascular permeability, dilates capillaries, and causes contraction of nonvascular smooth muscle. In some species, including rodents and domestic ruminants, serotonin may be the predominant vasoactive amine.

Cytokines, including interleukins 1–10, tumor necrosis factor α (TNF-α), and interferon γ (INF-γ) are produced predominantly by macrophages and lymphocytes but can be synthesized by other cell types as well. Their role in inflammation is complex. These polypeptides modulate the activity and function of other cells to coordinate and control the inflammatory response. Two of the more important cytokines, interleukin-1 (IL-1) and TNF-α, mobilize and activate leukocytes, enhance proliferation of B and T cells and natural killer cell cytotoxicity, and are involved in the biologic response to endotoxins. IL-1, IL-6, and TNF-α mediate the acute phase response and pyrexia that may accompany infection and can induce systemic clinical signs, including sleep and anorexia. In the acute phase response, interleukins stimulate the liver to synthesize acute-phase proteins, including complement components, coagulation factors, protease inhibitors, and metal-binding proteins. By increasing intracellular Ca^{2+} concentrations in leukocytes, cytokines are also important in the induction of PLA_2. Colony-stimulating factors (GM-CSF, G-CSF, and M-CSF) are cytokines that promote expansion of neutrophil, eosinophil, and macrophage colonies in bone marrow. In chronic inflammation, cytokines IL-1, IL-6, and TNF-α contribute to the activation of fibroblasts and osteoblasts and to the release of enzymes such as collagenase and stromelysin that can cause cartilage and bone resorption. Experimental evidence also suggests that cytokines stimulate synovial cells and chondrocytes to release pain-inducing mediators.

Lipid-derived autacoids play important roles in the inflammatory response and are a major focus of research into new anti-inflammatory drugs. These compounds include the eicosanoids such as prostaglandins, prostacyclin, leukotrienes, and thromboxane A and the modified phospholipids such as platelet activating factor (PAF). Eicosanoids are synthesized from 20-carbon polyunsaturated fatty acids by many cells, including activated leukocytes, mast cells, and platelets and are therefore widely distributed. Hormones and other inflammatory mediators (TNF-α, bradykinin) stimulate eicosanoid production either by direct activation of PLA_2, or indirectly by increasing intracellular Ca^{2+} concentrations, which in turn activate the enzyme. Cell membrane damage can also cause an increase in intracellular Ca^{2+}. Activated PLA_2 directly hydrolyzes AA, which is rapidly metabolized via one of two enzyme pathways—the cyclooxygenase (COX) pathway leading to the formation of prostaglandin and thromboxanes, or the 5-lipoxygenase (5-LOX) pathway that produces the leukotrienes.

Cyclooxygenase catalyzes the oxygenation of AA to form the cyclic endoperoxide PGG_2, which is converted to the closely related PGH_2. Both PGG_2 and PGH_2 are inherently unstable and rapidly converted to various prostaglandins, thromboxane A_2 (TXA_2), and prostacyclin (PGI_1). In the vascular beds of most animals, PGE_1, PGE_2, and PGI_1 are potent arteriolar dilators and enhance the effects of other mediators by increasing small-vein permeability. Other prostaglandins, including $PGF_{2\alpha}$ and thromboxane, cause smooth muscle contraction and vasoconstriction. Prostaglandins sensitize nociceptors to pain-provoking mediators such as bradykinin and histamine and, in high concentrations, can directly stimulate sensory nerve endings. TXA_2 is a potent platelet-aggregating agent involved in thrombus formation.

Found predominately in platelets, leukocytes, and the lungs, 5-LOX catalyzes the formation of unstable hydroxyperoxides from AA. These hydroxyperoxides are subsequently converted to peptide **leukotrienes**. Leukotriene B_4 (LTB_4) and 5-hydroxyeicosatetranoate (5-HETE) are strong chemoattractants stimulating polymorphonuclear leukocyte movement. LTB_4 also stimulates the production of cytokines in neutrophils, monocytes, and eosinophils and enhances the expression of C3b receptors. Other leukotrienes facilitate the release of histamine and other autacoids from mast cells and stimulate bronchiolar constriction and mucous secretion. In some species, leukotrienes C_4 and D_4 are more potent than histamine in contracting bronchial smooth muscle.

Platelet activating factor (PAF) is also derived from cell membrane phospholipids by the action of PLA_2. PAF, synthesized by mast cells, platelets, neutrophils, and eosinophils, induces platelet aggregation and stimulates platelets to release vasoactive amines and synthesize thromboxanes. PAF also increases vascular permeability and causes neutrophils to aggregate and degranulate.

The role of the free radical gas **nitric oxide** (NO) in inflammation is well established. NO is an important cell-signaling messenger in a wide range of physiologic and pathophysiologic processes. Small amounts of NO play a role in maintaining resting vascular tone, vasodilation, and antiaggregation of platelets. In response to certain cytokines (TNF-α, IL-1) and other inflammatory mediators, the production of relatively large quantities of NO is stimulated. In larger quantities, NO is a potent vasodilator, facilitates macrophage-induced cytotoxicity, and may contribute to joint destruction in some types of arthritis.

ANTIHISTAMINES

Antagonists that selectively block specific histamine receptors have been developed. H_1 antagonists block the actions of histamine responsible for increased capillary permeability and wheal and edema formation. However, because histamine is only one component of an incredibly complex inflammatory cascade, antihistamines have very weak anti-inflammatory activity. H_1 antihistamines may be useful to treat immediate hypersensitivity reactions such as anaphylaxis by blocking bronchoconstriction and vasodilation. H_1 antagonists may be less effective to treat allergic inflammatory diseases, such as atopy, primarily because mediators other than histamine play important roles in such conditions. H_2 (now classified as inverse agonists of the H_2 receptor, such as cimetidine and ranitidine) antagonists are routinely used to block the gastric secretory effects of histamine and have limited anti-inflammatory effects.

CORTICOSTEROIDS

Two classes of steroid hormones, mineralocorticoids and glucocorticoids, are naturally synthesized in the adrenal cortex from cholesterol. (*See also* THE ADRENAL GLANDS, p 573.)

Mineralocorticoids (aldosterone) are so named because they are important in maintaining electrolyte homeostasis. However, mineralocorticoids also trigger a broader range of functions in nonclassic target cellular sites, including some effects on wound healing after injury. In addition, a chronic and inappropriate (relative to intravascular volume and dietary sodium intake) increase in aldosterone secretion evokes a wound healing response in the absence of tissue injury. This can lead to antialdosterone (eg, spironolactone) drug treatment being recommended to prevent undesired heart remodeling and fibrosis.

Glucocorticoids suppress virtually every component of the inflammatory process; they inhibit PLA_2, decrease synthesis of interleukins and numerous other proinflammatory cytokines, suppress cell-mediated immunity, reduce complement synthesis, and decrease production and activity of leukocytes. Unsurprisingly then, glucocorticoids are by far the most efficacious anti-inflammatory drugs. They are also the most commonly used anti-inflammatory drugs. However, because their pharmacologic and physiologic effects are so broad, the potential for adverse effects is considerable.

Glucocorticoids play significant roles in carbohydrate, protein, and lipid metabolism; the immune response; and the response to stress. Natural glucocorticoids also have some mineralocorticoid activity and therefore affect fluid and electrolyte balance. While corticosteroids can be highly effective in suppressing or preventing inflammation, their physiologic and pharmacologic mechanisms of action are mediated by the same receptor. This explains why their pharmacologic and physiologic effects are inherently linked, and why supraphysiologic exposure to corticoids is potentially detrimental to several metabolic, hormonal, and immunologic functions.

All therapeutic corticosteroids have a 21-carbon steroid skeleton, similar to hydrocortisone (cortisol). Modifications to this skeleton selectively alter the degree of anti-inflammatory activity and the metabolic consequences and vary the duration of activity and protein-binding affinity of the resultant compound. The introduction of an additional double bond between C-1 and C-2 of cortisol in all synthetic corticosteroids selectivity increases glucocorticoid and anti-inflammatory activity. However, this single modification does not affect mineralocorticoid activity, resulting in an enhanced glucocorticoid/mineralocorticoid potency ratio, eg, prednisolone is ~4- to 5-fold more selective than cortisol. Additional fluorination at the C-9 position enhances both glucocorticoid and mineralocorticoid activity, as in 9α-fluorocortisol (fludrocortisone) and isoflupredone. Fludrocortisone (administered as fludrocortisone acetate) is 125-fold more potent than cortisol for mineralocorticoid effect and only 10-fold more for glucocorticoid effect. Thus, it is used in small animal medicine for its mineralocorticoid selectivity in the treatment of adrenocortical insufficiency.

Isoflupredone is used as an anti-inflammatory drug in cattle but lacks selectivity for mineralocortoid effects and increases the risk of severe hypokalemia. When a fluorinated derivative is substituted at the C-16 by an OH radical or a CH_3 group, the new C-16 substituted compound (eg, triamcinolone, dexamethasone, betamethasone) has virtually no mineralocorticoid effect but remains a potent anti-inflammatory glucocorticoid. This last substitution on C-16 yields a new property to these fluorocorticosteroids, enabling them to trigger parturition in various species, including cattle. Dexamethasone and flumethasone (short-acting formulations) can induce parturition when administered after 255 days of gestation in cattle, but induced calving is usually associated with a high incidence of adverse effects, including retained placenta.

Many corticoids are administered as esters. Esterification of the alcohol at C-21 determines the extent of water/lipid solubility and controls the in vivo disposition of the compound. Esterification with a monoacid, such as acetic acid, yields water-insoluble drugs (eg, methylprednisolone acetate) that can be used as long-acting formulations when administered by the IM,

SC, or intra-articular route. Other water-insoluble esters are diacetate, terbutate, and pivalate. By contrast, esterification of the same corticoid by a diacid such as succinic acid can yield a hydrosoluble ester, due to the second acid function (as for methylprednisolone sodium succinate) allowing a salt to be formed. Phosphate esters are also hydrosoluble. Solutions of free steroids or of hydrosoluble esters can be administered by the IV or IM route and are often used to treat life-threatening conditions such as heaves or hypersensitivity reaction. Esters may also be used PO, but hydrolysis occurs in the lumen of the digestive tract (pancreatic esterase) and the free active moiety is absorbed; thus, a formulation may be long-acting when administered parenterally but short-acting when given orally (eg, prednisolone acetate).

Nearly all esters are inactive prodrugs and require hydrolization to release their active moiety. Hydrolysis by esterases or pseudoesterases may occur either in body fluids such as blood or synovial fluid (acetate) or mainly in liver (succinate). Thus, for a local administration the choice of an appropriate ester is important. Hydrolysis may be only partial; for example, the bioavailability of methylprednisolone (the active moiety) from its hydrosoluble ester, methylprednisolone sodium succinate, is only 50% in dogs after IV administration, which must be considered when determining a dosage regimen.

Substances having a ketone radical in C-11, in lieu of an OH radical required for binding of the corticoid to its cellular receptors, are also prodrugs. Cortisone, prednisone, and methylprednisone are prodrugs of cortisol. These prodrugs are back transformed to their alcohol form in the liver by an 11-β-hydroxylase. There is no reason to administer them locally, because the activity of these prodrugs relies on hepatic metabolic activity. They are not recommended for use in animals with hepatic insufficiency. Prednisone is reported to have poor efficacy for treatment of heaves in horses because it is poorly absorbed, and its active metabolite, prednisolone, is rarely produced. By contrast, prednisolone has good bioavailability and is recommended in horses.

Other structural modifications allow more lipophilic substances to be obtained, such as the introduction of an acetonide between C-16 and C-17 (eg, triamcinolone acetonide). Triamcinolone acetonide, which is not a prodrug of triamcinolone, can be used for intra-articular administration in horses to treat osteoarthritis or as a topical formulation. Esterification at C-17 (valerate) produces a lipophilic compound with an enhanced topical:systemic potency ratio. Other approaches to achieve local glucocorticoid activity while minimizing systemic effects involve the formation of analogues that are rapidly inactivated after their systemic absorption. Fluticasone propionate, which is not a prodrug, is directly used to treat lung conditions. Similarly, beclomethasone dipropionate (a prodrug) locally yields an active metabolite (beclomethasone 17-monopropionate) that in turn yields beclomethasone, which has very weak anti-inflammatory activity.

Therapeutic corticosteroids are typically classified based on their relative glucocorticoid and mineralocorticoid potency (ie, the relative intensity of drug activity related to its concentration, a property that should not be confused with efficacy) as well as duration of effect (*see* TABLE 56). Compounds with the most potent glucocorticoid activity are also the most potent suppressors of the hypothalamic-pituitary-adrenal axis (HPAA).

Mode of Action: Glucocorticoids are capable of suppressing the inflammatory process through numerous pathways. They interact with specific intracellular receptor proteins in target tissues to alter the expression of corticosteroid-responsive genes. Glucocorticoid-specific receptors in the cell cytoplasm bind with steroid ligands to form hormone-receptor complexes that eventually translocate to the cell nucleus. There, these complexes bind to specific DNA sequences and alter their expression. The complexes may induce the transcription of mRNA, leading to synthesis of new proteins. Such proteins include lipocortin, a protein known to inhibit PLA_{2a} and thereby block the synthesis of prostaglandins, leukotrienes, and PAF. Glucocorticoids also inhibit the production of other mediators, including AA metabolites such as those produced via COX activation (both COX-1 and COX-2), cytokines, the interleukins, adhesion molecules, and enzymes such as collagenase.

Physiologic and Pharmacologic Effects: Peripherally and in the liver, glucocorticoids have important effects on carbohydrate, protein, and lipid metabolism. In the periphery, glucocorticoids stimulate lipolysis and protein breakdown, releasing glycerol and amino acids that act as substrates for gluconeogenesis. As a result, chronic exposure to excessive glucocorticoids may lead to muscle wasting

TABLE 56 RELATIVE POTENCIES OF COMMONLY USED CORTICOSTEROIDS

Compound	Relative Glucocorticoid Activity	Relative Mineralocorticoid Activity	Duration of Effect[a] (Alcohol Form)
Cortisol	1	1	S
Prednisone	5	0.8	I
Prednisolone	5	0.8	I
Methylprednisolone	5	0.5	I
Fludrocortisone	10	125	I
Isoflupredone	25	25	L
Triamcinolone	5	0	I
Triamcinolone acetonide	30	0	I
Dexamethasone	25	0	L
Betamethasone	25	0	L
Flumethasone	120	0	L

[a] S = short (~12 hr), I = intermediate (~24 hr), L = long (~48–72 hr)

and redistribution of body fat typical in animals with hyperadrenocorticism. In the liver, glucocorticoids stimulate hepatic gluconeogenesis and increase the hepatic synthesis and storage of glycogen. It is believed that gluconeogenesis is stimulated through the transcription of enzymes such as glucose-6-phosphatase and phosphoenolpyruvate carboxykinase. Glucocorticoids also decrease glucose uptake in peripheral tissues, including adipose tissue and mammary glands, further contributing to an increase in blood glucose. In dairy cattle, the reduction of milk yield is a major mechanism of the glucose-sparing effect of corticoids. In response to increased blood glucose, there is a compensatory increase in insulin. However, glucocorticoids inhibit the suppression of gluconeogenesis by insulin and cause insulin resistance in peripheral tissues, further contributing to hyperglycemia.

Although not as potent as the mineralocorticoid aldosterone, nonfluorinated glucocorticoids (prednisolone and methylprednisolone) do have some effects on water and electrolyte balance, enhancing potassium excretion and sodium retention primarily due to their activity in the kidneys. Fluorinated corticoids, provided that they are substituted at C-16 as in dexamethasone and triamcinolone, have no mineralocorticoid activity but rather exert a polyuric/polydipsic effect due to an inhibition of antidiuretic hormone (ADH) secretion and decreased renal sensitivity to ADH. Glucocorticoids can increase renal excretion and decrease the intestinal absorption of calcium, causing depletion of calcium stores. Glucocorticoids also inhibit osteoblasts, stimulate osteoclasts, and increase parathyroid secretion, which could affect bone healing.

A number of mechanisms are responsible for the anti-inflammatory and immunosuppressive actions of glucocorticoids. In homeostasis, glucocorticoids help maintain normal vascular permeability and microcirculation and stabilize cellular and lysosomal membranes. However, in acute inflammation, glucocorticoids decrease vascular permeability and inhibit the migration and egress of polymorphonuclear lymphocytes into tissues. Glucocorticoids suppress cell-mediated immunity by inducing apoptosis in normal lymphoid cells; inhibiting the clonal expansion of T and B lymphocytes; and reducing the number of circulating eosinophils, basophils, and monocytes. In contrast, glucocorticoids inhibit margination of neutrophils and increase the release of mature neutrophils from the bone marrow. Inflamed tissue, phagocytosis, and toxic oxygen-free radical production are inhibited in macrophages and monocytes. In the later stages of inflammation, glucocorticoids inhibit the activity of fibroblasts, reducing fibrosis and the formation of scar tissue. However, they may also slow wound healing.

Glucocorticoids modulate the synthesis and release of a number of chemical mediators of inflammation, including prostaglandins, leukotrienes, histamine, cytokines, complement, and PAF; they also suppress the production of inducible NO synthase and chondrodestructive enzymes such as collagenase.

Glucocorticoids have effects on other hormone systems. All anti-inflammatory glucocorticoid drugs in use today inhibit the HPAA, which can result in clinically significant adverse effects when stopping a prolonged corticoid treatment.

Administration and Pharmacokinetics: Steroid formulations are available for oral, parenteral, and topical use. Many, including prednisone, prednisolone, methylprednisolone, and dexamethasone are well absorbed when administered PO and are particularly useful when anti-inflammatory treatment is required for a period of one to several weeks. Other preparations are available for parenteral use. The sodium phosphate and succinate salts are highly water soluble, providing a rapid onset of action when given IV. Other injectable formulations include insoluble esters such as methylprednisolone acetate and triamcinolone acetate, which have limited water solubility. The systemic absorption from these preparations is very slow and may result in anti-inflammatory effects and associated HPAA suppression for several weeks. Corticosteroid preparations available for topical or intralesional administration can be effective in treating inflammation of the skin, eyes, or ears. Although controversial, intra-articular administration of glucocorticoids has been used in people and animals, particularly horses, to manage inflammatory joint disease. In horses, for intra-articular administration, triamcinolone acetonide is preferred over methylprednisolone acetate. Glucocorticoids are absorbed systemically from sites of local administration in amounts that may be sufficient to suppress the HPAA.

Following absorption, ~90% of cortisol is reversibly bound to plasma proteins, primarily corticosteroid-binding globulin (CBG) and albumin. Among synthetic corticoids, only prednisolone binds specifically and with high affinity to CBG. Prednisolone can displace cortisol from its CBG binding site, explaining the immediate decrease of plasma cortisol after prednisolone is administered IV, a decrease not associated with HPAA inhibition. Other synthetic corticoids are mainly bound to albumin. Only the unbound portion is available to exert physiologic and pharmacologic effects and to cross physiologic barriers such as the blood-brain barrier or the udder. Generally, glucocorticoids are metabolized in the liver, where they are reduced and conjugated, forming inactive water-soluble derivatives excreted by the kidney.

Adverse Effects: Adverse effects of glucocorticoids commonly result from the longterm use of supraphysiologic doses to control inflammatory or immunologic disorders. Longterm administration may lead to iatrogenic Cushing syndrome, characterized by polyuria, polydipsia, bilaterally symmetric alopecia, increased susceptibility to infection, muscle atrophy, and redistribution of body fat. The gluconeogenic and insulin antagonistic effects of glucocorticoids may precipitate the onset of diabetes mellitus or exacerbate diabetes in animals with existing disease. Longterm suppression of the HPAA may cause adrenal gland atrophy and resultant iatrogenic secondary hypoadrenocorticism. In affected animals, abrupt discontinuation of glucocorticoid therapy may lead to an Addisonian-like crisis characterized by lethargy, weakness, vomiting, and diarrhea. In severe cases, circulatory shock and death may result.

Glucocorticoids induce glycogen accumulation in hepatocytes, resulting in hepatopathy and hepatomegaly, and stimulate production of the steroid-specific isoenzyme of alkaline phosphatase. Slow turnover of enterocytes and inhibition of protective prostaglandins in the gut due to glucocorticoids may contribute to development of GI ulceration. Furthermore, glucocorticoids potentiate the ulcerogenic effects of NSAIDs. Glucocorticoids reduce collagen synthesis and may lead to thinning and increased fragility of the skin. Alterations in fluid and electrolyte balance may result in sodium and fluid retention and hypokalemic alkalosis. In horses, high doses of glucocorticoids may induce or exacerbate laminitis. Significant mood and behavioral changes have been described in people receiving corticosteroid therapy and may be seen in animals as well.

Although immunosuppression may be a desired effect of glucocorticoid therapy in autoimmune disease, susceptibility to infection may increase, or latent infections may be reactivated. Urinary tract infections are common in animals receiving glucocorticoids for longterm therapy of inflammatory or immunologic disease. In joints, glucocorticoids may reduce the formation of chondrocyte collagen and synovial fluid and contribute to the development of septic arthritis. Strict aseptic technique must be observed when administering intra-articular injections of steroids.

The adverse effects of longterm (>2 wk) glucocorticoid therapy can be diminished using an alternate-day treatment regimen. Once inflammation has been controlled using daily therapy with a drug that has intermediate duration of activity (eg, oral prednisolone or prednisone), a gradual change to alternate-day therapy can be made.

Therapeutic Uses: Short-acting soluble steroids such as the succinate esters have been routinely used in the treatment of septic shock, but this indication is controversial. The action of corticoids on hemorrhagic and cardiogenic shock is not established, even though product labeling includes this use as an adjunct to fluid therapy. Glucocorticoids are also routinely used in the treatment of cerebral edema, although controlled clinical trials supporting their effectiveness are lacking.

Glucocorticoids are used commonly to treat allergy and inflammation such as pruritic dermatoses and allergic lung and GI diseases. In acute cases of atopic or flea allergy dermatitis, anti-inflammatory dosages (prednisolone, 0.5–1 mg/kg/day) alleviate pruritus and limit self-trauma from scratching until the underlying cause can be addressed. Similar dosages are used in the management of chronic allergic bronchitis and feline asthma. Short-acting corticosteroids have also been used in treatment of acute respiratory distress syndrome in cattle and chronic obstructive pulmonary disease in horses. Historically, corticosteroids have been used to treat several musculoskeletal disorders, including osteoarthritis, myositis, and immune-mediated arthritis. More recently, the NSAIDs have become first-line therapy for musculoskeletal disorders, particularly in the treatment of osteoarthritis in companion animal species. In most inflammatory conditions, glucocorticoids should be used in conjunction with therapies that target the underlying cause.

NONSTEROIDAL ANTI-INFLAMMATORY DRUGS

The importance of pain management and the use of NSAIDs in animals has increased dramatically in recent decades, with use of NSAIDs in companion animals being routine. NSAIDs have the potential to relieve pain and inflammation without the myriad potential metabolic, hemodynamic, and immunosuppressive adverse effects associated with corticosteroids. However, all NSAIDs have the potential for other adverse effects that should be considered in overall management of the inflammatory process.

Mode of Action: Generally, the classification NSAID is applied to drugs that inhibit one or more steps in the metabolism of arachidonic acid (AA). Unlike corticosteroids, which inhibit numerous pathways, NSAIDs act primarily to reduce the biosynthesis of prostaglandins by inhibiting cyclooxygenase (COX). In general, NSAIDs do not inhibit the formation of 5-lipoxygenase (5-LOX) and hence leukotriene, or the formation of other inflammatory mediators. The novel NSAID tepoxalin is an exception in that it inhibits both COX and 5-LOX.

The discovery of the two isoforms of COX (COX-1 and COX-2) has led to greater understanding of the mechanism of action and potential adverse effects of NSAIDs. COX-1, expressed in virtually all tissues of the body (eg, gut and kidney), catalyzes the formation of constitutive prostaglandins, which mediate a variety of normal physiologic effects, including hemostasis, GI mucosal protection, and protection of the kidney from hypotensive insult. In contrast, COX-2 is activated in damaged and inflamed tissues and catalyzes the formation of inducible prostaglandin, including PGE_2, associated with intensifying the inflammatory response. COX-2 is also involved in thermoregulation and the pain response to injury. Therefore, COX-2 inhibition by NSAIDs is thought to be responsible for the antipyretic, analgesic, and anti-inflammatory actions of NSAIDs. However, concurrent inhibition of COX-1 may result in many of the unwanted effects of NSAIDs, including gastric ulceration and renal toxicity. Because NSAIDs vary in their ability to inhibit each COX isoform, a drug that inhibits COX-2 at a lower concentration than that necessary to inhibit COX-1 would be considered safer. This concept has propelled the development of the "COX-2 selective" NSAIDs. Although ratios of COX-1:COX-2 inhibition by various NSAIDs in people and animals have been reported, caution is advised when interpreting such ratios, because they vary greatly depending on the selectivity assay used. The COX selectivity of NSAIDs also varies by species; COX selectivity ratios reported for people cannot be directly extrapolated to other species.

In general, drugs with ratios suggesting preferential activity against COX-2 may have fewer adverse effects due to COX-1 inhibition. In dogs, favorable ratios have been reported for carprofen, meloxicam, deracoxib, firocoxib, and robenacoxib, whereas unfavorable ratios have been reported for aspirin, phenylbutazone, and vedaprofen. COX-1–sparing drugs are associated with less GI ulceration and less platelet inhibition; however, it may be an oversimplification to assume that complete COX-2 inhibition is without potential risk. Recent research has suggested that COX-2 can be induced constitutively in various organs, including the brain, spinal cord, ovary, and kidneys. In dogs, COX-2 mRNA is present in the loop of Henle and the maculae densa and may play an important role in the protective response to hypotension. However, a study that failed to demonstrate COX-2 expression in canine kidneys raised questions regarding its role. COX-2 also appears to be important in the healing of GI ulcers in people, and certain COX-2–specific inhibitors delay ulcer healing experimentally. Although COX-1 plays a primary role in regulating homeostasis, it may play a more significant role in inflammation than originally proposed.

NSAIDs enter the pocket of the COX enzyme, whereupon steric hindrance prevents entry of AA. Aspirin is unusual in that it irreversibly acetylates a serine residue of COX, resulting in a complete loss of COX activity. Thus, the duration of the aspirin effect depends on the turnover rate of COX; activity is lost for the life of the platelet (7–10 days) after aspirin administration, explaining the duration of aspirin's effect on hemostasis. Unlike aspirin, most other NSAIDs (including salicylic acid, an active metabolite of aspirin) are reversible competitive COX inhibitors; their duration of inhibition is primarily determined by the elimination pharmacokinetics of the drug.

Pharmacologic Effects: All NSAIDs, except for acetaminophen (also named paracetamol), are antipyretic, analgesic, and anti-inflammatory. They are routinely used for the relief of pain and inflammation associated with osteoarthritis in dogs and horses and for colic, navicular disease, and laminitis in horses. The use of NSAIDs for the relief of perioperative pain in companion animals is standard practice. In general, NSAIDs provide only symptomatic relief from pain and inflammation and do not significantly alter the course of pathologic damage. As analgesics, they are generally less effective than opioids and are therefore generally indicated only against mild to moderate pain in people. However, in veterinary medicine, NSAIDs also find use in management of severe pain, optimally in combination with an opioid.

As antipyretics, NSAIDs reduce body temperature in febrile states. Although the beneficial effects of the febrile response usually outweigh the negative effects, NSAID inhibition of PGE_2 activity in the hypothalamus may provide symptomatic relief and improve appetite. In Europe, NSAIDs have been used in conjunction with antibiotics for treatment of acute respiratory diseases in cattle. They may reduce morbidity through their antipyretic and anti-inflammatory effects and prevent development of irreversible lung lesions.

The effects of some NSAIDs on chondrocyte metabolism have been investigated. Some, including aspirin, naproxen, and ibuprofen, are considered chondrotoxic, because they inhibit the synthesis of cartilage proteoglycans. Others, including carprofen and meloxicam, may be considered chondroneutral, or depending on dose, actually stimulate the production of cartilage matrix. The potential beneficial or deleterious effects of NSAIDs on chondrocyte metabolism remain to be clarified.

A therapeutic area in which NSAID use may become important is in the treatment and prevention of cancer. Epidemiologic studies in people show that aspirin use is associated with a significant reduction in the incidence of colon cancer. Newer evidence suggests that the therapeutic effect of NSAIDs on colon cancer is mediated by inhibition of COX-2, which may be upregulated in many premalignant and malignant neoplasms. In veterinary medicine, piroxicam has been shown to reduce the size of tumors such as transitional cell carcinoma in dogs. Specific COX-2 inhibitors may prove useful as a primary or adjunctive therapy in the management of cancer.

Administration and Pharmacokinetics: Most NSAIDs are weak organic acids that are well absorbed after PO administration. However, food can impair the oral absorption of some NSAIDs (eg, phenylbutazone, meclofenamate, flunixin, and robenacoxib). Several NSAIDs are available as parenteral formulations for IV, IM, or SC administration. Some parenteral formulations are highly alkaline (eg, phenylbutazone) and may cause tissue necrosis if injected perivascularly. Once absorbed, most NSAIDs are extensively (up to 99%) bound to plasma proteins, with only a small proportion of unbound drug available to be active in the tissues. NSAIDs may also compete for binding sites with other highly protein-bound compounds, leading to some drug displacement; however, this displacement has little therapeutic consequence because it does not affect the concentration of the free drug. Because NSAIDs are highly protein bound and extravasation of protein occurs in inflammation, NSAIDs tend to concentrate in areas of inflammation. Consequently, their duration of action typically exceeds that predicted by elimination half-life.

Most NSAIDs are biotransformed in the liver to inactive metabolites that are excreted either by the kidney via glomerular filtration and tubular secretion or by the bile. Mavacoxib is an exception, mostly being excreted unchanged in the bile. Biotransformation and elimination half-lives vary significantly by species (and in some cases by breed or strain, as is the case for some COX-2 inhibitors in Beagles), so it is not possible to safely extrapolate dosages from one species or animal to another. Some NSAIDs, including naproxen, etodolac, and meclofenamic acid, undergo extensive enterohepatic recirculation in some species, resulting in prolonged elimination half-lives.

Adverse Effects: All NSAIDs have the potential to induce adverse reactions, some of which can be life threatening. Many reactions to NSAIDs are dose-related and are typically reversible with discontinuation of therapy and supportive care.

Vomiting is the most common adverse effect. GI ulceration is the most common life-threatening adverse effect. Loss of GI protective mechanisms results from inhibition of constitutive prostaglandins that regulate blood flow to the gastric mucosa and stimulate bicarbonate and mucus production. This disrupts the alkaline protective barrier of the gut, allowing diffusion of gastric acid back into the mucosa, injuring cells and blood vessels and causing gastritis and ulceration. As organic acids, NSAIDs, especially aspirin, may also cause direct chemical irritation of the GI mucosa. The enterohepatic recirculation of certain NSAIDs may result in high biliary concentrations that increase ulcerogenic potential in the gut. NSAID-induced GI bleeding may be occult, leading to iron-deficiency anemia, or be more severe, resulting in vomiting, hematemesis, and melena. Horses may develop oral, lingual, or colonic ulceration with accompanying signs of colic, weight loss, and diarrhea.

GI blood loss may be further complicated by impaired platelet function; NSAIDs, by inhibiting COX-1, prevent platelets from forming TXA_2, a potent aggregating agent. Because TXA_2 inhibition causes prolonged bleeding, evaluation of buccal mucosal bleeding time is advised in animals for which surgery is anticipated. Blood dyscrasias after longterm NSAID therapy have been reported in cats, dogs, and horses. Acetaminophen (paracetamol) administration in cats is associated with Heinz body anemia, methemoglobinemia, hepatic failure, and death. Bone marrow dyscrasias associated with phenylbutazone administration have also been reported.

Nephropathies associated with chronic NSAID use are common in people. Animals with underlying renal compromise receiving NSAIDs could experience exacerbation or decompensation of their disease. It is important to maintain hydration and renal perfusion in animals receiving NSAIDs, especially those undergoing anesthesia or surgery and in horses with colic.

Hepatopathies are relatively common in people and animals receiving NSAIDs. NSAID administration routinely induces mild hepatic changes characterized primarily by increases in liver enzymes without clinical signs or hepatic dysfunction. Rare reports of idiosyncratic reactions resulting in hepatic dysfunction or failure have been reported in people (acetaminophen and others), dogs (acetaminophen, carprofen, etodolac), and horses (phenylbutazone). Cytopathic (hepatocellular injury, necrosis), cholestatic, and mixed histopathologic patterns of injury have been documented. NSAIDs should be used with caution in animals with preexisting hepatic disease.

Specific Nonsteroidal Anti-inflammatory Drugs

Based on structure, most NSAIDs can be divided into two broad groups: carboxylic acid and enolic acid derivatives. The main subgroups of enolic acids are the pyrazolones (phenylbutazone) and the oxicams (meloxicam, piroxicam). Carboxylic acid subgroups include the salicylates (aspirin), propionic acids (ibuprofen, naproxen, carprofen, ketoprofen, and vedaprofen), fenemates (tolfenamic and meclofenamic acids), phenylacetic acids (acetaminophen), and aminonicotinic acids (flunixin). The newer coxib class of selective COX-2 inhibitors includes a diaryl-substituted pyrazole (celecoxib) and a diaryl-substituted isoxazole (valdecoxib), both available for human use. Four NSAIDs of the coxib class, deracoxib, firocoxib, robenacoxib, and mavacoxib have been introduced in veterinary medicine.

Aspirin: By far the most widely used NSAID in people, aspirin is primarily used in veterinary medicine for relief of mild to moderate pain associated with musculoskeletal inflammation or osteoarthritis. The salicylic ester of acetic acid, aspirin (acetylsalicylic acid) is available in several different dosage forms, including bolus (for cattle), oral paste (for horses), oral solution (for poultry), and tablets (for dogs). Enteric-coated products used in human medicine are not recommended in dogs, because gastric retention may lead to erratic plasma exposure. After PO administration, aspirin is rapidly absorbed from the stomach and upper small intestine. Aspirin is subjected to a large, first-pass effect in the liver to yield salicylic acid, its main active metabolite. In addition, the aspirin fraction that gains access to the systemic circulation is also rapidly hydrolyzed to salicylic acid with a half-life of ~15 min. After oral aspirin administration, salicylic acid is considered the main active substance in the systemic circulation. Aspirin primarily inhibits COX-1, whereas salicylic acid has more balanced COX-1/COX-2 activity. In addition, aspirin may irreversibly bind to COX-1 through acetylation of a serine residue near the enzyme active site. Because of this irreversible binding, the anticoagulant activity of aspirin lasts far longer than its anti-inflammatory effect; a single aspirin dose of 20 mg/kg in a horse may prolong bleeding for 48 hr. Depending on its route of administration, aspirin may have different pharmacologic effects. For irreversible platelet COX-1 inhibition (to treat a thromboembolic condition), aspirin given IV is more efficient than aspirin given PO because, for the same dose, aspirin exposure is greater for the IV route of administration.

After absorption, both aspirin and salicylate are widely distributed through most tissues and fluids and readily cross the placental barrier. Approximately 80%–90% of salicylate is bound to plasma proteins. Metabolism and elimination is via hepatic conjugation with glucuronic acid, followed by renal excretion. Cats, which lack glucuronyl transferase, metabolize salicylates slowly. In addition, salicylate metabolism is saturable and, if overexposure due to an aspirin overdose occurs, plasma salicylate elimination may follow a zero order and slower elimination kinetics. The elimination half-life of salicylic acid in cats approaches 40 hr, whereas it is ~7.5 hr in dogs.

Because aspirin is not approved for veterinary use, definitive efficacy studies have not been performed to establish effective dosages. Recommended dosages in dogs are 10–40 mg/kg, PO, bid-tid. Aspirin has been used for its anticlotting effect in the treatment of laminitis in horses at a dosage of 10 mg/kg/day, PO. In cats, aspirin may be used for its antiplatelet effects in thromboembolic disease at a dosage of 10 mg/kg, PO, every 48 hr, to allow for prolonged metabolism. Adverse effects are common after aspirin administration and appear to be dosage dependent. Even at therapeutic dosages of 25 mg/kg, plain aspirin may induce mucosal erosion and ulceration in dogs. Vomiting and melena may be seen at higher doses. The PGE_1 analogue misoprostol may decrease GI ulceration associated with aspirin and other NSAIDs. Aspirin overdose in any species can result in salicylate poisoning, characterized by severe acid-base abnormalities, hemorrhage, seizures, coma, and death.

Acetaminophen: Acetaminophen (paracetamol) is a para-aminophenol derivative with analgesic and antipyretic effects similar to those of aspirin, but it has weaker anti-inflammatory effects than does aspirin and other NSAIDs. The reason for this anomaly is that acetaminophen's selective COX-2 inhibition is via enzyme reduction; the high levels of peroxides in areas of inflammation are thought to interfere with COX-2 reduction peripherally, whereas the low peroxide levels in the brain and spinal cord account for any centrally mediated analgesia. Acetaminophen does not inhibit neutrophil activation, has little ulcerogenic potential, and has no effect on platelets or bleeding time. The recommended dosage of acetaminophen in dogs is 10–15 mg/kg, PO, tid. Dose-dependent adverse effects include depression, vomiting, and methemoglobinemia. Use in cats is contraindicated because of their deficiency of glucuronyl transferase, which makes them susceptible to methemoglobinemia and centrilobular hepatic necrosis.

Phenylbutazone: One of the earliest NSAIDs approved for use in horses and

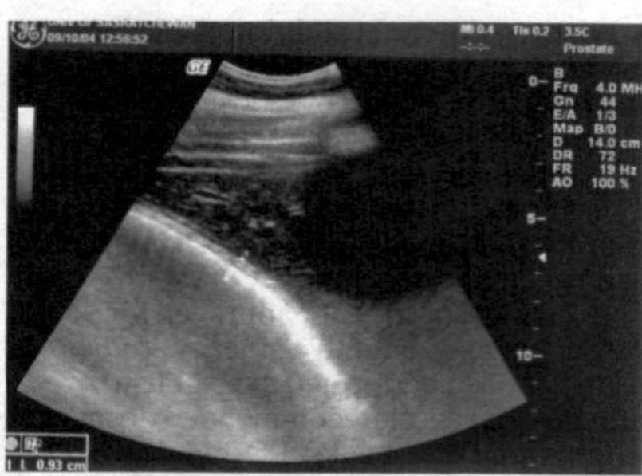

Phenylbutazone toxicity, right dorsal colitis in a horse (ultrasound). *Courtesy of Dr. Sameeh M. Abutarbush.*

dogs, phenylbutazone (PBZ) is a pyrazolone derivative available in tablet, paste, gel, and parenteral formulations. The plasma half-life of PBZ is 5–6 hr in horses and dogs and >30 hr in cattle (a reason that PBZ is not approved for use in cattle). When given PO, PBZ adsorbs to hay in the diet, to then be released during fermentation in the hindgut. Although this potentially may reduce GI absorption and bioavailability, the clinically relevant effect is a delay in absorption. Once absorbed, binding to plasma proteins is high (99% in horses). PBZ is metabolized by the liver to several active (oxyphenbutazone) and inactive metabolites, which are excreted in urine. One of the major therapeutic uses of PBZ is to treat acute laminitis in horses. Laminitis is treated initially with injectable PBZ at dosages up to 8.8 mg/kg, followed by therapy PO at 2.2–4.4 mg/kg, bid. Because the therapeutic index for PBZ is relatively narrow (PBZ exhibits zero order metabolism), the dosage should be adjusted to the minimum possible to maintain comfort and avoid toxicity. GI effects (eg, anorexia) and depression are the most frequent adverse effects associated with PBZ. Ulcers may develop in the mouth, stomach, cecum, and right dorsal colon. The ulcerogenic potential of PBZ in horses is greater than that of flunixin and ketoprofen. PBZ dosages of 3–7 mg/kg, PO, tid, are recommended in dogs. In dogs, PBZ has been associated with bleeding dyscrasias, hepatopathies, nephropathies, and rare cases of irreversible bone marrow suppression.

Meclofenamic Acid: Meclofenamic acid is a fenemate (anthranilic acid) NSAID available for horses as a granular preparation and for dogs as an oral tablet. The recommended dosage is 2.2 mg/kg/day for 5–7 days in horses and 1.1 mg/kg/day for 5–7 days in dogs. In cattle, administration of meclofenamic acid results in a biphasic pattern of absorption, with an initial peak plasma concentration reached at ~30 min and a secondary peak 4 hr after dosing. In horses, meclofenamic acid is rapidly absorbed, but feeding before dosing may delay absorption. The onset of action is slow, requiring 2–4 days of dosing for a clinical effect. Although it is effective in the treatment of chronic laminitis, meclofenamic acid has a therapeutic index that may be lower than that of other NSAIDs.

Tolfenamic Acid: Tolfenamic acid is an anthranilic (fenemate) NSAID class approved for use in Europe and other countries. It is used for fever, postoperative pain, and acute and chronic inflammatory conditions in cats, dogs, cattle, and pigs.

Flunixin: In the USA, the nicotinic acid derivative flunixin (as the meglumine salt) is approved for use in horses as PO and parenteral formulations. The recommended dosage is 1.1 mg/kg/day for 5 days, IV or PO. Flunixin is rapidly absorbed after PO or IM administration, and the elimination half-life is short (~2–3 hr). Elimination is primarily by renal excretion. Flunixin is effective for the treatment of visceral pain associated with colic in horses. It is also used to reduce the inflammatory-mediated hemodynamic response to endotoxin, although it is unlikely to reduce mortality associated with endotoxemic shock. The dosage recommended in horses is 1.1 mg/kg, bid, or 0.25 mg/kg, tid. Toxicity in horses is relatively uncommon, but GI ulceration and erosion may develop. Flunixin has been used to treat mastitis and acute pulmonary emphysema in cattle, although it is not approved for these indications. Chronic administration of flunixin to dogs may result in severe GI ulceration and renal damage. Flunixin is not marketed in the USA for dogs, but it is approved in Europe and other countries.

Carprofen: Carprofen is an NSAID of the arylpropionic acid class available in the USA in caplet and chewable tablet formulations. An injectable formulation is also available in the USA and Europe. Carprofen is approved by the FDA to manage pain and inflammation associated with osteoarthritis and acute pain associated with soft-tissue and orthopedic surgery in dogs. The recommended dosage is 4.4 mg/kg/day or divided bid, PO. In Europe and other countries, carprofen is also registered for use in horses and cattle and for short-term therapy in cats. In dogs, oral bioavailability is high (90%), and plasma concentrations peak ~2–3 hr after dosing. The elimination half-life is ~8 hr. As with other NSAIDs, carprofen is highly (99%) protein bound. Elimination is via hepatic biotransformation, with excretion of the resulting metabolites in feces and urine. Some enterohepatic recycling occurs. The exact mechanism of action of carprofen is unclear. Although it has greater selectivity for COX-2 over COX-1, carprofen is considered a weak COX inhibitor. In vitro assays with canine cell lines indicate that it is 129-fold more selective for COX-2, whereas in vitro assays with canine whole blood indicate that it is 7- to 17-fold more selective for COX-2. Equine whole blood assays indicate that it is 1.6-fold more selective for COX-2, and feline whole blood assays indicate it is >5.5-fold more selective for COX-2. Other mechanisms of action, including inhibition of PA_2, may be responsible for its anti-inflammatory effects. Carprofen has been used extensively in dogs since its introduction, and adverse events have been comparable to those of other NSAIDs (ie, ~2 events/1,000 dogs treated). Approximately one-fourth of the adverse reactions reported were GI signs, including vomiting, diarrhea, and GI ulceration. Renal and hepatic adverse effects are rare, as with other NSAIDs. Potentially serious idiosyncratic hepatopathies, characterized by acute hepatic necrosis, have been reported in some dogs. Approximately one-third of the dogs developing hepatopathies while receiving carprofen were Labrador Retrievers, although a true breed predisposition has not been established. As with any NSAID therapy, clinical laboratory monitoring for hepatic damage is advised, especially in geriatric animals that may be predisposed to more serious complications.

Ketoprofen: Ketoprofen is another propionic acid derivative available in the USA and other countries as a 10% injectable solution for horses, and in Europe and Canada as tablets and a 1% injectable solution for dogs and cats. Ketoprofen is recommended for acute pain (up to 5 days) in both dogs and cats. In horses, it is used for pain and inflammation associated with osteoarthritis and for visceral pain associated with colic. The recommended dosage is 1 mg/kg/day for up to 5 days, IV or PO, in dogs and cats; 2.2 mg/kg/day for up to 5 days, IV, in horses; and 3 mg/kg/day for 1–3 days, IV or IM, in cattle. Ketoprofen is a potent inhibitor of COX and bradykinin and may also inhibit some lipoxygenases. Its efficacy is comparable to that of opioids in the management of pain after orthopedic and soft-tissue surgery in dogs. After administration PO, ketoprofen is rapidly absorbed and has a terminal half-life in cats and dogs of 2–3 hr. As with other NSAIDs, ketoprofen is metabolized in the liver to inactive metabolites that are eliminated by renal excretion. Adverse effects, including GI upset, are similar to those of other NSAIDs. Other adverse effects, including hepatopathies and renal disease, have been reported in animals. Because of potential antiplatelet effects, care should be exercised when using ketoprofen perioperatively.

Etodolac: The pyranocarboxylic acid etodolac is approved for use in dogs in the USA. The elimination half-life is ~8–12 hr, allowing dosing at 10–15 mg/kg/day, PO. Extensive enterohepatic recirculation has been reported in dogs, followed by elimination of etodolac and its metabolites in the liver and feces. In in vitro studies, etodolac was more selective in inhibiting COX-2 than COX-1, although in vitro canine whole blood assays have also shown it to be nonselective. Etodolac has been shown to inhibit macrophage chemotaxis and has demonstrated efficacy for the treatment of lameness associated with hip dysplasia. Although the risk of GI ulceration is low at therapeutic doses, administration of three times the label dosage resulted in GI ulceration, vomiting, and weight loss in toxicity studies. GI, hepatic, and renal adverse reactions have been reported after administration of etodolac, similar to those of other NSAIDs.

Vedaprofen: The arylpropionic acid derivative vedaprofen is available in Europe in a gel formulation for horses and dogs and in an injectable formulation for horses. Vedaprofen is indicated for the treatment of pain and inflammation associated with musculoskeletal disorders in dogs (0.5 mg/kg/day) and horses (1 mg/kg, bid) and for the treatment of pain associated with colic in horses (2 mg/kg, IV, as a single injection). After administration PO, vedaprofen is rapidly absorbed. Bioavailability is generally high but may be reduced if the drug is administered with food. The terminal half-life is 10–13 hr in dogs and 6–8 hr in horses. Vedaprofen undergoes extensive biotransformation to hydroxylated metabolites, which are excreted in urine and feces.

Meloxicam: Meloxicam is an oxicam NSAID available as an oral syrup and injectable solution. It is approved for human use in the USA and Canada and for use in dogs in the USA. In Europe and other countries, it is approved for use in dogs, cats, cattle, and horses. A potent inhibitor of prostaglandin synthesis, meloxicam is used for the treatment of acute and chronic inflammation associated with musculoskeletal disease and for the management of postoperative pain. In dogs, a one-time loading dose of 0.2 mg/kg, PO, is recommended, followed by 0.1 mg/kg/day, PO. Once a therapeutic effect is seen, the dosage can be titrated to the lowest possible dose. COX-1:COX-2 ratios reported for meloxicam suggest the drug is COX-2 selective, with in vitro canine whole blood assays indicating it is 2.7- to 10-fold more selective for COX-2. Once absorbed, meloxicam is highly protein bound (97%) and has a relatively long elimination half-life (>12 hr). GI safety appears to be greater for meloxicam than for nonselective NSAIDs, and meloxicam has been shown to be chondroneutral in rodent studies.

Deracoxib: Deracoxib, the first NSAID of the coxib class approved for use in dogs, is available in a beef-flavored chewable tablet formulation in the USA. Deracoxib has been shown to inhibit COX-2–mediated PGE_2 production. COX-1:COX-2 ratios reported for deracoxib in in vitro cloned canine cell assays indicate it is 1,275-fold more selective for COX-2, whereas in vitro canine whole blood assays indicate it is 12- to 37-fold selective for COX-2. Deracoxib is indicated for the control of postoperative pain and inflammation associated with orthopedic surgery at a dosage of 3–4 mg/kg/day for up to 7 days, PO, and for the control of pain and inflammation associated with osteoarthritis at a dosage of 1–2 mg/kg/day, PO. Once absorbed, protein binding is >90%, and the elimination half-life is 3 hr.

Firocoxib: Firocoxib is a coxib-class NSAID approved in the USA and Europe for the control of pain and inflammation associated with osteoarthritis and for the control of postoperative pain and inflammation associated with soft-tissue and orthopedic surgery in dogs. In Canada, Australia, and New Zealand it is approved for use in osteoarthritis and soft-tissue and orthopedic surgery. It is available in a chewable *tablet* formulation. After administration PO, firocoxib is rapidly absorbed and then eliminated by hepatic metabolism and fecal excretion. The elimination half-life is ~8 hr, allowing dosing at 5 mg/kg/day, PO. COX-1:COX-2 ratios from in vitro canine whole blood assays indicate it is 384-fold more selective for COX-2. As with other NSAIDs, protein binding is high, at ~96%. GI safety appears to be greater than that of nonspecific NSAIDs.

Robenacoxib: Robenacoxib is a coxib-class highly selective COX-2 inhibitor, structurally related to the human NSAIDs diclofenac and lumiracoxib. Robenacoxib is used for the control of pain and inflammation associated with osteoarthritis, orthopedic and soft-tissue surgery in dogs (approved in Europe), and for musculoskeletal disorders and soft-tissue surgeries in cats (approved in the USA and Europe). Dosage is 2 mg/kg, PO, initially and then 1–2 mg/kg/day thereafter (for up to 6 days in cats). COX-1:COX-2 ratios from in vitro canine whole blood assays indicate it is 128-fold more selective for COX-2. As with other NSAIDs, protein binding is high, at ~98%. GI safety appears to be greater than that of nonselective NSAIDs. The elimination half-life is 1 hr after oral administration. Administration with food decreases bioavailability of robenacoxib.

Mavacoxib: Mavacoxib is a coxib-class COX-2 inhibitor approved in Europe and Australia for the control of pain and inflammation associated with degenerative joint disease in dogs. Mavacoxib is structurally related to the human NSAID celecoxib; however, substitution of a methyl group with a single fluorine atom has conferred great resistance to metabolism, resulting in an elimination half-life of 17 days in young Beagle dogs. Unlike the major route of elimination of other NSAIDs, that of mavacoxib is biliary excretion of the parent molecule. In field trials conducted in aged dogs with osteoarthritis, the half-life was found to be even longer at 44 days, and in these older dogs, approximately 1 in 20 exhibited a half-life of >80 days. These population pharmacokinetic studies in target patients were used to optimize the dose regimen. The long half-life means mavacoxib has a unique dose regimen: the initial dose is 2 mg/kg, PO, repeated 14 days later; thereafter, the dosing interval is 1 mo, with the total course not exceeding seven doses (6.5 mo). Food significantly increases bioavailability. COX-1:COX-2 ratios from in vitro canine whole blood assays indicate mavacoxib is 128-fold more selective for COX-2. As with other NSAIDs, protein binding is high, at ~98%. GI safety appears to be greater than that of nonselective NSAIDs.

The elimination half-life is 1 hr after oral administration.

Tepoxalin: Tepoxalin is a dual inhibitor of both cyclooxygenases (COX-1 and COX-2) and 5-lipoxygenase (5-LOX). From a mechanistic perspective, its LOX activity (reduction of leukotriene production) may reduce components of inflammation not controlled by COX isoenzyme inhibition. It is available for dogs as an oral tablet. The initial dosage is 20 mg/kg, followed by a maintenance dosage of 10 mg/kg/day. Tepoxalin is rapidly absorbed and reaches peak plasma concentration 2–3 hr after administration. Its plasma half-life is short (2 hr), but it is metabolized to a carboxylic active metabolite (tepoxalin pyrazol acid) that has a long half-life (12–15 hr). The metabolite, tepoxalin pyrazol acid, lacks the LOX activity of the parent molecule. Both tepoxalin and its active metabolite are highly bound to plasma protein (98%–99%). The most commonly reported adverse effects are GI related (eg, diarrhea and vomiting in ~20% of dogs treated for 4 wk).

Other NSAIDs: A large number of prescription and nonprescription NSAIDs are available for human use. However, because of species differences in metabolism, efficacy, and toxicity, many are not recommended for use in animals. For example, in dogs, indomethacin is highly toxic to the GI tract and may result in severe ulceration, hematemesis, and melena at therapeutic doses. Piroxicam undergoes extensive enterohepatic recycling in dogs, resulting in a prolonged plasma half-life. GI ulceration and bleeding and renal papillary necrosis have been seen in dogs receiving piroxicam at dosages of 0.3–1 mg/kg/day.

Ibuprofen is an arylpropionic acid derivative used in dogs as an anti-inflammatory agent. However, dogs are much more sensitive to the development of GI adverse effects from ibuprofen administration than are people. At therapeutic doses, adverse effects seen in dogs include vomiting, diarrhea, GI bleeding, and renal infection. Ibuprofen is not recommended for use in dogs or cats.

Naproxen has been used in horses at a dosage of 5–10 mg/kg, once to twice daily. Bioavailability is lower (~50%) for naproxen than for other NSAIDs, and the elimination half-life is ~5 hr in horses. In dogs, the elimination half-life of naproxen is 35–74 hr, presumably because of extensive enterohepatic recirculation. The pharmacokinetics in dogs also appear to be breed dependent. Because of the prolonged half-life of naproxen, dogs are extremely sensitive to its adverse effects.

Coxib class drugs, including celecoxib and valdecoxib, developed for use in human medicine are COX-2 selective. In clinical studies, the incidence of GI ulceration in patients receiving valdecoxib or celecoxib was significantly less than that of those receiving naproxen. The use of these drugs in animals has yet to be fully investigated. One pharmacokinetic study with celecoxib in Beagles demonstrated variability in drug elimination between dogs. In that study, one subgroup of Beagles metabolized celecoxib much more rapidly than the other, with elimination half-lives of ~2 and 18 hr, respectively. Until further data are available regarding the pharmacokinetics and safety of these drugs in animals, their use in veterinary medicine is not recommended.

CHONDROPROTECTIVE AGENTS

Polysulfated Glycosaminoglycan: Polysulfated glycosaminoglycan (PSGAG) is a semisynthetic glycosaminoglycan prepared from bovine tracheal cartilage and composed of a polymeric chain of repeating disaccharide units. The primary glycosaminoglycan in PSGAG is chondroitin sulfate. PSGAG is approved for IM use in dogs and intra-articular and IM use in horses for the control of signs associated with noninfectious degenerative or traumatic arthritis. In horses, the recommended dosage is 500 mg, IM, every 4 days for 28 days, or 250 mg by intra-articular injection once weekly for 5 wk. In dogs, the recommended dosage is 2 mg/lb, IM, twice weekly for up to 4 wk. After IM injection, PSGAG is absorbed into the systemic circulation and eventually incorporated into both healthy and damaged cartilage. The exact mechanism of action is unknown, but in vitro studies show that PSGAG inhibits PGE_2 and catabolic enzymes such as stromelysin, elastase, the metalloproteases, and others. PSGAG also increases the synthesis of hyaluronic acid, proteoglycan, and collagen in vitro. Toxicity associated with administration of PSGAG has been minimal. Because PSGAG is chemically similar to heparin, overdosage may inhibit coagulation, and concurrent use of aspirin may prolong bleeding times. The use of PSGAG is contraindicated in septic joints.

Pentosan Polysulfate Sodium: Pentosan polysulfate sodium (PPS) is a polysulfate ester of xylan, a polymer prepared semisynthetically from beechwood plant material. PPS is chemically and structurally similar to heparin and glycosaminoglycan. The compound is approved by the FDA for use as an oral capsule for the treatment of interstitial cystitis in people. An injectable product is available for use in people, dogs, and horses in Australia and other countries. The mechanism of action is unknown. PPS stimulates hyaluronic acid and GAG synthesis in damaged joints, inhibits proteolytic enzymes including metalloproteinases, and scavenges free radicals. PPS may also decrease cytokine activity. In canine models of osteoarthritis, IM administration of PPS significantly decreased overall cartilage damage. Because PPS has a heparin-like structure, coagulopathies may be seen. PPS is given once a week for 4 consecutive weeks, then once every 6 or 12 mo.

Hyaluronan: Hyaluronan (formerly hyaluronic acid), a polydisaccharide of glucuronic acid and glucosamine, is a component of synovial fluid and articular cartilage. In the USA, a purified fraction of the sodium salt of hyaluronic acid extracted from rooster combs is available for treatment of horses with osteoarthritis. Hyaluronan is responsible for the viscosity of the synovial fluid and contributes to its lubricating function in joint movement. As with other chondroprotective agents, the mode of action is unclear. However, because synovial fluid viscoelasticity is decreased in osteoarthritis, the intra-articular administration of hyaluronan may improve joint lubrication. Hyaluronan inhibits PGE_2 synthesis in vitro and in vivo and may inhibit inflammatory enzymes and reduce pain. Most clinical use has been in horses, in which it appears to have minimal adverse effects.

Orgotein: Orgotein is a water-soluble metalloprotein containing copper and zinc. Found in low concentrations throughout the body, orgotein has superoxide dismutase activity scavenging free oxygen radicals. Orgotein, available as an injectable formulation, has been used for treatment of soft-tissue inflammation in horses and of arthritis in dogs. Although it has been used as an IM or SC injection, orgotein is typically administered as an intra-articular injection, because its large molecular size may limit absorption via other routes. Intra-articular administration is effective in cases of acute lameness in horses, although the onset of therapeutic response may be slow (2–6 wk). Reports indicate that orgotein apparently has a wide safety margin.

ANTINEOPLASTIC AGENTS

Antineoplastic chemotherapy is an important component of small animal practice and is routinely used for selected tumors of horses and cattle. Effective use of antineoplastic chemotherapy depends on an understanding of basic principles of cancer biology, drug actions, toxicities, and drug handling safety.

Tumor Growth and Response to Chemotherapy: The fundamental biochemical and genetic differences between cancer cells and healthy cells are areas of intense investigation, because these divergences are not fully understood. None of the empirically developed conventional antineoplastic drugs appears to act on a process entirely unique to cancer cells. Newer therapies that specifically target markers or pathways unique to particular cancers are evolving. However, the mainstay of cancer therapy continues to be traditional chemotherapy. Clinically useful drugs achieve a degree of selectivity on the basis of certain characteristics of cancer cells that can be used as pharmacologic targets. These characteristics include rapid rate of division and growth, variations in the rate of drug uptake or in the sensitivity of different types of cells to particular drugs, and retention in the malignant cells of hormonal responses characteristic of the cells from which the cancer is derived, eg, estrogen responsiveness of certain breast carcinomas.

Aspects of normal cell growth and the cell cycle provide the rationale for and are of major importance in successful application of antineoplastic chemotherapy. In the S phase, DNA synthesis occurs; the M phase begins with mitosis and ends with cytokinesis; and the G_0 phase is a dormant or nonproliferative phase of the cell cycle. Tumor doubling time is related to the length of the cell cycle and the growth fraction (the proportion of a population of cells undergoing cell division). Antineoplastic agents can be classified according to a number of schemes relative to effects at different stages of the cell cycle. In the simplest sense, cycle-nonspecific agents are considered to be lethal to cells in all phases of the cell cycle. Cells are killed exponentially with increasing drug levels, and the dose-response curves follow first-order kinetics. Phase-specific agents exert their lethal effects exclusively or primarily during one phase of the cell cycle, usually S or M; the greater the rate of cell division, the more effective the drug. The G_0 phase of the cell cycle is important, not as a target for chemotherapeutic agents, but as a time during which dormant tumor cells can escape or repair the effects of drug therapy.

Principles of Antineoplastic Chemotherapy: The decision to use antineoplastic chemotherapy depends on the type of tumor to be treated, the stage of malignancy, the condition of the animal, and financial considerations. Chemotherapy can be used as an adjuvant to surgery and irradiation and can be administered immediately after or before the primary treatment. Neoadjuvant therapy is administered before surgery or irradiation and is intended to improve the effectiveness of the primary therapy by possibly decreasing tumor size, stage of malignancy, or presence of micrometastatic lesions. Responses to cancer chemotherapy can range from palliation (remission of secondary signs, generally without increase in survival time) to complete remission (in which clinically detectable tumor cells and all signs of malignancy are absent). The percentage and duration of complete remissions are criteria for the success of a particular chemotherapeutic protocol.

Effective clinical use of antineoplastic drugs depends on the ability to balance the killing of tumor cells against the inherent toxicity of many of these drugs to host cells. Because of the narrow therapeutic indices of antineoplastic agents, dosages are frequently calculated based on body surface area (BSA) rather than body mass. However, evidence suggests that small dogs and cats may best be treated based on body weight to avoid overdosage. This is especially true if the primary toxicity is bone marrow suppression. Evidently, BSA does not correlate well with either stem cell number in the bone marrow or resulting hematopoietic toxicity. Correlation is better between body weight and these toxicities. Antineoplastic agents can be administered by PO, IV, SC, IM, topical, intracavitary, intralesional, intravesicular, intrathecal, or intra-arterial routes. The route chosen depends on the individual agent and is determined by drug toxicity; location, size, and type of tumor; and physical constraints.

Antineoplastic agents are commonly administered in various combinations of dosages and timing; the specific regimen is referred to as a protocol. A protocol may use one or as many as five or six different antineoplastic agents. Selection of an appropriate protocol should be based on type of tumor, grade or degree of malignancy, stage of the disease, condition of the animal, and financial considerations. Preferences of individual clinicians for treatment of specific neoplastic conditions may also vary. Regardless of the protocol chosen, a thorough knowledge of the mechanism of action and toxicities of each therapeutic agent is essential.

Combination antineoplastic chemotherapy offers many advantages. Drugs with different target sites or mechanisms of action are used together to enhance destruction of tumor cells. If the adverse effects of the component agents are different, the combination may be no more toxic than the individual agents given separately. Combinations that include a cycle-nonspecific drug administered first, followed by a phase-specific drug, may offer the advantage that cells surviving treatment with the first drug are provoked into mitosis and, therefore, are more susceptible to the second drug. Another advantage of combination therapy is the decreased possibility of development of drug resistance.

Special considerations associated with administration of antineoplastic drugs include evaluation of the animal's quality of life, medical and nutritional support, control of pain, and psychologic comfort for the owner. Many owners who choose to treat neoplasia in their pets have experienced cancer themselves or have been involved with individuals or family members who have had cancer. Discussion of neoplasia in pets should be handled tactfully and should provide the owners with appropriate information for decision-making.

Resistance to Antineoplastic Agents: Failure to respond, or resistance, to antineoplastic agents can be seen for several reasons. Pharmacokinetic resistance is seen when the concentration of a drug in the target cell is below that required to kill the cell. This may be due to altered rates of drug absorption, distribution, biotransformation, or excretion. In addition, marginal blood flow to a tumor may not provide sufficient drug, resulting in inadequate therapeutic drug concentrations and the potential for creation of a population of quiescent, less susceptible cells. Cytokinetic resistance is seen when the tumor cell population is not completely eradicated; this may be a result of dormant tumor cells, dose-limiting host toxicity associated with drug therapy, or the inability to achieve a 100% kill rate even at therapeutic drug dosages. Resistance can also develop via biochemical mechanisms within the tumor cell itself that block transport mechanisms for drug uptake, alter target receptors or enzymes critical to drug action, increase concentrations of healthy metabolites antagonized by the antineoplastic drug, or cause genetic changes that result in protective gene amplification or altered patterns of DNA repair. Acquired multidrug resistance can result from amplification and overexpression of a multidrug resistance gene. This gene encodes a cell transmembrane protein that effectively pumps a variety of structurally unrelated antineoplastic agents out of the cell. As intracellular drug concentrations decline, tumor cell survival and resistance to therapy increase.

Patterns of Toxicity: Conventional antineoplastic agents that act primarily on rapidly dividing and growing cells produce multiple adverse effects or toxicities, including bone marrow or myelosuppression, GI complications, and immunosuppression. Patterns of toxicity may be either acute or delayed. Acute vomiting may develop during administration of an emetogenic drug or within 24 hr after administration of chemotherapy, probably from direct stimulation of the chemoreceptor trigger zone. Several drugs are available aimed at preventing these toxicities, including dolasetron, ondansetron, and maropitant citrate. Dolasetron and ondansetron act as serotonin receptor (5HT3) antagonists that work centrally on the brain to prevent emesis. Maropitant citrate is an oral or subcutaneous FDA-approved medication for acute nausea/vomiting in veterinary medicine. It works by inhibiting both central and peripheral vomiting pathways by blocking neurokinin-1 receptors to prevent activation of the emetic center.

Administration of oral antiemetics may be indicated for delayed GI toxicities, which can occur 3–5 days after chemotherapy administration. Neurokinin-1 receptor antagonists are used in human oncology to treat delayed emesis, and there is evidence they may work synergistically or at least in an additive fashion with 5HT3 inhibitors. In addition to the NK-1 inhibitor maropitant, common antiemetic therapy in veterinary oncology includes metoclopramide, which functions through direct antagonism of central and peripheral dopamine receptors. This drug has the added benefit of stimulating motility of the upper GI tract without stimulating gastric, biliary, or pancreatic secretions. This effect can be useful in dogs that develop ileus secondary to vincristine administration.

Allergic reactions and anaphylaxis may also be of immediate concern with selected drugs and can be treated with antihistamines or corticosteroids as needed. In more severe cases, epinephrine and IV fluids may be indicated.

Other delayed toxicities may develop days to weeks after antineoplastic therapy. Myelosuppression, a common delayed toxicity, can be life-threatening because of the increased risk of infection associated with neutropenia. Less commonly, increased risk of hemorrhage associated with thrombocytopenia and anemia may be seen.

Other important delayed toxicities include tissue damage associated with extravasation of selected drugs, and alopecia caused by hair follicle damage, particularly in nonshedding breeds with continuous hair growth. Adverse effects on spermatogenesis and teratogenesis may be of concern in breeding animals. Unlike in people, chemotherapy-induced stomatitis or ulcerative enteritis are rare events in dogs and cats.

Prevention and management of toxicities are crucial to successful antineoplastic therapy. Collection of an adequate database before treatment can identify potential problems so that contraindicated drugs can be avoided. Several antineoplastic agents should not be used in the presence of specific organ impairment. For example, doxorubicin should not be used in dogs with certain cardiac abnormalities that impair left ventricular function, and cisplatin is contraindicated in animals with impaired renal function.

When a drug is chosen, supportive or preventive therapy aimed at ameliorating toxic adverse effects may be required. Potential cardiotoxicity of doxorubicin may be abrogated with coadministration of dexrazoxane, an iron chelator that inhibits formation of free radicals implicated in myocardial injury. Active diuresis should accompany administration of nephrotoxic agents (eg, cisplatin). Administration or availability of appropriate antihistamines may be indicated with L-asparaginase and doxorubicin therapy.

The availability of recombinant products is an additional resource to manage myelosuppression and immunosuppression induced by antineoplastic chemotherapy. Recombinant human (rhG-CSF) and canine (rcG-CSF) granulocyte colony-stimulating factors have been used effectively to manage cytopenias induced by chemotherapy and radiation therapy. Administration of rcG-CSF results in a rapid, significant increase in neutrophil numbers that is sustainable as long as the factor is administered. Neutrophil counts drop quickly when therapy is discontinued. Neutrophil phagocytosis, superoxide generation, and antibody-dependent cellular cytotoxicity all increase with G-CSF treatment. Until rcG-CSF is commercially available, longterm (>2–3 wk) or repeated use of recombinant human products should be avoided in dogs and cats, because it can result in anti-factor antibody formation and a subsequent decline in targeted cell numbers.

Prophylactic antibiotics have been shown to reduce hospitalization rates and death in human cancer patients receiving chemotherapy. These are occasionally used in veterinary medicine to reduce the occurrence or severity of hematologic and nonhematologic complications that can result from administration of particular chemotherapy agents.

Safe Handling of Antineoplastic Chemotherapeutic Agents: Most antineoplastic chemotherapeutic agents are potentially toxic as mutagens, teratogens, or carcinogens. Handling of these agents can result in hazardous personal or environmental exposure in several ways.

A common route of exposure is inhalation due to aerosolization during mixing or administration of cytotoxic drugs. This may occur when a needle is withdrawn from a pressurized drug container or on expulsion of air from a drug-filled syringe. Transferring drugs between containers, opening drug-filled glass ampules, or crushing or splitting oral medications may also aerosolize drug residues.

The best way to prepare cytotoxic drugs to avoid aerosolization is in a biologic safety cabinet or hood; a Class II, type A vertical laminar air flow hood exhausted outside the building is recommended. Aerosol exposures can be further decreased through use of closed system transfer devices that limit escape of air from drug vials into the environment. Administration of chemotherapy should occur in dedicated areas, and meticulous attention to technique should be maintained. Intravenous lines used to administer chemotherapy should be primed with nontoxic solution whenever possible. Disposal of contaminated vials, syringes, needles, and gloves in this area should be anticipated, and the proper puncture-proof chemotherapy waste containers provided.

Personal protection equipment should be used for chemotherapy preparation, administration, cleanup, and disposal. This should include powder-free chemotherapy gloves, nonpermeable gowns, respiratory protection, plastic-backed underpads for the working surface, eye and/or splash protection, shoe covers, and a spill kit.

Another potential route of exposure to antineoplastic agents is by absorption of drug through the skin. This could occur during preparation or administration of drug, cleaning of the drug preparation area, or handling of excreta from animals that have received selected cytotoxic drugs. Conscientious wearing of disposable, powder-free gloves and careful handling of drug-contaminated needles or catheters may avoid most exposures of this type. Re-capping of needles containing drug residues is discouraged to avoid accidental self-inoculation. In addition, use of sprayers and pressure washers to clean cages, kennels, or stalls of treated animals should be avoided to minimize aerosolization of hazardous wastes.

Antineoplastic agents can be inadvertently ingested if food, drink, or tobacco products are allowed in the vicinity of drug preparation areas, treatment areas, or kennels housing treated animals. Any ingestible materials should be restricted to a separate area that is far enough away to avoid any possible contamination with these agents.

All personnel should handle antineoplastic agents with care. Women of child-bearing age should be particularly cautious, and women who are pregnant or breastfeeding should not handle antineoplastic drugs.

A source of exposure to cytotoxic drugs that is commonly overlooked is the handling of body fluids and excreta of treated patients. Uniform guidelines to handle these potentially dangerous substances have not been published. Nevertheless, simple measures can be taken to help minimize exposure of veterinary personnel and pet owners. Collection of biologic samples, such as blood, urine, or tissue, should be performed before chemotherapy administration. The duration and type of precautionary measures that should be taken after treatment depend on the half-life and routes of elimination of the drug administered. Pet owners and veterinary hospital personnel should be advised to allow dogs to urinate and defecate in a confined area outdoors, away from spaces where people may congregate or children play. A mask should be worn when cleaning litterboxes, and the contents placed in a sealed plastic bag. The use of low-dust kitty litter should be encouraged. Powder-free, disposable gloves should be used when cleaning up urine, feces, or vomitus. Veterinarians are encouraged to contact their local board of health and other federal, state, and local regulatory agencies for regulations regarding disposal of hazardous waste.

Classification of Antineoplastic Chemotherapeutic Agents: Conventional cytotoxic antineoplastic agents can be grouped by biochemical mechanism of action into the following general categories: alkylating agents, antimetabolites, mitotic inhibitors, antineoplastic antibiotics, hormonal agents, and miscellaneous. The clinically relevant drugs used in veterinary medicine are discussed below, and the indications, mechanism of action, and toxicities of selected agents are summarized in TABLE 57.

ALKYLATING AGENTS

Alkylating agents form highly reactive intermediate compounds that are able to transfer alkyl groups to DNA. Alkylation can result in miscoding of DNA strands, incomplete repair of alkylated segments (which leads to strand breakage or depurination), excessive cross-linking of DNA, and inhibition of strand separation at mitosis. Monofunctional alkylating agents transfer a single alkyl group and usually result in miscoding of DNA, strand breakage, or depurination. These reactions can result in cell death, mutagenesis, or carcinogenesis. Polyfunctional alkylating agents typically cause strand cross-linking and inhibition of mitosis with consequent cell death. Resistance to one alkylating agent often implies resistance to other drugs in the same class and can be caused by increased production of nucleophilic substances that compete with the target DNA for alkylation. Decreased permeation of alkylating agents and increased activity of DNA repair systems are also common mechanisms of resistance.

Individual alkylating agents are generally cell-cycle nonspecific and can be subgrouped according to chemical structure into nitrogen mustards, ethyleneamines, alkyl sulfonates, nitrosoureas, and triazene derivatives.

Nitrogen Mustards: The most common subgroup of alkylating agents used is the nitrogen mustard group. Mechlorethamine hydrochloride is the prototype of the nitrogen mustards and is commonly used in veterinary medicine to treat lymphoma in conjunction with other chemotherapeutics. Because of the highly unstable nature and extremely short duration of action of mechlorethamine, its use is somewhat limited in veterinary medicine. Derivatives of mechlorethamine commonly used for various neoplasias include cyclophosphamide, chlorambucil, and melphalan.

Cyclophosphamide is a cyclic phosphamide derivative of mechlorethamine that requires metabolic activation by the cytochrome P450 oxidation system in the liver. Cyclophosphamide is given PO or IV, and dose-limiting leukopenia associated with bone marrow suppression is the primary toxicity. However, among the alkylating chemotherapy agents, the myelosuppressive effect of cyclophosphamide is considered relatively sparing of platelets and progenitor cells. Sterile hemorrhagic cystitis may result from aseptic chemical inflammation of the bladder urothelium caused by acrolein, a metabolite of cyclophosphamide. Prevention of this toxicity is key to its management. Specifically, concurrent administration of a diuretic, such as furosemide, may be used when cyclophosphamide is given as a single dose to provide a dilutional effect. In addition, cyclophosphamide may be given in the morning so that patients can be provided several opportunities to urinate throughout the day to minimize contact time of acrolein with the bladder lining. In patients with evidence of sterile hemorrhagic cystitis, cyclophosphamide use should be discontinued. Although the signs may be self-limiting, treatment with fluids, NSAIDs, methylsulfonylmethane (MSM), and intravesicular DMSO may be considered. Mesna is a drug that binds and inactivates the urotoxic metabolites of cyclophosphamide within the bladder. Mesna coadministered with fluid diuresis is recommended when ifosfamide (an analogue of cyclophosphamide) or high-dose cyclophosphamide is used.

TABLE 57 MECHANISMS OF ACTION, INDICATIONS, AND TOXICITIES OF SELECTED ANTINEOPLASTIC AGENTS

Drug	Mechanism of Action	Major Indications	Toxicities
	ALKYLATING AGENTS		
Cyclophosphamide	Undergoes hepatic biotransformation to active metabolites that alkylate DNA; alkylation leads to miscoding of DNA and cross-linking of DNA strands	Lymphoma, mammary adenocarcinoma, sarcomas, lymphocytic leukemia	Nausea, vomiting (infrequent), moderate to severe myelosuppression, sterile hemorrhagic cystitis
Melphalan	Alkylates DNA causing miscoding and cross-linking of DNA strands	Multiple myeloma	Nausea, vomiting, anorexia, moderate myelosuppression (may be more myelosuppressive in cats)
Chlorambucil	Alkylates DNA causing miscoding and cross-linking of DNA strands; slowest-acting alkylating agent	Chronic lymphocytic leukemia, small-cell lymphoma	Nausea, vomiting, mild to moderate myelosuppression
Lomustine (CCNU)	Alkylates DNA causing miscoding and cross-linking of DNA strands; inhibits both DNA and RNA synthesis; not cross-resistant with other alkylating agents	Lymphoma, mast cell tumor, histiocytic sarcoma, CNS neoplasias, multiple myeloma	Nausea, vomiting, moderate to severe myelosuppression (may be delayed for 4–6 wk), hepatotoxicity, nephrotoxicity, pulmonary toxicity
Streptozotocin	Inhibits DNA synthesis; high affinity for pancreatic β cells	Insulinoma	Severe, potentially fatal nephrotoxicity (if given without diuresis) and hepatotoxicity, nausea (immediate and delayed), vomiting, mild myelosuppression
Dacarbazine (DTIC)	Undergoes hepatic biotransformation to active metabolites that alkylate DNA; inhibits RNA synthesis	Lymphoma, sarcomas	Severe acute nausea, vomiting, phlebitis, moderate myelosuppression, hepatotoxicity, anecdotal reports of pleural effusion in cats
Ifosfamide	Analogue of cyclophosphamide; undergoes hepatic biotransformation to active metabolites that alkylate DNA; alkylation leads to miscoding of DNA and cross-linking of DNA strands	Various sarcomas	Nausea, vomiting, myelosuppression, sterile hemorrhagic cystitis, possible nephrotoxicity

(continued)

TABLE 57 MECHANISMS OF ACTION, INDICATIONS, AND TOXICITIES OF SELECTED ANTINEOPLASTIC AGENTS *(continued)*

Drug	Mechanism of Action	Major Indications	Toxicities
ANTIMETABOLITES			
Methotrexate	Inhibition of dihydrofolate reductase that is required for formation of tetrahydrofolate, a necessary cofactor in thymidylate synthesis; thymidylate essential for DNA synthesis and repair	Lymphoma	Nausea, vomiting, moderate myelosuppression, GI ulceration, hepatotoxicity, pulmonary toxicity
5-Fluorouracil	Pyrimidine analogue; interferes with DNA synthesis and may be incorporated into RNA to cause toxic effects	Carcinomas (systemic); cutaneous carcinomas (topical)	Systemic: nausea, vomiting, moderate myelosuppression, neurotoxicity, GI ulceration, neurotoxicity, hepatotoxicity Topical: local irritation, pain, hyperpigmentation Cannot be given to cats (fatal neurotoxicity)
Cytarabine	Pyrimidine analogue; incorporates into DNA causing steric hindrance and inhibition of DNA synthesis	Lymphoma (including CNS), leukemias; no activity in solid tumors	Nausea, vomiting, moderate myelosuppression, nephrotoxicity, hepatotoxicity
Gemcitabine	Pyrimidine analogue; incorporates into DNA, causing steric hindrance and inhibition of DNA synthesis	Limited efficacy seen in lymphoma and various carcinomas	Mild nausea, vomiting, mild to moderate myelosuppression, pulmonary toxicity, nephrotoxicity
ANTIBIOTIC ANTINEOPLASTICS			
Doxorubicin	Intercalates and binds to DNA, disrupting helical structure and DNA template; inhibits RNA and DNA polymerases; causes DNA topoisomerase II–mediated chain scission; generates free radicals that cause DNA scission and cell membrane damage	Lymphoma, leukemias, multiple myeloma, osteosarcoma, hemangiosarcoma, and various other sarcomas and carcinomas	Nausea, vomiting, moderate myelosuppression, hemorrhagic colitis, severe cutaneous reactions if extravasated; red urine (not hematuria), transient ECG changes and arrhythmias, nephrotoxicity, anaphylactoid reactions Cumulative dose-related congestive heart failure in dogs; cumulative nephrotoxicity in cats

(continued)

TABLE 57 MECHANISMS OF ACTION, INDICATIONS, AND TOXICITIES OF SELECTED ANTINEOPLASTIC AGENTS *(continued)*

Drug	Mechanism of Action	Major Indications	Toxicities
Mitoxantrone	Topoisomerase II–mediated chain scission; DNA aggregation, oxidation, and strand breakage	Lymphoma, various carcinomas	Nausea, vomiting, moderate to severe myelosuppression, diarrhea, bluish discoloration to sclera; less severe adverse effects than others in this group
Bleomycin	Mixture of glycopeptides; generates oxygen radicals that cause chain scission and fragmentation of DNA	Carcinomas	Nausea, vomiting, myelosuppression, fever, allergic reactions including anaphylaxis, hyperpigmentation, skin ulceration, pneumonitis, pulmonary fibrosis
Dactinomycin (Actinomycin D)	Intercalates and binds to DNA, disrupting helical structure and DNA template; inhibits RNA and DNA polymerases; causes DNA topoisomerase II–mediated chain scission; generates free radicals that cause DNA scission and cell membrane damage	Lymphoma, various sarcomas	Nausea, vomiting, moderate to severe myelosuppression, phlebitis; severe tissue reaction if extravasated
MITOTIC INHIBITORS			
Vinblastine	Binds to tubulin, leading to disruption of mitotic spindle apparatus and arrest of cell cycle	Lymphoma and leukemias, mast cell tumors	Mild nausea, vomiting, severe myelosuppression, neurotoxicity with high doses, inappropriate secretion of antidiuretic hormone
Vincristine	Binds to tubulin, leading to disruption of mitotic spindle apparatus and arrest of cell cycle	Lymphoma and leukemias, transmissible venereal cell tumors, various sarcomas	Mild to moderate nausea, vomiting, mild to moderate myelosuppression, severe tissue reaction if extravasated, cumulative peripheral neuropathy, constipation, paralytic ileus, inappropriate secretion of antidiuretic hormone

(continued)

TABLE 57 MECHANISMS OF ACTION, INDICATIONS, AND TOXICITIES OF SELECTED ANTINEOPLASTIC AGENTS *(continued)*

Drug	Mechanism of Action	Major Indications	Toxicities
Vinorelbine	Binds to tubulin, leading to disruption of mitotic spindle apparatus and arrest of cell cycle	Primary lung tumors, limited efficacy in mast cell tumors	Mild nausea, vomiting, myelosuppression
Paclitaxel	Binds to tubulin, stabilizing microtubule polymer and arresting mitosis	Mammary carcinoma, squamous cell carcinoma	Myelosuppression, nausea, vomiting, hypersensitivity (when Cremor EL is used as vehicle)
MISCELLANEOUS			
Cisplatin	Reacts with proteins and nucleic acids; forms cross-links between DNA strands and between DNA and protein; disrupts DNA synthesis	Osteosarcoma, carcinomas, and mesothelioma	Intense nausea, vomiting, mild to moderate myelosuppression, potentially fatal nephrotoxicity if not given with diuresis, anaphylaxis, ototoxicity, peripheral neuropathy, hyperuricemia, hypermagnesemia Cannot be given to cats (fulminant pulmonary edema)
Carboplatin	Reacts with proteins and nucleic acids; forms cross-links between DNA strands and between DNA and protein; disrupts DNA synthesis	Osteosarcoma, carcinomas	Mild nausea, vomiting, diarrhea, moderate to severe myelosuppression
L-Asparaginase	Inhibits protein synthesis by hydrolyzing tumor cell supply of asparagine	Acute lymphoid leukemias and lymphoma	Hypersensitivity reactions, anaphylaxis especially after repeated doses, alteration in coagulation parameters, hepatotoxicity, pancreatitis (people), potential inhibition of immune responsiveness (B and T cells)
Mitotane (o,p′DDD)	Destroys adrenal zona fasciculata and zona reticularis	Pituitary hyperadrenocorticism, palliation of adrenal cortical tumors	Nausea, vomiting, anorexia, diarrhea, adrenal insufficiency, CNS depression, dermatitis

(continued)

TABLE 57 MECHANISMS OF ACTION, INDICATIONS, AND TOXICITIES OF SELECTED ANTINEOPLASTIC AGENTS *(continued)*

Drug	Mechanism of Action	Major Indications	Toxicities
Hydroxyurea	Inhibits conversion of ribonucleotides to deoxyribonucleotides by destroying ribonucleoside diphosphate reductase	Polycythemia vera, granulocytic and basophilic leukemia, thrombocythemia, investigational for meningiomas	Nausea, vomiting, mild myelosuppression, alopecia, sloughing of claws, dysuria
Procarbazine	Mechanism is unclear; inhibits DNA, RNA, and protein synthesis, perhaps through alkylation	Lymphoma, as part of MOPP chemotherapy protocol; brain tumors	Nausea, vomiting, myelosuppression, diarrhea
HORMONES			
Prednisone	Lympholytic; inhibits mitosis in lymphocytes	Lymphoma, mast cell tumors, multiple myeloma, palliative treatment of brain tumors	Sodium retention, GI ulceration, protein catabolism, muscle wasting, delayed wound healing, suppression of hypothalamic-pituitary-adrenal axis, immunosuppression

Chlorambucil, the slowest-acting nitrogen mustard, achieves effects gradually and often can be used in animals with compromised bone marrow. It can cause bone marrow suppression, which is usually mild; however, periodic monitoring is recommended with longterm administration. This drug is given PO and is most commonly used in treatment of chronic, well-differentiated cancers; it is considered ineffective in rapidly proliferating tumors.

Melphalan, an L-phenylalanine derivative of mechlorethamine, is given PO or IV and is primarily used in veterinary medicine to treat multiple myeloma.

Other Alkylating Agents: Of the other subgroups of alkylating agents, several have limited but specific uses. **Triethylenethiophosphoramide** (thiotepa), an ethylenimine, has been reported as an intravesicular treatment for transitional cell carcinoma of the bladder or as an intracavitary treatment for pleural and peritoneal effusions. **Busulfan**, an alkyl sulfonate, is used specifically in treatment of chronic myelocytic leukemia and polycythemia vera. **Streptozotocin**, a naturally occurring nitrosourea, is used for palliation of malignant pancreatic islet-cell tumors or insulinomas. Other nitrosoureas, such as **carmustine** and **lomustine**, readily cross the blood-brain barrier and have been useful in management of lymphoma (including epitheliotropic cutaneous lymphoma), mast cell tumors, histiocytic sarcomas, and CNS neoplasias. **Dacarbazine** (DTIC), a triazene derivative, has been used either in combination with doxorubicin or as a single-agent treatment for relapsed canine lymphoma and soft-tissue sarcomas.

Temozolomide is an oral imidazotetrazine derivative of dacarbazine and belongs to a class of chemotherapeutic agents that enter the CSF and do not require hepatic metabolism for activation. In people, it is used for refractory malignant gliomas and malignant melanomas. There have been reports in the veterinary literature of its use as a substitute for dacarbazine (DTIC).

ANTIMETABOLITES

Antimetabolites resemble normal cellular substances and so can subvert normal metabolic pathways in a toxic manner.

Three subgroups of antimetabolites are used: folic acid, pyrimidine, and purine analogues.

Folic Acid Analogues: The prototype folic acid analogue is methotrexate, an inhibitor of dihydrofolate reductase, the enzyme that catalyzes conversion of folic acid to tetrahydrofolate. Tetrahydrofolate deficiency blocks reactions requiring folate coenzymes, disrupting both DNA and RNA synthesis. Methotrexate is an S phase–specific drug that must be actively transported across cell membranes. It can be given PO, IV, IM, or intrathecally. Methotrexate is excreted in the urine, and at high doses may precipitate in renal tubules. Folinic acid can be used to bypass the metabolic blockade produced by folic acid analogues and thus result in rescue of treated cells. Because tumor cells appear less efficient at transport of folinic acid, some degree of selectivity is achieved in the rescue. Resistance to methotrexate may develop due to impaired transport of the drug into cells, production of altered forms, or increased concentrations of dihydrofolate reductase.

Pyrimidine Analogues: Two pyrimidine analogues, 5-fluorouracil and cytarabine, are commonly used.

5-Fluorouracil must be converted to an active 5-fluoro-2′-deoxyuridine-5′-phosphate form to bind the enzyme thymidylate synthetase and block or inhibit DNA and RNA synthesis. This drug is considered S phase–specific. It is used IV but is also available for topical use. Metabolism is via the liver, and the drug readily enters CSF. Occasional CNS reactions have been reported in dogs. Severe irreversible neurotoxicity and sudden death have been described in cats. In people, neurotoxicity is related to deficiency in the enzyme dihydropyrimidine dehydrogenase, but this has not been investigated in veterinary species. Resistance may develop by decreased activation of the drug or acquisition of altered thymidylate synthetase that is not inhibited.

Cytarabine (cytosine arabinoside) is an analogue of 2′-deoxycytidine and must be activated by conversion to a 5′-monophosphate nucleotide. The nucleotide analogue, AraCTP, inhibits DNA synthesis by substitution of arabinose for deoxyribose in the sugar moiety of DNA; cytarabine may also inhibit DNA repair enzymes. This drug is S phase–specific, and its effectiveness in hematopoietic neoplasms is directly proportional to exposure of cells to the drug; continuous infusion or repeated injections are usually required. Inhibition of conversion to AraCTP or increased degradation of AraCTP can account for development of resistance.

Gemcitabine is another nucleoside analogue of cytidine which, unlike cytarabine, has activity against solid tumors. The drug requires active carrier transport into the cytoplasm where it is terminally activated via phosphorylation; consequently, serum levels may not predict intracellular concentrations. By acting as a counterfeit nucleotide, coupled with the ability to inhibit multiple enzymes needed for pyridine biosynthesis and DNA repair, gemcitabine is capable of self-potentiation and synergism with other agents, particularly alkylators. Gemcitabine has also been used as a radiation sensitizer.

Purine Analogues: Two purine analogues, **6-mercaptopurine** (6-MP) and **6-thioguanine** (6-TG), are rarely used in veterinary medicine. In people, these drugs are occasionally used for acute leukemias or other autoimmune disorders.

MITOTIC INHIBITORS

Vinca Alkaloids: The vinca alkaloids are large, complex molecules derived from the periwinkle plant. Binding to tubulin, the major component of cellular microtubules, accounts for the antineoplastic effects of these drugs. Vinca alkaloids inhibit microtubule polymerization and increase microtubule disassembly. The mitotic spindle apparatus is disrupted, and segregation of chromosomes in metaphase is arrested. These effects account for the primary M-phase action of vinca alkaloids, although other antitubulin effects related to cytoskeletal maintenance and protein trafficking may be seen. The two drugs of importance in this class are **vincristine** and **vinblastine**. Both are given IV, and both cause severe local vesication if injected perivascularly. Drug extravasation may cause severe tissue reactions and promote exacerbation of self-trauma. The vinca alkaloids are metabolized primarily in the liver but may be partially excreted in an unchanged form in the urine. Although vinca alkaloids are related structurally, resistance to one does not imply resistance to all drugs in this category. Vincristine use is limited by neurologic toxicity that may include a slowly reversible sensorimotor peripheral neuropathy and muscle weakness. In comparison, the dose-limiting toxicity associated with vinblastine is related to myelosuppression and leukopenia; neurologic toxicity develops only at high doses.

Vinorelbine is a second-generation semisynthetic vinca alkaloid that is derived from vinblastine but with broader antitumor efficacy. According to studies in the veterinary literature, this drug may have efficacy in canine primary lung and cutaneous mast cell tumors.

Taxanes: Paclitaxel and **docetaxel** are antimicrotubule agents extracted from the Pacific and European yew trees, respectively. Taxanes bind to tubulin subunits, enhance microtubule polymerization, and inhibit microtubule depolymerization. Formation of stable microtubule bundles disrupts tubulin equilibrium and blocks normal progression through metaphase, and mitosis is arrested. These agents are actively used in human medicine, but hypersensitivity reactions related to the vehicle Cremophor EL have limited the drug's utility in veterinary medicine. A new water-soluble, micellar formulation of paclitaxel has received conditional approval by the FDA for treatment of canine mammary carcinoma and squamous cell carcinoma. Myelosuppression and GI effects (diarrhea, mucosal ulceration, and emesis) have been reported in dogs treated with paclitaxel.

ANTINEOPLASTIC ANTIBIOTICS

The antineoplastic antibiotics are products of *Streptomyces*. The important drugs in this group include actinomycin D (dactinomycin), doxorubicin, mitoxantrone, and bleomycin. Drugs less commonly used include daunorubicin, mithramycin, and mitomycin.

Actinomycin A was the first *Streptomyces* antibiotic isolated and was followed by related antibiotics, including actinomycin D. **Actinomycin D** binds with double-stranded DNA and blocks the action of RNA polymerase, which prevents DNA transcription. Actinomycin D is considered cell-cycle nonspecific and is given IV but does not cross the blood-brain barrier. Resistance may develop because of decreased cellular uptake of the drug. Occasionally, it is used as a substitute for doxorubicin in dogs with questionable cardiac function or for those dogs that have exceeded the cumulative cardiotoxic dose of doxorubicin.

The anthracycline antibiotics, particularly **doxorubicin**, have become important antineoplastic antibiotics. These drugs intercalate and bind to DNA between base pairs on adjacent strands. This causes the DNA helix to uncoil, which destroys the DNA template and inhibits RNA and DNA polymerases. Scission of DNA is thought to be mediated by either the enzyme topoisomerase II or by generation of free radicals. Intracellular interactions of anthracycline antibiotics result in the formation of semiquinone radical intermediates capable of generating hydrogen peroxide and hydroxyl radicals. Considered cell-cycle nonspecific because of the damage associated with radical formation, these drugs probably have their maximal effect during the S phase of the cell cycle. The anthracycline antibiotics are given IV; they are severe vesicants if administered perivascularly and may cause a severe, delayed phlebitis. Administration of a free radical scavenger, dexrazoxane, may limit the extent of tissue damage seen with extravasation of this drug. The anthracycline antibiotics are metabolized in the liver to a variety of less active and inactive products.

Doxorubicin toxicity can be manifested in a variety of acute and delayed reactions. Acute effects include hypersensitivity reactions (from nonspecific histamine release), extravasation injury, or transient cardiac arrhythmias. Delayed toxicities can be severe, with the major problem in dogs being cumulative, dose-related cardiac toxicity associated with binding of the drug to cardiac DNA and free radical damage to myocardial membranes. A nonspecific decrease in cardiac fibrils occurs, which leads to congestive heart failure unresponsive to digitalis. Because the cardiotoxic effects of doxorubicin are related to the peak plasma concentrations (rather than area under the curve), slow IV administration over 15–30 min is recommended to help lessen cardiac injury. Myocardial damage from doxorubicin also can be prevented by coadministration of dexrazoxane, at 10 times the dose of doxorubicin. In cats, cumulative doses of doxorubicin can result in nephrotoxicity and should be avoided or used judiciously in cats with preexisting renal insufficiency.

Dose-limiting toxicities of doxorubicin include severe myelosuppression and GI upset. Also, if doxorubicin is used in conjunction with radiation therapy, damage by radiation may be augmented. This radiation sensitization effect may necessitate reduction in radiation or drug dosages, or both. Because of the significant toxicity associated with use of doxorubicin, newer-generation drugs specifically aimed at reduction of cardiac toxicity have been developed and are available in human medicine. Two of these, idarubicin and epirubicin, have been studied, but neither is in common use in veterinary medicine.

A pegylated liposomal encapsulated form of doxorubicin, called doxorubicin HCL liposome injection, has been used effectively in both human and veterinary medicine. The liposomal formulation results in a longer drug circulation time and reduced myelosuppression and cardiotoxicity. In dogs, the dose-limiting toxicity of liposomal doxorubicin is a cutaneous reaction called palmar-plantar erythrodysesthesia. In cats, a delayed nephrotoxicity is the dose-limiting toxicity of both conventional and liposomal doxorubicin.

Mitoxantrone, an anthracenedione related to the anthracycline antibiotics, has shown promise in veterinary medicine for treatment of lymphoma and various carcinomas. The mechanism of action of mitoxantrone is similar to that of the anthracyclines, but most adverse effects are less severe than those of doxorubicin. An exception is myelosuppression, which is more profound with mitoxantrone than doxorubicin.

Bleomycin is actually a mixture of bleomycin glycopeptides that differ only in their terminal amine moiety. The cytotoxic action of these glycopeptides depends on their ability to cause chain scission and fragmentation of DNA molecules. Cells accumulate in the G_2 phase of the cell cycle, which accounts for the classification of bleomycin as a G_2 and M phase–specific agent. Bleomycin may also affect DNA repair enzymes. Given IV or SC, bleomycin does not cross the blood-brain barrier; a large portion is excreted via the kidneys. Bleomycin has minimal myelosuppressive and immunosuppressive activities but does have an unusual delayed pulmonary toxicity. Pulmonary toxicity, which is cumulative, may begin as a nonspecific pneumonitis that progresses to pulmonary fibrosis. Dangers from pulmonary complications are especially important in older animals with preexisting pulmonary disease.

HORMONAL AGENTS

Hormonal therapy for neoplasia commonly involves use of glucocorticoids. Direct antitumor effects are related to their lympholytic properties; glucocorticoids can inhibit mitosis, RNA synthesis, and protein synthesis in sensitive lymphocytes. Glucocorticoids are considered cell-cycle nonspecific and are often used in chemotherapeutic protocols after induction by another agent. Unfortunately, resistance to a given glucocorticoid may develop rapidly and typically extends to other glucocorticoids. Toxic effects of glucocorticoid therapy can include peptic ulceration, glucose intolerance, polydipsia and polyuria, immunosuppression, pancreatitis, osteopenia, hypokalemia, cataracts, and muscle wasting. Prednisone and prednisolone are commonly used to treat lymphoreticular neoplasms in combination with other drugs. Because they readily enter the CSF, dexamethasone, prednisone, and prednisolone are especially useful in treatment of leukemias and lymphomas of the CNS.

Indirect benefits of glucocorticoid therapy in cancer include symptomatic improvements in appetite and attitude, suppression of noninfectious fevers, management of hypercalcemia of malignancy (after a definitive diagnosis has been made), and relief of edema associated with spinal cord and brain tumors. However, evidence from several sources suggests that treatment of certain lymphomas with prednisone may increase resistance of neoplastic cells to subsequent cycles of antineoplastic chemotherapy through induction of MDR-1–related P-glycoprotein expression.

MISCELLANEOUS ANTINEOPLASTIC AGENTS

Several drugs used as antineoplastics do not fall into any of the categories mentioned thus far. These include L-asparaginase, cisplatin, mitotane (o,p′DDD), hydroxyurea, etoposide, and procarbazine.

L-Asparaginase is an enzyme derived from *Escherichia coli* that catalyzes hydrolysis of asparagine. Because some tumor cells have poor expression of asparagine synthetase and are unable to produce the amino acid asparagine, treatment with this drug deprives these cells of exogenously supplied asparagine and ultimately limits protein synthesis. Because protein synthesis is active in the G_1 phase of the cell cycle, L-asparaginase is considered to be a G_1 phase–specific drug. Preferred routes of administration for L-asparaginase include IM and SC. Anaphylaxis on repeated administration of L-asparaginase may occur as a result of host anti-asparaginase antibody production; pretreatment of animals with antihistamine helps to prevent this acute toxic reaction. Anti-asparaginase antibody production may also account for development of tumor resistance, as can a decreased tumor cell requirement for asparagine. A related drug, pegaspargase, is modified from L-asparaginase by covalent modification with monomethoxypolyethylene glycol. The conjugated drug produces fewer hypersensitivity reactions than does L-asparaginase.

Cisplatin (cis-diamine-dichloroplatinum) functions primarily as a bifunctional alkylator but is included in the miscellaneous category because of its unusual structure. It is a platinum ion complexed to two chloride ions and two ammonium molecules. Cisplatin causes inter- and intrastrand DNA cross-linking that disrupts DNA helices and prevents DNA synthesis. Cisplatin is cell-cycle nonspecific and has been used both for its direct antitumoral and radiation-sensitizing effects. It is administered by IV drip in combination with aggressive saline diuresis. Excretion is prolonged, with up to 50% of a dose still present in the body 5 days after administration. Extreme, dose-limiting, proximal tubular renal necrosis typifies the delayed adverse effects of cisplatin along with other responses that may include ototoxicity, moderate bone marrow suppression, peripheral neuropathy, and renal potassium and magnesium wasting. Cisplatin causes fatal pulmonary edema in cats and must not be used in this species.

Because of the extreme toxic adverse effects of cisplatin, newer generation derivatives such as **carboplatin** and others have been developed. Carboplatin is effective as an adjunct to surgery for treatment of osteosarcoma. Nausea and vomiting are less severe than with cisplatin, and carboplatin is not considered nephrotoxic. It is, however, myelosuppressive, with neutropenia being the dose-limiting toxicity. Carboplatin is excreted through the kidneys; consequently, dogs or cats with evidence of compromised renal function require dose adjustments to avoid excessive toxicity. Carboplatin is considered safe for administration to cats.

Mitotane (o,p′DDD), a derivative of the insecticides DDT and DDD, causes selective destruction of normal and neoplastic adrenal cortical cells. Mitotane may act by inhibiting production of steroids induced by adrenocorticotropic hormone, which causes atrophy of the inner zones of the adrenal cortex. Mitotane is administered PO, and plasma concentrations can be detected for several weeks.

Hydroxyurea, a simple hydroxylated derivative of urea, is most commonly used in treatment of polycythemia vera. Hydroxyurea inhibits ribonucleoside diphosphate reductase (RNDR), limits the conversion of ribonucleotides to deoxyribonucleotides, and blocks DNA synthesis. Cells are arrested in the G_1-S interface. Mechanisms of resistance include amplification of the RNDR gene or development of RNDR with reduced sensitivity to hydroxyurea. Loss of claws has been associated with hydroxyurea use in animals.

Epipodophyllotoxins are semisynthetic glycosides of podophyllotoxin derived from the mandrake plant. Although these toxins bind tubulin, their mechanism of action is unrelated to disruption of microtubules. Instead, they are thought to stimulate DNA cleavage mediated by topoisomerase II. Of the two drugs in this class, etoposide and teniposide, the former has been used primarily in treatment of testicular carcinoma.

Procarbazine is considered to function as an alkylating agent but is included in the miscellaneous category because the exact mechanism of action is not known. It is typically used as part of the MOPP protocol that includes mechlorethamine, vincristine (tradename Oncovin®), procarbazine, and prednisone for dogs with lymphoma. This drug is metabolized and activated in the liver. GI toxicity and myelosuppression are the primary concerns associated with the MOPP protocol.

Biologic Response Modifiers in Cancer Therapy: In recent years, a number of alternative modes of cancer therapy have become increasingly available in veterinary medicine. These novel forms of therapy work in myriad ways, including enhanced immune recognition, altered blood vessel formation, or by exploitation of specific pathways that are aberrant or overexpressed in neoplastic cells. The widespread use of these newer therapies alone or in combination with conventional chemotherapy has transformed the approach to treatment of many cancer patients.

NSAIDs represent one class of biologic response modifiers that work by inhibiting frequently overexpressed COX-2 enzyme activity present in many tumor types. Several studies have proposed that these drugs may work by reducing cell proliferation, increasing apoptosis, inhibiting angiogenesis, and modulating immune function. Piroxicam has been the drug most researched in dogs, but any of the newer NSAIDs with more COX-2 selective inhibition (such as deracoxib or meloxicam) theoretically may yield equal or improved effects. (*See also* NONSTEROIDAL ANTI-INFLAMMATORY DRUGS, p 2714.) The clinical usefulness of COX-2 inhibitors has been demonstrated in canine transitional cell carcinoma, squamous cell carcinoma, and other tumor types in dogs and cats. NSAIDs are often combined in antiangiogenic protocols.

Metronomic or antiangiogenic dosing of chemotherapy is a novel or nontraditional way to administer chemotherapy that consists of the administration of low doses of oral chemotherapy agents at very short intervals, often daily. This treatment approach targets the tumor neovasculature by leveraging the exquisite sensitivity of endothelial progenitor cells and immature endothelium to modest doses of alkylating agents. Studies indicate that antiangiogenic factors, such as thrombospondin-1, increase during metronomic chemotherapy. In addition, antitumor immunosuppression mediated through T regulatory cells may be mediated by metronomic protocols. Disease stabilization is considered a successful outcome of low-dose chemotherapy, because direct cytotoxicity to neoplastic cells is not the intent of metronomic chemotherapy. Preliminary studies in the veterinary literature suggest this is a promising alternative to maximally tolerated doses of conventional chemotherapy, particularly in a microscopic disease setting, and has the added benefit of limited adverse effects.

Targeting of specific pathways that are aberrant or dysregulated in cancers has yielded novel therapies in a variety of human cancers. An example of such a target is the receptor tyrosine kinases (RTKs), which mediate processes involved in tumor growth, progression, and metastasis. These drugs are competitive inhibitors of ATP, and so prevent receptor phosphorylation and subsequent downstream signal transduction. Mutations in c-kit, an RTK gene involved in mast cell differentiation and proliferation, has been reported in approximately a quarter of canine mast cell tumors. Toceranib has been approved by the FDA, and biologic response rates of 70%–90% have been reported in dogs that have mast cell tumors with recognized c-kit mutations. Moreover, toceranib has activity against other members of the split-kinase family of RTKs, such as vascular endothelial growth factor receptor, platelet-derived growth factor, and others. Preliminary evidence indicates that toceranib has activity against a variety of carcinomas and metastatic osteosarcoma, leading to tumor regression or more often to prolonged disease stabilization. Recent reports indicate that dosages of toceranib ranging from 2.4–2.9 mg/kg, PO, every 48 hr (below the label dosage of 3.25 mg/kg, PO, every 48 hr) result in sufficient target inhibition with substantially reduced toxicity.

Development of a therapeutic vaccine to stimulate active immunity against cancer has long been a goal in both human and veterinary oncology. This became a reality with introduction of a canine melanoma vaccine. The vaccine exploits the immune response induced by human tyrosinase, an enzyme in the pathway of melanin formation. The vaccine contains a human tyrosinase gene inserted into a bacterial plasmid, which is administered transdermally. The antibodies and T-cell responses produced by xenogeneic tyrosinase cross-react with the tyrosinase overexpressed on canine melanoma cells. Initial studies reported prolonged survival in dogs with advanced stage oral malignant melanoma treated with radiation therapy or surgery of the primary tumor, followed by vaccine administration.

Passive immunotherapy using monoclonal antibodies has grown substantially in human oncology in recent years. Monoclonal antibodies may attach to specific antigens on cancer cells, thereby either marking the cancer cells for destruction by the immune system or impairing functional pathways within the neoplastic cells. Furthermore, monoclonal antibodies may be conjugated to other antineoplastic agents (such as chemotherapy agents, radionuclides, or other toxins) to allow for more targeted delivery of cytotoxic therapy to cancer cells while sparing normal tissues. The introduction of anti-CD20 monoclonal antibodies in human oncology has revolutionized the treatment of B-cell lymphoma with significantly improved outcomes versus chemotherapy alone. In veterinary medicine, anti-CD20 and anti-CD52 monoclonal antibodies have received either USDA or conditional approval to treat canine B-cell and T-cell lymphoma, respectively. The mechanisms by which these antibodies work is not fully understood, but several potential mechanisms include antibody-dependent cell-mediated cytotoxicity, complement-dependent cytotoxicity, and direct signaling leading to inhibition of proliferation or to apoptosis. Field studies of each of these antibodies are underway.

Biologic response modifiers aimed at enhancing innate antitumor defense mechanisms of the host has been an area of active investigation. Nonspecific immunomodulators, including intact bacteria or bacterial cell components, acemannan, IL-2, IL-12, interferon alpha, levamisole, and cimetidine, have been reported with variable efficacy to enhance immune responsiveness and improve outcomes after surgery or antineoplastic chemotherapy. Liposome-encapsulated muramyl tripeptide phosphatidylethanolamine (L-MTP-PE) is perhaps the best studied nonspecific immunomodulator in veterinary medicine. This synthetic bacterial wall component has been used effectively with chemotherapy to confer a survival advantage in dogs with splenic hemangiosarcoma and osteosarcoma.

Development of immunomodulators such as lymphokines and cytokines (eg, interleukins, interferon, and tumor necrosis factor) for clinical use in cancer patients has not been fully realized, largely because of toxicity. Consequently, these agents are not commonly used in veterinary medicine.

Blocking angiogenesis is an attractive form of anticancer therapy, because tumors must develop their own vascular supply if they are to grow beyond a few millimeters in diameter. Various drugs, such as angiostatin, thrombospondin-1, and matrix metalloproteinase inhibitors, have been investigated with varying results. Specific angiogenesis inhibitors for veterinary patients are not yet commercially available. At present, metronomic chemotherapy combinations are the most practical approach to antiangiogenic therapy in clinical cases.

ANCILLARY ANTINEOPLASTIC AGENTS

Supplementary agents are occasionally used in veterinary oncology to either enhance the effect of certain chemotherapy treatments or support the well-being of the patient. Drugs in this category include antiemetic therapy, prophylactic antibiotics, COX-2 inhibitors (NSAIDs), and various pain medications.

Bisphosphonates are frequently used in veterinary oncology for a variety of reasons, including to treat bone pain from primary bone tumors or bone metastasis, and to effectively treat hypercalcemia of malignancy. Bisphosphonates belong to a class of drugs that directly inhibit osteoclast activity and the subsequent resorption of bone. In people, these drugs are used for various conditions that are characterized by bone resorption and bone fragility, such as osteoporosis. In addition to their inhibitory effects on osteoclasts, bisphosphonates are believed to exert direct cytotoxic effects on some cancer cells. These effects include induction of apoptosis, inhibition of new blood vessel formation, and reduction of tumor cell adhesion to bone matrix.

Retinoids are a class of compounds structurally related to vitamin A. In preclinical studies, all-trans retinoic acid (tretinoin), 13-cis retinoic acid (isotretinoin), and the aromatic retinoids etretinate and acitretin have preventive and therapeutic effects on carcinogen-induced premalignant and malignant lesions in both human and veterinary medicine. Isotretinoin and etretinate have been used with limited therapeutic success in superficial squamous cell carcinoma and cutaneous lymphoma. In people, dramatic therapeutic effects have been observed in treatment of acute promyelocytic leukemia with tretinoin. The mechanism of action of retinoids is thought to occur through modulation of cell proliferation and differentiation. Retinoids vary in their capacity to induce differentiation and to inhibit proliferation in a variety of human and veterinary cell lines.

TREATMENT OF CANINE LYMPHOMA

Lymphoma is the canine tumor most frequently treated with chemotherapy. It is the most common hematopoietic neoplasia of dogs (*see* p 40) and cats and is also among the most responsive to chemotherapy. Four antineoplastic agents, vincristine, cyclophosphamide, doxorubicin, and prednisone, form the basis for many lymphoma treatment protocols. Treatments based on these four drugs are often abbreviated as CHOP (cyclophosphamide, hydroxydaunorubicin [doxorubicin], Oncovin® [a trade name of vincristine], and prednisone) protocols. One commonly used CHOP protocol in veterinary medicine is shown in TABLE 58; nearly 40 protocols for management of lymphoma in dogs have been published.

The most common recommendation in veterinary oncology is to use a discontinuous chemotherapy protocol, as opposed to maintenance or continual chemotherapy. Discontinuous chemotherapy in dogs appears to have the same or similar remission and survival duration as a traditional maintenance protocol. For this treatment approach, all chemotherapy is discontinued for patients in a complete remission at the end of the treatment protocol. At the first signs of recurrence of lymphoma, reinduction using the original chemotherapy protocol should be used. Studies have suggested that dogs receiving a

TABLE 58 CHOP MULTIDRUG CHEMOTHERAPY FOR TREATMENT OF CANINE LYMPHOMA

Drug	Dosage	Schedule
L-Asparaginase	10,000 IU/m^2, SC	Wk 1
Vincristine	0.5–0.7 mg/m^2, IV	Wk 1, 3, 6, 8, 11, 13, 16, and 18
Cyclophosphamide	250 mg/m^2, IV or PO	Wk 2, 7, 12, and 17
Doxorubicin	30 mg/m^2, IV, for dogs >10 kg; 1 mg/kg for dogs <10 kg	Wk 4, 9, 14, and 19
Prednisone	2 mg/kg/day, PO	For first week, then 1.5 mg/kg/day, PO, for 7 days, then 1 mg/kg/day, PO, for 7 days, then 0.5 mg/kg/day, PO, for 7 days, then discontinue.

discontinuous protocol were more likely to achieve a second remission when they relapsed than dogs that received longterm or maintenance chemotherapy. If reinduction fails, then use of rescue protocols should be considered.

Other lymphoma protocols include a non-doxorubicin-based combination protocol (COP) or a protocol consisting of single-agent doxorubicin administered every 3 wk. These protocols are generally well tolerated, less expensive, and easy to administer but are considered to be less effective than a CHOP-based protocol.

CHOP-based chemotherapy protocols provide the basis for most lymphoma chemotherapy protocols in cats, although there is currently no consensus treatment protocol recommended for this species. In general, fewer studies document the clinical effectiveness of various CHOP combinations in cats than in dogs.

ANTISEPTICS AND DISINFECTANTS

Antiseptics and disinfectants are nonselective, anti-infective agents that are applied topically. Their activity ranges from simply reducing the number of microorganisms to within safe limits of public health interpretations (sanitization), to destroying all microorganisms (sterilization) on the applied surface. In general, antiseptics are applied on tissues to suppress or prevent microbial infection. Disinfectants are germicidal compounds usually applied to inanimate surfaces. Sometimes the same compound may act as an antiseptic and a disinfectant, depending on the drug concentration, conditions of exposure, number of organisms, etc. To achieve maximal efficiency, it is essential to use the proper concentration of the drug for the purpose intended. The logic that "if a little is good, twice as much is better" is not only uneconomical but often has toxicologic implications.

Topical anti-infective agents are extensively used in surgery for antisepsis of the surgical site and surgeon's hands and to disinfect surgical instruments, apparel, and hospital premises. Other common uses are as disinfectants for home and farm premises, food processing facilities, in water treatment, in public health sanitation, and as antiseptics in soaps, teat dips, dairy sanitizers, etc. Antiseptics also have been used to treat local infections. However, in most cases, systemic chemotherapeutic agents are preferred, because they often penetrate better into the foci of infection and are less likely than the topical anti-infectives to lose their potency when in contact with body fluids and debris in the infected area.

Ideally, antiseptics and disinfectants should have a broad spectrum and potent germicidal activity, with rapid onset and long-lasting effect. They should not be prone to development of resistance in target microorganisms. They should withstand a range of environmental factors (eg, pH, temperature, humidity) and must retain activity even in the presence of pus, necrotic tissue, soil, and other organic material. High lipid solubility and good dispersibility increase their effectiveness. Antiseptic preparations should not be toxic to the host tissues and should not impair healing. Disinfectants should be nondestructive to applied surfaces. They should be readily biodegradable, not accumulate in the environment, or react with other chemicals to produce toxic residues. Offensive odor, color, and staining properties should be absent or minimal.

Most of these compounds exert their antimicrobial effect by denaturation of intracellular protein, alteration of cellular membranes (often through extraction of membrane lipids), or enzyme inhibition. Although most classes of antiseptics and disinfectants have been in use for decades, the emergence of microbial resistance to some agents, especially in the hospital environment, has led to continued research into the development of new compounds.

ACIDS AND ALKALIES

Acids: Hydrogen ion is bacteriostatic at pH ~3–6 and bactericidal at pH <3. Strong mineral acids (HCl, H_2SO_4, etc) in concentrations of 0.1–1 N have been used as disinfectants; however, their corrosive action limits their usefulness. Un-ionized weak organic acids can readily penetrate and disrupt bacterial cell membranes. Acids are used as food preservatives (eg, benzoic acid), antiseptics (eg, boric acid, acetic acid), fungicides (eg, salicylic acid, benzoic acid), spermatocides (eg, acetic acid, lactic acid), and cauterizing agents (strong mineral acids).

Acetic acid, 1%, can be used in surgical dressings. At 5%, it is bactericidal to many bacteria and has been used to treat otitis externa produced by *Pseudomonas*, *Candida*, *Malassezia*, or *Aspergillus* spp. Skin and hides that have been contaminated by anthrax spores can be disinfected with 2.5% HCl.

Alkalies: Hydroxyl ion also exerts antimicrobial activity. At a pH >9, it inhibits most bacteria and many viruses. Hydroxides of sodium and calcium are used as disinfectants. Their irritant or caustic property usually precludes their application on tissues.

A 2% solution of soda lye (contains 94% sodium hydroxide [NaOH]) in hot water is used as a disinfectant against many common pathogens, such as those causing fowl cholera and pullorum disease. It is a potent caustic and must be handled with care.

Calcium oxide (CaO), ie, lime (hydrated or air-slaked lime), soaked in water produces $Ca(OH)_2$. Aqueous suspensions of slaked lime are used to disinfect premises.

ALCOHOLS

Primary aliphatic alcohols are germicidal. Their potency increases but water solubility decreases with chain length until amyl alcohol (6 carbons) is reached. Antimicrobial effect is related to their lipid solubility (damages bacterial membranes) and their ability to coagulate cytoplasmic proteins. However, they do not destroy bacterial spores. Ethyl alcohol (ethanol) and isopropyl alcohol (isopropanol) are the most widely used alcohols. They can be used in concentrations of 30%–90% in aqueous solutions; best results are usually obtained with 70% ethanol or 50% isopropanol. Higher concentrations tend to be less effective. Isopropanol is slightly more potent than ethanol because of its greater depression of surface tension. "Rubbing alcohol" is a mixture of alcohols, with isopropanol as its principal ingredient. It is used as a skin disinfectant and rubefacient. Alcohol-based hand rinses have rapid-acting antiseptic effects. This makes them useful in minimizing the transmission of transient flora acquired from infected patients and reducing nosocomial diseases.

BIGUANIDES

Chlorhexidine is the most popular antiseptic of this group. It has potent antimicrobial activity against most gram-positive and some gram-negative bacteria but not against spores. A 0.1% aqueous solution is bactericidal against *Staphylococcus aureus*, *Escherichia coli*, and *Pseudomonas aeruginosa* in 15 sec. However, it is relatively ineffective against other gram-negative organisms, spores, fungi, and most viruses. Nosocomial infections by *Pseudomonas* spp have developed from the use of contaminated chlorhexidine solutions in which the bacteria persisted. In susceptible organisms, chlorhexidine disrupts the cytoplasmic membrane. Its activity is unaffected or enhanced by alcohols, quaternary ammonium compounds, and alkaline pH, and is somewhat depressed by high concentrations of organic matter (pus, blood, etc), hard water, and contact with cork. It is incompatible with anionic compounds, including soap.

Chlorhexidine is one of the most commonly used surgical and dental antiseptics. A 4% emulsion of chlorhexidine gluconate is used as a skin cleanser, a 0.5% (w/v) solution in 70% isopropanol as a general antiseptic, and a 0.5% solution in 70% isopropanol with emollients as a hand rinse. Chlorhexidine soaps have good residual activity, which may be advantageous when applied as a presurgical scrub for prolonged surgical procedures. Chlorhexidine-alcohol mixtures are particularly effective in that they combine the antiseptic rapidity of alcohol with the persistence of chlorhexidine. Because of its antiseptic properties and low potential for systemic or dermal toxicity, chlorhexidine has been incorporated into shampoos, ointments, skin and wound cleansers, teat dips, and surgical scrubs. A 1% chlorhexidine acetate ointment is used as a topical antiseptic in treatment of external wounds in dogs, cats, and horses. Contact dermatitis has been reported in up to 8% of human patients after repeated topical exposure. Little data are available on hypersensitivity reactions in animals.

OXIDIZING AGENTS

Peroxides: These compounds generally exert a short-acting germicidal effect on most organisms through release of nascent oxygen, which irreversibly alters microbial proteins. Most have little or no action on bacterial spores. Nascent oxygen is rendered inactive when it combines with organic matter.

Hydrogen peroxide solution (3%) liberates oxygen when in contact with catalase present on wound surfaces and mucous membranes. One mL of 3% hydrogen peroxide liberates 10 mL of oxygen at standard temperature and pressure. The effervescent action mechanically helps remove pus and cellular debris from wounds and is useful to clean and deodorize infected tissue. The antimicrobial action is of short duration and is limited to the superficial layer of the applied surface because there is no penetration of the tissue. However, *the use of hydrogen peroxide in partially* closed spaces, such as operative wounds, may result in oxygen embolization due to dissection of gas under pressure into tissues. Although its usefulness as an antiseptic is limited, hydrogen peroxide is finding increased application as a disinfectant in water treatment and food processing facilities and for sterilization of dental and surgical instruments.

Accelerated hydrogen peroxide formulations are synergistic blends of 0.5%–2% hydrogen peroxide with anionic and nonionic surfactants and stabilizers that possess broad-spectrum antimicrobial activity. They are effective against bacteria, spores, mycobacteria, viruses, and fungi, with short contact times. Accelerated hydrogen peroxide formulations are nonirritating to eyes and skin and are biodegradable, decomposing to water and oxygen with no active chemical residues. They have become leading disinfectants in human hospitals and dental clinics. A disadvantage is the potential to damage soft metals, such as brass, copper, and aluminum, and carbon-tipped instruments.

Peracetic acid and the combination of peracetic acid (0.23%) and hydrogen peroxide (7.35%) have been recognized as useful sterilants and antiseptics, combining the broad antimicrobial spectrum and lack of harmful decomposition products of hydrogen peroxide with greater lipid solubility and freedom from inactivation by tissue catalase and peroxidase. They can be used over wide temperature (0°–40°C) and pH (3–7.5) ranges and are not affected by organic matter. They are effective against bacteria, yeasts, fungi, and viruses at concentrations of 0.001%–0.003% and are sporicidal at 0.25%–0.5%. Consequently, peracetic acid products have been accepted worldwide in the food industry, including meat and poultry processing plants and dairies, and are replacing traditional disinfectants for some medical devices. Solutions of 0.2% peracetic acid applied to compresses effectively reduce microbial populations in severely contaminated wounds.

Sodium perborate, used in antiseptic solutions and in mouthwashes, acts by decomposing into sodium metaborate and hydrogen peroxide, which then gradually liberates oxygen.

Benzoyl peroxide slowly releases oxygen to act as an antiseptic. However, it can cause skin irritation. It also has keratolytic and antiseborrheic activity, which makes it useful in treating pyoderma in dogs.

Potassium peroxymonosulfate is a broad-spectrum disinfectant with increasing use in barns and kennels. A 1% solution in water is highly effective against bacteria, viruses, and fungi, maintaining good activity in the presence of organic matter.

Potassium permanganate has broad antimicrobial properties, but its intense purple color in solution, which stains tissues and clothing brown, is a disadvantage. It is an effective algicide (0.01%) and virucide (1%) for disinfection, but concentrations >1:10,000 tend to irritate tissues. Old solutions turn chocolate brown and lose their activity.

Halogens and Halogen-containing Compounds: Iodine and chlorine are among the oldest topical antimicrobial agents. They owe their activity to high affinity for protoplasm, where they are believed to oxidize proteins and interfere with vital metabolic reactions.

Iodine: Elemental iodine is a potent germicide with a wide spectrum of activity and low toxicity to tissues. A solution containing 50 ppm iodine kills bacteria in 1 min and spores in 15 min. It is poorly soluble in water but readily dissolves in ethanol, which enhances its antibacterial activity.

Iodine tincture contains 2% iodine and 2.4% sodium iodide (NaI) dissolved in 50% ethanol; it is used as a skin disinfectant. Strong iodine tincture contains 7% iodine and 5% potassium iodide (KI) dissolved in 95% ethanol; it is more potent but also more irritating than tincture of iodine. Iodine solution contains 2% iodine and 2.4% NaI dissolved in aqueous solution; it is used as a nonirritant antiseptic on wounds and abrasions. Strong iodine solution (Lugol's solution) contains 5% iodine and 10% KI in aqueous solution.

Iodophores (eg, povidone-iodine and poloxamer-iodine) are combinations of iodine with a solubilizing agent or carrier; they are more stable and water soluble than older formulations. They slowly release iodine as an antimicrobial agent and are widely used as skin disinfectants, particularly before surgery. They do not sting or stain. Iodophores are nontoxic to tissues (although contact dermatitis can result from repeated exposure) but may be corrosive to metals. They are effective against bacteria, viruses, and fungi but less so against spores. Iodophor solutions retain good antibacterial activity at pH <4, even in the presence of organic matter, and often change color when the activity is lost. Phosphoric acid is often mixed with iodophores to maintain an acidic medium. They have been used in teat dips to control mastitis, as dairy sanitizers, and as a general antiseptic or disinfectant for various dermal and mucosal infections.

Chlorine: Chlorine exerts a potent germicidal effect against most bacteria, viruses, protozoa, and fungi through formation of undissociated hypochlorous acid (HOCl) in water at acid to neutral pH. It is effective against most organisms at a concentration of 0.1 ppm, but much higher concentrations are required in the presence of organic matter. Alkaline pH ionizes chlorine and decreases its activity by reducing its penetrability. Chlorine has a strong acid smell. It is irritating to the skin and mucous membranes, including the respiratory tract, and can cause severe bronchospasms and acute lung injury. It is widely used to disinfect water supplies and inanimate objects (eg, utensils, bottles, pipelines) in dairies, creameries, and milk houses. Chlorine dioxide has recently replaced chlorine as a disinfectant for drinking water in some jurisdictions, because it forms fewer by-products.

Inorganic chlorides include sodium hypochlorite solutions (bleach). A 2%–5% NaOCl solution is a commonly used and effective disinfectant. Calcium hypochlorite is used as a disinfectant.

Organic chlorides contain chlorine weakly bonded to nitrogen, which is slowly released for germicidal activity. They are generally less irritant, more stable, and more convenient to use than hypochlorite solutions.

METALS

Inorganic mercuric bichloride, one of the early antiseptics, was later replaced by the less irritant and less toxic organic mercurials, eg, merbromin, thimerosal (49% mercury), nitromersol, and phenylmercuric nitrate. At moderate concentrations, the organic mercurials are bacteriostatic and act by inhibiting bacterial enzymes through their affinity for sulfhydryl groups. This effect can be reversed by sulfur-containing compounds, eg, cysteine or glutathione. Mercurials are not effective against spores. Use of mercurial antiseptics or disinfectants has decreased, partly because of their environmental persistence and contaminant potential. Repeated application of topical mercurials can result in significant absorption and systemic toxicity.

Silver compounds can have caustic, astringent, and antibacterial effects. Silver ions combine with sulfhydryl, amino, phosphate, and carboxyl groups, and thus precipitate proteins, in addition to interfering with essential metabolic activities of microbial cells.

A 0.1% aqueous silver solution is bactericidal and somewhat irritating, whereas a 0.01% solution is bacteriostatic. A 0.5% solution is sometimes applied as a dressing on burns to reduce infection and induce rapid eschar formation. Colloidal silver compounds, which release silver ions slowly, are bacteriostatic and have a more sustained effect. They do not irritate the tissues and have little astringent or caustic effect. They are generally used as mild antiseptics and in ophthalmic preparations.

PHENOLS AND RELATED COMPOUNDS

Phenolic compounds used as antiseptics or disinfectants include pure phenol and substitution products with halogens and alkyl groups. They act to denature and coagulate proteins and are general protoplasmic poisons.

Phenol (carbolic acid) is one of the oldest antiseptic agents. It is bacteriostatic at concentrations of 0.1%–1% and is bactericidal/fungicidal at 1%–2%. A 5% solution kills anthrax spores in 48 hr. The bactericidal activity is enhanced by EDTA and warm temperatures; it is decreased by alkaline medium (through ionization), lipids, soaps, and cold temperatures. Concentrations >0.5% exert a local anesthetic effect, whereas a 5% solution is strongly irritating and corrosive to tissues. Oral ingestion or extensive application to skin can cause systemic toxicity, manifested primarily by CNS and cardiovascular effects; death may result.

Phenol has good penetrating power into organic matter and is mainly used for disinfection of equipment or organic materials that are to be destroyed (eg, infected food and excreta). Because of its irritant and corrosive properties and potential systemic toxicity, it is not used much as an antiseptic currently, except to cauterize infected areas, eg, the infected umbilicus of neonates. It is also incorporated into cutaneous applications for pruritus, stings, bites, burns, etc, because of its local anesthetic and antibacterial properties to relieve itching and control infections.

Cresol (cresylic acid) is a mixture of ortho-, meta-, and paracresols and their isomers. It is a colorless liquid; however, after exposure to light and air, it turns pink, then yellowish, and finally dark brown. A 2% solution of either pure or saponated cresol "lysol" in hot water is commonly used as a disinfectant for inanimate objects.

Hexachlorophene (a trichlorinated *bis*-phenol) has a strong bacteriostatic action against many gram-positive organisms (including staphylococci) but only a few gram-negative ones. It is used widely in medicated soaps. Frequent washings every day with hexachlorophene soaps lead to sufficient retention of residue on the skin to provide prolonged bacteriostatic action. Washing with other soaps promptly removes these residues. Repeated exposure of skin to high concentrations of hexachlorophene may lead to sufficient absorption of the antiseptic to cause spongiform degeneration of the white matter in the brain, cerebral edema, and nervous disorders. To prevent such neurotoxicity, products containing >0.75% hexachlorophene are available only by prescription. Accidental oral ingestion of hexachlorophene results in acute poisoning.

Pine tar is a viscid blackish brown liquid, used primarily for antiseptic bandaging of wounds of the hoof and horn. Pine tar contains phenol derivatives that provide antimicrobial properties.

Chloroxylenols are broad-spectrum bactericides with more activity against gram-positive than gram-negative bacteria. They are active in alkaline pH; however, contact with organic matter diminishes their activity. Streptococci are more susceptible than staphylococci. **Parachlorometaxylenol (PCMX)** and **dichlorometaxylenol (DCMX)** are the two most commonly used members of this group. DCMX is more active than PCMX. Strong solutions of these compounds can cause irritation and have a disagreeable odor. A 5% chloroxylenol (eg, PCMX) solution (in α-terpineol, soap, alcohol, and water) is diluted with water (1:4) for skin sterilization and (1:25 to 1:50) for wound cleansing and irrigation of the uterus and vagina. PCMX is also combined with hexachlorophene to enhance its antibacterial spectrum and to prevent contamination by gram-negative organisms.

REDUCING AGENTS

Formaldehyde is a gas, whereas **glutaraldehyde** is an oil at room temperature. However, both are readily soluble in water. Their solutions are irritating or caustic to tissues, causing coagulation necrosis and protein precipitation, but have potent germicidal properties against all organisms, including spores. Their solutions do not lose appreciable antimicrobial properties in the presence of organic matter and are noncorrosive to metals, paints, and fabric. Both are used as disinfectants. **Formalin** contains 37% formaldehyde gas in aqueous solution with variable amounts of methyl alcohol to prevent polymerization. A 1%–10% solution of formaldehyde is commonly used as a disinfectant. **Glutaral** (glutaraldehyde), a 1%–2% alkaline solution (pH 7.5–8.5) in 70% isopropanol, is a more potent germicide than 4% formaldehyde, effective against all microorganisms, including viruses and spores. It is often used to sterilize surgical and endoscopic instruments and plastic and rubber apparatus. It is a known sensitizer, causing occupational contact dermatitis, as well as bronchial and laryngeal mucous membrane irritation.

Orthophthaldehyde (OPA) is an aromatic aldehyde similar to glutaraldehyde but with several potential advantages. Typical 0.55% solutions have excellent stability over a wide pH range (3–9), are less toxic and irritating to eyes and nasal passages, and have a barely perceptible odor. They are compatible with most materials, including flexible endoscopes. OPA solutions are faster acting than glutaraldehyde against mycobacteria but have somewhat less sporicidal activity. A potential disadvantage of OPA is that it stains proteins (including unprotected skin) gray, so it must be handled with caution.

Sulfur dioxide, as a gaseous fumigant, is produced by burning sulfur in closed spaces. For maximal effect, the surface should be moist, because the gas dissolves in water to form sulfurous acid, which is bactericidal. However, this reducing effect of the acid can also corrode metals, rot fabrics, and bleach dyes.

SURFACE-ACTIVE COMPOUNDS

Surfactants lower the surface tension of an aqueous solution and are used as wetting agents, detergents, emulsifiers, antiseptics, and disinfectants. As antimicrobials, they alter the energy relationship at interfaces. Based on the position of the hydrophobic moiety in the molecule, surfactants are classified as anionic or cationic.

Anionic Surfactants: Soaps are dipolar anionic detergents with the general formula RCOONa/K, which dissociate in water into hydrophilic K^+ or Na^+ ions and lipophilic fatty acid ions. Because NaOH and KOH are strong bases (whereas most fatty acids are weak acids), most soap solutions are alkaline (pH 8–10) and may irritate sensitive skin and mucous membranes. Soaps emulsify lipoidal secretions of the skin and remove, along with most of the accompanying dirt, desquamated epithelium and bacteria, which are then rinsed away with the lather. The antibacterial potency of soaps is often enhanced by inclusion of certain antiseptics, eg, hexachlorophene, phenols, carbanilides, or potassium iodide. They are incompatible with cationic surfactants.

Cationic Surfactants: Cationic detergents are a group of alkyl- or aryl-substituted quaternary ammonium compounds (eg, benzalkonium chloride, benzathonium chloride, cetylpyridinium chloride) with an ionizable halogen, such as bromide, iodide, or chloride. The major site of action of these compounds appears to be the cell membrane, where they become adsorbed and cause changes in permeability. The activity of older quaternary ammonium compounds is reduced by hard water and by porous or fibrous materials (eg, fabrics, cellulose sponges) that adsorb them. They are also inactivated by anionic substances (eg, soaps, proteins, fatty acids, phosphates). Therefore, they are of limited value in the presence of blood and tissue debris. However, newer dialkyl quaternary ammonium compounds (fourth generation, including dodecyl dimethyl ammonium bromide, dioctyl dimethyl ammonium bromide, etc) purportedly remain active in hard water and are tolerant of anionic residues. Fifth-generation quaternaries are mixtures of the fourth generation with the second generation and demonstrate greater biocidal activity under conditions of high soil load, making them useful disinfectants in barns and footbaths. Quaternary ammonium compounds are effective against most bacteria, enveloped viruses, some fungi (including yeasts), and protozoa but not against nonenveloped viruses, mycobacteria, and spores. Aqueous solutions of 1:1,000 to 1:5,000 have good antimicrobial activity, especially at slightly alkaline pH, and are commonly used for disinfection of noncritical instruments and hard surface cleaning. When applied to skin, they may form a film under which microorganisms can survive, which limits their reliability as antiseptics. Concentrations >1% are injurious to mucous membranes.

Octenidine dihydrochloride is a cationic surfactant used increasingly in Europe as an alternative to quaternaries, chlorhexidine, and iodophores for skin, mucous membrane, and wound antisepsis.

OTHER ANTIBACTERIAL AGENTS

The antibacterial activity of **dyes** was first reported in 1913. Interestingly, the discovery of sulfonamides as chemotherapeutic agents ensued from the antibacterial activity observed in the dye prontosil.

Azo dyes (eg, scarlet red and phenazopyridine HCl) are most active in an acidic medium and are effective against gram-negative organisms. Scarlet red is often used as a 5% ointment on sores, ulcers, and wounds. Pyridium is often incorporated as an analgesic with sulfonamides to treat urinary tract infections.

Acridine dyes (eg, acriflavine, proflavine, aminacrine) are more active against gram-positive bacteria. Their activity is enhanced in alkaline medium and antagonized by hypochlorites. Impregnated bandages and gauze and acriflavine jelly have been used extensively for treatment of burns.

VAPOR-PHASE DISINFECTANTS

Alkylating agents such as formaldehyde, ethylene oxide, and propylene oxide are broad-spectrum biocides active against bacteria, viruses, and fungi, including spores.

Ethylene and propylene oxides are highly reactive gaseous fumigants used to sterilize animal feed, human food, surgical equipment that cannot be autoclaved (eg, endoscopes, gloves, syringes, catheters, tubing, implantable devices), laboratory equipment, etc. Both are noncorrosive. However, ethylene oxide has better penetrability than propylene oxide and, therefore, is more commonly used. For this application, ethylene oxide is mixed with chlorofluorocarbons or carbon dioxide and sold in gas cylinders.

Other gaseous disinfectants (eg, formaldehyde, sulfur dioxide, methylbromide) have been used infrequently because of their toxic or corrosive properties.

ANTIVIRAL AGENTS

The conventional approach to control of viral diseases is to develop effective vaccines, but this is not always possible. The objective of antiviral activity is to eradicate the virus while minimally impacting the host and to prevent further viral invasion. However, because of their method of replication, viruses present a greater therapeutic challenge than do bacteria.

Viruses comprise a core genome of nucleic acid surrounded by a protein shell or capsid. Some viruses are further surrounded by a lipoprotein membrane or envelope. Viruses cannot replicate independently and, as such, are obligate intracellular parasites. The host's pathways of energy generation, protein synthesis, and DNA or RNA replication provide the means of viral replication. Viral replication occurs in five sequential steps: host cell penetration, disassembly, control of host protein and nucleic acid synthesis such that viral components are made, assembly of viral proteins, and release of the virus.

Drugs that target viral processes must penetrate host cells; further, because viruses often assume direction of cell division, drugs that negatively impact a virus are also likely to negatively impact normal pathways of the host. For these reasons, particularly compared with antibacterial drugs, antiviral drugs are characterized by a narrow therapeutic margin. Nephrotoxicity is emerging as an adverse reaction to antiviral drugs in human medicine. Therapy is further complicated by viral latency, ie, the ability of the virus to incorporate its genome in the host genome, with clinical infection becoming evident without reexposure to the organism. In vitro susceptibility testing must depend on cell cultures, which are expensive. More importantly, in vitro inhibitory tests do not necessarily correlate with therapeutic efficacy of antiviral drugs. Part of the discrepancy between in vitro and in vivo testing occurs because some drugs require activation (metabolism) to be effective.

Only a few antiviral drugs are reasonably safe and effective against a limited number of viral diseases, and most of these have been developed in people. Few have been studied in animals, and widespread clinical use of antiviral drugs is not common in veterinary medicine. The advent of human immunodeficiency virus (HIV) and the development of the cat as a model of HIV infection has somewhat increased the animal knowledge base. Only a selection of the more promising agents and their purported attributes are briefly discussed.

Most antiviral drugs interfere with viral nucleic acid synthesis or regulation. Such drugs generally are nucleic acid analogues that interfere with RNA and DNA production. Other mechanisms of action include interference with viral cell binding or interruption of virus uncoating. Some viruses contain unique metabolic pathways that serve as a target of drug therapy. Drugs that simply inhibit single steps in the viral replication cycle are virustatic and only temporarily halt viral replication. Thus, optimal activity of some drugs depends on an adequate host immune response. Some antiviral drugs may enhance the immune system of the host. TABLE 59 lists the dosage rates for some commonly used antiviral drugs.

Pyrimidine Nucleosides: A variety of pyrimidine nucleosides (both halogenated and nonhalogenated) effectively inhibit the replication of herpes simplex viruses with limited host-cell toxicity. The exact mechanism of action of these compounds appears to reflect substitution of pyrimidine for thymidine, causing defective DNA molecules. Idoxuridine is effective for treatment of herpesvirus infection of the superficial layers of the cornea (herpesvirus keratitis) and of the skin but is toxic when administered systemically.

Trifluridine, also an analogue of deoxythymidine, is currently the agent of choice for treatment of herpesvirus keratitis in people. The other antiviral pyrimidine nucleosides have not been used clinically to any notable extent.

Purine Nucleosides: Certain purine nucleosides have proved to be effective antivirals and are used as systemic agents.

VIDARABINE

Vidarabine, or araA, is used topically for ocular herpesvirus and systemically for herpetic encephalitis and neonatal herpesviral infections. This drug is an adenosine derivative that is phosphorylated by cellular enzymes to a triphosphate compound that inhibits many viral and human DNA polymerases and thus DNA synthesis. Herpesviral enzymes are ~20-fold more susceptible to the drug than host DNA. Vidarabine is administered IV in large volumes of fluid and is rapidly inactivated. It may produce bone marrow suppression and CNS adverse effects when high blood levels are reached. An ophthalmic solution also is available.

ACYCLOVIR

Acyclovir (acycloguanosine) and its L-valyl ester prodrug valacyclovir, represent a new generation of antiviral agents, mainly because of the unique mechanism of action. This purine nucleoside is phosphorylated more efficiently by virus-induced thymidine kinase than host thymidine kinase. Once activated to the triphosphate form, it is a better substrate and inhibitor of viral, versus host, DNA polymerase. Binding to DNA polymerase is irreversible. Once acyclovir is incorporated into viral DNA, the DNA chain is terminated.

Acyclovir is relatively safe (probenecid renders the drug safer) and is useful against a variety of infections caused by DNA viruses, especially the herpesvirus family. However, resistance is increasing. Acyclovir is unable to eliminate latent infections. It is available as an ophthalmic ointment, a topical ointment and cream, an IV preparation, and various oral formulations. The prodrug deoxyacyclovir is more readily absorbed from the GI tract than acyclovir. Another similar antiviral purine nucleoside analogue is ganciclovir, a synthetic guanine effective against human cytomegalovirus. Its mechanism of action is similar to that of acyclovir.

PENCICLOVIR AND FAMCICLOVIR

Famciclovir is the prodrug form of penciclovir. Penciclovir is very similar to acyclovir in terms of mechanism of action and spectrum. Although it is much less potent than acyclovir, penciclovir accumulates to much higher concentrations inside the cell. Penciclovir has been studied in cats receiving famciclovir at 62.5 mg for 3 days; it appeared to be well tolerated.

RIBAVIRIN

Ribavirin is a synthetic triazole nucleoside (an analogue of guanosine) with a broad spectrum of activity against many RNA and DNA viruses, both in vitro and in vivo. Susceptible viruses include adenoviruses, herpesviruses, orthomyxoviruses, paramyxoviruses, poxviruses, picornaviruses, rhabdoviruses, rotaviruses, and retroviruses. Viral resistance to ribavirin is rare. The action of ribavirin involves specific inhibition of viral-associated enzymes, inhibition of the capping of viral mRNA, and inhibition of viral polypeptide synthesis. It is well absorbed, widely distributed in the body, eliminated by renal and biliary routes as both parent drug and

TABLE 59 DOSAGES OF ANTIVIRAL DRUGS

Drug	Preparation	Dose, Route, and Frequency	Indication
Idoxuridine	0.1% ophthalmic solution	1 drop, topical, every 5–6 hr	
	0.5% ophthalmic solution	1 drop, topical, every 1–2 hr	
Trifluridine	1% ophthalmic solution	1 drop, topical, every 2 hr initially (2 days), then 3–8 times daily	Ocular herpesvirus infection
Vidarabine	3% ophthalmic solution	0.4–1 cm ointment, topical, every 5–6 hr; 3–6 times daily	Ocular herpesvirus infection
	200 mg/mL suspension for injection	10–30 mg/kg/day, IV, as CRI for 12–24 hr	
Acyclovir	200-mg capsules or tablets	200 mg, PO, qid, every 4 hr, or 5 times daily	Feline herpesvirus
	5% cutaneous ointment	Cover lesion, topical, every 3 hr, 6 times daily	
	200 mg/5 mL suspension	80 mg/kg/day (mixed with peanut butter), PO, for 7–14 days	Pacheco's disease in birds
	500 mg/vial powder	250–500 mg/m^2, IV, tid, infused over at least 1 hr	
Ganciclovir	500 mg/vial powder	2–5 mg/kg, IV, bid-tid	
Ribavirin		11 mg/kg/day, IV, for 7 days	Susceptible viral infections
	6 g/100 mL vial powder	Using SPAC-2 nebulizer only, inhalation, 8–18 hr period daily	
Zidovudine	10 mg/mL syrup; 10 mg/mL injection	5–20 mg/kg (cats), PO or SC, bid-tid	FIV, FeLV
Amantadine	100- and 500-mg capsules	100 mg total (human), PO, once to twice daily	
	Syrup 10 mg/mL	100 mg/day total (juveniles), PO	
Rimantadine		200–300 mg/day total (human), PO	
Interferon α-2	3 × 10^6 IU/vial	3 × 10^6 IU/person/day, SC, IM; 0.5–5 U/kg/day, PO; 100,000 U/kg/day, SC	FeLV-associated disease
		1 U/day, PO	FeLV appetite stimulant
		15–30 U, PO, IM, SC, once daily on alternate weeks	FIP, FIV

CRI = constant-rate infusion; FeLV = feline leukemia virus; FIP = feline infectious peritonitis; FIV = *feline immunodeficiency virus* metabolites, and has a plasma half-life of 24 hr in people. It does not have a wide margin of safety in domestic animals. Toxicity is manifest by anorexia, weight loss, bone marrow depression and anemia, and GI disturbances. It has been successfully administered by topical, parenteral, oral, and aerosol routes. Efficacy depends on the site of infection, method of treatment, age of the animal, and infecting dose of virus. Results of human influenza studies with ribavirin have been equivocal.

ZIDOVUDINE

Zidovudine (azidothymidine, AZT) is a thymidine analogue. Within the virus-infected cell, the 3′-azido group is used by retroviral reverse transcriptase and incorporated into DNA transcription, preventing viral replication. The shared mechanism of action is inhibition of RNA-dependent DNA polymerase (reverse transcriptase). This enzyme is responsible for conversion of the viral RNA genome into double-stranded DNA before it is integrated into the cell genome. Because these actions occur early in replication, the drugs tend to be effective for acute infections but are relatively ineffective for chronically infected cells. Cellular α-DNA polymerases are inhibited only at concentrations 100-fold greater than those necessary to inhibit reverse transcriptase, thus rendering this drug relatively safe to host cells. Cellular γ-DNA polymerase, however, is inhibited at lower concentrations.

AZT is effective against a variety of retroviruses at low concentrations. Resistance to AZT is associated with point mutations resulting in amino acid substitutions in the reverse transcriptase. Prolonged use of AZT can facilitate viral resistance. The risk of resistance also appears to correlate with CD4 cell count and the state of infection. Viral susceptibility to AZT may return after the drug has been discontinued for a period of time.

Granulocytopenia and anemia are the major adverse effects of AZT in human patients. The risk of toxicity increases in human patients with low (CD4) lymphocyte counts, high doses, and prolonged therapy. Granulocyte colony-stimulating factor is indicated for management of granulocytopenia. CNS adverse effects are more likely as therapy is begun. The risk of myelosuppression is increased by drugs that inhibit glucuronidation or renal excretion and may be increased in cats.

After a single dose of AZT at 25 mg/kg in cats, bioavailability is ~75%–100%. The elimination half-life is ~1.5 hr, and volume of distribution is 0.82 L/kg. Drug concentrations remain above the effective concentration 50 (EC_{50}) of 0.19 mcg/mL for feline immunodeficiency virus for at least 24 hr after either IV or PO administration. Although this concentration is higher than that associated with myeloid suppression of human cells, adverse effects in cats are limited to transient restlessness, mild anxiety, and hemolysis.

Studies in cats regarding the efficacy of AZT (10–20 mg/kg, bid for 42 days) for feline leukemia virus infection indicated that AZT prevents retroviral infection if administered immediately after viral exposure and may reduce replication if administered to previously infected animals. Serum-neutralizing antibodies developed in some of the infected cats, and the cats became resistant to subsequent viral challenge. There was no altered progression of disease in cats when treatment was withheld until 28 days after infection, although the level of viremia was much lower than in untreated cats. AZT appeared to be nontoxic in uninfected cats, although 3 of 12 infected kittens became anorectic and icteric and were vomiting after 40 days of treatment. AZT may cause Heinz body anemia. CBCs should be performed on cats receiving AZT.

AMANTADINE

Amantadine, and its derivative rimantadine, are synthetic antiviral agents that appear to act on an early step of viral replication after attachment of virus to cell receptors. The effect seems to lead to inhibition or delay of the uncoating process that precedes primary transcription. Amantadine may also interfere with the early stages of viral mRNA transcription. Amantadine at usual concentrations inhibits replication of different strains of influenza A virus, influenza C virus, Sendai virus, and pseudorabies virus. It is almost completely absorbed from the GI tract, and ~90% of a dose administered PO is excreted unchanged in the urine over several days (human data). The main clinical use has been to prevent infection with various strains of influenza A viruses. However, in people, it also has been found to produce some therapeutic benefit if taken within 48 hr after the onset of illness. Amantadine and its derivatives may be given by the PO, intranasal, SC, IP, or aerosol routes. It produces few adverse effects, most of which are related to the CNS; stimulation of the CNS is evident at very high doses.

MISCELLANEOUS ANTIVIRAL AGENTS

Several drug classes continue to be investigated mainly because of their in vitro antiviral activities. Their potential clinical usefulness remains obscure in most instances. Included among these agents are thiosemicarbazones, guanidine, benzimidazoles, arildone, phosphonoacetic acid, rifamycins and other antibiotics, and several natural products.

Oseltamivir is a prodrug that, when hydrolyzed, yields the carboxylated metabolite that inhibits viral neuraminidases of human influenza viruses. Mature influenza viruses bud off from the cell in a sphere of host phospholipid membrane. The virus will adhere to the cell until neuraminidase has been cleaved from the sialic acid residues of the host cell membrane. Neuramidases allow separation and subsequent release of viral progeny. Hydrolysis, or activation, occurs in the GI tract and liver. The use of oseltamivir for treatment of viral diseases in dogs (parvovirus and parainfluenza) is thus far anecdotal.

ECTOPARASITICIDES

ECTOPARASITICIDES USED IN LARGE ANIMALS

Arthropod parasites (ectoparasites) are major causes of livestock production losses throughout the world. In addition, many arthropod species can act as vectors of disease agents for both animals and people. Treatment with various parasiticides to reduce or eliminate ectoparasites is often required to maintain health and to prevent economic loss in food animals. Some ectoparasiticides were derived from pesticides used to protect crops. The choice and use of ectoparasiticides depend to a large extent on husbandry and management practices, as well as on the type of ectoparasite causing the infestation. Endectocides are capable of killing both internal and external parasites. Accurate identification of the parasite or correct diagnosis based on clinical signs is necessary for selection of the appropriate parasiticide. The selected agent can be administered or applied directly to the animal, or introduced into the environment to reduce the arthropod population to a level that is no longer of economic or health consequence.

Parasites that live permanently on the skin, such as lice, keds, and mites, can be controlled by directly treating the host. Some mange mites burrow into the skin and are therefore more difficult to control with sprays than are lice and keds, which are found on the surface of the skin. However, once these obligate parasites are eradicated, reinfection occurs only from contact with other infected animals.

Ectoparasites with stages that live off the host (ticks, flies, etc) are less easily controlled. Only a small proportion of the ectoparasite population can be treated on the host at any one time, and other hosts may maintain them. Some tick species stay on the host only long enough to feed, which may be as short as 30 min or as long as 21 days. Biting flies, such as the horn fly, can be found continually on the backs and undersides of cattle, where they suck blood up to 20 times a day; other biting flies (such as stable flies and horse flies) and mosquitoes feed to repletion, then leave the animal to lay eggs. Nonbiting flies, such as the face fly or house fly, may visit infrequently but can be very annoying and may transmit disease agents. Larvae of certain blowflies live on the skin or in tissues of sheep and other animals and cause cutaneous myiasis. Larvae of other flies spend several months inside animals (eg, nasal bots in the nasal passages of sheep and goats, bots in the stomach of horses, and cattle grubs or warbles in the back or esophageal tissues). (*See also* FLIES, p 885.)

Many ectoparasite infestations are seasonal and predictable and can be countered by prophylactic use of ectoparasiticides. For example, in temperate countries, flies are seen predominantly from late spring to early autumn, tick populations often increase in the spring and autumn, and lice and mite infestations can be more common during the autumn and winter months. Treatments can be targeted at anticipated times of peak activity as a way to limit parasite populations and disease.

Products are available for parenteral administration or for topical application by various methods, including dips, sprays, pour-ons, spot-ons, dusting powders, and ear tags. The method used depends on the target parasite and host. (*See* ROUTES OF ADMINISTRATION AND DOSAGE FORMS, p 2508.) Importantly, most topical ectoparasiticides used in the USA are pesticides regulated by the U.S. Environmental Protection Agency (EPA). This is an important distinction from products regulated by the U.S. Food and Drug Administration (FDA), because it is illegal to use an EPA-regulated pesticide product inconsistent with its label directions (www.epa.gov). The regulating agency should be identifiable on the product label. The National Pesticide Information Retrieval System (NPIRS) is a searchable database of EPA-registered products (http://ppis.ceris.purdue.edu/).

Chemotherapeutic Agents

Most ectoparasiticides are neurotoxins, exerting their effect on the nervous system of the target parasite. Those used in large animals can be grouped according to structure and mode of action into the organochlorines, organophosphates and carbamates, pyrethrins and pyrethroids, macrocyclic lactones (avermectins and milbemycins), formamidines, insect growth regulators, and a number of miscellaneous compounds, including synergists (eg, piperonyl butoxide). There are also a number of useful compounds with repellent rather than insecticidal activity, including butoxypolypropylene-glycol and N,N-diethyl-3-methylbenzamide (DEET, previously called N,N-diethyl-metatoluamide).

Organochlorines: Organochlorine compounds have been withdrawn in many parts of the world because of concerns regarding environmental persistence.

Organochlorines fall into three main groups: 1) chlorinated ethane derivatives, such as DDT (dichlorodiphenyltrichloroethane), DDE (dichlorodiphenyldichloroethane), and DDD (dicofol, methoxychlor); 2) cyclodienes, including chlordane, aldrin, dieldrin, hepatochlor, endrin, and toxaphene; and 3) hexachlorocyclohexanes such as benzene hexachloride (BHC), which includes the γ-isomer, lindane.

Chlorinated ethanes cause inhibition of sodium conductance along sensory and motor nerve fibers by holding sodium channels open, resulting in delayed repolarization of the axonal membrane. This state renders the nerve vulnerable to repetitive discharge from small stimuli that would normally cause an action potential in a fully repolarized neuron.

The cyclodienes appear to have at least two component modes of action: inhibition of γ-aminobutyric acid (GABA)-stimulated Cl^- flux and interference with Ca^{2+} flux. The resultant inhibitory postsynaptic potential leads to a state of partial depolarization of the postsynaptic membrane and vulnerability to repeated discharge. A similar mode of action has been reported for lindane, which binds to the picrotoxin side of GABA receptors, resulting in an inhibition of GABA-dependent Cl^- ion flux into the neuron.

DDT and BHC were used extensively for flystrike control but subsequently replaced in many countries by more effective cyclodiene compounds, such as dieldrin and aldrin. Both the development of resistance and environmental concerns led to their withdrawal. DDT and lindane were widely used in dip formulations to control sheep scab, but they have mostly been replaced by the organophosphates and subsequently the synthetic pyrethroids.

Organophosphates and Carbamates: The organophosphates comprise a large group of chemicals, many of which are available for topical application and in ear tags as well as for premise control of parasites. There have been many products available worldwide for use in domestic animals, although only a few of the available compounds continue to be used for on-animal treatment.

Organophosphates are neutral esters of phosphoric acid or its thio analogue that inhibit the action of acetylcholinesterase (AChE) at cholinergic synapses and at muscle endplates. The compound mimics the structure of acetylcholine (ACh); when it binds to AChE, it causes transphosphorylation of the enzyme. The transphorylated AChE is unable to break down accumulating ACh at the postsynaptic membrane, leading to neuromuscular paralysis. The degree of transphorylation of the enzyme helps to determine the activity of the organophosphate. Eventually, the AChE is metabolized by oxidative and hydrolytic enzyme systems.

Organophosphates can be extremely toxic in animals and people, inhibiting AChE and other cholinesterases (*see* p 3064). Chronic toxicity results from inhibition of an enzyme known as neuropathy target esterase (NTE) or neurotoxic esterase and is associated with particular compounds. NTE hydrolyzes the fatty acids from the membrane lipid, phosphotidylcholine, and inhibition of NTE appears to cause structural changes in neuronal membranes and a reduction in conduction velocity, which may be manifest as posterior paralysis in some animals. Cases of organophosphate toxicity are treated with oximes or atropine.

Organophosphates used topically include coumaphos, diazinon, dichlorvos, malathion, tetrachlorvinphos,trichlorfon, phosmet, and pirimiphos. Ear tags containing chlorpyrifos, coumaphos, diazinon, or pirimiphos are available. These compounds are generally active against fly larvae, flies, lice, ticks, and mites on domestic livestock, although activity varies between compounds and differing formulations. Chlorpyrifos can be used in microencapsulated form for residual activity and improved safety. Diazinon and propetamphos have been available in dip formulations to control psoroptic mange in sheep. Both eliminate mites and protect in a single application when correctly applied. Diazinon provides longer residual protection than propetamphos. In cattle, a number of compounds have been used for systemic control of warble fly grubs and lice as pour-on applications or in hand sprays, spray races, or dips for tick control.

Carbamate insecticides are closely related to organophosphates and are anticholinesterases. Unlike organophosphates, they appear to cause a spontaneously reversible block on AChE without changing it. The main carbamate compound used in veterinary medicine is propoxur. Carbaryl, another carbamate previously used in veterinary medicine, has been withdrawn from the veterinary market.

Pyrethrins and Synthetic Pyrethroids: A number of pyrethroids are available in many countries as pour-on, spot-on, spray, and dip formulations with activity against biting and nuisance flies, lice, and ticks on domestic livestock. Flumethrin and high cis-cypermethrin are also active against mites and have been used to treat psoroptic mange of sheep.

Natural pyrethrins are derived from pyrethrum, a mixture of alkaloids from the *Chrysanthemum* plant. Pyrethrum extract, prepared from the pyrethrum flower head, contains several molecules collectively known as *pyrethrins* (*pyrethrin I and II*, cinerin I and II, and jasmolin I and II). Pyrethrins are lipophilic molecules that generally undergo rapid absorption, distribution, and excretion. They provide excellent knockdown (rapid kill) but have poor residual activity because of instability. Pyrethrin I is the most active ingredient for kill, and pyrethrin II for rapid insect knockdown.

Pyrethroids are synthesized chemicals modeled on the natural pyrethrin molecule. They are more stable, thus have longer residual activity, and have a higher potency than natural pyrethrins.

The mode of action of pyrethrins and synthetic pyrethroids appears to be interference with sodium channels of the parasite nerve axons, resulting in delayed repolarization and eventual paralysis. Synthetic pyrethroids can be divided into two groups (types I and II, depending on the presence or absence of an α-cyano moiety). Type I compounds have a mode of action similar to that of DDT, involving interference with the axonal Na^+ gate leading to delayed repolarization and repetitive discharge of the nerve. Type II compounds also act on the Na^+ gate but do so without causing repetitive discharge. The lethal activity of pyrethroids seems to involve action on both peripheral and central neurons, while peripheral neuronal effects alone probably produce the knockdown effect. Some preparations contain a synergist (eg, piperonyl butoxide), which inhibits breakdown of pesticides by microsomal mixed-function oxidase (cytochrome P450) systems in insects.

Pyrethroids are generally safe in mammals and birds but are highly toxic to fish and aquatic invertebrates. Concerns have been expressed over their environmental effects, particularly in relation to the aquatic environment, leading to their withdrawal as sheep dips in some countries.

Some of the more common pyrethroids used include β-cyfluthrin, bioallethrin, cyfluthrin, cypermethrin, deltamethrin, fenvalerate, flumethrin, lambda cyhalothrin, phenothrin, permethrin, prallethrin, and tetramethrin. The content of some synthetic pyrethroids is also expressed in terms of the drug isomers, eg, cypermethrin preparations may contain varying proportions of their cis and trans isomers. Thus, cypermethrin (cis:trans 60:40) 2.5% is equivalent to cypermethrin (cis:trans 80:20) 1.25%. In general, cis isomers are more active than the corresponding trans isomers.

Macrocyclic Lactones (Avermectins and Milbemycins): Avermectins and the structurally related milbemycins, collectively referred to as macrocyclic lactones, are fermentation products of *Streptomyces avermitilis* and *S cyanogriseus*, respectively. Avermectins differ from each other chemically in side chain substitutions on the lactone ring, whereas milbemycins differ from the avermectins through the absence of a sugar moiety from the lactone skeleton. A number of macrocyclic lactone compounds are available for use in animals and include the avermectins abamectin, doramectin, eprinomectin, ivermectin, and selamectin, and the milbemycins moxidectin and milbemycin oxime. These compounds are active against a wide range of nematodes and arthropods and are often referred to as endectocides.

Endectocidal activity, particularly against ectoparasites, is variable and depends on the active molecule, the product formulation, and the method of application. Macrocyclic lactones can be given PO, parenterally, or topically (as pour-ons and spot-ons). The method of application depends on the host and, to some degree, on the target parasites. In cattle, for example, available endectocide products can be given PO, by injection, or topically using pour-on formulations. The latter are generally more effective against lice (*Linognathus*, *Haematopinus*, and to some extent *Bovicola*) and headfly (*Haematobia/Lyperosia*) infestations than equivalent compounds administered parenterally. In sheep, PO administration of some endectocides has little effect against psoroptic mite infestations (*Psoroptes ovis*), but parenteral administration increases activity, providing both protection and control depending on the product used.

The route of administration and product formulation influence the rates of absorption, metabolism, excretion, and subsequent bioavailability and pharmacokinetics of individual compounds. Avermectins and milbemycins are highly lipophilic, a property that varies with only minor modifications in molecular structure or configuration. After administration, these compounds are stored in fat, from which they are slowly released, metabolized, and excreted. Ivermectin is absorbed systemically after PO, SC, or dermal administration; it is absorbed to a greater degree and has a longer half-life when given SC or dermally. Excretion of the unaltered molecule is mainly via the feces, with <2% excreted in urine of ruminants. In cattle, the reduced absorption and bioavailability of ivermectin given PO may be due to its metabolism in the rumen. The affinity of these compounds for fat explains their persistence in the body and the extended periods of protection afforded against some species of internal and external parasites. The prolonged half-life of these compounds also determines residue levels in meat and milk and the subsequent compulsory withdrawal periods after treatment in food-producing animals.

Macrocyclic lactones bind to glutamate receptors of glutamate-gated chloride channels, triggering Cl^- ion influx and hyperpolarization of parasite neurons, leading to flaccid paralysis. These molecules have low affinity for mammalian ligand-gated chloride channels and do not readily cross the blood-brain barrier.

Formamidines: Amitraz is the only formamidine used as an ectoparasiticide. It appears to act by inhibition of the enzyme monoamine oxidase and as an agonist at octopamine receptors. Monoamine oxidase metabolizes amine neurotransmitters in ticks and mites, and octopamine is thought to modify tonic contractions in parasite muscles. Amitraz has a relatively wide safety margin in mammals; the most frequently associated adverse effect is sedation, which may be associated with an agonist activity of amitraz on α_2-receptors in mammalian species.

Amitraz is available as a spray or dip for use against mites, lice, and ticks in domestic livestock. It controls lice and mange in pigs and psoroptic mange in sheep. In cattle, it has been used in dips, sprays, or pour-ons for control of single-host and multihost tick species. In dipping baths, amitraz can be stabilized by the addition of calcium hydroxide and maintained by standard replenishment methods for routine tick control. An alternative method involves the use of total replenishment formulations in which the dip bath is replenished with full concentration of amitraz at weekly intervals before use. Amitraz is contraindicated in horses.

Chloronicotinyls and Spinosyns: Imidacloprid is a chloronicotinyl insecticide, a synthesized chlorinated derivative of nicotine. Spinosad is a fermentation product of the soil actinomycete *Saccharopolyspora spinosa*. Both compounds bind to nicotinic acetylcholine receptors (but at different sites) in the insect's CNS, leading to inhibition of cholinergic transmission, paralysis, and death. Spinosad has been developed in some countries for use on sheep to control blowfly strike and lice.

Insect Growth Regulators: Insect growth regulators (IGRs) are used throughout the world and represent a relatively new category of insect control agents. They constitute a group of chemical compounds that do not directly kill the adult parasite but interfere with growth and development. Because they act mainly on immature parasite stages, IGRs are not usually suitable for rapid control of established adult parasite populations. Where parasites show a clear seasonal pattern, IGRs can be applied before any anticipated challenge as a preventive measure. They are widely used for blowfly control in sheep but have limited use in other livestock.

Based on their mode of action, IGRs can be divided into chitin synthesis inhibitors (benzoylphenyl ureas), chitin inhibitors (triazine/pyrimidine derivatives), and juvenile hormone analogues (S-methoprene, pyriproxyfen). Several benzoylphenyl ureas have been introduced to control ectoparasites. Chitin is a complex aminopolysaccharide and a major component of the insect's cuticle. During each molt, it has to be newly formed by polymerization of individual sugar molecules. The exact mode of action of the benzoylphenyl ureas is not fully understood. They inhibit chitin synthesis but have no effect on the enzyme chitin synthetase. It has been suggested that they interfere with the assembly of the chitin chains into microfibrils. When immature insect stages are exposed to these compounds, they are not able to complete ecdysis and die during molting. Benzoylphenyl ureas also appear to have a transovarial effect. Exposed adult female insects produce eggs in which the compound is incorporated into the egg nutrient. Egg development proceeds normally, but the newly developed larvae are incapable of hatching. Benzoylphenyl ureas show a broad spectrum of activity against insects but have relatively low efficacy against ticks and mites. The exception is fluazuron, which has greater activity against ticks and some mite species.

Benzoylphenyl ureas are highly lipophilic molecules. When administered to the host they build up in body fat, from which they are slowly released into the bloodstream and excreted largely unchanged. Diflubenzuron and flufenoxuron are used to prevent blowfly strike in sheep. Diflubenzuron is available in some countries as an emulsifiable concentrate for use as a dip or shower. It is more efficient against first-stage larvae than second and third instars and is therefore recommended as a preventive, providing protection for 12–14 wk. It may also have potential to control a number of major insect pests such as tsetse flies. Fluazuron is available in some countries for use in cattle as a tick development inhibitor. When applied as a pour-on, it provides longterm protection against the 1-host tick, *Rhipicephalus (Boophilus) microplus*.

Triazine and pyrimidine derivatives are closely related compounds that are also chitin inhibitors. They differ from the benzoylphenyl ureas both in chemical structure and mode of action, ie, they appear to alter the deposition of chitin into the cuticle rather than its synthesis.

Cyromazine, a triazine derivative, is effective against blowfly larvae on sheep and lambs and also against other *Diptera* such as houseflies and mosquitoes. At recommended dose rates, cyromazine shows only limited activity against established strikes and must therefore be used preventively. Blowflies usually lay eggs on damp fleece of treated sheep. Although larvae are able to hatch, the young larvae immediately come into contact with cyromazine, which prevents the molt to second instars. The efficacy of a pour-on preparation of cyromazine does not depend on factors such as weather, fleece length, and whether the fleece is wet or dry. Control can be maintained for up to 13 wk after a single pour-on application, or longer if cyromazine is applied by dip or shower.

Dicyclanil, a pyrimidine derivative, is highly active against dipteran larvae. A pour-on formulation, available in some countries for blowfly control in sheep, provides up to 20 wk of protection.

The juvenile hormone analogues mimic the activity of naturally occurring juvenile hormones and prevent metamorphosis to the adult stage. Once the larva is fully developed, enzymes within the insect's circulatory system destroy endogenous juvenile hormones, prompting development to the adult stage. The juvenile hormone analogues bind to juvenile hormone receptor sites, but because they are structurally different, are not destroyed by insect esterases. Metamorphosis and further development to the adult stage does not proceed. S-Methoprene is a terpenoid compound with very low mammalian toxicity that mimics a juvenile insect hormone and is used as a feed-through larvicide for hornfly (*Haematobia*) control on cattle.

Miscellaneous Compounds: Piperonyl butoxide and MGK 264 (N-octyl bicycloheptene dicarboximide) are used as synergistic additives in the control of arthropod pests. They are commonly formulated together with insecticides such as natural pyrethrins. The degree of potentiation of insecticidal activity is related to the ratio of components in the mixture; as the proportion of piperonyl butoxide or MGK 264 increases, the amount of natural pyrethrins required to evoke the same level of kill decreases. The insecticidal activity of other pyrethroids, particularly of knockdown agents, can also be enhanced by the addition of piperonyl butoxide or MGK 264. Piperonyl butoxide inhibits the microsomal enzyme system of some arthropods and is effective against some mites. In addition to having low mammalian toxicity and a long record of safety, it rapidly degrades in the environment.

Various products from natural sources, as well as synthetic compounds, have been used as insect repellents. Such compounds include cinerins, pyrethrins and jasmolins (*see* p 2750), citronella oil, di-N-propyl isocinchomeronate, butoxypolypropylene glycol, picaridin, DEET, and DMP (dimethylphthalate). The use of repellents is advantageous as legislative and regulatory authorities become more restrictive toward the use of conventional pesticides. They are used mainly to protect horses against blood-sucking arthropods, particularly midges (*Culicoides*).

Insecticides may be used to provide environmental control of some insects by application to premises. The insect pheromone (Z)-9-tricosene is incorporated into some products to attract insects to the site of application.

Other Control Methods

Biologic Control: The use of naturally occurring biologic pathogens, such as nematodes, bacteria, fungi, and viruses, offer an interesting approach to ectoparasite management. *Bacillus thuringiensis* has been used on sheep to prevent blowfly strike and body lice. The use of fungal pathogens such as *Metarhizium anisopliae* has also been investigated for control of ticks on livestock and mites on cattle and sheep.

Off-host Control: The control of populations of arthropod pest species using nonreturn traps and targets (screens), usually accompanied by semiochemical baits, has been considered widely for parasites such as ticks or flies. The aim is to attract and kill targeted pests in appropriate numbers during the stages in which they are off the host. This approach has been used as a component of the eradication of the primary screwworm fly, *Cochliomyia hominivorax*, from North America and for control of the horn fly, *Haematobia irritans*. Given the large numbers of adult females that must be attracted and killed to achieve effective population management, this is often not possible with the visual and olfactory baits available. One notable exception is in the control of the tsetse fly (*Glossina* spp), for which high levels of control can be achieved due to their very low rate of reproduction and the availability of highly effective baits and traps. In Australia, a nonreturn insecticide-free trap to catch *Lucilia cuprina* is commercially available. The ability of this trap and bait system to suppress fly populations and to reduce strike incidence has been investigated in the southern hemisphere with variable results, although reductions in strike incidence of up to 46% have been reported.

Safety Restrictions

It is important to be aware of and follow safety restrictions to prevent poisoning or injury to treated animals. All organophosphates available for use on animals are cholinesterase inhibitors. They should not be used simultaneously or within a few days before or after treatment or exposure to other cholinesterase-inhibiting drugs, pesticides, or chemicals. They should not be applied to young, sick, convalescent, or stressed animals.

Pyrethroid insecticides available for use on large animals are considered safe but have general precautionary statements on their labels, particularly in relation to disposal and their potential ecotoxicologic effects.

Some parasiticides may be used only by or under the supervision of a veterinarian; others are available via agricultural suppliers and pharmacists directly to the public. Approvals vary from country to country. Labels for pesticides contain explicit information on hazards to animals, people, and the environment; storage of unused insecticide; and disposal of the container. For each insecticide, the label is the primary source of information on uses and safety instructions, which should be carefully followed.

Restrictions are applied to many of the ectoparasiticides indicated for use in food-producing animals to ensure that unacceptable residues are not present in products intended for human consumption. These restrictions may require that animals are not slaughtered for prescribed periods after administration of the product or that the product is not used in animals producing milk for human consumption. Labels and data sheets on all products contain specific instructions on restrictions, including withdrawal periods, and must be followed.

ECTOPARASITICIDES USED IN SMALL ANIMALS

Flea and tick infestation is a major health problem in dogs and cats, and control presents an economic burden to owners. Traditionally, a wide array of ectoparasiticides has been available, and switching among brands was frequent, leading to problems in achieving acceptable external parasite control. Veterinarians are uniquely qualified to explain the host/parasite interrelationships and advise owners on selection of the most suitable control program. However, many pet owners still purchase flea and tick products in supermarkets or pet supply shops where professional advice is not available. Recent advances in product technology have greatly expanded the available options for veterinarians and pet owners. However, this wide array of available parasiticides can lead to confusion. Veterinarians should become familiar with these technologic improvements in both insecticidal chemistry and delivery systems and encourage client education by their staff.

Active Chemical Ingredients

Nomenclature can be confusing if the shorter approved name is not used and the full chemical name is written (eg, chlorpyrifos versus 0,0-diethyl 0-[3,5,6 trichloro 2] phosphorothioate). The use of trade names can cause added confusion. Although most commercial products contain only one active ingredient, it is not uncommon for two or more to be combined to provide enhanced efficacy or broader spectrum of activity. All labels should be read carefully for ingredients, age and species restrictions, and directions for use.

Macrocyclic Lactones: Currently, three macrocyclic lactones are used for control of internal and external parasites in dogs and cats: selamectin and aprinomectin, which are semisynthetic avermectins, and moxidectin, a semisynthetic milbemycin. Although the exact mode of action of macrocyclic lactones is not fully elucidated, it is believed that they bind to glutamate-gated chloride channels in the parasites' nervous system, increasing their permeability and allowing for the rapid and continued influx of Cl^- into the nerve cell. This inhibits nerve activity and causes paralysis of the parasite. Selamectin is presented as a single active ingredient; moxidectin is combined with imidacloprid (*see* NEONICOTINOIDS, below); and eprinomectin has been combined with fipronil (*see* PHENYLPYRAZOLES, p 2756), S-methoprene (*see* INSECT GROWTH REGULATORS, p 2756), and praziquantel. These macrocyclic lactones are applied topically, rapidly absorbed through the skin, and distributed via the blood. They have activity against a variety of internal and external parasites.

Cholinesterase Inhibitors: Two groups of compounds, organophosphates and carbamates, share the same mechanism of action—inhibition of acetylcholinesterase. This enzyme normally is responsible for acetylcholine (neurotransmitter) destruction. Applications of organophosphates or carbamates to insects produce spontaneous muscular contractions followed by paralysis. The binding of organophosphates to acetylcholinesterase is more persistent, if not permanent, whereas the interaction with carbamates is reversible. These compounds were once very popular for their prolonged action and potency. However, the use of organophosphates has declined because their low margin of safety and slight variance from approved use or continued use may lead to toxicity. When these compounds are used for flea or tick control, it should be determined before treatment whether any other cholinesterase inhibitor has been used on the animal or in its environment. Organophosphates for small animal therapy include chlorpyrifos, dichlorvos, malathion, diazinon, phosmet, fenthion, chlorfenvinphos, and cythioate. Carbamates include carbaryl and propoxur.

Chlorinated Hydrocarbons: These compounds are becoming less popular because of their persistence in the environment, although this factor brought the benefit of prolonged action. Lindane and methoxychlor are still occasionally used. (*See also* CHLORINATED HYDROCARBON COMPOUNDS, p 3060.)

Neonicotinoids: The neonicotinoids are a class of insecticides referred to as nitroquanidines, neonicotinyls, chloronicotines, and recently as chloronicotinyls. The neonicotinoids are modeled after natural nicotine. Three compounds in this category are currently available for veterinary use: dinotefuran, imidacloprid, and nitenpyram.

All neonicotinoids act as agonists on the postsynaptic acetylcholine receptors in insects. This inhibits cholinergic transmission, resulting in paralysis and death. Imidacloprid is applied as a spot-on topical product and is used primarily to control fleas on both dogs and cats. It also has excellent activity against lice. Although it has potent residual activity, it is readily soluble in water, so swimming and repeated bathing may compromise its duration of activity. Nitenpyram is administered PO in pill form to kill fleas in both dogs and cats. It is absorbed rapidly, with maximal blood concentrations reached within 1.2 hr in dogs and 0.6 hr in cats. Fleas begin to die within 20–30 min of administration, with 100% flea mortality within 3–4 hr. The compound is rapidly eliminated, with >90% excreted in the urine within 24–48 hr, primarily as unchanged nitenpyram. Even though imidacloprid and nitenpyram are classified similarly, their mechanisms of action appear to be different. Although imidacloprid is described as a paralytic, nitenpyram produces hyperexcitability in fleas before death.

The newest addition to the neonicotinoids is dinotefuran, considered a third-generation neonicotinoid. The structure of dinotefuran is unique in that it was derived from that of the acetylcholine molecule rather than nicotine. It has been proposed that dinotefuran does not bind to the same sites as imidacloprid and other neonicotinoids but at a different site in the nerve synapse. Dinotefuran is applied as a topical spot-on with different formulations for dogs and cats. The cat formulation is combined with the insect growth regulator pyriproxyfen and is used primarily to control fleas. The dog formulation contains pyriproxyfen and permethrin and is labeled for control of fleas, ticks, and mosquitoes.

Formamidines: This small group of acaricidal compounds has the proposed mode of action of binding to octopamine receptors, a specific group of receptors found in Acari. In veterinary medicine, the only approved formamidine is amitraz. It is used primarily as an acaricide to control ticks and mites. It is available as a dip for control of canine demodicosis, and it will also control scabies. An amitraz-impregnated collar is also marketed for control of ticks on dogs. Amitraz is not approved for use on cats.

Oxadiazines: Oxadiazine insecticides can control a broad spectrum of insects and were originally developed for use against a variety of insects infesting vegetables, fruit, and row crops. Indoxacarb is the only member of this group currently being used in veterinary medicine. It is considered a pro-insecticide that is metabolized within the insect to a more active form, which is an N-decarbomethoxylated metabolite that is at least 40 times more potent than parent indoxacarb. This metabolic conversion of indoxacarb, known as bioactivation, is attributed to actions of esterase and amidase enzymes within the insect. The active metabolite exerts its effect by blocking the voltage-gated sodium ion channels in insects. Indoxacarb is administered topically in a spot-on formulation for control of fleas on dogs and cats. Indoxacarb has also been combined with permethrin for control of ticks on dogs.

Isoxazolines: Isoxazolines are a new class of compounds that have both potent insecticidal and acaricidal activities. Isoxazolines have a novel mode of action and specifically block arthropod ligand-gated chloride channels. Afoxolaner and fluralaner are currently the only two compounds approved for use in veterinary medicine. Both are unique in that they were the first oral flea and tick products. The compounds are readily absorbed after oral administration and provide 4–12 wk of insecticide and acaricide activity.

Insect Growth Regulators: These compounds inhibit the development of immature stages of insects. They are generally classified as either juvenile hormone mimics (insect growth regulators) or as chitin synthesis inhibitors (insect development inhibitors). Methoprene, fenoxycarb, and pyriproxyfen are similar in structure to insect juvenile hormone and are classified as juvenile hormone mimics. When these compounds are applied to flea larvae or into their environment, they are absorbed by the larvae and act like natural insect juvenile hormone. Juvenile hormone analogues bind to juvenile hormone receptor sites; larvae are prevented from completing metamorphosis and subsequently die. These compounds also have ovicidal and embryocidal activity against flea eggs when applied topically to dogs and cats. Female fleas in the hair coat absorb the juvenile hormone analogue, which affects viability of developing eggs. These compounds are active against a wide range of insects, including mosquito larvae; methoprene is used as a larvicide in the strategic control of mosquito-borne diseases. For flea control, their outdoor use should be limited to specific flea habitats to avoid adverse effects on beneficial insect species.

Lufenuron, a benzoylphenyl urea, inhibits the formation of chitin (a polymer of *N*-acetyl glucosamine), which is a major component of insect exoskeletons. During each larval molt, chitin is reformed by polymerization. Lufenuron interferes with polymerization and deposition of chitin, killing developing larvae either within the egg or after hatching. Lufenuron is administered PO to dogs or cats or by injection to cats. Female fleas feeding on treated animals are prevented from producing viable eggs or larvae. Other insect development inhibitors, such as diflubenzuron (another chiton inhibitor) and cyromazine (a moulting disruptor), also have considerable activity against developing fleas. Insect growth regulators and insect development inhibitors affect many insect species that undergo complete metamorphosis, but they have little or no activity against ticks or other Acari, which undergo incomplete metamorphosis.

Phenylpyrazoles: This group of compounds has broad-spectrum activity that is both insecticidal and acaricidal. The members of this group currently available for use in veterinary medicine worldwide include fipronil and pyriprole. These compounds bind to γ-aminobutyric acid and glutamate-gated receptor sites of insect nervous systems, inhibiting the flux of Cl^- into nerve cells, which results in hyperexcitability. These compounds have broad-spectrum activity against fleas, ticks, mites, and lice. Numerous fipronil-containing formulations are available worldwide, including an alcohol-based fipronil-only spray, several spot-on formulations that contain only fipronil, a spot-on combination with the insect growth regulator methoprene, and numerous combination formulations that contain fipronil and various pyrethroids. Fipronil is very lipophilic; it accumulates in the sebaceous glands, has very low solubility in water, and has prolonged residual activity on both dogs and cats.

Pyrethrins and Pyrethroids: These compounds rapidly disrupt sodium and potassium ion transport in nerve membranes, resulting in spontaneous depolarizations, augmented neurotransmitter secretion, and neuromuscular blockade, causing paralysis. Although the activity is rapid, without sufficient exposure paralyzed insects can also recover rapidly. The synergists piperonyl butoxide and *N*-octyl bicycloheptene dicarboxymide interfere with the insect detoxification mechanism and can potentiate the activity of pyrethroids. Natural pyrethrum is extracted from chrysanthemum flowers and is notable for its rapid but brief action and relative lack of toxicity in dogs and cats.

Synthetic pyrethroids are pyrethrum-like compounds that generally have greater potency and residual effects but are less well tolerated in cats. Some pyrethroids, such as permethrin, can be highly toxic to cats. Pyrethroids are generally classified by developmental generation. First-generation pyrethroids are generally unstable in heat and sunlight (eg, allethrin); second-generation are more photostable, isomeric mixtures (eg, cypermethrin, permethrin); third-generation are photostable and more neurologically active isomers obtained by isomeric enrichment (eg, λ-cyhalothrin, β-cyfluthrin); and fourth-generation are nonester pyrethroids (eg, MTI 800, flufenprox, etofenprox).

Spinosyns: Spinosyns are a novel family of insecticides derived from the fermentation of the actinomycete, *Saccharopolyspora spinosa*. The two most abundant products derived from the fermentation process are spinosyns A and D, which are the major active components of spinosad. Spinosad is used to control a wide variety of insects, including flies and fleas. Spinosyns have a novel mode of action, primarily targeting binding sites on nicotinic acetylcholine receptors distinct from other insecticides such as neonicotinoids. Spinosyns also affect γ-aminobutyric acid receptor function, which may contribute further to their insecticidal activity. These actions cause excitation of the insect nervous system, leading to involuntary muscle contractions, prostration with tremors, and finally paralysis. Spinosad has activity against fleas and is formulated as a chewable tablet for dogs and cats. A topical spot-on spinosyn formulation called spinetoram has been developed for cats.

Repellents: N,N-diethyl-3-methylbenzamide (DEET, previously called N,N-diethyl-meta-toluamide) remains the most effective among currently available insect repellents for people. It is a broad-spectrum repellent effective against mosquitoes, biting flies, chiggers, fleas, and ticks.

However, the effectiveness of DEET formulations for dogs and cats has not been proved, and safety is a concern because concentrated formulations containing DEET have caused weakness, paralysis, liver disease, and seizures in pets. DEET should not be administered to dogs or cats.

The synthetic pyrethroid permethrin is a rapidly acting neurotoxicant that can produce what is termed a "hot-foot" effect and is often described as a repellency. Various permethrin formulations are labeled as repellents for ticks, mosquitoes, and fleas.

Synergists: Synergists are generally not considered toxic or insecticidal but are used with insecticides to enhance their activity. They are used primarily to potentiate the activity of pyrethrum or pyrethroids. Synergists inhibit cytochrome P450–dependent monooxygenases or glutathione S-transferases, enzymes produced by microsomes in insect tissues. They bind the oxidative enzymes that would normally break down the insecticide and prevent them from degrading the toxicant. Piperonyl butoxide and N-octyl bicycloheptene dicarboxamide are common synergists.

Target Parasite Efficacy

Because of specific formulation and drug delivery technology, certain insecticides are used in a wide variety of ectoparasite control products. Efficacy of specific compounds can vary against target species, and resistance to insecticides may develop in specific locations, especially with incorrect, prolonged, or repeated use. It cannot be assumed that ticks and fleas are controlled by the same active compounds; product labels should be carefully read. Products that contain compounds specifically active against the target parasite should be chosen, whether the concern is fleas, ticks, mites, or a combination of these parasites.

Duration of activity (ie, "knockdown" or sustained effects) can be the primary concern in product choices. Products should be evaluated based on both their immediate and residual speed of kill. A rapid residual speed of kill is critically important when attempting to manage flea allergy dermatitis and to reduce the chances of a tick transmitting a pathogen.

Modern parasiticides available for flea and tick control in companion animals provide superior parasite control, but an understanding of the life cycle of the parasites, along with the mode of action of the particular molecules, is also important. Often, perceived product failures are a result of massive reinfestation from the environment, incorrect product use, or unrealistic expectations.

Safety

Although LD_{50} data concerning the safety or toxicity of an insecticidal product is often helpful, LD_{50} values are not always the best indicator of the safety of specific insecticide formulations applied to pets or premises. Consideration must be given to the concentration of product (mg/mL), application rate (mg or g/m^2 for environmental products, and mcg or mg/kg for topicals), route of exposure (dermal or oral), total dose, and the species exposed. The actual risk of exposure during treatment, after treatment, or after accidental ingestion can be assessed only after evaluation of these criteria.

Because animal toxicity can be modified by formulation technology, active ingredients are not the sole guide to safety assessment of a product. Most commercially available products have undergone adequate safety evaluation for regulatory approval; the label noting such approval remains the best source of information. Cats are sensitive to many insecticides, and use of these insecticides on or near cats must be done with caution. Human and environmental safety also should be considered, especially when treating premises (eg, some compounds may break down into more toxic components; older products on the shelf might have been withdrawn because of safety concerns). Generalizations should not be made, because formulations generally safe for grass application may induce skin reactions, or even fatal reactions, in sensitive individuals and certain breeds of dogs and cats.

Delivery Systems

Consumer convenience is an important factor in product choice, especially for flea and tick control. An array of delivery systems has historically been available: powders, aerosols, sprays, shampoos, rinses, dips, spot-ons, mousses, injectables, oral tablets or liquids, and impregnated collars. However, the safety, efficacy, and ease of use of the newer spot-on and oral application systems have rendered many of the older application technologies essentially obsolete.

GROWTH PROMOTANTS AND PRODUCTION ENHANCERS

Achieving increased efficiency of conversion of feed into human food products of high quality, without posing any significant risk to the consumer, is an important goal of livestock producers worldwide. The physiologic mechanisms involved in converting feed into muscle, fat, and bone by animals are increasingly being elucidated. Recently, consumer concerns about additives for food production have focused on animal safety, organoleptic quality, and the potential human health hazards of the food we eat.

A number of approaches may be taken to improve conversion of animal feed into meat; two of the more practical approaches are hormonal treatments and antimicrobial feed additives. The hormonal approach includes administration of anabolic steroid hormones, use of growth hormone (GH) or insulin-like growth factor (IGF-1) to augment endogenous GH levels, and use of β-adrenergic agonists (βAAs) to preferentially increase nutrient partitioning to muscle (*see* TABLE 60). The antimicrobial feed additives approach includes feeding of antibiotics to decrease populations of pathologic bacteria in host GI tracts, use of compounds to manipulate ruminal fermentation by changing the ruminal microflora population in healthy animals, and use of probiotics to promote beneficial microflora in the GI tract.

The use of hormonal treatments and antimicrobial feed additives in production animals is currently under debate in many areas and is banned in some because of concerns surrounding their possible effects on people.

The EU has banned beef produced using growth-promotant implants since 1981. Despite subsequent findings by the European Economic Community's own panel of scientific experts, referred to as the "Lamming Committee," by the World Trade Organization, and by the international Codex Alimentarius Commission indicating that appropriate use of approved growth-promoting hormones poses no human health risk to consumers, the EU has continued its ban.

More recently, use of βAAs for growth promotion in swine and beef production has come under scrutiny in the international meat trade community. Some countries, including the EU, Russia, and China, have placed a total ban on beef and pork from nations that allow the use of βAAs, whereas other countries have adopted the maximum residue limits (MRLs) for the compounds as established by the Codex Alimentarius Commission. The FDA applies a greater MRL in the USA than the Codex standard.

The use of antimicrobial compounds specifically for growth-promotion purposes, as opposed to their use for control or treatment of bacterial infection, has also come under increased attention internationally because of rising concerns over antimicrobial resistance by pathogenic bacteria of concern in human medicine. Direct cause-effect evidence of antimicrobial use in livestock leading to bacterial resistance in human medicine is virtually nonexistent, requiring more complicated epidemiologic study. However, numerous studies have linked use of specific drugs in livestock, either for disease therapy or for growth-promotion purposes, to increased prevalence of drug resistance in target bacterial species. Results of these investigations are equivocal and have been the focal point of intense scrutiny and debate. In the absence of resoundingly clear cause-and-effect data, and because preservation of the continued efficacy of existing antimicrobial compounds is paramount, the cautionary principle has prevailed and will likely lead to greater restrictions on the use of antimicrobials for growth promotion in livestock and for therapeutic purposes as well.

STEROID HORMONES

In general, the principle that dictates which type of hormone to be used is the need to supplement or replace the particular hormone type that is deficient in the animals to be treated. Females produce estrogens normally, so better results are obtained from the administration of androgens, eg, trenbolone acetate (TBA). Estrogens should not be used in animals to be retained for breeding purposes.

Manufacturers' instructions must be followed to ensure proper implant placement and dose administration. Anabolic hormones should not be administered by IM injection for growth-promoting purposes. Additionally, steroid hormones must not be used for anabolic or other purposes unless the indication is specifically approved by the appropriate regulatory body. The EU has banned the use of hormonal growth promoters in meat production. Appropriate surveillance programs have been established to ensure compliance by producers.

Endogenous Steroids

The steroidal compounds used for anabolic purposes in food animals are estradiol, progesterone, and testosterone. Gender and maturity of an animal influence its growth rate and body composition. Bulls grow 8%–12% faster than steers, have better feed efficiencies, and produce leaner carcasses. Superior performance of bulls is due to the steroids produced in the testes (mainly testosterone but also estradiol, which in ruminants is also anabolic and is produced in relatively large quantities). Testosterone, or one of its physiologically active metabolites, binds to receptors in muscle and stimulates increased incorporation of amino acids into protein, thereby increasing muscle mass without a concomitant increase in adipose tissue. Estradiol, on the other hand, may act by stimulation of the somatotropic axis to increase growth hormone and thus IGF-1 production and

TABLE 60 NATURAL STEROID HORMONES FOR CONSIDERATION AS GROWTH PROMOTERS

Hormone	Form[a]	Dosage	Duration of Effect (days)	Growth Response	Potential Adverse Effects
Estradiol	1 - Pellet	20 mg EB[b] + 200 mg P4[c] (steers)	100–120	10%–15%	Transient increase in sexual behavior
	2 - Pellet	20 mg EB + 200 mg testosterone propionate (heifers, cull cows)	100–120	5%–15%	Udder development
	3 - Pellet	10 mg EB + 100 mg P4 (veal calves)	100–120	0–8%	
	4 - Silastic rubber	45 mg estradiol (steers)	365	10%–15%	Transient increase in sexual behavior
	5 - Silastic rubber	24 mg estradiol (steers)	200	10%–15%	Transient increase in sexual behavior
	6 - Polylactic acid	28 mg estradiol (steers)	365	10%–15%	Transient increase in sexual behavior
Progesterone	*See* 1 and 3 above				
Testosterone	*See* 2 above				

[a] Implants must be placed SC between the ear cartilage and skin to comply with label instructions so that consumption of residues may be avoided.

[b] Estradiol benzoate

[c] Progesterone

availability by modulation of the IGF binding proteins. Naturally produced endogenous steroids are not orally active, require picogram concentrations of estradiol and nanogram concentrations of testosterone in blood for physiologic effects, and can transiently affect the behavior of treated animals (*see* TABLE 60).

Estradiol: A potent anabolic agent in ruminants at blood concentrations of 5–100 pg/mL, estradiol is administered as an ear implant, either as compressed tablets or silastic rubber implants. When estradiol is formulated as compressed tablets, a second steroid (usually testosterone, TBA, or progesterone) is typically present when administered to feedlot cattle fed a high-energy diet, in a ratio of ~1 part estradiol to either 5 or 10 parts of the other, androgenic, steroid. The release of hormones from compressed pellets is biphasic, with a relatively rapid rate lasting 2–7 days after insertion (50–100 times greater than baseline), followed by a slower rate of release for the next 30–100 days (5–10 times greater than baseline). Hormone concentrations gradually decline up to day 80–100, when concentrations are no different from those in control animals.

Estradiol formulated in silastic rubber enhances the effective life span of the implant relative to pelleted formulations. The pattern of release includes a short-lived spike in plasma estrogen concentration for 2–5 days after insertion, followed by a stable but modest increase (5–10 times greater than baseline). Toward the end of the effective life span of the implant, there is a gradual decline to estradial concentrations found in control animals.

Estradiol, on its own, increases nitrogen retention, growth rate by 10%–20% in steers, lean meat content by 1%–3%, and feed efficiency by 5%–8%. It can be used in steers to best advantage, but it also has anabolic effects in heifers and veal calves. It works best in lambs in conjunction with androgens. It is not effective as an anabolic agent in pigs.

Testosterone: A potent anabolic agent at the relatively high concentrations of 1–5 ng/mL in peripheral circulation, testosterone is not used on its own as an anabolic agent in farm animals, because it is very difficult to achieve the effective physiologic concentrations for long periods (up to 100 days) with current delivery systems. It is generally used as a propionate formulation in conjunction with 20 mg estradiol benzoate (EB) in a compressed tablet implant; its major role in the compressed pellet may be to slow down the release rate of estradiol. In high concentrations in blood, testosterone induces male sexual behavior (eg, aggression and mounting), but this is not seen with the concentrations delivered by compressed pellets in the ear (1 ng/mL). Behavior resulting from use of 20 mg EB and 200 mg progesterone is not different from that seen after the use of 20 mg EB and 200 mg testosterone propionate.

Progesterone: Unambiguous data suggesting progesterone is anabolic in farm animals does not exist. Its major use is to slow the release of estradiol from compressed pellet implants.

Synthetic Steroids

Synthetic steroids are commercially available in some countries because of their efficacy, their relatively mild androgenicity, and because they cause few behavioral anomalies (*see* TABLE 61). Commercial synthetic steroids are androgenic (TBA) or progestogenic (melengestrol acetate [MGA]).

Synthetic steroidal androgens are not commonly used as anabolic agents except for TBA. TBA is currently the only synthetic androgen approved for use for growth promotion in cattle; it is used to a lesser extent in sheep and not in pigs or horses. It has weak androgenic activity but has greater anabolic activity than testosterone. When administered repeatedly during the feedlot phase when cattle are fed a high-energy diet, TBA can alter the physical appearance and behavior of steers, causing them to look and act like bulls. TBA has significant anabolic effects on its own in female cattle and sheep, but in castrated males it gives maximal response when used in conjunction with estrogens. It is administered as a pellet-type implant containing 140–200 mg TBA for heifers and cull cows, and it can be used with estradiol in doses ranging from 140–200 mg TBA as either combined or separate implants.

MGA is an orally active synthetic progestagen. It is fed at dosages of 0.25–0.5 mg/day per heifer in the feed. It suppresses recurrent estrus in feedlot heifers and increases growth rate and feed efficiency (*see* TABLE 61). It is not effective in pregnant or spayed heifers or in steers. Its mode of action is to suppress ovulation, presumably by suppressing luteinizing hormone (LH) pulse frequency; however, large follicles develop, which can increase concentrations of estradiol and growth hormone, and hence growth. MGA is permitted for use in the

TABLE 61 SYNTHETIC STEROID HORMONES FOR CONSIDERATION AS GROWTH PROMOTERS

Hormone[a]	Dosage	Duration of Effect (days)	Growth Response	Potential Adverse Effects
TBA	200 mg (heifers, cull cows)	60–90	5%–12%	
TBA + EB	200 mg TBA + 28 mg EB (steers, heifers)	90–120	10%–20%	Transient increase in sexual behavior
	100 mg TBA + 14 mg EB (steers)	90–120	10%–20%	Transient increase in sexual behavior
TBA + E	200 mg TBA + 20 mg E (steers, heifers)	90–120		
	120 mg TBA + 24 mg E (steers)	90–120		
	140 mg TBA + 14 mg E (heifers)	90–120		
	80 mg TBA + 16 mg E (steers)	90–120		
	80 mg TBA + 8 mg E (heifers)	90–120		
	40 mg TBA + 8 mg E (steers and heifers grazing pasture)	90–120		
TBA + E	200 mg TBA + 40 mg E (steers)	200		
Zeranol	36 mg zeranol	90–120	10%–15%	
	12 mg zeranol	90–120	10%–15%	
MGA	0.25–0.5 mg/day, PO	As long as it is given	3%–10%	Increased mammary development after longterm administration

[a] TBA = trenbolone acetate; EB = estradiol benzoate; E = estradiol 17β; MGA = melengestrol acetate

Note: All administered as pellet implants except MGA, which is administered in feed.

USA but not in the EU. When used in the absence of a growth-promoting implant, MGA increases growth rate through the increased estradiol released by the follicles; however, when used in conjunction with either estradiol or combination estradiol/TBA implants in the feedlot, the growth-promoting benefits of MGA are primarily derived from suppression of the excess, unproductive, and potentially harmful activities associated with recurrent estrus.

Synthetic Nonsteroidal Estrogens

Two major classes of synthetic nonsteroidal estrogens have been used as production enhancers in food animals. **Stilbene estrogens** (either diethylstilbestrol [DES] or hexestrol) have been banned in most countries as anabolic agents because of residue and food safety concerns.

The discovery of a naturally occurring estrogen, zearalenone (produced by the fungi *Fusarium* spp), led to the development of the synthetic analogue zeranol. **Zeranol** is estrogenic and has a weak affinity for the uterine estradiol receptor. It is used in animal production as a SC ear implant at a dose of 36 mg for cattle and 12 mg for sheep, with a duration of activity of 90–120 days. In steers, zeranol increases nitrogen retention, growth rate by 12%–15%, and feed conversion by 6%–10%. However, lower responses are seen in heifers. Its effects are additive to those of androgens (generally TBA).

Use in Cattle

Calves have a high conversion of feed into animal tissue compared with young growing swine or poultry. Therefore, their responses to anabolic agents are variable. Responses of 0–10% have been obtained when zeranol was given to 3-mo-old castrated male calves. Bull calves in an intensive bull beef system can be given an estrogen implant at 1–2 mo of age to suppress testicular development, which may lead to subsequent reduction in mounting and aggression. A growth response of ~5%–8% is also obtained from this implant. Reimplantation every 80–100 days is necessary if compressed pellet implants are used.

A major limitation to the use of anabolic agents in lightweight weaned calves is the low liveweight gain they may achieve because of poor nutritional status. Hence, anabolic agents should be considered only if the weanlings are expected to gain >0.25 kg/day. Zeranol, estradiol, and TBA can be used in male castrates. Dairy heifer replacements cannot be given steroid implants as weanlings.

Greater and more consistent responses are obtained in yearling and older cattle than in calves or weanlings, due primarily to greater intake and to the higher plane of nutrition. In the case of pellet-type implants with effectiveness of 90–120 days, consideration can be given to reimplanting cattle midway through the grazing season, provided gains >0.5 kg/day are maintained. Silastic implants of estradiol are effective for 200–400 days, depending on dose used. Daily gains in feedlot cattle fed a high-energy diet may be increased 20%–30% after implantation with an estrogen and an androgen; daily gain in pasture cattle is typically improved by 10%–15%.

Responses to growth promotion are good when animals are on a high plane of nutrition. Feed conversion efficiency is improved, and lean meat content of the carcass is generally increased. Although less clear, conformation of implanted cattle tends to improve. Negative impacts of implants on marbling content of the loin muscle can be minimized by finishing cattle to a fat-constant endpoint.

In steers and heifers in the feedlot and provided a high-energy diet, use of an androgen plus an estrogen hormone combination is common. Pellet-type implants are effective for as long as 150 days; reimplanting cattle after 70–100 days should be considered because of decreasing response from the pellet-type implants over time.

Results from large-pen studies (>25 animals/pen) show that heifers benefit from a combination of estradiol, TBA, and MGA. In small-pen research, however, when fed in combination with growth-promoting implants, MGA use results in reduced gain, feed efficiency, and ribeye area, as well as increased fatness. These contrary findings suggest that although progesterone may have an "anti-growth promoting" effect, the growth-promotion benefit realized from suppression of estrus overcomes the minor negative physiologic impact of progesterone in conventional large feedlot pens.

In some studies in which bulls were treated with estrogens, growth rate increased by 2%–10%, and testicular growth was suppressed with a subsequent reduction in mounting and aggression. This should make the bulls easier to manage on the farm and less subject to "dark cutting" after slaughter. The mechanism involved appears to be the reduction of the gonadotropic hormones LH and follicle-stimulating hormone (FSH) from the pituitary gland by estrogen, which has a strong negative feedback effect on LH and FSH secretion. This reduction in LH and FSH results in decreased testicular size and lower testosterone levels, with a consequent reduction in aggressive behavior. However, there appears to be sufficient testosterone secreted to maintain an anabolic effect. Therefore, the repeated use of estrogens in bulls beginning at 1–3 mo of age may lead to a hormonal castration effect with increased growth rate.

Use in Horses

The use of anabolic agents in horses is not recommended because of adverse effects on the reproductive system. Administration of a steroid hormonal androgen analogue decreases testicular size in stallions. Decreased hormonal concentrations, especially LH, testosterone, and inhibin, adversely affect testicular histology and spermatogenesis and transiently decrease sperm output and quality. One of the most commonly used compounds is 19-nortestosterone for therapy in debilitated and anemic horses. However, use of these compounds is contraindicated, and longterm treatment or large doses have serious adverse effects on reproductive tract function.

Use in Other Species

In **pigs**, the growth responses from the use of estradiol, progesterone, and zeranol are variable but generally low. TBA seems to increase lean meat content of pig carcasses.

In **sheep**, the responses to anabolic agents parallel those obtained in cattle. The most consistent responses have been obtained in lambs finished on high-concentrate diets; a 10%–15% increase in daily gain can be expected. Anabolic steroids should not be used in lambs to be retained for breeding. Also, implantation with zeranol reduces testicular development in ram lambs and delays the onset of puberty and reduces the ovulation rate in female sheep. Moreover, the short finishing period and the extensive nature of some production systems militate against widespread practical use of growth promotants in sheep on economic grounds.

In **poultry**, responses to estrogens include increased fat deposition. Androgens, however, have given conflicting responses. Hence, their use is of no practical significance at this time.

In **fish**, methyl testosterone can induce sex reversal in rainbow trout, thereby promoting growth and improved feed conversion efficiency.

Possible Complications

Any hormonal implant has a negative feedback effect on pituitary gonadotropins, thereby reducing LH and FSH secretion. Therefore, they can affect the onset of puberty and the regularity of estrous cycles, as well as reduce conception rate in females and testicular development (and thus sperm output) in males. Hormonal growth promotants should never be used in animals that are or may be used for breeding purposes, nor should they be used before puberty to increase growth in yearling thoroughbreds or young pedigree bulls for show purposes. If given to pregnant heifers, TBA results in increased incidence of severe dystocia, masculinization of female genitalia of the fetus, increased calf mortality, and reduced milk yield in the subsequent lactation.

The major problem thought to be associated with estrogenic implant use in the feedyard has been a transient increase in mounting behavior and aggression, commonly referred to as buller syndrome (*see* p 1552). However, it is also believed that the estrogen in the implant alone is not sufficient to cause bullers. The "buller" is the animal being pursued by one or more pen mates that repeatedly attempt to mount the buller throughout the day and several days. Buller syndrome generally affects 2%–3% of the feedyard steer population, but this rate can double or triple during the late summer and early fall months. An increase in yearling steers off native grass pasture (which are usually given a high-dose implant immediately on arrival), diurnal temperature fluctuations (hot days and cool nights that shift social activity to early evening hours), dusty pen conditions (exacerbated by evening social activity), feeding corn or hay that may be moldy, and incomplete fermentation on freshly harvested silage can also contribute to increases in buller syndrome. Feedlot pens with a greater number of animals experience a greater incidence of buller activity, and the incidence of bullers increases linearly with increasing number of animals within a pen above 80–100 animals per pen. This suggests the agonistic behavior is a population phenomenon, requiring a critical mass of both the dominant, mounting animals and the animals they are attempting to mount. Bullers have been shown to have greater circulating concentrations of monoamine oxidase and reduced circulating concentrations of progesterone than non-buller pen mates. These effects generally last for 1–10 days after implantation and then subside. However, there have been a few reports of undesirable behavior in steers that lasted for 4–10 wk. The cause of this unpredictable adverse behavior is not clear; it may be a function of rearing and socialization climate. It is generally more severe in dairy cattle used for beef production. If the problem is severe, the buller steers should be identified and removed; if very severe, removal of the implants or administration of 50–100 mg of progesterone in oil for a number of days to suppress behavior should be considered.

In addition to buller syndrome, estrogenic implants may increase the size of rudimentary teats.

Factors Affecting Response

A number of factors affect the response to growth-promoting implants, including genetic makeup, plane of nutrition, and the sex and age of the animal.

Animals should be gaining a minimum of 0.25 kg/day before an economic response is obtained. Implants are best used in animals on a high plane of nutrition and under good husbandry conditions. They are an aid to, but not a substitute for, good husbandry. Consequently, there is little economic incentive in implanting cattle destined for a 3- to 4-mo "store period," during which time animals are fed to gain little or no weight. Responses are reduced in calves (based on health condition and diet), and responses are good in yearlings.

Prior implantation does not affect the response to the next implantation. Also, once the implant effect has ceased, the rate of gain reverts to the rate that would be expected in nonimplanted animals, assuming the level of feeding is the same. Also, extra weight induced by implants in early life is transferred through to extra carcass weight at slaughter.

GROWTH HORMONE

The peptide most commonly used to enhance growth and production is growth hormone (GH). Its chemical structure is species-specific, and it has a short half-life (20–30 min). It is not orally active and is rapidly digested and cleared by the gut, liver, and kidney; thus, it must be administered via a parenteral route. Sustained-release (14–28 days) formulations have been developed for use in cattle to obviate the need for daily injections. When administered to cattle, GH increases growth rate (5%–10%), feed conversion efficiency, and the carcass lean:fat ratio. Gender has little effect on response in cattle. Response to GH is lower in older cattle with greater fat deposition. There is an interaction between magnitude of response and nutritional level; protein content and specific amino acid composition may be important to achieve maximal responses. The effects of GH are largely additive to those obtained from steroid implants. GH improves growth and feed efficiency in sheep but not in poultry. Recombinant GH in pigs has dramatic effects, resulting in an increase in daily gain (20%), decrease in feed intake (5%), and a decrease in the feed:gain ratio (20%). A 10% increase in lean content and a 35% decrease in adipose tissue may be realized in swine. Administration of bovine GH at 25 mg/day to lactating cattle increases milk yields of dairy cows by as much as 20%. GH has been approved for commercial use in some countries to increase milk production.

β-ADRENERGIC AGONISTS

As of 2015, there are two β-adrenergic agonists (βAAs) approved for use as growth promotants in feedlot cattle in the USA: ractopamine and zilpaterol. Phenethanolamine βAAs are chemically similar in structure to epinephrine and norepinephrine and have paracrine, neurotransmitter, and endocrine (hormonal) effects. There is a range of βAA compounds resulting from structural modifications and aromatic ring substitution. The βAAs bind to β-adrenergic receptors, which have been classified into β1, β2, and β3 subtypes based on the physiologic response obtained. β1 receptors are located primarily in cardiac muscle but also can be found in skeletal muscle, β2 receptors in tracheal and skeletal muscle, and β3 receptors in brown adipose tissue. In general, βAAs have specificity for receptor subtypes, thereby providing specificity regarding their physiologic actions. However, there are multiple receptor subclasses in most tissues, and the relative concentrations of β1 and β2 receptors in a tissue determine the physiologic response. Muscle and adipose cells have predominantly β2 receptors. βAA use leads to an increase in muscle mass caused by upregulation of mRNA transcription, resulting in increased protein synthesis, and a decrease in carcass fat due to decreased rates of lipid accretion. The exact proportion of receptor subtypes varies between tissues and also across species, resulting in species-specific responses to select βAAs. For example, swine are believed to have more β1 than β2 receptors in their skeletal muscle; ruminants are believed to have more β2 than β1 receptors. The physiologic activity of βAAs depends on the dose, receptor binding specificity, mode of administration, rate of absorption, and metabolic clearance rate in treated animals. Also, because tissue becomes refractory to exogenous βAA administration, βAAs are fed only during the final days of the finishing phase; extended feeding ultimately results in a complete loss of tissue response to βAAs.

The major use of βAAs in food animal production is to increase carcass leanness and lean tissue produced per animal. In cattle and sheep, weight gain, gain:feed ratio, and meat content are increased by 10%–20% and lipid content is decreased by 7%–20%. In swine and chickens, responses are much lower, with pigs responding better than chickens. Weight gain is increased by 2%–4%, and gain:feed ratio is slightly improved in chickens but not in pigs. Meat content is increased by 2%–4% and lipid content decreased by 7%–8% in chickens and pigs.

Adverse effects depend on compound administered, dose used, and species treated, but those selected for commercial use have minimal adverse effects. They are orally active. Dosage level of the compound used affects the response obtained; the optimal dose often varies for different production variables measured. The most consistent effects are increased proportion of lean meat, but the effects on meat quality vary with compound used, dosage given, duration of treatment, and species treated. Certain compounds have been reported to decrease tenderness of meat in cattle. The use of β-agonists as growth promoters is banned in the EU. Illegal use of clenbuterol in cattle and certain βAAs in poultry is a threat in some countries, requiring vigilance by regulatory authorities. The longterm accumulation of these compounds in hair and ocular tissue has been used to screen for their presence in some countries.

ANTIMICROBIAL FEED ADDITIVES

Maintenance of healthy animals requires prevention of infection by pathogenic organisms. In addition, specific alteration of a host's microflora may have beneficial effects on animal production by alteration of ruminal flora, resulting in changes in the proportions of volatile fatty acids produced during ruminal digestion. Thus, antimicrobial compounds may improve production efficiency of healthy animals fed optimal nutritional regimens. Production-enhancing antimicrobial compounds can be classified as ionophore or nonionophore antibiotics. This distinction is important, because ionophores have no use in human medicine and do not have any link or possible effect on antimicrobial resistance to therapeutic antibiotics in either people or food animals; to group all antimicrobials together for debate about the risk to therapeutic antibiotics is ill advised and overly simplistic. Antimicrobial compounds are administered in the feed at low dose rates relative to high doses required for therapeutic effects. Feed additives can be given once the rumen is functioning, although some antibiotic compounds can be fed to calves before this point.

Antimicrobial growth promotants commonly used in livestock are detailed in TABLE 62. Antimicrobials are used in male and female animals without adverse effects on ovarian and testicular development or function because they are poorly absorbed. Unlike anabolic steroids, they do not affect carcass composition. Antimicrobials are commonly used in conjunction with estradiol, zeranol, or TBA, and generally their combined effects are additive.

Ionophore Antibiotics

Ionophores (eg, monensin and lasalocid) modify the movement of monovalent (sodium and potassium) and divalent (calcium) ions across biologic membranes, modify the rumen microflora, decrease acetate and methane production, increase propionate, may improve nitrogen utilization, and can increase dry matter digestibility in ruminants. Their main effect is to increase feed efficiency, but they may also improve growth rates of ruminants on high-roughage diets. Administration of monensin to cattle results in 2%–10% improvement in liveweight gain (in animals on a high-roughage diet), 3%–7% increase in

TABLE 62 ANTIBACTERIAL GROWTH PROMOTERS FOR POTENTIAL USE IN LIVESTOCK PRODUCTION

Compound	Class	Absorption	Effects
Bambermycins	Phosphoglycolipid	Not absorbed	Increase FCE[a], growth promotion in poultry, cattle
Lasalocid sodium	Ionophore		Increase FCE in cattle
Monensin sodium	Ionophore	Poorly absorbed	Increase FCE, increase DLWG[b] in cattle and lambs
Salinomycin	Ionophore		Increase DLWG and FCE
Virginiamycin	Peptide	Not absorbed	Growth promotion in poultry
Zinc bacitracin	Peptide	Not absorbed	Growth promotion in poultry

[a] Feed conversion efficiency

[b] Daily liveweight gain

feed conversion efficiency, and up to a 6% decrease in food consumption. Initially, monensin was used only as a feed additive for ruminants fed in confinement, but its use has been extended to grazing animals. Other ionophores generally have similar effects. Doses range from 6–40 ppm in the diet. Ionophores are absorbed from the gut, rapidly metabolized by the liver, and reenter the gut from bile. Some ionophores also have a therapeutic use (eg, for prevention of coccidiosis in ruminants and poultry).

Although ionophore antibiotics are used for prevention of coccidiosis in ruminants and poultry, ionophores are not used in human medicine, and there are no medically important analogues of the ionophores used in human medicine. Therefore, there is no obvious relationship between ionophore use in livestock production and the concern regarding resistance of bacterial pathogens to antimicrobial compounds important in human medicine.

Nonionophore Antibiotics

These compounds are used to selectively modify microbial populations within animals to improve production efficiency and to maintain health by combating low-level infections, particularly in intensive systems. Phosphoglycolipid antibiotics (eg, flavophospholipol) alter ruminal flora by inhibiting the action of some gram-positive gut microorganisms and peptoglycan formation, yielding similar production responses to those produced by ionophores. In addition, flavophospholipol has been shown to influence the hindgut microflora populations, resulting in competitive exclusion of some harmful pathogens such as *Escherichia coli* and various species of *Salmonella*. A less understood effect of flavophospholipol is the reduction in plasmid transfer of antimicrobial resistance. Given the seemingly contradictory and highly charged interests of desire for a generalized reduction in the use of antibiotics for livestock production and the potential use of a specific antibiotic for reducing antimicrobial resistance, this potentially volatile topic has not been comprehensively assessed.

The means by which specific compounds exert their antimicrobial effect differ. Antibiotics may have a nitrogen-sparing effect, thereby increasing the availability of amino acids to the animal.

Most feeds for broiler and pig production in some countries contain antimicrobial *growth promoters*. These compounds can also be administered to calves, yearlings, and finishing cattle either in milk replacer or in supplementary concentrates. Antibiotic compounds, in general, increase growth rate by 2%–10% and feed conversion efficiency by 3%–9%. Their effects are greater in young animals, and production responses are reduced when production conditions are optimized (good housing, optimal health, and hygiene). They have minimal effects on carcass composition other than that because of improved growth rate.

The development of microbial resistance to antibiotics in treated animals, which can then be spread to people, is an important concern regarding the widespread use of antimicrobial feed additives in food production. There is circumstantial evidence that use of subtherapeutic doses of antimicrobials creates selective pressure for the emergence of antimicrobial resistance, which may be transmitted to the consumer from food or through contact with treated animals or animal manure. A ban on the use of antibiotics as feed additives decreased drug-resistant bacteria in a Danish study. Although overall mortality rates of chickens were not affected, more feed was consumed per kg of weight. Therapeutic use of antibiotics was increased, but the total volume of antibiotic use was significantly decreased. The EU has banned bacitracin, carbodox, olaquindox, tylosin, virginiamycin, avilamycin, flavophospholipol, lasalocid sodium, monensin sodium, and salinomycin as of 2009. There has been no reported evidence of any reduction in antimicrobial resistance in human bacterial pathogens as a result of the EU ban. This is understandable given that the most important and concerning cases of antimicrobial resistance in human medicine, namely methicillin-resistant *Staphylococcus aureus* (MRSA), vancomycin-resistant enterococcus (VRE), *Streptococcus pneumoniae*, and others, are not food-borne pathogens, are not found in food or companion animals, and the drugs of interest are not used and were not used before the ban in livestock. The issue of antimicrobial resistance is critical for the immediate and long-term future of human medicine; however, the complexity of the issue and the difficulty with which it must be assessed ensure that clear answers are not imminent and the debate over the most appropriate path forward in the USA and abroad will continue.

PROBIOTICS

Probiotics promote the establishment and development of a desirable intestinal microbial balance. There is a delicate balance between normal and pathogenic microorganisms. This balance can be upset by poor husbandry conditions, disease, or stressors (eg, transport). Bacteria that produce lactic acid can, in general, be beneficial to the animal; certain yeasts may also be beneficial. Their ability to increase growth and promote health are claimed to be due to one or more of the following factors: preventing colonization of the gut by pathogenic coliforms, altering GI absorption rate, and inhibiting bacterial growth and influencing the balance of bacteria in the gut. The probiotic feed additives consist of selected strains of lactobacilli and streptococci that alter the microbial species present in the GI system to the benefit of the treated animal. Unicellular yeasts are also used. The production benefits are variable, and positive responses are more likely when a stressful management change may result in a change in balance of gut microflora. Thus, they are useful in some cases to minimize GI upsets or to help overcome stress due to weaning or transport. The unicellular yeast fungus may also have beneficial effects on rumen fermentation, thereby improving digestion and feed efficiency. The effect of probiotics in older animals may be reduced because of the well-established, balanced population of microflora that is less sensitive to minor detrimental husbandry challenges.

VACCINES AND IMMUNOTHERAPY

The adaptive immune system responds to microbial invasion by producing protective antibodies or cell-mediated immunity, or both. Appropriate administration of specific microbial antigens, as in a vaccine, can provoke effective, longterm resistance to infection. Conserved microbial molecules can also stimulate the development of innate immune responses. This too enhances resistance to infection and may be clinically useful.

ACTIVE IMMUNIZATION

Active immunization involves administration of vaccines containing antigenic molecules (or genes for these molecules) derived from infectious agents. As a result, vaccinated animals mount acquired immune responses and develop prolonged, strong immunity to those agents. When properly used, vaccines are highly effective in controlling infectious diseases. Several criteria determine whether a vaccine can or should be used. First, the actual cause of the disease must be determined. Although this appears self-evident, it has not always been followed in practice. For example, *Mannheimia haemolytica* can be isolated consistently from the lungs of cattle with respiratory disease; however, these bacteria are not the sole cause of this syndrome, and vaccines against the primary viral pathogens are required for full protection. In some important viral diseases (eg, equine infectious anemia, feline infectious peritonitis, and Aleutian disease in mink), antibodies may contribute to the disease process, and vaccination can therefore increase disease severity.

An ideal vaccine for active immunization should confer prolonged, strong immunity in vaccinated animals, as well as rapid onset of immunity. It should not cause adverse effects and should be inexpensive, thermo- and genetically stable, and, for production animals, adaptable to mass administration. It should preferably stimulate immune responses distinguishable from those due to natural infection, so that vaccination and eradication may proceed simultaneously. Vaccination is not always an innocuous procedure; adverse effects can and do occur. Therefore, all vaccination must be governed by the principle of informed consent. The risks of vaccination must not exceed those caused by the disease itself.

Vaccines may contain either living or killed organisms or purified antigens from these organisms. Vaccines containing living organisms tend to trigger the best protective responses. Killed organisms or purified antigens may be less immunogenic than living ones. Because they are unable to grow and spread in the host, they are less likely to optimally stimulate the immune system. Living viruses from vaccines, for example, infect host cells and grow. The infected cells then process the viral antigens, triggering a response dominated by cytotoxic T cells, a Th1 response (*see* p 814). Killed organisms and purified antigens, in contrast, commonly stimulate responses dominated by antibodies, a Th2 response. This antibody response may not generate optimal protection against some organisms. As a result, vaccines that contain killed organisms or purified antigens usually require the use of adjuvants to maximize their effectiveness. Adjuvants may, however, cause local inflammation, and multiple doses or high doses of antigen increase the risks of producing hypersensitivity reactions.

Killed vaccines should resemble the living organisms as closely as possible. Chemical inactivation should cause minimal change to their antigens. Compounds used in this way include formaldehyde, ethylene oxide, ethyleneimine, acetylethyleneimine, and β-propiolactone.

Adjuvants

To maximize the effectiveness of vaccines, especially those containing poorly antigenic components or highly purified antigens, adjuvants are usually added. Adjuvants enhance response to vaccines and/or balance/shift the Th1/Th2 immune response. They can reduce the amount of antigen to be injected or the numbers of doses administered, and they may promote prolonged immunologic memory. It is believed that adjuvants work through three major mechanisms.

Depot adjuvants protect antigens from degradation and prolong immune responses as a result of the sustained release of antigen. Examples of depot-forming adjuvants include aluminum salts, such as aluminum hydroxide, aluminum phosphate, and aluminum potassium sulfate (alum), as well as calcium phosphate. These alum-based adjuvants also serve as very potent stimulators of toll-like receptors.

A second class of adjuvants consists of particles that effectively deliver antigen to antigen-presenting cells and so enhance antigen presentation. The immune system traps and processes particles such as bacteria or other microorganisms much more efficiently than soluble antigens. As a result, particulate antigens are much more effective than soluble ones. Examples of such adjuvants include emulsions, microparticles, immune-stimulating complexes (ISCOMs), and liposomes.

Immunostimulatory adjuvants consist of molecules that enhance cytokine production and so selectivity stimulate helper cell responses. Many contain microbial products that often represent pathogen-associated molecular patterns. As a result, they activate dendritic cells and macrophages through toll-like receptors and stimulate the secretion of critical cytokines such as IL-1 and IL-12. These cytokines in turn promote helper T-cell responses and drive and focus the adaptive immune responses. Depending on the specific microbial product used, they may enhance either Th1 or Th2 responses. Commonly used microbial immunostimulants include lipopolysaccharides (or their derivatives); killed anaerobic corynebacteria, especially *Propionibacterium acnes* and *Bordetella pertussis*; and saponins (triterpene glycosides) derived from the bark of the soapbark tree (*Quillaja saponaria*). Saponin-based adjuvants may selectively stimulate Th1 activity.

Adjuvants can be combined. For example, very effective adjuvants can be constructed by combining particulate or depot adjuvants with an immunostimulatory agent.

Types of Vaccines

Subunit Vaccines: Although vaccines containing whole killed organisms are economical to produce, they contain many antigens that do not contribute to protective immunity. They may also contain toxic components. Thus, it may be advantageous to identify, isolate, and purify the critical protective antigens. These can then be used in a vaccine by themselves. Thus, purified tetanus toxin, inactivated by treatment with formalin (tetanus toxoid), is used for active immunization against tetanus. Likewise, the attachment pili of enteropathogenic *Escherichia coli* can be purified and incorporated into vaccines. The antipilus antibodies protect animals by preventing bacterial attachment to the intestinal wall.

Antigens Generated by Gene Cloning: The cost of physically purifying a specific antigen may be prohibitive. In such cases, it may be appropriate to clone the genes coding for protective antigens. The DNA encoding the desired antigens may be inserted into a bacterium or yeast, which then expresses the protective antigen. The recombinant organism is propagated, and the antigens encoded by the inserted genes are harvested, purified, and administered as a vaccine. An example of such a vaccine is one directed against the cloned subunit of *E coli* enterotoxin. The cloned subunits are antigenic and function as effective toxoids. A purified subunit protein vaccine, called OspA, encoded by a gene from *Borrelia burgdorferi* effectively protects dogs against Lyme disease.

It is possible to clone viral antigen genes in plants. This has been successfully achieved for viruses such as transmissible gastroenteritis and Newcastle disease. The plants used include tobacco, potato, and corn. These plants contain very high concentrations of antigen, and successful vaccination may result from feeding the plants to animals.

Some recombinant vaccines contain viral structural proteins assembled into virus-like particles (VLPs). One or more viral proteins may be present in the VLP, and the particles may be either nonenveloped or enveloped. VLPs present viral antigen in a particulate form, and these antigens more closely resemble those of the infectious virus. VLPs are potent immunogens and may not require adjuvants. Because VLPs contain no viral genetic material, they cannot replicate in the vaccinee. The effectiveness of VLPs for animal vaccination has been shown in many experimental systems, but no veterinary VLP-based vaccines are commercially available at this time.

Attenuated Vaccines: The use of live organisms in vaccines presents many advantages. Most especially, they are usually more effective than inactivated vaccines in triggering cell-mediated immune responses. Their use, however, also presents certain hazards. Thus, the virulence of a live organism used for vaccination must be attenuated, so that it is able to replicate but is no longer pathogenic. The level of attenuation is critical to vaccine success. Underattenuation will result in residual virulence and disease (reversion to virulence); overattenuation will result in an ineffective vaccine. Rigorous reversion to virulence studies must be performed to demonstrate stability of the attenuation. Attenuated vaccines should not be used to vaccinate species for which they have neither been tested nor approved. Pathogens attenuated for one animal may be over- or under-attenuated in other animals. Thus, they may either cause disease or fail to provide adequate protection.

Attenuation has historically involved adapting organisms to growth in unusual conditions. Bacteria were attenuated by culture under abnormal conditions, and viruses were attenuated by growth in species to which they are not naturally adapted. Vaccine viruses may also be attenuated by growth in alternative media, such as tissue culture or eggs. This has been done for canine distemper, bluetongue, and rabies vaccines. Prolonged tissue culture was, for many years, the most usual method of attentuation.

For some diseases, related organisms normally adapted to another species may impart limited immunity. Examples include measles virus, which can protect dogs against distemper, and bovine viral diarrhea virus, which can protect pigs against classical swine fever.

Under rare circumstances, virulent organisms may be used for vaccination, eg, vaccination against contagious ecthyma (orf) of sheep. Lambs are vaccinated by rubbing dried, infected scab material into scratches made on the inner thigh, which produces local infection with only limited effects on the lambs; they become solidly immune. Because vaccinated animals may spread the disease, however, they must be separated from unvaccinated stock for a few weeks.

Considerable care must also be exercised in the preparation, storage, and handling of modified-live vaccines to avoid temperature extremes that can reduce viability of the organisms.

Gene-deleted Vaccines: Attenuation of viruses by prolonged tissue culture can be considered a primitive form of genetic engineering. Ideally, this resulted in the development of a strain of virus that was unable to cause disease. This was often difficult to achieve, and reversion to virulence was a constant hazard. Molecular genetic techniques now make it possible to modify the genes of an organism so that it becomes irreversibly attenuated. Deliberate deletion of the genes that code for proteins associated with virulence is an increasingly attractive procedure. For example, gene-deleted vaccines were first used against the pseudorabies herpesvirus in swine. In this case, the thymidine kinase gene was removed from the virus. Herpesvirus requires thymidine kinase to return from latency. Viruses from which this gene has been removed can infect neurons but cannot replicate and cause disease.

Similar genetic manipulation can be used to restrict the ability of bacteria to grow in vivo. For example, a modified-live vaccine is available that contains streptomycin-dependent *Mannheimia haemolytica* and *Pasteurella multocida*. These mutants depend on the presence of streptomycin for growth. When used in a vaccine, the absence of streptomycin will eventually result in the death of the bacteria, but not before a protective immune response has been stimulated.

Additionally, it is possible to alter the expression of other antigens so that a vaccine will induce an antibody response distinguishable from that caused by wild strains. This allows for a way to distinguish infected from vaccinated animals (referred to as DIVA).

Virus-vectored Vaccines: Another method to produce a highly effective living vaccine is to insert the genes that code for protection antigens into an avirulent "vector" organism. These vaccines are created by deleting genes from the vector and replacing them with genes coding for antigens from the pathogen. The recombinant vector is then administered as the vaccine, and the inserted genes express the antigens when body cells are infected by the vector virus. The vector may be attenuated so that it will not be shed from the vaccinate, or it may be host-restricted so that it will not replicate itself within the tissues of the vaccinate. Virus-vectored vaccines are well suited for use against organisms that are difficult or dangerous to grow in the laboratory.

The most widely used vaccine viral vectors are poxviruses such as fowlpox, canarypox, vaccinia, and herpesvirus. These viruses have a large genome that facilitates insertion of new genes. They also express relatively high levels of the recombinant antigen. In at least some cases, vectored vaccines appear able to induce immunity even when high levels of maternal antibody are present. Canarypox-vectored vaccines that incorporate genes obtained from canine distemper virus are now used to immunize dogs, and a similar vector containing the gene encoding rabies glycoprotein effectively protects dogs and cats against rabies.

An innovative example of a vectored vaccine involves the use of a yellow fever viral chimera to protect against West Nile virus. This technology uses the capsid and nonstructural genes of the attenuated yellow fever vaccine strain 17D to deliver the envelope genes of other flaviviruses such as West Nile virus. The resulting virus is a yellow fever/West Nile virus chimera that is much safer than either of the parent viruses. The margin of safety can be further increased by introducing targeted point mutations into the envelope genes.

Another example is a vaccine directed against Newcastle disease. The vector is fowlpox virus, into which Newcastle disease HA and F genes are incorporated. It has the benefit of conferring immunity against fowlpox as well.

Vectored vaccines are also commercially available for avian influenza, West Nile virus and influenza infection in horses, feline leukemia, and for vaccinating wildlife against rabies. These vaccines are stable and can work in the absence of an adjuvant, and like the gene-deleted vaccines, allow for DIVA. Some are adaptable to mass vaccination. Field data collected on these vaccines indicate strong immunity and limited adverse effects.

Polynucleotide (DNA) Vaccines: Animals may also be immunized by injection of DNA encoding viral antigens. This DNA can be inserted into a bacterial plasmid, a piece of circular DNA that acts as a vector. When the genetically engineered plasmid is injected, it can be taken up by host cells. The DNA is then transcribed, and mRNAs are translated to produce vaccine protein. Transfected host cells thus express the vaccine protein in association with major histocompatibility complex class I molecules. This can lead to the development of not only neutralizing antibodies but also cytotoxic T cells.

This type of DNA vaccine is used successfully to protect horses against West Nile virus infection. This approach has been applied experimentally to produce vaccines against the viruses that cause avian influenza, lymphocytic choriomeningitis, canine and feline rabies, canine parvovirus, bovine viral diarrhea, feline immunodeficiency virus–related disorders, feline leukemia, pseudorabies, foot-and-mouth disease, bovine herpesvirus-1 related disease, and Newcastle disease, among others. Because they can produce a response similar to that induced by attenuated live vaccines, these polynucleotide vaccines are ideally suited for use against organisms that are difficult or dangerous to grow in the laboratory. Some DNA vaccines appear to be able to induce immunity even in the presence of very high titers of maternal antibody. Immunization with purified DNA in this way allows presentation of viral antigens in their native form, because they are synthesized in the same way as antigens during a viral infection.

Administration of Vaccines

Route of Administration: The most common method of vaccine administration is by SC or IM injection. This approach is excellent for relatively small numbers of animals and for diseases in which systemic immunity is important. In addition, the veterinarian can be sure that an animal has received the appropriate dose of vaccine. However, local immunity is sometimes more important than systemic immunity, and in these cases, it is more appropriate to administer the vaccine at the site of microbial invasion. For example, intranasal vaccines are effective in protecting cattle against infectious bovine rhinotracheitis, cats against feline rhinotracheitis and calicivirus infections, and poultry against infectious bronchitis and Newcastle disease. Unfortunately, these techniques require handling each individual animal.

Aerosolization of vaccines enables them to be inhaled by all the animals in a herd, group, or flock—an obvious advantage when the unit is large. This method is commonly used in the poultry industry. Alternatively, a vaccine may be administered in feed or drinking water, eg, vaccination of poultry for Newcastle disease and avian encephalomyelitis. Fish and shrimp may be vaccinated by immersion in a solution of antigen, which is absorbed through their gills.

Combination Vaccines: Because of the complexity of many disease syndromes or to avoid giving animals multiple injections, it is common to use mixtures of organisms in single vaccines. For example, for bovine respiratory disease complex, combined vaccines are available for bovine respiratory syncytial virus, infectious bovine rhinotracheitis virus, bovine viral diarrhea virus, parainfluenza 3 virus, and *Mannheimia haemolytica*. Combination vaccines are also commonly used in dogs and cats.

When a mixture of different antigens is inoculated simultaneously, they may compete with one another. However, manufacturers have recognized this and modified vaccines accordingly. Vaccines should never be mixed indiscriminately, because one component may dominate and interfere with responses to the other components.

Some veterinarians and owners have expressed concern that the use of vaccine mixtures in this way may somehow "overwhelm" the immune system. This concern is unfounded. The immune system has evolved to respond to complex organisms and multiple simultaneous challenges. The simultaneous administration of multiple vaccines to an animal does not present difficulties to the immune system of normal, healthy animals.

Vaccination Schedules: Although it is not possible to devise precise schedules for each vaccine, certain principles are common to all methods of active immunization. Newborn animals are passively protected by maternal antibodies and, in general, cannot be vaccinated until maternal immunity has waned. If stimulation of immunity is deemed necessary at this stage, the mother may be vaccinated during late pregnancy, timing the doses so that peak antibody levels are reached at the time of colostrum formation. Neonatal animals with antibodies are protected against disease caused by that specific pathogen while maternal antibodies are present. However, passive antibody titers decrease exponentially. These maternal antibodies may drop below protective levels while, at the same time, preventing successful immunization. Inactivated vaccines are not very effective in conferring protective immunity in the face of maternal antibodies. Modified-live vaccines, however, may induce a protective primary immune response and some immunologic memory. Because the precise time of loss of maternal immunity cannot be predicted, young animals must usually be vaccinated multiple times to ensure successful immunization.

The interval between vaccine doses depends on an animal's immunologic memory. The duration of this memory depends on multiple factors, such as the nature of the antigen, the use of live or dead organisms, adjuvants used, and the route of administration. Some vaccines may induce immunity that persists for an animal's lifetime. Other vaccines may require boosting only once every 2–3 yr. Even killed viral vaccines may protect some animals against disease for many years. Unfortunately, the minimal duration of immunity has rarely been reliably measured. Annual revaccination has been the traditional rule, because this approach is administratively simple and has the advantage of ensuring that an animal is regularly seen by a veterinarian. It is likely that this is more than sufficient for most viral vaccines.

Individual animal and vaccine variability make it difficult to estimate the duration of protective immunity. Within a group of animals, there may be a great difference between the shortest and longest duration of protection. Vaccines may differ significantly in their composition, and although all may induce immunity in the short term, it cannot be assumed that they confer equal longterm immunity. A significant difference likely exists between the minimal level of immunity required to protect most animals and the level of immunity required to ensure protection of all animals.

A veterinarian should always assess the relative risks and benefits to an animal when determining the frequency of revaccination. Owners should be made aware that protection can be maintained reliably only when vaccines are used in accordance with the protocol approved by vaccine licensing authorities. The duration of immunity claimed by a vaccine manufacturer is the minimal duration supported by the data available at the time of approval.

It is common practice to rate vaccines according to their importance. Essential (or core) vaccines should be given to all animals of a species, and veterinarians should ensure that immunity is maintained throughout an animal's life by appropriate revaccination. Optional (or noncore) vaccines protect animals against sporadic, mild, or uncommon diseases and should be used only when circumstances warrant and when the benefits clearly outweigh the risks involved. For example, essential vaccines in dogs in the USA would normally include canine distemper, parvovirus, adenovirus, and rabies. Optional vaccines may include canine coronavirus, parainfluenza, *Bordetella*, leptospirosis, and Lyme disease.

Prime-boost Strategies: It has long been normal practice to use exactly the same vaccine for boosting an immune response as was used when first priming an animal. However, there is no reason why different forms of a vaccine should not be used for priming and for boosting. This approach is known as a prime-boost strategy. Under some circumstances, this may result in significantly improved vaccine effectiveness. Prime-boosting has been most widely investigated in attempts to improve the effectiveness of DNA vaccines. Combinations usually involve priming with a DNA vaccine and boosting with either a recombinant vaccine or with recombinant protein antigens.

Vaccine Failure

There are many reasons why vaccination may fail. In some cases, the vaccine may not be effective because it contains strains of organisms or antigens that are different from the disease-producing agent. In other cases, the method of manufacture may have destroyed the protective epitopes, or there may simply be insufficient antigen. Such problems are uncommon and can be avoided by using vaccines from reputable manufacturers. More commonly, an effective vaccine may fail because of unsatisfactory administration or storage. For example, a live bacterial vaccine may lose potency as a result of use of antibiotics. Route of administration may also affect efficacy. When vaccine is administered to poultry or mink by aerosol or in drinking water, the aerosol may not be evenly distributed throughout a building, or some animals may not drink adequate amounts. Also, chlorinated water may inactivate vaccines. If an animal is incubating the disease before vaccination, the vaccine may not be protective; vaccination against an already contracted disease is usually impossible.

The immune response, being a biologic process, never confers absolute protection nor is equal in all individuals of a vaccinated population. Because the response is influenced by many factors, the range in a random population tends to follow a normal distribution: the response will be average in most animals, excellent in a few, and poor in a few. An effective vaccine may not protect those with a poor response; it is difficult to protect 100% of a random population by vaccination. The size of this unresponsive population varies among vaccines, and its significance depends on the nature of the disease. For highly infectious diseases in which herd immunity is poor and infection is rapidly and efficiently transmitted (eg, foot-and-mouth disease), the presence of unprotected animals can permit the spread of disease and disrupt control programs. Problems also can arise if the unprotected animals are individually important, as in the case of companion animals or breeding stock. In contrast, for diseases that are inefficiently spread (eg, rabies), 60%–70% protection in a population may be sufficient to effectively block disease transmission within that population and therefore may be satisfactory from a public health perspective.

The most important cause of vaccination failure in young animals is the inability of a vaccine to immunize in the presence of maternal antibodies. Vaccines may also fail when the immune response is severely suppressed, eg, in heavily parasitized or malnourished animals. (Such animals should not be vaccinated.) Stress, including pregnancy, extremes of cold and heat, and fatigue or malnourishment, may reduce a normal immune response, probably due to increased glucocorticoid production.

Adverse Reactions

Modern, commercially produced, licensed vaccines are very safe. Nevertheless, they are not always innocuous. The more common risks associated with vaccines include residual virulence and toxicity, which may cause injection-site reactions, depression, allergic responses, disease in immunodeficient hosts (modified-live vaccines), neurologic complications, and rarely, contamination with other live agents. For example, lesions of mucosal disease may be seen in calves vaccinated against bovine viral diarrhea. Vaccines that contain killed gram-negative organisms may also contain bacterial cell-wall components that stimulate release of interleukin-1 and can cause fever and leukopenia and occasionally abortion. In general, it is prudent to avoid vaccinating pregnant animals unless the risks of not vaccinating are greater. Recent studies have indicated that vaccines are more likely to cause adverse effects in small dogs than in large. This is because both receive the same quantity of vaccine, and the smaller animals receive a relatively larger "dose." Certain modified-live virus bluetongue vaccines have been reported to cause congenital anomalies when given to pregnant ewes. The stress from a vaccination reaction may be sufficient to activate latent infections. For example, activation of equine herpesvirus has been demonstrated after vaccination against African horse sickness. Another adverse reaction is the "sting" that occurs when some vaccines are administered. This can cause problems for the vaccinator if the vaccinated animal objects strenuously. Some vaccines and vaccine mixtures may cause mild, transient immunosuppression.

In addition to potential toxicity, vaccines, like any antigen, may provoke hypersensitivity. For example, rapid allergic reactions (type I hypersensitivity) may occur in response to any of the antigens found in vaccines, including those from eggs or tissue-culture cells. All forms of hypersensitivity are more commonly associated with multiple injections of antigen; therefore, they tend to be associated with use of inactivated products. Immune complex (type III) reactions are also potential hazards of vaccination. These may cause an intense local inflammatory reaction or a generalized vascular disturbance such as purpura. An example of a type III reaction is clouding of the cornea in dogs vaccinated against canine adenovirus 1. Delayed (type IV) hypersensitivity reactions, expressed as granuloma formation, may develop at the site of inoculation in response to the use of depot adjuvants. Some chronic inflammatory reactions to long-acting feline vaccines may eventually lead to development of a fibrosarcoma at the injection site in cats.

Production of Vaccines

In most countries, government authorities regulate the production of biologics. In general, regulatory authorities license establishments that produce vaccines and inspect those premises to ensure that the facilities and the methods used are satisfactory. All vaccines are checked for safety, purity, potency, and efficacy. Safety tests include confirmation of the identity of the organism used, freedom of the vaccine from contamination with extraneous organisms, and host and non-host safety toxicity tests. Because the living organisms found in vaccines normally die over time, it is necessary to ensure that they will be effective even after storage (stability). Although properly stored vaccines may still be efficacious after the expiration of their designated shelf life, this should never be assumed; expired vaccines should not be used.

PASSIVE IMMUNIZATION

Passive immunization involves the production of antibodies in one animal by active immunization. These antibodies can be stored (as immunoglobulins) and then administered to susceptible animals to confer immediate but short-lived protection. The transfer of maternal antibody to offspring via the placenta or colostrum is the natural (and very important) form of passive immunization. Immunoglobulins may be produced in cattle against anthrax, in dogs against distemper, and in cats against panleukopenia. Their most important role is in protection against toxigenic organisms, eg, *Clostridium tetani* or *C perfringens*. These immunoglobulins are generally produced in young horses by a series of immunizing inoculations.

To check the potency of preparations of immunoglobulin, comparison is made with an international biological standard and expressed in international units (IUs). Tetanus immunoglobulin is given to animals to confer immediate protection against tetanus. At least 1,500–3,000 IUs of immunoglobulin should be given to horses and cattle; at least 500 IUs to calves, sheep, goats, and pigs; and at least 250 IUs to dogs. The exact amount varies with the amount of tissue damage, degree of wound contamination, and time elapsed since injury. Tetanus immunoglobulin is of little use once clinical signs appear, although massive doses of up to 300,000 IUs may help.

Monoclonal Antibodies: In a normal immune response, antibodies are produced by many different plasma cell populations and are thus said to be polyclonal. Although these antibodies all combine with a specific antigen, they are a heterogeneous mixture of proteins. Homogeneous antibodies can be generated through the use of cloned cell lines called hybridomas; these monoclonal antibodies represent an alternative source of passive immunization. Currently, however, these are mainly made by mouse hybridomas (and thus consist of mouse antibodies) and may sensitize other animal species.

Monoclonal antibodies are commonly used in diagnostic tests. Because they are homogeneous and specific, these antibodies can differentiate between closely related infectious agents in a manner impossible with conventional antibodies. For example, they can differentiate between the rabies viruses obtained from skunks, bats, or dogs.

NONSPECIFIC IMMUNOTHERAPY

Under some circumstances, it may be desirable to enhance the activity of an animal's immune system. This may include stimulation of the normal immune response to enhance protection and treatment of immunosuppressive conditions. Several types of immunostimulators have been used in veterinary medicine. They commonly contain microbial components, and many act by stimulating one or more toll-like receptors or related receptor systems.

POULTRY

CIRCULATORY SYSTEM

DIGESTIVE SYSTEM

GENERALIZED CONDITIONS

INTEGUMENTARY SYSTEM

MUSCULOSKELETAL SYSTEM

NERVOUS SYSTEM

REPRODUCTIVE SYSTEM

RESPIRATORY SYSTEM

NUTRITION AND MANAGEMENT

BLOODBORNE ORGANISMS

Avian blood may contain various disease agents, including viruses, bacteria, rickettsiae, protozoa, microfilariae, and rarely fungi. These organisms can be identified by microscopic examination of wet mounts, buffy coat, or blood smears or by appropriate culturing and molecular techniques. Microscopically, some are within blood cells (*Plasmodium*, *Haemoproteus*, *Leucocytozoon*, *Isospora [Atoxoplasma]*, *Hepatozoon*, *Babesia*, *Aegyptianella*), while others are free in the plasma (*Trypanosoma*, microfilariae, bacteria, spirochetes). None live exclusively in the blood; most are found in tissues but are present in blood during part of their life cycle. Some, such as microfilariae and *Plasmodium*, may have a periodicity when numbers or stages of parasites vary with time. In such cases, examining multiple smears at intervals will increase the likelihood of obtaining a diagnosis. Seasonal variations in infection rates relate to the activity of arthropod vectors. When possible, tissue cytology is also a useful adjunct to examination of blood. Most bloodborne organisms are either uncommonly or not associated with clinical disease. However, weakened or injured birds infected with hemoprotozoa may have higher mortality and slower recovery than uninfected birds. Examination for bloodborne organisms should be included in the clinical and diagnostic procedures for any ill bird.

Thin blood smears should be made with blood directly from the bird, if possible. Anticoagulants, storage, and cooling of the blood can distort protozoal morphology and introduce artifacts. A small drop of blood can be collected using a syringe and needle. The drop should be spread on a clean glass slide to make a thin smear. A Romanowsky-type stain that gives good polychromatic coloration (eg, Giemsa stain) should be used. At least 200 oil-immersion fields (~20,000 RBC) for single smears or 100 for multiple smears from the same bird should be examined. *Leucocytozoon* and microfilariae are found around the periphery of smears and can be easily seen on low-power magnification.

Bloodborne organisms in plasma or WBCs are concentrated in the buffy coat. The microhematocrit tube is cut just below the buffy coat above the packed RBCs. The buffy coat should be expressed from the cut end with a small amount of plasma to make a suspension, and a thin smear prepared. Stained buffy coat smears are recommended to detect bacteria, spirochetes, and chronic *Leucocytozoon*, *Trypanosoma*, or *Isospora (Atoxoplasma)* infections. An excellent technique to identify low numbers of motile organisms such as spirochetes and microfilariae is direct examination of the buffy coat by darkfield or phase contrast microscopy. The buffy coat and all of the plasma should be expressed onto a glass slide and covered with a coverglass, which is depressed slightly to spread the buffy coat. The buffy coat/plasma interface should be examined with darkfield or reduced light microscopy to detect motile organisms.

To make a diagnosis of infection with an intracellular blood protozoan on a thin blood film, it first should be determined that the "parasites" in question are neither normal structure nor artifact. The following should then be determined: the host cell and whether it is normal or deformed beyond identification, whether pigment granules (hemozoin) are present or absent, and whether merogony is occurring (*see* TABLE 1). Identification of an organism beyond genus is difficult and usually unnecessary for clinical purposes.

Serologic and molecular diagnostic methods have been developed for avian hemoparasites but are usually not available commercially. Molecular methods are very sensitive and can detect infection when parasite numbers are too low to be detected in blood or tissue smears or by histology. Hemoparasites can also be studied by subinoculation of infectious blood in birds of the same or a known susceptible avian species. Bacteria can usually be identified by blood culture and molecular methods.

AEGYPTIANELLOSIS

Aegyptianellosis is an acute, tickborne, febrile disease caused by *Aegyptianella* spp, a rickettsia in the family Anaplasmataceae. Infection of avian species, including chickens, turkeys, guineafowl, quail, pigeons, crows, waterfowl, ratites, falcons, passerines, and psittacines has been described. *A pullorum* is pathogenic in chickens. Ticks, especially *Argas* spp,

TABLE 1 CHARACTERISTICS OF PROTOZOA ENCOUNTERED IN AVIAN BLOOD

Protozoan	Host Cell	Pigment Present	Merogony in Blood
Plasmodium	RBC	Yes	Yes
Haemoproteus	RBC	Yes	No
Leucocytozoon	RBC or WBC; distorted and enlarged often beyond recognition	No	No
Isospora (*Atoxoplasma*)	WBC; in nuclear indentation	No	No[a]
Hepatozoon[b]	WBC, large, elongated oval shape	No	No
Babesia[b]	RBC	No	No[c]

[a] Multiple intracellular parasites may be seen in acute infections.
[b] Uncommon to rare.
[c] *Babesia* are pyriform and may be in a V, X, or fan pattern.

transmit the organism; infection can also be reproduced by blood inoculation. Organisms stain purple with Romanosky stain and appear as single or multiple, round, "signet-ring" (0.3–4 µm) or irregular oval bodies in RBCs often lateral to the nucleus. They must be differentiated from trophozoites of *Plasmodium* and gametocytes of *Haemoproteus*. Infections are most common in tropical and subtropical areas of Africa, Asia, and Europe; infection of wild turkeys in Texas has been reported.

In endemic areas, infection is mild or asymptomatic. Ruffled feathers, anorexia, droopiness, diarrhea, fever, and high mortality in younger birds can occur in introduced or otherwise susceptible birds. Anemia, which can lead to right-side heart failure and ascites, enlargement of the liver and spleen, enlarged discolored kidneys, and pinpoint serosal hemorrhages, can be seen. Infestation with larval argasid ticks and *Borrelia* infection (*see* p 2813) may accompany the disease.

Tetracyclines, especially doxycycline, effectively control the disease and possibly eliminate the organism from chronically infected birds. Tick control is an important adjunct to treatment.

ISOSPORIASIS

(Atoxoplasmosis, Lankesterellosis)

The taxonomic position of the Eimeriidae coccidia genera *Atoxoplasma* and *Isospora* has been subject to debate. It is currently suggested that *Atoxoplasma* be considered synonymous with *Isospora* and unified in a single group of coccidia with intra- and extra-intestinal forms.

Isosporiasis is a disease of passerine birds. Canaries, finches, sparrows, and species of the Sturnidae family (starlings, mynahs) are most often affected. Very rare cases of infection have also been reported in raptors. Poultry are not known to be affected.

Isospora has a direct life cycle that includes an intestinal and an extra-intestinal, systemic phase. Schizogony occurs in the intestinal epithelial cells as well as the circulating mononuclear cells. Gametogony and oocyst formation occur in the intestinal epithelial cells, and oocysts are passed in the feces. Transmission is fecal-oral.

Infection is most often not pathogenic, and high parasitemia may be seen in young birds. In susceptible species or weakened birds, mortality can be high (as much as 80%) and rapid, especially in fledglings. *Isospora* infection complicates management and is a threat to successful captive breeding of some species such as the endangered Bali mynahs. Clinical signs include listlessness, diarrhea, anorexia, and weight loss. In acutely affected birds, there is marked hepatomegaly and splenomegaly, often with multifocal necrosis. The enlarged liver and gallbladder can be seen through the abdominal wall, especially if it is moistened with alcohol, which provides the basis for the common name of black spot disease in passerine birds. Parasite-infected mononuclear cells are present in blood and organ impression smears or aspirates, especially in the liver and spleen. Oocysts are present in droppings. *Isospora* are pale-staining, nonpigmented, oval, intracytoplasmic bodies within mononuclear cells thought to be lymphocytes. Usually, cells contain a single parasite, but multiple organisms can be seen in severe, acute infections. Presence of the protozoan causes the nucleus to curve around it, giving the appearance that the organism is located within an indentation of the nucleus.

Diagnosis is difficult in chronically infected older birds. Very few parasites are present in blood and tissues, and oocysts are shed intermittently, sometimes in high numbers. A PCR test is available and can be performed on blood, tissues, or feces, although its sensitivity is poor in fecal samples. PCR is useful to determine the incidence and prevalence in a collection, confirming the diagnosis, and possibly evaluating the efficacy of treatment. PCR cannot be used to ascertain that a bird is free of *Isospora*, however. Buffy coat and organ smears are other but less sensitive diagnostic methods. Negative findings should not be interpreted to mean that infection is not present. In some chronically infected birds, hepatic and splenic enlargement persists because of infiltrations with high numbers of large lymphoid cells that serve as host cells for the parasite. Histopathologically, organisms are difficult to find and identify, and lesions may be mistaken for those of lymphoma.

Toltrazuril, sulfachlorpyridazine, and sulfachlorpyrazine have successfully reduced mortality and oocyst shedding. It is unlikely that these drugs clear the organism from the bird. Good management procedures, including isolation of age groups and scrupulous cleanliness (particularly daily cleaning before oocysts sporulate) help control the disease. Disinfectants have little effect on oocysts.

FILARIASIS

Microfilariae are commonly found in the blood of some wild bird species but are rare to absent in poultry except in southeast Asia where infections in chickens and waterfowl occur. Prevalence of microfilariae in wild birds varies from 3% to 6% but can be as high as 20% in some species such as ptarmigan, swans, and geese. When psittaciformes were commonly imported, it was not unusual to observe microfilariae in their peripheral blood, especially in imported cockatoos.

At least 16 genera of filarids are found in avian species. All have an indirect life cycle, with bloodsucking insects (eg, lice, mosquitoes, midges) serving as intermediate hosts. Adults mature in body cavities, including the eye and ventricles of the brain, respiratory system, cardiovascular system, or connective tissues; some produce characteristic subcutaneous nodules. Microfilariae may be numerous in circulation, especially in the skin vasculature. Microfilariae can be seen in blood smears. However, a buffy coat smear obtained from a microhematocrit tube is a more sensitive method of diagnosis. Increased numbers of microfilariae have been seen in stressed individuals, but they rarely cause clinical disease or mortality. A possible exception is infection of emus with *Chandlerella quiscali*, a common filarid of the brain of free-living grackles. Affected emus show signs of CNS disease (eg. torticollis, ataxia). *C quiscali* apparently does not produce microfilariae in emus. Treatment with ivermectin, fenbendazole, or levamisole, and surgical removal of adult parasites, have been used.

HAEMOPROTEUS INFECTION

Haemoproteus spp is the most common blood parasite in birds, especially nondomestic birds. More than 120 species have been reported. *Haemoproteus* spp are found in free-living ducks, quail, and turkeys but are rare to absent in commercial flocks, probably because of limited vector exposure or very specific feeding habits of *Culicoides* spp and hippoboscid flies, the invertebrate vectors. *Haemoproteus* is considered nonpathogenic in most avian species. Birds are usually asymptomatic; however, *Haemoproteus* infection may be more often significant than previously thought, based on increasing reports documenting decreased host fitness, nestling mortalities, fledging success, and delayed recovery in infected birds versus uninfected birds. Anemia, anorexia, weight loss, and depression have been reported. Rarely fatal disease occurs. Clinical disease is usually attributed to anemia, presence of megaloschizonts in the musculature, or host-cell destruction.

In poultry, infection with *H lophortyx* in bobwhite quail caused clinical disease and increased mortality with as much as 20% flock loss. Quail 5–10 wk old were usually affected, and clinical signs included reluctance to move, prostration, and death. Gross lesions included congested spleen and liver and hemorrhagic streaks in the muscles. Histology revealed myositis with megaloschizonts in the musculature, especially of the legs and back, and hemosiderin accumulation in the splenic macrophages. Experimental infection in turkeys with *H meleagridis* resulted in lameness, diarrhea, anorexia, and depression. Histologic lesions were associated mainly with megaloschizont development in the musculature. Infection in racing pigeons (called pigeon malaria) is commonly asymptomatic but often blamed for poor performances that are due to other diseases or inadequate housing and management. Clinical disease in Columbiformes is rare.

Diagnosis is made by examination of stained blood smears and observation of large, pigmented gametocytes in mature RBCs that partially or occasionally completely encircle the nucleus without displacing it. Merozoites are not seen in the peripheral blood. Schizogony within the endothelial cells of the lung, liver, and spleen may be seen histologically. PCR tests for *Haemoproteus* have been developed. Little is known about effective treatment. Antimalarial drugs reduce the parasitemia but do not eliminate the parasite. Chloroquine, primaquine, quinacrine, and buparvaquone have been used in pigeons. Combinations of chloroquine and primaquine or chloroquine and mefloquine have been used to treat owls. Treatment is not recommended in asymptomatic birds. Measures to control invertebrate vectors, such as screening of aviaries, help prevent transmission and heavy infections.

LEUCOCYTOZOONOSIS

Infections with *Leucocytozoon* spp are most often subclinical but can occasionally cause clinical and even fatal disease. Mortality varies greatly with the strain of parasite, species, degree of exposure, age, immune status, and other factors. Outbreaks of leucocytozoonosis have been reported in chickens (Asia, Africa), turkeys (North America), waterfowl (North America, Europe, Asia), and a number of free-living and captive avian species throughout the world. Species in domestic birds include *L simondi* in waterfowl; *L smithi* in turkeys; and *L caulleryi*, *L sabrazesi*, *L andrewsi*, and *L schoutedeni* in chickens. *L caulleryi* can be highly pathogenic, causing a lethal hemorrhagic disease of chickens in southeast Asia. *L simondi* causes mortality in ducks and geese. Numerous *Leucocytozoon* spp infect nondomestic birds. Clinical disease and mortality result from anemia caused by antierythrocytic factors produced by the parasite, high numbers of the large gametocytes blocking pulmonary capillaries, or parasites invading the endothelium of vessels in tissues (brain, heart, etc) where they form megaloschizonts that occlude vessels and result in multifocal necrosis.

Parasitemia often increases dramatically in late April and early May (called spring rise), just before arthropod vectors, black flies (*Simulium* spp), or biting midges (*Culicoides* spp) increase. Ducks that have recovered from infection with *L simondi* may relapse when light cycles are manipulated to increase egg production. Increased levels of prolactin have been suggested as a possible cause.

Acute disease is seen more often in the young with high parasitemia and when black flies or biting midges are most abundant. Subacute or chronic disease is seen in the young outside fly season and in older birds at any season; parasitemia is usually low. Recovered birds remain carriers and serve as a reservoir for young, susceptible birds.

Clinical Findings, Lesions, and Diagnosis: Ducklings or turkey poults are listless and show various combinations of the following signs: anemia, leukocytosis, tachypnea, anorexia, diarrhea with green droppings, and CNS signs. Mortality in ducklings can reach 70%. Mortality is low in adult ducks or turkeys. Egg production and hatchability is decreased. Signs are evident ~1 wk after infection and coincide with the onset of parasitemia. Visibly affected birds die after 7–20 days or may recover with sequelae of poor growth and egg production. Hemorrhages, splenomegaly, and hepatomegaly are seen. Grossly visible white dots in affected organs are megaloschizonts. Histologic lesions are associated with megaloschizont development in the spleen, liver, heart, and other organs. Infection with *L caulleryi* in chickens has a tropism for the

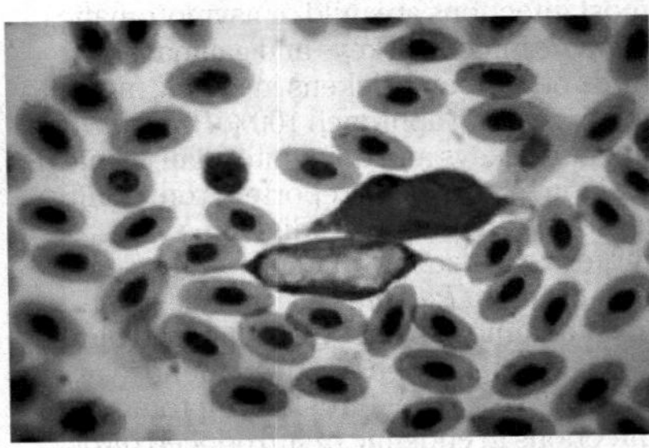

Leucocytozoon parasite in the peripheral blood of a turkey. *Courtesy of Dr. Jean Sander.*

reproductive tract and is associated with oviduct inflammation and edema and decreased egg production. Peritoneal, perirenal, and subdural hemorrhages are reported with severe disease.

In blood smears, gametocytes may be seen, especially along the edges and tail of the smear. *Leucocytozoon* is identified by large gametocytes that lack pigment and distort the host cell (RBC or WBC), making it no longer identifiable. The shape of gametocytes varies: some are elongated with long tapering extremities, whereas others are round. Serology may detect prior infection. PCR tests have been developed for diagnosis of leukocytozoonosis.

Treatment and Control: Treatment usually is not effective. Preventive medication using pyrimethamine (1 ppm) and sulfadimethoxine (10 ppm) combined in the feed controls *L caulleryi*. Clopidol (0.0125%–0.025%) controls *L smithi*. Measures to control invertebrate vectors are helpful. Humoral immunity resulting from vaccination will protect against *L caulleryi* infection. Treatments with quinacrine hydrochloride or trimethoprim/sulfamethoxazole solution have been used in raptors; parasitemia is reduced, but the infection is not cleared.

PLASMODIUM INFECTION

Plasmodium spp infect a wide variety of domestic and wild birds in most areas of the world. Infection is often not species specific. Thirty-five species of *Plasmodium* are considered valid species. *P gallinaceum*, *P juxtanucleare*, and *P durae* are the most pathogenic species found in poultry. *P gallinaceum* infects chickens in Asia and Africa and causes low mortality in indigenous chickens; however, rates may be as high as 80%–90% in commercial birds. *P juxtanucleare* infects chickens and turkeys in Asia, Africa, and South America; most infections are mild or asymptomatic. *P durae* infects turkeys and gallinaceous birds other than chickens in Africa; mortality in turkeys can approach 100%. *P hermani* infects turkeys and bobwhite quail. Clinical malaria has not been reported from poultry in North America, but indigenous wild turkeys can become infected with at least four different *Plasmodium* species. The most common species affecting wild birds is *P relictum*, which has been found in at least 360 species of birds. Asymptomatic infections in endemic or introduced birds can be spread via mosquitoes and cause fatal disease in introduced (eg, zoo birds) or resident (eg, Hawaiian avifauna) birds, respectively. Passerine birds commonly carry the organism asymptomatically. Cold-climate species held ouside their natural range are particularly susceptible to develop clinical disease (eg, penguins, snowy owls, and gyrfalcons in captivity). Invertebrate hosts are ornithophilic mosquitoes, usually *Culex*, *Culiseta*, or *Aedes* spp.

Clinical Findings, Lesions, and Diagnosis: Infection with *Plasmodium* spp may be nonclinical or cause illness characterized by weakness, lassitude, dyspnea, anemia, abdominal distention, increased right heart weight, ocular hemorrhage, biliverdinuria, and death. Death results from severe anemia or blockage of capillaries in the brain, lung, or other vital organs by exoerythrocytic meronts in endothelial cells. The liver and spleen are markedly enlarged and often discolored (dark brown to black). Pigmented parasites including meronts are found in both immature and mature RBCs. Infrequently, parasites are found in thrombocytes and WBCs. In birds that die acutely, organisms may be sparse or absent in blood, but numerous meronts can be found in capillaries by histology or examination of squash or impression smears of brain, lung, liver, and spleen. Serologic and molecular diagnostic methods exist but are not available commercially. Serology and PCR can detect infection when parasites are too few to be identified in blood smears.

Treatment and Control: Therapy is variably effective in treating infected birds or flocks. Persistent parasitemia or relapse may occur during and after treatment. Birds that survive initial infections may be refractory to subsequent infections. Prevention of exposure to mosquitoes by appropriate housing is essential.

No antimalarial drug is commercially available or approved to treat poultry flocks. However, a mixture of trimethoprim and sulfaquinoxaline in the feed for a 5-day period has been shown to be efficacious against experimentally induced *P gallinaceum* malaria in chickens. An experimental study on the pathogenicity and chemotherapy of *P durae* suggested that a combination of sulfamonomethoxine and sulfachloropyrazine could be an effective therapy; halofuginone was suggested for chemoprophylaxis in endemic areas. Chloroquine administered by gavage at 50 mg/kg in Leghorn chickens experimentally infected with *P juxtanucleare* may have reduced parasitemia.

In caged birds and penguins, chloroquine (10 mg/kg) and primaquine (0.3–1 mg/kg) is given orally and followed by administration of chloroquine (5 mg/kg) 6, 24, and 48 hr later. Chloroquine in drinking water (250 mg/120 mL) has also been used in songbirds. Grape or orange juice can disguise chloroquine's bitterness. Treatment including both primaquine and chloroquine is recommended over chloroquine alone, because only primaquine is active against the tissue schizonts. Chloroquine has activity against erythrocytic schizonts and gametocytes. Primaquine also has activity against erythrocytic gametocytes. When aliquoting the medications, note that a 500-mg tablet of chloroquine contains 300 mg of active base, and a 26-mg primaquine tablet contains 15 mg of active base.

In raptors, control of the disease has been achieved by oral administration of mefloquine (30 mg/kg) repeated 12, 24, and 48 hr after the initial dose. Alternatively, a combination of chloroquine (25 mg/kg) and primaquine (1.3 mg/kg) can be given orally and is followed by the administration of chloroquine (15 mg/kg) 12, 24, and 48 hr later. In endemic areas, mefloquine once a week (30 mg/kg) has been used successfully for chemoprophylaxis in large falcons.

In a DNA vaccine trial in captive African black-footed penguins, parasitemia and clinical disease were successfully reduced.

OTHER BLOODBORNE ORGANISMS

Trypanosomes have been described in several avian species but rarely if ever cause clinical disease. They are more commonly identified in organ smears, especially bone marrow, than in peripheral blood, and can be cultured. Invertebrate hosts are thought to be any of several bloodsucking insects. Treatment is not warranted.

Borreliae are tickborne (*Argas* spp) spirochetes that can cause fatal systemic disease. Penicillins, tertracyclines, tylosin, and tick control are used for prevention and treatment. (*See also* AVIAN SPIROCHETOSIS, p 2813.)

Babesia spp are uncommon, nonpigmented, pyriform-shaped, erythrocytic protozoan parasites of birds. Natural infections of penguins, falcons, cranes, and several other avian species occur. Ticks are considered to be the invertebrate hosts. V, X, or fan shapes characterize dividing forms. Knowledge regarding their significance, treatment, or control in birds is limited. Only *B shortti*, which rarely occurs in falconiformes, has been reported to be pathogenic. Reported treatment in infected falcons was IM administration of 2 or 3 doses of imidocarb dipropionate (5–13 mg/kg) 1 wk apart.

Hepatozoon is a protozoan parasite infrequently identified in birds. Prevalence in wild birds is 2%–5%. It produces relatively large, nonpigmented, elongated gametocytes with rounded ends that can be found in WBCs. Gametocytes are usually not located within an indentation of the nucleus, whereas *Isospora* is oval and partially encircled by the nucleus. The life cycle in birds is uncertain, but argasid ticks and fleas have been identified as probable vectors for *Hepatozoon* infecting swallows. *Ixodes* ticks, mites, and other arthropods may also be involved. *Hepatozoon* spp are not known to be pathogenic.

Zoites of other sporozoa (eg, *Toxoplasma*, *Sarcocystis*) and organisms normally in the digestive tract (eg, trichomonads, coccidia, histomonads) may be transiently found in blood. The latter often also produces liver lesions. (*See also* TRICHOMONOSIS, p 2804, and HISTOMONIASIS, p 2835.)

CHICKEN ANEMIA VIRUS INFECTION

(Chicken infectious anemia, Blue wing disease, Anemia dermatitis syndrome, Hemorrhagic aplastic anemia syndrome)

Etiology, Epidemiology, and Pathogenesis: Chicken anemia virus (CAV), a 25 nm, nonenveloped, icosahedral virus with a single-stranded, circular DNA genome, is the only member of the *Gyrovirus* genus of the Circoviridae family. The genome codes for three viral proteins (VP). VP1 is the capsid protein, but VP2 may be needed as a scaffold protein to allow proper folding of VP1. VP2 has also a dual-specificity protein phosphatase (DSP) activity, and mutations affecting the DSP activity resulted in attenuation of virus replication in vivo. VP3, or apoptin, is a nonstructural protein that induces apoptosis in infected cells. CAV infects only chickens, although antibodies have been detected in Japanese quail. The virus is present worldwide based on serology and virus isolation. The disease, chicken infectious anemia, has been described in most countries where chickens are raised commercially.

Horizontal transmission of CAV is by the fecal-oral route, perhaps by the respiratory route, and through infected feather follicle epithelium. Vertical transmission occurs when seronegative hens become infected and continues until neutralizing antibodies develop. Chicks hatched from these eggs are viremic, and CAV can rapidly spread horizontally from these chicks to susceptible, maternal antibody-negative hatchmates. Roosters shedding CAV in semen are another source of vertical transmission. Vaccination of seronegative flocks before the onset of egg production is recommended to prevent vertical transmission.

Maternal antibody–negative chicks are susceptible to infection and disease until 1–2 wk old. In contrast, maternal antibody–positive chicks are protected from disease and probably from infection. Age resistance to clinical disease, but not infection, begins at ~1 wk of age. The age resistance can be overcome by coinfection with viruses causing immunosuppression such as bursal disease virus (*see* p 2837), Marek's disease virus (*see* p 2849), and reticuloendotheliosis virus (*see* p 2854).

Many SPF flocks develop antibodies to CAV during or after onset of sexual development. Spread of infection by CAV-contaminated embryo- or cell-culture-derived vaccines is possible.

When day-old susceptible chicks are inoculated IM with CAV, viremia occurs within 24 hr. Virus can be recovered from most organs and rectal contents as long as 35 days after inoculation. The principal sites of CAV replication are hemocytoblasts in the bone marrow, precursor T cells in the cortex of the thymus, and dividing CD4 and CD8 cells in the spleen. Replication in the hemocytoblasts leads to anemia, while replication in the T cells causes immunosuppression. Neutralizing antibodies are detectable 21 days after infection, and clinical, hematologic, and pathologic parameters return to normal ~35 days after infection. CAV infection has adverse effects on proliferative responses of spleen lymphocytes and on the production of interleukin-2 and interferons by splenocytes. Infection can cause a marked decrease in generation of antigen-specific cytotoxic T cells and T-helper cells directed against other pathogens. In addition to T-cell defects, macrophage functions such as Fc-receptor expression, phagocytosis, and antimicrobial activity may be impaired. Subclinical, horizontally acquired infection with CAV in broiler progeny of seropositive parent flocks may be associated with impaired economic performance.

Clinical Findings: Signs of illness or adverse effects on egg production do not occur when seronegative adult chickens become infected. However, vertical transmission or infection of maternal antibody–negative chicks before 1 wk of age can cause clinical disease 12–17 days after hatching or infection. Chicks are anorectic, lethargic, depressed, and pale. PCV is low (in chicks, anemia is defined as a PCV ≤27), and blood smears often reveal anemia, leukopenia, or pancytopenia depending on the state of the disease. Blood may be watery and clot slowly. Mortality rates are variable but may be high with secondary complicating infections.

Lesions: Organs are pale; the thymus is generally atrophied, and the bursa of Fabricius may be small. Bone marrow is pale or yellow. Hemorrhages may be present in or under the skin, muscle, and other organs. Histologically, lymphoid cell populations are depleted in primary and secondary lymphoid organs. Granulocytic and erythrocytic compartments in the bone marrow are atrophic or hypoplastic.

Diagnosis: A tentative diagnosis is based on history, signs, and gross and histopathologic lesions. Confirmation requires detection of virus or viral DNA in the thymus or bone marrow. PCR and quantitative PCR techniques are commonly used to demonstrate the presence of CAV. Viral isolation can be used but is slow and expensive. To isolate CAV, chloroform-treated extracts of tissues are inoculated in MDCC-MSB1 or MDCC-147 cultures (both are lymphoblastoid cell lines derived from Marek's disease tumors) or into susceptible, immunocompromised and maternal antibody–negative day-old chicks. Commercial ELISA kits are available to detect serum antibodies to CAV and can be used to identify breeder flocks that are seronegative before egg production and to monitor the efficacy of vaccination.

Treatment and Prevention: There is no specific treatment. Secondary bacterial infections may be treated with antibiotics. Live vaccines are available for vaccination of antibody-negative breeder flocks before the start of egg production. Administration is by injection or by addition to the drinking water depending on the type of vaccine available in individual countries. A vaccine has been approved in the USA for use in broilers as young as 7 days old; administration is by addition to the drinking water. In some areas, transfer of litter to noncontaminated premises and the addition of crude homogenates of tissues from affected chickens to the drinking water have been used to ensure infection and seroconversion of parent flocks before they begin to lay eggs, thereby diminishing the risk of egg transmission. However, these procedures are extremely risky and not acceptable. Because of the synergism between CAV and other immunosuppressive viruses, control of the latter is also important.

DISSECTING ANEURYSM IN TURKEYS

(Aortic rupture, Internal hemorrhage)

Dissecting aneurysm is a fatal disease of turkeys. It is characterized by sudden death of rapidly growing birds with massive internal hemorrhage. The hemorrhage results from rupture of aneurysms formed in various parts of the vascular system. The frequency with which the posterior aorta is affected has given rise to the term "aortic rupture." The disease has been reported in North America, Europe, and Israel. Most breeds of turkeys are susceptible, and the largest and most rapidly growing males, 8–24 wk old, are affected most often; females are also affected but at a lower incidence.

Etiology: The cause is unknown. Likely, several factors contribute to the development of fatal cases. For the disease to occur, turkeys must be fed and managed in such a way that they grow rapidly, and they must have a genetic susceptibility. A prolonged lipemia generally develops during the period of rapid growth, and the period of greatest mortality typically corresponds to a sharp rise in blood pressure, with dissecting aneurysms developing at the site of arteriosclerotic plaques. The lipemia may result from a high dietary intake of fat or from the effects of hormonal factors, such as high dietary concentrations of estrogens. Although β-aminopropionitrile, the toxic agent in *Lathyrus odoratus*, is capable of producing the disease, there is no evidence that this or other nitriles are responsible for dissecting aneurysms in turkeys under natural conditions. The enzyme lysyloxidase, isolated from turkey aortas and active on tropelaston and collagen cross-linking, was found to be much lower in males than in females; this may be a factor in the development of spontaneous aortic aneurysms in male turkeys.

Clinical Findings: Affected turkeys that had shown no premonitory signs are found dead with marked pallor of the head and neck. Occasionally, a caretaker observes an apparently healthy turkey die within a few minutes. The incidence is usually <1% but may be as high as 10%. In the past, when male turkeys were implanted with stilbestrol, the incidence was as high as 20%.

Lesions: The carcass is markedly anemic, with large quantities of clotted blood in the peritoneal cavity and over the kidneys or in the pericardial sac. The rupture in the ventral wall of the posterior aorta at about the position of the testes, or in the cardiac atrium, can be located readily by carefully washing away the blood clot. The aortic lumen may contain an organized, adherent thrombus at the site of rupture. Ruptures in smaller blood vessels are more difficult to locate. Almost always, an intimal thickening or a large, fibrous plaque is present in the region of the rupture. The tunicas intima and media are thrown into deep folds and separated from the tunica adventitia. Marked accumulation of lipids in the thickened intima and in the fibrous plaques can be identified by stains. Fibers of the tunica media may show degenerative changes and infiltration with heterophils and macrophages.

Diagnosis: The diagnosis is made by finding large clots of blood in the coelomic cavity (aortic rupture) or within the pericardial sac (auricular rupture) of rapidly growing male turkeys. Dissecting aneurysm should be differentiated from hypertensive angiopathy (*see* p 2789), which is also seen in rapidly growing turkeys. In hypertensive angiopathy, the major lesions include pulmonary edema and supcapsular perirenal hemorrhage.

Treatment, Control, and Prevention: There is no known treatment. Coagulants and vitamin K are useless, because there is no defect in the clotting mechanism. Losses sometimes may be reduced during the critical period between 16 and 23 wk of age by limiting feed intake or slowing growth rate by reducing the energy level of the diet. High-fat diets should not be fed during this period. Some studies have indicated that the incidence of aortic rupture can be reduced by adding copper at 125–250 ppm to the diet from at least 4 wk of age until market.

INCLUSION BODY HEPATITIS/ HYDROPERICARDIUM SYNDROME

(Hepatitis hydropericardium)

Adenoviruses are widespread throughout all avian species. Studies have demonstrated the presence of antibodies in healthy poultry, and viruses have been isolated from normal birds. Despite their widespread distribution, most adenoviruses cause no or only mild disease; however, some are associated with specific clinical conditions. Avian adenoviruses (AAVs) in chickens are the etiologic agents of two important diseases known as inclusion body hepatitis (IBH) and hydropericardium syndrome (HP). Although in some cases each disease is observed separately, the two conditions have been frequently observed as a single entity; therefore, the name hepatitis hydropericardium has been widely used to describe the pathologic condition. The syndrome is an acute disease of young chickens associated with anemia, hemorrhagic disorders, and hydropericardium. It is a common disease in several countries, where broilers are severely affected, resulting in high mortality rates.

Etiology, Transmission, and Pathogenesis: The AAVs classified in the genus *Aviadenovirus* (formerly group I) are the etiologic agents of this condition. Although there are 12 different serotypes of AAV, the most common viruses isolated in cases of IBH/HP belong to serotypes 4 and 8. These AAVs are capable of producing the disease without the immunosuppressive effects of associated viruses such as infectious bursal disease (IBDV, *see* p 2837) or other immunosuppressive agents. However, the association with immunosuppressive viruses such as IBDV and chicken anemia virus (CAV, *see* p 2785) will result in a more severe disease.

Horizontal and vertical transmission play an important role in IBH/HP. Vertical transmission has been described in progeny from breeder flocks infected with AAV serotypes 4 and 8. Horizontal transmission has also been demonstrated; young chicks in contact with infected chicks can die of peracute IBH/HP. Infection with some strains of AAVs may result in minimal hepatic disease; however, if birds have been infected with immunosuppressive viruses (IBDV, CAV, Marek's disease), the clinical disease becomes evident.

Clinical Findings, Lesions, and Diagnosis: Sudden mortality usually is seen in chickens <6 wk old and as young as 4 days of age. Mortality normally ranges from 2%–40%, especially when birds are <3 wk old. However, in some outbreaks, mortality has reached 80%. Mortality rates also vary depending on the pathogenicity of the virus and infection with other viral or bacterial agents. Signs associated with diseases caused by other pathogens (eg, bacteria, fungi, or viruses) commonly occur if birds are immunosuppressed.

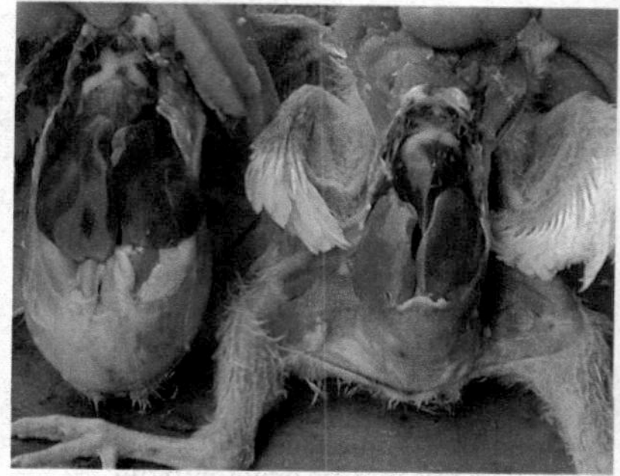

Hepatitis hydropericardium (right), normal liver on left. *Courtesy of Dr. Pedro Villegas.*

Flocks of 3- to 5-wk-old broilers with HP may not show specific clinical signs, but abrupt onset of mortality, lethargy, huddling with ruffled feathers, and yellow, mucoid droppings may be seen. The duration of the infection usually ranges from 9–14 days with morbidity of 10%–30% and a daily mortality of 3%–5%. Gross lesions include as much as 10 mL of a straw-colored transudate in the pericardial sac, generalized congestion, and an enlarged, pale, friable liver. Histopathologic lesions include myocardial edema in the heart with degeneration, necrosis, and mild mononuclear cell infiltration. Basophilic intranuclear inclusion bodies may be present in the liver. A tentative diagnosis is based on typical microscopic findings and confirmed by isolating adenoviruses from the liver. Serology, restriction enzyme analysis, and PCR are used to classify adenoviruses isolated from clinical cases. This information is used for epidemiologic studies.

Treatment and Prevention: As with many other viral diseases, there is no treatment. Antibiotics may help prevent secondary bacterial infections. Sulfonamides are contraindicated if evidence of hematologic disease or immunosuppression is seen.

Vaccines against IBH/HP are not commercially available in the USA; however, in other countries both live and inactivated vaccines are used to control the syndrome. The AAV serotypes most frequently used to prepare commercial vaccines are serotypes 4 and 8. Primary breeders with stringent biosecurity practices sometimes use autogenous inactivated vaccines to ensure the transfer of maternal immunity from breeding flocks to their progeny. In Australia, a live vaccine given via drinking water was developed for breeders between 10–14 wk of age. In other countries, including Mexico, Pakistan, and many countries in South America, inactivated vaccines are routinely used to vaccinate breeders and broilers. When breeders are properly vaccinated, antibodies generated by the vaccine are transmitted to the progeny, providing protection against field infections and clinical disease. Broilers are vaccinated at <10 days of age when their parents either do not have serotype-specific adenovirus antibodies or maternal antibody transmission is erratic because of improper vaccination procedures that result in a substantial number of unvaccinated birds.

PERIRENAL HEMORRHAGE SYNDROME OF TURKEYS

(Hypertensive angiopathy, Sudden death syndrome of turkeys)

Perirenal hemorrhage syndrome (PHS) is a noninfectious cardiovascular disorder usually affecting rapidly growing male turkeys 8–15 wk old. It is characterized by sudden death, perirenal hemorrhage, and hypertrophic cardiomyopathy. Mortality is usually 0.5%–2% but can be higher; there is no morbidity. Healthy, rapidly growing flocks are more likely to be affected.

The pathogenesis is unknown, but PHS is apparently unrelated to pulmonary function or hypertension. Inadequate or inappropriate cardiac response to exercise, resulting in systemic hypotension and vasodilation, ventricular arrhythmia, and sudden death, appears most likely. Acute congestive heart failure secondary to cardiac hypertrophy is also a potential cause. Renal hemorrhage may occur due to severe passive congestion; acute blood loss is likely not the primary cause of death because the extent of perirenal hemorrhage is variable and often mild.

Gross lesions include food in crop and stomach, enlarged dark red to purple spleen, variable retroperitoneal hemorrhage around one or both kidneys, generalized congestion, and pulmonary edema occasionally accompanied by hemorrhage. Body condition is usually good to excellent. Cardiac hypertrophy involving the left ventricle and intraventricular septum may also be seen. Microscopic changes are consistent with gross findings and include pulmonary congestion and edema with renal perivenous hemorrhage. Intimal vacuolation and medial hyperplasia of arteries and arterioles have been described in multiple organs, particularly the kidney, spleen, and lung of turkeys with PHS; however, similar lesions can be seen to a lesser extent in tissue of normal turkeys.

Diagnosis is based on history, typical gross lesions, and absence of infectious agents. PHS has several characteristics in common with aortic rupture (*see* p 2787) and sudden death syndrome of broilers (*see* p 2821). Extensive PHS lesions can resemble aortic rupture, and these two disorders can occur simultaneously in the same flock.

There is no specific treatment. Factors that decrease growth rate and activity also tend to decrease PHS. Reserpine (0.5 ppm feed) decreases PHS, but aspirin (0.005%) or increased calcium has no effect. Reserpine is not listed in the Feed Additive Compendium as approved for use in feed for turkeys. Increased room temperature and step up/step down lighting programs have also reduced PHS. Activities that increase cardiovascular stress (eg, moving birds, tilling litter, noise) should be minimized, especially between 7 and 15 wk of age. Lower ambient temperatures (55°F [13°C]), intermittent lighting, and leaving toes unclipped increase mortality from PHS. PHS may occur in commercial flocks of healthy male turkeys, regardless of management practices used to prevent its occurrence.

SPONTANEOUS CARDIOMYOPATHY OF TURKEYS

(Round heart disease)

Spontaneous cardiomyopathy of young turkeys is characterized by sudden death due to cardiac arrest and is not related to other cardiomyopathies of poultry.

The exact etiology of spontaneous cardiomyopathy in turkeys is unknown. However, studies using furazolidone to produce dilated cardiomyopathy in turkeys have indicated altered membrane transport resulting in myocardial failure. CK, glycolysis, glycogen, myofibril, Krebs cycle enzymes, fatty acid oxidation, and soluble proteins are all reduced. The calcium-transport ATPase activity of the sarcoplasmic reticulum is increased. This pattern of biochemical changes is consistent with ischemia playing a role in the pathogenesis of spontaneous cardiomyopathy in turkeys.

Although most deaths occur during the brooding period, the ratio of heart weight to body weight of affected birds is increased throughout the growing period. The chronic cardiac insufficiency causes reduced growth rate, resulting in attacks on affected birds by their healthy cohorts. In affected turkeys surviving to market age, body weights are reduced an average of 3 lb (1.4 kg). Some outbreaks of the condition have been associated with hypoxia during incubation of the eggs or during transportation of poults from the hatchery to the brood farm. It is possible that stratification of air in poorly ventilated facilities without *circulation* fans may similarly contribute to heart damage, with subsequent expression of this disease later in life.

Most deaths from spontaneous cardiomyopathy occur during the first 4 wk of life, with mortality peaking at 2–3 wk. Many poults die suddenly, but some may have ruffled feathers, drooping wings, and a general unthrifty appearance. They may show labored, gasping breathing before death. After 3 wk of age, mortality is sporadic. Characteristically, the affected poult in the first 4 wk of life has a greatly enlarged heart due to dilatation of both ventricles, congested lungs, and a swollen liver. Ascites, anasarca, pulmonary edema, and hydropericardium may be present. In older poults, enlarged hearts are due to marked hypertrophy of the ventricles in addition to dilatation. Histologically, lesions of abnormal hearts are nonspecific and include congestion, damage of the myofibrils of the cardiocytes, and focal infiltration by lymphocytes.

Generally, diagnosis is based on history and gross findings at necropsy; although an ECG can be used, it is of little practical use. Sodium and polychlorinated biphenyls or related compounds may produce similar syndromes.

No treatment is available. Hypoxia during incubation, transportation, or brooding has been associated with increased incidence, and enhanced ventilation during these periods appears to be critical. Practitioners have occasionally noted association of high levels of dietary (or drinking water) copper and increased incidence of spontaneous cardiomyopathy. Good brooding practices may reduce mortality, because overheating has also been postulated to increase the incidence of this disease.

CANDIDIASIS

(Thrush, Crop mycosis, Sour crop)

Candidiasis is a mycotic disease of the digestive tract of various avian species, including chickens, turkeys, and quail caused by *Candida albicans*. It commonly develops after use of therapeutic levels of various antibiotics or when using unsanitary drinking facilities. Lesions are most frequently found in the crop and consist of thickened mucosa and whitish, raised pseudomembranes. The same lesions may be seen in the mouth and esophagus. Occasionally, shallow ulcers and sloughing of necrotic epithelium may be present. Listlessness and inappetence may be the only signs. A presumptive diagnosis may be made on observation of gross lesions. Diagnosis can be confirmed by demonstrating tissue invasion histologically and by culture of the organism. However, culture alone is not diagnostic of disease, because the yeast-like fungus is commonly isolated from clinically normal birds. Young chicks and poults are most susceptible.

Improving sanitation and minimizing antibiotic use in poultry help reduce the incidence of candidiasis. Candidiasis can be treated or prevented with copper sulfate at 1:2,000 dilution in the drinking water, but its effectiveness is controversial. Nystatin, an antifungal medication, in the feed (220 mg/kg of diet) or drinking water (62.5–250 mg/L with sodium lauryl sulfate, a surfactant, at 7.8–25 mg/L) for 5 days may be effective for the treatment of affected turkeys.

COCCIDIOSIS

Coccidiosis is caused by protozoa of the phylum Apicomplexa, family Eimeriidae. In poultry, most species belong to the genus *Eimeria* and infect various sites in the intestine. The infectious process is rapid (4–7 days) and is characterized by parasite replication in host cells with extensive damage to the intestinal mucosa. Poultry coccidia are generally host-specific, and the different species parasitize specific parts of the intestine. However, in game birds, including quail, the coccidia may parasitize the entire intestinal tract. Coccidia are distributed worldwide in poultry, game birds reared in captivity, and wild birds. (*See also* CRYPTOSPORIDIOSIS, p 209.)

Etiology: Coccidia are almost universally present in poultry-raising operations, but clinical disease occurs only after ingestion of relatively large numbers of sporulated oocysts by susceptible birds. Both clinically infected and recovered birds shed oocysts in their droppings, which contaminate feed, dust, water, litter, and soil. Oocysts may be transmitted by mechanical carriers (eg, equipment, clothing, insects, farm workers, and other animals). Fresh oocysts are not infective until they sporulate; under optimal conditions (70°–90°F [21°–32°C] with adequate moisture and oxygen), this requires 1–2 days. The prepatent period is 4–7 days. Sporulated oocysts may survive for long periods, depending on environmental factors. Oocysts are resistant to some disinfectants commonly used around livestock but are killed by freezing or high environmental temperatures. (*See also* COCCIDIOSIS, p 203.)

Pathogenicity is influenced by host genetics, nutritional factors, concurrent diseases, age of the host, and species of the coccidium. *Eimeria necatrix* and *Eimeria tenella* are the most pathogenic in chickens, because schizogony occurs in the lamina propria and crypts of Lieberkühn of the small intestine and ceca, respectively, and causes extensive hemorrhage. *E kofoidi* and *E legionensis* are the most pathogenic in chukars, and *E lettyae* is most pathogenic in bobwhite quail. Several *Eimeria* species are pathogenic in pheasants, particularly *E phasiani* and *E colchici*. Most species develop in epithelial cells lining the villi. Protective immunity usually develops in response to moderate and continuing infection. True age-immunity does not occur, but older birds are usually more resistant than young birds because of earlier exposure to infection.

Clinical Findings: Signs of coccidiosis range from decreased growth rate to a high percentage of visibly sick birds, severe diarrhea, and high mortality. Feed and water consumption are depressed. Weight loss, development of culls, decreased egg production, and increased mortality may accompany outbreaks. Mild infections of intestinal species, which would otherwise be classed as subclinical, may cause depigmentation and potentially lead to secondary infection, particularly *Clostridium* spp infection. Survivors of severe infections recover in 10–14 days but may never recover lost performance.

The lesions are almost entirely in the intestinal tract and often have a distinctive location and appearance that is useful in diagnosis.

Chickens: *E tenella* infections are found only in the ceca and can be recognized by accumulation of blood in the ceca and by bloody droppings. Cecal cores, which are accumulations of clotted blood, tissue debris, and oocysts, may be found in birds surviving the acute stage.

E necatrix produces major lesions in the anterior and middle portions of the small intestine. Small white spots, usually intermingled with rounded, bright- or dull-red spots of various sizes, can be seen on the serosal surface. This appearance is sometimes described as "salt and pepper." The white spots are diagnostic for *E necatrix* if clumps of large schizonts can be demonstrated microscopically. In severe cases, the intestinal wall is thickened, and the infected area dilated to 2–2.5 times the normal diameter. The lumen may be filled with blood, mucus, and fluid. Fluid loss may result in marked dehydration. Although the damage is in the small intestine, the sexual phase of the life cycle is completed in the ceca. Oocysts of *E necatrix* are found only in the ceca. Because of concurrent infections, oocysts of other species may be found in the area of major lesions, misleading the diagnostician.

E acervulina is the most common cause of infection. Lesions include numerous whitish, oval or transverse patches in the upper half of the small intestine, which may be easily distinguished on gross examination. The clinical course in a flock is usually protracted and results in poor growth, an increase in culls, and slightly increased mortality.

E brunetti is found in the lower small intestine, rectum, ceca, and cloaca. In moderate infections, the mucosa is pale and disrupted but lacking in discrete foci, and may be thickened. In severe infections, coagulative necrosis and sloughing of the mucosa occurs throughout most of the small intestine.

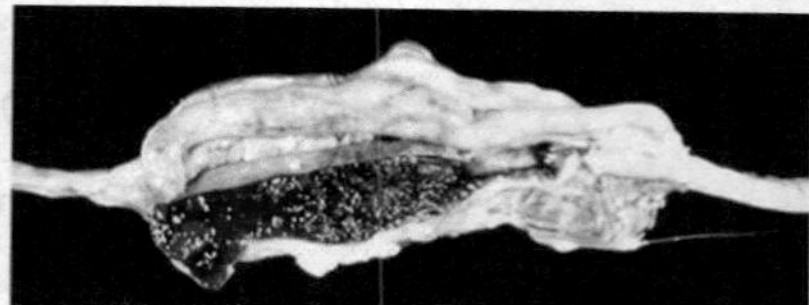

Gross lesions of *Eimeria tenella* with frank hemorrhaging into cecal pouches in a broiler chicken. *Courtesy of Dr. Jean Sander.*

E maxima develops in the small intestine, where it causes dilatation and thickening of the wall; petechial hemorrhage; and a reddish, orange, or pink viscous mucous exudate and fluid. The exterior of the midgut often has numerous whitish pinpoint foci, and the area may appear engorged. The oocysts and gametocytes (particularly macrogametocytes), which are present in the lesions, are distinctly large.

E mitis is recognized as pathogenic in the lower small intestine. Lesions are indistinct but may resemble moderate infections of *E brunetti*. *E mitis* can be distinguished from *E brunetti* by finding small, round oocysts associated with the lesion.

E praecox, which infects the upper small intestine, does not cause distinct lesions but may decrease rate of growth. The oocysts are larger than those of *E acervulina* and are numerous in affected areas. The intestinal contents may be watery. *E praecox* is considered to be of less economic importance than the other species.

E hagani and *E mivati* develop in the anterior part of the small intestine. The lesions of *E hagani* are indistinct and difficult to characterize. However, *E mivati* may cause severe lesions similar to those of *E acervulina*. In severe infections, *E mivati* may cause reddening of the duodenum because of denuding of the villi. Some consider these species to be of dubious provenance, but work with molecular diagnostics seems to support their validity.

Turkeys: Only four of the seven species of coccidia in turkeys are considered pathogenic: *E adenoides*, *E dispersa*, *E gallopavonis*, and *E meleagrimitis*. *E innocua*, *E meleagridis*, and *E subrotunda* are considered nonpathogenic. Oocysts sporulate within 1–2 days after expulsion from the host; the prepatent period is 4–6 days.

E adenoeides and *E gallopavonis* infect the lower ileum, ceca, and rectum. These species often cause mortality. The developmental stages are found in the epithelial cells of the villi and crypts. The affected portion of the intestine may be dilated and have a thickened wall. Thick, creamy material or caseous casts in the gut or excreta may contain enormous numbers of oocysts. *E meleagrimitis* chiefly infects the upper and mid small intestine. The lamina propria or deeper tissues may be parasitized, which may result in necrotic enteritis (*see* p 2802). *E dispersa* infects the upper small intestine and causes a creamy, mucoid enteritis that involves the entire intestine, including the ceca. Large numbers of gametocytes and oocysts are associated with the lesions.

Common signs in infected flocks include reduced feed consumption, rapid weight loss, droopiness, ruffled feathers, and severe diarrhea. Wet droppings with mucus are common. Clinical infections are seldom seen in poults >8 wk old. Morbidity and mortality may be high.

Game Birds: The Chinese ringneck pheasant, the chukar partridge, and the bobwhite quail, extremely popular as game birds, are reared in large numbers under conditions similar to those of chickens. Losses in these birds from coccidiosis often exceed 50% of a flock. In pheasants, the common species are *E phasiani*, *E colchici*, *E duodenalis*, *E tetartooimia*, and *E pacifica*. Chukars are infected by two species: *E kofoidi* and *E legionensis*. Bobwhite quail are infected mainly by *E lettyae*, *E dispersa*, and *E coloni*. Treatment and control of these coccidia are similar to that in poultry; however, amprolium appears to be of little use. Monensin and salinomycin are the approved drugs for quail, and lasalocid and sulfadimethoxine/ormetoprim are the approved drugs for chukars.

Ducks: A large number of specific coccidia have been reported in both wild and domestic ducks, but validity of some of the descriptions is questionable. Presence of *Eimeria*, *Wenyonella*, and *Tyzzeria* spp has been confirmed. *T perniciosa* is a known pathogen that balloons the entire small intestine with mucohemorrhagic or caseous material. *Eimeria* spp also have been described as pathogenic. Some species of coccidia of domestic ducks are considered relatively nonpathogenic. In wild ducks, infrequent but dramatic outbreaks of coccidiosis occur in ducklings 2–4 wk old; morbidity and mortality may be high.

Geese: The best known coccidial infection of geese is that produced by *E truncata*, in which the kidneys are enlarged and studded with poorly circumscribed, yellowish white streaks and spots. The tubules are dilated with masses of oocysts and urates. Mortality may be high. At least five other *Eimeria* spp have been reported to parasitize the intestine of geese, but these are of lesser importance.

Diagnosis: The location in the host, appearance of lesions, and the size of oocysts are used in determining the species present. Coccidial infections are readily confirmed by demonstration of oocysts in feces or intestinal scrapings; however, the number of oocysts present has little relationship to the extent of clinical disease. Severity of lesions as well as knowledge of flock appearance, morbidity, daily mortality, feed intake, growth rate, and rate of lay are important for diagnosis. Necropsy of several fresh specimens is advisable. Classic lesions of *E tenella* and *E necatrix* are pathognomonic, but infections of other species are more difficult to diagnose. Comparison of lesions and other signs with diagnostic charts allows a reasonably accurate differentiation of the coccidial species. Mixed coccidial infections are common.

A diagnosis of clinical coccidiosis is warranted if oocysts, merozoites, or schizonts are seen microscopically and if lesions are severe. Subclinical coccidial infections may be unimportant, and poor performance may be caused by other flock disorders.

Control: Practical methods of management cannot prevent coccidial infection. Poultry that are maintained at all times on wire floors to separate birds from droppings have fewer infections; clinical coccidiosis is seen only rarely under such circumstances. Other methods of control are vaccination or prevention with anticoccidial drugs.

Vaccination: A species-specific immunity develops after natural infection, the degree of which largely depends on the extent of infection and the number of reinfections. Protective immunity is primarily a T-cell response.

Commercial vaccines consist of live, sporulated oocysts of the various coccidial species administered at low doses. Modern anticoccidial vaccines should be given to day-old chicks, either at the hatchery or on

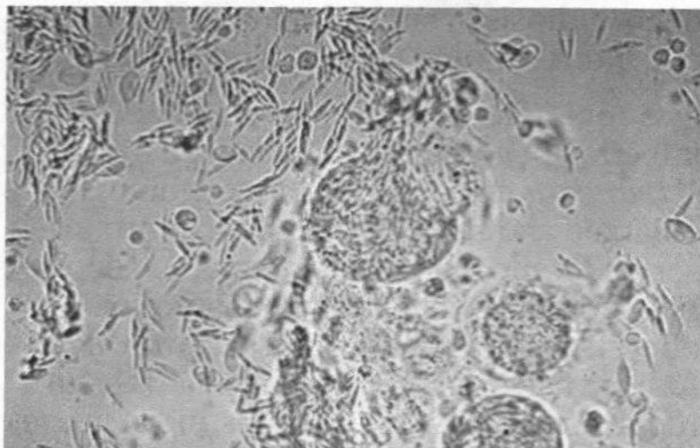

Release of merozoite from mature schizont, new methylene blue, 100×. *Courtesy of Dr. Jean Sander.*

the farm. Because the vaccine serves only to introduce infection, chickens are reinfected by progeny of the vaccine strain on the farm. Most commercial vaccines contain live oocysts of coccidia that are not attenuated. The self-limiting nature of coccidiosis is used as a form of attenuation for some vaccines, rather than biologic attenuation. Some vaccines sold in Europe and South America include attenuated lines of coccidia. Research has shown promise for vaccination in game birds.

Layers and breeders maintained on floor litter must have protective immunity. Historically, these birds were given a suboptimal dosage of an anticoccidial drug during early growth, with the expectation that immunity would continue to develop from repeated exposure to wild types of coccidia. This method has never been completely successful because of the difficulty in controlling all the factors affecting reproduction of coccidia under practical conditions. Although anticoccidial drugs have been preferred for protection of these birds, vaccination programs are gaining popularity. Better administration techniques and choice of coccidia strains in the product are improving the feasibility of vaccination in broilers.

Anticoccidial Drugs: Many products are available for prevention or treatment of coccidiosis in chickens and turkeys (*see* TABLES 1 and 2). Detailed instructions for use are provided by all manufacturers to help users with management considerations and to ensure compliance with regulatory approvals.

Anticoccidials are given in the feed to prevent disease and the economic loss often associated with subacute infection. Prophylactic use is preferred, because most of the damage occurs before signs become apparent and because drugs cannot completely stop an outbreak. Therapeutic treatments are usually given by water because of the logistical restraints of feed administration. Antibiotics and increased levels of vitamins A and K are sometimes used in the ration to improve rate of recovery and prevent secondary infections.

Continuous use of anticoccidial drugs promotes the emergence of drug-resistant strains of coccidia. Various programs are used in attempts to slow or stop selection of resistance. For instance, producers may use one anticoccidial continuously through succeeding flocks, change to alternative anticoccidials every 4–6 mo, or change anticoccidials during a single growout (ie, a shuttle program). While there is little cross-resistance to anticoccidials with different modes of action, there is widespread resistance to most drugs. Coccidia can be tested in the laboratory to determine which products are most effective. "Shuttle programs," in which one group of chickens is treated sequentially with different drugs (usually a change between the starter and grower rations), are common practice and offer some benefit in slowing the emergence of resistance. In the USA, the FDA considers shuttle programs as extra-label usage, but producers may use such programs on the recommendation of a veterinarian.

The effects of anticoccidial drugs may be coccidiostatic, in which growth of intracellular coccidia is arrested but development may continue after drug withdrawal, or coccidiocidal, in which coccidia are killed during their development. Some anticoccidial drugs may be coccidiostatic when given short-term but coccidiocidal when given longterm. Most anticoccidials currently used in poultry production are coccidiocidal.

The natural development of immunity to coccidiosis may proceed during the use of anticoccidials in the feed. However, in the production of broilers during a short growout of 37–44 days, this may be of little consequence. Natural immunity is important in replacement layer pullets, because they are likely to be exposed to coccidial infections for extended periods after termination of anticoccidial drugs. Anticoccidial programs for layer and breeder flocks are intended to allow immunizing infection while guarding against acute outbreaks.

Anticoccidials are commonly withdrawn from broilers 3–7 days before slaughter to meet regulatory requirements and to reduce production costs. Because broilers have varying susceptibility to infection at this point, the risk of coccidiosis outbreaks is increased with longer withdrawal.

Turkeys are given a preventive anticoccidial for confinement-reared birds up to 8–10 wk of age. Older birds are considered less susceptible to outbreaks.

The modes of action of anticoccidial drugs are poorly understood. Some that are better known are described below. Knowledge of mode of action is important in understanding toxicity and adverse effects.

Amprolium is an antagonist of thiamine (vitamin B_1). Rapidly dividing coccidia have a high requirement for thiamine. Amprolium has a safety margin of ~8:1 when used at

TABLE 2 DRUGS FOR PREVENTION OF COCCIDIOSIS IN POULTRY

Drug[a]	Use Level (% in feed) Chickens	Turkeys	Withdrawal Time (days)
Amprolium	0.0125–0.025	0.0125–0.025	0
Amprolium + ethopabate	0.0125–0.025 + 0.0004–0.004	—	0
Clopidol or meticlorpindol	0.0125–0.025	—	0
Decoquinate	0.003	—	0
Diclazuril	0.0001	0.0001	0
Dinitolmide (zoalene)	0.004–0.0125	0.0125–0.01875	0
Halofuginone hydrobromide	0.0003	0.00015–0.0003	4–7
Lasalocid sodium	0.0075–0.0125	0.0075–0.0125	3
Maduramicin ammonium	0.0005–0.0006	—	5
Monensin sodium	0.01–0.0121	0.006–0.01[b]	0
Narasin	0.006–0.008	—	0
Narasin + nicarbazin	0.003–0.005 (of the combination)	—	5
Nicarbazin	0.0125	—	4
Robenidine hydrochloride	0.0033	—	5
Salinomycin sodium	0.0044–0.0066	—	0
Semduramicin	0.0025	—	0
Sulfadimethoxine + ormetoprim	0.0125 + 0.0075	0.00625 + 0.00375	5

[a] Approved in the USA; compiled from various sources, including, with permission, the *Feed Additive Compendium*, The Miller Publishing Co., 2008. Anticoccidials not approved in the USA but available in various other countries include clazuril, a combination of clopidol plus methylbenzoquate, and various combinations of ionophores with nicarbazin.

[b] Up to 10 wk of age.

TABLE 3 DRUGS FOR TREATMENT OF COCCIDIOSIS IN CHICKENS

Drug[a]	Feed or Water	Use Level, Treatment Duration	Withdrawal Time (days)
Amprolium	Water	0.012%–0.024%, 3–5 days; 0.006%, 1–2 wk	0
Chlortetracycline	Feed	0.022% + 0.8% calcium, not more than 3 wk	0
Oxytetracycline	Feed	0.022% + 0.18%–0.55% calcium, not more than 5 days	3
Sodium sulfachloropyrazine monohydrate	Water	0.03%, 3 days	4
Sulfadimethoxine	Water	0.05%, 6 days	5
Sulfamethazine (sulfadimidine)	Water	0.1%, 2 days; 0.05%, 4 days	10
Toltrazuril	Water	25 ppm, 2 days	NA[b]

[a] Approved in the USA, except for toltrazuril
[b] Not applicable

the highest recommended level in feed (125–250 ppm). Because amprolium has poor activity against some *Eimeria* spp, its spectrum has been extended by using it in mixtures with the folic acid antagonists ethopabate and sulfaquinoxaline. The primary use of amprolium today is for water treatment during clinical outbreaks.

Clopidol and **quinolines** (eg, decoquinate, methylbenzoquate) are coccidiostatic against early development of *Eimeria* spp by inhibiting mitochondrial energy production. Clopidol and quinolines have a broad species spectrum and are sometimes mixed together for synergism. However, resistance may develop rapidly during extended use.

Folic acid antagonists include the sulfonamides, 2,4-diaminopyrimidines, and ethopabate. These compounds are structural antagonists of folic acid or of para-aminobenzoic acid (PABA), which is a precursor of folic acid. (The host does not synthesize folic acid and has no requirement for PABA.) Coccidia rapidly synthesize nucleic acids, accounting for activity of PABA antagonists. Although resistance to antifolate compounds is widespread, they are commonly used for water treatment when clinical signs are already evident. Diaveridine, ormetoprim, and pyrimethamine are active against the protozoan enzyme dihydrofolate reductase. They have synergistic activity with sulfonamides and often are used in mixtures with these compounds.

Halofuginone hydrobromide is related to the antimalarial drug febrifuginone and is effective against asexual stages of most species of *Eimeria*. It has both coccidiostatic and coccidiocidal effects, but coccidia may become resistant after extended exposure.

The **ionophores** (**monensin**, **salinomycin**, **lasalocid**, **narasin**, **maduramicin**, and **semduramicin**) form complexes with various ions, principally sodium, potassium, and calcium, and transport these into and through biologic membranes. The ionophores affect both extra- and intracellular stages of the parasite, especially during the early, asexual stages of parasite development. Drug tolerance was slow to emerge in chicken coccidia, probably because of the biochemically nonspecific way these fermentation products act on the parasite. Recent surveys suggest that drug tolerance is now widespread, but these products remain the most important class of anticoccidials.

Some ionophores may depress feed consumption when the dosage is above recommended levels. Primarily, this is the result of reduced feed consumption, but the reduced growth may be offset by improved feed conversion.

Nicarbazin was the first product to have truly broad-spectrum activity and has been in common use since 1955. Although not completely understood, the mode of action is thought to be via inhibition of succinate-linked nicotinamide adenine dinucleotide reduction and the energy-dependent transhydrogenase, and the accumulation of calcium in the presence of ATP. Nicarbazin is toxic for layers, causing mottling of egg yolks, decreased egg production, and blanching of brown egg shells. A 4-day withdrawal period is required in broilers. Medicated birds are at increased risk of heat stress in hot weather.

Nitrobenzamides (eg, dinitolmide) exert their greatest coccidiostatic activity against the asexual stages. Efficacy is limited to *E tenella* and *E necatrix* unless combined with other products.

Robenidine, a guanidine compound, allows initial intracellular development of coccidia but prevents formation of mature schizonts. It is coccidiostatic when given short term and coccidiocidal long term. Drug resistance may develop during use. A 5-day withdrawal period is needed to eliminate untoward flavor caused by residues in poultry meat.

Roxarsone is an organic arsenical compound. It has significant activity against *E tenella* and is used in combination with ionophores to improve control of that species. A withdrawal period is required.

Diclazuril and **toltrazuril** are highly effective against a broad spectrum of coccidia. Diclazuril is used mostly for prevention at 1 ppm in the feed, whereas toltrazuril is used primarily for treatment in the water.

CORONAVIRAL ENTERITIS OF TURKEYS

(Bluecomb, Mud fever, Transmissible enteritis)

Coronaviral enteritis is an acute, highly contagious disease of turkeys characterized by depression, anorexia, diarrhea, and decreased weight gain. Mortality may be high, particularly in young poults, but failure to gain body weight in adult birds may be more important economically. The causative agent is turkey coronavirus (TCV), but clinical disease usually is complicated by other enteric viral, bacterial, and protozoal infections.

Epidemiology: Coronaviral enteritis has been identified in turkeys in the USA, Canada, Brazil, Italy, UK, and Australia. The disease has been reported in most turkey-producing regions of the USA. Turkey coronavirus affects turkeys of all ages; however, clinical disease most commonly is seen in young turkeys during the first few weeks of life. Turkeys are believed to be the only natural host for TCV.

TCV is shed in feces of infected birds and spread horizontally through ingestion of feces and feces-contaminated materials. Virus is shed in droppings of turkeys for several weeks after recovery from clinical disease. Infection generally spreads rapidly through a flock and from flock to flock on the same or neighboring farms. Mechanical movement of the virus may occur by people, equipment, vehicles, and insects. Darkling beetle larvae and domestic house flies are potential mechanical vectors. Wild birds, rodents, and dogs also may serve as mechanical vectors. There is no evidence that TCV is egg transmitted; however, poults may become infected in the hatchery via contaminated personnel and fomites such as egg boxes from infected farms.

Clinical Findings: Clinical signs occur suddenly, usually with high morbidity. Birds exhibit depression, anorexia, decreased water consumption, watery diarrhea, dehydration, hypothermia, and weight loss. Droppings typically are green to brown, watery, and frothy, and may contain mucus and urates. Affected flocks have increased mortality, growth depression, and poor feed conversion. Morbidity generally approaches 100%, but mortality is variable; mortality may be high depending on the age of the birds, concurrent infection, management practices, and weather conditions.

In breeder hens, egg production drops rapidly. Egg quality also is affected; hens produce white, chalky eggs lacking normal pigmentation.

Lesions: Gross lesions are seen primarily in the intestines. The duodenum and jejunum generally are pale, thin-walled, and flaccid; ceca are distended with gas and watery contents. Emaciation, dehydration, and atrophy of the bursa of Fabricius also may be seen.

In the intestines, microscopic lesions consist of a decrease in villous length and increase in crypt depth; the columnar epithelium changes to a cuboidal epithelium, and these cells exhibit a loss of microvilli. There is a decrease in the number of goblet cells, separation of enterocytes from the lamina propria, and infiltration of the lamina propria with heterophils and lymphocytes.

In the bursa of Fabricius, the normal pseudostratified columnar epithelium is replaced by a stratified squamous epithelium, and intense heterophilic inflammation is seen within and underneath the epithelium.

Diagnosis: Diagnosis generally requires laboratory assistance, because other enteric pathogens of turkeys may cause similar clinical signs and lesions. Laboratory diagnosis is based on virus isolation, electron microscopy, serology, or detection of viral antigens or viral RNA in intestinal tissues, the bursa of Fabricius, or intestinal contents. Preferred clinical samples for diagnostic analyses include serum, intestinal contents, and fresh tissues (intestines and bursa of Fabricius); these samples should be kept cold (on ice at 4°C or frozen) at all times. Coronaviral enteritis must be distinguished from other enteric viral, bacterial, and parasitic infections, including those caused by astrovirus, rotavirus, reovirus, *Salmonella* spp, and crytosporidia.

Prevention and Treatment: Prevention is the preferred method to control TCV. No commercial vaccine is available. Infected turkeys shed virus in feces for prolonged periods after recovery; these turkeys, their feces, and the materials their feces contact are potential sources of infection for other susceptible turkeys. Feces from infected turkeys can be carried on a variety of fomites, including clothing, boots, equipment, feathers, and trucks. Other potential vectors, such as wild birds, rodents, dogs, and flies, also may be involved in transmission. Biosecurity measures must be instituted to prevent introduction of TCV via potentially contaminated personnel, fomites, animal and insect vectors, and infected turkeys.

TCV may be eliminated from contaminated premises by depopulation followed by thorough cleaning and disinfection of houses and equipment. After cleaning and disinfection procedures, premises should remain free of birds for a minimum of 3–4 wk.

There is no specific treatment for TCV enteritis. Antibiotic treatment reduces mortality but not growth depression, most likely by controlling secondary bacterial infections. No beneficial effect was seen when glucose, electrolytes, or calf milk replacer was added to drinking water. Effective management procedures to reduce mortality include raising brooder house temperatures and avoiding crowded conditions.

CRYPTOSPORIDIOSIS

Cryptosporidiosis is caused by protozoa (phylum Apicomplexa) that are members of the family Cryptosporidiidae and are related, but distinct, to coccidia of the genera *Eimeria*, *Isospora*, *Sarcocystis*, and *Toxoplasma*. Until recently, it was thought that there were 19 species in the genus *Cryptosporidium*, but research has shown that most are merely species that lack host specificity. Cryptosporidia are parasitic in the intestine of mammals (*see* p 209), but in birds they are commonly found in the bursa and in the respiratory tract. Cryptosporidiosis is more severe in turkeys than in chickens and is frequently fatal in quail.

The life cycle of *Cryptosporidium* involves asexual and sexual phases and culminates in oocyst production. In the host, the oocyst forms four sporozoites without sporocysts. The life cycle is not self-limiting, because some oocysts are thin-walled and release sporozoites (after trypsin/bile stimulation) that reinfect

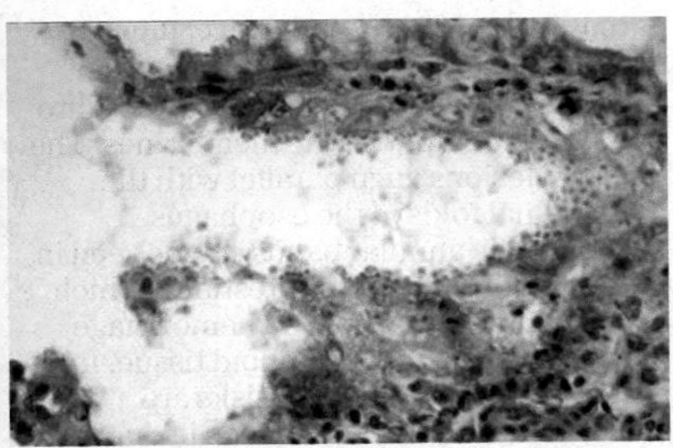
Cryptosporidium on tracheal mucosa of a turkey, H&E, 40×. *Courtesy of Dr. Jean Sander.*

adjacent tissues. The endogenous cycle is short (4–7 days), the endogenous stages are small (4–7 μm), and the parasites are just beneath the epithelial cell membranes.

In turkeys and chickens, *Cryptosporidium* have been found in the sinuses, trachea, bronchi, cloaca, and bursa. The most common clinical signs include diarrhea and dehydration. In addition to diarrhea, the parasites can infect the respiratory tract and lead to coughing, gasping, airsacculitis, and sometimes death. Lungs become gray and wet. Signs may last several weeks.

Diagnosis is by microscopic examination of tissue scrapings or histologic examination of tissues from the bursa, cloaca, and trachea. The small (5 μm) oocysts can be diagnostic but are difficult to see. Concentration of intestinal scrapings using saturated sugar solution and examination by phase-contrast or interference-contrast microscopy may improve visualization. Positive identification should be performed by trained researchers or diagnosticians.

There are no satisfactory control measures except isolation and good sanitation. None of the known anticoccidial drugs is effective against *Cryptosporidium* spp. Unlike *Cryptosporidium* spp of other mammals, the avian species are not infectious to people.

DUCK VIRAL ENTERITIS

(Duck plague, Anatid herpes, Eendenpest, Entenpest, Peste du canard)

Duck viral enteritis (DVE) is an acute, highly contagious disease of ducks, geese, and swans of all ages, characterized by sudden death, high mortality (particularly among older ducks), and hemorrhages and necrosis in internal organs. It has been reported in domestic and wild waterfowl in Europe, Asia, North America, and Africa, resulting in limited to serious economic losses on domestic duck farms and sporadic, limited to massive die-offs in wild waterfowl. In the USA, considerable losses due to DVE have been reported in the concentrated duck-producing areas located in Long Island, New York.

Members of the family Anatidae (ducks, geese, and swans) are the natural hosts for the virus. There are differences in susceptibility to the virus, with Muscovy ducks being the most susceptible. However, naturally occurring infections have been reported in a variety of domestic ducks such as Pekin, Khaki Campbell, Indian runners, and mixed breeds. The age at infection ranges from 7 days to maturity. The infection has not been reported in other avian species, mammals, or people and does not pose a zoonotic risk.

Etiology and Pathogenesis: The causative agent of DVE (species Anatid herpesvirus 1) is a member of the family Herpesviridae, subfamily Alphaherpesvirinae, and genus *Mardivirus*. Field strains of this virus display differences in virulence, but all seem to be immunologically identical. The virus is sensitive to lipid solvents and heat (10 min at 56°C [132.8°F]). Significant titer reduction is observed at pH 5, 6, and 10; rapid inactivation occurs at pH 3 and 11.

The virus induces vascular damage, especially in smaller blood vessels, venules, and capillaries. This results in the development of generalized hemorrhages and progressive degenerative changes of parenchymatous organs. Recently, it has been proposed that apoptosis and necrosis of lymphocytes induced by this virus may result in lymphoid depletion and possibly immunosuppression. An immunosuppressive state induced by DVE may also explain the presence of secondary infections by *Pasteurella multocida*, *Riemerella anatipestifer*, and *Escherichia coli*, which are frequently seen in natural outbreaks of DVE in ducklings.

Epidemiology and Transmission: The virus is mainly transmitted by direct contact from infected to susceptible ducks or by indirect contact with a contaminated environment. Water seems to be a natural route of viral transmission. Outbreaks are frequent in duck flocks with access to bodies of water cohabited with free-living waterfowl. Parenteral, intranasal, or oral administration of infected tissues can establish experimental infection. A carrier condition is suspected in wild birds. Recovered birds become latently infected carriers and may shed the virus periodically. DVE virus may undergo latency like other herpesviruses, and the trigeminal ganglion seems to be a latency site for the virus. Recovered birds may carry the virus in its latent form, and viral reactivation may be the cause of outbreaks in susceptible wild and domestic ducks.

Clinical Findings: The incubation period is 3–7 days. Sudden high and persistent mortality is often the first sign of the disease. Mortality varies and can be 5%–100%, depending on virulence of the infecting viral strain. Adult ducks usually die in higher proportions than young ones, increasing the economic significance of the disease. Sick birds are unable to stand and show indication of weakness and depression. Photophobia, inappetence, extreme thirst, droopiness, ataxia, nasal discharge, soiled vents, and watery or bloody diarrhea may be seen. Adult ducks may die in good flesh. In contrast, ducklings frequently show dehydration and weight loss, as well as blue beaks and blood-stained vents. Dead males may have prolapse of the penis. In laying flocks, egg production may drop sharply.

Lesions: The lesions are indicative of disseminated intravascular coagulopathy and necrosis of the mucosa and submucosa of the GI tract and lymphoid tissues. Damage of blood vessels throughout the body induces hemorrhages in various tissues or the presence of free blood in body cavities. Petechial and ecchymotic hemorrhages on the heart ("paint-brush" appearance), liver, pancreas, mesentery, and other organs are characteristic. Specific mucosal eruptions, found in the oral cavity, esophagus, ceca, rectum, and cloaca, undergo progressive alterations during the course of the disease. Macular hemorrhages initially develop into elevated, yellowish, crusted plaques and organize into green, superficial scabs, which may coalesce into large, patchy, diphtheritic membranes. The mucosal lesions align parallel with the longitudinal folds in the esophagus. Hemorrhagic annular bands can be seen in different portions of the intestines, which correspond to necrosis and hemorrhage of the gut-associated lymphoid tissue. In geese, intestinal lymphoid disks are analogous to the annular bands in ducks, and "button-like" ulcers may be seen. Diphtheritic esophagitis may be commonly seen in swans. Lumina of the intestines and gizzard are often filled with blood. The liver is enlarged, pale copper in color, and may have pinpoint surface hemorrhages mixed with white necrotic foci. The pancreas may have petechiation and multifocal necrosis.

The lymphoid organs are severely affected; the spleen may be normal or smaller in size and darkened due to congestion. The thymic lobes may be petechiated, and thymic atrophy has been reported with some strains. The bursa of Fabricius may be severely congested or hemorrhagic. In ducklings, the lesions of the lymphoid tissues are more evident than the lesions in other visceral organs. A lesion that can be easily detected on necropsy is a clear, yellow fluid that infiltrates and discolors the subcutaneous tissues from the thoracic inlet to the upper third of the neck. In mature hens, hemorrhages may be seen in deformed and discolored ovarian follicles, and ruptured yolk and free blood may be found in the abdominal cavity.

Microscopically, eosinophilic intranuclear inclusions may be seen in the epithelial cells of the GI tract and in the thymus, bursa, spleen, esophagus, cloaca, liver, conjunctiva, and Harderian gland. Occasional intracytoplasmic inclusions are also scattered in the epithelial cells of the conjunctiva, esophagus, bursa of Fabricius, and cloaca.

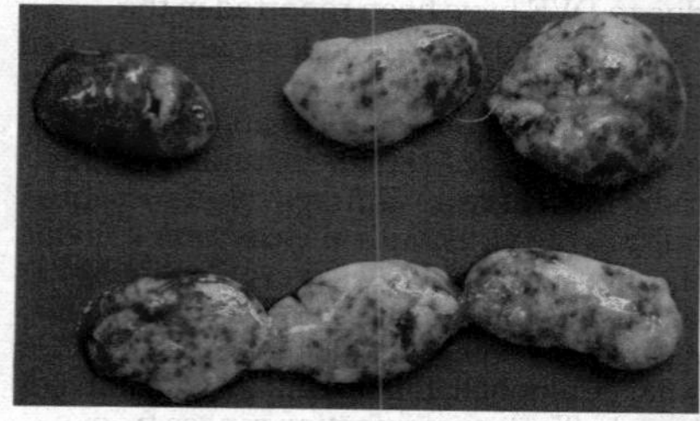

Duck viral enteritis, mottled thymus with multiple petechiae and necrotic focal areas. *Courtesy of Dr. Alejandro Banda.*

Diagnosis: Presumptive diagnosis is based on disease history and lesions. Definitive diagnosis may require viral isolation or identification of DVE. Different diagnostic protocols based on PCR are available, either by conventional or quantitative real-time PCR. These molecular techniques provide much more rapid and efficient diagnosis of this disease than other methods. The tissues to collect are liver, spleen, esophagus, and portions of small intestine that show suggestive lesions. Isolation of the virus from liver, spleen, or kidney tissues may be attempted in various cell cultures (preferably primary Muscovy duck embryo fibroblasts or Muscovy duck embryo liver cultures), duck embryos, or ducklings. Inoculating the chorioallantoic membrane of 9- to 14-day-old embryonated Muscovy duck eggs may result in isolation of the virus, but this method is not as sensitive as IM inoculation of day-old ducklings. Muscovy ducklings are more susceptible than White Pekin ducklings. Neutralization with specific antiserum in these systems confirms the identity of the virus. Fluorescent antibody testing can demonstrate DVE viral proteins. Serologic tests have little value in the diagnosis of acute infections. Serum neutralization tests have been used to monitor exposure to the virus in wildfowl.

Differential diagnoses include duck viral hepatitis, pasteurellosis, necrotic and hemorrhagic enteritis, trauma, drake damage, and various toxicoses. Newcastle disease, avian influenza, and fowlpox may cause similar lesions but are rarely reported in ducks. Established cases should be reported to the appropriate regulatory agency.

Prevention, Treatment, and Control: There is no treatment. Contact with wild, free-flying waterfowl and direct or indirect contact with contaminated birds or material (free-flowing water) should be avoided. Control is effected by depopulation, removal of birds from the infected environment, sanitation, and disinfection. Prevention is based on maintenance of susceptible birds in a disease-free environment or immunization. A chicken-embryo-adapted, modified-live virus vaccine has been approved in the USA to immunize domestic ducks in zoological aviaries and by private aviculturists. A 0.5-mL dose is administered SC or IM to domestic ducklings >2 wk old. Breeding flocks should be revaccinated annually. The vaccine can be used in an outbreak, because it elicits rapid protection after vaccination. It is not approved for use in wild ducks. An inactivated vaccine, which appears to be as efficacious as the modified-live vaccine, has not been tested on a large scale and is not currently licensed.

HEXAMITIASIS

Hexamitiasis is an acute, infectious, catarrhal enteritis of turkeys, pheasants, quail, chukar partridges, and peafowl. The highest mortality occurs in birds 1–9 wk old. Natural infection has not been observed in chickens. Pigeons are susceptible to another species of *Spironucleus* (*S columbae*). Hexamitiasis is rare in North America.

Etiology: The causative protozoan parasite in turkeys, *S meleagridis* (formerly *Hexamita meleagridis*) is spindle-shaped; averages 8 × 3 µm; and has four anterior, two anterolateral, and two posterior flagella. It has not yet been cultured in experimental media, although it has been grown in the allantoic cavity of developing chicken and turkey embryos. It is transmitted directly by ingestion of contaminated feces and water. Encysted hexamitids are resistant to environmental conditions outside the bird and, therefore, may be more important in the transmission of the disease. Up to ⅓ of the recovering birds become carriers and shed parasites in their droppings.

Clinical Findings and Lesions: Signs of hexamitiasis are nonspecific and include watery diarrhea that may be yellowish later in the disease, dry unkempt feathers, listlessness, and rapid weight loss despite the fact the birds continue to eat. Birds may die in coma or convulsions. Bulbous dilatations of the small intestine (especially duodenum and upper jejunum) filled with watery contents are characteristic. The crypts of Lieberkühn contain myriad *S meleagridis*, which attach to the epithelial cells by their posterior flagella.

Diagnosis: Diagnosis of hexamitiasis depends on finding the flagellates by microscopic examination of scrapings of the duodenal and jejunal mucosa. *Spironucleus* spp move with a rapid, darting motion (in contrast to the jerky motion of trichomonads). To avoid contamination of instruments with other cecal protozoa, the duodenum should be opened first. *Spironucleus* spp may be demonstrated in poults that have been dead for several hours if the scrapings are placed in a drop of warm (104°F [40°C]), isotonic saline solution on the slide. Presence of a few *Spironucleus* in birds >10 wk old may be unimportant in terms of the disease but still act as a reservoir of infection.

Prevention and Treatment: Because many birds remain carriers of *Spironucleus*, breeder turkeys and young poults should be raised on separate premises if possible, preferably with separate attendants. Wire platforms should be used under feeders and waterers. Pheasants and quail may also be carriers and should not be raised in the same location as poults. Indirect transmission can occur if affected fecal material is transferred to another location by contaminated equipment or clothing.

There is no effective treatment or vaccine for hexamitiasis, although oxytetracycline (0.011% in the feed for 2 wk) or chlortetracycline (0.022%–0.044% in the feed for 2 wk) may be of some benefit to control secondary infections.

NECROTIC ENTERITIS

Necrotic enteritis is an acute enterotoxemia. The clinical illness is usually very short, and often the only signs are a severe depression followed quickly by a sudden increase in flock mortality. The disease primarily affects broiler chickens (2–5 wk old) and turkeys (7–12 wk old) raised on litter but can also affect commercial layer pullets raised in cages. Early mortality is often related to coccidiosis vaccination programs, with *Eimeria* cycling in these flocks.

Etiology and Pathogenesis: The causative agent is the gram-positive, obligate, anaerobic bacteria *Clostridium perfringens*. It is usually isolated on blood agar, incubated anaerobically at 37°C (98.6°F), on which it produces a double zone of hemolysis. There are two primary *C perfringens* types, A and C, associated with necrotic enteritis in poultry. Toxins produced by the bacteria cause damage to the small intestine, liver lesions, and mortality.

C perfringens is a nearly ubiquitous bacteria readily found in soil, dust, feces, feed, and used poultry litter. It is also a normal inhabitant of the intestines of healthy chickens and turkeys. The enterotoxemia that results in clinical disease most often occurs either after a change in the intestinal microflora or from a condition that results in damage to the intestinal mucosa (eg, coccidiosis, mycotoxicosis, salmonellosis, ascarid larvae). High dietary levels of animal byproducts (eg, fishmeal), wheat, barley, oats, or rye predispose birds to the disease. Anything that promotes excessive bacterial growth and toxin production or slows feed passage rate in the small intestine could promote the occurrence of necrotic enteritis. In many cases, concurrent coccidiosis (especially *Eimeria maxima*, and *E acervulina* to a lesser extent) is associated with outbreaks in commercial broilers, although recent investigations with NetB-positive isolates have reportedly caused disease without predisposition from *Eimeria* infections.

Clinical Findings and Lesions: Most often the only sign of necrotic enteritis in a flock is a sudden increase in mortality. However, birds with depression, ruffled feathers, and diarrhea may also be seen. The gross lesions are primarily found in the small intestine (jejunum/ileum), which may be ballooned, friable, and contain a foul-smelling, brown fluid. The mucosa is usually covered with a tan to yellow pseudomembrane often referred to as a "Turkish towel" in appearance. This pseudomembrane may extend throughout the small intestine or be localized. The disease usually persists in a flock for 5–10 days, and mortality is 2%–50%.

Diagnosis: A presumptive diagnosis is based on gross lesions and a gram-stained smear of a mucosal scraping that exhibits large, gram-positive rods. Histologic

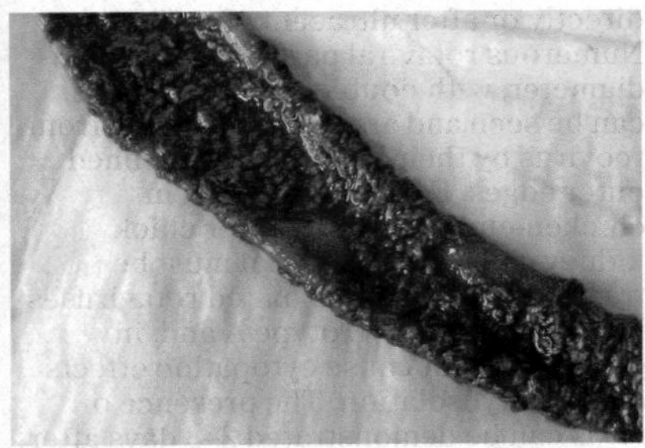

Mucosal surface of small intestine of a broiler chicken infected with *Clostridium perfringens* (necrotic enteritis). *Courtesy of Dr. Billy Hargis.*

findings consist of coagulative necrosis of one-third to one-half the thickness of the intestinal mucosa and masses of short, thick bacterial rods in the fibrinonecrotic debris. Isolation of large numbers of *C perfringens*, from intestinal contents that produce the double zone of hemolysis as described above, can confirm the diagnosis. Double zone hemolysis should not be used as the sole criterion for identification of *C perfringens*, because some strains do not produce both toxins responsible for the hemolysis characteristics. Differential media specifically designed for isolation of *C perfringens* is available and may be useful for diagnosis.

Necrotic enteritis must be differentiated from lesions produced by *Eimeria brunetti* and also from ulcerative enteritis. Uncomplicated coccidiosis rarely produces lesions as acute or severe as those seen with necrotic enteritis. Ulcerative enteritis caused by *C colinum* usually produces focal lesions from the distal portion of the small intestine (ileum) to the ceca and is almost always accompanied by hepatic necrosis.

Prevention, Control, and Treatment: Because *C perfringens* is nearly ubiquitous, it is important to prevent coccidiosis, especially *E acervulina* and *E maxima* infections, as well as changes in the intestinal microflora that would promote its growth. This has traditionally been accomplished by adding antibiotics in the feed such as virginiamycin (20 g/ton feed), bacitracin (50 g/ton feed), and lincomycin (2 g/ton feed), as well as ionophore-class anticoccidial treatments. The move to antibiotic-free feeds has also been associated with markedly increased use of coccidiosis vaccines, resulting in early circulation of mixed *Eimeria* infections that are associated with the resurgence in incidence of necrotic enteritis. Avoiding drastic changes in feed and minimizing the level of fishmeal, wheat, barley, or rye in the diet can also help prevent necrotic enteritis. When higher amounts of wheat, barley, or rye are necessary, use of enzymes for nonstarch polysaccharides in the feed has reduced the level of necrotic enteritis in flocks fed these cereals. Administration of selected probiotics or competitive exclusion cultures has been used successfully to both prevent and treat clinical necrotic enteritis (presumably by preventing proliferation of *C perfringens*).

Treatment for necrotic enteritis is most commonly administered in the drinking water, with bacitracin (200–400 mg/gal. for 5–7 days), penicillin (1,500,000 u/gal. for 5 days), and lincomycin (64 mg/gal. for 7 days) most often used. In each case, the medicated drinking water should be the sole source of water. Moribund birds should be removed promptly, because they can serve as a source of toxicosis or infection due to cannibalism.

ROTAVIRAL INFECTIONS IN CHICKENS, TURKEYS, AND PHEASANTS

Rotaviral infections are characterized by enteritis and diarrhea in young birds, but chickens have been infected without showing clinical signs.

Avian rotaviruses consist of four distinct serotypes (A–D). Group A rotaviruses share a common group antigen with mammalian rotaviruses. Group D rotaviruses have been identified only in avian species. The relationships of the other two avian serotypes to mammalian serotypes have not been established. Transmission is horizontally by the oral route. Egg transmission has not been reported.

Early signs of diarrhea (wet litter), depression, and poor or abnormal appetite can be seen 2–5 days after infection. Dehydration occurs rapidly, and mortality can be as high as 30%–50% in pheasants but is lower in turkeys and chickens. The survivors appear healthy but smaller than normal. Lesions consist of dilated intestines filled with yellowish, frothy, watery contents. Often, the carcass is dehydrated. Mortality is variable and is usually due to dehydration and emaciation or secondary bacterial infections.

Early diarrhea and inappetence that sometimes end with death are indicative but not pathognomonic of rotaviral infection. Fecal samples or intestinal contents can be examined by electron microscopy with negative staining, either directly or after ultracentrifugation. Numerous rotaviral particles ~70 nm in diameter, with double-shelled capsids, can be seen and are distinguishable from reovirus by their more sharply defined outer edges. For viral isolation in chicken-embryo liver cells or chick kidney cells, fecal material must be treated with trypsin. Isolated rotaviruses belong mostly to serotype A and, in general, do not cause cytopathic effects on primary isolation. The presence of virus can be demonstrated 2–3 days after inoculation by immunofluorescent staining. Reverse transcriptase PCR is currently used to detect the virus in gut contents.

No commercial vaccines are available. Thorough cleaning and disinfection of infected houses is advisable to limit infection. There is no specific treatment.

TRICHOMONOSIS

Trichomonosis in domestic fowl, pigeons, doves, songbirds, and hawks is characterized, in most cases, by caseous accumulations in the throat and usually by weight loss. It has been termed "canker," "roup," and, in hawks, "frounce."

Etiology: Both *Trichomonas gallinae* and a newly recognized species, *T stableri*, are the causative organisms of trichomonosis. These flagellated protozoa live in the sinuses, mouth, throat, esophagus, liver, and other organs. Trichomonosis is more prevalent among domestic pigeons and wild doves than among domestic fowl, although severe outbreaks have been reported in chickens and turkeys. Some trichomonad strains cause high mortality in pigeons and doves. Hawks may become diseased after eating infected birds and commonly show liver lesions, with or without throat involvement. Pigeons and doves transmit the infection to their offspring in contaminated pigeon milk. Contaminated water is probably the most important source of infection for chickens, turkeys, and songbirds, and the parasite has been shown to survive at least 20 min in distilled water.

Clinical Findings: The disease course of trichomonosis is rapid. The first lesions appear as small, yellowish areas on the oral mucosa. They grow rapidly and coalesce to form masses that frequently completely block the esophagus and may prevent the bird from closing its mouth. Much fluid may accumulate in the mouth. There is a watery ocular discharge and, in more advanced stages, exudate about the eyes that may result in blindness. Birds lose weight rapidly, become weak and listless, and sometimes die within 8–10 days. In chronic infections, birds appear healthy, although trichomonads can usually be demonstrated in scrapings from the mucous membranes of the throat.

Lesions: The bird may be riddled with caseous, necrotic foci. The mouth and esophagus contain a mass of necrotic material that may extend into the skull and sometimes through the surrounding tissues of the neck to involve the skin. In the esophagus and crop, the lesions may be yellow, rounded, raised areas, with a central conical caseous spur, often referred to as "yellow buttons." The crop may be covered by a yellowish, diphtheritic membrane that may extend to the proventriculus. The gizzard and intestine are not involved. Lesions of internal organs are most frequent in the liver; they vary from a few small, yellow areas of necrosis to almost complete replacement of liver tissue by caseous necrotic debris. Adhesions and involvement of other internal organs appear to be contact extensions of the liver lesions.

Diagnosis: Lesions of trichomonosis are characteristic but not pathognomonic; those of pox, fungal disease, *Salmonella*, and other infections can be similar. Trichomonosis has sometimes been confused with histomoniasis (*see* p 2835) because of the similarity in liver lesions. Diagnosis should be confirmed by microscopic examination of a smear of mucus or fluid from the throat to demonstrate the presence of trichomonads. Trichomonads can be cultured easily in various artificial media such as Diamond's media, 0.2% Loeffler's dried blood serum in Ringer's solution, or a 2% solution of pigeon serum in isotonic salt solution. Good growth is obtained at 98.6°F (37°C). Antibiotics may be used to reduce bacterial contamination.

Control: Because trichomonads in pigeons are so readily transmitted from parent to offspring in the normal feeding process, chronically infected birds should be separated from breeding birds. In pigeons, recovery from infection with a less virulent trichomonad strain appears to provide some protection against subsequent attack by a more virulent strain. Successful treatments include carnidazole (10 mg/kg body wt), metronidazole (60 mg/kg body wt), and dimetridazole (50 mg/kg body wt, PO; or in the drinking water at 0.05% for 5–6 days). None of these drugs is approved for use in birds in the USA, but they could be used in non-food-producing birds by veterinary prescription. Bird feeders and waterers should be cleaned regularly and if an outbreak of trichomonosis is documented or suspected, feeders and waterers should be removed for ~2 wk and cleaned with a 10% bleach solution.

ULCERATIVE ENTERITIS

(Quail disease)

Ulcerative enteritis was first diagnosed in bobwhite quail (*Colinus virginianus*). It also affects chickens, turkeys, pheasants, grouse, and other gallinaceous birds. The disease has also been reported in pigeons and psittacine birds. In Japanese quail (*Coturnix coturnix japonica*), only experimentally induced cases have been reported in highly inbred populations. An ulcerative enteritis–like disease is caused by *Clostridium perfringens* in *Coturnix* quail. Ulcerative enteritis occurs worldwide and may be acute or chronic.

Etiology, Epidemiology, and Pathogenesis: *Clostridium colinum* is the etiologic agent. It is an anaerobic, fastidious to culture, gram-positive, spore-forming, slightly curved rod, ~1 × 3–4 μm wide, with subterminal, oval spores. In chickens, the disease is a complex that is linked to stress, coccidiosis, infectious bursal disease, and other predisposing factors. To induce experimental disease in bobwhite quail, $>10^6$ viable bacterial cells must be administered PO; chickens inoculated at the same levels are not affected.

Birds that develop chronic ulcerative enteritis or that have recovered from the disease remain carriers. Infection can be introduced by flies feeding on contaminated fecal material or by recovered carrier birds. Infected birds shed the bacterium in their droppings. Bobwhite quail are the most susceptible to this highly contagious disease. Most cases are reported in captive populations of bobwhite quail, suggesting that management plays a role in the incidence. *C colinum* spores can survive in the premises for months. *Clostridium* spp have been isolated from water samples obtained from drinker pipes in which biofilm and mineral deposits were present.

After oral infection, the bacterium adheres to the intestinal villi, producing enteritis and ulcers in portions of the small intestine and upper large intestine. Bacilli migrate to the liver via portal circulation, producing necrotic foci that later coalesce into extensive hepatic necrosis. Infarcts of the spleen are common. Stained smears of the lesions reveal the rod-shaped *C colinum* microorganism. Although toxigenicity tests in mice have been negative, the role of an in situ-produced toxin in the pathogenesis has been suggested but not demonstrated.

Clinical Findings: In susceptible bobwhite quail, sudden death occurs without signs or weight loss and with up to 100% mortality in just 2–3 days. Acute lesions include hemorrhagic enteritis of the duodenum. In chickens and other game birds, the course of the disease is less severe and is accompanied by anorexia. Signs are similar to those seen in coccidiosis: depressed, listless birds with humped backs, ruffled feathers, diarrhea, and sometimes bloody or watery white droppings, especially in quail in the prolonged course. Chickens recover within 2–3 wk, and mortality rarely exceeds 10%.

Lesions: In early disease stages, the most common lesions include small, round ulcers surrounded by hemorrhages in the small intestine, ceca, and upper large intestine. Small ulcers later coalesce to form larger, sometimes perforating ulcers, producing local or diffuse peritonitis. The presence of blood in the gut resembles coccidiosis. Characteristic yellow to gray necrotic foci are the predominant lesions in the hepatic parenchyma. Splenomegaly with hemorrhages and necrotic areas may be present.

Diagnosis: Gross postmortem lesions, including intestinal ulcerations and yellow to gray necrotizing lesions in the liver, assist in diagnosis. *C colinum* can be seen in gram-stained smears of the liver and intestinal lesions. In bacteremic birds, the microorganism can also be found in blood and spleen smears. In chickens, differentiating ulcerative enteritis from coccidiosis (*see* p 2791) may be difficult, because both diseases may be present simultaneously. Necrotic enteritis (*see* p 2802) and histomoniasis (*see* p 2835) may also present a diagnostic problem, but the hepatic lesions of ulcerative enteritis help differentiate it from these diseases. *C colinum* can be isolated from liver samples cultured in strict anaerobic conditions in prereduced blood glucose-yeast horse plasma medium. A fluorescent antibody test has been used to accurately diagnose ulcerative enteritis. PCR assay has also been reported as an effective diagnostic test.

Prevention, Treatment, and Control: Bacitracin in the feed at 200 g/ton is used for prevention in quail. Streptomycin (0.006%) and furazolidone (0.02%) in the feed are effective to treat the disease. Prevention must start with good management practices (eg, avoiding the introduction of new birds into existing flocks). High population density is a predisposing factor. The use of cages is recommended in quail breeding. Sick and dead birds should be removed promptly. Total cleanup between flocks, pest control in and around the premises, and periodic treatment of watering systems with innocuous chemicals that dissolve mineral and or biofilm build-up are good preventive measures.

AVIAN *CAMPYLOBACTER* INFECTION

Campylobacteriosis is a significant enterocolitis of people frequently acquired through consumption of undercooked poultry meat contaminated with *Campylobacter jejuni*. It is the leading bacterial cause of sporadic enteritis in developed countries. It can also be acquired from handling backyard poultry as well as diarrheic companion animals and from contaminated water. The organism colonizes the intestine of chickens, turkeys, and waterfowl but is generally nonpathogenic in birds. Some strains of *C jejuni* have been reported to cause enteritis and death in newly hatched chicks and poults; however, it has not been possible to satisfy Koch's postulates and reproduce the syndrome previously termed "avian vibrionic hepatitis" by administering isolates of *C jejuni* to chickens.

Commercial poultry and free-living birds are natural reservoirs of the thermophilic campylobacters (*C jejuni*, *C coli*, and *C lari*) and other poorly defined species. It is estimated that more than half of all commercial broiler and turkey flocks harbor *C jejuni*, although the prevalence can vary from 0% to100% depending on season (lowest in fall and winter and highest in summer). The organism has been isolated from numerous birds, including Columbae and domestic and free-living Galliformes and Anseriformes.

C jejuni has been found in all areas of commercial poultry production. Isolation of the organism is a function of surveillance and ability of laboratory personnel to culture and identify *Campylobacter* spp.

Etiology and Epidemiology: *C jejuni* is the predominant species associated with foodborne infection derived from poultry. *C coli* and *C lari* can also be recovered from the intestinal tract of poultry and have also been implicated in foodborne infection.

Environmental contamination is probably the most common source of infection for poults, chicks, and ducklings. Litter can remain infective for long periods, subject to at least a 10% moisture level and neutral pH. Exposed chicks and poults become colonized and can continue to excrete *C jejuni* for their lifetimes. Contaminated water may introduce infection into poultry flocks, and nonchlorinated water derived from a dam, river, or shallow well should be regarded as a possible source. Rats, mice, wild birds, darkling beetles, and houseflies can infect flocks; equipment and footwear contaminated with feces from an infected source may also serve as a vehicle of transmission. Once *C jejuni* has been introduced into the environment, rapid transmission within the flock occurs, with subsequent colonization of a high proportion of exposed breeders, commercial-meat, or laying-strain poultry. Some strains of *Campylobacter* can be transmitted vertically, either on the surface of eggs or by transovarial transmission. It has been isolated from the reproductive tracts of hens and roosters.

Clinical Findings and Lesions: Many chicks are colonized with *Campylobacter* spp early in life with no associated clinical signs or pathology.

Most chicks display no lesions associated with *Campylobacter* infection. Some studies have reported that challenged chicks may exhibit distention of the jejunum, disseminated hemorrhagic enteritis, and in some cases, focal hepatic necrosis. Microscopic lesions of infected chicks include edema of the mucosa of the ileum and cecum with *C jejuni* in the brush border of enterocytes. Mononuclear infiltration of the submucosa and villous atrophy occur, with intraluminal accumulation of mucus, erythrocytes, and mononuclear and polymorphonuclear cells. However, infected flocks seldom exhibit increased mortality rates or decreased feed conversion. It is unclear whether these findings represent a true clinical syndrome in chicks, because challenge studies frequently result in no lesions.

Diagnosis: Fecal specimens should be collected using swabs, then placed in Cary-Blair transport medium. Alternatively, cecal droppings can be collected into sterile laboratory sampling bags and packed on ice. Enrichment culture of specimens in semisolid motility medium facilitates isolation when small numbers of *C jejuni* are present. *Campylobacter* can be cultured on many different selective media, but commonly available formulations contain *Brucella* agar base and bovine blood with as many as seven antibiotics that inhibit overgrowth of Enterobacteriaceae. They also can be cultured on blood agar by selective filtration; bacteria in a 1/10 diluted fecal sample are allowed to penetrate a filter (0.45 µm pores) placed on the surface of a blood agar plate. After the liquid is absorbed into the plate, the filter is removed. Thermophilic *Campylobacter* spp should be cultured at 42°C under humid, microaerophilic conditions (85% nitrogen, 10% carbon dioxide, and 5% oxygen) for 48 hr. Some strains require a hydrogen-enriched atmosphere (5%). *Campylobacter* spp of significance in poultry are oxidase- and catalase-positive, indole-negative, and reduce selenite. The thermophilic species may be characterized on the basis of hippurate hydrolysis; nalidixic acid sensitivity is no longer reliable because of the increasing prevalence of fluoroquinolone-resistant *C jejuni*. The Penner or Lior serotyping schemes can be used to classify *C jejuni* ribotyping, or pulsed-field gel analysis can distinguish among various *C jejuni* isolates.

Control and Prevention: Because *C jejuni* is not found as a specific pathogen under commercial conditions, treatment of poultry flocks is not a consideration. If *C jejuni* is considered a problem in companion bird aviaries or in exotic species, antibiotics such as erythromycin can be administered in drinking water. Galliformes should receive a dosage of 10–30 mg/kg for 4 consecutive days, and Psittaciformes and exotics should be medicated at 30–40 mg/kg. Because of the zoonotic risk associated with *C jejuni* and its ability to rapidly develop antibiotic resistance, antibiotics should be used with caution in companion birds. Fluoroquinolones and erythromycins are the classes of antimicrobials used to treat people for campylobacteriosis.

Preharvest prevention of *Campylobacter* infection in commercial species is based on strict biosecurity, decontamination of housing between successive flocks, exclusion of rodents and wild birds, and insect eradication. Chlorination of drinking water to 2 ppm and operation of farms on a strict "all-in/all-out" basis occasionally reduces the prevalence of infection. In the context of commercial production in the USA where earth-floored housing is used and litter is recycled, preharvest control of *C jejuni* is impractical. Innovative methods of prevention, such as competitive exclusion, bacteriophage therapy, bacteriocins, and the use of vaccines, are under intensive investigation. Withholding feed from broilers and turkeys for at least 12 hr before slaughter and thorough decontamination of transport coops and modules reduce fecal contamination and lower the level of *C jejuni* introduced into processing plants.

Zoonotic Risk: *C jejuni* is a major source of foodborne enteritis in people; contaminated, undercooked poultry is responsible for >50% of cases investigated. The condition was recognized in the mid-1970s, and the significance of the organism has become apparent with improved methods of isolation and identification. Nonchlorinated ground water, unpasteurized milk, young diarrheic pets, and contaminated beef and pork products are also responsible for infection of people.

Improved washing of carcasses, use of counter-flow scalding, elimination of immersion chillers, and reduction in manual handling by installation of advanced automated equipment can reduce *C jejuni* contamination on poultry meat. Chemical disinfectants, such as chlorine, peracetic acid with hydrogen peroxide, and trisodium phosphate, glutaraldehyde and succinic acid, and organic compounds, such as lactic and acetic acids, may effectively reduce *C jejuni* on poultry carcasses in the processing plant. Some research indicates that bacteriophages and bacteriocins may also be useful. However, the regulations regarding chemical or biological sanitizers that can be used in processing plants and the performance standards for *Campylobacter* in the plant are currently in flux.

Gamma irradiation at levels of 1–3 kGy effectively eliminates *C jejuni* from poultry carcasses and products. Irradiation has been endorsed by a number of international health agencies, but irradiated foods are not widely available in the USA because of consumer concerns. The risk of foodborne *C jejuni* infection can be reduced through cooking of poultry to achieve a core temperature of 74°C for 1 min. Concurrent hygienic storage, handling, and preparation are necessary to prevent contamination of prepared foods, work surfaces, and utensils by raw poultry and other meats.

AVIAN CHLAMYDIOSIS

(Psittacosis, Ornithosis, Parrot fever)

Avian chlamydiosis can be an inapparent subclinical infection or acute, subacute, or chronic disease of wild and domestic birds characterized by respiratory, digestive, or systemic infection. Infections occur worldwide and have been identified in at least 460 avian species, particularly caged birds (primarily psittacines), colonial nesting birds (eg, egrets, herons), ratites, raptors, and poultry. Among poultry, turkeys, ducks, and pigeons are most often affected. The disease is a significant cause of economic loss and human exposure in many parts of the world.

Etiology and Epidemiology: *Chlamydia psittaci*, formerly renamed *Chlamydophila psittaci*, is an obligate intracellular bacterium. All strains of chlamydia share an identical genus-specific antigen in their lipopolysaccharide but often differ in the composition of other cell-wall antigens, thus providing a basis for serotypic identification. Eight serotypes are recognized; of these, six (A–F) infect avian species and are distinct from mammalian *Chlamydia* serotypes. More recently, strains of *C psittaci* have been classified using genetic differences in the *omp1* gene into nine genotypes. Seven of these (A, B, C, D, E, F, and E/B) are found in avian species and usually correspond to the equivalent serotype. Each avian serotype/genotype tends to be associated with certain types of birds (*see* TABLE 4). The same serotype/genotype may cause mild disease or asymptomatic infection in one species but severe or fatal disease in another species. Serotype A and D are highly virulent for turkeys and can cause mortality of ≥30%. Serotypes B and E are most frequently recovered from wild birds. Avian serotypes are capable of infecting people and other mammals.

Transmission is by the fecal-oral route or by inhalation. Respiratory discharge or feces from infected birds contain elementary bodies that are resistant to drying and can remain infective for several months when protected by organic debris (eg, litter and feces). Airborne particles and dust spread the organism. After inhalation or ingestion, elementary bodies attach to mucosal epithelial cells and are internalized by endocytosis. Elementary bodies within endosomes in the cell cytoplasm inhibit phagolysosome formation and differentiate into metabolically active, noninfectious reticulate bodies that divide and multiply by binary fission, eventually forming numerous infectious, metabolically inactive elementary bodies. Newly formed elementary bodies are released from the host cell by lysis. The incubation period is typically 3–10 days but may be up to several months in older birds or after low exposure. Host and microbial factors, route and intensity of exposure, and treatment determine clinical course.

Possible sources of *C psittaci* include infected birds, asymptomatic carriers, vertical transmission from infected hens, infected mammals, and contaminated environments. Stressors (eg, transport, crowding, breeding, cold or wet weather, dietary changes, or reduced food availability) and concurrent infections, especially those causing immunosuppression, can initiate shedding in latently infected birds and cause recurrence of clinical disease. Carriers often shed the organism intermittently for extended periods. Persistence of *C psittaci* in the nasal glands of chronically infected birds may be an important source of organisms.

Longterm inapparent infections lasting for months to years are common and are considered the normal *Chlamydia*-host relationship. The prevalence of infection varies considerably between species and by geographic location. Infection is endemic in commercial turkey flocks; no clinical signs or mild respiratory signs and low mortality are the common presentations. Outbreaks are rare. Although chickens are relatively resistant to clinical disease, asymptomatic infection is frequent. Epidemiologic studies report prevalence varying from 10% to >90% using serology, culture, or PCR detection; 3%–50% of surveyed wild avian populations may be seropositive.

Clinical Findings and Lesions: Severity of clinical signs and lesions depends on the virulence of the organism, infectious dose, stress factors, and susceptibility of the bird species; asymptomatic infections are common. Nasal and ocular discharge, conjunctivitis, sinusitis, green to yellow-green droppings, fever, inactivity, ruffled feathers, weakness, inappetence, and weight loss can be seen in clinically affected birds. Clinical pathology test results vary with the organs most affected and severity of the disease. Hematologic changes most

TABLE 4 ASSOCIATIONS BETWEEN AVIAN GENOTYPES OF *CHLAMYDIA PSITTACI* AND TYPES OF BIRDS

	A	B	C	D	E	E/B	F
Psittacines	++	+			+		+
Pigeons, doves	+	++			++	+	
Waterfowl	+	+	++		+	++	
Turkeys	+	+	+	++	+	+	+
Chicken		++	+	++	+	+	
Passerines	+	++					
Ratites					++		
Wild birds		++			++		

++ = Genotype most commonly associated with this bird species or group.
+ = Genotype less commonly associated with this bird species or group.

often present are anemia and leukocytosis with heterophilia and monocytosis. Plasma bile acids, AST, LDH, and uric acid may be increased. A radiograph or a laparoscopy may reveal an enlarged liver and spleen and thickened airsacs. Necropsy findings in acute infections include serofibrinous polyserositis (airsacculitis, pericarditis, perihepatitis, peritonitis), pneumonia, hepatomegaly, and splenomegaly. Multiple tan to white to yellow foci and/or petechial hemorrhages can be seen in the liver and spleen. Similar lesions are seen in other systemic bacterial infections and are not specific for avian chlamydiosis. Multifocal necrosis in the liver and spleen is associated with small granular, basophilic intracytoplasmic bacterial inclusions in multiple cell types; occasional heterophils; and increased mononuclear cells (macrophages, lymphocytes, plasma cells) in hepatic sinusoids and splenic sinuses. Necrosis results from direct cell lysis or vascular damage. The latter is also the source of the generalized serofibrinous exudate. In chronic infections, enlargement and discoloration of the spleen or liver may be noted. Necrosis and bacterial inclusions are not seen, but the mononuclear cell response is present in these birds. Lesions are usually absent in latently infected birds, even though *C psittaci* is often being shed.

Diagnosis: Because of the variety of clinical presentations and common occurrence of latently infected carriers, no single diagnostic test can reliably determine infection. Procedures to detect the organism or antibodies are used. In general, the more acute the disease, the greater the number of infective organisms and the easier it is to make a diagnosis. When birds are acutely ill, clinical findings, including hematology, clinical chemistries, and radiology or typical gross lesions are adequate for a tentative diagnosis.

The combination of a serologic and an antigen detection test, especially PCR, or culture, is a practical diagnostic scheme to confirm chlamydiosis. In live birds, the preferred sample for bacterial culture or PCR is a single conjunctival, choanal, or cloacal swab. Multiple samples collected throughout 3–5 days are recommended for detection of intermittent shedding by asymptomatic birds.

Antibodies may or may not be detectable depending on the test used and on the level and stage of infection. Interpretation of titers from single serum samples is difficult. A 4-fold increase in titers between paired acute and convalescent samples is diagnostic, and high titers in a majority of samples from several birds in a population are sufficient for a presumptive diagnosis. Serologic methods include direct and modified direct complement fixation, elementary body agglutination, antibody ELISA, and indirect immunofluorescence. The elementary body agglutination test detects IgM and is useful to determine recent infection. The complement fixation methods are more sensitive than agglutination methods. High antibody titers may persist after treatment and complicate evaluation of subsequent tests.

Antigen detection methods include immunohistochemistry (eg, immunofluorescence, immunoperoxidase), ELISA, and PCR. ELISA kits developed for detection of *Chlamydia trachomatis* in people are available commercially and are relatively inexpensive. Their exact specificity and sensitivity for detection of *C psittaci* is most often unknown; they appear to have good specificity but somewhat low sensitivity. These kits are most useful when birds are clinically ill. PCR is the most sensitive and specific test, but results may differ between laboratories because of the lack of standardized PCR primers and laboratory method variations. False-positive results are a concern with PCR, because cross-contamination can occur relatively easily. The organism can also be identified in impression smears of affected tissues (eg, liver, spleen, and lung). Chlamydiae stain purple with Giemsa and red with Macchiavello and Gimenez stains.

Immunohistochemistry is usually more sensitive than the histochemical stains mentioned above for detecting bacteria in tissue.

Confirmation requires isolation and identification of *C psittaci* in chick embryo or cell cultures (BGM, L929, Vero) at a

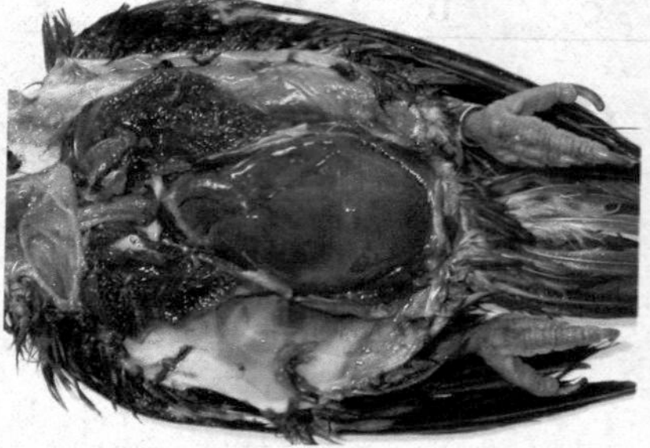

Marked hepatomegaly in an ornate lorikeet (*Trichoglossus ornatus*) with chlamydiosis. *Courtesy of Dr. A. J. Van Wettere.*

qualified laboratory. Cloacal, choanal, oropharyngeal, conjunctival, or fecal swabs (in a special *Chlamydia* transport media) from live birds, or tissues (liver and spleen preferred) from dead birds should be refrigerated and submitted promptly to the laboratory. Freezing, drying, improper handling, and improper transport media can affect viability. The laboratory should be contacted for directions to submit samples. Concurrent infections with other, more easily diagnosed diseases (eg, colibacillosis, pasteurellosis, herpesvirus infections, mycotic diseases) may mask chlamydial infection. Laboratory and clinical findings should be correlated. Chlamydiosis must be distinguished from other respiratory and systemic diseases of birds.

Prevention and Treatment: Human and avian chlamydiosis is a reportable disease; state and local governmental regulations should be followed wherever applicable. No effective vaccine for use in birds is available. Treatment prevents mortality and shedding but cannot be relied on to eliminate latent infection; shedding may recur. Tetracyclines (chlortetracycline, oxytetracycline, doxycycline) are the antibiotics of choice. Drug resistance to tetracyclines is rare, but reduced sensitivity requiring higher dosages is becoming more common. Tetracyclines are bacteriostatic and effective only against actively multiplying organisms, making extended treatment times (from 2–8 wk, during which minimum-inhibitory concentrations in blood must be consistently maintained) necessary. When tetracyclines are administered orally, additional sources of dietary calcium (eg, mineral block, supplement, cuttle bone) should be reduced to minimize interference with drug absorption.

Outbreaks of clinical disease in poultry flocks are not common. Treating infected flocks with chlortetracycline at 400–750 g/ton of feed for a minimum of 2 wk has effectively decreased potential risk of infection for plant employees. The medicated feed must be replaced by nonmedicated feed for 2 days before slaughter and processing. Calcium supplementation must be withheld during treatment with chlortetracycline, with calcium concentration in the feed reduced to ≤0.7%. Medicated feed should be provided for 45 days if elimination of the organism is attempted. Use of some tetracycline antibiotics and doxycycline in poultry is prohibited, and state regulations should be followed. Persistence of oxytetracycline residues in eggs of laying hens is 9 days, and persistance of doxycycline residues is 26 days after administration at 0.5 g/L for 7 days.

In pigeons and companion birds, use of chlortetracycline-medicated feeds for 45 days was historically a standard recommendation for imported birds (*see* p 1897). Difficulties in palatability of the feed itself or the high level of antibiotic necessary for adequate blood levels have limited its use. Doxycycline is the current drug of choice, because it is better absorbed, has less affinity for calcium, better tissue distribution, and a longer half-life than other tetracyclines. Doxycycline added to feed or water can also result in adequate blood levels and has less effect on normal intestinal flora than does chlortetracycline. The dosage and duration of the treatment varies between species. Protocols derived from controlled studies performed in the particular species treated should be used when available (*see* p 1897). *See also* information in the Compendium of Measures To Control *Chlamydophila psittaci* Infection Among Humans (Psittacosis) and Pet Birds (Avian Chlamydiosis), 2010, National Association of State Public Health Veterinarians (NASPHV). When specific information is lacking, an empiric starting dosage of 400 mg/L of water, or 25–50 mg/kg/day, PO, has been suggested.

Appropriate biosecurity practices are necessary to control the introduction and spread of chlamydiae in an avian population. Minimal standards include quarantine and examination of all new birds, prevention of exposure to wild birds, traffic control to minimize cross-contamination, isolation and treatment of affected and contact birds, thorough cleaning and disinfection of premises and equipment (preferably with small units managed on an all-in/all-out basis), provision of uncontaminated feed, maintenance of records on all bird movements, and continual monitoring for presence of chlamydial infection.

The organism is susceptible to heat (it may be destroyed in <5 min at 56°C) and most disinfectants (eg, 1:1,000 quaternary ammonium chloride, 1:100 bleach solution, 70% alcohol, etc) but is resistant to acid and alkali. It may persist for months in organic matter such as litter and nest material, but thorough cleaning before disinfection is necessary.

Zoonotic Risk: Avian chlamydiosis is a zoonotic disease that can affect people after exposure to aerosolized organisms shed from the digestive or respiratory tracts of infected live or dead birds or by direct contact with infected birds or tissues. Human disease most often results from exposure to pet psittacines and can occur even if there is only brief contact with a single infected bird. Other persons in close contact with birds such as pigeon fanciers, veterinarians, farmers, wildlife rehabilitators, zoo keepers, and employees in slaughtering and processing plants or hatcheries are also at risk. Recent studies showed that zoonotic transmission of *C psittaci* in poultry industry workers is likely underestimated. Precautions should be taken when examining live or dead infected birds to avoid exposure (eg, dust mask and plastic face shield or goggles, gloves, detergent disinfectant to wet feathers, and fan-exhausted examining hood).

Some individuals, especially pregnant women and those with impaired immunity, are more susceptible than others. The illness in people is usually respiratory and varies from flu-like symptoms to systemic disease with pneumonia and possibly endocarditis and encephalitis.

AVIAN NEPHRITIS VIRAL INFECTIONS

Avian nephritis viral infections are contagious infections of chickens characterized by renal damage and visceral urate deposits, growth retardation, and limited mortality (0–10%). They are seen mainly in chickens <7 days old, but interstitial nephritis can be seen in chicks as old as 4 wk. These infections have been reported worldwide. Subclinical infections are common and have been detected by serologic surveys in some SPF flocks and in turkeys.

Etiology and Transmission: The causal viruses are avian nephritis viruses (ANVs, which are astroviruses), some of which were previously recognized as enterovirus-like viruses (ELVs). There is some evidence that a taxonomically distinct astrovirus, chicken astrovirus (CAstV), also causes kidney disease and growth retardation. The descriptions below relate to ANV only. Strains of ANV vary in virulence and in antigenicity. Transmission occurs by direct or indirect contact. Indirect evidence suggests that egg transmission may occur. Infection can be transmitted by oral administration of virus to day-old birds. Virus is consistently isolated from the kidneys or feces during the first 10 days after infection.

Clinical Findings: Clinical signs vary from none to mortality resulting from kidney disease or severe growth retardation. Diarrhea and growth retardation are common in broilers. Outbreaks with mortality of 0–10% can occur in chicks newly hatched to as old as 7 days; cardinal necropsy findings are renal damage and visceral urate deposits (baby chick nephropathy).

Lesions: Nephritis is a common necropsy finding. Gross and microscopic lesions are often seen in the kidneys. Swelling, paleness, or yellowish discoloration with excessive urate deposition is frequent. Histologic lesions consist of a degeneration of the epithelial cells with infiltration of granulocytes, interstitial lymphocyte infiltration, and moderate fibrosis. In the latter stages, lymphoid follicles develop.

Some ANVs, formerly known as ELVs, induce only intestinal lesions varying from decreased length of the microvillus border to total desquamation of the intestinal epithelium.

Diagnosis: Nephropathogenic strains of infectious bronchitis virus (*see* p 2909) and CAstV isolates also cause interstitial nephritis. Therefore, when nephritis is diagnosed, it is necessary to isolate the causative agent.

ANV and related viruses may be isolated by inoculation of suspected material (kidney or rectal contents) in the yolk sac of SPF chick embryos and in chick kidney cells. However, many ANVs are difficult to isolate. The best way to detect ANV is by reverse transcriptase (RT)-PCR or real-time, quantitative RT-PCR of kidney or gut content samples. These tests are designed to detect multiple strains and allow quick differentiation from other viruses.

Serologic diagnosis can be made using direct or indirect immunofluorescence, seroneutralization, or ELISA tests, but these may detect only a limited number of strains of ANV because of its high antigenic diversity.

Treatment and Prevention: There is no effective treatment. General hygienic precautions are the only applicable preventive measures.

AVIAN SPIROCHETOSIS

(Avian borreliosis)

Avian spirochetosis is an acute, febrile, septicemic, bacterial disease that affects a wide variety of birds.

Etiology, Epidemiology, and Transmission: The causal organism, *Borrelia anserina*, is an actively motile spirochete, ~0.2–0.3 μm × 8–20 μm, and consists of 5–8 loosely arranged coils. Cultivation in vitro is difficult. *Borrelia* will grow on Barbour-Stoenner-Kelly medium but loses virulence after 12 passages. It can also be propagated in embryonating duck or chick embryos or in young ducks or chicks.

Spirochetosis is found in temperate or tropical regions, wherever the biologic vectors are found. The most common vector is *Argas persicus*, the "cosmopolitan" fowl tick, but other *Argas* spp transmit the bacteria in different geographic areas. In the western USA, a highly efficient vector is *A sanchezi*.

Diverse immunologic and serologic types of *B anserina* have been demonstrated in many areas. Recovery from one type confers solid immunity against the homologous types for ≥1 yr, but not against heterologous strains. Relapses, reported for some human *Borrelia* infections, are unknown in *B anserina* infection of birds. Therefore, any reinfection can be attributed to a heterologous type.

Generally, an infected *Argas* tick can transmit the bacteria at every feeding and maintains the infection throughout larval, nymphal, and adult stages. The ticks also transmit the infection transovarially, ie, the F_1 larvae are infective. Ticks remain infected despite feeding on chicks hyperimmune to *B anserina* or on chicks with high blood levels of chemotherapeutic agents effective against *Borrelia*. Other vectors (lice, mosquitoes, some species of ticks, inanimate objects) can transmit the spirochete mechanically to a susceptible host whenever the piercing apparatus becomes contaminated with blood that contains *Borrelia*. Ingestion of bile-stained fecal droppings containing the spirochete, contamination of feed or water, and cannibalism during spirochetemia can result in infection. After the bite of an infected tick, the incubation period is ~3–12 days.

Clinical Findings: Signs are highly variable, depending on the virulence of the spirochete, and may be absent. Signs include listlessness, depression, somnolence, moderate to marked shivering, and increased thirst. Ruffled feathers, anemia, and pale combs can be noticed as well, and inappetence can lead to reduced weight. Young birds are affected more severely than older ones. During the initial stages of the disease, there is usually a green or yellow diarrhea with increased urates. The course of the disease is 1–2 wk. Mild strains are common. However, in many tick-infested geographic areas, morbidity can approach 100% and mortality may be 33%–77%. Egg production in layers or breeders may be reduced by 5%–10%, with a higher number of small eggs.

Lesions: The spleen is enlarged, with petechial or ecchymotic hemorrhages, appearing dark or mottled. However, a contrasting situation may be seen in Mongolian pheasants, in which the spleen is reported to be small and pale. Occasionally, the liver may be swollen and contain focal areas of necrosis. Kidneys may be enlarged and pale. A green, catarrhal enteritis is common.

Diagnosis: Diagnosis depends on demonstration of *Borrelia* in the blood, either as actively motile during darkfield microscopy, as stained spirochetes in Giemsa-stained blood smears, or by PCR. In young birds, the *Borrelia* may reach vast numbers per oil-immersion field and persist for several days. Older birds usually have low numbers of *Borrelia* that are detected only with difficulty, or not at all, and that persist for only 1–2 days. Increased numbers of immature RBCs are noticed due to the anemia. Silver staining can be used to demonstrate the bacteria in tissues.

Agar-gel diffusion and various serologic tests have been described but are of questionable value because of the diverse serotypes that exist in some localities. Specific agglutinins clump the spirochetes in successively larger clumps during the terminal stages of the disease. Agglutination lysis then begins to disintegrate these clumps, and spirochetal degradation products are liberated, which may result in pyrexia. Death occurs most often 1–3 days after *Borrelia* disappear from the bloodstream. Spirochetal antibodies are readily detected in yolks of eggs laid by infected hens.

Treatment and Control: Several antibacterial agents are effective. The most widely used are penicillin derivatives, but streptomycins, tetracyclines, and tylosin are also effective. The antibiotics can be completely effective if begun when the number of spirochetes per oil-immersion field is low or moderate; however, if large numbers of spirochetes are present in the bloodstream, the sudden liberation of large quantities of spirochetal degradation products can result in higher mortality than with no treatment.

Control must be directed against the biologic vector. *Argas* ticks are notable for their long lifespan, ability to survive for extended periods without a blood meal, efficiency in transmitting the spirochete, and ability to remain securely hidden in cracks and crevices often beyond the effective reach of pesticides. Accordingly, control is difficult. A combination of tick eradication and immunization is the most effective means of control.

Immunization can be highly successful and, next to eradication of the biologic vector, is the preferred method of control. Bacterins prepared from local strains of *Borrelia* have been used with success. Vaccines may be prepared from formalin- or phenol-inactivated material from lysates of blood, tissues, embryos, or eggs infected with *B anserina*, and may be lyophilized or liquid. Whole-egg propagated bacterins are usually given in one or two IM injections. Little if any cross-protection is afforded to different serotypes. Birds normally have protective immunity after recovering from natural infection.

COLIBACILLOSIS

(Colisepticemia, *Escherichia coli* infection)

Colibacillosis occurs as an acute fatal septicemia or subacute pericarditis, airsacculitis, salpingitis, and peritonitis. It is a common disease of economic importance in poultry and is seen worldwide.

Etiology and Pathogenesis: *Escherichia coli* is a gram-negative, rod-shaped bacterium normally found in the intestine of poultry and most other animals. Although most serotypes are nonpathogenic, a limited number produce extraintestinal infections. Avian pathogenic *E coli* (APEC) strains are commonly of the O1, O2, and O78 serogroups, but many others have also been associated with cellulitis and colibacillosis. There is considerable diversity of serogroups among clinical isolates, with a high percentage of APEC isolates being untypeable. Therefore, no single *E coli* serogroup used as a bacterin can provide full protection against all of the serogroups that cause infections. Virulence factors include possession of large virulence plasmids and the abilities to resist phagocytosis and serum killing, acquire iron in low iron conditions, and adhere to host structures. APEC are generally nontoxigenic and poorly invasive.

Large numbers of *E coli* are maintained in the poultry house environment through fecal contamination. Initial exposure to APEC may occur in the hatchery from infected or contaminated eggs. Although most *E coli* isolated from colibacillosis are well equipped with virulence factors that distinguish them from fecal commensal strains, systemic infection often involves predisposing environmental factors or infectious causes. Thus, mycoplasmosis, infectious bronchitis, Newcastle disease, hemorrhagic enteritis, and turkey bordetellosis, or exposure to poor air quality and other environmental stresses, may precede colibacillosis.

Systemic infection occurs when large numbers of APEC gain access to the bloodstream from the respiratory tract or intestine. Bacteremia progresses to septicemia and death, or the infection extends to serosal surfaces, pericardium, joints, and other organs.

Clinical Findings and Lesions: Signs are nonspecific and vary with age, organs involved, and concurrent disease. Young birds dying of acute septicemia have few lesions except for an enlarged, hyperemic liver and spleen with increased fluid in body cavities. Birds that survive septicemia develop subacute fibrinopurulent airsacculitis, pericarditis, perihepatitis, and lymphocytic depletion of the bursa and thymus (unusually pathogenic salmonellae produce similar lesions in chicks). Although airsacculitis is a classic lesion of colibacillosis, it is unclear whether it results from primary respiratory exposure or from extension of serositis. Sporadic lesions include pneumonia, arthritis, osteomyelitis, peritonitis, and salpingitis.

Diagnosis: Unlike pathogenic *E coli* associated with illnesses in other animal species, avian isolates are generally nonhemolytic on sheep (5%) blood agar. Isolation of a pure culture of *E coli* from heart blood, liver, or typical visceral lesions in a fresh carcass indicates primary or secondary colibacillosis. Consideration should be given to predisposing infections and environmental factors. Pathogenicity of isolates is established using multiplex PCR panels for plasmid-mediated virulence genes or when parenteral inoculation of young chicks or poults results in fatal septicemia or typical lesions within 3 days. Pathogenicity can also be detected by inoculation of the allantoic sac of 12-day-old chicken embryos. Resulting gross lesions include cranial and skin hemorrhages in addition to encephalomalacia in embryos inoculated with virulent isolates.

Treatment and Control: Treatment strategies include attempts to control predisposing infections or environmental factors and early use of antibacterials indicated by susceptibility tests. Most isolates are resistant to tetracyclines, streptomycin, and sulfa drugs, although therapeutic success can sometimes be achieved with tetracycline. In fact, 90% of clinical isolates are resistant to tetracycline, with 60% of isolates resistant to five or more antibiotics. Fluoroquinolone use is now banned in many countries, including the USA. Commercial bacterins administered to breeder hens or chicks have provided some protection against homologous *E coli* serogroups.

DUCK VIRAL HEPATITIS

Duck viral hepatitis is an acute, highly contagious, viral disease of young ducklings characterized by a short incubation period, sudden onset, high mortality, and characteristic liver lesions. The disease is of economic importance in all duck-raising areas of the world. Three distinct types of duck hepatitis virus (DHV) have been isolated from diseased ducklings. A natural outbreak of DHV Type I has been reported in mallard ducklings; experimental DHV Type I infections have been produced in goslings, turkey poults, young pheasants, quail, and guinea fowl. In Muscovy ducks, DHV Type 1 has been reported to cause pancreatitis and encephalitis. The viruses that cause hepatitis in ducklings should not be confused with duck hepatitis B virus, a hepadnavirus infection of older ducks.

Etiology: The originally described, most widespread, and most virulent DHV Type I has been renamed duck hepatitis A virus type 1 (DHAV-1) and is now classified in the genus *Avihepatovirus* in the Picornaviridae family. It is readily propagated in chicken and duck embryos. Two new geno/serotypes, DHAV-2 and DHAV-3, have been identified in Mainland China, Taiwan,PRC, and Korea. They do not produce hemagglutinins. Field experience with DHAV-1 indicates that egg transmission does not occur. The disease can be transmitted experimentally by parenteral or oral administration of infected tissues.

Viruses that differ from classic DHAV-1 have been recognized as causes of hepatitis in ducklings. DHV Type II, now classified as duck astrovirus type 1 (DAstV-1), is difficult to propagate under laboratory conditions; DHV Type III is also now classified as an astrovirus (DAstV-2) and can be propagated in duck (but not chicken) embryos. Distinct serologic variants of DHAV-1, named DHV Type Ia and N-DHV, have also been described.

Clinical Findings: The incubation period for DHAV-1 is 18–48 hr. Affected ducklings become lethargic, lose balance, paddle spasmodically, and die within minutes, typically with opisthotonos. Although adults may become infected, clinical signs have not been seen in ducks >7 wk old. Mortality may be as high as 95% in ducklings. Practically all deaths occur within 1 wk after onset of signs.

The clinical course of DAstV-1 infection is similar to that of DHAV-1 and can be seen in ducklings immune to DHAV-1 infection. DAstV-2 infections are seen in ducklings despite immunity to DHAV-1. The clinical course of DAstV-2 infection is less severe, and mortality is rarely >30%.

Lesions: The lesions caused by all three types of DHV are similar. The liver is enlarged and covered with hemorrhagic foci up to 1 cm in diameter. The spleen may be enlarged and mottled. Kidneys may be swollen and renal blood vessels congested.

Diagnosis: A presumptive diagnosis can be based on the history and lesions. Sudden onset, rapid spread, and short course, together with characteristic liver lesions, are highly suggestive of duck viral hepatitis. DHAV-1 may be isolated in duck embryos, day-old ducklings, and duck-embryo liver cell cultures, or less easily in chicken embryos. The virus can be identified by neutralization with specific antisera or by inoculation into both susceptible and immune ducklings. DHAV-1 can also be identified by reverse transcriptase PCR. DAstV-1 and DAstV-2 are not neutralized by classic DHAV-1 antiserum.

Prevention and Treatment: Prevention is by strict isolation, particularly during the first 5 wk of age. Contact with wild waterfowl should be avoided. Rats have been reported as a reservoir host of the virus; therefore, pest control is indicated.

Immunization of breeder ducks with modified-live virus vaccines, using DHAV-1, DAstV-1, and DAstV-2 , provides parenteral immunity that effectively prevents high losses in young ducklings. The DHAV-1 vaccine is administered SC in the neck to breeder ducks at 16, 20, and 24 wk of age and every 12 wk thereafter throughout the laying period. Three immunizations are advisable for passive protection of ducklings.

An inactivated DHAV-1 vaccine for use in breeder ducks that have been previously primed with live DHAV-1 has been described. A single dose of the inactivated vaccine, given IM before the birds come into lay, provides passive immunity for a complete laying cycle to progeny ducklings.

The chick-embryo origin, modified-live DHAV-1 vaccine also can be used for early vaccination of ducklings susceptible to DHAV-1 (progeny of nonimmune breeders). This vaccine is administered SC or by foot web stab in a single dose to day-old ducklings. Vaccinated ducklings rapidly develop an active immunity within 3–4 days.

Antibody against DHAV-1, prepared from the eggs of hyperimmunized chickens and administered SC in the neck at the time of initial loss, is an effective flock treatment.

ENTEROCOCCOSIS

Enterococcosis has been reported in a variety of avian species worldwide. *Enterococcus* spp are normal microflora found in the intestinal tract of poultry and other bird species; infections are usually secondary to another disease. *Enterococcus* infections can result in either an acute or subacute/chronic form.

Etiology and Epidemiology: Enterococci are nonmotile, gram-positive, catalase-negative coccoid bacteria that appear singly, in pairs, or in short chains on stained smears. *Enterococcus* spp isolated from birds with clinical disease include *E avium*, *E durans*, *E faecalis*, *E faecium*, and *E hirae*. *E faecalis* affects birds of all ages, but infection is especially devastating for embryos and young chicks. *E cecorum* has been associated with arthritis in broiler chickens.

Transmission is via the oral and/or aerosol routes as well as from skin wounds. Infection may result in septicemia. Endocarditis can occur when the infection progresses to a subacute/chronic stage. Brain necrosis and encephalomalacia in young chickens have been reported in enterococcosis. Although enterococcosis has been reported in poultry species, it should also be noted that some strains of *Enterococcus* have a beneficial effect on growth and feed efficiency and are used as probiotics.

Clinical Findings: In the acute form of enterococcosis, clinical signs are related to septicemia and include depression, lethargy, ruffled feathers, diarrhea, and a decrease in egg production. In the subacute/chronic form, depression, lameness, and head tremors may be noted. If untreated, most affected birds die. Egg transmission or fecal contamination of hatching eggs can often lead to late embryo mortality, and an increased number of hatchlings are unable to "pip" through the shell at hatch.

Lesions: Acute enterococcosis lesions include splenomegaly, hepatomegaly, enlarged kidneys, and congestion of subcutaneous tissue. Multifocal, whitish-tan areas of necrosis may be observed on the liver and spleen. Omphalitis or enlarged yolk sacs may be seen in infected chicks or poults. In the subacute/chronic form, lesions include pericarditis, perihepatitis, airsacculitis, arthritis and/or tenosynovitis, osteomyelitis, myocarditis, and valvular endocarditis. An enlarged, flaccid heart with pale to hemorrhagic areas in the myocardium has also been reported along with infarcts throughout the internal organs. Focal granulomas can be found in many tissues as a result of septic emboli. Gram-positive bacterial colonies are readily seen in thrombosed vessels and within areas of necrosis.

Diagnosis: History, clinical signs, lesions, and demonstration of enterococci in blood or on impression smears are suggestive of enterococcosis. Isolation of *Enterococcus* spp from lesions will confirm the diagnosis. Enterococci are easily isolated on blood agar. Differential diagnoses includes bacterial septicemic diseases such as staphylococcosis, streptococcosis, colibacillosis, pasteurellosis, and erysipelas.

Treatment and Prevention: Antibiotics, including penicillin, erythromycin, novobiocin, oxytetracycline, chlortetracycline, or tetracycline, have been used to treat acute and subacute infections. Clinically affected birds respond well early in the course of the disease, but treatment efficacy decreases as the disease progresses. Antimicrobial susceptibility testing should be performed to ensure that the most efficacious antibiotic is used.

Prevention and control require preventing immunosuppressive diseases and conditions, because enterococcosis often occurs secondary to another disease. In addition, ensuring proper cleaning and disinfection of the facilities can reduce environmental sources.

Zoonotic Risk: A high percentage of ready-to-eat poultry products are contaminated with *Enterococcus* spp; however, food poisoning in people has not been reported.

ERYSIPELAS

Erysipelas is a bacterial disease caused by infection with *Erysipelothrix rhusiopathiae*. The disease is most often seen as septicemia, but urticarial and endocardial forms exist. *E rhusiopathiae* infects a wide range of both avian and mammalian hosts. The disease has been reported in domestic fowl, feral avian species, and captive wild birds and mammals. Infection in reptiles and amphibians has been reported. The organism has also been isolated from the surface slime on fish (without causing disease), which may serve as a source of infection for other species. From an economic standpoint, turkeys are the most important poultry species affected, but serious outbreaks have occurred in chickens, ducks, and geese. Among affected mammals, swine are the most economically important species, but *E rhusiopathiae* infection is also a cause of polyarthritis in lambs. (*See also* ERYSIPELOTHRIX RHUSIOPATHIAE INFECTION, p 625.)

Erysipelas in poultry is seen worldwide and, although considered a sporadic disease, endemic areas exist.

Etiology: *E rhusiopathiae* is a facultative, anaerobic bacterium. Two additional genomic species have been described: *E tonsillarum*, and most recently *E inopinata*, but neither is considered pathogenic for poultry. Morphologically, *E tonsillarum* and *E inopinata* cannot be distinguished from *E rhusiopathiae*. *E rhusiopathiae* stains gram-positive but tends to decolorize, particularly in older cultures. The organism is small, non-acid fast, nonmotile, does not form spores, and produces no known toxins. There is no flagellum, but a capsule has been demonstrated. The cellular morphology of *E rhusiopathiae* is variable. The presence of virulence factors such as neuraminidase play a role in bacterial attachment and invasion of host cells. Cells freshly isolated from tissues during acute infection or from smooth colonies are straight or slightly curved small rods that may occur in short chains. Cells from older cultures or rough colonies tend to become filamentous and may be confused with mycelia. The filamentous form occurs more frequently after repeated passages on artificial media.

E rhusiopathiae has three colony types and grows readily on ordinary culture media containing the blood or sera of various animals. Growth is enhanced by reducing the oxygen content or increasing the carbon dioxide level to 5%–10%. Optimal incubation temperature is 35°–37°C, and the optimal pH range is 7.4–7.8.

The organism is not readily destroyed by the usual laboratory disinfectants. It is quite resistant to dessication and can survive smoking and pickling processes. It may survive in litter or soil for various lengths of time. Infected carriers may shed the organism, seeding the environment and making disinfection of premises difficult. It is inactivated by a 1:1,000 concentration of bichloride of mercury, 0.5% sodium hydroxide solution, 3.5% liquid cresol, 5% solution of phenol, quaternary ammonium, chlorine, or 0.5% formalin as long as it is not in organic matter.

Although 26 different serotypes of *E rhusiopathiae* were described based on an agar gel diffusion test, some of these serotypes have been assigned to *E tonsillarum* after its confirmation as a separate species. *E rhusiopathiae* serotypes 1, 2, and 5 have been most frequently isolated from poultry.

Epidemiology: Erysipelas occurs sporadically in poultry of all ages. It is ubiquitous in nature and found where nitrogenous substances decompose. Turkeys are susceptible regardless of sex or age, although under field conditions it is more common in older birds. Recent evidence indicates there may be a genetically related resistance in turkeys. The incidence in males is reported to be higher, but this is not supported by experimental data. Erysipelas may affect the fertility of males and may contribute to downgrading and processing losses. Infection results from entrance of the organisms through breaks in the skin, through the mucous membranes such as during artificial insemination, by ingestion of contaminated foodstuffs (particularly cannibalism of infected carcasses), and possibly by mechanical transmission via biting insects. The poultry red mite (*see* p 2877) can harbor the organism and may serve as a mechanical vector. Fighting and cannibalism increase losses.

The organism is shed in feces from infected animals and contaminates the soil, in which it may survive for long periods depending on temperature and pH. Poultry, as well as other animals, may be carriers and shed the organism without showing clinical signs of disease. Carriers can shed from feces, urine, saliva, and nasal secretions. Transmission into poultry houses via rodents can occur.

In nonvaccinated flocks, morbidity and mortality rates may reach 40%–50%, but mortality is usually <15%. In vaccinated flocks, some birds may be depressed for a short period and recover. Mortality in vaccinated and nonvaccinated poultry is influenced by the virulence of the organism.

No correlation has been shown to exist between the serotype, chemical structure, or biochemical pattern and the manifestation of the septicemic, urticarial, or endocardial forms of erysipelas.

Clinical Findings: Erysipelas is primarily an acute infection that results in sudden death. In an affected flock, a few birds may be depressed but easily aroused; within 24 hr, a few birds will be dead. Just before death, some birds may be very droopy, with an unsteady gait. Chronic clinical disease in a flock is not usual but does occur; birds may have cutaneous lesions and swollen hocks. Turkeys with vegetative endocarditis usually do not have clinical signs and may die suddenly. Erysipelas should be suspected in flocks that have been artificially inseminated 4–5 days before an episode of death without clinical signs. Rainy, cold weather coinciding with the onset of sexual maturity increases risk of clinical disease. Clinical signs in chickens include general weakness, depression, diarrhea, and sudden death. Most sick birds die. In laying hens, egg production may drop markedly. Decreased egg production and conjunctival edema can be seen in organic, cage-free flocks.

Lesions: At necropsy, a generalized darkening of the skin or various sized areas of diffuse darkening is common. The liver and spleen are usually enlarged and friable and may be mottled. Other gross lesions such as peritonitis, pericarditis, petechiation of the heart, catarrhal exudate in the GI tract, and degeneration of fat associated with the thigh and heart may be noted. Vascular damage and fibrin thrombi are common findings on microscopic examination.

Diagnosis: A presumptive diagnosis can be based on an impression smear of the liver or spleen or on a smear of cardiac blood or bone marrow that shows gram-positive, slender, pleomorphic rods. Bone marrow is the tissue of choice in partially decomposed specimens. Isolation and identification of *E rhusiopathiae* is necessary for definitive diagnosis. Identification can be made by fluorescent antibody staining and PCR. PCR can distinguish *E rhusiopathiae* from *E tonsillarum*. A mouse ear scarification model has been described and is particularly helpful for mixed cultures. An indirect ELISA is available, but virtually all poultry are exposed, with antibody levels increasing with age. Caution must be used in attempting reisolation, because the organism produces pinpoint colonies that may be easily overlooked or masked by faster-growing bacteria. Highly selective media are available for reisolation.

Infections with *Escherichia coli* or *Pasteurella multocida*, as well as salmonellosis and peracute Newcastle disease, may be confused with the septicemic form of erysipelas. Urticaria and endocarditis may be caused by other miscellaneous bacterial or fungal pathogens. Noninfectious differential diagnoses include poisoning, stampede injuries, or predators.

Treatment, Control, and Prevention: The antibiotic of choice is a rapid-acting penicillin such as potassium or sodium penicillin. As soon as a presumptive diagnosis is made, penicillin should be administered IM at 22,000 U/kg body wt, simultaneously with a full dose of erysipelas bacterin. Injectable penicillin is warranted for an acute outbreak but may be an extra-label use. In situations in which it is impractical to handle every bird, administration of penicillin in the drinking water at 395,000 U/L for 4–5 days reduces losses. Sulfonamides and oral oxytetracycline are not effective; broad-spectrum antibiotics, eg, erythromycin, are effective. Antibiotic in feed or water treats only those in the flock that are still eating and drinking normally and may not have dramatic results. Recovered birds have a high degree of resistance. Vaccination with a bacterin helps protect those birds in the flock not yet infected. However, bacterin-derived immunity is not long-lasting and may require two or more injections at intervals of 2–4 wk. Antibiotic therapy or vaccination does not eliminate the carrier state. Antibiotic resistance to tetracycline has been reported.

Vaccination will control erysipelas. Both inactivated and live vaccines are available for use in turkeys; only vaccines approved for use in turkeys should be used. The use of bacterins in flocks used for meat is useful but labor intensive. For breeders, the bacterin should be given every 4 wk before onset of egg production. The use of live vaccines administered in the drinking water does not require handling each bird and, therefore, is less stressful. Live vaccines require two doses at intervals of 2–3 wk. Commercially available swine erysipelas vaccine can be used in layers and is given at up to two times the recommended dose for swine via injection. It does not interfere with egg production. Although the swine vaccine is safe, no challenge studies have been done.

There are no specific husbandry recommendations other than sound management practices for the control of erysipelas in poultry, particularly in endemic areas. After an outbreak, equipment should be thoroughly disinfected and dead birds removed from the premises.

Zoonotic Risks: *E rhusiopathiae* can infect people and causes three different syndromes: erysipeloid, a generalized cutaneous form, and a septicemic form with endocarditis. The organism usually enters through cuts in the skin, and those at risk include people who handle infected tissues, such as veterinarians, butchers, and fish handlers. There have been no reports of people becoming infected through the oral route.

FATTY LIVER HEMORRHAGIC SYNDROME

Fatty liver hemorrhagic syndrome (FLHS) was first described in the 1950s as excessive fat in the liver of prolific laying hens, associated with varying degrees of hemorrhage. The condition is almost universally confined to caged birds fed high-energy diets and is most often seen in white-egg layers in warm, summer months. The liver is usually enlarged, putty colored, and very friable, showing varying degrees of hemorrhage. The abdominal cavity often contains large amounts of oily, unsaturated fat. Affected birds often have pale combs, likely as a consequence of reduced egg production. The ovary is usually active, at least in the early stages of FLHS, and the metabolic and physical stress associated with oviposition may be factors that induce the final fatal hemorrhage.

Because FLHS seems to occur only when birds are in a positive energy balance, body weight monitoring is a good diagnostic tool, as is knowledge of daily feed intake and environmental temperature. Through force-feeding techniques, it has been shown that FLHS is caused by a surfeit of energy rather than an excess of any particular nutrients such as fat or carbohydrate. The condition can be induced experimentally in layers and even male birds by administration of estrogen. This supports the concept that FLHS occurs more frequently in high-producing birds that presumably are producing more estrogen from very active ovaries. Injecting immature pullets with testosterone also causes increased feed intake and liver fat accumulation, although without any major incidence of fatty liver.

FLHS is easy to recognize at necropsy because of the liver hemorrhage and the fact that the liver is enlarged and engorged with fat. This makes the liver friable, and it is difficult to remove each lobe in one piece. The pale yellow color of the liver, while characteristic, is not always specific to FLHS. Normal layers that are fed appreciable quantities of yellow corn or high levels of xanthophyll pigments will also have a yellow-colored liver but without associated hemorrhages. A number of specific diet ingredients can induce liver hemorrhage but without concomitant accumulation of excess fat. Likewise, feeding rancid fat can cause liver hemorrhage, again without fat accumulation. In birds with FLHS, the liver dry matter is characteristically at least 40% fat. The degree of FLHS can be described as a poultry liver hemorrhage score, which is usually based on a scale of 1–5, in which 1 = no hemorrhage; 2 = 1–5 hemorrhages; 3 = 6–15 hemorrhages; 4 = 16–25 hemorrhages; and 5 = >25 hemorrhages, as well as a massive, usually fatal, hemorrhage. There is some evidence that fatty liver disorder also impairs calcium metabolism in the bird, and hence skeletal integrity and eggshell quality. Layers with FLHS have increased blood levels of estrogen, osteocalcin, and leptin-like protein. There seems to be concomitant upregulation in bone turnover, which is a very significant occurrence for a laying hen that already relies on significant daily flux of calcium in and out of the skeleton.

Attempts have been made to prevent or treat the condition through dietary modification. Substituting carbohydrate with supplemental fat, while not increasing the energy content of the diet, seems to be beneficial. Presumably such modification means that the liver needs to synthesize less fat for yolk. Replacement of corn with other cereals, such as wheat and barley, is often beneficial. However, this substitution may involve reducing the dietary energy level or necessitate using additional fat to maintain isoenergetic conditions, two factors known to influence FLHS. FLHS has reportedly been reduced through the use of various byproduct feeds such as distiller's grains, fish meal, and alfalfa meal. Although such mode of action is unclear, unintentional supplementation of selenium may be involved. There are reports of layers having greater incidence of fatty liver when fed chelated trace minerals versus conventional inorganic minerals. However, the use of organic minerals in layer diets is increasing, and FLHS is not usually reported. There are also reports of association with *Mycoplasma* infection.

FLHS is best prevented by not allowing an excessive positive energy balance in older birds. Body weight can be monitored and, when potential problems are seen, remedial action taken to limit energy intake through the use of lower energy diets and/or change in feed management. A wide energy:protein ratio in the diet will aggravate FLHS. When a farm has a history of FLHS, the diet should contain at least 0.3 ppm selenium, ideally as organic selenium, up to 100 IU vitamin E/kg diet, and appropriate levels of an antioxidant such as ethoxyquin. These various additives collectively help to limit the occurrence of tissue rancidity, and hence hemorrhage of the excess fat in the liver.

SUDDEN DEATH SYNDROME OF BROILER CHICKENS

(Flip-over disease, Acute death syndrome, Dead in good condition)

A syndrome of sudden death has been reported in most areas of the world that raise broilers intensively. Young, healthy, fast-growing broiler chickens die suddenly with a short, terminal, wing-beating convulsion. Many affected broilers just "flip over" and die on their backs; 60%–80% are males. The condition is uncommon or unrecognized when low-density feed is used.

Etiology and Epidemiology: The cause is unknown, but it is thought to be a metabolic disease related to carbohydrate metabolism, lactic acidosis, loss of cell membrane integrity, and intracellular electrolyte imbalance. Recent studies link this disease to cardiac arrhythmias. The modern broiler, which has been selected for growth rate and feed conversion efficiency, has a predisposition to cardiac arrhythmias. One study found the prevalence of arrhythmias to be much higher in broilers (27%) than leghorns (1%), but it is not clear whether this predisposition is dietary or genetic. Stress is the most likely trigger of cardiac arrhythmias in broilers, which predisposes the bird to death from ventricular fibrillation. The prevalence in a rapidly growing healthy broiler flock is typically 0.5%–4%.

Clinical Findings: Broilers show no premonitory signs. They appear healthy and may be feeding, sparring, walking, or resting, but suddenly extend their necks, gasp or squawk, and die rapidly with a short period of wing beating and leg movement, during which they frequently flip onto their backs. They also may be found dead on their sides or breasts.

Sudden death syndrome may occur as early as day 3 and may continue until 10–12 wk in roaster flocks. Mortality usually peaks between days 12 and 28, although it may peak as early as day 9. If growth is restricted early, it may peak only after day 28. Mortality of 0.25%–0.5% per day can occur for 1–3 days.

Lesions: There are no specific gross lesions. Recent studies indicate that affected birds have characteristic microscopic lesions in cardiomyocytes and subendocardial Purkinje cells, and this may help in diagnosis. Dead birds are well fleshed, have an empty or partially filled crop, and feed in the gizzard. The abdomen is distended because the bird is fat and the intestines are filled with ingesta, indicating peracute death. The muscles are mottled red and white as a result of focal congestion, and the organs are moderately to severely congested. There may be small hemorrhages in the liver and kidney. Although the ventricles of the heart are contracted, there is no sign of hypertrophy, and the atria are dilated and blood filled. The lungs are congested and frequently edematous; however, pulmonary edema increases with time after death and is not prominent in broilers that are examined within a few minutes of death. The gallbladder may be small or empty, because feed intake is normal up until the time of death.

Diagnosis: Sudden death syndrome should be suspected in well grown and otherwise healthy-looking broilers found dead on their backs, because that position is rare in death from other causes except cardiac tamponade, asphyxia, and ascites syndrome (*see* p 2871). The syndrome is also the likely cause when dead birds that are otherwise in good condition are found lying on their sides or breasts randomly throughout the pen. Diagnosis is supported by necropsy findings if there is a lack of obvious pathology (ie, a digestive tract filled with ingesta, contracted ventricles, dilated and blood-filled atria, lung congestion, and edema). The presence of characteristic microscopic lesions in cardiomyocytes and subendocardial Purkinje cells is helpful in confirming the diagnosis. Affected cells have vacuolated sarcoplasm, cytoplasmic eosinophilia, and nuclear pyknosis.

The condition called sudden death syndrome in Australia in broiler breeders coming into production is a different disease; it is reported to be caused by potassium deficiency. Similar mortality caused by a combination of high environmental temperature and hypophosphatemia or by acute hypocalcemia has been reported in North America.

Sudden death in turkeys can be caused by choke, aortic rupture (*see* p 2787), focal (obstructive) granulomatous pneumonia, or by hypertrophic cardiomyopathy (*see* p 2790) with lung congestion and edema, splenomegaly, and perirenal hemorrhage (*see* p 2789).

Prevention and Control: The incidence of sudden death syndrome can be minimized by slowing the growth rate of broilers, particularly during the first 3 wk of life. Growth rate can be moderated by controlling nutrient intake. This can be accomplished by reducing the number of hours of light per day, reducing the energy and protein level in the diet, or limiting the amount of feed provided.

FOWL CHOLERA

Fowl cholera is a contagious, bacterial disease that affects domestic and wild birds worldwide. It usually occurs as a septicemia of sudden onset with high morbidity and mortality, but chronic and asymptomatic infections also occur.

Etiology and Transmission: *Pasteurella multocida*, the causal agent, is a small, gram-negative, nonmotile rod with a capsule that may exhibit pleomorphism after repeated subculture. *P multocida* is considered a single species although it includes three subspecies: *multocida*, *septica*, and *gallicida*. Subspecies *multocida* is the most common cause of disease, but *septica* and *gallicida* may also cause cholera-like disease.

In freshly isolated cultures or in tissues, the bacteria have a bipolar appearance when stained with Wright's stain. Although *P multocida* may infect a wide variety of animals, strains isolated from nonavian hosts generally do not produce fowl cholera. Strains that cause fowl cholera represent a number of immunotypes (or serotypes), which complicates efforts at widespread prevention using bacterins. The organism is susceptible to ordinary disinfectants, sunlight, drying, and heat. Turkeys and waterfowl are more susceptible than chickens, older chickens are more susceptible than young ones, and some breeds of chickens are more susceptible than others.

Chronically infected birds and asymptomatic carriers are considered to be major sources of infection. Wild birds may introduce the organism into a poultry flock, but mammals (including rodents, pigs, dogs, and cats) may also carry the infection. However, the role of these as a reservoir has not been thoroughly investigated. Dissemination of *P multocida* within a flock and between houses is primarily by excretions from the mouth, nose, and conjunctiva of diseased birds that contaminate their environment. In addition, *P multocida* survives long enough to be spread by contaminated crates, feed bags, shoes, and other equipment. The infection does not seem to be egg-transmitted.

Clinical Findings: Clinical findings vary greatly depending on the course of disease. In acute fowl cholera, finding a large number of dead birds without previous signs is usually the first indication of disease. Mortality often increases rapidly. In more protracted cases, depression, anorexia, mucoid discharge from the mouth, ruffled feathers, diarrhea, and increased respiratory rate are usually seen. Pneumonia is particularly common in turkeys.

In chronic fowl cholera, signs and lesions are generally related to localized infections of the sternal bursae, wattles, joints, tendon sheaths, and footpads, which often are swollen because of accumulated fibrinosuppurative exudate. There may be exudative conjunctivitis and pharyngitis. Torticollis may result when the meninges, middle ear, or cranial bones are infected.

Lesions: Lesions observed in peracute and acute forms of the disease are primarily vascular disturbances. These include general passive hyperemia and congestion throughout the carcass, accompanied by enlargement of the liver and spleen. Petechial and ecchymotic hemorrhages are common, particularly in subepicardial and subserosal locations. Increased amounts of peritoneal and pericardial fluids are frequently seen. In addition, acute oophoritis with hyperemic follicles may be observed. In subacute cases, multiple, small, necrotic foci may be disseminated throughout the liver and spleen.

In chronic forms of fowl cholera, suppurative lesions may be widely

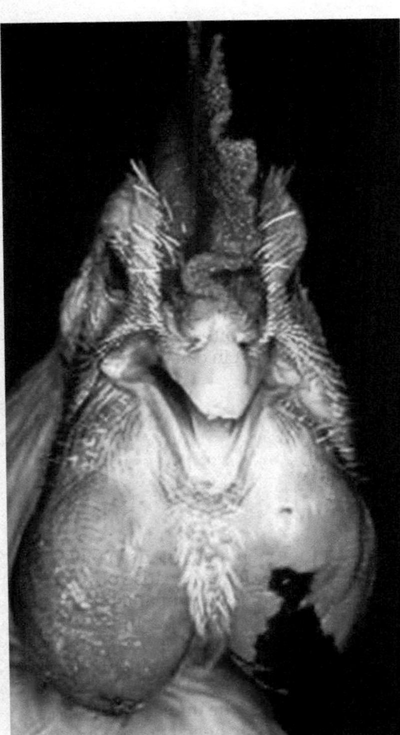

Swollen wattles in a broiler breeder male as the result of a chronic fowl cholera infection. *Courtesy of Dr. Jean Sander.*

distributed, often involving the respiratory tract, the conjunctiva, and adjacent tissues of the head. Caseous arthritis and productive inflammation of the peritoneal cavity and the oviduct are common in chronic infections. A fibrinonecrotic dermatitis that includes caudal parts of the dorsum, abdomen, and breast and involves the cutis, subcutis, and underlying muscle has been observed in turkeys and broilers. Sequestered necrotic lung lesions in poultry should always raise suspicion of cholera.

Diagnosis: Although the history, signs, and lesions may aid diagnosis, *P multocida* should be isolated, characterized, and identified for confirmation. Primary isolation can be accomplished using media such as blood agar, dextrose starch agar, or trypticase soy agar. Isolation may be improved by the addition of 5% heat-inactivated serum. *P multocida* can be readily isolated from viscera of birds dying from peracute/acute fowl cholera, whereas isolation from suppurative lesions of chronic cholera may be more difficult. At necropsy, bipolar microorganisms may be demonstrated by the use of Wright's or Giemsa stain of impression smears obtained from the liver in the case of acute cholera. In addition, immunofluorescent microscopy and in situ hybridization have been used to identify *P multocida* in infected tissues and exudates.

PCR has been used for the detection of *P multocida* in pure and mixed cultures and clinical samples. This method may help identify carrier animals within flocks. However, the specificity and sensitivity of the PCR must be improved. *P multocida* can be subgrouped by capsule serogroup antigens into five capsular types (A, B, D, E, and F) and into 16 somatic serotypes. Somatic serotyping is important to choose the right bacterins for prevention. However, conventional serotyping suffers from problems with reproducibility and reliability, and the methods are quite laborious. Recently, a multiplex PCR has been developed that can differentiate between different somatic serotypes. This will be of great value as a diagnostic tool and enable more efficient vaccine development in the future.

Serologic testing can be done by rapid whole blood agglutination, serum plate agglutination, agar diffusion tests, and ELISA. Serology may be used to evaluate vaccine responses but has very limited value for diagnostic purposes.

Several bacterial infections may be confused with fowl cholera based solely on the gross lesions. *Escherichia coli*, *Salmonella enterica*, *Ornithobacterium rhinotracheale*, gram-positive cocci, and *Erysipelothrix rhusiopathiae* (erysipelas) may all produce lesions indistinguishable from those caused by *P multocida*.

Prevention: Good management practices, including a high level of biosecurity, are essential to prevention. Rodents, wild birds, pets, and other animals that may be carriers of *P multocida* must be excluded from poultry houses. Adjuvant bacterins are widely used and generally effective; autogenous bacterins are recommended when polyvalent bacterins are found to be ineffective. Thus, it is important to know the most prevalent serotypes within an area to choose the right bacterins. Attenuated live vaccines are available for administration in drinking water to turkeys and by wing-web inoculation to chickens. These live vaccines can effectively induce immunity against different serotypes of *P multocida*. They are recommended for use in healthy flocks only.

Treatment: A number of drugs will lower mortality from fowl cholera; however, deaths may resume when treatment is discontinued, showing that treatment does not eliminate *P multocida* from a flock. Eradication of infection requires depopulation and cleaning and disinfection of buildings and equipment. The premise should then be kept free of poultry for a few weeks.

Sulfonamides and antibiotics are commonly used; early treatment and adequate dosages are important. Sensitivity testing often aids in drug selection and is important because of the emergence of multiresistant strains. Sulfaquinoxaline sodium in feed or water usually controls mortality, as do sulfamethazine and sulfadimethoxine. Sulfas should be used with caution in breeders because of potential toxicity. High levels of tetracycline antibiotics in the feed (0.04%), drinking water, or administered parenterally may be useful. Norfloxacin administered via drinking water is also effective against fowl cholera. However, many countries do not allow the use of quinolones in food-producing animals, including poultry, because of the risk of development of drug resistance. Penicillin is often effective for sulfa-resistant infections. In ducks, a combined injection of streptomycin and dihydrostreptomycin can be effective.

FOWLPOX

FOWLPOX IN CHICKENS AND TURKEYS

Fowlpox is a slow-spreading viral infection of chickens and turkeys characterized by proliferative lesions in the skin that progress to thick scabs (cutaneous form) and by lesions in the upper GI and respiratory tracts (diphtheritic form). Virulent strains may cause lesions in the internal organs (systemic form). Fowlpox is seen worldwide.

Etiology and Epidemiology: The large DNA virus (an avipoxvirus in the Poxviridae family) is resistant and may survive in the environment for extended periods in dried scabs. Photolyase and A-type inclusion body protein genes in the genome of fowlpox virus appear to protect the virus from environmental insults. Field and vaccine strains have only minor differences in their genomic profiles, although the strains can be differentiated to some extent by restriction endonuclease analysis and immunoblotting. Recently, molecular analyses of vaccine and field strains of fowlpox viruses have shown some significant differences. The virus is present in large numbers in the lesions and is usually transmitted by contact through abrasions of the skin. Skin lesions (scabs) shed from recovering birds in poultry houses can become a source of aerosol infection. Mosquitoes and other biting insects may serve as mechanical vectors. Transmission within flocks is rapid when mosquitoes are plentiful. The disease tends to persist for extended periods in multiple-age poultry complexes because of slow spread of the virus and availability of susceptible birds.

Clinical Findings: The cutaneous form of fowlpox is characterized by nodular lesions on various parts of the unfeathered skin of chickens and on the head and upper neck of turkeys. Generalized lesions of feathered skin may also be seen. In some cases, lesions are limited chiefly to the feet and legs. The lesion is initially a raised, blanched, nodular area that enlarges, becomes yellowish, and progresses to a thick, dark scab. Multiple lesions usually develop and often coalesce. Lesions in various stages of development may be found on the same bird. Localization around the nostrils may cause nasal discharge. Cutaneous lesions on the eyelids may cause complete closure of one or both eyes. Only a few birds develop cutaneous lesions at one time. Lesions are prominent in some birds and may significantly decrease flock performance.

In the diphtheritic form of fowlpox, lesions develop on the mucous membranes of the mouth, esophagus, pharynx, larynx, and trachea (wetpox or fowl diphtheria). Occasionally, lesions are seen almost exclusively in one or more of these sites. Caseous patches firmly adherent to the mucosa of the larynx and mouth or proliferative masses may develop. Mouth lesions interfere with feeding. Tracheal lesions cause difficulty in respiration. Laryngeal and tracheal lesions in chickens must be

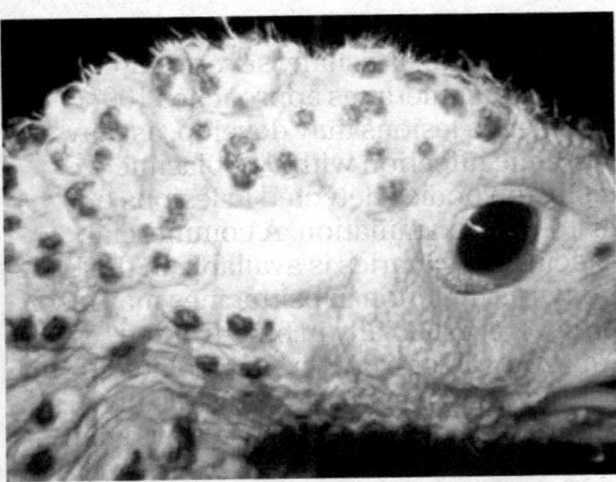

Scab-like lesion on the unfeathered portion of the skin due to fowlpox on a turkey.
Courtesy of Dr. Jean Sander.

differentiated from those of infectious laryngotracheitis (*see* p 2912), which is caused by a herpesvirus. In cases of systemic infection caused by virulent fowlpox virus strains, lesions may be seen in internal organs. More than one form of the disease, ie, cutaneous, diphtheritic, and/or systemic, may be seen in a single bird.

Often, the course of the disease in a flock is protracted. Extensive infection in a layer flock results in decreased egg production. Cutaneous infections alone ordinarily cause low or moderate mortality, and these flocks generally return to normal production after recovery. Mortality is usually high in diphtheritic or systemic infections.

Diagnosis: Cutaneous infections usually produce characteristic gross and microscopic lesions. When only small cutaneous lesions are present, it is often difficult to distinguish them from abrasions caused by fighting. Microscopic examination of affected tissues stained with H&E reveals eosinophilic cytoplasmic inclusion bodies. Cytoplasmic inclusions are also detectable by fluorescent antibody and immunohistochemical methods (using antibodies against fowlpox virus antigens). The elementary bodies in the inclusion bodies can be detected in smears from lesions stained by the Gimenez method. Viral particles with typical poxvirus morphology can be demonstrated by negative-staining electron microscopy as well as in ultrathin sections of the lesions. The virus can be isolated by inoculating chorioallantoic membrane of developing chicken embryos, susceptible birds, or cell cultures of avian origin. Chicken embryos (9–12 days old) from an SPF flock are the preferred and convenient host for virus isolation.

The genomic profiles of field isolates and vaccine strains of fowlpox virus can be compared by restriction fragment length polymorphism. This method is useful to compare closely related DNA genomes. However, because of the large size of the genome, minor differences are difficult to detect by this method. Detailed genetic analysis reveals differences between vaccine strains and field strains responsible for outbreaks of fowlpox in previously vaccinated chicken flocks. Whereas vaccine strains of fowlpox virus contain remnants of long terminal repeats of reticuloendotheliosis virus (REV), most field strains contain full-length REV in their genome.

Nucleic acid probes derived from cloned genomic fragments of fowlpox virus can also be used for diagnosis. This procedure is especially useful for differentiation of the diphtheritic form of fowlpox (involving the trachea) from infectious laryngotracheitis.

PCR can be used to amplify genomic DNA sequences of various sizes using specific primers. This procedure is useful when an extremely small amount of viral DNA is present in the sample. PCR has been used effectively to differentiate field and vaccine strains of the virus, whether full-length REV is present in those strains that are associated with outbreaks in vaccinated birds. DNA isolated from the formalin-fixed tissue sections of birds that are histologically positive for fowlpox can be used for PCR amplification of genomic fragments using specific primers. Because most outbreaks of fowlpox in previously vaccinated chickens are caused by strains with a genome that contains full-length REV, use of REV envelope-specific primers to determine the presence of full-length REV is helpful in such cases.

Two monoclonal antibodies that recognize different fowlpox virus antigens have been developed. These monoclonal antibodies are useful for strain differentiation by immunoblotting.

The complete nucleotide sequence of the fowlpox virus genome has been determined. It is useful in comparing the sequences of selected genes of other avian poxviruses.

Prevention and Treatment: Where fowlpox is prevalent, chickens and turkeys should be vaccinated with a live-embryo or cell-culture-propagated virus vaccine. The most widely used vaccines are attenuated fowlpox virus and pigeonpox virus isolates of high immunogenicity and low pathogenicity. In high-risk areas, vaccination with an attenuated vaccine of cell-culture origin in the first few weeks of life and revaccination at 12–16 wk is often sufficient. Health of birds, extent of exposure, and type of operation determine the timing of vaccinations. Because the infection spreads slowly, vaccination is often useful in limiting spread in affected flocks if administered when <20% of the birds have lesions. Passive immunity may interfere with multiplication of vaccine virus; progeny from recently vaccinated or recently infected flocks should be vaccinated only after passive immunity has declined. Vaccinated birds should be examined 1 wk later for swelling and scab formation ("take") at the site of vaccination. Absence of "take" indicates lack of potency of vaccine, passive or acquired immunity, or improper vaccination. Revaccination with another serial lot of vaccine may be indicated.

Naturally infected or vaccinated birds develop humoral as well as cell-mediated immune responses. Humoral immune responses can be measured by ELISA or virus neutralization tests.

Zoonotic Risk: There is no zoonotic risk associated with fowlpox virus. Avian poxviruses cause a productive infection in avian species but a nonproductive infection in mammalian hosts. Consequently, avianpox viruses have been used as vectors for expression of genes from mammalian pathogens in the development of safe recombinant vaccines.

POX IN OTHER AVIAN SPECIES

Infections with avian poxvirus have been seen in a variety of wild and pet birds. Some isolates are primarily infectious for only the homologous host, whereas others are infectious for one or more additional species. In the absence of genetic information on most of these viruses, classification has usually been based on host pathogenicity or cross-protection studies. The nucleotide sequence of canarypox virus genome has been determined. Canarypox virus infection is usually severe, and mortality sometimes approaches 100%. Cutaneous lesions may develop, as may systemic infection with cytoplasmic inclusion bodies detected in lesions on histologic examination. A commercial vaccine for canaries is available in the USA. Poxvirus infection in psittacines may also be severe, especially in blue-fronted Amazon parrots. Poxviruses isolated from psittacines appear to be antigenically different from poxviruses of other avian species.

Genomic profiles of canarypox, mynahpox, and quailpox viruses show marked differences from fowlpox virus when their DNA is compared by restriction fragment length polymorphism after restriction endonuclease digestion. Quailpox virus shows marked antigenic differences from fowlpox virus and, although some cross-reacting antigens are present, provides limited or no cross-protection against fowlpox virus. Avianpox virus infection has been considered as a population-limiting factor in endangered Hawaiian forest birds. Avianpox viruses isolated from Hawaiian crows (*Corvus hawaiiansis*), Hawaiian geese (*Branta sandvicensis*), Palila (*Loxiodes bailleui*), and Apapane species (*Himatione sanguinea*) are different from each other and from fowlpox virus. Similarly, a poxvirus isolated from an Andean condor (*Vultur gryphus*) at the San Diego Zoo is antigenically, genetically, and biologically different from fowlpox virus. Like fowlpox virus, these viruses appear to be suitable vectors for expression of foreign genes toward development of genetically modified virus vaccines for mammalian species. Several canarypox virus vectored vaccines expressing genes of mammalian pathogens are available commercially.

GOOSE PARVOVIRUS INFECTION

(Derzsy disease, Goose hepatitis, Goose plague)

Goose parvovirus infection is a highly contagious and fatal disease of goslings and Muscovy ducklings, often causing as much as 70%–100% mortality in goslings <4 wk old. Goose parvovirus has been reported from all the major goose-farming countries of Europe and the Far East, where the disease is of serious economic significance.

Muscovy ducks and several hybrid duck breeds are also susceptible to another parvovirus that has been shown to be antigenically related to goose parvovirus. This so-called Muscovy duck parvovirus has been isolated from an outbreak among Muscovy ducks in California. Goose parvovirus has not been detected in the USA.

Etiology: Goose parvovirus is a member of the family Parvoviridae and, based on phylogenetic analysis, has been shown to be related to the dependovirus genus. Apart from the Muscovy duck parvovirus, to which it is closely related, goose parvovirus shows no similarity to the other avian or mammalian parvoviruses. After primary infection, the virus replicates in the intestinal wall and, after a short viremic phase, reaches the heart, liver, and other organs.

Transmission and Epidemiology: The virus is excreted in large amounts in the feces of infected birds, resulting in rapid spread by direct and indirect means. Outbreaks are often initiated in susceptible goslings after transmission of the virus via eggs laid by infected breeder geese. Evidence suggests that older, subclinically infected geese may act as carriers. Infected eggs are often the source of the virus when outbreaks of goose parvovirus occur in countries or geographic locations formerly free of the disease. Serologic evidence suggests that the virus is present in several species of wild geese in Europe. No other avian or biologic vectors have been identified.

Clinical Findings: In susceptible goslings and ducklings, clinical signs vary according to the age of the birds. The course of the disease in birds <1 wk old is rapid, with anorexia and death occurring within 2–5 days. Mortality can reach 100% in birds infected in the hatchery. In older birds, the disease follows a more protracted course, characterized by ocular and nasal discharge, a profuse white diarrhea, and weakness. The eyelids and uropygial glands are red and swollen. Birds that survive the acute stage show profound growth retardation, with loss of feathers and reddening of the skin, particularly on the back. Birds may stand in a "penguin-like" posture due to accumulation of ascitic fluid in the abdomen. In 2- to 4-wk-old birds, mortality can reach 10%, but morbidity levels may be much higher. No clinical signs are seen in older birds, although adults will respond immunologically. An enteric form of goose parvovirus infection has been documented to exist.

Lesions: Gross lesions include the presence of a fibrinous pseudomembrane covering the tongue and oral cavity, perihepatitis, pericarditis, pulmonary edema, liver dystrophy, and catarrhal enteritis. In acute cases, the heart is characteristically rounded at the apex, with a pale myocardium. The main microscopic lesions are pronounced degenerative changes in the myocardial cells and the presence of Cowdry type-A intranuclear inclusion bodies.

Diagnosis: A presumptive diagnosis is based on the characteristic clinical course, age incidence, and gross and histologic lesions. Confirmation can be obtained after isolation of the parvovirus in cell cultures or embryonated eggs derived from susceptible geese and Muscovy ducks. Presence of the virus can be confirmed by electron microscopic examination of infected cultures and neutralization with specific goose parvovirus antiserum. Diagnosis can also be confirmed by direct detection of antigen or virus in tissues from infected birds, by immunofluorescence, or by the use of PCR. Serologic tests for goose parvovirus include virus neutralization, agar gel precipitation, immunofluorescence, and ELISA.

Although goose parvovirus causes disease in both geese and Muscovy ducks, Muscovy ducks are also infected with another antigenically related parvovirus. This virus causes serious disease in Muscovy ducklings, but not in goslings, and can be detected and differentiated using PCR combined with sequencing or restriction fragment length polymorphism. Differential diagnoses should also include duck viral enteritis (duck plague, *see* p 2799), which affects all types of waterfowl. Duck viral hepatitis (*see* p 2815) causes a fatal disease in ducklings but is not pathogenic for goslings or Muscovy ducklings. *Riemerella anatipestifer* and *Pasteurella multocida* may also cause high mortality in goslings and Muscovy ducklings but can be differentiated by bacterial isolation and identification.

Prevention and Treatment: Goslings should be hatched together only from flocks that are known to be free of goose parvovirus; many outbreaks are attributed to the practice of custom-hatching eggs from various sources. Eggs should be imported only from countries that can guarantee freedom from goose parvovirus. Geese that have survived an outbreak should not be used for breeding purposes. Both live, inactivated oil emulsion vaccines and baculovirus expressed VP2 capsid-based recombinant vaccines are available and are widely used in countries where the disease is endemic. Vaccination of breeding flocks induces high levels of maternal antibody in the progeny until ~2 wk of age.

HELMINTHIASIS

(Nematode and cestode infections)

Approximately 100 worm species have been recognized in wild and domestic birds in the USA. Nematodes (roundworms) are the most significant in number of species and in economic impact. Of species found in commercial poultry, the common roundworm (*Ascaridia galli*) is by far the most common. Field studies show that poultry maintained under free-range conditions may be heavily parasitized; therefore, control measures such as preventing infections or chemotherapy are likely to improve weight gain and egg production. In surveys of poultry raised under nonconfinement conditions throughout the world, an incidence of infection >80% is not uncommon.

Generally, nematodes have separate sexes that have morphologic differences; eg, males of *Tetrameres* spp are elongated and slender, whereas gravid females are globe-shaped. The size and shape of nematode species vary widely; ascarids are sturdy and long (up to 4.5 in. [116 mm]); capillarids are more delicate, slender, and long (2.3 in. [60 mm]); and other nematodes are much shorter (0.08–0.48 in. [2–12 mm]).

Cestodes (tapeworms) also vary in size. *Raillietina* spp may be >12 in. (30 cm), whereas *Davainea proglottina* often is <0.16 in. (4 mm). The proglottids of individual tapeworms are hermaphroditic. Tapeworms have been recovered in the thousands from individual chickens and turkeys.

See TABLE 5 for information on common nematodes and cestodes of poultry.

TABLE 5 COMMON HELMINTHS OF POULTRY

Parasite	Host	Intermediate Host or Life Cycle	Organ Infected	Pathogenicity
		NEMATODES		
Amidostomum anseri	Duck, goose, pigeon	Direct	Gizzard	Severe
Ascaridia dissimilis	Turkey	Direct	Small intestine	Moderate
Ascaridia galli	Chicken, turkey, duck, quail	Direct	Small intestine	Moderate
Capillaria caudinflata	Chicken, turkey, duck, game birds, pigeon	Earthworms	Small intestine	Moderate to severe
Capillaria contorta	Chicken, turkey, duck, game birds	None or earthworms	Mouth, esophagus, crop	Severe
Capillaria obsignata	Chicken, turkey, goose, pigeon, quail	Direct	Small intestine, ceca	Severe
Cheilospirura hamulosa	Chicken, turkey, game birds	Grasshoppers, beetles	Gizzard	Moderate
Cyathostoma bronchialis	Turkey, duck	Direct or earthworm	Trachea	Severe
Cyrnea colini	Turkey, game birds	Cockroaches	Proventriculus	Mild

(continued)

TABLE 5 COMMON HELMINTHS OF POULTRY *(continued)*

Parasite	Host	Intermediate Host or Life Cycle	Organ Infected	Pathogenicity
Dispharynx nasuta	Chicken, turkey, game birds, pigeon	Sowbugs	Proventriculus	Moderate to severe
Gongylonema ingluvicola	Chicken, game birds	Beetles, cockroaches	Crop, esophagus, proventriculus	Mild
Heterakis gallinarum	Chicken, turkey, duck, game birds	Direct	Ceca	Mild, but transmits agent of histomoniasis
Heterakis isolonche	Quail, duck, pheasant	Direct	Ceca	Severe
Ornithostrongylus quadriradiatus	Pigeon, dove	Direct	Small intestine	Severe
Oxyspirura mansoni	Chicken, turkey, guinea fowl, quail	Cockroaches	Eye	Moderate
Strongyloides avium	Chicken, turkey, quail, goose	Direct	Ceca	Moderate
Subulura brumpti	Chicken, turkey, duck, game birds	Earwigs, grasshoppers, beetles, cockroaches	Ceca	Mild
Syngamus trachea	Chicken, turkey, pheasant, quail	None or earthworm	Trachea	Severe
Tetrameres americana	Chicken, turkey, duck, game birds, pigeon	Grasshoppers, cockroaches	Proventriculus	Moderate to severe
Trichostrongylus tenuis	Chicken, turkey, duck, game birds, pigeon	Direct	Ceca	Severe
CESTODES				
Choanotaenia infundibulum	Chicken	House flies	Upper intestine	Moderate
Davainea proglottina	Chicken	Slugs, snails	Duodenum	Severe
Metroliasthes lucida	Turkey	Grasshoppers	Intestine	Unknown
Raillietina cesticillus	Chicken	Beetles	Duodenum, jejunum	Mild
Raillietina echinobothrida	Chicken	Ants	Lower intestine	Severe, nodules
Raillietina tetragona	Chicken	Ants	Lower intestine	Severe

Transmission: Modern confinement rearing of poultry has significantly reduced the frequency and variety of endoparasite infections, which are common in ranged birds and in backyard flocks. However, severe parasitism still may be seen in floor-reared layers, breeders, turkeys, or pen-reared game birds where management problems may exist. Contributing factors include the use of poorly managed built-up litter (which fosters the propagation of intermediate hosts and the accumulation of infective eggs) and resistance of the parasites to therapeutic drugs. Range infections of nematodes such as *Heterakis gallinarum* and *Syngamus trachea* may increase because of seasonal or climatic abundance of specific invertebrate intermediate hosts, eg, large numbers of earthworms brought to the surface by spring rains. Some species have been associated with large numbers of darkling beetles, which may act as mechanical vectors of infective eggs.

Nematodes have either a species-specific, direct life cycle with bird-to-bird transmission by ingestion of infective eggs or larvae, or an indirect cycle that requires an intermediate host (eg, insects, snails, or slugs). Eggs of many nematode species are resistant to low temperatures and disinfectants but may be more susceptible to heat and desiccation.

The life cycle of *A galli* is simple and direct. Eggs in the droppings become infective in 10–12 days under optimal conditions. The infective eggs are ingested and hatch in the proventriculus, and the larvae live free in the lumen of the duodenum for the first 9 days. They then penetrate the mucosa, causing hemorrhages, return to the lumen by 17–18 days, and reach maturity at 28–30 days. Levels of infection are often underestimated, because early larval stages are barely visible and can remain for long periods within intestinal tissues, whereas adult stages in the lumen are generally fewer in number. Maturation of larval stages can be hampered by adult worm numbers, thereby increasing the time larval stages remain in intestinal tissues and continue to cause damage.

The life cycle of *H gallinarum* is similar to that of *A galli*. The greatest production of eggs for each egg ingested occurs in the ring-necked pheasant, followed by the guinea fowl and chicken. The larvae are *closely associated* with the cecal tissue, but a true tissue phase rarely occurs. Most of the adult worms are found at the blind end of the ceca. Earthworms may ingest the eggs of the cecal worm and serve as a source of infection when ingested by poultry. Litter beetles may also serve as a mechanical vector.

The life cycle of *Capillaria* may be direct (*C obsignata*), require an intermediate host such as earthworms (*C caudinflata*), or be either direct or use earthworms (*C contorta*). Larval development in the egg takes 8–15 days depending on temperature. Worms reach maturity in 20–26 days after ingestion by the final host.

The gapeworm *Syngamus trachea* inhabits the trachea and lungs of many domestic and various wild birds. Infection may occur directly by ingestion of infective eggs or larvae; however, severe field infection is associated with ingestion of transport hosts such as earthworms, snails, slugs, and arthropods (eg, flies). Many gapeworm larvae may encyst and survive within a single invertebrate for years. Although gapeworms are not a problem in confinement-reared poultry, they cause serious economic losses in game-farm pens and in range-reared chickens, pheasants, turkeys, and peacocks. *Cyathostoma bronchialis* is the gapeworm of geese and ducks.

Eggs of *Oxyspirura mansoni*, Manson eyeworm, are deposited in the eye, reach the pharynx via the nasolacrimal duct, are swallowed, passed in the feces, and ingested by the Surinam cockroach, *Pycnoscelus surinamensis*. Larvae reach the infective stage in the cockroach. When infected intermediate hosts are eaten, liberated larvae migrate up the esophagus to the mouth and then through the nasolacrimal duct to the eye, where the cycle is completed. Other insect species may also serve as the intermediate host.

Cestodes require an intermediate host (eg, insects, crustaceans, earthworms, or snails). Floor layers, breeders, and broilers are infected with *Raillietina cesticillus* by

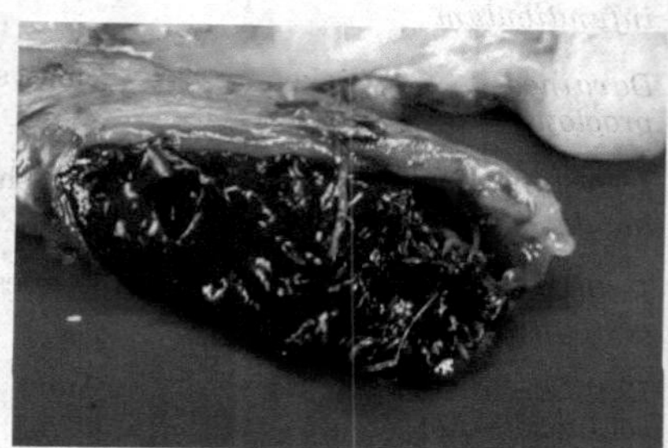

Heterakis gallinarum in the cecal pouches of a chicken. Courtesy of Dr. Jean Sander.

ingestion of the intermediate host, small beetles that breed in contaminated litter. Cage layers in unscreened houses may become infected with *Choanotaenia infundibulum* by eating its intermediate host, the house fly. Litter beetles in proximity may also serve as intermediate hosts.

More than 3,000 of the microscopic tapeworm *Davainea proglottina* have been recovered from a single bird. Several species of slugs and snails serve as intermediate hosts, and >1,500 infective parasites have been recovered from a single slug.

Pathogenesis and Clinical Findings: *Ascaridia*, *Heterakis*, and *Capillaria* spp are widely distributed and cause such nonspecific signs as general unthriftiness, inactivity, depressed appetite, and retarded growth; in severe cases, death may result. A mere few ascarids may depress weight, and larger numbers may block the intestinal tract. Ascarids may migrate up the oviduct (via the cloaca) to become enshelled later within the egg (an aesthetic, but not a public health, problem, avoidable by careful egg-candling before the release of eggs to market). *A dissimilis* (turkey roundworm) may also migrate out of the intestine, through the portal system, and into the liver, causing hepatic granulomas.

H gallinarum, a mild pathogen, in large numbers may cause thickening, inflammation, or nodulation in the cecal walls. Infection with *H gallinarum* has been associated with cecal and hepatic granulomas. *Heterakis isolonche*, highly pathogenic in pheasants, may cause 50% mortality. *H gallinarum* carries *Histomonas meleagridis*, the protozoan that causes histomoniasis (*see* p 2835).

C contorta in the mucosae of the crop and esophagus, and *C obsignata* in the wall of the small intestine, cause marked thickening and inflammation of the organs. Birds harboring large numbers of these threadlike worms become weak and emaciated and may die.

Young birds are the most severely affected by gapeworms. Sudden death and verminous pneumonia characterize early outbreaks. Signs of gasping, choking, shaking of the head, inanition, emaciation, and suffocation may follow. Necropsy reveals adult gapeworms obstructing the lumina of the trachea, bronchi, and lungs. Respiratory inflammation may be present. The blood-red, female gapeworm is usually found in copulation with a much smaller, paler male with its head embedded deep in the host tissue. The joined pair have a "Y"-shaped or forked appearance.

Oxyspirura mansoni is a slender nematode, 12–18 mm long, found beneath the nictitating membrane of chickens and other fowl in tropical and subtropical regions. The parasite causes various degrees of inflammation, lacrimation, corneal opacity, and disturbed vision.

Among other nematodes, *Amidostomum anseris* attacks the gizzard lining of ducks and geese and causes dark discoloration, necrosis, and sloughing at the parasitic loci. *Dispharynx nasuta* causes ulceration, thickening, and maceration of the proventriculus; heavily infected birds may die. *Tetrameres americana*, a bright red worm discernible through the proventricular wall, causes diarrhea, emaciation, and with heavy infection, death. *Trichostrongylus tenuis* causes inflamed ceca, weight loss, anemia, and death, especially in young birds. *Ornithostrongylus quadriradiatus*, a blood-sucking parasite, causes pigeons to regurgitate bile-stained fluid mixed with food; greenish mucoid diarrhea from hemorrhagic intestines, emaciation, and death follow.

Most pathogenic tapeworms are found in the small intestine; the scolex, usually buried in the mucosa, generally causes mild lesions. *Davainea proglottina* may cause weight loss. *Raillietina tetragona* causes weight loss and decreased egg production; *R echinobothrida* produces granulomas at its attachment sites ("nodular disease").

Diagnosis: A reliable diagnosis can be made only by accurate identification of the individually recovered parasites; careful and complete necropsy techniques are essential. Only by specific recognition of the parasite can meaningful recommendations for flock therapy and management be made.

Treatment and Control: Improvement of management and sanitation in confined operations will generally lower the parasite levels in the birds. In range birds, the only option is to move to new pastures, although the benefit that may result will be of short duration. Application of approved insecticides to soil and litter when premises are unoccupied may interrupt the life cycle of the parasite by destroying its intermediate host. When the premises are restocked, groups of birds of different species or ages should be widely separated to avoid spread of parasites. Migration of litter beetles or other insects may infect new or widely separated housing.

Approved compounds are very limited in the USA. Because of frequently changing regulations, the status of any medication should be checked before its administration. Approved drugs for the USA are listed online in the FDA's Green Book and in the commercially available Feed Compendium.

Only approved drugs may be used in birds producing eggs or meat for the commercial market. Label directions and recommended doses should be followed precisely, with scrupulous adherence to withdrawal times.

Piperazine compounds are relatively nontoxic and have been widely used against ascariasis. Because of this, drug resistance is widespread in many regions of the world. Several piperazine salts are available internationally. Because only the piperazine moiety is efficacious, doses should be calculated based on mg of active piperazine/bird. Piperazine should be completely consumed by birds within a few hours, because only relatively high concentrations of the drug eliminate worms. It may be given to chickens as a single dose, 50 mg/bird (<6 wk old), 100 mg/bird (≥6 wk old), in the feed at 0.2%–0.4% or in the drinking water at 0.1%–0.2%; it may be administered to turkeys at 100 mg/bird (<12 wk old) or 200 mg/bird (≥12 wk old). Some practitioners recommend the addition of molasses to unmedicated water after piperazine administration, so as to induce an osmotic flushing, theoretically removing any of the remaining worms from the intestinal tract. For severe cases, treatment can be repeated after 14 days. These medications must be withdrawn 14 days before slaughter. Piperazine is not approved in the USA for birds producing eggs for human consumption.

Fenbendazole is approved in the USA for use in growing turkeys at the rate of 14.5 g/ton of feed (16 ppm), fed continually as the sole ration for 6 days for the removal of *Ascaridia dissimilis* and *Heterakis gallinarum*. No withdrawal time is required. One study indicates a possible negative effect on sperm quality by the drug. It has been suggested that an alternative drug be used for treatment of breeding toms or that the sperm number and frequency of artificial inseminations be increased. Fenbendazole is not approved for use in other poultry in the USA but is effective against *Ascaris* when administered once at 10–50 mg/kg; if needed the treatment can be repeated after 10 days. At 10–50 mg/kg, fenbendazole when administered daily over 5 days is effective against *Capillaria*. Fenbendazole is also efffective against other nematodes when administered at 10–50 mg/kg/day for 3–5 days or as a single dosage of 20–100 mg/kg, or added to the drinking water at 125 mg/L for 5 days or to the feed at 100 mg/kg. Fenbendazole should not be administered during molt, because it may interfere with feather regrowth.

Hygromycin B given at 8–12 g/ton in feed is used to control ascarids, cecal worms, and capillarids in chickens. A withdrawal time of 3 days is required. Coumaphos, 0.004% in feed for 10–14 days for replacements, or 0.003% in feed for 14 days for layers, has been commonly used against capillarids. Chickens <8 wk old should not be given this medication, and it should not be used within 10 days of vaccination or other stress. In birds maintained on contaminated litter or exposed to infected birds, the medication regimen should be repeated using the same dosages as the first. There should be at least 3 wk between the first and second course of treatment. Hygromycin B is a cholinesterase inhibitor, and treated birds should not be exposed to other cholinesterase inhibitors (drugs, insecticides, pesticides, or chemicals) within 3 days before or after treatment.

As a treatment for Manson eyeworm, a local anesthetic can be applied to the eye, and the worms in the lacrimal sac exposed by lifting the nictitating membrane. A 5% cresol solution (1–2 drops) placed in the lacrimal sac kills the worms immediately. The eye should be irrigated with sterile water immediately to wash out the debris and excess solution. The eyes improve within 48–72 hr and gradually become clear if the destructive process caused by the parasite is not too far advanced.

The use of diatomaceous earth supplemented at 2% in feed and fed continuously lowers numbers of *Heterakis* and *Capillaria* in chickens. The efficacy of several essential oils have been measured, with inconsistent results.

Several compounds are reported to be effective against nematode infections but are not approved for use in poultry or other avian species in the USA. Three such compounds, tetramisole at 40 mg/kg, flubendazole at 30 ppm in feed, and ivermectin 1% at 10 mg/mL in water were effective in removing *A galli*, *H gallinarum*, and *Capillaria* in chickens. Pyrantel tartrate was more effective then pyrantel pamoate against the adult stage of *A galli*, and it was somewhat effective against *Capillaria* when administered at 15–25 mg/kg. Levamisole administered at 25–30 mg/kg appears to be effective against *A dissimilis*, *H gallinarum*, and *C obsignata*; it can also be given in the drinking water at 0.03%–0.06%. Phenothiazine has been used to treat cecal worms in chickens at 0.5 g/bird and in turkeys at 1 g/bird, given in 1 day. Combined in drinking water as a 1-day treatment, phenothiazine (0.5%–0.56%) and piperazine (0.11%) have been used to treat heterakids and ascarids; this drug combination is no longer approved for poultry in the USA. Methyridine injected SC at a dose of 25–45 mg/bird is effective in clearing *C obsignata*. In pigeons, a SC injection of 1 mL of 10% methyridine in the pectoral region or leg of pigeons removed *Capillaria*, but the drug must be handled with care because contact with skin may produce lesions. Coumaphos removes *Capillaria* in quail. Haloxon at 25 and 50 mg/kg, or at 750 ppm in the feed for 5–7 days, has good activity against *Capillaria* in chickens and quail.

Fenbendazole at 20 mg/kg for 3–4 days effectively removes gapeworms in pheasants. Toxicity has been reported in pigeons that received fenbendazole at the rate of 30 mg/kg for 5 days. Thiabendazole administered at 0.05% in the feed continually for 2 wk can be used for treatment of gapeworms in pheasants, and when given continually for ≥4 days is said to help prevent and control infections. Withdrawal of 21 days is required for meat consumption; specific precautions should be observed in feeds containing bentonite. Tetramisole at 3.6 mg/kg for 3 consecutive days in the drinking water removes gapeworms. Poultry treated while larvae are migrating in the body develop immunity to gapeworms, even though therapy may abort larval migration. Levamisole fed at a level of 0.04% for 2 days or at 2 g/gal. drinking water for 1 day each month has proved to be an effective control in game birds. Kiwis are reported to be acutely sensitive to levamisole at doses well within the safe range for domesticated poultry. Mebendazole fed prophylactically at 64 ppm or curatively at 125 ppm is effective in turkey poults. Cambendazole provided control when given in three treatments of 50 mg/kg for chickens and 20 mg/kg for turkeys. Albendazole administered as a single oral suspension (5 mg/kg bird weight) was reported effective against *A galli*, *H gallinarum*, and *C obsignata*. The drug also has been reported effective against cestodes if administered at 20 mg/kg. There are no published withdrawal times. Nitarsone at 170 g/ton (0.01875%) of feed has been reported to reduce *A dissimilis* fecundity and worm burden in chickens and turkeys.

There have been some reports of experimental drug treatment for other nematodes. Cambendazole (60 mg/kg), pyrantel (100 mg/kg), citarin (40 mg/kg), mebendazole (10 mg/kg for 3 days), and fenbendazole have been reported to be effective against *Amidostomum anseris*. *Trichostrongylus tenuis* is controlled by cambendazole (30 mg/kg), pyrantel (50 mg/kg), thiabendazole (75 mg/kg), mebendazole (10 mg/kg for 3 days), and citarin (40 mg/kg). At recommended levels for chickens, mebendazole has some reported effect against *Dispharynx nasuta*, tetramisole against *Subulura brumpti* and *Strongyloides avium*, and piperazine against *Tetrameres*.

Poultry producers wanting to treat for tapeworms should be aware that expulsion of the parasite will be a short-term remedy if the scolex is not removed or if the intermediate host is not eliminated as a source of reinfection. Butynorate in combination with piperazine and phenothiazine as a feed additive or individual tablets has shown some efficacy. Other promising experimental drugs include chlorophene and niclosamide. None is approved in the USA.

HEMORRHAGIC ENTERITIS/ MARBLE SPLEEN DISEASE

Hemorrhagic enteritis is an acute GI disorder affecting young turkeys ≥4 wk old. In its most severe form, it is characterized by depression and hemorrhagic droppings. Mortality may be increased; however, this is rare because of extensive use of vaccines. Marble spleen disease is an acute respiratory disease of pheasants characterized by depression, enlarged mottled spleens, pulmonary congestion, and death. Both diseases are caused by similar viruses. Species-specific differences in clinical response are thought to be related to differences in the target organs for anaphylaxis and variation in viral pathotype. Infection with less virulent pathotypes in either host often may go undetected until secondary bacterial infections begin to develop as a result of viral-induced immunosuppression.

Similar diseases have been seen sporadically in other species of birds such as chickens (splenomegaly), guinea fowl, peafowl, and chukar partridges.

Etiology and Epidemiology: The etiologic agent is a nonenveloped, icosahedral DNA virus, 70–90 nm in diameter. It is a member of the family Adenoviridae and the genus *Siadenovirus*. Based on differences in presentation within host species, numerous viral pathotypes appear to exist. These differ slightly at the DNA level but are indistinguishable serologically.

Both hemorrhagic enteritis and marble spleen disease are geographically widespread and considered endemic in areas where turkeys and pheasants are raised commercially. The usual route of infection is oral, and virus is often introduced onto previously uninfected premises via personnel or equipment contaminated with infectious feces. Turkey poults and pheasants 3–4 wk old are resistant to infection because of age-related resistance or, more commonly, the presence of maternal antibody. The virus may survive under moist conditions (ie, in litter) well beyond the refractory period. As infection begins to cycle through a flock, large quantities of virus are shed in the feces, which facilitates rapid spread through susceptible birds. Morbidity usually approaches 100% for both hemorrhagic enteritis and marble spleen disease.

Clinical Findings: In commercial operations, hemorrhagic enteritis typically affects turkeys 6–12 wk old but is most common between 7–9 wk of age. In outbreaks involving highly virulent pathotypes, clinical signs can include depression, pallor, and bloody droppings. Acute mortality can range from 1%–60%, with an average of 10%–15% throughout a 2-wk period. Birds that survive the acute phase experience a transient immunosuppression related to the lymphotrophic, lymphocytopathic nature of the virus. This often manifests itself in the form of secondary bacterial infections, eg, colibacillosis (*see* p 2814) ~10–14 days after exposure to the virus. Thus, a second peak in mortality, potentially overlapping the first, may be seen and, in less virulent outbreaks, may actually dominate the clinical picture. The second wave of mortality often lasts 2–4 wk and is characterized by lesions commonly associated with bacterial respiratory disease or septicemia, eg, fibrinopurulent pneumonia, airsacculitis, pericarditis, peritonitis, perihepatitis, hepatomegaly, and splenomegaly. Concomitant or prior exposure to necrotic enteritis (*see* p 2802), coccidiosis (*see* p 2791), Newcastle disease virus (*see* p 2856), *Bordetella avium* (*see* p 2907), or *Mycoplasma gallisepticum* and *M synoviae* (*see* p 2841) can exacerbate the problem. Similar multiple agent interactions have been implicated in mortality associated with the use of vaccines for hemorrhagic enteritis.

Marble spleen disease typically affects pheasants 3–8 mo old. Onset is acute, with dyspnea, asphyxiation, and sudden death occurring as a result of pulmonary congestion and edema. Mortality is commonly 2%–3% but can reach 15%. Secondary bacterial infections as a result of immunosuppression have also been noted.

Lesions: Necropsy of moribund or dead birds infected with hemorrhagic enteritis virus reveals gross congestion and occasional intraluminal hemorrhage in the proximal small intestine. The spleen is usually enlarged, friable, and mottled white, except in birds that have hemorrhaged extensively. Hemorrhage in the intestine is not common in field cases. Histopathologic changes in the duodenum include congestion, hemorrhage, and necrosis of the intestinal epithelium. This lesion in particular is thought to be the result of a virally induced, cytokine-mediated anaphylactic reaction, with the GI tract being considered the target shock organ in turkeys. Basophilic intranuclear inclusions can be found in lymphocytes and macrophages in a variety of tissues (eg, intestine, liver, and lungs) but predominantly in the spleen, where lymphoreticular hyperplasia and lymphoid necrosis are noted. Intranuclear inclusions in the renal tubular epithelial cells of the kidneys can be seen in turkeys that have recovered from hemorrhagic enteritis.

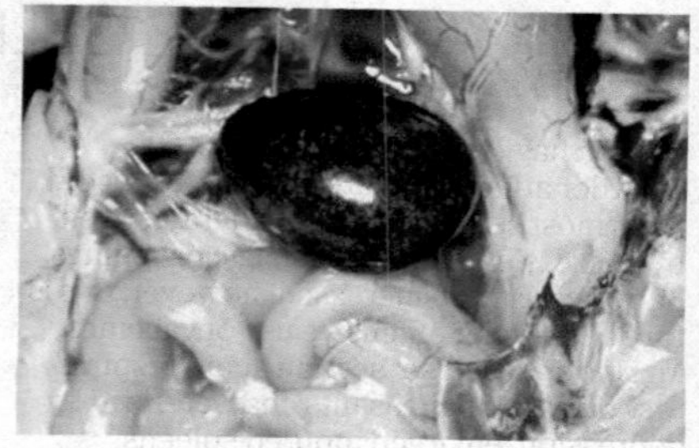

Enlarged, mottled spleen in a turkey with hemorrhagic enteritis. *Courtesy of Dr. Jean Sander.*

On histopathologic evaluation of pheasants with marble spleen disease, flooding of the atria and tertiary bronchi with fibrin and RBCs, as well as generalized vascular congestion and focal necrosis, are often seen in the lung. As with hemorrhagic enteritis, this response may be anaphylactic in nature, with the lung being considered the target shock organ in the pheasant. Splenomegaly with lymphoreticular hyperplasia and lymphoid necrosis also occur and are the characteristic lesions for which marble spleen disease is named. Basophilic or magenta-colored intranuclear inclusions may be found in a variety of tissues excluding the GI tract, with the highest concentration of virus found in the spleen.

Diagnosis: Diagnosis of virulent outbreaks of hemorrhagic enteritis or marble spleen disease can often be made based on clinical signs and gross lesions. Confirmation is by histopathology and the presence of seroprecipitating virus in the spleen as determined by agar gel immunodiffusion. PCR techniques to detect hemorrhagic enteritis viral DNA in tissue have also been described and are in regular use in select laboratories. To determine whether hemorrhagic enteritis or marble spleen disease is a predisposing factor in cases of bacterial respiratory disease or septicemia, or to verify a primary diagnosis, acute and convalescent sera (3 wk apart) can be tested using either agar gel immunodiffusion or ELISA. In turkeys, differential diagnoses include colibacillosis, pasteurellosis, paratyphoid, and erysipelas. Reticuloendotheliosis or lymphoproliferative disease should be considered when lymphoreticular hyperplasia is the predominant lesion. GI lesions without splenic involvement should evoke consideration of other viral, bacterial, parasitic, and toxic enteritides of turkeys. In pheasants with acute respiratory disease, differential diagnoses include Newcastle disease, avian influenza, and in the case of birds reared in confinement, gaseous toxins.

Treatment, Control, and Prevention: Virulent outbreaks of hemorrhagic enteritis have been successfully treated and controlled by SC injection of exposed birds with 0.5–1 mL of antiserum obtained from recovered flocks. It is presumed that a similar approach may be effective for pheasants. In anticipation of secondary bacterial complications, antibiotics may be used, but if possible, an informed choice should be made based on current antibiotic susceptibility profiles for locally obtained *Escherichia coli* isolates. In addition to good biosecurity, prevention hinges on the use of vaccines administered in the water at ~4–5 wk of age. Commercially available tissue culture products and crude splenic preparations containing avirulent isolates produce lifelong protection. Quality control on crude splenic preparations, such as examining them for bacteria, *Mycoplasma*, and other viruses, should be done before they are prepared. A subunit vaccine to prevent hemorrhagic enteritis in turkeys has been described in Europe.

Vaccines intended for use in turkeys should not be used in pheasants, and vice versa, because the avirulent isolates used for vaccinating one species are typically virulent in the other. Because of the potential for interaction with other agents, including live vaccines, regular disease monitoring and careful integration of hemorrhagic enteritis and marble spleen disease vaccines into flock vaccination protocols is encouraged. Intuitively, vaccines should not be administered to birds exhibiting signs of illness or within 2 wk of any other vaccination.

HISTOMONIASIS

(Blackhead, Infectious enterohepatitis)

Histomoniasis is caused by a protozoan that infects the ceca, and later the liver, of turkeys, chickens, and occasionally other galliform birds. In turkeys, most infections are fatal, whereas in other galliforms susceptibility varies between species and breeds.

Etiology: The causative agent of histomoniasis is the anaerobic, single cell protozoan parasite *Histomonas meleagridis* that can exist in flagellated (8–15 μm in diameter) and amoeboid (8–30 μm in diameter) forms. *Histomonas* is most often transmitted in embryonated eggs of the cecal nematode *Heterakis gallinarum*. A large percentage of chickens and other gallinaceous birds harbor this worm, which serves as a reservoir. Three species of earthworms can act as vectors for *H gallinarum* larvae containing *H meleagridis*, which are infective to both chickens and turkeys. *H meleagridis* survives for long periods within *Heterakis* eggs, which are resistant and may remain viable in the soil for years. Histomonads are released from *Heterakis* larvae in the ceca a few days after entry of the nematode and replicate rapidly in the ceca. The parasites migrate into the submucosa and muscularis mucosae and cause extensive and severe necrosis. Histomonads reach the liver either by the vascular system or via the peritoneal cavity, and rounded necrotic lesions quickly appear on the liver surface. Histomonads interact with other gut organisms, such as bacteria and coccidia, and depend on these for full virulence. In turkeys, transmission is by direct cloacal contact with infected birds or via fresh droppings, resulting in histomoniasis quickly spreading throughout the flock. Infection has not been shown to spread in this manner in chickens.

Traditionally, histomoniasis has been thought of as affecting turkeys, while doing little damage to chickens. However, outbreaks in chickens may cause high morbidity, moderate mortality, and extensive culling. Liver lesions tend to be less severe in chickens but often involve secondary bacterial infections. Morbidity can be especially high in young layer or breeder pullets. Layer flocks recover but lack uniformity. Experimental infections with *Histomonas* of 16-wk-old layers have demonstrated reduced egg production during infection. Tissue responses to infection may resolve in 4 wk, but birds may be carriers for another 6 wk.

Clinical Findings: Signs of histomoniasis are apparent in turkeys 7–12 days after infection and include listlessness, reduced appetite, drooping wings, unkempt feathers, and yellow droppings in the later stages of the disease. The origin of the name "blackhead" is obscure and misleading, with only a few birds displaying a cyanotic head. Young birds have a more acute disease and die within a few days after signs appear. Older birds may be sick for some time and become emaciated before death.

Lesions: The primary lesions of histomoniasis are in the ceca, which exhibit marked inflammatory changes and ulcerations, causing a thickening of the cecal wall. Occasionally, these ulcers erode the cecal wall, leading to peritonitis and involvement of other organs. The ceca contain a yellowish green, caseous exudate or, in later stages, a dry, cheesy core. Liver lesions are highly variable in appearance; in turkeys, they may be up to 4 cm in diameter and involve the entire organ. In some cases, the liver will appear green or tan. The liver and cecal lesions together are pathognomonic. However, the liver lesions must be differentiated from those of tuberculosis, leukosis, avian trichomonosis, and mycosis. Lesions are also seen in other organs, such as the kidneys, bursa of Fabricius, spleen, and pancreas. Studies by PCR show that *Histomonas* DNA can be found in the blood and in the tissues of most organs, whether lesions are present or not. Histopathologic examination is helpful for differentiation of diseases.

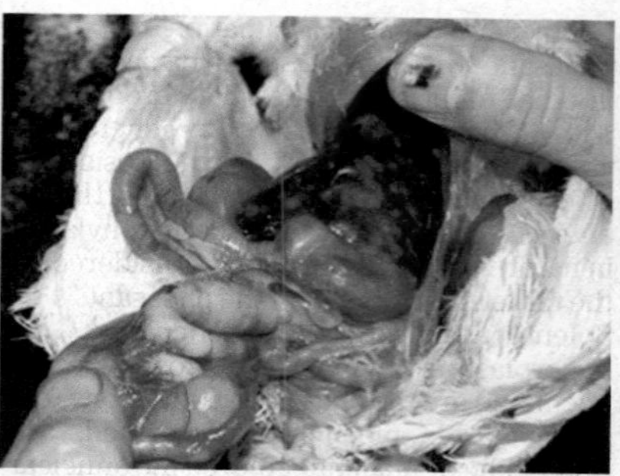

Liver lesions, an enlarged ceca with cores, and inflammation seen in multiple tissues of a turkey with histomoniasis. *Courtesy of Dr. Larry R. McDougald and Dr. Robert B. Beckstead.*

Histomonads are intercellular, although they may be so closely packed as to appear intracellular. The nuclei are much smaller than those of the host cells, and the cytoplasm less vacuolated. Scrapings from the liver lesions or ceca may be placed in isotonic saline solution for direct microscopic examination; *Histomonas* spp must be differentiated from other cecal flagellates. Molecular diagnosis is possible with published PCR primers.

Prevention and Treatment: Because healthy chickens and gamebirds often carry the cecal worm vector, any contact between turkeys and other galliforms should be avoided and care should be taken to reduce the worm population. Worm eggs, from contaminated soil, can be tracked inside by workers, causing infection. Arthropods such as flies may also serve as mechanical vectors. Because *H gallinarum* ova can survive in soil for many months or years, turkeys should not be put on ground contaminated by chickens. Once established in a turkey flock, infection spreads rapidly without a vector through direct contact. Dividing a facility into subunits using barriers can contain the outbreaks to specific units. Histomonads that are shed directly into the environment die quickly. Thus, in a turkey facility, where *Heterakis* is unable to complete its life cycle, decontamination is not required.

Immunization has only been partially successful in controlling histomoniasis, and reports differ on its effectiveness. The immune response of turkeys to live attenuated *Histomonas* requires 4 wk to develop. Vaccination of 18-wk-old pullets 5 wk before experimental infection has been shown to prevent a drop in egg production. Most workers have concluded that immunization of birds against this disease using live cultures is not practical. Killed organisms stimulate some immunity when given SC or IP but do not offer protection.

No drugs are currently approved for use as treatments for histomoniasis. Nitarsone is available for prophylaxis by feed medication. Nitarsone is mixed with the feed at 0.01875% and fed continually. A 5-day withdrawal period is required for animals slaughtered for human consumption. Under most conditions, nitarsone is effective, although some outbreaks in turkeys on medication have been reported. Historically, nitroimidazoles such as ronidazole, ipronidazole, and dimetridazole were used for prevention and treatment and were highly effective. Some of these products can be used by veterinary prescription in non-food-producing birds. Frequent worming of chickens with benzimidazole anthelmintics helps reduce exposure to heterakid worms that carry the infection.

INFECTIOUS BURSAL DISEASE

(Gumboro disease)

Infectious bursal disease (IBD) is seen in domestic chickens worldwide. It can present as a clinical or subclinical disease, but immunosuppression and related secondary infections are typically seen. Severity of the immunosuppression depends on the virulence of the infecting virus and age of the host.

Etiology and Transmission: IBD is caused by a birnavirus (infectious bursal disease virus; IBDV) that is most readily isolated from the bursa of Fabricius but may be isolated from other organs. It is shed in the feces and transferred from house to house by fomites. It is very stable and difficult to eradicate from premises.

Two serotypes of IBDV have been identified. The serotype 1 viruses cause disease in chickens and, within them, antigenic variation can exist between strains. Antigenic drift is largely responsible for this antigenic variation, but antigenic differences can also occur through genome homologous recombination. Serotype 2 strains of the virus infect chickens and turkeys but have not caused clinical disease or immunosuppression in these hosts. IBDVs have been identified in other avian species, including penguins, and antibodies to IBDV have been seen in several wild avian species. The contribution of IBDV to disease in these wild birds is unknown.

Clinical Findings: IBD is highly contagious; results of infection depend on age and breed of chicken and virulence of the virus. Infections may be subclinical or clinical. Infections before 3 wk of age are usually subclinical. Chickens are most susceptible to clinical disease at 3–6 wk of age when immature B cells populate the bursa and maternal immunity has waned, but severe infections have occurred in Leghorn chickens up to 18 wk of age.

Early subclinical infections are the most important form of the disease because of economic losses. They cause severe, long-lasting immunosuppression due to destruction of immature lymphocytes in the bursa of Fabricius, thymus, and spleen. The humoral (B cell) immune response is most severely affected; the cell-mediated (T cell) immune response is affected to a lesser extent. Chickens immunosuppressed by early IBDV infections do not respond well to vaccination and are predisposed to infections with normally nonpathogenic viruses and bacteria. Common diseases are usually exacerbated by IBDV infections.

Some strains of IBDV can cause subclinical infections in older birds (3–6 wk old), which leads to losses from poor feed efficiency and longer times to market. In these cases, the immunosuppression is usually transient, and convalescent birds may recover most or all of their humoral immune function. However, secondary infections that occur during the transient immunosuppression can cause significant economic losses.

In clinical infections, onset of the disease occurs after an incubation of 3–4 days. Chickens may exhibit severe prostration, incoordination, watery diarrhea, soiled vent feathers, vent picking, and inflammation of the cloaca. Flock morbidity is typically 100%, and mortality can range from 5%–20%. Recovery occurs in <1 wk, and broiler weight gain is delayed by 3–5 days. The presence of maternal antibody will modify the clinical course of the disease.

Virulence of field strains of the virus varies considerably. Viruses that range from naturally attenuated to very virulent (vv) have been observed. The vvIBDV strains that can cause high mortality (>20%) were first detected in Europe. They spread throughout the Middle East, Asia, and Africa, were detected in South and Central America in 1999, and in the USA in 2009.

Lesions: At necropsy, the lesions seen will depend on the strain of IBDV. For strains that cause a clinical disease, the cloacal bursa is swollen, edematous, yellowish, and occasionally hemorrhagic, especially in birds that died of the disease. Strains of vvIBDV cause similar cloacal bursa lesions, and congestion and hemorrhage of the pectoral and leg muscles can also occur. IBDV strains that cause subclinical disease (sometimes referred to as variant strains) cause atrophy of the cloacal bursa without inflammation. Chickens that have recovered from IBDV infections have small, atrophied, cloacal bursas due to the destruction and lack of regeneration of the bursal follicles.

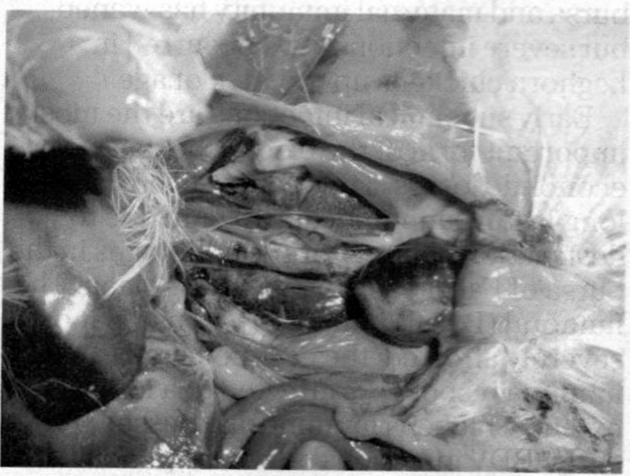

Enlarged, hemorrhagic bursa of Fabricius in a chicken infected with very virulent infectious bursal disease virus. *Courtesy of Dr. Daral J. Jackwood.*

Diagnosis: Molecular diagnostic assays are most often used to identify IBDV in diagnostic samples. They use reverse-transcriptase PCR to identify the viral genome in bursa tissue. Sequence analysis of the VP2 coding region has been used to further characterize the viruses. Samples for molecular diagnostic testing are typically collected after maternal antibodies have waned. IBDV may be isolated in 8- to 11-day-old, antibody-free chicken embryos with inocula from birds in the early stages of disease. The chorioallantoic membrane is more sensitive to inoculation than is the allantoic sac. Some strains of IBDV may also be isolated in cell cultures that include chicken embryo fibroblasts, cells from the cloacal bursa, and established avian and mammalian cell lines. Cell culture–adapted strains of IBDV produce a cytopathic effect and may be used for quantitative titration of the virus and virus-neutralization assays.

Control: There is no treatment. Rigorous disinfection of contaminated farms after depopulation has achieved limited success. Live vaccines of chicken embryo or cell-culture origin and of varying low pathogenicity can be administered by eye drop, drinking water, or SC routes at 1–21 days of age. Replication of these vaccines and thus the immune response can be altered by maternal antibody, although the more virulent vaccine strains can override higher levels of maternal antibody. Vectored vaccines that express the IBDV VP2 protein in herpesvirus of turkeys (HVT) can be used in ovo or at hatch. These HVT-IBD vaccines are not affected by maternal antibodies. Vaccines that use live-attenuated viruses bound to antibodies (immune-complex vaccines) are also available for in ovo or at hatch administration.

High levels of maternal antibody during early brooding of chicks in broiler flocks (and in some commercial layer operations) can minimize early infection, subsequent immunosuppression, or both. Breeder flocks should be vaccinated one or more times during the growing period, first with a live vaccine and again just before egg production with an oil-adjuvanted, inactivated vaccine. Inactivated vaccines of chicken embryo, bursa, or cell-culture origin are available. The latter vaccines induce higher, more uniform, and more persistent levels of antibody than do live vaccines. The immune status of breeder flocks should be monitored periodically with a quantitative serologic test such as virus neutralization or ELISA. If antibody levels decrease, hens should be revaccinated to maintain adequate immunity in the progeny.

The goal of any vaccination program for IBD should be to use vaccines that most closely match the antigenic profile of the field viruses. Diagnostic testing for the genomic sequences of field strains can be used to select the most appropriate vaccination program.

LISTERIOSIS

Listeriosis is caused by the bacterium *Listeria monocytogenes*. Although many species of birds, including chickens, turkeys, pigeons, ducks, geese, canaries, and cockatiels, are susceptible to infection, clinical disease in birds is rare. Generally, young birds are more susceptible to infection and more likely to develop clinical disease than older birds. In chickens, the disease occurs sporadically as either septicemia or encephalitis.

Etiology, Epidemiology, and Pathogenesis: *L monocytogenes* is a gram-positive, nonsporeforming, facultative intracellular, rod-shaped bacterium. It is widely distributed and commonly found in the environment. In temperate zones, the primary habitats of the organism are soil and decaying vegetation. The organism is common in poorly preserved stored corn silage. *L monocytogenes* has been isolated from the intestinal tract of healthy animals, including different species of mammals, birds, and fish. Transmission occurs via ingestion, inhalation, or wound contamination. In ruminants, the encephalitic form of listeriosis develops after entry of the organism through minor injuries in the conjunctiva or oral and nasal mucosa with subsequent migration along peripheral nerves to the brain. It is unknown if this same route of infection occurs in birds. Contamination of poultry farms with fecal material from nearby food animal farms (eg, cattle or swine farms) is an important source of infection, especially after a rain or flooding. Wounds from beak trimming and vaccine injection are possible sites of entry for the organism.

Clinical Findings: In the septicemic form of listeriosis, clinical signs are not specific and include depression, lethargy, and sudden death. In the encephalitic form, lateral recumbency, ataxia, torticollis, leg paddling, opsisthotonos, paresis, and paralysis have been seen.

Lesions: Birds affected with the septicemic form of listeriosis often have extensive degeneration and necrosis of the myocardium, with splenomegaly, necrotic foci in the liver, and pericarditis. Other lesions reported in broilers include ascites and petechial hemorrhages in the myocardium, liver, kidneys, and spleen. In the encephalitic form, no gross lesions are seen in the brain, but histopathologic lesions are remarkable and include disseminated microabscesses, extensive fibrinous thrombosis, foci of hemorrhages, necrosis (malacia) of the parenchyma, perivascular cuffs of lymphocytes and macrophages, and gliosis. Gram stain of tissues reveals typical gram-positive bacteria within the lesions. Lesions are found in the medulla oblongata, where they are generally most severe, and in the optic lobes and cerebellum.

Diagnosis: In the septicemic form, gross lesions should arouse suspicion, and histopathologic lesions should allow preliminary diagnosis of bacterial septicemia. Diagnosis is confirmed by immunohistochemistry to demonstrate *L monocytogenes* in the tissues or by isolation of the organism, usually from the liver and/or spleen in the septicemic form and brain in the encephalitic form. Direct culture of affected tissues, especially the brain, may not always be successful because of the low concentration of organisms in affected tissues. Recovery of *L monocytogenes* increases significantly if a portion of the specimen is refrigerated for 4–8 wk and subcultured weekly. Alternatively, tissue may be macerated or blended with a general nutrient broth (eg, trypticase soy broth, brain heart infusion) at a ratio of 1:10. The broth media is incubated at 35°C (95°F) for 5–7 days and examined daily for growth.

Differential diagnoses for septicemic listeriosis include other bacterial septicemias such as colibacillosis, pasteurellosis, and erysipelas. For encephalitic listeriosis, differential diagnoses include viral encephalitides, eg, Marek's disease and exotic Newcastle disease. With the latter, neurologic signs (torticollis, opisthotonos) typically follow high mortality in the flock, and lesions of the disease are present in visceral organs.

Treatment and Prevention: Antibiotics may be used successfully to treat the septicemic form of the disease. In vitro, *L monocytogenes* is susceptible to penicillin, tetracycline, erythromycin, gentamicin, and trimethoprim-sulfamethoxazole. Treatment of the encephalitic form is usually unsuccessful. Prevention should focus on identifying and eliminating potential sources of infection.

Zoonotic Risk: Listeriosis is a serious zoonotic disease. *L monocytogenes* is recognized as an important foodborne pathogen in people and is of great concern to the public and poultry industry. Outbreaks of listeriosis usually follow exposure to raw or uncooked poultry products but have also occurred after contaminated ready-to-eat poultry meat products were eaten.

MALABSORPTION SYNDROME

(Runting-stunting syndrome, Pale bird syndrome)

Malabsorption syndrome is a transmissible disease characterized by stunted growth and a lack of skin pigmentation in growing chickens, most commonly broiler breeds. Turkeys may also be affected; in these birds, it resembles poult enteritis mortality syndrome. The disease has been identified in virtually all countries in which intensive poultry production occurs. It has been associated with several different enteric viruses and appears to be multifactorial, although the true etiology remains to be identified. Poor management may contribute to the problem.

Etiology and Transmission: The disease has been reproduced with bacteria-free intestinal homogenates, suggesting a viral origin. Enteroviruses, parvoviruses, astroviruses, caliciviruses, arenaviruses, togaviruses, reoviruses, and rotaviruses have been implicated. Enteroviruses, reoviruses, and mycotoxins have been considered the most likely etiologic factors, although recent reports suggest an important role for astroviruses and unusual parvoviruses. A problem hampering the understanding of the etiology is the inability to isolate these viruses. Because the disease is seen in very young chicks, it is likely the viruses are vertically transmitted, although fecal/oral spread occurs after hatching. The involvement of feedborne mycotoxins is not well understood.

Clinical Findings: The disease is typically recognized in broiler chicks 1–3 wk old. It is characterized by uneven growth; temporary stunting; permanent runting; lack of pigmentation in the skin, feet, or beak; slow feathering; broken or twisted feathers ("helicopter wings"); undigested feed in the feces; and poor feed conversion ratios. Diarrhea is common during the initial phases, and eating feces is seen. Other signs include lameness, osteodystrophy, and secondary encephalomalacia. Severely affected birds do not respond immediately to changes in feed or management practices and are usually culled from flocks before processing. The number affected in a flock can vary from a few to 90%.

Lesions: The severity and type of lesions resulting from both field and laboratory infections vary with the particular agents or combinations of agents involved. Lesions often include enlarged proventriculi, small gizzards, pancreatic atrophy, and orange mucus in the small-intestinal lumen. No consistent microscopic lesions are found, although cystic lesions in the small intestine have been described, and sometimes changes are present in the bursa and thymus. Encephalomalacia or rickets may be seen occasionally, presumably as a result of malabsorption or malassimilation of nutrients.

Diagnosis: Clinical signs and postmortem lesions permit a presumptive diagnosis. Because of the complex etiology and the presence of enteric viruses in normal flocks, laboratory investigations may be difficult to interpret, particularly because virus culture may be difficult or impossible. Poor early management of flocks (especially feed and water supply and temperature control) may lead to a similar picture in the absence of specific infection.

Prevention and Control: There is no effective treatment for severely affected birds. Good broiler farm hygiene will reduce the burden of challenge caused by multiple infectious organisms. Good flock nutrition and sanitation and avoidance of intercurrent disease are beneficial. No vaccines prevent malabsorption syndrome. Some reovirus vaccines are marketed to prevent the stunting and poor feed conversions due to pathogenic reoviruses. Feeds should be analyzed for dietary toxins, and high levels of toxins should not knowingly be fed to commercial poultry. Antibiotics and vitamin supplements can be helpful.

Zoonotic Risks: There have been no reported zoonotic risks associated with malabsorption syndrome.

MYCOPLASMOSIS

Mycoplasmas are bacteria that lack a cell wall and are the smallest prokaryotes (0.2–0.8 μm in diameter). They have complex nutritional requirements but will grow on specialized artificial medium containing serum. Growth in broth and on agar media is slow (5–21 days), and the small (0.1–1 mm diameter) colony morphology typically has a "fried egg" appearance under low magnification. Mycoplasmas do not survive for more than a few days outside the host and are vulnerable to common disinfectants.

Several *Mycoplasma* species have been isolated from avian hosts; *M gallisepticum*, *M synoviae*, *M meleagridis*, and *M iowae* are the most important. Each has distinctive epidemiologic and pathologic characteristics.

MYCOPLASMA GALLISEPTICUM INFECTION

(Chronic respiratory disease, Infectious sinusitis)

M gallisepticum is commonly involved in the polymicrobial "chronic respiratory disease" of chickens; in turkeys, it frequently results in swollen infraorbital sinues and is called "infectious sinusitis." These diseases affect chickens and turkeys worldwide, causing the most significant economic losses in large commercial operations, and are commonly seen in noncommercial flocks. Infection also occurs in pheasants, chukar partridges, peafowl, pigeons, quail, ducks, geese, and psittacine birds. Songbirds are generally resistant, although *M gallisepticum* causes conjunctivitis in wild house finches (and some similar species) in North America.

M gallisepticum is the most pathogenic avian mycoplasma; however, considerable strain variability is manifest in a range of host susceptibility, virulence, clinical presentation, and immunologic response. Integral membrane surface proteins (adhesins) that attach to receptors on host cells, allowing for colonization and infection, are important virulence factors involved in antigenic variation and immune evasion.

Epidemiology and Transmission: *M gallisepticum* is transmitted vertically within some eggs (transovarian) from infected breeders to progeny, and horizontally via infectious aerosols and through contamination of feed, water, and the environment, and by human activity on fomites (shoes, equipment, etc). Infection may be latent in some birds for days to months, but when birds are stressed horizontal transmission may occur rapidly via aerosols and the respiratory route, after which infection and clinical disease spread through the flock. Flock-to-flock transmission occurs readily by direct or indirect contact from the movement of birds, people, or fomites from infected to susceptible flocks. Some potential reservoirs of *M gallisepticum* in the USA are noncommercial (backyard) flocks, multiple-age layer flocks, and some free-ranging songbird species. Good management and biosecurity practices are necessary to ensure that *M gallisepticum* infections are not introduced to commercial poultry from these and other sources. In many outbreaks, the source of infection is unknown. Cold weather, poor air quality or crowding, concurrent infections, and some live virus vaccinations may facilitate infection, disease, and transmission.

Epithelium of the conjunctiva, nasal passages, sinuses, and trachea are most susceptible to initial colonization and infection; however, in severe, acute disease, infection may also involve the bronchi, air sacs, and occasionally lungs. Once infected, birds may remain carriers for life. There is a marked interaction (polymicrobial disease) between respiratory viruses, *Escherichia coli*, and *M gallisepticum* in the pathogenesis and severity of chronic respiratory disease.

Clinical Findings and Lesions: In chickens, infection may be inapparent or result in varying degrees of respiratory distress, with slight to marked rales, difficulty breathing, coughing, and/or sneezing. Morbidity is high and mortality low in uncomplicated cases. Nasal discharge and conjunctivitis with frothiness about the eyes may be present. The disease is generally more severe in turkeys than in chickens, and swelling of the infraorbital sinuses is common. Feed efficiency and weight gains are reduced. Commercial broiler chickens and market turkeys may suffer high condemnations at processing due to airsacculitis. In laying flocks, birds may fail to reach peak egg production, and the overall production rate is lower than normal.

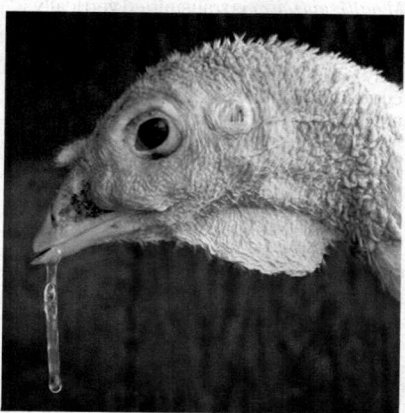

Turkey infected with *M gallisepticum* has clear-mucoid and dried nasal exudate and a swollen infraorbital sinus. *Courtesy of North Carolina State University Poultry Health Management.*

Uncomplicated *M gallisepticum* infections in chickens result in relatively mild catarrhal sinusitis, tracheitis, and airsacculitis. *E coli* infections are often concurrent and result in severe air sac thickening and turbidity, with exudative accumulations, adhesive pericarditis, and fibrinous perihepatitis. Turkeys develop severe mucopurulent sinusitis and varying degrees of tracheitis and airsacculitis. Microscopically, involved mucous membranes are thickened, hyperplastic, necrotic, and infiltrated with inflammatory cells. The mucosal lamina propria contains focal areas of lymphoid hypoplasia and germinal center formations.

Diagnosis: History, clinical signs, and typical gross lesions may be suggestive of *M gallisepticum* infection. Serology by agglutination and ELISA methods are commonly used for surveillance. Hemagglutination-inhibition is used as a confirmatory test, because nonspecific false agglutination reactions may occur, especially after injection of inactivated oil-emulsion vaccines or infection with *M synoviae*. *M gallisepticum* should be confirmed by isolation from swab samples of infraorbital sinuses, nasal turbinates, choanal cleft, trachea, air sacs, lungs, or conjunctiva. Primary isolation is made in mycoplasma medium containing 10%–15% serum. Colonies on agar medium are used for species identification by immunofluorescence with species-specific antibodies. PCR can also be used for detection of *M gallisepticum* DNA using swabs taken directly from infected sites (choana, sinuses, trachea, air sacs) or after growth in culture.

Mycoplasma isolates must be identified by species, because birds may also be infected with nonpathogenic mycoplasmas. *E coli* infection, Newcastle disease, avian influenza, and other respiratory diseases (eg, infectious bronchitis in chickens) should be considered in the differential diagnosis and can act as inciting or contributing pathogens.

Treatment, Control, and Prevention: Most strains of *M gallisepticum* are sensitive to a number of broad-spectrum antibiotics, including tylosin, tetracyclines, and others but not to penicillins or those that act on the cell wall. Tylosin or tetracyclines have been commonly used to reduce egg transmission or as prophylactic treatment to prevent respiratory disease in broilers and turkeys. Antibiotics may alleviate the clinical signs and lesions but do not eliminate infection. Regulations on the use of antibiotics in food animals are rapidly evolving and should be consulted before use.

Prevention is based largely on obtaining chicks or poults from *M gallisepticum*–free breeder flocks. Eradication of *M gallisepticum* from chicken and turkey commercial breeding stock is well advanced in the USA because of control programs coordinated by the National Poultry Improvement Plan. The most effective control program is to establish *M gallisepticum*–free breeder flocks, managed and maintained under good biosecurity to prevent introductions, and monitored regularly with serology to continually confirm infection-free status. In valuable breeding stock, treatment of eggs with antibiotics or heat has been used to eliminate egg transmission to progeny. Medication is not a good longterm control method but has been of value in treating individual infected flocks.

Laying chickens free of *M gallisepticum* are desirable, but infection in commercial multiple-age egg farms where depopulation is not feasible is a problem. Inactivated, oil-emulsion bacterins are available and help prevent egg production losses but not infection. Three live vaccines (F-strain, ts-11, and 6/85) have been licensed in the USA for use during the growing phase to provide some protection during lay and may be used in some areas with permission of the State Veterinarian. F-strain is of low virulence in chickens but is fully virulent for turkeys. Vaccinated chickens remain carriers of F-strain, and immunity lasts through the laying season. Vaccine strains ts-11 and 6/85 are less virulent, offer the advantage of improved safety for nontarget birds, and are widely used in commercial layers. A commercial recombinant fowlpox–*M gallisepticum* vaccine has been marketed.

MYCOPLASMA SYNOVIAE INFECTION

(Infectious synovitis)

M synoviae was first recognized as an acute to chronic infection of chickens and turkeys that produced an exudative tendinitis and synovitis (infectious synovitis); it now occurs most commonly as a subclinical infection of the upper respiratory tract, especially in multi-age layer flocks. *M synoviae* infection is also a complication of airsacculitis in association with Newcastle disease or infectious bronchitis. It is distributed worldwide and is seen primarily in chickens and turkeys, but ducks, geese, guinea fowl, parrots, pheasants, and quail may also be susceptible. Serum (preferably swine) and nicotinamide adenine dinucleotide (NAD) are required for growth in mycoplasma media.

M synoviae isolates vary widely in virulence, and suspected virulence factors include adhesins, sialidase, nitric oxide, cell invasion, and antigenic variation and immune evasion.

Epidemiology and Transmission: *M synoviae* is egg transmitted (transovarian), but the infection rate in breeder hens is low, and some hatches of progeny may be free of infection. Horizontal transmission is similar to that of *M gallisepticum* (*see* p 2841), primarily via the respiratory tract, with direct and indirect routes.

The incidence of *M synoviae* infection in commercial poultry in the USA has decreased because of the National Poultry Improvement Plan control programs implemented for chicken and turkey breeders. However, *M synoviae* infections of multiple-age layer flocks are common and may contribute to decreased egg production.

Clinical Findings and Lesions: Although slight rales may be present in birds with *M synoviae* respiratory infection, usually no signs are noticed. Birds under stress or with concurrent infections are more likely to be clinically affected. The first signs of infectious synovitis include pale-bluish head parts and lameness in many birds with a tendency to sit. The more severely affected birds are depressed and found resting around feeders and waterers. Hocks and footpads are swollen, and sternal bursitis (breast blisters) may be seen. Morbidity is usually low to moderate with mortality of 1%–10%. Effects on egg production are usually not apparent,

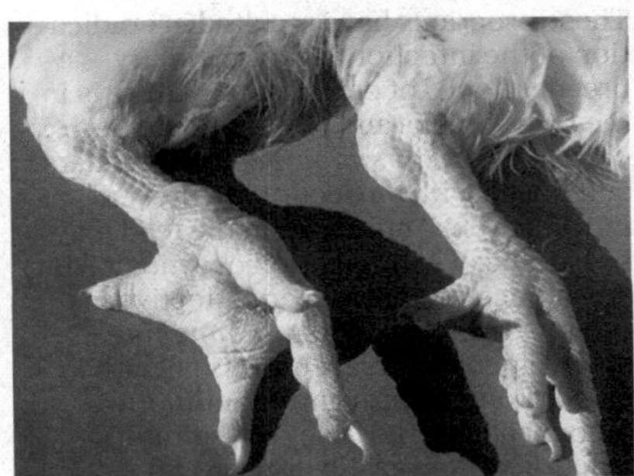

Swollen foot pad and swollen hock joint in chickens with infectious synovitis (*M synoviae* infection). *Courtesy of American Association of Avian Pathologists.*

but instances of transient egg production drops have occurred in layer flocks.

Respiratory lesions may be absent, or consist of mild mucoid tracheitis or sinusitis with airsacculitis when birds are stressed from poor air quality or challenged with Newcastle disease or infectious bronchitis. Early in infectious synovitis, a creamy to viscous yellow-gray exudate is present in most synovial structures but most commonly seen in swollen hock and wing joints. In chronic cases, this exudate may become inspissated; livers are enlarged and sometimes green, spleens are enlarged, kidneys are enlarged and pale, and birds may be weak and thin with breast blisters from sternal recumbency.

Diagnosis: Skeletal abnormalities and trauma must be eliminated as the cause of lameness. Differential diagnoses include viral tenosynovitis as well as staphylococcal and other bacterial joint infections.

A presumptive diagnosis based on clinical signs and gross lesions should be confirmed by laboratory tests. Serum plate agglutination or ELISA are used to detect *M synoviae* antibodies, but cross-reactions with *M gallisepticum* and other nonspecific reactions may occur. These reactors are confirmed as seropositive by hemagglutination-inhibition or by culture, isolation, and identification of the organism. PCR may be used to rapidly detect *M synoviae* DNA from pre- or postmortem specimens. In turkeys, the agglutination test for *M synoviae* may not be reliable, especially in birds with predominantly respiratory infection.

Treatment, Control, and Prevention: The National Poultry Improvement Plan coordinates control and serology-based surveillance programs for *M synoviae* similar to those for *M gallisepticum*. These programs have resulted in eradication of the infection in most primary breeder flocks of chickens and turkeys in the USA. Chicks and poults should be obtained from *M synoviae*–free breeders and raised with biosecurity to prevent introduction. Antibiotics in the feed may be beneficial in prevention of synovitis but are expensive and not very effective in established cases. When *M synoviae* involvement in airsacculitis is an anticipated problem, preventive antibiotic therapy during the time of respiratory reaction to Newcastle disease and infectious bronchitis vaccines may be helpful. A live temperature-sensitive vaccine (MS-H) is commercially available and permitted in some areas.

MYCOPLASMA MELEAGRIDIS INFECTION

M meleagridis causes an egg-transmitted (transovarian) disease of breeder turkeys that primarily impacts progeny with airsacculitis but has also been associated with decreased hatchability from infected breeder flocks and with poor growth and skeletal abnormalities in progeny. *M meleagridis* is strongly host-specific for turkeys (not for chickens), and with successful control programs (National Poultry Improvement Plan in the USA) major turkey primary breeders have eliminated the infection from their stocks, producing eggs and poults free of *M meleagridis*.

Epidemiology and Transmission: Before control programs, turkeys worldwide were commonly infected with *M meleagridis*. Infection of progeny occurs primarily through vertical (egg) transmission with rates that vary over the laying season. At the hatchery, organisms may be spread horizontally via aerosols from the respiratory tract or to the vent on contaminated hands during vent-sexing. Respiratory tract infection also leads to horizontal transmission among birds within young growing flocks and may be a factor in the spread to flocks previously free of infection (flock-to-flock transmission). In some infected turkeys, organisms localize in the reproductive tract; thus, the source of vertical transmission in hens is organisms incorporated in eggs. In toms, the phallus and adjacent tissues (cloaca) become infected and contaminate the semen. Artificial insemination of turkey hens with infected semen is an additional important method of transmission. Additionally, indirect transmission may result from management practices such as vaccination, whereby mycoplasmas are carried manually from infected to noninfected turkeys via contaminated hands, clothing, and equipment.

The marked difference in the pathogenicity of various strains of *M meleagridis* results in variable clinical manifestations, with airsacculitis in poults being the most common. High prevalence of airsacculitis with low mortality in poults suggests a highly evolved host-parasite relationship.

Clinical Findings and Lesions: Egg transmission and embryo infection reduces hatchability (due to late embryo mortality), poult quality, and growth rate. Only mild respiratory signs may be seen despite high rates of airsacculitis in poults from infected hens. Egg-borne infections may impact early rapid growth of hock joints, periarticular tissues, cervical vertebrae, and adjacent bone, producing skeletal abnormalities such as crooked (wry) necks or leg deformities. Adult breeders usually show no signs of venereal or respiratory infection.

Hatched poults may have airsacculitis with variable degrees of thickening, turbidity, foamy yellow exudate, and caseous flecks. These lesions recede with age. Poults with wry neck may have cervical airsacculitis and osteomyelitis of adjacent vertebrae. The generalized skeletal lesions that may develop in poults 1–6 wk old are characterized by chondrodystrophy or by varus deformities and perosis.

Microscopic lesions in hens consist of lymphocytic foci in the fimbria, uterus, and vagina, with plasma cells and heterophils in the lamina propria of the reproductive tract. Infected embryos and young poults show inflammatory lesions of pneumonia and exudative airsacculitis.

Diagnosis: A high prevalence of airsacculitis in day-old poults suggests *M meleagridis* infection. Serology by agglutination (tube or plate) or ELISA can demonstrate antibody. Confirmation was generally by hemagglutination-inhibition serology or by culture, isolation, and identification of the organism. PCR is now used to detect *M meleagridis* DNA from pre- or postmortem specimens. *M gallisepticum*, other *Mycoplasma* spp, and mixed infections (polymicrobial disease) must be considered in the differential diagnosis.

Treatment, Control, and Prevention: Turkey eggs or poults should be obtained from breeder flocks free of *M meleagridis* and monitored by serology and/or by examining pipped embryos or cull poults for airsacculitis. Semen used for insemination must be free of *M meleagridis*. Dipping eggs in tylosin or other antibiotic reduces the incidence of transmission in infected flocks. However, this practice has been generally eliminated with the eradication of *M meleagridis* from primary breeder flocks and is only used by multiplier breeders when there is an outbreak. Injection of a suitable antibiotic at 1 day of age or water medication for the first 5–10 days appeared to reduce infection and airsacculitis caused by *M meleagridis* and improve weight gain.

MYCOPLASMA IOWAE INFECTION

M iowae infection of turkey breeder hens has been most commonly associated with late embryo mortality and reduced hatchability and occasionally with a low prevalence of leg abnormalities in their young progeny. *M iowae* requires enriched media with cholesterol, similar to those used for other avian mycoplasmas for culture and isolation, but is resistant to bile salts.

Epidemiology and Transmission: *M iowae* is egg transmitted (transovarian) in turkeys, and horizontal transmission with slow spread within a flock may occur. Antigenicity and virulence vary considerably among *M iowae* strains. Infection rates in turkey flocks in Europe and North America have been reduced by intensive eradication efforts in certain primary breeding stocks, but *M iowae* is not currently included in the National Poultry Improvement Plan. It is a relatively uncommon infection of chickens and has been reported in geese.

Chickens and turkeys experimentally inoculated have shown airsacculitis, stunting, poor feathering, and leg lesions. These effects are rarely recognized in the field, except for some outbreaks in young turkeys with skeletal lesions.

Clinical Findings and Lesions: Affected turkey breeder flocks show no clinical signs other than reduced hatchability (usually

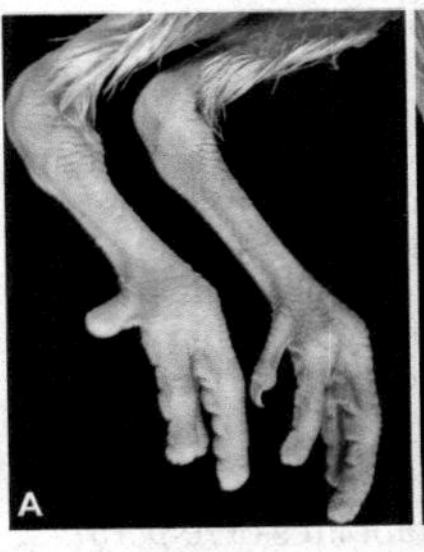

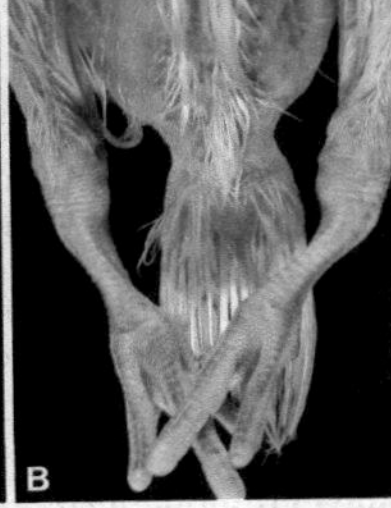

Mycoplasma iowae infection, turkeys. (A) Normal vs chondrodystrophic legs (left) of 28-day-old turkeys; note short, thick shanks and toes. (B) Legs of a 42-day-old turkey showing bilateral chondrodystrophy; note short, thick legs with enlarged hocks and marked medial bowing of both legs. *Courtesy of North Carolina State University Poultry Health Management.*

2%–5%) due to embryo mortality in the last 10 days of incubation. In many flocks, the hatchability returns to normal after 1–2 mo.

Dead turkey embryos are edematous, congested, and stunted; they may have "clubbed down." Poults experimentally challenged in ovo or at 1 day of age developed various skeletal deformities such as rotated tibia, deviated toes, chondrodystrophy, or erosion of the articular cartilage of the hock joint. Chicks experimentally challenged at 1 day of age developed tenosynovitis and ruptured tendons.

Natural infections in several young commercial turkey flocks were associated with skeletal lesions consistent with chondrodystrophy, characterized by leg and vertebral deformities. Microscopic skeletal lesions were characterized by excess cartilage matrix and disorganization of chondrocytes, features of osteochondrosis.

Diagnosis: In turkeys, *M iowae* infection should be considered in cases of late embryo mortality and decreased hatchability and in young turkeys with leg and vertebral chondrodystrophy. *M meleagridis* and nutrient deficiencies are the top differential diagnoses for these conditions, respectively.

Turkeys develop only a weak antibody response to *M iowae*, and no reliable serologic test is available. Diagnosis relies on culture, isolation, and identification of the organism, or on detection of *M iowae* DNA by PCR.

Treatment, Control, and Prevention: The best method of control and prevention is to establish and maintain turkey breeder flocks free of *M iowae*. Surveillance is challenging because serology is unreliable, but flock monitoring by PCR and strict biosecurity should help.

MYCOTOXICOSES

A mycotoxicosis is a disease caused by a natural toxin produced by a fungus. In poultry, this usually results when toxin-producing fungi grow in grain and feed. Hundreds of mycotoxins have been identified, and many are pathogenic. Mycotoxins may have additive or synergistic effects with other natural toxins, infectious agents, and nutritional deficiencies. Many are chemically stable and maintain toxicity over time. (*See also* MYCOTOXICOSES, p 3005.)

The significance of mycotoxin problems in poultry is probably considerable but yet insidious. The impact on poultry production may be best measured indirectly by the improvements in weight gain, feed efficiency, pigmentation, egg production, and reproductive performance that accompany effective control programs for mycotoxins.

Aflatoxicosis: The aflatoxins are toxic and carcinogenic metabolites of *Aspergillus flavus*, *A parasiticus*, and others. Aflatoxicosis in poultry primarily affects the liver but can involve immunologic, digestive, and hematopoietic functions. Aflatoxin can adversely affect weight gain, feed intake, feed conversion efficiency, pigmentation, processing yield, egg production, male and female fertility, and hatchability. Some effects are directly attributable to toxins, whereas others are indirect, such as reduced feed intake. Susceptibility to aflatoxins varies, but in general, ducklings, turkeys, and pheasants are susceptible, while chickens, Japanese quail, and guinea fowl are relatively resistant.

Clinical signs vary from general unthriftiness to high morbidity and mortality. At necropsy the lesions are found mainly in the liver, which can be reddened due to necrosis and congestion or yellow due to lipid accumulation. Hemorrhages may occur in liver and other tissues. In chronic aflatoxicosis, the liver becomes yellow to gray and atrophied. The aflatoxins are carcinogenic, but tumor formation is rare with the natural disease, probably because the birds do not live long enough for this to occur.

Fusariotoxicosis: The genus *Fusarium* produces many mycotoxins injurious to poultry. The trichothecene mycotoxins produce caustic and radiomimetic patterns of disease exemplified by T-2 toxin and diacetoxyscirpenol (DAS). Deoxynivalenol (vomitoxin, DON) and zearalenone are common trichothecene mycotoxins that are relatively nontoxic for poultry but may cause disease in pigs.

Fusariotoxicosis in poultry caused by the trichothecenes results in feed refusal, caustic injury of the oral mucosa and areas of the skin in contact with the mold, acute digestive disease, and injury to the bone marrow and immune system. Lesions include necrosis and ulceration of the oral mucosa, reddening of the GI mucosa, mottling of the liver, atrophy of the spleen and other lymphoid organs, and visceral hemorrhages. In laying hens, decreased egg production can be accompanied by depression, recumbency, feed refusal, and cyanosis evident in the comb and wattles. Ducks and geese develop necrosis and pseudomembranous inflammation of the esophagus, proventriculus, and gizzard.

Other *Fusarium* mycotoxins cause defective growth of long bones. The fumonisin mycotoxins produced by *F verticillioides* (formerly *F moniliforme*) impair feed conversion without causing specific lesions. Moniliformin is also produced by *F verticillioides* and is cardiotoxic and nephrotoxic in poultry. *F verticillioides* causes ear rot, kernel rot, and stalk rot of unharvested corn and is found in stored high-moisture shelled corn and on other grains that appear sound.

Ochratoxicosis: Ochratoxins are quite toxic to poultry. These nephrotoxins are produced chiefly by *Penicillium viridicatum* and *Aspergillus ochraceus* in grains and feed. Ochratoxicosis causes primarily renal disease but also affects the liver, immune system, and bone marrow. Severe intoxication causes reduced spontaneous activity, huddling, hypothermia, diarrhea, rapid weight loss, and death. Moderate intoxication impairs weight gain, feed conversion, pigmentation, carcass yield, egg production, fertility, and hatchability.

Ergotism: Toxic ergot alkaloids are produced by *Claviceps* spp, which are fungi that attack cereal grains. Rye is especially affected, but also wheat and other leading cereal grains. The mycotoxins form in the sclerotium, a visible, hard, dark mass of mycelium that displaces the grain tissue. Within the sclerotium are the ergot alkaloids, which affect the nervous system, causing convulsive and sensory neurologic disorders; the vascular system, causing vasoconstriction and gangrene of the extremities; and the endocrine system, including neuroendocrine control of the anterior pituitary gland.

In chicks, the toes become discolored due to vasoconstriction and ischemia. In older birds, vasoconstriction affects the comb, wattles, face, and eyelids, which become atrophied and disfigured. Vesicles and ulcers develop on the shanks of the legs and on the tops and sides of the toes. In laying hens, feed consumption and egg production are reduced.

Citrinin Mycotoxicosis: Citrinin is produced by *Penicillium* and *Aspergillus* and is a natural contaminant of corn, rice, and other cereal grains. Citrinin causes a diuresis that results in watery fecal droppings and reductions in weight gain. At necropsy, lesions are generally mild and involve the kidney.

Oosporein Mycotoxicosis: Oosporein is a mycotoxin produced by *Chaetomium* spp that causes gout and high mortality in poultry. *Chaetomium* are found on feeds and grains, including peanuts, rice, and corn. Oosporein mycotoxicosis is seen as visceral and articular gout related to impaired renal function and increased plasma concentrations of uric acid. Chickens are more sensitive to oosporein than turkeys. Water consumption increases during intoxication, and fecal droppings become unformed and fluid.

Cyclopiazonic Acid: Cyclopiazonic acid is a metabolite of *Aspergillus flavus*, which is the predominant producer of aflatoxin in feeds and grains. In chickens, cyclopiazonic acid causes impaired feed conversion, decreased weight gain, and mortality. Lesions develop in the proventriculus, gizzard, liver, and spleen. The proventriculus is dilated, and the mucosa is thickened and sometimes ulcerated.

Sterigmatocystin: Sterigmatocystin, a biogenic precursor to aflatoxin, is hepatotoxic and hepatocarcinogenic but is less common than aflatoxin.

Diagnosis:

Mycotoxicosis should be suspected when the history, signs, and lesions are suggestive of feed intoxication, and especially when moldy ingredients or feed are evident. Toxin exposure associated with consumption of a new batch of feed may result in subclinical or transient disease. Chronic or intermittent exposure can occur in regions where grain and feed ingredients are of poor quality or when feed storage is substandard or prolonged. Impaired production can be a clue to a mycotoxin problem, as can improvement because of correction of feed management deficiencies.

Definitive diagnosis involves detection and quantitation of the specific toxin(s). This can be difficult because of the rapid and high-volume use of feed and ingredients in poultry operations. Diagnostic laboratories differ in their respective capabilities to test for mycotoxins and should be contacted before sending samples. Feed and also birds that are sick or recently dead should be submitted for testing. A necropsy and related diagnostic tests should accompany feed analysis if mycotoxicosis is suspected. Concurrent diseases can adversely affect production and should be considered. Sometimes, a mycotoxicosis is suspected but not confirmed by feed analysis. In these situations, a complete laboratory evaluation can exclude other significant diseases.

Feed and ingredient samples should be properly collected and promptly submitted for analysis. Mycotoxin formation can be localized in a batch of feed or grain. Multiple samples taken from different sites increase the likelihood of confirming a mycotoxin formation zone (hot spot).

Samples should be collected at sites of ingredient storage, feed manufacture and transport, feed bins, and feeders. Fungal activity increases as feed is moved from the feed mill to the feeder pans. Samples of 500 g (1 lb) should be collected and submitted in separate containers. Clean paper bags, properly labeled, are adequate. Sealed plastic or glass containers are appropriate only for short-term storage and transport, because feed and grain rapidly deteriorate in airtight containers.

Treatment: The toxic feed should be removed and replaced with unadulterated feed. Concurrent diseases should be treated to alleviate disease interactions, and substandard management practices must be corrected. Some mycotoxins increase requirements for vitamins, trace minerals (especially selenium), protein, and lipids and can be compensated for by feed supplementation and water-based treatment. Nonspecific toxicologic therapies using activated charcoal (digestive tract adsorption) in the feed have a sparing effect but are not practical for larger production units.

Prevention: Prevention of mycotoxicoses should focus on using feed and ingredients free of mycotoxins and on management practices that prevent mold growth and mycotoxin formation during feed transport and storage. Regular inspection of feed storage and feeding systems can identify flow problems, which allow residual feed and enhance fungal activity and mycotoxin formation. Mycotoxins can form in decayed, crusted feed in feeders, feed mills, and storage bins; cleaning and correcting the problem can have immediate benefits. Temperature extremes cause moisture condensation and migration in bins and promote mycotoxin formation.

Ventilation of poultry houses to avoid high relative humidity also decreases the moisture available for fungal growth and toxin formation in the feed. Antifungal agents added to feeds to prevent fungal growth have no effect on toxin already formed but may be cost-effective in conjunction with other feed management practices. Organic acids (propionic acid, 500–1,500 ppm [0.5–1.5 g/kg]) are effective inhibitors, but the effectiveness may be reduced by the particle size of feed ingredients and the buffering effect of certain ingredients. Sorbent compounds such as hydrated sodium calcium aluminosilicate (HSCAS) effectively bind and prevent absorption of aflatoxin. Esterified glucomannan, derived from the cell wall of the yeast *Saccharomyces cerevisiae*, is protective against aflatoxin B_1 and ochratoxins. It reduces toxicity through the binding and reduction in bioavailability of fumonisins, zearalenone, and T-2 toxin. Various other fermentation products, algae and plant extracts, and microbial feed additives have demonstrated ability to bind or degrade mycotoxins and may be applicable and appropriate for the situation.

NEOPLASMS

Depending on whether the etiologic agent is known, neoplasms of poultry are divided into two main categories: virus-induced neoplasms and neoplasms of unknown etiology. There are three economically important virus-induced neoplastic diseases of poultry: Marek's disease, caused by a herpesvirus, and avian leukosis/sarcoma and reticuloendotheliosis, caused by retroviruses. While these neoplastic diseases cause economic losses from tumor mortality and poor performance, some of them have served as highly suitable models to study neoplasia.

A rare neoplastic disease of turkeys known as lymphoproliferative disease that has been reported in Europe and Israel is induced by a retrovirus that is distinct from both the leukosis/sarcoma and reticuloendotheliosis viruses. Although reports suggest that lymphoproliferative disease has recently been detected by PCR in a small number of wild turkeys in the USA, incidence of the disease has always been sporadic and therefore is not discussed in this chapter.

Neoplasms of unknown etiology are classified according to their morphologic characteristics; they include a wide variety of benign and malignant neoplasms. Of these tumors, only dermal squamous cell carcinoma (avian keratoacanthoma), multicentric histiocytosis, and adenocarcinoma are discussed in this chapter.

MAREK'S DISEASE

Chickens are the most important natural host for Marek's disease virus, a highly cell-associated but readily transmitted alphaherpesvirus with lymphotropic properties of gammaherpesviruses. Quail can be naturally infected, and turkeys can be infected experimentally. However, severe clinical outbreaks of Marek's disease in commercial turkey flocks, with mortality from tumors reaching 40%–80% between 8 and 17 wk of age, were reported in France, Israel, and Germany. In some of these cases, the affected turkey flocks were raised in proximity to broilers. Turkeys are also commonly infected with turkey herpesvirus (HVT), an avirulent strain related to Marek's disease virus that is commonly used as a Marek's disease vaccine in chickens. Other birds and mammals appear to be refractory to the disease or infection.

Marek's disease is one of the most ubiquitous avian infections; it is identified in chicken flocks worldwide. Every flock, except for those maintained under strict pathogen-free conditions, is presumed to be infected. Although clinical disease is not always apparent in infected flocks, a subclinical decrease in growth rate and egg production may be economically important.

Etiology: Marek's disease virus is a member of the genus *Mardivirus* within the subfamily Alphaherpesvirinae. Within the genus *Mardivirus* are three closely related species previously designated as three serotypes of Marek's disease virus. Gallid herpesvirus 2 (MDV-1) represents all virulent Marek's disease virus strains and is further divided into pathotypes, designated as mild (m), virulent (v), very virulent (vv), and very virulent plus (vv+). Gallid herpesvirus 3 (MDV-2) and Meleagrid herpesvirus 1 (turkey herpesvirus, MDV-3) represent avirulent virus strains isolated from chickens and turkeys, respectively, and are commonly used as vaccines against Marek's disease.

Transmission and Epidemiology: The disease is highly contagious and readily transmitted among chickens. The virus matures into a fully infective, enveloped form in the epithelium of the feather follicle, from which it is released into the environment. It may survive for months in poultry house litter or dust. Dust or dander from infected chickens is particularly effective in transmission. Once the virus is introduced into a chicken flock, regardless of vaccination status, infection spreads quickly from bird to bird. Infected chickens continue to be carriers for long periods and act as sources of infectious virus. Shedding of infectious virus can be reduced, but not prevented, by prior vaccination. Unlike virulent strains of Marek's disease virus, which are highly contagious, turkey herpesvirus is not readily transmissible among chickens (although it is easily transmitted among turkeys, its natural host). Attenuated Marek's disease virus strains vary greatly in their transmissibility among chickens; the most highly attenuated are not transmitted. Marek's disease virus is not vertically transmitted.

Pathogenesis: Currently, four phases of infection in vivo are recognized: 1) early productive-restrictive virus infection causing primarily degenerative changes, 2) latent infection, 3) a second phase of cytolytic, productive-restrictive infection coincident with permanent immunosuppression, and 4) a proliferative phase involving nonproductively infected lymphoid cells that may or may not progress to the point of lymphoma formation. Productive infection may occur transiently in B lymphocytes within a few days after infection with virulent Marek's disease virus strains and is characterized by antigen production, which leads to cell death. Because few if any virions are produced, this has also been termed a restrictive-productive infection. Productive infection also occurs in the feather follicle epithelium, in which enveloped virions are produced. Latent infection of activated T cells is responsible for the longterm carrier state. No antigens are expressed, but virus can be recovered from such lymphocytes by co-cultivation with susceptible cells in tissue cultures. Some T cells, latently infected with oncogenic Marek's disease virus strains, undergo neoplastic transformation. These transformed cells, provided they escape the immune system of the host, may multiply to form characteristic lymphoid neoplasms. Cell-mediated and humoral immune responses are both directed against viral antigens, with cell-mediated immunity probably being the most important.

Clinical Findings: The incidence of Marek's disease is quite variable in commercial flocks and depends on strain and dose of virus, age at exposure, maternal antibody, host gender and genetics, strain and dose of vaccine virus, and several environmental factors, including stress. In addition to lymphoid neoplasms, Marek's disease virus can also induce other clinically distinct disease syndromes, including transient paralysis, early mortality syndrome, cytolytic infection, atherosclerosis, and persistent neurologic disease. Typically, affected birds show only depression before death, but a transient paralysis syndrome has been associated with Marek's disease; chickens become ataxic for periods of several days and then recover. This syndrome is rare in immunized birds. Death is usually the result of paralysis, rendering the birds unable to reach food and water.

Lesions: Enlarged nerves are one of the most consistent gross lesions in affected birds. Various peripheral nerves, but particularly the vagus, brachial, and sciatic, become enlarged and lose their striations. Diffuse or nodular lymphoid tumors may be seen in various organs, particularly the liver, spleen, gonads, heart, lung, kidney, muscle, and proventriculus. Enlarged feather follicles (commonly termed skin leukosis) may be noted in broilers after defeathering during processing and are a cause for condemnation. The bursa is only rarely tumorous and more frequently is atrophic. Histologically, the lesions consist of a mixed population of small, medium, and large lymphoid cells plus plasma cells and large anaplastic lymphoblasts. These cell populations undoubtedly include tumor cells and reactive inflammatory cells. When the bursa is involved, the tumor cells typically appear in interfollicular areas.

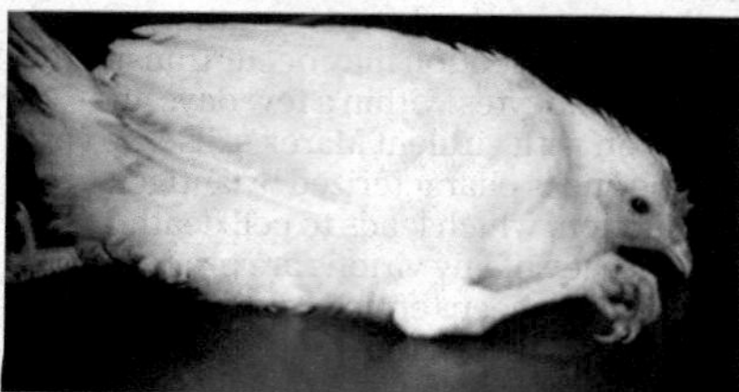

Typical presentation of leg paresis in a chicken with Marek's disease. *Courtesy of Dr. Jean Sander.*

Diagnosis: For the diagnosis of Marek's disease, it is critical to diagnose the tumors and not the infection because Marek's disease is considered ubiquitous within commercial poultry flocks. Usually, diagnosis is based on enlarged nerves and lymphoid tumors in various viscera. The absence of bursal tumors helps distinguish this disease from lymphoid leukosis (*see* below), although the presence of bursal tumors does not exclude Marek's disease. Marek's disease can develop in chickens as young as 3 wk old, whereas lymphoid leukosis typically is seen in chickens >14 wk old. Reticuloendotheliosis, although rare, can easily be confused with Marek's disease, because both diseases feature enlarged nerves and T-cell lymphomas in visceral organs. A diagnosis based on typical gross lesions may be confirmed histologically, or preferably by demonstration of predominant T-cell populations and Marek's viral DNA in lymphomas by histochemistry and PCR, respectively. There is a quantitative association between viral load and Marek's disease tumors; most tumor-bearing chickens have high viremia titers and are usually PCR positive. Thus, the demonstration of high quantities of virus, viral DNA, or viral antigens in tumor cells and the exclusion of other relevant tumor viruses should be sufficient for a specific diagnosis of Marek's disease. Furthermore, Marek's disease lymphomas usually lack evidence of clonally integrated avian retroviruses or alteration of the cellular oncogene c-*myc*.

Control: Vaccination is the central strategy for the prevention and control of Marek's disease. The efficacy of vaccines can be improved, however, by strict sanitation to reduce or delay exposure and by breeding for genetic resistance. Probably the most widely used vaccine consists of turkey herpesvirus (HVT), which has seen rapidly increased use as a backbone in recombinant vaccines featuring the insertion of genes from other poultry viruses, such as Newcastle disease virus (*see* p 2856), infectious bursal disease virus (*see* p 2837), or infectious laryngotracheitis virus (*see* p 2912). These recombinant vaccines offer protection against both Marek's disease virus and the inserted virus. Bivalent vaccines consisting of HVT and either the SB-1 or 301B/1 strains of Gallid herpesvirus 3 have been used to provide additional protection against challenge with virulent Marek's disease virus isolates. The most protective commercial vaccine currently available appears to be CVI988/Rispens, an attenuated Marek's disease virus strain that is also commonly mixed with HVT at vaccination. Because vaccines are administered at hatching and require 1–2 wk to produce an effective immunity, exposure of chickens to virus should be minimized during the first few days after hatching.

Vaccines are also effective when administered to embryos at the 18th day of incubation. In ovo vaccination is now performed by automated technology and is widely used for vaccination of commercial broiler chickens, mainly because of reduced labor costs and greater precision of vaccine administration.

Proper handling of vaccine during thawing and reconstitution is crucial to ensure that adequate doses are administered. Cell-associated vaccines are generally more effective than cell-free vaccines, because they are neutralized less by maternal antibodies. Under typical conditions, vaccine efficacy is usually >90%. Since the advent of vaccination, losses from Marek's disease have been reduced dramatically in broiler and layer flocks. However, disease may become a serious problem in individual flocks or in selected geographic areas (eg, the Delmarva broiler industry). Of the many causes proposed for these excessive losses, early exposure to very virulent virus strains appears to be among the most important.

LYMPHOID LEUKOSIS

(Avian leukosis)

Under natural conditions, lymphoid leukosis has been the most common form of the leukosis/sarcoma group of diseases seen in chicken flocks, although in the 1990s myeloid leukosis become prevalent in meat-type chickens. The International Committee on Taxonomy of Viruses placed viruses of the avian leukosis/sarcoma group in the *Alpharetrovirus* genus of the family Retroviridae.

Members of this RNA group of viruses have similar physical and molecular characteristics and share a common group-specific antigen. Detection of the major antigen (p27) present in the core of leukosis/sarcoma viruses forms the basis of several diagnostic tests. Lymphoid leukosis occurs naturally only in chickens. Experimentally, some of the viruses of the leukosis/sarcoma group can infect and produce tumors in other species of birds or even mammals. The infection is known to exist in virtually all chicken flocks except for some SPF flocks from which it has been eradicated. Tumor mortality commonly accounts for ~1%–2% of birds, with occasional losses of ≥20%. Subclinical infection, to which most flocks are subject, decreases several important performance traits, including egg production and quality. The frequency of infection has been reduced substantially in the primary breeding stocks of several commercial poultry breeding companies, particularly egg-type breeders. In recent years this control program has expanded, and infection has become infrequent or absent in certain commercial flocks. The frequency of lymphoid leukosis tumors even in heavily infected flocks is typically low (<4%), and disease is often inapparent. As much as 1.5% excess mortality per wk has been reported in commercial broiler-breeder flocks naturally infected with subgroup J avian leukosis virus.

Etiology: Lymphoid leukosis is caused by certain members of the leukosis/sarcoma group of avian retroviruses. Isolates that can induce lymphoid leukosis in chickens are commonly called avian leukosis viruses and are divided into subgroups A, B, C, D, and J, on the basis of differences in their viral envelope glycoproteins, which determine antigenicity, viral interference patterns with members of the same and different subgroups, and host range. Subgroups A and B are most prevalent in western countries. Since the initial isolation of subgroup J avian leukosis virus in England, the virus has been isolated from broiler-breeder stocks that experience myeloid neoplasms (myelocytoma) in many other countries. A sixth subgroup (E) designates nononcogenic endogenous viruses produced by viral genes integrated into the host cell DNA. All field strains of avian leukosis virus are oncogenic, although some differences in oncogenicity and replicative ability have been recognized. Recently, recombinant avian leukosis viruses with the envelope of subgroup B and long terminal repeat of subgroup J have been isolated from field cases of myeloid leukosis in commercial layers. Another recombinant avian leukosis virus with the envelope of subgroup A and long terminal repeat of subgroup E was shown to be a contaminant in commercial Marek's disease vaccines. Thus, recombination between two different subgroups of avian leukosis virus can occur in field conditions and cause economic losses.

Transmission and Epidemiology: Chickens are the natural hosts for all viruses of the leukosis/sarcoma group; these viruses have not been isolated from other avian species except pheasants, partridges, and quail. Avian leukosis virus is shed by the hen into the albumen or yolk, or both; infection probably occurs after the onset of incubation. Congenitally infected chickens fail to produce neutralizing antibodies and usually remain viremic for life. Horizontal infection after hatching is also important, especially when chicks are exposed immediately after hatching to high doses of virus, eg, in feces of congenitally infected chicks or in contaminated vaccines. Horizontally infected chickens have a transient viremia followed by antibody production. The earlier the infection, the more likely it is to lead to tolerance, persistent viremia, and tumors. Other factors known to increase the susceptibility of chickens to horizontal infection include the absence of maternal antibodies and the presence of endogenous retroviruses, especially those associated with the late feathering (K) gene. Tumors are more frequent in congenital than in horizontal infections, but many more chickens are exposed horizontally than congenitally. Rates of embryo transmission typically are 1%–10%; virtually all chicks in an infected flock are exposed by contact. Congenital and, in some cases, early horizontal infection can induce permanent carrier states characterized by shedding of virus or antigen into the environment and into eggs. Late infection (ie, inoculation at 12–20 wk of age) is unlikely to lead to viral shedding.

Four classes of avian leukosis virus infection are recognized in mature chickens: (1) no viremia, no antibody (V-A-); (2) no viremia, with antibody (V-A+); (3) with viremia, with antibody (V+A+); and (4) with viremia, no antibody (V+A-). Birds in an infection-free flock and genetically resistant birds in a susceptible flock fall into the category V-A-. Genetically susceptible birds in an infected flock fall into one of the other three categories. Most are V-A+, and a minority, usually <10%, are V+A-. Most V+A- hens transmit the virus to a varying but relatively high proportion of their progeny.

The virus is not highly contagious compared with other viral agents and is readily inactivated by disinfectants. Transmission can be reduced or eliminated by strict sanitation. After the infection is eradicated, standard disease control and sanitation practices can keep chicken flocks free of the disease. The role of males in transmission of avian leukosis virus is uncertain. Infected cocks apparently do not influence the rate of congenital infection of progeny but act only as virus carriers and sources of contact or venereal infection to other birds.

Pathogenesis: Lymphoid leukosis is a clonal malignancy of the bursal-dependent lymphoid system. Transformation invariably occurs in the intact bursa, often as early as 4–8 wk after infection. Tumors are often not detectable until ~14 wk of age. Death rarely occurs before 14 wk of age and is more frequent around the time of sexual maturity. The disease can be prevented, even up to 5 mo of age, by treatments that destroy the bursa. The tumors are composed almost entirely of B lymphocytes that, in many instances, have IgM on their surfaces. No antitumor immune response has been recognized. Antibodies are readily induced after infection, except when tolerance occurs.

The induction of lymphoid leukosis tumors can be enhanced in chickens coinfected with serotype 2 Marek's disease virus, a common vaccine virus. This enhancement requires a genetically susceptible chicken and early infection with lymphoid leukosis virus in addition to serotype 2 Marek's disease vaccination. Because most commercial chicken strains are resistant, and lymphoid leukosis virus infection has been largely eradicated from susceptible stocks, enhancement is not currently recognized as a field problem.

A subclinical disease syndrome characterized by depressed egg production in the absence of tumor formation is more important economically than are deaths from lymphoid leukosis. Chickens with subclinical disease usually shed virus or viral antigen into the albumen of eggs. The pathogenic mechanisms are poorly understood.

Clinical Findings and Lesions: Chickens with lymphoid leukosis have few typical clinical signs. These may include inappetence, weakness, diarrhea, dehydration, and emaciation. Infected chickens become depressed before death. Palpation often reveals an enlarged bursa and sometimes an enlarged liver. Infected birds may not necessarily develop tumors, but they may lay fewer eggs.

Diffuse or nodular lymphoid tumors are common in the liver, spleen, and bursa and are found occasionally in the kidneys, gonads, and mesentery. Involvement of the bursa has been considered virtually pathognomonic, although bursal lymphomas are also known to be induced by reticuloendotheliosis virus. Sometimes the bursal tumors are small and seen only after careful examination of the mucosal surface of the organ. Usually, no enlargement of peripheral nerves is apparent, although such lesions have been noted after experimental inoculation of subgroup J virus. Microscopically, the tumor cells are uniform, large lymphoblasts. Mitotic figures are frequent.

Outbreaks of neoplasms other than lymphoid leukosis such as myelocytomas, hemangiomas, and renal tumors have also been noted in meat-type chickens infected with subgroup J avian leukosis virus. Myelocytomatosis and skeletal myelocytomas may cause protuberances on the head, thorax, and shanks. Myelocytomas may occur in the orbit of the eye, causing hemorrhage and blindness. Hemangiomas may occur in the skin, appearing as "blood blisters," which may rupture and bleed. Renal tumors may cause paralysis due to pressure on the sciatic nerve. Microscopically, in cases of myelocytomas induced by subgroup J avian leukosis virus, the liver shows a massive intravascular and extravascular accumulation of myeloblasts characterized by the presence of cytoplasmic eosinophilic granules.

Most strains of leukosis/sarcoma viruses also induce nonlymphoid tumors (including sarcomas), erythroblastosis, myeloblastosis, myelocytomas, hemangiomas, nephroblastomas, osteopetrosis, and related neoplasms. The nature of the tumors and their frequency depend on virus strain, chicken strain, age, dose, and route of infection. Occasional outbreaks of predominantly one type of tumor are seen in the field. The Rous sarcoma virus, a member of this group, has been widely studied in the laboratory. Each strain usually causes a predominantly neoplastic disease and can be distinguished on the basis of pathogenicity. Some viruses (eg, Rous sarcoma and erythroblastosis viruses) contain a viral oncogene that enables the virus to induce neoplasms within a short incubation period, but such viruses are rare in the field. Others cannot replicate on their own and require a nondefective helper virus. In recent years, avian leukosis virus infection has been shown to be associated with the so-called "fowl glioma," characterized by cerebellar hypoplasia and myocarditis.

Diagnosis: Because avian leukosis virus is widespread among chickens, virus detection tests, including virus isolation and PCR and the demonstration of antigen or antibody, have limited or no value in diagnosing field cases of lymphomas. Gross characteristics of diagnostic significance include the tumorous involvement of the liver, spleen, or bursa in the absence of peripheral nerve lesions. The tumors are found in birds >14 wk old. Histologically, the lymphoid cells are uniform in character, large, and contain IgM and B-cell markers on their surface. Tumors can be differentiated from those of Marek's disease by gross and microscopic pathology and by molecular techniques that demonstrate the characteristic clonal integration of proviral DNA into the tumor cell genome with the associated disruption of the c-*myc* oncogene. Lymphoid leukosis cannot easily be differentiated from B-cell lymphomas caused by reticuloendotheliosis virus except by virologic assays; however, such tumors probably are extremely rare. Several PCR primers specific for detection of the most commonly isolated avian leukosis viruses, particularly subgroups A and J, have been developed. Other primers specific for endogenous, subgroup E avian leukosis virus have also been used. PCR has been used to detect and characterize avian leukosis virus strains contaminating commercial live virus vaccines of poultry. ELISA kits for detection of antibodies to avian leukosis virus subgroups A, B, and J are available commercially.

Control: Eradication of avian leukosis virus from primary breeding stocks is the most effective means to control avian leukosis virus infection and lymphoid leukosis in chickens. Breeder flocks are evaluated for viral shedding by testing for viral antigens in the albumen of eggs with enzyme immunoassays or by biologic assays for infectious virus. Eggs from shedder hens are discarded, so that progeny flocks typically have reduced levels of infection. If raised in small groups, infection-free flocks can be derived with relative ease. These control measures are applied only to primary breeder flocks. Voluntary programs to reduce viral infection have already reduced mortality from lymphoid leukosis and improved egg production in most layer strains; similar programs were equally successful in certain meat strains. Some breeders favor, and have virtually achieved, total eradication, while others favor a reduced level of viral infection. Some chickens have specific genetic resistance to infection with certain subgroups of virus. Although genetic cellular resistance is unlikely to replace the need for reduction or eradication of the virus, the cellular receptor gene has recently been cloned, and quick molecular assays for viral susceptibility could be developed. Thus far, vaccination for tumor prevention has not been promising.

RETICULOENDOTHELIOSIS

Reticuloendotheliosis designates a group of neoplastic and immunosuppressive syndromes in several avian species caused by reticuloendotheliosis virus, a member of the avian retrovirus group. The host range of reticuloendotheliosis virus is much broader than that of Marek's disease or avian leukosis. Natural infection and disease occurs in chickens, turkeys, ducks, geese, and quail; probably many species of birds can be infected. Mammals appear refractory, although certain mammalian cell cultures are susceptible.

Reticuloendotheliosis virus is not as ubiquitous as Marek's disease and avian leukosis viruses but is more widely distributed than once believed. Many recent cases have been attributed to accidental contamination of live virus poultry vaccines such as Marek's disease virus and fowlpox virus with reticuloendotheliosis virus. Although clinical outbreaks are not frequently seen, serologic surveys suggest that the virus is prevalent in both chicken and turkey flocks in many countries, including the USA.

Etiology: Reticuloendotheliosis virus is immunologically, morphologically, and structurally distinct from the leukosis/sarcoma group of avian retroviruses. The International Committee on Taxonomy of Viruses has classified reticuloendotheliosis viruses within the family Retroviridae, subfamily Orthoretrovirinae, genus *Gammaretrovirus*. Although all isolates belong to a single serotype, three subtypes of reticuloendotheliosis virus have been identified on the basis of neutralization tests and differential reactivity with monoclonal antibodies. Strains can be further classified by their ability to replicate in cell culture. Most field isolates appear to be nondefective for replication in cell cultures and contain no viral oncogene. One unique laboratory strain *(strain T) is defective for replication* in cell cultures and contains a viral oncogene, *v-rel*, that is responsible for an acute reticulum cell neoplasia in experimentally inoculated chicks; this neoplasm prompted the name reticuloendotheliosis but is not commonly seen in the field.

Transmission and Epidemiology: Horizontal transmission is probably more important than vertical, although both have been documented in chickens and turkeys. Transmission by mosquitoes and other blood-sucking insects is suspected. The virus has been isolated from litter. A high rate of congenital infection has been demonstrated in naturally infected turkeys, but such flocks are probably rare. The virus has been transmitted accidentally through use of contaminated vaccines. Most commonly, however, flocks seroconvert after 10 wk of age without clinical disease or viral shedding to progeny. Experimentally, contact transmission occurs, but the virus is neither highly contagious nor highly stable in the environment. Partial or complete genomic insertion of reticuloendotheliosis virus in the genome of other avian viruses, namely fowlpox and Marek's disease viruses, has been described. However, the significance of such insertion in transmission of reticuloendotheliosis virus is not known. Although semen from tolerantly infected turkeys contains infectious virus, the role of the tom in vertical transmission is not clear.

Pathogenesis: The nondefective strains of reticuloendotheliosis virus produce three distinct syndromes: non-neoplastic runting, acute neoplastic disease, and chronic neoplastic disease resulting in B and T lymphomas. Typically, the runting syndrome is seen 4–10 wk after administration of contaminated vaccines to day-old chicks, which can lead to dramatic economic losses. Chronic neoplastic disease has been induced experimentally in chickens, turkeys, and ducks; one type occurs in chickens after latent periods of >4 mo and appears identical to lymphoid leukosis. As in lymphoid leukosis, these tumors are composed of B cells, are bursal-dependent, and have IgM on their surface. Acute neoplasia, which occurs after a latent period of 6–8 wk, also has been seen in chickens, turkeys, ducks, and quail. This tumor in chickens involves T cells and may be confused with Marek's disease.

Clinical Findings and Lesions: The clinical findings for runting syndrome include weight loss, paleness, occasional paralysis, and abnormal feathering (Nakanuke disease). Death from acute or chronic neoplasia is preceded by depression and occasionally by some of the same clinical changes described for the runting syndrome.

The abnormal feather lesion, in which the barbules are compressed to the shaft over a small part of its length, may be of diagnostic value. Other lesions include bursal and thymic atrophy, enlarged nerves, and anemia. Neoplasms typically involve the liver, spleen, intestine, and heart. The bursa is involved in the chronic B-cell lymphomas of chickens in a manner similar to that of lymphoid leukosis. Nonbursal (T-cell) lymphomas with shorter latent periods and lesions superficially resembling those of Marek's disease also are recognized in chickens. In turkeys, prominent lesions include enlarged livers and nodular lesions on the intestines; the bursa is only rarely tumorous. The tumors, regardless of type or host species, are usually composed of uniform, large, lymphoreticular cells.

Diagnosis: Because lesions induced by reticuloendotheliosis virus are so diverse and resemble so closely those of other tumors, diagnosis at necropsy is difficult. A diagnosis of reticuloendotheliosis requires not only the presence of typical gross and microscopic lesions but also the demonstration of reticuloendotheliosis virus. Because reticuloendotheliosis virus is not yet as ubiquitous as avian leukosis and Marek's disease viruses, the demonstration of infectious virus, viral antigens, and proviral DNA in tumor cells has significant diagnostic value. The nerve lesions are usually less extensive and may contain more plasma cells than in Marek's disease, but in other cases are difficult to differentiate by histology. The runting syndrome is easily confused with immunosuppressive syndromes caused by other viral agents. The chronic B-cell lymphomas induced experimentally in chickens cannot easily be distinguished from those of lymphoid leukosis except by virus studies, including PCR. Similarly, the T-cell lymphomas of chickens cannot easily be distinguished from Marek's disease except by virus studies. However, both B- and T-cell lymphomas induced by reticuloendotheliosis virus contain a clonally integrated DNA provirus usually associated with the c-*myc* oncogene, which can be demonstrated by appropriate molecular methods. The chronic lymphomas that are seen in turkeys must be differentiated from lymphoproliferative disease of turkeys based on histology, virus isolation, and characterization of the virus-associated reverse transcriptase for activity in the presence of manganese or magnesium ions. Techniques based on immunocytochemistry with monoclonal antibodies to cellular, tumor, and viral antigens, or molecular hybridization can be used in the differential diagnosis of avian viral lymphomas, including reticuloendotheliosis.

Control: No control measures are currently practiced. An experimental recombinant fowlpox virus vaccine has been developed. Some breeder companies wish to avoid seroconversion of their primary breeder stocks to obviate restrictions on export of progeny to certain countries, but reliable techniques to prevent horizontal transmission have not been developed. Elimination of vertical transmission would presumably be possible by removing potential transmitter hens; rearing progeny under isolated conditions would prevent horizontal infection. Many of these principles have successfully been applied to the control of avian leukosis virus in chickens. Such control procedures could be considered if reticuloendotheliosis virus infection becomes endemic in especially valuable breeding stock, as was the case with reticuloendotheliosis virus infection in the endangered Attwater's prairie chickens.

NEOPLASMS OF UNKNOWN ETIOLOGY

Of the numerous tumors of unknown etiology in poultry, dermal squamous cell carcinoma (avian keratoacanthoma), multicentric histiocytosis, and adenocarcinomas are the most common but appear to be of limited economic importance.

Avian Keratoacanthoma: These neoplasms can occur at relatively high frequencies in some broiler flocks. Carcasses with extensive lesions are condemned at slaughter, while less affected birds undergo trimming. Condemnations of whole carcasses represent a significant economic loss. Typically, the lesions are seen during processing after the skin has been defeathered as crater-like ulcers with raised margins within feather tracts. In live chickens, the ulcers usually contain a mixture of keratin, cell debris, and bacteria. Histologically, lesions appear as proliferative expansion of feather follicle epithelium. An etiologic agent has not yet been identified, and the true neoplastic nature of the lesion has not been confirmed. Transmissibility of this tumor has neither been demonstrated nor excluded.

Multicentric Histiocytosis: This condition of young broiler chickens is characterized by both splenomegaly and hepatomegaly. Miliary (0.5–5 mm), white to yellow nodules can be seen in the spleen, liver, and kidneys. Microscopically, nodules of spindle-shaped cells diffusely expand periarteriolar lymphoid sheaths. These histiocytic cells contain elongated oval, fusiform, or more bizarrely configured nuclei. No definitive etiologic agent has been identified. A somewhat similar condition with lesions, termed "histiocytic sarcomatosis," has been described in meat-type chickens experimentally infected with subgroup J avian leukosis virus.

Adenocarcinomas: Adenocarcinomas of the ovary or oviduct are relatively common incidental tumors in mature chickens. These neoplasms often are characterized by multiple miliary implant tumors on the mesentery and other visceral surfaces, frequently accompanied by ascites. These tumors are not known to be virus-induced or to be transmissible.

NEWCASTLE DISEASE AND OTHER PARAMYXOVIRUS INFECTIONS

NEWCASTLE DISEASE

(Avian pneumoencephalitis, Exotic or velogenic Newcastle disease)

Newcastle disease is an infection of domestic poultry and other bird species with virulent Newcastle disease virus (NDV). It is a worldwide problem that presents primarily as an acute respiratory disease, but depression, nervous manifestations, or diarrhea may be the predominant clinical form. Severity depends on the virulence of the infecting virus and host susceptibility. Occurrence of the disease is reportable and may result in trade restrictions.

Etiology and Pathogenesis: NDV, synonymous with avian paramyxovirus serotype 1 (PMV-1), is an RNA virus and the most important of the 11 known PMV serotypes as a pathogen for poultry. The original classification of NDV isolates into one of three virulence groups by chicken embryo and chicken inoculation as virulent (velogenic), moderately virulent (mesogenic), or of low virulence (lentogenic) has been abbreviated for regulatory purposes. Velogens and mesogens are now classified as virulent NDV (vNDV), the cause of Newcastle disease and reportable infection, whereas infections with lentogens, the low virulence NDV (loNDV) widely used as live vaccines, are not reportable. Clinical manifestations vary from high morbidity and mortality to asymptomatic infections. Severity of infection depends on virus virulence and age, immune status, and susceptibility of the host species. Chickens are the most and waterfowl the least susceptible of domestic poultry; however, some differences may be seen if the NDV strain is adapted to a particular species.

Epidemiology and Transmission: Virulent NDV strains are endemic in poultry in most of Asia, Africa, and some countries of North and South America. Other countries, including the USA and Canada, are free of those strains in poultry and maintain that status with import restrictions and eradication by destroying infected poultry. Cormorants, pigeons, and imported psittacine species are more commonly infected with vNDV and have also been sources of vNDV infections of poultry. NDV strains of low virulence are prevalent in poultry and wild birds, especially waterfowl. Infection of domestic poultry with loNDV contributes to lower productivity.

Infected birds shed virus in exhaled air, respiratory discharges, and feces. Virus is shed during incubation, during the clinical stage, and for a varying but limited period during convalescence. Virus may also be present in eggs laid during clinical disease and in all parts of the carcass during acute vNDV infections. Chickens are readily infected by aerosols and by ingesting contaminated water or food. Infected chickens and other domestic and wild birds may be sources of NDV. Movement of infected birds and transfer of virus, especially in infective feces, by the movement of people and contaminated equipment or litter are the main methods of virus spread between poultry flocks.

Clinical Findings: Onset is rapid, and signs appear throughout the flock within 2–12 days (average 5) after aerosol exposure. Spread is slower if the fecal-oral route is the primary means of transmission, particularly for caged birds. Young birds are the most susceptible. Observed signs depend on whether the infecting virus has a predilection for respiratory, digestive, or nervous systems. Respiratory signs of gasping, coughing, sneezing, and rales predominate in infections with loNDV. Nervous signs of tremors, paralyzed wings and legs, twisted necks, circling, clonic spasms, and complete paralysis may accompany, but usually follow, the respiratory signs in neurotropic velogenic disease. Nervous signs with diarrhea are typical in pigeons, and nervous signs are frequently seen in cormorants and exotic bird species. Respiratory signs with depression, watery greenish diarrhea, and swelling of the tissues of the head and neck are typical of the most virulent form of the disease, viscerotropic velogenic Newcastle disease, although nervous signs are often seen, especially in vaccinated poultry. Varying degrees of depression and inappetence are seen. Partial or complete cessation of egg production may occur. Eggs may be abnormal in color, shape, or surface and have watery albumen. Mortality is variable but can be as high as 100% with vNDV infections. Well-vaccinated birds may not show any signs of being infected except for a decrease in egg production, but these birds will shed virus in saliva and feces. Poorly vaccinated birds may develop torticollis, ataxia, or body and head tremors 10–14 days after infection and may recover with supportive care.

Lesions: Remarkable gross lesions are usually seen only with viscerotropic velogenic Newcastle disease. Petechiae may be seen on the serous membranes; hemorrhages of the proventricular mucosa and intestinal serosa are accompanied by multifocal, necrotic hemorrhagic areas on the mucosal surface of the intestine, especially at lymphoid foci such as cecal tonsils. Splenic necrosis and hemorrhage and edema around the thymus may also be seen. In contrast, lesions in birds infected with loNDV strains may be limited to congestion and mucoid exudates seen in the respiratory tract with opacity and thickening of the air sacs. Secondary bacterial infections increase the severity of respiratory lesions.

Diagnosis: NDV can be isolated from oropharyngeal or cloacal swabs or tissues from infected birds by inoculation of the allantoic cavity of 9- to 11-day-old SPF embryonated chicken eggs. Infection is confirmed by recovery of a hemagglutinating virus that is inhibited with NDV antiserum or by detection of NDV RNA by reverse transcriptase PCR. A rise in NDV antibody titer by hemagglutination-inhibition or ELISA of paired serum samples indicates NDV infection. To confirm diagnosis, identification of an isolate such as vNDV is established by the rapidity of killing day-old SPF chicks inoculated by the intracerebral route, the intracerebral pathogenicity index, or by the presence of a specified amino acid motif at the cleavage site of the fusion protein (F) precursor (FO). Reference laboratories use nucleotide sequence analysis to detect genetic differences for comparison of isolates from different outbreaks and to identify the source of those infections. The acute form of ND should be differentiated from other diseases known to cause high mortality, such as highly pathogenic avian influenza (*see* p 2902).

Prevention: Vaccines are available for chickens, turkeys, and pigeons and are used to induce an antibody response, so vaccinated bids must be exposed to a larger dose of vNDV to be infected. Unfortunately, ND vaccines do not provide sterile immunity, and in many areas of the world vaccines are used to prevent losses from sickness and death. Live lentogenic vaccines, chiefly B1 and LaSota strains, are widely used and typically administered to poultry by mass application in drinking water or by spray. Mucosal immunity induced in birds vaccinated by live vaccines applied by these routes decreases the amount of vNDV the vaccinated birds will shed if infected with vNDV, compared with the immune response induced by an inactivated vaccine. Mass vaccination methods are less labor intensive but if not applied properly may lead to <85% of the flock being immunized, which is needed for herd immunity. Alternatively, individual administration of live vaccines is via the nares or conjunctival sac. Healthy chicks are vaccinated as early as day 1–4 of life. However, delaying vaccination until the second or third week avoids maternal antibody interference with an active immune response. *Mycoplasma*, some other bacteria, and other viruses affecting the respiratory tract, if present, may act synergistically with some vaccines to aggravate the vaccine reaction after spray administration.

Oil-adjuvanted inactivated vaccines are also used after live vaccine in breeders and layers and may be used alone in situations where use of live virus may be contraindicated (eg, in pigeons). In countries where vNDV is endemic, a combination of live virus and inactivated vaccine can be used; or alternatively, if permitted by law, a live mesogenic strain vaccine may be used in older birds. The frequency of revaccination to protect chickens throughout life largely depends on the risk of exposure and virulence of the field virus challenge. Administering inactivated vaccines is more labor intensive, because each bird has to be handled individually. Accidental inoculation of human tissues with oil-based vaccines requires prompt medical treatment.

Fowlpox or turkey herpesvirus–vectored NDV vaccines are commercially available for chickens and have the advantage of being able to be administered in ovo at the hatchery. These vaccines must be reconstituted as directed by the manufacturer and, because they take 3–4 wk to produce a protective level of immunity, biosecurity is even more important. A commercial kit to detect levels of antibodies induced by these vaccines is not yet available.

Zoonotic Risk: All NDV strains can produce a transitory conjunctivitis in people, but the condition has been limited primarily to laboratory workers and vaccination teams exposed to large quantities of virus. Before poultry vaccination was widely practiced, conjunctivitis from NDV infection occurred in crews eviscerating poultry in processing plants. The disease has not been reported in people who rear poultry or consume poultry products.

OTHER AVIAN PARAMYXOVIRUS INFECTIONS

Avian paramyxovirus infections have been reported in chickens and turkeys in association with respiratory disease or decreases in egg production.

Etiology and Epidemiology: There are 12 recognized serotypes of avian paramyxoviruses (PMV-1 to PMV-12). Newcastle disease virus (PMV-1, *see* p 2856) is the most important pathogen of this group for poultry, but PMV-2, -3, -6, and -7 are occasionally associated with disease in chickens and turkeys. The most recent serotypes (PMV-10, -11, and -12) were isolated from Rockhopper penguin (*Eudyptes chrysocome*) in the Falkland Islands, Common Snipe (*Gallinago gallinago*) in France, and Eurasian Widgeon (*Anas penelope*) in Italy, respectively, and were the first new serotypes in >30 yr.

PMV-2 has been isolated from wild birds, mainly passerines, and caged psittacine species. Primary infections in poultry are believed to be the result of contact with wild birds. The method of transmission to chickens or turkeys is unclear. PMV-3 has been isolated from imported exotic and other bird species held in captivity. Psittacines appear to be the primary host, although PMV-3 will spread among passerines in captivity. There are no reports of isolation of PMV-3 from wild birds. The method of transmission among turkeys is unclear, and spread within a flock is usually slow.

Clinical Findings: Infections by PMV-2, -3, -6, and -7 in turkeys have produced mild to severe respiratory disease, drops in egg production, reduced hatchability and infertility of eggs, and increased numbers of white-shelled eggs. Infection with PMV-2 has produced mild respiratory disease in chickens, but PMV-2 infection is usually most severe in turkeys, especially breeders. Infection is more severe when accompanied by secondary pathogens.

Diagnosis: Most diagnoses are made by clinical signs and confirmed by serology. PMV-2, -3, -6, and -7 can be isolated from oropharyngeal or cloacal swabs, or tissue samples from infected birds by inoculating the allantoic cavity of 8- to 10-day-old embryonating chicken eggs. Confirmation of the virus as PMV can be done by hemagglutination inhibition tests with specific antiserum to individual serotypes. However, PMV-1 (Newcastle disease virus) and PMV-3 may cross-react in hemagglutination inhibition tests (and in other serologic tests such as ELISA), which causes interpretation problems in vaccinated birds. Birds vaccinated against Newcastle disease show a rise in hemagglutination inhibition titers to both viruses if subsequently infected with PMV-3.

Prevention and Control: No vaccines are available for PMV-2, -6, and -7. Inactivated oil-emulsion vaccines against PMV-3 have been used in turkey breeder flocks. These are injected twice, 4 wk apart, before the birds begin to lay (usually when 20–24 wk old). The risk of introducing PMV-2 and other paramyxoviruses from wild birds may be minimized by bird-proofing poultry houses and using good hygiene and biosecurity practices. Treatment of secondary bacterial infections with antibiotics has had some success. PMV-3 appears to spread slowly.

Zoonotic Risk: No human infections have been reported for PMV-2 to PMV-12 viruses.

OMPHALITIS

(Navel ill, "Mushy chick" disease, Yolk sac infection)

Omphalitis is a condition characterized by infected yolk sacs, often accompanied by unhealed navels in young fowl. It is infectious but noncontagious and is associated with poor regulation of incubation temperature or humidity and marked contamination of the hatching eggs or incubator. If young poultry are placed in contaminated transportation boxes before their navels are completely closed, bacteria can migrate up the patent yolk stalk and infect the yolk sac.

The navel may be inflamed and fail to close, producing a wet spot on the abdomen; a scab may be present. Opportunistic bacteria (coliforms, staphylococci, *Pseudomonas* spp, and *Proteus* spp) are often involved, and mixed infections are common. Proteolytic bacteria are prevalent in outbreaks. The yolk sac is not absorbed and often is highly congested or may contain solidified pieces of yolk material; peritonitis may be extensive. Edema of the sternal subcutis may be seen. Affected chicks or poults usually appear normal until a few hours before death. They have little interest in food and water and are often found severely dehydrated. Depression, drooping of the head, and huddling near the heat source usually are the only signs. Mortality often begins at hatching and continues to 10–14 days of age, with losses of as much as 15% in chickens and 50% in turkeys. Chilling or overheating during shipment may increase losses. Persistent, unabsorbed, infected yolks often produce chicks or poults with reduced weight gain.

There is no specific treatment; antibiotic use is based on the prevalent bacterial type involved. Even then, treatment may not result in satisfactory outcomes, because severely affected chicks and poults often die, and unaffected birds are unlikely to be aided by antibiotic treatment. The disease is prevented by careful control of temperature, humidity, and sanitation in the incubator. Only clean, uncracked eggs should be set. If it is necessary to set dirty eggs, they should be segregated from clean eggs. Sanitizing detergents must be used according to directions if eggs are washed. Time, temperature, and frequent changes of water are as critical as the concentration of sanitizer in both wash and rinse water. The rinse should be warmer than the wash water (which should be warmer than the internal temperature of the egg) but should not be >60°C.

The incubator should be cleaned and disinfected thoroughly between hatches. If fumigation is to be done with formaldehyde, vents should be closed. Thirty mL of 40% formaldehyde/0.6 m^3, or paraformaldehyde (in the strength recommended by the manufacturer), should be allowed to evaporate in the closed incubator or hatcher. The machines are readily contaminated after fumigation unless the exterior of the machines and the rooms in which they are located are also cleaned and disinfected.

POISONINGS

See also TOXICOLOGY, p 2948 et seq.

When toxicosis in a poultry flock is suspected based on mortality, on decreased production/growth, or on other clinical signs such as paralysis, the flock owner or veterinarian should maintain and allow access to historical records. These records include use of disinfectants and rodenticides and insecticides on the premises, medications administered in feed and water, and nutritional additives to the feed. Samples to be collected for potential analysis in cases of suspected toxicosis include dead or recently euthanized birds that showed clinical signs, 2 lb (1 kg) of the feed available when the birds were showing clinical signs, and 500 mL of drinking water. For the safety of workers as well as poultry, the grower should have access to material safety data sheets for each chemical used on the premises. Carcasses should be refrigerated as soon as possible for examination by the veterinarian or laboratory diagnostician. Consultation with a toxicologist or laboratory diagnostician before collecting samples is highly recommended.

Aflatoxin: Aflatoxicosis is one of the most common intoxications in modern poultry production systems. Certain species of *Aspergillus* and *Penicillium* can produce aflatoxins in feedstuffs. The production of aflatoxins can occur either in the field where the crops are grown or during storage. Acute aflatoxicosis is characterized by inappetence, ataxia, convulsions, opisthotonos, depression, and death. A gross lesion often seen with acute aflatoxicosis is an enlarged yellow liver. All poultry are susceptible to aflatoxicosis; however, ducks and turkeys are particularly sensitive.

Ammonia (aerosolized): Ammonia gas is produced by the metabolism of uric acid by bacteria that can thrive in wet poultry litter. High ammonia levels often occur during the winter when ventilation is minimized to conserve heat and thus high litter moisture is common. Increased ammonia levels of 25–30 ppm can damage the mucociliary apparatus of the upper respiratory tract, and higher levels (50–75 ppm) can cause decreased feed intake as well as caustic burns to the cornea, which can result in blindness. These birds will often fail to find adequate food and water, resulting in death.

Anticoagulant Rodenticides: Rodenticides can be safely applied to poultry houses so that rodent baits are sequestered from the flock; however, careless application can result in rodent bait consumption by poultry with usually acute toxic effects. First-generation anticoagulant rodenticides, including warfarin, chlorphacinone, diphacinone, and coumtetralyl, require continual ingestion by rodents to induce toxic effects. Second-generation or single-feed anticoagulants, including brodifacoum, bromadialone, difenacoum, and difethialone, can be acutely fatal to rodents. Clinical signs in poultry are related to the anticoagulant effects and usually observed as sudden death with gross hemorrhagic lesions in one or more body sites, particularly lung, intestine, and peritoneal cavity. These lesions can be confused with flight injury (gamebirds) and trauma from wild animals and dogs. Definitive diagnosis of anticoagulant toxicosis should be based on gross lesions, history of anticoagulant application, and anticoagulant screen on liver of dead birds (available at several USA veterinary diagnostic laboratories).

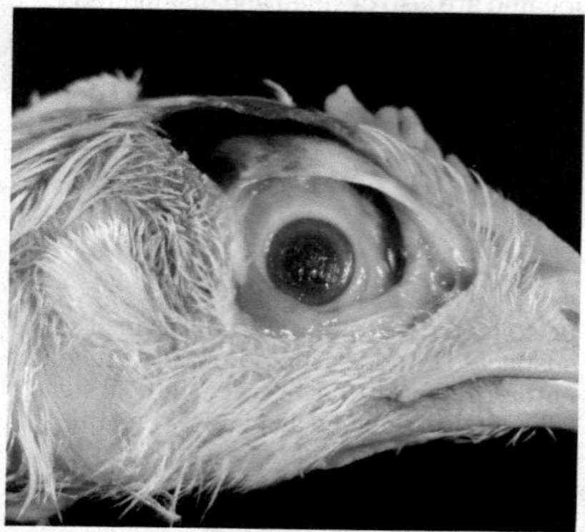

Pullets exposed to high levels of aerosolized ammonia in wet litter developed blindness as a result of corneal ulcers. *Courtesy of Dr. Robert Porter.*

Botulism: *Clostridium botulinum* bacteria produce several exotoxins that are among the most potent toxins known. In ducks and geese, botulism outbreaks commonly occur in the summer months in the vicinity of poorly aerated ponds and lakes. The waterfowl ingest the toxin by eating dead invertebrates from the margins of these lakes or eating maggots on the carcasses of ducks that have already succumbed to the intoxication. In pheasant and broiler flocks, where the timely removal of dead birds has not been practiced, carcasses can also become a source of toxin. The classic clinical sign of botulism intoxication in poultry is paralysis of the muscles of the neck or "limberneck." The toxin also causes paralysis affecting the legs, wings, and eyelids. Diagnosis of botulism is often based on exclusion of other possible causes, although intestinal contents and blood can be collected for botulism toxin analysis (mouse inoculation assay), which is available at several USA diagnostic laboratories.

Calcium: Excessive calcium intake in broiler chicks results in urolithiasis and visceral gout (hyperuricemia) with urate deposits on the abdominal viscera and in the joints. Tetanic convulsions can also be seen in chicks consuming excess calcium. Calcium levels >2% will induce these lesions in broilers. Feeding calcium in excess of 3% before the onset of egg production will induce the same lesions in egg-type or meat-type pullets.

Carbon Monoxide: This poisoning commonly arises from exhaust fumes when chicks are being transported by truck or from improper ventilation in hatchers. Mortality may be high unless fresh air is provided immediately. At necropsy, the beak and face are cyanotic, and a characteristic bright pink color is noted throughout the viscera, particularly the lungs. Diagnosis can be confirmed by a spectroscopic analysis of the blood.

Coffee Weed Seed: *Senna obtusifolia* seeds are frequently found in corn and soybeans. When present at ≥2%, they reduce feed intake and lower body weight, increase feed conversion in broilers, and significantly depress egg production in laying birds. Necropsy lesions are absent.

Copper: Copper sulfate has been used as a water additive for treatment of crop mycosis (*Candida* overgrowth) or nonspecific digestive tract disorders in poultry. Copper sulfate in a single dose of >1 g is fatal. The signs are watery diarrhea and listlessness. A catarrhal gastroenteritis and burns or erosions in the lining of the gizzard, accompanied by a greenish, seromucous exudate throughout the intestinal tract, are found at necropsy.

Crotalaria: Seeds of many species are toxic to chickens. Concentrations >0.05% in the feed produce signs of toxicosis. At 0.2%, weight gain is reduced markedly; 0.3% causes death in 18 days. Lesions consist of ascites, swelling or cirrhosis of the liver, and hemorrhages. Resistance to the toxin increases with age.

Diazinon: Diazinon is an organic phosphate and cholinesterase inhibitor commonly used to control a variety of insects around poultry houses. It should not be used inside poultry houses. Chickens will consume the diazinon crystals, which results in lacrimation, diarrhea, dyspnea, and death. Necropsy lesions include lung edema, fatty livers, and severe enteritis. The diazinon crystals might be seen in the crop and gizzard contents. Diagnosis can be confirmed by testing brain for cholinesterase activity.

Gossypol: Cottonseed meal contains appreciable amounts of gossypol, which produces severe cardiac edema that results in dyspnea, weakness, and anorexia. When fed to laying hens, gossypol also causes egg-yolk discoloration.

Lead: Lead poisoning usually is caused by paint or orchard-spray material. Metallic lead in amounts of 7.2 mg/kg body wt is lethal. Signs are depression, inappetence, emaciation, thirst, and weakness. Greenish droppings are commonly seen within 36 hr. As poisoning progresses, the wings may be extended downward. Young birds may die within 36 hr after ingestion. Acute lead poisoning may be diagnosed from the history and necropsy findings of a greenish brown gizzard mucosa, enteritis, and degeneration of the liver and kidney. Chronic poisoning results in emaciation and in atrophy of the liver and heart. The pericardium is distended with fluid, the gallbladder is thickened and enlarged, and urate deposits are usually found in the kidneys. Ingestion of lead shot often occurs in wild waterfowl on heavily gunned feeding grounds. Retention of only a few lead pellets in the gizzard can kill a duck.

Mercury: Poisoning occurs from mercurial disinfectants and fungicides, including mercurous chloride (calomel) and bichloride of mercury (corrosive sublimate). Clinical findings are progressive weakness and incoordination. Diarrhea may occur, depending on the amount ingested. The caustic action of the chemical may produce gray areas in the mouth and esophagus, which usually ulcerate if the bird lives >24 hr. Catarrhal inflammation of the proventriculus and intestines may occur; if a large amount of mercury is ingested, extensive hemorrhage may occur in these organs. The kidneys are pale and studded with small, white foci. The liver shows fatty degeneration.

Nicarbazin: This chemical coccidiostat is used in broilers. It should not be fed to layers, because it can cause discoloration and reduced hatchability of eggs (although the effect is reversible once the nicarbazin is withdrawn). It also may result in reduced heat tolerance in birds exposed to high temperature and humidity.

Nitrofurazone: This has been used to treat several bacterial diseases in poultry, but it is no longer approved for use in many countries, including the USA. When fed at 0.022%, it causes hyperexcitability manifest by rapid movements, loud squawking, and frequent falling forward. In turkeys, which are more sensitive to nitrofurazone than are chickens, it produces cardiac dilatation, ascites, and when fed at 0.033%, death.

3-Nitro-4-hydroxyphenylarsonic Acid: When this compound, widely used in feed to improve weight gain and feed efficiency, is improperly mixed or fed at a level 2–3 times higher than normal, it induces a high-pitched chirp and a "duck-walking" stance. Ataxia, neck extension, and paralysis can occur in chickens and turkeys that consume excessive amounts. Clinical signs are usually reversible in a few minutes. Chronic exposure may produce intrahepatic cholangitis.

Polychlorinated Biphenyls (PCBs): Residues have been reported in the fatty tissue of chickens and turkeys in excess of the 5 ppm permitted in edible tissue, and in egg products in excess of the permitted 0.5 ppm. PCBs depress egg production and hatchability, and levels of 50 ppm result in cirrhosis of the liver and ascites in broilers and a drop in egg production and hatchability in hens. (*See also* PERSISTENT HALOGENATED AROMATIC POISONING, p 3056.)

Polyether Ionophores: Polyether ionophores facilitate transport of divalent cations across cell membranes to interfere with osmoregulation, resulting in cell rupture. Toxicosis caused by ionophores is relatively common in poultry, because these compounds are commonly administered for the prevention and treatment of coccidiosis and are subject to overdosing and mixing errors. Additionally, these ionophores can interact with certain medications, such as sulfonamides, to cause toxicosis signs when the ionophore concentration in the feed is normal. Examples of ionophores used in poultry are described below.

Lasalocid: Lasalocid is an anticoccidial compound that has been used in hot summer months, because it increases water consumption. When used at other times of the year, the level of salt in the ration is reduced to prevent excessive water elimination and wet litter problems. If the salt level is reduced too much, it will result in stunting, increased lameness, and a characteristic clinical picture in broilers manifested by the bird walking on its toes. This clinical syndrome has been called lasalocid toxicity when, in reality, it is due to low levels of salt in the feed.

Monensin: This ionophore coccidiostat is widely used in the broiler industry. At levels >120 ppm it reduces feed intake and weight gain; in layers, egg production is reduced. Signs of toxicity include a characteristic paralysis in which the legs are extended backward. If naive turkeys are switched to a feed that contains monensin, they become paralyzed with the legs extended backward and mortality occurs; no lesions are seen at necropsy.

Narasin: This ionophore is often administered in combination with the chemical nicarbazone to prevent coccidiosis in broilers but can be particularly toxic in turkeys (often noted on product label), resulting in flaccid paralysis of the wings and legs. Toxic effects have also been described in broilers simultaneously treated with tiamulin or sulfonamides.

Salinomycin: Salinomycin is commonly used as an anticoccidial compound in the broiler industry. It is safe when used at 60 g/ton of feed. Toxicities occur when broiler feed containing salinomycin is accidentally fed to naive breeder hens. Clinical signs in these hen flocks include paralysis with the legs extended backward and decreased feed consumption, egg production, and hatchability. Levels of salinomycin >10 g/ton in breeder-hen feed are sufficient to produce these clinical signs. Necropsy lesions are absent in birds with this clinical picture.

Polytetrafluoroethylene (PTFE): PTFE is a synthetic fluoropolymer resin highly resistant to heat and chemically stable with low reactivity. PTFE has been used as nonstick coating for frying pans (Teflon®) and has been used to coat heat lamps and heater filaments that might be used in poultry houses. Although generally heat stable, PTFE heated above 280°C (536°F) can produce aerosolized hydrogen fluoride, carbon fluoride, carbon monoxide, and low-molecular-weight fluoropolymers. PTFE pyrolysis products can cause direct caustic damage to the lung, resulting in marked pulmonary edema and hemorrhage. Birds are often found dead with no premonitory signs. Diagnosis is based on gross lesions, history of using new heating lambs or filaments coated with PTFE, and excluding other possible causes of pulmonary hemorrhage.

Propane: Propane is commonly used in poultry facilities as a fuel source to provide heat for young poultry. Chicks are often surrounded by a cardboard brooder ring to provide a safe, warm environment during the first week of life. If a defective heater leaks propane into the brooder ring, the propane gas will displace the lighter air, resulting in asphyxiation of the chicks. On necropsy, these chicks have congested, edematous lungs that sink when placed in formalin.

Quaternary Ammonia: Quaternary-ammonia-based compounds are widely used as disinfectants. (*See also* ANTISEPTICS AND

DISINFECTANTS, p 2738.) Turkeys are very sensitive; levels of 150 ppm result in substantial mortality. Clinical signs include reduced water intake, nasal and ocular discharge, facial swelling, and gasping. Necropsy lesions include caseous ulcers at the base of the tongue and commissures of the mouth.

Selenium: Ingestion of feeds containing >5 ppm of selenium decreases the hatchability of eggs due to deformities of the embryos, which are unable to emerge from the shell because of beak anomalies. Eyes may be unilaterally hypoplastic or aplastic, and feet and wings may be deformed or underdeveloped. Selenium at 10 ppm, as in seleniferous grains in the laying ration, usually reduces hatchability to zero. Young laying hens entering egg production are more susceptible than older hens.

Mature birds seem to tolerate more selenium in their feed than do pigs, cattle, or horses and do not exhibit signs of poisoning other than poor hatchability of their eggs. Starting rations containing 8 ppm selenium have reduced the growth rate of chicks, but 4 ppm had no noticeable effect. Rations containing as little as 2.5 ppm have resulted in meat and eggs with concentrations of selenium in excess of the suggested tolerance limit in foods. Sodium arsenite and some of the organic arsenicals, when administered to laying hens with selenium, have increased hatchability.

Sodium (salt): The addition of 0.5% salt (NaCl) to the ration of chickens and turkeys is recommended, but amounts >2% are usually considered dangerous. Rations for chicks have contained as much as 8% without injurious effect, but in poults, rations containing 4% were harmful and levels of 6%–8% have resulted in mortality. The addition of 2% NaCl to the feed, or 4,000 ppm in the water, depresses growth in young ducks and lowers the fertility and hatchability of the eggs in breeding stock.

Salt levels high enough to produce poisoning may be reached when salty protein concentrates (eg, fish meal) are added to rations already fortified with salt or when the salt is poorly incorporated in the feed. Sporadic poisoning also has been reported from accidental ingestion of rock salt or salt provided for other livestock. Necropsy findings are not diagnostic; enteritis and ascites are common. Watery droppings and wet litter often are suggestive of a high salt intake. Edema of the testicle is pathognomonic of salt toxicity in young birds.

Sulfonamides: Sulfonamides are widely used for treatment of several bacterial and protozoal infections in poultry and are usually administered in drinking water. Sulfaquinoxaline, when fed at 0.25%, results in severe pancytopenia. Hemorrhages are common on the legs, breast muscle, and in virtually all abdominal organs. The bone marrow is pale, and the blood is slow to clot. Toxicity is frequently seen in hot weather when sulfaquinoxaline is provided in drinking water. Water consumption increases rapidly as the temperature increases, which leads to increased drug intake. This toxicity usually is responsive to vitamin K therapy.

Sulfur: Elemental sulfur is often used in broiler houses in an attempt to improve growth rate and feed conversion and to minimize bacterial disease. The compound is applied to the floor after the litter has been removed. Elemental sulfur is also used in dust baths for treatment of ectoparasites in adult layers. If the amount of new litter placed in the house is inadequate, young chicks will come in contact with the sulfur, resulting in conjunctivitis and cutaneous burns, especially under the wings and on the legs. Clinically, the birds appear cold and tend to huddle; in many instances, death will occur due to the birds piling up, causing overheating and suffocation. When sulfur comes into contact with moisture, sulfuric acid is produced, which results in the burns.

Thiram: Thiram is used to treat seed corn. It is toxic to chicks at 40 ppm and to goslings at 150 ppm; it causes leg deformities and weight loss. At 10 ppm, it causes soft-shelled eggs, and at 40 ppm, egg production and hatchability are reduced. Turkey poults tolerate up to 200 ppm.

Toxic Fat: A crystalline halogen has been identified as the "toxic fat" factor in some feeds. In young pullets, it reduces growth, retards sexual development, and increases mortality. Hatchability is decreased. Turkeys and ducks are less susceptible than chickens. Signs of intoxication include ruffled feathers, droopiness, and dyspnea. Lesions include ascites and hydropericardium, liver necrosis, subepicardial hemorrhage, and bile duct hyperplasia. Although the amount of toxin varies in feeds from different sources, 0.25%–0.5% fed for 35–150 days produces typical lesions.

RIEMERELLA ANATIPESTIFER INFECTION

(New duck disease, Infectious serositis, *Pasteurella anatipestifer* infection)

Infection with *Riemerella anatipestifer* is a contagious, widely distributed bacterial disease that primarily affects young ducks and less frequently turkeys and geese. Other waterfowl, chickens, and pheasants occasionally may be affected.

Etiology and Transmission: *R anatipestifer* is gram-negative, nonsporulating, catalase and oxidase positive, and non-motile. It grows microaerophilically in enriched media. *R anatipestifer* possesses few characteristic phenotypic properties, so isolation and identification procedures should be polyphasic. A definitive diagnosis should include genotypic identification (PCR amplification of a partial region of the *rpoB* or the 16S rRNA gene with subsequent sequencing is recommended). Just like *Pasteurella multocida*, *R anatipestifer* includes a number (>20) of immunotypes (or serotypes). This complicates efforts at widespread prevention using bacterins, because no cross-protection occurs between serotypes. However, currently, much effort is on the search for cross-protective vaccine candidates using an immunoproteomics approach.

The epidemiology and pathogenesis are poorly understood. Ducks are believed to be infected from the environment by the respiratory route or when *R anatipestifer* is introduced into lesions of the webbed foot. Turkeys may be infected by injuries or by the respiratory route when another pathogen disrupts the respiratory epithelium. Once the infection is established on a farm, it frequently becomes endemic.

Clinical Findings and Lesions: Signs usually develop after an incubation period of 2–5 days. Affected ducks, usually 1–7 wk old, often have ocular and nasal discharges, mild coughing and sneezing, tremors of the head and neck, and incoordination. In typical cases, affected ducklings lie on their backs, paddling their legs. Stunting may occur. Necrotic dermatitis on the lower back or around the vent may also be seen. Fibrinous exudate in the pericardial cavity and over the surface of the liver is the most characteristic lesion. Fibrinous airsacculitis is common, and infection of the CNS can result in fibrinous meningitis. The spleen and liver may be swollen. Pneumonia may be seen. Mortality is usually 2%–50%. A high proportion of affected birds develop mucopurulent or caseous salpingitis. Affected breeding stock should be slaughtered, because many become blind layers.

Affected turkeys, usually 5–15 wk old, often exhibit dyspnea, droopiness, hunched back, lameness, and a twisted neck. Fibrinous pericarditis and epicarditis are the most pronounced lesions. There may also be fibrinous perihepatitis, airsacculitis, and purulent synovitis. Osteomyelitis, meningitis, and focal pneumonia are seen occasionally. Mortality is 5%–60%, and condemnations are 3%–13%.

Diagnosis: Diagnosis is based on typical CNS signs (if present), lesions, and isolation and identification of the causative organism (using traditional biochemical characterization). Other diseases, eg, colibacillosis (*see* p 2814), salmonellosis (*see* p 195), and chlamydiosis (*see* p 2808), may produce similar lesions. Chocolate agar medium is recommended for isolation, although blood agar is also used, with incubation at 37°C in a candle jar or under 5% carbon dioxide. Several PCR-based diagnostic tests have been described, including assays for the *ompA* gene, 16S rRNA, *rpoB* gene, and an ERIC fragment. The published PCR tests are all able to detect *R anatipestifer*, but a high rate of false-positive reactions may occur. Consequently, PCR amplification of a partial region of the *rpoB* or the 16S rRNA gene with subsequent sequencing can be recommended to confirm identification. Recently, matrix-assisted laser desorption ionization time-of-flight mass spectrometry (MALDI-TOF MS) has been used successfully for identification. The isolate should be serotyped (only a few laboratories are capable), because the information may be needed for vaccine selection and epidemiologic studies. Plate agglutination is rapid and convenient for this purpose. However, unless titrations are carried out, only absorbed sera should be used because of the existence of multiple antigenic factors within a single strain. Biochemical characteristics can be used to differentiate this organism from other bacteria that cause important diseases of ducks and turkeys, particularly *Escherichia coli*, *P multocida*,

Salmonella enterica, *Coenonia anatine*, *Avibacterium gallinarum*, and *Bordetella avium*. Impression smears help to determine whether chlamydia is involved.

Prevention and Control: Careful management practices are important for prevention of infection. A high level of biosecurity is essential. Cleaning and disinfection between flocks and separation of flocks on multiple-age farms are other factors of major importance. Rigid sanitation and depopulation are necessary for elimination of the disease on endemically infected farms.

A bacterin and, more recently, a live vaccine, which include the three most common immunotypes of *R anatipestifer*, are available for use in ducks. An autogenous oil-emulsion bacterin can be used in turkeys. Breeder ducks can be vaccinated with a bacterin or live vaccine to provide protection to the ducklings that may last for up to 2–3 weeks of age. A combination of penicillin and streptomycin, or sulfaquinoxaline can be used for initial treatment, but an antibiotic sensitivity test should be performed, because multiresistant strains may develop. Enrofloxacin has also proved highly effective in preventing mortality in ducklings when administered in the drinking water. However, current legislation in many countries does not allow the use of quinolones in production animals.

SALMONELLOSES

Salmonella infections are classified as nonmotile serotypes (*S* Pullorum, *S* Gallinarum) and the many motile paratyphoid *Salmonella*. These *Salmonella* infections have a worldwide distribution. As a result of the institution of a testing and control program in the USA through the USDA-administered National Poultry Improvement Plan, the incidence of *S* Pullorum or *S* Gallinarum has decreased dramatically. Historically, *S* Arizonae was placed in its own category, but it is now included with the paratyphoid *Salmonella*. *S* Arizonae is an egg-transmiited disease primarily of young turkeys. In addition to the above nonmotile salmonellae, *Salmonella* paratyphoid infections in poultry are relatively common and have public health significance because of contaminated poultry product consumption.

S Pullorum and *S* Gallinarum are highly host-adapted to chickens and turkeys. There are >2,500 nonhost-adapted species (paratyphoid) that may be transmitted to almost all animals.

PULLORUM DISEASE

Etiology and Transmission: Infections with *Salmonella* Pullorum usually cause very high mortality (potentially approaching 100%) in young chickens and turkeys within the first 2–3 wk of age. In adult chickens, mortality may be high but frequently there are no clinical signs. Pullorum disease was once common but has been eradicated from most commercial chicken stock in the USA, although it may be seen in other avian species (eg, guinea fowl, quail, pheasants, sparrows, parrots, canaries, and bullfinches) and in small backyard or hobby flocks. Infection in mammals is rare, although experimental or natural infections have been reported (chimpanzees, rabbits, guinea pigs, chinchillas, pigs, kittens, foxes, dogs, swine, mink, cows, and wild rats).

Transmission can be vertical (transovarian) but also occurs via direct or indirect contact with infected birds (respiratory or fecal) or contaminated feed, water, or litter. Infection transmitted via egg or hatchery contamination usually results in death during the first few days of life up to 2–3 wk of age. Transmission between farms is due to poor biosecurity.

Clinical Findings and Lesions: The disease may be seen in all age groups, but birds <4 wk old are most commonly affected. Birds may die in the hatchery shortly after hatching. Affected birds huddle near a heat source, are anorectic, appear weak, and have whitish fecal pasting around the vent (diarrhea). Survivors are small in size and frequently become asymptomatic carriers with localized infection of the ovary. Some of the eggs laid by such hens hatch and produce infected progeny.

There may be no lesions due to an acute septicemia and death. Lesions in young birds usually include unabsorbed yolk sacs and classic gray nodules in the liver, spleen, lungs, heart, gizzard, and intestine. Firm, cheesy material in the ceca (cecal cores) and raised plaques in the mucosa of the lower intestine are sometimes seen. Occasionally, synovitis is prominent. Adult carriers usually have no gross lesions but may have nodular pericarditis; fibrinous peritonitis; or hemorrhagic, atrophic, regressing ovarian follicles with caseous contents. In mature chickens, chronic infections produce lesions indistinguishable from those of fowl typhoid (*see* below).

Diagnosis: Lesions may be highly suggestive, but diagnosis should be confirmed by isolation, identification, and serotyping of *S* Pullorum. Infections in mature birds can be identified by serologic tests, followed by necropsy evaluation complemented by microbiologic culture and typing for confirmation. Official testing recommendations for flocks in the USA are outlined in the National Poultry Improvement Plan.

Treatment and Control: Treatment of infected flocks to alleviate the perpetuation of the carrier state is not recommended. Control is based on routine serologic testing of breeding stock to assure freedom from infection. In addition, management and biosecurity measures should be taken to reduce the introduction of *S* Pullorum from feed, water, wild birds, rodents, insects, or people. Birds should be purchased from sources free of *S* Pullorum.

FOWL TYPHOID

Etiology and Epidemiology: The causal agent is *Salmonella* Gallinarum. The incidence of fowl typhoid is low in the USA, Canada, and some European countries but is much higher in other countries. Although *S* Gallinarum is egg-transmitted and produces lesions in chicks and poults similar to those produced by *S* Pullorum, there is a much greater tendency to spread among growing or mature flocks. Mortality in young birds is similar to that seen in *S* Pullorum infection but may be higher in older birds.

Clinical Findings and Lesions: The disease may be acute or chronic. Clinical signs and lesions in young birds are similar to those seen with *S* Pullorum infection. Older birds may be pale, dehydrated, and have diarrhea. Lesions in older birds may include a swollen, friable and often bile-stained liver, with or without necrotic foci; enlarged spleen and kidneys; anemia; and enteritis.

Diagnosis: Diagnosis should be confirmed by isolation, identification, and serotyping of *S* Gallinarum (National Poultry Improvement Plan testing procedure).

Treatment and Control: Treatment and control are as for pullorum disease (*see* above). There are no federally licensed vaccines in the USA. In other countries, vaccines (killed or modified live) made from a rough strain of *S* Gallinarum (9R) had variable results in controlling mortality. More recently, vaccines derived from outer membrane proteins, mutant strains, and a virulence-plasmid-cured derivative of *S* Gallinarum have shown promise in protecting birds against challenge. The standard serologic tests for pullorum disease are equally effective in detecting fowl typhoid.

PARATYPHOID INFECTIONS

Etiology: Paratyphoid infections can be caused by any one of the many non-host-adapted salmonellae. These *Salmonella* infect many types of birds, mammals, reptiles, and insects. Paratyphoid infections are of public health significance via contamination and mishandling of poultry products. *S* Typhimurium, *S* Enteritidis, *S* Kentucky, *S* Heidelberg, *S* Hadar, and *S* Saintpaul are among the most common *Salmonella* infections in poultry. Some serotypes are more pathogenic than others. The prevalence of other species varies widely by geographic location.

Transmission usually occurs horizontally from infected birds, contaminated environments, or infected rodents. Except for *S* Enteritidis and *S* Arizonae, transmission of most serotypes to progeny from infected breeders is mainly through fecal contamination of the eggshell. *S* Enteritidis and *S* Arizonae can infect the interior of the egg through transovarial transmission. Infected birds remain carriers.

Clinical Findings and Lesions: Although not common, clinical signs are sometimes seen in young birds. Mortality is most often limited to the first few weeks of age. Depression, poor growth, weakness, diarrhea, and dehydration are hallmarks of the disease, although these clinical signs are not distinctive.

Lesions may include an enlarged liver with focal necrosis, unabsorbed yolk sac, enteritis with necrotic lesions in the mucosa, and cecal cores. Infections occasionally localize in the eye or synovial tissues. Conversely, there may be no lesions due to acute death caused by septicemia. Isolation, identification, and serotyping of the causal agent are essential for diagnosis. Serology is not highly reliable.

Treatment and Control: General control measures for the paratyphoid *Salmonella* include strict sanitation in the hatchery, fumigation of hatching eggs, pelleting of feed, cleaning and disinfection of poultry houses, rodent control, and use of competitive exclusion products. Maintenance of poultry in confinement and exclusion of all pets, wild birds, and rodents help prevent introduction of infection. The use of antibiotics is highly debated. Several antibacterial agents help prevent mortality but cannot eliminate flock infection and may lead to drug resistance. Vaccination with live or killed products has been used. Complete protection is not afforded by vaccination, and it should be used in combination with other control measures to reduce the incidence of *Salmonella* infection.

S Enteritidis (a paratyphoid *Salmonella* serotype) is a major food safety concern primarily for the egg-laying industry. Possible sources in commercial layers include transmission from breeders, contaminated environments, infected rodents, and contaminated feed. Transmission to progeny from breeders is mainly through eggshell contamination, although, unlike other paratyphoid *Salmonella*, transovarial transmission may also occur. The National Poultry Improvement Plan includes *S* Enteritidis control measures in breeders, including depopulation of infected breeder flocks, cleaning and disinfection of pullet and layer houses, rodent control programs, pest management, feed management, use of competitive exclusion products, vaccination, biosecurity, and proper handling and refrigeration of eggs.

STAPHYLOCOCCOSIS

Staphylococcosis is a bacterial disease that can affect a wide range of avian species, including poultry, and is seen worldwide. *Staphylococcus aureus* is most commonly isolated from staphylococcosis cases, but species such as *S hyicus* have also been reported as the causative agent of osteomyelitis in turkey poults. The disease conditions associated with staphylococcosis vary with the site and route of inoculation and can involve the bones, joints, tendon sheaths, skin, sternal bursa, navel, and yolk sac. Economic losses may result from decreased weight gain, decreased egg production, lameness, mortality, and condemnation at slaughter.

Etiology: *S aureus* is a gram-positive, catalase-positive, coccoid bacteria that appears in grape-like clusters on stained smears. *S aureus* is the most common isolate recovered from clinical cases. Most pathogenic strains have been coagulase-positive; however, coagulase-negative *Staphylococcus*, including *S hyicus*, *S epidermidis*, and *S gallinarum* have been reported from clinical cases. Phage typing has been used to distinguish among the different strains. *Staphylococcus* toxins can enhance the pathogenicity of a strain.

Transmission, Epidemiology, and Pathogenesis: Because *Staphylococcus* is part of the normal skin and mucosal flora, many infections are the result of a wound, mucosal damage, or both. Infection can also occur in the hatchery as a result of contamination of an open navel. Birds that are immunocompromised are also more prone to staphylococcal infections. Once in the host, *S aureus* invades the metaphyseal area of the nearest joint, which leads to osteomyelitis and localization within that joint. Alternatively, the bacteria can invade the bloodstream and lead to a systemic infection in multiple organs.

Clinical Findings: Omphalitis, or infection of the yolk sac, caused by *S aureus* has been reported in young chicks and poults (*see* p 2859). Its prevalence depends on its presence in the breeder flock and the hatchery environment. Navel infections can occur in young hatchlings if the navel becomes infected with *Staphylococcus*. Gangrenous dermatitis can occur after skin trauma and subsequent contamination with *Staphylococcus*. Immunocompromised birds have a higher prevalence of gangrenous dermatitis. Because *Staphylococcus* is found on the skin, skin injuries can also lead to localized abscesses, such as on the foot (bumblefoot). Finally, *Staphylococcus* can be dispersed systemically and can cause arthritis, synovitis, osteomyelitis, and endocarditis. Most *Staphylococcus* infections in poultry cause synovitis, with lameness being the most common clinical presentation. The bones and associated joints most frequently affected are those of the leg, especially the stifle and tibiotarsus. In addition, septicemia can result in green livers or livers with multifocal necrosis and/or granulomas. In acute infections, a sudden increase in mortality may be noted.

Lesions: Chicks with omphalitis have navels that are moist and dark, and affected birds are often lethargic. Infected yolk sacs are retained longer than uninfected yolk sacs, which are normally resorbed by the developing chick within the first week of life. Infected yolks are abnormal in color (dark green to brown), have a doughy consistency, and are odorous. Gangrenous dermatitis is often reported in immunocompromised chickens and is often due to a combination of *S aureus* and *Clostridium septicum* and/or *Escherichia coli*. Affected areas are usually hemorrhagic and crepitant. Lesions associated with septicemia are most common. Within the musculoskeletal system, affected bones often have focal yellowish areas of necrosis, while lesions in the joints contain purulent exudate. At the processing plant, green liver has been reported in turkeys that have had osteomyelitis and synovitis. Liver spots and granulomas resulting from septicemia have been a cause of liver condemnation. In acute infections, necrosis and vascular congestion are seen in the liver, spleen, kidneys, and other internal organs. Vegetations on the heart valves have been reported.

Diagnosis: Although some lesions may be suggestive of a *Staphylococcus* infection, diagnosis is confirmed by identifying the organisms from stained smears of the lesion and by culture on blood agar plates. Phenotyping and genetic techniques have been used to classify strains of poultry *S aureus*. Differential diagnoses include *E coli* and *Pasteurella multocida* as well as other septicemic diseases of poultry.

Treatment and Prevention: Staphylococcosis can be successfully treated with antibiotics, but an antimicrobial susceptibility test should be performed because antibiotic resistance is common. Antibiotics used to treat *Staphylococcus* infections include penicillin, erythromycin, lincomycin, and spectinomycin. Proper management to prevent injury and immunocompromised poultry helps prevent staphylococcosis. Because wounds are the primary route by which *Staphylococcus* can enter the body, it is important to reduce all potential sources of injury to the bird. Wood splinters in litter, protruding wires from cages, and fighting/cannibalism have been associated with skin wounds and staphylococcosis. Because beak and toe trimming procedures in young chickens and turkeys could result in a staphylococcal septicemia, ensuring that equipment is sanitary will help to prevent outbreaks. Good litter management is important in controlling foot-pad injuries to prevent bumblefoot. Hatchery sanitation and good egg management practices are also important to reduce navel infections and omphalitis.

Zoonotic Risk: *S aureus* can cause food poisoning in people. Enterotoxin-producing strains are found on clinically healthy poultry, and proper precautions should be taken during the handling and cooking of poultry products. Methicillin-resistant *S aureus* (MRSA) has been isolated from poultry meat in a number of countries, but the prevalence and significance for human health are incompletely understood.

STREPTOCOCCOSIS

Streptococcosis has been reported in numerous bird species throughout the world. There are two forms of the disease, an acute septicemic form and a chronic form. Flock mortality can be as high as 50%. Because streptococci are part of the normal flora of the intestinal mucosa of most avian species, infections are often thought to occur secondarily to other diseases.

Etiology and Epidemiology: Streptococci are nonmotile, gram-positive, catalase-negative coccoid bacteria that occur singly, in pairs, or in short chains when observed on stained smears. *Streptococcus* spp commonly associated with disease in avian species include *S zooepidemicus* (*S gallinarum*), *S bovis*, *S dysgalactiae*, *S gallinaceus*, and *S mutans*. Streptococci have been associated with acute septicemia, joint infections, cellulitis, osteomyelitis, and endocarditis. Transmission is via oral or aerosol routes as well as through skin injuries.

Clinical Findings: Streptococcal infections can be localized or septicemic. Endocarditis and lameness occur during the subacute or chronic stage of the infection. In *S zooepidemicus* infections, clinical signs are typical of an acute septicemic infection, and lethargic birds are often prostrate. In affected layers, egg production may drop by 15%. In pigeons, *S bovis* infection produces acute mortality with lameness, inappetence, diarrhea, and the inability to fly. Acute fibrinopurulent conjunctivitis has been noted in infections caused by other *Streptococcus* spp.

Lesions: Lesions in the acute septicemic form include splenomegaly, hepatomegaly (with or without reddish tan to white multifocal necrotic foci), and enlarged kidneys. There may also be serosanguineous fluid in the subcutaneous space and in the pericardium. Bloodstained feathers around the mouth and head due to blood from the oral cavity have been reported occasionally. Cellulitis involving the skin and subcutaneous tissues has been associated with both *Escherichia coli* and *S dysgalactiae*.

Chronic streptococcal infections result in arthritis and/or tenosynovitis, osteomyelitis, salpingitis, pericarditis, myocarditis, and valvular endocarditis. Lesions on the heart valves appear as small yellowish white or tan raised areas on the valvular surface. Focal granulomas, as a result of septic emboli, can be found in many tissues. Gram-positive bacterial colonies are readily observed in thrombosed vessels and within necrotic foci microscopically.

Diagnosis: History, clinical signs, and lesions, along with demonstration of *Streptococcus*-like bacteria in blood films or impression smears of affected tissues, allows for a presumptive diagnosis of streptococcosis. Isolation of *Streptococcus* spp from lesions confirms the diagnosis. Streptococci can be cultured easily on blood agar.

Differential diagnoses include other bacterial septicemic diseases, including staphylococcosis, enterococcosis, colibacillosis, pasteurellosis, and erysipelas. Infectious laryngotracheitis, pasteurellosis, avian influenza, and exotic Newcastle disease should be considered as differential diagnoses when blood is noted coming from the mouth.

Treatment and Control: Antibiotics, including penicillin, erythromycin, novobiocin, oxytetracycline, chlortetracycline, and tetracycline, have been used to treat acute and subacute infections. Clinically affected birds respond well early in the course of the infection, but this response decreases as the disease progresses within a flock. Antimicrobial susceptibility testing should be performed to select a suitable antibiotic.

Because streptococcosis often occurs secondary to other diseases, it is important to prevent immunosuppressive diseases and conditions. In addition, because skin wounds can provide an entry for *Streptococcus*, it is important to reduce this risk factor. Proper cleaning and disinfection can reduce environmental sources of infection.

TUBERCULOSIS

Tuberculosis is a slowly spreading, chronic, granulomatous bacterial infection characterized by gradual weight loss. All birds appear to be susceptible, although to variable degrees; pheasants seem to be highly susceptible, whereas the disease is uncommon in turkeys. Tuberculosis is more prevalent in captive than in free-living wild birds. It is unlikely to be seen in commercial poultry because of the short life span and husbandry practices used. (*See also* TUBERCULOSIS AND OTHER MYCOBACTERIAL INFECTIONS, p 687.)

Etiology and Epidemiology: *Mycobacterium avium ss* is the most common cause, although *M genavense* has been isolated from some psittacine birds. Seroagglutination tests of isolates are recommended to differentiate strains of *M avium* that cause disease in chickens and birds from those that fail to produce disease in these species. *M tuberculosis*, the cause of tuberculosis in people, has infrequently been isolated from parrots and canaries. *M avium* is very resistant; it can survive in soil for ≥4 yr, in 3% hydrochloric acid for ≥2 hr, and in 2% sodium hydroxide for ≥30 min.

Tuberculosis is found worldwide, most commonly in small, barnyard flocks and in zoo aviaries; it is rarely found in young flocks. Wild birds, such as cranes, sparrows, starlings, and raptors, have been found to be infected. Tuberculosis has been found in emus and other ratites. The movement of ratites through sales and the long life of these animals have made tuberculosis a major concern for ratite producers. Isolation of ratites purchased at sales is essential to prevent the introduction of tuberculosis into established flocks.

Infected birds with advanced lesions often excrete the organism in their feces; therefore, ingestion of contaminated feces is the most common route of transmission. Carcasses and offal may infect predators and cannibalistic flock mates. Rabbits, pigs, nonhuman primates, and mink are readily infected. Cattle exposed to contaminated feces may develop granulomatous lesions in lymph nodes associated with the GI tract and respond to *M bovis* purified protein derivative (PPD) tuberculin and to PPD of *M avium*. *M avium* serovar 1 is often isolated from tuberculous free-living wild birds and birds in captivity. *M avium ss* and *M genavense* have been isolated from immunocompromised people; however, these organisms only rarely cause disease in nonimmunocompromised individuals.

Clinical Findings and Diagnosis: Signs usually do not develop until late in the infection, when birds become emaciated and sluggish and lameness may be seen. In chickens, granulomatous nodules of varying size are often found in the liver, spleen, bone marrow, and intestine. Some exotic species may have lesions in the liver and spleen without intestinal or bone marrow involvement. Small mesenteric nodules may be found. Lesions are not mineralized.

Live birds may be tested with *M avium* PPD tuberculin, although these tests are of limited value in birds that do not have wattles (it is often difficult to inject tuberculin intradermally because of skin thickness at other sites). A test conducted in skin on the underside of the wing has been used in Japanese quail exposed to *M avium*. The injection site is observed at 24 and 48 hr for induration and swelling. A positive test indicates exposure to *M avium*; however, a negative test is of little or no significance. Large numbers of acid-fast bacteria in smears from lesions provide a tentative diagnosis. Mycobacteriologic examination is required to confirm a diagnosis. Isolates can be identified based on biochemical, drug susceptibility, and seroagglutination tests and by restriction length polymorphism analyses.

Prevention and Control: Addition of exotic birds to an exhibit should originate from a closed collection with no history of tuberculosis, ie, tuberculosis has not been reported previously or diagnosed on necropsy during the past 5 yr. If no history is available, the birds should be quarantined or maintained in a separate exhibit away from the bird aviary. Transmission is by ingestion of food or water contaminated with *M avium ss*, ie, feces from contagious birds. Therefore, it is recommended that endangered and valuable species be housed in individual exhibits.

Chemotherapy is ineffective, because most *M avium* complex organisms are resistant to antituberculosis drugs. In commercial poultry flocks, relatively rapid turnover of populations, together with improved general sanitation, has largely eliminated this once common infection. Infected poultry should be destroyed, and housing facilities thoroughly cleaned and disinfected using cresylic compounds. Quaternary ammonium compounds and halogens (eg, chlorine) do not effectively kill mycobacteria. In exhibits with dirt floors, several inches of the floor should be removed and replaced with dirt from a place where poultry have not been maintained. All openings should be screened against wild birds.

Avian tuberculosis in zoos is difficult to eradicate. New additions to the aviary should be quarantined for ≥6 mo. Isolation and quarantine of birds of unknown status purchased at sales is essential to prevent introduction of tuberculosis into established flocks.

TURKEY VIRAL HEPATITIS

Turkey viral hepatitis is an acute, highly contagious, frequently subclinical disease of turkey poults 5 wk of age. The disease is widespread and common in some areas, with morbidity rates of as much as 100%. Mortality has been reported only in poults, is confined to a 4- to 8-day period, and may reach 25%.

Etiology: A picorna-like virus from poults with typical lesions has been reported, but its etiologic role has not been conclusively established. The causal virus has not been fully classified, but a picornavirus from turkeys with typical lesions of turkey viral hepatitis has been molecularly characterized and proposed as a new species in the order Picornavirales. It is isolated without difficulty from the liver and a variety of other tissues, including the pancreas, spleen, and kidney, as well as feces. The virus is isolated less consistently from older birds. It grows readily in the yolk sac of 5- to 7-day-old chicken or turkey embryos. It is thermostabile; resistant to ether, phenol, and creolin but not formalin; and susceptible to high, but not low, pH.

Clinical Findings: Disease is usually subclinical and becomes apparent only when the birds are stressed. Affected birds are stunted and unthrifty. Morbidity and mortality vary according to the severity of stress. In poults <5 wk old, morbidity may reach 100% and mortality 10%–25%. Breeder flocks may exhibit decreased production, fertility, and hatchability.

Lesions: Gross lesions are confined to the liver and pancreas. In the liver, foci of necrosis are 1–3 mm in diameter and may be confluent. Areas of hemorrhage or congestion are also present and frequently obscure the degenerative changes. Occasionally, the liver is diffusely bile-stained. Liver lesions may resemble those of bacterial infections, particularly from *Salmonella* spp, *Pasteurella multocida*, or *Escherichia coli*, and infections caused by Group 1 and Group 2 avian adenovirus and reovirus. The pancreas frequently exhibits relatively large, circular, gray areas of degeneration. In the subclinical form, lesions are less extensive, and hepatic hemorrhage or congestion is seldom prominent. Affected tissues return to normal in 3–4 wk.

Diagnosis: *Salmonella* spp and other bacterial infections produce necrotic areas in the liver that can be confused with those of viral hepatitis. Bacterial infections must be differentiated by appropriate culturing techniques. Liver lesions may resemble those of histomoniasis, but the absence of cecal lesions in turkey viral hepatitis helps to differentiate the two diseases. With histomoniasis, histologic examination or demonstration of the respective etiologic agents is necessary. Diagnosis is aided by demonstration of picornavirus by immunohistochemical or molecular techniques from poults with typical lesions.

Control: There is no known treatment. Secondary bacterial invasion does not appear to be important, but if it occurs, it should be treated on the basis of specific etiology. Although recovered birds demonstrate resistance to infection, neutralizing antibodies have not been detected. Improved sanitation may be of value in preventing dissemination of the agent.

MISCELLANEOUS CONDITIONS OF POULTRY

ASCITES SYNDROME

(Pulmonary hypertension syndrome, Waterbelly)

Ascites is an accumulation of noninflammatory transudate in one or more of the peritoneal cavities or potential spaces. The fluid, which accumulates most frequently in the two ventral hepatic, peritoneal, or pericardial spaces, may contain yellow protein clots. Ascites may result from increased vascular hydraulic pressure, vascular damage, increased tissue oncotic pressure, or decreased vascular oncotic (usually colloidal) pressure, but is most commonly associated with venous hypertension resulting from right heart failure in response to increased pulmonary resistance.

The most common cause of ascites is increased vascular hydraulic pressure in the venous system, which is most commonly caused by right ventricular failure (RVF), also associated with hepatic fibrosis. It is well documented that most cases are caused by a genetic predisposition to pulmonary hypertension, which progresses to congestive heart failure and terminal ascites in many cases.

Pulmonary hypertension occurs frequently in chickens secondary to high altitude-associated hypoxia with resultant polycythemia and increased blood viscosity. It also occurs frequently secondary to the RBC rigidity of sodium toxicity and less frequently from lung pathology. When ascites occurs at low altitudes in meat-type chickens, which have a high metabolic oxygen requirement, it is usually caused by primary or spontaneous pulmonary hypertension because of insufficient capacity of the pulmonary capillaries. Cold stress, even briefly, during the first 3 wk of life is known to markedly increase predisposition to ascites syndrome.

In poultry, liver damage may be caused by aflatoxin or by toxins from plants such as *Crotalaria*. In broiler chickens, obstructive cholangiohepatitis (caused by *Clostridium perfringens* infection) is the most common cause of the liver damage, which results in ascites. In both meat-type ducks and breeders, amyloidosis of the liver may also cause ascites.

Pathogenesis and Epidemiology: Pulmonary hypertension syndrome is caused by increased pressure in the pulmonary arteries when the heart tries to pump more blood through the lungs to meet the body's oxygen requirement. The resultant volume and pressure overload on the right ventricle cause dilatation and hypertrophy of the right ventricular wall, valvular insufficiency, RVF, and ascites.

Bird lungs are rigid and fixed in the thoracic cavity. The capillaries can expand very little to accommodate increased blood flow. Lung size in proportion to body weight, and particularly to muscle mass, decreases as meat-type chickens grow. Increased blood flow results in primary pulmonary *hypertension and cor pulmonale* with sporadic cases of RVF and ascites in fast-growing broilers. Predisposing factors that increase oxygen demand (eg, cold), reduce oxygen-carrying capacity of the blood (eg, acidosis, carbon monoxide), increase blood volume (eg, sodium), or interfere with blood flow through the lung (eg, lung pathology that narrows or occludes capillaries, increased RBC rigidity, or polycythemia with increased blood viscosity) may result in flock outbreaks of pulmonary hypertension syndrome with or without ascites.

The incidence of pulmonary hypertension syndrome is >2% in some broiler and many roaster flocks and is occasionally 15%–20% in other roaster flocks. Right ventricular hypertrophy is the response to an increased workload and eventually leads to RVF if the volume or pressure load persists. Hypertrophy and dilatation of the right ventricular wall is directly related to pulmonary hypertension, and the ratio of the right ventricle to the total ventricular mass can be used as a measure of the increased pressure load on the right ventricle.

Clinical Findings: Occasionally, young broilers develop pulmonary hypertension syndrome, particularly if increased sodium or lung pathology (eg, aspergillosis) is involved, but mortality is greatest after 5 wk of age. There are no signs until RVF occurs and ascites develops. Clinically affected broilers are cyanotic, the abdominal skin may be red, and peripheral vessels congested. Because growth stops as RVF develops, affected broilers may be smaller than their pen mates. However, rapid growth rate is a known predisposing factor, and sometimes the largest broilers are affected, with occurrence in males more frequent than in females. The ascites increases the respiratory rate and reduces exercise tolerance. Affected broilers frequently die on their backs. Not all broilers that die from pulmonary hypertension syndrome have ascites. Death may occur suddenly before signs are seen.

Lesions: Most lesions are the result of increased venous hydraulic pressure secondary to RVF. There is a variable amount of clear yellow fluid and clots of fibrin in the hepatoperitoneal spaces. The liver may be swollen and congested, or firm and irregular with edema, and have clotted protein adherent to the surface. It may be nodular or shrunken; it may be white with subcapsular edema and a thickened capsule or have large or small blebs of fluid between the capsule and the visceral peritoneum. Hydropericardium is mild to marked, and occasionally there is pericarditis with adhesions, usually from secondary infections. Right ventricular dilatation and mild to marked hypertrophy of the right ventricular wall may be noted. The right atrium and vena cava are markedly dilated in most cases. Occasionally, there is thinning of the left ventricle. The lungs are extremely congested and edematous. The intestine may or may not be empty.

Diagnosis: Broilers that die from ascites or suddenly as the result of RVF or pulmonary hypertension can be identified by the enlarged heart; enlarged, thickened right ventricle; or fluid in the body cavities and heart sac. If the wall of the right ventricle is enlarged or thickened, the broiler has probably died from pulmonary hypertension syndrome, even if there is no fluid in the body or heart sac.

Control: Reducing the birds' metabolic oxygen requirement by slowing growth or reducing feed density or availability can prevent ascites caused by pulmonary hypertension syndrome. Environmental temperature, humidity, and air movement should be controlled to prevent excessive loss of body heat, particularly in the early neonatal period. Even brief exposure to cold stress during the first weeks of life is known to predispose flocks to this condition. Ascites caused by other factors (eg, sodium, lung damage, liver damage, etc) can be prevented by avoiding the etiologic agents involved. Altitudes >3,000 ft (900 m) are unsatisfactory for meat-type chickens, and growth must be slowed to prevent mortality. More care to prevent chilling is also necessary at higher altitudes. Research has demonstrated that broilers can be genetically selected for both resistance and susceptibility to pulmonary hypertension syndrome and associated ascites.

BREAST BLISTERS

In chickens and turkeys, a bursa lined with synovial membrane is normally present over the anterior projection of the keel bone. When this bursa becomes inflamed by trauma or infection, fluid accumulates and appears as a fluid-filled blister 1–3 cm in diameter. Factors in trauma to the bursa include poor feathering, hard flooring, and leg weakness, which is associated with increased time of sitting on the keel (sternum). Coarse bedding materials or wet litter conditions are predisposing factors and should be corrected when identified. Infectious causes of sternal bursitis include *Mycoplasma synoviae*, *Staphylococcus*, and *Pasteurella* spp, either from local trauma (*Staphylococcus*) or as an extension of a systemic infection.

BREAST BUTTONS

Breast buttons develop in a location similar to that of breast blisters (*see* above). They have a localized, hard crust on the surface and a core of dead skin and chronic inflammation extending into the subcutis. The cause is not well defined, but a breast button may start as a chemical burn due to prolonged contact of poorly feathered skin with wet litter containing ammonia or toxins. The presence of good quality, dry litter is associated with a reduced number of affected turkeys.

CANNIBALISM

Cannibalism stems from aggressive behavior of chickens and turkeys that may begin by feather pecking by socially dominant birds. It may also involve vent pecking immediately after oviposition, or picking at skin on the head, comb, wattles, or toes. No single cause has been identified, but crowding, excessive light intensity, and nutritional imbalances are correlated with its occurrence. Additionally, in overweight pullets entering egg production or hens in production, mucosa will protrude from the vent during and after egg laying, and this red tissue attracts pecking. Other factors are insufficient feeder space, mineral and vitamin deficiencies, skin injuries, and failure to remove any dead birds daily. In addition to the loss of birds due to pecking trauma, cannibalism often leads to transmission of infectious diseases (eg, erysipelas) and botulism.

Control depends on correcting or reducing the above risk factors. Interventions include correcting an inadequate diet, replacing mash feed with pelleted feed, rearing birds on floor litter rather than slats, reducing light intensity, and providing perches as a refuge for targeted birds. Environmental enrichment such as hanging white or yellow strings may be beneficial. Trimming the sharp distal end (tip) of the upper beak will decrease skin trauma from pecking; this may be done at 1 day of age and repeated between 6 and 12 wk of age in maturing pullets or turkeys. The tip of the beak can also be treated by infrared heat on the day of hatching, which results in a shortened beak with minimal stress. Cauterization is required to provide hemostasis during beak trimming in older poultry.

FLUKE INFECTIONS

Modern poultry housed indoors are essentially free of flukes, because all flukes require a snail as an intermediate host and often require a third invertebrate host. However, these parasites persist in backyard poultry (*see* p 1815), which may have contact with snails or other hosts and wild birds. The trend toward free-range rearing of poultry may increase the exposure of poultry to this type of parasite, but flukes are mainly reported in wild birds with low prevalence.

Prosthogonimus macrorchis, the oviduct fluke of poultry, infects birds after they consume infective metacercariae in larval or mature dragonflies, the secondary host. The fluke matures in ~2 wk in the bursa of Fabricius or, in gallinaceous birds without a functional bursa (eg, chickens, turkeys, pheasants), in the oviduct.

Light infections without signs appear in ducks and other birds with a functional bursa. In gallinaceous birds, heavy infections in the oviduct cause inappetence, droopiness, weight loss, calcareous cloacal discharge, depressed egg production, and an increase in soft-shelled eggs. Lesions range from mild inflammation to distention or rupture of the oviduct; death may result. Diagnosis by fecal examination is unreliable, because fluke eggs are not consistently present. Adult flukes may appear in the bird's eggs or be found in the oviduct on necropsy.

To prevent fluke transmission, birds must be kept from feeding on dragonflies. There is no effective treatment approved for use in poultry. Carbon tetrachloride, a common remedy, is highly toxic to chickens and other birds.

Collyriclum faba, another common fluke in birds, appear as subcutaneous cysts 4–6 mm in diameter (usually containing two adults) anywhere on the body but more frequently near the vent in turkeys, chickens, and other birds. The cysts ooze an exudate, which attracts flies and predisposes to bacterial infection. Signs in young birds include locomotor difficulty and inappetence; heavy infections may cause death. The parasites can be removed surgically. The life cycle is unknown but probably involves snails and insects such as dragonflies or mayflies. Prevention of infection requires restricting birds from bodies of water and areas frequented by aquatic insects.

PENDULOUS CROP

Incidence of pendulous crop is low in flocks of chickens but appears to be increasing in turkeys. The crop is grossly distended and contains foul-smelling fluid, feed, and litter. Feed utilization is impaired, and severely affected birds become thin or emaciated. Survivors often are condemned or trimmed at processing to reduce contamination by crop contents.

The cause is not known, but a hereditary predisposition, potentially associated with hyperphagia, has been suggested in turkeys. Incidence may increase with erratic or excessive feed or water consumption. Vagus nerve damage has also been postulated as a cause in rare cases. There is no known efficacious treatment.

URATE DEPOSITION (GOUT)

Avian species excrete nitrogenous wastes as urates bound in colloidal form with mucus in their urine. Renal dysfunction decreases the clearance of uric acid from the blood, which results in hyperuricemia with precipitation of insoluble products within the kidney itself or other organs, leading to urate deposition or urolithiasis (gout). Urate deposits are white and semisolid and must be differentiated from yellow fibrinous or purulent inflammatory exudates that are secondary to infectious causes, such as synovitis, peritonitis, perihepatitis, and pericarditis.

Visceral urate deposition occurs after rapidly progressing renal failure, or as a terminal event with acute decompensation of chronic renal disease. Deposits develop most commonly on the pericardium, peritoneum, and liver capsule, and rarely on synovial surfaces of joints and tendons. Microscopically, urate deposits are often seen as feathery crystals or basophilic spherical masses, usually with little inflammation due to the rapid course. Visceral urate deposition may be secondary to **urolithiasis**, which is common in older laying chickens. Progressive obstruction of the ureters by uroliths causes kidney atrophy "upstream" of the site of ureteral obstruction and compensatory hypertrophy by the undamaged portions of the kidney. Distended ureters often contain brittle, white, staghorn calcium urate calculi or uroliths.

Predisposing factors for visceral urate deposition and urolithiasis in poultry include infectious bronchitis virus, avian nephritis virus, and cryptosporidiosis. Noninfectious causes include dehydration, ingestion of feed containing >3% calcium by nonlaying chickens, vitamin A deficiency, and exposure to myotoxins (eg, oosporein). Other avian species commonly develop visceral deposits secondary to nephrotoxin exposure, most commonly aminoglycoside antibiotics or heavy metals.

Articular urate deposition is less common and occurs after longterm increases in serum levels of uric acid. Deposits develop on synovial membranes in the toes and wing joints and incite a chronic granulomatous reaction to urate crystals (tophi). Articular urate deposition may be seen in birds that have hereditary defects in uric acid metabolism or that are fed excessive protein.

ECTOPARASITES

BEDBUGS

Cimex lectularius is a common bloodsucking parasite in temperate and subtropical climates that attacks poultry, people, and most other mammals. It is rare in modern laying operations, but breeding houses and pigeon lofts may become heavily infested. The life cycle may be completed in 2–6 wk or extend much longer, because nymphs can withstand fasting for ~70 days, and adults for as long as 12 mo. Feeding usually occurs at night. Bedbugs become engorged within 10 min, then hide in cracks and crevices. If attacked by large numbers of bedbugs, birds may become irritable and anemic. Bites are usually followed by swelling and itching due to injection of saliva into the wound. Signs of infestation include bug fecal droppings on eggs and nest boxes, breast and leg skin lesions, reduced egg production, and increased feed consumption.

Control is best accomplished by thoroughly cleaning the houses, reducing hiding places for the bedbugs, and fumigating the houses with organophosphates or pyrethroids that remain on surfaces providing access to hosts.

FLEAS

The **sticktight flea**, *Echidnophaga gallinacea*, is a major poultry pest in the subtropical and tropical New World. It is unique among poultry fleas in that the adults become sessile parasites and usually remain attached to the skin of the head or anus for days or weeks. The adult females forcibly eject their eggs so that they reach surrounding litter. The larvae develop best in sandy, well-drained litter. Hosts of the adult flea include chickens, turkeys, pigeons, pheasants, quail, people, and many other mammals. Fleas cause irritation, restlessness, and blood loss that results in anemia and death, particularly in young birds. Bites around the eyes can cause ulcerations, resulting in blindness.

The **Western chicken flea**, or **black hen flea**, *Ceratophyllus niger*, seems to be confined to the Pacific coast area of the USA and Canada. This flea breeds in droppings and feeds on birds only occasionally. The **European chicken flea**, *C gallinae*, is found worldwide. It breeds in nests and litter and is on the birds only to feed. In addition to chickens, it attacks many other birds as well as people and domestic pets. Heavy flea infestations cause host emaciation and reduced egg production.

The most important flea control measures are removing infested litter and dusting the litter surface with carbaryl, coumaphos, malathion, or pyrethroids to kill immature fleas. Insect growth regulators such as methoprene are also effective. Sticktight fleas can be controlled by topical application of pyrethrin.

FLIES AND GNATS

Biting Midge

Culicoides spp (Ceratopogonidae) feed on blood and transmit blood parasites to birds. They are vectors for transmission of *Haemoproteus* to ducks and geese in Canada and turkeys in North America, and of *Leucocytozoon* to chickens in Southeast Asia and Japan. They also transmit the skin mite *Myialges anchora* (Epidermoptidae). Bites are reddish and itch for as long as 3 days. Midges feed at twilight or night, and typical mesh screens do not keep them out. Pyrethroid insecticides can provide temporary control.

Black Fly

Simulium spp (Simuliidae), also known as buffalo gnats and turkey gnats, are bloodsuckers and transmit leucocytozoonosis (*see* p 2783) to ducks, turkeys, and other birds. They are most abundant in the north temperate and subarctic zones, but many species are found in tropical areas. They often attack in swarms and cause weight loss, reduced egg production, anemia, and death of birds either directly or through disease transmission. Control is extremely difficult because immature stages are restricted to running water, which is often some distance from the poultry farm. Larval control can be achieved with applications of *Bacillus thuringiensis israelensis* during early spring before adults emerge. Chemical larvicides such as temephos and methoxychlor can also be used. Screens of 24 mesh per in. (2.54 cm) or smaller are required for adult control. However, black flies rarely enter shelters.

Pigeon Fly

The pigeon fly, *Pseudolynchia canariensis* (Hippoboscidae), is an important bloodsucking parasite of pigeons in warm or tropical areas. It can transmit the blood parasites *Haemoproteus* and *Trypanosoma*, the skin mite *Myialges anchora* (Epidermoptidae), and pigeon lice (*Columbicola columbae*). It may also cause heavy losses in squabs. The pigeon loft should be cleaned every 20 days, and squabs can be dusted with permethrin or deltamethrin.

FOWL TICKS

The fowl tick, *Argas persicus*, is found worldwide in tropical and subtropical countries and is the vector of *Borrelia anserina* (avian spirochetosis, *see* p 2813) and the rickettsia *Aegyptianella pullorum*, which causes fowl disease (aegyptianellosis, *see* p 2780). In the USA, the *Argas persicus* complex has been divided to include *A miniatus*, *A sanchezi*, and *A radiatus* in addition to *A persicus*. These ticks are particularly active in poultry houses during warm, dry weather. All stages may be found hiding in cracks and crevices during the day. Larvae can be found on the birds, because they remain attached and feed for 2–7 days. Nymphs and adults feed at night for 15–30 min. Nymphs feed and molt several times before reaching the adult stage. Adults feed repeatedly, most commonly under the wings, and the females lay as many as 500 eggs after each feeding. Adult females may live >4 yr without a blood meal.

Fowl ticks produce anemia (most important), weight loss, depression, toxemia, and paralysis. Egg production decreases. Red spots can be seen on the skin where the ticks have fed. Because the ticks are nocturnal, the birds may show some uneasiness when roosting. Death is rare, but production may be severely depressed.

After houses are cleaned, walls, ceilings, cracks, and crevices should be treated thoroughly (using a high-pressure sprayer) with carbaryl, coumaphos, malathion, permethrin, stirofos, or a mixture of stirofos and dichlorvos. Cracks and crevices should be filled in.

LICE

Avian lice, which belong to the order Mallophaga, have a life cycle of ~3 wk and normally feed on bits of skin or feather products. Lice may live for several months on the host but only remain alive for ~1 wk off the host. People and other mammals may harbor avian lice, but only temporarily.

In intensive poultry systems, the most common and economically important louse to both chickens and turkeys is *Menacanthus stramineus*, the chicken body louse, which typically is found on the breast, vent, and thighs. It punctures soft quills near their base or gnaws the skin at the base of the feathers and feeds on the blood. Chickens are less commonly infested with *Menopon gallinae* (on feather shafts), *Lipeurus caponis* (mainly on the wing feathers), *Cuclotogaster heterographus* (mainly on the head and neck), *Goniocotes gallinae* (very small, in the fluff), *Goniodes gigas* (the large chicken louse), *Goniodes dissimilis* (the brown chicken louse), *Menacanthus cornutus* (the body louse), *Uchida pallidula* (the small body louse), or *Oxylipeurus dentatus*. Turkeys may also be infested with *Chelopistes meleagridis* (the large turkey louse), and *Oxylipeurus polytrapezius* (the slender turkey louse).

Because lice transfer from one bird species to another when the hosts are in close contact, other domestic and caged birds may be infested with species of Mallophaga that are usually host-specific. Lice also sometimes reach new bird hosts by using louse flies (Hippoboscidae) for transportation. Some lice of geese and swans are vectors of filarial nematodes.

Heavy populations of the chicken body louse decrease reproductive potential in males, egg production in females, and weight gain in growing chickens. The skin irritations are also sites for secondary bacterial infections. Other species of lice are not highly pathogenic to mature birds but may be fatal to chicks. Examination of birds, particularly around the vent and under the wings, reveals eggs or moving lice on the skin or feathers.

Lice are usually introduced to a farm through infested equipment (eg, crates or egg flats) or by galliform birds. Lice are best controlled on caged chickens or turkeys by spraying with pyrethroids, carbaryl, coumaphos, malathion, or stirofos. Birds on the floor are more easily treated by scattering carbaryl, coumaphos, malathion, or stirofos dust on the litter. Eggs are not killed, so insecticide treatment should be repeated after 10 days.

MITES

The most economically important of the many external parasites of poultry are mites of the families Dermanyssidae (chicken mite, northern fowl mite, and tropical fowl mite) and Trombiculidae (turkey chigger).

Chicken Mite

(Red mite, Roost mite, Poultry mite)

Dermanyssus gallinae infests chickens, turkeys, pigeons, canaries, and various wild birds worldwide. These bloodsucking mites will also bite people. While rare in modern commercial cage-layer operations, it is found in breeder and small farm flocks. Chicken mites are nocturnal feeders that hide during the day under manure, on roosts, and in cracks and crevices of the chicken house, where they deposit eggs. Populations develop rapidly during the warmer months and more slowly in cold weather; the life cycle may be completed in only 1 wk. A house may remain infested for 6 mo after birds are removed.

Transmission of the chicken mite, as well as the northern fowl mite and the tropical fowl mite (*see* below), is by mite dispersion or by contact with infested birds, animals, or inanimate objects. In the integrated poultry industry, mites are dispersed most frequently on inanimate objects such as egg flats, crates, or coops or by personnel going from house to house or farm to farm.

Heavy infestations of either chicken mites or northern fowl mites decrease reproductive potential in males, egg production in females, and weight gain in young birds; they can also cause anemia and death. Chicken mites may be found in the chicken houses during the day, particularly in cracks or where roost poles touch supports, or on birds at night. Their role as vectors of other pathogens in nature needs study, but experimental transmission of Eastern, Western, and Venezuelan equine encephalitis viruses, fowl poxvirus, and the bacteria *Salmonella* Enteritidis, *Pasteurella multocida*, *Coxiella burnetii*, and *Borrelia anserina* has been demonstrated.

Obtaining mite-free birds and using good sanitation practices are important to prevent a buildup of mite populations. Once poultry have been infested, control may be achieved by spraying or dusting the birds and litter with amitraz, carbaryl, coumaphos, malathion, stirofos, or a pyrethroid compound in areas where the parasites have not developed resistance to these chemicals. Miticide spray treatments must be applied with sufficient force to penetrate the feathers in the vent area. Nicotine sulfate is an effective fumigant for mites but is particularly hazardous. Pyrethrins and piperonyl butoxide are initially active but have poor residual killing power. For control of chicken mites, in addition to treating the birds, the inside of the house and all hiding places for the mite (such as roosts, behind nest boxes, and cracks and crevices) must be treated thoroughly using a high-pressure sprayer. Dimethoate and fenthion may be used as residual house sprays when poultry are not present. Inert dusts such as diatomaceous earth and pure synthetic amorphous silicas can be effective, but application rates need to be high when the humidity is very high. Systemic control with ivermectin (1.8–5.4 mg/kg) or moxidectin (8 mg/kg) is effective for short periods, but the high dosages are expensive, close to toxic levels, and require repeated use.

Common Chigger

The common chigger, *Trombicula alfreddugesi*, and other chigger species (harvest mites, red bugs) infest birds as well as people and other mammals, feeding on partially digested skin cells and lymph. Heavily parasitized birds become droopy, refuse to eat, and may die from starvation and exhaustion. Larvae may be found either singly or in clusters on the ventral portion of the birds. Control on the range is aided by keeping the grass cut short and dusting with sulfur, carbaryl, or malathion.

Depluming Mite

The depluming mite, *Neocnemidocoptes gallinae*, is found worldwide and burrows into the epidermis at the base of feather shafts, causing intense irritation and feather pulling and loss in chickens, pheasants, pigeons, and geese in spring and summer. Hyperkeratosis, skin lesions, and digit necrosis can result from the burrowing. Affected birds should be isolated and treated with ivermectin, malathion, or sevin dust.

Feather Mite

Most feather mites belong to the families Analgidae, Pterolichidae, and Proctophyllodidae. Surface feather mites feed mainly on feather oils, debris, fungi, and skin scales. More than 25 species, including *Megninia cubitalis*, *M ginglymura*, and *Pterolichus obtusus*, are found on domestic poultry, but they are rare on modern poultry ranches. Quill mites (Syringophilidae and Gaudoglyphidae) live in quills and feed on quill tissue or fluids obtained by piercing the calamus wall. *Syringophilus bipectinatus* is found in chicken and turkey feather quills worldwide, and *Columbiphilus polonica*, *Dermoglyphus elongatus*, and *Gaudoglyphus minor* live in chicken quills in Europe. Feather mites do little economic damage but may reduce egg production via malnutrition, feather loss, and dermatitis. Affected birds should be dusted with pyrethrin or carbaryl powder, or oral or topical ivermectin can be applied.

Northern Fowl Mite

The northern fowl mite, *Ornithonyssus sylviarum*, is the most important parasite of caged layers and breeding chickens in the USA and is a serious pest of chickens throughout the temperate zone of other countries. On turkeys, it is second in importance only to the turkey chigger in areas where the turkey chigger is found. It has been reported from many species of birds and from rats, mice, and people; however, fertile populations are reported only on birds. Northern fowl mites are obligate bloodsucking parasites that normally spend their entire life cycle (~1 wk) on the host. Off the host, mites may live as long as 2 mo, depending on temperature and relative humidity. Northern fowl mites are found on eggs or by parting feathers in the vent area, which may have thick, crusty skin, severe scabbing, and soiled feathers.

Western equine encephalomyelitis, St. Louis encephalitis, and Newcastle disease viruses, as well as fowlpox virus, have been isolated from these mites. However, the mites are not significant vectors of these viruses. For clinical findings and control, *see* above.

Scaly Leg Mite

The scaly leg mite, *Knemidocoptes mutans*, is a small, spherical, sarcoptic mite that usually tunnels into the tissue under the scales of the legs. It is rare in modern poultry facilities. When found, it is usually on older birds on which the irritation and exudation cause the legs to become thickened, encrusted, and unsightly. Feet and leg scales become raised, resulting in lameness. Birds stop feeding, and death can result after several months. This mite may occasionally attack the comb and wattles. The entire life cycle is in the skin; transmission is by contact. Infections can be latent for long periods until stress triggers a mite population increase.

For control, affected birds should be culled or isolated, and houses cleaned and sprayed frequently as recommended for the chicken mite (*see* above). Individual birds should be treated with oral or topical ivermectin or moxidectin (0.2 mg/kg), 10% sulphur solution, or 0.5% sodium fluoride.

Cyst Mite

Laminosioptes cysticola, the fowl cyst mite, is a small cosmopolitan parasite of chickens, turkeys, and pigeons that is most often diagnosed by observing white to yellowish caseocalcareous nodules ~1–3 mm in diameter in the subcutis, muscle, lungs, and abdominal viscera. Careful examination of the skin and subcutis of birds under a dissecting microscope frequently reveals the mites. Destroying the bird has been the best control for this parasite, but ivermectin may be effective.

Tropical Fowl Mite

The tropical fowl mite, *Ornithonyssus bursa*, is distributed throughout the warmer regions of the world and has been reported in Hawaii, Texas, Florida, Illinois, Indiana, Maryland, and New York. It closely resembles the northern fowl mite (*see* above) in its biology and habits but lays a greater proportion of its eggs in the nest. Hosts include chickens, turkeys, ducks, pigeons, sparrows, starlings, mynah birds, and people. Western equine encephalomyelitis virus has been recovered from this mite, but there is no evidence it transmits the virus.

For clinical findings and control, *see* above.

Turkey Chigger

The larvae of *Neoschongastia americana*, the turkey chigger, are parasitic on numerous birds. Across the southern USA, they are the major pest of turkeys ranged on heavy clay soils in the summer. The chiggers feed in groups of as many as 100 mites per lesion for 8–15 days. Turkeys may have 25–30 lesions each. One lesion, 3 mm in diameter, may cause significant downgrading at market time. To prevent downgrading, turkeys must be protected for at least 4 wk before marketing.

Sprays or dusts of carbaryl, malathion, or chlorpyrifos on turkey ranges control chiggers. A preventive measure now used in many turkey-growing areas includes a shift from range to confinement rearing, or use of sheds to provide shade.

MOSQUITOES

Mosquitoes that feed on poultry blood usually belong to the genera *Culex*, *Aedes*, or *Psorophora*. Large numbers can decrease egg production or cause death. Mosquitoes transmit *Plasmodium gallinaceum* (chicken malaria), *P hermani* (in turkeys), and other *Plasmodium* species causing avian malaria. They also transmit many viruses, including Eastern and Western equine encephalomyelitis, St. Louis encephalitis, fowlpox, and West Nile viruses. West Nile virus is transmitted from infected birds to other birds primarily by mosquitoes, particularly *Culex* spp in the USA, and has been found in >200 species of birds in America, including chickens, turkeys, pigeons, budgerigars, cockatiels, ducks, finches, and birds of prey. (*See also* WEST NILE VIRUS INFECTION, p 2893.)

Removal of mosquito-breeding habitats by emptying water-filled containers, clearing pool and pond edges of emergent vegetation, draining swampy areas, and filling low areas that collect water are the best physical control measures. Insecticidal control involves chemicals such as malathion, propoxur, permethrin, chlorpyrifos, or temephos. Insect growth regulators such as methoprene and diflubenzuron are also effective. Microbial control of mosquito larvae uses *Bacillus thuringiensis israelensis* and, against *Culex* spp, *Bacillus sphaericus*. Screening to prevent mosquito entry, residual wall sprays, and fogging within poultry houses also aid in control.

GANGRENOUS DERMATITIS

(Necrotic dermatitis, Clostridial dermatitis, Gangrenous cellulitis, Gangrenous dermatomyositis, Gas edema disease)

Gangrenous dermatitis is a disease of turkeys and chickens caused by *Clostridium septicum*, *C perfringens* type A, and *Staphylococcus aureus*, either singly or in combination. The condition is characterized by rapid onset of acute mortality. Birds succumbing to the infection have necrosis of the skin and subcutaneous tissue, usually involving the breast, abdomen, wing, or thigh.

Both clostridia and staphylococci are ubiquitous in the poultry house environment and in (intestine) or on (skin) the birds. The presence of these organisms, however, does not necessarily indicate a disease challenge. Other contributing factors are thought to play a major role in development of clinical disease within a flock. For example, gangrenous dermatitis often is believed to occur as a sequela of other diseases that produce immunosuppressive effects such as infectious bursal disease, chicken infectious anemia, reticuloendotheliosis, reovirus, and inclusion body hepatitis. Environmental conditions that promote poor litter conditions may also predispose flocks to gangrenous dermatitis, especially when present in conjunction with challenges from immunosuppressive viruses. Failing to remove moribund or dead birds may increase incidence of the disease, because such birds serve as a reservoir for the causative agent(s). Management practices that lead to scratching, such as overcrowding, feed outages, meal time feeding, and bird migration in tunnel-ventilated houses may increase incidence of infection. Affected farms tend to have repeat outbreaks if the environment is not treated. Incidence and severity of the disease depend on the bacterial strains involved in the infection, their ability to produce toxins, and the specific toxins produced.

Clinical Findings: The incubation period is relatively short (12–24 hr), with death occurring in well-fleshed birds. Other

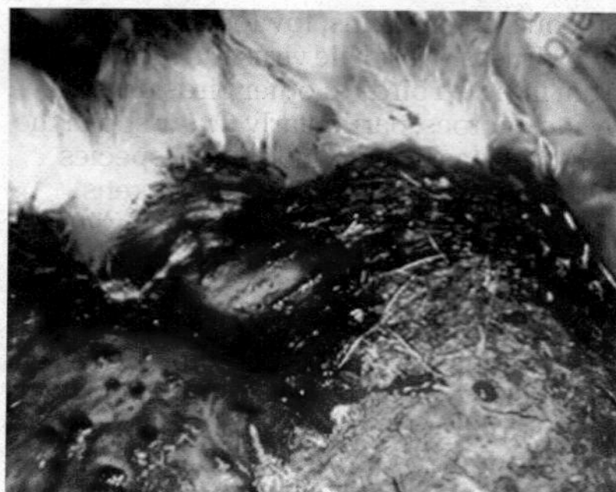

Necrotic area of the skin with serosanguineous exudate due to clostridial infection in a chicken with gangrenous dermatitis. *Courtesy of Dr. Jean Sander.*

clinical findings are general in nature and include depression, incoordination, inappetence, leg weakness, ataxia, and high fever.

Lesions: Gross lesions consist of dark reddish purple to green, weepy areas of the skin. Affected areas usually include abdomen, breast, wings, or legs. Areas of affected dermis and subcutis are characterized by extensive blood-tinged edema, with or without gas (crepitus). Infection may extend into underlying musculature, which may be discolored and contain edema and gas. Lesions in turkeys may be seen around the tail head, with blisters and tissue edema present around the tail.

Diagnosis: Presumptive diagnosis may be assigned based on an acute increase in mortality and characteristic gross lesions. Diagnostic confirmation is based on the presence of lesions and isolation of the causative agent(s) from affected tissue. Diagnosis of an underlying etiology is often necessary to fully understand the complexity of gangrenous dermatitis, because manifestation of the disease may be preceded by other immune-compromising infectious agents.

Treatment and Control: Total cleanout and disinfection of affected houses has reduced or eliminated gangrenous dermatitis infection on farms with historical problems. Salting of floors has also reduced bacterial challenge in subsequent flocks. Reducing excessive moisture and microbial levels in poultry house litter and minimizing trauma are useful adjuncts to other prevention and control measures. Where infection is secondary to predisposing viral infection, modification of vaccine programs directed at immunosuppressive agents may be used to control widespread gangrenous dermatitis.

Gangrenous dermatitis has historically been treated effectively with administration of many broad-spectrum and gram-positive antibiotics. Water acidifiers have been used in cases to reduce, but not eliminate, mortality where mortality rates are low or antibiotic efficacy has been poor.

Zoonotic Risk: The zoonotic potential and public health significance of gangrenous dermatitis is thought to be minimal, because nearly all affected birds succumb quickly to infection and do not survive to processing age.

DISORDERS OF THE SKELETAL SYSTEM

Production characteristics of modern poultry lines (eg, body weight in broiler chickens, egg production in laying hens) place high demands on the skeletal system, and inadequacies in nutrition or husbandry often result in skeletal diseases. Skeletal disorders may be primarily infectious or noninfectious; both may be seen concurrently within a flock. Skeletal disorders cause lameness from biomechanical dysfunction and in broiler chickens result in poor growth, culled birds, increased mortality (caused by starvation and dehydration), and carcass condemnation and downgrading. Bone fractures in spent hens may be a welfare issue. Before postmortem examination, flocks should be assessed; live, lame birds should be examined, and general flock health and management assessed. Serum samples may be collected for viral and mycoplasmal serology and/or biochemistry (eg, serum calcium). Gross pathology alone is often insufficient, and histopathology is usually necessary to reach a diagnosis. Bone ash measurement, feed nutritional analysis, and bacteriology are useful complementary investigations.

NONINFECTIOUS SKELETAL DISORDERS IN BROILERS

Rotational (Torsional) and Angular (Valgus/Varus) Deformities: These deformities often are seen as distinct flock problems. The most common abnormalities are seen in the distal limb and involve lateral or medial deviation and/or external rotation. Valgus or varus deviation of the intertarsal joint is the most common deformation in broiler chickens. Males are more commonly affected. The pathogenesis of the leg deformation is not well defined. Deformity may be a consequence of rickets at a younger age (*see* below). Poor mineralization of the bone, as in rickets, increases the potential for deformation and therefore the incidence and severity of deformities. Bone deformities may also be due to chondrodystrophy secondary to nutritional deficiencies (eg, choline, biotin, pyridoxine, folic acid). In breeds predisposed to deformities, the incidence may be reduced by slowing the growth rate via feed restriction or lighting programs. Rotated tibia has been a major problem in turkeys and a minor problem in Leghorns and guinea fowl. Excessive external tibial rotation occurs during development, but the pathogenesis is not well understood. Genetic, nutritional, and management factors are thought to be involved. The lack of bone angulation differentiates rotated tibia from valgus and varus deformation.

Spondylopathies: Vertebral deformities and/or displacements (spondylopathies) such as lordosis and kyphosis are common in thoracic vertebrae, particularly at the level of the free thoracic vertebra. Spondylolisthesis ("kinky back") is a developmental disorder resulting in rotation of the free thoracic vertebra with ventral displacement of the anterior end and over-riding of the posterior end, causing spinal cord compression and posterior paralysis. Spondylolisthesis is the most common vertebral column deformity, but incidence is low in most broiler flocks. Growth rate and conformation influence this developmental disorder.

Dyschondroplasia: Dyschondroplastic lesions are masses of avascular cartilage extending from the growth plate into the metaphysis and are attributed to the failure of chondrocyte differentiation. This results in a focal thickening of the growth plate and is most commonly seen in the proximal tibiotarsus (tibial dyschondroplasia). Dyschondroplasia can develop in other bones such as the proximal and distal femur and tarsometatarsus. The lesion in the proximal tibiotarsus can be associated with anterior bowing of the tibiotarsus and sometimes fractures distal to the plug of cartilage. Factors shown to influence the incidence and severity of dyschondroplasia include genetic selection, rapid growth, calcium:phosphorus ratio in feed, metabolic acidosis due to excess chloride in feed, acid/base imbalance, copper-deficient diet, *Fusarium* spp contamination of the feed, and exposure to dithiocarbamate fungicides and certain antibiotics such as salinomycin. The most common causes in modern broiler flocks may be marginal inadequacies in dietary calcium or a calcium:phosphorus imbalance. The disease is seen in broiler chickens, turkeys, and ducks.

Rickets: Rickets develops in growing birds due to deficiency of vitamin D, calcium, or phosphorus (*see* p 2930 and p 2937) or by calcium:phosphorus imbalance. Inadequate nutrition or intestinal disease with malabsorption can be the cause of the mineral or vitamin deficiency or imbalance. In rickets, abnormal endochondral ossification with failure of mineralization leads to defective bone formation, flexible long bones with subsequent bone deformities (eg, varus, valgus), and fractures. Lesions are most prominent at sites of rapid growth where cartilage contributes most significantly to skeletal growth (eg, long bones, ribs). Thick and pliable ribs and/or knobs at the costochondral junction (rachitic rosary) due to thickened and flared metaphyses are classic gross lesions. Beaks and claws can be soft and pliable. Hypertrophy and hyperplasia of the parathyroid glands are present. Subclinical rickets with only marginal thickening of the growth plates is fairly common and often associated with poor performance of broiler chickens. Bone pathology and bone ashing to estimate calcium and phosphorus content are useful diagnostic tools.

Degenerative Joint Disease: Degenerative joint disease is seen mainly in the coxofemoral, femorotibial, and intertarsal joints of broilers and male turkeys near market weight. Reluctance to move, abducted legs, and lameness can be observed. The pathogenesis is not well defined, but osteochondrosis or cartilage lesions and genetic factors may be involved.

NONINFECTIOUS SKELETAL DISORDERS IN BREEDERS

Osteopenia (Osteoporosis and Osteomalacia): Cage layer fatigue (*see* p 2897) describes a syndrome in which laying hens become paralyzed in their cages and have brittle bones. Layers 25–50 wk old are most severely affected. Osteopenia in cage layer fatigue is a consequence of osteoporosis, a deficiency in the quantity of normal fully mineralized structural bone, and osteomalacia, a reduction in bone density. The sternum is often deformed, and the ribs infolded at the junctions of the sternal and vertebral portions. Fractures occur in the long bones and vertebrae. Bone cortices are thin, and the medullary bone is osteomalacic. Parathyroid glands are hypertrophic and hyperplastic. This syndrome is due in part to a lack of exercise of hens held in cages and to selection for high egg production, but poor nutrition, with inadequate calcium, phosphorus, and/or vitamin D, exacerbates the condition. Although prevention of osteopenia in layers with nutritional management has not been successful, sources of calcium that enable the slow release of mineral, such as oyster shell, appear to give the best results to reduce development of osteopenia and improve eggshell quality.

Articular Gout: *See* p 2874.

INFECTIOUS SKELETAL DISORDERS

Coagulase-positive staphylococci (*see also* STAPHYLOCOCCOSIS, p 2867) are frequently responsible for bacterial infections in the bones and joints of broiler chickens. *Mycoplasma synoviae* (*see* p 2843) may also play a role in infectious bone disorders.

In broilers, bacterial infections are most common in the proximal femur and proximal tibiotarsus in birds >22 days old. In the proximal femur, the condition is also referred to as femoral head necrosis, which is reported to be the most common cause of lameness in broiler chickens. The etiology appears to be vertically transmitted staphylococci, often in combination with infection by immunosuppressive viruses (eg, INFECTIOUS BURSAL DISEASE, *see* p 2837). Floor eggs have been shown to be common carriers of staphylococci, so their use should be avoided. A high standard of hatchery hygiene can reduce this risk. Formaldehyde fumigation within the hatchers is also likely to help. In addition, hatchery fluff samples (ie, hatching debris such as down feather and egg shell remains) can be examined to monitor for contamination with staphylococci.

Staphylococcal infections in joints and tendons are also seen in breeders. Outbreaks are often due to bacterial infection subsequent to an existing tendinitis. A history of other diseases such as coccidiosis is often associated with an increase in staphylococcal infections in breeders. In some instances, reoviruses may also be isolated. (*See also* VIRAL ARTHRITIS, p 2886.) The virus is vertically transmitted. Vaccines against the condition have been developed.

Escherichia coli is often responsible for flock outbreaks of arthritis and osteomyelitis in broiler chickens and turkeys. Osteomyelitis and arthritis are sequelae of septicemia, and these outbreaks may be associated with enteric or respiratory disease. Infection of bones, joints, and periarticular tissues with *E coli*, *Staphylococcus aureus*, or *S hyicus* is referred to as turkey osteomyelitis complex (TOC) or green-liver osteomyelitis complex. Green discoloration of the liver is often associated with TOC and is mostly observed at the processing plant but is rare in birds that died or are euthanized in the field.

Enterococcus cecorum is a commensal enteric bacterium that can cause epidemics of osteomyelitis, arthritis, and spondylitis in broilers and broiler breeders. Enterococcal spondylitis is a defined clinical syndrome

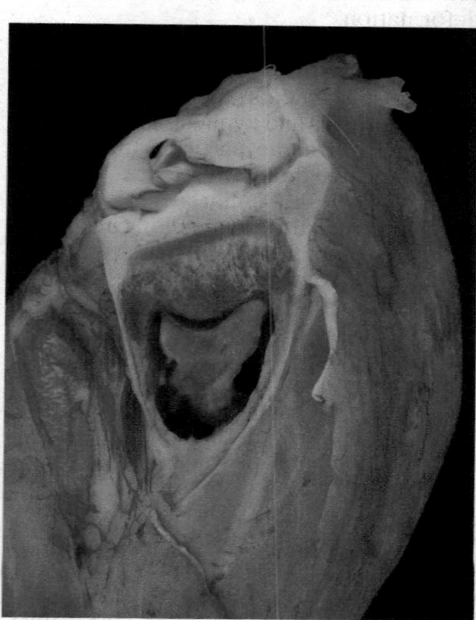

Osteomyelitis of the tibiotarsus in a 43-day-old broiler. *Courtesy of Dr. H. J. Barnes.*

with infection of the free thoracic and adjacent vertebrae, resulting in chronic osteomyelitis and spinal cord compression. Clinical signs of leg paresis often develop in broilers >35 days old.

Other sporadic causes of osteomyelitis and/or arthritis in poultry include *Pasteurella multocida*, *Ornithobacterium rhinotracheale*, *Trueperella (Arcanobacterium) pyogenes*, *Enterococcus* spp, *Streptococcus* spp, *Salmonella* spp, *Streptobacillus moniliformis*, and *Aspergillus* spp.

Osteomyelitis and arthritis are detected on gross examination by examination of articular surfaces and bone physes. Detection of subtle lesions requires histopathology. Affected joints are often swollen with fibrinous or caseous exudate. Bones have areas of lysis and/or replacement by caseous exudate, most often within the physeal region.

Response to treatment with antibiotics currently approved for use in poultry is often poor for bacterial bone and joint infections. Antibiotics may be used to control the bacteremia contributing to new cases and to modify the bacterial flora within a flock. When individual birds are of high value, long-term antibiotic therapy may improve some less severe cases. Control requires minimizing sources of infection and stock susceptibility.

Viral Arthritis: *See* p 2886.

Osteopetrosis: Osteopetrosis in chickens is due to infection with specific strains of avian leukosis virus (*see* p 2851). Growth and differentiation of osteoblasts is altered by the virus, resulting in diaphyseal and/or metaphyseal, periosteal, and circumferential accumulation of woven and lamellar bone. Osteopetrosis is bilaterally symmetrical and involves the long bones, especially the tibiotarsus and tarsometatarsus. Birds 8–12 wk old are most commonly affected. Lymphoid leukosis often occurs in chickens with osteopetrosis. Avian osteopetrosis differs from mammalian osteopetrosis in which a defect in osteoclast function results in abnormal bone resorption and accumulation of primary spongiosa in the marrow cavity.

Amyloid Arthropathy: Extensive amyloid arthropathy is primarily caused by *Enterococcus faecalis* or *Mycoplasma synoviae*. Clinical cases are seen only occasionally and most frequently affect the hock joint. Brown layer chickens are particularly susceptible. Some cases have been attributed to contamination of a previously sterile vaccine diluent with *E faecalis* during administration (eg, Marek's vaccine in day-old chicks). Joints may be enlarged by yellow-orange material in the articular space.

MYOPATHIES

EXERTIONAL MYOPATHY

Exertional myopathy results from overly strenuous muscular exercise and can be precipitated by preexisting conditions such as selenium deficiency. Inadequate energy metabolism and/or mechanical stresses occurring during contraction are thought to be the cause of myofiber degeneration. The lesions can be monophasic (resulting from a single event, eg, transport, capture, or restraint myopathy) or polyphasic (with repeated or ongoing events). Early gross lesions include muscle pallor with edema or bloodstained transudate. There is swelling, degeneration, necrosis, and mineralization of muscle fibers, with edema, hemorrhage, and infiltration of heterophils and macrophages. Deep pectoral myopathy and capture myopathy are the main examples of exertional myopathy in birds. Leg muscle myopathy after transport of poultry can also occur and is associated with increased body size and weight, increased transport time to processing plant, cool ambient temperatures, and valgus leg deformities.

Deep Pectoral Myopathy

(Degenerative myopathy, Green muscle disease)

Deep pectoral myopathy is characterized by degeneration, necrosis, and fibrosis of the deep pectoral (supracoracoideus) muscle in heavy meat birds (chickens, turkeys), secondary to excessive muscle activity (exertional myopathy and compartment syndrome).

The function of the deep pectoral muscle is to elevate the wing. Although well-developed in modern meat birds, the muscle is little used. After episodes of prolonged wing flapping (eg, handling, when a lame bird uses its wings to assist ambulation, or when a bird is placed on its back), deep pectoral muscle injury and swelling occurs. Because of the tight surrounding fascia, the swollen muscle cannot expand, which results in collapse of the blood vessles supplying the muscle. The decreased (or lack of) blood perfusion leads to ischemia, tissue hypoxia, and muscle necrosis (compartment syndrome). The lesion can be produced artificially by stimulating the deep pectoral muscle to contract and can be prevented by surgically opening the fascial sheath covering the muscle before exercise.

The myopathy may be unilateral or bilateral with the central ⅓ – ⅔ of the muscle most prominently affected. Early, the involved muscle is pale, swollen, and edematous. Later, it acquires a green coloration and becomes drier and sharply demarcated from adjacent, viable muscle. Eventually, the necrotic muscle becomes enclosed in a thick, fibrous capsule. The defect can be identified by a flattening or depression of the breast over affected muscles, by palpation, or by transillumination of carcasses at slaughter.

Flock prevalence is usually low, but prevalence as high as 25% has been reported, with few birds developing the disease before 24 wk of age. Deep pectoral myopathy occurs frequently in turkey breeder hens during artificial insemination. The disease is usually subclinical, and major loss is from downgrading or condemnation at processing. Deep pectoral myopathy is not easy to detect at processing when birds are marketed as whole carcasses.

Incidence can be decreased by careful handling of susceptible birds to prevent excessive wing flapping and, as a longterm method, by selective breeding because the condition has a genetic component. Supplementing rations with selenium, vitamin E, or methionine has not influenced incidence.

Capture Myopathy

Capture myopathy (exertional rhabdomyolysis) is mainly seen in zoo and wild birds and is rare in poultry. Long-legged wading birds are particularly susceptible. Capture myopathy results from exertion, struggle, or stress occurring during capture, handling, immobilization, or transport. Hyperthermia and metabolic acidosis due to anaerobic glycolysis are important factors. Pale skeletal muscle, especially muscle from the legs, or sometimes cardiac muscle, is seen grossly. However, no gross lesions are present in peracute cases. Ischemic and myoglobinuric nephrosis may be present in birds that survive for a few days. Prognosis of symptomatic birds is usually poor, but treatment of single, valuable birds can be attempted and may be successful. Such treatment may consist of a combination of corticosteroids, vitamin E, selenium, parenteral fluids, and forced feeding in conjunction with physiotherapy. Prevention is best. Well-planned and executed capture and restraint that minimizes pursuit time, struggling, noise, and visual stimulation is key. Sedation or anesthesia can be useful.

Transport Myopathy of Turkeys

(Leg edema syndrome)

Heavy toms are primarily affected by transport myopathy, although it also develops in hens. Transport myopathy is associated with increased body size and weight, increased transport time to processing plants, cool ambient temperatures, and valgus leg deformities. The pathogenesis is unknown but presumed to be similar to that of exertional myopathy. Often, only one leg is affected. No evidence of external trauma is seen. Skin over edematous subcutaneous tissue is pale, feather follicles are less visible, and the skin slips easily over underlying muscle when moved. Occasionally, there is crepitation. Affected areas are dark when the edematous areas contain blood. Typically, when lesions are cut, the edematous subcutis is a few to several millimeters thick and is amber, occasionally green, or rarely red. Purulent exudate is absent, which distinguishes transport myopathy from cellulitis. If hemorrhage is present, the adductor muscles usually are torn. Removal of affected legs at processing results in carcass downgrading. Microscopically, acute multifocal muscle necrosis is found, primarily in the adductor muscles. Sometimes subacute or chronic lesions are seen, suggesting earlier episodes of myopathy. Serum CK increases sharply between farm and processing. This is now a rare disease because of programs designed to improve leg strength and conformation, as well as improved handling and transportation conditions.

MECHANICALLY INDUCED MYOPATHY

Avascular necrosis caused by pressure in heavy birds that are down because of lameness or leg deformity is seen occasionally and occurs most frequently in the breast muscle. On gross examination, the tissue is firm and pale. Histologic examination reveals swelling, hyalinization, and necrosis of fibers with edema, heterophils, and macrophages at the periphery.

Rupture of the Gastrocnemius Tendon

Rupture of the gastrocnemius tendon is common in meat-type chickens, particularly roasters and breeders, and rare in turkeys. The rupture is due to application of excess weight to previously damaged tendons (most frequently by reoviral or staphylococcal tendinitis), or it can be spontaneous. The intra- and peritendinous fibroplasias that occur after infectious tendinitis make the tendon larger but weaker because of replacement of normal strong, dense tendon collagenous connective tissue with weaker, dense, irregular connective tissue. Synechiae between the tendon and its sheath may also develop, limiting the tendon's range of motion. Application of normal or excess weight to these previously damaged tendons results in partial or complete tearing or rupture. In noninfectious spontaneous tendon rupture, the cause of the rupture is uncertain but may be a combination of weaker tendons and heavier body weight in meat-type chickens. Rupture of the tendon of one leg puts stress on the other tendon, and bilateral rupture is frequent. Affected birds are lame or "down on their hocks" (creepers). Hemorrhage from the injury above the hock on the back of the leg is visible as red, blue, or green discoloration of the tissues, depending on the age of the lesion. No discoloration may be visible in chronic lesions. Tissue discoloration results in condemnation of the affected part at processing (red-leg, green-leg). The ruptured tendon can be palpated as a hard mass on the back of the leg above the hock. Broiler breeders >12 wk old are most commonly affected, and flock incidence may be as high as 20%.

Rupture of the Peroneus (Fibularis) Longus Muscle

The peroneus muscle originates on the proximal end of the tibiotarsus and patellar tissue, with attachments to other muscles in that area. In turkeys, the insertion appears to be in three places. A small band of tissue from the medial side of the muscle runs to the lateral tibial condyle. The main muscle tendon crosses the lateral side of the hock and joins other tendons that extend the hock and may affect foot and toe movement. The muscle is thin and wide, covering the anterior and lateral surface of the leg, and is covered by a heavy aponeurosis in which the tendon is embedded. Rupture of the aponeurosis and muscle occurs as a 1–2 cm horizontal wound on the anterior and/or lateral surface of the muscle. It occurs above the middle of the tibiotarsus at the top of the ossifying tendon where the tendon attaches to the muscle. Rupture usually occurs at 10–14 wk, the age at which turkey leg tendons become ossified, reducing the elasticity of the tissue in that location.

Rupture of the peroneus longus muscle is an uncommon muscle lesion. It is most frequent in females and may affect as much as 5% of the flock. The separation of the muscle likely occurs slowly, caused by activity such as repeated springing, in turkeys that are becoming heavier and maturing earlier. Affected birds are not lame, but the resulting hemorrhage causes a red, blue, or green discoloration under the skin around and ventral to the rupture site (drumstick). This results in downgrading of the carcass at processing. The affected portion can be trimmed.

NUTRITIONAL MYOPATHY

Nutritional myopathy in chickens, turkeys, waterfowl, and ostriches is attributed to vitamin E/selenium deficiency. However, as in mammals, selenium deficiency is most often the main cause of the myopathy. Vitamin E deficiency, when accompanied by a sulfur amino acid deficiency, causes nutritional myopathy in chicks by ~4 wk of age. Lesions of vitamin E/selenium deficiency have been reported in skeletal (especially breast muscle), heart, and smooth muscle (gizzard and intestine) of ducks, turkeys, and chickens. Arsenic, zinc, copper, and other metals are antagonistic to selenium, and exposure to these other metals may precipitate outbreaks. Gross lesions, with pale foci or streaking, are similar to those of nutritional myopathies in mammals. Microscopic changes include focal or widespread myofiber swelling, edema, hyalinization, mineralization, degeneration, and lysis with infiltration of macrophages and heterophils. Hypercellularity from proliferation of satellite cells may be prominent if regeneration is occurring. Poultry feeds in many parts of the world contain added selenium at 0.1–0.4 ppm to prevent this myopathy.

TOXIC MYOPATHY

Ionophores are toxic at increased doses. Ionophore toxicity causes muscle damage with incoordination, leg weakness, diarrhea, dyspnea, and reduced feed intake and weight. Stunting may also occur. Type I ("red muscle" or oxidative) fibers are most susceptible, and lesions are most prominent in the leg musculature. Lesions may also be found in heart and gizzard muscle. Adult birds (chickens, turkeys, ratites) and birds with no previous exposure are more sensitive to ionophore coccidiostats. Gross and histologic changes are similar to those of nutritional myopathy (*see* above). Ionophores promote movement of cations across the cell membrane, causing disruption of the ionic equilibrium, increased intracytoplasmic concentration of Ca^{2+}, and cell death. The toxic dose of ionophores is decreased if they are used in conjunction with tiamulin, erythromycin, or chloramphenicol. Salinomycin at the dose recommended for chickens (60 g/ton) is toxic for turkeys; doses >15 g/ton are toxic in turkeys. Monensin (100 g/ton) and lasalocid (100 g/ton) at the dose recommended for chickens are not toxic to turkeys.

Coffee senna (*Senna occidentalis*) toxicity can produce clinical signs and gross and histologic changes in muscles similar to those seen in ionophore toxicity.

INJECTION SITE INJURY

Injection of antibiotics and vaccines in any location can result in focal inflammatory myositis. Cellulitis and myositis in the neck region causing postural and/or neurologic signs can be seen in poultry after improper administration of vaccines. It is most commonly seen in broiler chicks. Affected birds may show ataxia, twisting of the neck, leg paralysis, and recumbency. Swelling of the subcutaneous and muscle tissue in the neck region at the injection site is seen grossly. Microscopically, a lymphocytic and/or granulomatous inflammatory infiltrate is present within the muscle and subcutis. The inflammatory infiltrate can extend to the epidural spaces. With oil-emulsion vaccines, empty spaces representing lipid droplets surrounded by a granulomatous inflammatory reaction can be seen.

MINIMAL MYOPATHY

A minimal myopathy is seen in otherwise normal meat-type poultry. Affected birds show no clinical signs, and their muscles are grossly normal, but microscopically there is mild myofiber degeneration and fat accumulation between myofibers. Focal or multifocal scattered myofibers are hyalinized and mineralized. More severe examples of this lesion contain individual myofiber necrosis, increased fat, and fibroplasia between fibers. No specific cause has been determined for these minimal changes, which have been observed by avian pathologists but are not described in the literature. Minimal myopathy is not an established name for this condition.

GENETIC MYOPATHY

Type II glycogen storage disease (acid maltase deficiency, Pompe disease) has been reported in Japanese quail. Symptoms start between 4 and 6 wk of age, and affected quail show progressive myopathy with reduced ability or inability to lift their wings, fly, or get back on their feet after being placed on their back (flip test). Glycogen deposition occurs in skeletal muscle, cardiac muscle, and smooth muscle, as well as in the brain and spinal cord. Both red and white muscle is affected, but lesions are more pronounced in the pectoralis superficialis (white muscle).

VIRAL ARTHRITIS

(Tenosynovitis, Reoviral arthritis)

Reovirus infections are ubiquitous in commercial poultry flocks. They are global in distribution, although the virulence of viruses appears to differ between regions. Most strains are nonpathogenic and appear to survive harmlessly in the intestine, whereas others have been associated with several disease conditions, including malabsorption and other enteric disorders, hydropericardium, and occasionally respiratory disease. In many instances, the association of the reovirus with disease is uncertain. An exception to this is viral arthritis, or tenosynovitis, because it can be reproduced experimentally by infecting birds with reovirus alone.

Viral arthritis results in severe lameness in heavy broiler breeds of chickens and occasionally in laying breeds. Although lameness in turkeys has sometimes been reported to be associated with avian reoviruses, experimental evidence in the past has been unable to confirm that turkeys are as susceptible to these viruses as chickens. However, recent field evidence from the USA indicates the presence of novel reoviruses causing arthritis and tendon rupture clinically identical to that in chickens. Reoviruses have been isolated from a range of other avian (including wild) species, and it is possible that cross-infection occurs, although ducks and geese have reoviruses that differ genetically from those of chickens.

Etiology and Pathogenesis: Viral arthritis is caused by avian reoviruses, which are RNA viruses related to but distinct from mammalian reoviruses. Strains differ in virulence, ranging from those causing arthritis and sometimes death to those that exist harmlessly in the gut. The mechanisms that determine whether a reovirus is pathogenic or harmless are poorly understood. Several antigenic types are known, and although some cross-protection occurs between types, it is rarely complete. Most infections are acquired by ingestion. After intestinal replication, the virus spreads via the bloodstream to all parts of the body. Pathogenic viruses localize in the hock joint, where they cause arthritis. Other organs, such as the liver, may be affected.

Transmission and Epidemiology: Avian reoviruses can be egg transmitted, so infected breeder hens pass virus to chicks. Transmission is short-lived, and only a small nucleus of chicks carry virus. Infection is spread locally to hatchmates by the fecal-oral route. The virus is quite resistant to inactivation and can persist on farm materials for many days or weeks. Fomites are important.

Serious outbreaks of viral arthritis are followed by a decreased incidence in later hatch groups of birds from the same parent flock and may be related to decreased egg transmission and development of maternal immunity. Day-old chicks are more susceptible than older birds when exposed by natural means. The younger the chick when infected, the more likely it is that disease will develop.

Clinical Findings: Viral arthritis usually is seen in broilers 4–8 wk old as unilateral or bilateral swellings of the tendons of the shank and above the hock. It can also be found in much older chickens, usually at peak of production or beyond, probably because of reactivation of persistent virus at sexual maturity. Affected birds walk with a stilted gait or prefer not to move. In the most severe form, rupture of the gastrocnemius tendon is common, although digital flexor tendons are sometimes affected and many cull birds are seen around the feeders and waterers. The most severely affected birds do not recover; less severely affected birds may recover in 4–6 wk. Infection is asymptomatic in many birds. Feed efficiency and rate of weight gain are decreased. Mortality is 2%–10% and morbidity 5%–50%.

Lesions: An acute, fulminating infection is occasionally seen in young chicks and embryos with cardiomegaly, hepatomegaly, and splenomegaly with necrotic foci. Edema around the tendons of the leg is marked, petechial hemorrhages develop in the synovial membranes above the hock, and fusion and calcification of the tendon bundles are common. Blood clots and hemorrhages are seen accompanying rupture of the gastrocnemius tendon. In the most severe cases, pitted erosions of the cartilage of the distal tibiotarsus are seen with flattening of the condyles. Histologically, the synovial cells are hypertrophied, hyperplastic, and infiltrated by lymphocytes and macrophages. The synovia contain lymphoid aggregates with heterophils and macrophages. In the heart, infiltration of heterophils or lymphocytes between myocardial fibers is a consistent finding.

Diagnosis: A presumptive diagnosis can be based on unilateral or bilateral swelling of the tendons of the shank and tendon bundle above the hock and on the inflammatory changes in the tendons and synovia described above. However, other causes of lameness such as *Mycoplasma synoviae* or *Escherichia coli* should be considered. Reovirus can be isolated from affected joints in primary chick embryo kidney, liver, or lung cell cultures, or via the yolk sac or chorioallantoic membrane of embryonated chicken eggs. In view of the widespread nature of reovirus infections without disease, isolation from the gut is not significant. In many laboratories, PCR is used for virus identification and is more rapid and sensitive than isolation. Avian reoviruses are now classified according to their sigma surface proteins, and the indications are that the novel USA turkey and European chicken viruses are different from the common ones associated with viral arthritis. The turkey isolates are genetically related to the turkey enteric reoviruses, but further molecular analysis is awaited. In view of the ability of avian reoviruses to recombine, it is possible these new arthritogenic variants in both species have evolved by this means. ELISA is the serologic test of choice, and most birds are positive early in infection. Virus neutralization tests and challenge of immunized chickens can be used to identify the specific serotype. However, serologic results can be difficult to interpret in view of the ubiquity of reovirus infections. Culture procedures should be used to differentiate mycoplasmal and other bacterial infections.

Treatment and Control: There is no treatment. Live and killed vaccines are available. Maternal antibodies prevent early infection in chicks and minimize or prevent egg transmission. In view of egg transmission and the greater susceptibility of baby chicks, the main objective of vaccination is to ensure good immunity in the parent flock. Vaccination programs should be directed to the serotype(s) present in local flocks. Adult birds are less susceptible to clinical disease if exposed by natural routes. Currently available commercial vaccines against viral arthritis are not effective against the newly encountered chicken viruses described in Europe or against those causing arthritis in turkeys.

Zoonotic Risk: There have been no reported zoonotic risks associated with avian reovirus infections.

AVIAN ENCEPHALOMYELITIS

(Epidemic tremor)

Avian encephalomyelitis (AE) is a viral disease of young chickens, turkeys, Japanese quail, pheasants, and pigeons. Turkeys are less susceptible to natural infection and generally develop a milder clinical disease than chickens. Ducklings and guinea fowl are susceptible to experimental infection. AE is characterized by neurologic signs that result from infection of the CNS with an RNA virus in the family Picornaviridae. Infection occurs via vertical and horizontal transmission. If a breeder flock becomes infected during egg production, the virus is vertically transmitted to the offspring and a major outbreak occurs. The disease often appears in a series of flocks hatched from the infected breeder flock. Field strains of the virus are enterotropic and multiply in the intestine. Infected birds shed the virus in their feces for a few days to a few weeks, which serves to spread the infection to hatchmates. There is no convincing evidence that the virus persists in infected birds. AE virus is resistant to environmental conditions and may remain infectious for long periods.

Clinical Findings: Vertically infected chicks commonly show clinical signs during the first week after hatching, although signs may be present in a few birds at hatching. Clinical signs appear later in hatchmates that are horizontally infected by the fecal-oral route. Vertical infection followed by horizontal infection causes a characteristic biphasic mortality pattern. The main clinical signs are ataxia and leg weakness that varies from sitting on hocks to paresis that progresses to paralysis and recumbency. Fine tremors of the head and neck are evident in some birds and are characteristic of the disease. They are responsible for the common name, epidemic tremors. Tremors vary in frequency and severity and are best seen after birds are disturbed or excited. This can easily be done by placing the bird on its back and letting it right itself. Cupping the bird in one's hands often results in a buzzing feeling because of rapid, fine tremors. Severely affected birds lay on their side and exhibit intermittent fine tremors of the head, neck, and legs. Horizontally infected chicks usually show clinical signs at 2–4 wk of age; thus, clinical disease progresses through the flock for the first few weeks, and the episode is usually over by the time the flock is ~4 wk old. Morbidity and mortality rates vary and depend on the level of egg transmission and degree of immunity in the flock. In severe outbreaks, both morbidity and mortality may exceed 50%.

After 4 wk of age, chickens are resistant to disease but not infection. An exception occurs occasionally in older chickens after vaccination with egg-embryo–adapted commercial vaccines. Affected birds exhibit typical CNS signs like those seen in younger chicks.

In laying chickens, there is a sudden, 5%–10% drop in egg production, which usually lasts for <2 wk, followed by a return to normal production. There is no deterioration in egg shell quality. Hatchability may drop as much as 5% during the decline in egg production due to late embryonic mortality. Infected eggs are laid during the period of viremia, which usually lasts 1–2 wk.

Lesions: No gross lesions are seen in the brain of infected birds. Gray to white foci may be visible on cut surfaces of the muscle of the gizzard. Weeks after infection, opacity of eye lenses (cataracts) may occur in a small percentage of chickens that survive the infection. Microscopic lesions in the CNS are found in the brain (cerebral peduncle, cerebellum, brain stem) and spinal cord and consist of degeneration and necrosis of neurons, perivascular lymphocytic cuffing, and gliosis with formation of glial nodules. In the cerebellum, there are areas of necrosis or loss of Purkinje cells and replacement by glial nodules that extend into the molecular layer of the gray matter. Neuronal lesions of central chromatolysis, shrinkage and increased basophilia, satellitosis, and neuronophagia are best found in neuron clusters (nuclei) in the brain stem, arbor vitae of the cerebellum, and lateral horn (gray matter) of the spinal cord. Central chromatolysis of neurons is characterized by rounding of the cell contour and displacement of Nissl granules to the periphery. Dorsal root ganglia have multifocal nodular collections of lymphocytes.

A common microscopic lesion outside the CNS is diffuse or nodular lymphocytic infiltrates in the gizzard muscle, muscular layer of the esophagus and proventriculus, myocardium, and pancreas. Except for cataracts, microscopic lesions generally are not found in infected adults unless they are showing nervous signs, in which case they will have CNS lesions similar to those in young birds.

Diagnosis: Diagnosis is based on history, clinical signs, and characteristic histopathologic lesions in the brain and spinal cord. The diagnosis is best confirmed by isolation and identification of the virus. Tissues collected for virus isolation must include the brain and duodenum with the pancreas. Demonstration of AE virus antigen in the brain, spinal cord, and other tissues by immunofluorescent and immunohistochemical staining is a reliable method of diagnosis. The major differential diagnosis for neurologic signs in very young chicks is bacterial or mycotic encephalitis. Rickets and nutritional encephalomalacia are next in the list of differential diagnoses, although the clinical manifestations of these diseases differ from those in AE. In adults, serologic testing of acute and convalescent sera to demonstrate an increase in antibody titers helps establish a diagnosis.

Prevention: Immunization of breeder pullets at 10–15 wk of age with a commercial live vaccine prevents vertical transmission of the virus and provides progeny with maternal immunity. Vaccination of table-egg flocks is also advisable to prevent decreases in egg production. AE vaccine is usually combined with fowlpox vaccine and given by wing-web inoculation. Also available is a live fowlpox-vectored infectious laryngotracheitis and AE combination vaccine. Affected chicks and poults are ordinarily destroyed because they rarely recover.

AE virus does not cause disease in people or other mammals.

BOTULISM

(Limberneck, Western duck sickness)

Botulism is an intoxication that results from ingestion of preformed exotoxin of *Clostridium botulinum*. The disease occurs worldwide and has been identified in at least 117 species of wild birds representing 22 families. There is concern that endangered avian species may be at risk of extinction because of the disease. Mammalian species affected by the toxin include people, mink, ferrets, cattle, pigs, dogs, horses, laboratory rodents, and various zoo animals. Intoxications are sporadic in poultry, but massive mortality has occurred in waterfowl. Ruminants fed poultry manure contaminated with *C botulinum* spores have developed the disease.

Etiology: *C botulinum* is a gram-positive, spore-forming, anaerobic bacterium. There are four genotypically distinct groups, designated by the Roman numerals I to IV. All strains of *C botulinum* can produce neurotoxins that cause flaccid paralysis. Seven immunologically distinct toxins, designated by the letters A to G, are produced by different strains, which are classified into toxinotypes (A-G) according to the type of toxin produced.

Botulinum toxins are the most potent naturally occurring toxins. They are neurotoxins with an affinity for motor neurons. After absorption, the toxin binds irreversibly to the presynaptic membrane of cholinergic nerve terminals. It enters the cell and blocks release of acetylcholine across the neuromuscular junctions, resulting in flaccid paralysis. Death results from cardiac and respiratory failure. Outbreaks in poultry and waterfowl are predominantly caused by type C toxin. Type A toxin occasionally causes botulism in domestic chickens. Type E toxin has been the cause of botulism in fish-eating birds such as gulls.

C botulinum is ubiquitous, inhabiting soils and freshwater wetland (lakes, marshes) sediments. It is commonly found in the intestine of wild birds, but its presence in the intestine of healthy poultry is questionable. Spore germination and cell multiplication with toxin production require an anaerobic environment that must also provide the necessary substrates and conditions required for multiplication. For toxinotype C, optimal growth occurs between 25°C and 40°C, which may explain why most outbreaks of botulism in waterfowl occur during the summer and fall.

Epizootiology: Wetlands are home to numerous invertebrates that can accumulate high levels of botulinum toxin. Carcasses and organic matter provide suitable substrates for multiplication of *C botulinum* and toxin production. Invertebrates, especially fly larvae (maggots), feed on carcasses that have died from botulism and thus consume botulinum toxin. They are resistant to the toxins and concentrate them in their bodies. Outbreaks in waterfowl and other water birds result from consumption of toxin-laden invertebrates. Birds that die from botulism become infested with maggots, which perpetuates the outbreak in what is known as a "carcass-maggot cycle." Evidence suggests that botulism may also result from direct ingestion of decaying organic matter that contains toxin.

Outbreaks in commercial poultry are rare and generally tend to recur on the same farm, often affecting the same houses or pens. The disease tends to be most severe in pen-reared pheasants with mortality up to 100%. Often, the source of the toxin in these outbreaks is difficult to find, leading to speculation that botulism in poultry is a "toxico-infection." Toxico-infection, also called "gut toxigenesis," results from proliferation of *C botulinum* in the intestine with subsequent production and absorption of the toxin. It is unclear what factors cause *C botulinum* to proliferate in the intestine and produce toxin. Studies have shown that healthy broilers do not harbor *C botulinum* type C in the ceca, and *C botulinum* was not recovered from the environment of poultry houses that did not have a history of botulism. These findings suggest that *C botulinum* is neither frequent nor widespread in broiler populations and that outbreaks result from infrequent and sporadic colonization of flocks with *C botulinum* introduced into a poultry house.

Clinical Findings: Clinical signs in poultry and wild birds are similar. Leg weakness and paresis that progress to flaccid paralysis of the legs, wings, neck, and eyelids are characteristic clinical signs. "Limberneck," the common name for botulism in birds, comes from the neck paralysis typically seen in affected birds. Signs in broiler chickens may also include ruffled or quivering feathers, feathers that are easily pulled out, labored breathing, and sometimes diarrhea with excess urates in loose droppings. Severely affected birds are in ventral recumbency on the floor with their eyes partially or completely closed and neck outstretched. They are unable to lift or hold their neck up and cannot raise their eyelids because of the flaccid paralysis that develops. Affected birds may have their legs extended behind them, because they are unable to pull them into a normal sitting position. Weakness is the earliest sign in waterfowl. Birds are initially reluctant to fly when approached and have weak wing-beats and difficulty taking flight. As the disease progresses, they lose their ability to fly and exhibit stumbling gaits and eventually paralysis. Birds in water can drown, because they cannot keep their heads above the water. The incubation period and time to onset of clinical signs is determined by the amount of toxin absorbed.

Lesions: *C botulinum* toxins do not cause lesions in affected birds, but maggots or other invertebrates may be found in the crop. Carcasses are usually in good condition and do not show evidence of a chronic or debilitating disease.

Diagnosis: Preliminary diagnosis is based on clinical signs and absence of gross or microscopic lesions that can explain the neurologic signs. Definitive diagnosis requires demonstration of the toxin in serum from sick birds. Liver, crop contents, gizzard contents, and intestinal washes from moribund or very freshly dead birds may also be collected for toxin detection. Samples from dead birds are unreliable, because *C botulinum* toxin can result from postmortem multiplication of the organism and toxin production. It is preferred to collect serum from birds with clinical signs of varying severity. A bioassay test in mice (mouse-protection test) used to be the standard method to detect *C botulinum* toxins, but molecular tests based on ELISA are now preferred. PCR can be used on a variety of samples to detect the genes responsible for toxin production and differentiate the different toxinotypes. Because botulinum toxins are heat labile and can be destroyed at 80°C for ≥10 min, sera must be refrigerated or frozen as soon as possible after collection and shipped with ice packs to the testing laboratory.

Leg weakness or paralysis may be the only sign in mild intoxications, which must be differentiated from Marek's disease, drug and chemical toxicosis (especially ionophore toxicity), or appendicular skeletal problems. In waterfowl, botulism must be differentiated from chemical toxicosis, especially lead poisoning, and acute, virulent infectious diseases (fowl cholera, duck viral enteritis, highly pathogenic avian influenza, etc).

Control and Prevention: Affected birds may recover without treatment. Antibiotics effective against clostridia may be useful if the disease is toxico-infectious. Collection and disposal of dead birds is critical to prevent and limit outbreaks, especially in pheasant and broiler chicken flocks. Fly control may reduce the risk of toxic maggots in the environment. Some, but not all, recurrent outbreaks in broiler flocks may be prevented by cleaning and disinfecting with products effective against spore-forming bacteria. Disinfection around poultry houses is suggested, because spores can be found outside of the houses and be reintroduced. In waterfowl outbreaks, ducks should be dispersed from affected areas and water levels stabilized. Elimination of large, shallow areas may prevent conditions favorable for decay of vegetation and die-off of invertebrates.

Active immunization with inactivated type C bacterin-toxoids has been successful in pheasant operations but is not cost-effective or feasible in commercial chickens and wild ducks. Treatment with type-specific antitoxin is effective but not practical.

Zoonotic Risk: The zoonotic potential of type C botulism is minimal. Botulism in people is caused mostly by toxin types A, B, and E. Furthermore, pathogenicity of toxin type C for people is questionable. However, botulism caused by type C toxin has been confirmed in several nonhuman primates.

VIRAL ENCEPHALITIDES

Encephalitis in poultry and farm-reared gamebirds may be caused by several different arboviruses. These include Eastern equine encephalitis (EEE) virus, Western equine encephalitis (WEE) virus, Highlands J (HJ) virus, Israel turkey meningoencephalitis virus, and West Nile virus (*See also* WEST NILE VIRUS INFECTION IN POULTRY, p 2893). The term "arbovirus," an abbreviation of arthropod-borne virus, is used to describe a virus that replicates in a hematophagous (bloodsucking) arthropod and is transmitted by bite to a vertebrate host.

Eastern Equine Encephalitis:

Eastern equine encephalitis (EEE) is most commonly a disease of horses (*see* p 1291); however, many outbreaks of EEE in farm-raised ringnecked pheasants and chukar partridges have been identified. EEE occurs only sporadically in other species of poultry (turkeys, ducks), game birds, and ratites (emus). EEE virus is found primarily in the eastern parts of North America, throughout Central America and the Caribbean, and in eastern parts of South America. In the USA, EEE has been identified in most states east of the

Mississippi River, as well as Louisiana and Texas; it is seen most often in Atlantic seaboard and Gulf Coast states. Reported isolations of the virus in Europe and Asia have not been confirmed.

EEE outbreaks generally occur in late summer and fall as a consequence of increasing numbers of mosquito vectors. *Culiseta melanura*, the principal mosquito vector, is likely responsible for transmission to poultry and game birds. Transmission to mammalian species most likely occurs by other mosquitoes such as *Aedes* and *Coquillettidia* spp, which feed on birds but also have a propensity to bite mammals. The virus has also been identified in a variety of other mosquitoes. Wild birds, primarily the smaller species of Passeriformes, are the principal vertebrate hosts of EEE virus. These birds rarely become ill but serve as maintenance and amplifying hosts for the virus in the transmission cycle.

Epornitics of EEE virus infection in pheasants are believed to be initiated by mosquito-borne infection of one or more birds in a flock, and subsequently spreading within the flock as a result of feather picking and cannibalism. In ratites, the virus may be transmitted by the fecal-oral route.

Clinical disease produced by EEE virus in poultry and game birds is usually attributed to CNS infection with or without visceral involvement. However, EEE also may produce visceral infections with little or no involvement of CNS tissues.

Pheasants develop incoordination, depression, leg paralysis, torticollis, and tremors. Mortality may be as high as 80%. Gross lesions are not observed; however, microscopic changes in the CNS consist of vasculitis, patchy necrosis, neuronal degeneration, and meningeal inflammation.

Chukar partridges exhibit clinical signs of depression, somnolence, and high mortality (30%–80%). Pale, focal areas generally are present on hearts of affected birds, and spleens are mottled and enlarged. Microscopic lesions consist of gliosis, satellitosis, perivascular lymphocytic infiltration in the brain, and myocardial necrosis with lymphocytic infiltration in the heart.

Turkeys with EEE virus infection may exhibit drowsiness, incoordination, progressive weakness, paralysis of legs and wings, and low mortality (<5%). In turkeys, EEE virus also has been identified as a cause of decreased egg production.

Ducklings infected with EEE virus develop a paralytic disease characterized by sudden onset, posterior paresis, and paralysis; mortality rates in affected flocks range from 2% to 60%. Microscopic lesions consist of edema of spinal cord white matter, lymphocytic meningitis, and microgliosis.

Ratites exhibit depression, hemorrhagic diarrhea, emesis of bloodstained ingesta, and high mortality (as much as 80%). Hemorrhagic enteritis is the principal lesion seen on postmortem examination. Microscopic lesions include necrosis of hepatocytes and intestinal mucosa.

Western Equine Encephalitis: Western equine encephalitis (WEE) virus has many characteristics in common with EEE virus; however, it is rarely associated with disease in avian species. WEE virus was identified as the cause of encephalitis and high mortality in turkeys; affected turkeys exhibited somnolence, tremors, and leg paralysis. WEE virus also has been identified as a cause of decreased egg production in turkeys.

WEE is seen mainly in western parts of the USA and Canada, Central America, and South America. In the USA and Canada, it is transmitted principally by *Culiseta tarsalis*, a mosquito vector that is relatively common west of the Mississippi River.

Highlands J Virus: Highlands J (HJ) virus is a cause of encephalitis in chukar partridges. Chukars exhibit somnolence, ruffled feathers, and recumbency before death. HJ virus infection in this species is associated with high mortality. Microscopic lesions primarily consist of nonpurulent meningoencephalitis and focal myocardial necrosis. HJ virus can cause decreased egg production in turkeys. The virus has been identified only in eastern parts of the USA.

Israel Turkey Meningoencephalitis: Israel turkey meningoencephalitis has been reported only in turkeys. It generally occurs only in birds >10 wk old. While the specific vector has not been identified, the seasonal incidence and sporadic occurrence in flocks on the same farms strongly suggest that it is transmitted by insect vectors, most likely mosquitoes and *Culicoides*. Turkeys exhibit neurologic dysfunction characterized by progressive paresis and paralysis, with variable mortality. Morbidity and mortality rates average 15%–30% but may be as high as 80%. In turkey breeder hens, egg production drops severely. Gross lesions in affected turkeys include splenomegaly or atrophy of the spleen, catarrhal enteritis, and myocarditis. The principal microscopic lesions are nonpurulent meningoencephalitis characterized by submeningeal and perivascular lymphocytic infiltration and focal myocardial necrosis.

Diagnosis: Diagnosis of EEE, WEE, and HJ virus infection or Israel turkey meningoencephalitis may be confirmed by isolation and identification of the virus, detection of viral antigens in tissues by ELISA, detection of viral RNA in tissues using reverse transcriptase PCR procedures, and serologic testing. Virus can be isolated by inoculation of newborn mice, day-old chickens, embryonated chicken eggs, or a variety of cell cultures. Brain, spleen, liver, and serum are the preferred materials for diagnostic analyses.

Arbovirus infections must be distinguished from other causes of neurologic disease in poultry and game birds such as Newcastle disease virus (*see* p 2856,) avian encephalomyelitis virus (*see* p 2888), botulism (*see* p 2889), and listeriosis (*see* p 2839).

Prevention and Control: EEE, WEE, and HJ virus infection and Israel turkey meningoencephalitis are best prevented by measures aimed at reducing vector populations. Such measures include reduction of vector habitats by modifying the environment or by chemical spraying. If feasible, farms that raise susceptible avian species should be located away from swamps and other areas that provide habitat for vectors.

Formalin-inactivated EEE virus vaccines, prepared for use in horses, have been used to protect pheasants against EEE, although their efficacy has been questioned. One-tenth the equine dose of either an eastern or bivalent eastern and western vaccine is injected into the pectoral muscle, preferably at 5–6 wk of age or when birds are released from the brooder house.

Israel turkey meningoencephalitis also can be controlled by vaccination. A live attenuated vaccine has been prepared by serial passage of virus in Japanese quail kidney cells; this vaccine is highly efficacious and commercially available.

Zoonotic Risk: EEE and WEE viruses are zoonotic agents and potential causes of significant human disease. These viruses result in neurologic disease that may progress to paralysis, convulsions, coma, and death. The case fatality rate for EEE virus in people is 50%–75%, and survivors often have permanent neurologic sequelae. WEE virus is less severe, with a case-fatality rate of ~3%–7%; most infections are subclinical. Human infection usually is acquired by mosquito bite; laboratory and clinically acquired infections are rare. However, care should be taken to avoid contact or droplet exposure when handling suspect infected birds or performing necropsies.

WEST NILE VIRUS INFECTION IN POULTRY

See also EQUINE ARBOVIRAL ENCEPHALOMYELITIS, p 1291.

West Nile virus (WNV), a flavivirus related to the St. Louis encephalitis/Japanese encephalitis complex, was first isolated from the blood of a febrile Ugandan woman in 1937. The virus was first described as the cause of a West Nile fever epidemic in people in Israel in 1951; in a later outbreak, severe meningoencephalitis was seen in elderly patients. The role of mosquitoes in viral transmission was clearly delineated in a series of field studies in Egypt in the 1950s. Wild birds were identified as the reservoir of the virus around the same time. Cases of West Nile fever in horses were reported several years later. WNV was first associated with disease in domestic avian species in 1997, when flocks of young geese in Israel were affected with a neuroparalytic disease. In August 1999, the disease appeared for the first time in the Western hemisphere when wild and zoo birds, horses, and people died in the northeast USA, notably in the New York City area.

Etiology and Epidemiology: WNV is considered to be endemic in many countries of Africa, Asia, southern Europe, and North America. Since 2001, serologic evidence of the spread of WNV into Latin America, the Caribbean, and South America has been reported. Epidemics appear in the human population at infrequent intervals in some of these countries, and there is evidence of viral transmission between Africa and Europe by migrating birds. Most outbreaks have occurred during the summer months and can continue until cold nights reduce mosquito vector activity, notably *Culex* spp.

Geese are the only known natural hosts of WNV among domestic avian species. Most of the flocks affected in the Israel outbreaks were 5–9 wk old, but goslings as young as 3 wk and as old as 11 wk were also affected.

Adult breeding flocks were clinically unaffected, but virus-neutralizing antibodies were found. Mortality of young Muscovy ducks but not young chickens or turkey poults was induced experimentally with a WNV isolate. While chickens are not killed by WNV, they do develop antibodies against the disease and have been used as sentinels to monitor WNV presence. Neither chickens nor turkeys develop high enough levels of viremia to infect mosquitoes or transmit the virus to other animals.

Transmission: The principal route of viral transmission is by the bite of a mosquito (primarily *Culex* spp). In the USA during 1999 and 2000, most of the viral isolates were made from *C pipiens* and *C restvans*. WNV has been isolated, RNA detected, or antibodies found in 62 mosquito species in North America. In Africa and the Middle East, the usual vector is *C univittatus*, and in Europe, *C pipiens* and *C modestus*. WNV has also been isolated from at least 10 tick species.

Clinical Findings: Affected geese show various degrees of neurologic involvement ranging from recumbency to leg and wing paralysis. Affected birds are either reluctant or unable to move when disturbed. Signs of incoordination are pronounced, and some birds flip over while attempting to stand. Naturally affected geese show torticollis and opisthotonos. Mortality rates of 20%–60% have been reported, probably due to horizontal spread of the virus.

Lesions: Pathologic changes include splenomegaly, hepatomegaly, and pallor of the myocardium and occasionally of the kidneys. The meningeal blood vessels are injected. Microscopic brain lesions consist of lymphocytic perivascular infiltration and neuronal degeneration. Small necrotic foci are present in the myocardium, but lymphocytic infiltration is minimal.

Diagnosis: The tissues of choice to isolate the virus from paralytic or dead birds are the brain, spleen, and kidneys. Homogenates are inoculated into the brain of newborn mice, into embryonated eggs by the yolk sac route, or into Vero and mosquito cell line cultures. Reverse transcriptase PCR with RNA extracted from either brain material or cell culture supernatant can also be performed. Gene expression assays/probes for rapid molecular diagnosis of field-collected mosquitoes and avian tissues are also available. Immunohistochemistry can be used on formalin-fixed paraffin-embedded tissues, in particular brain and kidney, to visualize viral antigens in infected birds. Several forms of ELISA have also been developed for flaviviruses.

Neurologic signs in young geese must be distinguished from those caused by *Riemerella* infections, especially *R anatipestifer*. Other bacteria include *Streptococcus gallolyticus*, and *Erysipelothrix*, *Listeria*, and *Salmonella* spp. Neurotropic viruses include Newcastle disease, which is rare in geese, and avian influenza. Ionophore intoxication can induce paralytic signs. *Aspergillus* also causes brain lesions and caseous nodules in the lungs.

Prevention and Control: Mosquito control is a mandatory component of any arboviral disease control program. Unfortunately, this is difficult to implement in a rural environment because of the distances that mosquitoes can fly or be carried by prevailing winds. Standing water and similar insect breeding sites in the vicinity of densely populated avian farms should be treated with larvicides. Poultry houses should be constructed to be insect free. Because many arboviral diseases are zoonoses, much can be achieved by cooperation with human disease surveillance agencies.

Control of WNV in geese is confined to vaccinating young flocks at risk, especially those raised during months when *Culex* spp are most numerous. Because of confounding factors such as possible horizontal transmission of virus, all birds in the flock should be vaccinated. Because of the age-related susceptibility to the virus, goslings should be immunized as young as possible, preferably at 3 wk old. Currently, WNV vaccines are not available commercially in North America, although several types have been developed and widely used in domestic geese in Israel. Laboratory trials have been performed with a formaldehyde-inactivated suckling mouse brain–derived product. More than 75% of geese vaccinated with a single dose of vaccine at 3 wk of age were protected, and 94% protection was achieved with 2 doses given 2 wk apart. Inactivated vaccines prepared from chick embryos or Vero cells are not protective because of their low antigenic mass. Other vaccines either approved for use in geese or under study include poxvirus vector vaccines and subunit vaccines that use WNV components such as membrane protein or envelope protein.

ARTIFICIAL INSEMINATION

Artificial insemination (AI) is widely used to overcome low fertility in commercial turkeys, which results from unsuccessful mating as a consequence of large, heavily muscled birds being unable to physically complete the mating process. This is a serious and costly problem in the production of commercial turkey hatching eggs. In most commercial chicken production systems in the USA, it has not been necessary to implement AI programs because natural mating results in adequate fertility levels, but AI is routinely used in special breeding work and research. However, as managing commercial broiler breeders to maximize fertility becomes more challenging, the use of AI in commercial poultry operations outside the USA is becoming more common. Certainly, the use of AI in chickens, as in turkeys, can improve fertility; however, the cost of implementing AI on a large scale is often cost prohibitive.

Collecting semen from a chicken or turkey is done by stimulating the copulatory organ (the phallus) to protrude by massaging the abdomen and the back over the testes. This is followed quickly by pushing the tail forward with one hand and, at the same time, using the thumb and forefinger of the same hand to apply pressure in the area and to "milk" semen from the ducts of this organ. Semen flow response is quicker and easier to stimulate in chickens than in turkeys. The semen may be collected with an aspirator (turkeys) or in a small tube or any cup-like container. In turkeys, the volume averages ~0.35–0.5 mL, with a spermatozoon concentration of 6 to >8 billion/mL. In chickens, volume is 1–2 times that of turkeys, but the concentration is about one-half. Collected semen is usually pooled and diluted with an extender before use.

Chicken and turkey semen begins to lose fertilizing ability when stored >1 hr. Liquid cold (4°C) storage of turkey and chicken semen can be used to transport semen and maintain spermatozoal viability for ~6–12 hr. This short-term storage of semen is common in turkeys, while not as common in chickens. When using liquid cold storage for >1 hr, turkey semen must be diluted with a semen extender at least 1:1 and then agitated slowly (150 rpm) to facilitate oxygenation; chicken semen should be diluted and then cooled—agitation is not necessary. Chicken and turkey semen may be frozen, but reduced fertility limits usage to special breeding projects. Under experimental conditions, fertility levels of 90% have been obtained in hens inseminated at 3-day intervals with 400–500 million frozen-thawed chicken spermatozoa.

Several commercial semen extenders are available and are routinely used, particularly for turkeys. Extenders enable more precise control over inseminating dose and facilitate filling of tubes. Results may be comparable to those using undiluted semen when product directions are followed. Dilution should result in an insemination dose containing ~300 million viable spermatozoa for turkeys. However, the number of spermatozoa inseminated will range from 150–300 million viable cells depending on the age of the turkey hens inseminated. In chickens, the number of diluted semen inseminated will range from ~100–200 million sperm cells per insemination. Producers usually determine the spermatozoa concentration and dilute the semen to obtain the appropriate sperm cell concentration for either the turkey or chicken.

For insemination, when holding the hen upright, pressure is applied to the abdomen around the vent, particularly on the left side. This causes the cloaca to evert and the oviduct to protrude, so that a syringe or plastic straw can be inserted ~1 in. (2.5 cm) into the oviduct and the appropriate amount of semen delivered. As the semen is expelled by the inseminator, pressure around the vent is released, which assists the hen in retaining sperm in the vagina or oviduct. When inseminating undiluted turkey semen, the high sperm cell concentration allows for 0.025 mL (~2 billion spermatozoa) to be inseminated at regular intervals of 7–10 days, yielding optimal fertility. In chickens, because of the lower spermatozoon concentration and shorter duration of fertility, 0.05 mL of undiluted pooled semen, at intervals of 7 days, is required. The hen's squatting behavior indicates receptivity and the time for the first insemination. For maximal fertility, inseminations may be started before the initial oviposition in turkeys, whereas this is not necessary in chickens. Fertility tends to decrease later in the season; therefore, it may be justified to inseminate more frequently or use more cells per insemination dose as hens age.

DISORDERS OF THE REPRODUCTIVE SYSTEM

CYSTIC RIGHT OVIDUCT

Fluid accumulation in the vestigial right oviduct is a common finding in hens. The abdominal cyst is filled with clear fluid and is attached to the right side of the cloacal wall. The cyst may vary in size from barely perceptible to 15–20 cm in diameter. An increased incidence has been seen in flocks after infectious bronchitis virus outbreaks. Oviductal cysts are a necropsy finding that rarely, if ever, affect flock performance.

DEFECTIVE OR ABNORMAL EGGS

Most "ridged," "sunburst," "slab-sided," soft-shelled, or double-shelled eggs are the result of eggs colliding in the shell gland region of the oviduct when an ovum (yolk) is released too soon after the previous one. Necropsy examinations have demonstrated that two full-sized eggs can be found in the shell gland pouch. As the second egg comes in contact with the first, pressure is exerted, disrupting the pattern of mineralization. The first egg acquires a white band and chalky appearance, while the second egg is flattened on its contiguous surface (ie, slab-sided). Pimpled or rough eggs may have been retained too long in the shell gland. Blood spots result when a follicle vessel along the stigma ruptures as the ovum is being released. Meat spots occur when a piece of follicle membrane or residual albumen from the previous day is incorporated into the developing egg.

Many abnormalities appear to have no specific cause, but the incidence is much higher in hens subjected to stressful management conditions, rough handling, or vaccination during production. A significant increase in the number of soft-shelled eggs is also common as a result of viral diseases such as infectious bronchitis, egg drop syndrome, and Newcastle disease.

Small eggs with no yolk form around a nidus of material (residual albumen) in the magnum of the oviduct. Small eggs with reduced albumen and eggs with defective shells may be the result of damage to the epithelium of the magnum or shell gland.

Very rarely, foreign material that enters the oviduct through the vagina (eg, a roundworm) may be incorporated into an egg.

EGG-BOUND OR IMPACTED OVIDUCTS

A fully formed egg may lodge in the shell gland or vagina because the egg is too big (eg, double-yolked) or because of hypocalcemia, calcium tetany, or previous trauma (usually pecking) to the vent and/or vagina that obstructs oviposition. This condition may be more prevalent in young hens that are brought into production before body development is adequate or in hens that are overweight or obese. It occurs more often during spring and summer months because of overstimulation of birds by increasing light intensity and day length, which can be compounded by rapid increases in the amount of feed and/or excessive protein (lysine). This is a medical emergency in pet birds but is usually recognized only during necropsy in commercial poultry. When impaction occurs, eggs that continue to form create layers of albumen and yolk material, and the oviduct becomes very large. Some eggs are refluxed to the abdominal cavity (abdominal laying), and affected hens assume a penguin-like posture.

EGG PERITONITIS

(Egg yolk peritonitis)

Egg peritonitis is characterized by fibrin or albumen-like material with a cooked appearance among the abdominal viscera. It is a common cause of sporadic death in layers or breeder hens, but in some flocks may become the major cause of death before or after reaching peak production and give the appearance of a contagious disease. It is diagnosed at necropsy. Peritonitis follows reverse movement of albumen and *Escherichia coli* bacteria from the oviduct into the abdomen. If the incidence is high, culture should be done to differentiate between *Pasteurella* (fowl cholera) or *Salmonella* infection. Antibiotic treatment of peritonitis caused by *E coli* infections is usually ineffective. Management of body weight and uniformity, reproductive development (ovary follicle growth and maturation), and drinking water sanitation are the best preventive strategies.

When hens have too many large ovarian follicles, a problem described as erratic oviposition and defective egg syndrome (EODES) is seen in broiler breeders. This condition is accompanied by a high incidence of double-yolked eggs, prolapses of the oviduct, internal ovulation, and/or internal laying that often results in egg peritonitis and mortality. EODES is prevented by avoiding light stimulation of underweight pullets too early and by following guidelines for body weight and uniformity, and lighting recommendations for each breeder strain. Overweight hens may also have a higher incidence of erratic ovulations and mortality associated with egg peritonitis.

FALSE LAYER

These hens ovulate normally, but the yolk is dropped into the abdominal cavity rather than being collected by the oviduct because of inflammation and resulting obstruction of the oviduct after infection with *Escherichia coli* or *Mycoplasma gallisepticum*. The yolk is absorbed from the abdominal cavity. The hen looks like a normal layer but does not produce eggs. Hypoplasia of the ovary and oviduct has been associated with infectious bronchitis virus infections (*see* p 2909) at an early age (1–2 wk). Atresia or even atrophy of the ovary are caused by severe stress, chronic infections, insufficient feed intake, inadequate feeder space, and feed refusal due to mycotoxins in the feed.

HYPOCALCEMIA, SUDDEN DEATH, OSTEOPOROSIS, OR CAGE LAYER FATIGUE

Pullets or hens with insufficient dietary calcium, phosphorus, or vitamin D_3 may die suddenly or be found paralyzed from hypocalcemia while shelling an egg. This may be associated with high production and withdrawal of calcium from bones for egg shell production, in which case the main lesion may be osteoporosis. At necropsy, there is an egg in the shell gland and the ova are active and fully developed. There are no other lesions, although medullary bone may be lacking. Paralyzed hens respond to calcium IV, and this response may be useful in diagnosis.

Osteoporosis is a major cause of death in high-production flocks. Hens with osteoporosis may show similar signs at necropsy, or the ova may be regressing with no egg in the oviduct. The femur is always fragile, and medullary bone is always absent in osteoporosis. These hens may also respond to calcium IV if there are no fractures of the legs or vertebrae. The use of large particle size calcium (limestone, oyster shell) in the diet may be beneficial. High rates of mortality due to fractures are common in birds affected with osteoporosis. This situation is more common in broiler breeder hens in slatted houses due to the trauma caused by jumping on and off the slats. Ruptured egg follicles indicating trauma can be found during necropsy examination of these birds.

A condition known as hypocalcemia or calcium tetany (paralysis) has been seen in modern or high-yielding broiler breeder hens. Signs such as panting, spread wings, and prostration may be seen in the early morning hours preceding paralysis and death by asphyxia. Careful postmortem examination reveals a fully active ovary and the presence of a partially or fully formed egg in the shell gland in the absence of other lesions. This indicates that the hen used all available calcium from the bloodstream in an effort to complete the egg shell. The condition is common in flocks with poor body weight uniformity that are fed high-calcium diets in the weeks before the onset of lay and brought into production by drastic increases in day length and feed allocation. Hypocalcemia can be prevented by management practices that promote body weight uniformity and avoid excessive/premature allocation of high-calcium diets and light stimulation. Mortality can be reduced by the administration ("topping of the feed") of 5 g of oyster shell per hen for 3 consecutive days, and addition of vitamin D_3 to the drinking water. This treatment should be suspended for 3 days and then repeated. Severe cases will require continual treatment for 2–3 wk (3 days of treatment followed by 3 days without). Feeding of recommended levels of calcium, using large-particle-size calcium, and providing adequate ventilation and cooling are helpful to prevent or reduce the incidence of this condition.

Mortality and the presence of an egg in the shell gland also can be caused by a condition referred to as sudden death syndrome, first reported in Australia. This is believed to be caused by marginal levels of potassium and phosphorus in the diet, resulting in cardiomyopathy.

INTERNAL LAYER

In these hens, partially or fully formed eggs are found in the abdominal cavity. Such eggs reach the cavity by reverse peristalsis of the oviduct. If they have no shell, they are often misshapen because of partial or complete absorption of the contents. Frequently, only empty shell membranes are present. No control or treatment is known. This condition is related to erratic ovulation and defective egg syndrome (*see* p 2896).

INFERTILITY

Infertility caused by male management problems is common. Problems may be caused by an inadequate number of healthy males or because males have reduced sperm production resulting from chronic disease, inadequate feed intake, or starvation (harsh feed restriction). However, obese females may be less efficient in transporting sperm to the infundibulum, resulting in reduced fertilization of the ovum as it is released from the ovary. The male must be dominant to the females, or mating will not occur. Commercial turkey hens are inseminated artificially with semen collected from the toms and used the same day (*see* p 2895). Parthenogenesis is responsible for some infertility in turkeys. There are host sperm glands in the oviduct of females, and live sperm can be retained for 3–4 wk. Waterfowl have a rudimentary penis, and prolapse of the penis is occasionally reported in drakes. There is no treatment.

NEOPLASIA

The most frequent tumor of the reproductive system is adenocarcinoma of the oviduct. Neoplastic cells are shed from tumors in the oviduct into the abdominal cavity. They implant on the ovary, pancreas, and other viscera and produce multiple, hard, yellow nodules. They may block lymph return and result in ascites. The incidence increases with age, and this tumor may be a frequent cause of death after 2 yr. Affected hens are condemned at processing.

Leiomyoma of the broad ligament is an estrogen-induced hypertrophy of the smooth muscle of the broad ligament. It is benign and is an incidental finding at necropsy or processing.

A variety of ovarian and testicular tumors has been described. Marek's disease (*see* p 2849) is a common cause of tumors of the ovary.

OOPHORITIS AND OVARY REGRESSION

Regression of the ovary may result in leakage of free yolk into the abdomen (yolk peritonitis); this rarely causes death except when yolk material migrates through the air sacs to the lung and causes foreign body pneumonia. Free yolk is seen in many cases of acute illness, injury, or forced molt. Regression of the ovary is frequently caused by low body weight, deliberate reduction of feed, overcrowding, or lack of feeder space. Infectious diseases such as Newcastle disease, fowl cholera, pullorum disease, and avian influenza are known to cause this condition. It can also result from severe stress, which is often accompanied by feather molt, emaciation, and dehydration.

PROLAPSE OF THE OVIDUCT

When an egg is laid, the vagina everts through the cloaca to deliver the egg. If there has been injury to the vagina, such as from a large or double-yolk egg, or if the hen is fat, the vagina may not retract immediately, leaving it exposed for a short time. This may result in cannibalism (*see* p 2873). When the protruding organ is pecked by other hens, the complete oviduct and parts of the adjacent intestinal tract may be pulled from the abdominal cavity ("peckout"). Bleeding from the vent is observed as a result of pecking. Alternatively, the vagina swells, cannot retract, and remains prolapsed ("blowout"). The hen dies from shock. Prolapse has been associated with excessive/premature photostimulation, poor body weight uniformity, early laying (inadequate body size), large eggs, double-yolked eggs, and obesity. Cannibalism may be prevented by beak trimming, managing light intensity, maintaining appropriate stocking density, and avoiding nutritional deficiencies.

SALPINGITIS

Salpingitis is an inflammation of the oviduct, which may contain liquid or caseous exudate. In young pullets, it is often due to *Mycoplasma gallisepticum*, *Escherichia coli*, *Salmonella* spp, or *Pasteurella multocida* (fowl cholera) infection and can result in reduced egg production. It is a frequent lesion in female broilers and ducks at processing. On gross examination, salpingitis may be difficult to differentiate from impacted oviduct in adults. As the oviduct becomes nonfunctional, the ovaries are usually atrophied. Unless associated with an infectious problem, this condition tends to be found sporadically during necropsy of cull hens.

SEX REVERSAL

If the normal left ovary of a hen is destroyed by infection, the vestigial right organ may develop as a testicle and the hen may develop male characteristics. Neoplasia in the adrenal glands or ovary that result in the production of testosterone could also cause the development of male secondary sexual characteristics (comb and wattles) in affected females.

EGG DROP SYNDROME '76

Egg drop syndrome '76 (EDS '76) is an atadenovirus-induced disease characterized by the production of pale, soft-shelled, and shell-less eggs by apparently healthy laying hens. The disease in laying hens has commonly been called "egg drop syndrome," but the full name (egg drop syndrome '76 [EDS '76]) should be used to distinguish it from the recently recognized flaviviral disease of ducks, which has been called "egg drop syndrome in ducks," and "duck egg drop syndrome," creating potential for confusion.

Etiology: EDS '76 is caused by a double-stranded DNA virus, duck adenovirus 1 (also known as EDSV), which belongs to the genus *Atadenovirus*. The virus commonly infects both wild and domestic ducks and geese, but evidence of infection has also been found in coots, grebes, herring gulls, owls, storks, swans, and quail. The adenovirus group antigen cannot be demonstrated by conventional means, and EDSV differs from other avian adenoviruses by strongly agglutinating avian RBCs, a fact that allows use of a hemagglutination-inhibition test for detection of antibodies to the virus. The virus grows to high titers in embryonated duck and goose eggs and in cell cultures of duck or goose origin. It replicates well in chick-embryo liver cells, less well in chick kidney cells, and comparatively poorly in chick-embryo fibroblasts. It does not grow in embryonated chicken eggs or in mammalian cells. The virus is resistant to pH range 3–10 and to heating for 3 hr at 56°C (132.8°F). Infectivity is lost after treatment with 0.5% formaldehyde or 0.5% glutaraldehyde.

Only one serotype of EDSV has been recognized to date.

Epidemiology and Pathogenesis: The natural hosts for EDSV are ducks and geese. It is thought that the virus was introduced to chickens through a vaccine that had been grown in contaminated duck-embryo fibroblasts. The virus became established in chickens, causing substantial problems with egg shell quality and loss of eggs. All ages and breeds of chickens are susceptible to infection. Disease tends to be most severe in heavy broiler-breeders and hens producing brown eggs. Japanese quail (*Coturnix coturnix japonica*) also develop disease. There are rare reports that the egg drop syndrome virus (EDSV) has caused either a drop in egg production or respiratory tract disease in other species, eg, turkeys, ducks, geese, and quail.

Three patterns of disease are recognized in chickens: 1) Classical EDS '76 occurs when primary breeding stock are infected and the virus is transmitted vertically through the egg. The virus often remains latent until the progeny chick reaches sexual maturity, at which time the virus is excreted in the eggs and droppings, infecting susceptible contacts. 2) Endemic EDS is the result of horizontal infection of the flock during lay. It is usually seen in commercial egg layers. Contaminated egg collection trays are one of the main vehicles of horizontal transmission between flocks, and outbreaks are often associated with a common egg-packing station. 3) Sporadic EDS '76 has been recognized occasionally in flocks. This is due either to direct contact with domestic ducks or geese or, more often, to use of a water supply contaminated with wildfowl droppings. Although infection by this route is uncommon, there is always a risk that these introductions of the virus could form a starting point for endemic disease.

The main method of horizontal spread is through contaminated eggs or equipment such as trays, crates, trucks, or personnel. Droppings are also infective. The virus can be transmitted by bleeding or vaccination needles. Insect transmission may be possible but has not been proved.

After horizontal infection, the virus grows to low titers in the nasal mucosa. This is followed by viremia, virus replication in lymphoid tissue, and then massive replication for ~5 days in the pouch shell gland. Changes in the egg shell coincide with viral replication in the shell gland. Both the exterior and interior of eggs produced between 8 and ~18 days after infection contain virus. Exudate and secretions from the oviduct are rich in virus and pass into the droppings, which may become mildly to moderately watery for 2–3 days. Unlike other fowl adenoviruses, there is little, if any, virus growth in the epithelial cells of the intestine. Interestingly, the massive viral replication in the pouch shell gland occurs after seroconversion, a fact that is useful diagnostically.

Chicks hatched from infected eggs may excrete virus and develop antibody. More often, the virus remains latent, and antibody does not develop until the bird starts to lay, at which time the virus reactivates and grows in the oviduct, repeating the cycle.

Clinical Findings: In flocks without antibody, the first sign of the disease is the production of pale-shelled eggs, quickly followed by production of soft-shelled and shell-less eggs. Internal quality of eggs is unaffected in experimentally induced disease. Transient dullness may be seen in the days before the shell changes are noticed. The thin-shelled and shell-less eggs are fragile, and the birds tend to eat them; these eggs also may get trampled into litter and may be overlooked unless a careful examination is made. Although it has been shown experimentally that eggs usually continue to be produced at a normal rate (so the disease name may be a misnomer), the number of useable eggs produced falls by 10%–40%. Egg production by the flock usually returns to normal. In flocks in which there has been some spread of virus and some of the birds have antibody (usually 10%–20%), the condition is seen as a failure to achieve predicted production targets; careful examination shows that these flocks experience a series of small group episodes of infection and disease. Birds with antibody slow the spread of virus.

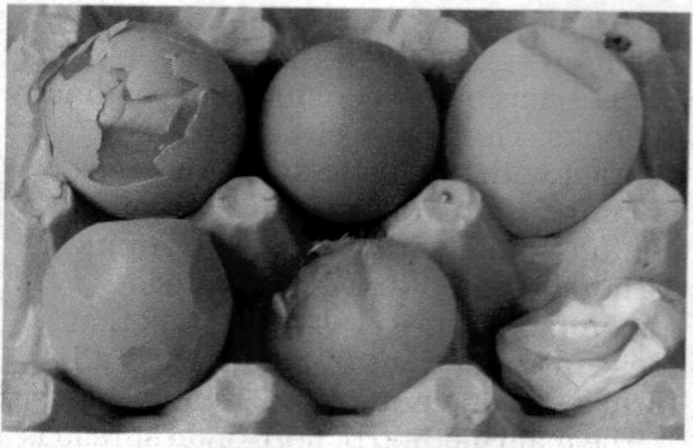

Eggs produced by hens in a flock with EDS'76. One normal egg is present (center, back row). Affected eggs include pale and thin-shelled eggs and shell-less eggs. The contents of the egg at the bottom right have been lost, leaving a thick, collapsed shell membrane. *Courtesy of Dr. Joan Smyth.*

There is no effect on fertility or hatchability of those eggs with a shell quality that is satisfactory for setting.

Diagnosis: Production of pale, thin-shelled and shell-less eggs by a flock that appears otherwise healthy should raise strong suspicion of EDS '76. Transient mild depression and/or mild watery droppings may be noted. Ridged eggs and poor internal quality are not features of EDS '76. Poor egg shell quality at peak production in healthy hens should also raise strong suspicion of classical EDS '76. With endemic or sporadic EDS '76, disease can develop in laying hens of any age. In cage units, spread can be slow, and the signs may be overlooked or perceived as a small depression (2%–4%) of egg yield.

Clinically, EDS '76 can be distinguished from Newcastle disease (*see* p 2856) and influenza virus infections (*see* p 2902) by the absence of illness, and from infectious bronchitis (*see* p 2909) by the absence of respiratory signs, the absence of ridged and malformed eggs, and the absence of poor internal egg quality. Confirmatory laboratory testing is needed for definitive diagnosis. Searching for evidence of seroconversion is the easiest diagnostic approach for nonvaccinated flocks. When selecting birds for diagnosis, especially in cage units, it is important to target hens that have produced affected eggs, because if the problem is due to EDSV infection, these hens will already have seroconverted. A hemagglutination-inhibition test using fowl RBCs, and ELISA, are the serologic tests of choice. In addition, the serum neutralization test can be used for confirmation. The double immunodiffusion test also has been used. PCR-based tests and antigen capture ELISA tests have been used to detect EDSV DNA and antigen, respectively. Again, appropriate selection of the hens to be examined is very important. EDSV can be isolated by inoculating embryonated duck or goose eggs or duck- or chick-embryo liver cell cultures. It is important to select recently infected birds for testing, but these can be difficult to identify, especially if the birds are on litter. An easier method is to feed affected eggs to antibody-free hens. These hens can then be tested for seroconversion after the first abnormal eggs are produced, or tested for evidence of EDSV DNA or antigen by PCR or antigen capture ELISA, respectively, or virus isolation can be attempted from the pouch shell gland of these hens.

Control: There is no treatment for EDS '76. The classic form has been eradicated from primary breeders. Use of dedicated equipment and egg trays for each farm, and/or washing and disinfecting plastic egg trays before use, can help to control the endemic form. The sporadic form can be prevented by separating chickens from other birds, especially waterfowl. General sanitary precautions are indicated, and potentially contaminated water should be chlorinated before use.

Inactivated vaccines with oil adjuvant are available and, if properly administered, successfully prevent the disease. They reduce but do not prevent virus shedding. These vaccines are given during the growing period, usually at 14–18 wk of age, and can be combined with other vaccines, such as those for Newcastle disease. Sentinel chickens may be placed along with vaccinated chickens and periodically checked for antibodies, which would allow detection of the presence of virus in the flock.

AIR SAC MITE

Cytodites nudus is a small cosmopolitan mite occasionally noticed as white spots on the bronchi, lungs, air sacs, and abdominal organs of chickens, turkeys, pheasants, pigeons, canaries, and mallards. (*See also* p 1906.) These mites are readily transmissible between birds through coughing. They are rarely found in commercial industries. The 14- to 21-day life cycle involves a larval and two nymphal stages. Infestation densities vary, and clinical signs range from none to weakness, weight loss, pneumonia, peritonitis, pulmonary edema, and death. Recommended treatments include ivermectin, a nearby dichlorvos pest strip (placed out of reach of the birds), topical moxidectin, or a pyrethrin/piperonyl butoxide spray.

ASPERGILLOSIS

(Brooder pneumonia, Mycotic pneumonia, Pneumomycosis)

Aspergillosis is a disease, usually of the respiratory system, of chickens, turkeys, and less frequently ducklings, pigeons, canaries, geese, and many other wild and pet birds. In chickens and turkeys, the disease may be endemic on some farms; in wild birds, it appears to be sporadic, frequently affecting only an individual bird. Severe outbreaks usually occur in birds 7–40 days old. (*See also* ASPERGILLOSIS in mammals, p 633, and in PET BIRDS, p 1899.)

Etiology and Epidemiology: *Aspergillus fumigatus* is a common cause of the disease. However, several other *Aspergillus* spp may be incriminated.

High mortality rates are seen in chicks and poults that inhale large numbers of spores during hatching in contaminated incubators or when placed on mold-bearing litter. In older birds, infection is caused primarily by inhalation of spore-laden dust from contaminated litter or feed or dusty range areas. Morbidity can be underestimated in finishing flocks until slaughter inspection reveals pulmonary lesions.

Clinical Findings and Lesions: Dyspnea, hyperpnea, somnolence and other signs of nervous system involvement, inappetence, emaciation, and increased thirst may be seen. In chicks or poults up to 6 wk old, the lungs are most frequently involved. Airsacculitis is a cause of postmortem condemnation in young mature turkeys intended for food supply. Pulmonary lesions are characterized by white to yellow plaques and nodules a few mm to several cm in diameter; occasionally, mycelial masses may be seen within the air passages on gross examination. The plaques and nodules also may be found in the syrinx, air sacs, liver, intestines, and occasionally the brain. The encephalitic form is most common in turkeys. An ocular form is seen in chickens and turkeys as mycotic keratitis, in which large plaques may be expressed from the medial canthus.

Diagnosis: The fungus can be demonstrated by culture or by microscopic examination of fresh preparations. One of the plaques is teased apart and placed on a suitable medium, usually resulting in a pure culture of the organism. Histopathologic examination using a special fungus stain reveals granulomas containing mycelia.

Differential diagnoses include infectious bronchitis, Newcastle disease, infectious laryngotracheitis, mycobacteriosis, colibacillosis, other mycoses (eg, ochroconosis, zygomycosis), and nutritional encephalomalacia.

Treatment and Control: Treatment of affected birds is generally ineffective. Spontaneous recovery from pulmonary aspergillosis can occur if reexposure to the mold is prevented. Strict adherence to sanitation procedures in the hatchery minimizes early outbreaks. Grossly contaminated or cracked eggs should not be set for incubation, because they enable bacterial and fungal growth and may explode and disseminate spores throughout the hatching machine. Contaminated hatchers should be thoroughly cleaned and fumigated with enilconazole or formaldehyde. Avoiding moldy litter or ranges serves to prevent outbreaks in older birds. Cleaned pens should be sprayed or fumigated with enilconazole following label directions, and all equipment should be cleaned and disinfected.

AVIAN INFLUENZA

Avian influenza (AI) viruses infect domestic poultry as well as pet, zoo, and wild birds. In domestic poultry, AI viruses are typically of low pathogenicity (LP), causing subclinical infections, respiratory disease, or drops in egg production. However, a few AI viruses cause severe systemic infections with high mortality. This highly pathogenic (HP) form of the disease has historically been called fowl plague. In most wild birds, AI viral infections are subclinical except for the recent H5N1 HP AI viruses of Eurasian lineage.

Etiology: AI viruses are type A orthomyxoviruses characterized by antigenically homologous nucleoprotein and matrix internal proteins, which are identified by serology in agar gel immunodiffusion (AGID) tests. AI viruses are further divided into 16 hemagglutinin (H1-16) and 9 neuraminidase (N1-9) subtypes based on hemagglutinin inhibition and neuraminidase inhibition tests, respectively. Most AI viruses (H1-16 subtypes) are of low pathogenicity, but some of the H5 and H7 AI viruses are highly pathogenic for chickens, turkeys, and related gallinaceous domestic poultry.

Epidemiology and Transmission: LP AI viruses are distributed worldwide and are recovered frequently from clinically normal shorebirds and migrating waterfowl. Occasionally, LP viruses are recovered from imported pet birds and ratites. The viruses may be present in village or backyard flocks and other birds sold through live-poultry markets, but most commercially raised poultry in developed countries are free of AI viruses. The HP viruses arise from mutation of some H5 and H7 LP viruses and cause devastating epidemics. Stamping-out programs are used to quickly eliminate the HP viruses in developed countries, but some developing countries may use vaccines to control HP viruses.

The incubation period is highly variable and ranges from a few days in individual birds to 2 wk in the flock. Transmission between individual birds is by ingestion or inhalation. Naturally and experimentally, cats and dogs have been infected with one strain of H5N1 Eurasian HP AI virus. Experimental infections occurred after respiratory exposure, ingestion of infected chickens, or contact exposure, but cats were more susceptible than dogs. Potentially, domestic pets could serve as a transmission vector between farms, but the ability of other AI viruses, including other H5N1 strains, to infect pets is unknown. Other mammals that have been experimentally infected include pigs, ferrets, rats, rabbits, guinea pigs, mice, mink, and nonhuman primates. Transmission between farms is the result of breaches in biosecurity practices, principally by movement of infected poultry or contaminated feces and respiratory secretions on fomites such as equipment or clothing. Airborne dissemination between farms may be important over limited distances. Limited spread by wild birds of the Eurasian H5N1 HP AI virus has been suggested but is not typical of other HP AI viruses. Other HP AI and all LP AI have minimal potential to infect dogs and cats.

Clinical Findings and Lesions: Clinical signs, severity of disease, and mortality rates vary depending on AI virus strain and host species.

Low Pathogenicity Avian Influenza Viruses: LP AI viruses typically produce respiratory signs such as sneezing, coughing, ocular and nasal discharge, and swollen infraorbital sinuses in poultry. Sinusitis is common in domestic ducks, quail, and turkeys. Lesions in the respiratory tract typically include congestion and inflammation of the trachea and lungs. In layers and breeders, there may be decreased egg production or fertility, ova rupture (evident as yolk in the abdominal cavity) or involution, or mucosal edema and inflammatory exudates in the lumen of the oviduct. A few layer and breeder chickens may have acute renal failure and visceral urate deposition (visceral gout). The morbidity and mortality is usually low unless accompanied by secondary bacterial or viral infections or aggravated by environmental stressors. Sporadic infections by any subtype of LP AI viruses can occur, but H9N2 LP AI is common in poultry in Asia, the Middle East, and North Africa.

High Pathogenicity Avian Influenza Viruses: Even in the absence of secondary pathogens, HP AI viruses cause severe, systemic disease with high mortality in chickens, turkeys, and other gallinaceous poultry; mortality can be as high as 100% in a few days. In peracute cases, clinical signs or gross lesions may be lacking before death. However, in acute cases, lesions may include cyanosis and edema of the head, comb, wattle, and snood (turkey); edema and red discoloration of the shanks and feet due to subcutaneous ecchymotic hemorrhages; petechial hemorrhages on visceral organs and in muscles; and blood-tinged oral and nasal discharges. In severely affected birds, greenish diarrhea is common. Birds that survive the peracute infection may develop CNS involvement evident as torticollis, opisthotonos, incoordination, paralysis, and drooping wings. The location and severity of microscopic lesions are highly variable and may consist of edema, hemorrhage, and necrosis in parenchymal cells of multiple visceral organs, skin, and CNS.

Diagnosis: LP and HP AI viruses can be readily isolated from oropharyngeal and cloacal swabs, and HP AI viruses from many internal organs. AI viruses grow well in the allantoic sac of 9- to 11-day-old embryonating chicken eggs, and they agglutinate RBCs. The hemagglutination is not inhibited by Newcastle disease or other paramyxoviral antiserum. AI viruses are identified by demonstrating the presence of 1) influenza A matrix or nucleoprotein antigens using AGID or other suitable immunoassays, or 2) viral RNA using an influenza A–specific reverse transcriptase-PCR test.

LP AI must be differentiated from other respiratory diseases or causes of decreased egg production, including 1) acute to subacute viral diseases such as infectious bronchitis, infectious laryngotracheitis, low virulent Newcastle disease, and infections by other paramyxoviruses; 2) bacterial diseases such as mycoplasmosis, infectious coryza, ornithobacteriosis, turkey coryza, and the respiratory form of fowl cholera; and 3) fungal diseases such as aspergillosis. HP AI must be differentiated from other causes of high mortality such as virulent Newcastle disease, peracute septicemic fowl cholera, heat exhaustion, and severe water deprivation.

Prevention and Treatment: Vaccines can prevent clinical signs and death. Further-

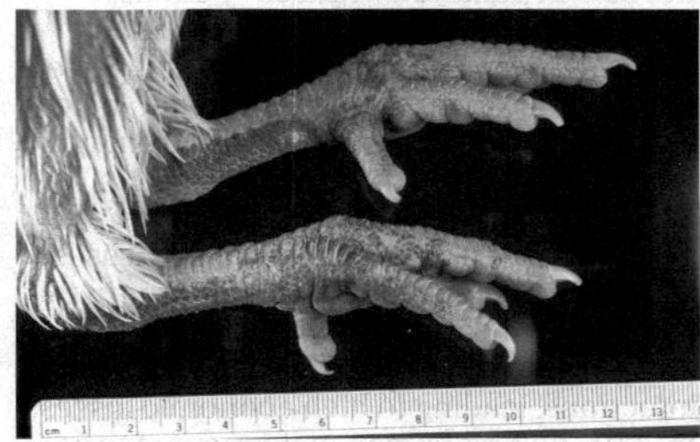

Hemorrhagic skin visible on the feet of a chicken with avian influenza. *Courtesy of Dr. David E. Swayne.*

more, viral replication and shedding from the respiratory and GI tracts may be reduced in vaccinated birds. Specific protection is achieved through autogenous virus vaccines or from vaccines prepared from AI virus of the same hemagglutinin subtype. Antibodies to the homologous viral neuraminidase antigens may provide partial protection. Currently, only inactivated whole AI virus, recombinant fowlpox-AI-H5, and recombinant herpesvirus-turkey-AI-H5 (rHVT-AI-H5) vaccines are licensed in the USA. The use of any licensed AI vaccine requires approval of the State Veterinarian. In addition, use of H5 and H7 AI vaccines in the USA requires USDA approval. Treating LP-affected flocks with broad-spectrum antibiotics to control secondary pathogens and increasing house temperatures may reduce morbidity and mortality. Treatment with antiviral compounds is not approved or recommended. Suspected outbreaks should be reported to appropriate regulatory authorities.

Zoonotic Risk: AI viruses exhibit host adaptation to birds. Human infections have occurred, usually as isolated, rare, individual cases. Most human cases have originated from infection with Eurasian H5N1 HP AI virus and, most recently, Chinese H7N9 LP AI virus. The total accumulated human cases of H5N1 HP AI virus in Asia and Africa from 2003–2013 is 648, of which 384 were fatal. The primary risk factor for human infection has been direct contact with live or dead infected poultry, but a few cases have resulted from consumption of uncooked poultry products, defeathering of infected wild swans, or close contact with human cases. Respiratory infection has been the most frequent presentation of human H5N1 cases. For H7N9 LP AI, total accumulated human cases in China for 2013 is 137, of which 45 were fatal. Most cases had exposure risk to live-poultry markets. Conjunctivitis was the most frequent symptom in human cases of H7N7 HP AI virus infection in the Netherlands during 2003, with 89 confirmed cases and 1 fatality. Other HP AI viruses and all LP AI viruses have produced very rare or no human infections.

AVIAN METAPNEUMOVIRUS

(Turkey rhinotracheitis, Avian pneumovirus, Swollen head syndrome)

Avian metapneumovirus (aMPV) causes turkey rhinotracheitis, an acute respiratory tract infection of turkeys. It is also associated with swollen head syndrome in broilers and broiler breeders, as well as egg production losses in layers. The virus was first detected in turkeys in South Africa in the late 1970s and has spread to all the major poultry-producing areas in the world except for Australia. aMPV has been detected not only in chickens and turkeys but also in pheasants, Muscovy ducks, and guinea fowl. Geese, most other duck species, and possibly pigeons are suggested to be refractory to disease. Epidemiologic studies provide evidence for the circulation of aMPV in wild birds, especially water-associated species. Some outbreaks have been attributed to vaccine-derived viruses, which may persist for several months in the environment. Infection with aMPV is often complicated by secondary bacterial *infections*, leading to high economic losses. In 2001 the first human metapneumovirus (hMPV) was isolated and classified as a member of the genus *Metapneumovirus*, which causes respiratory infections in people. Experimental studies suggest that turkeys also may be susceptible to hMPV. Complete genome sequencing confirmed that the genomic organization of hMPV is similar to that of aMPV. Overall, little is known about the cross-species pathogenicity of these two viruses.

Etiology: aMPV is a member of the family Paramyxoviridae and of subfamily Pneumovirinae, which consists of the genus *Pneumovirus* (including the human and bovine respiratory syncytial viruses) and the genus *Metapneumovirus*. Currently the genus *Metapneumovirus* comprises aMPV and hMPV.

Isolates of aMPV are grouped in subtypes A to D. The sequence of the attachment glycoprotein (G protein) can be used to subtype different strains. Based on the phylogenetic analysis of F protein sequences, it was suggested that the European subtypes A, B, and D are all more closely related to each other than to subtype C. More recently, aMPV subtype C isolates were also identified in pheasants in Korea and water-associated bird species in Europe. The latter was shown to be of a different genetic lineage than the USA subtype C isolates. Irrespective of the differences within subtype C, isolates of this subtype display a higher amino acid sequence homology to hMPV than to European aMPV subtypes A, B, and D.

Transmission and Epidemiology: The spread of aMPV appears to depend on the poultry population density, standard of hygiene, and biosecurity. Within or between poultry flocks, aMPV may spread rapidly horizontally by direct contact or by contact with contaminated material. aMPV is assumed to be highly contagious. The enveloped virus is rapidly destroyed after release from the host to the environment. Because aMPV affects mainly ciliated epithelial cells of the upper respiratory tract, transmission is most likely to be airborne, especially by aerosol. But ciliated cells of the reproductive tract and possibly macrophages also may be target cells of aMPV. Metapneumovirus subtype C was isolated from eggs of experimentally infected SPF turkeys, but it was suggested that the vertical route may be short-lived and may play only a minor role in viral transmission.

Birds appear to shed aMPV for only a few days after infection. This short period of shedding suggests that there is no latency or carrier status under experimental conditions. There is evidence that on farms aMPV may persist for longer periods. Reconvalescent flocks may be repeatedly reinfected with aMPV within one fattening period.

Clinical Findings: aMPV induces an acute, highly contagious infection of the upper respiratory tract of turkeys and chickens. The disease affects all age groups, although younger birds seem to be more susceptible. In fattening turkeys the upper respiratory tract is predominantly affected, while in laying hens only a mild respiratory infection with a drop in egg production and egg quality has been seen. Coughing associated with lower respiratory tract involvement may lead to prolapses of the uterus in laying turkeys.

Typical respiratory signs in young turkeys include serous, watery nasal and ocular discharge; frothy eyes; and conjunctivitis. At later stages, signs include mucopurulent, turbid nasal discharge; plugged nostrils; swollen infraorbital sinuses; and snicking, sneezing, coughing, or tracheal rales. These respiratory signs are accompanied by depression, anorexia, and ruffled feathers.

The incubation period is 3–7 days, and morbidity in birds of all ages may reach 100%. Mortality may be 1%–30% depending on age and constitution of the flock as well as secondary infections. Birds without secondary infections with good constitution may recover within 7–10 days. However, in birds with secondary infections and under poor management, the disease may be prolonged and exacerbated by airsacculitis, pericarditis, pneumonia, and perihepatitis.

Infection in chickens and pheasants is less clearly defined and may not always be associated with clinical signs. aMPV is associated with swollen head syndrome in chickens. This condition is characterized by swelling of the peri- and infraorbital sinuses, frothy eyes, nasal discharge, torticollis, and opisthotonos due to ear infection. Typically, <4% of the flock is affected, although respiratory signs may be widespread. Mortality is rarely >2%. In broiler breeders and commercial layers, egg production and quality are frequently affected.

Lesions: Macroscopic lesions depend on the course of infection, especially on secondary bacterial infections, and are most prominent on days 4–10 after infection. Gross lesions induced after experimental infection are due to rhinitis, tracheitis, sinusitis, and airsacculitis. Infected birds may be free of gross lesions. Serous to turbid mucus may be observed in the nasal cavity, nasal turbinates, trachea, and in infraorbital sinuses. During the course of infection, the secreted mucus turns from clear and serous to turbid and purulent. Nonspecific signs of inflammation, such as swelling and hyperemia of the mucosa and excessive mucus, can be seen in the upper respiratory tract and in the air sacs. If secondary bacterial infections are present, copious inflammatory exudates are found in the respiratory tract. In addition, pneumonia, pericarditis, perihepatitis, splenomegaly, and hepatomegaly are seen. In the reproductive tract of laying turkeys, lesions can include egg peritonitis, ovary and oviduct regression, folded shell membranes in the oviduct, and misshapen eggs. Microscopic examination of the upper respiratory tract, including the secondary bronchi during the first 2 days after aMPV infection, reveals loss of cilia, increased glandular activity, congestion, and mild mononuclear infiltration of the submucosa. The most pronounced microscopic lesions are found in the mucosa or the nasal turbinates, which may be the most suitable tissue for microscopic evaluation and diagnosis of aMPV infection. Harderian glands and lacrimal glands may also show infiltration of lymphocytes and formulation of lymphoid follicle-like structures in the interstitial tissue and around the secondary collecting ducts.

Diagnosis: Obtaining samples from the upper respiratory tract of birds in the early stages of the disease is extremely important when attempting virus isolation. Especially in broiler-type chickens, samples should be taken before the sixth day after infection. Once clinical signs are obvious, the isolation of replicating aMPV may not be successful. The most suitable samples for aMPV detection are tracheal and choanal swabs. Tracheal organ cultures prepared from turkey or chicken embryos, or 1- to 2-day-old chicks, are the most sensitive for primary isolation of aMPV. Ciliostasis may occur within 7 days of aMPV A and B but not subtype C inoculation or after passages. The virus has also been isolated after the inoculation of 6- to 8-day-old embryonated chicken or turkey eggs via the yolk sac route and identified by electron microscopy, virus neutralization test, or molecular techniques. Cell cultures have not proved successful for the primary isolation of the virus. However, once the virus has been isolated and adapted in the systems above, it will grow in a variety of avian and mammalian cultures.

Reverse transcriptase PCR (RT-PCR), as well as real-time RT-PCR, tests targeting the F, N, or G gene of aMPV have been developed and are widely used to detect the virus in clinical material, particularly respiratory swabs. Some nested RT-PCR tests have been constructed so that the subtype as well as the identity of virus can be determined from the clinical sample. Based on the growing amount of genome sequence data and access to sequencing techniques, detailed characterization and molecular differentiation of isolated aMPV strains is commonly done. Antigen detection tests have also been developed, including immunofluorescence and immunoperoxidase assays on both fixed and unfixed tissues.

Because of difficulties in isolation and identification of aMPV, serologic assays have been developed to confirm infection in commercial chickens and turkeys. A number of commercial ELISA kits are available and are commonly used, but other techniques, including virus neutralization and indirect *immunofluorescence tests*, have also been used. Both acute and convalescent serum samples should be submitted for analysis. Although ELISA systems that use either subgroup A or B strains as antigens detect antibodies to both of these subgroups because of some cross-reactivity, the homologous antigen should be used for the efficient detection of subgroup C. The subtype specificity of the applied test may result in limited or no detection of other subtypes or new emerging aMPV strains that do not cross-react.

Paramyxoviruses (particularly Newcastle disease and paramyxovirus 3 (*see* p 2856), infectious bronchitis virus (*see* p 2909), and influenza viruses (*see* p 2902) may cause respiratory disease and egg production problems in chickens and turkeys that closely resemble aMPV infection. These viruses can be differentiated on the basis of morphology, hemagglutinating and neuraminidase activity, and molecular characteristics. A wide range of bacteria and *Mycoplasma* spp can cause signs very similar to those of aMPV. These agents are frequently present as secondary opportunistic pathogens and may mask the presence of the aMPV.

Prevention and Treatment: Good management practices can significantly reduce the severity of infection, especially in turkeys; in particular, optimal ventilation, stocking densities, temperature control, litter quality, and biosecurity have a positive influence on the outcome of the disease. Some success in reducing disease severity by controlling secondary bacterial infections with antibiotics has also been reported.

Both live and inactivated vaccines are available for immunization of chickens and turkeys and are widely used in countries where the disease is endemic. Maternal antibodies do not provide sufficient protection against aMPV infection and do not interfere significantly with vaccination. Thus, a vaccination program should plan for the first immunization as soon as possible after hatching. It is crucial to achieve a homogenous state of immunization per flock and farm by application of an adequate vaccine dose to all birds.

Live vaccines, which may be applied by spray or drinking water in the field, stimulate both local respiratory and systemic immunity, and cross-protection between subtypes may occur. But live vaccines may induce only short-lived protection, especially for grow-out of toms, because of the fast decline of local immunity. Thus, repeated revaccination of turkeys is common practice. There is, however, a risk of reversion of the live vaccine stains to more virulent variants. Inactivated aMPV vaccines are often used for booster immunization of layer and breeder flocks after priming with live vaccines. While inactivated vaccines alone induce only partial protection against aMPV infection, the most efficient and long-lasting protection is achieved by a combined prime-boost vaccination program. This program comprises repeated priming with live attenuated vaccines and booster immunization with inactivated adjuvanted vaccines. As experimentally shown, in ovo vaccination may also be a promising strategy for effective, early induction of an immune response. Besides live attenuated and classical inactivated vaccines, some genetically engineered viruses, including recombinant vectored vaccines, have been designed and tested under experimental conditions. These have induced partial protection and need further development.

BORDETELLOSIS

(Turkey coryza, *Bordetella avium* rhinotracheitis)

Avian bordetellosis is a highly infectious, acute upper respiratory tract disease of turkeys characterized by high morbidity and usually low mortality. Other synonyms previously used for the disease include *Alcaligenes* rhinotracheitis, adenovirus-associated respiratory disease, acute respiratory disease syndrome, and turkey rhinotracheitis.

Although the disease primarily affects turkeys, quail are also susceptible, and it is an opportunistic infection in chickens. Damage to the upper respiratory tract from prior exposure to an upper respiratory disease agent or vaccine such as infectious bronchitis virus or Newcastle disease virus, or from an environmental irritant such as ammonia, is necessary to induce signs in chickens.

Bordetellosis has been identified in almost every area of the world where turkeys are intensively reared. Historically, it has been severe in focal areas and rare or nonapparent in other locations. The reasons for these epidemiologic differences are not known.

Etiology and Pathogenesis: The causative agent is *Bordetella avium*, a gram-negative, nonfermentative, motile, aerobic bacillus. It can be grown using many different media, including MacConkey agar, Bordet-Gengou agar, veal infusion broth, trypticase soy broth, blood agar, and brain-heart infusion broth. Strains of *B avium* typically produce small (0.2–1 mm diameter after 24 hr incubation), compact, translucent, glistening pearl-like colonies with smooth edges. After serial passage in the laboratory, a rough colony type with a dry appearance and a serrated, irregular edge can be observed for some isolates. Rough colonies represent a global suppression of virulence factors in *B avium* termed antigenic variation and are nonpathogenic. When the bacillus is grown in broth media high in nutrients, filamentous forms can be observed.

The mechanism of pathogenesis involves the ability of *B avium* to destroy ciliated epithelial cells in the trachea. Certain strains of the bacteria adhere to the ciliated pseudostratified columnar epithelium and produce toxins, some of which appear to be similar to those from other *Bordetella* spp. Toxins associated with pathogenic strains of *B avium* include a heat-labile toxin, tracheal cytotoxin, dermonecrotic toxin, and osteotoxin. Adherence factors associated with the bacterium include the hemagglutinin Baa1 autotransporter protein and possibly pili and components associated with lipopolysaccharide. Damage to the tracheal cartilage with distortion and discoloration of the tracheal rings is often observed and thought to be caused by the cytotoxin and/or the osteotoxin. Some mortality is due to suffocation from

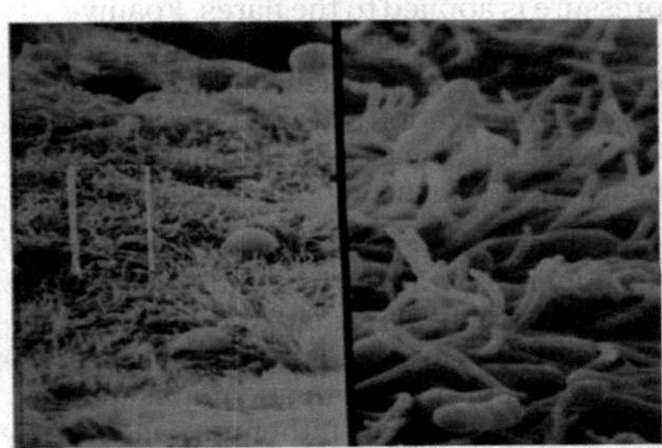

Scanning electron microscopy of a trachea from a poult 3 days after *Bordetella avium* infection; note numerous *B avium* cells attached to ciliated columnar epithelial cells. *Courtesy of Dr. Mark W. Jackwood.*

increased mucus production in the trachea and tracheal collapse. As with many bacterial infections, iron acquisition is necessary for colonization and spread of *B avium* in the host. Virulence factor expression is globally controlled by a virulence gene locus in response to environmental conditions that favor antigenic variation among *B avium* isolates.

Damage to the upper respiratory tract can lead to secondary infections with *Escherichia coli* or other agents, which can significantly increase the severity of the disease. In many cases, turkeys infected solely with *B avium* recover within 4–6 wk without serious consequences.

Epidemiology and Transmission: Morbidity is usually 80%–100% in young turkeys. Mortality can range from 0% in birds with uncomplicated disease to >40% if secondary invaders are present. Mortality can increase and signs can become severe if young turkeys infected with *B avium* also become infected with other agents (eg, *E coli*, Newcastle disease virus) or when environmental conditions in turkey barns are less than optimal. Bordetellosis is a major initiator of colibacillosis in turkeys. There is an age-related resistance to the disease. Turkeys >4–5 wk old are most often refractory to the disease but not infection, and thus can be a factor in spread of the bacterium.

B avium is highly contagious and easily transmitted from infected turkeys to susceptible birds by direct contact. It can also be transmitted through contaminated drinking water, feed, and litter, which can remain infectious for 1–6 mo.

Clinical Findings: Signs of the disease usually occur 7–10 days after infection and include sinusitis with a clear nasal discharge that can be observed when pressure is applied to the nares. Foamy-watery eyes, a snick or cough, mouth breathing, dyspnea, tracheal rales, and altered vocalization are also characteristic. Complicated disease can result in more exaggerated signs including airsacculitis.

Lesions: Lesions are primarily found in the upper respiratory tract and consist of nasal and tracheal exudates, collapse of cartilaginous rings, and progressive loss of ciliated epithelium. In uncomplicated disease, the tracheal epithelium can return to normal 4–6 wk after the onset of signs.

At necropsy, turkeys with characteristic bordetellosis have watery eyes and extensive mucus in the sinuses and trachea, which rarely extends below the tracheal bifurcation. The lining of the trachea may have extremely mild hemorrhage in some cases, and softening of the tracheal rings is usually felt. In addition, a dorsal/ventral flattening of the trachea can sometimes be observed. Pneumonia and airsacculitis are observed only when the disease is complicated by another disease agent.

Diagnosis: Diagnosis of infection is confirmed by isolation of *B avium* on MacConkey agar and identification using standard biochemical assays. Nonfermenting, small, slow-growing colonies from specimens from the anterior trachea are typical. The bacterium is best isolated from the anterior trachea; cultures taken from the sinuses frequently become overgrown with other, faster-replicating bacteria such as *Proteus* spp.

Serology is also important, and both microagglutination (detects IgM) and ELISA (detects IgG) tests are available. The microagglutination test can detect specific antibodies ~1 wk after infection. The ELISA test generally detects specific antibodies >2 wk after infection and has the added benefit of detecting maternal antibody. Monoclonal antibody-based agglutination and indirect immunofluorescent tests as well as PCR tests have also been used to identify *B avium*.

Other nonfermenters, *B bronchiseptica* and *B hinzii*, which are for the most part nonpathogenic, can sometimes be isolated from the trachea and must be differentiated from *B avium*. Pathogenic *B avium* can be differentiated by growth and colony morphology on MacConkey agar, no growth on minimal essential medium, a negative urease reaction, and hemagglutination of guinea pig erythrocytes. *B avium* also agglutinates chicken and turkey erythrocytes.

Treatment: Treatment with antimicrobial agents by aerosol, injection, or in the water has not been effective, even though *B avium* may be highly sensitive. The tracheal epithelium of the turkey is a difficult location to medicate even though blood levels of the antimicrobial appear to be adequate. Resistance to streptomycin, sulfonamides, and tetracycline can be carried on plasmids and has been observed for some strains of *B avium*. Antimicrobial therapy may be helpful for secondary colibacillosis.

Control and Prevention: Vaccination with bacterins and a live temperature-sensitive mutant vaccine have given mixed results depending on the age of the turkey and the method of administration.

Typically, turkeys >3 wk old respond positively to vaccination with the live temperature-sensitive vaccine. Vaccination is not widely practiced by turkey breeders, and the immunity that is passed to progeny generally comes from natural infections.

B avium is easily carried between farms. Thus, prevention should include a good biosecurity program. Rigorous cleanup and disinfection after field outbreaks is essential. Most of the commonly used disinfectants are effective.

Zoonotic Risk: *B avium* may be a rare opportunistic pathogen in people. In addition, a closely related organism, *B hinzii*, also isolated from poultry, has been associated with septicemia and bacteremia in older or immunocompromised people.

INFECTIOUS BRONCHITIS

Infectious bronchitis is an acute, highly contagious disease of major economic importance in commercial chicken flocks throughout the world. It is usually characterized by respiratory signs, although decreased egg production and poor egg quality are sometimes seen in breeders and layers. Some strains of the etiologic agent, infectious bronchitis virus (IBV), are nephropathogenic, causing interstitial nephritis, particularly in chicks. Associations with myopathy and proventriculitis have also been reported.

Etiology and Epidemiology: IBV is a coronavirus that only causes disease in chickens, although some other birds may be subclinically infected. Some serotypes are geographically restricted, but multiple serotypes commonly cocirculate in one geographic region. In recent years, a novel IBV genotype, the QX strain, has become increasingly common in Asia and Europe. IBV is shed by infected chickens in respiratory discharges and feces, and it can be spread by aerosol, ingestion of contaminated feed and water, and contact with contaminated equipment and clothing. Naturally infected chickens and those vaccinated with live IBV may shed virus intermittently for up to 20 wk after infection. The incubation period is generally 24–48 hr, with the peak in excretion of virus from the respiratory tract lasting 3–5 days after infection. The severity of disease and the body systems involved are influenced by the strain of the virus; the age, strain, immune status, and diet of the chickens; and cold stress. In addition, coinfection with *Mycoplasma gallisepticum*, *Mycoplasma synoviae*, *Escherichia coli*, and/or *Avibacterium paragallinarum* can exacerbate disease.

Clinical Findings: Morbidity is commonly close to 100%. Chicks may cough, sneeze, and have tracheal rales for 10–14 days. Conjunctivitis and dyspnea may be seen, and sometimes facial swelling, particularly with concurrent bacterial infection of the sinuses. Chicks may appear depressed and huddle under heat lamps. Feed consumption and weight gain are reduced. Infection with nephropathogenic strains can cause initial respiratory signs, then later depression, ruffled feathers, wet droppings, greater water intake, and death. In layers, egg production may drop by as much as 70%, and eggs are often misshapen, with thin, soft, rough, and/or pale shells, and can be smaller and have watery albumen. In most cases, egg production and egg quality return to normal, but this may take up to 8 wk. In most outbreaks mortality is 5%, although mortality rates are higher when disease is compli-cated by concurrent bacterial infection. Nephropathogenic strains can induce interstitial nephritis with high mortality (up to 60%) in young chicks. Infection of young chicks may cause permanent damage to the oviduct, resulting in layers or breeders that never reach normal levels of production.

Lesions: In the respiratory tract, the trachea, sinuses, and nasal passages may contain serous, catarrhal, or caseous exudates, and the air sacs a foamy exudate initially, progressing to cloudy thickening. If complicated by infection with *E coli*, there may be caseous airsacculitis, perihepatitis, and pericarditis. Birds infected when very young may have cystic oviducts, whereas those infected while in lay have an oviduct of reduced weight and length and regression of the ovaries. Infection with nephropathogenic strains results in swollen, pale kidneys, with the tubules and ureters distended with urates; in birds with urolithiasis, the ureters may be distended with urates and contain uroliths, and the kidneys may be atrophied.

Diagnosis: Laboratory confirmation is required for diagnosis of respiratory forms because of similarities to mild forms of disease caused by agents such as Newcastle disease virus, avian metapneumovirus, infectious laryngotracheitis virus, mycoplasmas, *A paragallinarum*, and *Ornithobacterium rhinotracheale*. Demonstration of seroconversion or a rise in antibody titer against IBV by ELISA, or hemagglutination inhibition or virus neutralization tests can be used for diagnosis when there is a history of respiratory disease or reduced egg production.

Definitive diagnosis is generally based on virus detection and identification. Virus can be isolated by inoculation of homogenates of tracheal, cecal tonsil, and/or kidney tissue into 9- to 11-day-old SPF chicken embryos, with growth of IBV indicated by embryo stunting and curling, and deposition of urates in the mesonephros, with variable mortality. Alternatively, IBV may be isolated in tracheal organ cultures, with growth of virus indicated by cessation of cilial motility. Several blind passages of the virus may be necessary for isolation of some field strains. More rapid diagnosis may be achieved using reverse transcriptase-polymerase chain reaction (RT-PCR) assays to detect viral RNA in nucleic acid extracts of tracheal, cecal tonsil, or kidney tissue.

Typing viruses can help distinguish vaccine and field strains and may help diagnose outbreaks caused by serotypes distinct from those of the vaccines used in a flock. Serotypes have been identified using sera from SPF chickens inoculated with known serotypes in virus neutralization tests. However, because this is expensive and time consuming, it is not readily available. A restricted range of serotype-specific monoclonal antibodies (MAb) have been developed for serotyping, but direct detection viral antigen using these MAbs to immunohistochemically stain tissue sections from diseased birds is of limited value because of the low concentration of antigen in tissues. The MAbs have been best used after propagation in chicken embryos, to detect viral antigen in the chorioallantoic membranes by immunofluorescence or immunoperoxidase staining, or in the allantoic fluid by ELISA. Analyses of the products of RT-PCR assays are now commonly used to identify the virus serotype and to identify individual strains within serotypes. The S1 region of the spike glycoprotein gene determines the serotype, and RT-PCR products derived from this region can be subjected to restriction fragment length polymorphism analysis, analyzed by nucleotide sequencing, or compared with reference strains using high-resolution melting curve analysis. Genotype determination based on the S1 region can be complemented by analyzing other regions of the viral genome, including the nucleocapsid gene and the 5′ untranslated region. These analyses can also aid in rapid detection of novel recombinant IBVs.

Control: No medication alters the course of IBV infection, although antimicrobial therapy may reduce mortalities caused by complicating bacterial infections. In cold weather, increasing the ambient temperature may reduce mortalities, and reducing the protein concentrations in feed and providing electrolytes in drinking water may assist in outbreaks caused by nephropathogenic strains.

The attenuated vaccines used for immunization may produce mild respiratory signs. These vaccines are initially given to 1- to 14-day-old chicks by spray, drinking water, or eye drop, and birds are commonly revaccinated. Revaccination with a virus from a distinct serotype can induce broader protection. Attenuated or adjuvanted inactivated vaccines can be used in breeders and layers to prevent egg production losses.

There are many distinct serotypes of IBV, and new or variant serotypes, which are not fully controlled by existing vaccines, are identified relatively frequently. Some variants may be derived from recombination between existing field strains and vaccine strains, whereas others result from point mutations in existing strains. Selection of vaccines should be based on knowledge of the most prevalent serotype(s) on the premises. The correlation between serotype and protection is imperfect, and definition of the most appropriate vaccine, or combination of vaccines, may require experimental assessment of several combinations of vaccines to identify the most effective regimen. The most commonly used live vaccines in the USA contain derivatives of the Massachusetts, Connecticut, and Arkansas strains, whereas in Australia, where the most prevalent serotypes are distinct from most other countries, vaccines are based on derivatives of the VicS and Armidale strains. In Europe, vaccines incorporating derivatives of the 4/91 strain and those derived from QX-like viruses are available. Vaccination with selected variant serotypes may be of use when these variants are the dominant strain in flocks, although regulatory authorities in some countries only permit use of vaccines derived from the Massachusetts strain.

INFECTIOUS CORYZA

Infectious coryza is an acute respiratory disease of chickens characterized by nasal discharge, sneezing, and swelling of the face under the eyes. It is found worldwide. The disease is seen only in chickens; reports of the disease in quail and pheasants probably describe a similar disease that is caused by a different etiologic agent.

In developed countries such as the USA, the disease is seen primarily in pullets and layers and occasionally in broilers. In the USA, it is most prevalent in commercial flocks in California and the southeast, although the northeastern USA has experienced significant outbreaks. In developing countries, the disease often is seen in very young chicks, even as young as 3 wk old. Poor biosecurity, poor environment, and the stress of other diseases are likely reasons why infectious coryza is more of a problem there. The disease has no public health significance.

Etiology: The causative bacterium is *Avibacterium paragallinarum*, a gram-negative, pleomorphic, nonmotile, catalase-negative, microaerophilic rod that requires nicotinamide adenine dinucleotide (V-factor) for in vitro growth. When grown on blood agar with a staphylococcal nurse colony that excretes the V-factor, the satellite colonies appear as dewdrops, growing adjacent to the nurse colony. V-factor–independent *Av paragallinarum* have been recovered in South Africa and Mexico. The most commonly used serotyping scheme is the Page scheme, which groups *Av paragallinarum* isolates into three serovars (A, B, and C) that correlate with immunotype specificity.

Epidemiology and Transmission: Chronically ill or healthy carrier birds are the reservoir of infection. Chickens of all ages are susceptible, but susceptibility increases with age. The incubation period is 1–3 days, and the disease duration is usually 2–3 wk. Under field conditions, the duration may be longer in the presence of concurrent diseases, eg, mycoplasmosis.

Infected flocks are a constant threat to uninfected flocks. Transmission is by direct contact, airborne droplets, and contamination of drinking water. "All-in/all-out" management has essentially eradicated infectious coryza from many commercial poultry establishments in the USA. Commercial farms that have multiple-age flocks tend to perpetuate the disease. Egg transmission does not occur. Molecular techniques such as restriction endonuclease analysis and ribotyping have been used to trace outbreaks of infectious coryza.

Clinical Findings: In the mildest form of the disease, the only signs may be depression, a serous nasal discharge, and occasionally slight facial swelling. In the more severe form, there is severe swelling of one or both infraorbital sinuses with edema of the surrounding tissue, which may close one or both eyes. In adult birds, especially males, the edema may extend to the intermandibular space and wattles. The swelling usually abates in 10–14 days; however, if secondary infection occurs, swelling can persist for months. There may be varying degrees of rales depending on the extent of infection. In Argentina, a septicemic form of the disease has been reported, probably due to concurrent infections. Egg production may be delayed in young pullets and severely reduced in producing hens. Birds may have diarrhea, and feed and water consumption usually is decreased during acute stages of the disease.

Lesions: In acute cases, lesions may be limited to the infraorbital sinuses. There is a copious, tenacious, grayish, semifluid exudate. As the disease becomes chronic or other pathogens become involved, the sinus exudate may become consolidated and turn yellowish. Other lesions may include conjunctivitis, tracheitis, bronchitis, and airsacculitis, particularly if other pathogens are involved. The histopathologic response of respiratory organs consists of disintegration and hyperplasia of mucosal and glandular epithelia and edema with infiltration of heterophils, macrophages, and mast cells.

Diagnosis: Isolation of a gram-negative, satellitic, catalase-negative organism from chickens in a flock with a history of a rapidly spreading coryza is diagnostic. The catalase test is essential, because nonpathogenic hemophilic organisms, which are catalase-positive, are present in both healthy and diseased chickens. A PCR test that can be used on the live chicken and that has proved superior to culture, even in developing countries, has been developed. A real-time version of the PCR is also available.

Production of typical signs after inoculation with nasal exudate from infected into susceptible chickens is also reliable diagnostically. No suitable serologic test exists; a hemagglutination-inhibition test is the best of those available. Swelling of the face and wattles must be differentiated from that seen in fowl cholera (*see* p 2822). Other diseases that must be considered are mycoplasmosis, laryngotracheitis, Newcastle disease, infectious bronchitis, avian influenza, swollen head syndrome (ornithobacterosis), and vitamin A deficiency.

While currently found only in South Africa and Mexico, the presence of a V-factor–independent *Av paragallinarum* must also be considered. The *Av paragallinarum* PCR is an ideal diagnostic tool in this situation.

Control and Treatment: Prevention is the only sound method of control. "All-in/all-out" farm programs with sound management and isolation methods are the best way to avoid infectious coryza. Replacements should be raised on the same farm or obtained from clean flocks. If replacement pullets are to be placed on a farm that has a history of infectious coryza, bacterins are available to help prevent and control the disease. USDA-licensed bacterins are available, and bacterins also are produced within states for intrastate use. Bacterins also are produced in many other countries. Because serovars A, B, and C are not cross-protective, it is essential that bacterins contain the serovars present in the target population. Vaccination should be completed ~4 wk before infectious coryza usually breaks out on the individual farm. Antibodies detected by the hemagglutination-inhibition test after bacterin administration do not necessarily correlate with protective immunity. Controlled exposure to live organisms also has been used to immunize layers in endemic areas.

Because early treatment is important, water medication is recommended immediately until medicated feed is available. Erythromycin and oxytetracycline are usually beneficial. Several new-generation antibiotics (eg, fluoroquinolones, macrolides) are active against infectious coryza. Various sulfonamides, sulfonamide-trimethoprim, and other combinations have been successful. Antibiotic use in chickens is subject to national regulations that vary from country to country, and use and efficacy of the various antibiotics must be reviewed in the light of the relevant national regulations. In more severe outbreaks, although treatment may result in improvement, the disease may recur when medication is discontinued.

Preventive medication may be combined with a vaccination program if started pullets are to be reared or housed on infected premises.

INFECTIOUS LARYNGOTRACHEITIS

Infectious laryngotracheitis (ILT) is an acute, highly contagious, herpesvirus infection of chickens and pheasants characterized by severe dyspnea, coughing, and rales. It can also be a subacute disease with nasal and ocular discharge, tracheitis, conjunctivitis, and mild rales. The disease is caused by *Gallid herpesvirus 1*, commonly known as infectious laryngotracheitis virus (ILTV). It has been reported from most areas of the USA in which poultry are intensively reared, as well as from many other countries.

Clinical Findings: In the acute form, gasping, coughing, rattling, and extension of the neck during inspiration are seen 5–12 days after natural exposure. Reduced productivity is a varying factor in laying flocks. Affected birds are anorectic and inactive. The mouth and beak may be bloodstained from the tracheal exudate. Mortality varies but may reach 50% in adults and is usually due to occlusion of the trachea by hemorrhage or exudate. Signs usually subside after ~2 wk, although some birds may show signs for longer periods. Strains of low virulence produce little or no mortality with mild respiratory signs and a slight decrease in egg production.

After recovery, birds remain carriers for life and become a source of infection for susceptible birds. The latent virus can be reactivated under stressful conditions. Infection also may be spread mechanically. Several epidemics have been traced to the transport of birds in contaminated crates, and the practice of litter spread in pastures is believed to be related to epidemics of the disease.

Diagnosis: The acute disease is characterized by the presence of blood, mucus, yellow caseous exudates, or a hollow caseous cast in the trachea. Microscopically, a desquamative, necrotizing tracheitis is characteristic of acute disease. In the subacute form, punctiform hemorrhagic areas in the trachea and larynx and mild conjunctivitis with lacrimation may be detected. A rapid diagnosis can be achieved by detection of intranuclear inclusion bodies in the tracheal epithelium early in the course of the disease; results of the microscopic examination can be rapidly confirmed by detection of viral DNA using virus-specific PCR assays. Isolation and identification of the virus is done in chicken embryos or tissue culture from embryo liver or kidney cells or from kidney cells from adult chickens. Chicken embryos are preferred for virus isolation. Chorioallantoic membrane of developing chicken embryos (9–12 days old) is inoculated with the specimen. Microscopic examination of the chorioallantoic membrane lesion shows intranuclear inclusions. On microscopic examination of the trachea, intranuclear inclusion lesions produced by ILTV infection must be differentiated from the diphtheritic form of fowlpox infection that produces intracytoplasmic inclusions.

Field isolates and vaccine strains of ILTV are routinely differentiated by PCR amplification of single or multiple ILTV genome areas, followed by sequencing of the PCR products and comparative analysis of the sequences obtained. More recently, field isolates and vaccines strains have been differentiated more accurately by full genome sequencing analysis.

Control: In endemic areas and on farms where a specific diagnosis is made, the disease is controlled by implementation of biosecurity measures and vaccination. Vaccination is done with live attenuated vaccines and viral vector recombinant vaccines. Live vaccines originated from virulent isolates that were attenuated by consecutive passages in embryos or tissue culture. These are applied via eye drop or through mass vaccination by water or spray. Viral vector recombinant vaccines in fowlpox and herpesvirus of turkeys have been designed to express ILTV immunogenic proteins and are administered to individual birds by in ovo, SC, or wing-web vaccination.

QUAIL BRONCHITIS

Quail bronchitis is a naturally occurring, highly contagious, often fatal respiratory disease of bobwhite quail, seen both in the wild and in captivity. The disease is of major economic significance to gamebird breeders and has a worldwide distribution. It is a serious disease on certain farms where quail are pen-raised, and particularly when quail of different ages are maintained on the same premises.

The causative agent, quail bronchitis virus, is a Group I serotype 1 avian adenovirus that can be readily isolated from the respiratory tract of acutely affected birds. The virus is also easily isolated from fecal samples, intestine, liver, and occasionally the bursa of Fabricius. It is highly contagious and spreads rapidly through multiple-age units. Other avian species, particularly chickens, may be carriers.

Clinical signs include respiratory distress, coughing, sneezing, rales, and nasal or ocular discharge. Loose, watery droppings are common in some acutely affected older birds. Conjunctivitis, mild to severe tracheitis (the trachea may be completely filled with mucus), airsacculitis, hepatitis, and gaseous distention of the intestines may be seen. Multiple pale, pinpoint (3 mm) foci of necrosis in the liver and mottling and enlargement of the spleen are common lesions in infected birds. Mortality may reach 100% in birds <2 wk old but is usually <25% in birds >4 wk old.

The disease is often self-limiting. Experimental vaccines have proved ineffective in preventing quail bronchitis. There is no specific treatment, but increasing the brooder temperature by 3°–5°F (1.5°–3°C), preventing "piling up," and avoiding contact between older and younger birds and other avian species are of value, as are strict isolation and sanitation. Immunity is long lasting, possibly for life, and recovered birds can be retained for breeders. New birds should not be introduced to premises without a 30-day quarantine.

NUTRITION AND MANAGEMENT: POULTRY

NUTRITIONAL REQUIREMENTS

Poultry convert feed into food products quickly, efficiently, and with relatively low environmental impact compared with other livestock. The high rate of productivity of poultry results in relatively high nutrient needs. Poultry require the presence of at least 38 dietary nutrients in appropriate concentrations and balance. The nutrient requirement figures published in *Nutrient Requirements of Poultry* (National Research Council, 1994) are the most recent available and should be viewed as minimal nutrient needs for poultry. They are derived from experimentally determined levels after an extensive review of the published data. Criteria used to determine the requirement for a given nutrient include growth, feed efficiency, egg production, prevention of deficiency symptoms, and quality of poultry product. These requirements assume the nutrients are in a highly bioavailable form, and they do not include a margin of safety. Consequently, adjustments should be made based on bioavailability of nutrients in various feedstuffs. A margin of safety should be added based on the length of time the diet will be stored before feeding, changes in rates of feed intake due to environmental temperature or dietary energy content, genetic strain, husbandry conditions (especially the level of sanitation), and the presence of stressors (such as diseases or mycotoxins).

Water: Water is an essential nutrient. Many factors influence water intake, including environmental temperature, relative humidity, salt and protein levels of the diet, birds' productivity (rate of growth or egg production), and the individual bird's ability to resorb water in the kidney. As a result, precise water requirements are highly variable. Water deprivation for ≥12 hr has an adverse effect on growth of young poultry and egg production of layers; water deprivation for ≥36 hr results in a marked increase in mortality of both young and mature poultry. Cool, clean water, uncontaminated by high levels of minerals or other potential toxic substances, must be available at all times.

Energy Requirements and Feed Intake: The energy requirements of poultry and the energy content of feedstuffs are expressed in kilocalories (1 kcal equals 4.1868 kilojoules). Two different measures of the bioavailable energy in feedstuffs are in use, metabolizable energy (AME_n) and the true metabolizable energy (TME_n). AME_n is the gross energy of the feed minus the gross energy of the excreta after a correction for the nitrogen retained in the body. Calculations of TME_n make an additional correction to account for endogenous losses of energy that are not directly attributable to the feedstuff and are usually a more useful measure. AME_n and TME_n are similar for many ingredients. However, the two values differ substantially for some ingredients such as feather meal, rice, wheat middlings, and corn distiller's grains with solubles.

Poultry can adjust their feed intake over a considerable range of feed energy levels to meet their daily energy needs. Energy needs and, consequently, feed intake also vary considerably with environmental temperature and amount of physical activity. A bird's daily need for amino acids, vitamins, and minerals are mostly independent of these factors. The nutrient requirement values in the following tables are based on typical rates of intake of birds in a thermoneutral environment consuming a diet that contains a specific energy content (eg, 3,200 kcal/kg for broilers). If a bird consumes a diet that has a higher energy content, it will decrease its feed intake; consequently, that diet must contain a proportionally higher amount of amino acids, vitamins, and minerals. Thus, nutrient density in the ration should be adjusted to provide appropriate nutrient intake based on requirements and the actual feed intake.

Because of the ability of poultry to adjust their feed intake to accommodate a wide range of diets with differing energy content, the energy values listed in the nutrient requirement tables in this section (*see* TABLES 6–15) should be regarded as guidelines rather than absolute requirements.

Appropriate body weight and fat deposition are important factors in rearing pullets for maximal egg production. Most strains of White Leghorn chickens have relatively low body weights and do not tend, under normal feeding, to become obese. Feed is normally provided for ad lib intake to this strain of pullets. For brown-egg strains of chickens, some degree of restriction is often practiced (~90% of ad lib feeding) to prevent precocial onset of lay. Broiler strains tend to become obese if fed ab lib; feed restriction is necessary for broiler pullets and broiler breeders. When feed restriction is practiced, the feed levels of amino acids, vitamins, and minerals must be proportionally increased to prevent deficiencies. Most large commercial breeders provide feed restriction and dietary nutrient guidelines specific for their strains.

Amino Acid Requirements: Poultry, like all animals, synthesize proteins that contain 20 L-amino acids. Birds are unable to synthesize 9 of these amino acids because of the lack of specific enzymes: arginine, isoleucine, leucine, lysine, methionine, phenylalanine, threonine, tryptophan, and

TABLE 6 NUTRIENT REQUIREMENTS OF GROWING PULLETS[a]

Age (wk)	0–6	6–12	12–18	18 to 1st Egg
WHITE-EGG LAYERS				
Body weight (g)[b]	**450**	**980**	**1,375**	**1,475**
Protein	18	16	15	17
Arginine	1.0	0.83	0.67	0.75
Lysine	0.85	0.60	0.45	0.52
Methionine	0.30	0.25	0.20	0.22
Methionine + cystine	0.62	0.52	0.42	0.47
Threonine	0.68	0.57	0.37	0.47
Tryptophan	0.17	0.14	0.11	0.12
Calcium	0.90	0.80	0.80	2.00
Phosphorus, available	0.40	0.35	0.30	0.32
BROWN-EGG LAYERS				
Body weight (g)[b]	**500**	**1,100**	**1,500**	**1,600**
Protein	17	15	14	16
Arginine	0.94	0.78	0.62	0.72
Lysine	0.80	0.56	0.42	0.49
Methionine	0.28	0.23	0.19	0.21
Methionine + cystine	0.59	0.49	0.39	0.44
Threonine	0.64	0.53	0.35	0.44
Tryptophan	0.16	0.13	0.10	0.11
Calcium	0.90	0.80	0.80	1.8
Phosphorus, available	0.40	0.35	0.30	0.35

[a] Requirements are listed as percentages of diet. Nutrient levels should be adjusted to meet specific strain requirements, level of feed intake, and body weight and skeletal development.

[b] Average body weight at end of each period.

TABLE 7 NUTRIENT REQUIREMENTS OF LAYING HENS AT DIFFERENT FEED INTAKES[a]

Pounds (approx.)/100 birds/day	**18**	**20**	**22**	**24**	**26**
Grams of feed/bird/day	**80**	**90**	**100**	**110**	**120**
WHITE-EGG LAYERS					
Protein	18.8	16.7	15.0	13.6	12.5
Arginine	0.88	0.78	0.70	0.64	0.58
Lysine	0.86	0.77	0.69	0.63	0.58
Methionine	0.38	0.33	0.30	0.27	0.25
Methionine + cystine	0.73	0.64	0.58	0.53	0.48
Threonine	0.59	0.52	0.47	0.43	0.39
Tryptophan	0.20	0.18	0.16	0.15	0.13
Calcium	4.12	3.67	3.30	3.00	2.75
Phosphorus, available	0.31	0.28	0.25	0.23	0.21
BROWN-EGG LAYERS					
Protein	22.5	20.0	18.0	16.4	15.0
Arginine	1.06	0.94	0.85	0.77	0.71
Lysine	1.05	0.93	0.84	0.76	0.70
Methionine	0.45	0.40	0.36	0.33	0.30
Methionine + cystine	0.89	0.79	0.71	0.65	0.59
Threonine	0.71	0.63	0.57	0.52	0.48
Tryptophan	0.24	0.21	0.19	0.17	0.16
Calcium	5.00	4.44	4.00	3.64	3.33
Phosphorus, available	0.38	0.33	0.30	0.27	0.25

[a] Requirements are listed as percentages of diet.

valine. Histidine, glycine, and proline can be synthesized by birds, but the rate is usually insufficient to meet metabolic needs and a dietary source is required. These 12 amino acids are referred to as the essential amino acids. Tyrosine and cysteine can be synthesized from phenylalanine and methionine, respectively, and are referred to as conditionally essential because they must be in the diet if phenylalanine or methionine levels are inadequate. The diet must also supply sufficient amounts of nitrogen to allow the synthesis of nonessential amino acids. Essential amino acids are often added to the diet in purified form (eg, DL-methionine and L-lysine) to minimize the total protein level as well as the cost of the diet. This has the added advantage of minimizing nitrogen excretion.

Vitamins: Requirements for vitamins A, D, and E are expressed in IU. For chickens, 1 IU of vitamin A activity is equivalent to 0.3 mcg of pure retinol, 0.344 mcg of retinyl acetate, or 0.6 mcg of β-carotene. However, young chicks use β-carotene less efficiently.

One IU of vitamin D is equal to 0.025 mcg of cholecalciferol (vitamin D_3). Ergocalciferol

TABLE 8 NUTRIENT REQUIREMENTS OF BROILERS[a]

Age[b]	**0–3 wk**	**3–6 wk**	**6–8 wk**
kcal AME_n/kg diet[c]	**3,200**	**3,200**	**3,200**
Crude protein[d]	23.00	20.00	18.00
Arginine	1.25	1.10	1.00
Glycine + serine	1.25	1.14	0.97
Histidine	0.35	0.32	0.27
Isoleucine	0.80	0.73	0.62
Leucine	1.20	1.09	0.93
Lysine[e]	1.10	1.00	0.85
Methionine	0.50	0.38	0.32
Methionine + cystine	0.90	0.72	0.60
Phenylalanine	0.72	0.65	0.56
Phenylalanine + tyrosine	1.34	1.22	1.04
Proline	0.60	0.55	0.46
Threonine	0.80	0.74	0.68
Tryptophan	0.20	0.18	0.16
Valine	0.90	0.82	0.70

[a] Requirements are listed as percentages of diet.

[b] The 0- to 3-, 3- to 6-, and 6- to 8-wk intervals for nutrient requirements are based on chronology for which research data were available; however, these nutrient requirements are often implemented at younger age intervals or on a weight-of-feed consumed basis.

[c] These are typical dietary energy concentrations. Different energy values may be appropriate depending on local ingredient prices and availability.

[d] Broiler chickens do not have a requirement for crude protein per se. However, there should be sufficient crude protein to ensure an adequate nitrogen supply for synthesis of nonessential amino acids. Suggested requirements for crude protein are typical of those derived with corn-soybean meal diets, and levels can be reduced when synthetic amino acids are used.

[e] Recent research has shown that higher levels of lysine are needed for maximal growth and efficiency of modern broilers.

(vitamin D_2) is used with an efficiency of <10% of vitamin D_3 in poultry.

One IU of vitamin E is equivalent to 1 mg of synthetic DL-α-tocopherol acetate. Vitamin E requirements vary with type and level of fat in the diet, the levels of selenium and trace minerals, and the presence or absence of other antioxidants. When diets high in long-chain highly polyunsaturated fatty acids are fed, vitamin E levels should be increased considerably.

Choline is required as an integral part of the body phospholipid, as a part of acetylcholine, and as a source of methyl groups. Growing chickens can also use betaine as a methylating agent. Betaine is widely distributed in practical feedstuffs and can spare the requirement for choline but cannot completely replace it in the diet.

All vitamins are subject to degradation over time, and this process is accelerated by moisture, oxygen, trace minerals, heat, and light. Stabilized vitamin preparations and generous margins of safety are often applied to account for these losses. This is especially true if diets are pelleted, extruded, or stored for long periods.

Minerals: Much of the phosphorus in feedstuffs of plant origin is complexed by phytate and is not absorbed efficiently by poultry. Consequently, it is critical that only

TABLE 9 PROTEIN AND AMINO ACID REQUIREMENTS OF TURKEYS[a]

	Age (wk)							
Male:	**0–4**	**4–8**	**8–12**	**12–16**	**16–20**	**20–24**		
Female:	**0–4**	**4–8**	**8–11**	**11–14**	**14–17**	**17–20**	**Holding**	**Breeding Hens**
Energy base kcal ME/kg diet[b]	**2,800**	**2,900**	**3,000**	**3,100**	**3,200**	**3,300**	**2,900**	**2,900**
Protein	28.0	26	22	19	16.5	14	12	14
Arginine	1.6	1.4	1.1	0.9	0.75	0.6	0.5	0.6
Glycine + serine	1.0	0.9	0.8	0.7	0.6	0.5	0.4	0.5
Histidine	0.58	0.5	0.4	0.3	0.25	0.2	0.2	0.3
Isoleucine	1.1	1.0	0.8	0.6	0.5	0.45	0.4	0.5
Leucine	1.9	1.75	1.5	1.25	1.0	0.8	0.5	0.5
Lysine	1.6	1.5	1.3	1.0	0.8	0.65	0.5	0.6
Methionine	0.55	0.45	0.4	0.35	0.25	0.25	0.2	0.2
Methionine + cystine	1.05	0.95	0.8	0.65	0.55	0.45	0.4	0.4
Phenylalanine	1.0	0.9	0.8	0.7	0.6	0.5	0.4	0.55
Phenylalanine + tyrosine	1.8	1.6	1.2	1.0	0.9	0.9	0.8	1.0
Threonine	1.0	0.95	0.8	0.75	0.6	0.5	0.4	0.45
Tryptophan	0.26	0.24	0.2	0.18	0.15	0.13	0.1	0.13
Valine	1.2	1.1	0.9	0.8	0.7	0.6	0.5	0.58

[a] Requirements are listed as percentages of diet.

[b] These are typical ME concentrations for corn-soya diets. Different ME values may be appropriate if other ingredients predominate.

Adapted, with permission, from *Nutrient Requirements of Poultry*, 1994, National Academy of Sciences, National Academy Press, Washington, DC.

the available phosphorus and not the total phosphorus levels be considered. Appropriate calcium nutrition depends on both the level of calcium and its ratio to that of available phosphorus. For growing poultry, this ratio should not deviate substantially from 2:1. The calcium requirement of laying hens is very high and increases with the rate of egg production and age of the hen.

Other Nutrients and Additives: The chick has requirements for 38 nutrients, together with an adequate level of metabolizable energy and water. Some additional nutrients may be necessary for growth and development under certain conditions. These include vitamin C, pyrroloquinoline quinone, and several heavy metals.

Non-nutrient antioxidants, such as ethoxyquin, are usually added to poultry diets to protect vitamins and unsaturated fatty acids from oxidation. Antibiotics at low levels (5–25 mg/kg of feed, depending on the antibiotic) and surfeit copper (150 ppm) are sometimes included to improve growth rate and feed efficiency. Enzymes

TABLE 10 NUTRIENT REQUIREMENTS OF PHEASANTS[a]

Energy base	0–4 wk	4–8 wk	9–17 wk	Breeding
kcal ME/kg diet[b]	**2,800**	**2,800**	**2,700**	**2,800**
Protein (%)	28	24	18	15
Glycine + serine (%)	1.8	1.55	1	0.5
Lysine (%)	1.5	1.40	0.8	0.68
Methionine + cystine (%)	1.0	0.93	0.6	0.6
Linoleic acid (%)	1	1	1	1
Calcium (%)	1.0	0.85	0.53	2.5
Phosphorus, available (%)	0.55	0.5	0.45	0.40
Sodium (%)	0.15	0.15	0.15	0.15
Chlorine (%)	0.11	0.11	0.11	0.11
Iodine (mg)	0.3	0.3	0.3	0.3
Riboflavin (mg)	3.4	3.4	3.0	4.0
Pantothenic acid (mg)	10	10	10	16
Niacin (mg)	70	70	40	30
Choline (mg)	1,430	1,300	1,000	1,000

[a] Requirements are listed as percentages or as mg/kg of diet. For values not listed, *see* requirements of turkeys (TABLE 9 and TABLE 15) as a guide.

[b] These are typical dietary energy concentrations.

Adapted, with permission, from *Nutrient Requirements of Poultry*, 1994, National Academy of Sciences, National Academy Press, Washington, DC.

that increase the bioavailability of dietary phosphorus, energy, and protein are often used in poultry diets when their costs are not prohibitive. In some cases, phytase enzymes are used to decrease the amount of phosphorus in the excreta to meet environmental regulations.

FEEDING AND MANAGEMENT PRACTICES

Success of the feeding program should be measured by how it achieves the breeder's goals for proper weight and development specific to each strain. Feed and the length of time required to attain certain weights in pullets and turkeys are presented in the growth and feed tables elsewhere in this chapter (*see* p 2914). The figures in these tables can be used as a guide to estimate the amount of feed required but will vary considerably because of differences in the nutrient density of feed, strain or breed of bird, amount of feed wasted, and environmental temperature.

Most diets used to feed poultry are nutritionally "complete" and commercially mixed, ie, prepared by feed manufacturing companies, most of which employ trained nutritionists. The formulation and mixing of poultry feeds requires knowledge and experience in purchasing ingredients, experimental testing of formulas, laboratory control of ingredient quality, and computer applications. Improper mixing can result in vitamin and mineral deficiencies, lack of protection against disease, or drug toxicity.

The physical form of the feed influences the expected results. Most feeds for starting and growing birds are produced as pellets or crumbles. In the pelleting process, the mash is treated with steam and then passed through a suitably sized die under pressure.

TABLE 11 NUTRIENT REQUIREMENTS OF BOBWHITE QUAIL[a]

Energy base kcal ME/kg diet[b]	Starting 2,800	Growing 2,800	Breeding 2,800
Protein (%)	26	20	24
Glycine + serine (%)	—	—	—
Lysine (%)	—	—	—
Methionine + cystine (%)	1.0	0.75	0.90
Linoleic acid (%)	1	1	1
Calcium (%)	0.65	0.65	2.4
Phosphorus, available (%)	0.45	0.30	0.7
Sodium (%)	0.15	0.15	0.15
Chlorine (%)	0.11	0.11	0.11
Iodine (mg)	0.3	0.3	0.3
Riboflavin (mg)	3.8	3.0	4.0
Pantothenic acid (mg)	12	9	15
Niacin (mg)	30	30	20
Choline (mg)	1,500	1,500	1,000

[a] Requirements are listed as percentages or as mg/kg of diet. For values not listed, *see* REQUIREMENTS OF LAYING HENS (TABLE 7) and LEGHORN-TYPE CHICKENS (TABLE 14) as a guide.

[b] These are typical dietary energy concentrations.

Adapted, with permission, from *Nutrient Requirements of Poultry*, 1994, National Academy of Sciences, National Academy Press, Washington, DC.

The pellets are then cooled quickly and dried by means of a forced air draft. The conditions under which pelleting occurs (eg, use of an expander rather than an extruder, exposure to high temperature, use of soft pellets) have an important effect on the nutritional quality of the pellets or of the crumbles produced by crushing the pellets.

FEEDING METHODS

For newly hatched birds of any species, a "complete" feed in crumble form is the program of choice, regardless of other considerations. A "complete" feed program for growing stock, particularly for laying and breeding stock, is also highly recommended. Advantages of the "complete" feed program over the "mash and grain" system include the simplicity of feeding, accuracy of medication, improved balance of dietary nutrients, and superior feed conversion efficiency.

Regardless of the system of feeding, recommendations of the feed manufacturer or the strain's breeder company should be followed with regard to the feeding of extra calcium, grit, or whole grain. Fresh, clean water should always be readily available.

VACCINATION PROGRAMS

See TABLES 16–21 for recommended vaccination programs for broilers, broiler-breeders, commercial layers, turkeys, duck breeders, and commercial ducklings.

MANAGEMENT OF GROWING CHICKENS

Broiler houses generally have specific areas designated for brooding. These areas could be throughout the whole house but with rings of cardboard (often referred to as chick guards) used to keep chicks around a heat source; more commonly, an area of the house is curtained off and preheated before chick placement. Either way, the brooder area floor temperature should be between

TABLE 12 NUTRIENT REQUIREMENTS OF PEKIN DUCKS[a]

Energy base kcal ME/kg diet[b]	Starting (0–2 wk) 2,900	Growing (2–7 wk) 3,000	Breeding 2,900
Protein (%)	22	16	15
Arginine (%)	1.1	1.0	—
Lysine (%)	0.9	0.65	0.6
Methionine + cystine (%)	0.7	0.55	0.5
Calcium (%)	0.65	0.6	2.75
Phosphorus, available (%)	0.40	0.30	0.30
Sodium (%)	0.15	0.15	0.15
Chlorine (%)	0.12	0.12	0.12
Magnesium (mg)	500	500	500
Manganese (mg)	50	?	?
Zinc (mg)	60	?	?
Selenium (mg)	0.2	?	?
Vitamin A (IU)	2,500	2,500	4,000
Vitamin D (IU)	400	400	900
Vitamin K (mg)	0.5	0.5	0.5
Riboflavin (mg)	4	4	4
Pantothenic acid (mg)	11	11	11
Niacin (mg)	55	55	55
Pyridoxine (mg)	2.5	2.5	3.0

[a] Requirements are listed as percentages or as units or mg/kg of diet. For nutrients not listed, *see* NUTRIENT REQUIREMENTS OF BROILERS (TABLE 8) as a guide.
[b] These are typical dietary energy concentrations.
Adapted, with permission, from *Nutrient Requirements of Poultry*, 1994, National Academy of Sciences, National Academy Press, Washington, DC.

85°–90°F (29.4°–32.2°C). As the birds become older, the brooder temperature is lowered 5°F (2.8°C) each week until it is 70°F (21.1°C). At ~1 wk of age, the chick guards are removed or the curtains are opened, and the chicks have access to the additional space in the house. In particularly large chicken houses, there may be a second area curtained off for several days (up to 10–14 days of age) before the chicks are given access to the complete house. Ample space should be provided for feeders and waterers, which should be well distributed in the house.

At least 3 in. (7.5 cm) of suitable litter, clean for each brood and spread to an even depth, should be provided at the start. Litter must be free of mold; it should absorb moisture without caking, be nontoxic, and of large enough particle size to discourage consumption. Chicks are started with 24 hr of light for several days; thereafter, light is reduced. Both length of day and intensity of light are important. Lighting programs vary widely, depending on whether housing is windowless or open-sided, and should comply with recommendations of major breeders in similar situations.

TABLE 13 NUTRIENT REQUIREMENTS OF GEESE[a]

Energy base kcal ME/kg diet[b]	Starting (0–4 wk) 2,900	Growing (after 4 wk) 3,000	Breeding 2,900
Protein (%)	20	15	15
Lysine (%)	1.0	0.85	0.6
Methionine + cystine (%)	0.6	0.5	0.5
Calcium (%)	0.65	0.6	2.25
Phosphorus, available (%)	0.3	0.3	0.3
Vitamin A (IU)	1,500	1,500	4,000
Vitamin D (IU)	200	200	200
Riboflavin (mg)	3.8	2.5	4.0
Pantothenic acid (mg)	15	10	10
Niacin (mg)	65	35	20

[a] Requirements are listed as percentages or as units or mg/kg of diet. For nutrients not listed, *see* NUTRIENT REQUIREMENTS OF BROILERS (TABLE 8) as a guide.

[b] These are typical dietary energy concentrations.

Adapted, with permission, from *Nutrient Requirements of Poultry*, 1994, National Academy of Sciences, National Academy Press, Washington, DC.

When rearing pullets to be used as commercial egg laying or meat type breeding hens, feeding systems are often combined with day-length control during rearing to influence the rate at which birds mature. Under certain conditions, pullets may be beak trimmed at the hatchery or, in rare cases, within the first 7 days after hatch. In controlled environment housing, day lengths are controlled more precisely; with dim lights, beak trimming may be delayed until later in the growing period.

Pullets should be treated for external and internal parasites as required. Vaccination should be used to control problem diseases of the geographic area (*see* p 2920).

Many commercial egg laying type pullets are reared in cages. The cage manufacturer usually supplies specific instructions regarding heating, bird density, and feeding space. Most commercial rations are fortified with sufficient nutrients to meet the requirements of cage-reared birds.

MANAGEMENT OF LAYING CHICKENS

Most laying pullets are housed in cages and should be moved to these facilities at least 1 wk before egg production begins. Breeders moved from a growing house to an adult house should also be given at least 1 wk to adjust to their new environment before the stress of egg production begins. Beaks should be retrimmed as necessary, and cull birds removed at the time of rehousing.

Feeders and waterers should be of the proper type, size, and height for the stock and management system. Feeders that are too shallow, too narrow, or lacking a lip or flange on the upper edge may permit excess feed waste. Uneven distribution of waterers or lack of water space results in reduced intake and thus reduced performance.

Artificial Lights: Day length should be increased gradually as the pullets come into egg production and should reach a 14- to 16-hr light period/day at peak production for both market-egg and hatching-egg layers. An intensity of at least 1 foot-candle of light (10 lux) at the feed trough should be provided; this is about equal to one 60-watt light bulb to each 100 sq ft (~9 sq m), hanging 7 ft (2.1 m) above the birds. Production may decrease if day length or light intensity is reduced during the laying period. With cage systems of all types, illumination is more even if smaller wattage bulbs placed closer together are used, rather than large bulbs suspended over the center of each aisle. With

TABLE 14 LINOLEIC ACID, MINERAL, AND VITAMIN REQUIREMENTS OF LEGHORN-TYPE CHICKENS[a]

Age	0–6 wk	6–18 wk	18 wk to 1st egg	Layers	Breeders
Linoleic acid (%)	1.00	1.00	1.00	1.00	1.00
Potassium (%)	0.25	0.25	0.25	0.15	0.15
Sodium (%)	0.15	0.15	0.15	0.15	0.15
Chlorine (%)	0.15	0.15	0.15	0.13	0.13
Magnesium (mg)	600	500	400	500	500
Manganese (mg)	60	30	30	20	20
Zinc (mg)	40	35	35	35	45
Iron (mg)	80	60	60	45	60
Copper (mg)	5	4	4	?	?
Iodine (mg)	0.35	0.35	0.35	0.035	0.01
Selenium (mg)	0.15	0.1	0.1	0.06	0.06
Vitamin A (IU)	1,500	1,500	1,500	3,000	3,000
Vitamin D_3 (IU)	200	200	300	300	300
Vitamin E (IU)	10	5	5	5	10
Vitamin K (mg)	0.5	0.5	0.5	0.5	1.0
Riboflavin (mg)	3.6	1.8	2.2	2.5	3.6
Pantothenic acid (mg)	10	10	10	2	7
Niacin (mg)	27	10	10	10	10
Vitamin B_{12} (mg)	0.009	0.003	0.004	0.004	0.08
Choline (mg)	1,300	900	500	1,050	1,050
Biotin (mg)	0.15	0.1	0.1	0.1	0.1
Folacin (mg)	0.55	0.25	0.25	0.25	0.35
Thiamine (mg)	1.0	1.0	0.8	0.7	0.7
Pyridoxine (mg)	3	3	3	2.5	4.5

[a] Requirements are listed as percentages or as units or mg/kg of diet. Assumes an average daily intake of 110 g of feed/hen/day.

Adapted, with permission, from *Nutrient Requirements of Poultry*, 1994, National Academy of Sciences, National Academy Press, Washington, DC.

tiered cages, the bulbs are suspended 6–7 in. (15–18 cm) above the level of the top cage.

Record Keeping: Successful intensive poultry keeping requires good records of all flock activities, including hatch date, regular body weights (to ensure that the pullets will have reached optimal body weight when they are brought into egg production), lighting program, house temperatures,

TABLE 15 LINOLEIC ACID, MINERAL, AND VITAMIN REQUIREMENTS OF TURKEYS[a]

	Age (wk)							
	Male: 0–4	4–8	8–12	12–16	16–20	20–24		
	Female: 0–4	4–8	8–11	11–14	14–17	17–20	Holding	Breeding Hens
Energy base kcal ME/kg diet[b]	2,800	2,900	3,000	3,100	3,200	3,300	2,900	2,900
Linoleic acid (%)	1.0	1.0	0.8	0.8	0.8	0.8	0.8	1.1
Calcium (%)	1.2	1.0	0.85	0.75	0.65	0.55	0.5	2.25
Phosphorus, available (%)	0.6	0.5	0.42	0.38	0.32	0.28	0.25	0.35
Potassium (%)	0.7	0.6	0.5	0.5	0.4	0.4	0.4	0.6
Sodium (%)	0.17	0.15	0.12	0.12	0.12	0.12	0.12	0.12
Chlorine (%)	0.15	0.14	0.14	0.12	0.12	0.12	0.12	0.12
Magnesium (mg)	500	500	500	500	500	500	500	500
Manganese (mg)	60	60	60	60	60	60	60	60
Zinc (mg)	70	65	50	40	40	40	40	65
Iron (mg)	80	60	60	60	50	50	50	60
Copper (mg)	8	8	6	6	6	6	6	8
Iodine (mg)	0.4	0.4	0.4	0.4	0.4	0.4	0.4	0.4
Selenium (mg)	0.2	0.2	0.2	0.2	0.2	0.2	0.2	0.2
Vitamin A (IU)	5,000	5,000	5,000	5,000	5,000	5,000	5,000	5,000
Vitamin D[c] (IU)	1,100	1,100	1,100	1,100	1,100	1,100	1,100	1,100
Vitamin E (IU)	12	12	10	10	10	10	10	25
Vitamin K (mg)	1.75	1.5	1.0	0.75	0.75	0.5	0.5	1.0
Riboflavin (mg)	4.0	3.6	3.0	3.0	2.5	2.5	2.5	4.0
Pantothenic acid (mg)	10	9	9	9	9	9	9	16
Niacin (mg)	60	60	50	50	40	40	40	40
Vitamin B_{12} (mg)	0.003	0.003	0.003	0.003	0.003	0.003	0.003	0.003
Choline (mg)	1,600	1,400	1,100	1,100	950	800	800	1,000
Biotin (mg)	0.2	0.2	0.125	0.125	0.100	0.100	0.100	0.2
Folacin (mg)	1.0	1.0	0.8	0.8	0.7	0.7	0.7	1.0
Thiamine (mg)	2	2	2	2	2	2	2	2
Pyridoxine (mg)	4.5	4.5	3.5	3.5	3.0	3.0	3.0	4.0

[a] Requirements are listed as percentages or as units or mg/kg of diet.

[b] These are typical ME concentrations for corn-soya diets. Different ME values may be appropriate if other ingredients predominate.

[c] These concentrations of vitamin D are satisfactory when the dietary concentrations of calcium and available phosphorus conform with those in this table.

Adapted, with permission, from *Nutrient Requirements of Poultry*, 1994, National Academy of Sciences, National Academy Press, Washington, DC.

TABLE 16 VACCINATION PROGRAM FOR BROILERS[a]

Vaccine	Age	Route	Type
Marek's disease[b]	1 day	SC	Turkey herpesvirus and SB-1 or Rispens strain for high-challenge areas
Newcastle disease	1 day or	Coarse spray	B1
	14–21 days	Water or coarse spray	B1 or LaSota
Infectious bronchitis	1 day or	Coarse spray	Massachusetts
	14–21 days	Water or coarse spray	Massachusetts
Infectious bursal disease	14–21 days	Water	Intermediate

[a] This is an example of a typical vaccination program. Individual programs are highly variable and reflect local conditions, disease prevalence, severity of challenge, and individual preferences.

[b] Most USA commercial broiler hatcheries use an in ovo vaccination system for Marek's disease at 17–19 days of embryonation. Infectious bursal disease vaccine (mild strain) may be combined with Marek's disease vaccines. Vectored vaccines in which Marek's and fowlpox vaccines have been safely modified to carry immunizing antigens for laryngotracheitis, Newcastle disease, or infectious bursal disease are also commonly used in ovo or day-old chicks. Connecticut strain is often combined with Massachusetts. Bronchitis vaccine is usually combined with Newcastle. Other bronchitis strains such as Arkansas 99 and Florida 88 are included in some areas. Vaccinations at 14–21 days are optional. A single drinking water application for Newcastle disease/bronchitis is also common.

disease history, medication and vaccination dates, quantity and type of feed given (important in calculating efficiency of feed utilization), and mortality.

Floor Space, Feeding, and Water Requirements: Egg-production birds usually spend their entire lives in cages. Although some broiler breeders are similarly housed, most are reared on litter floors or in pens in which as much as two-thirds of the floor is slatted. For egg-strain pullets reared in cages, there is little chance of altering the feeding and watering space available, but periodic checks are necessary to ensure that feed and water are being continuously supplied. With the success of nipple- and cup-waterers and the various types of automatic feeding systems, it becomes more difficult to give specific recommendations for feeding and watering space. Decisions must be made about optimal floor space and feeding and watering requirements based on advice from equipment manufacturers, primary breeders, careful observation, and past experience as to productivity. *See* TABLE 22 and TABLE 23 for space requirements for egg-strain and meat-strain birds. Environmental housing and various types of ventilation may alter these specifications.

Layers per Cage: Within the guidelines indicated in TABLE 22 and TABLE 23, most colony cages house 5–10 layers. The ideal flock size depends on several factors, including labor and cost, and is best determined by the individual poultry manager or producer.

ORGANIC PRODUCTION PRACTICES

Organic Poultry: According to livestock standards, birds for slaughter designated as organic must be raised under organic management starting no later than the second day of life. Preventive management practices, including the use of vaccines to keep animals healthy, are used; however, antibiotics cannot be used for any reason, and federal regulations prohibit the use of hormones in all poultry. Organic management standards prohibit producers from withholding treatment from a sick or injured animal, but animals treated with a prohibited medication may not be sold as organic. All organically raised animals must have access to the outdoors; they may be temporarily confined only for reasons of health, safety, or to protect soil or water quality.

For a product to be labeled with the "USDA organic" seal, it must comply with

TABLE 17 VACCINATION PROGRAM FOR BROILER BREEDERS[a]

Age	Vaccine	Route	Type
1 day	Marek's disease	SC	Turkey herpesvirus
6–7 days	Tenosynovitis	SC	Live (Mild)
14–21 days	Newcastle/infectious bronchitis	Water	B1/Mass
14–28 days	Infectious bursal disease	Water	Intermediate
4 wk	Newcastle/infectious bronchitis	Water or coarse spray	B1/Mass
6–8 wk	Tenosynovitis	SC	Live (Mild)
8–10 wk	Infectious bursal disease	Water or coarse spray	Live
8–10 wk	Newcastle/infectious bronchitis	Water or coarse spray	B1 or LaSota/Mass
10–12 wk	Encephalomyelitis	Wing web	Live, chick-embryo origin
10–12 wk	Fowlpox	Wing web	Modified live
10–12 wk	Chicken infectious anemia	Wing web	Modified live
10–12 wk	Laryngotracheitis	Intraocular	Modified live
10–12 wk	Tenosynovitis	Parenteral	Inactivated
10–12 wk	Fowl cholera	Parenteral *or* Wing web	Inactivated Live CU, PM-1, or M9
12–14 wk	Newcastle/infectious bronchitis	Water or aerosol	B1 or LaSota/Mass
14–18 wk	Fowl cholera	Parenteral *or* Wing web	Inactivated Live CU, PM-1, or M9
16–18 wk	Infectious bursal disease	Parenteral	Inactivated
16–18 wk	Tenosynovitis	Parenteral	Inactivated
16–18 wk	Newcastle/infectious bronchitis	Water or aerosol	B1 or LaSota/Mass
Every 60–90 days or 18 wk	Newcastle/infectious bronchitis	Parenteral	Inactivated

[a] This is an example of a vaccination program. Individual programs are highly variable and reflect local conditions, disease prevalence, severity of challenge, and individual preferences. SB-1, MDV301, or Rispens strain may be combined with turkey herpesvirus in some areas. Vaccination for fowlpox and laryngotracheitis depends on local requirements. Other strains of infectious bronchitis (Connecticut, Arkansas 99, Florida 88, etc) are included in some areas.

TABLE 18 VACCINATION PROGRAM FOR COMMERCIAL LAYERS[a]

Age	Vaccine	Route	Type
1 day	Marek's disease	SC	Turkey herpesvirus and SB-1
14–21 days	Newcastle/infectious bronchitis	Water	B1/Mass
14–21 days	Infectious bursal disease	Water	Intermediate
5 wk	Newcastle/infectious bronchitis	Water or coarse spray	B1/Mass
8–10 wk	Newcastle/infectious bronchitis	Water or coarse spray	B1 or LaSota/Mass
10–12 wk	Encephalomyelitis	Wing web	Live, chick-embryo origin
10–12 wk	Fowlpox	Wing web	Modified live
10–12 wk	Laryngotracheitis	Intraocular	Modified live
10–14 wk	*Mycoplasma gallisepticum*[b]	Intraocular or spray	Mild live strain
or 18 wk		Parenteral	Inactivated
12–14 wk	Newcastle/infectious bronchitis	Water or aerosol	B1 or LaSota/Mass
16–18 wk	Newcastle/infectious bronchitis	Water or aerosol	B1 or LaSota/Mass
Every 60–90 days or 18 wk	Newcastle/infectious bronchitis	Parenteral	Inactivated

[a] This is an example of a vaccination program. Individual programs are highly variable and reflect local conditions, disease prevalence, severity of challenge, and individual preferences.

[b] The use of *M gallisepticum* vaccine is regulated or prohibited in some states. SB-1 or MDV301 may be combined with turkey herpesvirus in some areas, or Rispens strain may be used in high-challenge areas. Vaccination for infectious bursal disease, laryngotracheitis, and fowlpox depends on local requirements. Other strains of infectious bronchitis (Connecticut, Arkansas 99, Florida 88, etc) are included in some areas. *M gallisepticum* and *Haemophilus gallinarum* (coryza) are used only on infected, multiage premises in some areas.

USDA National Organic Standards. Congress passed the Organic Foods Production Act in 1990, and the USDA established national organic standards in 2002. As of 2011, the organic layer flock in the USA was approximately 6.5 million hens, and the average number of organic broilers processed each week was approximately 0.5 million birds. This represents approximately 2.3% of the layer population and 0.3% of the broiler production. In the years from 2001 to 2011, the organic layer flock has grown 400%, and broilers processed as organic has grown 900%. However, it is important to realize that there are years in the past 10 when both layer and broiler organic numbers have shrunk from one year to the next. Growth of these areas is not a straight and predictable line.

The first step toward organic certification for a poultry producer is to select a third-party certifier. The USDA keeps an actively updated list of accredited certification agencies, all of which follow the same USDA National Organic Standards. The producer then submits an application and Organic System Plan (OSP) to the selected certification agency. In livestock production, this plan includes information on the animal source, feeding practices, management practices, health care, recordkeeping, and product labeling. The certifier then reviews the OSP and, if it is deemed adequate, assigns a qualified organic inspector to the livestock facility. The inspector conducts a detailed evaluation of the OSP and the actual farm practices, provides a written exit interview

TABLE 19 VACCINATION PROGRAM FOR TURKEYS[a]

Age (wk)[b]	Market Turkeys	Breeder Hens	Breeder Toms
2–3	ND[c] B1-B1[d] or LaSota, DW[e] or spray	ND, B1-B1 or LaSota, DW or spray	ND, B1-B1 or LaSota, DW or spray
4	Hemorrhagic enteritis, DW	Hemorrhagic enteritis, DW	Hemorrhagic enteritis, DW
6	Fowl cholera,[f] DW (live) or SC (inactivated)	Fowl cholera, DW (live) or SC (inactivated)	Fowl cholera, DW (live) or SC (inactivated)
9–10	ND, LaSota, DW or spray	ND, LaSota, DW or spray	ND, LaSota, DW or spray
12	Fowl cholera, DW (live) or SC (inactivated)	Fowl cholera, DW (live) or SC (inactivated)	Fowl cholera, DW (live) or SC (inactivated)
15	ND, LaSota, DW or spray	ND, LaSota, DW or spray	ND, LaSota, DW or spray
18	—	Fowl cholera, DW (live) or SC (inactivated)	Fowl cholera, DW (live) or SC (inactivated)
21	—	ND, LaSota, DW or spray	ND, LaSota, DW or spray
24	—	Fowl cholera, DW (live) or SC (inactivated)	Fowl cholera, DW (live) or SC (inactivated)
26	—	Erysipelas, DW (live) or SC (inactivated) Pox, WW[e]	Erysipelas, DW (live) or SC (inactivated) Pox, WW
28	—	ND, SC (inactivated) Fowl cholera, DW (live) or SC (inactivated) Encephalomyelitis, DW	ND, SC (inactivated) Fowl cholera, DW (live) or SC (inactivated) Encephalomyelitis, DW

[a] Recommendations are for production areas where the diseases listed are common. In addition, other vaccinations may be advisable if previous experience indicates prevalence of certain diseases in the area. These may include turkey bordetellosis eye drop vaccine at 1 day old and in water or spray at 14 days old, or bacterin; paramyxovirus 3 and influenza A (prevalent hemagglutinin) at 26–28 and 40 wk old; erysipelas—live or killed products might be required for market turkeys, and repeated vaccinations might be required for breeders; and salmonellosis bacterins at 24 and 28 wk old.

[b] Recommended age at vaccination is an approximation.

[c] ND = Newcastle disease

[d] Spray ND vaccines should not be used for birds suffering from respiratory disease; in such cases and at that age, the mild B1-B1 strain vaccine could be used in water. Timing of vaccination depends on maternal antibody levels.

[e] DW = drinking water; WW = wing web stab

[f] Live fowl cholera vaccines should be used only in healthy flocks.

of findings to the producer, and prepares a report to the certifier. If the farm is found to meet all National Organic Program standards, an organic certificate may be issued. The livestock product must be labeled with information identifying both the producer and certifier ("Certified organic by . . ."). The use of the USDA organic seal on packaging is optional. Organic certification requires annual inspections of the poultry farm.

Animal Production Claims and "Natural" Claims: The USDA Food Safety and Inspection Service (FSIS) permits the use of animal production claims and the term "natural." FSIS permits the application of "animal production claims" (ie, truthful statements about the raising of animals from which meat and poultry products are derived) on the labeling of meat and poultry products. For many years,

TABLE 20 VACCINATION PROGRAM FOR DUCK BREEDERS

Age	Vaccine	Route	Type
1 day old	*Riemerella anatipestifer*	Aerosol	Live vaccine[a]
10–14 days	*R anatipestifer*	Drinking water	Live vaccine[a]
3 wk	*R anatipestifer*	SC	Bacterin[b]
4 wk	Duck viral hepatitis	SC	Live vaccine[c] (Type 1)
4 wk	Duck viral enteritis	SC	Live vaccine[c]
10 and 20 wk[d]	*R anatipestifer*	SC	Bacterin[b]
10 and 20 wk	Duck viral hepatitis	SC	Killed virus vaccine (Type 1)

[a] A live, avirulent vaccine consisting of the three major serotypes (1, 2, and 5) of *R anatipestifer*

[b] A formalin-inactivated cell suspension of the three major serotypes (1, 2, and 5) of *R anatipestifer*. Bacterins and killed virus vaccines are administered SC in the neck.

[c] A modified-live virus vaccine of chick embryo origin.

[d] White Pekin breeder ducks normally start egg production at 24 wk of age. Egg production can be accelerated or delayed and breeder vaccination should be completed before the onset of egg production to optimize the passage of parental immunity to the progeny.

animal production claims have served as an alternative to the use of the term “organic” on the labeling of meat and poultry products in the absence of a uniformly accepted definition. Thus, producers may wish to continue the use of animal production claims (eg, “Raised Without Added Hormones,” “Free Range,” “No Antibiotics Ever,” “All Vegetarian Diet”) on meat and poultry labeling. The system FSIS has in place to evaluate the necessary supporting documentation to ensure the accuracy of animal production claims, such as producer affidavits of specific raising protocols or independent third-party programs with audits, will continue to be used whenever these types of claims are made.

The term “natural” may be used when products contain no artificial ingredients and are no more than minimally processed in accordance with FSIS Policy Memo 055. This term may be used in combination with the claim “certified organic by (a certifying entity)” when these requirements are met. The definition of “naturally raised” is being reviewed by the USDA and may result in changes to these definitions.

NUTRITIONAL DEFICIENCIES

A nutritional deficiency may be due to a nutrient being omitted from the diet, adverse interaction between nutrients in otherwise apparently well-fortified diets, or

TABLE 21 VACCINATION PROGRAM FOR COMMERCIAL DUCKLINGS

Age	Vaccine	Route	Type
1 day old	*Riemerella anatipestifer*	Aerosol	Live vaccine[a]
10–14 days	*R anatipestifer*	Drinking water	Live vaccine[a]
3 wk	*R anatipestifer*	SC	Bacterin[b]

[a] A live, avirulent vaccine consisting of the three major serotypes (1, 2, and 5) of *R anatipestifer*

[b] A formalin-inactivated cell suspension of the three major serotypes (1, 2, and 5) of *R anatipestifer* is recommended for preventive immunization on farms where the disease is endemic or epidemic. An *Escherichia coli* bacterin can also be used where field challenge warrants. Ducklings should not be vaccinated within 21 days of slaughter.

the overriding effect of specific antinutrients. The latter two scenarios are difficult to diagnose, because diet analysis suggests a normal level of the nutrient(s) under investigation. Micronutrients such as vitamins and trace minerals are usually added to diets in the form of stand-alone micro premixes, so it is rare to see classic symptoms of deficiency of individual nutrients—rather, the effect seen is more commonly a compilation of many individual metabolic conditions. In many instances, a correct diagnosis can be made only by obtaining complete information about diet and management, clinical signs in the affected living birds, necropsies, and tissue analyses. Unfortunately, tissue, and especially liver and serum analysis, can be misleading, because relative to the time of initial occurrence of any deficiency, the bird often sequesters nutrients in the liver, and so even with deficient diets, liver assays show erroneously high values. This latter effect is most significant for minerals such as copper.

A diet that, by analysis, appears to contain just enough of one or more nutrients may actually be deficient to some degree in those nutrients. Stress (bacterial, parasitic, or viral infections; high or low temperatures; etc) may either interfere with absorption of a nutrient or increase the quantity required. Thus, a toxin or microorganism, for example, may destroy or render unavailable to the bird a particular nutrient that is present in the diet at apparently adequate levels according to conventional chemical or physical assay procedures.

PROTEIN, AMINO ACID, AND ENERGY DEFICIENCIES

The optimal level of balanced protein intake for growing chicks is ~18%–23% of the diet; for growing poults and gallinaceous upland game birds, ~26%–30%; and for growing ducklings and goslings, ~20%–22%. If the protein and component amino acid content of the diet is below these levels, birds tend to grow more slowly. Even when a diet contains the recommended quantities of protein, optimal growth also requires sufficient quantities and proper balance of all the essential amino acids.

Few specific signs are associated with a deficiency of the various amino acids, except for a peculiar, cup-shaped appearance of the feathers in chickens with arginine deficiency and loss of pigment in some of the wing feathers in bronze turkeys with lysine deficiency. All deficiencies of essential amino acids result in retarded growth or reduced egg size or egg production. If a diet is deficient in protein or certain amino acids, the bird may initially consume more feed in an attempt to resolve the deficiency. After a few days, this transient increase in feed intake shifts to a situation of reduced feed intake. Consequently, there will be inferior feed efficiency, and the birds are invariably fatter as a consequence of overconsuming energy.

All commercial breeds of poultry have an amazing ability to consume energy to requirement regardless of dietary energy concentration, assuming they can physically eat enough feed in extreme situations. A deficiency of energy can therefore occur only if the diet is so low in energy concentration that the bird physically cannot eat a sufficient quantity of feed to normalize energy intake. With a deficiency of energy, the bird will grow slowly or stop ovulating. As sources of energy, protein and amino acids will be deaminated, and any lipids will undergo β-oxidation. The latter condition can lead to ketosis, which more commonly occurs in mammals, yet the classic signs are similar.

MINERAL DEFICIENCIES

Calcium and Phosphorus Imbalances

A deficiency of either calcium or phosphorus in the diet of young growing birds results in abnormal bone development, even when the diet contains adequate vitamin D_3 (*see* p 2937). A deficiency of either calcium or phosphorus results in lack of normal skeletal calcification. Rickets is seen mainly in growing birds, whereas calcium deficiency in laying hens results in reduced shell quality and subsequently osteoporosis. This depletion of bone structure causes a disorder commonly referred to as "cage layer fatigue." When calcium is mobilized from bone to overcome a dietary deficiency, the cortical bone erodes and is unable to support the weight of the hen.

Rickets: Rickets occurs most commonly in young meat birds; the main characteristic is inadequate bone mineralization. Calcium deficiency at the cellular level is the main cause, although feeding a diet deficient or imbalanced in calcium, phosphorus, or vitamin D_3 can also induce this problem. Young broilers and turkey poults can exhibit lameness at ~10–14 days of age. Their bones are rubbery, and the rib cage is flattened and beaded at the attachment of the vertebrae. Rachitic birds exhibit a disorganized cartilage matrix, with an irregular vascular

TABLE 22 MINIMUM SPACE REQUIREMENTS FOR WHITE LEGHORN EGG-STRAIN BIRDS[a]

	Age (wk)		
	0–6	7–17	18 onward
CAGES			
Floor area per bird (sq in.)	25	45	60
Straight trough feeder space per bird, not less than (in.)	2	2.5	3
Waterers			
Birds per nipple	15	10	8
Birds per cup	25	15	12
Trough space per bird (in.)	1	1	2
LITTER AND SLATS			
Floor area—litter only or combined with slats (sq ft/bird)	0.5	1	1–1.5
Straight trough feeder space per bird (in.)	1	2	3.5
Pans (15 in. [38 cm] diameter) per 100 birds			
Full fed	3	4	5
Restricted	—	5	—
Waterers			
Birds per fount	100	50	25
Trough space per bird (in.)	1	1	2

[a] Requirements for White Leghorns and brown-egg layers are different.

penetration. There is an indication of impaired metabolism of collagen precursors such as hyaluronic acid and desmosine. Rickets is not caused by a failure in the initiation of bone mineralization but rather by impairment of the early maturation of this process. There is often an enlargement of the ends of the long bones, with a widening of the epiphyseal plate. A determination of whether rickets is due to deficiencies of calcium, phosphorus, or vitamin D_3, or to an excess of calcium (which induces a phosphorus deficiency) may require analysis of blood phosphorus levels and investigation of parathyroid activity.

In most field cases of rickets, a deficiency of vitamin D_3 is suspected. This can be due to simple dietary deficiency, inadequate potency of the D_3 supplement, or other factors that reduce the absorption of vitamin D_3. Rickets can best be prevented by providing adequate levels and potency of vitamin D_3 supplements, and by ensuring that the diet is formulated to ensure optimal utilization of all fat-soluble compounds. Young birds have limited ability to digest saturated fats, and these undigested compounds can complex with calcium to form insoluble soaps, leading to an induced deficiency of calcium. Again, this situation cannot be diagnosed through diet assay for calcium but rather through excreta assay of this mineral. Diets must also provide a correct balance of calcium to available phosphorus. For this reason, ingredients notoriously variable in their content of these minerals, such as animal proteins, should be used with extra caution. In recent years, the use of $25(OH)D_3$ has become very popular as a partial replacement for vitamin D_3, with reports of greatly reduced incidence of rickets, especially in poults.

TABLE 23 SPACE REQUIREMENTS FOR MEAT-STRAIN BIRDS

Age	Floor Space[a]	Feeder Space[b]	Cups or Founts[b] (per 1,000 birds)
From day 1	Heated area 5 sq ft brooder/100 chicks	10 trays/1,000 (feed little and often)	8
From wk 1	1 sq ft/bird	2 in./bird	20
From wk 8	2 sq ft/bird	4 in./bird	30
Mated adults	All litter: 3 sq ft/bird ½ to ⅔ slats: 2¼ sq ft/bird	4 in./bird	30 (60 in hot weather)

[a] Welfare programs in broiler production are relatively proscriptive on space requirements and should be appropriately referenced; the below listings are general guidelines.

[b] For feeder and drinking trough space, both sides of the trough should be counted. Drinking trough space (all ages) is 1 in. (2.5 cm) per bird but doubled for adults in hot weather.

This metabolite is similar to that naturally produced in the liver of birds in the first step of conversion of vitamin D_3 to $1,25(OH)_2D_3$, the active form of the vitamin. The commercial form of $25(OH)D_3$ is therefore especially useful if normal liver metabolism is compromised in any way, such as occurs with mycotoxins or other "natural" toxins in the feed that potentially impair liver metabolism.

Tibial Dyschondroplasia (Osteochondrosis): Tibial dyschondroplasia is characterized by an abnormal cartilage mass in the proximal head of the tibiotarsus. It has been seen in all fast-growing types of meat birds but is most common in broiler chickens. Regardless of diet or environmental conditions, fast versus slow growth rate seems to at least double the incidence of tibial dyschondroplasia. Signs can occur early but more usually are not initially seen until 14–25 days of age. Birds are reluctant to move, and when forced to walk, do so with a swaying motion or stiff gait. Tibial dyschondroplasia results from disruption of the normal metaphyseal blood supply in the proximal tibiotarsal growth plate, where the disruption in nutrient supply means the normal process of ossification does not occur. The abnormal cartilage is composed of severely degenerated cells, with cytoplasm and nuclei appearing shrunken. Affected cartilage contains less protein and less DNA.

The exact cause of tibial dyschondroplasia is unknown. Incidence can quickly be altered through genetic selection and is likely affected by a major sex-linked recessive gene. Imbalance of dietary electrolyte, and particularly high levels of chloride relative to other dietary cations, seem to be a major contributor in many field outbreaks. More tibial dyschondroplasia is also seen when the level of dietary calcium is low relative to that of available phosphorus, or more commonly when diet phosphorus is high relative to calcium. Treatment involves dietary adjustment of the calcium:phosphorus ratio and by achieving a dietary electrolyte balance of ~250 mEq/kg. Dietary changes rarely result in complete recovery. Tibial dyschondroplasia can be prevented by tempering growth rate; however, programs of light or feed restriction must be considered in relation to economic consequences of reduced growth rate. There is evidence that replacement of some of the dietary vitamin D_3 with metabolites such as $1,25(OH)D_3$ improves chondrocyte differentiation and hence limits occurrence of this skeletal disorder.

Cage Layer Fatigue: High-producing laying hens maintained in cages sometimes show paralysis during and just after the period of peak egg production due to a fracture of the vertebrae that subsequently affects the spinal cord. The fracture is caused by an impaired calcium flux related to the high output of calcium in the eggshell. Layers are capable of early egg production exceeding 95% for at least 6 mo, which places even more pressure on maintenance of adequate calcium flux between the diet, the skeleton, and the oviduct. Because medullary bone reserves become depleted, the bird uses cortical bone as a source of calcium for the eggshell. The condition is rarely seen in floor-housed birds, suggesting that reduced activity within the cage is a predisposing or associated factor. Affected birds are invariably found on their sides in the back of the cage. At the time of initial paralysis, birds appear healthy and often have a shelled egg in the oviduct and an active ovary. Death occurs from starvation or dehydration, because the birds simply cannot reach feed or water.

Affected birds will recover if moved to the floor. A high incidence of cage layer fatigue can be prevented by ensuring the normal weight-for-age of pullets at sexual maturity and by giving pullets a high-calcium diet (minimum 4% calcium) for at least 7 days before first oviposition. Older caged layers are also susceptible to bone breakage during removal from the cage and transport to processing. It is not known whether cage layer fatigue and bone breakage are related. However, bone strength cannot practically be improved without adverse consequences to other economically important traits such as eggshell quality. Cage layer fatigue is undoubtedly related to high, sustained egg output and associated clutch lengths of 200–230 eggs laid on successive days.

Diets must provide adequate quantities of calcium and phosphorus to prevent deficiencies. However, feeding diets that contain >2.5% calcium during the immature growing period (<16 wk) produces a high incidence of nephritis, visceral gout, calcium urate deposits in the ureters, and sometimes high mortality, especially in the presence of infectious bronchitis virus. Eggshell strength and bone strength can both be improved by feeding ~50% of the dietary calcium supplement in the form of coarse limestone, with the remaining half as fine particle limestone. Offering the coarse supplement permits the birds to satisfy their requirements when they need it most, allowing the coarse material to be retained in the gizzard where the calcium can be absorbed continually and especially at night-time when the bird is not feeding. A readily available calcium and/or calcium phosphate supplement is often effective if started very soon after paralysis is first observed. Although these supplements may be advantageous to afflicted layers, they are not ideal for the regular birds in the flock; therefore, decisions regarding treatment are often influenced by the severity of the condition and the proportion of the flock affected.

Manganese Deficiency

A deficiency of manganese in the diet of immature chickens and turkeys is one of the potential causes of perosis and chondrodystrophy, and also the production of thin-shelled eggs and poor hatchability in mature birds (*see also* CALCIUM AND PHOSPHORUS IMBALANCES, p 2930).

The most dramatic classic effect of manganese deficiency syndrome is perosis, characterized by enlargement and malformation of the tibiometatarsal joint, twisting and bending of the distal end of the tibia and the proximal end of the tarsometatarsus, thickening and shortening of the leg bones, and slippage of the gastrocnemius tendon from its condyles. Increased intakes of calcium and/or phosphorus will aggravate the condition because of reduced absorption of manganese via the action of precipitated calcium phosphate in the intestinal tract. In laying hens, reduced egg production, markedly reduced hatchability, and eggshell thinning are often noted.

A manganese-deficient breeder diet can result in chondrodystrophy in chick embryos. This condition is characterized by shortened, thickened legs and shortened wings. Other signs can include a parrot beak brought about by a disproportionate shortening of the lower mandible, globular contour of the head due to anterior bulging of the skull, edema occurring just above the atlas joint of the neck and extending posteriorly, and protruding of the abdomen due to unassimilated yolk. Growth is also reduced, and development of down and feathers is retarded. A manganese-deficient chick has a characteristic star-gazing posture, because the physiology of the inner ear becomes defective.

Deformities cannot be corrected by feeding more manganese. Effects of manganese deficiency on egg production are fully corrected by feeding a diet that contains at least 30–40 mg of manganese/kg, provided the diet does not contain excess calcium and/or phosphorus. There is an indication of the need for Fe^{2+} ions as well as manganese to correct the deficiency, although most commercial poultry diets contain a surfeit of iron.

Iron and Copper Deficiencies

Deficiencies of both iron and copper can lead to anemia. Iron deficiency causes a severe anemia with a reduction in PCV. In color-feathered strains, there is also loss of pigmentation in the feathers. The birds' requirements for RBC synthesis take precedence over metabolism of feather pigments, although if a fortified diet is introduced, all subsequent feather growth is normal and lines of demarcation on the feathers are part of diagnosis. Iron may be needed not only for the red feather pigments, which are known to contain iron, but also to function in an enzyme system involved in the pigmentation process. Ochratoxin at 4–8 mcg/g diet also causes an iron deficiency characterized by hypochromic microcytic anemia. Aflatoxin also reduces iron absorption.

Young chicks become lame within 2–4 wk when fed a copper-deficient diet. Bones are fragile and easily broken, the epiphyseal cartilage becomes thickened, and vascular penetration of the thickened cartilage is markedly reduced. These bone lesions resemble the changes noted in birds with a vitamin A deficiency. Copper is required for cartilage formation, and certain antinutrients such as some grain fumigants have been shown to impact skeletal development, likely via interaction with copper metabolism. Copper-deficient chickens may also display ataxia and spastic paralysis.

Copper deficiency in birds, and especially in turkeys, can lead to rupture of the aorta. The biochemical lesion in the copper-deficient aorta is likely related to failure to synthesize desmosine, the cross-link precursor of elastin. The lysine content of copper-deficient elastin is three times that seen in control birds, suggesting failure to incorporate lysine into the desmosine molecule. In field cases of naturally occurring aortic rupture, many birds have <10 ppm copper in the liver, compared with 15–30 ppm normally seen in birds of comparable age. High levels of sulfate ions, molybdenum, and also ascorbic acid can reduce liver copper levels. A high incidence of aortic rupture has been seen in turkeys fed 4-nitrophenylarsonic acid. The problem can be resolved by feeding higher levels of copper, suggesting that products such as 4-nitro may physically complex with copper.

Iodine Deficiency

Iodine deficiency results in a decreased output of thyroxine from the thyroid gland, which in turn stimulates the anterior pituitary to produce and release increased amounts of thyroid stimulating hormone (TSH). This increased production of TSH results in subsequent enlargement of the thyroid gland, usually termed goiter. The enlarged gland results from hypertrophy and hyperplasia of the thyroid follicles, which increases the secretory surface of the follicles.

Lack of thyroid activity or inhibition of the thyroid by administration of thiouracil or thiourea causes hens to cease laying and become obese. It also results in the growth of abnormally long, lacy feathers. Administration of thyroxine or iodinated casein reverses the effects on egg production, with eggshell quality returning to normal. The iodine content of an egg is markedly influenced by the hen's intake of iodine. Eggs from a breeder fed an iodine-deficient diet will exhibit reduced hatchability and delayed yolk sac absorption. Rapeseed meal and, to a lesser extent, canola meal contain goitrogens that cause thyroid enlargement in young birds. Iodine deficiency in poultry can be avoided by supplementing the feed with as little as 0.5 mg of iodine/kg, although a level of 2–3 mg/kg is more commonly provided to sustain good feathering in fast-growing birds.

Magnesium Deficiency

Natural feed ingredients are rich in magnesium; thus, deficiency is rare and magnesium is never specifically used as a supplement to poultry diets. Newly hatched chicks fed a diet totally devoid of magnesium live only a few days. They grow slowly, are lethargic, and often pant and gasp. When disturbed, they exhibit brief convulsions and become comatose, which is sometimes temporary but often fatal. Mortality is quite high on diets only marginally deficient in magnesium, even though growth of survivors may approach that of control birds.

A magnesium deficiency in laying hens results in a rapid decline in egg production, hypomagnesemia, and a marked withdrawal of magnesium from bones. Egg size, shell weight, and the magnesium content of yolk and shell are decreased. Increasing the dietary calcium of laying hens accentuates these effects. Magnesium seems to play a central role in eggshell formation, although it is not clear whether there is a structural need or whether magnesium simply gets deposited as a cofactor along with calcium.

Magnesium requirements for most classes of chickens seem to be ~500–600 ppm, a level that is usually achieved with contributions by natural feed ingredients.

Potassium, Sodium, and Chloride Deficiencies

Although requirements for potassium, sodium, and chloride have been clearly defined, it is also important to maintain a balance of these and all other electrolytes in the body. Often termed electrolyte balance or acid-base balance, the effects of deficiency of any one element are often a consequence of alteration to this important balance as it affects osmoregulation.

Simple Deficiency: A deficiency of chloride causes ataxia with classic signs of nervousness, often induced by sudden noise or fright. The main sign of hypokalemia is an overall muscle weakness characterized by weak extremities, poor intestinal tone with intestinal distention, cardiac weakness, and weakness and ultimately failure of the respiratory muscles. Hypokalemia is apt to occur during severe stress. Plasma protein is increased, causing the kidney, under the influence of adrenocortical hormone, to discharge potassium into the urine. During adaptation to the stress, blood flow to the muscle gradually improves and the muscle begins uptake of potassium. As liver glycogen is restored, potassium returns to the liver.

Birds fed a diet low in both protein and potassium or that are starving grow slowly but do not show a potassium deficiency. Potassium derived from catabolized tissue protein replaces that lost in the urine. The ratio of potassium to nitrogen in urine is relatively constant and is the same as that found in muscle. Thus, tissue nitrogen and potassium are released together from the catabolized tissue.

A deficiency of sodium leads to a lowering of osmotic pressure and a change in acid-base balance in the body. Cardiac output and blood pressure both decrease, PCV increases, elasticity of subcutaneous tissues decreases, and adrenal function is impaired. This leads to an increase in blood uric acid levels, which can result in shock and death. A less severe sodium deficiency in chicks can result in retarded growth, soft bones, corneal keratinization, impaired food utilization, and a decrease in plasma volume. In layers, reduced egg production, poor growth, and cannibalism may be noted. A number of diseases can result in sodium depletion from the body, such as GI losses from diarrhea or urinary losses due to renal or adrenal damage.

Electrolyte Imbalance: Electrolyte balance is commonly described by the simple formula of Na + K – Cl expressed as mEq/kg of diet. An overall dietary balance of 250–300 mEq/kg is generally considered optimal for normal physiologic function. The buffering systems in the body ensure the maintenance of near normal physiologic pH, preventing electrolyte imbalance. The primary role of electrolytes is in maintenance of body water and ionic balance. Thus, requirements for elements such as sodium, potassium, and chloride cannot be considered individually, because it is the overall balance that is important. Electrolyte balance, also referred to as acid-base balance, is affected by three factors: the balance and proportion of these electrolytes in the diet, endogenous acid production, and the rate of renal clearance.

In most situations, the body maintains a normal balance between cations and anions in the body such that physiologic pH is maintained. If there is a shift toward acid or base conditions, metabolic processes return the body to a normal pH. Actual electrolyte imbalances are rare, because regulatory mechanisms must sustain optimal cellular pH and osmolarity. Electrolyte balance can therefore more correctly be described as the changes that necessarily occur in the body processes to achieve normal pH. In extreme situations, such modifications in regulatory mechanisms seem to adversely affect other physiologic systems, and they produce or accentuate potentially debilitating conditions.

Electrolyte imbalance causes a number of metabolic disorders in birds, most notably tibial dyschondroplasia and respiratory alkalosis in layers. Tibial dyschondroplasia in young broiler chickens can be affected by the electrolyte balance of the diet. The unusual development of the cartilage plug at the growth plate of the tibia can be induced by a number of factors, although its incidence can be greatly increased by metabolic acidosis induced by feeding products such as NH_4Cl. Tibial dyschondroplasia seems to occur more frequently when the diet contains an excess of sodium relative to potassium, along with very high chloride levels. The latter situation is most easily remedied by substitution of sodium bicarbonate for sodium chloride in the diet.

Overall electrolyte balance is always important but is most critical when chloride or sulfur levels are high. With low dietary chloride levels, there is often little response to the manipulation of electrolyte balance; however, when dietary chloride levels are high, it is critical to make adjustments to the dietary cations to maintain overall balance. Alternatively, chloride levels can be reduced, although chickens have requirements of ~0.12%–0.15% of the diet, and deficiency signs will develop with dietary levels <0.12%. Sodium content of drinking water can have a meaningful impact on total sodium intake of the bird. When drinking water contains >300 ppm of sodium, it may be necessary to reduce sodium levels in the diet. A recent innovation in poultry nutrition that impacts electrolyte balance is the use of phytase enzyme. This commonly used exogenous enzyme supplement is intended to reduce dependence on supplemental phosphorus, but it has been shown to concomitantly reduce renal excretion of sodium. Diets therefore need less supplemental sodium when they contain phytase enzyme.

Selenium Deficiency

A deficiency of selenium in growing chickens causes exudative diathesis. Early signs of unthriftiness and ruffled feathers usually occur at 3–6 wk of age, depending on the degree of deficiency. The edema results in weeping of the skin, which is often seen on the inner surface of the thighs and wings. The birds bruise easily, and large scabs often form on old bruises. In laying hens, such tissue damage is unusual, but egg production, hatchability, and feed conversion are adversely affected.

The metabolism of selenium is closely linked to that of vitamin E, and signs of deficiency can sometimes be treated with either the mineral or the vitamin. Vitamin E can spare selenium in its role as an antioxidant, and so some selenium-responsive conditions can also be treated by supplemental vitamin E. In most countries, there are limits to the quantity of selenium that can be added to a diet; the upper limit is usually 0.3 ppm.

The commonly used forms are sodium selenite and, more recently, organic selenium chelates. Feeds grown on high-selenium soils are sometimes necessarily used in poultry rations and are good sources of selenium. Fish meal and dried brewer's yeast are also rich in available selenium.

Zinc Deficiency

Zinc requirements and signs of deficiency are influenced by dietary ingredients. In semipurified diets, it is difficult to show a response to zinc levels much above 25–30 mg/kg diet, whereas in practical corn-soybean meal diets, requirement values are increased to 60–80 mg/kg. Such variable zinc needs likely relate to phytic acid content of the diet, because this ligand is a potent zinc chelator. If phytase enzyme is used in diets, the need for supplemental zinc is reduced by up to 10 mg/kg diet.

In young chicks, signs of zinc deficiency include retarded growth, shortening and thickening of leg bones and enlargement of the hock joint, scaling of the skin (especially on the feet), very poor feathering, loss of appetite, and in severe cases, mortality. Although zinc deficiency can reduce egg production in aging hens, the most striking effects are seen in developing embryos. Chicks hatched from zinc-deficient hens are weak and cannot stand, eat, or drink. They have accelerated respiratory rates and labored breathing. If the chicks are disturbed, the signs are aggravated and the chicks often die. Retarded feathering and frizzled feathers are also found. However, the major defect is grossly impaired skeletal development. Zinc-deficient embryos show micromelia, curvature of the spine, and shortened, fused thoracic and lumbar vertebrae. Toes often are missing and, in extreme cases, the embryos have no lower skeleton or limbs. Some embryos are rumpless, and occasionally the eyes are absent or not developed.

VITAMIN DEFICIENCIES

Vitamin deficiencies are most commonly due to inadvertent omission of a complete vitamin premix from the birds' diet. Multiple signs are therefore seen, although in general, signs of B vitamin deficiencies appear first. Because there are some stores of fat-soluble vitamins in the body, it often takes longer for these deficiencies to affect the bird, and it may take months for vitamin A deficiency to affect adult birds.

Treatment and prevention rely on an adequate dietary supply, usually microencapsulated in gelatin or starch along with an antioxidant. Vitamin destruction in feeds is a factor of time, temperature, and humidity. For most feeds, efficacy of vitamins is little affected over 2-mo storage within mixed feed.

Vitamin A Deficiency

Depending on liver stores, adult birds could be fed a vitamin A–deficient diet for 2–5 mo before signs of deficiency develop. Eventually, birds become emaciated and weak with ruffled feathers. Egg production drops markedly, hatchability decreases, and embryonic mortality increases. As egg production declines, there will likely be only small follicles in the ovary, some of which show signs of hemorrhage. A watery discharge from the eyes may also be noted. As the deficiency continues, milky white, cheesy material accumulates in the eyes, making it impossible for birds to see (xerophthalmia). The eye, in many cases, may be destroyed.

The first lesion usually noted in adult birds is in the mucous glands of the upper alimentary tract. The normal epithelium is replaced by a stratified squamous, keratinized layer. This blocks the ducts of the mucous glands, resulting in necrotic secretions. Small, white pustules may be found in the nasal passages, mouth, esophagus, and pharynx, and these may extend into the crop. Breakdown of the mucous membrane usually allows pathogenic microorganisms to invade these tissues and cause secondary infections.

Depending on the quantity of vitamin A passed on from the breeder hen, day-old chicks reared on a vitamin A–deficient diet may show signs within 7 days. However, chicks with a good reserve of maternal vitamin A may not show signs of a deficiency for up to 7 wk. Gross signs in chicks include anorexia, growth retardation, drowsiness, weakness, incoordination, emaciation, and ruffled feathers. If the deficiency is severe, the chicks may become ataxic, which is also seen with vitamin E deficiency (*see* below). The yellow pigment in the shanks and beaks is usually lost, and the comb and wattles are pale. A cheesy material may be noted in the eyes, but xerophthalmia is seldom seen because chicks usually die before the eyes become affected. Secondary infection may play a role in many of the deaths noted with acute vitamin A deficiency.

Young chicks with chronic vitamin A deficiency may also develop pustules in the mucous membrane of the esophagus that usually affect the respiratory tract. Kidneys may be pale and the tubules distended because of uric acid deposits, and in extreme cases, the ureters may be plugged with urates. Blood levels of uric acid can rise from a normal level of ~5 mg to as high as 40 mg/100 mL. Vitamin A deficiency does not interfere with uric acid metabolism but does prevent normal excretion of uric acid from the kidney. Histologic findings include atrophy of the cytoplasm and a loss of the cilia in the columnar, ciliated epithelium.

Although vitamin A–deficient chicks can be ataxic, similar to those with vitamin E deficiency, no gross lesions are found in the brain of vitamin A–deficient chicks as compared with degeneration of the Purkinje cells in the cerebellum of vitamin E–deficient chicks (*see* below). The livers of ataxic vitamin A–deficient chicks contain little or no vitamin A.

Because stabilized vitamin A supplements are almost universally used in poultry diets, it is unlikely that a deficiency will be encountered. However, if a deficiency does develop because of either inadvertent omission of the vitamin A supplement or inadequate feed preparation, up to 2 times the normally recommended level, should be fed for ~2 wk. Vitamin A can be administered through the drinking water, and such treatment usually results in faster recovery than supplemtation via the feed.

Vitamin D_3 Deficiency

Vitamin D_3 is required for the normal absorption and metabolism of calcium and phosphorus. A deficiency can result in rickets in young growing chickens or in osteoporosis and/or poor eggshell quality in laying hens, even though the diet may be well supplied with calcium and phosphorus. Abnormal skeletal development is discussed under calcium and phosphorus imbalances (*see* p 2930) and manganese deficiency (*see* p 2933).

Laying hens fed a vitamin D_3–deficient diet show loss of egg production within 2–3 wk, and depending on the degree of deficiency, shell quality deteriorates almost instantly. Using a corn-soybean meal diet with no supplemental vitamin D_3, shell weight decreases dramatically by ~150 mg/day throughout the first 7 days of deficiency. The less obvious decline in shell quality with suboptimal, rather than deficient, supplements is more difficult to diagnose, especially because it is very difficult to assay vitamin D_3 in complete feeds.

There is a significant increase in plasma $1,25(OH)_2D_3$ of birds producing good versus poor eggshells. Feeding purified $1,25(OH)_2D_3$ improves the shell quality of these inferior layers, suggesting a potential inherent problem with metabolism of cholecalciferol.

Retarded growth and severe leg weakness are the first signs noted when chicks are deficient in vitamin D_3. Beaks and claws become soft and pliable. Chicks may have trouble walking and will take a few steps before squatting on their hocks. While resting, they often sway from side to side, suggesting loss of equilibrium. Feathering is usually poor, and an abnormal banding of feathers may be seen in colored breeds. With chronic vitamin D_3 deficiency, marked skeletal disorders are noted. The spinal column may bend downward and the sternum may deviate to one side. These structural changes reduce the size of the thorax, with subsequent crowding of the internal organs, especially the air sacs. A characteristic finding in chicks is a beading of the ribs at the junction of the spinal column along with a downward and posterior bending. Poor calcification can also be seen at the epiphysis of the tibia and femur. By immersing the split bone in a silver nitrate solution and allowing it to stand under incandescent light for a few minutes, the calcified areas are easily distinguished from the areas of cartilage. Adding synthetic 1,25$(OH)_2D_3$ to the diet of susceptible chicks reduces the incidence of this condition. Although response is variable, results suggest that some leg abnormalities may be a consequence of inefficient metabolism of cholecalciferol.

In laying hens, signs of gross pathology are usually confined to the bones and parathyroid glands. Bones are soft and easily broken, and the ribs may become beaded. The ribs may also show spontaneous fractures in the sternovertebral region. Histologic examination shows decreased calcification in the long bones, with excess of osteoid tissue and parathyroid enlargement.

Dry, stabilized forms of vitamin D_3 are recommended to treat deficiencies. In cases of severe mycotoxicosis, a water-miscible form of vitamin D_3 is administered in the drinking water to provide the amount normally supplied in the diet. In cases of impaired liver function, metabolites of vitamin D are the usual choice for treatment.

Vitamin E Deficiency

The three main disorders seen in chicks deficient in vitamin E are encephalomalacia, exudative diathesis, and muscular dystrophy. The occurrence of these conditions depends on various other dietary and environmental factors.

Encephalomalacia is seen in commercial flocks if diets are very low in vitamin E, if an antioxidant is either omitted or is not present in sufficient quantities, or if the diet contains a reasonably high level of an unstable and unsaturated fat. For exudative diathesis to occur, the diet must be deficient in both vitamin E and selenium. Signs of muscular dystrophy are rare in chicks, because the diet must be deficient in both sulfur amino acids and vitamin E. Because the sulfur amino acids are necessary for growth, a deficiency severe enough to induce muscular dystrophy is unlikely to occur under commercial conditions. Signs of exudative diathesis and muscular dystrophy can be reversed in chicks by supplementing the diet with liberal amounts of vitamin E, assuming the deficiency is not too advanced. Encephalomalacia may respond to vitamin E supplementation, depending on the extent of the damage to the cerebellum.

The classic sign of encephalomalacia is ataxia. The results from hemorrhage and edema within the granular layers of the cerebellum, with pyknosis and eventual disappearance of the Purkinje cells and separation of the granular layers of the cerebellar folia. Because of its inherently low level of vitamin E, the cerebellum is particularly susceptible to lipid peroxidation. In prevention of encephalomalacia, vitamin E functions as a biologic antioxidant. The quantitative need for vitamin E for this function depends on the amount of linoleic acid and polyunsaturated fatty acids in the diet. Over prolonged periods, antioxidants have been shown to prevent encephalomalacia in chicks when added to diets with very low levels of vitamin E or in chicks fed vitamin E–depleted purified diets. Chicks hatched from breeders that are given additional dietary vitamin E seem less susceptible to lipid peroxidation in the brain. The fact that antioxidants can help prevent encephalomalacia, but fail to prevent exudative diathesis or muscular dystrophy in chicks, strongly suggests that vitamin E is acting as an antioxidant in this situation. Exudative diathesis results in a severe edema caused by a marked increase in capillary permeability. Electrophoretic patterns of the blood show a decrease in albumin levels, whereas exudative fluids contained a protein pattern similar to that of normal blood plasma.

Vitamin E deficiency accompanied by sulfur amino acid deficiency results in severe muscular dystrophy in chicks by ~4 wk of age. This condition is characterized by degeneration of the muscle fibers, usually in the breast but sometimes also in the leg muscles. Histologic examination shows Zenker's degeneration, with perivascular infiltration and marked accumulation of infiltrated eosinophils, lymphocytes, and histocytes. Accumulation of these cells in dystrophic tissue results in an increase in lysosomal enzymes, which appear to function in the breakdown and removal of the products of dystrophic degeneration. Initial studies involving the effects of dietary vitamin E on muscular dystrophy show that the addition of selenium at 1–5 mg/kg diet reduced the incidence of muscular dystrophy in chicks receiving a vitamin E–deficient diet that was also low in methionine and cysteine, but did not completely prevent the disease. However, selenium was completely effective in preventing muscular dystrophy in chicks when the diet contained a low level of vitamin E, which alone had been shown to have no effect on the disease. Throughout the past few years, the incidence of "muscular dystrophy–type" lesions in the breast muscle of older (>35 day) broilers has increased. Characteristic parallel white striations on the muscle are similar to those seen in chicks with muscular dystrophy, yet on analysis the diet of these birds seems adequate in vitamin E as well as selenium.

Studies with chicks on the interrelationships between antioxidants, linoleic acid, selenium, and sulfur amino acids have shown that selenium and vitamin E play supportive roles in several processes, one of which involves cysteine metabolism and its role in prevention of muscular dystrophy in chickens. Glutathione peroxidase is soluble and located in the aqueous portions of the cell, whereas vitamin E is located mainly in the hydrophobic environments of membranes and in adipose tissue and other lipid storage cells. The overlapping manner in which vitamin E and selenium function in the cellular antioxidant system suggest that they spare one another in prevention of deficiency signs.

Only stabilized fat should be used in feeds. Adequate levels of stabilized vitamin E should be used in conjunction with a commercial antioxidant and at least 0.3 ppm selenium. Signs of exudative diathesis and muscular dystrophy due to vitamin E deficiency can be reversed if treatment is begun early by administering vitamin E through the feed or drinking water. Oral administration of a single dose of vitamin E (300 IU per bird) usually causes remission.

Vitamin K Deficiency

Impairment of blood coagulation is the major clinical sign of vitamin K deficiency. With a severe deficiency, subcutaneous and internal hemorrhages can prove fatal. Vitamin K deficiency results in a reduction in prothrombin content of the blood, and in the young chick, plasma levels are as low as 2% of normal. Because the prothrombin content of newly hatched chicks is only ~40% that of adult birds, young chicks are readily affected by a vitamin K–deficient diet. A carryover of vitamin K from the hen to eggs, and subsequently to hatched chicks, has been demonstrated, so breeder diets should be well fortified. Hemorrhagic syndrome in day-old chicks has been attributed to a deficiency of vitamin K in the diet of the breeder hens. Gross deficiency of vitamin K results in such prolonged blood clotting that severely deficient chicks may bleed to death from a slight bruise or other injury. Borderline deficiencies often cause small hemorrhagic blemishes. Hemorrhages may appear on the breast, legs, wings, in the abdominal cavity, and on the surface of the intestine. Chicks are anemic, which may be due in part to loss of blood but also to development of hypoplastic bone marrow. Although blood-clotting time is a reasonable measure of the degree of vitamin K deficiency, a more accurate measure is obtained by determining the prothrombin time. Prothrombin times in severely deficient chicks may be extended from a normal of 17–20 sec to 5–6 min or longer. No major heart lesions are seen in vitamin K–deficient chicks such as those that occur in pigs.

A vitamin K deficiency in poultry may be related to low dietary levels of the vitamin, low levels in the maternal diet, lack of intestinal synthesis, extent of coprophagy, or the presence of sulfur drugs and other feed additives in the diet. Chicks with coccidiosis can have severe damage to their intestinal wall and can bleed excessively. Antimicrobial agents can suppress intestinal synthesis of vitamin K, rendering the bird completely dependent on the diet for its supply of the vitamin. Synthesis of vitamin K does occur in the bacteria resident in the bird's digestive tract; however, such vitamin K remains inside the bacterial cell, so the only benefit to the bird arises from the bacterial cell digestion or via coprophagy.

The inclusion of menadione at 1–4 mg/ton of feed is an effective and common practice to prevent vitamin K deficiency. If signs of deficiency are seen, the level should be doubled. A number of stress factors (eg, coccidiosis and other intestinal parasitic diseases) increase the requirements for vitamin K. Dicumarol, sulfaquinoxaline, and warfarin are antimetabolites of vitamin K.

Vitamin B_{12} Deficiency

Vitamin B_{12} is an essential part of several enzyme systems, with most reactions involving the transfer or synthesis of methyl groups. Although the most important function of vitamin B_{12} is in the metabolism of nucleic acids and proteins, it also functions in carbohydrate and fat metabolism.

In growing chickens, a deficiency of vitamin B_{12} results in reduced weight gain and feed intake, along with poor feathering and nervous disorders. Although deficiency may lead to perosis, this is probably a secondary effect due to a dietary deficiency of methionine or choline as sources of methyl groups. Vitamin B_{12} may alleviate perosis because of its effect on the synthesis of methyl groups. Other signs reported in poultry are anemia, gizzard erosion, and fatty infiltration of the heart, liver, and kidneys. Laying hens initially appear to be able to maintain body weight and egg production; however, egg size is reduced. In breeders, hatchability can be markedly reduced, although several weeks may be needed for signs of deficiency to appear. Changes noted in embryos from B_{12}-deficient breeders include a general hemorrhagic condition, fatty liver, fewer myelinated fibers in the spinal cord, and high incidence of mid-term embryo deaths.

Deficiency of vitamin B_{12} is highly unlikely, especially for birds grown on litter or where animal-based ingredients are used. Treatment involves feeding up to 20 mcg/g feed for 1–2 wk.

Choline Deficiency

In addition to poor growth, the classic sign of choline deficiency in chicks and poults is perosis. Perosis is first characterized by pinpoint hemorrhages and a slight puffiness about the hock joint, followed by an apparent flattening of the tibiometatarsal joint caused by a rotation of the metatarsus. The metatarsus continues to twist and may become bent or bowed so that it is out of alignment with the tibia. When this condition exists, the leg cannot adequately support the weight of the bird. The articular cartilage is displaced, and the Achilles tendon slips from its condyles. Perosis is not a specific deficiency sign; it appears with several nutrient deficiencies.

Although choline deficiency readily develops in chicks fed diets low in choline, a deficiency in laying hens is not easily produced. Eggs contain ~12–13 mg of choline/g of dried whole egg. A large egg contains ~170 mg of choline, found almost entirely in the phospholipids. Thus, there appears to be a considerable need for choline to produce an egg. In spite of this, producing a marked choline deficiency in laying hens has been difficult, even when highly purified diets essentially devoid of choline are provided for a prolonged period. Under these conditions, the choline content of eggs is not reduced, suggesting possible intestinal synthesis by the bird.

Diets that contain appreciable quantities of soybean meal, wheat bran, and wheat shorts are unlikely to be deficient in choline. Soybean meal is a good source of choline, and wheat byproducts are good sources of betaine, which can perform the methyl-donor function of choline. Other good sources of choline are distiller's grains, fishmeal, liver meal, meat meals, distiller's solubles, and yeast. A number of commercial choline supplements are available, and supplemental choline is routinely used in most poultry feeds.

Niacin (Nicotinic Acid) Deficiency

There is considerable evidence that poultry, and even chick and turkey embryos, can synthesize niacin but at a rate too slow for optimal growth. It has been claimed that a marked deficiency of niacin cannot occur in chickens unless there is a concomitant deficiency of the amino acid tryptophan, which is a niacin precursor.

Niacin deficiency is characterized by severe disorders in the skin and digestive organs. The first signs are usually loss of appetite, retarded growth, general weakness, and diarrhea. Deficiency produces enlargement of the tibiotarsal joint, valgus-varus bowing of the legs, poor feathering, and dermatitis on the head and feet.

Niacin deficiency in chicks can also result in "black tongue." At ~2 wk of age, the tongue, oral cavity, and esophagus become distinctly inflamed. In the niacin-deficient hen, weight loss, reduced egg production, and a marked decrease in hatchability can result. Turkeys, ducks, pheasants, and goslings are much more severely affected by niacin deficiency than are chickens. Their apparently higher requirements are likely related to their less efficient conversion of tryptophan to niacin. Ducks and turkeys with a niacin deficiency show a severe bowing of the legs and an enlargement of the hock joint. The main difference between the leg seen in niacin deficiency and perosis as seen in manganese and choline deficiency is that with niacin deficiency the Achilles tendon seldom slips from its condyles.

Niacin deficiency in chickens may be prevented by feeding a diet that contains niacin at ≥30 mg/kg; however, many nutritionists recommend 2–2.5 times as much. An allowance of 55–70 mg/kg of feed appears to be satisfactory for ducks, geese, and turkeys. Ample niacin should be provided in poultry diets so as to spare the utilization of tryptophan.

Pantothenic Acid Deficiency

Pantothenic acid is the prosthetic group within coenzyme A, an important coenzyme involved in many reversible acetylation reactions in carbohydrate, fat, and amino acid metabolism. Signs of deficiency therefore relate to general avian metabolism.

The major lesions of pantothenic acid deficiency involve the nervous system, the adrenal cortex, and the skin. Deficiency may result in reduced egg production; however, a marked drop in hatchability is usually noted before this event. Embryos from hens with pantothenic acid deficiency can have subcutaneous hemorrhages and severe edema, with most mortality showing up during the later part of the incubation period. In chicks, the first signs are reduced growth and feed consumption, poor feathering with feathers becoming ruffled and brittle, and a rapidly developing dermatitis. The corners of the beak and the area below the beak are usually the worst affected regions for dermatitis, but the condition is also noted on the feet. In severe cases, the skin of the feet may cornify, and wart-like lumps occur on the balls of the feet. The foot problem often leads to bacterial infection.

Liver concentration of pantothenic acid is reduced during a deficiency, with the liver becoming atrophied, with a faint dirty yellow color developing. Nerve fibers of the spinal cord may show myelin degeneration. Pantothenic acid–deficient chicks show lymphoid cell necrosis in the bursa of Fabricius and thymus, together with lymphocytic paucity in the spleen. The foot condition in chicks and the poor feathering are difficult to differentiate from signs of a biotin deficiency. In a pantothenic acid deficiency, dermatitis of the feet is usually noted first on the toes; in contrast, a biotin deficiency primarily affects the foot pads and is usually more severe. Ducks do not show the usual signs noted for chickens and turkeys, except for retarded growth, but mortality can be quite high.

Most poultry diets contain supplements of calcium pantothenate. Periodically, growing chickens fed practical diets develop a scaly condition of the skin, the exact cause of which is not known. Treatment with both calcium pantothenate (2 g) and riboflavin (0.5 g) in the drinking water (50 gal [190 L]) for a few days has been successful in some instances. Diets usually contain supplemental pantothenic acid at 12 mg/kg.

Riboflavin Deficiency

Many tissues may be affected by riboflavin deficiency, although the epithelium and the myelin sheaths of some of the main nerves are major targets. Changes in the sciatic nerves produce "curled-toe" paralysis in growing chickens. Egg production is affected, and riboflavin-deficient eggs do not hatch. When the diet is inadvertently devoid of the entire spectrum of vitamins, it is signs of riboflavin deficiency that first appear. When chicks are fed a diet deficient in riboflavin, their appetite is fairly good but they grow slowly, become weak and emaciated, and develop diarrhea between the first and second weeks. Deficient chicks are reluctant to move unless forced and then frequently walk on their hocks with the aid of their wings. The leg muscles are atrophied and flabby, and the skin is dry and harsh. In advanced stages of deficiency, the chicks lie prostrate with their legs extended, sometimes in opposite directions. The characteristic sign of riboflavin deficiency is a marked enlargement of the sciatic and brachial nerve sheaths; sciatic nerves usually show the most pronounced effects. Histologic examination of the affected nerves shows degenerative changes in the myelin sheaths that, when severe, pinch the nerve. This produces a permanent stimulus, which causes the curled-toe paralysis.

Signs of riboflavin deficiency in hens are decreased egg production, increased embryonic mortality, and an increase in size and fat content of the liver. Hatchability declines within 2 wk when hens are fed a riboflavin-deficient diet but returns to near normal when riboflavin is restored. Affected embryos are dwarfed and show characteristically defective "clubbed" down. The nervous system of these embryos shows degenerative changes much like those described in riboflavin-deficient chicks. Clubbed down is periodically seen in cases of poor hatchability, when the "reject" chicks or dead embryos show this condition, even though the breeder diet is apparently adequate in riboflavin. Anecdotal evidence suggests greater occurrence of this clubbed-down condition in farms that select "floor-eggs" for incubation.

Signs of riboflavin deficiency first appear at 10 days of incubation, when embryos become hypoglycemic and accumulate intermediates of fatty acid oxidation. Although flavin-dependent enzymes are depressed with riboflavin deficiency, the main effect seems to be impaired fatty acid oxidation, which is a critical function in the developing embryo. An autosomal recessive trait blocks the formation of the riboflavin-binding protein needed for transport of riboflavin to the egg. Although the adults appear normal, their eggs fail to hatch regardless of dietary riboflavin content. As eggs become deficient in riboflavin, the egg albumen loses its characteristic yellow color. In fact, albumen color score has been used to assess riboflavin status of birds.

Chicks receiving diets only partially deficient in riboflavin may recover spontaneously, indicating that the requirement rapidly decreases with age. A 100-mcg dose should be sufficient for treatment of riboflavin-deficient chicks, followed by incorporation of an adequate level in the diet. However, when the curled-toe deformity is longstanding, irreparable damage occurs in the sciatic nerve, and the administration of riboflavin is no longer curative.

Most diets contain up to 10 mg of riboflavin/kg. Treatment can be given as two sequential daily 100-mcg doses for chicks or poults, followed by an adequate amount of riboflavin in feed.

Folic Acid (Folacin) Deficiency

A folacin deficiency results in a macrocytic (megaloblastic) anemia and leukopenia. Tissues with a rapid turnover, such as epithelial linings, GI tract, epidermis, and bone marrow, as well as cell growth and tissue regeneration, are principally affected.

Poultry seem more susceptible to folacin deficiency than other farm animals. Deficiency results in poor feathering, slow growth, an anemic appearance, and sometimes perosis. As anemia develops, the comb becomes a waxy-white color, and pale mucous membranes in the mouth are noted. Increased erythrocyte phosphoribosylpyrophosphate concentration can be used as a diagnostic tool in folacin-deficient chicks. There may also be damage to liver parenchyma and depleted glycogen reserves. Although turkey poults show some of the same signs as chickens, mortality is usually higher and the birds develop a spastic type of cervical paralysis that results in the neck becoming stiff and extended.

The abnormal feather condition in chickens leads to weak and brittle shafts, and depigmentation develops in colored feathers. Although a folacin deficiency can result in reduced egg production, the main sign noted with breeders is a marked decrease in hatchability associated with an increase in embryonic mortality, usually during the last few days of incubation. Embryos have deformed beaks and bending of the tibiotarsus. Birds may exhibit perosis, but the lesions seen differ histologically from those that develop due to choline or manganese deficiency. Abnormal structure of the hyaline cartilage and retardation of ossification are noted with folacin deficiency. Increasing the protein content of the diet has been shown to increase the severity of perosis in chicks receiving diets low in folic acid, because there is an increased folacin demand for uric acid synthesis.

Signs of folic acid deficiency in poultry can be prevented by ensuring diets contain supplements of up to 1 mg/kg.

Biotin Deficiency

Biotin deficiency results in dermatitis of the feet and the skin around the beak and eyes similar to that described for pantothenic acid deficiency (*see* p 2940). Perosis and footpad dermatitis are also characteristic signs. Although signs of classic biotin deficiency are rare, occurrence of fatty liver and kidney syndrome (FLKS) is important to commercial poultry producers. FLKS was first described in Denmark in 1958 but was not a major concern until the late 1960s, when the condition became more prevalent and especially so in Europe and Australia. Chicks ~3 wk old become lethargic and unable to stand, then die within hours. Mortality is usually quite low at 1%–2% but can reach 20%–30%. Postmortem examination reveals pale liver and kidney with accumulation of fat.

The condition as described in the 1960s was usually confined to wheat-fed birds and was most problematic in low-fat, high-energy diets. High vitamin supplementation in general corrected the problem, and biotin was isolated as the causative agent. It is now known that biotin in wheat has exceptionally low availability. The trigger of high-energy diets led to investigation of biotin in carbohydrate metabolism. Chicks with FLKS are invariably hypoglycemic, emphasizing the importance of biotin in two key enzymes, namely pyruvate carboxylase and acetyl Co-A carboxylase. Acetyl Co-A carboxylase appears to preferentially sequester biotin, such that with low biotin availability and need for high de novo fat synthesis (high-energy, low-fat diet), pyruvate carboxylase activity is severely compromised. Even with this imbalance, birds are able to grow. However, with a concurrent deprivation in feed intake or increased demand for glucose, hypoglycemia develops, leading to adipose catabolism and the characteristic accumulation of fat in both liver and kidneys. Birds with FLKS rarely show signs of classic biotin deficiency.

Plasma biotin levels <100 ng/100 mL have been reported as a sign of deficiency. However, recent evidence suggests that plasma biotin levels are quite insensitive to the birds' biotin status, and that biotin levels in the liver or kidneys are more useful indicators. Plasma pyruvic carboxylase is positively correlated with dietary biotin concentration, and levels plateau much later than does the growth response to supplemental biotin.

Embryos are also sensitive to biotin status. Congenital perosis, ataxia, and characteristic skeletal deformities may be seen in embryos and newly hatched chicks when hens are fed a deficient diet. Embryonic deformities include a shortened tibiotarsus that is bent posteriorly, a much shortened tarsometatarsus, shortening of the bones of the wing and skull, and shortening and bending of the anterior end of the scapula. Syndactyly, which is an extensive webbing between the third and fourth toes, is seen in biotin-deficient embryos. Such embryos are chondrodystrophic and characterized by reduced size, parrot beak, crooked tibia, and shortened or twisted tarsometatarsus.

A number of factors increase biotin requirements, including oxidative rancidity of any feed fat, competition by intestinal microorganisms, and lack of carryover into the newly hatched chick or poult. It is good practice to add 150 mg biotin/tonne of feed, especially when significant amounts of wheat or wheat byproducts are used in the diet.

Pyridoxine (Vitamin B_6) Deficiency

A vitamin B_6 deficiency causes retarded growth, dermatitis, and anemia. Because a major role of the vitamin is in protein metabolism, deficiency can result in reduced nitrogen retention. Dietary protein is not well utilized, and thus nitrogen excretion increases. Increased iron levels and decreased copper levels are noted in the serum, and iron utilization appears to be markedly decreased. The resulting anemia is likely due to a disturbance in the synthesis of protoporphyrins. Anemia is often noted in ducks but is seldom seen in chickens and turkeys. Young chicks may show nervous movements of the legs when walking and often undergo spasmodic convulsions, leading to death. During convulsions, the chicks may run about aimlessly, flapping their wings and falling with jerking motions. The greater intensity of activity, resulting from vitamin B_6 deficiency, distinguishes these signs from those of encephalomalacia. Gizzard erosion has been noted in vitamin B_6–deficient chicks. It can be prevented by inclusion of 1% taurocholic acid in the diet, leading to the speculation that pyridoxine is involved in taurine synthesis and is important for gizzard integrity. In pyridoxine deficiency, collagen maturation is incomplete, suggesting that this vitamin is essential for integrity of the connective tissue matrix. A chronic deficiency can result in perosis, with one leg usually being crippled and one or both middle toes bent inward at the first joint.

In adult birds, pyridoxine deficiency results in reduced appetite, leading to reduced egg production and a decline in hatchability. Severe deficiency can cause rapid involution of the ovary, oviduct, comb, and wattles, and of the testis in cockerels. Feed consumption in vitamin B_6–deficient hens and cockerels declines sharply. Although a partial molt is seen in some hens, normal egg production returns within 2 wk after provision of a normal dietary level of pyridoxine.

Deficiency can be prevented by adding pyridoxine at 3–4 mg/kg feed.

Thiamine Deficiency

Polyneuritis in birds represents the later stages of a thiamine deficiency, probably caused by buildup of the intermediates of carbohydrate metabolism. Because the brain's immediate source of energy results from the degradation of glucose, it depends on biochemical reactions involving thiamine. In the initial stages of deficiency, lethargy and head tremors may be noted. A marked decrease in appetite is seen in birds fed a thiamine-deficient diet. Poultry are also susceptible to neuromuscular problems, resulting in impaired digestion, general weakness, star-gazing, and frequent convulsions.

Polyneuritis may be seen in mature birds ~3 wk after they are fed a thiamine-deficient diet. As the deficiency progresses, birds may sit on flexed legs and draw back their heads in a star-gazing position. Retraction of the head is due to paralysis of the anterior neck muscles. Soon after this stage, chickens lose the ability to stand or sit upright and topple to the floor, where they may lie with heads still retracted. Thiamine deficiency may also lead to a decrease in body temperature and respiratory rate. Testicular degeneration may be noted, and the heart may show slight atrophy. Birds consuming a thiamine-deficient diet soon show severe anorexia. They lose all interest in feed and will not resume eating unless given thiamine. If a severe deficiency has developed, thiamine must be force-fed or injected to induce the chickens to resume eating.

Thiamine deficiency is most common when poorly processed fish meals are used, because they contain thiaminase enzyme. In such situations, adding extra thiamine may be ineffective. There is no good evidence suggesting that, unlike in some mammalian species, certain *Fusarium* mycotoxins can increase the need for supplemental thiamine. In otherwise adequate diets, deficiency is prevented by supplements of thiamine up to 4 mg/kg.

TOXICOLOGY

FEED CONTAMINANTS

INDUSTRIAL TOXICANTS

INSECTICIDES, ACARICIDES, AND MOLLUSCICIDES

METALS AND MICRONUTRIENTS

PLANTS AND FUNGI

POISONOUS AND VENOMOUS ORGANISMS

RODENTICIDES

TOXICOLOGY INTRODUCTION

For a discussion of common poisonings in poultry, *see* p 2859.

Veterinary toxicology involves the evaluation of toxicosis and deficiencies, identification and characterization of toxins and determination of their fate in the body, and treatment of toxicosis. Toxicology has been receiving even more attention in the general public with the widespread interest in crime scene investigator (CSI) television shows. The recent worldwide melamine contamination in pet and swine feed, pet jerky treats causing illness and death, and concerns with use of β-agonists in food animals demonstrates the relevancy of veterinary toxicology to current animal health and food safety. Veterinary toxicology can be challenging because of the low frequency of cases observed in a practice setting. When a toxicosis occurs, it often involves a large number of animals and may also involve litigation. A current veterinary toxicology reference book is helpful to ensure the correct samples are obtained and submitted for diagnosis.

A toxic agent is referred to as a toxicant or poison. The term **toxin** refers to a poison produced by a biologic source (eg, venoms, plant toxins); the redundant term biotoxin is occasionally used. **Toxicosis**, **poisoning**, and **intoxication** are synonymous terms for the disease produced by a toxicant. **Toxicity** (sometimes incorrectly used instead of poisoning) refers to the amount of a toxicant necessary to produce a detrimental effect.

Acute toxicosis refers to effects during the first 24-hr period. Effects produced by prolonged exposure (≥3 mo) are referred to as **chronic toxicosis**. Terms such as subacute and subchronic are used to cover the large gap between acute and chronic.

All toxic effects are dose dependent. A dose may cause undetectable, therapeutic, toxic, or lethal effects. A dose is expressed as the amount of compound per unit of body weight, and toxicant concentration as part per million or part per billion. These quantitative expressions are also used for feedstuffs, water, and air, as well as for tissue levels.

LD_{50} is the dose that is lethal to 50% of a test sample. It is an estimator of lethality and the most common expression used to rate the potency of toxicants. Other terms used for prediction of illness or lethality include no observed effect level (NOEL), maximum nontoxic dose (MNTD), and maximum tolerated dose or minimum toxic dose (MTD).

ABSORPTION, DISTRIBUTION, METABOLISM, AND EXCRETION

The basis of toxicology involves the absorption, distribution, metabolism, and excretion (ADME) of a toxicant. Knowledge of these processes is important to evaluate risk of exposure to toxins. (*See also* DISPOSITION AND FATE OF DRUGS, p 2492.)

Absorption: Absorption may occur through the alimentary tract, skin, lungs, via the eye, mammary gland, or uterus, as well as from sites of injection. Toxic effects may be local, but the toxicant must be dissolved and absorbed to some extent to affect the cell. Solubility is the primary factor affecting absorption. Insoluble salts and ionized compounds are poorly absorbed, whereas lipid-soluble substances are generally readily absorbed, even through intact skin. For example, barium is toxic, but barium sulfate can be used for intestinal contrast radiography because of low absorption.

Distribution: Distribution or translocation of a toxicant is via the bloodstream to reactive sites, including storage depots. The liver receives the portal circulation and is the organ most commonly involved with intoxication (and detoxification). The selective deposit of foreign chemicals in various tissues depends on receptor sites. Ease of chemical distribution depends largely on its water solubility. Polar or aqueous-soluble agents tend to be excreted by the kidneys; lipid-soluble chemicals are more likely to be excreted via the bile and accumulate in fat depots. The highest concentration of a toxin within an animal is not necessarily found in the organ or tissue on which it exerts its maximal effect (the target organ). Lead may be found in highest concentrations in bone, which is neither a site for toxic effects nor a reliable tissue for toxicologic interpretation. Knowledge of the translocation characteristics of toxicants is necessary for proper selection of organs for analysis.

Metabolism: Metabolism or biotransformation of toxicants by the body is an "attempt to detoxify." In some instances, metabolized xenobiotic agents are more toxic than the original compound. This is referred to as lethal synthesis. Metabolism of many organophosphorous insecticides produces metabolites more toxic than the initial (or parent) compounds (eg, parathion to paroxan).

There are two phases of metabolism. Phase I includes oxidation, reduction, and hydrolysis mechanisms. These reactions, catalyzed by hepatic enzymes, generally convert foreign compounds to derivatives for Phase II reactions. Products of Phase I, however, may be excreted as such, if polar solubility permits translocation. Phase II principally involves conjugation or synthesis reactions. Common conjugates include glucuronides, acetylation products, and combinations with glycine. Metabolism of xenobiotic agents seldom follows a single pathway. Usually, a fraction is excreted unchanged, and the rest is excreted or stored as metabolites. Significant differences in metabolic mechanisms exist between species. For example, because cats lack forms of glucuronyl transferase, their ability to conjugate compounds such as morphine and phenols is compromised. Increased tolerance to subsequent exposures of a toxicant, in some instances, is due to enzyme induction initiated by the previous exposure.

Excretion: Excretion of most toxicants and their metabolites is by way of the kidneys. Some excretion occurs in the digestive tract and some via milk. Many polar and high-molecular-weight compounds are excreted into the bile. An enterohepatic cycle occurs when these compounds are excreted from the liver via bile, reabsorbed from the intestine, and returned to the liver. Milk is also an excretion pathway for some toxicants. The excretion rate may be of primary concern, because some toxicants can cause violative residues in food-producing animals. The route of administration, dose, and condition of the animal—to name a few factors—can have a profound effect on excretion rates. Toxicants are removed in the kidney by glomerular filtration, tubular excretion by passive diffusion, and active tubular secretion. The damage to the kidney from the excretion of xenobiotics is specific to the anatomic location where the excretion occurs. Excretion sites are proximal tubules, glomeruli, medulla, papilla, and loop of Henle. The proximal convoluted tubule is the most common site of toxicant-induced injury.

The important Phase I enzymes present in the kidney are cytochrome P450, prostaglandin synthase, and prostaglandin reductase. The Phase I enzyme cytochrome P450 is present in the kidney at 10% of the level of the liver. Important Phase II enzymes present in the kidneys are UDP-glucuronosyltransferases (UGT), sulfotransferases, and glutathione-S-transferase.

The medulla and papilla are the target sites for phenylbutazone, the tubules are targets for many plant toxins, the loop of Henle is the target site for fluoride, and the glomeruli for immune complexes.

The elimination or disappearance (by metabolic change) of a chemical from an organ or the body is expressed in terms of **half-life (t½)**, defined as the amount of time required for the disappearance of half of the compound. The rate of elimination usually depends on the concentration of the compound. A constant fraction (eg, ½) eliminated per unit of time is referred to as first-order kinetics. A metabolic reaction may dictate the rate of elimination. A constant amount eliminated per unit of time is referred to as zero-order kinetics. Different body compartments will likely have different elimination rates. A two-compartment system describes elimination that is initially rapid (eg, from the central or plasma component) and subsequently slower from the peripheral component (eg, liver, kidney, or fat).

FACTORS AFFECTING THE ACTIVITY OF TOXICANTS

Toxicosis potential is usually determined more by the multitude of related factors than by actual toxicity of the toxicant. Exposure-related, biologic, or chemical factors regulate absorption, metabolism, and elimination, and thus, influence observed clinical consequences.

Factors Related to Exposure: Dose is the primary concern; however, the exact intake of a toxicant is seldom known. Duration and frequency of exposure are important. The route of exposure affects absorption, translocation, and perhaps metabolic pathways. Exposure of a toxicant relative to periods of stress or food intake may also be a factor. After ingestion of some toxicants, emesis may occur if the stomach is empty, but if partly filled, the toxicant is retained and toxicosis can occur. Environmental factors, such as temperature, humidity, and barometric pressure, affect rates of consumption and even the occurrence of some toxic agents. Many mycotoxins and poisonous plants are correlated with seasonal or climatic changes. For example, the ischemic effects of ergot toxicosis are more often seen during the winter cold, and plant nitrate levels are affected by rainfall amounts.

Biologic Factors: Various species and strains within species react differently to a particular toxicant because of variations in absorption, metabolism, or elimination. Functional differences in species may also affect the likelihood of toxicosis, eg, species unable to vomit can be intoxicated with a lower dose of some agents.

Age and size of the animal are primary factors in toxicosis. Metabolism and translocation of xenobiotic agents are compromised by the underdeveloped microsomal enzyme system in young animals. Membrane permeability and hepatic and renal clearance capabilities vary with age, species, and health. The amount of toxicant required to cause pathology is generally correlated to body weight, but with greater body weight, a disproportionate increase in toxicity (per unit body weight) of a compound often occurs. Body surface area may correlate more closely with the toxic dose. No measurement parameter is consistent for every situation.

Nutritional and dietary factors, hormonal and health status, organ pathology, stress, and sex all affect toxicosis. Nutritional factors may directly affect the toxicant (ie, by altering absorption) or indirectly affect the metabolic processes or availability of receptor sites. The copper-molybdenum-sulfate interaction is an example of both.

Chemical Factors: The chemical nature of a toxicant determines solubility, which in turn influences absorption. Nonpolar or lipid-soluble substances tend to be more readily absorbed than polar or ionized substances. The vehicle or carrier of the toxic compound also affects its availability for absorption. Isomers, including optical isomers, vary in toxicity. For example, the γ isomer of hexachlorocyclohexane (lindane) is more toxic than other isomers.

Adjuvants are formulation factors used to alter the toxicologic effect of the active ingredient (eg, piperonyl butoxide enhances the insecticidal activity of pyrethrins). Binding agents, enteric coating, and sustained-release preparations influence absorption of the active ingredient. As absorption is delayed, toxicity decreases. Flavoring agents affect palatability and thus the amount ingested.

DIAGNOSIS

Diagnosis of a toxicosis, as with any disease, is based on history, clinical signs, lesions, laboratory examinations, and in some cases, analytical procedures. Circumstantial evidence is valuable and should be noted but does not replace a thorough clinical and postmortem examination. Histories from animal owners may stress obvious factors and omit subtle, important details. "Sudden death" is often actually "tardy observation," or sometimes the animal is simply found dead.

Pertinent data and samples should be submitted to the diagnostic laboratory. A complete history is necessary to develop the scheme of laboratory investigation and may be valuable in case of litigation. Information should be detailed. For example, a notation of CNS signs is insufficient; most animals exhibit some type of CNS signs before death. Exact actions and signs should be described. Examples of pertinent information include the following: 1) number of animals exposed/sick/dead, age, weight, and a chronology of morbidity and mortality; 2) clinical signs and course of the disease; 3) any prior disease conditions; 4) lesions seen at necropsy, with careful examination of ingesta; 5) response to treatment (medication should be listed to avoid analytic confusion); 6) related events, eg, feed change, water source, other medications, feed additives, pesticide applications; 7) description of facilities (a drawing or digital photograph may be helpful), access to refuse, machinery, etc; and 8) recent past locations and when moved. The diagnostic laboratory should be contacted if there are questions regarding the appropriate sample, amount, or container. (*See also* COLLECTION AND SUBMISSION OF LABORATORY SAMPLES, p 1584, and TABLE 1, GUIDELINES FOR SUBMITTING SAMPLES FOR TOXICOLOGIC EXAMINATION, p 1586.)

PRINCIPLES OF THERAPY

At initial examination, certain immediate, life-saving measures may be needed. Beyond this, treatment for toxicosis includes three basic principles: 1) prevention of further absorption, 2) supportive/symptomatic treatment, and 3) specific antidotes.

Prevention of Further Absorption: Topically applied toxicants usually can be removed by thorough washing with soap and water; clipping of the hair or wool may be necessary. Emesis is of value in dogs, cats, and pigs if done within a few hours of ingestion. Emesis is contraindicated when the swallowing reflex is absent; the animal is convulsing; corrosive agents, volatile hydrocarbons, or petroleum distillates are involved; or risk of aspiration pneumonia is imminent. Oral emetics include syrup of ipecac (10–20 mL, PO in dogs) and hydrogen peroxide (2 mL/kg, PO). Apomorphine can be used in dogs parenterally at a dosage of 0.05–0.1 mg/kg.

Gastric lavage, using an endotracheal tube and the largest bore stomach tube possible, is done on the unconscious or anesthetized animal. The head is lowered to a 30° angle, and 10 mL of lavage fluid (water or saline) per kg of body weight is gently flushed into the stomach and then removed. This process is repeated until returned fluid is clear. Cathartics and laxatives may be indicated in some instances for more rapid elimination of the toxicant from the GI tract. A gastrotomy or rumenotomy may be necessary when lavage techniques are insufficient (or too slow in ruminants).

When the toxicant cannot be physically removed, certain agents administered orally can adsorb it and prevent its absorption from the alimentary tract. Activated charcoal (1–2 g/kg) effectively adsorbs a wide variety of compounds and usually is the adsorbent and detoxicant of choice when toxicosis is suspected. The maximum amount of a drug adsorbed by activated charcoal is ~100–1,000 mg/g of charcoal. Sorbitol is sometimes added to activated charcoal to increase its palatability (in people) and to increase the GI transit time and flush out charcoal-bound toxins more rapidly. Activated charcoal should not be used in animals with known hypersensitivity or allergy to the drug. With administration of high doses, vomiting, constipation, or diarrhea may occur, and feces will appear black.

Supportive Therapy: Supportive therapy is often necessary until the toxicant can be metabolized and eliminated. The type of support required depends on the animal's clinical condition. Supportive efforts may include control of convulsive seizures, maintenance of respiration, treatment for shock, correction of electrolyte imbalance and fluid loss, and control of cardiac dysfunction, as well as alleviation of pain.

Specific Antidotes: Specific antidotes for various toxicants work by various mechanisms. Some complex with the toxicant (eg, the oximes bind with organophosphorous insecticides, and EDTA chelates lead). Others block or compete for receptor sites (eg, vitamin K competes with the receptor for coumarin anticoagulants). A few affect metabolism of the toxicant (eg, nitrite and thiosulfate ions release and bind cyanide).

TOXICOLOGIC HAZARDS IN THE WORKPLACE

Veterinarians are potentially exposed to myriad potent pharmaceuticals and other hazardous materials as part of their work environment, and particularly during patient decontamination procedures (most notably dermal decontamination). Therefore, knowledge of important toxicologic workplace hazards and basic personal protective equipment (PPE) is important. It is critical to recognize that PPE is the "last line of defense" and not a panacea for toxicologic hazards. The overarching principle is to avoid exposure if at all possible. Over-reliance on inadequately fitted or inappropriate types of PPE continues to be a substantial cause of human casualties because of the feeling of overconfidence these devices can provide. In particular, respirators should be selected, fitted, and tested by persons qualified to do this.

The following general PPE principles apply: The general minimum assumed PPE is long pants, a long-sleeved shirt, socks, closed footwear, and eye protection. Gloves with appropriate chemical resistance characteristics for a given situation should be used; gloves should be changed regularly, and double gloving done if necessary. If there is any risk of significant inhalation and eye exposure, a properly fitted full-face respirator and appropriate filters/cartridges should be used. If there is any doubt regarding air quality, it should be tested before entry into a potentially contaminated space (particularly if it is a potentially contaminated closed space). Anyone entering into a confined space should be able to be extracted/rescued without others needing to enter the space. If there is any question regarding the safety of the work environment, one should not work alone. Appropriate antidote kits (eg, cyanide antidote kit) should be readily available if relevant to the situation. Relevant human exposure guidelines and limits are set by local regulatory agencies.

Although this chapter is not meant to be a comprehensive discussion of every possible toxicologic workplace hazard faced by veterinarians, some common, important, and potentially lethal agents known to have caused injuries and fatalities to veterinarians are briefly discussed.

CARBON MONOXIDE

Carbon monoxide (CO) will most commonly be encountered by veterinarians working in enclosed spaces (eg, intensive animal production facilities) being heated by combustion sources (eg, gas space heating). Accordingly, this exposure most commonly occurs during cold weather and winter. Indeed, epidemics of fatal CO poisoning notoriously occur during extreme winter weather conditions, especially in conjunction with electrical power failures (ie, use of combustion heaters, electrical generators, combustion engines, combustion power tools, wood heaters, etc, in enclosed spaces without adequate ventilation). Like cyanide, CO is also a component of smoke inhalation poisoning. Inhalation is the main route of exposure to CO. CO poisoning is the most common form of fatal air poisoning in many countries.

CO is colorless and tasteless and has no odor, making it especially hazardous in occupational settings, particularly in enclosed spaces with inadequate ventilation. The use of CO monitors and/or testing of breathing air with a Dräger tube apparatus or similar test method are strongly recommended before entry into any environment where CO might be present. The use of CO monitors in animal production facilities being heated by combustion sources is strongly recommended.

CO binds to hemoglobin, forming carboxyhemoglobin and disrupting blood oxygen transport. The development of impaired hemoglobin oxygen transport can cumulatively progress over time because of the relatively slow reversal of carboxyhemoglobin to normal hemoglobin. Thus, CO poisoning can "creep up unexpectedly and without being noticed" over time. The signs and symptoms of CO poisoning in people are relatively nonspecific. One of the early and important indicators of exposure to excessive amounts of CO is development of a severe and persistent headache. Other common early clinical signs include dizziness, weakness, nausea, vomiting, chest pain, shortness of breath, irritability, and altered mental status. Loss of consciousness, coma, and death can occur. Other signs and symptoms include tachycardia, tachypnea, hypotension, various neurologic findings (including impaired memory and cognitive and sensory disturbances), metabolic acidosis, arrhythmias, myocardial ischemia or infarction, and noncardiogenic pulmonary edema; any organ system can be involved. Many survivors of severe CO poisoning have hypoxic brain injuries, which can be associated with personality changes, memory deficits, disturbances in voluntary muscle movements, and the appearance of involuntary movements (extrapyramidal syndromes).

Persons with significant CO poisoning have been described as having a "healthy" red complexion and mucous membranes because of the presence of high levels of carboxyhemoglobin. Normal pulse oximeters will not detect the presence of carboxyhemoglobin; pulse co-oximetry is required. Additionally, blood carboxyhemoglobin levels correlate poorly with the clinical severity of the poisoning.

There is no specific antidote for CO poisoning. Resuscitation combined with oxygen is the only known effective approach to treatment. Rescue and treatment of individuals with CO poisoning is a matter for properly equipped and trained professionals.

CYANIDE

Important sources of exposure in veterinary medicine include rumen contents of grazing animals that have consumed or been poisoned with plant cyanogenic glycosides (eg, during necropsy/sample collection procedures), handling or exposure to cyanide vertebrate pesticide agents (or animals poisoned by them), and combustion sources (particularly of nitrogen-containing materials such as plastics, wool, silk). Aqueous solutions of cyanide are commonly referred to as prussic acid, and hydrocyanic acid and formonitrile are commonly used synonyms. (*See also* CYANIDE POISONING, p 2959.)

Solutions of hydrogen cyanide are colorless or pale-blue liquid at room temperature. Cyanide is very volatile and highly toxic, and flammable/explosive concentrations can rapidly develop at normal temperatures and pressures, especially in enclosed spaces.

Hydrogen cyanide gas has a distinctive, bitter almond smell; however, the ability of people to detect the odor is genetically determined. Anosmic individuals (20%–40% of the human population) are not able to detect it. Accordingly, odor detection cannot be relied on in terms of detection and warning in relation to exposure. The wearing of cyanide detection devices and/or testing of breathing air with a Dräger tube apparatus or similar test method is strongly recommended before entry into any environment where cyanide might be present.

The major potential route of workplace exposure in veterinary medicine is by inhalation. Substantial skin absorption can occur if the atmospheric concentration is high or if the skin comes into contact with cyanide solutions. High ambient temperatures and high humidity appear to increase skin absorption. Skin or clothing contamination with cyanide-containing materials can result in off-gassing of cyanide vapor and inhalation. Exposure by any route can cause systemic toxicity. Cyanide is also a skin and eye irritant. Children are more susceptible to poisoning because of their higher minute ventilation per kg body wt.

Significant cyanide exposures result in death within a few minutes because of the arrest of mitochondrial oxidative phosphorylation, histotoxic hypoxia, and severe metabolic acidosis, which results in rapid onset CNS, cardiovascular, and respiratory effects. CNS signs and symptoms in people develop very quickly and are nonspecific: excitement, dizziness, nausea, vomiting, headache, and weakness, which progresses to drowsiness, tetanic spasm, lockjaw, convulsions, hallucinations, loss of consciousness, and terminal coma. Cardiovascular signs include arrhythmias and intractable hypotension. Respiratory signs typically include shortness of breath and chest tightness, rapid breathing, and increased depth of respirations progressing to agonal respiration. Pulmonary edema and cyanosis of the skin may or may not be present. Severe, intractable anion-gap metabolic acidosis due to lactic acidosis typically develops rapidly. Cyanide poisoning survivors usually develop some form of hypoxic brain damage, and this can be associated with personality changes, memory deficits, disturbances in voluntary muscle movements, and appearance of involuntary movements (extrapyramidal syndromes).

Victims exposed only to hydrogen cyanide gas do not pose secondary contamination risks to rescuers, but resuscitation without a barrier should not be attempted. Victims whose clothing or skin is contaminated with hydrogen cyanide liquid or solution can secondarily contaminate response personnel by direct contact or through off-gassing vapor. Dermal contact with cyanide-contaminated victims or with gastric contents of victims who may have ingested cyanide-containing materials should be avoided.

Veterinarians poisoned by cyanide require speedy treatment, rapid administration of antidotes, and specialist care. Great care should be taken by rescuers who plan to enter a contamination "hot zone." Many human casualties have occurred because of well-intentioned but misguided attempts at rescue from hydrogen cyanide–contaminated hot zones. Rescue and emergency treatment is best left to those with specialized training in these areas.

HYDROGEN SULFIDE

Veterinarians are most likely to encounter hydrogen sulfide emanating from concentrated decaying organic matter (eg, septic/sewage ponds/manure handling facilities in intensive animal production facilities, rotting feed stores, carcass pits, etc). When near sewage ponds, it is particularly important not to disturb the surface of the pond or to cause mixing of the contents, because this will trigger degassing of dissolved hydrogen sulfide.

Hydrogen sulfide is a colorless, flammable, and very rapidly toxic gas. Hydrogen sulfide is slightly heavier than air, tends to accumulate in low-lying, poorly ventilated spaces, and is highly flammable and explosive. It has a characteristic rotten-egg odor that can be sensed at concentrations as low as 0.5 ppb. However, the sensitivity to hydrogen sulfide odor is genetically determined, and a significant proportion of the human population has poor odor detection ability to this gas; additionally, extended exposure (2–15 min at 100 ppm) to hydrogen sulfide results in paralysis of the olfactory nerve, resulting in a loss of ability to detect the gas. Therefore, odor is not a reliable indicator of the presence of hydrogen sulfide and cannot be relied on to provide a warning of hazardous concentrations. The use of hydrogen sulfide monitors and/or testing of breathing air with a Dräger tube apparatus or similar test method are strongly recommended before entry into any environment where hydrogen sulfide might be present.

Veterinarians are typically exposed to hydrogen sulfide via inhalation. Children are more susceptible because of their high minute volume to weight ratio and higher lung surface area to body weight ratio. Prolonged exposure to hydrogen sulfide is notably irritating to the skin and eyes. Hydrogen sulfide is also a notable mucous membrane and respiratory tract irritant, and the acute and/or delayed (up to 72 hr after exposure) respiratory distress syndromes are common sequela of prolonged inhalation exposure to nonacutely fatal levels of hydrogen sulfide.

Hydrogen sulfide acts by inactivating mitochondrial cytochrome oxidase, resulting in the failure of oxidative metabolism, histotoxic hypoxia, and acute anion-gap metabolic acidosis. Its mode of action resembles that of cyanide. Acute exposure to high concentrations of hydrogen sulfide will result in sudden collapse and death due to central respiratory failure (hydrogen sulfide knock-down effect) caused by its peracute effects on the brain. Signs and symptoms of acute exposure include initial CNS stimulation, nausea, headaches, impaired gait, dizziness, disturbed equilibrium, tremors, convulsions, skin and eye irritation, coma, respiratory paralysis, and death. Many survivors of acute hydrogen sulfide poisoning have hypoxic brain and cardiac injuries. Hypoxic brain damage can be associated with personality changes, memory deficits, disturbances in voluntary muscle movements, and appearance of involuntary movements (extrapyramidal syndromes).

Low concentrations of hydrogen sulfide (~50 ppm) rapidly produce upper respiratory tract irritation, and prolonged exposure can result in pulmonary irritation (cough, shortness of breath, and bronchial or lung hemorrhage, bronchitis, and immediate or delayed pulmonary edema). Cyanosis may be present. Hydrogen sulfide inhalation is associated with cardiac arrhythmias. Nausea and vomiting are also common.

Chronic, repeated, lower-level hydrogen sulfide exposure is associated with hypotension, headache, nausea, loss of appetite, weight loss, ataxia, conjunctivitis, chronic cough, and neuropsychological disorders.

Ill-advised and poorly equipped attempts at rescuing victims from hydrogen sulfide–contaminated hot zones have resulted in large numbers of hydrogen sulfide–associated human casualties. There is currently no effective antidote for hydrogen sulfide poisoning. Resuscitation combined with oxygen is the only known effective approach to treatment. Rescue and treatment of individuals with hydrogen sulfide poisoning is a matter for properly equipped and trained professionals.

NITROGEN DIOXIDE

(Silo filler's disease)

Veterinarians are most likely to encounter nitrogen dioxide in association with grain silos, grain silo chutes in intensive animal production facilities, silage, silage bags, and silage pit vents. When a silo or pit is filled with fresh organic material (grain, grass etc), nitrogen dioxide is formed by anaerobic fermentation. High levels can develop at the top of grain in silos or at the top of silage pits within hours of their filling. Veterinarians working in or around silo chutes and hatches or silage pits or silage bags during the first 10 days or so after fill will be exposed to nitrogen dioxide. Silo chutes and other nearby structures exposed to significant levels of nitrogen dioxide are often stained yellow to red by the gas.

Nitrogen dioxide is a reddish, water-insoluble, reactive gas with a characteristic pungent odor. Because of its low water solubility, it is not scrubbed by the upper respiratory tract. It penetrates deeply into the lung, where it is reactive with lung surface fluids and acts as a pulmonary irritant. When nitrogen dioxide contacts the lung surface fluids, it slowly hydrolyzes to nitrous and nitric acid, producing chemical pneumonitis and pulmonary edema.

Acute, high-level exposures to nitrogen dioxide result in acute respiratory distress syndrome in people, which is characterized by rapid or delayed onset (up to 72 hr after exposure) progressive pulmonary edema and respiratory failure. Nitrogen dioxide acute respiratory distress syndrome is less common than other toxic injuries, because the pungent odor and other effects of nitrogen dioxide usually trigger an escape from the source of exposure. This type of severe effect is more likely if the affected person cannot escape.

More common acute signs and symptoms include cough, light-headedness, dyspnea, chest tightness, choking, sweating, chest pain, and wheezing. Because of nitrogen dioxide's low water solubility, mucous membrane and eye irritation are relatively uncommon signs.

Usually of greater concern is the capacity of nitrogen dioxide inhalation to induce sometimes severe delayed effects, including bronchiolitis obliterans (fever, cough, and dyspnea), respiratory insufficiency new-onset asthma, COPD, and hypoxia/cyanosis.

There is no specific antidote for nitrogen dioxide poisoning. Treatment requires specialist medical care.

PHOSPHINE GAS SOURCES

Phosphide salts (commonly zinc and aluminum) release phosphine gas in the presence of acids and have been extensively used as vertebrate pesticides. Veterinarians are most commonly exposed to phosphine via inhalation when attempting to decontaminate and treat animals that have been poisoned with zinc or aluminum phosphide rodenticides or during necropsy/sample collection procedures on animals that died from these poisonings. Phosphine gas is also used as a fumigant for grain and other agricultural products.

Phosphine is a colorless, flammable, and explosive gas. Technical grade phosphine (the type most commonly encountered by veterinarians) has an unpleasant, garlic-like, rotting fish-like smell, due to the presence of substituted phosphine and diphosphane. The human odor threshold for phosphine is below relevant exposure limits; the implication is that persons who can smell phosphine are being exposed to a hazardous level.

Phosphine is described as a "general protoplasmic poison," and it is extremely and acutely toxic after inhalation. Acute inhalation exposure to phosphine can result in respiratory, neurologic, and GI effects. Signs and symptoms may include headaches, dizziness, fatigue, drowsiness, burning substernal pain, nausea, vomiting, GI distress, cough with fluorescent green sputum, labored breathing, chest tightness, pulmonary irritation, pulmonary edema, tremors, and convulsions (may occur after apparent recovery). Skin contact with phosphides may result in numbness and paresthesia. Chronic occupational exposure effects include upper respiratory tract inflammation, weakness, dizziness, nausea, jaundice, liver effects, increased bone density, and symptoms referable to the GI, cardiorespiratory, and central nervous systems.

Veterinarians are very strongly encouraged to use respiratory and eye protection when dealing with patients poisoned by zinc or aluminum phosphide; emergency room staff casualties have occurred during treatment of human patients poisoned with these agents.

There is no antidote for phosphine poisoning, and emergency treatment requires specialist care.

LACK OF OXYGEN

Veterinarians commonly encounter low-oxygen environments in enclosed spaces that contain biologically respiring materials. Freshly cut plant material will continue to be metabolically active, and thus potentially consume oxygen from the air, for surprisingly long periods of time. If such materials (eg, grains, hays, freshly cut timber, etc) are stored in sealed confined spaces (eg, silos, ship holds, etc) with little ventilation, a low-oxygen atmosphere will develop. Such circumstances have resulted in significant human casualties and deaths. Such environments should always be treated with suspicion, and their atmosphere tested for the presence of breathable air; testing with a flame is not an adequate method. It is strongly recommended that individuals do not work alone in such environments and that a method of safe extraction of a person entering into such environments is immediately available.

Entry into low-oxygen environments can result in rapid loss of consciousness and death. Typical signs and symptoms of hypoxia include lightheadedness, fatigue, numbness, tingling of extremities, nausea, ataxia, confusion, disorientation, hallucinations, behavioral change, severe headaches, reduced consciousness, papilledema, breathlessness, pallor, tachycardia, and tachypnea, with eventual progression to cyanosis, slow heart rate/cor pulmonale and low blood pressure, and death.

Ill-considered and poorly equipped rescue attempts from low-oxygen environments have resulted in many human casualties. Rescue operations under such circumstances are best performed by properly equipped and trained professionals.

ALGAL POISONING

Algal poisoning is an acute, often fatal condition caused by high concentrations of toxic blue-green algae (more commonly known as cyanobacteria—literally blue-green bacteria) in drinking water as well as in water used for agriculture, recreation, and aquaculture. Fatalities and severe illness of livestock, pets, wildlife, birds, and fish from heavy growths of cyanobacteria waterblooms occur in almost all countries of the world. Acute lethal poisonings have also been documented in people. Poisoning usually occurs during warm seasons when the waterblooms are more intense and of longer duration. Most poisonings occur among animals drinking cyanobacteria-infested freshwater, but aquatic animals, especially maricultured fish and shrimp, are also affected. The toxins of cyanobacteria comprise six distinct chemical classes collectively called cyanotoxins.

Etiology, Epidemiology, and Pathogenesis: Although toxic strains within species of *Anabaena*, *Aphanizomenon*, *Cylindrospermopsis*, *Microcystis*, *Nodularia*, *Nostoc*, *Oscillatoria*, and *Planktothrix* are responsible for most cases of toxicity, there are >30 species of cyanobacteria that can be associated with toxic waterblooms. Neurotoxic alkaloids (called anatoxins) can be produced by *Anabaena*, *Aphanizomenon*, and *Planktothrix*, while saxitoxins (also called paralytic shellfish toxins) can be produced by *Anabaena*, *Aphanizomenon*, and *Lyngbya*. Hepatotoxic heptapeptides called microcystins can be produced by *Anabaena*, *Microcystis*, *Nostoc*, and *Planktothrix*. The brackish water genus *Nodularia* produces a hepatotoxic pentapeptide related, in both structure and function, to microcystins. *Cylindrospermopsis*, *Anabaena*, *Aphanizomenon*, *Raphidiopsis*, and *Umezakia* can produce a potent hepatotoxic alkaloid called cylindrospermopsin. Some genera, especially *Anabaena*, can produce both neuro- and hepatotoxins. If a toxic waterbloom contains both types of toxins, the neurotoxin signs are seen first, because their effects occur much sooner (minutes) than those of the hepatotoxins (1 to a few hours). Other noncyclic peptides and amino acids produced by cyanobacteria can also have biological activity. One recent amino acid with neurologic degenerative activity is BMAA (ß-methylamino alanine). BMAA has been implicated as the causative agent of amyotrophic lateral sclerosis or parkinsonism dementia.

Poisoning usually does not occur unless there is a heavy waterbloom that forms a dense surface scum. Factors that contribute to heavy waterblooms are nutrient-rich eutrophic to hypereutrophic water and warm, sunny weather. Evidence supports the observation that global climate change causes earlier, more intense, and longer-lasting warm weather that leads to more extensive waterblooms of cyanobacteria. Agriculture practices (eg, runoff of fertilizers and animal wastes) that promote nutrient enrichment also contribute to and intensify waterbloom formation. The problem is augmented by light winds or wind conditions that lead to areas of very high (scum) concentrations of cyanobacteria, especially leeward shoreline locations where livestock drink. Experiments with both toxin groups have revealed a steep dose-response curve, with as much as 90% of the lethal dose being ingested without measurable effect. Animal size and species sensitivity influence the degree of intoxication. Monogastric animals are less sensitive than ruminants and birds. Depending on waterbloom densities and toxin content, animals may need to ingest only a few ounces to be affected. However, if the waterbloom is less dense or cyanotoxin content is low, as much as several gallons may be needed to cause acute or lethal toxicity. Among domestic animals, dogs are most susceptible to a toxic waterbloom. This is due to their preference for swimming and drinking in dense waterblooms and a greater species sensitivity to the cyanotoxins, especially the neurotoxins.

Although the species sensitivity and signs of poisoning can vary depending on the type of exposure, the gross and histopathologic lesions are quite similar among species poisoned by the hepatotoxic peptides and neurotoxic alkaloids. Death from hepatotoxicosis induced by cyclic peptides is generally accepted as being the result of intrahepatic hemorrhage and hypovolemic shock. This conclusion is based on large increases in liver weight as well as in hepatic hemoglobin and iron content that account for blood loss sufficient to induce irreversible shock. In animals that live more than a few hours, hyperkalemia or hypoglycemia, or both, may lead to death from liver failure within a few days to a few weeks.

Neurotoxicosis, with death occurring in minutes to a few hours from respiratory arrest, may result from ingestion of the cyanobacteria that produce neurotoxic alkaloids. Species and strains of *Anabaena*, *Aphanizomenon*, *Oscillatoria*, and *Planktothrix* can produce a potent, postsynaptic cholinergic (nicotinic) agonist called anatoxin-a that causes a depolarizing neuromuscular blockade. Strains of *Anabaena* can produce an irreversible organophosphate anticholinesterase called anatoxin-a(s). *Anabaena*, *Aphanizomenon*, *Cylindrospermopsis*, and *Lyngbya* can produce the potent, presynaptic sodium channel blockers called saxitoxins.

Clinical Findings and Lesions: One of the earliest effects (15–30 min) of microcystin poisoning is increased serum concentrations of bile acids, alkaline phosphatase, γ-glutamyltransferase, and AST. The WBC count and clotting times increase. Death may occur within a few hours (usually within 4–24 hr), up to a few days. Death may be preceded by coma, muscle tremors, paddling, and dyspnea. Watery or bloody diarrhea may also be seen. Gross lesions include hepatomegaly due mostly to intrahepatic hemorrhage. Intact clumps of greenish cyanobacteria can be found in the stomach and GI tract, and there is a greenish stain on the mouth, nose, legs, and feet. Hepatic necrosis begins centrilobularly and proceeds to the periportal regions. Hepatocytes are disassociated and rounded. After death, debris from disassociated hepatocytes can be found in the pulmonary vessels and kidneys. Clinical signs of neurotoxicosis progress from muscle fasciculations to decreased movement, abdominal breathing, cyanosis, convulsions, and death. Signs in birds are similar but include opisthotonos. In smaller animals, death is often preceded by leaping movements. Cattle and horses that survive acute poisoning may have signs of photosensitization in areas exposed to light (nose, ears, and back), followed by hair loss and sloughing of the skin.

Diagnosis: Diagnosis is based primarily on history (recent contact with cyanobacteria waterbloom), signs of poisoning, and necropsy findings. Samples of the waterbloom should be taken as soon as possible for microscopic examination to confirm the presence of the toxigenic cyanobacteria and for cyanotoxin analysis. Although there are nontoxic and toxic strains of all the known toxic species, it is not possible to identify a toxic strain by visual examination. Cyanobacteria are detected by light microscopy, identified using morphologic characteristics, and counted per standard volume of water. Standard protocols to sample and monitor cyanobacteria as well as practical keys for the identification of toxic species are available.

Some laboratories can analyze for the cyanotoxins either by chemical or biologic assay. Animal bioassays (mouse tests) have traditionally been used to detect the presence of the entire range of cyanotoxins based on survival times and signs of poisoning. These tests provide a definitive indication of toxicity, although they cannot be used for precise quantification of compounds in water or to determine compliance with standards for environmental levels. A number of analytic techniques are available to determine microcystins in water. These techniques must provide for quantitative comparison to the guideline or regulatory value in terms of toxicity equivalents. The method most suitable in this regard is high-performance liquid chromatography (HPLC) or HPLC coupled with mass spectrometry. These methods still involve estimation of the concentration and therefore provide only an estimate of toxicity. This is largely due to the limited availability of certified reference standards for the cyanotoxins. Commercial reference materials, purified from laboratory cultures or waterbloom material, for some microcystins, nodularin, cylindrospermopsin, and saxitoxins are available. A synthetic reference material for anatoxin-a is also available. No known commercial reference material is available for anatoxin-a(s). Newer methods of immunoassay, for quantification purposes, are also available. These include commercial ELISA kits in both laboratory and field formats for microcystins/nodularin, cylindrospermopsin, and saxitoxins. Also available is a receptor-binding assay colorimetric plate kit for anatoxin-a.

Treatment: After removal from the contaminated water supply, affected animals should be placed in a protected area out of direct sunlight. Ample quantities of water and good quality feed should be made available. Because the toxins have a steep dose-response curve, surviving animals have a good chance for recovery. Although therapies for cyanobacterial poisonings have not been investigated in detail, activated charcoal slurry is likely to be of benefit. In laboratory studies, an ion-exchange resin such as cholestyramine has proved useful to absorb the toxins from the GI tract, and certain bile acid transport blockers such as cyclosporin A, rifampin, and silymarin injected before dosing of microcystin have effectively prevented hepatotoxicity. No therapeutic antagonist has been found effective against anatoxin-a, cylindrospermopsin, or the saxitoxins, but atropine and activated charcoal reduce the muscarinic effects of the anticholinesterase anatoxin-a(s).

Prevention: Removal of animals from the affected water supply is essential. If no other water supply is available, animals should be allowed to drink only from shore areas kept free (by prevailing winds) of dense surface scums of cyanobacteria. Some efforts have been made to erect surface barriers (logs or floating plastic booms) to keep shore areas free of surface scum, but these are not very successful. Cyanobacteria can be controlled by adding copper sulfate ($CuSO_4$) or other copper-based algicidal treatments to the water. The usual treatment for $CuSO_4$ is 0.2–0.4 ppm, equivalent to 0.65–1.3 oz/10,000 gal. of water or 1.4–2.8 lb/acre-foot of water. Livestock (especially sheep) should not be watered for at least 5 days after the last visible evidence of the cyanobacteria waterbloom. $CuSO_4$ is best used to prevent waterbloom formation, and care should be taken to avoid water that has dead cyanobacteria cells, either from treatment with algicide or natural aging of the bloom, because most toxin is released in the water only after breakdown of the intact cyanobacteria cells. A chemical control method receiving attention are compounds to bind and remove phosphorus from eutrophic waters. This has the potential to minimize one of the more important nutrients responsible for cyanobacteria waterblooms. Common phosphorus treatments include lime, aluminum sulfate, ferric chloride, and some types of clay particles. These treatments also act as flocculating agents and form particulates with algae cells and other debris that settle out and remove the bloom from the water column. For example, when alum (potassium aluminum sulfate) is used in a water supply, a precipitate (floc) forms that carries algae cells, dirt, and bacteria to the bottom, but charged items such as phosphate and colloids are bound by the same precipitate through their charges. A newer, effective phosphorus-binding compound product available in the USA since 2010 uses a patented phosphorus-locking technology containing lanthanum (5%), a naturally occurring earth element, embedded inside a clay matrix (~95%).

Source water management techniques for control of cyanobacterial growth include flow maintenance in regulated rivers, water mixing techniques both to eliminate stratification and reduce nutrient release from sediments in reservoirs, and the use of algicides in dedicated water supply storages. Algicides disrupt cells and liberate intracellular toxins. Algicide use should be in accordance with local environment and chemical registration regulations. In situations where multiple offtakes are available, the selective withdrawal of water from different depths can minimize the intake of high surface accumulations of cyanobacterial cells.

Water treatment techniques can be highly effective to remove both cyanobacterial cells and cyanotoxins (especially microcystins) with the appropriate technology. Most cyanotoxins remain intracellular, unless the cells are lysed or damaged from age or stress from water conditions or chemical treatment. The one exception is cylindrospermopsin, which is actively secreted from even healthy cells. This makes it possible to remove cells and cyanotoxins (especially microcystins) by coagulation and filtration in a conventional treatment plant. Treatment of water containing cyanobacterial cells with oxidants such as chlorine or ozone, while killing cells, will result in the release of free cyanotoxin. Therefore, the practice of prechlorination or preozonation is not recommended without a subsequent step to remove dissolved cyanotoxins.

Microcystins are readily oxidized by a range of oxidants, including ozone and chlorine. Adequate contact time and pH control are needed to achieve optimal removal of these compounds, which is more difficult in the presence of whole cells. Microcystins, anatoxin-a, cylindrospermopsin, and some saxitoxins are also adsorbed from solution by both granular activated carbon and, less efficiently, by powdered activated carbon. The effectiveness of the process should be determined by monitoring cyanotoxin in the product water.

CYANIDE POISONING

In acute cyanide poisoning, cyanide ions (CN^-) bind to, and inhibit, the ferric (Fe^{3+}) heme moeity form of mitochondrial cytochrome c oxidase (synonyms: aa_3, complex IV, cytochrome A3, EC 1.9.3.1). This blocks the fourth step in the mitochondrial electron transport chain (reduction of O_2 to H_2O), resulting in the arrest of aerobic metabolism and death from histotoxic anoxia. Tissues that heavily depend on aerobic metabolism such as the heart and brain are particularly susceptible to these effects. Cyanide also binds to other heme-containing enzymes, such as members of the cytochrome p450 family, and to myoglobin. However, these tissue cyanide "sinks" do not provide sufficient protection from histotoxic anoxia. The acute lethal dosage of hydrogen cyanide (HCN) in most animal species is ~2 mg/kg. Plant materials containing ≥200 ppm of cyanogenic glycosides are dangerous.

There are at least two forms of chronic cyanide poisoning in domestic animals: 1) hypothyroidism due to disruption of iodide uptake by the follicular thyroid cell sodium-iodide symporter by thiocyanate, a metabolite in the detoxification of cyanide, and 2) chronic cyanide and plant cyanide metabolite (eg, various glutamyl β-cyanoalanines) –associated neuropathy toxidromes (eg, equine sorghum cystitis ataxia syndrome, cystitis ataxia syndromes in cattle, sheep, and goats).

Etiology: Various chemical forms of cyanides are found in plants, fumigants, soil sterilizers, fertilizers (eg, cyanamide), pesticides/rodenticides (eg, calcium cyanomide) and salts used in industrial processes, such as gold mining, metal cleaning and electroplating, photographic processes, and others. Hydrogen cyanide is also known as prussic acid, and cyanide salts liberate cyanide gas in the presence of acids (eg, in the stomach). Cyanide preparations are still used as vertebrate pest control agents for control of feral pigs, fox, Australian brush-tailed possums, and other pest or predator species in a number of countries. Cyanide salts are still used as killing agents in entomology and (illegally) as a method of fishing and/or collection of aquarium fish species (ie, cyanide fishing). Combustion of common polyacrylonitriles (plastics), wool, silk, keratin, polyurethane (insulation/upholstery), melamine resins (household goods), and synthetic rubber results in the release of cyanide gas. Car fires are notorious sources of cyanide exposure, and cyanide is also a notable component of internal combustion engine exhaust and tobacco smoke. Carbon monoxide poisoning with cyanide gas is thus an extremely common component of smoke inhalation toxidromes.

Toxicity can result from accidental, improper, or malicious use or exposure. However, in livestock species, the most frequent cause of acute and chronic cyanide poisoning is ingestion of plants that either constitutively contain cyanogenic glycosides or are induced to produce cyanogenic glycosides and cyanolipids as a protective response to environmental conditions (plant cyanogenesis). Plant cyanogenesis is a common process and has been documented in >3,000 different plant species distributed over ~110 different families of ferns, gymnosperms, and angiosperms. Of these plants, ~300 species are potential causes of acute and chronic cyanogenic glycoside poisoning, and there are ~75 different cyanogenic glycosides (all of which are *O*-β-glycosidic derivatives of α-hydroxynitriles). Plant species of notable veterinary importance include *Sorghum* spp (Johnson grass, Sudan grass, and *S bicolor*, the common cereal grain crop referred to as "sorghum" or the synonyms durra, jowari, milo), *Acacia greggii* (guajillo), *Amelanchier alnifolia* (western service berry), *Linum* spp (linseeds and flaxes), *Sambucus nigra* (elderberry), *Suckley suckleyana* (poison suckleya), *Triglochin maritima* and *T palustris* (marsh arrow grasses), *Mannihot esculentum* (cassava), all members of the *Prunus* genus until proved otherwise (apricot, peach, chokecherry, pincherry, wild black cherry, ornamental cherry, peaches, nectarines, apricots, almonds, bird cherries, black thorn, cherry laurels [commercial orchard species are often specifically bred for low cyanide content; however, ornamental members of this genus are often highly poisonous]), *Nandina domestica* (heavenly or sacred bamboo), *Phaseolus lunatus* (lima beans), members of the *Vicia* genus until proved otherwise (vetches; often, pasture species have been bred for low cyanogenesis), *Lotus* spp (bird's-foot treefoils; often, pasture species have been bred for low cyanogenesis), *Trifolium* sp (clovers; often, pasture species have been bred for low cyanide content), *Zea mays* (corn), *Eucalyptus* spp (gum trees), *Hydrangea* spp (hydrangeas), *Pteridium aquilinum* (bracken fern), *Bahia oppositifolia* (bahia), and *Chaenomales* spp (flowering quince) (*See also* SORGHUM POISONING, p 3155). A number of insect species are also able to synthesize hydrogen cyanide and/or sequester hydrogen cyanide that is derived from the cyanogenic glycosides of their plant hosts (notably the USA eastern tent caterpillar *Malacosoma americanum* that is associated with mare reproductive loss syndrome (*see also* MARE REPRODUCTIVE LOSS SYNDROME, p 1343); however, cyanide is *not* the cause of mare reproductive loss syndrome. Invertebrates such as Burnet moths (*Zygaena* spp) that feed on bird's-foot trefoils), as well as certain centipede and millipedes, are potentially hazardous food sources for exotic pet species.

Plant cyanogenesis in response to environmental stressors is an important part of the etiology and risk of acute cyanogenic glycoside poisoning. Within plants, amino acids that are not used for protein synthesis can be metabolized to α-hydroxynitriles and then to cyanogenic glycosides. Plants are protected from the potential adverse effects of cyanogenic glycosides by two features: cyanogenic glycosides are largely found within cell vacuoles, and the presence of the detoxifying enzyme β-cyanoalanine synthase (which is responsible for production of some of the cyanide derivatives putatively involved in the chronic cyanide-associated neurologic toxidromes). Even so-called "acyanogenic" plants can become toxic under appropriate environmental circumstances. Environmental conditions that damage relevant plant species, reduce protein synthesis, enhance the conversion of nitrate to amino acids in the presence of reduced protein synthesis, and/or inhibit β-cyanoalanine synthase potentially increase the risk of cyanogenesis. Relevant environmental factors include crushing, wilting, freezing, high environmental temperatures, herbicide treatment, water stress, cool moist growing conditions, nitrate fertilization, high soil nitrogen:phosphorus ratios, soil phosphorus deficiency, low soil sulfur (decreases detoxification of cyanogenic glycosides to thiocyanates within plants), insect attack, and various plant diseases. Herbicide treatment of plants is important in that it may also increase plant palatability. Crushing and/or mastication of potentially cyanogenic plants is important in development of the acute toxidrome, because this releases cyanogenic glycosides from plant cell vacuoles and exposes them to catabolism by β-glucosidase and hydroxynitrile lyase present in the plant cell cytosol. Young, rapidly growing areas of plants and areas of regrowth after cutting often have high cyanogenic glycoside content. As a rough approximation, rapidly growing *Sorghum* spp are often hazardous until they reach ~60 cm in height; however, this is no guarantee of safety, and if there is any doubt regarding cyanogenic potential, samples of potential forage should be tested. Plant seeds and leaves typically have higher cyanogenic potential, while the fleshy parts of fruits generally have low levels. Drying often increases the cyanogenic potential of plants, whereas ensiling may reduce cyanide content by ~50%.

β-glucosidase and hydroxynitrile lyase are also present in the rumen microflora, and a rumen pH of ~6.5–7 favors conversion of cyanogenic glycosides to cyanide. Ruminants on high-energy grain rations are somewhat less susceptible, because their lower rumen pH (~4–6) reduces the formation of cyanide. Consumption of water before grazing on cyanogenic pastures appears to increase the risk. Monogastric animals with low stomach pH are also somewhat less susceptible to cyanogenic glycoside poisoning. However, these factors do not guarantee immunity from poisoning.

Under conditions of low-level exposure, mammals detoxify ~80% of ingested cyanide to thiocyanate via mitochondrial rhodanese. Thiocyanate is then largely excreted in urine. Often, the rate of the rhodanese pathway is limited by the availability of thiosulfate; also notably, dogs have lower overall rhodanese activity than other species. Minor, but toxicologically important, pathways of detoxification in mammals include the combination of cyanide with hydroxycobalamin (vitamin B_{12a}) to yield cyanocobalamin (vitamin B_{12}), and the nonenzymatic combination of cyanide with cysteine to form β-thiocyanoalanine, which is converted to 2-iminothiazolidine-4-carboxylic acid and subsequently excreted. Small amounts of β-thiocyanoalanine are also excreted in saliva. Dietary levels of sulfur amino acids (L-cysteine and L-methionine) strongly influence the rate of detoxification of cyanide, and low dietary intakes are associated with higher blood cyanide levels, particularly under conditions of chronic, low level exposure. Dietary sulfur and sulfur amino acid intake are known to strongly affect the neurologic toxidromes associated with chronic cyanide/cyanogenic glycoside exposure in people.

Chronic low-level cyanide/cyanogenic glycoside exposure is associated with increased exposure to the cyanide metabolite thiocyanate. Under conditions of thiocyanate overload, thiocyanate acts as a competitive inhibitor of thyroid follicular cell iodine uptake by the sodium/iodide symporter. This results in reduced iodination of tyrosine, reduced T_3 synthesis, increased blood TSH, goiter, and hypothyroidism. Similar effects occur with some plant glucosinolates (goitrogenic glycosides). Selenium deficiency appears to enhance these effects.

Chronic, low-level cyanide/cyanogenic glycoside exposure (often in combination with low dietary sulfur and/or sulfur amino acid intake) is associated with neuropathy syndromes in horses and ruminants. Sorghum cystitis ataxia syndrome of horses is associated with diffuse nerve fiber degeneration in the lateral and ventral funiculi of the spinal cord and brain stem. Similar syndromes have been described in ruminants. Comparisons between these syndromes as chronic cyanogenic glycoside–associated human myeloneuropathies such as Konzo and tropical ataxic neuropathy have been made; however, the precise toxins and modes of action are yet to be fully defined. All of these toxidromes appear to be related to a combination of chronic cyanide/cyanogenic glycoside exposure combined with low dietary sulfur and/or sulfur amino acid intake and possibly other nutritional deficiencies. Lathyrogenic plant cyanide metabolites such as β-cyanoalanine have been implicated as causative or at least contributory agents.

Chronic, low-level cyanogenic glycoside exposure (notably from *Sorghum* spp) has been associated with musculoskeletal teratogenesis (ankyloses or arthrogryposes) and abortion.

Clinical Findings: *Acute cyanide poisoning:* Signs generally occur within 15–20 min to a few hours after animals consume toxic forage, and survival after onset of clinical signs is rarely >2 hr. Excitement can be displayed initially, accompanied by rapid respiration rate. Dyspnea follows shortly, with tachycardia. The classic "bitter almond" breath smell may be present; however, the ability to detect this smell is genetically determined in people, and anosmic people (a significant proportion of the population) cannot detect it. Salivation, excess lacrimation, and voiding of urine and feces may occur. Vomiting may occur, especially in pigs. Muscle fasciculation is common and progresses to generalized spasms and coma before death. Animals may stagger and struggle before collapse. In other cases, sudden unexpected death may ensue. Mucous membranes are bright red but may become cyanotic terminally. Venous blood is classically described as "cherry red" because of the presence of high venous blood pO_2; however, this color rapidly changes after death. Serum ammonia and neutral and aromatic amino acids are typically increased. Cardiac arrhythmias are common due to myocardial histotoxic hypoxia. Death occurs during severe asphyxial convulsions. The heart may continue to beat for several minutes after struggling, and breathing stops. The elimination half-life of cyanide in dogs is reported to be 19 hr, so prognosis of recovery without therapeutic intervention is grave: it would take more than 4 days to eliminate >95% of the cyanide present.

Chronic cyanide poisoning: Chronic cyanogenic glycoside hypothyroidism will present as hypothyroidism with or without goiter. Cystitis ataxia toxidromes are typically associated with posterior ataxia or incoordination that may progress to irreversible flaccid paralysis, cystitis secondary to urinary incontinence, and hindlimb urine scalding and alopecia. Death, although uncommon, is often associated with pyelonephritis. Late-term abortion and musculoskeletal teratogenesis may also occur.

Lesions: *Acute cyanide poisoning:* Necropsy personnel may require appropriate personal protective equipment, including respirators with suitable cartridges. Venous blood is classically described as being "bright cherry red"; however, this color rapidly fades after death or if the blood is exposed to the atmosphere. Whole blood clotting may be slow or not occur. Mucous membranes may also be pink initially, then become cyanotic after respiration ceases. The rumen may be distended with gas; in some cases the odor of "bitter almonds" may be detected after opening. Rumen contents may provide a positive sodium picrate paper test (or positive results on other rapid cyanide test strip systems). Rumen gases may provide positive results in cyanide Draeger tube rapid test systems. Agonal hemorrhages of the heart may be seen. Liver, serosal surfaces, tracheal mucosa, and lungs may be congested or hemorrhagic; some froth may be seen in respiratory passages. Cyanide also binds to iron (both Fe^{2+} and Fe^{3+}) present in myoglobin (although this occurs more slowly than the binding to cytochrome c oxidase and, hence, is not protective); this may result in a generalized dark coloration of skeletal muscle. Neither gross nor histologic lesions are consistently seen.

Multiple foci of degeneration or necrosis may be seen in the CNS of dogs chronically exposed to sublethal amounts of cyanide. These lesions have not been reported in livestock.

Chronic cyanide poisoning: Goiter may be present. Cystitis ataxia toxidromes are characterized by opportunistic bacterial cystitis with or without pyelonephritis and diffuse nerve fiber degeneration in the lateral and ventral funiculi of the spinal cord and brain stem. Hindlimb urine scalding and alopecia may be present.

Diagnosis: Appropriate history, clinical signs, postmortem findings, and demonstration of HCN in rumen (stomach) contents or other diagnostic specimens support a diagnosis of cyanide poisoning. Veterinarians should be aware of the possible need to use appropriate personal protective equipment, including a respirator, when collecting samples that may liberate cyanide gas (eg, rumen contents and rumen gas cap). A rapid qualitative and presumptive diagnosis can be made by testing representative plant samples or stomach contents using the picric acid paper test or by collecting rumen gas cap samples by trocarization and testing with a Draeger cyanide gas detection tube or other cyanide gas detection system. Negative results with such rapid presumptive tests do not completely exclude the possibility of cyanide poisoning. Suitable specimens for more sophisticated testing include the suspected food source, rumen/stomach contents, samples of the rumen gas cap, heparinized whole blood, liver, and muscle. Antemortem whole blood is preferred; other specimens should be collected as soon as possible after death, preferably within 4 hr. Specimens should be sealed in an airtight container, refrigerated or frozen, and submitted to the laboratory without delay. When cold storage is unavailable, immersion of specimens in 1%–3% mercuric chloride has been satisfactory. The rationale for using liver as a diagnostic sample is that cyanide binds to the Fe^{3+} form of cytochrome p450 and other heme-containing metabolic enzymes. The rationale for using skeletal muscle is that cyanide will bind to the iron moiety in myoglobin.

Where available, measurement of the urinary metabolite of cyanide, thiocyanate, may reveal increased concentrations after cyanide poisoning.

Hay, green chop, silage, or growing plants containing >220 ppm cyanide as HCN on a wet-weight (as is) basis are very dangerous as animal feed. Forage containing <100 ppm HCN, wet weight, is usually safe to pasture. Analyses performed on a dry-weight basis have the following criteria: >750 ppm HCN is hazardous, 500–750 ppm HCN is doubtful, and <500 ppm HCN is considered safe.

Normally expected cyanide concentrations in blood of most animal species are usually <0.5 mcg/mL. Minimal lethal blood concentrations are ~3 mcg/mL or less. Cyanide concentrations in muscle are similar to those in blood, but concentrations in liver are generally lower than those in blood. In dogs, whole blood cyanide concentrations may be 4–5 times greater than serum concentrations because of binding to ferric ions and sequestration in RBCs.

Differential diagnoses include poisonings by nitrate or nitrite, urea, organophosphate, carbamate, chlorinated hydrocarbon pesticides, and toxic gases (carbon monoxide and hydrogen sulfide), as well as infectious or noninfectious diseases and other toxidromes that cause sudden death.

Treatment, Control, and Prevention: Immediate treatment is necessary. The goal of treatment is to break the cyanide-cytochrome c oxidase bond and reestablish the mitochondrial electron transport chain. One way to accomplish this is by using Fe^{3+} in hemoglobin (ie, inducing methemoglobinemia), which then acts as a high-affinity decoy chemical receptor for cyanide and forms cyanmethemoglobin. Classically, various nitrites have been used for this purpose; eg, inhaled amyl nitrite followed by IV injection of a nitrite salt (typically sodium nitrite) has been used to rapidly induce methemoglobinemia. Cyanide bound to methemoglobin can then be detoxified by rhodanese to thiocyanate. Because the rhodanese-mediated detoxification of cyanide to thiocyanate is usually capacity and rate limited by the availability of sulfur donors, treatment with nitrites is usually followed up by injection of sodium thiosulfate. Oral dosing with sodium thiosulfate into the rumen and/or stomach has also been suggested because the reaction between thiosulfate and cyanide can also occur nonenzymatically, and this may reduce any ongoing production of cyanide in the rumen/stomach environments.

If possible, the contents of one 0.3-mL vial of amyl nitrite should be inhaled by the animal as soon as possible after exposure, followed by an IV infusion of sodium nitrite (10 g/100 mL of distilled water or isotonic saline; 20 mg/kg body wt) over 3–4 min. Nitrite treatment is then followed by a slow IV injection of sodium thiosulfate (20% w/w) at ≥500 mg/kg. Thiosulfate is generally well tolerated; however, vomiting and hypotension can occur. The thiosulfate injection can be repeated if necessary. Oral administration of thiosulfate can also be considered in an attempt to convert any cyanide in the stomach/rumen into thiocyanate. Sodium nitrite therapy may be carefully repeated at 10 mg/kg, every 2–4 hr or as needed. Ideally, decisions regarding repeated treatment with nitrites should consider the degree of methemoglobinemia present.

Notably, thiosulfate treatment alone has been successful in some cases. However, thiosulfate treatment should ideally be preceded by nitrite induction of methemoglobinemia in cases of confirmed cyanide poisoning. However, because thiosulfate is generally well tolerated, it is often administered alone in situations when cyanide exposure is likely but unconfirmed (eg, smoke inhalation or exposure to fires).

Hydroxocobalamin (vitamin B_{12a}) is also used as a cyanide antidote. Hydroxocobalamin detoxifies cyanide by binding to it and forming cyanocobalamin (ie, another decoy receptor approach), which is then excreted in urine. It has the advantages that it is relatively well tolerated, does not compromise blood oxygen-carrying capacity, and does not produce hypotension. Hydroxocobalamin does produce chromaturia (which may result in false urinalysis results), as well as infusion site reactions, GI upset, pruritus, and dysphagia. The suggested dosage is 70 mg/kg, infused IV over 15 min, repeated as necessary.

Sulfanegen (as the sodium or triethanolamine salt) has been developed for treatment of cyanide mass poisoning incidents. This approach has the advantage that sulfanegen is water soluble and can be administered IM. Sulfanegen is a prodrug that generates 3-mercaptopyruvic acid (3-MP), an intermediate in cysteine metabolism, which again acts as a decoy receptor for cyanide. By itself, the half-life of 3-MP is too short to be effective against cyanide poisoning. For this reason, prodrugs such as sulfanegen have been developed to increase the duration of action of 3-MP in vivo.

Alternative inducers of methemoglobinemia such as 4-dimethyl-aminophenol (DMAP; IM at 5 mg/kg) or hydroxylamine hydrochlorine (IM at 50 mg/kg) have been suggested, because they produce methemoglobinemia more quickly than the nitrites currently in use. However, these hemoglobin-oxidizing agents are also relatively toxic to RBCs and can induce severe effects such as hemolysis and renal damage. These "rapid agents" still have the disadvantage of reducing blood oxygen-carrying capacity.

Other alternative antidotes in clinical development and use worldwide include dicobalt-ethylenediaminetetraacetic acid (EDTA) and α-ketoglutaric acid. Although hydroxycobalamin has been approved by the FDA for use in the USA, none of the others is readily available. Dicobalt-EDTA releases cobalt ions that react with cyanide ions; highly stable cyanide-cobalt complexes are then excreted by the kidneys. This drug is very potent and has immediate action but is reported to have numerous, severe adverse effects in people. The investigational antidote α-ketoglutaric acid has a molecular configuration that renders it amenable to nucleophilic binding of cyanide without generation of methemoglobin. Pretreatment with this drug reduced lethal outcomes and increased efficacy of sodium thiosulfate, but postexposure efficacy in animals is unknown.

Sodium thiosulfate alone is also an effective antidotal therapy at ≥500 mg/kg, IV, plus 30 g/cow, PO, to detoxify any remaining HCN in the rumen. When available, oxygen should be used to supplement nitrite or thiosulfate therapy, especially in small animals. Hyperbaric oxygen therapy (100% oxygen breathed intermittently at a pressure >1 atmosphere absolute) causes an above-normal partial pressure of oxygen (PO_2) in arterial blood and markedly increases the amount of oxygen dissolved in plasma. Oxygen-dependent cellular metabolic processes benefit from heightened oxygen tension in capillaries and enhanced oxygen diffusion from capillaries to critical tissues. Activated charcoal does not effectively absorb cyanide and thus is not recommended PO for antidotal therapy.

Caution is indicated in treatment. All cyanide antidotes are toxic by themselves. Many clinical signs of nitrate and prussic acid poisoning are similar, and injecting sodium nitrite induces methemoglobinemia identical to that produced by nitrite poisoning. If in doubt of the diagnosis, methylene blue, IV, at 4–22 mg/kg, may be used to induce methemoglobin. Because methylene blue can serve as both a donor and acceptor of electrons, it can reduce methemoglobin in the presence of excess methemoglobin or induce methemoglobin when only hemoglobin is present (but sodium nitrate is the more effective treatment for cyanide poisoning if the diagnosis is certain).

The best preventive step is to test suspect feed and/or pastures before allowing consumption. Pasture and forage sorghums (eg, Sudan grass and sorghum-Sudan grass hybrids) should not be grazed until they are >60 cm tall or have been proved by testing to have acceptable cyanide levels, to reduce danger from prussic acid poisoning. Animals should be fed before first turning out to pasture; hungry animals may consume forage too rapidly to detoxify HCN released in the rumen. Animals should be turned out to new pasture later in the day; potential for prussic acid release is reported to be highest during early morning hours. Free-choice salt and mineral with added sulfur may help protect against prussic acid toxicity. Grazing should be monitored closely during periods of environmental stress, eg, drought or frost. Abundant regrowth of sorghum can be dangerous; these shoots should be frozen and wilted before grazing.

Green chop forces livestock to eat both stems and leaves, thereby reducing problems caused by selective grazing. Cutting height can be raised to minimize inclusion of regrowth.

Sorghum hay and silage usually lose ≥50% of prussic acid content during curing and ensiling processes. Free cyanide is released by enzyme activity and escapes as a gas. Although a rare occurrence, hazardous concentrations of prussic acid may still remain in the final product, especially if the forage had an extremely high cyanide content before cutting. Hay has been dried at oven temperatures for up to 4 days with no significant loss of cyanide potential. These feeds should be analyzed before use whenever high prussic acid concentrations are suspected. Potentially toxic feed should be diluted or mixed with grain or forage that is low in prussic acid content to achieve safe concentrations in the final product. At least in theory, the risk of chronic cyanide poisoning syndromes may be reduced by iodine supplementation in the case of hypothyroidism and by sulfur-containing amino acids in the case of chronic neurologic toxidromes. Great care must be taken when providing supplemental elemental sulfur sources in ruminants because of the possible risk of polioencephalomalacia (*see* p 1281).

FOOD HAZARDS

AVOCADO

Ingestion of avocado (*Persea americana*) has been associated with myocardial necrosis in mammals and birds and with sterile mastitis in lactating mammals. Cattle, goats, horses, mice, rabbits, guinea pigs, rats, sheep, budgerigars, canaries, cockatiels, ostriches, chickens, turkeys, and fish are susceptible. Caged birds appear more sensitive to the effects of avocado, while chickens and turkeys appear more resistant. Although an old case report exists of two dogs developing myocardial damage after avocado ingestion, dogs appear to be relatively resistant compared with other species.

Etiology: Ingestion of fruit, leaves, stems, and seeds of avocado has been associated with toxicosis in animals; leaves are the most toxic part. The Guatemalan varieties of avocado have been most commonly associated with toxicosis.

When purified, the toxic principle in avocado, persin, causes mastitis in lactating mice at 60–100 mg/kg, and dosages >100 mg/kg result in myocardial necrosis. Goats develop severe mastitis when ingesting 20 g of leaves/kg, whereas 30 g of leaves/kg results in cardiac injury. Acute cardiac failure developed in sheep fed avocado leaves at 25 g/kg for 5 days; 5.5 g/kg of leaves fed for 21 days or 2.5 g/kg for 32 days caused chronic cardiac insufficiency. Budgerigars fed 1 g of avocado fruit developed agitation and feather pulling, while 8.7 g of mashed avocado fruit resulted in death within 48 hr. Myocardial injury, mastitis, and colic have been reported in horses ingesting avocado fruit and/or leaves.

Pathogenesis: Avocado causes necrosis and hemorrhage of mammary gland epithelium of lactating mammals and myocardial necrosis in birds and mammals. Persin isolated from avocado leaves has caused lesions similar to those reported in natural cases.

Clinical Findings: In lactating animals, sterile mastitis occurs within 24 hr of exposure to avocado, accompanied by a 75% decrease in milk production. Affected mammary glands are firm, swollen, and produce watery, curdled milk. Lactation may provide a degree of protection against myocardial injury when avocado is ingested at lower doses. In nonlactating mammals, or at higher doses, myocardial insufficiency may develop within 24–48 hr of ingestion and is characterized by lethargy, respiratory distress, subcutaneous edema, cyanosis, cough, exercise intolerance, and death. Horses may develop edema of the head, tongue, and brisket. Birds develop lethargy, dyspnea, anorexia, subcutaneous edema of the neck and pectoral regions, and may die.

Lesions: Mammary glands are edematous and reddened, with watery, curdled milk. In animals with cardiac insufficiency, there is congestion of lungs and liver, often with dependent subcutaneous edema. There may be pulmonary edema and free fluid within the abdominal cavity, pericardial sac, and thoracic cavity. The heart may contain pale streaks. Histopathologic lesions in the mammary gland include degeneration and necrosis of secretory epithelium, with interstitial edema and hemorrhage. Myocardial lesions include degeneration and necrosis of myocardial fibers, which are most pronounced in ventricular walls and septum; interstitial hemorrhage and/or edema may be present. In horses, symmetric ischemic myopathy of the head muscles and tongue, as well as ischemic myelomalacia of the lumbar spinal cord, have been described.

Diagnosis: Diagnosis of avocado toxicosis relies on history of exposure and clinical signs. There are no readily available specific tests that will confirm diagnosis. Differential diagnoses include other causes of mastitis (eg, infectious) and other myocardial disorders, including ionophore toxicosis, yew toxicosis, vitamin E/selenium deficiency, gossypol, cardiac glycoside toxicosis (eg, oleander), cardiomyopathy, and infectious myocarditis.

Treatment: NSAIDs and analgesics may benefit animals with mastitis. Treatment for congestive heart failure (eg, diuretics, antiarrhythmic drugs) may be of benefit but may not be economically feasible in livestock.

BREAD DOUGH

Raw bread dough made with yeast poses mechanical and biochemical hazards when ingested, including gastric distention, metabolic acidosis, and CNS depression. Although any species is susceptible, dogs are most commonly involved because of their indiscriminate eating habits.

Pathogenesis: The warm, moist environment of the stomach serves as an efficient incubator for the replication of yeast within the dough. The expanding dough mass causes the stomach to distend, resulting in vascular compromise to the gastric wall similar to that seen in gastric dilatation/volvulus. With sufficient gastric distention, respiratory compromise occurs. Yeast fermentation products include ethanol, which is absorbed into the bloodstream, resulting in inebriation and metabolic acidosis.

Clinical Findings: Early clinical signs may include unproductive attempts at emesis, abdominal distention, and depression. As ethanol intoxication develops, the animal becomes ataxic and disoriented. Eventually, profound CNS depression, weakness, recumbency, coma, hypothermia, or seizures may be seen. Death is usually due to the effects of the alcohol rather than from gastric distention; however, the potential for dough to trigger gastric dilatation/volvulus in susceptible dog breeds should not be overlooked.

Diagnosis: A presumptive diagnosis can be based on history of exposure and clinical signs. Blood ethanol levels are consistently increased in cases of bread dough toxicosis. Differential diagnoses include gastric dilatation/volvulus, foreign body obstruction, ethylene glycol toxicosis, and ingestion of other CNS depressants (eg, benzodiazepines).

Treatment: With recent ingestions in asymptomatic animals, emesis may be attempted, although the glutinous nature of bread dough may make removal via emesis difficult. In animals in which emesis (whether induced or spontaneous) has been unsuccessful, gastric lavage may be attempted. Cold water introduced into the stomach may slow the rate of yeast fermentation and aid in dough removal. In rare cases, surgical removal of the dough mass may be required. Animals presenting with signs of alcohol toxicosis should be stabilized and any life-threatening conditions corrected before attempts to remove the dough are made. Alcohol toxicosis is managed by correcting acid-base abnormalities, managing cardiac arrhythmias as needed, and maintaining normal body temperature. Providing fluid diuresis to enhance alcohol elimination may be helpful. Anecdotally, yohimbine (0.1 mg/kg, IV) has been used to stimulate severely comatose dogs with alcohol toxicosis.

CHOCOLATE

Chocolate toxicosis may result in potentially life-threatening cardiac arrhythmias and CNS dysfunction. Chocolate poisoning occurs most commonly in dogs, although many species are susceptible. Contributing factors include indiscriminate eating habits and readily available sources of chocolate. Deaths have also been reported in livestock fed cocoa by-products and in animals consuming mulch from cocoa-bean hulls.

Etiology: Chocolate is derived from the roasted seeds of *Theobroma cacao*. The primary toxic principles in chocolate are the methylxanthines theobromine (3,7-dimethylxanthine) and caffeine (1,3,7-trimethylxanthine). Although the concentration of theobromine in chocolate is 3–10 times that of caffeine, both constituents contribute to the clinical syndrome seen in chocolate toxicosis. The exact amount of methylxanthines in chocolate varies because of the natural variation of cocoa beans and variation within brands of chocolate products. However, in general, the total methylxanthine concentration of dry cocoa powder is ~800 mg/oz (28.5 mg/g), unsweetened (baker's) chocolate is ~450 mg/oz (16 mg/g), semisweet chocolate and sweet dark chocolate is ~150–160 mg/oz (5.4–5.7 mg/g), and milk chocolate is ~64 mg/oz (2.3 mg/g). Chocolate bars labeled as a percentage of cocoa/cacao are based on unsweetened chocolate, ie, a 65% cacao bar would contain ~293 mg (450 mg × 0.65) of methylxanthines per oz (10.4 mg/g). White chocolate is an insignificant source of methylxanthines. Cocoa bean hulls contain ~255 mg/oz (9.1 mg/g) methylxanthines.

The LD_{50} of both caffeine and theobromine is reportedly 100–200 mg/kg, but severe signs and deaths may occur at much lower dosages, and individual sensitivity to methylxanthines varies. In general, mild signs (vomiting, diarrhea, polydipsia) may be seen in dogs ingesting 20 mg/kg, cardiotoxic effects may be seen at 40–50 mg/kg, and seizures may occur at dosages ≥60 mg/kg. One ounce of milk chocolate per pound of body weight is a potentially lethal dose in dogs.

Pathogenesis: Theobromine and caffeine are readily absorbed from the GI tract and widely distributed throughout the body. They are metabolized in the liver and undergo enterohepatic recycling. Methylxanthines are excreted in the urine as both metabolites and unchanged parent compounds. The half-lives of theobromine and caffeine in dogs are 17.5 hr and 4.5 hr, respectively.

Theobromine and caffeine competitively inhibit cellular adenosine receptors, resulting in CNS stimulation, diuresis, and tachycardia. Methylxanthines also increase intracellular calcium levels by increasing cellular calcium entry and inhibiting intracellular sequestration of calcium by the sarcoplasmic reticulum of striated muscle. The net effect is increased strength and contractility of skeletal and cardiac muscle. Methylxanthines may also compete for benzodiazepine receptors within the CNS and inhibit phosphodiesterase, resulting in increased cyclic AMP levels. Methylxanthines may also increase circulating levels of epinephrine and norepinephrine.

Clinical Findings: Clinical signs of chocolate toxicosis usually occur within 6–12 hr of ingestion. Initial signs may include polydipsia, vomiting, diarrhea, abdominal distention, and restlessness. Signs may progress to hyperactivity, polyuria, ataxia, rigidity, tremors, and seizures. Tachycardia, premature ventricular contractions, tachypnea, cyanosis, hypertension, hyperthermia, bradycardia, hypotension, or coma may occur. Hypokalemia may occur late in the course of the toxicosis, contributing to cardiac dysfunction. Death is generally due to cardiac arrhythmias, hyperthermia, or respiratory failure. The high fat content of chocolate products may trigger pancreatitis in susceptible animals.

Lesions: No specific lesions may be found in animals succumbing to chocolate toxicosis. Hyperemia, hemorrhages, or congestion of multiple organs may occur as agonal changes. Severe arrhythmias may result in pulmonary edema or congestion. Chocolate or cocoa bean hulls may be present in the GI tract at necropsy.

Diagnosis: Diagnosis is based on history of exposure, along with clinical signs. Amphetamine toxicosis, ma huang/guarana (ephedra/caffeine) toxicosis, pseudoephedrine toxicosis, cocaine toxicosis, and ingestion of antihistamines, antidepressants, or other CNS stimulants should be considered in the differential diagnosis.

Treatment: Stabilization of symptomatic animals is a priority in treating chocolate toxicosis. Methocarbamol (50–220 mg/kg, slow IV; no more than 330 mg/kg/day) or diazepam (0.5–2 mg/kg, slow IV) may be used for tremors and/or mild seizures; barbiturates may be required for severe seizures. Arrhythmias should be treated as needed: propranolol (0.02–0.06 mg/kg, slow IV) or metoprolol (0.2–0.4 mg/kg, slow IV) for tachyarrhythmias, atropine (0.01–0.02 mg/kg) for bradyarrhythmias, and lidocaine (1–2 mg/kg, IV, followed by 25–80 mg/kg/min infusion) for refractory ventricular tachyarrhythmias. Fluid diuresis may assist in stabilizing cardiovascular function and hastening urinary excretion of methylxanthines.

Once animals have stabilized, or in animals presenting before clinical signs have developed (eg, within 1 hr of ingestion), decontamination should be performed. Induction of emesis using apomorphine or hydrogen peroxide should be initiated; in animals that have been sedated because of seizure activity, gastric lavage may be considered. Activated charcoal (1–4 g/kg, PO) should be administered; because of the enterohepatic recirculation of methylxanthines, repeated doses should be administered every 12 hr in symptomatic animals for as long as signs are present (control vomiting with metoclopramide, 0.2–0.4 mg/kg, SC or IM, qid as needed).

Other treatment for symptomatic animals includes maintaining thermoregulation, correcting acid-base and electrolyte abnormalities, monitoring cardiac status via electrocardiography, and placing a urinary catheter (methylxanthines and their metabolites can be reabsorbed across the bladder wall). Clinical signs may persist up to 72 hr in severe cases.

MACADAMIA NUTS

Ingestion of macadamia nuts by dogs has been associated with a nonfatal syndrome characterized by vomiting, ataxia, weakness, hyperthermia, and depression. Dogs are the only species in which signs have been reported.

Etiology: Macadamia nuts are cultivated from *Macadamia integrifolia* in the continental USA and *M tetraphylla* in Hawaii and Australia. The mechanism of toxicity is not known. Dogs have shown signs after ingesting 2.4 g of nuts/kg body weight. Dogs experimentally dosed with commercially prepared macadamia nuts at 20 g/kg developed clinical signs within 12 hr and were clinically normal without treatment within 48 hr.

Clinical Findings: Within 12 hr of ingestion, dogs develop weakness, depression, vomiting, ataxia, tremors, and/or hyperthermia. Tremors may be secondary to muscle weakness. Macadamia nuts may be identified in vomitus or feces. Mild transient increases in serum triglycerides, lipases, and alkaline phosphatase were reported in some dogs experimentally dosed with macadamia nuts; these values quickly returned to baseline. Signs generally resolve within 12–48 hr.

Diagnosis: Diagnosis is based on history of exposure and clinical signs. Differential diagnoses include ethylene glycol toxicosis, ingestion of hypotensive agents, and infectious diseases (eg, viral enteritis).

Treatment: For asymptomatic dogs with recent ingestion of more than 1–2 g/kg, emesis should be induced; activated charcoal may be of benefit with large ingestions. Fortunately, most symptomatic dogs recover without any specific treatment. Severely affected dogs may be given supportive treatment such as fluids, analgesics, or antipyretics.

RAISINS AND GRAPES

Ingestion of grapes or raisins has resulted in development of anuric renal failure in some dogs. Cases reported to date have been in dogs; anecdotal reports exist of renal failure in cats and ferrets after ingestion of grapes or raisins. It is not known why many dogs can ingest grapes or raisins with impunity while others develop renal failure after ingestion. The condition has not been reproduced experimentally, although raisin extracts have been shown to cause damage to canine kidney cells in vitro.

Pathogenesis: The exact mechanism of toxicity is unknown, although the primary injury appears to be in the proximal renal tubular epithelium. Affected dogs develop anuric renal failure within 72 hr of ingestion of grapes or raisins. A clear dose-response relationship has not been determined, but as few as 4–5 grapes were implicated in the death of an 18-lb (8.2-kg) dog.

Clinical Findings: Most affected dogs develop vomiting and/or diarrhea within 6–12 hr of ingestion of grapes or raisins. Other signs include lethargy, anorexia, abdominal pain, weakness, dehydration, polydipsia, and tremors (shivering). Serum creatinine levels tend to rise early and disproportionately compared with serum urea nitrogen levels. Oliguric or anuric renal failure develops within 24–72 hr of exposure; once anuric renal failure develops, most dogs die or are euthanized. Transient increases in serum glucose, liver enzymes, pancreatic enzymes, serum calcium, or serum phosphorus develop in some dogs.

Diagnosis: Diagnosis is based on history of exposure, along with clinical signs. Other causes of renal failure (eg, ethylene glycol, cholecalciferol) should be considered in the differential diagnosis.

Treatment: Prompt decontamination of significant ingestion of grapes or raisins is recommended. Emesis may be induced with 3% hydrogen peroxide (2 mL/kg; no more than 45 mL), followed by activated charcoal. With large ingestions or in cases in which vomiting and/or diarrhea has spontaneously developed within 12 hr of ingestion of grapes or raisins, aggressive fluid diuresis for a minimum of 48 hr is recommended. Renal function and fluid balance should be monitored during fluid administration. For oliguric dogs, urine production may be stimulated by using dopamine (0.5–3 mcg/kg/min, IV) and/or furosemide (2 mg/kg, IV). Anuric dogs are unlikely to survive unless peritoneal dialysis or hemodialysis is performed; even then, the prognosis is guarded.

XYLITOL

Xylitol is a sugar alcohol used to sweeten sugar-free products such as gums, candies, and baked goods. Ingestion of xylitol or xylitol-containing products by dogs has resulted in development of hypoglycemia and, less commonly, hepatic injury and/or failure. Dogs are the only species in which xylitol toxicosis has been reported.

Pathogenesis: In most mammals, xylitol has no significant effect on insulin levels, but in dogs, xylitol stimulates a rapid, dose-dependent insulin release that can result in profound hypoglycemia. Dosages of xylitol over ~75–100 mg/kg (34–45 mg/lb) have been associated with hypoglycemia in dogs. Some dogs ingesting xylitol at dosages >500 mg/kg (227 mg/lb) may develop severe hepatic insufficiency or failure, the mechanism of which is unknown.

Clinical Findings: Signs of hypoglycemia can develop within 30 min of ingestion or may be delayed up to 12–18 hr if the xylitol is in a substrate that slows its absorption (eg, some gum products). Clinical signs of hypoglycemia include vomiting, weakness, ataxia, depression, hypokalemia, seizures, and coma. Signs of liver injury may not occur until ≥24-48 hr after ingestion of xylitol, although increases in liver enzymes are often detectable within 8–12 hr of ingestion. Clinical signs of liver injury include depression, vomiting, icterus, and coagulopathy; other findings include hyperbilirubinemia, thrombocytopenia, and hyperphosphatemia. Hyperphosphatemia is considered a poor prognostic indicator, because it was present in 4 of 5 dogs that died of liver failure after xylitol ingestion (phosphorus was not measured in the fifth dog). Not all dogs that develop xylitol-induced liver injury develop hypoglycemia.

Diagnosis: Diagnosis is based on clinical findings and history of exposure. Other causes of hypoglycemia include hypoglycemic drugs, juvenile hypoglycemia, hunting dog hypoglycemia, insulinoma, and parenteral insulin overdose. Differential diagnoses for liver insufficiency include infectious (eg, leptospirosis, viral hepatitis), environmental (eg, heat stroke, trauma), and toxic (eg, iron, acetaminophen, mushroom, blue-green algae, cycad palms) causes. Lesions of dogs succumbing to liver injury have included hepatic necrosis with loss of normal hepatic architecture.

Treatment: Because of the potential for rapid onset of clinical signs of hypoglycemia, emesis should ideally be attempted only under veterinary supervision and in asymptomatic animals. Activated charcoal does not appreciably bind xylitol and is not recommended. If >75–100 mg/kg (227 mg/lb) of xylitol has been ingested, animals should be hospitalized and baseline blood glucose values measured; dogs ingesting >500 mg/kg (227 mg/lb) of xylitol should have baseline liver values measured. Blood glucose should be monitored every 1–2 hr for at least 12 hr, while liver values should be evaluated every 24 hr for at least 72 hr. If hypoglycemia develops, it should be managed with dextrose IV boluses and/or constant-rate infusions. Hypoglycemia may persist as long as 24 hr or more, so treatment should be continued until the dog can maintain a normal blood glucose level without supplemental dextrose. Dextrose should be administered to dogs ingesting xylitol at >500 mg/kg (227 mg/lb), even though normoglycemic, and hepatoprotectants such as *N*-acetylcysteine, *S*-adenosylmethionine, and silymarin should be considered. Treatment of coagulopathy or other manifestations of liver insufficiency should be performed as needed. The prognosis for uncomplicated hypoglycemia is good, if prompt treatment is obtained. Mild increases in liver enzyme usually resolve within a few days. Severe increases in liver enzymes and/or signs of liver insufficiency indicate a more guarded prognosis; in one study, 62.5% of dogs with signs of liver injury died or were euthanized despite aggressive veterinary intervention.

HERBICIDE POISONING

Herbicides are used routinely to control noxious plants. Most of these chemicals, particularly the more recently developed synthetic organic herbicides, are quite selective for specific plants and have low toxicity for mammals; other, less-selective compounds (eg, sodium arsenite, arsenic trioxide, sodium chlorate, ammonium sulfamate, borax, and many others) were formerly used on a large scale and are more toxic to animals.

Vegetation treated with herbicides at proper rates normally will not be hazardous to animals, including people. Particularly after the herbicides have dried on the vegetation, only small amounts can be dislodged. When herbicide applications have been excessive, damage to lawns, crops, or other foliage is often evident.

The residue potential for most of these agents is low. However, runoff from agricultural applications and entrance into drinking water cannot be excluded. The possibility of residues should be explored if significant exposure of food-producing animals occurs. The time recommended before treated vegetation is grazed or used as animal feed is available for a number of products.

Most health problems in animals result from exposure to excessive quantities of herbicides because of improper or careless use or disposal of containers. When herbicides are used properly, poisoning problems in veterinary practice are rare. With few exceptions, it is only when animals gain direct access to the product that acute poisoning occurs. Acute signs usually will not lead to a diagnosis, although acute GI signs are frequent. All common differential diagnoses should be excluded in animals showing signs of a sudden onset of disease or sudden death. The case history is critical. Sickness after feeding, spraying of pastures or crops adjacent to pastures, a change in housing, or direct exposure may lead to a tentative diagnosis of herbicide poisoning. Generally, the nature of exposure is hard to identify because of storage of herbicides in mis- or unlabeled containers. Unidentified spillage of liquid from containers or powder from torn or damaged bags near a feed source, or visual confusion with a dietary ingredient or supplement, may cause the exposure. Once a putative chemical source has been identified, an animal poison control center should be contacted for information on treatments, laboratory tests, and likely outcome.

Chronic disease caused by herbicides is even more difficult to diagnose. It may include a history of herbicide use in proximity to the animals or animal feed or water source, or a gradual change in the animals' performance or behavior over a period of weeks, months, or even years. Occasionally, it involves manufacture or storage of herbicides nearby. Samples of possible sources (ie, contaminated feed and water) for residue analysis, as well as tissues from exposed animals taken at necropsy, are essential. Months or even years may be required to successfully identify a problem of chronic exposure.

To recognize whether an animal has been exposed to herbicides or accidental poisoning, standardized analytical procedures for diagnostic investigation of biologic materials have become established and are subsumed under the term "biomonitoring." Accurate biomonitoring is an important tool to evaluate human or animal exposure to such herbicides by measuring the levels of these chemicals, their metabolites, or altered biologic structures or functions in biologic materials such as urine, blood or blood components, exhaled air, hair or nails, and tissues. The use of urine is advantageous because of ready availability. As such, urine has been used for biomonitoring of several herbicides, including 2,4-D, 2,4,5-T, MCPA (2-methyl-4-chlorophenoxyacetic acid), atrazine, diuron, alachlor, metolachlor, paraquat, diquat, imazapyr, imazapic, imazethapyr, imazamox, imazaquin, and imazamethabenz-methyl herbicides, with the objective to assess exposure and health risk to exposed animals.

If poisoning is suspected, the first step in management is to halt further exposure. Animals should be separated from any possible source before attempting to stabilize and support them. If there are life-threatening signs, efforts to stabilize animals by general mitigation methods should be started. Specific antidotal treatments, when available, may help to confirm the diagnosis. As time permits, a

TABLE 1 HERBICIDE POISONING

Compound	Acute Oral LD_{50}—Rat	NOAEL[a] (oral)	Acute Dermal LD_{50}
Acetochlor	2,148–2,950 mg/kg	Dog, 1 yr 12 mg/kg/day	Rabbit 4,166 mg/kg
Acifluorfen	1,300 mg/kg (F)	Rat, 2 yr 180 ppm	Rabbit >2,000 mg/kg
Acrolein	29 mg/kg	Rat, 13 wk 150 mg/L in drinking water	Rabbit 231 mg/kg
Alachlor	930–1,200 mg/kg	Dog, 90 days <200 mg/kg/day	Rabbit 13,300 mg/kg
Ametryn	1,009–1,405 mg/kg	Rat reproduction, 50 ppm	Rabbit 2,020 mg/kg
α-Metolachlor	2,675–2,952 mg/kg	Dog, 90 days 0.0125 mg/kg/day	Rat 2,020 mg/kg

more detailed history and investigation should be completed. The owner should be made aware of the need for full disclosure of facts to successfully determine the source of poisoning, eg, unapproved use or failure to properly store a chemical.

Toxicity and Management of Poisoning

There are >200 active ingredients used as herbicides; however, some of them are believed to be obsolete or no longer in use. Of these, several have been evaluated for their toxic potential and are discussed below. More specific information is available on the label and from the manufacturer, cooperative extension service, or poison control center. Selected information on herbicides, such as the acute oral toxic dose (LD_{50}) in rats, the amount an animal can be exposed to without being affected (no adverse effect level), the likelihood of problems caused by dermal contact in rabbits (dermal LD_{50}, eye and skin irritation), deleterious effects on avian species, and toxicity to fish in water, is included for some commonly used herbicides (*see* TABLE 1). Comparative toxic doses (TD) and lethal doses (LD) of selected herbicides in domesticated species, such as monkeys, cattle, sheep, pigs, cats, dogs, and chickens, is also summarized (*see* TABLE 2). The information is only a guideline, because the toxicity of herbicides may be altered by the presence of other ingredients (eg, impurities, surfactants, stabilizers, emulsifiers) present in the compound. With a few exceptions, most of the newly developed chemicals have a low order of toxicity to mammals. However, some herbicides, such as atrazine, buturon, butiphos, chloridazon, chlorpropham, cynazine, 2,4-D and 2,4,5-T alone or in combination, dichlorprop, dinoseb, dinoterb, linuron, mecoprop, monolinuron, MCPA (2-methyl-4-chlorophenoxyacetic acid), prometryn, propachlor, nitrofen, silvex, TCDD (a common contaminant during manufacturing process of some herbicides such as 2,4-D and 2,4,5-T), and tridiphane, are known to have adverse effects on development of embryos and reproduction abnormalities in experimental animals. A list of such chemicals is summarized in TABLE 3.

TABLE 1 HERBICIDE POISONING *(continued)*

Avian Toxicity/NOAEC[b]	Toxicity to Fish in Water	Skin and Eye Irritation
LC_{50} 5 day Bobwhite quail and Mallard duck 5,620 mg/kg	LC_{50} 96 hr Rainbow trout 0.45 mg/L	Skin–mild Eye–mild
LC_{50} 8 day Mallard duck > 10,000 mg/kg	LC_{50} 96 hr Rainbow trout 31 mg/L	Skin–moderate Eye–severe
LD_{50} (oral) Bobwhite quail 19 mg/kg Mallard duck 9.1 mg/kg	LC_{50} 24 hr Bluegill and Rainbow trout 0.024 mg/L	Skin–severe Eye–severe
		Skin–mild
LD_{50} (oral) Birds >2,250 mg/kg LC_{50} 5 day Birds >5,620 ppm		Skin–irritation Guinea pig–dermal sensitization Eye–mild
LC_{50} 8 day Bobwhite quail and Mallard duck >10,000 ppm	LC_{50} 96 hr Bluegill and Rainbow trout 3.9–10 ppm	Skin–slight Eye–mild

(continued)

TABLE 1 HERBICIDE POISONING *(continued)*

Compound	Acute Oral LD_{50}—Rat	NOAEL[a] (oral)	Acute Dermal LD_{50}
Atrazine	2,000–3,080 mg/kg	Dog, 1 yr 150 ppm Rat, 2 yr 10 ppm	Rabbit 7,500 mg/kg
Amitrole	4,080 mg/kg (M)	Rat, 13 wk 2 mg/kg/day	Rat >5,000 mg/kg
Ammonium sulfamate	3,900 mg/kg	Rat, 105 days 10,000 mg/kg/day	
Bensulfron methyl	>5,000 mg/kg	Rat, dog, 2 yr 750 ppm in diet	Rat >2,000 mg/kg
Bensulide[c]	271–770 mg/kg	Dog, 90 days 12.5 mg/kg/day	Rabbit 3,950 mg/kg
Bentazon	1,100 mg/kg (cat 500 mg/kg)	Rat, 90 days 3.5 mg/kg/day Dog, 90 days 7.5 mg/kg/day	Rat >2,500 mg/kg
Bispyribac sodium		Rat, 2 yr 1.1 mg/kg/day (M) 1.4 mg/kg/day (F)	
Borax	2,000–6,000 mg/kg		
Bromacil	5,200 mg/kg	Rat, dog, 2 yr 250 mg/kg/day	Rabbit >5,000 mg/kg
Bromoxynil	190–779 mg/kg	Rat, 90 days 50 mg/kg/day	Rabbit >2,000 mg/kg
Butachlor[c]	2,000–3,300 mg/kg	Rabbits maternal and fetal effects, 50 mg/kg/day	Rat >13.3 g/kg
Butylate[c]	>5,431 mg/kg (M) 4,659 mg/kg (F)	Rat, 2 yr 20 mg/kg/day Dog, 1 yr 25 mg/kg/day	Rabbit >4,640 mg/kg
Carfentrazone ethyl	>5,000 mg/kg	Rat, 2 yr 9 mg/kg/day (M) 3 mg/kg/day (F)	Rat >5,000 mg/kg

TABLE 1 HERBICIDE POISONING *(continued)*

Avian Toxicity/NOAEC[b]	Toxicity to Fish in Water	Skin and Eye Irritation
LC_{50} 8 day Mallard duck >10,000 ppm in diet	LC_{50} 96 hr Rainbow trout 8.8 mg/L	Skin–slight
LD_{50} Mallard duck 2,000 mg/kg		Skin–mild Eye–mild
LD_{50} Bobwhite quail 3,000 mg/kg	LC_{50} 48 hr Crucian carp 1,000–2,000 mg/L	Skin–none
	LC_{50} 96 hr Bluegill and Rainbow trout >150 ppm	Skin–none Eye–serious
LD_{50} Bobwhite quail 3 wk 50 mg/kg, poor hatchability	LC_{50} 96 hr Bluegill 1.4 mg/L Rainbow trout 0.7 mg/L	Eye–none
LD_{50} Japanese quail 720 mg/kg Mallard duck 2,000 mg/kg	LC_{50} 96 hr Bluegill 616 mg/L Rainbow trout 1,060 mg/L	Slight irritant
LC_{50} Bobwhite quail and Mallard duck >5,620 ppm	LC_{50} 96 hr Bluegill and Rainbow trout >100 ppm	Skin–minor Eye–minor
LC_{50} 8 day Bobwhite quail and Mallard duck >10,000 mg/kg	LC_{50} 48 hr Bluegill 71 mg/L Rainbow trout 56 mg/L	Skin–irritating Eye–irritating
Acute LD_{50} Bobwhite quail 100 mg/kg Mallard duck 200 mg/kg	LC_{50} 96 hr Rainbow trout 0.05 mg/L	Skin–none Eye–none
		Skin–none Eye–moderate Guinea pig–dermal sensitization
LC_{50} 8 day Bobwhite quail 40,000 mg/kg Mallard duck 46,400 ppm in diet	LC_{50} 96 hr Bluegill 6.9 mg/L Rainbow trout 4.2 mg/L	Skin–moderate Eye–mild
LC_{50} Bobwhite quail and Mallard duck >5,620 ppm	LC_{50} 96 hr Bluegill 2 ppm Rainbow trout 16 ppm	Skin–none to slight Eye–minimum

(continued)

TABLE 1 HERBICIDE POISONING *(continued)*

Compound	Acute Oral LD_{50}—Rat	NOAEL[a] (oral)	Acute Dermal LD_{50}
Chloramben	5,620 mg/kg		Rabbit >3,160 mg/kg
Chlorotoluron	>10,000 mg/kg		
Chlorpropham	4,100–7,000 mg/kg	Rat, dog, 2 yr 100–350 mg/kg/day	
Chlorsulfuron	5,545 mg/kg (M) 6,293 mg/kg (F)	Rat, 2 yr 100 ppm in diet	Rabbit >3,400 mg/kg
Chlorthal dimethyl	3,000–12,000 mg/kg	Rat, 2 yr <50 mg/kg/day	Rabbit >2,000 mg/kg
Clethodim	1,630 mg/kg (M) 1,360 mg/kg (F)	Dog, 1 yr >1 mg/kg/day	Rabbit >5,000 mg/kg
Clodinafop-propargyl	1,392 mg/kg (M) 2,271 mg/kg (F)	Dog, 90 days 0.346 mg/kg/day (M) 1.89 mg/kg/day (F)	Rabbit >2,000 mg/kg
Clomazone	2,077 mg/kg (M) 1,369 mg/kg (F)	Dog, 1 yr <2.5 mg/kg/day	Rabbit >2,000 mg/kg
Clopyralid	>4,300 mg/kg	Rat, 2 yr 50 mg/kg/day	Rabbit >2,000 mg/kg
Cloransulam-methyl	>5,000 mg/kg	Dog, 1 yr 10 mg/kg/day	Rabbit >2,000 mg/kg
Copper chelate	498 mg/kg		Rabbit >2,000 mg/kg
Copper sulfate	470 mg/kg		Rabbit >8,000 mg/kg
Cyanazine[d]	182–334 mg/kg	Dog, 2 yr <225 mg/kg/day	Rabbit >2,000 mg/kg
Cycloate	2,000–3,190 mg/kg	Dog, 240 mg/kg/day	Rabbit >4,640 mg/kg

TABLE 1 HERBICIDE POISONING *(continued)*

Avian Toxicity/NOAEC[b]	Toxicity to Fish in Water	Skin and Eye Irritation
LC_{50} 8 day Mallard duck >4,640 mg/kg	Not toxic to fish	Skin–mild Eye–mild
	LC_{50} 96 hr Rainbow trout >100 mg/L	
LD_{50} 8 day Mallard duck >2,000 mg/kg	LC_{50} 48 hr Bluegill 6.3–6.8 mg/L Rainbow trout 3–6 mg/L	Skin–moderate Eye–moderate
LC_{50} 8 day Mallard duck >5,000 mg/kg	LC_{50} 96 hr Rainbow trout >250 mg/L	Skin–none Eye–mild
LD_{50} young Bobwhite quail 5,500 mg/kg	Not toxic to fish	Skin–none Eye–mild
LC_{50} 8 day Bobwhite quail 4,270 ppm Mallard duck 3,978 ppm in diet	LC_{50} Bluegill 13 ppm Rainbow trout 18 ppm	Skin–none Eye–moderate
LC_{50} Birds >5,000 ppm	LC_{50} Freshwater fish 0.3 ppm	Skin–none Eye–slight to severe
LD_{50} 8 day Bobwhite quail and Mallard duck 5,620 ppm in diet	LC_{50} 96 hr Bluegill 34 mg/L Rainbow trout 19 mg/L	Skin–mild Eye–moderate
LC_{50} Bobwhite quail and Mallard duck >4,640 ppm in diet	LC_{50} 96 hr Bluegill 125 mg/L Rainbow trout 103.5 mg/L	Skin–mild Eye–severe
LC_{50} 5 day Bobwhite quail and Mallard duck >5,620 ppm	LC_{50} 96 hr Bluegill >154 ppm Rainbow trout >86 ppm	Skin–none Eye–slight
LC_{50} 8 day Mallard duck >1,000 ppm in diet	LC_{50} 96 hr Bluegill 1.2–7.5 mg/L Rainbow trout <0.2–4 mg/L	Skin–slight Eye–moderate
LD_{50} (oral) Pheasant 1,000 ppm in diet (estimated)	LC_{50} 96 hr Bluegill 4.4–7.3 mg/L Rainbow trout 0.135 mg/L	Skin–moderate Eye–severe
LD_{50} Bobwhite quail 400 mg/kg Mallard duck >2,000 mg/kg	LC_{50} 96 hr Bluegill 23 mg/L Rainbow trout 9 mg/L	Skin–none Eye–mild
LC_{50} 7 day Bobwhite quail >56,000 mg/kg	LC_{50} 96 hr Rainbow trout 5.6 mg/L	Skin–none Eye–none

(continued)

TABLE 1 HERBICIDE POISONING *(continued)*

Compound	Acute Oral LD_{50}—Rat	NOAEL[a] (oral)	Acute Dermal LD_{50}
Cyhalofopbutyl	>5,000 mg/kg	Dog 46.7 mg/kg/day (M) 45.9 mg/kg/day (F)	Rat >5,000 mg/kg
Dalapon	6,600–9,330 mg/kg		
Di-allate[d]	340–460 mg/kg		
2,4-D	370–700 mg/kg	Rat, 2 yr 50 mg/kg/day	Rabbit >2,000 mg/kg
2,4-D dimethyl-amine	949–4,650 mg/kg	Dog, 1 yr 1 mg/kg/day	Rabbit >2,000 mg/kg
2,4-D isooctyl ester	500–700 mg/kg	Dog, 1 yr 1 mg/kg/day	Rabbit >2,000 mg/kg
Dazomet	551–646 mg/kg (M) 335–562 mg/kg (F)	Rat, 2 yr 1.6 mg/kg/day	Rabbit >2,000 mg/kg
Dicamba	1,707 mg/kg	Rat, 2 yr 125 mg/kg/day Dog, 2 yr 50 mg/kg day	Rabbit >2,000 mg/kg
Dichlobenil	>3,160 mg/kg	Rat, 2 yr >20 ppm in diet Pig, 6 mo >50 ppm in diet	Rabbit >1,350 mg/kg
Dichlorprop or 2,4-DP	700 mg/kg (M) 500 mg/kg (F)	Rat, 4 mg/kg	Mouse 1,400 mg/kg
Diclosulam	>5,000 mg/kg	Rat, 0.05 mg/kg	Rabbit >2,000 mg/kg
Difenzoquat (methylsulfate)	617 mg/kg (M) 373 mg/kg (F)	Dog, 1 yr 20 mg/kg/day	Rabbit >2,000 mg/kg
Diflufenzopyr	1,600 to >5,000 mg/kg	Dog, 1 yr 28 mg/kg/day (M) 26 mg/kg/day (F)	Rabbit >5,000 mg/kg

TABLE 1 HERBICIDE POISONING *(continued)*

Avian Toxicity/NOAEC[b]	Toxicity to Fish in Water	Skin and Eye Irritation
	LC_{50} 96 hr Bluegill >99.2 mg/L Rainbow trout >1.65 mg/L	Skin–none Eye–minimal
	LC_{50} 96 hr Fish 210–340 mg/L	
	LC_{50} 96 hr Fish 8.2 mg/L	
LC_{50} 8 day Mallard duck >4,640 mg/kg	LC_{50} 96 hr Bluegill >300 mg/L Rainbow trout 800 mg/L	Skin–none Eye–moderate
LC_{50} 8 day Mallard duck >5,600 ppm	LC_{50} 96 hr Bluegill 524 mg/L Rainbow trout 250 mg/L	Skin–minimal Eye–severe
As for 2,4-D (above)		Skin–none Eye–severe
LD_{50} Bobwhite quail 415 ppm in diet	LC_{50} Rainbow trout 2.4–16.2 mg/L	Skin–mild Eye–severe
LC_{50} 8 day Bobwhite quail and Mallard duck >4,600 mg/kg	LC_{50} 96 hr Bluegill and Rainbow trout >1,000 mg/L	Skin–moderate Eye–extreme
LC_{50} 8 day Mallard duck >5,200 ppm in diet	LC_{50} 96 hr Bluegill and Rainbow trout 7 mg/L	Skin–none Eye–mild to moderate
LC_{50} Upland birds, waterfowl >10,000 ppm in diet	LC_{50} Bluegill 1.1 mg/L Rainbow trout 100–200 mg/L	Skin–none Eye–none
	LC_{50} Most sensitive aquatic species 10-100 mg/L	Skin–moderate Eye–moderate
LC_{50} 8 day Bobwhite quail and Mallard duck 4,640 ppm in diet	LC_{50} 96 hr Bluegill 696 mg/L Rainbow trout 711 mg/L	Skin–mild Eye–mild
LC_{50} Mallard duck >5,620 ppm	LC_{50} Bluegill 135 ppm Rainbow trout 106 ppm	Skin–very slight Eye–mild to slight

(continued)

TABLE 1 HERBICIDE POISONING *(continued)*

Compound	Acute Oral LD_{50}—Rat	NOAEL[a] (oral)	Acute Dermal LD_{50}
Dimethenamid	429–1,293 mg/kg	Dog, 1 yr 50–250 ppm in diet	Rabbit >2,000 mg/kg
Dinoterb	25 mg/kg		
Diquat	231–440 mg/kg	Rat reproduction, 1 mg/kg/day	Rabbit >400 mg/kg
Dithiopyr	>5,000 mg/kg	Dog, 1 yr <0.5 mg/kg/day	Rabbit >5,000 mg/kg
Diuron	3,400 mg/kg	Dog, 2 yr 25 mg/kg	Rat >2,000 mg/kg
DNOC	25–85 mg/kg	Rat, 2 yr 0.59 mg/kg/day	Rat 600–2,000 mg/kg Rabbit 1,000 mg/kg
EPTC (s-ethyldipropylthiocarbamate)	1,630 mg/kg	Dog, 90 days 20 mg/kg	Rabbit 2,750–5,000 mg/kg
Ethalfluralin	Rat >5,000 mg/kg (dog, cat >200 mg/kg)	Rat, mouse, 90 days 68 mg/kg	Rabbit >2,000 mg/kg
Ethephon	1,600–4,229 mg/kg	Rat, 2 yr 375 mg/kg/day Mouse, 78 wk 4.5 mg/kg/day	Rabbit >5,000 mg/kg
Fenoxaprop[d]	2,357 mg/kg (M) 2,500 mg/kg (F)	Dog, 2 yr 0.375 mg/kg/day	Rabbit >1,000 mg/kg
Fenoxaprop-ethyl[d]	4,430 mg/kg	Dog, 2 yr 0.9 mg/kg/day	Rat >5,000 mg/kg
Flamprop-methyl	1,210 mg/kg	Dog, 2 yr 10 mg/kg/day	Rat >294 mg/kg

TABLE 1 HERBICIDE POISONING *(continued)*

Avian Toxicity/NOAEC[b]	Toxicity to Fish in Water	Skin and Eye Irritation
LC_{50} Bobwhite quail and Mallard duck >5,620 ppm in diet	LC_{50} Bluegill 6.4 mg/L Rainbow trout 2.6 mg/L	Skin–mild Eye–moderate
LC_{50} Partridges 3–5 ppm in diet	Toxic to fish	
LC_{50} Partridges 270–300 ppm in diet	LC_{50} Fish 80–210 mg/L	Skin–none Eye–mild
LC_{50} Bobwhite quail and Mallard duck >5,260 ppm in diet	LC_{50} Bluegill 0.7 mg/L Rainbow trout 0.5 mg/L	Skin–slight Eye–moderate
LC_{50} Bobwhite quail 1,730 ppm Mallard duck >5,000 ppm in diet	LC_{50} Bluegill 7.4 mg/L Rainbow trout 4.3 mg/L	Skin–none Eye–mild
LD_{50} Japanese quail 10–25 mg/kg	LC_{50} Fish 0.2–13 mg/L	Skin–erythema and edema Eyes–corrosive Guinea pig–dermal sensitization
LC_{50} 7 day Bobwhite quail 20,000 ppm in diet	LC_{50} Bluegill 27 mg/L Rainbow trout 19 mg/L	Skin–mild Eye–severe
LC_{50} 8 day Bobwhite quail and Mallard duck >5,000 ppm	LC_{50} Bluegill 0.03–0.1 mg/L Rainbow trout 0.037–0.136 mg/L	Skin–slight to moderate Eye–slight
LC_{50} 8 day Mallard duck >10,000 ppm	LC_{50} 96 hr Bluegill 222–300 mg/L Rainbow trout 254–350 mg/L	Skin–corrosive Eye–corrosive
LD_{50} Japanese quail >5,000 mg/kg	LC_{50} Bluegill 3.3 mg/L Rainbow trout 3.4 mg/L	Skin–slight Eye–serious nonreversible corneal opacity
LC_{50} 8 day Bobwhite quail and Mallard duck 5,620 ppm	LC_{50} Bluegill 0.31 mg/L Rainbow trout 0.46 mg/L	Skin–slight Eye–moderate
LD_{50} Bobwhite quail 4,640 mg/kg Mallard duck >1,000 mg/kg	LC_{50} 96 hr Rainbow trout 4.7 mg/L	Skin–none Eye–none

(continued)

TABLE 1 HERBICIDE POISONING *(continued)*

Compound	Acute Oral LD_{50}—Rat	NOAEL[a] (oral)	Acute Dermal LD_{50}
Florasulam	>6,000 mg/kg	Dog, 1 yr 5 mg/kg/day	Rabbit >2,000 mg/kg
Fluazifop-p-butyl	3,680– 4,096 mg/kg (M) 2,451– 2,721 mg/kg (F)[e]	Rat, 90 days >10 mg/kg/day	Rabbit >2,400 mg/kg
Flucarbazone-sodium	>5,000 mg/kg	Dog, 1 yr 35.9 mg/kg/day	Rat >5,000 mg/kg
Flufenacet	1,617 mg/kg (M) 589 mg/kg (F)	Dog, 1 yr 1.29 mg/kg/day	Rat >2,000 mg/kg
Flumetsulam	>5,000 mg/kg		Rat >2,000 mg/kg
Flumiclorac	3,200 to >5,000 mg/kg	Dog, 1 yr 100 mg/kg/day	Rat >2,000 mg/kg
Fluometuron	>8,000 mg/kg	Rat, 103 wk 125 mg/kg/day	Rat >2 g/kg Rabbit 10 g/kg
Fluroxypyr	>5,000 mg/kg	Dog, 1 yr 150 mg/kg/day	Rat >2,000 mg/kg
Fluthiacet	>5,000 mg/kg	Dog, 1 yr 57.6 mg/kg/day (M) 30.3 mg/kg/day (F)	Rat >2,000 mg/kg
Foramsulfuron	>3,881 mg/kg	Rat, 2 yr 849 mg/kg/day (M) 1,135 mg/kg/day (F)	Rat >5,000 mg/kg
Fosamine ammonium	24,000 mg/kg	Rat, 90 days 1,000 mg/kg	Rabbit >1,683 mg/kg
Glufosinate (ammonium salt)	1,510–2,030 mg/kg	Dog, 1 yr 5 mg/kg/day	Rat >1,390 mg/kg
Glyphosate	4,230–5,600 mg/kg	Dog, 2 yr >500 mg/kg/day	Rabbit >5,000 mg/kg

TABLE 1 HERBICIDE POISONING *(continued)*

Avian Toxicity/NOAEC[b]	Toxicity to Fish in Water	Skin and Eye Irritation
LD_{50} 14 day Japanese quail 175 mg/kg	LC_{50} 96 hr Rainbow trout >100 mg/L	Skin–none Eye–none
LD_{50} 5 day Bobwhite quail >4,659 ppm Mallard duck >4,321 ppm	LC_{50} 96 hr Bluegill 0.5 mg/L Rainbow trout 1.4 mg/L	Skin–slight Eye–mild
NOAEC (reproduction) Mallard duck 233 mg/kg/day	NOAEL (chronic) Rainbow trout 2.75 mg/L	Skin–none Eye–minimal
LC_{50} 5 day Bobwhite quail >5,317 ppm Mallard duck >4,970 ppm	LC_{50} Bluegill 2.26–2.4 ppm Rainbow trout 3.49–5.84 ppm	Skin–none Eye–minimal
LC_{50} Mallard duck >5,620 ppm	LC_{50} Bluegill >300 ppm Rainbow trout >293 ppm	Skin–none Eye–slight
LC_{50} Mallard duck >5,620 ppm	LC_{50} 96 hr Bluegill 17.4 mg/L Rainbow trout 1.1 mg/L	Skin–severe Eye–moderate
	LC_{50} 96 hr Bluegill 96 mg/L Rainbow trout 47 mg/L Crucian carp 17 mg/L	
LC_{50} 5 day Mallard duck >5,000 ppm	LC_{50} 96 hr Bluegill 14.3 mg/L Rainbow trout 13.4–100 mg/L	Skin–none Eye–slight
LC_{50} 5 day Bobwhite quail and Mallard duck >5,620 ppm	LC_{50} 96 hr Bluegill 140 mcg/L Rainbow trout 43 mcg/L	Skin–none Eye–minimal
LC_{50} Bobwhite quail and Mallard duck >5,000 ppm		Skin–moderate Eye–mild
LD_{50} Mallard duck >10,000 ppm in diet	LC_{50} Bluegill 670 mg/L Rainbow trout 1,000 mg/L	Skin–none Eye–moderate to severe
LC_{50} 5 day Japanese quail >5,000 mg/kg	LC_{50} 96 hr Bluegill 56–75 mg/L Rainbow trout >26.7 mg/L	Skin–slight Eye–moderate to severe
LC_{50} 8 day Bobwhite quail and Mallard duck 4,500 ppm in diet	LC_{50} 96 hr Bluegill 120 mg/L Rainbow trout 86 mg/L	Skin–none Eye–slight to moderate

(continued)

TABLE 1 HERBICIDE POISONING *(continued)*

Compound	Acute Oral LD_{50}—Rat	NOAEL[a] (oral)	Acute Dermal LD_{50}
Halosulfuron	1,287 mg/kg	Dog, 13 wk 10 mg/kg/day	Rat >5,000 mg/kg
Hexazinone	1,690 mg/kg	Rat, 2 yr 250 mg/kg in diet	Rabbit >5,278 mg/kg
Imazamethabenz-methyl	>5,000 mg/kg	Dog, 1 yr 1,000 ppm	Rabbit >2,000 mg/kg
Imazaquin	>5,000 mg/kg	Dog, 1 yr 1,000 ppm	Rabbit >2,000 mg/kg
Imazamox	>5,000 mg/kg	Dog, 1 yr 40,000 ppm	Rat >4,000 mg/kg
Imazapic	>5,000 mg/kg	Dog, 1 yr 5,000 ppm	Rabbit >2,000 mg/kg
Imazapyr	>5,000 mg/kg	Dog, 1 yr feeding 1,000 ppm Rat 300 mg/kg/day (teratology)	Rabbit >2,000 mg/kg
Imazethapyr	>5,000 mg/kg	Dog, 1 yr 25 mg/kg/day	Rabbit >2,000 mg/kg
Isoproturon	1,800–2,400 mg/kg	Dog, 90 days Rat, 2 yr 3 mg/kg/day	Rat >3.2 g/kg
Isoxaflutole	>5,000 mg/kg	Dog, 1 yr 1,200 ppm	Rat >2,000 mg/kg
Linuron	1,200–4,000 mg/kg	Dog, 2 yr 6.25 mg/kg/day (observed anemia)	Rabbit >5,000 mg/kg
Maleic hydrazide	>5,000 mg/kg (acid) >6,950 mg/kg (Na^+ salt) >3,900 mg/kg (K^+ salt)	Dog, 1 yr 25 mg/kg	Rabbit >20,000 mg/kg
MCPA	700–1,160 mg/kg	Rat, 7 mo 100 mg/kg/day (lowers wt gain)	Rabbit 3,400– 4,800 mg/kg

TABLE 1 HERBICIDE POISONING *(continued)*

Avian Toxicity/NOAEC[b]	Toxicity to Fish in Water	Skin and Eye Irritation
LC_{50} 5 day Bobwhite quail and Mallard duck >5,620 ppm	LC_{50} 96 hr Bluegill >118 mg/L Rainbow trout >131 mg/L	Skin–slight Eye–slight
LC_{50} 5–8 day Bobwhite quail and Mallard duck >10,000 ppm in diet	LC_{50} 96 hr Bluegill 370–420 mg/L Rainbow trout 320–420 mg/L	Skin–none Eye–severe but reversible
		Skin–none Eye–slight
		Skin–slight
LC_{50} Mallard duck >5,672 ppm	LC_{50} 96 hr Bluegill >119 ppm Rainbow trout >122 ppm	Skin–none Eye–none
		Skin–slight Eye–moderate
LC_{50} 8 day Bobwhite quail and Mallard duck >5,000 ppm in diet	LC_{50} 96 hr Bluegill and Rainbow trout >100 mg/L	Skin–mild Eye–more severe
LD_{50} Bobwhite quail and Mallard duck >2,150 ppm in diet	LC_{50} 96 hr Bluegill 420 mg/L Rainbow trout 340 mg/L	Skin–mild Eye–irritation reversible
	LC_{50} 96 hr Crucian carp 193 mg/L Rainbow trout 240 mg/L	Skin–none Eye–none
LC_{50} 5 day Bobwhite quail and Mallard duck >4,255 ppm	LC_{50} 96 hr Bluegill >4.5 mg/L Rainbow trout >1.7 mg/L	Skin–minimal Eye–minimal
LC_{50} 5–8 day Japanese quail >5,000 ppm Mallard duck 3,083 ppm in diet	LC_{50} 96 hr Bluegill and Rainbow trout 16 mg/L	Skin–mild Eye–moderate
LD_{50} Bobwhite quail and Mallard duck >10,000 mg/kg	LC_{50} 96 hr Bluegill 1,608 mg/L Rainbow trout 1,435 mg/L	Skin–slight Eye–severe
LD_{50} Bobwhite quail 377 mg/kg	LC_{50} 96 hr Bluegill and Rainbow trout 90 mg/L	Skin–slight Eye–moderate

(continued)

TABLE 1 HERBICIDE POISONING *(continued)*

Compound	Acute Oral LD_{50}—Rat	NOAEL[a] (oral)	Acute Dermal LD_{50}
MCPB	4,700 mg/kg	Rat, 6 mo 1.6 mg/kg/day	Rat >2,000 mg/kg
Mecoprop	930–1,210 mg/kg	Rat, 90 days 3.8 mg/kg/day Dog, 90 days 15 mg/kg/day	Rabbit 900 mg/kg
Mesotrione	>5,050 mg/kg		Rat >5,050 mg/kg
Metam (sodium and isothiocyanate)	1,800 mg/kg (M) 1,700 mg/kg (F) 97 mg/kg (isothio-cyanate)	Rat, 65 days (inhalation, in inspired air) 6 hr/day for 5 days/wk at 0.045 mg/L	Rabbit 10,000 mg/kg
Methyl bromide	Acute LC_{50} (inhalation) 4.5 mg/L air	Safe threshold for people 0.065 mg/L air	
Methyl isothio-cyanate	82 mg/kg (M)	Dog, 2 yr 10 mg/L in drinking water	Rabbit 202 mg/kg (F) 145 mg/kg (M)
Metobromuron	2,450–2,500 mg/kg	Rat, 2 yr 250 mg/kg/day Dog, 100 mg/kg/day	Rabbit >2,000 mg/kg
Metolachlor[c]	800–2,780 mg/kg	Rat, 90 days 1,000 mg/kg Dog, 90 days 500 mg/kg	Rabbit >5,000 mg/kg Rat >10 g/kg
Metosulam	>5,000 mg/kg	Dog, 1 yr 10 mg/kg/day	Rabbit >2,000 mg/kg
Metribuzin	1,090–2,300 mg/kg	Rat, 2 yr 5 mg/kg Dog, 2 yr 2.5 mg/kg	Rat, rabbit >20,000 mg/kg
Napropamide	>5,000 mg/kg	Dog, 13 wk <100 mg/kg	Rabbit >4,640 mg/kg

TABLE 1 HERBICIDE POISONING *(continued)*

Avian Toxicity/NOAEC[b]	Toxicity to Fish in Water	Skin and Eye Irritation
LC_{50} 8 day Bobwhite quail and Mallard duck >5,000 ppm in diet	LC_{50} 96 hr Bluegill 14 mg/L Rainbow trout 4.3 mg/L	Skin–moderate Eye–moderate
LC_{50} Bobwhite quail and Mallard duck 5,000–5,500 ppm in diet	LC_{50} 96 hr Bluegill >100 mg/L Rainbow trout 124 mg/L	Skin–slight Eye–intense
LD_{50} Bobwhite quail >2,000 mg/kg Mallard duck >5,200 mg/kg	LC_{50} 96 hr Bluegill and Rainbow trout >120 mg/L	Skin–slight Eye–moderate
LC_{50} Bobwhite quail >10,000 Mallard duck >5,000 ppm in diet	LC_{50} 96 hr Bluegill 0.047 mg/L Rainbow trout 0.029 mg/L	Skin–corrosive Eye–corrosive
	Acute toxicity Bluegill 11 mg/L	Skin–severe Eye–severe
LC_{50} 5 day Mallard duck 10,936 mg/kg	LC_{50} 96 hr Bluegill 0.13 mg/L Rainbow trout 0.37 mg/L	Skin–corrosive Eye–severe
LC_{50} 8 day Bobwhite quail >20,000 ppm Mallard duck >4,640 ppm in diet	LC_{50} 96 hr Bluegill 4 mg/L Rainbow trout 3 mg/L	Skin–moderate Eye–moderate
LC_{50} 5 day Bobwhite quail and Mallard duck >10,000 ppm in diet	LC_{50} 96 hr Bluegill 15 mg/L Rainbow trout 3 mg/L	Skin–none Eye–none
		Skin–none Eye–slight
LC_{50} Bobwhite quail and Mallard duck >4,000 ppm in diet	LC_{50} 96 hr Bluegill 80 mg/L Rainbow trout 64–76 mg/L	Skin–none Eye–none
LC_{50} 5 day Bobwhite quail >5,600 ppm Mallard duck 7,200 ppm in diet	LC_{50} 96 hr Bluegill 20–30 mg/L Rainbow trout 9–16 mg/L	Skin–none Eye–none

(continued)

TABLE 1 HERBICIDE POISONING *(continued)*

Compound	Acute Oral LD_{50}—Rat	NOAEL[a] (oral)	Acute Dermal LD_{50}
Naptalam	>5,000 mg/kg 1,770 mg/kg (Na^+ salt)	Rat, dog, 90 days 1,000 mg/kg (Na^+ salt)	Rabbit >20,000 mg/kg
Nicosulfuron	Mouse >5,000 mg/kg	Dog, 1 yr >5,000 ppm in diet (M)	Rat, rabbit >2,000 mg/kg
Oxadiazon	>5,000 mg/kg	Rat, dog, 2 yr 100 mg/kg	Rabbit >2,000 mg/kg
Oxyfluorfen	Rat, dog >5,000 mg/kg	Rat, 2 yr 2 mg/kg Dog, 2.5 mg/kg	Rabbit >5,000 mg/kg
Paraquat (dichloride)	150–283 mg/kg	Rat, 2 yr 1.25 mg/kg Dog, 1 yr 0.45 mg/kg	Rat >2,000 mg/kg (finished product)
Pebulate	1,120 mg/kg	Rat, 2 yr 15 ppm in diet (eye lesions)	Rabbit 4,640 mg/kg
Pendimethalin	1,050 to >5,000 mg/kg	Dog, 2 yr 12.5 mg/kg/day	Rabbit >5,000 mg/kg
Phenmedipham	8,000 mg/kg	Dog, 2 yr >1,000 ppm in diet	Rat >2,000 mg/kg Rabbit >10,000 mg/kg
Picloram	5,000–8,200 mg/kg	Rat, 2 yr 150 mg/kg/day	Rabbit >4,000 mg/kg
Prometryn	3,750–5,235 mg/kg	Dog, 90 days <200 ppm in diet	Rabbit >2,000 mg/kg
Propanil	1,080 to >2,500 mg/kg	Dog, 2 yr <85 ppm in diet	Rabbit >5,000 mg/kg
Propoxycarbazone	>5,000 mg/kg	Dog, 1 yr 258 mg/kg (M) 55.7 mg/kg (F)	Rat >5,000 mg/kg

TABLE 1 HERBICIDE POISONING *(continued)*

Avian Toxicity/NOAEC[b]	Toxicity to Fish in Water	Skin and Eye Irritation
LC_{50} 8 day Bobwhite quail 5,600 ppm Mallard duck >10,000 ppm in diet	LC_{50} 96 hr Bluegill 354 mg/L Rainbow trout 76 mg/L	Skin–mild Eye–moderate
LC_{50} Bobwhite quail and Mallard duck >5,620 ppm in diet	LC_{50} 96 hr Bluegill and Rainbow trout >1,000 mg/L	Skin–none Eye–moderate
LC_{50} Bobwhite quail and Mallard duck >5,620 ppm in diet	LC_{50} 96 hr Bluegill 12.5 mg/L Rainbow trout 2 mg/L	Skin–moderate Eye–mild
LC_{50} Bobwhite quail >5,000 Mallard duck >4,000 ppm in diet	LC_{50} 96 hr Bluegill 0.2 mg/L Rainbow trout 0.41 mg/L	Skin–none Eye–moderate
LC_{50} 5 day Bobwhite quail 981 ppm Mallard duck 4,048 ppm in diet	LC_{50} 96 hr Rainbow trout 26 mg/L	Skin–slight Eye–moderate
LC_{50} Bobwhite quail and Mallard duck >2,400 ppm in diet	LC_{50} 96 hr Bluegill and Rainbow trout 7.4 mg/L	Skin–slight Eye–mild
LC_{50} 8 day Bobwhite quail 3,149 ppm Mallard duck 10,900 ppm in diet	LC_{50} 96 hr Bluegill 0.199 mg/L Rainbow trout 0.138 mg/L	Skin–none Eye–mild
LC_{50} 4 day Bobwhite quail >2,480 ppm in diet	LC_{50} 96 hr Bluegill 760 mg/L LC_{50} 21 day Rainbow trout >210 mg/L	Skin–moderate Eye–severe
LD_{50} 8 day Bobwhite quail >2,500 Mallard duck >5,000 mg/kg	LC_{50} 96 hr Bluegill 14.5 mg/L Rainbow trout 19.3 mg/L	Skin–mild Eye–moderate
LC_{50} 5–7 day Bobwhite quail and Mallard duck >10,000 ppm in diet	LC_{50} 96 hr Bluegill 10 mg/kg Rainbow trout 2.5–2.9 mg/L	Skin–none Eye–slight
LC_{50} 8 day Bobwhite quail 2,861 ppm Mallard duck 5,627 ppm in diet	LC_{50} 96 hr Bluegill 2.3 mg/L Rainbow trout 4.6 mg/L	Skin–moderate Eye–serious
		Skin–slight Eye–minimal

(continued)

TABLE 1 HERBICIDE POISONING *(continued)*

Compound	Acute Oral LD_{50}—Rat	NOAEL[a] (oral)	Acute Dermal LD_{50}
Propyzamide	5,620–8,350 mg/kg	Dog, 2 yr >7.5 ppm in diet	Rabbit 3,160 mg/kg
Pyrazon	3,030–3,600 mg/kg	Dog, 2 yr 1,500 ppm in diet	Rat >2,000 mg/kg
Pyridate	1,285–1,412 mg/kg	Dog, 1 yr 30 mg/kg/day	Rabbit >2,000 mg/kg
Pyrithiobac-sodium	4,000 mg/kg	Rat (longterm), 59 mg/kg	Rat >2,000 mg/kg
Quinclorac	3,060 mg/kg (M) 2,190 mg/kg (F)	Dog, 1 yr 142 mg/kg/day (M) 140 mg/kg/day (F)	Rat >2,000 mg/kg
Quizalofop-p-ethyl	1,210– 1,670 mg/kg (M) 1,182– 1,480 mg/kg (F)	Dog, 1 yr <10 mg/kg/day	Rat, mouse, rabbit >10,000 mg/kg
Rimsulfuron	>5,000 mg/kg	Dog, 1 yr 50 ppm in diet	Rabbit >2,000 mg/kg
Sethoxydim	3,200 mg/kg (M) 2,676 mg/kg (F)	Dog, 1 yr >8.86 mg/kg (M) >9.41 mg/kg (F)	Rat, mouse >5,000 mg/kg
Siduron	>7,500 mg/kg	Rat, 2 yr 500 ppm in diet	Rabbit >5,500 mg/kg
Simazine	>5,000 mg/kg	Rat, 2 yr >5 mg/kg/day	Rabbit >10,200 mg/kg
Sodium chlorate	1,200–7,000 mg/kg		Rabbit 500 mg/kg
Sulfentrazone	2,416–3,297 mg/kg	Rat, 10 mg/kg/day (oral developmental studies)	Rat >5,000 mg/kg
Sulfosulfuron	>5,000 mg/kg	Mouse, 90 days 7,000 mg/kg of diet	Rat >5,000 mg/kg

TABLE 1 HERBICIDE POISONING *(continued)*

Avian Toxicity/NOAEC[b]	Toxicity to Fish in Water	Skin and Eye Irritation
LC_{50} 8 day Bobwhite quail and Mallard duck >10,000 ppm in diet	LC_{50} 96 hr Bluegill 100 mg/L Rainbow trout 72 mg/L	Skin–slight Eye–moderate
	LC_{50} Bluegill 40 mg/L	Skin–slight Eye–slight
LC_{50} 8 day Bobwhite quail >5,000 ppm in diet	LC_{50} 96 hr Rainbow trout >1.2 mg/L	Skin–none Eye–slight
LC_{50} Bobwhite quail and Mallard duck >6,300 ppm	LC_{50} 96 hr Bluegill 5.8 mg/L Rainbow trout 8.2 mg/L	Skin–mild Eye–moderate
LD_{50} Bobwhite quail and Mallard duck >5,000 mg/kg	LC_{50} 96 hr Bluegill and Rainbow trout >100 mg/L	Skin–irritating Eye–moderate
LC_{50} 8 day Bobwhite quail and Mallard duck >5,000 ppm in diet	LC_{50} 96 hr Bluegill 0.46–2.8 mg/L Rainbow trout 10.7 mg/L	Skin–none Eye–slight
LC_{50} 8 day Bobwhite quail >5,620 ppm Mallard duck >2,510 ppm in diet	LC_{50} 96 hr Bluegill 100 mg/L Rainbow trout 32 mg/L	Skin–mild Eye–mild
LC_{50} 8 day Bobwhite quail and Mallard duck >5,600 ppm in diet	LC_{50} 96 hr Bluegill and Rainbow trout >1,000 mg/L	Skin–none Eye–moderate
LC_{50} Bobwhite quail and Mallard duck >10,000 mg/kg	LC_{50} 48 hr Crucian carp 18 mg/L	Skin–slight Eye–slight
LC_{50} 8 day Bobwhite quail >5,260 ppm Mallard duck 10,000 ppm in diet	LC_{50} 96 hr Bluegill and Rainbow trout >100 mg/L	Skin–none Eye–none
	LC_{50} 48 hr Fish 10,000 mg/L	Skin–moderate Eye–moderate
LD_{50} Bobwhite quail and Mallard duck >5,620 ppm	LC_{50} 96 hr Bluegill 93.8 mg/L Rainbow trout >130 mg/L	Skin–mild Eye–moderate
LD_{50} Bobwhite quail and Mallard duck 5,620 ppm	LC_{50} 96 hr Rainbow trout >97 mg/L	Skin–slight Eye–slight

(continued)

TABLE 1 HERBICIDE POISONING *(continued)*

Compound	Acute Oral LD$_{50}$—Rat	NOAEL[a] (oral)	Acute Dermal LD$_{50}$
Tebuthiuron	644 mg/kg	Dog, 1 yr >25 mg/kg/day	Rabbit >200 mg/kg
Thiazopyr	>5,000 mg/kg	Dog, 1 yr 0.8 mg/kg/day	Rat >5,000 mg/kg
Thifensulfuron-methyl	>5,000 mg/kg	Rat, 2 yr 25 ppm in diet	Rabbit >2,000 mg/kg
Tralkoxydim	1,258 mg/kg (M) 934 mg/kg (F)	Rat (teratogen), 30 mg/kg	Rat >2,000 mg/kg
Triallate	800–2,165 mg/kg	Dog, 2 yr 15 mg/kg/day (highest tested)	Rabbit 8,200 mg/kg
Triasulfuron	>5,000 mg/kg	Dog, 1 yr 129 mg/kg/day	Rat >2,000 mg/kg
Tribenuron-methyl	>5,000 mg/kg	Dog, 1 yr 875 ppm in diet	Rabbit >2,000 mg/kg
Trichloracetic acid	3,200–5,000 mg/kg		Rat >2,000 mg/kg
Triclopyr	630–729 mg/kg	Rat, 2 yr 3 mg/kg/day	Rabbit >2,000 mg/kg
Trifluralin	>5,000 mg/kg	Dog, 2 yr 18.75 mg/kg/day	Rabbit >2,000 mg/kg
Vernolate	1,200–1,900 mg/kg	Dog, 90 days >38 mg/kg/day	Rabbit >1,955 mg/kg

[a] NOAEL = No observable adverse effect level, daily dosage or ppm concentration in the diet

[b] NOAEC = No observable adverse effect concentration

[c] Liquid

[d] *Obsolete or no active registration*

[e] Technical grade chemical

TABLE 1 HERBICIDE POISONING *(continued)*

Avian Toxicity/NOAEC[b]	Toxicity to Fish in Water	Skin and Eye Irritation
LD_{50} Bobwhite quail and Mallard duck >2,500 mg/kg	LC_{50} 96 hr Bluegill 112 mg/L Rainbow trout 144 mg/L	Skin–slight Eye–slight
LD_{50} Bobwhite quail and Mallard duck 5,328 mg/kg	LC_{50} Bluegill and Rainbow trout 3.5 mg/L	Skin–slight Eye–slight
LC_{50} 8 day Bobwhite quail and Mallard duck >5,620 mg/kg	LC_{50} 96 hr Bluegill and Rainbow trout 100 mg/L	Skin–none Eye–moderate
LD_{50} Mallard duck >3,020 mg/kg	LC_{50} 96 hr Bluegill >6.1 mg/L Rainbow trout >7.2 mg/L	Skin–mild Eye–mild
LC_{50} 8 day Bobwhite quail and Mallard duck >5,000 mg/kg	LC_{50} 96 hr Bluegill 1.3 mg/L Rainbow trout 1.2 mg/L	Skin–moderate Eye–slight
LC_{50} 8 day Bobwhite quail and Mallard duck >5,000 ppm	LC_{50} 96 hr Bluegill and Rainbow trout >100 ppm	Skin–none Eye–none
LC_{50} Bobwhite quail and Mallard duck >5,620 ppm	LC_{50} 96 hr Bluegill 760 mg/L Rainbow trout 730 mg/L	Skin–none Eye–mild to moderate
LD_{50} Chicken 4,280 mg/kg	Not toxic to fish	Skin–severe Eye–severe
LC_{50} 8 day Bobwhite quail 2,935 ppm Mallard duck >5,401 ppm in diet	LC_{50} 96 hr Bluegill 148 mg/L Rainbow trout 117 mg/L	Skin–none Eye–slight
LC_{50} 8 day Bobwhite quail and Mallard duck >5,000 ppm in diet	LC_{50} 96 hr Bluegill 0.05–0.07 mg/L Rainbow trout 0.02–0.06 mg/L	Skin–none Eye–moderate
LC_{50} 7 day Bobwhite quail 12,000 ppm in diet	LC_{50} 96 hr Bluegill 8.4 mg/L Rainbow trout 9.6 mg/L	Skin–none Eye–none

TABLE 2 ORAL TOXIC DOSES (TD) AND LETHAL DOSES (LD) OF HERBICIDES IN DOMESTIC SPECIES

Compound	TD/LD	Species	Dosage (mg/kg)
Phenoxy acid derivatives			
Phenoxy acid and its sodium salt	LD_{50}	Chickens	547
		Dogs	100–800
	LD	Pigs	500
		Hens	380–765
	TD	Pigs	100
		Calves	200
Butyl glycol ester	TD	Cattle	250 for 3 days
		Sheep	250 for 2 days
Amine salts	TD	Cattle	250 for 10 days
		Sheep	250 for 10 days or 500 for 7 days
Bipyridyl compounds or quaternary ammonium			
Paraquat	LD_{50}	Dogs	25–50
		Cats	35
		Monkeys	50–70
		Cattle	35–50
		Chickens	110–360
	LD	Sheep	8–10
		Pigs	75
Diquat	LD_{50}	Dogs	100–200
		Cats	35–50
		Cattle	20–40
		Chickens	200–400
Ureas and thioureas			
Diuron	TD	Cattle	100 for 10 days
		Sheep	250 or 100 for 2 days
		Chickens	50 for 10 days
Linuron	TD	Dogs	100–200
		Cats	35–50

(*continued*)

TABLE 2 ORAL TOXIC DOSES (TD) AND LETHAL DOSES (LD) OF HERBICIDES IN DOMESTIC SPECIES *(continued)*

Compound	TD/LD	Species	Dosage (mg/kg)
		Cattle	20–40
		Chickens	200–400
Tebuthiuron	LD_{50}	Cats	>200
	TD	Cats	200
	LD_{50}	Dogs	>500
	TD	Dogs	50/day for 3 mo[a]
		Chickens, quail, or ducks	No deaths were reported at a dosage of 500 mg/kg body wt.
Protoporphyrinogen oxidase inhibitors			
Metribuzin	LD_{50}	Cats	>500
Anilide, acetamides, or amide compounds			
Propanil	LD_{50}	Dogs	1,217
Propyzamide	LD_{50}	Dogs	>10,000
Dinitrophenolic compounds			
DNOC	LD_{50}	Hens	26
		Dogs	50
		Pigs	50
		Goats	100
	TD	Cattle	2–50
		Sheep	20–50
	LD	Sheep	25 for 5 days
Dinoseb	LD_{50}	Hens	26
	TD	Cattle	25 for 8 days
		Sheep	25 for 10 days
Dinitroaniline			
Trifluralin	LD_{50}	Dogs	>2,000
Bromacil			
	TD	Cattle	250
		Chickens	500 for 10 days

(continued)

TABLE 2 ORAL TOXIC DOSES (TD) AND LETHAL DOSES (LD) OF HERBICIDES IN DOMESTIC SPECIES *(continued)*

Compound	TD/LD	Species	Dosage (mg/kg)
		Sheep	50 for 10 days or 250 for 8 days
Carbamates and thiocarbamate compounds			
Asulam	LD_{50}	Rabbits	>2,000
		Chickens	>2,000
		Dogs	>5,000
Di-allate	LD_{50}	Dogs	510
	TD	Chickens	150 for 10 days or 250 for 7 days
		Cattle	25 for 5 days or 50 for 3 days
		Sheep	25 for 5 days or 50 for 3 days
Phenmedipham	LD_{50}	Dogs	>4,000
	LD_{50}	Chickens	>3,000
Picrolinic acid derivative			
Picloram	LD_{50}	Cattle	>750
		Sheep	>1,000

[a] Anorexia and weight loss reported. No deaths were reported in dogs at a tebuthiuron dosage of 500 mg/kg body wt.

INORGANIC HERBICIDES AND ORGANIC ARSENICALS

Substances such as inorganic arsenicals (sodium arsenite, arsenic trioxide), organic arsenicals (methyl arsonate, methyl arsonic acid), sodium chlorate, ammonium sulfamate, borax, and many others were formerly used on a large scale. These older herbicides are nonselective, generally cheaper, more toxic, and more likely to cause problems than newer compounds. Their use has been mostly curtailed in developed countries.

Arsenicals: The use of inorganic arsenicals as herbicides has been reduced greatly because of livestock losses, environmental persistence, and their carcinogenic potential. These compounds can be hazardous to animals when used as recommended. Ruminants (including deer) are apparently attracted to and lick plants poisoned with arsenite.

The highly soluble organic arsenicals can concentrate in pools in toxic quantities after a rain has washed them from recently treated plants. Arsenicals are used as desiccants or defoliants on cotton, and residues of cotton harvest fed to cattle may contain toxic amounts of arsenic. Signs and lesions caused by organic arsenical herbicides resemble those of inorganic arsenical poisoning. Single toxic oral doses for cattle and sheep are 22–55 mg/kg. Poisoning may be expected from smaller doses if consumed on successive days.

Dimercaprol (3 mg/kg for large animals, and 2.5–5 mg/kg for small animals, IM, every 4–6 hr) is the recommended therapy. Sodium thiosulfate also has been used (20–30 g, PO, in ~300 mL of water for cattle; one-fourth this dose for sheep); however, a

TABLE 3 HERBICIDES WITH POTENTIAL TO CAUSE DEVELOPMENTAL TOXICITY IN EXPERIMENTAL ANIMALS

Compound	Effects
Atrizine	Disruption of ovarian cycle and induced repetitive pseudopregnancy (rats, at high doses)
Buturon	Cleft palate, increased fetal mortality (mice)
Butiphos	Teratogenic (rabbit)
Chloridazon	Malformations
Chlorpropham	Malformations or other developmental toxicity (mice)
Cynazine	Malformations such as cyclopia and diaphragmatic hernia (rabbits); skeletal variations in rats
2,4-D[a] or 2,4,5-T[a] alone or in combination	Malformations such as cleft palate, hydronephrosis; teratogenic (mice, rats)
Dichlorprop	Teratogenic (mice); affect postnatal behavior (rats)
Dinoseb[b]	Multiple defects (mice, rabbits)
Dinoterb	Skeletal malformations (rats); skeletal, jaw, head, and visceral (rabbits)
Linuron	Malformations (rats)
Mecoprop	Malformations (mice only)
Monolinuron	Cleft palate (mice)
MCPA[c]	Teratogenic and embryotoxic (rats), teratogenic (mice)
Prometryn	Head, limbs, and tail defects (rat)
Propachlor	Slightly teratogenic (rats)
Nitrofen[b]	Malformations (mice, rats, hamsters)
Silvex	Teratogenic (mice)
TCDD[a]	Malformations/teratogenic (fetotoxicity in chickens, rats, mice, rabbits, guinea pigs, hamsters, and monkeys)
Tridiphane	Malformations such as cleft palate (mice); skeletal variations (rats)

[a] TCDD is a common contaminant during the manufacturing process of some herbicides such as 2,4-D and 2,4,5-T.
[b] Obsolete
[c] 2-methyl-4-chlorophenoxyacetic acid

rationale for its use is not established, and it may be unrewarding. (*See also* ARSENIC POISONING, p 3071.)

Ammonium Sulfamate: Ruminants apparently can metabolize ammonium sulfamate to some extent and, in some studies, exposed animals made better gains than did control animals. However, sudden deaths have occurred in cattle and deer that consumed treated plants. Large doses (>1.5 g/kg) induce ammonia poisoning in ruminants. Treatment is designed to lower rumen pH by dilution with copious amounts of water to which weak acetic acid (vinegar) has been added.

Borax: Borax is toxic to animals if consumed in moderate to large doses (>0.5 g/kg). Poisoning has not been reported when borax was used properly but has occurred when it was accidentally added to livestock feed and when borax powder was scattered in the open for cockroach control. Principal signs of acute poisoning are diarrhea, rapid prostration, and perhaps convulsions. An effective antidote is not known. Balanced electrolyte fluid therapy with supportive care is indicated.

Sodium Chlorate: Many cases of chlorate poisoning of livestock have occurred both from ingestion of treated plants and from accidental consumption of feed to which it was mistakenly added as salt. Cattle sometimes are attracted to foliage treated with sodium chlorate. Considerable quantities must be consumed before signs of toxicity appear. The minimum lethal dose is 1.1 g/kg for cattle, 1.54–2.86 g/kg for sheep, and 5.06 g/kg for poultry. Ingestion results in hemolysis of RBCs and conversion of Hgb to methemoglobin. Treatment with methylene blue (10 mg/kg) must be repeated frequently because, unlike the nitrites, the chlorate ion is not inactivated during conversion of Hgb to methemoglobin and is capable of producing an unlimited quantity of methemoglobin as long as it is present in the body. Blood transfusions may reduce some of the tissue anoxia caused by methemoglobin; IV isotonic saline can hasten elimination of the chlorate ion. Mineral oil containing 1% sodium thiosulfate will inhibit further absorption of chlorate in monogastric animals.

ORGANIC HERBICIDES

Anilide, Acetamides, or Amide Compounds: These herbicides (propanil, cypromid, clomiprop, bensulide, dimethenamid) are plant growth regulators, and some members of this group are more toxic than others. Hemolysis, methemoglobinemia, and immunotoxicity have occurred after experimental exposure to propanil. (For discussion of bensulide, *see* p 2997.)

Bipyridyl Compounds or Quaternary *Ammonium Herbicides:* The bipyridyl compounds (diquat, paraquat) produce toxic effects in the tissues of exposed animals by development of free radicals. Tissues can be irritated after contact. For example, mouth lesions have been seen after contact with recently sprayed pastures. Skin irritation and corneal opacity occur on external exposure to these chemicals, and inhalation is dangerous. Animals, including people, have died as a result of drinking from contaminated containers.

Paraquat and diquat have somewhat different mechanisms of action. Diquat exerts most of its harmful effects in the GI tract. Animals drinking from an old diquat container showed anorexia, gastritis, GI distention, and severe loss of water into the lumen of the GI tract. Signs of renal impairment, CNS excitement, and convulsions occur in severely affected individuals. Lung lesions are uncommon.

Paraquat has a biphasic toxic action after ingestion. Immediate effects include excitement, convulsions or depression and incoordination, gastroenteritis with anorexia, and possibly renal involvement and respiratory difficulty. Eye, nasal, and skin irritation can be caused by direct contact, followed within days to 2 wk by pulmonary lesions as a result of lipid-membrane peroxidation and thus destruction of the type I alveolar pneumocytes. This is reflected in progressive respiratory distress and is evident on necropsy as pulmonary edema, hyaline membrane deposition, and alveolar fibrosis.

There is no specific treatment. Because these chemicals are absorbed slowly, intensive oral administration of adsorbents in large quantities and cathartics is advised. Bentonite or Fuller's earth is preferred, but activated charcoal will suffice. Toxicity of paraquat is enhanced by deficiency of vitamin E or selenium, oxygen, and low tissue activity of glutathione peroxidase. Therefore, vitamin E and selenium with supportive therapy may be useful in early stages of intoxication. Excretion may be accelerated by forced diuresis induced by mannitol and furosemide. Oxygen therapy and fluid therapy are contraindicated.

Carbamate and Thiocarbamate Compounds: These herbicides (terbucarb, asulam, carboxazole, EPTC, pebulate, triallate, vernolate, butylate, thiobencarb) are moderately toxic; however, they are used at low concentrations, and poisoning problems would not be expected from normal use. Massive overdosage, as seen with accidental exposure, produces signs similar to those induced by the insecticide carbamates, with lack of appetite, depression, respiratory difficulty, mouth watering, diarrhea, weakness, and seizures. Thiobencarb has induced toxic neuropathies in neonatal and adult laboratory rats. It appears to increase permeability of the blood-brain barrier. There is no suitable antidote. Supportive and symptomatic treatment is recommended.

Aromatic/Benzoic Acid Compounds: The herbicides in this group (chloramben, dicamba, and naptalam) have a low order of toxicity to domestic animals, and poisoning after normal use has not been reported. Environmental persistence and toxicity to wildlife is also low. The signs and lesions are similar to those described for the phenoxy acid derivatives (*see* below). There is no suitable antidote. Supportive and symptomatic treatment is recommended.

Phenoxy Acid Derivatives: These acids and their salts and esters (2,4-D [2-4-dichlorophenoxyacetic acid], dalapon, dichlorprop [2,4-DP], 2,4,5-T [2,4,5-trichlorophenoxyacetic acid], 2,4-DB, MCPA, MCPB, mecoprop, and silvex) are commonly used to control undesirable plants. As a group, they are essentially nontoxic to animals, except silvex which is unusually very toxic. When large doses are fed experimentally, general depression, anorexia, weight loss, tenseness, and muscular weakness (particularly of the hindquarters) are noted. Large doses in cattle may interfere with rumen function. Dogs may develop myotonia, ataxia, posterior weakness, vomiting, diarrhea, and metabolic acidosis. The oral LD_{50} for 2,4-D and 2,4,5-T in dogs is 100–800 mg/kg. Even large doses, up to 2 g/kg, have not been shown to leave residues in the fat of animals. These compounds are plant growth regulators, and treatment may result in increased palatability of some poisonous plants as well as increased nitrate and cyanide content.

The use of 2,4,5-T was curtailed because extremely toxic contaminants, collectively called dioxins (TCDD and HCDD), were found in technical grade material (*see* p 3056). TCDD is considered carcinogenic, mutagenic, teratogenic, and fetotoxic, and is able to cause reproductive damage and other toxic effects. Although manufacturing methods have reduced the level of the contaminants, use of this herbicide is very limited worldwide.

Treatment is usually symptomatic and supportive. IV fluids should be given to promote diuresis. Adsorbents and drugs that aid in restoration of liver function are recommended.

Dinitrophenolic Compounds: Several substituted dinitrophenols alone or as salts such as dinitrophenol, dinitrocresol, dinoseb, and binapacryl are highly toxic to all classes of animals (LD_{50} 20–100 mg/kg body wt). Poisoning can occur if animals are sprayed accidentally or have immediate access to forage that has been sprayed, because these compounds are readily absorbed through skin or lungs. Dinitrophenolic herbicides markedly increase oxygen consumption and deplete glycogen reserves. Clinical signs include fever, dyspnea, acidosis, tachycardia, and convulsions, followed by coma and death with a rapid onset of rigor mortis. Cataracts can occur in animals with chronic dinitrophenol intoxication. In cattle and other ruminants, methemoglobinemia, intravascular hemolysis, and hemoproteinemia have been seen. Exposure to these compounds may cause yellow staining of the skin, conjunctiva, or hair.

An effective antidote for dinitrophenol compounds is not known. Affected animals should be cooled and sedated to help control hyperthermia. Use of physical cooling measures (eg, cool baths or sponging and keeping the animal in a shaded area) are recommended. Atropine sulfate, aspirin, and antipyretics should not be used. Dextrose-saline infusions in combination with diuretics and tranquilizers such as diazepam (not barbiturates) are very useful. Phenothiazine tranquilizers are contraindicated. IV administration of large doses of sodium bicarbonate (in carnivores), parenteral vitamin A, and oxygen therapy may be useful. If the toxin was ingested and the animal is alert, emetics should be administered; if the animal is depressed, gastric lavage and treatment with activated charcoal should be performed.

In ruminants with methemoglobinemia, methylene blue solution (2%–4%, 10 mg/kg, IV, tid, during the first 24–48 hr) and ascorbic acid (5–10 mg/kg, IV) are useful.

Organophosphate Compounds: Organophosphate compounds such as glyphosate, glufosinate, and bensulide are broad-spectrum, nonselective systemic herbicides. Glyphosate and glufosinate exist as free acids, but because of their slow solubility they are marketed as the isopropyl amine or trimethylsulfonium salts of glyphosate and the ammonium salt of glufosinate. These are widely used herbicides with low toxicity. However, they are toxic to fish. Sprayed forage appears to be preferred by cattle for 5–7 days after application, but this causes little or no problem.

Dogs and cats show eye, skin, and upper respiratory tract signs when exposed during or subsequent to an application to weeds or grass. Nausea, vomiting, staggering, and hindleg weakness have been seen in dogs and cats exposed to fresh chemical on treated foliage. The signs usually disappear when exposure ceases, and minimal symptomatic treatment is needed. However, formulations of these compounds may lead to hemolysis and GI, cardiovascular, and CNS effects due to presence of the surfactant polyoxyethyleneamine. Treatment should include washing the chemical off the skin, evacuating the stomach, and tranquilizing the animal. Massive exposure with acute signs due to accidental poisoning should be handled as an organophosphate poisoning (*see* p 3064).

Bensulide, listed as a plant growth regulator, has an oral LD_{50} in rats of 271–770 mg/kg; in dogs, the lethal dose is >200 mg/kg. The most prominent clinical sign is anorexia, but other signs are similar to those caused by 2,4-D poisoning.

Triazolopyrimidine Compounds: Triazolopyrimidine herbicides include cloransulam-methyl, diclosulam, florasulam-methyl, flumetsulam, and metosulam. The acute oral toxicity is very low. There is no suitable antidote. Supportive and symptomatic treatment is recommended.

Ureas and Thiourea Compounds: The ureas and thioureas (polyureas) are available under different names such as diuron, fluometuron, isoproturon, linuron, buturon, chlorbromuron, chlortoluron, chloroxuron, difenoxuron, fenuron, methiuron, metobromuron, metoxuron, monuron, neburon, parafluron, siduron, tebuthiuron, tetrafluron, and thidiazuron. Of these, diuron and fluometuron are the most commonly used in the USA, whereas isoproturon is mostly used in other countries. In general, these compounds have low acute toxicity and are unlikely to present any hazard in normal use, except tebuthiuron, which may be slightly hazardous. Cattle are more sensitive to polyurea herbicides than sheep, cats, and dogs.

Signs and lesions are similar to those described for the phenoxyacetic herbicides (*see* above). The substituted urea herbicides induce hepatic microsomal enzymes and may alter metabolism of other xenobiotic agents. Altered calcium metabolism and bone morphology have been seen in laboratory animals. Recovery from diuron intoxication is quick (within 72 hr), and no signs of skin irritation or dermal sensitization have been reported in guinea pigs. After repeated administration, hemoglobin levels and RBC counts are significantly reduced, while methemoglobin concentration and WBC counts are increased. Increased pigmentation (hemosiderin) in the spleen is seen histopathologically. Linuron in sheep causes erythrocytosis and leukocytosis with hypohemoglobinemia and hypoproteinemia, hematuria, ataxia, enteritis, degeneration of the liver, and muscular dystrophy. In chickens, it leads to weight loss, dyspnea, cyanosis, and diarrhea. It is nontoxic to fish. Fluometuron is less toxic than diuron. In sheep, depression, salivation, grinding of teeth, chewing movements of the jaws, mydriasis, dyspnea, incoordination of movements, and drowsiness are commonly seen. On histopathology, severe congestion of the red pulp with corresponding atrophy of the white pulp of the spleen and depletion of the lymphocyte elements have been reported. The acute LD_{50} of isoproturon in rats is similar to that of diuron.

Polyurea herbicides have been suspected to have some mutagenic effects but do not have carcinogenic potential. In general, these compounds do not cause developmental and reproductive toxicity, except for monolinuron, linuron, and buturon, which are known to cause some teratogenic abnormalities in experimental animals. There is no suitable antidote. Supportive and symptomatic treatment is recommended.

Polycyclic Alkanoic Acids or Aryloxyphenoxypropionic Compounds: Members of this group (diclofop, fenoxaprop, fenthiaprop, fluazifop, haloxyfop) have moderately low toxicity (acute oral LD_{50} in rats 950 mg/kg to >4,000 mg/kg), except for haloxyfop-methyl (LD_{50} ~400 mg/kg). These compounds are more toxic if exposure is dermal. The dermal LD_{50} of diclofop in rabbits is only 180 mg/kg. There is no suitable antidote. Supportive and symptomatic treatment is recommended.

Triazinylsulfonylurea or Sulfonylurea Compounds: Toxicity of this group of herbicides (chlorsulfuron, sulfometuron, ethametsulfuron, chloremuron) appears to be quite low. The oral acute LD_{50} in rats is in the range of 4,000–5,000 mg/kg. The dermal acute LD_{50} in rabbits is ~2,000 mg/kg. There is no suitable antidote. Supportive and symptomatic treatment is recommended.

Triazines and Triazoles: Triazines and triazoles have been used extensively as selective herbicides. These herbicides are inhibitors of photosynthesis and include both the asymmetric and symmetric triazines. Examples of symmetric triazines are chlorostriazines (simazine, atrazine, propazine, and cyanazine), the thiomethyl-s-triazines (ametryn, prometryn, terbutryn), and methoxy-s-triazine (prometon). The commonly used asymmetric triazine is metribuzin.

These herbicides have low oral toxicity and are unlikely to pose acute hazards in normal use, except ametryn and metribuzin, which may be slightly to moderately hazardous. They do not irritate the skin or eyes and are not skin sensitizers. The exceptions are atrazine, which is a skin sensitizer, and cyanazine, which is toxic by the oral route. Sensitivity of sheep and cattle to these herbicides is appreciably high. The main signs are anorexia, hemotoxia, hypothermia, locomotor disturbances, irritability, tachypnea, and hypersensitivity. Simazine is excreted in milk, so it is of public health concern. Atrazine is more toxic to rats but comparatively less toxic to sheep and cattle than simazine. When cultured human cells are exposed to atrazine, splenocytes are damaged; bone marrow cells are not affected. Atrazine induces liver microsomal enzymes and is converted to *N*-dealkylated derivatives. In contrast to simazine, it is not excreted in milk. There is no suitable antidote. Supportive and symptomatic treatment is recommended.

Protoporphyrinogen Oxidase Inhibitors: Protox inhibitors may be diphenyl ether (DPE) or non-diphenyl ether (non-DPE) such as nitrofen and oxadiazon. In the past few years, numerous other non-oxygen-bridged compounds (non-DPE protox inhibitors) with the same site of action (carfentrazone, JV 485, and oxadiargyl) have been marketed. Protox inhibitors have little acute toxicity and are unlikely to pose an acute hazard in normal use. These compounds increase porphyrin levels in animals when administered orally; the porphyrin levels return to normal within a few days. There is no suitable antidote. Supportive and symptomatic treatment is recommended.

Substituted Anilines: The most commonly used herbicides of this group are alachlor, acetochlor, butachlor, metolachlor, and propachlor. Low doses in rats and dogs do not produce any adverse effects, but longterm exposure in dogs causes liver toxicity and affects the spleen. Ocular lesions produced by alachlor are considered to be unique to the Long-Evans rat, because the response has not been seen in other strains of rats or in mice or dogs.

Compared with other substituted anilines, propachlor is severely irritating to the eye and slightly irritating to the skin. Propachlor produces skin sensitization in guinea pigs. High doses of propachlor produce erosion, ulceration, and hyperplasia of the mucosa and herniated mucosal glands in the pyloric region of stomach and hypertrophy and necrosis of the liver in rats. In dogs, there is poor diet palatability, which results in poor feed consumption and weight loss. There is no suitable antidote. Supportive and symptomatic treatment is recommended.

Imidazolinones: Imidazolinone herbicides include imazapyr, imazamethabenz-methyl, imazapic, imazethapyr, imazamox, and imazaquin. These are selective broad-spectrum herbicides. Imidazolinone herbicides caused slight to moderate skeletal myopathy and/or slight anemia in dogs during 1-yr dietary toxicity studies with three structurally similar imidazolinones (imazapic, imazaquin, and imazethapyr). There is no evidence of any adverse effect on reproductive performance or of fetal abnormalities in rats or rabbits. There is no suitable antidote. Supportive and symptomatic treatment is recommended.

Other Herbicides: Bromacil and terbacil are commonly used methyluracil compounds. Toxic doses of bromacil can be hazardous, especially for sheep, but no field case of toxicity has been reported. The nitrile herbicides, ioxynil and bromoxynil, may uncouple and/or inhibit oxidative phosphorylation. Ioxynil, presumably because of its iodine content, causes enlargement of the thyroid gland in rats.

A number of substances are used as defoliants in agriculture. For example, sulfuric acid is used to destroy potato haulms and two closely related trialkylphosphorothioates (DEF and merphos) to defoliate cotton. A notable feature of the latter is that it produces organophosphate-induced delayed neuropathy in hens. Chlomequat is used as a growth regulator on fruit trees. The signs of toxicity in experimental animals indicate that it is a partial cholinergic agonist.

HOUSEHOLD HAZARDS

See also RODENTICIDE POISONING, p 3165; TOXICITIES FROM HUMAN DRUGS, p 3024; POISONOUS PLANTS, p 3103; and FOOD HAZARDS, p 2964.

Household chemicals (eg, products containing alcohols, bleaches, or corrosives) found in the home represent a risk of toxicosis if companion animals are exposed to concentrates or undiluted products, but casual exposure to areas in which these compounds have been used appropriately rarely causes any serious problems.

ALCOHOLS

Alcohol toxicosis results in metabolic acidosis, hypothermia, and CNS depression. All species are susceptible.

Etiology: Ethanol, methanol, and isopropanol are the alcohols most frequently associated with toxicosis in companion animals. Ethanol is present in a variety of alcoholic beverages, some rubbing alcohols, drug elixirs, and fermenting bread dough (*see* p 2965). Methanol is most commonly found in windshield washer fluids (windshield "antifreeze"). The lethal oral dose of methanol in dogs is 4–8 mL/kg, although significant clinical signs may be seen at lower dosages. Isopropanol is twice as toxic as ethanol and is found in rubbing alcohols and in alcohol-based flea sprays for pets. Oral dosages of isopropanol ≥0.5 mL/kg may result in significant clinical signs in dogs.

Pathogenesis: All alcohols are rapidly absorbed via the GI tract and most are well absorbed dermally; toxicosis from overspraying pets with alcohol-based flea sprays is not uncommon. Alcohols reach peak plasma levels within 1.5–2 hr and are widely distributed throughout the body. They are metabolized in the liver to acetaldehyde (ethanol), formaldehyde (methanol), and acetone (isopropanol); these intermediate metabolites are then further converted to acetic acid, formic acid, and/or carbon dioxide. (In people and some other primates, accumulation of *formic acid after methanol ingestion* results in retinal and neuronal damage; nonprimates are efficient at eliminating formic acid and therefore do not develop the blindness and cerebral necrosis seen in primates.) Alcohols are eliminated via the urine as parent compound as well as metabolites. In dogs, up to 50% of a dose of methanol may be eliminated unchanged via the lungs.

Alcohols are GI irritants, and ingestion may result in vomiting and hypersalivation. Alcohols and their metabolites are potent CNS depressants, affecting a variety of neurotransmitters within the nervous system. Metabolites such as acetaldehyde may stimulate the release of catecholamines, which can affect myocardial function. Metabolic acidosis results from the formation of acidic intermediates, and both parent compounds and metabolites contribute to increases in osmolal gap. Hypothermia may develop due to peripheral vasodilation, CNS depression, and interference with thermoregulatory mechanisms. Hypoglycemia develops secondary to alcohol-induced depletion of pyruvate, resulting in inhibition of gluconeogenesis.

Clinical Findings and Diagnosis: Signs generally begin within 30–60 min of ingestion and include vomiting, diarrhea, ataxia, disorientation (inebriation), depression, tremors, and dyspnea. Severe cases may progress to coma, hypothermia, seizures, bradycardia, and respiratory depression. Death is generally due to respiratory failure, hypothermia, hypoglycemia, and/or metabolic acidosis. Pneumonia secondary to aspiration of vomitus is possible.

The determination of blood alcohol levels may help to confirm the diagnosis of alcohol intoxication.

Treatment: Stabilization of severely symptomatic animals is a priority. Adequate ventilation should be maintained, and cardiovascular and acid-base abnormalities should be corrected. Seizures can be controlled with diazepam (0.5–2 mg/kg, IV) as needed. For asymptomatic animals, induction of emesis may be of benefit in the first 20–40 min after ingestion. Activated charcoal is not thought to appreciably bind small-chain alcohols and is not often recommended. Bathing with mild shampoo is recommended for significant dermal exposures. Supportive care, including thermoregulation and fluid diuresis to enhance alcohol elimination, should be administered. Anecdotally, yohimbine (0.1 mg/kg, IV) has been used to stimulate respiration in severely comatose dogs with alcohol toxicosis.

CHLORINE BLEACHES

Exposure to undiluted chlorine bleaches may result in GI, dermal, and ocular irritation or ulceration as well as significant respiratory irritation. All species are susceptible. Because of the countercurrent anatomy and physiology of the avian lung, caged birds are at increased risk of succumbing to fumes from bleaches and other cleaning agents.

Etiology: Chlorine bleaches are primarily used as household cleaners and pool sanitizers. Household bleaches tend to contain sodium hypochlorite at 3%–10%, and pH of these products may range from 9 (mildly irritating) to >11 (corrosive). Pool treatments may contain lithium, calcium, or sodium hypochlorites at concentrations up to 70%–80%, with pH that may range from acidic to alkaline. Pets may be exposed by chewing on containers of undiluted product, drinking from buckets containing product diluted in water, or swimming in recently treated pools.

Pathogenesis: The relative hazard of a particular bleach product depends on the concentration of hypochlorite, pH, and dilution of the product. In general, levels of hypochlorite <10% tend to be mild irritants; however, if the product has a pH >11 or <3.5, alkaline or acid corrosive injury may occur. Dilution of bleaches with water per label directions will often reduce the corrosive potential of these products and make them little more than mild GI or ocular irritants. Mixing of hypochlorite and ammonia produces highly toxic chloramine gas that can cause acute respiratory distress or delayed onset of pulmonary edema within 12–24 hr of exposure.

Clinical Findings and Lesions: Ingestion of dilute or moderate pH household bleach products rarely causes more than mild vomiting, hypersalivation, depression, anorexia, and/or diarrhea. Concentrated (>10%) bleach products or products with pH >11 may cause significant GI corrosive injury. Ingestion or inhalation of significant amounts of chlorine bleach occasionally results in hypernatremia, hyperchloremia, and/or metabolic acidosis. Acute inhalation may result in immediate coughing, gagging, sneezing, or retching. In addition to the immediate respiratory signs, animals exposed to concentrated chlorine fumes may develop pulmonary edema 12–24 hr after exposure. Ocular exposures may result in epiphora, blepharospasm, eyelid edema, and/or corneal ulceration. Dermal exposure may result in mild dermal irritation and bleaching of the hair coat. Oral, dermal, and ocular irritation or ulceration are possible. Respiratory lesions may include tracheitis, bronchitis, alveolitis, and pulmonary edema.

Treatment: For oral exposures, emesis and activated charcoal are contraindicated; instead, dilution with milk or water is recommended. Any spontaneous vomiting should be managed, and animals should be monitored for development of GI irritation/ulceration (*see* below). In cases when protracted vomiting causes electrolyte or hydration abnormalities, fluid therapy may be of benefit. For respiratory exposures, the animal should be moved to an area with fresh air and monitored for dyspnea. Stabilization of severely dyspneic animals is a must; pulmonary edema should be treated as needed. Bathing with mild shampoo and thorough rinsing is recommended for significant dermal exposures. Ocular exposures should be treated with 10–20 min of ocular irrigation with physiologic saline, followed by fluorescein staining of the cornea to detect corneal injury.

CORROSIVES

Acid or alkaline corrosives produce significant local tissue injury that can result in full-thickness burns of skin, cornea, and the mucosa of the oral cavity, esophagus, and stomach. All species are susceptible. Heavy coats may provide some protection from dermal exposure.

Etiology: Corrosives are divided into acid and alkaline corrosives. Acidic household products include anti-rust compounds, toilet bowl cleaners, gun-cleaning fluids, automotive batteries, swimming pool cleaning agents, and etching compounds. Alkaline corrosive agents include drain openers, automatic dishwasher detergents, toilet bowl cleaners, radiator cleaning agents, and swimming pool algicides and “shock” agents. In general, alkaline products with pH >11 pose risk of significant corrosive injury.

Pathogenesis: Acids produce immediate coagulative necrosis of tissue and impart significant pain on contact, which may limit exposure. Alkaline agents produce immediate, penetrating liquefactive necrosis of tissue; the lack of significant discomfort on contact with alkaline products may result in prolonged exposure. For these reasons, burns from alkaline products tend to be deeper and more extensive than burns from acidic agents. Burns from alkaline agents may take up to 12 hr after exposure to become fully apparent, whereas the extent of acid burns is usually evident shortly after contact. Esophageal burns are more common with alkaline agents, and the absence of significant oral burns does not necessarily indicate that no esophageal damage has developed. Full-thickness ulceration of the esophagus may result in pleuritis or peritonitis due to leakage of ingesta into body cavities. Esophageal burns may result in stricture formation during healing, resulting in dysphagia, megaesophagus, and aspiration pneumonia. Additionally, although the contents of the stomach may serve to buffer and dilute corrosive agents, gastric ulceration and possibly perforation may occur with significant exposures. Respiratory exposure to corrosives (especially acids) may result in respiratory distress, tracheobronchitis, or pneumonitis. Dermal or ocular exposures may result in severe ulceration of dermis or cornea.

Clinical Findings and Lesions: Clinical signs that may occur after ingestion of corrosive agents include vocalization, hypersalivation, lethargy, polydipsia, vomiting (with or without blood), abdominal pain, dysphagia, pharyngeal edema, dyspnea, and oral, esophageal, and/or gastric ulceration. In severe cases, shock may develop rapidly after exposure. Lesions are initially milky white to gray but gradually turn black as eschar formation occurs. Necrotic tissue may slough within days of exposure. Dyspnea, cyanosis, and pulmonary edema may occur secondary to inhaled corrosive agents. Dermal exposure may result in significant burns, with local pain, erythema, and tissue sloughing. Ocular exposure may cause blepharospasm, epiphora, eyelid edema, conjunctivitis, or corneal ulceration. Burns of skin, cornea, and GI mucosa range from mild ulceration to full-thickness necrosis with extensive tissue sloughing. Peritonitis or pleuritis may develop secondary to perforating ulcers of esophagus or stomach. Respiratory lesions may include tracheitis, bronchitis, pneumonitis, pulmonary edema, or aspiration pneumonia.

Treatment: Because of the rapid action of corrosive agents, much of the damage from exposure occurs before treatment can be started. Stabilization of animals presenting as dyspneic, in shock, or with severe electrolyte abnormalities is always a priority. For recent oral exposures, immediate dilution with water or milk should be done. Under no circumstances should emesis be attempted because of the risk of further mucosal exposure to corrosive material. Likewise, gastric lavage is contraindicated because of the risk of perforation of weakened esophageal/gastric walls and the risk of further exposure of mucosa to the corrosive material as it is removed. Attempts to chemically neutralize an acid with weak alkali (or alkali with weak acid) are also contraindicated because of the production of exothermic reactions that can result in thermal burns. Activated charcoal is ineffective in cases involving ingestion of corrosives, and the presence of charcoal on damaged mucosa may impede wound healing.

After dilution, general supportive care should be instituted, including monitoring for respiratory difficulty, pain management, antibiotics (if ulcers are present), and anti-inflammatories as needed. Endoscopic evaluation of the esophagus and stomach for ulceration should be performed ~12 hr after exposure; this time frame will allow the full extent of tissue injury to become apparent. The use of corticosteroids in cases with significant esophageal mucosal injury is controversial. Corticosteroids decrease inflammation and may aid in minimizing stricture formation, but they also suppress the immune system and may enhance susceptibility to secondary infection. In animals with significant oral and/or esophageal burns, gastrostomy tubes may be necessary to provide nutrition while affected tissues heal.

Dermal or ocular exposures should be managed by flushing with copious amounts of water or physiologic saline; eyes should be flushed for a minimum of 20 min, followed by fluorescein staining. Standard topical treatments for dermal or ocular burns should be instituted as needed.

Alkaline Batteries

Ingestion of alkaline batteries poses a risk of GI tract corrosive injury and foreign body obstruction. Dogs are most commonly involved.

Etiology: Alkaline batteries are present in many household electronic products, including remote controls, hearing aids, toys, watches, computers, and calculators. Most alkaline dry cell batteries use potassium hydroxide or sodium hydroxide to generate currents. Nickel-cadmium and lithium batteries also tend to contain alkaline material.

Pathogenesis: The alkaline gel in batteries causes liquefactive necrosis of tissues on contact, resulting in burns that can penetrate deeply into tissue. Lithium disk or "button" batteries may lodge in the esophagus and generate a current against the esophageal walls, resulting in circular ulcers that have the potential to be perforating. Some battery casings may contain metals such as zinc or mercury, posing hazards of foreign body obstruction and metal toxicosis if they remain in the stomach for prolonged periods. Additionally, small batteries (especially disk batteries) may be inhaled and pose a choking hazard.

Clinical Findings and Lesions: For discussion of alkaline burns, *see* p 3001. Foreign body obstruction may present as vomiting, anorexia, abdominal discomfort, or tenesmus. Respiratory obstruction due to battery inhalation may present with acute onset of dyspnea and cyanosis. Mucosal burns may occur within the oral cavity, esophagus, and less commonly, stomach. Perforation of the esophagus may lead to secondary pyothorax, while gastric perforation may result in acute blood loss and/or peritonitis.

Diagnosis: Radiographs may help to confirm the diagnosis as well as the location of the battery; however, some disk batteries do not show up well on radiographs. Differential diagnoses include GI or respiratory foreign bodies and other oral, dermal, or ocular corrosive agents.

Treatment: For batteries swallowed intact without any chewing, induction of emesis may result in expulsion. Because of the risk of leakage of alkaline gel onto oral and esophageal mucosa during vomiting, emesis should not be induced if there is any possibility that the battery casing has been punctured. When disk batteries have been ingested, 20 mL boluses of tap water every 15 min will decrease the severity and delay the development of current-induced esophageal ulceration. The decision on whether to remove a battery from the stomach depends on the size of the animal, battery size, and evidence of battery puncture. Radiography may be performed to determine the location of the battery casing; generally, batteries that have passed through the pylorus will pass through the intestinal tract uneventfully (adding bulk to the diet and judicious use of cathartics may facilitate passage). Serial radiography to verify battery location is recommended until the battery is expelled. Batteries that do not pass through the pylorus within 48 hr of ingestion are unlikely to pass on their own and may require surgical or endoscopic removal. Batteries that have obviously been punctured should be removed surgically to prevent gastric or intestinal ulceration due to leakage of alkaline gel. Endoscopic removal is not recommended in cases in which it is suspected that the battery casing has been punctured. Treatment of cases with suspected oral, esophageal, or gastric ulceration is the same as for other alkaline corrosive injuries (*see* p 3001). Dermal or ocular exposures to alkaline gels should be managed by copious rinsing of the area with tap water (skin) or physiologic saline solution (eyes). The affected areas should be monitored for development of ulcers, and topical therapy administered as needed.

Cationic Detergents

Exposure to cationic detergents may result in local corrosive tissue injury as well as severe systemic effects. All species are susceptible. Cats are at increased risk of oral exposure because of grooming habits.

Etiology: Cationic detergents are present in a variety of algicides, germicides (including quaternary ammonium compounds), sanitizers, fabric softeners (including dryer softener sheets), and liquid potpourris. Concentrations of cationic detergents ≤2% have been associated with oral mucosal ulcers in cats.

Pathogenesis: Cationic detergents are locally corrosive agents, causing dermal, ocular, and mucosal injury similar to that of alkaline corrosive agents. Additionally, exposure to cationic detergents may result in systemic effects ranging from CNS depression to pulmonary edema. The mechanism for these systemic effects is not known.

Clinical Findings and Lesions: Signs of oral exposure include oral ulceration, stomatitis, pharyngitis, hypersalivation, swollen tongue, depression, vomiting, abdominal discomfort, and increased upper respiratory noises within 6–12 hr of ingestion. Affected animals frequently have significant fever and increases in WBC counts. Systemic effects include metabolic acidosis, CNS depression, hypotension, coma, seizures, muscular weakness and fasciculation, collapse, and pulmonary edema. Dermal irritation, erythema, ulceration, and pain are possible with dermal contact. Conjunctivitis, blepharospasm, eyelid edema, lacrimation, and corneal ulceration may be seen secondary to ocular exposure. Lesions can include GI, ocular, or dermal irritation or ulceration.

Treatment: Systemic signs should be treated symptomatically, eg, diazepam (0.5–2 mg/kg, slow IV) for seizures, fluid therapy for hypotension, etc. Because of the potential for corrosive mucosal injury, induction of emesis and administration of activated charcoal are contraindicated with cationic detergents. For recent oral exposures, milk or water can be given for dilution, and the animal monitored for development of oral or esophageal burns. Oral burns should be treated the same as other corrosive injuries (*see* p 3001). Dermal and ocular exposures should be managed by thorough flushing of the affected area with tepid water or physiologic saline, followed by monitoring for development of dermal or ocular irritation or ulceration. Topical treatment for dermal or ocular burns should be instituted as needed; in severe cases, analgesics may be indicated.

DETERGENTS, SOAPS, AND SHAMPOOS

Exposures to products containing anionic and nonionic detergents generally cause mild GI irritation that responds well to symptomatic care. All animals are susceptible.

Etiology: Mild detergents, soaps, and shampoos contain anionic and nonionic detergents; products included in this group include human and pet shampoos, liquid hand dishwashing soaps, bar bath soaps (except homemade soaps, which may contain lye), many laundry detergents, and many household all-purpose cleaners. Most are of moderate pH, but agents with pH >11 (eg, electric dishwasher detergents) are alkaline corrosives and should be treated as such (*see* p 3001).

Pathogenesis: Anionic and nonionic detergents are mild irritants; many have been pH adjusted to have minimal dermal irritation, although ocular and mucosal irritation is possible. There is no appreciable systemic absorption of these agents, and toxicity is limited to ocular, oral, or GI irritation, which is usually mild and self-limiting. Cats exposed to undiluted shampoos or other products containing sodium lauryl sulfate may develop significant respiratory compromise after inhalation during grooming, including dyspnea, increased bronchial secretions, and mild pulmonary edema. Although the exact mechanism of this syndrome is not known, it may relate to interference by the detergent with normal pulmonary surfactants.

Clinical Findings: Nausea, vomiting, and diarrhea are the most common signs. Secondary dehydration and electrolyte imbalance may develop in rare instances due to protracted vomiting or diarrhea. Mild ocular irritation is possible, with lacrimation and blepharospasm. No significant lesions beyond mild local irritation are seen. Cats grooming after application of sodium lauryl sulfate–containing products may develop moist respiratory sounds, cyanosis, and dyspnea within 1–3 hr of exposure.

Treatment: Dilution with milk or water may reduce the risk of spontaneous vomiting. Vomiting is usually self-limiting and responds to short periods of food and water restriction. In severe cases or in animals with sensitive stomachs, antiemetics may be required (eg, metoclopramide, 0.2–0.4 mg/kg, PO, SC, or IM, qid). Rarely, parenteral fluid therapy is required to correct electrolyte or hydration abnormalities due to protracted vomiting or diarrhea. For ocular exposures, irrigation of eyes using tepid water or physiologic saline for 5 min will usually suffice. For cats that have respiratory compromise, supplemental oxygen and general supportive care are recommended; in most cases, signs resolve within 24 hr.

MYCOTOXICOSES

For discussion of mycotoxicoses in poultry, *see* p 2846.

Acute or chronic toxicoses can result from exposure to feed or bedding contaminated with toxins produced during growth of various saprophytic or phytopathogenic fungi or molds on cereals, hay, straw, pastures, or any other fodder. These toxins are not consistently produced by specific molds and are known as secondary (not essential) metabolites that are formed under conditions of stress to the fungus or its plant host.

A few principles characterize mycotoxic diseases: 1) The cause may not be immediately identified. 2) They are not transmissible from one animal to another. 3) Treatment with drugs or antibiotics has little effect on the course of the disease. 4) Outbreaks are often seasonal, because particular climatic sequences may favor fungal growth and toxin production. 5) Study indicates specific association with a particular feed. 6) Large numbers of fungi or their spores found on examination of feedstuffs does not necessarily indicate that toxin production has occurred. However, absence of molds does not exclude mycotoxicosis, because feed storage or preparation conditions, eg, acid treatment or high pelleting, can destroy molds while the heat-tolerant mycotoxin persists.

Diagnosis of mycotoxic disease requires a combination of information. Most veterinary mycotoxicoses are found in large animal species, but important outbreaks can happen in pets and exotic animals. Especially important in diagnosis is the presence of a disease documented to be caused by a known mycotoxin, combined with detection of the mycotoxin in either feedstuffs or animal tissues.

Sometimes more than one mycotoxin may be present in feedstuffs, and their different toxicologic properties may cause clinical signs and lesions inconsistent with those seen when animals are dosed experimentally with pure, single mycotoxins. Some mycotoxins are immunosuppressive, which may allow viruses, bacteria, or parasites to create a secondary disease that is more obvious than the primary. When immunosuppression by a mycotoxin is suspected, differential diagnoses must be carefully established by thorough clinical and historical evaluation, examination of production records, and appropriate diagnostic testing.

Mycotoxicoses are generally not successfully treated with medical therapy after diagnosis. A preventive approach with recognition of risk factors and avoiding or reducing exposure is preferred. Best management practices are aimed at prevention of the occurrence of mycotoxins, inactivation of the preformed toxin in grain or feed, and adsorption or inactivation of the toxin in the GI tract. Testing of suspect grain at harvest, maintaining clean and dry storage facilities, using acid additives (eg, propionic acid) to control mold growth in storage, ensuring effective air exclusion in silage storage, and reducing storage time of prepared feeds are established procedures to prevent mycotoxin formation. Acidic additives control mold growth but do not destroy preformed toxins.

There are no specific antidotes for mycotoxins; removal of the source of the toxin (ie, the moldy feedstuff) eliminates further exposure. The absorption of some mycotoxins (eg, aflatoxin) has been effectively prevented by aluminosilicates. If financial circumstances do not allow for disposal of the moldy feed, it can be blended with unspoiled feed just before feeding to reduce the toxin concentration. This approach should be monitored by follow-up toxin analysis and may not be acceptable to regulatory agencies. Alternatively, feed with known mycotoxin concentrations can be fed to less susceptible species, remembering that some mycotoxins such as aflatoxin could result in violative food residues in the absence of illness. When contaminated feed is blended with good feed, care must be taken to prevent further mold growth by the toxigenic contaminants. This may be accomplished by thorough drying or by addition of organic acids (eg, propionic acid).

Important mycotoxic diseases occur in domestic animals worldwide (*see* TABLE 1).

TABLE 4 MYCOTOXICOSES IN DOMESTIC ANIMALS

Disease	Toxins (When Known)	Fungi or Molds	Regions Where Reported
Aflatoxicosis	Aflatoxins	*Aspergillus flavus*, *A parasiticus*	Widespread (warmer climatic zones)
Diplodiosis	Unknown	*Diplodia zeae*	South Africa
Ergotism	Ergot alkaloids	*Claviceps purpurea*	Widespread
	Paspalinine and paspalitrems, tremorgens	*C paspali*, *C cinerea*	Widespread
Estrogenism and vulvovaginitis	Zearalenone	*Fusarium graminearum* Perfect state: *Gibberella zeae*	Widespread
Facial eczema (Pithomycotoxicosis)	Sporidesmins	*Pithomyces chartarum*	Widespread
Fescue foot	Ergovaline	*Neotyphodium coenophialum*	USA, Australia, New Zealand, Italy
Fusariotoxicosis, vomiting and feed refusal in pigs	Nonmacrocyclic trichothecenes (deoxynivalenol, T-2 toxin, diacetoxyscirpenol [DAS], many other trichothecenes)	*Fusarium sporotrichioides*, *F culmorum*, *F graminearum*, *F nivale*; other fungal species	Widespread (except for deoxynivalenol, more likely in temperate to colder climates)
Leukoencephalomalacia	Fumonisin B_1	*Fusarium verticilloides*	Egypt, USA, South Africa, Greece
Mycotoxic lupinosis (as distinct from *alkaloid poisoning)*	Phomopsins	*Phomopsis leptostromiformis*	Widespread

TABLE 4 MYCOTOXICOSES IN DOMESTIC ANIMALS *(continued)*

Contaminated Toxic Foodstuff	Animals Affected	Signs and Lesions
Moldy peanuts, soybeans, cottonseeds, rice, sorghum, corn (maize), other cereals	All poultry, pigs, cattle, sheep, dogs	Major effects in all species are slow growth and hepatotoxicosis. *See also* AFLATOXICOSIS, p 3011, and MYCOTOXICOSES IN POULTRY, p 2846.
Moldy corn (maize)	Cattle, sheep	Nervous system disorders, cold and insensitive limbs. Recovery usual on removal of source.
Seed heads of many grasses, grains	Cattle, horses, pigs, poultry	Peripheral gangrene, late gestation suppression of lactation initiation. *See* p 3012.
Seed heads of paspalum grasses	Cattle, horses, sheep	Acute tremors and ataxia. *See* PASPALUM STAGGERS, p 3019.
Moldy corn (maize) and pelleted cereal feeds, standing corn, corn silage, other grains	Pigs, cattle, sheep, poultry	Vulvovaginitis in pigs, anestrus or pseudopregnancy in mature sows, early embryonic death of swine embryos, estrogenism in cattle and sheep, reduced egg production in poultry. *See also* p 3014.
Toxic spores on pasture litter	Sheep, cattle, farmed deer	*See also* p 3015.
Tall fescue grass (*Lolium arundinacea*)	Cattle, horses	Lameness, weight loss, hyperthermia, heat intolerance, dry gangrene of extremities, agalactia, thickened fetal membranes. *See also* p 3016.
Cereal crops, moldy roughage	Pigs, cattle, horses, poultry	Vomiting and feed refusal (deoxynivalenol), loss of appetite and milk production, diarrhea, staggers, skin irritation, immunosuppression; recovery (from T-2, DAS) on removal of contaminated feed. *See also* p 3020.
Moldy corn (maize)	Horses, other Equidae, pigs	Depends on degree and specific site of brain lesion. *See also* p 3017.
Moldy seed, pods, stubble, and haulm of several *Lupinus* spp affected by *Phomopsis* stem blight	Sheep, occasionally cattle, horses, pigs	Lassitude, inappetence, stupor, icterus, marked liver injury. Usually fatal. *See also* p 3018.

(continued)

TABLE 4 MYCOTOXICOSES IN DOMESTIC ANIMALS *(continued)*

Disease	Toxins (When Known)	Fungi or Molds	Regions Where Reported
Myrotheciotoxicosis, dendrodochiotoxicosis	Macrocyclic trichothecenes (verrucarins, roridins, etc)	*Myrothecium verrucaria*, *M roridum*	Southeast Europe, former USSR
	Macrocyclic trichothecenes (baccharinoids)	*M verrucaria*	Brazil
Ochratoxicosis	Ochratoxin, also citrinin	*Aspergillus ochraceus* and others, *Penicillium viridicatum*, *P citrinum*	Widespread
Penicillium-associated tremorgens	Penitrem A	*P crustosum*, *P cyclopium*, *P commune*	Widespread
	Roquefortine	*P roqueforti*	
Perennial ryegrass staggers	Lolitrems	*Lolium perenne*, *Neotyphodium lolii*, an endophyte fungus confined to *L perenne*	Australia, New Zealand, Europe, USA
Poultry hemorrhagic syndrome	Probably aflatoxins and rubratoxins	Probably *Aspergillus flavus*, *A clavatus*, *Penicillium purpurogenum*, *Alternaria* sp	USA
Pulmonary edema, emphysema	4-Ipomeanol	*Fusarium solani*	USA
Porcine pulmonary edema	Fumonisin B_1 and Fumonisin B_2	*Fusarium verticilloides*	USA, South Africa
Slobbers syndrome	Slaframine (and swainsonine)	*Rhizoctonia leguminicola*	USA

TABLE 4 MYCOTOXICOSES IN DOMESTIC ANIMALS *(continued)*

Contaminated Toxic Foodstuff	Animals Affected	Signs and Lesions
Moldy rye stubble, straw	Sheep, cattle, horses	Acute—diarrhea, respiratory distress, hemorrhagic gastroenteritis, immunosuppression, death. Chronic—ulceration of GI tract, unthriftiness, gradual recovery. *See also* p 3020.
Plants of *Baccharis* spp that contain the toxins	Cattle, other herbivores	Epithelial necrosis of GI tract. *See also* p 3020.
Moldy barley, corn (maize), wheat	Pigs, poultry	Perirenal edema, enlarged pale kidneys with cortical cysts, and tubular degeneration and fibrosis; immunosuppression, polyuria and polydipsia.
Cereal grains, cheese, fruit, meats, nuts, refrigerated foods; compost	Cattle, dogs, horses, sheep	Neurotoxic signs, including continual tremors, seizures, hyperexcitability, ataxia. Vomiting and CNS signs in dogs.
As above, and in silage		
Endophyte-infected ryegrass pastures	Sheep, cattle, horses, deer	Tremors, incoordination, collapse, convulsive spasms. *See also* RYEGRASS STAGGERS, p 3153.
Moldy grain and meal	Growing chickens	Depression, anorexia, no weight gain, widespread internal hemorrhages, sometimes aplastic anemia, death. *See* MYCOTOXICOSES IN POULTRY, p 2846.
Moldy sweet potatoes	Cattle	Acute pulmonary edema, leading to interstitial pneumonia and emphysema.
Corn	Swine	Acute interlobular pulmonary edema and hydrothorax cause anoxia and cyanosis. Survivors may develop icterus and chronic hepatotoxicosis.
Black patch disease, legumes (notably red clover) eaten as forage or hay	Horses, sheep, cattle	Salivation, bloat, diarrhea, sometimes death. Recovery usual when removed from clover. *See also* SLAFRAMINE TOXICOSIS, p 3019.

(continued)

TABLE 4 MYCOTOXICOSES IN DOMESTIC ANIMALS *(continued)*

Disease	Toxins (When Known)	Fungi or Molds	Regions Where Reported
Stachybotryo-toxicosis	Macrocyclic trichothecenes (satratoxin, roridin, verrucarin)	*Stachybotrys atra* (*S alternans*)	Former USSR, southeast Europe
Sweet clover poisoning	Dicumarol	*Penicillium* spp, *Mucor* spp, *Aspergillus* spp	North America
Tremorgen ataxia syndrome	Penitrems, verruculogen, paxilline, fumitremorgens, aflatrems, roquefortine	*Penicillium crustosum*, *P puberulum*, *P verruculosum*, *P roqueforti*, *Aspergillus flavus*, *A fumigatus*, *A clavatus*, and others	USA, South Africa, probably worldwide

Managing a Suspected Mycotoxicosis

When mycotoxicosis is suspected, corrective actions could include the following: 1) Change the feed even when a specific mycotoxin is not identified. 2) Thoroughly inspect storage bins, mixing equipment, and feeders for caking, molding, or musty odors. 3) Remove contaminated feed and clean equipment and sanitize with hypochlorite (laundry bleach) to reduce contaminating fungi. 4) Analyze for known mycotoxins. 5) Use spore counts or fungal cultures for some indication of potential mycotoxin production. 6) If storage conditions or grain moisture are adverse, use a mold inhibitor to reduce or delay mold growth. Remember, mold inhibitors do not destroy preformed toxins. 7) Use a mycotoxin adsorbent if appropriate for the mycotoxin suspected. 8) Save a representative sample of each diet mixed until animals are at 1 mo beyond when the feed was consumed. 9) Take a representative sample of suspect feed after milling by passing a cup through a moving auger stream at frequent intervals, mixing samples thoroughly, and saving a 4.5-kg (10-lb) sample for analysis. *Alternatively*, use probe sampling of recently blended grain in bins or trucks at five locations in each structure for each 6 feet of depth. Freeze or dry samples, and submit for analysis in a paper bag (not plastic). Dry samples are preferable in a paper bag to prevent condensation during transport and storage. Samples should be dried at 176°–194°F (80°–90°C) for ~3 hr to reduce moisture to 12%–13%. If mold studies are to be done, dry at 140°F (60°C) for 6–12 hr to preserve fungal activity.

Mycotoxin Adsorbents

Adsorption of mycotoxins in contaminated feeds is an area of active research. Aflatoxins are effectively adsorbed by the aluminosilicate feed additives (*see* below). However, this group of adsorbents are of little or limited use for other mycototoxins. Trichothecene mycotoxins, including deoxynivalenol, are not readily adsorbed by common feed additives. The aluminosilicate adsorbents that are effective against aflatoxins have limited or no benefits against trichothecenes. Sodium bentonite is an effective adsorbent for aflatoxins in cattle and poultry but appears ineffective for trichothecenes and zearalenone. The polymeric glucomannan adsorbents (GM) are useful for poultry growth and feed consumption with low natural concentrations of aflatoxin, ochratoxin, T-2 toxin, and zearalenone. When added to *Fusarium*-contaminated diets, GM reduced the number of stillborn piglets compared with controls. GM adsorbent efficacy for ruminants has been

TABLE 4 MYCOTOXICOSES IN DOMESTIC ANIMALS *(continued)*

Contaminated Toxic Foodstuff	Animals Affected	Signs and Lesions
Moldy roughage, other contaminated feed	Horses, cattle, sheep, pigs	Stomatitis and ulceration, anorexia, leukopenia, extensive hemorrhages in many organs, inflammation and necrosis in the gut, immunosuppression. *See also* TRICHOTHECENE TOXICOSIS, p 3020.
Sweet clover (*Melilotus* spp)	Cattle, horses, sheep	Vitamin K antagonism with coagulopathy and hemorrhage. *See also* p 3156.
Moldy feed; high-protein food products, even under refrigeration, eg, cream cheese, walnuts	All species, but dogs are quite susceptible	Tremors, polypnea, ataxia, collapse, convulsive spasms.

variable in different studies. Cholestyramine has been an effective binder of fumonisins and zearalenone in vitro and for fumonisins in animal experiments, but response in cattle is unknown. Although various adsorbents are allowed for animal feed in various countries, none is FDA approved in the USA.

AFLATOXICOSIS

Aflatoxins are produced by toxigenic strains of *Aspergillus flavus* and *A parasiticus* on peanuts, soybeans, corn (maize), and other cereals either in the field or during storage when moisture content and temperatures are sufficiently high for mold growth. Usually, this means consistent day and night temperatures >70°F. The toxic response and disease in mammals and poultry varies in relation to species, sex, age, nutritional status, and the duration of intake and level of aflatoxins in the ration. Earlier recognized disease outbreaks called "moldy corn toxicosis," "poultry hemorrhagic syndrome," and "*Aspergillus* toxicosis" may have been caused by aflatoxins.

Aflatoxicosis occurs in many parts of the world and affects growing poultry (especially ducklings and turkey poults), young pigs, pregnant sows, calves, and dogs. Adult cattle, sheep, and goats are relatively resistant to the acute form of the disease but are susceptible if toxic diets are fed over long periods. Experimentally, all species of animals tested have shown some degree of susceptibility. Dietary levels of aflatoxin (in ppb) generally tolerated are ≤50 in young poultry, ≤100 in adult poultry, ≤50 in weaner pigs, ≤200 in finishing pigs, <50 in dogs, <100 in calves, and <300 in cattle. Approximately two times the tolerable levels stated is likely to cause clinical disease, including some mortality. Dietary levels as low as 10–20 ppb result in measurable metabolites of aflatoxin (aflatoxin M_1 and M_2) being excreted in milk; feedstuffs that contain aflatoxins should not be fed to dairy cows. Acceptable regulatory values in milk may range from 0.05 ppb to 0.5 ppb in different countries; individual state or federal regulatory agencies should be consulted when contamination occurs.

Aflatoxins are metabolized in the liver to an epoxide that binds to macromolecules, especially nucleic acids and nucleoproteins. Their toxic effects include mutagenesis due to alkylation of nuclear DNA, carcinogenesis, teratogenesis, reduced protein synthesis, and immunosuppression. Reduced protein synthesis results in reduced production of essential metabolic enzymes and structural proteins for growth. The liver is the principal organ affected. High dosages of aflatoxins result in hepatocellular necrosis; prolonged low dosages result in reduced growth rate, immunosuppression, and liver enlargement.

Clinical Findings: In acute outbreaks, deaths occur after a short period of inappetence; other acute signs include vomiting, depression, hemorrhage, and icterus. Subacute outbreaks are more usual, with unthriftiness, weakness, anorexia, reduced growth and feed efficiency, and occasional sudden deaths. Laboratory changes in most species are related to liver damage, coagulopathy, and impaired protein synthesis. Specific laboratory changes include increased AST, ALT, and alkaline phosphatase; hypothrombinemia, prolonged prothrombin and activated partial thromboplastin times, hyperbilirubinemia, hypocholesterolemia, hypoalbuminemia, and variable thrombocytopenia. Generally, aflatoxin concentrations in feed twice the tolerable levels given above are associated with acute aflatoxicosis. Recently, acute and fatal aflatoxicosis with many of these signs and laboratory changes has been documented in dogs. Frequently, there is a high incidence of concurrent infectious disease, often respiratory, that responds poorly to the usual drug therapy. Dairy cattle experience inappetence, and ruminants may have decreased ruminal contractions at high concentrations (>1,000 ppb) of aflatoxins. Liver damage can lead to reduced clotting factor synthesis with acute to chronic hemorrhage. Subclinical effects are reduced growth rate and feed efficiency, hypoproteinemia, and reduced resistance to some infectious diseases despite vaccination.

Lesions: In acute cases, there are widespread hemorrhages and icterus. The liver is the major target organ. Microscopically, the liver is enlarged and shows marked fatty accumulations and massive centrilobular necrosis and hemorrhage. In subacute cases, the hepatic changes are not so pronounced, but the liver is somewhat enlarged and firmer than usual. There may be edema of the gallbladder. Microscopically, the liver shows periportal inflammatory response and proliferation and fibrosis of the bile ductules; the hepatocytes and their nuclei (megalocytosis) are enlarged. The GI mucosa may show glandular atrophy and associated inflammation. Rarely, there may be tubular degeneration and regeneration in the kidneys. Prolonged feeding of low concentrations of aflatoxins may result in diffuse liver *fibrosis* (cirrhosis) and, rarely, carcinoma of the bile ducts or liver.

Diagnosis: Disease history, laboratory data, necropsy findings, and microscopic examination of the liver should indicate the nature of the hepatotoxin, but hepatic changes are somewhat similar in *Senecio* poisoning (*see* p 3150). The presence and levels of aflatoxins in the feed should be determined. Acutely affected animals have increases in liver enzymes (alkaline phosphatase, AST, or ALT), bilirubin, serum bile acids, and prothrombin time. Chronic exposure can cause hypoproteinemia (including decrease in both albumin and globulin). Aflatoxin M_1 (principal metabolite of aflatoxin B_1) can be detected in urine, liver, kidney, or milk of lactating animals if toxin intakes are high. Aflatoxin residues in organs and dairy products generally are eliminated within 1–3 wk after exposure ends.

Control: Contaminated feeds can be avoided by monitoring batches for aflatoxin content. Local crop conditions (drought, insect infestation) should be monitored as predictors of aflatoxin formation. Young, newly weaned, pregnant, and lactating animals require special protection from suspected toxic feeds. Dilution with noncontaminated feedstuffs is one possibility, but this may not be acceptable on a regulatory basis. Cleaning to remove lightweight or broken grains will often substantially reduce mycotoxin concentration in remaining grain. Ammoniation reduces aflatoxin contamination in grain but is not currently approved by the FDA for use in food animals in the USA because of uncertainty about by-products produced.

Numerous products are marketed as anticaking agents to sequester or "bind" aflatoxins and reduce absorption from the GI tract. One effective binder for aflatoxins is hydrated sodium calcium aluminosilicates (HSCAS), which reduce the effects of aflatoxin when fed to pigs or poultry at 10 lb/ton (5 kg/tonne). They also provide substantial protection against dietary aflatoxin. HSCAS reduce aflatoxin M_1 in milk by ~50% but do not eliminate residues of aflatoxin M_1 in milk from dairy cows fed aflatoxin B_1. Other adsorbents (sodium bentonites, polymeric glucomannans) have shown variable but partial efficacy in reducing low-level aflatoxin residues in poultry and dairy cattle. To date, the FDA has not licensed any product for use as a "mycotoxin binder" in animal feeds.

ERGOTISM

Ergotism is a worldwide disease of farm animals that results from ingestion of sclerotia of the parasitic fungus *Claviceps purpurea*, which replaces the grain or seed of rye and other small grains or forage plants, such as the bromes, bluegrasses, fescues, and ryegrasses. The hard, black, elongated sclerotia may contain varying quantities of ergot alkaloids, of which ergotamine and ergonovine (ergometrine) are pharmacologically most important. Cattle, pigs, sheep, and poultry are involved in sporadic outbreaks, and most other species are susceptible. Poisoning can come from grazing seed heads or from infected grains in concentrate rations.

Etiology: Ergot causes vasoconstriction by direct action on the muscles of the arterioles, and repeated doses injure the vascular endothelium. These actions initially reduce blood flow and eventually lead to complete stasis with terminal necrosis of the extremities due to thrombosis. A cold environment predisposes the extremities to gangrene. In addition, ergot also causes stimulation of the CNS, followed by depression. Ergot alkaloids inhibit pituitary release of prolactin in many mammalian species, with failure of both mammary development in late gestation and delayed initiation of milk secretion, resulting in agalactia at parturition. Ergot alkaloids have also been associated with heat intolerance, dyspnea, and reduced milk production in dairy cattle, similar to the "summer syndrome" described for fescue toxicosis.

Clinical Findings and Lesions: Cattle may be affected by eating ergotized hay or grain or occasionally by grazing seeded pastures infested with ergot. Lameness, the first sign, may appear 2–6 wk or more after initial ingestion, depending on the concentration of alkaloids in the ergot and the quantity of ergot in the feed. Hindlimbs are affected before forelimbs, but the extent of involvement of a limb and the number of limbs affected depends on the daily intake of ergot. Body temperature and pulse and respiration rates are increased. **Epidemic hyperthermia** and hypersalivation may also occur in cattle poisoned with *C purpurea* (*see also* FESCUE POISONING, p 3016). Ergot alkaloids may interfere with embryonic development in pregnant females.

Associated with the lameness are swelling and tenderness of the fetlock joint and pastern. Within ~1 wk, sensation is lost in the affected part, an indented line appears at the limit of normal tissue, and dry gangrene affects the distal part. Eventually, one or both claws or any part of the limbs up to the hock or knee may be sloughed. In a similar way, the tip of the tail or ears may become necrotic and slough. Exposed skin areas, such as teats and udder, appear unusually pale or anemic. Abortion is not seen.

The most consistent lesions at necropsy are in the skin and subcutaneous parts of the extremities. The skin is normal to the indented line, but beyond, it is cyanotic and hardened in advanced cases. Subcutaneous hemorrhage and some edema occur proximal to the necrotic area.

In pigs, ingestion of ergot-infested grains may result in reduced feed intake and reduced weight gain. Occasionally, swine may show necrosis of the tips of ears or tail. If fed to pregnant sows, ergotized grains result in lack of udder development with agalactia at parturition, and the piglets born may be smaller than normal. Most of the litter die within a few days because of starvation. No other clinical signs or lesions are seen.

Clinical signs in sheep are similar to those in cattle. Additionally, the mouth may be ulcerated, and marked intestinal inflammation may be seen at necropsy. A convulsive syndrome has been associated with ergotism in sheep.

Diagnosis: Diagnosis is based on finding the causative fungus (ergot sclerotia) in grains, hay, or pastures provided to livestock showing signs of ergotism. Ergot alkaloids may be extracted and detected in suspect ground grain meals. At 200–600 ppb, ergot alkaloids may cause clinical signs and effects; however, this is influenced by the relative amounts of various ergot alkaloids in the grain.

Identical signs and lesions of lameness, and sloughing of the hooves and tips of ears and tail, are seen in fescue foot in cattle grazing in winter on tall fescue grass infected with an endophyte fungus, in which the ergot alkaloid ergovaline is considered a major toxic principle. In gilts and sows, lactation failure not associated with ergot alkaloids must be differentiated from prolactin inhibition due to ergot.

Treatment: In horses, parenteral use of the dopamine D2 antagonist domperidone (1.1 mg/kg, PO, bid for 10–14 days) is effective in prevention of agalactia from ergot alkaloids in fescue. Use against the same alkaloids produced by *C purpurea* could be medically logical (*see* p 3016).

Control: Intake of ergot bodies should be <0.1% of the total diet, and concentrations of ergot alkaloids should be <100 ppm in the total diet. Ergotism can be controlled by an immediate change to an ergot-free diet. In pregnant sows, however, removal of ergot in late gestation (<1 wk before parturition) may not correct the agalactia syndrome, and animals with clinical peripheral gangrene will not likely recover. Under pasture feeding conditions, frequent grazing or topping of pastures prone to ergot infestation during the summer months reduces flower-head production and helps control the disease. Grain that contains even small amounts of ergot should not be fed to pregnant or lactating sows.

ESTROGENISM AND VULVOVAGINITIS

(*Fusarium* estrogenism)

Fusarium spp molds are extremely common and often contaminate growing plants and stored feeds. Corn (maize), wheat, and barley are commonly contaminated. In moderate climates under humid weather conditions, *F graminearum* may produce zearalenone, one of the resorcyclic acid lactones (RALs). Zearalenone (formerly called F_2 toxin) is a potent nonsteroidal estrogen and is the only known mycotoxin with primarily estrogenic effects. Often, zearalenone is produced concurrently with deoxynivalenol. Depending on the ratio of these two mycotoxins, signs of reduced feed intake or reproductive dysfunction may predominate, but presence of deoxynivalenol may limit exposure to zearalenone, thus reducing its practical effect.

Zearalenone binds to receptors for 17β-estradiol, and this complex binds to estradiol sites on DNA. Specific RNA synthesis leads to signs of estrogenism. Zearalenone is a weak estrogen with potency 2–4 times less than estradiol. Under controlled administration, zearalanol, a closely related RAL, is widely used in cattle as an anabolic agent.

Estrogenism due to zearalenone was first clinically recognized as vulvovaginitis in prepubertal gilts fed moldy corn (maize), but zearalenone is occasionally reported as a suspected disease-causing agent for sporadic outbreaks in dairy cattle, sheep, chickens, and turkeys. High dietary concentrations (>20–30 ppm) are required to produce infertility in cattle and sheep, and extremely high dosages are required to affect poultry.

Etiology: Zearalenone has been detected in corn, oats, barley, wheat, and sorghum (both fresh and stored); in rations compounded for cattle and pigs; in corn ensiled at the green stage; and very rarely in hay. It has been detected occasionally in samples from pastures in temperate climates at levels believed sufficient to cause reproductive failure of grazing herbivores.

Clinical Findings: Clinical effects cannot be distinguished from excessive estrogen administration. Physical and behavioral signs of estrus are induced in young gilts by as little as 1 ppm dietary zearalenone. In pigs, zearalenone primarily affects weaned and prepubertal gilts, causing hyperemia and enlargement of the vulva (known as vulvovaginitis). There is hypertrophy of the mammary glands and uterus, and abdominal straining results in prolapse of the uterus in severe cases. Removal of affected grain results in return to normal in ~1 wk.

Zearalenone causes reproductive toxicosis in sexually mature sows by inhibiting secretion and release of follicle-stimulating hormone (FSH), resulting in arrest of preovulatory ovarian follicle maturation. Reproductive effects in sexually mature sows depend on time of consumption. Zearalenone fed at 3–10 ppm on days 12–14 of the estrous cycle in open gilts results in retention of corpora lutea and prolonged anestrus (pseudopregnancy) for up to 40–60 days. Zearalenone fed at ≥30 ppm in early gestation (7–10 days after breeding) may prevent implantation and cause early embryonic death. Zearalenone metabolites can be excreted in milk of exposed sows, resulting in hyperestrogenic effects in their nursing piglets.

In cattle, dietary concentrations >10 ppm may cause reproductive dysfunction in dairy heifers, although mature cows may tolerate up to 20 ppm.

Young males, both swine and cattle, may become infertile, with atrophy of the testes. However, mature boars appear unaffected by as much as 200 ppm dietary zearalenone.

Ewes may show reduced reproductive performance (reduced ovulation rates and numbers of fertilized ova, and markedly increased duration of estrus) and abortion or premature live births.

Lesions: Lesions in pigs include ovarian atrophy and follicular atresia, uterine edema, cellular hypertrophy in all layers of the uterus, and a cystic appearance in degenerative endometrial glands. The mammary glands show ductal hyperplasia and epithelial proliferation. Squamous metaplasia is seen in the cervix and vagina. Sexually mature sows will have retained corpora lutea for 40–70 days after exposure, consistent with signs of pseudopregnancy.

Diagnosis: Diagnosis is based on reproductive performance in the herd or flock, clinical signs, history of diet-related occurrence, and excluding other known causes of infertility. Chemical analysis of suspect feed for zearalenone and careful examination of reproductive organs at necropsy are required. As a bioassay, virgin prepubertal mice fed diets or extracts of zearalenone-contaminated feed demonstrate enlarged uteri and vaginal cornification typical of estrogens.

Differential diagnoses include reproductive tract infections and other causes of impaired fertility such as diethylstilbestrol in the diet of housed stock. In grazing herbivores, especially sheep, the plant estrogens (eg, isoflavones associated with some varieties of subterranean and red clovers, and coumestans in certain fodders [eg, alfalfa]) should be considered.

Control: Unless stock are severely or chronically affected, usually reproductive functions recover and signs regress 1–4 wk after intake of zearalenone stops. However, multiparous sows may remain anestrous up to 8–10 wk.

Management of swine with hyperestrogenism should include changing the grain immediately. Signs should stop within 1 wk. Animals should be treated symptomatically for vaginal or rectal prolapse and physical damage to external genitalia. For sexually mature sows with anestrus, one 10-mg dose of prostaglandin $F_2\alpha$, or two 5-mg doses on successive days, has corrected anestrus caused by retained corpora. Alfalfa and alfalfa meal fed to swine at 25% of the ration may reduce absorption and increase fecal excretion of zearalenone, but this is often not considered practical. Feeding activated charcoal, cholestyramine, or alfalfa meal may reduce zearalenone absorption and retention, but the high concentrations needed generally render this impractical.

FACIAL ECZEMA

(Pithomycotoxicosis)

In this mycotoxic disease of grazing livestock, the toxic liver injury commonly results in photodynamic dermatitis. In sheep, the face is the only site of the body readily exposed to ultraviolet light, hence the common name. The disease is most common in New Zealand but also occurs in Australia, France, South Africa, several South American countries, and probably North America. Sheep, cattle, and farmed deer of all ages can contract the disease, but it is most severe in young animals.

Etiology and Pathogenesis: Sporidesmins are secondary metabolites of the saprophytic fungus *Pithomyces chartarum*, which grows on dead pasture litter. The warm ground temperatures and high humidity required for rapid growth of this fungus restrict disease occurrence to hot summer and autumn periods shortly after warm rains. By observing weather conditions and estimating toxic spore numbers on pastures, danger periods can be predicted and farmers alerted.

The sporidesmins are excreted via the biliary system, in which they produce severe cholangitis and pericholangitis as a result of tissue necrosis. Biliary obstruction may be seen, which restricts excretion of bile pigments and results in jaundice. Similarly, failure to excrete phylloerythrin in bile leads to photosensitization.

Previous ingestion of toxic spores causes potentiation; thus, a succession of small intakes of the spores can lead to subsequent severe outbreaks.

Clinical Findings, Lesions, and Diagnosis: Few signs are apparent until photosensitization and jaundice appear ~10–14 days after intake of the toxins. Animals frantically seek shade. Even short exposure to the sun rapidly produces the typical erythema and edema of photodermatitis in nonpigmented skin. The animals suffer considerably, and deaths occur from one to several weeks after photodermatitis appears.

Characteristic liver and bile duct lesions are seen in all affected animals whether photosensitized or not. In acute cases showing photodermatitis, livers are initially enlarged, icteric, and have a marked lobular pattern. Later, there is atrophy and marked fibrosis. The shape is distorted, and large nodules of regenerated tissue appear on the surface. In subclinical cases, livers often develop extensive areas in which the tissue is depressed and shrunken below the normal contour, which distorts and roughens the capsule. Generally, these areas are associated with fibrosis and thickening of corresponding bile ducts. The bladder mucosa commonly shows hemorrhagic or bile pigment–stained ulcerative erosions with circumscribed edema.

The clinical signs together with characteristic liver lesions are pathognomonic. In live animals, high levels of hepatic enzymes may reflect the extensive injury to the liver.

Control: To minimize intake of pasture litter and toxic spores, short grazing should be avoided. Other feedstuffs should be fed during danger periods; encouraging clover dominance in pastures helps to provide a milieu unsuited to growth and sporulation of *P chartarum* on litter.

The application of benzimidazole fungicides to pastures considerably restricts the buildup of *P chartarum* spores and reduces pasture toxicity. A pasture area calculated at 1 acre (0.45 hectare)/15 cows or 100 sheep should be sprayed in midsummer with a suspension of thiabendazole. When danger periods of fungal activity are predicted, animals should be allowed only on the sprayed areas. The fungicide is effective within 4 days after spraying, provided that no more than 1 in. (2.5 cm) of rain falls within 24 hr during the 4-day period. After this time, heavy rainfall does little to reduce the effectiveness of spraying, because the thiabendazole becomes incorporated within the plants. Pastures will then remain safe for ~6 wk, after which spraying should be repeated to ensure protection over the entire dangerous season.

Sheep and cattle can be protected from the effects of sporidesmin if given adequate amounts of zinc. Zinc may be administered by drenching with zinc oxide slurry, by spraying pastures with zinc oxide, or by adding zinc sulfate to drinking water.

Sheep may be selectively bred for natural resistance to the toxic effects of sporidesmin. The heritable trait for resistance is high. Ram sires are now being selected in stud and commercial flocks for resistance either by natural field challenge or by low-level, controlled dosage of ram lambs with sporidesmin.

FESCUE POISONING

Fescue Lameness

(Fescue foot)

Fescue lameness, which resembles ergot poisoning, is believed to be caused by ergot alkaloids, especially ergovaline, produced by the endophyte fungus *Neotyphodium coenophialum* in tall fescue grass (*Lolium arundinaceum*, formerly *Festuca arundinacea*). It begins with lameness in one or both hindfeet and may progress to necrosis of the distal part of the affected limb(s). The tail and ears also may be affected independently of the lameness. In addition to gangrene of these extremities, animals may show loss of body mass, an arched back, and a rough coat. Outbreaks have been confirmed in cattle, and similar lesions have been reported in sheep.

Tall fescue is a cool-season perennial grass adapted to a wide range of soil and climatic conditions; it is used in Australia and New Zealand for stabilizing the banks of watercourses. It is the predominant pasture grass in the transition zone in the eastern and central USA. Fescue lameness has been reported in Kentucky, Tennessee, Florida, California, Colorado, and Missouri, as well as in New Zealand, Australia, and Italy.

The causative toxic substance, ergovaline, has actions similar to those produced by sclerotia of *Claviceps purpurea*. However, ergot poisoning (*see* p 3012) is not the cause of fescue lameness. Ergotism is most prevalent in late summer when the seed heads of grass mature. Fescue lameness is most common in late fall and winter and has been reproduced in cattle by feeding dried fescue free of seed heads and ergot. However, occasionally, ergotized fescue seed produced in early summer may inadvertently be baled and result in ergot toxicosis instead of or in addition to fescue toxicosis.

The endophyte fungus *N coenophialum* growing within the fescue plant can synthesize ergot alkaloids. The ergot alkaloid ergovaline has been detected in toxic fescue and constitutes ~90% of the ergopeptide alkaloids produced. Ergovaline content of infected tall fescue often ranges from 100 to 500 ppb, and >200 ppb is considered a toxic concentration. Susceptible species from most to least sensitive are horses, cattle, and sheep. Endophyte-infected fescue that does not produce ergovaline has not caused fescue toxicosis. In cattle, >90% of ergovaline metabolites are found in urine. Removal of animals from infected fescue pasture reduces urinary ergovaline below detectable concentrations within 48 hr.

Ergovaline is an agonist for dopamine D2 receptors, which initiate several physiologic abnormalities. First, inhibition of prolactin secretion causes agalactia in horses and swine and reduced lactation in cattle. The dopaminergic effect also causes imbalances of progesterone and estrogen, associated with early parturition for cattle and prolonged gestation with oversized fetuses in mares. Finally, inadequate prolactin disturbs the hypothalamic thermoregulatory center, leading to temperature intolerance when environmental temperature exceeds 31°C (88°F).

Some reports indicate an increased incidence of fescue lameness as plants age and after severe droughts. Strains of tall fescue vary in their toxicity (eg, Kentucky-31 is more toxic than Fawn) because of variation in infection level with the fungus and to high variability within a strain. In some Kentucky-31 fescues, infection levels cannot be detected. High nitrogen applications appear to enhance toxicity. Susceptibility of cattle is subject to individual variation.

Low environmental temperature may exacerbate the lesions of fescue lameness; however, high temperatures increase the severity of a toxic problem known as **epidemic hyperthermia** or "summer syndrome," in which a high proportion of a herd of cattle exhibits hypersalivation and hyperthermia. The toxin appears to be a vasoconstrictor acting as an α_2-adrenergic agonist on blood vessels; this promotes hyperthermia in hot weather and results in cold extremities during cold weather. Another cause of this is poisoning with *C purpurea* (ergot alkaloids).

Erythema and swelling of the coronary region occur, and cattle are alert but lose weight and may be seen "paddling" or weight-shifting. The back is slightly arched, and knuckling of a hind pastern may be an initial sign. There is progressive lameness, anorexia, depression, and later, dry gangrene of the distal limbs (hindlimbs first). Signs usually develop within 10–21 days after turnout into a fescue-contaminated pasture in fall. A period of frost tends to increase the incidence.

For control, all infected forage should be removed.

Summer Fescue Toxicosis

Summer fescue toxicosis is a warm season condition characterized by reduced feed intake and weight gains or milk production. The toxin(s) affects cattle, sheep, and horses during the summer when they are grazing or being fed tall fescue forage or seed contaminated with the endophytic fungus *Neotyphodium coenophialum*. The severity of the condition varies from field to field and year to year.

Signs other than reduced performance, which may appear within 1–2 wk after fescue feeding is started, include fever, tachypnea, rough coat, lower serum prolactin levels, and excessive salivation. The animals seek wet spots or shade. Lowered reproductive performance also has been reported. Agalactia has been reported for both horses and cattle. Thickened placentas, delayed parturition, and birth of weak foals have been reported in horses. The severity increases when environmental temperatures are >75°–80°F (24°–27°C) and if high nitrogen fertilizer has been applied to the grass.

Medical treatment for equine agalactia/reproductive syndrome is domperidone administered at 1.1 mg/kg, PO, bid for 10–14 days. For control and prevention, toxic tall fescue pastures must either be destroyed and reseeded with seed that does not contain endophytic fungus, or infected fields must be managed to avoid the high risk factor. Transfer of the fungus from plant to plant is primarily, if not solely, through infected seed. Not using pastures during hot weather, diluting tall fescue pastures with interseeded legumes, clipping or close grazing of pastures to reduce seed formation, or offering other feedstuffs help reduce severity. Removing pregnant horses or cattle 1 mo before parturition will usually prevent parturition- and lactation-related problems. Specific feed additives may provide some protection against contaminated hay. Yeast cell derivatives known as glucomannans are reported to improve performance by preventing toxin absorption in cattle; a seaweed product is reported to lessen the immunosuppressive effects of toxic tall fescue. (*See also* ABDOMINAL FAT NECROSIS, p 360.)

FUMONISIN TOXICOSIS

Fumonisins are responsible for two well-described diseases of livestock, equine leukoencephalomalacia and porcine pulmonary edema.

Equine leukoencephalomalacia is a mycotoxic disease of the CNS that affects horses, mules, and donkeys. It occurs sporadically in North and South America, South Africa, Europe, and China. It is associated with the feeding of moldy corn (maize), usually over a period of several weeks. Fumonisins are produced worldwide primarily by *Fusarium verticillioides* (previously *F moniliforme* Sheldon) and *F proliferatum*. Conditions favoring fumonisin production appear to include a period of drought during the growing season with subsequent cool, moist conditions during pollination and kernel formation. Three toxins produced by the fungi have been classified as fumonisin B_1 (FB_1), B_2 (FB_2), and B_3 (FB_3). Current evidence suggests that FB_1 and FB_2 are of similar toxicity, whereas FB_3 is relatively nontoxic. Corn grain may commonly contain 1–3 ppm fumonisins, but occasionally some years as much as 20–100 ppm. The toxins are concentrated primarily in molded, damaged, or light test weight corn. Major health effects are seen in Equidae and swine.

Signs in Equidae include apathy, drowsiness, pharyngeal paralysis, blindness, circling, staggering, and recumbency. The clinical course is usually 1–2 days but may be as short as several hours or as long as several weeks. Icterus may be present when the liver is involved. The characteristic lesion is liquefactive necrosis of the white matter of the cerebrum; the necrosis is usually unilateral but may be asymmetrically bilateral. Some horses may have hepatic necrosis similar to that seen in aflatoxicosis. Horses may develop leukoencephalomalacia from prolonged exposure to as little as 8–10 ppm fumonisins in the diet, and onset of neurologic signs almost invariably leads to death.

Fumonisins have also been reported to cause acute epidemics of disease in weanling or adult pigs, characterized by pulmonary edema and hydrothorax. **Porcine pulmonary edema** (PPE) is usually an acute, fatal disease and appears to be caused by pulmonary hypertension with transudation of fluids in the thorax, resulting in interstitial pulmonary edema and hydrothorax. Acute PPE results after consumption of fumonisins for 3–6 days at dietary concentrations >100 ppm. Morbidity within a herd may be >50%, and mortality among affected pigs is 50%–100%. Signs include acute onset of dyspnea, cyanosis of mucous membranes, weakness, recumbency, and death, often within 24 hr after the first clinical signs. Affected sows in late gestation that survive acute PPE may abort within 2–3 days, presumably as a result of fetal anoxia. Prolonged exposure of pigs to sublethal concentrations of fumonisins results in hepatotoxicosis characterized by reduced growth; icterus; and increased serum levels of cholesterol, bilirubin, AST, lactate dehydrogenase, and γ-glutamyltransferase.

The biochemical mechanism of action for PPE or liver toxicosis is believed to be due to the ability of fumonisins to interrupt sphingolipid synthesis in many animal species, and fatalities result from disturbances in cardiopulmonary dynamics leading to acute pulmonary edema.

Cattle, sheep, and poultry are considerably less susceptible to fumonisins than are horses or swine. Cattle and sheep tolerate fumonisin concentrations of 100 ppm with little effect. Dietary concentrations of 150–200 ppm cause inappetence, weight loss, and mild liver damage. Poultry are affected by concentrations of >200–400 ppm and may develop inappetence, weight loss, and skeletal abnormalities.

No effective treatment is available. Avoidance of moldy corn is the only prevention, although this is difficult because the corn may not be grossly moldy or may be contained in a mixed feed. However, most of the toxin is present in broken or small, poorly formed kernels. Cleaning grain to remove the screenings markedly reduces fumonisin concentration. Corn suspected of containing fumonisins should not be given to horses. Binding of fumonisins with glucose has been demonstrated to alleviate or eliminate toxicosis in pigs, but development of the process on a commercial scale has not yet been accomplished. Advisory exposure guidelines by the FDA have recommended total dietary concentrations (ppm) as follows: horses <1, swine <10, ruminants <30, poultry <50, breeding ruminants and poultry <15 ppm.

MYCOTOXIC LUPINOSIS

Lupines (*Lupinus* spp) cause two distinct forms of poisoning in livestock: lupine poisoning and lupinosis. The former is a nervous syndrome caused by alkaloids present in bitter lupines; the latter is a mycotoxic disease characterized by liver injury and jaundice, which results mainly from the feeding of sweet lupines. Lupinosis is important in Australia and South Africa and also has been reported from New Zealand and Europe. There is increasing use of sweet lupines, either as forage crops or through feeding of their residues after grain harvest, as strategic feed for sheep in Mediterranean climate zones. Sheep, and occasionally cattle and horses, are affected, and pigs are also susceptible.

Etiology and Pathogenesis: The causal fungus is *Phomopsis leptostromiformis*, which causes *Phomopsis* stem-blight, especially in white and yellow lupines; blue varieties are resistant. It produces sunken, linear stem lesions that contain black, stromatic masses, and it also affects the pods and seeds. The fungus is also a saprophyte and grows well on dead lupine material (eg, haulm, pods, stubble) under favorable conditions. It produces phomopsins as secondary metabolites on infected lupine material, especially after rain.

Clinical Findings, Lesions, and Diagnosis: Clinical changes are mainly attributable to toxic hepatocyte injury, which causes mitotic arrest in metaphase, isolated cell necrosis, and hepatic enzyme leakage, with loss of metabolic and excretory function.

Early signs in sheep and cattle are inappetence and listlessness. Complete anorexia and jaundice follow, and ketosis is common. Cattle may show lacrimation and salivation. Ketosis is a common sequela in pregnant cattle or recently calved cows. Survivors may develop hepatic cirrhosis. Sheep may become photosensitive, and a skeletal muscle myopathy can develop. As disease progresses, liver failure may cause hepatoencephalopathy characterized by stumbling, disorientation, and recumbency before death. In acute outbreaks, deaths occur in 2–14 days.

In acute disease, icterus is marked. Livers are enlarged, orange-yellow, and fatty. More chronic cases show bronze- or tan-colored livers that are firm, contracted in size, and fibrotic. Copious amounts of transudates may be found in the abdominal and thoracic cavities and in the pericardial sac. Some animals may have spongiform lesions in the brain.

Feeding of moldy lupine material, together with clinical signs and increased levels of serum liver enzymes, strongly indicate lupinosis.

Control: Frequent surveillance of sheep and of lupine fodder material for characteristic black spot fungal infestation, especially after rains, is advised. The utilization of lupine cultivars, bred and developed for resistance to *P leptostromiformis*, is advocated. Oral doses of zinc (≥0.5 g/day) have protected sheep against liver injury induced by phomopsins.

PASPALUM STAGGERS

This incoordination results from eating paspalum grasses (*Paspalum* spp) infested by *Claviceps paspali*. The life cycle of this fungus is similar to that of *C purpurea* (see p 3012). Toxic infestations are most likely after humid, wet summers. The yellow-gray sclerotia, which mature in the seed heads in autumn, are round, roughened, and 2–4 mm in diameter. Ingestion of sclerotia causes nervous signs in cattle most commonly, but horses and sheep also are susceptible. Guinea pigs can be affected experimentally. The toxicity is not ascribed to ergot alkaloids; the toxic principles are thought to be paspalinine and paspalitrem A and B, tremorgenic compounds from the sclerotia.

A sufficiently large single dose causes signs that persist for several days. Animals display continuous trembling of the large muscle groups; movements are jerky and incoordinated. If they attempt to run, they fall over in awkward positions. Appetite remains good, and animals will eat if feed is provided. Affected animals may be belligerent and dangerous to approach or handle. After prolonged exposure, condition is lost and complete paralysis can occur. The time of onset of signs depends on the degree of the infestation of seed heads and the grazing habits of the animals. Experimentally, early signs appear in cattle after sclerotia at ~100 g/day has been administered for >2 days. Although the mature ergots are toxic, they are most dangerous just when they are maturing to the hard, black (sclerotic) stage.

Medical treatment is usually not necessary, unless animals have physical injuries or are compromised from dehydration or lack of eating. Recovery follows removal of the animals to feed not contaminated with sclerotia of *C paspali*. Animals are less affected if left alone and provided readily available nutritious forages. Care should be taken to prevent accidental access to ponds or rough terrain where accidental trauma or drowning could occur. Topping of the pasture to remove affected seed heads has been effective in control.

SLAFRAMINE TOXICOSIS

Trifolium pratense (red clover) may become infected with the fungus *Rhizoctonia leguminicola* (black patch disease), especially in wet, cool years. Rarely, other legumes (white clover, alsike, alfalfa) may be infected. Slaframine is an indolizidine alkaloid recognized as the toxic principle, and it is stable in dried hay and probably in silage. Horses are highly sensitive to slaframine, but clinical cases occur in cattle as well. Profuse salivation (salivary syndrome) develops within hours after first consumption of contaminated hay; signs also include mild lacrimation, diarrhea, mild bloat, and frequent urination. Morbidity can be high, but death is not expected, and removal of contaminated hay allows recovery and return of appetite within 24–48 hr. A related alkaloid, swainsonine, produced by *R leguminicola*, has caused a lysosomal storage disease from prolonged exposure, but its importance in the salivary syndrome is not confirmed. Diagnosis is tentatively based on recognition of the characteristic clinical signs and the presence of "black patch" on the forages. Chemical detection of slaframine or swainsonine in forages helps to confirm the diagnosis. There is no specific antidote to slaframine toxicosis, although atropine may control at least some of the prominent salivary and GI signs. Removal of animals from the contaminated hay is essential. Prevention of *Rhizoctonia* infection of clovers has been difficult. Some clover varieties may be relatively resistant to black patch disease. Reduced usage of red clover for forages or dilution with other feeds is helpful.

TRICHOTHECENE TOXICOSIS

The trichothecene mycotoxins are a group of closely related secondary metabolic products of several families of imperfect or plant pathogenic fungi. Those of most importance in much of the world are produced species of *Fusarium*, but also from genera of *Trichothecium*, *Myrothecium*, *Cephalosporium*, *Stachybotrys*, *Trichodesma*, *Cylindrocarpon*, and *Verticimonosporium*. Trichothecenes are classified as nonmacrocyclic (eg, deoxynivalenol [DON] or vomitoxin, T-2 toxin, diacetoxyscirpenol [DAS], and others) or macrocyclic (eg, satratoxin, roridin, verrucarin). For livestock, the most important trichothecene mycotoxin is DON, which is commonly a contaminant of corn, wheat, and other commodity grains. Lesser amounts of T-2 toxin and DAS are found sporadically in the same sources.

The trichothecene mycotoxins are highly toxic at the subcellular, cellular, and organic system level. Trichothecenes inhibit protein synthesis by affecting ribosomes to interfere with protein synthesis and covalently bond to sulfhydryl groups.

Toxicity of T-2 toxin and DAS is based on direct cytotoxicity and is often referred to as a radiomimetic effect (eg, bone marrow hypoplasia, gastroenteritis, diarrhea, hemorrhages). Direct contact with skin and oral cavity causes irritation and ulceration. Stomatitis, hyperkeratosis with ulceration of the esophageal portion of the gastric mucosa, and necrosis of the GI tract have been seen after ingestion of trichothecenes. Systemic effects of T-2 and DAS are often self-limiting because of oral irritation and feed refusal.

Given in sublethal toxic doses via any route, the trichothecenes are immunosuppressive in mammals; however, longterm feeding of high levels of T-2 toxin does not seem to activate latent viral or bacterial infections. The toxins may affect function of helper T cells, B cells, or macrophages, or the interaction among these cells.

Irritation of the skin and mucous membranes and gastroenteritis are another set of signs typical of trichothecene toxicosis. Hemorrhagic diathesis can occur, and the radiomimetic injury (damage to dividing cells) is expressed as lymphopenia or pancytopenia. Eventually, hypotension may lead to death. Many of the severe effects described for experimental trichothecene toxicosis are due to dosing by gavage. From a practical perspective, high concentrations of trichothecenes often cause feed refusal and therefore are often self-limiting as a toxic problem.

Because of the immunosuppressive action of trichothecenes, secondary bacterial, viral, or parasitic infections may mask the primary injury. The lymphatic organs are smaller than normal and may be difficult to find on necropsy.

Refusal to consume contaminated feedstuffs is the typical sign, which limits development of other signs. If no other food is offered, animals may eat reluctantly, but in some instances, excessive salivation and vomiting may occur. In the past, the ability to cause vomiting had been ascribed to DON only (hence the common name vomitoxin). However, other members of the trichothecene family also can induce vomiting.

In North America and many other parts of the world, DON is a substantial concern because of its common occurrence in feed grains and its well-known ability to cause feed refusal. Swine appear to be most sensitive to feed refusal, with greater tolerance by horses and dogs and even higher acceptance by ruminants.

In swine, reduced feed intake may occur at dietary concentrations as low as 1 ppm, and refusal may be complete at 10 ppm. Ruminants generally will readily consume as much as 10 ppm dietary vomitoxin, and beef cattle have tolerated 12–20 ppm in some circumstances. Poultry may tolerate as much as 100 ppm. Horses may accept as much as 35–45 ppm dietary DON without feed refusal or adverse clinical effects. Dogs also will refuse foods containing DON, usually at concentrations >5 ppm. Related effects of weight loss, hypoproteinemia, and weakness may follow prolonged feed refusal. There is little evidence that DON causes reproductive dysfunction in domestic animals. Experimental studies suggest that DON may cause variable effects of immunosuppression or immunostimulation, but research is continuing to define whether DON has a practical role in disease susceptibility in field conditions.

Feed refusal caused by DON is a learned response known as taste aversion. The major effect of DON is feed refusal; it is rarely if ever a cause of the trichothecene effects described above. It appears related to brain neurochemical changes in serotonin, dopamine, and 5-hydroxyindoleacetic acid. Feed refusal response to DON varies widely among species. DON in swine causes conditioned taste aversion, and swine appear to recognize new flavors (eg, flavoring agents) added to DON-containing feed and thus develop aversion to the new taste as well. Once uncontaminated feed is provided, animals usually resume eating within 1–2 days. A less well-known mycotoxin, fusaric acid, appears to interact with DON in the neurochemical response, leading to feed refusal.

Confirmation of increased levels of DON by analysis in a ration is often used to confirm DON-related feed refusal or to judge the fitness of a feed ingredient. However, some mycotoxins may be "masked" or undetected by routine assay methods. These conjugated mycotoxins may escape detection and not provide adequate warning of feed refusal levels. Use of binders for DON mycotoxin is currently an active area of research. Currently, the aluminosilicates effective for aflatoxins appear not to be useful against DON. Glucomannan yeast-derived adsorbents may have potential to improve some aspects of DON feed refusal in swine, but work is ongoing to clarify use of this category of detoxicants. DON has been removed from barley by an abrasive pearling procedure, which removed two-thirds of DON with loss of only 15% of the grain mass. This and other forms of cleaning grain may prove useful to decrease DON when alternative grain is not available. In addition, diverting grain from swine to the more tolerable ruminants is an alternative as well.

Macrocyclic trichothecene–related diseases have received a number of specific names. The best known is **stachybotryotoxicosis** of horses, cattle, sheep, pigs, and poultry, first diagnosed in the former USSR but occurring also in Europe and South Africa. Cutaneous and mucocutaneous lesions, panleukopenia, nervous signs, and abortions have been seen. Death may occur in 2–12 days.

Myrotheciotoxicosis and **dendrodochiotoxicosis** have been reported from the former USSR and New Zealand. The signs resemble those of stachybotryotoxicosis, but death may occur in 1–5 days.

Diagnosis: Because the clinical signs are nonspecific, or masked by secondary infections and disease, diagnosis is difficult. Analysis of feed is often costly and time consuming but ideally should be attempted. Interim measures are carefully examining feedstuffs for signs of mold growth or caking of feed particles and switching to an alternative feed supply. Change of feed supply often results in improvement and thus may provide one more clue that the original feed was contaminated.

Control: Symptomatic treatment and feeding of uncontaminated feed are recommended. Steroidal antishock and anti-inflammatory agents, such as methylprednisolone, prednisolone, and dexamethasone, have been used successfully in experimental trials. Poultry and cattle are more tolerant of trichothecenes than are pigs. Pigs exposed to DON often recover appetite promptly when uncontaminated feed is offered.

DON-contaminated feed treated with various adsorbents, including calcium aluminosilicates, bentonite, sodium bisulfite, and yeast-based glucomannans have not been helpful to correct feed refusal in swine. Addition of 0.2% glucomannan mycotoxin adsorbent to DON-contaminated diet for pregnant sows increased percentage of pigs born live but did not correct reduced feed intake. Physical seed treatment (abrasive pearling procedure) has removed two-thirds of DON from barley. In general, cleaning and removal of damaged grain (screenings) improves feed quality and acceptance of mycotoxin-contaminated grains.

SMOKE INHALATION

Smoke inhalation caused by fires is a major cause of fatalities in animals. It usually involves inhalation of a complex mixture of toxicologic agents and pyrolysis products. Injury typically results from a combination of thermal injury to the upper airways, oxygen deprivation, and toxicity from inhaled materials. Smaller animals and in particular birds are usually more susceptible to inhaled toxicants because of their greater respiratory minute volume per unit mass and relatively larger respiratory surface area per unit mass.

Etiology: Important agents involved in smoke inhalation include thermal injury, soot, carbon monoxide, cyanide gas, nitrogen, methane, oxides of nitrogen (NO_x), zinc oxide, phosphorus, sulfur trioxide, titanium tetrachloride, oil fog, Teflon® particles, and Teflon® pyrolysis products (polymer fume fever). Nitrogen and methane are not especially toxic; however, they are important in fires because they dilute oxygen in the breathable atmosphere.

Inhalation thermal injury can occur without obvious external injuries and be relatively slow to manifest, so it is often clinically underestimated. Airway compromise generally peaks 12–24 hr after initial injury. Except for steam inhalation and possibly inhalation of particles with continuing pyrolysis, inhalation thermal injuries are usually confined to the upper airways because of their large heat capacitance. Burns of the upper airway typically induce upper airway edema. Loss of oncotic pressure and fluid resuscitation can exacerbate these effects. Inhalation of steam typically produces severe lung injuries.

Carbonaceous soot particles are not especially toxic in themselves. However, they act as carriers of other toxicants adsorbed onto the surfaces of soot particles. This results in increased toxicant exposure and, depending on particle size, deeper penetration of toxicants into the respiratory system. The degree and site of damage depends on particle size, particle surface area, solubility, concentration, duration of exposure, and rate of particle clearance. Large, chemically reactive and irritating particles tend to affect the upper airways and are cleared quickly, whereas smaller, low-solubility particles tend to affect the deeper respiratory structures and are cleared more slowly.

Important inhaled blood agents/asphyxiants that disrupt tissue oxygen delivery or utilization include cyanide, carbon monoxide, nitrogen, and methane. Cyanide inhalation is extremely common with smoke inhalation. Essentially, pyrolysis of most nitrogen-containing materials (eg, nitrocellulose, nylon, wool, silk, asphalt, polyurethane, and many plastics) will liberate cyanide. Cyanide is a rapidly acting histotoxic agent that inhibits mitochondrial cytochrome c oxidase, resulting in the arrest of aerobic metabolism. (*See also* CYANIDE POISONING, p 2959.)

Carbon monoxide poisoning is ubiquitous after smoke inhalation. Carbon monoxide is produced by the incomplete combustion of any organic material. Carbon monoxide binds to hemoglobin to form carboxyhemoglobin, which cannot carry oxygen and, therefore, results in tissue hypoxia. A visible flame is not necessary for carbon monoxide poisoning, and gas appliances can liberate large amounts of it. Epizootics of fatal carbon monoxide poisoning classically occur during periods of cold weather, particularly after an electrical outage.

NO_X have low water solubility, and low concentrations generally cause delayed pulmonary irritation. Also, compared with other agents, the NO_2 present in NO_X reacts relatively slowly with respiratory secretions, forming nitrous (HNO_2) and nitric (HNO_3) acid. The end result is delayed chemical pneumonitis and pulmonary edema. These features often result in delayed clinical recognition of NO_X injuries.

Zinc oxide fumes are a classical cause of metal fume fever and are formed when zinc or zinc alloys (eg, galvanized metals, brass) are heated. Metal fume fever is a classical cytokine cascade acute phase–like response. Notably, tolerance to zinc oxide fumes develops rapidly but is also quickly lost.

Phosphorous, titanium tetrachloride, and sulfur trioxide fumes are notoriously irritating. Titanium tetrachloride releases hydrochloric acid in contact with water in respiratory secretions. Inhaled sulfur trioxide forms sulfuric acid when it contacts respiratory secretions. Smoke machines that atomize mineral oils can produce an oil mist that is mildly irritating to the respiratory system and may trigger underlying respiratory conditions.

Inhalation of PTFE (Teflon®) fumes triggers acute malaise, fever, and respiratory irritation (polymer fume fever). It can result in severe chemical pneumonitis and is notoriously lethal for caged birds. In addition to overheated cooking ware, Teflon® fume fever has been caused by burning of hair spray, dry lubricants, and water-proofing sprays.

Clinical Findings: The most important aspects of the history are duration of exposure, the circumstances of exposure (eg, enclosed versus open spaces), amount of smoke inhaled, severity of injury to other animals, and the sources of the smoke (ie, what toxicants are likely to have been present in the smoke). Unfortunately, this type of information is rarely available. Exposure to smoke in an enclosed space, prolonged entrapment, carbonaceous oculonasal discharges, a history of resuscitation, evidence of respiratory distress, and altered consciousness all indicate a higher risk of serious lung damage. Preexisting respiratory diseases (eg, COPD) will likely increase the severity of injury.

Clinically serious smoke inhalation often occurs in the absence of obvious external physical injury. However, facial burns, oropharyngeal blistering and/or edema, changed voice, stridor, coughing, upper airway mucosal lesions, and carbonaceous discharges may be present. Evidence of lower respiratory tract injury such as tachypnea, dyspnea, cough, decreased breath sounds, wheezing, rales, rhonchi, and retractions may be present. Both upper and lower respiratory injury may be relatively slow to develop and may peak 12–24 hr or even later after exposure. There is always a substantial risk of delayed airway obstruction secondary to upper airway edema for at least 24–48 hr after initial injury. Lack of apparent injury immediately after smoke inhalation should not reduce the level of clinical suspicion.

In general, evidence of asphyxiant exposure commonly includes CNS depression, changes in affect, lethargy, generalized muscle weakness, and obtundation. Neurologic injury secondary to hypoxia, often permanent, is common under these circumstances. Coma after smoke inhalation is most commonly caused by severe carbon monoxide poisoning and the ensuing hypoxia. The prognosis is poor.

The onset of zinc oxide fume fever is typically delayed by 4–8 hr after exposure. Common clinical signs include general malaise, cough, sternal pain, voice changes, and fever. Typically, these signs are self-limiting, and recovery is rapid unless high levels of exposure have occurred. In these cases, there is often an apparent period of recovery followed by onset of dyspnea and respiratory distress 24–36 hr later.

Polymer (Teflon®) fume fever typically presents as general malaise, cough, sternal pain, voice changes, and fever. Severe lung injuries are common in birds, and sudden death is a common outcome.

Diagnosis: Important diagnostic techniques include laryngoscopy/bronchoscopy, pulse oximetry/co-oximetry, arterial blood gases, carboxyhemoglobin level determination, lactate level determination, CBCs, chest imaging, electrocardiography, and pulmonary function testing.

Bronchoscopy and laryngoscopy are the gold standard methods to diagnose and assess smoke inhalation. Bronchoscopy is the single most reliable method to establish the diagnosis and extent/severity of injury. It is generally superior to and more accurate than other diagnostic methods (including clinical examination). Classic findings include severe subglottic injury, erythema, charring, deposition of soot, edema, and/or mucosal ulceration.

Ordinary pulse oximetry (two wavelengths) is inaccurate when carboxyhemoglobin and/or methemoglobin are present. Both situations will generate falsely high pulse oximetry readings that are not reflective of the degree of underlying disease. Pulse co-oximetry (four or five wavelengths) is more reliable in these situations.

PaO_2 is a poor indicator of carbon monoxide poisoning and/or cellular hypoxia, because it reflects the amount of oxygen dissolved in blood. This is not altered in carbon monoxide poisoning, because the dissolved oxygen is a small fraction of total arterial blood oxygen content. Because blood gas machines usually calculate oxygen saturation based on PaO_2, this measurement will also be inaccurate.

Blood carboxyhemoglobin measurements may underestimate the actual level of exposure if oxygen has been administered before sample collection. Additionally, there is a poor correlation between carboxyhemoglobin level and the ultimate neurologic outcome in cases of significant poisoning.

Metabolic acidosis and increased lactate is common when hypoxia, carboxyhemoglobin, cyanide poisoning, methemoglobinemia, and trauma are present. Very high blood lactate levels are typical in acute cyanide poisoning. Given the usually slow turnaround time associated with cyanide measurements, high levels of blood lactate combined with a history of smoke inhalation provide a strong index of suspicion of cyanide poisoning. Cyanide measurements are strongly correlated with exposure and toxicity levels.

Clinically significant smoke inhalation is often associated with declines in hemoglobin and PCV approximately 1 wk after exposure.

Pulmonary radiographic changes after smoke inhalation typically develop 24–36 hr after exposure. An initially clear chest radiograph does not exclude significant lung injury after smoke inhalation. Repeat imaging at 24–36 hr after exposure typically demonstrates radiographic signs consistent with atelectasis, pulmonary edema, and hyperinflation. Depending on the agents involved, late radiographic changes may reflect fibrosis and bronchiolitis obliterans.

CT changes typically develop earlier than chest radiographic changes and classically consist of peribronchial ground-glass opacities and peribronchial consolidations. Brain CT findings may demonstrate cerebral hypoxia–associated ischemia and injuries to the globus pallidus, which are nearly pathognomonic for carbon monoxide poisoning.

Treatment, Control, and Prevention: Treatment involves maintenance of the airway, aggressive management of acute respiratory distress, antidote treatment if warranted, suppression of inflammation, and prevention of secondary infections with broad spectrum antibiotics. Severe carbon monoxide poisoning combined with significant smoke inhalation is almost uniformly fatal in people; thus, euthanasia should be considered early in the treatment and assessment processes.

Maintenance of the airway either by endotracheal intubation or tracheostomy is often critical given that severe upper airway edema may occur. It is often better to intubate earlier in the disease progression, because delayed airway edema may subsequently make intubation difficult or impossible.

Carbon monoxide poisoning should always be assumed to have occurred in all individuals with smoke inhalation. The mainstay of treatment is oxygen supplementation.

Some degree of cyanide poisoning should also be assumed in almost all cases of smoke inhalation. Induction of methemoglobinemia is not recommended in cases of smoke inhalation because of the risk of further reducing oxygen-carrying capacity of the blood in the presence of carboxyhemoglobinemia. Because of its efficacy, ease of administration, and low toxicity, hydroxocobalamin administration is currently recommended in cases of smoke inhalation. Hydroxocobalamin can be combined with thiosulfate administration. Data are limited on the effectiveness of thiosulfate alone; however, it is useful in cyanide poisoning and will not compromise oxygen-carrying capacity of the blood (ie, unlikely to cause harm and may be beneficial).

Methemoglobinemia after smoke inhalation is uncommon and can be managed with methylene blue treatment if required.

Notably, *N*-acetylcysteine has been effective for the treatment of polymer fume fever. Chest physiotherapy is regarded as being beneficial. Low tidal volume positive-pressure ventilation (PEEP) and high-frequency percussive ventilation (HFPV) have been demonstrated to increase short-term survival in people but are rarely available in veterinary practice.

Bronchodilation with a β_2-agonist (eg, albuterol, terbutaline, epinephrine) is an important aspect of treatment, because smoke induces bronchospasm and bronchoconstriction. When combined with airway edema, these effects contribute to airway obstruction.

The effectiveness of corticosteroids after smoke inhalation is contentious. Corticosteroids are notably beneficial in cases of metal fume fever.

Control and prevention of smoke inhalation involves avoidance of exposure, adequate ventilation if smoke is likely to be present, and use of smoke detection systems.

TOXICITIES FROM HUMAN DRUGS

TOXICITIES FROM OVER-THE-COUNTER DRUGS

Human drugs or nutritional supplements available without a prescription are known as over-the-counter (OTC) medications. Exposures to OTC drugs in pets can be accidental or intentional. A valid client-patient-veterinarian relationship must exist for veterinarians to recommend extra-label use of these drugs to their clients. Most are not approved for veterinary use by the FDA, and safety of most OTC drugs has not been determined in animals. Veterinarians should understand the potential risks of using OTC medications and communicate these risks to their clients.

COLD AND COUGH MEDICATIONS

Antihistamines

Antihistamines are H_1-receptor antagonists that provide symptomatic relief of allergic signs caused by histamine release, including pruritus and anaphylactic reactions. They are also used as sedatives and antiemetics. Antihistamines belong to different classes and are categorized as first- or second-generation (also called nonsedating) antihistamines. First-generation antihistamines may cause adverse effects because of their cholinergic activity and ability to cross the blood-brain barrier. Second-generation antihistamines are more lipophobic than first-generation antihistamines and are thought to lack CNS and cholinergic effects at therapeutic doses. Antihistamines are often found in combination with other ingredients (eg, decongestants, analgesics like acetaminophen or NSAIDs) in many OTC cold, sinus, and allergy medications.

Chlorpheniramine is a first-generation propylamine-derivative antihistamine. Oral absorption of chlorpheniramine in dogs is rapid and complete, reaching peak plasma concentrations in 30–60 min. Chlorpheniramine maleate undergoes substantial first-pass effect. Chlorpheniramine and its metabolites are primarily excreted in urine. The recommended dose in cats and dogs is 1–2 mg and 2–8 mg respectively, PO, bid-tid. Mild clinical signs such as depression and GI upset have been reported for dosages <1 mg/kg. Significant clinical signs such as ataxia, tremors, depression or hyperactivity, hyperthermia, and seizures may be seen within 6 hr of ingestion of large amounts.

Clemestine, because of its low oral bioavailability in dogs (3% vs 20%–70% in people), may have limited effectiveness at the recommended dosages of 0.05–0.1 mg/kg, PO, bid; 1.34 mg of clemestine fumerate is equivalent to 1 mg of clemestine. Common adverse effects of clemestine may include sedation, lethargy, and anticholinergic signs (dry mouth, tachycardia, agitation, decreased intestinal secretions/motility).

Dimenhydrinate and **diphenhydramine** are first-generation ethanolamine-derivative antihistamines. Dimenhydrinate is used for its antiemetic effects and for prevention of motion sickness in dogs and cats. Diphenhydramine is well absorbed orally in people but undergoes first-pass metabolism in the liver with only 40%–60% of the drug reaching the systemic circulation. Peak plasma concentrations of ethanolamine-derivative antihistamines occur within 1–5 hr; elimination half-lives vary from 2.4–10 hr. A recommended dosage of dimenhydrinate and diphenhydramine in cats and dogs is 4–8 mg/kg and 2–4 mg/kg, respectively. Hyperactivity or depression, hypersalivation, tachypnea, and tachycardia are the most common adverse effects reported with these antihistamines, generally within 1 hr of exposure.

Promethazine hydrochloride is an ethylamino derivative of phenothiazine and first-generation antihistamine used to manage motion sickness. Promethazine is widely distributed in body tissues and readily crosses the placenta. Overdoses may result in CNS depression or excitation. CNS depression was reported in a dog 30 min after ingesting promethazine at 1 mg/kg.

Meclizine is a first-generation piperazine-derivative antihistamine commonly used as an antiemetic. Peak plasma concentrations occur within 2–3 hr of oral administration. Meclizine is primarily excreted as metabolites in urine, with a reported serum half-life of 6 hr. The recommended dose in dogs is 25 mg/day (per dog). When dogs have received meclizine at <33 mg/kg, only mild hyperactivity or depression has been reported.

Loratadine is a tricyclic, long-acting antihistamine with selective peripheral histamine H_1-receptor antagonist activity. In people, loratadine is well absorbed orally and extensively metabolized to an active metabolite. Most of the parent drug is excreted unchanged in the urine. The mean elimination half-life in people is 8.4 hr. Loratadine appears to have a large margin of safety in animals. The suggested dose in dogs is 5–10 mg, PO, once to twice daily (per dog). No deaths were reported at oral dosages up to 5 g/kg in rats and mice. In rats, mice, and monkeys, no clinical signs were seen at 10 times the maximum recommended human daily oral dose.

Cetirizine, a major metabolite of hydroxyzine, is a piperazine derivative nonsedating antihistamine. It selectively inhibits peripheral H_1 receptors and does not have significant anticholinergic or antiserotonergic effects when used at the recommended dosage. The recommended dosage for histamine-mediated pruritic conditions in dogs is 1 mg/kg, PO, once to twice daily, and 5 mg, PO, bid for cats. The drug appears to be well tolerated in dogs and cats. The minimum lethal dosage is 237 mg/kg in mice and 562 mg/kg in rats. Adverse reactions include vomiting, hypersalivation, sedation, drowsiness, and occasionally hyperactivity.

Treatment: Treatment of antihistamine toxicosis is primarily symptomatic and supportive. Emesis should only be considered in asymptomatic patients. Activated charcoal may be useful for recent ingestion. Symptomatic patients should be watched for anticholinergic signs (agitation, mydriasis, tachycardia, decreased intestinal motility) and treated as needed. Cardiovascular functions (heart rate and blood pressure) and body temperature should be closely monitored. Propranolol (0.02-0.06 mg/kg, IV) can be helpful to treat consistent tachycardia in normotensive patients. Diazepam can be used to control seizures or seizure-type activity. Physostigmine is recommended to counteract the CNS anticholinergic effects of antihistamine overdoses in people, although the risk of seizures associated with this drug may limit its use. IV fluids should be given as needed.

Dextromethorphan

Dextromethorphan is a nonsedating, nonaddictive, centrally acting opioid cough suppressant. It is available in many OTC cold and cough medications. At the recommended dosage, it enhances the threshold for coughing. It is rapidly absorbed orally and converts to the active metabolite dextrorphan in the liver. Cough suppressant activity can last 3–12 hr, depending on the formulation. Overdoses can cause CNS and GI effects such as agitation, hallucination, nervousness, mydriasis, shaking, vomiting, or diarrhea. Some clinical signs may be similar to those of serotonin syndrome (agitation, disorientation, hyperthermia, nervousness, shaking). Treatment is mainly supportive care. Diazepam can be used to control some of the CNS effects. Phenothiazine tranquilizers (acepromazine or chlorpromazine) or cyproheptadine (1.1 mg/kg, PO or per rectum, for dogs, and 2–4 mg per cat; repeat once in 6–8 hr if needed) can be given for serotonin syndrome.

DECONGESTANTS

Imidazoline Decongestants

The imidazoline derivatives, **oxymetazoline**, **xylometazoline**, **tetrahydrozoline**, and **naphazoline**, are found in topical ophthalmic and nasal decongestants available OTC. They are generally used as *topical* vasoconstrictors in the nose and eyes for temporary relief of nasal congestion due to colds, hay fever or other upper respiratory allergies, or sinusitis.

Imidazolines are sympathomimetic agents, with primary effects on α-adrenergic receptors and little if any effect on β-adrenergic receptors. Oxymetazoline is readily absorbed orally. Effects on α-receptors from systemically absorbed oxymetazoline hydrochloride may persist for up to 7 hr after a single dose. The elimination half-life in people is 5–8 hr. It is excreted unchanged both by the kidneys (30%) and in feces (10%).

Clinical Findings: In dogs, signs of intoxication may include vomiting, bradycardia, cardiac arrhythmias, poor capillary refill time, hypotension or hypertension, panting, increased upper respiratory sounds, depression, weakness, collapse, nervousness, hyperactivity, or shaking. These signs usually appear within 30 min to 4 hr after exposure. In general, imidazoline decongestant exposure may affect the GI, cardiopulmonary, and nervous systems.

Treatment: Decontamination (induction of emesis and administration of activated charcoal) may not be practical because of the rapid absorption and onset of clinical signs. Heart rate and rhythm and blood pressure should be assessed, and an ECG obtained if needed. IV fluids should be given, along with atropine at 0.02 mg/kg, IV, if bradycardia is present. Diazepam (0.25–0.5 mg/kg, IV) can be given if CNS signs (eg, apprehension, shaking) are present. Serum electrolytes (ie, potassium, sodium, chloride) should be assessed and corrected as needed. Yohimbine, a specific α_2-adrenergic antagonist, can also be used at 0.1 mg/kg, IV, and repeated in 2–3 hr if needed. If yohimbine is not available, atipamezole can be used at 50 mcg/kg, one-fourth IV and the rest IM; it can be repeated in 30–60 min if there is no improvement.

Phenylephrine

Phenylephrine is a sympathomimetic amine with mainly an α_1-adrenergic receptor agonist effect, available OTC as a decongestant in oral formulations (5–10 mg tablets), nasal sprays, or eye drops (0.25%–1%). It has poor oral bioavailability (38%) in people because of a significant first-pass effect and extensive metabolism by monoamine oxidases in the GI tract and liver. The oral LD_{50} in rats and mice is 350 mg/kg and 120 mg/kg, respectively. The half-life is 2–3 hr. CNS stimulation, agitation, nervousness, and hypertension are possible but less frequent with phenylephrine than with pseudoephedrine. Treatment is mainly symptomatic care and is similar to that for pseudoephedrine toxicosis (*see* below).

Pseudoephedrine and Ephedrine

Pseudoephedrine is a sympathomimetic drug found naturally in plants of the genus *Ephedra*. Several states in the USA have limited the availability and use of pseudoephedrine as an OTC decongestant because of its use as a precursor in illegal amphetamine synthesis. It is being replaced with other decongestants such as phenylephrine.

Pseudoephedrine is a stereoisomer of ephedrine and is available as the hydrochloride or sulfate salt. Both ephedrine and pseudoephedrine have α- and β-adrenergic agonist effects. The pharmacologic effects of the drugs are due to direct stimulation of adrenergic receptors and the release of norepinephrine.

In people, pseudoephedrine is rapidly absorbed orally. The onset of action is 15–30 min, with peak effects within 30–60 min. With extended-release preparations (12–24 hr), onset of clinical signs can be delayed (2–8 hr) and duration of clinical signs can be longer than with regular preparations. It is incompletely metabolized in the liver. Approximately 90% of the drug is eliminated through the kidneys. Renal excretion is accelerated in acidic urine. Elimination half-life varies between 2–21 hr, depending on urinary pH.

Clinical Findings: Pseudoephedrine and ephedrine overdose can result in mainly sympathomimetic effects, including agitation, hyperactivity, mydriasis, tachycardia, hypertension, sinus arrhythmias, anxiety, tremors, hyperthermia, head bobbing, hiding, and vomiting. Clinical signs can be seen at dosages of 5–6 mg/kg, and death may occur at 10–12 mg/kg.

Treatment: Treatment of pseudoephedrine toxicosis consists of decontamination, controlling the CNS and cardiovascular effects, and supportive care. Vomiting should be induced only in asymptomatic patients, followed by administration of activated charcoal with a cathartic. If the animal's condition contraindicates induction of emesis, a gastric lavage with a cuffed endotracheal tube should be performed. Hyperactivity, nervousness, or seizures can be controlled with acepromazine (0.05–1 mg/kg, IM, IV, or SC), chlorpromazine (0.5–1 mg/kg, IV), phenobarbital (3–4 mg/kg, IV), or pentobarbital to effect. Diazepam should be avoided, because it can exaggerate hyperactivity. Phenothiazines should be used with caution because they can lower the seizure threshold, lower blood pressure, and cause bizarre behavioral changes. Tachycardia can be controlled with propranolol at 0.02–0.04 mg/kg, IV, repeated if needed, or with esmolol at 0.2–0.5 mg/kg, given slowly IV or as a constant-rate infusion at 25–200 mcg/kg/min. IV fluids should be given. Acidifying the urine with ammonium chloride (50 mg/kg, PO, qid) or ascorbic acid (20–30 mg/kg, IM or IV, tid) may enhance urinary excretion of pseudoephedrine. Acid-base status should be monitored if ammonium chloride or ascorbic acid is given. Electrolytes, heart rate and rhythm, and blood pressure should be monitored. Excessive trembling or shaking can cause myoglobinuria; if this occurs, kidney function should be monitored. Significant and persistent hyperthermia due to severe hyperactivity and CNS excitation could result in disseminated intravascular coagulation. Clinical signs of toxicosis can last 1–4 days. The presence of pseudoephedrine in urine can support the diagnosis.

ANALGESICS

Over-the-Counter Nonsteroidal Anti-inflammatory Drugs

NSAIDs are the most commonly used class of human medications in the world. Because of their widespread availability and use, acute accidental ingestion of human NSAIDs in dogs and cats is quite common. Ibuprofen, aspirin, and naproxen are some of the most commonly encountered NSAIDs in pet animals.

NSAIDs inhibit the enzyme cyclooxygenase (COX; also referred to as prostaglandin synthetase), blocking the production of prostaglandins. It is believed that most NSAIDs act through COX inhibition, although they may also have other mechanisms of action. (*See also* p 2714.)

Ibuprofen, 2-(4-isobutylphenyl) propionic acid, is used for its anti-inflammatory, antipyretic, and analgesic properties in animals and people. It is rapidly absorbed orally in dogs, with peak plasma concentrations seen in 30 min to 3 hr. Presence of food can delay absorption and the time to reach peak plasma concentration. The mean elimination half-life is ~4.6 hr. Ibuprofen is metabolized in the liver to several metabolites, which are mainly excreted in the urine within 24 hr. The major metabolic pathway is via conjugation with glucuronic acid, sometimes preceded by oxidation and hydroxylation.

Ibuprofen has been recommended in dogs at 5 mg/kg. However, prolonged use at this dosage may cause gastric ulcers and perforations. GI irritation or ulceration, GI hemorrhage, and renal damage are the most commonly reported toxic effects of ibuprofen ingestion in dogs. In addition, CNS depression, hypotension, ataxia, cardiac effects, and seizures can be seen. Ibuprofen has a narrow margin of safety in dogs. Dogs dosed with ibuprofen at 8–16 mg/kg/day, PO for 30 days, showed gastric ulceration or erosions, along with other clinical signs of GI disturbances. An acute single ingestion of 100–125 mg/kg can lead to vomiting, diarrhea, nausea, abdominal pain, and anorexia. Renal failure may follow dosages of 175–300 mg/kg. CNS effects (ie, seizures, ataxia, depression, coma) in addition to renal and GI signs can be seen at dosages >400 mg/kg. Dosages >600 mg/kg are potentially lethal in dogs.

Cats are susceptible to ibuprofen toxicosis at approximately half the dosage required to cause toxicosis in dogs. Cats are especially sensitive, because they have limited glucuronyl-conjugating capacity. Ibuprofen toxicity is more severe in ferrets than in dogs that consume similar dosages. Typical toxic effects of ibuprofen in ferrets involve the CNS, GI, and renal systems.

Aspirin (acetylsalicylic acid), the salicylate ester of acetic acid, is the prototype of salicylate drugs. It is a weak acid derived from phenol. The oral bioavailability of aspirin may vary because of differences in drug formulation. Aspirin reduces prostaglandin and thromboxane synthesis by COX inhibition. Salicylates also uncouple mitochondrial oxidative phosphorylation and inhibit specific dehydrogenases. Platelets are incapable of synthesizing new cyclooxgenase, leading to an effect on platelet aggregation.

Aspirin is rapidly absorbed from the stomach and proximal small intestine in monogastric animals. The rate of absorption depends on gastric emptying, tablet disintegration rates, and gastric pH. Peak salicylate levels are reached 0.5–3 hr after ingestion. Topically applied salicylic acid can be absorbed systemically.

Aspirin is hydrolyzed to salicylic acid by esterases in the liver and, to a lesser extent, in the GI mucosa, plasma, RBCs, and synovial fluid. Salicylic acid is 50%–70% protein bound, especially to albumin. Salicylic acid readily distributes to extracellular fluids and to the kidneys, liver, lungs, and heart. Salicylic acid is eliminated by hepatic conjugation with glucuronide and glycine. Renal clearance is enhanced by an alkaline urinary pH. There are significant differences in the elimination and biotransformation of salicylates among different species. Plasma half-lives vary from 1–37.6 hr in animals.

Aspirin toxicosis is usually characterized by depression, fever, hyperpnea, seizures, respiratory alkalosis, metabolic acidosis, coma, gastric irritation or ulceration, liver necrosis, or increased bleeding time. Seizures may occur as a consequence of severe intoxication, although the exact cause is unknown.

Cats are deficient in glucuronyl transferase and have a prolonged excretion of aspirin (half-life 37.5 hr). No clinical signs of toxicosis occurred when cats were given aspirin at 25 mg/kg every 48 hr for up to 4 wk. Dosages of 5 grains (325 mg), bid, can be lethal to cats.

Dogs tolerate aspirin better than cats; however, prolonged use can lead to development of gastric ulcers. Regular aspirin at dosages of 25 mg/kg, tid, has caused mucosal erosions in 50% of dogs after 2 days. Gastric ulcers were seen by day 30 in 66% of dogs given aspirin at 35 mg/kg, PO, tid. Similarly, 43% of dogs given aspirin at 50 mg/kg, PO, bid, showed gastric ulcers after 5–6 wk of dosing. Acute ingestion of 450–500 mg/kg can cause GI disturbances, hyperthermia, panting, seizures, or coma. Alkalosis due to stimulation of the respiratory center can occur early in the course of intoxication. Metabolic acidosis with an increased anion gap usually develops later.

Naproxen, a propionic acid–derivative NSAID, is available OTC as an acid or the sodium salt. It is available as tablets or gel caps (200–550 mg) or as a suspension (125 mg/5 mL). Structurally and pharmacologically, naproxen is similar to carprofen and ibuprofen. In people and dogs, it is used for its anti-inflammatory, analgesic, and antipyretic properties.

Oral absorption of naproxen in dogs is rapid, with peak plasma concentration reached in 0.5–3 hr. The reported elimination half-life in dogs is 34–72 hr. Naproxen is highly protein bound (>99%). In dogs, naproxen is primarily eliminated through the bile, whereas in other species, the primary route of elimination is through the kidneys. The long half-life of naproxen in dogs appears to be because of its extensive enterohepatic recirculation.

Several cases of naproxen toxicosis in dogs have been reported. Dosages of

5.6–11.1 mg/kg, PO, for 3–7 days have caused melena, frequent vomiting, abdominal pain, perforating duodenal ulcer, weakness, stumbling, pale mucous membranes, regenerative anemia, neutrophilia with a left shift, increased BUN and creatinine, and decreased total protein. Acute toxicity from a single oral dose of 35 mg/kg has been reported. Cats may be more sensitive to naproxen toxicity than dogs because of their limited glucuronyl-conjugating capacity.

Treatment: Treatment of NSAID toxicosis consists of early decontamination, protection of the GI tract and kidneys, and supportive care. Vomiting should be induced in recent exposures, followed by administration of activated charcoal with a cathartic. Activated charcoal can be repeated in 6–8 hr to prevent NSAID reabsorption from enterohepatic recirculation. Use of H_2-receptor antagonists (ranitidine, famotidine, cimetidine) may not prevent GI ulcers but can be useful in treating them. Omeprazole, a proton-pump inhibitor used to inhibit gastric acid secretions, can be used instead of an H_2 blocker at 0.5–1 mg/kg/day, PO, in dogs. Sucralfate (dogs: 0.5–1 g, PO, bid-tid; cats: 0.25–0.5 tablet, PO, bid-tid) reacts with hydrochloric acid in the stomach and forms a paste-like complex that binds to the proteins in ulcers and protects them from further damage. Because sucralfate requires an acidic environment, it should be given ≥30 min before administering H_2 antagonists. Misoprostol (dogs: 1–3 mcg/kg, PO, tid) has been shown to prevent GI ulceration when used concomitantly with aspirin and other NSAIDs.

IV fluids should be given at a diuretic rate if the potential for renal damage exists. Alkalinization of the urine with sodium bicarbonate results in ion trapping of salicylates in kidney tubules and can increase their excretion. However, ion trapping should be used judiciously and only in cases when the acid-base balance can be monitored closely. Baseline renal function should be monitored and rechecked at 24, 48, and 72 hr. Prognosis depends on the dose ingested and how soon the animal receives treatment after exposure.

Acetaminophen

Acetaminophen is a synthetic nonopiate derivative of p-aminophenol widely used in people for its antipyretic and analgesic properties. Its use has largely replaced salicylates because of the reduced risk of gastric ulceration.

Acetaminophen is rapidly absorbed from the GI tract. Peak plasma concentrations are usually seen within an hour but can be delayed with extended-release formulations. It is uniformly distributed into most body tissues. Protein binding varies from 5%–20%. The metabolism of acetaminophen involves two major conjugation pathways in most species. Both involve cytochrome P450 metabolism, followed by glucuronidation or sulfation.

Cats are more sensitive to acetaminophen toxicosis, because they are deficient in glucuronyl transferase and therefore have limited capacity to glucuronidate this drug. In cats, acetaminophen is primarily metabolized via sulfation; when this pathway is saturated, toxic metabolites are produced. In dogs, signs of acute toxicity are usually not seen unless the dosage of acetaminophen exceeds 100 mg/kg. Clinical signs of methemoglobinemia have been reported in 3 of 4 dogs at 200 mg/kg. Toxicity can be seen at lower dosages with repeated exposures. In cats, toxicity can occur with 10–40 mg/kg.

Methemoglobinemia and hepatotoxicity characterize acetaminophen toxicosis. Renal injury is also possible. Acute keratoconjunctivitis sicca has been reported in some dogs after acetaminophen ingestion. Cats primarily develop methemoglobinemia within a few hours, followed by Heinz body formation. Methemoglobinemia makes mucous membranes brown or muddy in color and is usually accompanied by tachycardia, hyperpnea, weakness, and lethargy. Other clinical signs of acetaminophen toxicity include depression, weakness, hyperventilation, icterus, vomiting, hypothermia, facial or paw edema, cyanosis, dyspnea, hepatic necrosis, and death. Liver necrosis is more common in dogs than in cats. Liver damage in dogs is usually seen 24–36 hr after ingestion. Centrilobular necrosis is the most common form of hepatic necrosis seen with acetaminophen toxicity.

Treatment: The objectives of treating acetaminophen toxicosis are early decontamination, prevention or treatment of methemoglobinemia and hepatic damage, and provision of supportive care. A Schirmer tear test (to confirm keratoconjunctivitis) can be used if necessary. Induction of emesis is useful when performed early. This should be followed by administration of activated charcoal with a cathartic. Activated charcoal may be repeated, because acetaminophen undergoes some enterohepatic recirculation.

Administration of *N*-acetylcysteine (NAC), a sulfur-containing amino acid, can reduce the extent of liver injury or methemoglobinemia. NAC provides sulfhydryl groups, directly binds with acetaminophen metabolites to enhance their elimination, and serves as a glutathione precursor. It is available as a 10% or 20% solution. The loading dose is 140 mg/kg of a 5% solution IV or PO (diluted in 5% dextrose or sterile water), followed by 70 mg/kg, PO, qid for generally seven or more treatments (some authors recommend up to 17 doses). Vomiting can occur with oral NAC. NAC is not labeled for IV use; however, it can be administered as a slow IV (over 15–20 min) with a 0.2-micron bacteriostatic filter. Activated charcoal and oral NAC should be administered 2 hr apart, because activated charcoal could adsorb NAC.

Liver enzymes should be monitored and rechecked at 24 and 48 hr. The animal should also be monitored for methemoglobinemia, Heinz body anemia, and hemolysis. Fluids and blood transfusions should be given as needed. Ascorbic acid (30 mg/kg, PO or injectable, bid-qid) may further reduce methemoglobin levels. Cimetidine (5–10 mg/kg, PO, IM, or IV), a cytochrome P450 inhibitor, may help reduce formation of toxic metabolites and prevent liver damage in dogs only. Cimetidine should not be used in cats. In vitro evidence indicates that use of cimetidine in cats can produce more toxic metabolites of acetaminophen. *S*-Adenosyl methionine has been suggested as an adjunct to manage acute or chronic hepatic injury at 18 mg/kg, PO, for 1–3 mo in dogs and cats.

GASTROINTESTINAL DRUGS

H_2-Receptor Antagonists

H_2-receptor antagonists are structural analogues of histamine, commonly used to treat GI ulcers, erosive gastritis, esophagitis, and gastric reflux. They act at the H_2 receptors of parietal cells to competitively inhibit histamine, reducing gastric acid secretions during basal conditions and when stimulated by food, amino acids, pentagastrin, histamine, or insulin. Cimetidine, famotidine, nizatidine, and *ranitidine* are examples of this group, also commonly referred to as H_2 blockers. These drugs are rapidly absorbed, reaching peak plasma concentrations within 1–3 hr. Ranitidine is widely distributed throughout the body. H_2 blockers are primarily metabolized in the liver. Nizatidine, famotidine, and ranitidine are excreted in the urine as metabolites and unchanged drug, whereas cimetidine is eliminated in feces. The elimination half-life for these drugs is short (~2.2 hr). Because cimetidine may inhibit the hepatic microsomal enzyme system, ingestion of an H_2 blocker may result in reduced metabolism of certain drugs, including β blockers, calcium channel blockers, diazepam, metronidazole, and theophylline.

H_2 blockers have a wide margin of safety, with acute oral overdoses typically resulting in minor effects such as vomiting, diarrhea, anorexia, and dry mouth. Serious adverse effects, such as tremors, hypotension, and bradycardia, are more likely to occur with IV H_2-blocker overdoses. The minimum lethal dose of famotidine in dogs is >2 g/kg, PO, and 300 mg/kg, IV. Single oral doses of nizatidine at 800 mg/kg in dogs were not lethal. Most exposures require only monitoring for development of GI signs and supportive care, although massive overdoses may also warrant decontamination.

Antacids

Antacids come in pill and liquid forms and are frequently used to treat GI upset. Common antacids include calcium carbonate, aluminum hydroxide, and magnesium hydroxide (milk of magnesia). These agents are poorly absorbed orally. Calcium- and aluminum-containing antacids generally cause constipation, whereas magnesium-containing antacids tend to cause diarrhea. Some products contain both aluminum and magnesium salts in an attempt to balance their constipating and laxative effects. Acute single ingestion of calcium salts may cause transient hypercalcemia but is unlikely to be associated with significant systemic effects. Induction of emesis within 2–3 hr of exposure may help prevent severe GI upset.

MULTIVITAMINS AND IRON

The common ingredients in multivitamins include ascorbic acid (vitamin C), cyanocobalamin (vitamin B_{12}), folic acid, thiamine (vitamin B_1), riboflavin (vitamin B_2), niacin (vitamin B_3), biotin, pantothenic acid, pyridoxine (vitamin B_6), calcium, phosphorus, iodine, iron, magnesium, copper, zinc, and vitamins A, D, and E. Among these ingredients, iron and vitamins

A and D may cause significant systemic signs. Acute ingestion of other listed ingredients in companion animals can result in self-limiting GI upset (eg, vomiting, diarrhea, anorexia, lethargy). However, toxicity is typically rare in pets.

Multivitamin preparations contain varying amounts of **iron**. Unless otherwise listed, iron should be assumed to be elemental iron. Various iron salts may contain 12%–48% elemental iron. Iron has direct caustic or irritant effects on the GI mucosa. It can also be a direct mitochondrial poison. Once the iron-carrying capacity of serum has been exceeded, free iron is deposited in the liver, where it damages mitochondria and leads to necrosis of periportal hepatocytes. Signs of iron toxicosis usually develop within 6 hr. Initial vomiting and diarrhea, with or without blood, may be followed by hypovolemic shock, depression, fever, acidosis, and liver failure 12–24 hr later, often with a period of apparent recovery in between. Oliguria and anuria secondary to shock-induced renal failure may also occur. Ingestion of elemental iron at >20 mg/kg generally warrants decontamination (emesis) and administration of GI protectants. Activated charcoal does not bind iron well. Additional treatment and monitoring is necessary for patients that have ingested elemental iron at >60 mg/kg. Milk of magnesia (magnesium hydroxide; 5–30 mL once or twice daily, per dog) can complex with iron to decrease its absorption from the GI tract. Serum iron levels and the total serum iron binding capacity should be checked at 3 hr and again at 8–10 hr after exposure. If serum iron is >300 mcg/dL along with clinical signs such as repeated vomiting and shock, or greater than the total iron binding capacity, chelation therapy may be needed. Deferoxamine (40 mg/kg, IM, every 4–8 hr) is a specific iron chelator and is most effective within 24 hr of ingestion, before iron has been distributed from blood to tissues. Other signs should be treated symptomatically.

Vitamin A toxicity after consumption of large amounts of fish oil or bear's liver has been well documented, but it is less likely to occur after acute ingestion of multivitamins. The amount of vitamin A needed to cause toxic effects is 10–1,000 times the dietary requirements for most species. The vitamin A requirement for cats is 10,000 IU/kg of diet fed, with levels up to 100,000 IU/kg of diet considered to be safe. For dogs, the requirement is 3,333 IU/kg of diet fed, with up to 333,300 IU/kg of diet considered to be safe. Signs associated with acute vitamin A toxicity include general malaise, anorexia, nausea, peeling skin, weakness, tremors, convulsions, paralysis, and death.

Vitamin D is included in many calcium supplements to aid the absorption of the calcium. Most vitamins contain cholecalciferol (vitamin D_3). After consumption, cholecalciferol is converted into 25-hydroxycholecalciferol (calcifediol) in the liver, which is subsequently converted to the active metabolite 1,25-dihydroxycholecalciferol (calcitriol) in the kidneys. One IU of vitamin D_3 is equivalent to 0.025 mcg of cholecalciferol. Even though the oral LD_{50} of cholecalciferol in dogs has been reported as 88 mg/kg, signs have been seen at dosages as low as 0.5 mg/kg. Vomiting, depression, polyuria and polydipsia, and hyperphosphatemia may be seen within 12 hr of a significant vitamin D exposure, followed by hypercalcemia and acute renal failure in 24–48 hr. In addition to renal failure, the kidneys, heart, and GI tract may show signs of necrosis and mineralization. Initial treatment should include decontamination and assessment of baseline calcium, phosphorus, BUN, and creatinine. Multiple doses of activated charcoal with a cathartic should be administered. If clinical signs of toxicosis and significant hypercalcemia/hyperphosphatemia develop, treatment consists of saline diuresis and the use of furosemide, corticosteroids, and phosphate binders. Specific agents such as (salmon) calcitonin or pamidronate may be needed for animals that remain hypercalcemic despite symptomatic treatment. Stabilization of serum calcium may require days of treatment because of the long half-life of calcifediol (16–30 days).

TOPICAL PREPARATIONS

Zinc Oxide

Zinc oxide ointments or creams are commonly used as topical skin protectants, astringents, and bactericidal agents. Most ointments contain 10%–40% zinc oxide. Acute ingestion of zinc oxide–containing products usually results in gastric irritation (vomiting) and diarrhea, without the intravascular hemolysis and liver and renal damage associated with ingestion of elemental zinc. Signs are usually seen within 2–4 hr of a significant exposure. Vomiting animals should be managed symptomatically and supportively. Some dogs show hypersensitivity-type reactions manifested by facial and ocular edema. Such cases can be treated with diphenhydramine or other antiallergic medications.

HERBAL SUPPLEMENTS

Ma Huang (Ephedrine) and Guarana (Caffeine)

Several herbal supplements, sold with the claim of providing weight loss and energy, contain guarana (*Paullinia cupana*), a natural source of caffeine, and ma huang (*Ephedra sinica*), a natural source of ephedrine. The amount of ma huang and guarana present in herbal products may vary considerably (labels should be read for amounts). In people, use of herbal supplements containing guarana and ma huang have been linked to acute hepatitis, nephrolithiasis, hypersensitivity myocarditis, and sudden death. In dogs, accidental ingestion of herbal supplements containing ma huang and guarana can have synergistic effects when ingested together and can lead to severe hyperactivity, tremors, seizures, vomiting, tachycardia, hyperthermia, and death within a few hours of exposure. The use of ephedra-containing supplements has been banned by the FDA. For treatment, *see* p 3027.

5-Hydroxytryptophan

Several OTC herbal supplements containing 5-hydroxytryptophan (5-HTP) or *Griffonia* seed extracts claim to treat depression, headaches, insomnia, and obesity. Orally, 5-HTP is rapidly absorbed and constitutively converted to serotonin (5-hydroxytryptamine). In cases of 5-HTP overdose, excessive concentrations of serotonin at target cells (GI, CNS, cardiovascular, and respiratory systems) can lead to a serotonin-like syndrome in dogs (eg, seizures, depression, tremors, ataxia, vomiting, diarrhea, hyperthermia, transient blindness, and death). Clinical signs can develop within 4 hr after ingestion and last up to 36 hr. Treatment consists of early decontamination, control of CNS signs (diazepam, barbiturates, phenothiazines such as acepromazine or chlorpromazine), thermoregulation (cool water bath, fans), fluid therapy, and administration of a serotonin antagonist such as cyproheptadine (1.1 mg/kg, PO or rectally for dogs, and 2–4 mg per cat, once or twice at an 8-hr interval).

TOXICITIES FROM PRESCRIPTION DRUGS

Pets commonly ingest prescription medications from countertops, pill minders, mail-order packages, or other sources. Veterinarians also can prescribe certain human drugs for animals. Safety data for human prescription drugs in certain animal species may not be available—most are not approved for veterinary use by the FDA. A valid client-patient-veterinarian relationship must exist for veterinarians to recommend extra-label use of human prescription medications to their clients.

CARDIOVASCULAR MEDICATIONS

See also SYSTEMIC PHARMACOTHERAPEUTICS OF THE CARDIOVASCULAR SYSTEM, p 2525.

Angiotensin-converting Enzyme (ACE) Inhibitors

Several angiotensin-converting enzyme (ACE) inhibitors (eg, enalapril, captopril, lisinopril, benazepril) are used therapeutically to treat congestive heart failure in dogs and cats. The primary concern in cases of acute ACE inhibitor overdose is usually marked hypotension. If hypotension is severe, secondary renal damage may result. Onset occurs within a few hours of exposure, depending on the agent (extended-release formulations may have a delayed onset of action). Other clinical signs of overdose may include vomiting, poor mucous membrane color, weakness, and tachycardia or bradycardia. Activated charcoal is effective in binding the drug from the GI tract if administered within 1–2 hr of ingestion. Blood pressure should be monitored and IV fluids given at twice the maintenance rate if hypotension develops. Renal function should be monitored if severe or persistent hypotension develops.

Calcium Channel Blockers

Calcium channel blockers (eg, diltiazem, amlodipine, nifedipine, verapamil) inhibit movement of calcium from extracellular sites through cell membrane–based calcium channels. The most common signs seen with overdoses of calcium channel blockers are hypotension, bradycardia, GI upset, noncardiogenic pulmonary edema, and heart block. Reflex tachycardia may develop in response to the drop in blood pressure.

Management of an acute overdose includes correcting hypotension and rhythm disturbances. In general, emesis is induced within 2 hr of ingestion only if the animal is showing no clinical signs. Induction of emesis in animals with signs can increase vagal tone and worsen the bradycardia. Activated charcoal binds unabsorbed drug in the GI tract and is most useful when administered within the first few hours after ingestion; if a sustained-release product was ingested, repeat doses of activated charcoal every 4–6 hr for a total of 2–4 doses can provide additional benefit. Specific therapies should be instituted based on blood pressure, heart rate, ECG, and blood chemistry profiles. IV fluids are recommended; calcium gluconate (10% solution at 0.5–1.5 mL/kg, slow IV) should be added while monitoring the ECG closely. Atropine (0.02–0.04 mg/kg) can be given for bradycardia; isoproterenol can be used if the ECG indicates atrioventricular block. For persistent hypotension not corrected by administration of IV fluids, synthetic colloids (Hetastarch), dopamine (1–20 mcg/kg/min), or dobutamine (2–20 mcg/kg/min) can be given via continuous IV infusion. A temporary cardiac pacemaker may be needed in cases of severe cardiac conduction disturbances unresponsive to medical therapy. Calcium channel blockers may interact with almost any other cardioactive medication, resulting in more profound bradycardia, hypotension, and depression of cardiac contractility. Because of the lipophilic nature of calcium channel blockers, using IV lipid emulsion solution (Intralipid™ 20% solution) may help sequester calcium channel blockers in overdose situations and prevent them from reaching their site of action. The recommended dose of 20% lipid emulsion solution in dogs is 1.5 mL/kg, IV, as an initial bolus followed by 0.25 mL/kg/min for 30–60 min. This dose can be repeated in 6 hr for a total of three treatments. Serum color and response should be monitored. If serum color is yellow, repeating the dose should be delayed until it becomes clear. If no response is seen after three doses, lipid emulsion should be discontinued. Hyperlipidemia, infection, intravascular hemolysis, lack of efficacy, and embolism are potential adverse effects associated with IV lipid emulsion therapy. The use of IV lipid emulsion for the treatment of some lipophilic drug overdoses is experimental and should be considered only if other conventional treatment options fail. Efficacy and safety of IV lipid emulsion has not been studied.

β Blockers

Drugs in this class (eg, propanolol, metoprolol, atenolol, timolol, esmolol) act by competitively inhibiting catecholamine binding to β-adrenergic receptor sites. The most common signs of overdose are bradycardia and hypotension; respiratory depression, coma, seizures, hyperkalemia, and hypoglycemia may occur. It is also possible to precipitate congestive heart failure. Significant clinical signs may arise even at therapeutic (published) doses—no approved veterinary products are on the market.

Because of rapid absorption, emesis should only be induced in asymptomatic animals within 2 hr of ingestion. Administration of activated charcoal should be considered if either multiple tablets or capsules or sustained-release formulation tablets are ingested. Heart rate, blood pressure, and clinical condition should be monitored for several hours, because extended-release pills can lead to delayed onset of clinical signs. If clinical signs do develop, blood chemistries should also be measured. Hypotension should be treated with IV fluids; atropine can be used for bradycardia. Glucagon or isoproterenol can also be used if needed (*see* above). If hyperkalemia is confirmed, administration of insulin, followed by IV glucose, may drive the excess potassium back into the cells.

Phenylpropanolamine

Phenylpropanolamine (PPA) is a sympathomimetic amine used primarily for treating urinary incontinence in dogs and cats. PPA is believed to indirectly stimulate both α- and β-adrenergic receptors, causing the release of norepinephrine. It is rapidly absorbed orally and distributes to various tissues, including the CNS. PPA is mainly excreted through the kidneys as a parent drug. Overdose of PPA can result in CNS effects (restlessness, agitation, nervousness) and cardiovascular signs (hypertension or hypotension, tachycardia or bradycardia, premature ventricular contractions, cardiovascular collapse). Dogs can also show piloerection, hyperemia, vomiting, hyperthermia or hypothermia, and mydriasis. Treatment consists of early decontamination (emesis in asymptomatic animals within a couple of hours of ingestion, followed by administration of activated charcoal). CNS effects and mild hypertension can be managed with acepromazine (0.02 mg/kg, IV or IM, repeated as needed). A nitroprusside constant-rate infusion can be tried for hypertension not responsive to acepromazine. Lidocaine can be considered for treating premature ventricular contractions. IV fluids should be given to promote excretion. Other signs should be treated symptomatically.

Diuretics

Oral diuretic agents include thiazides (eg, chlorothiazide, hydrochlorothiazide), loop diuretics such as furosemide, and potassium-sparing agents such as spironolactone (an aldosterone antagonist) and triamterene. Osmotic diuretics, administered by injection, include mannitol and urea. The most common signs of diuretic overdose include vomiting, depression, polyuria and polydipsia, and electrolyte changes. Electrolytes, especially potassium, may shift subsequent to a large ingestion of a diuretic. Management should include monitoring hydration and electrolytes, with correction as needed.

TRANQUILIZERS, ANTIDEPRESSANTS, SLEEP AIDS, AND ANTICONVULSANTS

See also SYSTEMIC PHARMACOTHERAPEUTICS OF THE NERVOUS SYSTEM, p 2590.

Benzodiazepines

Benzodiazepines bind γ-aminobutyric acid (inhibitory neurotransmitter) receptors and are used for seizure control and as anxiolytics. Whereas diazepam is probably best known in the veterinary field, alprazolam, chlordiazepoxide, clonazepam, lorazepam, oxazepam, and triazolam are all commonly prescribed medications. In general, all are rapidly and fairly completely absorbed, lipophilic, and highly protein bound. Metabolism is mostly by glucuronidation, so cats may be more sensitive to adverse effects. Several have active metabolites (eg, diazepam, clorazepate) and consequently have much longer duration of signs.

The most common signs seen, at a wide range of dosages, are CNS depression, respiratory depression, ataxia, weakness, disorientation, nausea, and vomiting. Some animals, especially at high doses, may show CNS excitation instead of depression (paradoxical reaction), which may be followed by CNS depression. Other common signs are hypothermia, hypotension, tachycardia, muscle hypotonia, and meiosis. Some cats develop signs of acute, potentially fatal hepatic failure after repeated oral administration of diazepam for several days.

Emesis can be induced if ingestion is recent and no clinical signs are present. Gastric lavage, followed by administration of activated charcoal, can be performed if the ingested amount is very high. The animal should be kept warm and quiet and closely monitored for responsiveness to stimuli and adequate breathing. IV fluids will help support blood pressure. If the affected animal is recumbent and severe respiratory depression has developed, the reversal agent flumazenil can be given at a dosage of 0.01 mg/kg, slow IV, in both cats and dogs. Flumazenil has a short half-life, so it may need to be repeated. Benzodiazepines should not be used to control CNS excitation, because a paradoxical reaction may occur. In such situations, low doses of acepromazine or barbiturates may be useful to control initial CNS excitation.

Antidepressants

Antidepressants fall into several classes. An overdose of almost any of them can result in development of serotonin syndrome (*see* below).

Selective Serotonin Reuptake Inhibitors: Selective serotonin reuptake inhibitors (SSRIs) include sertraline, fluoxetine, paroxetine, and fluvoxamine. They block the activity of serotonin receptors at presynaptic membranes and have little effect on other neurotransmitters. In veterinary medicine, these SSRIs are sometimes used to control aggression, obsessive-compulsive disorder, separation anxiety, pruritus, and inappropriate elimination in dogs and cats. Overdosage of SSRIs in dogs and cats is manifested by vomiting, lethargy, mydriasis, ataxia, shaking, seizures, hyperactivity, tachycardia or bradycardia, and vocalization (*see* below).

Tricyclic Antidepressants: Tricyclic antidepressants (eg, amitriptyline, clomipramine, nortriptyline) are commonly used psychoactive agents. They are structurally similar to the phenothiazines, with similar anticholinergic, adrenergic, and α-blocking properties. After absorption, these agents are extensively bound to plasma proteins and also bind to tissue and cellular sites, including the mitochondria. Cyclic antidepressants block the amine pump and stop neuronal reuptake of norepinephrine, serotonin, and dopamine. These agents also appear to have a slight α-adrenergic blocking effect. Tricyclics may exert their major toxicity via a nonspecific membrane-stabilizing effect, similar to chlorpromazine and the β blockers. Tricyclics also have central and peripheral anticholinergic activity, along with antihistaminic effects. Clinical signs of toxicosis include CNS stimulation (agitation, confusion, pyrexia), cardiac arrhythmias, hypertension, myoclonus, nystagmus, seizures, metabolic acidosis, urinary retention, dry mouth, mydriasis, and constipation. This may be followed by CNS depression (lethargy), ataxia, hypothermia, respiratory depression, cyanosis, hypotension, and coma.

Monoamine Oxidase Inhibitors: Monoamine oxidase inhibitors are antidepressants used mainly to treat atypical depression in people. In dogs, selegiline, a monoamine oxidase-B inhibitor, is used to treat Cushing disease and cognitive dysfunction (canine dementia). Selegiline is absorbed rapidly orally. Metabolites of selegiline include amphetamine and methamphetamine. Its half-life in dogs is ~1 hr.

Miscellaneous (Atypical) Antidepressants: These antidepressants have nonselective receptor-blocking effects and are used when SSRIs or tricyclic antidepressants have not been effective. Examples include bupropion, trazodone, and mirtazapine.

Treatment: Emesis should be induced in cases of recent exposure if the animal is asymptomatic. This can be followed by activated charcoal (even several hours after ingestion) plus a cathartic such as sorbitol or sodium sulfate (magnesium sulfate is contraindicated, because it can add to CNS depression). Diazepam can be given to control seizures. Serotonin syndrome signs should be managed as needed. Heart rate and rhythm should be monitored, and cardiac arrhythmias treated. Atropine should not be used to control bradycardia, because it can aggravate anticholinergic effects of tricyclic antidepressants.

Serotonin Syndrome: This group of clinical signs usually includes three of the following features: altered mental status, agitation, nervousness, myoclonus, hyperreflexia, tremors, diarrhea, incoordination, cardiovascular changes (heart rate and blood pressure), and fever. It often occurs because of repeated use or overdose or ingestion of substances that result in increased free levels of serotonin, such as antidepressants or profound stimulants (eg, amphetamines). Cyproheptadine is a serotonin antagonist often used for treatment. It is available only as a tablet but can be dissolved in a small amount of saline and administered per rectum at 1.1 mg/kg in dogs or 2 mg/dose in cats. If there is a good response to the initial dose, it can be repeated only if signs recur. Phenothiazines such as acepromazine or chlorpromazine also have antiserotonergic effects and can be used to control hyperactivity. Benzodiazepines such as diazepam can be used to control CNS effects. β blockers such as propranolol (0.02–0.04 mg/kg, IV) can be used to control tachycardia. Other treatment measures may include induction of emesis in asymptomatic animals within 2 hr of exposure, followed by administration of activated charcoal and IV fluids.

Barbiturates

Both long-acting and short-acting barbiturates may be encountered. The long-acting group includes phenobarbital, mephobarbital, and primidone—all commonly used as anticonvulsants or sedatives. The short-acting (butabarbital, pentobarbital, secobarbital) and ultra short-acting (thiamylal and thiopental) barbiturates are used mainly for induction of anesthesia and seizure control. All are readily absorbed from the gut and have extensive liver metabolism; metabolites are primarily excreted via the kidneys. The onset of clinical signs varies from 15 min to several hours, and duration can be up to several days for the long-acting class. The most common signs are sedation, ataxia, respiratory depression, coma, loss of reflexes, hypotension, and hypothermia.

Management is aimed at life support while attempting to remove unmetabolized drug from the body. Emesis should be induced if the exposure is very recent and the animal is asymptomatic. Gastric lavage while protecting the airway can remove much of the drug still in the stomach. Activated charcoal readily adsorbs barbiturates; small doses repeated every 4–6 hr can further decrease the body burden, even if overdose has resulted from use of an injectable product. IV fluids can be given to support blood pressure. Respiratory effort and effectiveness needs to be closely monitored; treatment may require positive-pressure ventilation or oxygen. Doxapram (1–5 mg/kg, slow IV in dogs, and 5–10 mg/cat) may help to stimulate respiration. Support to maintain body temperature may be necessary. Comatose animals should be intubated with a cuffed endotracheal tube, because aspiration is a common complication. Depending on the dose, aggressive supportive treatment may be necessary for 1–3 days.

Sleep Aids

Zolpidem, zaleplon, and eszopiclone are drugs used as sleep aids and have a mechanism of action similar to that of the benzodiazepines. These agents have a very rapid onset (usually <30 min) and a similarly short half-life. While the expected result from ingestion would be marked sedation, paradoxical excitement also occurs. Dosages as low as 0.22 mg/kg have resulted in sedation and ataxia, and dogs have developed tremors, vocalizing, and pacing at dosages as low as 0.6 mg/kg.

GI decontamination can be performed if the ingestion was recent and no signs are seen. For mild signs, keeping the pet quiet and in a safe place may suffice. If paradoxical excitement develops, symptomatic treatment should be given and will vary with the signs and their intensity. Hyperexcitation may be controlled with low doses of acepromazine or other phenothiazines. Use of diazepam may aggravate signs of CNS depression. Flumazenil (0.01 mg/kg, IV) can be used if clinical signs of toxicosis are severe.

Phenothiazine Tranquilizers

The most commonly used phenothiazines in veterinary medicine are acepromazine, chlorpromazine, and promazine. In domestic animals, they are used as tranquilizers, preanesthetic agents, antiemetics, and for treatment of CNS agitation after specific drug overdoses (amphetamines, cocaine). The most common signs of overdose are sedation, weakness, ataxia, collapse, behavioral changes, hypothermia, hypotension, tachycardia, and bradycardia.

Treatment consists of symptomatic and supportive care. Because of the rapid onset of CNS signs, emesis should only be attempted in a recent exposure and should be followed by administration of activated charcoal and a cathartic. Repeated doses of activated charcoal may be helpful, especially for large ingestions. Hypotension should be treated with IV fluids. Dopamine may be used if fluid administration does not correct hypotension. Body temperature, heart rate, and blood pressure should be monitored and treated symptomatically.

MUSCLE RELAXANTS

The most commonly encountered centrally acting muscle relaxants include baclofen, carisoprodol, methocarbamol, tizanidine, and cyclobenzaprine. Baclofen is rapidly absorbed orally. The onset of clinical signs of toxicosis may be <30 min to 2 hr after ingestion. The most common signs of toxicosis are vocalization, salivation, vomiting, ataxia, weakness, tremors, shaking, coma, seizures, bradycardia, hypothermia, and blood pressure abnormalities. Cyclobenzaprine, often used in management of acute muscle spasms, is almost completely absorbed after an oral dose, with peak plasma levels in 3–8 hr. It has extensive liver metabolism and undergoes enterohepatic recirculation. The most common signs seen in dogs and cats include depression and ataxia.

Treatment of muscle relaxant overdose consists of symptomatic and supportive care. Vomiting should be induced if the exposure is recent and no clinical signs are present, followed by administration of activated charcoal. Respiratory support (ie, ventilator) should be provided if needed. Recumbent or comatose animals should be monitored for hypothermia and aspiration. Seizures can be controlled with diazepam. Cyproheptadine (1.1 mg/kg, PO, once or twice every 8 hr) seems to work well for vocalization in dogs. IV fluids should be given as needed. Treatment with IV lipid emulsion solution may be beneficial (*see* p 3032).

TOPICAL AGENTS

Pets ingest many topical preparations, often resulting in only mild gastroenteritis. For example, ingestion of most corticosteroid-containing creams or ointments usually results in only mild to moderate stomach upset, polydipsia, and polyphagia. However, ingestion of certain topical agents in pet animals, such as 5-fluorouracil and calcipotriene, can be fatal even at low doses.

5-Fluorouracil

5-Fluorouracil (5-FU) is available as an ointment (1% or 5%) or topical solution (1%, 2%, or 5%). It is used in the treatment of skin cancers and solar keratoses in people. Most exposures result from accidental ingestion, although occasionally 5-FU is used extra-label in pets. Ingestion in dogs and cats leads to the onset of signs within a few hours. In dogs, signs have been seen at dosages as low as 8.6 mg/kg, with the minimum lethal dose reported as 20 mg/kg. Initial signs include severe vomiting, which may progress to bloody vomiting and diarrhea. Signs often progress to severe tremors, ataxia, and seizures. In cats and dogs, 5-FU may be converted to fluorocitrate and interfere with the Kreb's cycle, which may be one cause of seizures and ataxia. Generally, 5-FU destroys rapidly dividing cells, affecting the GI tract, liver, kidneys, CNS, and bone marrow. The mortality rate among dogs ingesting 5-FU is high.

All 5-FU exposures in pets should be treated aggressively. Treatment consists primarily of symptomatic and supportive care. Emesis should be induced, and the animal given activated charcoal and a cathartic if it is asymptomatic and the ingestion has occurred within 1 hr. Symptomatic animals (eg, vomiting or seizuring) should be stabilized first. The GI tract should be protected with sucralfate (1 g in large dogs, 0.5 g in small dogs, PO, tid) and inhibitors of gastric acid secretion such as cimetidine. Diazepam may be used initially to control seizures and tremors, but in severe cases it is usually not effective, and other anticonvulsants such as pentobarbital (3–15 mg/kg, IV slowly to effect) or phenobarbital (3–30 mg/kg, slowly IV to effect) can be used. Constant-rate infusion using diazepam or barbiturates has successfully controlled severe seizures. If this also fails to control CNS signs, gas anesthetics (eg, isoflurane) and propofol (4–6 mg/kg, IV, or as a continuous drip at 0.6 mg/kg/min) can be tried. IV fluids should be given, and body temperature monitored. Monitoring electrolytes, serum chemistries (liver-specific enzymes and renal function), and CBC is usually required for ~2 wk. Surviving dogs may show evidence of bone marrow suppression later. For severe neutropenia in dogs, administration of filgrastim or granulocyte colony-stimulating factor at 4–6 mcg/kg, SC, may be useful.

Calcipotriene

Calcipotriene, used to treat psoriasis in people, is available as an ointment or cream (0.005% or 50 mcg/g). Calcipotriene is a novel structural analogue of calcitriol (1,25-dihydroxycholecalciferol), the most active metabolite of cholecalciferol (vitamin D_3). Accidental ingestion of 40–60 mcg/kg of calcipotriene in dogs has been associated with life-threatening hypercalcemia. Clinical signs usually occur within 24–72 hr of ingestion and include anorexia, vomiting, diarrhea, polyuria and polydipsia, depression, and weakness. Serum calcium is usually increased within 12–24 hr and may remain above normal for weeks. This is usually accompanied by an increase in serum phosphorus concentration and calcium phosphorus product and soft-tissue mineralization. Acute renal failure as evidenced by increased BUN and creatinine levels, coma, and death occur in severe or untreated cases.

Treatment of calcipotriene toxicosis involves standard decontamination (emesis induction, administration of activated charcoal and a cathartic) and reduction of serum calcium concentrations by saline diuresis, furosemide, and corticosteroids, with or without salmon calcitonin treatment (*see* p 568). Concurrent use of pamidronate (1.3–2 mg/kg diluted in saline and given IV over 2 hr) in dogs may be a useful adjunctive therapy. Calcipotriene toxicosis cases usually require monitoring of serum calcium, phosphorus, BUN, and creatinine for several days or even weeks. Signs of renal failure are managed with ongoing supportive fluids.

PRESCRIPTION NONSTEROIDAL ANTI-INFLAMMATORY DRUGS

For a general discussion of commonly seen adverse effects and treatment of NSAID toxicosis, *see* p 3027.

Etodolac

Etodolac is an indole acetic acid–derivative NSAID labeled for use in dogs to treat pain and inflammation associated with osteoarthritis. It is rapidly absorbed orally, with peak serum concentrations seen 2 hr after dosing. It is primarily eliminated through the bile. The elimination half-life is 8–12 hr. Etodolac appears to be well tolerated by dogs when used at the labeled dosage (10–15 mg/kg/day, PO) for 1 yr. With multiple doses, clinical signs of toxicity such as GI ulcers, vomiting, diarrhea, and weight loss can be seen at 40 mg/kg. Six of 8 dogs died or became moribund because of GI ulceration at 80 mg/kg.

Meloxicam

Meloxicam is an enolic acid–derivative NSAID approved for use in dogs and cats for controlling pain and inflammation. Meloxicam is available as a solution for injection (5 mg/mL) and as an oral suspension. In cats, it has been approved for use as a single SC injection at 0.3 mg/kg. In dogs, the recommended initial dosage is 0.2 mg/kg, followed by 0.1 mg/kg, PO. Meloxicam has a good margin of safety in dogs. Oral administration at 0.1 mg/kg for 26 weeks was well tolerated in dogs. Some dogs at 0.3 or 0.5 mg/kg, PO, for 42 days have shown clinical signs consistent with NSAID toxicity (vomiting, diarrhea, renal effects). In cats, the margin of safety appears to be narrow; extra-label dosing at 0.1–0.2 mg/kg, PO, for a few days has caused adverse effects.

Deracoxib

Deracoxib is a coxib COX-2 inhibitor (in vitro) used to treat osteoarthritis in dogs. It is not approved for use in cats. The recommended dosage is 1–2 mg/kg/day or 3–4 mg/kg/day as needed for postoperative pain, not to exceed 7 days of therapy. Oral bioavailability in dogs is > 90%; the time to peak serum concentration is ~2 hr. In a 14-day study of dogs that received 10 mg/kg, no clinically observable adverse effects were seen. Dogs that received 25 mg/kg/day, 50 mg/kg/day, or 100 mg/kg/day for 10–11 days showed vomiting and melena; no hepatic or renal lesions were seen in these dogs. Dogs ingesting >100 mg/kg should be aggressively decontaminated and treated with IV fluids to prevent renal damage.

Piroxicam

Piroxicam is an oxicam derivative. It is not approved in dogs and cats but has been used at 0.3 mg/kg, PO, every other day. Piroxicam in dogs and people has a long half-life (40 hr and 50 hr, respectively) likely due to extensive enterohepatic recirculation. The LD_{50} of piroxicam in dogs is >700 mg/kg. Adverse GI effects were seen in 18% of dogs given piroxicam at 0.3 mg/kg/day, PO, for several months.

Diclofenac

Diclofenac is a phenylacetic acid derivative structurally related to meclofenamate sodium and mefenamic acid. After a single injection of diclofenac sodium at 1 mg/kg in dogs, 35%–40% is excreted in the urine. The reported oral LD_{50} of diclofenac sodium in dogs is 500 mg/kg.

Indomethacin

Indomethacin is an indole acetic acid derivative available as the base and as the sodium trihydrate salt. The drug is structurally and pharmacologically related to another NSAID, sulindac. The reported oral LD_{50} of indomethacin in rats is 12 mg/kg. Administration of indomethacin to dogs at 2 mg/kg for 30 days resulted in GI ulcers in 60% of dogs and perforation in 20%.

Etodolac

Etodolac, an indole acetic acid derivative, is used for pain relief, osteoarthritis, and rheumatoid arthritis in people. It is approved in the USA for use in dogs (>12 mo old) to manage pain and inflammation associated with osteoarthritis. The suggested dosage in dogs is 10–15 mg/kg. Etodolac is well absorbed orally in dogs, with peak plasma concentration seen in 2 hr. It is primarily excreted through bile, and the half-life in dogs is 8–12 hr. In dogs, etodolac at 40 mg/kg/day was associated with GI ulcers, weight loss, emesis, and local occult blood loss. Dosages of 80 mg/kg/day caused 6 of 8 dogs to die or become moribund because of GI ulceration.

Nabumetone

Nabumetone differs from other NSAIDs in that it is neutral as opposed to acidic. The risk of GI ulcers from nabumetone is considered less than that of other NSAIDs. Nabumetone is primarily excreted in the urine in most species. However, in dogs, when nabumetone was administered at 20 mg/kg, only 27% of the dose was found in the urine. The reported oral LD_{50} of nabumetone in rats is >2 g/kg. At a dosage of >300 mg/kg, the lower GI tract and the kidneys were affected in rats, mice, rabbits, and rhesus monkeys.

TOXICITIES FROM ILLICIT AND ABUSED DRUGS

Exposures to illicit or abused drugs in pet animals can be accidental, intentional, or malicious. Occasionally, drug-sniffing dogs also ingest these substances. Because of the illegal nature of illicit or abused drugs, owners may provide inaccurate, incomplete, or misleading exposure histories. Illicit drugs are often adulterated with other pharmacologically active substances, making the diagnosis even more difficult.

In suspected cases of exposure to illicit or abused drugs, an attempt should be made to gather information about the animal's environment; amount of exposure; and time of onset of clinical signs and their type, severity, and duration. These questions will help include or exclude possible exposure to an illicit or abused drug. Illicit and abused drugs are often known by street names that vary from area to area. A call to a local police station, or animal or human poison control center, may help identify the illicit substance if its street name is known. Most human hospitals, emergency clinics, and some veterinary diagnostic laboratories have illicit drug screens available and can check for the presence of illicit drugs or their metabolites in different body fluids. The presence of a parent drug or its metabolites in blood or urine may help confirm exposure in suspect cases. The laboratories should be contacted for information on the types of samples needed and time required to complete the screens or tests.

Commonly available over-the-counter drug test kits may help exclude a suspected case of illicit drug toxicosis. They are designed to detect drug metabolites in the urine and can detect most commonly available illicit or recreational drugs such as amphetamines, cocaine, marijuana, opiates, and barbiturates. The sensitivities and specificities of these test kits may vary. The kits are inexpensive, efficient, and easy to use, but the instructions provided with each kit should be followed carefully for best results.

Amphetamines and Related Drugs

Amphetamines and their derivatives are CNS and cardiovascular system stimulants commonly used in people for suppression of appetite, narcolepsy, attention deficit disorder, parkinsonism, and some behavior disorders. Some commonly encountered amphetamines or related drugs are benzphetamine, dextroamphetamine, lisdexamfetamine, pemoline, methylphenidate, phentermine, diethylpropion, phendimetrazine, methamphetamine, and phenmetrazine. Amphetamines sold on the street have common names such as speed, bennies, or uppers. Commonly used adulterants are caffeine, ephedrine, or phenylpropanolamine.

Pharmacokinetics and Toxicity: Amphetamines are rapidly absorbed in the GI tract, reaching peak plasma concentrations in 1–2 hr. Sustained-release formulations have a delayed absorption and relatively longer half-life. The plasma half-life of amphetamines depends on the urinary pH. With an alkaline pH, the half-life is 15–30 hr; with an acidic pH, the half-life is 8–10 hr. The acute oral LD_{50} of amphetamine in rats and mice is 10–30 mg/kg. In people, deaths have been reported after ingestion of methamphetamine at 1.3 mg/kg.

Pathogenesis: Amphetamine stimulates the release of norepinephrine, affecting both α- and β-adrenergic receptor sites. Amphetamine also stimulates catecholamine release centrally in the cerebral cortex, medullary respiratory center, and reticular activating system. It increases the amount of catecholamine at nerve endings by increasing release and inhibiting reuptake and metabolism. The neurotransmitters affected in the CNS are norepinephrine, dopamine, and serotonin.

Clinical Findings and Diagnosis: Clinical signs of amphetamine and cocaine toxicosis are similar and difficult to differentiate clinically. The only difference may be the longer duration of clinical signs of amphetamine toxicosis because the half-life of amphetamine is longer than that of cocaine. The most commonly reported signs are hyperactivity, aggression, hyperthermia, tremors, ataxia, tachycardia, hypertension, mydriasis, circling, head bobbing, and death.

Diagnosis is as for cocaine (*see* below) and relies mostly on owner knowledge of exposure. Most amphetamines and related drugs or their metabolites are detectable in the stomach contents and urine. They are difficult to detect in plasma unless large amounts have been ingested.

Treatment: Phenothiazines are preferred to control CNS signs in amphetamine toxicosis (*see* below for cocaine toxicosis). Other anticonvulsants, such as diazepam, barbiturates, or isoflurane, may be used if needed. Acidifying the urine with ammonium chloride (25–50 mg/kg/day, PO, qid) or ascorbic acid (20–30 mg/kg, PO, SC, IM, or IV) may enhance amphetamine elimination in the urine. However, this should be done only if acid-base status can be monitored. Cyproheptadine (1.1 mg/kg, PO or per rectum) may also be given once or twice (6–8 hr apart) for serotonin syndrome (disorientation, muscle stiffness, agitation). Heart rate and rhythm (*see* p 3040 for using β blockers to treat tachycardia), body temperature, and electrolytes should be monitored and treated as needed.

Cocaine

Cocaine (benzoylmethylecgonine) alkaloid is obtained from the leaves of the coca plant, *Erythroxylon coca* and *E monogymnum*. Some common street names for cocaine are coke, gold dust, stardust, snow, C, white girl, white lady, baseball, and speedball (cocaine and heroin). Cocaine alkaloid from coca leaves is processed into cocaine hydrochloride salt, then reprocessed to form cocaine alkaloid or free base (a process called free-basing or base balling), which is colorless, odorless, transparent, and more heat stable. Free-base cocaine is also called crack, rock, or flake. Cocaine is cut (diluted) several times before it reaches the user. Xanthine alkaloids, local anesthetics, and decongestants are some of the most common adulterants.

Cocaine is a schedule II drug approved for human use. Its medical uses are restricted to topical administration as a local anesthetic on mucous membranes of the oral, laryngeal, and nasal cavities. However, it is mostly used as a recreational drug.

Pharmacokinetics and Toxicity: Cocaine is absorbed from most routes. Orally, it is better absorbed in an alkaline medium (ie, intestine). In people, ~20% of an oral dose is absorbed. The reported plasma half-life is 0.9–2.8 hr. Cocaine is extensively metabolized by liver and plasma cholinesterases to several inactive metabolites that are primarily excreted in the urine. The acute LD_{50} of cocaine hydrochloride administered IV in dogs is 13 mg/kg; the LD_{100} is 12 mg/kg in dogs and 15 mg/kg in cats. The oral LD_{50} in dogs is believed to be 2–4 times more than the IV dose.

Pathogenesis: Cocaine acts on the sympathetic division of the autonomic nervous system. It blocks the reuptake of dopamine and norepinephrine in the CNS, leading to feelings of euphoria, restlessness, and increased motor activity. Cocaine can also decrease concentrations of serotonin or its metabolites. Topical use of cocaine causes vasoconstriction of small vessels. Hyperthermia in cocaine toxicosis may develop either due to increased heat production from muscular activity or due to decreased heat loss from vasoconstriction.

Clinical Findings and Diagnosis: CNS excitation, hyperactivity, shaking, ataxia, panting, agitation, mydriasis, nervousness, seizures, tachycardia, hypertension, acidosis, or hyperthermia characterize cocaine toxicosis. CNS depression and coma may follow CNS excitation. Death may be due to hyperthermia, cardiac arrest, or respiratory arrest. Some nonspecific chemistry changes may include hyperglycemia and increased CK and liver-specific enzymes.

Diagnosis is based on a history of exposure and the presence of characteristic clinical signs. Identification of cocaine in plasma, stomach contents, or urine can confirm exposure. Differential diagnoses include amphetamines, pseudoephedrine, ephedrine, caffeine, chocolate, metaldehyde, strychnine, tremorgenic mycotoxins, lead, nicotine, permethrin (cats) and other pesticides, and encephalitis.

Treatment: The objectives of treatment are GI decontamination, stabilization of CNS and cardiovascular effects, thermoregulation, and supportive care. Animals with clinical signs should be stabilized first before attempting decontamination. Emesis can be induced in a recent exposure if the animal is asymptomatic and has the ability to guard its airway via a gag reflex. This should be followed by administration of activated charcoal with a cathartic. If the animal's condition contraindicates induction of emesis (eg, presence of CNS signs or extreme tachycardia), a gastric lavage with a cuffed endotracheal tube to reduce the risk of aspiration should be performed. A dose of activated charcoal with a cathartic should be left in the stomach after the lavage.

Controlling the CNS signs may require use of more than one anticonvulsant. Clinical signs of CNS excitation can be controlled with diazepam; however, the effects of diazepam are short-lived, and repeated administration may be needed. Phenothiazine tranquilizers such as acepromazine (0.05–1 mg/kg, IV, IM, or SC, repeated as needed) or chlorpromazine (0.5–1 mg/kg, IV or IM) also usually work well to control the CNS effects. However, phenothiazines should be used cautiously, because they may lower the seizure threshold. If phenothiazines are ineffective, phenobarbital at 3–4 mg/kg, IV, or pentobarbital, IV to effect, could be used. If CNS signs are uncontrolled by the preceding measures, a gas anesthetic such as isoflurane may be useful.

Blood pressure, heart rate and rhythm, ECG, and body temperature should be monitored frequently and treated as needed. Propranolol at 0.02–0.06 mg/kg, IV, tid-qid, or other β-blocking agents such as esmolol (0.2–0.5 mg/kg, slow IV over 1 min, or 25–200 mcg/kg/min as a constant-rate infusion) can be used to control tachycardia. After CNS and cardiovascular effects have been stabilized, IV fluids should be administered, and electrolyte changes and acid-base status monitored and corrected as needed. Treatment and monitoring should continue until all clinical signs have resolved.

Ecstasy (MDMA or 3,4-Methylenedioxymethamphetamine)

Ecstasy is a semisynthetic psychoactive designer drug (developed by street chemists with minor structural changes in parent compounds) with hallucinogenic and amphetamine-like properties. Street names include Adam, XTC, E, Roll, X, or Love Drug. A typical dose may be 75–150 mg. MDMA is believed to cause excessive release of serotonin. It also binds to serotonin transporter (a protein), which is responsible for removing serotonin from the synapse. The overall effect is increased serotonin and serotonergic effects. MDMA also affects dopamine and norepinephrine. Studies in rodents indicate that use of MDMA can lead to permanent serotonergic neuronal injury.

In pets, MDMA toxicosis is not common. It is usually acute and occurs from accidental ingestion (powder, pills, or capsules). Clinical signs develop within 30 min to 2 hr after ingestion and may consist of sympathomimetic effects (CNS excitation, agitation, hyperactivity, pacing, hyperthermia, tachycardia, hypertension, seizures [just like amphetamines]), sedation, or signs thought to be related to hallucination (vocalization, disorientation, muscle rigidity). The half-life in people is 7.6–8.7 hr. Treatment is similar to that for amphetamine toxicosis (*see* p 3039). For serotonergic effects (agitation, muscle rigidity, nervousness), antiserotonergic drugs such as cyproheptadine can be tried (1.1 mg/kg, PO, repeated once in 6–8 hr).

Marijuana

Marijuana refers to a mixture of cut, dried, and ground flowers, leaves, and stems of the leafy green hemp plant *Cannabis sativa*. Several cannabinoids are present in the plant resin, but delta-9-tetrahydrocannabinol (THC) is considered the most active and main psychoactive agent. The concentration of THC in marijuana varies between 1%–8%. Hashish is the resin extracted from the top of the flowering plant and is higher in THC concentration than marijuana. Street names for marijuana include pot, Mary Jane, hashish, weed, grass, THC, ganja, bhang, and charas. Pure THC is available by prescription under the generic name dronabinol. A synthetic cannabinoid, nabilone, is also available. Marijuana or hashish sold on the streets may be contaminated with phencyclidine, LSD, or other drugs.

Marijuana is a schedule I controlled substance mostly used by people as a recreational drug. It is also used as an antiemetic for chemotherapy patients and to decrease intraocular pressure in glaucoma patients. Some clinicians advocate the use of dronabinol as an appetite stimulant, but the dysphoric effects of this drug outweigh any benefit of appetite stimulation.

Synthetic marijuana is a designer drug in which different herbs or incense or other leafy materials are sprayed with laboratory-synthesized chemicals. The use of synthetic marijuana produces psychoactive effects similar to those of THC. It is often claimed to be natural, safe, and legal. Spice, K-2, skunk, and moon rocks are some of the common street names. Clinical signs of toxicosis from ingestion of synthetic marijuana in dogs can be more severe and last longer than those of THC.

Pharmacokinetics and Toxicity: The most common route of exposure is oral. After ingestion, THC goes through a substantial first-pass effect. It is metabolized by liver microsomal hydroxylation and nonmicrosomal oxidation. In dogs, clinical signs begin within 30–90 min and can last up to 72 hr. THC is highly lipophilic and readily distributes to the brain and other fatty tissues after absorption. The oral LD_{50} of pure THC is 666 mg/kg in rats and 482 mg/kg in mice. However, clinical effects of marijuana are seen at much lower doses than this.

Pathogenesis: THC is believed to act on a unique receptor in the brain that is selective for cannabinoids and is responsible for the CNS effects. Cannabinoids can enhance the formation of norepinephrine, dopamine, and serotonin. They can also stimulate release of dopamine and enhance γ-aminobutyric acid turnover.

Clinical Findings and Diagnosis: The most common signs of marijuana toxicosis are depression, ataxia, bradycardia, hypothermia, vocalization, hypersalivation, vomiting, diarrhea, urinary incontinence, seizures, and coma.

Diagnosis is based on a history of exposure and typical clinical signs. THC is difficult to detect in body fluids because of the low levels found in the plasma. Urine testing at human hospitals or using an over-the-counter marijuana drug test kit in the early course of exposure may help confirm the diagnosis. Marijuana toxicosis can be confused with ethylene glycol (antifreeze, *see* p 3046) or ivermectin toxicosis; hypoglycemia; benzodiazepine, barbiturate, or opioid overdose; intervertebral disc problems; or head trauma.

Treatment: Treatment consists of supportive care. If the exposure is recent and there are no contraindications, emesis should be induced and activated charcoal administered. Comatose animals should be monitored for aspiration pneumonia, given IV fluids, treated for hypothermia, and rotated frequently to prevent dependent edema or decubital ulceration. Diazepam can be given for sedation or to control seizures. Treatment and monitoring should continue until all clinical signs have resolved (up to 72 hr in dogs). For cases of synthetic marijuana toxicosis, in addition to the preceding treatment options, use of IV lipid emulsion solution may be considered.

Opiates

The term opiate initially referred to all naturally occurring alkaloids obtained from the sap of the opium poppy (*Papaver somniferum*). Opium sap contains morphine, codeine, and several other alkaloids. Currently, opioid refers to all drugs, natural or synthetic, that have morphine-like actions or actions mediated through opioid receptors. Structurally, opioids can be divided into five classes. Some of the common agents within each class are 1) phenanthrenes—morphine, heroin, hydromorphone, oxymorphone, hydrocodone, codeine, and oxycodone; 2) morphinan—butorphanol; 3) diphenylheptanes—methadone and propoxyphene; 4) phenylpiperidines—meperidine, diphenoxylate, fentanyl, loperamide, and profadol; and 5) benzomorphans—pentazocine and buprenorphine. Some of the widely used opioids in veterinary medicine include tramadol, buprenorphine, fentanyl, loperamide (antidiarrheal), and hydromorphone. The use of meperidine is no longer common.

Opioids are used primarily for analgesia. In addition, they are used as cough suppressants and to treat diarrhea. Occasionally, opioids are used for sedation before surgery and as a supplement to anesthesia.

Pharmacokinetics and Toxicity: Opioids are generally well absorbed after oral, rectal, or parenteral administration. Some more lipophilic opioids are also absorbed through nasal, buccal, respiratory (heroin, fentanyl, buprenorphine), or transdermal (fentanyl) routes. For some opioids, there is variable reduction in bioavailability because of a first-pass effect when given orally. Opioids generally undergo hepatic metabolism with some form of conjugation, hydrolysis, oxidation, dealkylation, or glucuronidation. Because cats are deficient in glucuronidase, the half-life of some opioids in cats may be prolonged. After absorption, opioids are rapidly cleared from blood and stored in kidney, liver, brain, lung, spleen, skeletal muscle, and placental tissue. Most of the opioid metabolites are excreted through the kidneys.

Toxicity of opioids in animals is highly variable. In dogs, morphine administered at 100–200 mg/kg, SC or IV, is considered lethal. The estimated lethal dose of codeine in human adults is 7–14 mg/kg; in infants, 2.5 mg of hydrocodone has been lethal.

Pathogenesis: The effects of opioids are due to their interaction with opiate receptors (μ, κ, δ, σ, and ε) found in the limbic system, spinal cord, thalamus, hypothalamus, striatum, and midbrain. Opioids may be agonists, mixed agonist-antagonists, or antagonists at these receptors. Agonists bind and activate a receptor, whereas antagonists bind without causing activation.

Clinical Findings: The primary effects of opioids are on the CNS, respiratory, cardiovascular, and GI systems. Commonly reported clinical signs of toxicosis include CNS depression, drowsiness, ataxia, vomiting, seizures, miosis, coma, respiratory depression, hypotension, constipation/defecation, and death. Some animals—especially cats, horses, cattle, and swine—can show CNS excitation instead of CNS depression.

Diagnosis: Diagnosis of opioid toxicosis is based on history of exposure and the types of clinical signs (CNS and respiratory depression) present. Plasma opioid levels are usually not clinically useful. Urine may be used to determine exposure to opioids using some of the over-the-counter illicit drug kits (manufacturer's instructions should be followed). Opioid toxicosis should be differentiated from ethylene glycol, ivermectin, benzodiazepine, barbiturate, and marijuana toxicosis, as well as hypoglycemia-inducing conditions.

Treatment: Clinical signs can be reversed with the opiate antagonist naloxone. The dosages in different species are dog and cat, 0.04–0.16 mg/kg, IV, IM, or SC; rabbit and rodent, 0.01–0.1 mg/kg, SC or IP; horse, 0.01–0.02 mg/kg, IV. Administration of naloxone should be repeated as needed (hourly), because its duration of action may be shorter than that of the opioid toxicity being treated. Animals should be closely monitored for respiratory depression and ventilatory support provided if needed. Other signs should be treated symptomatically. Dysphoric reactions (vocalization, agitation, restlessness, and excitation) can be treated with diazepam or other benzodiazepines. For serotonin-like syndrome (disorientation, muscle rigidity, agitation) induced by some opioids, cyproheptadine (1.1 mg/kg, PO or per rectum) once or twice (6–8 hr apart) can be tried.

NONPROTEIN NITROGEN POISONING

(Ammonia toxicosis)

Poisoning by ingestion of excess urea or other sources of nonprotein nitrogen (NPN) is usually acute, rapidly progressive, and highly fatal. NPN is any source of nitrogen not present in a polypeptide (precipitable protein) form. Sources of NPN have different toxicities in various species, but mature ruminants are affected most commonly. After ingestion, NPN undergoes hydrolysis and releases excess ammonia (NH_3) into the GI tract, which is absorbed and leads to hyperammonemia.

Etiology: Ruminants use NPN by converting it via the ruminal microflora to ammonia, which is then combined with carbohydrate-derived keto acids to form amino acids. The most common sources of NPN in feeds are urea, urea phosphate, ammonia (anhydrous), and salts such as monoammonium and diammonium phosphate. Because feed-grade urea is unstable, it is formulated (usually pelleted) to prevent degradation to NH_3. Biuret, a less toxic source of NPN, is being used less frequently than in the past. Natural protein sources such as rice hulls, beet or citrus pulp, cottonseed meal, and straw or other low-quality forages may be treated with anhydrous ammonia to increase available nitrogen in supplemented livestock diets. Fermentation byproducts from alcohol (ethanol) manufacture are a source of NPN that comes from incomplete proteins, and these products are commonly used in liquid or feed supplements. Most sources of NPN are provided to ruminants by direct addition of dry supplement to a complete mixed or blended diet, by free-choice access to NPN-containing range blocks or cubes, or by lick tank systems combined with molasses as a supplement. Ammonia or NPN poisoning is a common sequela of abrupt change to urea or other NPN in the diet when only natural protein was previously fed; animals have to be gradually acclimated to NPN so that rumen microflora can increase in numbers to use the NH_3 produced. Also, farm animals sometimes drink liquid fertilizers or ingest dry granular fertilizers that contain ammonium salts or urea.

Ruminants are most sensitive, because urease is normally present in the functional rumen after 50 days of age. Dietary exposure of unacclimated ruminants to 0.3–0.5 g of urea/kg body wt may cause adverse effects; dosages of 1–1.5 g/kg are usually lethal. Urease activity in the equine cecum is ~25% that of the rumen, and horses may receive NPN as a feed additive; however, horses are more sensitive to urea than other monogastrics, and dosages ≥4 g/kg can be lethal. Ammonium salts at 0.3–0.5 g/kg may be toxic in all species and ages of farm animals; dosages ≥1.5 g/kg usually are fatal. Pigs and neonatal calves are generally unaffected by ingestion of urea except for a transient diuresis. Wild birds (silver gulls) reportedly have been poisoned after consuming water contaminated with urea fertilizer spillage.

Livestock may require days or weeks for total adaptation before rumen microflora can utilize the gradually increasing amounts of urea or other NPN in the diets; however, adaptation is lost relatively quickly (1–3 days) once NPN is removed from the diet.

Diets low in energy and high in fiber are more commonly associated with NPN toxicosis, even in acclimated animals. Highly palatable supplements (such as liquid molasses or large protein blocks crumbled by precipitation), range cubes, or improperly maintained lick tanks may lead to consumption of lethal amounts of NPN.

A related CNS disorder in cattle fed ammoniated high-quality hay, silage, molasses, and protein blocks is thought to be caused by formation of 4-methylimidazole (4-MI) through the action of NH_3 on soluble carbohydrates (reducing sugars) in these feedstuffs. Cattle fed dietary components containing 4-MI develop a syndrome known as the "bovine bonkers syndrome," named for the wildly aberrant behavior exhibited. Signs relate to CNS effects, with stampeding, ear twitching, trembling, champing, salivating, and convulsions. Because nursing calves are affected, the toxic principle apparently is excreted in milk. Ammoniated low-quality forages do not have sufficient concentrations of reducing sugars to form 4-MI, and thus serve as a relatively safe nitrogen source for acclimated animals.

Another related disorder involves accidental excessive exposure of ruminants (cattle and sheep) to raw soybeans. Soybeans have high concentrations of both carbohydrates and proteins, as well as urease. Overconsumption can cause acute carbohydrate fermentation and excessive ammonia release, resulting in ammonia toxicosis and lactic acidosis. Affected animals have engorged rumens with a gray, amorphous mass inside.

Clinical Findings: The period from urea ingestion to onset of clinical signs is 20–60 min in cattle, 30–90 min in sheep, and longer in horses. Early signs include muscle tremors (especially of face and ears), exophthalmia, abdominal pain, frothy salivation, polyuria, and bruxism. Tremors progress to incoordination and weakness. Pulmonary edema leads to marked salivation, dyspnea, and gasping.

Horses may exhibit head pressing; cattle are often agitated, hyperirritable, aggressive, and belligerent as toxicosis progresses; sheep usually appear depressed. An early sign in cattle is ruminal atony; as toxicosis progresses, ruminal tympany is usually evident, and violent struggling and bellowing, a marked jugular pulse, severe twitching, tetanic spasms, and convulsions may be seen. Affected cattle with belligerent aberrant behavior may have produced some 4-MI in vivo through reaction of excessive NH_3, released from NPN, with carbohydrates and reducing sugars in the rumen. The PCV and serum concentrations of NH_3, glucose, lactate, potassium, phosphorus, AST, ALT, and BUN usually are significantly increased.

As death nears, animals become cyanotic, dyspneic, anuric, and hyperthermic, and blood pH decreases from 7.4 to 7.0. Regurgitation may occur, especially in sheep. Death related to excess NPN usually occurs within 2 hr in cattle, 4 hr in sheep, and 3–12 hr in horses. Survivors recover in 12–24 hr with no sequelae.

Carcasses of animals dying of NPN poisoning appear to bloat and decompose rapidly, with no specific characteristic lesions. Gross brain lesions are not usually reported in NPN-induced ammonia toxicosis, but histopathologic lesions may include neuronal degeneration, spongy degeneration of the neuropil, and congestion and hemorrhage in the pia mater. Frequently, pulmonary edema, congestion, and petechial hemorrhages may be seen. Mild bronchitis and catarrhal gastroenteritis are often reported. Regurgitated and inhaled rumen contents are commonly found in the trachea and bronchi, especially in sheep. The odor of NH_3 may or may not be apparent in ingesta from a freshly opened rumen or cecum. A ruminal or cecal pH ≥7.5 from a recently dead animal is highly suggestive of NPN poisoning. The ruminal pH remains stable for several hours after death under most circumstances but continues to rise in NPN toxicosis.

Diagnosis: Ammonia or NPN poisoning is suggested by signs, lesions, history of acute illness, and dietary exposure. Exposure to excess NPN may be evaluated through laboratory analysis for the ammonia nitrogen (NH_3-N) in both antemortem and postmortem specimens and for urea or other NPN in suspected feeds and other dietary sources. Specimens for NH_3-N analysis include ruminal-reticular fluid, serum, whole blood, and urine. All specimens should be frozen immediately after collection and thawed only for analysis; alternatively, ruminal-reticular fluid may be preserved with a few drops of saturated mercuric chloride solution added to each 100 mL of specimen.

Animals dead more than a few hours in hot ambient temperatures or 12 hr in moderate climates probably have undergone too much autolysis to be of diagnostic value.

The amount of urea or the equivalent NPN in biologic specimens is meaningless; however, urea and NPN should be determined in representative feeds and other dietary sources. Values for urea and NPN in feed permit calculation of the protein equivalent (1 part protein = 0.36 parts urea; 1 part urea = 2.92 parts protein) in feed as well as the total estimated dose of NPN ingested.

NH_3-N concentrations of ≥2 mg/100 mL in blood, serum, or vitreous humor indicate excess NPN exposure. Clinical signs usually appear at ~1 mg/100 mL. The concentration of NH_3-N in ruminal-reticular fluid is >80 mg/100 mL in most cases of NPN poisoning and may be >200 mg/100 mL. Acclimated ruminants fed diets high in legume hay, soybean meal, cottonseed meal, linseed meal, fish meal, or milk byproducts may have NH_3-N concentrations in rumen fluid approaching 60 mg/100 mL with no apparent toxicity. The pH of ruminal-reticular fluid should also be determined; a pH of 7.5–8 (at time of death) is indicative of NPN toxicity.

Differential diagnoses include poisonings by nitrate/nitrite, cyanide, organophosphate/carbamate pesticides, raw soybean overload, 4-methylimidazole, lead, chlorinated hydrocarbon pesticides, and toxic gases (carbon monoxide, hydrogen sulfide, nitrogen dioxide); acute infectious diseases; and noninfectious diseases such as encephalopathies (eg, leukoencephalomalacia, hepatic encephalopathy, polioencephalomalacia), enterotoxemia or rumen autointoxication, protein engorgement, grain engorgement, ruminal tympany, and pulmonary adenomatosis. Nutritional and metabolic disorders related to hypocalcemia, hypomagnesemia, and other elemental aberrations should also be considered.

Treatment: Examination and treatment may be difficult because of sudden and violent behavior. Animals that are recumbent and moribund usually do not respond favorably to treatment.

If possible, affected animals should be treated by ruminal infusion of 5% acetic acid (vinegar, 0.5–2 L in sheep and goats and 2–8 L in cattle). Ruminal-reticular fluid specimens for analysis should be taken before acetic acid therapy. Concomitant infusion of iced (0–4°C) water (up to 40 L in adult cattle, proportionally less in sheep and goats) is also recommended. Acetic acid lowers rumen pH and prevents further absorption of NH_3 by converting uncharged NH_3 to the charged ammonium ion (NH_4^+); administration may have to be repeated if affected animals again show clinical signs. Acetic acid inactivates existing NH_3 in the GI tract and rapidly forms ammonium acetate, which can be used by rumen microflora but does not release NH_3. Cold water lowers the rumen temperature and dilutes the reacting media, which slows urease activity. In severely affected valuable animals, removed rumen contents should be replaced with a hay slurry, and a transfer of some rumen contents from a healthy animal may serve as an inoculum to restore normal function. Ruminal tympany should be corrected if indicated, and a trocar may be installed to prevent recurrence.

Supportive therapy is indicated and includes IV isotonic saline solutions to correct dehydration, and IV calcium gluconate and magnesium solutions to relieve tetanic seizures. Convulsions may also be controlled with sodium pentobarbital or other injectable anesthetic agents.

Prevention and Control: Urea should not be fed at a rate exceeding 2%–3% of the concentrate or grain portion of ruminant diets and should be limited to ≤1% of the total diet. Additionally, NPN should constitute no more than one-third of the total nitrogen in the ruminant diet. Once the decision is made to feed NPN, animals must be slowly adapted to, and maintained on, a consistent dietary NPN content with no significant deviation; cows fed range cubes with NPN must receive the cubes daily with no interruptions. Temporary absences of NPN from the diet should be avoided at all costs. Overconsumption of palatable liquid supplements can be controlled by the addition of phosphoric acid; 1% phosphorus from phosphoric acid should restrict consumption of liquid supplement to ~2 lb/animal/day. Although properly adapted adult cattle can tolerate urea at a rate of up to 1 g/kg body wt/day, a safer feeding rate is no more than half that amount.

COAL-TAR PRODUCTS POISONING

A variety of coal-tar derivatives induce acute to chronic disease in animals, with clinical signs that vary based on the constituents. Clinical effects are acute to chronic hepatic damage with signs of icterus, ascites, anemia, and death. Phenolic components may cause renal tubular damage. Coal tar–related poisoning has been reported in farm animals and pets.

Etiology: The distillation of coal tar yields a variety of compounds, three of which are notably toxic: cresols (phenolic compounds), crude creosote (composed of cresols, heavy oils, and anthracene), and pitch. Tars are also produced from crude petroleum or wood. Creosote contains less volatile liquid and solid aromatic hydrocarbons of coal tar and some phenols. They have been used for restricted applications as wood preservatives. Cresols, composed mainly of hydroxytoluenes, are used in soaps and disinfectants. Coal-tar and pine-tar pitch are the brown to black, amorphous, polynuclear hydrocarbon residues left after coal tar is redistilled. Access of animals to coal tars is often by direct chewing on or consumption of product, rather than inclusion in feed or water. Clay pigeons (older products), tar paper, creosote-treated wood, and bitumen-based flooring are typical sources.

Phenol is the most important toxicant in coal-tar products and is found in antiseptics, creosote, germicides, cleaners, and disinfectants. The approximate oral acute LD_{50} of phenol for most species is 0.5 g/kg, except for cats, which are more susceptible because of limited ability to form glucuronides and excrete phenols. Phenols are directly corrosive, and ingestion results in oral and upper gastroenteric necrosis. After oral or dermal absorption, phenols accumulate in the liver and kidneys, commonly resulting in liver damage and renal tubular necrosis.

Cresols are readily absorbed orally and through the skin. The oral lethal dose is 100–200 mg/kg, except in cats, which are more sensitive. Sows in creosote-treated wooden farrowing crates delivered stillborn pigs. Coal tars may reduce absorption of vitamin A by sows. Other species are less susceptible (eg, the lethal dose of creosote in calves is 4 g/kg). Pitch is no longer used as a binder in clay pigeons, but road asphalt, some insulation, and tar paper and roofing compounds may still contain cresols. Flooring with lignite pitch or asphalt can reduce growth rate and/or cause liver damage in pigs.

Clinical Findings: The cresols and phenols are locally corrosive, causing necrosis and scarring of skin, mouth, and esophagus; CNS stimulation, tremors, and incoordination; and cardiovascular depression and shock. Capillary damage and hepatic or renal damage can occur. Icterus can result from intravascular hemolysis and hepatic damage. Death can occur from 15 min to several days after exposure. The first sign of pitch poisoning often is several dead animals. Signs may progress to weakness, ataxia, sternal recumbency, icterus, coma, and death. Secondary anemia may develop. Other problems have included stillbirths in pigs and hyperkeratosis in calves.

Lesions: Phenols, cresols, and creosote produce contact irritation of skin, mouth, and esophagus and nonspecific liver and kidney lesions. The liver is markedly swollen with a diffuse, mottled appearance. There is centrilobular liver necrosis, with blood replacing the lost cells and filling the center of the lobule. Renal tubular degeneration and necrosis also can be present. The blood clots slowly or not at all. The carcass is icteric. Excessive fluid is found in the peritoneal cavity.

Diagnosis: Differential diagnoses include toxic plant poisonings (*Crotalaria*, *Senecio*, cocklebur), aflatoxicosis, blue-green algae poisoning, fumonisin toxicosis, gossypol toxicosis, yellow phosphorus poisoning, and vitamin E or selenium deficiency. Fragments of tar paper or other sources of coal tars found in the GI tract, or chemical detection of coal-tar products in liver, kidney, serum, or urine, aid in confirming the diagnosis. Laboratory changes include hypoglycemia, and increases in serum liver enzymes, thymol turbidity, chloride, and phosphorus. Proteinuria, hematuria, and urinary cells and casts reflect kidney damage from phenolic fractions of coal tars.

A rapid presumptive test is to mix 1 mL of urine with 0.1 mL of 20% ferric chloride; purple color indicates phenol, but results should be confirmed by a laboratory.

Treatment: There is no specific antidote for coal-tar product poisoning. Emetics and gastric lavage are not recommended for recent oral exposure, but activated charcoal and saline cathartics may reduce absorption. Owners may reduce acute exposure by administration of egg whites to dilute and bind the phenols. Dermal exposures are mitigated by bathing with glycerol followed by liquid dish soap. Supportive therapy for shock, liver and kidney damage, respiratory failure, and acidosis are important supportive measures for individual animals. *N*-acetylcysteine (140 mg/kg, IV, loading dosage, followed by 70 mg/kg, qid for another 3 days) has been recommended. Oral antibiotics, B vitamins, vitamin E, and high-quality–protein diets may aid recovery.

ETHYLENE GLYCOL TOXICITY

All animals are susceptible to ethylene glycol (EG) toxicity, but it is most common in dogs and cats. Most intoxications are associated with ingestion of antifreeze, which is typically 95% EG. These 95% commercial antifreeze preparations are diluted ~50% with water when used in vehicle cooling systems. The widespread availability of antifreeze, its sweet taste and small minimum lethal dose, and the lack of public awareness of the toxicity (ie, improper storage and disposal) contribute to the frequency of this intoxication. In addition, antifreeze may be ingested by way of intentional poisoning or because it is the only available liquid in cold weather. Other sources of EG include some heat-exchange fluids used in solar collectors and ice-rink freezing equipment and some brake and transmission fluids. Cutaneous absorption from topical products that contain EG has been reported to cause toxicity in cats.

EG intoxication occurs most commonly in temperate and cold climates, because antifreeze is used both to decrease the freezing point and to increase the boiling point of radiator fluid. In colder climates, the incidence of EG intoxications is seasonal, with most cases occurring in the fall, winter, and early spring, when antifreeze is added to radiator fluid or when cooling systems are flushed.

The minimum lethal dose of undiluted EG is 1.4 mL/kg body wt in cats, 4.4 mL/kg in dogs, 7–8 mL/kg in poultry, and 2–10 mL/kg in cattle. Younger animals may be more susceptible.

Pathogenesis: EG is rapidly absorbed from the GI tract; in dogs, blood concentrations of EG peak within 3 hr of ingestion. Approximately 50% of ingested EG is excreted unchanged by the kidneys; however, a series of oxidation reactions in the liver and kidneys metabolize the remaining EG. Toxic metabolites of EG cause severe metabolic acidosis and renal tubular epithelial damage.

The first of two rate-limiting biotransformation steps is the production of glycoaldehyde from EG by the enzyme alcohol dehydrogenase. Glycolaldehyde is then rapidly metabolized to glycolic acid. The oxidation of glycolic acid to glyoxylic acid is the second rate-limiting step, which allows glycolic acid to accumulate, resulting in acidosis and nephrotoxicosis. Glyoxylic acid is rapidly metabolized to formic acid, carbon dioxide, glycine, serine, and oxalate. Oxalate is not further metabolized and is cytotoxic to the renal tubular epithelium and exacerbates the metabolic acidosis. Glycolic acid and oxalate are the metabolites thought to be most responsible for acute tubular necrosis associated with EG ingestion. Oxalate also combines with calcium to form a soluble complex that is excreted via glomerular filtration. Calcium oxalate crystals form within the lumina of tubules as water is reabsorbed from the glomerular filtrate and the pH decreases (smaller numbers of calcium oxalate crystals may also be observed in the adventitia of blood vessel walls throughout the body).

Clinical Findings: Clinical signs are dose- and time-dependent and can be divided into those caused by unmetabolized EG and those caused by its toxic metabolites. The onset of clinical signs is almost immediate and resembles alcohol (ethanol) intoxication. Dogs and cats exhibit vomiting due to GI irritation, polydipsia and polyuria, and neurologic signs (CNS depression, stupor, ataxia, knuckling, decreased withdrawal and righting reflexes). Polydipsia occurs due to osmotic stimulation of the thirst center, and polyuria occurs due to an osmotic diuresis and decreased production and release of antidiuretic hormone. As CNS depression increases in severity, dogs and cats drink less; however, the osmotic diuresis continues and results in dehydration. Dogs may appear to transiently recover from these CNS signs ~12 hr after ingestion.

Oliguric acute renal failure usually develops between 12 and 24 hr in cats and between 36 and 72 hr in dogs. Signs include lethargy, anorexia, dehydration, vomiting, diarrhea, oral ulcers, salivation, tachypnea, and possibly seizures or coma. The kidneys are often swollen and painful on abdominal palpation.

Pigs ingesting EG are usually depressed, weak, and reluctant to move; knuckling, posterior ataxia, trembling, collapse, abdominal distention, pulmonary edema, and muffled heart sounds are common sequelae. Poultry may become drowsy, ataxic, dyspneic, and recumbent; torticollis, ruffled feathers, and watery droppings are also seen. Cattle may become depressed, tachypneic, and ataxic, and develop paraparesis or recumbency. Epistaxis and hemoglobinuria have also been seen in cattle that have ingested large doses of EG.

Lesions: Renal tubular epithelial necrosis with calcium oxalate crystals in the tubular lumina is the characteristic finding of EG intoxication. Calcium oxalate crystals appear birefringent when viewed with polarized light. Pulmonary edema and hemorrhagic gastroenteritis are common secondary findings in dogs and cats. Pigs and cattle often develop renal and perirenal edema. Pigs may also have pulmonary edema with tan fluid in the pleural and peritoneal cavities. Poultry usually do not develop gross lesions.

Diagnosis: Diagnosis is often difficult because the nonspecific multisystemic signs may appear similar to other types of CNS disease or trauma, gastroenteritis, pancreatitis, ketoacidotic diabetes mellitus, and acute renal failure due to renal ischemia or other nephrotoxicants. If ingestion of EG is not witnessed, diagnosis is usually based on a combination of history, physical examination, and laboratory data.

Within 3 hr of ingestion of toxic doses of EG, dogs and cats develop normochloremic metabolic acidosis with an increased anion gap, minimally concentrated or isosthenuric urine with an acidic pH, and marked serum hyperosmolality with an increased osmolal gap. Serum osmolality can be increased as much as 100 mOsm/kg above normal (280–310 mOsm/kg) within 3 hr of EG ingestion. The difference between measured and calculated (1.86 [Na^+ + K^+] + glucose/18 + BUN/2.8 + 9) osmolality is referred to as the osmolal gap. The gap is caused by the presence of osmotically active particles (eg, ethylene glycol) in the serum that are not factored into the above equation. Calcium oxalate crystalluria may be observed as early as 3 and 6 hr after ingestion in cats and dogs, respectively. Monohydrate calcium oxalate crystals (clear, 6-sided prisms) are more common than dihydrate calcium oxalate crystals (maltese cross or envelope-shaped). EG concentrations in serum and urine are detectable by 1–2 hr after ingestion. Commercial test kits can detect serum EG concentrations of ≥50 mg/dL. Some antifreeze preparations contain fluorescein, which appears bright yellow-green when viewed under a Wood's lamp. Urine fluorescence has been used as a qualitative adjunctive test in suspected EG ingestions in people and may be of value in veterinary medicine. Hyperphosphatemia has been seen in dogs within 3 hr of ingestion of commercial antifreeze solutions that contain phosphate rust inhibitors. This hyperphosphatemia resolves before the onset of EG-induced acute renal failure and azotemia, then recurs when the animal becomes azotemic.

Treatment: The prognosis varies inversely with the amount of time that elapses between ingestion and initiation of treatment. Treatment is aimed at decreasing absorption of ingested EG, increasing excretion of unmetabolized EG, preventing metabolism of EG, and correcting the metabolic acidosis that occurs with EG metabolism. Further absorption of EG is prevented by induction of emesis or gastric lavage (or both) within 1–2 hr of ingestion, although the rapidity of EG absorption from the GI tract suggests these procedures may not be beneficial. Vomiting should not be induced in a dog or cat exhibiting neurologic signs because of increased risk of aspiration. Activated charcoal is not likely to reduce absorption of EG from the GI tract. Once absorption has occurred, excretion of EG is increased by fluid therapy designed to correct dehydration and increase urine production. To prevent metabolism of EG, the activity of alcohol dehydrogenase is decreased by direct inactivation or by competitive inhibition. 4-Methylpyrazole (4-MP, fomepizole) effectively inactivates alcohol dehydrogenase in dogs without the adverse effects of ethanol and is the treatment of choice. The dose of 4-MP (5% solution [50 mg/mL]) is 20 mg/kg body wt, IV, initially, followed by 15 mg/kg, IV, at 12 and 24 hr, and 5 mg/kg, IV, at 36 hr. Commercial formulations of 4-MP are available. If 4-MP is not available, an ethanol regimen (5.5 mL of 20% ethanol/kg body wt, IV, every 4 hr for five treatments and then every 6 hr for four additional treatments) is recommended.

In cats, 4-MP is ineffective at the canine dosage, and either a higher, extra-label dosage (125 mg/kg initially, followed by 31.3 mg/kg at 12, 24, and 36 hr after the initial dose) or ethanol is used. The recommended dosage is 5 mL of 20% ethanol/kg body wt diluted in IV fluids and given as a drip over 6 hr for five treatments, and then over 8 hr for four more treatments.

The metabolic acidosis associated with metabolism of EG is corrected by administration of sodium bicarbonate. The formula 0.3 – (0.5 × kg body wt) × (24 – plasma bicarbonate) is used to determine the dose, in mEq of bicarbonate. One-half of this dose should be given IV slowly to prevent overdose, and plasma bicarbonate concentrations should be monitored every 4–6 hr. Additional doses of bicarbonate based on the above formula are frequently necessary. Monitoring urine pH may also be helpful, with a goal of maintaining the urine pH between 7.0 and 7.5.

In dogs and cats with azotemia or in oliguric acute renal failure, inhibition of alcohol dehydrogenase is of little benefit, because almost all of the EG has already been metabolized. The prognosis for these animals is guarded to poor. Treatment should include correction of fluid, electrolyte, and acid-base disorders and, if possible, induction of diuresis.

PROPYLENE GLYCOL TOXICOSIS

Although less toxic than EG, ingestion of propylene glycol (PG) may be associated with a toxic syndrome similar to the acute phase of EG toxicosis. The oral LD_{50} of PG in dogs is ~9 mL/kg. In cats, ingestion of a diet containing 6%–12% PG can result in Heinz body formation and decreased RBC survival. Treatment of PG toxicosis is largely supportive—the use of alcohol dehydrogenase inhibitors is not indicated. Ingestion of PG may result in false-positive EG test kit results.

NITRATE AND NITRITE POISONING

Many species are susceptible to nitrate and nitrite poisoning, but cattle are affected most frequently. Ruminants are especially vulnerable because the ruminal flora reduces nitrate to ammonia, with nitrite (~10 times more toxic than nitrate) as an intermediate product. Nitrate reduction (and nitrite production) occurs in the cecum of equids but not to the same extent as in ruminants. Young pigs also have GI microflora capable of reducing nitrate to nitrite, but mature monogastric animals (except equids) are more resistant to nitrate toxicosis because this pathway is age-limited.

Acute intoxication is manifested primarily by methemoglobin formation (nitrite ion in contact with RBCs oxidizes ferrous iron in Hgb to the ferric state, forming stable methemoglobin incapable of oxygen transport) and resultant anoxia. Secondary effects due to vasodilatory action of the nitrite ion on vascular smooth muscle may occur. The nitrite ion may also alter metabolic protein enzymes. Ingested nitrates may directly irritate the GI mucosa and produce abdominal pain and diarrhea.

Although usually acute, the effects of nitrite or nitrate toxicity may be subacute or chronic and are reported to include retarded growth, lowered milk production, vitamin A deficiency, minor transitory goitrogenic effects, abortions and fetotoxicity, and increased susceptibility to infection. Chronic nitrate toxicosis remains a controversial issue and is not as yet well characterized, but most current evidence does not support assertions of lowered milk production in dairy cows due to excessive dietary nitrate exposure alone.

Etiology: Nitrates and nitrites are used in pickling and curing brines to preserve meats, and in certain machine oils and antirust tablets, gunpowder and explosives, and fertilizers. They may also serve as therapeutic agents for certain noninfectious diseases, eg, cyanide poisoning. Toxicoses occur in unacclimated domestic animals, most commonly from ingestion of plants that contain excess nitrate, especially by hungry animals engorging themselves and taking in an enormous body burden of nitrate. Confounding interactions with nonprotein nitrogen, monensin, and other feed components may exacerbate effects of excessive nitrate content in livestock diets, especially when coupled with management errors.

Nitrate toxicosis can also result from accidental ingestion of fertilizer or other chemicals. Nitrate concentrations may be hazardous in ponds that receive extensive feedlot or fertilizer runoff; these types of nitrate sources may also contaminate shallow, poorly cased wells. Although nitrate concentrations are increasing in groundwater in the USA, well water is rarely the sole cause of excess nitrate exposure.

Water with both high nitrate content and significant coliform contamination has greater potential to adversely affect health and productivity than does either nitrate or bacteria alone. Livestock losses have occurred during cold weather due to the concentrating effect of freezing, which increases nitrate content of remaining water in stock tanks.

Crops that readily concentrate nitrate include cereal grasses (especially oats, millet, and rye), corn (maize), sunflower, and sorghums. Weeds that commonly have high nitrate concentrations are pigweed, lamb's-quarter, thistle, Jimson weed, fireweed (*Kochia*), smartweed, dock, and Johnson grass. Anhydrous ammonia and nitrate fertilizers and soils naturally high in nitrogen tend to increase nitrate content in forage.

Excess nitrate in plants is generally associated with damp weather conditions and cool temperatures (55°F [13°C]), although high concentrations are also likely to develop when growth is rapid during hot, humid weather. Drought conditions, particularly if occurring when plants are immature, may leave the vegetation with high nitrate content. Decreased light, cloudy weather, and shading associated with crowding conditions can also cause increased concentrations of nitrates within plants. Well-aerated soil with a low pH, and low or deficient amounts of molybdenum, sulfur, or phosphorus in soil tend to enhance nitrate uptake, whereas soil deficiencies of copper, cobalt, or manganese tend to have opposing effects. Anything that stunts growth increases nitrate accumulation in the lower part of the plant. Phenoxy acid derivative herbicides (eg, 2,4-D and 2,4,5-T), applied to nitrate-accumulating plants during early stages, cause increased growth and a high nitrate residual (10%–30%) in surviving plants, which are lush and eaten with apparent relish even though previously avoided.

Nitrate, which does not selectively accumulate in fruits or grain, is found chiefly in the lower stalk with lesser amounts in the upper stalk and leaves. Nitrate in plants can be converted to nitrite under the proper conditions of moisture, heat, and microbial activity after harvesting.

Clinical Findings: Signs of nitrite poisoning usually appear suddenly because of tissue hypoxia and low blood pressure as a consequence of vasodilation. Rapid, weak heartbeat with subnormal body temperature, muscular tremors, weakness, and ataxia are early signs of toxicosis when methemoglobinemia reaches 30%–40%. Brown, cyanotic mucous membranes develop rapidly as methemoglobinemia exceeds 50%. Dyspnea, tachypnea, anxiety, and frequent urination are common. Some monogastric animals, usually because of excess nitrate exposure from nonplant sources, exhibit salivation, vomiting, diarrhea, abdominal pain, and gastric hemorrhage. Affected animals may die suddenly without appearing ill, in terminal anoxic convulsions within 1 hr, or after a clinical course of 12–24 hr or longer. Acute lethal toxicoses almost always are due to development of ≥80% methemoglobinemia.

Under certain conditions, adverse effects may not be apparent until animals have been eating nitrate-containing forages for days to weeks. Some animals that develop marked dyspnea recover but then develop interstitial pulmonary emphysema and have continued respiratory distress; most of these recover fully within 10–14 days. Abortion and stillbirths may be seen in some cattle 5–14 days after excessive nitrate/nitrite exposure but likely only in cows that have survived a ≥50% methemoglobinemia for 6–12 hr or longer. Prolonged exposure to excess nitrate coupled with cold stress and inadequate nutrition may lead to the alert downer cow syndrome (*see* p 1188) in pregnant beef cattle; sudden collapse and death can result.

Lesions: Blood that contains methemoglobin usually has a chocolate-brown color, although dark red hues may also be seen. There may be pinpoint or larger hemorrhages on serosal surfaces. Hydroperitoneum and ascites have been reported in stillborn calves, as well as edema and hemorrhage in the lungs and digestive system of perinatal calves with excessive maternal nitrate exposure. However, dark brown discoloration evident in moribund or recently dead animals is not pathognomonic, and other methemoglobin inducers must be considered. If necropsy is postponed too long, the brown discoloration may disappear with conversion of methemoglobin back to Hgb.

Diagnosis: Excess nitrate exposure can be assessed by laboratory analysis for nitrate in both pre- and postmortem specimens. High nitrate and nitrite values in postmortem specimens may be an incidental finding, indicative only of exposure and not toxicity. Plasma is the preferred premortem specimen, because some plasma protein–bound nitrite could be lost in the clot if serum was collected. Nitrite present in whole blood also continues to react with Hgb in vitro, so these specimens must be centrifuged immediately and plasma separated to prevent erroneous values of both. Additional postmortem specimens from either toxicoses or abortions include ocular fluids, fetal pleural or thoracic fluids, fetal stomach contents, and maternal uterine fluid. All specimens should be frozen in clean plastic or glass containers before submission, except when whole blood is collected for methemoglobin analysis. Because the amount of nitrate in rumen contents is not representative of concentrations in the diet, evaluation of rumen contents is not indicated.

Bacterial contamination of postmortem specimens, especially ocular fluid, is likely to cause conversion of nitrate to nitrite at room temperature or higher; such specimens may have abnormally high nitrite concentrations with reduced to absent nitrate concentrations. Endogenous biosynthesis of nitrate and nitrite by macrophages stimulated by lipopolysaccharide or other bacterial products may also complicate interpretation of analytical findings; this should be considered as a possible maternal or fetal response to an infection.

Methemoglobin analysis alone is not a reliable indicator of excess nitrate or nitrite exposure except in acute toxicosis, because 50% of methemoglobin present will be converted back to Hgb in ~2 hr, and alternative forms of nonoxygenated Hgb that may be formed by reaction with nitrite are not detected by methemoglobin analysis. Nitrate and nitrite concentrations >20 mcg NO_3/mL and >0.5 mcg NO_2/mL, respectively, in maternal and perinatal serum, plasma, ocular fluid, and other similar biologic fluids are usually indicative of excessive nitrate or nitrite exposure in most domestic animal species; nitrate concentrations of up to 40 mcg NO_3/mL have been present in the plasma of healthy calves at birth but are reduced rapidly as normal neonatal renal function eliminates nitrate in the urine. In acutely poisoned ruminant livestock, nitrate and nitrite concentrations as high as 300 mcg NO_3/mL and 25–50 mcg NO_2/mL, respectively, can be found in plasma or serum, with ~ ⅓ less in postmortem ocular fluid because of diffusion equilibrium delay. However, postmortem ocular fluid nitrate concentrations are relatively stable and remain diagnostically significant for up to 60 hr after death. Once collected, plasma, serum, and ocular fluid specimens have stable nitrate concentration for at least 1 mo at –20°C.

Normally expected nitrate and nitrite concentrations in similar diagnostic specimens are usually <10 mcg NO_3/mL and <0.2 mcg NO_2/mL, respectively. Nitrate and nitrite concentrations >10 but <20 mcg NO_3/mL and >0.2 but <0.5 mcg NO_2/mL, respectively, are suspect and indicate nitrate or nitrite exposure of unknown duration, extent, or origin. The possible contribution of endogenous nitrate or nitrite synthesis by activated macrophages must also be considered. The biologic half-life of nitrate in beef cattle, sheep, and ponies was determined to be 7.7, 4.2, and 4.8 hr, respectively, so it will be at least five biologic half-lives (24–36 hr) before increased nitrate concentrations from excessive nitrate exposure diminish to normally expected values, allowing additional time for valid premortem specimen collection.

A latent period may exist between excessive maternal dietary nitrate exposure and equilibrium in perinatal ocular fluids. Aqueous humor is actively secreted into the anterior chamber at a rate of ~0.1/mL/hr, and nitrate and nitrite are thought to enter the globe of the eye by this mechanism. Equilibrium between aqueous and vitreous humor is by passive diffusion rather than by active secretion, so nitrate or nitrite may be present in comparatively lesser concentrations in vitreous humor after acute exposure.

Field tests for nitrate are presumptive and should be confirmed by standard analytical methods at a qualified laboratory. The diphenylamine blue test (1% in concentrated sulfuric acid) is more suitable to determine the presence or absence of nitrate in suspected forages. Nitrate test strips (dipsticks) are effective in determining nitrate values in water supplies and can be used to evaluate nitrate and nitrite content in serum, plasma, ocular fluid, and urine.

Differential diagnoses include poisonings by cyanide, urea, pesticides, toxic gases (eg, carbon monoxide, hydrogen sulfide), chlorates, aniline dyes, aminophenols, or drugs (eg, sulfonamides, phenacetin, and acetaminophen), as well as infectious or noninfectious diseases (eg, grain overload, hypocalcemia, hypomagnesemia, pulmonary adenomatosis, or emphysema) and any other cause of sudden unexplained deaths.

Treatment: Slow IV injection of 1% methylene blue in distilled water or isotonic saline should be given at 4–22 mg/kg or more, depending on severity of exposure. Lower dosages may be repeated in 20–30 min if the initial response is not satisfactory. Lower dosages of methylene blue can be used in all species, but only ruminants can safely tolerate higher dosages. If additional exposure or absorption occurs during therapy, re-treating with methylene blue every 6–8 hr should be considered. Rumen lavage with cold water and antibiotics may stop the continuing microbial production of nitrite.

Control: Animals may adapt to higher nitrate content in feeds, especially when grazing summer annuals such as sorghum-Sudan hybrids. Multiple, small feedings help animals adapt. Trace mineral supplements and a balanced diet may help prevent nutritional or metabolic disorders associated with longterm excess dietary nitrate consumption. Feeding grain with high-nitrate forages may reduce nitrite production. However, caution is advised when combining other feed additives/components, including nonprotein nitrogen, ionophores (such as monensin) and other growth and performance enhancers, with high-nitrate diets in ruminants. Proper management, especially regarding acclimation, is critical. Forage nitrate concentrations >1% nitrate dry-weight basis (10,000 ppm NO_3) may cause acute toxicoses in unacclimated animals, and forage nitrate concentrations ≤5,000 ppm NO_3 (dry-weight basis) are recommended for pregnant beef cows. However, even forage concentrations of 1,000 ppm NO_3 dry-weight basis have been lethal to hungry cows engorging themselves in a single feeding within an hour, so the total dose of nitrate ingested is a deciding factor.

High-nitrate forages may also be harvested and stored as ensilage rather than dried hay or green chop; this may reduce the nitrate content in forages by up to 50%. Raising cutter heads of machinery during harvesting operations selectively leaves the more hazardous stalk bases in the field.

Hay appears to be more hazardous than fresh green chop or pasture with similar nitrate content. Heating may assist bacterial conversion of nitrate to nitrite; feeding high-nitrate hay, straw, or fodder that has been damp or wet for several days, or stockpiled, green-chopped forage should be avoided. Large round bales with excess nitrate are especially dangerous if stored uncovered outside; rain or snow can leach and subsequently concentrate most of the total nitrate present into the lower third of these bales.

Water transported in improperly cleaned liquid fertilizer tanks may be extremely high in nitrate. Young, unweaned livestock, especially neonatal pigs, can be more sensitive to nitrate in water.

PENTACHLOROPHENOL POISONING

(Penta poisoning)

Pentachlorophenol (PCP), commonly known as penta, has been used as a fungicide, molluscicide, insecticide, and wood preservative. Its use is now permitted only for industrial purposes; agricultural and domestic uses are prohibited, because it is classified as a highly hazardous pesticide.

The oral LD_{50} of penta in rats is 150–210 mg/kg body wt. Common signs of poisoning include nervousness, rapid pulse and respiratory rate, weakness, fever, muscle tremors, convulsions, loss in righting reflexes, and asphyxial spasms followed by death. Corneal injury may result from splashes or vapor overexposure. Chronic poisoning results in emaciation, fatty liver, nephrosis, and weight loss.

The persistence of penta in soil and water and apparent widespread use has resulted in significant exposure to animals. Young swine have died after dermal exposure to freshly penta-treated wood used in farrowing crates or farrowing houses. In vivo studies in swine demonstrated that exposure to penta-contaminated soil can result in significant dermal absorption of the pesticide. Penta can be absorbed through intact skin and lungs and is an intense irritant to the skin and mucous membranes. Penta absorption in skin was greater in water or water-based mixtures than in 100% ethanol. Because animals typically have access to water at all times, this hydrophilic characteristic of penta suggests enhanced dermal absorption.

When absorbed, penta increases metabolism by uncoupling cellular phosphorylation. Animals fed in troughs made of lumber treated with PCP may salivate and have irritated oral mucosa. Both penta and its major metabolite, tetrachlorohydroquinone (TCHQ), can induce epidermal hyperplasia in mice.

Poultry have been exposed to sawdust and shavings from penta-treated wood. Associated adverse effects include reduced growth rates, kidney hypertrophy, and decreased humoral immune response. Penta exposure can also result in an off-taste to eggs and meat as a result of degradation of chlorophenols to chloroanisols. Vaporization or leaching of penta in pens, enclosures, homes, and barns has caused illness and death.

Cattle and pigs exposed to wood treated with commercial grade penta had increased mortality, possibly decreased fertility in boars, and reduced productivity (milk, meat, etc). The lethal dose in cattle and sheep is ~120–140 mg/kg body wt.

Commercial lots of technical-grade penta contain small but biologically significant amounts of highly toxic impurities such as chlorinated dioxins and dibenzofurans, tetrachlorophenols, and hydroxychlorodiphenyl ethers; these compounds can exert their own effects such as early fetotoxicity. Commercial-grade penta causes hepatic porphyria, increased microsomal monooxygenase activity, and increased liver weight. Pure penta was not teratogenic in rats.

Penta can cause residues in animal tissues. Also, a significant amount of hexachlorobenzene is metabolized in animal tissues to penta. Pentachlorophenol is considered to be a carcinogen and a tumor promoter, although studies have shown that the pure material does not increase the incidence of tumors in rats and mice. The technical-grade material has also been shown to be immunotoxic in laboratory studies. Penta must be handled very carefully and kept away from animal contact.

Whole blood analysis for penta may aid in the diagnosis of poisoning; diagnosis is usually made on the basis of the signs and the proximity of treated lumber in the animal's environment.

There is no known antidote. Termination of exposure, bathing dermally exposed animals, oral administration of activated charcoal, and supportive therapy may be indicated. Bathing should be done gently with cold water and detergent so as not to cause vasodilation and increased absorption. Antipyretics, eg, aspirin and acetaminophen, should not be used. Treatment involves cooling the animal and administering fluids, electrolytes, and anticonvulsants.

PETROLEUM PRODUCT POISONING

Ingestion or inhalation of, or skin contact with, petroleum, petroleum condensate, gasoline, diesel fuel, kerosene, crude oil, or other hydrocarbon mixtures may cause illness and occasionally death in domestic and wild animals. Dogs and cats both may ingest petroleum products during grooming of contaminated fur or directly from open containers. Inhalation may occur in poorly ventilated areas where these chemicals have been used or stored. Ruminants may ingest such products in large amounts because they are thirsty, curious, or seeking salt or other nutrients, or if food or water is contaminated.

Small quantities of petroleum product used as carriers for insecticides have few or no harmful effects, but large quantities and prolonged exposure can induce severe reactions. Pipeline breaks, accidental release from storage, tank car accidents, and open or leaky containers are potential sources. Physical properties can affect exposure and toxicity. Volatility increases at lower molecular weight and lower saturation or aromaticity. Absorption is greater with highly volatile, lower molecular weight hydrocarbons (eg, hexane, gasoline) as well as aromatic hydrocarbons (benzene, toluene) because of greater lipid solubility. Crude petroleum that has lost much of its lighter, more volatile components through weathering may still be hazardous.

Crude oil and gasoline contain varying amounts of aromatic hydrocarbons, including benzene (2%–5% in gasoline), toluene, ethylbenzene, and xylene. These compounds ingested or inhaled in sufficient amounts can have acute and chronic effects different from those of other hydrocarbons that make up most oil and gas products. Benzene is hemotoxic and a known carcinogen at high levels of exposure. Toluene causes neurologic signs and damage at high dosages. Central nervous signs occur when sufficient petroleum product is absorbed into the brain or peripheral nerves. Toxicosis generally occurs rapidly after exposure.

Variation in composition of petroleum and petroleum-derived hydrocarbon mixtures explains some of the differences in toxic effects. Mixtures of low viscosity/high volatility (eg, gasoline, naphtha, kerosene, xylene) have a high aspiration hazard and irritant activity on pulmonary tissues. Gasoline and naphtha fractions may induce vomiting, which contributes to aspiration hazard. Fractions more viscous than kerosene (asphalt, mineral oil, waxes) are less likely to be inhaled and, even if aspirated, are somewhat less damaging to lung tissue. Older formulations of lubricating oils and greases can be particularly hazardous because of toxic additives or contaminants (eg, lead).

Comparative toxicity of petroleum hydrocarbons can be considered high (oral LD_{50} <10 mL/kg, eg, acetone, benzene, carbon disulfide, diesel fuel, toluene, xylene), moderate (oral LD_{50} 10–20 mL/kg, eg, diesel fuel, gasoline, heating oil, isopropanol, turpentine), or limited (oral LD_{50} >20 mL/kg, eg, motor oil, jet fuel, lighter fluid). Toxicity of crude oil depends on the relative content of kerosene, naphtha, and gasoline. Sweet crude oil (high gasoline, naphtha, and kerosene content) at ~50 mL/kg and sour crude oil (low fractions of gasoline, naphtha, and kerosene) at 75 mL/kg exposure for 1 wk have caused aspiration pneumonia.

Clinical Findings: Petroleum hydrocarbon toxicity may involve the respiratory, GI, or integumentary systems or the CNS. In most cases of ingestion, no clinical signs are seen, but small animals are reported to show oral irritation, salivation, and champing of jaws, followed by coughing, choking, and vomiting. Pneumonia due to aspiration of hydrocarbons into the lungs is usually the most serious consequence of ingestion of these materials. Aspiration can occur during vomiting by monogastrics or eructation of rumen contents. Pulmonary damage can occur from a combination of volatility, viscosity, and surface tension. Higher volatility promotes access of vapors to the lung and airways and displaces alveolar oxygen. Risk of pulmonary toxicity is increased by products of lower viscosity and surface tension, with increased penetration into smaller airways and spread of product to a larger lung surface area.

Acute bloat from petroleum products in ruminants has been reported after consumption of highly volatile hydrocarbons such as gasoline or naphtha. CNS signs may be a result of the anesthetic-like action of low-molecular-weight aliphatic hydrocarbons and/or cerebral anoxia that can result from lung damage or displacement of oxygen by the more volatile hydrocarbons. Some compounds when absorbed in high doses may sensitize the myocardium to endogenous catecholamines. Anorexia, decreased rumen motility, and mild depression may begin in ~24 hr and last 3–14 days depending on dose and content. Hypoglycemia may be seen several days after ingestion. These signs and weight loss may be the only responses seen in animals that do not bloat or aspirate oil. Some animals do not reestablish normal rumen function after ingestion and can develop a chronic wasting condition.

After ingestion of oil, the feces may not be affected until several days later, when they become dry and formed, in the case of kerosene or lighter hydrocarbon fractions; in contrast, heavier hydrocarbon mixtures (eg, motor oil) *tend to be cathartic. Oil* may be found in feces and rumen contents as long as 2 wk after ingestion. Regurgitated or vomited oil may be seen on the muzzle and lips.

CNS signs attributable to pulmonary, dermal, or GI absorption of hydrocarbons or cerebral anoxia include excitability (associated with aromatic fractions—benzene, toluene, etc), depression (aliphatic or saturated low-molecular-weight hydrocarbons), shivering, head tremors, visual dysfunction (sometimes associated with lead contamination), and incoordination. Acute pneumonia and possibly pleuritis (coughing, tachypnea, shallow respiration, reluctance to move, head held low, weakness, oily nasal discharge, and dehydrated appearance) are seen in some animals that aspirate highly volatile mixtures; deaths usually are seen within days. Respiratory signs may be limited to dyspnea shortly before death in animals that aspirate heavier hydrocarbons. Increased PCV, Hgb, and BUN, indicating mild to moderate hemoconcentration, are associated with development of pneumonia. Neutropenia, lymphopenia, and eosinopenia occur initially and are followed by a relative increase in neutrophils.

There are a few anecdotal reports of abortion after exposure. Laboratory data in rodents support the occurrence of increased fetal loss and decreased fetal growth. However, the doses necessary to affect the fetus were also sufficient to profoundly affect maternal health and weight.

Lesions: Aspiration pneumonia is the most consistent postmortem finding in animals that do not die of bloat. This may be accompanied by tracheitis, pleuritis, and hydrothorax if highly volatile fractions such as gasoline or naphtha are involved. Lung lesions are usually bilateral and found in the caudoventral apical, cardiac, cranioventral diaphragmatic, and intermediate lobes. Affected portions are dark red and consolidated and may contain multiple abscesses. Encapsulated pulmonary abscesses may be found in cattle surviving up to several months after aspiration. Skin lesions may be obvious after repeated topical application or severe exposure and include drying, cracking, or blistering.

Diagnosis: A hydrocarbon odor may be detected in lungs, ruminal contents, and feces. Even if ingested in large doses, hydrocarbons may not be visible in ruminal contents after ~4 days. Adding warm water to the GI contents may cause any oily contents to collect at the surface, but finding oil in the GI tract does not in itself justify a diagnosis of poisoning; most oils have low toxicity if not aspirated. Samples of GI contents, lung, liver, kidney, and the suspected source should be collected for chemical analysis to demonstrate presence of hydrocarbons in tissue (particularly lung) and GI contents and to match those found in tissues and ingesta with the suspected source. Samples must be carefully protected from cross-contamination during necropsy and transportation to the laboratory. Instructions from the receiving diagnostic laboratory should be checked to ensure collection equipment and transport containers are appropriate to prevent evaporative loss of important components and contamination. Positive chemical findings together with appropriate clinical and pathologic findings are confirmatory. Diagnosis in oil-field situations has historically been complicated by involvement of other toxicants, eg, explosives, lead from grease and "pipe dope," arsenicals, organophosphate esters, caustics (acids or alkalis), and saltwater.

Treatment: Bloat pressure should be released by passing a stomach tube if absolutely necessary to save the life of the animal; using a trocar risks forcing oil into the peritoneal cavity, which results in peritonitis. Passing a stomach tube dramatically increases the risk of aspiration, and extreme caution is necessary. In the absence of bloat, the prime objectives are to prevent aspiration and to mitigate GI dysfunction. Rumenotomy to remove ruminal contents and replace them with healthy ruminal material is safer. More chronic cases involving primarily hypofunction of the rumen may also respond to this procedure. Cathartics, if used, should be of the saline or sorbitol type; however, there is no evidence that they improve prognosis. Recent information no longer supports use of oil-based cathartics for petroleum ingestion.

Activated charcoal has occasionally been suggested for use in small animals. Although it does not effectively adsorb petroleum distillates, it may be given if necessary to adsorb additives and other contaminants. Gastric lavage is generally contraindicated for petroleum and volatile hydrocarbon ingestions. Care should be taken to avoid inducing vomiting and aspiration. Small animals with acute respiratory distress may require supplemental oxygen and positive-pressure ventilation, used cautiously because of existing physical pulmonary damage. Frequent purging of ventilators is necessary to eliminate volatile hydrocarbons.

Animals with evidence of bacterial respiratory infection may require broad-spectrum antibiotic treatment. Pathogens can be introduced into the lungs from aspirated rumen or stomach contents mixed with the hydrocarbons. However, the use of steroids in hydrocarbon aspiration may further reduce the chance of recovery and are generally contraindicated. Treatment of aspiration pneumonia (*see* p 1417) is rarely effective, and the prognosis is poor. However, because signs of aspiration may not appear for several days, prognosis based on initial clinical findings may be misleading.

Most high-molecular-weight compounds pass through the GI tract unchanged. Most of the petroleum hydrocarbons are highly lipophilic and will be stored for varying times in tissues with high lipid content, including fat, nervous tissue, and the liver. Some of the absorbed compounds are metabolized into more toxic by-products (eg, benzene, toluene, and n-hexane). Although most of these compounds do not remain in the body for prolonged periods, little is known about exactly how long tissue levels persist in highly exposed animals. The potential for tissue residues must be considered before the slaughter of animals intended for human consumption.

In poisoning or damage due to cutaneous exposure, the material should be removed from the skin with the aid of soap or mild detergents and copious amounts of cool water. The skin should not be brushed or abraded. Further treatment depends on the clinical signs and is largely restricted to supportive therapy.

Petroleum hydrocarbon poisoning can be avoided only by preventing access to these materials through proper storage of home and farm chemicals and well-maintained fencing around high-risk petroleum facilities.

Effects of Oil and Gas Fields on Cattle Health and Production: Anecdotal reports in the literature have documented producer concerns about the effect of oil fields on cattle health and production. Some observational studies have suggested that exposure to emissions from sour gas processing plants and sour gas flares (natural gas containing hydrogen sulfide) may be associated with an increased risk of certain reproductive losses in cattle. Researchers are currently reexamining these findings and exploring the impact of oil and gas field emissions on the immune system.

PERSISTENT HALOGENATED AROMATIC POISONING

Persistent halogenated hydrocarbons (PHAs) are manmade chemicals and can be products of incomplete combustion. PHAs are a complex mixture of chemicals with differing molecular composition. Some PHAs are added to consumer products to provide unique properties and have been/are used as pesticides and disinfection agents. Most PHAs persist in the environment and are classified as persistent organic pollutants. PHAs cause acute and chronic toxicity. There is evidence that lifetime chronic toxicity can be expressed differently during life stages from embryogenesis to senility. Exposure at early life stages may not be expressed until a later life stage. PHAs can be biomagnified in body fat and liver, translocated to the fetus, and secreted in milk and eggs. Biomagnification is a process wherein PHAs are concentrated in fat and liver at a factor higher than dietary levels and is a food safety issue. Important groups of PHAs include polybrominated diphenyl ethers (PBDEs), polychlorinated dibenzo-p-dioxins, dibenzofurans (PCDD/Fs), polychlorinated biphenyls (PCBs), DDT, and triclosan.

Etiology: Exposure to PHAs results from contamination of the indoor environment, especially house dust, atmospheric deposition of PHAs, amending agricultural lands with sewage sludge and industrial wastes, industrial incidents, and feed contamination including byproduct ingredients. Indoor dust is an important route of exposure of companion animals to PBDE fire retardants. For the other PHAs, diet is generally considered the primary route of exposure. Atmospheric PHAs, dispersed worldwide, tend to have higher concentrations in the arctic and antarctic regions. Atmospheric PHAs are deposited on soil and forages. Consumption of contaminated forage and soil by ruminants is a significant source of PCDD/Fs and other PHAs in the food web. Animal by-products containing PHAs, previously biomagnified in fat and liver by other animals in the food web, are also an important source of PHAs in animal diets. Ball clay contaminated with PCDDs has been incorporated in the diets of food-producing animals, and contaminated clay has been used in human food processing. Exposure assessments must include all sources of PHAs. Human dietary exposure to PHAs is generally from ingestion of ruminant products and farmed and wild fish. Cats, like small children, are also exposed in the indoor environment.

Soil can be contaminated by industrial activity and spreading of waste materials on land. For example, spreading sewage sludge on soil can cause a 50× increase in the soil levels of PCDDs. Levels of PBDEs in sewage sludge have been reported as high as 2.3 ppm (dry), and the most consistent PBDE in sewage sludge is the penta-PDE. The primary source of the PCDD/Fs in forages harvested from contaminated soils is incorporated soil. Grass silages generally contain more PCDD/Fs than corn (maize) silage. The congener profile in forages can be used to chemically "fingerprint" the sources. Birds and other animals consume soil by geophagy when feeding. Grazing cattle and sheep can consume up to 17% and 30%, respectively, of the dry matter intake as soil. Ruminants and horses can also be exposed to PHAs by direct atmospheric deposition on vegetation. Atmospheric levels of PHAs generally vary with the season.

Companion animals have indoor environmental exposures to PHAs, especially the PBDEs, and cats are studied as a model to assess infant/toddler exposure. The PBDEs are a chemical mixture of congeners solubilized in plastics, carpets and other synthetic fabrics and foams, and electronic equipment to retard combustion. They contaminate indoor air as a vapor, migrate from carpets and other synthetic fibers, and are a component of house dust. PBDEs can also leach from products after disposal. The PBDEs with a lower bromination number generally are more environmentally persistent in food webs. The higher brominated PBDEs can be debrominated by biota to lower brominated PBDEs. Burning plastics containing PBDEs forms polybrominated dibenzo-p-dioxins (PBDDs) and dibenzofurans (PBDFs). The PBDD/Fs have toxicity similar to that of their chlorinated analogues and have been measured in adipose tissue. Triclosan, a polychlorinated hydroxydiphenyl ether, is widely used as a broad-spectrum bactericide and is an ingredient in many cleaning agents and hygiene products. Surfaces of products such as cutting boards, food wrappers, refrigerator linings, and cat litter can be impregnated with triclosan for bactericidal action and to reduce odors. PHAs can be present in feedstuffs fed to dogs and cats. For example, fish oil, which may be used in formulated diets, generally is 2-fold higher in PCDD/Fs than in meat and bone meal.

Biomagnification, Translocation, and Food Safety: PHAs are readily absorbed from the gut, lungs, and through the skin. After absorption, they can be biomagnified in body fat and the liver, translocated to the fetus, and excreted in milk and eggs. Food-producing animals can relay PHAs in foods and animal by-products. PHAs are in rendered animal products, including fat, bone, and meat meals. After absorption, the congener profile can be altered by biotransformation, with the congener profile in tissues and edible animal products different from the PHAs absorbed. The congeners translocated to the fetus can be different from the congeners deposited in fat. Toxicity can vary with the congener profile. Biomagnification of PHAs has been estimated for chickens and pigs. PHAs analyzed in chicken fat had biomagnification factors ranging from 7 to 35. For pigs, biomagnification factors ranging from <7 to 15 were observed. Lactating and egg-laying females generally have a lower body burden of PHAs. The PHA levels in milk generally are higher during the early part of the first lactation. In rainbow trout, ~30% of the dietary PCDD/Fs are transferred to fat located in muscle tissue. The biomagnification factor generally varies between PHAs, animal species, and food webs.

Toxicology: Studies have shown that people and domestic and wild animals are exposed to a chemical soup of PHAs throughout a lifetime. The possible antagonistic, additive, synergistic, and potentiating interactions of the PHAs in the mixture are not well known.

PHA groups and individual PHAs are potent up- and down-regulators of enzyme systems by interaction with immunotoxic nuclear receptors; some PHAs interact with an assortment of endocrine receptors. Cell signaling can also be disrupted. Exposure begins during embryologic development and continues with possible differing toxic effects occurring during development, maturation, and aging. For some effects, toxicity occurring at one life stage may not be expressed until the next life stage. The general toxicology includes disruption of the immune and endocrine systems and associated organs/functions. Immunotoxicity is considered a sensitive parameter for some PCBs and TCDD/Fs congeners. The overall immune effect is reduced native resistance to infectious disease and a likely increased risk of neoplasia. The best-studied immunotoxic effect of PHAs is on the lymphocytes and acquired immunity. An abnormal increase in occurrences of infectious diseases can be observed in affected animals.

PHAs can alter endocrine functions. The US National Toxicology Program Workshop Review concluded there is evidence to support an association between selected exposure to PHAs and type 2 diabetes in people. Studies suggest that some PHAs may act as obesogens. There is growing general consensus that increased diagnosis of obesity in companion animals cannot be fully explained by genetics, lifestyle, and nutrition. Cats with lower capacity to metabolize PCBs have increased risk of acromegaly. In cats, an association between diabetes and PHA exposure has not been demonstrated in the studies published. Some PHAs are known to have an effect on thyroid endocrinology. The PHAs that induce hepatic uridine diphospho-glucuronosyltransferase or sulfotransferase isozymes increase biliary excretion of conjugated thyroid hormones. Some PCBs or their metabolites may interfere with binding of thyroid hormones to transporter proteins and the nuclear receptor. Exposure in utero to PCBs can increase brain deiodinases and may be a compensatory response to maintain tissue T_3 concentrations due to decreased fetal circulating and brain concentrations of T_4. There is an association between high levels of PBDEs in house dust and hyperthyroidism in cats. Blood levels of PHAs have not been associated with hyperthyroidism in cats. The PBDEs have been shown in laboratory studies to disrupt thyroid function in mice and American kestrels. One mechanism appears to be competitive displacement of T_4 from its carrier protein by hydroxylated PBDE metabolites. Tetrabromobisphenol A has been shown to alter the thyroid hormone receptor. There is evidence that triclosan disrupts thyroid function.

PHAs can be steroid hormonal agonists and antagonists and can disrupt endocrine homeostasis. These disruptions can cause reproductive dysfunctions. A study on PCBs in cattle tissues showed that the stimulatory effects of follicle-stimulating hormone and luteinizing hormone on luteal, granulosa, and thecal cells were decreased for secretion of progesterone, estradiol, and testosterone, respectively. Using cattle uterine strips, PCBs have been shown to increase the force of myometrial contractions and increase endometrial section of prostaglandin $F_2\alpha$. Exposure to PCBs and brominated biphenyls can delay onset of parturition in cattle.

There is increasing concern that some PHAs can alter hormonal function in utero. Exposure to PHAs in utero may alter body mass index and sexual functions later in life. Pre- and postnatal exposure to PHAs, through endocrine disruption mechanisms, may alter mammary gland development and function and increase the risk of mammary diseases. Goats exposed to PCBs in utero had altered adenyl function that varied with age and sex. The goats had lower basal cortisol levels during prepubertal development, and this effect persisted during their first breeding season. Male goats at 9 mo of age had a greater and prolonged rise in plasma cortisol levels when subjected to moderate stress.

PHAs can up-regulate the activities of cytochrome CYP (P450) and other enzymes. Changes in drug metabolism can occur. Changes in CYP activity can increase the formation of the ultimate toxicant of a variety of toxic substances. PHAs can also be promoters of carcinogens.

Clinical Findings, Lesions, and Diagnosis: In chickens, acute exposure to PHAs may cause a sudden drop in egg production followed by reduced egg hatchability. Ascites and edema may be seen, together with ataxia. Lesions include degenerative changes in skeletal and cardiac muscle. Altered thyroid function is associated with anomalous development in birds and mammals.

In cats, acromegaly appears to be linked to a decreased ability to metabolize PCB congeners. Hyperthyroidism in cats is associated with high levels of PBDEs in house dust. Feeding mink or whale blubber, naturally contaminated with PHAs and other pollutants, to sled dogs was shown to increase occurrences of diffuse thickening of the glomerular capillary wall and Bowman's basement membranes. Tubular hyalinization-degeneration and increased chronic interstitial nephritis were also noted.

Blood, plasma, serum, body fat, and liver can be assayed for PHAs. These levels can be linked to exposure and clinical and pathologic findings to establish a putative diagnosis.

Treatment and Control: There is no known treatment for intoxication by PHAs. Supportive care is recommended. Attention should be given to the indoor environment, the use of nonplastic feeding and watering utensils, and feed sources to prevent exposures to PBDEs. Avoiding contact with materials impregnated with PBDEs reduces the percutaneous exposure of companion animals. Avoiding household furnishings and plastics that contain PBDEs generally reduces the levels of PBDEs in the indoor environment. Allowing a companion animal more access to the outdoors reduces the indoor exposure to PBDEs. The PHAs in body fat are excreted in milk fat and contribute to the body burden of the neonate. The levels in milk are higher in the first lactation.

INSECTICIDE AND ACARICIDE (ORGANIC) TOXICITY

Insecticides are any substance or a mixture of substances intended to prevent, destroy, repel, or mitigate insects. Similarly, acaricides are substances that can destroy mites. A chemical can exert both insecticidal and acaricidal effects. Based on their properties, these chemicals can be classified into four groups: 1) organophosphates, 2) carbamates, 3) organochlorines, and 4) pyrethrins and pyrethroids. Because of worldwide use, these chemicals pose health risks to nontarget species, including people, domestic and companion animals, wildlife, and aquatic species. In large animals, poisoning is often due to inadvertent or accidental use, whereas in small animals (particularly dogs) poisoning is often due to malicious intent.

Pesticide labels must carry warnings against use on unapproved species or under untested circumstances. These warnings may pertain to acute or chronic toxicity, or to residues in meat, milk, or other animal products. Because labels change to meet current government regulations, it is important to always read and follow all label directions accompanying the product.

Each exposure, no matter how brief or small, results in some of the compound being absorbed and perhaps stored. Repeated short exposures may eventually result in intoxication because of cumulative effect. Every precaution should be taken to minimize human exposure. This may include frequent changes of clothing with bathing at each change, or if necessary, the use of respirators, rain gear, and gloves impervious to pesticides. Respirators must have filters approved for the type of insecticide being used (eg, ordinary dust filters will not protect the operator from organophosphorus insecticide fumes). Such measures are generally sufficient to guard against intoxication. Overexposure to chlorinated hydrocarbon insecticides is difficult to measure except by the occurrence of overt signs of poisoning.

Organophosphate and carbamate insecticides produce their toxicity by inactivation of acetylcholinesterase (AChE) enzyme at the synapses in nervous tissue and neuromuscular junctions, and in RBCs. Therefore, the cholinesterase-inhibiting property of organophosphates or carbamates may be used to indicate degree of exposure if the activity of the blood/RBC-AChE is determined during an early period of exposure.

Organic pesticides are known to exert deleterious effects on fish and wildlife as well as on domestic species. In no event should amounts greater than those specifically recommended be used, and maximal precautions should be taken to prevent drift or drainage to adjoining fields, pastures, ponds, streams, or other premises outside the treatment area.

The safety and exposure level of these compounds in target species has been carefully established, and application recommendations and regulations must be followed. Individuals, including veterinarians, have been prosecuted for failure to follow label directions or to heed label warnings and for failure to warn animal owners of the necessary precautions.

An ideal insecticide or acaricide should be efficacious without risk to livestock or persons making the application and without leaving residues in tissues, eggs, or milk. Only a few compounds may meet all these requirements.

Poisoning by organic insecticides and acaricides may be caused by direct application, by ingestion of contaminated feed or forage treated for control of plant parasites, or by accidental exposure. This discussion is limited to only those insecticides or acaricides most frequently hazardous to livestock or likely to leave residues in animal products.

Chemical synthesis rarely yields 100% of the product of interest, and normally there are, in variable proportions, structurally related compounds that have biologic effects different from those of the compound sought. A prime example is dichlorodiphenylethane (DDD): the p,p′-isomer is an effective insecticide of low toxicity for most mammals; the o,p′-isomer causes necrosis of the adrenal glands of people and dogs and is used to treat certain adrenal malfunctions.

In general, products stored under temperature extremes or held in partially emptied containers for long periods may deteriorate. But during storage, malathion produces isomalathion, which is many times more toxic than malathion. In addition to isomalathion, two other technical impurities of malathion (malaoxon and trimethyl phosphorodithioate) can be formed and can potentiate the toxicity of malathion by several fold. Similar impurities can be formed and potentiate the toxicity of another organophosphate insecticide, phenthoate. Storing a chemical in anything but the original container is hazardous, because in time its identity may be forgotten. Accidental contact with animals or people may then have disastrous consequences. Consumer-mixed and unapproved combinations can be very dangerous and should never be used. For example, simultaneous administration of two organophosphate insecticides can result in potentiation of malathion toxicity by a hundredfold.

A number of cholinesterase-inhibiting carbamate and organophosphate insecticides (eg, carbaryl, dichlorvos, methiocarb, carbofuran, paraoxon, mevinophos, aldicarb, and monocrotophos) are also immunotoxic. Impaired macrophage signaling through interleukins 1 and 2 appears to be involved, and the insecticide levels that cause this effect are very low. This can lead to subtle but damaging influences on the health of exposed animals.

CARBAMATE INSECTICIDES

The carbamates are esters of carbamic acid. Unlike organophosphates, carbamates are not structurally complex. Presently, the volume of carbamates used exceeds that of organophosphates, because carbamates are considered to be safer than organophosphates.

Aldicarb: The oral LD_{50} in rats is 0.9 mg/kg, and the dermal LD_{50} in rabbits is 5 mg/kg. Dogs are frequently poisoned with malicious intent.

Carbaryl: The oral LD_{50} in rats is 307 mg/kg, and the dermal LD_{50} in rabbits is 2,000 mg/kg. A 2% spray is nontoxic to calves; 4% is nontoxic to mature cattle when applied dermally.

Carbofuran: The oral LD_{50} in rats, dogs, chickens, ducks, pheasants, quails, and wild birds is 8, 19, 6.3, 0.415, 4.2, 5, and 0.42 mg/kg, respectively. Dogs are commonly poisoned with malicious intent by tainting food. The minimum toxic dose in cattle and sheep is 4.5 mg/kg, becoming lethal at 18 and 9 mg/kg, respectively. Cattle and other domestic animals are often poisoned by accidental exposure. Pigs have been poisoned after drinking water contaminated by this compound. In Africa, wildlife populations (including deer, lions, and birds) are declining because of malicious use of carbofuran. The dermal LD_{50} in rabbits is 2,550 mg/kg.

Methomyl: The oral LD_{50} in rats is 17 mg/kg, and the dermal LD_{50} in rabbits is >2,000 mg/kg. Dogs have been commonly poisoned with malicious intent by tainting food. Cattle have been reported to be poisoned after consumption of forage inadvertently sprayed with methomyl.

Propoxur: The oral LD_{50} is 95 mg/kg in rats and >800 mg/kg in goats. The dermal LD_{50} in rabbits is >1,000 mg/kg.

Clinical Findings: The carbamate insecticides act similarly to the organophosphates (*see* p 3064) in that they inhibit acetylcholinesterase (AChE) at nerve synapses and neuromuscular junctions. This inhibition is reversible because the inhibiting bond is much less durable; thus, the inhibition of blood AChE frequently is not evident at the laboratory. Signs include hypersalivation, GI hypermotility, abdominal cramping, vomiting, diarrhea, sweating, dyspnea, cyanosis, miosis, muscle fasciculations (in extreme cases, tetany followed by weakness and paralysis), and convulsions. In brief, the acronym SLUD (salivation, lacrimation, urination, and diarrhea) describes the overall clinical features of carbamate poisoning. Death usually results from respiratory failure and hypoxia due to bronchoconstriction leading to tracheobronchial secretion and pulmonary edema.

Diagnosis: Diagnosis of carbamate poisoning usually depends on history of exposure to a particular carbamate and response to atropine therapy. However, when a history of carbamate poisoning is not provided, but cholinergic signs and a clear positive response to atropine suggest carbamate or organophosphate poisoning, AChE activity levels should be determined in RBCs or whole blood (live animals), or in brain cortex (dead animals). Enzyme activity that is significantly inhibited (>50%) is confirmatory. Signs of hypercholinergic activity are usually seen with AChE inhibition >70%. Screening GI contents for carbamate insecticides by gas chromatography coupled with mass spectrometry is helpful in identification, confirmation, and quantitation of a particular carbamate and aids in differential diagnosis if an organophosphate insecticide is also involved.

Treatment: Treatment of carbamate poisoning is similar to that of organophosphate poisoning in that atropine sulfate injections readily reverse the effects. Recommended dosages for atropine are as follows: dogs and cats—dosed to effect (repeated as needed), usually 0.2–2 mg/kg, parenterally, one-fourth of the dose given IV and the remainder given SC (cats should be dosed at the lower end of the range); cattle and sheep—0.6–1 mg/kg, one-fourth of the dose IV and the remainder SC, repeated as needed; horses and pigs—0.1–0.2 mg/kg, IV, repeated as needed.

Pralidoxime (2-PAM) should not be used to treat carbamate poisoning. 2-PAM can be beneficial if poisoning is caused by a mixture of organophosphates and carbamates. Signs of excessive cholinergic activity may warrant its use, in case the cause is organophosphate exposure. 2-PAM can be fatal if given too rapidly; it must be administered slowly (ie, in 5% saline over a 10-min period). *See also* ORGANOPHOSPHATES, p 3064. Also, 2-PAM solution should be prepared freshly, because old solutions are known to produce cyanide. Use of morphine or barbiturates is contraindicated.

CHLORINATED HYDROCARBON COMPOUNDS

Because of persistent tissue residues and chronic toxicity, use of chlorinated hydrocarbon compounds has been drastically curtailed. Only lindane and methoxychlor are approved for use on or around livestock. Detectable residues of some chlorinated hydrocarbon insecticides, including BHC, heptachlor, heptachlor epoxide, lindane, and oxychlordane, can be found in fatty tissue after acute or chronic exposure.

Aldrin: Aldrin is a potent insecticide similar to dieldrin with the same order of toxicity (*see* below). It is no longer registered in the USA but was used for termite control. The oral LD_{50} in rats is 39 mg/kg, and the dermal LD_{50} in rabbits is 65 mg/kg. In farm animals, the toxic dose is ~15–30 mg/kg.

Benzene Hexachloride (BHC, HCH, Hexachlorocyclohexane): Benzene hexachloride (BHC) is composed of 12%–45% γ isomer. BHC was a useful insecticide for large animals and dogs but is highly toxic to cats in the concentrations necessary for parasite control. Only the γ isomer (γ–BHC, lindane) is a useful insecticidal agent; the other isomers are stored for excessively long periods in body tissues. Lindane, which contains >99% of the γ isomer, should be used in preference to the technical grade of BHC, which contains several isomers. The oral LD_{50} of lindane in rats is 76 mg/kg, and the dermal LD_{50} in rabbits is 500 mg/kg. Presently, BHC is not sold in the USA.

Cattle in good condition have tolerated 0.2% lindane applications, but stressed, emaciated cattle have been poisoned from spraying or dipping in 0.075% lindane. Horses and pigs appear to tolerate 0.2%–0.5%, and sheep and goats ordinarily tolerate 0.5% applications. Emaciation and lactation increase the susceptibility of animals to poisoning by lindane; such animals should be treated with extreme caution. Young calves are very susceptible to lindane and are poisoned by a single oral dose of 4.4 mg/kg. Mild signs appear in sheep given 22 mg/kg, and death occurs at 100 mg/kg. Adult cattle have tolerated 13 mg/kg without signs. BHC is stored in body fat and excreted in milk.

Chlordane: Chlordane is no longer registered as an insecticide in the USA. Exposure occurs when livestock consume treated plants or when they come in direct contact through carelessness and accidents. The lethal dose of chlordane for most species is in the range of 200–300 mg/kg. Very young calves have been killed by doses of 44 mg/kg, and the minimum toxic dose for cattle is ~88 mg/kg. Cattle fed chlordane at 25 ppm of their diet for 56 days showed 19 ppm in their fat at the end of the feeding. Topical emulsions and suspensions have been used safely on dogs at concentrations up to 0.25%, provided freshly diluted materials were used; dry powders up to 5% have been safe. The no-effect level in dogs in a 2-yr feeding study was 3 mg/kg. Pigeons and Leghorn cockerels and pullets suffered no effects after 1–2 mo exposure to vapors emanating from chlordane-treated surfaces. The oral LD_{50} in rats is 283 mg/kg, and the dermal LD_{50} in rabbits is 580 mg/kg.

Dieldrin: Dieldrin is not a registered pesticide in the USA. Residues limit its application, and it is one of the most toxic chlorinated hydrocarbon insecticides. The oral LD_{50} in rats is 40 mg/kg, and the dermal LD_{50} in rabbits is 65 mg/kg. Young dairy calves are poisoned by 8.8 mg/kg, PO, but tolerate 4.4 mg/kg, whereas adult cattle tolerate 8.8 mg/kg and are poisoned by 22 mg/kg. Pigs tolerate 22 mg/kg and are poisoned by 44 mg/kg. Horses are poisoned by 22 mg/kg. Because of its effectiveness against insect pests on crops and pasture and the low dosage per acre, dieldrin is not likely to poison livestock grazing the treated areas. Diets containing 25 ppm of dieldrin have been fed to cattle and sheep for 16 wk without harmful effects other than residues in fat, which are slow to disappear. Great care must be exercised in marketing animals that have grazed treated areas or consumed products from previously treated areas. There is a zero tolerance level for residues in edible tissues.

Statements pertaining to dieldrin also apply, in general, to **endrin**, the most toxic of the three chlorinated cyclodiene insecticides.

Endosulfan: Endosulfan is widely used to control insect and mite pests on a variety of crops and orchards. It is heavily used on tobacco. Endosulfan is very toxic to mammalian species. The oral LD_{50} in rats is 18 mg/kg, and the dermal LD_{50} in rabbits is 74 mg/kg. The LD_{50} of endosulfan in dogs is 77 mg/kg. Its lethal dose in cattle is 8 g. Generally, cattle are poisoned by accidental exposure, and dogs are poisoned by malicious intent. Exposure of cattle to endosulfan produces residues in the liver, kidneys, muscle, and milk.

Heptachlor: Heptachlor is not currently registered in the USA and is not recommended for use on livestock in the USA. Among its few agricultural applications, heptachlor is used for residual control of subterranean termites. The oral LD_{50} in rats is 40 mg/kg, and the dermal LD_{50} in rabbits is 119 mg/kg. Because it is very effective against certain plant-feeding insects, it is encountered from time to time in some geographic areas grazed by livestock. Young dairy calves tolerate dosages as high as 13 mg/kg but are poisoned by 22 mg/kg. Sheep tolerate 22 mg/kg but are poisoned by 40 mg/kg. Diets containing 60 ppm of heptachlor have been fed to cattle for 16 wk without harmful effects other than residues in fat. Heptachlor is converted to heptachlor epoxide by animals and stored in body fat. For this reason, a specific analysis performed for heptachlor usually yields negative results, while that for epoxide is positive.

Methoxychlor: Methoxychlor is one of the safest chlorinated hydrocarbon insecticides and one of the few with active registration in the USA. The oral LD_{50} in rats is 5,000 mg/kg, and the dermal LD_{50} in rabbits is 2,820 mg/kg. Young dairy calves tolerate 265 mg/kg; 500 mg/kg is mildly toxic. While 1 g/kg produces rather severe poisoning in young calves, sheep are not affected. One dog was given 990 mg/kg/day for 30 days without showing signs. Six applications to cattle of a 0.5% spray at 3-wk intervals produced fat residues of 2.4 ppm; ~0.4 ppm of methoxychlor is found in milk 1 day after spraying a cow with a 0.5% concentration. Methoxychlor sprays are not approved for use on animals producing milk for human consumption. Cattle and sheep store essentially no methoxychlor when fed 25 ppm in the total diet for 112 days. If methoxychlor is used as recommended, the established tolerance in fat will not be exceeded. Commercial products are available for garden, orchard, and field crops, and for horses and ponies.

Numerous reports suggest that methoxychlor has negative reproductive effects in laboratory animal experiments, but this has not been seen in the field.

Toxaphene: Toxaphene is no longer under active registration in the USA. It has been used with reasonable safety if recommendations were followed, but it can cause poisoning when applied or ingested in excessive quantities. The oral LD_{50} in rats is 40 mg/kg, and the dermal LD_{50} in rabbits is 600 mg/kg. Dogs and cats are particularly susceptible. Young calves have been poisoned by 1% toxaphene sprays, while all other farm animals except poultry can withstand 1% or more as sprays or dips. Chickens have been poisoned by dipping in 0.1% emulsions, and turkeys have been poisoned by spraying with 0.5% material. Toxaphene is primarily an acute toxicant and does not persist long in the tissues. Adult cattle have been mildly intoxicated by 4% sprays and severely affected by 8%. Adult cattle have been poisoned from being dipped in emulsions that contained only 0.5% toxaphene (an amount ordinarily safe) because the emulsions had begun to break down, allowing the fine droplets to coalesce into larger droplets that readily adhere to the hair of cattle. The resultant dosage becomes equivalent to that obtained by spray treatments of much higher concentrations. Toxaphene is lethal to young calves at 8.8 mg/kg but not at 4.4 mg/kg. The minimum toxic dose for cattle is ~33 mg/kg, and for sheep between 22 and 33 mg/kg. Spraying Hereford cattle 12 times at 2-wk intervals with 0.5% toxaphene produced a *maximum residue* of 8 ppm in fat. Cattle fed 10 ppm of toxaphene in the diet for 30 days had no detectable toxaphene tissue residues, whereas steers fed 100 ppm for 112 days stored only 40 ppm in their fat (this amount was eliminated 2 mo after the toxaphene was discontinued).

Clinical Findings: The chlorinated hydrocarbon insecticides are general CNS stimulants. They produce a great variety of signs—the most obvious are neuromuscular tremors and convulsions—and there may be obvious behavioral changes common to other poisonings and CNS infections. Body temperature may be very high. Affected animals are generally first noted to be more alert or apprehensive. Muscle fasciculation occurs, becoming visible in the facial region and extending backward until the whole body is involved. Large doses of DDT, DDD, endosulfan, lindane, and methoxychlor cause progressive involvement leading to trembling or shivering, followed by convulsions and death. With the other chlorinated hydrocarbons, muscular twitching is followed by convulsions, usually without the intermediate trembling. Convulsions may be clonic or tonic lasting from a few minutes to several hours, or intermittent and leading to the animal becoming comatose. High fever may accompany convulsions, particularly in warm environments.

Behavioral changes such as abnormal postures (eg, resting the sternum on the ground while remaining upright in the rear, keeping the head down between the forelegs, "head pressing" against a wall or fence, or continual chewing movements) may be seen. Occasionally, an affected animal becomes belligerent and attacks other animals, people, or moving objects. Vocalization is common. Some animals are depressed, almost oblivious to their surroundings, and do not eat or drink; they may last longer than those showing more violent symptoms. Usually, there is a copious flow of thick saliva and urinary incontinence. In certain cases, the clinical signs alternate, with the animal first being extremely excited, then severely depressed.

The severity of the signs seen at a given time is not a sure prognostic index. Some animals have only a single convulsion and die, whereas others suffer innumerable convulsions but subsequently recover. Animals showing acute excitability often have a fever >106°F (41°C). The signs of poisoning by these insecticides are highly suggestive but not diagnostic; other poisons and encephalitis or meningitis must be considered.

Signs of acute intoxication by chlordane in birds are nervous chirping, excitability, collapse on hocks or side, and mucous exudates in the nasal passages. Signs of subacute and chronic intoxication are molting, dehydration and cyanosis of the comb, weight loss, and cessation of egg production.

Lesions: If death has occurred suddenly, there may be nothing more than cyanosis. More definite lesions occur as the duration of intoxication increases. Usually, there is congestion of various organs (particularly the lungs, liver, and kidneys) and a blanched appearance of all organs if the body temperature was high before death. The heart generally stops in systole, and there may be many hemorrhages of varying size on the epicardium. The appearance of the heart and lungs may suggest a peracute pneumonia and, if the animal was affected for more than a few hours, there may be pulmonary edema. The trachea and bronchi may contain a blood-tinged froth. In many cases, the CSF volume is excessive, and the brain and spinal cord frequently are congested and edematous.

Diagnosis: Chemical analysis of brain, liver, kidney, fat, and stomach or rumen contents is necessary to confirm chlorinated hydrocarbon compound poisoning. The suspected source, if identified, should also be analyzed. Brain levels of the insecticide are the most useful. Whole blood, serum, and urine from live animals may be analyzed to evaluate exposure in the rest of the herd or flock. In food animal poisoning, if exposure is more than just the animals visibly affected, fat biopsies from survivors may be necessary to estimate the potential residue. Identification, confirmation, and quantitation of organochlorine insecticides are usually done by gas chromatography coupled with mass spectrometry.

Treatment: There are no known specific antidotes to chlorinated hydrocarbon compound poisoning. When exposure is by spraying, dipping, or dusting, a thorough bathing without irritating the skin (no brushes), using detergents and copious quantities of cool water, is recommended. If exposure is by ingestion, gastric lavage and saline purgatives are indicated. The use of digestible oils such as corn oil is contraindicated; however, heavy-grade mineral oil plus a purgative hastens the removal of the chemical from the intestine. Activated charcoal appears to be useful in preventing absorption from the GI tract. When signs are excitatory, a sedative anticonvulsant such as a barbiturate or diazepam is indicated. Anything in the environment that stresses the animal (eg, noise, handling) should be reduced or removed if possible. If the animal shows marked depression, anorexia, and dehydration, therapy should be directed toward rehydration and nourishment either IV or by stomach tube. Residues in exposed animals may be reduced by giving a slurry of activated charcoal or providing charcoal in feed. Feeding phenobarbital, 5 g/day, may hasten residue removal.

INSECTICIDES DERIVED FROM PLANTS

Most insecticides derived from plants (eg, rotenone from *Derris* and pyrethrins from *Chrysanthemum* or *Pyrethrum*) have traditionally been considered safe for use on animals. **Nicotine** in the form of nicotine sulfate is an exception. Unless it is carefully used, poisoning may result. Pets are exposed to tobacco by ingesting commercial tobacco products (eg, cigarettes or chewing tobacco), whereas livestock may consume discarded tobacco stalks or hay contaminated with tobacco plant drippings in the barn. The minimum lethal dose of nicotine is 1 g in cattle, 0.2–0.3 g in horses, 0.1–0.2 g in sheep, and 0.02–0.1 g in dogs and cats. Affected animals show tremors, incoordination, nausea, disturbed respiration, muscle paralysis, and finally coma and death. Nicotine and related alkaloids from tobacco can cross the placenta and produce teratogenic effects. Recovery from sublethal doses is usually complete within 3 hr. Death occurs within a matter of hours from paralysis of thoracic respiratory muscles and cardiac arrest. Necropsy may reveal parts of tobacco leaves or stalks in the rumen contents. Lesions include pale mucous membranes, dark blood, hemorrhages on the heart and in the lungs, and congestion of the brain. Treatment consists of removing the material by washing or by gastric lavage with tannic acid, administering activated charcoal, providing artificial respiration, and treating for cardiac arrest and shock.

Pyrethrins: Pyrethrins are insecticides obtained from the flowers of *C cinerariaefolium* and have been used as insecticides for many years. Pyrethrins and pyrethroids produce toxicity affecting primarily the sodium channel, but also chloride and calcium channels of nerve cells. These insecticides also interact with nicotinic acetylcholine receptors. Synergists, such as piperonyl butoxide, sesamex, piperonyl cyclonene, etc, are added to increase stability and effectiveness. This is accomplished by inhibiting mixed function oxidases, enzymes that detoxify pyrethrins and pyrethroids; unfortunately, this also potentiates mammalian toxicity.

Pyrethroids: Pyrethroids are synthetic derivatives of natural pyrethrins. There are two types of pyrethroids. Type I compounds that lack an α-cyano substituent include pyrethrin I, allethrin, tetramethrin, kadethrin, resmethrin, phenothrin, and permethrin. Type II compounds that contain a stabilizing α-cyano-3-phenoxybenzyl component include cyfluthrin, cypermethrin, fenpropanthrin, deltamethrin, cyphenothrin, fenvalerate, and fluvalinate. Type I pyrethroids produce a neurologic syndrome through their effects on both the central and peripheral nervous systems, with signs including tremors, incoordination, prostration, seizures, and death. Type II pyrethroids work primarily by CNS mechanisms to exert the choreoathetosis/salivation syndrome, characterized by hyperactivity, hunched back, salivation, tremors, and incoordination progressing to sinuous writhing movements.

Diagnosis of pyrethrin/pyrethroid poisoning is based on clinical signs, history of exposure, and determination of insecticide residue in body tissues and fluids. These insecticides do not produce characteristic pathologic lesions.

Generally, symptomatic and supportive treatment is required after ingestion of a dilute pyrethrin or pyrethroid preparation. Toxicity may also be due to the solvent. Induction of emesis may be contraindicated. A slurry of activated charcoal at 2–8 g/kg may be administered, followed by a saline cathartic (magnesium or sodium sulfate [10% solution] at 0.5 mg/kg). Vegetable oils and fats, which promote the intestinal absorption of pyrethrum, should be avoided. If dermal exposure occurs, the animal should be bathed with a mild detergent and cool water. The area should be washed very gently so as not to stimulate the circulation and enhance skin absorption. Initial assessment of the animal's respiratory and cardiovascular integrity is important. Further treatment involves continuing symptomatic and supportive care. Seizures should be controlled with either diazepam (administered to effect at 0.2–2 mg/kg, IV) or methocarbamol (55–220 mg/kg, IV, not exceeding 200 mg/min). Phenobarbital or pentobarbital (IV), to effect, can be used if diazepam or methocarbamol are too short-acting.

D-Limonene: D-Limonene is the major component of the oil extracted from citrus rind. It is used for the control of fleas on cats and for other insect pests. Adult fleas and eggs appear to be most sensitive to D-limonene, which is more effective if combined with the synergist piperonyl butoxide. At recommended dosages, the solution containing D-limonene appears to be safe, but increasing the concentration 5–10 fold in sprays or dips increases the severity of toxic signs, which include hypersalivation, muscle tremors, ataxia, and mild to severe hypothermia. The inclusion of piperonyl butoxide in the formulation potentiates the toxicity in cats. Allergies have also been reported in people in contact with D-limonene, and it appears to increase dermal absorption of some chemicals. When orally administered to dogs, D-limonene causes vomiting (median effective dose 1.6 mL/kg). No antidote is available.

ORGANOPHOSPHATES

The organophosphates (OPs) are derivatives of phosphoric or phosphonic acid. OPs have replaced the banned organochlorine compounds and are a major cause of animal poisoning. They vary greatly in toxicity, residue levels, and excretion. Many have been developed for plant and animal protection, and in general, they offer a distinct advantage by producing little tissue and environmental residue. Some of the OPs developed initially as pesticides are also used as anthelmintics. Five such compounds include dichlorvos, trichlorfon, haloxon, naphthalophos, and crufomate. The first two are primarily used against parasitic infestations in horses, dogs, and pigs; the latter three are used against parasites in ruminants.

Many of the OPs now used as pesticides (eg, chlorpyrifos, diazinon, fenitrothion, malathion, parathion, etc) are not potent inhibitors of cholinesterase until activated in the liver by microsomal oxidation enzymes; they are generally less toxic, and intoxication occurs more slowly. Certain OP preparations are microencapsulated, and the active compound is released slowly; this increases the duration of activity and reduces toxicity, but the toxic properties are still present.

Organophosphate Insecticides

Azinphos-methyl (or -ethyl): The maximum nontoxic oral dose is 0.44 mg/kg for calves, 2.2 mg/kg for cattle and goats, and 4.8 mg/kg for sheep. The oral LD_{50} in rats is 5 mg/kg, and the dermal LD_{50} in rabbits is 220 mg/kg.

Carbophenothion: Carbophenothion has been used as a spray for fruit trees and as a dip or spray for sheep blowfly, keds, and lice. Dairy calves <2 wk old sprayed with water-based formulations showed poisoning at concentrations ≥0.05%, and adult cattle were poisoned by spraying with 1%. Sheep and goats have been poisoned by 22 mg/kg, PO, but not by 8 mg/kg. In sheep, 0.1% as a dip produces no signs of poisoning. The LD_{50} for rats is ~31 mg/kg; a daily dosage of 2.2 mg/kg for 90 days produced poisoning. Dogs tolerated a diet containing 32 ppm for 90 days. A single application of a powder containing 1% of carbophenothion is lethal to cats.

Chlorfenvinphos: Adult cattle were poisoned by 5% or higher sprays, whereas young calves were poisoned at concentrations of 2%. The minimum oral toxic dose appears to be ~22 mg/kg for cattle of all ages. The acute oral LD_{50} for rats is 12 mg/kg, and the dermal LD_{50} in rabbits is 3,200 mg/kg.

Chlorpyrifos: The oral LD_{50} is 500 mg/kg in goats and 941 mg/kg in rats. In comparison with calves, steers, and cows, bulls (particularly of the exotic breeds) are highly susceptible to a single dose of chlorpyrifos. The maximum tolerated dose of chlorpyrifos in sheep is 750 mg/kg. Sheep given 850 mg/kg died 5 days after dosing, those given 900 mg/kg died on the third day, and a dose of 1,000 mg/kg was lethal within 30 hours. Onset of poisoning signs is usually delayed compared with that of many other commonly used organophosphates because of the conversion of chlorpyrifos to the active cholinesterase inhibitor chlorpyrifos-oxon. Chlorpyrifos produces reproductive and developmental toxicity.

Coumaphos: Coumaphos is used against cattle grubs and a number of other ectoparasites and for treatment of premises. The maximum concentration that may be safely used on adult cattle, horses, and pigs is 0.5%. Young calves and all ages of sheep and goats must not be sprayed with concentrations >0.25%; 0.5% concentrations may be lethal. Adult cattle may show mild toxicity at 1% concentrations. The minimum lethal dose for calves appears to be between 10 and 40 mg/kg. A dose of 25 mg/kg is usually fatal in sheep. The oral LD_{50} in rats is 13 mg/kg.

Crotoxyphos: Crotoxyphos is used as a spray or powder for the control of ectoparasites on cattle and pigs. Crotoxyphos is of rather low toxicity; however, Brahman cattle are markedly more susceptible than European breeds. Cattle (except as above), sheep, goats, and pigs all tolerate sprays containing crotoxyphos at 0.5% levels or higher. Crotoxyphos is safe at a level of 1%, although skin lesions have been found in pigs. Toxic doses appears to be in the 2% range, except for in Brahman cattle, in which 0.144%–0.3% may be toxic.

Demeton: Demeton is used as a systemic insecticide against sucking insects and mites. Demeton is used mainly as a foliage spray and has a relatively long residual life. It is a mixture of demeton-O and demeton-S and is highly toxic to mammals. The oral LD_{50} is 8 mg/kg in goats and 2 mg/kg in rats; the dermal LD_{50} in rats and rabbits is 8 mg/kg. Demeton-O poisoning developed in several hundred cattle grazing near cotton treated with this insecticide. The corresponding analogues of demeton (demeton-O-methyl and demeton-S-methyl) are also used for similar purposes but are less toxic than demeton.

Diazinon: Young calves appear to tolerate 0.05% spray but are poisoned by 0.1% concentrations. Adult cattle may be sprayed at weekly intervals with 0.1% concentrations without inducing poisoning. Young calves tolerate 0.44 mg/kg, PO, but are poisoned by 0.88 mg/kg. Cattle tolerate 8.8 mg/kg, PO, but are poisoned by 22 mg/kg. Sheep tolerate 17.6 mg/kg but are poisoned by 26 mg/kg. The oral LD_{50} in rats is 300 mg/kg, and the dermal LD_{50} in rabbits is 379 mg/kg.

Dichlorvos: Dichlorvos has many uses on both plants and animals. It is rapidly metabolized and excreted, and residues in meat and milk are not a problem if label directions are followed. It is of moderate toxicity, with a minimum toxic dose of 10 mg/kg in young calves and 25 mg/kg in horses and sheep. The oral LD_{50} in rats is 25 mg/kg, PO, and the dermal LD_{50} in rabbits is 59 mg/kg. A 1% dust was not toxic to cattle. Flea collars containing dichlorvos may cause skin reactions in some pets. Cats wearing dichlorvos-impregnated collars can develop signs of ataxia-depression syndrome, followed by death.

Dimethoate: Dimethoate is used extensively in horticulture as a systemic insecticide, but it also kills insects by contact. When administered PO, the minimum toxic dose for young dairy calves was ~48 mg/kg, while 22 mg/kg was lethal for cattle 1 yr old. Daily doses of 10 mg/kg for 5 days in adult cattle lowered blood cholinesterase activity to 20% of normal but did not produce poisoning. Horses have been poisoned by doses of 60–80 mg/kg, PO. When applied topically, 1% sprays have been tolerated by calves, cattle, and adult sheep. The oral LD_{50} in rats is 215 mg/kg, and the dermal LD_{50} in rabbits is 400 mg/kg.

Dioxathion: Dioxathion is a nonsystemic acaricide and insecticide for the control of ticks. Dioxathion is a mixture of cis- and trans-isomers, usually in the ratio of 1:2. The cis-isomer is more toxic than the trans-isomer. Used on both plants and animals, it is rapidly metabolized and not likely to produce residues in meat greater than the 1 ppm official tolerance. Concentrations of ≥0.15% are generally used on animals. The minimum toxic dose in calves is 5 mg/kg. Sprays of 0.5%

in cattle and sheep or 0.25% in goats and pigs are nontoxic. Sprays at concentrations up to 0.1% are usually safe for calves and lambs. Twice this concentration may produce signs of poisoning. Dioxathion at 8.8 mg/kg, PO, has killed young calves, and it produced intoxication at 4.4 mg/kg. Emaciated cattle with severe tick infestation are more frequently poisoned than healthy animals. Maximum residues of dioxathion in adipose tissue of cattle occur 2–4 days after dipping. The elimination half-life, after obtaining maximum concentrations, is ~16 days.

Disulfoton: The maximum nontoxic oral dose is 0.88 mg/kg for young calves, 2.2 mg/kg for cattle and goats, and 4.8 mg/kg for sheep. Poisoning has occurred in cattle after consuming harvested forages previously sprayed with this insecticide. The oral LD_{50} in rats is 2 mg/kg, and the dermal LD_{50} in rabbits is 6 mg/kg. Chronic exposure to disulfoton may result in tolerance to toxicity.

Ethyl 4-Nitrophenyl Phenylphosphonothioate (EPN): EPN is a nonsystemic insecticide and acaricide structurally related to parathion. The acute oral LD_{50} in rats is 8–36 mg/kg. EPN at a dosage of 10 mg/kg was found to be nontoxic to adult cattle and sheep. The minimum oral toxic dose of EPN is 2.5 mg/kg in calves and 25 mg/kg in sheep and yearling cattle. Sprays containing 0.025%–0.05% EPN are toxic to young calves, and 0.25% EPN is lethal. Dogs were not poisoned at dosages >100 mg/kg.

Famphur: The oral LD_{50} in rats is 35 mg/kg, and the dermal LD_{50} in rabbits is 2,730 mg/kg. The maximum nontoxic dose is 10 mg/kg in calves and 50 mg/kg in cattle, sheep, and horses. In general, Brahman cattle are especially susceptible to famphur toxicity. This compound is effective against warbles in cattle, but (as for all grubicides) directions must be followed as to time of application; larvae killed while migrating and the resultant local reaction can cause serious problems. In several instances, famphur poisoning occurred in birds (mainly magpies and robins) shortly after cattle had been treated with a pour-on preparation containing famphur.

Fenitrothion: Fenitrothion, also known as sumithion, is used as a contact insecticide in agriculture and horticulture. The oral LD_{50} in rats is 250 mg/kg, and the dermal LD_{50} in rabbits is 1,300 mg/kg. When applied to cattle, its metabolites are excreted at low levels in milk and urine. Fenitrothion produces reproductive and developmental toxicity in chickens.

Fenthion: Fenthion is commonly applied topically to control warble infestation in cattle and fleas in dogs. The minimum toxic dose, PO, is 25 mg/kg for cattle; 50 mg/kg is lethal to sheep. The oral LD_{50} in rats is 255 mg/kg, and the dermal LD_{50} in rabbits is 330 mg/kg.

Malathion: Malathion is one of the safest organophosphates because of its selective toxicity; it is highly toxic to insects but much less toxic to mammalian species. The oral LD_{50} in rats is 885 mg/kg, and the dermal LD_{50} in rabbits is 4,000 mg/kg. The oral acute toxic dose in calves is 10–20 mg/kg and in adult cattle and sheep is 50–100 mg/kg. In a chronic study in buffalo calves (6–9 mo old), daily oral administration of malathion at 0.5 mg/kg for 1 yr produced no biochemical or clinical effects. Dosages >1 mg/kg inhibited blood acetylcholinesterase (AChE) activity and increased liver enzymes (ALT and AST). A 20 mg/kg dose produced clinical signs after 10 days. The acute oral LD_{50} in buffalo calves is 53 mg/kg. Dermal application by spray containing 0.5% or 1% of malathion had no apparent effect on calves, but 5% spray caused death within 75 hr. Malathion at 0.5% or 1% should not be sprayed on calves for more than 3 consecutive days. Malathion is excreted in cow's milk.

Methyl Parathion: Methyl parathion is less toxic than parathion (diethyl parathion). The LD_{50} in rats from a single oral dose is 9–25 mg/kg, and the dermal LD_{50} in rabbits is 63 mg/kg. Methyl parathion at 2.5 mg/kg had no ill effect, but 10 mg/kg daily quickly led to toxic signs. The lethal dose in cattle is 100 mg/kg. Methyl parathion is excreted in cow's milk. Methyl parathion produces reproductive and developmental toxicity.

Mevinphos: The LD_{50} in rats is 3 mg/kg, and the dermal LD_{50} in rabbits is 16 mg/kg. Mevinphos has been commonly used to control the population of birds, and thereby caused poisoning in nontarget species. Mevinphos at 200 ppm in the diet is lethal in dogs.

Naled: Naled is essentially a dibrominated dichlorvos, which has the ability to act as a contact insecticide. It has a broad spectrum of insecticidal action. Because it has a short residual life, it poses relatively little hazard to fish and wildlife. The oral LD_{50} in rats is 191 mg/kg, and the dermal LD_{50} in rabbits is 390 mg/kg.

Oxydemeton-methyl: The maximum nontoxic oral dose is 0.88 mg/kg for young calves, 2.2 mg/kg for cattle, and 4.8 mg/kg for sheep and goats.

Parathion: Parathion (diethyl parathion) is widely used for control of plant pests and is approximately one-half as toxic as tetraethyl pyrophosphate (*see* below). The oral LD_{50} in rats is 3 mg/kg, and the dermal LD_{50} in rabbits is 6.8 mg/kg. It is used as a dip and spray for cattle in some countries (not in the USA). Most cases of occupational insecticide poisonings in people have been attributed to parathion or its degradation products. The minimum toxic dose in calves is 0.25–0.5 mg/kg and in cattle is 25–50 mg/kg. The minimum oral lethal dose in sheep is 20 mg/kg and in goats is 50 mg/kg. The LD_{50} in dogs is 23–35 mg/kg and in cats is 15 mg/kg. Dermal sprays containing 0.02%, 1%, and 1% of parathion are lethal to calves, sheep, and goats, respectively. Parathion is used extensively to control mosquitoes and insects in orchards and on market garden crops. Normally, because so little is used per acre, it presents no hazard to livestock. However, because of the potency of parathion, care should be taken to prevent accidental exposure. Parathion does not produce significant residues in animal tissues.

Phorate: Phorate is closely related to demeton (*see* above). It is a systemic insecticide and miticide. The oral LD_{50} in rats is 1.6 mg/kg, and the dermal LD_{50} in rabbits is 2.5 mg/kg. The minimum toxic dose PO is 0.25 mg/kg in calves, 0.75 mg/kg in sheep, and 1 mg/kg in cattle.

Phosmet: Phosmet is a nonsystemic acaricide and insecticide. The minimum oral toxic dose is 25 mg/kg in cattle and calves and 50 mg/kg in sheep. Spraying with a 0.5% solution has no toxic effect, but a 1% solution of phosmet produces intoxication in cattle. Phosmet is not excreted in milk.

Ronnel (Fenchlorphos): Ronnel is an excellent oral systemic insecticide. It is effective against many ecto- and endoparasitic arthropods, including cattle grubs, screw worms, and sucking lice. Ronnel is also used as a residual spray insecticide to control flies, fleas, and cockroaches. The oral LD_{50} in rats is 1,250 mg/kg, and the dermal LD_{50} in rabbits is 2,000 mg/kg. Ronnel produces mild signs of poisoning in cattle at 132 mg/kg, but severe signs do not appear until the dosage is >400 mg/kg. The minimum toxic dose in sheep is 400 mg/kg. Concentrations as high as 2.5% in sprays have failed to produce poisoning of cattle, young dairy calves, or sheep. Poisoning usually occurs in two stages. The animal first becomes weak and, although able to move about normally, may be placid. Diarrhea, often flecked with blood, may also be seen. Salivation and dyspnea then appear if the dose was high enough. Blood cholinesterase activity declines slowly over 5–7 days. Ronnel produces residues in meat and milk; strict adherence to label restrictions is essential. The residues may be removed by giving the animal activated charcoal for several days.

Ruelene: Ruelene is active both as a systemic and contact insecticide in livestock, has some anthelmintic activity, and has rather low toxicity. Dairy calves have been poisoned by 44 mg/kg, PO, while adult cattle require 88 mg/kg for the same effect. Sheep are moderately intoxicated by 176 mg/kg; Angora goats are about twice as sensitive. Pigs have been poisoned by 11 mg/kg and horses by 44 mg/kg. Most livestock tolerate a 2% topical spray.

Temephos: Temephos is used as an insecticide against mosquitoes and midges. It is of low toxicity to mammalian species. The oral LD_{50} for rats is 1 g (or more)/kg, while the dermal LD_{50} is >4 g/kg. Daily exposure of cattle for 1 yr at 1–1.5 mg/kg is known to produce clinical signs of poisoning and affect fertility in heifers.

Terbufos: This soil insecticide is used to control corn rootworms. The oral LD_{50} in rats is 1.6 mg/kg. The minimum oral toxic dose is ~1.5 mg/kg for sheep and cattle. Cases of intoxication in cattle have occurred. Ingestion of 7.5 mg/kg was lethal to heifers.

Tetrachlorvinphos: Tetrachlorvinphos has low toxicity in dogs; chronic feeding studies indicate the lowest effect level was 50 mg/kg/day, and the no observed effect level (NOEL) was 3.13 mg/kg/day. The minimum toxic dose in pigs is 100 mg/kg.

Tetraethylpyrophosphate (TEPP): Tetraethyl pyrophosphate (TEPP) is one of the most acutely toxic insecticides. Although not used on animals, accidental exposure occurs occasionally. One herd of 29 cattle (including calves and adults) was accidentally sprayed with 0.33% TEPP emulsion; all died within 40 min.

Trichlorfon: Trichlorfon is used as a systemic insecticide and anthelmintic in domestic animals. It is also used as an acaricide in sheep at the dose rate of 80 mg/kg at weekly intervals for not more than 4 wk. The oral LD_{50} in rats is 630 mg/kg, and the dermal LD_{50} in rabbits is >2,000 mg/kg. As a spray, trichlorfon at a 1% concentration is tolerated by adult cattle; given PO, it is tolerated by young dairy calves at 4.4 mg/kg but produces poisoning at 8.8 mg/kg. Adult cattle, sheep, and horses appear to tolerate 44 mg/kg, while 88 mg/kg produces poisoning. Dogs were unaffected when fed 1,000 ppm of trichlorfon for 4 mo. Administration of trichlorfon at 75 mg/kg, PO, produces adverse clinical signs in dogs. Trichlorfon is metabolized rapidly.

Clinical Findings: In general, OP pesticides have a narrow margin of safety, and the dose-response curve is quite steep. Signs of OP poisoning are those of cholinergic overstimulation, which can be grouped into three categories: muscarinic, nicotinic, and central. Muscarinic signs, which are usually first to appear, include hypersalivation, miosis, frequent urination, diarrhea, vomiting, colic, and dyspnea due to increased bronchial secretions and bronchoconstriction. Nicotinic effects include muscle fasciculations and weakness. The central effects include nervousness, ataxia, apprehension, and seizures. Cattle and sheep commonly show severe depression. CNS stimulation in dogs and cats usually progresses to convulsions. Some OPs (eg, amidothioates) do not enter the brain easily, so that CNS signs are mild. Onset of signs after exposure is usually within minutes to hours but may be delayed for >2 days in some cases. Severity and course of intoxication is influenced principally by the dosage and route of exposure. In acute poisoning, the primary clinical signs may be respiratory distress and collapse followed by death due to respiratory muscle paralysis. In addition to brain and skeletal muscles, OPs are known to adversely affect other organ systems, including the cardiovascular, respiratory, hepatic, reproductive and developmental, and immune systems.

Diagnosis: An important diagnostic aid for OP poisoning is the determination of acetylcholinesterase (AChE) activity in blood and brain. Unfortunately, the depression of blood cholinesterase does not necessarily correlate with the severity of poisoning; signs are seen when brain AChE activity is inhibited >70%, and the enzyme in blood reflects, only in a general way, the levels in nervous tissue. The key factors appear to be the degree and rate at which the enzyme activity is reduced. Analyses performed after exposure may be negative, because OPs do not remain long in tissues as the parent compounds. Chlorinated OP compounds have greater potential for tissue residue. Frozen stomach and rumen contents should be analyzed for the pesticide, using GC-MS for identification, confirmation, and quantitation. Blood/serum and urine can also be analyzed for residue of OPs or their metabolites. More than 70% of OPs produce one or more of the six dialkylphosphates (dimethyl phosphate, diethyl phosphate, dimethyl thiophosphate, diethyl thiophosphate, dimethyl dithiophosphate, and diethyl dithiophosphate).

Lesions: Animals with acute OP poisoning have nonspecific or no lesions. Pulmonary edema and congestion, hemorrhages, and edema of the bowel and other organs may be found. Animals surviving >1 day may become emaciated and dehydrated.

Treatment: Three categories of drugs are used to treat OP poisoning: 1) muscarinic receptor–blocking agents, 2) cholinesterase reactivators, and 3) emetics, cathartics, and adsorbents to decrease further absorption. Atropine sulfate blocks the central and peripheral muscarinic receptor–associated effects of OPs; it is administered to effect in dogs and cats, usually at a dosage of 0.2–2 mg/kg (cats at the lower end of the range), every 3–6 hr or as often as clinical signs indicate. For horses and pigs, the dosage is 0.1–0.2 mg/kg, IV, repeated every 10 min as needed; for cattle and sheep, the dosage is 0.6–1 mg/kg, one-third given IV, the remainder IM or SC, and repeated as needed. Atropinization is adequate when the pupils are dilated, salivation ceases, and the animal appears more alert. Animals initially respond well to atropine sulfate; however, the response diminishes after repeated treatments. Overtreatment with atropine should be avoided. Atropine does not alleviate the nicotinic cholinergic effects, such as muscle fasciculations and muscle paralysis, so death from massive overdoses of OPs can still occur. Including diazepam in the treatment reduced the incidence of seizures and increased survival of nonhuman primates experimentally.

An improved treatment combines atropine with the cholinesterase-reactivating oxime, 2-pyridine aldoxime methochloride (2-PAM, pralidoxime chloride). The dosage of 2-PAM is 20–50 mg/kg, given as a 5% solution IM or by slow IV (over 5–10 min), repeated at half the dose as needed. IV 2-PAM must be given very slowly to avoid musculoskeletal paralysis and respiratory arrest. Response to cholinesterase reactivators decreases with time after exposure; therefore, treatment with oximes must be instituted as soon as possible (within 24–48 hr). The rate at which the enzyme/organophosphate complex becomes unresponsive to reactivators (due to ageing phenomenon) varies with the particular pesticide.

Removal of the poison from the animal also should be attempted. If exposure was dermal, the animal should be washed with detergent and water (about room temperature) but without scrubbing and irritating the skin. Emesis should be induced if oral exposure occurred <2 hr previously; emesis is contraindicated if the animal is depressed. Oral administration of mineral oil decreases absorption of pesticide from the GI tract. Activated charcoal (1–2 g/kg as a water slurry) adsorbs OPs and helps elimination in the feces. This is particularly recommended in cattle. Continued absorption of OPs from the large amount of ingesta in the rumen has caused prolonged toxicosis in cattle. Artificial respiration or administration of oxygen may be required. Phenothiazine tranquilizers, barbiturates, and morphine are contraindicated.

Intermediate Syndrome

Organophosphate-induced intermediate syndrome (IMS) has been seen in people and animals (particularly dogs and cats) acutely poisoned with a massive dose of an OP insecticide. OPs known to cause IMS include bromophos, chlorpyrifos, diazinon, dicrotophos, dimethoate, disulfoton, fenthion, malathion, merphos, methamidophos, methyl parathion, monocrotophos, omethoate, parathion, phosmet, and trichlorfon. Clinically, IMS is characterized by acute paralysis and weakness in the areas of several cranial motor nerves, neck flexors, and facial, extraocular, palatal, nuchal, proximal limb, and respiratory muscles 24–96 hr after poisoning. IMS is a separate clinical entity from acute toxicity and delayed neuropathy. Generalized weakness, depressed deep tendon reflexes, ptosis, and diplopia are also evident. These symptoms may last for several days or weeks depending on the OP involved. Although the exact mechanism of action involved in IMS in unclear, the defect occurs at the neuromuscular junction (decreased AChE activity and expression of nicotinic receptors). Despite AChE inhibition, muscle fasciculations and hypersecretory activities are absent. There is no specific treatment; therapy relies on atropine sulfate and 2-PAM and should be continued for weeks.

DELAYED NEUROTOXICITY FROM TRIARYL PHOSPHATES

For some time, compounds known as triaryl phosphates (eg, triorthocresyl phosphate) have been used as flame retardants, plasticizers, lubricating oils, and hydraulic fluids. They are weak cholinesterase inhibitors but do inhibit "neurotoxic esterase" (NTE) present in the brain and spinal cord. A form of delayed neurotoxicity results from the inhibition and aging of NTE, often referred to as OP-induced delayed neuropathy (OPIDN). Triaryl phosphates have caused accidental poisonings in people and other species (mostly cattle). Some other OPs, including EPN, leptophos, parathion, haloxon, diisopropylphosphorofluoridate, and tetraethyl pyrophosphate, are known to cause OPIDN, and field cases have been seen. The lesions associated with delayed neurotoxicity include demyelination of peripheral and spinal motor tracts due to loss of neurotoxic esterase function. Clinical signs associated with delayed neurotoxicity include muscle weakness and ataxia that progresses to flaccid paralysis. Signs are usually not manifest until 10–14 days after exposure to a neurotoxic triaryl phosphate. There are no specific antidotes.

PESTICIDE POTENTIATING AGENTS

Piperonyl butoxide is used as a potentiator or synergist in many pesticide formulations, including carbamates, organophosphates, organochlorines, pyrethrins, pyrethroids, and D-limonene. It decreases breakdown of these pesticides in the animal or insect's body by inhibiting mixed function oxidase enzymes and makes the pesticide more toxic to the insect—and the host. Animals that are debilitated or have decreased drug-metabolizing capability become more susceptible to the pesticide. However, toxins that must be activated in the body to a toxic form are frequently less toxic when piperonyl butoxide exposure occurs at the same time. This potentiating or synergistic effect has been seen in many species, including cats, dogs, rats, and people. Cimetidine, a drug that reduces stomach acid secretion by blocking gastric H_2 receptors, and the antibiotic chloramphenicol have the same effect.

SOLVENTS AND EMULSIFIERS

Solvents and emulsifiers are required in most liquid insecticide preparations. Usually they have low toxicity, but like the petroleum products (which many are), they must be considered as possible causes of poisoning. In direct treatment with pesticides, emulsification must be thorough, with an average droplet size of 5 microns (preferably smaller), or excessive amounts may stick to treated animals. Treatment should be as for petroleum product poisoning (*see* p 3053).

Acetone: GI irritation, narcosis, and kidney and liver damage are the main signs of acetone poisoning. Treatment consists of gastric lavage, oxygen, and a low-fat diet. Additional supportive treatment to alleviate clinical signs may be given.

Isopropyl Alcohol: Isopropyl alcohol poisoning signs are GI pain, cramps, vomiting, diarrhea, and CNS depression (dizziness, stupor, coma, and death from respiratory paralysis). The liver and kidneys are reversibly affected. Dehydration and pneumonia may occur. Treatment consists of emetics, gastric lavage, milk, oxygen, and artificial respiration.

Methanol: Typical signs of methanol poisoning include nausea, vomiting, gastric pain, reflex hyperexcitability, opisthotonos, convulsions, fixed pupils, and acute peripheral neuritis. Large overdoses can lead to blindness. Toxic effects are due in part to the alcohol itself, and in part to formic acid produced by its oxidation. Treatment should include emetics (apomorphine) followed by gastric lavage with 4% sodium bicarbonate, saline laxative, oxygen therapy, sodium bicarbonate solution IV, and analgesics; however, the prognosis is poor. Intensive and prolonged alkalinization is the mainstay of treatment. Ethanol retards the oxidation of methanol and may be given as an adjunct therapy.

SULFUR AND LIME-SULFUR

Sulfur and lime-sulfur are two of the oldest insecticides. Elemental sulfur is practically devoid of toxicity, although poisoning has occurred occasionally when large amounts were mixed in cattle feed. Specific toxic dosages are not known but probably exceed 4 g/kg. Lime-sulfur, which is a complex of sulfides, may cause irritation, discomfort, or blistering but rarely causes death. Treatment consists of removing residual material and applying bland protective ointments, plus any supportive measures that may be indicated.

METALDEHYDE POISONING

Metaldehyde, a cyclic polymer of acetaldehyde, is the active component in molluscicides used to control slugs and snails. It is commonly used in wet coastal areas worldwide. This neurotoxicant has been associated with poisoning in a variety of domestic and wildlife species, although most poisonings have been reported in dogs and are related to careless placement of bait. Metaldehyde may be combined with other agents such as carbamate insecticides to enhance efficacy. It is not considered to be a persistent chemical. Under typical application circumstances, metaldehyde may remain effective for as long as 10 days.

Etiology and Pathogenesis: Metaldehyde may be purchased in liquid, dust, granular, or pelleted formulations. The active ingredient may vary from 1.5%–5% in the formulation. The bait is highly palatable and potentially addictive, which often results in consumption of large quantities. Most avian and mammalian species are susceptible. The lethal oral dose ranges from ~100–600 mg/kg in various species.

After ingestion, metaldehyde undergoes partial hydrolysis in the stomach to produce acetaldehyde. Both metaldehyde and acetaldehyde are readily absorbed from the GI tract. The nature of the stomach contents and the rate of gastric emptying influence the rate of absorption and the onset of the clinical syndrome. After absorption, metaldehyde is rapidly metabolized. Enterohepatic circulation may prolong retention of metaldehyde in the animal, but ultimately, both metaldehyde and acetaldehyde are excreted in the urine. Clinical manifestations are attributed primarily to metaldehyde, although acetaldehyde does play a role in the clinical syndrome. Metaldehyde exposure alters a variety of neurotransmitter concentrations and enzyme activities. Metaldehyde reduces concentrations of γ-aminobutyric acid, an inhibitory neurotransmitter that causes CNS excitation. Reduced concentrations of brain serotonin (5-hydroxytryptamine) and norepinephrine decrease the threshold for convulsions. Monoamine oxidase activity is increased after metaldehyde exposure. Increased muscle activity and the production of acidic metaldehyde metabolites cause severe electrolyte disturbances and metabolic acidosis.

Clinical Signs and Lesions: The clinical syndrome is similar in most species. Neurologic manifestations, which predominate, develop within 1–3 hr after ingestion. Severe muscle tremors, anxiety, hyperesthesia, ataxia, tachycardia, and hyperthermia may be evident initially. As the acidosis becomes more severe, depression and hyperpnea may become more evident. As the syndrome progresses, opisthotonos and continuous tonic convulsions that are unresponsive to external stimuli (in contrast to those in strychnine poisoning) are typical manifestations. Emesis, diarrhea, hypersalivation, colic, cyanosis, sweating (horses), mydriasis, and nystagmus (cats) are often reported.

No consistent pathognomonic gross or histologic lesions are seen with metaldehyde poisoning. Hepatic, renal, and pulmonary congestion and intestinal ecchymotic and petechial hemorrhages, which may be associated with prolonged hyperthermia, are common. Neuronal degeneration in the brain and hepatic degeneration with cellular swelling are often present histologically.

Diagnosis: A history of exposure plus the presence of typical clinical disease is suggestive of metaldehyde poisoning. Stomach contents often have a distinctive acetaldehyde or apple cider–like odor. Rapid analysis of stomach contents submitted frozen for metaldehyde and acetaldehyde may be useful to confirm the diagnosis. Analysis of urine, blood, or liver may be useful but is often unreliable.

Neurologic, GI, and pulmonary disease caused by other agents may be confused with metaldehyde poisoning. Potential differential diagnoses include poisonings by strychnine, roquefortine, sodium fluoroacetate, zinc phosphide, bromethalin, organophosphate, carbamate, organochlorine or pyrethroid insecticides, cyanide, blue-green algae, or compost (tremorgonic mycotoxins). Nontoxic conditions such as epilepsy, various encephalitic infections, lysosomal storage diseases, or metabolic diseases such as hypocalcemia also may resemble metaldehyde poisoning.

Treatment: There is no specific treatment for metaldehyde poisoning, although aggressive symptomatic treatment during the first 24 hr will enable most affected animals to make a full recovery within 2–3 days. Activated charcoal and cathartics may be administered to assist in decontamination and to reduce enterohepatic cycling of metaldehyde. Diazepam (2–5 mg/kg, IV, to effect) may be used to control neurologic manifestations. Barbiturate treatment should be considered with caution, because barbiturates compete with acetaldehyde metabolism and induce cytochrome P450 enzymes involved in metaldehyde metabolism. Gas anesthesia may also be a useful alternative. Administration of IV fluids containing sodium lactate or sodium bicarbonate is essential to correct the metabolic acidosis and electrolyte imbalance. Cold water to correct the hyperthermia, methocarbamol (150 mg/kg, IV) to produce muscle relaxation, and dextrose (IV) or calcium borogluconate (IV) to minimize liver damage may be helpful. Xylazine is an effective treatment in horses to reduce neurologic manifestations. Treatment options, dosages, and duration of treatment vary considerably from species to species.

Metaldehyde and acetaldehyde are rapidly eliminated. Consequently, tissue residues in food-producing animals are not a major concern. Withdrawal times, if established, will be relatively short.

ARSENIC POISONING

The ubiquitous element arsenic (As) is a nonmetal or metalloid in group V on the periodic chart. It is often referred to as arsenic metal and for toxicologic purposes is classified as a metal. It exists in several forms and has a long history of various uses, including insecticides for animals, wood preservatives, herbicides, and even some medicinal uses. It is responsible for many poisonings in people and animals.

Arsenic poisoning is caused by several different forms of the element; the form may determine the toxicity. Arsenic is found as inorganic and organic forms with valences of +3 and +5. Arsenite (As^{+3}) is more toxic than arsenate (As^{+5}). Toxicity varies with factors such as oxidation state of the arsenic, solubility, species of animal involved, and duration of exposure. Therefore, the toxic effects produced by phenylarsonic feed additives and other inorganic and organic compounds must be distinguished. (*See also* HERBICIDE POISONING, p 2969.)

INORGANIC ARSENICALS

Trivalent arsenicals, or arsenites, are more soluble and therefore more toxic than the pentavalent, or arsenate, compounds. These include arsenic trioxide, arsenic pentoxide, sodium and potassium arsenate, sodium and potassium arsenite, and lead or calcium arsenate. The lethal oral dose of sodium arsenite in most species is from 1–25 mg/kg.

Cats may be more sensitive. In livestock, arsenates are 5–10 times less toxic than arsenites. Decreased use of these compounds as pesticides, ant baits, and wood preservatives has made poisonings less frequent. Arsenites were used to some extent as dips for tick control. Lead arsenate was sometimes used as a taeniacide in sheep. Many of these compounds are no longer used in the USA but may still be available in other countries.

Toxicokinetics and Mechanism of Action: Soluble forms of arsenic compounds are well absorbed orally. After absorption, most of the arsenic is bound to RBCs; it distributes to several tissues, with the highest levels found in liver, kidneys, heart, and lungs. In subchronic or chronic exposures, arsenic accumulates in skin, nails, hooves, sweat glands, and hair. Most of the absorbed arsenic is excreted in the urine as inorganic arsenic or in methylated form.

The mechanism of action of arsenic toxicosis varies with the type of arsenical compound. Generally, tissues rich in oxidative enzymes, such as the GI tract, liver, kidneys, lungs, endothelium, and epidermis, are considered more vulnerable to arsenic damage. Trivalent inorganic and aliphatic organic arsenic compounds exert their toxicity by interacting with sulfhydryl enzymes, resulting in disruption of cellular metabolism. Arsenate can uncouple oxidative phosphorylation.

Clinical Findings: Poisoning is usually acute, with major effects on the GI tract and cardiovascular system. Arsenic has a direct effect on the capillaries, causing damage to microvascular integrity, transudation of plasma, loss of blood, and hypovolemic shock. Profuse watery diarrhea, sometimes tinged with dark blood, is characteristic, as are severe colic, dehydration, weakness, depression, weak pulse, and cardiovascular collapse. Onset is rapid, and signs are usually seen within a few hours (or up to 24 hr). The course may run from hours to several days, depending on the quantity ingested. In peracute poisoning, most animals may simply be found dead, and a few will be found dead without any lesions.

Lesions: In peracute toxicosis, there are usually some lesions in the GI tract. Inflammation and reddening of GI mucosa (local or diffuse) may be seen, followed by edema, rupture of blood vessels, and necrosis of epithelial and subepithelial tissue. In ruminants, hyperemic "paint-brush" lesions may be seen on the serosal surface of the omasum, and the abomasal mucosa may be hyperemic. Necrosis may progress to perforation of the gastric or intestinal wall. GI contents are often fluid, foul smelling, and blood tinged; they may contain shreds of epithelial tissue. There is diffuse inflammation of the liver, kidneys, and other visceral organs. The liver may have fatty degeneration and necrosis, and the kidneys have tubular damage. In cases of cutaneous exposure, the skin may exhibit necrosis and be dry or leathery.

Diagnosis: Chemical determination of arsenic in tissues (liver or kidney) or stomach contents provides confirmation. Liver and kidneys of healthy animals rarely contain >0.1 ppm arsenic (wet wt); toxicity is associated with tissue concentrations >3 ppm (wet wt). The determination of arsenic in stomach contents is of value usually within the first 24–48 hr after ingestion. The concentration of arsenic in urine can be high for several days after ingestion. Drinking water containing >0.25 ppm arsenic is considered potentially toxic, especially for large animals.

Treatment: In animals with recent exposure and no clinical signs, emesis should be induced (in capable species), followed by activated charcoal with a cathartic (efficacy of charcoal in arsenic toxicosis remains to be determined) and then oral administration of GI protectants (small animals, 1–2 hr after charcoal) such as kaolin-pectin, and fluid therapy as needed. In animals already showing clinical signs, aggressive fluid therapy, blood transfusion (if needed), and administration of dimercaprol (British anti-lewisite, 4–7 mg/kg, IM, tid for 2–3 days or until recovery) is recommended. In large animals, thioctic acid (lipoic acid or α-lipoic acid) may be used alone (50 mg/kg, IM, tid, as a 20% solution) or in combination with dimercaprol (3 mg/kg, IM, every 4 hr for the first 2 days, qid for the third day, and bid for the next 10 days or until recovery). In large animals, the efficacy of dimercaprol alone is questionable. Sodium thiosulfate has also been used, PO, at 20–30 g in 300 mL of water in horses and cattle, one-fourth this dose in sheep and goats, and 0.5–3 g in small animals or as a 20% solution, IV, at 30–40 mg/kg, bid-tid for 3–4 days or until recovery. The water-soluble analogues of dimercaprol, 2,3-dimercaptopropane-1-sulfonate (DMPS) and dimercaptosuccinic acid (DMSA), are considered to be less toxic and more effective and could be given orally. D-Penicillamine is reportedly an effective arsenic chelator in people. It has a wide margin of safety and could be used in animals at 10–50 mg/kg, PO, tid-qid for 3–4 days. Supportive therapy may be of even greater value, particularly when cardiovascular collapse is imminent, and should involve IV fluids to restore blood volume and correct dehydration. Kidney and liver function should be monitored during treatment.

ORGANIC ARSENICALS

Phenylarsonic organic arsenicals are relatively less toxic than inorganic compounds or aliphatic and other aromatic organic compounds.

Aliphatic organic arsenicals include cacodylic acid and acetarsonic acid. These were historically used as stimulants in large animals, but their use is now uncommon. Some aliphatic arsenicals such as monosodium methanearsonate (MSMA) and disodium methanearsonate (DSMA) are occasionally used as herbicides or grassburr and crabgrass killers. Ruminants, especially cattle, are very sensitive to MSMA and DSMA. Clinical signs, lesions, and treatment of aliphatic organic arsenicals are similar to those of inorganic arsenicals, except that ruminants may have necrosis of the mucosa of the rumen and omasum and gelatinous serosal edema of the omasum and abomasum.

Aromatic organic arsenicals include trivalent phenylorganics, such as thiacetarsamide and arsphenamine for the treatment of adult heartworms in dogs, and pentavalent compounds such as phenylarsonic acids and their salts. Thiacetarsamide and arsphenamine are no longer used commonly, especially since the introduction of melarsomine dihydrochloride (*see also* HEARTWORM DISEASE, p 127).

Phenylarsonic compounds were widely used as feed additives to improve production in swine and poultry rations and to treat dysentery in pigs. The three major compounds in this class are arsanilic acid, roxarsone (4-hydroxy-3-nitrophenylarsonic acid), and nitarsone (4-nitro-phenylarsonic acid).

Etiology: Toxicosis results from an excess of arsenic-containing additives in pig or poultry diets. Severity and rapidity of onset are dose-dependent. Signs may be delayed for weeks after incorporation of 2–3 times the recommended (100 ppm) levels or may occur within days when the excess is >10 times the recommended levels. Chickens are tolerant of arsanilic acid; however, roxarsone can produce toxicosis in turkeys at only twice the recommended dose (50 ppm). In pigs, roxarsone also has a higher toxicity than other phenylarsonics.

Clinical Findings and Diagnosis: The earliest sign in pigs may be reduced weight gain, followed by incoordination, posterior paralysis, and eventually quadriplegia. Animals remain alert and maintain good appetite. Blindness is characteristic of arsanilic acid intoxication but not of other organic arsenicals. In ruminants, phenylarsonic toxicosis is similar to inorganic arsenic poisoning. There are usually no specific lesions present in phenylarsonic poisoning. Demyelination and gliosis of peripheral nerves, the optic tract, and optic nerves are usually seen on histopathology. Analyses of feed for the presence of high levels of phenylarsonics confirm the diagnosis.

Phenylarsonic poisoning in pigs should be differentiated from salt poisoning, insecticide poisoning, and pseudorabies. In cattle, arsenic poisoning should be differentiated from other heavy metal poisoning, insecticide poisoning, and infectious diseases such as bovine viral diarrhea.

Treatment and Prognosis: There is no specific treatment, but the neurotoxic effects are usually reversible if the offending feed is withdrawn within 2–3 days of onset of ataxia. Once paralysis occurs, the nerve damage is irreversible. Blindness is usually irreversible, but animals retain their appetite, and weight gain is good if competition for food is eliminated. Recovery may be doubtful when the exposure is long and the onset of intoxication slow.

COPPER POISONING

Acute or chronic copper poisoning is encountered in most parts of the world. Sheep are affected most often, although other species are also susceptible. In various breeds of dogs, especially Bedlington Terriers, an inherited sensitivity to copper toxicosis similar to Wilson disease in people has been identified. Chronic copper poisoning has been reported in other breeds of dogs, including Labrador Retrievers, West

Highland White Terriers, Skye Terriers, Keeshonds, American Cocker Spaniels, and Doberman Pinschers. Acute poisoning is usually seen after accidental administration of excessive amounts of soluble copper salts, which may be present in anthelmintic drenches, mineral mixes, or improperly formulated rations.

Many factors that alter copper metabolism influence chronic copper poisoning by enhancing the absorption or retention of copper. Low levels of molybdenum or sulfate in the diet are important examples. Primary chronic poisoning is seen most commonly in sheep when excessive amounts of copper are ingested over a prolonged period. The toxicosis remains subclinical until the copper that is stored in the liver is released in massive amounts. Increased liver enzymes may provide an early warning of the pending crisis. Blood copper concentrations increase suddenly, causing lipid peroxidation and intravascular hemolysis. The hemolytic crisis may be precipitated by many factors, including transportation, handling, weather conditions, pregnancy, lactation, strenuous exercise, or a deteriorating plane of nutrition.

Phytogenous and hepatogenous factors influence secondary chronic copper poisoning. Phytogenous chronic poisoning is seen after ingestion of plants, such as subterranean clover (*Trifolium subterraneum*), that produce a mineral imbalance and result in excessive copper retention. The plants that are not hepatotoxic contain normal amounts of copper and low levels of molybdenum. The ingestion of plants such as *Heliotropium europaeum* or *Senecio* spp (*see* p 3150) for several months may cause hepatogenous chronic copper poisoning. These plants contain hepatotoxic alkaloids, which result in retention of excessive copper in the liver. In dogs with liver diseases such as chronic active hepatitis (CAH), the primary clinical signs may resemble those of chronic copper poisoning, which can be attributed to the liver damage and subsequent retention of excessive copper; however, it is not clear whether CAH causes the accumulation of copper in the liver or is the result of accumulation.

Acute poisoning may follow intakes of 20–100 mg of copper/kg in sheep and young calves and of 200–800 mg/kg in mature cattle. Chronic poisoning of sheep may occur with daily intakes of 3.5 mg of copper/kg when grazing pastures that contain 15–20 ppm (dry matter) of copper and low levels of molybdenum. Clinical disease may occur in sheep or camelid species that ingest cattle rations, which normally contain higher levels of copper, or when their water is supplied via copper plumbing; cattle and goats are more resistant to copper poisoning than sheep and thus are not affected in these instances. Species-specific diets with respect to copper are recommended to minimize the occurrence of chronic copper poisoning. Breed differences related to the suceptibility to chronic copper poisoning have been reported in sheep and goats. Young calves or sheep injected with soluble forms of copper may develop acute clinical signs of toxicity without evidence of a hemolytic crisis. Copper is used as a feed additive for pigs at 125–250 ppm; levels >250 ppm are dangerous—although as for sheep, other factors may be protective, eg, high levels of protein, zinc, or iron. Chronic copper toxicosis is more likely to occur with low dietary intake of molybdenum and sulfur. Reduced formation of copper molybdate or copper sulfide complexes in tissues impairs the excretion of copper in urine or feces.

Clinical Findings: Acute copper poisoning causes severe gastroenteritis characterized by abdominal pain, diarrhea, anorexia, dehydration, and shock. Hemolysis and hemoglobinuria may develop after 3 days if the animal survives the GI disturbances. The sudden onset of clinical signs in chronic copper poisoning is associated with the hemolytic crisis. The time of onset is influenced by the concentration of copper in the diet. Signs in affected animals include depression, lethargy, weakness, recumbency, rumen stasis, anorexia, thirst, dyspnea, pale mucous membranes, hemoglobinuria, and jaundice. Several days or weeks before the hemolytic crisis, liver enzymes, including ALT and AST, are usually increased. During the hemolytic crisis, methemoglobinemia, hemoglobinemia, and decreases in PCV and blood glutathione are usually seen. In camelid species such as alpacas or llamas, no hemolytic crisis is seen, although extensive liver necrosis remains a consistent manifestation. Morbid animals often die within 1–2 days. Herd morbidity is often <5%, although usually >75% of affected animals die. Losses may continue for several months after the dietary problem has been rectified. Severe hepatic insufficiency is responsible for early deaths. Animals that survive the acute episode may die of subsequent renal failure. Photosensitization may occur in association with chronic copper poisoning, reflecting the hepatotoxicity common to both syndromes. Cirrhosis of the liver is also associated with the syndrome in dogs.

Lesions: Acute copper poisoning produces severe gastroenteritis with erosions and ulcerations in the abomasum of ruminants. Icterus develops in animals that survive >24 hr. Tissues discolored by icterus and methemoglobin are characteristic of chronic poisoning. Swollen, gunmetal-colored kidneys, port-wine-colored urine, and an enlarged spleen with dark brown-black parenchyma are manifestations of the hemolytic crisis. The liver is enlarged and friable. Histologically, there is centrilobular hepatic and renal tubular necrosis.

Diagnosis: Evidence of blue-green ingesta and increased fecal (8,000–10,000 ppm) and kidney (>15 ppm, wet wt) copper levels are considered significant in acute copper poisoning. In chronic poisoning, blood and liver copper concentrations are increased during the hemolytic period. Blood concentrations often rise to 5–20 mcg/mL, as compared with normal levels of ~1 mcg/mL. Liver concentrations >150 ppm (wet wt) are significant in sheep. The concentration of copper in the tissue must be determined to eliminate other causes of hemolytic disease. Molybdenum tissue concentrations should be evaluated to determine whether the syndrome is due to primary or secondary chronic copper poisoning.

Treatment and Control: Often, treatment is not successful. The prognosis is poor in all species. GI sedatives and symptomatic treatment for shock may be useful in acute toxicity. Penicillamine (50 mg/kg/day, PO, for 6 days) or calcium versenate may be useful if administered in the early stages of disease to enhance copper excretion. Vitamin C (500 mg/day/sheep, SC) has been shown to reduce oxidative damage to RBCs during the hemolytic crisis. Ammonium tetrathiomolybdate (1.7 mg/kg, IV, every other day for 6 days) is effective for the treatment and prevention of copper poisoning. This treatment, which reduces copper absorption and enhances copper elimination, should be used conservatively. A withdrawal period of ~10 days is required for this medication. Daily oral administration of ammonium molybdate (100 mg) and sodium thiosulfate (1 g) for 3 wk reduces losses in affected lambs. Dietary supplementation with zinc acetate (250 ppm) may be useful to reduce the absorption of copper. Plant eradication or reducing access to plants that cause phytogenous or hepatogenous copper poisoning is desirable. Primary chronic or phytogenous poisoning may be prevented by top-dressing pastures with 1 oz of molybdenum per acre (70 g/hectare) in the form of molybdenized superphosphate or by molybdenum supplementation or restriction of copper intake. High-risk flocks of sheep may be supplemented with sodium thiosulfate in the diet to prevent or control chronic copper poisoning. In dogs, genetic testing is available to identify carriers of the autosomal recessive gene associated with abnormal copper accumulation, although the mode of inheritance is not known for all susceptible breeds. Periodic liver biopsies, tissue copper determination, and liver enzyme assessment may also be useful to evaluate disease status. In addition to previously described treatments, zinc supplementation and prednisone or prednisolone administration enhance copper excretion and limit development of liver disease.

FLUORIDE POISONING

(Fluorosis)

Fluoride exposure from the environment has been associated with natural contamination of rock, soil, and water or from industrial waste or smelting processes. Fluoride compounds have been added to human water supplies at concentrations of ~1 mg/kg to reduce dental caries. This recommendation is not universally accepted. Both acute and chronic toxicoses are reported with fluoride ingestion. Maximum tolerance levels in animal feeds range from ~20–50 mg/kg (dry weight) in most species. In poultry, as much as 200 mg/kg can be tolerated. These tolerances may vary depending on age, duration of exposure, and nutritional status. Animals with a long, productive life span such as dairy cattle are more susceptible.

Etiology and Pathogenesis: Fluorides are found naturally in rock phosphates and limestone. Industrial wastes associated with fertilizer and mineral supplement production are frequent sources of fluoride exposure. Metal ores associated with steel and aluminum processing are common industrial sources. Fluoride dusts dispersed downwind from these sources may contaminate forage crops for many kilometers. Forage crops grown on contaminated soil may contain increased concentrations of fluoride associated with physical contamination with soil particulates. There is minimal direct uptake of fluoride by the plant. With the potential of fluoride contamination in many feed and water sources, it is recommended that feed-grade phosphates contain <1% fluoride. Acute fluoride exposure at high concentrations will cause corrosive damage to tissues. In contrast, chronic exposure, which is seen more frequently, causes delayed or impaired mineralization of bones and teeth. The solubility of fluoride correlates generally with the degree of toxicity. Fluoride is known to interact with various elements, including aluminum, calcium, phosphorus, and iodine. Fluoride is a cellular poison that interferes with the metabolism of essential metals such as magnesium, manganese, iron, copper, and zinc. Because bacterial metabolism may be affected in a similar manner, this attribute accounts for the use of fluoride in dental hygiene products. Soluble fluoride is rapidly absorbed; ~50% is excreted by glomerular filtration. More than 95% of the fluoride that is retained is deposited in the bones and teeth, forming hydroxyapatite after the interference with calcium metabolism and replacement of hydroxyl ions. At low levels of fluoride exposure, the solubility of the enamel is reduced, resulting in protection. At higher levels of exposure, the enamel becomes dense and brittle. If exposure occurs during pregnancy, developing bones and teeth are severely affected. Faulty, irregular mineralization of the matrix associated with altered ameloblastic, odontoblastic, or osteoblastic activity ultimately results in poor enamel formation, exostosis, sclerosis, and osteoporosis.

Clinical Findings: Acute poisoning associated with massive ingestion of ascaricides (sodium fluoride), rodenticides (sodium fluorosilicate), or oral dental products will produce clinical disease within 2 hr. The fatal dosage of sodium fluoride is ~5–10 mg/kg. Toxic manifestations may be evident after consumption of ~1 mg/kg. Serum calcium and magnesium concentrations decline rapidly after the onset of the clinical syndrome. Severe gastroenteritis, salivation, restlessness, sweating, anorexia, muscle weakness, stiffness, dyspnea, ventricular tachycardia, and clonic convulsions followed by depression and death are typically seen. Chronic fluorosis is characterized by unthrifty animals with skeletal and dental abnormalities. Reduced feed and water intake accompanied by poor weight gain and milk production reflect dental lesions and impaired mastication. Mottled, chalky, pitted and stained enamel, and uneven and excessive wear on the teeth are frequently seen. Dental pain manifested by lapping of drinking water may be apparent. Skeletal abnormalities associated with increased bone resorption and remodeling produces severe lameness, stiffness, abnormal hoof growth, and exostoses. In later stages of the syndrome, severely affected cattle may be forced to move on their knees because of spurring and bridging of joints. Periosteal hyperostosis is seen on ribs. Metabolically active and growing bones of young animals are more severely affected. Anemia and hypothyroidism manifested by reduced T_3 and T_4 levels plus reduced serum calcium concentrations are often present.

Lesions: Severe GI inflammation and degenerative changes in other organs such as the liver, kidney, and lungs reflect the cytotoxic effects of acute fluorosis. After chronic exposure during pregnancy, offspring are more severely affected. Bilateral and symmetrical skeletal abnormalities are present. The bones are chalky white with disrupted osteogenesis, accelerated bone remodeling, and resorption in association with production of abnormal bone osteoid that results in exostoses, sclerosis, and osteoporosis. The mandible, ribs, metacarpals, and metatarsals are most often affected. Exostoses are most evident in the long bones. In addition to the mottled, chalky, stained teeth exhibiting uneven wear, eruption of permanent incisor teeth may be delayed.

Diagnosis: A diagnosis of acute fluoride poisoning should be based on a history of exposure and typical clinical or pathologic manifestations. Confirmation with urine or serum measurements should be interpreted with caution, because rapid, time-dependent elimination of fluoride occurs. The measurement of serum calcium and magnesium concentrations may provide supportive evidence. Chronic fluorosis may require many months to develop. Fluoride concentrations in tissues must be considered in association with history, clinical disease, and necropsy findings. Animals exhibiting skeletal and dental abnormalities manifested by lameness, osteoporosis, anorexia, or reduced productivity should be evaluated for chronic fluorosis. Other disease syndromes such as arthritis; calcium, phosphorous, or vitamin D deficiency; metal toxicities such as molybdenum, selenium, or arsenic; and ergotism may be confused with chronic poisoning. In addition to tissue analysis, radiographs and histologic evaluation may provide useful information. In livestock, normal fluoride concentrations in the diet range from ~20–50 mg/kg. Depending on the duration of exposure and species susceptibility, concentrations in the diet ranging from 100–300 mg/kg may produce chronic poisoning. Water concentrations >30 mg/L are considered toxic. In young dairy cattle with a lengthy lifetime production potential, tolerance levels should be reduced by at least 2-fold. Because fluoride does not accumulate in soft tissue, analysis of liver and kidney has limited usefulness. In livestock, normal plasma concentrations are <0.2 mg/L, whereas concentrations ranging from 0.7–1.9 mg/L are consistent with poisoning. Corresponding urinary concentrations <0.5 mg/L are normal. Toxic concentrations based on recent exposure range from 14–120 mg/L. Fluoride concentrations in bones and teeth may reach levels as high as 1,500 mg/kg and 1,000 mg/kg, respectively, without adverse effects. Concentrations ranging from 6,000–13,000 mg/kg and 7,500–11,000 mg/kg, respectively, are consistent with a diagnosis of chronic fluorosis in livestock. Plasma concentrations may rise substantially once the skeletal concentrations of fluoride approach saturation.

Treatment and Control: Animals developing acute poisoning may be administered calcium gluconate (IV) and magnesium hydroxide or milk orally to minimize fluoride absorption, although the prognosis may remain poor if massive amounts of fluoride were ingested. Once manifestations of chronic fluorosis develop, treatment is ineffective. The primary objective should be directed toward prevention. In many instances, it may be difficult or impractical to remove livestock from contaminated areas. Supplementation with calcium carbonate, aluminum salts, magnesium metasilicate, or boron will reduce absorption or enhance excretion. It is recommended that livestock consume supplements and mineral mixes containing <1% fluoride content. If it is impractical to limit fluoride exposure, raising species with a relatively short production life, such as poultry, pigs, or sheep, should be considered. Reducing fluoride exposure of young or pregnant animals may limit the development of chronic fluorosis.

IRON TOXICITY IN NEWBORN PIGS

Reports of toxicity after SC or IM injection of iron preparations in newborn piglets are sporadic, and the risk is not high; however, toxicity does occur occasionally. In some litters, death occurs quickly, from 30 min to 6 hr after injection; in others, death is delayed for 2–4 days. (*See also* NONREGENERATIVE ANEMIAS, p 12.)

Toxicity may be seen in three forms. In the first form, damage to the muscles around the injection site causes potassium, among other substances, to be released; the blood potassium level rises and interferes with cardiac function. Usually, the whole litter is affected. Piglets may appear anemic, become weak, cannot stand, and have muscle tremors followed by convulsions. Respiratory distress may be seen. There is swelling at the injection site. On necropsy, skin and muscles may appear pale, and there is edema and a brownish black discoloration at the injection site. Waxy degeneration of skeletal and heart muscle may be seen; there may be hemorrhages in the heart and necrosis of the liver and kidneys.

In the second, less acute form of toxicity, the excess iron appears to block the body's defense mechanisms by overwhelming the phagocytic cells, which increases the likelihood of infection. Death occurs in ~2–4 days. In young piglets, the most likely infection is an *Escherichia coli* enteritis and, although some of the changes seen in the first form may be seen at necropsy, they are less obvious, and the enteritis contributes markedly to death.

The most important precipitating factor of iron toxicosis in pigs is a low vitamin E or selenium status of the sow. If either nutrient is low in the sow, pigs will either be born deficient in vitamin E or selenium or the colostrum will not be able to provide adequate amounts of these nutrients to meet the antioxidant needs of nursing piglets. Supplementing the sow's diet with 50 IU of vitamin E/kg and 0.15 mg of selenium/kg will improve the status of the sow and prevent iron toxicity in the piglets. Injections of vitamin E/selenium during late gestation may also help prevent iron toxicity in piglets.

A third, more rare form of toxicity is associated with **calciphylaxis**, the massive mobilization of calcium after injection of iron preparations, both in the presence and absence of supplementary vitamin D. It occurs within several days of iron injection and is associated with development of hard swellings at injection sites. Death may occur, and calcification in other parts of the body may be seen at necropsy.

LEAD POISONING

Lead poisoning in animals and people is a major concern worldwide. Poisoning in animal populations may serve as a sentinel to assess the extent of environmental contamination and human health problems related to lead. In veterinary medicine, lead poisoning is most common in dogs and cattle. Lead poisoning in other species is limited by reduced accessibility, more selective eating habits, or lower susceptibility. In cattle, many cases are associated with seeding and harvesting activities when used oil and battery disposal from machinery is handled improperly. With the elimination of tetraethyl lead from gasoline in many countries, the number of lead poisoning cases attributed to oil consumption has declined. Other sources of lead include paint, linoleum, grease, lead weights, lead shot, and contaminated foliage growing near smelters or along roadsides. To prevent future occurrences of lead poisoning, it is crucial to identify the source. Lead poisoning is also encountered in urban environments and during the renovation of old houses that have been painted with lead-based paint, leading to exposure of small animals and children. The consumption, through grooming, of dust containing lead has been reported in cats. Improper disposal of lead-poisoned animal carcasses may result in toxicoses in nontarget scavenger animals. Scavenging by endangered species such as the condor raises unique concerns.

Pathogenesis: Absorbed lead enters the blood and soft tissues and eventually redistributes to the bone. The degree of absorption and retention is influenced by dietary factors such as calcium or iron levels. In ruminants, particulate lead lodged in the reticulum slowly dissolves and releases significant quantities of lead. Lead has a profound effect on sulfhydryl-containing enzymes, the thiol content of erythrocytes, antioxidant defenses, and tissues rich in mitochondria, which is reflected in the clinical syndrome. In addition to the cerebellar hemorrhage and edema associated with capillary damage, lead is also irritating, immunosuppressive, gametotoxic, teratogenic, nephrotoxic, and toxic to the hematopoietic system.

Clinical Findings: Acute lead poisoning is more common in young animals. The prominent clinical signs are associated with the GI and nervous systems. In cattle, signs that appear within 24–48 hr of exposure include ataxia, blindness, salivation, spastic twitching of eyelids, jaw champing, bruxism, muscle tremors, and convulsions.

Subacute lead poisoning, usually seen in sheep or older cattle, is characterized by anorexia, rumen stasis, colic, dullness, and transient constipation, frequently followed by diarrhea, blindness, head pressing, bruxism, hyperesthesia, and incoordination.

Chronic lead poisoning, occasionally seen in cattle, may produce a syndrome that has many features in common with acute or subacute lead poisoning. Impairment of the swallowing reflexes frequently contributes to development of aspiration pneumonia. Embryotoxicity and poor semen quality may contribute to infertility.

GI abnormalities, including anorexia, colic, emesis, and diarrhea or constipation are predominant manifestations in dogs. Anxiety, hysterical barking, jaw champing, salivation, blindness, ataxia, muscle spasms, opisthotonos, and convulsions may develop. CNS depression rather than CNS excitation may be evident in some dogs. In horses, lead poisoning usually produces a chronic syndrome characterized by weight loss, depression, weakness, colic, diarrhea, laryngeal or pharyngeal paralysis (roaring), and dysphagia that frequently results in aspiration pneumonia.

In birds, anorexia, ataxia, loss of condition, wing and leg weakness, and anemia are the most notable signs.

Lesions: Animals that die from acute lead poisoning may have few observable gross lesions. Oil or flakes of paint or battery may be evident in the GI tract. The caustic action of lead salts causes gastroenteritis. In the nervous system, edema, congestion of the cerebral cortex, and flattening of the cortical gyri are present. Histologically, endothelial swelling, laminar cortical necrosis, and edema of the white matter may be evident. Tubular necrosis and degeneration and intranuclear acid-fast inclusion bodies may be seen in the kidneys. Osteoporosis has been described in lambs. Placentitis and accumulation of lead in the fetus may result in abortion.

Diagnosis: Lead concentrations in various tissues may be useful to evaluate excessive accumulation and to reflect the level or duration of exposure, severity, and prognosis and the success of treatment. Concentrations of lead in the blood at 0.35 ppm, liver at 10 ppm, or kidney cortex at 10 ppm are consistent with a diagnosis of lead poisoning in most species. Many countries have deemed blood lead concentrations >0.05–0.10 ppm to be a notifiable disease in food-producing animals. Inspection or clearance by a regulatory veterinary officer or biosecurity inspector is mandatory before shipment for food consumption is permitted.

Hematologic abnormalities, which may be indicative but not confirmatory of lead poisoning, include anemia, anisocytosis, poikilocytosis, polychromasia, basophilic stippling, metarubricytosis, and hypochromia. Blood or urinary δ-aminolevulinic acid and free erythrocyte protoporphyrin levels are sensitive indicators of lead exposure but may not be reliable indicators of clinical disease. Radiologic examination may be useful to determine the magnitude of lead exposure.

Lead poisoning may be confused with other diseases that cause nervous or GI abnormalities. In cattle, such diseases may include polioencephalomalacia, nervous coccidiosis, tetanus, hypovitaminosis A, hypomagnesemic tetany, nervous acetonemia, organochlorine insecticide poisoning, arsenic or mercury poisoning, brain abscess or neoplasia, rabies, listeriosis, and *Haemophilus* infections.

In dogs, rabies, distemper, and hepatitis may appear similar to lead poisoning.

Treatment: If tissue damage is extensive, particularly to the nervous system, treatment may not be successful. In livestock, calcium disodium edetate (Ca-EDTA) is given IV or SC (110 mg/kg/day) divided bid for 3 days; this treatment should be repeated 2 days later. In dogs, a similar dose divided qid is administered SC in 5% dextrose for 2–5 days. After a 1-wk rest period, an additional 5-day treatment may be required if clinical signs persist. No approved veterinary product containing Ca-EDTA is currently commercially available.

Thiamine (2–4 mg/kg/day, SC) alleviates clinical manifestations and reduces tissue deposition of lead. Combined Ca-EDTA and thiamine treatment appears to produce the most beneficial response.

D-Penicillamine can be administered PO to dogs (110 mg/kg/day) for 2 wk. However, undesirable adverse effects such as emesis and anorexia have been associated with this treatment. D-Penicillamine is not recommended for livestock. Succimer (meso 2,3-dimercaptosuccinic acid [DMSA]) is a chelating agent that has proved to be effective in dogs (10 mg/kg, PO, tid for 10 days) and is also useful in birds. Fewer adverse effects have been associated with DMSA than with Ca-EDTA.

Cathartics such as magnesium sulfate (400 mg/kg, PO) or a rumenotomy may be useful to remove lead from the GI tract. In cattle, surgery to remove particulate lead material from the reticulum after the ingestion of batteries is rarely successful. Barbiturates or tranquilizers may be indicated to control convulsions. Chelation therapy, in combination with antioxidant treatment, may limit oxidative damage associated with acute lead poisoning. Antioxidants such as *N*-acetylcysteine (50 mg/kg/day, PO) have been used in combination with DMSA.

Mobilization of lead at parturition, excretion of lead into milk, and lengthy withdrawal times in food-producing animals raise considerable controversy regarding the rationale for treatment from both public health and animal management perspectives. The half-life of lead in the blood of cattle ingesting particulate lead is usually >9 wk. Withdrawal times, which may be >1 yr, should be estimated by periodic monitoring of blood lead concentrations. In a herd of cattle with confirmed cases of lead poisoning, all potentially exposed cattle should be evaluated. A small but significant portion of the asymptomatic cattle may have concentrations of lead in tissues that exceed recognized food safety standards.

MERCURY POISONING

Historically, mercury poisoning was a common occurrence in both human and animal populations. The replacement of mercury products used for medicinal, agricultural, or industrial purposes has resulted in a decline in acute and chronic poisoning, although many wildlife species remain at risk. Predator species considered to be near the top of the food chain, such as fish, seals, polar bears, and various bird species, bioaccumulate significant quantities of mercury from dietary sources. Commercial fish products such as tuna have been associated with chronic poisoning in human and animal (cats) populations. Mercury exists in a variety of chemical forms, including elemental mercury (eg, thermometers, light bulbs), inorganic mercurial (mercuric or mercurous) salts (eg, batteries, latex paints), and organic mercury (aryl, methyl, or ethyl). Fossil fuels represent an important environmental source of mercury. In the environment, inorganic forms of mercury are converted to methylmercury under anaerobic conditions in the sediment of most water bodies. Similar conversions may also occur in the body.

Pathogenesis: The physical, chemical, and kinetic properties of the various forms of mercury play an important role influencing the clinical manifestations, the extent and nature of lesions, and the tissue distribution of mercury. The organic forms of mercury, primarily methylmercury, are lipid soluble and well absorbed orally. Consequently, bioaccumulation is extensive in tissues such as the brain, kidney, and fetus. Methylmercury interferes with metabolic activity, resulting in degeneration and necrosis in many tissues, although the brain and fetus are more susceptible. In the brain, histologically, neuronal degeneration and perivascular cuffing is evident in the cerebrocortical grey matter. Cerebellar atrophy or hypoplasia and Purkinje cell degeneration are seen. Encephalomalacia, the loss of myelin, and necrosis of axons may also be evident. Methylmercury is mutagenic, carcinogenic, embryotoxic, and highly teratogenic. The inorganic forms of mercury, including elemental mercury, are poorly absorbed after dermal exposure. Elemental mercury vapors are inhaled and rapidly absorbed. This highly toxic form of mercury produces corrosive bronchitis and interstitial pneumonia. All forms of mercury cross the placenta. Inorganic forms of mercury bind to sulfhydryl groups in enzymes and other thiol-containing molecules such as cysteine and glutathione. Tissues rich in these components, such as the renal cortex, accumulate significant concentrations of mercury. Inorganic forms of mercury are cytotoxic and highly corrosive. Consequently, these forms of mercury cause severe inflammation, ulcers, and direct tissue necrosis in the GI tract. Pale, swollen kidneys manifested histologically by tubular necrosis and interstitial nephritis are consistent findings.

Clinical Findings: The inhalation of corrosive elemental mercury vapors that produces severe dyspnea and compromised respiratory function is usually fatal at high levels of exposure. Neurologic manifestations may eventually develop if exposure is not excessive. Inorganic mercury, related to its corrosive nature, produces primarily GI manifestations, including colic, anorexia, stomatitis, pharyngitis, vomiting, diarrhea, shock, dyspnea, and dehydration. Death often occurs within hours at high levels of exposure. Animals that survive may exhibit eczema, skin keratinization, anuria, polydypsia, hematuria, or melena. Neurologic manifestations, including CNS depression or excitation similar to that which occurs in organic mercury poisoning, may develop after chronic exposure. Depending on the level of exposure to organic mercury compounds such as methylmercury, clinical manifestations may require days to develop. Because these compounds are not corrosive, GI signs are not seen. Neurologic manifestations that predominate include blindness, ataxia, incoordination, tremors, abnormal behavior, hypermetria, nystagmus (cats), and tonic-clonic convulsions. Advanced stages may be characterized by depression, anorexia, proprioceptive defects, total blindness, paralysis, and high mortality. The nervous system of young, developing animals is particularly susceptible to organic mercury exposure, which is frequently manifested by cerebellar ataxia and death.

Diagnosis: The considerable variation associated with the clinical manifestations related to the form of mercury and the duration of exposure accentuates the need for multiple tissue analyses. Because inorganic forms of mercury are excreted in the urine, urinary mercury concentrations are the most reliable indicator of exposure. In contrast, organic mercury compounds, which bioaccumulate in soft tissues, are most appropriately assessed in the liver, kidney, or brain tissues. In most species, blood, kidney, brain, and feed concentrations of mercury <0.1 mg/kg (wet weight) are considered normal. In poisoned species, concentrations >6 mg/kg (blood), 10 mg/kg (kidney), 0.5 mg/kg (brain), and 4 mg/kg (feed, dry weight) are consistent with a diagnosis of mercury poisoning. Generally, the kidney is considered to be the most useful tissue diagnostically. Concentrations in all tissues may be substantially higher after chronic exposure. Marine mammals and fish often contain substantially increased concentrations of mercury that may not be associated with clinical disease (as such concentrations would be associated in traditional livestock or companion animal species), but they may be a potential source of exposure for more susceptible species, particularly the fetus or younger animals. Other measurements, including the presence of proteinuria, azotemia, or a nonregenerative anemia, may provide useful evidence to support a diagnosis of mercury poisoning. The diagnosis may be made on the basis of tissue analysis in association with appropriate histopathology, clinical pathology, clinical manifestations, and history. Differential diagnoses may include conditions that produce GI disturbances, renal disease, or neurologic dysfunction manifested by tremors, ataxia, or convulsions. Metals such as lead, arsenic, thallium, or cadmium; insecticides, including organophosphate, carbamate, or organochlorine compounds; oxalates; vitamin D; or mycotoxins such as T-2 toxin should be considered. Infectious diseases, including hog cholera, erysipelas, and feline parvovirus, may resemble mercury poisoning.

Treatment and Control: Because the neurologic and renal damage is irreversible, treatment alternatives may be ineffective. Consequently, the prognosis for a complete recovery is very poor. In food-producing animals, significant mercury accumulation in edible tissues and profound effects on reproduction limit treatment options. Euthanasia and disposal, in consultation with regulatory officials, is recommended. Oral administration of activated charcoal (1–3 g/kg) and sodium thiosulfate (0.5–1 g/kg) will bind mercury and limit absorption. Vitamin E and selenium, which are antioxidants, may limit oxidative damage. Chelation therapy may be useful if treatment is started soon after exposure before nephrotoxic effects become severe. The lipid-soluble chelator dimercaprol (3 mg/kg body wt, IM, every 4 hr for 2 days, followed by qid treatment on day 3 and bid treatment for 10 days) may be beneficial. For organic mercury poisoning, 2.3-dimercaptosuccinic acid (10 mg/kg, PO, tid for 10 days) has been useful in dogs. If the GI tract has been decontaminated for mercury, administration of penicillamine (50–100 mg/kg/day, PO, for 2 wk) may reduce clinical signs.

MOLYBDENUM POISONING

Molybdenum is an essential element associated with a variety of metalloenzymes and corresponding metabolic functions. Excessive dietary intake of molybdenum induces a secondary copper deficiency. The syndrome, predominately reported in ruminants (versus nonruminant species) is seen worldwide. Cattle and sheep are ~10-fold more susceptible than other species. Acute toxicity associated with massive doses is rarely encountered.

Etiology: The interactions associated with copper, molybdenum, and sulfate metabolism related to the utilization, bioavailability, and kinetics of copper are among the most biologically significant interrelationships in veterinary medicine. The complexity of the interactions is not fully understood. In ruminants, various molybdates react with sulfides to produce thiomolybdate compounds, which react with copper to form an insoluble complex that is poorly absorbed. The reduced copper absorption impairs copper utilization and the synthesis of a variety of copper-dependent proteins. The reduced bioavailability of copper ultimately induces secondary copper deficiency. Excessive molybdenum intake also enhances the excretion of copper. Based on this observation, the administration of tetrathiomolybdates may be a useful treatment for chronic copper poisoning (*see* p 3073). The limited bacterial formation of thiomolybdates in monogastric animals is primarily responsible for the tolerance to molybdenum encountered in these species. Excessive molybdenum exposure may also impair a variety of enzymes involved in collagen and elastin maintenance and stability, which has been associated with cardiovascular disorders. Molybdenum exposure may reduce phospholipid synthesis in nervous tissue, resulting in demyelination and neurologic disorders clinically.

The susceptibility to molybdenum toxicity in ruminants depends on a number of factors, including 1) dietary copper content—susceptibility increases as the copper content decreases; 2) dietary sulfate content—susceptibility increases with high sulfate levels by impairing copper utilization, whereas low sulfate content enhances susceptibility by reducing molybdenum excretion; 3) the chemical form of molybdenum—water-soluble forms found in fresh feed are more toxic; 4) sulfur-containing amino acids may alter copper utilization or molybdenum excretion; 5) animal species—cattle are more susceptible; 6) age—young animals are more susceptible, and excretion of molybdenum into milk may produce toxicoses in nursing calves; 7) season of year—molybdenum concentrations in plants increase in the fall; 8) plant species—legumes bioaccumulate more molybdenum; and 9) breed differences—seen in sheep and goats.

Molybdenum toxicity has been encountered in regions of the world containing peat, muck, or shale soil types that are naturally contaminated with molybdenum. Industrial contamination associated with mining or metal production or areas using molybdenum-contaminated fertilizers result in enhanced uptake of molybdenum by plants used as a feed source.

Clinical Findings: The manifestations of molybdenum toxicity are related primarily to impaired copper metabolism and utilization, resulting in secondary copper deficiency. Typically, the syndrome is a herd problem, with morbidity as high as 80%. In cattle, clinical disease is characterized by severe, persistent diarrhea with the presence of green, liquid feces containing gas bubbles, often referred to as peat or teart scours. Depigmentation, resulting in fading achromotrichia of the hair coat, is evident in black animals associated with impaired tyrosinase activity and reduced melanin synthesis. Pica, unthriftiness, microcytic hypochromic anemia, emaciation, joint pain characterized by lameness, and osteoporosis often manifested by bone fractures are seen. Molybdenum competes with phosphorus utilization, resulting in reduced mineralization of bone. In heifers, fertility is reduced. Delayed puberty, poor conception rates, decreased weight at puberty, and decreased milk production are common. Reduced libido has been reported in bulls. In sheep, particularly in lambs <30 days old, the animals exhibit stiffness of the back and legs and have difficulty rising. The syndrome in sheep is known as enzootic ataxia, or swayback. Abnormal development of connective tissue and growth plates are apparent in affected animals. Manifestations appear within 1–2 wk if molybdenum levels are excessive.

Occasionally, acute toxicity may be encountered in cattle or sheep. Anorexia and lethargy may be evident within 3 days. Deaths begin within 1 wk and may continue for many months. Neonates frequently exhibit hindlimb ataxia that often progresses to the forelimbs. Salivation and scant mucoid feces are common.

At necropsy, hemosiderosis, periacinar to severe hepatic necrosis, and nephrosis are evident. In affected sheep, neuronal degeneration, demyelination, and lysis of white matter are seen in nervous tissue.

Diagnosis: Distinguishing between primary copper deficiency and secondary copper deficiency related to excessive molybdenum exposure is important. Often with molybdenum toxicity, there is a poor correlation between tissue concentrations of copper and clinical disease. Clinical improvement after copper sulfate administration provides valuable support for the diagnosis. Analysis of the ration for copper and molybdenum concentrations is recommended. In cattle rations, a copper:molybdenum ratio of 6:1 is optimal. If the ratio is less than 2:1, molybdenum toxicity will occur. Ratios exceeding 15:1 may cause chronic copper poisoning. Absolute molybdenum concentrations in the diet >10 mg/kg will cause poisoning independent of copper consumption. Massive molybdenum exposure in the ration >2,000 mg/kg will result in death. Analysis of the liver and plasma for molybdenum provides useful insight to confirm the diagnosis, but the concentrations must be interpreted in association with the comparable tissue concentrations of copper. In cattle, liver concentrations >2 ppm (wet weight) and plasma concentrations >0.1 ppm are consistent with a diagnosis of molybdenum poisoning in the presence of a low copper status. Other disease syndromes characterized by emaciation or unthriftiness (parasite infections, selenosis, fluorosis, ergotism), diarrhea (metal poisonings, GI infections), and lameness or bone abnormalities (fluorosis, selenosis, ergotism, lead poisoning) may resemble molybdenum poisoning and should be investigated as possible etiologies.

Treatment and Prevention: Most treatment options are associated with the biological interactions associated with copper, molybdenum, and sulfate. Under circumstances in which dietary exposure is difficult to eliminate, simple treatment with copper products may be futile. If the source of molybdenum can be removed, excess molybdenum is rapidly eliminated and food products are safe for consumption within a relatively short time. If the dietary exposure cannot be reduced, elimination of molybdenum in the milk may produce toxicosis in nursing calves. Dietary supplementation with copper sulfate will reduce the bioavailability of molybdenum in the GI tract, ultimately reducing absorption and enhancing excretion. In feed containing molybdenum at >5 mg/kg, supplementation with 1% copper sulfate in salt will control development of the syndrome. In recovered mining areas, the supplementation may need to be increased to as much as 5% copper sulfate in the salt. When the consumption of mineral supplements is impractical, the treatment may be administered as a weekly drench. Injectable products such as copper glycinate or copper edetate (Cu-EDTA) may be given at a dose of 120 mg/cow. These products are approved only in some jurisdictions.

SALT TOXICITY

Excessive salt (sodium chloride, NaCl) intake can lead to the condition known as salt poisoning, salt toxicity, hypernatremia, or water deprivation–sodium ion intoxication. The last term is the most descriptive, giving the result (sodium ion intoxication) as well as the most common predisposing factor (water deprivation.) Salt poisoning is unlikely to occur as long as sodium-regulating mechanisms are intact and fresh drinking water is available.

Salt poisoning has been reported in virtually all species of animals all over the world. Although salt poisoning has historically been more common in swine (the most sensitive species), cattle, and poultry, there are increasing reports of adverse effects in dogs from acute excess salt consumption. The acute oral lethal dose of salt in swine, horses, and cattle is ~2.2 g/kg; in dogs, it is ~4 g/kg. Sheep appear to be the most resistant species, with an acute oral lethal dose of 6 g/kg.

Etiology: In general, animals can tolerate high concentrations of salt or sodium in the diet if they have continuous access to fresh water. Salt poisoning is often directly related to water consumption and can be reduced significantly or abolished completely by appropriate management of factors such as mechanical failure of waterers, overcrowding, unpalatable medicated water, new surroundings, or frozen water sources. Both swine and poultry on normal diets can be severely affected when water intake is completely restricted or when consuming high-salt diets with moderate water restriction. Increased water requirements increase the susceptibility of lactating cows and sows to salt poisoning, especially in response to sudden restrictions in water.

High concentrations of salt in the diet (up to 13%) have been used to limit feed intake of cattle. Salt-deprived animals or those not acclimated to high-salt diets can overconsume these feeds, making the animals prone to salt poisoning. Improperly formulated or mixed feed can be sources of excess salt. The use of whey as a feed or as a component of wet mash can add to sodium intake. Additional sources of excess sodium can include high-saline ground water, brine, or seawater.

Chickens can tolerate up to 0.25% salt in drinking water but are susceptible to salt poisoning when water intake is restricted. Wet mash containing 2% salt has caused salt poisoning in ducklings. High salt content in wet mash is more likely to cause poisoning than in dry feed, probably because birds eat more wet mash.

Sheep can tolerate 1% salt in drinking water; however, 1.5% may be toxic. It is generally recommended that drinking water contain <0.5% total salt for all species of livestock.

Companion animal exposures to excess salt have included the use of salt as an emetic (no longer recommended) and the ingestion of various salt-containing materials including rock salt and dough-salt mixtures. Dogs have been reported to develop hypernatremia after swimming/playing in the ocean (which contains 3.5% sodium) without having access to fresh water. Horses appear to be rarely affected with classic salt poisoning but can develop it under conditions of increased salt intake and sudden water restriction.

Clinical Findings: In pigs, early signs (rarely seen) may be increased thirst, pruritus, and constipation. Affected pigs may be blind, deaf, and oblivious to their surroundings; they will not eat, drink, or respond to external stimuli. They may wander aimlessly, bump into objects, circle, or pivot around a single limb. After 1–5 days of limited water intake, intermittent seizures occur with the pig sitting on its haunches, jerking its head backward and upward, and finally falling on its side in clonic-tonic seizures and opisthotonos. Terminally, pigs may lie on their sides, paddling in a coma, and die within a few to 48 hr.

In cattle, signs of acute salt poisoning involve the GI tract and CNS. Salivation, increased thirst, vomiting (regurgitation), abdominal pain, and diarrhea are followed by ataxia, circling, blindness, seizures, and partial paralysis. Cattle sometimes manifest belligerent and aggressive behavior. A sequela of salt poisoning in cattle is dragging of hindfeet while walking or, in more severe cases, knuckling of the fetlock joint.

In poultry and other birds, clinical signs include increased thirst, dyspnea, fluid discharge from the beak, weakness, diarrhea, and leg paralysis.

Excess salt intake in dogs results in vomiting within several hours of ingestion. The clinical signs can progress to weakness, diarrhea, muscle tremors, and seizures.

Lesions: Postmortem examination may reveal some degree of gastric irritation, including ulceration and hemorrhages. The content of the GI tract may be abnormally dry. Histopathologic lesions may be limited to the brain and include cerebral edema and inflammation of the meninges. During the first 48 hr, swine develop eosinopenia, eosinophilic cuffs around vessels in the cerebral cortex and adjacent meninges, and cerebral edema or necrosis. After 3–4 days, eosinophilic cuffs are usually no longer present. Cattle do not develop eosinophilic cuffs but can have edema of the skeletal muscles as well as hydropericardium. Chickens can also have hydropericardium.

In acute cases, no gross lesions may be present in any species.

Diagnosis: Serum and CSF concentrations of sodium >160 mEq/L, especially when CSF has a greater sodium concentration than serum, indicate salt poisoning. Brain sodium concentrations >2,000 ppm (wet weight) are considered diagnostic in cattle and swine. There is a lack of data on normal brain sodium concentrations in other common domestic species, making interpretations of brain sodium concentrations difficult. Characteristic history and clinical signs, along with clinical pathology, postmortem findings, and analyses of feed or water for sodium content are essential for establishing a diagnosis.

In swine, differential diagnoses include insecticide poisoning (organochlorine, organophosphorus, and carbamate), phenylarsonic poisoning, and pseudorabies. In cattle, differential diagnoses include insecticide and lead poisoning, polioencephalomalacia, hypomagnesemic tetany, and the nervous form of ketosis.

Treatment: There is no specific treatment for salt poisoning. Immediate removal of offending feed or water is imperative. Fresh water must be provided to all animals, initially in small amounts at frequent intervals to avoid exacerbation of clinical signs. On a herd basis with large animals, water intake should be limited to 0.5% of body weight at hourly intervals until normal hydration is accomplished, usually taking several days. Severely affected animals can be given water via stomach tube. The mortality rate may be >50% in affected animals regardless of treatment. In small animals before the onset of clinical signs, the acute ingestion of salt can best be treated by allowing the animal access to water and closely observing it for several hours. Emetics may be used in dogs if known ingestions occur and the dog is not yet showing clinical signs.

For all affected animals, the treatment should slowly return the animal to normal water and electrolyte balance over 2–3 days. Quickly lowering the serum sodium concentration will increase the osmotic gradient between the serum and the brain, with water following the gradient into the brain and increasing the likelihood of severe cerebral edema.

Monitoring serum sodium concentration is the first step in treating individual animals. Serum sodium levels should be lowered at a rate of 0.5–1 mEq/L/hr. The use of slightly hypertonic IV fluids has been recommended to reduce the likelihood of cerebral edema. IV fluids can be made to approximate the serum sodium concentration of the animal, or a solution containing sodium at 170 mEq/L can be used initially, with the concentration decreased as clinical signs improve. In dogs, a series of warm water enemas given at intervals of several hours has helped reduce acutely increased sodium levels. If brain edema is suspected, mannitol, dexamethasone, or DMSO may be helpful.

SELENIUM TOXICOSIS

Selenium is an essential element that has a narrow margin of safety, with the difference between adequate and potentially toxic concentrations in the diet being approximately 10- to 20-fold. Feed supplements, resulting in final selenium content of 0.2–0.3 ppm, are added to diets to prevent deficiency and resultant diseases such as white muscle disease in cattle and sheep, exertional myopathy in horses, hepatosis dietetica in pigs, and exudative diathesis in chickens. The maximum tolerable concentrations for selenium in most livestock feed is considered to be 2–5 ppm, although some believe 4–5 ppm can inhibit growth.

Selenium is an essential component of >25 selenoenzymes and selenoproteins. The most recognized of these are the glutathione peroxidase enzymes that act as antioxidants in the body. In excess, selenium potentially has three general toxic effects: the direct inhibition of cellular oxidation/reduction reactions by depleting glutathione and *S*-adenosylmethionine reserves, the production of free radicals that cause oxidative tissue damage, and the replacement of sulfur/sulfur-containing amino acids in the body with selenium/seleno-amino acids. The inhibition of numerous cellular functions by high concentrations of selenium results in acute generalized cytotoxicity. The replacement of sulfur-containing amino acids with seleno-amino acids leads to altered structure and function of cellular components and enzymes due to loss of the disulfide bonds that commonly occur between sulfur-containing amino acids. Loss of these disulfide bonds can alter the three-dimensional configuration of proteins, potentially resulting in loss of or diminished enzyme activity. The most commonly altered sulfur-containing amino acids are methionine and cysteine, which are replaced with selenomethionine and selenocysteine, respectively. Replacement of these amino acids with selenium-containing amino acids also affects cell division and growth. Especially susceptible are the cells that form keratin (keratinocytes) and the sulfur-containing keratin molecule. Selenium therefore weakens the hooves and hair, which tend to fracture when subjected to mechanical stress.

Etiology: All animal species are susceptible to selenium toxicosis. However, poisoning is more common in forage-eating animals such as cattle, sheep, horses, and other herbivores that may graze selenium-containing plants. Plants may accumulate selenium when the element is found at high concentrations in the soil, but pH and moisture content of the soil play roles in the relative bioavailability of selenium to plants. Generally, selenium is most bioavailable to plants when they grow on more alkaline soils with low rainfall (<50 cm). The alkalinity and low moisture content of the soil tend to allow more of the selenium to be retained as the oxidized form of selenate, which is the most readily available for plant uptake. Because low moisture in the soil decreases the anaerobic environments to greater depths, drought conditions could allow for more/deeper selenium in the soil to be oxidized into plant-available forms, resulting in year-to-year variability in available selenium for plant uptake.

Selenium-accumulating plants have been categorized based on their relative requirements and ability to accumulate selenium. Obligate indicator plants require large amounts of selenium for growth and contain high selenium concentrations (often >1,000 to 10,000 ppm). Obligate indicators include species of *Astragalus*, *Stanleya*,

Machaeranthera, *Oonopsis*, and *Xylorhiza*. Facultative indicator plants absorb and tolerate higher concentrations of soil selenium, with accumulations ranging from trace amounts to a few thousand ppm, but they do not require selenium for growth. Facultative indicators include species of *Aster*, *Castilleja*, *Grindelia*, *Atriplex*, *Gatierreaia*, and *Comandra*. Nonaccumulator plants, such as most grasses, passively absorb much lower amounts of selenium from the soil, resulting in trace amounts to a few hundred ppm.

Numerous organic and inorganic chemical forms of selenium are potentially present in plants. Nonaccumulator plants primarily contain selenomethionine, while indicator plants contain more selenate and methylselenocysteine. In comparison, most supplemental dietary sources are in the form of selenite, but selenomethionine supplements are becoming more commonly used in marketed products.

Poisoning may also occur in swine, poultry, and other species consuming grain raised on seleniferous soils or, more commonly, due to errors in feed formulation. Selenium toxicosis after ingestion of selenium-containing shampoos or selenium supplement tablets is rare in small animal pets but can occur. Several factors are known to alter selenium toxicity; however, in general, a single acute oral dose of selenium in the range of 1–10 mg/kg may be lethal in most animals. Parenteral selenium products are also quite toxic, especially to young animals, and have caused deaths in piglets, calves, lambs, and dogs at dosages as low as 1 mg/kg. Younger animals tend to be more susceptible to selenium poisoning, and the chemical forms can result in some differences in relative toxicity.

Diagnosis: Severity of clinical signs of selenium toxicosis depends on the quantity and duration of exposure. Poisoning in animals is characterized as acute, subchronic, or chronic. Diagnosis is based on clinical signs, necropsy findings, and laboratory confirmation of the presence of high selenium content in an animal's diet (feed, forage, grains, or water), serum, blood, or tissues (eg, kidney, liver). Selenium in the diet at >5 ppm may produce mild clinical effects after prolonged exposure of ≥30 days. Concentrations of 10–25 ppm would be expected to produce severe clinical signs with prolonged exposure. Environmental exposure potential should be based on forage, feed, or water content, not on soil selenium content, because some chemical forms in soil are not available for uptake by plants and would not result in high exposure potential.

Tissue selenium content is the basis for diagnosing selenium poisoning in animals. Organic chemical forms of selenium have greater bioavailability and are retained in the tissues for much longer periods. Thus, timing of the exposure in relation to the collection of tissue, blood, or serum, as well as the chemical form of the selenium exposure, must be taken into account when interpreting the selenium content. In addition, some species variability in regard to concentrations also occurs. In acute toxicosis, the blood and serum selenium concentrations are generally >3–4 ppm, and in chronic toxicosis, it is generally >1–2 ppm. Liver generally contains >3–5 ppm selenium in acute cases, whereas in chronic cases it should be >1.5 ppm. Kidney of selenium-poisoned animals generally contains >1–5 ppm. Hair and hoof wall may have >1.5–5 ppm selenium in chronic poisoning. A "garlicky" odor on the animal's breath may be noted; this finding is more prominent with acute poisoning but can be seen with chronic poisoning as well. The odor is due to elimination pathways producing methylated selenium metabolites that are volatile and expired but may last for only 1–2 days after an acute poisoning incident.

CHRONIC SELENIUM TOXICOSIS

(Alkali disease)

Chronic selenium poisoning usually develops when livestock consume seleniferous forages and grains containing 5–50 ppm of selenium for many weeks or months, although chronic exposure to high concentrations of inorganic selenium can also produce chronic selenosis. Naturally occurring seleno-amino acids in plants are readily absorbed and inserted into proteins in place of their corresponding sulfur-containing amino acids (ie, selenomethionine in place of methionine or selenocysteine in place of cysteine). Until recently, two types of chronic selenium poisoning were discussed in the literature: alkali disease and blind staggers. Blind staggers is no longer believed to be caused by selenium but by sulfate toxicity due to consumption of high-sulfate alkali water and/or high sulfur-containing forages. Excess sulfate (>1% of diet) leads to polioencephalomalacia and the classical signs of blind staggers. Animals consuming milk vetch (*Astragalus bisulcatus*) have demonstrated clinical signs similar to those of blind staggers. Although milk vetch contains high levels of selenium, evidence now indicates that the alkaloid swainsonine in milk vetch is responsible for locoism and produces the neurologic clinical signs.

Clinical Findings: Alkali disease has been reported in cattle, sheep, and horses. Affected animals are inactive, weak, anorexic, lame, emaciated, anemic, and lack vitality. In addition, the most distinctive lesions are those produced by damage of the keratin of the hair and hooves. For horses, the predominant clinical manifestation is lameness due to founder. The animal has a rough hair coat, and the long hairs of the mane and tail break off, giving a "bob" tail and "roached" mane appearance. Abnormal growth and structure of horns and hooves result in circular ridges and cracking of the hoof wall at the coronary band. Extremely long, deformed hooves that turn upward at the ends also may be seen. Subsequent lameness is compounded by degeneration of joint cartilage and bone. Reduced fertility and reproductive performance occurs, especially in sheep and cattle. Reproductive performance may be impaired with a dietary selenium content lower than that required to produce the other typical signs of alkali disease. Other lesions may include liver cirrhosis, ascites, and myocardial necrosis/scarring.

Birds also may be affected with chronic selenium toxicosis. Eggs with >2.5 ppm selenium from birds in high selenium areas have low hatchability and embryos that are usually deformed. Teratologic effects include underdeveloped feet and legs, malformed eyes, crooked beaks, and ropy feathers. This has been a problem with waterfowl in southern California, where selenium was concentrated in lakes by runoff.

In selenium-poisoned animals, some alterations in blood chemistries occur. These changes include decreased prothrombin activity, fibrinogen, and glutathione, as well as increased serum alkaline phosphatase, ALT, AST, and succinic dehydrogenase.

Treatment and Control: There is no specific treatment for selenium toxicosis. Eliminating the source and exposure, as well as symptomatic and supportive care of the animal, should be started as soon as possible. Addition of substances that antagonize or inhibit the toxic effects of selenium in the diet may help reduce the risk of selenium toxicosis. A high-protein diet, linseed oil meal, sulfur, arsenic, silver, copper, cadmium, and mercury have reduced selenium toxicity in laboratory animals, but their use under field conditions is limited. However, some of the poor reproductive performance associated with selenium poisoning can be decreased by copper supplementation. Addition of arsenic salt at 0.00375% to enhance biliary excretion of selenium or a high-protein diet to bind free selenium has historically been used to reduce incidence of selenium poisoning in cattle. However, this has minimal to poor overall efficacy. Chronically selenium-poisoned animals are less likely to thrive than herdmates, even after exposure has been stopped.

Forages should be tested regularly in high-selenium areas to evaluate year-to-year risk.

SUBCHRONIC SELENIUM TOXICOSIS

Pigs fed a diet supplemented with selenium >20–50 ppm for >3 days develop a subchronic selenium toxicosis characterized by neurologic abnormalities. Animals are initially ataxic and uncoordinated, followed by anterior paresis, then quadriplegia. Even though neurologic impairment is occurring, the pigs continue to eat, which would indicate neurologic damage that is not centrally mediated. The hooves show breaks and impaired growth similar to those seen in cattle. Alopecia may also be seen. In sows, conception rate decreases and the number of stillborn pigs increases. Lesions of subchronic toxicosis include focal symmetric poliomyelomalacia, which is most prominent in the cervical and thoracic spinal cord. Death may result from complications of permanent paralysis. Hoof and hair damage is similar to but in most cases less severe than that seen in chronic selenium toxicosis. Treatment is similar to that for chronic toxicosis, but spinal lesions are usually permanent.

ACUTE SELENIUM TOXICOSIS

Acute oral selenium poisoning due to consumption of plants or mis-mixed diets with concentrations >50 ppm (dosages 1–10 mg/kg or greater, depending on the species, age, and chemical form of selenium) is not common but has caused large losses in cattle, sheep, and pigs. Animals usually avoid plants with high selenium content because of their offensive odor; however, when pasture is limited, accumulator plants may be the only food available. In some cases, plants may not have the profound offensive odor. Young animals are most susceptible to acute parenteral selenium toxicosis with dosages of 0.2–0.5 mg/kg. Clinical signs are different from those of chronic selenosis and are characterized by abnormal behavior, respiratory difficulty, GI upset, and sudden death. Abnormal posture and depression, anorexia, unsteady gait, diarrhea, colic, increased pulse and respiration rates, frothy nasal discharge, moist rales, and cyanosis may be noted. Sheep usually show these signs to a much lesser degree or just become depressed and die suddenly.

Most deaths usually follow within a few hours to 2 days after an acutely toxic consumption or injection of selenium. The major lesions are pulmonary edema, pulmonary congestion, pulmonary hemorrhage, hepatic necrosis, myocardial necrosis, myocardial hemorrhage, and potentially renal necrosis.

Blood or serum selenium concentration in acute poisoning is often higher than in chronic poisoning. Treatment consists of symptomatic and supportive care. Acetylcysteine to boost systemic glutathione concentrations may be beneficial.

ZINC TOXICOSIS

Zinc is an essential trace metal that plays an important role in many of the body's enzymatic processes. It is ubiquitous in nature and exists in many forms. The ingestion of some forms of zinc causes the creation of toxic zinc salts in the acidic environment of the stomach. Zinc toxicity has been documented in people as well as in a wide range of large, small, exotic, and wild animals. Exposure typically stems from dietary indiscretion. Household sources of zinc include paint, batteries, automotive parts, zinc oxide creams, vitamin and mineral supplements, zipper pulls, board-game pieces, pet carrier screws and nuts, and the coating on certain types of pipes and cookware. One of the most well-known sources of zinc that causes toxicity after ingestion is the USA Lincoln penny. Some pennies minted during 1983, and all pennies minted since, are 97.5% zinc by weight (~2,440 mg of elemental zinc per coin).

Pathogenesis: The low pH in the stomach causes the release of free zinc, which then forms soluble, caustic zinc salts. These salts are absorbed from the duodenum and rapidly distributed to the liver, kidneys, prostate, muscles, bones, and pancreas. Zinc salts have direct irritant and corrosive effects on tissue, interfere with the metabolism of other ions such as copper, calcium, and iron, and inhibit erythrocyte production and function. The mechanisms by which zinc exerts these toxic effects are not completely understood. The LD_{50} of zinc salts in cases of acute toxicity has been reported to be ~100 mg/kg. Also, diets containing high levels of zinc (>2,000 ppm) have been reported to cause chronic zinc toxicosis in large animals.

Clinical Findings and Lesions: Clinical signs vary based on the duration and degree of exposure. Signs progress from anorexia, vomiting, diarrhea, and lethargy to more advanced signs such as intravascular hemolysis, icterus, hemoglobinuria, cardiac arrhythmias, and seizures. Large animals often show decreases in weight gain and milk production, and lameness has been reported in foals secondary to epiphyseal swelling.

Major histopathologic findings include hepatocellular centrilobular necrosis with hemosiderosis and vacuolar degeneration, renal tubular necrosis with hemoglobin casts, and pancreatic duct necrosis with fibrosis of the interlobular fat.

Diagnosis: Radiodense foreign bodies are easily seen on radiographs of the GI tract and should raise suspicion of potential zinc toxicosis in animals with correlating clinical signs. Changes in the CBC, chemistry profile, urinalysis, and coagulation profile reflect the degree of toxicity to various organ systems. The hemogram can reveal anemia characterized by changes in erythrocyte morphology such as spherocytosis and Heinz body formation. (It has been suggested that zinc's interference with enzymes such as glutathione reductase leads to erythrocyte fragility due to oxidative damage.) The leukogram often shows a mature neutrophilic leukocytosis secondary to stress, pancreatitis, and a regenerative response by the bone marrow. Serum chemistry changes that are seen secondary to hepatic damage include increases in bilirubin, the transaminases, and alkaline phosphatase.

As zinc accumulates in the pancreas, increases in amylase and lipase can be seen following pancreatitis and pancreatic necrosis. Glomerular damage and renal tubular epithelial necrosis result in increases in BUN, creatinine, amylase, and urine protein. Hemoglobinuria can be differentiated from hematuria during urinalysis; the urine color will not clear after centrifugation in the presence of hemoglobinuria. Prolongation of prothrombin time and activated partial thromboplastin time can also result from toxic effects on the synthesis or function of coagulation factors and the loss of clotting proteins through the glomerulus of the kidneys.

The hematologic and clinical findings in animals with zinc toxicosis are similar to the changes in animals with immune-mediated hemolytic anemia (IMHA). Zinc toxicosis can cause the direct antiglobulin test (direct Coombs' test) to be positive in the absence of a primary autoimmune disorder, so the direct Coombs' test is not a reliable method to differentiate zinc intoxication from IMHA.

Zinc levels can be measured in blood to confirm toxicosis, although this is usually unnecessary to diagnose zinc poisoning in the clinical setting. In dogs and cats, the normal serum zinc level is 0.7–2 mcg/mL. Reference laboratories usually request that samples be submitted in green-top heparinized tubes, royal blue–top trace element tubes, or purple-top EDTA tubes. Methods to quantify zinc levels from saliva and hair have not been validated in domestic animals, and measuring zinc in urine is unreliable because elimination of zinc through the kidneys is variable.

Treatment and Prevention: After stabilizing the animal with fluids, oxygen, and blood products as necessary, removal of the source of zinc as early as possible is paramount. This often requires surgery or endoscopy. Inducing emesis to remove chronic gastric zinc foreign bodies may be tried within the first hour or two of exposure but may not be rewarding in advanced cases because zinc objects can adhere to the gastric mucosa.

Proton pump inhibitors and H_2-blockers can be used to decrease the formation of zinc salts in the stomach before removal of the source of zinc, and gastroprotectant therapy with sucralfate can later be considered to help address gastric ulceration.

Diuresis with a balanced crystalloid solution is indicated to promote renal excretion of zinc and prevent hemoglobinuric nephrosis.

There is debate regarding the necessity of chelation therapy in cases of zinc toxicosis. Animals often recover from zinc intoxication after only supportive care and removal of the source. Chelation therapy can enhance elimination of zinc and thus accelerate recovery, but there is some concern that chelation treatment may actually increase zinc absorption from the intestines. Chelation can be achieved through the use of specific compounds. Ca-EDTA chelates zinc when given at 100 mg/kg/day, IV or SC, for 3 days (diluted and divided into four doses) but may exacerbate zinc-induced nephrotoxicity. Although they have been used to treat animals with zinc toxicity, D-penicillamine and dimercaprol (British anti-lewisite) have not been specifically validated for this purpose. Reported dosages are 110 mg/kg/day for 7–14 days for D-penicillamine, and 3–6 mg/kg, tid, for 3–5 days for dimercaprol. Chelation therapy with any of these agents should be performed only after careful consideration and should be monitored with serial serum zinc levels to help determine the appropriate duration of treatment.

With early diagnosis and treatment, the outcome is usually favorable for animals with zinc toxicosis. Eliminating exposure to zinc in the environment is essential to prevent recurrence.

BRACKEN FERN POISONING

Bracken fern (*Pteridium aquilinum*) is found throughout the world and is among the five most numerous vascular plants. The species includes numerous subspecies and varieties, and plant size varies with frond lengths of 0.5–4.5 m. Bracken fern is perennial, with erect deciduous fronds that remain green until they are killed by frost or drought. It spreads primarily through dense rhizome networks and can dominate plant communities, especially those burned or disturbed. Bracken fern may be found in a diversity of sites but is most common in semishaded, well-drained, open woodlands.

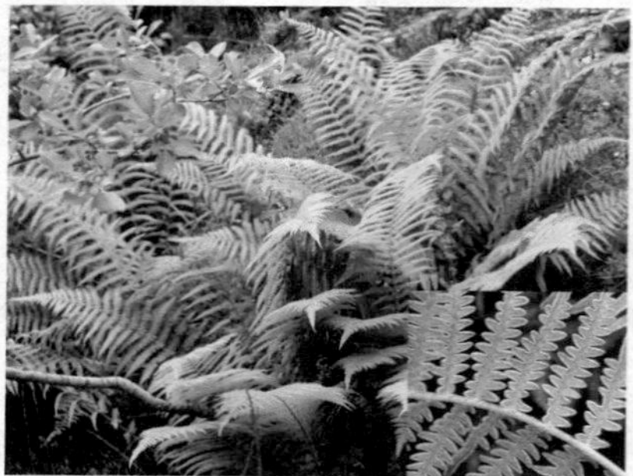

Bracken fern (*Pteridium aquilinum*), growing from large dense woody rhizomes, forms deciduous, stipitate, erect to spreading fronds with nonanastomosing veins. The pinnae are stalked, opposite or subopposite (inset). *Courtesy of Dr. Bryan Stegelmeier.*

Syndromes: A variety of syndromes have been associated with bracken fern poisoning. These syndromes are largely determined by the dose and duration, and also by the species of the poisoned animal.

Enzootic Hematuria: Enzootic hematuria is the most common result of bracken fern poisoning. It primarily affects cattle and, less frequently, sheep. It is characterized by intermittent hematuria and anemia. Poisoning most often occurs during late summer when other feed is scarce, or when animals are fed hay containing bracken fern. Poisoning requires prolonged exposures; affected livestock must ingest bracken fern for several weeks to years before disease develops.

Affected cattle are weak, rapidly lose weight, and develop pyrexia (106°–110°F [41°–43°C]) once clinical effects manifest. Calves often have difficulty breathing, with pale mucous membranes. Hemorrhages vary from minor mucosal petechia to effusive bleeding, and at times large blood clots form that may be passed in the feces. Coagulation is prolonged, and bleeding may be pronounced and excessive even at small wounds such as small insect bites or minor scratches.

Once animals develop clinical disease, poisoning is almost always fatal. Postmortem examinations usually reveal multiple hemorrhages or bruises throughout the carcass. Necrotic ulcers in the GI tract may be noted. The bladder mucosa often contains small hemorrhages; dilated vessels; or vascular, fibrous, or epithelial neoplasms. Other neoplasms in the upper GI tract of cattle and other species have also been reported. In most cases, mixtures of hemorrhagic and neoplastic lesions are found.

Although not all bracken fern toxins have been completely characterized, the primary cause of enzootic hematuria has been attributed to norsesquiterpene glycosides (ptaquiloside, ptesculentoside, and caudatoside). Ptaquiloside is a potent radiomimetic that initially damages the bone marrow and later is carcinogenic (producing urinary tract neoplasia in ruminants). Both the hemorrhagic syndrome and uroepithelial neoplasms have been reproduced experimentally with bracken fern and ptaquiloside. Although less well characterized, the other norsesquiterpene glycosides, which predominate in some bracken fern populations, probably have similar toxicity and carcinogenicity.

Acute Brackenism (Hemorrhagic Disease): Acute brackenism occurs when animals ingest high doses over relatively short durations of weeks or months. It is characterized by bleeding. This toxicity is attributed to ptaquiloside's radiomimetic damage to proliferating bone marrow stem cells. This is seen as depletion of bone marrow megakaryocytes followed by panhypoplasia. The leukogram often shows a mixed response. In the initial phases, monocytosis may be pronounced and followed by granulocytopenia and thrombocytopenia. Final phases include marked thrombocytopenia with anemia, leukopenia, and hypergammaglobulinemia. Urinalysis generally shows hematuria and proteinuria. Affected animals have both an increased susceptibility to infection and a tendency for spontaneous hemorrhage.

Lower doses of bracken fern for longer duration are more likely to be carcinogenic. The effects seem cumulative, as animals are exposed repeatedly for years. Often the onset of clinical disease can be delayed for weeks, or even months, after animals have been removed from bracken fern–infested ranges and pastures. The carcinogenic potential of bracken fern and ptaquiloside has been confirmed not only in livestock but also in rats, mice, guinea pigs, quail, and Egyptian toads.

Ptaquiloside is excreted in the urine and milk, and small amounts have also been identified in skeletal muscle and liver of poisoned animals even after a 15-day withdrawal period. Contaminated milk retains toxicity; it has been shown to produce GI neoplasms in rats. Several investigators have suggested ptaquiloside neoplastic transformation may be promoted or enhanced by bovine papillomavirus infection. However, this may be a secondary change due to bracken fern–associated myelodysplasia and subsequent immunosuppression that are likely to promote papillomavirus infection.

Bright Blindness: A less common manifestation of ptaquiloside toxicity is called bright blindness. It is seen clinically as tapetal hyperreflectivity that is most commonly reported in sheep in parts of England and Wales. Affected sheep are permanently blind and adopt a characteristic alert attitude. The pupils respond poorly to light, and ophthalmoscopic examination of sheep with advanced disease reveals narrowing of arteries and veins and a pale tapetum nigrum with fine cracks and spots of gray. Histologically, the lesion is seen as severe atrophy of the retinal rods, cones, and outer nuclear layer that is most pronounced in the tapetal portion of the retina. Affected animals often have many of the other bracken fern–associated lesions such as bone marrow suppression, hemorrhage, immunosuppression, and urinary tract neoplasia.

Bracken Staggers: Bracken fern poisoning in monogastric animals was first recognized as a neurologic disease when horses consumed contaminated hay. Ingestion at a rate of 20%–25% bracken fern for ≥3 mo may result in bracken staggers. Clinical signs in horses include anorexia, weight loss, incoordination, and a crouching stance while arching the back and neck with the feet placed wide apart. When the horse is forced to move, trembling muscles are noted. In severe cases, tachycardia and arrhythmias are present; death (usually 2–10 days after onset) is preceded by convulsions, clonic spasms, and opisthotonos. These changes are due to bracken fern thiaminases. The resulting disease is similar to vitamin B_1 deficiency, and therefore most animals respond to thiamine therapy. Horses seem to be particularly susceptible, whereas disease in pigs is rare. In pigs, the signs of thiamine deficiency are less distinct and may resemble heart failure. Affected pigs become anorectic and lose weight. Death can occur suddenly after recumbency and dyspnea. Thiamine deficiency is generally not a problem in ruminants, because the vitamin is synthesized in the rumen; however, polioencephalomalacia (*see* p 1281) associated with impaired thiamine metabolism in sheep has been attributed to consumption of bracken fern and rock or mulga fern (*Cheilanthes sieberi*) in Australia.

Treatment: Initial treatment for all species is to discontinue exposure to bracken fern; however, disease can appear weeks after livestock are removed from the fern-infested area. In acutely affected cattle, mortality is usually >90%. Measurement of the platelet count is recommended, because it is the best prognostic indicator for poisoned animals.

Treatment of thiamine deficiency in horses is highly effective if diagnosis is made early. Injection of a thiamine solution at 5 mg/kg is suggested, given initially IV every 3 hr, then IM for several days. Oral supplementation may be required for an additional 1–2 wk, although SC injection of 100–200 mg/day for 6 days has been successful in some cases. Thiamine treatment should also include animals similarly exposed but not yet showing clinical disease, because signs can develop days or weeks after removal from the source of bracken.

Antibiotics may be useful to prevent secondary infections. Blood or even platelet transfusions may be appropriate but require large volumes (2–4 L blood) to effectively treat cattle. Though untested, treatment with granulocyte-macrophage colony-stimulating factor (used to treat aplastic anemia in people) may also be considered.

Prevention: Poisoning, apart from thiamine deficiency, is essentially untreatable; however, it is most easily controlled by preventing exposure. Bracken fern is usually grazed for want of alternative forages. Most commonly, animals are forced to eat bracken fern when other forage is exhausted in late summer, although some animals may develop a taste for the young tender shoots and leaves. Poisoning can be avoided by improving pasture management to increase production of alternative forage. It has been suggested that alternating bracken fern–contaminated and noncontaminated pastures at 3-wk intervals can minimize poisoning.

Bracken fern growth can be retarded by close grazing or trampling in alternative grazing pasture systems. Bracken fern density can be reduced by regular cutting of the mature plant or, if the land is suitable, by deep plowing. Herbicide treatment using asulam or glyphosate can be an effective method of control, especially if combined with cutting before treatment. Some bracken fern populations contain very low or no ptaquiloside. More work is needed to identify these populations, determine why they are not toxic, and use this information to predict or reduce toxicity.

Human Poisoning: Initial epidemiologic studies suggest that consumption of milk from cattle with access to bracken increases risk of human esophageal or gastric cancer. Certainly the greater risk to people is direct consumption of bracken fern. Rhizomes have been used to make flour, and the young shoots or croziers are considered a delicacy in many parts of the world. Although preparing and cooking lessens the toxicity of ptaquiloside, it has been identified in these foods. Japanese scientists have shown an association between consumption of bracken crozier and esophageal cancer. Additionally, ptaquiloside has been found as an environmental contaminant in soil and water, and air-borne spores may also present a risk of human exposure. Human exposure through any means should be of concern, because ptaquiloside is a proven carcinogen.

GOSSYPOL POISONING

Gossypol poisoning, usually chronic, cumulative, and sometimes insidious, follows consumption of cottonseed or cottonseed products that contain excess free gossypol. It is of most concern in domestic livestock, especially preruminants or immature ruminants and pigs; mature ruminants are more resistant to gossypol's toxic effects. However, gossypol toxicosis can affect high-producing dairy cows with high feed intake, dairy goats, and other mature ruminants fed excess gossypol for long periods. It has also been reported in dogs fed cottonseed meal in diets or housed on cottonseed bedding.

Etiology: Gossypol, the predominant pigment and probably the major toxic ingredient in the cotton plant (*Gossypium* spp), and other polyphenolic pigments are contained within small, discrete structures called pigment glands found in various parts of the cotton plant. Gossypol is found in cottonseed as both protein-bound and free forms; only the free form is toxic. Gossypol content of cottonseeds varies from a trace to >6% and is affected by plant species and variety and by environmental factors such as climate, soil type, and fertilization. Gossypol is a natural component of all but the rarely produced "glandless" variety of cotton.

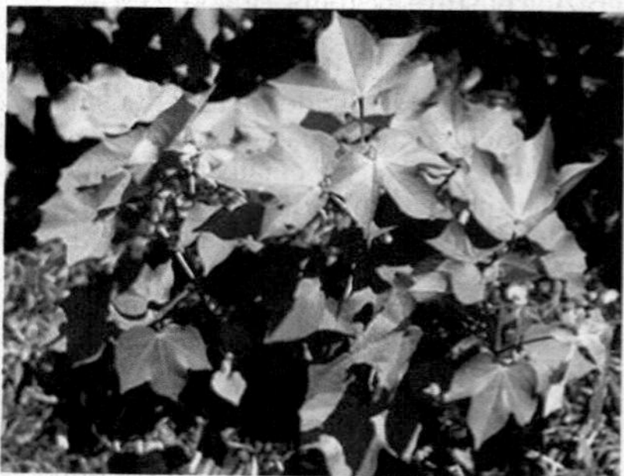

Gossypium spp (cotton plant), young plant.
Courtesy of Dr. Cecil Brownie.

Cottonseed is processed into edible oil, meal, linters (short fibers), and hulls. Cottonseed meal is marketed with 50%–90% protein, depending on intended use. Cottonseed and cottonseed meal are widely used as protein supplements in animal feed. Cottonseed oil soapstock (foots) is the principal by-product of cottonseed oil refining. Cottonseed soapstocks are being increasingly used as animal feed additives; cottonseed hulls are used as a source of additional fiber in animal feeds and contain much lower gossypol concentrations than do whole cottonseeds.

Lipid-soluble gossypol is readily absorbed from the GI tract. It is highly protein-bound to amino acids, especially lysine, and to dietary iron. The precise mechanism of action is not known, but gossypol renders many amino acids unavailable by the formation of a Schiff's base-type derivative as well as additional protein/gossypol interactions. Gossypol also affects enzymatic reactions critical for many biologic processes, including the ability of cells to respond to oxidative stress and inhibition of oxygen release from hemoglobin. Conjugation, metabolism, and urinary excretion of gossypol is limited; most is eliminated in the feces.

All animals are susceptible, but monogastrics, preruminants, immature ruminants, and poultry appear to be affected most frequently. Adult ruminants are able to detoxify gossypol by formation of stable complexes with soluble proteins in the rumen, thus preventing absorption, something lacking in swine, preruminants, and young ruminants with only a partially functioning rumen. Pigs, guinea pigs, and rabbits are reported to be sensitive. Dogs and cats appear to have intermediate sensitivity. Goats may be more sensitive to gossypol than are cattle. Horses appear relatively resistant but caution is still advised. Toxic effects usually occur only after longterm exposure to gossypol, often weeks to months.

Clinical Findings: Signs may relate to effects on the cardiac, hepatic, renal, reproductive, or other systems. Prolonged exposure can cause acute heart failure resulting from cardiac necrosis. Also, a form of cardiac conduction failure similar to hyperkalemic heart failure can result in sudden death. Pulmonary effects, labored breathing, and chronic dyspnea are most likely secondary to cardiotoxicity from congestive heart failure.

Hepatotoxicity can be a primary effect from direct damage to hepatocytes or metabolism of phenolic compounds to reactive intermediates, or liver necrosis may be secondary to congestive heart failure. Gossypol inhibits glutathione-S-transferase, impairing the liver's ability to metabolize xenobiotic compounds. Hematologic effects include anemia with reduced numbers of RBCs and increased RBC fragility, decreased oxygen release from oxyhemoglobin, and reduced oxygen-carrying capacity of blood with lowered Hgb and PCV values due to complexing of iron by gossypol.

Reproductive effects include reduced libido with decreased spermatogenesis and sperm motility, as well as sperm abnormalities (which are reversible) resulting from enzyme inhibition of steroid synthesis in testicular Leydig cells. Specific mitochondrial damage in spermatozoa appears to cause immobility and depressed sperm counts. Extensive damage to germinal epithelium in both rams and bulls fed excessive gossypol may be responsible for depressed spermatogenesis. Effects in females may include irregular cycling, luteolytic disruption of pregnancy, and direct embryotoxicity; probable mechanisms include an endocrine effect on the ovary as well as a direct cytotoxic effect on the uterus or embryo. Green discoloration of egg yolks and decreased egg hatchability have been reported in poultry. However, antifertility and reproductive effects in many nonruminant species are secondary to the more toxic effects, particularly in females.

Signs of prolonged excess gossypol exposure in many animals are reduced growth rate, weight loss, weakness, anorexia, and increased susceptibility to stress. Young lambs, goats, and calves may suffer cardiomyopathy and sudden death; if the course is more chronic, they may be depressed, anorectic, and have pronounced dyspnea. Adult dairy cattle may show weakness, depression, anorexia, edema of the brisket, and dyspnea, and also have gastroenteritis, hemoglobinuria, and reproductive problems. In monogastric animals, acute exposure may result in sudden circulatory failure, whereas subacute exposure may result in pulmonary edema secondary to congestive heart failure; anemia may be another common sequela. Violent dyspnea ("thumping") is the outstanding clinical sign in pigs. In dogs, gossypol poisoning is primarily reflected by cardiotoxic effects; condition deteriorates progressively, and ascites may be marked. Affected dogs may show polydipsia and have serum electrolyte imbalances, most notably hyperkalemia, with pronounced ECG abnormalities.

Lesions: An enlarged, flabby, pale, streaked, and mottled heart with pale myocardial streaking, enlarged and dilated ventricles, and valvular edema may be evident. Skeletal muscles may also be pale. A froth-filled trachea and edematous, congested lungs are common, with interstitial pulmonary edema and markedly edematous interlobular septa. Generalized icterus and an enlarged, congested, mottled or golden, friable "nutmeg" liver with distinct lobular patterns may be seen. The kidneys, spleen, and other splanchnic organs may be congested, possibly with petechiae; mild renal tubular nephrosis may be present. Hemoglobinuria and edema and hyperemia of the visceral mucosa may develop. Cardiomyopathy in affected dogs has been characterized as focal or general, granular myocardial degeneration with edema between and within myofibers; severe abnormalities in contractility have resulted in right-side congestive heart failure without pronounced dilatation, and pulmonary or hepatic changes can be minimal.

Diagnosis: Diagnosis is based on the following: 1) a history of dietary exposure to cottonseed meal or cottonseed products over a relatively long period; 2) signs, especially sudden death or chronic dyspnea, affecting multiple animals within a group; 3) lesions consistent with the reported syndrome and associated cardiomyopathy and hepatopathy, with increased amounts of fluids in various body cavities; 4) no response to antibiotic therapy; and 5) the presence of significant concentrations of free gossypol in the diet. Analyses of dietary components for free gossypol must be correlated with history, clinical signs, and postmortem findings. However, as with many feed-induced toxicoses, the responsible feed may be already completely consumed and not available for analysis. Free gossypol at >100 mg/kg (100 ppm) of feed in the diet of pigs or young ruminants <4 mo old supports a presumptive diagnosis. Adult ruminants can detoxify higher concentrations of gossypol, but intake should still be <1,000 ppm in the diet. Gossypol toxicosis developed in mature dairy goats each fed an estimated 350–400 mg gossypol/day for 3 mo in a diet containing ~400 ppm free gossypol. Adverse effects on semen quality (decreased sperm motility and morphologic abnormalities) occurred in young bulls fed a concentrate containing 1,500 ppm free gossypol (providing 8.2 g free gossypol/head/day). Cottonseed meal containing 26.6% (266,000 ppm) total gossypol and 0.175% (1,750 ppm) free gossypol was toxic when fed to adult dogs for an unspecified length of time; however, the equivalent oral dosage of free gossypol fed was <6 mg/kg/day.

Gossypol can gradually accumulate in the kidneys and liver, which are additional specimens for postmortem analyses. In sheep, gossypol concentrations (free or bound) >10 ppm in the kidneys and >20 ppm in the liver suggest excess gossypol exposure. However, background and significantly increased tissue gossypol concentrations have not been determined in all animal species, so tissue analyses may be of limited diagnostic value.

Differential diagnoses include poisonings by cardiotoxic ionophoric antibiotics (eg, monensin, lasalocid, salinomycin, narasin) and ammonia, nutritional or metabolic disorders (eg, selenium, vitamin E, or copper deficiency), infectious diseases, noninfectious diseases (eg, pulmonary adenomatosis, emphysema), mycotoxicoses caused by *Fusarium*-contaminated grain, and toxicoses caused by plants with cardiotoxic and other effects. Cardiotoxic plants (*see* p 3103), which may cause confusing or similar clinical signs and postmortem lesions, include English yew (*Taxus baccata*), Japanese yew (*T cuspidata*), laurel (*Kalmia* spp), azalea (*Rhododendron* spp), oleander (*Nerium oleander*), yellow oleander or yellow-be-still tree (*Thevetia peruviana*), purple foxglove (*Digitalis purpurea*), lily-of-the-valley (*Convallaria majalis*), dogbane (*Apocynum* spp), coffee senna (*Senna occidentalis*), bracken fern (*Pteridium aquilinum*), white snakeroot (*Eupatorium rugosum*), death camas (*Zygadenus* spp), lantana (*Lantana camara*), monkshood (*Aconitum napellum*), and milkweed (*Asclepias* spp).

Prevention, Treatment, and Control: There is no effective treatment for gossypol poisoning. Adsorbents such as activated charcoal and saline cathartics are of little value because of the chronic exposure and cumulative nature of gossypol. If gossypol toxicity is suspected, all cottonseed products should be removed from the diet immediately. However, severely affected animals may still die up to 4 wk after withdrawal of gossypol from the diet. Recovery depends primarily on the extent of toxic cardiopathy. Because exposure is usually chronic, and life-threatening lesions may be advanced before a diagnosis is made, a favorable prognosis for complete recovery may be unrealistic. Mild to moderate myocardial lesions may be reversible with time if stress is minimized and animals are carefully handled. However, poor weight gains in affected livestock and increased susceptibility to stress may persist for several weeks after cottonseed products are removed from the diet. A high-quality diet supplemented with lysine, methionine, and fat-soluble vitamins should be included in supportive therapy. Selenium or copper deficiencies may potentiate gossypol toxicosis.

A high intake of protein, calcium hydroxide, or iron salts appears to be protective in cattle. Mature cattle should also be given ≥40% of dry-matter intake from a forage source, and dietary gossypol concentrations should be limited to ≤1,000 ppm, because 1,500 ppm may cause anemia, poor growth, or decreased milk production. Swine and young ruminants are affected by dietary gossypol concentrations >100 ppm. Added iron of up to 400 ppm in swine diets and up to 600 ppm in poultry diets was reported to be effective in preventing signs and tissue residues of dietary gossypol exposure when used in ratios of 1:1 to 4:1 of iron to free gossypol. Poultry are affected by dietary gossypol concentrations >200 ppm.

POISONOUS MUSHROOMS

Mushrooms are the fruiting bodies of a variety of fleshy fungi that are found worldwide. They typically appear suddenly from growing vegetative (mycelium) portions, and they contain spores as reproductive units. Fungi lack chlorophyll; their nutritional requirements are met by utilizing organic material from a saprophytic, parasitic, and/or mycorrhizal life cycle.

Exposure is by ingestion. Although most mushrooms are edible and safe, a few contain diverse secondary metabolites (cyclopeptides, monomethylhydrazine, orelline/orellanin, muscarine, ibotenic acid and muscimol, psilocybin, and unknowns) that on ingestion/absorption result in mild to severe illness and even death. The mushroom species most frequently implicated in human/animal mushroom fatalities globally is *Amanita phalloides*. Most *Amanita* species are typically identified by their physical characteristics: veil (universal/partial), cap or pileus (with scales—remnants of universal veil), lamellae (gill-like, spore-bearing structure under surface of pileus), spores (reproductive structure—white to black and other shades of color), stipe/stalk (cap support), annulus or ring (remnant of partial veil on stipe below pileus), volva (remnant of universal veil at base of bulb), and mycelium. Other characteristics helpful in the identification of some poisonous mushrooms are listed in TABLE 5.

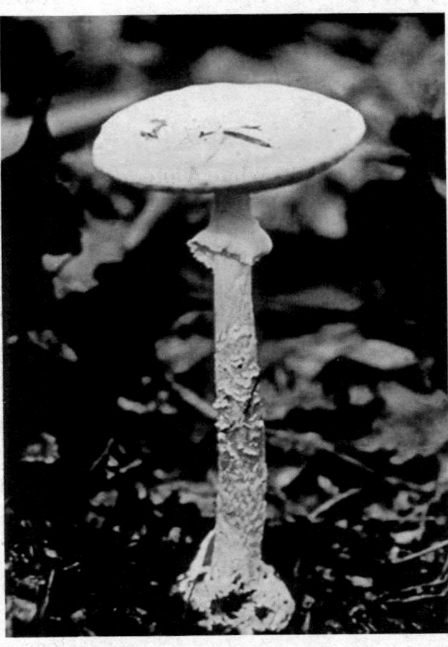

Amanita phalloides. Courtesy of Dr. Cecil Brownie.

The time lapse (latent period) between mushroom ingestion and observed clinical signs in exposed animals largely dictates the prognosis. A long delay time is synonymous with fatality (TABLE 6). However, short latent periods do not always indicate survival, because the animal may have ingested a

TABLE 5 PHYSICAL CHARACTERISTICS OF COMMON POISONOUS MUSHROOMS

Genus and Species	Color of Cap/ Spores	Habitat	Season	Range
Amanita muscaria	Red-tan to yellow/ orange/ white	Ground-pine, spruce, birch, poplar, and oak trees	Autumn/winter: June–Nov	Widespread, common in East and California
A pantherina	White with whitish patches; dark to yellow-brown/white at margin	Ground under conifers (Douglas fir)	Autumn/winter: June, Sept–Oct, Nov–Feb (California)	Rocky Mountains/ West coast; rare in East

(continued)

TABLE 5 PHYSICAL CHARACTERISTICS OF COMMON POISONOUS MUSHROOMS *(continued)*

Genus and Species	Color of Cap/ Spores	Habitat	Season	Range
A phalloides	Yellow/green or green/white	Ground under conifers, hardwoods; junipers and oaks	Autumn: late Sept–Nov, Nov–Jan	Massachusetts to Virginia west to Ohio; Pacific northwest to California
A virosa	White/white	Ground; mixed woods; grass, near trees	Autumn: late June–early Nov	North America
Chlorophyllum molybdites	White/green or grayish white	Lawn, pastures, meadows, fairy rings	Summer: Aug–Sept	Florida to California, common in Denver, reported in New York and New Jersey
Clitocybe spp	White/white	Ground	Perennial	Widespread in North America
Cortinarius orellanus	Orange/brown	Ground under conifers	July–Aug; Sept–Oct (Rocky Mountains)	Widespread in North America
Galerina spp	Brown-orange/ rust-brown	Ground-wood, well-decayed conifers and logs	Autumn/spring: Oct–Nov, May–June	Throughout North America
Gyromitra esculenta	Brown-rust/ yellow to buff	Ground under conifers	Spring: April–early June	Throughout North America
Inocybe spp	Brown/bright rust/orange-brown or dull gray-brown	Ground	Autumn: May–Nov	Widespread in North America
Lepiota spp	White with brownish scales/ white	Ground conifers, grass, leaf litter, oak and mixed woods	July–Oct (Michigan, Ohio); July–Nov (Florida); Nov–Feb (California)	Throughout North America
Paxillus involutus	Brown/sienna (clay-brown)	Ground: single/ numerous on wood in mixed woods	July–Nov	Widespread in North America
Psilocybe cubensis	Brown/lilac brown to dark purple brown	Ground/wood/ dung (cattle, horses)	Year round	Gulf Coast
Russula emetica	Reddish/white to yellowish white/ whitish	Single/group; on sphagnum moss, rarely on very rotten wood, conifers, or mixed woods	July–Sept	Widespread in North America

TABLE 6 POISONOUS MUSHROOMS: ONSET OF ACTION AND ORGANS TARGETED

Mushrooms	Toxin	Onset Time	Organ/System
LATENT PERIOD >6 HR AFTER INGESTION; LIFE-THREATENING			
Amanita phalloides; *A virosa*	Cyclopeptides, α and β amanitins, phallotoxins, virotoxins	6–24 hr, rarely >24 hr	Primarily liver, kidney secondary
Conocybe filaris	α and β amanitins	6–14 hr, rarely >24 hr	Primarily liver
Cortinarius gentilis	Orellanin, orelline	3–14 days (days/weeks)	Primarily renal[a]
Galerina autumnalis; *G venenata*	α and β amanitins	6–14 hr, rarely >24 hr	Primarily liver
Gyromitra esculenta	Monomethyl-hydrazine	6–24 hr	CNS
Lepiota spp	α and β amanitins	6–14 hr, rarely >24 hr	Primarily liver
LATENT PERIOD ≤3 HR AFTER INGESTION; NOT LIFE-THREATENING			
Amanita muscaria; *A pantherina*	Isoxazoles: ibotenic acid muscimol	30 min–2 hr; recovery 4–24 hr	CNS
Chlorophyllum molybdites	Unknown	30 min–3 hr; recovery 1–2 days	GI
Clitocybe dealbata; *Clitocybe* spp; *Inocybe* spp	Muscarine	30 min–2 hr; recovery 6–24 hr	Autonomic nervous system
Paxillus involutus	Unknown	1–3 hr; recovery 2–4 days	Immune system
Psilocybe spp; *Conocybe smithii*; *Gymnopilus spectabilis*; *Panaeolus subbalteatus*	Psilocybin and psilocin	30–60 min; rarely 6 hr	CNS
Russula emetica	Unknown	30 min–3 hr; recovery 1–2 days	GI

[a] No reported veterinary cases

combination of non-lethal/lethal mushroom species growing in the same location (dilution effect, or dose determines toxicity). In mushroom species with clinical signs that appear <3 hr after ingestion, effects are generally self-limiting and not life-threatening. Those with clinical signs that appear >6 hr after ingestion are life-threatening.

The sudden appearance of mushrooms and their short lifespan within the environment, coupled with the indiscriminate eating habits of many animals, creates diagnostic challenges. History and time after ingestion at which clinical signs are seen determine the treatment approach and prognosis. Establishing the time of ingestion may be difficult to impossible. With no proven antidotes to treat mushroom poisonings, treatment is primarily directed at decontamination, mushroom identification when possible, and intensive supportive care.

TOXIN LATENT PERIOD <3 HR AFTER INGESTION

Clitocybe dealbata, C dilatata, and *Inocybe* spp

Clitocybe are fleshy, small mushrooms with white-tan-grey caps, gills that are attached and that descend the stalk, and white spore print. They are widely distributed and usually grow on the ground in open woods, parks, and lawns. *Inocybe* are small, brown mushrooms that grow on conifers or broad-leafed trees and oak woods (mycorrhizal). They have a cap with a knob, ringless stalk, veil covered immature gills, no remnant of universal veil, and a spore print that is bright rust/orange-brown or gray-brown.

The toxin in these mushrooms is muscarine, a quaternary ammonium compound that is poorly absorbed orally and does not cross the blood-brain barrier. Its cholinergic effects are therefore peripheral. The absorbed portion is quickly distributed throughout the body and undergoes urinary excretion. Muscarine is structurally similar to acetylcholine, a cholinergic neurotransmitter. Whereas the acetylcholine-muscarine receptor complex is susceptible to acetycholinesterase inactivation, the muscarine-muscarine receptor complex is not. Muscarine competes with acetylcholine at cholinergic receptor binding sites, leading to excessive stimulation of postganglionic cholinergic fibers and the subsequent observed clinical signs (cholinergic excess).

Clinical Findings: Within 30–120 min of ingestion, there is mild to excessive cholinergic stimulation—ataxia, vomiting, abdominal pain, salivation, lacrimation, watery diarrhea, miosis, bronchoconstriction, bradycardia, arrhythmias, hypotension/hypertension, and shock.

Diagnosis: Diagnosis may be based on a history of mushroom ingestion, identification of suspected mushroom and consistent clinical signs, response to supportive care, and atropine therapy. Tests used to evaluate fluid and electrolyte status in severe gastroenteritis cases, together with a liver profile, may be useful.

Treatment: Other than offering supportive care (fluid and electrolyte replacement), treatment is unnecessary in most cases. In life-threatening cases, atropine therapy (0.2–2 mg/kg, a portion of the calculated dose given IV and the remaining portion IM or SC), repeated as necessary, is the treatment of choice. Efficacy of treatment should be based on lack of respiratory difficulties and respiratory secretions and not on mydriasis. Excessive atropine therapy can lead to anticholinergic effects (eg, tachycardia, GI stasis, behavioral changes, and hyperthermia); therefore, animals should be monitored.

Amanita muscaria and *A pantherina*

Amanita muscaria have an orange-red cap with distinctive white to yellow warts, gills that are somewhat attached, white spore print, ring stalk, and bulbous base (cup). *A pantherina* have a tan to yellow-brown/dark brown cap with white patches, a ringed stalk with basal bulb, and white spore print. Both of these mushrooms are found in coniferous and deciduous forests of the Pacific northwest.

The toxins in these mushrooms are isoxazole derivatives: ibotenic acid, which is structurally similar to the stimulatory neurotransmitter glutamic acid, and its decarboxylated metabolite muscimol, which is stereochemically similar to the inhibitory neurotransmitter γ-aminobutyric acid (GABA). They both cross the blood-brain barrier and effect functional changes within the CNS. The toxic dose of ibotenic acid is reported to be 30–60 mg, and that of muscimol is 6 mg (ingestion of more than two mushrooms).

Ibotenic acid undergoes spontaneous decarboxylation (stomach, liver, and brain), forming muscimol, which is a GABA-receptor agonist. Both are analogues of γ-aminobutyric acid and act as weak, noncompetitive inhibitors of GABA (inhibits neuronal and glial GABA uptake). This reduces the inhibitory effect of the Purkinje cells in the cerebellum, increases brain serotonin, and decreases catecholamine levels.

Clinical Findings: Both compounds are rapidly absorbed from the GI tract. The onset of clinical signs (tachycardia, hypotension, ataxia, seizures, hyperthermia, vomiting, muscle fasciculation, mydriasis, incoordination, hyperactivity [paddling, chewing movements], opisthotonos, respiratory depression, coma, and death) are reportedly seen within 30–120 min after ingestion. Duration of signs is ~24 hr.

Diagnosis: Diagnosis is based on a history of ingestion, clinical presentation, and response to treatment (symptomatic, supportive, and specific drugs, eg, benzodiazepine).

Treatment: Symptomatic and supportive treatment includes maintaining hydration (IV fluids), keeping airways free of respiratory secretions, and frequent positional changes. Seizures may be controlled with diazepam (0.5 mg/kg, IV to effect; repeated as needed), phenobarbital (6 mg/kg, IV), or pentobarbital (5–15 mg/kg, IV). Benzodiazepines and barbiturates are GABA-receptor agonists and may potentiate CNS and respiratory depression. Muscarine concentrations in *A muscaria* are very low, and peripheral effects are more anticholinergic than cholinergic. Therefore, atropine therapy is contraindicated.

Chlorophyllum molybdites and *Russula emetica*

Chlorophyllum molybdites mushrooms have caps that are large, white to brown, egg-shaped, convex knobbed to flat, with numerous cinnamon or buff scales. They have unattached white gills, green or grayish-olive spores, and a ring on the stalk. They are common in the southern and central USA. *Russula emetica* mushrooms have a reddish, slimy cap with short whitish stalk and gills; no veils; and a white to yellowish-white spore print. They grow singly or in a group and are found throughout the USA. The toxins in these mushrooms are varied and unknown GI irritants that are thought to be high-molecular-weight proteins found throughout the mushroom.

Clinical Findings: Within minutes to hours (0.5–3 hr) after exposure, clinical signs become evident. These include vomiting, bloody diarrhea, abdominal pain, muscle cramps, liver injury, and circulatory disturbances that are self-limiting. Although recovery generally occurs within 6–24 hr, it could be prolonged or become life threatening (rare) in cases of hypovolemic shock, oliguria, and/or transient increased BUN secondary to dehydration. Death is rare.

Diagnosis: A tentative diagnosis may be based on history and early onset of reported clinical signs (gastroenteritis—vomiting and bloody diarrhea). Except for dehydration, there are no systemic signs. If the mushroom is available, the gills (light green) and spore print (green) color may be used to distinguish *C molybdites*, the most common GI irritant mushroom species, from others.

Treatment: There are no specific antidotes. Dehydration and electrolyte imbalance should be addressed. Gastric lavage and activated charcoal therapy may be considered. Analgesics are useful in some cases, but caution should be exercised in administering acetaminophen (inherently hepatotoxic) to hepatic insult cases. Phenothiazines interact adversely with toxins to induce CNS and/or GI effects. Fluids and vasopressors should be administered in hypovolemic shock cases. Liver and kidney functions should be monitored.

Psilocybe cubensis, *Conocybe cyanopus*, *Gymnopilus spectabilis*, and *Panaeolus subbalteatus*

Psilocybe cubensis are small, brown, slender-stalked mushrooms. They commonly grow in piles of dung and fertilized grasses in moist areas throughout the USA, especially in the southeastern and northwest regions. The mushrooms develop a blue-green color in handled and injured areas. They have yellowish, sticky to moist caps with brown gills; a persistent ring on the stalk; and a purple-brown spore print. *Conocybe cyanopus* are small and fragile, with brown caps, brown gills, and a large ring midway down the long, thin stalk. The spore print is cinnamon brown. They are widely distributed in North America. *Gymnopilus spectabilis* are large yellow-orange mushrooms with an orange to rust orange spore print. They are found in clusters on wood, stumps, or on the ground over buried wood. *Panaeolus subbalteatus* have broadly conical to flat caps with a dark belt around margin, brown gills, hairy reddish stalks, and a blackish spore print. They are widely distributed in North America.

These hallucinogenic mushrooms contain psilocybin and psilocin, which are indole alkaloids similar to lysergic acid diethylamide (LSD). Psilocybin undergoes rapid dephosphorylation (plasma, kidneys, and liver), forming psilocin, which is structurally similar to serotonin (stimulatory to serotonin receptors in the central and peripheral nervous systems). Metabolites cross the blood-brain barrier and concentrate in brain tissue. Growth conditions, geographic location, storage conditions, and mushroom species are factors that influence toxin concentrations. Ingestion of five or six dried mushroom caps is reported to be toxic.

Clinical Findings: Clinical signs occur within 0.5–1 hr; they are rarely delayed as long as 3 hr after ingestion. Signs include vocalization, aggression, nystagmus, ataxia, tachycardia, vomiting, urinary incontinence, dyspnea, mydriasis, weakness, hyperthermia, mild methemoglobinemia, and hallucination, with recovery within 6 hr of observed clinical signs.

Diagnosis: A history of mushroom ingestion, identification of suspected mushroom(s), consistent clinical presentation, and response to supportive and symptomatic care are critical for diagnosis. With isoxazole-induced toxicity, coma is distinctly expressed; however, the opposite is true in psilocin-induced toxicity. Tests detecting psilocin and its glucuronide metabolite in urine, serum, and blood, although confirmatory, are not widely available clinically.

Treatment: Treatment is primarily symptomatic and supportive. Diazepam (0.5–1 mg/kg, IV, with incremental dose increase of 5–10 mg to effect) or phenobarbital (6 mg/kg to effect) may be given. Body temperature should be monitored. In some cases, leaving the animal untreated in a quiet, dark environment might be all that is necessary.

TOXIN LATENT PERIOD >6 HR AFTER INGESTION

Amanita phalloides, A virosa, Lepiota helveola, Galerina autumnalis, G venenata, and *Conocybe filaris*

These mushroom species account for >95% of the reported mushroom-induced deaths. They are common throughout North America and are associated with oaks and birch trees.

Amanita phalloides and *A virosa* have olive to green caps with veil patches, gills that are unattached to the stalk, a white spore print, and stalks with a ring (often but not always) and a cup (volva) or remnants at the base. The features of *Lepiota helveola* are similar to those of *Amanita* spp but without volva; they have scaly caps with a knob in the center and stalks with a movable ring. *Galerina autumnalis* (autumn galerina), *G venenata*, and *Conocybe filaris* have brownish, tacky caps with yellowish gills becoming rust and a ring on their brownish stalks. They have no volva, and their spore print is brown to rust-brown. These species are abundant on well-decayed coniferous and deciduous logs throughout North America.

Toxin present in these mushrooms include cyclopeptide amatoxins (bicyclic octapeptides), phallotoxins, and virotoxins (bicyclic heptapeptides). Amatoxins (α and β amanitin derivatives) are the most potent; they are not found in all *Amanita* spp. An estimated reported lethal dose is 0.1 mg/kg (equivalent to the concentrations in one cap of *A phalloides*) across animal species. Whereas the amatoxins are reported to be well absorbed orally, phallotoxins and virotoxins are not. Amanitins are not protein bound and are excreted in urine (80%–90%), feces, and bile (7%). Amatoxins bind to nuclear RNA polymerase-11 (transcription phase), thus preventing the formation of phosphodiesterase bonds and subsequent RNA, DNA, and protein synthesis. High-protein synthesis cells are most sensitive. Amatoxins are primarily liver toxins, but they also affect many organ systems, resulting in hypoglycemia, blood clotting defects, thyroid/parathyroid functional anomalies, renal failure, and intestinal damage (enterohepatic recirculation of the toxin).

Clinical Findings: Signs can be characterized in four phases: 1) latent (6–12 hr after ingestion), in which the animal shows no clinical signs; 2) GI signs (as long as 24 hr after ingestion); 3) remission (as long as 72 hr after ingestion), in which the animal appears to have recovered; and 4) hepatic/renal (3–6 days after ingestion), leading to recovery or death throughout the next 7–14 days. The reported long latent phase is of diagnostic importance. The GI phase, indicated by vomiting, abdominal discomfort, hepatitis, and pancreatitis follows and signals initial hepatic, hematologic, cardiovascular, endocrine, CNS, and renal changes. The remission phase follows, only to enter a fulminant hepatic/renal phase, indicated by icterus, hypoglycemia, and coma, 3–4 days after ingestion. Recovery or death (>50%) from hepatic and/or renal failure occurs 7–14 days after mushroom ingestion.

Diagnosis: Mushroom identification characteristics, coupled with consistent clinical signs as stated above, is diagnostic. Meixner test results (time taken, and color intensity of suspected mushroom specimen—fresh, vomited fragments) would be diagnostic. During the GI phase, animals should be monitored for decreased serum thyroxine levels, hypoglycemia, and/or increased insulin, calcitonin, and parathyroid levels. Routine blood and serum chemistry profiles are unremarkable until liver/kidney damage. Because the toxin is primarily hepatotoxic, changes in clotting factor V, fibrinogen, and kidney and liver profiles would also be helpful. Amanitins can be detected in urine from animals not showing clinical signs. They are also detectable in liver and kidney specimens as long as 22 days after ingestion.

Treatment: There are no specific antidotes. Silibinin (not FDA approved), penicillin G (high levels), combined silibinin/penicillin, cimetidine, *N*-acetylcysteine, or vitamin C therapies have been used with some success in people and could therefore be tried, although animal study data are not readily available. Hypoglycemia remains an adverse effect with or without treatment. Supportive care (IV fluids, dextrose, and antibiotics) counters the effects of severe liver and kidney damage. Early institution of treatment is essential to save the animal; the prognosis is poor after hepatic/renal pathology. Activated charcoal (1 g/kg with cathartic) during the first 24 hr after ingestion absorbs amanitin undergoing enterohepatic recirculation and thus may be helpful.

Gyromitra esculenta

These mushrooms have a non-gilled, yellow-brown to dark-red, deeply wrinkled, honeycomb (unlike true morels that are hallowed and not chambered), saddle-shaped cap on a short stalk. They are found on the ground under conifers throughout North America. The toxin involved is the hydrazone gyromitrin, which on ingestion is hydrolyzed to N-methyl-N-formylhydrazine (depletes hepatic cytochrome P-450) and monomethylhydrazine (inhibitor of the coenzyme pyridoxal phosphate and γ-aminobutyric acid in the CNS 6–12 hr after ingestion. The concentration of gyromitrin varies with environmental conditions.

Clinical Findings: Vomiting, watery diarrhea, abdominal discomfort, convulsions, and coma may be noted 6–24 hr after ingestion of a toxic dose. Methemoglobinemia and hemolytic anemia, hepatitis, jaundice, nephritis, and death develop some time later. Death appears to be due to hepatorenal failure.

Treatment: Activated charcoal (1 g/kg) may be helpful if given early after ingestion. IV fluids should be given as needed. IV pyridoxine controls neurologic signs, and methylene blue can be given in cyanotic and methemoglobin cases. Pyridoxine-induced peripheral neuropathy from administering high doses should be avoided. For the induced hepatic encephalopathy, supportive therapy is essential. In addition to monitoring methemoglobin levels, hepatic and renal functions should also be monitored.

TOXIN LATENT PERIOD >24 HR AFTER INGESTION

Cortinarius orellanus and *C rainierensis*

These mushrooms have a colorful but mostly brownish cap, stalk, and young gills; the matured gills are orange-rust in color. The spore print is bright rust/orange-brown/gray-brown but not purple-brown. Stalks may or may not have a ring-like zone.

The toxins involved are orelline and orellanine, which are chemically related to the herbicide diquat (bipyridyl derivatives). Thin-layer chromatography can detect orellanine in renal biopsy material long after clinical exposure but not in urine and/or blood during clinically active states. Ingestion of three to ten caps is reported to be lethal. There have been no reported cases from ingestion of species grown in North America.

Clinical Findings: The onset of clinical signs is delayed (17 days after ingestion). Signs include anorexia, vomiting, diarrhea/constipation, gastritis, thirst, and polyuria progressing to oliguric renal failure in 3–14 days after initial clinical signs. The kidney seems to be the target organ; lesions include interstitial nephritis, tubular damage, and fibrosis. Hepatic damage is infrequently reported. In most cases, marked improvement over an extended period (6 mo) is seen; however, chronic renal failure occurs in some cases.

Diagnosis: Urinalysis indicates concentrated urine, hematuria, protein, and RBC casts early in the latent period, followed by diluted urine with protein and few casts later. It therefore becomes necessary to monitor renal function. Renal pathology without hepatic involvement after a long latent period (days) has been reported in people. Blood, urinalysis, and kidney profile testing would be supportive. Mushroom identification can differentiate *Cortinarius* spp from *Paxillus involutus*, a mushroom reported to cause hypersensitivity leading to renal failure.

Treatment: Treatment should be focused on decontamination, mushroom identification (often difficult), and intensive supportive care. Hemodialysis should be instituted until normal kidney function returns. Pentobarbital and/or furosemide usage should be avoided or limited, because these drugs increase toxicity.

MISCELLANEOUS POISONOUS MUSHROOMS

Ramaria flavo-brunnescens

Ramaria flavo-brunnescens is found exclusively in eucalyptus woods in North America, Australia, Brazil, and Uruguay, and is easily identified from the spore print color of pale buff to brownish yellow. It is reported to be poisonous to ruminants (cattle and sheep). The toxin is an unknown, volatile compound or compounds found throughout the plant that is reported to interfere with sulfur-containing amino acid incorporation. Drying decreases toxicity.

Clinical Findings: Signs may appear as early as 3 days but as long as 6 days after exposure and include anorexia, diarrhea, salivation, hyperthermia, depression, hyperemic coronary band, hemorrhage (anterior chamber of eyes), oral ulceration, altered keratinization (hair/hoof loss, similar to selenium poisoning), and recumbency. Death or recovery may be expected in 3–15 days.

Diagnosis: These mushrooms grow exclusively among eucalyptus plants, so history of exposure to eucalyptus is key. Selenium exposure and toxicity causes similar signs. The duration and outcome of the clinical expression helps to confirm diagnosis.

Treatment: Treatment involves removing the affected animal from the source and offering supportive care. Recovery requires time.

Paxillus involutus

Paxillus involutus has a dry or slimy, brownish cap with an in-rolled margin and yellowish gills descending a short distance on the brown, smooth stalk. The spore print is clay-brown. *P involutus* is widely distributed in North America. It may appear singly or in groups of several, near or on wood in mixed woods in the spring/autumn. The toxin is unknown, but it may cause hypersensitivity over time, leading to kidney failure.

Clinical Findings: Vomiting, diarrhea, cardiovascular irregularity, and RBC destruction may be noted 1–3 hr after ingestion. Recovery generally takes 2–4 days but could be longer. Acquired sensitivity develops over time.

Diagnosis and Treatment: A diagnosis can be made based on mushroom identification, consistent clinical signs, and response to supportive care. Treatment involves symptomatic and supportive measures.

POISONOUS PLANTS

HOUSEPLANTS AND ORNAMENTALS

Plants are an important part of the decor of homes; pets having access to these plants often chew on or ingest them, with toxicity a possible outcome (*see* TABLE 7). Inquiries to poison control centers on plants ingested by children <5 yr old are estimated at 5%–10% of all inquiries. Similar estimates (although not documented) could be made for pets.

Little research has been done on the toxicity of houseplants. Most are hybrids, and selecting for growth outside their natural environment could affect their degree of toxicity. Age of the pet, boredom, and changes in the surroundings are factors that may affect the incidence of poisoning. Puppies and kittens are very inquisitive, and mouth or chew almost any and everything. Pets (especially single household pets) of all ages may become bored or restless if left alone or confined for too long at any one time, and chewing on objects for relief is common. Pets of all ages also explore changes in their environment (eg, pets commonly chew the leaves or ripe berries of potentially poisonous plants placed in the home during holidays).

RANGE PLANTS OF TEMPERATE NORTH AMERICA

Poisonous plants are among the important causes of economic loss to the livestock industry and should be considered when evaluating illness and decreased productivity (*see* TABLE 8). Poisonous plants can affect animals in many ways, including death, chronic illness and debilitation, decreased weight gain, abortion, birth defects, increased parturition interval, and photosensitization. In addition to these more obvious losses, other considerations include loss of forage, additional fencing, increased labor and management costs, and frequently interference with proper harvesting of forage.

Most poisonous range plants fall into two general categories: those that are indigenous to a range and increase with heavy grazing, and those that invade after overgrazing or disturbance of the land. Among those not in these categories are certain locoweeds and larkspurs, both of which form part of the normal range plant community. Poisonous plants can be found in most plant communities and should be considered in most grazing situations.

Livestock poisoning by plants often can be traced to problems of management or range condition, rather than simply to the presence of poisonous plants. Usually, animals are poisoned because hunger or other conditions cause them to graze abnormally. Overgrazing, trucking, trailing, corralling, or introducing animals onto a new range tend to induce hunger or change behavior, and poisoning may occur.

Not all poisonous plants are unpalatable, and they are not restricted to overgrazed ranges and pastures. Furthermore, poisonous plants do not always kill or otherwise harm animals when consumed; the dose determines toxicity. Many plants can be either useful forage or toxic. For example, plants such as lupine and greasewood may be part of an animal's diet, and the animal is poisoned only when it consumes too much of the plant too fast. To prevent poisoning, it is important to understand the factors involved when a useful forage becomes a poisonous plant.

Definitive diagnosis of suspect plant poisonings is difficult. It is important to be familiar with the poisonous plants growing in the specific area and the conditions under which livestock may be poisoned. A tentative diagnosis is possible if the following information is available: 1) any local soil deficiencies or excesses (which may complicate plant toxicities or simply confuse as to cause of a syndrome), 2) the syndromes associated with each of the poisonous plants in the area, 3) the time of year during which each is most likely to cause problems, 4) the detailed history of the animal(s) over the last 6–8 mo, and 5) any change of management or environmental condition that may cause an animal to change its diet or grazing habits (in some cases, eg, locoism, this may be all that is required in addition to identification of the plant involved). Identification of the plant is important, whatever its stage of growth, and is especially useful if it can be identified in the stomach contents of the poisoned animal. Chemical analysis of toxicants often is not useful. Metabolic profiles are useful for some toxicities, and in some, the necropsy lesions are distinctive (*see* TABLE 8).

TABLE 7 POISONOUS HOUSEPLANTS AND ORNAMENTALS[a]

Scientific Name (Family)	Common Name	Important Characteristics
Abrus precatorius (Fabaceae)	Rosary pea, Precatory bean, Prayer beads, Crab's eye	Climbing/twining vine on other objects as substratum. Compound leaves/light sensitive, pale reddish purple flowers, pea-shaped pods with 3–5 red seeds with black spots. Jewelry handicrafts as souvenir gifts in homes.
Adenium obesum (Apocynaceae)	Desert rose, Mock azalea, Desert azalea	Succulent shrubs or small trees. Perennials, milky viscous sap with fleshy swollen stems. Simple, fleshy to leathery, lanceolate, dark leaves. Showy flower clusters—red petals with pink or white centers at tip of branch. Fruits—follicles with many seeds. Houseplant grown outside in dry, hot locations.
Agapanthus orientalis (Liliaceae)	African blue lily, Blue African lily	Grows to a height of ~2 ft in large containers. Perennial herbs with simple, heart-shaped, thin, highlighted veins, variegated leaves; yellow-green spathe; grown from rhizomes.
Agave americana (Agavaceae)	Century plant, American aloe	Clumps of thick, long strap-shaped blue/green leaves with hook (margin) and pointed spines (tip). Central flower stalk with small tubular flowers in clusters.
Aglaonema modestum (Araceae)	Chinese evergreen, Painted drop tongue	Central stem with solid medium green or splotched gray/green leaves; small greenish flowers.
Allamanda cathartica (Apocynaceae)	Allamanda, Yellow allamanda	Ornamental, sprawling, woody climbing shrub with large yellow flowers: opposite lance-shaped leaves: fruitless.
Alocasia spp (Araceae)	Elephant's ear	Erect perennials from running rhizomes; single, long-stemmed, spear-headed varicolored leaves; prominent veins.
Aloe barbadensis (Liliaceae)	Barbados aloe, Curacao aloe	Succulent herb with cluster of narrow fleshy, spinous or coarsely serrated margin leaves, with hook spines on leaf margin. Dense spiked tubular yellow flowers at end of single stalk.

TABLE 7 POISONOUS HOUSEPLANTS AND ORNAMENTALS[a] *(continued)*

Comments and Toxic Principles and Effects	Treatment
Abrin, a plant lectin (taxalbumin) related to ricin in hard seed coat, released when chewed on or otherwise broken. Toxin inhibits cellular protein synthesis.	Ingested whole intact seeds nontoxic in most cases. GI clinical signs; assess dehydration and electrolyte status. Electrolyte replacement therapy in severe cases.
Cardioactive steroids and cardiac glycosides throughout entire plant. Na^+/K^+ ATPase inhibition, increased intracellular Ca^{2+} leading to myocardial excitation, bradycardia, ventricular tachycardia/fibrillation and heart block, hyperkalemia, abdominal distress, vomiting, anorexia, and inactivity.	Symptomatic
Unknown toxin(s) but thought to be a sticky, acrid, irritant latex rather than allergens. Calcium oxalate crystals and unknowns found in all parts, especially rhizomes. Ingestion causes immediate intense pain, local irritation to mucous membranes, excess salivation, swollen tongue and pharynx, diarrhea, and dyspnea. Pets' access to plant associated with rhizomes brought indoors for winter storage.	Symptomatic
Sap contains calcium oxalate crystals; saponins and acrid volatile oil in leaves and seeds. On ingestion, causes dermal and oral mucosal irritation and edema.	Symptomatic
The entire plant contains calcium oxalate crystals. On ingestion, causes oral mucosal irritation and edema.	Symptomatic
Contains plumericin, a GI irritant found in the bark, leaves, fruit, seeds, and sap.	Based on exposure dose (abdominal discomfort, diarrhea, dehydration, and electrolyte imbalance). Symptomatic therapy (rehydration and electrolyte replacement) in severe cases.
Water-insoluble calcium oxalate and possible proteinaceous toxins (raphides) in leaves, stems, and tubers.	Burning/painful/inflammatory reaction in mouth on ingestion. Analgesics and/or demulcents may be indicated. Systemic reaction to insoluble calcium oxalate not reported.
Contains anthraquinone glycosides (barbaloin, emodin) and chrysophanic acid in the latex of the leaves; higher concentrations in younger leaves. On ingestion, causes abrupt, severe diarrhea and/or hypoglycemia, with vomiting in some cases.	Symptomatic; control diarrhea and fluid loss.

(continued)

TABLE 7 POISONOUS HOUSEPLANTS AND ORNAMENTALS[a] *(continued)*

Scientific Name (Family)	Common Name	Important Characteristics
Anthurium spp (Araceae)	Anthurium, Flamingo lily, Flamingo flower, Tail flower	Dark green or shiny broad heart-shaped, leathery leaves; a persistent white/scarlet/green spike; flowering, colorful berries.
Arum spp (Araceae)	Italian arum, Black calla, Starch root, Cuckoopint	Stemless plant with large ovate leaves and tuberous roots; showy flower, purple enclosing a spike having red fruits; common houseplant of Europe/Near East origin.
Aucuba japonica (Cornaceae)	Japanese aucuba, Japanese laurel, Spotted laurel	Cultivated as an ornamental and house-plant (large bush) with coarsely toothed, large opposite leaves; purple flowers in panicle at end of branches; scarlet berry, single seed fruit; matures in early winter.
Brunfelsia pauciflora floribunda (Solanaceae)	Yesterday-today-and-tomorrow, Lady-of-the-night	Evergreen shrubs to small trees with alternate, undivided, toothless, thick, rather leathery, lustrous leaves. Winter-blooming; large showy sometimes fragrant flowers, clustered or solitary at the branch ends, with 5-lobed tubular calyx, 5 petals, and funnel-shaped corolla. Fruits berry-like capsules.
Caladium spp (Araceae)	Caladium, Fancy leaf caladium, Angel wings	Perennial herbs with simple, heart-shaped, thin, highlighted veins, variegated leaves; yellow-green spathe; grown from rhizomes.
Cannabis sativa (Cannabaceae)	Mary Jane, Marijuana, Grass, Pot, Hashish, Indian hemp, Reefer, Weed	Annual herb, grown from seeds, ≥6 ft tall. Leaves opposite or alternate, palmately compound with 5–7 linear, coarsely dentate leaflets; small green flowers at tip (male) or along entire length (female) of branch; fruits achenes. Grown for its fiber; legally cultivated under federal license only in most states.
Capsicum annuum (Solanaceae)	Cherry pepper, Chili pepper, Ornamental pepper, Capsicum	Annual shrub; branched, erect stem; dark, glossy, ovate, entire margin leaves; white flowers. Fruits are shiny berries of various colors, shapes, sizes.

TABLE 7 POISONOUS HOUSEPLANTS AND ORNAMENTALS[a] *(continued)*

Comments and Toxic Principles and Effects	Treatment
Native to tropical America (common houseplant); raphides (water-insoluble calcium oxalate and proteinaceous toxins) in leaves and stems.	On ingestion, painful/burning sensation and inflammation of oral cavity. Remove from source; symptomatic treatment helpful, but clinical signs subside over time.
Entire plant contains yet to be identified GI toxin (once thought to be calcium oxalate); dose-dependent mucous membrane irritation, ulcerations, abdominal discomfort, vomiting, diarrhea, and dehydration.	Analgesics for oral mucosal irritation and pain, rehydration, antiemetics, and electrolyte replacement as needed.
Aucubin (acid labile glycoside) found throughout the plant (concentrated in fruit, which is colorful and to which pets are attracted). Large exposure dose required for toxicity (GI discomfort).	None in small dose exposure cases. Rehydration, antiemetics, and electrolyte replacement may be necessary in severely affected cases.
Alkaloid components (atropine, scopolamine, hyoscyamine) found in the flowers, leaves, bark, and roots. On ingestion, animals show tachycardia, dry mouth, dilated pupils, ataxia, tremors, depression, urinary retention, and sometimes coma (deep sedation). Not reported to cause death.	In severely depressed animals, stimulants (respiratory and cardiac), along with supportive therapy recommended.
Calcium oxalate crystals and unknowns found in all parts, especially rhizomes. Ingestion causes immediate intense pain, local irritation to mucous membranes, excess salivation, swollen tongue and pharynx, diarrhea, and dyspnea. Pets' access to plant associated with rhizomes brought indoors for winter storage.	Symptomatic
Leaves, stems, and flower buds of mature plants contain tetrahydrocannabinol (THC) and related compounds. THC concentrations vary with plant variety (1%–6%), parts (female flowers have highest concentrations), processing (extracts have as much as 28%), sex, and growing conditions. Lethal dose for dogs >3 g/kg body wt. Pets' exposure usually from accidental access to this plant being used for in-home treatment of cancer patient or for illegal (in most states) recreational uses by owner. Pets (dogs primarily) show ataxia, vomiting, mydriasis, prolonged depression, tachycardia or bradycardia, salivation, hyperexcitability, tremors, and hypothermia. Death results when vital CNS regulatory centers are severely depressed.	Remove animal from source. Effectiveness of emetics limited by antiemetic effect of THC. Oral tannic acid, activated charcoal, followed by saline cathartics have been recommended. Stimulants (cardiac and respiratory) along with supportive therapy essential in severely depressed animals. Recovery slow at best. *See also* p 3041.
Capsaicinoids (capsaicin) in the mature fruits, solanine and scopoletin in foliage; irritating to the GI tract, with vomiting and diarrhea. Not likely to be lethal.	Symptomatic; irritation relief—cool water irrigation, topical or oral mineral or vegetable oil. Rarely topical anesthetics.

(continued)

TABLE 7 POISONOUS HOUSEPLANTS AND ORNAMENTALS[a] *(continued)*

Scientific Name (Family)	Common Name	Important Characteristics
Catharanthus reseus (Apocynaceae)	Madagascar periwinkle, Bigleaf periwinkle, Vinca, Large periwinkle	Perennial herb with milky sap; erect stems with glossy green opposite leaves; solitary rose-pink to white flowers. Cultivated as an ornamental.
Chlorophytum spp (Liliaceae)	Spider plant, St. Bernard's lily, Airplane plant	Rhizomatous herbs with leaves slightly glossy, succulent, narrow, strap-like, green—some with a broad, yellow, or white band down the middle; long, cream, hanging stems with small, white flowers developing into plantlets. Often grown in hanging baskets.
Colchicum autumnale (Liliaceae, Colchicaceae)	Autumn crocus, Crocus, Fall crocus, Meadow saffron, Wonder bulb	Popular house or yard plant, perennial herb, ovoid underground corm covered with brown membrane or scales. Leaves large, lanceolate, basal, ovate, smooth, ribbed, appear in spring and die back before flowering. Flowers tubular, solitary, pale purple or white appearing in fall; fruit a 3-celled ovoid capsule with numerous seeds.
Convallaria majalis (Liliaceae)	Lily-of-the-valley, Conval lily, Mayflower	Herbaceous perennial from slender running rhizome; stem leafless, bearing a 1-sided raceme of nodding white, aromatic, bell-shaped flowers; leaves 2 or 3, basal to 1 ft long. Fruit a red berry but seldom formed.
Cyclamen spp (Primulaceae)	Cyclamen, Snowbread, Shooting star	Herbaceous plants, grown from rhizomes or tubers. Petioled, heart-shaped, deep green intermixed with lighter green coloration (same leaf), serrated leaves; stems upright, with a terminal pink or white butterfly-like flower.
Dieffenbachia spp (Araceae)	Dumbcane	Fairly tall, erect, unbranched, fleshy plant; stem girdled with leaf scars; leaves large, thickly veined, sheath-like petioles, white or yellow spots on blade.

TABLE 7 POISONOUS HOUSEPLANTS AND ORNAMENTALS[a] *(continued)*

Comments and Toxic Principles and Effects	Treatment
Vinca alkaloids (vincristine/vinblastine) throughout the plant inhibit microtubule formation. Toxic exposures lead to pharyngeal pain, GI signs (abdominal pain, severe diarrhea), dehydration, peripheral nerve damage, bone marrow suppression/depression, and cardiovascular damage.	Aggressive supportive and symptomatic therapy essential, with extended monitoring.
More commonly grown for its filtering ability. Pets (especially cats) reach these plants either by climbing or when plantlets fall from mature stems. Unknown toxin(s) found in leaves and plantlets. Vomiting, salivation, retching, and transient anorexia seen in cats within hours of ingestion. Deaths and diarrhea not reported.	Symptomatic
Colchicine and related alkaloids found throughout plant. These alkaloids are heat stable and not affected by drying. Colchicine is used experimentally in genetic investigations, and medically in the treatment of gout in people. It is cumulative and slowly excreted. Milk of lactating animals is a major excretory pathway. Clinical signs include thirst, difficult swallowing, abdominal pain, profuse vomiting and diarrhea, weakness, and shock within hours of ingestion. Death from respiratory failure.	Prolonged course due to slow excretion of colchicine. Gastric lavage; supportive care for dehydration and electrolyte losses (fluid therapy); CNS, circulatory, and respiratory disturbances. Analgesics and atropine recommended for abdominal pain and diarrhea.
Cardiac glycosides (convallarin, convallamarin, convallatoxin), irritant saponins found in leaves, flowers, rhizome, and water in which flowers have been kept. Variable latent period depending on dose. GI signs (vomiting, trembling, abdominal pain, diarrhea), progressive cardiac irregularities (irregular heart beats, AV block), and death. Hyperkalemia in acute cases. Gastroenteritis, petechial hemorrhages throughout.	Aimed at gut decontamination (gastric lavage) and at correcting bradycardia (atropine), conduction defects (phenytoin), and electrolyte imbalance such as hyperkalemia (IV electrolytes). Electrocardiographic and serum potassium monitoring necessary.
Triterpinoid saponins found in tuberous rhizomes cause GI irritation, thereby increasing systemic absorption and severe toxicity. Anorexia, diarrhea, convulsions, and paralysis are observed clinical signs. Pets have greater access to these plants over winter months (both pets and plants are indoors).	Symptomatic
Calcium oxalate crystals and unknown toxic proteins (possibly asparagine or protoanemonin) in all parts, including sap. On ingestion, immediate intense pain, burning, and inflammation of mouth and throat, anorexia, vomiting, and possibly diarrhea, with tongue extended, head shaking, excessive salivation, and dyspnea. Immediate pain limits amount consumed. Death infrequent.	Symptomatic

(continued)

TABLE 7 POISONOUS HOUSEPLANTS AND ORNAMENTALS[a] *(continued)*

Scientific Name (Family)	Common Name	Important Characteristics
Digitalis purpurea (Scrophulariac)	Foxglove	Erect biennial with simple, petioled (long on lower, short or sessile on upper), alternate, toothed, hairy, ovate to lanceolate leaves. Purple, pink, red, white, or yellow tubular flowers (with spots) in terminal racemes; fruit is a capsule with many seeds.
Dracaena spp (Agavaceae)	Dragon tree	Robust, palm-like houseplant with lance-shaped, thin, variegated, alternate, non-petioled leaves. Yellow, red, or green stripes along leaf margins in some species. Lower leaves are lost, leaf scars remain and clearly demarcated, terminal leaves retained as plant matures.
Epipremnum aureum (Araceae)	Golden pathos, Hunter's robe, Taro vine, Amarillo	Climbing vine with large heart-shaped yellow streaked leaves. Outdoor plants in the tropics, indoor potted plant (leaves are much smaller).
Euphorbia pulcherrima (Euphorbiaceae)	Poinsettia, Christmas flower, Christmas star	Perennial shrub with milky, white sap throughout. Leaves alternate, petioled, distinctly veined, entire or lobed, and conspicuously bright red, pink, or white (terminal leaves), lower leaves remain green. Flowers small and inconspicuous.
Ficus spp (Moraceae)	Weeping fig, Rubber tree, Climbing fig	Numerous species (trees/shrubs/ vines) within the family. Milky sap (leaves, stems) in all. Commonly cultivated as potted and/or indoor landscape houseplants.
Hedera spp (Araliaceae)	Canary ivy, English ivy, Common ivy	Climbing vine (wall cover); leaves with 5 lobes on young and root-free stems; non-lobed leaves (mature sections and root-free stems). Fruits are black berries when mature. Plant escapes cultivation; common houseplants.
Hyacinthus spp (Liliaceae)	Hyacinths	Garden ornamentals that grow from bulbs (close resemblance to onion bulbs) and flower in early spring. Bulbs harvested and stored in fall for replanting in spring.
Ilex aquifolium (Aquifoliaceae)	English holly, European holly	Evergreen shrub with leaves leathery, glossy upper surface, spiny toothed, alternate, and petioled; fruits red to yellow berries with many seeds and aromatic taste.

TABLE 7 POISONOUS HOUSEPLANTS AND ORNAMENTALS[a] *(continued)*

Comments and Toxic Principles and Effects	Treatment
Cardiac glycosides (digitoxin, digitalin, digoxin, and others), saponins, and alkaloids found throughout plant. Potency not affected by drying. Generally, acute abdominal pain, vomiting, bloody diarrhea, frequent urination, irregular slow pulse, tremors, convulsions, and rarely death.	Symptomatic
Alkaloids, saponins, and resin found in leaves. Vomiting and severe diarrhea indicative of GI irritation expected. Clinical cases have not been reported.	Symptomatic, to correct fluid and electrolyte imbalance.
Entire plant is poisonous. Contains water-insoluble calcium oxalate raphides and unknown proteinaceous toxins throughout. Causes immediate intense pain (oral cavity) on chewing any portion of plant.	Oral pain resolves slowly without treatment. In severe cases, demulcents and analgesics may be indicated. Systemic involvement, if any, is not associated with raphide chewing and release of insoluble calcium oxalate.
Milky sap contains unknown toxic principle(s); irritates mucous membranes and causes excessive salivation and vomiting but not death. Toxicity (hybrid species) not supported experimentally. Toxic diterpenes (ingenol derivatives) found in other *Euphorbia* spp have not been found in this species.	Symptomatic; gastric lavage, activated charcoal, and saline cathartics should be considered.
Furocoumarins, psoralens, ficin, sesquiterpinoid glycoside, and triterpines are found in sap and implicated (although not clear) in dermatologic toxicity (contact dermatitis) in pets/people.	Symptomatic and supportive care as needed.
Hederin, a saponin found in berries and leaves. Toxin poorly absorbed on ingestion; therefore, limited toxic effects observed. Large exposure dose results in GI effects (abdominal discomfort, diarrhea). Allergic sensitization common in people (contact dermatitis).	Concerns GI-associated problems (dehydration, vomiting, and electrolyte disturbances). Correct dehydration; antiemetics and electrolyte supplementation.
Calcium oxalate crystals and alkaloids (toxic potential yet to be defined) found in bulbs. After ingestion of toxic dose (bulbs), vomiting, diarrhea, and rare deaths reported. Bulbs in storage may be accessible to pets.	Symptomatic
Saponins; an alkaloid (theobromine), triterpene compounds, and unknown compounds with digitalis-like cardiotonic activity have been found in leaves, fruits, and seeds. Abdominal pain, vomiting, and diarrhea seen after ingestion of ≥2 berries. Death rare.	Symptomatic (at best)

(continued)

TABLE 7 POISONOUS HOUSEPLANTS AND ORNAMENTALS[a] *(continued)*

Scientific Name (Family)	Common Name	Important Characteristics
Kalanchoe spp (Crassulaceae)	Kalanchoe, Air plant, Cathedral bells	Winter flowering, herbaceous, succulent, nonhardy annuals or perennials. Fleshy, serrate or crenate, opposite, petioled leaves. Bright red, orange, or pink flowers in umbel. Stems become woody and untidy with age.
Lilium longiflorum, L tigrinum (Liliaceae)	Easter lily, Trumpet lily	Plants grown from bulbs; leaves alternate or whorled, sessile, linear or lanceolate blades; large showy funnel-form flowers. Fruits capsules with numerous, flat seeds.
Narcissus spp (Amaryllidaceae)	Daffodils, Amaryllis, Naked lady lily	Plant grown from bulb with leaves arising from ground. Flower(s) white or yellow arising from stalk. Plant grows from bulb (extends partially above ground). Flowers of various colors, red, pink, and white most common.
Persea americana (Lauraceae)	Avocado pear, Alligator pear	Trees or shrubs with long branches arising from terminal buds, widely cultivated for its fruits. Three commonly cultivated races (Mexican, Guatemalan, and West Indies). Leaves ovate-elliptical, entire, alternate, veined, dark-green above and paler below, papery to the feel. Flowers inconspicuous, yellow-green in axillary or terminal panicles; fruit berry, ovoid to pyriform in shape with thick, leathery, glossy dark green skin over lime-green to yellow flesh and a smooth, ovoid, solitary seed.
Philodendron spp (Araceae)	Philodendron	Climbing vines with aerial roots; leaves (major attraction as a houseplant) are large, unlobed or pinnately lobed and heart-shaped; rarely flowering.
Phoradendron flavescens (Viscaceae)	Mistletoe	Perennial parasitic shrub that grows on deciduous trees. Evergreen, ovoid, opposite leaves on round, highly branched, green stem. White berries with single seed. Brought into homes during Christmas season.
Rhododendron spp (Ericaceae)	Azalea, Rhododendron	Evergreen or deciduous shrub with simple, alternate, entire leaves; funnel-shaped flowers in terminal umbel-like clusters or solitary and of various colors; fruits are capsules with many seeds.

TABLE 7 POISONOUS HOUSEPLANTS AND ORNAMENTALS[a] *(continued)*

Comments and Toxic Principles and Effects	Treatment
Cardiac glycosides found in leaves. Within hours of ingesting toxic dose, depression, rapid breathing, teeth grinding, ataxia, paralysis, opisthotonos (rabbit), and death (rat).	Symptomatic; atropine has been effective in rabbits.
Unknown toxin found throughout plants. Renal failure in cats 2–4 days after ingestion. Not reported toxic to other species. Vomiting, depression, loss of appetite within 12 hr after ingestion. Increased creatinine, BUN, phosphorus, and potassium indicate toxicity.	Emetics, activated charcoal, saline cathartic, and nursing care—as for renal failure—within hours of ingestion. Delayed treatment is associated with poor prognosis.
Bulbs are poisonous; contain lycorine and related phenanthridine alkaloids. If small dose ingested, few or no clinical signs; if large-dose exposure, vomiting, abdominal discomfort, diarrhea, dehydration, and electrolyte imbalance.	Most exposures result in limited toxic responses and resolve without treatment. In large-dose exposure, symptomatic treatment with rehydration, antiemetics, electrolyte replacement.
All above-ground parts (leaves in particular) reported toxic to cattle, horses, goats, rabbits, canaries, ostriches, and fish. Responsible toxin a monoglyceride. Oil found in fruits used for cosmetic purposes. Toxicity associated with noninfectious agalactia (cattle, rabbits, goats), pulmonary congestion, cardiac arrhythmia, submandibular edema, acute death (rabbits, caged birds, goats), respiratory distress, generalized congestion, subcutaneous edema, and hydropericardium (suggestive of cardiac failure [caged birds]). In caged birds, clinical signs may be seen within 24 hr (usually after ≥12 hr), with death 1–2 days after exposure.	Primarily symptomatic and supportive (*see* p 2964).
Calcium oxalate crystals and unidentified proteins throughout entire plant. On ingestion, immediate pain, local irritation to mucous membranes, excessive salivation, edematous tongue and pharynx, dyspnea, and renal failure. Excitability, nervous spasms, convulsions, and occasional encephalitis reported in cats.	Symptomatic
Amines (β-phenylethylamine, acetylcholine, choline, and tyramine), toxic proteins (viscotoxins), and unknowns in all parts. Vomiting, profuse diarrhea, dilated pupils, rapid labored breathing, shock, and death from cardiovascular collapse within hours of ingesting toxic dose.	Symptomatic
Andromedotoxins (grayanotoxins) found in all parts, including pollen and nectar. Within hours of ingestion of toxic dose (1 g/kg), salivation, lacrimation, vomiting, diarrhea, dyspnea, muscle weakness, convulsions, coma, and death. Signs may last several days, but toxin is not cumulative.	Symptomatic; gastric lavage, activated charcoal, saline cathartics, calcium injection, and antibiotics to control possible pneumonia suggested.

(continued)

TABLE 7 POISONOUS HOUSEPLANTS AND ORNAMENTALS[a] *(continued)*

Scientific Name (Family)	Common Name	Important Characteristics
Sansevieria spp (Agavaceae)	Sansevieria, Snake plant, Mother-in-law's tongue	Hardy, succulent houseplant. Leaves erect, elongate, lanceolate, and flat or cylindrical, dark green with or without a yellow stripe along the margins, and horizontal gray bands throughout; many yellow star-like flowers on tall central raceme or spike.
Schefflera spp (Araliaceae)	Schefflera, Umbrella tree	Fast-growing evergreen with glossy, palmately compound leaves that hang and spread, appearing like an umbrella. Depending on the species, leaflets increase with plant maturity and become more compact; veins pronounced; margins entire to slightly crenate.
Solanum pseudocapsicum (Solanaceae)	Jerusalem cherry	Shrub with simple, lanceolate, entire or slightly serrated leaves. Small, star-shaped white flowers. Ripe fruits are red, shiny berries with many white seeds.
Taxus spp (Taxaceae)	Yew	Evergreen tree or small erect shrub with alternate, needle-like, glossy (upper surface), dull (lower surface) leaves. Seeds (generally one per fruit) black-brown or green, nearly enclosed in a cup-shaped, fleshy, red covering (aril).
Zamia pumila (Zamiaceae)	Coontie, Florida arrowroot, Seminole bread, Cycad	Palm-like plant with thick underground fleshy, tuberous stem from which grow few pinnately compound, palm-like leaves ~2 ft long; cones containing inch-long, shiny, orange-red seeds.

[a] Images for many of the plants described here, as well as for plants of Australia, the Caribbean, and South Africa, are available online at www.merckvetmanual.com.

TABLE 7 POISONOUS HOUSEPLANTS AND ORNAMENTALS[a] *(continued)*

Comments and Toxic Principles and Effects	Treatment
Hemolytic saponin and organic acids found in leaves and flowers. Vomiting, salivation, diarrhea, and hemolysis related to GI activity of these compounds.	Symptomatic; fluids and electrolytes may be necessary.
Oxalate found in the leaves. Mucous membrane irritation, salivation, anorexia, vomiting, and if severe enough, diarrhea.	Symptomatic
Solanocapsine and related alkaloids found in leaves and fruits. Anorexia, abdominal pain, vomiting, hemorrhagic diarrhea, salivation, progressive weakness or paralysis, dyspnea, bradycardia, circulatory collapse, dilated pupils, and convulsions reported.	Symptomatic; gastric lavage, activated charcoal, electrolytes and fluids, and anticonvulsants suggested.
The alkaloids (taxines and ephedrine), cyanide, and volatile oils found throughout plant except the fleshy aril. Nervousness, trembling, ataxia, dyspnea, collapse; bradycardia progressing to cardiac standstill and death without struggle. Empty right side of heart; dark, tarry blood in left side of heart; limited nonspecific postmortem lesions.	Symptomatic at best; usually futile once clinical signs appear. Atropine may be helpful.
The glucoside cycasin and its aglycone methylazoxymethanol (a colon-specific carcinogen in mice) found in leaves, seeds, and stem. Ingestion associated with hepatic and GI disturbances and ataxia. Clinical signs are persistent vomiting, diarrhea, abdominal pain, depression, and muscular paralysis. A neurologic condition characterized by hindleg paralysis (hyperextension followed by incomplete extension) has been reported in cattle.	No specific therapy; IV fluids and symptomatic care recommended.

TABLE 8 POISONOUS RANGE PLANTS OF TEMPERATE NORTH AMERICA[a]

Scientific and Common Names	Habitat and Distribution	Affected Animals
DANGEROUS SEASON: SPRING AND FALL		
Allamanda cathartica, A blanchetti (Apocynaceae) Allamanda, Yellow allamanda, Golden trumpet, Purple allamanda	Native to tropical America (2 cultivated taxa in North America); indoors and as ornamentals.	Sheep, cattle, and goats
Cicuta spp Water hemlock	Open, moist to wet environments; throughout North America	All
Hymenoxys odorata Bitterweed	Roadways, lakebeds, flooded areas, overgrazed range; southwest	Sheep, rarely cattle
Hymenoxys richardsonii Pingue, Colorado rubber weed	Arid foothills (6,000–8,000 ft [1,800–2,400 m]); western	Sheep, cattle, goats
Oxalis spp, *O corniculata* (Oxalidaceae) Wood sorrel, Creeping lady's sorrel, Creeping yellow wood sorrel	Herb/ornamentals found as weeds, growing from rhizomes/bulbs in fields and/or grazing pasture; worldwide	Sheep, rarely cattle

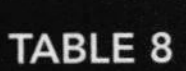

TABLE 8 POISONOUS RANGE PLANTS OF TEMPERATE NORTH AMERICA[a] *(continued)*

Important Characteristics	Toxic Principle and Effects	Comments and Treatment
DANGEROUS SEASON: SPRING AND FALL		
Perennial, evergreen shrub, climbing; leaves simple, whorled; leathery, margins entire, axillary glands at base; large showy, yellow or purple petal flowers; fruit is spiny capsule with numerous winged seeds.	The entire plant contains alkyliridoid-type terpinoids (allamandin, qallamandin, allamandacin), iridioids plumericin and plumieride, and little cardiotoxin. GI irritants in all parts (highest concentrations in the sap and roots). On ingestion, causes excess salivation, ruminal atony, abdominal cramps, diarrhea, dehydration, and electrolyte imbalance. Little cardiotoxic effects and no deaths. Lethal dose (fresh foliage) in cattle is 30 g/kg body wt.	Supportive, antidiarrheals
White flower, umbels. Veins of leaflets ending at notches. Stems hollow except at nodes. Tuberous roots from chambered rootstock.	Resinoids (cicutoxin, cicutol) in roots, stem base, young leaves. Toxicity retained when dry, except in hay. Rapid onset of clinical signs, with death in 15–30 min. Salivation, muscular twitching, dilated pupils. Violent convulsions, coma, death. Poisoning in people common.	Sedatives to control spasm and heart action. Prognosis good if alive 2 hr after ingestion.
Multibranched annual or perennial up to 2 ft high. Yellow flower head. Leaves divided into narrow glandular segments.	Sesquiterpene lactone (hymenovin) in fresh or dry plant. Salivation, vomiting, green nasal discharge, depression, anorexia, abdominal pain. Lesions include inflammation of GI tract, foreign body pneumonia, renal degeneration.	Toxin cumulative. Avoid overgrazing. Remove from pasture.
Perennial herb. Leaves bright green, divided into narrow glandular segments.	Same as for *H odorata* (above).	Same as for *H odorata*.
Annual/perennial with palmately compound leaves with 3 leaflets on erect or ascending stem. Inflorescence cymes or umbel or solitary flower; fruits are capsules with many seeds and basal ariels.	High oxalate contents throughout. Acute, subacute, or chronic manifestation after chronic ingestion. Clinical signs—progression from depression, weakness, labored respiration to prostration, coma, and death in 1–2 days in acute cases. Chronic cases—weight loss, anorexia, polyuria, edema, increased BUN and creatinine levels, failure to concentrate urine, presence of oxalate crystals in urine sediments, and renal failure.	Parenteral calcium solution. Supportive care to allow for tubular regeneration.

(continued)

TABLE 8 POISONOUS RANGE PLANTS OF TEMPERATE NORTH AMERICA[a] *(continued)*

Scientific and Common Names	Habitat and Distribution	Affected Animals
DANGEROUS SEASON: SPRING AND FALL (continued)		
Zephyranthes atamasco (Amaryllidaceae) Atamasco lily, Rain lily, Zephyr lily, Easter lily	Ornamental, commonly grows from bulbs in low woods and wet meadow areas.	Horses, cattle, and indoor pets (cats)
DANGEROUS SEASON: SPRING		
Baptisia spp (Papilionoideae, Leguminosae, Fabaceae) False indigo, Wild indigo, Rattle weed, Yellow indigo, Indigo weed	Open woods in Eastern North America on clay, loam, and sandy soils	Horses, cattle, goats
Caesalpinia spp (Leguminosae) Nikals, Grey nicker bean	Grown in the tropics in dry, open shrub or lowland rain forest. Found in southwestern USA. Ornamentals cultivated in warmer areas.	Cattle, sheep, probably horses
Nolina texana Sacahuista, Beargrass	Open areas on rolling hills and slopes; southwest USA and Mexico	Cattle, sheep, goats

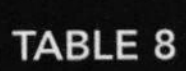

TABLE 8 POISONOUS RANGE PLANTS OF TEMPERATE NORTH AMERICA[a] *(continued)*

Important Characteristics	Toxic Principle and Effects	Comments and Treatment
DANGEROUS SEASON: SPRING AND FALL (continued)		
Basal leaves with star-shaped white flowers turning pink on fading.	Phenanthridine (lycorine, tazettine) and other alkaloids primarily in the bulbs but also in the leaves and flowers. Anticholinergic-type effects (inhibitor of protein synthesis, decreases heart rate, and cardiac abnormalities) in cats. Vomiting, excess salivation, bloody diarrhea (dehydration and electrolyte imbalance), seizures, cardiac function changes, and dermatitis.	Prompt resolution of dermatologic signs with discontinued exposure. Supportive care—antiemetics, antidiarrheals, and electrolyte replacement. Rarely lethal.
DANGEROUS SEASON: SPRING		
Herbaceous perennials, branched solitary stem, palmately compound sessile/short petiole, 3-leaflet leaves; terminal or axillary raceme inflorescence. Flowers with variably colored petals; legumes stipitate with one to many seeds. Plants black-gray or silvery gray when dry in the field or as hay.	Contains quinolizidine alkaloid cystisine, pyridine alkaloids anagyrine and baptifoline, and other related nicotine-like alkaloids. Interact with nicotinic, muscarinic, and acetylcholinergic receptors. On ingestion, causes severe diarrhea in cattle, decreased appetite, excess salivation, incoordination, and tremors. Fetal anomalies can be produced.	Remove animals from plant source. Symptomatic and supportive care.
Perennial tree, shrub, or herb armed with thorns, erect or climbing stem, 2 pinnately compound leaves, terminal racemes, showy yellow to orange or red flowers, legumes ovate with 2 to many seeds.	Gallotannins (30%–50%), phytohemagglutinins in fruit and flowers and diterpenoids pulcherralpin and caesalpin in the leaves. Within a few hours of ingestion, animals show vomiting, ± bloody diarrhea, abdominal discomfort, and dehydration. Not reported to cause death.	Supportive care—IV fluids, electrolytes, antiemetics, and antidiarrheals.
Perennial with many clustered, long narrow leaves. Stem mostly underground. Several flower stems with many small, white flowers in clusters.	Unidentified hepatotoxin (buds, flowers, fruit). Photosensitization, anorexia, icterus, prostration. Dark urine, yellowish discharge from eyes, nostrils. Lesions include hepatic and renal degeneration, GI inflammation.	Remove animals from area where plant grows during blooming season. Oral daily zinc oxide (not zinc sulfate) supplementation at 30 mg/kg body wt appears promising. (*See also* PHOTOSENSITIZATION, p 976).

(continued)

TABLE 8 POISONOUS RANGE PLANTS OF TEMPERATE NORTH AMERICA[a] *(continued)*

Scientific and Common Names	Habitat and Distribution	Affected Animals
DANGEROUS SEASON: SPRING (continued)		
Peganum harmala African rue	Arid to semiarid ranges; western USA	Cattle, sheep, probably horses and camels
Phytolacca americana Pokeweed, Poke	Disturbed rich soils such as recent clearings, pastures, waste areas; eastern half of USA	Pigs, cattle, sheep, horses, people
Quercus spp Oaks	Most deciduous woods; throughout North America	All grazing animals, mostly cattle
Sarcobatus vermiculatus Greasewood, Black greasewood	Alkaline or saline bottom soils, not in higher mountains; arid west. Dangerous season spring; may be year-round.	Sheep, cattle
Xanthium spp Cocklebur	Fields, waste places, exposed shores of ponds or rivers; throughout North America. Dangerous season spring and occasionally fall.	All animals, more common in pigs

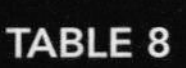

TABLE 8 POISONOUS RANGE PLANTS OF TEMPERATE NORTH AMERICA[a] *(continued)*

Important Characteristics	Toxic Principle and Effects	Comments and Treatment
DANGEROUS SEASON: SPRING (continued)		
Multibranched, leafy, perennial, bright green, succulent herb. Leaves divided. Flowers white, single.	Related β-carboline indole alkaloids (seeds, leaves, stems; seeds more toxic). Anorexia, hindleg weakness, knuckling of fetlock, listlessness, excess salivation, subnormal temperature, pollakiuria. Lesions include gastroenteritis, with hemorrhages on heart and under liver capsule.	Unpalatable. Eaten only under drought conditions. General supportive care most helpful.
Tall (to 9 ft), glabrous, green, red-purple, perennial herbs. Berries black-purple, staining, in drooping racemes.	Oxalic acid, a saponin (phytolacca-toxin), and an alkaloid (phytolaccin) in all parts; roots most toxic. Vomiting, abdominal pain, bloody diarrhea, hemolytic anemia, drop in production (dairy cattle). Terminal convulsions, death from respiratory failure. Lesions include ulcerative gastritis, mucosal hemorrhage, dark liver.	No specific remedy for intoxication. Supportive and symptomatic care helpful. Monitor for hypotension and other cardiac effects. Oils and protectants (GI tract). Dilute acetic acid PO, stimulants. Blood transfusion (hemolytic anemia).
Mostly deciduous trees, rarely shrubs, with 2–4 leaves clustered at tips of all twigs. Diverse leaf shape. Acorn fruiting body.	Gallotannin thought to be the toxin (young leaves and swollen or sprouting acorn). Anorexia, rumen stasis, constipation, followed by dark tarry diarrhea, dry muzzle, frequent urination, rapid weak pulse, death. Lesions include perirenal edema, nephrosis, gastroenteritis.	Diet must consist of >50% oak buds and young leaves for a period of time. Increased BUN with diet history diagnostic. Treatment symptomatic. Oral ruminatorics helpful. *See also* p 3152.
Large deciduous shrub with spiny stems. Fleshy, alternate, round in cross-section. Flowers inconspicuous.	Oxalates (sodium and potassium) 10%–15% dry weight (leaves primarily, less so in stems and fruits). Dyspnea, weakness, depression, some salivation, atony of GI tract, coma, death (neurologic effects and renal failure). Hyperkalemia, hypocalcemia, increased BUN. Lesions include hemorrhage and edema of rumen wall, ascites, swollen kidneys (renal tubular necrosis and dilation).	Toxic when large quantity consumed in short time. Do not allow hungry animals to graze plant. Parenteral calcium solution offers temporary relief but relapses.
Coarse annual herb. Fruit covered with spines, 2-beaked, with 2 compartments.	Carboxyatractyloside (seeds and young seedlings). Anorexia, depression, nausea, vomiting, weakness, rapid weak pulse, dyspnea, muscle spasms, convulsions. Lesions include GI inflammation, acute hepatitis, nephritis.	Seedlings or grain contaminated with seeds. Oils and fats PO may be beneficial; parenteral glucose and bicarbonate are reported helpful; warmth, stimulants IM.

(continued)

TABLE 8 POISONOUS RANGE PLANTS OF TEMPERATE NORTH AMERICA[a] (continued)

Scientific and Common Names	Habitat and Distribution	Affected Animals
DANGEROUS SEASON: SPRING (continued)		
Zygadenus spp Death camas, Meadow death camas, Grassy death camas	Foothill grazing lands, occasionally boggy grasslands, low open woods; throughout North and Central America	Sheep, cattle, horses
DANGEROUS SEASON: SPRING AND SUMMER		
Aesculus spp Buckeye	Woods and thickets; eastern USA and California	All grazing animals
Amianthium muscaetoxicum Fly poison, Stagger-grass, Crow poison, Gray fly poison	Open woods, fields, and acid bogs; eastern USA	All grazing animals
Delphinium spp Larkspurs	Either cultivated or wild, usually in open foothills or meadows and among aspen; mostly western USA. Dangerous season spring and summer, also seeds in fall.	All grazing animals, mostly cattle; sheep are somewhat resistant.
Descurainia pinnata Tansy mustard	Dense stands especially in wet years; arid southwest	Cattle

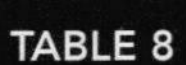

TABLE 8 POISONOUS RANGE PLANTS OF TEMPERATE NORTH AMERICA[a] *(continued)*

Important Characteristics	Toxic Principle and Effects	Comments and Treatment
	DANGEROUS SEASON: SPRING (continued)	
Perennial, bulbous, unbranched herbs with basal, flat, grass-like leaves. Flowers greenish, yellow, or pink; in racemes or panicles. No onion odor.	Cevanine-type veratrum azasteroid alkaloids, steroidal alkaloids, glycoalkaloids, and ester alkaloids (all parts). Salivation, vomiting, muscle weakness, ataxia or prostration, fast weak pulse, coma, death (central respiratory depression). No distinctive lesions.	Seeds most toxic. Leaves and stems lose toxicity as plant matures. Atropine sulfate and picrotoxin SC.
	DANGEROUS SEASON: SPRING AND SUMMER	
Trees or shrubs. Leaves opposite and palmately compound. Seeds large, glossy brown, with large white scar.	Glycoside, aesculin; also alkaloids and saponins in all parts, especially seeds and leaves. Depression, incoordination, twitching, paralysis, inflammation of mucous membranes.	Young shoots and seeds especially poisonous. Treatment only in severe cases. Stimulants and purgatives. Prevent access to toxic plant. Recovery in days. Rarely fatal.
Bulbous perennial herb. Leaves basal, linear. White flowers in a compact raceme, the pedicels subtended by short, brownish bracts.	Unidentified alkaloid, similar to those with *Zygadenus* (all parts). Salivation, vomiting, rapid and irregular respiration, weakness, death from respiratory failure.	No practical treatment. Especially dangerous for animals new to pasture. Keep animals well fed.
Annual or perennial erect herbs. Flowers each with 1 spur, in racemes. Perennial with tuberous roots. Leaves palmately lobed or divided.	Polycyclic diterpenoid alkaloids (eg, delphinine) in all parts, fresh or dry. Straddled stance, arched back, repeated falling, forelegs first. Constipation, bloat, salivation, vomiting. Death from respiratory and cardiac failure. Most often no lesions.	Young plants and seeds more toxic. Toxicity decreases with maturity. Antidote physostigmine rather than atropine.
Annual to 2 ft tall, stem and leaves covered with fine pubescence. Leaves alternate, deeply pinnately dissected. Inflorescence on elongated raceme. Flower small with 4 spreading yellow to yellow-green petals. Fruit is copula with 2 carpels and long waxy seeds in 2 rows.	Toxic principle unknown; must be grazed over relatively long period. Partial or complete blindness, inability to use tongue or swallow, "paralyzed tongue," "blind staggers," wandering, head pressing, emaciation, death if not treated.	Administer 2–3 gal. (8–12 L) water bid with stomach tube. Include nourishment if animal weak. Prognosis good if treatment started early. Possibly mustards cause same condition.

(continued)

TABLE 8 POISONOUS RANGE PLANTS OF TEMPERATE NORTH AMERICA[a] (continued)

Scientific and Common Names	Habitat and Distribution	Affected Animals
DANGEROUS SEASON: SPRING AND SUMMER (continued)		
Lantana spp Lantana	Ornamentals and wild; in lower coastal plain of southeast USA, and southern California	All grazing animals except horses
Senna obtusifolia Coffeepod, Sicklepod	Found in cultivated (corn, soybean, or sorghum) and abandoned fields, along fences, roadsides; naturalized in eastern USA	All grazing animals, mostly cattle, and poultry (*see* p 2861)
Senna occidentalis Coffee senna, Coffee weed, Styptic weed, Wild coffee	Common along roadsides, waste areas and pastures; naturalized in eastern USA	Cattle, horses, chickens, goats, sheep, rabbits
Tetradymia spp Horsebrush	Arid foothills and higher desert and sagebrush ranges, dense stands along trails; western USA	Sheep

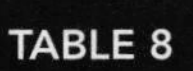

TABLE 8 POISONOUS RANGE PLANTS OF TEMPERATE NORTH AMERICA[a] *(continued)*

Important Characteristics	Toxic Principle and Effects	Comments and Treatment
DANGEROUS SEASON: SPRING AND SUMMER (continued)		
Shrubs. Young stems 4-angled. Leaves opposite. Flowers in flat-topped clusters, yellow, pink, orange, or red. Berries black.	Triterpenes (lantadene A and B) and unknowns in all parts, especially leaves and green berries. Anorexia, jaundice, watery feces, photosensitization. Lesions include degenerative changes in liver and kidneys. Death due to liver insufficiency, renal failure, myocardial damage.	Remove plants from pasture (herbicide 2,4-D susceptible). Keep animals out of light sources after eating plant.
Annual shrub frequently found in same fields as *S occidentalis*. Distinguishing features include leaflets fewer in number and more rounded. Seed pods long, round to 4-sided and more curved. Seeds shiny, brown, and rhomboid.	Toxic principles thought to be same as in *S occidentalis*. Clinical signs, although similar, less severe with *S obtusifolia*.	Treatment ineffective in down animals; salvaging most economic. Heat labile toxins not known to persist as residue. Meat from affected animals should be safe for human consumption.
Annual herb >3 ft tall, with glandular, alternate pinnately compound leaves (8–12 ovate to lanceolate leaflets, terminal pair largest). Flowers are yellow, axillary, solitary, or in short racemes. Long, flat, straight to slightly curved pods with clearly outlined seed contents. Of the pods, seeds, and wilted foliage, seeds are most toxic.	Anthraquinones (emodinglycosides and oxymethylanthraquinone), chrysarobin and lectin (toxalbumins), and alkaloids are associated with GI dysfunction and myodegeneration. Afebrile, ataxic, with diarrhea and coffee-color urine, recumbent but eat and are alert shortly before death. Increased serum CK and isocitric dehydrogenase activities; hyperkalemia and myoglobinuria frequent. Lesions include cardiac and skeletal muscle degeneration. Congestion, fatty degeneration, and centrilobular necrosis (liver) in addition to tubular degeneration (kidneys) also reported. Death probably due to hyperkalemic heart failure.	No specific treatment known. Symptomatic and supportive care essential. Although gross lesions similar to those of vitamin E/selenium deficiency, this therapy is contraindicated. Mineralocorticoid therapy may facilitate potassium excretion. Remove animals from source. Salvaging for economic reasons (*see Senna obtusifolia*, above).
Shrubs with yellow flowers in spring, not later. Leaves spiny, silvery white. Early deciduous.	Furanoeremophilanes (tetradymol and others). Photosensitization, "bighead," loss of hair and wool, skin ulcerations, blindness, secondary infections. Lesions include dermal necrosis and edema, hepatic and renal degeneration. Abortions may occur.	Photosensitization seen with concurrent ingestion of other green forages. Remove animals from plant source and sunlight. Antihistamines, topical antibiotics, and parenteral corticosteroids beneficial. Recovery slow and possibly incomplete.

(continued)

TABLE 8 POISONOUS RANGE PLANTS OF TEMPERATE NORTH AMERICA[a] *(continued)*

Scientific and Common Names	Habitat and Distribution	Affected Animals
DANGEROUS SEASON: SPRING AND SUMMER (continued)		
Veratrum spp False hellebore, Skunk cabbage	Low, moist woods and pastures, and high mountain valleys; western USA	Sheep, cattle
DANGEROUS SEASON: SUMMER AND FALL		
Acer rubrum Red maple	Moist land and swamps; eastern	Horses
Apocynum spp Dogbanes	Open woods, roadsides, fields; throughout North America	All
Centaurea repens Russian knapweed	Waste areas, roadsides, railroads, and overgrazed rangeland; not common in cultivated or irrigated pastures; mostly western and upper midwestern USA	Horses

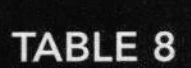

TABLE 8 POISONOUS RANGE PLANTS OF TEMPERATE NORTH AMERICA[a] *(continued)*

Important Characteristics	Toxic Principle and Effects	Comments and Treatment
DANGEROUS SEASON: SPRING AND SUMMER (continued)		
Erect herbs. Leafy throughout, leaves large and plaited. Flowers small and white or greenish.	Steroidal alkaloids. Vomiting, excess salivation, cardiac arrhythmia, bradycardia, dyspnea, muscle weakness and paralysis, coma, congenital cyclops in lambs from ewes exposed to *V californicum*.	Respiratory and heart stimulants.
DANGEROUS SEASON: SUMMER AND FALL		
A large tree at maturity. Leaves opposite, 2–6 in. across, palmately 3- or 5-lobed each, roughly triangular, and coarsely toothed. Red to yellow polygamous flowers. Fruit, a pair of 1-seeded winged units connected at base.	Unknown toxic principle(s) in wilted leaves. Methemoglobinemia, Heinz body anemia, and intravascular hemolysis; weakness, polypnea, tachycardia, depression, icterus, cyanosis, brownish discoloration of blood and urine.	Not common. Methemoglobinemia a prognostic indicator. Isotonic fluids, oxygen, and blood transfusion can be helpful. Methylene blue therapy not rewarding. Early ascorbic acid treatment essential for recovery.
Erect, branching, perennial herb with milky sap arising from creeping underground root stock. Leaves opposite. Flowers white to greenish white in terminal clusters. Fruit long, slender, paired, with silky-haired seeds.	A resinoid and glucoside with some cardioactivity found in leaves and stems of green or dry plants. Increased temperature and pulse, dilated pupils, anorexia, discolored mucous membranes, cold extremities, death.	Symptomatic (cardiotoxin) IV fluids and gastric protectants suggested.
Perennial weed with slender rhizomes. Stems erect and well branched. Leaves pinnately lobed to entire, not spiny, narrowed basally but not petioled and of decreasing length up the plant. Thinly pubescent or glabrous. Blue, pink, or white flowers. One-seeded fruit with whitish, slightly ridged attachment scar.	Unidentified alkaloid in fresh or dried plant. Chronic exposure, acute onset of signs. Inability to eat or drink, facial dystonia, chewing, yawning, standing with head down, severe facial edema, gait normal, head pressing, aimless walking or excitement most severe the first 2 days, become static thereafter. Death from starvation, dehydration, aspiration pneumonia.	More toxic than *C solstitialis* (below) but with similar pathology and prognosis. Some relief with massive doses of atropine but not an effective treatment. Euthanasia recommended.

(continued)

TABLE 8 POISONOUS RANGE PLANTS OF TEMPERATE NORTH AMERICA[a] *(continued)*

Scientific and Common Names	Habitat and Distribution	Affected Animals
DANGEROUS SEASON: SUMMER AND FALL (continued)		
Centaurea solstitialis Yellow star thistle, Yellow knapweed	Waste areas, roadsides, pastures; mostly western	Horses
Eupatorium rugosum White snakeroot	Woods, cleared areas, waste places, usually the moister and richer soils; eastern USA	Sheep, cattle, horses
Hypochaeris radicata Flatweed, Cat's-ear, Gosmore	Native to the Mediterranean and South America; widely distributed in the USA—Pacific states, eastern/southeastern USA	Horses
Oxytenia acerosa, *Iva acerosa* Copperweed	Arid, alkaline soils in foothills, sagebrush plains; western USA	Cattle, sheep
Perilla frutescens Perilla mint, Beefsteak plant	Ornamental originally from India, escaped to moist pastures, fields, roadsides, and waste places; southeastern USA	Cattle primarily, horses and other livestock susceptible

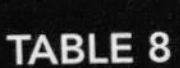

TABLE 8 POISONOUS RANGE PLANTS OF TEMPERATE NORTH AMERICA[a] *(continued)*

Important Characteristics	Toxic Principle and Effects	Comments and Treatment
DANGEROUS SEASON: SUMMER AND FALL (continued)		
Annual weed. Leaves densely covered with cottony hair. Terminal spreading cluster of bright yellow flowers with spines below. Branches winged.	Unidentified alkaloid. Involuntary chewing movements, twitching of lips, flicking of tongue. Mouth commonly held open. Unable to eat; death from dehydration, starvation, aspiration pneumonia.	Horses graze because of lack of other forage. Extended period of consumption essential for toxicity. Liquefactive necrosis of substantia nigra and globus pallidus (brain) pathognomonic. No treatment. Euthanasia recommended.
Erect perennial herb. Tremetol leaves, opposite, simple, serrated. Flowers small, white, and many. Often grows in large patches.	Complex benzyl alcohol (tremetol in leaves and stems). Excreted via milk; cumulative. Weight loss, weakness, trembling (muzzle and legs) prominent after exercise, constipation, acetone odor, fatty degeneration of liver, partial paralysis of throat, death in 1–3 days.	"Milk sickness" or "trembles." Treatment nonspecific and symptomatic. Heart and respiratory stimulants and laxative may be necessary. Remove animal from access to plant, discard milk (hazardous to people).
Perennial herb with viscid sap, stemless. Simple, serrated to lobed, basal, alternate leaves. One to several bright yellow flowers per plant.	Unknown; associated with but not proven cause of a neurologic condition in horses—stringhalt (hypermetria/hyperflexion of pelvic limb) in dry years. Sudden onset of abnormal gait; flexion/delayed extension of hocks, knuckling of carpal joints, laryngeal hemiplasia; spontaneous recovery possible, but condition could be permanent.	Tranquilizers, sedatives, mephenesin, and thiamine (questionable effectiveness); longterm phenytoin therapy seems helpful. Treatment with baclofen also reported helpful. Surgery (pelvic tenotomy of the lateral digital extensors) reported helpful.
Tall, annual/perennial herb with narrow leaflets. Flowers in many heads resembling goldenrod.	Unknown (pseudoguaianolide sesquiterpene lactones found in species—consistent clinical signs with these toxins); all above-ground parts, green or dry. Metabolic disease, anorexia, marked depression, weakness, coma; death without struggle within 1–3 days.	No specific treatment. Supplement diet or change pasture.
Annual, freely branched, squared stems. Opposite, purple or green, coarsely serrated leaves. White to purple flowers. Strong pungent odor when crushed.	Green or dry, 3-substituted furans (perilla ketone, egomaketone, isoegomaketone). Signs 2–10 days after exposure include dyspnea (especially on exhaling), open-mouth breathing, lowered head, reluctance to move, death on exertion. Lesions include pulmonary emphysema and edema.	Treatment ineffective once clinical signs severe. Parenteral steroids, antihistamines, and antibiotics may help. Handle gently (prevents exertion and death). Avoid/limit grazing during flowering and fruiting period.

(continued)

TABLE 8 POISONOUS RANGE PLANTS OF TEMPERATE NORTH AMERICA[a] *(continued)*

Scientific and Common Names	Habitat and Distribution	Affected Animals
DANGEROUS SEASON: SUMMER AND FALL (continued)		
Prosopis glandulosa Mesquite	Dry ranges, washes, draws; southwest	Primarily cattle, also goats; sheep resistant
Robinia pseudoacacia Black locust, False acacia, Locust tree	Open woods, roadsides, pinelands, on clay soils preferably; eastern USA	All grazing animals, mostly horses
Rumex crispus Curly dock, Dock, Sorrel	Commonly found on acid or sterile, graveled, seasonally moist soils of waste places, pastures, and fields throughout USA	Cattle, sheep
Solanum spp Nightshades, Jerusalem cherry, Potato, Horse nettle, Buffalo bur	Fence rows, waste areas, grain and hay fields; throughout North America	All

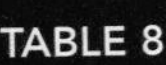

TABLE 8 POISONOUS RANGE PLANTS OF TEMPERATE NORTH AMERICA[a] *(continued)*

Important Characteristics	Toxic Principle and Effects	Comments and Treatment
DANGEROUS SEASON: SUMMER AND FALL (continued)		
Perennials, deciduous shrub or small tree with smooth or furrowed gray bark, paired spines. Leaves divided. Legume pod long, constricted between seeds.	Unknown principle in the beans. Chronic wasting with rumen atony, excess salivation, continual chewing. Partial paralysis of tongue, facial muscle tremor, submandibular edema, anemia. Lesions include emaciation, small firm kidneys and liver, gastroenteritis, filled rumen.	High sucrose content of beans alters rumen microflora, inhibiting cellulose digestion and B vitamin synthesis if grazed for extended period.
Tree or shrub. Deciduous, alternate, pinnately compound (>10 elliptic to ovate leaflets) leaves. Pair of spines at base of each leaf. Flowers in loose, fragrant, white to cream, drooping racemes. Flattened, brown pods containing 4–8 seeds.	The glycoside robitin, a lectin (hemagglutinin), and the phytotoxins robin and phasin found throughout plant, although flowers have been suggested as the toxic principles. Diarrhea, anorexia, weakness, posterior paralysis, depression, mydriasis, cold extremities; frequently laminitis and weak pulse. Death infrequent; recovery period extensive. Postmortem lesions restricted to GI tract.	Laxatives and stimulants suggested. Treatment symptomatic.
Perennial herb with erect stems, 3–4 ft tall. Leaves alternate, lanceolate to elliptic, finely crisped margins, base obtuse to cuneate, petioles form sheath around stem. Flowers small, numerous, greenish, in long terminal panicles; fruit an achene, papery 3-winged, with lustrous brown seeds.	Oxalic acid and soluble oxalate in leaves, stem, and seeds. Acute course (hypocalcemia, labored breathing, anorexia, depression, muscle fasciculation, tremor, weakness, teeth grinding, pulmonary edema, tetany, seizure, recumbency, and prostration); subacute (hypocalcemia, altered kidney function) or chronic course (renal fibrosis, renal insufficiency, and urolithiasis). Hemorrhage, edema (rumen and abomasal walls), and ascites (intestinal mucosa) seen in toxic cases. Death resulting from shock and hemorrhagic rumenitis.	In acute cases, death is too rapid for any treatment. Symptomatic and supportive care can be helpful. Remove animals from source. Calcium IV to correct hypocalcemia is ineffective. Give lime water to precipitate oxalate and prevent absorption. Allow animals to develop tolerance to oxalate by exposure to small amounts over time. Do not allow animals to graze pasture or offer hay highly contaminated with oxalate-producing plants.
Fruits small; yellow, red, or black when ripe; structurally like tomatoes; clustered on stalk arising from stem between leaves.	Glycoalkaloid solanine (leaves, shoots, unripe berries). Acute hemorrhagic gastroenteritis, weakness, excess salivation, dyspnea, trembling, progressive paralysis, prostration, death.	Pilocarpine, physostigmine, GI protectants. Seeds may contaminate grain.

(continued)

TABLE 8 POISONOUS RANGE PLANTS OF TEMPERATE NORTH AMERICA[a] (continued)

Scientific and Common Names	Habitat and Distribution	Affected Animals
DANGEROUS SEASON: FALL AND WINTER		
Allium cepa, A canadense Onions (cultivated and wild)	Cultivated and grown on rich soils throughout USA	Cattle, horses, sheep, dogs
Astrolepis sinuata cochisensis Jimmy fern, Cloak fern	Dry rocky slopes and crevices, chiefly limestone areas; southwest	Sheep, goats, cattle
Daubentonia punicea Rattlebox, Purple sesbane	Cultivated and escaped, in waste places; southeastern USA coastal plain	All
Glottidium vesicarium Bladderpod, Rattlebox, Sesbane, Coffeebean	Mostly open, low ground, abandoned cultivated fields; southeastern USA coastal plain	All

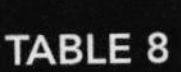

TABLE 8 POISONOUS RANGE PLANTS OF TEMPERATE NORTH AMERICA[a] *(continued)*

Important Characteristics	Toxic Principle and Effects	Comments and Treatment
DANGEROUS SEASON: FALL AND WINTER		
Biennials and perennials, bulb plants, onion odor. Leaves basal, green, hollow, cylindrical (*A cepa*), lustrous green, flat (*A canadense*); flowers on hollow flowering stalks, terminal umbels of many small blooms; fruits 3-celled capsules with many seeds.	N-propyl disulfide, an oxidant, in all parts. Anemia develops within days of exposure. Toxicosis in cattle associated with prolonged ingestion of large amounts of onions. N-propyl disulfide inhibits RBC glucose-6-phosphate dehydrogenase, leading to hemolysis and formation of Heinz bodies. Clinical signs are hemoglobinuria, diarrhea, loss of appetite, jaundice, ataxia, collapse, and possible death if untreated. Hemolytic anemia reported in livestock ingesting wild onions. Heinz body anemia; swollen, pale, necrotic liver; hemosiderin in liver, kidneys, and spleen are reported pathologic lesions.	Clinical signs similar to toxicity induced by S-methylcysteine sulfoxide (a rare toxic amino acid in *Brassica* spp) in livestock. Susceptibility to onion poisoning varies across animal species: cattle more susceptible than horses and dogs, which are more susceptible than sheep and goats. Remove animals from source and prevent future access to cull onions. Symptomatic and supportive care essential.
Evergreen from rhizomes, perennial, erect fern with divided leaves, folding when dry. Leaflets about as wide as long, scaly on back.	Unknown (excreted in milk). Nervous syndrome, incoordination, arched back, trembling, increased respiratory rate and pulse. Death when not allowed to rest.	No specific treatment. Supportive and general nursing care helps. Avoid driving during danger period. Provide ample watering, placed to avoid long walks. Allow rest if signs occur.
Annuals or perennials, shrub. Leaves pinnately compound with ≥20 leaflets. Flowers orange-red, rose, or purple. Legume pods (≥5 seeds) longitudinally 4-winged.	*S punicea* most toxic species (0.1% body wt toxic to sheep and cattle). Toxin(s) not fully characterized, but saponins are primary suspects; 12–24 hr delay in clinical signs after ingestion. Rapid pulse, weak respiration, diarrhea, death.	Symptomatic treatment; specific cause unknown. Seeds poisonous. Remove animal from source. Fluids and electrolytes for dehydration.
Tall annual. Legume pods flat, tapered at both ends, 2-seeded. Leaves pinnate, divided. Flowers yellow.	Unknown (green plant and seeds). In ruminants, hemorrhagic diarrhea, shallow rapid respiration, fast irregular pulse, coma, death. Lesions include hemorrhages in abomasum and intestines, dark tarry blood.	Green seeds are more toxic. Remove animal from source immediately. Symptomatic, general supportive treatment—saline purgatives, rumen stimulants, IV fluids.

(continued)

TABLE 8 POISONOUS RANGE PLANTS OF TEMPERATE NORTH AMERICA[a] *(continued)*

Scientific and Common Names	Habitat and Distribution	Affected Animals
DANGEROUS SEASON: FALL AND WINTER (continued)		
Halogeton glomeratus Halogeton	Deserts, overgrazed areas, winter ranges, alkaline soils; western USA	Sheep, cattle
Isocoma pluriflora (*Haplopappus heterophyllus*) Rayless goldenrod, Burroweed, Jimmy-weed	Dry plains, grasslands, open woodlands, and along irrigation canals; alkaline soils; southwestern USA and northern Mexico	Cattle, sheep, horses
Juglans nigra Black walnut	Native to eastern USA; now from eastern seacoast, west to Michigan and most of the Midwest, south to Georgia and Texas	Horses
Melilotus officinalis and *M alba* Sweet clover, White sweet clover	Commonly found on alkaline soils, fields, roadsides, and waste places; forage crop in southern and northern USA	Most commonly cattle, also horses and sheep
Sophora secundiflora Mescal bean, Coral bean, Sophora, Frijolito, Texas mountain laurel	Hills and canyons, limestone soils; southwestern Texas into Mexico	Cattle, sheep, goats

TABLE 8 **POISONOUS RANGE PLANTS OF TEMPERATE NORTH AMERICA**[a] *(continued)*

Important Characteristics	Toxic Principle and Effects	Comments and Treatment
DANGEROUS SEASON: FALL AND WINTER (continued)		
Annual herb. Leaves fleshy, round in cross-section, tip with stiff hair. Axillary flowers inconspicuous. Fruits bracted and conspicuous.	Oxalic acid, oxalate. Acute course. Rapid labored respiration, depression, weakness, coma, death. Lesions include hemorrhages and edema of rumen wall, swollen kidneys, oxalate crystals in kidneys and rumen wall.	Toxic dose consumed over short period. Increase water consumption. Standard therapy IV calcium borogluconate (helpful in cattle, delay deaths in sheep). Calcium supplement (83% alfalfa, 15% calcium carbonate, 2% molasses) in feed before grazing. Halogeton forage can be helpful. Herbicide 2,4-D control.
Bushy perennial 2–4 ft tall, with many yellow flowerheads. Leaves alternate, linear, sticky.	Complex benzyl alcohol (tremetol); resin acid; primarily nursing young and nonlactating animals. Reluctance to move, trembling, weakness, vomiting, dyspnea, constipation, prostration, coma, death.	"Milk sickness." Similar treatment to *E rugosum* intoxication. Prevent access to plants (growing season). Remove young and discard milk (hazardous to people).
Tree with deciduous, alternate, pinnately compound leaves (numerous lanceolate leaflets with serrated margins); leaflets in middle are largest. Male and female flowers on same tree but different inflorescences. Thick husked nut does not open when ripe. Twigs have chambered pith.	Juglone, phenolic derivative of naphthoquinone. Shavings with as little as 20% black walnut toxic within 24 hr of exposure. Reluctance to move; depression; increased temperature, pulse, respiration rate, abdominal sounds, digital pulse, hoof temperature; distal limb edema; lameness. Severe laminitis with continued exposure.	Nonfatal; laminitis and edema of lower limbs. Remove shavings promptly (relief signs). Treat for limb edema and laminitis. Improvement in 24–48 hr with no sequelae. NSAIDs are mainstay; prazosin, nifedipine are promising. Avoid corticosteroids (worsen existing vasoconstriction).
Annual or biennial herb 3–6 ft tall. Leaves alternate, pinnately compound with 3 obovate leaflets, serrated margins. Yellow or white flowers on racemes. Small 1-seeded pods.	*See* SWEET CLOVER POISONING, p 3156.	*See* p 3156.
Evergreen shrub or small tree. Leaves alternate, divided, and leathery. Flowers violet-blue, fragrant. Seeds large and bright red with hard seed coat, in legume pod.	Quinolizidine alkaloid (seeds and probably leaves). Violent trembling, stiff gait, falling on exercise, recumbent for a few minutes, becoming alert and eating.	Symptomatic. Toxic effect not cumulative, consume large amounts quickly. Seeds more dangerous when crushed.

(continued)

TABLE 8 POISONOUS RANGE PLANTS OF TEMPERATE NORTH AMERICA[a] (continued)

Scientific and Common Names	Habitat and Distribution	Affected Animals
DANGEROUS SEASON: FALL, WINTER, AND SPRING		
Melia azedarach Chinaberry	Fence rows, brush, waste places; southern USA	Pigs and sheep, others (dogs) less susceptible
DANGEROUS SEASON: ALL SEASONS		
Acacia berlandieri Guajillo, Catclaw, Blackbrush, Acacia	Semiarid rangelands; southwestern Texas into Mexico	Sheep, goats
Agave lechuguilla Lechuguilla	Low limestone hills, dry valleys, and canyons; southwest. Dangerous all seasons, especially spring.	Sheep, goats, cattle, usually during drought
Agrostemma githago Corn cockle	Weed, grainfields, and waste areas; throughout North America	All
Asclepias spp Milkweeds	Dry areas, usually waste places, roadsides, streambeds, western USA	All
Astragalus spp, *Oxytropis* spp (certain species only) Locoweed	Mostly western	All grazing animals

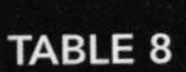

TABLE 8 POISONOUS RANGE PLANTS OF TEMPERATE NORTH AMERICA[a] *(continued)*

Important Characteristics	Toxic Principle and Effects	Comments and Treatment
DANGEROUS SEASON: FALL, WINTER, AND SPRING		
Small to medium deciduous tree. Fruit cream or yellow with a furrowed globose stone, persisting on tree through winter. Large amount required for intoxication.	Several alkaloids and a saponin (all parts), fruit most toxic. Restlessness, vomiting, constipation, cyanosis, rapid pulse, dyspnea, death within 24 hr.	Gastroenteritis usual. Recovery may be spontaneous. Laxatives and GI protectants suggested.
DANGEROUS SEASON: ALL SEASONS		
Deciduous shrub or small tree. Leaf divided. Flowers white to yellowish in dense heads. Fruit a legume with margins thickened.	Amine, N-methyl-β-phenylethylamine. Chronic course. Ataxia of hindquarters (limberleg), marked excitation, prostration, remain alert, death from starvation.	Dominates vegetation in some areas. Valuable to sheep industry due to high nutritive value and dominance. Supplement during drought to reduce possibility of poisoning.
Perennial, stemless, with thick, fleshy, tapered leaves having sharply serrated margins. Flowers infrequently with tall terminal panicle.	Unidentified hepatotoxin (causing photosensitivity) and a toxic saponin (abortifacient action). Subacute course. Listlessness, anorexia, icterus, yellow discharge from eyes and nostrils, photosensitization, coma, death.	Remove animals from range and provide shade. *See* PHOTOSENSITIZATION, p 976.
Green winter annual with silky-white hairs, opposite leaves, purple flowers, black seeds.	Saponin (githagenin) in seeds. Acute course. Profuse watery diarrhea, vomiting, dullness, general weakness, tachypnea, hemoglobinuria, death.	Maintain hydration (fluids and electrolytes) and control diarrhea. Oils and GI protectants. Neutralize toxin (dilute acetic acid PO). Blood transfusions may be necessary.
Perennial erect herbs, shrubs, vines, or small trees with milky sap. Leaves simple, opposite/whorled with entire margins. Seeds silky-hairy from elongated pods.	Steroid glycosides and toxic resinous substances (all parts), green or dry. Staggering, tetanic convulsions, bloating, dyspnea, dilated pupils, rapid and weak pulse, coma, death.	Sedatives, laxatives, and IV fluids suggested. Prevent plant consumption. Do not feed milkweed-contaminated hay.
Stemmed or stemless perennial herbs. Leaves alternate and pinnately compound. Flowers leguminous. Chronic intoxication.	Swainsonine. Depression, emaciation, incoordination, dry lusterless hair. Abortions. Neurovisceral cytoplasmic vacuolation, congestive right heart failure in cattle grazing at high altitudes.	Avoid grazing of source. Both green and dry plants toxic.

(continued)

TABLE 8 POISONOUS RANGE PLANTS OF TEMPERATE NORTH AMERICA[a] *(continued)*

Scientific and Common Names	Habitat and Distribution	Affected Animals
DANGEROUS SEASON: ALL SEASONS (continued)		
Astragalus spp (certain species only) Milk vetch, etc (many common names)	Nearly all	All grazing animals
Astragalus spp (certain species only— selenium accumulators) Many common names	Seleniferous areas, mostly western and midwestern	All grazing animals
Baccharis spp Silverling, Baccharis, Yerba-de-pasmo	Open areas, often moist; southeastern and southwestern USA	Cattle
Brassica spp, *Raphanus* spp, *Descurainia* spp, *Berteroa incana* Mustards, Crucifers, Cress; and for *B incana*, Hoary alyssum, Hoary false alyssum	Fields, waste areas, hay meadows, roadsides; throughout North America	Cattle, horses, pigs
Cestrum diurnum, C nocturnum Day-blooming jessamine and night-blooming jessamine, respectively	Open woods and fields; Gulf Coast states (Florida, Texas) and California	Cattle, horses, and dogs (ingesting cholecalciferol-based rodenticides)

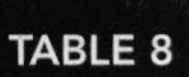

TABLE 8 POISONOUS RANGE PLANTS OF TEMPERATE NORTH AMERICA[a] *(continued)*

Important Characteristics	Toxic Principle and Effects	Comments and Treatment
DANGEROUS SEASON: ALL SEASONS (continued)		
As above.	Miserotoxin, other aliphatic nitro compounds. Posterior paralysis, goose-stepping, depression, rough coat, pulmonary emphysema, acute death, cord demyelination.	Avoid grazing of preflower stage.
As above.	Selenium (chronic). Slow growth, reproductive failure, loss of hair, sore feet, acute death.	Avoid grazing seleniferous plants for extended periods. *See* SELENIUM TOXICOSIS, p 3085.
Shrubs. Numerous small, whitish flowers. Leaves resin-dotted and persistent southward.	Unidentified. Acute course. Rumen stasis, bloat, anorexia, excess salivation, diarrhea, staggering, trembling, restlessness, polypnea, tachycardia, death.	Most dangerous in early growing stage. Toxin concentrated in leaves and flowers. No specific treatment. Treatment toward relief of diarrhea is best.
Annuals/biennials herbaceous weeds with terminal clusters of yellowish flowers and slender, elongated seed pods.	Glucosinolates (isothiocyanate, thiocyanates, nitrites) in seeds and vegetative parts, fresh or dry. Acute/chronic course. Anorexia, severe gastroenteritis, salivation, diarrhea, paralysis, photosensitization, hemoglobinuria. Unknown toxin(s) in *B incana* cause rapid onset of transient distal limb edema, laminitis (horses), and severe GI disturbances with continued exposure. Late abortions and/or weak, premature foals at birth.	No specific treatment (*B incana* disease in horses). Phenylbutazone, flunixin, furosemide or other diuretics helpful in relieving pain, inflammation, and edema. Remove from source. Administer GI protectants (mineral oil).
Evergreen shrubs or tall bush; leaves alternate, ovate smooth-edged; flowers white, tubular, small clusters, fragrant by day; fruit, a greenish-white to lavender (immature), becoming dark purple to black (mature), fleshy berry, with several small, black, oblong seeds, dispersed by birds in droppings. Leaves longer, night fragrant flowers, white fruits at maturity (*C nocturnum*).	Atropine-like alkaloids (fruit), saponins (fruit and sap), and glycosides of 1,25-dihydroxycholecalciferol (leaves primarily, stem, fruits, and roots) are found. Gastroenteritis develops on ingestion of fruits. Vomiting, depression, anorexia, chronic weight loss with normal appetite, choppy stiff gait, increased pulse, persistent hypercalcemia and hyperphosphatemia, calcinosis (aorta, carotid and pulmonary arteries, tendons, ligaments, and kidneys). Parathyroid atrophy, thyroid (C-cell) hypertrophy, and osteopetrosis reported with chronic ingestion of leaves.	Prevent further access of animals to plants. In early stages, treatment might be effective and cost-effective. Correct fluid and electrolyte imbalances in cases with persistent vomiting or diarrhea. Reduce or prevent hypercalcemia (calciuresis, diuretics, steroids, calcitonin). Maintenance therapy of diuretics and steroids may be necessary.

(continued)

TABLE 8 POISONOUS RANGE PLANTS OF TEMPERATE NORTH AMERICA[a] *(continued)*

Scientific and Common Names	Habitat and Distribution	Affected Animals
DANGEROUS SEASON: ALL SEASONS (continued)		
Conium maculatum Poison hemlock	Roadside ditches, damp waste areas; throughout North America	All
Crotalaria spp Crotalaria, Rattlebox	Fields and roadsides; eastern and central USA	All
Cynoglossum officinale Hound's tongue	Common in waste places, roadsides, and pastured areas throughout USA	Cattle, sheep, horses
Datura stramonium Jimson weed, Thorn apple	Fields, barn lots, trampled pastures, and waste places on rich bottom soils; throughout North America	All

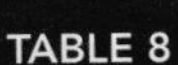

TABLE 8 POISONOUS RANGE PLANTS OF TEMPERATE NORTH AMERICA[a] *(continued)*

Important Characteristics	Toxic Principle and Effects	Comments and Treatment
DANGEROUS SEASON: ALL SEASONS (continued)		
Purple-spotted hollow stem. Leaves resemble parsley, parsnip odor when crushed. Taproot. Flowers white, in umbels.	Piperidine alkaloids (coniine and others) in vegetative parts. Acute course. Dilated pupils; weakness; staggering gait; slow pulse, progressing to rapid and thready. Slow, irregular breathing; death from respiratory failure. Teratogenic in cattle.	Coniine excreted via lungs and kidneys, mousy odor of breath and urine diagnostic. Administer saline cathartics; neutralize alkaloids with tannic acid, together with stimulants.
Annual or perennial legume. Yellow flowers in racemes, pods inflated. Bracts at base of pedicels of flowers and fruits persistent. Leaves simple or divided. Seeds in harvested grain.	Pyrrolizidine alkaloid (monocrotaline) and other unidentified alkaloids (all parts, especially seeds). Chronic course. Chickens—diarrhea, pale comb, ruffled feathers; horses—unthriftiness, ataxic, walking in circles, icterus; cattle—bloody diarrhea, icterus, rough coat, edema, weakness. Death may occur from a few weeks to months after ingestion.	Cumulative, fresh or dry. No treatment.
Annual or biennial herbaceous plant, rough hairy stem and foliage, 3–4 ft tall. Leaves alternate, oblanceolate, narrowed to petiole (lower), lanceolate, sessile, clasping (upper). Flowers numerous in coiled racemes, without bracts, blue, purple, or white blooms. Fruit, burr-like from 4 nutlets, thickly covered with hooked prickles.	Pyrrolizidine alkaloids (0.6%–2.1% of dry matter) including heliosupine and echinatine in the foliage. Unpleasant odor discourages consumption when fresh, becomes palatable in hay and is readily consumed. Toxic insult primarily hepatic and chronic in nature. Pyrrolizidine alkaloids (inactive) undergo hepatic metabolization to active intermediates—pyrroles (alkylating agent), which are toxic. Clinical signs are anorexia, depression, rough hair coat, hemorrhage, tenesmus, bloody feces, ataxia, jaundice, death. Hepatic lesions of necrosis, edema, megalocytosis, bile duct hyperplasia, and cytoplasmic vacuolation reported.	Know source and quality of hay. Treatment symptomatic and supportive at best. Affected animals seldom recover.
Leaves wavy. Flower large (4 in.), white, tubular. Fruit a spiny pod, 2 in. (5 cm) long.	Tropane alkaloids (atropine, scopolamine, hyoscyamine) in all parts, seeds in particular. Acute course. Weak rapid pulse and heartbeat, dilated pupils, dry mouth, incoordination, convulsions, coma.	All parts, mainly in hay or silage. Urine from animal dilates pupils of laboratory animals (diagnostic). Treatment nonspecific; cardiac and respiratory stimulants (physostigmine, pilocarpine, arecoline).

(continued)

TABLE 8 POISONOUS RANGE PLANTS OF TEMPERATE NORTH AMERICA[a] *(continued)*

Scientific and Common Names	Habitat and Distribution	Affected Animals
DANGEROUS SEASON: ALL SEASONS (continued)		
Drymaria pachyphylla Inkweed, Thickleaf drymary	Heavy alkaline clay soil in low areas or dry, overgrazed pastures; southwestern USA	Cattle, sheep, goats
Festuca arundinacea Tall fescue	A coarse, hardy, drought-resistant grass; Pacific Northwest, Missouri, Oklahoma, and Kentucky; major pasture grass in southeastern USA	Mostly cattle and horses
Gelsemium sempervirens, G rankinii Yellow jessamine, Evening trumpet flower, Carolina jessamine	Open woods, thickets, swamps, low areas, and open fields; southeastern USA	All
Gutierrezia microcephala Threadleaf, Snakeweed, Small-head matchweed, Sticky snakeweed	Widespread over dry range and desert; primarily southwestern USA	Cattle, sheep, goats, pigs
Helenium hoopesii Orange sneezeweed	Moist slopes and well-drained mountain meadows; abundant in overgrazed areas; western USA	Sheep, rarely cattle
Helenium microcephalum Small head sneezeweed	Moist ground; southern USA	Cattle, sheep, goats

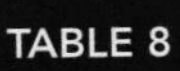

TABLE 8 POISONOUS RANGE PLANTS OF TEMPERATE NORTH AMERICA[a] *(continued)*

Important Characteristics	Toxic Principle and Effects	Comments and Treatment
DANGEROUS SEASON: ALL SEASONS (continued)		
Multibranched, succulent, prostrate annual. Opposite or whorled appearing leaves. Small white flowers.	Problem in heavily overgrazed areas. Unknown toxin. Sudden onset of diarrhea, restlessness, depression, coma, death. Lesions include gastroenteritis with congestion of liver, kidneys, spleen. Petechial hemorrhages on heart.	Dangerous during drought, after rain, or at night. Avoid overstocking to improve range. In well-fed and watered animals, little or no problem observed. Poor response to treatment.
Coarse, deeply rooted perennial grass. Broad, dark-green, ribbed, rough upper surface, and smooth sheathed leaves. Grows in clumps.	*See* FESCUE POISONING, p 3016.	*See* p 3016.
Climbing or trailing vines. Evergreen, entire, opposite leaves. Yellow tubular flowers, very fragrant.	Potent neurotoxic alkaloids (gelsemine and others, related to strychnine) in all parts. Gelsemine the most toxic. Acute course. Weakness, incoordination, dilated pupils, convulsions, coma, death within 48 hr. Limberneck in fowl. Clinical signs indicative of a poor prognosis.	No specific treatment. Relaxants and sedatives suggested. PO administration of strong tea/ coffee or poison hemlock suggested on early exposure (before observation of clinical signs) seems helpful in reducing further toxin absorption (more basic stomach pH).
Multibranched, perennial (toxicologically significant), resinous shrub. Simple leaves, alternate; yellow-flowered heads.	Unknown. Steroidal effect of saponins, mono- and diterpene acids. Acute poisoning, anorexia, listlessness, hematuria, diarrhea followed by constipation. In cattle, abortions with retained placenta, stillbirths, or premature and weak calves.	No specific treatment. Supplementing diet will help but not entirely prevent abortion in cattle.
Annuals, biennials, perennial herb. Orange sunflower-like heads or yellow flowers. Leaves alternate.	Sesquiterpene lactones (helenalin, hymenoxin). Subacute course (spewing sickness). Depression, weakness, restlessness, stiff gait, salivation, pronounced vomiting, emaciation, eventual death.	Cumulative. Aspiration pneumonia frequent. Remove from access to plant. Graze sneezeweed areas for only short periods of time. Can graze intermittently with some success.
Annual, erect herb, simple-stemmed below, bushy above. Stem winged. Narrow leaves throughout. Flowers in small heads; disk pale red-brown, rays yellow.	Sesquiterpene lactone (helenalin) in flowering stage. Depression, weakness, restlessness, stiff gait, salivation, vomiting.	Cumulative. Remove from pasture. Cathartics may help.

(continued)

TABLE 8 POISONOUS RANGE PLANTS OF TEMPERATE NORTH AMERICA[a] *(continued)*

Scientific and Common Names	Habitat and Distribution	Affected Animals
DANGEROUS SEASON: ALL SEASONS (continued)		
Hypericum perforatum St. John's-wort, Goatweed, Klamath weed	Dry soil, roadsides, pastures, ranges; throughout North America	Sheep, cattle, horses, goats
Kalmia spp Laurel, Ivybush, Lambkill	Rich moist woods, meadows, or acid bogs; eastern and northwestern. Dangerous all seasons, especially winter and spring.	All, often sheep
Kochia scoparia Kochia, Burning bush, Fireball, Fireweed, Poor man's alfalfa	Throughout North America	Cattle, sheep
Ligustrum spp Privet, Ligustrum, Hedge plant	An ornamental; common as hedge; found at abandoned farm home sites, along fences, and in bottomlands; eastern USA	All livestock
Lupinus spp Lupines, Silky lupine, Sink lupine, Bluebonnet	Dry to moist soils, roadsides, fields, and mountains; throughout, but poisoning mostly western USA	Sheep, cattle, goats, horses, pigs

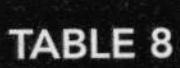

TABLE 8 POISONOUS RANGE PLANTS OF TEMPERATE NORTH AMERICA[a] *(continued)*

Important Characteristics	Toxic Principle and Effects	Comments and Treatment
DANGEROUS SEASON: ALL SEASONS (continued)		
Perennial herb or woody below. Leaves simple, opposite or whorled, dotted. Flowers many, yellow, with many stamens.	Photodynamic pigment (hypericin). Subacute course. Photosensitization, pruritus and erythema, blindness, convulsions, diarrhea, hypersensitivity to cold water contact, death.	Remove animals from source and sunlight. Corticosteroids parenterally, topical broad-spectrum antibiotics.
Woody shrub. Evergreen, glossy leaves. Flowers pink to rose, showy.	Resinoid (andromedotoxin) and a glucoside (arbutin) in vegetative parts. Acute course. Incoordination, excess salivation, vomiting, bloat, weakness, muscular spasms, coma, death.	Undigested rumen contents and ingesta in lungs at necropsy. Laxatives, demulcents, nerve stimulants, atropine.
Annual to 5 ft tall. Many branched stems give bushy appearance. Leaves petiolate, lanceolate, thin, and flat; alternate. Fruit has 5 wedge-shaped wings.	An alkaloid has been suggested. This plant may also accumulate nitrate and oxalate. Disease syndromes: photosensitization, weight loss, and polioencephalomalacia, which seems intensified by slow growth and sulfates.	Harvested foliage is source of toxin. Protect from sun in case of photosensitization; treat polioencephalomalacia with vitamin B. Supplement with copper (preventive against polioencephalomalacia).
Shrubs up to 15 ft tall. Simple, opposite, short-petioled, evergreen or deciduous leaves. Numerous small, white flowers in panicles. Fruit is 1- to 2-seeded, black or dark blue berry that persists throughout winter.	Ligustrin, ligustron, syringin, syringopicrin, and other unknown compounds in leaves and fruit. Primarily GI irritants. Diarrhea, abdominal pain, incoordination, paresis, weak pulse, hypothermia, convulsions, sometimes death.	Treatment symptomatic and supportive; correct dehydration.
Perennials. Leaves simple or palmately divided. Flowers blue, white, red, or yellow in terminal raceme.	Quinolizidine alkaloids (20 known) concentrated in seeds (fresh and dry); some piperidine alkaloids. Acute course. Inappetence, dyspnea, struggle, convulsions, death from respiratory paralysis. Lupinosis (hepatotoxicosis) not a reported problem in the USA. Some species teratogenic in cattle (crooked calf disease, weak and deformed calves, stillbirths).	Do not disturb sick animals; remove from source as they begin to recover. No effective treatment, but survivors recover completely. *See also* p 3018.

(continued)

TABLE 8 POISONOUS RANGE PLANTS OF TEMPERATE NORTH AMERICA[a] *(continued)*

Scientific and Common Names	Habitat and Distribution	Affected Animals
DANGEROUS SEASON: ALL SEASONS (continued)		
Nandina domestica Nandina, Heavenly bamboo, Chinese sacred bamboo	Common ornamental in southern USA	All grazing animals, especially ruminants
Nerium oleander Oleander, Laurel rosa, Laurel blanco	Common ornamental in southern regions	All
Photinia fraseri, P serrulata, P glabra Fraser's photinia, Chinese photinia, Red leaf photinia, Red tip photinia	Common ornamental (hedge or screen) in southern USA	All grazing animals, mostly ruminants
Pinus ponderosa Ponderosa pine, Western yellow pine	Coniferous forests of Rocky Mountains at moderate elevations; western USA. Dangerous all seasons, especially winter.	Cattle. Sheep and deer seem not to be affected.
Prunus caroliniana Laurel cherry, Cherry laurel, Mock orange	Woods, fence rows, and often escaped from cultivation; southern regions. Dangerous all seasons, especially winter and spring.	All grazing animals

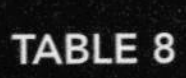

POISONOUS RANGE PLANTS OF TEMPERATE NORTH AMERICA[a] *(continued)*

Important Characteristics	Toxic Principle and Effects	Comments and Treatment
DANGEROUS SEASON: ALL SEASONS (continued)		
Upright, unbranched, and multistemmed, evergreen shrub, 3–7 ft tall. Alternate, bi- to tripinnately compound leaves; leaflets subsessile, elliptic-lanceolate, half as wide as long, entire, leathery, metallic bluish-green becoming purple in fall. Small, white flowers; 2-seeded, bright red berries in large panicles persist throughout fall and winter.	Cyanogenic glycosides in foliage and fruits, hydrolyzed in GI tract to free cyanide, thereby affecting cellular respiration. *See* CYANIDE POISONING, p 2959. Prognosis good if animal survives for 1 hr after signs begin.	Acute outcome precludes effective treatment for most; IV sodium nitrite/sodium thiosulfate treatment of choice. Picrate test indicates toxic potential of the plant. *See* CYANIDE POISONING, p 2959.
Evergreen shrub or tree. Leaves whorled and prominently, finely, pinnately veined beneath. Flowers showy, white to deep pink.	Digitoxin-type glycosides (oleandroside, nerioside, and others) in all parts, fresh or dry. Acute course. Severe gastroenteritis, vomiting, diarrhea, increased pulse rate, weakness, death.	No specific treatment. Atropine in conjunction with propranolol reported helpful.
Evergreen shrubs, 10–15 ft tall. Alternate, oblong-ovate serrated leaves, copper-red (when young) turning dark green in 2–4 wk. Prominent, whitish flowers in spring; showy, red berries in fall.	Same as for *N domestica* (above).	Same as for *N domestica*.
Evergreen tree, 150–180 ft. Leaves in groups of 3, yellowish green, 7–11 in. long. Small soft cones, seeds mature in 2–3 yr. Bark platy, reddish orange.	Unknown toxin (diterpene esters of isocupressic acid are suspected). Chronic course. Abortions in late gestation, stillbirths or weak calves, depressed, edema of vulva and udder, retained placenta.	Pine-needle ingestion during last half of gestation—may abort after single exposure. Supportive care, remove retained placenta, treat metritis, provide good nutrition. Keep pregnant cows away from source.
Leaves evergreen, shiny, leathery. Broken twigs with strong cherry bark odor. Fruit black.	Hydrocyanic acid (wilted leaves, bark, and twigs). Peracute course. Difficult breathing, bloat, staggering, convulsions, followed by prostration and death. Mucous membranes and blood bright red.	*See* CYANIDE POISONING, p 2959.

(continued)

TABLE 8 POISONOUS RANGE PLANTS OF TEMPERATE NORTH AMERICA[a] *(continued)*

Scientific and Common Names	Habitat and Distribution	Affected Animals
DANGEROUS SEASON: ALL SEASONS (continued)		
Prunus spp Chokecherries, Wild cherries, Peaches	Waste areas, fence rows, woods, orchards, prairies, dry slopes	All grazing animals, mostly cattle and sheep
Psilostrophe spp Paperflowers	Open range lands and pastures; southwestern USA	Sheep primarily; cattle and goats less susceptible and less likely to eat the plant.
Pteridium aquilinum Bracken fern, Bracken, Brake fern	Dry poor soil, open woods, sandy ridges, throughout North America	All grazing animals
Ricinus communis Castor bean	Cultivated in southern regions	All
Senecio spp Groundsel, Senecio	Grassland areas; mostly western USA	Cattle, horses, sheep to a limited extent in USA
Sorghum halepense Johnson grass	Weed of open fields and waste places; southern and scattered north to New York and Iowa	All grazing animals
Sorghum vulgare Sorghum, Sudan grass, Kafir, Durra, Milo, Broomcorn, Schrock, etc	Forage crops and escapes; throughout North America	All

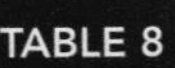

TABLE 8 POISONOUS RANGE PLANTS OF TEMPERATE NORTH AMERICA[a] *(continued)*

Important Characteristics	Toxic Principle and Effects	Comments and Treatment
DANGEROUS SEASON: ALL SEASONS (continued)		
Large shrubs or trees. Flowers white or pink. Cherries or peaches. Crushed twigs with strong odor.	Glycoside-yielding cyanide (rumen hydrolysis). Excitement leading to depression, dyspnea, incoordination, convulsions, prostration. Death may occur in 15 min from asphyxiation.	Mucous membranes, bright pink color; blood, bright red color. *See* CYANIDE POISONING, p 2959.
Perennial composite. Erect, woolly stems branching from base. Leaves simple, alternate, petioled. Many small heads of yellow flowers.	Sesquiterpene lactone. Depression, incoordination, anorexia, weakness, trembling, rapid irregular pulse and respiration, coughing, vomiting, aspiration pneumonia, death.	Antimicrobial actions of sesquiterpene lactone in rumen affect metabolism. Supplement diet with sodium sulfate and high protein.
Leaves firm, leathery, 3-pinnate.	*See* BRACKEN FERN POISONING, p 3089.	*See* p 3089.
Large, palmately lobed leaves. Seeds resembling engorged ticks, usually 3 in somewhat spiny pod.	Phytotoxin—ricin in all parts (seeds especially toxic). Acute to chronic course (death or recovery). Violent purgation, straining with bloody diarrhea, weakness, salivation, trembling, incoordination.	Diagnosis based on presence of seeds, RBC agglutination, precipitin test. Specific antiserum, ideal antidote; sedatives, arecoline hydrobromide, followed by saline cathartics suggested.
Perennial or annual herbs. Heads of yellow flowers with whorl of bracts below.	Pyrrolizidine alkaloids, volatile oils, and nitrogen oxides (fresh or dry). Acute poisoning not common. Dullness, aimless walking, increased pulse, rapid respiration, weakness, colic, delayed death (days to months). In cattle, prolapsed rectum from persistent straining. In horses, nervous signs evident in later stages.	Effects are cumulative. Liver biopsy diagnostic in early stages. Liver function test of value for subclinical condition in cattle. No general treatment. *See also* p 3150.
Coarse grass with large rhizomes and white midvein on leaf. Topped by large, open panicle.	Same as for *S vulgare* (below).	Same as for *S vulgare*.
Coarse grasses with terminal flower cluster. Some to 8 ft tall.	Hydrocyanic acid (drought, trampling, frost, second growth) and nitrate (heavy in vegetative parts). Acute course. Difficult breathing, bloat, staggering, convulsions, death. Blood bright red (cyanide) or chocolate brown (nitrate).	Hay safe for cyanide (volatile), not safe for nitrate (analyze). *See* CYANIDE POISONING, p 2959, and NITRATE AND NITRITE POISONING, p 3049.

(continued)

TABLE 8 POISONOUS RANGE PLANTS OF TEMPERATE NORTH AMERICA[a] *(continued)*

Scientific and Common Names	Habitat and Distribution	Affected Animals
DANGEROUS SEASON: ALL SEASONS (continued)		
Taxus spp Yew	Most of North America; Japanese and English yew common ornamentals	All except deer
Triglochin spp Arrowgrass	Salt marshes, wet alkaline soils, lake shores; dangerous all seasons, especially dry season; northern half of North America	Sheep, cattle

[a] Images for many of the plants described here, as well as for plants of Australia, the Caribbean, and South Africa, are available online at www.merckvetmanual.com.

PYRROLIZIDINE ALKALOIDOSIS

(Seneciosis, *Senecio* poisoning, Ragwort toxicity)

Typically, pyrrolizidine alkaloidosis is a chronic poisoning that results in hepatic failure. It is caused by many toxic plants, most commonly of the genera *Senecio*, *Crotalaria*, *Heliotropium*, *Amsinckia*, *Echium*, *Cynoglossum*, and *Trichodesma*. These plants grow mainly in temperate climates, but some (eg, *Crotalaria* spp) require tropical or subtropical climates. The plants most often implicated include ragwort (*S jacobea*), groundsel (*S riddellii*, *S longilobus*), rattleweed (*Crotalaria retusa*), and seeds of yellow tarweed (*A intermedia*).

Cattle, horses, farmed deer, and pigs are most susceptible; sheep and goats require ~20 times more plant material than cattle. Individual susceptibility varies greatly within species; young growing animals are most susceptible.

Etiology and Pathogenesis: More than 300 toxic factors (alkaloids with a pyrrolizidine base) have been found in plants, with some plants containing a mixture of several different pyrrolizidine alkaloid toxins. *S jacobea* contains jacobine; retrorsine, seneciphylline, and monocrotaline are other pyrrolizidine alkaloids frequently incriminated in toxicities.

These plants, which under normal conditions are avoided by grazing animals, may be eaten during drought conditions. Some animals may eat these plants preferentially as roughage when they are available on extremely lush pasture. Animals are also poisoned by eating the plant material in hay, silage, or pellets. Seeds from *Crotalaria*, *Amsinckia*, and *Heliotropium* spp, which have been harvested with grain, have caused disease in horses, cattle, pigs, and poultry.

TABLE 8 POISONOUS RANGE PLANTS OF TEMPERATE NORTH AMERICA[a] *(continued)*

Important Characteristics	Toxic Principle and Effects	Comments and Treatment
DANGEROUS SEASON: ALL SEASONS (continued)		
Evergreen perennial tree or shrub. Bark reddish brown then flaking in scales. Leaves linear, 0.5–1 in. (1.5–2.5 cm) long, 2-ranked on twig, upper surface dark green, lower yellow-green, midribs prominent. Flowers unisexual, inconspicuous. Fruit single stony seed. Bright scarlet color.	Toxic alkaloids in bark, leaves, seeds. Gaseous distress, diarrhea, vomiting, tremors, dyspnea, dilated pupils, respiratory difficulty, weakness, fatigue, collapse, coma, convulsions, bradycardia, circulatory failure, death. Death may be rapid.	Poisoning usually results when branches and trimmings fed to livestock.
Grasslike, except leaves are thick. Heads of fruits globular on erect raceme. Flowers inconspicuous.	Hydrocyanic acid in leaves. Salivation, dyspnea, excitement followed by depression, incoordination, prostration, convulsions followed by death from anoxia.	Often, animals found dead. *See* CYANIDE POISONING, p 2959.

The alkaloids are metabolized in the liver to highly reactive pyrroles, which produce cytotoxic effects on target sites, most commonly the nuclei of hepatocytes. Other target sites may include the epithelial and vascular tissues of the kidneys and lungs. These toxic pyrroles cross-link DNA strands and also unite DNA with nucleoproteins such as actin. These molecular alterations are presumed to create the cytotoxic, antimitotic, and megalocytic effects characteristic of pyrrolizidine alkalosis.

Clinical Findings: Hepatic pathology with associated clinical signs is the most common manifestation of pyrrolizidine alkalosis in domestic animal species. Acute intoxication is characterized by sudden death from hemorrhagic hepatic necrosis and visceral hemorrhages. This is a rare event, because the poor palatability of these plants makes rapid ingestion of large quantities of the toxins uncommon. More chronic exposure is typical, and the liver reflects the cumulative and progressive effects of repeated ingestion of small doses of toxin. Clinical signs may not be seen for several weeks or months after initial exposure. Consumption of the offending plant may even have ceased months earlier. The ongoing hepatic damage in these instances is suspected to be due to the recycling of toxic pyrroles as they are released from one dying cell and taken up by another. Clinical progression may also be altered by concurrent hepatic pathology; a hemolytic crisis may be precipitated in sheep with excessive hepatic copper stores (*see* p 3073).

In horses and cattle, signs include loss of condition, anorexia, dullness, and constipation or diarrhea. Tenesmus and passing of bloodstained feces may be followed by rectal prolapse, especially in cattle. Ascites and icterus may be present, and cattle and sheep sometimes show intermittent photosensitization (*see* p 976). Some animals become progressively weaker and reluctant to move. Others exhibit signs of hepatic encephalopathy such as head-pressing, yawning, aimless wandering, or even frenzied and aggressive behavior. Pica may be seen. Death may occur suddenly or after prolonged recumbency with hepatic coma and high levels of ammonia in the blood.

Less common clinical signs that have been described with pyrrolizidine toxicoses include inspiratory dyspnea in ponies due to laryngeal and pharyngeal paralysis, dyspnea due to interstitial pneumonia in horses, and renal disease in pigs.

Lesions: In acute cases, the liver may be enlarged, hemorrhagic, and icteric. In chronic cases, it is atrophied, fibrous, finely nodular, and usually pale with a glistening surface due to fibrous thickening of the capsule. Other livers are markedly icteric. The gallbladder is often edematous and grossly distended with thick, mucoid bile. Edema of the abomasum and segments of the bowel, mesentery, and associated lymph nodes is common, and there may be ascites. In some cases, numerous small hemorrhages are present in the abdominal serous membranes. The lungs of some severely affected horses may be emphysematous and fail to collapse (often due to ingestion of *Crotalaria* spp).

Characteristic histologic changes occur in the liver. Irreversible enlargement of individual hepatocytes (megalocytosis) is often seen; it is conspicuous in horses and sheep but less pronounced in cattle. In cattle, marked perivenous fibrosis of sublobular veins is usually present, but this is not a consistent finding in horses and sheep. In all species, increases in connective tissue, both within and around the lobules, are marked. Bile duct hyperplasia is variable but may be the most striking microscopic change seen in some livers. Pulmonary changes seen in horses exposed to some *Crotalaria* spp may include hyperplasia of bronchoalveolar epithelium, congestion, septal fibrosis, and emphysema. Renal tubular lining cells and glomerular epithelial cells also may be individually enlarged in pigs.

Diagnosis: Chemical analysis of whole blood for toxic metabolites can confirm recent exposure but depends on the half-life of RBCs to which these pyrroles are bound. An ELISA that recognizes riddelliine and closely related pyrrolizidine alkaloids present in whole blood has also been described but is not widely available. More commonly, a presumptive diagnosis is made based on clinical signs, compatible changes in biochemical parameters, and a history of exposure. When hepatic cirrhosis is extensive, hypoalbuminemia and hyperglobulinemia develop. Serum levels of fibrinogen, bilirubin, γ-glutamyltransferase, and glutamate dehydrogenase may be increased, but it should be recognized that the insidious nature of this disease can result in surprisingly mild serum biochemical changes. Hepatic biopsy is often useful, especially if megalocytic change is seen. Other hepatotoxins, such as copper or aflatoxin, as well as infections such as chronic fascioliasis, must be considered before making the diagnosis. At necropsy the diagnosis can often be made based on gross findings, together with characteristic histologic changes in hepatic, pulmonary, and/or renal tissues. Hepatic assay for pyrrolic metabolites can also be performed.

Treatment and Control: Further intake of toxic plant material must be prevented. Animals showing signs rarely recover, and lesions present in asymptomatic animals may progress and result in further losses over several months. Because high protein intake may precipitate clinical signs, rations high in carbohydrates are indicated. Supportive treatment for dehydration and photosensitization may be needed.

Preventing further outbreaks by reducing exposure should be stressed.

Sheep are commonly used for grazing control of these plants, but this practice carries risks unless sheep destined for early slaughter are used. Biologic control of plants with predator moths, flea beetles, and seed flies has met with variable success. *Senecio* and related toxic species in pastures have been controlled satisfactorily by annual herbicide applications, preferably in spring before hay or silage conservation.

QUERCUS POISONING

(Oak bud poisoning, Acorn poisoning)

Most animals are susceptible to *Quercus* poisoning, although cattle and sheep are affected most often. Most species of oak (*Quercus* spp) found in Europe and North America are considered toxic. Clinical signs occur 3–7 days after consumption of large quantities of young oak leaves in the spring or green acorns in the fall. Fallen trees associated with a recent storm are often reported with outbreaks. Feed restriction before exposure plays a crucial role enhancing susceptibility. Mortality as high as 70% may be seen. Malformed calves and abortions have been reported in dams consuming acorns during the second trimester of pregnancy. The toxic principle, which appears to be pyrogallol, gallotannins, polyhydroxyphenolic compounds, or their metabolites produced by microbial hydrolysis in the rumen, binds and precipitates proteins, which results in GI and renal dysfunction.

Signs include anorexia, depression, emaciation, brisket edema, dehydration, rumen stasis, tenesmus, smell of ammonia on the breath, serous ocular or nasal discharge, polydipsia, polyuria, hematuria, icterus, and constipation followed by mucoid to hemorrhagic diarrhea. Renal insufficiency, which is evident 4–6 days after exposure, may be characterized by increased BUN and creatinine, proteinuria, glucosuria, hyperbilirubinuria, hyperphosphatemia, hypocalcemia, and urine with a low specific gravity. Pale swollen kidneys characterized by coagulative necrosis of the proximal convoluted tubular cells, perirenal edema, subcutaneous edema, ascites, and hydrothorax are common necropsy findings. Edema and subserosal petechial or ecchymotic hemorrhage of intestinal mucosa and ulceration of the esophagus and rumen may be seen. Evidence of hepatotoxicity characterized by increased liver enzymes may also be present.

Diagnosis is based on clinical findings, necropsy, history, and histopathologic examination of the kidney (ie, nephrosis). Other common diseases that resemble oak poisoning include pigweed (*Amaranthus* spp) poisoning, aminoglycoside antibiotic poisoning, oxalate poisoning, and ochratoxicosis.

Consumption of a pelleted ration supplement (1 kg/head/day) containing 10%–15% calcium hydroxide plus access to more palatable feeds may be used as a preventive measure if exposure to acorns or oak leaves cannot be avoided. Calcium hydroxide, activated charcoal, ruminatorics, and purgatives (such as mineral oil [1 L/500 kg], sodium sulfate [1 kg/400 kg], or magnesium sulfate [450 g/400 kg]) may be effective antidotes if administered early in the course of disease. Polyethylene glycol (1 g/kg/day) administered in the feed or water will bind tannins and reduce tissue damage. Fluid therapy to correct dehydration and acidosis and transplantation of ruminal microflora may be beneficial. Clinical recovery usually occurs within 60 days but is rare if renal dysfunction is severe. Improved range management to limit grazing in immature oak stands will prevent development of the syndrome.

RYEGRASS TOXICITY

ANNUAL RYEGRASS STAGGERS

This often fatal neurotoxic disease occurs in livestock of any age that graze pastures in which annual ryegrass (*Lolium rigidum*) is present and in the seedhead stage of growth. It is seen in western and southern Australia and in South Africa from November to March. Hay of *Festuca rubra commutata* (Chewing's fescue) with *Rathayibacter toxicus*–infected seedhead galls has caused a similar disease in cattle and horses in Oregon. Outbreaks of ergot alkaloid toxicity in cattle on *L rigidum* have been reported in South Africa and should not be confused with annual ryegrass staggers.

In Australia, the responsible corynetoxins (members of the tunicaminyluracil group) are produced in seedhead galls induced by the nematode *Anguina funesta* and colonized by *R toxicus*. These bacteria-infected galls are present in infected annual ryegrass pastures from early spring onward, but they are most toxic when the plants senesce. Hence, animals show no sign of toxicity until late spring and summer. Spread of bacteria-infested nematodes to adjacent healthy annual ryegrass pastures is slow.

The corynetoxins are highly toxic glycolipids that inhibit specific glycosylation enzymes and therefore deplete or reduce activity of essential glycoproteins. Experimentally, the corynetoxins deplete fibronectins and cause failure of the hepatic reticuloendothelial system. Cardiovascular function and vascular integrity are consequently impaired, and peripheral circulation and oxygen distribution is compromised. Tunicamycin irreversibly downregulates the expression of specific γ-aminobutyric acid receptors and causes cell death in cultured brain neurons. Hence, the clinical expression of the disorder is nervous.

Outbreaks occur 2–6 days after animals graze a pasture that contains annual ryegrass infected at a toxic level. Deaths occur within hours, or as long as 1 wk after onset of signs. Characteristic neurologic signs are similar to those of perennial ryegrass staggers (*see* p 3154). However, mortality from annual ryegrass toxicity is commonly 40%–50% and occasionally higher. The lesions include congestion, edema, hemorrhage of the brain and lungs, and degeneration of the liver and kidneys.

Diagnosis is based on the characteristic neurologic signs of tremors, incoordination, rigidity, and collapse when stressed, with animals often becoming apparently normal again when left undisturbed. When animals are severely affected, nervous spasms supervene, and convulsions could be precipitated by either forced exercise or high ambient temperatures. A thorough history and evaluation of the pastures will assist in differentiation of staggers caused by other grasses such as perennial ryegrass, phalaris, and the ergots of paspalum and other grasses. Polioencephalomalacia and enterotoxemia are other differential diagnoses.

Clinical signs identical to those of annual ryegrass toxicity have been described in Australia in animals grazing *Agrostis avenacea* (annual blown grass), *Polypogon monspeliensis* (annual beard grass), or *Ehrharta longiflora* (annual veldtgrass) infected with nematode galls containing *R toxicus*. These diseases have been called flood plain staggers, Stewart range syndrome, and veldtgrass staggers, respectively. Although the same bacterium is responsible for all the diseases, the *Anguina* nematode vectors of *R toxicus* for these three grasses are different species than the *A funesta* associated with annual ryegrass toxicity. Whereas the inflorescences of annual ryegrass infected with *A funesta* usually appear normal, nematode-infested inflorescences of these other grasses show distinctive signs.

A significant increase in survival of sheep experimentally poisoned with tunicamycin was observed after treatment with derivatives of β-cyclodextrin. The promising result with this toxin-binding agent offers hope for treatment of animals once they have become affected with annual ryegrass staggers. Losses from the disorder can be minimized by early recognition of signs and removal to safe grazing or by reducing grazing pressure. Gall identification is difficult in annual ryegrass pastures, and in south Australia the bacterium in emerging seedheads is detected and quantified by ELISA. Early detection of toxic fields enables farmers to mow the heads off grass or to allow grazing before the grass becomes too toxic. Grazing of hay aftermath from toxic pastures should be avoided. Burning annual ryegrass pastures in the fall destroys most of the galls colonized by bacteria and minimizes the risk of toxicity in the following season.

PERENNIAL RYEGRASS STAGGERS

This neurotoxic condition of grazing livestock of all ages occurs only in late spring, summer, and fall and only in pastures in which perennial ryegrass (*Lolium perenne*) or hybrid ryegrass are the major components. Sheep, cattle, horses, farmed deer, and llamas are susceptible. In New Zealand, a high incidence most years causes considerable loss and seriously disrupts management procedures and stock movement. Perennial ryegrass staggers occurs sporadically in parts of North and South America, Europe, and Australia.

The tremorgenic neurotoxins responsible are lolitrems, mainly lolitrem B. These indole diterpene alkaloids are produced in perennial and hybrid ryegrasses infected with the endophytic fungus *Neotyphodium lolii*. The amounts of fungal hyphae and lolitrem B in infected plants increase to toxic levels as the temperature rises in late spring and decrease again to safe levels in the cooler seasons. Mycelia of the fungus are present in all above-ground parts of infected plants but are especially concentrated in leaf sheaths, flower stalks, and seed. Infected plants exhibit no signs, and the fungus is spread only through infected seed. Viability of the endophyte gradually declines when infected seed is stored at ambient temperatures and moderate to high humidity, so that few seeds contain viable endophyte after 2 yr. Lolitrem B acts as a potent large conductance calcium-activated potassium (BK) channel inhibitor. It is thought that the incoordination observed when animals are exposed to lolitrem B is caused by interference with neuronal transmission in the cerebellum; no specific histologic lesion is recognized. *N lolii* also produces the ergopeptine alkaloid ergovaline, which is the alkaloid responsible for fescue toxicosis. Ergovaline raises the temperature of animals in the warmer months of the year, inducing heat stress. It also depresses prolactin levels, and reduced milk yield in cows has been recorded in New Zealand and Australia.

Signs develop gradually over a few days. Fine tremors of the head and nodding movements are the first signs noted in animals approached quietly and watched carefully. Noise, sudden exercise, or fright elicits more severe signs of head nodding with jerky movements and incoordination when first moved. Running movements are stiff and bounding with marked incoordination and often result in collapse in lateral recumbency with opisthotonos, nystagmus, and flailing of stiffly extended limbs. In less severe cases, the attack soon subsides, and the animal regains its feet within minutes. If the animal is again forced to run, the episode is repeated. Signs are most severe when the animal is heat stressed.

Within flocks and herds, individual susceptibility varies greatly, and this trait is heritable. In outbreaks, morbidity may reach 80%–90%, but mortality is low (0–5%). Deaths are usually accidental, often by drowning when drinking from ponds or streams, or due to the inability to forage for food and water.

The strict seasonal occurrence of characteristic tremors, incoordination, and collapse in several or many animals grazing predominantly perennial ryegrass pastures strongly implicates this disease. Reference to the botanical composition of the pastures will exclude annual ryegrass toxicity (*see* p 3153) and paspalum staggers (*see* p 3019), which have similar clinical signs and seasonality. Microscopic examination of the leaf sheaths of the ryegrass sward will reveal the extent of endophyte infection.

Because movement and handling of animals exacerbates signs, individual treatment is generally impractical. Recovery is spontaneous in 1–2 wk if animals are moved to nontoxic pastures or crops.

Because the endophyte and the lolitrems and ergovaline are not uniformly distributed within ryegrass plants, control by grazing management can help reduce or prevent the disease. Lolitrems and ergovaline are concentrated in the leaf sheath and inflorescences. If pastures are not overgrazed down into the leaf sheath zone or grazed when the plants are flowering, then animals should be relatively safe even when a high proportion of the ryegrass plants are infected with endophytes. Encouragement of growth of other grass species and legumes in established swards also reduces the intake of toxic grass.

Safe new pastures can be established using ryegrass seed with little or no endophyte infection. Alternatively, seed that has been stored at ambient temperatures for 18–24 mo probably contains few viable endophytes and would produce nontoxic pastures. However, the presence of endophyte in grasses makes the plants resistant to attack from many insects; thus, infected pastures are more persistent than endophyte-free pastures. Cultivars of ryegrass artificially infected with a strain of endophyte that does not produce lolitrem B or ergovaline are available in New Zealand. Signs of ryegrass staggers have not been seen in animals grazing these grasses. A strain of *Neotyphodium* that produces compounds known as epoxy janthetrems has been developed that offers an extended range of pasture insect resistance with the trade-off of sporadic occurrence of low-level staggers.

SORGHUM POISONING

(Sudan grass poisoning)

Sorghum species are drought-tolerant plants that may produce neuropathic and teratogenic manifestations. Sorghum poisoning has been seen primarily in the southwestern USA and Australia. The syndrome is reported almost exclusively in horses, although a similar disease has been reported in sheep and cattle. Lathyrogenic nitriles such as β-cyanoalanine, cyanogenic glycosides, and nitrates have been suggested as causative agents. The syndrome develops in horses after they have grazed hybrid Sudan pastures for weeks to months and produces axonal degeneration and myelomalacia in the spinal cord and cerebellum. (*See also* CYANIDE POISONING, p 2959.) Consumption of the seed will not produce the syndrome.

Sorghum poisoning is characterized by posterior ataxia or incoordination, cystitis, urinary incontinence (which predisposes both male and female horses to cystitis), and alopecia on the hindlegs due to urine scald. The loss of urinary bladder function is related to degeneration of spinal cord neurons. The incoordination may progress to irreversible flaccid paralysis. Deformities of the fetal musculoskeletal system (ankylosis or arthrogryposis) and abortion may occur during late pregnancy. The diagnosis is based on the analysis of urine for evidence of cystitis, characterization of spinal cord lesions, and analysis of forage for cyanide. Although fatal poisoning is infrequent, the impact on reproduction is the primary concern. Consumption of sorghum hybrids with low cyanogenic potential or restriction of access to sorghum grasses may limit the incidence. Dietary supplementation with sulfur may be beneficial. Affected horses often die from pyelonephritis. Treatment with antibiotics may be helpful, but a full recovery is rare if ataxia has developed. Consumption of pastures containing sorghum plant species is not recommended for horses.

SWEET CLOVER POISONING

Sweet clover poisoning, an insidious hemorrhagic disease, is seen in animals that consume toxic quantities of spoiled sweet clover (*Melilotus officinalis* and *M alba*) hay or silage.

Etiology: During the process of spoiling, the coumarins in sweet clover are converted to toxic dicumarol, a potent vitamin K antagonist and anticoagulant. Any method of hay storage that allows molding of sweet clover promotes the likelihood of formation of dicumarol in the hay. Weathered, large round bales, particularly the outer portions, usually contain the highest concentrations of dicumarol. When toxic hay or silage is consumed for several weeks, dicumarol alters proenzymes required for synthesis of prothrombin, resulting in hypoprothrombinemia (by preventing formation of the active enzyme). It probably also interferes with synthesis of factor VII and other vitamin K–dependent coagulation factors (*see* p 44). Dicumarol concentrations of 20–30 mg/kg of hay ingested throughout several weeks are usually required to cause poisoning in cattle. The toxic agent crosses the placenta in pregnant animals, and newborn animals may be affected at birth. All species of animals studied are susceptible, but instances of poisoning involve cattle and, to a limited extent, sheep, pigs, and horses.

Clinical Findings and Lesions: Clinical signs are referable to hemorrhages that result from faulty blood coagulation. The time between consumption of toxic sweet clover and appearance of clinical disease varies greatly and depends on the dicumarol content of the particular sweet clover variety being fed, age of the animals, and amount of feed consumed. If the dicumarol content of the ration is low or variable, animals may consume it for months before signs of disease appear.

The first indication of dicumarol poisoning may be the death of one or more animals. In affected animals, the first signs may be stiffness and lameness, due to bleeding into the muscles and joints. Hematomas, epistaxis, or GI bleeding may also be seen. Death is generally caused by massive hemorrhage or bleeding after injury, surgery, or parturition. Neonatal deaths rarely occur without signs in the dam.

Diagnosis: Poisoning occurs when sweet clover hay or silage is consumed continually for relatively long periods. Diagnosis is made by identifying compatible signs and lesions and markedly prolonged blood clotting time or demonstration of reduced plasma prothrombin concentrations. The nature of the coagulopathy can be confirmed in the laboratory when the prothrombin time is prolonged. Sweet clover poisoning is normally a herd problem, making conditions that affect individual animals,such as blackleg, pasteurellosis, bracken fern poisoning, and aplastic anemia, less likely causes.

Rodenticide poisoning (*see* p 3165) is the primary differential diagnosis in which such large hemorrhages are also likely to occur. Congenital or inherited diseases affecting coagulation factors or blood platelets (eg, hemophilia A) may produce similar large hemorrhages but with largely different morbidity.

Treatment: The hypoprothrombinemia, hemorrhages, and anemia can be immediately corrected, to a degree, by IV administration of whole blood. This may be difficult in large animals, because effective dosages range from 2–10 L of fresh blood per 1,000 lb (450 kg) body wt. Care should be taken to ensure that donor animals are not receiving sweet clover feed. All clinically affected animals should receive a transfusion, which can be repeated if necessary. In addition, all severely affected animals should receive parenteral administration of synthetic vitamin K_1 (phytonadione). SC or IM injection is recommended to avoid the substantial risk of anaphylaxis; SC vitamin K_1 may not be as effective as IM treatment. The usual dosage recommended for cattle is 1 mg/kg, bid-tid for 2 days. Although it is more costly, vitamin K_1 is more effective than K_3 (menadione). Because reversal of the dicumarol by vitamin K_1 requires synthesis of coagulation proteins, several hours are required for significant improvement in homeostasis, and >24 hr is required to completely restore coagulation. Either vitamin K_1 or a blood transfusion is sufficient to correct mild cases if additional exposure is stopped.

Prevention: Cultivars of sweet clover low in coumarin and safe to feed (eg, Polara) have been developed. If one of these is not available, the only certain method of prevention is to avoid feeding sweet clover hay or silage. Although well-cured sweet clover is not dangerous, the absence of visible spoilage is insufficient evidence of safety.

Alternating sweet clover hay suspected of containing dicumarol with other roughage such as alfalfa or a grass-legume hay mixture can be used to avoid severe poisoning. A 7- to 10-day period on the sweet clover hay, followed by an equal time on the alternative hay, can prevent poisoning, but it will not completely prevent prolonged bleeding times. Because some animals have higher risks of serious hemorrhage (surgical candidates or pending parturition), they should not receive sweet clover hay for a minimum of 2–3 wk, and preferably ≥4 wk, before surgery or parturition.

CANTHARIDIN POISONING

(Blister beetle poisoning)

In nature, cantharidin is found in beetles belonging to the Meloidae family. More than 200 species of these beetles are found throughout the continental USA, but members of the genus *Epicauta* are most frequently associated with toxicosis in horses. The striped blister beetles (*E occidentalis*, *E temexia*, and *E vittata*) are particularly troublesome in the southwestern USA. The black blister beetle, *E pennsylvanica*, has caused toxicosis in horses in Illinois. Cantharidin is the sole toxin, but its concentration in beetles varies widely.

Blister beetles usually feed on various weeds and occasionally move into alfalfa fields in large swarms. These insects are gregarious and may be found in hay in large numbers when it is baled. One flake of alfalfa may contain several hundred beetles, but a flake from the other end of the same bale may have none. Animals are usually exposed by eating alfalfa hay or alfalfa products that have been contaminated with blister beetles.

Pathogenesis: Cantharidin is an odorless, colorless compound that is soluble in various organic solvents but only slightly soluble in water. It is highly irritating and causes acantholysis and vesicle formation when in contact with skin or mucous membranes. After ingestion, it is absorbed from the GI tract and rapidly excreted by the kidneys. The minimum lethal oral dose in horses has not been established, but it appears to be <1 mg/kg body wt. As little as 4–6 g of dried beetles may be fatal to a horse. The toxicity of cantharidin does not decrease in stored hay, and cantharidin is also toxic to people, cattle, sheep, goats, dogs, cats, rabbits, and rats.

Clinical Findings: The severity of clinical signs associated with cantharidin toxicosis varies according to dose. Signs may range from mild depression or discomfort to severe pain, shock, and death. Typical signs are related to GI and urinary tract irritation, endotoxemia and shock, hypocalcemia, and myocardial dysfunction. The onset and duration of signs can vary from hours to days. The signs seen most frequently include varying degrees of abdominal pain, depression, anorexia, and frequent attempts to drink small amounts of water or submerge the muzzle in water. Some horses show only signs of depression or make frequent attempts to urinate. Urine may be blood-tinged or contain blood clots but frequently appears normal. A striking feature is that affected horses invariably have dark, congested mucous membranes, even if other systemic signs of toxicosis are minimal. Sweating, delayed capillary refill time, increased heart and respiratory rates, and increased rectal temperature are other common signs. Less frequent signs include oral erosions; salivation; synchronous diaphragmatic flutter; a stiff, short-strided gait; and diarrhea that may contain blood. Horses that ingest a massive amount of toxin may show signs of severe shock and die within hours.

Diagnosis: Both high-performance liquid chromatography and gas chromatography or mass spectrometry analyses are sensitive, reliable methods of detecting cantharidin in gastric contents or in urine. The concentration of cantharidin in urine becomes negligible in 3–4 days, so urine should be collected early in the course of disease if it is to be analyzed. Microscopic evaluation of stomach contents (and often cecal contents) of fatally poisoned horses may reveal fragments of the insect, which can be positively identified if from one of the three striped species.

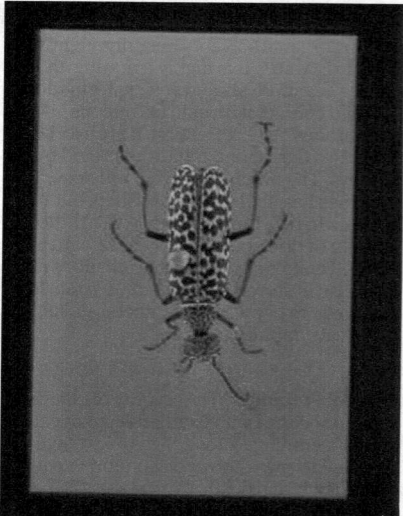

Epicauta pardalis blister beetle. *Courtesy of Dr. D. G. Schmitz.*

Certain laboratory findings are particularly helpful in differentiating cantharidin toxicosis from other causes of acute abdominal crisis. Serum calcium concentration is usually markedly decreased and may remain low for a prolonged time. Serum magnesium concentration is also typically low, and concentration of serum CK usually increases markedly within 24 hr of onset. In acutely affected horses, urinalysis typically reveals markedly decreased specific gravity (usually <1.010) and varying degrees of hematuria. Peritoneal fluid usually contains increased protein (>4 g/dL) but normal numbers of WBCs and normal fibrinogen concentration. Other laboratory abnormalities may include mild increases of serum urea nitrogen and creatinine and development of hypoproteinemia. Acutely affected horses are almost always hyperglycemic.

Treatment: There is no specific antidote for cantharidin poisoning, but prompt, vigorous symptomatic therapy is necessary for a good outcome. Oral administration of mineral oil aids in evacuation of the GI tract, and repeated dosing may be indicated. Activated charcoal, PO, may be helpful if given early. Other oral adsorbents containing ditrioctahedral smectite might be helpful as well, but their efficacy has not been evaluated. Calcium and magnesium supplementation for prolonged periods is almost always indicated. Other symptomatic therapy includes administration of fluids, analgesics, and diuretics and maintenance of normal blood pH and serum electrolyte concentrations. The prognosis for affected horses improves daily if no complications occur.

Prevention: Prevention is by feeding beetle-free hay. The hay field must be scouted before it is cut and during baling, because the insects can be crushed in the cutting and crimping process as well as during baling. Areas of the field that contain swarms of beetles must be avoided for a few days because most of the insects will leave. Once the beetles have left, these areas can be harvested.

First-cutting hay is almost always free of blister beetles, because the insects overwinter as subadults and usually do not emerge until late May or June in the southwestern USA. Likewise, the last cutting of hay is often safe, because it is usually harvested after the adult insects are no longer active.

SNAKEBITE

Venomous snakes of North America are members of either of two families: 1) the Elapidae or coral snakes (*Micrurus* spp); or 2) the Crotalidae, or pit vipers (rattlesnakes [*Crotalus* spp], cottonmouth moccasin [*Agkistrodon piscivorus*], and copperhead [*A cortotrix*]). Elapids are generally restricted to southern edges of the USA, whereas crotalids are dispersed across the continent. Because of their wider distribution and less secluded natures, bites by crotalids are much more common than elapid bites. Rattlesnakes account for most snakebite-related deaths in people and domestic animals in the USA. Although Australia is home to a large number of venomous snakes from the families Colubridae, Hydrophiidae, and Elapidae, the most clinically significant venomous species are elapids, particularly the black (*Pseudechis*), brown (*Pseudonaja textilis*), Taipan (*Oxyuranus* sp), and tiger (*Notechis scutatus*) snakes.

Crotalids have long, hinged, tubular fangs with which they strike, inject venom (a voluntary action), and withdraw. Many bites by vipers reportedly do not result in injection of substantial quantities of venom and are therefore termed "dry bites." Crotalid venom is typically hemotoxic, necrotizing, and anticoagulant, although a neurotoxic component is present in the venom of some species, eg, the Mojave rattlesnake (*C scutulatus scutulatus*). North American elapids have short fangs that deliver a neurotoxic venom that paralyzes the respiratory center. Except for death adders (*Acanthophis* spp), the venom delivery system of which resembles that of crotalids, Australian elapids tend to have relatively short, grooved to tubular fangs. The venoms of Australian elapids may have neurotoxic, myotoxic, procoagulant, anticoagulant, and/or hemolytic properties; pronounced cardiovascular abnormalities have been associated with envenomation by tiger and brown snakes.

Fatal snakebites are more common in dogs than in other domestic animals. Because of the relatively small size of some dogs in proportion to the amount of venom injected, the bite of even a small snake may be fatal. In dogs and cats, mortality is generally higher in bites to the thorax or abdomen than bites to the head or extremities. Because of their larger sizes, horses and cattle seldom die as a direct result of snakebite, but deaths may follow bites on the muzzle, head, or neck when dyspnea results from excessive swelling. Serious secondary damage sometimes occurs; livestock bitten near the coronary band may slough a hoof.

Snakebite with envenomation is a true emergency. Rapid examination and appropriate treatment are paramount. Owners should not spend time on first aid other than to keep the animal quiet and limit its activity. The following commonly touted measures are ineffective and can be potentially harmful: use of ice, cold packs, or sprays; incision and suction; tourniquets; electric shock; hot packs; and delay in presentation for medical treatment (waiting until problems develop).

Diagnosis: In many instances, the bite has been witnessed, and diagnosis is not a problem. However, fractures, abscesses, spider envenomations (*see* p 3162), or allergic reactions to insect bites or stings could all potentially be confused with a snakebite by the inexperienced eye. When possible, the *dead* snake should be brought along with the bitten animal; mutilation of the snake's head should be avoided, because this may hinder proper identification. Some bites do not result in envenomation or have been made by nonvenomous snakes. In Australia, venom detection test kits have been developed to detect the various snake venoms and determine the appropriate antivenom to use, but these appear to be infrequently used for veterinary patients.

Typical crotalid bites are characterized by severe local tissue damage that spreads from the bite site. The tissue becomes markedly discolored within a few minutes, and dark, bloody fluid may ooze from the fang wounds if not prevented by swelling. The epidermis may slough when the overlying hair is clipped or parted. Hair may hide the typical fang marks. Sometimes, only one fang mark or multiple punctures are present. Neurologic signs, including muscle fasciculations, are possible if neurotoxic crotalid venom is involved. In elapid snakebites, pain and swelling are minimal, and systemic neurologic signs predominate. Signs of coral snake envenomation include tetraparesis, ptyalism, tachypnea, shallow/abdominal breathing, depressed gag reflex, ataxia, muscle fasciculation, decreased spinal reflexes, and quiet mentation. Australian elapid bite victims may show collapse, vomiting, ptyalism, tremors, tachypnea, urinary and/or fecal incontinence, tetraparesis, hemolysis, coagulopathy, rhabdomyolysis, swelling at the bite site, renal failure, and/or delayed immune-mediated hemolytic anemia (red-bellied black snake).

Treatment: Intensive therapy should be instituted as soon as possible, because irreversible effects of venom begin immediately after envenomation. The bite site(s) should be shaved, and the wounds cleansed thoroughly with germicidal soap. For animals bitten by crotalids, the leading edge of tissue swelling should be marked on the skin with a magic marker at frequent intervals to monitor the spread of tissue injury. All snakebite victims should be monitored closely for a minimum of 24 (crotalid) to 48 (elapid) hr for the development of clinical signs.

Treatment for crotalid envenomation should be directed toward preventing or controlling shock, neutralizing venom, preventing or controlling coagulopathy, minimizing necrosis, and preventing secondary infection. Any dog or cat presented within 24 hr of a snakebite showing signs of crotalid envenomation requires intensive treatment, starting with IV crystalloids to combat hypotension. Rapid-acting corticosteroids may be of benefit in the first 24 hr to help control shock, protect against tissue damage, and minimize the likelihood of allergic reactions to antivenin; however, prolonged use of corticosteroids is not recommended. Monitoring for the development of echinocytes or coagulopathy is recommended, because these are often early signs of severe envenomation.

Antivenom is the only direct and specific means of neutralizing snake venom. Antivenoms available against North American pit vipers include equine-derived polyvalent antivenin, ovine-origin polyvalent F(ab) fragment antivenin, and equine-origin polyvalent F(ab)^2 fragment antivenin. The F(ab) antivenins use the F(ab) components of the immunoglobulin molecule, resulting in an antivenin that has lower risk of allergic reaction, faster reconstitution, and potency similar to that of the polyvalent immunoglobulin. Antivenin is most effective if administered in the first 6 hr after the bite, although improvement in clinical condition may be seen after antivenin administered ≥24 hr after the bite. In the unlikely event of an anaphylactic reaction to the antivenin, 0.5–1 mL of 1:1,000 epinephrine, with or without antihistamines such as diphenhydramine, should be administered SC. In severe envenomations, multiple vials of antivenom/antivenin may be required, although this is frequently cost-prohibitive in veterinary patients.

Antivenin generally helps significantly in managing the pain of a crotalid bite, but opioid analgesics may be used as needed for residual pain. If coagulopathy (thrombocytopenia, disseminated intravascular coagulation, etc) occurs, appropriate treatment, including blood replacement products and heparin sodium (in mini dose at 5–10 U/kg/hr or low dose at 50–100 U/kg, SC, tid), should be administered. Hemoglobin glutamer-200 (bovine) or hetastarch may be helpful to manage hypovolemia; however, colloids should be used with caution because of their potential to leak out of damaged vessels and pull fluids into tissue beds.

Several potential pathogens, including *Pseudomonas aeruginosa*, *Clostridium* spp, *Corynebacterium* spp, and staphylococci have been isolated from the mouth of rattlesnakes. However, the incidence of wound infection after snake bites is low, and many clinicians use antibiotics only when significant tissue necrosis is present. Broad-spectrum antibiotics such as amoxicillin/clavulanate or cephalosporins are preferred.

Tetanus antitoxin also should be considered, especially in horses, and other supportive treatment should be administered as needed (eg, blood or plasma transfusions in the case of hemolytic or anticoagulant venoms). In most cases, surgical excision of tissue is impractical or unwarranted. Antihistamines have been reported to be contraindicated, but diphenhydramine hydrochloride (10–50 mg, SC or IV) has been shown to be helpful to manage fractious patients and may possibly assist in minimizing risk of allergic reactions to antivenin.

Animals bitten by elapids may be treated with supportive care as needed (IV fluids, ventilatory support, anticonvulsants, etc) and antivenom/antivenin, if available. Ventilatory support is frequently required for 6–8 hr in animals experiencing Australian elapid envenomation; additional vials of antivenom can reduce ventilator time. Antivenom against coral snake venoms is no longer being manufactured in the USA, although some practitioners have received special permission to import coral snake antivenom from Mexico. In Australia, several antivenoms/antivenins are available for use in veterinary patients. A polyvalent antivenin is available for use when the identity of the snake cannot be ascertained, and many clinicians prefer to use the polyvalent antivenin for all envenomations. Additionally, animals bitten by Australian elapids should be monitored for development of coagulopathy, hemolysis, renal injury, cardiovascular abnormalities, or rhabdomyolysis; appropriate treatment should be instituted as needed. As with crotalid bites, broad-spectrum antibiotics may be indicated if there is risk of infection of the bite wound.

Prognosis: The prognosis of snakebite depends on the type and species of snake, location of the bite, size of the victim, degree of envenomation, and the time interval between the bite and the institution of treatment. Animals that survive elapid bites generally make full recoveries, but crotalid bites can result in longterm sequelae due to tissue necrosis (amputation, loss of function, etc), depending on the severity of the bite and the promptness and aggressiveness of treatment instituted.

TOAD POISONING

Dogs and, less frequently, cats may be poisoned by oral exposure to many types of toads. Severity varies greatly, depending on extent of contact and type of toad. Toxins are produced by all toads, but potency varies with species and apparently between geographic locations within individual species. Toad toxin, a defensive mechanism, is secreted by large glands located dorsal and posterior to the eyes and by smaller glands distributed throughout the skin. The toxin, a thick, creamy white, highly irritating substance, can be expelled quickly by the contraction of periglandular muscles in the skin. Its many components include bufagenins, which have digitalis-like effects, and bufotoxins, which block sodium channels in nerves similar to the actions of local anesthetics, catecholamines, and serotonin. The most toxic species in the USA is the giant or marine toad, *Rhinella marina* (formerly *Bufo marinus*), an introduced species that is established in Florida, Hawaii, and Texas. *R marina* is also known as the cane toad in Australia, where its range extends across the northeastern half of the continent. Mortality ranges from 20%–100% in untreated cases, depending on exposure circumstances. The Colorado River toad, *Incillus* (formerly *Bufo*) *alvarius*, found in the southwestern USA and northern Mexico, is another toad of sufficient size to have potentially lethal levels of toxins in its skin secretions.

Clinical Findings and Diagnosis: Encounters with toads are most common in warm or mild weather. Signs of poisoning are variable and range from local effects to convulsions and death. Severity depends on host factors, extent of exposure, length of time since exposure, and species of toad. Local effects (profuse, sometimes frothy salivation, accompanied by vigorous head shaking, pawing at the mouth, and retching) are immediate, probably because the toxin is extremely irritating. Vomiting is not unusual, especially in severe cases, and although it may persist for several hours, no further signs may develop in poisoning by common indigenous toads. With more severe intoxication, as from *R marina* or *I alvarius*, cardiac arrhythmias, dyspnea, cyanosis, and seizures are characteristic. Cardiac and CNS involvement can be life-threatening.

Treatment: A specific antidote for toad toxins is not available. Therapy is directed at minimizing toxin absorption and controlling associated clinical signs. Minimal treatment may be required after exposure to toxins in areas where less toxic toads are found. The mouth should be immediately and thoroughly flushed with copious amounts of water. Affected animals should be prevented from inhaling aerosols of saliva or water that contain toad toxin. Atropine may reduce the volume of saliva and the risk of aspiration but should not be used until cardiovascular status is assessed. More severely affected animals require more extensive therapy. Cardiac arrhythmias should be identified and controlled using standard treatment protocols (*see also* ARRHYTHMIAS, p 90). If bradyarrhythmias exist, atropine or dopamine should be considered;

tachyarrhythmias should be treated with lidocaine, phenytoin, propranolol, or procainamide hydrochloride. Digoxin-specific Fab may be considered in cases of severe arrhythmias refractory to standard antiarrhythmic therapy. CNS excitation, if present, should be controlled by benzodiazepines, barbiturates, or a combination of the two. Anesthetics that predispose to ventricular fibrillation (eg, halothane) should be avoided. Supplemental oxygen and mechanical ventilation may also be needed if cyanosis and dyspnea are prominent.

VENOMOUS ARTHROPODS

Envenomation of animals by poisonous arthropods is relatively uncommon and difficult to recognize. It may be suspected relative to presenting clinical signs, but confirmatory evidence is rare because of the inability to capture the offending arthropod.

SPIDERS AND SCORPIONS

Spiders of medical importance in the USA do not inflict particularly painful bites, so it is unusual for a spider bite to be suspected until clinical signs appear. It is also unlikely that the spider will remain in close proximity to the victim for the time required for signs to develop (30 min to 6 hr). Almost all spiders are venomous, but few possess the attributes necessary to cause clinical envenomation in mammals—mouth parts of sufficient size to allow penetration of the skin and toxin of sufficient quantity or potency to result in morbidity.

The spiders in the USA that are capable of causing clinical envenomation belong to two groups: widow spiders (*Latrodectus* spp) and brown spiders (mostly *Loxosceles* spp).

Widow Spiders: Widow spiders usually bite only when accidental skin contact occurs. The most common species is the black widow spider, *Latrodectus mactans*, characterized by a red hourglass shape on its ventral abdomen. In the western USA, the western black widow, *L hesperus*, predominates, while the brown widow, *L bishopi*, is found in the south, and the red widow, *L geometricus*, is found in Florida.

Venom from these spiders is one of the most potent biologic toxins. The most important of its five or six components is a neurotoxin that causes release of the neurotransmitters norepinephrine and acetylcholine at synaptic junctions, which continues until neurotransmitters are depleted. The resulting severe, painful cramping of all large muscle groups accounts for most of the clinical signs attributed to envenomation.

Unless there is visual confirmation of a widow spider bite, diagnosis must be based on clinical signs, which include restlessness with apparent anxiety or apprehension; rapid, shallow, irregular respiration; shock; abdominal rigidity or tenderness; and painful muscle rigidity, sometimes accompanied by intermittent relaxation (which may progress to clonus and eventually to respiratory paralysis). Partial paresis also has been described.

An antivenin (equine origin) is commercially available but is usually reserved for confirmed bites of high-risk individuals (very young or very old). Symptomatic treatment is usually sufficient but may require a combination of therapeutic agents. Calcium gluconate IV (10 mL of a 10% solution is the usual human dose) is reportedly helpful. Meperidine hydrochloride or morphine, also given IV, provides relief from pain and produces muscle relaxation. Muscle relaxants and diazepam are also beneficial. Tetanus antitoxin also should be administered. Recovery may be prolonged; weakness and even partial paralysis may persist for several days.

Brown Recluse Spiders: There are at least 10 species of *Loxosceles* spiders in the USA, but the brown recluse spider, *L reclusa*, is the most common, and envenomation by it is typical for the genus. These spiders have a violin-shaped marking (or "fiddleback") on the spider's dorsum, the cephalothorax, although it may be indistinct or absent in some species. In the northwestern USA, the unrelated spider *Tegenaria* *agrestis* reportedly causes a clinically indistinguishable dermonecrosis in people and presumably in domesticated animals. Brown recluse spider venom has vasoconstrictive, thrombotic, hemolytic, and necrotizing properties. It contains several enzymes, including a phospholipase (sphingomylinase D) that attacks cell membranes. Pathogenetic mechanisms of the characteristic dermal necrosis are poorly understood, but activation of complement, chemotaxis, and accumulations of neutrophils affect (or amplify) the process.

A history of a bite by a brown recluse spider is useful but rare. A presumptive diagnosis may be based on the presence of a discrete, erythematous, intensely pruritic skin lesion that may have irregular ecchymoses. Within 4–8 hr, a vesicle develops at the bite wound, and sometimes a blanched zone surrounds the erythematous area, producing a "bull's-eye" appearance to the lesion. The central area sometimes appears pale or cyanotic. The vesicle may degenerate to an ulcer that, unless treated in a timely manner, may enlarge and extend to underlying tissues, including muscle. Sometimes, a pustule follows the vesicle and, on its breakdown, a black eschar remains. The final tissue defect may be extensive and indolent and require months to heal. However, medical authorities claim that not all brown recluse spider bites result in severe, localized dermal necrosis.

Systemic signs sometimes accompany brown recluse spider envenomation and may not appear for 3–4 days after the bite. Hemolysis, thrombocytopenia, and disseminated intravascular coagulation are more likely to occur in cases with severe dermal necrosis. Fever, vomiting, edema, hemoglobinuria, hemolytic anemia, renal failure, and shock may result from systemic loxoscelism.

In known spider bites, early treatment can be successful, but unfortunately, many cases are not recognized until cutaneous necrosis has become extensive; treatment at that stage is less rewarding but is still of value. Immediate application of cold packs is beneficial, and if administered early, corticosteroids protect against cutaneous necrosis by stabilizing cell membranes and suppressing chemotaxis. Corticosteroids also tend to protect against systemic involvement. Radical excision has been advocated, but its value is questionable. Dapsone, an inhibitor of leukocyte function, which is frequently used in the treatment of leprosy, is currently considered the drug of choice for brown recluse spider bites. In people, it is administered at 100 mg, bid, for 14–25 days. Broad-spectrum antibiotics are useful in preventing secondary infection, and tetanus immunoprophylaxis should be considered.

Tarantulas: Tarantulas (many assorted genera and species) are common throughout the USA and South America. They are increasingly being kept as household pets throughout the world. Along with many other exotic arthropods, they are frequently sold in exotic pet stores.

Tarantulas should not be mixed with or allowed contact with other domesticated pets. Fine hairs (setae), present over much of the tarantula's abdomen, may be discharged (or cast off) by the tarantula as a defense mechanism against larger creatures. If these fine hairs make contact with unprotected skin, they can produce contact allergic reactions. Care must be taken to keep these fine hairs from entering the eye, particularly the cornea, because they can be quite difficult to remove. In addition, the bite of the tarantula can be fatal to dogs or cats, which are very susceptible to tarantula venom. Safety of the tarantula is another reason to keep these spiders separated from other pets, because a dog or cat can easily injure or kill a pet tarantula.

Scorpions: Most of the scorpions found throughout the USA possess posterior abdominal stingers that connect to venom glands. The stinger and its associated venom can be used both as mechanisms of self-defense and of predation. For the most part, the stings of these scorpions are considered to be innocuous in most domesticated mammalian species, because the amount of venom is too minute or the venom has very little pharmacologic potency. The sting of these arthropods is analogous to an insect sting/bite, with pain and swelling at the site of the injury.

Relative to pharmacologically potent scorpion stings in domesticated animals, there are two geographic scenarios of veterinary clinical importance. The first involves *Centruroides sculpturatus*, commonly known as the Arizona bark scorpion. This venomous arthropod can be found in all counties of Arizona, into western New Mexico, southern Utah, southern Nevada to the Las Vegas vicinity, California along the Colorado River (where it is rare), and down to the area of the state of Sonora, Mexico. It has been reported to produce envenomation in dogs; however, its sting is similar to that of the venomous hymenopterans, producing local pain and swelling with the possibility of associated hypertension. Most animals recover without a problem, but more severe reactions are possible.

The second scenario involves myriad geographic locales (eg, desert-like and jungle ecosystems) throughout the world where many venomous scorpions abound. People with penchants for hiking the world should be warned to be wary of visits to these areas, and traveling with canine companions in such scenarios should be strongly discouraged.

HYMENOPTERA

Honey Bees, Wasps, Hornets, and Yellow Jackets: There are many venomous hymenopterans (eg, honey bees, wasps, hornet, yellow jackets), in which the female drone possesses a barbed ovipositor on the tip of the abdomen that connects to paired venom glands. Bees possess a barbed stinging apparatus; after stinging the victim, bees die because the stinger and its associated venom sac are pulled out of the abdomen. Wasps, hornets, and yellow jackets possess a stinging apparatus that is not barbed; they are capable of stinging multiple times. The venom glands of honeybees contain a hydrolyzing protein, mast cell degranulating peptides, a phospholipase, hyaluronidase, vasoactive amines, and a neurotoxin apamin.

A single bee sting will produce pain, swelling, erythema, edema, and local induration, which can be followed by pruritus at the injection site. The incidence of anaphylactic reactions is not known in companion animals—if a severe systemic reaction has not occurred within 30 min, it is not likely to occur. In dogs, bee and wasp stings cause only local redness, erythema, and transient pain. Dogs may vocalize when stung and may rub their mouth and eyes on the ground. Usually cutaneous reactions appear quickly and regress spontaneously. With repeated stings, anaphylaxis, with salivation, vomiting, diarrhea, circulatory collapse, pallor, or cyanosis, may result (*see* p 823).

The stinger/ovipositor (if present) with accompanying venom glands should be removed, if it can be located. In severe cases with urticaria, epinephrine should be given IM. In cases of anaphylaxis, epinephrine should be immediately administered, SC, at a dosage of 1:1,000 (0.1–0.5 mL) for dogs or cats. This dosage can be repeated every 10–20 min. When given IV, it must be diluted to 1:10,000, and 0.5–1 mL is administered with vigilant monitoring of heart rate, heart rhythm, and blood pressure. IV fluids are indicated to prevent vascular collapse. Antihistamines and corticosteroids should also be given. The animal may require intubation to provide supplemental oxygen.

Africanized Honeybees ("Killer Bees"): The common honeybees in America were brought to the New World by European settlers; as a result, the European varieties of honeybees established themselves throughout North and South America. In the 1950s, African colonies of bees were crossed with the docile European varieties of honeybees in laboratories in Brazil, but their offspring managed to escape from the laboratory environment. These hybridized offspring were characterized by excitability, aggressive defense of the hive, and frequent swarming activity. Since their escape in 1957, these "killer bees" have spread throughout most of South America, through Central America and Mexico, and into the southern regions of the USA; their range is expected to expand northward.

Africanized bees are difficult to distinguish morphologically from their European counterparts. Their stinging behavior is primarily defensive, eg, in response to a perceived threat to the colony. These bees habitually sting en masse. Once initiated, stinging recruitment within the colony can result in hundreds or thousands of stings; bees may pursue their victim for as far as 1 km. Hives are generally found in exposed locations such as on tree branches or in old tires or boxes where domesticated animals may come in contact with them. Stings occur generally in the vicinity of the hive. Smaller pets are particularly susceptible to the effects of multiple stings, because they receive a larger dose of venom/kg body wt. It is the cumulative dose of venom that becomes fatal.

Animals that receive massive envenomations are visibly depressed and usually febrile. They may exhibit facial paralysis, ataxia, seizures, and neurologic signs. The urine may be dark brown or red, and the feces are bloody. Bloody or dark brown vomitus may be seen. Leukocytosis may be present. The animal may be thrombocytopenic; disseminated intravascular coagulation may be imminent. Urinalysis may reveal granular casts due to renal tubular damage. The animal may develop acute renal failure caused by acute tubular necrosis or direct toxic effect of massive envenomation. Dogs may develop a secondary immune-mediated hemolytic anemia.

Access to cardiac monitoring, supplemental oxygen, "crash cart" drugs, and airway intubation must be readily available. Any animal that receives massive, multiple stings must be hospitalized, treated aggressively, and hospitalized for 24 hr after cessation of clinical signs.

Fire Ants: Fire ants (red imported fire ants and black imported fire ants) are not native to North America but were introduced into the USA in the early years of the 20th century. Since their introduction, red imported fire ants (*Solenopsis invicta*) have colonized more than 310 million acres in 12 southern states, whereas black imported fire ants (*S richteri*) have been contained in a small area in Alabama and Mississippi. Fire ants attack domestic animals and native wildlife. The ant anchors onto its victim with its prominent mandibles, tucks its abdomen under its body, and stings with its nonbarbed stinger, a modified ovipositor with an associated venom gland. It retracts its stinger, rotates its body to the side, and stings again. This act is repeated in a circular pattern. Unlike bees, wasps, and hornets, fire ants inject their venom slowly. Each ant can deliver 0.11 μL with a total of 20 consecutive stings before the venom gland is depleted.

The typical reaction to a fire ant sting is a wheal and flare, which usually resolves within an hour. Pain and inflammation begin immediately. A papule will form at the sting site and develop into a sterile pustule. These pustules are pruritic and may become secondarily infected due to self-inflicted trauma. Regional reactions can occur and may be erythematous, indurated, and quite pruritic. Regional edema may be severe enough to impede blood flow to a limb. Systemic or anaphylactic reactions can produce clinical signs removed from the site of the initial sting, including urticaria, cutaneous edema, laryngeal edema, bronchospasm, vascular collapse, and death. Deaths due to systemic anaphylaxis occur within minutes of the sting, whereas deaths due to venom toxicity occur >24 hr after the sting.

There are no treatments to prevent or resolve localized reactions to fire ant stings; however, symptomatic therapy might be beneficial. Local reactions may be treated with antihistamines, topical corticosteroids, water or alcohol compresses, ice, and topical treatment with menthol and camphor. Warm baths may provide some relief for dogs. Regional reactions occur less frequently and should be treated with antihistamines, corticosteroids, analgesics, and fluid therapy. Antibiotics are indicated for secondary infections. Anaphylactic reactions to fire ant stings are treated similarly to those from honeybees, wasps, and yellow jackets (*see* above).

RODENTICIDE POISONING

Many poisons have been used against rodent pests. If baits are not well secured, they may be ingested directly by nontarget animal species (farm animals, pets, and wildlife). Sometimes, nontarget species may ingest recently poisoned rodent pests and develop relay or secondary poisoning. Occasionally, baits may be used maliciously or intentionally to kill either domestic animals or wildlife. This chapter discusses only the most commonly used rodenticides currently available in the market: anticoagulants, bromethalin, cholecalciferol, and zinc phosphide. Strychnine poisoning (*see* p 3170) is discussed separately.

Whenever a rodenticide exposure is suspected, owners should be asked history questions to determine the day and time of exposure, brand name and manufacturer of rodenticide, active ingredients and their concentration, package size, and the potential amount missing. The Environmental Protection Agency (EPA) registration number is the most accurate way to confirm identity of an active ingredient. There is no way to identify differing class by color, shape, or size of a bait.

ANTICOAGULANT RODENTICIDES (WARFARIN AND CONGENERS)

Anticoagulant rodenticides inhibit the enzyme vitamin K epoxide reductase, which normally reactivates vitamin K, a crucial component in a number of normal clotting factors, after those factors are consumed in normal maintenance. Potentially dangerous to all mammals and birds, anticoagulant rodenticides are a common cause of poisoning in pets and wildlife. Intoxications in domestic animals have resulted from contamination of feed with anticoagulant concentrate, malicious use of these chemicals, and feed mixed in equipment used to prepare rodent bait.

All anticoagulants have the basic coumarin or indanedione nucleus. The "first-generation" anticoagulants (warfarin, pindone, coumafuryl, coumachlor, isovaleryl indanedione, and others less frequently used) require multiple feedings to result in toxicity. The "intermediate" anticoagulants (chlorophacinone and in particular diphacinone) require fewer feedings than "first-generation" chemicals, and thus are more toxic to nontarget species. The "second-generation" anticoagulants (brodifacoum, bromadiolone, difethiolone) are highly toxic to nontarget species (dogs, cats, livestock, or wildlife) after a single feeding. Secondary poisoning in nontarget animal species from anticoagulants has also been documented. The concentration of brodifacoum and bromadiolone in the bait available as pellets or blocks is usually 0.005% and that of difethiolone 0.0025%.

Anticoagulants antagonize vitamin K, which interferes with the normal synthesis of coagulation proteins (factors I, II, VII, IX, and X) in the liver; thus, adequate amounts are not available to convert prothrombin into thrombin. A latent period, dependent on species, dose, and activity, is required, during which clotting factors already present are used up. New products have a longer biologic half-life and therefore prolonged effects (which require prolonged treatment). For example, the half-life in canine plasma of warfarin is 15 hr, diphacinone is 5 days, and

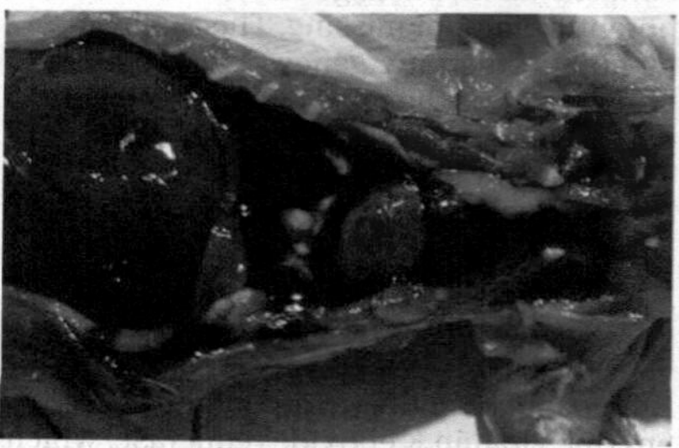

Anticoagulant rodenticide poisoning, thorax hemorrhage. *Courtesy of Dr. Frederick W. Oehme.*

bromadiolone is 6 days, with maximum effects estimated at 12–15 days. Brodifacoum may continue to be detectable in serum for up to 24 days. All of these may be detected in liver even after serum levels drop.

Clinical signs generally reflect some manifestation of hemorrhage, including anemia, hematomas, melena, hemothorax, hyphema, epistaxis, hemoptysis, and hematuria, any of which may lead to weakness, ataxia, colic, polypnea, etc. Petechiae rarely develop until after repeated small bleeds have consumed too many platelets. Depression and anorexia may be seen in all species even before bleeding occurs. Typically, the onset of clinical signs is delayed (due to consumption of vitamin K–dependent clotting factors) for 3-7 days after exposure (can be a little earlier with a fairly large dose). Dogs can also show nonspecific clinical signs, such as limping or swollen joints (due to hemorrhage in the joints), coughing or wheezing (bleeding in the lungs), bulging of eyes (retrobulbar hemorrhages), and pale mucous membrane color. Sudden death with no obvious clinical signs is also possible.

Anticoagulant rodenticide toxicosis may be diagnosed based on history of availability of the bait in the animal's environment and evidence of exposure (missing or chewed up package/bait, passing of greenish blue feces [color of the bait]) but cannot be discounted if there is no known history of exposure. Differential diagnoses when hemorrhage is encountered include disseminated intravascular coagulation, congenital factor deficiencies, von Willebrand disease, platelet deficiencies, and canine ehrlichiosis. A prolonged prothrombin time (PT), activated partial thromboplastin time (APTT), or thrombin time in the presence of normal fibrinogen, fibrin degradation products, and platelet counts is strongly suggestive of anticoagulant rodenticide toxicosis, as is a positive therapeutic response to vitamin K_1. Stomach contents, serum, or plasma can be analyzed for the presence of anticoagulant to confirm a diagnosis. Most veterinary diagnostic laboratories have an "anticoagulant screen" to detect most of the anticoagulants available in the market in the serum, plasma, liver, or kidney.

Vitamin K_1 is antidotal. Because the vast majority of exposures are to the second-generation agents, recommended dosages are generally 3–5 mg/kg/day, PO, for 3–4 wk. Treating for an extra week will not be harmful, whereas discontinuing treatment too soon can be lethal. The best way to know when to stop vitamin K_1 treatment is by checking the PT time 72 hr after the last dose of vitamin K_1 has been given. If PT at that point is normal, treatment with vitamin K_1 can be stopped; if it is still prolonged, treatment with vitamin K_1 for 1 more week is warranted. The doses should be administered with small amounts of fatty food (milk, meat, or cheese), because fat will enhance vitamin K_1 absorption. Administering half of the daily dose every 12 hr will provide more constant levels of vitamin K_1. In animals exhibiting clinical signs when coagulation factors are abnormal, it is probably safer to avoid injections (unless the animal is unable to take vitamin K_1 orally) because of the risk of bleeding and hematoma formation at the injection site. Also, the possibility of anaphylactoid reaction cannot be excluded when vitamin K_1 injection is administered parentally.

Fresh or frozen plasma (9 mL/kg) or whole blood (20 mL/kg) IV may be indicated to replace needed clotting factors and RBCs immediately if bleeding is present. Administration of oxygen may be very useful. Activity should be limited as much as possible during the first week of therapy to minimize bleeds due to trauma to tissues. Oral vitamin K_1 alone (3–5 mg/kg, PO) can be used to prevent coagulopathy after a known exposure to an anticoagulant.

If a coagulopathy has developed, rechecking the PT and APTT every 24 hr until normalized should be considered. At the end of a course of vitamin K_1 supplementation, a coagulation profile is needed ~48–72 hr after the last dose to confirm that no indication of coagulopathy remains.

Vitamin K_3 given as a feed supplement is ineffective in treatment of anticoagulant rodenticide toxicosis. Administration of vitamin K_3 by injection in horses has been associated with acute renal failure and is never an appropriate treatment.

To increase protection to nontarget animal species and children, the US EPA has promulgated new rules on packaging and availability of anticoagulants. Some of the highlights of these new rules include the following: 1) Consumer products available in retail, hardware, grocery, or convenient stores with under a pound of bait can no longer contain second-generation anticoagulants (brodifacoum, difethialone, bromadiolone, or difenacoum). 2) Only first-generation anticoagulants (warfarin, diphacinone, chlorophacinone) or rodenticides other than anticoagulants (bromethalin, cholecalciferol) are allowed for sale in retail stores for use by consumers. 3) All outdoor, above-ground use must be in a bait station intended to be resistant to children and pets. 4) Loose poison baits (pellets, meals) are prohibited. 5) All outdoor products are to be placed within 50 feet of a building. 6) Professional use products are available in quantities of at least 8 or 16 pounds (second-generation anticoagulants) or at least 4 pounds (first-generation anticoagulants); they are to be placed in bait stations. 7) Professional class anticoagulants (second-generation) are not to be marketed in "consumer" stores (grocery, hardware, or club stores).

The possible unintended end result of these new EPA regulations is likely to be a higher incidence of exposure to rodent baits that contain either bromethalin or cholecalciferol (vitamin D_3).

BROMETHALIN

Bromethalin, a nonanticoagulant, single-dose rodenticide, is a neurotoxin available as bars (blocks), pellets, seed, and worm. Mole baits are sold as worm containing 0.025% bromethalin, whereas rat and mouse baits contain 0.01% bromethalin. Bromethalin and its main metabolite desmobromethalin are strong uncouplers of oxidative phosphorylation. This results in intra-myelin fluid accumulation, leading to long nerve demyelination and intra-myelin cerebral edema. The net result is cerebral and spinal edema and increased CSF pressure, leading to neurologic dysfunction. In toxicity trials, the oral toxic dose of bromethalin when used as part of bait appears to be much lower than the dose administered as a technical grade agent. For example, in dogs, an average lethal dose of technical grade bromethalin is reported to be 4.7 mg/kg but 2.38 mg/kg in bait. Young dogs (<1 yr old) appear more sensitive; death has been reported at dosages of ~1 mg/kg in bait. Dogs are more commonly involved. Cats are 2–3 times more sensitive than dogs.

Bromethalin can cause either an acute or a subacute/chronic syndrome, depending on the dose ingested. At doses equivalent to or more than the average lethal dose, dogs may develop an acute convulsant (or high-dose) syndrome resulting in clinical signs within 4–36 hr of exposure; such signs include hyperexcitability, muscle tremors, grand mal seizures, hindlimb hyperreflexia, CNS depression, hyperthermia, and death. The paralytic (subacute or chronic) syndrome is seen at lower doses, and clinical signs may not appear for several days (up to 7 days) after exposure. Initial signs may include depression, hindlimb weakness or paresis, decreased propioception, ataxia, and possible tremors. Muscle weakness often progresses from posterior to anterior muscles. Cats typically develop paralytic syndrome irrespective of dose of bromethalin.

Presumptive diagnosis of bromethalin toxicosis is made based on known or suspected history of exposure to the bait, followed by development of neurologic signs within 1–7 days of exposure. Diagnosis can be confirmed by detecting the presence of bromethalin or its major metabolite in liver, kidney, brain, or fat; this analysis is available only in some veterinary diagnostic laboratories in the USA.

Based on the history of exposure, bromethalin toxicosis should be considered when there is moderate to acute onset of weakness, hindlimb paralysis, tremors, and seizures. Some other toxicologic and nontoxicologic differential diagnoses should include ethylene glycol toxicosis, marijuana ingestion, 2,4-D and other phenoxyacetic acid herbicide toxicosis, copper head snake envenomation (cats), intervertebral disc problems, spinal cord and CNS trauma, and tick paralysis.

Treatment of bromethalin toxicosis is aimed at early decontamination (induction of emesis and administration of activated charcoal) in an asymptomatic animal and controlling CNS signs (seizures) and providing supportive care in a symptomatic animal. Emesis using 3% hydrogen peroxide solution or apomorphine in dogs and xylazine in cats within 4 hr of ingestion may remove some bait from the gut. Depending on the ingested dose of bromethalin, administration of activated charcoal is considered an effective method to prevent toxicosis. Bromethalin undergoes enterohepatic recirculation, so administration of repeated doses of activated charcoal may be helpful.

The following can be used as a guideline to treat bromethalin exposure in dogs and cats:

At a bromethalin dosage of 0.1–0.49 mg/kg in dogs, or 0.05-0.1 mg/kg in cats, emesis alone within 4 hr of exposure may be adequate. If emesis is not successful, or if > 4 hr have elapsed since ingestion, a single dose of activated charcoal at 1–2 g/kg body wt is indicated. Whenever administering activated charcoal, the clinician must remain aware of the risk of aspiration or hypernatremia secondary to fluid shift into the gut. The clinical signs of acute hypernatremia may mimic those seen with bromethalin toxicosis.

At a bromethalin dosage of 0.5–0.75 mg/kg in dogs, or 0.1–0.3 mg/kg in cats, an initial dose of activated charcoal at 1–2 g/kg body wt should be considered. A repeat dose at half the original dose at 8-hr intervals for a total of three doses can be administered, again being aware of and monitoring for possible hypernatremia.

At a bromethalin dosage of ≥0.75 mg/kg in dogs, or ≥0.3 mg/kg in cats, administration of six doses of activated charcoal over 48 hr (repeat every 8 hr) can be considered to reduce the body burden by interrupting enterohepatic recirculation.

Use of mannitol and corticosteroids has been suggested to treat clinical signs, because they may help manage cerebral edema due to other causes. However, this has not been shown to be very helpful, likely because of the presence of intra-myelin edema. Diazepam, barbiturates, and other anticonvulsant medications should be used to control seizures and other CNS signs. Full recovery may require days to weeks of treatment.

CHOLECALCIFEROL

Cholecalciferol (vitamin D_3) is used both as a dietary supplement and a rodenticide. It appears to be toxic at a much lower dose when consumed in a bait form than when ingested as a technical grade agent. Most rodenticide baits contain 0.075% cholecalciferol. Incidence of vitamin D_3 toxicosis in animals is relatively less than that of anticoagulant and bromethalin toxicosis. Relay toxicosis from vitamin D_3 has not been documented. One international unit (1 IU) of vitamin D_3 in nutritional supplement is equivalent to 0.025 mcg of cholecalciferol.

Cholecalciferol toxicosis is characterized by hyperphosphatemia and hypercalcemia, leading to renal failure, cardiac abnormalities, hypertension, CNS depression, anorexia, vomiting, diarrhea, and lethargy. The increased calcium and phosphorus can lead to calcification of soft tissue, notably the highly vascular areas of kidneys and lungs, as well as within the walls of the great blood vessels.

Clinical signs generally develop within 18–36 hr of ingestion; initial signs can include depression, anorexia, polyuria, and polydipsia. The serum phosphorus more commonly rises first, at ~12–24 hr after ingestion, with serum calcium levels rising within another 12–24 hr. Nausea, vomiting, hematemesis, and depression are common as the clinical signs progress. It is important to obtain a baseline biochemistry profile as early as possible after the exposure, so that each animal can be monitored based on individual values.

Ingestion of vitamin D_3 at >0.1 mg/kg may require decontamination (induction of emesis and administration of activated charcoal) and monitoring of serum calcium, phosphorus, and renal values. Emesis can be induced within 2 hr of exposure with 3% hydrogen peroxide or apomorphine in dogs and xylazine in cats. Activated charcoal at 1–2 g/kg is an appropriate initial dose for decontamination, and a second half dose after ~6–8 hr may be helpful. In addition, use of cholestyramine, a bile acid sequestrant, may be useful to decrease the body burden of vitamin D_3 that undergoes enterohepatic recirculation with bile acids. However, the efficacy of cholestyramine to reduce vitamin D_3 levels in dogs has not been determined. The recommended dosage is 0.3–0.5 g/kg, dissolved in liquid and administered orally every 6–8 hr for 3–5 days, depending on the initial dose of cholecalciferol ingested. Premature initiation of calciuresis (*see* below) may disrupt normal calcium-phosphorus metabolism, triggering osteoclasts to move additional calcium into the blood stream, artificially increasing serum calcium and phosphorus levels and mimicking vitamin D_3 toxicosis.

Once the biochemical values begin to increase, there are two approaches to management. The first is to promote calciuresis by administering normal (0.9%) saline at 2–3 times normal rates. Furosemide at 2.5–4.5 mg/kg, PO, every 6–8 hr promotes calcium excretion but can also increase fluid loss (so hydration status should be monitored). Prednisolone at 1–3 mg/kg, PO, bid-tid, can reduce bone resorption as well as decrease calcium absorption from the intestine. Treatment with a phosphate binder (aluminum hydroxide 30–90 mg/kg, PO, in divided doses) to decrease phosphorus absorption and feeding a diet low in calcium should also be considered.

The preferred treatment for persistent significant hypercalcemia is pamidronate, an injectable bisphosphonate that inhibits osteoclastic bone resorption. It is administered at 1.3–2 mg/kg via slow IV infusion in saline over 2 hr. After administration, as the calcium and phosphorus levels start to decrease, supportive therapies (furosemide, prednisolone) should be tapered. A repeat dose may be required if significant hypercalcemia redevelops.

In the past, use of salmon calcitonin (administered at 4–6 IU/kg, SC, every 2–3 hr) has been suggested to decrease calcium and phosphorus levels, but this treatment is no longer used commonly. The two major disadvantages are that some animals may become refractory to calcitonin, and that once this therapy is instituted the use of pamidronate is not helpful.

Calcium and phosphorus levels should be monitored and treated until they return to baseline. Treatment may have to be continued for days or weeks because of the lipophilic nature of vitamin D_3. Renal function should be monitored, and other clinical signs treated as needed.

ZINC PHOSPHIDE

Zinc phosphide is a component in a number of mole, gopher, ground squirrel, and vole baits intended for outdoor use only. It is a dark gray powder, not soluble in water, and is commonly sold in 2%–5% bait pellets, paste, or tracking powder. In the past several years, an oat-based bait labeled for killing prairie voles has been marketed. There is evidently no way to identify this grain mixture, and bait ingestion has resulted in lethal exposure to a number of horses. The clinical effects of aluminum phosphide, used as a grain fumigator, are similar to those of zinc phosphide.

Lethal doses of zinc phosphide vary markedly between species and are much more toxic to species unable to vomit. The phosphide salts are unstable in an acid environment. At gastric pH, they degrade rapidly to form phosphine gas. Presence of food in the stomach, which will trigger release of gastric acid, increases the rate of this transition. Phosphine gas, when inhaled, results in acute noncardiogenic pulmonary edema. Vomiting, often hemorrhagic, is a common presenting sign in animals capable of vomiting. Tachypnea, ataxia, weakness, trembling, collapse, seizures, and death may ensue.

If there is no food in the stomach, undegraded zinc phosphide can be absorbed systemically. An animal surviving for 48 hr can then have liver and/or renal failure within 5–14 days due to absorption of intact zinc phosphide. Zinc phosphide is thought to block cytochrome C oxidase, leading to formation of highly reactive oxygen compounds, which cause most of the tissue injury; the most severe damage is in tissues with the highest oxygen demand, ie, brain, lungs, liver, and kidney.

Phosphine gas is a public health hazard. Animal owners and veterinary staff members must be cautious while inducing emesis, because they can be exposed to phosphine gas from the presence of zinc phosphide bait in the stomach contents after vomiting. The gas is reported to have a garlic-like or fishy odor.

Management of zinc phosphide ingestion relies on effective decontamination. If the animal has not already vomited, emesis can be induced by use of apomorphine. Decreasing gastric acid may be beneficial, via oral magnesium hydroxide antacid or using famotidine at 1 mg/kg, SC. IV fluid support is recommended while the animal is under observation. Use of activated charcoal may be considered; although metals are poorly bound by activated charcoal, the larger zinc phosphide molecule may be. If vomiting is ongoing, administration of activated charcoal should be avoided because of the aspiration risk. Obtaining a baseline biochemical profile, with repeat evaluation of liver and renal values at 24, 48, and possibly 72 hr, is recommended. Use of *N*-acetylcysteine may be beneficial, with a loading dose of 140 mg/kg, followed by 70 mg/kg every 6 hr for six total doses. Administration of *S*-adenosyl methionine (SAM-e) may also be beneficial. Seizures should be controlled with diazepam or barbiturates, and other signs treated symptomatically.

STRYCHNINE POISONING

Strychnine is an indole alkaloid obtained from the seeds of the Indian tree *Strychnos nux-vomica*. Strychnine-containing baits are currently labelled for below-ground use and are intended for the control of pocket gophers. Their use as indoor pesticides has been eliminated since 1989. In the past, strychnine has been used as a pesticide to control rats, moles, gophers, and coyotes. Strychnine is highly toxic to most domestic animals. Its oral LD_{50} in dogs, cattle, horses, and pigs is 0.5–1 mg/kg, and in cats is 2 mg/kg. Strychnine is considered a restricted-use pesticide. Its sale is forbidden in a number of states. Grain-laced or pelleted commercial baits (usually <0.5%) are often dyed red or green. Malicious or accidental strychnine poisoning, although not very common in the USA, occurs mainly in small animals, especially dogs and occasionally cats, and rarely in livestock. Most poisonings occur when nontarget species consume commercial baits. Young and large-breed, intact male dogs are more likely to be involved. Most poisonings are reported from the western USA.

Pathogenesis: Strychnine is ionized in an acidic pH and then rapidly and completely absorbed in the small intestine. It is metabolized in the liver by microsomal enzymes. The highest concentrations of strychnine are found in the blood, liver, and kidneys. Strychnine and its metabolites are excreted in the urine. Depending on the quantity ingested and treatment measures taken, most of the toxic dose is eliminated within 24–48 hr.

Strychnine inhibits competitively and reversibly the inhibitory neurotransmitter glycine at postsynaptic neuronal sites in the spinal cord and medulla. This results in unchecked reflex stimulation of motor neurons affecting all the striated muscles. Because the extensor muscles are relatively more powerful than the flexor muscles, they predominate to produce generalized rigidity and tonic-clonic seizures. Death results from anoxia and exhaustion.

Clinical Findings: The onset of strychnine poisoning is fast. After oral exposure, clinical signs may appear within 30–60 min. Presence of food in the stomach can delay onset. Early signs, which may often be overlooked, consist of apprehension, nervousness, tenseness, and stiffness. Vomiting is possible but uncommon. Severe tetanic seizures may appear spontaneously or may be initiated by stimuli such as touch, sound, or a sudden bright light. An extreme and overpowering extensor rigidity causes the animal to assume a "sawhorse" stance. Hyperthermia (104°–106°F [40°–41°C]) due to stiffness and seizures is often present in dogs. The tetanic convulsions may last from a few seconds to ~1 min. Respiration may stop momentarily. Intermittent periods of relaxation are seen during convulsions but become less frequent as the clinical course progresses. The mucous membranes become cyanotic and the pupils dilated. Frequency of the seizures increases, and death eventually occurs from exhaustion or asphyxiation during seizures. If untreated, the entire syndrome may last only 1–2 hr. There are no characteristic necropsy lesions. Sometimes, because of prolonged convulsions before death, agonal hemorrhages of heart and lungs and cyanotic congestion from anoxia may be seen. Animals dying from strychnine poisoning have rapid rigor mortis.

Diagnosis: Tentative diagnosis of strychnine poisoning is usually based on history of exposure and clinical signs. Recovery of strychnine alkaloid from the stomach contents, vomitus, liver, kidneys, or urine should be considered diagnostic. Sometimes, urine may not have a detectable amount of strychnine present if analyzed 1–2 days after exposure; therefore, multiple samples should be collected and analyzed. Occasionally, poisoned animals may show presence of undigested grain-laced red or green strychnine bait in the stomach.

Strychnine poisoning can be confused with poisonings by several other seizurigenic substances such as metaldehyde; tremorgenic mycotoxins (penitrem a); organochlorine, organophosphate, or carbamate insecticides; fluoroacetate (1080); zinc phosphide; nicotine; 4-aminopyridine; caffeine; or human medications (tricyclic antidepressants, 5-fluorouracil, metronidazole, isoniazid). Acute, massive hepatic necrosis (hepatic encephalopathy) can also produce clinical signs that resemble those of strychnine poisoning.

Treatment: Strychnine poisoning is an emergency, and treatment should be instituted quickly. Treatment should be aimed at decontamination, control of seizures, prevention of asphyxiation, and supportive care. Seizures should be controlled, and symptomatic animals stabilized before decontamination is attempted.

Decontamination consists of removal of gastric contents by inducing emesis or gastric lavage, and binding of remaining bait in the GI tract with activated charcoal. Because of the rapid onset of clinical signs, emesis may be of limited value in most cases. If exposure is recent and no clinical signs are present, emesis should be induced with 3% hydrogen peroxide (small animals and pigs) at 1–2 mL/kg, PO, maximum 3 tbsp, repeated once after 30 min if vomiting has not occurred; apomorphine (dogs only) at 0.03 mg/kg, IV, or 0.04 mg/kg, IM; or xylazine (dogs or cats) at 0.5–1 mg/kg, IV or IM. If emesis cannot be induced, gastric lavage should be performed with tepid water. Animals already seizuring should be anesthetized first (with pentobarbital), and an endotracheal tube passed before gastric lavage. After emesis or gastric lavage, activated charcoal should be administered at 2–3 g/kg in small animals and 0.5–1 g/kg in large animals with a cathartic such as magnesium sulfate at 250 mg/kg, PO, or sorbitol at 1–3 mL/kg, PO.

Seizures should be controlled in small animals with pentobarbital, IV to effect, repeated as necessary. Muscle relaxants such as methocarbamol at 100–200 mg/kg, IV, also work well; they should be repeated as needed with a maximal dose of 330 mg/kg/day. In large animals, chloral hydrate or xylazine can be used to control seizures. Other medications such as glyceryl guaiacolate (5%, 110 mg/kg), diazepam, and xylazine have been used in dogs to control seizures with variable success. Propofol (3–6 mg/kg, IV, or 0.1–0.6 mg/kg/min as a constant-rate IV infusion) can also be tried to control seizures in dogs or cats. Isoflurane inhalation anesthesia can be used in small animals if preceding measures to control seizures do not work.

Severely affected dogs should be intubated, and artificial respiration provided. Acidification of urine with ammonium chloride (100 mg/kg, bid, PO) may be useful for ion trapping and urinary excretion of the alkaloid. IV fluids should be administered to force diuresis and maintain normal kidney function. Hyperthermia treatment (fans, cool bath) should be given if necessary. Acid-base balance should be monitored and corrected as needed. Most clinical cases may require 1–3 days of treatment.

REFERENCE GUIDES

TABLE 1 NORMAL RECTAL TEMPERATURE RANGES

Species	°C	°F
Cattle		
Beef cow	36.7–39.1	98.0–102.4
Dairy cow	38.0–39.3	100.4–102.8
Cat	38.1–39.2	100.5–102.5
Chicken (daylight)	40.6–43.0	105.0–109.4
Dog	37.9–39.9	100.2–103.8
Goat	38.5–39.7	101.3–103.5
Horse		
Mare	37.3–38.2	99.1–100.8
Stallion	37.2–38.1	99.0–100.6
Pig	38.7–39.8	101.6–103.6
Rabbit	38.6–40.1	101.5–104.2
Sheep	38.3–39.9	100.9–103.8

Adapted from Robertshaw D. Temperature Regulation and Thermal Environment, in *Dukes' Physiology of Domestic Animals*, 12th ed., Reece WO, Ed. Copyright 2004 by Cornell University.

TABLE 2 RESTING HEART RATES

Species	bpm (range)
Cat	120–140
Chick	350–450
Chicken (adult)	250–300
Dairy cow	48–84
Dog	70–120
Elephant	25–35
Goat	70–80
Guinea Pig	200–300
Hamster	300–600
Horse	28–40
Mouse	450–750
Ox	36–60
Pig	70–120
Rabbit	180–350
Rat	250–400
Rhesus monkey (anesthetized)	160–330
Sheep	70–80

Adapted from Detweiler DK and Erickson HH, Regulation of the Heart, in *Dukes' Physiology of Domestic Animals*, 12th ed., Reece WO, Ed. Copyright 2004 by Cornell University.

TABLE 3 RESTING RESPIRATORY RATES

Species	Breaths/min (range)
Cat	16–40
Dairy cow	26–50
Dog	18–34
Horse	10–14
Pig	32–58
Sheep	16–34

Adapted from Reece WO, Respiration in Mammals, in *Dukes' Physiology of Domestic Animals*, 12th ed., Reece WO, Ed. Copyright 2004 by Cornell University.

TABLE 4 URINE VOLUME AND SPECIFIC GRAVITY

Species	Volume (mL/kg body wt/day)	Specific Gravity (range)
Cat	10–20	1.020–1.040
Cow	17–45	1.030–1.045
Dog	20–100	1.016–1.060
Goat	10–40	1.015–1.045
Horse	3–18	1.025–1.060
Pig	5–30	1.010–1.050
Sheep	10–40	1.015–1.045

Adapted from Reece WO, Kidney Function in Mammals, in *Dukes' Physiology of Domestic Animals*, 12th ed., Reece WO, Ed. Copyright 2004 by Cornell University.

TABLE 5 BLOOD-GAS REFERENCE RANGES

Measure	Units	Dog	Cat	Cow	Horse
IN CONVENTIONAL (USA) UNITS					
pH		7.31–7.42	7.24–7.40	7.35–7.50	7.32–7.44
HCO_3	mEq/L	17–24	17–24	20–30	24–30
pCO_2	mmHg	29–42	29–42	35–44	36–46
pO_2	mmHg	85–95	85–95	92	94
IN SI UNITS					
HCO_3	μmol/L	17–24	17–24	20–30	24–30
pCO_2	kPa	3.86–5.60	3.86–5.60	2.67–3.99	4.67–6.13
pO_2	kPa	11.3–12.66	11.3–12.66	12.26	12.53

TABLE 6 HEMATOLOGIC REFERENCE RANGES

	Conventional (USA) Units	SI Units	Dog	Cat	Cow
PCV	%	$\times 10^{-2}$ L/L	35–57	30–45	24–46
Hgb	g/dL	$\times 10$ g/L	11.9–18.9	9.8–15.4	8–15
RBCs	$\times 10^{6}$/µL	$\times 10^{12}$/L	4.95–7.87	5.0–10.0	5.0–10.0
Reticulocytes	%	%	0–1.0	0–0.6	
Absolute reticulocyte count	$\times 10^{3}$/µL	$\times 10^{9}$/L	<80	<60	
MCV	fL	fL	66–77	39–55	40–60
MCH	pg	pg	21.0–26.2	13–17	11–17
MCHC	g/dL	$\times 10$ g/L	32.0–36.3	30–36	30–36
Platelets	$\times 10^{3}$/µL	$\times 10^{9}$/L	211–621	300–800	100–800
MPV	fL	fL	6.1–10.1	12–18	3.5–6.5
WBCs	$\times 10^{3}$/µL	$\times 10^{9}$/L	5.0–14.1	5.5–19.5	4.0–12.0
Neutrophils	%	%	58–85	45–64	15–33
(segmented)	$\times 10^{3}$/µL	$\times 10^{9}$/L	2.9–12.0	2.5–12.5	0.6–4.0
Neutrophils	%	%	0–3	0–2	0–2
(band)	$\times 10^{3}$/µL	$\times 10^{9}$/L	0–0.45	0–0.3	0–0.1
Lymphocytes	%	%	8–21	27–36	45–75
	$\times 10^{3}$/µL	$\times 10^{9}$/L	0.4–2.9	1.5–7.0	2.5–7.5
Monocytes	%	%	2–10	0–5	0–8
	$\times 10^{3}$/µL	$\times 10^{9}$/L	0.1–1.4	0–0.9	0–0.9
Eosinophils	%	%	0–9	0–4	0–20
	$\times 10^{3}$/µL	$\times 10^{9}$/L	0–1.3	0–0.8	0–2.4
Basophils	%	%	0–1	0–1	0–2
	$\times 10^{3}$/µL	$\times 10^{9}$/L	0–0.14	0–0.2	0–0.2
M:E			0.75–2.5	0.6–3.9	0.3–1.8
Plasma proteins	g/dL	10 g/L	6.0–7.5	6.0–7.5	6.0–8.0
Plasma fibrinogen	mg/dL	g/L	150–300	150–300	100–600

TABLE 6 HEMATOLOGIC REFERENCE RANGES *(continued)*

Horse	Pig	Sheep	Goat	Rabbit	Llama	Vietnamese Potbellied Pig	Ostrich
27–43	36–43	27–45	22–38	33–50	29–39	22–50	32
10.1–16.1	10–16	9–15	8–12	10–17	12.8–17.7	7.8–16.2	12.2
6.0–10.4	5–8	9–15	8–18	5–8	11.3–17.7	3.6–7.8	1.7
	0–0.1						
37–49	50–68	28–40	16–25	58–67	20.9–28	55–71	174
13.7–18.2	17–21	8–12	5.2–8			18–24	61
35.3–39.3	30–34	31–34	30–36	29–37	43.1–46.6	31–36	33
117–256	200–500	800–1,100	300–600	250–650		204–518	
4.0–6.0							
5.6–12.1	11–22	4–8	4–13	5.2–12.5	7.5–21.5	5.2–17.9	5.5
52–70	28–47	10–50	30–48	20–75	60–74	0–63	63[a]
2.9–8.5	2–15	0.7–6.0	1.0–7.2	1–9.4	4.6–16	0–11.4	3.4
0–1	0–4	0	rare		0–1	0–1	
0–0.1	0–0.8				0–0.35	0–0.19	
21–42	39–62	40–55	50–70	30–85	13–35	15–55	34
1.2–5.1	3.8–16.5	2–9	2–9	1.6–10.6	1–7.5	0.8–9.8	1.87
0–6	2–10	0–6	0–4	1–4	1–4	0–13	2.8
0–0.7	0–1	0–0.75	0–0.55	0.05–0.5	0.05–0.8	0–0.67	0.15
0–7	0.5–11	0–10	1–8	1–4	0–15	0–12	0.3
0–0.8	0–1.5	0–1	0.05–0.65	0.05–0.5	0–3.3	0–0.73	0.02
0–2	0–2	0–3	0–1	1–7	0–2	0	0.2
0–0.3	0–0.5	0–0.3	0–0.12	0.05–0.9	0–0.4	0–0.61	0.01
0.5–1.5	1.2–2.2	0.77–1.7	0.7–1.0				
6.0–8.5	6–8	6–7.5	6–7.5	5.4–8.3		5.4–7.5	
100–500	200–400	100–500	100–400	200–400	100–400	100–400	

Data on various species compiled and adapted in part from multiple sources, including Latimer KS, *Duncan & Prasse's Veterinary Laboratory Medicine: Clinical Pathology*, 5th ed., Wiley-Blackwell, 2011; and Weiss DJ, Wardrop KJ, *Schalm's Veterinary Hematology*, 6th Ed., Wiley-Blackwell, 2010. Reference ranges vary between laboratories. Values provided by the reference laboratory should be used.

MCV = mean corpuscular volume
MCH = mean corpuscular hemoglobin
MCHC = mean corpuscular hemoglobin concentration
MPV = mean platelet volume
M:E = myeloid:erythroid ratio

[a] Heterophil

TABLE 7 SERUM BIOCHEMICAL REFERENCE RANGES

Measure	Units	Dog	Cat	Cow	Horse
IN CONVENTIONAL (USA) UNITS					
ALT	U/L	10–109	25–97		
Amylase	U/L	226–1,063	550–1,458		
Alk phos[a]	U/L	1–114	0–45		
AST	U/L	13–15	7–38	60–125	160–412
CK	U/L	52–368	69–214	0–350	60–330
GGT[a]	U/L			6–17.4	6–32
LDH	U/L	0–236	58–120		112–456
SDH[a]	U/L			4.3–15.3	1–8
Bicarbonate	mEq/L	17–24	17–24	20–30	24–30
Bilirubin	mg/dL	0–0.3	0–0.1	0–1.6	0–3.2
Calcium	mg/dL	9.1–11.7	8.7–11.7	8.0–11.4	10.2–13.4
Chloride	mEq/L	110–124	115–130	99–107	98–109
Cholesterol	mg/dL	135–278	71–156		
Creatinine	mg/dL	0.5–1.7	0.9–2.2	0.5–2.2	0.4–2.2
Glucose	mg/dL	76–119	60–120	40–100	62–134
Magnesium	mg/dL	1.6–2.4	1.7–2.6	1.5–2.9	1.4–2.3
Phosphorus	mg/dL	2.9–5.3	3.0–6.1	5.6–8.0	1.5–4.7
Potassium	mEq/L	3.9–5.1	3.7–6.1	3.6–4.9	2.9–4.6
Protein	g/dL	5.4–7.5	6.0–7.9	6.7–7.5	5.6–7.6
Albumin	g/dL	2.3–3.1	2.8–3.9	2.5–3.8	2.6–4.1
Globulin	g/dL	2.7–4.4	2.6–5.1	3.0–3.5	2.6–4.0
Sodium	mEq/L	142–152	146–156	136–144	128–142
Urea nitrogen	mg/dL	8–28	19–34	10–25	11–27
IN SI UNITS					
Bicarbonate	mmol/L	17–24	17–24	20–30	24–30
Bilirubin	μmol/L	0–5.1	0–1.7	0–27.4	0–54.7
Calcium	mmol/L	2.3–2.9	2.2–2.9	2.0–2.8	2.5–3.3
Chloride	mmol/L	110–124	115–130	99–107	98–109
Cholesterol	mmol/L	3.5–7.2	1.8–4.0		
Creatinine	μmol/L	44–150	80–194	44–194	35–194
Glucose	mmol/L	4.2–6.6	3.3–6.7	2.2–5.6	3.4–7.4

TABLE 7 SERUM BIOCHEMICAL REFERENCE RANGES *(continued)*

Pig	Sheep	Goat	Rabbit	Llama	Vietnamese Potbellied Pig	Ostrich
IN CONVENTIONAL (USA) UNITS						
31–58	26–34	6–19	45–80	6–14	10.9–95.1	
			200–400			
118–395	68–387	93–387	12–96	41–92	27–160	
32–84	60–280	167–513	35–130	216–378	16–64	252–401
2.4–22.5	8.1–12.9	0.8–8.9	140–372	17–101	212.5–2,851.5	1,655–4,246
10–60	20–52	20–56	0–7	7–29	14.5–56.2	0–1
380–634	238–440	123–392		88–487		869–2,047
1.0–5.8	5.8–27.9	14.0–23.6		1–17		
18–27	20–25					
0–10.0	0.1–0.5	0–0.1	0–0.7	0–0.1	0.2–0.45	
7.1–11.6	11.5–12.8	8.9–11.7	11–14	8.0–10.3		10.0–18.4
94–106	95–103	99–110.3		102–109	106–113	94–105
36–54	52–76	80–130	10–80	35–113		
1.0–2.7	1.2–1.9	1.0–1.8	0.5–2.5	1.1–2.5	1.0–2.3	
85–150	50–80	50–75	75–155	103–160	59.8–175.2	187–247
2.7–3.7	2.2–2.8	2.8–3.6		1.82–3.77		
5.3–9.6	5.0–7.3	4.2–9.1	4.0–6.5	3.1–10.8		4.0–6.8
4.4–6.7	3.9–5.4	3.5–6.7	3.5–6.9	4.6–7.1	3.7–5.0	4.5–5.9
7.9–8.9	6.0–7.9	6.4–7.0	5.4–7.5	5.8–7.5	6.6–8.9	4–5.4
1.9–3.9	2.4–3.0	2.7–3.9	2.7–5.0	3.6–4.8	3.6–5.0	
5.3–6.4	3.5–5.7	2.7–4.1	1.5–2.7	1.6–2.9		
135–150	139–152	142–155	138–150	148–155	139–148.8	147–157
10–30	8–20	10–20	20–45	12–34	4.2–15.1	1.4–2.2
IN SI UNITS						
18–27	20–25					
0–17.1	1.71–8.55	0–1.71	0–12	0–17.1	3.4–7.7	
1.78–2.9	2.88–3.2	2.23–2.93	2.7–3.5	2.2–2.58		2.5–4.6
94–106	95–103	99–110.3		102–109	106–113	94–105
0.93–1.40	1.35–1.97	2.07–3.37	0.3–2.1	0.91–2.93		
141–239	106–168	88.4–159	44.2–221	97.2–221	88.4–203.3	
4.72–8.33	2.78–4.44	2.78–4.16	4.1–8.6	5.72–8.89	3.3–9.9	10.4–13.7

TABLE 7 SERUM BIOCHEMICAL REFERENCE RANGES *(continued)*

Measure	Units	Dog	Cat	Cow	Horse
Magnesium	mmol/L	0.7–1.0	0.7–1.1	0.6–1.2	0.6–0.9
Phosphorus	mmol/L	0.9–1.7	1.0–2.0	1.8–2.6	0.5–1.5
Potassium	mmol/L	3.9–5.1	3.7–6.1	3.6–4.9	2.9–4.6
Protein	g/L	54–75	60–79	67–75	56–76
Albumin	g/L	23–31	28–39	25–38	26–41
Globulin	g/L	27–44	26–51	30–35	26–40
Sodium	mmol/L	142–152	146–156	136–144	128–142
Urea nitrogen	mmol urea/L	2.9–10.0	6.8–12.1	3.6–8.9	3.9–9.6

TABLE 8 CLINICAL CHEMISTRY SI CONVERSION FACTORS

Measure	Conventional (USA) Units	Conversion Factor (×)	SI Units
Alkaline phosphatase	IU/L	1.0	U/L
ALT	U/L	1.0	U/L
Albumin	g/dL	10.0	g/L
Ammonia (NH_4)	mcg/dL	0.5872	µmol/L
Amylase	Somogyi units	1.85	U/L
AST	U/L	1.0	U/L
Bilirubin	mg/dL	17.10	µmol/L
Calcium	mg/dL	0.25	mmol/L
Carbon dioxide	mEq/L	1.0	mmol/L
Chloride	mEq/L	1.0	mmol/L
Cholesterol	mg/dL	0.026	mmol/L
Copper	mcg/dL	0.16	µmol/L
Cortisol	mcg/dL	27.6	nmol/L
CK	IU/L	1.0	U/L
Creatinine	mg/dL	88.40	µmol/L
Fibrinogen	mg/dL	0.01	g/L
Glucose	mg/dL	0.055	mmol/L
Iron, binding	mcg/dL	0.179	µmol/L
Iron, total	mcg/dL	0.179	µmol/L

TABLE 7 SERUM BIOCHEMICAL REFERENCE RANGES *(continued)*

Pig	Sheep	Goat	Rabbit	Llama	Vietnamese Potbellied Pig	Ostrich
1.11–1.52	0.9–1.31	0.31–1.48		0.75–1.55		
1.71–3.10	1.62–2.36	1.4–2.9	1.3–2.1	1.0–3.49		1.3–2.2
4.4–6.7	3.9–5.4	3.5–6.7	3.5–6.9	4.6–7.1	3.7–5.0	4.5–5.9
79–89	60–79	64–70	54–75	58–75	66–89	40–54
19–39	24–30	27–39	27–50	36–48	36–50	
53–64	35–57	27–41	15–27	16–29		
135–150	139–152	142–155	138–150	148–155	139–148.8	147–157
3.6–10.7	2.8–7.1	3.6–7.1	7.1–16.1	4.3–12.1	1.5–5.4	0.5–0.8

Data on various species compiled and adapted in part from multiple sources, including Latimer KS, *Duncan & Prasse's Veterinary Laboratory Medicine: Clinical Pathology*, 5th Ed., Wiley-Blackwell, 2011; and Kaneko JJ, Harvey JW, Bruss ML, *Clinical Biochemistry of Domestic Animals*, 6th Ed., Academic Press, 2008. Reference ranges vary between laboratories. Values provided by the reference laboratory should be used.

[a] Alk phos = alkaline phosphatase; GGT = gamma glutamyltransferase; SDH = sorbitol dehydrogenase

TABLE 8 CLINICAL CHEMISTRY SI CONVERSION FACTORS *(continued)*

Measure	Conventional (USA) Units	Conversion Factor (×)	SI Units
Lipase	IU/L	1	U/L
	Cherry-Crandall U	278	U/L
Magnesium	mEq/L	0.5	mmol/L
Osmolality	Osm/kg	1.0	mmol/L
Phosphorus	mg/dL	0.323	mmol/L
Potassium	mEq/L	1.0	mmol/L
Protein, total	g/dL	10.0	g/L
Sodium	mEq/L	1.0	mmol/L
Triglycerides	mg/dL	0.011	mmol/L
Triiodothyronine (T_3)	mcg/dL	15.6	nmol/L
Thyroxine (T_4)	mcg/dL	12.87	nmol/L
Urea nitrogen	mg/dL	0.357	mmol/L
Uric acid	mg/dL	0.059	mmol/L
Urine protein/creatinine ratio	g/g	0.113	g/mmol
Xylose absorption	mg/dL	0.067	mmol/L

Adapted from *Veterinary Laboratory Medicine: Interpretation and Diagnosis*, Meyer DH, Harvey JW, 3rd ed., Copyright 2004, with permission from Elsevier.

TABLE 9 WEIGHT TO BODY SURFACE AREA CONVERSION

Dogs				Cats	
Body wt (kg)	BSA (m^2)	Body wt (kg)	BSA (m^2)	Body wt (kg)	BSA (m^2)
0.5	0.064	26	0.886	0.5	0.063
1.0	0.101	27	0.909	1.0	0.100
1.5	0.132	28	0.931	1.5	0.131
2.0	0.160	29	0.953	2.0	0.159
2.5	0.186	30	0.975	2.5	0.184
3.0	0.210	31	0.997	3.0	0.208
3.5	0.233	32	1.018	3.5	0.231
4.0	0.255	33	1.039	4.0	0.252
4.5	0.275	34	1.060	4.5	0.273
5	0.295	35	1.081	5.0	0.292
6	0.333	36	1.101	5.5	0.312
7	0.370	37	1.121	6.0	0.330
8	0.404	38	1.142	6.5	0.348
9	0.437	39	1.162	7.0	0.366
10	0.469	40	1.181	7.5	0.383
11	0.500	41	1.201	8.0	0.400
12	0.529	42	1.220	8.5	0.416
13	0.558	43	1.240	9.0	0.433
14	0.587	44	1.259	9.5	0.449
15	0.614	45	1.278	10.0	0.464
16	0.641	46	1.297		
17	0.668	47	1.315		
18	0.694	48	1.334		
19	0.719	49	1.352		
20	0.744	50	1.371		
21	0.769	51	1.389		
22	0.793	52	1.407		
23	0.817	53	1.425		
24	0.840	54	1.443		
25	0.864	55	1.461		

Note: body surface area (BSA) in square meters = K × (body wt in grams$^{2/3}$) × 10^{-4}

K = constant (10.1 for dogs and 10.0 for cats)

TABLE 10 TEMPERATURE EQUIVALENTS AND CONVERSIONS

Celsius (°C)	°C = (°F – 32) × 5/9 °F = (°C × 9/5) + 32	Fahrenheit (°F)
0	Freezing	32
36.0		96.8
36.5		97.7
37.0		98.6
37.5		99.5
38.0		100.4
38.5		101.3
39.0		102.2
39.5		103.1
40.0		104.0
40.5		104.9
41.0		105.8
41.5		106.7
42.0		107.6
100	Boiling	212

TABLE 11 METRIC SYSTEM PREFIXES AND SYMBOLS

Factor	Prefix	Symbol	Factor	Prefix	Symbol
10^{18}	exa	E	10^{-1}	deci	d
10^{15}	peta	P	10^{-2}	centi	c
10^{12}	tera	T	10^{-3}	milli	m
10^{9}	giga	G	10^{-6}	micro	µ
10^{6}	mega	M	10^{-9}	nano	n
10^{3}	kilo	k	10^{-12}	pico	p
10^{2}	hecto	h	10^{-15}	femto	f
10	deka	da	10^{-18}	atto	a

TABLE 12 WEIGHTS AND MEASURES EQUIVALENTS AND CONVERSIONS

Length	1 m = 39.37 in.	1 ft = 30.48 cm
	1 yd = 91.44 cm	1 in. = 2.54 cm
Weight[a]	1 kg = 2.205 lb	1 lb = 0.454 kg
	1 g = 0.035 oz	1 oz = 28.35 g
	1 mg = 0.015 grain	1 grain = 64.8 mg
	1 ton = 2,000 lb	1 metric ton = 1,000 kg = 2,205 lb
Capacity		*Imperial system*:
	1 gal. = 3.785 L	1 gal. = 4.55 L
	1 quart = 0.946 L	1 quart = 1.136 L
	1 pint = 473.2 mL	1 pint = 568.26 mL
	1 oz = 29.57 mL	
	1 tablespoon = 15 mL	
	1 teaspoon = 5 mL	

[a] Avoirdupois (used in the USA as the common system of measuring weight) unless otherwise specified

TABLE 13 PERCENTAGE, PPM, AND PPB CONVERSIONS

ppm	ppb	Percentage
0.001	1	0.0000001
0.01	10	0.000001
0.1	100	0.00001
1	1,000	0.0001
10		0.001
100		0.01
1,000		0.1
10,000		1

Other useful conversions: 1 mg/kg = 1 ppm; 1 g/ton = 1.1 ppm; 100 g/ton = 110 ppm

TABLE 14 MILLIGRAM-MILLIEQUIVALENT CONVERSIONS AND ATOMIC WEIGHTS

Ion	Atomic Weight	Valence
Hydrogen (H)	1	1
Carbon (C)	12	4
Nitrogen (N)	14	3
Oxygen (O)	16	2
Sodium (Na)	23	1
Magnesium (Mg)	24	2
Phosphate (P)[a]	31	3, 5
Chlorine (Cl)	35.5	1
Potassium (K)	39	1
Calcium (Ca)	40	2

Note: The milliequivalent (mEq) is the unit of measure often used for electrolytes. It indicates the chemical activity, or combining power, of an element relative to the activity of 1 mg of hydrogen. Thus, 1 mEq is represented by 1 mg of hydrogen (1 mole) or 23 mg of Na+, 39 mg of K+, etc.

$$\text{mEq/L} = \frac{(\text{mg/L}) \times \text{valence}}{\text{molecular weight}}$$

$$\text{mg/L} = \frac{(\text{mEq/L}) \times \text{molecular weight}}{\text{valence}}$$

[a] As phosphorus, inorganic

INDEX

Page numbers in **bold type** indicate principal references.

A

IN.

C

E

F

G

J

K

M

O

P

T

U

W